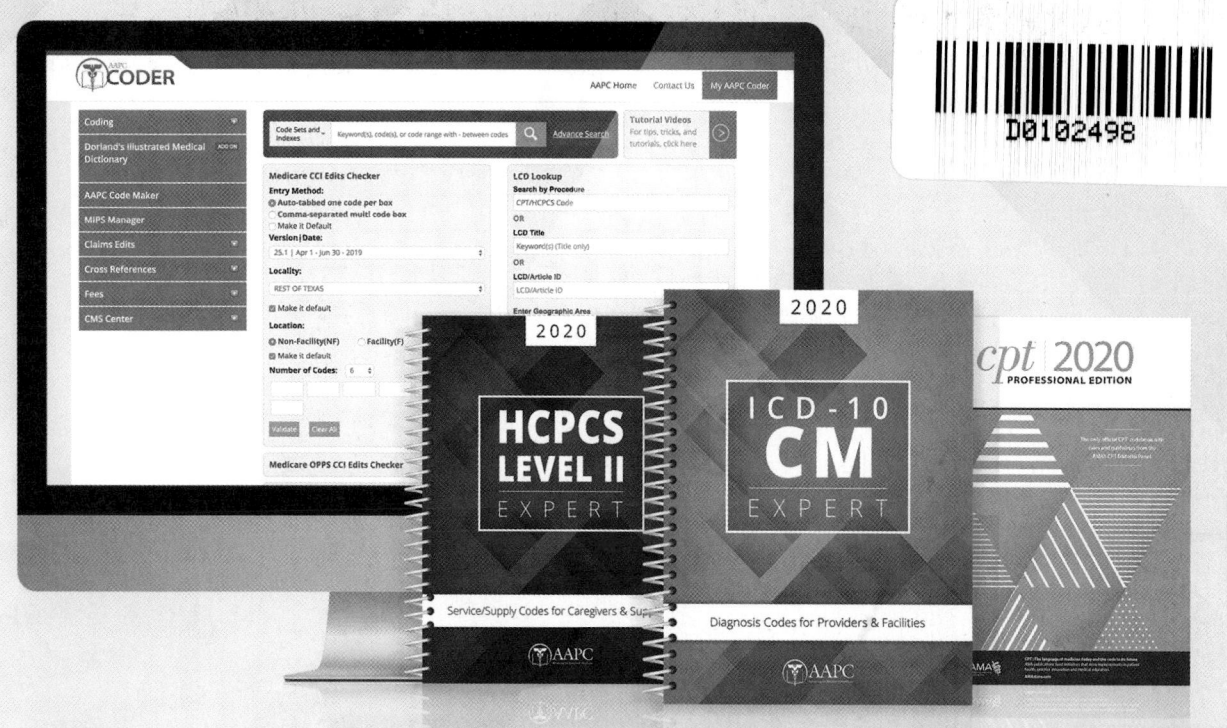
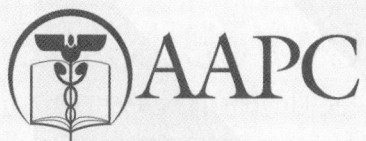

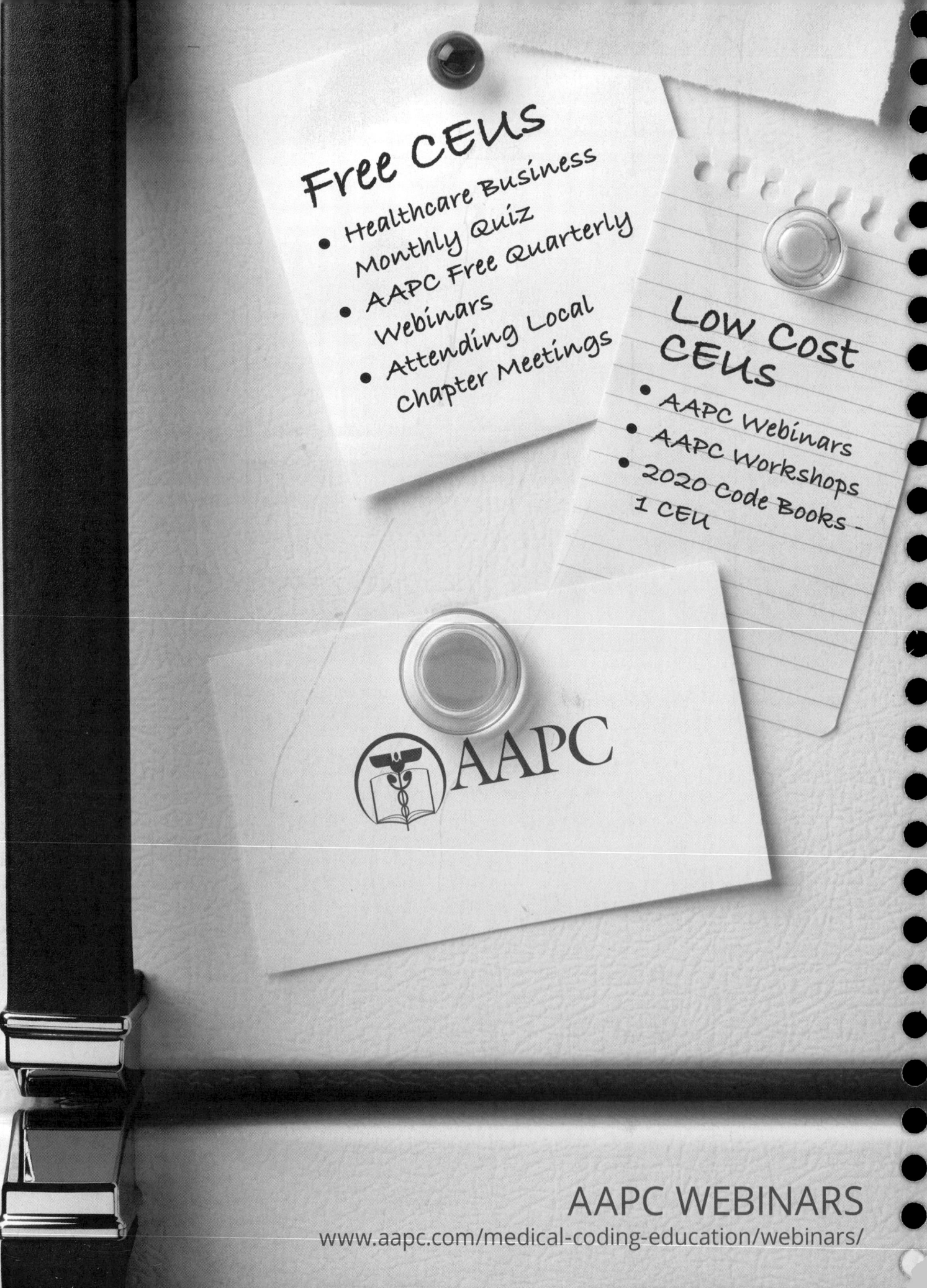

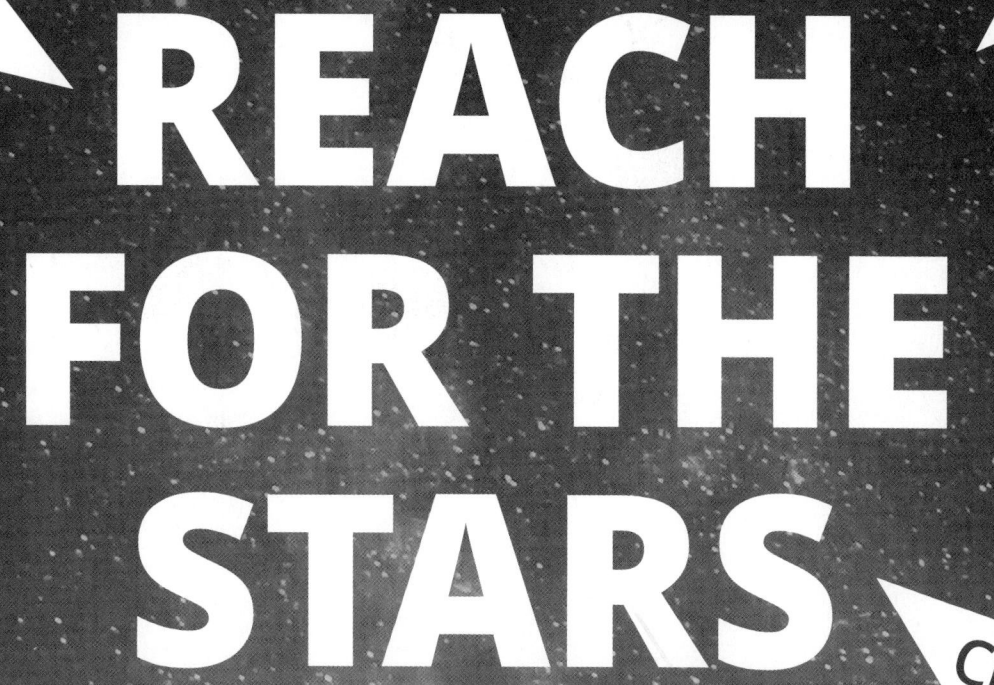
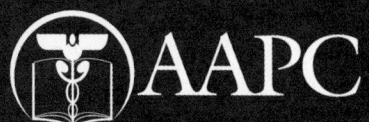

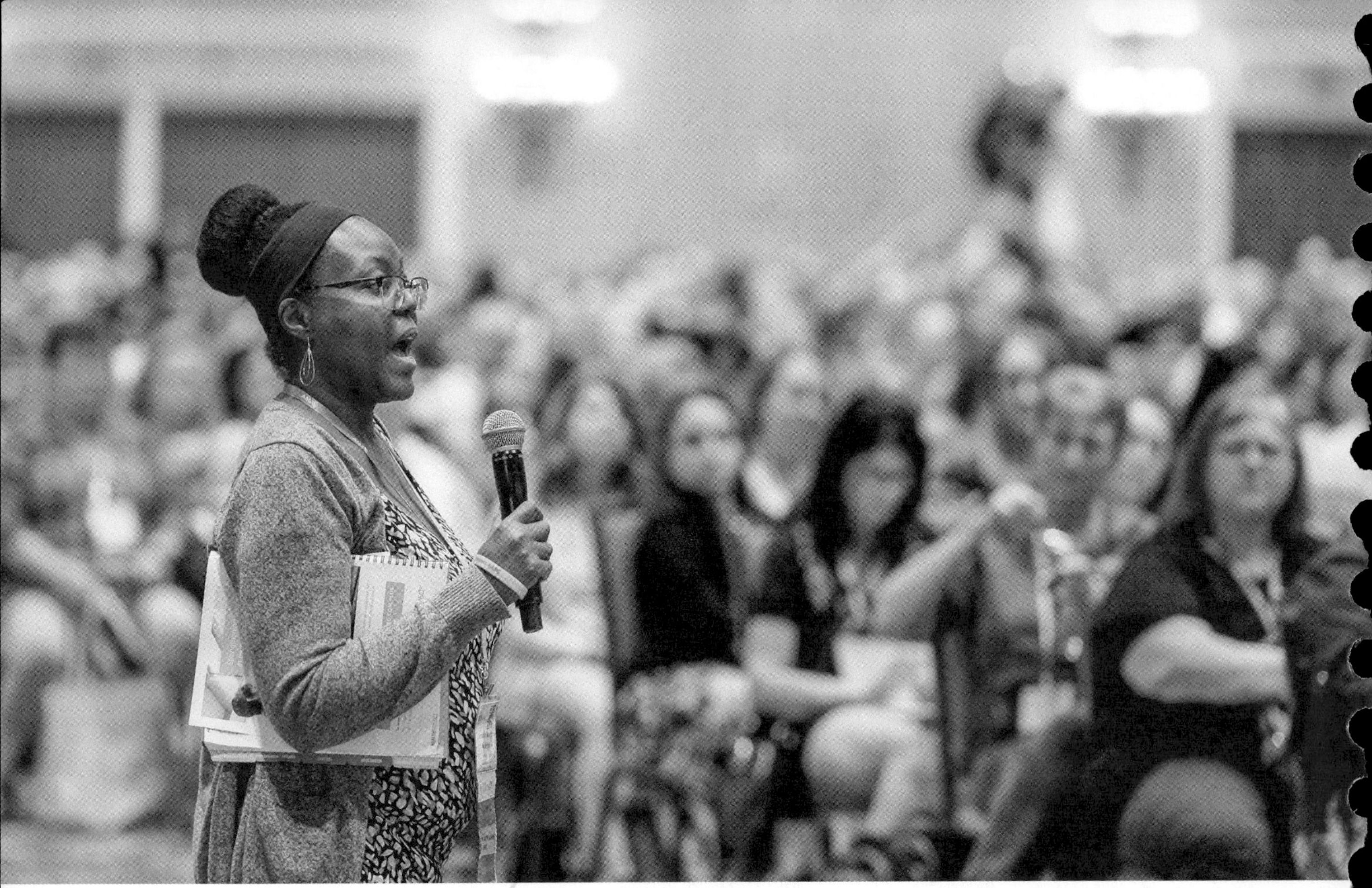

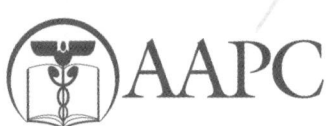

2020

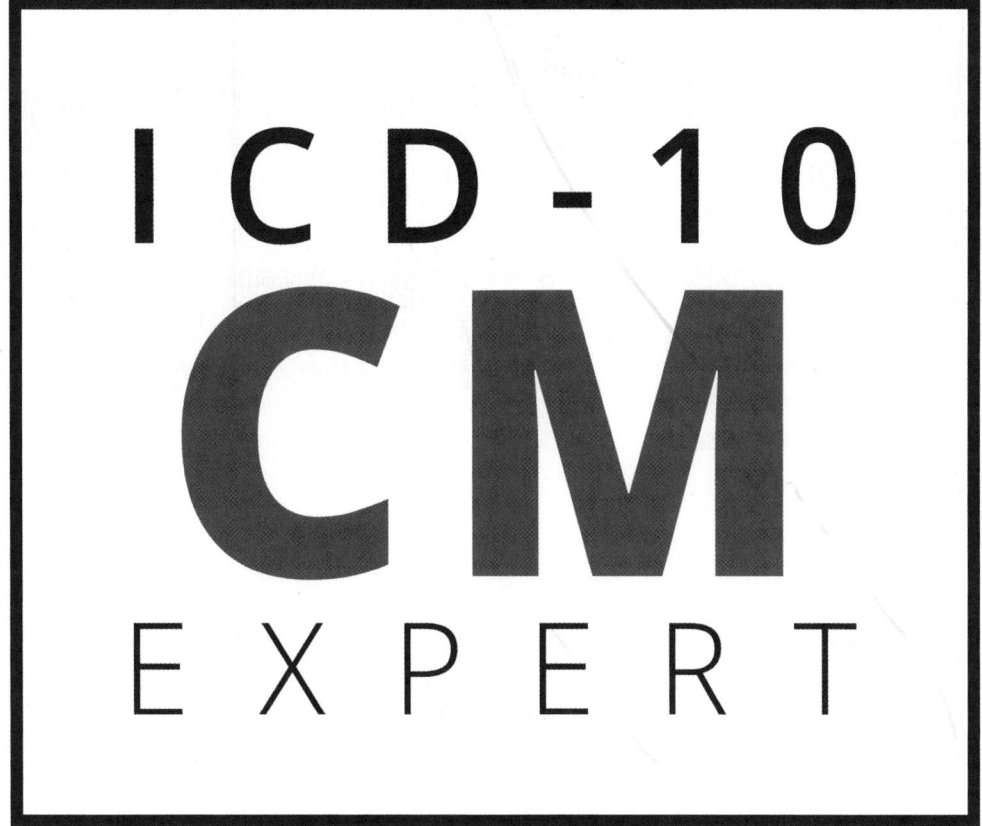

ICD-10
CM
EXPERT

The Official CMS Code Set

Diagnosis Codes for Providers & Facilities

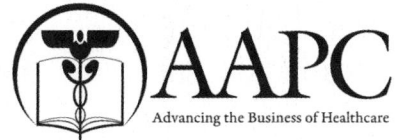
AAPC
Advancing the Business of Healthcare

PUBLISHER'S NOTICE

Coding, billing, and reimbursement decisions should not be made based solely upon information within this ICD-10-CM code book. Application of the information in this book does not imply or guarantee claims payment. Make inquiries of your local carriers' bulletins, policy announcements, etc., to resolve local billing requirements. Finally, the law, applicable regulations, payers' instructions, interpretations, enforcement, etc., of ICD-10-CM codes may change at any time in any particular area. Information in this book is solely based on ICD-10-CM rules and regulations.

This ICD-10-CM is designed to be an accurate and authoritative source regarding coding, and every reasonable effort has been made to ensure accuracy and completeness of content. However, this publisher makes no guarantee, warranty, or representation that this publication is complete, accurate, or without errors. It is understood that this publisher is not rendering any legal or professional services or advice in this code book and bears no liability for any results or consequences arising from use of this ICD-10-CM book.

Code edit symbols and colors in this book are based on the Medicare Code Editor (MCE), Medicare's Integrated Outpatient Code Editor (I/OCE), and MS-DRG v36.0 Definitions Manual. The code edit information in this book is based on MCE v36 with the addition of FY 2020 Inpatient Prospective Payment System (IPPS) Proposed Rule updates, the most current information available at the time of printing.

AAPC'S COMMITMENT TO ACCURACY

This publisher is committed to providing our members accurate and reliable materials. However, codes and the guidelines by which they are applied change or are reinterpreted through the year. Check www.aapc.com periodically for updates. To report corrections and updates, please contact AAPC Customer Service via 1-800-626-2633 or, via email to code.books@aapc.com.

ACKNOWLEDGEMENT

Jaspal Singh Arora, Operations

Brad Ericson, MPC, CPC, COSC

Rahul Jain, MDSE

Prashant Kumar, MBA

Sabyasachi Nath, MS

Rajendra Sharma, RN, CPC

Chandrashekhar Boreda, CPC

Amit Gupta

Melissa L. Kirshner, MPH, CPC, CRC, CPC-I, AAPC Fellow

Beth Martin, BS, COC, CSM

Ganesh Prasad Sahoo

Patricia Zubritzky, BS, CRCE-I

Sushanta Das, MBA

Leesa Israel, CPC, CUC, CEMC, CPPM, CMBS

Sandra Krokaugger

Lisa Meaney, BS

Harshita Sharma, PT, PhD

Get Updates, Coding Tips, and Corrections for this book at www.aapc.com/codebook_updates.

Images/Illustrations by the following artists at shutterstock.com

stockshoppe - 180896807, 99671552, 180896810, 187162193, 180896855, 180896738, 177790997, 177791516, 180896873 | Blamb - 24129706, 105550307, 101583709, 23557609, 104886824, 24764461, 786347626 | Alila Medical Media - 125581517, 149230217, 228843253, 155445671, 147789479, 228843103, 88094230, 106263560, 72231811, 149230337, 155445686, 101696095, 96426923, 97755608, 147943922, 147943910, 155445662, 147943874, 106263593, 125891585, 228843262, 91093100, 116411527, 101205484, 127006943, 128044649, 77803252, 76386163, 79593496, 79592488, 78688351, 75043309, 97190072, 74674165, 73140514, 113164513, 120439864, 127500677, 112082045, 75512560, 147789395, 74226295, 75043312, 88937434, 117587797, 89870971, 128669354, 147789407, 89870962, 110902643, 88241464, 101419795, 101056498, 89144548, 119184292, 128044655, 117983611, 75515092, 120437533, 75923548, 125899337, 127507436, 74586256, 125581514, 125899361, 122081125, 129469667, 88937437, 88094233, 89870968, 121363498, 118506328, 90428200, 88241755, 90181153 | Designua - 430118209, 180938618, 135935735, 165084413, 138357839, 118528180 | Suwin - 405537832 | Vecton - 661087531 | Sakurra - 676139677 | stihii - 129969767, 124562680, 121824442, 129804629, 109588457, 225637774, 505306105, 505306069, 135303347 | DeryaDraws - 557609659 | Naeblys - 650014342 | NatthapongSachan - 416973331 452997697 | udaix - 109311614, 1336924949, 502058023, 108531449, 108605000 | ducu59us - 104022683, 125200733, 94324789 | BlueRingMedia - 141161404, 141162229, 141161560 | joshya - 261971498 | Della_Liner - 324447776 | snapgalleria - 142194094 | okili77 - 156466463 | lotan - 186878060 | Alexander_P - 404964388 | Marochkina Anastasiia - 496840036 | logika600 - 501771241 | Athanasia Nomikou -113340007 | Sergii Chepulskyi - 137806217 | Suzanne Tucker - 88023844 | Beneda Miroslav - 125238926 | olavs - 127188179 | somersault1824 - 80995972 | Carolina K. Smith MD - 87546805 | D. Kucharski K. Kucharska - 147360692 | Arkela - 131740481 | Gromovataya - 147818714 | ARZTSAMUI - 150573029 | konmesa - 122366692 | dr OX - 129535535

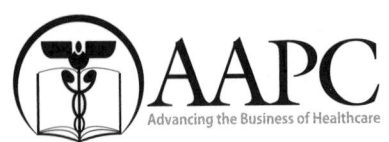

Table of Contents

This page intentionally left blank

ICD-10-CM Official Guidelines for Coding and Reporting FY 2020
(October 1, 2019 - September 30, 2020)

Narrative changes appear in bold text

Items <u>underlined</u> have been moved within the guidelines since the FY 2019 version

Italics **are used to indicate revisions to heading changes**

The Centers for Medicare and Medicaid Services (CMS) and the National Center for Health Statistics (NCHS), two departments within the U.S. Federal Government's Department of Health and Human Services (DHHS) provide the following guidelines for coding and reporting using the International Classification of Diseases, 10th Revision, Clinical Modification (ICD-10-CM). These guidelines should be used as a companion document to the official version of the ICD-10-CM as published on the NCHS website. The ICD-10-CM is a morbidity classification published by the United States for classifying diagnoses and reason for visits in all health care settings. The ICD-10-CM is based on the ICD-10, the statistical classification of disease published by the World Health Organization (WHO).

These guidelines have been approved by the four organizations that make up the Cooperating Parties for the ICD-10-CM: the American Hospital Association (AHA), the American Health Information Management Association (AHIMA), CMS, and NCHS.

These guidelines are a set of rules that have been developed to accompany and complement the official conventions and instructions provided within the ICD-10-CM itself. The instructions and conventions of the classification take precedence over guidelines. These guidelines are based on the coding and sequencing instructions in the Tabular List and Alphabetic Index of ICD-10-CM, but provide additional instruction. Adherence to these guidelines when assigning ICD-10-CM diagnosis codes is required under the Health Insurance Portability and Accountability Act (HIPAA). The diagnosis codes (Tabular List and Alphabetic Index) have been adopted under HIPAA for all healthcare settings. A joint effort between the healthcare provider and the coder is essential to achieve complete and accurate documentation, code assignment, and reporting of diagnoses and procedures. These guidelines have been developed to assist both the healthcare provider and the coder in identifying those diagnoses that are to be reported. The importance of consistent, complete documentation in the medical record cannot be overemphasized. Without such documentation accurate coding cannot be achieved. The entire record should be reviewed to determine the specific reason for the encounter and the conditions treated.

The term encounter is used for all settings, including hospital admissions. In the context of these guidelines, the term provider is used throughout the guidelines to mean physician or any qualified health care practitioner who is legally accountable for establishing the patient's diagnosis. Only this set of guidelines, approved by the Cooperating Parties, is official.

The guidelines are organized into sections. Section I includes the structure and conventions of the classification and general guidelines that apply to the entire classification, and chapter-specific guidelines that correspond to the chapters as they are arranged in the classification. Section II includes guidelines for selection of principal diagnosis for non-outpatient settings. Section III includes guidelines for reporting additional diagnoses in non-outpatient settings. Section IV is for outpatient coding and reporting. It is necessary to review all sections of the guidelines to fully understand all of the rules and instructions needed to code properly.

Section I Conventions, general coding guidelines and chapter specific guidelines

The conventions, general guidelines and chapter-specific guidelines are applicable to all health care settings unless otherwise indicated. The conventions and instructions of the classification take precedence over guidelines.

A. Conventions for the ICD-10-CM

The conventions for the ICD-10-CM are the general rules for use of the classification independent of the guidelines. These conventions are incorporated within the Alphabetic Index and Tabular List of the ICD-10-CM as instructional notes.

1. The Alphabetic Index and Tabular List

The ICD-10-CM is divided into the Alphabetic Index, an alphabetical list of terms and their corresponding code, and the Tabular List, a structured list of codes divided into chapters based on body system or condition. The Alphabetic Index consists of the following parts: the Index of Diseases and Injury, the Index of External Causes of Injury, the Table of Neoplasms and the Table of Drugs and Chemicals.

See Section I.C2. General guidelines

See Section I.C.19. Adverse effects, poisoning, underdosing and toxic effects

2. Format and Structure:

The ICD-10-CM Tabular List contains categories, subcategories and codes. Characters for categories, subcategories and codes may be either a letter or a number. All categories are 3 characters. A three-character category that has no further subdivision is equivalent to a code. Subcategories are either 4 or 5 characters. Codes may be 3, 4, 5, 6 or 7 characters. That is, each level of subdivision after a category is a subcategory. The final level of subdivision is a code. Codes that have applicable 7th characters are still referred to as codes, not subcategories. A code that has an applicable 7th character is considered invalid without the 7th character.

The ICD-10-CM uses an indented format for ease in reference.

3. Use of codes for reporting purposes

For reporting purposes only codes are permissible, not categories or subcategories, and any applicable 7th character is required.

4. Placeholder character

The ICD-10-CM utilizes a placeholder character "X". The "X" is used as a placeholder at certain codes to allow for future expansion. An example of this is at the poisoning, adverse effect and underdosing codes, categories T36-T50.

Where a placeholder exists, the X must be used in order for the code to be considered a valid code.

5. 7th Characters

Certain ICD-10-CM categories have applicable 7th characters. The applicable 7th character is required for all codes within the category, or as the notes in the Tabular List instruct. The 7th character must always be the 7th character in the data field. If a code that requires a 7th character is not 6 characters, a placeholder X must be used to fill in the empty characters.

6. Abbreviations

a. Alphabetic Index abbreviations

NEC	"Not elsewhere classifiable"
	This abbreviation in the Alphabetic Index represents "other specified." When a specific code is not available for a condition, the Alphabetic Index directs the coder to the "other specified" code in the Tabular List.
NOS	"Not otherwise specified"
	This abbreviation is the equivalent of unspecified.

b. Tabular List abbreviations

NEC	"Not elsewhere classifiable"
	This abbreviation in the Tabular List represents "other specified". When a specific code is not available for a condition, the Tabular List includes an NEC entry under a code to identify the code as the "other specified" code.
NOS	"Not otherwise specified"
	This abbreviation is the equivalent of unspecified.

7. Punctuation

[ ] Brackets are used in the Tabular List to enclose synonyms, alternative wording or explanatory phrases. Brackets are used in the Alphabetic Index to identify manifestation codes.

( ) Parentheses are used in both the Alphabetic Index and Tabular List to enclose supplementary words that may be present or absent in the statement of a disease or procedure without affecting the code number to which it is assigned. The terms within the parentheses are referred to as nonessential modifiers. The nonessential modifiers in the Alphabetic Index to Diseases apply to sub terms following a main term except when a nonessential modifier and a sub entry are mutually exclusive, the sub entry takes precedence. For example, in the ICD-10-CM Alphabetic Index under the main term Enteritis, "acute" is a nonessential modifier and "chronic" is a sub entry. In this case, the nonessential modifier "acute" does not apply to the sub entry "chronic".

: Colons are used in the Tabular List after an incomplete term which needs one or more of the modifiers following the colon to make it assignable to a given category.

8. Use of "and".

See Section I.A.14. Use of the term "And"

9. Other and Unspecified codes (*See* **Fig. I.A.9**)

a. "Other" codes

Codes titled "other" or "other specified" are for use when the information in the medical record provides detail for which a specific code does not exist. Alphabetic Index entries with NEC in the line designate "other" codes in the Tabular List. These Alphabetic Index entries represent specific disease entities for which no specific code exists so the term is included within an "other" code.

b. "Unspecified" codes

Codes titled "unspecified" are for use when the information in the medical record is insufficient to assign a more specific code. For those categories for which an unspecified code is not provided, the "other specified" code may represent both other and unspecified.

See Section I.B.18 Use of Signs/Symptom/Unspecified Codes

10. Includes Notes

This note appears immediately under a three character code title to further define, or give examples of, the content of the category.

11. Inclusion terms

List of terms is included under some codes. These terms are the conditions for which that code is to be used. The terms may be synonyms of the code title, or, in the case of "other specified" codes, the terms are a list of the various conditions assigned to that code. The inclusion terms are not necessarily exhaustive. Additional terms found only in the Alphabetic Index may also be assigned to a code.

12. Excludes Notes

The ICD-10-CM has two types of excludes notes. Each type of note has a different definition for use but they are all similar in that they indicate that codes excluded from each other are independent of each other.

a. Excludes1

A type 1 Excludes note is a pure excludes note. It means "NOT CODED HERE!" An Excludes1 note indicates that the code excluded should never be used at the same time as the code above the Excludes1 note. An Excludes1 is used when two conditions cannot occur together, such as a congenital form versus an acquired form of the same condition.

An exception to the Excludes1 definition is the circumstance when the two conditions are unrelated to each other. If it is not clear whether the

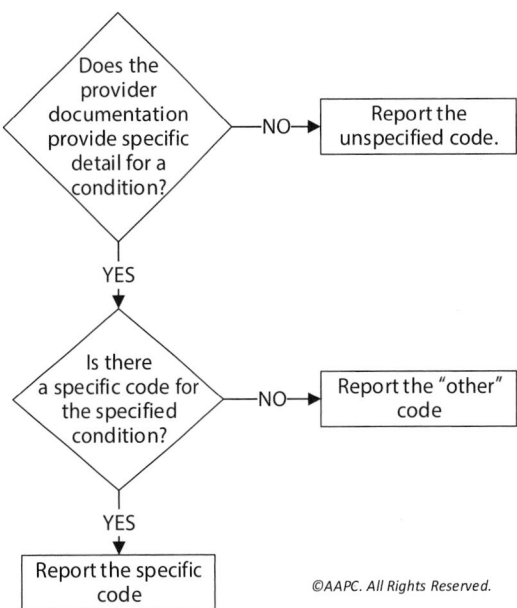

Figure I.A.9: Other and Unspecified codes

two conditions involving an Excludes1 note are related or not, query the provider. For example, code F45.8, Other somatoform disorders, has an Excludes1 note for "sleep related teeth grinding (G47.63)" because "teeth grinding" is an inclusion term under F45.8. Only one of these two codes should be assigned for teeth grinding. However psychogenic dysmenorrhea is also an inclusion term under F45.8, and a patient could have both this condition and sleep related teeth grinding. In this case, the two conditions are clearly unrelated to each other, and so it would be appropriate to report F45.8 and G47.63 together.

b. Excludes2

A type 2 Excludes note represents "Not included here." An excludes2 note indicates that the condition excluded is not part of the condition represented by the code, but a patient may have both conditions at the same time. When an Excludes2 note appears under a code, it is acceptable to use both the code and the excluded code together, when appropriate.

13. Etiology/manifestation convention ("code first", "use additional code" and "in diseases classified elsewhere" notes)

Certain conditions have both an underlying etiology and multiple body system manifestations due to the underlying etiology. For such conditions, the ICD-10-CM has a coding convention that requires the underlying condition be sequenced first, if applicable, followed by the manifestation. Wherever such a combination exists, there is a "use additional code" note at the etiology code, and a "code first" note at the manifestation code. These instructional notes indicate the proper sequencing order of the codes, etiology followed by manifestation.

In most cases the manifestation codes will have in the code title, "in diseases classified elsewhere." Codes with this title are a component of the etiology/manifestation convention. The code title indicates that it is a manifestation code. "In diseases classified elsewhere" codes are never permitted to be used as first-listed or principal diagnosis codes. They must be used in conjunction with an underlying condition code and they must be listed following the underlying condition. *See* category F02, Dementia in other diseases classified elsewhere, for an example of this convention.

There are manifestation codes that do not have "in diseases classified elsewhere" in the title. For such codes, there is a "use additional code" note at the etiology code and a "code first" note at the manifestation code, and the rules for sequencing apply.

In addition to the notes in the Tabular List, these conditions also have a specific Alphabetic Index entry structure. In the Alphabetic Index both conditions are listed together with the etiology code first followed by the manifestation codes in brackets. The code in brackets is always to be sequenced second.

An example of the etiology/manifestation convention is dementia in Parkinson's disease. In the Alphabetic Index, code G20 is listed first, followed by code F02.80 or F02.81 in brackets. Code G20 represents the underlying etiology, Parkinson's disease, and must be sequenced first, whereas code F02.80 and F02.81 represent the manifestation of dementia in diseases classified elsewhere, with or without behavioral disturbance.

"Code first" and "Use additional code" notes are also used as sequencing rules in the classification for certain codes that are not part of an etiology/manifestation combination.

See Section I.B.7. Multiple coding for a single condition.

14. "And"

The word "and" should be interpreted to mean either "and" or "or" when it appears in a title.

For example, cases of "tuberculosis of bones", "tuberculosis of joints" and "tuberculosis of bones and joints" are classified to subcategory A18.0, Tuberculosis of bones and joints.

15. "With"

The word "with" or "in" should be interpreted to mean "associated with" or "due to" when it appears in a code title, the Alphabetic Index (either under a main term or subterm), or an instructional note in the Tabular List. The classification presumes a causal relationship between the two conditions linked by these terms in the Alphabetic Index or Tabular List. These conditions should be coded as related even in the absence of provider documentation explicitly linking them, unless the documentation clearly states the conditions are unrelated or when another guideline exists that specifically requires a documented linkage between two conditions (e.g., sepsis guideline for "acute organ dysfunction that is not clearly associated with the sepsis").

For conditions not specifically linked by these relational terms in the classification or when a guideline requires that a linkage between two conditions be explicitly documented, provider documentation must link the conditions in order to code them as related.

The word "with" in the Alphabetic Index is sequenced immediately following the main term **or subterm,** not in alphabetical order.

16. "See" and "See Also"

The "*see*" instruction following a main term in the Alphabetic Index indicates that another term should be referenced. It is necessary to go to the main term referenced with the "*see*" note to locate the correct code.

A "*see also*" instruction following a main term in the Alphabetic Index instructs that there is another main term that may also be referenced that may provide additional Alphabetic Index entries that may be useful. It is not necessary to follow the "*see also*" note when the original main term provides the necessary code.

17. "Code also" note

A "code also" note instructs that two codes may be required to fully describe a condition, but this note does not provide sequencing direction. The sequencing depends on the circumstances of the encounter.

18. Default codes

A code listed next to a main term in the ICD-10-CM Alphabetic Index is referred to as a default code. The default code represents that condition that is most commonly associated with the main term, or is the unspecified code for the condition. If a condition is documented in a medical record (for example, appendicitis) without any additional information, such as acute or chronic, the default code should be assigned.

19. Code assignment and Clinical Criteria

The assignment of a diagnosis code is based on the provider's diagnostic statement that the condition exists. The provider's statement that the patient has a particular condition is sufficient. Code assignment is not based on clinical criteria used by the provider to establish the diagnosis.

B. General Coding Guidelines

1. Locating a code in the ICD-10-CM (*See* **Fig. I.B.1**)

To select a code in the classification that corresponds to a diagnosis or reason for visit documented in a medical record, first locate the term in the Alphabetic Index, and then verify the code in the Tabular List. Read and be guided by instructional notations that appear in both the Alphabetic Index and the Tabular List.

It is essential to use both the Alphabetic Index and Tabular List when locating and assigning a code. The Alphabetic Index does not always provide the full code. Selection of the full code, including laterality and any applicable 7th character can only be done in the Tabular List. A dash (-) at the end of an Alphabetic Index entry indicates that additional characters are required. Even if a dash is not included at the Alphabetic Index entry, it is necessary to refer to the Tabular List to verify that no 7th character is required.

2. Level of Detail in Coding

Diagnosis codes are to be used and reported at their highest number of characters available.

ICD-10-CM diagnosis codes are composed of codes with 3, 4, 5, 6 or 7 characters. Codes with three characters are included in ICD-10-CM as the heading of a category of codes that may be further subdivided by the use of fourth and/or fifth characters and/or sixth characters, which provide greater detail.

A three-character code is to be used only if it is not further subdivided.

A code is invalid if it has not been coded to the full number of characters required for that code, including the 7th character, if applicable.

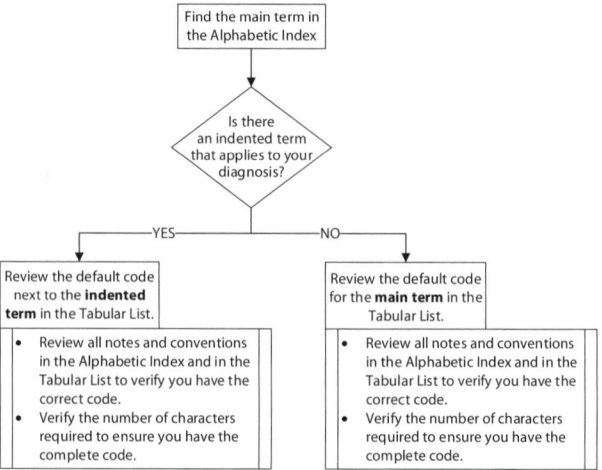

©AAPC. All Rights Reserved.

Figure I.B.1: Locating a code in the ICD-10-CM

3. Code or codes from A00.0 through T88.9, Z00-Z99.8

The appropriate code or codes from A00.0 through T88.9, Z00-Z99.8 must be used to identify diagnoses, symptoms, conditions, problems, complaints or other reason(s) for the encounter/visit.

4. Signs and symptoms

Codes that describe symptoms and signs, as opposed to diagnoses, are acceptable for reporting purposes when a related definitive diagnosis has not been established (confirmed) by the provider. Chapter 18 of ICD-10-CM, Symptoms, Signs, and Abnormal Clinical and Laboratory Findings, Not Elsewhere Classified (codes R00.0 - R99) contains many, but not all, codes for symptoms.

See Section I.B.18 Use of Signs/Symptom/Unspecified Codes

5. Conditions that are an integral part of a disease process

Signs and symptoms that are associated routinely with a disease process should not be assigned as additional codes, unless otherwise instructed by the classification.

6. Conditions that are not an integral part of a disease process

Additional signs and symptoms that may not be associated routinely with a disease process should be coded when present.

7. Multiple coding for a single condition

In addition to the etiology/manifestation convention that requires two codes to fully describe a single condition that affects multiple body systems, there are other single conditions that also require more than one code. "Use additional code" notes are found at codes that are not part of an etiology/manifestation pair where a secondary code is useful to fully describe a condition. The sequencing rule is the same as the etiology/manifestation pair, "use additional code" indicates that a secondary code should be added, if known.

For example, for bacterial infections that are not included in chapter 1, a secondary code from category B95, Streptococcus, Staphylococcus, and Enterococcus, as the cause of diseases classified elsewhere, or B96, Other bacterial agents as the cause of diseases classified elsewhere, may be required to identify the bacterial organism causing the infection. A "use additional code" note will normally be found at the infectious disease code, indicating a need for the organism code to be added as a secondary code.

"Code first" notes are also under certain codes that are not specifically manifestation codes but may be due to an underlying cause. When there is a "code first" note and an underlying condition is present, the underlying condition should be sequenced first, if known.

"Code, if applicable, any causal condition first" notes indicate that this code may be assigned as a principal diagnosis when the causal condition is unknown or not applicable. If a causal condition is known, then the code for that condition should be sequenced as the principal or first-listed diagnosis.

Multiple codes may be needed for sequela, complication codes and obstetric codes to more fully describe a condition. See the specific guidelines for these conditions for further instruction.

8. Acute and Chronic Conditions

If the same condition is described as both acute (subacute) and chronic, and separate subentries exist in the Alphabetic Index at the same indentation level, code both and sequence the acute (subacute) code first.

9. Combination Code

A combination code is a single code used to classify: Two diagnoses, or

A diagnosis with an associated secondary process (manifestation) A diagnosis with an associated complication

Combination codes are identified by referring to subterm entries in the Alphabetic Index and by reading the inclusion and exclusion notes in the Tabular List.

Assign only the combination code when that code fully identifies the diagnostic conditions involved or when the Alphabetic Index so directs. Multiple coding should not be used when the classification provides a combination code that clearly identifies all of the elements documented in the diagnosis. When the combination code lacks necessary specificity in describing the manifestation or complication, an additional code should be used as a secondary code.

10. Sequela (Late Effects)

A sequela is the residual effect (condition produced) after the acute phase of an illness or injury has terminated. There is no time limit on when a sequela code can be used. The residual may be apparent early, such as in cerebral infarction, or it may occur months or years later, such as that due to a previous injury.

Examples of sequela include: scar formation resulting from a burn, deviated septum due to a nasal fracture, and infertility due to tubal occlusion from old tuberculosis. Coding of sequela generally requires two codes sequenced in the following order: the condition or nature of the sequela is sequenced first. The sequela code is sequenced second.

An exception to the above guidelines are those instances where the code for the sequela is followed by a manifestation code identified in the Tabular List and title, or the sequela code has been expanded (at the fourth, fifth or sixth character levels) to include the manifestation(s). The code for the acute phase of an illness or injury that led to the sequela is never used with a code for the late effect.

See Section I.C.9. Sequelae of cerebrovascular disease

See Section I.C.15. Sequelae of complication of pregnancy, childbirth and the puerperium

See Section I.C.19. Application of 7th characters for Chapter 19

11. Impending or Threatened Condition (*See* **Fig. I.B.11**)

Code any condition described at the time of discharge as "impending" or "threatened" as follows:

If it did occur, code as confirmed diagnosis.

If it did not occur, reference the Alphabetic Index to determine if the condition has a subentry term for "impending" or "threatened" and also reference main term entries for "Impending" and for "Threatened."

If the subterms are listed, assign the given code.

If the subterms are not listed, code the existing underlying condition(s) and not the condition described as impending or threatened.

12. Reporting Same Diagnosis Code More than Once

Each unique ICD-10-CM diagnosis code may be reported only once for an encounter. This applies to bilateral conditions when there are no distinct codes identifying laterality or two different conditions classified to the same ICD-10-CM diagnosis code.

13. Laterality

Some ICD-10-CM codes indicate laterality, specifying whether the condition occurs on the left, right or is bilateral. If no bilateral code is provided and the condition is bilateral, assign separate codes for both the left and right

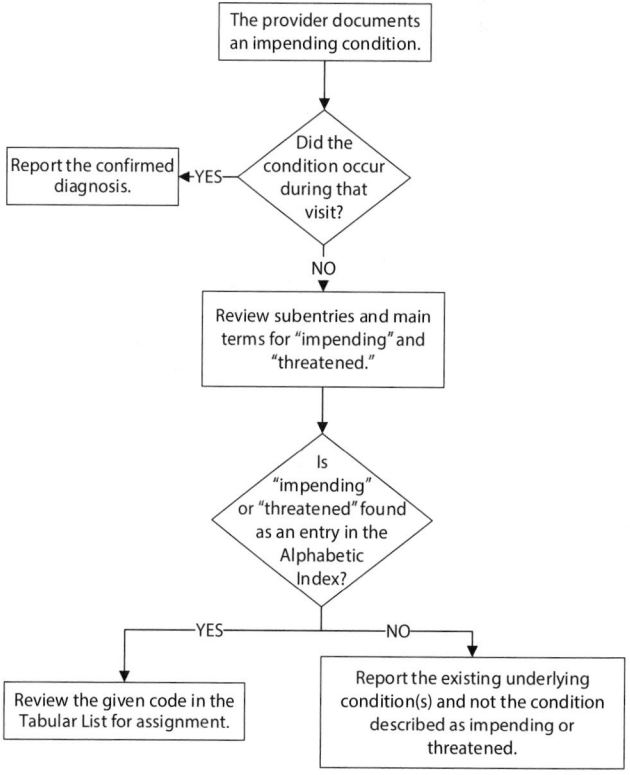

Figure I.B.11: Impending or Threatened Condition

side. If the side is not identified in the medical record, assign the code for the unspecified side.

When a patient has a bilateral condition and each side is treated during separate encounters, assign the "bilateral" code (as the condition still exists on both sides), including for the encounter to treat the first side. For the second encounter for treatment after one side has previously been treated and the condition no longer exists on that side, assign the appropriate unilateral code for the side where the condition still exists (e.g., cataract surgery performed on each eye in separate encounters). The bilateral code would not be assigned for the subsequent encounter, as the patient no longer has the condition in the previously-treated site. If the treatment on the first side did not completely resolve the condition, then the bilateral code would still be appropriate.

14. Documentation *by Clinicians Other than the Patient's Provider*

Code assignment is based on the documentation by patient's provider (i.e., physician or other qualified healthcare practitioner legally accountable for establishing the patient's diagnosis). There are a few exceptions, such as codes for the Body Mass Index (BMI), depth of non-pressure chronic ulcers, pressure ulcer stage, coma scale, and NIH stroke scale (NIHSS) codes, code assignment may be based on medical record documentation from clinicians who are not the patient's provider (i.e., physician or other qualified healthcare practitioner legally accountable for establishing the patient's diagnosis), since this information is typically documented by other clinicians involved in the care of the patient (e.g., a dietitian often documents the BMI, a nurse often documents the pressure ulcer stages, and an emergency medical technician often documents the coma scale). However, the associated diagnosis (such as overweight, obesity, acute stroke, or pressure ulcer) must be documented by the patient's provider. If there is conflicting medical record documentation, either from the same clinician or different clinicians, the patient's attending provider should be queried for clarification.

For social determinants of health, such as information found in categories Z55-Z65, Persons with potential health hazards related to socioeconomic and psychosocial circumstances, code assignment may be based on medical record documentation from clinicians involved in the care of the patient who are not the patient's provider since this information represents social information, rather than medical diagnoses.

The BMI, coma scale, NIHSS codes and categories Z55-Z65 should only be reported as secondary diagnoses.

15. Syndromes

Follow the Alphabetic Index guidance when coding syndromes. In the absence of Alphabetic Index guidance, assign codes for the documented manifestations of the syndrome. Additional codes for manifestations that are not an integral part of the disease process may also be assigned when the condition does not have a unique code.

16. Documentation of Complications of Care

Code assignment is based on the provider's documentation of the relationship between the condition and the care or procedure, unless otherwise instructed by the classification. The guideline extends to any complications of care, regardless of the chapter the code is located in. It is important to note that not all conditions that occur during or following medical care or surgery are classified as complications. There must be a cause-and-effect relationship between the care provided and the condition, and an indication in the documentation that it is a complication. Query the provider for clarification, if the complication is not clearly documented.

17. Borderline Diagnosis

If the provider documents a "borderline" diagnosis at the time of discharge, the diagnosis is coded as confirmed, unless the classification provides a specific entry (e.g., borderline diabetes). If a borderline condition has a specific index entry in ICD-10-CM, it should be coded as such. Since borderline conditions are not uncertain diagnoses, no distinction is made between the care setting (inpatient versus outpatient). Whenever the documentation is unclear regarding a borderline condition, coders are encouraged to query for clarification.

18. Use of Sign/Symptom/Unspecified Codes

Sign/symptom and "unspecified" codes have acceptable, even necessary, uses. While specific diagnosis codes should be reported when they are supported by the available medical record documentation and clinical knowledge of the patient's health condition, there are instances when signs/symptoms or unspecified codes are the best choices for accurately reflecting the healthcare encounter. Each healthcare encounter should be coded to the level of certainty known for that encounter.

If a definitive diagnosis has not been established by the end of the encounter, it is appropriate to report codes for sign(s) and/or symptom(s) in lieu of a definitive diagnosis. When sufficient clinical information isn't known or available about a particular health condition to assign a more specific code, it is acceptable to report the appropriate "unspecified" code (e.g., a diagnosis of pneumonia has been determined, but not the specific type). Unspecified codes should be reported when they are the codes that most accurately reflect what is known about the patient's condition at the time of that

particular encounter. It would be inappropriate to select a specific code that is not supported by the medical record documentation or conduct medically unnecessary diagnostic testing in order to determine a more specific code.

19. Coding for Healthcare Encounters in Hurricane Aftermath

a. Use of External Cause of Morbidity Codes

An external cause of morbidity code should be assigned to identify the cause of the injury (ies) incurred as a result of the hurricane. The use of external cause of morbidity codes is supplemental to the application of ICD-10-CM codes. External cause of morbidity codes are never to be recorded as a principal diagnosis (first-listed in non-inpatient settings). The appropriate injury code should be sequenced before any external cause codes. The external cause of morbidity codes capture how the injury or health condition happened (cause), the intent (unintentional or accidental; or intentional, such as suicide or assault), the place where the event occurred, the activity of the patient at the time of the event, and the person's status (e.g., civilian, military). They should not be assigned for encounters to treat hurricane victims' medical conditions when no injury, adverse effect or poisoning is involved.

External cause of morbidity codes should be assigned for each encounter for care and treatment of the injury. External cause of morbidity codes may be assigned in all health care settings. For the purpose of capturing complete and accurate ICD-10-CM data in the aftermath of the hurricane, a healthcare setting should be considered as any location where medical care is provided by licensed healthcare professionals.

b. Sequencing of External Causes of Morbidity Codes

Codes for cataclysmic events, such as a hurricane, take priority over all other external cause codes except child and adult abuse and terrorism and should be sequenced before other external cause of injury codes. Assign as many external cause of morbidity codes as necessary to fully explain each cause. For example, if an injury occurs as a result of a building collapse during the hurricane, external cause codes for both the hurricane and the building collapse should be assigned, with the external causes code for hurricane being sequenced as the first external cause code. For injuries incurred as a direct result of the hurricane, assign the appropriate code(s) for the injuries, followed by the code X37.0-, Hurricane (with the appropriate 7th character), and any other applicable external cause of injury codes.

Code X37.0- also should be assigned when an injury is incurred as a result of flooding caused by a levee breaking related to the hurricane. Code X38.-, Flood (with the appropriate 7th character), should be assigned when an injury is from flooding resulting directly from the storm. Code X36.0.-, Collapse of dam or man-made structure, should not be assigned when the cause of the collapse is due to the hurricane. Use of code X36.0- is limited to collapses of man-made structures due to earth surface movements, not due to storm surges directly from a hurricane.

c. Other External Causes of Morbidity Code Issues

For injuries that are not a direct result of the hurricane, such as an evacuee that has incurred an injury as a result of a motor vehicle accident, assign the appropriate external cause of morbidity code(s) to describe the cause of the injury, but do not assign code X37.0-, Hurricane. If it is not clear whether the injury was a direct result of the hurricane, assume the injury is due to the hurricane and assign code X37.0-, Hurricane, as well as any other applicable external cause of morbidity codes. In addition to code X37.0-, Hurricane, other possible applicable external cause of morbidity codes include:

> W54.0-, Bitten by dog
>
> X30-, Exposure to excessive natural heat
>
> X31-, Exposure to excessive natural cold X38-, Flood

d. Use of Z codes

Z codes (other reasons for healthcare encounters) may be assigned as appropriate to further explain the reasons for presenting for healthcare services, including transfers between healthcare facilities. The ICD-10-CM Official Guidelines for Coding and Reporting identify which codes maybe assigned as principal or first-listed diagnosis only, secondary diagnosis only, or principal/first-listed or secondary (depending on the circumstances). Possible applicable Z codes include:

> Z59.0, Homelessness Z59.1, Inadequate housing Z59.5, Extreme poverty
>
> Z75.1, Person awaiting admission to adequate facility elsewhere
>
> Z75.3, Unavailability and inaccessibility of healthcare facilities
>
> Z75.4, Unavailability and inaccessibility of other helping agencies
>
> Z76.2, Encounter for health supervision and care of other healthy infant and child
>
> Z99.12, Encounter for respirator [ventilator] dependence during power failure

The external cause of morbidity codes and the Z codes listed above are not an all-inclusive list. Other codes may be applicable to the encounter based upon the documentation. Assign as many codes as necessary to fully explain each healthcare encounter. Since patient history information may be very limited, use any available documentation to assign the appropriate external cause of morbidity and Z codes.

C. Chapter-Specific Coding Guidelines

In addition to general coding guidelines, there are guidelines for specific diagnoses and/or conditions in the classification. Unless otherwise indicated, these guidelines apply to all health care settings. Please refer to Section II for guidelines on the selection of principal diagnosis.

1. Chapter 1: Certain Infectious and Parasitic Diseases (A00-B99)

a. Human Immunodeficiency Virus (HIV) Infections

1) Code only confirmed cases

Code only confirmed cases of HIV infection/illness. This is an exception to the hospital inpatient guideline Section II, H.

In this context, "confirmation" does not require documentation of positive serology or culture for HIV; the provider's diagnostic statement that the patient is HIV positive, or has an HIV-related illness is sufficient.

2) Selection and sequencing of HIV codes

(a) **Patient admitted for HIV-related condition**

If a patient is admitted for an HIV-related condition, the principal diagnosis should be B20, Human immunodeficiency virus [HIV] disease followed by additional diagnosis codes for all reported HIV-related conditions.

(b) **Patient with HIV disease admitted for unrelated condition**

If a patient with HIV disease is admitted for an unrelated condition (such as a traumatic injury), the code for the unrelated condition (e.g., the nature of injury code) should be the principal diagnosis. Other diagnoses would be B20 followed by additional diagnosis codes for all reported HIV-related conditions.

(c) **Whether the patient is newly diagnosed**

Whether the patient is newly diagnosed or has had previous admissions/encounters for HIV conditions is irrelevant to the sequencing decision.

(d) **Asymptomatic human immunodeficiency virus** (*See* **Fig. I.C.1.a.2.d**)

Z21, Asymptomatic human immunodeficiency virus [HIV] infection status, is to be applied when the patient without any documentation of symptoms is listed as being "HIV positive", "known HIV", "HIV test positive", or similar terminology. Do not use this code if the term "AIDS" is used or if the patient is treated for any HIV-related illness or is described as having any condition(s) resulting from his/her HIV positive status; use B20 in these cases.

(e) **Patients with inconclusive HIV serology**

Patients with inconclusive HIV serology, but no definitive diagnosis or manifestations of the illness, may be assigned code R75, Inconclusive laboratory evidence of human immunodeficiency virus [HIV].

(f) **Previously diagnosed HIV-related illness**

Patients with any known prior diagnosis of an

HIV-related illness should be coded to B20. Once a patient has developed an HIV-related illness, the patient should always be assigned code B20 on every subsequent admission/encounter. Patients previously diagnosed with any HIV illness (B20) should never be assigned to R75 or Z21, Asymptomatic human immunodeficiency virus [HIV] infection status.

(g) **HIV Infection in Pregnancy, Childbirth and the Puerperium**

During pregnancy, childbirth or the puerperium, a patient admitted (or presenting for a health care encounter) because of an HIV-related illness should receive a principal diagnosis code of O98.7-, Human immunodeficiency [HIV] disease complicating pregnancy, childbirth and the puerperium, followed by B20 and the code(s) for the HIV-related illness(es).

Codes from Chapter 15 always take sequencing priority.

Patients with asymptomatic HIV infection status admitted (or presenting for a health care encounter) during pregnancy, childbirth, or the puerperium should receive codes of O98.7- and Z21.

(h) **Encounters for testing for HIV**

If a patient is being seen to determine his/her HIV status, use code Z11.4, Encounter for screening for human immunodeficiency virus [HIV]. Use additional codes for any associated high risk behavior.

If a patient with signs or symptoms is being seen for HIV testing, code the signs and symptoms. An additional counseling code Z71.7, Human immunodeficiency virus [HIV] counseling, may be used if counseling is provided during the encounter for the test.

When a patient returns to be informed of his/her HIV test results and the test result is negative, use code Z71.7, Human immunodeficiency virus [HIV] counseling.

If the results are positive, see previous guidelines and assign codes as appropriate.

b. Infectious agents as the cause of diseases classified to other chapters

Certain infections are classified in chapters other than Chapter 1 and no organism is identified as part of the infection code. In these instances, it is necessary to use an additional code from Chapter 1 to identify the organism. A code from category B95, Streptococcus, Staphylococcus, and Enterococcus as the cause of diseases classified to other chapters, B96, Other bacterial agents as the cause of diseases classified to other chapters, or B97, Viral agents as the cause of diseases classified to other chapters, is to be used as an additional code to identify the organism. An instructional note will be found at the infection code advising that an additional organism code is required.

c. Infections resistant to antibiotics

Many bacterial infections are resistant to current antibiotics. It is necessary to identify all infections documented as antibiotic resistant. Assign a code from category Z16, Resistance to antimicrobial drugs, following the infection code only if the infection code does not identify drug resistance.

d. Sepsis, Severe Sepsis, and Septic Shock (*See* **Fig. 1.C.1.d**)

1) Coding of Sepsis and Severe Sepsis

(a) **Sepsis**

For a diagnosis of sepsis, assign the appropriate code for the underlying systemic infection. If the type of infection or causal organism is not further specified, assign code A41.9, Sepsis, unspecified organism.

A code from subcategory R65.2, Severe sepsis, should not be assigned unless severe sepsis or an associated acute organ dysfunction is documented.

(i) **Negative or inconclusive blood cultures and sepsis**

Negative or inconclusive blood cultures do not preclude a diagnosis of sepsis in patients with clinical evidence of the condition; however, the provider should be queried.

(ii) **Urosepsis**

The term urosepsis is a nonspecific term. It is not to be considered synonymous with sepsis. It has no default code in the Alphabetic Index.

Should a provider use this term, he/she must be queried for clarification.

(iii) **Sepsis with organ dysfunction**

If a patient has sepsis and associated acute organ dysfunction or multiple organ dysfunction (MOD), follow the instructions for coding severe sepsis.

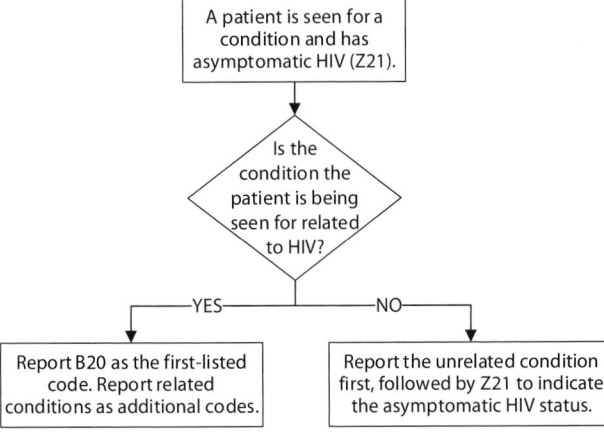

A patient is seen for a condition and has asymptomatic HIV (Z21).

Is the condition the patient is being seen for related to HIV?

YES → Report B20 as the first-listed code. Report related conditions as additional codes.

NO → Report the unrelated condition first, followed by Z21 to indicate the asymptomatic HIV status.

Figure I.C.1.a.2.d: Asymptomatic human immunodeficiency virus

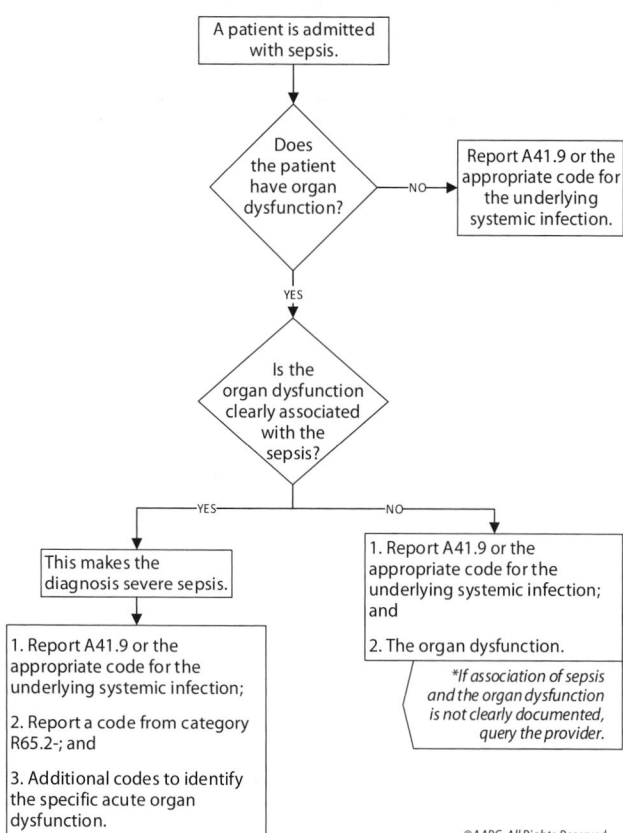

Figure I.C.1.d: Sepsis, Severe Sepsis, and Septic Shock

(iv) Acute organ dysfunction that is not clearly associated with the sepsis

If a patient has sepsis and an acute organ dysfunction, but the medical record documentation indicates that the acute organ dysfunction is related to a medical condition other than the sepsis, do not assign a code from subcategory R65.2, Severe sepsis. An acute organ dysfunction must be associated with the sepsis in order to assign the severe sepsis code. If the documentation is not clear as to whether an acute organ dysfunction is related to the sepsis or another medical condition, query the provider.

(b) Severe sepsis

The coding of severe sepsis requires a minimum of 2 codes: first a code for the underlying systemic infection, followed by a code from subcategory R65.2, Severe sepsis. If the causal organism is not documented, assign code A41.9, Sepsis, unspecified organism, for the infection. Additional code(s) for the associated acute organ dysfunction are also required.

Due to the complex nature of severe sepsis, some cases may require querying the provider prior to assignment of the codes.

2) Septic shock

(a) Septic shock generally refers to circulatory failure associated with severe sepsis, and therefore, it represents a type of acute organ dysfunction.

For cases of septic shock, the code for the systemic infection should be sequenced first, followed by code R65.21, Severe sepsis with septic shock or code T81.12, Postprocedural septic shock. Any additional codes for the other acute organ dysfunctions should also be assigned. As noted in the sequencing instructions in the Tabular List, the code for septic shock cannot be assigned as a principal diagnosis.

3) Sequencing of severe sepsis

If severe sepsis is present on admission, and meets the definition of principal diagnosis, the underlying systemic infection should be assigned as principal diagnosis followed by the appropriate code from subcategory R65.2 as required by the sequencing rules in the Tabular List. A code from subcategory R65.2 can never be assigned as a principal diagnosis.

When severe sepsis develops during an encounter (it was not present on admission), the underlying systemic infection and the appropriate code from subcategory R65.2 should be assigned as secondary diagnoses.

Severe sepsis may be present on admission, but the diagnosis may not be confirmed until sometime after admission. If the documentation is not clear whether severe sepsis was present on admission, the provider should be queried.

4) Sepsis *or* severe sepsis with a localized infection

If the reason for admission is sepsis or severe sepsis and a localized infection, such as pneumonia or cellulitis, a code(s) for the underlying systemic infection should be assigned first and the code for the localized infection should be assigned as a secondary diagnosis. If the patient has severe sepsis, a code from subcategory R65.2 should also be assigned as a secondary diagnosis. If the patient is admitted with a localized infection, such as pneumonia, and sepsis/severe sepsis doesn't develop until after admission, the localized infection should be assigned first, followed by the appropriate sepsis/severe sepsis codes.

5) Sepsis due to a postprocedural infection

(a) Documentation of causal relationship

As with all postprocedural complications, code assignment is based on the provider's documentation of the relationship between the infection and the procedure.

(b) Sepsis due to a postprocedural infection

For infections following a procedure, a code from T81.40, to T81.43 Infection following a procedure, or a code from O86.00 to O86.03, Infection of obstetric surgical wound, that identifies the site of the infection should be coded first, if known. Assign an additional code for sepsis following a procedure (T81.44) or sepsis following an obstetrical procedure (O86.04). Use an additional code to identify the infectious agent. If the patient has severe sepsis, the appropriate code from subcategory R65.2 should also be assigned with the additional code(s) for any acute organ dysfunction.

For infections following infusion, transfusion, therapeutic injection, or immunization, a code from subcategory T80.2, Infections following infusion, transfusion, and therapeutic injection, or code T88.0-, Infection following immunization, should be coded first, followed by the code for the specific infection. If the patient has severe sepsis, the appropriate code from subcategory R65.2 should also be assigned, with the additional codes(s) for any acute organ dysfunction.

(c) Postprocedural infection and postprocedural septic shock

If a postprocedural infection has resulted in postprocedural septic shock, assign the codes indicated above for sepsis due to a postprocedural infection, followed by code T81.12-, Postprocedural septic shock. Do not assign code R65.21, Severe sepsis with septic shock. Additional code(s) should be assigned for any acute organ dysfunction.

6) Sepsis and severe sepsis associated with a noninfectious process (condition)

In some cases a noninfectious process (condition), such as trauma, may lead to an infection which can result in sepsis or severe sepsis. If sepsis or severe sepsis is documented as associated with a noninfectious condition, such as a burn or serious injury, and this condition meets the definition for principal diagnosis, the code for the noninfectious condition should be sequenced first, followed by the code for the resulting infection. If severe sepsis is present, a code from subcategory R65.2 should also be assigned with any associated organ dysfunction(s) codes. It is not necessary to assign a code from subcategory R65.1, Systemic inflammatory response syndrome (SIRS) of non-infectious origin, for these cases.

If the infection meets the definition of principal diagnosis, it should be sequenced before the non-infectious condition. When both the associated non-infectious condition and the infection meet the definition of principal diagnosis, either may be assigned as principal diagnosis.

Only one code from category R65, symptoms and signs specifically associated with systemic inflammation and infection, should be assigned. Therefore, when a non-infectious condition leads to an infection resulting in severe sepsis, assign the appropriate code from subcategory R65.2, Severe sepsis. Do not additionally assign a code from subcategory R65.1, Systemic inflammatory response syndrome (SIRS) of non- infectious origin.

See Section I.C.18. SIRS due to non-infectious process

7) Sepsis and septic shock complicating abortion, pregnancy, childbirth, and the puerperium

See Section I.C.15. Sepsis and septic shock complicating abortion, pregnancy, childbirth and the puerperium

8) Newborn sepsis

See Section I.C.16. f. Bacterial sepsis of Newborn

e. Methicillin Resistant Staphylococcus aureus (MRSA) Conditions

1) Selection and sequencing of MRSA codes

(a) Combination codes for MRSA infection

When a patient is diagnosed with an infection that is due to methicillin resistant Staphylococcus aureus (MRSA), and that infection has a combination code that includes the causal organism (e.g., sepsis, pneumonia) assign the appropriate combination code for the condition (e.g., code A41.02, Sepsis due to Methicillin resistant Staphylococcus aureus or code J15.212, Pneumonia due to Methicillin resistant Staphylococcus aureus). Do not assign code B95.62, Methicillin resistant Staphylococcus aureus infection as the cause of diseases classified elsewhere, as an additional code, because the combination code includes the type of infection and the MRSA organism. Do not assign a code from subcategory Z16.11, Resistance to penicillins, as an additional diagnosis.

See Section C.1. for instructions on coding and sequencing of sepsis and severe sepsis.

(b) Other codes for MRSA infection

When there is documentation of a current infection (e.g., wound infection, stitch abscess, urinary tract infection) due to MRSA, and that infection does not have a combination code that includes the causal organism, assign the appropriate code to identify the condition along with code B95.62, Methicillin resistant Staphylococcus aureus infection as the cause of diseases classified elsewhere for the MRSA infection. Do not assign a code from subcategory Z16.11, Resistance to penicillins.

(c) Methicillin susceptible Staphylococcus aureus (MSSA) and MRSA colonization

The condition or state of being colonized or carrying MSSA or MRSA is called colonization or carriage, while an individual person is described as being colonized or being a carrier.

Colonization means that MSSA or MSRA is present on or in the body without necessarily causing illness. A positive MRSA colonization test might be documented by the provider as "MRSA screen positive" or "MRSA nasal swab positive".

Assign code Z22.322, Carrier or suspected carrier of Methicillin resistant Staphylococcus aureus, for patients documented as having MRSA colonization. Assign code Z22.321, Carrier or suspected carrier of Methicillin susceptible Staphylococcus aureus, for patients documented as having MSSA colonization. Colonization is not necessarily indicative of a disease process or as the cause of a specific condition the patient may have unless documented as such by the provider.

(d) MRSA colonization and infection

If a patient is documented as having both MRSA colonization and infection during a hospital admission, code Z22.322, Carrier or suspected carrier of Methicillin resistant Staphylococcus aureus, and a code for the MRSA infection may both be assigned.

f. Zika virus infections

1) Code only confirmed cases

Code only a confirmed diagnosis of Zika virus (A92.5, Zika virus disease) as documented by the provider. This is an exception to the hospital inpatient guideline Section II, H. In this context, "confirmation" does not require documentation of the type of test performed; the **provider's** diagnostic statement that the condition is confirmed is sufficient. This code should be assigned regardless of the stated mode of transmission.

If the provider documents "suspected", "possible" or "probable" Zika, do not assign code A92.5. Assign a code(s) explaining the reason for encounter (such as fever, rash, or joint pain) or Z20.821, Contact with and (suspected) exposure to Zika virus.

2. Chapter 2: Neoplasms (C00-D49)

General guidelines

Chapter 2 of the ICD-10-CM contains the codes for most benign and all malignant neoplasms. Certain benign neoplasms, such as prostatic adenomas, may be found in the specific body system chapters. To properly code a neoplasm it is necessary to determine from the record if the neoplasm is benign, in-situ, malignant, or of uncertain histologic behavior. If malignant, any secondary (metastatic) sites should also be determined.

Primary malignant neoplasms overlapping site boundaries

A primary malignant neoplasm that overlaps two or more contiguous (next to each other) sites should be classified to the subcategory/code .8 ('overlapping lesion'), unless the combination is specifically indexed elsewhere. For multiple neoplasms of the same site that are not contiguous such as tumors in different quadrants of the same breast, codes for each site should be assigned.

Malignant neoplasm of ectopic tissue

Malignant neoplasms of ectopic tissue are to be coded to the site of origin mentioned, e.g., ectopic pancreatic malignant neoplasms involving the stomach are coded to malignant neoplasm of pancreas, unspecified (C25.9).

The neoplasm table in the Alphabetic Index should be referenced first. However, if the histological term is documented, that term should be referenced first, rather than going immediately to the Neoplasm Table, in order to determine which column in the Neoplasm Table is appropriate. For example, if the documentation indicates "adenoma," refer to the term in the Alphabetic Index to review the entries under this term and the instructional note to "see also neoplasm, by site, benign." The table provides the proper code based on the type of neoplasm and the site. It is important to select the proper column in the table that corresponds to the type of neoplasm. The Tabular List should then be referenced to verify that the correct code has been selected from the table and that a more specific site code does not exist.

See Section I.C.21. Factors influencing health status and contact with health services, Status, for information regarding Z15.0, codes for genetic susceptibility to cancer.

a. Treatment directed at the malignancy

If the treatment is directed at the malignancy, designate the malignancy as the principal diagnosis.

The only exception to this guideline is if a patient admission/encounter is solely for the administration of chemotherapy, immunotherapy or external beam radiation therapy, assign the appropriate Z51.- code as the first-listed or principal diagnosis, and the diagnosis or problem for which the service is being performed as a secondary diagnosis.

b. Treatment of secondary site

When a patient is admitted because of a primary neoplasm with metastasis and treatment is directed toward the secondary site only, the secondary neoplasm is designated as the principal diagnosis even though the primary malignancy is still present.

c. Coding and sequencing of complications (*See* **Table I.C.2.c.i**)

Coding and sequencing of complications associated with the malignancies or with the therapy thereof are subject to the following guidelines:

1) Anemia associated with malignancy

When admission/encounter is for management of an anemia associated with the malignancy, and the treatment is only for anemia, the appropriate code for the malignancy is sequenced as the principal or first-listed diagnosis followed by the appropriate code for the anemia (such as code D63.0, Anemia in neoplastic disease).

Table I.C.2.c.i: Coding and sequencing of complications

Reason for Encounter	Sequencing
Treatment of primary malignancy	1. Primary site 2. Metastatic sites
Treatment of secondary malignancy	1. Metastatic site(s) 2. Primary site
Malignant neoplasm in a pregnant patient	1. A code from subcategory 09A.1- 2. Neoplasm code(s)
Complication (except anemia) associated with neoplasm, treatment is only for the complication	1. Complication 2. Neoplasm code(s)
Anemia associated with neoplasm, treatment is only for anemia	1. Neoplasm code(s) 2. D63.0, Anemia in neoplastic disease
Complication from a surgical procedure for treatment of a neoplasm	1. Complication 2. Current neoplasm code(s) or personal history of malignancy (See I.C.2.m)
Pathologic fracture due to a neoplasm, focus of treatment is the fracture	1. M84.5- Pathological fracture in neoplastic disease 2. Neoplasm code(s)
Pathologic fracture due to a neoplasm, focus of treatment is the neoplasm	1. Neoplasm code(s) 2. M84.5- Pathological fracture in neoplastic disease

2) Anemia associated with chemotherapy, immunotherapy and radiation therapy

When the admission/encounter is for management of an anemia associated with an adverse effect of the administration of chemotherapy or immunotherapy and the only treatment is for the anemia, the anemia code is sequenced first followed by the appropriate codes for the neoplasm and the adverse effect (T45.1X5-, Adverse effect of antineoplastic and immunosuppressive drugs).

When the admission/encounter is for management of an anemia associated with an adverse effect of radiotherapy, the anemia code should be sequenced first, followed by the appropriate neoplasm code and code Y84.2, Radiological procedure and radiotherapy as the cause of abnormal reaction of the patient, or of later complication, without mention of misadventure at the time of the procedure.

3) Management of dehydration due to the malignancy

When the admission/encounter is for management of dehydration due to the malignancy and only the dehydration is being treated (intravenous rehydration), the dehydration is sequenced first, followed by the code(s) for the malignancy.

4) Treatment of a complication resulting from a surgical procedure

When the admission/encounter is for treatment of a complication resulting from a surgical procedure, designate the complication as the principal or first-listed diagnosis if treatment is directed at resolving the complication.

d. Primary malignancy previously excised

When a primary malignancy has been previously excised or eradicated from its site and there is no further treatment directed to that site and there is no evidence of any existing primary malignancy at that site, a code from category Z85, Personal history of malignant neoplasm, should be used to indicate the former site of the malignancy. Any mention of extension, invasion, or metastasis to another site is coded as a secondary malignant neoplasm to that site. The secondary site may be the principal or first-listed **diagnosis** with the Z85 code used as a secondary code.

e. Admissions/Encounters involving chemotherapy, immunotherapy and radiation therapy

1) Episode of care involves surgical removal of neoplasm

When an episode of care involves the surgical removal of a neoplasm, primary or secondary site, followed by adjunct chemotherapy or radiation treatment during the same episode of care, the code for the neoplasm should be assigned as principal or first-listed diagnosis.

2) Patient admission/encounter solely for administration of chemotherapy, immunotherapy and radiation therapy

If a patient admission/encounter is solely for the administration of chemotherapy, immunotherapy or external beam radiation therapy assign code Z51.0, Encounter for antineoplastic radiation therapy, or Z51.11, Encounter for antineoplastic chemotherapy, or Z51.12, Encounter for antineoplastic immunotherapy as the first-listed or principal diagnosis. If a patient receives more than one of these therapies during the same admission more than one of these codes may be assigned, in any sequence.

The malignancy for which the therapy is being administered should be assigned as a secondary diagnosis.

If a patient admission/encounter is for the insertion or implantation of radioactive elements (e.g., brachytherapy) the appropriate code for the malignancy is sequenced as the principal or first-listed diagnosis. Code Z51.0 should not be assigned.

3) Patient admitted for radiation therapy, chemotherapy or immunotherapy and develops complications

When a patient is admitted for the purpose of external beam radiotherapy, immunotherapy or chemotherapy and develops complications such as uncontrolled nausea and vomiting or dehydration, the principal or first-listed diagnosis is Z51.0, Encounter for antineoplastic radiation therapy, or Z51.11, Encounter for antineoplastic chemotherapy, or Z51.12,

Encounter for antineoplastic immunotherapy followed by any codes for the complications.

When a patient is admitted for the purpose of insertion or implantation of radioactive elements (e.g., brachytherapy) and develops complications such as uncontrolled nausea and vomiting or dehydration, the principal or first-listed diagnosis is the appropriate code for the malignancy followed by any codes for the complications.

f. Admission/encounter to determine extent of malignancy

When the reason for admission/encounter is to determine the extent of the malignancy, or for a procedure such as paracentesis or thoracentesis, the primary malignancy or appropriate metastatic site is designated as the principal or first-listed diagnosis, even though chemotherapy or radiotherapy is administered.

g. Symptoms, signs, and abnormal findings listed in Chapter 18 associated with neoplasms

Symptoms, signs, and ill-defined conditions listed in Chapter 18 characteristic of, or associated with, an existing primary or secondary site malignancy cannot be used to replace the malignancy as principal or first-listed diagnosis, regardless of the number of admissions or encounters for treatment and care of the neoplasm.

See section I.C.21. Factors influencing health status and contact with health services, Encounter for prophylactic organ removal.

h. Admission/encounter for pain control/management

See Section I.C.6. for information on coding admission/encounter for pain control/management.

i. Malignancy in two or more noncontiguous sites

A patient may have more than one malignant tumor in the same organ. These tumors may represent different primaries or metastatic disease, depending on the site. Should the documentation be unclear, the provider should be queried as to the status of each tumor so that the correct codes can be assigned.

j. Disseminated malignant neoplasm, unspecified

Code C80.0, Disseminated malignant neoplasm, unspecified, is for use only in those cases where the patient has advanced metastatic disease and no known primary or secondary sites are specified. It should not be used in place of assigning codes for the primary site and all known secondary sites.

k. Malignant neoplasm without specification of site

Code C80.1, Malignant (primary) neoplasm, unspecified, equates to Cancer, unspecified. This code should only be used when no determination can be made as to the primary site of a malignancy. This code should rarely be used in the inpatient setting.

l. Sequencing of neoplasm codes

1) Encounter for treatment of primary malignancy

If the reason for the encounter is for treatment of a primary malignancy, assign the malignancy as the principal/first-listed diagnosis. The primary site is to be sequenced first, followed by any metastatic sites.

2) Encounter for treatment of secondary malignancy

When an encounter is for a primary malignancy with metastasis and treatment is directed toward the metastatic (secondary) site(s) only, the metastatic site(s) is designated as the principal/first-listed diagnosis. The primary malignancy is coded as an additional code.

3) Malignant neoplasm in a pregnant patient

When a pregnant woman has a malignant neoplasm, a code from subcategory O9A.1-, Malignant neoplasm complicating pregnancy, childbirth, and the puerperium, should be sequenced first, followed by the appropriate code from Chapter 2 to indicate the type of neoplasm.

4) Encounter for complication associated with a neoplasm

When an encounter is for management of a complication associated with a neoplasm, such as dehydration, and the treatment is only for the complication, the complication is coded first, followed by the appropriate code(s) for the neoplasm.

The exception to this guideline is anemia. When the admission/encounter is for management of an anemia associated with the malignancy, and the treatment is only for anemia, the appropriate code for the malignancy is sequenced as the principal or first-listed diagnosis followed by code D63.0, Anemia in neoplastic disease.

5) Complication from surgical procedure for treatment of a neoplasm

When an encounter is for treatment of a complication resulting from a surgical procedure performed for the treatment of the neoplasm, designate the complication as the principal/first-listed diagnosis. See **the** guideline regarding the coding of a current malignancy versus personal history to determine if the code for the neoplasm should also be assigned.

6) Pathologic fracture due to a neoplasm

When an encounter is for a pathological fracture due to a neoplasm, and the focus of treatment is the fracture, a code from subcategory M84.5, Pathological fracture in neoplastic disease, should be sequenced first, followed by the code for the neoplasm.

If the focus of treatment is the neoplasm with an associated pathological fracture, the neoplasm code should be sequenced first, followed by a code from M84.5 for the pathological fracture.

m. Current malignancy versus personal history of malignancy

When a primary malignancy has been excised but further treatment, such as an additional surgery for the malignancy, radiation therapy or

chemotherapy is directed to that site, the primary malignancy code should be used until treatment is completed.

When a primary malignancy has been previously excised or eradicated from its site, there is no further treatment (of the malignancy) directed to that site, and there is no evidence of any existing primary malignancy at that site, a code from category Z85, Personal history of malignant neoplasm, should be used to indicate the former site of the malignancy.

Subcategories Z85.0 – Z85.7 should only be assigned for the former site of a primary malignancy, not the site of a secondary malignancy. Codes from subcategory Z85.8-, may be assigned for the former site(s) of either a primary or secondary malignancy included in this subcategory.

See Section I.C.21. Factors influencing health status and contact with health services, History (of)

n. Leukemia, Multiple Myeloma, and Malignant Plasma Cell Neoplasms in remission versus personal history

The categories for leukemia, and category C90, Multiple myeloma and malignant plasma cell neoplasms, have codes indicating whether or not the leukemia has achieved remission. There are also codes Z85.6, Personal history of leukemia, and Z85.79, Personal history of other malignant neoplasms of lymphoid, hematopoietic and related tissues. If the documentation is unclear as to whether the leukemia has achieved remission, the provider should be queried.

See Section I.C.21. Factors influencing health status and contact with health services, History (of)

o. Aftercare following surgery for neoplasm

See Section I.C.21. Factors influencing health status and contact with health services, Aftercare

p. Follow-up care for completed treatment of a malignancy

See Section I.C.21. Factors influencing health status and contact with health services,Follow-up

q. Prophylactic organ removal for prevention of malignancy

See Section I.C. 21, Factors influencing health status and contact with health services, Prophylactic organ removal

r. Malignant neoplasm associated with transplanted organ

A malignant neoplasm of a transplanted organ should be coded as a transplant complication. Assign first the appropriate code from category T86.-, Complications of transplanted organs and tissue, followed by code C80.2, Malignant neoplasm associated with transplanted organ. Use an additional code for the specific malignancy.

3. Chapter 3: Disease of the blood and blood-forming organs and certain disorders involving the immune mechanism (D50-D89)

Reserved for future guideline expansion

4. Chapter 4: Endocrine, Nutritional, and Metabolic Diseases (E00-E89)

a. Diabetes mellitus (*See* Fig. I.C.4.a)

The diabetes mellitus codes are combination codes that include the type of diabetes mellitus, the body system affected, and the complications affecting that body system. As many codes within a particular category as are necessary to describe all of the complications of the disease may be used. They should be sequenced based on the reason for a particular encounter. Assign as many codes from categories E08 – E13 as needed to identify all of the associated conditions that the patient has.

1) Type of diabetes

The age of a patient is not the sole determining factor, though most type 1 diabetics develop the condition before reaching puberty. For this reason type 1 diabetes mellitus is also referred to as juvenile diabetes.

2) Type of diabetes mellitus not documented (*See* Fig. I.C.4.a.2)

If the type of diabetes mellitus is not documented in the medical record the default is E11.-, Type 2 diabetes mellitus.

3) Diabetes mellitus and the use of insulin and oral hypoglycemics

If the documentation in a medical record does not indicate the type of diabetes but does indicate that the patient uses insulin, code E11-, Type 2 diabetes mellitus, should be assigned. An additional code should be assigned from category Z79 to identify the long-term (current) use of insulin or oral hypoglycemic drugs. If the patient is treated with both oral medications and insulin, only the code for long-term (current) use of insulin should be assigned. Code Z79.4 should not be assigned if insulin is given temporarily to bring a type 2 patient's blood sugar under control during an encounter.

4) Diabetes mellitus in pregnancy and gestational diabetes

See Section I.C.15. Diabetes mellitus in pregnancy.

See Section I.C.15. Gestational (pregnancy induced) diabetes

5) Complications due to insulin pump malfunction

(a) Underdose of insulin due to insulin pump failure

An underdose of insulin due to an insulin pump failure should be assigned to a code from subcategory T85.6, Mechanical complication of other specified internal and external prosthetic devices, implants and grafts, that specifies the type of pump malfunction, as the principal or first-listed code, followed by code T38.3X6-, Underdosing of insulin and oral hypoglycemic [antidiabetic] drugs. Additional codes for the type of diabetes mellitus and any associated complications due to the underdosing should also be assigned.

(b) Overdose of insulin due to insulin pump failure

The principal or first-listed code for an encounter due to an insulin pump malfunction resulting in an overdose of insulin, should also be T85.6-, Mechanical complication of other specified internal and external prosthetic devices, implants and grafts, followed by code

T38.3X1-, Poisoning by insulin and oral hypoglycemic [antidiabetic] drugs, accidental (unintentional).

6) Secondary diabetes mellitus

Codes under categories E08, Diabetes mellitus due to underlying condition, E09, Drug or chemical induced diabetes mellitus, and E13, Other specified diabetes mellitus, identify complications/manifestations associated with secondary diabetes mellitus. Secondary diabetes is always caused by another condition or event (e.g., cystic fibrosis, malignant neoplasm of pancreas, pancreatectomy, adverse effect of drug, or poisoning).

(a) Secondary diabetes mellitus and the use of insulin or oral hypoglycemic drugs

For patients with secondary diabetes mellitus who routinely use insulin or oral hypoglycemic drugs, an additional code from category Z79 should be assigned to identify the long-term (current) use of insulin or oral hypoglycemic drugs. If the patient is treated with both oral medications and insulin, only the code for long-term (current) use of insulin should be assigned. Code Z79.4 should not be assigned if insulin is given temporarily to bring a secondary diabetic patient's blood sugar under control during an encounter.

(b) Assigning and sequencing secondary diabetes codes and its causes

The sequencing of the secondary diabetes codes in relationship to codes for the cause of the diabetes is based on the Tabular List instructions for categories E08, E09 and E13.

(i) Secondary diabetes mellitus due to pancreatectomy

For postpancreatectomy diabetes mellitus (lack of insulin due to the surgical removal of all or part of the pancreas), assign code E89.1, Postprocedural hypoinsulinemia. Assign a code from category E13 and a code from subcategory Z90.41, Acquired absence of pancreas, as additional codes.

(ii) Secondary diabetes due to drugs

Secondary diabetes may be caused by an adverse effect of correctly administered medications, poisoning or sequela of poisoning.

See section I.C.19.e for coding of adverse effects and poisoning, and section I.C.20 for external cause code reporting.

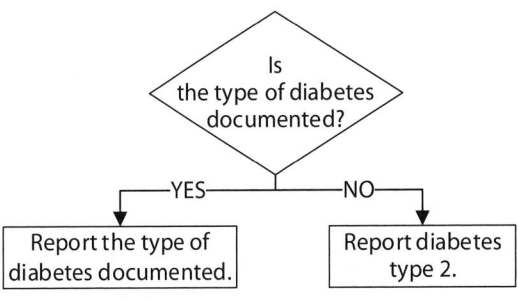

Is the type of diabetes documented?

─YES─ │ ─NO─

| Report the type of diabetes documented. | Report diabetes type 2. |

Figure I.C.4.a.2: Type of diabetes mellitus not documented

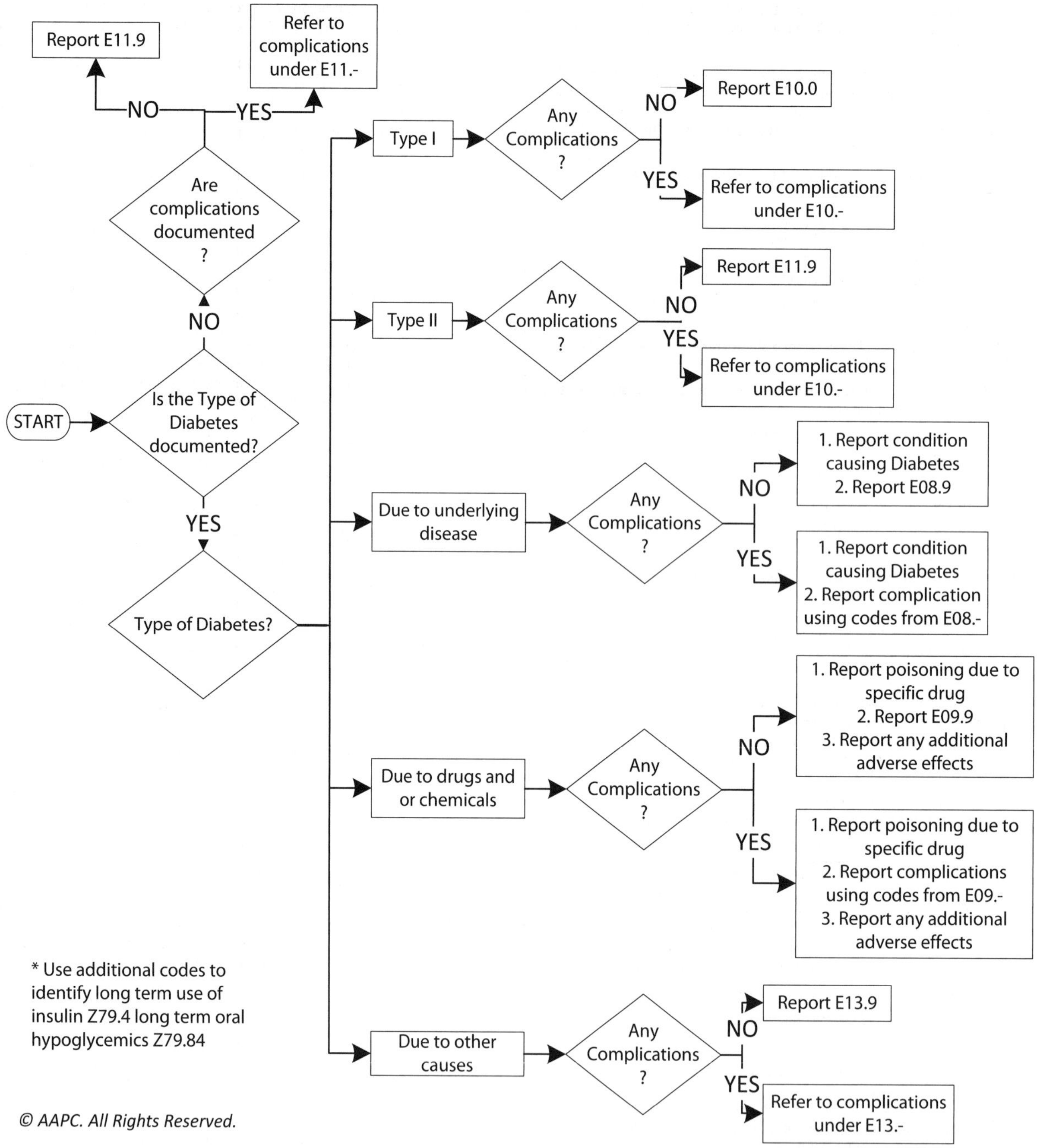

Report E11.9

Refer to complications under E11.-

NO — YES

Type I → Any Complications? — NO → Report E10.0

YES → Refer to complications under E10.-

Are complications documented?

NO

Type II → Any Complications? — NO → Report E11.9

YES → Refer to complications under E10.-

START → Is the Type of Diabetes documented?

YES

Due to underlying disease → Any Complications? — NO → 1. Report condition causing Diabetes 2. Report E08.9

YES → 1. Report condition causing Diabetes 2. Report complication using codes from E08.-

Type of Diabetes?

Due to drugs and or chemicals → Any Complications? — NO → 1. Report poisoning due to specific drug 2. Report E09.9 3. Report any additional adverse effects

YES → 1. Report poisoning due to specific drug 2. Report complications using codes from E09.- 3. Report any additional adverse effects

* Use additional codes to identify long term use of insulin Z79.4 long term oral hypoglycemics Z79.84

Due to other causes → Any Complications? — NO → Report E13.9

YES → Refer to complications under E13.-

Figure I.C.4.a: Diabetes Mellitus (DM)

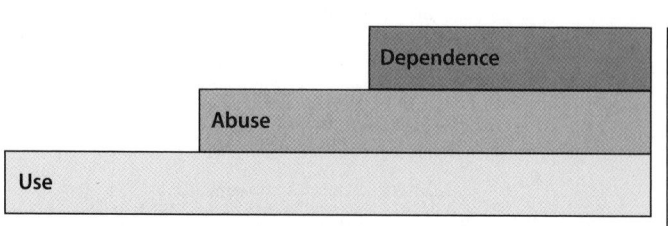

When provider documentation refers to use, abuse, and dependence of the same substance (e.g., alcohol, opioid, cannabis, etc.), only one code should be assigned to identify the pattern of use based on the highest step. Example: The provider documents tobacco use and abuse. Report only tobacco abuse. If alcohol use and dependence is documented, report alcohol dependence.

Figure I.C.5.b.2: Psychoactive Substance Use, Abuse and Dependence

5. **Chapter 5: Mental, Behavioral and Neurodevelopmental disorders (F01–F99)**

   a. **Pain disorders related to psychological factors**

   Assign code F45.41, for pain that is exclusively related to psychological disorders. As indicated by the Excludes 1 note under category G89, a code from category G89 should not be assigned with code F45.41.

   Code F45.42, Pain disorders with related psychological factors, should be used with a code from category G89, Pain, not elsewhere classified, if there is documentation of a psychological component for a patient with acute or chronic pain.

   See Section I.C.6. Pain

   b. **Mental and behavioral disorders due to psychoactive substance use**

   1) **In Remission**

   Selection of codes for "in remission" for categories F10-F19, Mental and behavioral disorders due to psychoactive substance use (categories F10-F19 with -.11, -.21) requires the provider's clinical judgment. The appropriate codes for "in remission" are assigned only

on the basis of provider documentation (as defined in the Official Guidelines for Coding and Reporting), unless otherwise instructed by the classification.

Mild substance use disorders in early or sustained remission are classified to the appropriate codes for substance abuse in remission, and moderate or severe substance use disorders in early or sustained remission are classified to the appropriate codes for substance dependence in remission.

2) Psychoactive Substance Use, Abuse and Dependence (*See* **Fig. I.C.5.b.2**)

When the provider documentation refers to use, abuse and dependence of the same substance (e.g. alcohol, opioid, cannabis, etc.), only one code should be assigned to identify the pattern of use based on the following hierarchy:

- ❑ If both use and abuse are documented, assign only the code for abuse
- ❑ If both abuse and dependence are documented, assign only the code for dependence
- ❑ If use, abuse and dependence are all documented, assign only the code for dependence
- ❑ If both use and dependence are documented, assign only the code for dependence.

3) Psychoactive Substance Use, Unspecified

As with all other unspecified diagnoses, the codes for unspecified psychoactive substance use (F10.9-, F11.9-, F12.9-, F13.9-, F14.9-, F15.9-, F16.9-, F18.9-, F19.9-) should only be assigned based on provider documentation and when they meet the definition of a reportable diagnosis (*see* Section III, Reporting Additional Diagnoses). These codes are to be used only when the psychoactive substance use is associated with a physical, mental or behavioral disorder, and such a relationship is documented by the provider.

c. Factitious Disorder

Factitious disorder imposed on self or Munchausen's syndrome is a disorder in which a person falsely reports or causes his or her own physical or psychological signs or symptoms. For patients with documented factitious disorder on self or Munchausen's syndrome, assign the appropriate code from subcategory F68.1-, Factitious disorder imposed on self.

Munchausen's syndrome by proxy (MSBP) is a disorder in which a caregiver (perpetrator) falsely reports or causes an illness or injury in another person (victim) under his or her care, such as a child, an elderly adult, or a person who has a disability. The condition is also referred to as "factitious disorder imposed on another" or "factitious disorder by proxy." The perpetrator, not the victim, receives this diagnosis. Assign code F68.A, Factitious disorder imposed on another, to the perpetrator's record. For the victim of a patient suffering from MSBP, assign the appropriate code from categories T74, Adult and child abuse, neglect and other maltreatment, confirmed, or T76, Adult and child abuse, neglect and other maltreatment, suspected.

See Section I.C.19.f. Adult and child abuse, neglect and other maltreatment

6. Chapter 6: Diseases of the Nervous System (G00-G99)

a. Dominant/nondominant side

Codes from category G81, Hemiplegia and hemiparesis, and subcategories G83.1, Monoplegia of lower limb, G83.2, Monoplegia of upper limb, and G83.3, Monoplegia, unspecified, identify whether the dominant or nondominant side is affected. Should the affected side be documented, but not specified as dominant or nondominant, and the classification system does not indicate a default, code selection is as follows:

- ❑ For ambidextrous patients, the default should be dominant.
- ❑ If the left side is affected, the default is non-dominant.
- ❑ If the right side is affected, the default is dominant.

b. Pain - Category G89

1) General coding information

Codes in category G89, Pain, not elsewhere classified, may be used in conjunction with codes from other categories and chapters to provide more detail about acute or chronic pain and neoplasm-related pain, unless otherwise indicated below.

If the pain is not specified as acute or chronic, post- thoracotomy, postprocedural, or neoplasm-related, do not assign codes from category G89.

A code from category G89 should not be assigned if the underlying (definitive) diagnosis is known, unless the reason for the encounter is pain control/ management and not management of the underlying condition.

When an admission or encounter is for a procedure aimed at treating the underlying condition (e.g., spinal fusion, kyphoplasty), a code for the underlying condition (e.g., vertebral fracture, spinal stenosis) should be assigned as the principal diagnosis. No code from category G89 should be assigned.

(a) Category G89 Codes as Principal or First-Listed Diagnosis

Category G89 codes are acceptable as principal diagnosis or the first-listed code:

- ❑ When pain control or pain management is the reason for the admission/encounter (e.g., a patient with displaced intervertebral disc, nerve impingement and severe back pain presents for injection of steroid into the spinal canal). The underlying cause of the pain should be reported as an additional diagnosis, if known.
- ❑ When a patient is admitted for the insertion of a neurostimulator for pain control, assign the appropriate pain code as the principal or first-listed diagnosis. When an admission or encounter is for a procedure aimed at treating the underlying condition and a neurostimulator is inserted for pain control during the same admission/encounter, a code for the underlying condition should be assigned as the principal diagnosis and the appropriate pain code should be assigned as a secondary diagnosis.

(b) Use of Category G89 Codes in Conjunction with Site Specific Pain Codes

(i) Assigning Category G89 and Site-Specific Pain Codes

Codes from category G89 may be used in conjunction with codes that identify the site of pain (including codes from chapter 18) if the category G89 code provides additional information. For example, if the code describes the site of the pain, but does not fully describe whether the pain is acute or chronic, then both codes should be assigned.

(ii) Sequencing of Category G89 Codes with Site- Specific Pain Codes

The sequencing of category G89 codes with site- specific pain codes (including chapter 18 codes), is dependent on the circumstances of the encounter/admission as follows:

- ❑ If the encounter is for pain control or pain management, assign the code from category G89 followed by the code identifying the specific site of pain (e.g., encounter for pain management for acute neck pain from trauma is assigned code G89.11, Acute pain due to trauma, followed by code M54.2, Cervicalgia, to identify the site of pain).
- ❑ If the encounter is for any other reason except pain control or pain management, and a related definitive diagnosis has not been established (confirmed) by the provider, assign the code for the specific site of pain first, followed by the appropriate code from categoryG89.

2) Pain due to devices, implants and grafts

See Section I.C.19. Pain due to medical devices

3) Postoperative Pain

The provider's documentation should be used to guide the coding of postoperative pain, as well as *Section III. Reporting Additional Diagnoses* and *Section IV. Diagnostic Coding and Reporting in the Outpatient Setting*.

The default for post-thoracotomy and other postoperative pain not specified as acute or chronic is the code for the acute form.

Routine or expected postoperative pain immediately after surgery should not be coded.

(a) Postoperative pain not associated with specific postoperative complication

Postoperative pain not associated with a specific postoperative complication is assigned to the appropriate postoperative pain code in category G89.

(b) Postoperative pain associated with specific postoperative complication

Postoperative pain associated with a specific postoperative complication (such as painful wire sutures) is assigned to the appropriate code(s) found in Chapter 19, Injury, poisoning, and certain other consequences of external causes. If appropriate, use additional code(s) from category G89 to identify acute or chronic pain (G89.18 or G89.28).

4) Chronic pain

Chronic pain is classified to subcategory G89.2. There is no time frame defining when pain becomes chronic pain. The provider's documentation should be used to guide use of these codes.

5) Neoplasm Related Pain

Code G89.3 is assigned to pain documented as being related, associated or due to cancer, primary or secondary malignancy, or tumor. This code is assigned regardless of whether the pain is acute or chronic.

This code may be assigned as the principal or first-listed code when the stated reason for the admission/encounter is documented as pain control/pain management. The underlying neoplasm should be reported as an additional diagnosis.

When the reason for the admission/encounter is management of the neoplasm and the pain associated with the neoplasm is also documented, code G89.3 may be assigned as an additional diagnosis. It is not necessary to assign an additional code for the site of the pain.

See Section I.C.2 for instructions on the sequencing of neoplasms for all other stated reasons for the admission/encounter (except for pain control/ pain management).

6) Chronic pain syndrome

Central pain syndrome (G89.0) and chronic pain syndrome (G89.4) are different than the term "chronic pain," and therefore codes should only be used when the provider has specifically documented this condition.

See Section I.C.5. Pain disorders related to psychological factors

7. Chapter 7: Diseases of the Eye and Adnexa (H00-H59)

a. Glaucoma

1) Assigning Glaucoma Codes

Assign as many codes from category H40, Glaucoma, as needed to identify the type of glaucoma, the affected eye, and the glaucoma stage.

2) Bilateral glaucoma with same type and stage

When a patient has bilateral glaucoma and both eyes are documented as being the same type and stage, and there is a code for bilateral glaucoma, report only the code for the type of glaucoma, bilateral, with the seventh character for the stage.

When a patient has bilateral glaucoma and both eyes are documented as being the same type and stage, and the classification does not provide a code for bilateral glaucoma (i.e. subcategories H40.10, and H40.20) report only one code for the type of glaucoma with the appropriate seventh character for the stage.

3) Bilateral glaucoma stage with different types or stages

When a patient has bilateral glaucoma and each eye is documented as having a different type or stage, and the classification distinguishes laterality, assign the appropriate code for each eye rather than the code for bilateral glaucoma.

When a patient has bilateral glaucoma and each eye is documented as having a different type, and the classification does not distinguish laterality (i.e., subcategories H40.10, and H40.20), assign one code for each type of glaucoma with the appropriate seventh character for the stage.

When a patient has bilateral glaucoma and each eye is documented as having the same type, but different stage, and the classification does not distinguish laterality (i.e., subcategories H40.10 and H40.20), assign a code for the type of glaucoma for each eye with the seventh character for the specific glaucoma stage documented for each eye.

4) Patient admitted with glaucoma and stage evolves during the admission

If a patient is admitted with glaucoma and the stage progresses during the admission, assign the code for highest stage documented.

5) Indeterminate stage glaucoma

Assignment of the seventh character "4" for "indeterminate stage" should be based on the clinical documentation. The seventh character "4" is used for glaucomas whose stage cannot be clinically determined. This seventh character should not be confused with the seventh character "0", unspecified, which should be assigned when there is no documentation regarding the stage of the glaucoma.

b. Blindness

If "blindness" or "low vision" of both eyes is documented but the visual impairment category is not documented, assign code H54.3, Unqualified visual loss, both eyes. If "blindness" or "low vision" in one eye is documented but the visual impairment category is not documented, assign a code from H54.6-, Unqualified visual loss, one eye. If "blindness" or "visual loss" is documented without any information about whether one or both eyes are affected, assign code H54.7, Unspecified visual loss.

8. Chapter 8: Diseases of the Ear and Mastoid Process (H60-H95)

Reserved for future guideline expansion

9. Chapter 9: Diseases of the Circulatory System (I00-I99)

a. Hypertension (*See* **Figure I.C.9.a)**

The classification presumes a causal relationship between hypertension and heart involvement and between hypertension and kidney involvement, as the two conditions are linked by the term "with" in the Alphabetic Index. These conditions should be coded as related even in the absence of provider documentation explicitly linking them, unless the documentation clearly states the conditions are unrelated.

For hypertension and conditions not specifically linked by relational terms such as "with," "associated with" or "due to" in the classification,provider documentation must link the conditions in order to code them as related.

1) Hypertension with Heart Disease

Hypertension with heart conditions classified to I50.- or I51.4- I51.7, I51.89, I51.9, are assigned to a code from category I11, Hypertensive heart disease. Use additional code(s) from category I50, Heart failure, to identify the type(s) of heart failure in those patients with heart failure.

The same heart conditions (I50.-, I51.4-I51.7, I51.89, I51.9) with hypertension are coded separately if the provider has documented they are unrelated to the hypertension. Sequence according to the circumstances of the admission/encounter.

2) Hypertensive Chronic Kidney Disease

Assign codes from category I12, Hypertensive chronic kidney disease, when both hypertension and a condition classifiable to category N18, Chronic kidney disease (CKD), are present. CKD should not be coded as hypertensive if the provider indicates the CKD is not related to the hypertension.

The appropriate code from category N18 should be used as a secondary code with a code from category I12 to identify the stage of chronic kidney disease.

See Section I.C.14. Chronic kidney disease.

If a patient has hypertensive chronic kidney disease and acute renal failure, an additional code for the acute renal failure is required.

3) Hypertensive Heart and Chronic Kidney Disease

Assign codes from combination category I13, Hypertensive heart and chronic kidney disease, when there is hypertension with both heart and kidney involvement. If heart failure is present, assign an additional code from category I50 to identify the type of heart failure.

The appropriate code from category N18, Chronic kidney disease, should be used as a secondary code with a code from category I13 to identify the stage of chronic kidney disease.

See Section I.C.14. Chronic kidney disease.

The codes in category I13, Hypertensive heart and chronic kidney disease, are combination codes that include hypertension, heart disease and chronic kidney disease. The Includes note at I13 specifies that the conditions included at I11 and I12 are included together in I13. If a patient has hypertension, heart disease and chronic kidney disease, then a code from I13 should be used, not individual codes for hypertension, heart disease and chronic kidney disease, or codes from I11 orI12.

For patients with both acute renal failure and chronic kidney disease, an additional code for acute renal failure is required.

4) Hypertensive Cerebrovascular Disease

For hypertensive cerebrovascular disease, first assign the appropriate code from categories I60-I69, followed by the appropriate hypertension code.

5) Hypertensive Retinopathy

Subcategory H35.0, Background retinopathy and retinal vascular changes, should be used with a code from category I10– I15, Hypertensive disease to include the systemic hypertension. The sequencing is based on the reason for the encounter.

6) Hypertension, Secondary

Secondary hypertension is due to an underlying condition. Two codes are required: one to identify the underlying etiology and one from category I15 to identify the hypertension. Sequencing of codes is determined by the reason for admission/encounter.

7) Hypertension, Transient

Assign code R03.0, Elevated blood pressure reading without diagnosis of hypertension, unless patient has an established diagnosis of hypertension. Assign code O13.-, Gestational [pregnancy-induced] hypertension without significant proteinuria, or O14.-, Pre-eclampsia, for transient hypertension of pregnancy.

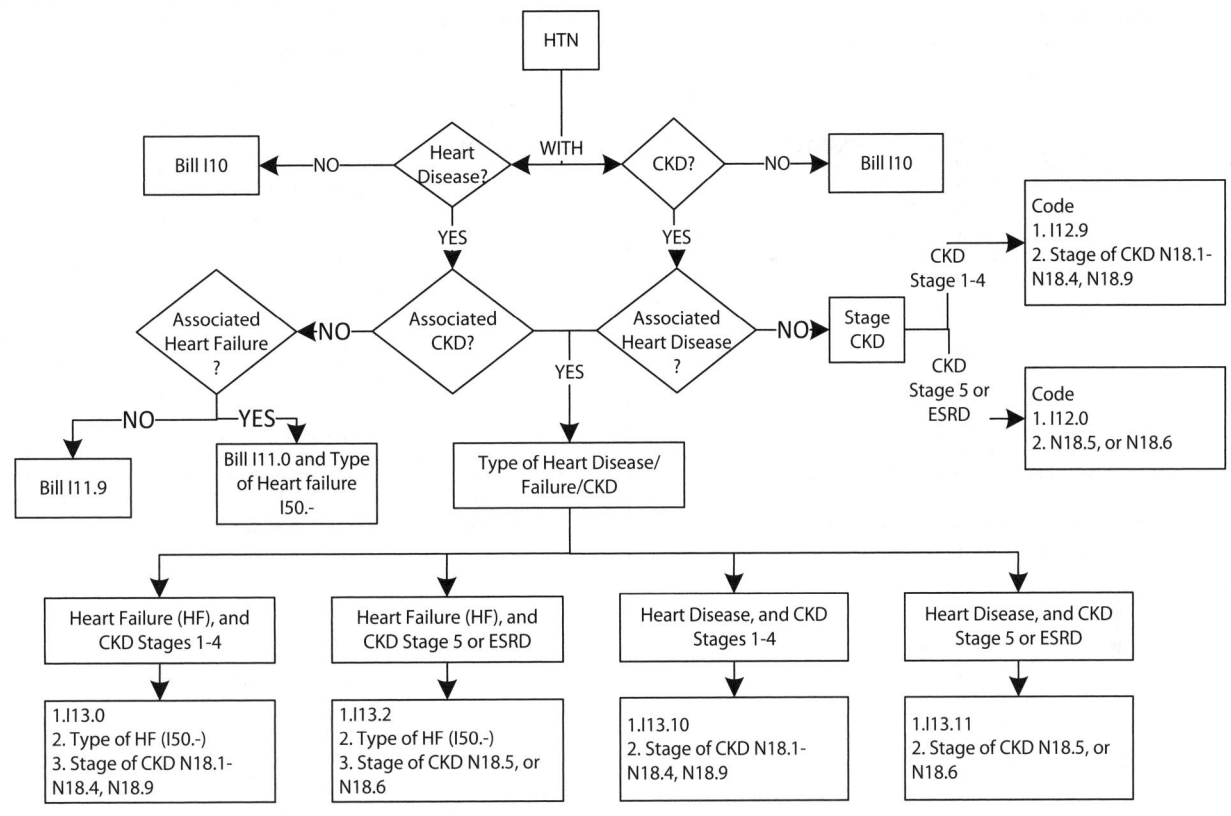

©AAPC. All Rights Reserved.

Figure I.C.9.a: Hypertension (HTN)

8) Hypertension, Controlled

This diagnostic statement usually refers to an existing state of hypertension under control by therapy. Assign the appropriate code from categories I10-I15, Hypertensive diseases.

9) Hypertension, Uncontrolled

Uncontrolled hypertension may refer to untreated hypertension or hypertension not responding to current therapeutic regimen. In either case, assign the appropriate code from categories I10- I15, Hypertensive diseases.

10) Hypertensive Crisis

Assign a code from category I16, Hypertensive crisis, for documented hypertensive urgency, hypertensive emergency or unspecified hypertensive crisis. Code also any identified hypertensive disease (I10-I15). The sequencing is based on the reason for the encounter.

11) Pulmonary Hypertension

Pulmonary hypertension is classified to category I27, Other pulmonary heart diseases. For secondary pulmonary hypertension (I27.1, I27.2-), code also any associated conditions or adverse effects of drugs or toxins. The sequencing is based on the reason for the encounter, except for adverse effects of drugs (*See Section I.C.19.e.*).

b. Atherosclerotic Coronary Artery Disease and Angina

ICD-10-CM has combination codes for atherosclerotic heart disease with angina pectoris. The subcategories for these codes areI25.11, Atherosclerotic heart disease of native coronary artery with angina pectoris and I25.7, Atherosclerosis of coronary artery bypass graft(s) and coronary artery of transplanted heart with angina pectoris.

When using one of these combination codes it is not necessary to use an additional code for angina pectoris. A causal relationship can be assumed in a patient with both atherosclerosis and angina pectoris, unless the documentation indicates the angina is due to something other than the atherosclerosis.

If a patient with coronary artery disease is admitted due to an acute myocardial infarction (AMI), the AMI should be sequenced before the coronary artery disease.

See Section I.C.9. Acute myocardial infarction (AMI)

c. Intraoperative and Postprocedural Cerebrovascular Accident

Medical record documentation should clearly specify the cause-and- effect relationship between the medical intervention and the cerebrovascular accident in order to assign a code for intraoperative or postprocedural cerebrovascular accident.

Proper code assignment depends on whether it was an infarction or hemorrhage and whether it occurred intraoperatively or postoperatively. If it was a cerebral hemorrhage, code assignment depends on the type of procedure performed.

d. Sequelae of Cerebrovascular Disease

1) Category I69, Sequelae of Cerebrovascular disease

Category I69 is used to indicate conditions classifiable to categories I60-I67 as the causes of sequela (neurologic deficits), themselves classified elsewhere. These "late effects" include neurologic deficits that persist after initial onset of conditions classifiable to categories I60-I67. The neurologic deficits caused by cerebrovascular disease may be present from the onset or may arise at any time after the onset of the condition classifiable to categories I60-I67.

Codes from category I69, Sequelae of cerebrovascular disease, that specify hemiplegia, hemiparesis and monoplegia identify whether the dominant or nondominant side is affected. Should the affected side be documented, but not specified as dominant or nondominant, and the classification system does not indicate a default, code selection is as follows:

- ❏ For ambidextrous patients, the default should be dominant.
- ❏ If the left side is affected, the default is non-dominant.
- ❏ If the right side is affected, the default is dominant.

2) Codes from category I69 with codes from I60-I67

Codes from category I69 may be assigned on a health care record with codes from I60-I67, if the patient has a current cerebrovascular disease and deficits from an old cerebrovascular disease.

3) Codes from category I69 and Personal history of transient ischemic attack (TIA) and cerebral infarction (Z86.73)

Codes from category I69 should not be assigned if the patient does not have neurologic deficits.

See Section I.C.21. 4. History (of) for use of personal history codes

e. Acute myocardial infarction (AMI)

1) Type 1 ST elevation myocardial infarction (STEMI) and non-ST elevation myocardial infarction (NSTEMI)

The ICD-10-CM codes for type 1 acute myocardial infarction (AMI) identify the site, such as anterolateral wall or true posterior wall. Subcategories I21.0-I21.2 and code I21.3 are used for type 1 ST elevation myocardial infarction (STEMI). Code I21.4, Non-ST elevation (NSTEMI) myocardial infarction, is used for type 1 non ST elevation myocardial infarction (NSTEMI) and nontransmural MIs.

If a type 1 NSTEMI evolves to STEMI, assign the STEMI code. If a type 1 STEMI converts to NSTEMI due to thrombolytic therapy, it is still coded as STEMI.

For encounters occurring while the myocardial infarction is equal to, or less than, four weeks old, including transfers to another acute setting or a postacute setting, and the myocardial infarction meets the definition for "other diagnoses" (see Section III, Reporting Additional Diagnoses), codes from category I21 may continue to be reported. For encounters after the 4 week time frame and the patient is still receiving care related to the myocardial infarction, the appropriate aftercare code should be assigned, rather than a code from category I21. For old or healed myocardial infarctions not requiring further care, code I25.2, Old myocardial infarction, may be assigned.

2) Acute myocardial infarction, unspecified

Code I21.9, Acute myocardial infarction, unspecified, is the default for unspecified acute myocardial infarction or unspecified type. If only type 1 STEMI or transmural MI without the site is documented, assign code I21.3, ST elevation (STEMI) myocardial infarction of unspecified site.

3) AMI documented as nontransmural or subendocardial but site provided

If an AMI is documented as nontransmural or subendocardial, but the site is provided, it is still coded as a subendocardial AMI.

See Section I.C.21.3 for information on coding status post administration of tPA in a different facility within the last 24 hours.

4) Subsequent acute myocardial infarction

A code from category I22, Subsequent ST elevation (STEMI) and non-ST elevation (NSTEMI) myocardial infarction, is to be used when a patient who has suffered a type 1 or unspecified AMI has a new AMI within the 4 week time frame of the initial AMI. A code from category I22 must be used in conjunction with a code from category I21. The sequencing of the I22 and I21 codes depends on the circumstances of the encounter.

Do not assign code I22 for subsequent myocardial infarctions other than type 1 or unspecified. For subsequent type 2 AMI assign only code I21.A1. For subsequent type 4 or type 5 AMI, assign only code I21.A9.

If a subsequent myocardial infarction of one type occurs within 4 weeks of a myocardial infarction of a different type, assign the appropriate codes from category I21 to identify each type. Do not assign a code from I22. Codes from category I22 should only be assigned if both the initial and subsequent myocardial infarctions are type 1 or unspecified.

5) Other Types of Myocardial Infarction

The ICD-10-CM provides codes for different types of myocardial infarction. Type 1 myocardial infarctions are assigned to codes I21.0-I21.4.

Type 2 myocardial infarction (myocardial infarction due to demand ischemia or secondary to ischemic **im**balance) is assigned to code I21.A1, Myocardial infarction type 2 with the underlying cause **coded first.** Do not assign code I24.8, Other forms of acute ischemic heart disease, for the demand ischemia.

If a type 2 AMI is described as NSTEMI or STEMI, only assign code I21.A1.

Codes I21.01-I21.4 should only be assigned for type 1 AMIs.

Acute myocardial infarctions type 3, 4a, 4b, 4c and 5 are assigned to code I21.A9, Other myocardial infarction type.

The "Code also" and "Code first" notes should be followed related to complications, and for coding of postprocedural myocardial infarctions during or following cardiac surgery.

10. Chapter 10: Diseases of the Respiratory System (J00-J99)

a. Chronic Obstructive Pulmonary Disease [COPD] and Asthma

1) Acute exacerbation of chronic obstructive bronchitis and asthma

The codes in categories J44 and J45 distinguish between uncomplicated cases and those in acute exacerbation. An acute exacerbation is a worsening or a decompensation of a chronic condition. An acute exacerbation is not equivalent to an infection superimposed on a chronic condition, though an exacerbation may be triggered by an infection.

b. Acute Respiratory Failure (See Fig. 1.C.10.b)

1) Acute respiratory failure as principal diagnosis

A code from subcategory J96.0, Acute respiratory failure, or subcategory J96.2, Acute and chronic respiratory failure, may be assigned as a principal diagnosis when it is the condition established after study to be chiefly responsible for occasioning the admission to the hospital, and the selection is supported by the Alphabetic Index and Tabular List. However, chapter- specific coding guidelines (such as obstetrics, poisoning, HIV, newborn) that provide sequencing direction take precedence.

2) Acute respiratory failure as secondary diagnosis

Respiratory failure may be listed as a secondary diagnosis if it occurs after admission, or if it is present on admission, but does not meet the definition of principal diagnosis.

3) Sequencing of acute respiratory failure and another acute condition

When a patient is admitted with respiratory failure and another acute condition, (e.g., myocardial infarction, cerebrovascular accident, aspiration pneumonia), the principal diagnosis will not be the same in every situation. This applies whether the other acute condition is a respiratory or nonrespiratory condition.

Selection of the principal diagnosis will be dependent on the circumstances of admission. If both the respiratory failure and the other acute condition are equally responsible for occasioning the admission to the hospital, and there are no chapter-specific sequencing rules, the guideline regarding two or more diagnoses that equally meet the definition for principal diagnosis (Section II, C.) may be applied in these situations.

If the documentation is not clear as to whether acute respiratory failure and another condition are equally responsible for occasioning the admission, query the provider for clarification.

c. Influenza due to certain identified influenza viruses

Code only confirmed cases of influenza due to certain identified influenza viruses (category J09), and due to other identified influenza virus (category J10). This is an exception to the hospital inpatient guideline Section II, H. (Uncertain Diagnosis).

In this context, "confirmation" does not require documentation of positive laboratory testing specific for avian or other novel influenza A or other identified influenza virus. However, coding should be based on the provider's diagnostic statement that the patient has avian influenza, or other novel influenza A, for category J09, or has another particular identified strain of influenza, such as H1N1 or H3N2, but not identified as novel or variant, for category J10.

If the provider records "suspected" or "possible" or "probable" avian influenza, or novel influenza, or other identified influenza, then the appropriate influenza code from category J11, Influenza due to unidentified influenza virus, should be assigned. A code from category J09, Influenza due to certain identified influenza viruses, should not be assigned nor should a code from category J10, Influenza due to other identified influenza virus.

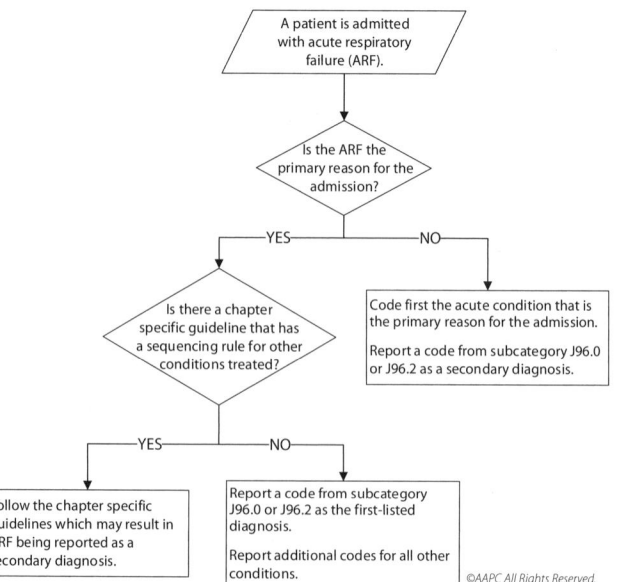

Figure I.C.10.b: Acute Respiratory Failure

d. Ventilator associated Pneumonia

1) Documentation of Ventilator associated Pneumonia

As with all procedural or postprocedural complications, code assignment is based on the provider's documentation of the relationship between the condition and the procedure.

Code J95.851, Ventilator associated pneumonia, should be assigned only when the provider has documented ventilator associated pneumonia (VAP). An additional code to identify the organism (e.g., Pseudomonas aeruginosa, code B96.5) should also be assigned. Do not assign an additional code from categories J12-J18 to identify the type of pneumonia.

Code J95.851 should not be assigned for cases where the patient has pneumonia and is on a mechanical ventilator and the provider has not specifically stated that the pneumonia is ventilator-associated pneumonia. If the documentation is unclear as to whether the patient has a pneumonia that is a complication attributable to the mechanical ventilator, query the provider.

2) Ventilator associated Pneumonia Develops after Admission

A patient may be admitted with one type of pneumonia (e.g., code J13, Pneumonia due to Streptococcus pneumonia) and subsequently develop VAP. In this instance, the principal diagnosis would be the appropriate code from categories J12- J18 for the pneumonia diagnosed at the time of admission. Code J95.851, Ventilator associated pneumonia, would be assigned as an additional diagnosis when the provider has also documented the presence of ventilator associated pneumonia.

11. Chapter 11: Diseases of the Digestive System (K00-K95)

Reserved for future guideline expansion

12. Chapter 12: Diseases of the Skin and Subcutaneous Tissue (L00-L99)

a. Pressure ulcer stage codes (*See* **Fig. I.C.12.a**)

1) Pressure ulcer stages

Codes **in** category L89, Pressure ulcer, identify the site **and stage** of the pressure ulcer.

The ICD-10-CM classifies pressure ulcer stages based on severity, which is designated by stages 1-4, **deep tissue pressure injury,** unspecified stage, and unstageable.

Assign as many codes from category L89 as needed to identify all the pressure ulcers the patient has, if applicable.

See Section I.B.14 for pressure ulcer stage documentation by clinicians other than patient's provider.

2) Unstageable pressure ulcers

Assignment of the code for unstageable pressure ulcer (L89.--0) should be based on the clinical documentation. These codes are used for pressure ulcers whose stage cannot be clinically determined (e.g., the ulcer is covered by eschar or has been treated with a skin or muscle graft). This code should not be confused with the codes

for unspecified stage (L89.--9). When there is no documentation regarding the stage of the pressure ulcer, assign the appropriate code for unspecified stage (L89.-- 9).

3) Documented pressure ulcer stage

Assignment of the pressure ulcer stage code should be guided by clinical documentation of the stage or documentation of the terms found in the Alphabetic Index. For clinical terms describing the stage that are not found in the Alphabetic Index, and there is no documentation of the stage, the provider should be queried.

4) Patients admitted with pressure ulcers documented as healed

No code is assigned if the documentation states that the pressure ulcer is completely healed **at the time of admission.**

5) Pressure ulcers documented as healing

Pressure ulcers described as healing should be assigned the appropriate pressure ulcer stage code based on the documentation in the medical record. If the documentation does not provide information about the stage of the healing pressure ulcer, assign the appropriate code for unspecified stage.

If the documentation is unclear as to whether the patient has a current (new) pressure ulcer or if the patient is being treated for a healing pressure ulcer, query the provider.

For ulcers that were present on admission but healed at the time of discharge, assign the code for the site and stage of the pressure ulcer at the time of admission.

6) Patient admitted with pressure ulcer evolving into another stage during the admission

If a patient is admitted to an inpatient hospital with a pressure ulcer at one stage and it progresses to a higher stage, two separate codes should be assigned: one code for the site and stage of the ulcer on admission and a second code for the same ulcer site and the highest stage reported during the stay.

7) Pressure-induced deep tissue damage

For pressure-induced deep tissue damage or deep tissue pressure injury, assign only the appropriate code for pressure-induced deep tissue damage (L89.--6).

b. Non-Pressure Chronic Ulcers

1) Patients admitted with non-pressure ulcers documented as healed

No code is assigned if the documentation states that the nonpressure ulcer is completely healed **at the time of admission.**

2) Non-pressure ulcers documented as healing

Non-pressure ulcers described as healing should be assigned the appropriate non-pressure ulcer code based on the documentation in the medical record. If the documentation does not provide information about the severity of the healing non-pressure ulcer, assign the appropriate code for unspecified severity.

If the documentation is unclear as to whether the patient has a current (new) non-pressure ulcer or if the patient is being treated for a healing non-pressure ulcer, query the provider.

For ulcers that were present on admission but healed at the time of discharge, assign the code for the site and severity of the non-pressure ulcer at the time of admission.

3) Patient admitted with non-pressure ulcer that progresses to another severity level during the admission

If a patient is admitted to an inpatient hospital with a non- pressure ulcer at one severity level and it progresses to a higher severity level, two separate codes should be assigned: one code for the site and severity level of the ulcer on admission and a second code for the same ulcer site and the highest severity level reported during the stay.

See Section I.B.14 for pressure ulcer stage documentation by clinicians other than patient's provider

13. Chapter 13: Diseases of the Musculoskeletal System and Connective Tissue (M00-M99)

a. Site and laterality

Most of the codes within Chapter 13 have site and laterality designations. The site represents the bone, joint or the muscle involved. For some conditions where more than one bone, joint or muscle is usually involved, such as osteoarthritis, there is a "multiple sites" code available. For categories where no multiple site code is provided and more than one bone, joint or muscle is involved, multiple codes should be used to indicate the different sites involved.

1) Bone versus joint

For certain conditions, the bone may be affected at the upper or lower end, (e.g., avascular necrosis of bone, M87, Osteoporosis, M80, M81). Though the portion of the bone affected may be at the joint, the site designation will be the bone, not the joint.

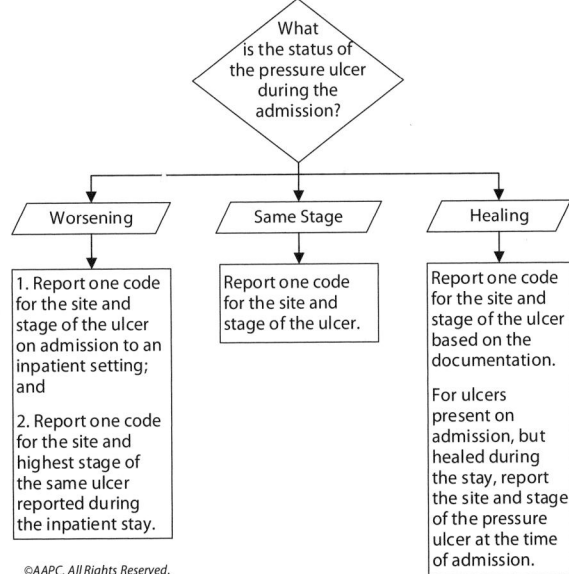

©AAPC. All Rights Reserved.

Figure I.C.12.a: Pressure ulcer stage codes

b. **Acute traumatic versus chronic or recurrent musculoskeletal conditions**

Many musculoskeletal conditions are a result of previous injury or trauma to a site, or are recurrent conditions. Bone, joint or muscle conditions that are the result of a healed injury are usually found in chapter 13. Recurrent bone, joint or muscle conditions are also usually found in chapter 13. Any current, acute injury should be coded to the appropriate injury code from chapter 19. Chronic or recurrent conditions should generally be coded with a code from chapter 13. If it is difficult to determine from the documentation in the record which code is best to describe a condition, query the provider.

c. **Coding of Pathologic Fractures** (*See* **Fig. I.C.13.c**)

7th character A is for use as long as the patient is receiving active treatment for the fracture. While the patient may be seen by a new or different provider over the course of treatment for a pathological fracture, assignment of the 7th character is based on whether the patient is undergoing active treatment and not whether the provider is seeing the patient for the first time.

7th character D is to be used for encounters after the patient has completed active treatment for the fracture and is receiving routine care for the fracture during the healing or recovery phase. The other 7th characters, listed under each subcategory in the Tabular List, are to be used for subsequent encounters for treatment of problems associated with the healing, such as malunions, nonunions, and sequelae.

Care for complications of surgical treatment for fracture repairs during the healing or recovery phase should be coded with the appropriate complication codes.

See Section I.C.19. Coding of traumatic fractures.

d. **Osteoporosis**

Osteoporosis is a systemic condition, meaning that all bones of the musculoskeletal system are affected. Therefore, site is not a component of the codes under category M81, Osteoporosis without current pathological fracture. The site codes under category M80, Osteoporosis with current pathological fracture, identify the site of the fracture, not the osteoporosis.

1) **Osteoporosis without pathological fracture**

Category M81, Osteoporosis without current pathological fracture, is for use for patients with osteoporosis who do not currently have

a pathologic fracture due to the osteoporosis, even if they have had a fracture in the past. For patients with a history of osteoporosis fractures, status code Z87.310, Personal history of (healed) osteoporosis fracture, should follow the code from M81.

2) **Osteoporosis with current pathological fracture**

Category M80, Osteoporosis with current pathological fracture, is for patients who have a current pathologic fracture at the time of an encounter. The codes under M80 identify the site of the fracture. A code from category M80, not a traumatic fracture code, should be used for any patient with known osteoporosis who suffers a fracture, even if the patient had a minor fall or trauma, if that fall or trauma would not usually break a normal, healthy bone.

14. **Chapter 14: Diseases of Genitourinary System (N00-N99)**

a. **Chronic kidney disease**

1) **Stages of chronic kidney disease (CKD)**

The ICD-10-CM classifies CKD based on severity. The severity of CKD is designated by stages 1-5. Stage 2, code N18.2, equates to mild CKD; stage 3, code N18.3, equates to moderate CKD; and stage 4, code N18.4, equates to severe CKD. Code N18.6, End stage renal disease (ESRD), is assigned when the provider has documented end-stage renal disease (ESRD).

If both a stage of CKD and ESRD are documented, assign codeN18.6 only.

2) **Chronic kidney disease and kidney transplant status**

Patients who have undergone kidney transplant may still have some form of chronic kidney disease (CKD) because the kidney transplant may not fully restore kidney function. Therefore, the presence of CKD alone does not constitute a transplant complication. Assign the appropriate N18 code for the patient's stage of CKD and code Z94.0, Kidney transplant status. If a transplant complication such as failure or rejection or other transplant complication is documented, see section I.C.19.g for information on coding complications of a kidney transplant. If the documentation is unclear as to whether the patient has a complication of the transplant, query the provider.

3) **Chronic kidney disease with other conditions**

Patients with CKD may also suffer from other serious conditions, most commonly diabetes mellitus and hypertension. The sequencing of the CKD code in relationship to codes for other contributing conditions is based on the conventions in the Tabular List.

See I.C.9. Hypertensive chronic kidney disease.

See I.C.19. Chronic kidney disease and kidney transplant complications.

15. **Chapter 15: Pregnancy, Childbirth, and the Puerperium (O00-O9A)**

a. **General Rules for Obstetric Cases**

1) **Codes from chapter 15 and sequencing priority** (*See* **Fig. I.C.15.a.1**)

Obstetric cases require codes from chapter 15, codes in the range O00-O9A, Pregnancy, Childbirth, and the Puerperium.

Chapter 15 codes have sequencing priority over codes from

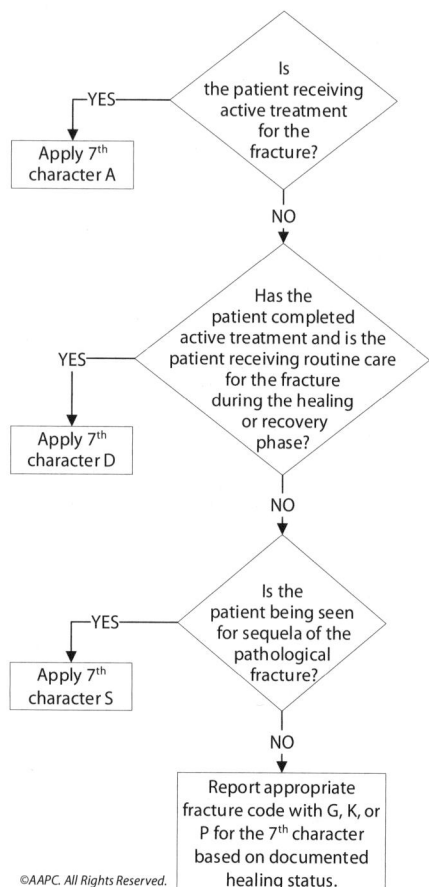

Figure I.C.13.c: Coding of Pathologic Fractures

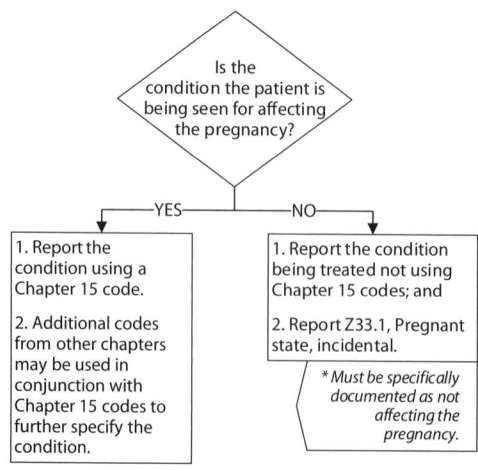

Figure I.C.15.a.1: Codes from chapter 15 and sequencing priority (Coding for Pregnancy)

other chapters. Additional codes from other chapters may be used in conjunction with chapter 15 codes to further specify conditions.

Should the provider document that the pregnancy is incidental to the encounter, then code Z33.1, Pregnant state, incidental, should be used in place of any chapter 15 codes. It is the provider's responsibility to state that the condition being treated is not affecting the pregnancy.

2) **Chapter 15 codes used only on the maternal record**

Chapter 15 codes are to be used only on the maternal record, never on the record of the newborn.

3) **Final character for trimester**

The majority of codes in Chapter 15 have a final character indicating the trimester of pregnancy. The time frames for the trimesters are indicated at the beginning of the chapter. If trimester is not a component of a code, it is because the condition always occurs in a specific trimester, or the concept of trimester of pregnancy is not applicable. Certain codes have characters for only certain trimesters because the condition does not occur in all trimesters, but it may occur in more than just one.

Assignment of the final character for trimester should be based on the provider's documentation of the trimester (or number of weeks) for the current admission/encounter. This applies to the assignment of trimester for pre-existing conditions as well as those that develop during or are due to the pregnancy. The provider's documentation of the number of weeks may be used to assign the appropriate code identifying the trimester.

Whenever delivery occurs during the current admission, and there is an "in childbirth" option for the obstetric complication being coded, the "in childbirth" code should be assigned.

4) **Selection of trimester for inpatient admissions that encompass more than one trimester**

In instances when a patient is admitted to a hospital for complications of pregnancy during one trimester and remains in the hospital into a subsequent trimester, the trimester character for the antepartum complication code should be assigned on the basis of the trimester when the complication developed, not the trimester of the discharge. If the condition developed prior to the current admission/encounter or represents a pre-existing condition, the trimester character for the trimester at the time of the admission/encounter should be assigned.

5) **Unspecified trimester**

Each category that includes codes for trimester has a code for "unspecified trimester." The "unspecified trimester" code should rarely be used, such as when the documentation in the record is insufficient to determine the trimester and it is not possible to obtain clarification.

6) **7th character for Fetus Identification**

Where applicable, a 7th character is to be assigned for certain categories (O31, O32, O33.3 - O33.6, O35, O36, O40, O41, O60.1, O60.2, O64, and O69) to identify the fetus for which the complication code applies.

Assign 7th character "0":

❑ For single gestations

❑ When the documentation in the record is insufficient to determine the fetus affected and it is not possible to obtain clarification.

❑ When it is not possible to clinically determine which fetus is affected.

b. **Selection of OB Principal or First-listed Diagnosis**

1) **Routine outpatient prenatal visits**

For routine outpatient prenatal visits when no complications are present, a code from category Z34, Encounter for supervision of normal pregnancy, should be used as the first-listed diagnosis. These codes should not be used in conjunction with chapter 15 codes.

2) **Supervision of High-Risk Pregnancy**

Codes from category O09, Supervision of high-risk pregnancy, are intended for use only during the prenatal period. For complications during the labor or delivery episode as a result of a high-risk pregnancy, assign the applicable complication codes from Chapter 15. If there are no complications during the labor or delivery episode, assign code O80, Encounter for full-term uncomplicated delivery.

For routine prenatal outpatient visits for patients with high-risk pregnancies, a code from category O09, Supervision of high-risk pregnancy, should be used as the first-listed diagnosis. Secondary chapter 15 codes may be used in conjunction with these codes if appropriate.

3) **Episodes when no delivery occurs**

In episodes when no delivery occurs, the principal diagnosis should correspond to the principal complication of the pregnancy which

necessitated the encounter. Should more than one complication exist, all of which are treated or monitored, any of the complication codes may be sequenced first.

4) **When a delivery occurs**

When an obstetric patient is admitted and delivers during that admission, the condition that prompted the admission should be sequenced as the principal diagnosis. If multiple conditions prompted the admission, sequence the one most related to the delivery as the principal diagnosis. A code for any complication of the delivery should be assigned as an additional diagnosis. In cases of cesarean delivery, if the patient was admitted with a condition that resulted in the performance of a cesarean procedure, that condition should be selected as the principal diagnosis. If the reason for the admission was unrelated to the condition resulting in the cesarean delivery, the condition related to the reason for the admission should be selected as the principal diagnosis.

5) **Outcome of delivery**

A code from category Z37, Outcome of delivery, should be included on every maternal record when a delivery has occurred. These codes are not to be used on subsequent records or on the newborn record.

c. **Pre-existing conditions versus conditions due to the pregnancy**

Certain categories in Chapter 15 distinguish between conditions of the mother that existed prior to pregnancy (pre-existing) and those that are a direct result of pregnancy. When assigning codes from Chapter 15, it is important to assess if a condition was pre-existing prior to pregnancy or developed during or due to the pregnancy in order to assign the correct code.

Categories that do not distinguish between pre-existing and pregnancy-related conditions may be used for either. It is acceptable to use codes specifically for the puerperium with codes complicating pregnancy and childbirth if a condition arises postpartum during the delivery encounter.

d. **Pre-existing hypertension in pregnancy**

Category O10, Pre-existing hypertension complicating pregnancy, childbirth and the puerperium, includes codes for hypertensive heart and hypertensive chronic kidney disease. When assigning one of the O10 codes that includes hypertensive heart disease or hypertensive chronic kidney disease, it is necessary to add a secondary code from the appropriate hypertension category to specify the type of heart failure or chronic kidney disease.

See Fig. I.C.15.g.

e. **Fetal Conditions Affecting the Management of the Mother**

1) **Codes from categories O35 and O36**

Codes from categories O35, Maternal care for known or suspected fetal abnormality and damage, and O36, Maternal care for other fetal problems, are assigned only when the fetal condition is actually responsible for modifying the management of the mother, i.e., by requiring diagnostic studies, additional observation, special care, or termination of pregnancy. The fact that the fetal condition exists does not justify assigning a code from this series to the mother's record.

2) **Inutero surgery**

In cases when surgery is performed on the fetus, a diagnosis code from category O35, Maternal care for known or suspected fetal abnormality and damage, should be assigned identifying the fetal condition. Assign the appropriate procedure code for the procedure performed.

No code from Chapter 16, the perinatal codes, should be used on the mother's record to identify fetal conditions. Surgery performed in utero on a fetus is still to be coded as an obstetric encounter.

f. **HIV Infection in Pregnancy, Childbirth and the Puerperium**

During pregnancy, childbirth or the puerperium, a patient admitted because of an HIV-related illness should receive a principal diagnosis from subcategory O98.7-, Human immunodeficiency [HIV] disease complicating pregnancy, childbirth and the puerperium, followed by the code(s) for the HIV-related illness(es).

Patients with asymptomatic HIV infection status admitted during pregnancy, childbirth, or the puerperium should receive codes of O98.7- and Z21, Asymptomatic human immunodeficiency virus [HIV]infection status.

g. **Diabetes mellitus in pregnancy (*See* Fig. I.C.15.g)**

Diabetes mellitus is a significant complicating factor in pregnancy. Pregnant women who are diabetic should be assigned a code from category O24, Diabetes mellitus in pregnancy, childbirth, and the puerperium, first, followed by the appropriate diabetes code(s) (E08-E13) from Chapter 4.

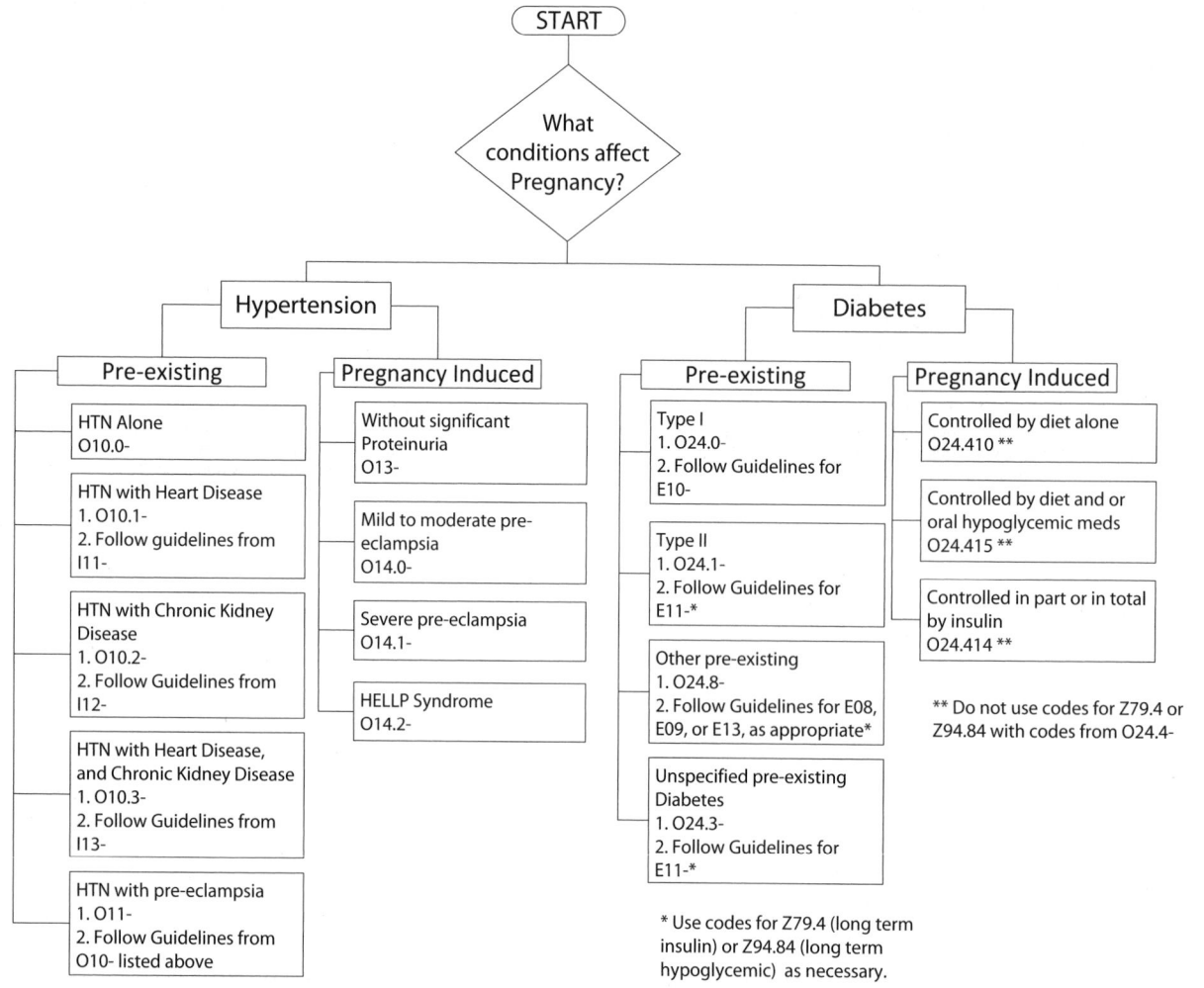

© AAPC. All Rights Reserved.

Figure I.C.15.g: Conditions Affecting Pregnancy

h. Long term use of insulin and oral hypoglycemics

See section I.C.4.a.3 for information on the long term use of insulin and oral hypoglycemic.

i. Gestational (pregnancy induced)diabetes (*See* **Fig. I.C.15.g**)

Gestational (pregnancy induced) diabetes can occur during the second and third trimester of pregnancy in women who were not diabetic prior to pregnancy. Gestational diabetes can cause complications in the pregnancy similar to those of pre-existing diabetes mellitus. It also puts the woman at greater risk of developing diabetes after the pregnancy.

Codes for gestational diabetes are in subcategory O24.4, Gestational diabetes mellitus. No other code from category O24, Diabetes mellitus in pregnancy, childbirth, and the puerperium, should be used with a code from O24.4.

The codes under subcategory O24.4 include diet controlled, insulin controlled, and controlled by oral hypoglycemic drugs. If a patient with gestational diabetes is treated with both diet and insulin, only the code for insulin-controlled is required. If a patient with gestational diabetes is treated with both diet and oral hypoglycemic medications, only the code for "controlled by oral hypoglycemic drugs" is required. Code Z79.4, Long-term (current) use of insulin or code Z79.84, Long-term (current) use of oral hypoglycemic drugs, should not be assigned with codes from subcategory O24.4.

An abnormal glucose tolerance in pregnancy is assigned a code from subcategory O99.81, Abnormal glucose complicating pregnancy, childbirth, and the puerperium.

j. Sepsis and septic shock complicating abortion, pregnancy, childbirth and the puerperium

When assigning a chapter 15 code for sepsis complicating abortion, pregnancy, childbirth, and the puerperium, a code for the specific type of infection should be assigned as an additional diagnosis. If severe sepsis is present, a code from subcategory R65.2, Severe sepsis, and code(s) for associated organ dysfunction(s) should also be assigned as additional diagnoses.

k. Puerperal sepsis

Code O85, Puerperal sepsis, should be assigned with a secondary code to identify the causal organism (e.g., for a bacterial infection, assign a code from category B95-B96, Bacterial infections in conditions classified elsewhere). A code from category A40, Streptococcal sepsis, or A41, Other sepsis, should not be used for puerperal sepsis. If applicable, use additional codes to identify severe sepsis (R65.2-) and any associated acute organ dysfunction.

l. Alcohol, tobacco and drug use during pregnancy, childbirth and the puerperium

1) Alcohol use during pregnancy, childbirth and the puerperium

Codes under subcategory O99.31, Alcohol use complicating pregnancy, childbirth, and the puerperium, should be assigned for any pregnancy case when a mother uses alcohol during the pregnancy or postpartum. A secondary code from category F10, Alcohol related disorders, should also be assigned to identify manifestations of the alcohol use.

2) Tobacco use during pregnancy, childbirth and the puerperium

Codes under subcategory O99.33, Smoking (tobacco) complicating pregnancy, childbirth, and the puerperium, should be assigned for any pregnancy case when a mother uses any type of tobacco product during the pregnancy or postpartum.

A secondary code from category F17, Nicotine dependence, should also be assigned to identify the type of nicotine dependence.

3) Drug use during pregnancy, childbirth and the puerperium

Codes under subcategory O99.32, Drug use complicating pregnancy, childbirth, and the puerperium, should be assigned for any pregnancy case when a mother uses drugs during the pregnancy or postpartum. This can involve illegal drugs, or inappropriate use or abuse of prescription drugs. Secondary code(s) from categories F11-F16 and F18-F19 should also be assigned to identify manifestations of the drug use.

m. Poisoning, toxic effects, adverse effects and underdosing in a pregnant patient

A code from subcategory O9A.2, Injury, poisoning and certain other consequences of external causes complicating pregnancy, childbirth, and the puerperium, should be sequenced first, followed by the appropriate injury, poisoning, toxic effect, adverse effect or underdosing code, and then the additional code(s) that specifies the condition caused by the poisoning, toxic effect, adverse effect or underdosing.

See Section I.C.19. Adverse effects, poisoning, underdosing and toxic effects.

n. Normal Delivery, Code O80

1) Encounter for full term uncomplicated delivery

Code O80 should be assigned when a woman is admitted for a full-term normal delivery and delivers a single, healthy infant without any complications antepartum, during the delivery, or postpartum during the delivery episode. Code O80 is always a principal diagnosis. It is not to be used if any other code from chapter 15 is needed to describe a current complication of the antenatal, delivery, or **postnatal** period. Additional codes from other chapters may be used with code O80 if they are not related to or are in any way complicating the pregnancy.

2) Uncomplicated delivery with resolved antepartum complication

Code O80 may be used if the patient had a complication at some point during the pregnancy, but the complication is not present at the time of the admission for delivery.

3) Outcome of delivery for O80

Z37.0, Single live birth, is the only outcome of delivery code appropriate for use with O80.

o. The Peripartum and Postpartum Periods

1) Peripartum and Postpartum periods

The postpartum period begins immediately after delivery and continues for six weeks following delivery. The peripartum period is defined as the last month of pregnancy to five months postpartum.

2) Peripartum and postpartum complication

A postpartum complication is any complication occurring within the six-week period.

3) Pregnancy-related complications after 6 week period

Chapter 15 codes may also be used to describe pregnancy-related complications after the peripartum or postpartum period if the provider documents that a condition is pregnancy related.

4) Admission for routine postpartum care following delivery outside hospital

When the mother delivers outside the hospital prior to admission and is admitted for routine postpartum care and no complications are noted, code Z39.0, Encounter for care and examination of mother immediately after delivery, should be assigned as the principal diagnosis.

5) Pregnancy associated cardiomyopathy

Pregnancy associated cardiomyopathy, code O90.3, is unique in that it may be diagnosed in the third trimester of pregnancy but may continue to progress months after delivery. For this reason, it is referred to as peripartum cardiomyopathy. Code O90.3 is only for use when the cardiomyopathy develops as a result of pregnancy in a woman who did not have pre-existing heart disease.

p. Code O94, Sequelae of complication of pregnancy, childbirth, and the puerperium

1) CodeO94

Code O94, Sequelae of complication of pregnancy, childbirth, and the puerperium, is for use in those cases when an initial complication of a pregnancy develops a sequelae requiring care or treatment at a future date.

2) After the initial postpartum period

This code may be used at any time after the initial postpartum period.

3) Sequencing of Code O94

This code, like all sequela codes, is to be sequenced following the code describing the sequelae of the complication.

q. Termination of Pregnancy and Spontaneous abortions

1) Abortion with Liveborn Fetus

When an attempted termination of pregnancy results in a liveborn fetus, assign code Z33.2, Encounter for elective termination of pregnancy and a code from category Z37,Outcome of Delivery.

2) Retained Products of Conception following an abortion

Subsequent encounters for retained products of conception following a spontaneous abortion or elective termination of pregnancy, without complications are assigned O03.4, Incomplete spontaneous abortion without complication, or code O07.4, Failed attempted termination of pregnancy without complication. This advice is appropriate even when the patient was discharged previously with a discharge diagnosis of complete abortion. If the patient has a specific complication associated with the spontaneous abortion or elective termination of pregnancy in addition to retained products of conception, assign the appropriate complication **code (e.g., O03.-, O04.-, O07.-)** instead of code O03.4 or O07.4.

3) Complications leading to abortion

Codes from Chapter 15 may be used as additional codes to identify any documented complications of the pregnancy in conjunction with codes in categories in O04, O07 and O08.

r. Abuse in a pregnant patient

For suspected or confirmed cases of abuse of a pregnant patient, a code(s) from subcategories O9A.3, Physical abuse complicating pregnancy, childbirth, and the puerperium, O9A.4, Sexual abuse complicating pregnancy, childbirth, and the puerperium, and O9A.5, Psychological abuse complicating pregnancy, childbirth, and the puerperium, should be sequenced first, followed by the appropriate codes (if applicable) to identify any associated current injury due to physical abuse, sexual abuse, and the perpetrator of abuse.

See Section I.C.19. Adult and child abuse, neglect and other maltreatment.

16. Chapter 16: Certain Conditions Originating in the Perinatal Period (P00-P96)

For coding and reporting purposes the perinatal period is defined as before birth through the 28th day following birth. The following guidelines are provided for reporting purposes.

a. General Perinatal Rules

1) Use of Chapter 16 Codes

Codes in this chapter are never for use on the maternal record. Codes from Chapter 15, the obstetric chapter, are never permitted on the newborn record. Chapter 16 codes may be used throughout the life of the patient if the condition is still present.

2) Principal Diagnosis for Birth Record

When coding the birth episode in a newborn record, assign a code from category Z38, Liveborn infants according to place of birth and type of delivery, as the principal diagnosis. A code from category Z38 is assigned only once, to a newborn at the time of birth. If a newborn is transferred to another institution, a code from category Z38 should not be used at the receiving hospital.

A code from category Z38 is used only on the newborn record, not on the mother's record.

3) Use of Codes from other Chapters with Codes from Chapter 16

Codes from other chapters may be used with codes from chapter 16 if the codes from the other chapters provide more specific detail. Codes for signs and symptoms may be assigned when a definitive diagnosis has not been established. If the reason for the encounter is a perinatal condition, the code from chapter 16 should be sequenced first.

4) Use of Chapter 16 Codes after the Perinatal Period

Should a condition originate in the perinatal period, and continue throughout the life of the patient, the perinatal code should continue to be used regardless of the patient's age.

5) Birth process or community acquired conditions

If a newborn has a condition that may be either due to the birth process or community acquired and the documentation does not indicate which it is, the default is due to the birth process and the code from Chapter 16 should be used. If the condition is community-acquired, a code from Chapter 16 should not be assigned.

6) Code all clinically significant conditions

All clinically significant conditions noted on routine newborn examination should be coded. A condition is clinically significant if it requires:

❑ clinical evaluation; or

❑ therapeutic treatment; or

❑ diagnostic procedures; or

❑ extended length of hospital stay; or

❑ increased nursing care and/or monitoring; or

❑ has implications for future health care needs

Note: The perinatal guidelines listed above are the same as the general coding guidelines for "additional diagnoses," except for the

final point regarding implications for future health care needs. Codes should be assigned for conditions that have been specified by the provider as having implications for future health care needs.

b. Observation and Evaluation of Newborns for Suspected Conditions not Found

1) Use of Z05 codes

Assign a code from category Z05, Observation and evaluation of newborns and infants for suspected conditions ruled out, to identify those instances when a healthy newborn is evaluated for a suspected condition that is determined after study not to be present. Do not use a code from category Z05 when the patient has identified signs or symptoms of a suspected problem; in such cases code the sign or symptom.

2) Z05 on other than the birth record

A code from category Z05 may also be assigned as a principal or first-listed code for readmissions or encounters when the code from category Z38 code no longer applies. Codes from category Z05 are for use only for healthy newborns and infants for which no condition after study is found to be present.

3) Z05 on a birth record

A code from category Z05 is to be used as a secondary code after the code from category Z38, Liveborn infants according to place of birth and type of delivery.

c. Coding Additional Perinatal Diagnoses

1) Assigning codes for conditions that require treatment

Assign codes for conditions that require treatment or further investigation, prolong the length of stay, or require resource utilization.

2) Codes for conditions specified as having implications for future health care needs

Assign codes for conditions that have been specified by the provider as having implications for future health care needs.

Note: This guideline should not be used for adult patients.

d. Prematurity and Fetal Growth Retardation

Providers utilize different criteria in determining prematurity. A code for prematurity should not be assigned unless it is documented.

Assignment of codes in categories P05, Disorders of newborn related to slow fetal growth and fetal malnutrition, and P07, Disorders of newborn related to short gestation and low birth weight, not elsewhere classified, should be based on the recorded birth weight and estimated gestational age.

When both birth weight and gestational age are available, two codes from category P07 should be assigned, with the code for birth weight sequenced before the code for gestational age.

e. Low birth weight and immaturity status

Codes from category P07, Disorders of newborn related to short gestation and low birth weight, not elsewhere classified, are for use for a child or adult who was premature or had a low birth weight as a newborn and this is affecting the patient's current health status.

See Section I.C.21. Factors influencing health status and contact with health services, Status.

f. Bacterial Sepsis of Newborn

Category P36, Bacterial sepsis of newborn, includes congenital sepsis. If a perinate is documented as having sepsis without documentation of congenital or community acquired, the default is congenital and a code from category P36 should be assigned. If the P36 code includes the causal organism, an additional code from category B95, Streptococcus, Staphylococcus, and Enterococcus as the cause of diseases classified elsewhere, or B96, Other bacterial agents as the cause of diseases classified elsewhere, should not be assigned. If the P36 code does not include the causal organism, assign an additional code from category B96. If applicable, use additional codes to identify severe sepsis (R65.2-) and any associated acute organ dysfunction.

g. Stillbirth

Code P95, Stillbirth, is only for use in institutions that maintain separate records for stillbirths. No other code should be used with P95.Code P95 should not be used on the mother's record.

17. Chapter 17: Congenital malformations, deformations, and chromosomal abnormalities (Q00-Q99)

Assign an appropriate code(s) from categories Q00-Q99, Congenital malformations, deformations, and chromosomal abnormalities when a malformation/deformation or chromosomal abnormality is documented. A malformation/deformation/or chromosomal abnormality may be the principal/first-listed diagnosis on a record or a secondary diagnosis.

When a malformation/deformation or chromosomal abnormality does not have a unique code assignment, assign additional code(s) for any manifestations that may be present.

When the code assignment specifically identifies the malformation/deformation or chromosomal abnormality, manifestations that are an inherent component of the anomaly should not be coded separately.

Additional codes should be assigned for manifestations that are not an inherent component.

Codes from Chapter 17 may be used throughout the life of the patient. If a congenital malformation or deformity has been corrected, a personal history code should be used to identify the history of the malformation or deformity. Although present at birth, **a** malformation/deformation/or chromosomal abnormality may not be identified until later in life. Whenever the condition is diagnosed by the **provider**, it is appropriate to assign a code from codes Q00- Q99. For the birth admission, the appropriate code from category Z38, Liveborn infants, according to place of birth and type of delivery, should be sequenced as the principal diagnosis, followed by any congenital anomaly codes, Q00- Q99.

18. Chapter 18: Symptoms, signs, and abnormal clinical and laboratory findings, not elsewhere classified (R00-R99)

Chapter 18 includes symptoms, signs, abnormal results of clinical or other investigative procedures, and ill-defined conditions regarding which no diagnosis classifiable elsewhere is recorded. Signs and symptoms that point to a specific diagnosis have been assigned to a category in other chapters of the classification.

a. Use of symptom codes

Codes that describe symptoms and signs are acceptable for reporting purposes when a related definitive diagnosis has not been established (confirmed) by the provider.

b. Use of a symptom code with a definitive diagnosis code

Codes for signs and symptoms may be reported in addition to a related definitive diagnosis when the sign or symptom is not routinely associated with that diagnosis, such as the various signs and symptoms associated with complex syndromes. The definitive diagnosis code should be sequenced before the symptom code.

Signs or symptoms that are associated routinely with a disease process should not be assigned as additional codes, unless otherwise instructed by the classification.

c. Combination codes that include symptoms

ICD-10-CM contains a number of combination codes that identify both the definitive diagnosis and common symptoms of that diagnosis.

When using one of these combination codes, an additional code should not be assigned for the symptom.

d. Repeated falls

Code R29.6, Repeated falls, is for use for encounters when a patient has recently fallen and the reason for the fall is being investigated.

Code Z91.81, History of falling, is for use when a patient has fallen in the past and is at risk for future falls. When appropriate, both codes R29.6 and Z91.81 may be assigned together.

e. Coma scale

The coma scale codes (R40.2-) can be used in conjunction with traumatic brain injury codes, acute cerebrovascular disease or sequelae of cerebrovascular disease codes. These codes are primarily for use by trauma registries, but they may be used in any setting where this information is collected. The coma scale may also be used to assess the status of the central nervous system for other non-trauma conditions, such as monitoring patients in the intensive care unit regardless of medical condition. The coma scale codes should be sequenced after the diagnosis code(s).

These codes, one from each subcategory, are needed to complete the scale. The 7th character indicates when the scale was recorded. The 7th character should match for all three codes.

At a minimum, report the initial score documented on presentation at your facility. This may be a score from the emergency medicine technician (EMT) or in the emergency department. If desired, a facility may choose to capture multiple coma scale scores.

Assign code R40.24, Glasgow coma scale, total score, when only the total score is documented in the medical record and not the individual score(s).

Do not report codes for individual or total Glasgow coma scale scores for a patient with a medically induced coma or a sedated patient.

See Section I.B.14 for coma scale documentation by clinicians other than patient's provider

f. Functional quadriplegia

GUIDELINE HAS BEEN DELETED EFFECTIVE OCTOBER 1, 2017

g. SIRS due to Non-Infectious Process

The systemic inflammatory response syndrome (SIRS) can develop as a result of certain non-infectious disease processes, such as trauma, malignant neoplasm, or pancreatitis. When SIRS is documented with a noninfectious

condition, and no subsequent infection is documented, the code for the underlying condition, such as an injury, should be assigned, followed by code R65.10, Systemic inflammatory response syndrome (SIRS) of non-infectious origin without acute organ dysfunction, or code R65.11, Systemic inflammatory response syndrome (SIRS) of non-infectious origin with acute organ dysfunction. If an associated acute organ dysfunction is documented, the appropriate code(s) for the specific type of organ dysfunction(s) should be assigned in addition to code R65.11. If acute organ dysfunction is documented, but it cannot be determined if the acute organ dysfunction is associated with SIRS or due to another condition (e.g., directly due to the trauma), the provider should be queried.

h. Death NOS

Code R99, Ill-defined and unknown cause of mortality, is only for use in the very limited circumstance when a patient who has already died is brought into an emergency department or other healthcare facility and is pronounced dead upon arrival. It does not represent the discharge disposition of death.

i. NIHSS Stroke Scale

The NIH stroke scale (NIHSS) codes (R29.7- -) can be used in conjunction with acute stroke codes (I63) to identify the patient's neurological status and the severity of the stroke. The stroke scale codes should be sequenced after the acute stroke diagnosis code(s).

At a minimum, report the initial score documented. If desired, a facility may choose to capture multiple stroke scale scores.

See Section I.B.14 for NIHSS stroke scale documentation by clinicians other than patient's provider

19. Chapter 19: Injury, poisoning, and certain other consequences of external causes (S00-T88)

a. Application of 7th Characters in Chapter 19

Most categories in chapter 19 have a 7th character requirement for each applicable code. Most categories in this chapter have three 7th character values (with the exception of fractures): A, initial encounter, D, subsequent encounter and S, sequela. Categories for traumatic fractures have additional 7th character values. While the patient may be seen by a new or different provider over the course of treatment for an injury, assignment of the 7th character is based on whether the patient is undergoing active treatment and not whether the provider is seeing the patient for the first time.

For complication codes, active treatment refers to treatment for the condition described by the code, even though it may be related to an earlier precipitating problem. For example, code T84.50XA, Infection and inflammatory reaction due to unspecified internal joint prosthesis, initial encounter, is used when active treatment is provided for the infection, even though the condition relates to the prosthetic device, implant or graft that was placed at a previous encounter.

7th character "A", initial encounter is used for each encounter where the patient is receiving active treatment for the condition.

7th character "D" subsequent encounter is used for encounters after the patient has completed active treatment of the condition and is receiving routine care for the condition during the healing or recovery phase.

The aftercare Z codes should not be used for aftercare for conditions such as injuries or poisonings, where 7th characters are provided to identify subsequent care. For example, for aftercare of an injury, assign the acute injury code with the 7th character "D" (subsequent encounter).

7th character "S", sequela, is for use for complications or conditions that arise as a direct result of a condition, such as scar formation after a burn. The scars are sequelae of the burn. When using 7th character "S", it is necessary to use both the injury code that precipitated the sequela and the code for the sequela itself. The "S" is added only to the injury code, not the sequela code. The 7th character "S" identifies the injury responsible for the sequela. The specific type of sequela (e.g. scar) is sequenced first, followed by the injury code.

See Section I.B.10 Sequelae, (Late Effects)

b. Coding of Injuries

When coding injuries, assign separate codes for each injury unless a combination code is provided, in which case the combination code is assigned. Codes from category T07, Unspecified multiple injuries should not be assigned in the inpatient setting unless information for a more specific code is not available. Traumatic injury codes (S00- T14.9) are not to be used for normal, healing surgical wounds or to identify complications of surgical wounds.

The code for the most serious injury, as determined by the provider and the focus of treatment, is sequenced first.

1) Superficial injuries

Superficial injuries such as abrasions or contusions are not coded when associated with more severe injuries of the same site.

2) Primary injury with damage to nerves/blood vessels

When a primary injury results in minor damage to peripheral nerves or blood vessels, the primary injury is sequenced first with additional code(s) for injuries to nerves and spinal cord (such as category S04), and/or injury to blood vessels (such as category S15). When the primary injury is to the blood vessels or nerves, that injury should be sequenced first.

3) Iatrogenic injuries

Injury codes from Chapter 19 should not be assigned for injuries that occur during, or as a result of, a medical intervention. Assign the appropriate complication code(s).

c. Coding of Traumatic Fractures (*See* **Fig. I.C.19.c**)

The principles of multiple coding of injuries should be followed in coding fractures. Fractures of specified sites are coded individually by site in accordance with both the provisions within categories S02, S12, S22, S32, S42, S49, S52, S59, S62, S72, S79, S82, S89, S92 and the level of detail furnished by medical record content.

A fracture not indicated as open or closed should be coded to closed. A fracture not indicated whether displaced or not displaced should be coded to displaced.

More specific guidelines are as follows:

1) Initial vs. subsequent encounter for fractures

Traumatic fractures are coded using the appropriate 7th character for initial encounter (A, B, C) for each encounter where the patient is receiving active treatment for the fracture. The appropriate 7th character for initial encounter should also be assigned for a patient who delayed seeking treatment for the fracture or nonunion.

Fractures are coded using the appropriate 7th character for subsequent care for encounters after the patient has completed active treatment of the fracture and is receiving routine care for the fracture during the healing or recovery phase.

Care for complications of surgical treatment for fracture repairs during the healing or recovery phase should be coded with the appropriate complication codes.

Care of complications of fractures, such as malunion and nonunion, should be reported with the appropriate 7th character for subsequent care with nonunion (K, M, N,) or subsequent care with malunion (P, Q, R).

Malunion/nonunion: The appropriate 7th character for initial encounter should also be assigned for a patient who delayed seeking treatment for the fracture or nonunion.

The open fracture designations in the assignment of the 7th character for fractures of the forearm, femur and lower leg, including ankle are based on the Gustilo open fracture classification. When the Gustilo classification type is not specified for an open fracture, the 7th character for open fracture type I or II should be assigned (B, E, H, M, Q).

A code from category M80, not a traumatic fracture code, should be used for any patient with known osteoporosis who suffers a fracture, even if the patient had a minor fall or trauma, if that fall or trauma would not usually break a normal, healthy bone.

See Section I.C.13.Osteoporosis.

The aftercare Z codes should not be used for aftercare for traumatic fractures. For aftercare of a traumatic fracture, assign the acute fracture code with the appropriate 7th character.

2) Multiple fractures sequencing

Multiple fractures are sequenced in accordance with the severity of the fracture.

3) Physeal fractures

For physeal fractures, assign only the code identifying the type of physeal fracture. Do not assign a separate code to identify the specific bone that is fractured.

d. Coding of Burns and Corrosions

The ICD-10-CM makes a distinction between burns and corrosions. The burn codes are for thermal burns, except sunburns, that come from a heat source, such as a fire or hot appliance. The burn codes are also for burns resulting from electricity and radiation. Corrosions are burns due to chemicals. The guidelines are the same for burns and corrosions.

Current burns (T20-T25) are classified by depth, extent and by agent (X code). Burns are classified by depth as first degree (erythema), second degree (blistering), and third degree (full-thickness involvement).

Burns of the eye and internal organs (T26-T28) are classified by site, but not by degree.

1) Sequencing of burn and related condition codes

Sequence first the code that reflects the highest degree of burn when more than one burn is present.

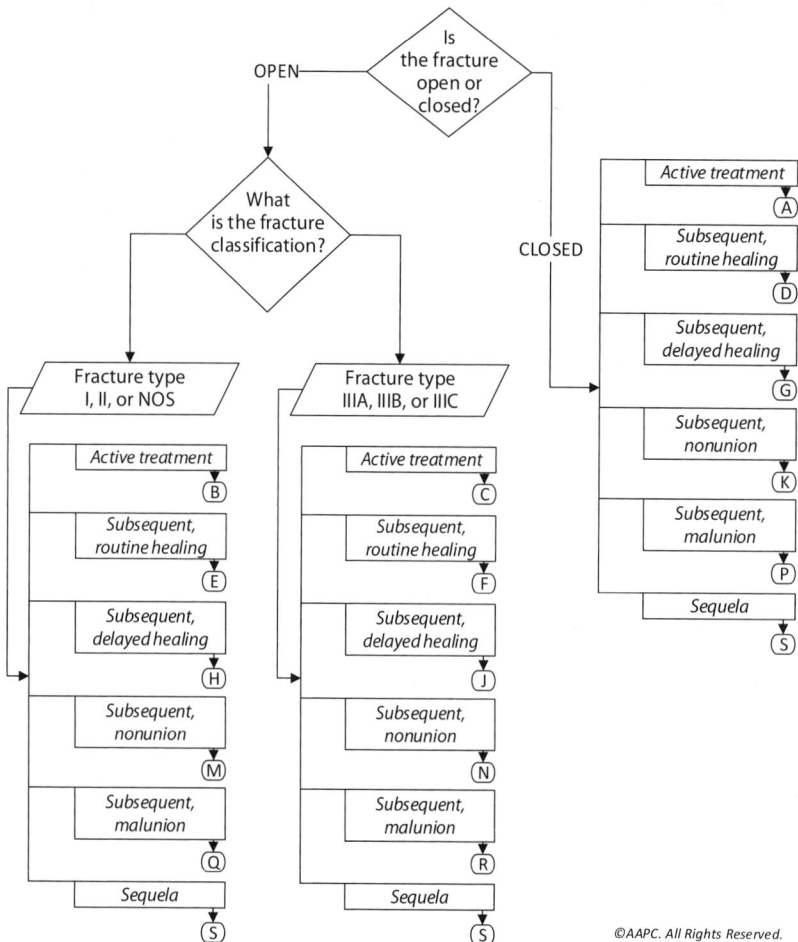

Figure I.C.19.c: Coding of Traumatic Fractures

(a) When the reason for the admission or encounter is for treatment of external multiple burns, sequence first the code that reflects the burn of the highest degree.

(b) When a patient has both internal and external burns, the circumstances of admission govern the selection of the principal diagnosis or first-listed diagnosis.

(c) When a patient is admitted for burn injuries and other related conditions such as smoke inhalation and/or respiratory failure, the circumstances of admission govern the selection of the principal or first-listed diagnosis.

2) Burns of the same *anatomic* site

Classify burns of the same anatomic site and on the same side but of different degrees to the subcategory identifying the highest degree recorded in the diagnosis (e.g., for second and third degree burns of right thigh, assign only code T24.311-).

3) Non-healing burns

Non-healing burns are coded as acute burns.

Necrosis of burned skin should be coded as a non-healed burn.

4) Infected burn

For any documented infected burn site, use an additional code for the infection.

5) Assign separate codes for each burn site

When coding burns, assign separate codes for each burn site. Category T30, Burn and corrosion, body region unspecified is extremely vague and should rarely be used.

Codes for burns of "multiple sites" should only be assigned when the medical record documentation does not specify the individual sites.

6) Burns and corrosions classified according to extent of body surface involved

Assign codes from category T31, Burns classified according to extent of body surface involved, or T32, Corrosions classified according to extent of body surface involved, when the site of the burn is not specified or when there is a need for additional data. It is advisable to use category T31 as additional coding when needed to provide data for evaluating burn mortality, such as that needed by burn units. It is also advisable to use category T31 as an additional code for reporting purposes when there is mention of a third-degree burn involving 20 percent or more of the body surface.

Categories T31 and T32 are based on the classic "rule of nines" in estimating body surface involved: head and neck are assigned nine percent, each arm nine percent, each leg 18 percent, the anterior trunk 18 percent, posterior trunk 18 percent, and genitalia one percent. Providers may change these percentage assignments where necessary to accommodate infants and children who have proportionally larger heads than adults, and patients who have large buttocks, thighs, or abdomen that involve burns.

7) Encounters for treatment of sequela of burns

Encounters for the treatment of the late effects of burns or corrosions (i.e., scars or joint contractures) should be coded with a burn or corrosion code with the 7th character "S" for sequela.

8) Sequelae with a late effect code and current burn

When appropriate, both a code for a current burn or corrosion with 7th character "A" or "D" and a burn or corrosion code with 7th character "S" may be assigned on the same record (when both a current burn and sequelae of an old burn exist). Burns and corrosions do not heal at the same rate and a current healing wound may still exist with sequela of a healed burn or corrosion.

See Section I.B.10 Sequela (Late Effects)

9) Use of an external cause code with burns and corrosions

An external cause code should be used with burns and corrosions to identify the source and intent of the burn, as well as the place where it occurred.

e. Adverse Effects, Poisoning, Underdosing and Toxic Effects

Codes in categories T36-T65 are combination codes that include the substance that was taken as well as the intent. No additional external cause code is required for poisonings, toxic effects, adverse effects and underdosing codes.

1) Do not code directly from the Table of Drugs

Do not code directly from the Table of Drugs and Chemicals. Always refer back to the Tabular List.

2) Use as many codes as necessary to describe

Use as many codes as necessary to describe completely all drugs, medicinal or biological substances.

3) If the same code would describe the causative agent

If the same code would describe the causative agent for more than one adverse reaction, poisoning, toxic effector underdosing, assign the code only once.

4) If two or more drugs, medicinal or biological substances

If two or more drugs, medicinal or biological substances are **taken**, code each individually unless a combination code is listed in the Table of Drugs and Chemicals.

If multiple unspecified drugs, medicinal or biological substances were taken, assign the appropriate code from subcategory T50.91, Poisoning by, adverse effect of and underdosing of multiple unspecified drugs, medicaments and biological substances.

5) The occurrence of drug toxicity is classified in ICD-10-CM as follows (*See* **Table I.C.19.e.5**):

(a) Adverse Effect

When coding an adverse effect of a drug that has been correctly prescribed and properly administered, assign the appropriate code for the nature of the adverse effect followed by the appropriate code for the adverse effect of the drug (T36-T50). The code for the drug should have a 5th or 6th character "5" (for example T36.0X5-) Examples of the nature of an adverse effect are tachycardia, delirium, gastrointestinal hemorrhaging, vomiting, hypokalemia, hepatitis, renal failure, or respiratory failure.

(b) Poisoning

When coding a poisoning or reaction to the improper use of a medication (e.g., overdose, wrong substance given or taken in error, wrong route of administration), first assign the appropriate code from categories T36-T50.

The poisoning codes have an associated intent as their 5th or 6th character (accidental, intentional self-harm, assault and undetermined. If the intent of the poisoning is unknown or unspecified, code the intent as accidental intent. The undetermined intent is only for use if the documentation in the record specifies that the intent cannot be determined. Use additional code(s) for all manifestations of poisonings.

If there is also a diagnosis of abuse or dependence of the substance, the abuse or dependence is assigned as an additional code.

Examples of poisoning include:

(i) Error was made in drug prescription Errors made in drug prescription or in the administration of the drug by provider, nurse, patient, or other person.

(ii) Overdose of a drug intentionally taken

If an overdose of a drug was intentionally taken or administered and resulted in drug toxicity, it would be coded as a poisoning.

(iii) Nonprescribed drug taken with correctly prescribed and properly administered drug

If a nonprescribed drug or medicinal agent was taken in combination with a correctly prescribed and properly administered drug, any drug toxicity or other reaction resulting from the interaction of the two drugs would be classified as a poisoning.

(iv) Interaction of drug(s) and alcohol

When a reaction results from the interaction of a drug(s) and alcohol, this would be classified as poisoning.

See Section I.C.4. if poisoning is the result of insulin pump malfunctions.

(c) Underdosing

Underdosing refers to taking less of a medication than is prescribed by a provider or a manufacturer's instruction. Discontinuing the use of a prescribed medication on the patient's own initiative (not directed by the patient's provider) is also classified as an underdosing. For underdosing, assign the code from categories T36-T50 (fifth or sixth character "6").

Codes for underdosing should never be assigned as principal or first-listed codes. If a patient has a relapse or exacerbation of the medical condition for which the drug is prescribed because of the reduction in dose, then the medical condition itself should be coded.

Noncompliance (Z91.12-, Z91.13- and Z91.14-) or complication of care (Y63.6-Y63.9) codes are to be used with an underdosing code to indicate intent, if known.

(d) Toxic Effects

When a harmful substance is ingested or comes in contact with a person, this is classified as a toxic effect. The toxic effect codes are in categories T51-T65.

Toxic effect codes have an associated intent: accidental, intentional self-harm, assault and undetermined.

f. Adult and child abuse, neglect and other maltreatment

Sequence first the appropriate code from categories T74, Adult and child abuse, neglect and other maltreatment, confirmed) or T76, Adult and child abuse, neglect and other maltreatment, suspected) for abuse, neglect and other maltreatment, followed by any accompanying mental health or injury code(s).

If the documentation in the medical record states abuse or neglect it is coded as confirmed (T74.-). It is coded as suspected if it is documented as suspected (T76.-).

For cases of confirmed abuse or neglect an external cause code from the assault section (X92-Y09) should be added to identify the cause of any physical injuries. A perpetrator code (Y07) should be added when the perpetrator of the abuse is known. For suspected cases of abuse or neglect, do not report external cause or perpetrator code.

If a suspected case of abuse, neglect or mistreatment is ruled out during an encounter code Z04.71, Encounter for examination and observation following alleged physical adult abuse, ruled out, or code Z04.72, Encounter for examination and observation following alleged child physical abuse, ruled out, should be used, not a code from T76.

If a suspected case of alleged rape or sexual abuse is ruled out during an encounter code Z04.41, Encounter for examination and observation following alleged adult rape or code Z04.42, Encounter for examination and observation following alleged child rape, should be used, not a code from T76.

If a suspected case of forced sexual exploitation or forced labor exploitation is ruled out during an encounter, code Z04.81, Encounter for examination and observation of victim following forced sexual exploitation, or code Z04.82, Encounter for examination and observation of victim following forced labor exploitation, should be used, not a code from T76.

See Section I.C.15. Abuse in a pregnant patient.

g. Complications of care

1) General guidelines for complications of care

(a) Documentation of complications of care

See Section I.B.16. for information on documentation of complications of care.

2) Pain due to medical devices

Pain associated with devices, implants or grafts left in a surgical site (for example painful hip prosthesis) is assigned to the appropriate

Table I.C.19.e.5: Adverse Effect, Poisoning, Underdosing, and Toxic Effects

Condition and Definition	Coding
Adverse Effect – drug has been correctly prescribed and properly administered.	1. Nature of the adverse effect (tachycardia, delirium, etc.); and 2. Adverse effect (T36-T50 with 5th or 6th character 5).
Poisoning – Improper use of a drug.	1. Poisoning code (T36-T50). The 5th or 6th character identifies the associated intent; and 2. All manifestations of poisoning; and 3. Abuse or dependence of the substance (if applicable).
Underdosing – taking less of a medication than is prescribed by a provider or a manufacturer's instruction.	1. Condition caused by the underdosing; and 2. Underdosing code (T36-T50 with 5th or 6th character 6); and 3. Noncompliance (Z91.12-, Z91.13-) or complication of care (Y63.6-Y63.9) codes, if known.
Toxic Effects – when a harmful substance is ingested or comes in contact with a person.	1. Toxic effect code (T51-T65). These codes include associated intent.

code(s) found in Chapter 19, Injury, poisoning, and certain other consequences of external causes. Specific codes for pain due to medical devices are found in the T code section of the ICD-10-CM. Use additional code(s) from category G89 to identify acute or chronic pain due to presence of the device, implant or graft (G89.18 or G89.28).

3) Transplant complications

(a) Transplant complications other than kidney

Codes under category T86, Complications of transplanted organs and tissues, are for use for both complications and rejection of transplanted organs. A transplant complication code is only assigned if the complication affects the function of the transplanted organ. Two codes are required to fully describe a transplant complication: the appropriate code from category T86 and a secondary code that identifies the complication.

Pre-existing conditions or conditions that develop after the transplant are not coded as complications unless they affect the function of the transplanted organs.

See I.C.21. for transplant organ removal status

See I.C.2. for malignant neoplasm associated with transplanted organ.

(b) Kidney transplant complications

Patients who have undergone kidney transplant may still have some form of chronic kidney disease (CKD) because the kidney transplant may not fully restore kidney function. Code T86.1- should be assigned for documented complications of a kidney transplant, such as transplant failure or rejection or other transplant complication. Code T86.1- should not be assigned for post kidney transplant patients who have chronic kidney (CKD) unless a transplant complication such as transplant failure or rejection is documented. If the documentation is unclear as to whether the patient has a complication of the transplant, query the provider.

Conditions that affect the function of the transplanted kidney, other than CKD, should be assigned a code from subcategory T86.1, Complications of transplanted organ, Kidney, and a secondary code that identifies the complication.

For patients with CKD following a kidney transplant, but who do not have a complication such as failure or rejection, *see section I.C.14. Chronic kidney disease and kidney transplant status.*

4) Complication codes that include the external cause

As with certain other T codes, some of the complications of care codes have the external cause included in the code. The code includes the nature of the complication as well as the type of procedure that caused the complication. No external cause code indicating the type of procedure is necessary for these codes.

5) Complications of care codes within the body system chapters

Intraoperative and postprocedural complication codes are found within the body system chapters with codes specific to the organs and structures of that body system. These codes should be sequenced first, followed by a code(s) for the specific complication, if applicable.

Complication codes from the body system chapters should be assigned for intraoperative and postprocedural complications (e.g., the appropriate complication code from chapter 9 would be assigned for a vascular intraoperative or postprocedural complication) unless the complication is specifically indexed to a T code in chapter 19.

20. Chapter 20: External Causes of Morbidity (V00-Y99)

The external causes of morbidity codes should never be sequenced as the first- listed or principal diagnosis.

External cause codes are intended to provide data for injury research and evaluation of injury prevention strategies. These codes capture how the injury or health condition happened (cause), the intent (unintentional or accidental; or intentional, such as suicide or assault), the place where the event occurred the activity of the patient at the time of the event, and the person's status (e.g., civilian, military).

There is no national requirement for mandatory ICD-10-CM external cause code reporting. Unless a provider is subject to a state-based external cause code reporting mandate or these codes are required by a particular payer, reporting of ICD-10-CM codes in Chapter 20, External Causes of Morbidity, is not required. In the absence of a mandatory reporting requirement, providers

are encouraged to voluntarily report external cause codes, as they provide valuable data for injury research and evaluation of injury prevention strategies.

a. General External Cause Coding Guidelines

1) Used with any code in the range of A00.0-T88.9, Z00-Z99

An external cause code may be used with any code in the range of A00.0-T88.9, Z00-Z99, classification that represents a health condition due to an external cause. Though they are most applicable to injuries, they are also valid for use with such things as infections or diseases due to an external source, and other health conditions, such as a heart attack that occurs during strenuous physical activity.

2) External cause code used for length of treatment

Assign the external cause code, with the appropriate 7th character (initial encounter, subsequent encounter or sequela) for each encounter for which the injury or condition is being treated.

Most categories in chapter 20 have a 7th character requirement for each applicable code. Most categories in this chapter have three 7th character values: A, initial encounter, D, subsequent encounter and S, sequela. While the patient may be seen by a new or different provider over the course of treatment for an injury or condition, assignment of the 7th character for external cause should match the 7th character of the code assigned for the associated injury or condition for the encounter.

3) Use the full range of external cause codes

Use the full range of external cause codes to completely describe the cause, the intent, the place of occurrence, and if applicable, the activity of the patient at the time of the event, and the patient's status, for all injuries, and other health conditions due to an external cause.

4) Assign as many external cause codes as necessary

Assign as many external cause codes as necessary to fully explain each cause. If only one external code can be recorded, assign the code most related to the principal diagnosis.

5) The selection of the appropriate external cause code

The selection of the appropriate external cause code is guided by the Alphabetic Index of External Causes and by Inclusion and Exclusion notes in the Tabular List.

6) External cause code can never be a principal diagnosis

An external cause code can never be a principal (first-listed) diagnosis.

7) Combination external cause codes

Certain of the external cause codes are combination codes that identify sequential events that result in an injury, such as a fall which results in striking against an object. The injury may be due to either event or both. The combination external cause code used should correspond to the sequence of events regardless of which caused the most serious injury.

8) No external cause code needed in certain circumstances

No external cause code from Chapter 20 is needed if the external cause and intent are included in a code from another chapter (e.g. T36.0X1- Poisoning by penicillin, accidental (unintentional)).

b. Place of Occurrence Guideline

Codes from category Y92, Place of occurrence of the external cause, are secondary codes for use after other external cause codes to identify the location of the patient at the time of injury or other condition.

Generally, a place of occurrence code is assigned only once, at the initial encounter for treatment. However, in the rare instance that a new injury occurs during hospitalization, an additional place of occurrence code may be assigned. No 7th characters are used for Y92.

Do not use place of occurrence code Y92.9 if the place is not stated oris not applicable.

c. Activity Code

Assign a code from category Y93, Activity code, to describe the activity of the patient at the time the injury or other health condition occurred.

An activity code is used only once, at the initial encounter for treatment. Only one code from Y93 should be recorded on a medical record.

The activity codes are not applicable to poisonings, adverse effects, misadventures or sequela.

Do not assign Y93.9, Unspecified activity, if the activity is not stated.

A code from category Y93 is appropriate for use with external cause and intent codes if identifying the activity provides additional information about the event.

d. Place of Occurrence, Activity, and Status Codes Used with other External Cause Code

When applicable, place of occurrence, activity, and external cause status codes are sequenced after the main external cause code(s). Regardless of the number of external cause codes assigned, generally there should be only one place of occurrence code, one activity code, and one external cause status code assigned to an encounter. However, in the rare instance that a new injury occurs during hospitalization, an additional place of occurrence code may be assigned.

e. If the Reporting Format Limits the Number of External Cause Codes

If the reporting format limits the number of external cause codes that can be used in reporting clinical data, report the code for the cause/intent most related to the principal diagnosis. If the format permits capture of additional external cause codes, the cause/intent, including medical misadventures, of the additional events should be reported rather than the codes for place, activity, or external status.

f. Multiple External Cause Coding Guidelines

More than one external cause code is required to fully describe the external cause of an illness or injury. The assignment of external cause codes should be sequenced in the following priority:

If two or more events cause separate injuries, an external cause code should be assigned for each cause. The first-listed external cause code will be selected in the following order:

External codes for child and adult abuse take priority over all other external cause codes.

See Section I.C.19., Child and Adult abuse guidelines.

External cause codes for terrorism events take priority over all other external cause codes except child and adult abuse.

External cause codes for cataclysmic events take priority over all other external cause codes except child and adult abuse and terrorism.

External cause codes for transport accidents take priority over all other external cause codes except cataclysmic events, child and adult abuse and terrorism.

Activity and external cause status codes are assigned following all causal (intent) external cause codes.

The first-listed external cause code should correspond to the cause of the most serious diagnosis due to an assault, accident, or self-harm, following the order of hierarchy listed above.

g. Child and Adult Abuse Guideline

Adult and child abuse, neglect and maltreatment are classified as assault. Any of the assault codes may be used to indicate the external cause of any injury resulting from the confirmed abuse.

For confirmed cases of abuse, neglect and maltreatment, when the perpetrator is known, a code from Y07, Perpetrator of maltreatment and neglect, should accompany any other assault codes.

See Section I.C.19. Adult and child abuse, neglect and other maltreatment

h. Unknown or Undetermined Intent Guideline

If the intent (accident, self-harm, assault) of the cause of an injury or other condition is unknown or unspecified, code the intent as accidental intent. All transport accident categories assume accidental intent.

1) Use of undetermined intent

External cause codes for events of undetermined intent are only for use if the documentation in the record specifies that the intent cannot be determined.

i. Sequelae (Late Effects) of External Cause Guidelines

1) Sequelae external cause codes

Sequela are reported using the external cause code with the 7th character "S" for sequela. These codes should be used with any report of a late effect or sequela resulting from a previous injury.

See Section I.B.10 Sequela (Late Effects)

2) Sequela external cause code with a related current injury

A sequela external cause code should never be used with a related current nature of injury code.

3) Use of sequela external cause codes for subsequent visits

Use a late effect external cause code for subsequent visits when a late effect of the initial injury is being treated. Do not use a late effect external cause code for subsequent visits for follow-up care (e.g., to assess healing, to receive rehabilitative therapy) of the injury when no late effect of the injury has been documented.

j. Terrorism Guidelines

1) Cause of injury identified by the Federal Government (FBI) as terrorism

When the cause of an injury is identified by the Federal Government (FBI) as terrorism, the first-listed external cause code should be a code from category Y38, Terrorism. The definition of terrorism employed by the FBI is found at the inclusion note at the beginning of category Y38. Use additional code for place of occurrence (Y92.-). More than one Y38 code may be assigned if the injury is the result of more than one mechanism of terrorism.

2) Cause of an injury is suspected to be the result of terrorism

When the cause of an injury is suspected to be the result of terrorism a code from category Y38 should not be assigned. Suspected cases should be classified as assault.

3) Code Y38.9, Terrorism, secondary effects

Assign code Y38.9, Terrorism, secondary effects, for conditions occurring subsequent to the terrorist event. This code should not be assigned for conditions that are due to the initial terrorist act.

It is acceptable to assign code Y38.9 with another code from Y38 if there is an injury due to the initial terrorist event and an injury that is a subsequent result of the terrorist event.

k. External Cause Status

A code from category Y99, External cause status, should be assigned whenever any other external cause code is assigned for an encounter, including an Activity code, except for the events noted below. Assign a code from category Y99, External cause status, to indicate the work status of the person at the time the event occurred. The status code indicates whether the event occurred during military activity, whether a non-military person was at work, whether an individual including a student or volunteer was involved in a non-work activity at the time of the causal event.

A code from Y99, External cause status, should be assigned, when applicable, with other external cause codes, such as transport accidents and falls. The external cause status codes are not applicable to poisonings, adverse effects, misadventures or late effects.

Do not assign a code from category Y99 if no other external cause codes (cause, activity) are applicable for the encounter.

An external cause status code is used only once, at the initial encounter for treatment. Only one code from Y99 should be recorded on a medical record.

Do not assign code Y99.9, Unspecified external cause status, if the status is not stated.

21. Chapter 21: Factors influencing health status and contact with health services (Z00-Z99)

Note: The chapter specific guidelines provide additional information about the use of Z codes for specified encounters.

a. Use of Z Codes in Any Healthcare Setting

Z codes are for use in any healthcare setting. Z codes may be used as either a first-listed (principal diagnosis code in the inpatient setting) or secondary code, depending on the circumstances of the encounter.

Certain Z codes may only be used as first-listed or principal diagnosis.

b. Z Codes Indicate a Reason for an Encounter

Z codes are not procedure codes. A corresponding procedure code must accompany a Z code to describe any procedure performed.

c. Categories of Z Codes

1) Contact/Exposure

Category Z20 indicates contact with, and suspected exposure to, communicable diseases. These codes are for patients who do not show any sign or symptom of a disease but are suspected to have been exposed to it by close personal contact with an infected individual or are in an area where a disease is epidemic.

Category Z77, Other contact with and (suspected) exposures hazardous to health, indicates contact with and suspected exposures hazardous to health.

Contact/exposure codes may be used as a first-listed code to explain an encounter for testing, or, more commonly, as a secondary code to identify a potential risk.

2) Inoculations and vaccinations

Code Z23 is for encounters for inoculations and vaccinations. It indicates that a patient is being seen to receive a prophylactic inoculation against a disease. Procedure codes are required to identify the actual administration of the injection and the type(s) of immunizations given. Code Z23 may be used as a secondary code if the inoculation is given as a routine part of preventive health care, such as a well-baby visit.

3) Status

Status codes indicate that a patient is either a carrier of a disease or has the sequelae or residual of a past disease or condition.

This includes such things as the presence of prosthetic or mechanical devices resulting from past treatment. A status code is informative, because the status may affect the course of treatment and its outcome. A status code is distinct from a history code. The history code indicates that the patient no longer has the condition.

A status code should not be used with a diagnosis code from one of the body system chapters, if the diagnosis code includes the information provided by the status code. For example, code Z94.1, Heart transplant status, should not be used with a code from subcategory T86.2, Complications of heart transplant. The status code does not provide additional information. The complication code indicates that the patient is a heart transplant patient.

For encounters for weaning from a mechanical ventilator, assign a code from subcategory J96.1, Chronic respiratory failure, followed by code Z99.11, Dependence on respirator [ventilator] status.

The status Z codes/categories are:

Z14   Genetic carrier

Genetic carrier status indicates that a person carries a gene, associated with a particular disease, which may be passed to offspring who may develop that disease. The person does not have the disease and is not at risk of developing the disease.

Z15   Genetic susceptibility to disease

Genetic susceptibility indicates that a person has a gene that increases the risk of that person developing the disease.

Codes from category Z15 should not be used as principal or first-listed codes. If the patient has the condition to which he/she is susceptible, and that condition is the reason for the encounter, the code for the current condition should be sequenced first. If the patient is being seen for follow-up after completed treatment for this condition, and the condition no longer exists, a follow-up code should be sequenced first, followed by the appropriate personal history and genetic susceptibility codes. If the purpose of the encounter is genetic counseling associated with procreative management, code Z31.5, Encounter for genetic counseling, should be assigned as the first-listed code, followed by a code from category Z15. Additional codes should be assigned for any applicable family or personal history.

Z16   Resistance to antimicrobial drugs

This code indicates that a patient has a condition that is resistant to antimicrobial drug treatment. Sequence the infection code first.

Z17   Estrogen receptor status

Z18   Retained foreign body fragments

Z19   Hormone sensitivity malignancy status

Z21   Asymptomatic HIV infection status

This code indicates that a patient has tested positive for HIV but has manifested no signs or symptoms of the disease.

Z22   Carrier of infectious disease

Carrier status indicates that a person harbors the specific organisms of a disease without manifest symptoms and is capable of transmitting the infection.

Z28.3   Under immunization status

Z33.1   Pregnant state, incidental

This code is a secondary code only for use when the pregnancy is in no way complicating the reason for visit. Otherwise, a code from the obstetric chapter is required.

Z66   Do not resuscitate

This code may be used when it is documented by the provider that a patient is on do not resuscitate status at any time during the stay.

Z67   Blood type

Z68   Body mass index (BMI)

BMI codes should only be assigned when **there is an associated, reportable diagnosis (such as obesity).** Do not assign BMI codes during pregnancy.

See Section I.B.14 for BMI documentation by clinicians other than the patient's provider.

Z74.01   Bed confinement status

Z76.82   Awaiting organ transplant status

Z78   Other specified health status

Code Z78.1, Physical restraint status, may be used when it is documented by the provider that a patient has been put in restraints during the current encounter. Please note that this code should not be reported when it is documented by the provider that a patient is temporarily restrained during a procedure.

Z79   Long-term (current) drug therapy

Codes from this category indicate a patient's continuous use of a prescribed drug (including such things as aspirin therapy) for the long-term treatment of a condition or for prophylactic use. It is not for use for patients who have addictions to drugs. This subcategory is not for use of medications for detoxification or maintenance programs to prevent withdrawal symptoms in patients with drug dependence (e.g., methadone maintenance for opiate dependence). Assign the appropriate code for the drug dependence instead.

Assign a code from Z79 if the patient is receiving a medication for an extended period as a prophylactic measure (such as for the prevention of deep vein thrombosis) or as treatment of a chronic condition (such as arthritis) or a disease requiring a lengthy course of treatment (such as cancer). Do not assign a code from category Z79 for medication being administered for a brief period of time to treat an acute illness or injury (such as a course of antibiotics to treat acute bronchitis).

Z88   Allergy status to drugs, medicaments and biological substances

Except: Z88.9, Allergy status to unspecified drugs, medicaments and biological substances status

Z89   Acquired absence of limb

Z90   Acquired absence of organs, not elsewhere classified

Z91.0-   Allergy status, other than to drugs and biological substances

Z92.82   Status post administration of tPA (rtPA) in a different facility within the last 24 hours prior to admission to a current facility.

Assign code Z92.82, Status post administration of tPA (rtPA) in a different facility within the last 24 hours prior to admission to current facility, as a secondary diagnosis when a patient is received by transfer into a facility and documentation indicates they were administered tissue plasminogen activator (tPA) within the last 24 hours prior to admission to the current facility.

This guideline applies even if the patient is still receiving the tPA at the time they are received into the current facility.

The appropriate code for the condition for which the tPA was administered (such as cerebrovascular disease or myocardial infarction) should be assigned first.

Code Z92.82 is only applicable to the receiving facility record and not to the transferring facility record.

Z93   Artificial opening status

Z94   Transplanted organ and tissue status

Z95   Presence of cardiac and vascular implants and grafts

Z96   Presence of other functional implants

Z97   Presence of other devices

Z98   Other postprocedural states

Assign code Z98.85, Transplanted organ removal status, to indicate that a transplanted organ has been previously removed. This code should not be assigned for the encounter in which the transplanted organ is removed. The complication necessitating removal of the transplant organ should be assigned for that encounter.

See section I.C19. for information on the coding of organ transplant complications.

Z99   Dependence on enabling machines and devices, not elsewhere classified

Note: Categories Z89-Z90 and Z93-Z99 are for use only if there are no complications or malfunctions of the organ or tissue replaced, the amputation site or the equipment on which the patient is dependent.

4)   **History (of)**

There are two types of history Z codes, personal and family. Personal history codes explain a patient's past medical condition that no longer exists and is not receiving any treatment, but that has the potential for recurrence, and therefore may require continued monitoring.

Family history codes are for use when a patient has a family member(s) who has had a particular disease that causes the patient to be at higher risk of also contracting the disease.

Personal history codes may be used in conjunction with follow-up codes and family history codes may be used in conjunction with screening codes to explain the need for a test or procedure. History codes are also acceptable on any medical record regardless of the reason for visit. A history of an illness, even if no longer present, is important information that may alter the type of treatment ordered.

The history Z code categories are:

Z80   Family history of primary malignant neoplasm

Z81   Family history of mental and behavioral disorders

Z82   Family history of certain disabilities and chronic diseases (leading to disablement)

Z83   Family history of other specific disorders

Z84   Family history of other conditions

Z85   Personal history of malignant neoplasm

Z86   Personal history of certain other diseases

Z87   Personal history of other diseases and conditions

Z91.4- Personal history of psychological trauma, not elsewhere classified

Z91.5   Personal history of self-harm

Z91.81 History of falling

Z91.82 Personal history of military deployment

Z92   Personal history of medical treatment

    Except: Z92.0, Personal history of contraception Except: Z92.82, Status post administration of tPA (rtPA) in a different facility within the last 24 hours prior to admission to a current facility

5) Screening (*See* **Fig. I.C.21.c.5**)

Screening is the testing for disease or disease precursors in seemingly well individuals so that early detection and treatment can be provided for those who test positive for the disease (e.g., screening mammogram).

The testing of a person to rule out or confirm a suspected diagnosis because the patient has some sign or symptom is a diagnostic examination, not a screening. In these cases, the sign or symptom is used to explain the reason for the test.

A screening code may be a first-listed code if the reason for the visit is specifically the screening exam. It may also be used as an additional code if the screening is done during an office visit for other health problems. A screening code is not necessary if the screening is inherent to a routine examination, such as a pap smear done during a routine pelvic examination.

Should a condition be discovered during the screening then the code for the condition may be assigned as an additional diagnosis.

The Z code indicates that a screening exam is planned. A procedure code is required to confirm that the screening was performed.

The screening Z codes/categories:

Z11   Encounter for screening for infectious and parasitic diseases

Z12   Encounter for screening for malignant neoplasms

Z13   Encounter for screening for other diseases and disorders

    Except: Z13.9, Encounter for screening, unspecified

Z36   Encounter for antenatal screening for mother

6) Observation

There are three observation Z code categories. They are for use in very limited circumstances when a person is being observed for a suspected condition that is ruled out. The observation codes are not for use if an injury or illness or any signs or symptoms related to the suspected condition are present. In such cases the diagnosis/symptom code is used with the corresponding external cause code.

The observation codes are to be used as principal diagnosis only. The only exception to this is when the principal diagnosis

is required to be a code from category Z38, Liveborn infants according to place of birth and type of delivery. Then a code from category Z05, Encounter for observation and evaluation of newborn for suspected diseases and conditions ruled out, is sequenced after the Z38 code. Additional codes may be used in addition to the observation code, but only if they are unrelated to the suspected condition being observed.

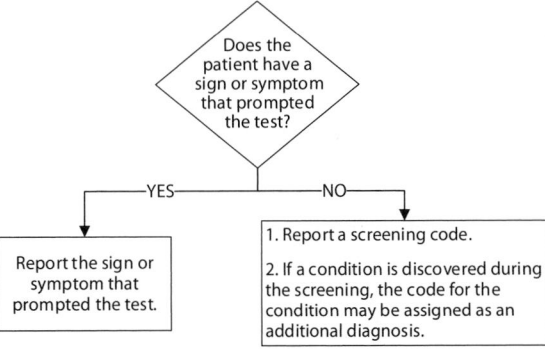

Figure I.C.21.c.5: Screening vs therapeutic

Codes from subcategory Z03.7, Encounter for suspected maternal and fetal conditions ruled out, may either be used as a first-listed or as an additional code assignment depending on the case. They are for use in very limited circumstances on a maternal record when an encounter is for a suspected maternal or fetal condition that is ruled out during that encounter (for example, a maternal or fetal condition may be suspected due to an abnormal test result). These codes should not be used when the condition is confirmed. In those cases, the confirmed condition should be coded. In addition, these codes are not for use if an illness or any signs or symptoms related to the suspected condition or problem are present. In such cases the diagnosis/symptom code is used.

Additional codes may be used in addition to the code from subcategory Z03.7, but only if they are unrelated to the suspected condition being evaluated.

Codes from subcategory Z03.7 may not be used for encounters for antenatal screening of mother. *See* Section I.C.21.

Screening.

For encounters for suspected fetal condition that are inconclusive following testing and evaluation, assign the appropriate code from category O35, O36, O40 or O41.

The observation Z code categories:

Z03   Encounter for medical observation for suspected diseases and conditions ruled out

Z04   Encounter for examination and observation for other reasons

    Except: Z04.9, Encounter for examination and observation for unspecified reason

Z05   Encounter for observation and evaluation of newborn for suspected diseases and conditions ruled out

7) Aftercare

Aftercare visit codes cover situations when the initial treatment of a disease has been performed and the patient requires continued care during the healing or recovery phase, or for the long-term consequences of the disease. The aftercare Z code should not be used if treatment is directed at a current, acute disease. The diagnosis code is to be used in these cases.

Exceptions to this rule are codes Z51.0, Encounter for antineoplastic radiation therapy, and codes from subcategory Z51.1, Encounter for antineoplastic chemotherapy and immunotherapy. These codes are to be first-listed, followed by the diagnosis code when a patient's encounter is solely to receive radiation therapy, chemotherapy, or immunotherapy for the treatment of a neoplasm. If the reason for the encounter is more than one type of antineoplastic therapy, code Z51.0 and a code from subcategory Z51.1 may be assigned together, in which case one of these codes would be reported as a secondary diagnosis.

The aftercare Z codes should also not be used for aftercare for injuries. For aftercare of an injury, assign the acute injury code with the appropriate 7th character (for subsequent encounter).

The aftercare codes are generally first-listed to explain the specific reason for the encounter. An aftercare code may be used as an additional code when some type of aftercare is provided in addition to the reason for admission and no diagnosis code is applicable. An example of this would be the closure of a colostomy during an encounter for treatment of another condition.

Aftercare codes should be used in conjunction with other aftercare codes or diagnosis codes to provide better detail on the specifics of an aftercare encounter visit, unless otherwise directed by the classification. The sequencing of multiple aftercare codes depends on the circumstances of the encounter.

Certain aftercare Z code categories need a secondary diagnosis code to describe the resolving condition or sequelae. For others, the condition is included in the code title.

Additional Z code aftercare category terms include fitting and adjustment, and attention to artificial openings.

Status Z codes may be used with aftercare Z codes to indicate the nature of the aftercare. For example, code Z95.1, Presence of aortocoronary bypass graft, may be used with code Z48.812, Encounter for surgical aftercare following surgery on the circulatory system, to indicate the surgery for which the aftercare is being performed. A status code should not be used when the aftercare code indicates the type of status, such as using Z43.0, Encounter for attention to tracheostomy, with Z93.0, Tracheostomy status.

The aftercare Z category/codes:

Z42   Encounter for plastic and reconstructive surgery following medical procedure or healed injury

Z43   Encounter for attention to artificial openings

Z44	Encounter for fitting and adjustment of external prosthetic device
Z45	Encounter for adjustment and management of implanted device
Z46	Encounter for fitting and adjustment of other devices
Z47	Orthopedic aftercare
Z48	Encounter for other post-procedural aftercare
Z49	Encounter for care involving renal dialysis
Z51	Encounter for other aftercare and medical care

8) Follow-up

The follow-up codes are used to explain continuing surveillance following completed treatment of a disease, condition, or injury. They imply that the condition has been fully treated and no longer exists. They should not be confused with aftercare codes, or injury codes with a 7th character for subsequent encounter, that explain ongoing care of a healing condition or its sequelae. Follow-up codes may be used in conjunction with history codes to provide the full picture of the healed condition and its treatment. The follow-up code is sequenced first, followed by the history code.

A follow-up code may be used to explain multiple visits. Should a condition be found to have recurred on the follow-up visit, then the diagnosis code for the condition should be assigned in place of the follow-up code.

The follow-up Z code categories:

Z08	Encounter for follow-up examination after completed treatment for malignant neoplasm
Z09	Encounter for follow-up examination after completed treatment for conditions other than malignant neoplasm
Z39	Encounter for maternal postpartum care and examination

9) Donor

Codes in category Z52, Donors of organs and tissues, are used for living individuals who are donating blood or other body tissue. These codes are only for individuals donating for others, not for self-donations. They are not used to identify cadaveric donations.

10) Counseling

Counseling Z codes are used when a patient or family member receives assistance in the aftermath of an illness or injury, or when support is required in coping with family or social problems.

The counseling Z codes/categories:

Z30.0-	Encounter for general counseling and advice on contraception
Z31.5	Encounter for procreative genetic counseling
Z31.6-	Encounter for general counseling and advice on procreation
Z32.2	Encounter for child-birth instruction
Z32.3	Encounter for child-care instruction
Z69	Encounter for mental health services for victim and perpetrator of abuse
Z70	Counseling related to sexual attitude, behavior and orientation
Z71	Persons encountering health services for other counseling and medical advice, not elsewhere classified

Note: Code Z71.84, Encounter for health counseling related to travel, is to be used for health risk and safety counseling for future travel purposes.

Z76.81	Expectant mother prebirth pediatrician visit

11) Encounters for Obstetrical and Reproductive Services

See Section I.C.15. Pregnancy, Child-birth, and the Puerperium, for further instruction on the use of these codes.

Z codes for pregnancy are for use in those circumstances when none of the problems or complications included in the codes from the Obstetrics chapter exist (a routine prenatal visit or postpartum care). Codes in category Z34, Encounter for supervision of normal pregnancy, are always first-listed and are not to be used with any other code from the OB chapter.

Codes in category Z3A, Weeks of gestation, may be assigned to provide additional information about the pregnancy. Category Z3A codes should not be assigned for pregnancies with abortive outcomes (categories O00-O08), elective termination of pregnancy (code Z33.2), nor for postpartum conditions, as category Z3A is not applicable to these conditions. The date of the admission should be used to determine weeks of gestation for inpatient admissions that encompass more than one gestational week.

The outcome of delivery, category Z37, should be included on all maternal delivery records. It is always a secondary code. Codes in category Z37 should not be used on the newborn record.

Z codes for family planning (contraceptive) or procreative management and counseling should be included on an obstetric record either during the pregnancy or the postpartum stage, if applicable.

Z codes/categories for obstetrical and reproductive services:

Z30	Encounter for contraceptive management
Z31	Encounter for procreative management
Z32.2	Encounter for childbirth instruction
Z32.3	Encounter for childcare instruction
Z33	Pregnant state
Z34	Encounter for supervision of normal pregnancy
Z36	Encounter for antenatal screening of mother
Z3A	Weeks of gestation
Z37	Outcome of delivery
Z39	Encounter for maternal postpartum care and examination
Z76.81	Expectant mother prebirth pediatrician visit

12) Newborns and Infants

See Section I.C.16. Newborn (Perinatal) Guidelines, for further instruction on the use of these codes.

Newborn Z codes/categories:

Z76.1	Encounter for health supervision and care of foundling
Z00.1-	Encounter for routine child health examination
Z38	Liveborn infants according to place of birth and type of delivery

13) Routine and Administrative Examinations

The Z codes allow for the description of encounters for routine examinations, such as, a general check-up, or, examinations for administrative purposes, such as, a pre-employment physical. The codes are not to be used if the examination is for diagnosis of a suspected condition or for treatment purposes. In such cases the diagnosis code is used. During a routine exam, should a diagnosis or condition be discovered, it should be coded as an additional code. Pre-existing and chronic conditions and history codes may also be included as additional codes as long as the examination is for administrative purposes and not focused on any particular condition.

Some of the codes for routine health examinations distinguish between "with" and "without" abnormal findings. Code assignment depends on the information that is known at the time the encounter is being coded. For example, if no abnormal findings were found during the examination, but the encounter is being coded before test results are back, it is acceptable to assign the code for "without abnormal findings." When assigning a code for "with abnormal findings," additional code(s) should be assigned to identify the specific abnormal finding(s).

Pre-operative examination and pre-procedural laboratory examination Z codes are for use only in those situations when a patient is being cleared for a procedure or surgery and no treatment is given.

The Z codes/categories for routine and administrative examinations:

Z00	Encounter for general examination without complaint, suspected or reported diagnosis
Z01	Encounter for other special examination without complaint, suspected or reported diagnosis
Z02	Encounter for administrative examination Except: Z02.9, Encounter for administrative examinations, unspecified
Z32.0-	Encounter for pregnancy test

14) Miscellaneous Z Codes

The miscellaneous Z codes capture a number of other health care encounters that do not fall into one of the other categories. Certain of these codes identify the reason for the encounter; others are for use as additional codes that provide useful information on circumstances that may affect a patient's care and treatment.

Prophylactic Organ Removal

For encounters specifically for prophylactic removal of an organ (such as prophylactic removal of breasts due to a genetic susceptibility to cancer or a family history of cancer), the principal or first-listed code should be a code from category Z40, Encounter for prophylactic surgery, followed by the appropriate codes to identify the associated risk factor (such as genetic susceptibility or family history).

If the patient has a malignancy of one site and is having prophylactic removal at another site to prevent either a new primary malignancy

or metastatic disease, a code for the malignancy should also be assigned in addition to a code from subcategory Z40.0, Encounter for prophylactic surgery for risk factors related to malignant neoplasms. A Z40.0 code should not be assigned if the patient is having organ removal for treatment of a malignancy, such as the removal of the testes for the treatment of prostate cancer.

Miscellaneous Z codes/categories:

Z28	Immunization not carried out
	Except: Z28.3, Under immunization status
Z29	Encounter for other prophylactic measures
Z40	Encounter for prophylactic surgery
Z41	Encounter for procedures for purposes other than remedying health state
	Except: Z41.9, Encounter for procedure for purposes other than remedying health state, unspecified
Z53	Persons encountering health services for specific procedures and treatment, not carried out
Z55	Problems related to education and literacy
Z56	Problems related to employment and unemployment
Z57	Occupational exposure to risk factors
Z58	Problems related to physical environment
Z59	Problems related to housing and economic circumstances
Z60	Problems related to social environment
Z62	Problems related to upbringing
Z63	Other problems related to primary support group, including family circumstances
Z64	Problems related to certain psychosocial circumstances
Z65	Problems related to other psychosocial circumstances
Z72	Problems related to lifestyle

Note: These codes should be assigned only when the documentation specifies that the patient has an associated problem

Z73	Problems related to life management difficulty
Z74	Problems related to care provider dependency
	Except: Z74.01, Bed confinement status
Z75	Problems related to medical facilities and other healthcare
Z76.0	Encounter for issue of repeat prescription
Z76.3	Healthy person accompanying sick person
Z76.4	Other boarder to healthcare facility
Z76.5	Malingerer [conscious simulation]
Z91.1-	Patient's noncompliance with medical treatment and regimen
Z91.83	Wandering in diseases classified elsewhere
Z91.84-	Oral health risk factors
Z91.89	Other specified personal risk factors, not elsewhere classified

See Section I.B.14 for Z55-Z65 Persons with potential health hazards related to socioeconomic and psychosocial circumstances, documentation by clinicians other than the patient's provider

15) Nonspecific Z Codes

Certain Z codes are so non-specific, or potentially redundant with other codes in the classification, that there can be little justification for their use in the inpatient setting. Their use in the outpatient setting should be limited to those instances when there is no further documentation to permit more precise coding. Otherwise, any sign or symptom or any other reason for visit that is captured in another code should be used.

Non-specific Z codes/categories:

Z02.9	Encounter for administrative examinations, unspecified
Z04.9	Encounter for examination and observation for unspecified reason
Z13.9	Encounter for screening, unspecified
Z41.9	Encounter for procedure for purposes other than remedying health state, unspecified
Z52.9	Donor of unspecified organ or tissue
Z86.59	Personal history of other mental and behavioral disorders
Z88.9	Allergy status to unspecified drugs, medicaments and biological substances status
Z92.0	Personal history of contraception

16) Z Codes That May Only be Principal/First-Listed Diagnosis

The following Z codes/categories may only be reported as the principal/first-listed diagnosis, except when there are multiple encounters on the same day and the medical records for the encounters are combined:

Z00	Encounter for general examination without complaint, suspected or reported diagnosis Except: Z00.6
Z01	Encounter for other special examination without complaint, suspected or reported diagnosis
Z02	Encounter for administrative examination
Z03	Encounter for medical observation for suspected diseases and conditions ruled out
Z04	Encounter for examination and observation for other reasons
Z33.2	Encounter for elective termination of pregnancy
Z31.81	Encounter for male factor infertility in female patient
Z31.83	Encounter for assisted reproductive fertility procedure cycle
Z31.84	Encounter for fertility preservation procedure
Z34	Encounter for supervision of normal pregnancy
Z39	Encounter for maternal postpartum care and examination
Z38	Liveborn infants according to place of birth and type of delivery
Z40	Encounter for prophylactic surgery
Z42	Encounter for plastic and reconstructive surgery following medical procedure or healed injury
Z51.0	Encounter for antineoplastic radiation therapy
Z51.1-	Encounter for antineoplastic chemotherapy and immunotherapy
Z52	Donors of organs and tissues
	Except: Z52.9, Donor of unspecified organ or tissue
Z76.1	Encounter for health supervision and care of foundling
Z76.2	Encounter for health supervision and care of other healthy infant and child
Z99.12	for respirator [ventilator] dependence during power failure

Section II. Selection of Principal Diagnosis

The circumstances of inpatient admission always govern the selection of principal diagnosis. The principal diagnosis is defined in the Uniform Hospital Discharge Data Set (UHDDS) as "that condition established after study to be chiefly responsible for occasioning the admission of the patient to the hospital for care."

The UHDDS definitions are used by hospitals to report inpatient data elements in a standardized manner. These data elements and their definitions can be found in the July 31, 1985, Federal Register (Vol. 50, No, 147), pp. 31038-40.

Since that time the application of the UHDDS definitions has been expanded to include all non- outpatient settings (acute care, short term, long term care and psychiatric hospitals; home health agencies; rehab facilities; nursing homes, etc). The UHDDS definitions also apply to hospice services (all levels of care).

In determining principal diagnosis, coding conventions in the ICD-10-CM, the Tabular List and Alphabetic Index take precedence over these official coding guidelines.

(*See* Section I.A., Conventions for the ICD-10-CM)

The importance of consistent, complete documentation in the medical record cannot be overemphasized. Without such documentation the application of all coding guidelines is a difficult, if not impossible, task.

A. Codes for symptoms, signs, and ill-defined conditions

Codes for symptoms, signs, and ill-defined conditions from Chapter 18 are not to be used as principal diagnosis when a related definitive diagnosis has been established.

B. Two or more interrelated conditions, each potentially meeting the definition for principal diagnosis.

When there are two or more interrelated conditions (such as diseases in the same ICD-10-CM chapter or manifestations characteristically associated with a certain disease) potentially meeting the definition of principal diagnosis, either condition may be sequenced first, unless the circumstances of the admission, the therapy provided, the Tabular List, or the Alphabetic Index indicate otherwise.

C. Two or more diagnoses that equally meet the definition for principal diagnosis

In the unusual instance when two or more diagnoses equally meet the criteria for principal diagnosis as determined by the circumstances of admission, diagnostic workup and/or therapy provided, and the Alphabetic Index, Tabular List, or another coding guidelines does not provide sequencing direction, any one of the diagnoses may be sequenced first.

D. Two or more comparative or contrasting conditions

In those rare instances when two or more contrasting or comparative diagnoses are documented as "either/or" (or similar terminology), they are coded as if the diagnoses were confirmed and the diagnoses are sequenced according to the circumstances of the admission. If no further determination can be made as to which diagnosis should be principal, either diagnosis may be sequenced first.

E. Asymptom(s) followed by contrasting/comparative diagnoses

GUIDELINE HAS BEEN DELETED EFFECTIVE OCTOBER 1, 2014

F. Original treatment plan not carried out

Sequence as the principal diagnosis the condition, which after study occasioned the admission to the hospital, even though treatment may not have been carried out due to unforeseen circumstances.

G. Complications of surgery and other medical care

When the admission is for treatment of a complication resulting from surgery or other medical care, the complication code is sequenced as the principal diagnosis. If the complication is classified to the T80-T88 series and the code lacks the necessary specificity in describing the complication, an additional code for the specific complication should be assigned.

H. Uncertain Diagnosis

If the diagnosis documented at the time of discharge is qualified as "probable," "suspected," "likely," "questionable," "possible," or "still to be ruled out," **"compatible with," "consistent with,"** or other similar terms indicating uncertainty, code the condition as if it existed or was established. The bases for these guidelines are the diagnostic workup, arrangements for further workup or observation, and initial therapeutic approach that correspond most closely with the established diagnosis.

Note: This guideline is applicable only to inpatient admissions to short-term, acute, long-term care and psychiatric hospitals.

I. Admission from Observation Unit

1. Admission Following Medical Observation

When a patient is admitted to an observation unit for a medical condition, which either worsens or does not improve, and is subsequently admitted as an inpatient of the same hospital for this same medical condition, the principal diagnosis would be the medical condition which led to the hospital admission.

2. Admission Following Post-Operative Observation

When a patient is admitted to an observation unit to monitor a condition (or complication) that develops following outpatient surgery, and then is subsequently admitted as an inpatient of the same hospital, hospitals should apply the Uniform Hospital Discharge Data Set (UHDDS) definition of principal diagnosis as "that condition established after study to be chiefly responsible for occasioning the admission of the patient to the hospital for care."

J. Admission from Outpatient Surgery

When a patient receives surgery in the hospital's outpatient surgery department and is subsequently admitted for continuing inpatient care at the same hospital, the following guidelines should be followed in selecting the principal diagnosis for the inpatient admission:

❑ If the reason for the inpatient admission is a complication, assign the complication as the principal diagnosis.

❑ If no complication, or other condition, is documented as the reason for the inpatient admission, assign the reason for the outpatient surgery as the principal diagnosis.

❑ If the reason for the inpatient admission is another condition unrelated to the surgery, assign the unrelated condition as the principal diagnosis.

K. Admissions/Encounters for Rehabilitation

When the purpose for the admission/encounter is rehabilitation, sequence first the code for the condition for which the service is being performed. For example, for an admission/encounter for rehabilitation for right-sided dominant hemiplegia following a cerebrovascular infarction, report code I69.351, Hemiplegia and hemiparesis following cerebral infarction affecting right dominant side, as the first-listed or principal diagnosis.

If the condition for which the rehabilitation service is being provided is no longer present, report the appropriate aftercare code as the first-listed or principal diagnosis, unless the rehabilitation service is being provided following an injury. For rehabilitation services following active treatment of an injury, assign the injury code with the appropriate seventh character for subsequent encounter as the first-listed or principal diagnosis. For example, if a patient with severe degenerative osteoarthritis of the hip, underwent hip replacement and the current encounter/admission is for rehabilitation, report code Z47.1, Aftercare following joint replacement surgery, as the first-listed or principal diagnosis. If the patient requires rehabilitation post hip replacement for right intertrochanteric femur fracture, report code S72.141D,

Displaced intertrochanteric fracture of right femur, subsequent encounter for closed fracture with routine healing, as the first-listed or principal diagnosis.

See Section I.C.21.c.7, Factors influencing health states and contact with health services, Aftercare.

See Section I.C.19.a for additional information about the use of 7th characters for injury codes.

Section III. Reporting Additional Diagnoses (*See* **Fig. Sec III**)

GENERAL RULES FOR OTHER (ADDITIONAL) DIAGNOSES

For reporting purposes the definition for "other diagnoses" is interpreted as additional conditions that affect patient care in terms of requiring:

    clinical evaluation; or

    therapeutic treatment; or

    diagnostic procedures; or

    extended length of hospital stay; or

    increased nursing care and/or monitoring.

The UHDDS item #11-b defines Other Diagnoses as "all conditions that coexist at the time of admission, that develop subsequently, or that affect the treatment received and/or the length of stay. Diagnoses that relate to an earlier episode which have no bearing on the current hospital stay are to be excluded." UHDDS definitions apply to inpatients in acute care, short-term, long term care and psychiatric hospital setting. The UHDDS definitions are used by acute care short- term hospitals to report inpatient data elements in a standardized manner. These data elements and their definitions can be found in the July 31, 1985, Federal Register (Vol. 50, No, 147), pp. 31038-40.

Since that time the application of the UHDDS definitions has been expanded to include all non- outpatient settings (acute care, short term, long term care and psychiatric hospitals; home health agencies; rehab facilities; nursing homes, etc). The UHDDS definitions also apply to hospice services (all levels of care).

The following guidelines are to be applied in designating "other diagnoses" when neither the Alphabetic Index nor the Tabular List in ICD-10-CM provide direction. The listing of the diagnoses in the patient record is the responsibility of the attending provider.

A. Previous conditions

If the provider has included a diagnosis in the final diagnostic statement, such as the discharge summary or the face sheet, it should ordinarily be coded. Some providers include in the diagnostic statement resolved conditions or diagnoses and status-post procedures from previous admission that have no bearing on the current stay. Such conditions are not to be reported and are coded only if required by hospital policy.

However, history codes (categories Z80-Z87) may be used as secondary codes if the historical condition or family history has an impact on current care or influences treatment.

B. Abnormal findings

Abnormal findings (laboratory, x-ray, pathologic, and other diagnostic results) are not coded and reported unless the provider indicates their clinical significance. If the findings are outside the normal range and the attending provider has ordered other tests to evaluate the condition or prescribed treatment, it is appropriate to ask the provider whether the abnormal finding should be added.

Please note: This differs from the coding practices in the outpatient setting for coding encounters for diagnostic tests that have been interpreted by a provider.

Previous Conditions	Abnormal Findings	Uncertain Diagnosis
• Code conditions included in the discharge summary if pertinent to current stay • Code history of codes if relevant to the current stay	• Code abnormal findings only if documented as clinically significant by the provider • Query the provider if ordering additional tests and there is no documentation of clinical significance	• Uncertain diagnoses present on inpatient discharge are coded as if they exist • This guideline differs from outpatient coding. *See* IV.H.

Figure Sec III: Reporting Additional Diagnoses

C. Uncertain Diagnosis

If the diagnosis documented at the time of discharge is qualified as "probable," "suspected," "likely," "questionable," "possible," or "still to be ruled out," **"compatible with," "consistent with,"** or other similar terms indicating uncertainty, code the condition as if it existed or was established. The bases for these guidelines are the diagnostic workup, arrangements for further workup or observation, and initial therapeutic approach that correspond most closely with the established diagnosis.

Note: This guideline is applicable only to inpatient admissions to short-term, acute, long-term care and psychiatric hospitals.

Section IV. Diagnostic Coding and Reporting Guidelines for Outpatient Services

These coding guidelines for outpatient diagnoses have been approved for use by hospitals/ providers in coding and reporting hospital-based outpatient services and provider-based office visits. Guidelines in Section I, Conventions, general coding guidelines and chapter-specific guidelines, should also be applied for outpatient services and office visits.

Information about the use of certain abbreviations, punctuation, symbols, and other conventions used in the ICD-10-CM Tabular List (code numbers and titles), can be found in Section IA of these guidelines, under "Conventions Used in the Tabular List." Section I.B. contains general guidelines that apply to the entire classification. Section I.C. contains chapter-specific guidelines that correspond to the chapters as they are arranged in the classification. Information about the correct sequence to use in finding a code is also described in Section I.

The terms encounter and visit are often used interchangeably in describing outpatient service contacts and, therefore, appear together in these guidelines without distinguishing one from the other.

Though the conventions and general guidelines apply to all settings, coding guidelines for outpatient and provider reporting of diagnoses will vary in a number of instances from those for inpatient diagnoses, recognizing that:

The Uniform Hospital Discharge Data Set (UHDDS) definition of principal diagnosis does not apply to hospital-based outpatient services and provider-based office visits.

Coding guidelines for inconclusive diagnoses (probable, suspected, rule out, etc.) were developed for inpatient reporting and do not apply to outpatients.

A. Selection of first-listed condition

In the outpatient setting, the term first-listed diagnosis is used in lieu of principal diagnosis.

In determining the first-listed diagnosis the coding conventions of ICD-10-CM, as well as the general and disease specific guidelines take precedence over the outpatient guidelines.

Diagnoses often are not established at the time of the initial encounter/visit. It may take two or more visits before the diagnosis is confirmed.

The most critical rule involves beginning the search for the correct code assignment through the Alphabetic Index. Never begin searching initially in the Tabular List as this will lead to coding errors.

1. Outpatient Surgery

When a patient presents for outpatient surgery (same day surgery), code the reason for the surgery as the first-listed diagnosis (reason for the encounter), even if the surgery is not performed due to a contraindication.

2. Observation Stay

When a patient is admitted for observation for a medical condition, assign a code for the medical condition as the first-listed diagnosis.

When a patient presents for outpatient surgery and develops complications requiring admission to observation, code the reason for the surgery as the first reported diagnosis (reason for the encounter), followed by codes for the complications as secondary diagnoses.

B. Codes from A00.0 through T88.9, Z00-Z99

The appropriate code(s) from A00.0 through T88.9, Z00-Z99 must be used to identify diagnoses, symptoms, conditions, problems, complaints, or other reason(s) for the encounter/visit.

C. Accurate reporting of ICD-10-CM diagnosis codes

For accurate reporting of ICD-10-CM diagnosis codes, the documentation should describe the patient's condition, using terminology which includes specific diagnoses as well as symptoms, problems, or reasons for the encounter. There are ICD-10-CM codes to describe all of these.

D. Codes that describe symptoms and signs

Codes that describe symptoms and signs, as opposed to diagnoses, are acceptable for reporting purposes when a diagnosis has not been established (confirmed) by the provider. Chapter 18 of ICD-10-CM, Symptoms, Signs, and Abnormal Clinical and Laboratory Findings Not Elsewhere Classified (codes R00-R99) contain many, but not all codes for symptoms.

E. Encounters for circumstances other than a disease or injury

ICD-10-CM provides codes to deal with encounters for circumstances other than a disease or injury. The Factors Influencing Health Status and Contact with Health Services codes (Z00-Z99) are provided to deal with occasions when circumstances other than a disease or injury are recorded as diagnosis or problems.

See Section I.C.21. Factors influencing health status and contact with health services.

F. Level of Detail in Coding

1. ICD-10-CM codes with 3, 4, 5, 6 or 7 characters

ICD-10-CM is composed of codes with 3, 4, 5, 6 or 7 characters. Codes with three characters are included in ICD-10-CM as the heading of a category of codes that may be further subdivided by the use of fourth, fifth, sixth or seventh characters to provide greater specificity.

2. Use of full number of characters required for a code

A three-character code is to be used only if it is not further subdivided. A code is invalid if it has not been coded to the full number of characters required for that code, including the 7th character, if applicable.

G. ICD-10-CM code for the diagnosis, condition, problem, or other reason for encounter/visit

List first the ICD-10-CM code for the diagnosis, condition, problem, or other reason for encounter/visit shown in the medical record to be chiefly responsible for the services provided. List additional codes that describe any coexisting conditions. In some cases, the first-listed diagnosis may be a symptom when a diagnosis has not been established (confirmed) by the **provider**.

H. Uncertain diagnosis (*See* **Fig. IV. H**)

Do not code diagnoses documented as "probable", "suspected," "questionable," "rule out," **"compatible with," "consistent with,"** or "working diagnosis" or other similar terms indicating uncertainty. Rather, code the condition(s) to the highest degree of certainty for that encounter/visit, such as symptoms, signs, abnormal test results, or other reason for the visit.

Please note: This differs from the coding practices used by short-term, acute care, long-term care and psychiatric hospitals.

I. Chronic diseases

Chronic diseases treated on an ongoing basis may be coded and reported as many times as the patient receives treatment and care for the condition(s)

J. Code all documented conditions that coexist

Code all documented conditions that coexist at the time of the encounter/visit, and require or affect patient care treatment or management. Do not code conditions that were previously treated and no longer exist. However, history codes (categories Z80-Z87) may be used as secondary codes if the historical condition or family history has an impact on current care or influences treatment.

K. Patients receiving diagnostic services only

For patients receiving diagnostic services only during an encounter/visit, sequence first the diagnosis, condition, problem, or other reason for encounter/visit shown in the medical record to be chiefly responsible for the outpatient services provided

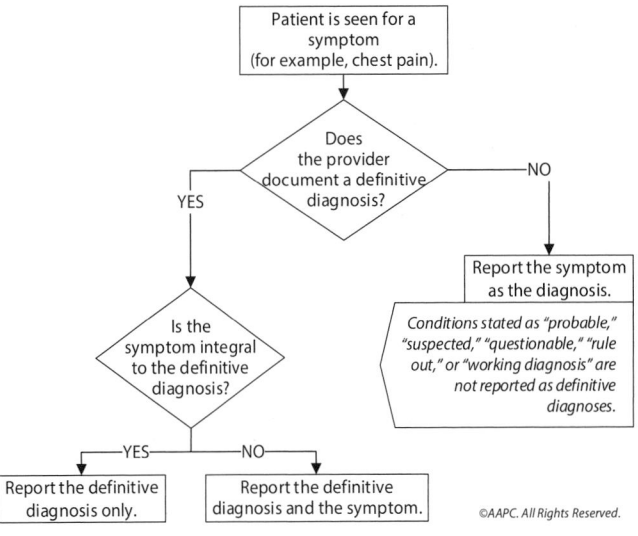

Figure IV.H: Uncertain diagnosis

during the encounter/visit. Codes for other diagnoses (e.g., chronic conditions) may be sequenced as additional diagnoses.

For encounters for routine laboratory/radiology testing in the absence of any signs, symptoms, or associated diagnosis, assign Z01.89, Encounter for other specified special examinations. If routine testing is performed during the same encounter as a test to evaluate a sign, symptom, or diagnosis, it is appropriate to assign both the Z code and the code describing the reason for the non-routine test.

For outpatient encounters for diagnostic tests that have been interpreted by a physician, and the final report is available at the time of coding, code any confirmed or definitive diagnosis(es) documented in the interpretation. Do not code related signs and symptoms as additional diagnoses.

Please note: This differs from the coding practice in the hospital inpatient setting regarding abnormal findings on test results.

L. Patients receiving therapeutic services only

For patients receiving therapeutic services only during an encounter/visit, sequence first the diagnosis, condition, problem, or other reason for encounter/visit shown in the medical record to be chiefly responsible for the outpatient services provided during the encounter/visit. Codes for other diagnoses (e.g., chronic conditions) may be sequenced as additional diagnoses.

The only exception to this rule is that when the primary reason for the admission/encounter is chemotherapy or radiation therapy, the appropriate Z code for the service is listed first, and the diagnosis or problem for which the service is being performed listed second.

M. Patients receiving preoperative evaluations only (*See* **Fig. IV. M**)

For patients receiving preoperative evaluations only, sequence first a code from subcategory Z01.81, Encounter for pre-procedural examinations, to describe the pre-op consultations. Assign a code for the condition to describe the reason for the surgery as an additional diagnosis. Code also any findings related to the pre-op evaluation.

N. Ambulatory surgery

For ambulatory surgery, code the diagnosis for which the surgery was performed. If the postoperative diagnosis is known to be different from the preoperative diagnosis at the time the diagnosis is confirmed, select the postoperative diagnosis for coding, since it is the most definitive.

O. Routine outpatient prenatal visits

See Section I.C.15. Routine outpatient prenatal visits.

P. Encounters for general medical examinations with abnormal findings

The subcategories for encounters for general medical examinations, Z00.0- and encounter for routine child health examination, Z00.12-, provide codes for with and without abnormal findings. Should a general medical examination result in an abnormal finding, the code for general medical examination with abnormal finding should be assigned as the first-listed diagnosis. An examination with abnormal findings refers to a condition/diagnosis that is newly identified or a change in severity of a chronic condition (such as uncontrolled hypertension, or an acute exacerbation of chronic obstructive pulmonary disease) during a routine physical examination. A secondary code for the abnormal finding should also be coded.

Q. Encounters for routine health screenings

See Section I.C.21. Factors influencing health status and contact with health services, Screening

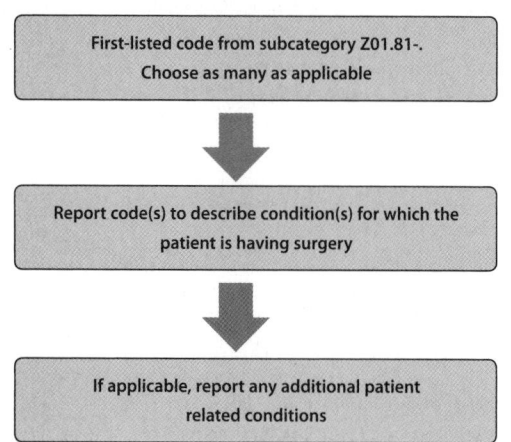

Figure IV.M: Patients receiving preoperative evaluations only

Appendix I Present on Admission Reporting Guidelines (*See* **Fig. Appendix I**)

Introduction

These guidelines are to be used as a supplement to the *ICD-10-CM Official Guidelines for Coding and Reporting* to facilitate the assignment of the Present on Admission (POA) indicator for each diagnosis and external cause of injury code reported on claim forms (UB-04 and 837 Institutional).

These guidelines are not intended to replace any guidelines in the main body of the *ICD-10-CM Official Guidelines for Coding and Reporting*. The POA guidelines are not intended to provide guidance on when a condition should be coded, but rather, how to apply the POA indicator to the final set of diagnosis codes that have been assigned in accordance with Sections I, II, and III of the official guidelines. Subsequent to the assignment of the ICD-10-CM codes, the POA indicator should then be assigned to those conditions that have been coded.

As stated in the Introduction to the ICD-10-CM Official Guidelines for Coding and Reporting, a joint effort between the healthcare provider and the coder is essential to achieve complete and accurate documentation, code assignment, and reporting of diagnoses and procedures. The importance of consistent, complete documentation in the medical record cannot be overemphasized. Medical record documentation from any provider involved in the care and treatment of the patient may be used to support the determination of whether a condition was present on admission or not. In the context of the official coding guidelines, the term "provider" means a physician or any qualified healthcare practitioner who is legally accountable for establishing the patient's diagnosis.

These guidelines are not a substitute for the provider's clinical judgment as to the determination of whether a condition was/was not present on admission. The provider should be queried regarding issues related to the linking of signs/symptoms, timing of test results, and the timing of findings.

Please see the CDC website for the detailed list of ICD-10-CM codes that do not require the use of a POA indicator (https://www.cdc.gov/nchs/icd/icd10cm.htm). The codes and categories on this exempt list are for circumstances regarding the healthcare encounter or factors influencing health status that do not represent a current disease or injury or that describe conditions that are always present on admission.

General Reporting Requirements

All claims involving inpatient admissions to general acute care hospitals or other facilities that are subject to a law or regulation mandating collection of present on admission information.

Present on admission is defined as present at the time the order for inpatient admission occurs -- conditions that develop during an outpatient encounter, including emergency department, observation, or outpatient surgery, are considered as present on admission.

POA indicator is assigned to principal and secondary diagnoses (as defined in Section II of the Official Guidelines for Coding and Reporting) and the external cause of injury codes.

Issues related to inconsistent, missing, conflicting or unclear documentation must still be resolved by the provider.

If a condition would not be coded and reported based on UHDDS definitions and current official coding guidelines, then the POA indicator would not be reported.

Reporting Options

Y - Yes N - No

U - Unknown

W – Clinically undetermined

Unreported/Not used – (Exempt from POA reporting)

Reporting Definitions

Y = present at the time of inpatient admission

N = not present at the time of inpatient admission

U = documentation is insufficient to determine if condition is present on admission

W = provider is unable to clinically determine whether condition was present on admission or not

Timeframe for POA Identification and Documentation

There is no required timeframe as to when a provider (per the definition of "provider" used in these guidelines) must identify or document a condition to be present on admission. In some clinical situations, it may not be possible for a provider to make a definitive diagnosis (or a condition may not be recognized or reported by the patient) for a period of time after admission. In some cases it may be several days before the provider arrives at a definitive diagnosis. This does not mean that the condition was not present on admission. Determination of whether the condition was present on admission or not will be based on the applicable POA guideline as identified in this document, or on the provider's best clinical judgment.

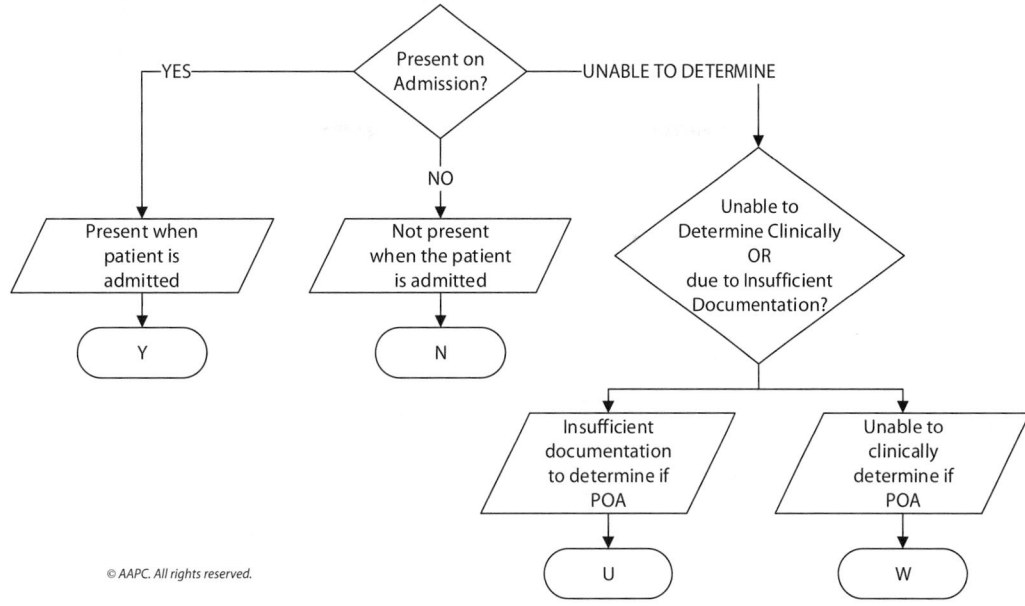

Figure Appendix I: Present on Admission Reporting Guidelines

If at the time of code assignment the documentation is unclear as to whether a condition was present on admission or not, it is appropriate to query the provider for clarification.

Assigning the POA Indicator

Condition is on the "Exempt from Reporting" list

Leave the "present on admission" field blank if the condition is on the list of ICD-10-CM codes for which this field is not applicable. This is the only circumstance in which the field may be left blank.

POA Explicitly Documented

Assign Y for any condition the provider explicitly documents as being present on admission.

Assign N for any condition the provider explicitly documents as not present at the time of admission.

Conditions diagnosed prior to inpatient admission

Assign "Y" for conditions that were diagnosed prior to admission (example: hypertension, diabetes mellitus, asthma)

Conditions diagnosed during the admission but clearly present before admission Assign "Y" for conditions diagnosed during the admission that were clearly present but not diagnosed until after admission occurred.

Diagnoses subsequently confirmed after admission are considered present on admission if at the time of admission they are documented as suspected, possible, rule out, differential diagnosis, or constitute an underlying cause of a symptom that is present at the time of admission.

Condition develops during outpatient encounter prior to inpatient admission

Assign Y for any condition that develops during an outpatient encounter prior to a written order for inpatient admission.

Documentation does not indicate whether condition was present on admission

Assign "U" when the medical record documentation is unclear as to whether the condition was present on admission. "U" should not be routinely assigned and used only in very limited circumstances. Coders are encouraged to query the providers when the documentation is unclear.

Documentation states that it cannot be determined whether the condition was or was not present on admission

Assign "W" when the medical record documentation indicates that it cannot be clinically determined whether or not the condition was present on admission.

Chronic condition with acute exacerbation during the admission

If a single code identifies both the chronic condition and the acute exacerbation, see POA guidelines pertaining to codes that contain multiple clinical concepts.

If a single code only identifies the chronic condition and not the acute exacerbation (e.g., acute exacerbation of chronic leukemia), assign "Y."

Conditions documented as possible, probable, suspected, or rule out at the time of discharge

If the final diagnosis contains a possible, probable, suspected, or rule out diagnosis, and this diagnosis was based on signs, symptoms or clinical findings suspected at the time of inpatient admission, assign "Y."

If the final diagnosis contains a possible, probable, suspected, or rule out diagnosis, and this diagnosis was based on signs, symptoms or clinical findings that were not present on admission, assign "N".

Conditions documented as impending or threatened at the time of discharge

If the final diagnosis contains an impending or threatened diagnosis, and this diagnosis is based on symptoms or clinical findings that were present on admission, assign "Y".

If the final diagnosis contains an impending or threatened diagnosis, and this diagnosis is based on symptoms or clinical findings that were not present on admission, assign "N".

Acute and Chronic Conditions

Assign "Y" for acute conditions that are present at time of admission and N for acute conditions that are not present at time of admission.

Assign "Y" for chronic conditions, even though the condition may not be diagnosed until after admission.

If a single code identifies both an acute and chronic condition, see the POA guidelines for codes that contain multiple clinical concepts.

Codes That Contain Multiple Clinical Concepts

Assign "N" if at least one of the clinical concepts included in the code was not present on admission (e.g., COPD with acute exacerbation and the exacerbation was not present on admission; gastric ulcer that does not start bleeding until after admission; asthma patient develops status asthmaticus after admission).

Assign "Y" if all of the clinical concepts included in the code were present on admission (e.g., duodenal ulcer that perforates prior to admission).

For infection codes that include the causal organism, assign "Y" if the infection (or signs of the infection) were present on admission, even though the culture results may not be known until after admission (e.g., patient is admitted with pneumonia and the provider documents Pseudomonas as the causal organism a few days later).

Same Diagnosis Code for Two or More Conditions

When the same ICD-10-CM diagnosis code applies to two or more conditions during the same encounter (e.g. two separate conditions classified to the same ICD-10-CM diagnosis code).

Assign "Y" if all conditions represented by the single ICD-10-CM code were present on admission (e.g. bilateral unspecified age-related cataracts).

Assign "N" if any of the conditions represented by the single ICD-10-CM code was not present on admission (e.g. traumatic secondary and recurrent hemorrhage and seroma is assigned to a single code T79.2, but only one of the conditions was present on admission).

Obstetrical conditions

Whether or not the patient delivers during the current hospitalization does not affect assignment of the POA indicator. The determining factor for POA assignment is whether the pregnancy complication or obstetrical condition described by the code was present at the time of admission or not.

If the pregnancy complication or obstetrical condition was present on admission (e.g., patient admitted in preterm labor), assign "Y".

If the pregnancy complication or obstetrical condition was not present on admission (e.g., 2nd degree laceration during delivery, postpartum hemorrhage that occurred during current hospitalization, fetal distress develops after admission), assign "N".

If the obstetrical code includes more than one diagnosis and any of the diagnoses identified by the code were not present on admission assign "N".

(e.g., Category O11, Pre-existing hypertension with pre-eclampsia)

Perinatal conditions

Newborns are not considered to be admitted until after birth. Therefore, any condition present at birth or that developed in utero is considered present at admission and should be assigned "Y". This includes conditions that occur during delivery (e.g., injury during delivery, meconium aspiration, exposure to streptococcus B in the vaginal canal).

Congenital conditions and anomalies

Assign "Y" for congenital conditions and anomalies except for categories Q00-Q99, Congenital anomalies, which are on the exempt list. Congenital conditions are always considered present on admission.

External cause of injury codes

Assign "Y" for any external cause code representing an external cause of morbidity that occurred prior to inpatient admission (e.g., patient fell out of bed at home, patient fell out of bed in emergency room prior to admission).

Assign "N" for any external cause code representing an external cause of morbidity that occurred during inpatient hospitalization (e.g., patient fell out of hospital bed during hospital stay, patient experienced an adverse reaction to a medication administered after inpatient admission).

Preface

ICD-10-CM Official Preface

This FY 2020 update of the International Statistical Classification of Diseases and Related Health Problems, 10th revision, Clinical Modification (ICD-10-CM) is being published by the United States government in recognition of its responsibility to promulgate this classification throughout the United States for morbidity coding. The International Statistical Classification of Diseases and Related Health Problems, 10th Revision ICD-10, published by the World Health Organization (WHO), is the foundation of ICD-10-CM. ICD-10 continues to be the classification used in cause-of-death coding in the United States. The ICD-10-CM is comparable with the ICD-10. The WHO Collaborating Center for the Family of International Classifications in North America, housed at the Centers for Disease Control and Prevention's National Center for Health Statistics (NCHS), has responsibility for the implementation of ICD and other WHO-FIC classifications and serves as a liaison with the WHO, fulfilling international obligations for comparable classifications and the national health data needs of the United States. The historical background of ICD and ICD-10 can be found in the Introduction to the International Classification of Diseases and Related Health Problems (ICD-10), 2010, World Health Organization, Geneva, Switzerland.

ICD-10-CM is the United States' clinical modification of the World Health Organization's ICD-10. The term "clinical" is used to emphasize the modification's intent: to serve as a useful tool in the area of classification of morbidity data for indexing of health records, medical care review, and ambulatory and other health care programs, as well as for basic health statistics. To describe the clinical picture of the patient the codes must be more precise than those needed only for statistical groupings and trend analysis.

Characteristics of ICD-10-CM

ICD-10-CM far exceeds its predecessors in the number of concepts and codes provided. The disease classification has been expanded to include health-related conditions and to provide greater specificity at the sixth and seventh character level.

The sixth and seventh characters are not optional and are intended for use in recording the information documented in the clinical record. ICD-10-CM extensions, interpretations, modifications, addenda, or errata other than those approved by the Centers for Disease Control and Prevention are not to be considered official and should not be utilized. Continuous maintenance of the ICD-10-CM is the responsibility of the aforementioned agencies. However, because the ICD-10-CM represents the best in contemporary thinking of clinicians, nosologists, epidemiologists, and statisticians from both public and private sectors, when future modifications are considered, advice will be sought from all stakeholders. All official authorized addenda since the last complete update have been included in this revision. For more detailed information please see the complete official authorized addenda to ICD-10-CM, including the "ICD-10-CM Official Guidelines for Coding and Reporting," and a description of the ICD-10-CM updating and maintenance process at www.cms.gov.

2020 ICD-10-CM

This 2020 ICD-10-CM edition includes the following features, designed in consultation with coding consultants and ICD-10 trainers, to provide a comprehensive and easy-to-use reference manual:

- A table of contents page
- The complete 2020 ICD-10-CM code set
- Full code descriptions
- Special color coding throughout to highlight instructional notes, bilateral and unilateral indicators, and other features
- Color coding and symbols for Medicare code edits to highlight age, sex, manifestation, other specified and unspecified codes, and MACRA codes required for quality and cost measures reporting under the Merit-based Incentive Payment System (MIPS)
- Illustrations at the beginning of the book and throughout the Tabular List
- ICD-10-CM conventions
- ICD-10-CM Official Guidelines for Coding and Reporting
- Official Index to Diseases and Injuries
- Official Index to External Causes of Injuries
- Table of Drugs and Chemicals
- Table of Neoplasms
- Extension "X" symbol to alert readers to the ICD-10-CM placeholder "x" convention
- **New:** "Eye" symbol to alert readers that a specific code has a guideline reference
- Anatomy and physiology for various body systems, including illustrations and pathologies
- Trimester icon for applicable codes
- HCC and RxHCC icons
- Coding tips and terminology definitions throughout the Tabular List
- Vertical yellow rule in the Alphabetic Index to Diseases and Injuries and Index to External Causes of Injuries
- A section on coding certification exam preparation

List of Features

ICD-10-CM is essential to documenting medical necessity for services rendered, and accurate codes mean better outcomes for the patient, your claims, and your practice or facility.

Count on this manual to help you choose and report the right ICD-10-CM code. Unique features, intuitive design, and expert features that coders developed assure this manual will keep your coding on target.

This manual includes the ICD-10-CM complete code set for 2020, including the Tabular List, Alphabetic Index to Diseases and Injuries, Table of Neoplasms, Table of Drugs and Chemicals, and Index to External Causes of Injuries, effective October 1, 2019.

To help you make the most of this manual, we also include the following features:

- ICD-10-CM Official Guidelines for Coding and Reporting for 2020 located at the front of the book for quick reference. The Health Insurance Portability and Accountability Act (HIPAA) requires all entities assigning ICD-10-CM codes to follow these guidelines.

- Guideline Tips for each chapter of the relevant ICD-10-CM Official Guidelines in easy-to-understand lay language are located on the publisher's website

- A chapter dedicated to preparation tips for AAPC's national coding exam

- Anatomy and physiology descriptions before Tabular List chapters containing codes pertaining to specific body anatomy

- Enhanced full illustrations of body systems at the front of the book so you don't have to search the manual for these large color images

- Illustrations of anatomy and conditions throughout the Tabular List to help you to better understand how to assign specific codes

- AHA *Coding Clinic®* article references from the quarterly publication of the American Hospital Association

- Symbols indicating "Additional character required" so you know when a code requires an additional character for code specificity and validity (provided in both the Alphabetic Index and Tabular List)

- Red font for Code first, Code also, and Use additional code notes

- Bold coding tips and definitions of medical terms appear throughout the Tabular List

- Symbols identify adult, pediatric, newborn, maternity, trimester, male, and female codes

- Age and sex edits showing which codes have restrictions on use based on age or sex of the patient

- Highlighted coding instructional and informational notes help you recognize important code usage guidance for specific sections including Includes, Excludes1, and Excludes2 notes

- Z code as first-listed diagnosis symbol to alert you when you can only assign a Z code as the first-listed diagnosis

- HCC and RxHCC symbols to alert you to HCC and RxHCC diagnoses

- New "eye" symbol to alert you that more information about a specific code can be found in the Official Guidelines

- Intuitive color-coded symbols and alerts identify critical coding and reimbursement issues quickly, such as "Other Specified" and "Unspecified" diagnosis alerts, along with MACRA codes shown in pink

- Manifestation code alerts, highlighted in blue, so you properly use codes that represent manifestations of an underlying disease and know when you must use two codes

- Symbols for unacceptable principal diagnosis, code exempt from diagnosis present on admission requirement, complication or comorbidity, CC/MCC exclusion, questionable admission, and HAC alert

- A user-friendly page design, including dictionary-style headers, color bleed tabs, and legend keys

- Key word green font is used to differentiate key words that appear in similar code descriptions in a given category

- Symbols indicating new code, revised code, or revised text

- Updated stick-on tabs to use for main sections of the book, including each Tabular List chapter

- Updated and enhanced Appendix including Z codes for long-term use of drugs organized alphabetically by brand and generic drug name

- Appendix including 7-character codes for symbols throughout the book

- Notes pages throughout Tabular List chapters to record important coding information

Practical Steps for Using the ICD-10-CM Book

This manual includes the diagnosis code set from the International Classification of Diseases, 10th Revision, Clinical Modification (ICD-10-CM) 2020.

Understand Code Structure to Choose the Most Specific Code

ICD-10-CM codes are made up of a minimum of three characters and a maximum of seven characters:

- Character 1 – capital letter A-Z, except the letter U, which is not used
- Character 2 – number
- Character 3 – number
- Character 4 – number or letter – capital or lowercase
- Character 5 – number or letter – capital or lowercase
- Character 6 – number or letter – capital or lowercase
- Character 7 – number or letter – capital or lowercase; character 7 is only used in specific chapters, including pregnancy, musculoskeletal, injuries, and external causes of morbidity

Each Tabular List chapter is divided into subchapters, which are also called blocks.

Subchapters are divided into:
Categories (3 characters) – Represent one disease or a group of diseases or related conditions. If a category does not have a further subdivision, it is called a code.

Categories are divided into:
Subcategories (4-5 characters) – Represent greater specificity of one disease or a group of diseases.

Subcategories are divided into:
Codes (4-7 characters) – Codes are the final level which cannot be subdivided further. Codes that are 7 characters are always called "codes" because 7 is the maximum number of characters in a code.

Review the ICD-10-CM Volumes Included in This Manual

This manual includes the:

- **ICD-10-CM Volume 1 Tabular List of Diseases and Injuries,** which includes diagnosis codes in numerical order, and their official descriptors, for 21 chapters

- **ICD-10-CM Volume 2 Alphabetic Index,** consisting of:
  o Index of Diseases and Injuries
  o Index of External Causes of Injury
  o Table of Neoplasms
  o Table of Drugs and Chemicals

This manual follows the industry standard of placing the Alphabetic Index before the Tabular List because when you search for a code, you should always check the Index first to make a preliminary code choice and then check the Tabular List for confirmation.

Code Diagnoses With Confidence Following This Approach

➤ The first step in choosing the proper ICD-10-CM code is reading the medical documentation to identify the diagnosis the provider documents and confirms. If there is no confirmed diagnosis, look for the sign or symptom that brought the patient in or other reason for the encounter.
  - Be sure to check online or hard copy references, such as medical dictionaries and anatomy resources to look up unfamiliar terms.

➤ Next, decide which main term you will search in the Index based on the patient's specific case. ICD-10-CM doesn't use body sites as main terms. Instead, look for the disease, sign, symptom, etc. You can find the body site as a subterm. For neoplasm diagnoses, review the Table of Neoplasms for the appropriate diagnosis. Search for the neoplasm histology as a main term (carcinoma, leukemia, glioblastoma) and the body site as a subterm. The histology will take you to a code to cross-reference to the Tabular or direct you to the Table of Neoplasms. If you cannot find the histology as a main term, or cannot find a code to cross-reference for the histology and body site, then go directly to the Table of Neoplasms to search for the body site of the neoplasm. You will also need to go directly to the Table of Neoplasms if the provider does not document the histology.

➤ Once you find the main term in the Index, note the recommended code. Start with the main term and review any available subterms. Also note whether the Index offers any other clues to proper coding, such as the need for additional characters or the need for an additional code.

➤ Turn to that code in the Tabular List, and read the full code descriptor. Keep in mind that you may need to read the subcategory and category titles as well as the code descriptor to get the full meaning of the code.

➤ Check to see whether ICD-10-CM requires additional characters for that code. If so, review the code definitions of any available categories and subcategories.
  - Remember, if a code has seven characters available, you must report all seven characters, both to comply with coding rules and to prevent insurers from denying your claim. Similarly, if a code has four characters, with no fifth character available, you must report all four characters rather than a three-character code. This manual will alert you to the need for an additional character using easily identifiable symbols.

➤ If the Index points you to a code that includes the terms other, unspecified, NOS (not otherwise specified), or NEC (not elsewhere classifiable), double check that a more specific code isn't available. Always report the most specific code the medical record supports.

➤ Before making your final code decision, review all applicable notes and instructions to be sure they don't affect your choice. You'll find these notes and instructions on every level, from the chapter to the code itself. You will find many notes highlighted and color coded for easy reference in the Tabular List. You can find the meaning of the highlights in the legend at the bottom of each page in the Tabular List. Also review the surrounding codes to be sure there isn't a more appropriate code available.

➤ Finally, take a moment to confirm that your code choice complies with the philosophy of ethical coding. Never report an ICD-10-CM code simply because it will support reimbursement from a payer. Report only those codes the documentation supports.

Factor In the Other Resources in This Manual

In addition to the Alphabetic Index and Tabular List, you'll find the following materials in this manual:

Symbols and Conventions Specific to This ICD-10-CM Manual: Read this section to make the most of all of the resources and instructional symbols this manual includes.

ICD-10-CM Official Guidelines for Coding and Reporting: No coder should let a year go by without reviewing the Official Guidelines. These authoritative rules provide many instructions not available in the Tabular List.

Additional Content in Tabular List Chapters: At the beginning of specific Tabular List chapters, you'll find anatomy descriptions, and the publisher's website also includes a useful breakdown of the relevant Official Guidelines specific to codes in that chapter, called Guideline Tips.

Symbols and Conventions

Additional Characters Required

Indexes

☑ Additional character required after the symbol

This symbol appears after codes throughout the Alphabetic Index to Diseases and Injuries and the Index to External Causes of Injuries to remind you that a code requires one or more additional characters.

Tabular List

- [4th] This red symbol cautions that the code requires an additional fourth character.
- [5th] This red symbol cautions that the code requires an additional fifth character.
- [6th] This red symbol cautions that the code requires an additional sixth character.
- [7th] This red symbol cautions that the code requires an additional seventh character.

Extension "X" Alert

- [7th] This blue symbol cautions that the code requires an additional seventh character following the placeholder X.

Medicare Code Edits Symbols and Colors

Code edit symbols and colors in this manual are based on the Medicare Code Editor (MCE) and Medicare's Integrated Outpatient Code Editor (I/OCE). The code edit information in this manual is based on MCE v36 with the addition of FY 2020 Inpatient Prospective Payment System (IPPS) Proposed Rule updates for the most current information available at the time of printing.

Age Conflict

Medicare's MCE and I/OCE code editors detect inconsistencies between a patient's age and any diagnosis on the patient's record. Examples include: a five-year-old patient with benign prostatic hypertrophy or a 78-year-old patient coded with a delivery.

[N] Newborn	Age of 0 years; a subset of diagnoses intended only for newborns and neonates (e.g., fetal distress, perinatal jaundice).
[P] Pediatric	Age range is 0–17 years inclusive (e.g., Reye's syndrome, routine child health exam).
[M] Maternity	Age range is 12–55 years inclusive (e.g., diabetes in pregnancy, antepartum pulmonary complication).
[A] Adult	Age range is 18–124 years inclusive (e.g., senile delirium, mature cataract).

Sex Conflict

Medicare's MCE and I/OCE code editors detect inconsistencies between a patient's sex and any diagnosis or procedure on the patient's record. Examples include: a male patient with cervical cancer (diagnosis) or a female patient with a prostatectomy (procedure).

In both instances, the indicated diagnosis or the procedure conflicts with the stated sex of the patient. Therefore, either the patient's diagnosis, procedure or sex is presumed to be incorrect.

♂ Male code symbol

♀ Female code symbol

Other Symbols and Color Coding

Manifestation Codes

The code description is highlighted with a light blue color. Manifestation codes describe the manifestation of an underlying disease, not the disease itself, and therefore should not be used as a primary diagnosis.

Key Terms

Bold green font is used in code descriptions throughout the Tabular List to quickly identify key terms in a given category.

MACRA code

MACRA codes are identified in pink.

Other Specified Codes

The code description is highlighted with gray color. These codes are assigned when the documentation indicates a specified diagnosis, but the ICD-10-CM code set does not have a specific code that describes the condition.

Unspecified Codes

The code description is highlighted with yellow color. These codes are assigned when neither the diagnostic statement nor the documentation provides enough information to assign a more specific code.

TIP Coding guidance	Coding tips appear throughout the Tabular List to help you to choose the correct code.
DEFINITION Describes condition/terminology	Definitions of medical terms and conditions appear throughout the Tabular List to improve your understanding of terminology.
[1st]	The 1st trimester symbol appears with applicable codes that apply to the first trimester.
[2nd]	The 2nd trimester symbol appears with applicable codes that apply to the second trimester.
[3rd]	The 3rd trimester symbol appears with applicable codes that apply to the third trimester.
● New Code	The new code symbol appears with a code that is new for the current year.
▲ Revised Code Title	A revised code title symbol appears with a code title that is revised for the current year.
▶◀ Revised Text	The revised text facing triangles symbol appears before and after text that is revised for the current year.

Sequencing, Admission, Complication, and Comorbidity

When relevant, you'll see the following symbols to the right of the code descriptor:

[PDx]	Unacceptable principal diagnosis; based on Medicare code edits
[POA]	Code exempt from diagnosis present on admission requirement
[CC]	Complication or comorbidity; based on CMS data
[MCC]	Major complication or comorbidity; based on CMS data
[CC/MCC Exc]	Complications or comorbidities/Major complications or comorbidities (CC/MCC) exclusions; based on CMS data

HAC	Hospital-acquired condition (HAC) alert; based on CMS data
?	Questionable admission when used as principal diagnosis symbol; based on Medicare code edits
HCC	HCC diagnosis codes
RxHCC	RxHCC diagnosis codes
Z-1	Z code as first-listed diagnosis; certain codes may only be reported as the primary/first-listed diagnosis, except when there are multiple encounters on the same day and the medical records for the encounters are combined.

This data is based on 2019 CMS data which was the most current available at the time of printing.

Official Guideline Reference

👁 This eye symbol indicates that more information about this code can be found in the Official Guidelines.

These references are based on 2019 ICD-10-CM Official Guidelines, which were the most current available at the time of printing.

Instructional Notes

| EXCLUDES1 | Not coded here Excludes1 notes are highlighted in black to alert you to NEVER assign codes listed under Excludes1 along with the code that you cross-referenced, with some exceptions. |
| EXCLUDES2 | Not included here Excludes2 notes are highlighted in gray to alert you that you most likely will not assign codes listed under Excludes2 along with the code that you cross-referenced. However, you could assign both an Excludes2 code with the cross-referenced code, as long as the provider documents both conditions. |

INCLUDES	The word "Includes" appears immediately under certain categories to further define, or give examples of, the content of the category.
NOTES	Notes appear throughout the Tabular List to provide additional coding information.
🖝 Code first alert	Code first notes appear throughout the Tabular List to provide the code to assign first.
Use additional code	Use additional code notes appear on etiology codes throughout the Tabular List to identify when to assign a manifestation code in addition to the principal or primary etiology diagnosis.
Code also	Code also notes indicate that two codes may be necessary to capture a condition. Sequencing of these codes will depend upon the actual encounter.

Citations to AHA's *Coding Clinic®* for ICD-10-CM

AHA's *Coding Clinic®*, a quarterly newsletter, is the official publication for coding guidelines and advice as designated by the four Cooperating Parties (American Hospital Association, American Health Information Management Association, Centers for Medicare and Medicaid Services (CMS), and National Center for Health Statistics) and the Editorial Advisory Board.

AHA We've marked codes with related *Coding Clinic®* articles with a citation that includes the quarter and year of the issue.

Using ICD-10-CM Toward Your Credentialing Exam

The ICD-10-CM is an essential book for all AAPC certification examinations. Other code books required for most exams include the American Medical Association's (AMA's) *CPT® Professional,* which is the only official CPT® manual published, and HCPCS Level II (any publisher).

Until December 31, 2019, AAPC examinations require the 2019 code books. Beginning January 1, 2020, examinees are tested using 2020 codes, descriptions, and guidelines. AAPC offers several examination preparation resources, such as distance learning programs, study guides, practice examinations, and Practicode.

Studying for Your Exam

AAPC exams are open book. Read your code books from cover to cover, including all coding guidelines found within each section and subsection of the CPT®, the Official Coding Guidelines in the ICD-10-CM, and all coding guidelines in the HCPCS Level II code books. Know how to locate the codes, guidelines, tables, and instructions within them easily.

Go through your books to mark them, tab and label them, and make notes in them for easy reference. You may highlight, circle, or "bubble" parts of the page to help you easily find information. Tab or mark any information you feel would provide extra help. DO NOT glue, tape, staple, or add any other information to the books. Highlight certain guidelines in your code books. Notes in your code books should be relevant to a coder, although an occasional note of encouragement can make the exam easier. Add to or modify tabs to help you pass your exam.

AAPC's online practice tests are excellent test simulation tools. The practice tests are available at www.aapc.com/training/practice-exams.aspx. Attend local chapter meetings, and don't be afraid to let your colleagues know your credentialing aspirations. Local chapters have credentialing exam classes and workshops, and you can find study buddies for the exam.

Taking Your Exam

You must be a member of AAPC to register for your credentialing examination. Begin registration on the AAPC website at https://www.aapc.com/certification/locate-examination.aspx.

CPC®, CIC™, and COC™ examinees must have two years of experience to avoid Apprentice status. Contact AAPC about removing an Apprenticeship status. You will have 5 hours, 40 minutes to complete the exam. Most credentials have 150 questions in the exam, and you will not have time to research and learn new guidelines or ideas.

Here are some more tips, once you've received confirmation:

- Confirm what exam materials are allowed during the examination. Please view our exam instructions at www.aapc.com/documents/exm-instructions.pdf to see what code books and supportive material are acceptable for each exam.
- Practice quickly locating the codes, guidelines, tables, and instructions within them.
- Plan to leave your phone in your car. Electronic devices with an on/off switch (cell phones, smart phones, tablets, etc.) aren't allowed into the examination room. Failure to comply with this policy may result in disqualification of your exam.

Gather the following supplies the week before your examination:

- Clothing layers in case the room temperature fluctuates.
- Light, quiet snacks such as hard candy and peppermint.
- Cough drops if you are coughing.
- A water bottle.
- Ear plugs in case the noise in the room disturbs you.
- No. 2 pencils with erasers.
- Don't forget code books and any errata!

Verify the start time and examination address at least two days prior to your test date. Map your driving directions in advance. Factor potential construction, traffic, or possible inclement weather during your commute and plan to arrive 10 to 15 minutes early.

Get a good night's sleep before your exam. Cramming at the last minute won't help. Relax instead. Stick to your morning routine, but make sure you leave for your examination to get there early. **Proctors will examine your books before the examination begins.** You won't be able to bring your books into the exam if they find the following:

- Glued, taped, and stapled notes or scratch sheets
- Post-It™ notes
- Study guide questions or cases
- Examination questions
- Notes on full page tabs (i.e., in Optum's code books)

Here are some recommendations for while you're taking your exam:

- Listen carefully while the proctor reads the instructions. Ask questions before the examination begins if you do not understand the instructions given.
- Be especially careful about marking your answer sheet. Fill out the bubbles as shown on the example on your test grid.
- Scan the entire test when you begin.
- Remember to pace yourself. Stay relaxed. You will have time to finish.
- Read each question carefully. Note such words in the question as "not, except, most, least and greatest." These words are often crucial in determining the correct answer.
- Answer every question. If you do not know the right answer, eliminate as many wrong answers as possible, then select among the remaining answers. If you don't have a clue, guess.
- If you finish with some additional time, go back and review any questions for which you were not fully sure you had the correct answer. Use the code books again to confirm.
- Don't talk to others who've also finished their exam until you are all finished.
- If you find the exam environment too distracting, discontinue testing, but it will be YOUR responsibility to contact AAPC to address your concerns on the first business day after your exam date. AAPC will review your concerns, and if any portion of the exam has been completed, AAPC reserves the right to still grade the exam.

AAPC grades examinations within seven to 10 business days of receipt; however, grading may take longer. Keep checking your AAPC website and your mailbox for your results.

Should you fail, you may take another exam for the same credential within 12 months at no cost. AAPC will let you know what sections to work on before that exam.

Go to www.aapc.com for more information about your examination or call AAPC at 800-626-2633 if you have any questions. We wish you the best of luck on passing your exam!

Anatomical Illustrations

Circulatory System — Arteries and Veins

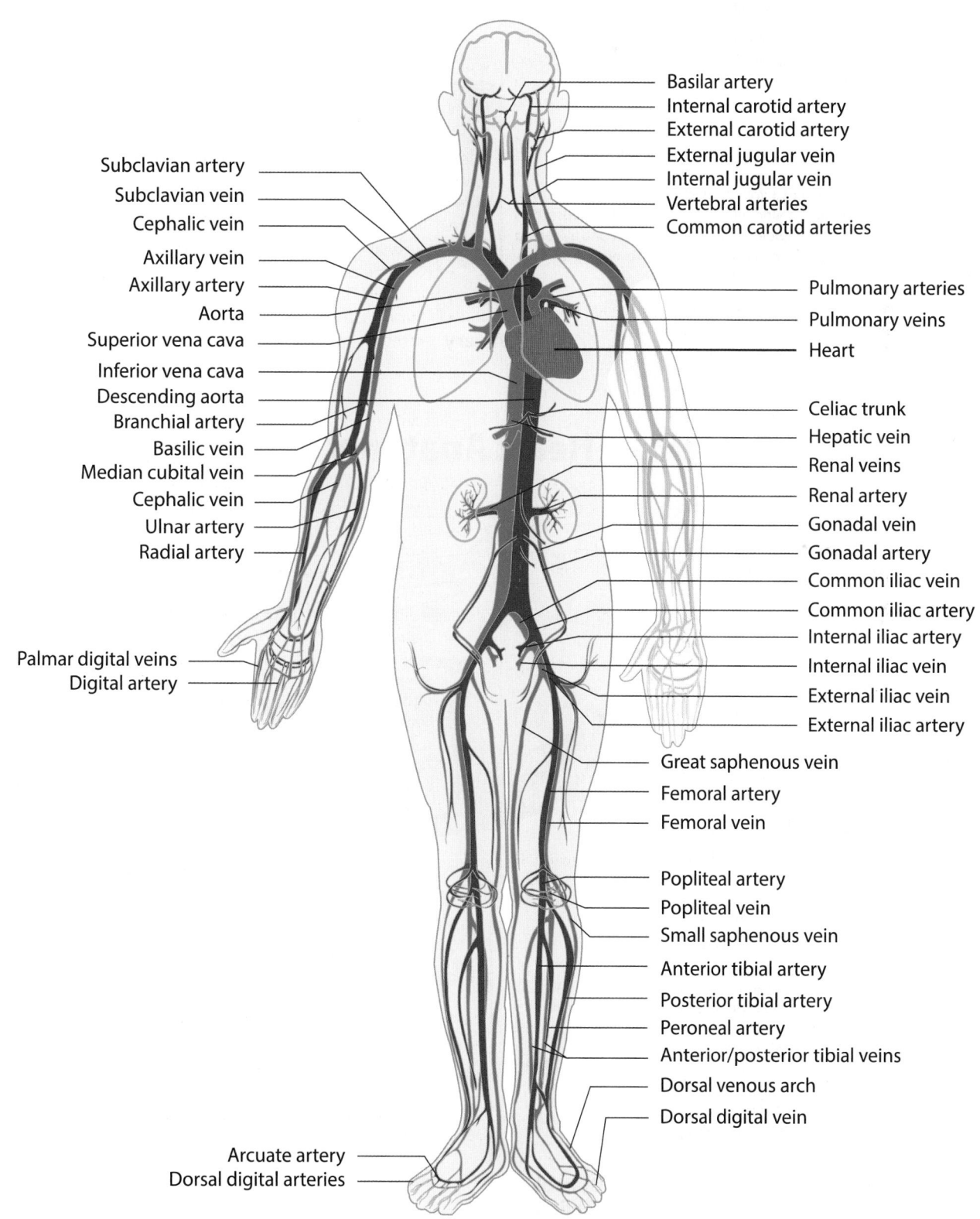

Subclavian artery
Subclavian vein
Cephalic vein
Axillary vein
Axillary artery
Aorta
Superior vena cava
Inferior vena cava
Descending aorta
Branchial artery
Basilic vein
Median cubital vein
Cephalic vein
Ulnar artery
Radial artery

Palmar digital veins
Digital artery

Arcuate artery
Dorsal digital arteries

Basilar artery
Internal carotid artery
External carotid artery
External jugular vein
Internal jugular vein
Vertebral arteries
Common carotid arteries

Pulmonary arteries
Pulmonary veins
Heart

Celiac trunk
Hepatic vein
Renal veins
Renal artery
Gonadal vein
Gonadal artery
Common iliac vein
Common iliac artery
Internal iliac artery
Internal iliac vein
External iliac vein
External iliac artery

Great saphenous vein
Femoral artery
Femoral vein

Popliteal artery
Popliteal vein
Small saphenous vein
Anterior tibial artery
Posterior tibial artery
Peroneal artery
Anterior/posterior tibial veins
Dorsal venous arch
Dorsal digital vein

Circulatory System — Artery and Vein Anatomy

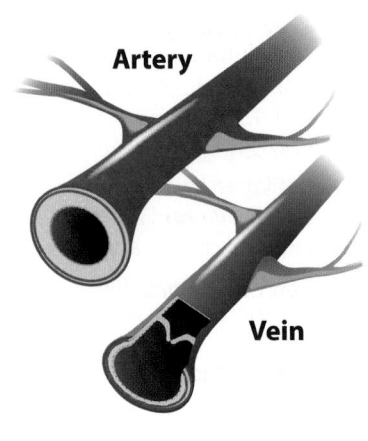

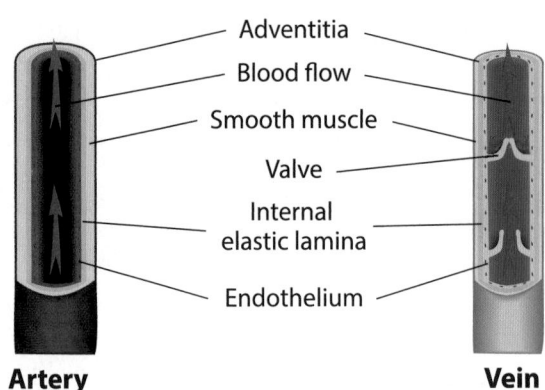

Circulatory System — Heart Anatomy and Cardiac Cycle

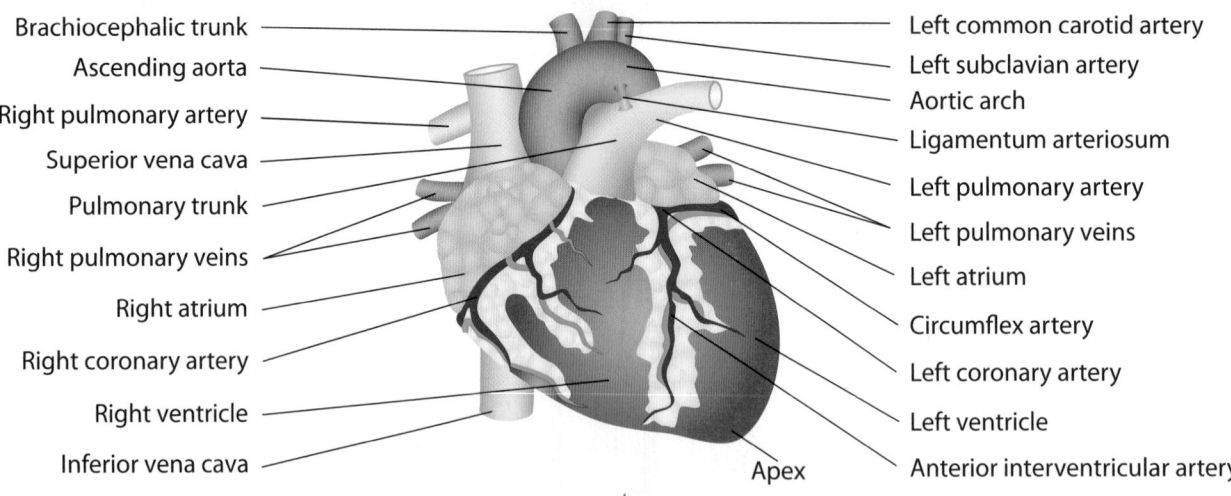

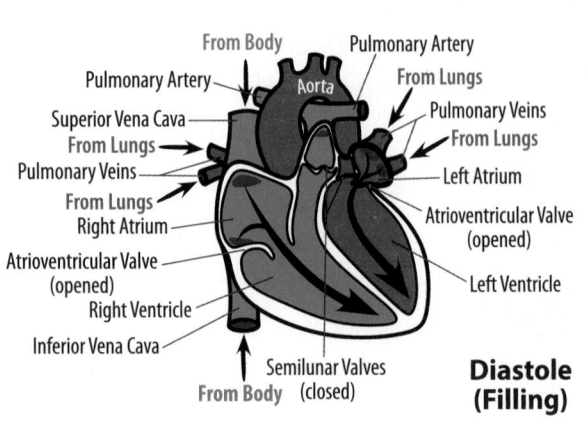

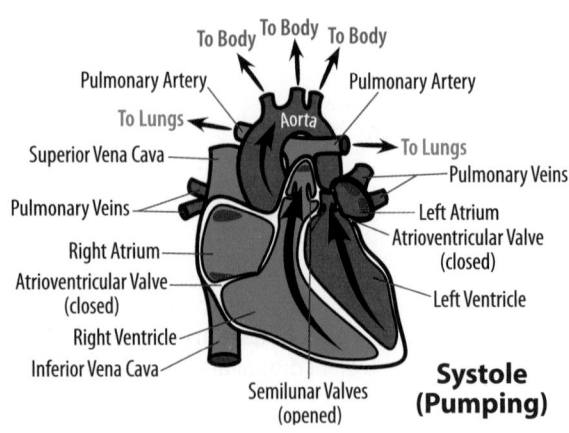

Electrical Conducting System of the Heart

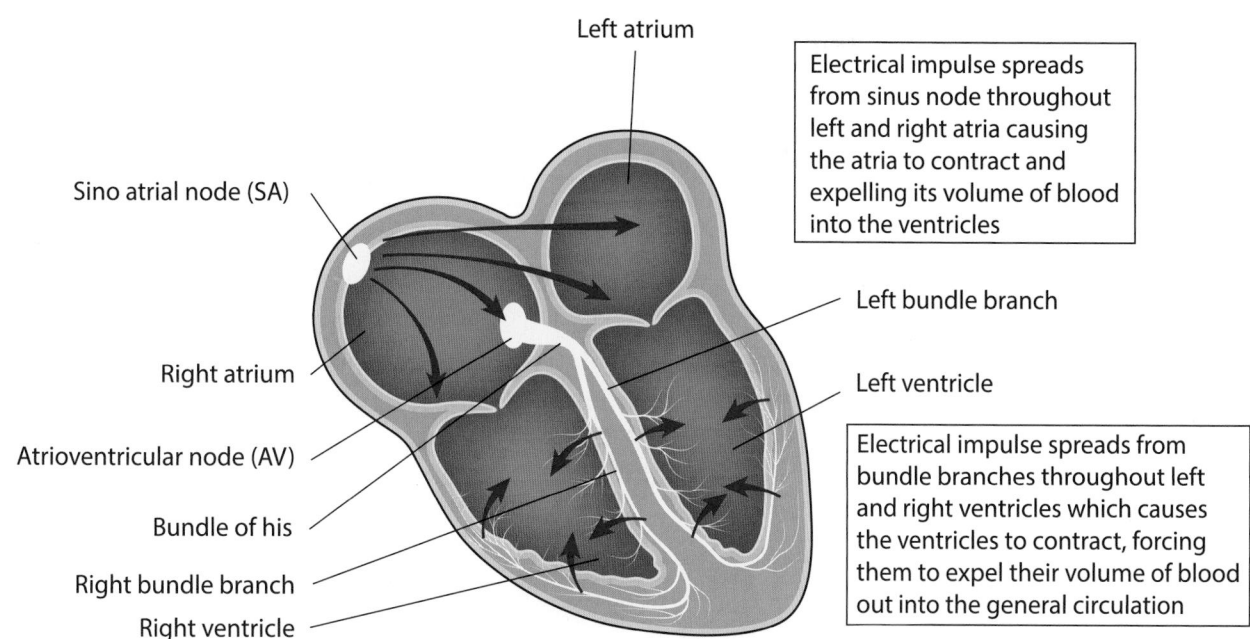

Left atrium

Electrical impulse spreads from sinus node throughout left and right atria causing the atria to contract and expelling its volume of blood into the ventricles

Sino atrial node (SA)

Left bundle branch

Right atrium

Left ventricle

Atrioventricular node (AV)

Electrical impulse spreads from bundle branches throughout left and right ventricles which causes the ventricles to contract, forcing them to expel their volume of blood out into the general circulation

Bundle of his

Right bundle branch

Right ventricle

The Pathway of Blood Flow Through the Heart

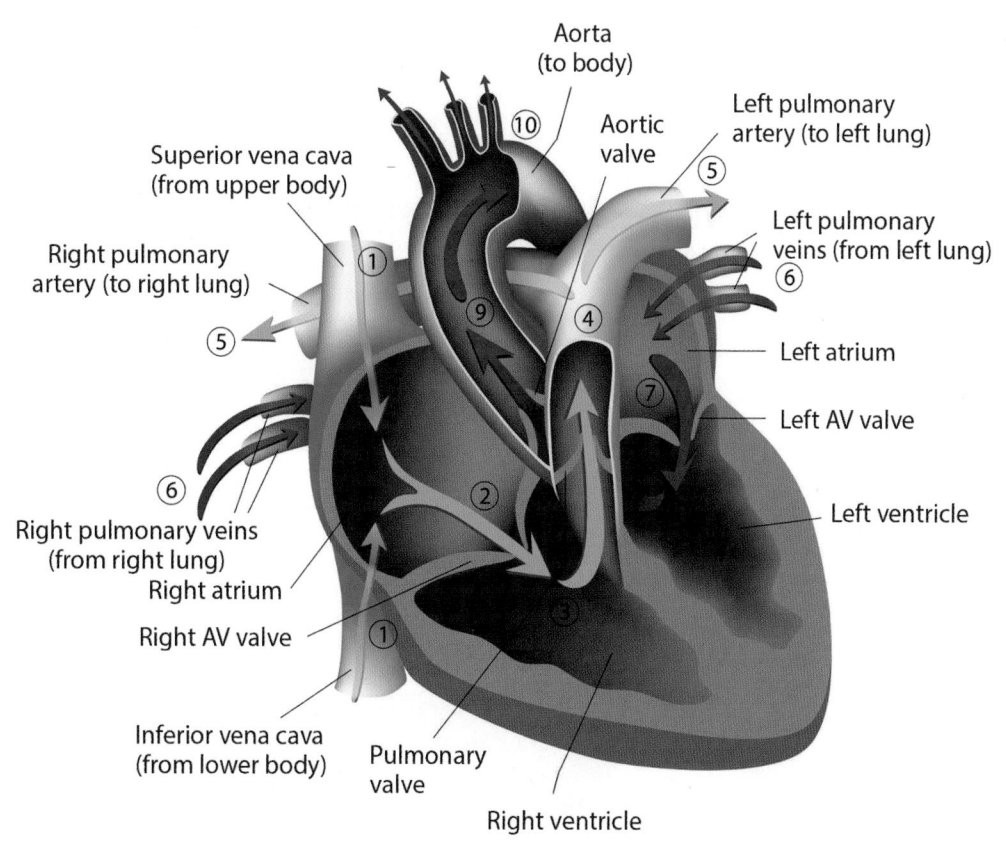

Aorta (to body)

Aortic valve

Left pulmonary artery (to left lung)

Superior vena cava (from upper body)

Right pulmonary artery (to right lung)

Left pulmonary veins (from left lung)

Left atrium

Left AV valve

Left ventricle

Right pulmonary veins (from right lung)

Right atrium

Right AV valve

Inferior vena cava (from lower body)

Pulmonary valve

Right ventricle

Digestive System Anatomy

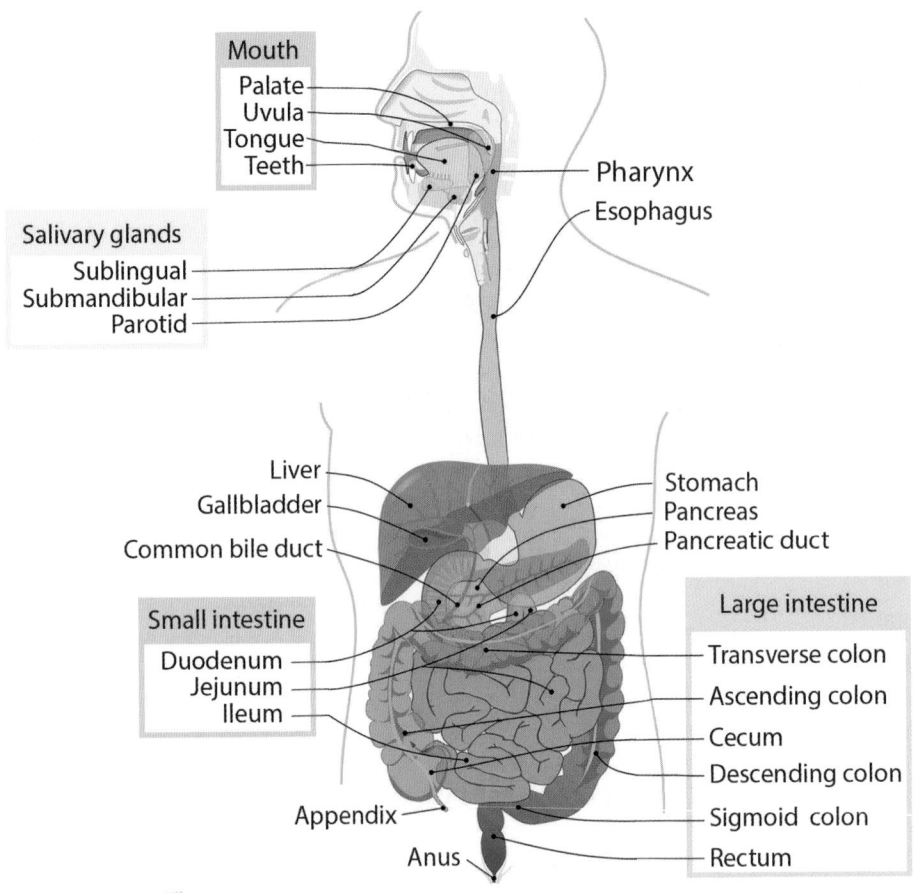

Title: Diagram of the gastrointestinal tract, **Author:** Mariana Ruiz (Lady of Hats), Jmarchn, **Source:** Own work, **License:** Public domain, **URL link:** https://en.wikiversity.org/wiki/File:Digestive_system_diagram_en.svg

Digestive System — Liver, Gallbladder, Pancreas

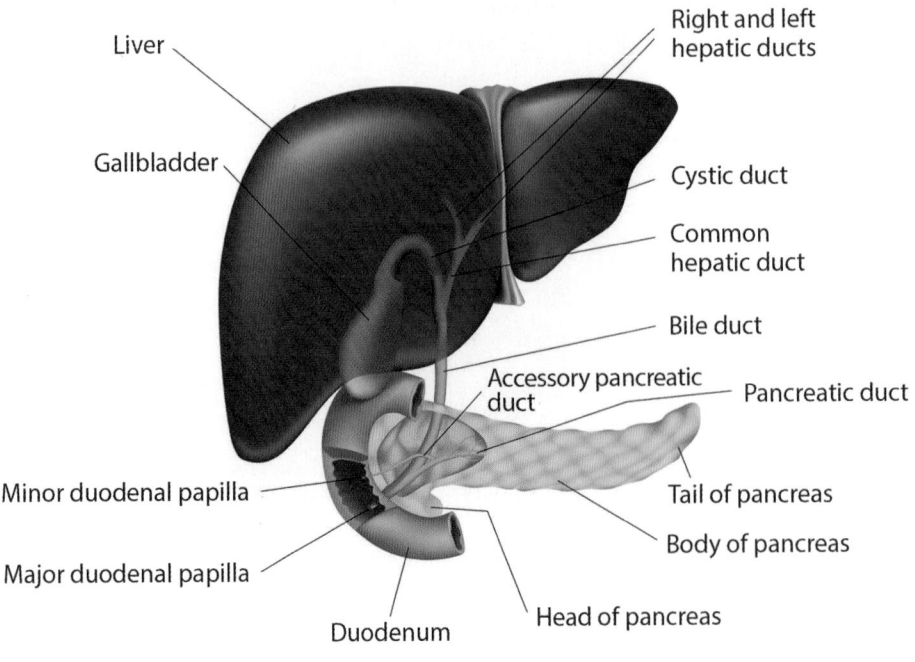

Digestive System — Mouth Anatomy

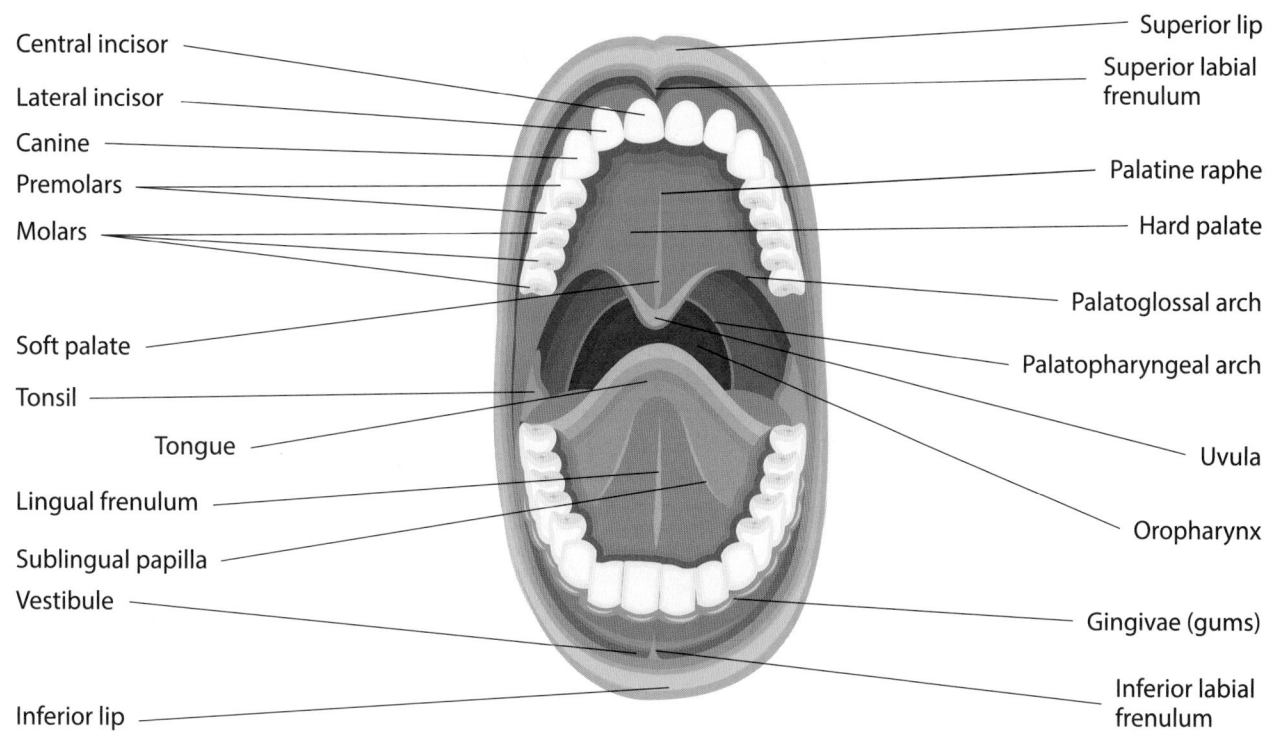

Central incisor
Lateral incisor
Canine
Premolars
Molars
Soft palate
Tonsil
Tongue
Lingual frenulum
Sublingual papilla
Vestibule
Inferior lip

Superior lip
Superior labial frenulum
Palatine raphe
Hard palate
Palatoglossal arch
Palatopharyngeal arch
Uvula
Oropharynx
Gingivae (gums)
Inferior labial frenulum

Digestive System — Tongue Anatomy

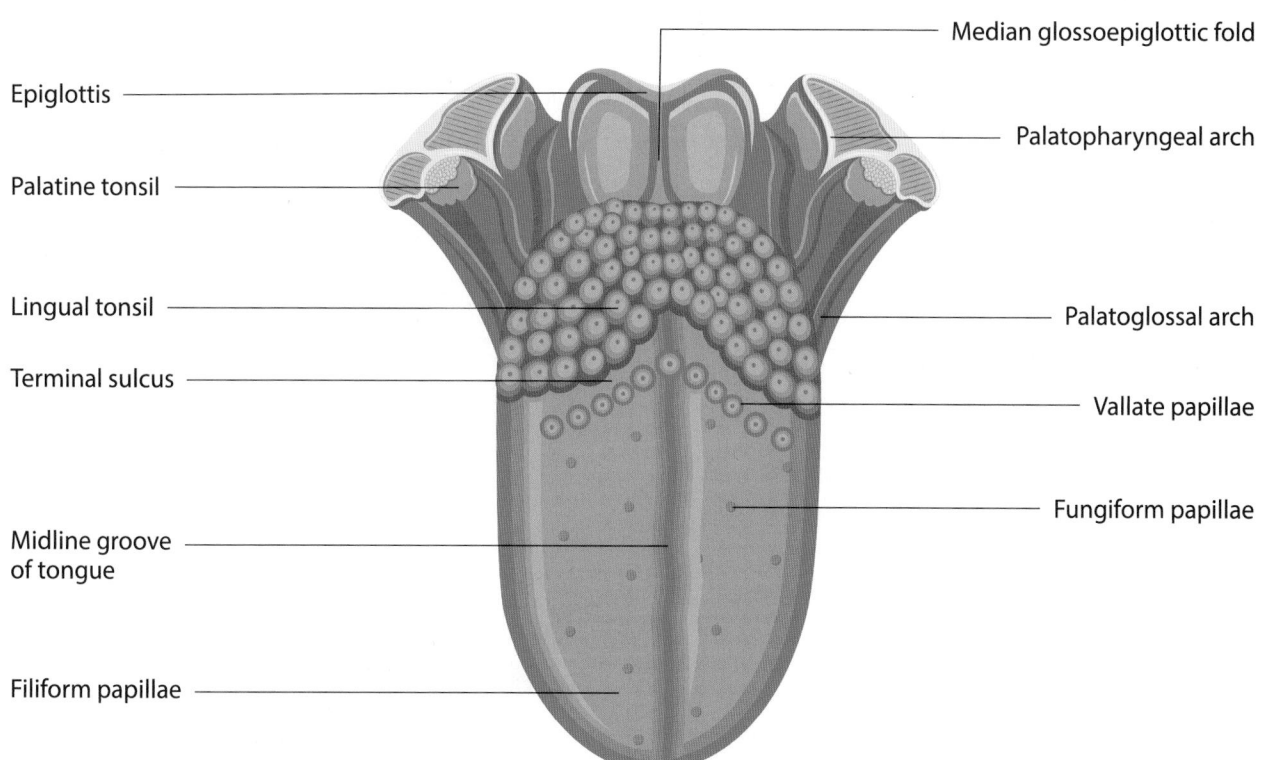

Epiglottis
Palatine tonsil
Lingual tonsil
Terminal sulcus
Midline groove of tongue
Filiform papillae

Median glossoepiglottic fold
Palatopharyngeal arch
Palatoglossal arch
Vallate papillae
Fungiform papillae

Digestive System — Stomach Anatomy

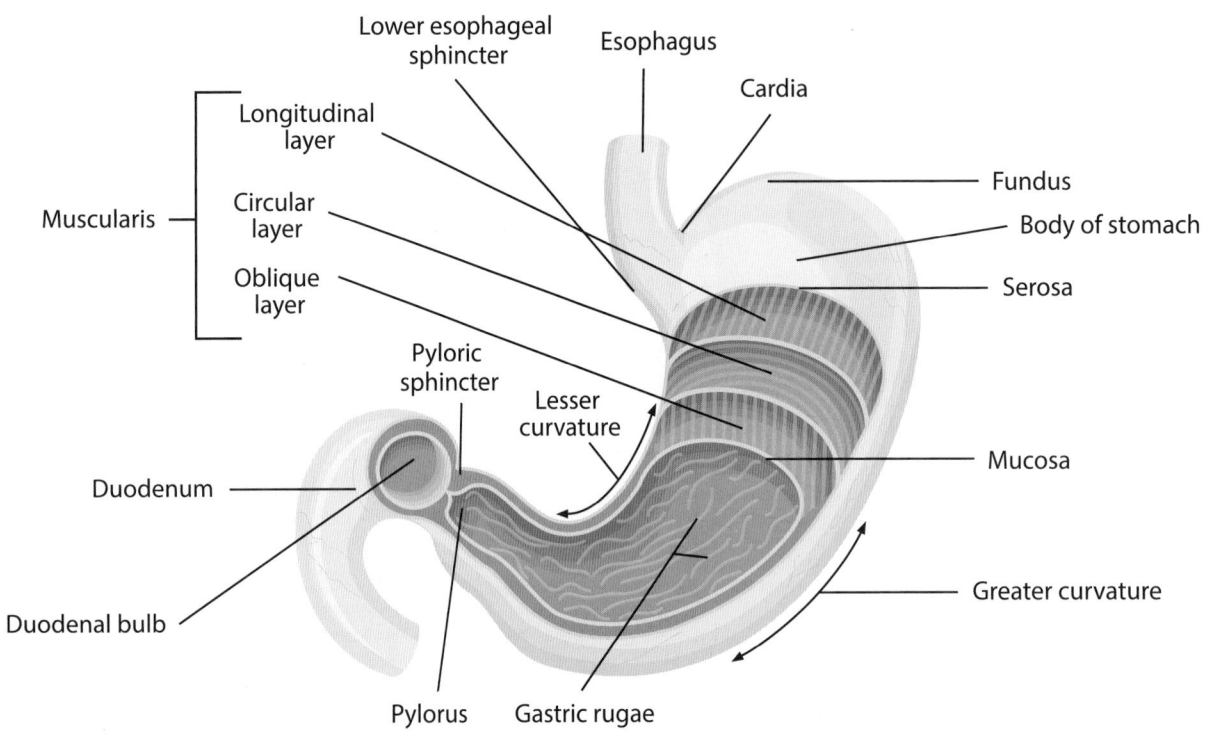

Digestive System — Small Intestine Anatomy

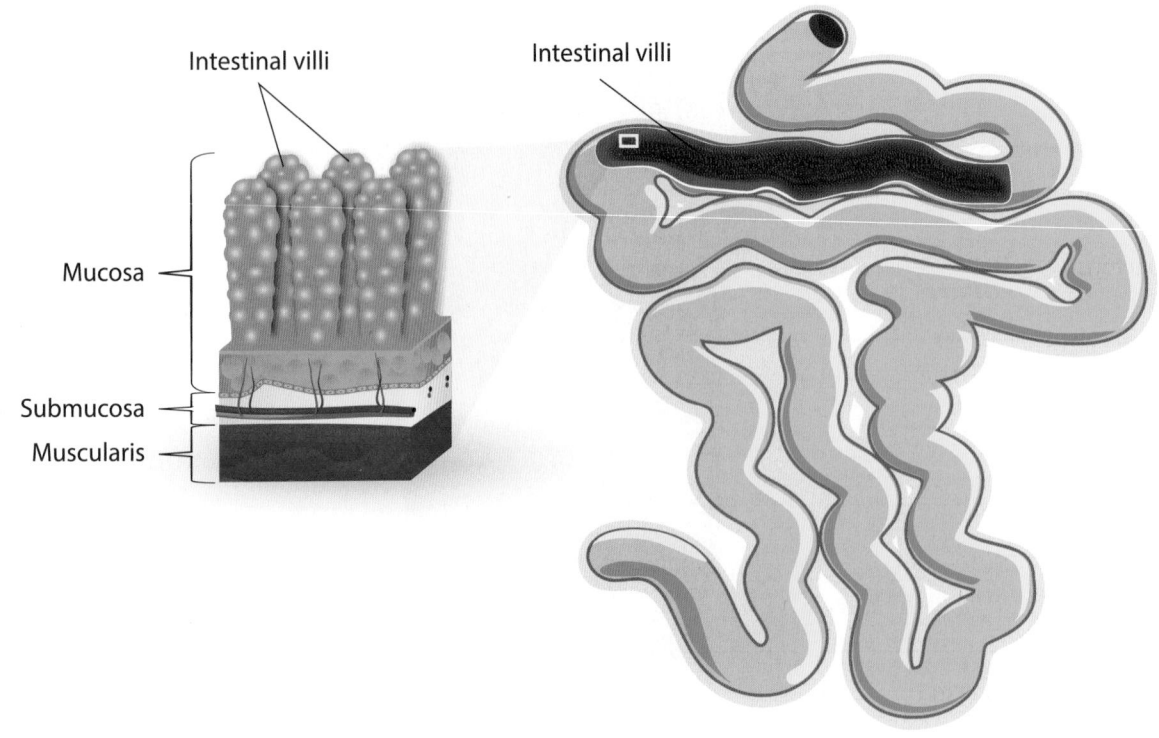

Digestive System — Large Intestine Anatomy

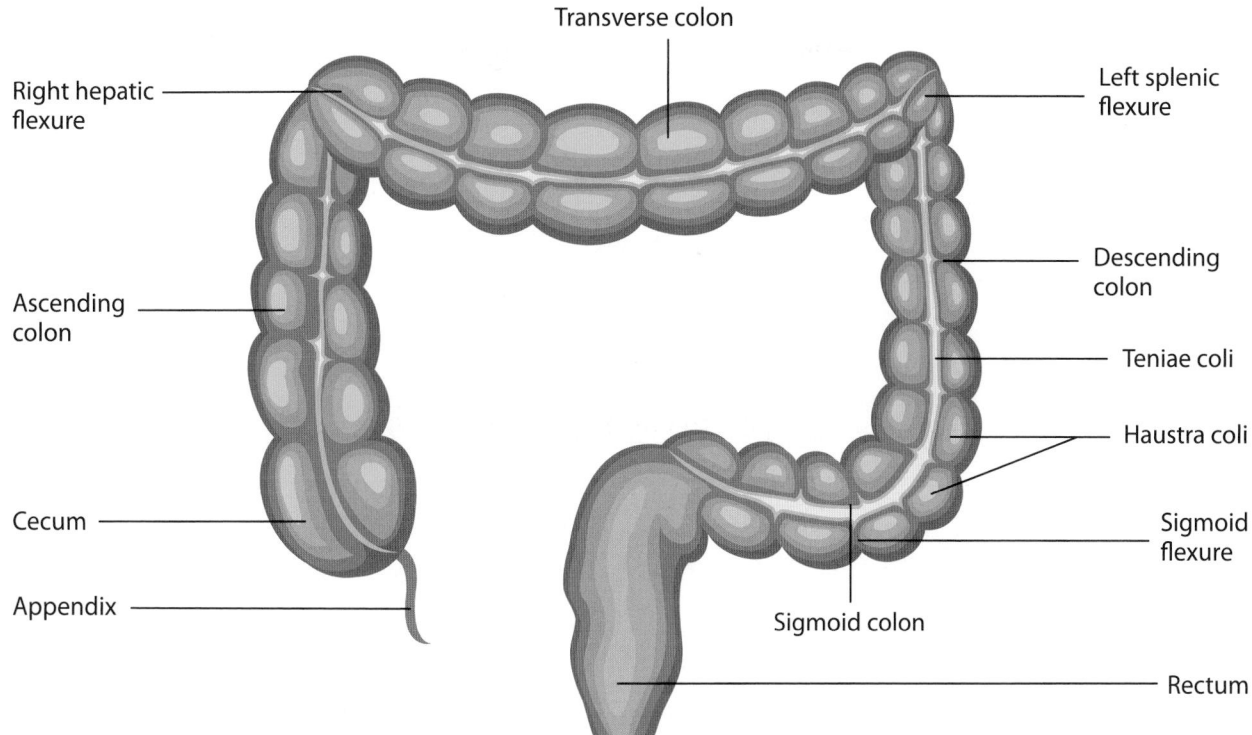

Transverse colon

Right hepatic flexure

Left splenic flexure

Ascending colon

Descending colon

Teniae coli

Haustra coli

Cecum

Sigmoid flexure

Appendix

Sigmoid colon

Rectum

Digestive System — Rectum Anatomy

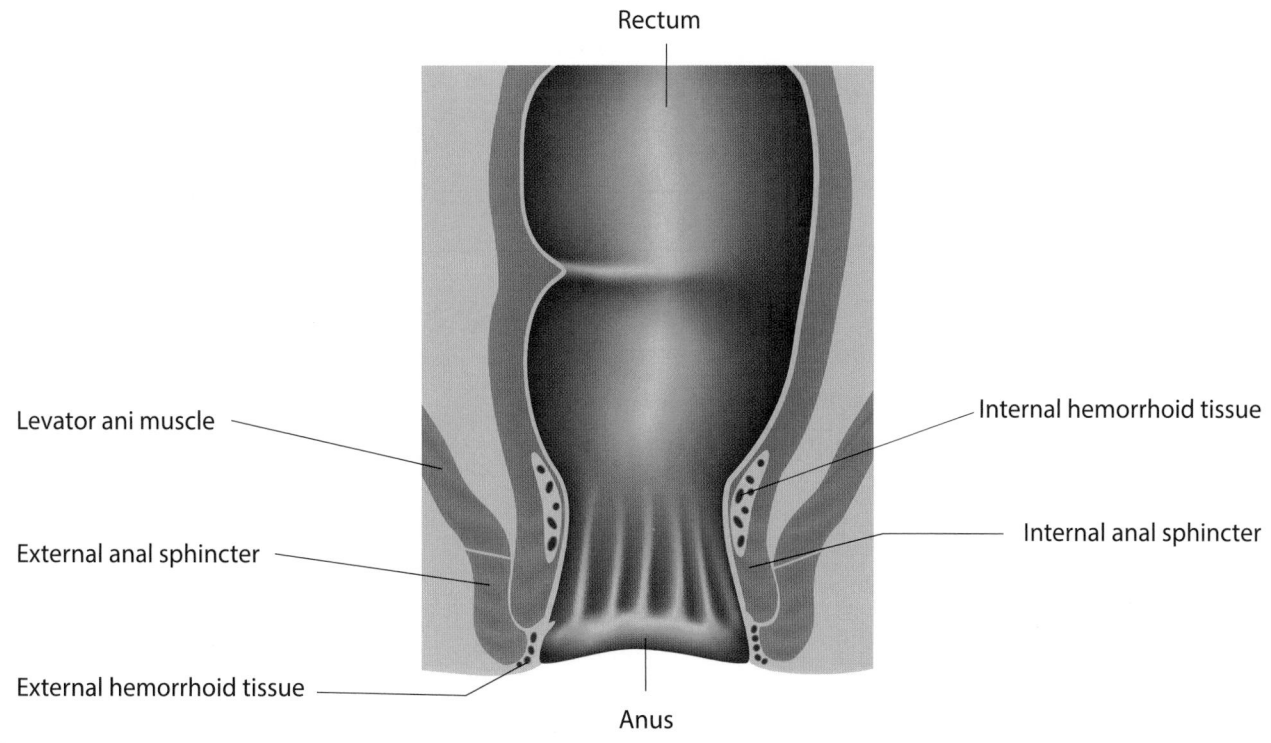

Rectum

Levator ani muscle

Internal hemorrhoid tissue

External anal sphincter

Internal anal sphincter

External hemorrhoid tissue

Anus

Ear Anatomy

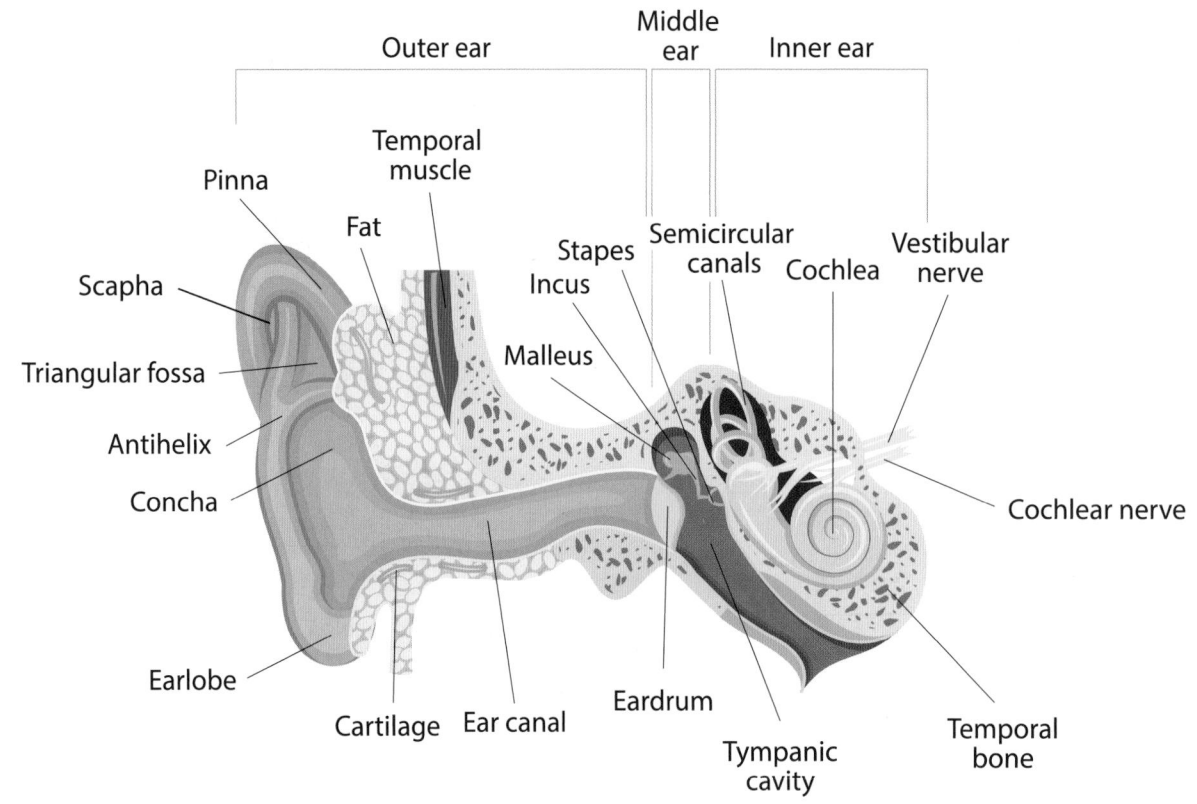

Ear Anatomy - Cochlea (Inner Ear)

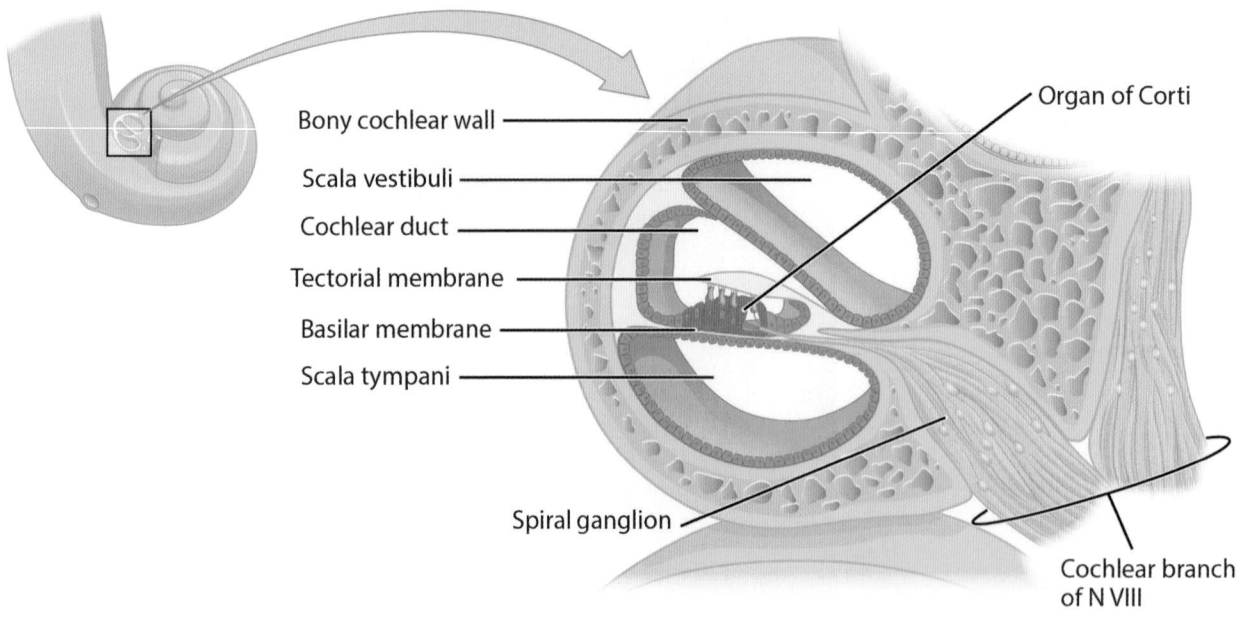

Endocrine System Anatomy and Hormones

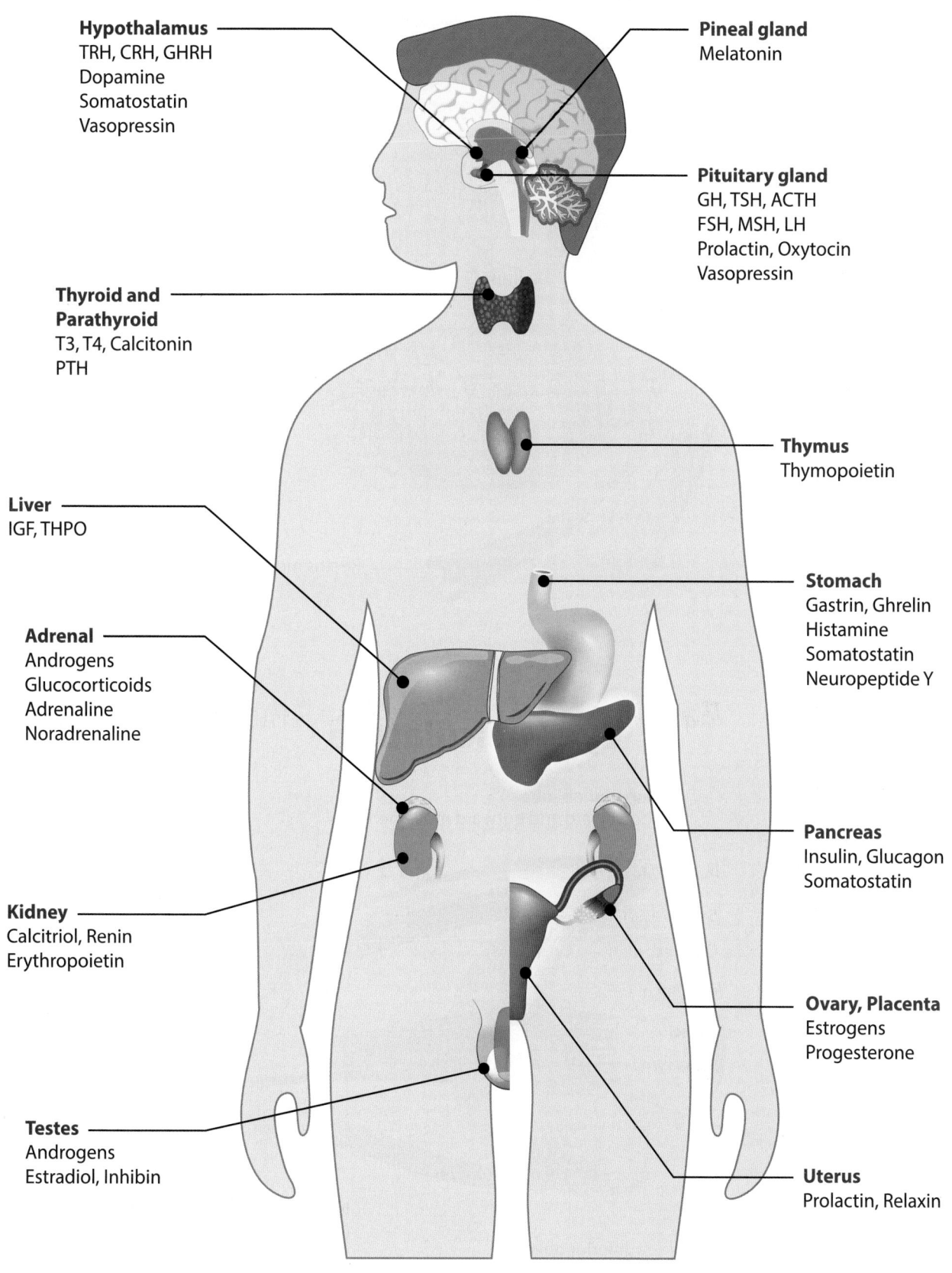

Hypothalamus
TRH, CRH, GHRH
Dopamine
Somatostatin
Vasopressin

Pineal gland
Melatonin

Pituitary gland
GH, TSH, ACTH
FSH, MSH, LH
Prolactin, Oxytocin
Vasopressin

Thyroid and Parathyroid
T3, T4, Calcitonin
PTH

Thymus
Thymopoietin

Liver
IGF, THPO

Stomach
Gastrin, Ghrelin
Histamine
Somatostatin
Neuropeptide Y

Adrenal
Androgens
Glucocorticoids
Adrenaline
Noradrenaline

Pancreas
Insulin, Glucagon
Somatostatin

Kidney
Calcitriol, Renin
Erythropoietin

Ovary, Placenta
Estrogens
Progesterone

Testes
Androgens
Estradiol, Inhibin

Uterus
Prolactin, Relaxin

Eye Anatomy

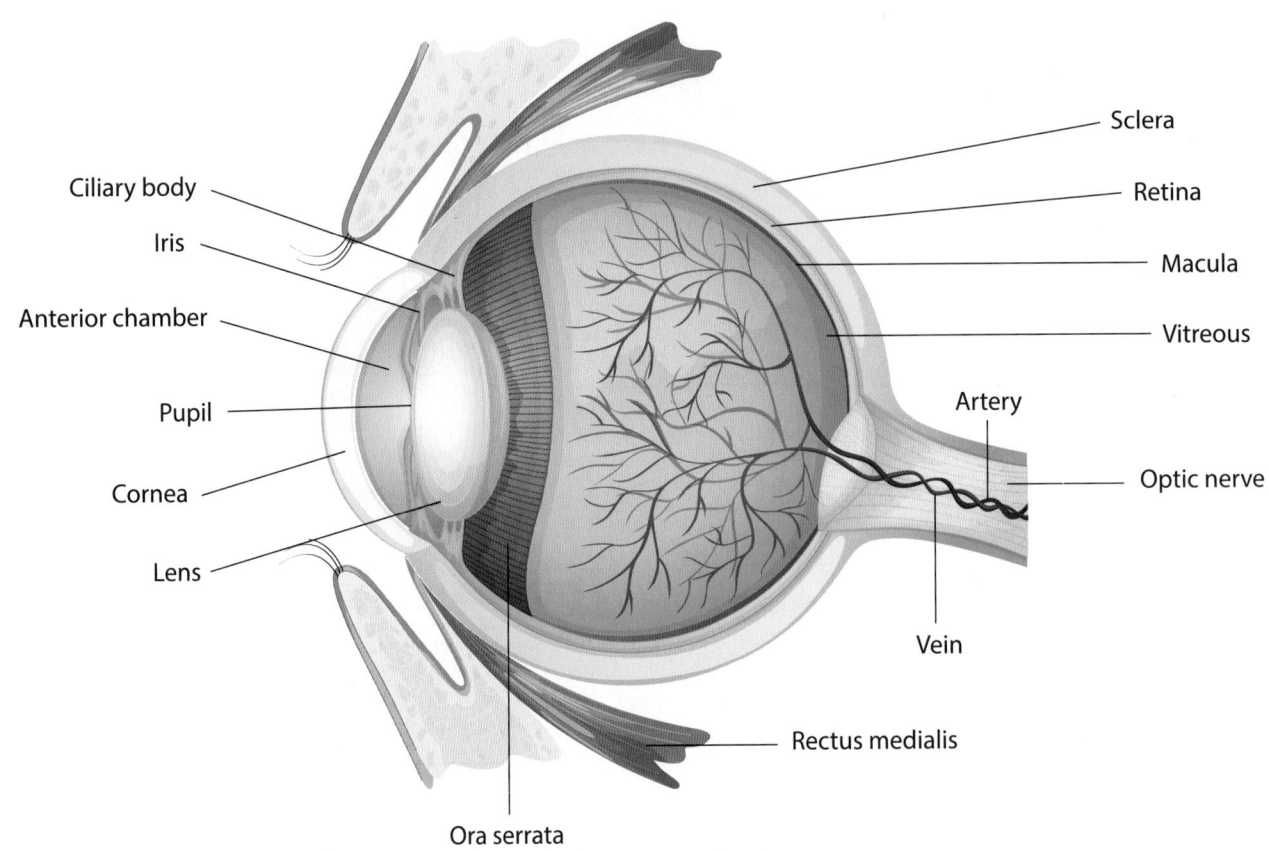

Ciliary body

Iris

Anterior chamber

Pupil

Cornea

Lens

Ora serrata

Sclera

Retina

Macula

Vitreous

Artery

Optic nerve

Vein

Rectus medialis

Eye Musculature

Superior oblique
(downward and outward movement)

Superior rectus
(upward movement)

Lateral rectus
(outward movement)

Inferior oblique
(upward and outward movement)

Inferior rectus
(downward movement)

Medial rectus
(inward movement)

Female Reproductive System Anatomy

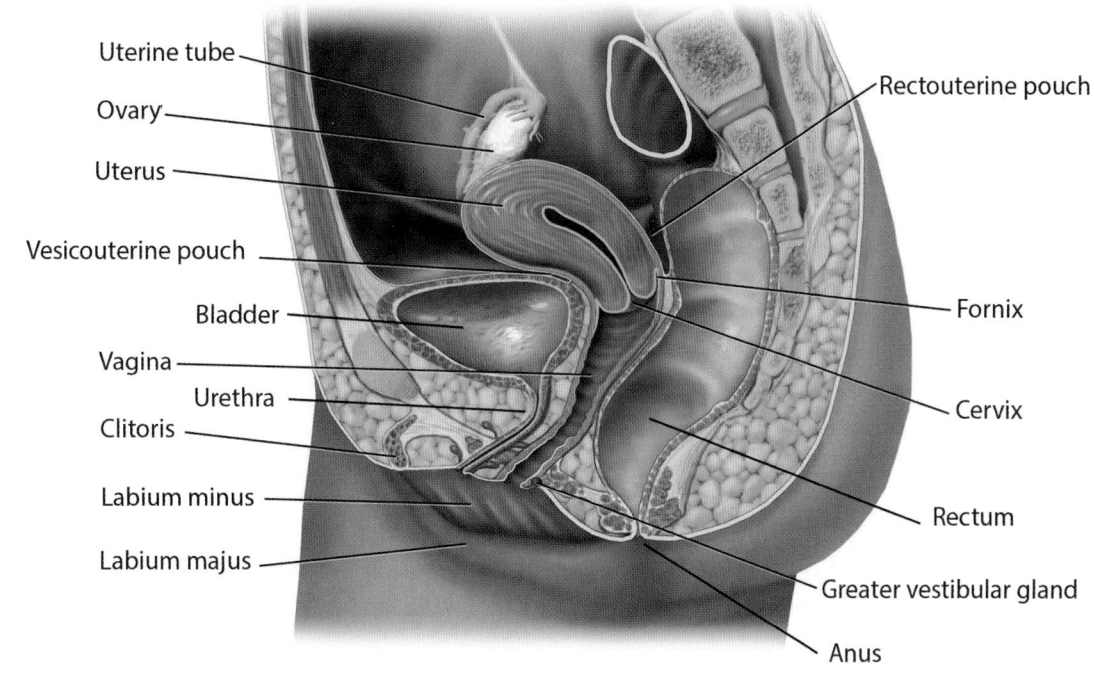

- Uterine tube
- Ovary
- Uterus
- Vesicouterine pouch
- Bladder
- Vagina
- Urethra
- Clitoris
- Labium minus
- Labium majus
- Rectouterine pouch
- Fornix
- Cervix
- Rectum
- Greater vestibular gland
- Anus

Title: Blausen 0400 FemaleReproSystem 02b.png, **Author:** BruceBlaus., **Source:** Blausen.com staff (2014). "Medical gallery of Blausen Medical 2014". *WikiJournal of Medicine* **1** (2). DOI:10.15347/wjm/2014.010. ISSN 2002-4436.Modified by User:ArnoldReinhold who released mods under CC0, **License/Permission:** This file is licensed under the Creative Commons Attribution 3.0 Unported license., **URL link:** https://commons.wikimedia.org/wiki/File:Blausen_0400_FemaleReproSystem_02b.png

Female Reproductive System — Uterus and Adnexa Anatomy

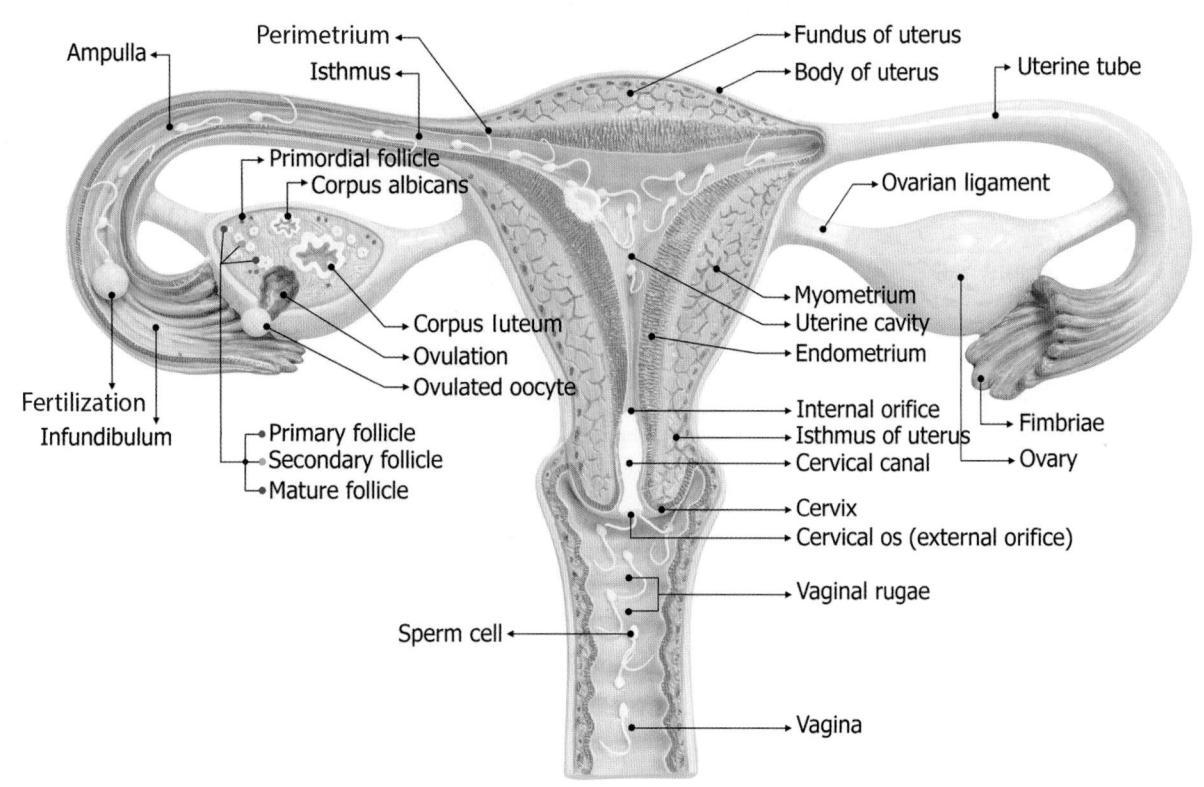

- Ampulla
- Perimetrium
- Isthmus
- Fundus of uterus
- Body of uterus
- Uterine tube
- Primordial follicle
- Corpus albicans
- Ovarian ligament
- Corpus luteum
- Ovulation
- Ovulated oocyte
- Myometrium
- Uterine cavity
- Endometrium
- Fertilization
- Infundibulum
- Primary follicle
- Secondary follicle
- Mature follicle
- Internal orifice
- Isthmus of uterus
- Cervical canal
- Fimbriae
- Ovary
- Cervix
- Cervical os (external orifice)
- Vaginal rugae
- Sperm cell
- Vagina

Female Reproductive System — Breast Anatomy

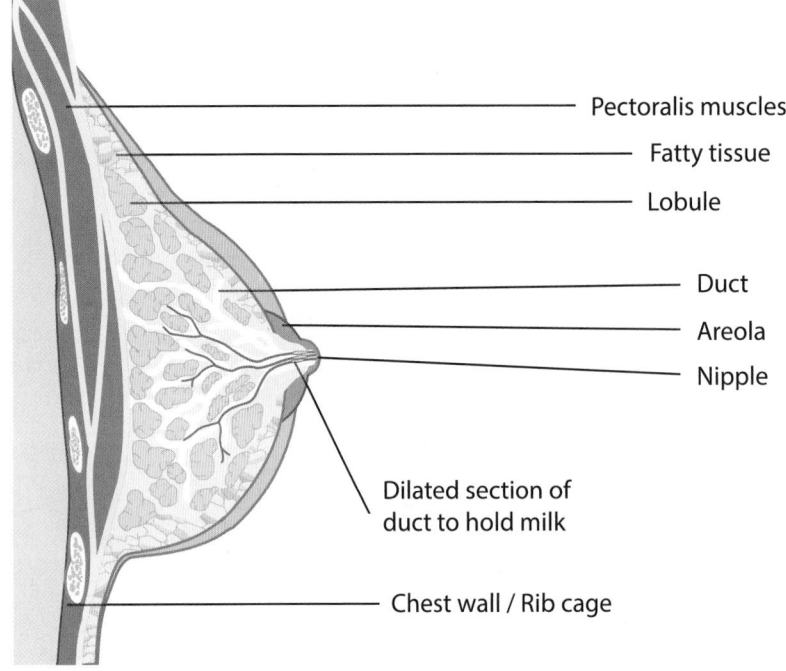

- Pectoralis muscles
- Fatty tissue
- Lobule
- Duct
- Areola
- Nipple
- Dilated section of duct to hold milk
- Chest wall / Rib cage

Female Reproductive System — Perineum Anatomy

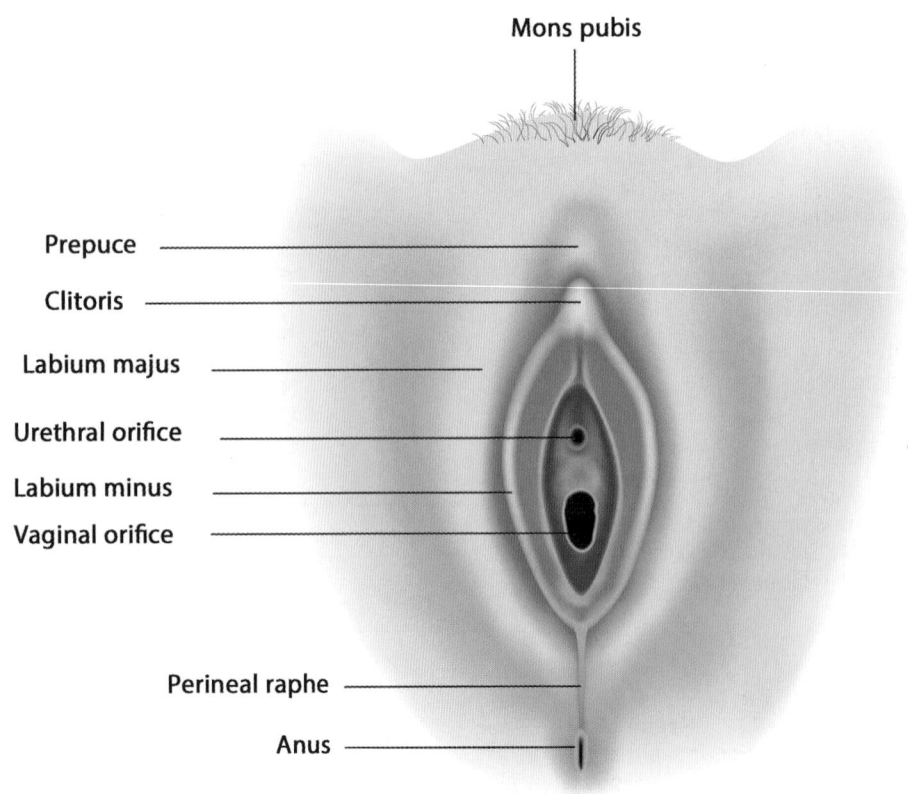

Mons pubis

- Prepuce
- Clitoris
- Labium majus
- Urethral orifice
- Labium minus
- Vaginal orifice
- Perineal raphe
- Anus

Integumentary System Anatomy

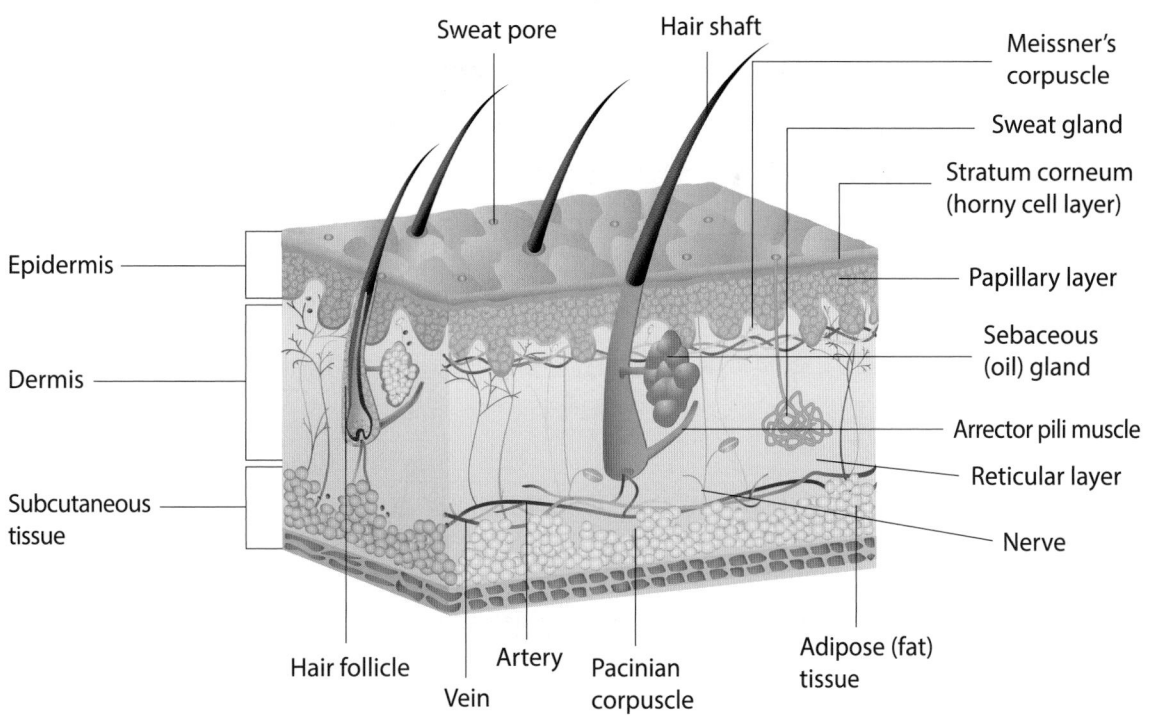

- Sweat pore
- Hair shaft
- Meissner's corpuscle
- Sweat gland
- Stratum corneum (horny cell layer)
- Epidermis
- Papillary layer
- Dermis
- Sebaceous (oil) gland
- Arrector pili muscle
- Reticular layer
- Subcutaneous tissue
- Nerve
- Hair follicle
- Artery
- Vein
- Pacinian corpuscle
- Adipose (fat) tissue

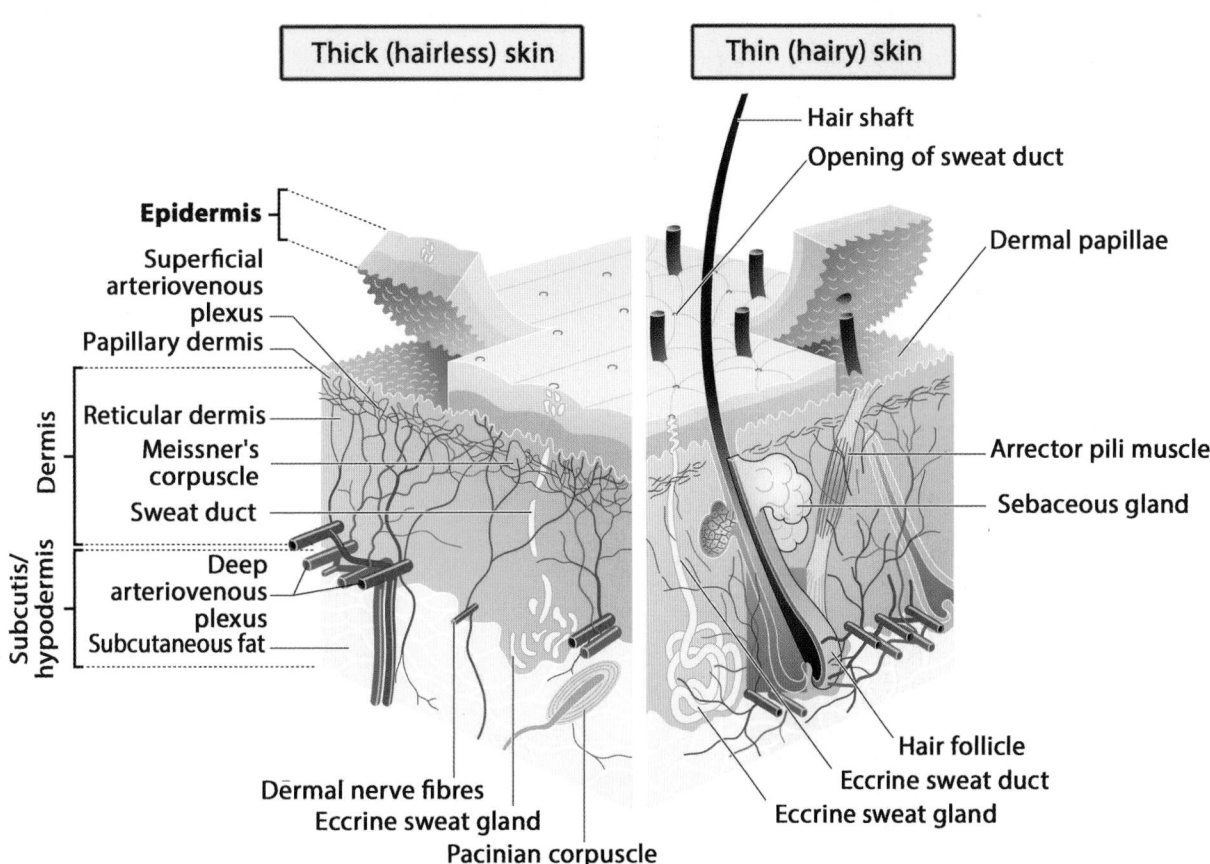

Thick (hairless) skin

Thin (hairy) skin

- Hair shaft
- Opening of sweat duct
- Epidermis
- Dermal papillae
- Superficial arteriovenous plexus
- Papillary dermis
- Dermis
  - Reticular dermis
  - Meissner's corpuscle
  - Sweat duct
- Arrector pili muscle
- Sebaceous gland
- Subcutis/hypodermis
  - Deep arteriovenous plexus
  - Subcutaneous fat
- Dermal nerve fibres
- Eccrine sweat gland
- Pacinian corpuscle
- Hair follicle
- Eccrine sweat duct
- Eccrine sweat gland

Lymphatic System Anatomy

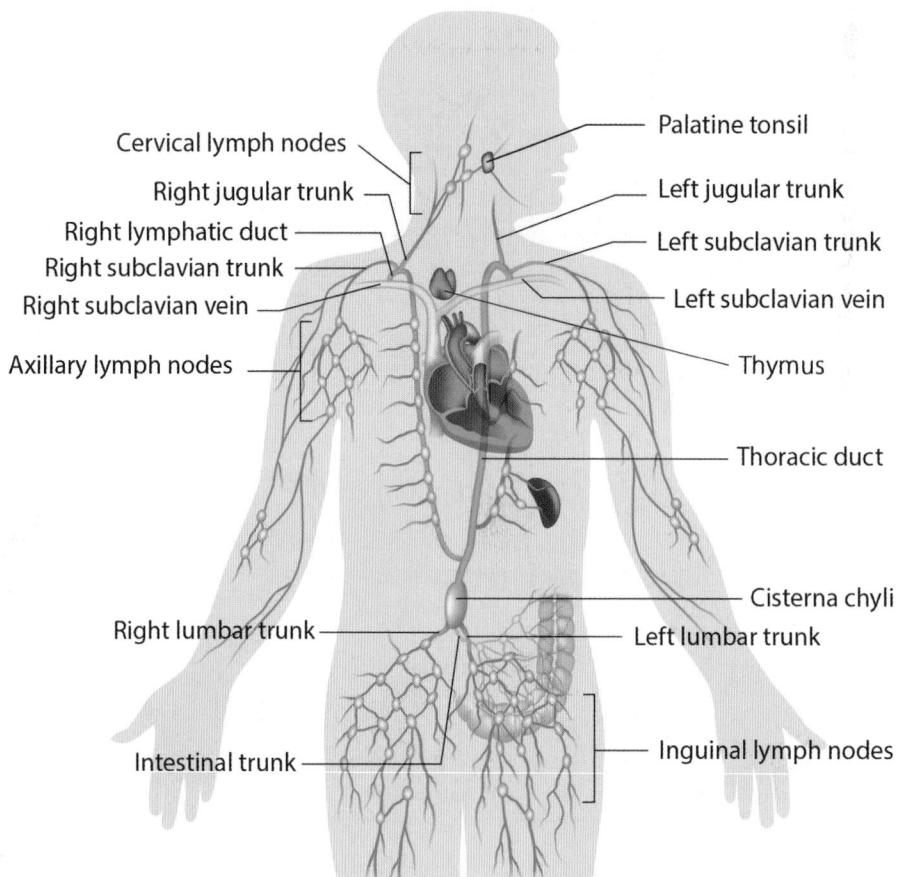

Cervical lymph nodes
Right jugular trunk
Right lymphatic duct
Right subclavian trunk
Right subclavian vein
Axillary lymph nodes

Palatine tonsil
Left jugular trunk
Left subclavian trunk
Left subclavian vein
Thymus

Thoracic duct

Cisterna chyli
Right lumbar trunk
Left lumbar trunk

Intestinal trunk
Inguinal lymph nodes

Lymphatic System — Lymph Nodes of the Head and Neck

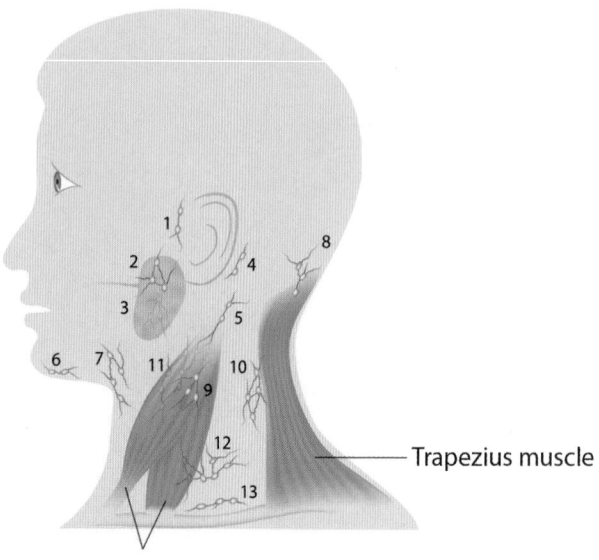

1. Preauricular
2. Superficial parotid
3. Deep parotid
4. Posterior auricular
5. Mastoid
6. Submental
7. Submandibular
8. Occipital
9. Superficial anterior cervical
10. Superficial posterior cervical
11. Superior deep cervical
12. Inferior deep cervical
13. Supraclavicular

Trapezius muscle

Sternocleidomastoid muscle

Lymphatic System — Humoral Immunity

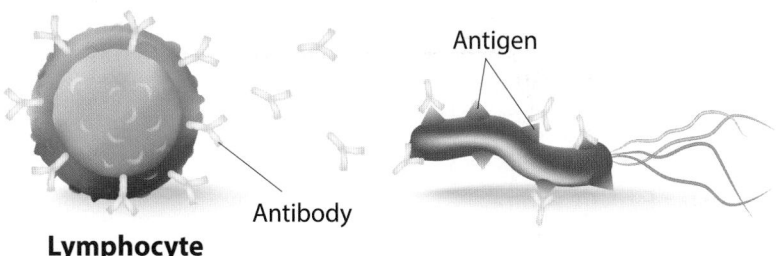

Antigen

Antibody

Lymphocyte

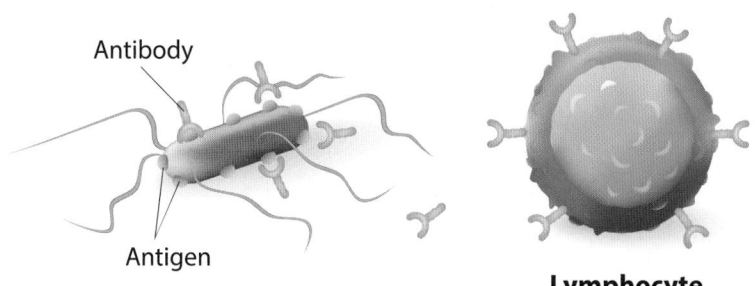

Antibody

Antigen

Lymphocyte

Lymphatic System — Lymph Node Anatomy

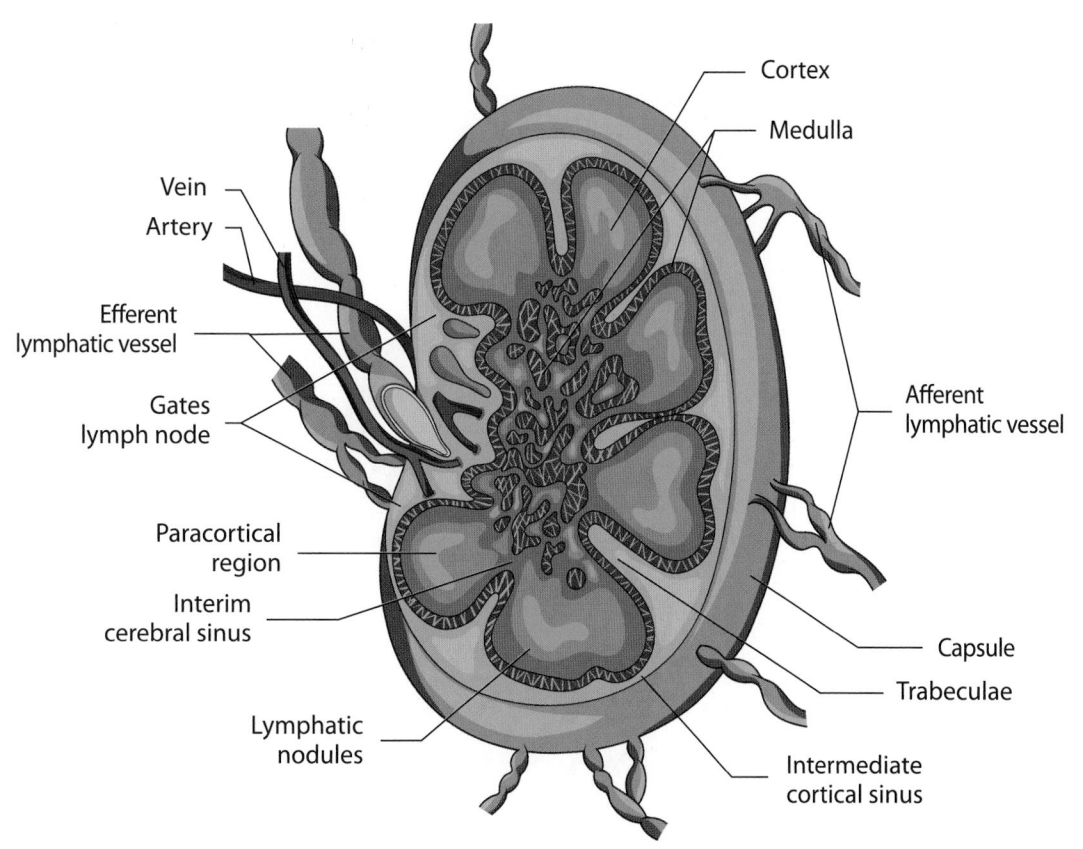

Cortex

Medulla

Vein

Artery

Efferent
lymphatic vessel

Afferent
lymphatic vessel

Gates
lymph node

Paracortical
region

Interim
cerebral sinus

Capsule

Trabeculae

Lymphatic
nodules

Intermediate
cortical sinus

Male Reproductive System Anatomy

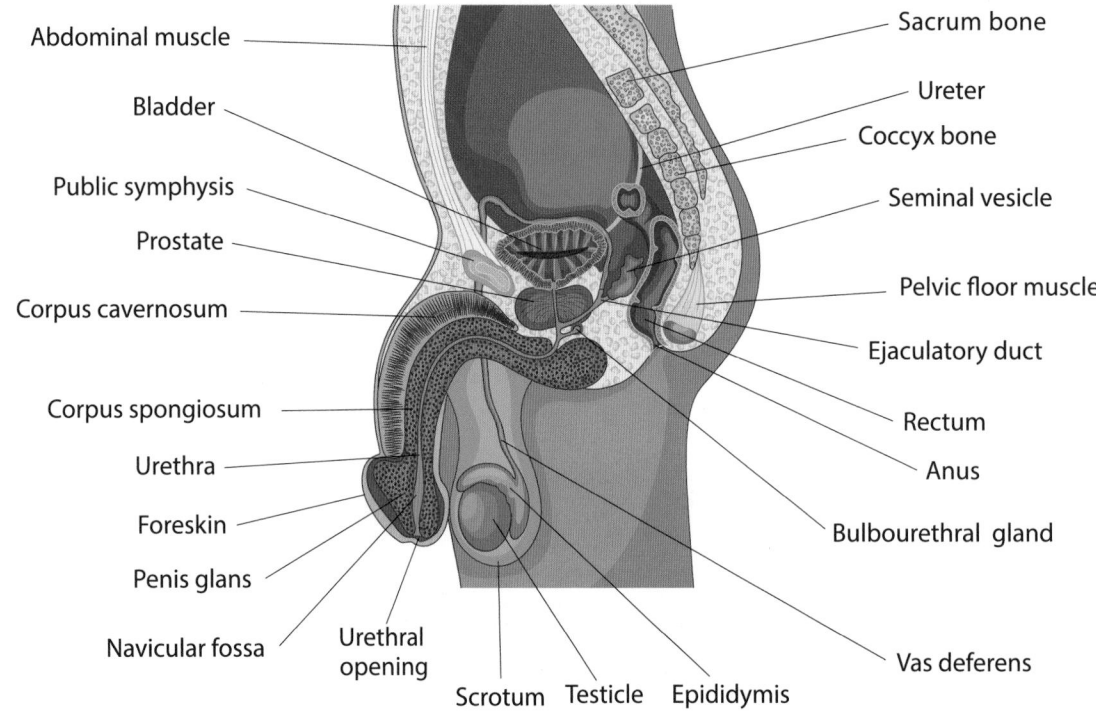

Abdominal muscle
Bladder
Public symphysis
Prostate
Corpus cavernosum
Corpus spongiosum
Urethra
Foreskin
Penis glans
Navicular fossa
Urethral opening
Scrotum
Testicle
Epididymis
Sacrum bone
Ureter
Coccyx bone
Seminal vesicle
Pelvic floor muscle
Ejaculatory duct
Rectum
Anus
Bulbourethral gland
Vas deferens

Male Reproductive System — Testicle

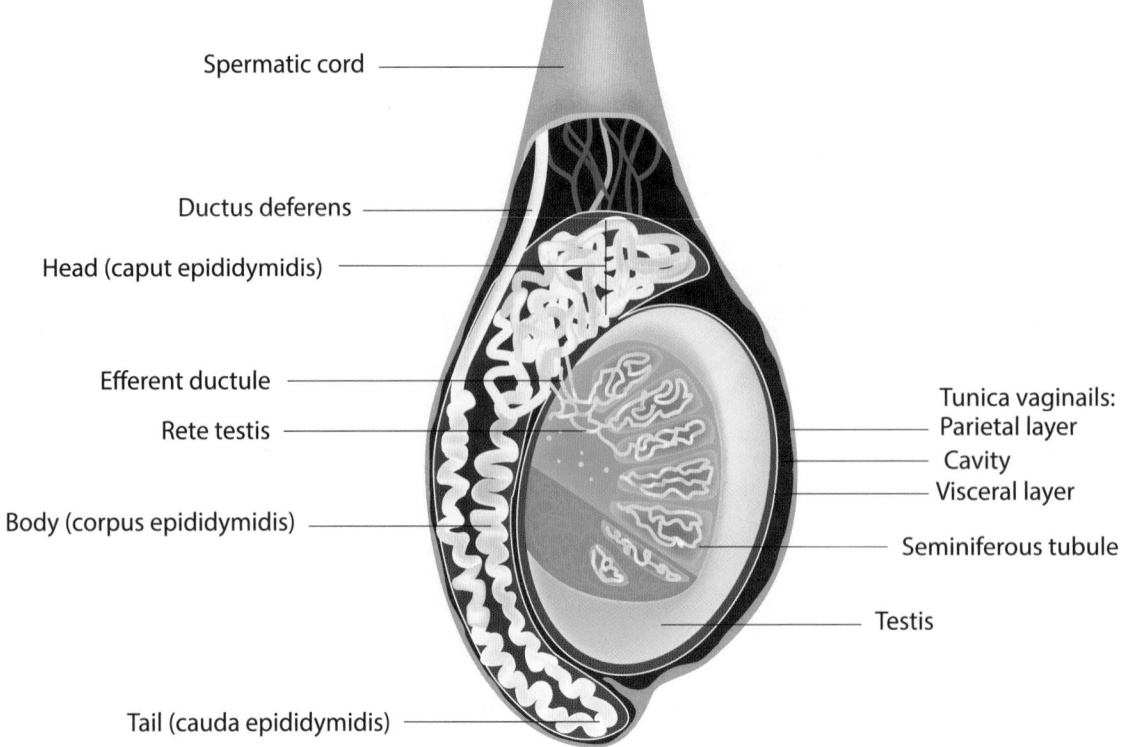

Spermatic cord
Ductus deferens
Head (caput epididymidis)
Efferent ductule
Rete testis
Body (corpus epididymidis)
Tail (cauda epididymidis)
Tunica vaginails:
Parietal layer
Cavity
Visceral layer
Seminiferous tubule
Testis

Male Reproductive System — Penis Anatomy

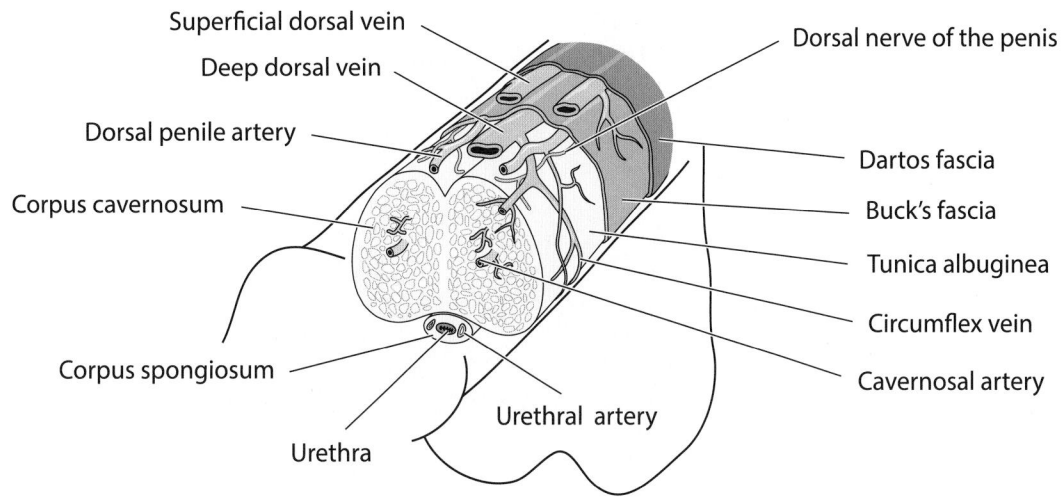

Superficial dorsal vein
Deep dorsal vein
Dorsal penile artery
Corpus cavernosum
Corpus spongiosum
Urethra
Urethral artery
Dorsal nerve of the penis
Dartos fascia
Buck's fascia
Tunica albuginea
Circumflex vein
Cavernosal artery

Muscular System Anatomy

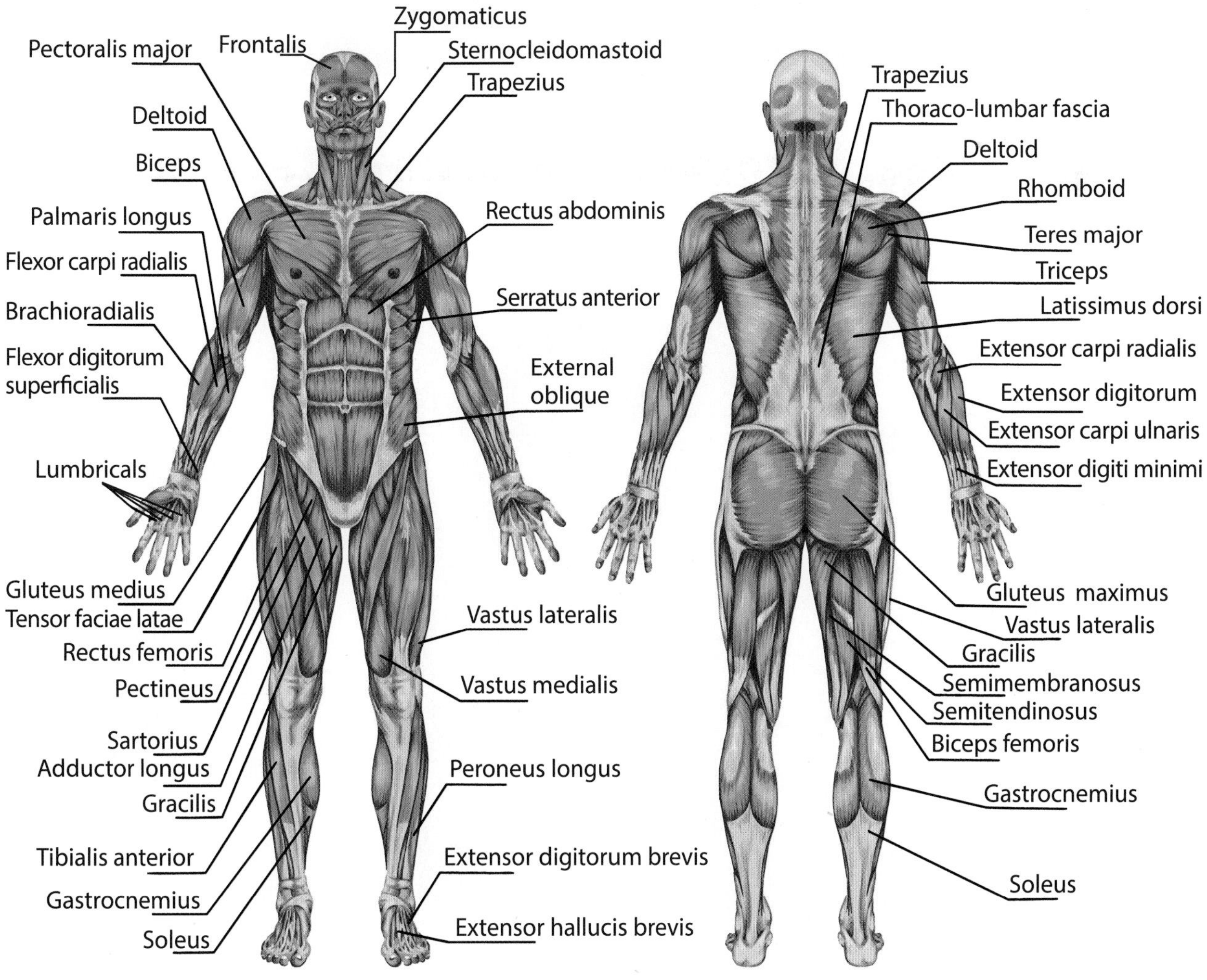

Pectoralis major
Frontalis
Zygomaticus
Sternocleidomastoid
Trapezius
Deltoid
Biceps
Palmaris longus
Flexor carpi radialis
Brachioradialis
Flexor digitorum superficialis
Rectus abdominis
Serratus anterior
External oblique
Lumbricals
Gluteus medius
Tensor faciae latae
Rectus femoris
Pectineus
Sartorius
Adductor longus
Gracilis
Tibialis anterior
Gastrocnemius
Soleus
Vastus lateralis
Vastus medialis
Peroneus longus
Extensor digitorum brevis
Extensor hallucis brevis

Trapezius
Thoraco-lumbar fascia
Deltoid
Rhomboid
Teres major
Triceps
Latissimus dorsi
Extensor carpi radialis
Extensor digitorum
Extensor carpi ulnaris
Extensor digiti minimi
Gluteus maximus
Vastus lateralis
Gracilis
Semimembranosus
Semitendinosus
Biceps femoris
Gastrocnemius
Soleus

Muscular System — Face Muscles

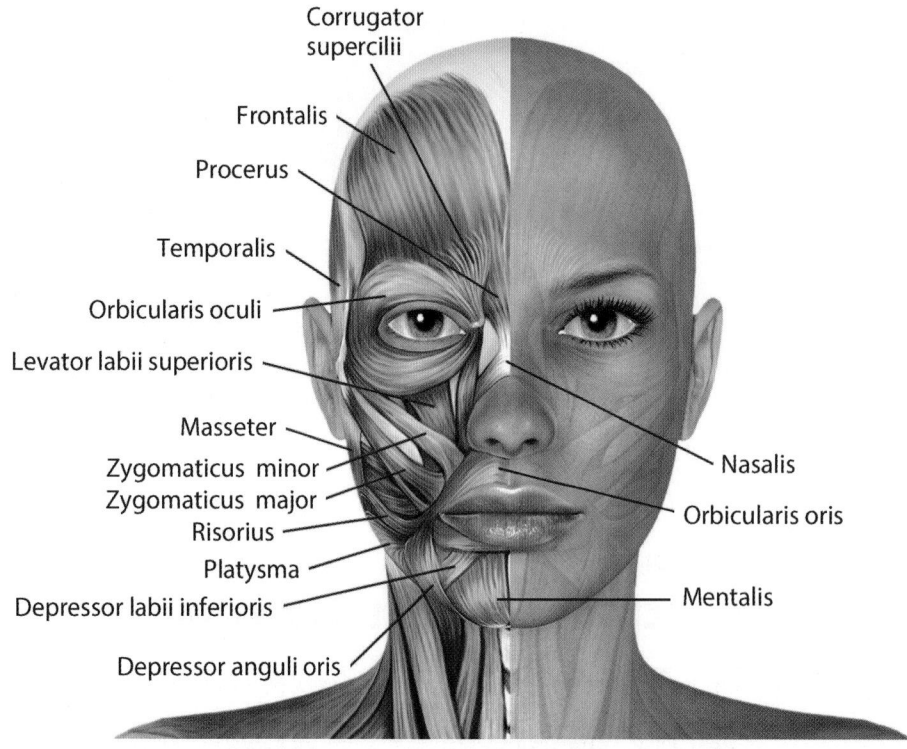

Corrugator supercilii

Frontalis

Procerus

Temporalis

Orbicularis oculi

Levator labii superioris

Masseter

Zygomaticus minor

Zygomaticus major

Risorius

Platysma

Depressor labii inferioris

Depressor anguli oris

Nasalis

Orbicularis oris

Mentalis

Muscular System — Neck, Chest, Thorax Muscles

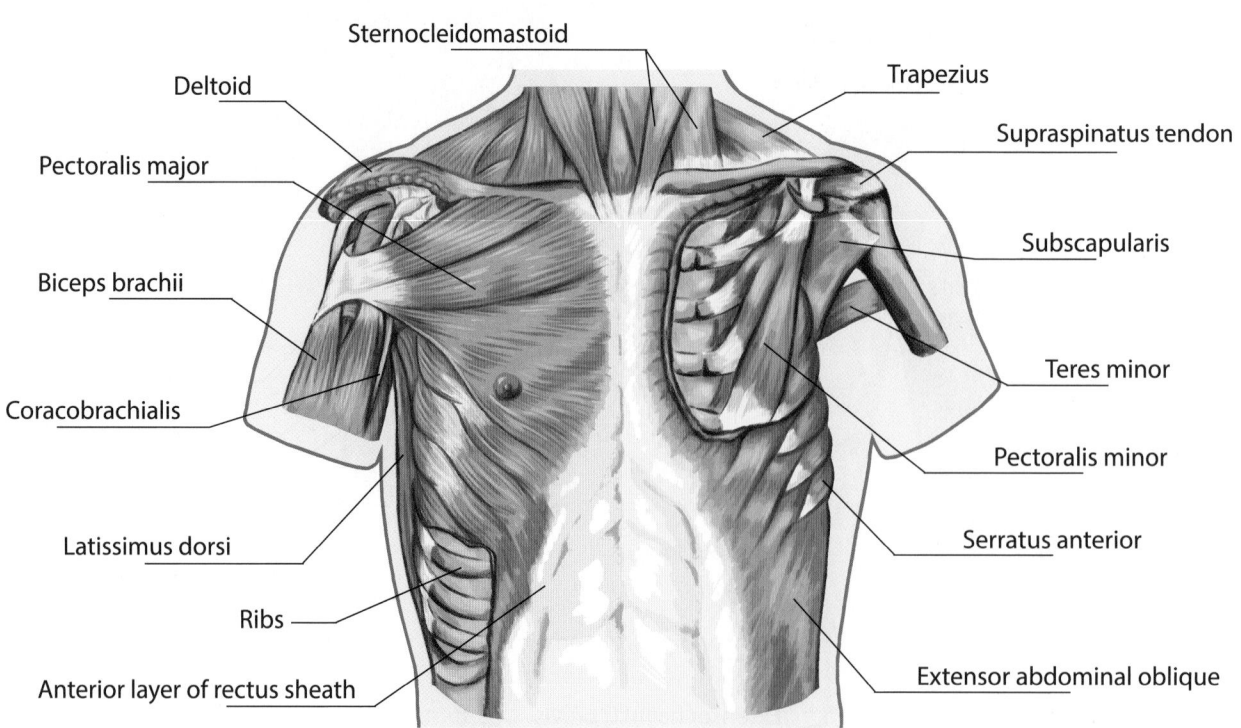

Sternocleidomastoid

Deltoid

Pectoralis major

Biceps brachii

Coracobrachialis

Latissimus dorsi

Ribs

Anterior layer of rectus sheath

Trapezius

Supraspinatus tendon

Subscapularis

Teres minor

Pectoralis minor

Serratus anterior

Extensor abdominal oblique

Muscular System — Shoulder (Rotator Cuff) Muscles

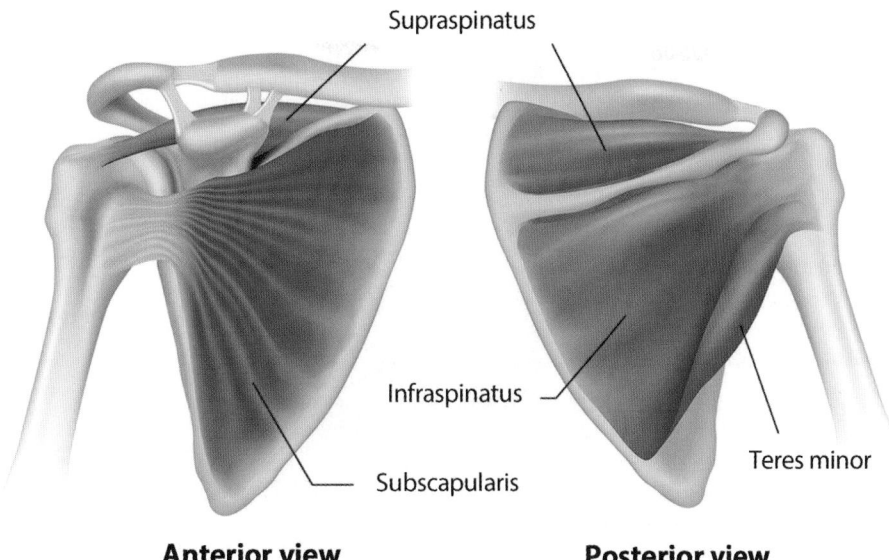

Supraspinatus

Infraspinatus

Subscapularis

Teres minor

Anterior view   **Posterior view**

Muscular System — Forearm Muscles (Right Arm, Posterior Compartment)

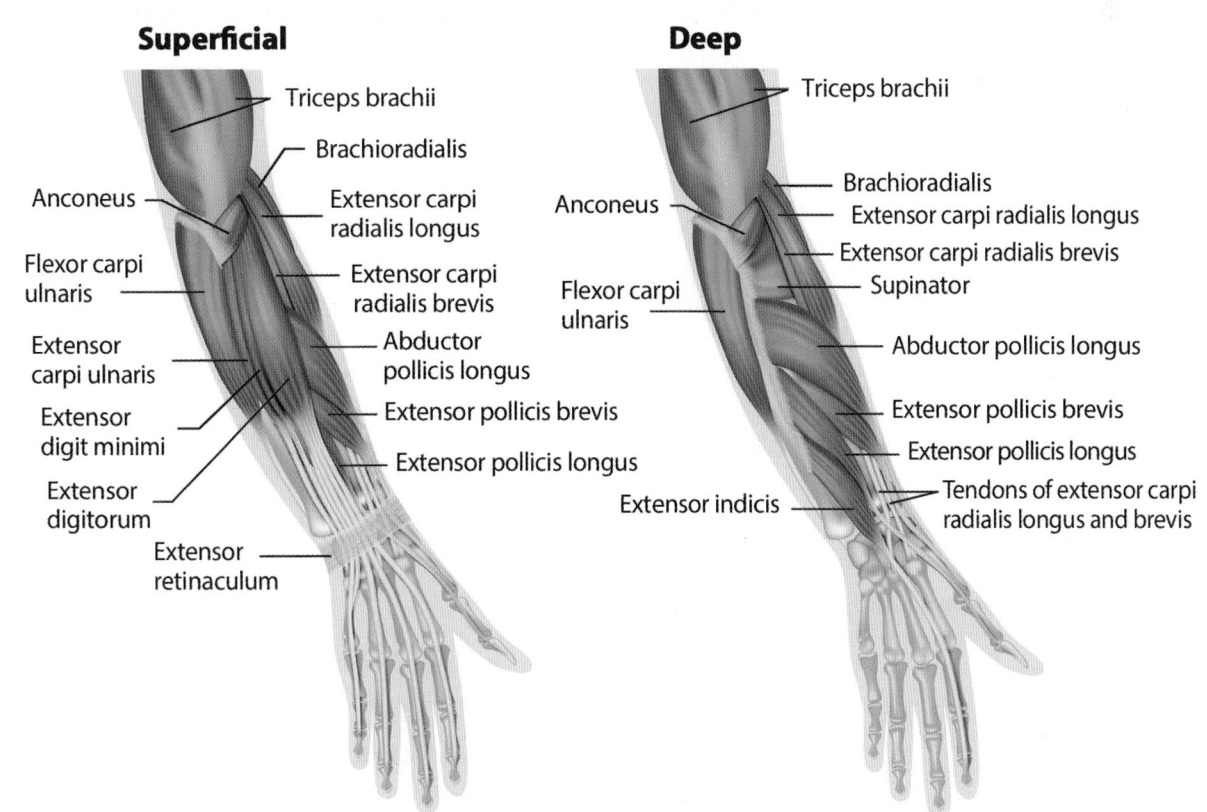

Superficial

Triceps brachii

Brachioradialis

Anconeus

Extensor carpi radialis longus

Flexor carpi ulnaris

Extensor carpi radialis brevis

Extensor carpi ulnaris

Abductor pollicis longus

Extensor digit minimi

Extensor pollicis brevis

Extensor digitorum

Extensor pollicis longus

Extensor retinaculum

Deep

Triceps brachii

Brachioradialis

Anconeus

Extensor carpi radialis longus

Extensor carpi radialis brevis

Flexor carpi ulnaris

Supinator

Abductor pollicis longus

Extensor pollicis brevis

Extensor pollicis longus

Extensor indicis

Tendons of extensor carpi radialis longus and brevis

Muscular System — Muscles of the Hand
(right hand, dorsal view)

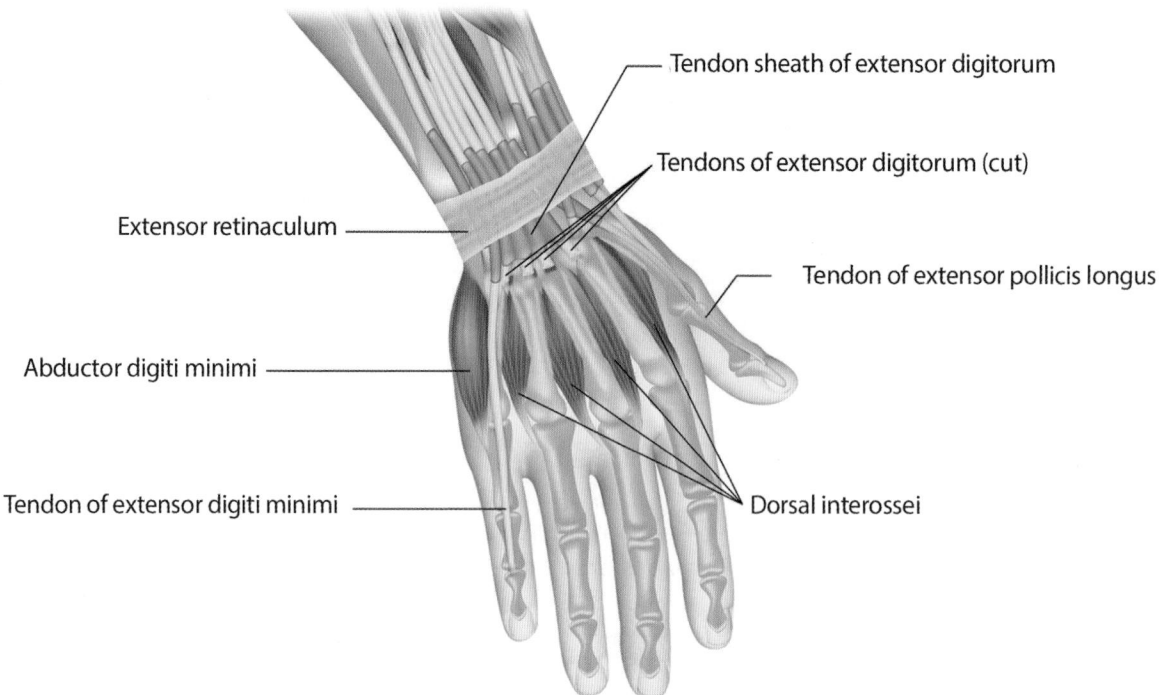

Tendon sheath of extensor digitorum

Tendons of extensor digitorum (cut)

Extensor retinaculum

Tendon of extensor pollicis longus

Abductor digiti minimi

Tendon of extensor digiti minimi

Dorsal interossei

Muscular System — Muscles of the Hand
(right hand, palmar view)

Deep

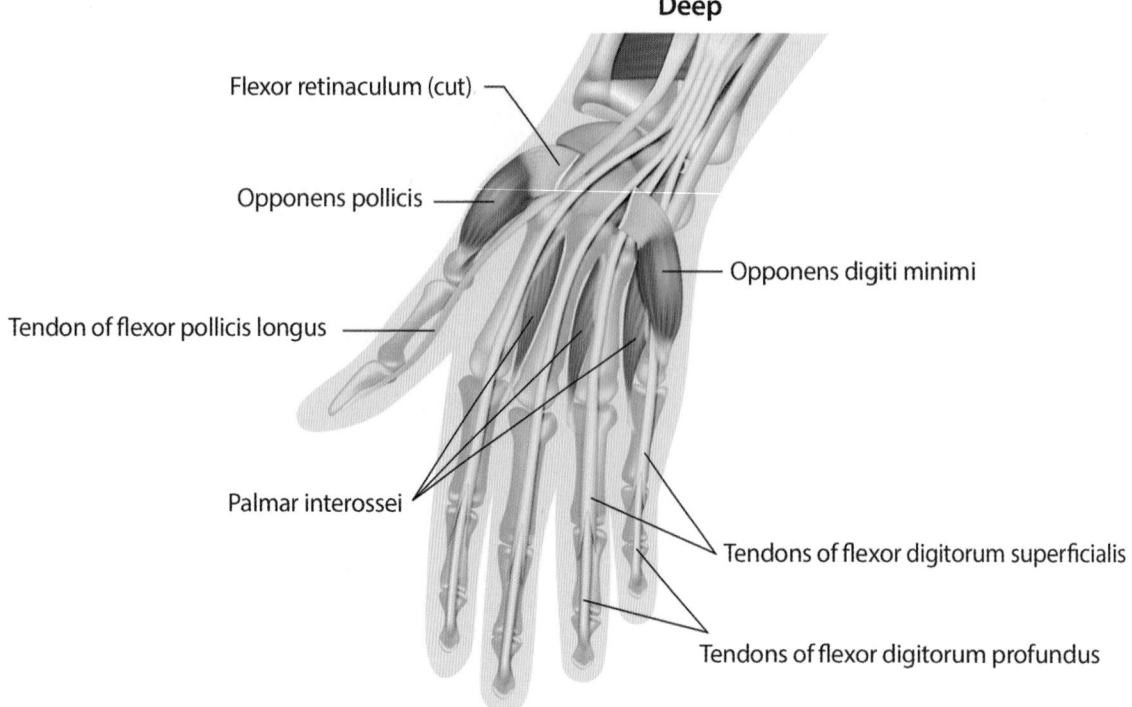

Flexor retinaculum (cut)

Opponens pollicis

Opponens digiti minimi

Tendon of flexor pollicis longus

Palmar interossei

Tendons of flexor digitorum superficialis

Tendons of flexor digitorum profundus

Muscular System — Leg Muscles

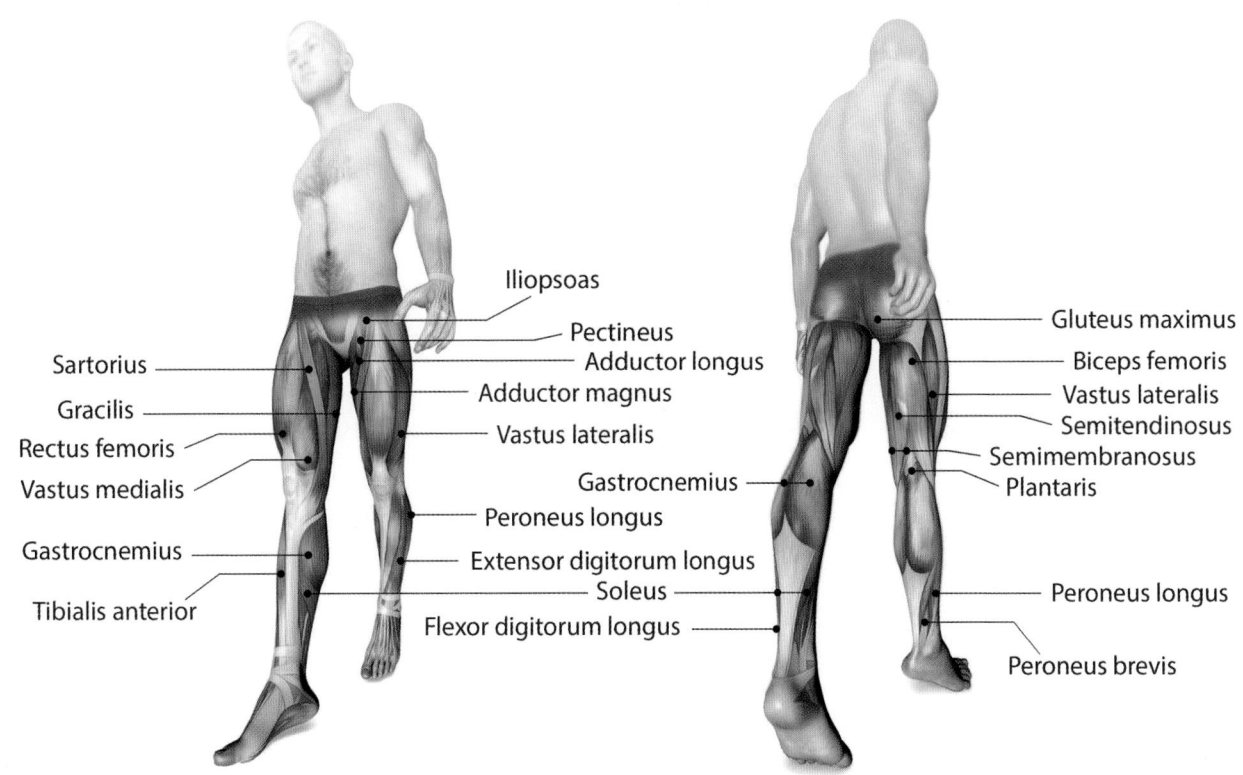

Iliopsoas
Pectineus
Adductor longus
Adductor magnus
Vastus lateralis
Gastrocnemius
Peroneus longus
Extensor digitorum longus
Soleus
Flexor digitorum longus

Sartorius
Gracilis
Rectus femoris
Vastus medialis
Gastrocnemius
Tibialis anterior

Gluteus maximus
Biceps femoris
Vastus lateralis
Semitendinosus
Semimembranosus
Plantaris
Peroneus longus
Peroneus brevis

Muscular System — Knee and Leg

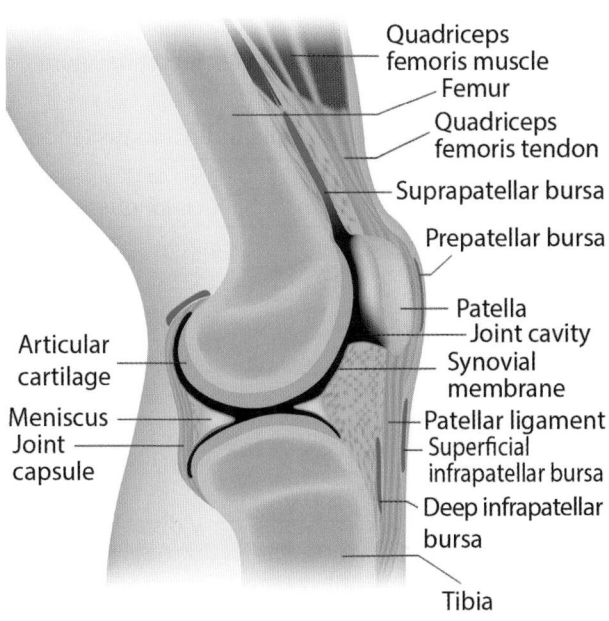

Quadriceps femoris muscle
Femur
Quadriceps femoris tendon
Suprapatellar bursa
Prepatellar bursa
Patella
Joint cavity
Synovial membrane
Patellar ligament
Superficial infrapatellar bursa
Deep infrapatellar bursa
Tibia

Articular cartilage
Meniscus
Joint capsule

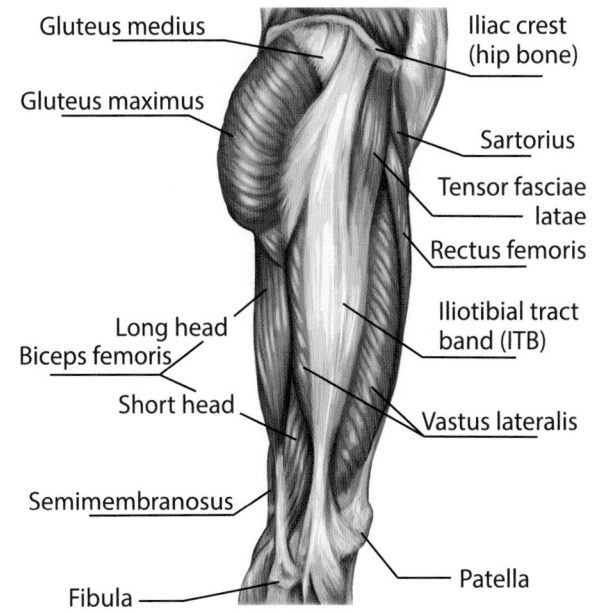

Gluteus medius
Gluteus maximus
Iliac crest (hip bone)
Sartorius
Tensor fasciae latae
Rectus femoris
Iliotibial tract band (ITB)
Vastus lateralis
Patella

Long head
Biceps femoris
Short head
Semimembranosus
Fibula

Muscular System — Foot Muscles

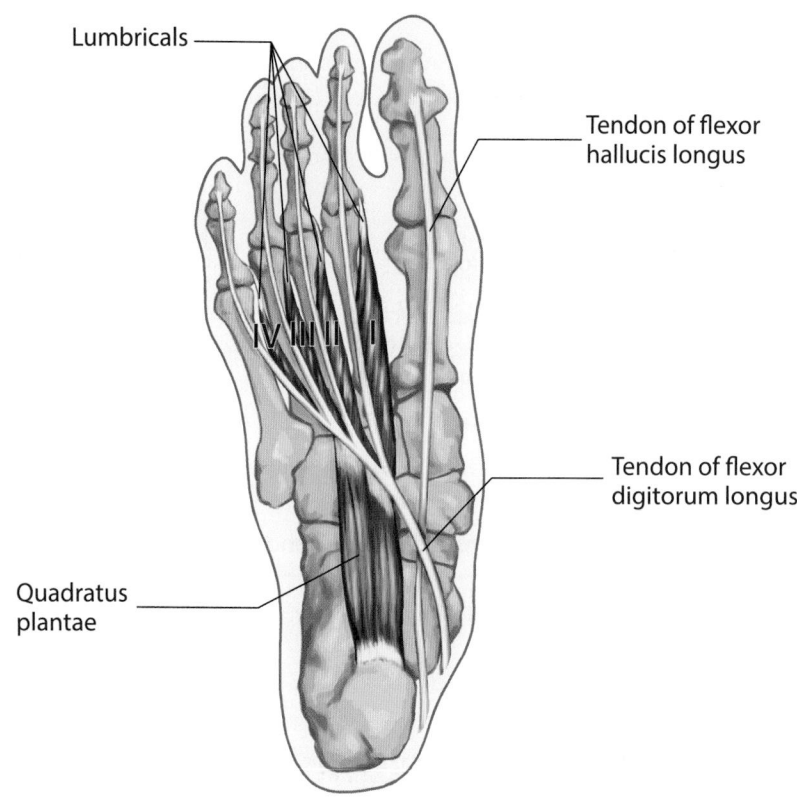

Lumbricals

Tendon of flexor hallucis longus

Tendon of flexor digitorum longus

Quadratus plantae

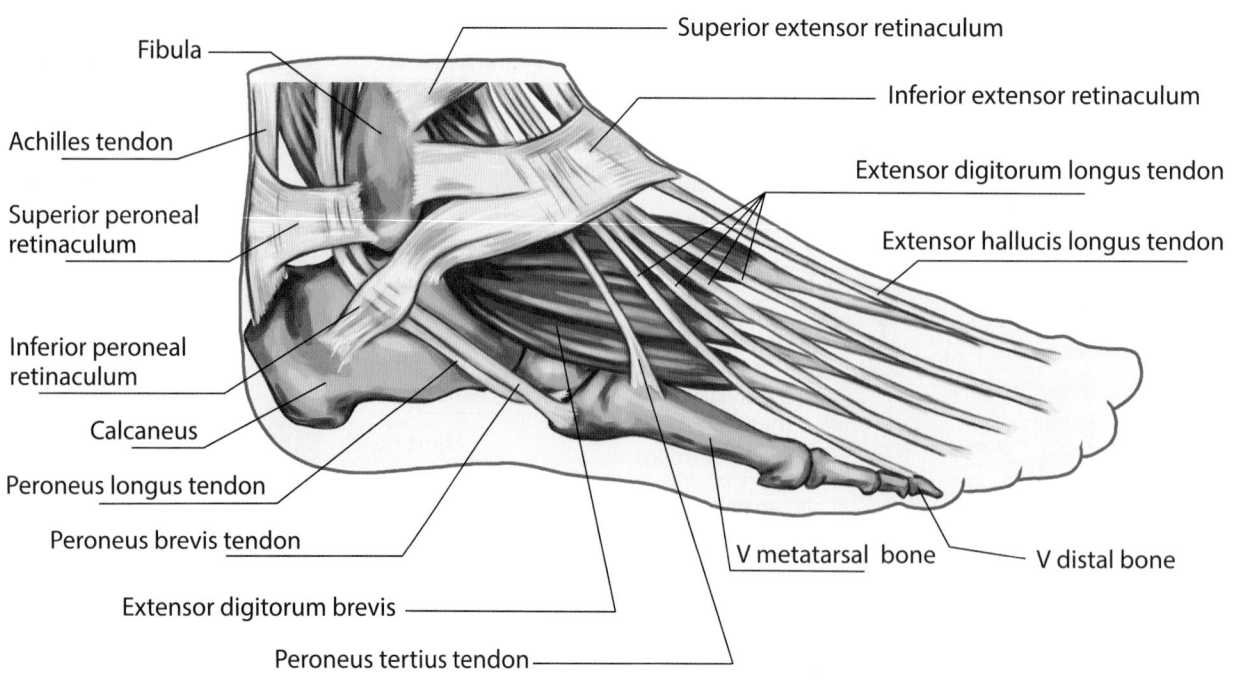

Fibula

Superior extensor retinaculum

Inferior extensor retinaculum

Achilles tendon

Extensor digitorum longus tendon

Superior peroneal retinaculum

Extensor hallucis longus tendon

Inferior peroneal retinaculum

Calcaneus

Peroneus longus tendon

Peroneus brevis tendon

V metatarsal bone

V distal bone

Extensor digitorum brevis

Peroneus tertius tendon

Musculoskeletal System — Shoulder Joint Structure

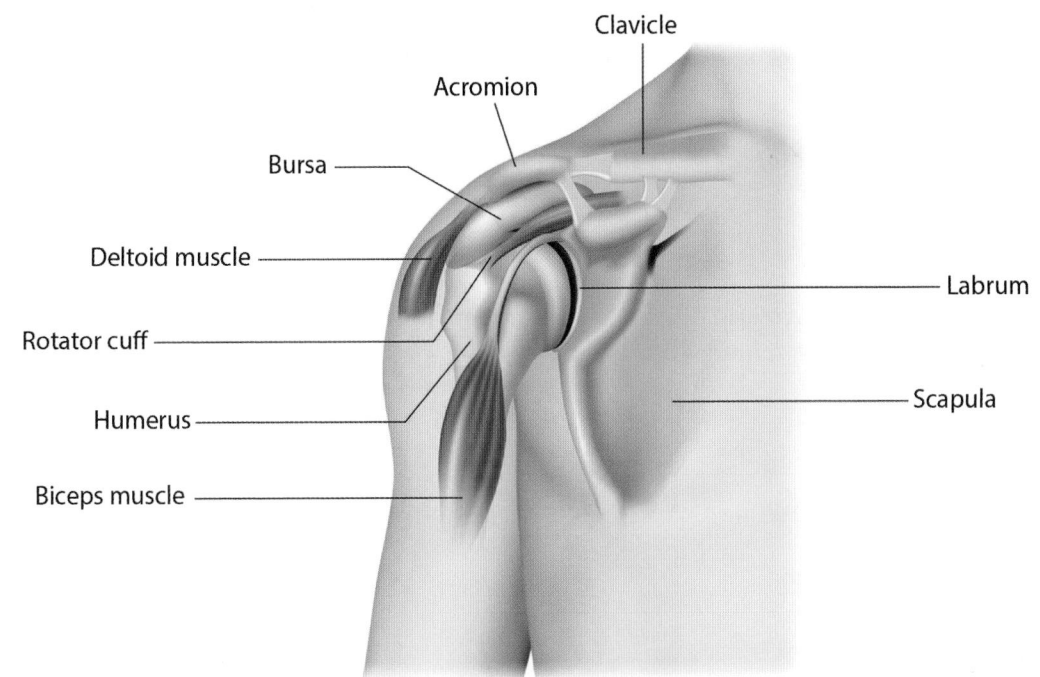

Clavicle

Acromion

Bursa

Deltoid muscle

Rotator cuff

Humerus

Biceps muscle

Labrum

Scapula

Nervous System Anatomy

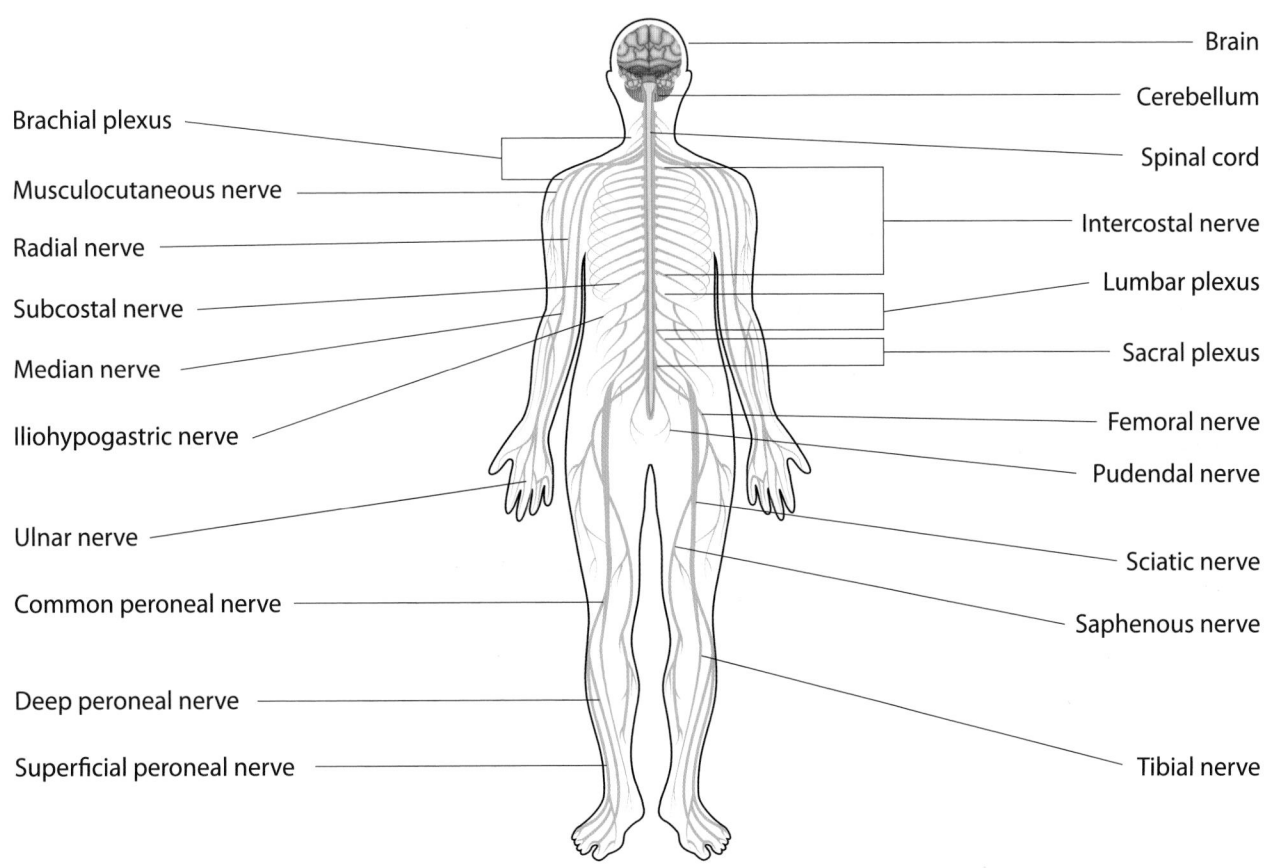

Brachial plexus

Musculocutaneous nerve

Radial nerve

Subcostal nerve

Median nerve

Iliohypogastric nerve

Ulnar nerve

Common peroneal nerve

Deep peroneal nerve

Superficial peroneal nerve

Brain

Cerebellum

Spinal cord

Intercostal nerve

Lumbar plexus

Sacral plexus

Femoral nerve

Pudendal nerve

Sciatic nerve

Saphenous nerve

Tibial nerve

Nervous System — Brain Anatomy

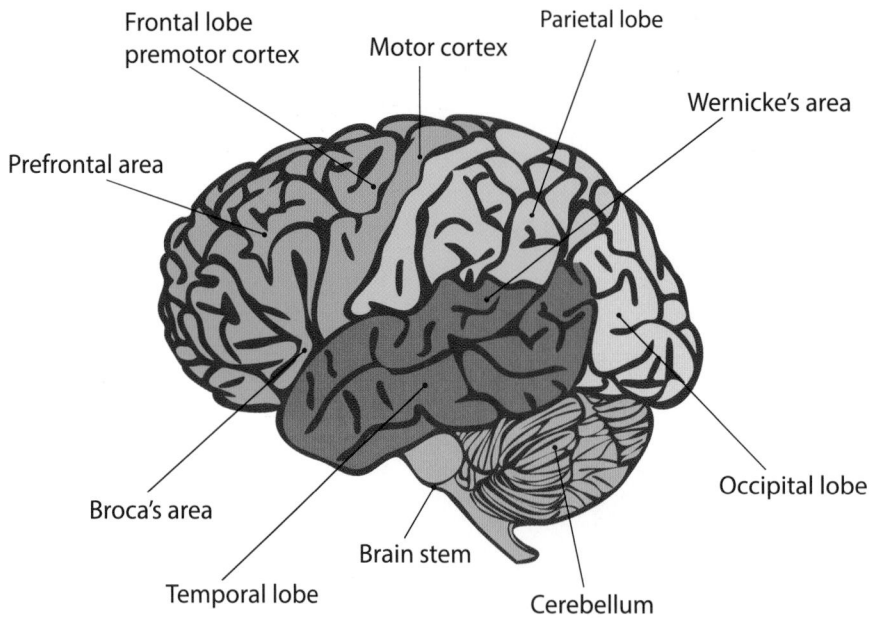

Frontal lobe premotor cortex

Motor cortex

Parietal lobe

Wernicke's area

Prefrontal area

Broca's area

Temporal lobe

Brain stem

Cerebellum

Occipital lobe

Nervous System — Median Section of the Brain

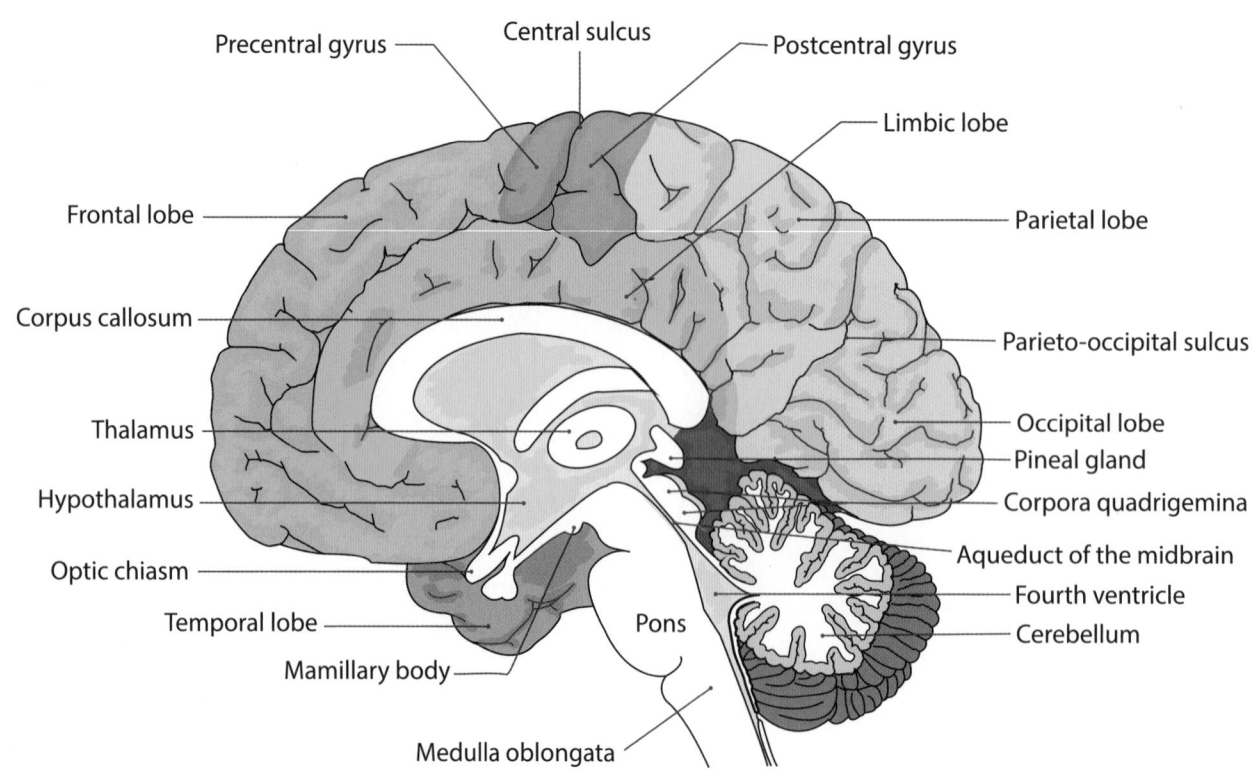

Precentral gyrus

Central sulcus

Postcentral gyrus

Limbic lobe

Frontal lobe

Parietal lobe

Corpus callosum

Parieto-occipital sulcus

Thalamus

Occipital lobe

Hypothalamus

Pineal gland

Corpora quadrigemina

Optic chiasm

Aqueduct of the midbrain

Temporal lobe

Pons

Fourth ventricle

Cerebellum

Mamillary body

Medulla oblongata

Nervous System — Cranial Nerves

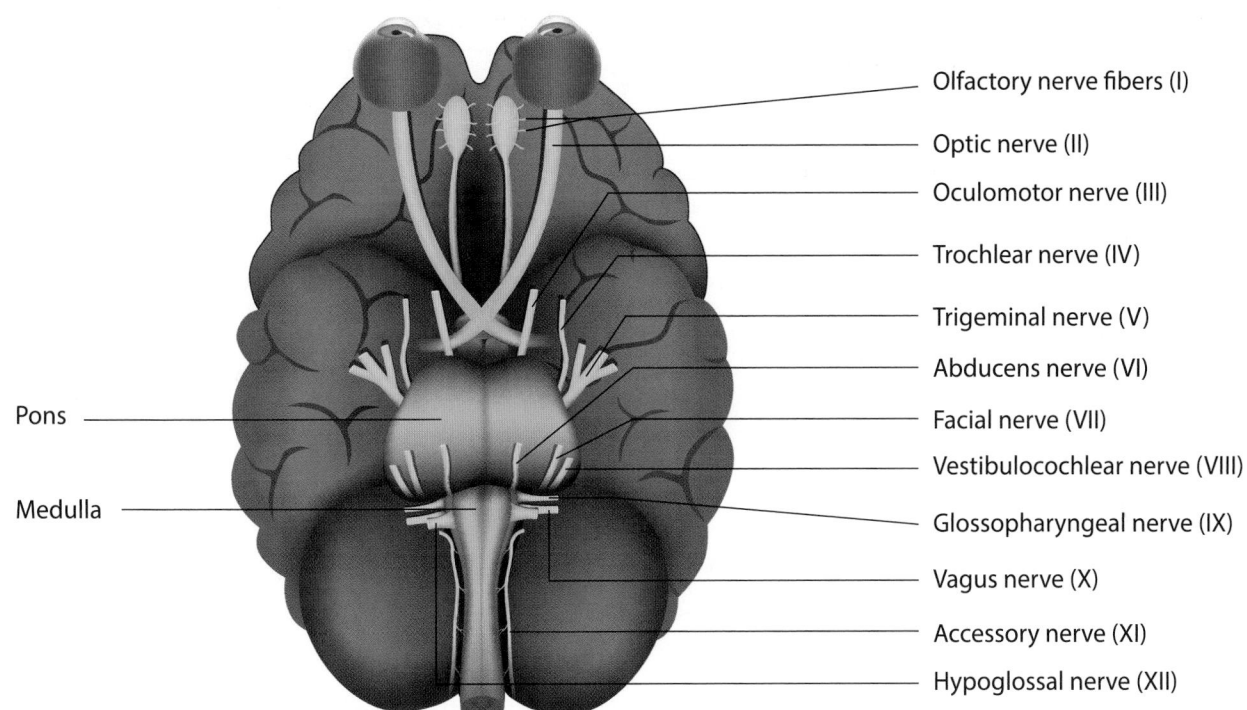

Olfactory nerve fibers (I)

Optic nerve (II)

Oculomotor nerve (III)

Trochlear nerve (IV)

Trigeminal nerve (V)

Abducens nerve (VI)

Pons

Facial nerve (VII)

Vestibulocochlear nerve (VIII)

Medulla

Glossopharyngeal nerve (IX)

Vagus nerve (X)

Accessory nerve (XI)

Hypoglossal nerve (XII)

Nervous System — Nerve Anatomy

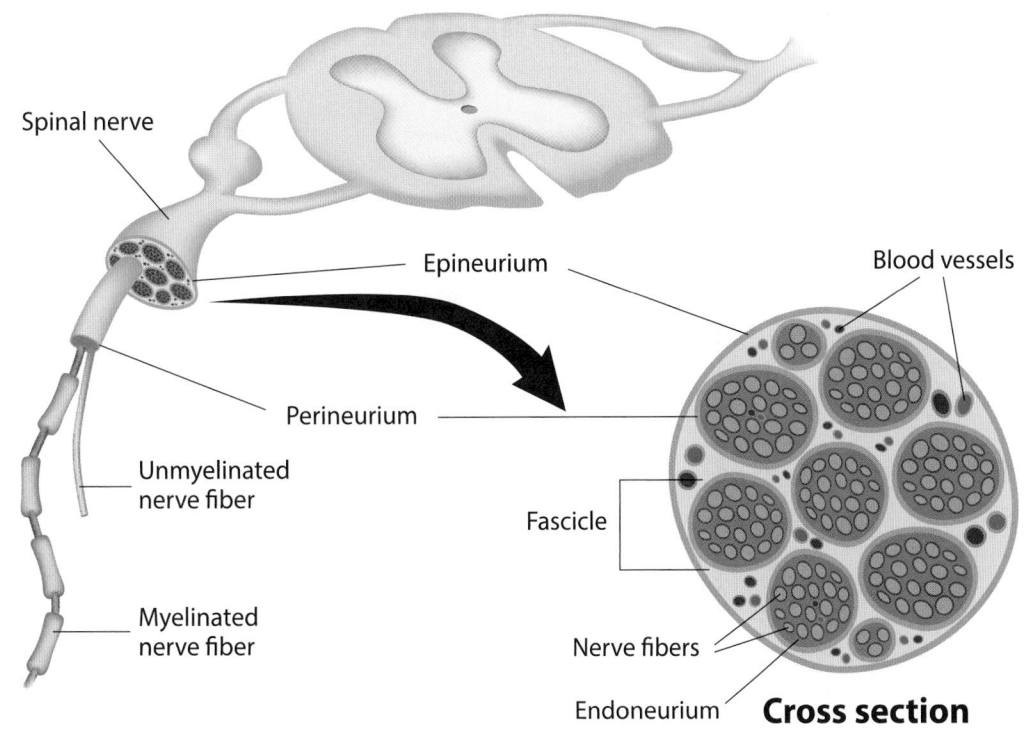

Spinal nerve

Epineurium

Blood vessels

Perineurium

Unmyelinated nerve fiber

Fascicle

Myelinated nerve fiber

Nerve fibers

Endoneurium

Cross section

Nervous System — Parasympathetic System Anatomy

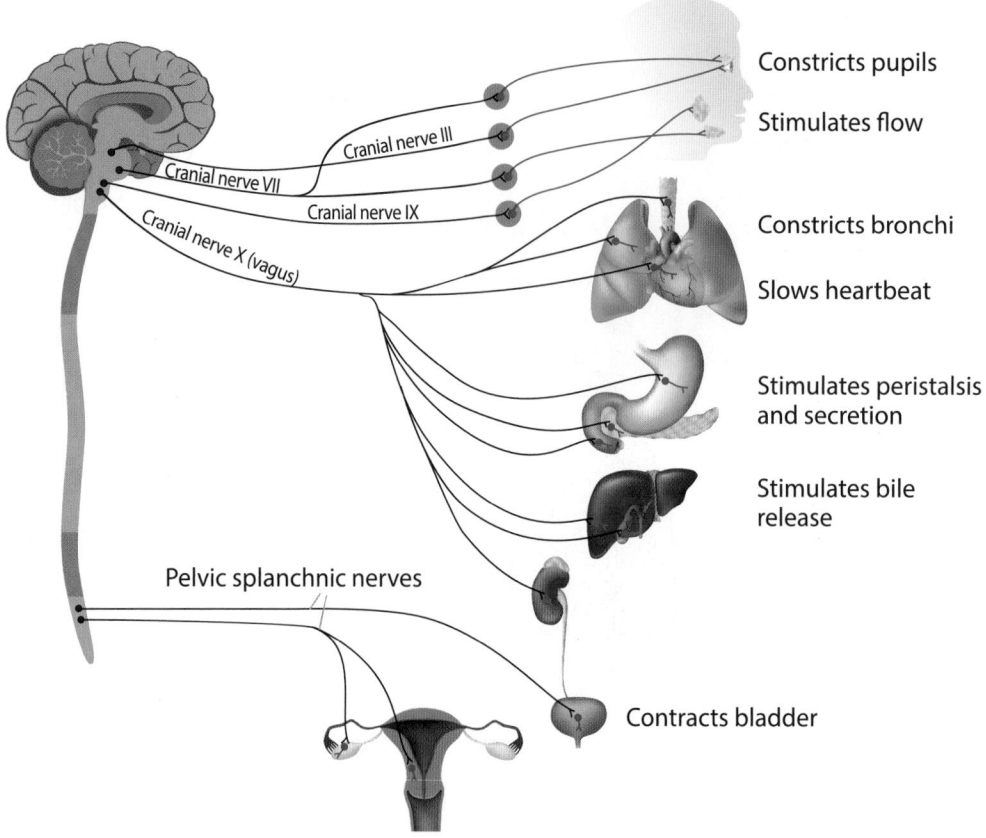

Cranial nerve III

Cranial nerve VII

Cranial nerve IX

Cranial nerve X (vagus)

Pelvic splanchnic nerves

Constricts pupils

Stimulates flow

Constricts bronchi

Slows heartbeat

Stimulates peristalsis and secretion

Stimulates bile release

Contracts bladder

Nervous System — Sympathetic System Anatomy

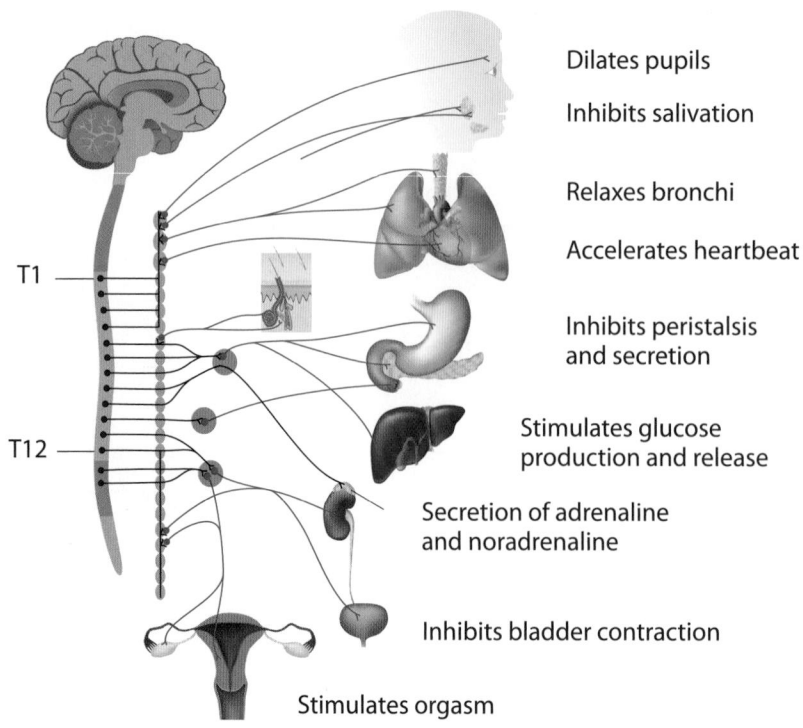

T1

T12

Dilates pupils

Inhibits salivation

Relaxes bronchi

Accelerates heartbeat

Inhibits peristalsis and secretion

Stimulates glucose production and release

Secretion of adrenaline and noradrenaline

Inhibits bladder contraction

Stimulates orgasm

Respiratory System Anatomy

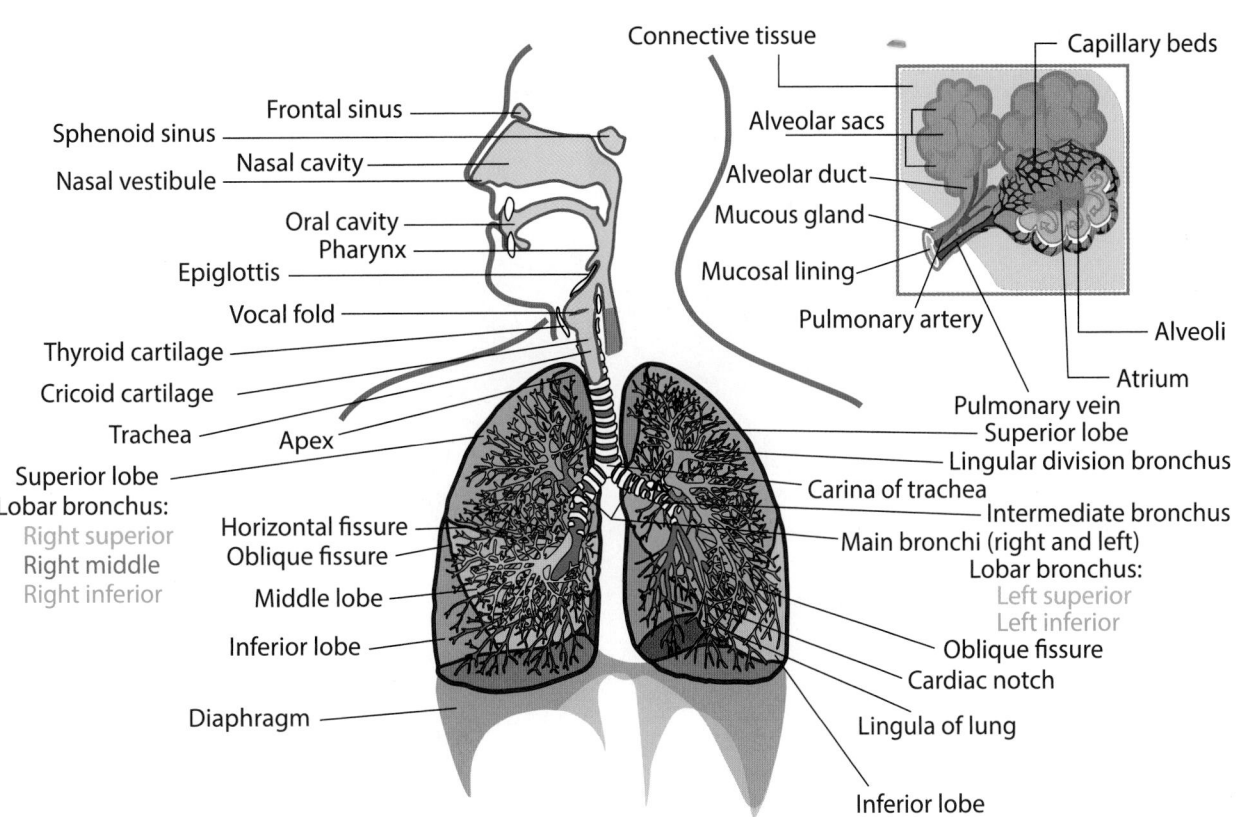

Respiratory System — Larynx Anatomy

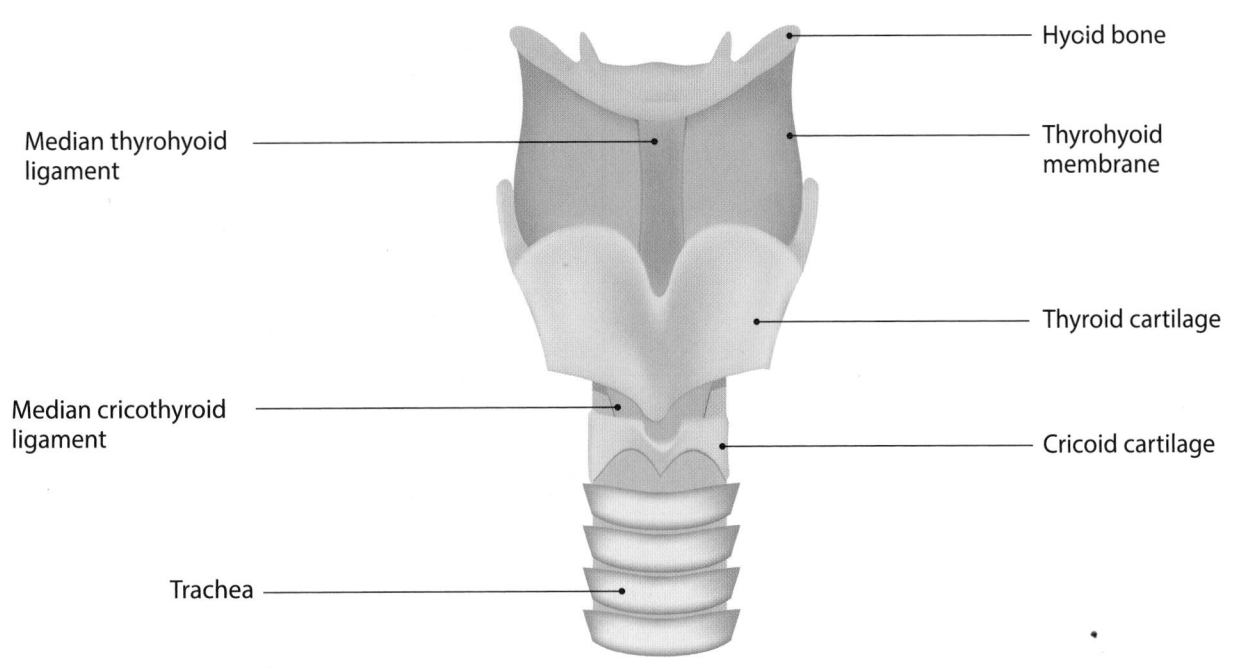

Respiratory System — Lung Anatomy

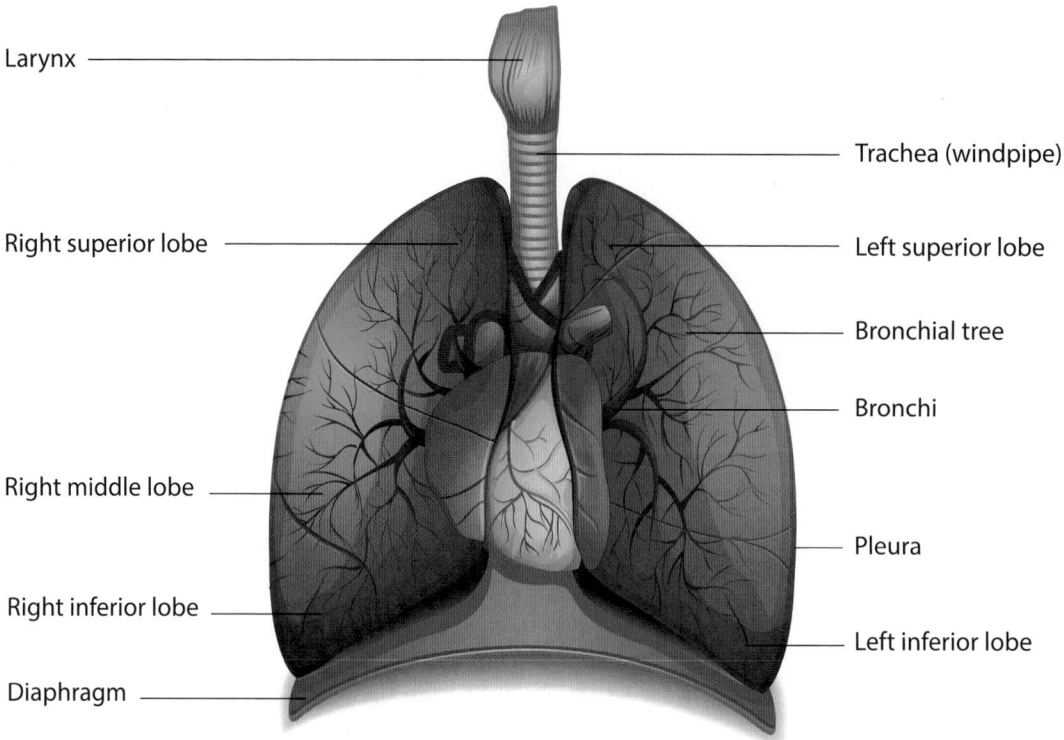

Larynx

Trachea (windpipe)

Right superior lobe

Left superior lobe

Bronchial tree

Bronchi

Right middle lobe

Pleura

Right inferior lobe

Left inferior lobe

Diaphragm

Respiratory System Function

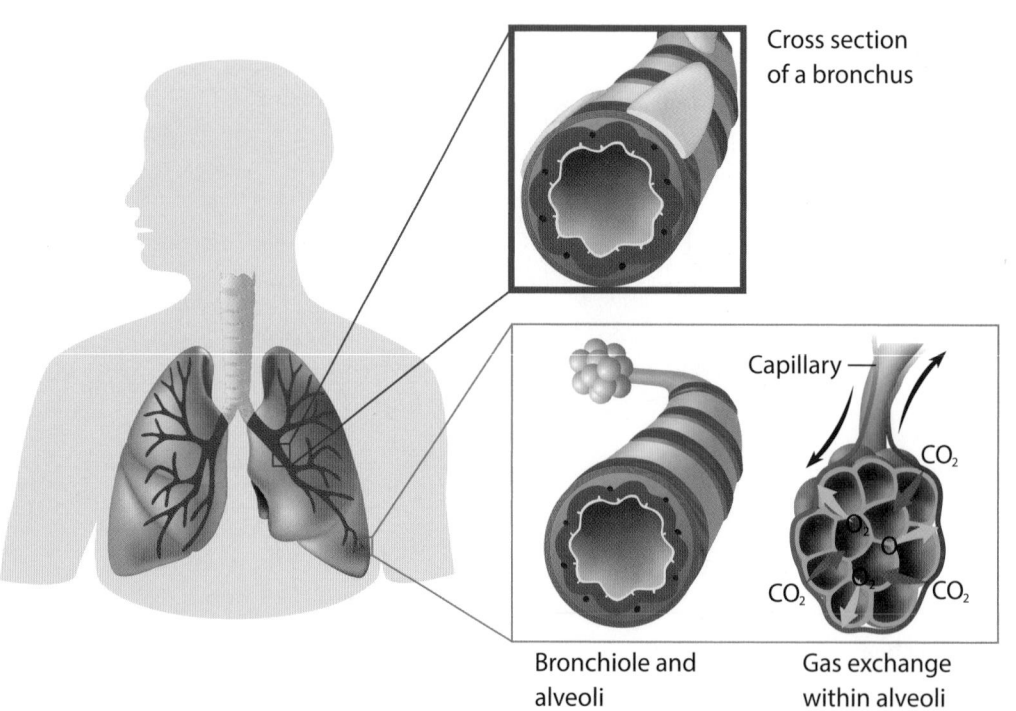

Cross section
of a bronchus

Capillary

CO_2

CO_2

CO_2

Bronchiole and
alveoli

Gas exchange
within alveoli

Respiratory System — Nose Anatomy

Respiratory System — Sinus Anatomy

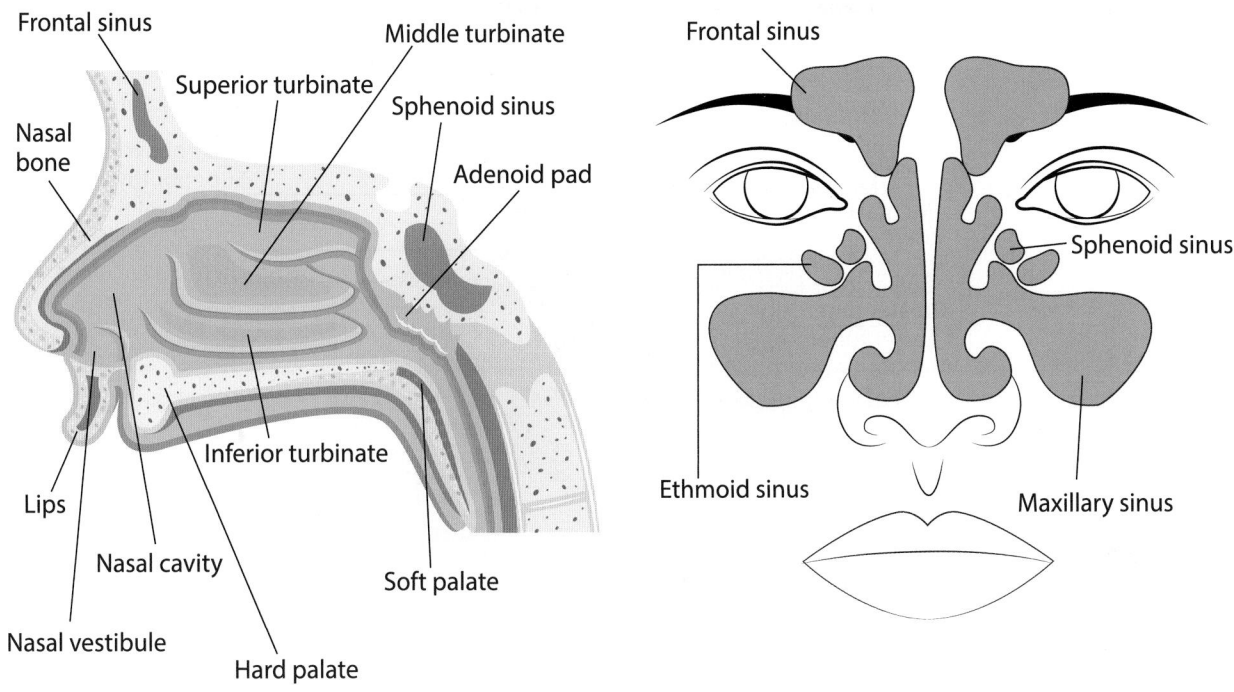

- Frontal sinus
- Middle turbinate
- Superior turbinate
- Sphenoid sinus
- Nasal bone
- Adenoid pad
- Inferior turbinate
- Lips
- Nasal cavity
- Soft palate
- Nasal vestibule
- Hard palate

- Frontal sinus
- Sphenoid sinus
- Ethmoid sinus
- Maxillary sinus

Respiratory System — Throat Anatomy

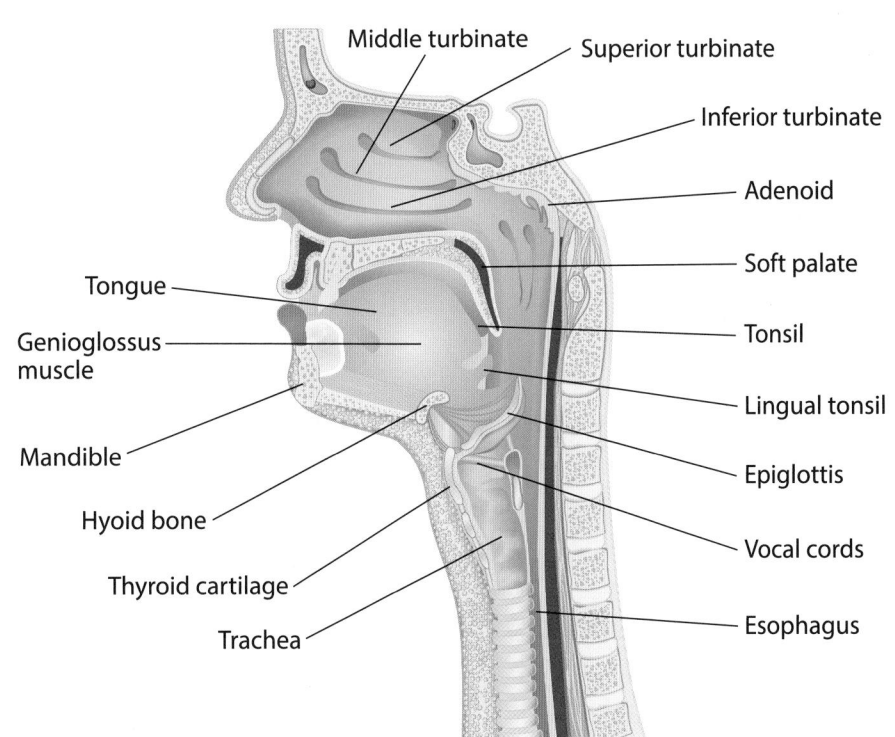

- Middle turbinate
- Superior turbinate
- Inferior turbinate
- Adenoid
- Soft palate
- Tongue
- Tonsil
- Genioglossus muscle
- Lingual tonsil
- Mandible
- Epiglottis
- Hyoid bone
- Vocal cords
- Thyroid cartilage
- Esophagus
- Trachea

Skeletal System Anatomy

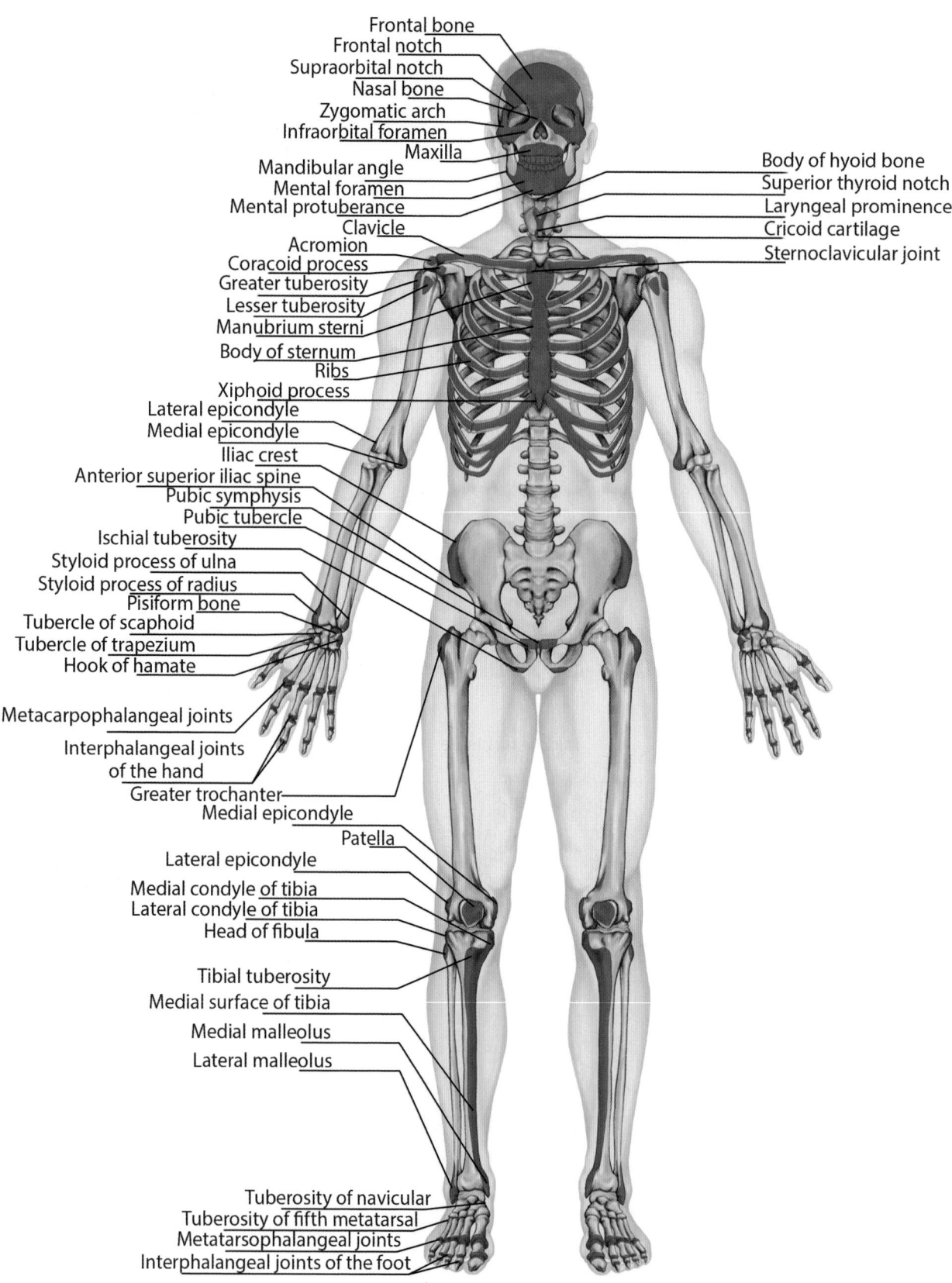

Frontal bone
Frontal notch
Supraorbital notch
Nasal bone
Zygomatic arch
Infraorbital foramen
Maxilla
Mandibular angle
Mental foramen
Mental protuberance
Clavicle
Acromion
Coracoid process
Greater tuberosity
Lesser tuberosity
Manubrium sterni
Body of sternum
Ribs
Xiphoid process
Lateral epicondyle
Medial epicondyle
Iliac crest
Anterior superior iliac spine
Pubic symphysis
Pubic tubercle
Ischial tuberosity
Styloid process of ulna
Styloid process of radius
Pisiform bone
Tubercle of scaphoid
Tubercle of trapezium
Hook of hamate

Metacarpophalangeal joints

Interphalangeal joints
of the hand
Greater trochanter
Medial epicondyle
Patella
Lateral epicondyle
Medial condyle of tibia
Lateral condyle of tibia
Head of fibula

Tibial tuberosity
Medial surface of tibia

Medial malleolus

Lateral malleolus

Tuberosity of navicular
Tuberosity of fifth metatarsal
Metatarsophalangeal joints
Interphalangeal joints of the foot

Body of hyoid bone
Superior thyroid notch
Laryngeal prominence
Cricoid cartilage
Sternoclavicular joint

Skeletal System — Bone Structure

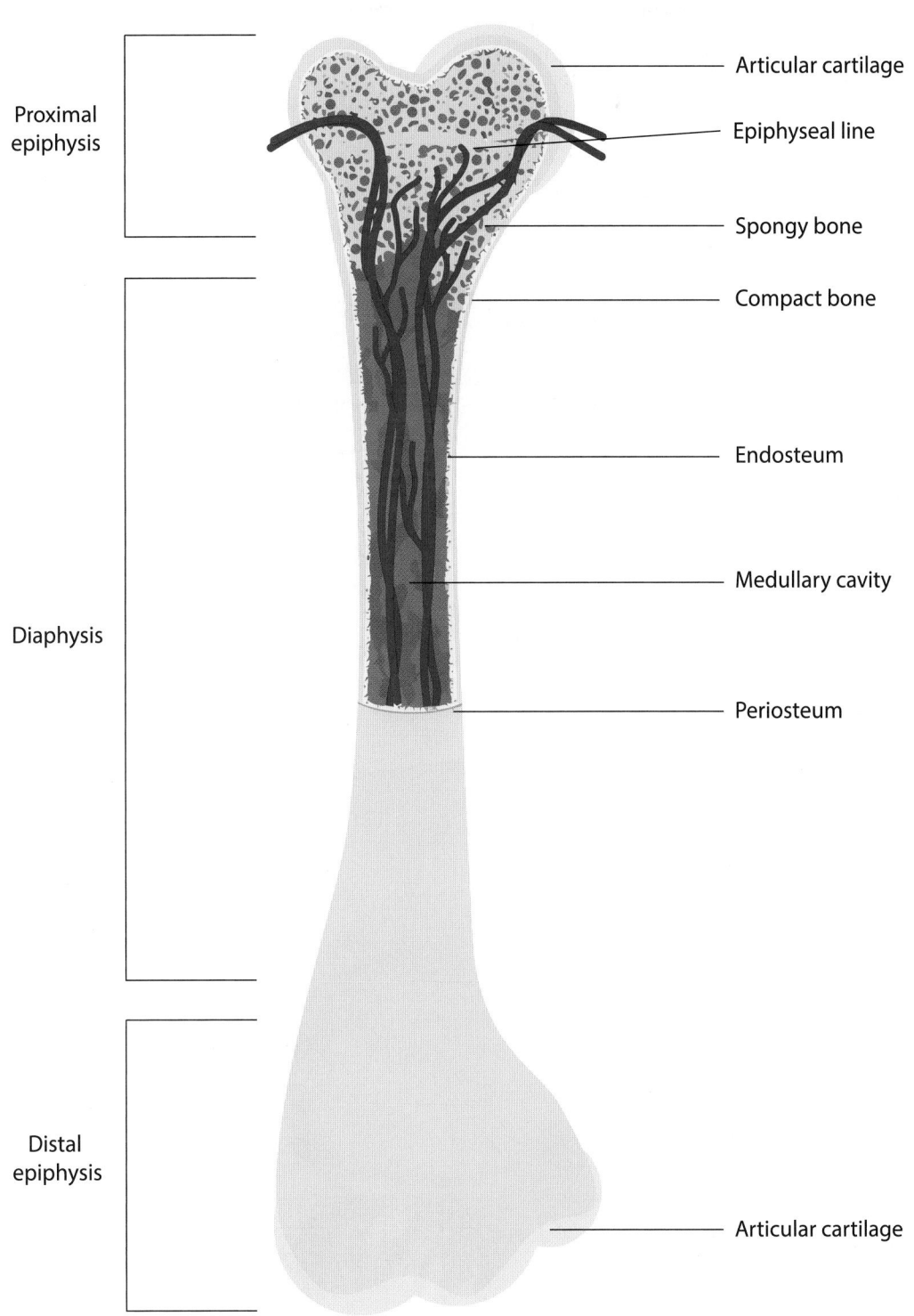

Proximal epiphysis

Diaphysis

Distal epiphysis

Articular cartilage

Epiphyseal line

Spongy bone

Compact bone

Endosteum

Medullary cavity

Periosteum

Articular cartilage

Skeletal System — Skull

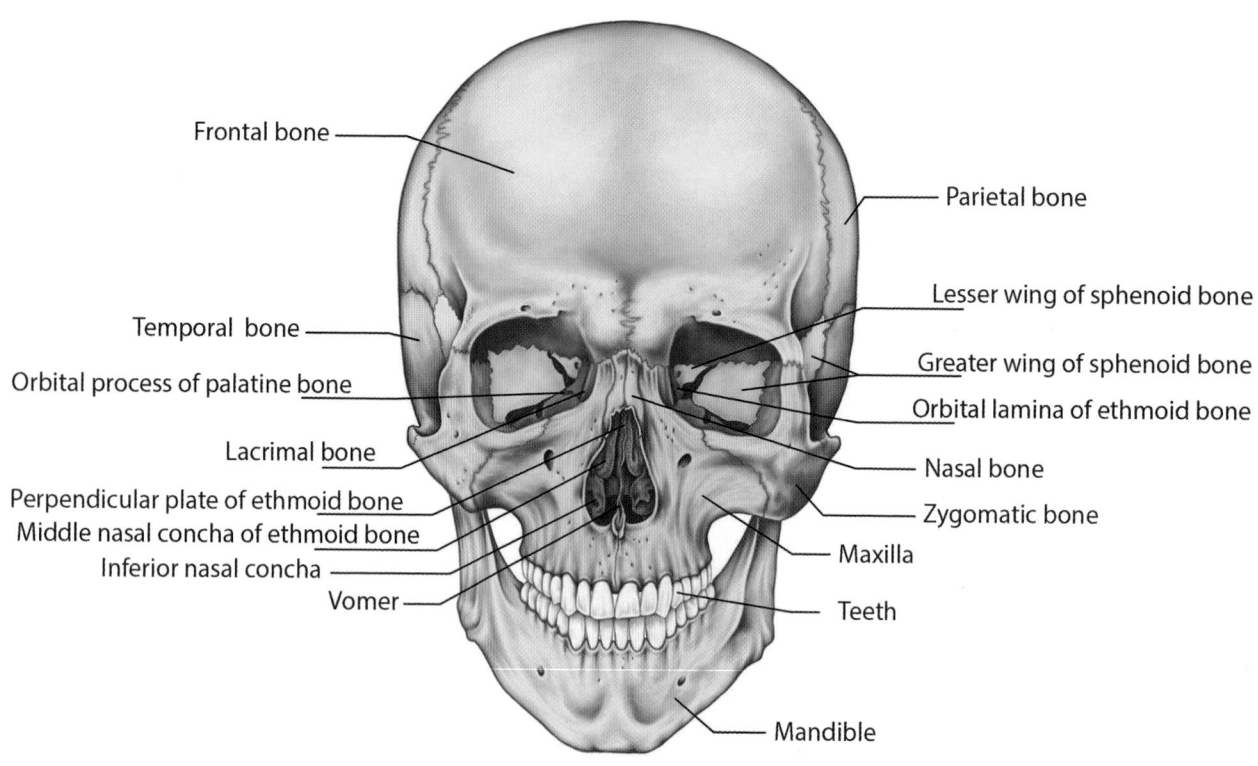

Frontal bone

Parietal bone

Temporal bone

Lesser wing of sphenoid bone

Orbital process of palatine bone

Greater wing of sphenoid bone

Orbital lamina of ethmoid bone

Lacrimal bone

Nasal bone

Perpendicular plate of ethmoid bone

Zygomatic bone

Middle nasal concha of ethmoid bone

Inferior nasal concha

Maxilla

Vomer

Teeth

Mandible

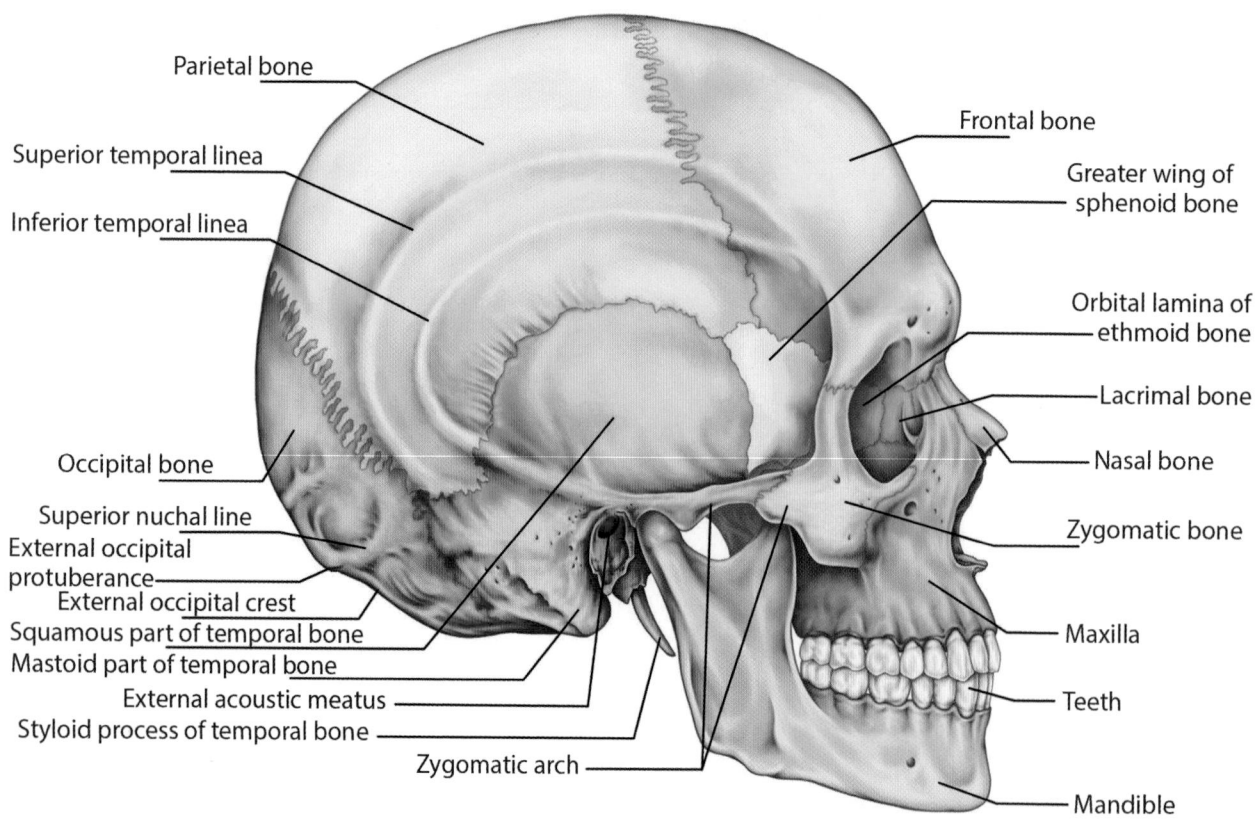

Parietal bone

Frontal bone

Superior temporal linea

Greater wing of sphenoid bone

Inferior temporal linea

Orbital lamina of ethmoid bone

Lacrimal bone

Nasal bone

Occipital bone

Zygomatic bone

Superior nuchal line

External occipital protuberance

External occipital crest

Maxilla

Squamous part of temporal bone

Mastoid part of temporal bone

Teeth

External acoustic meatus

Styloid process of temporal bone

Zygomatic arch

Mandible

Skeletal System — Cervical, Thoracic, and Lumbar Spine

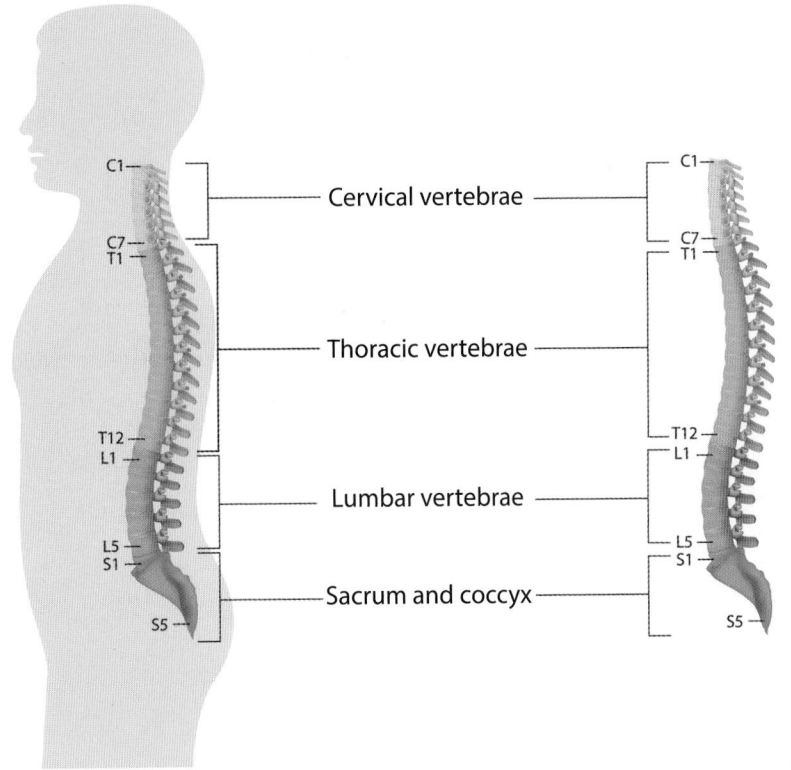

Cervical vertebrae

Thoracic vertebrae

Lumbar vertebrae

Sacrum and coccyx

Skeletal System — Pelvic Girdle

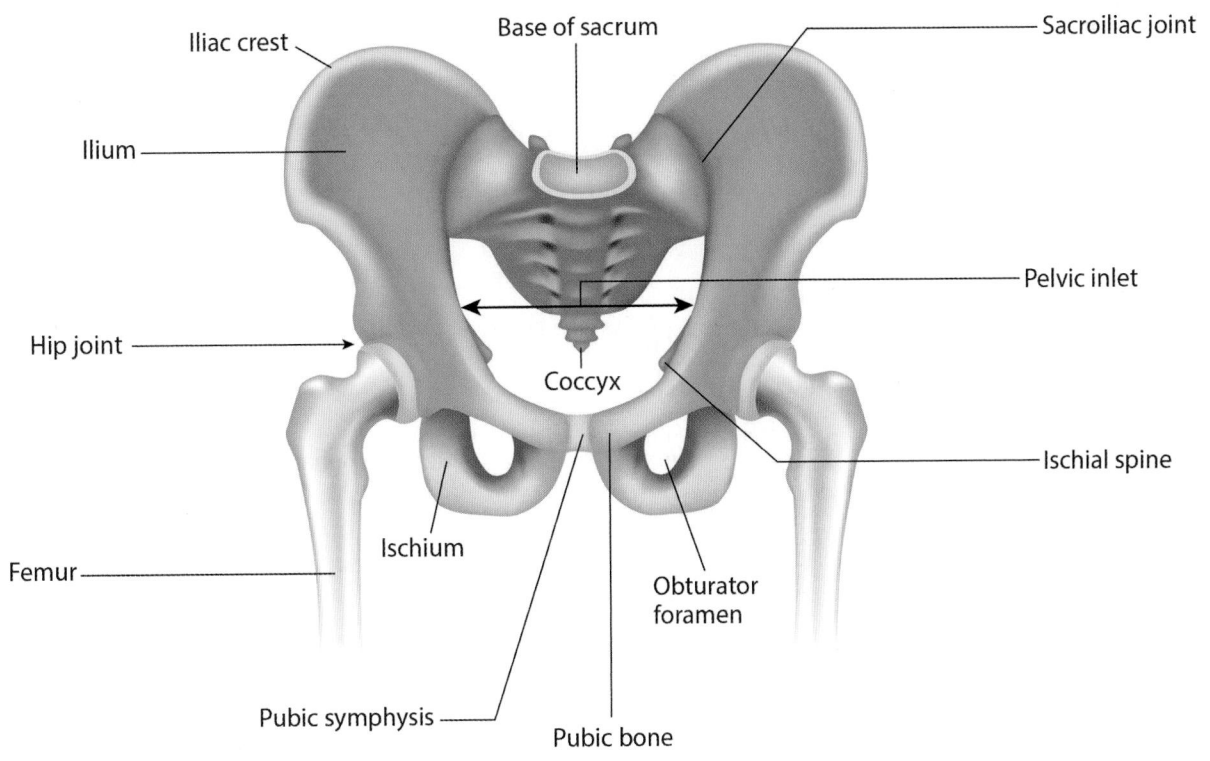

Iliac crest

Base of sacrum

Sacroiliac joint

Ilium

Hip joint

Pelvic inlet

Coccyx

Ischial spine

Ischium

Femur

Obturator foramen

Pubic symphysis

Pubic bone

Skeletal System — Elbow Joint Structure

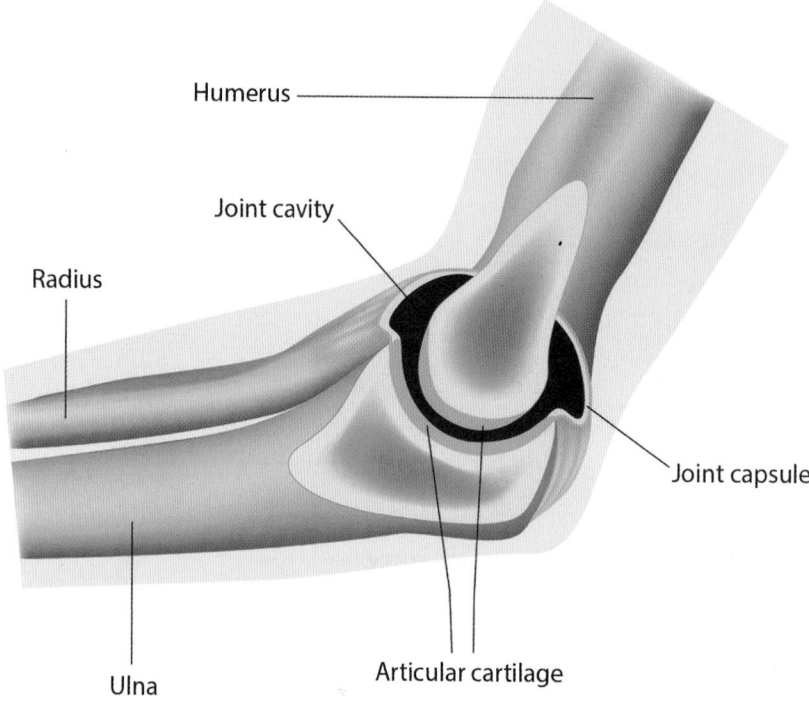

Humerus

Joint cavity

Radius

Joint capsule

Ulna

Articular cartilage

Skeletal System — Hand Bones

Bones

Joints

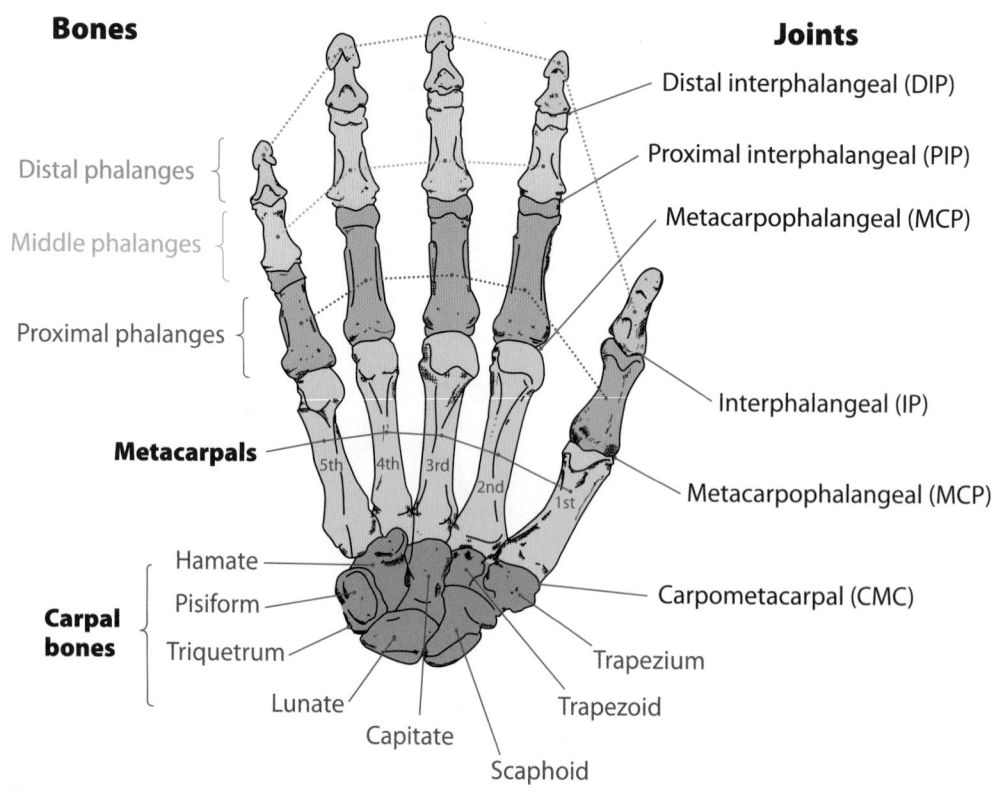

Distal phalanges

Middle phalanges

Proximal phalanges

Distal interphalangeal (DIP)

Proximal interphalangeal (PIP)

Metacarpophalangeal (MCP)

Interphalangeal (IP)

Metacarpals

5th 4th 3rd 2nd 1st

Metacarpophalangeal (MCP)

Hamate

Pisiform

Triquetrum

Carpal bones

Carpometacarpal (CMC)

Trapezium

Lunate

Trapezoid

Capitate

Scaphoid

Skeletal System — Foot Bones
(Right Foot, Lateral View)

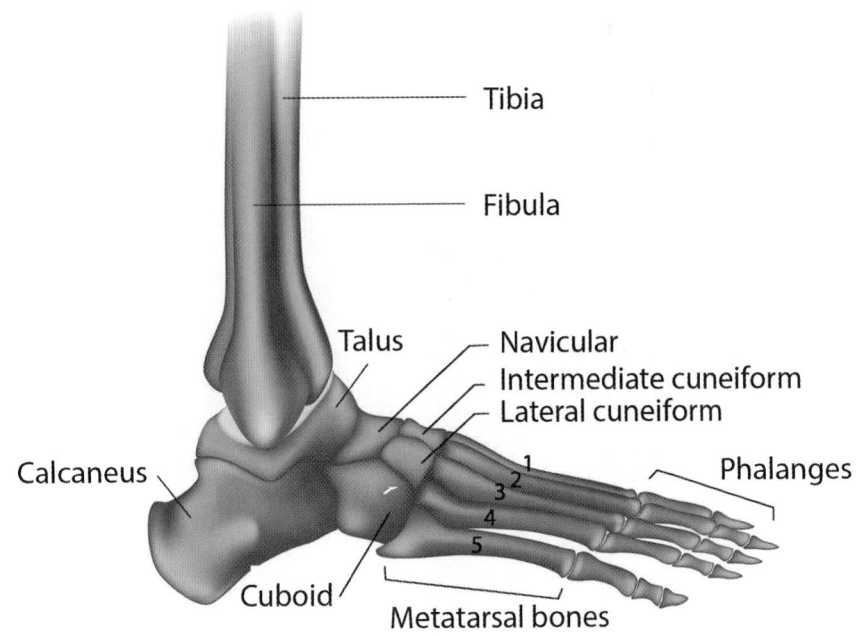

Tibia

Fibula

Talus

Navicular
Intermediate cuneiform
Lateral cuneiform

Calcaneus

1
2
3
4
5

Phalanges

Cuboid

Metatarsal bones

Urinary System Anatomy

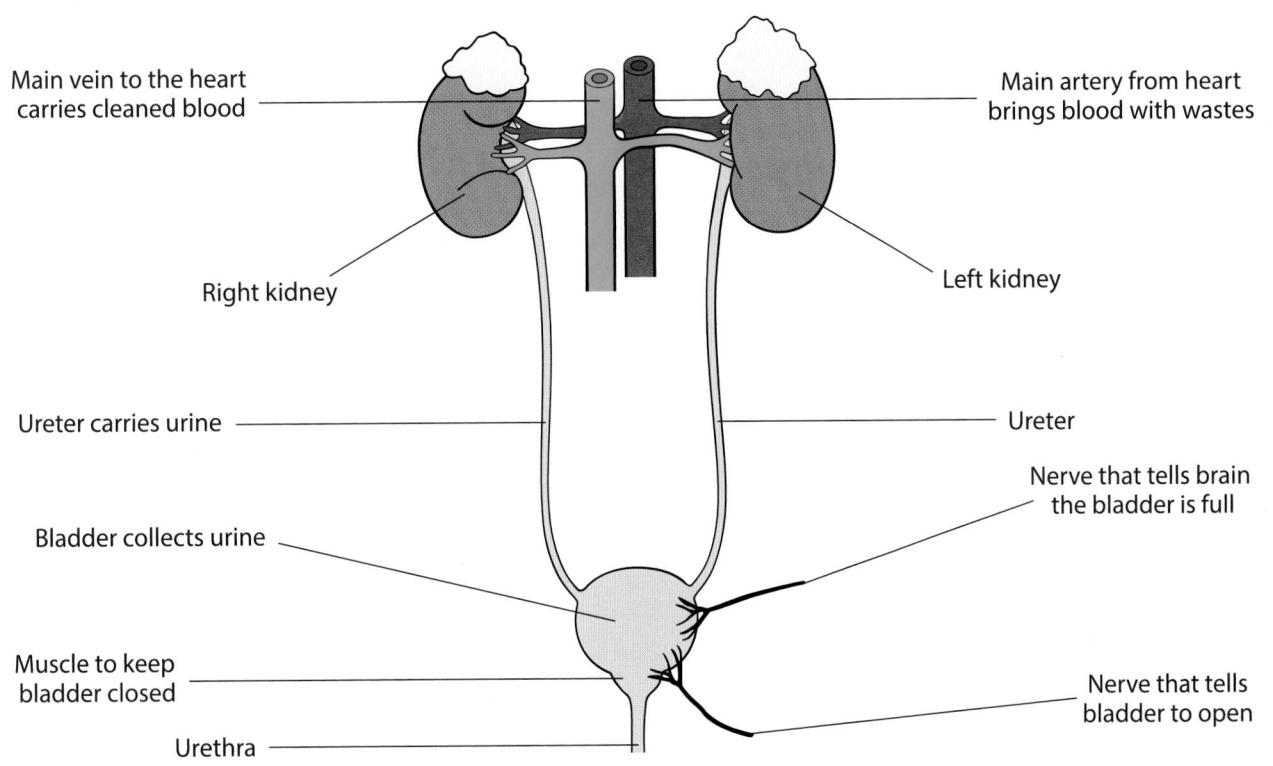

Main vein to the heart carries cleaned blood

Main artery from heart brings blood with wastes

Right kidney

Left kidney

Ureter carries urine

Ureter

Nerve that tells brain the bladder is full

Bladder collects urine

Muscle to keep bladder closed

Nerve that tells bladder to open

Urethra

Urinary System — Kidney Anatomy

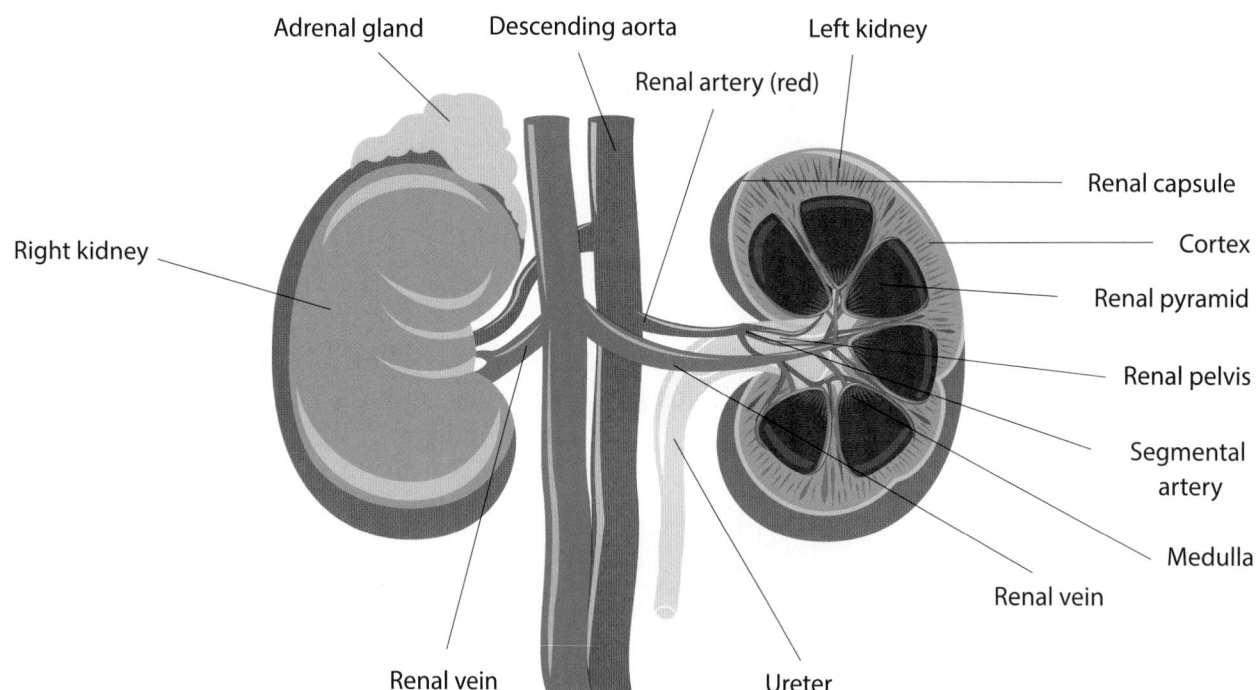

ICD-10-CM Index to Diseases and Injuries

The vertical yellow line appears at the 2nd and 4th indentations throughout the index.

A

Aarskog's syndrome Q87.19
Abandonment — *see* Maltreatment
Abasia (-astasia) (hysterical) F44.4
Abderhalden-Kaufmann-Lignac syndrome (cystinosis) E72.04
Abdomen, abdominal (*see also* condition)
    acute R10.0
    angina K55.1
    muscle deficiency syndrome Q79.4
Abdominalgia — *see* Pain, abdominal
Abduction contracture, hip or other joint — *see* Contraction, joint
Aberrant (congenital) (*see also* Malposition, congenital)
    adrenal gland Q89.1
    artery (peripheral) Q27.8
        basilar NEC Q28.1
        cerebral Q28.3
        coronary Q24.5
        digestive system Q27.8
        eye Q15.8
        lower limb Q27.8
        precerebral Q28.1
        pulmonary Q25.79
        renal Q27.2
        retina Q14.1
        specified site NEC Q27.8
        subclavian Q27.8
        upper limb Q27.8
        vertebral Q28.1
    breast Q83.8
    endocrine gland NEC Q89.2
    hepatic duct Q44.5
    pancreas Q45.3
    parathyroid gland Q89.2
    pituitary gland Q89.2
    sebaceous glands, mucous membrane, mouth, congenital Q38.6
    spleen Q89.09
    subclavian artery Q27.8
    thymus (gland) Q89.2
    thyroid gland Q89.2
    vein (peripheral) NEC Q27.8
        cerebral Q28.3
        digestive system Q27.8
        lower limb Q27.8
        precerebral Q28.1
        specified site NEC Q27.8
        upper limb Q27.8
Aberration
    distantial — *see* Disturbance, visual
    mental F99
Abetalipoproteinemia E78.6
Abiotrophy R68.89
Ablatio, ablation
    retinae — *see* Detachment, retina
Ablepharia, ablepharon Q10.3
Abnormal, abnormality, abnormalities (*see also* Anomaly)
    acid-base balance (mixed) E87.4
    albumin R77.0
    alphafetoprotein R77.2
    alveolar ridge K08.9
    anatomical relationship Q89.9
    apertures, congenital, diaphragm Q79.1
    auditory perception H93.29 ☑
        diplacusis — *see* Diplacusis
        hyperacusis — *see* Hyperacusis
        recruitment — *see* Recruitment, auditory
        threshold shift — *see* Shift, auditory threshold
    autosomes Q99.9
        fragile site Q95.5
    basal metabolic rate R94.8
    biosynthesis, testicular androgen E29.1
    bleeding time R79.1
    blood-gas level R79.81
    blood level (of)
        cobalt R79.0
        copper R79.0
        iron R79.0
        lithium R78.89
        magnesium R79.0
        mineral NEC R79.0
        zinc R79.0

Abnormal — *continued*
    blood pressure
        elevated R03.0
        low reading (nonspecific) R03.1
    blood sugar R73.09
    bowel sounds R19.15
        absent R19.11
        hyperactive R19.12
    brain scan R94.02
    breathing R06.9
    caloric test R94.138
    cerebrospinal fluid R83.9
        cytology R83.6
        drug level R83.2
        enzyme level R83.0
        hormones R83.1
        immunology R83.4
        microbiology R83.5
        nonmedicinal level R83.3
        specified type NEC R83.8
    chemistry, blood R79.9
        C-reactive protein R79.82
        drugs — *see* Findings, abnormal, in blood
        gas level R79.81
        minerals R79.0
        pancytopenia D61.818
        PTT R79.1
        specified NEC R79.89
        toxins — *see* Findings, abnormal, in blood
    chest sounds (friction) (rales) R09.89
    chromosome, chromosomal Q99.9
        with more than three X chromosomes, female Q97.1
        analysis result R89.8
            bronchial washings R84.8
            cerebrospinal fluid R83.8
            cervix uteri NEC R87.89
            nasal secretions R84.8
            nipple discharge R89.8
            peritoneal fluid R85.89
            pleural fluid R84.8
            prostatic secretions R86.8
            saliva R85.89
            seminal fluid R86.8
            sputum R84.8
            synovial fluid R89.8
            throat scrapings R84.8
            vagina R87.89
            vulva R87.89
            wound secretions R89.8
        dicentric replacement Q93.2
        ring replacement Q93.2
        sex Q99.8
            female phenotype Q97.9
                specified NEC Q97.8
            male phenotype Q98.9
                specified NEC Q98.8
            structural male Q98.6
        specified NEC Q99.8
    clinical findings NEC R68.89
    coagulation D68.9
        newborn, transient P61.6
        profile R79.1
        time R79.1
    communication — *see* Fistula
    conjunctiva, vascular H11.41 ☑
    coronary artery Q24.5
    cortisol-binding globulin E27.8
    course, eustachian tube Q17.8
    creatinine clearance R94.4
    cytology
        anus R85.619
            atypical squamous cells cannot exclude high grade squamous intraepithelial lesion (ASC-H) R85.611
            atypical squamous cells of undetermined significance (ASC-US) R85.610
            cytologic evidence of malignancy R85.614
            high grade squamous intraepithelial lesion (HGSIL) R85.613
            human papillomavirus (HPV) DNA test
                high risk positive R85.81
                low risk positive R85.82
            inadequate smear R85.615
            low grade squamous intraepithelial lesion (LGSIL) R85.612

Abnormal — *continued*
    cytology — *continued*
        satisfactory anal smear but lacking transformation zone R85.616
        specified NEC R85.618
        unsatisfactory smear R85.615
        female genital organs — *see* Abnormal, Papanicolaou (smear)
    dark adaptation curve H53.61
    dentofacial NEC — *see* Anomaly, dentofacial
    development, developmental Q89.9
        central nervous system Q07.9
    diagnostic imaging
        abdomen, abdominal region NEC R93.5
        biliary tract R93.2
        bladder R93.41
        breast R92.8
        central nervous system NEC R90.89
        cerebrovascular NEC R90.89
        coronary circulation R93.1
        digestive tract NEC R93.3
        gastrointestinal (tract) R93.3
        genitourinary organs R93.89
        head R93.0
        heart R93.1
        intrathoracic organ NEC R93.89
        kidney R93.42 ☑
        limbs R93.6
        liver R93.2
        lung (field) R91.8
        musculoskeletal system NEC R93.7
        renal pelvis R93.41
        retroperitoneum R93.5
        site specified NEC R93.89
        skin and subcutaneous tissue R93.89
        skull R93.0
        testis R93.81 ☑
        urinary organs specified NEC R93.49
        ureter R93.41
    direction, teeth, fully erupted M26.30
    ear ossicles, acquired NEC H74.39 ☑
        ankylosis — *see* Ankylosis, ear ossicles
        discontinuity — *see* Discontinuity, ossicles, ear
        partial loss — *see* Loss, ossicles, ear (partial)
    Ebstein Q22.5
    echocardiogram R93.1
    echoencephalogram R90.81
    echogram — *see* Abnormal, diagnostic imaging
    electrocardiogram [ECG] [EKG] R94.31
    electroencephalogram [EEG] R94.01
    electrolyte — *see* Imbalance, electrolyte
    electromyogram [EMG] R94.131
    electro-oculogram [EOG] R94.110
    electrophysiological intracardiac studies R94.39
    electroretinogram [ERG] R94.111
    erythrocytes
        congenital, with perinatal jaundice D58.9
    feces (color) (contents) (mucus) R19.5
    finding — *see* Findings, abnormal, without diagnosis
    fluid
        amniotic — *see* Abnormal, specimen, specified
        cerebrospinal — *see* Abnormal, cerebrospinal fluid
        peritoneal — *see* Abnormal, specimen, digestive organs
        pleural — *see* Abnormal, specimen, respiratory organs
        synovial — *see* Abnormal, specimen, specified
        thorax (bronchial washings) (pleural fluid) — *see* Abnormal, specimen, respiratory organs
        vaginal — *see* Abnormal, specimen, female genital organs
    form
        teeth K00.2
        uterus — *see* Anomaly, uterus
    function studies
        auditory R94.120
        bladder R94.8
        brain R94.09
        cardiovascular R94.30
        ear R94.128
        endocrine NEC R94.7
        eye NEC R94.118
        kidney R94.4
        liver R94.5

Abnormal

Abnormal — *continued*
    function studies — *continued*
        nervous system
            central NEC R94.09
            peripheral NEC R94.138
        pancreas R94.8
        placenta R94.8
        pulmonary R94.2
        special senses NEC R94.128
        spleen R94.8
        thyroid R94.6
        vestibular R94.121
    gait — *see* Gait
        hysterical F44.4
    gastrin secretion E16.4
    globulin R77.1
        cortisol-binding E27.8
        thyroid-binding E07.89
    glomerular, minor (*see also* N00-N07 with fourth
            character .0) N05.0
    glucagon secretion E16.3
    glucose tolerance (test) (non-fasting) R73.09
    gravitational (G) forces or states (effect of) T75.81 ☑
    hair (color) (shaft) L67.9
        specified NEC L67.8
    hard tissue formation in pulp (dental) K04.3
    head movement R25.0
    heart
        rate R00.9
            specified NEC R00.8
        shadow R93.1
        sounds NEC R01.2
    hemoglobin (disease) (*see also* Disease,
            hemoglobin) D58.2
        trait — *see* Trait, hemoglobin, abnormal
    histology NEC R89.7
    immunological findings R89.4
        in serum R76.9
            specified NEC R76.8
    increase in appetite R63.2
    involuntary movement — *see* Abnormal,
            movement, involuntary
    jaw closure M26.51
    karyotype R89.8
    kidney function test R94.4
    knee jerk R29.2
    leukocyte (cell) (differential) NEC D72.9
    liver function test R94.5
    loss of
        height R29.890
        weight R63.4
    mammogram NEC R92.8
        calcification (calculus) R92.1
        microcalcification R92.0
    Mantoux test R76.11
    movement (disorder) (*see also* Disorder, movement)
        head R25.0
        involuntary R25.9
            fasciculation R25.3
            of head R25.0
            spasm R25.2
            specified type NEC R25.8
            tremor R25.1
    myoglobin (Aberdeen) (Annapolis) R89.7
    neonatal screening P09
    oculomotor study R94.113
    palmar creases Q82.8
    Papanicolaou (smear)
        anus R85.619
            atypical squamous cells cannot exclude high
                    grade squamous intraepithelial lesion
                    (ASC-H) R85.611
            atypical squamous cells of undetermined
                    significance (ASC-US) R85.610
            cytologic evidence of malignancy R85.614
            high grade squamous intraepithelial lesion
                    (HGSIL) R85.613
            human papillomavirus (HPV) DNA test
                high risk positive R85.81
                low risk positive R85.82
            inadequate smear R85.615
            low grade squamous intraepithelial lesion
                    (LGSIL) R85.612
            satisfactory anal smear but lacking
                    transformation zone R85.616
            specified NEC R85.618
            unsatisfactory smear R85.615
        bronchial washings R84.6
        cerebrospinal fluid R83.6
        cervix R87.619

Abnormal — *continued*
    Papanicolaou — *continued*
        atypical squamous cells cannot exclude high
                grade squamous intraepithelial lesion
                (ASC-H) R87.611
        atypical squamous cells of undetermined
                significance (ASC-US) R87.610
        cytologic evidence of malignancy R87.614
        high grade squamous intraepithelial lesion
                (HGSIL) R87.613
        inadequate smear R87.615
        low grade squamous intraepithelial lesion
                (LGSIL) R87.612
        non-atypical endometrial cells R87.618
        satisfactory cervical smear but lacking
                transformation zone R87.616
        specified NEC R87.618
        thin preparation R87.619
        unsatisfactory smear R87.615
    nasal secretions R84.6
    nipple discharge R89.6
    peritoneal fluid R85.69
    pleural fluid R84.6
    prostatic secretions R86.6
    saliva R85.69
    seminal fluid R86.6
    sites NEC R89.6
    sputum R84.6
    synovial fluid R89.6
    throat scrapings R84.6
    vagina R87.629
        atypical squamous cells cannot exclude high
                grade squamous intraepithelial lesion
                (ASC-H) R87.621
        atypical squamous cells of undetermined
                significance (ASC-US) R87.620
        cytologic evidence of malignancy R87.624
        high grade squamous intraepithelial lesion
                (HGSIL) R87.623
        inadequate smear R87.625
        low grade squamous intraepithelial lesion
                (LGSIL) R87.622
        specified NEC R87.628
        thin preparation R87.629
        unsatisfactory smear R87.625
    vulva R87.69
    wound secretions R89.6
partial thromboplastin time (PTT) R79.1
pelvis (bony) — *see* Deformity, pelvis
percussion, chest (tympany) R09.89
periods (grossly) — *see* Menstruation
phonocardiogram R94.39
plantar reflex R29.2
plasma
    protein R77.9
        specified NEC R77.8
    viscosity R70.1
pleural (folds) Q34.0
posture R29.3
product of conception O02.9
    specified type NEC O02.89
prothrombin time (PT) R79.1
pulmonary
    artery, congenital Q25.79
    function, newborn P28.89
    test results R94.2
pulsations in neck R00.2
pupillary H21.56 ☑
    function (reaction) (reflex) — *see* Anomaly, pupil,
            function
radiological examination — *see* Abnormal,
        diagnostic imaging
red blood cell(s) (morphology) (volume) R71.8
reflex — *see* Reflex
renal function test R94.4
response to nerve stimulation R94.130
retinal correspondence H53.31
retinal function study R94.111
rhythm, heart (*see also* Arrhythmia)
saliva — *see* Abnormal, specimen, digestive organs
scan
    kidney R94.4
    liver R93.2
    thyroid R94.6
secretion
    gastrin E16.4
    glucagon E16.3
semen, seminal fluid — *see* Abnormal, specimen,
        male genital organs
serum level (of)
    acid phosphatase R74.8
    alkaline phosphatase R74.8

Abnormal — *continued*
    serum level — *continued*
        amylase R74.8
        enzymes R74.9
            specified NEC R74.8
        lipase R74.8
        triacylglycerol lipase R74.8
    shape
        gravid uterus — *see* Anomaly, uterus
    sinus venosus Q21.1
    size, tooth, teeth K00.2
    spacing, tooth, teeth, fully erupted M26.30
    specimen
        digestive organs (peritoneal fluid) (saliva) R85.9
            cytology R85.69
            drug level R85.2
            enzyme level R85.0
            histology R85.7
            hormones R85.1
            immunology R85.4
            microbiology R85.5
            nonmedicinal level R85.3
            specified type NEC R85.89
        female genital organs (secretions) (smears) R87.9
            cytology R87.69
                cervix R87.619
                    human papillomavirus (HPV) DNA test
                        high risk positive R87.810
                        low risk positive R87.820
                    inadequate (unsatisfactory) smear R87.615
                    non-atypical endometrial cells R87.618
                    specified NEC R87.618
                vagina R87.629
                    human papillomavirus (HPV) DNA test
                        high risk positive R87.811
                        low risk positive R87.821
                    inadequate (unsatisfactory) smear
                            R87.625
                vulva R87.69
            drug level R87.2
            enzyme level R87.0
            histological R87.7
            hormones R87.1
            immunology R87.4
            microbiology R87.5
            nonmedicinal level R87.3
            specified type NEC R87.89
        male genital organs (prostatic secretions) (semen)
                R86.9
            cytology R86.6
            drug level R86.2
            enzyme level R86.0
            histological R86.7
            hormones R86.1
            immunology R86.4
            microbiology R86.5
            nonmedicinal level R86.3
            specified type NEC R86.8
        nipple discharge — *see* Abnormal, specimen,
                specified
        respiratory organs (bronchial washings) (nasal
                secretions) (pleural fluid) (sputum) R84.9
            cytology R84.6
            drug level R84.2
            enzyme level R84.0
            histology R84.7
            hormones R84.1
            immunology R84.4
            microbiology R84.5
            nonmedicinal level R84.3
            specified type NEC R84.8
        specified organ, system and tissue NOS R89.9
            cytology R89.6
            drug level R89.2
            enzyme level R89.0
            histology R89.7
            hormones R89.1
            immunology R89.4
            microbiology R89.5
            nonmedicinal level R89.3
            specified type NEC R89.8
        synovial fluid — *see* Abnormal, specimen,
                specified
        thorax (bronchial washings) (pleural fluids) — *see*
                Abnormal, specimen, respiratory organs
        vagina (secretion) (smear) R87.629
        vulva (secretion) (smear) R87.69
        wound secretion — *see* Abnormal, specimen,
                specified
    spermatozoa — *see* Abnormal, specimen, male
            genital organs
    sputum (amount) (color) (odor) R09.3

☑ **Additional character required**

Abnormal — *continued*
- stool (color) (contents) (mucus) R19.5
  - bloody K92.1
  - guaiac positive R19.5
- synchondrosis Q78.8
- thermography (*see also* Abnormal, diagnostic imaging) R93.89
- thyroid-binding globulin E07.89
- tooth, teeth (form) (size) K00.2
- toxicology (findings) R78.9
- transport protein E88.09
- tumor marker NEC R97.8
- ultrasound results — *see* Abnormal, diagnostic imaging
- umbilical cord complicating delivery O69.9 ☑
- urination NEC R39.198
- urine (constituents) R82.90
  - bile R82.2
  - cytological examination R82.89
  - drugs R82.5
  - fat R82.0
  - glucose R81
  - heavy metals R82.6
  - hemoglobin R82.3
  - histological examination R82.89
  - ketones R82.4
  - microbiological examination (culture) R82.79
  - myoglobin R82.1
  - positive culture R82.79
  - protein — *see* Proteinuria
  - specified substance NEC R82.998
    - chromoabnormality NEC R82.91
  - substances nonmedical R82.6
- uterine hemorrhage — *see* Hemorrhage, uterus
- vectorcardiogram R94.39
- visually evoked potential (VEP) R94.112
- white blood cells D72.9
  - specified NEC D72.89
- X-ray examination — *see* Abnormal, diagnostic imaging

Abnormity (any organ or part) — *see* Anomaly

Abocclusion M26.29
- hemolytic disease (newborn) P55.1
- incompatibility reaction ABO — *see* Complication(s), transfusion, incompatibility reaction, ABO

Abolition, language R48.8

Aborter, habitual or recurrent — *see* Loss (of), pregnancy, recurrent

Abortion (complete) (spontaneous) O03.9
- with
  - retained products of conception — *see* Abortion, incomplete
- attempted (elective) (failed) O07.4
  - complicated by O07.30
    - afibrinogenemia O07.1
    - cardiac arrest O07.36
    - chemical damage of pelvic organ(s) O07.34
    - circulatory collapse O07.31
    - cystitis O07.38
    - defibrination syndrome O07.1
    - electrolyte imbalance O07.33
    - embolism (air) (amniotic fluid) (blood clot) (fat) (pulmonary) (septic) (soap) O07.2
    - endometritis O07.0
    - genital tract and pelvic infection O07.0
    - hemolysis O07.1
    - hemorrhage (delayed) (excessive) O07.1
    - infection
      - genital tract or pelvic O07.0
      - urinary tract O07.38
    - intravascular coagulation O07.1
    - laceration of pelvic organ(s) O07.34
    - metabolic disorder O07.33
    - oliguria O07.32
    - oophoritis O07.0
    - parametritis O07.0
    - pelvic peritonitis O07.0
    - perforation of pelvic organ(s) O07.34
    - renal failure or shutdown O07.32
    - salpingitis or salpingo-oophoritis O07.0
    - sepsis O07.37
    - shock O07.31
    - specified condition NEC O07.39
    - tubular necrosis (renal) O07.32
    - uremia O07.32
    - urinary tract infection O07.38
    - venous complication NEC O07.35
      - embolism (air) (amniotic fluid) (blood clot) (fat) (pulmonary) (septic) (soap) O07.2
- complicated (by) (following) O03.80
  - afibrinogenemia O03.6
  - cardiac arrest O03.86

Abortion — *continued*
- complicated — *continued*
  - chemical damage of pelvic organ(s) O03.84
  - circulatory collapse O03.81
  - cystitis O03.88
  - defibrination syndrome O03.6
  - electrolyte imbalance O03.83
  - embolism (air) (amniotic fluid) (blood clot) (fat) (pulmonary) (septic) (soap) O03.7
  - endometritis O03.5
  - genital tract and pelvic infection O03.5
  - hemolysis O03.6
  - hemorrhage (delayed) (excessive) O03.6
  - infection
    - genital tract or pelvic O03.5
    - urinary tract O03.88
  - intravascular coagulation O03.6
  - laceration of pelvic organ(s) O03.84
  - metabolic disorder O03.83
  - oliguria O03.82
  - oophoritis O03.5
  - parametritis O03.5
  - pelvic peritonitis O03.5
  - perforation of pelvic organ(s) O03.84
  - renal failure or shutdown O03.82
  - salpingitis or salpingo-oophoritis O03.5
  - sepsis O03.87
  - shock O03.81
  - specified condition NEC O03.89
  - tubular necrosis (renal) O03.82
  - uremia O03.82
  - urinary tract infection O03.88
  - venous complication NEC O03.85
    - embolism (air) (amniotic fluid) (blood clot) (fat) (pulmonary) (septic) (soap) O03.7
- failed — *see* Abortion, attempted
- habitual or recurrent N96
  - with current abortion — *see* categories O03-O04
  - without current pregnancy N96
  - care in current pregnancy O26.2 ☑
- incomplete (spontaneous) O03.4
  - complicated (by) (following) O03.30
    - afibrinogenemia O03.1
    - cardiac arrest O03.36
    - chemical damage of pelvic organ(s) O03.34
    - circulatory collapse O03.31
    - cystitis O03.38
    - defibrination syndrome O03.1
    - electrolyte imbalance O03.33
    - embolism (air) (amniotic fluid) (blood clot) (fat) (pulmonary) (septic) (soap) O03.2
    - endometritis O03.0
    - genital tract and pelvic infection O03.0
    - hemolysis O03.1
    - hemorrhage (delayed) (excessive) O03.1
    - infection
      - genital tract or pelvic O03.0
      - urinary tract O03.38
    - intravascular coagulation O03.1
    - laceration of pelvic organ(s) O03.34
    - metabolic disorder O03.33
    - oliguria O03.32
    - oophoritis O03.0
    - parametritis O03.0
    - pelvic peritonitis O03.0
    - perforation of pelvic organ(s) O03.34
    - renal failure or shutdown O03.32
    - salpingitis or salpingo-oophoritis O03.0
    - sepsis O03.37
    - shock O03.31
    - specified condition NEC O03.39
    - tubular necrosis (renal) O03.32
    - uremia O03.32
    - urinary infection O03.38
    - venous complication NEC O03.35
      - embolism (air) (amniotic fluid) (blood clot) (fat) (pulmonary) (septic) (soap) O03.2
- induced (encounter for) Z33.2
  - complicated by O04.80
    - afibrinogenemia O04.6
    - cardiac arrest O04.86
    - chemical damage of pelvic organ(s) O04.84
    - circulatory collapse O04.81
    - cystitis O04.88
    - defibrination syndrome O04.6
    - electrolyte imbalance O04.83
    - embolism (air) (amniotic fluid) (blood clot) (fat) (pulmonary) (septic) (soap) O04.7
    - endometritis O04.5
    - genital tract and pelvic infection O04.5
    - hemolysis O04.6
    - hemorrhage (delayed) (excessive) O04.6

Abortion — *continued*
- induced — *continued*
  - infection
    - genital tract or pelvic O04.5
    - urinary tract O04.88
  - intravascular coagulation O04.6
  - laceration of pelvic organ(s) O04.84
  - metabolic disorder O04.83
  - oliguria O04.82
  - oophoritis O04.5
  - parametritis O04.5
  - pelvic peritonitis O04.5
  - perforation of pelvic organ(s) O04.84
  - renal failure or shutdown O04.82
  - salpingitis or salpingo-oophoritis O04.5
  - sepsis O04.87
  - shock O04.81
  - specified condition NEC O04.89
  - tubular necrosis (renal) O04.82
  - uremia O04.82
  - urinary tract infection O04.88
  - venous complication NEC O04.85
    - embolism (air) (amniotic fluid) (blood clot) (fat) (pulmonary) (septic) (soap) O04.7
- missed O02.1
- spontaneous — *see* Abortion (complete) (spontaneous)
  - threatened O20.0
- threatened (spontaneous) O20.0
- tubal O00.10 ☑
  - with intrauterine pregnancy O00.11 ☑

Abortus fever A23.1

Aboulomania F60.7

Abrami's disease D59.8

Abramov-Fiedler myocarditis (acute isolated myocarditis) I40.1

Abrasion T14.8 ☑
- abdomen, abdominal (wall) S30.811 ☑
- alveolar process S00.512 ☑
- ankle S90.51 ☑
- antecubital space — *see* Abrasion, elbow
- anus S30.817 ☑
- arm (upper) S40.81 ☑
- auditory canal — *see* Abrasion, ear
- auricle — *see* Abrasion, ear
- axilla — *see* Abrasion, arm
- back, lower S30.810 ☑
- breast S20.11 ☑
- brow S00.81 ☑
- buttock S30.810 ☑
- calf — *see* Abrasion, leg
- canthus — *see* Abrasion, eyelid
- cheek S00.81 ☑
  - internal S00.512 ☑
- chest wall — *see* Abrasion, thorax
- chin S00.81 ☑
- clitoris S30.814 ☑
- cornea S05.0 ☑
- costal region — *see* Abrasion, thorax
- dental K03.1
- digit(s)
  - foot — *see* Abrasion, toe
  - hand — *see* Abrasion, finger
- ear S00.41 ☑
- elbow S50.31 ☑
- epididymis S30.813 ☑
- epigastric region S30.811 ☑
- epiglottis S10.11 ☑
- esophagus (thoracic) S27.818 ☑
  - cervical S10.11 ☑
- eyebrow — *see* Abrasion, eyelid
- eyelid S00.21 ☑
- face S00.81 ☑
- finger(s) S60.41 ☑
  - index S60.41 ☑
  - little S60.41 ☑
  - middle S60.41 ☑
  - ring S60.41 ☑
- flank S30.811 ☑
- foot (except toe(s) alone) S90.81 ☑
  - toe — *see* Abrasion, toe
- forearm S50.81 ☑
  - elbow only — *see* Abrasion, elbow
- forehead S00.81 ☑
- genital organs, external
  - female S30.816 ☑
  - male S30.815 ☑
- groin S30.811 ☑
- gum S00.512 ☑
- hand S60.51 ☑
- head S00.91 ☑
  - ear — *see* Abrasion, ear

Abrasion - Abscess

Abrasion — *continued*
head — *continued*
eyelid — *see* Abrasion, eyelid
lip S00.511 ☑
nose S00.31 ☑
oral cavity S00.512 ☑
scalp S00.01 ☑
specified site NEC S00.81 ☑
heel — *see* Abrasion, foot
hip S70.21 ☑
inguinal region S30.811 ☑
interscapular region S20.419 ☑
jaw S00.81 ☑
knee S80.21 ☑
labium (majus) (minus) S30.814 ☑
larynx S10.11 ☑
leg (lower) S80.81 ☑
knee — *see* Abrasion, knee
upper — *see* Abrasion, thigh
lip S00.511 ☑
lower back S30.810 ☑
lumbar region S30.810 ☑
malar region S00.81 ☑
mammary — *see* Abrasion, breast
mastoid region S00.81 ☑
mouth S00.512 ☑
nail
finger — *see* Abrasion, finger
toe — *see* Abrasion, toe
nape S10.81 ☑
nasal S00.31 ☑
neck S10.91 ☑
specified site NEC S10.81 ☑
throat S10.11 ☑
nose S00.31 ☑
occipital region S00.01 ☑
oral cavity S00.512 ☑
orbital region — *see* Abrasion, eyelid
palate S00.512 ☑
palm — *see* Abrasion, hand
parietal region S00.01 ☑
pelvis S30.810 ☑
penis S30.812 ☑
perineum
female S30.814 ☑
male S30.810 ☑
periocular area — *see* Abrasion, eyelid
phalanges
finger — *see* Abrasion, finger
toe — *see* Abrasion, toe
pharynx S10.11 ☑
pinna — *see* Abrasion, ear
popliteal space — *see* Abrasion, knee
prepuce S30.812 ☑
pubic region S30.810 ☑
pudendum
female S30.816 ☑
male S30.815 ☑
sacral region S30.810 ☑
scalp S00.01 ☑
scapular region — *see* Abrasion, shoulder
scrotum S30.813 ☑
shin — *see* Abrasion, leg
shoulder S40.21 ☑
skin NEC T14.8 ☑
sternal region S20.319 ☑
submaxillary region S00.81 ☑
submental region S00.81 ☑
subungual
finger(s) — *see* Abrasion, finger
toe(s) — *see* Abrasion, toe
supraclavicular fossa S10.81 ☑
supraorbital S00.81 ☑
temple S00.81 ☑
temporal region S00.81 ☑
testis S30.813 ☑
thigh S70.31 ☑
thorax, thoracic (wall) S20.91 ☑
back S20.41 ☑
front S20.31 ☑
throat S10.11 ☑
thumb S60.31 ☑
toe(s) (lesser) S90.416 ☑
great S90.41 ☑
tongue S00.512 ☑
tooth, teeth (dentifrice) (habitual) (hard tissues) (occupational) (ritual) (traditional) K03.1
trachea S10.11 ☑
tunica vaginalis S30.813 ☑
tympanum, tympanic membrane — *see* Abrasion, ear
uvula S00.512 ☑

Abrasion — *continued*
vagina S30.814 ☑
vocal cords S10.11 ☑
vulva S30.814 ☑
wrist S60.81 ☑
Abrism — *see* Poisoning, food, noxious, plant
Abruptio placentae O45.9 ☑
with
afibrinogenemia O45.01 ☑
coagulation defect O45.00 ☑
specified NEC O45.09 ☑
disseminated intravascular coagulation O45.02 ☑
hypofibrinogenemia O45.01 ☑
specified NEC O45.8 ☑
Abruption, placenta — *see* Abruptio placentae
Abscess (connective tissue) (embolic) (fistulous) (infective) (metastatic) (multiple) (pernicious) (pyogenic) (septic) L02.91
with
diverticular disease (intestine) K57.80
with bleeding K57.81
large intestine K57.20
with
bleeding K57.21
small intestine K57.40
with bleeding K57.41
small intestine K57.00
with
bleeding K57.01
large intestine K57.40
with bleeding K57.41
lymphangitis - code by site under Abscess
abdomen, abdominal
cavity K65.1
wall L02.211
abdominopelvic K65.1
accessory sinus — *see* Sinusitis
adrenal (capsule) (gland) E27.8
alveolar K04.7
with sinus K04.6
amebic A06.4
brain (and liver or lung abscess) A06.6
genitourinary tract A06.82
liver (without mention of brain or lung abscess) A06.4
lung (and liver) (without mention of brain abscess) A06.5
specified site NEC A06.89
spleen A06.89
anerobic A48.0
ankle — *see* Abscess, lower limb
anorectal K61.2
antecubital space — *see* Abscess, upper limb
antrum (chronic) (Highmore) — *see* Sinusitis, maxillary
anus K61.0
apical (tooth) K04.7
with sinus (alveolar) K04.6
appendix K35.33
areola (acute) (chronic) (nonpuerperal) N61.1
puerperal, postpartum or gestational — *see* Infection, nipple
arm (any part) — *see* Abscess, upper limb
artery (wall) I77.89
atheromatous I77.2
auricle, ear — *see* Abscess, ear, external
axilla (region) L02.41 ☑
lymph gland or node L04.2
back (any part, except buttock) L02.212
Bartholin's gland N75.1
with
abortion — *see* Abortion, by type complicated by, sepsis
ectopic or molar pregnancy O08.0
following ectopic or molar pregnancy O08.0
Bezold's — *see* Mastoiditis, acute
bilharziasis B65.1
bladder (wall) — *see* Cystitis, specified type NEC
bone (subperiosteal) (see also Osteomyelitis, specified type NEC)
accessory sinus (chronic) — *see* Sinusitis
chronic or old — *see* Osteomyelitis, chronic
jaw (lower) (upper) M27.2
mastoid — *see* Mastoiditis, acute, subperiosteal
petrous — *see* Petrositis
spinal (tuberculous) A18.01
nontuberculous — *see* Osteomyelitis, vertebra
bowel K63.0
brain (any part) (cystic) (otogenic) G06.0
amebic (with abscess of any other site) A06.6
gonococcal A54.82
pheomycotic (chromomycotic) B43.1
tuberculous A17.81

Abscess — *continued*
breast (acute) (chronic) (nonpuerperal) N61.1
newborn P39.0
puerperal, postpartum, gestational — *see* Mastitis, obstetric, purulent
broad ligament N73.2
acute N73.0
chronic N73.1
Brodie's (localized) (chronic) M86.8X ☑
bronchi J98.09
buccal cavity K12.2
bulbourethral gland N34.0
bursa M71.00
ankle M71.07 ☑
elbow M71.02 ☑
foot M71.07 ☑
hand M71.04 ☑
hip M71.05 ☑
knee M71.06 ☑
multiple sites M71.09
pharyngeal J39.1
shoulder M71.01 ☑
specified site NEC M71.08
wrist M71.03 ☑
buttock L02.31
canthus — *see* Blepharoconjunctivitis
cartilage — *see* Disorder, cartilage, specified type NEC
cecum K35.33
cerebellum, cerebellar G06.0
sequelae G09
cerebral (embolic) G06.0
sequelae G09
cervical (meaning neck) L02.11
lymph gland or node L04.0
cervix (stump) (uteri) — *see* Cervicitis
cheek (external) L02.01
inner K12.2
chest J86.9
with fistula J86.0
wall L02.213
chin L02.01
choroid — *see* Inflammation, chorioretinal
circumtonsillar J36
cold (lung) (tuberculous) (see also Tuberculosis, abscess, lung)
articular — *see* Tuberculosis, joint
colon (wall) K63.0
colostomy K94.02
conjunctiva — *see* Conjunctivitis, acute
cornea H16.31 ☑
corpus
cavernosum N48.21
luteum — *see* Oophoritis
Cowper's gland N34.0
cranium G06.0
cul-de-sac (Douglas') (posterior) — *see* Peritonitis, pelvic, female
cutaneous — *see* Abscess, by site
dental K04.7
with sinus (alveolar) K04.6
dentoalveolar K04.7
with sinus K04.6
diaphragm, diaphragmatic K65.1
Douglas' cul-de-sac or pouch — *see* Peritonitis, pelvic, female
Dubois A50.59
ear (middle) (see also Otitis, media, suppurative)
acute — *see* Otitis, media, suppurative, acute
external H60.0 ☑
entamebic — *see* Abscess, amebic
enterostomy K94.12
epididymis N45.4
epidural G06.2
brain G06.0
spinal cord G06.1
epiglottis J38.7
epiploon, epiploic K65.1
erysipelatous — *see* Erysipelas
esophagus K20.8
ethmoid (bone) (chronic) (sinus) J32.2
external auditory canal — *see* Abscess, ear, external
extradural G06.2
brain G06.0
sequelae G09
spinal cord G06.1
extraperitoneal K68.19
eye — *see* Endophthalmitis, purulent
eyelid H00.03 ☑
face (any part, except ear, eye and nose) L02.01
fallopian tube — *see* Salpingitis
fascia M72.8

☑ **Additional character required**

Abscess — *continued*
  fauces J39.1
  fecal K63.0
  femoral (region) — *see* Abscess, lower limb
  filaria, filarial — *see* Infestation, filarial
  finger (any) (*see also* Abscess, hand)
    nail — *see* Cellulitis, finger
  foot L02.61 ☑
  forehead L02.01
  frontal sinus (chronic) J32.1
  gallbladder K81.0
  genital organ or tract
    female (external) N76.4
    male N49.9
      multiple sites N49.8
      specified NEC N49.8
  gestational mammary O91.11 ☑
  gestational subareolar O91.11 ☑
  gingival — *see* Periodontitis, localized
  gland, glandular (lymph) (acute) — *see*
    Lymphadenitis, acute
  gluteal (region) L02.31
  gonorrheal — *see* Gonococcus
  groin L02.214
  gum — *see* Periodontitis, localized
  hand L02.51 ☑
  head NEC L02.811
    face (any part, except ear, eye and nose) L02.01
  heart — *see* Carditis
  heel — *see* Abscess, foot
  helminthic — *see* Infestation, helminth
  hepatic (cholangitic) (hematogenic) (lymphogenic)
    (pylephlebitic) K75.0
    amebic A06.4
  hip (region) — *see* Abscess, lower limb
  horseshoe K61.31
  ileocecal K35.33
  ileostomy (bud) K94.12
  iliac (region) L02.214
    fossa K35.33
  infraclavicular (fossa) — *see* Abscess, upper limb
  inguinal (region) L02.214
    lymph gland or node L04.1
  intersphincteric K61.4
  intestine, intestinal NEC K63.0
    rectal K61.1
  intra-abdominal (*see also* Abscess, peritoneum)
    K65.1
    following procedure T81.43 ☑
      obstetrical O86.03
    postprocedural T81.49 ☑
      retroperitoneal K68.11
  intracranial G06.0
  intramammary — *see* Abscess, breast
  intramuscular, following procedure T81.42 ☑
    obstetrical O86.02
  intraorbital — *see* Abscess, orbit
  intraperitoneal K65.1
  intrasphincteric (anus) K61.4
  intraspinal G06.1
  intratonsillar J36
  ischiorectal (fossa) (specified NEC) K61.39
  jaw (bone) (lower) (upper) M27.2
  joint — *see* Arthritis, pyogenic or pyemic
    spine (tuberculous) A18.01
      nontuberculous — *see* Spondylopathy, infective
  kidney N15.1
    with calculus N20.0
      with hydronephrosis N13.6
    puerperal (postpartum) O86.21
  knee (*see also* Abscess, lower limb)
    joint M00.9
  labium (majus) (minus) N76.4
  lacrimal
    caruncle — *see* Inflammation, lacrimal, passages,
      acute
    gland — *see* Dacryoadenitis
    passages (duct) (sac) — *see* Inflammation,
      lacrimal, passages, acute
  lacunar N34.0
  larynx J38.7
  lateral (alveolar) K04.7
    with sinus K04.6
  leg (any part) — *see* Abscess, lower limb
  lens H27.8
  lingual K14.0
    tonsil J36
  lip K13.0
  Littre's gland N34.0
  liver (cholangitic) (hematogenic) (lymphogenic)
    (pylephlebitic) (pyogenic) K75.0

Abscess — *continued*
  liver — *continued*
    amebic (due to Entamoeba histolytica)
      (dysenteric) (tropical) A06.4
      with
        brain abscess (and liver or lung abscess) A06.6
        lung abscess A06.5
  loin (region) L02.211
  lower limb L02.41 ☑
  lumbar (tuberculous) A18.01
    nontuberculous L02.212
  lung (miliary) (putrid) J85.2
    with pneumonia J85.1
      due to specified organism (*see* Pneumonia, in
        (due to))
    amebic (with liver abscess) A06.5
      with
        brain abscess A06.6
        pneumonia A06.5
  lymph, lymphatic, gland or node (acute) (*see also*
    Lymphadenitis, acute)
    mesentery I88.0
  malar M27.2
  mammary gland — *see* Abscess, breast
  marginal, anus K61.0
  mastoid — *see* Mastoiditis, acute
  maxilla, maxillary M27.2
    molar (tooth) K04.7
      with sinus K04.6
    premolar K04.7
    sinus (chronic) J32.0
  mediastinum J85.3
  meibomian gland — *see* Hordeolum
  meninges G06.2
  mesentery, mesenteric K65.1
  mesosalpinx — *see* Salpingitis
  mons pubis L02.215
  mouth (floor) K12.2
  muscle — *see* Myositis, infective
  myocardium I40.0
  nabothian (follicle) — *see* Cervicitis
  nasal J32.9
  nasopharyngeal J39.1
  navel L02.216
    newborn P38.9
      with mild hemorrhage P38.1
      without hemorrhage P38.9
  neck (region) L02.11
    lymph gland or node L04.0
  nephritic — *see* Abscess, kidney
  nipple N61.1
    associated with
      lactation — *see* Pregnancy, complicated by
      pregnancy — *see* Pregnancy, complicated by
  nose (external) (fossa) (septum) J34.0
    sinus (chronic) — *see* Sinusitis
  omentum K65.1
  operative wound T81.49 ☑
  orbit, orbital — *see* Cellulitis, orbit
  otogenic G06.0
  ovary, ovarian (corpus luteum) — *see* Oophoritis
  oviduct — *see* Oophoritis
  palate (soft) K12.2
    hard M27.2
  palmar (space) — *see* Abscess, hand
  pancreas (duct) — *see* Pancreatitis, acute
  parafrenal N48.21
  parametric, parametrium N73.2
    acute N73.0
    chronic N73.1
  paranephric N15.1
  parapancreatic — *see* Pancreatitis, acute
  parapharyngeal J39.0
  pararectal K61.1
  parasinus — *see* Sinusitis
  parauterine (*see also* Disease, pelvis, inflammatory)
    N73.2
  paravaginal — *see* Vaginitis
  parietal region (scalp) L02.811
  parodontal — *see* Periodontitis, aggressive,
    localized
  parotid (duct) (gland) K11.3
    region K12.2
  pectoral (region) L02.213
  pelvis, pelvic
    female — *see* Disease, pelvis, inflammatory
    male, peritoneal K65.1
  penis N48.21
    gonococcal (accessory gland) (periurethral) A54.1
  perianal K61.0
  periapical K04.7
    with sinus (alveolar) K04.6

Abscess — *continued*
  periappendicular K35.33
  pericardial I30.1
  pericecal K35.33
  pericemental — *see* Periodontitis, aggressive,
    localized
  pericholecystic — *see* Cholecystitis, acute
  pericoronal — *see* Periodontitis, aggressive,
    localized
  peridental — *see* Periodontitis, aggressive, localized
  perimetric (*see also* Disease, pelvis, inflammatory)
    N73.2
  perinephric, perinephritic — *see* Abscess, kidney
  perineum, perineal (superficial) L02.215
    urethra N34.0
  periodontal (parietal) — *see* Periodontitis,
    aggressive, localized
    apical K04.7
  periosteum, periosteal (*see also* Osteomyelitis,
    specified type NEC)
    with osteomyelitis (*see also* Osteomyelitis,
      specified type NEC)
      acute — *see* Osteomyelitis, acute
      chronic — *see* Osteomyelitis, chronic
  peripharyngeal J39.0
  peripleuritic J86.9
    with fistula J86.0
  periprostatic N41.2
  perirectal K61.1
  perirenal (tissue) — *see* Abscess, kidney
  perisinuous (nose) — *see* Sinusitis
  peritoneum, peritoneal (perforated) (ruptured) K65.1
    with appendicitis (*see also* Appendicitis) K35.33
    pelvic
      female — *see* Peritonitis, pelvic, female
      male K65.1
    postoperative T81.49 ☑
    puerperal, postpartum, childbirth O85
    tuberculous A18.31
  peritonsillar J36
  perityphlic K35.33
  periureteral N28.89
  periurethral N34.0
    gonococcal (accessory gland) (periurethral) A54.1
  periuterine (*see also* Disease, pelvis, inflammatory)
    N73.2
  perivesical — *see* Cystitis, specified type NEC
  petrous bone — *see* Petrositis
  phagedenic NOS L02.91
    chancroid A57
  pharynx, pharyngeal (lateral) J39.1
  pilonidal L05.01
  pituitary (gland) E23.6
  pleura J86.9
    with fistula J86.0
  popliteal — *see* Abscess, lower limb
  postcecal K35.33
  postlaryngeal J38.7
  postnasal J34.0
  postoperative (any site) (*see also* Infection,
    postoperative wound) T81.49 ☑
    retroperitoneal K68.11
  postpharyngeal J39.0
  posttonsillar J36
  post-typhoid A01.09
  pouch of Douglas — *see* Peritonitis, pelvic, female
  premammary — *see* Abscess, breast
  prepatellar — *see* Abscess, lower limb
  prostate N41.2
    gonococcal (acute) (chronic) A54.22
  psoas muscle K68.12
  puerperal - code by site under Puerperal, abscess
  pulmonary — *see* Abscess, lung
  pulp, pulpal (dental) K04.01
    irreversible K04.02
    reversible K04.01
  rectovaginal septum K63.0
  rectovesical — *see* Cystitis, specified type NEC
  rectum K61.1
  renal — *see* Abscess, kidney
  retina — *see* Inflammation, chorioretinal
  retrobulbar — *see* Abscess, orbit
  retrocecal K65.1
  retrolaryngeal J38.7
  retromammary — *see* Abscess, breast
  retroperitoneal NEC K68.19
    postprocedural K68.11
  retropharyngeal J39.0
  retrouterine — *see* Peritonitis, pelvic, female
  retrovesical — *see* Cystitis, specified type NEC
  root, tooth K04.7
    with sinus (alveolar) K04.6

Abscess - Absence

Abscess — *continued*
round ligament (*see also* Disease, pelvis, inflammatory) N73.2
rupture (spontaneous) NOS L02.91
sacrum (tuberculous) A18.01
nontuberculous M46.28
salivary (duct) (gland) K11.3
scalp (any part) L02.811
scapular — *see* Osteomyelitis, specified type NEC
sclera — *see* Scleritis
scrofulous (tuberculous) A18.2
scrotum N49.2
seminal vesicle N49.0
septal, dental K04.7
with sinus (alveolar) K04.6
serous — *see* Periostitis
shoulder (region) — *see* Abscess, upper limb
sigmoid K63.0
sinus (accessory) (chronic) (nasal) (*see also* Sinusitis)
intracranial venous (any) G06.0
Skene's duct or gland N34.0
skin — *see* Abscess, by site
specified site NEC L02.818
spermatic cord N49.1
sphenoidal (sinus) (chronic) J32.3
spinal cord (any part) (staphylococcal) G06.1
tuberculous A17.81
spine (column) (tuberculous) A18.01
epidural G06.1
nontuberculous — *see* Osteomyelitis, vertebra
spleen D73.3
amebic A06.89
stitch T81.41 ☑
following an obstetrical procedure O86.01
subarachnoid G06.2
brain G06.0
spinal cord G06.1
subareolar — *see* Abscess, breast
subcecal K35.33
subcutaneous (*see also* Abscess, by site)
following procedure T81.41 ☑
obstetrical O86.01
pheomycotic (chromomycotic) B43.2
subdiaphragmatic K65.1
subdural G06.2
brain G06.0
sequelae G09
spinal cord G06.1
sub-fascial, following an obstetrical procedure O86.02
subgaleal L02.811
subhepatic K65.1
sublingual K12.2
gland K11.3
submammary — *see* Abscess, breast
submandibular (region) (space) (triangle) K12.2
gland K11.3
submaxillary (region) L02.01
gland K11.3
submental L02.01
gland K11.3
subperiosteal — *see* Osteomyelitis, specified type NEC
subphrenic K65.1
following an obstetrical procedure O86.03
postoperative T81.43 ☑
suburethral N34.0
sudoriparous L75.8
supraclavicular (fossa) — *see* Abscess, upper limb
supralevator K61.5
suprapelvic, acute N73.0
suprarenal (capsule) (gland) E27.8
sweat gland L74.8
tear duct — *see* Inflammation, lacrimal, passages, acute
temple L02.01
temporal region L02.01
temporosphenoidal G06.0
tendon (sheath) M65.00
ankle M65.07 ☑
foot M65.07 ☑
forearm M65.03 ☑
hand M65.04 ☑
lower leg M65.06 ☑
pelvic region M65.05 ☑
shoulder region M65.01 ☑
specified site NEC M65.08
thigh M65.05 ☑
upper arm M65.02 ☑
testis N45.4
thigh — *see* Abscess, lower limb
thorax J86.9
with fistula J86.0

Abscess — *continued*
throat J39.1
thumb (*see also* Abscess, hand)
nail — *see* Cellulitis, finger
thymus (gland) E32.1
thyroid (gland) E06.0
toe (any) (*see also* Abscess, foot)
nail — *see* Cellulitis, toe
tongue (staphylococcal) K14.0
tonsil(s) (lingual) J36
tonsillopharyngeal J36
tooth, teeth (root) K04.7
with sinus (alveolar) K04.6
supporting structures NEC — *see* Periodontitis, aggressive, localized
trachea J39.8
trunk L02.219
abdominal wall L02.211
back L02.212
chest wall L02.213
groin L02.214
perineum L02.215
umbilicus L02.216
tubal — *see* Salpingitis
tuberculous — *see* Tuberculosis, abscess
tubo-ovarian — *see* Salpingo-oophoritis
tunica vaginalis N49.1
umbilicus L02.216
upper
limb L02.41 ☑
respiratory J39.8
urethral (gland) N34.0
urinary N34.0
uterus, uterine (wall) (*see also* Endometritis)
ligament (*see also* Disease, pelvis, inflammatory) N73.2
neck — *see* Cervicitis
uvula K12.2
vagina (wall) — *see* Vaginitis
vaginorectal — *see* Vaginitis
vas deferens N49.1
vermiform appendix K35.33
vertebra (column) (tuberculous) A18.01
nontuberculous — *see* Osteomyelitis, vertebra
vesical — *see* Cystitis, specified type NEC
vesico-uterine pouch — *see* Peritonitis, pelvic, female
vitreous (humor) — *see* Endophthalmitis, purulent
vocal cord J38.3
von Bezold's — *see* Mastoiditis, acute
vulva N76.4
vulvovaginal gland N75.1
web space — *see* Abscess, hand
wound T81.49 ☑
wrist — *see* Abscess, upper limb
Absence (of) (organ or part) (complete or partial)
adrenal (gland) (congenital) Q89.1
acquired E89.6
albumin in blood E88.09
alimentary tract (congenital) Q45.8
upper Q40.8
alveolar process (acquired) — *see* Anomaly, alveolar
ankle (acquired) Z89.44 ☑
anus (congenital) Q42.3
with fistula Q42.2
aorta (congenital) Q25.41
appendix, congenital Q42.8
arm (acquired) Z89.20 ☑
above elbow Z89.22 ☑
congenital (with hand present) — *see* Agenesis, arm, with hand present
and hand — *see* Agenesis, forearm, and hand
below elbow Z89.21 ☑
congenital (with hand present) — *see* Agenesis, arm, with hand present
and hand — *see* Agenesis, forearm, and hand
congenital — *see* Defect, reduction, upper limb
shoulder (following explantation of shoulder joint prosthesis) (joint) (with or without presence of antibiotic-impregnated cement spacer) Z89.23 ☑
congenital (with hand present) — *see* Agenesis, arm, with hand present
artery (congenital) (peripheral) Q27.8
brain Q28.3
coronary Q24.5
pulmonary Q25.79
specified NEC Q27.8
umbilical Q27.0
atrial septum (congenital) Q21.1
auditory canal (congenital) (external) Q16.1
auricle (ear), congenital Q16.0

Absence — *continued*
bile, biliary duct, congenital Q44.5
bladder (acquired) Z90.6
congenital Q64.5
bowel sounds R19.11
brain Q00.0
part of Q04.3
breast(s) (and nipple(s)) (acquired) Z90.1 ☑
congenital Q83.8
broad ligament Q50.6
bronchus (congenital) Q32.4
canaliculus lacrimalis, congenital Q10.4
cerebellum (vermis) Q04.3
cervix (acquired) (with uterus) Z90.710
with remaining uterus Z90.712
congenital Q51.5
chin, congenital Q18.8
cilia (congenital) Q10.3
acquired — *see* Madarosis
clitoris (congenital) Q52.6
coccyx, congenital Q76.49
cold sense R20.8
congenital
lumen — *see* Atresia
organ or site NEC — *see* Agenesis
septum — *see* Imperfect, closure
corpus callosum Q04.0
cricoid cartilage, congenital Q31.8
diaphragm (with hernia), congenital Q79.1
digestive organ(s) or tract, congenital Q45.8
acquired NEC Z90.49
upper Q40.8
ductus arteriosus Q28.8
duodenum (acquired) Z90.49
congenital Q41.0
ear, congenital Q16.9
acquired H93.8 ☑
auricle Q16.0
external Q16.0
inner Q16.5
lobe, lobule Q17.8
middle, except ossicles Q16.4
ossicles Q16.3
ossicles Q16.3
ejaculatory duct (congenital) Q55.4
endocrine gland (congenital) NEC Q89.2
acquired E89.89
epididymis (congenital) Q55.4
acquired Z90.79
epiglottis, congenital Q31.8
esophagus (congenital) Q39.8
acquired (partial) Z90.49
eustachian tube (congenital) Q16.2
extremity (acquired) Z89.9
congenital Q73.0
knee (following explantation of knee joint prosthesis) (joint) (with or without presence of antibiotic-impregnated cement spacer) Z89.52 ☑
lower (above knee) Z89.619
below knee Z89.51 ☑
upper — *see* Absence, arm
eye (acquired) Z90.01
congenital Q11.1
muscle (congenital) Q10.3
eyeball (acquired) Z90.01
eyelid (fold) (congenital) Q10.3
acquired Z90.01
face, specified part NEC Q18.8
fallopian tube(s) (acquired) Z90.79
congenital Q50.6
family member (causing problem in home) NEC (*see also* Disruption, family) Z63.32
femur, congenital — *see* Defect, reduction, lower limb, longitudinal, femur
fibrinogen (congenital) D68.2
acquired D65
finger(s) (acquired) Z89.02 ☑
congenital — *see* Agenesis, hand
foot (acquired) Z89.43 ☑
congenital — *see* Agenesis, foot
forearm (acquired) — *see* Absence, arm, below elbow
gallbladder (acquired) Z90.49
congenital Q44.0
gamma globulin in blood D80.1
hereditary D80.0
genital organs
acquired (female) (male) Z90.79
female, congenital Q52.8
external Q52.71
internal NEC Q52.8
male, congenital Q55.8

☑ **Additional character required**

Absence — *continued*
  genitourinary organs, congenital NEC
    female Q52.8
    male Q55.8
  globe (acquired) Z90.01
    congenital Q11.1
  glottis, congenital Q31.8
  hand and wrist (acquired) Z89.11 ☑
    congenital — *see* Agenesis, hand
  head, part (acquired) NEC Z90.09
  heat sense R20.8
  hip (following explantation of hip joint
      prosthesis) (joint) (with or without presence
      of antibiotic-impregnated cement spacer)
      Z89.62 ☑
  hymen (congenital) Q52.4
  ileum (acquired) Z90.49
    congenital Q41.2
  immunoglobulin, isolated NEC D80.3
    IgA D80.2
    IgG D80.3
    IgM D80.4
  incus (acquired) — *see* Loss, ossicles, ear
    congenital Q16.3
  inner ear, congenital Q16.5
  intestine (acquired) (small) Z90.49
    congenital Q41.9
      specified NEC Q41.8
    large Z90.49
      congenital Q42.9
        specified NEC Q42.8
  iris, congenital Q13.1
  jejunum (acquired) Z90.49
    congenital Q41.1
  joint
    acquired
      hip (following explantation of hip joint
          prosthesis) (with or without presence of
          antibiotic-impregnated cement spacer)
          Z89.62 ☑
      knee (following explantation of knee joint
          prosthesis) (with or without presence of
          antibiotic-impregnated cement spacer)
          Z89.52 ☑
      shoulder (following explantation of shoulder
          joint prosthesis) (with or without presence
          of antibiotic-impregnated cement spacer)
          Z89.23 ☑
    congenital NEC Q74.8
  kidney(s) (acquired) Z90.5
    congenital Q60.2
      bilateral Q60.1
      unilateral Q60.0
  knee (following explantation of knee joint
      prosthesis) (joint) (with or without presence
      of antibiotic-impregnated cement spacer)
      Z89.52 ☑
  labyrinth, membranous Q16.5
  larynx (congenital) Q31.8
    acquired Z90.02
  leg (acquired) (above knee) Z89.61 ☑
    below knee (acquired) Z89.51 ☑
    congenital — *see* Defect, reduction, lower limb
  lens (acquired) (*see also* Aphakia)
    congenital Q12.3
    post cataract extraction Z98.4 ☑
  limb (acquired) — *see* Absence, extremity
  lip Q38.6
  liver (congenital) Q44.7
  lung (fissure) (lobe) (bilateral) (unilateral)
      (congenital) Q33.3
    acquired (any part) Z90.2
  menstruation — *see* Amenorrhea
  muscle (congenital) (pectoral) Q79.8
    ocular Q10.3
  neck, part Q18.8
  neutrophil — *see* Agranulocytosis
  nipple(s) (with breast(s)) (acquired) Z90.1 ☑
    congenital Q83.2
  nose (congenital) Q30.1
    acquired Z90.09
  organ
    of Corti, congenital Q16.5
    or site, congenital NEC Q89.8
      acquired NEC Z90.89
  osseous meatus (ear) Q16.4
  ovary (acquired)
    bilateral Z90.722
    congenital
      bilateral Q50.02
      unilateral Q50.01
    unilateral Z90.721

Absence — *continued*
  oviduct (acquired)
    bilateral Z90.722
    congenital Q50.6
    unilateral Z90.721
  pancreas (congenital) Q45.0
    acquired Z90.410
      complete Z90.410
      partial Z90.411
      total Z90.410
  parathyroid gland (acquired) E89.2
    congenital Q89.2
  patella, congenital Q74.1
  penis (congenital) Q55.5
    acquired Z90.79
  pericardium (congenital) Q24.8
  pituitary gland (congenital) Q89.2
    acquired E89.3
  prostate (acquired) Z90.79
    congenital Q55.4
  pulmonary valve Q22.0
  punctum lacrimale (congenital) Q10.4
  radius, congenital — *see* Defect, reduction, upper
      limb, longitudinal, radius
  rectum (congenital) Q42.1
    with fistula Q42.0
    acquired Z90.49
  respiratory organ NOS Q34.9
  rib (acquired) Z90.89
    congenital Q76.6
  sacrum, congenital Q76.49
  salivary gland(s), congenital Q38.4
  scrotum, congenital Q55.29
  seminal vesicles (congenital) Q55.4
    acquired Z90.79
  septum
    atrial (congenital) Q21.1
    between aorta and pulmonary artery Q21.4
    ventricular (congenital) Q20.4
  sex chromosome
    female phenotype Q97.8
    male phenotype Q98.8
  skull bone (congenital) Q75.8
    with
      anencephaly Q00.0
      encephalocele — *see* Encephalocele
      hydrocephalus Q03.9
        with spina bifida — *see* Spina bifida, by site,
            with hydrocephalus
      microcephaly Q02
  spermatic cord, congenital Q55.4
  spine, congenital Q76.49
  spleen (congenital) Q89.01
    acquired Z90.81
  sternum, congenital Q76.7
  stomach (acquired) (partial) Z90.3
    congenital Q40.2
  superior vena cava, congenital Q26.8
  teeth, tooth (congenital) K00.0
    acquired (complete) K08.109
      class I K08.101
      class II K08.102
      class III K08.103
      class IV K08.104
      due to
        caries K08.139
          class I K08.131
          class II K08.132
          class III K08.133
          class IV K08.134
        periodontal disease K08.129
          class I K08.121
          class II K08.122
          class III K08.123
          class IV K08.124
        specified NEC K08.199
          class I K08.191
          class II K08.192
          class III K08.193
          class IV K08.194
        trauma K08.119
          class I K08.111
          class II K08.112
          class III K08.113
          class IV K08.114
      partial K08.409
        class I K08.401
        class II K08.402
        class III K08.403
        class IV K08.404
        due to
          caries K08.439

Absence — *continued*
  teeth, tooth — *continued*
          class I K08.431
          class II K08.432
          class III K08.433
          class IV K08.434
        periodontal disease K08.429
          class I K08.421
          class II K08.422
          class III K08.423
          class IV K08.424
        specified NEC K08.499
          class I K08.491
          class II K08.492
          class III K08.493
          class IV K08.494
        trauma K08.419
          class I K08.411
          class II K08.412
          class III K08.413
          class IV K08.414
  tendon (congenital) Q79.8
  testis (congenital) Q55.0
    acquired Z90.79
  thumb (acquired) Z89.01 ☑
    congenital — *see* Agenesis, hand
  thymus gland Q89.2
  thyroid (gland) (acquired) E89.0
    cartilage, congenital Q31.8
    congenital E03.1
  toe(s) (acquired) Z89.42 ☑
    with foot — *see* Absence, foot and ankle
    congenital — *see* Agenesis, foot
    great Z89.41 ☑
  tongue, congenital Q38.3
  trachea (cartilage), congenital Q32.1
  transverse aortic arch, congenital Q25.49
  tricuspid valve Q22.4
  umbilical artery, congenital Q27.0
  upper arm and forearm with hand present,
      congenital — *see* Agenesis, arm, with hand
      present
  ureter (congenital) Q62.4
    acquired Z90.6
  urethra, congenital Q64.5
  uterus (acquired) Z90.710
    with cervix Z90.710
    with remaining cervical stump Z90.711
    congenital Q51.0
  uvula, congenital Q38.5
  vagina, congenital Q52.0
  vas deferens (congenital) Q55.4
    acquired Z90.79
  vein (peripheral) congenital NEC Q27.8
    cerebral Q28.3
    digestive system Q27.8
    great Q26.8
    lower limb Q27.8
    portal Q26.5
    precerebral Q28.1
    specified site NEC Q27.8
    upper limb Q27.8
  vena cava (inferior) (superior), congenital Q26.8
  ventricular septum Q20.4
  vertebra, congenital Q76.49
  vulva, congenital Q52.71
  wrist (acquired) Z89.12 ☑
Absorbent system disease I87.8
Absorption
  carbohydrate, disturbance K90.49
  chemical — *see* Table of Drugs and Chemicals
    through placenta (newborn) P04.9
      environmental substance P04.6
      nutritional substance P04.5
      obstetric anesthetic or analgesic drug P04.0
  drug NEC — *see* Table of Drugs and Chemicals
    addictive
      through placenta (newborn) (*see also* Newborn,
          affected by, maternal, use of) P04.40
        cocaine P04.41
        hallucinogens P04.42
        specified drug NEC P04.49
    medicinal
      through placenta (newborn) P04.19
    through placenta (newborn) P04.19
      obstetric anesthetic or analgesic drug P04.0
  fat, disturbance K90.49
    pancreatic K90.3
  noxious substance — *see* Table of Drugs and
      Chemicals
  protein, disturbance K90.49
  starch, disturbance K90.49

Absorption — *continued*
- toxic substance — *see* Table of Drugs and Chemicals
- uremic — *see* Uremia

Abstinence symptoms, syndrome
- alcohol F10.239
  - with delirium F10.231
- cocaine F14.23
- neonatal P96.1
- nicotine — *see* Dependence, drug, nicotine, with, withdrawal
- opioid F11.93
  - with dependence F11.23
- psychoactive NEC F19.939
  - with
    - delirium F19.931
    - dependence F19.239
      - with
        - delirium F19.231
        - perceptual disturbance F19.232
      - uncomplicated F19.230
    - perceptual disturbance F19.932
    - uncomplicated F19.930
- sedative F13.939
  - with
    - delirium F13.931
    - dependence F13.239
      - with
        - delirium F13.231
        - perceptual disturbance F13.232
      - uncomplicated F13.230
    - perceptual disturbance F13.932
    - uncomplicated F13.930
- stimulant NEC F15.93
  - with dependence F15.23

Abulia R68.89
Abulomania F60.7
Abuse
- adult — *see* Maltreatment, adult
- as reason for
  - couple seeking advice (including offender) Z63.0
- alcohol (non-dependent) F10.10
  - with
    - anxiety disorder F10.180
    - intoxication F10.129
      - with delirium F10.121
      - uncomplicated F10.120
    - mood disorder F10.14
    - other specified disorder F10.188
    - psychosis F10.159
      - delusions F10.150
      - hallucinations F10.151
    - sexual dysfunction F10.181
    - sleep disorder F10.182
    - unspecified disorder F10.19
  - counseling and surveillance Z71.41
  - in remission (early) (sustained) F10.11
- amphetamine (or related substance) (*see also* Abuse, drug, stimulant NEC)
  - stimulant NEC F15.10
    - with
      - anxiety disorder F15.180
      - intoxication F15.129
        - with
          - delirium F15.121
          - perceptual disturbance F15.122
- analgesics (non-prescribed) (over the counter) F55.8
- antacids F55.0
- antidepressants — *see* Abuse, drug, psychoactive NEC
- anxiolytic — *see* Abuse, drug, sedative
- barbiturates — *see* Abuse, drug, sedative
- caffeine — *see* Abuse, drug, stimulant NEC
- cannabis, cannabinoids — *see* Abuse, drug, cannabis
- child — *see* Maltreatment, child
- cocaine — *see* Abuse, drug, cocaine
- drug NEC (non-dependent) F19.10
  - with sleep disorder F19.182
  - amphetamine type — *see* Abuse, drug, stimulant NEC
  - analgesics (non-prescribed) (over the counter) F55.8
  - antacids F55.0
  - antidepressants — *see* Abuse, drug, psychoactive NEC
  - anxiolytics — *see* Abuse, drug, sedative
  - barbiturates — *see* Abuse, drug, sedative
  - caffeine — *see* Abuse, drug, stimulant NEC
  - cannabis F12.10
    - with

Abuse — *continued*
- drug NEC — *continued*
  - anxiety disorder F12.180
  - intoxication F12.129
    - with
      - delirium F12.121
      - perceptual disturbance F12.122
    - uncomplicated F12.120
  - other specified disorder F12.188
  - psychosis F12.159
    - delusions F12.150
    - hallucinations F12.151
  - unspecified disorder F12.19
  - in remission (early) (sustained) F12.11
- cocaine F14.10
  - with
    - anxiety disorder F14.180
    - intoxication F14.129
      - with
        - delirium F14.121
        - perceptual disturbance F14.122
      - uncomplicated F14.120
    - mood disorder F14.14
    - other specified disorder F14.188
    - psychosis F14.159
      - delusions F14.150
      - hallucinations F14.151
    - sexual dysfunction F14.181
    - sleep disorder F14.182
    - unspecified disorder F14.19
  - in remission (early) (sustained) F14.11
- counseling and surveillance Z71.51
- hallucinogen F16.10
  - with
    - anxiety disorder F16.180
    - flashbacks F16.183
    - intoxication F16.129
      - with
        - delirium F16.121
        - perceptual disturbance F16.122
      - uncomplicated F16.120
    - mood disorder F16.14
    - other specified disorder F16.188
    - perception disorder, persisting F16.183
    - psychosis F16.159
      - delusions F16.150
      - hallucinations F16.151
    - unspecified disorder F16.19
  - in remission (early) (sustained) F16.11
- hashish — *see* Abuse, drug, cannabis
- herbal or folk remedies F55.1
- hormones F55.3
- hypnotics — *see* Abuse, drug, sedative
- inhalant F18.10
  - with
    - anxiety disorder F18.180
    - dementia, persisting F18.17
    - intoxication F18.129
      - with delirium F18.121
      - uncomplicated F18.120
    - mood disorder F18.14
    - other specified disorder F18.188
    - psychosis F18.159
      - delusions F18.150
      - hallucinations F18.151
    - unspecified disorder F18.19
  - in remission (early) (sustained) F18.11
- in remission (early) (sustained) F19.11
- laxatives F55.2
- LSD — *see* Abuse, drug, hallucinogen
- marihuana — *see* Abuse, drug, cannabis
- morphine type (opioids) — *see* Abuse, drug, opioid
- opioid F11.10
  - with
    - intoxication F11.129
      - with
        - delirium F11.121
        - perceptual disturbance F11.122
      - uncomplicated F11.120
    - mood disorder F11.14
    - other specified disorder F11.188
    - psychosis F11.159
      - delusions F11.150
      - hallucinations F11.151
    - sexual dysfunction F11.181
    - sleep disorder F11.182
    - unspecified disorder F11.19
  - in remission (early) (sustained) F11.11
- PCP (phencyclidine) (or related substance) — *see* Abuse, drug, hallucinogen
- psychoactive NEC F19.10

Abuse — *continued*
- drug NEC — *continued*
  - with
    - amnestic disorder F19.16
    - anxiety disorder F19.180
    - dementia F19.17
    - intoxication F19.129
      - with
        - delirium F19.121
        - perceptual disturbance F19.122
      - uncomplicated F19.120
    - mood disorder F19.14
    - other specified disorder F19.188
    - psychosis F19.159
      - delusions F19.150
      - hallucinations F19.151
    - sexual dysfunction F19.181
    - sleep disorder F19.182
    - unspecified disorder F19.19
  - sedative, hypnotic or anxiolytic F13.10
    - with
      - anxiety disorder F13.180
      - intoxication F13.129
        - with delirium F13.121
        - uncomplicated F13.120
      - mood disorder F13.14
      - other specified disorder F13.188
      - psychosis F13.159
        - delusions F13.150
        - hallucinations F13.151
      - sexual dysfunction F13.181
      - sleep disorder F13.182
      - unspecified disorder F13.19
    - in remission (early) (sustained) F13.11
  - solvent — *see* Abuse, drug, inhalant
  - steroids F55.3
  - stimulant NEC F15.10
    - with
      - anxiety disorder F15.180
      - intoxication F15.129
        - with
          - delirium F15.121
          - perceptual disturbance F15.122
        - uncomplicated F15.120
      - mood disorder F15.14
      - other specified disorder F15.188
      - psychosis F15.159
        - delusions F15.150
        - hallucinations F15.151
      - sexual dysfunction F15.181
      - sleep disorder F15.182
      - unspecified disorder F15.19
    - in remission (early) (sustained) F15.11
  - tranquilizers — *see* Abuse, drug, sedative
  - vitamins F55.4
- hallucinogens — *see* Abuse, drug, hallucinogen
- hashish — *see* Abuse, drug, cannabis
- herbal or folk remedies F55.1
- hormones F55.3
- hypnotic — *see* Abuse, drug, sedative
- inhalant — *see* Abuse, drug, inhalant
- laxatives F55.2
- LSD — *see* Abuse, drug, hallucinogen
- marihuana — *see* Abuse, drug, cannabis
- morphine type (opioids) — *see* Abuse, drug, opioid
- non-psychoactive substance NEC F55.8
  - antacids F55.0
  - folk remedies F55.1
  - herbal remedies F55.1
  - hormones F55.3
  - laxatives F55.2
  - steroids F55.3
  - vitamins F55.4
- opioids — *see* Abuse, drug, opioid
- PCP (phencyclidine) (or related substance) — *see* Abuse, drug, hallucinogen
- physical (adult) (child) — *see* Maltreatment
- psychoactive substance — *see* Abuse, drug, psychoactive NEC
- psychological (adult) (child) — *see* Maltreatment
- sedative — *see* Abuse, drug, sedative
- sexual — *see* Maltreatment
- solvent — *see* Abuse, drug, inhalant
- steroids F55.3
- vitamins F55.4

Acalculia R48.8
- developmental F81.2
Acanthamebiasis (with) B60.10
- conjunctiva B60.12
- keratoconjunctivitis B60.13
- meningoencephalitis B60.11
- other specified B60.19

☑ **Additional character required**

Acanthocephaliasis B83.8
Acanthocheilonemiasis B74.4
Acanthocytosis E78.6
Acantholysis L11.9
Acanthosis (acquired) (nigricans) L83
 benign Q82.8
 congenital Q82.8
 seborrheic L82.1
  inflamed L82.0
 tongue K14.3
Acapnia E87.3
Acarbia E87.2
Acardia, acardius Q89.8
Acardiacus amorphus Q89.8
Acardiotrophia I51.4
Acariasis B88.0
 scabies B86
Acarodermatitis (urticarioides) B88.0
Acarophobia F40.218
Acatalasemia, acatalasia E80.3
Acathisia (drug induced) G25.71
Accelerated atrioventricular conduction I45.6
Accentuation of personality traits (type A) Z73.1
Accessory (congenital)
 adrenal gland Q89.1
 anus Q43.4
 appendix Q43.4
 atrioventricular conduction I45.6
 auditory ossicles Q16.3
 auricle (ear) Q17.0
 biliary duct or passage Q44.5
 bladder Q64.79
 blood vessels NEC Q27.9
  coronary Q24.5
 bone NEC Q79.8
 breast tissue, axilla Q83.1
 carpal bones Q74.0
 cecum Q43.4
 chromosome(s) NEC (nonsex) Q92.9
  with complex rearrangements NEC Q92.5
   seen only at prometaphase Q92.8
  partial Q92.9
  sex
   female phenotype Q97.8
  13 — see Trisomy, 13
  18 — see Trisomy, 18
  21 — see Trisomy, 21
 coronary artery Q24.5
 cusp(s), heart valve NEC Q24.8
  pulmonary Q22.3
 cystic duct Q44.5
 digit(s) Q69.9
 ear (auricle) (lobe) Q17.0
 endocrine gland NEC Q89.2
 eye muscle Q10.3
 eyelid Q10.3
 face bone(s) Q75.8
 fallopian tube (fimbria) (ostium) Q50.6
 finger(s) Q69.0
 foreskin N47.8
 frontonasal process Q75.8
 gallbladder Q44.1
 genital organ(s)
  female Q52.8
   external Q52.79
   internal NEC Q52.8
  male Q55.8
 genitourinary organs NEC Q89.8
  female Q52.8
  male Q55.8
 hallux Q69.2
 heart Q24.8
  valve NEC Q24.8
   pulmonary Q22.3
 hepatic ducts Q44.5
 hymen Q52.4
 intestine (large) (small) Q43.4
 kidney Q63.0
 lacrimal canal Q10.6
 leaflet, heart valve NEC Q24.8
 ligament, broad Q50.6
 liver Q44.7
  duct Q44.5
 lobule (ear) Q17.0
 lung (lobe) Q33.1
 muscle Q79.8
 navicular of carpus Q74.0
 nervous system, part NEC Q07.8
 nipple Q83.3
 nose Q30.8
 organ or site not listed — see Anomaly, by site
 ovary Q50.31

Accessory — continued
 oviduct Q50.6
 pancreas Q45.3
 parathyroid gland Q89.2
 parotid gland (and duct) Q38.4
 pituitary gland Q89.2
 preauricular appendage Q17.0
 prepuce N47.8
 renal arteries (multiple) Q27.2
 rib Q76.6
  cervical Q76.5
 roots (teeth) K00.2
 salivary gland Q38.4
 sesamoid bones Q74.8
  foot Q74.2
  hand Q74.0
 skin tags Q82.8
 spleen Q89.09
 sternum Q76.7
 submaxillary gland Q38.4
 tarsal bones Q74.2
 teeth, tooth K00.1
 tendon Q79.8
 thumb Q69.1
 thymus gland Q89.2
 thyroid gland Q89.2
 toes Q69.2
 tongue Q38.3
 tooth, teeth K00.1
 tragus Q17.0
 ureter Q62.5
 urethra Q64.79
 urinary organ or tract NEC Q64.8
 uterus Q51.28
 vagina Q52.10
 valve, heart NEC Q24.8
  pulmonary Q22.3
 vertebra Q76.49
 vocal cords Q31.8
 vulva Q52.79
Accident
 birth — see Birth, injury
 cardiac — see Infarct, myocardium
 cerebral I63.9
 cerebrovascular (embolic) (ischemic) (thrombotic)
   I63.9
  aborted I63.9
  hemorrhagic — see Hemorrhage, intracranial,
   intracerebral
  old (without sequelae) Z86.73
   with sequelae (of) — see Sequelae, infarction,
    cerebral
  coronary — see Infarct, myocardium
  craniovascular I63.9
  vascular, brain I63.9
Accidental — see condition
Accommodation (disorder) (see also condition)
 hysterical paralysis of F44.89
 insufficiency of H52.4
 paresis — see Paresis, of accommodation
 spasm — see Spasm, of accommodation
Accouchement — see Delivery
Accreta placenta O43.21 ☑
Accretio cordis (nonrheumatic) I31.0
Accretions, tooth, teeth K03.6
Acculturation difficulty Z60.3
Accumulation secretion, prostate N42.89
Acephalia, acephalism, acephalus, acephaly Q00.0
Acephalobrachia monster Q89.8
Acephalochirus monster Q89.8
Acephalogaster Q89.8
Acephalostomus monster Q89.8
Acephalothorax Q89.8
Acerophobia F40.298
Acetonemia R79.89
 in Type 1 diabetes E10.10
  with coma E10.11
Acetonuria R82.4
Achalasia (cardia) (esophagus) K22.0
 congenital Q39.5
 pylorus Q40.0
 sphincteral NEC K59.8
Ache(s) — see Pain
Acheilia Q38.6
Achillobursitis — see Tendinitis, Achilles
Achillodynia — see Tendinitis, Achilles
Achlorhydria, achlorhydric (neurogenic) K31.83
 anemia D50.8
 diarrhea K31.83
 psychogenic F45.8
 secondary to vagotomy K91.1
Achluophobia F40.228

Acholia K82.8
Acholuric jaundice (familial) (splenomegalic) (see also
  Spherocytosis)
 acquired D59.8
Achondrogenesis Q77.0
Achondroplasia (osteosclerosis congenita) Q77.4
Achroma, cutis L80
Achromat (ism), achromatopsia (acquired) (congenital)
  H53.51
Achromia, congenital — see Albinism
Achromia parasitica B36.0
Achylia gastrica K31.89
 psychogenic F45.8
Acid
 burn — see Corrosion
 deficiency
  amide nicotinic E52
  ascorbic E54
  folic E53.8
  nicotinic E52
  pantothenic E53.8
 intoxication E87.2
 peptic disease K30
 phosphatase deficiency E83.39
 stomach K30
  psychogenic F45.8
Acidemia E87.2
 argininosuccinic E72.22
 isovaleric E71.110
 metabolic (newborn) P19.9
  first noted before onset of labor P19.0
  first noted during labor P19.1
  noted at birth P19.2
 methylmalonic E71.120
 pipecolic E72.3
 propionic E71.121
Acidity, gastric (high) K30
 psychogenic F45.8
Acidocytopenia — see Agranulocytosis
Acidocytosis D72.1
Acidopenia — see Agranulocytosis
Acidosis (lactic) (respiratory) E87.2
 in Type 1 diabetes E10.10
  with coma E10.11
 kidney, tubular N25.89
 lactic E87.2
 metabolic NEC E87.2
  with respiratory acidosis E87.4
  hyperchloremic, of newborn P74.421
  late, of newborn P74.0
 mixed metabolic and respiratory, newborn P84
 newborn P84
 renal (hyperchloremic) (tubular) N25.89
 respiratory E87.2
  complicated by
   metabolic
    acidosis E87.4
    alkalosis E87.4
Aciduria
 4-hydroxybutyric E72.81
 argininosuccinic E72.22
 gamma-hydroxybutyric E72.81
 glutaric (type I) E72.3
  type II E71.313
  type III E71.5 ☑
 orotic (congenital) (hereditary) (pyrimidine
   deficiency) E79.8
  anemia D53.0
Acladiosis (skin) B36.0
Aclasis, diaphyseal Q78.6
Acleistocardia Q21.1
Aclusion — see Anomaly, dentofacial, malocclusion
Acne L70.9
 artificialis L70.8
 atrophica L70.2
 cachecticorum (Hebra) L70.8
 conglobata L70.1
 cystic L70.0
 decalvans L66.2
 excoriée (des jeunes filles) L70.5
 frontalis L70.2
 indurata L70.0
 infantile L70.4
 keloid L73.0
 lupoid L70.2
 necrotic, necrotica (miliaris) L70.2
 neonatal L70.4
 nodular L70.0
 occupational L70.8
 picker's L70.5
 pustular L70.0
 rodens L70.2

Acne - Adenocarcinoma

Acne — *continued*
  rosacea L71.9
  specified NEC L70.8
  tropica L70.3
  varioliformis L70.2
  vulgaris L70.0
Acnitis (primary) A18.4
Acosta's disease T70.29 ☑
Acoustic — *see* condition
Acousticophobia F40.298
Acquired (*see also* condition)
  immunodeficiency syndrome (AIDS) B20
Acrania Q00.0
Acroangiodermatitis I78.9
Acroasphyxia, chronic I73.89
Acrobystitis N47.7
Acrocephalopolysyndactyly Q87.0
Acrocephalosyndactyly Q87.0
Acrocephaly Q75.0
Acrochondrohyperplasia — *see* Syndrome, Marfan's
Acrocyanosis I73.89
  newborn P28.2
    meaning transient blue hands and feet - omit code
Acrodermatitis L30.8
  atrophicans (chronica) L90.4
  continua (Hallopeau) L40.2
  enteropathica (hereditary) E83.2
  Hallopeau's L40.2
  infantile papular L44.4
  perstans L40.2
  pustulosa continua L40.2
  recalcitrant pustular L40.2
Acrodynia — *see* Poisoning, mercury
Acromegaly, acromegalia E22.0
Acromelalgia I73.81
Acromicria, acromikria Q79.8
Acronyx L60.0
Acropachy, thyroid — *see* Thyrotoxicosis
Acroparesthesia (simple) (vasomotor) I73.89
Acropathy, thyroid — *see* Thyrotoxicosis
Acrophobia F40.241
Acroposthitis N47.7
Acroscleriasis, acroscleroderma, acrosclerosis — *see* Sclerosis, systemic
Acrosphacelus I96
Acrospiroma, eccrine — *see* Neoplasm, skin, benign
Acrostealgia — *see* Osteochondropathy
Acrotrophodynia — *see* Immersion
ACTH ectopic syndrome E24.3
Actinic — *see* condition
Actinobacillosis, actinobacillus A28.8
  mallei A24.0
  muris A25.1
Actinomyces israelii (infection) — *see* Actinomycosis
Actinomycetoma (foot) B47.1
Actinomycosis, actinomycotic A42.9
  with pneumonia A42.0
  abdominal A42.1
  cervicofacial A42.2
  cutaneous A42.89
  gastrointestinal A42.1
  pulmonary A42.0
  sepsis A42.7
  specified site NEC A42.89
Actinoneuritis G62.82
Action, heart
  disorder I49.9
  irregular I49.9
    psychogenic F45.8
Activated protein C resistance D68.51
Activation
  mast cell (disorder) (syndrome) D89.40
    idiopathic D89.42
    monoclonal D89.41
    secondary D89.43
    specified type NEC D89.49
Active — *see* condition
Acute (*see also* condition)
  abdomen R10.0
  gallbladder — *see* Cholecystitis, acute
Acyanotic heart disease (congenital) Q24.9
Acystia Q64.5
Adair-Dighton syndrome (brittle bones and blue sclera, deafness) Q78.0
Adamantinoblastoma — *see* Ameloblastoma
Adamantinoma (*see also* Cyst, calcifying odontogenic)
  long bones C40.90
    lower limb C40.2 ☑
    upper limb C40.0 ☑
  malignant C41.1
    jaw (bone) (lower) C41.1
      upper C41.0

Adamantinoma — *continued*
  tibial C40.2 ☑
Adamantoblastoma — *see* Ameloblastoma
Adams-Stokes (-Morgagni) disease or syndrome I45.9
Adaption reaction — *see* Disorder, adjustment
Addiction (*see also* Dependence) F19.20
  alcohol, alcoholic (ethyl) (methyl) (wood) (without remission) F10.20
    with remission F10.21
  drug — *see* Dependence, drug
  ethyl alcohol (without remission) F10.20
    with remission F10.21
  heroin — *see* Dependence, drug, opioid
  methyl alcohol (without remission) F10.20
    with remission F10.21
  methylated spirit (without remission) F10.20
    with remission F10.21
  morphine (-like substances) — *see* Dependence, drug, opioid
  nicotine — *see* Dependence, drug, nicotine
  opium and opioids — *see* Dependence, drug, opioid
  tobacco — *see* Dependence, drug, nicotine
Addisonian crisis E27.2
Addison's
  anemia (pernicious) D51.0
  disease (bronze) or syndrome E27.1
    tuberculous A18.7
  keloid L94.0
Addison-Biermer anemia (pernicious) D51.0
Addison-Schilder complex E71.528
Additional (*see also* Accessory)
  chromosome(s) Q99.8
    sex — *see* Abnormal, chromosome, sex
    21 — *see* Trisomy, 21
Adduction contracture, hip or other joint — *see* Contraction, joint
Adenitis (*see also* Lymphadenitis)
  acute, unspecified site L04.9
  axillary I88.9
    acute L04.2
    chronic or subacute I88.1
  Bartholin's gland N75.8
  bulbourethral gland — *see* Urethritis
  cervical I88.9
    acute L04.0
    chronic or subacute I88.1
  chancroid (Hemophilus ducreyi) A57
  chronic, unspecified site I88.1
  Cowper's gland — *see* Urethritis
  due to Pasteurella multocida (P. septica) A28.0
  epidemic, acute B27.09
  gangrenous L04.9
  gonorrheal NEC A54.89
  groin I88.9
    acute L04.1
    chronic or subacute I88.1
  infectious (acute) (epidemic) B27.09
  inguinal I88.9
    acute L04.1
    chronic or subacute I88.1
  lymph gland or node, except mesenteric I88.9
    acute — *see* Lymphadenitis, acute
    chronic or subacute I88.1
  mesenteric (acute) (chronic) (nonspecific) (subacute) I88.0
  parotid gland (suppurative) — *see* Sialoadenitis
  salivary gland (any) (suppurative) — *see* Sialoadenitis
  scrofulous (tuberculous) A18.2
  Skene's duct or gland — *see* Urethritis
  strumous, tuberculous A18.2
  subacute, unspecified site I88.1
  sublingual gland (suppurative) — *see* Sialoadenitis
  submandibular gland (suppurative) — *see* Sialoadenitis
  submaxillary gland (suppurative) — *see* Sialoadenitis
  tuberculous — *see* Tuberculosis, lymph gland
  urethral gland — *see* Urethritis
  Wharton's duct (suppurative) — *see* Sialoadenitis
Adenoacanthoma — *see* Neoplasm, malignant, by site
Adenoameloblastoma — *see* Cyst, calcifying odontogenic
Adenocarcinoid (tumor) — *see* Neoplasm, malignant, by site
Adenocarcinoma (*see also* Neoplasm, malignant, by site)
  acidophil
    specified site — *see* Neoplasm, malignant, by site
    unspecified site C75.1
  adrenal cortical C74.0 ☑
  alveolar — *see* Neoplasm, lung, malignant

Adenocarcinoma — *continued*
  apocrine
    breast — *see* Neoplasm, breast, malignant
    in situ
      breast D05.8 ☑
      specified site NEC — *see* Neoplasm, skin, in situ
      unspecified site D04.9
    specified site NEC — *see* Neoplasm, skin, malignant
    unspecified site C44.99
  basal cell
    specified site — *see* Neoplasm, skin, malignant
    unspecified site C08.9
  basophil
    specified site — *see* Neoplasm, malignant, by site
    unspecified site C75.1
  bile duct type C22.1
    liver C22.1
    specified site NEC — *see* Neoplasm, malignant, by site
    unspecified site C22.1
  bronchiolar — *see* Neoplasm, lung, malignant
  bronchioloalveolar — *see* Neoplasm, lung, malignant
  ceruminous C44.29 ☑
  cervix, in situ (*see also* Carcinoma, cervix uteri, in situ) D06.9
  chromophobe
    specified site — *see* Neoplasm, malignant, by site
    unspecified site C75.1
  diffuse type
    specified site — *see* Neoplasm, malignant, by site
    unspecified site C16.9
  duct
    infiltrating
      with Paget's disease — *see* Neoplasm, breast, malignant
      specified site — *see* Neoplasm, malignant, by site
      unspecified site (female) C50.91 ☑
        male C50.92 ☑
    specified site — *see* Neoplasm, malignant, by site
    unspecified site
      female C56.9
      male C61
  eosinophil
    specified site — *see* Neoplasm, malignant, by site
    unspecified site C75.1
  follicular
    with papillary C73
    moderately differentiated C73
    specified site — *see* Neoplasm, malignant, by site
    trabecular C73
    unspecified site C73
    well differentiated C73
  Hurthle cell C73
  in
    adenomatous
      polyposis coli C18.9
  infiltrating duct
    with Paget's disease — *see* Neoplasm, breast, malignant
    specified site — *see* Neoplasm, by site, malignant
    unspecified site (female) C50.91 ☑
      male C50.92 ☑
  inflammatory
    specified site — *see* Neoplasm, by site, malignant
    unspecified site (female) C50.91 ☑
      male C50.92 ☑
  intestinal type
    specified site — *see* Neoplasm, malignant, by site
    unspecified site C16.9
  intracystic papillary
  intraductal
    breast D05.1 ☑
    noninfiltrating
      breast D05.1 ☑
    papillary
      with invasion
        specified site — *see* Neoplasm, by site, malignant
        unspecified site (female) C50.91 ☑
          male C50.92 ☑
      breast D05.1 ☑
      specified site NEC — *see* Neoplasm, in situ, by site
      unspecified site D05.1 ☑
    specified site NEC — *see* Neoplasm, in situ, by site
    unspecified site D05.1 ☑
  papillary
    with invasion

☑ **Additional character required**

Adenocarcinoma — *continued*
  intraductal — *continued*
      specified site — *see* Neoplasm, malignant, by site
      unspecified site (female) C50.91 ☑
        male C50.92 ☑
    breast D05.1 ☑
    specified site — *see* Neoplasm, in situ, by site
    unspecified site D05.1 ☑
    specified site NEC — *see* Neoplasm, in situ, by site
    unspecified site D05.1 ☑
  islet cell
    with exocrine, mixed
      specified site — *see* Neoplasm, malignant, by site
      unspecified site C25.9
    pancreas C25.4
    specified site NEC — *see* Neoplasm, malignant, by site
    unspecified site C25.4
  lobular
    in situ
      breast D05.0 ☑
      specified site NEC — *see* Neoplasm, in situ, by site
      unspecified site D05.0 ☑
    specified site — *see* Neoplasm, malignant, by site
    unspecified site (female) C50.91 ☑
      male C50.92 ☑
  mucoid (*see also* Neoplasm, malignant, by site)
    cell
      specified site — *see* Neoplasm, malignant, by site
      unspecified site C75.1
  nonencapsulated sclerosing C73
  papillary
    with follicular C73
    follicular variant C73
    intraductal (noninfiltrating)
      with invasion
        specified site — *see* Neoplasm, malignant, by site
        unspecified site (female) C50.91 ☑
          male C50.92 ☑
      breast D05.1 ☑
      specified site NEC — *see* Neoplasm, in situ, by site
      unspecified site D05.1 ☑
  serous
    specified site — *see* Neoplasm, malignant, by site
    unspecified site C56.9
  papillocystic
    specified site — *see* Neoplasm, malignant, by site
    unspecified site C56.9
  pseudomucinous
    specified site — *see* Neoplasm, malignant, by site
    unspecified site C56.9
  renal cell C64 ☑
  sebaceous — *see* Neoplasm, skin, malignant
  serous (*see also* Neoplasm, malignant, by site)
    papillary
      specified site — *see* Neoplasm, malignant, by site
      unspecified site C56.9
  sweat gland — *see* Neoplasm, skin, malignant
  water-clear cell C75.0
Adenocarcinoma-in-situ (*see also* Neoplasm, in situ, by site)
  breast D05.9 ☑
Adenofibroma
  clear cell — *see* Neoplasm, benign, by site
  endometrioid D27.9
    borderline malignancy D39.10
    malignant C56 ☑
  mucinous
    specified site — *see* Neoplasm, benign, by site
    unspecified site D27.9
  papillary
    specified site — *see* Neoplasm, benign, by site
    unspecified site D27.9
  prostate — *see* Enlargement, enlarged, prostate
  serous
    specified site — *see* Neoplasm, benign, by site
    unspecified site D27.9
  specified site — *see* Neoplasm, benign, by site
  unspecified site D27.9
Adenofibrosis
  breast — *see* Fibroadenosis, breast
  endometrioid N80.0
Adenoiditis (chronic) J35.02
  with tonsillitis J35.03

Adenoiditis — *continued*
  acute J03.90
    recurrent J03.91
    specified organism NEC J03.80
      recurrent J03.81
    staphylococcal J03.80
      recurrent J03.81
    streptococcal J03.00
      recurrent J03.01
Adenoids — *see* condition
Adenolipoma — *see* Neoplasm, benign, by site
Adenolipomatosis, Launois-Bensaude E88.89
Adenolymphoma
  specified site — *see* Neoplasm, benign, by site
  unspecified site D11.9
Adenoma (*see also* Neoplasm, benign, by site)
  acidophil
    specified site — *see* Neoplasm, benign, by site
    unspecified site D35.2
  acidophil-basophil, mixed
    specified site — *see* Neoplasm, benign, by site
    unspecified site D35.2
  adrenal (cortical) D35.00
    clear cell D35.00
    compact cell D35.00
    glomerulosa cell D35.00
    heavily pigmented variant D35.00
    mixed cell D35.00
  alpha-cell
    pancreas D13.7
    specified site NEC — *see* Neoplasm, benign, by site
    unspecified site D13.7
  alveolar D14.30
  apocrine
    breast D24 ☑
    specified site NEC — *see* Neoplasm, skin, benign, by site
    unspecified site D23.9
  basal cell D11.9
  basophil
    specified site — *see* Neoplasm, benign, by site
    unspecified site D35.2
  basophil-acidophil, mixed
    specified site — *see* Neoplasm, benign, by site
    unspecified site D35.2
  beta-cell
    pancreas D13.7
    specified site NEC — *see* Neoplasm, benign, by site
    unspecified site D13.7
  bile duct D13.4
    common D13.5
    extrahepatic D13.5
    intrahepatic D13.4
    specified site NEC — *see* Neoplasm, benign, by site
    unspecified site D13.4
  black D35.00
  bronchial D38.1
    cylindroid type — *see* Neoplasm, lung, malignant
  ceruminous D23.2 ☑
  chief cell D35.1
  chromophobe
    specified site — *see* Neoplasm, benign, by site
    unspecified site D35.2
  colloid
    specified site — *see* Neoplasm, benign, by site
    unspecified site D34
  duct
  eccrine, papillary — *see* Neoplasm, skin, benign
  endocrine, multiple
    single specified site — *see* Neoplasm, uncertain behavior, by site
    two or more specified sites D44 ☑
    unspecified site D44.9
  endometrioid (*see also* Neoplasm, benign)
    borderline malignancy — *see* Neoplasm, uncertain behavior, by site
  eosinophil
    specified site — *see* Neoplasm, benign, by site
    unspecified site D35.2
  fetal
    specified site — *see* Neoplasm, benign, by site
    unspecified site D34
  follicular
    specified site — *see* Neoplasm, benign, by site
    unspecified site D34
  hepatocellular D13.4
  Hurthle cell D34
  islet cell
    pancreas D13.7

Adenoma — *continued*
  islet cell — *continued*
    specified site NEC — *see* Neoplasm, benign, by site
    unspecified site D13.7
  liver cell D13.4
  macrofollicular
    specified site — *see* Neoplasm, benign, by site
    unspecified site D34
  malignant, malignum — *see* Neoplasm, malignant, by site
  microcystic
    pancreas D13.6
    specified site NEC — *see* Neoplasm, benign, by site
    unspecified site D13.6
  microfollicular
    specified site — *see* Neoplasm, benign, by site
    unspecified site D34
  mucoid cell
    specified site — *see* Neoplasm, benign, by site
    unspecified site D35.2
  multiple endocrine
    single specified site — *see* Neoplasm, uncertain behavior, by site
    two or more specified sites D44 ☑
    unspecified site D44.9
  nipple D24 ☑
  papillary (*see also* Neoplasm, benign, by site)
    eccrine — *see* Neoplasm, skin, benign, by site
  Pick's tubular
    specified site — *see* Neoplasm, benign, by site
    unspecified site
      female D27.9
      male D29.20
  pleomorphic
    carcinoma in — *see* Neoplasm, salivary gland, malignant
    specified site — *see* Neoplasm, malignant, by site
    unspecified site C08.9
  polypoid (*see also* Neoplasm, benign)
    adenocarcinoma in — *see* Neoplasm, malignant, by site
    adenocarcinoma in situ — *see* Neoplasm, in situ, by site
  prostate — *see* Neoplasm, benign, prostate
  rete cell D29.20
  sebaceous — *see* Neoplasm, skin, benign
  Sertoli cell
    specified site — *see* Neoplasm, benign, by site
    unspecified site
      female D27.9
      male D29.20
  skin appendage — *see* Neoplasm, skin, benign
  sudoriferous gland — *see* Neoplasm, skin, benign
  sweat gland — *see* Neoplasm, skin, benign
  testicular
    specified site — *see* Neoplasm, benign, by site
    unspecified site
      female D27.9
      male D29.20
  tubular (*see also* Neoplasm, benign, by site)
    adenocarcinoma in — *see* Neoplasm, malignant, by site
    adenocarcinoma in situ — *see* Neoplasm, in situ, by site
    Pick's
      specified site — *see* Neoplasm, benign, by site
      unspecified site
        female D27.9
        male D29.20
  tubulovillous (*see also* Neoplasm, benign, by site)
    adenocarcinoma in — *see* Neoplasm, malignant, by site
    adenocarcinoma in situ — *see* Neoplasm, in situ, by site
  villous — *see* Neoplasm, uncertain behavior, by site
    adenocarcinoma in — *see* Neoplasm, malignant, by site
    adenocarcinoma in situ — *see* Neoplasm, in situ, by site
  water-clear cell D35.1
Adenomatosis
  endocrine (multiple) E31.20
    single specified site — *see* Neoplasm, uncertain behavior, by site
  erosive of nipple D24 ☑
  pluriendocrine — *see* Adenomatosis, endocrine
  pulmonary D38.1
    malignant — *see* Neoplasm, lung, malignant
  specified site — *see* Neoplasm, benign, by site
  unspecified site D12.6

Adenomatous - Admission

Adenomatous
  goiter (nontoxic) E04.9
    with hyperthyroidism — *see* Hyperthyroidism,
      with, goiter, nodular
    toxic — *see* Hyperthyroidism, with, goiter,
      nodular
Adenomyoma (*see also* Neoplasm, benign, by site)
  prostate — *see* Enlarged, prostate
Adenomyometritis N80.0
Adenomyosis N80.0
Adenopathy (lymph gland) R59.9
  generalized R59.1
  inguinal R59.0
  localized R59.0
  mediastinal R59.0
  mesentery R59.0
  syphilitic (secondary) A51.49
  tracheobronchial R59.0
    tuberculous A15.4
      primary (progressive) A15.7
  tuberculous (*see also* Tuberculosis, lymph gland)
    tracheobronchial A15.4
      primary (progressive) A15.7
Adenosalpingitis — *see* Salpingitis
Adenosarcoma — *see* Neoplasm, malignant, by site
Adenosclerosis I88.8
Adenosis (sclerosing) breast — *see* Fibroadenosis,
  breast
Adenovirus, as cause of disease classified elsewhere
  B97.0
Adentia (complete) (partial) — *see* Absence, teeth
Adherent (*see also* Adhesions)
  labia (minora) N90.89
  pericardium (nonrheumatic) I31.0
    rheumatic I09.2
  placenta (with hemorrhage) O72.0
    without hemorrhage O73.0
  prepuce, newborn N47.0
  scar (skin) L90.5
  tendon in scar L90.5
Adhesions, adhesive (postinfective) K66.0
  with intestinal obstruction K56.50
    complete K56.52
    incomplete K56.51
    partial K56.51
  abdominal (wall) — *see* Adhesions, peritoneum
  appendix K38.8
  bile duct (common) (hepatic) K83.8
  bladder (sphincter) N32.89
  bowel — *see* Adhesions, peritoneum
  cardiac I31.0
    rheumatic I09.2
  cecum — *see* Adhesions, peritoneum
  cervicovaginal N88.1
    congenital Q52.8
    postpartal O90.89
      old N88.1
  cervix N88.1
  ciliary body NEC — *see* Adhesions, iris
  clitoris N90.89
  colon — *see* Adhesions, peritoneum
  common duct K83.8
  congenital (*see also* Anomaly, by site)
    fingers — *see* Syndactylism, complex, fingers
    omental, anomalous Q43.3
    peritoneal Q43.3
    tongue (to gum or roof of mouth) Q38.3
  conjunctiva (acquired) H11.21 ☑
    congenital Q15.8
  cystic duct K82.8
  diaphragm — *see* Adhesions, peritoneum
  due to foreign body — *see* Foreign body
  duodenum — *see* Adhesions, peritoneum
  ear
    middle H74.1 ☑
  epididymis N50.89
  epidural — *see* Adhesions, meninges
  epiglottis J38.7
  eyelid H02.59
  female pelvis N73.6
  gallbladder K82.8
  globe H44.89
  heart I31.0
    rheumatic I09.2
  ileocecal (coil) — *see* Adhesions, peritoneum
  ileum — *see* Adhesions, peritoneum
  intestine (*see also* Adhesions, peritoneum)
    with obstruction K56.50
      complete K56.52
      incomplete K56.51
      partial K56.51
  intra-abdominal — *see* Adhesions, peritoneum

Adhesions — *continued*
  iris H21.50 ☑
    anterior H21.51 ☑
    goniosynechiae H21.52 ☑
    posterior H21.54 ☑
    to corneal graft T85.898 ☑
  joint — *see* Ankylosis
    knee M23.8X ☑
    temporomandibular M26.61 ☑
  labium (majus) (minus), congenital Q52.5
  liver — *see* Adhesions, peritoneum
  lung J98.4
  mediastinum J98.59
  meninges (cerebral) (spinal) G96.12
    congenital Q07.8
    tuberculous (cerebral) (spinal) A17.0
  mesenteric — *see* Adhesions, peritoneum
  nasal (septum) (to turbinates) J34.89
  ocular muscle — *see* Strabismus, mechanical
  omentum — *see* Adhesions, peritoneum
  ovary N73.6
    congenital (to cecum, kidney or omentum)
      Q50.39
  paraovarian N73.6
  pelvic (peritoneal)
    female N73.6
      postprocedural N99.4
    male — *see* Adhesions, peritoneum
    postpartal (old) N73.6
    tuberculous A18.17
  penis to scrotum (congenital) Q55.8
  periappendiceal (*see also* Adhesions, peritoneum)
  perigastric (nonrheumatic) I31.0
    focal I31.8
    rheumatic I09.2
    tuberculous A18.84
  pericholecystic K82.8
  perigastric — *see* Adhesions, peritoneum
  periovarian N73.6
  periprostatic N42.89
  perirectal — *see* Adhesions, peritoneum
  perirenal N28.89
  peritoneum, peritoneal (postinfective) K66.0
    with obstruction (intestinal) K56.50
      complete K56.52
      incomplete K56.51
      partial K56.51
    congenital Q43.3
    pelvic, female N73.6
      postprocedural N99.4
    postpartal, pelvic N73.6
    postprocedural K66.0
    to uterus N73.6
  peritubal N73.6
  periureteral N28.89
  periuterine N73.6
  perivesical N32.89
  perivesicular (seminal vesicle) N50.89
  pleura, pleuritic J94.8
    tuberculous NEC A15.6
  pleuropericardial J94.8
  postoperative (gastrointestinal tract) K66.0
    with obstruction (*see also* Obstruction, intestine,
      postoperative) K91.30
    due to foreign body accidentally left in wound
      — *see* Foreign body, accidentally left during
      a procedure
    pelvic peritoneal N99.4
    urethra — *see* Stricture, urethra, postprocedural
    vagina N99.2
  postpartal, old (vulva or perineum) N90.89
  preputial, prepuce N47.5
  pulmonary J98.4
  pylorus — *see* Adhesions, peritoneum
  sciatic nerve — *see* Lesion, nerve, sciatic
  seminal vesicle N50.89
  shoulder (joint) — *see* Capsulitis, adhesive
  sigmoid flexure — *see* Adhesions, peritoneum
  spermatic cord (acquired) N50.89
    congenital Q55.4
  spinal canal G96.12
  stomach — *see* Adhesions, peritoneum
  subscapular — *see* Capsulitis, adhesive
  temporomandibular M26.61 ☑
  tendinitis (*see also* Tenosynovitis, specified type
    NEC)
    shoulder — *see* Capsulitis, adhesive
  testis N44.8
  tongue, congenital (to gum or roof of mouth) Q38.3
    acquired K14.8
  trachea J39.8
  tubo-ovarian N73.6

Adhesions — *continued*
  tunica vaginalis N44.8
  uterus N73.6
    internal N85.6
    to abdominal wall N73.6
  vagina (chronic) N89.5
    postoperative N99.2
  vitreomacular H43.82 ☑
  vitreous H43.89
  vulva N90.89
Adiaspiromycosis B48.8
Adie (-Holmes) pupil or syndrome — *see* Anomaly,
  pupil, function, tonic pupil
Adiponecrosis neonatorum P83.88
Adiposis (*see also* Obesity)
  cerebralis E23.6
  dolorosa E88.2
Adiposity (*see also* Obesity)
  heart — *see* Degeneration, myocardial
  localized E65
Adiposogenital dystrophy E23.6
Adjustment
  disorder — *see* Disorder, adjustment
  implanted device — *see* Encounter (for), adjustment
    (of)
  prosthesis, external — *see* Fitting
  reaction — *see* Disorder, adjustment
Administration of tPA (rtPA) in a different facility
  within the last 24 hours prior to admission to current
  facility Z92.82
Admission (for) (*see also* Encounter (for))
  adjustment (of)
    artificial
      arm Z44.00 ☑
        complete Z44.01 ☑
        partial Z44.02 ☑
      eye Z44.2 ☑
      leg Z44.10 ☑
        complete Z44.11 ☑
        partial Z44.12 ☑
    brain neuropacemaker Z46.2
      implanted Z45.42
    breast
      implant Z45.81 ☑
      prosthesis (external) Z44.3 ☑
    colostomy belt Z46.89
    contact lenses Z46.0
    cystostomy device Z46.6
    dental prosthesis Z46.3
    device NEC
      abdominal Z46.89
      implanted Z45.89
        cardiac Z45.09
          defibrillator (with synchronous cardiac
            pacemaker) Z45.02
          pacemaker (cardiac resynchronization
            therapy (CRT-P)) Z45.018
          pulse generator Z45.010
          resynchronization therapy defibrillator
            (CRT-D) Z45.02
        hearing device Z45.328
          bone conduction Z45.320
          cochlear Z45.321
        infusion pump Z45.1
        nervous system Z45.49
          CSF drainage Z45.41
          hearing device — *see* Admission,
            adjustment, device, implanted, hearing
            device
          neuropacemaker Z45.42
          visual substitution Z45.31
        specified NEC Z45.89
        vascular access Z45.2
        visual substitution Z45.31
    nervous system Z46.2
      implanted — *see* Admission, adjustment,
        device, implanted, nervous system
    orthodontic Z46.4
    prosthetic Z44.9
      arm — *see* Admission, adjustment, artificial,
        arm
      breast Z44.3 ☑
      dental Z46.3
      eye Z44.2 ☑
      leg — *see* Admission, adjustment, artificial,
        leg
      specified type NEC Z44.8
    substitution
      auditory Z46.2
        implanted — *see* Admission, adjustment,
          device, implanted, hearing device
      nervous system Z46.2

☑ **Additional character required**

Admission — *continued*
  adjustment — *continued*
      implanted — *see* Admission, adjustment, device, implanted, nervous system
      visual Z46.2
        implanted Z45.31
    urinary Z46.6
    hearing aid Z46.1
      implanted — *see* Admission, adjustment, device, implanted, hearing device
    ileostomy device Z46.89
    intestinal appliance or device NEC Z46.89
    neuropacemaker (brain) (peripheral nerve) (spinal cord) Z46.2
      implanted Z45.42
    orthodontic device Z46.4
    orthopedic (brace) (cast) (device) (shoes) Z46.89
    pacemaker (cardiac resynchronization therapy (CRT-P))
      cardiac Z45.018
        pulse generator Z45.010
      nervous system Z46.2
        implanted Z45.42
    portacath (port-a-cath) Z45.2
    prosthesis Z44.9
      arm — *see* Admission, adjustment, artificial, arm
      breast Z44.3 ☑
      dental Z46.3
      eye Z44.2 ☑
      leg — *see* Admission, adjustment, artificial, leg
      specified NEC Z44.8
    spectacles Z46.0
  aftercare (*see also* Aftercare) Z51.89
    postpartum
      immediately after delivery Z39.0
      routine follow-up Z39.2
    radiation therapy (antineoplastic) Z51.0
  attention to artificial opening (of) Z43.9
    artificial vagina Z43.7
    colostomy Z43.3
    cystostomy Z43.5
    enterostomy Z43.4
    gastrostomy Z43.1
    ileostomy Z43.2
    jejunostomy Z43.4
    nephrostomy Z43.6
    specified site NEC Z43.8
      intestinal tract Z43.4
      urinary tract Z43.6
    tracheostomy Z43.0
    ureterostomy Z43.6
    urethrostomy Z43.6
  breast augmentation or reduction Z41.1
  breast reconstruction following mastectomy Z42.1
  change of
    dressing (nonsurgical) Z48.00
    neuropacemaker device (brain) (peripheral nerve) (spinal cord) Z46.2
      implanted Z45.42
    surgical dressing Z48.01
  circumcision, ritual or routine (in absence of diagnosis) Z41.2
  clinical research investigation (control) (normal comparison) (participant) Z00.6
  contraceptive management Z30.9
  cosmetic surgery NEC Z41.1
  counseling (*see also* Counseling)
    dietary Z71.3
    gestational carrier Z31.7
    HIV Z71.7
    human immunodeficiency virus Z71.7
    nonattending third party Z71.0
    procreative management NEC Z31.69
  delivery, full-term, uncomplicated O80
    cesarean, without indication O82
  desensitization to allergens Z51.6
  dietary surveillance and counseling Z71.3
  ear piercing Z41.3
  examination at health care facility (adult) (*see also* Examination) Z00.00
    with abnormal findings Z00.01
    clinical research investigation (control) (normal comparison) (participant) Z00.6
    dental Z01.20
      with abnormal findings Z01.21
    donor (potential) Z00.5
    ear Z01.10
      with abnormal findings NEC Z01.118
    eye Z01.00
      with abnormal findings Z01.01
      following failed vision screening Z01.020
        with abnormal findings Z01.021

Admission — *continued*
  examination at health care facility — *continued*
    general, specified reason NEC Z00.8
    hearing Z01.10
      with abnormal findings NEC Z01.118
      infant or child (over 28 days old) Z00.129
        with abnormal findings Z00.121
    postpartum checkup Z39.2
    psychiatric (general) Z00.8
      requested by authority Z04.6
    vision Z01.00
      with abnormal findings Z01.01
      following failed vision screening Z01.020
        with abnormal findings Z01.021
      infant or child (over 28 days old) Z00.129
        with abnormal findings Z00.121
  fitting (of)
    artificial
      arm — *see* Admission, adjustment, artificial, arm
      eye Z44.2 ☑
      leg — *see* Admission, adjustment, artificial, leg
    brain neuropacemaker Z46.2
      implanted Z45.42
    breast prosthesis (external) Z44.3 ☑
    colostomy belt Z46.89
    contact lenses Z46.0
    cystostomy device Z46.6
    dental prosthesis Z46.3
    dentures Z46.3
    device NEC
      abdominal Z46.89
      nervous system Z46.2
        implanted — *see* Admission, adjustment, device, implanted, nervous system
      orthodontic Z46.4
      prosthetic Z44.9
        breast Z44.3 ☑
        dental Z46.3
        eye Z44.2 ☑
      substitution
        auditory Z46.2
          implanted — *see* Admission, adjustment, device, implanted, hearing device
        nervous system Z46.2
          implanted — *see* Admission, adjustment, device, implanted, nervous system
        visual Z46.2
          implanted Z45.31
    hearing aid Z46.1
    ileostomy device Z46.89
    intestinal appliance or device NEC Z46.89
    neuropacemaker (brain) (peripheral nerve) (spinal cord) Z46.2
      implanted Z45.42
    orthodontic device Z46.4
    orthopedic device (brace) (cast) (shoes) Z46.89
    prosthesis Z44.9
      arm — *see* Admission, adjustment, artificial, arm
      breast Z44.3 ☑
      dental Z46.3
      eye Z44.2 ☑
      leg — *see* Admission, adjustment, artificial, leg
      specified type NEC Z44.8
    spectacles Z46.0
  follow-up examination Z09
  intrauterine device management Z30.431
    initial prescription Z30.014
  mental health evaluation Z00.8
    requested by authority Z04.6
  observation — *see* Observation
  Papanicolaou smear, cervix Z12.4
    for suspected malignant neoplasm Z12.4
  plastic and reconstructive surgery following medical procedure or healed injury NEC Z42.8
  plastic surgery, cosmetic NEC Z41.1
  postpartum observation
    immediately after delivery Z39.0
    routine follow-up Z39.2
  poststerilization (for restoration) Z31.0
    aftercare Z31.42
  procreative management Z31.9
  prophylactic (measure) (*see also* Encounter, prophylactic measures)
    organ removal Z40.00
      breast Z40.01
      fallopian tube(s) Z40.03
        with ovary(s) Z40.02
      ovary(s) Z40.02
      specified organ NEC Z40.09
      testes Z40.09
  vaccination Z23

Admission — *continued*
  psychiatric examination (general) Z00.8
    requested by authority Z04.6
  radiation therapy (antineoplastic) Z51.0
  reconstructive surgery following medical procedure or healed injury NEC Z42.8
  removal of
    cystostomy catheter Z43.5
    drains Z48.03
    dressing (nonsurgical) Z48.00
    implantable subdermal contraceptive Z30.46
    intrauterine contraceptive device Z30.432
    neuropacemaker (brain) (peripheral nerve) (spinal cord) Z46.2
      implanted Z45.42
    staples Z48.02
    surgical dressing Z48.01
    sutures Z48.02
    ureteral stent Z46.6
  respirator [ventilator] use during power failure Z99.12
  restoration of organ continuity (poststerilization) Z31.0
    aftercare Z31.42
  sensitivity test (*see also* Test, skin)
    allergy NEC Z01.82
    Mantoux Z11.1
  tuboplasty following previous sterilization Z31.0
    aftercare Z31.42
  vasoplasty following previous sterilization Z31.0
    aftercare Z31.42
  vision examination Z01.00
    with abnormal findings Z01.01
    following failed vision screening Z01.020
      with abnormal findings Z01.021
    infant or child (over 28 days old) Z00.129
      with abnormal findings Z00.121
  waiting period for admission to other facility Z75.1
Adnexitis (suppurative) — *see* Salpingo-oophoritis
Adolescent X-linked adrenoleukodystrophy E71.521
Adrenal (gland) — *see* condition
Adrenalism, tuberculous A18.7
Adrenalitis, adrenitis E27.8
  autoimmune E27.1
  meningococcal, hemorrhagic A39.1
Adrenarche, premature E27.0
Adrenocortical syndrome — *see* Cushing's, syndrome
Adrenogenital syndrome E25.9
  acquired E25.8
  congenital E25.0
  salt loss E25.0
Adrenogenitalism, congenital E25.0
Adrenoleukodystrophy E71.529
  neonatal E71.511
  X-linked E71.529
    Addison only phenotype E71.528
    Addison-Schilder E71.528
    adolescent E71.521
    adrenomyeloneuropathy E71.522
    childhood cerebral E71.520
    other specified E71.528
Adrenomyeloneuropathy E71.522
Adventitious bursa — *see* Bursopathy, specified type NEC
Adverse effect — *see* Table of Drugs and Chemicals, categories T36-T50, with 6th character 5
Advice — *see* Counseling
Adynamia (episodica) (hereditary) (periodic) G72.3
Aeration lung imperfect, newborn — *see* Atelectasis
Aerobullosis T70.3 ☑
Aerocele — *see* Embolism, air
Aerodermectasia
  subcutaneous (traumatic) T79.7 ☑
Aerodontalgia T70.29 ☑
Aeroembolism T70.3 ☑
Aerogenes capsulatus infection A48.0
Aero-otitis media T70.0 ☑
Aerophagy, aerophagia (psychogenic) F45.8
Aerophobia F40.228
Aerosinusitis T70.1 ☑
Aerotitis T70.0 ☑
Affection — *see* Disease
Afibrinogenemia (*see also* Defect, coagulation) D68.8
  acquired D65
  congenital D68.2
  following ectopic or molar pregnancy O08.1
  in abortion — *see* Abortion, by type, complicated by, afibrinogenemia
  puerperal O72.3
African
  sleeping sickness B56.9
  tick fever A68.1

African - Agenesis

African — *continued*
- trypanosomiasis B56.9
  - gambian B56.0
  - rhodesian B56.1
- **Aftercare** (*see also* Care) Z51.89
  - following surgery (for) (on)
    - amputation Z47.81
    - attention to
      - drains Z48.03
      - dressings (nonsurgical) Z48.00
        - surgical Z48.01
      - sutures Z48.02
    - circulatory system Z48.812
    - delayed (planned) wound closure Z48.1
    - digestive system Z48.815
    - explantation of joint prosthesis (staged procedure)
      - hip Z47.32
      - knee Z47.33
      - shoulder Z47.31
    - genitourinary system Z48.816
    - joint replacement Z47.1
    - neoplasm Z48.3
    - nervous system Z48.811
    - oral cavity Z48.814
    - organ transplant
      - bone marrow Z48.290
      - heart Z48.21
      - heart-lung Z48.280
      - kidney Z48.22
      - liver Z48.23
      - lung Z48.24
      - multiple organs NEC Z48.288
      - specified NEC Z48.298
    - orthopedic NEC Z47.89
    - planned wound closure Z48.1
    - removal of internal fixation device Z47.2
    - respiratory system Z48.813
    - scoliosis Z47.82
    - sense organs Z48.810
    - skin and subcutaneous tissue Z48.817
    - specified body system
      - circulatory Z48.812
      - digestive Z48.815
      - genitourinary Z48.816
      - nervous Z48.811
      - oral cavity Z48.814
      - respiratory Z48.813
      - sense organs Z48.810
      - skin and subcutaneous tissue Z48.817
      - teeth Z48.814
    - specified NEC Z48.89
    - spinal Z47.89
    - teeth Z48.814
  - fracture - code to fracture with seventh character D
  - involving
    - removal of
      - drains Z48.03
      - dressings (nonsurgical) Z48.00
      - staples Z48.02
      - surgical dressings Z48.01
      - sutures Z48.02
  - neuropacemaker (brain) (peripheral nerve) (spinal cord) Z46.2
    - implanted Z45.42
  - orthopedic NEC Z47.89
  - postprocedural — *see* Aftercare, following surgery
- **After-cataract** — *see* Cataract, secondary
- **Agalactia** (primary) O92.3
  - elective, secondary or therapeutic O92.5
- **Agammaglobulinemia** (acquired (secondary)) (nonfamilial) D80.1
  - with
    - immunoglobulin-bearing B-lymphocytes D80.1
    - lymphopenia D81.9
  - autosomal recessive (Swiss type) D80.0
  - Bruton's X-linked D80.0
  - common variable (CVAgamma) D80.1
  - congenital sex-linked D80.0
  - hereditary D80.0
  - lymphopenic D81.9
  - Swiss type (autosomal recessive) D80.0
  - X-linked (with growth hormone deficiency) (Bruton) D80.0
- **Aganglionosis** (bowel) (colon) Q43.1
- **Age** (old) — *see* Senility
- **Agenesis**
  - adrenal (gland) Q89.1
  - alimentary tract (complete) (partial) NEC Q45.8
    - upper Q40.8
  - anus, anal (canal) Q42.3
    - with fistula Q42.2

Agenesis — *continued*
- aorta Q25.41
- appendix Q42.8
- arm (complete) Q71.0 ☑
  - with hand present Q71.1 ☑
- artery (peripheral) Q27.9
  - brain Q28.3
  - coronary Q24.5
  - pulmonary Q25.79
  - specified NEC Q27.8
  - umbilical Q27.0
- auditory (canal) (external) Q16.1
- auricle (ear) Q16.0
- bile duct or passage Q44.5
- bladder Q64.5
- bone Q79.9
- brain Q00.0
  - part of Q04.3
- breast (with nipple present) Q83.8
  - with absent nipple Q83.0
- bronchus Q32.4
- canaliculus lacrimalis Q10.4
- carpus — *see* Agenesis, hand
- cartilage Q79.9
- cecum Q42.8
- cerebellum Q04.3
- cervix Q51.5
- chin Q18.8
- cilia Q10.3
- circulatory system, part NOS Q28.9
- clavicle Q74.0
- clitoris Q52.6
- coccyx Q76.49
- colon Q42.9
  - specified NEC Q42.8
- corpus callosum Q04.0
- cricoid cartilage Q31.8
- diaphragm (with hernia) Q79.1
- digestive organ(s) or tract (complete) (partial) NEC Q45.8
  - upper Q40.8
- ductus arteriosus Q28.8
- duodenum Q41.0
- ear Q16.9
  - auricle Q16.0
  - lobe Q17.8
- ejaculatory duct Q55.4
- endocrine (gland) NEC Q89.2
- epiglottis Q31.8
- esophagus Q39.8
- eustachian tube Q16.2
- eye Q11.1
  - adnexa Q15.8
- eyelid (fold) Q10.3
- face
  - bones NEC Q75.8
  - specified part NEC Q18.8
- fallopian tube Q50.6
- femur — *see* Defect, reduction, lower limb, longitudinal, femur
- fibula — *see* Defect, reduction, lower limb, longitudinal, fibula
- finger (complete) (partial) — *see* Agenesis, hand
- foot (and toes) (complete) (partial) Q72.3 ☑
- forearm (with hand present) — *see* Agenesis, arm, with hand present
  - and hand Q71.2 ☑
- gallbladder Q44.0
- gastric Q40.2
- genitalia, genital (organ(s))
  - female Q52.8
    - external Q52.71
    - internal NEC Q52.8
  - male Q55.8
- glottis Q31.8
- hair Q84.0
- hand (and fingers) (complete) (partial) Q71.3 ☑
- heart Q24.8
  - valve NEC Q24.8
    - pulmonary Q22.0
- hepatic Q44.7
- humerus — *see* Defect, reduction, upper limb
- hymen Q52.4
- ileum Q41.2
- incus Q16.3
- intestine (small) Q41.9
  - large Q42.9
    - specified NEC Q42.8
- iris (dilator fibers) Q13.1
- jaw M26.09
- jejunum Q41.1
- kidney(s) (partial) Q60.2

Agenesis — *continued*
- kidney(s) — *continued*
  - bilateral Q60.1
  - unilateral Q60.0
- labium (majus) (minus) Q52.71
- labyrinth, membranous Q16.5
- lacrimal apparatus Q10.4
- larynx Q31.8
- leg (complete) Q72.0 ☑
  - with foot present Q72.1 ☑
  - lower leg (with foot present) — *see* Agenesis, leg, with foot present
    - and foot Q72.2 ☑
- lens Q12.3
- limb (complete) Q73.0
  - lower — *see* Agenesis, leg
  - upper — *see* Agenesis, arm
- lip Q38.0
- liver Q44.7
- lung (fissure) (lobe) (bilateral) (unilateral) Q33.3
- mandible, maxilla M26.09
- metacarpus — *see* Agenesis, hand
- metatarsus — *see* Agenesis, foot
- muscle Q79.8
  - eyelid Q10.3
  - ocular Q15.8
- musculoskeletal system NEC Q79.8
- nail(s) Q84.3
- neck, part Q18.8
- nerve Q07.8
- nervous system, part NEC Q07.8
- nipple Q83.2
- nose Q30.1
- nuclear Q07.8
- organ
  - of Corti Q16.5
  - or site not listed — *see* Anomaly, by site
- osseous meatus (ear) Q16.1
- ovary
  - bilateral Q50.02
  - unilateral Q50.01
- oviduct Q50.6
- pancreas Q45.0
- parathyroid (gland) Q89.2
- parotid gland(s) Q38.4
- patella Q74.1
- pelvic girdle (complete) (partial) Q74.2
- penis Q55.5
- pericardium Q24.8
- pituitary (gland) Q89.2
- prostate Q55.4
- punctum lacrimale Q10.4
- radioulnar — *see* Defect, reduction, upper limb
- radius — *see* Defect, reduction, upper limb, longitudinal, radius
- rectum Q42.1
  - with fistula Q42.0
- renal Q60.2
  - bilateral Q60.1
  - unilateral Q60.0
- respiratory organ NEC Q34.8
- rib Q76.6
- roof of orbit Q75.8
- round ligament Q52.8
- sacrum Q76.49
- salivary gland Q38.4
- scapula Q74.0
- scrotum Q55.29
- seminal vesicles Q55.4
- septum
  - atrial Q21.1
  - between aorta and pulmonary artery Q21.4
  - ventricular Q20.4
- shoulder girdle (complete) (partial) Q74.0
- skull (bone) Q75.8
  - with
    - anencephaly Q00.0
    - encephalocele — *see* Encephalocele
    - hydrocephalus Q03.9
      - with spina bifida — *see* Spina bifida, by site, with hydrocephalus
    - microcephaly Q02
- spermatic cord Q55.4
- spinal cord Q06.0
- spine Q76.49
- spleen Q89.01
- sternum Q76.7
- stomach Q40.2
- submaxillary gland(s) (congenital) Q38.4
- tarsus — *see* Agenesis, foot
- tendon Q79.8
- testicle Q55.0

☑ **Additional character required**

Agenesis — *continued*
  thymus (gland) Q89.2
  thyroid (gland) E03.1
    cartilage Q31.8
  tibia — *see* Defect, reduction, lower limb,
    longitudinal, tibia
  tibiofibular — *see* Defect, reduction, lower limb,
    specified type NEC
  toe (and foot) (complete) (partial) — *see* Agenesis,
    foot
  tongue Q38.3
  trachea (cartilage) Q32.1
  ulna — *see* Defect, reduction, upper limb,
    longitudinal, ulna
  upper limb — *see* Agenesis, arm
  ureter Q62.4
  urethra Q64.5
  urinary tract NEC Q64.8
  uterus Q51.0
  uvula Q38.5
  vagina Q52.0
  vas deferens Q55.4
  vein(s) (peripheral) Q27.9
    brain Q28.3
    great NEC Q26.8
    portal Q26.5
  vena cava (inferior) (superior) Q26.8
  vermis of cerebellum Q04.3
  vertebra Q76.49
  vulva Q52.71
Ageusia R43.2
Agitated — *see* condition
Agitation R45.1
Aglossia (congenital) Q38.3
Aglossia-adactylia syndrome Q87.0
Aglycogenosis E74.00
Agnosia (body image) (other senses) (tactile) R48.1
  developmental F88
  verbal R48.1
    auditory R48.1
      developmental F80.2
    developmental F80.2
  visual (object) R48.3
Agoraphobia F40.00
  with panic disorder F40.01
  without panic disorder F40.02
Agrammatism R48.8
Agranulocytopenia — *see* Agranulocytosis
Agranulocytosis (chronic) (cyclical) (genetic) (infantile)
  (periodic) (pernicious) (*see also* Neutropenia) D70.9
  congenital D70.0
  cytoreductive cancer chemotherapy sequela D70.1
  drug-induced D70.2
    due to cytoreductive cancer chemotherapy D70.1
  due to infection D70.3
  secondary D70.4
    drug-induced D70.2
      due to cytoreductive cancer chemotherapy
        D70.1
Agraphia (absolute) R48.8
  with alexia R48.0
  developmental F81.81
Ague (dumb) — *see* Malaria
Agyria Q04.3
Ahumada-del Castillo syndrome E23.0
Aichomophobia F40.298
AIDS (related complex) B20
Ailment heart — *see* Disease, heart
Ailurophobia F40.218
Ainhum (disease) L94.6
AIN — *see* Neoplasia, intraepithelial, anal
AIPHI (acute idiopathic pulmonary hemorrhage in
  infants (over 28 days old)) R04.81
Air
  anterior mediastinum J98.2
  compressed, disease T70.3 ☑
  conditioner lung or pneumonitis J67.7
  embolism (artery) (cerebral) (any site) T79.0 ☑
    with ectopic or molar pregnancy O08.2
    due to implanted device NEC — *see*
      Complications, by site and type, specified
      NEC
    following
      abortion — *see* Abortion by type, complicated
        by, embolism
      ectopic or molar pregnancy O08.2
    infusion, therapeutic injection or transfusion
      T80.0 ☑
    in pregnancy, childbirth or puerperium — *see*
      Embolism, obstetric
    traumatic T79.0 ☑
  hunger, psychogenic F45.8

Air — *continued*
  rarefied, effects of — *see* Effect, adverse, high
    altitude
    sickness T75.3 ☑
Airplane sickness T75.3 ☑
Akathisia (drug-induced) (treatment-induced)
  G25.71
  neuroleptic induced (acute) G25.71
  tardive G25.71
Akinesia R29.898
Akinetic mutism R41.89
Akureyri's disease G93.3
Alactasia, congenital E73.0
Alagille's syndrome Q44.7
Alastrim B03
Albers-Schönberg syndrome Q78.2
Albert's syndrome — *see* Tendinitis, Achilles
Albinism, albino E70.30
  with hematologic abnormality E70.339
    Chédiak-Higashi syndrome E70.330
    Hermansky-Pudlak syndrome E70.331
    other specified E70.338
  I E70.320
  II E70.321
  ocular E70.319
    autosomal recessive E70.311
    other specified E70.318
    X-linked E70.310
  oculocutaneous E70.329
    other specified E70.328
    tyrosinase (ty) negative E70.320
    tyrosinase (ty) positive E70.321
  other specified E70.39
Albinismus E70.30
Albright (-McCune)(-Sternberg) syndrome Q78.1
Albuminous — *see* condition
Albuminuria, albuminuric (acute) (chronic) (subacute)
  (*see also* Proteinuria) R80.9
  complicating pregnancy — *see* Proteinuria,
    gestational
  with
    gestational hypertension — *see* Pre-eclampsia
    pre-existing hypertension — *see* Hypertension,
      complicating pregnancy, pre-existing, with,
      pre-eclampsia
  gestational — *see* Proteinuria, gestational
  with
    gestational hypertension — *see* Pre-eclampsia
    pre-existing hypertension — *see* Hypertension,
      complicating pregnancy, pre-existing, with,
      pre-eclampsia
  orthostatic R80.2
  postural R80.2
  pre-eclamptic — *see* Pre-eclampsia
  scarlatinal A38.8
Albuminurophobia F40.298
Alcaptonuria E70.29
Alcohol, alcoholic, alcohol-induced
  addiction (without remission) F10.20
    with remission F10.21
  amnestic disorder, persisting F10.96
    with dependence F10.26
  anxiety disorder F10.980
  bipolar and related disorder F10.94
  depressive disorder F10.94
  major neurocognitive disorder, amnestic-
    confabulatory type F10.96
  major neurocognitive disorder, nonamnestic-
    confabulatory type F10.97
  mild neurocognitive disorder F10.988
  psychotic disorder F10.959
  sexual dysfunction F10.981
  sleep disorder F10.982
  brain syndrome, chronic F10.97
    with dependence F10.27
  cardiopathy I42.6
  counseling and surveillance Z71.41
    family member Z71.42
  delirium (acute) (tremens) (withdrawal) F10.231
    with intoxication F10.921
    in
      abuse F10.121
      dependence F10.221
  dementia F10.97
    with dependence F10.27
  deterioration F10.97
    with dependence F10.27
  hallucinosis (acute) F10.951
    in
      abuse F10.151
      dependence F10.251
  insanity F10.959

Alcohol — *continued*
  intoxication (acute) (without dependence) F10.129
    with
      delirium F10.121
      dependence F10.229
        with delirium F10.221
        uncomplicated F10.220
    uncomplicated F10.120
  jealousy F10.988
  Korsakoff's, Korsakov's, Korsakow's F10.26
  liver K70.9
    acute — *see* Disease, liver, alcoholic, hepatitis
  mania (acute) (chronic) F10.959
  paranoia, paranoid (type) psychosis F10.950
  pellagra E52
  poisoning, accidental (acute) NEC — *see* Table of
    Drugs and Chemicals, alcohol, poisoning
  psychosis — *see* Psychosis, alcoholic
  withdrawal (without convulsions) F10.239
    with delirium F10.231
Alcoholism (chronic) (without remission) F10.20
  with
    psychosis — *see* Psychosis, alcoholic
  remission F10.21
  Korsakov's F10.96
    with dependence F10.26
Alder (-Reilly) anomaly or syndrome (leukocyte
  granulation) D72.0
Aldosteronism E26.9
  familial (type I) E26.02
  glucocorticoid-remediable E26.02
  primary (due to (bilateral) adrenal hyperplasia)
    E26.09
  primary NEC E26.09
  secondary E26.1
  specified NEC E26.89
Aldosteronoma D44.10
Aldrich (-Wiskott) syndrome (eczema-
  thrombocytopenia) D82.0
Alektorophobia F40.218
Aleppo boil B55.1
Aleukemic — *see* condition
Aleukia
  congenital D70.0
  hemorrhagica D61.9
    congenital D61.09
  splenica D73.1
Alexia R48.0
  developmental F81.0
  secondary to organic lesion R48.0
Algoneurodystrophy M89.00
  ankle M89.07 ☑
  foot M89.07 ☑
  forearm M89.03 ☑
  hand M89.04 ☑
  lower leg M89.06 ☑
  multiple sites M89.0 ☑
  shoulder M89.01 ☑
  specified site NEC M89.08
  thigh M89.05 ☑
  upper arm M89.02 ☑
Algophobia F40.298
Alienation, mental — *see* Psychosis
Alkalemia E87.3
Alkalosis E87.3
  metabolic E87.3
    with respiratory acidosis E87.4
    of newborn P74.41
  respiratory E87.3
Alkaptonuria E70.29
Allen-Masters syndrome N83.8
Allergy, allergic (reaction) (to) T78.40 ☑
  air-borne substance NEC (rhinitis) J30.89
  alveolitis (extrinsic) J67.9
    due to
      Aspergillus clavatus J67.4
      Cryptostroma corticale J67.6
      organisms (fungal, thermophilic actinomycete)
        growing in ventilation (air conditioning)
        systems J67.7
      specified type NEC J67.8
  anaphylactic reaction or shock T78.2 ☑
  angioneurotic edema T78.3 ☑
  animal (dander) (epidermal) (hair) (rhinitis) J30.81
  bee sting (anaphylactic shock) — *see* Toxicity,
    venom, arthropod, bee
  biological — *see* Allergy, drug
  colitis (*see also* Colitis, allergic) K52.29
  dander (animal) (rhinitis) J30.81
  dandruff (rhinitis) J30.81
  dental restorative material (existing) K08.55
  dermatitis — *see* Dermatitis, contact, allergic

Allergy — *continued*
  diathesis — *see* History, allergy
  drug, medicament & biological (any) (external) (internal) T78.40 ☑
    correct substance properly administered — *see* Table of Drugs and Chemicals, by drug, adverse effect
    wrong substance given or taken NEC (by accident) — *see* Table of Drugs and Chemicals, by drug, poisoning
  due to pollen J30.1
  dust (house) (stock) (rhinitis) J30.89
    with asthma — *see* Asthma, allergic extrinsic
  eczema — *see* Dermatitis, contact, allergic
  epidermal (animal) (rhinitis) J30.81
  feathers (rhinitis) J30.89
  food (any) (ingested) NEC T78.1 ☑
    anaphylactic shock — *see* Shock, anaphylactic, due to food
    dermatitis — *see* Dermatitis, due to, food
    dietary counseling and surveillance Z71.3
    in contact with skin L23.6
    rhinitis J30.5
    status (without reaction) Z91.018
      eggs Z91.012
      milk products Z91.011
      peanuts Z91.010
      seafood Z91.013
      specified NEC Z91.018
  gastrointestinal (*see also* specific type of allergic reaction)
    meaning colitis (*see also* Colitis, allergic) K52.29
    meaning gastroenteritis (*see also* Gastroenteritis, allergic) K52.29
    meaning other adverse food reaction not elsewhere classified T78.1 ☑
  grain J30.1
  grass (hay fever) (pollen) J30.1
    asthma — *see* Asthma, allergic extrinsic
  hair (animal) (rhinitis) J30.81
  history (of) — *see* History, allergy
  horse serum — *see* Allergy, serum
  inhalant (rhinitis) J30.89
    pollen J30.1
  kapok (rhinitis) J30.89
  medicine — *see* Allergy, drug
  milk protein (*see also* Allergy, food) Z91.011
    anaphylactic reaction T78.07 ☑
    dermatitis L27.2
    enterocolitis syndrome K52.21
    enteropathy K52.22
    gastroenteritis K52.29
    gastroesophageal reflux (*see also* Reaction, adverse, food) K21.9
      with esophagitis K21.0
    proctocolitis K52.82
  nasal, seasonal due to pollen J30.1
  pneumonia J82
  pollen (any) (hay fever) J30.1
    asthma — *see* Asthma, allergic extrinsic
  primrose J30.1
  primula J30.1
  proctocolitis K52.82
  purpura D69.0
  ragweed (hay fever) (pollen) J30.1
    asthma — *see* Asthma, allergic extrinsic
  rose (pollen) J30.1
  seasonal NEC J30.2
  Senecio jacobae (pollen) J30.1
  serum (*see also* Reaction, serum) T80.69 ☑
    anaphylactic shock T80.59 ☑
  shock (anaphylactic) T78.2 ☑
    due to
      administration of blood and blood products T80.51 ☑
      adverse effect of correct medicinal substance properly administered T88.6 ☑
      immunization T80.52 ☑
      serum NEC T80.59 ☑
      vaccination T80.52 ☑
  specific NEC T78.49 ☑
  tree (any) (hay fever) (pollen) J30.1
    asthma — *see* Asthma, allergic extrinsic
  upper respiratory J30.9
  urticaria L50.0
  vaccine — *see* Allergy, serum
  wheat — *see* Allergy, food
Allescheriasis B48.2
Alligator skin disease Q80.9
Allocheiria, allochiria R20.8
Almeida's disease — *see* Paracoccidioidomycosis

Alopecia (hereditaria) (seborrheica) L65.9
  androgenic L64.9
    drug-induced L64.0
    specified NEC L64.8
  areata L63.9
    ophiasis L63.2
    specified NEC L63.8
    totalis L63.0
    universalis L63.1
  cicatricial L66.9
    specified NEC L66.8
  circumscripta L63.9
  congenital, congenitalis Q84.0
  due to cytotoxic drugs NEC L65.8
  mucinosa L65.2
  postinfective NEC L65.8
  postpartum L65.0
  premature L64.8
  specific (syphilitic) A51.32
  specified NEC L65.8
  syphilitic (secondary) A51.32
  totalis (capitis) L63.0
  universalis (entire body) L63.1
  X-ray L58.1
Alpers' disease G31.81
Alpine sickness T70.29 ☑
Alport syndrome Q87.81
ALTE (apparent life threatening event) in newborn and infant R68.13
Alteration (of), Altered
  awareness
    transient R40.4
    unintended under general anesthesia, during procedure T88.53 ☑
  mental status R41.82
  pattern of family relationships affecting child Z62.898
  sensation
    following
      cerebrovascular disease I69.998
        cerebral infarction I69.398
        intracerebral hemorrhage I69.198
        nontraumatic intracranial hemorrhage NEC I69.298
        specified disease NEC I69.898
        subarachnoid hemorrhage I69.098
Alternating — *see* condition
Altitude, high (effects) — *see* Effect, adverse, high altitude
Aluminosis (of lung) J63.0
Alveolitis
  allergic (extrinsic) — *see* Pneumonitis, hypersensitivity
  due to
    Aspergillus clavatus J67.4
    Cryptostroma corticale J67.6
  fibrosing (cryptogenic) (idiopathic) J84.112
  jaw M27.3
  sicca dolorosa M27.3
Alveolus, alveolar — *see* condition
Alymphocytosis D72.810
  thymic (with immunodeficiency) D82.1
Alymphoplasia, thymic D82.1
Alzheimer's disease or sclerosis — *see* Disease, Alzheimer's
Amastia (with nipple present) Q83.8
  with absent nipple Q83.0
Amathophobia F40.228
Amaurosis (acquired) (congenital) (*see also* Blindness)
  fugax G45.3
  hysterical F44.6
  Leber's congenital H35.50
  uremic — *see* Uremia
Amaurotic idiocy (infantile) (juvenile) (late) E75.4
Amaxophobia F40.248
Ambiguous genitalia Q56.4
Amblyopia (congenital) (ex anopsia) (partial) (suppression) H53.00 ☑
  anisometropic — *see* Amblyopia, refractive
  deprivation H53.01 ☑
  hysterical F44.6
  nocturnal (*see also* Blindness, night)
    vitamin A deficiency E50.5
  refractive H53.02 ☑
  strabismic H53.03 ☑
  suspect H53.04 ☑
  tobacco H53.8
  toxic NEC H53.8
  uremic — *see* Uremia
Ameba, amebic (histolytica) (*see also* Amebiasis)
  abscess (liver) A06.4
Amebiasis A06.9
  with abscess — *see* Abscess, amebic

Amebiasis — *continued*
  acute A06.0
  chronic (intestine) A06.1
    with abscess — *see* Abscess, amebic
  cutaneous A06.7
  cutis A06.7
  cystitis A06.81
  genitourinary tract NEC A06.82
  hepatic — *see* Abscess, liver, amebic
  intestine A06.0
  nondysenteric colitis A06.2
  skin A06.7
  specified site NEC A06.89
Ameboma (of intestine) A06.3
Amelia Q73.0
  lower limb — *see* Agenesis, leg
  upper limb — *see* Agenesis, arm
Ameloblastoma (*see also* Cyst, calcifying odontogenic)
  long bones C40.9 ☑
    lower limb C40.2 ☑
    upper limb C40.0 ☑
  malignant C41.1
    jaw (bone) (lower) C41.1
      upper C41.0
  tibial C40.2 ☑
Amelogenesis imperfecta K00.5
  nonhereditaria (segmentalis) K00.4
Amenorrhea N91.2
  hyperhormonal E28.8
  primary N91.0
  secondary N91.1
Amentia — *see* Disability, intellectual
  Meynert's (nonalcoholic) F04
American
  leishmaniasis B55.2
  mountain tick fever A93.2
Ametropia — *see* Disorder, refraction
AMH (asymptomatic microscopic hematuria) R31.21
Amianthosis J61
Amimia R48.8
Amino-acid disorder E72.9
  anemia D53.0
Aminoacidopathy E72.9
Aminoaciduria E72.9
Amnes (t)ic syndrome (post-traumatic) F04
  induced by
    alcohol F10.96
      with dependence F10.26
    psychoactive NEC F19.96
      with
        abuse F19.16
        dependence F19.26
    sedative F13.96
      with dependence F13.26
Amnesia R41.3
  anterograde R41.1
  auditory R48.8
  dissociative F44.0
    with dissociative fugue F44.1
  hysterical F44.0
  postictal in epilepsy — *see* Epilepsy
  psychogenic F44.0
  retrograde R41.2
  transient global G45.4
Amnion, amniotic — *see* condition
Amnionitis — *see* Pregnancy, complicated by
Amok F68.8
Amoral traits F60.89
Amphetamine (or other stimulant)-induced
  anxiety disorder F15.980
  bipolar and related disorder F15.94
  delirium F15.921
  depressive disorder F15.94
  obsessive-compulsive and related disorder F15.988
  psychotic disorder F15.959
  sexual dysfunction F15.981
  sleep disorder F15.982
  stimulant withdrawal F15.23
Ampulla
  lower esophagus K22.8
  phrenic K22.8
Amputation (*see also* Absence, by site, acquired)
  neuroma (postoperative) (traumatic) — *see* Complications, amputation stump, neuroma
  stump (surgical)
    abnormal, painful, or with complication (late) — *see* Complications, amputation stump
    healed or old NOS Z89.9
  traumatic (complete) (partial)
    arm (upper) (complete) S48.91 ☑
      at
        elbow S58.01 ☑

☑ **Additional character required**

Amputation — *continued*
  traumatic — *continued*
      partial S58.02 ☑
     shoulder joint (complete) S48.01 ☑
      partial S48.02 ☑
    between
     elbow and wrist (complete) S58.11 ☑
      partial S58.12 ☑
     shoulder and elbow (complete) S48.11 ☑
      partial S48.12 ☑
    partial S48.92 ☑
   breast (complete) S28.21 ☑
    partial S28.22 ☑
   clitoris (complete) S38.211 ☑
    partial S38.212 ☑
   ear (complete) S08.11 ☑
    partial S08.12 ☑
   finger (complete) (metacarpophalangeal) S68.11 ☑
    index S68.11 ☑
    little S68.11 ☑
    middle S68.11 ☑
    partial S68.12 ☑
     index S68.12 ☑
     little S68.12 ☑
     middle S68.12 ☑
     ring S68.12 ☑
    ring S68.11 ☑
    thumb — *see* Amputation, traumatic, thumb
    transphalangeal (complete) S68.61 ☑
     index S68.61 ☑
     little S68.61 ☑
     middle S68.61 ☑
     partial S68.62 ☑
      index S68.62 ☑
      little S68.62 ☑
      middle S68.62 ☑
      ring S68.62 ☑
     ring S68.61 ☑
   foot (complete) S98.91 ☑
    at ankle level S98.01 ☑
     partial S98.02 ☑
    midfoot S98.31 ☑
     partial S98.32 ☑
    partial S98.92 ☑
   forearm (complete) S58.91 ☑
    at elbow level (complete) S58.01 ☑
     partial S58.02 ☑
    between elbow and wrist (complete) S58.11 ☑
     partial S58.12 ☑
    partial S58.92 ☑
   genital organ(s) (external)
    female (complete) S38.211 ☑
     partial S38.212 ☑
    male
     penis (complete) S38.221 ☑
      partial S38.222 ☑
     scrotum (complete) S38.231 ☑
      partial S38.232 ☑
     testes (complete) S38.231 ☑
      partial S38.232 ☑
   hand (complete) (wrist level) S68.41 ☑
    finger(s) alone — *see* Amputation, traumatic, finger
    partial S68.42 ☑
    thumb alone — *see* Amputation, traumatic, thumb
    transmetacarpal (complete) S68.71 ☑
     partial S68.72 ☑
   head
    ear — *see* Amputation, traumatic, ear
    nose (partial) S08.812 ☑
     complete S08.811 ☑
    part S08.89 ☑
     scalp S08.0 ☑
   hip (and thigh) (complete) S78.91 ☑
    at hip joint (complete) S78.01 ☑
     partial S78.02 ☑
    between hip and knee (complete) S78.11 ☑
     partial S78.12 ☑
    partial S78.92 ☑
   labium (majus) (minus) (complete) S38.21 ☑
    partial S38.21 ☑
   leg (lower) S88.91 ☑
    at knee level S88.01 ☑
     partial S88.02 ☑
    between knee and ankle S88.11 ☑
     partial S88.12 ☑
    partial S88.92 ☑
   nose (partial) S08.812 ☑
    complete S08.811 ☑
   penis (complete) S38.221 ☑
    partial S38.222 ☑

Amputation — *continued*
  traumatic — *continued*
   scrotum (complete) S38.231 ☑
    partial S38.232 ☑
   shoulder — *see* Amputation, traumatic, arm
    at shoulder joint — *see* Amputation, traumatic, arm, at shoulder joint
   testes (complete) S38.231 ☑
    partial S38.232 ☑
   thigh — *see* Amputation, traumatic, hip
   thorax, part of S28.1 ☑
    breast — *see* Amputation, traumatic, breast
   thumb (complete) (metacarpophalangeal) S68.01 ☑
    partial S68.02 ☑
    transphalangeal (complete) S68.51 ☑
     partial S68.52 ☑
   toe (lesser) S98.13 ☑
    great S98.11 ☑
     partial S98.12 ☑
    more than one S98.21 ☑
     partial S98.22 ☑
    partial S98.14 ☑
   vulva (complete) S38.211 ☑
    partial S38.212 ☑
Amputee (bilateral) (old) Z89.9
Amsterdam dwarfism Q87.19
Amusia R48.8
  developmental F80.89
Amyelencephalus, amyelencephaly Q00.0
Amyelia Q06.0
Amygdalitis — *see* Tonsillitis
Amygdalolith J35.8
Amyloid heart (disease) E85.4 *[I43]*
Amyloidosis (generalized) (primary) E85.9
  with lung involvement E85.4 *[J99]*
  familial E85.2
  genetic E85.2
  heart E85.4 *[I43]*
  hemodialysis-associated E85.3
  light chain (AL) E85.81
  liver E85.4 *[K77]*
  localized E85.4
  neuropathic heredofamilial E85.1
  non-neuropathic heredofamilial E85.0
  organ limited E85.4
  Portuguese E85.1
  pulmonary E85.4 *[J99]*
  secondary systemic E85.3
  senile systemic (SSA) E85.82
  skin (lichen) (macular) E85.4 *[L99]*
  specified NEC E85.89
  subglottic E85.4 *[J99]*
  wild-type transthyretin-related (ATTR) E85.82
Amylopectinosis (brancher enzyme deficiency) E74.03
Amylophagia — *see* Pica
Amyoplasia congenita Q79.8
Amyotonia M62.89
  congenita G70.2
Amyotrophia, amyotrophy, amyotrophic G71.8
  congenita Q79.8
  diabetic — *see* Diabetes, amyotrophy
  lateral sclerosis G12.21
  neuralgic G54.5
  spinal progressive G12.25
Anacidity, gastric K31.83
  psychogenic F45.8
Anaerosis of newborn P28.89
Analbuminemia E88.09
Analgesia — *see* Anesthesia
Analphalipoproteinemia E78.6
Anaphylactic
  purpura D69.0
  shock or reaction — *see* Shock, anaphylactic
Anaphylactoid shock or reaction — *see* Shock, anaphylactic
Anaphylactoid syndrome of pregnancy O88.01 ☑
Anaphylaxis — *see* Shock, anaphylactic
Anaplasia cervix (*see also* Dysplasia, cervix) N87.9
Anaplasmosis, human A77.49
Anarthria R47.1
Anasarca R60.1
  cardiac — *see* Failure, heart, congestive
  lung J18.2
  newborn P83.2
  nutritional E43
  pulmonary J18.2
  renal N04.9
Anastomosis
  aneurysmal — *see* Aneurysm
  arteriovenous ruptured brain I60.8
   intracerebral I61.8

Anastomosis — *continued*
  arteriovenous ruptured brain — *continued*
   intraparenchymal I61.8
   intraventricular I61.5
   subarachnoid I60.8
  intestinal K63.89
   complicated NEC K91.89
    involving urinary tract N99.89
  retinal and choroidal vessels (congenital) Q14.8
Anatomical narrow angle H40.03 ☑
Ancylostoma, ancylostomiasis (braziliense) (caninum) (ceylanicum) (duodenale) B76.0
  Necator americanus B76.1
Andersen's disease (glycogen storage) E74.09
Anderson-Fabry disease E75.21
Andes disease T70.29 ☑
Andrews' disease (bacterid) L08.89
Androblastoma
  benign
   specified site — *see* Neoplasm, benign, by site
   unspecified site
    female D27.9
    male D29.20
  malignant
   specified site — *see* Neoplasm, malignant, by site
   unspecified site
    female C56.9
    male C62.90
  specified site — *see* Neoplasm, uncertain behavior, by site
  tubular
   with lipid storage
    specified site — *see* Neoplasm, benign, by site
    unspecified site
     female D27.9
     male D29.20
   specified site — *see* Neoplasm, benign, by site
   unspecified site
    female D27.9
    male D29.20
  unspecified site
   female D39.10
   male D40.10
Androgen insensitivity syndrome (*see also* Syndrome, androgen insensitivity) E34.50
Androgen resistance syndrome (*see also* Syndrome, androgen insensitivity) E34.50
Android pelvis Q74.2
  with disproportion (fetopelvic) O33.3 ☑
   causing obstructed labor O65.3
Andro phobia F40.290
Anectasis, pulmonary (newborn) — *see* Atelectasis
Anemia (essential) (general) (hemoglobin deficiency) (infantile) (primary) (profound) D64.9
  with (due to) (in)
   disorder of
    anaerobic glycolysis D55.2
    pentose phosphate pathway D55.1
   koilonychia D50.9
  achlorhydric D50.8
  achrestic D53.1
  Addison (-Biermer) (pernicious) D51.0
  agranulocytic — *see* Agranulocytosis
  amino-acid-deficiency D53.0
  aplastic D61.9
   congenital D61.09
   drug-induced D61.1
   due to
    drugs D61.1
    external agents NEC D61.2
    infection D61.2
    radiation D61.2
   idiopathic D61.3
   red cell (pure) D60.9
    chronic D60.0
    congenital D61.01
    specified type NEC D60.8
    transient D60.1
   specified type NEC D61.89
   toxic D61.2
  aregenerative
   congenital D61.09
  asiderotic D50.9
  atypical (primary) D64.9
  Baghdad spring D55.0
  Balantidium coli A07.0
  Biermer's (pernicious) D51.0
  blood loss (chronic) D50.0
   acute D62
  bothriocephalus B70.0 *[D63.8]*
  brickmaker's B76.9 *[D63.8]*
  cerebral I67.89

Anemia

Anemia — *continued*
- childhood D58.9
- chlorotic D50.8
- chronic
  - blood loss D50.0
  - hemolytic D58.9
    - idiopathic D59.9
  - simple D53.9
- chronica congenita aregenerativa D61.09
- combined system disease NEC D51.0 *[G32.0]*
  - due to dietary vitamin B12 deficiency D51.3 *[G32.0]*
- complicating pregnancy, childbirth or puerperium — *see* Pregnancy, complicated by (management affected by), anemia
- congenital P61.4
  - aplastic D61.09
  - due to isoimmunization NOS P55.9
  - dyserythropoietic, dyshematopoietic D64.4
  - following fetal blood loss P61.3
  - Heinz body D58.2
  - hereditary hemolytic NOS D58.9
  - pernicious D51.0
  - spherocytic D58.0
- Cooley's (erythroblastic) D56.1
- cytogenic D51.0
- deficiency D53.9
  - 2, 3 diphosphoglycerate mutase D55.2
  - 2, 3 PG D55.2
  - 6 phosphogluconate dehydrogenase D55.1
  - 6-PGD D55.1
  - amino-acid D53.0
  - combined B12 and folate D53.1
  - enzyme D55.9
    - drug-induced (hemolytic) D59.2
    - glucose-6-phosphate dehydrogenase (G6PD) D55.0
    - glycolytic D55.2
    - nucleotide metabolism D55.3
    - related to hexose monophosphate (HMP) shunt pathway NEC D55.1
    - specified type NEC D55.8
  - erythrocytic glutathione D55.1
  - folate D52.9
    - dietary D52.0
    - drug-induced D52.1
  - folic acid D52.9
    - dietary D52.0
    - drug-induced D52.1
  - G SH D55.1
  - GGS-R D55.1
  - glucose-6-phosphate dehydrogenase D55.0
  - glutathione reductase D55.1
  - glyceraldehyde phosphate dehydrogenase D55.2
  - G6PD D55.0
  - hexokinase D55.2
  - iron D50.9
    - secondary to blood loss (chronic) D50.0
  - nutritional D53.9
    - with
      - poor iron absorption D50.8
      - specified deficiency NEC D53.8
  - phosphofructo-aldolase D55.2
  - phosphoglycerate kinase D55.2
  - PK D55.2
  - protein D53.0
  - pyruvate kinase D55.2
  - transcobalamin II D51.2
  - triose-phosphate isomerase D55.2
  - vitamin B12 NOS D51.9
    - dietary D51.3
    - due to
      - intrinsic factor deficiency D51.0
      - selective vitamin B12 malabsorption with proteinuria D51.1
    - pernicious D51.0
    - specified type NEC D51.8
- Diamond-Blackfan (congenital hypoplastic) D61.01
- dibothriocephalus B70.0 *[D63.8]*
- dimorphic D53.1
- diphasic D53.1
- Diphyllobothrium (Dibothriocephalus) B70.0 *[D63.8]*
- due to (in) (with)
  - antineoplastic chemotherapy D64.81
  - blood loss (chronic) D50.0
    - acute D62
  - chemotherapy, antineoplastic D64.81
  - chronic disease classified elsewhere NEC D63.8
  - chronic kidney disease D63.1
  - deficiency
    - amino-acid D53.0

Anemia — *continued*
- due to — *continued*
  - copper D53.8
  - folate (folic acid) D52.9
    - dietary D52.0
    - drug-induced D52.1
  - molybdenum D53.8
  - protein D53.0
  - zinc D53.8
  - dietary vitamin B12 deficiency D51.3
  - disorder of
    - glutathione metabolism D55.1
    - nucleotide metabolism D55.3
  - drug — *see* Anemia, by type (*see also* Table of Drugs and Chemicals)
  - end stage renal disease D63.1
  - enzyme disorder D55.9
  - fetal blood loss P61.3
  - fish tapeworm (D.latum) infestation B70.0 *[D63.8]*
  - hemorrhage (chronic) D50.0
    - acute D62
  - impaired absorption D50.9
  - loss of blood (chronic) D50.0
    - acute D62
  - myxedema E03.9 *[D63.8]*
  - Necator americanus B76.1 *[D63.8]*
  - prematurity P61.2
  - selective vitamin B12 malabsorption with proteinuria D51.1
  - transcobalamin II deficiency D51.2
- Dyke-Young type (secondary) (symptomatic) D59.1
- dyserythropoietic (congenital) D64.4
- dyshematopoietic (congenital) D64.4
- Egyptian B76.9 *[D63.8]*
- elliptocytosis — *see* Elliptocytosis
- enzyme-deficiency, drug-induced D59.2
- epidemic (*see also* Ancylostomiasis) B76.9 *[D63.8]*
- erythroblastic
  - familial D56.1
  - newborn (*see also* Disease, hemolytic) P55.9
  - of childhood D56.1
- erythrocytic glutathione deficiency D55.1
- erythropoietin-resistant anemia (EPO resistant anemia) D63.1
- Faber's (achlorhydric anemia) D50.9
- factitious (self-induced bloodletting) D50.0
- familial erythroblastic D56.1
- Fanconi's (congenital pancytopenia) D61.09
- favism D55.0
- fish tapeworm (D. latum) infestation B70.0 *[D63.8]*
- folate (folic acid) deficiency D52.9
- glucose-6-phosphate dehydrogenase (G6PD) deficiency D55.0
- glutathione-reductase deficiency D55.1
- goat's milk D52.0
- granulocytic — *see* Agranulocytosis
- Heinz body, congenital D58.2
- hemolytic D58.9
  - acquired D59.9
    - with hemoglobinuria NEC D59.6
    - autoimmune NEC D59.1
    - infectious D59.4
    - specified type NEC D59.8
    - toxic D59.4
  - acute D59.9
    - due to enzyme deficiency specified type NEC D55.8
    - Lederer's D59.1
  - autoimmune D59.1
    - drug-induced D59.0
  - chronic D58.9
    - idiopathic D59.9
  - cold type (secondary) (symptomatic) D59.1
  - congenital (spherocytic) — *see* Spherocytosis
  - due to
    - cardiac conditions D59.4
    - drugs (nonautoimmune) D59.2
      - autoimmune D59.0
    - enzyme disorder D55.9
      - drug-induced D59.2
    - presence of shunt or other internal prosthetic device D59.4
  - familial D58.9
  - hereditary D58.9
    - due to enzyme disorder D55.9
      - specified type NEC D55.8
    - specified type NEC D58.8
  - idiopathic (chronic) D59.9
  - mechanical D59.4
  - microangiopathic D59.4
  - nonautoimmune D59.4
    - drug-induced D59.2

Anemia — *continued*
- hemolytic — *continued*
  - nonspherocytic
    - congenital or hereditary NEC D55.8
      - glucose-6-phosphate dehydrogenase deficiency D55.0
      - pyruvate kinase deficiency D55.2
      - type
        - I D55.1
        - II D55.2
    - type
      - I D55.1
      - II D55.2
  - secondary D59.4
    - autoimmune D59.1
  - specified (hereditary) type NEC D58.8
  - Stransky-Regala type (*see also* Hemoglobinopathy) D58.8
  - symptomatic D59.4
    - autoimmune D59.1
  - toxic D59.4
  - warm type (secondary) (symptomatic) D59.1
- hemorrhagic (chronic) D50.0
  - acute D62
- Herrick's D57.1
- hexokinase deficiency D55.2
- hookworm B76.9 *[D63.8]*
- hypochromic (idiopathic) (microcytic) (normoblastic) D50.9
  - due to blood loss (chronic) D50.0
    - acute D62
  - familial sex-linked D64.0
  - pyridoxine-responsive D64.3
  - sideroblastic, sex-linked D64.0
- hypoplasia, red blood cells D61.9
  - congenital or familial D61.01
- hypoplastic (idiopathic) D61.9
  - congenital or familial (of childhood) D61.01
- hypoproliferative (refractive) D61.9
- idiopathic D64.9
  - aplastic D61.3
  - hemolytic, chronic D59.9
- in (due to) (with)
  - chronic kidney disease D63.1
  - end stage renal disease D63.1
  - failure, kidney (renal) D63.1
  - neoplastic disease (*see also* Neoplasm) D63.0
- intertropical (*see also* Ancylostomiasis) D63.8
- iron deficiency D50.9
  - secondary to blood loss (chronic) D50.0
    - acute D62
  - specified type NEC D50.8
- Joseph-Diamond-Blackfan (congenital hypoplastic) D61.01
- Lederer's (hemolytic) D59.1
- leukoerythroblastic D61.82
- macrocytic D53.9
  - nutritional D52.0
  - tropical D52.8
- malarial (*see also* Malaria) B54 *[D63.8]*
- malignant (progressive) D51.0
- malnutrition D53.9
- marsh (*see also* Malaria) B54 *[D63.8]*
- Mediterranean (with other hemoglobinopathy) D56.9
- megaloblastic D53.1
  - combined B12 and folate deficiency D53.1
  - hereditary D51.1
  - nutritional D52.0
  - orotic aciduria D53.0
  - refractory D53.1
  - specified type NEC D53.1
- megalocytic D53.1
- microcytic (hypochromic) D50.9
  - due to blood loss (chronic) D50.0
    - acute D62
  - familial D56.8
- microdrepanocytosis D57.40
- microelliptopoikilocytic (Rietti-Greppi- Micheli) D56.9
- miner's B76.9 *[D63.8]*
- myelodysplastic D46.9
- myelofibrosis D75.81
- myelogenous D64.89
- myelopathic D64.89
- myelophthisic D61.82
- myeloproliferative D47.Z9
- newborn P61.4
  - due to
    - ABO (antibodies, isoimmunization, maternal/fetal incompatibility) P55.1

☑ **Additional character required**

Anemia — *continued*
newborn — *continued*
Rh (antibodies, isoimmunization, maternal/fetal incompatibility) P55.0
following fetal blood loss P61.3
posthemorrhagic (fetal) P61.3
nonspherocytic hemolytic — *see* Anemia, hemolytic, nonspherocytic
normocytic (infectional) D64.9
due to blood loss (chronic) D50.0
acute D62
myelophthisic D61.82
nutritional (deficiency) D53.9
with
poor iron absorption D50.8
specified deficiency NEC D53.8
megaloblastic D52.0
of prematurity P61.2
orotaciduric (congenital) (hereditary) D53.0
osteosclerotic D64.89
ovalocytosis (hereditary) — *see* Elliptocytosis
paludal (*see also* Malaria) B54 [D63.8]
pernicious (congenital) (malignant) (progressive) D51.0
pleochromic D64.89
of sprue D52.8
posthemorrhagic (chronic) D50.0
acute D62
newborn P61.3
postoperative (postprocedural)
due to (acute) blood loss D62
chronic blood loss D50.0
specified NEC D64.9
postpartum O90.81
pressure D64.89
progressive D64.9
malignant D51.0
pernicious D51.0
protein-deficiency D53.0
pseudoleukemica infantum D64.89
pure red cell D60.9
congenital D61.01
pyridoxine-responsive D64.3
pyruvate kinase deficiency D55.2
refractory D46.4
with
excess of blasts D46.20
1 (RAEB 1) D46.21
2 (RAEB 2) D46.22
in transformation (RAEB T) — *see* Leukemia, acute myeloblastic
hemochromatosis D46.1
sideroblasts (ring) (RARS) D46.1
megaloblastic D53.1
sideroblastic D46.1
sideropenic D50.9
without ring sideroblasts, so stated D46.0
without sideroblasts without excess of blasts D46.0
Rietti-Greppi-Micheli D56.9
scorbutic D53.2
secondary to
blood loss (chronic) D50.0
acute D62
hemorrhage (chronic) D50.0
acute D62
semiplastic D61.89
sickle-cell — *see* Disease, sickle-cell
sideroblastic D64.3
hereditary D64.0
hypochromic, sex-linked D64.0
pyridoxine-responsive NEC D64.3
refractory D46.1
secondary (due to)
disease D64.1
drugs and toxins D64.2
specified type NEC D64.3
sideropenic (refractory) D50.9
due to blood loss (chronic) D50.0
acute D62
simple chronic D53.9
specified type NEC D64.89
spherocytic (hereditary) — *see* Spherocytosis
splenic D64.89
splenomegalic D64.89
stomatocytosis D58.8
syphilitic (acquired) (late) A52.79 [D63.8]
target cell D64.89
thalassemia D56.9
thrombocytopenic — *see* Thrombocytopenia
toxic D61.2
tropical B76.9 [D63.8]
macrocytic D52.8

Anemia — *continued*
tuberculous A18.89 [D63.8]
vegan D51.3
vitamin
B6-responsive D64.3
B12 deficiency (dietary) pernicious D51.0
von Jaksch's D64.89
Witts' (achlorhydric anemia) D50.8
Anemophobia F40.228
Anencephalus, anencephaly Q00.0
Anergasia — *see* Psychosis, organic
Anesthesia, anesthetic R20.0
complication or reaction NEC (*see also* Complications, anesthesia) T88.59 ☑
due to
correct substance properly administered — *see* Table of Drugs and Chemicals, by drug, adverse effect
overdose or wrong substance given — *see* Table of Drugs and Chemicals, by drug, poisoning
unintended awareness under general anesthesia during procedure T88.53 ☑
personal history of Z92.84
cornea H18.81 ☑
dissociative F44.6
functional (hysterical) F44.6
hyperesthetic, thalamic G89.0
hysterical F44.6
local skin lesion R20.0
sexual (psychogenic) F52.1
shock (due to) T88.2 ☑
skin R20.0
testicular N50.9
Anetoderma (maculosum) (of) L90.8
Jadassohn-Pellizzari L90.2
Schweninger-Buzzi L90.1
Aneurin deficiency E51.9
Aneurysm (anastomotic) (artery) (cirsoid) (diffuse) (false) (fusiform) (multiple) (saccular) I72.9
abdominal (aorta) I71.4
ruptured I71.3
syphilitic A52.01
aorta, aortic (nonsyphilitic) I71.9
abdominal I71.4
ruptured I71.3
arch I71.2
ruptured I71.1
arteriosclerotic I71.9
ruptured I71.8
ascending I71.2
ruptured I71.1
congenital Q25.43
descending I71.9
abdominal I71.4
ruptured I71.3
ruptured I71.8
thoracic I71.2
ruptured I71.1
root Q25.43
ruptured I71.8
sinus, congenital Q25.43
syphilitic A52.01
thoracic I71.2
ruptured I71.1
thoracoabdominal I71.6
ruptured I71.5
thorax, thoracic (arch) I71.2
ruptured I71.1
transverse I71.2
ruptured I71.1
valve (heart) (*see also* Endocarditis, aortic) I35.8
arteriosclerotic I72.9
cerebral I67.1
ruptured — *see* Hemorrhage, intracranial, subarachnoid
arteriovenous (congenital) (*see also* Malformation, arteriovenous)
acquired I77.0
brain I67.1
ruptured — *see* Aneurysm, arteriovenous, brain, ruptured
coronary I25.41
pulmonary I28.0
brain Q28.2
ruptured I60.8
intracerebral I61.8
intraparenchymal I61.8
intraventricular I61.5
subarachnoid I60.8
peripheral — *see* Malformation, arteriovenous, peripheral

Aneurysm — *continued*
arteriovenous — *continued*
precerebral vessels Q28.0
specified site NEC (*see also* Malformation, arteriovenous)
acquired I77.0
basal — *see* Aneurysm, brain
basilar (trunk) I72.5
berry (congenital) (nonruptured) I67.1
ruptured I60.7
brain I67.1
arteriosclerotic I67.1
ruptured — *see* Hemorrhage, intracranial, subarachnoid
arteriovenous (congenital) (nonruptured) Q28.2
acquired I67.1
ruptured — *see* Aneurysm, arteriovenous, brain, ruptured I60.8
ruptured — *see* Aneurysm, arteriovenous, brain, ruptured I60.8
berry (congenital) (nonruptured) I67.1
ruptured (*see also* Hemorrhage, intracranial, subarachnoid) I60.7
congenital Q28.3
ruptured I60.7
meninges I67.1
ruptured I60.8
miliary (congenital) (nonruptured) I67.1
ruptured (*see also* Hemorrhage, intracranial, subarachnoid) I60.7
mycotic I33.0
ruptured — *see* Hemorrhage, intracranial, subarachnoid
syphilitic (hemorrhage) A52.05
cardiac (false) (*see also* Aneurysm, heart) I25.3
carotid artery (common) (external) I72.0
internal (intracranial) I67.1
extracranial portion I72.0
ruptured into brain I60.0 ☑
syphilitic A52.09
intracranial A52.05
cavernous sinus I67.1
arteriovenous (congenital) (nonruptured) Q28.3
ruptured I60.8
celiac I72.8
central nervous system, syphilitic A52.05
cerebral — *see* Aneurysm, brain
chest — *see* Aneurysm, thorax
circle of Willis I67.1
congenital Q28.3
ruptured I60.6
ruptured I60.6
common iliac artery I72.3
congenital (peripheral) Q27.8
aorta (root) (sinus) Q25.43
brain Q28.3
ruptured I60.7
coronary Q24.5
digestive system Q27.8
lower limb Q27.8
pulmonary Q25.79
retina Q14.1
specified site NEC Q27.8
upper limb Q27.8
conjunctiva — *see* Abnormality, conjunctiva, vascular
conus arteriosus — *see* Aneurysm, heart
coronary (arteriosclerotic) (artery) I25.41
arteriovenous, congenital Q24.5
congenital Q24.5
ruptured — *see* Infarct, myocardium
syphilitic A52.06
vein I25.89
cylindroid (aorta) I71.9
ruptured I71.8
syphilitic A52.01
ductus arteriosus Q25.0
endocardial, infective (any valve) I33.0
femoral (artery) (ruptured) I72.4
gastroduodenal I72.8
gastroepiploic I72.8
heart (wall) (chronic or with a stated duration of over 4 weeks) I25.3
valve — *see* Endocarditis
hepatic I72.8
iliac (common) (artery) (ruptured) I72.3
infective I72.9
endocardial (any valve) I33.0
innominate (nonsyphilitic) I72.8
syphilitic A52.09
interauricular septum — *see* Aneurysm, heart
interventricular septum — *see* Aneurysm, heart

Aneurysm — *continued*
  intrathoracic (nonsyphilitic) I71.2
    ruptured I71.1
    syphilitic A52.01
  lower limb I72.4
  lung (pulmonary artery) I28.1
  mediastinal (nonsyphilitic) I72.8
    syphilitic A52.09
  miliary (congenital) I67.1
    ruptured — *see* Hemorrhage, intracerebral,
      subarachnoid, intracranial
  mitral (heart) (valve) I34.8
  mural — *see* Aneurysm, heart
  mycotic I72.9
    endocardial (any valve) I33.0
    ruptured, brain — *see* Hemorrhage, intracerebral,
      subarachnoid
  myocardium — *see* Aneurysm, heart
  neck I72.0
  pancreaticoduodenal I72.8
  patent ductus arteriosus Q25.0
  peripheral NEC I72.8
    congenital Q27.8
      digestive system Q27.8
      lower limb Q27.8
      specified site NEC Q27.8
      upper limb Q27.8
  popliteal (artery) (ruptured) I72.4
  precerebral
    congenital (nonruptured) Q28.1
    specified site, NEC I72.5
  pulmonary I28.1
    arteriovenous Q25.72
      acquired I28.0
    syphilitic A52.09
    valve (heart) — *see* Endocarditis, pulmonary
  racemose (peripheral) I72.9
    congenital — *see* Aneurysm, congenital
  radial I72.1
  Rasmussen NEC A15.0
  renal (artery) I72.2
  retina (*see also* Disorder, retina, microaneurysms)
    congenital Q14.1
    diabetic — *see* E08-E13 with .3 ☑
  sinus of Valsalva Q25.49
  specified NEC I72.8
  spinal (cord) I72.8
    syphilitic (hemorrhage) A52.09
  splenic I72.8
  subclavian (artery) (ruptured) I72.8
    syphilitic A52.09
  superior mesenteric I72.8
  syphilitic (aorta) A52.01
    central nervous system A52.05
    congenital (late) A50.54 [*I79.0*]
    spine, spinal A52.09
  thoracoabdominal (aorta) I71.6
    ruptured I71.5
    syphilitic A52.01
  thorax, thoracic (aorta) (arch) (nonsyphilitic) I71.2
    ruptured I71.1
    syphilitic A52.01
  traumatic (complication) (early), specified site — *see*
    Injury, blood vessel
  tricuspid (heart) (valve) I07.8
  ulnar I72.1
  upper limb (ruptured) I72.1
  valve, valvular — *see* Endocarditis
  venous (*see also* Varix) I86.8
    congenital Q27.8
      digestive system Q27.8
      lower limb Q27.8
      specified site NEC Q27.8
      upper limb Q27.8
  ventricle — *see* Aneurysm, heart
  vertebral artery I72.6
  visceral NEC I72.8
Angelman syndrome Q93.51
Anger R45.4
Angiectasis, angiectopia I99.8
Angiitis I77.6
  allergic granulomatous M30.1
  hypersensitivity M31.0
  necrotizing M31.9
    specified NEC M31.8
  nervous system, granulomatous I67.7
Angina (attack) (cardiac) (chest) (heart) (pectoris)
  (syndrome) (vasomotor) I20.9
  with
    atherosclerotic heart disease — *see*
      Arteriosclerosis, coronary (artery),
      documented spasm I20.1

Angina — *continued*
  abdominal K55.1
  accelerated — *see* Angina, unstable
  agranulocytic — *see* Agranulocytosis
  angiospastic — *see* Angina, with documented
    spasm
  aphthous B08.5
  crescendo — *see* Angina, unstable
  croupous J05.0
  cruris I73.9
  de novo effort — *see* Angina, unstable
  diphtheritic, membranous A36.0
  equivalent I20.8
  exudative, chronic J37.0
  following acute myocardial infarction I23.7
  gangrenous diphtheritic A36.0
  intestinal K55.1
  Ludovici K12.2
  Ludwig's K12.2
  malignant diphtheritic A36.0
  membranous J05.0
    diphtheritic A36.0
    Vincent's A69.1
  mesenteric K55.1
  monocytic — *see* Mononucleosis, infectious
  of effort — *see* Angina, specified NEC
  phlegmonous J36
    diphtheritic A36.0
  post-infarctional I23.7
  pre-infarctional — *see* Angina, unstable
  Prinzmetal — *see* Angina, with documented spasm
  progressive — *see* Angina, unstable
  pseudomembranous A69.1
  pultaceous, diphtheritic A36.0
  spasm-induced — *see* Angina, with documented
    spasm
  specified NEC I20.8
  stable I20.8
  stenocardia — *see* Angina, specified NEC
  stridulous, diphtheritic A36.2
  tonsil J36
  trachealis J05.0
  unstable I20.0
  variant — *see* Angina, with documented spasm
  Vincent's A69.1
  worsening effort — *see* Angina, unstable
Angioblastoma — *see* Neoplasm, connective tissue,
  uncertain behavior
Angiocholecystitis — *see* Cholecystitis, acute
Angiocholitis (*see also* Cholecystitis, acute) K83.09
Angiodysgenesis spinalis G95.19
Angiodysplasia (cecum) (colon) K55.20
  with bleeding K55.21
  duodenum (and stomach) K31.819
    with bleeding K31.811
  stomach (and duodenum) K31.819
    with bleeding K31.811
Angioedema (allergic) (any site) (with urticaria)
  T78.3 ☑
  hereditary D84.1
Angioendothelioma — *see* Neoplasm, uncertain
  behavior, by site
  benign D18.00
    intra-abdominal D18.03
    intracranial D18.02
    skin D18.01
    specified site NEC D18.09
  bone — *see* Neoplasm, bone, malignant
  Ewing's — *see* Neoplasm, bone, malignant
Angioendotheliomatosis C85.8 ☑
Angiofibroma (*see also* Neoplasm, benign, by site)
  juvenile
    specified site — *see* Neoplasm, benign, by site
    unspecified site D10.6
Angiohemophilia (A) (B) D68.0
Angioid streaks (choroid) (macula) (retina) H35.33
Angiokeratoma — *see* Neoplasm, skin, benign
  corporis diffusum E75.21
Angioleiomyoma — *see* Neoplasm, connective tissue,
  benign
Angiolipoma (*see also* Lipoma)
  infiltrating — *see* Lipoma
Angioma (*see also* Hemangioma, by site)
  capillary I78.1
  hemorrhagicum hereditaria I78.0
  intra-abdominal D18.03
  intracranial D18.02
  malignant — *see* Neoplasm, connective tissue,
    malignant
  plexiform D18.00
    intra-abdominal D18.03
    intracranial D18.02

Angioma — *continued*
  plexiform — *continued*
    skin D18.01
    specified site NEC D18.09
  senile I78.1
  serpiginosum L81.7
  skin D18.01
  specified site NEC D18.09
  spider I78.1
  stellate I78.1
  venous Q28.3
Angiomatosis Q82.8
  bacillary A79.89
  encephalotrigeminal Q85.8
  hemorrhagic familial I78.0
  hereditary familial I78.0
  liver K76.4
Angiomyolipoma — *see* Lipoma
Angiomyoliposarcoma — *see* Neoplasm, connective
  tissue, malignant
Angiomyoma — *see* Neoplasm, connective tissue,
  benign
Angiomyosarcoma — *see* Neoplasm, connective
  tissue, malignant
Angiomyxoma — *see* Neoplasm, connective tissue,
  uncertain behavior
Angioneurosis F45.8
Angioneurotic edema (allergic) (any site) (with
  urticaria) T78.3 ☑
  hereditary D84.1
Angiopathia, angiopathy I99.9
  cerebral I67.9
    amyloid E85.4 [*I68.0*]
  diabetic (peripheral) — *see* Diabetes, angiopathy
  peripheral I73.9
    diabetic — *see* Diabetes, angiopathy
    specified type NEC I73.89
  retinae syphilitica A52.05
  retinalis (juvenilis)
    diabetic — *see* Diabetes, retinopathy
    proliferative — *see* Retinopathy, proliferative
Angiosarcoma (*see also* Neoplasm, connective tissue,
  malignant)
  liver C22.3
Angiosclerosis — *see* Arteriosclerosis
Angiospasm (peripheral) (traumatic) (vessel) I73.9
  brachial plexus G54.0
  cerebral G45.9
  cervical plexus G54.2
  nerve
    arm — *see* Mononeuropathy, upper limb
      axillary G54.0
      median — *see* Lesion, nerve, median
      ulnar — *see* Lesion, nerve, ulnar
    axillary G54.0
    leg — *see* Mononeuropathy, lower limb
    median — *see* Lesion, nerve, median
    plantar — *see* Lesion, nerve, plantar
    ulnar — *see* Lesion, nerve, ulnar
Angiospastic disease or edema I73.9
Angiostrongyliasis
  due to
    Parastrongylus
      cantonensis B83.2
      costaricensis B81.3
  intestinal B81.3
Anguillulosis — *see* Strongyloidiasis
Angulation
  cecum — *see* Obstruction, intestine
  coccyx (acquired) (*see also* subcategory) M43.8 ☑
    congenital NEC Q76.49
  femur (acquired) (*see also* Deformity, limb, specified
    type NEC, thigh)
    congenital Q74.2
  intestine (large) (small) — *see* Obstruction, intestine
  sacrum (acquired) (*see also* subcategory) M43.8 ☑
    congenital NEC Q76.49
  sigmoid (flexure) — *see* Obstruction, intestine
  spine — *see* Dorsopathy, deforming, specified NEC
  tibia (acquired) (*see also* Deformity, limb, specified
    type NEC, lower leg)
    congenital Q74.2
  ureter N13.5
    with infection N13.6
  wrist (acquired) (*see also* Deformity, limb, specified
    type NEC, forearm)
    congenital Q74.0
Angulus infectiosus (lips) K13.0
Anhedonia R45.84
  sexual F52.0
Anhidrosis L74.4
Anhydration E86.0

Anhydremia E86.0
Anidrosis L74.4
Aniridia (congenital) Q13.1
Anisakiasis (infection) (infestation) B81.0
Anisakis larvae infestation B81.0
Aniseikonia H52.32
Anisocoria (pupil) H57.02
   congenital Q13.2
Anisocytosis R71.8
Anisometropia (congenital) H52.31
Ankle — *see* condition
Ankyloblepharon (eyelid) (acquired) (*see also* Blepharophimosis)
   filiforme (adnatum) (congenital) Q10.3
   total Q10.3
Ankyloglossia Q38.1
Ankylosis (fibrous) (osseous) (joint) M24.60
   ankle M24.67 ☑
   arthrodesis status Z98.1
   cricoarytenoid (cartilage) (joint) (larynx) J38.7
   dental K03.5
   ear ossicles H74.31 ☑
   elbow M24.62 ☑
   foot M24.67 ☑
   hand M24.64 ☑
   hip M24.65 ☑
   incostapedial joint (infectional) — *see* Ankylosis, ear ossicles
   jaw (temporomandibular) M26.61 ☑
   knee M24.66 ☑
   lumbosacral (joint) M43.27
   postoperative (status) Z98.1
   produced by surgical fusion, status Z98.1
   sacro-iliac (joint) M43.28
   shoulder M24.61 ☑
   spine (joint) (*see also* Fusion, spine)
     spondylitic — *see* Spondylitis, ankylosing
   surgical Z98.1
   temporomandibular M26.61 ☑
   tooth, teeth (hard tissues) K03.5
   wrist M24.63 ☑
Ankylostoma — *see* Ancylostoma
Ankylostomiasis — *see* Ancylostomiasis
Ankylurethria — *see* Stricture, urethra
Annular (*see also* condition)
   detachment, cervix N88.8
   organ or site, congenital NEC — *see* Distortion
   pancreas (congenital) Q45.1
Anodontia (complete) (partial) (vera) K00.0
   acquired K08.10 ☑
Anomaly, anomalous (congenital) (unspecified type) Q89.9
   abdominal wall NEC Q79.59
   acoustic nerve Q07.8
   adrenal (gland) Q89.1
   Alder (-Reilly) (leukocyte granulation) D72.0
   alimentary tract Q45.9
     upper Q40.9
   alveolar M26.70
     hyperplasia M26.79
       mandibular M26.72
       maxillary M26.71
     hypoplasia M26.79
       mandibular M26.74
       maxillary M26.73
     ridge (process) M26.79
     specified NEC M26.79
   ankle (joint) Q74.2
   anus Q43.9
   aorta (arch) NEC Q25.40
     coarctation (preductal) (postductal) Q25.1
   aortic cusp or valve Q23.9
   appendix Q43.8
   apple peel syndrome Q41.1
   aqueduct of Sylvius Q03.0
     with spina bifida — *see* Spina bifida, with hydrocephalus
   arm Q74.0
   arteriovenous NEC
     coronary Q24.5
     gastrointestinal Q27.33
       acquired — *see* Angiodysplasia
   artery (peripheral) Q27.9
     basilar NEC Q28.1
     cerebral Q28.3
     coronary Q24.5
     digestive system Q27.8
     eye Q15.8
     great Q25.9
       specified NEC Q25.8
     lower limb Q27.8
     peripheral Q27.9

Anomaly — *continued*
   artery — *continued*
     specified NEC Q27.8
     pulmonary NEC Q25.79
     renal Q27.2
     retina Q14.1
     specified site NEC Q27.8
     subclavian Q27.8
       origin Q25.48
     umbilical Q27.0
     upper limb Q27.8
     vertebral NEC Q28.1
   aryteno-epiglottic folds Q31.8
   atrial
     bands or folds Q20.8
     septa Q21.1
   atrioventricular
     excitation I45.6
     septum Q21.0
   auditory canal Q17.8
   auricle
     ear Q17.8
       causing impairment of hearing Q16.9
     heart Q20.8
   Axenfeld's Q15.0
   back Q89.9
   band
     atrial Q20.8
     heart Q24.8
     ventricular Q24.8
   Bartholin's duct Q38.4
   biliary duct or passage Q44.5
   bladder Q64.70
     absence Q64.5
     diverticulum Q64.6
     exstrophy Q64.10
       cloacal Q64.12
       extroversion Q64.19
       specified type NEC Q64.19
       supravesical fissure Q64.11
     neck obstruction Q64.31
     specified type NEC Q64.79
   bone Q79.9
     arm Q74.0
     face Q75.9
     leg Q74.2
     pelvic girdle Q74.2
     shoulder girdle Q74.0
     skull Q75.9
       with
         anencephaly Q00.0
         encephalocele — *see* Encephalocele
         hydrocephalus Q03.9
           with spina bifida — *see* Spina bifida, by site, with hydrocephalus
         microcephaly Q02
   brain (multiple) Q04.9
     vessel Q28.3
   breast Q83.9
   broad ligament Q50.6
   bronchus Q32.4
   bulbus cordis Q21.9
   bursa Q79.9
   canal of Nuck Q52.4
   canthus Q10.3
   capillary Q27.9
   cardiac Q24.9
     chambers Q20.9
       specified NEC Q20.8
     septal closure Q21.9
       specified NEC Q21.8
     valve NEC Q24.8
       pulmonary Q22.3
   cardiovascular system Q28.8
   carpus Q74.0
   caruncle, lacrimal Q10.6
   cascade stomach Q40.2
   cauda equina Q06.3
   cecum Q43.9
   cerebral Q04.9
     vessels Q28.3
   cervix Q51.9
   Chédiak-Higashi (-Steinbrinck) (congenital gigantism of peroxidase granules) E70.330
   cheek Q18.9
   chest wall Q67.8
     bones Q76.9
   chin Q18.9
   chordae tendineae Q24.8
   choroid Q14.3
     plexus Q07.8

Anomaly — *continued*
   chromosomes, chromosomal Q99.9
     D (1) — *see* condition, chromosome 13
     E (3) — *see* condition, chromosome 18
     G — *see* condition, chromosome 21
     sex
       female phenotype Q97.8
       gonadal dysgenesis (pure) Q99.1
       Klinefelter's Q98.4
       male phenotype Q98.9
       Turner's Q96.9
     specified NEC Q99.8
   cilia Q10.3
   circulatory system Q28.9
   clavicle Q74.0
   clitoris Q52.6
   coccyx Q76.49
   colon Q43.9
   common duct Q44.5
   communication
     coronary artery Q24.5
     left ventricle with right atrium Q21.0
   concha (ear) Q17.3
   connection
     portal vein Q26.5
     pulmonary venous Q26.4
       partial Q26.3
       total Q26.2
     renal artery with kidney Q27.2
   cornea (shape) Q13.4
   coronary artery or vein Q24.5
   cranium — *see* Anomaly, skull
   cricoid cartilage Q31.8
   cystic duct Q44.5
   dental
     alveolar — *see* Anomaly, alveolar
     arch relationship M26.20
       specified NEC M26.29
   dentofacial M26.9
     alveolar — *see* Anomaly, alveolar
     dental arch relationship M26.20
       specified NEC M26.29
     functional M26.50
       specified NEC M26.59
     jaw-cranial base relationship M26.10
       asymmetry M26.12
         maxillary M26.11
       specified type NEC M26.19
     jaw size M26.00
       macrogenia M26.05
       mandibular
         hyperplasia M26.03
         hypoplasia M26.04
       maxillary
         hyperplasia M26.01
         hypoplasia M26.02
       microgenia M26.06
       specified type NEC M26.09
     malocclusion M26.4
       dental arch relationship NEC M26.29
       jaw-cranial base relationship — *see* Anomaly, dentofacial, jaw-cranial base relationship
       jaw size — *see* Anomaly, dentofacial, jaw size
       specified type NEC M26.89
     temporomandibular joint M26.60 ☑
       adhesions M26.61 ☑
       ankylosis M26.61 ☑
       arthralgia M26.62 ☑
       articular disc M26.63 ☑
       specified type NEC M26.69
     tooth position, fully erupted M26.30
       specified NEC M26.39
   dermatoglyphic Q82.8
   diaphragm (apertures) NEC Q79.1
   digestive organ(s) or tract Q45.9
     lower Q43.9
     upper Q40.9
   distance, interarch (excessive) (inadequate) M26.25
   distribution, coronary artery Q24.5
   ductus
     arteriosus Q25.0
     botalli Q25.0
   duodenum Q43.9
   dura (brain) Q04.9
     spinal cord Q06.9
   ear (external) Q17.9
     causing impairment of hearing Q16.9
     inner Q16.5
     middle (causing impairment of hearing) Q16.4
       ossicles Q16.3
   Ebstein's (heart) (tricuspid valve) Q22.5
   ectodermal Q82.9

Anomaly

Anomaly — *continued*
- Eisenmenger's (ventricular septal defect) Q21.8
- ejaculatory duct Q55.4
- elbow Q74.0
- endocrine gland NEC Q89.2
- epididymis Q55.4
- epiglottis Q31.8
- esophagus Q39.9
- eustachian tube Q17.8
- eye Q15.9
  - anterior segment Q13.9
    - specified NEC Q13.89
  - posterior segment Q14.9
    - specified NEC Q14.8
  - ptosis (eyelid) Q10.0
  - specified NEC Q15.8
- eyebrow Q18.8
- eyelid Q10.3
  - ptosis Q10.0
- face Q18.9
  - bone(s) Q75.9
- fallopian tube Q50.6
- fascia Q79.9
- femur NEC Q74.2
- fibula NEC Q74.2
- finger Q74.0
- fixation, intestine Q43.3
- flexion (joint) NOS Q74.9
  - hip or thigh Q65.89
- foot NEC Q74.2
  - varus (congenital) Q66.3 ☑
- foramen
  - Botalli Q21.1
  - ovale Q21.1
- forearm Q74.0
- forehead Q75.8
- form, teeth K00.2
- fovea centralis Q14.1
- frontal bone — *see* Anomaly, skull
- gallbladder (position) (shape) (size) Q44.1
- Gartner's duct Q52.4
- gastrointestinal tract Q45.9
- genitalia, genital organ(s) or system
  - female Q52.9
    - external Q52.70
    - internal NOS Q52.9
  - male Q55.9
    - hydrocele P83.5
    - specified NEC Q55.8
- genitourinary NEC
  - female Q52.9
  - male Q55.9
- Gerbode Q21.0
- glottis Q31.8
- granulation or granulocyte, genetic (constitutional) (leukocyte) D72.0
- gum Q38.6
- gyri Q07.9
- hair Q84.2
- hand Q74.0
- hard tissue formation in pulp K04.3
- head — *see* Anomaly, skull
- heart Q24.9
  - auricle Q20.8
  - bands or folds Q24.8
  - fibroelastosis cordis I42.4
  - obstructive NEC Q22.6
  - patent ductus arteriosus (Botalli) Q25.0
  - septum Q21.9
    - auricular Q21.1
    - interatrial Q21.1
    - interventricular Q21.0
      - with pulmonary stenosis or atresia, dextraposition of aorta and hypertrophy of right ventricle Q21.3
    - specified NEC Q21.8
    - ventricular Q21.0
      - with pulmonary stenosis or atresia, dextraposition of aorta and hypertrophy of right ventricle Q21.3
  - tetralogy of Fallot Q21.3
  - valve NEC Q24.8
    - aortic
      - bicuspid valve Q23.1
      - insufficiency Q23.1
      - stenosis Q23.0
        - subaortic Q24.4
    - mitral
      - insufficiency Q23.3
      - stenosis Q23.2
    - pulmonary Q22.3
      - atresia Q22.0

Anomaly — *continued*
- heart — *continued*
    - insufficiency Q22.2
    - stenosis Q22.1
      - infundibular Q24.3
      - subvalvular Q24.3
    - tricuspid
      - atresia Q22.4
      - stenosis Q22.4
    - ventricle Q20.8
- heel NEC Q74.2
- Hegglin's D72.0
- hemianencephaly Q00.0
- hemicephaly Q00.0
- hemicrania Q00.0
- hepatic duct Q44.5
- hip NEC Q74.2
- hourglass stomach Q40.2
- humerus Q74.0
- hydatid of Morgagni
  - female Q50.5
  - male (epididymal) Q55.4
  - testicular Q55.29
- hymen Q52.4
- hypersegmentation of neutrophils, hereditary D72.0
- hypophyseal Q89.2
- ileocecal (coil) (valve) Q43.9
- ileum Q43.9
- ilium NEC Q74.2
- integument Q84.9
  - specified NEC Q84.8
- interarch distance (excessive) (inadequate) M26.25
- intervertebral cartilage or disc Q76.49
- intestine (large) (small) Q43.9
  - with anomalous adhesions, fixation or malrotation Q43.3
- iris Q13.2
- ischium NEC Q74.2
- jaw — *see* Anomaly, dentofacial
  - alveolar — *see* Anomaly, alveolar
- jaw-cranial base relationship — *see* Anomaly, dentofacial, jaw-cranial base relationship
- jejunum Q43.8
- joint Q74.9
  - specified NEC Q74.8
- Jordan's D72.0
- kidney(s) (calyx) (pelvis) Q63.9
  - artery Q27.2
  - specified NEC Q63.8
- Klippel-Feil (brevicollis) Q76.1
- knee Q74.1
- labium (majus) (minus) Q52.70
- labyrinth, membranous Q16.5
- lacrimal apparatus or duct Q10.6
- larynx, laryngeal (muscle) Q31.9
  - web (bed) Q31.0
- lens Q12.9
- leukocytes, genetic D72.0
  - granulation (constitutional) D72.0
- lid (fold) Q10.3
- ligament Q79.9
  - broad Q50.6
  - round Q52.8
- limb Q74.9
  - lower NEC Q74.2
    - reduction deformity — *see* Defect, reduction, lower limb
  - upper Q74.0
- lip Q38.0
- liver Q44.7
  - duct Q44.5
- lower limb NEC Q74.2
- lumbosacral (joint) (region) Q76.49
  - kyphosis — *see* Kyphosis, congenital
  - lordosis — *see* Lordosis, congenital
- lung (fissure) (lobe) Q33.9
- mandible — *see* Anomaly, dentofacial
- maxilla — *see* Anomaly, dentofacial
- May (-Hegglin) D72.0
- meatus urinarius NEC Q64.79
- meningeal bands or folds Q07.9
  - constriction of Q07.8
  - spinal Q06.9
- meninges Q07.9
  - cerebral Q04.8
  - spinal Q06.9
- meningocele Q05.9
- mesentery Q45.9
- metacarpus Q74.0
- metatarsus NEC Q74.2
- middle ear Q16.4
  - ossicles Q16.3

Anomaly — *continued*
- mitral (leaflets) (valve) Q23.9
  - insufficiency Q23.3
  - specified NEC Q23.8
  - stenosis Q23.2
- mouth Q38.6
- Müllerian (*see also* Anomaly, by site)
  - uterus NEC Q51.818
- multiple NEC Q89.7
- muscle Q79.9
  - eyelid Q10.3
- musculoskeletal system, except limbs Q79.9
- myocardium Q24.8
- nail Q84.6
- narrowness, eyelid Q10.3
- nasal sinus (wall) Q30.8
- neck (any part) Q18.9
- nerve Q07.9
  - acoustic Q07.8
  - optic Q07.8
- nervous system (central) Q07.9
- nipple Q83.9
- nose, nasal (bones) (cartilage) (septum) (sinus) Q30.9
  - specified NEC Q30.8
- ocular muscle Q15.8
- omphalomesenteric duct Q43.0
- opening, pulmonary veins Q26.4
- optic
  - disc Q14.2
  - nerve Q07.8
- opticociliary vessels Q13.2
- orbit (eye) Q10.7
- organ Q89.9
  - of Corti Q16.5
- origin
  - artery
    - innominate Q25.8
    - pulmonary Q25.79
    - renal Q27.2
    - subclavian Q25.48
- osseous meatus (ear) Q16.1
- ovary Q50.39
- oviduct Q50.6
- palate (hard) (soft) NEC Q38.5
- pancreas or pancreatic duct Q45.3
- papillary muscles Q24.8
- parathyroid gland Q89.2
- paraurethral ducts Q64.79
- parotid (gland) Q38.4
- patella Q74.1
- Pelger-Huët (hereditary hyposegmentation) D72.0
- pelvic girdle NEC Q74.2
- pelvis (bony) NEC Q74.2
  - rachitic E64.3
- penis (glans) Q55.69
- pericardium Q24.8
- peripheral vascular system Q27.9
- Peter's Q13.4
- pharynx Q38.8
- pigmentation L81.9
  - congenital Q82.8
- pituitary (gland) Q89.2
- pleural (folds) Q34.0
- portal vein Q26.5
  - connection Q26.5
- position, tooth, teeth, fully erupted M26.30
  - specified NEC M26.39
- precerebral vessel Q28.1
- prepuce Q55.69
- prostate Q55.4
- pulmonary Q33.9
  - artery NEC Q25.79
  - valve Q22.3
    - atresia Q22.0
    - insufficiency Q22.2
    - specified type NEC Q22.3
    - stenosis Q22.1
      - infundibular Q24.3
      - subvalvular Q24.3
  - venous connection Q26.4
    - partial Q26.3
    - total Q26.2
- pupil Q13.2
  - function H57.00
    - anisocoria H57.02
    - Argyll Robertson pupil H57.01
    - miosis H57.03
    - mydriasis H57.04
    - specified type NEC H57.09
    - tonic pupil H57.05 ☑
- pylorus Q40.3

☑ **Additional character required**

Anomaly — *continued*
radius Q74.0
rectum Q43.9
reduction (extremity) (limb)
  femur (longitudinal) — *see* Defect, reduction,
    lower limb, longitudinal, femur
  fibula (longitudinal) — *see* Defect, reduction,
    lower limb, longitudinal, fibula
  lower limb — *see* Defect, reduction, lower limb
  radius (longitudinal) — *see* Defect, reduction,
    upper limb, longitudinal, radius
  tibia (longitudinal) — *see* Defect, reduction, lower
    limb, longitudinal, tibia
  ulna (longitudinal) — *see* Defect, reduction, upper
    limb, longitudinal, ulna
  upper limb — *see* Defect, reduction, upper limb
refraction — *see* Disorder, refraction
renal Q63.9
  artery Q27.2
  pelvis Q63.9
    specified NEC Q63.8
respiratory system Q34.9
  specified NEC Q34.8
retina Q14.1
rib Q76.6
  cervical Q76.5
Rieger's Q13.81
rotation — *see* Malrotation
  hip or thigh Q65.89
round ligament Q52.8
sacroiliac (joint) NEC Q74.2
sacrum NEC Q76.49
  kyphosis — *see* Kyphosis, congenital
  lordosis — *see* Lordosis, congenital
saddle nose, syphilitic A50.57
salivary duct or gland Q38.4
scapula Q74.0
scrotum — *see* Malformation, testis and scrotum
sebaceous gland Q82.9
seminal vesicles Q55.4
sense organs NEC Q07.8
sex chromosomes NEC (*see also* Anomaly,
  chromosomes)
  female phenotype Q97.8
  male phenotype Q98.9
shoulder (girdle) (joint) Q74.0
sigmoid (flexure) Q43.9
simian crease Q82.8
sinus of Valsalva Q25.49
skeleton generalized Q78.9
skin (appendage) Q82.9
skull Q75.9
  with
    anencephaly Q00.0
    encephalocele — *see* Encephalocele
    hydrocephalus Q03.9
      with spina bifida — *see* Spina bifida, by site,
        with hydrocephalus
    microcephaly Q02
specified organ or site NEC Q89.8
spermatic cord Q55.4
spine, spinal NEC Q76.49
  column NEC Q76.49
    kyphosis — *see* Kyphosis, congenital
    lordosis — *see* Lordosis, congenital
  cord Q06.9
  nerve root Q07.8
spleen Q89.09
  agenesis Q89.01
stenonian duct Q38.4
sternum NEC Q76.7
stomach Q40.3
submaxillary gland Q38.4
tarsus NEC Q74.2
tendon Q79.9
testis — *see* Malformation, testis and scrotum
thigh NEC Q74.2
thorax (wall) Q67.8
  bony Q76.9
throat Q38.8
thumb Q74.0
thymus gland Q89.2
thyroid (gland) Q89.2
  cartilage Q31.8
tibia NEC Q74.2
  saber A50.56
toe Q74.2
tongue Q38.3
tooth, teeth K00.9
  eruption K00.6
  position, fully erupted M26.30
  spacing, fully erupted M26.30

Anomaly — *continued*
trachea (cartilage) Q32.1
tragus Q17.9
tricuspid (leaflet) (valve) Q22.9
  atresia or stenosis Q22.4
  Ebstein's Q22.5
Uhl's (hypoplasia of myocardium, right ventricle)
  Q24.8
ulna Q74.0
umbilical artery Q27.0
union
  cricoid cartilage and thyroid cartilage Q31.8
  thyroid cartilage and hyoid bone Q31.8
  trachea with larynx Q31.8
upper limb Q74.0
urachus Q64.4
ureter Q62.8
  obstructive NEC Q62.39
    cecoureterocele Q62.32
    orthotopic ureterocele Q62.31
urethra Q64.70
  absence Q64.5
  double Q64.74
  fistula to rectum Q64.73
  obstructive Q64.39
    stricture Q64.32
  prolapse Q64.71
  specified type NEC Q64.79
urinary tract Q64.9
uterus Q51.9
  with only one functioning horn Q51.4
uvula Q38.5
vagina Q52.4
valleculae Q31.8
valve (heart) NEC Q24.8
  coronary sinus Q24.5
  inferior vena cava Q24.8
  pulmonary Q22.3
  sinus coronario Q24.5
  venae cavae inferioris Q24.8
vas deferens Q55.4
vascular Q27.9
  brain Q28.3
  ring Q25.45
vein(s) (peripheral) Q27.9
  brain Q28.3
  cerebral Q28.3
  coronary Q24.5
  developmental Q28.3
  great Q26.9
    specified NEC Q26.8
vena cava (inferior) (superior) Q26.9
venous — *see* Anomaly, vein(s)
venous return Q26.8
ventricular
  bands or folds Q24.8
  septa Q21.0
vertebra Q76.49
  kyphosis — *see* Kyphosis, congenital
  lordosis — *see* Lordosis, congenital
vesicourethral orifice Q64.79
vessel(s) Q27.9
  optic papilla Q14.2
  precerebral Q28.1
vitelline duct Q43.0
vitreous body or humor Q14.0
vulva Q52.70
wrist (joint) Q74.0
Anomia R48.8
Anonychia (congenital) Q84.3
  acquired L60.8
Anophthalmos, anophthalmus (congenital) (globe)
  Q11.1
  acquired Z90.01
Anopia, anopsia H53.46 ☑
  quadrant H53.46 ☑
Anorchia, anorchism, anorchidism Q55.0
Anorexia R63.0
  hysterical F44.89
  nervosa F50.00
    atypical F50.9
    binge-eating type F50.2
      with purging F50.02
    restricting type F50.01
Anorgasmy, psychogenic (female) F52.31
  male F52.32
Anosmia R43.0
  hysterical F44.6
  postinfectional J39.8
Anosognosia R41.89
Anosteoplasia Q78.9
Anovulatory cycle N97.0

Anoxemia R09.02
  newborn P84
Anoxia (pathological) R09.02
  altitude T70.29 ☑
  cerebral G93.1
    complicating
      anesthesia (general) (local) or other sedation
        T88.59 ☑
        in labor and delivery O74.3
        in pregnancy O29.21 ☑
        postpartum, puerperal O89.2
      delivery (cesarean) (instrumental) O75.4
    during a procedure G97.81
    newborn P84
    resulting from a procedure G97.82
  due to
    drowning T75.1 ☑
    high altitude T70.29 ☑
  heart — *see* Insufficiency, coronary
  intrauterine P84
  myocardial — *see* Insufficiency, coronary
  newborn P84
  spinal cord G95.11
  systemic (by suffocation) (low content in
    atmosphere) — *see* Asphyxia, traumatic
Anteflexion — *see* Anteversion
Antenatal
  care (normal pregnancy) Z34.90
  screening (encounter for) of mother (*see also*
    Encounter, antenatal screening) Z36.9
Antepartum — *see* condition
Anterior — *see* condition
Antero-occlusion M26.220
Anteversion
  cervix — *see* Anteversion, uterus
  femur (neck), congenital Q65.89
  uterus, uterine (cervix) (postinfectional) (postpartal,
    old) N85.4
    congenital Q51.818
    in pregnancy or childbirth — *see* Pregnancy,
      complicated by
Anthophobia F40.228
Anthracosilicosis J60
Anthracosis (lung) (occupational) J60
  lingua K14.3
Anthrax A22.9
  with pneumonia A22.1
  cerebral A22.8
  colitis A22.2
  cutaneous A22.0
  gastrointestinal A22.2
  inhalation A22.1
  intestinal A22.2
  meningitis A22.8
  pulmonary A22.1
  respiratory A22.1
  sepsis A22.7
  specified manifestation NEC A22.8
Anthropoid pelvis Q74.2
  with disproportion (fetopelvic) O33.0
Anthropophobia F40.10
  generalized F40.11
Antibodies, maternal (blood group) — *see*
  Isoimmunization, affecting management of
  pregnancy
  anti-D — *see* Isoimmunization, affecting
    management of pregnancy, Rh
  newborn P55.0
Antibody
  anticardiolipin R76.0
    with
      hemorrhagic disorder D68.312
      hypercoagulable state D68.61
  antiphosphatidylglycerol R76.0
    with
      hemorrhagic disorder D68.312
      hypercoagulable state D68.61
  antiphosphatidylinositol R76.0
    with
      hemorrhagic disorder D68.312
      hypercoagulable state D68.61
  antiphosphatidylserine R76.0
    with
      hemorrhagic disorder D68.312
      hypercoagulable state D68.61
  antiphospholipid R76.0
    with
      hemorrhagic disorder D68.312
      hypercoagulable state D68.61
Anticardiolipin syndrome D68.61
Anticoagulant, circulating (intrinsic) (*see also* -
  Disorder, hemorrhagic) D68.318

Anticoagulant - Apraxia

Anticoagulant — *continued*
  drug-induced (extrinsic) (*see also* - Disorder,
    hemorrhagic) D68.32
  iatrogenic D68.32
Antidiuretic hormone syndrome E22.2
Antimonial cholera — *see* Poisoning, antimony
Antiphospholipid
  antibody
    with hemorrhagic disorder D68.312
    syndrome D68.61
Antisocial personality F60.2
Antithrombinemia — *see* Circulating anticoagulants
Antithromboplastinemia D68.318
Antithromboplastinogenemia D68.318
Antitoxin complication or reaction — *see*
  Complications, vaccination
Antlophobia F40.228
Antritis J32.0
  maxilla J32.0
    acute J01.00
      recurrent J01.01
  stomach K29.60
    with bleeding K29.61
Antrum, antral — *see* condition
Anuria R34
  calculous (impacted) (recurrent) (*see also* Calculus,
    urinary) N20.9
  following
    abortion — *see* Abortion by type complicated by,
      renal failure
    ectopic or molar pregnancy O08.4
  newborn P96.0
  postprocedural N99.0
  postrenal N13.8
  traumatic (following crushing) T79.5 ☑
Anus, anal — *see* condition
Anusitis K62.89
Anxiety F41.9
  depression F41.8
  episodic paroxysmal F41.0
  generalized F41.1
  hysteria F41.8
  neurosis F41.1
  panic type F41.0
  reaction F41.1
  separation, abnormal (of childhood) F93.0
  specified NEC F41.8
  state F41.1
Aorta, aortic — *see* condition
Aortectasia — *see* Ectasia, aorta
  with aneurysm — *see* Aneurysm, aorta
Aortitis (nonsyphilitic) (calcific) I77.6
  arteriosclerotic I70.0
  Doehle-Heller A52.02
  luetic A52.02
  rheumatic — *see* Endocarditis, acute, rheumatic
  specific (syphilitic) A52.02
  syphilitic A52.02
    congenital A50.54 *[I79.1]*
Apathetic thyroid storm — *see* Thyrotoxicosis
Apathy R45.3
Apeirophobia F40.228
Apepsia K30
  psychogenic F45.8
Aperistalsis, esophagus K22.0
Apertognathia M26.29
Apert's syndrome Q87.0
Aphagia R13.0
  psychogenic F50.9
Aphakia (acquired) (postoperative) H27.0 ☑
  congenital Q12.3
Aphasia (amnestic) (global) (nominal) (semantic)
  (syntactic) R47.01
  acquired, with epilepsy (Landau-Kleffner syndrome)
    — *see* Epilepsy, specified NEC
  auditory (developmental) F80.2
  developmental (receptive type) F80.2
    expressive type F80.1
    Wernicke's F80.2
  following
    cerebrovascular disease I69.920
      cerebral infarction I69.320
      intracerebral hemorrhage I69.120
      nontraumatic intracranial hemorrhage NEC
        I69.220
      specified disease NEC I69.820
      subarachnoid hemorrhage I69.020
  primary progressive G31.01 *[F02.80]*
    with behavioral disturbance G31.01 *[F02.81]*
  progressive isolated G31.01 *[F02.80]*
    with behavioral disturbance G31.01 *[F02.81]*
  sensory F80.2

Aphasia — *continued*
  syphilis, tertiary A52.19
  Wernicke's (developmental) F80.2
Aphonia (organic) R49.1
  hysterical F44.4
  psychogenic F44.4
Aphthae, aphthous (*see also* condition)
  Bednar's K12.0
  cachectic K14.0
  epizootic B08.8
  fever B08.8
  oral (recurrent) K12.0
  stomatitis (major) (minor) K12.0
  thrush B37.0
  ulcer (oral) (recurrent) K12.0
    genital organ(s) NEC
      female N76.6
      male N50.89
    larynx J38.7
Apical — *see* condition
Apiphobia F40.218
Aplasia (*see also* Agenesis)
  abdominal muscle syndrome Q79.4
  alveolar process (acquired) — *see* Anomaly, alveolar
    congenital Q38.6
  aorta (congenital) Q25.41
  axialis extracorticalis (congenita) E75.29
  bone marrow (myeloid) D61.9
    congenital D61.01
  brain Q00.0
    part of Q04.3
  bronchus Q32.4
  cementum K00.4
  cerebellum Q04.3
  cervix (congenital) Q51.5
  congenital pure red cell D61.01
  corpus callosum Q04.0
  cutis congenita Q84.8
  erythrocyte congenital D61.01
  extracortical axial E75.29
  eye Q11.1
  fovea centralis (congenital) Q14.1
  gallbladder, congenital Q44.0
  iris Q13.1
  labyrinth, membranous Q16.5
  limb (congenital) Q73.8
    lower — *see* Defect, reduction, lower limb
    upper — *see* Agenesis, arm
  lung, congenital (bilateral) (unilateral) Q33.3
  pancreas Q45.0
  parathyroid-thymic D82.1
  Pelizaeus-Merzbacher E75.29
  penis Q55.5
  prostate Q55.4
  red cell (with thymoma) D60.9
    acquired D60.9
      due to drugs D60.9
    adult D60.9
    chronic D60.0
    congenital D61.01
    constitutional D61.01
    due to drugs D60.9
    hereditary D61.01
    of infants D61.01
    primary D61.01
    pure D61.01
      due to drugs D60.9
    specified type NEC D60.8
    transient D60.1
  round ligament Q52.8
  skin Q84.8
  spermatic cord Q55.4
  spleen Q89.01
  testicle Q55.0
  thymic, with immunodeficiency D82.1
  thyroid (congenital) (with myxedema) E03.1
  uterus Q51.0
  ventral horn cell Q06.1
Apnea, apneic (of) (spells) R06.81
  newborn NEC P28.4
    obstructive P28.4
    sleep (central) (obstructive) (primary) P28.3
  prematurity P28.4
  sleep G47.30
    central (primary) G47.31
      idiopathic G47.31
      in conditions classified elsewhere G47.37
    obstructive (adult) (pediatric) G47.33
      hypopnea G47.33
    primary central G47.31
    specified NEC G47.39
Apneumatosis, newborn P28.0

Apocrine metaplasia (breast) — *see* Dysplasia,
  mammary, specified type NEC
Apophysitis (bone) (*see also* Osteochondropathy)
  calcaneus M92.8
  juvenile M92.9
Apoplectiform convulsions (cerebral ischemia) I67.82
Apoplexia, apoplexy, apoplectic
  adrenal A39.1
  heart (auricle) (ventricle) — *see* Infarct, myocardium
  heat T67.01 ☑
  hemorrhagic (stroke) — *see* Hemorrhage,
    intracranial
  meninges, hemorrhagic — *see* Hemorrhage,
    intracranial, subarachnoid
  uremic N18.9 *[I68.8]*
Appearance
  bizarre R46.1
  specified NEC R46.89
  very low level of personal hygiene R46.0
Appendage
  epididymal (organ of Morgagni) Q55.4
  intestine (epiploic) Q43.8
  preauricular Q17.0
  testicular (organ of Morgagni) Q55.29
Appendicitis (pneumococcal) (retrocecal) K37
  with
    gangrene K35.891
    perforation NOS K35.32
    peritoneal abscess K35.33
    peritonitis NEC K35.33
      generalized (with perforation or rupture) K35.20
        with abscess K35.21
      localized K35.30
        with
          gangrene K35.31
          perforation K35.32
            and abscess K35.33
      rupture (with localized peritonitis) K35.32
  acute (catarrhal) (fulminating) (gangrenous)
    (obstructive) (retrocecal) (suppurative) K35.80
    with
      gangrene K35.891
      peritoneal abscess K35.33
      peritonitis NEC K35.33
        generalized (with perforation or rupture)
          K35.20
          with abscess K35.21
        localized K35.30
          with
            gangrene K35.31
            perforation K35.32
              and abscess K35.33
      specified NEC K35.890
        with gangrene K35.891
  amebic A06.89
  chronic (recurrent) K36
  exacerbation — *see* Appendicitis, acute
  gangrenous — *see* Appendicitis, acute
  healed (obliterative) K36
  interval K36
  neurogenic K36
  obstructive K36
  recurrent K36
  relapsing K36
  ruptured NOS (with localized peritonitis) K35.32
  subacute (adhesive) K36
  subsiding K36
  suppurative — *see* Appendicitis, acute
  tuberculous A18.32
Appendicopathia oxyurica B80
Appendix, appendicular (*see also* condition)
  epididymis Q55.4
  Morgagni
    female Q50.5
    male (epididymal) Q55.4
      testicular Q55.29
  testis Q55.29
Appetite
  depraved — *see* Pica
  excessive R63.2
  lack or loss (*see also* Anorexia) R63.0
    nonorganic origin F50.89
    psychogenic F50.89
  perverted (hysterical) — *see* Pica
Apple peel syndrome Q41.1
Apprehension state F41.1
Apprehensiveness, abnormal F41.9
Approximal wear K03.0
Apraxia (classic) (ideational) (ideokinetic) (ideomotor)
  (motor) (verbal) R48.2
  following
    cerebrovascular disease I69.990

☑ **Additional character required**

Apraxia — continued
  following — continued
    cerebral infarction I69.390
    intracerebral hemorrhage I69.190
    nontraumatic intracranial hemorrhage NEC
      I69.290
    specified disease NEC I69.890
    subarachnoid hemorrhage I69.090
  oculomotor, congenital H51.8
Aptyalism K11.7
Apudoma — see Neoplasm, uncertain behavior, by site
Aqueous misdirection H40.83 ☑
Arabicum elephantiasis — see Infestation, filarial
Arachnitis — see Meningitis
Arachnodactyly — see Syndrome, Marfan's
Arachnoiditis (acute) (adhesive) (basal) (brain)
  (cerebrospinal) — see Meningitis
Arachnophobia F40.210
Arboencephalitis, Australian A83.4
Arborization block (heart) I45.5
ARC (AIDS-related complex) B20
Arch
  aortic Q25.49
  bovine Q25.49
Arches — see condition
Arcuate uterus Q51.810
Arcuatus uterus Q51.810
Arcus (cornea) senilis — see Degeneration, cornea,
  senile
Arc-welder's lung J63.4
Areflexia R29.2
Areola — see condition
Argentaffinoma (see also Neoplasm, uncertain
  behavior, by site)
  malignant — see Neoplasm, malignant, by site
  syndrome E34.0
Argininemia E72.21
Arginosuccinic aciduria E72.22
Argyll Robertson phenomenon, pupil or syndrome
  (syphilitic) A52.19
  atypical H57.09
  nonsyphilitic H57.09
Argyria, argyriasis
  conjunctival H11.13 ☑
  from drug or medicament — see Table of Drugs and
    Chemicals, by substance
Argyrosis, conjunctival H11.13 ☑
Arhinencephaly Q04.1
Ariboflavinosis E53.0
Arm — see condition
Arnold-Chiari disease, obstruction or syndrome (type
  II) Q07.00
  with
    hydrocephalus Q07.02
      with spina bifida Q07.03
    spina bifida Q07.01
      with hydrocephalus Q07.03
  type III — see Encephalocele
  type IV Q04.8
Aromatic amino-acid metabolism disorder E70.9
  specified NEC E70.8
Arousals, confusional G47.51
Arrest, arrested
  cardiac I46.9
    complicating
      abortion — see Abortion, by type, complicated
        by, cardiac arrest
      anesthesia (general) (local) or other sedation —
        see Table of Drugs and Chemicals, by drug,
        in labor and delivery O74.2
        in pregnancy O29.11 ☑
        postpartum, puerperal O89.1
      delivery (cesarean) (instrumental) O75.4
    due to
      cardiac condition I46.2
      specified condition NEC I46.8
    intraoperative I97.71 ☑
    newborn P29.81
    personal history, successfully resuscitated Z86.74
    postprocedural I97.12 ☑
      obstetric procedure O75.4
  cardiorespiratory — see Arrest, cardiac
  circulatory — see Arrest, cardiac
  deep transverse O64.0 ☑
  development or growth
    bone — see Disorder, bone, development or
      growth
    child R62.50
    tracheal rings Q32.1
  epiphyseal
    complete
      femur M89.15 ☑

Arrest — continued
  epiphyseal — continued
    humerus M89.12 ☑
    tibia M89.16 ☑
    ulna M89.13 ☑
    forearm M89.13 ☑
      specified NEC M89.13 ☑
    ulna — see Arrest, epiphyseal, by type, ulna
    lower leg M89.16 ☑
      specified NEC M89.168
      tibia — see Arrest, epiphyseal, by type, tibia
    partial
      femur M89.15 ☑
      humerus M89.12 ☑
      tibia M89.16 ☑
      ulna M89.13 ☑
    specified NEC M89.18
  granulopoiesis — see Agranulocytosis
  growth plate — see Arrest, epiphyseal
  heart — see Arrest, cardiac
  legal, anxiety concerning Z65.3
  physeal — see Arrest, epiphyseal
  respiratory R09.2
    newborn P28.81
  sinus I45.5
  spermatogenesis (complete) — see Azoospermia
    incomplete — see Oligospermia
  transverse (deep) O64.0 ☑
Arrhenoblastoma
  benign
    specified site — see Neoplasm, benign, by site
    unspecified site
      female D27.9
      male D29.20
  malignant
    specified site — see Neoplasm, malignant, by site
    unspecified site
      female C56.9
      male C62.90
  specified site — see Neoplasm, uncertain behavior,
    by site
  unspecified site
    female D39.10
    male D40.10
Arrhythmia (auricle)(cardiac)(juvenile)(nodal) (reflex)
  (sinus)(supraventricular)(transitory)(ventricle) I49.9
  block I45.9
  extrasystolic I49.49
  newborn
    bradycardia P29.12
    occurring before birth P03.819
      before onset of labor P03.810
      during labor P03.811
    tachycardia P29.11
  psychogenic F45.8
  specified NEC I49.8
  vagal R55
  ventricular re-entry I47.0
Arrillaga-Ayerza syndrome (pulmonary sclerosis with
  pulmonary hypertension) I27.0
Arsenical pigmentation L81.8
  from drug or medicament — see Table of Drugs and
    Chemicals
Arsenism — see Poisoning, arsenic
Arterial — see condition
Arteriofibrosis — see Arteriosclerosis
Arteriolar sclerosis — see Arteriosclerosis
Arteriolith — see Arteriosclerosis
Arteriolitis I77.6
  necrotizing, kidney I77.5
  renal — see Hypertension, kidney
Arteriolosclerosis — see Arteriosclerosis
Arterionephrosclerosis — see Hypertension, kidney
Arteriopathy I77.9
  cerebral autosomal dominant, with subcortical
    infarcts and leukoencephalopathy (CADASIL)
    I67.850
Arteriosclerosis, arteriosclerotic (diffuse) (obliterans)
  (of) (senile) (with calcification) I70.90
  aorta I70.0
  arteries of extremities — see Arteriosclerosis,
    extremities
  brain I67.2
  bypass graft
    coronary — see Arteriosclerosis, coronary, bypass
      graft
    extremities — see Arteriosclerosis, extremities,
      bypass graft
  cardiac — see Disease, heart, ischemic,
    atherosclerotic
  cardiopathy — see Disease, heart, ischemic,
    atherosclerotic

Arteriosclerosis — continued
  cardiorenal — see Hypertension, cardiorenal
  cardiovascular — see Disease, heart, ischemic,
    atherosclerotic
  carotid (see also Occlusion, artery, carotid) I65.2 ☑
  central nervous system I67.2
  cerebral I67.2
  cerebrovascular I67.2
  coronary (artery) I25.10
    due to
      calcified coronary lesion (severely) I25.84
      lipid rich plaque I25.83
    bypass graft I25.810
      with
        angina pectoris I25.709
          with documented spasm I25.701
          specified type NEC I25.708
          unstable I25.700
        ischemic chest pain I25.709
      autologous artery I25.810
        with
          angina pectoris I25.729
            with documented spasm I25.721
            specified type I25.728
            unstable I25.720
          ischemic chest pain I25.729
      autologous vein I25.810
        with
          angina pectoris I25.719
            with documented spasm I25.711
            specified type I25.718
            unstable I25.710
          ischemic chest pain I25.719
      nonautologous biological I25.810
        with
          angina pectoris I25.739
            with documented spasm I25.731
            specified type I25.738
            unstable I25.730
          ischemic chest pain I25.739
      specified type NEC I25.810
        with
          angina pectoris I25.799
            with documented spasm I25.791
            specified type I25.798
            unstable I25.790
          ischemic chest pain I25.799
    native vessel
      with
        angina pectoris I25.119
          with documented spasm I25.111
          specified type NEC I25.118
          unstable I25.110
        ischemic chest pain I25.119
    transplanted heart I25.811
      bypass graft I25.812
        with
          angina pectoris I25.769
            with documented spasm I25.761
            specified type I25.768
            unstable I25.760
          ischemic chest pain I25.769
      native coronary artery I25.811
        with
          angina pectoris I25.759
            with documented spasm I25.751
            specified type I25.758
            unstable I25.750
          ischemic chest pain I25.759
  extremities (native arteries) I70.209
    bypass graft I70.309
      autologous vein graft I70.409
        leg I70.409
          with
            gangrene (and intermittent claudication,
              rest pain and ulcer) I70.469
            intermittent claudication I70.419
            rest pain (and intermittent claudication)
              I70.429
        bilateral I70.403
          with
            gangrene (and intermittent
              claudication, rest pain and ulcer)
              I70.463
            intermittent claudication I70.413
            rest pain (and intermittent
              claudication) I70.423
          specified type NEC I70.493
        left I70.402
          with

Arteriosclerosis

Arteriosclerosis — *continued*
  extremities — *continued*
    gangrene (and intermittent claudication, rest pain and ulcer) I70.462
    intermittent claudication I70.412
    rest pain (and intermittent claudication) I70.422
    ulceration (and intermittent claudication and rest pain) I70.449
      ankle I70.443
      calf I70.442
      foot site NEC I70.445
      heel I70.444
      lower leg NEC I70.448
      midfoot I70.444
      thigh I70.441
    specified type NEC I70.492
   right I70.401
    with
      gangrene (and intermittent claudication, rest pain and ulcer) I70.461
      intermittent claudication I70.411
      rest pain (and intermittent claudication) I70.421
      ulceration (and intermittent claudication and rest pain) I70.439
        ankle I70.433
        calf I70.432
        foot site NEC I70.435
        heel I70.434
        lower leg NEC I70.438
        midfoot I70.434
        thigh I70.431
      specified type NEC I70.491
   specified type NEC I70.499
  specified NEC I70.408
   with
    gangrene (and intermittent claudication, rest pain and ulcer) I70.468
    intermittent claudication I70.418
    rest pain (and intermittent claudication) I70.428
    ulceration (and intermittent claudication and rest pain) I70.45
   specified type NEC I70.498
 leg I70.309
  with
    gangrene (and intermittent claudication, rest pain and ulcer) I70.369
    intermittent claudication I70.319
    rest pain (and intermittent claudication) I70.329
   bilateral I70.303
    with
      gangrene (and intermittent claudication, rest pain and ulcer) I70.363
      intermittent claudication I70.313
      rest pain (and intermittent claudication) I70.323
    specified type NEC I70.393
   left I70.302
    with
      gangrene (and intermittent claudication, rest pain and ulcer) I70.362
      intermittent claudication I70.312
      rest pain (and intermittent claudication) I70.322
      ulceration (and intermittent claudication and rest pain) I70.349
        ankle I70.343
        calf I70.342
        foot site NEC I70.345
        heel I70.344
        lower leg NEC I70.348
        midfoot I70.344
        thigh I70.341
      specified type NEC I70.392
   right I70.301
    with
      gangrene (and intermittent claudication, rest pain and ulcer) I70.361
      intermittent claudication I70.311
      rest pain (and intermittent claudication) I70.321
      ulceration (and intermittent claudication and rest pain) I70.339
        ankle I70.333
        calf I70.332
        foot site NEC I70.335
        heel I70.334

Arteriosclerosis — *continued*
  extremities — *continued*
        lower leg NEC I70.338
        midfoot I70.334
        thigh I70.331
      specified type NEC I70.391
    specified type NEC I70.399
  nonautologous biological graft I70.509
   leg I70.509
    with
      gangrene (and intermittent claudication, rest pain and ulcer) I70.569
      intermittent claudication I70.519
      rest pain (and intermittent claudication) I70.529
    bilateral I70.503
     with
       gangrene (and intermittent claudication, rest pain and ulcer) I70.563
       intermittent claudication I70.513
       rest pain (and intermittent claudication) I70.523
      specified type NEC I70.593
    left I70.502
     with
       gangrene (and intermittent claudication, rest pain and ulcer) I70.562
       intermittent claudication I70.512
       rest pain (and intermittent claudication) I70.522
       ulceration (and intermittent claudication and rest pain) I70.549
         ankle I70.543
         calf I70.542
         foot site NEC I70.545
         heel I70.544
         lower leg NEC I70.548
         midfoot I70.544
         thigh I70.541
       specified type NEC I70.592
    right I70.501
     with
       gangrene (and intermittent claudication, rest pain and ulcer) I70.561
       intermittent claudication I70.511
       rest pain (and intermittent claudication) I70.521
       ulceration (and intermittent claudication and rest pain) I70.539
         ankle I70.533
         calf I70.532
         foot site NEC I70.535
         heel I70.534
         lower leg NEC I70.538
         midfoot I70.534
         thigh I70.531
       specified type NEC I70.591
    specified type NEC I70.599
   specified NEC I70.508
    with
      gangrene (and intermittent claudication, rest pain and ulcer) I70.568
      intermittent claudication I70.518
      rest pain (and intermittent claudication) I70.528
      ulceration (and intermittent claudication and rest pain) I70.55
    specified type NEC I70.598
  nonbiological graft I70.609
   leg I70.609
    with
      gangrene (and intermittent claudication, rest pain and ulcer) I70.669
      intermittent claudication I70.619
      rest pain (and intermittent claudication) I70.629
    bilateral I70.603
     with
       gangrene (and intermittent claudication, rest pain and ulcer) I70.663
       intermittent claudication I70.613
       rest pain (and intermittent claudication) I70.623
      specified type NEC I70.693
    left I70.602
     with

Arteriosclerosis — *continued*
  extremities — *continued*
    gangrene (and intermittent claudication, rest pain and ulcer) I70.662
    intermittent claudication I70.612
    rest pain (and intermittent claudication) I70.622
    ulceration (and intermittent claudication and rest pain) I70.649
      ankle I70.643
      calf I70.642
      foot site NEC I70.645
      heel I70.644
      lower leg NEC I70.648
      midfoot I70.644
      thigh I70.641
    specified type NEC I70.692
   right I70.601
    with
      gangrene (and intermittent claudication, rest pain and ulcer) I70.661
      intermittent claudication I70.611
      rest pain (and intermittent claudication) I70.621
      ulceration (and intermittent claudication and rest pain) I70.639
        ankle I70.633
        calf I70.632
        foot site NEC I70.635
        heel I70.634
        lower leg NEC I70.638
        midfoot I70.634
        thigh I70.631
      specified type NEC I70.691
   specified NEC I70.608
    with
      gangrene (and intermittent claudication, rest pain and ulcer) I70.668
      intermittent claudication I70.618
      rest pain (and intermittent claudication) I70.628
      ulceration (and intermittent claudication and rest pain) I70.65
    specified type NEC I70.698
  specified graft NEC I70.709
   leg I70.709
    with
      gangrene (and intermittent claudication, rest pain and ulcer) I70.769
      intermittent claudication I70.719
      rest pain (and intermittent claudication) I70.729
    bilateral I70.703
     with
       gangrene (and intermittent claudication, rest pain and ulcer) I70.763
       intermittent claudication I70.713
       rest pain (and intermittent claudication) I70.723
      specified type NEC I70.793
    left I70.702
     with
       gangrene (and intermittent claudication, rest pain and ulcer) I70.762
       intermittent claudication I70.712
       rest pain (and intermittent claudication) I70.722
       ulceration (and intermittent claudication and rest pain) I70.749
         ankle I70.743
         calf I70.742
         foot site NEC I70.745
         heel I70.744
         lower leg NEC I70.748
         midfoot I70.744
         thigh I70.741
       specified type NEC I70.792
    right I70.701
     with
       gangrene (and intermittent claudication, rest pain and ulcer) I70.761
       intermittent claudication I70.711
       rest pain (and intermittent claudication) I70.721
       ulceration (and intermittent claudication and rest pain) I70.739

☑ **Additional character required**

Arteriosclerosis — *continued*
  extremities — *continued*
    ankle I70.733
    calf I70.732
    foot site NEC I70.735
    heel I70.734
    lower leg NEC I70.738
    midfoot I70.734
    thigh I70.731
    specified type NEC I70.791
    specified type NEC I70.799
   specified NEC I70.708
    with
     gangrene (and intermittent claudication, rest pain and ulcer) I70.768
     intermittent claudication I70.718
     rest pain (and intermittent claudication) I70.728
     ulceration (and intermittent claudication and rest pain) I70.75
     specified type NEC I70.798
  specified NEC I70.308
   with
    gangrene (and intermittent claudication, rest pain and ulcer) I70.368
    intermittent claudication I70.318
    rest pain (and intermittent claudication) I70.328
    ulceration (and intermittent claudication and rest pain) I70.35
    specified type NEC I70.398
  leg I70.209
   with
    gangrene (and intermittent claudication, rest pain and ulcer) I70.269
    intermittent claudication I70.219
    rest pain (and intermittent claudication) I70.229
   bilateral I70.203
    with
     gangrene (and intermittent claudication, rest pain and ulcer) I70.263
     intermittent claudication I70.213
     rest pain (and intermittent claudication) I70.223
     specified type NEC I70.293
   left I70.202
    with
     gangrene (and intermittent claudication, rest pain and ulcer) I70.262
     intermittent claudication I70.212
     rest pain (and intermittent claudication) I70.222
     ulceration (and intermittent claudication and rest pain) I70.249
      ankle I70.243
      calf I70.242
      foot site NEC I70.245
      heel I70.244
      lower leg NEC I70.248
      midfoot I70.244
      thigh I70.241
     specified type NEC I70.292
   right I70.201
    with
     gangrene (and intermittent claudication, rest pain and ulcer) I70.261
     intermittent claudication I70.211
     rest pain (and intermittent claudication) I70.221
     ulceration (and intermittent claudication and rest pain) I70.239
      ankle I70.233
      calf I70.232
      foot site NEC I70.235
      heel I70.234
      lower leg NEC I70.238
      midfoot I70.234
      thigh I70.231
     specified type NEC I70.291
    specified type NEC I70.299
  specified site NEC I70.208
   with
    gangrene (and intermittent claudication, rest pain and ulcer) I70.268
    intermittent claudication I70.218
    rest pain (and intermittent claudication) I70.228
    ulceration (and intermittent claudication and rest pain) I70.25
    specified type NEC I70.298
  generalized I70.91

Arteriosclerosis — *continued*
  heart (disease) — *see* Arteriosclerosis, coronary (artery),
  kidney — *see* Hypertension, kidney
  medial — *see* Arteriosclerosis, extremities
  mesenteric (artery) K55.1
  Mönckeberg's — *see* Arteriosclerosis, extremities
  myocarditis I51.4
  peripheral (of extremities) — *see* Arteriosclerosis, extremities
  pulmonary (idiopathic) I27.0
  renal (arterioles) (*see also* Hypertension, kidney)
   artery I70.1
  retina (vascular) I70.8 *[H35.0 ☑]*
  specified artery NEC I70.8
  spinal (cord) G95.19
  vertebral (artery) I67.2
Arteriospasm I73.9
Arteriovenous — *see* condition
Arteritis I77.6
  allergic M31.0
  aorta (nonsyphilitic) I77.6
   syphilitic A52.02
  aortic arch M31.4
  brachiocephalic M31.4
  brain I67.7
   syphilitic A52.04
  cerebral I67.7
   in
    diseases classified elsewhere I68.2
    systemic lupus erythematosus M32.19
   listerial A32.89
   syphilitic A52.04
   tuberculous A18.89
  coronary (artery) I25.89
   rheumatic I01.8
    chronic I09.89
   syphilitic A52.06
  cranial (left) (right), giant cell M31.6
  deformans — *see* Arteriosclerosis
  giant cell NEC M31.6
   with polymyalgia rheumatica M31.5
  necrosing or necrotizing M31.9
   specified NEC M31.8
  nodosa M30.0
  obliterans — *see* Arteriosclerosis
  pulmonary I28.8
  rheumatic — *see* Fever, rheumatic
  senile — *see* Arteriosclerosis
  suppurative I77.2
  syphilitic (general) A52.09
   brain A52.04
   coronary A52.06
   spinal A52.09
  temporal, giant cell M31.6
  young female aortic arch syndrome M31.4
Artery, arterial (*see also* condition)
  abscess I77.89
  single umbilical Q27.0
Arthralgia (allergic) (*see also* Pain, joint)
  in caisson disease T70.3 ☑
  temporomandibular M26.62 ☑
Arthritis, arthritic (acute) (chronic) (nonpyogenic) (subacute) M19.90
  allergic — *see* Arthritis, specified form NEC
  ankylosing (crippling) (spine) (*see also* Spondylitis, ankylosing)
   sites other than spine — *see* Arthritis, specified form NEC
  atrophic — *see* Osteoarthritis
   spine — *see* Spondylitis, ankylosing
  back — *see* Spondylopathy, inflammatory
  blennorrhagic (gonococcal) A54.42
  Charcot's — *see* Arthropathy, neuropathic
   diabetic — *see* Diabetes, arthropathy, neuropathic
   syringomyelic G95.0
  chylous (filarial) (*see also* category M01 ☑) B74.9
  climacteric (any site) NEC — *see* Arthritis, specified form NEC
  crystal (-induced) — *see* Arthritis, in, crystals
  deformans — *see* Osteoarthritis
  degenerative — *see* Osteoarthritis
  due to or associated with
   acromegaly E22.0
   brucellosis — *see* Brucellosis
   caisson disease T70.3 ☑
   diabetes — *see* Diabetes, arthropathy
   dracontiasis (*see also* category M01 ☑) B72
   enteritis NEC
    regional — *see* Enteritis, regional
   erysipelas (*see also* category M01 ☑) A46
   erythema

Arthritis — *continued*
  due to or associated with — *continued*
   epidemic A25.1
   nodosum L52
   filariasis NOS B74.9
   glanders A24.0
   helminthiasis (*see also* category M01 ☑) B83.9
   hemophilia D66 *[M36.2]*
   Henoch- (Schönlein) purpura D69.0 *[M36.4]*
   human parvovirus (*see also* category M01 ☑) B97.6
   infectious disease NEC — *see* category M01 ☑
   leprosy (*see also* category M01 ☑) (*see also* Leprosy) A30.9
   Lyme disease A69.23
   mycobacteria (*see also* category M01 ☑) A31.8
   parasitic disease NEC (*see also* category M01 ☑) B89
   paratyphoid fever (*see also* category M01 ☑) (*see also* Fever, paratyphoid) A01.4
   rat bite fever (*see also* category M01 ☑) A25.1
   regional enteritis — *see* Enteritis, regional
   respiratory disorder NOS J98.9
   serum sickness (*see also* Reaction, serum) T80.69 ☑
   syringomyelia G95.0
   typhoid fever A01.04
  epidemic erythema A25.1
  febrile — *see* Fever, rheumatic
  gonococcal A54.42
  gouty (acute) — *see* Gout
  in (due to)
   acromegaly (*see also* subcategory M14.8 ☑) E22.0
   amyloidosis (*see also* subcategory M14.8 ☑) E85.4
   bacterial disease (*see also* subcategory M01 ☑) A49.9
   Behçet's syndrome M35.2
   caisson disease (*see also* subcategory M14.8 ☑) T70.3 ☑
   coliform bacilli (Escherichia coli) — *see* Arthritis, in, pyogenic organism NEC
   crystals M11.9
    dicalcium phosphate — *see* Arthritis, in, crystals, specified type NEC
    hydroxyapatite M11.0 ☑
    pyrophosphate — *see* Arthritis, in, crystals, specified type NEC
    specified type NEC M11.80
     ankle M11.87 ☑
     elbow M11.82 ☑
     foot joint M11.87 ☑
     hand joint M11.84 ☑
     hip M11.85 ☑
     knee M11.86 ☑
     multiple sites M11.8 ☑
     shoulder M11.81 ☑
     vertebrae M11.88
     wrist M11.83 ☑
   dermatoarthritis, lipoid E78.81
   dracontiasis (dracunculiasis) (*see also* category M01 ☑) B72
   endocrine disorder NEC (*see also* subcategory M14.8 ☑) E34.9
   enteritis, infectious NEC (*see also* category M01 ☑) A09
    specified organism NEC (*see also* category M01 ☑) A08.8
   erythema
    multiforme (*see also* subcategory M14.8 ☑) L51.9
    nodosum (*see also* subcategory M14.8 ☑) L52
   gout — *see* Gout
   helminthiasis NEC (*see also* category M01 ☑) B83.9
   hemochromatosis (*see also* subcategory M14.8 ☑) E83.118
   hemoglobinopathy NEC D58.2 *[M36.3]*
   hemophilia NEC D66 *[M36.2]*
   Hemophilus influenzae M00.8 ☑ *[B96.3]*
   Henoch (-Schönlein) purpura D69.0 *[M36.4]*
   hyperparathyroidism NEC (*see also* subcategory M14.8 ☑) E21.3
   hypersensitivity reaction NEC T78.49 ☑ *[M36.4]*
   hypogammaglobulinemia (*see also* subcategory M14.8 ☑) D80.1
   hypothyroidism NEC (*see also* subcategory M14.8 ☑) E03.9
   infection — *see* Arthritis, pyogenic or pyemic
    spine — *see* Spondylopathy, infective
   infectious disease NEC — *see* category M01 ☑
   leprosy (*see also* category M01 ☑) A30.9
   leukemia NEC C95.9 ☑ *[M36.1]*

☑ **Additional character required**

Arthritis

Arthritis — *continued*
  in — *continued*
    lipoid dermatoarthritis E78.81
    Lyme disease A69.23
    Mediterranean fever, familial (*see also* subcategory M14.8 ☑) M04.1
    Meningococcus A39.83
    metabolic disorder NEC (*see also* subcategory M14.8 ☑) E88.9
    multiple myelomatosis C90.0 ☑ [M36.1]
    mumps B26.85
    mycosis NEC (*see also* category M01 ☑) B49
    myelomatosis (multiple) C90.0 ☑ [M36.1]
    neurological disorder NEC G98.0
    ochronosis (*see also* subcategory M14.8 ☑) E70.29
    O'nyong-nyong (*see also* category M01 ☑) A92.1
    parasitic disease NEC (*see also* category M01 ☑) B89
    paratyphoid fever (*see also* category M01 ☑) A01.4
    Pseudomonas — *see* Arthritis, pyogenic, bacterial NEC
    psoriasis L40.50
    pyogenic organism NEC — *see* Arthritis, pyogenic, bacterial NEC
    Reiter's disease — *see* Reiter's disease
    respiratory disorder NEC (*see also* subcategory M14.8 ☑) J98.9
    reticulosis, malignant (*see also* subcategory M14.8 ☑) C86.0
    rubella B06.82
    Salmonella (arizonae) (cholerae-suis) (enteritidis) (typhimurium) A02.23
    sarcoidosis D86.86
    specified bacteria NEC — *see* Arthritis, pyogenic, bacterial NEC
    sporotrichosis B42.82
    syringomyelia G95.0
    thalassemia NEC D56.9 [M36.3]
    tuberculosis — *see* Tuberculosis, arthritis
    typhoid fever A01.04
    urethritis, Reiter's — *see* Reiter's disease
    viral disease NEC (*see also* category M01 ☑) B34.9
  infectious or infective (*see also* Arthritis, pyogenic or pyemic)
    spine — *see* Spondylopathy, infective
  juvenile M08.90
    with systemic onset — *see* Still's disease
    ankle M08.97 ☑
    elbow M08.92 ☑
    foot joint M08.97 ☑
    hand joint M08.94 ☑
    hip M08.95 ☑
    knee M08.96 ☑
    multiple site M08.99
    pauciarticular M08.40
      ankle M08.47 ☑
      elbow M08.42 ☑
      foot joint M08.47 ☑
      hand joint M08.44 ☑
      hip M08.45 ☑
      knee M08.46 ☑
      shoulder M08.41 ☑
      vertebrae M08.48
      wrist M08.43 ☑
    psoriatic L40.54
    rheumatoid — *see* Arthritis, rheumatoid, juvenile
    shoulder M08.91 ☑
    vertebra M08.98
    specified type NEC M08.80
      ankle M08.87 ☑
      elbow M08.82 ☑
      foot joint M08.87 ☑
      hand joint M08.84 ☑
      hip M08.85 ☑
      knee M08.86 ☑
      multiple site M08.89
      shoulder M08.81 ☑
      specified joint NEC M08.88
      vertebrae M08.88
      wrist M08.83 ☑
    wrist M08.93 ☑
  meaning osteoarthritis — *see* Osteoarthritis
  meningococcal A39.83
  menopausal (any site) NEC — *see* Arthritis, specified form NEC
  mutilans (psoriatic) L40.52
  mycotic NEC (*see also* category M01 ☑) B49
  neuropathic (Charcot) — *see* Arthropathy, neuropathic
    diabetic — *see* Diabetes, arthropathy, neuropathic
    nonsyphilitic NEC G98.0
    syringomyelic G95.0

Arthritis — *continued*
  ochronotic (*see also* subcategory M14.8 ☑) E70.29
  palindromic (any site) — *see* Rheumatism, palindromic
  pneumococcal M00.10
    ankle M00.17 ☑
    elbow M00.12 ☑
    foot joint — *see* Arthritis, pneumococcal, ankle
    hand joint M00.14 ☑
    hip M00.15 ☑
    knee M00.16 ☑
    multiple site M00.19
    shoulder M00.11 ☑
    vertebra M00.18
    wrist M00.13 ☑
  postdysenteric — *see* Arthropathy, postdysenteric
  postmeningococcal A39.84
  postrheumatic, chronic — *see* Arthropathy, postrheumatic, chronic
  primary progressive (*see also* Arthritis, specified form NEC)
    spine — *see* Spondylitis, ankylosing
  psoriatic L40.50
  purulent (any site except spine) — *see* Arthritis, pyogenic or pyemic
    spine — *see* Spondylopathy, infective
  pyogenic or pyemic (any site except spine) M00.9
    bacterial NEC M00.80
      ankle M00.87 ☑
      elbow M00.82 ☑
      foot joint — *see* Arthritis, pyogenic, bacterial NEC, ankle
      hand joint M00.84 ☑
      hip M00.85 ☑
      knee M00.86 ☑
      multiple site M00.89
      shoulder M00.81 ☑
      vertebra M00.88
      wrist M00.83 ☑
    pneumococcal — *see* Arthritis, pneumococcal
    spine — *see* Spondylopathy, infective
    staphylococcal — *see* Arthritis, staphylococcal
    streptococcal — *see* Arthritis, streptococcal NEC
    pneumococcal — *see* Arthritis, pneumococcal
  reactive — *see* Reiter's disease
  rheumatic (*see also* Arthritis, rheumatoid)
    acute or subacute — *see* Fever, rheumatic
  rheumatoid M06.9
    with
      carditis — *see* Rheumatoid, carditis
      endocarditis — *see* Rheumatoid, carditis
      heart involvement NEC — *see* Rheumatoid, carditis
      lung involvement — *see* Rheumatoid, lung
      myocarditis — *see* Rheumatoid, carditis
      myopathy — *see* Rheumatoid, myopathy
      pericarditis — *see* Rheumatoid, carditis
      polyneuropathy — *see* Rheumatoid, polyneuropathy
      rheumatoid factor — *see* Arthritis, rheumatoid, seropositive
      splenoadenomegaly and leukopenia — *see* Felty's syndrome
      vasculitis — *see* Rheumatoid, vasculitis
      visceral involvement NEC — *see* Rheumatoid, arthritis, with involvement of organs NEC
    juvenile (with or without rheumatoid factor) M08.00
      ankle M08.07 ☑
      elbow M08.02 ☑
      foot joint M08.07 ☑
      hand joint M08.04 ☑
      hip M08.05 ☑
      knee M08.06 ☑
      multiple site M08.09
      shoulder M08.01 ☑
      vertebra M08.08
      wrist M08.03 ☑
    seronegative M06.00
      ankle M06.07 ☑
      elbow M06.02 ☑
      foot joint M06.07 ☑
      hand joint M06.04 ☑
      hip M06.05 ☑
      knee M06.06 ☑
      multiple site M06.09
      shoulder M06.01 ☑
      vertebra M06.08
      wrist M06.03 ☑
    seropositive M05.9
      specified NEC M05.80
        ankle M05.87 ☑

Arthritis — *continued*
  rheumatoid — *continued*
    elbow M05.82 ☑
    foot joint M05.87 ☑
    hand joint M05.84 ☑
    hip M05.85 ☑
    knee M05.86 ☑
    multiple sites M05.89
    shoulder M05.81 ☑
    vertebra — *see* Spondylitis, ankylosing
    wrist M05.83 ☑
    without organ involvement M05.70
      ankle M05.77 ☑
      elbow M05.72 ☑
      foot joint M05.77 ☑
      hand joint M05.74 ☑
      hip M05.75 ☑
      knee M05.76 ☑
      multiple sites M05.79
      shoulder M05.71 ☑
      vertebra — *see* Spondylitis, ankylosing
      wrist M05.73 ☑
    specified type NEC M06.80
      ankle M06.87 ☑
      elbow M06.82 ☑
      foot joint M06.87 ☑
      hand joint M06.84 ☑
      hip M06.85 ☑
      knee M06.86 ☑
      multiple site M06.89
      shoulder M06.81 ☑
      vertebra M06.88
      wrist M06.83 ☑
    spine — *see* Spondylitis, ankylosing
  rubella B06.82
  scorbutic (*see also* subcategory M14.8 ☑) E54
  senile or senescent — *see* Osteoarthritis
  septic (any site except spine) — *see* Arthritis, pyogenic or pyemic
    spine — *see* Spondylopathy, infective
  serum (nontherapeutic) (therapeutic) — *see* Arthropathy, postimmunization
  specified form NEC M13.80
    ankle M13.87 ☑
    elbow M13.82 ☑
    foot joint M13.87 ☑
    hand joint M13.84 ☑
    hip M13.85 ☑
    knee M13.86 ☑
    multiple site M13.89
    shoulder M13.81 ☑
    specified joint NEC M13.88
    wrist M13.83 ☑
  spine (*see also* Spondylopathy, inflammatory)
    infectious or infective NEC — *see* Spondylopathy, infective
    Marie-Strümpell — *see* Spondylitis, ankylosing
    pyogenic — *see* Spondylopathy, infective
    rheumatoid — *see* Spondylitis, ankylosing
    traumatic (old) — *see* Spondylopathy, traumatic
    tuberculous A18.01
  staphylococcal M00.00
    ankle M00.07 ☑
    elbow M00.02 ☑
    foot joint — *see* Arthritis, staphylococcal, ankle
    hand joint M00.04 ☑
    hip M00.05 ☑
    knee M00.06 ☑
    multiple site M00.09
    shoulder M00.01 ☑
    vertebra M00.08
    wrist M00.03 ☑
  streptococcal NEC M00.20
    ankle M00.27 ☑
    elbow M00.22 ☑
    foot joint — *see* Arthritis, streptococcal, ankle
    hand joint M00.24 ☑
    hip M00.25 ☑
    knee M00.26 ☑
    multiple site M00.29
    shoulder M00.21 ☑
    vertebra M00.28
    wrist M00.23 ☑
  suppurative — *see* Arthritis, pyogenic or pyemic
  syphilitic (late) A52.16
    congenital A50.55 [M12.80]
  syphilitica deformans (Charcot) A52.16
  temporomandibular M26.69
  toxic of menopause (any site) — *see* Arthritis, specified form NEC
  transient — *see* Arthropathy, specified form NEC
  traumatic (chronic) — *see* Arthropathy, traumatic

☑ **Additional character required**

Arthritis — *continued*
  tuberculous A18.02
    spine A18.01
  uratic — *see* Gout
  urethritica (Reiter's) — *see* Reiter's disease
  vertebral — *see* Spondylopathy, inflammatory
  villous (any site) — *see* Arthropathy, specified form
    NEC
Arthrocele — *see* Effusion, joint
Arthrodesis status Z98.1
Arthrodynia (*see also* Pain, joint)
Arthrodysplasia Q74.9
Arthrofibrosis, joint — *see* Ankylosis
Arthrogryposis (congenital) Q68.8
  multiplex congenita Q74.3
Arthrokatadysis M24.7
Arthropathy (*see also* Arthritis) M12.9
  Charcot's — *see* Arthropathy, neuropathic
    diabetic — *see* Diabetes, arthropathy, neuropathic
    syringomyelic G95.0
  cricoarytenoid J38.7
  crystal (-induced) — *see* Arthritis, in, crystals
  diabetic NEC — *see* Diabetes, arthropathy
  distal interphalangeal, psoriatic L40.51
  enteropathic M07.60
    ankle M07.67 ☑
    elbow M07.62 ☑
    foot joint M07.67 ☑
    hand joint M07.64 ☑
    hip M07.65 ☑
    knee M07.66 ☑
    multiple site M07.69
    shoulder M07.61 ☑
    vertebra M07.68
    wrist M07.63 ☑
  following intestinal bypass M02.00
    ankle M02.07 ☑
    elbow M02.02 ☑
    foot joint M02.07 ☑
    hand joint M02.04 ☑
    hip M02.05 ☑
    knee M02.06 ☑
    multiple site M02.09
    shoulder M02.01 ☑
    vertebra M02.08
    wrist M02.03 ☑
  gouty (*see also* Gout)
    in (due to)
      Lesch-Nyhan syndrome E79.1 *[M14.8 ☑]*
      sickle-cell disorders D57 ☑ *[M14.8 ☑]*
  hemophilic NEC D66 *[M36.2]*
    in (due to)
      hyperparathyroidism NEC E21.3 *[M14.8 ☑]*
      metabolic disease NOS E88.9 *[M14.8 ☑]*
  in (due to)
    acromegaly E22.0 *[M14.8 ☑]*
    amyloidosis E85.4 *[M14.8 ☑]*
    blood disorder NOS D75.9 *[M36.3]*
    diabetes — *see* Diabetes, arthropathy
    endocrine disease NOS E34.9 *[M14.8 ☑]*
    erythema
      multiforme L51.9 *[M14.8 ☑]*
      nodosum L52 *[M14.8 ☑]*
    hemochromatosis E83.118 *[M14.8 ☑]*
    hemoglobinopathy NEC D58.2 *[M36.3]*
    hemophilia NEC D66 *[M36.2]*
    Henoch-Schönlein purpura D69.0 *[M36.4]*
    hyperthyroidism E05.90 *[M14.8 ☑]*
    hypothyroidism E03.9 *[M14.8 ☑]*
    infective endocarditis I33.0 *[M12.80]*
    leukemia NEC C95.9 ☑ *[M36.1]*
    malignant histiocytosis C96.A *[M36.1]*
    metabolic disease NOS E88.9 *[M14.8 ☑]*
    multiple myeloma C90.0 ☑ *[M36.1]*
    neoplastic disease NOS (*see also* Neoplasm) D49.9
      [M36.1]
    nutritional deficiency (*see also* subcategory
      M14.8 ☑) E63.9
    psoriasis NOS L40.50
    sarcoidosis D86.86
    syphilis (late) A52.77
      congenital A50.55 *[M12.80]*
    thyrotoxicosis (*see also* subcategory M14.8 ☑)
      E05.90
    ulcerative colitis K51.90 *[M07.60]*
    viral hepatitis (postinfectious) NEC B19.9 *[M12.80]*
    Whipple's disease (*see also* subcategory M14.8 ☑)
      K90.81
  Jaccoud — *see* Arthropathy, postrheumatic, chronic
  juvenile — *see* Arthritis, juvenile
    psoriatic L40.54
  mutilans (psoriatic) L40.52

Arthropathy — *continued*
  neuropathic (Charcot) M14.60
    ankle M14.67 ☑
    diabetic — *see* Diabetes, arthropathy, neuropathic
    elbow M14.62 ☑
    foot joint M14.67 ☑
    hand joint M14.64 ☑
    hip M14.65 ☑
    knee M14.66 ☑
    multiple site M14.69
    nonsyphilitic NEC G98.0
    shoulder M14.61 ☑
    syringomyelic G95.0
    vertebra M14.68
    wrist M14.63 ☑
  osteopulmonary — *see* Osteoarthropathy,
    hypertrophic, specified NEC
  postdysenteric M02.10
    ankle M02.17 ☑
    elbow M02.12 ☑
    foot joint M02.17 ☑
    hand joint M02.14 ☑
    hip M02.15 ☑
    knee M02.16 ☑
    multiple site M02.19
    shoulder M02.11 ☑
    vertebra M02.18
    wrist M02.13 ☑
  postimmunization M02.20
    ankle M02.27 ☑
    elbow M02.22 ☑
    foot joint M02.27 ☑
    hand joint M02.24 ☑
    hip M02.25 ☑
    knee M02.26 ☑
    multiple site M02.29
    shoulder M02.21 ☑
    vertebra M02.28
    wrist M02.23 ☑
  postinfectious NEC B99 ☑ *[M12.80]*
    in (due to)
      enteritis due to Yersinia enterocolitica A04.6
        [M12.80]
      syphilis A52.77
      viral hepatitis NEC B19.9 *[M12.80]*
  postrheumatic, chronic (Jaccoud) M12.00
    ankle M12.07 ☑
    elbow M12.02 ☑
    foot joint M12.07 ☑
    hand joint M12.04 ☑
    hip M12.05 ☑
    knee M12.06 ☑
    multiple site M12.09
    shoulder M12.01 ☑
    specified joint NEC M12.08
    vertebrae M12.08
    wrist M12.03 ☑
  psoriatic NEC L40.59
    interphalangeal, distal L40.51
  reactive M02.9
    in (due to)
      infective endocarditis I33.0 *[M02.9]*
    specified type NEC M02.80
      ankle M02.87 ☑
      elbow M02.82 ☑
      foot joint M02.87 ☑
      hand joint M02.84 ☑
      hip M02.85 ☑
      knee M02.86 ☑
      multiple site M02.89
      shoulder M02.81 ☑
      vertebra M02.88
      wrist M02.83 ☑
  specified form NEC M12.80
    ankle M12.87 ☑
    elbow M12.82 ☑
    foot joint M12.87 ☑
    hand joint M12.84 ☑
    hip M12.85 ☑
    knee M12.86 ☑
    multiple site M12.89
    shoulder M12.81 ☑
    specified joint NEC M12.88
    vertebrae M12.88
    wrist M12.83 ☑
  syringomyelic G95.0
  tabes dorsalis A52.16
  tabetic A52.16
  transient — *see* Arthropathy, specified form NEC
  traumatic M12.50
    ankle M12.57 ☑
    elbow M12.52 ☑

Arthropathy — *continued*
  traumatic — *continued*
    foot joint M12.57 ☑
    hand joint M12.54 ☑
    hip M12.55 ☑
    knee M12.56 ☑
    multiple site M12.59
    shoulder M12.51 ☑
    specified joint NEC M12.58
    vertebrae M12.58
    wrist M12.53 ☑
Arthropyosis — *see* Arthritis, pyogenic or pyemic
Arthrosis (deformans) (degenerative) (localized)
  (*see also* Osteoarthritis) M19.90
  spine — *see* Spondylosis
Arthus' phenomenon or reaction T78.41 ☑
  due to
    drug — *see* Table of Drugs and Chemicals, by
      drug
Articular — *see* condition
Articulation, reverse (teeth) M26.24
Artificial
  insemination complication — *see* Complications,
    artificial, fertilization
  opening status (functioning) (without
    complication) Z93.9
    anus (colostomy) Z93.3
    colostomy Z93.3
    cystostomy Z93.50
      appendico-vesicostomy Z93.52
      cutaneous Z93.51
      specified NEC Z93.59
    enterostomy Z93.4
    gastrostomy Z93.1
    ileostomy Z93.2
    intestinal tract NEC Z93.4
    jejunostomy Z93.4
    nephrostomy Z93.6
    specified site NEC Z93.8
    tracheostomy Z93.0
    ureterostomy Z93.6
    urethrostomy Z93.6
    urinary tract NEC Z93.6
    vagina Z93.8
  vagina status Z93.8
Arytenoid — *see* condition
Asbestosis (occupational) J61
ASC-H (atypical squamous cells cannot exclude high
  grade squamous intraepithelial lesion on cytologic
  smear)
  anus R85.611
  cervix R87.611
  vagina R87.621
ASC-US (atypical squamous cells of undetermined
  significance on cytologic smear)
  anus R85.610
  cervix R87.610
  vagina R87.620
Ascariasis B77.9
  with
    complications NEC B77.89
    intestinal complications B77.0
    pneumonia, pneumonitis B77.81
Ascaridosis, ascaridiasis — *see* Ascariasis
Ascaris (infection) (infestation) (lumbricoides) — *see*
  Ascariasis
Ascending — *see* condition
Aschoff's bodies — *see* Myocarditis, rheumatic
Ascites (abdominal) R18.8
  cardiac (*see also* Failure, heart, right) I50.810
  chylous (nonfilarial) I89.8
    filarial — *see* Infestation, filarial
  due to
    cirrhosis, alcoholic K70.31
    hepatitis
      alcoholic K70.11
      chronic active K71.51
    S. japonicum B65.2
  heart (*see also* Failure, heart, right) I50.810
  malignant R18.0
  pseudochylous R18.8
  syphilitic A52.74
  tuberculous A18.31
Aseptic — *see* condition
Asherman's syndrome N85.6
Asialia K11.7
Asiatic cholera — *see* Cholera
Asimultagnosia (simultanagnosia) R48.3
Askin's tumor — *see* Neoplasm, connective tissue,
  malignant
Asocial personality F60.2
Asomatognosia R41.4

Aspartylglucosaminuria - Asthma

Aspartylglucosaminuria E77.1
Asperger's disease or syndrome F84.5
Aspergilloma — *see* Aspergillosis
Aspergillosis (with pneumonia) B44.9
  bronchopulmonary, allergic B44.81
  disseminated B44.7
  generalized B44.7
  pulmonary NEC B44.1
    allergic B44.81
    invasive B44.0
  specified NEC B44.89
  tonsillar B44.2
Aspergillus (flavus) (fumigatus) (infection) (terreus) —
  see Aspergillosis
Aspermatogenesis — *see* Azoospermia
Aspermia (testis) — *see* Azoospermia
Asphyxia, asphyxiation (by) R09.01
  antenatal P84
  birth P84
  bunny bag — *see* Asphyxia, due to, mechanical
    threat to breathing, trapped in bed clothes
  crushing S28.0 ☑
  drowning T75.1 ☑
  gas, fumes, or vapor — *see* Table of Drugs and
    Chemicals
  inhalation — *see* Inhalation
  intrauterine P84
  local I73.00
    with gangrene I73.01
  mucus (*see also* Foreign body, respiratory tract,
    causing asphyxia)
  newborn P84
  pathological R09.01
  postnatal P84
    mechanical — *see* Asphyxia, due to, mechanical
      threat to breathing
  prenatal P84
  reticularis R23.1
  strangulation — *see* Asphyxia, due to, mechanical
    threat to breathing
  submersion T75.1 ☑
  traumatic T71.9 ☑
    due to
      crushed chest S28.0 ☑
      foreign body (in) — *see* Foreign body,
        respiratory tract, causing asphyxia
      low oxygen content of ambient air T71.20 ☑
        due to
          being trapped in
            low oxygen environment T71.29 ☑
            in car trunk T71.221 ☑
              circumstances undetermined
                T71.224 ☑
              done with intent to harm by
                another person T71.223 ☑
                self T71.222 ☑
            in refrigerator T71.231 ☑
              circumstances undetermined
                T71.234 ☑
              done with intent to harm by
                another person T71.233 ☑
                self T71.232 ☑
          cave-in T71.21 ☑
      mechanical threat to breathing (accidental)
        T71.191 ☑
        circumstances undetermined T71.194 ☑
        done with intent to harm by
          another person T71.193 ☑
          self T71.192 ☑
      hanging T71.161 ☑
        circumstances undetermined T71.164 ☑
        done with intent to harm by
          another person T71.163 ☑
          self T71.162 ☑
      plastic bag T71.121 ☑
        circumstances undetermined T71.124 ☑
        done with intent to harm by
          another person T71.123 ☑
          self T71.122 ☑
      smothering
        in furniture T71.151 ☑
          circumstances undetermined T71.154 ☑
          done with intent to harm by
            another person T71.153 ☑
            self T71.152 ☑
        under
          another person's body T71.141 ☑
            circumstances undetermined
              T71.144 ☑
            done with intent to harm T71.143 ☑
          pillow T71.111 ☑

Asphyxia — *continued*
  traumatic — *continued*
      circumstances undetermined
        T71.114 ☑
      done with intent to harm by
        another person T71.113 ☑
        self T71.112 ☑
      trapped in bed clothes T71.131 ☑
        circumstances undetermined T71.134 ☑
        done with intent to harm by
          another person T71.133 ☑
          self T71.132 ☑
  vomiting, vomitus — *see* Foreign body, respiratory
    tract, causing asphyxia
Aspiration
  amniotic (clear) fluid (newborn) P24.10
    with
      pneumonia (pneumonitis) P24.11
      respiratory symptoms P24.11
  blood
    newborn (without respiratory symptoms) P24.20
      with
        pneumonia (pneumonitis) P24.21
        respiratory symptoms P24.21
    specified age NEC — *see* Foreign body, respiratory
      tract
  bronchitis J69.0
  food or foreign body (with asphyxiation) — *see*
    Asphyxia, food
  liquor (amnii) (newborn) P24.10
    with
      pneumonia (pneumonitis) P24.11
      respiratory symptoms P24.11
  meconium (newborn) (without respiratory
    symptoms) P24.00
      with
        pneumonitis (pneumonitis) P24.01
        respiratory symptoms P24.01
  milk (newborn) (without respiratory symptoms)
    P24.30
      with
        pneumonia (pneumonitis) P24.31
        respiratory symptoms P24.31
    specified age NEC — *see* Foreign body, respiratory
      tract
  mucus (*see also* Foreign body, by site, causing
    asphyxia)
    newborn P24.10
      with
        pneumonia (pneumonitis) P24.11
        respiratory symptoms P24.11
  neonatal P24.9
    specific NEC (without respiratory symptoms)
      P24.80
      with
        pneumonia (pneumonitis) P24.81
        respiratory symptoms P24.81
  newborn P24.9
    specific NEC (without respiratory symptoms)
      P24.80
      with
        pneumonia (pneumonitis) P24.81
        respiratory symptoms P24.81
  pneumonia J69.0
  pneumonitis J69.0
  syndrome of newborn — *see* Aspiration, by
    substance, with pneumonia
  vernix caseosa (newborn) P24.80
    with
      pneumonia (pneumonitis) P24.81
      respiratory symptoms P24.81
  vomitus (*see also* Foreign body, respiratory tract)
    newborn (without respiratory symptoms) P24.30
      with
        pneumonia (pneumonitis) P24.31
        respiratory symptoms P24.31
Asplenia (congenital) Q89.01
  postsurgical Z90.81
Assam fever B55.0
Assault, sexual — *see* Maltreatment
Assmann's focus NEC A15.0
Astasia (-abasia) (hysterical) F44.4
Asteatosis cutis L85.3
Astereognosia, astereognosis R48.1
Asterixis R27.8
  in liver disease K71.3
Asteroid hyalitis — *see* Deposit, crystalline
Asthenia, asthenic R53.1
  cardiac (*see also* Failure, heart) I50.9
    psychogenic F45.8
  cardiovascular (*see also* Failure, heart) I50.9
    psychogenic F45.8

Asthenia — *continued*
  heart (*see also* Failure, heart) I50.9
    psychogenic F45.8
  hysterical F44.4
  myocardial (*see also* Failure, heart) I50.9
    psychogenic F45.8
  nervous F48.8
  neurocirculatory F45.8
  neurotic F48.8
  psychogenic F48.8
  psychoneurotic F48.8
  psychophysiologic F48.8
  reaction (psychophysiologic) F48.8
  senile R54
Asthenopia (*see also* Discomfort, visual)
  hysterical F44.6
  psychogenic F44.6
Asthenospermia — *see* Abnormal, specimen, male
  genital organs
Asthma, asthmatic (bronchial) (catarrh) (spasmodic)
  J45.909
  with
    chronic obstructive bronchitis J44.9
      with
        acute lower respiratory infection J44.0
        exacerbation (acute) J44.1
    chronic obstructive pulmonary disease J44.9
      with
        acute lower respiratory infection J44.0
        exacerbation (acute) J44.1
    exacerbation (acute) J45.901
    hay fever — *see* Asthma, allergic extrinsic
    rhinitis, allergic — *see* Asthma, allergic extrinsic
    status asthmaticus J45.902
  allergic extrinsic J45.909
    with
      exacerbation (acute) J45.901
      status asthmaticus J45.902
  atopic — *see* Asthma, allergic extrinsic
  cardiac — *see* Failure, ventricular, left
  cardiobronchial I50.1
  childhood J45.909
    with
      exacerbation (acute) J45.901
      status asthmaticus J45.902
  chronic obstructive J44.9
    with
      acute lower respiratory infection J44.0
      exacerbation (acute) J44.1
  collier's J60
  cough variant J45.991
  detergent J69.8
  due to
    detergent J69.8
    inhalation of fumes J68.3
  eosinophilic J82
  extrinsic, allergic — *see* Asthma, allergic extrinsic
  grinder's J62.8
  hay — *see* Asthma, allergic extrinsic
  heart I50.1
  idiosyncratic — *see* Asthma, nonallergic
  intermittent (mild) J45.20
    with
      exacerbation (acute) J45.21
      status asthmaticus J45.22
  intrinsic, nonallergic — *see* Asthma, nonallergic
  Kopp's E32.8
  late-onset J45.909
    with
      exacerbation (acute) J45.901
      status asthmaticus J45.902
  mild intermittent J45.20
    with
      exacerbation (acute) J45.21
      status asthmaticus J45.22
  mild persistent J45.30
    with
      exacerbation (acute) J45.31
      status asthmaticus J45.32
  Millar's (laryngismus stridulus) J38.5
  miner's J60
  mixed J45.909
    with
      exacerbation (acute) J45.901
      status asthmaticus J45.902
  moderate persistent J45.40
    with
      exacerbation (acute) J45.41
      status asthmaticus J45.42
  nervous — *see* Asthma, nonallergic
  nonallergic (intrinsic) J45.909
    with

☑ **Additional character required**

Asthma — *continued*
  nonallergic — *continued*
    exacerbation (acute) J45.901
    status asthmaticus J45.902
  persistent
    mild J45.30
      with
        exacerbation (acute) J45.31
        status asthmaticus J45.32
    moderate J45.40
      with
        exacerbation (acute) J45.41
        status asthmaticus J45.42
    severe J45.50
      with
        exacerbation (acute) J45.51
        status asthmaticus J45.52
  platinum J45.998
  pneumoconiotic NEC J64
  potter's J62.8
  predominantly allergic J45.909
  psychogenic F54
  pulmonary eosinophilic J82
  red cedar J67.8
  Rostan's I50.1
  sandblaster's J62.8
  sequoiosis J67.8
  severe persistent J45.50
    with
      exacerbation (acute) J45.51
      status asthmaticus J45.52
  specified NEC J45.998
  stonemason's J62.8
  thymic E32.8
  tuberculous — *see* Tuberculosis, pulmonary
  Wichmann's (laryngismus stridulus) J38.5
  wood J67.8
Astigmatism (compound) (congenital) H52.20 ☑
  irregular H52.21 ☑
  regular H52.22 ☑
Astraphobia F40.220
Astroblastoma
  specified site — *see* Neoplasm, malignant, by site
  unspecified site C71.9
Astrocytoma (cystic)
  anaplastic
    specified site — *see* Neoplasm, malignant, by site
    unspecified site C71.9
  fibrillary
    specified site — *see* Neoplasm, malignant, by site
    unspecified site C71.9
  fibrous
    specified site — *see* Neoplasm, malignant, by site
    unspecified site C71.9
  gemistocytic
    specified site — *see* Neoplasm, malignant, by site
    unspecified site C71.9
  juvenile
    specified site — *see* Neoplasm, malignant, by site
    unspecified site C71.9
  pilocytic
    specified site — *see* Neoplasm, malignant, by site
    unspecified site C71.9
  piloid
    specified site — *see* Neoplasm, malignant, by site
    unspecified site C71.9
  protoplasmic
    specified site — *see* Neoplasm, malignant, by site
    unspecified site C71.9
  specified site NEC — *see* Neoplasm, malignant, by site
  subependymal D43.2
    giant cell
      specified site — *see* Neoplasm, uncertain behavior, by site
      unspecified site D43.2
    specified site — *see* Neoplasm, uncertain behavior, by site
    unspecified site D43.2
  unspecified site C71.9
Astroglioma
  specified site — *see* Neoplasm, malignant, by site
  unspecified site C71.9
Asymbolia R48.8
Asymmetry (*see also* Distortion)
  between native and reconstructed breast N65.1
  face Q67.0
  jaw (lower) — *see* Anomaly, dentofacial, jaw-cranial base relationship, asymmetry
Asynergia, asynergy R27.8
  ventricular I51.89
Asystole (heart) — *see* Arrest, cardiac

At risk
  for
    dental caries Z91.849
      high Z91.843
      low Z91.841
      moderate Z91.842
    falling Z91.81
Ataxia, ataxy, ataxic R27.0
  acute R27.8
  brain (hereditary) G11.9
  cerebellar (hereditary) G11.9
    with defective DNA repair G11.3
    alcoholic G31.2
    early-onset G11.1
    in
      alcoholism G31.2
      myxedema E03.9 *[G13.2]*
      neoplastic disease (*see also* Neoplasm) D49.9 *[G32.81]*
      specified disease NEC G32.81
    late-onset (Marie's) G11.2
  cerebral (hereditary) G11.9
  congenital nonprogressive G11.0
  family, familial — *see* Ataxia, hereditary
  following
    cerebrovascular disease I69.993
      cerebral infarction I69.393
      intracerebral hemorrhage I69.193
      nontraumatic intracranial hemorrhage NEC I69.293
      specified disease NEC I69.893
      subarachnoid hemorrhage I69.093
  Friedreich's (heredofamilial) (cerebellar) (spinal) G11.1
  gait R26.0
    hysterical F44.4
  general R27.8
  gluten M35.9 *[G32.81]*
    with celiac disease K90.0 *[G32.81]*
  hereditary G11.9
    with neuropathy G60.2
    cerebellar — *see* Ataxia, cerebellar
    spastic G11.4
    specified NEC G11.8
    spinal (Friedreich's) G11.1
  heredofamilial — *see* Ataxia, hereditary
  Hunt's G11.1
  hysterical F44.4
  locomotor (progressive) (syphilitic) (partial) (spastic) A52.11
    diabetic — *see* Diabetes, ataxia
  Marie's (cerebellar) (heredofamilial) (late- onset) G11.2
  nonorganic origin F44.4
  nonprogressive, congenital G11.0
  psychogenic F44.4
  Roussy-Lévy G60.0
  Sanger-Brown's (hereditary) G11.2
  spastic hereditary G11.4
  spinal
    hereditary (Friedreich's) G11.1
    progressive (syphilitic) A52.11
  spinocerebellar, X-linked recessive G11.1
  telangiectasia (Louis-Bar) G11.3
Ataxia-telangiectasia (Louis-Bar) G11.3
Atelectasis (massive) (partial) (pressure) (pulmonary) J98.11
  newborn P28.10
    due to resorption P28.11
    partial P28.19
    primary P28.0
    secondary P28.19
  primary (newborn) P28.0
  tuberculous — *see* Tuberculosis, pulmonary
Atelocardia Q24.9
Atelomyelia Q06.1
Atheroembolism
  of
    extremities
      lower I75.02 ☑
      upper I75.01 ☑
    kidney I75.81
    specified NEC I75.89
Atheroma, atheromatous (*see also* Arteriosclerosis) I70.90
  aorta, aortic I70.0
    valve (*see also* Endocarditis, aortic) I35.8
  aorto-iliac I70.0
  artery — *see* Arteriosclerosis
  basilar (artery) I67.2
  carotid (artery) (common) (internal) I67.2
  cerebral (arteries) I67.2

Atheroma — *continued*
  coronary (artery) I25.10
    with angina pectoris — *see* Arteriosclerosis, coronary (artery),
  degeneration — *see* Arteriosclerosis
  heart, cardiac — *see* Disease, heart, ischemic, atherosclerotic
  mitral (valve) I34.8
  myocardium, myocardial — *see* Disease, heart, ischemic, atherosclerotic
  pulmonary valve (heart) (*see also* Endocarditis, pulmonary) I37.8
  tricuspid (heart) (valve) I36.8
  valve, valvular — *see* Endocarditis
  vertebral (artery) I67.2
Atheromatosis — *see* Arteriosclerosis
Atherosclerosis (*see also* Arteriosclerosis)
  coronary
    artery I25.10
      with angina pectoris — *see* Arteriosclerosis, coronary (artery),
      due to
        calcified coronary lesion (severely) I25.84
        lipid rich plaque I25.83
    transplanted heart I25.811
      bypass graft I25.812
        with angina pectoris — *see* Arteriosclerosis, coronary (artery),
      native coronary artery I25.811
        with angina pectoris — *see* Arteriosclerosis, coronary (artery),
Athetosis (acquired) R25.8
  bilateral (congenital) G80.3
  congenital (bilateral) (double) G80.3
  double (congenital) G80.3
  unilateral R25.8
Athlete's
  foot B35.3
  heart I51.7
Athrepsia E41
Athyrea (acquired) (*see also* Hypothyroidism)
  congenital E03.1
Atonia, atony, atonic
  bladder (sphincter) (neurogenic) N31.2
  capillary I78.8
  cecum K59.8
    psychogenic F45.8
  colon — *see* Atony, intestine
  congenital P94.2
  esophagus K22.8
  intestine K59.8
    psychogenic F45.8
  stomach K31.89
    neurotic or psychogenic F45.8
  uterus (during labor) O62.2
    with hemorrhage (postpartum) O72.1
    postpartum (with hemorrhage) O72.1
      without hemorrhage O75.89
Atopy — *see* History, allergy
Atransferrinemia, congenital E88.09
Atresia, atretic
  alimentary organ or tract NEC Q45.8
    upper Q40.8
  ani, anus, anal (canal) Q42.3
    with fistula Q42.2
  aorta (ring) Q25.29
  aortic (orifice) (valve) Q23.0
    arch Q25.21
    congenital with hypoplasia of ascending aorta and defective development of left ventricle (with mitral stenosis) Q23.4
    in hypoplastic left heart syndrome Q23.4
  aqueduct of Sylvius Q03.0
    with spina bifida — *see* Spina bifida, with hydrocephalus
  artery NEC Q27.8
    cerebral Q28.3
    coronary Q24.5
    digestive system Q27.8
    eye Q15.8
    lower limb Q27.8
    pulmonary Q25.5
    specified site NEC Q27.8
    umbilical Q27.0
    upper limb Q27.8
  auditory canal (external) Q16.1
  bile duct (common) (congenital) (hepatic) Q44.2
    acquired — *see* Obstruction, bile duct
  bladder (neck) Q64.39
    obstruction Q64.31
  bronchus Q32.4
  cecum Q42.8

Atresia — *continued*
  cervix (acquired) N88.2
    congenital Q51.828
    in pregnancy or childbirth — *see* Anomaly, cervix,
      in pregnancy or childbirth
    causing obstructed labor O65.5
  choana Q30.0
  colon Q42.9
    specified NEC Q42.8
  common duct Q44.2
  cricoid cartilage Q31.8
  cystic duct Q44.2
    acquired K82.8
      with obstruction K82.0
  digestive organs NEC Q45.8
  duodenum Q41.0
  ear canal Q16.1
  ejaculatory duct Q55.4
  epiglottis Q31.8
  esophagus Q39.0
    with tracheoesophageal fistula Q39.1
  eustachian tube Q17.8
  fallopian tube (congenital) Q50.6
    acquired N97.1
  follicular cyst N83.0 ☑
  foramen of
    Luschka Q03.1
      with spina bifida — *see* Spina bifida, with
        hydrocephalus
    Magendie Q03.1
      with spina bifida — *see* Spina bifida, with
        hydrocephalus
  gallbladder Q44.1
  genital organ
    external
      female Q52.79
      male Q55.8
    internal
      female Q52.8
      male Q55.8
  glottis Q31.8
  gullet Q39.0
    with tracheoesophageal fistula Q39.1
  heart valve NEC Q24.8
    pulmonary Q22.0
    tricuspid Q22.4
  hymen Q52.3
    acquired (postinfective) N89.6
  ileum Q41.2
  intestine (small) Q41.9
    large Q42.9
      specified NEC Q42.8
  iris, filtration angle Q15.0
  jejunum Q41.1
  lacrimal apparatus Q10.4
  larynx Q31.8
  meatus urinarius Q64.33
  mitral valve Q23.2
    in hypoplastic left heart syndrome Q23.4
  nares (anterior) (posterior) Q30.0
  nasopharynx Q34.8
  nose, nostril Q30.0
    acquired J34.89
  organ or site NEC Q89.8
  osseous meatus (ear) Q16.1
  oviduct (congenital) Q50.6
    acquired N97.1
  parotid duct Q38.4
    acquired K11.8
  pulmonary (artery) Q25.5
    valve Q22.0
  pulmonic Q22.0
  pupil Q13.2
  rectum Q42.1
    with fistula Q42.0
  salivary duct Q38.4
    acquired K11.8
  sublingual duct Q38.4
    acquired K11.8
  submandibular duct Q38.4
    acquired K11.8
  submaxillary duct Q38.4
    acquired K11.8
  thyroid cartilage Q31.8
  trachea Q32.1
  tricuspid valve Q22.4
  ureter Q62.10
    pelvic junction Q62.11
    vesical orifice Q62.12
  ureteropelvic junction Q62.11
  ureterovesical orifice Q62.12

Atresia — *continued*
  urethra (valvular) Q64.39
    stricture Q64.32
  urinary tract NEC Q64.8
  uterus Q51.818
    acquired N85.8
  vagina (congenital) Q52.4
    acquired (postinfectional) (senile) N89.5
  vas deferens Q55.3
  vascular NEC Q27.8
    cerebral Q28.3
    digestive system Q27.8
    lower limb Q27.8
    specified site NEC Q27.8
    upper limb Q27.8
  vein NEC Q27.8
    digestive system Q27.8
    great Q26.8
    lower limb Q27.8
    portal Q26.5
    pulmonary Q26.4
      partial Q26.3
      total Q26.2
    specified site NEC Q27.8
    upper limb Q27.8
    vena cava (inferior) (superior) Q26.8
  vesicourethral orifice Q64.31
  vulva Q52.79
    acquired N90.5
Atrichia, atrichosis — *see* Alopecia
Atrophia (*see also* Atrophy)
  cutis senilis L90.8
    due to radiation L57.8
  gyrata of choroid and retina H31.23
  senilis R54
    dermatological L90.8
      due to radiation (nonionizing) (solar) L57.8
  unguium L60.3
    congenita Q84.6
Atrophie blanche (en plaque) (de Milian) L95.0
Atrophoderma, atrophodermia (of) L90.9
  diffusum (idiopathic) L90.4
  maculatum L90.8
    et striatum L90.8
      due to syphilis A52.79
    syphilitic A51.39
  neuriticum L90.8
  Pasini and Pierini L90.3
  pigmentosum Q82.1
  reticulatum symmetricum faciei L66.4
  senile L90.8
    due to radiation (nonionizing) (solar) L57.8
  vermiculata (cheeks) L66.4
Atrophy, atrophic (of)
  adrenal (capsule) (gland) E27.49
    primary (autoimmune) E27.1
  alveolar process or ridge (edentulous) K08.20
  anal sphincter (disuse) N81.84
  appendix K38.8
  arteriosclerotic — *see* Arteriosclerosis
  bile duct (common) (hepatic) K83.8
  bladder N32.89
    neurogenic N31.8
  blanche (en plaque) (of Milian) L95.0
  bone (senile) NEC (*see also* Disorder, bone, specified
      type NEC)
    due to
      tabes dorsalis (neurogenic) A52.11
  brain (cortex) (progressive) G31.9
    frontotemporal circumscribed G31.01 *[F02.80]*
      with behavioral disturbance G31.01 *[F02.81]*
    senile NEC G31.1
  breast N64.2
    obstetric — *see* Disorder, breast, specified type
      NEC
  buccal cavity K13.79
  cardiac — *see* Degeneration, myocardial
  cartilage (infectional) (joint) — *see* Disorder,
      cartilage, specified NEC
  cerebellar — *see* Atrophy, brain
  cerebral — *see* Atrophy, brain
  cervix (mucosa) (senile) (uteri) N88.8
    menopausal N95.8
  Charcot-Marie-Tooth G60.0
  choroid (central) (macular) (myopic) (retina)
      H31.10 ☑
    diffuse secondary H31.12 ☑
    gyrate H31.23
    senile H31.11 ☑
  ciliary body — *see* Atrophy, iris
  conjunctiva (senile) H11.89
  corpus cavernosum N48.89

Atrophy — *continued*
  cortical — *see* Atrophy, brain
  cystic duct K82.8
  Déjérine-Thomas G23.8
  disuse NEC — *see* Atrophy, muscle
  Duchenne-Aran G12.21
  ear H93.8 ☑
  edentulous alveolar ridge K08.20
  endometrium (senile) N85.8
    cervix N88.8
  enteric K63.89
  epididymis N50.89
  eyeball — *see* Disorder, globe, degenerated
      condition, atrophy
  eyelid (senile) — *see* Disorder, eyelid, degenerative
  facial (skin) L90.9
  fallopian tube (senile) N83.32 ☑
    with ovary N83.33 ☑
  fascioscapulohumeral (Landouzy- Déjérine) G71.02
  fatty, thymus (gland) E32.8
  gallbladder K82.8
  gastric K29.40
    with bleeding K29.41
  gastrointestinal K63.89
  glandular I89.8
  globe H44.52 ☑
  gum — *see* Recession, gingival
  hair L67.8
  heart (brown) — *see* Degeneration, myocardial
  hemifacial Q67.4
    Romberg G51.8
  infantile E41
    paralysis, acute — *see* Poliomyelitis, paralytic
  intestine K63.89
  iris (essential) (progressive) H21.26 ☑
    specified NEC H21.29
  kidney (senile) (terminal) (*see also* Sclerosis, renal)
      N26.1
    congenital or infantile Q60.5
      bilateral Q60.4
      unilateral Q60.3
    hydronephrotic — *see* Hydronephrosis
  lacrimal gland (primary) H04.14 ☑
    secondary H04.15 ☑
  Landouzy-Déjérine G71.02
  laryngitis, infective J37.0
  larynx J38.7
  Leber's optic (hereditary) H47.22
  lip K13.0
  liver (yellow) K72.90
    with coma K72.91
    acute, subacute K72.00
      with coma K72.01
    chronic K72.10
      with coma K72.11
  lung (senile) J98.4
  macular (dermatological) L90.8
    syphilitic, skin A51.39
    striated A52.79
  mandible (edentulous) K08.20
    minimal K08.21
    moderate K08.22
    severe K08.23
  maxilla K08.20
    minimal K08.24
    moderate K08.25
    severe K08.26
  muscle, muscular (diffuse) (general) (idiopathic)
      (primary) M62.50
    ankle M62.57 ☑
    Duchenne-Aran G12.21
    foot M62.57 ☑
    forearm M62.53 ☑
    hand M62.54 ☑
    infantile spinal G12.0
    lower leg M62.56 ☑
    multiple sites M62.59
    myelopathic — *see* Atrophy, muscle, spinal
    myotonic G71.11
    neuritic G58.9
    neuropathic (peroneal) (progressive) G60.0
    pelvic (disuse) N81.84
    peroneal G60.0
    progressive (bulbar) G12.21
      adult G12.1
      infantile (spinal) G12.0
      spinal G12.25
        adult G12.1
        infantile G12.0
    pseudohypertrophic G71.02
    shoulder region M62.51 ☑
    specified site NEC M62.58

☑ **Additional character required**

Atrophy — *continued*
  muscle, muscular — *continued*
    spinal G12.9
      adult form G12.1
      Aran-Duchenne G12.21
      childhood form, type II G12.1
      distal G12.1
      hereditary NEC G12.1
      infantile, type I (Werdnig-Hoffmann) G12.0
      juvenile form, type III (Kugelberg- Welander) G12.1
      progressive G12.25
      scapuloperoneal form G12.1
      specified NEC G12.8
    syphilitic A52.78
    thigh M62.55 ☑
    upper arm M62.52 ☑
  myocardium — *see* Degeneration, myocardial
  myometrium (senile) N85.8
    cervix N88.8
  myopathic NEC — *see* Atrophy, muscle
  myotonia G71.11
  nail L60.3
  nasopharynx J31.1
  nerve (*see also* Disorder, nerve)
    abducens — *see* Strabismus, paralytic, sixth nerve
    accessory G52.8
    acoustic or auditory — *see* subcategory H93.3 ☑
    cranial G52.9
      eighth (auditory) — *see* subcategory H93.3 ☑
      eleventh (accessory) G52.8
      fifth (trigeminal) G50.8
      first (olfactory) G52.0
      fourth (trochlear) — *see* Strabismus, paralytic, fourth nerve
      second (optic) H47.20
      sixth (abducens) — *see* Strabismus, paralytic, sixth nerve
      tenth (pneumogastric) (vagus) G52.2
      third (oculomotor) — *see* Strabismus, paralytic, third nerve
      twelfth (hypoglossal) G52.3
    hypoglossal G52.3
    oculomotor — *see* Strabismus, paralytic, third nerve
    olfactory G52.0
    optic (papillomacular bundle)
      syphilitic (late) A52.15
        congenital A50.44
    pneumogastric G52.2
    trigeminal G50.8
    trochlear — *see* Strabismus, paralytic, fourth nerve
    vagus (pneumogastric) G52.2
  neurogenic, bone, tabetic A52.11
  nutritional E41
  old age R54
  olivopontocerebellar G23.8
  optic (nerve) H47.20
    glaucomatous H47.23 ☑
    hereditary H47.22
    primary H47.21 ☑
    specified type NEC H47.29 ☑
    syphilitic (late) A52.15
      congenital A50.44
  orbit H05.31 ☑
  ovary (senile) N83.31 ☑
    with fallopian tube N83.33 ☑
  oviduct (senile) — *see* Atrophy, fallopian tube
  palsy, diffuse (progressive) G12.22
  pancreas (duct) (senile) K86.89
  parotid gland K11.0
  pelvic muscle N81.84
  penis N48.89
  pharynx J39.2
  pluriglandular E31.8
    autoimmune E31.0
  polyarthritis M15.9
  prostate N42.89
  pseudohypertrophic (muscle) G71.02
  renal (*see also* Sclerosis, renal) N26.1
  retina, retinal (postinfectional) H35.89
  rhinitis J31.0
  salivary gland K11.0
  scar L90.5
  sclerosis, lobar (of brain) G31.09 *[F02.80]*
    with behavioral disturbance G31.09 *[F02.81]*
  scrotum N50.89
  seminal vesicle N50.89
  senile R54
    due to radiation (nonionizing) (solar) L57.8

Atrophy — *continued*
  skin (patches) (spots) L90.9
    degenerative (senile) L90.8
    due to radiation (nonionizing) (solar) L57.8
    senile L90.8
  spermatic cord N50.89
  spinal (acute) (cord) G95.89
    muscular — *see* Atrophy, muscle, spinal
    paralysis G12.20
      acute — *see* Poliomyelitis, paralytic
      meaning progressive muscular atrophy G12.25
  spine (column) — *see* Spondylopathy, specified NEC
  spleen (senile) D73.0
  stomach K29.40
    with bleeding K29.41
  striate (skin) L90.6
    syphilitic A52.79
  subcutaneous L90.9
  sublingual gland K11.0
  submandibular gland K11.0
  submaxillary gland K11.0
  Sudeck's — *see* Algoneurodystrophy
  suprarenal (capsule) (gland) E27.49
    primary E27.1
  systemic affecting central nervous system in
    myxedema E03.9 *[G13.2]*
    neoplastic disease (*see also* Neoplasm) D49.9 *[G13.1]*
    specified disease NEC G13.8
  tarso-orbital fascia, congenital Q10.3
  testis N50.0
  thenar, partial — *see* Syndrome, carpal tunnel
  thymus (fatty) E32.8
  thyroid (gland) (acquired) E03.4
    with cretinism E03.1
    congenital (with myxedema) E03.1
  tongue (senile) K14.8
    papillae K14.4
  trachea J39.8
  tunica vaginalis N50.89
  turbinate J34.89
  tympanic membrane (nonflaccid) H73.82 ☑
    flaccid H73.81 ☑
  upper respiratory tract J39.8
  uterus, uterine (senile) N85.8
    cervix N88.8
    due to radiation (intended effect) N85.8
      adverse effect or misadventure N99.89
  vagina (senile) N95.2
  vas deferens N50.89
  vascular I99.8
  vertebra (senile) — *see* Spondylopathy, specified NEC
  vulva (senile) N90.5
  Werdnig-Hoffmann G12.0
  yellow — *see* Failure, hepatic
Attack, attacks
  with alteration of consciousness (with automatisms) — *see* Epilepsy, localization- related, symptomatic, with complex partial seizures
  Adams-Stokes I45.9
  akinetic — *see* Epilepsy, generalized, specified NEC
  angina — *see* Angina
  atonic — *see* Epilepsy, generalized, specified NEC
  benign shuddering G25.83
  cataleptic — *see* Catalepsy
  coronary — *see* Infarct, myocardium
  cyanotic, newborn P28.2
  drop NEC R55
  epileptic — *see* Epilepsy
  heart — *see* Infarct, myocardium
  hysterical F44.9
  jacksonian — *see* Epilepsy, localization-related, symptomatic, with simple partial seizures
  myocardium, myocardial — *see* Infarct, myocardium
  myoclonic — *see* Epilepsy, generalized, specified NEC
  panic F41.0
  psychomotor — *see* Epilepsy, localization-related, symptomatic, with complex partial seizures
  salaam — *see* Epilepsy, spasms
  schizophreniform, brief F23
  shuddering, benign G25.83
  Stokes-Adams I45.9
  syncope R55
  transient ischemic (TIA) G45.9
    specified NEC G45.8
  unconsciousness R55
    hysterical F44.89

Attack — *continued*
  vasomotor R55
  vasovagal (paroxysmal) (idiopathic) R55
  without alteration of consciousness — *see* Epilepsy, localization-related, symptomatic, with simple partial seizures
Attention (to)
  artificial
    opening (of) Z43.9
      digestive tract NEC Z43.4
        colon Z43.3
        ilium Z43.2
        stomach Z43.1
      specified NEC Z43.8
      trachea Z43.0
      urinary tract NEC Z43.6
        cystostomy Z43.5
        nephrostomy Z43.6
        ureterostomy Z43.6
        urethrostomy Z43.6
      vagina Z43.7
  colostomy Z43.3
  cystostomy Z43.5
  deficit disorder or syndrome F98.8
    with hyperactivity — *see* Disorder, attention- deficit hyperactivity
  gastrostomy Z43.1
  ileostomy Z43.2
  jejunostomy Z43.4
  nephrostomy Z43.6
  surgical dressings Z48.01
  sutures Z48.02
  tracheostomy Z43.0
  ureterostomy Z43.6
  urethrostomy Z43.6
Attrition
  gum — *see* Recession, gingival
  tooth, teeth (excessive) (hard tissues) K03.0
Atypical, atypism (*see also* condition)
  cells (on cytolgocial smear) (endocervical) (endometrial) (glandular)
    cervix R87.619
    vagina R87.629
  cervical N87.9
  endometrium N85.9
    hyperplasia N85.00
  parenting situation Z62.9
Auditory — *see* condition
Aujeszky's disease B33.8
Aurantiasis, cutis E67.1
Auricle, auricular (*see also* condition)
  cervical Q18.2
Auriculotemporal syndrome G50.8
Austin Flint murmur (aortic insufficiency) I35.1
Australian
  Q fever A78
  X disease A83.4
Autism, autistic (childhood) (infantile) F84.0
  atypical F84.9
  spectrum disorder F84.0
Autodigestion R68.89
Autoerythrocyte sensitization (syndrome) D69.2
Autographism L50.3
Autoimmune
  disease (systemic) M35.9
  inhibitors to clotting factors D68.311
  lymphoproliferative syndrome [ALPS] D89.82
  thyroiditis E06.3
Autointoxication R68.89
Automatism G93.89
  with temporal sclerosis G93.81
  epileptic — *see* Epilepsy, localization-related, symptomatic, with complex partial seizures
  paroxysmal, idiopathic — *see* Epilepsy, localization- related, symptomatic, with complex partial seizures
Autonomic, autonomous
  bladder (neurogenic) N31.2
  hysteria seizure F44.5
Autosensitivity, erythrocyte D69.2
Autosensitization, cutaneous L30.2
Autosome — *see* condition by chromosome involved
Autotopagnosia R48.1
Autotoxemia R68.89
Autumn — *see* condition
Avellis' syndrome G46.8
Aversion
  oral R63.3
    newborn P92. ☑
    nonorganic origin F98.2 ☑
  sexual F52.1

Aviator's
  disease or sickness — *see* Effect, adverse, high altitude
  ear T70.0 ☑
Avitaminosis (multiple) (*see also* Deficiency, vitamin) E56.9
  B E53.9
    with
      beriberi E51.11
      pellagra E52
    B2 E53.0
    B6 E53.1
    B12 E53.8
    D E55.9
      with rickets E55.0
    G E53.0
    K E56.1
    nicotinic acid E52
AVNRT (atrioventricular nodal re-entrant tachycardia) I47.1
AVRT (atrioventricular nodal re-entrant tachycardia) I47.1
Avulsion (traumatic)
  blood vessel — *see* Injury, blood vessel
  bone — *see* Fracture, by site
  cartilage (*see also* Dislocation, by site)
    symphyseal (inner), complicating delivery O71.6
  external site other than limb — *see* Wound, open, by site
  eye S05.7 ☑
  head (intracranial)
    external site NEC S08.89 ☑
    scalp S08.0 ☑
  internal organ or site — *see* Injury, by site
  joint (*see also* Dislocation, by site)
    capsule — *see* Sprain, by site
  kidney S37.06 ☑
  ligament — *see* Sprain, by site
  limb (*see also* Amputation, traumatic, by site)
    skin and subcutaneous tissue — *see* Wound, open, by site
  muscle — *see* Injury, muscle
  nerve (root) — *see* Injury, nerve
  scalp S08.0 ☑
  skin and subcutaneous tissue — *see* Wound, open, by site
  spleen S36.032 ☑
  symphyseal cartilage (inner), complicating delivery O71.6
  tendon — *see* Injury, muscle
  tooth S03.2 ☑
Awareness of heart beat R00.2
Axenfeld's
  anomaly or syndrome Q15.0
  degeneration (calcareous) Q13.4
Axilla, axillary (*see also* condition)
  breast Q83.1
Axonotmesis — *see* Injury, nerve
Ayerza's disease or syndrome (pulmonary artery sclerosis with pulmonary hypertension) I27.0
Azoospermia (organic) N46.01
  due to
    drug therapy N46.021
    efferent duct obstruction N46.023
    infection N46.022
    radiation N46.024
    specified cause NEC N46.029
    systemic disease N46.025
Azotemia R79.89
  meaning uremia N19
Aztec ear Q17.3
Azygos
  continuation inferior vena cava Q26.8
  lobe (lung) Q33.1

B

Baastrup's disease — *see* Kissing spine
Babesiosis B60.0
Babington's disease (familial hemorrhagic telangiectasia) I78.0
Babinski's syndrome A52.79
Baby
  crying constantly R68.11
  floppy (syndrome) P94.2
Bacillary — *see* condition
Bacilluria R82.71
Bacillus (*see also* Infection, bacillus)
  abortus infection A23.1
  anthracis infection A22.9

Bacillus — *continued*
  coli infection (*see also* Escherichia coli) B96.20
  Flexner's A03.1
  mallei infection A24.0
  Shiga's A03.0
  suipestifer infection — *see* Infection, salmonella
Back — *see* condition
Backache (postural) M54.9
  sacroiliac M53.3
  specified NEC M54.89
Backflow — *see* Reflux
Backward reading (dyslexia) F81.0
Bacteremia R78.81
  with sepsis — *see* Sepsis
Bactericholia — *see* Cholecystitis, acute
Bacterid, bacteride (pustular) L40.3
Bacterium, bacteria, bacterial
  agent NEC, as cause of disease classified elsewhere B96.89
  in blood — *see* Bacteremia
  in urine — *see* Bacteriuria
Bacteriuria, bacteruria R82.71
  asymptomatic R82.71
Bacteroides
  fragilis, as cause of disease classified elsewhere B96.6
Bad
  heart — *see* Disease, heart
  trip
    due to drug abuse — *see* Abuse, drug, hallucinogen
    due to drug dependence — *see* Dependence, drug, hallucinogen
Baelz's disease (cheilitis glandularis apostematosa) K13.0
Baerensprung's disease (eczema marginatum) B35.6
Bagasse disease or pneumonitis J67.1
Bagassosis J67.1
Baker's cyst — *see* Cyst, Baker's
Bakwin-Krida syndrome (metaphyseal dysplasia) Q78.5
Balancing side interference M26.56
Balanitis (circinata) (erosiva) (gangrenosa) (phagedenic) (vulgaris) N48.1
  amebic A06.82
  candidal B37.42
  due to Haemophilus ducreyi A57
  gonococcal (acute) (chronic) A54.23
  xerotica obliterans N48.0
Balanoposthitis N47.6
  gonococcal (acute) (chronic) A54.23
  ulcerative (specific) A63.8
Balanorrhagia — *see* Balanitis
Balantidiasis, balantidiosis A07.0
Bald tongue K14.4
Baldness (*see also* Alopecia)
  male-pattern — *see* Alopecia, androgenic
Balkan grippe A78
Balloon disease — *see* Effect, adverse, high altitude
Balo's disease (concentric sclerosis) G37.5
Bamberger-Marie disease — *see* Osteoarthropathy, hypertrophic, specified type NEC
Bancroft's filariasis B74.0
Band(s)
  adhesive — *see* Adhesions, peritoneum
  anomalous or congenital (*see also* Anomaly, by site)
    heart (atrial) (ventricular) Q24.8
    intestine Q43.3
    omentum Q43.3
  cervix N88.1
  constricting, congenital Q79.8
  gallbladder (congenital) Q44.1
  intestinal (adhesive) — *see* Adhesions, peritoneum
  obstructive
    intestine K56.50
      complete K56.52
      incomplete K56.51
      partial K56.51
    peritoneum K56.50
      complete K56.52
      incomplete K56.51
      partial K56.51
  periappendiceal, congenital Q43.3
  peritoneal (adhesive) — *see* Adhesions, peritoneum
  uterus N73.6
    internal N85.6
  vagina N89.5
Bandemia D72.825
Bandl's ring (contraction), complicating delivery O62.4
Bangkok hemorrhagic fever A91
Bang's disease (brucella abortus) A23.1
Bankruptcy, anxiety concerning Z59.8
Bannister's disease T78.3 ☑
  hereditary D84.1

Banti's disease or syndrome (with cirrhosis) (with portal hypertension) K76.6
Bar, median, prostate — *see* Enlargement, enlarged, prostate
Barcoo disease or rot — *see* Ulcer, skin
Barlow's disease E54
Barodontalgia T70.29 ☑
Baron Münchausen syndrome — *see* Disorder, factitious
Barosinusitis T70.1 ☑
Barotitis T70.0 ☑
Barotrauma T70.29 ☑
  odontalgia T70.29 ☑
  otitic T70.0 ☑
  sinus T70.1 ☑
Barraquer (-Simons) disease or syndrome (progressive lipodystrophy) E88.1
Barré-Guillain disease or syndrome G61.0
Barré-Liéou syndrome (posterior cervical sympathetic) M53.0
Barrel chest M95.4
Barrett's
  disease — *see* Barrett's, esophagus
  esophagus K22.70
    with dysplasia K22.719
      high grade K22.711
      low grade K22.710
    without dysplasia K22.70
  syndrome — *see* Barrett's, esophagus
  ulcer K22.10
    with bleeding K22.11
    without bleeding K22.10
Bársony (-Polgár) (-Teschendorf) syndrome (corkscrew esophagus) K22.4
Bartholinitis (suppurating) N75.8
  gonococcal (acute) (chronic) (with abscess) A54.1
Barth syndrome E78.71
Bartonellosis A44.9
  cutaneous A44.1
  mucocutaneous A44.1
  specified NEC A44.8
  systemic A44.0
Barton's fracture S52.56 ☑
Bartter's syndrome E26.81
Basal — *see* condition
Basan's (hidrotic) ectodermal dysplasia Q82.4
Baseball finger — *see* Dislocation, finger
Basedow's disease (exophthalmic goiter) — *see* Hyperthyroidism, with, goiter
Basic — *see* condition
Basilar — *see* condition
Bason's (hidrotic) ectodermal dysplasia Q82.4
Basopenia — *see* Agranulocytosis
Basophilia D72.824
Basophilism (cortico-adrenal) (Cushing's) (pituitary) E24.0
Bassen-Kornzweig disease or syndrome E78.6
Bat ear Q17.5
Bateman's
  disease B08.1
  purpura (senile) D69.2
Bathing cramp T75.1 ☑
Bathophobia F40.248
Batten (-Mayou) disease E75.4
  retina E75.4 *[H36]*
Batten-Steinert syndrome G71.11
Battered — *see* Maltreatment
Battey Mycobacterium infection A31.0
Battle exhaustion F43.0
Battledore placenta O43.19 ☑
Baumgarten-Cruveilhier cirrhosis, disease or syndrome K74.69
Bauxite fibrosis (of lung) J63.1
Bayle's disease (general paresis) A52.17
Bazin's disease (primary) (tuberculous) A18.4
Beach ear — *see* Swimmer's, ear
Beaded hair (congenital) Q84.1
Béal conjunctivitis or syndrome B30.2
Beard's disease (neurasthenia) F48.8
Beat(s)
  atrial, premature I49.1
  ectopic I49.49
  elbow — *see* Bursitis, elbow
  escaped, heart I49.49
  hand — *see* Bursitis, hand
  knee — *see* Bursitis, knee
  premature I49.40
    atrial I49.1
    auricular I49.1
    supraventricular I49.1
Beau's
  disease or syndrome — *see* Degeneration, myocardial
  lines (transverse furrows on fingernails) L60.4

Bechterev's syndrome — *see* Spondylitis, ankylosing
Beck's syndrome (anterior spinal artery occlusion) I65.8
Becker's
  cardiomyopathy I42.8
  disease
    idiopathic mural endomyocardial disease I42.3
    myotonia congenita, recessive form G71.12
  dystrophy G71.01
  pigmented hairy nevus D22.5
Beckwith-Wiedemann syndrome Q87.3
Bed confinement status Z74.01
Bed sore — *see* Ulcer, pressure, by site
Bedbug bite(s) — *see* Bite(s), by site, superficial, insect
Bedclothes, asphyxiation or suffocation by — *see*
  Asphyxia, traumatic, due to, mechanical, trapped
Bednar's
  aphthae K12.0
  tumor — *see* Neoplasm, malignant, by site
Bedridden Z74.01
Bedsore — *see* Ulcer, pressure, by site
Bedwetting — *see* Enuresis
Bee sting (with allergic or anaphylactic shock) — *see*
  Toxicity, venom, arthropod, bee
Beer drinker's heart (disease) I42.6
Begbie's disease (exophthalmic goiter) — *see*
  Hyperthyroidism, with, goiter
Behavior
  antisocial
    adult Z72.811
    child or adolescent Z72.810
  disorder, disturbance — *see* Disorder, conduct
  disruptive — *see* Disorder, conduct
  drug seeking Z76.5
  inexplicable R46.2
  marked evasiveness R46.5
  obsessive-compulsive R46.81
  overactivity R46.3
  poor responsiveness R46.4
  self-damaging (life-style) Z72.89
  sleep-incompatible Z72.821
  slowness R46.4
  specified NEC R46.89
  strange (and inexplicable) R46.2
  suspiciousness R46.5
  type A pattern Z73.1
  undue concern or preoccupation with stressful
    events R46.6
  verbosity and circumstantial detail obscuring
    reason for contact R46.7
Behçet's disease or syndrome M35.2
Behr's disease — *see* Degeneration, macula
Beigel's disease or morbus (white piedra) B36.2
Bejel A65
Bekhterev's syndrome — *see* Spondylitis, ankylosing
Belching — *see* Eructation
Bell's
  mania F30.8
  palsy, paralysis G51.0
    infant or newborn P11.3
  spasm G51.3 ☑
Bence Jones albuminuria or proteinuria NEC R80.3
Bends T70.3 ☑
Benedikt's paralysis or syndrome G46.3
Benign (*see also* condition)
  prostatic hyperplasia — *see* Hyperplasia, prostate
Bennett's fracture (displaced) S62.21 ☑
Benson's disease — *see* Deposit, crystalline
Bent
  back (hysterical) F44.4
  nose M95.0
    congenital Q67.4
Bereavement (uncomplicated) Z63.4
Bergeron's disease (hysterical chorea) F44.4
Berger's disease — *see* Nephropathy, IgA
Beriberi (dry) E51.11
  heart (disease) E51.12
  polyneuropathy E51.11
  wet E51.12
    involving circulatory system E51.11
Berlin's disease or edema (traumatic) S05.8X ☑
Berlock (berloque) dermatitis L56.2
Bernard-Horner syndrome G90.2
Bernard-Soulier disease or thrombopathia D69.1
Bernhardt (-Roth) disease — *see* Mononeuropathy,
  lower limb, meralgia paresthetica
Bernheim's syndrome — *see* Failure, heart, right
Bertielliasis B71.8
Berylliosis (lung) J63.2
Besnier-Boeck (-Schaumann) disease — *see* Sarcoidosis
Besnier's
  lupus pernio D86.3
  prurigo L20.0

Bestiality F65.89
Best's disease H35.50
Beta-mercaptolactate-cysteine disulfiduria E72.09
Betalipoproteinemia, broad or floating E78.2
Betting and gambling Z72.6
  pathological (compulsive) F63.0
Bezoar T18.9 ☑
  intestine T18.3 ☑
  stomach T18.2 ☑
Bezold's abscess — *see* Mastoiditis, acute
Bianchi's syndrome R48.8
Bicornate or bicornis uterus Q51.3
  in pregnancy or childbirth O34.00
    causing obstructed labor O65.5
Bicuspid aortic valve Q23.1
Biedl-Bardet syndrome Q87.89
Bielschowsky (-Jansky) disease E75.4
Biermer's (pernicious) anemia or disease D51.0
Biett's disease L93.0
Bifid (congenital)
  apex, heart Q24.8
  clitoris Q52.6
  kidney Q63.8
  nose Q30.2
  patella Q74.1
  scrotum Q55.29
  toe NEC Q74.2
  tongue Q38.3
  ureter Q62.8
  uterus Q51.3
  uvula Q35.7
Biforis uterus (suprasimplex) Q51.3
Bifurcation (congenital)
  gallbladder Q44.1
  kidney pelvis Q63.8
  renal pelvis Q63.8
  rib Q76.6
  tongue, congenital Q38.3
  trachea Q32.1
  ureter Q62.8
  urethra Q64.74
  vertebra Q76.49
Big spleen syndrome D73.1
Bigeminal pulse R00.8
Bilateral — *see* condition
Bile
  duct — *see* condition
  pigments in urine R82.2
Bilharziasis (*see also* Schistosomiasis)
  chyluria B65.0
  cutaneous B65.3
  galacturia B65.0
  hematochyluria B65.0
  intestinal B65.1
  lipemia B65.9
  lipuria B65.0
  oriental B65.2
  piarhemia B65.9
  pulmonary NOS B65.9 *[J99]*
    pneumonia B65.9 *[J17]*
  tropical hematuria B65.0
  vesical B65.0
Biliary — *see* condition
Bilirubin metabolism disorder E80.7
  specified NEC E80.6
Bilirubinemia, familial nonhemolytic E80.4
Bilirubinuria R82.2
Biliuria R82.2
Bilocular stomach K31.2
Binswanger's disease I67.3
Biparta, biparite
  carpal scaphoid Q74.0
  patella Q74.1
  vagina Q52.10
Bird
  face Q75.8
  fancier's disease or lung J67.2
Birt-Hogg-Dube syndrome Q87.89
Birth
  complications in mother — *see* Delivery,
    complicated
  compression during NOS P15.9
  defect — *see* Anomaly
  immature (less than 37 completed weeks) — *see*
    Preterm, newborn
    extremely (less than 28 completed weeks) — *see*
      Immaturity, extreme
  inattention, at or after — *see* Maltreatment, child,
    neglect
  injury NOS P15.9
    basal ganglia P11.1
    brachial plexus NEC P14.3

Birth — *continued*
  injury — *continued*
    brain (compression) (pressure) P11.2
    central nervous system NOS P11.9
    cerebellum P11.1
    cerebral hemorrhage P10.1
    external genitalia P15.5
    eye P15.3
    face P15.4
    fracture
      bone P13.9
        specified NEC P13.8
      clavicle P13.4
      femur P13.2
      humerus P13.3
      long bone, except femur P13.3
      radius and ulna P13.3
      skull P13.0
      spine P11.5
      tibia and fibula P13.3
    intracranial P11.2
      laceration or hemorrhage P10.9
        specified NEC P10.8
    intraventricular hemorrhage P10.2
    laceration
      brain P10.1
      by scalpel P15.8
      peripheral nerve P14.9
    liver P15.0
    meninges
      brain P11.1
      spinal cord P11.5
    nerve
      brachial plexus P14.3
      cranial NEC (except facial) P11.4
      facial P11.3
      peripheral P14.9
      phrenic (paralysis) P14.2
    paralysis
      facial nerve P11.3
      spinal P11.5
    penis P15.5
    rupture
      spinal cord P11.5
    scalp P12.9
    scalpel wound P15.8
    scrotum P15.5
    skull NEC P13.1
      fracture P13.0
    specified type NEC P15.8
    spinal cord P11.5
    spine P11.5
    spleen P15.1
    sternomastoid (hematoma) P15.2
    subarachnoid hemorrhage P10.3
    subcutaneous fat necrosis P15.6
    subdural hemorrhage P10.0
    tentorial tear P10.4
    testes P15.5
    vulva P15.5
  lack of care, at or after — *see* Maltreatment, child,
    neglect
  neglect, at or after — *see* Maltreatment, child,
    neglect
  palsy or paralysis, newborn, NOS (birth injury) P14.9
  premature (infant) — *see* Preterm, newborn
  shock, newborn P96.89
  trauma — *see* Birth, injury
  weight
    low (2499 grams or less) — *see* Low, birthweight
      extremely (999 grams or less) — *see* Low,
        birthweight, extreme
    4000 grams to 4499 grams P08.1
    4500 grams or more P08.0
Birthmark Q82.5
Bisalbuminemia E88.09
Biskra's button B55.1
Bite(s) (animal) (human)
  abdomen, abdominal
    wall S31.159 ☑
      with penetration into peritoneal cavity
        S31.659 ☑
      epigastric region S31.152 ☑
        with penetration into peritoneal cavity
          S31.652 ☑
      left
        lower quadrant S31.154 ☑
          with penetration into peritoneal cavity
            S31.654 ☑
        upper quadrant S31.151 ☑
          with penetration into peritoneal cavity
            S31.651 ☑

Bite(s)

Bite(s) — *continued*
  abdomen — *continued*
    periumbilic region S31.155 ☑
      with penetration into peritoneal cavity
        S31.655 ☑
      right
        lower quadrant S31.153 ☑
          with penetration into peritoneal cavity
            S31.653 ☑
        upper quadrant S31.150 ☑
          with penetration into peritoneal cavity
            S31.650 ☑
      superficial NEC S30.871 ☑
        insect S30.861 ☑
  alveolar (process) — *see* Bite, oral cavity
  amphibian (venomous) — *see* Venom, bite,
      amphibian
  animal (*see also* Bite, by site)
    venomous — *see* Venom
  ankle S91.05 ☑
    superficial NEC S90.57 ☑
      insect S90.56 ☑
  antecubital space — *see* Bite, elbow
  anus S31.835 ☑
    superficial NEC S30.877 ☑
      insect S30.867 ☑
  arm (upper) S41.15 ☑
    lower — *see* Bite, forearm
    superficial NEC S40.87 ☑
      insect S40.86 ☑
  arthropod NEC — *see* Venom, bite, arthropod
  auditory canal (external) (meatus) — *see* Bite, ear
  auricle, ear — *see* Bite, ear
  axilla — *see* Bite, arm
  back (*see also* Bite, thorax, back)
    lower S31.050 ☑
      with penetration into retroperitoneal space
        S31.051 ☑
      superficial NEC S30.870 ☑
        insect S30.860 ☑
  bedbug — *see* Bite(s), by site, superficial, insect
  breast S21.05 ☑
    superficial NEC S20.17 ☑
      insect S20.16 ☑
  brow — *see* Bite, head, specified site NEC
  buttock S31.805 ☑
    left S31.825 ☑
    right S31.815 ☑
    superficial NEC S30.870 ☑
      insect S30.860 ☑
  calf — *see* Bite, leg
  canaliculus lacrimalis — *see* Bite, eyelid
  canthus, eye — *see* Bite, eyelid
  centipede — *see* Toxicity, venom, arthropod,
      centipede
  cheek (external) S01.45 ☑
    superficial NEC S00.87 ☑
      insect S00.86 ☑
    internal — *see* Bite, oral cavity
  chest wall — *see* Bite, thorax
  chigger B88.0
  chin — *see* Bite, head, specified site NEC
  clitoris — *see* Bite, vulva
  costal region — *see* Bite, thorax
  digit(s)
    hand — *see* Bite, finger
    toe — *see* Bite, toe
  ear (canal) (external) S01.35 ☑
    superficial NEC S00.47 ☑
      insect S00.46 ☑
  elbow S51.05 ☑
    superficial NEC S50.37 ☑
      insect S50.36 ☑
  epididymis — *see* Bite, testis
  epigastric region — *see* Bite, abdomen
  epiglottis — *see* Bite, neck, specified site NEC
  esophagus, cervical S11.25 ☑
    superficial NEC S10.17 ☑
      insect S10.16 ☑
  eyebrow — *see* Bite, eyelid
  eyelid S01.15 ☑
    superficial NEC S00.27 ☑
      insect S00.26 ☑
  face NEC — *see* Bite, head, specified site NEC
  finger(s) S61.259 ☑
    with
      damage to nail S61.359 ☑
    index S61.258 ☑
      with
        damage to nail S61.358 ☑
      left S61.251 ☑
        with

Bite(s) — *continued*
  finger(s) — *continued*
      damage to nail S61.351 ☑
    right S61.250 ☑
      with
        damage to nail S61.350 ☑
    superficial NEC S60.478 ☑
      insect S60.46 ☑
    little S61.25 ☑
      with
        damage to nail S61.35 ☑
      superficial NEC S60.47 ☑
        insect S60.46 ☑
    middle S61.25 ☑
      with
        damage to nail S61.35 ☑
      superficial NEC S60.47 ☑
        insect S60.46 ☑
    ring S61.25 ☑
      with
        damage to nail S61.35 ☑
      superficial NEC S60.47 ☑
        insect S60.46 ☑
    superficial NEC S60.479 ☑
      insect S60.469 ☑
    thumb — *see* Bite, thumb
  flank — *see* Bite, abdomen, wall
  flea — *see* Bite, by site, superficial, insect
  foot (except toe(s) alone) S91.35 ☑
    superficial NEC S90.87 ☑
      insect S90.86 ☑
    toe — *see* Bite, toe
  forearm S51.85 ☑
    elbow only — *see* Bite, elbow
    superficial NEC S50.87 ☑
      insect S50.86 ☑
  forehead — *see* Bite, head, specified site NEC
  genital organs, external
    female S31.552 ☑
      superficial NEC S30.876 ☑
        insect S30.866 ☑
      vagina and vulva — *see* Bite, vulva
    male S31.551 ☑
      penis — *see* Bite, penis
      scrotum — *see* Bite, scrotum
      superficial NEC S30.875 ☑
        insect S30.865 ☑
      testes — *see* Bite, testis
  groin — *see* Bite, abdomen, wall
  gum — *see* Bite, oral cavity
  hand S61.45 ☑
    finger — *see* Bite, finger
    superficial NEC S60.57 ☑
      insect S60.56 ☑
    thumb — *see* Bite, thumb
  head S01.95 ☑
    cheek — *see* Bite, cheek
    ear — *see* Bite, ear
    eyelid — *see* Bite, eyelid
    lip — *see* Bite, lip
    nose — *see* Bite, nose
    oral cavity — *see* Bite, oral cavity
    scalp — *see* Bite, scalp
    specified site NEC S01.85 ☑
      superficial NEC S00.87 ☑
        insect S00.86 ☑
    superficial NEC S00.97 ☑
      insect S00.96 ☑
    temporomandibular area — *see* Bite, cheek
  heel — *see* Bite, foot
  hip S71.05 ☑
    superficial NEC S70.27 ☑
      insect S70.26 ☑
  hymen S31.45 ☑
  hypochondrium — *see* Bite, abdomen, wall
  hypogastric region — *see* Bite, abdomen, wall
  inguinal region — *see* Bite, abdomen, wall
  insect — *see* Bite, by site, superficial, insect
  instep — *see* Bite, foot
  interscapular region — *see* Bite, thorax, back
  jaw — *see* Bite, head, specified site NEC
  knee S81.05 ☑
    superficial NEC S80.27 ☑
      insect S80.26 ☑
  labium (majus) (minus) — *see* Bite, vulva
  lacrimal duct — *see* Bite, eyelid
  larynx S11.015 ☑
    superficial NEC S10.17 ☑
      insect S10.16 ☑
  leg (lower) S81.85 ☑
    ankle — *see* Bite, ankle
    foot — *see* Bite, foot

Bite(s) — *continued*
  leg — *continued*
    knee — *see* Bite, knee
    superficial NEC S80.87 ☑
      insect S80.86 ☑
    toe — *see* Bite, toe
    upper — *see* Bite, thigh
  lip S01.551 ☑
    superficial NEC S00.571 ☑
      insect S00.561 ☑
  lizard (venomous) — *see* Venom, bite, reptile
  loin — *see* Bite, abdomen, wall
  lower back — *see* Bite, back, lower
  lumbar region — *see* Bite, back, lower
  malar region — *see* Bite, head, specified site NEC
  mammary — *see* Bite, breast
  marine animals (venomous) — *see* Toxicity, venom,
      marine animal
  mastoid region — *see* Bite, head, specified site NEC
  mouth — *see* Bite, oral cavity
  nail
    finger — *see* Bite, finger
    toe — *see* Bite, toe
  nape — *see* Bite, neck, specified site NEC
  nasal (septum) (sinus) — *see* Bite, nose
  nasopharynx — *see* Bite, head, specified site NEC
  neck S11.95 ☑
    involving
      cervical esophagus — *see* Bite, esophagus,
          cervical
      larynx — *see* Bite, larynx
      pharynx — *see* Bite, pharynx
      thyroid gland S11.15 ☑
      trachea — *see* Bite, trachea
    specified site NEC S11.85 ☑
      superficial NEC S10.87 ☑
        insect S10.86 ☑
    superficial NEC S10.97 ☑
      insect S10.96 ☑
    throat S11.85 ☑
      superficial NEC S10.17 ☑
        insect S10.16 ☑
  nose (septum) (sinus) S01.25 ☑
    superficial NEC S00.37 ☑
      insect S00.36 ☑
  occipital region — *see* Bite, scalp
  oral cavity S01.552 ☑
    superficial NEC S00.572 ☑
      insect S00.562 ☑
  orbital region — *see* Bite, eyelid
  palate — *see* Bite, oral cavity
  palm — *see* Bite, hand
  parietal region — *see* Bite, scalp
  pelvis S31.050 ☑
    with penetration into retroperitoneal space
      S31.051 ☑
    superficial NEC S30.870 ☑
      insect S30.860 ☑
  penis S31.25 ☑
    superficial NEC S30.872 ☑
      insect S30.862 ☑
  perineum
    female — *see* Bite, vulva
    male — *see* Bite, pelvis
  periocular area (with or without lacrimal passages)
      — *see* Bite, eyelid
  phalanges
    finger — *see* Bite, finger
    toe — *see* Bite, toe
  pharynx S11.25 ☑
    superficial NEC S10.17 ☑
      insect S10.16 ☑
  pinna — *see* Bite, ear
  poisonous — *see* Venom
  popliteal space — *see* Bite, knee
  prepuce — *see* Bite, penis
  pubic region — *see* Bite, abdomen, wall
  rectovaginal septum — *see* Bite, vulva
  red bug B88.0
  reptile NEC (*see also* Venom, bite, reptile)
    nonvenomous — *see* Bite, by site
    snake — *see* Venom, bite, snake
  sacral region — *see* Bite, back, lower
  sacroiliac region — *see* Bite, back, lower
  salivary gland — *see* Bite, oral cavity
  scalp S01.05 ☑
    superficial NEC S00.07 ☑
      insect S00.06 ☑
  scapular region — *see* Bite, shoulder
  scrotum S31.35 ☑
    superficial NEC S30.873 ☑
      insect S30.863 ☑

☑ **Additional character required**

Bite(s) — *continued*
sea-snake (venomous) — *see* Toxicity, venom,
   snake, sea snake
shin — *see* Bite, leg
shoulder S41.05 ☑
  superficial NEC S40.27 ☑
   insect S40.26 ☑
snake (*see also* Venom, bite, snake)
  nonvenomous — *see* Bite, by site
spermatic cord — *see* Bite, testis
spider (venomous) — *see* Toxicity, venom, spider
  nonvenomous — *see* Bite, by site, superficial,
   insect
sternal region — *see* Bite, thorax, front
submaxillary region — *see* Bite, head, specified
  site NEC
submental region — *see* Bite, head, specified site
  NEC
subungual
  finger(s) — *see* Bite, finger
  toe — *see* Bite, toe
superficial — *see* Bite, by site, superficial
supraclavicular fossa S11.85 ☑
supraorbital — *see* Bite, head, specified site NEC
temple, temporal region — *see* Bite, head, specified
  site NEC
temporomandibular area — *see* Bite, cheek
testis S31.35 ☑
  superficial NEC S30.873 ☑
   insect S30.863 ☑
thigh S71.15 ☑
  superficial NEC S70.37 ☑
   insect S70.36 ☑
thorax, thoracic (wall) S21.95 ☑
  back S21.25 ☑
   with penetration into thoracic cavity S21.45 ☑
  breast — *see* Bite, breast
  front S21.15 ☑
   with penetration into thoracic cavity S21.35 ☑
  superficial NEC S20.97 ☑
   back S20.47 ☑
   front S20.37 ☑
   insect S20.96 ☑
    back S20.46 ☑
    front S20.36 ☑
throat — *see* Bite, neck, throat
thumb S61.05 ☑
  with
   damage to nail S61.15 ☑
  superficial NEC S60.37 ☑
   insect S60.36 ☑
thyroid S11.15 ☑
  superficial NEC S10.87 ☑
   insect S10.86 ☑
toe(s) S91.15 ☑
  with
   damage to nail S91.25 ☑
  great S91.15 ☑
   with
    damage to nail S91.25 ☑
  lesser S91.15 ☑
   with
    damage to nail S91.25 ☑
  superficial NEC S90.47 ☑
   great S90.47 ☑
   insect S90.46 ☑
    great S90.46 ☑
tongue S01.552 ☑
trachea S11.025 ☑
  superficial NEC S10.17 ☑
   insect S10.16 ☑
tunica vaginalis — *see* Bite, testis
tympanum, tympanic membrane — *see* Bite, ear
umbilical region S31.155 ☑
uvula — *see* Bite, oral cavity
vagina — *see* Bite, vulva
venomous — *see* Venom
vocal cords S11.035 ☑
  superficial NEC S10.17 ☑
   insect S10.16 ☑
vulva S31.45 ☑
  superficial NEC S30.874 ☑
   insect S30.864 ☑
wrist S61.55 ☑
  superficial NEC S60.87 ☑
   insect S60.86 ☑
Biting, cheek or lip K13.1
Biventricular failure (heart) I50.82
Björck (-Thorson) syndrome (malignant carcinoid)
  E34.0
Black
  death A20.9

Black — *continued*
eye S00.1 ☑
hairy tongue K14.3
heel (foot) S90.3 ☑
lung (disease) J60
palm (hand) S60.22 ☑
Blackfan-Diamond anemia or syndrome (congenital
  hypoplastic anemia) D61.01
Blackhead L70.0
Blackout R55
Bladder — *see* condition
Blast (air) (hydraulic) (immersion) (underwater)
  blindness S05.8X ☑
  injury
   abdomen or thorax — *see* Injury, by site
   ear (acoustic nerve trauma) — *see* Injury, nerve,
    acoustic, specified type NEC
   syndrome NEC T70.8 ☑
Blastoma — *see* Neoplasm, malignant, by site
  pulmonary — *see* Neoplasm, lung, malignant
Blastomycosis, blastomycotic B40.9
  Brazilian — *see* Paracoccidioidomycosis
  cutaneous B40.3
  disseminated B40.7
  European — *see* Cryptococcosis
  generalized B40.7
  keloidal B48.0
  North American B40.9
  primary pulmonary B40.0
  pulmonary B40.2
   acute B40.0
   chronic B40.1
  skin B40.3
  South American — *see* Paracoccidioidomycosis
  specified NEC B40.89
Bleb(s) R23.8
  emphysematous (lung) (solitary) J43.9
  endophthalmitis H59.43
  filtering (vitreous), after glaucoma surgery Z98.83
  inflamed (infected), postprocedural H59.40
   stage 1 H59.41
   stage 2 H59.42
   stage 3 H59.43
  lung (ruptured) J43.9
   congenital — *see* Atelectasis
   newborn P25.8
  subpleural (emphysematous) J43.9
Blebitis, postprocedural H59.40
  stage 1 H59.41
  stage 2 H59.42
  stage 3 H59.43
Bleeder (familial) (hereditary) — *see* Hemophilia
Bleeding (*see also* Hemorrhage)
  anal K62.5
  anovulatory N97.0
  atonic, following delivery O72.1
  capillary I78.8
   puerperal O72.2
  contact (postcoital) N93.0
  due to uterine subinvolution N85.3
  ear — *see* Otorrhagia
  excessive, associated with menopausal onset N92.4
  familial — *see* Defect, coagulation
  following intercourse N93.0
  gastrointestinal K92.2
  hemorrhoids — *see* Hemorrhoids
  intermenstrual (regular) N92.3
   irregular N92.1
  intraoperative — *see* Complication, intraoperative,
   hemorrhage
  irregular N92.6
  menopausal N92.4
  newborn, intraventricular — *see* Newborn, affected
   by, hemorrhage, intraventricular
  nipple N64.59
  nose R04.0
  ovulation N92.3
  perimenopausal N92.4
  postclimacteric N95.0
  postcoital N93.0
  postmenopausal N95.0
  postoperative — *see* Complication, postprocedural,
   hemorrhage
  preclimacteric N92.4
  pre-pubertal vaginal N93.1
  puberty (excessive, with onset of menstrual
   periods) N92.2
  rectum, rectal K62.5
   newborn P54.2
  tendencies — *see* Defect, coagulation
  throat R04.1
  tooth socket (post-extraction) K91.840

Bleeding — *continued*
  umbilical stump P51.9
  uterus, uterine NEC N93.9
   climacteric N92.4
   dysfunctional or functional N93.8
   menopausal N92.4
   preclimacteric or premenopausal N92.4
   unrelated to menstrual cycle N93.9
  vagina, vaginal (abnormal) N93.9
   dysfunctional or functional N93.8
   newborn P54.6
   pre-pubertal N93.1
  vicarious N94.89
Blennorrhagia, blennorrhagic — *see* Gonorrhea
Blennorrhea (acute) (chronic) (*see also* Gonorrhea)
  inclusion (neonatal) (newborn) P39.1
  lower genitourinary tract (gonococcal) A54.00
  neonatorum (gonococcal ophthalmia) A54.31
Blepharelosis — *see* Entropion
Blepharitis (angularis) (ciliaris) (eyelid) (marginal)
  (nonulcerative) H01.009
  herpes zoster B02.39
  left H01.006
   lower H01.005
   upper H01.004
   upper and lower H01.00B
  right H01.003
   lower H01.002
   upper H01.001
   upper and lower H01.00A
  squamous H01.029
   left H01.026
    lower H01.025
    upper H01.024
    upper and lower H01.02B
   right H01.023
    lower H01.022
    upper H01.021
    upper and lower H01.02A
  ulcerative H01.019
   left H01.016
    lower H01.015
    upper H01.014
    upper and lower H01.01B
   right H01.013
    lower H01.012
    upper H01.011
    upper and lower H01.01A
Blepharochalasis H02.30
  congenital Q10.0
  left H02.36
   lower H02.35
   upper H02.34
  right H02.33
   lower H02.32
   upper H02.31
Blepharoclonus H02.59
Blepharoconjunctivitis H10.50 ☑
  angular H10.52 ☑
  contact H10.53 ☑
  ligneous H10.51 ☑
Blepharophimosis (eyelid) H02.529
  congenital Q10.3
  left H02.526
   lower H02.525
   upper H02.524
  right H02.523
   lower H02.522
   upper H02.521
Blepharoptosis H02.40 ☑
  congenital Q10.0
  mechanical H02.41 ☑
  myogenic H02.42 ☑
  neurogenic H02.43 ☑
  paralytic H02.43 ☑
Blepharopyorrhea, gonococcal A54.39
Blepharospasm G24.5
  drug induced G24.01
Blighted ovum O02.0
Blind (*see also* Blindness)
  bronchus (congenital) Q32.4
  loop syndrome K90.2
   congenital Q43.8
  sac, fallopian tube (congenital) Q50.6
  spot, enlarged — *see* Defect, visual field, localized,
   scotoma, blind spot area
  tract or tube, congenital NEC — *see* Atresia, by site
Blindness (acquired) (congenital) (both eyes)
  H54.0X ☑
  blast S05.8X ☑
  color — *see* Deficiency, color vision
  concussion S05.8X ☑

Blindness — *continued*
  cortical H47.619
    left brain H47.612
    right brain H47.611
  day H53.11
  due to injury (current episode) S05.9 ☑
    sequelae - code to injury with seventh character S
  eclipse (total) — *see* Retinopathy, solar
  emotional (hysterical) F44.6
  face H53.16
  hysterical F44.6
  legal (both eyes) (USA definition) H54.8
  mind R48.8
  night H53.60
    abnormal dark adaptation curve H53.61
    acquired H53.62
    congenital H53.63
    specified type NEC H53.69
    vitamin A deficiency E50.5
  one eye (other eye normal) H54.40
    left (normal vision on right) H54.42 ☑
      low vision on right H54.12 ☑
    low vision, other eye H54.10
    right (normal vision on left) H54.41 ☑
      low vision on left H54.11 ☑
  psychic R48.8
  river B73.01
  snow — *see* Photokeratitis
  sun, solar — *see* Retinopathy, solar
  transient — *see* Disturbance, vision, subjective, loss, transient
  traumatic (current episode) S05.9 ☑
  word (developmental) F81.0
    acquired R48.0
    secondary to organic lesion R48.0
Blister (nonthermal)
  abdominal wall S30.821 ☑
  alveolar process S00.522 ☑
  ankle S90.52 ☑
  antecubital space — *see* Blister, elbow
  anus S30.827 ☑
  arm (upper) S40.82 ☑
  auditory canal — *see* Blister, ear
  auricle — *see* Blister, ear
  axilla — *see* Blister, arm
  back, lower S30.820 ☑
  beetle dermatitis L24.89
  breast S20.12 ☑
  brow S00.82 ☑
  calf — *see* Blister, leg
  canthus — *see* Blister, eyelid
  cheek S00.82 ☑
    internal S00.522 ☑
  chest wall — *see* Blister, thorax
  chin S00.82 ☑
  costal region — *see* Blister, thorax
  digit(s)
    foot — *see* Blister, toe
    hand — *see* Blister, finger
  due to burn — *see* Burn, by site, second degree
  ear S00.42 ☑
  elbow S50.32 ☑
  epiglottis S10.12 ☑
  esophagus, cervical S10.12 ☑
  eyebrow — *see* Blister, eyelid
  eyelid S00.22 ☑
  face S00.82 ☑
  fever B00.1
  finger(s) S60.429 ☑
    index S60.42 ☑
    little S60.42 ☑
    middle S60.42 ☑
    ring S60.42 ☑
  foot (except toe(s) alone) S90.82 ☑
    toe — *see* Blister, toe
  forearm S50.82 ☑
    elbow only — *see* Blister, elbow
  forehead S00.82 ☑
  fracture - omit code
  genital organ
    female S30.826 ☑
    male S30.825 ☑
  gum S00.522 ☑
  hand S60.52 ☑
  head S00.92 ☑
    ear — *see* Blister, ear
    eyelid — *see* Blister, eyelid
    lip S00.521 ☑
    nose S00.32 ☑
    oral cavity S00.522 ☑
    scalp S00.02 ☑
    specified site NEC S00.82 ☑

Blister — *continued*
  heel — *see* Blister, foot
  hip S70.22 ☑
  interscapular region S20.429 ☑
  jaw S00.82 ☑
  knee S80.22 ☑
  larynx S10.12 ☑
  leg (lower) S80.82 ☑
    knee — *see* Blister, knee
    upper — *see* Blister, thigh
  lip S00.521 ☑
  malar region S00.82 ☑
  mammary — *see* Blister, breast
  mastoid region S00.82 ☑
  mouth S00.522 ☑
  multiple, skin, nontraumatic R23.8
  nail
    finger — *see* Blister, finger
    toe — *see* Blister, toe
  nasal S00.32 ☑
  neck S10.92 ☑
    specified site NEC S10.82 ☑
    throat S10.12 ☑
  nose S00.32 ☑
  occipital region S00.02 ☑
  oral cavity S00.522 ☑
  orbital region — *see* Blister, eyelid
  palate S00.522 ☑
  palm — *see* Blister, hand
  parietal region S00.02 ☑
  pelvis S30.820 ☑
  penis S30.822 ☑
  periocular area — *see* Blister, eyelid
  phalanges
    finger — *see* Blister, finger
    toe — *see* Blister, toe
  pharynx S10.12 ☑
  pinna — *see* Blister, ear
  popliteal space — *see* Blister, knee
  scalp S00.02 ☑
  scapular region — *see* Blister, shoulder
  scrotum S30.823 ☑
  shin — *see* Blister, leg
  shoulder S40.22 ☑
  sternal region S20.329 ☑
  submaxillary region S00.82 ☑
  submental region S00.82 ☑
  subungual
    finger(s) — *see* Blister, finger
    toe(s) — *see* Blister, toe
  supraclavicular fossa S10.82 ☑
  supraorbital S00.82 ☑
  temple S00.82 ☑
  temporal region S00.82 ☑
  testis S30.823 ☑
  thermal — *see* Burn, second degree, by site
  thigh S70.32 ☑
  thorax, thoracic (wall) S20.92 ☑
    back S20.42 ☑
    front S20.32 ☑
  throat S10.12 ☑
  thumb S60.32 ☑
  toe(s) S90.42 ☑
    great S90.42 ☑
  tongue S00.522 ☑
  trachea S10.12 ☑
  tympanum, tympanic membrane — *see* Blister, ear
  upper arm — *see* Blister, arm (upper)
  uvula S00.522 ☑
  vagina S30.824 ☑
  vocal cords S10.12 ☑
  vulva S30.824 ☑
  wrist S60.82 ☑
Bloating R14.0
Bloch-Sulzberger disease or syndrome Q82.3
Block, blocked
  alveolocapillary J84.10
  arborization (heart) I45.5
  arrhythmic I45.9
  atrioventricular (incomplete) (partial) I44.30
    with atrioventricular dissociation I44.2
    complete I44.2
      congenital Q24.6
    congenital Q24.6
    first degree I44.0
    second degree (types I and II) I44.1
    specified NEC I44.39
    third degree I44.2
    types I and II I44.1
  auriculoventricular — *see* Block, atrioventricular
  bifascicular (cardiac) I45.2

Block — *continued*
  bundle-branch (complete) (false) (incomplete) I45.4
    bilateral I45.2
    left I44.7
      with right bundle branch block I45.2
      hemiblock I44.60
        anterior I44.4
        posterior I44.5
      incomplete I44.7
        with right bundle branch block I45.2
    right I45.10
      with
        left bundle branch block I45.2
        left fascicular block I45.2
      specified NEC I45.19
    Wilson's type I45.19
  cardiac I45.9
  conduction I45.9
    complete I44.2
  fascicular (left) I44.60
    anterior I44.4
    posterior I44.5
    right I45.0
    specified NEC I44.69
  foramen Magendie (acquired) G91.1
    congenital Q03.1
      with spina bifida — *see* Spina bifida, by site, with hydrocephalus
  heart I45.9
    bundle branch I45.4
      bilateral I45.2
    complete (atrioventricular) I44.2
    congenital Q24.6
    first degree (atrioventricular) I44.0
    second degree (atrioventricular) I44.1
    specified type NEC I45.5
    third degree (atrioventricular) I44.2
  hepatic vein I82.0
  intraventricular (nonspecific) I45.4
    bundle branch
      bilateral I45.2
  kidney N28.9
    postcystoscopic or postprocedural N99.0
  Mobitz (types I and II) I44.1
  myocardial — *see* Block, heart
  nodal I45.5
  organ or site, congenital NEC — *see* Atresia, by site
  portal (vein) I81
  second degree (types I and II) I44.1
  sinoatrial I45.5
  sinoauricular I45.5
  third degree I44.2
  trifascicular I45.3
  tubal N97.1
  vein NOS I82.90
  Wenckebach (types I and II) I44.1
Blockage — *see* Obstruction
Blocq's disease F44.4
Blood
  constituents, abnormal R78.9
  disease D75.9
  donor — *see* Donor, blood
  dyscrasia D75.9
    with
      abortion — *see* Abortion, by type, complicated by, hemorrhage
      ectopic pregnancy O08.1
      molar pregnancy O08.1
    following ectopic or molar pregnancy O08.1
    newborn P61.9
    puerperal, postpartum O72.3
  flukes NEC — *see* Schistosomiasis
  in
    feces K92.1
      occult R19.5
    urine — *see* Hematuria
  mole O02.0
  occult in feces R19.5
  pressure
    decreased, due to shock following injury T79.4 ☑
    examination only Z01.30
    fluctuating I99.8
    high — *see* Hypertension
      borderline R03.0
      incidental reading, without diagnosis of hypertension R03.0
    low (*see also* Hypotension)
      incidental reading, without diagnosis of hypotension R03.1
  spitting — *see* Hemoptysis
  staining cornea — *see* Pigmentation, cornea, stromal

Blood — *continued*
  transfusion
    reaction or complication — *see* Complications, transfusion
    type
      A (Rh positive) Z67.10
        Rh negative Z67.11
      AB (Rh positive) Z67.30
        Rh negative Z67.31
      B (Rh positive) Z67.20
        Rh negative Z67.21
      O (Rh positive) Z67.40
        Rh negative Z67.41
      Rh (positive) Z67.90
        negative Z67.91
    vessel rupture — *see* Hemorrhage
    vomiting — *see* Hematemesis
Blood-forming organs, disease D75.9
Bloodgood's disease — *see* Mastopathy, cystic
Bloom (-Machacek)(-Torre) syndrome Q82.8
Blount's disease or osteochondrosis — *see* Osteochondrosis, juvenile, tibia
Blue
  baby Q24.9
  diaper syndrome E72.09
  dome cyst (breast) — *see* Cyst, breast
  dot cataract Q12.0
  nevus D22.9
  sclera Q13.5
    with fragility of bone and deafness Q78.0
  toe syndrome I75.02 ☑
Blueness — *see* Cyanosis
Blues, postpartal O90.6
  baby O90.6
Blurring, visual H53.8
Blushing (abnormal) (excessive) R23.2
BMI — *see* Body, mass index
Boarder, hospital NEC Z76.4
  accompanying sick person Z76.3
  healthy infant or child Z76.2
  foundling Z76.1
Bockhart's impetigo L01.02
Bodechtel-Guttman disease (subacute sclerosing panencephalitis) A81.1
Boder-Sedgwick syndrome (ataxia-telangiectasia) G11.3
Body, bodies
  Aschoff's — *see* Myocarditis, rheumatic
  asteroid, vitreous — *see* Deposit, crystalline
  cytoid (retina) — *see* Occlusion, artery, retina
  drusen (degenerative) (macula) (retinal) (*see also* Degeneration, macula, drusen)
    optic disc — *see* Drusen, optic disc
  foreign — *see* Foreign body
  loose
    joint, except knee — *see* Loose, body, joint
      knee M23.4 ☑
    sheath, tendon — *see* Disorder, tendon, specified type NEC
  mass index (BMI)
    adult
      19.9 or less Z68.1
      20.0-20.9 Z68.20
      21.0-21.9 Z68.21
      22.0-22.9 Z68.22
      23.0-23.9 Z68.23
      24.0-24.9 Z68.24
      25.0-25.9 Z68.25
      26.0-26.9 Z68.26
      27.0-27.9 Z68.27
      28.0-28.9 Z68.28
      29.0-29.9 Z68.29
      30.0-30.9 Z68.30
      31.0-31.9 Z68.31
      32.0-32.9 Z68.32
      33.0-33.9 Z68.33
      34.0-34.9 Z68.34
      35.0-35.9 Z68.35
      36.0-36.9 Z68.36
      37.0-37.9 Z68.37
      38.0-38.9 Z68.38
      39.0-39.9 Z68.39
      40.0-44.9 Z68.41
      45.0-49.9 Z68.42
      50.0-59.9 Z68.43
      60.0-69.9 Z68.44
      70 and over Z68.45
    pediatric
      5th percentile to less than 85th percentile for age Z68.52
      85th percentile to less than 95th percentile for age Z68.53

Body — *continued*
  mass index — *continued*
    greater than or equal to ninety-fifth percentile for age Z68.54
    less than fifth percentile for age Z68.51
  Mooser's A75.2
  rice (*see also* Loose, body, joint)
    knee M23.4 ☑
  rocking F98.4
Boeck's
  disease or sarcoid — *see* Sarcoidosis
  lupoid (miliary) D86.3
Boerhaave's syndrome (spontaneous esophageal rupture) K22.3
Boggy
  cervix N88.8
  uterus N85.8
Boil (*see also* Furuncle, by site)
  Aleppo B55.1
  Baghdad B55.1
  Delhi B55.1
  lacrimal
    gland — *see* Dacryoadenitis
    passages (duct) (sac) — *see* Inflammation, lacrimal, passages, acute
  Natal B55.1
  orbit, orbital — *see* Abscess, orbit
  tropical B55.1
Bold hives — *see* Urticaria
Bombé, iris — *see* Membrane, pupillary
Bone — *see* condition
Bonnevie-Ullrich syndrome (*see also* Turner's syndrome) Q87.19
Bonnier's syndrome — *see* subcategory H81.8 ☑
Bonvale dam fever T73.3 ☑
Bony block of joint — *see* Ankylosis
BOOP (bronchiolitis obliterans organized pneumonia) J84.89
Borderline
  diabetes mellitus R73.03
  hypertension R03.0
  osteopenia M85.8 ☑
  pelvis, with obstruction during labor O65.1
  personality F60.3
Borna disease A83.9
Bornholm disease B33.0
Boston exanthem A88.0
Botalli, ductus (patent) (persistent) Q25.0
Bothriocephalus latus infestation B70.0
Botulism (foodborne intoxication) A05.1
  infant A48.51
  non-foodborne A48.52
  wound A48.52
Bouba — *see* Yaws
Bouchard's nodes (with arthropathy) M15.2
Bouffée délirante F23
Bouillaud's disease or syndrome (rheumatic heart disease) I01.9
Bourneville's disease Q85.1
Boutonniere deformity (finger) — *see* Deformity, finger, boutonniere
Bouveret (-Hoffmann) syndrome (paroxysmal tachycardia) I47.9
Bovine heart — *see* Hypertrophy, cardiac
Bowel — *see* condition
Bowen's
  dermatosis (precancerous) — *see* Neoplasm, skin, in situ
  disease — *see* Neoplasm, skin, in situ
  epithelioma — *see* Neoplasm, skin, in situ
  type
    epidermoid carcinoma-in-situ — *see* Neoplasm, skin, in situ
    intraepidermal squamous cell carcinoma — *see* Neoplasm, skin, in situ
Bowing
  femur (*see also* Deformity, limb, specified type NEC, thigh)
    congenital Q68.3
  fibula (*see also* Deformity, limb, specified type NEC, lower leg)
    congenital Q68.4
  forearm — *see* Deformity, limb, specified type NEC, forearm
  leg(s), long bones, congenital Q68.5
  radius — *see* Deformity, limb, specified type NEC, forearm
  tibia (*see also* Deformity, limb, specified type NEC, lower leg)
    congenital Q68.4
Bowleg(s) (acquired) M21.16 ☑
  congenital Q68.5
  rachitic E64.3

Boyd's dysentery A03.2
Brachial — *see* condition
Brachycardia R00.1
Brachycephaly Q75.0
Bradley's disease A08.19
Bradyarrhythmia, cardiac I49.8
Bradycardia (sinoatrial) (sinus) (vagal) R00.1
  neonatal P29.12
  reflex G90.09
  tachycardia syndrome I49.5
Bradykinesia R25.8
Bradypnea R06.89
Bradytachycardia I49.5
Brailsford's disease or osteochondrosis — *see* Osteochondrosis, juvenile, radius
Brain (*see also* condition)
  death G93.82
  syndrome — *see* Syndrome, brain
Branched-chain amino-acid disorder E71.2
Branchial — *see* condition
  cartilage, congenital Q18.2
Branchiogenic remnant (in neck) Q18.0
Brandt's syndrome (acrodermatitis enteropathica) E83.2
Brash (water) R12
Bravais-jacksonian epilepsy — *see* Epilepsy, localization-related, symptomatic, with simple partial seizures
Braxton Hicks contractions — *see* False, labor
Brazilian leishmaniasis B55.2
BRBPR K62.5
Break, retina (without detachment) H33.30 ☑
  with retinal detachment — *see* Detachment, retina
  horseshoe tear H33.31 ☑
  multiple H33.33 ☑
  round hole H33.32 ☑
Breakdown
  device, graft or implant (*see also* Complications, by site and type, mechanical) T85.618 ☑
    arterial graft NEC — *see* Complication, cardiovascular device, mechanical, vascular
    breast (implant) T85.41 ☑
    catheter NEC T85.618 ☑
      cystostomy T83.010 ☑
      Hopkins T83.018 ☑
      ileostomy T83.018 ☑
      dialysis (renal) T82.41 ☑
        intraperitoneal T85.611 ☑
      infusion NEC T82.514 ☑
        cranial T85.610 ☑
        epidural T85.610 ☑
        intrathecal T85.610 ☑
        spinal T85.610 ☑
        subarachnoid T85.610 ☑
        subdural T85.610 ☑
      nephrostomy T83.012 ☑
      urethral indwelling T83.011 ☑
      urinary NEC T83.018 ☑
      urostomy T83.018 ☑
    electronic (electrode) (pulse generator) (stimulator)
      bone T84.310 ☑
      cardiac T82.119 ☑
        electrode T82.110 ☑
        pulse generator T82.111 ☑
        specified type NEC T82.118 ☑
      nervous system — *see* Complication, prosthetic device, mechanical, electronic nervous system stimulator
      urinary — *see* Complication, genitourinary, device, urinary, mechanical
    fixation, internal (orthopedic) NEC — *see* Complication, fixation device, mechanical
    gastrointestinal — *see* Complications, prosthetic device, mechanical, gastrointestinal device
    genital NEC T83.418 ☑
      intrauterine contraceptive device T83.31 ☑
      penile prosthesis (cylinder) (implanted) (pump) (reservoir) T83.410 ☑
      testicular prosthesis T83.411 ☑
    heart NEC — *see* Complication, cardiovascular device, mechanical
    intrathecal infusion pump T85.615 ☑
    joint prosthesis — *see* Complications..., joint prosthesis, internal, mechanical, by site
    nervous system, specified device NEC T85.615 ☑
    ocular NEC — *see* Complications, prosthetic device, mechanical, ocular device
    orthopedic NEC — *see* Complication, orthopedic, device, mechanical
    specified NEC T85.618 ☑
    subcutaneous device pocket

Breakdown — *continued*
  device, graft or implant — *continued*
    nervous system prosthetic device, implant, or graft T85.890 ☑
    other internal prosthetic device, implant, or graft T85.898 ☑
    sutures, permanent T85.612 ☑
      used in bone repair — *see* Complications, fixation device, internal (orthopedic), mechanical
    urinary NEC T83.118 ☑
      graft T83.21 ☑
      sphincter, implanted T83.111 ☑
      stent (ileal conduit) (nephroureteral) T83.113 ☑
      ureteral indwelling T83.112 ☑
    vascular NEC — *see* Complication, cardiovascular device, mechanical
    ventricular intracranial shunt T85.01 ☑
  nervous F48.8
  perineum O90.1
  respirator J95.850
    specified NEC J95.859
  ventilator J95.850
    specified NEC J95.859
Breast (*see also* condition)
  buds E30.1
    in newborn P96.89
  dense R92.2
  nodule (*see also* Lump, breast) N63.0
Breath
  foul R19.6
  holder, child R06.89
  holding spell R06.89
  shortness R06.02
Breathing
  labored — *see* Hyperventilation
  mouth R06.5
    causing malocclusion M26.5 ☑
  periodic R06.3
    high altitude G47.32
Breathlessness R06.81
Breda's disease — *see* Yaws
Breech presentation (mother) O32.1 ☑
  causing obstructed labor O64.1 ☑
  footling O32.8 ☑
    causing obstructed labor O64.8 ☑
  incomplete O32.8 ☑
    causing obstructed labor O64.8 ☑
Breisky's disease N90.4
Brennemann's syndrome I88.0
Brenner
  tumor (benign) D27.9
    borderline malignancy D39.1 ☑
    malignant C56 ☑
    proliferating D39.1 ☑
Bretonneau's disease or angina A36.0
Breus' mole O02.0
Brevicollis Q76.49
Brickmakers' anemia B76.9 *[D63.8]*
Bridge, myocardial Q24.5
Bright red blood per rectum (BRBPR) K62.5
Bright's disease (*see also* Nephritis)
  arteriosclerotic — *see* Hypertension, kidney
Brill (-Zinsser) disease (recrudescent typhus) A75.1
Brill-Symmers' disease C82.90
Brion-Kayser disease — *see* Fever, parathyroid
Briquet's disorder or syndrome F45.0
Brissaud's
  infantilism or dwarfism E23.0
  motor-verbal tic F95.2
Brittle
  bones disease Q78.0
  nails L60.3
    congenital Q84.6
Broad (*see also* condition)
  beta disease E78.2
  ligament laceration syndrome N83.8
Broad- or floating-betalipoproteinemia E78.2
Brock's syndrome (atelectasis due to enlarged lymph nodes) J98.19
Brocq-Duhring disease (dermatitis herpetiformis) L13.0
Brodie's abscess or disease M86.8X ☑
Broken
  arches (*see also* Deformity, limb, flat foot)
  arm (meaning upper limb) — *see* Fracture, arm
  back — *see* Fracture, vertebra
  bone — *see* Fracture
  implant or internal device — *see* Complications, by site and type, mechanical
  leg (meaning lower limb) — *see* Fracture, leg
  nose S02.2 ☑
  tooth, teeth — *see* Fracture, tooth

Bromhidrosis, bromidrosis L75.0
Bromidism, bromism G92
  due to
    correct substance properly administered — *see* Table of Drugs and Chemicals, by drug, adverse effect
    overdose or wrong substance given or taken — *see* Table of Drugs and Chemicals, by drug, poisoning
  chronic (dependence) F13.20
Bromidrosiphobia F40.298
Bronchi, bronchial — *see* condition
Bronchiectasis (cylindrical) (diffuse) (fusiform) (localized) (saccular) J47.9
  with
    acute
      bronchitis J47.0
      lower respiratory infection J47.0
    exacerbation (acute) J47.1
  congenital Q33.4
  tuberculous NEC — *see* Tuberculosis, pulmonary
Bronchiolectasis — *see* Bronchiectasis
Bronchiolitis (acute) (infective) (subacute) J21.9
  with
    bronchospasm or obstruction J21.9
    influenza, flu or grippe — *see* Influenza, with, respiratory manifestations NEC
  chemical (chronic) J68.4
    acute J68.0
  chronic (fibrosing) (obliterative) J44.9
  due to
    external agent — *see* Bronchitis, acute, due to
    human metapneumovirus J21.1
    respiratory syncytial virus (RSV) J21.0
    specified organism NEC J21.8
  fibrosa obliterans J44.9
  influenzal — *see* Influenza, with, respiratory manifestations NEC
  obliterans J42
    with organizing pneumonia (BOOP) J84.89
  obliterative (chronic) (subacute) J44.9
    due to fumes or vapors J68.4
    due to chemicals, gases, fumes or vapors (inhalation) J68.4
  respiratory, interstitial lung disease J84.115
Bronchitis (diffuse) (fibrinous) (hypostatic) (infective) (membranous) J40
  with
    influenza, flu or grippe — *see* Influenza, with, respiratory manifestations NEC
    obstruction (airway) (lung) J44.9
    tracheitis (15 years of age and above) J40
      acute or subacute J20.9
      chronic J42
      under 15 years of age J20.9
  acute or subacute (with bronchospasm or obstruction) J20.9
    with
      bronchiectasis J47.0
      chronic obstructive pulmonary disease J44.0
    chemical (due to gases, fumes or vapors) J68.0
    due to
      fumes or vapors J68.0
      Haemophilus influenzae J20.1
      Mycoplasma pneumoniae J20.0
      radiation J70.0
      specified organism NEC J20.8
      Streptococcus J20.2
      virus
        coxsackie J20.3
        echovirus J20.7
        parainfluenzae J20.4
        respiratory syncytial (RSV) J20.5
        rhinovirus J20.6
    viral NEC J20.8
  allergic (acute) J45.909
    with
      exacerbation (acute) J45.901
      status asthmaticus J45.902
  arachidic T17.528 ☑
  aspiration (due to fumes or vapors) J68.0
  asthmatic J45.9 ☑
    chronic J44.9
      with
        acute lower respiratory infection J44.0
        exacerbation (acute) J44.1
  capillary — *see* Pneumonia, broncho
  caseous (tuberculous) A15.5
  Castellani's A69.8
  catarrhal (15 years of age and above) J40
    acute — *see* Bronchitis, acute
    chronic J41.0

Bronchitis — *continued*
  catarrhal — *continued*
    under 15 years of age J20.9
  chemical (acute) (subacute) J68.0
    chronic J68.4
    due to fumes or vapors J68.0
      chronic J68.4
  chronic J42
    with
      airways obstruction J44.9
      tracheitis (chronic) J42
    asthmatic (obstructive) J44.9
    catarrhal J41.0
    chemical (due to fumes or vapors) J68.4
    due to
      chemicals, gases, fumes or vapors (inhalation) J68.4
      radiation J70.1
      tobacco smoking J41.0
    emphysematous J44.9
    mucopurulent J41.1
    non-obstructive J41.0
    obliterans J44.9
    obstructive J44.9
    purulent J41.1
    simple J41.0
  croupous — *see* Bronchitis, acute
  due to gases, fumes or vapors (chemical) J68.0
  emphysematous (obstructive) J44.9
  exudative — *see* Bronchitis, acute
  fetid J41.1
  grippal — *see* Influenza, with, respiratory manifestations NEC
  in those under 15 years age — *see* Bronchitis, acute
    chronic — *see* Bronchitis, chronic
  influenzal — *see* Influenza, with, respiratory manifestations NEC
  mixed simple and mucopurulent J41.8
  moulder's J62.8
  mucopurulent (chronic) (recurrent) J41.1
    acute or subacute J20.9
    simple (mixed) J41.8
  obliterans (chronic) J44.9
  obstructive (chronic) (diffuse) J44.9
  pituitous J41.1
  pneumococcal, acute or subacute J20.2
  pseudomembranous, acute or subacute — *see* Bronchitis, acute
  purulent (chronic) (recurrent) J41.1
    acute or subacute — *see* Bronchitis, acute
  putrid J41.1
  senile (chronic) J42
  simple and mucopurulent (mixed) J41.8
  smokers' J41.0
  spirochetal NEC A69.8
  subacute — *see* Bronchitis, acute
  suppurative (chronic) J41.1
    acute or subacute — *see* Bronchitis, acute
  tuberculous A15.5
  under 15 years of age — *see* Bronchitis, acute
    chronic — *see* Bronchitis, chronic
  viral NEC, acute or subacute (*see also* Bronchitis, acute) J20.8
Bronchoalveolitis J18.0
Bronchoaspergillosis B44.1
Bronchocele meaning goiter E04.0
Broncholithiasis J98.09
  tuberculous NEC A15.5
Bronchomalacia J98.09
  congenital Q32.2
Bronchomycosis NOS B49 *[J99]*
  candidal B37.1
Bronchopleuropneumonia — *see* Pneumonia, broncho
Bronchopneumonia — *see* Pneumonia, broncho
Bronchopneumonitis — *see* Pneumonia, broncho
Bronchopulmonary — *see* condition
Bronchopulmonitis — *see* Pneumonia, broncho
Bronchorrhagia (*see* Hemoptysis)
Bronchorrhea J98.09
  acute J20.9
  chronic (infective) (purulent) J42
Bronchospasm (acute) J98.01
  with
    bronchiolitis, acute J21.9
    bronchitis, acute (conditions in J20 ☑) — *see* Bronchitis, acute
  due to external agent — *see* condition, respiratory, acute, due to
  exercise induced J45.990
Bronchospirochetosis A69.8
  Castellani A69.8

☑ **Additional character required**

Bronchostenosis J98.09
Bronchus — *see* condition
Brontophobia F40.220
Bronze baby syndrome P83.88
Bronze baby syndrome P83.88
Brooke's tumor — *see* Neoplasm, skin, benign
Brown enamel of teeth (hereditary) K00.5
Brown's sheath syndrome H50.61 ☑
Brown-Séquard disease, paralysis or syndrome G83.81
Bruce sepsis A23.0
Brucellosis (infection) A23.9
    abortus A23.1
    canis A23.3
    dermatitis A23.9
    melitensis A23.0
    mixed A23.8
    sepsis A23.9
      melitensis A23.0
      specified NEC A23.8
    suis A23.2
Bruck-de Lange disease Q87.19
Bruck's disease — *see* Deformity, limb
BRUE (brief resolved unexplained event) R68.13
Brugsch's syndrome Q82.8
Bruise (skin surface intact) (*see also* Contusion)
    with
      open wound — *see* Wound, open
    internal organ — *see* Injury, by site
    newborn P54.5
    scalp, due to birth injury, newborn P12.3
    umbilical cord O69.5 ☑
Bruit (arterial) R09.89
    cardiac R01.1
Brush burn — *see* Abrasion, by site
Bruton's X-linked agammaglobulinemia D80.0
Bruxism
    psychogenic F45.8
    sleep related G47.63
Bubbly lung syndrome P27.0
Bubo I88.9
    blennorrhagic (gonococcal) A54.89
    chancroidal A57
    climatic A55
    due to Haemophilus ducreyi A57
    gonococcal A54.89
    indolent (nonspecific) I88.8
    inguinal (nonspecific) I88.8
      chancroidal A57
      climatic A55
      due to H. ducreyi A57
      infective I88.8
    scrofulous (tuberculous) A18.2
    soft chancre A57
    suppurating — *see* Lymphadenitis, acute
    syphilitic (primary) A51.0
      congenital A50.07
    tropical A55
    virulent (chancroidal) A57
Bubonic plague A20.0
Bubonocele — *see* Hernia, inguinal
Buccal — *see* condition
Buchanan's disease or osteochondrosis M91.0
Buchem's syndrome (hyperostosis corticalis) M85.2
Bucket-handle fracture or tear (semilunar cartilage) — *see* Tear, meniscus
Budd-Chiari syndrome (hepatic vein thrombosis) I82.0
Budgerigar fancier's disease or lung J67.2
Buds
    breast E30.1
      in newborn P96.89
Buerger's disease (thromboangiitis obliterans) I73.1
Bulbar — *see* condition
Bulbus cordis (left ventricle) (persistent) Q21.8
Bulimia (nervosa) F50.2
    atypical F50.9
    normal weight F50.9
Bulky
    stools R19.5
    uterus N85.2
Bulla (e) R23.8
    lung (emphysematous) (solitary) J43.9
      newborn P25.8
Bullet wound (*see also* Wound, open)
    fracture - code as Fracture, by site
    internal organ — *see* Injury, by site
Bundle
    branch block (complete) (false) (incomplete) — *see* Block, bundle-branch
    of His — *see* condition
Bunion M21.61 ☑
    tailor's M21.62 ☑
Bunionette M21.62 ☑
Buphthalmia, buphthalmos (congenital) Q15.0

Burdwan fever B55.0
Bürger-Grütz disease or syndrome E78.3
Buried
    penis (congenital) Q55.64
      acquired N48.83
    roots K08.3
Burke's syndrome K86.89
Burkitt
    cell leukemia C91.0 ☑
    lymphoma (malignant) C83.7 ☑
      small noncleaved, diffuse C83.7 ☑
      spleen C83.77
      undifferentiated C83.7 ☑
    tumor C83.7 ☑
    type
      acute lymphoblastic leukemia C91.0 ☑
      undifferentiated C83.7 ☑
Burn (electricity) (flame) (hot gas, liquid or hot object) (radiation) (steam) (thermal) T30.0
    abdomen, abdominal (muscle) (wall) T21.02 ☑
      first degree T21.12 ☑
      second degree T21.22 ☑
      third degree T21.32 ☑
    above elbow T22.039 ☑
      first degree T22.139 ☑
      left T22.032 ☑
        first degree T22.132 ☑
        second degree T22.232 ☑
        third degree T22.332 ☑
      right T22.031 ☑
        first degree T22.131 ☑
        second degree T22.231 ☑
        third degree T22.331 ☑
      second degree T22.239 ☑
      third degree T22.339 ☑
    acid (caustic) (external) (internal) — *see* Corrosion, by site
    alimentary tract NEC T28.2 ☑
      esophagus T28.1 ☑
      mouth T28.0 ☑
      pharynx T28.0 ☑
    alkaline (caustic) (external) (internal) — *see* Corrosion, by site
    ankle T25.019 ☑
      first degree T25.119 ☑
      left T25.012 ☑
        first degree T25.112 ☑
        second degree T25.212 ☑
        third degree T25.312 ☑
      multiple with foot — *see* Burn, lower, limb, multiple, ankle and foot
      right T25.011 ☑
        first degree T25.111 ☑
        second degree T25.211 ☑
        third degree T25.311 ☑
      second degree T25.219 ☑
      third degree T25.319 ☑
    anus — *see* Burn, buttock
    arm (lower) (upper) — *see* Burn, upper, limb
    axilla T22.049 ☑
      first degree T22.149 ☑
      left T22.042 ☑
        first degree T22.142 ☑
        second degree T22.242 ☑
        third degree T22.342 ☑
      right T22.041 ☑
        first degree T22.141 ☑
        second degree T22.241 ☑
        third degree T22.341 ☑
      second degree T22.249 ☑
      third degree T22.349 ☑
    back (lower) T21.04 ☑
      first degree T21.14 ☑
      second degree T21.24 ☑
      third degree T21.34 ☑
      upper T21.03 ☑
        first degree T21.13 ☑
        second degree T21.23 ☑
        third degree T21.33 ☑
    blisters - code as Burn, second degree, by site
    breast(s) — *see* Burn, chest wall
    buttock(s) T21.05 ☑
      first degree T21.15 ☑
      second degree T21.25 ☑
      third degree T21.35 ☑
    calf T24.039 ☑
      first degree T24.139 ☑
      left T24.032 ☑
        first degree T24.132 ☑
        second degree T24.232 ☑
        third degree T24.332 ☑
      right T24.031 ☑

Burn — *continued*
    calf — *continued*
      first degree T24.131 ☑
      second degree T24.231 ☑
      third degree T24.331 ☑
      second degree T24.239 ☑
      third degree T24.339 ☑
    canthus (eye) — *see* Burn, eyelid
    caustic acid or alkaline — *see* Corrosion, by site
    cervix T28.3 ☑
    cheek T20.06 ☑
      first degree T20.16 ☑
      second degree T20.26 ☑
      third degree T20.36 ☑
    chemical (acids) (alkalines) (caustics) (external) (internal) — *see* Corrosion, by site
    chest wall T21.01 ☑
      first degree T21.11 ☑
      second degree T21.21 ☑
      third degree T21.31 ☑
    chin T20.03 ☑
      first degree T20.13 ☑
      second degree T20.23 ☑
      third degree T20.33 ☑
    colon T28.2 ☑
    conjunctiva (and cornea) — *see* Burn, cornea
    cornea (and conjunctiva) T26.1 ☑
      chemical — *see* Corrosion, cornea
    corrosion (external) (internal) — *see* Corrosion, by site
    deep necrosis of underlying tissue - code as Burn, third degree, by site
    dorsum of hand T23.069 ☑
      first degree T23.169 ☑
      left T23.062 ☑
        first degree T23.162 ☑
        second degree T23.262 ☑
        third degree T23.362 ☑
      right T23.061 ☑
        first degree T23.161 ☑
        second degree T23.261 ☑
        third degree T23.361 ☑
      second degree T23.269 ☑
      third degree T23.369 ☑
    due to ingested chemical agent — *see* Corrosion, by site
    ear (auricle) (external) (canal) T20.01 ☑
      first degree T20.11 ☑
      second degree T20.21 ☑
      third degree T20.31 ☑
    elbow T22.029 ☑
      first degree T22.129 ☑
      left T22.022 ☑
        first degree T22.122 ☑
        second degree T22.222 ☑
        third degree T22.322 ☑
      right T22.021 ☑
        first degree T22.121 ☑
        second degree T22.221 ☑
        third degree T22.321 ☑
      second degree T22.229 ☑
      third degree T22.329 ☑
    epidermal loss - code as Burn, second degree, by site
    erythema, erythematous - code as Burn, first degree, by site
    esophagus T28.1 ☑
    extent (percentage of body surface)
      less than 10 percent T31.0
      10-19 percent T31.10
        with 0-9 percent third degree burns T31.10
        with 10-19 percent third degree burns T31.11
      20-29 percent T31.20
        with 0-9 percent third degree burns T31.20
        with 10-19 percent third degree burns T31.21
        with 20-29 percent third degree burns T31.22
      30-39 percent T31.30
        with 0-9 percent third degree burns T31.30
        with 10-19 percent third degree burns T31.31
        with 20-29 percent third degree burns T31.32
        with 30-39 percent third degree burns T31.33
      40-49 percent T31.40
        with 0-9 percent third degree burns T31.40
        with 10-19 percent third degree burns T31.41
        with 20-29 percent third degree burns T31.42
        with 30-39 percent third degree burns T31.43
        with 40-49 percent third degree burns T31.44
      50-59 percent T31.50
        with 0-9 percent third degree burns T31.50
        with 10-19 percent third degree burns T31.51
        with 20-29 percent third degree burns T31.52
        with 30-39 percent third degree burns T31.53

Burn — *continued*
- extent — *continued*
  - with 40-49 percent third degree burns T31.54
  - with 50-59 percent third degree burns T31.55
  - 60-69 percent T31.60
    - with 0-9 percent third degree burns T31.60
    - with 10-19 percent third degree burns T31.61
    - with 20-29 percent third degree burns T31.62
    - with 30-39 percent third degree burns T31.63
    - with 40-49 percent third degree burns T31.64
    - with 50-59 percent third degree burns T31.65
    - with 60-69 percent third degree burns T31.66
  - 70-79 percent T31.70
    - with 0-9 percent third degree burns T31.70
    - with 10-19 percent third degree burns T31.71
    - with 20-29 percent third degree burns T31.72
    - with 30-39 percent third degree burns T31.73
    - with 40-49 percent third degree burns T31.74
    - with 50-59 percent third degree burns T31.75
    - with 60-69 percent third degree burns T31.76
    - with 70-79 percent third degree burns T31.77
  - 80-89 percent T31.80
    - with 0-9 percent third degree burns T31.80
    - with 10-19 percent third degree burns T31.81
    - with 20-29 percent third degree burns T31.82
    - with 30-39 percent third degree burns T31.83
    - with 40-49 percent third degree burns T31.84
    - with 50-59 percent third degree burns T31.85
    - with 60-69 percent third degree burns T31.86
    - with 70-79 percent third degree burns T31.87
    - with 80-89 percent third degree burns T31.88
  - 90 percent or more T31.90
    - with 0-9 percent third degree burns T31.90
    - with 10-19 percent third degree burns T31.91
    - with 20-29 percent third degree burns T31.92
    - with 30-39 percent third degree burns T31.93
    - with 40-49 percent third degree burns T31.94
    - with 50-59 percent third degree burns T31.95
    - with 60-69 percent third degree burns T31.96
    - with 70-79 percent third degree burns T31.97
    - with 80-89 percent third degree burns T31.98
    - with 90 percent or more third degree burns T31.99
- extremity — *see* Burn, limb
- eye(s) and adnexa T26.4 ☑
  - with resulting rupture and destruction of eyeball T26.2 ☑
  - conjunctival sac — *see* Burn, cornea
  - cornea — *see* Burn, cornea
  - lid — *see* Burn, eyelid
  - periocular area — *see* Burn, eyelid
  - specified site NEC T26.3 ☑
- eyeball — *see* Burn, eye
- eyelid(s) T26.0 ☑
  - chemical — *see* Corrosion, eyelid
- face — *see* Burn, head
- finger T23.029 ☑
  - first degree T23.129 ☑
  - left T23.022 ☑
    - first degree T23.122 ☑
    - second degree T23.222 ☑
    - third degree T23.322 ☑
  - multiple sites (without thumb) T23.039 ☑
    - with thumb T23.049 ☑
      - first degree T23.149 ☑
      - left T23.042 ☑
        - first degree T23.142 ☑
        - second degree T23.242 ☑
        - third degree T23.342 ☑
      - right T23.041 ☑
        - first degree T23.141 ☑
        - second degree T23.241 ☑
        - third degree T23.341 ☑
      - second degree T23.249 ☑
      - third degree T23.349 ☑
    - first degree T23.139 ☑
    - left T23.032 ☑
      - first degree T23.132 ☑
      - second degree T23.232 ☑
      - third degree T23.332 ☑
    - right T23.031 ☑
      - first degree T23.131 ☑
      - second degree T23.231 ☑
      - third degree T23.331 ☑
    - second degree T23.239 ☑
    - third degree T23.339 ☑
  - right T23.021 ☑
    - first degree T23.121 ☑
    - second degree T23.221 ☑
    - third degree T23.321 ☑
  - second degree T23.229 ☑
  - third degree T23.329 ☑

Burn — *continued*
- flank — *see* Burn, abdominal wall
- foot T25.029 ☑
  - first degree T25.129 ☑
  - left T25.022 ☑
    - first degree T25.122 ☑
    - second degree T25.222 ☑
    - third degree T25.322 ☑
  - multiple with ankle — *see* Burn, lower, limb, multiple, ankle and foot
  - right T25.021 ☑
    - first degree T25.121 ☑
    - second degree T25.221 ☑
    - third degree T25.321 ☑
  - second degree T25.229 ☑
  - third degree T25.329 ☑
- forearm T22.019 ☑
  - first degree T22.119 ☑
  - left T22.012 ☑
    - first degree T22.112 ☑
    - second degree T22.212 ☑
    - third degree T22.312 ☑
  - right T22.011 ☑
    - first degree T22.111 ☑
    - second degree T22.211 ☑
    - third degree T22.311 ☑
  - second degree T22.219 ☑
  - third degree T22.319 ☑
- forehead T20.06 ☑
  - first degree T20.16 ☑
  - second degree T20.26 ☑
  - third degree T20.36 ☑
- fourth degree - code as Burn, third degree, by site
- friction — *see* Burn, by site
- from swallowing caustic or corrosive substance NEC — *see* Corrosion, by site
- full thickness skin loss - code as Burn, third degree, by site
- gastrointestinal tract NEC T28.2 ☑
  - from swallowing caustic or corrosive substance T28.7 ☑
- genital organs
  - external
    - female T21.07 ☑
      - first degree T21.17 ☑
      - second degree T21.27 ☑
      - third degree T21.37 ☑
    - male T21.06 ☑
      - first degree T21.16 ☑
      - second degree T21.26 ☑
      - third degree T21.36 ☑
  - internal T28.3 ☑
    - from caustic or corrosive substance T28.8 ☑
- groin — *see* Burn, abdominal wall
- hand(s) T23.009 ☑
  - back — *see* Burn, dorsum of hand
  - finger — *see* Burn, finger
  - first degree T23.109 ☑
  - left T23.002 ☑
    - first degree T23.102 ☑
    - second degree T23.202 ☑
    - third degree T23.302 ☑
  - multiple sites with wrist T23.099 ☑
    - first degree T23.199 ☑
    - left T23.092 ☑
      - first degree T23.192 ☑
      - second degree T23.292 ☑
      - third degree T23.392 ☑
    - right T23.091 ☑
      - first degree T23.191 ☑
      - second degree T23.291 ☑
      - third degree T23.391 ☑
    - second degree T23.299 ☑
    - third degree T23.399 ☑
  - palm — *see* Burn, palm
  - right T23.001 ☑
    - first degree T23.101 ☑
    - second degree T23.201 ☑
    - third degree T23.301 ☑
  - second degree T23.209 ☑
  - third degree T23.309 ☑
  - thumb — *see* Burn, thumb
- head (and face) (and neck) T20.00 ☑
  - cheek — *see* Burn, cheek
  - chin — *see* Burn, chin
  - ear — *see* Burn, ear
  - eye(s) only — *see* Burn, eye
  - first degree T20.10 ☑
  - forehead — *see* Burn, forehead
  - lip — *see* Burn, lip
  - multiple sites T20.09 ☑
    - first degree T20.19 ☑

Burn — *continued*
- head — *continued*
  - second degree T20.29 ☑
  - third degree T20.39 ☑
  - neck — *see* Burn, neck
  - nose — *see* Burn, nose
  - scalp — *see* Burn, scalp
  - second degree T20.20 ☑
  - third degree T20.30 ☑
- hip(s) — *see* Burn, thigh
- inhalation — *see* Burn, respiratory tract
  - caustic or corrosive substance (fumes) — *see* Corrosion, respiratory tract
- internal organ(s) T28.40 ☑
  - alimentary tract T28.2 ☑
    - esophagus T28.1 ☑
  - eardrum T28.41 ☑
  - esophagus T28.1 ☑
  - from caustic or corrosive substance (swallowing) NEC — *see* Corrosion, by site
  - genitourinary T28.3 ☑
  - mouth T28.0 ☑
  - pharynx T28.0 ☑
  - respiratory tract — *see* Burn, respiratory tract
  - specified organ NEC T28.49 ☑
- interscapular region — *see* Burn, back, upper
- intestine (large) (small) T28.2 ☑
- knee T24.029 ☑
  - first degree T24.129 ☑
  - left T24.022 ☑
    - first degree T24.122 ☑
    - second degree T24.222 ☑
    - third degree T24.322 ☑
  - right T24.021 ☑
    - first degree T24.121 ☑
    - second degree T24.221 ☑
    - third degree T24.321 ☑
  - second degree T24.229 ☑
  - third degree T24.329 ☑
- labium (majus) (minus) — *see* Burn, genital organs, external, female
- lacrimal apparatus, duct, gland or sac — *see* Burn, eye, specified site NEC
- larynx T27.0 ☑
  - with lung T27.1 ☑
- leg(s) (lower) (upper) — *see* Burn, lower, limb
- lightning — *see* Burn, by site
- limb(s)
  - lower (except ankle or foot alone) — *see* Burn, lower, limb
  - upper — *see* Burn, upper limb
- lip(s) T20.02 ☑
  - first degree T20.12 ☑
  - second degree T20.22 ☑
  - third degree T20.32 ☑
- lower
  - back — *see* Burn, back
  - limb T24.009 ☑
    - ankle — *see* Burn, ankle
    - calf — *see* Burn, calf
    - first degree T24.109 ☑
    - foot — *see* Burn, foot
    - hip — *see* Burn, thigh
    - knee — *see* Burn, knee
    - left T24.002 ☑
      - first degree T24.102 ☑
      - second degree T24.202 ☑
      - third degree T24.302 ☑
    - multiple sites, except ankle and foot T24.099 ☑
      - ankle and foot T25.099 ☑
        - first degree T25.199 ☑
        - left T25.092 ☑
          - first degree T25.192 ☑
          - second degree T25.292 ☑
          - third degree T25.392 ☑
        - right T25.091 ☑
          - first degree T25.191 ☑
          - second degree T25.291 ☑
          - third degree T25.391 ☑
        - second degree T25.299 ☑
        - third degree T25.399 ☑
      - first degree T24.199 ☑
      - left T24.092 ☑
        - first degree T24.192 ☑
        - second degree T24.292 ☑
        - third degree T24.392 ☑
      - right T24.091 ☑
        - first degree T24.191 ☑
        - second degree T24.291 ☑
        - third degree T24.391 ☑
      - second degree T24.299 ☑
      - third degree T24.399 ☑

☑ **Additional character required**

Burn — *continued*
- lower — *continued*
  - right T24.001 ☑
    - first degree T24.101 ☑
      - second degree T24.201 ☑
      - third degree T24.301 ☑
    - second degree T24.209 ☑
    - thigh — *see* Burn, thigh
    - third degree T24.309 ☑
    - toe — *see* Burn, toe
- lung (with larynx and trachea) T27.1 ☑
- mouth T28.0 ☑
- neck T20.07 ☑
  - first degree T20.17 ☑
  - second degree T20.27 ☑
  - third degree T20.37 ☑
- nose (septum) T20.04 ☑
  - first degree T20.14 ☑
  - second degree T20.24 ☑
  - third degree T20.34 ☑
- ocular adnexa — *see* Burn, eye
- orbit region — *see* Burn, eyelid
- palm T23.059 ☑
  - first degree T23.159 ☑
  - left T23.052 ☑
    - first degree T23.152 ☑
    - second degree T23.252 ☑
    - third degree T23.352 ☑
  - right T23.051 ☑
    - first degree T23.151 ☑
    - second degree T23.251 ☑
    - third degree T23.351 ☑
  - second degree T23.259 ☑
  - third degree T23.359 ☑
- partial thickness - code as Burn, degree, by site
- pelvis — *see* Burn, trunk
- penis — *see* Burn, genital organs, external, male
- perineum
  - female — *see* Burn, genital organs, external, female
  - male — *see* Burn, genital organs, external, male
- periocular area — *see* Burn, eyelid
- pharynx T28.0 ☑
- rectum T28.2 ☑
- respiratory tract T27.3 ☑
  - larynx — *see* Burn, larynx
  - specified part NEC T27.2 ☑
  - trachea — *see* Burn, trachea
- sac, lacrimal — *see* Burn, eye, specified site NEC
- scalp T20.05 ☑
  - first degree T20.15 ☑
  - second degree T20.25 ☑
  - third degree T20.35 ☑
- scapular region T22.069 ☑
  - first degree T22.169 ☑
  - left T22.062 ☑
    - first degree T22.162 ☑
    - second degree T22.262 ☑
    - third degree T22.362 ☑
  - right T22.061 ☑
    - first degree T22.161 ☑
    - second degree T22.261 ☑
    - third degree T22.361 ☑
  - second degree T22.269 ☑
  - third degree T22.369 ☑
- sclera — *see* Burn, eye, specified site NEC
- scrotum — *see* Burn, genital organs, external, male
- shoulder T22.059 ☑
  - first degree T22.159 ☑
  - left T22.052 ☑
    - first degree T22.152 ☑
    - second degree T22.252 ☑
    - third degree T22.352 ☑
  - right T22.051 ☑
    - first degree T22.151 ☑
    - second degree T22.251 ☑
    - third degree T22.351 ☑
  - second degree T22.259 ☑
  - third degree T22.359 ☑
- stomach T28.2 ☑
- temple — *see* Burn, head
- testis — *see* Burn, genital organs, external, male
- thigh T24.019 ☑
  - first degree T24.119 ☑
  - left T24.012 ☑
    - first degree T24.112 ☑
    - second degree T24.212 ☑
    - third degree T24.312 ☑
  - right T24.011 ☑
    - first degree T24.111 ☑
    - second degree T24.211 ☑
    - third degree T24.311 ☑

Burn — *continued*
- thigh — *continued*
  - second degree T24.219 ☑
  - third degree T24.319 ☑
- thorax (external) — *see* Burn, trunk
- throat (meaning pharynx) T28.0 ☑
- thumb(s) T23.019 ☑
  - first degree T23.119 ☑
  - left T23.012 ☑
    - first degree T23.112 ☑
    - second degree T23.212 ☑
    - third degree T23.312 ☑
  - multiple sites with fingers T23.049 ☑
    - first degree T23.149 ☑
    - left T23.042 ☑
      - second degree T23.242 ☑
      - third degree T23.342 ☑
    - right T23.041 ☑
      - first degree T23.141 ☑
      - second degree T23.241 ☑
      - third degree T23.341 ☑
    - second degree T23.249 ☑
    - third degree T23.349 ☑
  - right T23.011 ☑
    - first degree T23.111 ☑
    - second degree T23.211 ☑
    - third degree T23.311 ☑
  - second degree T23.219 ☑
  - third degree T23.319 ☑
- toe T25.039 ☑
  - first degree T25.139 ☑
  - left T25.032 ☑
    - first degree T25.132 ☑
    - second degree T25.232 ☑
    - third degree T25.332 ☑
  - right T25.031 ☑
    - first degree T25.131 ☑
    - second degree T25.231 ☑
    - third degree T25.331 ☑
  - second degree T25.239 ☑
  - third degree T25.339 ☑
- tongue T28.0 ☑
- tonsil(s) T28.0 ☑
- trachea T27.0 ☑
  - with lung T27.1 ☑
- trunk T21.00 ☑
  - abdominal wall — *see* Burn, abdominal wall
  - anus — *see* Burn, buttock
  - axilla — *see* Burn, upper limb
  - back — *see* Burn, back
  - breast — *see* Burn, chest wall
  - buttock — *see* Burn, buttock
  - chest wall — *see* Burn, chest wall
  - first degree T21.10 ☑
  - flank — *see* Burn, abdominal wall
  - genital
    - female — *see* Burn, genital organs, external, female
    - male — *see* Burn, genital organs, external, male
  - groin — *see* Burn, abdominal wall
  - interscapular region — *see* Burn, back, upper
  - labia — *see* Burn, genital organs, external, female
  - lower back — *see* Burn, back
  - penis — *see* Burn, genital organs, external, male
  - perineum
    - female — *see* Burn, genital organs, external, female
    - male — *see* Burn, genital organs, external, male
  - scapula region — *see* Burn, scapular region
  - scrotum — *see* Burn, genital organs, external, male
  - second degree T21.20 ☑
  - specified site NEC T21.09 ☑
    - first degree T21.19 ☑
    - second degree T21.29 ☑
    - third degree T21.39 ☑
  - testes — *see* Burn, genital organs, external, male
  - third degree T21.30 ☑
  - upper back — *see* Burn, back, upper
  - vulva — *see* Burn, genital organs, external, female
- unspecified site with extent of body surface involved specified
  - less than 10 percent T31.0
  - 10-19 percent (0-9 percent third degree) T31.10
    - with 10-19 percent third degree T31.11
  - 20-29 percent (0-9 percent third degree) T31.20
    - with
      - 10-19 percent third degree T31.21
      - 20-29 percent third degree T31.22
  - 30-39 percent (0-9 percent third degree) T31.30
    - with

Burn — *continued*
- unspecified site — *continued*
  - 10-19 percent third degree T31.31
  - 20-29 percent third degree T31.32
  - 30-39 percent third degree T31.33
  - 40-49 percent (0-9 percent third degree) T31.40
    - with
      - 10-19 percent third degree T31.41
      - 20-29 percent third degree T31.42
      - 30-39 percent third degree T31.43
      - 40-49 percent third degree T31.44
  - 50-59 percent (0-9 percent third degree) T31.50
    - with
      - 10-19 percent third degree T31.51
      - 20-29 percent third degree T31.52
      - 30-39 percent third degree T31.53
      - 40-49 percent third degree T31.54
      - 50-59 percent third degree T31.55
  - 60-69 percent (0-9 percent third degree) T31.60
    - with
      - 10-19 percent third degree T31.61
      - 20-29 percent third degree T31.62
      - 30-39 percent third degree T31.63
      - 40-49 percent third degree T31.64
      - 50-59 percent third degree T31.65
      - 60-69 percent third degree T31.66
  - 70-79 percent (0-9 percent third degree) T31.70
    - with
      - 10-19 percent third degree T31.71
      - 20-29 percent third degree T31.72
      - 30-39 percent third degree T31.73
      - 40-49 percent third degree T31.74
      - 50-59 percent third degree T31.75
      - 60-69 percent third degree T31.76
      - 70-79 percent third degree T31.77
  - 80-89 percent (0-9 percent third degree) T31.80
    - with
      - 10-19 percent third degree T31.81
      - 20-29 percent third degree T31.82
      - 30-39 percent third degree T31.83
      - 40-49 percent third degree T31.84
      - 50-59 percent third degree T31.85
      - 60-69 percent third degree T31.86
      - 70-79 percent third degree T31.87
      - 80-89 percent third degree T31.88
  - 90 percent or more (0-9 percent third degree) T31.90
    - with
      - 10-19 percent third degree T31.91
      - 20-29 percent third degree T31.92
      - 30-39 percent third degree T31.93
      - 40-49 percent third degree T31.94
      - 50-59 percent third degree T31.95
      - 60-69 percent third degree T31.96
      - 70-79 percent third degree T31.97
      - 80-89 percent third degree T31.98
      - 90-99 percent third degree T31.99
- upper limb T22.00 ☑
  - above elbow — *see* Burn, above elbow
  - axilla — *see* Burn, axilla
  - elbow — *see* Burn, elbow
  - first degree T22.10 ☑
  - forearm — *see* Burn, forearm
  - hand — *see* Burn, hand
  - interscapular region — *see* Burn, back, upper
  - multiple sites T22.099 ☑
    - first degree T22.199 ☑
    - left T22.092 ☑
      - first degree T22.192 ☑
      - second degree T22.292 ☑
      - third degree T22.392 ☑
    - right T22.091 ☑
      - first degree T22.191 ☑
      - second degree T22.291 ☑
      - third degree T22.391 ☑
    - second degree T22.299 ☑
    - third degree T22.399 ☑
  - scapular region — *see* Burn, scapular region
  - second degree T22.20 ☑
  - shoulder — *see* Burn, shoulder
  - third degree T22.30 ☑
  - wrist — *see* Burn, wrist
- uterus T28.3 ☑
- vagina T28.3 ☑
- vulva — *see* Burn, genital organs, external, female
- wrist T23.079 ☑
  - first degree T23.179 ☑
  - left T23.072 ☑
    - first degree T23.172 ☑
    - second degree T23.272 ☑
    - third degree T23.372 ☑
  - multiple sites with hand T23.099 ☑

Burn - Calcification

Burn — *continued*
 wrist — *continued*
  first degree T23.199 ☑
  left T23.092 ☑
   first degree T23.192 ☑
   second degree T23.292 ☑
   third degree T23.392 ☑
  right T23.091 ☑
   first degree T23.191 ☑
   second degree T23.291 ☑
   third degree T23.391 ☑
  second degree T23.299 ☑
  third degree T23.399 ☑
  right T23.071 ☑
   first degree T23.171 ☑
   second degree T23.271 ☑
   third degree T23.371 ☑
  second degree T23.279 ☑
  third degree T23.379 ☑
Burnett's syndrome E83.52
Burning
 feet syndrome E53.9
 sensation R20.8
 tongue K14.6
Burn-out (state) Z73.0
Burns' disease or osteochondrosis — *see*
 Osteochondrosis, juvenile, ulna
Bursa — *see* condition
Bursitis M71.9
 Achilles — *see* Tendinitis, Achilles
 adhesive — *see* Bursitis, specified NEC
 ankle — *see* Enthesopathy, lower limb, ankle,
  specified type NEC
 calcaneal — *see* Enthesopathy, foot, specified type
  NEC
 collateral ligament, tibial — *see* Bursitis, tibial
  collateral
 due to use, overuse, pressure (*see also* Disorder, soft
  tissue, due to use, specified type NEC)
  specified NEC — *see* Disorder, soft tissue, due to
   use, specified NEC
 Duplay's M75.0 ☑
 elbow NEC M70.3 ☑
  olecranon M70.2 ☑
 finger — *see* Disorder, soft tissue, due to use,
  specified type NEC, hand
 foot — *see* Enthesopathy, foot, specified type NEC
 gonococcal A54.49
 gouty — *see* Gout
 hand M70.1 ☑
 hip NEC M70.7 ☑
  trochanteric M70.6 ☑
 infective NEC M71.10
  abscess — *see* Abscess, bursa
  ankle M71.17 ☑
  elbow M71.12 ☑
  foot M71.17 ☑
  hand M71.14 ☑
  hip M71.15 ☑
  knee M71.16 ☑
  multiple sites M71.19
  shoulder M71.11 ☑
  specified site NEC M71.18
  wrist M71.13 ☑
 ischial — *see* Bursitis, hip
 knee NEC M70.5 ☑
  prepatellar M70.4 ☑
 occupational NEC (*see also* Disorder, soft tissue, due
  to, use)
 olecranon — *see* Bursitis, elbow, olecranon
 pharyngeal J39.1
 popliteal — *see* Bursitis, knee
 prepatellar M70.4 ☑
 radiohumeral M77.8
 rheumatoid M06.20
  ankle M06.27 ☑
  elbow M06.22 ☑
  foot joint M06.27 ☑
  hand joint M06.24 ☑
  hip M06.25 ☑
  knee M06.26 ☑
  multiple site M06.29
  shoulder M06.21 ☑
  vertebra M06.28
  wrist M06.23 ☑
 scapulohumeral — *see* Bursitis, shoulder
 semimembranous muscle (knee) — *see* Bursitis,
  knee
 shoulder M75.5 ☑
  adhesive — *see* Capsulitis, adhesive
 specified NEC M71.50
  ankle M71.57 ☑

Bursitis — *continued*
 specified NEC — *continued*
  due to use, overuse or pressure — *see* Disorder,
   soft tissue, due to, use
  elbow M71.52 ☑
  foot M71.57 ☑
  hand M71.54 ☑
  hip M71.55 ☑
  knee M71.56 ☑
  shoulder — *see* Bursitis, shoulder
  specified site NEC M71.58
  tibial collateral M76.4 ☑
  wrist M71.53 ☑
 subacromial — *see* Bursitis, shoulder
 subcoracoid — *see* Bursitis, shoulder
 subdeltoid — *see* Bursitis, shoulder
 syphilitic A52.78
 Thornwaldt, Tornwaldt J39.2
 tibial collateral M76.4 ☑
 toe — *see* Enthesopathy, foot, specified type NEC
 trochanteric (area) — *see* Bursitis, hip, trochanteric
 wrist — *see* Bursitis, hand
Bursopathy M71.9
 specified type NEC M71.80
  ankle M71.87 ☑
  elbow M71.82 ☑
  foot M71.87 ☑
  hand M71.84 ☑
  hip M71.85 ☑
  knee M71.86 ☑
  multiple sites M71.89
  shoulder M71.81 ☑
  specified site NEC M71.88
  wrist M71.83 ☑
Burst stitches or sutures (complication of surgery)
 T81.31 ☑
  external operation wound T81.31 ☑
  internal operation wound T81.32 ☑
Buruli ulcer A31.1
Bury's disease L95.1
Buschke's
 disease B45.3
 scleredema — *see* Sclerosis, systemic
Busse-Buschke disease B45.3
Buttock — *see* condition
Button
 Biskra B55.1
 Delhi B55.1
 oriental B55.1
Buttonhole deformity (finger) — *see* Deformity, finger,
 boutonniere
Bwamba fever A92.8
Byssinosis J66.0
Bywaters' syndrome T79.5 ☑

C

Cachexia R64
 cancerous R64
 cardiac — *see* Disease, heart
 dehydration E86.0
 due to malnutrition R64
 exophthalmic — *see* Hyperthyroidism
 heart — *see* Disease, heart
 hypophyseal E23.0
 hypopituitary E23.0
 lead — *see* Poisoning, lead
 malignant R64
 marsh — *see* Malaria
 nervous F48.8
 old age R54
 paludal — *see* Malaria
 pituitary E23.0
 renal N28.9
 saturnine — *see* Poisoning, lead
 senile R54
 Simmonds' E23.0
 splenica D73.0
 strumipriva E03.4
 tuberculous NEC — *see* Tuberculosis
CADASIL (cerebral autosomal dominant arteriopathy
 with subcortical infarcts and leukoencephalopathy)
 I67.850
Café, au lait spots L81.3
Caffeine-induced
 anxiety disorder F15.980
 sleep disorder F15.982
Caffey's syndrome Q78.8
Caisson disease T70.3 ☑
Cake kidney Q63.1

Caked breast (puerperal, postpartum) O92.79
Calabar swelling B74.3
Calcaneal spur — *see* Spur, bone, calcaneal
Calcaneo-apophysitis M92.8
Calcareous — *see* condition
Calcicosis J62.8
Calciferol (vitamin D) deficiency E55.9
 with rickets E55.0
Calcification
 adrenal (capsule) (gland) E27.49
  tuberculous E35 *[B90.8]*
 aorta I70.0
 artery (annular) — *see* Arteriosclerosis
 auricle (ear) — *see* Disorder, pinna, specified type
  NEC
 basal ganglia G23.8
 bladder N32.89
  due to Schistosoma hematobium B65.0
 brain (cortex) — *see* Calcification, cerebral
 bronchus J98.09
 bursa M71.40
  ankle M71.47 ☑
  elbow M71.42 ☑
  foot M71.47 ☑
  hand M71.44 ☑
  hip M71.45 ☑
  knee M71.46 ☑
  multiple sites M71.49
  shoulder M75.3 ☑
  specified site NEC M71.48
  wrist M71.43 ☑
 cardiac — *see* Degeneration, myocardial
 cerebral (cortex) G93.89
  artery I67.2
 cervix (uteri) N88.8
 choroid plexus G93.89
 conjunctiva — *see* Concretion, conjunctiva
 corpora cavernosa (penis) N48.89
 cortex (brain) — *see* Calcification, cerebral
 dental pulp (nodular) K04.2
 dentinal papilla K00.4
 fallopian tube N83.8
 falx cerebri G96.19
 gallbladder K82.8
 general E83.59
 heart (*see also* Degeneration, myocardial)
  valve — *see* Endocarditis
 idiopathic infantile arterial (IIAC) Q28.8
 intervertebral cartilage or disc (postinfective) — *see*
  Disorder, disc, specified NEC
 intracranial — *see* Calcification, cerebral
 joint — *see* Disorder, joint, specified type NEC
 kidney N28.89
  tuberculous N29 *[B90.1]*
 larynx (senile) J38.7
 lens — *see* Cataract, specified NEC
 lung (active) (postinfectional) J98.4
  tuberculous B90.9
 lymph gland or node (postinfectional) I89.8
  tuberculous (*see also* Tuberculosis, lymph gland)
   B90.8
 mammographic R92.1
 massive (paraplegic) — *see* Myositis, ossificans, in,
  quadriplegia
 medial — *see* Arteriosclerosis, extremities
 meninges (cerebral) (spinal) G96.19
 metastatic E83.59
 Mönckeberg's — *see* Arteriosclerosis, extremities
 muscle M61.9
  due to burns — *see* Myositis, ossificans, in, burns
  paralytic — *see* Myositis, ossificans, in,
   quadriplegia
  specified type NEC M61.40
   ankle M61.47 ☑
   foot M61.47 ☑
   forearm M61.43 ☑
   hand M61.44 ☑
   lower leg M61.46 ☑
   multiple sites M61.49
   pelvic region M61.45 ☑
   shoulder region M61.41 ☑
   specified site NEC M61.48
   thigh M61.45 ☑
   upper arm M61.42 ☑
 myocardium, myocardial — *see* Degeneration,
  myocardial
 ovary N83.8
 pancreas K86.89
 penis N48.89
 periarticular — *see* Disorder, joint, specified type
  NEC
 pericardium (*see also* Pericarditis) I31.1

☑ **Additional character required**

Calcification — *continued*
pineal gland E34.8
pleura J94.8
postinfectional J94.8
tuberculous NEC B90.9
pulpal (dental) (nodular) K04.2
sclera H15.89
spleen D73.89
subcutaneous L94.2
suprarenal (capsule) (gland) E27.49
tendon (sheath) (*see also* Tenosynovitis, specified
type NEC)
with bursitis, synovitis or tenosynovitis — *see*
Tendinitis, calcific
trachea J39.8
ureter N28.89
uterus N85.8
vitreous — *see* Deposit, crystalline
Calcified — *see* Calcification
Calcinosis (interstitial) (tumoral) (universalis) E83.59
with Raynaud's phenomenon, esophageal
dysfunction, sclerodactyly, telangiectasia
(CREST syndrome) M34.1
circumscripta (skin) L94.2
cutis L94.2
Calciphylaxis (*see also* Calcification, by site) E83.59
Calcium
deposits — *see* Calcification, by site
metabolism disorder E83.50
salts or soaps in vitreous — *see* Deposit, crystalline
Calciuria R82.994
Calculi — *see* Calculus
Calculosis, intrahepatic — *see* Calculus, bile duct
Calculus, calculi, calculous
ampulla of Vater — *see* Calculus, bile duct
anuria (impacted) (recurrent) (*see also* Calculus,
urinary) N20.9
appendix K38.1
bile duct (common) (hepatic) K80.50
with
calculus of gallbladder — *see* Calculus,
gallbladder and bile duct
cholangitis K80.30
with
cholecystitis — *see* Calculus, bile duct, with
cholecystitis
obstruction K80.31
acute K80.32
with
chronic cholangitis K80.36
with obstruction K80.37
obstruction K80.33
chronic K80.34
with
acute cholangitis K80.36
with obstruction K80.37
obstruction K80.35
cholecystitis (with cholangitis) K80.40
with obstruction K80.41
acute K80.42
with
chronic cholecystitis K80.46
with obstruction K80.47
obstruction K80.43
chronic K80.44
with
acute cholecystitis K80.46
with obstruction K80.47
obstruction K80.45
obstruction K80.51
biliary (*see also* Calculus, gallbladder)
specified NEC K80.80
with obstruction K80.81
bilirubin, multiple — *see* Calculus, gallbladder
bladder (encysted) (impacted) (urinary)
(diverticulum) N21.0
bronchus J98.09
calyx (kidney) (renal) — *see* Calculus, kidney
cholesterol (pure) (solitary) — *see* Calculus,
gallbladder
common duct (bile) — *see* Calculus, bile duct
conjunctiva — *see* Concretion, conjunctiva
cystic N21.0
duct — *see* Calculus, gallbladder
dental (subgingival) (supragingival) K03.6
diverticulum
bladder N21.0
kidney N20.0
epididymis N50.89
gallbladder K80.20
with

Calculus — *continued*
gallbladder — *continued*
bile duct calculus — *see* Calculus, gallbladder
and bile duct
cholecystitis K80.10
with obstruction K80.11
acute K80.00
with
chronic cholecystitis K80.12
with obstruction K80.13
obstruction K80.01
chronic K80.10
with
acute cholecystitis K80.12
with obstruction K80.13
obstruction K80.11
specified NEC K80.18
with obstruction K80.19
obstruction K80.21
gallbladder and bile duct K80.70
with
cholecystitis K80.60
with obstruction K80.61
acute K80.62
with
chronic cholecystitis K80.66
with obstruction K80.67
obstruction K80.63
chronic K80.64
with
acute cholecystitis K80.66
with obstruction K80.67
obstruction K80.65
obstruction K80.71
hepatic (duct) — *see* Calculus, bile duct
hepatobiliary K80.80
with obstruction K80.81
ileal conduit N21.8
intestinal (impaction) (obstruction) K56.49
kidney (impacted) (multiple) (pelvis) (recurrent)
(staghorn) N20.0
with calculus, ureter N20.2
congenital Q63.8
lacrimal passages — *see* Dacryolith
liver (impacted) — *see* Calculus, bile duct
lung J98.4
mammographic R92.1
nephritic (impacted) (recurrent) — *see* Calculus,
kidney
nose J34.89
pancreas (duct) K86.89
parotid duct or gland K11.5
pelvis, encysted — *see* Calculus, kidney
prostate N42.0
pulmonary J98.4
pyelitis (impacted) (recurrent) N20.0
with hydronephrosis N13.6
pyelonephritis (impacted) (recurrent) — *see*
category N20 ☑
with hydronephrosis N13.6
renal (impacted) (recurrent) — *see* Calculus,
kidney
salivary (duct) (gland) K11.5
seminal vesicle N50.89
staghorn — *see* Calculus, kidney
Stensen's duct K11.5
stomach K31.89
sublingual duct or gland K11.5
congenital Q38.4
submandibular duct, gland or region K11.5
submaxillary duct, gland or region K11.5
suburethral N21.8
tonsil J35.8
tooth, teeth (subgingival) (supragingival) K03.6
tunica vaginalis N50.89
ureter (impacted) (recurrent) N20.1
with calculus, kidney N20.2
with hydronephrosis N13.2
with infection N13.6
urethra (impacted) N21.1
urinary (duct) (impacted) (passage) (tract) N20.9
with hydronephrosis N13.2
with infection N13.6
in (due to)
lower N21.9
specified NEC N21.8
vagina N89.8
vesical (impacted) N21.0
Wharton's duct K11.5
xanthine E79.8 *[N22]*
Caliectasis N28.89
Caliectasis N28.89

California
disease B38.9
encephalitis A83.5
Caligo cornea — *see* Opacity, cornea, central
Callositas, callosity (infected) L84
Callus (infected) L84
bone — *see* Osteophyte
excessive, following fracture - code as Sequelae
of fracture
CALME (childhood asymmetric labium majus
enlargement) N90.61
Calorie deficiency or malnutrition (*see also*
Malnutrition) E46
Calvé-Perthes disease — *see* Legg-Calvé-Perthes
disease
Calvé's disease — *see* Osteochondrosis, juvenile, spine
Calvities — *see* Alopecia, androgenic
Cameroon fever — *see* Malaria
Camptocormia (hysterical) F44.4
Camurati-Engelmann syndrome Q78.3
Canal (*see also* condition)
atrioventricular common Q21.2
Canaliculitis (lacrimal) (acute) (subacute) H04.33 ☑
Actinomyces A42.89
chronic H04.42 ☑
Canavan's disease E75.29
Canceled procedure (surgical) Z53.9
because of
contraindication Z53.09
smoking Z53.01
left against medical advice (AMA) Z53.29
patient's decision Z53.20
for reasons of belief or group pressure Z53.1
specified reason NEC Z53.29
specified reason NEC Z53.8
Cancer (*see also* Neoplasm, by site, malignant)
bile duct type liver C22.1
blood — *see* Leukemia
breast (*see also* Neoplasm, breast, malignant)
C50.91 ☑
hepatocellular C22.0
lung (*see also* Neoplasm, lung, malignant) C34.90
ovarian (*see also* Neoplasm ovary, malignant)
C56.9
unspecified site (primary) C80.1
Cancer (o)phobia F45.29
Cancerous — *see* Neoplasm, malignant, by site
Cancrum oris A69.0
Candidiasis, candidal B37.9
balanitis B37.42
bronchitis B37.1
cheilitis B37.83
congenital P37.5
cystitis B37.41
disseminated B37.7
endocarditis B37.6
enteritis B37.82
esophagitis B37.81
intertrigo B37.2
lung B37.1
meningitis B37.5
mouth B37.0
nails B37.2
neonatal P37.5
onychia B37.2
oral B37.0
osteomyelitis B37.89
otitis externa B37.84
paronychia B37.2
perionyxis B37.2
pneumonia B37.1
proctitis B37.82
pulmonary B37.1
pyelonephritis B37.49
sepsis B37.7
skin B37.2
specified site NEC B37.89
stomatitis B37.0
systemic B37.7
urethritis B37.41
urogenital site NEC B37.49
vagina B37.3
vulva B37.3
vulvovaginitis B37.3
Candidid L30.2
Candidosis — *see* Candidiasis
Candiru infection or infestation B88.8
Canities (premature) L67.1
congenital Q84.2
Canker (mouth) (sore) K12.0
rash A38.9
Cannabinosis J66.2

Cannabis - Carcinoma

Cannabis induced
- anxiety disorder F12.980
- psychotic disorder F12.959
- sleep disorder F12.988

Canton fever A75.9
Cantrell's syndrome Q87.89
Capillariasis (intestinal) B81.1
- hepatic B83.8

Capillary — *see* condition
Caplan's syndrome — *see* Rheumatoid, lung
Capsule — *see* condition
Capsulitis (joint) (*see also* Enthesopathy)
- adhesive (shoulder) M75.0 ☑
- hepatic K65.8
- labyrinthine — *see* Otosclerosis, specified NEC
- thyroid E06.9

Caput
- crepitus Q75.8
- medusae I86.8
- succedaneum P12.81

Car sickness T75.3 ☑
Carapata (disease) A68.0
Carate — *see* Pinta
Carbon lung J60
Carbuncle L02.93
- abdominal wall L02.231
- anus K61.0
- auditory canal, external — *see* Abscess, ear, external
- auricle ear — *see* Abscess, ear, external
- axilla L02.43 ☑
- back (any part) L02.232
- breast N61.1
- buttock L02.33
- cheek (external) L02.03
- chest wall L02.233
- chin L02.03
- corpus cavernosum N48.21
- ear (any part) (external) (middle) — *see* Abscess, ear, external
- external auditory canal — *see* Abscess, ear, external
- eyelid — *see* Abscess, eyelid
- face NEC L02.03
- femoral (region) — *see* Carbuncle, lower limb
- finger — *see* Carbuncle, hand
- flank L02.231
- foot L02.63 ☑
- forehead L02.03
- genital — *see* Abscess, genital
- gluteal (region) L02.33
- groin L02.234
- hand L02.53 ☑
- head NEC L02.831
- heel — *see* Carbuncle, foot
- hip — *see* Carbuncle, lower limb
- kidney — *see* Abscess, kidney
- knee — *see* Carbuncle, lower limb
- labium (majus) (minus) N76.4
- lacrimal
  - gland — *see* Dacryoadenitis
  - passages (duct) (sac) — *see* Inflammation, lacrimal, passages, acute
- leg — *see* Carbuncle, lower limb
- lower limb L02.43 ☑
- malignant A22.0
- navel L02.236
- neck L02.13
- nose (external) (septum) J34.0
- orbit, orbital — *see* Abscess, orbit
- palmar (space) — *see* Carbuncle, hand
- partes posteriores L02.33
- pectoral region L02.233
- penis N48.21
- perineum L02.235
- pinna — *see* Abscess, ear, external
- popliteal — *see* Carbuncle, lower limb
- scalp L02.831
- seminal vesicle N49.0
- shoulder — *see* Carbuncle, upper limb
- specified site NEC L02.838
- temple (region) L02.03
- thumb — *see* Carbuncle, hand
- toe — *see* Carbuncle, foot
- trunk L02.239
  - abdominal wall L02.231
  - back L02.232
  - chest wall L02.233
  - groin L02.234
  - perineum L02.235
  - umbilicus L02.236
- umbilicus L02.236
- upper limb L02.43 ☑

Carbuncle — *continued*
- urethra N34.0
- vulva N76.4

Carbunculus — *see* Carbuncle
Carcinoid (tumor) — *see* Tumor, carcinoid
Carcinoidosis E34.0
Carcinoma (malignant) (*see also* Neoplasm, by site, malignant)
- acidophil
  - specified site — *see* Neoplasm, malignant, by site
  - unspecified site C75.1
- acidophil-basophil, mixed
  - specified site — *see* Neoplasm, malignant, by site
  - unspecified site C75.1
- adnexal (skin) — *see* Neoplasm, skin, malignant
- adrenal cortical C74.0 ☑
- alveolar — *see* Neoplasm, lung, malignant
  - cell — *see* Neoplasm, lung, malignant
- ameloblastic C41.1
  - upper jaw (bone) C41.0
- apocrine
  - breast — *see* Neoplasm, breast, malignant
  - specified site NEC — *see* Neoplasm, skin, malignant
  - unspecified site C44.99
- basal cell (pigmented) (*see also* Neoplasm, skin, malignant) C44.91
  - fibro-epithelial — *see* Neoplasm, skin, malignant
  - morphea — *see* Neoplasm, skin, malignant
  - multicentric — *see* Neoplasm, skin, malignant
- basaloid
- basal-squamous cell, mixed — *see* Neoplasm, skin, malignant
- basophil
  - specified site — *see* Neoplasm, malignant, by site
  - unspecified site C75.1
- basophil-acidophil, mixed
  - specified site — *see* Neoplasm, malignant, by site
  - unspecified site C75.1
- basosquamous — *see* Neoplasm, skin, malignant
- bile duct
  - with hepatocellular, mixed C22.0
  - liver C22.1
  - specified site NEC — *see* Neoplasm, malignant, by site
  - unspecified site C22.1
- branchial or branchiogenic C10.4
- bronchial or bronchogenic — *see* Neoplasm, lung, malignant
- bronchiolar — *see* Neoplasm, lung, malignant
- bronchioloalveolar — *see* Neoplasm, lung, malignant
- C cell
  - specified site — *see* Neoplasm, malignant, by site
  - unspecified site C73
- ceruminous C44.29 ☑
- cervix uteri
  - in situ D06.9
    - endocervix D06.0
    - exocervix D06.1
    - specified site NEC D06.7
- chorionic
  - specified site — *see* Neoplasm, malignant, by site
  - unspecified site
    - female C58
    - male C62.90
- chromophobe
  - specified site — *see* Neoplasm, malignant, by site
  - unspecified site C75.1
- cloacogenic
  - specified site — *see* Neoplasm, malignant, by site
  - unspecified site C21.2
- diffuse type
  - specified site — *see* Neoplasm, malignant, by site
  - unspecified site C16.9
- duct (cell)
  - with Paget's disease — *see* Neoplasm, breast, malignant
  - infiltrating
    - with lobular carcinoma (in situ)
      - specified site — *see* Neoplasm, malignant, by site
      - unspecified site (female) C50.91 ☑
        - male C50.92 ☑
    - specified site — *see* Neoplasm, malignant, by site
    - unspecified site (female) C50.91 ☑
      - male C50.92 ☑
- ductal
  - with lobular
    - specified site — *see* Neoplasm, malignant, by site

Carcinoma — *continued*
- ductal — *continued*
  - unspecified site (female) C50.91 ☑
    - male C50.92 ☑
- ductular, infiltrating
  - specified site — *see* Neoplasm, malignant, by site
  - unspecified site (female) C50.91 ☑
    - male C50.92 ☑
- embryonal
  - liver C22.7
- endometrioid
  - specified site — *see* Neoplasm, malignant, by site
  - unspecified site
    - female C56.9
    - male C61
- eosinophil
  - specified site — *see* Neoplasm, malignant, by site
  - unspecified site C75.1
- epidermoid (*see also* Neoplasm, skin malignant)
  - in situ, Bowen's type — *see* Neoplasm, skin, in situ
- fibroepithelial, basal cell — *see* Neoplasm, skin, malignant
- follicular
  - with papillary (mixed) C73
  - moderately differentiated C73
  - pure follicle C73
  - specified site — *see* Neoplasm, malignant, by site
  - trabecular C73
  - unspecified site C73
  - well differentiated C73
- generalized, with unspecified primary site C80.0
- glycogen-rich — *see* Neoplasm, breast, malignant
- granulosa cell C56 ☑
- hepatic cell C22.0
- hepatocellular C22.0
  - with bile duct, mixed C22.0
  - fibrolamellar C22.0
- hepatocholangiolitic C22.0
- Hurthle cell C73
- in
  - adenomatous
    - polyposis coli C18.9
  - pleomorphic adenoma — *see* Neoplasm, salivary glands, malignant
  - situ — *see* Carcinoma-in-situ
- infiltrating
  - duct
    - with lobular
      - specified site — *see* Neoplasm, malignant, by site
      - unspecified site (female) C50.91 ☑
        - male C50.92 ☑
    - with Paget's disease — *see* Neoplasm, breast, malignant
    - specified site — *see* Neoplasm, malignant
    - unspecified site (female) C50.91 ☑
      - male C50.92 ☑
  - ductular
    - specified site — *see* Neoplasm, malignant
    - unspecified site (female) C50.91 ☑
      - male C50.92 ☑
  - lobular
    - specified site — *see* Neoplasm, malignant
    - unspecified site (female) C50.91 ☑
      - male C50.92 ☑
- inflammatory
  - specified site — *see* Neoplasm, malignant
  - unspecified site (female) C50.91 ☑
    - male C50.92 ☑
- intestinal type
  - specified site — *see* Neoplasm, malignant, by site
  - unspecified site C16.9
- intracystic
  - noninfiltrating — *see* Neoplasm, in situ, by site
- intraductal (noninfiltrating)
  - with Paget's disease — *see* Neoplasm, breast, malignant
  - breast D05.1 ☑
  - papillary
    - with invasion
      - specified site — *see* Neoplasm, malignant, by site
      - unspecified site (female) C50.91 ☑
        - male C50.92 ☑
    - breast D05.1 ☑
    - specified site NEC — *see* Neoplasm, in situ, by site
    - unspecified site (female) D05.1 ☑
  - specified site NEC — *see* Neoplasm, in situ, by site
  - unspecified site (female) D05.1 ☑

Carcinoma — *continued*
  intraepidermal — *see* Neoplasm, in situ
    squamous cell, Bowen's type — *see* Neoplasm, skin, in situ
  intraepithelial — *see* Neoplasm, in situ, by site
    squamous cell — *see* Neoplasm, in situ, by site
  intraosseous C41.1
    upper jaw (bone) C41.0
  islet cell
    with exocrine, mixed
      specified site — *see* Neoplasm, malignant, by site
      unspecified site C25.9
    pancreas C25.4
    specified site NEC — *see* Neoplasm, malignant, by site
    unspecified site C25.4
  juvenile, breast — *see* Neoplasm, breast, malignant
  large cell
    small cell
      specified site — *see* Neoplasm, malignant, by site
      unspecified site C34.90
  Leydig cell (testis)
    specified site — *see* Neoplasm, malignant, by site
    unspecified site
      female C56.9
      male C62.90
  lipid-rich (female) C50.91 ☑
    male C50.92 ☑
  liver cell C22.0
  liver NEC C22.7
  lobular (infiltrating)
    with intraductal
      specified site — *see* Neoplasm, malignant, by site
      unspecified site (female) C50.91 ☑
        male C50.92 ☑
    noninfiltrating
      breast D05.0 ☑
      specified site NEC — *see* Neoplasm, in situ, by site
      unspecified site D05.0 ☑
    specified site — *see* Neoplasm, malignant, by site
    unspecified site (female) C50.91 ☑
      male C50.92 ☑
  medullary
    with
      amyloid stroma
        specified site — *see* Neoplasm, malignant, by site
        unspecified site C73
      lymphoid stroma
        specified site — *see* Neoplasm, malignant, by site
        unspecified site (female) C50.91 ☑
          male C50.92 ☑
  Merkel cell C4A.9
    anal margin C4A.51
    anal skin C4A.51
    canthus C4A.1 ☑
    ear and external auricular canal C4A.2 ☑
    external auricular canal C4A.2 ☑
    eyelid, including canthus C4A.1 ☑
    face C4A.30
      specified NEC C4A.39
    hip C4A.7 ☑
    lip C4A.0
    lower limb, including hip C4A.7 ☑
    neck C4A.4
    nodal presentation C7B.1
    nose C4A.31
    overlapping sites C4A.8
    perianal skin C4A.51
    scalp C4A.4
    secondary C7B.1
    shoulder C4A.6 ☑
    skin of breast C4A.52
    trunk NEC C4A.59
    upper limb, including shoulder C4A.6 ☑
    visceral metastatic C7B.1
  metastatic — *see* Neoplasm, secondary, by site
  metatypical — *see* Neoplasm, skin, malignant
  morphea, basal cell — *see* Neoplasm, skin, malignant
  mucoid
    cell
      specified site — *see* Neoplasm, malignant, by site
      unspecified site C75.1
  neuroendocrine (*see also* Tumor, neuroendocrine)
    high grade, any site C7A.1
    poorly differentiated, any site C7A.1

Carcinoma — *continued*
  nonencapsulated sclerosing C73
  noninfiltrating
    intracystic — *see* Neoplasm, in situ, by site
    intraductal
      breast D05.1 ☑
      papillary
        breast D05.1 ☑
        specified site NEC — *see* Neoplasm, in situ, by site
        unspecified site D05.1 ☑
      specified site — *see* Neoplasm, in situ, by site
      unspecified site D05.1 ☑
    lobular
      breast D05.0 ☑
      specified site NEC — *see* Neoplasm, in situ, by site
      unspecified site (female) D05.0 ☑
  oat cell
    specified site — *see* Neoplasm, malignant, by site
    unspecified site C34.90
  odontogenic C41.1
    upper jaw (bone) C41.0
  papillary
    with follicular (mixed) C73
    follicular variant C73
    intraductal (noninfiltrating)
      with invasion
        specified site — *see* Neoplasm, malignant, by site
        unspecified site (female) C50.91 ☑
          male C50.92 ☑
      breast D05.1 ☑
      specified site NEC — *see* Neoplasm, in situ, by site
      unspecified site D05.1 ☑
    serous
      specified site — *see* Neoplasm, malignant, by site
      surface
        specified site — *see* Neoplasm, malignant, by site
        unspecified site C56.9
      unspecified site C56.9
  papillocystic
    specified site — *see* Neoplasm, malignant, by site
    unspecified site C56.9
  parafollicular cell
    specified site — *see* Neoplasm, malignant, by site
    unspecified site C73
  pilomatrix — *see* Neoplasm, skin, malignant
  pseudomucinous
    specified site — *see* Neoplasm, malignant, by site
    unspecified site C56.9
  renal cell C64
  Schmincke — *see* Neoplasm, nasopharynx, malignant
  Schneiderian
    specified site — *see* Neoplasm, malignant, by site
    unspecified site C30.0
  sebaceous — *see* Neoplasm, skin, malignant
  secondary (*see also* Neoplasm, secondary, by site)
    Merkel cell C7B.1
  secretory, breast — *see* Neoplasm, breast, malignant
  serous
    papillary
      specified site — *see* Neoplasm, malignant, by site
      unspecified site C56.9
    surface, papillary
      specified site — *see* Neoplasm, malignant, by site
      unspecified site C56.9
  Sertoli cell
    specified site — *see* Neoplasm, malignant, by site
    unspecified site C62.90
      female C56.9
      male C62.90
  skin appendage — *see* Neoplasm, skin, malignant
  small cell
    fusiform cell
      specified site — *see* Neoplasm, malignant, by site
      unspecified site C34.90
    intermediate cell
      specified site — *see* Neoplasm, malignant, by site
      unspecified site C34.90
    large cell
      specified site — *see* Neoplasm, malignant, by site
      unspecified site C34.90

Carcinoma — *continued*
  solid
    with amyloid stroma
      specified site — *see* Neoplasm, malignant, by site
      unspecified site C73
    microinvasive
      specified site — *see* Neoplasm, malignant, by site
      unspecified site C53.9
  sweat gland — *see* Neoplasm, skin, malignant
  theca cell C56. ☑
  thymic C37
  unspecified site (primary) C80.1
  water-clear cell C75.0
Carcinoma-in-situ (*see also* Neoplasm, in situ, by site)
  breast NOS D05.9 ☑
    specified type NEC D05.8 ☑
  epidermoid (*see also* Neoplasm, in situ, by site)
    with questionable stromal invasion
      cervix D06.9
      specified site NEC — *see* Neoplasm, in situ, by site
      unspecified site D06.9
    Bowen's type — *see* Neoplasm, skin, in situ
  intraductal
    breast D05.1 ☑
    specified site NEC — *see* Neoplasm, in situ, by site
    unspecified site D05.1 ☑
  lobular
    with
      infiltrating duct
        breast (female) C50.91 ☑
          male C50.92 ☑
        specified site NEC — *see* Neoplasm, malignant
        unspecified site (female) C50.91 ☑
          male C50.92 ☑
      intraductal
        breast D05.8 ☑
        specified site NEC — *see* Neoplasm, in situ, by site
        unspecified site (female) D05.8 ☑
    breast D05.0 ☑
    specified site NEC — *see* Neoplasm, in situ, by site
    unspecified site D05.0 ☑
  squamous cell (*see also* Neoplasm, in situ, by site)
    with questionable stromal invasion
      cervix D06.9
      specified site NEC — *see* Neoplasm, in situ, by site
      unspecified site D06.9
Carcinomaphobia F45.29
Carcinomatosis C80.0
  peritonei C78.6
  unspecified site (primary) (secondary) C80.0
Carcinosarcoma — *see* Neoplasm, malignant, by site
  embryonal — *see* Neoplasm, malignant, by site
Cardia, cardial — *see* condition
Cardiac (*see also* condition)
  death, sudden — *see* Arrest, cardiac
  pacemaker
    in situ Z95.0
    management or adjustment Z45.018
  tamponade I31.4
Cardialgia — *see* Pain, precordial
Cardiectasis — *see* Hypertrophy, cardiac
Cardiochalasia K21.9
Cardiomalacia I51.5
Cardiomegalia glycogenica diffusa E74.02 *[I43]*
Cardiomegaly (*see also* Hypertrophy, cardiac)
  congenital Q24.8
  glycogen E74.02 *[I43]*
  idiopathic I51.7
Cardiomyoliposis I51.5
Cardiomyopathy (familial) (idiopathic) I42.9
  alcoholic I42.6
  amyloid E85.4 *[I43]*
    transthyretin-related (ATTR) familial E85.4 *[I43]*
  arteriosclerotic — *see* Disease, heart, ischemic, atherosclerotic
  beriberi E51.12
  cobalt-beer I42.6
  congenital I42.4
  congestive I42.0
  constrictive NOS I42.5
  dilated I42.0
  due to
    alcohol I42.6
    beriberi E51.12
    cardiac glycogenosis E74.02 *[I43]*
    drugs I42.7

Cardiomyopathy - Cataract

Cardiomyopathy — *continued*
  due to — *continued*
    external agents NEC I42.7
    Friedreich's ataxia G11.1
    myotonia atrophica G71.11 *[I43]*
    progressive muscular dystrophy G71.09 *[I43]*
  glycogen storage E74.02 *[I43]*
  hypertensive — *see* Hypertension, heart
  hypertrophic (nonobstructive) I42.2
    obstructive I42.1
      congenital Q24.8
  in
    Chagas' disease (chronic) B57.2
      acute B57.0
    sarcoidosis D86.85
  ischemic I25.5
  metabolic E88.9 *[I43]*
    thyrotoxic E05.90 *[I43]*
      with thyroid storm E05.91 *[I43]*
  newborn I42.8
    congenital I42.4
  non-ischemic (*see also* by cause) I42.8
  nutritional E63.9 *[I43]*
    beriberi E51.12
  obscure of Africa I42.8
  peripartum O90.3
  postpartum O90.3
  restrictive NEC I42.5
  rheumatic I09.0
  secondary I42.9
  specified NEC I42.8
  stress induced I51.81
  takotsubo I51.81
  thyrotoxic E05.90 *[I43]*
    with thyroid storm E05.91 *[I43]*
  toxic NEC I42.7
  transthyretin-related (ATTR) familial amyloid E85.4
  tuberculous A18.84
  viral B33.24
Cardionephritis — *see* Hypertension, cardiorenal
Cardionephropathy — *see* Hypertension, cardiorenal
Cardionephrosis — *see* Hypertension, cardiorenal
Cardiopathia nigra I27.0
Cardiopathy (*see also* Disease, heart) I51.9
  idiopathic I42.9
  mucopolysaccharidosis E76.3 *[I52]*
Cardiopericarditis — *see* Pericarditis
Cardiophobia F45.29
Cardiorenal — *see* condition
Cardiorrhexis — *see* Infarct, myocardium
Cardiosclerosis — *see* Disease, heart, ischemic, atherosclerotic
Cardiosis — *see* Disease, heart
Cardiospasm (esophagus) (reflex) (stomach) K22.0
  congenital Q39.5
    with megaesophagus Q39.5
Cardiostenosis — *see* Disease, heart
Cardiosymphysis I31.0
Cardiovascular — *see* condition
Carditis (acute) (bacterial) (chronic) (subacute) I51.89
  meningococcal A39.50
  rheumatic — *see* Disease, heart, rheumatic
  rheumatoid — *see* Rheumatoid, carditis
  viral B33.20
Care (of) (for) (following)
  child (routine) Z76.2
  family member (handicapped) (sick)
    creating problem for family Z63.6
    provided away from home for holiday relief Z75.5
    unavailable, due to
      absence (person rendering care) (sufferer) Z74.2
      inability (any reason) of person rendering care Z74.2
  foundling Z76.1
  holiday relief Z75.5
  improper — *see* Maltreatment
  lack of (at or after birth) (infant) — *see* Maltreatment, child, neglect
  lactating mother Z39.1
  palliative Z51.5
  postpartum
    immediately after delivery Z39.0
    routine follow-up Z39.2
  respite Z75.5
  unavailable, due to
    absence of person rendering care Z74.2
    inability (any reason) of person rendering care Z74.2
  well-baby Z76.2
Caries
  bone NEC A18.03

Caries — *continued*
  dental (dentino enamel junction) (early childhood) (of dentine) (pre-eruptive) (recurrent) (to the pulp) K02.9
    arrested (coronal) (root) K02.3
    chewing surface
      limited to enamel K02.51
      penetrating into dentin K02.52
      penetrating into pulp K02.53
    coronal surface
      chewing surface
        limited to enamel K02.51
        penetrating into dentin K02.52
        penetrating into pulp K02.53
      pit and fissure surface
        limited to enamel K02.51
        penetrating into dentin K02.52
        penetrating into pulp K02.53
      smooth surface
        limited to enamel K02.61
        penetrating into dentin K02.62
        penetrating into pulp K02.63
    pit and fissure surface
      limited to enamel K02.51
      penetrating into dentin K02.52
      penetrating into pulp K02.53
    primary, cervical origin K02.52
    root K02.7
    smooth surface
      limited to enamel K02.61
      penetrating into dentin K02.62
      penetrating into pulp K02.63
  external meatus — *see* Disorder, ear, external, specified type NEC
  hip (tuberculous) A18.02
  initial (tooth)
    chewing surface K02.51
    pit and fissure surface K02.51
    smooth surface K02.61
  knee (tuberculous) A18.02
  labyrinth — *see* subcategory H83.8 ☑
  limb NEC (tuberculous) A18.03
  mastoid process (chronic) — *see* Mastoiditis, chronic
    tuberculous A18.03
  middle ear — *see* subcategory H74.8 ☑
  nose (tuberculous) A18.03
  orbit (tuberculous) A18.03
  ossicles, ear — *see* Abnormal, ear ossicles
  petrous bone — *see* Petrositis
  root (dental) (tooth) K02.7
  sacrum (tuberculous) A18.01
  spine, spinal (column) (tuberculous) A18.01
  syphilitic A52.77
    congenital (early) A50.02 *[M90.80]*
  tooth, teeth — *see* Caries, dental
  tuberculous A18.03
  vertebra (column) (tuberculous) A18.01
Carious teeth — *see* Caries, dental
Carneous mole O02.0
Carnitine insufficiency E71.40
Carotid body or sinus syndrome G90.01
Carotidynia G90.01
Carotenemia (dietary) E67.1
Carotenosis (cutis) (skin) E67.1
Carpal tunnel syndrome — *see* Syndrome, carpal tunnel
Carpenter's syndrome Q87.0
Carpopedal spasm — *see* Tetany
Carr-Barr-Plunkett syndrome Q97.1
Carrier (suspected) of
  amebiasis Z22.1
  bacterial disease NEC Z22.39
    diphtheria Z22.2
    intestinal infectious NEC Z22.1
      typhoid Z22.0
    meningococcal Z22.31
    sexually transmitted Z22.4
    specified NEC Z22.39
    staphylococcal (Methicillin susceptible) Z22.321
      Methicillin resistant Z22.322
    streptococcal Z22.338
      group B Z22.330
        complicating pregnancy or delivery O99.82 ☑
    typhoid Z22.0
  cholera Z22.1
  diphtheria Z22.2
  gastrointestinal pathogens NEC Z22.1
  genetic Z14.8
    cystic fibrosis Z14.1
    hemophilia A (asymptomatic) Z14.01
      symptomatic Z14.02

Carrier — *continued*
  gestational, pregnant Z33.1
  gonorrhea Z22.4
  HAA (hepatitis Australian-antigen) B18.8
  HB (c)(s)-AG B18.1
  hepatitis (viral) B18.9
    Australia-antigen (HAA) B18.8
    B surface antigen (HBsAg) B18.1
      with acute delta- (super)infection B17.0
    C B18.2
    specified NEC B18.8
  human T-cell lymphotropic virus type-1 (HTLV-1) infection Z22.6
  infectious organism Z22.9
    specified NEC Z22.8
  meningococci Z22.31
  Salmonella typhosa Z22.0
  serum hepatitis — *see* Carrier, hepatitis
  staphylococci (Methicillin susceptible) Z22.321
    Methicillin resistant Z22.322
  streptococci Z22.338
    group B Z22.330
      complicating pregnancy or delivery O99.82 ☑
  syphilis Z22.4
  typhoid Z22.0
  venereal disease NEC Z22.4
Carrion's disease A44.0
Carter's relapsing fever (Asiatic) A68.1
Cartilage — *see* condition
Caruncle (inflamed)
  conjunctiva (acute) — *see* Conjunctivitis, acute
  labium (majus) (minus) N90.89
  lacrimal — *see* Inflammation, lacrimal, passages
  myrtiform N89.8
  urethral (benign) N36.2
Cascade stomach K31.2
Caseation lymphatic gland (tuberculous) A18.2
Cassidy (-Scholte) syndrome (malignant carcinoid) E34.0
Castellani's disease A69.8
Castration, traumatic, male S38.231 ☑
Casts in urine R82.998
Cat
  cry syndrome Q93.4
  ear Q17.3
  eye syndrome Q92.8
Catabolism, senile R54
Catalepsy (hysterical) F44.2
  schizophrenic F20.2
Cataplexy (idiopathic) — *see -* Narcolepsy
Cataract (cortical) (immature) (incipient) H26.9
  with
    neovascularization — *see* Cataract, complicated
  age-related — *see* Cataract, senile
  anterior
    and posterior axial embryonal Q12.0
    pyramidal Q12.0
  associated with
    galactosemia E74.21 *[H28]*
    myotonic disorders G71.19 *[H28]*
  blue Q12.0
  central Q12.0
  cerulean Q12.0
  complicated H26.20
    with
      neovascularization H26.21 ☑
      ocular disorder H26.22 ☑
    glaucomatous flecks H26.23 ☑
  congenital Q12.0
  coraliform Q12.0
  coronary Q12.0
  crystalline Q12.0
  diabetic — *see* Diabetes, cataract
  drug-induced H26.3 ☑
  due to
    ocular disorder — *see* Cataract, complicated
    radiation H26.8
  electric H26.8
  extraction status Z98.4 ☑
  glass-blower's H26.8
  heat ray H26.8
  heterochromic — *see* Cataract, complicated
  hypermature — *see* Cataract, senile, morgagnian type
  in (due to)
    chronic iridocyclitis — *see* Cataract, complicated
    diabetes — *see* Diabetes, cataract
    endocrine disease E34.9 *[H28]*
    eye disease — *see* Cataract, complicated
    hypoparathyroidism E20.9 *[H28]*
    malnutrition-dehydration E46 *[H28]*
    metabolic disease E88.9 *[H28]*

Cataract — *continued*
  in — *continued*
    myotonic disorders G71.19 *[H28]*
    nutritional disease E63.9 *[H28]*
  infantile — *see* Cataract, presenile
  irradiational — *see* Cataract, specified NEC
  juvenile — *see* Cataract, presenile
  malnutrition-dehydration E46 *[H28]*
  morgagnian — *see* Cataract, senile, morgagnian type
  myotonic G71.19 *[H28]*
  myxedema E03.9 *[H28]*
  nuclear
    embryonal Q12.0
    sclerosis — *see* Cataract, senile, nuclear
  presenile H26.00 ☑
    combined forms H26.06 ☑
    cortical H26.01 ☑
    lamellar — *see* Cataract, presenile, cortical
    nuclear H26.03 ☑
    specified NEC H26.09
    subcapsular polar (anterior) H26.04 ☑
      posterior H26.05 ☑
    zonular — *see* Cataract, presenile, cortical
  secondary H26.40
    Soemmering's ring H26.41 ☑
    specified NEC H26.49 ☑
    to eye disease — *see* Cataract, complicated
  senile H25.9
    brunescens — *see* Cataract, senile, nuclear
    combined forms H25.81 ☑
    coronary — *see* Cataract, senile, incipient
    cortical H25.01 ☑
    hypermature — *see* Cataract, senile, morgagnian type
    incipient (mature) (total) H25.09 ☑
      cortical — *see* Cataract, senile, cortical
      subcapsular — *see* Cataract, senile, subcapsular
    morgagnian type (hypermature) H25.2 ☑
    nuclear (sclerosis) H25.1 ☑
    polar subcapsular (anterior) (posterior) — *see* Cataract, senile, incipient
    punctate — *see* Cataract, senile, incipient
    specified NEC H25.89
    subcapsular polar (anterior) H25.03 ☑
      posterior H25.04 ☑
  snowflake — *see* Diabetes, cataract
  specified NEC H26.8
  toxic — *see* Cataract, drug-induced
  traumatic H26.10 ☑
    localized H26.11 ☑
    partially resolved H26.12 ☑
    total H26.13 ☑
  zonular (perinuclear) Q12.0
Cataracta (*see also* Cataract)
  brunescens — *see* Cataract, senile, nuclear
  centralis pulverulenta Q12.0
  cerulea Q12.0
  complicata — *see* Cataract, complicated
  congenita Q12.0
  coralliformis Q12.0
  coronaria Q12.0
  diabetic — *see* Diabetes, cataract
  membranacea
    accreta — *see* Cataract, secondary
    congenita Q12.0
  nigra — *see* Cataract, senile, nuclear
  sunflower — *see* Cataract, complicated
Catarrh, catarrhal (acute) (febrile) (infectious) (inflammation) (*see also* condition) J00
  bronchial — *see* Bronchitis
  chest — *see* Bronchitis
  chronic J31.0
  due to congenital syphilis A50.03
  enteric — *see* Enteritis
  eustachian H68.009
  fauces — *see* Pharyngitis
  gastrointestinal — *see* Enteritis
  gingivitis K05.00
    nonplaque induced K05.01
    plaque induced K05.00
  hay — *see* Fever, hay
  intestinal — *see* Enteritis
  larynx, chronic J37.0
  liver B15.9
    with hepatic coma B15.0
  lung — *see* Bronchitis
  middle ear, chronic — *see* Otitis, media, nonsuppurative, chronic, serous
  mouth K12.1
  nasal (chronic) — *see* Rhinitis
  nasobronchial J31.1

Catarrh — *continued*
  nasopharyngeal (chronic) J31.1
    acute J00
  pulmonary — *see* Bronchitis
  spring (eye) (vernal) — *see* Conjunctivitis, acute, atopic
  summer (hay) — *see* Fever, hay
  throat J31.2
  tubotympanal (*see also* Otitis, media, nonsuppurative)
    chronic — *see* Otitis, media, nonsuppurative, chronic, serous
Catatonia (schizophrenic) F20.2
Catatonic
  disorder due to known physiologic condition F06.1
  schizophrenia F20.2
  stupor R40.1
Cat-scratch (*see also* Abrasion)
  disease or fever A28.1
Cauda equina — *see* condition
Cauliflower ear M95.1 ☑
Causalgia (upper limb) G56.4 ☑
  lower limb G57.7 ☑
Cause
  external, general effects T75.89 ☑
Caustic burn — *see* Corrosion, by site
Cavare's disease (familial periodic paralysis) G72.3
Cave-in, injury
  crushing (severe) — *see* Crush
  suffocation — *see* Asphyxia, traumatic, due to low oxygen, due to cave-in
Cavernitis (penis) N48.29
Cavernositis N48.29
Cavernous — *see* condition
Cavitation of lung (*see also* Tuberculosis, pulmonary)
  nontuberculous J98.4
Cavities, dental — *see* Caries, dental
Cavity
  lung — *see* Cavitation of lung
  optic papilla Q14.2
  pulmonary — *see* Cavitation of lung
Cavovarus foot, congenital Q66.1 ☑
Cavus foot (congenital) Q66.7 ☑
  acquired — *see* Deformity, limb, foot, specified NEC
Cazenave's disease L10.2
Cecitis K52.9
  with perforation, peritonitis, or rupture K65.8
Cecoureterocele Q62.32
Cecum — *see* condition
Celiac
  artery compression syndrome I77.4
  disease (with steatorrhea) K90.0
  infantilism K90.0
Cell(s), cellular (*see also* condition)
  in urine R82.998
Cellulitis (diffuse) (phlegmonous) (septic) (suppurative) L03.90
  abdominal wall L03.311
  anaerobic A48.0
  ankle — *see* Cellulitis, lower limb
  anus K61.0
  arm — *see* Cellulitis, upper limb
  auricle (ear) — *see* Cellulitis, ear
  axilla L03.11 ☑
  back (any part) L03.312
  breast (acute) (nonpuerperal) (subacute) N61.0
    nipple N61.0
  broad ligament
    acute N73.0
  buttock L03.317
  cervical (meaning neck) L03.221
  cervix (uteri) — *see* Cervicitis
  cheek (external) L03.211
    internal K12.2
  chest wall L03.313
  chronic L03.90
  clostridial A48.0
  corpus cavernosum N48.22
  digit
    finger — *see* Cellulitis, finger
    toe — *see* Cellulitis, toe
  Douglas' cul-de-sac or pouch
    acute N73.0
  drainage site (following operation) T81.49 ☑
  ear (external) H60.1 ☑
  eosinophilic (granulomatous) L98.3
  erysipelatous — *see* Erysipelas
  external auditory canal — *see* Cellulitis, ear
  eyelid — *see* Abscess, eyelid
  face NEC L03.211
  finger (intrathecal) (periosteal) (subcutaneous) (subcuticular) L03.01 ☑

Cellulitis — *continued*
  foot — *see* Cellulitis, lower limb
  gangrenous — *see* Gangrene
  genital organ NEC
    female (external) N76.4
    male N49.9
      multiple sites N49.8
      specified NEC N49.8
  gluteal (region) L03.317
  gonococcal A54.89
  groin L03.314
  hand — *see* Cellulitis, upper limb
  head NEC L03.811
    face (any part, except ear, eye and nose) L03.211
  heel — *see* Cellulitis, lower limb
  hip — *see* Cellulitis, lower limb
  jaw (region) L03.211
  knee — *see* Cellulitis, lower limb
  labium (majus) (minus) — *see* Vulvitis
  lacrimal passages — *see* Inflammation, lacrimal, passages
  larynx J38.7
  leg — *see* Cellulitis, lower limb
  lip K13.0
  lower limb L03.11 ☑
    toe — *see* Cellulitis, toe
  mouth (floor) K12.2
  multiple sites, so stated L03.90
  nasopharynx J39.1
  navel L03.316
    newborn P38.9
      with mild hemorrhage P38.1
      without hemorrhage P38.9
  neck (region) L03.221
  nipple (acute) (nonpuerperal) (subacute) N61.0
  nose (septum) (external) J34.0
  orbit, orbital H05.01 ☑
  palate (soft) K12.2
  pectoral (region) L03.313
  pelvis, pelvic (chronic)
    female (*see also* Disease, pelvis, inflammatory) N73.2
      acute N73.0
      following ectopic or molar pregnancy O08.0
    male K65.0
  penis N48.22
  perineal, perineum L03.315
  periorbital L03.213
  perirectal K61.1
  peritonsillar J36
  periurethral N34.0
  periuterine (*see also* Disease, pelvis, inflammatory) N73.2
    acute N73.0
  pharynx J39.1
  preseptal L03.213
  rectum K61.1
  retroperitoneal K68.9
  round ligament
    acute N73.0
  scalp (any part) L03.811
  scrotum N49.2
  seminal vesicle N49.0
  shoulder — *see* Cellulitis, upper limb
  specified site NEC L03.818
  submandibular (region) (space) (triangle) K12.2
    gland K11.3
  submaxillary (region) K12.2
    gland K11.3
  thigh — *see* Cellulitis, lower limb
  thumb (intrathecal) (periosteal) (subcutaneous) (subcuticular) — *see* Cellulitis, finger
  toe (intrathecal) (periosteal) (subcutaneous) (subcuticular) L03.03 ☑
  tonsil J36
  trunk L03.319
    abdominal wall L03.311
    back (any part) L03.312
    buttock L03.317
    chest wall L03.313
    groin L03.314
    perineal, perineum L03.315
    umbilicus L03.316
  tuberculous (primary) A18.4
  umbilicus L03.316
  upper limb L03.11 ☑
    axilla — *see* Cellulitis, axilla
    finger — *see* Cellulitis, finger
    thumb — *see* Cellulitis, finger
  vaccinal T88.0 ☑
  vocal cord J38.3
  vulva — *see* Vulvitis
  wrist — *see* Cellulitis, upper limb

Cementoblastoma - Chemotherapy

Cementoblastoma, benign — see Cyst, calcifying
  odontogenic
Cementoma — see Cyst, calcifying odontogenic
Cementoperiostitis — see Periodontitis
Cementosis K03.4
Central auditory processing disorder H93.25
Central pain syndrome G89.0
Cephalematocele, cephal (o)hematocele
  newborn P52.8
    birth injury P10.8
  traumatic — see Hematoma, brain
Cephalematoma, cephalhematoma (calcified)
  newborn (birth injury) P12.0
  traumatic — see Hematoma, brain
Cephalgia, cephalalgia (see also Headache)
  histamine G44.009
    intractable G44.001
    not intractable G44.009
  trigeminal autonomic (TAC) NEC G44.099
    intractable G44.091
    not intractable G44.099
Cephalic — see condition
Cephalitis — see Encephalitis
Cephalocele — see Encephalocele
Cephalomenia N94.89
Cephalopelvic — see condition
Cerclage (with cervical incompetence) in pregnancy —
  see Incompetence, cervix, in pregnancy
Cerebellitis — see Encephalitis
Cerebellum, cerebellar — see condition
Cerebral — see condition
Cerebritis — see Encephalitis
Cerebro-hepato-renal syndrome Q87.89
Cerebromalacia — see Softening, brain
  sequelae of cerebrovascular disease I69.398
Cerebroside lipidosis E75.22
Cerebrospasticity (congenital) G80.1
Cerebrospinal — see condition
Cerebrum — see condition
Ceroid-lipofuscinosis, neuronal E75.4
Cerumen (accumulation) (impacted) H61.2 ☑
Cervical (see also condition)
  auricle Q18.2
  dysplasia in pregnancy — see Abnormal, cervix, in
    pregnancy or childbirth
  erosion in pregnancy — see Abnormal, cervix, in
    pregnancy or childbirth
  fibrosis in pregnancy — see Abnormal, cervix, in
    pregnancy or childbirth
  fusion syndrome Q76.1
  rib Q76.5
  shortening (complicating pregnancy) O26.87 ☑
Cervicalgia M54.2
Cervicitis (acute) (chronic) (nonvenereal) (senile
  (atrophic)) (subacute) (with ulceration) N72
  with
    abortion — see Abortion, by type complicated by
      genital tract and pelvic infection
    ectopic pregnancy O08.0
    molar pregnancy O08.0
  chlamydial A56.09
  gonococcal A54.03
  herpesviral A60.03
  puerperal (postpartum) O86.11
  syphilitic A52.76
  trichomonal A59.09
  tuberculous A18.16
Cervicocolpitis (emphysematosa) (see also Cervicitis)
  N72
Cervix — see condition
Cesarean delivery, previous, affecting management of
  pregnancy O34.219
  classical (vertical) scar O34.212
  low transverse scar O34.211
Céstan (-Chenais) paralysis or syndrome G46.3
Céstan-Raymond syndrome I65.8
Cestode infestation B71.9
  specified type NEC B71.8
Cestodiasis B71.9
Chabert's disease A22.9
Chacaleh E53.8
Chafing L30.4
Chagas' (-Mazza) disease (chronic) B57.2
  with
    cardiovascular involvement NEC B57.2
    digestive system involvement B57.30
      megacolon B57.32
      megaesophagus B57.31
      other specified B57.39
      megacolon B57.32
      megaesophagus B57.31
      myocarditis B57.2

Chagas — continued
  with — continued
    nervous system involvement B57.40
      meningitis B57.41
      meningoencephalitis B57.42
      other specified B57.49
    specified organ involvement NEC B57.5
  acute (with) B57.1
    cardiovascular NEC B57.0
    myocarditis B57.0
Chagres fever B50.9
Chairridden Z74.09
Chalasia (cardiac sphincter) K21.9
Chalazion H00.19
  left H00.16
    lower H00.15
    upper H00.14
  right H00.13
    lower H00.12
    upper H00.11
Chalcosis (see also Disorder, globe, degenerative,
  chalcosis)
  cornea — see Deposit, cornea
  crystalline lens — see Cataract, complicated
  retina H35.89
Chalicosis (pulmonum) J62.8
Chancre (any genital site) (hard) (hunterian) (mixed)
  (primary) (seronegative) (seropositive) (syphilitic)
  A51.0
  congenital A50.07
  conjunctiva NEC A51.2
  Ducrey's A57
  extragenital A51.2
  eyelid A51.2
  lip A51.2
  nipple A51.2
  Nisbet's A57
  of
    carate A67.0
    pinta A67.0
    yaws A66.0
  palate, soft A51.2
  phagedenic A57
  simple A57
  soft A57
    bubo A57
    palate A51.2
  urethra A51.0
  yaws A66.0
Chancroid (anus) (genital) (penis) (perineum) (rectum)
  (urethra) (vulva) A57
Chandler's disease (osteochondritis dissecans, hip) —
  see Osteochondritis, dissecans, hip
Change(s) (in) (of) (see also Removal)
  arteriosclerotic — see Arteriosclerosis
  bone (see also Disorder, bone)
    diabetic — see Diabetes, bone change
  bowel habit R19.4
  cardiorenal (vascular) — see Hypertension,
    cardiorenal
  cardiovascular — see Disease, cardiovascular
  circulatory I99.9
  cognitive (mild) (organic) R41.89
  color, tooth, teeth
    during formation K00.8
    posteruptive K03.7
  contraceptive device Z30.433
  corneal membrane H18.30
    Bowman's membrane fold or rupture H18.31 ☑
    Descemet's membrane
      fold H18.32 ☑
      rupture H18.33 ☑
  coronary — see Disease, heart, ischemic
  degenerative, spine or vertebra — see Spondylosis
  dental pulp, regressive K04.2
  dressing (nonsurgical) Z48.00
    surgical Z48.01
  heart — see Disease, heart
  hip joint — see Derangement, joint, hip
  hyperplastic larynx J38.7
  hypertrophic
    nasal sinus J34.89
    turbinate, nasal J34.3
    upper respiratory tract J39.8
  indwelling catheter Z46.6
  inflammatory (see also Inflammation)
    sacroiliac M46.1
  job, anxiety concerning Z56.1
  joint — see Derangement, joint
  life — see Menopause
  mental status R41.82

Change(s) — continued
  minimal (glomerular) (see also N00-N07 with fourth
    character .0) N05.0
  myocardium, myocardial — see Degeneration,
    myocardial
  of life — see Menopause
  pacemaker Z45.018
    pulse generator Z45.010
  personality (enduring) F68.8
    due to (secondary to)
      general medical condition F07.0
    secondary (nonspecific) F60.89
  regressive, dental pulp K04.2
  renal — see Disease, renal
  retina H35.9
    myopic (see also Myopia, degenerative) H44.2 ☑
  sacroiliac joint M53.3
  senile (see also condition) R54
  sensory R20.8
  skin R23.9
    acute, due to ultraviolet radiation L56.9
      specified NEC L56.8
    chronic, due to nonionizing radiation L57.9
      specified NEC L57.8
    cyanosis R23.0
    flushing R23.2
    pallor R23.1
    petechiae R23.3
    specified change NEC R23.8
    swelling — see Mass, localized
    texture R23.4
  trophic
    arm — see Mononeuropathy, upper limb
    leg — see Mononeuropathy, lower limb
  vascular I99.9
  vasomotor I73.9
  voice R49.9
    psychogenic F44.4
    specified NEC R49.8
Changing sleep-work schedule, affecting sleep G47.26
Changuinola fever A93.1
Chapping skin T69.8 ☑
Charcot-Marie-Tooth disease, paralysis or syndrome
  G60.0
Charcot's
  arthropathy — see Arthropathy, neuropathic
  cirrhosis K74.3
  disease (tabetic arthropathy) A52.16
  joint (disease) (tabetic) A52.16
    diabetic — see Diabetes, with, arthropathy
    syringomyelic G95.0
  syndrome (intermittent claudication) I73.9
CHARGE association Q89.8
Charley-horse (quadriceps) M62.831
  traumatic (quadriceps) S76.11 ☑
Charlouis' disease — see Yaws
Cheadle's disease E54
Checking (of)
  cardiac pacemaker (battery) (electrode(s)) Z45.018
    pulse generator Z45.010
  implantable subdermal contraceptive Z30.46
  intrauterine contraceptive device Z30.431
  wound Z48.0 ☑
    due to injury - code to Injury, by site, using
      appropriate seventh character for
      subsequent encounter
Check-up — see Examination
Chédiak-Higashi (-Steinbrinck) syndrome (congenital
  gigantism of peroxidase granules) E70.330
Cheek — see condition
Cheese itch B88.0
Cheese-washer's lung J67.8
Cheese-worker's lung J67.8
Cheilitis (acute) (angular) (catarrhal) (chronic)
  (exfoliative) (gangrenous) (glandular) (infectional)
  (suppurative) (ulcerative) (vesicular) K13.0
  actinic (due to sun) L56.8
    other than from sun L59.8
  candidal B37.83
Cheilodynia K13.0
Cheiloschisis — see Cleft, lip
Cheilosis (angular) K13.0
  with pellagra E52
  due to
    vitamin B2 (riboflavin) deficiency E53.0
Cheiromegaly M79.89
Cheiropompholyx L30.1
Cheloid — see Keloid
Chemical burn — see Corrosion, by site
Chemodectoma — see Paraganglioma, nonchromaffin
Chemosis, conjunctiva — see Edema, conjunctiva
Chemotherapy (session) (for)

☑ **Additional character required**

Chemotherapy — *continued*
  cancer Z51.11
  neoplasm Z51.11
Cherubism M27.8
Chest — *see* condition
Cheyne-Stokes breathing (respiration) R06.3
Chiari's
  disease or syndrome (hepatic vein thrombosis)
    I82.0
  malformation
    type I G93.5
    type II — *see* Spina bifida
  net Q24.8
Chicago disease B40.9
Chickenpox — *see* Varicella
Chiclero ulcer or sore B55.1
Chigger (infestation) B88.0
Chignon (disease) B36.8
  newborn (from vacuum extraction) (birth injury)
    P12.1
Chilaiditi's syndrome (subphrenic displacement,
  colon) Q43.3
Chilblain(s) (lupus) T69.1 ☑
Child
  custody dispute Z65.3
Childbirth — *see* Delivery
Childhood
  cerebral X-linked adrenoleukodystrophy E71.520
  period of rapid growth Z00.2
Chill(s) R68.83
  with fever R50.9
  congestive in malarial regions B54
  without fever R68.83
Chilomastigiasis A07.8
Chimera 46,XX/46,XY Q99.0
Chin — *see* condition
Chinese dysentery A03.9
Chionophobia F40.228
Chitral fever A93.1
Chlamydia, chlamydial A74.9
  cervicitis A56.09
  conjunctivitis A74.0
  cystitis A56.01
  endometritis A56.11
  epididymitis A56.19
  female
    pelvic inflammatory disease A56.11
    pelviperitonitis A56.11
  orchitis A56.19
  peritonitis A74.81
  pharyngitis A56.4
  proctitis A56.3
  psittaci (infection) A70
  salpingitis A56.11
  sexually-transmitted infection NEC A56.8
  specified NEC A74.89
  urethritis A56.01
  vulvovaginitis A56.02
Chlamydiosis — *see* Chlamydia
Chloasma (skin) (idiopathic) (symptomatic) L81.1
  eyelid H02.719
    hyperthyroid E05.90 *[H02.719]*
      with thyroid storm E05.91 *[H02.719]*
    left H02.716
      lower H02.715
      upper H02.714
    right H02.713
      lower H02.712
      upper H02.711
Chloroma C92.3 ☑
Chlorosis D50.9
  Egyptian B76.9 *[D63.8]*
  miner's B76.9 *[D63.8]*
Chlorotic anemia D50.8
Chocolate cyst (ovary) N80.1
Choked
  disc or disk — *see* Papilledema
  on food, phlegm, or vomitus NOS — *see* Foreign
    body, by site
  while vomiting NOS — *see* Foreign body, by site
Chokes (resulting from bends) T70.3 ☑
Choking sensation R09.89
Cholangiectasis K83.8
Cholangiocarcinoma
  with hepatocellular carcinoma, combined C22.0
  liver C22.1
  specified site NEC — *see* Neoplasm, malignant, by
    site
  unspecified site C22.1
Cholangiohepatitis K83.8
  due to fluke infestation B66.1
Cholangiohepatoma C22.0

Cholangiolitis (acute) (chronic) (extrahepatic)
  (gangrenous) (intrahepatic) K83.09
  paratyphoidal — *see* Fever, paratyphoid
  typhoidal A01.09
Cholangioma D13.4
  malignant — *see* Cholangiocarcinoma
Cholangitis (ascending) (recurrent) (secondary)
  (stenosing) (suppurative) K83.09
  with calculus, bile duct — *see* Calculus, bile duct,
    with cholangitis
  chronic nonsuppurative destructive K74.3
  primary K83.09
    sclerosing K83.01
  sclerosing K83.09
Cholecystectasia K82.8
Cholecystitis K81.9
  with
    calculus, stones in
      bile duct (common) (hepatic) — *see* Calculus,
        bile duct, with cholecystitis
      cystic duct — *see* Calculus, gallbladder, with
        cholecystitis
      gallbladder — *see* Calculus, gallbladder, with
        cholecystitis
    choledocholithiasis — *see* Calculus, bile duct,
      with cholecystitis
    cholelithiasis — *see* Calculus, gallbladder, with
      cholecystitis
    gangrene of gallbladder K82.A1
    perforation of gallbladder K82.A2
  acute (emphysematous) (gangrenous)
    (suppurative) K81.0
    with
      calculus, stones in
        cystic duct — *see* Calculus, gallbladder, with
          cholecystitis, acute
        gallbladder — *see* Calculus, gallbladder, with
          cholecystitis, acute
      choledocholithiasis — *see* Calculus, bile duct,
        with cholecystitis, acute
      cholelithiasis — *see* Calculus, gallbladder, with
        cholecystitis, acute
    chronic cholecystitis K81.2
      with gallbladder calculus K80.12
        with obstruction K80.13
  chronic K81.1
    with acute cholecystitis K81.2
      with gallbladder calculus K80.12
        with obstruction K80.13
  emphysematous (acute) — *see* Cholecystitis, acute
  gangrenous — *see* Cholecystitis, acute
  paratyphoidal, current A01.4
  suppurative — *see* Cholecystitis, acute
  typhoidal A01.09
Cholecystolithiasis — *see* Calculus, gallbladder
Choledochitis (suppurative) K83.09
Choledocholith — *see* Calculus, bile duct
Choledocholithiasis (common duct) (hepatic duct) —
  see Calculus, bile duct
  cystic — *see* Calculus, gallbladder
  typhoidal A01.09
Cholelithiasis (cystic duct) (gallbladder) (impacted)
  (multiple) — *see* Calculus, gallbladder
  bile duct (common) (hepatic) — *see* Calculus, bile
    duct
  hepatic duct — *see* Calculus, bile duct
  specified NEC K80.80
    with obstruction K80.81
Cholemia (*see also* Jaundice)
  familial (simple) (congenital) E80.4
  Gilbert's E80.4
Choleperitoneum, choleperitonitis K65.3
Cholera (Asiatic) (epidemic) (malignant) A00.9
  antimonial — *see* Poisoning, antimony
  classical A00.0
  due to Vibrio cholerae 01 A00.9
    biovar cholerae A00.0
    biovar eltor A00.1
    el tor A00.1
  el tor A00.1
Cholerine — *see* Cholera
Cholestasis NEC K83.1
  with hepatocyte injury K71.0
  due to total parenteral nutrition (TPN) K76.89
  pure K71.0
Cholesteatoma (ear) (middle) (with reaction) H71.9 ☑
  attic H71.0 ☑
  external ear (canal) H60.4 ☑
  mastoid H71.2 ☑
  postmastoidectomy cavity (recurrent) — *see*
    Complications, postmastoidectomy, recurrent
    cholesteatoma

Cholesteatoma — *continued*
  recurrent (postmastoidectomy) — *see*
    Complications, postmastoidectomy, recurrent
    cholesteatoma
  tympanum H71.1 ☑
Cholesteatosis, diffuse H71.3 ☑
Cholesteremia E78.00
Cholesterin in vitreous — *see* Deposit, crystalline
Cholesterol
  deposit
    retina H35.89
    vitreous — *see* Deposit, crystalline
  elevated (high) E78.00
    with elevated (high) triglycerides E78.2
    screening for Z13.220
  imbibition of gallbladder K82.4
Cholesterolemia (essential) (pure) E78.00
  familial E78.01
  hereditary E78.01
Cholesterolosis, cholesterosis (gallbladder) K82.4
  cerebrotendinous E75.5
Cholocolic fistula K82.3
Choluria R82.2
Chondritis M94.8X9
  auricle H61.03 ☑
  costal (Tietze's) M94.0
  external ear H61.03 ☑
  patella, posttraumatic — *see* Chondromalacia,
    patella
  pinna H61.03 ☑
  purulent M94.8X ☑
  tuberculous NEC A18.02
    intervertebral A18.01
Chondroblastoma (*see also* Neoplasm, bone, benign)
  malignant — *see* Neoplasm, bone, malignant
Chondrocalcinosis M11.20
  ankle M11.27 ☑
  elbow M11.22 ☑
  familial M11.10
    ankle M11.17 ☑
    elbow M11.12 ☑
    foot joint M11.17 ☑
    hand joint M11.14 ☑
    hip M11.15 ☑
    knee M11.16 ☑
    multiple site M11.19
    shoulder M11.11 ☑
    vertebrae M11.18
    wrist M11.13 ☑
  foot joint M11.27 ☑
  hand joint M11.24 ☑
  hip M11.25 ☑
  knee M11.26 ☑
  multiple site M11.29
  shoulder M11.21 ☑
  vertebrae M11.28
  specified type NEC M11.20
    ankle M11.27 ☑
    elbow M11.22 ☑
    foot joint M11.27 ☑
    hand joint M11.24 ☑
    hip M11.25 ☑
    knee M11.26 ☑
    multiple site M11.29
    shoulder M11.21 ☑
    vertebrae M11.28
    wrist M11.23 ☑
  wrist M11.23 ☑
Chondrodermatitis nodularis helicis or anthelicis —
  see Perichondritis, ear
Chondrodysplasia Q78.9
  with hemangioma Q78.4
  calcificans congenita Q77.3
  fetalis Q77.4
  metaphyseal (Jansen's) (McKusick's) (Schmid's)
    Q78.8
  punctata Q77.3
Chondrodystrophy, chondrodystrophia (familial)
  (fetalis) (hypoplastic) Q78.9
  calcificans congenita Q77.3
  myotonic (congenital) G71.13
  punctata Q77.3
Chondroectodermal dysplasia Q77.6
Chondrogenesis imperfecta Q77.4
Chondrolysis M94.35 ☑
Chondroma (*see also* Neoplasm, cartilage, benign)
  juxtacortical — *see* Neoplasm, bone, benign
  periosteal — *see* Neoplasm, bone, benign
Chondromalacia (systemic) M94.20
  acromioclavicular joint M94.21 ☑
  ankle M94.27 ☑
  elbow M94.22 ☑

Chondromalacia - Cirrhosis

Chondromalacia — *continued*
- foot joint M94.27 ☑
- glenohumeral joint M94.21 ☑
- hand joint M94.24 ☑
- hip M94.25 ☑
- knee M94.26 ☑
  - patella M22.4 ☑
- multiple sites M94.29
- patella M22.4 ☑
- rib M94.28
- sacroiliac joint M94.259
- shoulder M94.21 ☑
- sternoclavicular joint M94.21 ☑
- vertebral joint M94.28
- wrist M94.23 ☑

Chondromatosis (*see also* Neoplasm, cartilage, uncertain behavior)
- internal Q78.4

Chondromyxosarcoma — *see* Neoplasm, cartilage, malignant

Chondro-osteodysplasia (Morquio-Brailsford type) E76.219

Chondro-osteodystrophy E76.29

Chondro-osteoma — *see* Neoplasm, bone, benign

Chondropathia tuberosa M94.0

Chondrosarcoma — *see* Neoplasm, cartilage, malignant
- juxtacortical — *see* Neoplasm, bone, malignant
- mesenchymal — *see* Neoplasm, connective tissue, malignant
- myxoid — *see* Neoplasm, cartilage, malignant

Chordee (nonvenereal) N48.89
- congenital Q54.4
- gonococcal A54.09

Chorditis (fibrinous) (nodosa) (tuberosa) J38.2

Chordoma — *see* Neoplasm, vertebral (column), malignant

Chorea (chronic) (gravis) (posthemiplegic) (senile) (spasmodic) G25.5
- with
  - heart involvement I02.0
    - active or acute (conditions in I01 ☑) I02.0
      - rheumatic I02.9
        - with valvular disorder I02.0
    - rheumatic heart disease (chronic) (inactive) (quiescent) - code to rheumatic heart condition involved
- drug-induced G25.4
- habit F95.8
- hereditary G10
- Huntington's G10
- hysterical F44.4
- minor I02.9
  - with heart involvement I02.0
- progressive G25.5
  - hereditary G10
- rheumatic (chronic) I02.9
  - with heart involvement I02.0
- Sydenham's I02.9
  - with heart involvement — *see* Chorea, with rheumatic heart disease
  - nonrheumatic G25.5

Choreoathetosis (paroxysmal) G25.5

Chorioadenoma (destruens) D39.2

Chorioamnionitis O41.12 ☑

Chorioangioma D26.7

Choriocarcinoma — *see* Neoplasm, malignant, by site
- combined with
  - embryonal carcinoma — *see* Neoplasm, malignant, by site
  - other germ cell elements — *see* Neoplasm, malignant, by site
  - teratoma — *see* Neoplasm, malignant, by site
- specified site — *see* Neoplasm, malignant, by site
- unspecified site
  - female C58
  - male C62.90

Chorioencephalitis (acute) (lymphocytic) (serous) A87.2

Chorioepithelioma — *see* Choriocarcinoma

Choriomeningitis (acute) (lymphocytic) (serous) A87.2

Chorionepithelioma — *see* Choriocarcinoma

Chorioretinitis (*see also* Inflammation, chorioretinal)
- disseminated (*see also* Inflammation, chorioretinal, disseminated)
  - in neurosyphilis A52.19
- Egyptian B76.9 *[D63.8]*
- focal (*see also* Inflammation, chorioretinal, focal)
- histoplasmic B39.9 *[H32]*
- in (due to)
  - histoplasmosis B39.9 *[H32]*
  - syphilis (secondary) A51.43
    - late A52.71

Chorioretinitis — *continued*
- in — *continued*
  - toxoplasmosis (acquired) B58.01
    - congenital (active) P37.1 *[H32]*
  - tuberculosis A18.53
- juxtapapillary, juxtapapillaris — *see* Inflammation, chorioretinal, focal, juxtapapillary
- leprous A30.9 *[H32]*
- miner's B76.9 *[D63.8]*
- progressive myopia (degeneration) (*see also* Myopia, degenerative) H44.2 ☑
- syphilitic (secondary) A51.43
  - congenital (early) A50.01 *[H32]*
  - late A50.32
  - late A52.71
- tuberculous A18.53

Chorioretinopathy, central serous H35.71 ☑

Choroid — *see* condition

Choroideremia H31.21

Choroiditis — *see* Chorioretinitis

Choroidopathy — *see* Disorder, choroid

Choroidoretinitis — *see* Chorioretinitis

Choroidoretinopathy, central serous — *see* Chorioretinopathy, central serous

Christian-Weber disease M35.6

Christmas disease D67

Chromaffinoma (*see also* Neoplasm, benign, by site)
- malignant — *see* Neoplasm, malignant, by site

Chromatopsia — *see* Deficiency, color vision

Chromhidrosis, chromidrosis L75.1

Chromoblastomycosis — *see* Chromomycosis

Chromoconversion R82.91

Chromomycosis B43.9
- brain abscess B43.1
- cerebral B43.1
- cutaneous B43.0
- skin B43.0
- specified NEC B43.8
- subcutaneous abscess or cyst B43.2

Chromophytosis B36.0

Chromosome — *see* condition by chromosome
- involved
  - D (1) — *see* condition, chromosome 13
  - E (3) — *see* condition, chromosome 18
  - G — *see* condition, chromosome 21

Chromotrichomycosis B36.8

Chronic — *see* condition
- fracture — *see* Fracture, pathological

Churg-Strauss syndrome M30.1

Chyle cyst, mesentery I89.8

Chylocele (nonfilarial) I89.8
- filarial (*see also* Infestation, filarial) B74.9 *[N51]*
- tunica vaginalis N50.89
  - filarial (*see also* Infestation, filarial) B74.9 *[N51]*

Chylomicronemia (fasting) (with hyperprebetalipoproteinemia) E78.3

Chylopericardium I31.3
- acute I30.9

Chylothorax (nonfilarial) I89.8
- filarial (*see also* Infestation, filarial) B74.9 *[J91.8]*

Chylous — *see* condition

Chyluria (nonfilarial) R82.0
- due to
  - bilharziasis B65.0
  - Brugia (malayi) B74.1
    - timori B74.2
  - schistosomiasis (bilharziasis) B65.0
  - Wuchereria (bancrofti) B74.0
- filarial — *see* Infestation, filarial

Cicatricial (deformity) — *see* Cicatrix

Cicatrix (adherent) (contracted) (painful) (vicious) (*see also* Scar) L90.5
- adenoid (and tonsil) J35.8
- alveolar process M26.79
- anus K62.89
- auricle — *see* Disorder, pinna, specified type NEC
- bile duct (common) (hepatic) K83.8
- bladder N32.89
- bone — *see* Disorder, bone, specified type NEC
- brain G93.89
- cervix (postoperative) (postpartal) N88.1
- common duct K83.8
- cornea H17.9
  - tuberculous A18.59
- duodenum (bulb), obstructive K31.5
- esophagus K22.2
- eyelid — *see* Disorder, eyelid function
- hypopharynx J39.2
- lacrimal passages — *see* Obstruction, lacrimal
- larynx J38.7
- lung J98.4
- middle ear — *see* subcategory H74.8 ☑

Cicatrix — *continued*
- mouth K13.79
- muscle M62.89
  - with contracture — *see* Contraction, muscle NEC
- nasopharynx J39.2
- palate (soft) K13.79
- penis N48.89
- pharynx J39.2
- prostate N42.89
- rectum K62.89
- retina — *see* Scar, chorioretinal
- semilunar cartilage — *see* Derangement, meniscus
- seminal vesicle N50.89
- skin L90.5
  - infected L08.89
  - postinfective L90.5
  - tuberculous B90.8
- specified site NEC L90.5
- throat J39.2
- tongue K14.8
- tonsil (and adenoid) J35.8
- trachea J39.8
- tuberculous NEC B90.9
- urethra N36.8
- uterus N85.8
- vagina N89.8
  - postoperative N99.2
- vocal cord N48.8
- wrist, constricting (annular) L90.5

CIDP (chronic inflammatory demyelinating polyneuropathy) G61.81

CIN — *see* Neoplasia, intraepithelial, cervix

CINCA (chronic infantile neurological, cutaneous and articular syndrome) M04.2

Cinchonism — *see* Deafness, ototoxic
- correct substance properly administered — *see* Table of Drugs and Chemicals, by drug, adverse effect
- overdose or wrong substance given or taken — *see* Table of Drugs and Chemicals, by drug, poisoning

Circle of Willis — *see* condition

Circular — *see* condition

Circulating anticoagulants (*see also* - Disorder, hemorrhagic) D68.318
- due to drugs (*see also* - Disorder, hemorrhagic) D68.32
- following childbirth O72.3

Circulation
- collateral, any site I99.8
- defective (lower extremity) I99.9
  - congenital Q28.9
  - embryonic Q28.9
  - failure (peripheral) R57.9
    - newborn P29.89
  - fetal, persistent P29.38
  - heart, incomplete Q28.9

Circulatory system — *see* condition

Circulus senilis (cornea) — *see* Degeneration, cornea, senile

Circumcision (in absence of medical indication) (ritual) (routine) Z41.2

Circumscribed — *see* condition

Circumvallate placenta O43.11 ☑

Cirrhosis, cirrhotic (hepatic) (liver) K74.60
- alcoholic K70.30
  - with ascites K70.31
- atrophic — *see* Cirrhosis, liver
- Baumgarten-Cruveilhier K74.69
- biliary (cholangiolitic) (cholangitic) (hypertrophic) (obstructive) (pericholangiolitic) K74.5
  - due to
    - Clonorchiasis B66.1
    - flukes B66.3
    - primary K74.3
    - secondary K74.4
- cardiac (of liver) K76.1
- Charcot's K74.3
- cholangiolitic, cholangitic, cholostatic (primary) K74.3
- congestive K76.1
- Cruveilhier-Baumgarten K74.69
- cryptogenic (liver) K74.69
- due to
  - hepatolenticular degeneration E83.01
  - Wilson's disease E83.01
  - xanthomatosis E78.2
- fatty K76.0
  - alcoholic K70.0
- Hanot's (hypertrophic) K74.3
- hepatic — *see* Cirrhosis, liver
- hypertrophic K74.3

☑ **Additional character required**

Cirrhosis — *continued*
  Indian childhood K74.69
  kidney — *see* Sclerosis, renal
  Laennec's K70.30
    with ascites K70.31
    alcoholic K70.30
      with ascites K70.31
    nonalcoholic K74.69
  liver K74.60
    alcoholic K70.30
      with ascites K70.31
      fatty K70.0
    congenital P78.81
    syphilitic A52.74
  lung (chronic) J84.10
  macronodular K74.69
    alcoholic K70.30
      with ascites K70.31
  micronodular K74.69
    alcoholic K70.30
      with ascites K70.31
  mixed type K74.69
  monolobular K74.3
  nephritis — *see* Sclerosis, renal
  nutritional K74.69
    alcoholic K70.30
      with ascites K70.31
  obstructive — *see* Cirrhosis, biliary
  ovarian N83.8
  pancreas (duct) K86.89
  pigmentary E83.110
  portal K74.69
    alcoholic K70.30
      with ascites K70.31
  postnecrotic K74.69
    alcoholic K70.30
      with ascites K70.31
  pulmonary J84.10
  renal — *see* Sclerosis, renal
  spleen D73.2
  stasis K76.1
  Todd's K74.3
  unilobar K74.3
  xanthomatous (biliary) K74.5
    due to xanthomatosis (familial) (metabolic)
      (primary) E78.2
Cistern, subarachnoid R93.0
Citrullinemia E72.23
Citrullinuria E72.23
Civatte's disease or poikiloderma L57.3
Clam digger's itch B65.3
Clammy skin R23.1
Clap — *see* Gonorrhea
Clarke-Hadfield syndrome (pancreatic infantilism) K86.89
Clark's paralysis G80.9
Clastothrix L67.8
Claude Bernard-Horner syndrome G90.2
    traumatic — *see* Injury, nerve, cervical sympathetic
Claude's disease or syndrome G46.3
Claudication (intermittent) I73.9
  cerebral (artery) G45.9
  spinal cord (arteriosclerotic) G95.19
    syphilitic A52.09
  venous (axillary) I87.8
Claudicatio venosa intermittens I87.8
Claustrophobia F40.240
Clavus (infected) L84
Clawfoot (congenital) Q66.89
  acquired — *see* Deformity, limb, clawfoot
Clawhand (acquired) (*see also* Deformity, limb, clawhand)
  congenital Q68.1
Clawtoe (congenital) Q66.89
  acquired — *see* Deformity, toe, specified NEC
Clay eating — *see* Pica
Cleansing of artificial opening — *see* Attention to, artificial, opening
Cleft (congenital) (*see also* Imperfect, closure)
  alveolar process M26.79
  branchial (persistent) Q18.2
    cyst Q18.0
      fistula Q18.0
      sinus Q18.0
  cricoid cartilage, posterior Q31.8
  foot Q72.7 ☑
  hand Q71.6 ☑
  lip (unilateral) Q36.9
    with cleft palate Q37.9
      hard Q37.1
        with soft Q37.5
      soft Q37.3
        with hard Q37.5

Cleft — *continued*
  lip — *continued*
    bilateral Q36.0
      with cleft palate Q37.8
        hard Q37.0
          with soft Q37.4
        soft Q37.2
          with hard Q37.4
    median Q36.1
  nose Q30.2
  palate Q35.9
    with cleft lip (unilateral) Q37.9
      bilateral Q37.8
    hard Q35.1
      with
        cleft lip (unilateral) Q37.1
          bilateral Q37.0
        soft Q35.5
          with cleft lip (unilateral) Q37.5
            bilateral Q37.4
    medial Q35.5
    soft Q35.3
      with
        cleft lip (unilateral) Q37.3
          bilateral Q37.2
        hard Q35.5
          with cleft lip (unilateral) Q37.5
            bilateral Q37.4
  penis Q55.69
  scrotum Q55.29
  thyroid cartilage Q31.8
  uvula Q35.7
Cleidocranial dysostosis Q74.0
Cleptomania F63.2
Clicking hip (newborn) R29.4
Climacteric (female) (*see also* Menopause)
  arthritis (any site) NEC — *see* Arthritis, specified form NEC
  depression (single episode) F32.89
    recurrent episode F33.8
  melancholia (single episode) F32.89
    recurrent episode F33.8
  male (symptoms) (syndrome) NEC N50.89
  paranoid state F22
  polyarthritis NEC — *see* Arthritis, specified form NEC
  symptoms (female) N95.1
Clinical research investigation (clinical trial) (control subject) (normal comparison) (participant) Z00.6
Clitoris — *see* condition
Cloaca (persistent) Q43.7
Clonorchiasis, clonorchis infection (liver) B66.1
Clonus R25.8
Closed bite M26.29
Clostridium (C.) perfringens, as cause of disease classified elsewhere B96.7
Closure
  congenital, nose Q30.0
  cranial sutures, premature Q75.0
  defective or imperfect NEC — *see* Imperfect, closure
  fistula, delayed — *see* Fistula
  foramen ovale, imperfect Q21.1
  hymen N89.6
  interauricular septum, defective Q21.1
  interventricular septum, defective Q21.0
  lacrimal duct (*see also* Stenosis, lacrimal, duct)
    congenital Q10.5
  nose (congenital) Q30.0
    acquired M95.0
  of artificial opening — *see* Attention to, artificial, opening
  primary angle, without glaucoma damage H40.06 ☑
  vagina N89.5
  valve — *see* Endocarditis
  vulva N90.5
Clot (blood) (*see also* Embolism)
  artery (obstruction) (occlusion) — *see* Embolism
  bladder N32.89
  brain (intradural or extradural) — *see* Occlusion, artery, cerebral
  circulation I74.9
  heart (*see also* Infarct, myocardium)
    not resulting in infarction I51.3
  vein — *see* Thrombosis
Clouded state R40.1
  epileptic — *see* Epilepsy, specified NEC
  paroxysmal — *see* Epilepsy, specified NEC
Cloudy antrum, antra J32.0
Clouston's (hidrotic) ectodermal dysplasia Q82.4
Clubbed nail pachydermoperiostosis M89.40 *[L62]*
Clubbing of finger(s) (nails) R68.3
Clubfinger R68.3
  congenital Q68.1

Clubfoot (congenital) Q66.89
  acquired — *see* Deformity, limb, clubfoot
  equinovarus Q66.0 ☑
  paralytic — *see* Deformity, limb, clubfoot
Clubhand (congenital) (radial) Q71.4 ☑
  acquired — *see* Deformity, limb, clubhand
Clubnail R68.3
  congenital Q84.6
Clump, kidney Q63.1
Clumsiness, clumsy child syndrome F82
Cluttering F80.81
Clutton's joints A50.51 *[M12.80]*
Coagulation, intravascular (diffuse) (disseminated) (*see also* Defibrination syndrome)
  complicating abortion — *see* Abortion, by type, complicated by, intravascular coagulation
  following ectopic or molar pregnancy O08.1
Coagulopathy (*see also* Defect, coagulation)
  consumption D65
  intravascular D65
    newborn P60
Coalition
  calcaneo-scaphoid Q66.89
  tarsal Q66.89
Coalminer's
  elbow — *see* Bursitis, elbow, olecranon
  lung or pneumoconiosis J60
Coalworker's lung or pneumoconiosis J60
Coarctation
  aorta (preductal) (postductal) Q25.1
  pulmonary artery Q25.71
Coated tongue K14.3
Coats' disease (exudative retinopathy) — *see* Retinopathy, exudative
Cocaine-induced
  anxiety disorder F14.980
  bipolar and related disorder F14.94
  depressive disorder F14.94
  obsessive-compulsive and related disorder F14.988
  psychotic disorder F14.959
  sleep disorder F14.982
  sexual dysfunction F14.981
Cocainism — *see* Disorder, cocaine use
Coccidioidomycosis B38.9
  cutaneous B38.3
  disseminated B38.7
  generalized B38.7
  meninges B38.4
  prostate B38.81
  pulmonary B38.2
    acute B38.0
    chronic B38.1
  skin B38.3
  specified NEC B38.89
Coccidioidosis — *see* Coccidioidomycosis
Coccidiosis (intestinal) A07.3
Coccyx — *see* condition
Coccydynia, coccygodynia M53.3
Cochin-China diarrhea K90.1
Cockayne's syndrome Q87.19
Cocked up toe — *see* Deformity, toe, specified NEC
Cock's peculiar tumor L72.3
Codman's tumor — *see* Neoplasm, bone, benign
Coenurosis B71.8
Coffee-worker's lung J67.8
Cogan's syndrome H16.32 ☑
  oculomotor apraxia H51.8
Coitus, painful (female) N94.10
  male N53.12
  psychogenic F52.6
Cold J00
  with influenza, flu, or grippe — *see* Influenza, with, respiratory manifestations NEC
  agglutinin disease or hemoglobinuria (chronic) D59.1
  bronchial — *see* Bronchitis
  chest — *see* Bronchitis
  common (head) J00
  effects of T69.9 ☑
    specified effect NEC T69.8 ☑
  excessive, effects of T69.9 ☑
    specified effect NEC T69.8 ☑
  exhaustion from T69.8 ☑
  exposure to T69.9 ☑
    specified effect NEC T69.8 ☑
  head J00
  injury syndrome (newborn) P80.0
  on lung — *see* Bronchitis
  rose J30.1
  sensitivity, auto-immune D59.1
  symptoms J00
  virus J00

Coldsore - Coma

Coldsore B00.1
Colibacillosis A49.8
  as the cause of other disease (*see also* Escherichia coli) B96.20
  generalized A41.50
Colic (bilious) (infantile) (intestinal) (recurrent) (spasmodic) R10.83
  abdomen R10.83
    psychogenic F45.8
  appendix, appendicular K38.8
  bile duct — *see* Calculus, bile duct
  biliary — *see* Calculus, bile duct
  common duct — *see* Calculus, bile duct
  cystic duct — *see* Calculus, gallbladder
  Devonshire NEC — *see* Poisoning, lead
  gallbladder — *see* Calculus, gallbladder
  gallstone — *see* Calculus, gallbladder
    gallbladder or cystic duct — *see* Calculus, gallbladder
  hepatic (duct) — *see* Calculus, bile duct
  hysterical F45.8
  kidney N23
  lead NEC — *see* Poisoning, lead
  mucous K58.9
    with diarrhea K58.0
    psychogenic F54
  nephritic N23
  painter's NEC — *see* Poisoning, lead
  pancreas K86.89
  psychogenic F45.8
  renal N23
  saturnine NEC — *see* Poisoning, lead
  ureter N23
  urethral N36.8
    due to calculus N21.1
  uterus NEC N94.89
    menstrual — *see* Dysmenorrhea
  worm NOS B83.9
Colicystitis — *see* Cystitis
Colitis (acute) (catarrhal) (chronic) (noninfective) (hemorrhagic) (*see also* Enteritis) K52.9
  allergic K52.29
    with
      food protein-induced enterocolitis syndrome K52.21
      proctocolitis K52.82
  amebic (acute) (*see also* Amebiasis) A06.0
    nondysenteric A06.2
  anthrax A22.2
  bacillary — *see* Infection, Shigella
  balantidial A07.0
  Clostridium difficile
    not specified as recurrent A04.72
    recurrent A04.71
  coccidial A07.3
  collagenous K52.831
  cystica superficialis K52.89
  dietary counseling and surveillance (for) Z71.3
  dietetic (*see also* Colitis, allergic) K52.29
  drug-induced K52.1
  due to radiation K52.0
  eosinophilic K52.82
  food hypersensitivity (*see also* Colitis, allergic) K52.29
  giardial A07.1
  granulomatous — *see* Enteritis, regional, large intestine
  indeterminate, so stated K52.3
  infectious — *see* Enteritis, infectious
  ischemic K55.9
    acute (subacute) (*see also* Ischemia, intestine, acute) K55.039
    chronic K55.1
    due to mesenteric artery insufficiency K55.1
    fulminant (acute) (*see also* Ischemia, intestine, acute) K55.039
  left sided K51.50
    with
      abscess K51.514
      complication K51.519
        specified NEC K51.518
      fistula K51.513
      obstruction K51.512
      rectal bleeding K51.511
  lymphocytic K52.832
  membranous
    psychogenic F54
  microscopic K52.839
    specified NEC K52.838
  mucous — *see* Syndrome, irritable, bowel
    psychogenic F54
  noninfective K52.9
    specified NEC K52.89

Colitis — *continued*
  polyposa — *see* Polyp, colon, inflammatory
  protozoal A07.9
  pseudomembranous
    not specified as recurrent A04.72
    recurrent A04.71
  pseudomucinous — *see* Syndrome, irritable, bowel
  regional — *see* Enteritis, regional, large intestine
    infectious A09
  segmental — *see* Enteritis, regional, large intestine
  septic — *see* Enteritis, infectious
  spastic K58.9
    with diarrhea K58.0
    psychogenic F54
  staphylococcal A04.8
    foodborne A05.0
  subacute ischemic (*see also* Ischemia, intestine, acute) K55.039
  thromboulcerative (*see also* Ischemia, intestine, acute) K55.039
  toxic NEC K52.1
    due to Clostridium difficile
      not specified as recurrent A04.72
      recurrent A04.71
  transmural — *see* Enteritis, regional, large intestine
  trichomonal A07.8
  tuberculous (ulcerative) A18.32
  ulcerative (chronic) K51.90
    with
      complication K51.919
        abscess K51.914
        fistula K51.913
        obstruction K51.912
        rectal bleeding K51.911
        specified complication NEC K51.918
    enterocolitis — *see* Enterocolitis, ulcerative
    ileocolitis — *see* Ileocolitis, ulcerative
    mucosal proctocolitis — *see* Proctocolitis, mucosal
    proctitis — *see* Proctitis, ulcerative
    pseudopolyposis — *see* Polyp, colon, inflammatory
    psychogenic F54
    rectosigmoiditis — *see* Rectosigmoiditis, ulcerative
    specified type NEC K51.80
      with
        complication K51.819
          abscess K51.814
          fistula K51.813
          obstruction K51.812
          rectal bleeding K51.811
          specified complication NEC K51.818
Collagenosis, collagen disease (nonvascular) (vascular) M35.9
  cardiovascular I42.8
  reactive perforating L87.1
  specified NEC M35.8
Collapse R55
  adrenal E27.2
  cardiorespiratory R57.0
  cardiovascular R57.0
    newborn P29.89
  circulatory (peripheral) R57.9
    during or after labor and delivery O75.1
    following ectopic or molar pregnancy O08.3
    newborn P29.89
  during or
    after labor and delivery O75.1
    resulting from a procedure, not elsewhere classified T81.10 ☑
  external ear canal — *see* Stenosis, external ear canal
  general R55
  heart — *see* Disease, heart
  heat T67.1 ☑
  hysterical F44.89
  labyrinth, membranous (congenital) Q16.5
  lung (massive) (*see also* Atelectasis) J98.19
    pressure due to anesthesia (general) (local) or other sedation T88.2 ☑
      during labor and delivery O74.1
      in pregnancy O29.02 ☑
      postpartum, puerperal O89.09
  myocardial — *see* Disease, heart
  nervous F48.8
  neurocirculatory F45.8
  nose M95.0
  postoperative T81.10 ☑
  pulmonary (*see also* Atelectasis) J98.19
    newborn — *see* Atelectasis
  trachea J39.8
  tracheobronchial J98.09

Collapse — *continued*
  valvular — *see* Endocarditis
  vascular (peripheral) R57.9
    during or after labor and delivery O75.1
    following ectopic or molar pregnancy O08.3
    newborn P29.89
  vertebra M48.50 ☑
    cervical region M48.52 ☑
    cervicothoracic region M48.53 ☑
    in (due to)
      metastasis — *see* Collapse, vertebra, in, specified disease NEC
      osteoporosis (*see also* Osteoporosis) M80.88 ☑
        cervical region M80.88 ☑
        cervicothoracic region M80.88 ☑
        lumbar region M80.88 ☑
        lumbosacral region M80.88 ☑
        multiple sites M80.88 ☑
        occipito-atlanto-axial region M80.88 ☑
        sacrococcygeal region M80.88 ☑
        thoracic region M80.88 ☑
        thoracolumbar region M80.88 ☑
      specified disease NEC M48.50 ☑
        cervical region M48.52 ☑
        cervicothoracic region M48.53 ☑
        lumbar region M48.56 ☑
        lumbosacral region M48.57 ☑
        occipito-atlanto-axial region M48.51 ☑
        sacrococcygeal region M48.58 ☑
        thoracic region M48.54 ☑
        thoracolumbar region M48.55 ☑
    lumbar region M48.56 ☑
    lumbosacral region M48.57 ☑
    occipito-atlanto-axial region M48.51 ☑
    sacrococcygeal region M48.58 ☑
    thoracic region M48.54 ☑
    thoracolumbar region M48.55 ☑
Collateral (*see also* condition)
  circulation (venous) I87.8
  dilation, veins I87.8
Colles' fracture S52.53 ☑
Collet (-Sicard) syndrome G52.7
Collier's asthma or lung J60
Collodion baby Q80.2
Colloid nodule (of thyroid) (cystic) E04.1
Coloboma (iris) Q13.0
  eyelid Q10.3
  fundus Q14.8
  lens Q12.2
  optic disc (congenital) Q14.2
    acquired H47.31 ☑
Coloenteritis — *see* Enteritis
Colon — *see* condition
Colonization
  MRSA (Methicillin resistant Staphylococcus aureus) Z22.322
  MSSA (Methicillin susceptible Staphylococcus aureus) Z22.321
  status — *see* Carrier (suspected) of
Coloptosis K63.4
Color blindness — *see* Deficiency, color vision
Colostomy
  attention to Z43.3
  fitting or adjustment Z46.89
  malfunctioning K94.03
  status Z93.3
Colpitis (acute) — *see* Vaginitis
Colpocele N81.5
Colpocystitis — *see* Vaginitis
Colpospasm N94.2
Column, spinal, vertebral — *see* condition
Coma R40.20
  with
    motor response (none) R40.231 ☑
      abnormal R40.233 ☑
      abnormal extensor posturing to pain or noxious stimuli (< 2 years of age) R40.232 ☑
      abnormal flexure posturing to pain or noxious stimuli (0-5 years of age) R40.233 ☑
      extension R40.232 ☑
      extensor posturing to pain or noxious stimuli (2-5 years of age) R40.232 ☑
      flexion/decorticate posturing (< 2 years of age) R40.233 ☑
      flexion withdrawal R40.234 ☑
      localizes pain (2-5 years of age) R40.235 ☑
      normal or spontaneous movement (< 2 years of age) R40.236 ☑
      obeys commands (2-5 years of age) R40.236 ☑
    score of
      1 R40.231 ☑

☑ **Additional character required**

Coma — *continued*
  with — *continued*
    2 R40.232 ☑
    3 R40.233 ☑
    4 R40.234 ☑
    5 R40.235 ☑
    6 R40.236 ☑
    withdraws from pain or noxious stimuli (0-5 years of age) R40.234 ☑
    withdraws to touch (< 2 years of age) R40.235 ☑
    opening of eyes (never) R40.211 ☑
      in response to
        pain R40.212 ☑
        sound R40.213 ☑
      score of
        1 R40.211 ☑
        2 R40.212 ☑
        3 R40.213 ☑
        4 R40.214 ☑
      spontaneous R40.214 ☑
    verbal response (none) R40.221 ☑
      confused conversation R40.224 ☑
      cooing or babbling or crying appropriately (< 2 years of age) R40.225 ☑
      inappropriate crying or screaming (< 2 years of age) R40.223 ☑
      inappropriate words R40.223 ☑
      inappropriate words (2-5 years of age) R40.224 ☑
      incomprehensible sounds (2-5 years of age) R40.222 ☑
      incomprehensible words R40.222 ☑
      irritable cries (< 2 years of age) R40.224 ☑
      moans/grunts to pain; restless (< 2 years old) R40.222 ☑
      oriented R40.225 ☑
      score of
        1 R40.221 ☑
        2 R40.222 ☑
        3 R40.223 ☑
        4 R40.224 ☑
        5 R40.225 ☑
      screaming (2-5 years of age) R40.223 ☑
      uses appropriate words (2- 5 years of age) R40.225 ☑
  eclamptic — *see* Eclampsia
  epileptic — *see* Epilepsy
  Glasgow, scale score — *see* Glasgow coma scale
  hepatic — *see* Failure, hepatic, by type, with coma
  hyperglycemic (diabetic) — *see* Diabetes, by type, with hyperosmolarity, with coma
  hyperosmolar (diabetic) — *see* Diabetes, by type, with hyperosmolarity, with coma
  hypoglycemic (diabetic) — *see* Diabetes, by type, with hypoglycemia, with coma
    nondiabetic E15
  in diabetes — *see* Diabetes, coma
  insulin-induced — *see* Coma, hypoglycemic
  ketoacidotic (diabetic) — *see* Diabetes, by type, with ketoacidosis, with coma
  myxedematous E03.5
  newborn P91.5
  persistent vegetative state R40.3
  specified NEC, without documented Glasgow coma scale score, or with partial Glasgow coma scale score reported R40.244 ☑
Comatose — *see* Coma
Combat fatigue F43.0
Combined — *see* condition
Comedo, comedones (giant) L70.0
Comedocarcinoma (*see also* Neoplasm, breast, malignant)
  noninfiltrating
    breast D05.8 ☑
    specified site — *see* Neoplasm, in situ, by site
    unspecified site D05.8 ☑
Comedomastitis — *see* Ectasia, mammary duct
Comminuted fracture - code as Fracture, closed
Common
  arterial trunk Q20.0
  atrioventricular canal Q21.2
  atrium Q21.1
  cold (head) J00
  truncus (arteriosus) Q20.0
  variable immunodeficiency — *see* Immunodeficiency, common variable
  ventricle Q20.4
Commotio, commotion (current)
  brain — *see* Injury, intracranial, concussion
  cerebri — *see* Injury, intracranial, concussion
  retinae S05.8X ☑

Commotio — *continued*
  spinal cord — *see* Injury, spinal cord, by region
  spinalis — *see* Injury, spinal cord, by region
Communication
  between
    base of aorta and pulmonary artery Q21.4
    left ventricle and right atrium Q20.5
    pericardial sac and pleural sac Q34.8
    pulmonary artery and pulmonary vein, congenital Q25.72
  congenital between uterus and digestive or urinary tract Q51.7
Compartment syndrome (deep) (posterior) (traumatic) T79.A0 ☑
  abdomen T79.A3 ☑
  lower extremity (hip, buttock, thigh, leg, foot, toes) T79.A2 ☑
  nontraumatic
    abdomen M79.A3
    lower extremity (hip, buttock, thigh, leg, foot, toes) M79.A2 ☑
    specified site NEC M79.A9
    upper extremity (shoulder, arm, forearm, wrist, hand, fingers) M79.A1 ☑
  specified site NEC T79.A9 ☑
  upper extremity (shoulder, arm, forearm, wrist, hand, fingers) T79.A1 ☑
Compensation
  failure — *see* Disease, heart
  neurosis, psychoneurosis — *see* Disorder, factitious
Complaint (*see also* Disease)
  bowel, functional K59.9
    psychogenic F45.8
  intestine, functional K59.9
    psychogenic F45.8
  kidney — *see* Disease, renal
  miners' J60
Complete — *see* condition
Complex
  Addison-Schilder E71.528
  cardiorenal — *see* Hypertension, cardiorenal
  Costen's M26.69
  disseminated mycobacterium avium- intracellulare (DMAC) A31.2
  Eisenmenger's (ventricular septal defect) I27.83
  hypersexual F52.8
  jumped process, spine — *see* Dislocation, vertebra
  primary, tuberculous A15.7
  Schilder-Addison E71.528
  subluxation (vertebral) M99.19
    abdomen M99.19
    acromioclavicular M99.17
    cervical region M99.11
    cervicothoracic M99.11
    costochondral M99.18
    costovertebral M99.18
    head region M99.10
    hip M99.15
    lower extremity M99.16
    lumbar region M99.13
    lumbosacral M99.13
    occipitocervical M99.10
    pelvic region M99.15
    pubic M99.15
    rib cage M99.18
    sacral region M99.14
    sacrococcygeal M99.14
    sacroiliac M99.14
    specified NEC M99.19
    sternochondral M99.18
    sternoclavicular M99.17
    thoracic region M99.12
    thoracolumbar M99.12
    upper extremity M99.17
  Taussig-Bing (transposition, aorta and overriding pulmonary artery) Q20.1
Complication(s) (from) (of)
  accidental puncture or laceration during a procedure (of) — *see* Complications, intraoperative (intraprocedural), puncture or laceration
  amputation stump (surgical) (late) NEC T87.9
    dehiscence T87.81
    infection or inflammation T87.40
      lower limb T87.4 ☑
      upper limb T87.4 ☑
    necrosis T87.50
      lower limb T87.5 ☑
      upper limb T87.5 ☑
    neuroma T87.30
      lower limb T87.3 ☑
      upper limb T87.3 ☑

Complication(s) — *continued*
  amputation stump — *continued*
    specified type NEC T87.89
  anastomosis (and bypass) (*see also* Complications, prosthetic device or implant)
    intestinal (internal) NEC K91.89
      involving urinary tract N99.89
    urinary tract (involving intestinal tract) N99.89
    vascular — *see* Complications, cardiovascular device or implant
  anesthesia, anesthetic (*see also* Anesthesia, complication) T88.59 ☑
    brain, postpartum, puerperal O89.2
    cardiac
      in
        labor and delivery O74.2
        pregnancy O29.19 ☑
      postpartum, puerperal O89.1
    central nervous system
      in
        labor and delivery O74.3
        pregnancy O29.29 ☑
      postpartum, puerperal O89.2
    difficult or failed intubation T88.4 ☑
      in pregnancy O29.6 ☑
    failed sedation (conscious) (moderate) during procedure T88.52 ☑
    general, unintended awareness during procedure T88.53 ☑
    hyperthermia, malignant T88.3 ☑
    hypothermia T88.51 ☑
    intubation failure T88.4 ☑
    malignant hyperthermia T88.3 ☑
    pulmonary
      in
        labor and delivery O74.1
        pregnancy NEC O29.09 ☑
      postpartum, puerperal O89.09
    shock T88.2 ☑
    spinal and epidural
      in
        labor and delivery NEC O74.6
          headache O74.5
        pregnancy NEC O29.5X ☑
      postpartum, puerperal NEC O89.5
        headache O89.4
    unintended awareness under general anesthesia during procedure T88.53 ☑
  anti-reflux device — *see* Complications, esophageal anti-reflux device
  aortic (bifurcation) graft — *see* Complications, graft, vascular
  aortocoronary (bypass) graft — *see* Complications, coronary artery (bypass) graft
  aortofemoral (bypass) graft — *see* Complications, extremity artery (bypass) graft
  arteriovenous
    fistula, surgically created T82.9 ☑
      embolism T82.818 ☑
      fibrosis T82.828 ☑
      hemorrhage T82.838 ☑
      infection or inflammation T82.7 ☑
      mechanical
        breakdown T82.510 ☑
        displacement T82.520 ☑
        leakage T82.530 ☑
        malposition T82.520 ☑
        obstruction T82.590 ☑
        perforation T82.590 ☑
        protrusion T82.590 ☑
      pain T82.848 ☑
      specified type NEC T82.898 ☑
      stenosis T82.858 ☑
      thrombosis T82.868 ☑
    shunt, surgically created T82.9 ☑
      embolism T82.818 ☑
      fibrosis T82.828 ☑
      hemorrhage T82.838 ☑
      infection or inflammation T82.7 ☑
      mechanical
        breakdown T82.511 ☑
        displacement T82.521 ☑
        leakage T82.531 ☑
        malposition T82.521 ☑
        obstruction T82.591 ☑
        perforation T82.591 ☑
        protrusion T82.591 ☑
      pain T82.848 ☑
      specified type NEC T82.898 ☑
      stenosis T82.858 ☑
      thrombosis T82.868 ☑
  arthroplasty — *see* Complications, joint prosthesis

☑ **Additional character required**

Complication(s)

Complication(s) — *continued*
  artificial
    fertilization or insemination N98.9
      attempted introduction (of)
        embryo in embryo transfer N98.3
        ovum following in vitro fertilization N98.2
      hyperstimulation of ovaries N98.1
      infection N98.0
      specified NEC N98.8
    heart T82.9 ☑
      embolism T82.817 ☑
      fibrosis T82.827 ☑
      hemorrhage T82.837 ☑
      infection or inflammation T82.7 ☑
      mechanical
        breakdown T82.512 ☑
        displacement T82.522 ☑
        leakage T82.532 ☑
        malposition T82.522 ☑
        obstruction T82.592 ☑
        perforation T82.592 ☑
        protrusion T82.592 ☑
      pain T82.847 ☑
      specified type NEC T82.897 ☑
      stenosis T82.857 ☑
      thrombosis T82.867 ☑
  opening
    cecostomy — *see* Complications, colostomy
    colostomy — *see* Complications, colostomy
    cystostomy — *see* Complications, cystostomy
    enterostomy — *see* Complications, enterostomy
    gastrostomy — *see* Complications, gastrostomy
    ileostomy — *see* Complications, enterostomy
    jejunostomy — *see* Complications, enterostomy
    nephrostomy — *see* Complications, stoma,
      urinary tract
    tracheostomy — *see* Complications,
      tracheostomy
    ureterostomy — *see* Complications, stoma,
      urinary tract
    urethrostomy — *see* Complications, stoma,
      urinary tract
  balloon implant or device
    gastrointestinal T85.9 ☑
      embolism T85.818 ☑
      fibrosis T85.828 ☑
      hemorrhage T85.838 ☑
      infection and inflammation T85.79 ☑
      pain T85.848 ☑
      specified type NEC T85.898 ☑
      stenosis T85.858 ☑
      thrombosis T85.868 ☑
    vascular (counterpulsation) T82.9 ☑
      embolism T82.818 ☑
      fibrosis T82.828 ☑
      hemorrhage T82.838 ☑
      infection or inflammation T82.7 ☑
      mechanical
        breakdown T82.513 ☑
        displacement T82.523 ☑
        leakage T82.533 ☑
        malposition T82.523 ☑
        obstruction T82.593 ☑
        perforation T82.593 ☑
        protrusion T82.593 ☑
      pain T82.848 ☑
      specified type NEC T82.898 ☑
      stenosis T82.858 ☑
      thrombosis T82.868 ☑
  bariatric procedure
    gastric band procedure K95.09
      infection K95.01
    specified procedure NEC K95.89
      infection K95.81
  bile duct implant (prosthetic) T85.9 ☑
    embolism T85.818 ☑
    fibrosis T85.828 ☑
    hemorrhage T85.838 ☑
    infection and inflammation T85.79 ☑
    mechanical
      breakdown T85.510 ☑
      displacement T85.520 ☑
      malfunction T85.510 ☑
      malposition T85.520 ☑
      obstruction T85.590 ☑
      perforation T85.590 ☑
      protrusion T85.590 ☑
      specified NEC T85.590 ☑
    pain T85.848 ☑
    specified type NEC T85.898 ☑
    stenosis T85.858 ☑
    thrombosis T85.868 ☑

Complication(s) — *continued*
  bladder device (auxiliary) — *see* Complications,
    genitourinary, device or implant, urinary
    system
  bleeding (postoperative) — *see* Complication,
    postoperative, hemorrhage
    intraoperative — *see* Complication,
      intraoperative, hemorrhage
  blood vessel graft — *see* Complications, graft,
    vascular
  bone
    device NEC T84.9 ☑
      embolism T84.81 ☑
      fibrosis T84.82 ☑
      hemorrhage T84.83 ☑
      infection or inflammation T84.7 ☑
      mechanical
        breakdown T84.318 ☑
        displacement T84.328 ☑
        malposition T84.328 ☑
        obstruction T84.398 ☑
        perforation T84.398 ☑
        protrusion T84.398 ☑
      pain T84.84 ☑
      specified type NEC T84.89 ☑
      stenosis T84.85 ☑
      thrombosis T84.86 ☑
    graft — *see* Complications, graft, bone
    growth stimulator (electrode) — *see*
      Complications, electronic stimulator device,
      bone
    marrow transplant — *see* Complications,
      transplant, bone, marrow
  brain neurostimulator (electrode) — *see*
    Complications, electronic stimulator device,
    brain
  breast implant (prosthetic) T85.9 ☑
    capsular contracture T85.44 ☑
    embolism T85.818 ☑
    fibrosis T85.828 ☑
    hemorrhage T85.838 ☑
    infection and inflammation T85.79 ☑
    mechanical
      breakdown T85.41 ☑
      displacement T85.42 ☑
      leakage T85.43 ☑
      malposition T85.42 ☑
      obstruction T85.49 ☑
      perforation T85.49 ☑
      protrusion T85.49 ☑
      specified NEC T85.49 ☑
    pain T85.848 ☑
    specified type NEC T85.898 ☑
    stenosis T85.858 ☑
    thrombosis T85.868 ☑
  bypass (*see also* Complications, prosthetic device
    or implant)
    aortocoronary — *see* Complications, coronary
      artery (bypass) graft
    arterial (*see also* Complications, graft, vascular)
      extremity — *see* Complications, extremity
        artery (bypass) graft
  cardiac (*see also* Disease, heart)
    device, implant or graft T82.9 ☑
      embolism T82.817 ☑
      fibrosis T82.827 ☑
      hemorrhage T82.837 ☑
      infection or inflammation T82.7 ☑
        valve prosthesis T82.6 ☑
      mechanical
        breakdown T82.519 ☑
          specified device NEC T82.518 ☑
        displacement T82.529 ☑
          specified device NEC T82.528 ☑
        leakage T82.539 ☑
          specified device NEC T82.538 ☑
        malposition T82.529 ☑
          specified device NEC T82.528 ☑
        obstruction T82.599 ☑
          specified device NEC T82.598 ☑
        perforation T82.599 ☑
          specified device NEC T82.598 ☑
        protrusion T82.599 ☑
          specified device NEC T82.598 ☑
      pain T82.847 ☑
      specified type NEC T82.897 ☑
      stenosis T82.857 ☑
      thrombosis T82.867 ☑
  cardiovascular device, graft or implant T82.9 ☑
    aortic graft — *see* Complications, graft, vascular
    arteriovenous

Complication(s) — *continued*
  cardiovascular device — *continued*
    fistula, artificial — *see* Complication,
      arteriovenous, fistula, surgically created
    shunt — *see* Complication, arteriovenous,
      shunt, surgically created
  artificial heart — *see* Complication, artificial, heart
  balloon (counterpulsation) device — *see*
    Complication, balloon implant, vascular
  carotid artery graft — *see* Complications, graft,
    vascular
  coronary bypass graft — *see* Complication,
    coronary artery (bypass) graft
  dialysis catheter (vascular) — *see* Complication,
    catheter, dialysis
  electronic T82.9 ☑
    electrode T82.9 ☑
      embolism T82.817 ☑
      fibrosis T82.827 ☑
      hemorrhage T82.837 ☑
      infection T82.7 ☑
      mechanical
        breakdown T82.110 ☑
        displacement T82.120 ☑
        leakage T82.190 ☑
        obstruction T82.190 ☑
        perforation T82.190 ☑
        protrusion T82.190 ☑
        specified type NEC T82.190 ☑
      pain T82.847 ☑
      specified NEC T82.897 ☑
      stenosis T82.857 ☑
      thrombosis T82.867 ☑
    embolism T82.817 ☑
    fibrosis T82.827 ☑
    hemorrhage T82.837 ☑
    infection T82.7 ☑
    mechanical
      breakdown T82.119 ☑
      displacement T82.129 ☑
      leakage T82.199 ☑
      obstruction T82.199 ☑
      perforation T82.199 ☑
      protrusion T82.199 ☑
      specified type NEC T82.199 ☑
    pain T82.847 ☑
    pulse generator T82.9 ☑
      embolism T82.817 ☑
      fibrosis T82.827 ☑
      hemorrhage T82.837 ☑
      infection T82.7 ☑
      mechanical
        breakdown T82.111 ☑
        displacement T82.121 ☑
        leakage T82.191 ☑
        obstruction T82.191 ☑
        perforation T82.191 ☑
        protrusion T82.191 ☑
        specified type NEC T82.191 ☑
      pain T82.847 ☑
      specified NEC T82.897 ☑
      stenosis T82.857 ☑
      thrombosis T82.867 ☑
    specified condition NEC T82.897 ☑
    specified device NEC T82.9 ☑
      embolism T82.817 ☑
      fibrosis T82.827 ☑
      hemorrhage T82.837 ☑
      infection T82.7 ☑
      mechanical
        breakdown T82.118 ☑
        displacement T82.128 ☑
        leakage T82.198 ☑
        obstruction T82.198 ☑
        perforation T82.198 ☑
        protrusion T82.198 ☑
        specified type NEC T82.198 ☑
      pain T82.847 ☑
      specified NEC T82.897 ☑
      stenosis T82.857 ☑
      thrombosis T82.867 ☑
    stenosis T82.857 ☑
    thrombosis T82.867 ☑
  extremity artery graft — *see* Complication,
    extremity artery (bypass) graft
  femoral artery graft — *see* Complication,
    extremity artery (bypass) graft
  heart-lung transplant — *see* Complication,
    transplant, heart, with lung
  heart
    transplant — *see* Complication, transplant,
      heart

☑ **Additional character required**

Complication(s) — *continued*
cardiovascular device — *continued*
valve — *see* Complication, prosthetic device, heart valve
graft — *see* Complication, heart, valve, graft
infection or inflammation T82.7 ☑
umbrella device — *see* Complication, umbrella device, vascular
vascular graft (or anastomosis) — *see* Complication, graft, vascular
carotid artery (bypass) graft — *see* Complications, graft, vascular
catheter (device) NEC (*see also* Complications, prosthetic device or implant)
cranial infusion
infection and inflammation T85.735 ☑
mechanical
breakdown T85.610 ☑
displacement T85.620 ☑
leakage T85.630 ☑
malfunction T85.690 ☑
malposition T85.620 ☑
obstruction T85.690 ☑
perforation T85.690 ☑
protrusion T85.690 ☑
specified NEC T85.690 ☑
cystostomy T83.9 ☑
embolism T83.81 ☑
fibrosis T83.82 ☑
hemorrhage T83.83 ☑
infection and inflammation T83.510 ☑
mechanical
breakdown T83.010 ☑
displacement T83.020 ☑
leakage T83.030 ☑
malposition T83.020 ☑
obstruction T83.090 ☑
perforation T83.090 ☑
protrusion T83.090 ☑
specified NEC T83.090 ☑
pain T83.84 ☑
specified type NEC T83.89 ☑
stenosis T83.85 ☑
thrombosis T83.86 ☑
dialysis (vascular) T82.9 ☑
embolism T82.818 ☑
fibrosis T82.828 ☑
hemorrhage T82.838 ☑
infection and inflammation T82.7 ☑
intraperitoneal — *see* Complications, catheter, intraperitoneal
mechanical
breakdown T82.41 ☑
displacement T82.42 ☑
leakage T82.43 ☑
malposition T82.42 ☑
obstruction T82.49 ☑
perforation T82.49 ☑
protrusion T82.49 ☑
pain T82.848 ☑
specified type NEC T82.898 ☑
stenosis T82.858 ☑
thrombosis T82.868 ☑
epidural infusion T85.9 ☑
embolism T85.810 ☑
fibrosis T85.820 ☑
hemorrhage T85.830 ☑
infection and inflammation T85.735 ☑
mechanical
breakdown T85.610 ☑
displacement T85.620 ☑
leakage T85.630 ☑
malfunction T85.610 ☑
malposition T85.620 ☑
obstruction T85.690 ☑
perforation T85.690 ☑
protrusion T85.690 ☑
specified NEC T85.690 ☑
pain T85.840 ☑
specified type NEC T85.890 ☑
stenosis T85.850 ☑
thrombosis T85.860 ☑
intraperitoneal dialysis T85.9 ☑
embolism T85.818 ☑
fibrosis T85.828 ☑
hemorrhage T85.838 ☑
infection and inflammation T85.71 ☑
mechanical
breakdown T85.611 ☑
displacement T85.621 ☑
leakage T85.631 ☑
malfunction T85.611 ☑

Complication(s) — *continued*
catheter — *continued*
malposition T85.621 ☑
obstruction T85.691 ☑
perforation T85.691 ☑
protrusion T85.691 ☑
specified NEC T85.691 ☑
pain T85.848 ☑
specified type NEC T85.898 ☑
stenosis T85.858 ☑
thrombosis T85.868 ☑
intrathecal infusion
infection and inflammation T85.735 ☑
mechanical
breakdown T85.610 ☑
displacement T85.620 ☑
leakage T85.630 ☑
malfunction T85.690 ☑
malposition T85.620 ☑
obstruction T85.690 ☑
perforation T85.690 ☑
protrusion T85.690 ☑
specified NEC T85.690 ☑
intravenous infusion T82.9 ☑
embolism T82.818 ☑
fibrosis T82.828 ☑
hemorrhage T82.838 ☑
infection or inflammation T82.7 ☑
mechanical
breakdown T82.514 ☑
displacement T82.524 ☑
leakage T82.534 ☑
malposition T82.524 ☑
obstruction T82.594 ☑
perforation T82.594 ☑
protrusion T82.594 ☑
pain T82.848 ☑
specified type NEC T82.898 ☑
stenosis T82.858 ☑
thrombosis T82.868 ☑
spinal infusion
infection and inflammation T85.735 ☑
mechanical
breakdown T85.610 ☑
displacement T85.620 ☑
leakage T85.630 ☑
malfunction T85.690 ☑
malposition T85.620 ☑
obstruction T85.690 ☑
perforation T85.690 ☑
protrusion T85.690 ☑
specified NEC T85.690 ☑
subarachnoid infusion
infection and inflammation T85.735 ☑
mechanical
breakdown T85.610 ☑
displacement T85.620 ☑
leakage T85.630 ☑
malfunction T85.690 ☑
malposition T85.620 ☑
obstruction T85.690 ☑
perforation T85.690 ☑
protrusion T85.690 ☑
specified NEC T85.690 ☑
subdural infusion T85.9 ☑
embolism T85.810 ☑
fibrosis T85.820 ☑
hemorrhage T85.830 ☑
infection and inflammation T85.735 ☑
mechanical
breakdown T85.610 ☑
displacement T85.620 ☑
leakage T85.630 ☑
malfunction T85.610 ☑
malposition T85.620 ☑
obstruction T85.690 ☑
perforation T85.690 ☑
protrusion T85.690 ☑
specified NEC T85.690 ☑
pain T85.840 ☑
specified type NEC T85.890 ☑
stenosis T85.850 ☑
thrombosis T85.860 ☑
urethral T83.9 ☑
displacement T83.028 ☑
embolism T83.81 ☑
fibrosis T83.82 ☑
hemorrhage T83.83 ☑
indwelling
breakdown T83.011 ☑
displacement T83.021 ☑
infection and inflammation T83.511 ☑

Complication(s) — *continued*
catheter — *continued*
leakage T83.031 ☑
specified complication NEC T83.091 ☑
infection and inflammation T83.511 ☑
leakage T83.038 ☑
malposition T83.028 ☑
mechanical
breakdown T83.011 ☑
obstruction (mechanical) T83.091 ☑
pain T83.84 ☑
perforation T83.091 ☑
protrusion T83.091 ☑
specified type NEC T83.091 ☑
stenosis T83.85 ☑
thrombosis T83.86 ☑
urinary NEC
breakdown T83.018 ☑
displacement T83.028 ☑
infection and inflammation T83.518 ☑
leakage T83.038 ☑
specified complication NEC T83.098 ☑
cecostomy (stoma) — *see* Complications, colostomy
cesarean delivery wound NEC O90.89
disruption O90.0
hematoma O90.2
infection (following delivery) O86.00
chemotherapy (antineoplastic) NEC T88.7 ☑
chin implant (prosthetic) — *see* Complication, prosthetic device or implant, specified NEC
circulatory system I99.8
intraoperative I97.88
postprocedural I97.89
following cardiac surgery (*see also* Infarct, myocardium, associated with revascularization procedure) I97.19 ☑
postcardiotomy syndrome I97.0
hypertension I97.3
lymphedema after mastectomy I97.2
postcardiotomy syndrome I97.0
specified NEC I97.89
colostomy (stoma) K94.00
hemorrhage K94.01
infection K94.02
malfunction K94.03
mechanical K94.03
specified complication NEC K94.09
contraceptive device, intrauterine — *see* Complications, intrauterine, contraceptive device
cord (umbilical) — *see* Complications, umbilical cord
corneal graft — *see* Complications, graft, cornea
coronary artery (bypass) graft T82.9 ☑
atherosclerosis — *see* Arteriosclerosis, coronary (artery),
embolism T82.818 ☑
fibrosis T82.828 ☑
hemorrhage T82.838 ☑
infection and inflammation T82.7 ☑
mechanical
breakdown T82.211 ☑
displacement T82.212 ☑
leakage T82.213 ☑
malposition T82.212 ☑
obstruction T82.218 ☑
perforation T82.218 ☑
protrusion T82.218 ☑
specified NEC T82.218 ☑
pain T82.848 ☑
specified type NEC T82.898 ☑
stenosis T82.858 ☑
thrombosis T82.868 ☑
counterpulsation device (balloon), intra- aortic — *see* Complications, balloon implant, vascular
cystostomy (stoma) N99.518
catheter — *see* Complications, catheter, cystostomy
hemorrhage N99.510
infection N99.511
malfunction N99.512
specified type NEC N99.518
delivery (*see also* Complications, obstetric) O75.9
procedure (instrumental) (manual) (surgical) O75.4
specified NEC O75.89
dialysis (peritoneal) (renal) (*see also* Complications, infusion)
catheter (vascular) — *see* Complication, catheter, dialysis
peritoneal, intraperitoneal — *see* Complications, catheter, intraperitoneal

Complication(s)

Complication(s) — *continued*
  dorsal column (spinal) neurostimulator — *see* Complications, electronic stimulator device, spinal cord
  drug NEC T88.7 ☑
  ear procedure (*see also* Disorder, ear)
    intraoperative H95.88
      hematoma — *see* Complications, intraoperative, hemorrhage (hematoma) (of), ear
      hemorrhage — *see* Complications, intraoperative, hemorrhage (hematoma) (of), ear
      laceration — *see* Complications, intraoperative, puncture or laceration..., ear
      specified NEC H95.88
    postoperative H95.89
      external ear canal stenosis H95.81 ☑
      hematoma — *see* Complications, postprocedural, hematoma (of), ear
      hemorrhage — *see* Complications, postprocedural, hemorrhage (of), ear
      postmastoidectomy — *see* Complications, postmastoidectomy
      seroma — *see* Complications, postprocedural, seroma (of), mastoid process
      specified NEC H95.89
  ectopic pregnancy O08.9
    damage to pelvic organs O08.6
    embolism O08.2
    genital infection O08.0
    hemorrhage (delayed) (excessive) O08.1
    metabolic disorder O08.5
    renal failure O08.4
    shock O08.3
    specified type NEC O08.0
    venous complication NEC O08.7
  electronic stimulator device
    bladder (urinary) — *see* Complications, electronic stimulator device, urinary
    bone T84.9 ☑
      breakdown T84.310 ☑
      displacement T84.320 ☑
      embolism T84.81 ☑
      fibrosis T84.82 ☑
      hemorrhage T84.83 ☑
      infection or inflammation T84.7 ☑
      malfunction T84.310 ☑
      malposition T84.320 ☑
      mechanical NEC T84.390 ☑
      obstruction T84.390 ☑
      pain T84.84 ☑
      perforation T84.390 ☑
      protrusion T84.390 ☑
      specified type NEC T84.89 ☑
      stenosis T84.85 ☑
      thrombosis T84.86 ☑
    brain T85.9 ☑
      embolism T85.810 ☑
      fibrosis T85.820 ☑
      hemorrhage T85.830 ☑
      infection and inflammation T85.731 ☑
      mechanical
        breakdown T85.110 ☑
        displacement T85.120 ☑
        leakage T85.190 ☑
        malposition T85.120 ☑
        obstruction T85.190 ☑
        perforation T85.190 ☑
        protrusion T85.190 ☑
        specified NEC T85.190 ☑
      pain T85.840 ☑
      specified type NEC T85.890 ☑
      stenosis T85.850 ☑
      thrombosis T85.860 ☑
    cardiac (defibrillator) (pacemaker) — *see* Complications, cardiovascular device or implant, electronic
    generator (brain) (gastric) (peripheral) (sacral) (spinal)
      breakdown T85.113 ☑
      displacement T85.123 ☑
      leakage T85.193 ☑
      malposition T85.123 ☑
      obstruction T85.193 ☑
      perforation T85.193 ☑
      protrusion T85.193 ☑
      specified type NEC T85.193 ☑
    muscle T84.9 ☑
      breakdown T84.418 ☑
      displacement T84.428 ☑
      embolism T84.81 ☑
      fibrosis T84.82 ☑

Complication(s) — *continued*
  electronic stimulator device — *continued*
      hemorrhage T84.83 ☑
      infection or inflammation T84.7 ☑
      mechanical NEC T84.498 ☑
      pain T84.84 ☑
      specified type NEC T84.89 ☑
      stenosis T84.85 ☑
      thrombosis T84.86 ☑
    nervous system T85.9 ☑
      brain — *see* Complications, electronic stimulator device, brain
      cranial nerve — *see* Complications, electronic stimulator device, peripheral nerve
      embolism T85.810 ☑
      fibrosis T85.820 ☑
      gastric nerve — *see* Complications, electronic stimulator device, peripheral nerve
      hemorrhage T85.830 ☑
      infection and inflammation T85.738 ☑
      mechanical
        breakdown T85.118 ☑
        displacement T85.128 ☑
        leakage T85.199 ☑
        malposition T85.128 ☑
        obstruction T85.199 ☑
        perforation T85.199 ☑
        protrusion T85.199 ☑
        specified NEC T85.199 ☑
      pain T85.840 ☑
      peripheral nerve — *see* Complications, electronic stimulator device, peripheral nerve
      sacral nerve — *see* Complications, electronic stimulator device, peripheral nerve
      specified type NEC T85.890 ☑
      spinal cord — *see* Complications, electronic stimulator device, spinal cord
      stenosis T85.850 ☑
      thrombosis T85.860 ☑
      vagal nerve — *see* Complications, electronic stimulator device, peripheral nerve
    peripheral nerve T85.9 ☑
      embolism T85.810 ☑
      fibrosis T85.820 ☑
      hemorrhage T85.830 ☑
      infection and inflammation T85.732 ☑
      mechanical
        breakdown T85.111 ☑
        displacement T85.121 ☑
        leakage T85.191 ☑
        malposition T85.121 ☑
        obstruction T85.191 ☑
        perforation T85.191 ☑
        protrusion T85.191 ☑
        specified NEC T85.191 ☑
      pain T85.840 ☑
      specified type NEC T85.890 ☑
      stenosis T85.850 ☑
      thrombosis T85.860 ☑
    spinal cord T85.9 ☑
      embolism T85.810 ☑
      fibrosis T85.820 ☑
      hemorrhage T85.830 ☑
      infection and inflammation T85.733 ☑
      mechanical
        breakdown T85.112 ☑
        displacement T85.122 ☑
        leakage T85.192 ☑
        malposition T85.122 ☑
        obstruction T85.192 ☑
        perforation T85.192 ☑
        protrusion T85.192 ☑
        specified NEC T85.192 ☑
      pain T85.840 ☑
      specified type NEC T85.890 ☑
      stenosis T85.850 ☑
      thrombosis T85.860 ☑
    urinary T83.9 ☑
      embolism T83.81 ☑
      fibrosis T83.82 ☑
      hemorrhage T83.83 ☑
      infection and inflammation T83.598 ☑
      mechanical
        breakdown T83.110 ☑
        displacement T83.120 ☑
        malposition T83.120 ☑
        perforation T83.190 ☑
        protrusion T83.190 ☑
        specified NEC T83.190 ☑
      pain T83.84 ☑
      specified type NEC T83.89 ☑

Complication(s) — *continued*
  electronic stimulator device — *continued*
      stenosis T83.85 ☑
      thrombosis T83.86 ☑
  electroshock therapy T88.9 ☑
    specified NEC T88.8 ☑
  endocrine E34.9
    postprocedural
      adrenal hypofunction E89.6
      hypoinsulinemia E89.1
      hypoparathyroidism E89.2
      hypopituitarism E89.3
      hypothyroidism E89.0
      ovarian failure E89.40
        asymptomatic E89.40
        symptomatic E89.41
      specified NEC E89.89
      testicular hypofunction E89.5
  endodontic treatment NEC M27.59
  enterostomy (stoma) K94.10
    hemorrhage K94.11
    infection K94.12
    malfunction K94.13
    mechanical K94.13
    specified complication NEC K94.19
  episiotomy, disruption O90.1
  esophageal anti-reflux device T85.9 ☑
    embolism T85.818 ☑
    fibrosis T85.828 ☑
    hemorrhage T85.838 ☑
    infection and inflammation T85.79 ☑
    mechanical
      breakdown T85.511 ☑
      displacement T85.521 ☑
      malfunction T85.511 ☑
      malposition T85.521 ☑
      obstruction T85.591 ☑
      perforation T85.591 ☑
      protrusion T85.591 ☑
      specified NEC T85.591 ☑
    pain T85.848 ☑
    specified type NEC T85.898 ☑
    stenosis T85.858 ☑
    thrombosis T85.868 ☑
  esophagostomy K94.30
    hemorrhage K94.31
    infection K94.32
    malfunction K94.33
    mechanical K94.33
    specified complication NEC K94.39
  extracorporeal circulation T80.90 ☑
  extremity artery (bypass) graft T82.9 ☑
    arteriosclerosis — *see* Arteriosclerosis, extremities, bypass graft
    embolism T82.818 ☑
    fibrosis T82.828 ☑
    hemorrhage T82.838 ☑
    infection and inflammation T82.7 ☑
    mechanical
      breakdown T82.318 ☑
        femoral artery T82.312 ☑
      displacement T82.328 ☑
        femoral artery T82.322 ☑
      leakage T82.338 ☑
        femoral artery T82.332 ☑
      malposition T82.328 ☑
        femoral artery T82.322 ☑
      obstruction T82.398 ☑
        femoral artery T82.392 ☑
      perforation T82.398 ☑
        femoral artery T82.392 ☑
      protrusion T82.398 ☑
        femoral artery T82.392 ☑
    pain T82.848 ☑
    specified type NEC T82.898 ☑
    stenosis T82.858 ☑
    thrombosis T82.868 ☑
  eye H57.9
    corneal graft — *see* Complications, graft, cornea
    implant (prosthetic) T85.9 ☑
      embolism T85.818 ☑
      fibrosis T85.828 ☑
      hemorrhage T85.838 ☑
      infection and inflammation T85.79 ☑
      mechanical
        breakdown T85.318 ☑
        displacement T85.328 ☑
        leakage T85.398 ☑
        malposition T85.328 ☑
        obstruction T85.398 ☑
        perforation T85.398 ☑
        protrusion T85.398 ☑

☑ **Additional character required**

Complication(s) — *continued*
 eye — *continued*
   specified NEC T85.398 ☑
   pain T85.848 ☑
   specified type NEC T85.898 ☑
   stenosis T85.858 ☑
   thrombosis T85.868 ☑
  intraocular lens — *see* Complications, intraocular
   lens
  orbital prosthesis — *see* Complications, orbital
   prosthesis
 female genital N94.9
  device, implant or graft NEC — *see* Complications,
   genitourinary, device or implant, genital tract
 femoral artery (bypass) graft — *see* Complication,
  extremity artery (bypass) graft
 fixation device, internal (orthopedic) T84.9 ☑
  infection and inflammation T84.60 ☑
   arm T84.61 ☑
    humerus T84.61 ☑
    radius T84.61 ☑
    ulna T84.61 ☑
   leg T84.629 ☑
    femur T84.62 ☑
    fibula T84.62 ☑
    tibia T84.62 ☑
   specified site NEC T84.69 ☑
   spine T84.63 ☑
  mechanical
   breakdown
    limb T84.119 ☑
     carpal T84.210 ☑
     femur T84.11 ☑
     fibula T84.11 ☑
     humerus T84.11 ☑
     metacarpal T84.210 ☑
     metatarsal T84.213 ☑
     phalanx
      foot T84.213 ☑
      hand T84.210 ☑
     radius T84.11 ☑
     tarsal T84.213 ☑
     tibia T84.11 ☑
     ulna T84.11 ☑
    specified bone NEC T84.218 ☑
    spine T84.216 ☑
   displacement
    limb T84.129 ☑
     carpal T84.220 ☑
     femur T84.12 ☑
     fibula T84.12 ☑
     humerus T84.12 ☑
     metacarpal T84.220 ☑
     metatarsal T84.223 ☑
     phalanx
      foot T84.223 ☑
      hand T84.220 ☑
     radius T84.12 ☑
     tarsal T84.223 ☑
     tibia T84.12 ☑
     ulna T84.12 ☑
    specified bone NEC T84.228 ☑
    spine T84.226 ☑
   malposition — *see* Complications, fixation
    device, internal, mechanical, displacement
   obstruction — *see* Complications, fixation
    device, internal, mechanical, specified
    type NEC
   perforation — *see* Complications, fixation
    device, internal, mechanical, specified
    type NEC
   protrusion — *see* Complications, fixation
    device, internal, mechanical, specified
    type NEC
   specified type NEC
    limb T84.199 ☑
     carpal T84.290 ☑
     femur T84.19 ☑
     fibula T84.19 ☑
     humerus T84.19 ☑
     metacarpal T84.290 ☑
     metatarsal T84.293 ☑
     phalanx
      foot T84.293 ☑
      hand T84.290 ☑
     radius T84.19 ☑
     tarsal T84.293 ☑
     tibia T84.19 ☑
     ulna T84.19 ☑
    specified bone NEC T84.298 ☑
    vertebra T84.296 ☑
  specified type NEC T84.89 ☑

 fixation device — *continued*
   embolism T84.81 ☑
   fibrosis T84.82 ☑
   hemorrhage T84.83 ☑
   pain T84.84 ☑
   specified complication NEC T84.89 ☑
   stenosis T84.85 ☑
   thrombosis T84.86 ☑
 following
  acute myocardial infarction NEC I23.8
   aneurysm (false) (of cardiac wall) (of heart wall)
    (ruptured) I23.3
   angina I23.7
   atrial
    septal defect I23.1
    thrombosis I23.6
   cardiac wall rupture I23.3
   chordae tendinae rupture I23.4
   defect
    septal
     atrial (heart) I23.1
     ventricular (heart) I23.2
   hemopericardium I23.0
   papillary muscle rupture I23.5
   rupture
    cardiac wall I23.3
     with hemopericardium I23.0
    chordae tendineae I23.4
    papillary muscle I23.5
   specified NEC I23.8
   thrombosis
    atrium I23.6
    auricular appendage I23.6
    ventricle (heart) I23.6
   ventricular
    septal defect I23.2
    thrombosis I23.6
  ectopic or molar pregnancy O08.9
   cardiac arrest O08.81
   sepsis O08.82
   specified type NEC O08.89
   urinary tract infection O08.83
  termination of pregnancy — *see* Abortion
 gastrointestinal K92.9
  bile duct prosthesis — *see* Complications, bile
   duct implant
  esophageal anti-reflux device — *see*
   Complications, esophageal anti-reflux device
  postoperative
   colostomy — *see* Complications, colostomy
   dumping syndrome K91.1
   enterostomy — *see* Complications, enterostomy
   gastrostomy — *see* Complications, gastrostomy
   malabsorption NEC K91.2
   obstruction (*see also* Obstruction, intestine,
    postoperative) K91.30
   postcholecystectomy syndrome K91.5
   specified NEC K91.89
   vomiting after GI surgery K91.0
  prosthetic device or implant
   bile duct prosthesis — *see* Complications, bile
    duct implant
   esophageal anti-reflux device — *see*
    Complications, esophageal anti-reflux
    device
   specified type NEC
    embolism T85.818 ☑
    fibrosis T85.828 ☑
    hemorrhage T85.838 ☑
    mechanical
     breakdown T85.518 ☑
     displacement T85.528 ☑
     malfunction T85.518 ☑
     malposition T85.528 ☑
     obstruction T85.598 ☑
     perforation T85.598 ☑
     protrusion T85.598 ☑
     specified NEC T85.598 ☑
    pain T85.848 ☑
    specified complication NEC T85.898 ☑
    stenosis T85.858 ☑
    thrombosis T85.868 ☑
 gastrostomy (stoma) K94.20
  hemorrhage K94.21
  infection K94.22
  malfunction K94.23
  mechanical K94.23
  specified complication NEC K94.29
 genitourinary
  device or implant T83.9 ☑
   genital tract T83.9 ☑

 genitourinary — *continued*
    infection or inflammation T83.69 ☑
    intrauterine contraceptive device —
     see Complications, intrauterine,
     contraceptive device
    mechanical — *see* Complications, by device,
     mechanical
    mesh — *see* Complications, prosthetic device
     or implant, mesh
    penile prosthesis — *see* Complications,
     prosthetic device, penile
    specified type NEC T83.89 ☑
     embolism T83.81 ☑
     fibrosis T83.82 ☑
     hemorrhage T83.83 ☑
     pain T83.84 ☑
     specified complication NEC T83.89 ☑
     stenosis T83.85 ☑
     thrombosis T83.86 ☑
    vaginal mesh — *see* Complications, prosthetic
     device or implant, mesh
   urinary system T83.9 ☑
    cystostomy catheter — *see* Complication,
     catheter, cystostomy
    electronic stimulator — *see* Complications,
     electronic stimulator device, urinary
    indwelling urethral catheter — *see*
     Complications, catheter, urethral,
     indwelling
    infection or inflammation T83.598 ☑
     indwelling urethral catheter T83.511 ☑
    kidney transplant — *see* Complication,
     transplant, kidney
    organ graft — *see* Complication, graft, urinary
     organ
    specified type NEC T83.89 ☑
     embolism T83.81 ☑
     fibrosis T83.82 ☑
     hemorrhage T83.83 ☑
     mechanical T83.198 ☑
      breakdown T83.118 ☑
      displacement T83.128 ☑
      malfunction T83.118 ☑
      malposition T83.128 ☑
      obstruction T83.198 ☑
      perforation T83.198 ☑
      protrusion T83.198 ☑
      specified NEC T83.198 ☑
     sphincter, implanted T83.191 ☑
     stent (ileal conduit) (nephroureteral) T83.193 ☑
     ureteral indwelling T83.192 ☑
     pain T83.84 ☑
     specified complication NEC T83.89 ☑
     stenosis T83.85 ☑
     thrombosis T83.86 ☑
    sphincter implant — *see* Complications,
     implant, urinary sphincter
  postprocedural
   pelvic peritoneal adhesions N99.4
   renal failure N99.0
   specified NEC N99.89
   stoma — *see* Complications, stoma, urinary
    tract
   urethral stricture — *see* Stricture, urethra,
    postprocedural
   vaginal
    adhesions N99.2
    vault prolapse N99.3
 graft (bypass) (patch) (*see also* Complications,
  prosthetic device or implant)
  aorta — *see* Complications, graft, vascular
  arterial — *see* Complication, graft, vascular
  bone T86.839
   failure T86.831
   infection T86.832
   mechanical T84.318 ☑
    breakdown T84.318 ☑
    displacement T84.328 ☑
    protrusion T84.398 ☑
    specified type NEC T84.398 ☑
   rejection T86.830
   specified type NEC T86.838
  carotid artery — *see* Complications, graft, vascular
  cornea T86.849
   failure T86.841
   infection T86.842
   mechanical T85.398 ☑
    breakdown T85.318 ☑
    displacement T85.328 ☑
    protrusion T85.398 ☑
    specified type NEC T85.398 ☑

Complication(s)

Complication(s) — *continued*
  graft — *continued*
    rejection T86.840
    retroprosthetic membrane T85.398 ☑
    specified type NEC T86.848
  femoral artery (bypass) — *see* Complication, extremity artery (bypass) graft
  genital organ or tract — *see* Complications, genitourinary, device or implant, genital tract
  muscle T84.9 ☑
    breakdown T84.410 ☑
    displacement T84.420 ☑
    embolism T84.81 ☑
    fibrosis T84.82 ☑
    hemorrhage T84.83 ☑
    infection and inflammation T84.7 ☑
    mechanical NEC T84.490 ☑
    pain T84.84 ☑
    specified type NEC T84.89 ☑
    stenosis T84.85 ☑
    thrombosis T84.86 ☑
  nerve — *see* Complication, prosthetic device or implant, specified NEC
  skin — *see* Complications, prosthetic device or implant, skin graft
  tendon T84.9 ☑
    breakdown T84.410 ☑
    displacement T84.420 ☑
    embolism T84.81 ☑
    fibrosis T84.82 ☑
    hemorrhage T84.83 ☑
    infection and inflammation T84.7 ☑
    mechanical NEC T84.490 ☑
    pain T84.84 ☑
    specified type NEC T84.89 ☑
    stenosis T84.85 ☑
    thrombosis T84.86 ☑
  urinary organ T83.9 ☑
    embolism T83.81 ☑
    fibrosis T83.82 ☑
    hemorrhage T83.83 ☑
    infection and inflammation T83.598 ☑
      indwelling urethral catheter T83.511 ☑
    mechanical
      breakdown T83.21 ☑
      displacement T83.22 ☑
      erosion T83.24 ☑
      exposure T83.25 ☑
      leakage T83.23 ☑
      malposition T83.22 ☑
      obstruction T83.29 ☑
      perforation T83.29 ☑
      protrusion T83.29 ☑
      specified NEC T83.29 ☑
    pain T83.84 ☑
    specified type NEC T83.89 ☑
    stenosis T83.85 ☑
    thrombosis T83.86 ☑
  vascular T82.9 ☑
    embolism T82.818 ☑
    femoral artery — *see* Complication, extremity artery (bypass) graft
    fibrosis T82.828 ☑
    hemorrhage T82.838 ☑
    mechanical
      breakdown T82.319 ☑
        aorta (bifurcation) T82.310 ☑
        carotid artery T82.311 ☑
        specified vessel NEC T82.318 ☑
      displacement T82.329 ☑
        aorta (bifurcation) T82.320 ☑
        carotid artery T82.321 ☑
        specified vessel NEC T82.328 ☑
      leakage T82.339 ☑
        aorta (bifurcation) T82.330 ☑
        carotid artery T82.331 ☑
        specified vessel NEC T82.338 ☑
      malposition T82.329 ☑
        aorta (bifurcation) T82.320 ☑
        carotid artery T82.321 ☑
        specified vessel NEC T82.328 ☑
      obstruction T82.399 ☑
        aorta (bifurcation) T82.390 ☑
        carotid artery T82.391 ☑
        specified vessel NEC T82.398 ☑
      perforation T82.399 ☑
        aorta (bifurcation) T82.390 ☑
        carotid artery T82.391 ☑
        specified vessel NEC T82.398 ☑
      protrusion T82.399 ☑
        aorta (bifurcation) T82.390 ☑
        carotid artery T82.391 ☑

Complication(s) — *continued*
  graft — *continued*
      specified vessel NEC T82.398 ☑
    pain T82.848 ☑
    specified complication NEC T82.898 ☑
    stenosis T82.858 ☑
    thrombosis T82.868 ☑
  heart I51.9
    assist device
      infection and inflammation T82.7 ☑
    following acute myocardial infarction — *see* Complications, following, acute myocardial infarction
    postoperative — *see* Complications, circulatory system
    transplant — *see* Complication, transplant, heart and lung(s) — *see* Complications, transplant, heart, with lung
  valve
    graft (biological) T82.9 ☑
      embolism T82.817 ☑
      fibrosis T82.827 ☑
      hemorrhage T82.837 ☑
      infection and inflammation T82.7 ☑
      mechanical T82.228 ☑
        breakdown T82.221 ☑
        displacement T82.222 ☑
        leakage T82.223 ☑
        malposition T82.222 ☑
        obstruction T82.228 ☑
        perforation T82.228 ☑
        protrusion T82.228 ☑
      pain T82.847 ☑
      specified type NEC T82.897 ☑
      stenosis T82.857 ☑
      thrombosis T82.867 ☑
    prosthesis T82.9 ☑
      embolism T82.817 ☑
      fibrosis T82.827 ☑
      hemorrhage T82.837 ☑
      infection or inflammation T82.6 ☑
      mechanical T82.09 ☑
        breakdown T82.01 ☑
        displacement T82.02 ☑
        leakage T82.03 ☑
        malposition T82.02 ☑
        obstruction T82.09 ☑
        perforation T82.09 ☑
        protrusion T82.09 ☑
      pain T82.847 ☑
      specified type NEC T82.897 ☑
        mechanical T82.09 ☑
      stenosis T82.857 ☑
      thrombosis T82.867 ☑
  hematoma
    intraoperative — *see* Complication, intraoperative, hemorrhage
    postprocedural — *see* Complication, postprocedural, hematoma
  hemodialysis — *see* Complications, dialysis
  hemorrhage
    intraoperative — *see* Complication, intraoperative, hemorrhage
    postprocedural — *see* Complication, postprocedural, hemorrhage
  ileostomy (stoma) — *see* Complications, enterostomy
  immunization (procedure) — *see* Complications, vaccination
  implant (*see also* Complications, by site and type)
    urinary sphincter T83.9 ☑
      embolism T83.81 ☑
      fibrosis T83.82 ☑
      hemorrhage T83.83 ☑
      infection and inflammation T83.591 ☑
      mechanical
        breakdown T83.111 ☑
        displacement T83.121 ☑
        leakage T83.191 ☑
        malposition T83.121 ☑
        obstruction T83.191 ☑
        perforation T83.191 ☑
        protrusion T83.191 ☑
        specified NEC T83.191 ☑
      pain T83.84 ☑
      specified type NEC T83.89 ☑
      stenosis T83.85 ☑
      thrombosis T83.86 ☑
  infusion (procedure) T80.90 ☑
    air embolism T80.0 ☑
    blood — *see* Complications, transfusion
    catheter — *see* Complications, catheter

Complication(s) — *continued*
  infusion — *continued*
    infection T80.29 ☑
    pump — *see* Complications, cardiovascular, device or implant
    sepsis T80.29 ☑
    serum reaction (*see also* Reaction, serum) T80.69 ☑
      anaphylactic shock (*see also* Shock, anaphylactic) T80.59 ☑
    specified type NEC T80.89 ☑
  inhalation therapy NEC T81.81 ☑
  injection (procedure) T80.90 ☑
    drug reaction — *see* Reaction, drug
    infection T80.29 ☑
    sepsis T80.29 ☑
    serum (prophylactic) (therapeutic) — *see* Complications, vaccination
    specified type NEC T80.89 ☑
    vaccine (any) — *see* Complications, vaccination
  inoculation (any) — *see* Complications, vaccination
  insulin pump
    infection and inflammation T85.72 ☑
    mechanical
      breakdown T85.614 ☑
      displacement T85.624 ☑
      leakage T85.633 ☑
      malposition T85.624 ☑
      obstruction T85.694 ☑
      perforation T85.694 ☑
      protrusion T85.694 ☑
      specified NEC T85.694 ☑
  intestinal pouch NEC K91.858
  intraocular lens (prosthetic) T85.9 ☑
    embolism T85.818 ☑
    fibrosis T85.828 ☑
    hemorrhage T85.838 ☑
    infection and inflammation T85.79 ☑
    mechanical
      breakdown T85.21 ☑
      displacement T85.22 ☑
      malposition T85.22 ☑
      obstruction T85.29 ☑
      perforation T85.29 ☑
      protrusion T85.29 ☑
      specified NEC T85.29 ☑
    pain T85.848 ☑
    specified type NEC T85.898 ☑
    stenosis T85.858 ☑
    thrombosis T85.868 ☑
  intraoperative (intraprocedural)
    cardiac arrest (*see also* Infarct, myocardium, associated with revascularization procedure)
      during cardiac surgery I97.710
      during other surgery I97.711
    cardiac functional disturbance NEC (*see also* Infarct, myocardium, associated with revascularization procedure)
      during cardiac surgery I97.790
      during other surgery I97.791
    hemorrhage (hematoma) (of)
      circulatory system organ or structure
        during cardiac bypass I97.411
        during cardiac catheterization I97.410
        during other circulatory system procedure I97.418
        during other procedure I97.42
      digestive system organ
        during procedure on digestive system K91.61
        during procedure on other organ K91.62
      ear
        during procedure on ear and mastoid process H95.21
        during procedure on other organ H95.22
      endocrine system organ or structure
        during procedure on endocrine system organ or structure E36.01
        during procedure on other organ E36.02
      eye and adnexa
        during ophthalmic procedure H59.11 ☑
        during other procedure H59.12 ☑
      genitourinary organ or structure
        during procedure on genitourinary organ or structure N99.61
        during procedure on other organ N99.62
      mastoid process
        during procedure on ear and mastoid process H95.21
        during procedure on other organ H95.22
      musculoskeletal structure
        during musculoskeletal surgery M96.810
        during non-orthopedic surgery M96.811
        during orthopedic surgery M96.810

☑ **Additional character required**

Complication(s) — *continued*
  intraoperative — *continued*
    nervous system
      during a nervous system procedure G97.31
      during other procedure G97.32
    respiratory system
      during other procedure J95.62
      during procedure on respiratory system
        organ or structure J95.61
    skin and subcutaneous tissue
      during a dermatologic procedure L76.01
      during a procedure on other organ L76.02
    spleen
      during a procedure on other organ D78.02
      during a procedure on the spleen D78.01
  puncture or laceration (accidental)
      (unintentional) (of)
    brain
      during a nervous system procedure G97.48
      during other procedure G97.49
    circulatory system organ or structure
      during circulatory system procedure I97.51
      during other procedure I97.52
    digestive system
      during procedure on digestive system K91.71
      during procedure on other organ K91.72
    ear
      during procedure on ear and mastoid process
        H95.31
      during procedure on other organ H95.32
    endocrine system organ or structure
      during procedure on endocrine system organ
        or structure E36.11
      during procedure on other organ E36.12
    eye and adnexa
      during ophthalmic procedure H59.21 ☑
      during other procedure H59.22 ☑
    genitourinary organ or structure
      during procedure on genitourinary organ or
        structure N99.71
      during procedure on other organ N99.72
    mastoid process
      during procedure on ear and mastoid process
        H95.31
      during procedure on other organ H95.32
    musculoskeletal structure
      during musculoskeletal surgery M96.820
      during non-orthopedic surgery M96.821
      during orthopedic surgery M96.820
    nervous system
      during a nervous system procedure G97.48
      during other procedure G97.49
    respiratory system
      during other procedure J95.72
      during procedure on respiratory system
        organ or structure J95.71
    skin and subcutaneous tissue
      during a dermatologic procedure L76.11
      during a procedure on other organ L76.12
    spleen
      during a procedure on other organ D78.12
      during a procedure on the spleen D78.11
  specified NEC
    circulatory system I97.88
    digestive system K91.81
    ear H95.88
    endocrine system E36.8
    eye and adnexa H59.88
    genitourinary system N99.81
    mastoid process H95.88
    musculoskeletal structure M96.89
    nervous system G97.81
    respiratory system J95.88
    skin and subcutaneous tissue L76.81
    spleen D78.81
  intraperitoneal catheter (dialysis) (infusion) — *see*
      Complications, catheter, intraperitoneal
  intrathecal infusion pump
    infection and inflammation T85.738 ☑
    mechanical
      breakdown T85.615 ☑
      displacement T85.625 ☑
      leakage T85.635 ☑
      malfunction T85.695 ☑
      malposition T85.625 ☑
      obstruction T85.695 ☑
      perforation T85.695 ☑
      protrusion T85.695 ☑
      specified NEC T85.695 ☑
  intrauterine
    contraceptive device
      embolism T83.81 ☑

Complication(s) — *continued*
  intrauterine — *continued*
    fibrosis T83.82 ☑
    hemorrhage T83.83 ☑
    infection and inflammation T83.69 ☑
    mechanical
      breakdown T83.31 ☑
      displacement T83.32 ☑
      malposition T83.32 ☑
      obstruction T83.39 ☑
      perforation T83.39 ☑
      protrusion T83.39 ☑
      specified NEC T83.39 ☑
    pain T83.84 ☑
    specified type NEC T83.89 ☑
    stenosis T83.85 ☑
    thrombosis T83.86 ☑
  procedure (fetal), to newborn P96.5
  jejunostomy (stoma) — *see* Complications,
      enterostomy
  joint prosthesis, internal T84.9 ☑
    breakage (fracture) T84.01 ☑
    dislocation T84.02 ☑
    fracture T84.01 ☑
    infection or inflammation T84.50 ☑
      hip T84.5 ☑
      knee T84.5 ☑
      specified joint NEC T84.59 ☑
    instability T84.02 ☑
    malposition — *see* Complications, joint
        prosthesis, mechanical, displacement
    mechanical
      breakage, broken T84.01 ☑
      dislocation T84.02 ☑
      fracture T84.01 ☑
      instability T84.02 ☑
      leakage — *see* Complications, joint prosthesis,
          mechanical, specified NEC
      loosening T84.039 ☑
        hip T84.03 ☑
        knee T84.03 ☑
        specified joint NEC T84.038 ☑
      obstruction — *see* Complications, joint
          prosthesis, mechanical, specified NEC
      perforation — *see* Complications, joint
          prosthesis, mechanical, specified NEC
      osteolysis T84.059 ☑
        hip T84.05 ☑
        knee T84.05 ☑
        other specified joint T84.058 ☑
      periprosthetic T84.059 ☑
      protrusion — *see* Complications, joint
          prosthesis, mechanical, specified NEC
      specified complication NEC T84.099 ☑
        hip T84.09 ☑
        knee T84.09 ☑
        other specified joint T84.098 ☑
      subluxation T84.02 ☑
      wear of articular bearing surface T84.069 ☑
        hip T84.06 ☑
        knee T84.06 ☑
        other specified joint T84.068 ☑
    specified joint NEC T84.89 ☑
      embolism T84.81 ☑
      fibrosis T84.82 ☑
      hemorrhage T84.83 ☑
      pain T84.84 ☑
      specified complication NEC T84.89 ☑
      stenosis T84.85 ☑
      thrombosis T84.86 ☑
      subluxation T84.02 ☑
  kidney transplant — *see* Complications, transplant,
      kidney
  labor O75.9
    specified NEC O75.89
  liver transplant (immune or nonimmune) — *see*
      Complications, transplant, liver
  lumbar puncture G97.1
    cerebrospinal fluid leak G97.0
    headache or reaction G97.1
  lung transplant — *see* Complications, transplant,
      lung
    and heart — *see* Complications, transplant, lung,
        with heart
  male genital N50.9
    device, implant or graft — *see* Complications,
        genitourinary, device or implant, genital tract
    postprocedural or postoperative — *see*
        Complications, genitourinary, postprocedural
      specified NEC N99.89
  mastoid (process) procedure
    intraoperative H95.88

Complication(s) — *continued*
  mastoid — *continued*
    hematoma — *see* Complications, intraoperative,
        hemorrhage (hematoma) (of), mastoid
        process
    hemorrhage — *see* Complications,
        intraoperative, hemorrhage (hematoma)
        (of), mastoid process
    laceration — *see* Complications, intraoperative,
        puncture or laceration..., mastoid process
    specified NEC H95.88
    postmastoidectomy — *see* Complications,
        postmastoidectomy
    postoperative H95.89
      external ear canal stenosis H95.81 ☑
      hematoma — *see* Complications...,
          postprocedural, hematoma (of), mastoid
          process
      hemorrhage — *see* Complications...,
          postprocedural, hemorrhage (of), mastoid
          process
      postmastoidectomy — *see* Complications,
          postmastoidectomy
      seroma — *see* Complications, postprocedural,
          seroma (of), mastoid process
      specified NEC H95.89
  mastoidectomy cavity — *see* Complications,
      postmastoidectomy
  mechanical — *see* Complications, by site and type,
      mechanical
  medical procedures (*see also* Complication(s),
      intraoperative) T88.9 ☑
  metabolic E88.9
    postoperative E89.89
    specified NEC E89.89
  molar pregnancy NOS O08.9
    damage to pelvic organs O08.6
    embolism O08.2
    genital infection O08.0
    hemorrhage (delayed) (excessive) O08.1
    metabolic disorder O08.5
    renal failure O08.4
    shock O08.3
    specified type NEC O08.0
    venous complication NEC O08.7
  musculoskeletal system (*see also* Complication,
      intraoperative (intraprocedural), by site)
    device, implant or graft NEC — *see* Complications,
        orthopedic, device or implant
    internal fixation (nail) (plate) (rod) — *see*
        Complications, fixation device, internal
    joint prosthesis — *see* Complications, joint
        prosthesis
    postoperative (postprocedural) M96.89
      with osteoporosis — *see* Osteoporosis
      fracture following insertion of device — *see*
          Fracture, following insertion of orthopedic
          implant, joint prosthesis or bone plate
      joint instability after prosthesis removal M96.89
      lordosis M96.4
      postlaminectomy syndrome NEC M96.1
        kyphosis M96.3
      pseudarthrosis M96.0
      specified complication NEC M96.89
    post radiation M96.89
      kyphosis M96.2
      scoliosis M96.5
      specified complication NEC M96.89
  nephrostomy (stoma) — *see* Complications, stoma,
      urinary tract, external NEC
  nervous system G98.8
    central G96.9
    device, implant or graft (*see also* Complication,
        prosthetic device or implant, specified NEC)
      electronic stimulator (electrode(s)) — *see*
          Complications, electronic stimulator device
      specified NEC
        infection and inflammation T85.738 ☑
        mechanical T85.695 ☑
          breakdown T85.615 ☑
          displacement T85.625 ☑
          leakage T85.635 ☑
          malfunction T85.695 ☑
          malposition T85.625 ☑
          obstruction T85.695 ☑
          perforation T85.695 ☑
          protrusion T85.695 ☑
          specified NEC T85.695 ☑
      ventricular shunt — *see* Complications,
          ventricular shunt
      electronic stimulator (electrode(s)) — *see*
          Complications, electronic stimulator device

Complication(s)

Complication(s) — *continued*
  nervous system — *continued*
    postprocedural G97.82
      intracranial hypotension G97.2
      specified NEC G97.82
      spinal fluid leak G97.0
  newborn, due to intrauterine (fetal) procedure P96.5
  nonabsorbable (permanent) sutures — *see* Complication, sutures, permanent
  obstetric O75.9
    procedure (instrumental) (manual) (surgical) specified NEC O75.4
    specified NEC O75.89
    surgical wound NEC O90.89
      hematoma O90.2
      infection O86.00
  ocular lens implant — *see* Complications, intraocular lens
  ophthalmologic
    postprocedural bleb — *see* Blebitis
  orbital prosthesis T85.9 ☑
    embolism T85.818 ☑
    fibrosis T85.828 ☑
    hemorrhage T85.838 ☑
    infection and inflammation T85.79 ☑
    mechanical
      breakdown T85.31 ☑
      displacement T85.32 ☑
      malposition T85.32 ☑
      obstruction T85.39 ☑
      perforation T85.39 ☑
      protrusion T85.39 ☑
      specified NEC T85.39 ☑
    pain T85.848 ☑
    specified type NEC T85.898 ☑
    stenosis T85.858 ☑
    thrombosis T85.868 ☑
  organ or tissue transplant (partial) (total) — *see* Complications, transplant
  orthopedic (*see also* Disorder, soft tissue)
    device or implant T84.9 ☑
      bone
        device or implant — *see* Complication, bone, device NEC
        graft — *see* Complication, graft, bone
      breakdown T84.418 ☑
      displacement T84.428 ☑
      electronic bone stimulator — *see* Complications, electronic stimulator device, bone
      embolism T84.81 ☑
      fibrosis T84.82 ☑
      fixation device — *see* Complication, fixation device, internal
      hemorrhage T84.83 ☑
      infection or inflammation T84.7 ☑
      joint prosthesis — *see* Complication, joint prosthesis, internal
      malfunction T84.418 ☑
      malposition T84.428 ☑
      mechanical NEC T84.498 ☑
      muscle graft — *see* Complications, graft, muscle
      obstruction T84.498 ☑
      pain T84.84 ☑
      perforation T84.498 ☑
      protrusion T84.498 ☑
      specified complication NEC T84.89 ☑
      stenosis T84.85 ☑
      tendon graft — *see* Complications, graft, tendon
      thrombosis T84.86 ☑
    fracture (following insertion of device) — *see* Fracture, following insertion of orthopedic implant, joint prosthesis or bone plate
    postprocedural M96.89
      fracture — *see* Fracture, following insertion of orthopedic implant, joint prosthesis or bone plate
      postlaminectomy syndrome NEC M96.1
        kyphosis M96.3
        lordosis M96.4
      postradiation
        kyphosis M96.2
        scoliosis M96.5
      pseudarthrosis post-fusion M96.0
      specified type NEC M96.89
  pacemaker (cardiac) — *see* Complications, cardiovascular device or implant, electronic
  pancreas transplant — *see* Complications, transplant, pancreas

Complication(s) — *continued*
  penile prosthesis (implant) — *see* Complications, prosthetic device, penile
  perfusion NEC T80.90 ☑
  perineal repair (obstetrical) NEC O90.89
    disruption O90.1
    hematoma O90.2
    infection (following delivery) O86.09
  phototherapy T88.9 ☑
    specified NEC T88.8 ☑
  postmastoidectomy NEC H95.19 ☑
    cyst, mucosal H95.13 ☑
    granulation H95.12 ☑
    inflammation, chronic H95.11 ☑
    recurrent cholesteatoma H95.0 ☑
  postoperative — *see* Complications, postprocedural
    circulatory — *see* Complications, circulatory system
    ear — *see* Complications, ear
    endocrine — *see* Complications, endocrine
    eye — *see* Complications, eye
    lumbar puncture G97.1
      cerebrospinal fluid leak G97.0
    nervous system (central) (peripheral) — *see* Complications, nervous system
    respiratory system — *see* Complications, respiratory system
  postprocedural (*see also* Complications, surgical procedure)
    cardiac arrest (*see also* Infarct, myocardium, associated with revascularization procedure)
      following cardiac surgery I97.120
      following other surgery I97.121
    cardiac functional disturbance NEC (*see also* Infarct, myocardium, associated with revascularization procedure)
      following cardiac surgery I97.190
      following other surgery I97.191
    cardiac insufficiency
      following cardiac surgery I97.110
      following other surgery I97.111
    chorioretinal scars following retinal surgery H59.81 ☑
    following cataract surgery
      cataract (lens) fragments H59.02 ☑
      cystoid macular edema H59.03 ☑
      specified NEC H59.09 ☑
      vitreous (touch) syndrome H59.01 ☑
    heart failure
      following cardiac surgery I97.130
      following other surgery I97.131
    hematoma (of)
      circulatory system organ or structure
        following cardiac bypass I97.631
        following cardiac catheterization I97.630
        following other circulatory system procedure I97.638
        following other procedure I97.621
      digestive system
        following procedure on digestive system K91.870
        following procedure on other organ K91.871
      ear
        following other procedure H95.52
        following procedure on ear and mastoid process H95.51
      endocrine system
        following endocrine system procedure E89.820
        following other procedure E89.821
      eye and adnexa
        following ophthalmic procedure H59.33 ☑
        following other procedure H59.34 ☑
      genitourinary organ or structure
        following procedure on genitourinary organ or structure N99.840
        following procedure on other organ N99.841
      mastoid process
        following other procedure H95.52
        following procedure on ear and mastoid process H95.51
      musculoskeletal structure
        following musculoskeletal surgery M96.840
        following non-orthopedic surgery M96.841
        following orthopedic surgery M96.840
      nervous system
        following nervous system procedure G97.61
        following other procedure G97.62
      respiratory system
        following other procedure J95.861
        following procedure on respiratory system organ or structure J95.860

Complication(s) — *continued*
  postprocedural — *continued*
    skin and subcutaneous tissue
      following dermatologic procedure L76.31
      following procedure on other organ L76.32
    spleen
      following procedure on other organ D78.32
      following procedure on the spleen D78.31
    hemorrhage (of)
      circulatory system organ or structure
        following cardiac bypass I97.611
        following cardiac catheterization I97.610
        following other circulatory system procedure I97.618
        following other procedure I97.620
      digestive system
        following procedure on digestive system K91.840
        following procedure on other organ K91.841
      ear
        following other procedure H95.42
        following procedure on ear and mastoid process H95.41
      endocrine system
        following endocrine system procedure E89.810
        following other procedure E89.811
      eye and adnexa
        following ophthalmic procedure H59.31 ☑
        following other procedure H59.32 ☑
      genitourinary organ or structure
        following procedure on genitourinary organ or structure N99.820
        following procedure on other organ N99.821
      mastoid process
        following other procedure H95.42
        following procedure on ear and mastoid process H95.41
      musculoskeletal structure
        following musculoskeletal surgery M96.830
        following non-orthopedic surgery M96.831
        following orthopedic surgery M96.830
      nervous system
        following nervous system procedure G97.51
        following other procedure G97.52
      respiratory system
        following other procedure J95.831
        following procedure on respiratory system organ or structure J95.830
      skin and subcutaneous tissue
        following dermatologic procedure L76.21
        following a procedure on other organ L76.22
      spleen
        following procedure on other organ D78.22
        following procedure on the spleen D78.21
    seroma (of)
      circulatory system organ or structure
        following cardiac bypass I97.641
        following cardiac catheterization I97.640
        following other circulatory system procedure I97.648
        following other procedure I97.622
      digestive system
        following procedure on digestive system K91.872
        following procedure on other organ K91.873
      ear
        following other procedure H95.54
        following procedure on ear and mastoid process H95.53
      endocrine system
        following endocrine system procedure E89.822
        following other procedure E89.823
      eye and adnexa
        following ophthalmic procedure H59.35 ☑
        following other procedure H59.36 ☑
      genitourinary organ or structure
        following procedure on genitourinary organ or structure N99.842
        following procedure on other organ N99.843
      mastoid process
        following other procedure H95.54
        following procedure on ear and mastoid process H95.53
      musculoskeletal structure
        following musculoskeletal surgery M96.842
        following non-orthopedic surgery M96.843
        following orthopedic surgery M96.842
      nervous system
        following nervous system procedure G97.63
        following other procedure G97.64

☑ **Additional character required**

Complication(s) — *continued*
  postprocedural — *continued*
    respiratory system
      following other procedure J95.863
      following procedure on respiratory system
        organ or structure J95.862
    skin and subcutaneous tissue
      following dermatologic procedure L76.33
      following procedure on other organ L76.34
    spleen
      following procedure on other organ D78.34
      following procedure on the spleen D78.33
    specified NEC
      circulatory system I97.89
      digestive K91.89
      ear H95.89
      endocrine E89.89
      eye and adnexa H59.89
      genitourinary N99.89
      mastoid process H95.89
      metabolic E89.89
      musculoskeletal structure M96.89
      nervous system G97.82
      respiratory system J95.89
      skin and subcutaneous tissue L76.82
      spleen D78.89
  pregnancy NEC — *see* Pregnancy, complicated by
  prosthetic device or implant T85.9 ☑
    bile duct — *see* Complications, bile duct implant
    breast — *see* Complications, breast implant
    bulking agent
      ureteral
        erosion T83.714 ☑
        exposure T83.724 ☑
      urethral
        erosion T83.713 ☑
        exposure T83.723 ☑
    cardiac and vascular NEC — *see* Complications,
      cardiovascular device or implant
    corneal transplant — *see* Complications, graft,
      cornea
    electronic nervous system stimulator — *see*
      Complications, electronic stimulator device
    epidural infusion catheter — *see* Complications,
      catheter, epidural
    esophageal anti-reflux device — *see*
      Complications, esophageal anti-reflux device
    genital organ or tract — *see* Complications,
      genitourinary, device or implant, genital tract
      specified NEC T83.79 ☑
    heart valve — *see* Complications, heart, valve,
      prosthesis
    infection or inflammation T85.79 ☑
      intestine transplant T86.892
      liver transplant T86.43
      lung transplant T86.812
      pancreas transplant T86.892
      skin graft T86.822
    intraocular lens — *see* Complications, intraocular
      lens
    intraperitoneal (dialysis) catheter — *see*
      Complications, catheter, intraperitoneal
    joint — *see* Complications, joint prosthesis,
      internal
    mechanical NEC T85.698 ☑
      dialysis catheter (vascular) (*see also*
        Complication, catheter, dialysis,
        mechanical)
        peritoneal — *see* Complication, catheter,
          intraperitoneal, mechanical
      gastrointestinal device T85.598 ☑
      ocular device T85.398 ☑
      subdural (infusion) catheter T85.690 ☑
      suture, permanent T85.692 ☑
        that for bone repair — *see* Complications,
          fixation device, internal (orthopedic),
          mechanical
      ventricular shunt
        breakdown T85.01 ☑
        displacement T85.02 ☑
        leakage T85.03 ☑
        malposition T85.02 ☑
        obstruction T85.09 ☑
        perforation T85.09 ☑
        protrusion T85.09 ☑
        specified NEC T85.09 ☑
    mesh
      erosion (to surrounding organ or tissue)
        T83.718 ☑
      urethral (into pelvic floor muscles) T83.712 ☑
      vaginal (into pelvic floor muscles) T83.711 ☑

Complication(s) — *continued*
  prosthetic device — *continued*
    exposure (into surrounding organ or tissue)
      T83.728 ☑
      urethral (through urethral wall) T83.722 ☑
      vaginal (into vagina) (through vaginal wall)
        T83.721 ☑
    orbital — *see* Complications, orbital prosthesis
    penile T83.9 ☑
      embolism T83.81 ☑
      fibrosis T83.82 ☑
      hemorrhage T83.83 ☑
      infection and inflammation T83.61 ☑
      mechanical
        breakdown T83.410 ☑
        displacement T83.420 ☑
        leakage T83.490 ☑
        malposition T83.420 ☑
        obstruction T83.490 ☑
        perforation T83.490 ☑
        protrusion T83.490 ☑
        specified NEC T83.490 ☑
      pain T83.84 ☑
      specified type NEC T83.89 ☑
      stenosis T83.85 ☑
      thrombosis T83.86 ☑
    prosthetic materials NEC
      erosion (to surrounding organ or tissue)
        T83.718 ☑
      exposure (into surrounding organ or tissue)
        T83.728 ☑
    skin graft T86.829
      artificial skin or decellularized allodermis
        embolism T85.818 ☑
        fibrosis T85.828 ☑
        hemorrhage T85.838 ☑
        infection and inflammation T85.79 ☑
        mechanical
          breakdown T85.613 ☑
          displacement T85.623 ☑
          malfunction T85.613 ☑
          malposition T85.623 ☑
          obstruction T85.693 ☑
          perforation T85.693 ☑
          protrusion T85.693 ☑
          specified NEC T85.693 ☑
        pain T85.848 ☑
        specified type NEC T85.898 ☑
        stenosis T85.858 ☑
        thrombosis T85.868 ☑
      failure T86.821
      infection T86.822
      rejection T86.820
      specified NEC T86.828
    sling
      urethral (female) (male)
        erosion T83.712 ☑
        exposure T83.722 ☑
    specified NEC T85.9 ☑
      embolism T85.818 ☑
      fibrosis T85.828 ☑
      hemorrhage T85.838 ☑
      infection and inflammation T85.79 ☑
      mechanical
        breakdown T85.618 ☑
        displacement T85.628 ☑
        leakage T85.638 ☑
        malfunction T85.618 ☑
        malposition T85.628 ☑
        obstruction T85.698 ☑
        perforation T85.698 ☑
        protrusion T85.698 ☑
        specified NEC T85.698 ☑
      pain T85.848 ☑
      specified type NEC T85.898 ☑
      stenosis T85.858 ☑
      thrombosis T85.868 ☑
    subdural infusion catheter — *see* Complications,
      catheter, subdural
    sutures — *see* Complications, sutures
    urinary organ or tract NEC — *see* Complications,
      genitourinary, device or implant, urinary
      system
    vascular — *see* Complications, cardiovascular
      device or implant
    ventricular shunt — *see* Complications,
      ventricular shunt (device)
  puerperium — *see* Puerperal
  puncture, spinal G97.1
    cerebrospinal fluid leak G97.0
    headache or reaction G97.1
  pyelogram N99.89

Complication(s) — *continued*
  radiation
    kyphosis M96.2
    scoliosis M96.5
  reattached
    extremity (infection) (rejection)
      lower T87.1X ☑
      upper T87.0X ☑
    specified body part NEC T87.2
  reconstructed breast
    asymmetry between native and reconstructed
      breast N65.1
    deformity N65.0
    disproportion between native and reconstructed
      breast N65.1
    excess tissue N65.0
    misshapen N65.0
  reimplant NEC (*see also* Complications, prosthetic
    device or implant)
    limb (infection) (rejection) — *see* Complications,
      reattached, extremity
    organ (partial) (total) — *see* Complications,
      transplant
    prosthetic device NEC — *see* Complications,
      prosthetic device
  renal N28.9
    allograft — *see* Complications, transplant, kidney
    dialysis — *see* Complications, dialysis
  respirator
    mechanical J95.850
      specified NEC J95.859
  respiratory system J98.9
    device, implant or graft — *see* Complication,
      prosthetic device or implant, specified NEC
    lung transplant — *see* Complications, prosthetic
      device or implant, lung transplant
    postoperative J95.89
      air leak J95.812
      Mendelson's syndrome (chemical pneumonitis)
        J95.4
      pneumothorax J95.811
      pulmonary insufficiency (acute) (after
        nonthoracic surgery) J95.2
      chronic J95.3
      following thoracic surgery J95.1
      respiratory failure (acute) J95.821
        acute and chronic J95.822
      specified NEC J95.89
      subglottic stenosis J95.5
      tracheostomy complication — *see*
        Complications, tracheostomy
    therapy T81.89 ☑
  sedation during labor and delivery O74.9
    cardiac O74.2
    central nervous system O74.3
    pulmonary NEC O74.1
  shunt (*see also* Complications, prosthetic device or
    implant)
    arteriovenous — *see* Complications,
      arteriovenous, shunt
    ventricular (communicating) — *see*
      Complications, ventricular shunt
  skin
    graft T86.829
      failure T86.821
      infection T86.822
      rejection T86.820
      specified type NEC T86.828
  spinal
    anesthesia — *see* Complications, anesthesia,
      spinal
    catheter (epidural) (subdural) — *see*
      Complications, catheter
    puncture or tap G97.1
      cerebrospinal fluid leak G97.0
      headache or reaction G97.1
  stent
    bile duct — *see* Complications, bile duct
      prosthesis
    ureteral indwelling
      breakdown T83.112 ☑
      displacement T83.122 ☑
      leakage T83.192 ☑
      malposition T83.122 ☑
      obstruction T83.192 ☑
      perforation T83.192 ☑
      protrusion T83.192 ☑
      specified NEC T83.192 ☑
    urinary NEC (ileal conduit) (nephroureteral)
      T83.193 ☑
      embolism T83.81 ☑
      fibrosis T83.82 ☑

Complication(s)

Complication(s) — *continued*
  stent — *continued*
    hemorrhage T83.83 ☑
    infection and inflammation T83.593 ☑
    mechanical
      breakdown T83.113 ☑
      displacement T83.123 ☑
      leakage T83.193 ☑
      malposition T83.123 ☑
      obstruction T83.193 ☑
      perforation T83.193 ☑
      protrusion T83.193 ☑
      specified NEC T83.193 ☑
    pain T83.84 ☑
    specified type NEC T83.89 ☑
    stenosis T83.85 ☑
    thrombosis T83.86 ☑
    vascular
      end stent stenosis — *see* Restenosis, stent
      in stent stenosis — *see* Restenosis, stent
  stoma
    digestive tract
      colostomy — *see* Complications, colostomy
      enterostomy — *see* Complications, enterostomy
      esophagostomy — *see* Complications, esophagostomy
      gastrostomy — *see* Complications, gastrostomy
    urinary tract N99.528
      continent N99.538
        hemorrhage N99.530
        herniation N99.533
        infection N99.531
        malfunction N99.532
        specified type NEC N99.538
        stenosis N99.534
      cystostomy — *see* Complications, cystostomy
      external NOS N99.528
      hemorrhage N99.520
      herniation N99.523
      incontinent N99.528
        hemorrhage N99.520
        herniation N99.523
        infection N99.521
        malfunction N99.522
        specified type NEC N99.528
        stenosis N99.524
      infection N99.521
      malfunction N99.522
      specified type NEC N99.528
      stenosis N99.524
  stomach banding — *see* Complication(s), bariatric procedure
  stomach stapling — *see* Complication(s), bariatric procedure
  surgical material, nonabsorbable — *see* Complication, suture, permanent
  surgical procedure (on) T81.9 ☑
    amputation stump (late) — *see* Complications, amputation stump
    cardiac — *see* Complications, circulatory system
    cholesteatoma, recurrent — *see* Complications, postmastoidectomy, recurrent cholesteatoma
    circulatory (early) — *see* Complications, circulatory system
    digestive system — *see* Complications, gastrointestinal
    dumping syndrome (postgastrectomy) K91.1
    ear — *see* Complications, ear
    elephantiasis or lymphedema I97.89
      postmastectomy I97.2
    emphysema (surgical) T81.82 ☑
    endocrine — *see* Complications, endocrine
    eye — *see* Complications, eye
    fistula (persistent postoperative) T81.83 ☑
    foreign body inadvertently left in wound (sponge) (suture) (swab) — *see* Foreign body, accidentally left during a procedure
    gastrointestinal — *see* Complications, gastrointestinal
    genitourinary NEC N99.89
    hematoma
      intraoperative — *see* Complication, intraoperative, hemorrhage
      postprocedural — *see* Complication, postprocedural, hematoma
    hemorrhage
      intraoperative — *see* Complication, intraoperative, hemorrhage
      postprocedural — *see* Complication, postprocedural, hemorrhage
    hepatic failure K91.82
    hyperglycemia (postpancreatectomy) E89.1

Complication(s) — *continued*
  surgical procedure — *continued*
    hypoinsulinemia (postpancreatectomy) E89.1
    hypoparathyroidism (postparathyroidectomy) E89.2
    hypopituitarism (posthypophysectomy) E89.3
    hypothyroidism (post-thyroidectomy) E89.0
    intestinal obstruction (*see also* Obstruction, intestine, postoperative) K91.30
    intracranial hypotension following ventricular shunting (ventriculostomy) G97.2
    lymphedema I97.89
      postmastectomy I97.2
    malabsorption (postsurgical) NEC K91.2
      osteoporosis — *see* Osteoporosis, postsurgical malabsorption
    mastoidectomy cavity NEC — *see* Complications, postmastoidectomy
    metabolic E89.89
      specified NEC E89.89
    musculoskeletal — *see* Complications, musculoskeletal system
    nervous system (central) (peripheral) — *see* Complications, nervous system
    ovarian failure E89.40
      asymptomatic E89.40
      symptomatic E89.41
    peripheral vascular — *see* Complications, surgical procedure, vascular
    postcardiotomy syndrome I97.0
    postcholecystectomy syndrome K91.5
    postcommissurotomy syndrome I97.0
    postgastrectomy dumping syndrome K91.1
    postlaminectomy syndrome NEC M96.1
      kyphosis M96.3
    postmastectomy lymphedema syndrome I97.2
    postmastoidectomy cholesteatoma — *see* Complications, postmastoidectomy, recurrent cholesteatoma
    postvagotomy syndrome K91.1
    postvalvulotomy syndrome I97.0
    pulmonary insufficiency (acute) J95.2
      chronic J95.3
      following thoracic surgery J95.1
    reattached body part — *see* Complications, reattached
    respiratory — *see* Complications, respiratory system
    shock (hypovolemic) T81.19 ☑
    spleen (postoperative) D78.89
      intraoperative D78.81
    stitch abscess T81.41 ☑
    subglottic stenosis (postsurgical) J95.5
    testicular hypofunction E89.5
    transplant — *see* Complications, organ or tissue transplant
    urinary NEC N99.89
    vaginal vault prolapse (posthysterectomy) N99.3
    vascular (peripheral)
      artery T81.719 ☑
        mesenteric T81.710 ☑
        renal T81.711 ☑
        specified NEC T81.718 ☑
      vein T81.72 ☑
    wound infection T81.49 ☑
  suture, permanent (wire) NEC T85.9 ☑
    with repair of bone — *see* Complications, fixation device, internal
    embolism T85.818 ☑
    fibrosis T85.828 ☑
    hemorrhage T85.838 ☑
    infection and inflammation T85.79 ☑
    mechanical
      breakdown T85.612 ☑
      displacement T85.622 ☑
      malfunction T85.612 ☑
      malposition T85.622 ☑
      obstruction T85.692 ☑
      perforation T85.692 ☑
      protrusion T85.692 ☑
      specified NEC T85.692 ☑
    pain T85.848 ☑
    specified type NEC T85.898 ☑
    stenosis T85.858 ☑
    thrombosis T85.868 ☑
  tracheostomy J95.00
    granuloma J95.09
    hemorrhage J95.01
    infection J95.02
    malfunction J95.03
    mechanical J95.03
    obstruction J95.03

Complication(s) — *continued*
  tracheostomy — *continued*
    specified type NEC J95.09
    tracheo-esophageal fistula J95.04
  transfusion (blood) (lymphocytes) (plasma) T80.92 ☑
    air embolism T80.0 ☑
    circulatory overload E87.71
    febrile nonhemolytic transfusion reaction R50.84
    hemolysis T80.89 ☑
    hemochromatosis E83.111
    hemolytic reaction (antigen unspecified) T80.919 ☑
    incompatibility reaction (antigen unspecified) T80.919 ☑
      ABO T80.30 ☑
        delayed serologic (DSTR) T80.39 ☑
        hemolytic transfusion reaction (HTR) (unspecified time after transfusion) T80.319 ☑
          acute (AHTR) (less than 24 hours after transfusion) T80.310 ☑
          delayed (DHTR) (24 hours or more after transfusion) T80.311 ☑
        specified NEC T80.39 ☑
      acute (antigen unspecified) T80.910 ☑
      delayed (antigen unspecified) T80.911 ☑
      delayed serologic (DSTR) T80.89 ☑
      Non-ABO (minor antigens (Duffy) (K) (Kell) (Kidd) (Lewis) (M) (N) (P)(s)) T80.A0 ☑
        delayed serologic (DSTR) T80.A9 ☑
        hemolytic transfusion reaction (HTR) (unspecified time after transfusion) T80.A19 ☑
          acute (AHTR) (less than 24 hours after transfusion) T80.A10 ☑
          delayed (DHTR) (24 hours or more after transfusion) T80.A11 ☑
        specified NEC T80.A9 ☑
      Rh (antigens (C) (c) (D) (E) (e)) (factor) T80.40 ☑
        delayed serologic (DSTR) T80.49 ☑
        hemolytic transfusion reaction (HTR) (unspecified time after transfusion) T80.419 ☑
          acute (AHTR) (less than 24 hours after transfusion) T80.410 ☑
          delayed (DHTR) (24 hours or more after transfusion) T80.411 ☑
        specified NEC T80.49 ☑
    infection T80.29 ☑
      acute T80.22 ☑
    reaction NEC T80.89 ☑
    sepsis T80.29 ☑
    shock T80.89 ☑
  transplant T86.90
    bone T86.839
      failure T86.831
      infection T86.832
      rejection T86.830
      specified type NEC T86.838
    bone marrow T86.00
      failure T86.02
      infection T86.03
      rejection T86.01
      specified type NEC T86.09
    cornea T86.849
      failure T86.841
      infection T86.842
      rejection T86.840
      specified type NEC T86.848
    failure T86.92
    heart T86.20
      with lung T86.30
      cardiac allograft vasculopathy T86.290
        failure T86.32
        infection T86.33
        rejection T86.31
        specified type NEC T86.39
      failure T86.22
      infection T86.23
      rejection T86.21
      specified type NEC T86.298
    infection T86.93
    intestine T86.859
      failure T86.851
      infection T86.852
      rejection T86.850
      specified type NEC T86.858
    kidney T86.10
      failure T86.12
      infection T86.13
      rejection T86.11
      specified type NEC T86.19

☑ **Additional character required**

Complication(s) — *continued*
  transplant — *continued*
    liver T86.40
      failure T86.42
      infection T86.43
      rejection T86.41
      specified type NEC T86.49
    lung T86.819
      with heart T86.30
        failure T86.32
        infection T86.33
        rejection T86.31
        specified type NEC T86.39
      failure T86.811
      infection T86.812
      rejection T86.810
      specified type NEC T86.818
    malignant neoplasm C80.2
    pancreas T86.899
      failure T86.891
      infection T86.892
      rejection T86.890
      specified type NEC T86.898
    peripheral blood stem cells T86.5
    post-transplant lymphoproliferative disorder (PTLD) D47.Z1
    rejection T86.91
    skin T86.829
      failure T86.821
      infection T86.822
      rejection T86.820
      specified type NEC T86.828
    specified
      tissue T86.899
        failure T86.891
        infection T86.892
        rejection T86.890
        specified type NEC T86.898
      type NEC T86.99
    stem cell (from peripheral blood) (from umbilical cord) T86.5
    umbilical cord stem cells T86.5
  trauma (early) T79.9 ☑
    specified NEC T79.8 ☑
  ultrasound therapy T88.9 ☑
  umbilical cord NEC
    complicating delivery O69.9 ☑
      specified NEC O69.89 ☑
  umbrella device, vascular T82.9 ☑
    embolism T82.818 ☑
    fibrosis T82.828 ☑
    hemorrhage T82.838 ☑
    infection or inflammation T82.7 ☑
    mechanical
      breakdown T82.515 ☑
      displacement T82.525 ☑
      leakage T82.535 ☑
      malposition T82.525 ☑
      obstruction T82.595 ☑
      perforation T82.595 ☑
      protrusion T82.595 ☑
    pain T82.848 ☑
    specified type NEC T82.898 ☑
    stenosis T82.858 ☑
    thrombosis T82.868 ☑
  urethral catheter — *see* Complications, catheter, urethral, indwelling
  vaccination T88.1 ☑
    anaphylaxis NEC T80.52 ☑
    arthropathy — *see* Arthropathy, postimmunization
    cellulitis T88.0 ☑
    encephalitis or encephalomyelitis G04.02
    infection (general) (local) NEC T88.0 ☑
    meningitis G03.8
    myelitis G04.02
    protein sickness T80.62 ☑
    rash T88.1 ☑
    reaction (allergic) T88.1 ☑
      serum T80.62 ☑
    sepsis T88.0 ☑
    serum intoxication, sickness, rash, or other serum reaction NEC T80.62 ☑
      anaphylactic shock T80.52 ☑
    shock (allergic) (anaphylactic) T80.52 ☑
    vaccinia (generalized) (localized) T88.1 ☑
  vas deferens device or implant — *see* Complications, genitourinary, device or implant, genital tract
  vascular I99.9
    device or implant T82.9 ☑
      embolism T82.818 ☑

Complication(s) — *continued*
  vascular — *continued*
    fibrosis T82.828 ☑
    hemorrhage T82.838 ☑
    infection or inflammation T82.7 ☑
    mechanical
      breakdown T82.519 ☑
        specified device NEC T82.518 ☑
      displacement T82.529 ☑
        specified device NEC T82.528 ☑
      leakage T82.539 ☑
        specified device NEC T82.538 ☑
      malposition T82.529 ☑
        specified device NEC T82.528 ☑
      obstruction T82.599 ☑
        specified device NEC T82.598 ☑
      perforation T82.599 ☑
        specified device NEC T82.598 ☑
      protrusion T82.599 ☑
        specified device NEC T82.598 ☑
    pain T82.848 ☑
    specified type NEC T82.898 ☑
    stenosis T82.858 ☑
    thrombosis T82.868 ☑
  dialysis catheter — *see* Complication, catheter, dialysis
  following infusion, therapeutic injection or transfusion T80.1 ☑
  graft T82.9 ☑
    embolism T82.818 ☑
    fibrosis T82.828 ☑
    hemorrhage T82.838 ☑
    mechanical
      breakdown T82.319 ☑
        aorta (bifurcation) T82.310 ☑
        carotid artery T82.311 ☑
        specified vessel NEC T82.318 ☑
      displacement T82.329 ☑
        aorta (bifurcation) T82.320 ☑
        carotid artery T82.321 ☑
        specified vessel NEC T82.328 ☑
      leakage T82.339 ☑
        aorta (bifurcation) T82.330 ☑
        carotid artery T82.331 ☑
        specified vessel NEC T82.338 ☑
      malposition T82.329 ☑
        aorta (bifurcation) T82.320 ☑
        carotid artery T82.321 ☑
        specified vessel NEC T82.328 ☑
      obstruction T82.399 ☑
        aorta (bifurcation) T82.390 ☑
        carotid artery T82.391 ☑
        specified vessel NEC T82.398 ☑
      perforation T82.399 ☑
        aorta (bifurcation) T82.390 ☑
        carotid artery T82.391 ☑
        specified vessel NEC T82.398 ☑
      protrusion T82.399 ☑
        aorta (bifurcation) T82.390 ☑
        carotid artery T82.391 ☑
        specified vessel NEC T82.398 ☑
    pain T82.848 ☑
    specified complication NEC T82.898 ☑
    stenosis T82.858 ☑
    thrombosis T82.868 ☑
  postoperative — *see* Complications, postoperative, circulatory
  vena cava device (filter) (sieve) (umbrella) — *see* Complications, umbrella device, vascular
  ventilation therapy NEC T81.81 ☑
  ventilator
    mechanical J95.850
    specified J95.859
  ventricular (communicating) shunt (device) T85.9 ☑
    embolism T85.810 ☑
    fibrosis T85.820 ☑
    hemorrhage T85.830 ☑
    infection and inflammation T85.730 ☑
    mechanical
      breakdown T85.01 ☑
      displacement T85.02 ☑
      leakage T85.03 ☑
      malposition T85.02 ☑
      obstruction T85.09 ☑
      perforation T85.09 ☑
      protrusion T85.09 ☑
      specified NEC T85.09 ☑
    pain T85.840 ☑
    specified type NEC T85.890 ☑
    stenosis T85.850 ☑
    thrombosis T85.860 ☑

Complication(s) — *continued*
  wire suture, permanent (implanted) — *see* Complications, suture, permanent
Compressed air disease T70.3 ☑
Compression
  with injury - code by Nature of injury
  artery I77.1
    celiac, syndrome I77.4
  brachial plexus G54.0
  brain (stem) G93.5
    due to
      contusion (diffuse) — *see* Injury, intracranial, diffuse
      focal — *see* Injury, intracranial, focal
      injury NEC — *see* Injury, intracranial, diffuse
      traumatic — *see* Injury, intracranial, diffuse
  bronchus J98.09
  cauda equina G83.4
  celiac (artery) (axis) I77.4
  cerebral — *see* Compression, brain
  cervical plexus G54.2
  cord
    spinal — *see* Compression, spinal
    umbilical — *see* Compression, umbilical cord
  cranial nerve G52.9
    eighth — *see* subcategory H93.3 ☑
    eleventh G52.8
    fifth G50.8
    first G52.0
    fourth — *see* Strabismus, paralytic, fourth nerve
    ninth G52.1
    second — *see* Disorder, nerve, optic
    seventh G51.8
    sixth — *see* Strabismus, paralytic, sixth nerve
    tenth G52.2
    third — *see* Strabismus, paralytic, third nerve
    twelfth G52.3
  diver's squeeze T70.3 ☑
  during birth (newborn) P15.9
  esophagus K22.2
  eustachian tube — *see* Obstruction, eustachian tube, cartilaginous
  facies Q67.1
  fracture
    nontraumatic NOS — *see* Collapse, vertebra
    pathological — *see* Fracture, pathological
    traumatic — *see* Fracture, traumatic
  heart — *see* Disease, heart
  intestine — *see* Obstruction, intestine
  laryngeal nerve, recurrent G52.2
    with paralysis of vocal cords and larynx J38.00
      bilateral J38.02
      unilateral J38.01
  lumbosacral plexus G54.1
  lung J98.4
  lymphatic vessel I89.0
  medulla — *see* Compression, brain
  nerve (*see also* Disorder, nerve) G58.9
    arm NEC — *see* Mononeuropathy, upper limb
    axillary G54.0
    cranial — *see* Compression, cranial nerve
    leg NEC — *see* Mononeuropathy, lower limb
    median (in carpal tunnel) — *see* Syndrome, carpal tunnel
    optic — *see* Disorder, nerve, optic
    plantar — *see* Lesion, nerve, plantar
    posterior tibial (in tarsal tunnel) — *see* Syndrome, tarsal tunnel
    root or plexus NOS (in) G54.9
      intervertebral disc disorder NEC — *see* Disorder, disc, with, radiculopathy
      with myelopathy — *see* Disorder, disc, with, myelopathy
      neoplastic disease (*see also* Neoplasm) D49.9 [G55]
      spondylosis — *see* Spondylosis, with radiculopathy
    sciatic (acute) — *see* Lesion, nerve, sciatic
    sympathetic G90.8
    traumatic — *see* Injury, nerve
    ulnar — *see* Lesion, nerve, ulnar
    upper extremity NEC — *see* Mononeuropathy, upper limb
  spinal (cord) G95.20
    by displacement of intervertebral disc NEC (*see also* Disorder, disc, with, myelopathy)
    nerve root NOS G54.9
      due to displacement of intervertebral disc NEC — *see* Disorder, disc, with, radiculopathy
      with myelopathy — *see* Disorder, disc, with, myelopathy
    specified NEC G95.29

Compression - Constipation

Compression — *continued*
  spinal — *continued*
    spondylogenic (cervical) (lumbar, lumbosacral)
        (thoracic) — *see* Spondylosis, with
        myelopathy NEC
      anterior — *see* Syndrome, anterior, spinal artery,
          compression
    traumatic — *see* Injury, spinal cord, by region
  subcostal nerve (syndrome) — *see*
      Mononeuropathy, upper limb, specified NEC
  sympathetic nerve NEC G90.8
  syndrome T79.5 ☑
  trachea J39.8
  ulnar nerve (by scar tissue) — *see* Lesion, nerve, ulnar
  umbilical cord
    complicating delivery O69.2 ☑
      cord around neck O69.1 ☑
      prolapse O69.0 ☑
      specified NEC O69.2 ☑
  ureter N13.5
  vein I87.1
  vena cava (inferior) (superior) I87.1
Compulsion, compulsive
  gambling F63.0
  neurosis F42.8
  personality F60.5
  states F42.8
  swearing F42.8
    in Gilles de la Tourette's syndrome F95.2
  tics and spasms F95.9
Concato's disease (pericardial polyserositis) A19.9
  nontubercular I31.1
  pleural — *see* Pleurisy, with effusion
Concavity chest wall M95.4
Concealed penis Q55.64
Concern (normal) about sick person in family Z63.6
Concrescence (teeth) K00.2
Concretio cordis I31.1
  rheumatic I09.2
Concretion (*see also* Calculus)
  appendicular K38.1
  canaliculus — *see* Dacryolith
  clitoris N90.89
  conjunctiva H11.12 ☑
  eyelid — *see* Disorder, eyelid, specified type NEC
  lacrimal passages — *see* Dacryolith
  prepuce (male) N47.8
  salivary gland (any) K11.5
  seminal vesicle N50.89
  tonsil J35.8
Concussion (brain) (cerebral) (current) S06.0X9 ☑
  with
    loss of consciousness of 30 minutes or less S06.0X1 ☑
    loss of consciousness of unspecified duration
        S06.0X9 ☑
  blast (air) (hydraulic) (immersion) (underwater)
    abdomen or thorax — *see* Injury, blast, by site
    ear with acoustic nerve injury — *see* Injury, nerve,
        acoustic, specified type NEC
  cauda equina S34.3 ☑
  conus medullaris S34.02 ☑
  ocular S05.8X ☑
  spinal (cord)
    cervical S14.0 ☑
    lumbar S34.01 ☑
    sacral S34.02 ☑
    thoracic S24.0 ☑
  syndrome F07.81
  without loss of consciousness S06.0X0 ☑
Condition — *see* Disease
Conditions arising in the perinatal period — *see*
    Newborn, affected by
Conduct disorder — *see* Disorder, conduct
Condyloma A63.0
  acuminatum A63.0
  gonorrheal A54.09
  latum A51.31
  syphilitic A51.31
    congenital A50.07
  venereal, syphilitic A51.31
Conflagration (*see also* Burn)
  asphyxia (by inhalation of gases, fumes or vapors)
      (*see also* Table of Drugs and Chemicals) T59.9 ☑
Conflict (with) (*see also* Discord)
  family Z73.9
  marital Z63.0
    involving divorce or estrangement Z63.5
  parent-child Z62.820
    parent-adopted child Z62.821
    parent-biological child Z62.820
    parent-foster child Z62.822
  social role NEC Z73.5

Confluent — *see* condition
Confusion, confused R41.0
  epileptic F05
  mental state (psychogenic) F44.89
  psychogenic F44.89
  reactive (from emotional stress, psychological
      trauma) F44.89
Confusional arousals G47.51
Congelation T69.9 ☑
Congenital (*see also* condition)
  aortic septum Q25.49
  intrinsic factor deficiency D51.0
  malformation — *see* Anomaly
Congestion, congestive
  bladder N32.89
  bowel K63.89
  brain G93.89
  breast N64.59
  bronchial J98.09
  catarrhal J31.0
  chest R09.89
  chill, malarial — *see* Malaria
  circulatory NEC I99.8
  duodenum K31.89
  eye — *see* Hyperemia, conjunctiva
  facial, due to birth injury P15.4
  general R68.89
  glottis J37.0
  heart — *see* Failure, heart, congestive
  hepatic K76.1
  hypostatic (lung) — *see* Edema, lung
  intestine K63.89
  kidney N28.89
  labyrinth — *see* subcategory H83.8 ☑
  larynx J37.0
  liver K76.1
  lung R09.89
    active or acute — *see* Pneumonia
  malaria, malarial — *see* Malaria
  nasal R09.81
  nose R09.81
  orbit, orbital (*see also* Exophthalmos)
    inflammatory (chronic) — *see* Inflammation, orbit
  ovary N83.8
  pancreas K86.89
  pelvic, female N94.89
  pleural J94.8
  prostate (active) N42.1
  pulmonary — *see* Congestion, lung
  renal N28.89
  retina H35.81
  seminal vesicle N50.1
  spinal cord G95.19
  spleen (chronic) D73.2
  stomach K31.89
  trachea — *see* Tracheitis
  urethra N36.8
  uterus N85.8
    with subinvolution N85.3
  venous (passive) I87.8
  viscera R68.89
Congestive — *see* Congestion
Conical
  cervix (hypertrophic elongation) N88.4
  cornea — *see* Keratoconus
  teeth K00.2
Conjoined twins Q89.4
Conjugal maladjustment Z63.0
  involving divorce or estrangement Z63.5
Conjunctiva — *see* condition
Conjunctivitis (staphylococcal) (streptococcal) NOS
    H10.9
  Acanthamoeba B60.12
  acute H10.3 ☑
    atopic H10.1 ☑
    mucopurulent H10.02 ☑
      follicular H10.01 ☑
    chemical (*see also* Corrosion, cornea) H10.21 ☑
    pseudomembranous H10.22 ☑
    serous except viral H10.23 ☑
      viral — *see* Conjunctivitis, viral
    toxic H10.21 ☑
  adenoviral (acute) (follicular) B30.1
  allergic (acute) — *see* Conjunctivitis, acute, atopic
    chronic H10.45
      vernal H10.44
  anaphylactic — *see* Conjunctivitis, acute, atopic
  Apollo B30.3
  atopic (acute) — *see* Conjunctivitis, acute, atopic
  Béal's B30.2
  blennorrhagic (gonococcal) (neonatorum) A54.31

Conjunctivitis — *continued*
  chemical (acute) (*see also* Corrosion, cornea)
      H10.21 ☑
  chlamydial A74.0
    due to trachoma A71.1
    neonatal P39.1
  chronic (nodosa) (petrificans) (phlyctenular)
      H10.40
    allergic H10.45
      vernal H10.44
    follicular H10.43 ☑
    giant papillary H10.41 ☑
    simple H10.42 ☑
    vernal H10.44
  coxsackievirus 24 B30.3
  diphtheritic A36.86
  due to
    dust — *see* Conjunctivitis, acute, atopic
    filariasis B74.9
    mucocutaneous leishmaniasis B55.2
  enterovirus type 70 (hemorrhagic) B30.3
  epidemic (viral) B30.9
    hemorrhagic B30.3
  gonococcal (neonatorum) A54.31
  granular (trachomatous) A71.1
    sequelae (late effect) B94.0
  hemorrhagic (acute) (epidemic) B30.3
  herpes zoster B02.31
  in (due to)
    Acanthamoeba B60.12
    adenovirus (acute) (follicular) B30.1
    Chlamydia A74.0
    coxsackievirus 24 B30.3
    diphtheria A36.86
    enterovirus type 70 (hemorrhagic) B30.3
    filariasis B74.9
    gonococci A54.31
    herpes (simplex) virus B00.53
      zoster B02.31
    infectious disease NEC B99 ☑
    meningococci A39.89
    mucocutaneous leishmaniasis B55.2
    rosacea H10.82 ☑
    syphilis (late) A52.71
    zoster B02.31
  inclusion A74.0
  infantile P39.1
    gonococcal A54.31
  Koch-Weeks' — *see* Conjunctivitis, acute,
      mucopurulent
  light — *see* Conjunctivitis, acute, atopic
  ligneous — *see* Blepharoconjunctivitis, ligneous
  meningococcal A39.89
  mucopurulent — *see* Conjunctivitis, acute,
      mucopurulent
  neonatal P39.1
    gonococcal A54.31
  Newcastle B30.8
  of Béal B30.2
  parasitic
    filariasis B74.9
    mucocutaneous leishmaniasis B55.2
  Parinaud's H10.89
  petrificans H10.89
  rosacea H10.82 ☑
  specified NEC H10.89
  swimming-pool B30.1
  trachomatous A71.1
    acute A71.0
    sequelae (late effect) B94.0
  traumatic NEC H10.89
  tuberculous A18.59
  tularemic A21.1
  tularensis A21.1
  viral B30.9
    due to
      adenovirus B30.1
      enterovirus B30.3
      specified NEC B30.8
Conjunctivochalasis H11.82 ☑
Connective tissue — *see* condition
Conn's syndrome E26.01
Conradi (-Hunermann) disease Q77.3
Consanguinity Z84.3
  counseling Z71.89
Conscious simulation (of illness) Z76.5
Consecutive — *see* condition
Consolidation lung (base) — *see* Pneumonia, lobar
Constipation (atonic) (neurogenic) (simple) (spastic)
    K59.00
  chronic K59.09
    idiopathic K59.04

Constipation — *continued*
drug-induced K59.03
functional K59.04
outlet dysfunction K59.02
psychogenic F45.8
slow transit K59.01
specified NEC K59.09
Constitutional (*see also* condition)
substandard F60.7
Constitutionally substandard F60.7
Constriction (*see also* Stricture)
auditory canal — *see* Stenosis, external ear canal
bronchial J98.09
duodenum K31.5
esophagus K22.2
external
abdomen, abdominal (wall) S30.841 ☑
alveolar process S00.542 ☑
ankle S90.54 ☑
antecubital space — *see* Constriction, external, forearm
arm (upper) S40.84 ☑
auricle — *see* Constriction, external, ear
axilla — *see* Constriction, external, arm
back, lower S30.840 ☑
breast S20.14 ☑
brow S00.84 ☑
buttock S30.840 ☑
calf — *see* Constriction, external, leg
canthus — *see* Constriction, external, eyelid
cheek S00.84 ☑
internal S00.542 ☑
chest wall — *see* Constriction, external, thorax
chin S00.84 ☑
clitoris S30.844 ☑
costal region — *see* Constriction, external, thorax
digit(s)
foot — *see* Constriction, external, toe
hand — *see* Constriction, external, finger
ear S00.44 ☑
elbow S50.34 ☑
epididymis S30.843 ☑
epigastric region S30.841 ☑
esophagus, cervical S10.14 ☑
eyebrow — *see* Constriction, external, eyelid
eyelid S00.24 ☑
face S00.84 ☑
finger(s) S60.44 ☑
index S60.44 ☑
little S60.44 ☑
middle S60.44 ☑
ring S60.44 ☑
flank S30.841 ☑
foot (except toe(s) alone) S90.84 ☑
toe — *see* Constriction, external, toe
forearm S50.84 ☑
elbow only — *see* Constriction, external, elbow
forehead S00.84 ☑
genital organs, external
female S30.846 ☑
male S30.845 ☑
groin S30.841 ☑
gum S00.542 ☑
hand S60.54 ☑
head S00.94 ☑
ear — *see* Constriction, external, ear
eyelid — *see* Constriction, external, eyelid
lip S00.541 ☑
nose S00.34 ☑
oral cavity S00.542 ☑
scalp S00.04 ☑
specified site NEC S00.84 ☑
heel — *see* Constriction, external, foot
hip S70.24 ☑
inguinal region S30.841 ☑
interscapular region S20.449 ☑
jaw S00.84 ☑
knee S80.24 ☑
labium (majus) (minus) S30.844 ☑
larynx S10.14 ☑
leg (lower) S80.84 ☑
knee — *see* Constriction, external, knee
upper — *see* Constriction, external, thigh
lip S00.541 ☑
lower back S30.840 ☑
lumbar region S30.840 ☑
malar region S00.84 ☑
mammary — *see* Constriction, external, breast
mastoid region S00.84 ☑
mouth S00.542 ☑
nail
finger — *see* Constriction, external, finger

Constriction — *continued*
external — *continued*
toe — *see* Constriction, external, toe
nasal S00.34 ☑
neck S10.94 ☑
specified site NEC S10.84 ☑
throat S10.14 ☑
nose S00.34 ☑
occipital region S00.04 ☑
oral cavity S00.542 ☑
orbital region — *see* Constriction, external, eyelid
palate S00.542 ☑
palm — *see* Constriction, external, hand
parietal region S00.04 ☑
pelvis S30.840 ☑
penis S30.842 ☑
perineum
female S30.844 ☑
male S30.840 ☑
periocular area — *see* Constriction, external, eyelid
phalanges
finger — *see* Constriction, external, finger
toe — *see* Constriction, external, toe
pharynx S10.14 ☑
pinna — *see* Constriction, external, ear
popliteal space — *see* Constriction, external, knee
prepuce S30.842 ☑
pubic region S30.840 ☑
pudendum
female S30.846 ☑
male S30.845 ☑
sacral region S30.840 ☑
scalp S00.04 ☑
scapular region — *see* Constriction, external, shoulder
scrotum S30.843 ☑
shin — *see* Constriction, external, leg
shoulder S40.24 ☑
sternal region S20.349 ☑
submaxillary region S00.84 ☑
submental region S00.84 ☑
subungual
finger(s) — *see* Constriction, external, finger
toe(s) — *see* Constriction, external, toe
supraclavicular fossa S10.84 ☑
supraorbital S00.84 ☑
temple S00.84 ☑
temporal region S00.84 ☑
testis S30.843 ☑
thigh S70.34 ☑
thorax, thoracic (wall) S20.94 ☑
back S20.44 ☑
front S20.34 ☑
throat S10.14 ☑
thumb S60.34 ☑
toe(s) (lesser) S90.44 ☑
great S90.44 ☑
tongue S00.542 ☑
trachea S10.14 ☑
tunica vaginalis S30.843 ☑
uvula S00.542 ☑
vagina S30.844 ☑
vulva S30.844 ☑
wrist S60.84 ☑
gallbladder — *see* Obstruction, gallbladder
intestine — *see* Obstruction, intestine
larynx J38.6
congenital Q31.8
specified NEC Q31.8
subglottic Q31.1
organ or site, congenital NEC — *see* Atresia, by site
prepuce (acquired) (congenital) N47.1
pylorus (adult hypertrophic) K31.1
congenital or infantile Q40.0
newborn Q40.0
ring dystocia (uterus) O62.4
spastic (*see also* Spasm)
ureter N13.5
ureter N13.5
with infection N13.6
urethra — *see* Stricture, urethra
visual field (peripheral) (functional) — *see* Defect, visual field
Constrictive — *see* condition
Consultation
medical — *see* Counseling, medical
religious Z71.81
specified reason NEC Z71.89
spiritual Z71.81
without complaint or sickness Z71.9
feared complaint unfounded Z71.1
specified reason NEC Z71.89

Consumption — *see* Tuberculosis
Contact (with) (*see also* Exposure (to))
acariasis Z20.7
AIDS virus Z20.6
air pollution Z77.110
algae and algae toxins Z77.121
algae bloom Z77.121
anthrax Z20.810
aromatic amines Z77.020
aromatic (hazardous) compounds NEC Z77.028
aromatic dyes NOS Z77.028
arsenic Z77.010
asbestos Z77.090
bacterial disease NEC Z20.818
benzene Z77.021
blue-green algae bloom Z77.121
body fluids (potentially hazardous) Z77.21
brown tide Z77.121
chemicals (chiefly nonmedicinal) (hazardous) NEC Z77.098
cholera Z20.09
chromium compounds Z77.018
communicable disease Z20.9
bacterial NEC Z20.818
specified NEC Z20.89
viral NEC Z20.828
Zika virus Z20.821
cyanobacteria bloom Z77.121
dyes Z77.098
Escherichia coli (E. coli) Z20.01
fiberglass — *see* Table of Drugs and Chemicals, fiberglass
German measles Z20.4
gonorrhea Z20.2
hazardous metals NEC Z77.018
hazardous substances NEC Z77.29
hazards in the physical environment NEC Z77.128
hazards to health NEC Z77.9
HIV Z20.6
HTLV-III/LAV Z20.6
human immunodeficiency virus (HIV) Z20.6
infection Z20.9
specified NEC Z20.89
infestation (parasitic) NEC Z20.7
intestinal infectious disease NEC Z20.09
Escherichia coli (E. coli) Z20.01
lead Z77.011
meningococcus Z20.811
mold (toxic) Z77.120
nickel dust Z77.018
noise Z77.122
parasitic disease Z20.7
pediculosis Z20.7
pfiesteria piscicida Z77.121
poliomyelitis Z20.89
pollution
air Z77.110
environmental NEC Z77.118
soil Z77.112
water Z77.111
polycyclic aromatic hydrocarbons Z77.028
rabies Z20.3
radiation, naturally occurring NEC Z77.123
radon Z77.123
red tide (Florida) Z77.121
rubella Z20.4
sexually-transmitted disease Z20.2
smallpox (laboratory) Z20.89
syphilis Z20.2
tuberculosis Z20.1
uranium Z77.012
varicella Z20.820
venereal disease Z20.2
viral disease NEC Z20.828
viral hepatitis Z20.5
water pollution Z77.111
Zika virus Z20.821
Contamination, food — *see* Intoxication, foodborne
Contraception, contraceptive
advice Z30.09
counseling Z30.09
device (intrauterine) (in situ) Z97.5
causing menorrhagia T83.83 ☑
checking Z30.431
complications — *see* Complications, intrauterine, contraceptive device
in place Z97.5
initial prescription Z30.014
reinsertion Z30.433
removal Z30.432
replacement Z30.433
emergency (postcoital) Z30.012

Contraception - Contusion

Contraception — *continued*
  initial prescription Z30.019
    barrier Z30.018
    diaphragm Z30.018
    injectable Z30.013
    intrauterine device Z30.014
    pills Z30.011
    postcoital (emergency) Z30.012
    specified type NEC Z30.018
    subdermal implantable Z30.017
    transdermal patch hormonal Z30.016
    vaginal ring hormonal Z30.015
  maintenance Z30.40
    barrier Z30.49
    diaphragm Z30.49
    examination Z30.8
    injectable Z30.42
    intrauterine device Z30.431
    pills Z30.41
    specified type NEC Z30.49
    subdermal implantable Z30.46
    transdermal patch hormonal Z30.45
    vaginal ring hormonal Z30.44
  management Z30.9
    specified NEC Z30.8
  postcoital (emergency) Z30.012
  prescription Z30.019
    repeat Z30.40
  sterilization Z30.2
  surveillance (drug) — *see* Contraception,
      maintenance
Contraction(s), contracture, contracted
  Achilles tendon (*see also* Short, tendon, Achilles)
    congenital Q66.89
  amputation stump (surgical) (flexion) (late) (next
      proximal joint) T87.89
  anus K59.8
  bile duct (common) (hepatic) K83.8
  bladder N32.89
    neck or sphincter N32.0
  bowel, cecum, colon or intestine, any part — *see*
      Obstruction, intestine
  Braxton Hicks — *see* False, labor
  breast implant, capsular T85.44 ☑
  bronchial J98.09
  burn (old) — *see* Cicatrix
  cervix — *see* Stricture, cervix
  cicatricial — *see* Cicatrix
  conjunctiva, trachomatous, active A71.1
    sequelae (late effect) B94.0
  Dupuytren's M72.0
  eyelid — *see* Disorder, eyelid function
  fascia (lata) (postural) M72.8
    Dupuytren's M72.0
    palmar M72.0
    plantar M72.2
  finger NEC (*see also* Deformity, finger)
    congenital Q68.1
    joint — *see* Contraction, joint, hand
  flaccid — *see* Contraction, paralytic
  gallbladder K82.0
  heart valve — *see* Endocarditis
  hip — *see* Contraction, joint, hip
  hourglass
    bladder N32.89
      congenital Q64.79
    gallbladder K82.0
      congenital Q44.1
    stomach K31.89
      congenital Q40.2
      psychogenic F45.8
    uterus (complicating delivery) O62.4
  hysterical F44.4
  internal os — *see* Stricture, cervix
  joint (abduction) (acquired) (adduction) (flexion)
      (rotation) M24.50
    ankle M24.57 ☑
    congenital NEC Q68.8
      hip Q65.89
    elbow M24.52 ☑
    foot joint M24.57 ☑
    hand joint M24.54 ☑
    hip M24.55 ☑
      congenital Q65.89
    hysterical F44.4
    knee M24.56 ☑
    shoulder M24.51 ☑
    wrist M24.53 ☑
  kidney (granular) (secondary) N26.9
    congenital Q63.8
    hydronephritic — *see* Hydronephrosis
    Page N26.2

Contraction(s) — *continued*
  kidney — *continued*
    pyelonephritic — *see* Pyelitis, chronic
    tuberculous A18.11
  ligament (*see also* Disorder, ligament)
    congenital Q79.8
  muscle (postinfective) (postural) NEC M62.40
    with contracture of joint — *see* Contraction, joint
    ankle M62.47 ☑
    congenital Q79.8
      sternocleidomastoid Q68.0
    extraocular — *see* Strabismus
    eye (extrinsic) — *see* Strabismus
    foot M62.47 ☑
    forearm M62.43 ☑
    hand M62.44 ☑
    hysterical F44.4
    ischemic (Volkmann's) T79.6 ☑
    lower leg M62.46 ☑
    multiple sites M62.49
    pelvic region M62.45 ☑
    posttraumatic — *see* Strabismus, paralytic
    psychogenic F45.8
      conversion reaction F44.4
    shoulder region M62.41 ☑
    specified site NEC M62.48
    thigh M62.45 ☑
    upper arm M62.42 ☑
  neck — *see* Torticollis
  ocular muscle — *see* Strabismus
  organ or site, congenital NEC — *see* Atresia, by site
  outlet (pelvis) — *see* Contraction, pelvis
  palmar fascia M72.0
  paralytic
    joint — *see* Contraction, joint
    muscle (*see also* Contraction, muscle NEC)
      ocular — *see* Strabismus, paralytic
  pelvis (acquired) (general) M95.5
    with disproportion (fetopelvic) O33.1
      causing obstructed labor O65.1
      inlet O33.2
      mid-cavity O33.3 ☑
      outlet O33.3 ☑
  plantar fascia M72.2
  premature
    atrium I49.1
    auriculoventricular I49.49
    heart I49.49
    junctional I49.2
    supraventricular I49.1
    ventricular I49.3
  prostate N42.89
  pylorus NEC (*see also* Pylorospasm)
    psychogenic F45.8
  rectum, rectal (sphincter) K59.8
  ring (Bandl's) (complicating delivery) O62.4
  scar — *see* Cicatrix
  spine — *see* Dorsopathy, deforming
  sternocleidomastoid (muscle), congenital Q68.0
  stomach K31.89
    hourglass K31.89
      congenital Q40.2
      psychogenic F45.8
    psychogenic F45.8
  tendon (sheath) M62.40
    with contracture of joint — *see* Contraction, joint
    Achilles — *see* Short, tendon, Achilles
    ankle M62.47 ☑
      Achilles — *see* Short, tendon, Achilles
    foot M62.47 ☑
    forearm M62.43 ☑
    hand M62.44 ☑
    lower leg M62.46 ☑
    multiple sites M62.49
    neck M62.48
    pelvic region M62.45 ☑
    shoulder region M62.41 ☑
    specified site NEC M62.48
    thigh M62.45 ☑
    thorax M62.48
    trunk M62.48
    upper arm M62.42 ☑
  toe — *see* Deformity, toe, specified NEC
  ureterovesical orifice (postinfectional) N13.5
    with infection N13.6
  urethra (*see also* Stricture, urethra)
    orifice N32.0
  uterus N85.8
    abnormal NEC O62.9
    clonic (complicating delivery) O62.4
    dyscoordinate (complicating delivery) O62.4
    hourglass (complicating delivery) O62.4

Contraction(s) — *continued*
  uterus — *continued*
    hypertonic O62.4
    hypotonic NEC O62.2
    inadequate
      primary O62.0
      secondary O62.1
    incoordinate (complicating delivery) O62.4
    poor O62.2
    tetanic (complicating delivery) O62.4
  vagina (outlet) N89.5
  vesical N32.89
    neck or urethral orifice N32.0
  visual field — *see* Defect, visual field, generalized
  Volkmann's (ischemic) T79.6 ☑
Contusion (skin surface intact) T14.8 ☑
  abdomen, abdominal (muscle) (wall) S30.1 ☑
  adnexa, eye NEC S05.8X ☑
  adrenal gland S37.812 ☑
  alveolar process S00.532 ☑
  ankle S90.0 ☑
  antecubital space — *see* Contusion, forearm
  anus S30.3 ☑
  arm (upper) S40.02 ☑
    lower (with elbow) — *see* Contusion, forearm
  auditory canal — *see* Contusion, ear
  auricle — *see* Contusion, ear
  axilla — *see* Contusion, arm, upper
  back (*see also* Contusion, thorax, back)
    lower S30.0 ☑
  bile duct S36.13 ☑
  bladder S37.22 ☑
  bone NEC T14.8 ☑
  brain (diffuse) — *see* Injury, intracranial, diffuse
    focal — *see* Injury, intracranial, focal
  brainstem S06.38 ☑
  breast S20.0 ☑
  broad ligament S37.892 ☑
  brow S00.83 ☑
  buttock S30.0 ☑
  canthus, eye S00.1 ☑
  cauda equina S34.3 ☑
  cerebellar, traumatic S06.37 ☑
  cerebral S06.33 ☑
    left side S06.32 ☑
    right side S06.31 ☑
  cheek S00.83 ☑
    internal S00.532 ☑
  chest (wall) — *see* Contusion, thorax
  chin S00.83 ☑
  clitoris S30.23 ☑
  colon — *see* Injury, intestine, large, contusion
  common bile duct S36.13 ☑
  conjunctiva S05.1 ☑
    with foreign body (in conjunctival sac) — *see*
      Foreign body, conjunctival sac
  conus medullaris (spine) S34.139 ☑
  cornea — *see* Contusion, eyeball
    with foreign body — *see* Foreign body, cornea
  corpus cavernosum S30.21 ☑
  cortex (brain) (cerebral) — *see* Injury, intracranial,
      diffuse
    focal — *see* Injury, intracranial, focal
  costal region — *see* Contusion, thorax
  cystic duct S36.13 ☑
  diaphragm S27.802 ☑
  duodenum S36.420 ☑
  ear S00.43 ☑
  elbow S50.0 ☑
    with forearm — *see* Contusion, forearm
  epididymis S30.22 ☑
  epigastric region S30.1 ☑
  epiglottis S10.0 ☑
  esophagus (thoracic) S27.812 ☑
    cervical S10.0 ☑
  eyeball S05.1 ☑
  eyebrow S00.1 ☑
  eyelid (and periocular area) S00.1 ☑
  face NEC S00.83 ☑
  fallopian tube S37.529 ☑
    bilateral S37.522 ☑
    unilateral S37.521 ☑
  femoral triangle S30.1 ☑
  finger(s) S60.00 ☑
    with damage to nail (matrix) S60.10 ☑
    index S60.02 ☑
      with damage to nail S60.12 ☑
    little S60.05 ☑
      with damage to nail S60.15 ☑
    middle S60.03 ☑
      with damage to nail S60.13 ☑
    ring S60.04 ☑

☑ **Additional character required**

Contusion — *continued*
    finger(s) — *continued*
        with damage to nail S60.14 ☑
      thumb — *see* Contusion, thumb
    flank S30.1 ☑
    foot (except toe(s) alone) S90.3 ☑
      toe — *see* Contusion, toe
    forearm S50.1 ☑
      elbow only — *see* Contusion, elbow
    forehead S00.83 ☑
    gallbladder S36.122 ☑
    genital organs, external
      female S30.202 ☑
      male S30.201 ☑
    globe (eye) — *see* Contusion, eyeball
    groin S30.1 ☑
    gum S00.532 ☑
    hand S60.22 ☑
      finger(s) — *see* Contusion, finger
      wrist — *see* Contusion, wrist
    head S00.93 ☑
      ear — *see* Contusion, ear
      eyelid — *see* Contusion, eyelid
      lip S00.531 ☑
      nose S00.33 ☑
      oral cavity S00.532 ☑
      scalp S00.03 ☑
      specified part NEC S00.83 ☑
    heart (*see also* Injury, heart) S26.91 ☑
    heel — *see* Contusion, foot
    hepatic duct S36.13 ☑
    hip S70.0 ☑
    ileum S36.428 ☑
    iliac region S30.1 ☑
    inguinal region S30.1 ☑
    interscapular region S20.229 ☑
    intra-abdominal organ S36.92 ☑
      colon — *see* Injury, intestine, large, contusion
      liver S36.112 ☑
      pancreas — *see* Contusion, pancreas
      rectum S36.62 ☑
      small intestine — *see* Injury, intestine, small, contusion
      specified organ NEC S36.892 ☑
      spleen — *see* Contusion, spleen
      stomach S36.32 ☑
    iris (eye) — *see* Contusion, eyeball
    jaw S00.83 ☑
    jejunum S36.428 ☑
    kidney S37.01 ☑
      major (greater than 2 cm) S37.02 ☑
      minor (less than 2 cm) S37.01 ☑
    knee S80.0 ☑
    labium (majus) (minus) S30.23 ☑
    lacrimal apparatus, gland or sac S05.8X ☑
    larynx S10.0 ☑
    leg (lower) S80.1 ☑
      knee — *see* Contusion, knee
    lens — *see* Contusion, eyeball
    lip S00.531 ☑
    liver S36.112 ☑
    lower back S30.0 ☑
    lumbar region S30.0 ☑
    lung S27.329 ☑
      bilateral S27.322 ☑
      unilateral S27.321 ☑
    malar region S00.83 ☑
    mastoid region S00.83 ☑
    membrane, brain — *see* Injury, intracranial, diffuse
      focal — *see* Injury, intracranial, focal
    mesentery S36.892 ☑
    mesosalpinx S37.892 ☑
    mouth S00.532 ☑
    muscle — *see* Contusion, by site
    nail
      finger — *see* Contusion, finger, with damage to nail
      toe — *see* Contusion, toe, with damage to nail
    nasal S00.33 ☑
    neck S10.93 ☑
      specified site NEC S10.83 ☑
      throat S10.0 ☑
    nerve — *see* Injury, nerve
    newborn P54.5
    nose S00.33 ☑
    occipital
      lobe (brain) — *see* Injury, intracranial, diffuse
        focal — *see* Injury, intracranial, focal
      region (scalp) S00.03 ☑
    orbit (region) (tissues) S05.1 ☑
    ovary S37.429 ☑
      bilateral S37.422 ☑
      unilateral S37.421 ☑

Contusion — *continued*
    palate S00.532 ☑
    pancreas S36.229 ☑
      body S36.221 ☑
      head S36.220 ☑
      tail S36.222 ☑
    parietal
      lobe (brain) — *see* Injury, intracranial, diffuse
        focal — *see* Injury, intracranial, focal
      region (scalp) S00.03 ☑
    pelvic organ S37.92 ☑
      adrenal gland S37.812 ☑
      bladder S37.22 ☑
      fallopian tube — *see* Contusion, fallopian tube
      kidney — *see* Contusion, kidney
      ovary — *see* Contusion, ovary
      prostate S37.822 ☑
      specified organ NEC S37.892 ☑
      ureter S37.12 ☑
      urethra S37.32 ☑
      uterus S37.62 ☑
    pelvis S30.0 ☑
    penis S30.21 ☑
    perineum
      female S30.23 ☑
      male S30.0 ☑
    periocular area S00.1 ☑
    peritoneum S36.81 ☑
    periurethral tissue — *see* Contusion, urethra
    pharynx S10.0 ☑
    pinna — *see* Contusion, ear
    popliteal space — *see* Contusion, knee
    prepuce S30.21 ☑
    prostate S37.822 ☑
    pubic region S30.1 ☑
    pudendum
      female S30.202 ☑
      male S30.201 ☑
    quadriceps femoris — *see* Contusion, thigh
    rectum S36.62 ☑
    retroperitoneum S36.892 ☑
    round ligament S37.892 ☑
    sacral region S30.0 ☑
    scalp S00.03 ☑
      due to birth injury P12.3
    scapular region — *see* Contusion, shoulder
    sclera — *see* Contusion, eyeball
    scrotum S30.22 ☑
    seminal vesicle S37.892 ☑
    shoulder S40.01 ☑
    skin NEC T14.8 ☑
    small intestine — *see* Injury, intestine, small, contusion
    spermatic cord S30.22 ☑
    spinal cord — *see* Injury, spinal cord, by region
      cauda equina S34.3 ☑
      conus medullaris S34.139 ☑
    spleen S36.029 ☑
      major S36.021 ☑
      minor S36.020 ☑
    sternal region S20.219 ☑
    stomach S36.32 ☑
    subconjunctival S05.1 ☑
    subcutaneous NEC T14.8 ☑
    submaxillary region S00.83 ☑
    submental region S00.83 ☑
    subperiosteal NEC T14.8 ☑
    subungual
      finger — *see* Contusion, finger, with damage to nail
      toe — *see* Contusion, toe, with damage to nail
    supraclavicular fossa S10.83 ☑
    supraorbital S00.83 ☑
    suprarenal gland S37.812 ☑
    temple (region) S00.83 ☑
    temporal
      lobe (brain) — *see* Injury, intracranial, diffuse
        focal — *see* Injury, intracranial, focal
      region S00.83 ☑
    testis S30.22 ☑
    thigh S70.1 ☑
    thorax (wall) S20.20 ☑
      back S20.22 ☑
      front S20.21 ☑
    throat S10.0 ☑
    thumb S60.01 ☑
      with damage to nail S60.11 ☑
    toe(s) (lesser) S90.12 ☑
      with damage to nail S90.22 ☑
      great S90.11 ☑
        with damage to nail S90.21 ☑
    tongue S00.532 ☑

Contusion — *continued*
    trachea (cervical) S10.0 ☑
      thoracic S27.52 ☑
    tunica vaginalis S30.22 ☑
    tympanum, tympanic membrane — *see* Contusion, ear
    ureter S37.12 ☑
    urethra S37.32 ☑
    urinary organ NEC S37.892 ☑
    uterus S37.62 ☑
    uvula S00.532 ☑
    vagina S30.23 ☑
    vas deferens S37.892 ☑
    vesical S37.22 ☑
    vocal cord(s) S10.0 ☑
    vulva S30.23 ☑
    wrist S60.21 ☑
Conus (congenital) (any type) Q14.8
    cornea — *see* Keratoconus
    medullaris syndrome G95.81
Conversion hysteria, neurosis or reaction F44.9
Converter, tuberculosis (test reaction) R76.11
Conviction (legal), anxiety concerning Z65.0
    with imprisonment Z65.1
Convulsions (idiopathic) (*see also* Seizure(s)) R56.9
    apoplectiform (cerebral ischemia) I67.82
    dissociative F44.5
    epileptic — *see* Epilepsy
    epileptiform, epileptoid — *see* Seizure, epileptiform
    ether (anesthetic) — *see* Table of Drugs and Chemicals, by drug
    febrile R56.00
      with status epilepticus G40.901
      complex R56.01
        with status epilepticus G40.901
      simple R56.00
    hysterical F44.5
    infantile P90
      epilepsy — *see* Epilepsy
    jacksonian — *see* Epilepsy, localization-related, symptomatic, with simple partial seizures
    myoclonic G25.3
    newborn P90
    obstetrical (nephritic) (uremic) — *see* Eclampsia
    paretic A52.17
    post traumatic R56.1
    psychomotor — *see* Epilepsy, localization-related, symptomatic, with complex partial seizures
    recurrent R56.9
    reflex R25.8
    scarlatinal A38.8
    tetanus, tetanic — *see* Tetanus
    thymic E32.8
Convulsive (*see also* Convulsions)
Cooley's anemia D56.1
Coolie itch B76.9
Cooper's
    disease — *see* Mastopathy, cystic
    hernia — *see* Hernia, abdomen, specified site NEC
Copra itch B88.0
Coprophagy F50.89
Coprophobia F40.298
Coproporphyria, hereditary E80.29
Cor
    biloculare Q20.8
    bovis, bovinum — *see* Hypertrophy, cardiac
    pulmonale (chronic) I27.81
      acute I26.09
    triatriatum, triatrium Q24.2
    triloculare Q20.8
      biatrium Q20.4
      biventriculare Q21.1
Corbus' disease (gangrenous balanitis) N48.1
Cord (*see also* condition)
    around neck
      complicating delivery O69.81 ☑
        with compression O69.1 ☑
    bladder G95.89
      tabetic A52.19
Cordis ectopia Q24.8
Corditis (spermatic) N49.1
Corectopia Q13.2
Cori's disease (glycogen storage) E74.03
Corkhandler's disease or lung J67.3
Corkscrew esophagus K22.4
Corkworker's disease or lung J67.3
Corn (infected) L84
Cornea (*see also* condition)
    donor Z52.5
    plana Q13.4
Cornelia de Lange syndrome Q87.19
Cornu cutaneum L85.8

Cornual gestation or pregnancy - Corrosion

Cornual gestation or pregnancy O00.80
  with intrauterine pregnancy O00.81
Coronary (artery) — *see* condition
Coronavirus, as cause of disease classified elsewhere
  B97.29
  SARS-associated B97.21
Corpora (*see also* condition)
  amylacea, prostate N42.89
  cavernosa — *see* condition
Corpulence — *see* Obesity
Corpus — *see* condition
Corrected transposition Q20.5
Corrosion (injury) (acid) (caustic) (chemical) (lime)
  (external) (internal) T30.4
  abdomen, abdominal (muscle) (wall) T21.42 ☑
    first degree T21.52 ☑
    second degree T21.62 ☑
    third degree T21.72 ☑
  above elbow T22.439 ☑
    first degree T22.539 ☑
    left T22.432 ☑
      first degree T22.532 ☑
      second degree T22.632 ☑
      third degree T22.732 ☑
    right T22.431 ☑
      first degree T22.531 ☑
      second degree T22.631 ☑
      third degree T22.731 ☑
    second degree T22.639 ☑
    third degree T22.739 ☑
  alimentary tract NEC T28.7 ☑
  ankle T25.419 ☑
    first degree T25.519 ☑
    left T25.412 ☑
      first degree T25.512 ☑
      second degree T25.612 ☑
      third degree T25.712 ☑
    multiple with foot — *see* Corrosion, lower, limb,
      multiple, ankle and foot
    right T25.411 ☑
      first degree T25.511 ☑
      second degree T25.611 ☑
      third degree T25.711 ☑
    second degree T25.619 ☑
    third degree T25.719 ☑
  anus — *see* Corrosion, buttock
  arm(s) (meaning upper limb(s)) — *see* Corrosion,
    upper limb
  axilla T22.449 ☑
    first degree T22.549 ☑
    left T22.442 ☑
      first degree T22.542 ☑
      second degree T22.642 ☑
      third degree T22.742 ☑
    right T22.441 ☑
      first degree T22.541 ☑
      second degree T22.641 ☑
      third degree T22.741 ☑
    second degree T22.649 ☑
    third degree T22.749 ☑
  back (lower) T21.44 ☑
    first degree T21.54 ☑
    second degree T21.64 ☑
    third degree T21.74 ☑
    upper T21.43 ☑
      first degree T21.53 ☑
      second degree T21.63 ☑
      third degree T21.73 ☑
  blisters - code as Corrosion, second degree, by site
  breast(s) — *see* Corrosion, chest wall
  buttock(s) T21.45 ☑
    first degree T21.55 ☑
    second degree T21.65 ☑
    third degree T21.75 ☑
  calf T24.439 ☑
    first degree T24.539 ☑
    left T24.432 ☑
      first degree T24.532 ☑
      second degree T24.632 ☑
      third degree T24.732 ☑
    right T24.431 ☑
      first degree T24.531 ☑
      second degree T24.631 ☑
      third degree T24.731 ☑
    second degree T24.639 ☑
    third degree T24.739 ☑
  canthus (eye) — *see* Corrosion, eyelid
  cervix T28.8 ☑
  cheek T20.46 ☑
    first degree T20.56 ☑
    second degree T20.66 ☑
    third degree T20.76 ☑

Corrosion — *continued*
  chest wall T21.41 ☑
    first degree T21.51 ☑
    second degree T21.61 ☑
    third degree T21.71 ☑
  chin T20.43 ☑
    first degree T20.53 ☑
    second degree T20.63 ☑
    third degree T20.73 ☑
  colon T28.7 ☑
  conjunctiva (and cornea) — *see* Corrosion, cornea
  cornea (and conjunctiva) T26.6 ☑
  deep necrosis of underlying tissue - code as
    Corrosion, third degree, by site
  dorsum of hand T23.469 ☑
    first degree T23.569 ☑
    left T23.462 ☑
      first degree T23.562 ☑
      second degree T23.662 ☑
      third degree T23.762 ☑
    right T23.461 ☑
      first degree T23.561 ☑
      second degree T23.661 ☑
      third degree T23.761 ☑
    second degree T23.669 ☑
    third degree T23.769 ☑
  ear (auricle) (external) (canal) T20.41 ☑
    drum T28.91 ☑
    first degree T20.51 ☑
    second degree T20.61 ☑
    third degree T20.71 ☑
  elbow T22.429 ☑
    first degree T22.529 ☑
    left T22.422 ☑
      first degree T22.522 ☑
      second degree T22.622 ☑
      third degree T22.722 ☑
    right T22.421 ☑
      first degree T22.521 ☑
      second degree T22.621 ☑
      third degree T22.721 ☑
    second degree T22.629 ☑
    third degree T22.729 ☑
  entire body — *see* Corrosion, multiple body regions
  epidermal loss - code as Corrosion, second degree,
    by site
  epiglottis T27.4 ☑
  erythema, erythematous - code as Corrosion, first
    degree, by site
  esophagus T28.6 ☑
  extent (percentage of body surface)
    less than 10 percent T32.0
    10-19 percent (0-9 percent third degree) T32.10
      with 10-19 percent third degree T32.11
    20-29 percent (0-9 percent third degree) T32.20
      with
        10-19 percent third degree T32.21
        20-29 percent third degree T32.22
    30-39 percent (0-9 percent third degree) T32.30
      with
        10-19 percent third degree T32.31
        20-29 percent third degree T32.32
        30-39 percent third degree T32.33
    40-49 percent (0-9 percent third degree) T32.40
      with
        10-19 percent third degree T32.41
        20-29 percent third degree T32.42
        30-39 percent third degree T32.43
        40-49 percent third degree T32.44
    50-59 percent (0-9 percent third degree) T32.50
      with
        10-19 percent third degree T32.51
        20-29 percent third degree T32.52
        30-39 percent third degree T32.53
        40-49 percent third degree T32.54
        50-59 percent third degree T32.55
    60-69 percent (0-9 percent third degree) T32.60
      with
        10-19 percent third degree T32.61
        20-29 percent third degree T32.62
        30-39 percent third degree T32.63
        40-49 percent third degree T32.64
        50-59 percent third degree T32.65
        60-69 percent third degree T32.66
    70-79 percent (0-9 percent third degree) T32.70
      with
        10-19 percent third degree T32.71
        20-29 percent third degree T32.72
        30-39 percent third degree T32.73
        40-49 percent third degree T32.74
        50-59 percent third degree T32.75
        60-69 percent third degree T32.76

Corrosion — *continued*
  extent — *continued*
        70-79 percent third degree T32.77
    80-89 percent (0-9 percent third degree) T32.80
      with
        10-19 percent third degree T32.81
        20-29 percent third degree T32.82
        30-39 percent third degree T32.83
        40-49 percent third degree T32.84
        50-59 percent third degree T32.85
        60-69 percent third degree T32.86
        70-79 percent third degree T32.87
        80-89 percent third degree T32.88
    90 percent or more (0-9 percent third degree)
      T32.90
      with
        10-19 percent third degree T32.91
        20-29 percent third degree T32.92
        30-39 percent third degree T32.93
        40-49 percent third degree T32.94
        50-59 percent third degree T32.95
        60-69 percent third degree T32.96
        70-79 percent third degree T32.97
        80-89 percent third degree T32.98
        90-99 percent third degree T32.99
  extremity — *see* Corrosion, limb
  eye(s) and adnexa T26.9 ☑
    with resulting rupture and destruction of eyeball
      T26.7 ☑
    conjunctival sac — *see* Corrosion, cornea
    cornea — *see* Corrosion, cornea
    lid — *see* Corrosion, eyelid
    periocular area — *see* Corrosion eyelid
    specified site NEC T26.8 ☑
  eyeball — *see* Corrosion, eye
  eyelid(s) T26.5 ☑
  face — *see* Corrosion, head
  finger T23.429 ☑
    first degree T23.529 ☑
    left T23.422 ☑
      first degree T23.522 ☑
      second degree T23.622 ☑
      third degree T23.722 ☑
    multiple sites (without thumb) T23.439 ☑
      with thumb T23.449 ☑
        first degree T23.549 ☑
        left T23.442 ☑
          first degree T23.542 ☑
          second degree T23.642 ☑
          third degree T23.742 ☑
        right T23.441 ☑
          first degree T23.541 ☑
          second degree T23.641 ☑
          third degree T23.741 ☑
      second degree T23.649 ☑
      third degree T23.749 ☑
    first degree T23.539 ☑
    left T23.432 ☑
      first degree T23.532 ☑
      second degree T23.632 ☑
      third degree T23.732 ☑
    right T23.431 ☑
      first degree T23.531 ☑
      second degree T23.631 ☑
      third degree T23.731 ☑
    second degree T23.639 ☑
    third degree T23.739 ☑
    right T23.421 ☑
      first degree T23.521 ☑
      second degree T23.621 ☑
      third degree T23.721 ☑
    second degree T23.629 ☑
    third degree T23.729 ☑
  flank — *see* Corrosion, abdomen
  foot T25.429 ☑
    first degree T25.529 ☑
    left T25.422 ☑
      first degree T25.522 ☑
      second degree T25.622 ☑
      third degree T25.722 ☑
    multiple with ankle — *see* Corrosion, lower, limb,
      multiple, ankle and foot
    right T25.421 ☑
      first degree T25.521 ☑
      second degree T25.621 ☑
      third degree T25.721 ☑
    second degree T25.629 ☑
    third degree T25.729 ☑
  forearm T22.419 ☑
    first degree T22.519 ☑
    left T22.412 ☑
      first degree T22.512 ☑

☑ **Additional character required**

Corrosion — *continued*
  forearm — *continued*
    second degree T22.612 ☑
    third degree T22.712 ☑
    right T22.411 ☑
      first degree T22.511 ☑
      second degree T22.611 ☑
      third degree T22.711 ☑
    second degree T22.619 ☑
    third degree T22.719 ☑
  forehead T20.46 ☑
    first degree T20.56 ☑
    second degree T20.66 ☑
    third degree T20.76 ☑
  fourth degree - code as Corrosion, third degree, by site
  full thickness skin loss - code as Corrosion, third degree, by site
  gastrointestinal tract NEC T28.7 ☑
  genital organs
    external
      female T21.47 ☑
        first degree T21.57 ☑
        second degree T21.67 ☑
        third degree T21.77 ☑
      male T21.46 ☑
        first degree T21.56 ☑
        second degree T21.66 ☑
        third degree T21.76 ☑
    internal T28.8 ☑
  groin — *see* Corrosion, abdominal wall
  hand(s) T23.409 ☑
    back — *see* Corrosion, dorsum of hand
    finger — *see* Corrosion, finger
    first degree T23.509 ☑
    left T23.402 ☑
      first degree T23.502 ☑
      second degree T23.602 ☑
      third degree T23.702 ☑
    multiple sites with wrist T23.499 ☑
      first degree T23.599 ☑
      left T23.492 ☑
        first degree T23.592 ☑
        second degree T23.692 ☑
        third degree T23.792 ☑
      right T23.491 ☑
        first degree T23.591 ☑
        second degree T23.691 ☑
        third degree T23.791 ☑
      second degree T23.699 ☑
      third degree T23.799 ☑
    palm — *see* Corrosion, palm
    right T23.401 ☑
      first degree T23.501 ☑
      second degree T23.601 ☑
      third degree T23.701 ☑
    second degree T23.609 ☑
    third degree T23.709 ☑
    thumb — *see* Corrosion, thumb
  head (and face) (and neck) T20.40 ☑
    cheek — *see* Corrosion, cheek
    chin — *see* Corrosion, chin
    ear — *see* Corrosion, ear
    eye(s) only — *see* Corrosion, eye
    first degree T20.50 ☑
    forehead — *see* Corrosion, forehead
    lip — *see* Corrosion, lip
    multiple sites T20.49 ☑
      first degree T20.59 ☑
      second degree T20.69 ☑
      third degree T20.79 ☑
    neck — *see* Corrosion, neck
    nose — *see* Corrosion, nose
    scalp — *see* Corrosion, scalp
    second degree T20.60 ☑
    third degree T20.70 ☑
  hip(s) — *see* Corrosion, lower, limb
  inhalation — *see* Corrosion, respiratory tract
  internal organ(s) (*see also* Corrosion, by site) T28.90 ☑
    alimentary tract T28.7 ☑
      esophagus T28.6 ☑
    esophagus T28.6 ☑
    genitourinary T28.8 ☑
    mouth T28.5 ☑
    pharynx T28.5 ☑
    specified organ NEC T28.99 ☑
  interscapular region — *see* Corrosion, back, upper
  intestine (large) (small) T28.7 ☑
  knee T24.429 ☑
    first degree T24.529 ☑
    left T24.422 ☑

Corrosion — *continued*
  knee — *continued*
    first degree T24.522 ☑
    second degree T24.622 ☑
    third degree T24.722 ☑
    right T24.421 ☑
      first degree T24.521 ☑
      second degree T24.621 ☑
      third degree T24.721 ☑
    second degree T24.629 ☑
    third degree T24.729 ☑
  labium (majus) (minus) — *see* Corrosion, genital organs, external, female
  lacrimal apparatus, duct, gland or sac — *see* Corrosion, eye, specified site NEC
  larynx T27.4 ☑
    with lung T27.5 ☑
  leg(s) (meaning lower limb(s)) — *see* Corrosion, lower limb
  limb(s)
    lower — *see* Corrosion, lower, limb
    upper — *see* Corrosion, upper limb
  lip(s) T20.42 ☑
    first degree T20.52 ☑
    second degree T20.62 ☑
    third degree T20.72 ☑
  lower
    back — *see* Corrosion, back
    limb T24.409 ☑
      ankle — *see* Corrosion, ankle
      calf — *see* Corrosion, calf
      first degree T24.509 ☑
      foot — *see* Corrosion, foot
      knee — *see* Corrosion, knee
      left T24.402 ☑
        first degree T24.502 ☑
        second degree T24.602 ☑
        third degree T24.702 ☑
      multiple sites, except ankle and foot T24.499 ☑
        ankle and foot T25.499 ☑
          first degree T25.599 ☑
          left T25.492 ☑
            first degree T25.592 ☑
            second degree T25.692 ☑
            third degree T25.792 ☑
          right T25.491 ☑
            first degree T25.591 ☑
            second degree T25.691 ☑
            third degree T25.791 ☑
          second degree T25.699 ☑
          third degree T25.799 ☑
        first degree T24.599 ☑
        left T24.492 ☑
          first degree T24.592 ☑
          second degree T24.692 ☑
          third degree T24.792 ☑
        right T24.491 ☑
          first degree T24.591 ☑
          second degree T24.691 ☑
          third degree T24.791 ☑
        second degree T24.699 ☑
        third degree T24.799 ☑
      right T24.401 ☑
        first degree T24.501 ☑
        second degree T24.601 ☑
        third degree T24.701 ☑
      second degree T24.609 ☑
      hip — *see* Corrosion, thigh
      thigh — *see* Corrosion, thigh
      third degree T24.709 ☑
  lung (with larynx and trachea) T27.5 ☑
  mouth T28.5 ☑
  neck T20.47 ☑
    first degree T20.57 ☑
    second degree T20.67 ☑
    third degree T20.77 ☑
  nose (septum) T20.44 ☑
    first degree T20.54 ☑
    second degree T20.64 ☑
    third degree T20.74 ☑
  ocular adnexa — *see* Corrosion, eye
  orbit region — *see* Corrosion, eyelid
  palm T23.459 ☑
    first degree T23.559 ☑
    left T23.452 ☑
      first degree T23.552 ☑
      second degree T23.652 ☑
      third degree T23.752 ☑
    right T23.451 ☑
      first degree T23.551 ☑
      second degree T23.651 ☑
      third degree T23.751 ☑

Corrosion — *continued*
  palm — *continued*
    second degree T23.659 ☑
    third degree T23.759 ☑
  partial thickness - code as Corrosion, unspecified degree, by site
  pelvis — *see* Corrosion, trunk
  penis — *see* Corrosion, genital organs, external, male
  perineum
    female — *see* Corrosion, genital organs, external, female
    male — *see* Corrosion, genital organs, external, male
  periocular area — *see* Corrosion, eyelid
  pharynx T28.5 ☑
  rectum T28.7 ☑
  respiratory tract T27.7 ☑
    larynx — *see* Corrosion, larynx
    specified part NEC T27.6 ☑
    trachea — *see* Corrosion, larynx
  sac, lacrimal — *see* Corrosion, eye, specified site NEC
  scalp T20.45 ☑
    first degree T20.55 ☑
    second degree T20.65 ☑
    third degree T20.75 ☑
  scapular region T22.469 ☑
    first degree T22.569 ☑
    left T22.462 ☑
      first degree T22.562 ☑
      second degree T22.662 ☑
      third degree T22.762 ☑
    right T22.461 ☑
      first degree T22.561 ☑
      second degree T22.661 ☑
      third degree T22.761 ☑
    second degree T22.669 ☑
    third degree T22.769 ☑
  sclera — *see* Corrosion, eye, specified site NEC
  scrotum — *see* Corrosion, genital organs, external, male
  shoulder T22.459 ☑
    first degree T22.559 ☑
    left T22.452 ☑
      first degree T22.552 ☑
      second degree T22.652 ☑
      third degree T22.752 ☑
    right T22.451 ☑
      first degree T22.551 ☑
      second degree T22.651 ☑
      third degree T22.751 ☑
    second degree T22.659 ☑
    third degree T22.759 ☑
  stomach T28.7 ☑
  temple — *see* Corrosion, head
  testis — *see* Corrosion, genital organs, external, male
  thigh T24.419 ☑
    first degree T24.519 ☑
    left T24.412 ☑
      first degree T24.512 ☑
      second degree T24.612 ☑
      third degree T24.712 ☑
    right T24.411 ☑
      first degree T24.511 ☑
      second degree T24.611 ☑
      third degree T24.711 ☑
    second degree T24.619 ☑
    third degree T24.719 ☑
  thorax (external) — *see* Corrosion, trunk
  throat (meaning pharynx) T28.5 ☑
  thumb(s) T23.419 ☑
    first degree T23.519 ☑
    left T23.412 ☑
      first degree T23.512 ☑
      second degree T23.612 ☑
      third degree T23.712 ☑
    multiple sites with fingers T23.449 ☑
      first degree T23.549 ☑
      left T23.442 ☑
        first degree T23.542 ☑
        second degree T23.642 ☑
        third degree T23.742 ☑
      right T23.441 ☑
        first degree T23.541 ☑
        second degree T23.641 ☑
        third degree T23.741 ☑
      second degree T23.649 ☑
      third degree T23.749 ☑
    right T23.411 ☑
      first degree T23.511 ☑
      second degree T23.611 ☑
      third degree T23.711 ☑

Corrosion — *continued*
  thumb(s) — *continued*
    second degree T23.619 ☑
    third degree T23.719 ☑
  toe T25.439 ☑
    first degree T25.539 ☑
    left T25.432 ☑
      first degree T25.532 ☑
      second degree T25.632 ☑
      third degree T25.732 ☑
    right T25.431 ☑
      first degree T25.531 ☑
      second degree T25.631 ☑
      third degree T25.731 ☑
    second degree T25.639 ☑
    third degree T25.739 ☑
  tongue T28.5 ☑
  tonsil(s) T28.5 ☑
  total body — *see* Corrosion, multiple body regions
  trachea T27.4 ☑
    with lung T27.5 ☑
  trunk T21.40 ☑
    abdominal wall — *see* Corrosion, abdominal wall
    anus — *see* Corrosion, buttock
    axilla — *see* Corrosion, upper limb
    back — *see* Corrosion, back
    breast — *see* Corrosion, chest wall
    buttock — *see* Corrosion, buttock
    chest wall — *see* Corrosion, chest wall
    first degree T21.50 ☑
    flank — *see* Corrosion, abdominal wall
    genital
      female — *see* Corrosion, genital organs, external, female
      male — *see* Corrosion, genital organs, external, male
    groin — *see* Corrosion, abdominal wall
    interscapular region — *see* Corrosion, back, upper
    labia — *see* Corrosion, genital organs, external, female
    lower back — *see* Corrosion, back
    penis — *see* Corrosion, genital organs, external, male
    perineum
      female — *see* Corrosion, genital organs, external, female
      male — *see* Corrosion, genital organs, external, male
    scapular region — *see* Corrosion, upper limb
    scrotum — *see* Corrosion, genital organs, external, male
    second degree T21.60 ☑
    shoulder — *see* Corrosion, upper limb
    specified site NEC T21.49 ☑
      first degree T21.59 ☑
      second degree T21.69 ☑
      third degree T21.79 ☑
    testes — *see* Corrosion, genital organs, external, male
    third degree T21.70 ☑
    upper back — *see* Corrosion, back, upper
    vagina T28.8 ☑
    vulva — *see* Corrosion, genital organs, external, female
  unspecified site with extent of body surface involved specified
    less than 10 percent T32.0
    10-19 percent (0-9 percent third degree) T32.10
      with 10-19 percent third degree T32.11
    20-29 percent (0-9 percent third degree) T32.20
      with
        10-19 percent third degree T32.21
        20-29 percent third degree T32.22
    30-39 percent (0-9 percent third degree) T32.30
      with
        10-19 percent third degree T32.31
        20-29 percent third degree T32.32
        30-39 percent third degree T32.33
    40-49 percent (0-9 percent third degree) T32.40
      with
        10-19 percent third degree T32.41
        20-29 percent third degree T32.42
        30-39 percent third degree T32.43
        40-49 percent third degree T32.44
    50-59 percent (0-9 percent third degree) T32.50
      with
        10-19 percent third degree T32.51
        20-29 percent third degree T32.52
        30-39 percent third degree T32.53
        40-49 percent third degree T32.54
        50-59 percent third degree T32.55
    60-69 percent (0-9 percent third degree) T32.60

Corrosion — *continued*
  unspecified site — *continued*
    with
      10-19 percent third degree T32.61
      20-29 percent third degree T32.62
      30-39 percent third degree T32.63
      40-49 percent third degree T32.64
      50-59 percent third degree T32.65
      60-69 percent third degree T32.66
    70-79 percent (0-9 percent third degree) T32.70
      with
        10-19 percent third degree T32.71
        20-29 percent third degree T32.72
        30-39 percent third degree T32.73
        40-49 percent third degree T32.74
        50-59 percent third degree T32.75
        60-69 percent third degree T32.76
        70-79 percent third degree T32.77
    80-89 percent (0-9 percent third degree) T32.80
      with
        10-19 percent third degree T32.81
        20-29 percent third degree T32.82
        30-39 percent third degree T32.83
        40-49 percent third degree T32.84
        50-59 percent third degree T32.85
        60-69 percent third degree T32.86
        70-79 percent third degree T32.87
        80-89 percent third degree T32.88
    90 percent or more (0-9 percent third degree) T32.90
      with
        10-19 percent third degree T32.91
        20-29 percent third degree T32.92
        30-39 percent third degree T32.93
        40-49 percent third degree T32.94
        50-59 percent third degree T32.95
        60-69 percent third degree T32.96
        70-79 percent third degree T32.97
        80-89 percent third degree T32.98
        90-99 percent third degree T32.99
  upper limb (axilla) (scapular region) T22.40 ☑
    above elbow — *see* Corrosion, above elbow
    axilla — *see* Corrosion, axilla
    elbow — *see* Corrosion, elbow
    first degree T22.50 ☑
    forearm — *see* Corrosion, forearm
    hand — *see* Corrosion, hand
    interscapular region — *see* Corrosion, back, upper
    multiple sites T22.499 ☑
      first degree T22.599 ☑
      left T22.492 ☑
        first degree T22.592 ☑
        second degree T22.692 ☑
        third degree T22.792 ☑
      right T22.491 ☑
        first degree T22.591 ☑
        second degree T22.691 ☑
        third degree T22.791 ☑
      second degree T22.699 ☑
      third degree T22.799 ☑
    scapular region — *see* Corrosion, scapular region
    second degree T22.60 ☑
    shoulder — *see* Corrosion, shoulder
    third degree T22.70 ☑
    wrist — *see* Corrosion, hand
  uterus T28.8 ☑
  vagina T28.8 ☑
  vulva — *see* Corrosion, genital organs, external, female
  wrist T23.479 ☑
    first degree T23.579 ☑
    left T23.472 ☑
      first degree T23.572 ☑
      second degree T23.672 ☑
      third degree T23.772 ☑
    multiple sites with hand T23.499 ☑
      first degree T23.599 ☑
      left T23.492 ☑
        first degree T23.592 ☑
        second degree T23.692 ☑
        third degree T23.792 ☑
      right T23.491 ☑
        first degree T23.591 ☑
        second degree T23.691 ☑
        third degree T23.791 ☑
      second degree T23.699 ☑
      third degree T23.799 ☑
    right T23.471 ☑
      first degree T23.571 ☑
      second degree T23.671 ☑
      third degree T23.771 ☑
    second degree T23.679 ☑
    third degree T23.779 ☑

Corrosive burn — *see* Corrosion
Corsican fever — *see* Malaria
Cortical — *see* condition
Cortico-adrenal — *see* condition
Coryza (acute) J00
  with grippe or influenza — *see* Influenza, with, respiratory manifestations NEC
  syphilitic
    congenital (chronic) A50.05
Costen's syndrome or complex M26.69
Costiveness — *see* Constipation
Costochondritis M94.0
Cotard's syndrome F22
Cot death R99
Cotia virus B08.8
Cotton wool spots (retinal) H35.81
Cotungo's disease — *see* Sciatica
Cough (affected) (chronic) (epidemic) (nervous) R05
  with hemorrhage — *see* Hemoptysis
  bronchial R05
    with grippe or influenza — *see* Influenza, with, respiratory manifestations NEC
  functional F45.8
  hysterical F45.8
  laryngeal, spasmodic R05
  psychogenic F45.8
  smokers' J41.0
  tea taster's B49
Counseling (for) Z71.9
  abuse NEC
    perpetrator Z69.82
    victim Z69.81
  alcohol abuser Z71.41
    family Z71.42
  child abuse
    nonparental
      perpetrator Z69.021
      victim Z69.020
    parental
      perpetrator Z69.011
      victim Z69.010
  consanguinity Z71.89
  contraceptive Z30.09
  dietary Z71.3
  drug abuser Z71.51
    family member Z71.52
  exercise Z71.82
  family Z71.89
  fertility preservation (prior to cancer therapy) (prior to removal of gonads) Z31.62
  for non-attending third party Z71.0
    related to sexual behavior or orientation Z70.2
  genetic
    nonprocreative Z71.83
    procreative NEC Z31.5
  gestational carrier Z31.7
  health (advice) (education) (instruction) — *see* Counseling, medical
    risk for travel (international) Z71.84
  human immunodeficiency virus (HIV) Z71.7
  impotence Z70.1
  insulin pump use Z46.81
  medical (for) Z71.9
    boarding school resident Z59.3
    consanguinity Z71.89
    feared complaint and no disease found Z71.1
    human immunodeficiency virus (HIV) Z71.7
    institutional resident Z59.3
    on behalf of another Z71.0
      related to sexual behavior or orientation Z70.2
    person living alone Z60.2
    specified reason NEC Z71.89
  natural family planning
    procreative Z31.61
    to avoid pregnancy Z30.02
  perpetrator (of)
    abuse NEC Z69.82
    child abuse
      non-parental Z69.021
      parental Z69.011
    rape NEC Z69.82
    spousal abuse Z69.12
  procreative NEC Z31.69
    fertility preservation (prior to cancer therapy) (prior to removal of gonads) Z31.62
    using natural family planning Z31.61
  promiscuity Z70.1
  rape victim Z69.81
  religious Z71.81
  safety for travel (international) Z71.84
  sex, sexual (related to) Z70.9
    attitude(s) Z70.0

Counseling — *continued*
  sex — *continued*
    behavior or orientation Z70.1
    combined concerns Z70.3
    non-responsiveness Z70.1
    on behalf of third party Z70.2
    specified reason NEC Z70.8
  specified reason NEC Z71.89
  spiritual Z71.81
  spousal abuse (perpetrator) Z69.12
    victim Z69.11
  substance abuse Z71.89
    alcohol Z71.41
    drug Z71.51
    tobacco Z71.6
  tobacco use Z71.6
  travel (international) Z71.84
  use (of)
    insulin pump Z46.81
  victim (of)
    abuse Z69.81
    child abuse
      by parent Z69.010
      non-parental Z69.020
    rape NEC Z69.81
Coupled rhythm R00.8
Couvelaire syndrome or uterus (complicating delivery) O45.8X ☑
Cowperitis — *see* Urethritis
Cowper's gland — *see* condition
Cowpox B08.010
  due to vaccination T88.1 ☑
Coxa
  magna M91.4 ☑
  plana M91.2 ☑
  valga (acquired) (*see also* Deformity, limb, specified type NEC, thigh)
    congenital Q65.81
    sequelae (late effect) of rickets E64.3
  vara (acquired) (*see also* Deformity, limb, specified type NEC, thigh)
    congenital Q65.82
    sequelae (late effect) of rickets E64.3
Coxalgia, coxalgic (nontuberculous) (*see also* Pain, joint, hip)
  tuberculous A18.02
Coxitis — *see* Monoarthritis, hip
Coxsackie (virus) (infection) B34.1
  as cause of disease classified elsewhere B97.11
  carditis B33.20
  central nervous system NEC A88.8
  endocarditis B33.21
  enteritis A08.39
  meningitis (aseptic) A87.0
  myocarditis B33.22
  pericarditis B33.23
  pharyngitis B08.5
  pleurodynia B33.0
  specific disease NEC B33.8
Crabs, meaning pubic lice B85.3
Crack baby P04.41
Cracked nipple N64.0
  associated with
    lactation O92.13
    pregnancy O92.11 ☑
    puerperium O92.12
Cracked tooth K03.81
Cradle cap L21.0
Craft neurosis F48.8
Cramp(s) R25.2
  abdominal — *see* Pain, abdominal
  bathing T75.1 ☑
  colic R10.83
    psychogenic F45.8
  due to immersion T75.1 ☑
  fireman T67.2 ☑
  heat T67.2 ☑
  immersion T75.1 ☑
  intestinal — *see* Pain, abdominal
    psychogenic F45.8
  leg, sleep related G47.62
  limb (lower) (upper) NEC R25.2
    sleep related G47.62
  linotypist's F48.8
    organic G25.89
  muscle (limb) (general) R25.2
    due to immersion T75.1 ☑
    psychogenic F45.8
  occupational (hand) F48.8
    organic G25.89
  salt-depletion E87.1
  sleep related, leg G47.62

Cramp(s) — *continued*
  stoker's T67.2 ☑
  swimmer's T75.1 ☑
  telegrapher's F48.8
    organic G25.89
  typist's F48.8
    organic G25.89
  uterus N94.89
    menstrual — *see* Dysmenorrhea
  writer's F48.8
    organic G25.89
Cranial — *see* condition
Craniocleidodysostosis Q74.0
Craniofenestria (skull) Q75.8
Craniolacunia (skull) Q75.8
Craniopagus Q89.4
Craniopathy, metabolic M85.2
Craniopharyngeal — *see* condition
Craniopharyngioma D44.4
Craniorachischisis (totalis) Q00.1
Cranioschisis Q75.8
Craniostenosis Q75.0
Craniosynostosis Q75.0
Craniotabes (cause unknown) M83.8
  neonatal P96.3
  rachitic E64.3
  syphilitic A50.56
Cranium — *see* condition
Craw-craw — *see* Onchocerciasis
Creaking joint — *see* Derangement, joint, specified type NEC
Creeping
  eruption B76.9
  palsy or paralysis G12.22
Crenated tongue K14.8
Creotoxism A05.9
Crepitus
  caput Q75.8
  joint — *see* Derangement, joint, specified type NEC
Crescent or conus choroid, congenital Q14.3
CREST syndrome M34.1
Cretin, cretinism (congenital) (endemic) (nongoitrous) (sporadic) E00.9
  pelvis
    with disproportion (fetopelvic) O33.0
      causing obstructed labor O65.0
  type
    hypothyroid E00.1
    mixed E00.2
    myxedematous E00.1
    neurological E00.0
Creutzfeldt-Jakob disease or syndrome (with dementia) A81.00
  familial A81.09
  iatrogenic A81.09
  specified NEC A81.09
  sporadic A81.09
  variant (vCJD) A81.01
Crib death R99
Cribriform hymen Q52.3
Cri-du-chat syndrome Q93.4
Crigler-Najjar disease or syndrome E80.5
Crime, victim of Z65.4
Crimean hemorrhagic fever A98.0
Criminalism F60.2
Crisis
  abdomen R10.0
  acute reaction F43.0
  addisonian E27.2
  adrenal (cortical) E27.2
  celiac K90.0
  Dietl's N13.8
  emotional (*see also* Disorder, adjustment)
    acute reaction to stress F43.0
    specific to childhood and adolescence F93.8
  glaucomatocyclitic — *see* Glaucoma, secondary, inflammation
  heart — *see* Failure, heart
  nitritoid I95.2
    correct substance properly administered — *see* Table of Drugs and Chemicals, by drug, adverse effect
    overdose or wrong substance given or taken — *see* Table of Drugs and Chemicals, by drug, poisoning
  oculogyric H51.8
    psychogenic F45.8
  Pel's (tabetic) A52.11
  psychosexual identity F64.2
  renal N28.0

Crisis — *continued*
  sickle-cell D57.00
    with
      acute chest syndrome D57.01
      splenic sequestration D57.02
  state (acute reaction) F43.0
  tabetic A52.11
  thyroid — *see* Thyrotoxicosis with thyroid storm
  thyrotoxic — *see* Thyrotoxicosis with thyroid storm
Crocq's disease (acrocyanosis) I73.89
Crohn's disease — *see* Enteritis, regional
Crooked septum, nasal J34.2
Cross syndrome E70.328
Crossbite (anterior) (posterior) M26.24
Cross-eye — *see* Strabismus, convergent concomitant
Croup, croupous (catarrhal) (infectious) (inflammatory) (nondiphtheritic) J05.0
  bronchial J20.9
  diphtheritic A36.2
  false J38.5
  spasmodic J38.5
    diphtheritic A36.2
  stridulous J38.5
    diphtheritic A36.2
Crouzon's disease Q75.1
Crowding, tooth, teeth, fully erupted M26.31
CRST syndrome M34.1
Cruchet's disease A85.8
Cruelty in children (*see also* Disorder, conduct)
Crural ulcer — *see* Ulcer, lower limb
Crush, crushed, crushing T14.8 ☑
  abdomen S38.1 ☑
  ankle S97.0 ☑
  arm (upper) (and shoulder) S47. ☑
  axilla — *see* Crush, arm
  back, lower S38.1 ☑
  buttock S38.1 ☑
  cheek S07.0 ☑
  chest S28.0 ☑
  cranium S07.1 ☑
  ear S07.0 ☑
  elbow S57.0 ☑
  extremity
    lower
      ankle — *see* Crush, ankle
      below knee — *see* Crush, leg
      foot — *see* Crush, foot
      hip — *see* Crush, hip
      knee — *see* Crush, knee
      thigh — *see* Crush, thigh
      toe — *see* Crush, toe
    upper
      below elbow S67.9 ☑
      elbow — *see* Crush, elbow
      finger — *see* Crush, finger
      forearm — *see* Crush, forearm
      hand — *see* Crush, hand
      thumb — *see* Crush, thumb
      upper arm — *see* Crush, arm
      wrist — *see* Crush, wrist
  face S07.0 ☑
  finger(s) S67.1 ☑
    with hand (and wrist) — *see* Crush, hand, specified site NEC
    index S67.19 ☑
    little S67.19 ☑
    middle S67.19 ☑
    ring S67.19 ☑
    thumb — *see* Crush, thumb
  foot S97.8 ☑
    toe — *see* Crush, toe
  forearm S57.8 ☑
  genitalia, external
    female S38.002 ☑
      vagina S38.03 ☑
      vulva S38.03 ☑
    male S38.001 ☑
      penis S38.01 ☑
      scrotum S38.02 ☑
      testis S38.02 ☑
  hand (except fingers alone) S67.2 ☑
    with wrist S67.4 ☑
  head S07.9 ☑
    specified NEC S07.8 ☑
  heel — *see* Crush, foot
  hip S77.0 ☑
    with thigh S77.2 ☑
  internal organ (abdomen, chest, or pelvis) NEC T14.8 ☑
  knee S87.0 ☑
  labium (majus) (minus) S38.03 ☑
  larynx S17.0 ☑

Crush - Cyst

Crush — *continued*
  leg (lower) S87.8 ☑
    knee — *see* Crush, knee
  lip S07.0 ☑
  lower
    back S38.1 ☑
    leg — *see* Crush, leg
  neck S17.9 ☑
  nerve — *see* Injury, nerve
  nose S07.0 ☑
  pelvis S38.1 ☑
  penis S38.01 ☑
  scalp S07.8 ☑
  scapular region — *see* Crush, arm
  scrotum S38.02 ☑
  severe, unspecified site T14.8 ☑
  shoulder (and upper arm) — *see* Crush, arm
  skull S07.1 ☑
  syndrome (complication of trauma) T79.5 ☑
  testis S38.02 ☑
  thigh S77.1 ☑
    with hip S77.2 ☑
  throat S17.8 ☑
  thumb S67.0 ☑
    with hand (and wrist) — *see* Crush, hand,
      specified site NEC
  toe(s) S97.10 ☑
    great S97.11 ☑
    lesser S97.12 ☑
  trachea S17.0 ☑
  vagina S38.03 ☑
  vulva S38.03 ☑
  wrist S67.3 ☑
    with hand S67.4 ☑
Crusta lactea L21.0
Crusts R23.4
Crutch paralysis — *see* Injury, brachial plexus
Cruveilhier-Baumgarten cirrhosis, disease or
  syndrome K74.69
Cruveilhier's atrophy or disease G12.8
Crying (constant) (continuous) (excessive)
  child, adolescent, or adult R45.83
  infant (baby) (newborn) R68.11
Cryofibrinogenemia D89.2
Cryoglobulinemia (essential) (idiopathic) (mixed)
  (primary) (purpura) (secondary) (vasculitis) D89.1
    with lung involvement D89.1 *[J99]*
Cryptitis (anal) (rectal) K62.89
Cryptococcosis, cryptococcus (infection) (neoformans)
  B45.9
  bone B45.3
  cerebral B45.1
  cutaneous B45.2
  disseminated B45.7
  generalized B45.7
  meningitis B45.1
  meningocerebralis B45.1
  osseous B45.3
  pulmonary B45.0
  skin B45.2
  specified NEC B45.8
Cryptopapillitis (anus) K62.89
Cryptophthalmos Q11.2
  syndrome Q87.0
Cryptorchid, cryptorchism, cryptorchidism Q53.9
  bilateral Q53.20
    abdominal Q53.211
    perineal Q53.22
  unilateral Q53.10
    abdominal Q53.111
    perineal Q53.12
Cryptosporidiosis A07.2
  hepatobiliary B88.8
  respiratory B88.8
Cryptostromosis J67.6
Crystalluria R82.998
Cubitus
  congenital Q68.8
  valgus (acquired) M21.0 ☑
    congenital Q68.8
    sequelae (late effect) of rickets E64.3
  varus (acquired) M21.1 ☑
    congenital Q68.8
    sequelae (late effect) of rickets E64.3
Cultural deprivation or shock Z60.3
Curling esophagus K22.4
Curling's ulcer — *see* Ulcer, peptic, acute
Curschmann (-Batten) (-Steinert) disease or syndrome
  G71.11
Curse, Ondine's — *see* Apnea, sleep
Curvature
  organ or site, congenital NEC — *see* Distortion

Curvature — *continued*
  penis (lateral) Q55.61
  Pott's (spinal) A18.01
  radius, idiopathic, progressive (congenital) Q74.0
  spine (acquired) (angular) (idiopathic) (incorrect)
    (postural) — *see* Dorsopathy, deforming
    congenital Q67.5
    due to or associated with
      Charcot-Marie-Tooth disease (*see also*
        subcategory M49.8 ☑) G60.0
      osteitis
        deformans M88.88
        fibrosa cystica (*see also* subcategory
          M49.8 ☑) E21.0
    tuberculosis (Pott's curvature) A18.01
  sequelae (late effect) of rickets E64.3
  tuberculous A18.01
Cushingoid due to steroid therapy E24.2
  correct substance properly administered — *see* Table
    of Drugs and Chemicals, by drug, adverse effect
  overdose or wrong substance given or taken —
    see Table of Drugs and Chemicals, by drug,
    poisoning
Cushing's
  syndrome or disease E24.9
    drug-induced E24.2
    iatrogenic E24.2
    pituitary-dependent E24.0
    specified NEC E24.8
  ulcer — *see* Ulcer, peptic, acute
Cusp, Carabelli - omit code
Cut (external) (*see also* Laceration)
  muscle — *see* Injury, muscle
Cutaneous (*see also* condition)
  hemorrhage R23.3
  larva migrans B76.9
Cutis (*see also* condition)
  hyperelastica Q82.8
    acquired L57.4
  laxa (hyperelastica) — *see* Dermatolysis
  marmorata R23.8
  osteosis L94.2
  pendula — *see* Dermatolysis
  rhomboidalis nuchae L57.2
  verticis gyrata Q82.8
    acquired L91.8
Cyanosis R23.0
  due to
    patent foramen botalli Q21.1
    persistent foramen ovale Q21.1
  enterogenous D74.8
  paroxysmal digital — *see* Raynaud's disease
    with gangrene I73.01
  retina, retinal H35.89
Cyanotic heart disease I24.9
  congenital Q24.9
Cycle
  anovulatory N97.0
  menstrual, irregular N92.6
Cyclencephaly Q04.9
Cyclical vomiting, in migraine, (*see also* Vomiting,
  cyclical) G43.A0
  psychogenic F50.89
Cyclitis (*see also* Iridocyclitis) H20.9
  chronic — *see* Iridocyclitis, chronic
  Fuchs' heterochromic H20.81 ☑
  granulomatous — *see* Iridocyclitis, chronic
  lens-induced — *see* Iridocyclitis, lens-induced
  posterior H30.2 ☑
Cycloid personality F34.0
Cyclophoria H50.54
Cyclopia, cyclops Q87.0
Cyclopism Q87.0
Cyclosporiasis A07.4
Cyclothymia F34.0
Cyclothymic personality F34.0
Cyclotropia H50.41 ☑
Cylindroma (*see also* Neoplasm, malignant, by site)
  eccrine dermal — *see* Neoplasm, skin, benign
  skin — *see* Neoplasm, skin, benign
Cylindruria R82.998
Cynanche
  diphtheritic A36.2
  tonsillaris J36
Cynophobia F40.218
Cynorexia R63.2
Cyphosis — *see* Kyphosis
Cyprus fever — *see* Brucellosis
Cyst (colloid) (mucous) (simple) (retention)
  adenoid (infected) J35.8
  adrenal gland E27.8
    congenital Q89.1

Cyst — *continued*
  air, lung J98.4
  allantoic Q64.4
  alveolar process (jaw bone) M27.40
  amnion, amniotic O41.8X ☑
  aneurysmal M27.49
  anterior
    chamber (eye) — *see* Cyst, iris
    nasopalatine K09.1
  antrum J34.1
  anus K62.89
  apical (tooth) (periodontal) K04.8
  appendix K38.8
  arachnoid, brain (acquired) G93.0
    congenital Q04.6
  arytenoid J38.7
  Baker's M71.2 ☑
    ruptured M66.0
    tuberculous A18.02
  Bartholin's gland N75.0
  bile duct (common) (hepatic) K83.5
  bladder (multiple) (trigone) N32.89
  blue dome (breast) — *see* Cyst, breast
  bone (local) NEC M85.60
    aneurysmal M85.50
      ankle M85.57 ☑
      foot M85.57 ☑
      forearm M85.53 ☑
      hand M85.54 ☑
      jaw M27.49
      lower leg M85.56 ☑
      multiple site M85.59
      neck M85.58
      rib M85.58
      shoulder M85.51 ☑
      skull M85.58
      specified site NEC M85.58
      thigh M85.55 ☑
      toe M85.57 ☑
      upper arm M85.52 ☑
      vertebra M85.58
    solitary M85.40
      ankle M85.47 ☑
      fibula M85.46 ☑
      foot M85.47 ☑
      hand M85.44 ☑
      humerus M85.42 ☑
      jaw M27.49
      neck M85.48
      pelvis M85.45 ☑
      radius M85.43 ☑
      rib M85.48
      shoulder M85.41 ☑
      skull M85.48
      specified site NEC M85.48
      tibia M85.46 ☑
      toe M85.47 ☑
      ulna M85.43 ☑
      vertebra M85.48
    specified type NEC M85.60
      ankle M85.67 ☑
      foot M85.67 ☑
      forearm M85.63 ☑
      hand M85.64 ☑
      jaw M27.40
        developmental (nonodontogenic) K09.1
        odontogenic K09.0
        latent M27.0
      lower leg M85.66 ☑
      multiple site M85.69
      neck M85.68
      rib M85.68
      shoulder M85.61 ☑
      skull M85.68
      specified site NEC M85.68
      thigh M85.65 ☑
      toe M85.67 ☑
      upper arm M85.62 ☑
      vertebra M85.68
  brain (acquired) G93.0
    congenital Q04.6
    hydatid B67.99 *[G94]*
    third ventricle (colloid), congenital Q04.6
  branchial (cleft) Q18.0
  branchiogenic Q18.0
  breast (benign) (blue dome) (pedunculated)
    (solitary) N60.0
    involution — *see* Dysplasia, mammary, specified
      type NEC
    sebaceous — *see* Dysplasia, mammary, specified
      type NEC
  broad ligament (benign) N83.8

☑ **Additional character required**

Cyst — *continued*
- bronchogenic (mediastinal) (sequestration) J98.4
  - congenital Q33.0
- buccal K09.8
- bulbourethral gland N36.8
- bursa, bursal NEC M71.30
  - with rupture — *see* Rupture, synovium
  - ankle M71.37 ☑
  - elbow M71.32 ☑
  - foot M71.37 ☑
  - hand M71.34 ☑
  - hip M71.35 ☑
  - multiple sites M71.39
  - pharyngeal J39.2
  - popliteal space — *see* Cyst, Baker's
  - shoulder M71.31 ☑
  - specified site NEC M71.38
  - wrist M71.33 ☑
- calcifying odontogenic D16.5
  - upper jaw (bone) (maxilla) D16.4
- canal of Nuck (female) N94.89
  - congenital Q52.4
- canthus — *see* Cyst, conjunctiva
- carcinomatous — *see* Neoplasm, malignant, by site
- cauda equina G95.89
- cavum septi pellucidi — *see* Cyst, brain
- celomic (pericardium) Q24.8
- cerebellopontine (angle) — *see* Cyst, brain
- cerebellum — *see* Cyst, brain
- cerebral — *see* Cyst, brain
- cervical lateral Q18.0
- cervix NEC N88.8
  - embryonic Q51.6
  - nabothian N88.8
- chiasmal optic NEC — *see* Disorder, optic, chiasm
- chocolate (ovary) N80.1
- choledochus, congenital Q44.4
- chorion O41.8X ☑
- choroid plexus G93.0
  - congenital Q04.6
- ciliary body — *see* Cyst, iris
- clitoris N90.7
- colon K63.89
- common (bile) duct K83.5
- congenital NEC Q89.8
  - adrenal gland Q89.1
  - epiglottis Q31.8
  - esophagus Q39.8
  - fallopian tube Q50.4
  - kidney Q61.00
    - more than one (multiple) Q61.02
      - specified as polycystic Q61.3
        - adult type Q61.2
        - infantile type NEC Q61.19
          - collecting duct dilation Q61.11
    - solitary Q61.01
  - larynx Q31.8
  - liver Q44.6
  - lung Q33.0
  - mediastinum Q34.1
  - ovary Q50.1
  - oviduct Q50.4
  - periurethral (tissue) Q64.79
  - prepuce Q55.69
  - salivary gland (any) Q38.4
  - sublingual Q38.6
  - submaxillary gland Q38.6
  - thymus (gland) Q89.2
  - tongue Q38.3
  - ureterovesical orifice Q62.8
  - vulva Q52.79
- conjunctiva H11.44 ☑
- cornea H18.89 ☑
- corpora quadrigemina G93.0
- corpus
  - albicans N83.29 ☑
  - luteum (hemorrhagic) (ruptured) N83.1 ☑
- Cowper's gland (benign) (infected) N36.8
- cranial meninges G93.0
- craniobuccal pouch E23.6
- craniopharyngeal pouch E23.6
- cystic duct K82.8
- Cysticercus — *see* Cysticercosis
- Dandy-Walker Q03.1
  - with spina bifida — *see* Spina bifida
- dental (root) K04.8
  - developmental K09.0
  - eruption K09.0
  - primordial K09.0
- dentigerous (mandible) (maxilla) K09.0
- dermoid — *see* Neoplasm, benign, by site
  - with malignant transformation C56. ☑

Cyst — *continued*
- dermoid — *continued*
  - implantation
    - external area or site (skin) NEC L72.0
    - iris — *see* Cyst, iris, implantation
    - vagina N89.8
    - vulva N90.7
  - mouth K09.8
  - oral soft tissue K09.8
  - sacrococcygeal (*see also* Cyst, pilonidal)
- developmental K09.1
  - odontogenic K09.0
  - oral region (nonodontogenic) K09.1
  - ovary, ovarian Q50.1
- dura (cerebral) G93.0
  - spinal G96.19
- ear (external) Q18.1
- echinococcal — *see* Echinococcus
- embryonic
  - cervix uteri Q51.6
  - fallopian tube Q50.4
  - vagina Q52.4
- endometrium, endometrial (uterus) N85.8
  - ectopic — *see* Endometriosis
- enterogenous Q43.8
- epidermal, epidermoid (inclusion) (*see also* Cyst, skin) L72.0
  - mouth K09.8
  - oral soft tissue K09.8
- epididymis N50.3
- epiglottis J38.7
- epiphysis cerebri E34.8
- epithelial (inclusion) L72.0
- epoophoron Q50.5
- eruption K09.0
- esophagus K22.8
- ethmoid sinus J34.1
- external female genital organs NEC N90.7
- eye NEC H57.89
  - congenital Q15.8
- eyelid (sebaceous) H02.829
  - infected — *see* Hordeolum
  - left H02.826
    - lower H02.825
    - upper H02.824
  - right H02.823
    - lower H02.822
    - upper H02.821
- fallopian tube N83.8
  - congenital Q50.4
- fimbrial (twisted) Q50.4
- fissural (oral region) K09.1
- follicle (graafian) (hemorrhagic) N83.0 ☑
  - nabothian N88.8
- follicular (atretic) (hemorrhagic) (ovarian) N83.0 ☑
  - dentigerous K09.0
  - odontogenic K09.0
  - skin L72.9
    - specified NEC L72.8
- frontal sinus J34.1
- gallbladder K82.8
- ganglion — *see* Ganglion
- Gartner's duct Q52.4
- gingiva K09.0
- gland of Moll — *see* Cyst, eyelid
- globulomaxillary K09.1
- graafian follicle (hemorrhagic) N83.0 ☑
- granulosal lutein (hemorrhagic) N83.1 ☑
- hemangiomatous D18.00
  - intra-abdominal D18.03
  - intracranial D18.02
  - skin D18.01
  - specified site NEC D18.09
- hemorrhagic M27.49
- hydatid (*see also* Echinococcus) B67.90
  - brain B67.99 *[G94]*
  - liver (*see also* Cyst, liver, hydatid) B67.8
  - lung NEC B67.99 *[J99]*
  - Morgagni
    - female Q50.5
    - male (epididymal) Q55.4
      - testicular Q55.29
  - specified site NEC B67.99
- hymen N89.8
  - embryonic Q52.4
- hypopharynx J39.2
- hypophysis, hypophyseal (duct) (recurrent) E23.6
  - cerebri E23.6
- implantation (dermoid)
  - external area or site (skin) NEC L72.0
  - iris — *see* Cyst, iris, implantation
  - vagina N89.8

Cyst — *continued*
- implantation — *continued*
  - vulva N90.7
- incisive canal K09.1
- inclusion (epidermal) (epithelial) (epidermoid) (squamous) L72.0
  - not of skin - code under Cyst, by site
- intestine (large) (small) K63.89
- intracranial — *see* Cyst, brain
- intraligamentous (*see also* Disorder, ligament)
  - knee — *see* Derangement, knee
- intrasellar E23.6
- iris H21.309
  - exudative H21.31 ☑
  - idiopathic H21.30 ☑
  - implantation H21.32 ☑
  - parasitic H21.33 ☑
  - pars plana (primary) H21.34 ☑
    - exudative H21.35 ☑
- jaw (bone) M27.40
  - aneurysmal M27.49
  - hemorrhagic M27.49
  - traumatic M27.49
  - developmental (odontogenic) K09.0
  - fissural K09.1
- joint NEC — *see* Disorder, joint, specified type NEC
- kidney (acquired) N28.1
  - calyceal — *see* Hydronephrosis
  - congenital Q61.00
  - more than one (multiple) Q61.02
    - specified as polycystic Q61.3
      - adult type (autosomal dominant) Q61.2
      - infantile type (autosomal recessive) NEC Q61.19
        - collecting duct dilation Q61.11
  - pyelogenic — *see* Hydronephrosis
  - simple N28.1
  - solitary (single) Q61.01
    - acquired N28.1
- labium (majus) (minus) N90.7
  - sebaceous N90.7
- lacrimal (*see also* Disorder, lacrimal system, specified NEC)
  - gland H04.13 ☑
  - passages or sac — *see* Disorder, lacrimal system, specified NEC
- larynx J38.7
- lateral periodontal K09.0
- lens H27.8
  - congenital Q12.8
- lip (gland) K13.0
- liver (idiopathic) (simple) K76.89
  - congenital Q44.6
  - hydatid B67.8
    - granulosus B67.0
    - multilocularis B67.5
- lung J98.4
  - congenital Q33.0
  - giant bullous J43.9
- lutein N83.1 ☑
- lymphangiomatous D18.1
- lymphoepithelial, oral soft tissue K09.8
- macula — *see* Degeneration, macula, hole
- malignant — *see* Neoplasm, malignant, by site
- mammary gland — *see* Cyst, breast
- mandible M27.40
  - dentigerous K09.0
  - radicular K04.8
- maxilla M27.40
  - dentigerous K09.0
  - radicular K04.8
- medial, face and neck Q18.8
- median
  - anterior maxillary K09.1
  - palatal K09.1
- mediastinum, congenital Q34.1
- meibomian (gland) — *see* Chalazion
  - infected — *see* Hordeolum
- membrane, brain G93.0
- meninges (cerebral) G93.0
  - spinal G96.19
- meniscus, knee — *see* Derangement, knee, meniscus, cystic
- mesentery, mesenteric K66.8
  - chyle I89.8
- mesonephric duct
  - female Q50.5
  - male Q55.4
- milk N64.89
- Morgagni (hydatid)
  - female Q50.5
  - male (epididymal) Q55.4
    - testicular Q55.29

Cyst - Cystadenocarcinoma

Cyst — *continued*
  mouth K09.8
  Müllerian duct Q50.4
    appendix testis Q55.29
    cervix Q51.6
    fallopian tube Q50.4
    female Q50.4
    male Q55.29
    prostatic utricle Q55.4
    vagina (embryonal) Q52.4
  multilocular (ovary) D39.10
    benign — *see* Neoplasm, benign, by site
  myometrium N85.8
  nabothian (follicle) (ruptured) N88.8
  nasoalveolar K09.1
  nasolabial K09.1
  nasopalatine (anterior) (duct) K09.1
  nasopharynx J39.2
  neoplastic — *see* Neoplasm, uncertain behavior,
      by site
    benign — *see* Neoplasm, benign, by site
  nervous system NEC G96.8
  neuroenteric (congenital) Q06.8
  nipple — *see* Cyst, breast
  nose (turbinates) J34.1
    sinus J34.1
  odontogenic, developmental K09.0
  omentum (lesser) K66.8
    congenital Q45.8
  ora serrata — *see* Cyst, retina, ora serrata
  oral
    region K09.9
      developmental (nonodontogenic) K09.1
      specified NEC K09.8
    soft tissue K09.9
      specified NEC K09.8
  orbit H05.81 ☑
  ovary, ovarian (twisted) N83.20 ☑
    adherent N83.20 ☑
    chocolate N80.1
    corpus
      albicans N83.29 ☑
      luteum (hemorrhagic) N83.1 ☑
    dermoid D27.9
    developmental Q50.1
    due to failure of involution NEC N83.20 ☑
    endometrial N80.1
    follicular (graafian) (hemorrhagic) N83.0 ☑
    hemorrhagic N83.20 ☑
    in pregnancy or childbirth O34.8 ☑
      with obstructed labor O65.5
    multilocular D39.10
    pseudomucinous D27.9
    retention N83.29 ☑
    serous N83.20 ☑
    specified NEC N83.29 ☑
    theca lutein (hemorrhagic) N83.1 ☑
    tuberculous A18.18
  oviduct N83.8
  palate (median) (fissural) K09.1
  palatine papilla (jaw) K09.1
  pancreas, pancreatic (hemorrhagic) (true) K86.2
    congenital Q45.2
    false K86.3
  paralabral
    hip M24.85 ☑
    shoulder S43.43 ☑
  paramesonephric duct Q50.4
    female Q50.4
    male Q55.29
  paranephric N28.1
  paraphysis, cerebri, congenital Q04.6
  parasitic B89
  parathyroid (gland) E21.4
  paratubal N83.8
  paraurethral duct N36.8
  paroophoron Q50.5
  parotid gland K11.6
  parovarian Q50.5
  pelvis, female N94.89
    in pregnancy or childbirth O34.8 ☑
      causing obstructed labor O65.5
  penis (sebaceous) N48.89
  periapical K04.8
  pericardial (congenital) Q24.8
    acquired (secondary) I31.8
  pericoronal K09.0
  periodontal K04.8
    lateral K09.0
  peripelvic (lymphatic) N28.1
  peritoneum K66.8
    chylous I89.8

Cyst — *continued*
  periventricular, acquired, newborn P91.1
  pharynx (wall) J39.2
  pilar L72.11
  pilonidal (infected) (rectum) L05.91
    with abscess L05.01
    malignant C44.59 ☑
  pituitary (duct) (gland) E23.6
  placenta O43.19 ☑
  pleura J94.8
  popliteal — *see* Cyst, Baker's
  porencephalic Q04.6
    acquired G93.0
  postanal (infected) — *see* Cyst, pilonidal
  postmastoidectomy cavity (mucosal) — *see*
      Complications, postmastoidectomy, cyst
  preauricular Q18.1
  prepuce N47.4
    congenital Q55.69
  primordial (jaw) K09.0
  prostate N42.83
  pseudomucinous (ovary) D27.9
  pupillary, miotic H21.27 ☑
  radicular (residual) K04.8
  radiculodental K04.8
  ranular K11.8
  Rathke's pouch E23.6
  rectum (epithelium) (mucous) K62.89
  renal — *see* Cyst, kidney
  residual (radicular) K04.8
  retention (ovary) N83.29 ☑
    salivary gland K11.6
  retina H33.19 ☑
    ora serrata H33.11 ☑
    parasitic H33.12 ☑
  retroperitoneal K68.9
  sacrococcygeal (dermoid) — *see* Cyst, pilonidal
  salivary gland or duct (mucous extravasation or
      retention) K11.6
  Sampson's N80.1
  sclera H15.89
  scrotum L72.9
    sebaceous L72.3
  sebaceous (duct) (gland) L72.3
    breast — *see* Dysplasia, mammary, specified type
      NEC
    eyelid — *see* Cyst, eyelid
    genital organ NEC
      female N94.89
      male N50.89
    scrotum L72.3
  semilunar cartilage (knee) (multiple) — *see*
      Derangement, knee, meniscus, cystic
  seminal vesicle N50.89
  serous (ovary) N83.20 ☑
  sinus (accessory) (nasal) J34.1
  Skene's gland N36.8
  skin L72.9
    breast — *see* Dysplasia, mammary, specified type
      NEC
    epidermal, epidermoid L72.0
    epithelial L72.0
    eyelid — *see* Cyst, eyelid
    genital organ NEC
      female N90.7
      male N50.89
    inclusion L72.0
    scrotum L72.9
    sebaceous L72.3
    sweat gland or duct L74.8
  solitary
    bone — *see* Cyst, bone, solitary
    jaw M27.40
    kidney N28.1
  spermatic cord N50.89
  sphenoid sinus J34.1
  spinal meninges G96.19
  spleen NEC D73.4
    congenital Q89.09
    hydatid (*see also* Echinococcus) B67.99 *[D77]*
  Stafne's M27.0
  subarachnoid intrasellar R93.0
  subcutaneous, pheomycotic (chromomycotic)
      B43.2
  subdural (cerebral) G93.0
    spinal cord G96.19
  sublingual gland K11.6
  submandibular gland K11.6
  submaxillary gland K11.6
  suburethral N36.8
  suprarenal gland E27.8
  suprasellar — *see* Cyst, brain

Cyst — *continued*
  sweat gland or duct L74.8
  synovial (*see also* Cyst, bursa)
    ruptured — *see* Rupture, synovium
  tarsal — *see* Chalazion
  tendon (sheath) — *see* Disorder, tendon, specified
      type NEC
  testis N44.2
    tunica albuginea N44.1
  theca lutein (ovary) N83.1 ☑
  Thornwaldt's J39.2
  thymus (gland) E32.8
  thyroglossal duct (infected) (persistent) Q89.2
  thyrolingual duct (infected) (persistent) Q89.2
  thyroid (gland) E04.1
  tongue K14.8
  tonsil J35.8
  tooth — *see* Cyst, dental
  Tornwaldt's J39.2
  trichilemmal (proliferating) L72.12
  trichodermal L72.12
  tubal (fallopian) N83.8
    inflammatory — *see* Salpingitis, chronic
  tubo-ovarian N83.8
    inflammatory N70.13
  tunica
    albuginea testis N44.1
    vaginalis N50.89
  turbinate (nose) J34.1
  Tyson's gland N48.89
  urachus, congenital Q64.4
  ureter N28.89
  ureterovesical orifice N28.89
  urethra, urethral (gland) N36.8
  uterine ligament N83.8
  uterus (body) (corpus) (recurrent) N85.8
    embryonic Q51.818
      cervix Q51.6
  vagina, vaginal (implantation) (inclusion)
      (squamous cell) (wall) N89.8
    embryonic Q52.4
  vallecula, vallecular (epiglottis) J38.7
  vesical (orifice) N32.89
  vitreous body H43.89
  vulva (implantation) (inclusion) N90.7
    congenital Q52.79
    sebaceous gland N90.7
  vulvovaginal gland N90.7
  wolffian
    female Q50.5
    male Q55.4
Cystadenocarcinoma — *see* Neoplasm, malignant,
    by site
  bile duct C22.1
  endometrioid — *see* Neoplasm, malignant, by site
    specified site — *see* Neoplasm, malignant, by site
    unspecified site
      female C56.9
      male C61
  mucinous
    papillary
      specified site — *see* Neoplasm, malignant, by
        site
      unspecified site C56.9
    specified site — *see* Neoplasm, malignant, by site
    unspecified site C56.9
  papillary
    mucinous
      specified site — *see* Neoplasm, malignant, by
        site
      unspecified site C56.9
    pseudomucinous
      specified site — *see* Neoplasm, malignant, by
        site
      unspecified site C56.9
    serous
      specified site — *see* Neoplasm, malignant, by
        site
      unspecified site C56.9
    specified site — *see* Neoplasm, malignant, by site
    unspecified site C56.9
  pseudomucinous
    papillary
      specified site — *see* Neoplasm, malignant, by
        site
      unspecified site C56.9
    specified site — *see* Neoplasm, malignant, by site
    unspecified site C56.9
  serous
    papillary
      specified site — *see* Neoplasm, malignant, by site
      unspecified site C56.9

☑ **Additional character required**

Cystadenocarcinoma — *continued*
  serous — *continued*
    specified site — *see* Neoplasm, malignant, by site
    unspecified site C56.9
Cystadenofibroma
  clear cell — *see* Neoplasm, benign, by site
  endometrioid D27.9
    borderline malignancy D39.1 ☑
    malignant C56. ☑
  mucinous
    specified site — *see* Neoplasm, benign, by site
    unspecified site D27.9
  serous
    specified site — *see* Neoplasm, benign, by site
    unspecified site D27.9
  specified site — *see* Neoplasm, benign, by site
  unspecified site D27.9
Cystadenoma (*see also* Neoplasm, benign, by site)
  bile duct D13.4
  endometrioid — *see* Neoplasm, benign, by site
    borderline malignancy — *see* Neoplasm, uncertain behavior, by site
  malignant — *see* Neoplasm, malignant, by site
  mucinous
    borderline malignancy
      ovary C56. ☑
      specified site NEC — *see* Neoplasm, uncertain behavior, by site
      unspecified site C56.9
    papillary
      borderline malignancy
        ovary C56. ☑
        specified site NEC — *see* Neoplasm, uncertain behavior, by site
        unspecified site C56.9
      specified site — *see* Neoplasm, benign, by site
      unspecified site D27.9
    specified site — *see* Neoplasm, benign, by site
    unspecified site D27.9
  papillary
    borderline malignancy
      ovary C56. ☑
      specified site NEC — *see* Neoplasm, uncertain behavior, by site
      unspecified site C56.9
    lymphomatosum
      specified site — *see* Neoplasm, benign, by site
      unspecified site D11.9
    mucinous
      borderline malignancy
        ovary C56. ☑
        specified site NEC — *see* Neoplasm, uncertain behavior, by site
        unspecified site C56.9
      specified site — *see* Neoplasm, benign, by site
      unspecified site D27.9
    pseudomucinous
      borderline malignancy
        ovary C56. ☑
        specified site NEC — *see* Neoplasm, uncertain behavior, by site
        unspecified site C56.9
      specified site — *see* Neoplasm, benign, by site
      unspecified site D27.9
    serous
      borderline malignancy
        ovary C56. ☑
        specified site NEC — *see* Neoplasm, uncertain behavior, by site
        unspecified site C56.9
      specified site — *see* Neoplasm, benign, by site
      unspecified site D27.9
    specified site — *see* Neoplasm, benign, by site
    unspecified site D27.9
  pseudomucinous
    borderline malignancy
      ovary C56. ☑
      specified site NEC — *see* Neoplasm, uncertain behavior, by site
      unspecified site C56.9
    papillary
      borderline malignancy
        ovary C56. ☑
        specified site NEC — *see* Neoplasm, uncertain behavior, by site
        unspecified site C56.9
      specified site — *see* Neoplasm, benign, by site
      unspecified site D27.9
    specified site — *see* Neoplasm, benign, by site
    unspecified site D27.9
  serous
    borderline malignancy

Cystadenoma — *continued*
  serous — *continued*
    ovary C56. ☑
    specified site NEC — *see* Neoplasm, uncertain behavior, by site
    unspecified site C56.9
    papillary
      borderline malignancy
        ovary C56. ☑
      specified site NEC — *see* Neoplasm, uncertain behavior, by site
      unspecified site C56.9
      specified site — *see* Neoplasm, benign, by site
      unspecified site D27.9
    specified site — *see* Neoplasm, benign, by site
    unspecified site D27.9
Cystathionine synthase deficiency E72.11
Cystathioninemia E72.19
Cystathioninuria E72.19
Cystic (*see also* condition)
  breast (chronic) — *see* Mastopathy, cystic
  corpora lutea (hemorrhagic) N83.1 ☑
  duct — *see* condition
  eyeball (congenital) Q11.0
  fibrosis — *see* Fibrosis, cystic
  kidney (congenital) Q61.9
    adult type Q61.2
    infantile type NEC Q61.19
      collecting duct dilatation Q61.11
    medullary Q61.5
  liver, congenital Q44.6
  lung disease J98.4
    congenital Q33.0
  mastitis, chronic — *see* Mastopathy, cystic
  medullary, kidney Q61.5
  meniscus — *see* Derangement, knee, meniscus, cystic
  ovary N83.20 ☑
Cysticercosis, cysticerciasis B69.9
  with
    epileptiform fits B69.0
    myositis B69.81
  brain B69.0
  central nervous system B69.0
  cerebral B69.0
  ocular B69.1
  specified NEC B69.89
Cysticercus cellulose infestation — *see* Cysticercosis
Cystinosis (malignant) E72.04
Cystinuria E72.01
Cystitis (exudative) (hemorrhagic) (septic) (suppurative) N30.90
  with
    fibrosis — *see* Cystitis, chronic, interstitial
    hematuria N30.91
    leukoplakia — *see* Cystitis, chronic, interstitial
    malakoplakia — *see* Cystitis, chronic, interstitial
    metaplasia — *see* Cystitis, chronic, interstitial
    prostatitis N41.3
  acute N30.00
    with hematuria N30.01
    of trigone N30.30
      with hematuria N30.31
  allergic — *see* Cystitis, specified type NEC
  amebic A06.81
  bilharzial B65.9 *[N33]*
  blennorrhagic (gonococcal) A54.01
  bullous — *see* Cystitis, specified type NEC
  calculous N21.0
  chlamydial A56.01
  chronic N30.20
    with hematuria N30.21
    interstitial N30.10
      with hematuria N30.11
    of trigone N30.30
      with hematuria N30.31
    specified NEC N30.20
      with hematuria N30.21
  cystic (a) — *see* Cystitis, specified type NEC
  diphtheritic A36.85
  echinococcal
    granulosus B67.39
    multilocularis B67.69
  emphysematous — *see* Cystitis, specified type NEC
  encysted — *see* Cystitis, specified type NEC
  eosinophilic — *see* Cystitis, specified type NEC
  follicular — *see* Cystitis, of trigone
  gangrenous — *see* Cystitis, specified type NEC
  glandularis — *see* Cystitis, specified type NEC
  gonococcal A54.01
  incrusted — *see* Cystitis, specified type NEC
  interstitial (chronic) — *see* Cystitis, chronic, interstitial

Cystitis — *continued*
  irradiation N30.40
    with hematuria N30.41
  irritation — *see* Cystitis, specified type NEC
  malignant — *see* Cystitis, specified type NEC
  of trigone N30.30
    with hematuria N30.31
  panmural — *see* Cystitis, chronic, interstitial
  polyposa — *see* Cystitis, specified type NEC
  prostatic N41.3
  puerperal (postpartum) O86.22
  radiation — *see* Cystitis, irradiation
  specified type NEC N30.80
    with hematuria N30.81
  subacute — *see* Cystitis, chronic
  submucous — *see* Cystitis, chronic, interstitial
  syphilitic (late) A52.76
  trichomonal A59.03
  tuberculous A18.12
  ulcerative — *see* Cystitis, chronic, interstitial
Cystocele (-urethrocele)
  female N81.10
    with prolapse of uterus — *see* Prolapse, uterus
    lateral N81.12
    midline N81.11
    paravaginal N81.12
  in pregnancy or childbirth O34.8 ☑
    causing obstructed labor O65.5
  male N32.89
Cystolithiasis N21.0
Cystoma (*see also* Neoplasm, benign, by site)
  endometrial, ovary N80.1
  mucinous
    specified site — *see* Neoplasm, benign, by site
    unspecified site D27.9
  serous
    specified site — *see* Neoplasm, benign, by site
    unspecified site D27.9
  simple (ovary) N83.29 ☑
Cystoplegia N31.2
Cystoptosis N32.89
Cystopyelitis — *see* Pyelonephritis
Cystorrhagia N32.89
Cystosarcoma phyllodes D48.6 ☑
  benign D24 ☑
  malignant — *see* Neoplasm, breast, malignant
Cystostomy
  attention to Z43.5
  complication — *see* Complications, cystostomy
  status Z93.50
    appendico-vesicostomy Z93.52
    cutaneous Z93.51
    specified NEC Z93.59
Cystourethritis — *see* Urethritis
Cystourethrocele (*see also* Cystocele)
  female N81.10
    with uterine prolapse — *see* Prolapse, uterus
    lateral N81.12
    midline N81.11
    paravaginal N81.12
  male N32.89
Cytomegalic inclusion disease
  congenital P35.1
Cytomegalovirus infection B25.9
Cytomycosis (reticuloendothelial) B39.4
Cytopenia D75.9
  refractory
    with multilineage dysplasia D46.A
      and ring sideroblasts (RCMD RS) D46.B
Czerny's disease (periodic hydrarthrosis of the knee) — *see* Effusion, joint, knee

D

Daae (-Finsen) disease (epidemic pleurodynia) B33.0
Da Costa's syndrome F45.8
Dabney's grip B33.0
Dacryoadenitis, dacryadenitis H04.00 ☑
  acute H04.01 ☑
  chronic H04.02 ☑
Dacryocystitis H04.30 ☑
  acute H04.32 ☑
  chronic H04.41 ☑
  neonatal P39.1
  phlegmonous H04.31 ☑
  syphilitic A52.71
    congenital (early) A50.01
  trachomatous, active A71.1
    sequelae (late effect) B94.0

Dacryocystoblenorrhea - Defect

Dacryocystoblenorrhea — *see* Inflammation, lacrimal, passages, chronic
Dacryocystocele — *see* Disorder, lacrimal system, changes
Dacryolith, dacryolithiasis H04.51 ☑
Dacryoma — *see* Disorder, lacrimal system, changes
Dacryopericystitis — *see* Dacryocystitis
Dacryops H04.11 ☑
Dacryostenosis (*see also* Stenosis, lacrimal)
  congenital Q10.5
Dactylitis
  bone — *see* Osteomyelitis
  sickle-cell D57.00
    Hb C D57.219
    Hb SS D57.00
    specified NEC D57.819
  skin L08.9
  syphilitic A52.77
  tuberculous A18.03
Dactylolysis spontanea (ainhum) L94.6
Dactylosymphysis Q70.9
  fingers — *see* Syndactylism, complex, fingers
  toes — *see* Syndactylism, complex, toes
Damage
  arteriosclerotic — *see* Arteriosclerosis
  brain (nontraumatic) G93.9
    anoxic, hypoxic G93.1
      resulting from a procedure G97.82
    child NEC G80.9
    due to birth injury P11.2
  cardiorenal (vascular) — *see* Hypertension, cardiorenal
  cerebral NEC — *see* Damage, brain
  coccyx, complicating delivery O71.6
  coronary — *see* Disease, heart, ischemic
  deep tissue, pressure-induced (*see also* L89 ☑ with final character .6)
  eye, birth injury P15.3
  liver (nontraumatic) K76.9
    alcoholic K70.9
    due to drugs — *see* Disease, liver, toxic
    toxic — *see* Disease, liver, toxic
  medication T88.7 ☑
  pelvic
    joint or ligament, during delivery O71.6
    organ NEC
      during delivery O71.5
      following ectopic or molar pregnancy O08.6
  renal — *see* Disease, renal
  subendocardium, subendocardial — *see* Degeneration, myocardial
  vascular I99.9
Dana-Putnam syndrome (subacute combined sclerosis with pernicious anemia) — *see* Degeneration, combined
Danbolt (-Cross) syndrome (acrodermatitis enteropathica) E83.2
Dandruff L21.0
Dandy-Walker syndrome Q03.1
  with spina bifida — *see* Spina bifida
Danlos' syndrome (*see also* Syndrome, Ehlers-Danlos) Q79.60
Darier (-White) disease (congenital) Q82.8
  meaning erythema annulare centrifugum L53.1
Darier-Roussy sarcoid D86.3
Darling's disease or histoplasmosis B39.4
Darwin's tubercle Q17.8
Dawson's (inclusion body) encephalitis A81.1
De Beurmann (-Gougerot) disease B42.1
De la Tourette's syndrome F95.2
De Lange's syndrome Q87.19
De Morgan's spots (senile angiomas) I78.1
De Quervain's
  disease (tendon sheath) M65.4
  syndrome E34.51
  thyroiditis (subacute granulomatous thyroiditis) E06.1
De Toni-Fanconi (-Debré) syndrome E72.09
  with cystinosis E72.04
Dead
  fetus, retained (mother) O36.4 ☑
    early pregnancy O02.1
  labyrinth — *see* subcategory H83.2 ☑
  ovum, retained O02.0
Deaf nonspeaking NEC H91.3
Deaf mutism (acquired) (congenital) NEC H91.3
  hysterical F44.6
  syphilitic, congenital (*see also* subcategory H94.8 ☑) A50.09
Deafness (acquired) (complete) (hereditary) (partial) H91.9 ☑
  with blue sclera and fragility of bone Q78.0

Deafness — *continued*
  auditory fatigue — *see* Deafness, specified type NEC
  aviation T70.0 ☑
    nerve injury — *see* Injury, nerve, acoustic, specified type NEC
  boilermaker's — *see* subcategory H83.3 ☑
  central — *see* Deafness, sensorineural
  conductive H90.2
    and sensorineural
      mixed H90.8
        bilateral H90.6
    bilateral H90.0
    unilateral H90.1 ☑
      with restricted hearing on the contralateral side H90.A ☑
  congenital H90.5
    with blue sclera and fragility of bone Q78.0
  due to toxic agents — *see* Deafness, ototoxic
  emotional (hysterical) F44.6
  functional (hysterical) F44.6
  high frequency H91.9 ☑
  hysterical F44.6
  low frequency H91.9 ☑
  mental R48.8
  mixed conductive and sensorineural H90.8
    bilateral H90.6
    unilateral H90.7 ☑
  nerve — *see* Deafness, sensorineural
  neural — *see* Deafness, sensorineural
  noise-induced (*see also* subcategory) H83.3 ☑
    nerve injury — *see* Injury, nerve, acoustic, specified type NEC
  nonspeaking H91.3
  ototoxic — *see* subcategory H91.0 ☑
  perceptive — *see* Deafness, sensorineural
  psychogenic (hysterical) F44.6
  sensorineural H90.5
    and conductive
      mixed H90.8
        bilateral H90.6
    bilateral H90.3
    unilateral H90.4 ☑
      with restricted hearing on the contralateral side H90.A ☑
  sensory — *see* Deafness, sensorineural
  specified type NEC — *see* subcategory H91.8 ☑
  sudden (idiopathic) H91.2 ☑
  syphilitic A52.15
  transient ischemic H93.01 ☑
  traumatic — *see* Injury, nerve, acoustic, specified type NEC
  word (developmental) H93.25
Death (cause unknown) (of) (unexplained) (unspecified cause) R99
  brain G93.82
  cardiac (sudden) (with successful resuscitation) - code to underlying disease
    family history of Z82.41
    personal history of Z86.74
  family member (assumed) Z63.4
Debility (chronic) (general) (nervous) R53.81
  congenital or neonatal NOS P96.9
  nervous R53.81
  old age R54
  senile R54
Débove's disease (splenomegaly) R16.1
Decalcification
  bone — *see* Osteoporosis
  teeth K03.89
Decapsulation, kidney N28.89
Decay
  dental — *see* Caries, dental
  senile R54
  tooth, teeth — *see* Caries, dental
Deciduitis (acute)
  following ectopic or molar pregnancy O08.0
Decline (general) — *see* Debility
  cognitive, age-associated R41.81
Decompensation
  cardiac (acute) (chronic) — *see* Disease, heart
  cardiovascular — *see* Disease, cardiovascular
  heart — *see* Disease, heart
  hepatic — *see* Failure, hepatic
  myocardial (acute) (chronic) — *see* Disease, heart
  respiratory J98.8
Decompression sickness T70.3 ☑
Decrease (d)
  absolute neutrophil count — *see* Neutropenia
  blood
    platelets — *see* Thrombocytopenia
    pressure R03.1
      due to shock following

Decrease — *continued*
  blood — *continued*
      injury T79.4 ☑
      operation T81.19 ☑
  estrogen E28.39
    postablative E89.40
      asymptomatic E89.40
      symptomatic E89.41
  fragility of erythrocytes D58.8
  function
    lipase (pancreatic) K90.3
    ovary in hypopituitarism E23.0
    parenchyma of pancreas K86.89
    pituitary (gland) (anterior) (lobe) E23.0
      posterior (lobe) E23.0
  functional activity R68.89
  glucose R73.09
  hematocrit R71.0
  hemoglobin R71.0
  leukocytes D72.819
    specified NEC D72.818
  libido R68.82
  lymphocytes D72.810
  platelets D69.6
  respiration, due to shock following injury T79.4 ☑
  sexual desire R68.82
  tear secretion NEC — *see* Syndrome, dry eye
  tolerance
    fat K90.49
    glucose R73.09
    pancreatic K90.3
    salt and water E87.8
  vision NEC H54.7
  white blood cell count D72.819
    specified NEC D72.818
Decubitus (ulcer) — *see* Ulcer, pressure, by site
  cervix N86
Deepening acetabulum — *see* Derangement, joint, specified type NEC, hip
Defect, defective Q89.9
  3-beta-hydroxysteroid dehydrogenase E25.0
  11-hydroxylase E25.0
  21-hydroxylase E25.0
  abdominal wall, congenital Q79.59
  antibody immunodeficiency D80.9
  aorticopulmonary septum Q21.4
  atrial septal (ostium secundum type) Q21.1
    following acute myocardial infarction (current complication) I23.1
    ostium primum type Q21.2
  atrioventricular
    canal Q21.2
    septum Q21.2
  auricular septal Q21.1
  bilirubin excretion NEC E80.6
  biosynthesis, androgen (testicular) E29.1
  bulbar septum Q21.0
  catalase E80.3
  cell membrane receptor complex (CR3) D71
  circulation I99.9
    congenital Q28.9
    newborn Q28.9
  coagulation (factor) (*see also* Deficiency, factor) D68.9
    with
      ectopic pregnancy O08.1
      molar pregnancy O08.1
    acquired D68.4
    antepartum with hemorrhage — *see* Hemorrhage, antepartum, with coagulation defect
    due to
      liver disease D68.4
      vitamin K deficiency D68.4
    hereditary NEC D68.2
    intrapartum O67.0
    newborn, transient P61.6
    postpartum O99.13
      with hemorrhage O72.3
    specified type NEC D68.8
  complement system D84.1
  conduction (heart) I45.9
    bone — *see* Deafness, conductive
  congenital, organ or site not listed — *see* Anomaly, by site
  coronary sinus Q21.1
  cushion, endocardial Q21.2
  degradation, glycoprotein E77.1
  dental bridge, crown, fillings — *see* Defect, dental restoration
  dental restoration K08.50
    specified NEC K08.59

☑ **Additional character required**

Defect — *continued*
 dentin (hereditary) K00.5
 Descemet's membrane, congenital Q13.89
 developmental (*see also* Anomaly)
  cauda equina Q06.3
 diaphragm
  with elevation, eventration or hernia — *see*
    Hernia, diaphragm
  congenital Q79.1
   with hernia Q79.0
   gross (with hernia) Q79.0
 ectodermal, congenital Q82.9
 Eisenmenger's Q21.8
 enzyme
  catalase E80.3
  peroxidase E80.3
 esophagus, congenital Q39.9
 extensor retinaculum M62.89
 fibrin polymerization D68.2
 filling
  bladder R93.41
  kidney R93.42 ☑
  renal pelvis R93.41
  stomach R93.3
  ureter R93.41
  urinary organs, specified NEC R93.49
 GABA (gamma aminobutyric acid) metabolic E72.81
 Gerbode Q21.0
 glycoprotein degradation E77.1
 Hageman (factor) D68.2
 hearing — *see* Deafness
 high grade F70
 interatrial septal Q21.1
 interauricular septal Q21.1
 interventricular septal Q21.0
  with dextroposition of aorta, pulmonary stenosis
    and hypertrophy of right ventricle Q21.3
  in tetralogy of Fallot Q21.3
 learning (specific) — *see* Disorder, learning
 lymphocyte function antigen-1 (LFA-1) D84.0
 lysosomal enzyme, post-translational modification
    E77.0
 major osseous M89.70
  ankle M89.77 ☑
  carpus M89.74 ☑
  clavicle M89.71 ☑
  femur M89.75 ☑
  fibula M89.76 ☑
  fingers M89.74 ☑
  foot M89.77 ☑
  forearm M89.73 ☑
  hand M89.74 ☑
  humerus M89.72 ☑
  lower leg M89.76 ☑
  metacarpus M89.74 ☑
  metatarsus M89.77 ☑
  multiple sites M89.79
  pelvic region M89.75 ☑
  pelvis M89.75 ☑
  radius M89.73 ☑
  scapula M89.71 ☑
  shoulder region M89.71 ☑
  specified NEC M89.78
  tarsus M89.77 ☑
  thigh M89.75 ☑
  tibia M89.76 ☑
  toes M89.77 ☑
  ulna M89.73 ☑
 mental — *see* Disability, intellectual
 modification, lysosomal enzymes, post-translational
    E77.0
 obstructive, congenital
  renal pelvis Q62.39
  ureter Q62.39
   atresia — *see* Atresia, ureter
   cecoureterocele Q62.32
   megaureter Q62.2
   orthotopic ureterocele Q62.31
 osseous, major M89.70
  ankle M89.77 ☑
  carpus M89.74 ☑
  clavicle M89.71 ☑
  femur M89.75 ☑
  fibula M89.76 ☑
  fingers M89.74 ☑
  foot M89.77 ☑
  forearm M89.73 ☑
  hand M89.74 ☑
  humerus M89.72 ☑
  lower leg M89.76 ☑
  metacarpus M89.74 ☑
  metatarsus M89.77 ☑

Defect — *continued*
 osseous — *continued*
  multiple sites M89.9
  pelvic region M89.75 ☑
  pelvis M89.75 ☑
  radius M89.73 ☑
  scapula M89.71 ☑
  shoulder region M89.71 ☑
  specified NEC M89.78
  tarsus M89.77 ☑
  thigh M89.75 ☑
  tibia M89.76 ☑
  toes M89.77 ☑
  ulna M89.73 ☑
 osteochondral NEC (*see also* Deformity) M95.8
 ostium
  primum Q21.2
  secundum Q21.1
 peroxidase E80.3
 placental blood supply — *see* Insufficiency,
    placental
 platelets, qualitative D69.1
  constitutional D68.0
 postural NEC, spine — *see* Dorsopathy, deforming
 reduction
  limb Q73.8
   lower Q72.9 ☑
    absence — *see* Agenesis, leg
    foot — *see* Agenesis, foot
    longitudinal
     femur Q72.4 ☑
     fibula Q72.6 ☑
     tibia Q72.5 ☑
    specified type NEC Q72.89 ☑
    split foot Q72.7 ☑
   specified type NEC Q73.8
   upper Q71.9 ☑
    absence — *see* Agenesis, arm
    forearm — *see* Agenesis, forearm
    hand — *see* Agenesis, hand
    lobster-claw hand Q71.6 ☑
    longitudinal
     radius Q71.4 ☑
     ulna Q71.5 ☑
    specified type NEC Q71.89 ☑
 renal pelvis Q63.8
  obstructive Q62.39
 respiratory system, congenital Q34.9
 restoration, dental K08.50
  specified NEC K08.59
 retinal nerve bundle fibers H35.89
 septal (heart) NOS Q21.9
  acquired (atrial) (auricular) (ventricular) (old) I51.0
  atrial Q21.1
   concurrent with acute myocardial infarction —
     see Infarct, myocardium
   following acute myocardial infarction (current
     complication) I23.1
  ventricular (*see also* Defect, ventricular septal)
    Q21.0
 sinus venosus Q21.1
 speech R47.9
  developmental F80.9
  specified NEC R47.89
 Taussig-Bing (aortic transposition and overriding
    pulmonary artery) Q20.1
 teeth, wedge K03.1
 vascular (local) I99.9
  congenital Q27.9
 ventricular septal Q21.0
  concurrent with acute myocardial infarction —
    see Infarct, myocardium
  following acute myocardial infarction (current
    complication) I23.2
  in tetralogy of Fallot Q21.3
 vision NEC H54.7
 visual field H53.40
  bilateral
   heteronymous H53.47
   homonymous H53.46 ☑
  generalized contraction H53.48 ☑
  localized
   arcuate H53.43 ☑
   scotoma (central area) H53.41 ☑
    blind spot area H53.42 ☑
   sector H53.43 ☑
   specified type NEC H53.45 ☑
 voice R49.9
  specified NEC R49.8
 wedge, tooth, teeth (abrasion) K03.1
Deferentitis N49.1
 gonorrheal (acute) (chronic) A54.23

Defibrination (syndrome) D65
 antepartum — *see* Hemorrhage, antepartum, with
   coagulation defect, disseminated intravascular
   coagulation
 following ectopic or molar pregnancy O08.1
 intrapartum O67.0
 newborn P60
 postpartum O72.3
Deficiency, deficient
 3-beta hydroxysteroid dehydrogenase E25.0
 5-alpha reductase (with male
   pseudohermaphroditism) E29.1
 11-hydroxylase E25.0
 21-hydroxylase E25.0
 abdominal muscle syndrome Q79.4
 accelerator globulin (Ac G) (blood) D68.2
 AC globulin (congenital) (hereditary) D68.2
  acquired D68.4
 acid phosphatase E83.39
 activating factor (blood) D68.2
 ADA2 (adenosine deaminase 2) D81.32
 adenosine deaminase (ADA) D81.30
  with severe combined immunodeficiency (SCID)
    D81.31
  partial (type 1) D81.39
  specified NEC D81.39
  type 1 (without SCID) (without severe combined
    immunodeficiency) D81.39
  type 2 D81.32
 aldolase (hereditary) E74.19
 alpha-1-antitrypsin E88.01
 amino-acids E72.9
 anemia — *see* Anemia
 aneurin E51.9
 antibody with
  hyperimmunoglobulinemia D80.6
  near-normal immunoglobins D80.6
 antidiuretic hormone E23.2
 anti-hemophilic
  factor (A) D66
   B D67
   C D68.1
  globulin (AHG) NEC D66
 antithrombin (antithrombin III) D68.59
 ascorbic acid E54
 attention (disorder) (syndrome) F98.8
  with hyperactivity — *see* Disorder, attention-
    deficit hyperactivity
 autoprothrombin
  I D68.2
  II D67
  C D68.2
 beta-glucuronidase E76.29
 biotin E53.8
 biotin-dependent carboxylase D81.819
 biotinidase D81.810
 brancher enzyme (amylopectinosis) E74.03
 calciferol E55.9
  with
   adult osteomalacia M83.8
   rickets — *see* Rickets
 calcium (dietary) E58
 calorie, severe E43
  with marasmus E41
   and kwashiorkor E42
 cardiac — *see* Insufficiency, myocardial
 carnitine E71.40
  due to
   hemodialysis E71.43
   inborn errors of metabolism E71.42
   Valproic acid therapy E71.43
  iatrogenic E71.43
  muscle palmityltransferase E71.314
  primary E71.41
  secondary E71.448
 carotene E50.9
 central nervous system G96.8
 ceruloplasmin (Wilson) E83.01
 choline E53.8
 Christmas factor D67
 chromium E61.4
 clotting (blood) (*see also* Deficiency, coagulation
   factor) D68.9
 clotting factor NEC (hereditary) (*see also* Deficiency,
   factor) D68.2
 coagulation NOS D68.9
  with
   ectopic pregnancy O08.1
   molar pregnancy O08.1
  acquired (any) D68.4
  antepartum hemorrhage — *see* Hemorrhage,
    antepartum, with coagulation defect

Defect - Deficiency

ICD-10-CM INDEX TO DISEASES AND INJURIES

Deficiency

Deficiency — *continued*

coagulation NOS — *continued*
clotting factor NEC (*see also* Deficiency, factor) D68.2
due to
hyperprothrombinemia D68.4
liver disease D68.4
vitamin K deficiency D68.4
newborn, transient P61.6
postpartum O72.3
specified NEC D68.8
cognitive F09
color vision H53.50
achromatopsia H53.51
acquired H53.52
deuteranomaly H53.53
protanomaly H53.54
specified type NEC H53.59
tritanomaly H53.55
combined glucocorticoid and mineralocorticoid E27.49
contact factor D68.2
copper (nutritional) E61.0
corticoadrenal E27.40
primary E27.1
craniofacial axis Q75.0
cyanocobalamin E53.8
C1 esterase inhibitor (C1-INH) D84.1
debrancher enzyme (limit dextrinosis) E74.03
dehydrogenase
long chain/very long chain acyl CoA E71.310
medium chain acyl CoA E71.311
short chain acyl CoA E71.312
diet E63.9
dihydropyrimidine dehydrogenase (DPD) E88.89
disaccharidase E73.9
edema — *see* Malnutrition, severe
endocrine E34.9
energy-supply — *see* Malnutrition
enzymes, circulating NEC E88.09
ergosterol E55.9
with
adult osteomalacia M83.8
rickets — *see* Rickets
essential fatty acid (EFA) E63.0
factor (*see also* Deficiency, coagulation)
Hageman D68.2
I (congenital) (hereditary) D68.2
II (congenital) (hereditary) D68.2
IX (congenital) (functional) (hereditary) (with functional defect) D67
multiple (congenital) D68.8
acquired D68.4
V (congenital) (hereditary) D68.2
VII (congenital) (hereditary) D68.2
VIII (congenital) (functional) (hereditary) (with functional defect) D66
with vascular defect D68.0
X (congenital) (hereditary) D68.2
XI (congenital) (hereditary) D68.1
XII (congenital) (hereditary) D68.2
XIII (congenital) (hereditary) D68.2
femoral, proximal focal (congenital) — *see* Defect, reduction, lower limb, longitudinal, femur
fibrin-stabilizing factor (congenital) (hereditary) D68.2
acquired D68.4
fibrinase D68.2
fibrinogen (congenital) (hereditary) D68.2
acquired D65
folate E53.8
folic acid E53.8
foreskin N47.3
fructokinase E74.11
fructose 1,6-diphosphatase E74.19
fructose-1-phosphate aldolase E74.19
GABA (gamma aminobutyric acid) transaminase E72.81
GABA-T (gamma aminobutyric acid transaminase) E72.81
galactokinase E74.29
galactose-1-phosphate uridyl transferase E74.29
gammaglobulin in blood D80.1
hereditary D80.0
glass factor D68.2
glucocorticoid E27.49
mineralocorticoid E27.49
glucose-6-phosphatase E74.01
glucose-6-phosphate dehydrogenase
anemia D55.0
without anemia D75.A
glucuronyl transferase E80.5

Deficiency — *continued*
glycogen synthetase E74.09
gonadotropin (isolated) E23.0
growth hormone (idiopathic) (isolated) E23.0
Hageman factor D68.2
hemoglobin D64.9
hepatophosphorylase E74.09
homogentisate 1,2-dioxygenase E70.29
hormone
anterior pituitary (partial) NEC E23.0
growth E23.0
growth (isolated) E23.0
pituitary E23.0
testicular E29.1
hypoxanthine- (guanine)- phosphoribosyltransferase (HG- PRT) (total H-PRT) E79.1
immunity D84.9
cell-mediated D84.8
with thrombocytopenia and eczema D82.0
combined D81.9
humoral D80.9
IgA (secretory) D80.2
IgG D80.3
IgM D80.4
immuno — *see* Immunodeficiency
immunoglobulin, selective
A (IgA) D80.2
G (IgG) (subclasses) D80.3
M (IgM) D80.4
inositol (B complex) E53.8
intrinsic
factor (congenital) D51.0
sphincter N36.42
with urethral hypermobility N36.43
iodine E61.8
congenital syndrome — *see* Syndrome, iodine-deficiency, congenital
iron E61.1
anemia D50.9
kalium E87.6
kappa-light chain D80.8
labile factor (congenital) (hereditary) D68.2
acquired D68.4
lacrimal fluid (acquired) (*see also* Syndrome, dry eye)
congenital Q10.6
lactase
congenital E73.0
secondary E73.1
Laki-Lorand factor D68.2
lecithin cholesterol acyltransferase E78.6
lipocaic K86.89
lipoprotein (familial) (high density) E78.6
liver phosphorylase E74.09
lysosomal alpha-1, 4 glucosidase E74.02
magnesium E61.2
major histocompatibility complex
class I D81.6
class II D81.7
manganese E61.3
menadione (vitamin K) E56.1
newborn P53
mental (familial) (hereditary) — *see* Disability, intellectual
methylenetetrahydrofolate reductase (MTHFR) E72.12
mevalonate kinase M04.1
mineral NEC E61.8
mineralocorticoid E27.49
with glucocorticoid E27.49
molybdenum (nutritional) E61.5
moral F60.2
multiple nutrient elements E61.7
multiple sulfatase (MSD) E75.26
muscle
carnitine (palmityltransferase) E71.314
phosphofructokinase E74.09
myoadenylate deaminase E79.2
myocardial — *see* Insufficiency, myocardial
myophosphorylase E74.04
NADH diaphorase or reductase (congenital) D74.0
NADH-methemoglobin reductase (congenital) D74.0
natrium E87.1
niacin (amide) (-tryptophan) E52
nicotinamide E52
nicotinic acid E52
number of teeth — *see* Anodontia
nutrient element E61.9
multiple E61.7
specified NEC E61.8

Deficiency — *continued*
nutrition, nutritional E63.9
sequelae — *see* Sequelae, nutritional deficiency
specified NEC E63.8
of interleukin 1 receptor antagonist [DIRA] M04.8
ornithine transcarbamylase E72.4
ovarian E28.39
oxygen — *see* Anoxia
pantothenic acid E53.8
parathyroid (gland) E20.9
perineum (female) N81.89
phenylalanine hydroxylase E70.1
phosphoenolpyruvate carboxykinase E74.4
phosphofructokinase E74.19
phosphomannomutase E74.8
phosphomannose isomerase E74.8
phosphomannosyl mutase E74.8
phosphorylase kinase, liver E74.09
pituitary hormone (isolated) E23.0
plasma thromboplastin
antecedent (PTA) D68.1
component (PTC) D67
plasminogen (type 1) (type 2) E88.02
platelet NEC D69.1
constitutional D68.0
polyglandular E31.8
autoimmune E31.0
potassium (K) E87.6
prepuce N47.3
proaccelerin (congenital) (hereditary) D68.2
acquired D68.4
proconvertin factor (congenital) (hereditary) D68.2
acquired D68.4
protein (*see also* Malnutrition) E46
anemia D53.0
C D68.59
S D68.59
prothrombin (congenital) (hereditary) D68.2
acquired D68.4
Prower factor D68.2
pseudocholinesterase E88.09
PTA (plasma thromboplastin antecedent) D68.1
PTC (plasma thromboplastin component) D67
purine nucleoside phosphorylase (PNP) D81.5
pyracin (alpha) (beta) E53.1
pyridoxal E53.1
pyridoxamine E53.1
pyridoxine (derivatives) E53.1
pyruvate
carboxylase E74.4
dehydrogenase E74.4
riboflavin (vitamin B2) E53.0
salt E87.1
secretion
ovary E28.39
salivary gland (any) K11.7
urine R34
selenium (dietary) E59
serum antitrypsin, familial E88.01
short stature homeobox gene (SHOX)
with
dyschondrosteosis Q78.8
short stature (idiopathic) E34.3
Turner's syndrome Q96.9
sodium (Na) E87.1
SPCA (factor VII) D68.2
sphincter, intrinsic N36.42
with urethral hypermobility N36.43
stable factor (congenital) (hereditary) D68.2
acquired D68.4
Stuart-Prower (factor X) D68.2
succinic semialdehyde dehydrogenase E72.81
sucrase E74.39
sulfatase E75.26
sulfite oxidase E72.19
thiamin, thiaminic (chloride) E51.9
beriberi (dry) E51.11
wet E51.12
thrombokinase D68.2
newborn P53
thyroid (gland) — *see* Hypothyroidism
tocopherol E56.0
tooth bud K00.0
transcobalamine II (anemia) D51.2
vanadium E61.6
vascular I99.9
vasopressin E23.2
vertical ridge K06.8
viosterol — *see* Deficiency, calciferol
vitamin (multiple) NOS E56.9
A E50.9
with

☑ **Additional character required**

Deficiency — *continued*
  vitamin — *continued*
    Bitot's spot (corneal) E50.1
    follicular keratosis E50.8
    keratomalacia E50.4
    manifestations NEC E50.8
    night blindness E50.5
    scar of cornea, xerophthalmic E50.6
    xeroderma E50.8
    xerophthalmia E50.7
    xerosis
      conjunctival E50.0
        and Bitot's spot E50.1
      cornea E50.2
        and ulceration E50.3
    sequelae E64.1
  B (complex) NOS E53.9
    with
      beriberi (dry) E51.11
        wet E51.12
      pellagra E52
    B1 NOS E51.9
      beriberi (dry) E51.11
        with circulatory system manifestations E51.11
        wet E51.12
    B12 E53.8
    B2 (riboflavin) E53.0
    B6 E53.1
    C E54
      sequelae E64.2
    D E55.9
      with
        adult osteomalacia M83.8
        rickets — *see* Rickets
      25-hydroxylase E83.32
    E E56.0
    folic acid E53.8
    G E53.0
    group B E53.9
      specified NEC E53.8
    H (biotin) E53.8
    K E56.1
      of newborn P53
    nicotinic E52
    P E56.8
    PP (pellagra-preventing) E52
    specified NEC E56.8
    thiamin E51.9
      beriberi — *see* Beriberi
  zinc, dietary E60
Deficit (*see also* Deficiency)
  attention and concentration R41.840
    following
      cerebral infarction I69.310
      cerebrovascular disease I69.910
        specified disease NEC I69.810
      nontraumatic
        intracerebral hemorrhage I69.110
        specified intracranial hemorrhage NEC I69.210
        subarachnoid hemorrhage I69.010
  disorder — *see* Attention, deficit
  cognitive
    communication R41.841
    emotional
      following
        cerebral infarction I69.315
        cerebrovascular disease I69.915
          specified disease NEC I69.815
        nontraumatic
          intracerebral hemorrhage I69.115
          specified intracranial hemorrhage NEC I69.215
          subarachnoid hemorrhage I69.015
      following
        cerebral infarction I69.319
        cerebrovascular disease I69.919
          specified disease NEC I69.819
        nontraumatic
          intracerebral hemorrhage I69.119
          specified intracranial hemorrhage NEC I69.219
          subarachnoid hemorrhage I69.019
    social
      following
        cerebral infarction I69.315
        cerebrovascular disease I69.915
          specified disease NEC I69.815
        nontraumatic
          intracerebral hemorrhage I69.115
          specified intracranial hemorrhage NEC I69.215
          subarachnoid hemorrhage I69.015

Deficit — *continued*
  cognitive NEC R41.89
    following
      cerebral infarction I69.318
      cerebrovascular disease I69.918
        specified disease NEC I69.818
      nontraumatic
        intracerebral hemorrhage I69.118
        specified intracranial hemorrhage NEC I69.218
        subarachnoid hemorrhage I69.018
  concentration R41.840
  executive function R41.844
    following
      cerebral infarction I69.314
      cerebrovascular disease I69.914
        specified disease NEC I69.814
      nontraumatic
        intracerebral hemorrhage I69.114
        specified intracranial hemorrhage NEC I69.214
        subarachnoid hemorrhage I69.014
  frontal lobe R41.844
    following
      cerebral infarction I69.314
      cerebrovascular disease I69.914
        specified disease NEC I69.814
      nontraumatic
        intracerebral hemorrhage I69.114
        specified intracranial hemorrhage NEC I69.214
        subarachnoid hemorrhage I69.014
  memory
    following
      cerebral infarction I69.311
      cerebrovascular disease I69.911
        specified disease NEC I69.811
      nontraumatic
        intracerebral hemorrhage I69.111
        specified intracranial hemorrhage NEC I69.211
        subarachnoid hemorrhage I69.011
  neurologic NEC R29.818
    ischemic
      reversible (RIND) I63.9
        prolonged (PRIND) I63.9
  oxygen R09.02
  prolonged reversible ischemic neurologic (PRIND) I63.9
  psychomotor R41.843
    following
      cerebral infarction I69.313
      cerebrovascular disease I69.913
        specified disease NEC I69.813
      nontraumatic
        intracerebral hemorrhage I69.113
        specified intracranial hemorrhage NEC I69.213
        subarachnoid hemorrhage I69.013
  visuospatial R41.842
    following
      cerebral infarction I69.312
      cerebrovascular disease I69.912
        specified disease NEC I69.812
      nontraumatic
        intracerebral hemorrhage I69.112
        specified intracranial hemorrhage NEC I69.212
        subarachnoid hemorrhage I69.012
Deflection
  radius — *see* Deformity, limb, specified type NEC, forearm
  septum (acquired) (nasal) (nose) J34.2
  spine — *see* Curvature, spine
  turbinate (nose) J34.2
Defluvium
  capillorum — *see* Alopecia
  ciliorum — *see* Madarosis
  unguium L60.8
Deformity Q89.9
  abdomen, congenital Q89.9
  abdominal wall
    acquired M95.8
    congenital Q79.59
  acquired (unspecified site) M95.9
  adrenal gland Q89.1
  alimentary tract, congenital Q45.9
    upper Q40.9
  ankle (joint) (acquired) (*see also* Deformity, limb, lower leg)
    abduction — *see* Contraction, joint, ankle
    congenital Q68.8

Deformity — *continued*
  ankle — *continued*
    contraction — *see* Contraction, joint, ankle
    specified type NEC — *see* Deformity, limb, foot, specified NEC
  anus (acquired) K62.89
    congenital Q43.9
  aorta (arch) (congenital) Q25.40
    acquired I77.89
  aortic
    arch, acquired I77.89
    cusp or valve (congenital) Q23.8
      acquired (*see also* Endocarditis, aortic) I35.8
  arm (acquired) (upper) (*see also* Deformity, limb, upper arm)
    congenital Q68.8
    forearm — *see* Deformity, limb, forearm
  artery (congenital) (peripheral) NOS Q27.9
    acquired I77.89
    coronary (acquired) I25.9
      congenital Q24.5
    umbilical Q27.0
  atrial septal Q21.1
  auditory canal (external) (congenital) (*see also* Malformation, ear, external)
    acquired — *see* Disorder, ear, external, specified type NEC
  auricle
    ear (congenital) (*see also* Malformation, ear, external)
      acquired — *see* Disorder, pinna, deformity
  back — *see* Dorsopathy, deforming
  bile duct (common) (congenital) (hepatic) Q44.5
    acquired K83.8
  biliary duct or passage (congenital) Q44.5
    acquired K83.8
  bladder (neck) (trigone) (sphincter) (acquired) N32.89
    congenital Q64.79
  bone (acquired) NOS M95.9
    congenital Q79.9
    turbinate M95.0
  brain (congenital) Q04.9
    acquired G93.89
    reduction Q04.3
  breast (acquired) N64.89
    congenital Q83.9
    reconstructed N65.0
  bronchus (congenital) Q32.4
    acquired NEC J98.09
  bursa, congenital Q79.9
  canaliculi (lacrimalis) (acquired) (*see also* Disorder, lacrimal system, changes)
    congenital Q10.6
  canthus, acquired — *see* Disorder, eyelid, specified type NEC
  capillary (acquired) I78.8
  cardiovascular system, congenital Q28.9
  caruncle, lacrimal (acquired) (*see also* Disorder, lacrimal system, changes)
    congenital Q10.6
  cascade, stomach K31.2
  cecum (congenital) Q43.9
    acquired K63.89
  cerebral, acquired G93.89
    congenital Q04.9
  cervix (uterus) (acquired) NEC N88.8
    congenital Q51.9
  cheek (acquired) M95.2
    congenital Q18.9
  chest (acquired) (wall) M95.4
    congenital Q67.8
    sequelae (late effect) of rickets E64.3
  chin (acquired) M95.2
    congenital Q18.9
  choroid (congenital) Q14.3
    acquired H31.8
    plexus Q07.8
      acquired G96.19
  cicatricial — *see* Cicatrix
  cilia, acquired — *see* Disorder, eyelid, specified type NEC
  clavicle (acquired) M95.8
    congenital Q68.8
  clitoris (congenital) Q52.6
    acquired N90.89
  clubfoot — *see* Clubfoot
  coccyx (acquired) — *see* subcategory M43.8 ☑
  colon (congenital) Q43.9
    acquired K63.89
  concha (ear), congenital (*see also* Malformation, ear, external)
    acquired — *see* Disorder, pinna, deformity

Deformity

Deformity — *continued*
cornea (acquired) H18.70
  congenital Q13.4
  descemetocele — *see* Descemetocele
  ectasia — *see* Ectasia, cornea
  specified NEC H18.79 ☑
  staphyloma — *see* Staphyloma, cornea
coronary artery (acquired) I25.9
  congenital Q24.5
cranium (acquired) — *see* Deformity, skull
cricoid cartilage (congenital) Q31.8
  acquired J38.7
cystic duct (congenital) Q44.5
  acquired K82.8
Dandy-Walker Q03.1
  with spina bifida — *see* Spina bifida
diaphragm (congenital) Q79.1
  acquired J98.6
digestive organ NOS Q45.9
ductus arteriosus Q25.0
duodenal bulb K31.89
duodenum (congenital) Q43.9
  acquired K31.89
dura — *see* Deformity, meninges
ear (acquired) (*see also* Disorder, pinna, deformity)
  congenital (external) Q17.9
   internal Q16.5
   middle Q16.4
    ossicles Q16.3
   ossicles Q16.3
ectodermal (congenital) NEC Q84.9
ejaculatory duct (congenital) Q55.4
  acquired N50.89
elbow (joint) (acquired) (*see also* Deformity, limb, upper arm)
  congenital Q68.8
  contraction — *see* Contraction, joint, elbow
endocrine gland NEC Q89.2
epididymis (congenital) Q55.4
  acquired N50.89
epiglottis (congenital) Q31.8
  acquired J38.7
esophagus (congenital) Q39.9
  acquired K22.8
eustachian tube (congenital) NEC Q17.8
eye, congenital Q15.9
eyebrow (congenital) Q18.8
eyelid (acquired) (*see also* Disorder, eyelid, specified type NEC)
  congenital Q10.3
face (acquired) M95.2
  congenital Q18.9
fallopian tube, acquired N83.8
femur (acquired) — *see* Deformity, limb, specified type NEC, thigh
fetal
  with fetopelvic disproportion O33.7 ☑
  causing obstructed labor O66.3
finger (acquired) M20.00 ☑
  boutonniere M20.02 ☑
  congenital Q68.1
  flexion contracture — *see* Contraction, joint, hand
  mallet finger M20.01 ☑
  specified NEC M20.09 ☑
  swan-neck M20.03 ☑
flexion (joint) (acquired) (*see also* Deformity, limb, flexion) M21.20
  congenital NOS Q74.9
   hip Q65.89
foot (acquired) (*see also* Deformity, limb, lower leg)
  cavovarus (congenital) Q66.1 ☑
  congenital NOS Q66.9 ☑
   specified type NEC Q66.89
  specified type NEC — *see* Deformity, limb, foot, specified NEC
  valgus (congenital) Q66.6
   acquired — *see* Deformity, valgus, ankle
  varus (congenital) NEC Q66.3 ☑
   acquired — *see* Deformity, varus, ankle
forearm (acquired) (*see also* Deformity, limb, forearm)
  congenital Q68.8
forehead (acquired) M95.2
  congenital Q75.8
frontal bone (acquired) M95.2
  congenital Q75.8
gallbladder (congenital) Q44.1
  acquired K82.8
gastrointestinal tract (congenital) NOS Q45.9
  acquired K63.89
genitalia, genital organ(s) or system NEC
  female (congenital) Q52.9

Deformity — *continued*
genitalia — *continued*
  acquired N94.89
  external Q52.70
  male (congenital) Q55.9
   acquired N50.89
globe (eye) (congenital) Q15.8
  acquired H44.89
gum, acquired NEC K06.8
hand (acquired) — *see* Deformity, limb, hand
  congenital Q68.1
head (acquired) M95.2
  congenital Q75.8
heart (congenital) Q24.9
  septum Q21.9
   auricular Q21.1
   ventricular Q21.0
  valve (congenital) NEC Q24.8
   acquired — *see* Endocarditis
heel (acquired) — *see* Deformity, foot
hepatic duct (congenital) Q44.5
  acquired K83.8
hip (joint) (acquired) (*see also* Deformity, limb, thigh)
  congenital Q65.9
  due to (previous) juvenile osteochondrosis — *see* Coxa, plana
  flexion — *see* Contraction, joint, hip
hourglass — *see* Contraction, hourglass
humerus (acquired) M21.82 ☑
  congenital Q74.0
hypophyseal (congenital) Q89.2
ileocecal (coil) (valve) (acquired) K63.89
  congenital Q43.9
ileum (congenital) Q43.9
  acquired K63.89
ilium (acquired) M95.5
  congenital Q74.2
integument (congenital) Q84.9
intervertebral cartilage or disc (acquired) — *see* Disorder, disc, specified NEC
intestine (large) (small) (congenital) NOS Q43.9
  acquired K63.89
intrinsic minus or plus (hand) — *see* Deformity, limb, specified type NEC, forearm
iris (acquired) H21.89
  congenital Q13.2
ischium (acquired) M95.5
  congenital Q74.2
jaw (acquired) (congenital) M26.9
joint (acquired) NEC M21.90
  congenital Q68.8
  elbow M21.92 ☑
  hand M21.94 ☑
  hip M21.95 ☑
  knee M21.96 ☑
  shoulder M21.92 ☑
  wrist M21.93 ☑
kidney(s) (calyx) (pelvis) (congenital) Q63.9
  acquired N28.89
  artery (congenital) Q27.2
   acquired I77.89
Klippel-Feil (brevicollis) Q76.1
knee (acquired) NEC (*see also* Deformity, limb, lower leg)
  congenital Q68.2
labium (majus) (minus) (congenital) Q52.79
  acquired N90.89
lacrimal passages or duct (congenital) NEC Q10.6
  acquired — *see* Disorder, lacrimal system, changes
larynx (muscle) (congenital) Q31.8
  acquired J38.7
  web (glottic) Q31.0
leg (upper) (acquired) NEC (*see also* Deformity, limb, thigh)
  congenital Q68.8
  lower leg — *see* Deformity, limb, lower leg
lens (acquired) H27.8
  congenital Q12.9
lid (fold) (acquired) (*see also* Disorder, eyelid, specified type NEC)
  congenital Q10.3
ligament (acquired) — *see* Disorder, ligament
  congenital Q79.9
limb (acquired) M21.90
  clawfoot M21.53 ☑
  clawhand M21.51 ☑
  clubfoot M21.54 ☑
  clubhand M21.52 ☑
  congenital, except reduction deformity Q74.9
  flat foot M21.4 ☑
  flexion M21.20

Deformity — *continued*
limb — *continued*
  ankle M21.27 ☑
  elbow M21.22 ☑
  finger M21.24 ☑
  hip M21.25 ☑
  knee M21.26 ☑
  shoulder M21.21 ☑
  toe M21.27 ☑
  wrist M21.23 ☑
  foot
   claw — *see* Deformity, limb, clawfoot
   club — *see* Deformity, limb, clubfoot
   drop M21.37 ☑
   flat — *see* Deformity, limb, flat foot
   specified NEC M21.6X ☑
  forearm M21.93 ☑
  hand M21.94 ☑
  lower leg M21.96 ☑
  specified type NEC M21.80
   forearm M21.83 ☑
   lower leg M21.86 ☑
   thigh M21.85 ☑
   upper arm M21.82 ☑
  thigh M21.95 ☑
  unequal length M21.70
   short site is
    femur M21.75 ☑
    fibula M21.76 ☑
    humerus M21.72 ☑
    radius M21.73 ☑
    tibia M21.76 ☑
    ulna M21.73 ☑
  upper arm M21.92 ☑
  valgus — *see* Deformity, valgus
  varus — *see* Deformity, varus
  wrist drop M21.33 ☑
lip (acquired) NEC K13.0
  congenital Q38.0
liver (congenital) Q44.7
  acquired K76.89
lumbosacral (congenital) (joint) (region) Q76.49
  acquired — *see* subcategory M43.8 ☑
  kyphosis — *see* Kyphosis, congenital
  lordosis — *see* Lordosis, congenital
lung (congenital) Q33.9
  acquired J98.4
lymphatic system, congenital Q89.9
Madelung's (radius) Q74.0
mandible (acquired) (congenital) M26.9
maxilla (acquired) (congenital) M26.9
meninges or membrane (congenital) Q07.9
  cerebral Q04.8
   acquired G96.19
  spinal cord (congenital) G96.19
   acquired G96.19
metacarpus (acquired) — *see* Deformity, limb, forearm
  congenital Q74.0
metatarsus (acquired) — *see* Deformity, foot
  congenital Q66.9 ☑
middle ear (congenital) Q16.4
  ossicles Q16.3
mitral (leaflets) (valve) I05.8
  parachute Q23.2
  stenosis, congenital Q23.2
mouth (acquired) K13.79
  congenital Q38.6
multiple, congenital NEC Q89.7
muscle (acquired) M62.89
  congenital Q79.9
   sternocleidomastoid Q68.0
musculoskeletal system (acquired) M95.9
  congenital Q79.9
  specified NEC M95.8
nail (acquired) L60.8
  congenital Q84.6
nasal — *see* Deformity, nose
neck (acquired) M95.3
  congenital Q18.9
   sternocleidomastoid Q68.0
nervous system (congenital) Q07.9
nipple (congenital) Q83.9
  acquired N64.89
nose (acquired) (cartilage) M95.0
  bone (turbinate) M95.0
  congenital Q30.9
   bent or squashed Q67.4
  saddle M95.0
   syphilitic A50.57
  septum (acquired) J34.2
   congenital Q30.8

Deformity — *continued*
  nose — *continued*
    sinus (wall) (congenital) Q30.8
      acquired M95.0
    syphilitic (congenital) A50.57
      late A52.73
  ocular muscle (congenital) Q10.3
    acquired — *see* Strabismus, mechanical
  opticociliary vessels (congenital) Q13.2
  orbit (eye) (acquired) H05.30
    atrophy — *see* Atrophy, orbit
    congenital Q10.7
    due to
      bone disease NEC H05.32 ☑
      trauma or surgery H05.33 ☑
    enlargement — *see* Enlargement, orbit
    exostosis — *see* Exostosis, orbit
  organ of Corti (congenital) Q16.5
  ovary (congenital) Q50.39
    acquired N83.8
  oviduct, acquired N83.8
  palate (congenital) Q38.5
    acquired M27.8
    cleft (congenital) — *see* Cleft, palate
  pancreas (congenital) Q45.3
    acquired K86.89
  parathyroid (gland) Q89.2
  parotid (gland) (congenital) Q38.4
    acquired K11.8
  patella (acquired) — *see* Disorder, patella, specified
    NEC
  pelvis, pelvic (acquired) (bony) M95.5
    with disproportion (fetopelvic) O33.0
      causing obstructed labor O65.0
    congenital Q74.2
    rachitic sequelae (late effect) E64.3
  penis (glans) (congenital) Q55.69
    acquired N48.89
  pericardium (congenital) Q24.8
    acquired — *see* Pericarditis
  pharynx (congenital) Q38.8
    acquired J39.2
  pinna, acquired (*see also* Disorder, pinna, deformity)
    congenital Q17.9
  pituitary (congenital) Q89.2
  posture — *see* Dorsopathy, deforming
  prepuce (congenital) Q55.69
    acquired N47.8
  prostate (congenital) Q55.4
    acquired N42.89
  pupil (congenital) Q13.2
    acquired — *see* Abnormality, pupillary
  pylorus (congenital) Q40.3
    acquired K31.89
  rachitic (acquired), old or healed E64.3
  radius (acquired) (*see also* Deformity, limb, forearm)
    congenital Q68.8
  rectum (congenital) Q43.9
    acquired K62.89
  reduction (extremity) (limb), congenital (*see also*
    condition and site) Q73.8
    brain Q04.3
    lower — *see* Defect, reduction, lower limb
    upper — *see* Defect, reduction, upper limb
  renal — *see* Deformity, kidney
  respiratory system (congenital) Q34.9
  rib (acquired) M95.4
    congenital Q76.6
    cervical Q76.5
  rotation (joint) (acquired) — *see* Deformity, limb,
    specified site NEC
    congenital Q74.9
    hip — *see* Deformity, limb, specified type NEC,
      thigh
    congenital Q65.89
  sacroiliac joint (congenital) Q74.2
    acquired — *see* subcategory M43.8 ☑
  sacrum (acquired) — *see* subcategory M43.8 ☑
  saddle
    back — *see* Lordosis
    nose M95.0
      syphilitic A50.57
  salivary gland or duct (congenital) Q38.4
    acquired K11.8
  scapula (acquired) M95.8
    congenital Q68.8
  scrotum (congenital) (*see also* Malformation, testis
    and scrotum)
    acquired N50.89
  seminal vesicles (congenital) Q55.4
    acquired N50.89
  septum, nasal (acquired) J34.2

Deformity — *continued*
  shoulder (joint) (acquired) — *see* Deformity, limb,
    upper arm
    congenital Q74.0
    contraction — *see* Contraction, joint, shoulder
  sigmoid (flexure) (congenital) Q43.9
    acquired K63.89
  skin (congenital) Q82.9
  skull (acquired) M95.2
    congenital Q75.8
      with
        anencephaly Q00.0
        encephalocele — *see* Encephalocele
        hydrocephalus Q03.9
          with spina bifida — *see* Spina bifida, by site,
            with hydrocephalus
        microcephaly Q02
  soft parts, organs or tissues (of pelvis)
    in pregnancy or childbirth NEC O34.8 ☑
      causing obstructed labor O65.5
  spermatic cord (congenital) Q55.4
    acquired N50.89
    torsion — *see* Torsion, spermatic cord
  spinal — *see* Dorsopathy, deforming
    column (acquired) — *see* Dorsopathy, deforming
    congenital Q67.5
    cord (congenital) Q06.9
      acquired G95.89
    nerve root (congenital) Q07.9
  spine (acquired) (*see also* Dorsopathy, deforming)
    congenital Q67.5
    rachitic E64.3
    specified NEC — *see* Dorsopathy, deforming,
      specified NEC
  spleen
    acquired D73.89
    congenital Q89.09
  Sprengel's (congenital) Q74.0
  sternocleidomastoid (muscle), congenital Q68.0
  sternum (acquired) M95.4
    congenital NEC Q76.7
  stomach (congenital) Q40.3
    acquired K31.89
  submandibular gland (congenital) Q38.4
  submaxillary gland (congenital) Q38.4
    acquired K11.8
  talipes — *see* Talipes
  testis (congenital) (*see also* Malformation, testis and
    scrotum)
    acquired N44.8
    torsion — *see* Torsion, testis
  thigh (acquired) (*see also* Deformity, limb, thigh)
    congenital NEC Q68.8
  thorax (acquired) (wall) M95.4
    congenital Q67.8
    sequelae of rickets E64.3
  thumb (acquired) (*see also* Deformity, finger)
    congenital NEC Q68.1
  thymus (tissue) (congenital) Q89.2
  thyroid (gland) (congenital) Q89.2
    cartilage Q31.8
      acquired J38.7
  tibia (acquired) (*see also* Deformity, limb, specified
    type NEC, lower leg)
    congenital NEC Q68.8
    saber (syphilitic) A50.56
  toe (acquired) M20.6 ☑
    congenital Q66.9 ☑
    hallux rigidus M20.2 ☑
    hallux valgus M20.1 ☑
    hallux varus M20.3 ☑
    hammer toe M20.4 ☑
    specified NEC M20.5X ☑
  tongue (congenital) Q38.3
    acquired K14.8
  tooth, teeth K00.2
  trachea (rings) (congenital) Q32.1
    acquired J39.8
  transverse aortic arch (congenital) Q25.49
  tricuspid (leaflets) (valve) I07.8
    atresia or stenosis Q22.4
    Ebstein's Q22.5
  trunk (acquired) M95.8
    congenital Q89.9
  ulna (acquired) (*see also* Deformity, limb, forearm)
    congenital NEC Q68.8
  urachus, congenital Q64.4
  ureter (opening) (congenital) Q62.8
    acquired N28.89
  urethra (congenital) Q64.79
    acquired N36.8

Deformity — *continued*
  urinary tract (congenital) Q64.9
    urachus Q64.4
  uterus (congenital) Q51.9
    acquired N85.8
  uvula (congenital) Q38.5
  vagina (acquired) N89.8
    congenital Q52.4
  valgus NEC M21.00
    ankle M21.07 ☑
    elbow M21.02 ☑
    hip M21.05 ☑
    knee M21.06 ☑
  valve, valvular (congenital) (heart) Q24.8
    acquired — *see* Endocarditis
  varus NEC M21.10
    ankle M21.17 ☑
    elbow M21.12 ☑
    hip M21.15 ☑
    knee M21.16 ☑
  tibia — *see* Osteochondrosis, juvenile, tibia
  vas deferens (congenital) Q55.4
    acquired N50.89
  vein (congenital) Q27.9
    great Q26.9
  vertebra — *see* Dorsopathy, deforming
  vertical talus (congenital) Q66.80
    left foot Q66.82
    right foot Q66.81
  vesicourethral orifice (acquired) N32.89
    congenital NEC Q64.79
  vessels of optic papilla (congenital) Q14.2
  visual field (contraction) — *see* Defect, visual field
  vitreous body, acquired H43.89
  vulva (congenital) Q52.79
    acquired N90.89
  wrist (joint) (acquired) (*see also* Deformity, limb,
    forearm)
    congenital Q68.8
    contraction — *see* Contraction, joint, wrist
Degeneration, degenerative
  adrenal (capsule) (fatty) (gland) (hyaline)
    (infectional) E27.8
  amyloid (*see also* Amyloidosis) E85.9
  anterior cornua, spinal cord G12.29
  anterior labral S43.49 ☑
  aorta, aortic I70.0
    fatty I77.89
  aortic valve (heart) — *see* Endocarditis, aortic
  arteriovascular — *see* Arteriosclerosis
  artery, arterial (atheromatous) (calcareous) (*see also*
    Arteriosclerosis)
    cerebral, amyloid E85.4 *[I68.0]*
    medial — *see* Arteriosclerosis, extremities
  articular cartilage NEC — *see* Derangement, joint,
    articular cartilage, by site
  atheromatous — *see* Arteriosclerosis
  basal nuclei or ganglia G23.9
    specified NEC G23.8
  bone NEC — *see* Disorder, bone, specified type
    NEC
  brachial plexus G54.0
  brain (cortical) (progressive) G31.9
    alcoholic G31.2
    arteriosclerotic I67.2
    childhood G31.9
      specified NEC G31.89
    cystic G31.89
      congenital Q04.6
    in
      alcoholism G31.2
      beriberi E51.2
      cerebrovascular disease I67.9
      congenital hydrocephalus Q03.9
        with spina bifida (*see also* Spina bifida)
      Fabry-Anderson disease E75.21
      Gaucher's disease E75.22
      Hunter's syndrome E76.1
      lipidosis
        cerebral E75.4
        generalized E75.6
      mucopolysaccharidosis — *see*
        Mucopolysaccharidosis
      myxedema E03.9 *[G32.89]*
      neoplastic disease (*see also* Neoplasm) D49.6
        [G32.89]
      Niemann-Pick disease E75.249 *[G32.89]*
      sphingolipidosis E75.3 *[G32.89]*
      vitamin B12 deficiency E53.8 *[G32.89]*
    senile NEC G31.1
  breast N64.89
  Bruch's membrane — *see* Degeneration, choroid

Degeneration

Degeneration — *continued*
- capillaries (fatty) I78.8
  - amyloid E85.89 [I79.8]
- cardiac (*see also* Degeneration, myocardial)
  - valve, valvular — *see* Endocarditis
- cardiorenal — *see* Hypertension, cardiorenal
- cardiovascular (*see also* Disease, cardiovascular)
  - renal — *see* Hypertension, cardiorenal
- cerebellar NOS G31.9
  - alcoholic G31.2
  - primary (hereditary) (sporadic) G11.9
- cerebral — *see* Degeneration, brain
- cerebrovascular I67.9
  - due to hypertension I67.4
- cervical plexus G54.2
- cervix N88.8
  - due to radiation (intended effect) N88.8
    - adverse effect or misadventure N99.89
- chamber angle H21.21 ☑
- changes, spine or vertebra — *see* Spondylosis
- chorioretinal (*see also* Degeneration, choroid)
  - hereditary H31.20
- choroid (colloid) (drusen) H31.10 ☑
  - atrophy — *see* Atrophy, choroidal
  - hereditary — *see* Dystrophy, choroidal, hereditary
- ciliary body H21.22 ☑
- cochlear — *see* subcategory H83.8 ☑
- combined (spinal cord) (subacute) E53.8 [G32.0]
  - with anemia (pernicious) D51.0 [G32.0]
    - due to dietary vitamin B12 deficiency D51.3 [G32.0]
  - in (due to)
    - vitamin B12 deficiency E53.8 [G32.0]
      - anemia D51.9 [G32.0]
- conjunctiva H11.10
  - concretions — *see* Concretion, conjunctiva
  - deposits — *see* Deposit, conjunctiva
  - pigmentations — *see* Pigmentation, conjunctiva
  - pinguecula — *see* Pinguecula
  - xerosis — *see* Xerosis, conjunctiva
- cornea H18.40
  - calcerous H18.43
    - band keratopathy H18.42 ☑
  - familial, hereditary — *see* Dystrophy, cornea
  - hyaline (of old scars) H18.49
  - keratomalacia — *see* Keratomalacia
  - nodular H18.45 ☑
  - peripheral H18.46 ☑
  - senile H18.41 ☑
  - specified type NEC H18.49
- cortical (cerebellar) (parenchymatous) G31.89
  - alcoholic G31.2
  - diffuse, due to arteriopathy I67.2
- corticobasal G31.85
- cutis L98.8
  - amyloid E85.4 [L99]
- dental pulp K04.2
- disc disease — *see* Degeneration, intervertebral disc NEC
- dorsolateral (spinal cord) — *see* Degeneration, combined
- extrapyramidal G25.9
- eye, macular (*see also* Degeneration, macula)
  - congenital or hereditary — *see* Dystrophy, retina
- facet joints — *see* Spondylosis
- fatty
  - liver NEC K76.0
    - alcoholic K70.0
- grey matter (brain) (Alpers') G31.81
- heart (*see also* Degeneration, myocardial)
  - amyloid E85.4 [I43]
  - atheromatous — *see* Disease, heart, ischemic, atherosclerotic
  - ischemic — *see* Disease, heart, ischemic
- hepatolenticular (Wilson's) E83.01
- hepatorenal K76.7
- hyaline (diffuse) (generalized)
  - localized — *see* Degeneration, by site
- infrapatellar fat pad M79.4
- intervertebral disc NOS
  - with
    - myelopathy — *see* Disorder, disc, with, myelopathy
    - radiculitis or radiculopathy — *see* Disorder, disc, with, radiculopathy
  - cervical, cervicothoracic — *see* Disorder, disc, cervical, degeneration
    - with
      - myelopathy — *see* Disorder, disc, cervical, with myelopathy
      - neuritis, radiculitis or radiculopathy — *see* Disorder, disc, cervical, with neuritis

Degeneration — *continued*
- intervertebral disc NOS — *continued*
  - lumbar region M51.36
    - with
      - myelopathy M51.06
      - neuritis, radiculitis, radiculopathy or sciatica M51.16
  - lumbosacral region M51.37
    - with
      - neuritis, radiculitis, radiculopathy or sciatica M51.17
  - sacrococcygeal region M53.3
  - thoracic region M51.34
    - with
      - myelopathy M51.04
      - neuritis, radiculitis, radiculopathy M51.14
  - thoracolumbar region M51.35
    - with
      - myelopathy M51.05
      - neuritis, radiculitis, radiculopathy M51.15
- intestine, amyloid E85.4
- iris (pigmentary) H21.23 ☑
- ischemic — *see* Ischemia
- joint disease — *see* Osteoarthritis
- kidney N28.89
  - amyloid E85.4 [N29]
  - cystic, congenital Q61.9
  - fatty N28.89
  - polycystic Q61.3
    - adult type (autosomal dominant) Q61.2
    - infantile type (autosomal recessive) NEC Q61.19
      - collecting duct dilatation Q61.11
- Kuhnt-Junius (*see also* Degeneration, macula) H35.32 ☑
- lens — *see* Cataract
- lenticular (familial) (progressive) (Wilson's) (with cirrhosis of liver) E83.01
- liver (diffuse) NEC K76.89
  - amyloid E85.4 [K77]
  - cystic K76.89
    - congenital Q44.6
  - fatty NEC K76.0
    - alcoholic K70.0
  - hypertrophic K76.89
  - parenchymatous, acute or subacute K72.00
    - with coma K72.01
  - pigmentary K76.89
  - toxic (acute) K71.9
- lung J98.4
- lymph gland I89.8
  - hyaline I89.8
- macula, macular (acquired) (age-related) (senile) H35.30
  - angioid streaks H35.33
  - atrophic age-related H35.31 ☑
  - congenital or hereditary — *see* Dystrophy, retina
  - cystoid H35.35 ☑
  - drusen H35.36 ☑
  - dry age-related H35.31 ☑
  - exudative H35.32 ☑
  - hole H35.34 ☑
  - nonexudative H35.31 ☑
  - puckering H35.37 ☑
  - toxic H35.38 ☑
  - wet age-related H35.32 ☑
- membranous labyrinth, congenital (causing impairment of hearing) Q16.5
- meniscus — *see* Derangement, meniscus
- mitral — *see* Insufficiency, mitral
- Mönckeberg's — *see* Arteriosclerosis, extremities
- motor centers, senile G31.1
- multi-system G90.3
- mural — *see* Degeneration, myocardial
- muscle (fatty) (fibrous) (hyaline) (progressive) M62.89
  - heart — *see* Degeneration, myocardial
- myelin, central nervous system G37.9
- myocardial, myocardium (fatty) (hyaline) (senile) I51.5
  - with rheumatic fever (conditions in I00) I09.0
    - active, acute or subacute I01.2
      - with chorea I02.0
    - inactive or quiescent (with chorea) I09.0
  - hypertensive — *see* Hypertension, heart
  - rheumatic — *see* Degeneration, myocardial, with rheumatic fever
  - syphilitic A52.06
- nasal sinus (mucosa) J32.9
  - frontal J32.1
  - maxillary J32.0
- nerve — *see* Disorder, nerve

Degeneration — *continued*
- nervous system G31.9
  - alcoholic G31.2
  - amyloid E85.4 [G99.8]
  - autonomic G90.9
  - fatty G31.89
  - specified NEC G31.89
- nipple N64.89
- olivopontocerebellar (hereditary) (familial) G23.8
- osseous labyrinth — *see* subcategory H83.8 ☑
- ovary N83.8
  - cystic N83.20 ☑
  - microcystic N83.20 ☑
- pallidal pigmentary (progressive) G23.0
- pancreas K86.89
  - tuberculous A18.83
- penis N48.89
- pigmentary (diffuse) (general)
  - localized — *see* Degeneration, by site
  - pallidal (progressive) G23.0
- pineal gland E34.8
- pituitary (gland) E23.6
- popliteal fat pad M79.4
- posterolateral (spinal cord) — *see* Degeneration, combined
- pulmonary valve (heart) I37.8
- pulp (tooth) K04.2
- pupillary margin H21.24 ☑
- renal — *see* Degeneration, kidney
- retina H35.9
  - hereditary (cerebroretinal) (congenital) (juvenile) (macula) (peripheral) (pigmentary) — *see* Dystrophy, retina
  - Kuhnt-Junius (*see also* Degeneration, macula) H35.32 ☑
  - macula (cystic) (exudative) (hole) (nonexudative) (pseudohole) (senile) (toxic) — *see* Degeneration, macula
  - peripheral H35.40
    - lattice H35.41 ☑
    - microcystoid H35.42 ☑
    - paving stone H35.43 ☑
    - secondary
      - pigmentary H35.45 ☑
      - vitreoretinal H35.46 ☑
    - senile reticular H35.44 ☑
  - pigmentary (primary) (*see also* Dystrophy, retina)
    - secondary — *see* Degeneration, retina, peripheral, secondary
  - posterior pole — *see* Degeneration, macula
- saccule, congenital (causing impairment of hearing) Q16.5
- senile R54
  - brain G31.1
  - cardiac, heart or myocardium — *see* Degeneration, myocardial
  - motor centers G31.1
  - vascular — *see* Arteriosclerosis
- sinus (cystic) (*see also* Sinusitis)
  - polypoid J33.1
- skin L98.8
  - amyloid E85.4 [L99]
  - colloid L98.8
- spinal (cord) G31.89
  - amyloid E85.4 [G32.89]
  - combined (subacute) — *see* Degeneration, combined
  - dorsolateral — *see* Degeneration, combined
  - familial NEC G31.89
  - fatty G31.89
  - funicular — *see* Degeneration, combined
  - posterolateral — *see* Degeneration, combined
  - subacute combined — *see* Degeneration, combined
  - tuberculous A17.81
- spleen D73.0
  - amyloid E85.4 [D77]
- stomach K31.89
- striatonigral G23.2
- suprarenal (capsule) (gland) E27.8
- synovial membrane (pulpy) — *see* Disorder, synovium, specified type NEC
- tapetoretinal — *see* Dystrophy, retina
- thymus (gland) E32.8
  - fatty E32.8
- thyroid (gland) E07.89
- tricuspid (heart) (valve) I07.9
- tuberculous NEC — *see* Tuberculosis
- turbinate J34.89
- uterus (cystic) N85.8
- vascular (senile) — *see* Arteriosclerosis
  - hypertensive — *see* Hypertension

☑ **Additional character required**

Degeneration — *continued*
    vitreoretinal, secondary — *see* Degeneration, retina,
        peripheral, secondary, vitreoretinal
    vitreous (body) H43.81 ☑
    Wallerian — *see* Disorder, nerve
    Wilson's hepatolenticular E83.01
Deglutition
    paralysis R13.0
        hysterical F44.4
    pneumonia J69.0
Degos' disease I77.89
Dehiscence (of)
    amputation stump T87.81
    cesarean wound O90.0
    closure of
        cornea T81.31 ☑
        craniotomy T81.32 ☑
        fascia (muscular) (superficial) T81.32 ☑
        internal organ or tissue T81.32 ☑
        laceration (external) (internal) T81.33 ☑
        ligament T81.32 ☑
        mucosa T81.31 ☑
        muscle or muscle flap T81.32 ☑
        ribs or rib cage T81.32 ☑
        skin and subcutaneous tissue (full-thickness)
            (superficial) T81.31 ☑
        skull T81.32 ☑
        sternum (sternotomy) T81.32 ☑
        tendon T81.32 ☑
        traumatic laceration (external) (internal) T81.33 ☑
    episiotomy O90.1
    operation wound NEC T81.31 ☑
        external operation wound (superficial) T81.31 ☑
        internal operation wound (deep) T81.32 ☑
    perineal wound (postpartum) O90.1
    traumatic injury wound repair T81.33 ☑
    wound T81.30 ☑
        traumatic repair T81.33 ☑
Dehydration E86.0
    newborn P74.1
Déjérine-Roussy syndrome G89.0
Déjérine-Sottas disease or neuropathy (hypertrophic)
    G60.0
Déjérine-Thomas atrophy G23.8
Delay, delayed
    any plane in pelvis
        complicating delivery O66.9
    birth or delivery NOS O63.9
    closure, ductus arteriosus (Botalli) P29.38
    coagulation — *see* Defect, coagulation
    conduction (cardiac) (ventricular) I45.9
    delivery, second twin, triplet, etc., O63.2
    development R62.50
        global F88
        intellectual (specific) F81.9
        language F80.9
            due to hearing loss F80.4
        learning F81.9
        pervasive F84.9
        physiological R62.50
            specified stage NEC R62.0
        reading F81.0
        sexual E30.0
        speech F80.9
            due to hearing loss F80.4
        spelling F81.81
    ejaculation F52.32
    gastric emptying K30
    menarche E30.0
    menstruation (cause unknown) N91.0
    milestone R62.0
    passage of meconium (newborn) P76.0
    primary respiration P28.9
    puberty (constitutional) E30.0
    separation of umbilical cord P96.82
    sexual maturation, female E30.0
    sleep phase syndrome G47.21
    union, fracture — *see* Fracture, by site
    vaccination Z28.9
Deletion(s)
    autosome Q93.9
        identified by fluorescence in situ hybridization
            (FISH) Q93.89
        identified by in situ hybridization (ISH) Q93.89
    chromosome
        with complex rearrangements NEC Q93.7
        part of NEC Q93.59
        seen only at prometaphase Q93.89
        short arm
            4 Q93.3
            5p Q93.4
            22q11.2 Q93.81

Deletion(s) — *continued*
    chromosome — *continued*
        specified NEC Q93.89
        long arm chromosome 18 or 21 Q93.89
            with complex rearrangements NEC Q93.7
        microdeletions NEC Q93.88
Delhi boil or button B55.1
Delinquency (juvenile) (neurotic) F91.8
    group Z72.810
Delinquent immunization status Z28.3
Delirium, delirious (acute or subacute) (not alcohol- or
    drug-induced) (with dementia) R41.0
    alcoholic (acute) (tremens) (withdrawal) F10.921
        with intoxication F10.921
        in
            abuse F10.121
            dependence F10.221
    due to (secondary to)
        alcohol
            intoxication F10.921
            in
                abuse F10.121
                dependence F10.221
            withdrawal F10.231
        amphetamine intoxication F15.921
            in
                abuse F15.121
                dependence F15.221
        anxiolytic
            intoxication F13.921
            in
                abuse F13.121
                dependence F13.221
            withdrawal F13.231
        cannabis intoxication (acute) F12.921
            in
                abuse F12.121
                dependence F12.221
        cocaine intoxication (acute) F14.921
            in
                abuse F14.121
                dependence F14.221
        general medical condition F05
        hallucinogen intoxication F16.921
            in
                abuse F16.121
                dependence F16.221
        hypnotic
            intoxication F13.921
            in
                abuse F13.121
                dependence F13.221
            withdrawal F13.231
        inhalant intoxication (acute) F18.921
            in
                abuse F18.121
                dependence F18.221
        multiple etiologies F05
        opioid intoxication (acute) F11.921
            in
                abuse F11.121
                dependence F11.221
        other (or unknown) substance F19.921
        phencyclidine intoxication (acute) F16.921
            in
                abuse F16.121
                dependence F16.221
        psychoactive substance NEC intoxication (acute)
            F19.921
            in
                abuse F19.121
                dependence F19.221
        sedative
            intoxication F13.921
            in
                abuse F13.121
                dependence F13.221
            withdrawal F13.231
        unknown etiology R41.0
    exhaustion F43.0
    hysterical F44.89
    postprocedural (postoperative) F05
    puerperal F05
    thyroid — *see* Thyrotoxicosis with thyroid storm
    traumatic — *see* Injury, intracranial
    tremens (alcohol-induced) F10.231
        sedative-induced F13.231
Delivery (childbirth) (labor)
    arrested active phase O62.1
    cesarean (for)
        abnormal

Delivery — *continued*
    cesarean — *continued*
        pelvis (bony) (deformity) (major) NEC with
            disproportion (fetopelvic) O33.0
            with obstructed labor O65.0
        presentation or position O32.9 ☑
    abruptio placentae (*see also* Abruptio placentae)
        O45.9 ☑
    acromion presentation O32.2 ☑
    atony, uterus O62.2
    breech presentation O32.1 ☑
        incomplete O32.8 ☑
    brow presentation O32.3 ☑
    cephalopelvic disproportion O33.9
    cerclage O34.3 ☑
    chin presentation O32.3 ☑
    cicatrix of cervix O34.4 ☑
    contracted pelvis (general)
        inlet O33.2
        outlet O33.3 ☑
    cord presentation or prolapse O69.0 ☑
    cystocele O34.8 ☑
    deformity (acquired) (congenital)
        pelvic organs or tissues NEC O34.8 ☑
        pelvis (bony) NEC O33.0
    disproportion NOS O33.9
    eclampsia — *see* Eclampsia
    face presentation O32.3 ☑
    failed
        forceps O66.5
        induction of labor O61.9
            instrumental O61.1
            mechanical O61.1
            medical O61.0
            specified NEC O61.8
            surgical O61.1
        trial of labor NOS O66.40
            following previous cesarean delivery O66.41
        vacuum extraction O66.5
        ventouse O66.5
    fetal-maternal hemorrhage O43.01 ☑
    hemorrhage (intrapartum) O67.9
        with coagulation defect O67.0
        specified cause NEC O67.8
    high head at term O32.4 ☑
    hydrocephalic fetus O33.6 ☑
    incarceration of uterus O34.51 ☑
    incoordinate uterine action O62.4
    increased size, fetus O33.5 ☑
    inertia, uterus O62.2
        primary O62.0
        secondary O62.1
    lateroversion, uterus O34.59 ☑
    mal lie O32.9 ☑
    malposition
        fetus O32.9 ☑
        pelvic organs or tissues NEC O34.8 ☑
        uterus NEC O34.59 ☑
    malpresentation NOS O32.9 ☑
    oblique presentation O32.2 ☑
    occurring after 37 completed weeks of gestation
        but before 39 completed weeks gestation
        due to (spontaneous) onset of labor O75.82
    oversize fetus O33.5 ☑
    pelvic tumor NEC O34.8 ☑
    placenta previa O44.0 ☑
        complete O44.0 ☑
            with hemorrhage O44.1 ☑
    placental insufficiency O36.51 ☑
    planned, occurring after 37 completed weeks of
        gestation but before 39 completed weeks
        gestation due to (spontaneous) onset of
        labor O75.82
    polyp, cervix O34.4 ☑
        causing obstructed labor O65.5
    poor dilatation, cervix O62.0
    pre-eclampsia O14.94
        mild O14.04
        moderate O14.04
        severe O14.14
            with hemolysis, elevated liver enzymes and
                low platelet count (HELLP) O14.24
    previous
        cesarean delivery O34.219
            classical (vertical) scar O34.212
            low transverse scar O34.211
        surgery (to)
            cervix O34.4 ☑
            gynecological NEC O34.8 ☑
            rectum O34.7 ☑
            uterus O34.29
            vagina O34.6 ☑

Delivery

Delivery — *continued*
 cesarean — *continued*
  prolapse
   arm or hand O32.2 ☑
   uterus O34.52 ☑
  prolonged labor NOS O63.9
  rectocele O34.8 ☑
  retroversion
   uterus O34.53 ☑
  rigid
   cervix O34.4 ☑
   pelvic floor O34.8 ☑
   perineum O34.7 ☑
   vagina O34.6 ☑
   vulva O34.7 ☑
  sacculation, pregnant uterus O34.59 ☑
  scar(s)
   cervix O34.4 ☑
   cesarean delivery O34.219
    classical (vertical) O34.212
    low transverse O34.211
    transmural uterine O34.29
    uterus O34.29
  Shirodkar suture in situ O34.3 ☑
  shoulder presentation O32.2 ☑
  stenosis or stricture, cervix O34.4 ☑
  streptococcus group B (GBS) carrier state O99.824
  transmural uterine scar O34.29
  transverse presentation or lie O32.2 ☑
  tumor, pelvic organs or tissues NEC O34.8 ☑
   cervix O34.4 ☑
  umbilical cord presentation or prolapse O69.0 ☑
  without indication O82
 completely normal case O80
 complicated O75.9
  by
   abnormal, abnormality (of)
    forces of labor O62.9
     specified type NEC O62.8
    glucose O99.814
    uterine contractions NOS O62.9
   abruptio placentae (*see also* Abruptio
    placentae) O45.9 ☑
   abuse
    physical O9A.32
    psychological O9A.52
    sexual O9A.42
   adherent placenta O72.0
    without hemorrhage O73.0
   alcohol use O99.314
   anemia (pre-existing) O99.02
   anesthetic death O74.8
   annular detachment of cervix O71.3
   atony, uterus O62.2
   attempted vacuum extraction and forceps
    O66.5
   Bandl's ring O62.4
   bariatric surgery status O99.844
   biliary tract disorder O26.62
   bleeding — *see* Delivery, complicated by,
    hemorrhage
   blood disorder NEC O99.12
   cervical dystocia (hypotonic) O62.2
    primary O62.0
    secondary O62.1
   circulatory system disorder O99.42
   compression of cord (umbilical) NEC O69.2 ☑
   condition NEC O99.89
   contraction, contracted ring O62.4
   cord (umbilical)
    around neck
     with compression O69.1 ☑
     without compression O69.81 ☑
    bruising O69.5 ☑
    complication O69.9 ☑
     specified NEC O69.89 ☑
    compression NEC O69.2 ☑
    entanglement O69.2 ☑
     without compression O69.82 ☑
    hematoma O69.5 ☑
    presentation O69.0 ☑
    prolapse O69.0 ☑
    short O69.3 ☑
    thrombosis (vessels) O69.5 ☑
    vascular lesion O69.5 ☑
   Couvelaire uterus O45.8X ☑
   damage to (injury to) NEC
    perineum O71.82
    periurethral tissue O71.82
    vulva O71.82
   delay following rupture of membranes
    (spontaneous) — *see* Pregnancy,

Delivery — *continued*
 complicated — *continued*
   complicated by, premature rupture of
    membranes
   depressed fetal heart tones O76
   diabetes O24.92
    gestational O24.429
     diet controlled O24.420
     insulin controlled O24.424
     oral drug controlled (antidiabetic)
      (hypoglycemic) O24.425
    pre-existing O24.32
     specified NEC O24.82
     type 1 O24.02
     type 2 O24.12
   diastasis recti (abdominis) O71.89
   dilatation
    bladder O66.8
    cervix incomplete, poor or slow O62.0
   disease NEC O99.89
   disruptio uteri — *see* Delivery, complicated by,
    rupture, uterus
   drug use O99.324
   dysfunction, uterus NOS O62.9
    hypertonic O62.4
    hypotonic O62.2
     primary O62.0
     secondary O62.1
    incoordinate O62.4
   eclampsia O15.1
   embolism (pulmonary) — *see* Embolism,
    obstetric
   endocrine, nutritional or metabolic disease NEC
    O99.284
   failed
    attempted vaginal birth after previous
     cesarean delivery O66.41
    induction of labor O61.9
     instrumental O61.1
     mechanical O61.1
     medical O61.0
     specified NEC O61.8
     surgical O61.1
    trial of labor O66.40
   female genital mutilation O65.5
   fetal
    abnormal acid-base balance O68
    acidemia O68
    acidosis O68
    alkalosis O68
    death, early O02.1
    deformity O66.3
    heart rate or rhythm (abnormal) (non-
     reassuring) O76
    hypoxia O77.8
    stress O77.9
     due to drug administration O77.1
     electrocardiographic evidence of O77.8
     specified NEC O77.8
     ultrasound evidence of O77.8
   fever during labor O75.2
   gastric banding status O99.844
   gastric bypass status O99.844
   gastrointestinal disease NEC O99.62
   gestational
    diabetes O24.429
     diet controlled O24.420
     insulin (and diet) controlled O24.424
     oral drug controlled (antidiabetic)
      (hypoglycemic) O24.425
    edema O12.04
     with proteinuria O12.24
    proteinuria O12.14
   gonorrhea O98.22
   hematoma O71.7
    ischial spine O71.7
    pelvic O71.7
    vagina O71.7
    vulva or perineum O71.7
   hemorrhage (uterine) O67.9
    associated with
     afibrinogenemia O67.0
     coagulation defect O67.0
     hyperfibrinolysis O67.0
     hypofibrinogenemia O67.0
    due to
     low implantation of placenta O44.5 ☑
     low lying placenta O44.5 ☑
     placenta previa O44.1 ☑
      marginal O44.3 ☑
      partial O44.3 ☑

Delivery — *continued*
 complicated — *continued*
   premature separation of placenta
    (normally implanted) (*see also* Abruptio
    placentae) O45.9 ☑
   retained placenta O72.0
    uterine leiomyoma O67.8
   placenta NEC O67.8
   postpartum NEC (atonic) (immediate) O72.1
    with retained or trapped placenta O72.0
    delayed O72.2
    secondary O72.2
    third stage O72.0
   hourglass contraction, uterus O62.4
   hypertension, hypertensive (pre-existing) — *see*
    Hypertension, complicated by, childbirth
    (labor)
   hypotension O26.5 ☑
   incomplete dilatation (cervix) O62.0
   incoordinate uterus contractions O62.4
   inertia, uterus O62.2
    during latent phase of labor O62.0
    primary O62.0
    secondary O62.1
   infection (maternal) O98.92
    carrier state NEC O99.834
    gonorrhea O98.22
    human immunodeficiency virus (HIV) O98.72
    sexually transmitted NEC O98.32
    specified NEC O98.82
    syphilis O98.12
    tuberculosis O98.02
    viral hepatitis O98.42
    viral NEC O98.52
   injury (to mother) (*see also* Delivery,
    complicated, by, damage to) O71.9
    nonobstetric O9A.22
     caused by abuse — *see* Delivery,
      complicated by, abuse
   intrauterine fetal death, early O02.1
   inversion, uterus O71.2
   laceration (perineal) O70.9
    anus (sphincter) O70.4
     with third degree laceration (*see also*
      Delivery, complicated, by, laceration,
      perineum, third degree) O70.20
      with mucosa O70.3
     without third degree laceration O70.4
    bladder (urinary) O71.5
    bowel O71.5
    cervix (uteri) O71.3
    fourchette O70.0
    hymen O70.0
    labia O70.0
    pelvic
     floor O70.1
     organ NEC O71.5
    perineum, perineal O70.9
     first degree O70.0
     fourth degree O70.3
     muscles O70.1
     second degree O70.1
     skin O70.0
     slight O70.0
     third degree O70.20
      with
       both external anal sphincter (EAS) and
        internal anal sphincter (IAS) torn
        (IIIc) O70.23
       less than 50% of external anal
        sphincter (EAS) thickness torn (IIIa)
        O70.21
       more than 50% external anal sphincter
        (EAS) thickness torn (IIIb) O70.22
      IIIa O70.21
      IIIb O70.22
      IIIc O70.23
    peritoneum (pelvic) O71.5
    rectovaginal (septum) (without perineal
     laceration) O71.4
     with perineum (*see also* Delivery,
      complicated, by, laceration, perineum,
      third degree) O70.20
      with anal or rectal mucosa O70.3
    specified NEC O71.89
    sphincter ani — *see* Delivery, complicated, by,
     laceration, anus (sphincter)
    urethra O71.5
    uterus O71.81
     before labor O71.81
    vagina, vaginal (deep) (high) (without
     perineal laceration) O71.4

☑ **Additional character required**

Delivery — *continued*
  complicated — *continued*
    with perineum O70.0
      muscles, with perineum O70.1
    vulva O70.0
  liver disorder O26.62
  malignancy O9A.12
  malnutrition O25.2
  malposition, malpresentation
    placenta O44.0 ☑
      with hemorrhage O44.1 ☑
    uterus or cervix O65.5
    without obstruction (*see also* Delivery,
        complicated by, obstruction) O32.9 ☑
      breech O32.1 ☑
      compound O32.6 ☑
      face (brow) (chin) O32.3 ☑
      footling O32.8 ☑
      high head O32.4 ☑
      oblique O32.2 ☑
      specified NEC O32.8 ☑
      transverse O32.2 ☑
      unstable lie O32.0 ☑
  meconium in amniotic fluid O77.0
  mental disorder NEC O99.344
  metrorrhexis — *see* Delivery, complicated by,
      rupture, uterus
  nervous system disorder O99.354
  obesity (pre-existing) O99.214
  obesity surgery status O99.844
  obstetric trauma O71.9
    specified NEC O71.89
  obstructed labor
    due to
      breech (complete) (frank) presentation
          O64.1 ☑
        incomplete O64.8 ☑
      brow presentation O64.3 ☑
      buttock presentation O64.1 ☑
      chin presentation O64.2 ☑
      compound presentation O64.5 ☑
      contracted pelvis O65.1
      deep transverse arrest O64.0 ☑
      deformed pelvis O65.0
      dystocia (fetal) O66.9
        due to
          conjoined twins O66.3
          fetal
            abnormality NEC O66.3
            ascites O66.3
            hydrops O66.3
            meningomyelocele O66.3
            sacral teratoma O66.3
            tumor O66.3
          hydrocephalic fetus O66.3
        shoulder O66.0
      face presentation O64.2 ☑
      fetopelvic disproportion O65.4
      footling presentation O64.8 ☑
      impacted shoulders O66.0
      incomplete rotation of fetal head O64.0 ☑
      large fetus O66.2
      locked twins O66.1
      malposition O64.9 ☑
        specified NEC O64.8 ☑
      malpresentation O64.9 ☑
        specified NEC O64.8 ☑
      multiple fetuses NEC O66.6
      pelvic
        abnormality (maternal) O65.9
          organ O65.5
          specified NEC O65.8
        contraction
          inlet O65.2
          mid-cavity O65.3
          outlet O65.3
        persistent (position)
          occipitoiliac O64.0 ☑
          occipitoposterior O64.0 ☑
          occipitosacral O64.0 ☑
          occipitotransverse O64.0 ☑
        prolapsed arm O64.4 ☑
        shoulder presentation O64.4 ☑
      specified NEC O66.8
  pathological retraction ring, uterus O62.4
  penetration, pregnant uterus by instrument
      O71.1
  perforation — *see* Delivery, complicated by,
      laceration
  placenta, placental
    ablatio (*see also* Abruptio placentae) O45.9 ☑
    abnormality O43.9 ☑

Delivery — *continued*
  complicated — *continued*
    specified NEC O43.89 ☑
    abruptio (*see also* Abruptio placentae)
        O45.9 ☑
    accreta O43.21 ☑
    adherent (with hemorrhage) O72.0
      without hemorrhage O73.0
    detachment (premature) (*see also* Abruptio
        placentae) O45.9 ☑
    disorder O43.9 ☑
      specified NEC O43.89 ☑
    hemorrhage NEC O67.8
    increta O43.22 ☑
    low (implantation) (lying) O44.4 ☑
      with hemorrhage O44.5 ☑
    malformation O43.10 ☑
    malposition O44.0 ☑
      without hemorrhage O44.1 ☑
    percreta O43.23 ☑
    previa (central) (complete) (lateral) (total)
        O44.0 ☑
      with hemorrhage O44.1 ☑
      marginal O44.2 ☑
        with hemorrhage O44.3 ☑
      partial O44.2 ☑
        with hemorrhage O44.3 ☑
    retained (with hemorrhage) O72.0
      without hemorrhage O73.0
    separation (premature) O45.9 ☑
      specified NEC O45.8X ☑
    vicious insertion O44.1 ☑
  precipitate labor O62.3
  premature rupture, membranes (*see also*
      Pregnancy, complicated by, premature
      rupture of membranes) O42.90
  prolapse
    arm or hand O32.2 ☑
    cord (umbilical) O69.0 ☑
    foot or leg O32.8 ☑
    uterus O34.52 ☑
  prolonged labor O63.9
    first stage O63.0
    second stage O63.1
  protozoal disease (maternal) O98.62
  respiratory disease NEC O99.52
  retained membranes or portions of placenta
      O72.2
    without hemorrhage O73.1
  retarded birth O63.9
  retention of secundines (with hemorrhage)
      O72.0
    without hemorrhage O73.0
    partial O72.2
      without hemorrhage O73.1
  rupture
    bladder (urinary) O71.5
    cervix O71.3
    pelvic organ NEC O71.5
    urethra O71.5
    uterus (during or after labor) O71.1
      before labor O71.0 ☑
  separation, pubic bone (symphysis pubis)
      O71.6
  shock O75.1
  shoulder presentation O64.4 ☑
  skin disorder NEC O99.72
  spasm, cervix O62.4
  stenosis or stricture, cervix O65.5
  streptococcus group B (GBS) carrier state
      O99.824
  subluxation of symphysis (pubis) O26.72
  syphilis (maternal) O98.12
  tear — *see* Delivery, complicated by, laceration
  tetanic uterus O62.4
  trauma (obstetrical) (*see also* Delivery,
      complicated, by, damage to) O71.9
    non-obstetric O9A.22
    periurethral O71.82
    specified NEC O71.89
  tuberculosis (maternal) O98.02
  tumor, pelvic organs or tissues NEC O65.5
  umbilical cord around neck
    with compression O69.1 ☑
    without compression O69.81 ☑
  uterine inertia O62.2
    during latent phase of labor O62.0
    primary O62.0
    secondary O62.1
  vasa previa O69.4 ☑
  velamentous insertion of cord O43.12 ☑
specified complication NEC O75.89

Delivery — *continued*
  delayed NOS O63.9
    following rupture of membranes
      artificial O75.5
    second twin, triplet, etc., O63.2
  forceps, low following failed vacuum extraction
      O66.5
  missed (at or near term) O36.4 ☑
  normal O80
  obstructed — *see* Delivery, complicated by,
      obstructed labor
  precipitate O62.3
  preterm (*see also* Pregnancy, complicated by,
      preterm labor) O60.10 ☑
  spontaneous O80
  term pregnancy NOS O80
  uncomplicated O80
  vaginal, following previous cesarean delivery O34.219
    classical (vertical) scar O34.212
    low transverse scar O34.211
Delusions (paranoid) — *see* Disorder, delusional
Dementia (degenerative (primary)) (old age)
    (persisting) F03.90
  with
    aggressive behavior F03.91
    behavioral disturbance F03.91
    combative behavior F03.91
    Lewy bodies G31.83 *[F02.80]*
      with behavioral disturbance G31.83 *[F02.81]*
    Parkinsonism G31.83 *[F02.80]*
      with behavioral disturbance G31.83 *[F02.81]*
    Parkinson's disease G20 *[F02.80]*
      with behavioral disturbance G20 *[F02.81]*
    violent behavior F03.91
  alcoholic F10.97
    with dependence F10.27
  Alzheimer's type — *see* Disease, Alzheimer's
  arteriosclerotic — *see* Dementia, vascular
  atypical, Alzheimer's type — *see* Disease,
      Alzheimer's, specified NEC
  congenital — *see* Disability, intellectual
  frontal (lobe) G31.09 *[F02.80]*
    with behavioral disturbance G31.09 *[F02.81]*
  frontotemporal G31.09 *[F02.80]*
    with behavioral disturbance G31.09 *[F02.81]*
    specified NEC G31.09 *[F02.80]*
      with behavioral disturbance G31.09 *[F02.81]*
  in (due to)
    alcohol F10.97
      with dependence F10.27
    Alzheimer's disease — *see* Disease, Alzheimer's
    arteriosclerotic brain disease — *see* Dementia,
        vascular
    cerebral lipidoses E75. ☑ *[F02.80]*
      with behavioral disturbance E75. ☑ *[F02.81]*
    Creutzfeldt-Jakob disease (*see also* Creutzfeldt-
        Jakob disease or syndrome (with dementia))
        A81.00
    epilepsy G40. ☑ *[F02.80]*
      with behavioral disturbance G40. ☑ *[F02.81]*
    hepatolenticular degeneration E83.01 *[F02.80]*
      with behavioral disturbance E83.01 *[F02.81]*
    human immunodeficiency virus (HIV) disease B20
        [F02.80]
      with behavioral disturbance B20 *[F02.81]*
    Huntington's disease or chorea G10 *[F02.80]*
      with behavioral disturbance G10 *[F02.81]*
    hypercalcemia E83.52 *[F02.80]*
      with behavioral disturbance E83.52 *[F02.81]*
    hypothyroidism, acquired E03.9 *[F02.80]*
      with behavioral disturbance E03.9 *[F02.81]*
      due to iodine deficiency E01.8 *[F02.80]*
        with behavioral disturbance E01.8 *[F02.81]*
    inhalants F18.97
      with dependence F18.27
    multiple
      etiologies F03 ☑
      sclerosis G35 *[F02.80]*
        with behavioral disturbance G35 *[F02.81]*
    neurosyphilis A52.17 *[F02.80]*
      with behavioral disturbance A52.17 *[F02.81]*
      juvenile A50.49 *[F02.80]*
        with behavioral disturbance A50.49 *[F02.81]*
    niacin deficiency E52 *[F02.80]*
      with behavioral disturbance E52 *[F02.81]*
    paralysis agitans G20 *[F02.80]*
      with behavioral disturbance G20 *[F02.81]*
    Parkinson's disease G20 *[F02.80]*
    pellagra E52 *[F02.80]*
      with behavioral disturbance E52 *[F02.81]*
    Pick's G31.01 *[F02.80]*
      with behavioral disturbance G31.01 *[F02.81]*

Dementia - Dependence

Dementia — *continued*
  in — *continued*
    polyarteritis nodosa M30.0 *[F02.80]*
      with behavioral disturbance M30.0 *[F02.81]*
    psychoactive drug F19.97
      with dependence F19.27
      inhalants F18.97
        with dependence F18.27
      sedatives, hypnotics or anxiolytics F13.97
        with dependence F13.27
    sedatives, hypnotics or anxiolytics F13.97
      with dependence F13.27
    systemic lupus erythematosus M32. ☑ *[F02.80]*
      with behavioral disturbance M32. ☑ *[F02.81]*
    trypanosomiasis
      African B56.9 *[F02.80]*
        with behavioral disturbance B56.9 *[F02.81]*
    unknown etiology F03 ☑
    vitamin B12 deficiency E53.8 *[F02.80]*
      with behavioral disturbance E53.8 *[F02.81]*
    volatile solvents F18.97
      with dependence F18.27
    with behavioral disturbance G31.83 *[F02.81]*
  infantile, infantilis F84.3
  Lewy body G31.83 *[F02.80]*
    with behavioral disturbance G31.83 *[F02.81]*
  multi-infarct — *see* Dementia, vascular
  paralytica, paralytic (syphilitic) A52.17 *[F02.80]*
    with behavioral disturbance A52.17 *[F02.81]*
    juvenilis A50.45
  paretic A52.17
  praecox — *see* Schizophrenia
  presenile F03 ☑
    Alzheimer's type — *see* Disease, Alzheimer's, early onset
  primary degenerative F03 ☑
  progressive, syphilitic A52.17
  senile F03 ☑
    with acute confusional state F05
    Alzheimer's type — *see* Disease, Alzheimer's, late onset
    depressed or paranoid type F03 ☑
  vascular (acute onset) (mixed) (multi-infarct) (subcortical) F01.50
    with behavioral disturbance F01.51
Demineralization, bone — *see* Osteoporosis
Demodex folliculorum (infestation) B88.0
Demophobia F40.248
Demoralization R45.3
Demyelination, demyelinization
  central nervous system G37.9
    specified NEC G37.8
  corpus callosum (central) G37.1
  disseminated, acute G36.9
    specified NEC G36.8
  global G35
  in optic neuritis G36.0
Dengue (classical) (fever) A90
  hemorrhagic A91
  sandfly A93.1
Dennie-Marfan syphilitic syndrome A50.45
Dens evaginatus, in dente or invaginatus K00.2
Dense breasts R92.2
Density
  increased, bone (disseminated) (generalized) (spotted) — *see* Disorder, bone, density and structure, specified type NEC
  lung (nodular) J98.4
Dental (*see also* condition)
  examination Z01.20
    with abnormal findings Z01.21
  restoration
    aesthetically inadequate or displeasing K08.56
    defective K08.50
      specified NEC K08.59
    failure of marginal integrity K08.51
    failure of periodontal anatomical integrity K08.54
Dentia praecox K00.6
Denticles (pulp) K04.2
Dentigerous cyst K09.0
Dentin
  irregular (in pulp) K04.3
  opalescent K00.5
  secondary (in pulp) K04.3
  sensitive K03.89
Dentinogenesis imperfecta K00.5
Dentinoma — *see* Cyst, calcifying odontogenic
Dentition (syndrome) K00.7
  delayed K00.6
  difficult K00.7
  precocious K00.6

Dentition — *continued*
  premature K00.6
  retarded K00.6
Dependence (on) (syndrome) F19.20
  with remission F19.21
  alcohol (ethyl) (methyl) (without remission) F10.20
    with
      amnestic disorder, persisting F10.26
      anxiety disorder F10.280
      dementia, persisting F10.27
      intoxication F10.229
        with delirium F10.221
        uncomplicated F10.220
      mood disorder F10.24
      psychotic disorder F10.259
        with
          delusions F10.250
          hallucinations F10.251
      remission F10.21
      sexual dysfunction F10.281
      sleep disorder F10.282
      specified disorder NEC F10.288
      withdrawal F10.239
        with
          delirium F10.231
          perceptual disturbance F10.232
        uncomplicated F10.230
    counseling and surveillance Z71.41
  amobarbital — *see* Dependence, drug, sedative
  amphetamine(s) (type) — *see* Dependence, drug, stimulant NEC
  amytal (sodium) — *see* Dependence, drug, sedative
  analgesic NEC F55.8
  anesthetic (agent) (gas) (general) (local) NEC — *see* Dependence, drug, psychoactive NEC
  anxiolytic NEC — *see* Dependence, drug, sedative
  barbital(s) — *see* Dependence, drug, sedative
  barbiturate(s) (compounds) (drugs classifiable to T42 ☑) — *see* Dependence, drug, sedative
  benzedrine — *see* Dependence, drug, stimulant NEC
  bhang — *see* Dependence, drug, cannabis
  bromide(s) NEC — *see* Dependence, drug, sedative
  caffeine — *see* Dependence, drug, stimulant NEC
  cannabis (sativa) (indica) (resin) (derivatives) (type) — *see* Dependence, drug, cannabis
  chloral (betaine) (hydrate) — *see* Dependence, drug, sedative
  chlordiazepoxide — *see* Dependence, drug, sedative
  coca (leaf) (derivatives) — *see* Dependence, drug, cocaine
  cocaine — *see* Dependence, drug, cocaine
  codeine — *see* Dependence, drug, opioid
  combinations of drugs F19.20
  dagga — *see* Dependence, drug, cannabis
  demerol — *see* Dependence, drug, opioid
  dexamphetamine — *see* Dependence, drug, stimulant NEC
  dexedrine — *see* Dependence, drug, stimulant NEC
  dextromethorphan — *see* Dependence, drug, opioid
  dextromoramide — *see* Dependence, drug, opioid
  dextro-nor-pseudo-ephedrine — *see* Dependence, drug, stimulant NEC
  dextrorphan — *see* Dependence, drug, opioid
  diazepam — *see* Dependence, drug, sedative
  dilaudid — *see* Dependence, drug, opioid
  D-lysergic acid diethylamide — *see* Dependence, drug, hallucinogen
  drug NEC F19.20
    with sleep disorder F19.282
    cannabis F12.20
      with
        anxiety disorder F12.280
        intoxication F12.229
          with
            delirium F12.221
            perceptual disturbance F12.222
          uncomplicated F12.220
        other specified disorder F12.288
        psychosis F12.259
          delusions F12.250
          hallucinations F12.251
        unspecified disorder F12.29
        withdrawal F12.23
      in remission F12.21
    cocaine F14.20
      with
        anxiety disorder F14.280
        intoxication F14.229
          with

Dependence — *continued*
  drug NEC — *continued*
        delirium F14.221
        perceptual disturbance F14.222
        uncomplicated F14.220
      mood disorder F14.24
      other specified disorder F14.288
      psychosis F14.259
        delusions F14.250
        hallucinations F14.251
      sexual dysfunction F14.281
      sleep disorder F14.282
      unspecified disorder F14.29
      withdrawal F14.23
    in remission F14.21
    withdrawal symptoms in newborn P96.1
  counseling and surveillance Z71.51
  hallucinogen F16.20
    with
      anxiety disorder F16.280
      flashbacks F16.283
      intoxication F16.229
        with delirium F16.221
        uncomplicated F16.220
      mood disorder F16.24
      other specified disorder F16.288
      perception disorder, persisting F16.283
      psychosis F16.259
        delusions F16.250
        hallucinations F16.251
      unspecified disorder F16.29
    in remission F16.21
  in remission F19.21
  inhalant F18.20
    with
      anxiety disorder F18.280
      dementia, persisting F18.27
      intoxication F18.229
        with delirium F18.221
        uncomplicated F18.220
      mood disorder F18.24
      other specified disorder F18.288
      psychosis F18.259
        delusions F18.250
        hallucinations F18.251
      unspecified disorder F18.29
    in remission F18.21
  nicotine F17.200
    with disorder F17.209
    in remission F17.201
    specified disorder NEC F17.208
    withdrawal F17.203
    chewing tobacco F17.220
      with disorder F17.229
      in remission F17.221
      specified disorder NEC F17.228
      withdrawal F17.223
    cigarettes F17.210
      with disorder F17.219
      in remission F17.211
      specified disorder NEC F17.218
      withdrawal F17.213
    specified product NEC F17.290
      with disorder F17.299
      remission F17.291
      specified disorder NEC F17.298
      withdrawal F17.293
  opioid F11.20
    with
      intoxication F11.229
        with
          delirium F11.221
          perceptual disturbance F11.222
        uncomplicated F11.220
      mood disorder F11.24
      other specified disorder F11.288
      psychosis F11.259
        delusions F11.250
        hallucinations F11.251
      sexual dysfunction F11.281
      sleep disorder F11.282
      unspecified disorder F11.29
      withdrawal F11.23
    in remission F11.21
  psychoactive NEC F19.20
    with
      amnestic disorder F19.26
      anxiety disorder F19.280
      dementia F19.27
      intoxication F19.229
        with
          delirium F19.221

☑ **Additional character required**

Dependence — *continued*
  drug NEC — *continued*
        perceptual disturbance F19.222
        uncomplicated F19.220
      mood disorder F19.24
      other specified disorder F19.288
      psychosis F19.259
        delusions F19.250
        hallucinations F19.251
      sexual dysfunction F19.281
      sleep disorder F19.282
      unspecified disorder F19.29
      withdrawal F19.239
        with
          delirium F19.231
          perceptual disturbance F19.232
        uncomplicated F19.230
    sedative, hypnotic or anxiolytic F13.20
      with
        amnestic disorder F13.26
        anxiety disorder F13.280
        dementia, persisting F13.27
        intoxication F13.229
          with delirium F13.221
          uncomplicated F13.220
        mood disorder F13.24
        other specified disorder F13.288
        psychosis F13.259
          delusions F13.250
          hallucinations F13.251
        sexual dysfunction F13.281
        sleep disorder F13.282
        unspecified disorder F13.29
        withdrawal F13.239
          with
            delirium F13.231
            perceptual disturbance F13.232
          uncomplicated F13.230
      in remission F13.21
    stimulant NEC F15.20
      with
        anxiety disorder F15.280
        intoxication F15.229
          with
            delirium F15.221
            perceptual disturbance F15.222
          uncomplicated F15.220
        mood disorder F15.24
        other specified disorder F15.288
        psychosis F15.259
          delusions F15.250
          hallucinations F15.251
        sexual dysfunction F15.281
        sleep disorder F15.282
        unspecified disorder F15.29
        withdrawal F15.23
      in remission F15.21
  ethyl
    alcohol (without remission) F10.20
      with remission F10.21
    bromide — *see* Dependence, drug, sedative
    carbamate F19.20
    chloride F19.20
    morphine — *see* Dependence, drug, opioid
  ganja — *see* Dependence, drug, cannabis
  glue (airplane) (sniffing) — *see* Dependence, drug, inhalant
  glutethimide — *see* Dependence, drug, sedative
  hallucinogenics — *see* Dependence, drug, hallucinogen
  hashish — *see* Dependence, drug, cannabis
  hemp — *see* Dependence, drug, cannabis
  heroin (salt) (any) — *see* Dependence, drug, opioid
  hypnotic NEC — *see* Dependence, drug, sedative
  Indian hemp — *see* Dependence, drug, cannabis
  inhalants — *see* Dependence, drug, inhalant
  khat — *see* Dependence, drug, stimulant NEC
  laudanum — *see* Dependence, drug, opioid
  LSD (-25) (derivatives) — *see* Dependence, drug, hallucinogen
  luminal — *see* Dependence, drug, sedative
  lysergic acid — *see* Dependence, drug, hallucinogen
  maconha — *see* Dependence, drug, cannabis
  marihuana — *see* Dependence, drug, cannabis
  meprobamate — *see* Dependence, drug, sedative
  mescaline — *see* Dependence, drug, hallucinogen
  methadone — *see* Dependence, drug, opioid
  methamphetamine(s) — *see* Dependence, drug, stimulant NEC
  methaqualone — *see* Dependence, drug, sedative

Dependence — *continued*
  methyl
    alcohol (without remission) F10.20
      with remission F10.21
    bromide — *see* Dependence, drug, sedative
    morphine — *see* Dependence, drug, opioid
    phenidate — *see* Dependence, drug, stimulant NEC
    sulfonal — *see* Dependence, drug, sedative
  morphine (sulfate) (sulfite) (type) — *see* Dependence, drug, opioid
  narcotic (drug) NEC — *see* Dependence, drug, opioid
  nembutal — *see* Dependence, drug, sedative
  neraval — *see* Dependence, drug, sedative
  neravan — *see* Dependence, drug, sedative
  neurobarb — *see* Dependence, drug, sedative
  nicotine — *see* Dependence, drug, nicotine
  nitrous oxide F19.20
  nonbarbiturate sedatives and tranquilizers with similar effect — *see* Dependence, drug, sedative
  on
    artificial heart (fully implantable) (mechanical) Z95.812
    aspirator Z99.0
    care provider (because of) Z74.9
      impaired mobility Z74.09
      need for
        assistance with personal care Z74.1
        continuous supervision Z74.3
      no other household member able to render care Z74.2
      specified reason NEC Z74.8
    machine Z99.89
      enabling NEC Z99.89
      specified type NEC Z99.89
    renal dialysis (hemodialysis) (peritoneal) Z99.2
    respirator Z99.11
    ventilator Z99.11
    wheelchair Z99.3
  opiate — *see* Dependence, drug, opioid
  opioids — *see* Dependence, drug, opioid
  opium (alkaloids) (derivatives) (tincture) — *see* Dependence, drug, opioid
  oxygen (long-term) (supplemental) Z99.81
  paraldehyde — *see* Dependence, drug, sedative
  paregoric — *see* Dependence, drug, opioid
  PCP (phencyclidine) (or related substance) — *see* Dependence, drug, hallucinogen
  pentobarbital — *see* Dependence, drug, sedative
  pentobarbitone (sodium) — *see* Dependence, drug, sedative
  pentothal — *see* Dependence, drug, sedative
  peyote — *see* Dependence, drug, hallucinogen
  phencyclidine (PCP) (or related substance) — *see* Dependence, drug, hallucinogen
  phenmetrazine — *see* Dependence, drug, stimulant NEC
  phenobarbital — *see* Dependence, drug, sedative
  polysubstance F19.20
  psilocibin, psilocin, psilocyn, psilocyline — *see* Dependence, drug, hallucinogen
  psychostimulant NEC — *see* Dependence, drug, stimulant NEC
  secobarbital — *see* Dependence, drug, sedative
  seconal — *see* Dependence, drug, sedative
  sedative NEC — *see* Dependence, drug, sedative
  specified drug NEC — *see* Dependence, drug
  stimulant NEC — *see* Dependence, drug, stimulant NEC
  substance NEC — *see* Dependence, drug
  supplemental oxygen Z99.81
  tobacco — *see* Dependence, drug, nicotine
    counseling and surveillance Z71.6
  tranquilizer NEC — *see* Dependence, drug, sedative
  vitamin B6 E53.1
  volatile solvents — *see* Dependence, drug, inhalant
Dependency
  care-provider Z74.9
  passive F60.7
  reactions (persistent) F60.7
Depersonalization (in neurotic state) (neurotic) (syndrome) F48.1
Depletion
  extracellular fluid E86.9
  plasma E86.1
  potassium E87.6
    nephropathy N25.89
  salt or sodium E87.1
    causing heat exhaustion or prostration T67.4 ☑
    nephropathy N28.9
  volume NOS E86.9

Deployment (current) (military) status Z56.82
  in theater or in support of military war, peacekeeping and humanitarian operations Z56.82
  personal history of Z91.82
    military war, peacekeeping and humanitarian deployment (current or past conflict) Z91.82
  returned from Z91.82
Depolarization, premature I49.40
  atrial I49.1
  junctional I49.2
  specified NEC I49.49
  ventricular I49.3
Deposit
  bone in Boeck's sarcoid D86.89
  calcareous, calcium — *see* Calcification
  cholesterol
    retina H35.89
    vitreous (body) (humor) — *see* Deposit, crystalline
  conjunctiva H11.11 ☑
  cornea H18.00 ☑
    argentous H18.02 ☑
    due to metabolic disorder H18.03 ☑
    Kayser-Fleischer ring H18.04 ☑
    pigmentation — *see* Pigmentation, cornea
  crystalline, vitreous (body) (humor) H43.2 ☑
  hemosiderin in old scars of cornea — *see* Pigmentation, cornea, stromal
  metallic in lens — *see* Cataract, specified NEC
  skin R23.8
  tooth, teeth (betel) (black) (green) (materia alba) (orange) (tobacco) K03.6
  urate, kidney — *see* Calculus, kidney
Depraved appetite — *see* Pica
Depressed
  HDL cholesterol E78.6
Depression (acute) (mental) F32.9
  agitated (single episode) F32.2
  anaclitic — *see* Disorder, adjustment
  anxiety F41.8
    persistent F34.1
  arches (*see also* Deformity, limb, flat foot)
  atypical (single episode) F32.89
    recurrent episode F33.8
  basal metabolic rate R94.8
  bone marrow D75.89
  central nervous system R09.2
  cerebral R29.818
    newborn P91.4
  cerebrovascular I67.9
  chest wall M95.4
  climacteric (single episode) F32.89
    recurrent episode F33.8
  endogenous (without psychotic symptoms) F33.2
    with psychotic symptoms F33.3
  functional activity R68.89
  hysterical F44.89
  involutional (single episode) F32.89
    recurrent episode F33.8
  major F32.9
    with psychotic symptoms F32.3
    recurrent — *see* Disorder, depressive, recurrent
  manic-depressive — *see* Disorder, depressive, recurrent
  masked (single episode) F32.89
  medullary G93.89
  menopausal (single episode) F32.89
    recurrent episode F33.8
  metatarsus — *see* Depression, arches
  monopolar F33.9
  nervous F34.1
  neurotic F34.1
  nose M95.0
  postnatal (NOS) F53.0
  postpartum (NOS) F53.0
  post-psychotic of schizophrenia F32.89
  post-schizophrenic F32.89
  psychogenic (reactive) (single episode) F32.9
  psychoneurotic F34.1
  psychotic (single episode) F32.3
    recurrent F33.3
  reactive (psychogenic) (single episode) F32.9
    psychotic (single episode) F32.3
  recurrent — *see* Disorder, depressive, recurrent
  respiratory center G93.89
  seasonal — *see* Disorder, depressive, recurrent
  senile F03 ☑
  severe, single episode F32.2
  situational F43.21
  skull Q67.4
  specified NEC (single episode) F32.89
  sternum M95.4

Depression — *continued*
  visual field — *see* Defect, visual field
  vital (recurrent) (without psychotic symptoms)
    F33.2
    with psychotic symptoms F33.3
    single episode F32.2
Deprivation
  cultural Z60.3
  effects NOS T73.9 ☑
    specified NEC T73.8 ☑
  emotional NEC Z65.8
    affecting infant or child — *see* Maltreatment,
      child, psychological
  food T73.0 ☑
  protein — *see* Malnutrition
  sleep Z72.820
  social Z60.4
    affecting infant or child — *see* Maltreatment,
      child, psychological
  specified NEC T73.8 ☑
  vitamins — *see* Deficiency, vitamin
  water T73.1 ☑
Derangement
  ankle (internal) — *see* Derangement, joint, ankle
  cartilage (articular) NEC — *see* Derangement, joint,
    articular cartilage, by site
    recurrent — *see* Dislocation, recurrent
  cruciate ligament, anterior, current injury — *see*
    Sprain, knee, cruciate, anterior
  elbow (internal) — *see* Derangement, joint, elbow
  hip (joint) (internal) (old) — *see* Derangement,
    joint, hip
  joint (internal) M24.9
    ankylosis — *see* Ankylosis
    articular cartilage M24.10
      ankle M24.17 ☑
      elbow M24.12 ☑
      foot M24.17 ☑
      hand M24.14 ☑
      hip M24.15 ☑
      knee NEC M23.9 ☑
      loose body — *see* Loose, body
      shoulder M24.11 ☑
      wrist M24.13 ☑
    contracture — *see* Contraction, joint
    current injury (*see also* Dislocation)
      knee, meniscus or cartilage — *see* Tear,
        meniscus
    dislocation
      pathological — *see* Dislocation, pathological
      recurrent — *see* Dislocation, recurrent
    knee — *see* Derangement, knee
    ligament — *see* Disorder, ligament
    loose body — *see* Loose, body
    recurrent — *see* Dislocation, recurrent
    specified type NEC M24.80
      ankle M24.87 ☑
      elbow M24.82 ☑
      foot joint M24.87 ☑
      hand joint M24.84 ☑
      hip M24.85 ☑
      shoulder M24.81 ☑
      wrist M24.83 ☑
    temporomandibular M26.69
  knee (recurrent) M23.9 ☑
    ligament disruption, spontaneous M23.60 ☑
      anterior cruciate M23.61 ☑
      capsular M23.67 ☑
      instability, chronic M23.5 ☑
      lateral collateral M23.64 ☑
      medial collateral M23.63 ☑
      posterior cruciate M23.62 ☑
    loose body M23.4 ☑
    meniscus M23.30 ☑
      cystic M23.00 ☑
        lateral M23.002
          anterior horn M23.04 ☑
          posterior horn M23.05 ☑
          specified NEC M23.06 ☑
        medial M23.005
          anterior horn M23.01 ☑
          posterior horn M23.02 ☑
          specified NEC M23.03 ☑
      degenerate — *see* Derangement, knee,
        meniscus, specified NEC
      detached — *see* Derangement, knee, meniscus,
        specified NEC
      due to old tear or injury M23.20 ☑
        lateral M23.20 ☑
          anterior horn M23.24 ☑
          posterior horn M23.25 ☑
          specified NEC M23.26 ☑

Derangement — *continued*
  knee — *continued*
      medial M23.20 ☑
        anterior horn M23.21 ☑
        posterior horn M23.22 ☑
        specified NEC M23.23 ☑
      retained — *see* Derangement, knee, meniscus,
        specified NEC
      specified NEC M23.30 ☑
        lateral M23.30 ☑
          anterior horn M23.34 ☑
          posterior horn M23.35 ☑
          specified NEC M23.36 ☑
        medial M23.30 ☑
          anterior horn M23.31 ☑
          posterior horn M23.32 ☑
          specified NEC M23.33 ☑
      old M23.8X ☑
    specified NEC — *see* subcategory M23.8 ☑
    low back NEC — *see* Dorsopathy, specified NEC
    meniscus — *see* Derangement, knee, meniscus
    mental — *see* Psychosis
    patella, specified NEC — *see* Disorder, patella,
      derangement NEC
    semilunar cartilage (knee) — *see* Derangement,
      knee, meniscus, specified NEC
    shoulder (internal) — *see* Derangement, joint, shoulder
Dercum's disease E88.2
Derealization (neurotic) F48.1
Dermal — *see* condition
Dermaphytid — *see* Dermatophytosis
Dermatitis (eczematous) L30.9
  ab igne L59.0
  acarine B88.0
  actinic (due to sun) L57.8
    other than from sun L59.8
  allergic — *see* Dermatitis, contact, allergic
  ambustionis, due to burn or scald — *see* Burn
  amebic A06.7
  ammonia L22
  arsenical (ingested) L27.8
  artefacta L98.1
    psychogenic F54
  atopic L20.9
    psychogenic F54
    specified NEC L20.89
  autoimmune progesterone L30.8
  berlock, berloque L56.2
  blastomycotic B40.3
  blister beetle L24.89
  bullous, bullosa L13.9
    mucosynechial, atrophic L12.1
    seasonal L30.8
    specified NEC L13.8
  calorica L59.0
    due to burn or scald — *see* Burn
  caterpillar L24.89
  cercarial B65.3
  combustionis L59.0
    due to burn or scald — *see* Burn
  congelationis T69.1 ☑
  contact (occupational) L25.9
    allergic L23.9
      due to
        adhesives L23.1
        cement L23.5
        chemical products NEC L23.5
        chromium L23.0
        cosmetics L23.2
        dander (cat) (dog) L23.81
        drugs in contact with skin L23.3
        dyes L23.4
        food in contact with skin L23.6
        hair (cat) (dog) L23.81
        insecticide L23.5
        metals L23.0
        nickel L23.0
        plants, non-food L23.7
        plastic L23.5
        rubber L23.5
        specified agent NEC L23.89
    due to
      cement L25.3
      chemical products NEC L25.3
      cosmetics L25.0
      dander (cat) (dog) L23.81
      drugs in contact with skin L25.1
      dyes L25.2
      food in contact with skin L25.4
      hair (cat) (dog) L23.81
      plants, non-food L25.5
      specified agent NEC L25.8

Dermatitis — *continued*
  contact — *continued*
    irritant L24.9
      due to
        cement L24.5
        chemical products NEC L24.5
        cosmetics L24.3
        detergents L24.0
        drugs in contact with skin L24.4
        food in contact with skin L24.6
        oils and greases L24.1
        plants, non-food L24.7
        solvents L24.2
        specified agent NEC L24.89
  contusiformis L52
  diabetic — *see* E08-E13 with .620
  diaper L22
  diphtheritica A36.3
  dry skin L85.3
  due to
    acetone (contact) (irritant) L24.2
    acids (contact) (irritant) L24.5
    adhesive(s) (allergic) (contact) (plaster) L23.1
      irritant L24.5
    alcohol (irritant) (skin contact) (substances in
      category T51 ☑) L24.2
      taken internally L27.8
    alkalis (contact) (irritant) L24.5
    arsenic (ingested) L27.8
    carbon disulfide (contact) (irritant) L24.2
    caustics (contact) (irritant) L24.5
    cement (contact) L25.3
    cereal (ingested) L27.2
    chemical(s) NEC L25.3
      taken internally L27.8
    chlorocompounds L24.2
    chromium (contact) (irritant) L24.81
    coffee (ingested) L27.2
    cold weather L30.8
    cosmetics (contact) L25.0
      allergic L23.2
      irritant L24.3
    cyclohexanes L24.2
    dander (cat) (dog) L23.81
    Demodex species B88.0
    Dermanyssus gallinae B88.0
    detergents (contact) (irritant) L24.0
    dichromate L24.81
    drugs and medicaments (generalized) (internal
      use) L27.0
      external — *see* Dermatitis, due to, drugs, in
        contact with skin
      in contact with skin L25.1
        allergic L23.3
        irritant L24.4
      localized skin eruption L27.1
      specified substance — *see* Table of Drugs and
        Chemicals
    dyes (contact) L25.2
      allergic L23.4
      irritant L24.89
    epidermophytosis — *see* Dermatophytosis
    esters L24.2
    external irritant NEC L24.9
    fish (ingested) L27.2
    flour (ingested) L27.2
    food (ingested) L27.2
      in contact with skin L25.4
    fruit (ingested) L27.2
    furs (allergic) (contact) L23.81
    glues — *see* Dermatitis, due to, adhesives
    glycols L24.2
    greases NEC (contact) (irritant) L24.1
    hair (cat) (dog) L23.81
    hot
      objects and materials — *see* Burn
      weather or places L59.0
    hydrocarbons L24.2
    infrared rays L59.8
    ingestion, ingested substance L27.9
      chemical NEC L27.8
      drugs and medicaments — *see* Dermatitis, due
        to, drugs
      food L27.2
      specified NEC L27.8
    insecticide in contact with skin L24.5
    internal agent L27.9
      drugs and medicaments (generalized) — *see*
        Dermatitis, due to, drugs
      food L27.2
    irradiation — *see* Dermatitis, due to, radioactive
      substance

Dermatitis — *continued*
   due to — *continued*
      ketones L24.2
      lacquer tree (allergic) (contact) L23.7
      light (sun) NEC L57.8
         acute L56.8
         other L59.8
      Liponyssoides sanguineus B88.0
      low temperature L30.8
      meat (ingested) L27.2
      metals, metal salts (contact) (irritant) L24.81
      milk (ingested) L27.2
      nickel (contact) (irritant) L24.81
      nylon (contact) (irritant) L24.5
      oils NEC (contact) (irritant) L24.1
      paint solvent (contact) (irritant) L24.2
      petroleum products (contact) (irritant)
         (substances in T52.0 ☑) L24.2
      plants NEC (contact) L25.5
         allergic L23.7
         irritant L24.7
      plasters (adhesive) (any) (allergic) (contact) L23.1
         irritant L24.5
      plastic (contact) L25.3
      preservatives (contact) — *see* Dermatitis, due to,
         chemical, in contact with skin
      primrose (allergic) (contact) L23.7
      primula (allergic) (contact) L23.7
      radiation L59.8
         nonionizing (chronic exposure) L57.8
         sun NEC L57.8
            acute L56.8
      radioactive substance L58.9
         acute L58.0
         chronic L58.1
      radium L58.9
         acute L58.0
         chronic L58.1
      ragweed (allergic) (contact) L23.7
      Rhus (allergic) (contact) (diversiloba) (radicans)
         (toxicodendron) (venenata) (verniciflua) L23.7
      rubber (contact) L24.5
      Senecio jacobaea (allergic) (contact) L23.7
      solvents (contact) (irritant) (substances in
         categories T52 ☑) L24.2
      specified agent NEC (contact) L25.8
         allergic L23.89
         irritant L24.89
      sunshine NEC L57.8
         acute L56.8
      tetrachlorethylene (contact) (irritant) L24.2
      toluene (contact) (irritant) L24.2
      turpentine (contact) L24.2
      ultraviolet rays (sun NEC) (chronic exposure)
         L57.8
         acute L56.8
      vaccine or vaccination L27.0
         specified substance — *see* Table of Drugs and
            Chemicals
      varicose veins — *see* Varix, leg, with, inflammation
      X-rays L58.9
         acute L58.0
         chronic L58.1
   dyshydrotic L30.1
   dysmenorrheica N94.6
   escharotica — *see* Burn
   exfoliative, exfoliativa (generalized) L26
      neonatorum L00
   eyelid (*see also* Dermatosis, eyelid)
      allergic H01.119
         left H01.116
            lower H01.115
            upper H01.114
         right H01.113
            lower H01.112
            upper H01.111
      contact — *see* Dermatitis, eyelid, allergic
      due to
         Demodex species B88.0
         herpes (zoster) B02.39
            simplex B00.59
      eczematous H01.139
         left H01.136
            lower H01.135
            upper H01.134
         right H01.133
            lower H01.132
            upper H01.131
   facta, factitia, factitial L98.1
      psychogenic F54
   flexural NEC L20.82
   friction L30.4

Dermatitis — *continued*
   fungus B36.9
      specified type NEC B36.8
   gangrenosa, gangrenous infantum L08.0
   harvest mite B88.0
   heat L59.0
   herpesviral, vesicular (ear) (lip) B00.1
   herpetiformis (bullous) (erythematosus) (pustular)
      (vesicular) L13.0
      juvenile L12.2
      senile L12.0
   hiemalis L30.8
   hypostatic, hypostatica — *see* Varix, leg, with,
      inflammation
   infectious eczematoid L30.3
   infective L30.3
   irritant — *see* Dermatitis, contact, irritant
   Jacquet's (diaper dermatitis) L22
   Leptus B88.0
   lichenified NEC L28.0
   medicamentosa (generalized) (internal use) — *see*
      Dermatitis, due to drugs
   mite B88.0
   multiformis L13.0
      juvenile L12.2
   napkin L22
   neurotica L13.0
   nummular L30.0
   papillaris capillitii L73.0
   pellagrous E52
   perioral L71.0
   photocontact L56.2
   polymorpha dolorosa L13.0
   pruriginosa L13.0
   pruritic NEC L30.8
   psychogenic F54
   purulent L08.0
   pustular
      contagious B08.02
      subcorneal L13.1
   pyococcal L08.0
   pyogenica L08.0
   repens L40.2
   Ritter's (exfoliativa) L00
   Schamberg's L81.7
   schistosome B65.3
   seasonal bullous L30.8
   seborrheic L21.9
      infantile L21.1
      specified NEC L21.8
   sensitization NOS L23.9
   septic L08.0
   solare L57.8
   specified NEC L30.8
   stasis I87.2
      with
         varicose ulcer — *see* Varix, leg, with ulcer, with
            inflammation
         varicose veins — *see* Varix, leg, with,
            inflammation
      due to postthrombotic syndrome — *see*
         Syndrome, postthrombotic
   suppurative L08.0
   traumatic NEC L30.4
   trophoneurotica L13.0
   ultraviolet (sun) (chronic exposure) L57.8
      acute L56.8
   varicose — *see* Varix, leg, with, inflammation
   vegetans L10.1
   verrucosa B43.0
   vesicular, herpesviral B00.1
Dermatoarthritis, lipoid E78.81
Dermatochalasis, eyelid H02.839
   left H02.836
      lower H02.835
      upper H02.834
   right H02.833
      lower H02.832
      upper H02.831
Dermatofibroma (lenticulare) — *see* Neoplasm, skin,
   benign
   protuberans — *see* Neoplasm, skin, uncertain
      behavior
Dermatofibrosarcoma (pigmented) (protuberans) —
   see Neoplasm, skin, malignant
Dermatographia L50.3
Dermatolysis (exfoliativa) (congenital) Q82.8
   acquired L57.4
   eyelids — *see* Blepharochalasis
   palpebrarum — *see* Blepharochalasis
   senile L57.4
Dermatomegaly NEC Q82.8

Dermatomucosomyositis M33.10
   with
      myopathy M33.12
      respiratory involvement M33.11
      specified organ involvement NEC M33.19
Dermatomycosis B36.9
   furfuracea B36.0
   specified type NEC B36.8
Dermatomyositis (acute) (chronic) (*see also*
   Dermatopolymyositis)
   adult (*see also* Dermatomyositis, specified NEC)
      M33.10
   in (due to) neoplastic disease (*see also* Neoplasm)
      D49.9 *[M36.0]*
   juvenile M33.00
      with
         myopathy M33.02
         respiratory involvement M33.01
         specified organ involvement NEC M33.09
      without myopathy M33.03
   specified NEC M33.10
      with
         myopathy M33.12
         respiratory involvement M33.11
         specified organ involvement NEC M33.19
      without myopathy M33.13
Dermatoneuritis of children — *see* Poisoning, mercury
Dermatophilosis A48.8
Dermatophytid L30.2
Dermatophytide — *see* Dermatophytosis
Dermatophytosis (epidermophyton) (infection)
   (Microsporum) (tinea) (Trichophyton) B35.9
   beard B35.0
   body B35.4
   capitis B35.0
   corporis B35.4
   deep-seated B35.8
   disseminated B35.8
   foot B35.3
   granulomatous B35.8
   groin B35.6
   hand B35.2
   nail B35.1
   perianal (area) B35.6
   scalp B35.0
   specified NEC B35.8
Dermatopolymyositis M33.90
   with
      myopathy M33.92
      respiratory involvement M33.91
      specified organ involvement NEC M33.99
   in neoplastic disease (*see also* Neoplasm) D49.9 *[M36.0]*
   juvenile M33.00
      with
         myopathy M33.02
         respiratory involvement M33.01
         specified organ involvement NEC M33.09
      specified NEC M33.10
         myopathy M33.12
         respiratory involvement M33.11
         specified organ involvement NEC M33.19
      without myopathy M33.93
Dermatopolyneuritis — *see* Poisoning, mercury
Dermatorrhexis (*see also* Syndrome, Ehlers-Danlos)
   Q79.60
   acquired L57.4
Dermatosclerosis (*see also* Scleroderma)
   localized L94.0
Dermatosis L98.9
   Andrews' L08.89
   Bowen's — *see* Neoplasm, skin, in situ
   bullous L13.9
      specified NEC L13.8
   exfoliativa L26
   eyelid (noninfectious)
      dermatitis — *see* Dermatitis, eyelid
      discoid lupus erythematosus — *see* Lupus,
         erythematosus, eyelid
      xeroderma — *see* Xeroderma, acquired, eyelid
   factitial L98.1
   febrile neutrophilic L98.2
   gonococcal A54.89
   herpetiformis L13.0
      juvenile L12.2
   linear IgA L13.8
   menstrual NEC L98.8
   neutrophilic, febrile L98.2
   occupational — *see* Dermatitis, contact
   papulosa nigra L82.1
   pigmentary L81.9
      progressive L81.7
      Schamberg's L81.7

Dermatosis — *continued*
  psychogenic F54
  purpuric, pigmented L81.7
  pustular, subcorneal L13.1
  transient acantholytic L11.1
Dermographia, dermographism L50.3
Dermoid (cyst) (*see also* Neoplasm, benign, by site)
  with malignant transformation C56 ☑
  due to radiation (nonionizing) L57.8
Dermopathy
  infiltrative with thyrotoxicosis — *see* Thyrotoxicosis
  nephrogenic fibrosing L90.8
Dermophytosis — *see* Dermatophytosis
Descemetocele H18.73 ☑
Descemet's membrane — *see* condition
Descending — *see* condition
Descensus uteri — *see* Prolapse, uterus
Desert
  rheumatism B38.0
  sore — *see* Ulcer, skin
Desertion (newborn) — *see* Maltreatment
Desmoid (extra-abdominal) (tumor) — *see* Neoplasm, connective tissue, uncertain behavior
  abdominal D48.1
Despondency F32.9
Desquamation, skin R23.4
Destruction, destructive (*see also* Damage)
  articular facet (*see also* Derangement, joint, specified type NEC)
    knee M23.8X ☑
    vertebra — *see* Spondylosis
  bone (*see also* Disorder, bone, specified type NEC)
    syphilitic A52.77
  joint (*see also* Derangement, joint, specified type NEC)
    sacroiliac M53.3
  rectal sphincter K62.89
  septum (nasal) J34.89
  tuberculous NEC — *see* Tuberculosis
  tympanum, tympanic membrane (nontraumatic) — *see* Disorder, tympanic membrane, specified NEC
  vertebral disc — *see* Degeneration, intervertebral disc
Destructiveness (*see also* Disorder, conduct)
  adjustment reaction — *see* Disorder, adjustment
Desultory labor O62.2
Detachment
  cartilage — *see* Sprain
  cervix, annular N88.8
    complicating delivery O71.3
  choroid (old) (postinfectional) (simple) (spontaneous) H31.40 ☑
    hemorrhagic H31.41 ☑
    serous H31.42 ☑
  ligament — *see* Sprain
  meniscus (knee) (*see also* Derangement, knee, meniscus, specified NEC)
    current injury — *see* Tear, meniscus
    due to old tear or injury — *see* Derangement, knee, meniscus, due to old tear
  retina (without retinal break) (serous) H33.2 ☑
    with retinal:
      break H33.00 ☑
        giant H33.03 ☑
        multiple H33.02 ☑
        single H33.01 ☑
      dialysis H33.04 ☑
    pigment epithelium — *see* Degeneration, retina, separation of layers, pigment epithelium detachment
    rhegmatogenous — *see* Detachment, retina, with retinal, break
    specified NEC H33.8
    total H33.05 ☑
    traction H33.4 ☑
  vitreous (body) H43.81 ☑
Detergent asthma J69.8
Deterioration
  epileptic F06.8
  general physical R53.81
  heart, cardiac — *see* Degeneration, myocardial
  mental — *see* Psychosis
  myocardial, myocardium — *see* Degeneration, myocardial
  senile (simple) R54
Deuteranomaly (anomalous trichromat) H53.53
Deuteranopia (complete) (incomplete) H53.53
Development
  abnormal, bone Q79.9
  arrested R62.50
    bone — *see* Arrest, development or growth, bone

Development — *continued*
  arrested — *continued*
    child R62.50
    due to malnutrition E45
  defective, congenital (*see also* Anomaly, by site)
    cauda equina Q06.3
    left ventricle Q24.8
      in hypoplastic left heart syndrome Q23.4
    valve Q24.8
      pulmonary Q22.3
  delayed (*see also* Delay, development) R62.50
    arithmetical skills F81.2
    language (skills) (expressive) F80.1
    learning skill F81.9
    mixed skills F88
    motor coordination F82
    reading F81.0
    specified learning skill NEC F81.89
    speech F80.9
    spelling F81.81
    written expression F81.81
  imperfect, congenital (*see also* Anomaly, by site)
    heart Q24.9
    lungs Q33.6
  incomplete
    bronchial tree Q32.4
    organ or site not listed — *see* Hypoplasia, by site
    respiratory system Q34.9
  sexual, precocious NEC E30.1
  tardy, mental (*see also* Disability, intellectual) F79
Developmental — *see* condition
  testing, infant or child — *see* Examination, child
Devergie's disease (pityriasis rubra pilaris) L44.0
Deviation (in)
  conjugate palsy (eye) (spastic) H51.0
  esophagus (acquired) K22.8
  eye, skew H51.8
  midline (jaw) (teeth) (dental arch) M26.29
    specified site NEC — *see* Malposition
  nasal septum J34.2
    congenital Q67.4
  opening and closing of the mandible M26.53
  organ or site, congenital NEC — *see* Malposition, congenital
  septum (nasal) (acquired) J34.2
    congenital Q67.4
  sexual F65.9
    bestiality F65.89
    erotomania F52.8
    exhibitionism F65.2
    fetishism, fetishistic F65.0
      transvestism F65.1
    frotteurism F65.81
    masochism F65.51
    multiple F65.89
    necrophilia F65.89
    nymphomania F52.8
    pederosis F65.4
    pedophilia F65.4
    sadism, sadomasochism F65.52
    satyriasis F52.8
    specified type NEC F65.89
    transvestism F64.1
    voyeurism F65.3
  teeth, midline M26.29
  trachea J39.8
  ureter, congenital Q62.61
Device
  cerebral ventricle (communicating) in situ Z98.2
  contraceptive — *see* Contraceptive, device
  drainage, cerebrospinal fluid, in situ Z98.2
Devic's disease G36.0
Devil's
  grip B33.0
  pinches (purpura simplex) D69.2
Devitalized tooth K04.99
Devonshire colic — *see* Poisoning, lead
Dextraposition, aorta Q20.3
  in tetralogy of Fallot Q21.3
Dextrinosis, limit (debrancher enzyme deficiency) E74.03
Dextrocardia (true) Q24.0
  with
    complete transposition of viscera Q89.3
    situs inversus Q89.3
Dextrotransposition, aorta Q20.3
d-glycericacidemia E72.59
Dhat syndrome F48.8
Dhobi itch B35.6
Di George's syndrome D82.1
Di Guglielmo's disease C94.0 ☑

Diabetes, diabetic (mellitus) (sugar) E11.9
  with
    amyotrophy E11.44
    arthropathy NEC E11.618
    autonomic (poly)neuropathy E11.43
    cataract E11.36
    Charcot's joints E11.610
    chronic kidney disease E11.22
    circulatory complication NEC E11.59
    complication E11.8
      specified NEC E11.69
    dermatitis E11.620
    foot ulcer E11.621
    gangrene E11.52
    gastroparalysis E11.43
    gastroparesis E11.43
    glomerulonephrosis, intracapillary E11.21
    glomerulosclerosis, intercapillary E11.21
    hyperglycemia E11.65
    hyperosmolarity E11.00
      with coma E11.01
    hypoglycemia E11.649
      with coma E11.641
    ketoacidosis E11.10
      with coma E11.11
    kidney complications NEC E11.29
    Kimmelstiel-Wilson disease E11.21
    loss of protective sensation (LOPS) — *see* Diabetes, by type, with neuropathy
    mononeuropathy E11.41
    myasthenia E11.44
    necrobiosis lipoidica E11.620
    nephropathy E11.21
    neuralgia E11.42
    neurologic complication NEC E11.49
    neuropathic arthropathy E11.610
    neuropathy E11.40
    ophthalmic complication NEC E11.39
    oral complication NEC E11.638
    osteomyelitis E11.69
    periodontal disease E11.630
    peripheral angiopathy E11.51
      with gangrene E11.52
    polyneuropathy E11.42
    renal complication NEC E11.29
    renal tubular degeneration E11.29
    retinopathy E11.319
      with macular edema E11.311
        resolved following treatment E11.37 ☑
      nonproliferative E11.329 ☑
        with macular edema E11.321 ☑
        mild E11.329 ☑
          with macular edema E11.321 ☑
        moderate E11.339 ☑
          with macular edema E11.331 ☑
        severe E11.349 ☑
          with macular edema E11.341 ☑
      proliferative E11.359 ☑
        with
          combined traction retinal detachment and rhegmatogenous retinal detachment E11.354 ☑
          macular edema E11.351 ☑
          stable proliferative diabetic retinopathy E11.355 ☑
          traction retinal detachment involving the macula E11.352 ☑
          traction retinal detachment not involving the macula E11.353 ☑
    skin complication NEC E11.628
    skin ulcer NEC E11.622
  brittle — *see* Diabetes, type 1
  bronzed E83.110
  complicating pregnancy — *see* Pregnancy, complicated by, diabetes
  dietary counseling and surveillance Z71.3
  due to
    autoimmune process — *see* Diabetes, type 1
    immune mediated pancreatic islet beta-cell destruction — *see* Diabetes, type 1
  due to drug or chemical E09.9
    with
      amyotrophy E09.44
      arthropathy NEC E09.618
      autonomic (poly)neuropathy E09.43
      cataract E09.36
      Charcot's joints E09.610
      chronic kidney disease E09.22
      circulatory complication NEC E09.59
      complication E09.8
        specified NEC E09.69
      dermatitis E09.620

☑ **Additional character required**

Diabetes — *continued*
  due to drug or chemical — *continued*
    foot ulcer E09.621
    gangrene E09.52
    gastroparalysis E09.43
    gastroparesis E09.43
    glomerulonephrosis, intracapillary E09.21
    glomerulosclerosis, intercapillary E09.21
    hyperglycemia E09.65
    hyperosmolarity E09.00
      with coma E09.01
    hypoglycemia E09.649
      with coma E09.641
    ketoacidosis E09.10
      with coma E09.11
    kidney complications NEC E09.29
    Kimmelstiel-Wilson disease E09.21
    mononeuropathy E09.41
    myasthenia E09.44
    necrobiosis lipoidica E09.620
    nephropathy E09.21
    neuralgia E09.42
    neurologic complication NEC E09.49
    neuropathic arthropathy E09.610
    neuropathy E09.40
    ophthalmic complication NEC E09.39
    oral complication NEC E09.638
    periodontal disease E09.630
    peripheral angiopathy E09.51
      with gangrene E09.52
    polyneuropathy E09.42
    renal complication NEC E09.29
    renal tubular degeneration E09.29
    retinopathy E09.319
      with macular edema E09.311
      resolved following treatment E09.37 ☑
      nonproliferative E09.329 ☑
        with macular edema E09.321 ☑
        mild E09.329 ☑
          with macular edema E09.321 ☑
        moderate E09.339 ☑
          with macular edema E09.331 ☑
        severe E09.349 ☑
          with macular edema E09.341 ☑
      proliferative E09.359 ☑
        with
          combined traction retinal detachment
            and rhegmatogenous retinal
            detachment E09.354 ☑
          macular edema E09.351 ☑
          stable proliferative diabetic retinopathy
            E09.355 ☑
          traction retinal detachment involving the
            macula E09.352 ☑
          traction retinal detachment not involving
            the macula E09.353 ☑
    skin complication NEC E09.628
    skin ulcer NEC E09.622
  due to underlying condition E08.9
    with
      amyotrophy E08.44
      arthropathy NEC E08.618
      autonomic (poly)neuropathy E08.43
      cataract E08.36
      Charcot's joints E08.610
      chronic kidney disease E08.22
      circulatory complication NEC E08.59
      complication E08.8
        specified NEC E08.69
      dermatitis E08.620
      foot ulcer E08.621
      gangrene E08.52
      gastroparalysis E08.43
      gastroparesis E08.43
      glomerulonephrosis, intracapillary E08.21
      glomerulosclerosis, intercapillary E08.21
      hyperglycemia E08.65
      hyperosmolarity E08.00
        with coma E08.01
      hypoglycemia E08.649
        with coma E08.641
      ketoacidosis E08.10
        with coma E08.11
      kidney complications NEC E08.29
      Kimmelstiel-Wilson disease E08.21
      mononeuropathy E08.41
      myasthenia E08.44
      necrobiosis lipoidica E08.620
      nephropathy E08.21
      neuralgia E08.42
      neurologic complication NEC E08.49
      neuropathic arthropathy E08.610

Diabetes — *continued*
  due to underlying condition — *continued*
    neuropathy E08.40
    ophthalmic complication NEC E08.39
    oral complication NEC E08.638
    periodontal disease E08.630
    peripheral angiopathy E08.51
      with gangrene E08.52
    polyneuropathy E08.42
    renal complication NEC E08.29
    renal tubular degeneration E08.29
    retinopathy E08.319
      with macular edema E08.311
      resolved following treatment E08.37 ☑
      nonproliferative E08.329 ☑
        with macular edema E08.321 ☑
        mild E08.329 ☑
          with macular edema E08.321 ☑
        moderate E08.339 ☑
          with macular edema E08.331 ☑
        severe E08.349 ☑
          with macular edema E08.341 ☑
      proliferative E08.359 ☑
        with
          combined traction retinal detachment
            and rhegmatogenous retinal
            detachment E08.354 ☑
          macular edema E08.351 ☑
          stable proliferative diabetic retinopathy
            E08.355 ☑
          traction retinal detachment involving the
            macula E08.352 ☑
          traction retinal detachment not involving
            the macula E08.353 ☑
    skin complication NEC E08.628
    skin ulcer NEC E08.622
  gestational (in pregnancy) O24.419
    affecting newborn P70.0
    diet controlled O24.410
    in childbirth O24.429
      diet controlled O24.420
      insulin (and diet) controlled O24.424
      oral drug controlled (antidiabetic)
        (hypoglycemic) O24.425
    insulin (and diet) controlled O24.414
    oral drug controlled (antidiabetic) (hypoglycemic)
      O24.415
    puerperal O24.439
      diet controlled O24.430
      insulin (and diet) controlled O24.434
      oral drug controlled (antidiabetic)
        (hypoglycemic) O24.435
  hepatogenous E13.9
  idiopathic — *see* Diabetes, type 1
  inadequately controlled - code to Diabetes, by type,
    with hyperglycemia
  insipidus E23.2
    nephrogenic N25.1
    pituitary E23.2
    vasopressin resistant N25.1
  insulin dependent - code to type of diabetes
  juvenile-onset — *see* Diabetes, type 1
  ketosis-prone — *see* Diabetes, type 1
  latent R73.03
  neonatal (transient) P70.2
  non-insulin dependent - code to type of diabetes
  out of control - code to Diabetes, by type, with
    hyperglycemia
  phosphate E83.39
  poorly controlled - code to Diabetes, by type, with
    hyperglycemia
  postpancreatectomy — *see* Diabetes, specified
    type NEC
  postprocedural — *see* Diabetes, specified type NEC
  secondary diabetes mellitus NEC — *see* Diabetes,
    specified type NEC
  specified type NEC E13.9
    with
      amyotrophy E13.44
      arthropathy NEC E13.618
      autonomic (poly)neuropathy E13.43
      cataract E13.36
      Charcot's joints E13.610
      chronic kidney disease E13.22
      circulatory complication NEC E13.59
      complication E13.8
        specified NEC E13.69
      dermatitis E13.620
      foot ulcer E13.621
      gangrene E13.52
      gastroparalysis E13.43
      gastroparesis E13.43

Diabetes — *continued*
  specified type NEC — *continued*
    glomerulonephrosis, intracapillary E13.21
    glomerulosclerosis, intercapillary E13.21
    hyperglycemia E13.65
    hyperosmolarity E13.00
      with coma E13.01
    hypoglycemia E13.649
      with coma E13.641
    ketoacidosis E13.10
      with coma E13.11
    kidney complications NEC E13.29
    Kimmelsteil-Wilson disease E13.21
    mononeuropathy E13.41
    myasthenia E13.44
    necrobiosis lipoidica E13.620
    nephropathy E13.21
    neuralgia E13.42
    neurologic complication NEC E13.49
    neuropathic arthropathy E13.610
    neuropathy E13.40
    ophthalmic complication NEC E13.39
    oral complication NEC E13.638
    periodontal disease E13.630
    peripheral angiopathy E13.51
      with gangrene E13.52
    polyneuropathy E13.42
    renal complication NEC E13.29
    renal tubular degeneration E13.29
    retinopathy E13.319
      with macular edema E13.311
      resolved following treatment E13.37 ☑
      nonproliferative E13.329 ☑
        with macular edema E13.321 ☑
        mild E13.329 ☑
          with macular edema E13.321 ☑
        moderate E13.339 ☑
          with macular edema E13.331 ☑
        severe E13.349 ☑
          with macular edema E13.341 ☑
      proliferative E13.359 ☑
        with
          combined traction retinal detachment
            and rhegmatogenous retinal
            detachment E13.354 ☑
          macular edema E13.351 ☑
          stable proliferative diabetic retinopathy
            E13.355 ☑
          traction retinal detachment involving the
            macula E13.352 ☑
          traction retinal detachment not involving
            the macula E13.353 ☑
    skin complication NEC E13.628
    skin ulcer NEC E13.622
  steroid-induced — *see* Diabetes, due to, drug or
    chemical
  type 1 E10.9
    with
      amyotrophy E10.44
      arthropathy NEC E10.618
      autonomic (poly)neuropathy E10.43
      cataract E10.36
      Charcot's joints E10.610
      chronic kidney disease E10.22
      circulatory complication NEC E10.59
      complication E10.8
        specified NEC E10.69
      dermatitis E10.620
      foot ulcer E10.621
      gangrene E10.52
      gastroparalysis E10.43
      gastroparesis E10.43
      glomerulonephrosis, intracapillary E10.21
      glomerulosclerosis, intercapillary E10.21
      hyperglycemia E10.65
      hypoglycemia E10.649
        with coma E10.641
      ketoacidosis E10.10
        with coma E10.11
      kidney complications NEC E10.29
      Kimmelstiel-Wilson disease E10.21
      mononeuropathy E10.41
      myasthenia E10.44
      necrobiosis lipoidica E10.620
      nephropathy E10.21
      neuralgia E10.42
      neurologic complication NEC E10.49
      neuropathic arthropathy E10.610
      neuropathy E10.40
      ophthalmic complication NEC E10.39
      oral complication NEC E10.638
      osteomyelitis E10.69

Diabetes — *continued*
  type 1 — *continued*
    periodontal disease E10.630
    peripheral angiopathy E10.51
      with gangrene E10.52
    polyneuropathy E10.42
    renal complication NEC E10.29
    renal tubular degeneration E10.29
    retinopathy E10.319
      with macular edema E10.311
      resolved following treatment E10.37 ☑
      nonproliferative E10.329 ☑
        with macular edema E10.321 ☑
        mild E10.329 ☑
          with macular edema E10.321 ☑
        moderate E10.339 ☑
          with macular edema E10.331 ☑
        severe E10.349 ☑
          with macular edema E10.341 ☑
      proliferative E10.359 ☑
        with
          combined traction retinal detachment
            and rhegmatogenous retinal
            detachment E10.354 ☑
          macular edema E10.351 ☑
          stable proliferative diabetic retinopathy
            E10.355 ☑
          traction retinal detachment involving the
            macula E10.352 ☑
          traction retinal detachment not involving
            the macula E10.353 ☑
    skin complication NEC E10.628
    skin ulcer NEC E10.622
  type 2 E11.9
    with
      amyotrophy E11.44
      arthropathy NEC E11.618
      autonomic (poly)neuropathy E11.43
      cataract E11.36
      Charcot's joints E11.610
      chronic kidney disease E11.22
      circulatory complication NEC E11.59
      complication E11.8
        specified NEC E11.69
      dermatitis E11.620
      foot ulcer E11.621
      gangrene E11.52
      gastroparalysis E11.43
      gastroparesis E11.43
      glomerulonephrosis, intracapillary E11.21
      glomerulosclerosis, intercapillary E11.21
      hyperglycemia E11.65
      hyperosmolarity E11.00
        with coma E11.01
      hypoglycemia E11.649
        with coma E11.641
      ketoacidosis E11.10
        with coma E11.11
      kidney complications NEC E11.29
      Kimmelstiel-Wilson disease E11.21
      mononeuropathy E11.41
      myasthenia E11.44
      necrobiosis lipoidica E11.620
      nephropathy E11.21
      neuralgia E11.42
      neurologic complication NEC E11.49
      neuropathic arthropathy E11.610
      neuropathy E11.40
      ophthalmic complication NEC E11.39
      oral complication NEC E11.638
      osteomyelitis E11.69
      periodontal disease E11.630
      peripheral angiopathy E11.51
        with gangrene E11.52
      polyneuropathy E11.42
      renal complication NEC E11.29
      renal tubular degeneration E11.29
      retinopathy E11.319
        with macular edema E11.311
        resolved following treatment E11.37 ☑
        nonproliferative E11.329 ☑
          with macular edema E11.321 ☑
          mild E11.329 ☑
            with macular edema E11.321 ☑
          moderate E11.339 ☑
            with macular edema E11.331 ☑
          severe E11.349 ☑
            with macular edema E11.341 ☑
        proliferative E11.359 ☑
          with

Diabetes — *continued*
  type 2 — *continued*
    with
      combined traction retinal detachment
        and rhegmatogenous retinal
        detachment E11.354 ☑
      macular edema E11.351 ☑
      stable proliferative diabetic retinopathy
        E11.355 ☑
      traction retinal detachment involving the
        macula E11.352 ☑
      traction retinal detachment not involving
        the macula E11.353 ☑
    skin complication NEC E11.628
    skin ulcer NEC E11.622
  uncontrolled
    meaning
      hyperglycemia — *see* Diabetes, by type, with,
        hyperglycemia
      hypoglycemia — *see* Diabetes, by type, with,
        hypoglycemia
Diacyclothrombopathia D69.1
Diagnosis deferred R69
Dialysis (intermittent) (treatment)
  noncompliance (with) Z91.15
  renal (hemodialysis) (peritoneal), status Z99.2
  retina, retinal — *see* Detachment, retina, with
    retinal, dialysis
Diamond-Blackfan anemia (congenital hypoplastic)
  D61.01
Diamond-Gardener syndrome (autoerythrocyte
  sensitization) D69.2
Diaper rash L22
Diaphoresis (excessive) R61
Diaphragm — *see* condition
Diaphragmalgia R07.1
Diaphragmatitis, diaphragmitis J98.6
Diaphysial aclasis Q78.6
Diaphysitis — *see* Osteomyelitis, specified type NEC
Diarrhea, diarrheal (disease) (infantile) (inflammatory)
  R19.7
  achlorhydric K31.83
  allergic K52.29
    due to
      colitis — *see* Colitis, allergic
      enteritis — *see* Enteritis, allergic
  amebic (*see also* Amebiasis) A06.0
    with abscess — *see* Abscess, amebic
    acute A06.0
    chronic A06.1
    nondysenteric A06.2
  bacillary — *see* Dysentery, bacillary
  balantidial A07.0
  cachectic NEC K52.89
  Chilomastix A07.8
  choleriformis A00.1
  chronic (noninfectious) K52.9
  coccidial A07.3
  Cochin-China K90.1
    strongyloidiasis B78.0
  Dientamoeba A07.8
  dietetic (*see also* Diarrhea, allergic) K52.29
  drug-induced K52.1
  due to
    bacteria A04.9
      specified NEC A04.8
    Campylobacter A04.5
    Capillaria philippinensis B81.1
    Clostridium difficile
      not specified as recurrent A04.72
      recurrent A04.71
    Clostridium perfringens (C) (F) A04.8
    Cryptosporidium A07.2
    drugs K52.1
    Escherichia coli A04.4
      enteroaggregative A04.4
      enterohemorrhagic A04.3
      enteroinvasive A04.2
      enteropathogenic A04.0
      enterotoxigenic A04.1
      specified NEC A04.4
    food hypersensitivity (*see also* Diarrhea, allergic)
      K52.29
    Necator americanus B76.1
    S. japonicum B65.2
    specified organism NEC A08.8
      bacterial A04.8
      viral A08.39
    Staphylococcus A04.8
    Trichuris trichiuria B79
    virus — *see* Enteritis, viral
    Yersinia enterocolitica A04.6
  dysenteric A09

Diarrhea — *continued*
  endemic A09
  epidemic A09
  flagellate A07.9
  Flexner's (ulcerative) A03.1
  functional K59.1
    following gastrointestinal surgery K91.89
    psychogenic F45.8
  Giardia lamblia A07.1
  giardial A07.1
  hill K90.1
  infectious A09
  malarial — *see* Malaria
  mite B88.0
  mycotic NEC B49
  neonatal (noninfectious) P78.3
  nervous F45.8
  neurogenic K59.1
  noninfectious K52.9
  postgastrectomy K91.1
  postvagotomy K91.1
  protozoal A07.9
    specified NEC A07.8
  psychogenic F45.8
  specified
    bacterium NEC A04.8
    virus NEC A08.39
  strongyloidiasis B78.0
  toxic K52.1
  trichomonal A07.8
  tropical K90.1
  tuberculous A18.32
  viral — *see* Enteritis, viral
Diastasis
  cranial bones M84.88
  congenital NEC Q75.8
  joint (traumatic) — *see* Dislocation
  muscle M62.00
    ankle M62.07 ☑
    congenital Q79.8
    foot M62.07 ☑
    forearm M62.03 ☑
    hand M62.04 ☑
    lower leg M62.06 ☑
    pelvic region M62.05 ☑
    shoulder region M62.01 ☑
    specified site NEC M62.08
    thigh M62.05 ☑
    upper arm M62.02 ☑
  recti (abdomen)
    complicating delivery O71.89
    congenital Q79.59
Diastema, tooth, teeth, fully erupted M26.32
Diastematomyelia Q06.2
Diataxia, cerebral G80.4
Diathesis
  allergic — *see* History, allergy
  bleeding (familial) D69.9
  cystine (familial) E72.00
  gouty — *see* Gout
  hemorrhagic (familial) D69.9
    newborn NEC P53
  spasmophilic R29.0
Diaz's disease or osteochondrosis (juvenile) (talus) —
  see Osteochondrosis, juvenile, tarsus
Dibothriocephalus, dibothriocephaliasis (latus)
  (infection) (infestation) B70.0
    larval B70.1
Dicephalus, dicephaly Q89.4
Dichotomy, teeth K00.2
Dichromat, dichromatopsia (congenital) — *see*
  Deficiency, color vision
Dichuchwa A65
Dicroceliasis B66.2
Didelphia, didelphys — *see* Double uterus
Didymytis N45.1
  with orchitis N45.3
Dietary
  inadequacy or deficiency E63.9
  surveillance and counseling Z71.3
Dietl's crisis N13.8
Dieulafoy lesion (hemorrhagic)
  duodenum K31.82
  esophagus K22.8
  intestine (colon) K63.81
  stomach K31.82
Difficult, difficulty (in)
  acculturation Z60.3
  feeding R63.3
    newborn P92.9
      breast P92.5
      specified NEC P92.8

Difficult — *continued*
  feeding — *continued*
    nonorganic (infant or child) F98.29
  intubation, in anesthesia T88.4 ☑
  mechanical, gastroduodenal stoma K91.89
    causing obstruction (*see also* Obstruction, intestine, postoperative) K91.30
  micturition
    need to immediately re-void R39.191
    position dependent R39.192
    specified NEC R39.198
  reading (developmental) F81.0
    secondary to emotional disorders F93.9
  spelling (specific) F81.81
    with reading disorder F81.89
    due to inadequate teaching Z55.8
  swallowing — *see* Dysphagia
  walking R26.2
  work
    conditions NEC Z56.5
    schedule Z56.3
Diffuse — *see* condition
DiGeorge's syndrome (thymic hypoplasia) D82.1
Digestive — *see* condition
Dihydropyrimidine dehydrogenase disease (DPD) E88.89
Diktyoma — *see* Neoplasm, malignant, by site
Dilaceration, tooth K00.4
Dilatation
  anus K59.8
    venule — *see* Hemorrhoids
  aorta (focal) (general) — *see* Ectasia, aorta
    with aneurysm — *see* Aneurysm, aorta
    congenital Q25.44
  artery — *see* Aneurysm
  bladder (sphincter) N32.89
    congenital Q64.79
  blood vessel I99.8
  bronchial J47.9
    with
      exacerbation (acute) J47.1
      lower respiratory infection J47.0
  calyx (due to obstruction) — *see* Hydronephrosis
  capillaries I78.8
  cardiac (acute) (chronic) (*see also* Hypertrophy, cardiac)
    congenital Q24.8
      valve NEC Q24.8
        pulmonary Q22.3
    valve — *see* Endocarditis
  cavum septi pellucidi Q06.8
  cervix (uteri) (*see also* Incompetency, cervix)
    incomplete, poor, slow complicating delivery O62.0
  colon K59.39
    congenital Q43.1
    psychogenic F45.8
    toxic K59.31
  common duct (acquired) K83.8
    congenital Q44.5
  cystic duct (acquired) K82.8
    congenital Q44.5
  duct, mammary — *see* Ectasia, mammary duct
  duodenum K59.8
  esophagus K22.8
    congenital Q39.5
    due to achalasia K22.0
  eustachian tube, congenital Q17.8
  gallbladder K82.8
  gastric — *see* Dilatation, stomach
  heart (acute) (chronic) (*see also* Hypertrophy, cardiac)
    congenital Q24.8
    valve — *see* Endocarditis
  ileum K59.8
    psychogenic F45.8
  jejunum K59.8
    psychogenic F45.8
  kidney (calyx) (collecting structures) (cystic) (parenchyma) (pelvis) (idiopathic) N28.89
  lacrimal passages or duct — *see* Disorder, lacrimal system, changes
  lymphatic vessel I89.0
  mammary duct — *see* Ectasia, mammary duct
  Meckel's diverticulum (congenital) Q43.0
    malignant — *see* Table of Neoplasms, small intestine, malignant
  myocardium (acute) (chronic) — *see* Hypertrophy, cardiac
  organ or site, congenital NEC — *see* Distortion
  pancreatic duct K86.89
  pericardium — *see* Pericarditis

Dilatation — *continued*
  pharynx J39.2
  prostate N42.89
  pulmonary
    artery (idiopathic) I28.8
    valve, congenital Q22.3
  pupil H57.04
  rectum K59.39
  saccule, congenital Q16.5
  salivary gland (duct) K11.8
  sphincter ani K62.89
  stomach K31.89
    acute K31.0
    psychogenic F45.8
  submaxillary duct K11.8
  trachea, congenital Q32.1
  ureter (idiopathic) N28.82
    congenital Q62.2
    due to obstruction N13.4
  urethra (acquired) N36.8
  vasomotor I73.9
  vein I86.8
  ventricular, ventricle (acute) (chronic) (*see also* Hypertrophy, cardiac)
    cerebral, congenital Q04.8
  venule NEC I86.8
  vesical orifice N32.89
Dilated, dilation — *see* Dilatation
Diminished, diminution
  hearing (acuity) — *see* Deafness
  sense or sensation (cold) (heat) (tactile) (vibratory) R20.8
  vision NEC H54.7
  vital capacity R94.2
Diminuta taenia B71.0
Dimitri-Sturge-Weber disease Q85.8
Dimple
  congenital sacral Q82.6
  parasacral Q82.6
  pilonidal or postanal — *see* Cyst, pilonidal
Dioctophyme renalis (infection) (infestation) B83.8
Dipetalonemiasis B74.4
Diphallus Q55.69
Diphtheria, diphtheritic (gangrenous) (hemorrhagic) A36.9
  carrier (suspected) Z22.2
  cutaneous A36.3
  faucial A36.0
  infection of wound A36.3
  laryngeal A36.2
  myocarditis A36.81
  nasal, anterior A36.89
  nasopharyngeal A36.1
  neurological complication A36.89
  pharyngeal A36.0
  specified site NEC A36.89
  tonsillar A36.0
Diphyllobothriasis (intestine) B70.0
  larval B70.1
Diplacusis H93.22 ☑
Diplegia (upper limbs) G83.0
  congenital (cerebral) G80.8
  facial G51.0
  lower limbs G82.20
  spastic G80.1
Diplococcus, diplococcal — *see* condition
Diplopia H53.2
Dipsomania F10.20
  with
    psychosis — *see* Psychosis, alcoholic
    remission F10.21
Dipylidiasis B71.1
DIRA (deficiency of interleukin 1 receptor antagonist) M04.8
Direction, teeth, abnormal, fully erupted M26.30
Dirofilariasis B74.8
Dirt-eating child F98.3
Disability, disabilities
  heart — *see* Disease, heart
  intellectual F79
    with
      autistic features F84.9
    mild (I.Q.50-69) F70
    moderate (I.Q.35-49) F71
    profound (I.Q. under 20) F73
    severe (I.Q.20-34) F72
    specified level NEC F78
  knowledge acquisition F81.9
  learning F81.9
  limiting activities Z73.6
  spelling, specific F81.81
Disappearance of family member Z63.4

Disarticulation — *see* Amputation
  meaning traumatic amputation — *see* Amputation, traumatic
Discharge (from)
  abnormal finding in — *see* Abnormal, specimen
  breast (female) (male) N64.52
  diencephalic autonomic idiopathic — *see* Epilepsy, specified NEC
  ear (*see also* Otorrhea)
    blood — *see* Otorrhagia
  excessive urine R35.8
  nipple N64.52
  penile R36.9
  postnasal R09.82
  prison, anxiety concerning Z65.2
  urethral R36.9
    without blood R36.0
    hematospermia R36.1
  vaginal N89.8
Discitis, diskitis M46.40
  cervical region M46.42
  cervicothoracic region M46.43
  lumbar region M46.46
  lumbosacral region M46.47
  multiple sites M46.49
  occipito-atlanto-axial region M46.41
  pyogenic — *see* Infection, intervertebral disc, pyogenic
  sacrococcygeal region M46.48
  thoracic region M46.44
  thoracolumbar region M46.45
Discoid
  meniscus (congenital) Q68.6
  semilunar cartilage (congenital) — *see* Derangement, knee, meniscus, specified NEC
Discoloration
  nails L60.8
  teeth (posteruptive) K03.7
    during formation K00.8
Discomfort
  chest R07.89
  visual H53.14 ☑
Discontinuity, ossicles, ear H74.2 ☑
Discord (with)
  boss Z56.4
  classmates Z55.4
  counselor Z64.4
  employer Z56.4
  family Z63.8
  fellow employees Z56.4
  in-laws Z63.1
  landlord Z59.2
  lodgers Z59.2
  neighbors Z59.2
  probation officer Z64.4
  social worker Z64.4
  teachers Z55.4
  workmates Z56.4
Discordant connection
  atrioventricular (congenital) Q20.5
  ventriculoarterial Q20.3
Discrepancy
  centric occlusion maximum intercuspation M26.55
  leg length (acquired) — *see* Deformity, limb, unequal length
    congenital — *see* Defect, reduction, lower limb
  uterine size date O26.84 ☑
Discrimination
  ethnic Z60.5
  political Z60.5
  racial Z60.5
  religious Z60.5
  sex Z60.5
Disease, diseased (*see also* Syndrome)
  absorbent system I87.8
  acid-peptic K30
  Acosta's T70.29 ☑
  Adams-Stokes (-Morgagni) (syncope with heart block) I45.9
  Addison's anemia (pernicious) D51.0
  adenoids (and tonsils) J35.9
  adrenal (capsule) (cortex) (gland) (medullary) E27.9
    hyperfunction E27.0
    specified NEC E27.8
  ainhum L94.6
  airway
    obstructive, chronic J44.9
    due to
      cotton dust J66.0
      specific organic dusts NEC J66.8
    reactive — *see* Asthma
  akamushi (scrub typhus) A75.3

Disease

Disease — *continued*

Albers-Schönberg (marble bones) Q78.2
Albert's — *see* Tendinitis, Achilles
alimentary canal K63.9
alligator-skin Q80.9
  acquired L85.0
alpha heavy chain C88.3
alpine T70.29 ☑
altitude T70.20 ☑
alveolar ridge
  edentulous K06.9
    specified NEC K06.8
alveoli, teeth K08.9
Alzheimer's G30.9 *[F02.80]*
  with behavioral disturbance G30.9 *[F02.81]*
  early onset G30.0 *[F02.80]*
    with behavioral disturbance G30.0 *[F02.81]*
  late onset G30.1 *[F02.80]*
    with behavioral disturbance G30.1 *[F02.81]*
  specified NEC G30.8 *[F02.80]*
    with behavioral disturbance G30.8 *[F02.81]*
amyloid — *see* Amyloidosis
Andersen's (glycogenosis IV) E74.09
Andes T70.29 ☑
Andrews' (bacterid) L08.89
angiospastic I73.9
  cerebral G45.9
  vein I87.8
anterior
  chamber H21.9
  horn cell G12.29
antiglomerular basement membrane (anti- GBM)
    antibody M31.0
  tubulo-interstitial nephritis N12
antral — *see* Sinusitis, maxillary
anus K62.9
  specified NEC K62.89
aorta (nonsyphilitic) I77.9
  syphilitic NEC A52.02
aortic (heart) (valve) I35.9
  rheumatic I06.9
Apollo B30.3
aponeuroses — *see* Enthesopathy
appendix K38.9
  specified NEC K38.8
aqueous (chamber) H21.9
Arnold-Chiari — *see* Arnold-Chiari disease
arterial I77.9
  occlusive — *see* Occlusion, by site
    due to stricture or stenosis I77.1
  peripheral I73.9
arteriocardiorenal — *see* Hypertension, cardiorenal
arteriolar (generalized) (obliterative) I77.9
arteriorenal — *see* Hypertension, kidney
arteriosclerotic (*see also* Arteriosclerosis)
  cardiovascular — *see* Disease, heart, ischemic,
    atherosclerotic
  coronary (artery) — *see* Disease, heart, ischemic,
    atherosclerotic
  heart — *see* Disease, heart, ischemic, atherosclerotic
artery I77.9
  cerebral I67.9
  coronary I25.10
    with angina pectoris — *see* Arteriosclerosis,
      coronary (artery)
  peripheral I73.9
arthropod-borne NOS (viral) A94
  specified type NEC A93.8
atticoantral, chronic H66.20
  left H66.22
    with right H66.23
  right H66.21
    with left H66.23
auditory canal — *see* Disorder, ear, external
auricle, ear NEC — *see* Disorder, pinna
Australian X A83.4
autoimmune (systemic) NOS M35.9
  hemolytic (cold type) (warm type) D59.1
    drug-induced D59.0
  thyroid E06.3
autoinflammatory M04.9
  NOD2-associated M04.8
  specified type NEC M04.8
aviator's — *see* Effect, adverse, high altitude
Ayerza's (pulmonary artery sclerosis with
    pulmonary hypertension) I27.0
Babington's (familial hemorrhagic telangiectasia)
    I78.0
bacterial A49.9
  specified NEC A48.8
  zoonotic A28.9
    specified type NEC A28.8

Disease — *continued*

Baelz's (cheilitis glandularis apostematosa) K13.0
bagasse J67.1
balloon — *see* Effect, adverse, high altitude
Bang's (brucella abortus) A23.1
Bannister's T78.3 ☑
barometer makers' — *see* Poisoning, mercury
Barraquer (-Simons') (progressive lipodystrophy)
    E88.1
Barrett's — *see* Barrett's, esophagus
Bartholin's gland N75.9
basal ganglia G25.9
  degenerative G23.9
    specified NEC G23.8
  specified NEC G25.89
Basedow's (exophthalmic goiter) — *see*
    Hyperthyroidism, with, goiter (diffuse)
Bateman's B08.1
Batten-Steinert G71.11
Battey A31.0
Beard's (neurasthenia) F48.8
Becker
  idiopathic mural endomyocardial I42.3
  myotonia congenita G71.12
Begbie's (exophthalmic goiter) — *see*
    Hyperthyroidism, with, goiter (diffuse)
behavioral, organic F07.9
Beigel's (white piedra) B36.2
Benson's — *see* Deposit, crystalline
Bernard-Soulier (thrombopathy) D69.1
Bernhardt (-Roth) — *see* Mononeuropathy, lower
    limb, meralgia paresthetica
Biermer's (pernicious anemia) D51.0
bile duct (common) (hepatic) K83.9
  with calculus, stones — *see* Calculus, bile duct
  specified NEC K83.8
biliary (tract) K83.9
  specified NEC K83.8
Billroth's — *see* Spina bifida
bird fancier's J67.2
black lung J60
bladder N32.9
  in (due to)
    schistosomiasis (bilharziasis) B65.0 *[N33]*
  specified NEC N32.89
bleeder's D66
blood D75.9
  forming organs D75.9
  vessel I99.9
Bloodgood's — *see* Mastopathy, cystic
Bodechtel-Guttmann (subacute sclerosing
    panencephalitis) A81.1
bone (*see also* Disorder, bone)
  aluminum M83.4
  fibrocystic NEC
    jaw M27.49
bone-marrow D75.9
Borna A83.9
Bornholm (epidemic pleurodynia) B33.0
Bouchard's (myopathic dilatation of the stomach)
    K31.0
Bouillaud's (rheumatic heart disease) I01.9
Bourneville (-Brissaud) (tuberous sclerosis) Q85.1
Bouveret (-Hoffmann) (paroxysmal tachycardia)
    I47.9
bowel K63.9
  functional K59.9
    psychogenic F45.8
brain G93.9
  arterial, artery I67.9
  arteriosclerotic I67.2
  congenital Q04.9
  degenerative — *see* Degeneration, brain
  inflammatory — *see* Encephalitis
  organic G93.9
    arteriosclerotic I67.2
  parasitic NEC B71.9 *[G94]*
  senile NEC G31.1
  specified NEC G93.89
breast (*see also* Disorder, breast) N64.9
  cystic (chronic) — *see* Mastopathy, cystic
  fibrocystic — *see* Mastopathy, cystic
  Paget's
    female, unspecified side C50.91 ☑
    male, unspecified side C50.92 ☑
  specified NEC N64.89
Breda's — *see* Yaws
Bretonneau's (diphtheritic malignant angina) A36.0
Bright's — *see* Nephritis
  arteriosclerotic — *see* Hypertension, kidney
Brill's (recrudescent typhus) A75.1
Brill-Zinsser (recrudescent typhus) A75.1

Disease — *continued*

Brion-Kayser — *see* Fever, paratyphoid
broad
  beta E78.2
  ligament (noninflammatory) N83.9
    inflammatory — *see* Disease, pelvis,
      inflammatory
    specified NEC N83.8
Brocq-Duhring (dermatitis herpetiformis) L13.0
Brocq's
  meaning
    dermatitis herpetiformis L13.0
    prurigo L28.2
bronchopulmonary J98.4
bronchus NEC J98.09
bronze Addison's E27.1
  tuberculous A18.7
budgerigar fancier's J67.2
bullous L13.9
  chronic of childhood L12.2
  specified NEC L13.8
Buerger's (thromboangiitis obliterans) I73.1
Bürger-Grütz (essential familial hyperlipemia)
    E78.3
bursa — *see* Bursopathy
caisson T70.3 ☑
California — *see* Coccidioidomycosis
capillaries I78.9
  specified NEC I78.8
Carapata A68.0
cardiac — *see* Disease, heart
cardiopulmonary, chronic I27.9
cardiorenal (hepatic) (hypertensive) (vascular) —
    see Hypertension, cardiorenal
cardiovascular (atherosclerotic) I25.10
  with angina pectoris — *see* Arteriosclerosis,
    coronary (artery),
  congenital Q28.9
  newborn P29.9
    specified NEC P29.89
  hypertensive — *see* Hypertension, heart
  renal (hypertensive) — *see* Hypertension,
    cardiorenal
  syphilitic (asymptomatic) A52.00
cartilage — *see* Disorder, cartilage
Castellani's A69.8
Castleman (unicentric) (multicentric) D47.Z2
  HHV-8-associated (*see also* Herpesvirus, human,
    8) D47.Z2
cat-scratch A28.1
Cavare's (familial periodic paralysis) G72.3
cecum K63.9
celiac (adult) (infantile) (with steatorrhea) K90.0
cellular tissue L98.9
central core G71.2
cerebellar, cerebellum — *see* Disease, brain
cerebral (*see also* Disease, brain)
  degenerative — *see* Degeneration, brain
cerebrospinal G96.9
cerebrovascular I67.9
  acute I67.89
    embolic I63.4 ☑
    thrombotic I63.3 ☑
  arteriosclerotic I67.2
  hereditary NEC I67.858
  specified NEC I67.89
cervix (uteri) (noninflammatory) N88.9
  inflammatory — *see* Cervicitis
  specified NEC N88.8
Chabert's A22.9
Chandler's (osteochondritis dissecans, hip) — *see*
    Osteochondritis, dissecans, hip
Charlouis — *see* Yaws
Chédiak-Steinbrinck (-Higashi) (congenital
    gigantism of peroxidase granules) E70.330
chest J98.9
Chiari's (hepatic vein thrombosis) I82.0
Chicago B40.9
Chignon B36.8
chigo, chigoe B88.1
childhood granulomatous D71
Chinese liver fluke B66.1
chlamydial A74.9
  specified NEC A74.89
cholecystic K82.9
choroid H31.9
  specified NEC H31.8
Christmas D67
chronic bullous of childhood L12.2
chylomicron retention E78.3
ciliary body H21.9
  specified NEC H21.89

☑ **Additional character required**

Disease — *continued*
  circulatory (system) NEC I99.8
    newborn P29.9
    syphilitic A52.00
      congenital A50.54
  coagulation factor deficiency (congenital) — *see*
    Defect, coagulation
  coccidioidal — *see* Coccidioidomycosis
  cold
    agglutinin or hemoglobinuria D59.1
      paroxysmal D59.6
    hemagglutinin (chronic) D59.1
  collagen NOS (nonvascular) (vascular) M35.9
    specified NEC M35.8
  colon K63.9
    functional K59.9
      congenital Q43.2
    ischemic (*see also* Ischemia, intestine, acute)
      K55.039
  colonic inflammatory bowel, unclassified (IBDU)
    K52.3
  combined system — *see* Degeneration, combined
  compressed air T70.3 ☑
  Concato's (pericardial polyserositis) A19.9
    nontubercular I31.1
    pleural — *see* Pleurisy, with effusion
  conjunctiva H11.9
    chlamydial A74.0
    specified NEC H11.89
    viral B30.9
      specified NEC B30.8
  connective tissue, systemic (diffuse) M35.9
    in (due to)
      hypogammaglobulinemia D80.1 [M36.8]
      ochronosis E70.29 [M36.8]
    specified NEC M35.8
  Conor and Bruch's (boutonneuse fever) A77.1
  Cooper's — *see* Mastopathy, cystic
  Cori's (glycogenosis III) E74.03
  corkhandler's or corkworker's J67.3
  cornea H18.9
    specified NEC H18.89 ☑
  coronary (artery) — *see* Disease, heart, ischemic,
    atherosclerotic
    congenital Q24.5
    ostial, syphilitic (aortic) (mitral) (pulmonary)
      A52.03
  corpus cavernosum N48.9
    specified NEC N48.89
  Cotugno's — *see* Sciatica
  coxsackie (virus) NEC B34.1
  cranial nerve NOS G52.9
  Creutzfeldt-Jakob — *see* Creutzfeldt-Jakob disease
    or syndrome
  Crocq's (acrocyanosis) I73.89
  Crohn's — *see* Enteritis, regional
  Curschmann G71.11
  cystic
    breast (chronic) — *see* Mastopathy, cystic
    kidney, congenital Q61.9
    liver, congenital Q44.6
    lung J98.4
      congenital Q33.0
  cytomegalic inclusion (generalized) B25.9
    with pneumonia B25.0
    congenital P35.1
  cytomegaloviral B25.9
    specified NEC B25.8
  Czerny's (periodic hydrarthrosis of the knee) — *see*
    Effusion, joint, knee
  Daae (-Finsen) (epidemic pleurodynia) B33.0
  Darling's — *see* Histoplasmosis capsulati
  Débove's (splenomegaly) R16.1
  deer fly — *see* Tularemia
  Degos' I77.89
  demyelinating, demyelinizating (nervous system)
    G37.9
    multiple sclerosis G35
    specified NEC G37.8
  dense deposit (*see also* N00-N07 with fourth
    character .6) N05.6
  deposition, hydroxyapatite — *see* Disease,
    hydroxyapatite deposition
  de Quervain's (tendon sheath) M65.4
    thyroid (subacute granulomatous thyroiditis) E06.1
  Devergie's (pityriasis rubra pilaris) L44.0
  Devic's G36.0
  diaphorase deficiency D74.0
  diaphragm J98.6
  diarrheal, infectious NEC A09
  digestive system K92.9
    specified NEC K92.89

Disease — *continued*
  disc, degenerative — *see* Degeneration,
    intervertebral disc
  discogenic (*see also* Displacement, intervertebral
    disc NEC)
    with myelopathy — *see* Disorder, disc, with,
      myelopathy
  diverticular — *see* Diverticula
  Dubois (thymus) A50.59 [E35]
  Duchenne-Griesinger G71.01
  Duchenne's
    muscular dystrophy G71.01
    pseudohypertrophy, muscles G71.01
  ductless glands E34.9
  duodenum K31.9
    specified NEC K31.89
  Dupré's (meningism) R29.1
  Dupuytren's (muscle contracture) M72.0
  Durand-Nicholas-Favre (climatic bubo) A55
  Duroziez's (congenital mitral stenosis) Q23.2
  ear — *see* Disorder, ear
  Eberth's — *see* Fever, typhoid
  Ebola (virus) A98.4
  Ebstein's heart Q22.5
  Echinococcus — *see* Echinococcus
  echovirus NEC B34.1
  Eddowes' (brittle bones and blue sclera) Q78.0
  edentulous (alveolar) ridge K06.9
    specified NEC K06.8
  Edsall's T67.2 ☑
  Eichstedt's (pityriasis versicolor) B36.0
  Eisenmenger's (irreversible) I27.83
  Ellis-van Creveld (chondroectodermal dysplasia)
    Q77.6
  end stage renal (ESRD) N18.6
    due to hypertension I12.0
  endocrine glands or system NEC E34.9
  endomyocardial (eosinophilic) I42.3
  English (rickets) E55.0
  enteroviral, enterovirus NEC B34.1
    central nervous system NEC A88.8
  epidemic B99.9
    specified NEC B99.8
  epididymis N50.9
  Erb (-Landouzy) G71.02
  Erdheim-Chester (ECD) E88.89
  esophagus K22.9
    functional K22.4
    psychogenic F45.8
    specified NEC K22.8
  Eulenburg's (congenital paramyotonia) G71.19
  eustachian tube — *see* Disorder, eustachian tube
  external
    auditory canal — *see* Disorder, ear, external
    ear — *see* Disorder, ear, external
  extrapyramidal G25.9
    specified NEC G25.89
  eye H57.9
    anterior chamber H21.9
    inflammatory NEC H57.89
    muscle (external) — *see* Strabismus
    specified NEC H57.89
    syphilitic — *see* Oculopathy, syphilitic
  eyeball H44.9
    specified NEC H44.89
  eyelid — *see* Disorder, eyelid
    specified NEC — *see* Disorder, eyelid, specified
      type NEC
  eyeworm of Africa B74.3
  facial nerve (seventh) G51.9
    newborn (birth injury) P11.3
  Fahr (of brain) G23.8
  Fahr Volhard (of kidney) I12. ☑
  fallopian tube (noninflammatory) N83.9
    inflammatory — *see* Salpingo-oophoritis
    specified NEC N83.8
  familial periodic paralysis G72.3
  Fanconi's (congenital pancytopenia) D61.09
  fascia NEC (*see also* Disorder, muscle)
    inflammatory — *see* Myositis
    specified NEC M62.89
  Fauchard's (periodontitis) — *see* Periodontitis
  Favre-Durand-Nicolas (climatic bubo) A55
  Fede's K14.0
  Feer's — *see* Poisoning, mercury
  female pelvic inflammatory (*see also* Disease, pelvis,
    inflammatory) N73.9
    syphilitic (secondary) A51.42
    tuberculous A18.17
  Fernels' (aortic aneurysm) I71.9
  fibrocaseous of lung — *see* Tuberculosis, pulmonary

Disease — *continued*
  fibrocystic — *see* Fibrocystic disease
  Fiedler's (leptospiral jaundice) A27.0
  fifth B08.3
  file-cutter's — *see* Poisoning, lead
  fish-skin Q80.9
    acquired L85.0
  Flajani (-Basedow) (exophthalmic goiter) — *see*
    Hyperthyroidism, with, goiter (diffuse)
  flax-dresser's J66.1
  fluke — *see* Infestation, fluke
  foot and mouth B08.8
  foot process N04.9
  Forbes' (glycogenosis III) E74.03
  Fordyce-Fox (apocrine miliaria) L75.2
  Fordyce's (ectopic sebaceous glands) (mouth)
    Q38.6
  Forestier's (rhizomelic pseudopolyarthritis) M35.3
    meaning ankylosing hyperostosis — *see*
      Hyperostosis, ankylosing
  Fothergill's
    neuralgia — *see* Neuralgia, trigeminal
    scarlatina anginosa A38.9
  Fournier (gangrene) N49.3
    female N76.89
  fourth B08.8
  Fox (-Fordyce) (apocrine miliaria) L75.2
  Francis' — *see* Tularemia
  Franklin C88.2
  Frei's (climatic bubo) A55
  Friedreich's
    combined systemic or ataxia G11.1
    myoclonia G25.3
  frontal sinus — *see* Sinusitis, frontal
  fungus NEC B49
  Gaisböck's (polycythemia hypertonica) D75.1
  gallbladder K82.9
    calculus — *see* Calculus, gallbladder
    cholecystitis — *see* Cholecystitis
    cholesterolosis K82.4
    fistula — *see* Fistula, gallbladder
    hydrops K82.1
    obstruction — *see* Obstruction, gallbladder
    perforation K82.2
    specified NEC K82.8
  gamma heavy chain C88.2
  Gamna's (siderotic splenomegaly) D73.2
  Gamstorp's (adynamia episodica hereditaria) G72.3
  Gandy-Nanta (siderotic splenomegaly) D73.2
  ganister J62.8
  gastric — *see* Disease, stomach
  gastroesophageal reflux (GERD) K21.9
    with esophagitis K21.0
  gastrointestinal (tract) K92.9
    amyloid E85.4
    functional K59.9
      psychogenic F45.8
    specified NEC K92.89
  Gee (-Herter) (-Heubner) (-Thaysen) (nontropical
    sprue) K90.0
  genital organs
    female N94.9
    male N50.9
  Gerhardt's (erythromelalgia) I73.81
  Gibert's (pityriasis rosea) L42
  Gierke's (glycogenosis I) E74.01
  Gilles de la Tourette's (motor-verbal tic) F95.2
  gingiva K06.9
    plaque induced K05.00
    specified NEC K06.8
  gland (lymph) I89.9
  Glanzmann's (hereditary hemorrhagic
    thrombasthenia) D69.1
  glass-blower's (cataract) — *see* Cataract, specified
    NEC
  salivary gland hypertrophy K11.1
  Glisson's — *see* Rickets
  globe H44.9
    specified NEC H44.89
  glomerular (*see also* Glomerulonephritis)
    with edema — *see* Nephrosis
    acute — *see* Nephritis, acute
    chronic — *see* Nephritis, chronic
    minimal change N05.0
    rapidly progressive N01.9
  glycogen storage E74.00
    Andersen's E74.09
    Cori's E74.03
    Forbes' E74.03
    generalized E74.00
    glucose-6-phosphatase deficiency E74.01
    heart E74.02 [I43]

Disease

Disease — *continued*
  glycogen storage — *continued*
    hepatorenal E74.09
    Hers' E74.09
    liver and kidney E74.09
    McArdle's E74.04
    muscle phosphofructokinase E74.09
    myocardium E74.02 *[I43]*
    Pompe's E74.02
    Tauri's E74.09
    type 0 E74.09
    type I E74.01
    type II E74.02
    type III E74.03
    type IV E74.09
    type V E74.04
    type VI-XI E74.09
    Von Gierke's E74.01
  Goldstein's (familial hemorrhagic telangiectasia) I78.0
  gonococcal NOS A54.9
  graft-versus-host (GVH) D89.813
    acute D89.810
    acute on chronic D89.812
    chronic D89.811
  grainhandler's J67.8
  granulomatous (childhood) (chronic) D71
  Graves' (exophthalmic goiter) — *see*
    Hyperthyroidism, with, goiter (diffuse)
  Griesinger's — *see* Ancylostomiasis
  Grisel's M43.6
  Gruby's (tinea tonsurans) B35.0
  Guillain-Barré G61.0
  Guinon's (motor-verbal tic) F95.2
  gum K06.9
  gynecological N94.9
  H (Hartnup's) E72.02
  Haff — *see* Poisoning, mercury
  Hageman (congenital factor XII deficiency) D68.2
  hair (color) (shaft) L67.9
    follicles L73.9
      specified NEC L73.8
  Hamman's (spontaneous mediastinal emphysema) J98.2
  hand, foot and mouth B08.4
  Hansen's — *see* Leprosy
  Hantavirus, with pulmonary manifestations B33.4
    with renal manifestations A98.5
  Harada's H30.81 ☑
  Hartnup (pellagra-cerebellar ataxia-renal aminoaciduria) E72.02
  Hart's (pellagra-cerebellar ataxia-renal aminoaciduria) E72.02
  Hashimoto's (struma lymphomatosa) E06.3
  Hb — *see* Disease, hemoglobin
  heart (organic) I51.9
    with
      pulmonary edema (acute) (*see also* Failure, ventricular, left) I50.1
      rheumatic fever (conditions in I00)
        active I01.9
          with chorea I02.0
          specified NEC I01.8
        inactive or quiescent (with chorea) I09.9
          specified NEC I09.89
    amyloid E85.4 *[I43]*
    aortic (valve) I35.9
    arteriosclerotic or sclerotic (senile) — *see* Disease, heart, ischemic, atherosclerotic
    artery, arterial — *see* Disease, heart, ischemic, atherosclerotic
    beer drinkers' I42.6
    beriberi (wet) E51.12
    black I27.0
    congenital Q24.9
      cyanotic Q24.9
      specified NEC Q24.8
    coronary — *see* Disease, heart, ischemic
    cryptogenic I51.9
    fibroid — *see* Myocarditis
    functional I51.89
      psychogenic F45.8
    glycogen storage E74.02 *[I43]*
    gonococcal A54.83
    hypertensive — *see* Hypertension, heart
    hyperthyroid (*see also* Hyperthyroidism) E05.90 *[I43]*
      with thyroid storm E05.91 *[I43]*
    ischemic (chronic or with a stated duration of over 4 weeks) I25.9
      atherosclerotic (of) I25.10
        with angina pectoris — *see* Arteriosclerosis, coronary (artery)

Disease — *continued*
  heart — *continued*
    coronary artery bypass graft — *see* Arteriosclerosis, coronary (artery),
    cardiomyopathy I25.5
    diagnosed on ECG or other special investigation, but currently presenting no symptoms I25.6
    silent I25.6
    specified form NEC I25.89
    kyphoscoliotic I27.1
    meningococcal A39.50
      endocarditis A39.51
      myocarditis A39.52
      pericarditis A39.53
    mitral I05.9
      specified NEC I05.8
    muscular — *see* Degeneration, myocardial
    psychogenic (functional) F45.8
    pulmonary (chronic) I27.9
      in schistosomiasis B65.9 *[I52]*
      specified NEC I27.89
    rheumatic (chronic) (inactive) (old) (quiescent) (with chorea) I09.9
      active or acute I01.9
        with chorea (acute) (rheumatic) (Sydenham's) I02.0
      specified NEC I09.89
    senile — *see* Myocarditis
    syphilitic A52.06
      aortic A52.03
        aneurysm A52.01
      congenital A50.54 *[I52]*
    thyrotoxic (*see also* Thyrotoxicosis) E05.90 *[I43]*
      with thyroid storm E05.91 *[I43]*
    valve, valvular (obstructive) (regurgitant) (*see also* Endocarditis)
      congenital NEC Q24.8
        pulmonary Q22.3
    vascular — *see* Disease, cardiovascular
  heavy chain NEC C88.2
    alpha C88.3
    gamma C88.2
    mu C88.2
  Hebra's
    pityriasis
      maculata et circinata L42
      rubra pilaris L44.0
    prurigo L28.2
  hematopoietic organs D75.9
  hemoglobin or Hb
    abnormal (mixed) NEC D58.2
      with thalassemia D56.9
    AS genotype D57.3
    Bart's D56.0
    C (Hb-C) D58.2
      with other abnormal hemoglobin NEC D58.2
      elliptocytosis D58.1
      Hb-S D57.2 ☑
      sickle-cell D57.2 ☑
      thalassemia D56.8
    Constant Spring D58.2
    D (Hb-D) D58.2
    E (Hb-E) D58.2
    E-beta thalassemia D56.5
    elliptocytosis D58.1
    H (Hb-H) (thalassemia) D56.0
      with other abnormal hemoglobin NEC D56.9
      Constant Spring D56.0
    I thalassemia D56.9
    M D74.0
    S or SS D57.1
    SC D57.2 ☑
    SD D57.8 ☑
    SE D57.8 ☑
    spherocytosis D58.0
    unstable, hemolytic D58.2
  hemolytic (newborn) P55.9
    autoimmune (cold type) (warm type) D59.1
    drug-induced D59.0
    due to or with
      incompatibility
        ABO (blood group) P55.1
        blood (group) (Duffy) (K) (Kell) (Kidd) (Lewis) (M)(s) NEC P55.8
        Rh (blood group) (factor) P55.0
        Rh negative mother P55.0
    specified type NEC P55.8
    unstable hemoglobin D58.2
  hemorrhagic D69.9
    newborn P53
  Henoch (-Schönlein) (purpura nervosa) D69.0

Disease — *continued*
  hepatic — *see* Disease, liver
  hepatobiliary K83.9
    toxic K71.9
  hepatolenticular E83.01
  heredodegenerative NEC
    spinal cord G95.89
  herpesviral, disseminated B00.7
  Hers' (glycogenosis VI) E74.09
  Herter (-Gee) (-Heubner) (nontropical sprue) K90.0
  Heubner-Herter (nontropical sprue) K90.0
  high fetal gene or hemoglobin thalassemia D56.9
  Hildenbrand's — *see* Typhus
  hip (joint) M25.9
    congenital Q65.89
    suppurative M00.9
    tuberculous A18.02
  His (-Werner) (trench fever) A79.0
  Hodgson's I71.2
    ruptured I71.1
  Holla — *see* Spherocytosis
  hookworm B76.9
    specified NEC B76.8
  host-versus-graft D89.813
    acute D89.810
    acute on chronic D89.812
    chronic D89.811
  human immunodeficiency virus (HIV) B20
  Huntington's G10
    with dementia G10 *[F02.80]*
  Hutchinson's (cheiropompholyx) — *see* Hutchinson's disease
  hyaline (diffuse) (generalized)
    membrane (lung) (newborn) P22.0
      adult J80
  hydatid — *see* Echinococcus
  hydroxyapatite deposition M11.00
    ankle M11.07 ☑
    elbow M11.02 ☑
    foot joint M11.07 ☑
    hand joint M11.04 ☑
    hip M11.05 ☑
    knee M11.06 ☑
    multiple site M11.09
    shoulder M11.01 ☑
    vertebra M11.08
    wrist M11.03 ☑
  hyperkinetic — *see* Hyperkinesia
  hypertensive — *see* Hypertension
  hypophysis E23.7
  Iceland G93.3
  I-cell E77.0
  immune D89.9
  immunoproliferative (malignant) C88.9
    small intestinal C88.3
    specified NEC C88.8
  inclusion B25.9
    salivary gland B25.9
  infectious, infective B99.9
    congenital P37.9
      specified NEC P37.8
      viral P35.9
        specified type NEC P35.8
    specified NEC B99.8
  inflammatory
    penis N48.29
      abscess N48.21
      cellulitis N48.22
    prepuce N47.7
      balanoposthitis N47.6
    tubo-ovarian — *see* Salpingo-oophoritis
  intervertebral disc (*see also* Disorder, disc)
    with myelopathy — *see* Disorder, disc, with, myelopathy
    cervical, cervicothoracic — *see* Disorder, disc, cervical
    with
      myelopathy — *see* Disorder, disc, cervical, with myelopathy
      neuritis, radiculitis or radiculopathy — *see* Disorder, disc, cervical, with neuritis
      specified NEC — *see* Disorder, disc, cervical, specified type NEC
    lumbar (with)
      myelopathy M51.06
      neuritis, radiculitis, radiculopathy or sciatica M51.16
      specified NEC M51.86
    lumbosacral (with)
      neuritis, radiculitis, radiculopathy or sciatica M51.17
      specified NEC M51.87

Disease — *continued*
- intervertebral disc — *continued*
  - specified NEC — *see* Disorder, disc, specified NEC
  - thoracic (with)
    - myelopathy M51.04
    - neuritis, radiculitis or radiculopathy M51.14
    - specified NEC M51.84
  - thoracolumbar (with)
    - myelopathy M51.05
    - neuritis, radiculitis or radiculopathy M51.15
    - specified NEC M51.85
- intestine K63.9
  - functional K59.9
    - psychogenic F45.8
    - specified NEC K59.8
  - organic K63.9
  - protozoal A07.9
  - specified NEC K63.89
- iris H21.9
  - specified NEC H21.89
- iron metabolism or storage E83.10
- island (scrub typhus) A75.3
- itai-itai — *see* Poisoning, cadmium
- Jakob-Creutzfeldt — *see* Creutzfeldt-Jakob disease or syndrome
- jaw M27.9
  - fibrocystic M27.49
  - specified NEC M27.8
- jigger B88.1
- joint (*see also* Disorder, joint)
  - Charcot's — *see* Arthropathy, neuropathic (Charcot)
  - degenerative — *see* Osteoarthritis
    - multiple M15.9
    - spine — *see* Spondylosis
  - hypertrophic — *see* Osteoarthritis
  - sacroiliac M53.3
  - specified NEC — *see* Disorder, joint, specified type NEC
  - spine NEC — *see* Dorsopathy
  - suppurative — *see* Arthritis, pyogenic or pyemic
- Jourdain's (acute gingivitis) K05.00
  - nonplaque induced K05.01
  - plaque induced K05.00
- Kaschin-Beck (endemic polyarthritis) M12.10
  - ankle M12.17 ☑
  - elbow M12.12 ☑
  - foot joint M12.17 ☑
  - hand joint M12.14 ☑
  - hip M12.15 ☑
  - knee M12.16 ☑
  - multiple site M12.19
  - shoulder M12.11 ☑
  - vertebra M12.18
  - wrist M12.13 ☑
- Katayama B65.2
- Kedani (scrub typhus) A75.3
- Keshan E59
- kidney (functional) (pelvis) N28.9
  - chronic N18.9
    - hypertensive — *see* Hypertension, kidney
    - stage 1 N18.1
    - stage 2 (mild) N18.2
    - stage 3 (moderate) N18.3
    - stage 4 (severe) N18.4
    - stage 5 N18.5
  - complicating pregnancy — *see* Pregnancy, complicated by, renal disease
  - cystic (congenital) Q61.9
  - diabetic — *see* E08-E13 with .22
  - fibrocystic (congenital) Q61.8
  - hypertensive — *see* Hypertension, kidney
  - in (due to)
    - schistosomiasis (bilharziasis) B65.9 [*N29*]
  - multicystic Q61.4
  - polycystic Q61.3
    - adult type Q61.2
    - childhood type NEC Q61.19
      - collecting duct dilatation Q61.11
- Kimmelstiel (-Wilson) (intercapillary polycystic (congenital) glomerulosclerosis) — *see* E08-E13 with .21
- Kimura D21.9
  - specified site (*see* Neoplasm, connective tissue benign)
- Kinnier Wilson's (hepatolenticular degeneration) E83.01
- kissing — *see* Mononucleosis, infectious
- Klebs' (*see also* Glomerulonephritis) N05. ☑
- Klippel-Feil (brevicollis) Q76.1
- Köhler-Pellegrini-Stieda (calcification, knee joint) — *see* Bursitis, tibial collateral

Disease — *continued*
- Kok Q89.8
- König's (osteochondritis dissecans) — *see* Osteochondritis, dissecans
- Korsakoff's (nonalcoholic) F04
  - alcoholic F10.96
    - with dependence F10.26
- Kostmann's (infantile genetic agranulocytosis) D70.0
- kuru A81.81
- Kyasanur Forest A98.2
- labyrinth, ear — *see* Disorder, ear, inner
- lacrimal system — *see* Disorder, lacrimal system
- Lafora's — *see* Epilepsy, generalized, idiopathic
- Lancereaux-Mathieu (leptospiral jaundice) A27.0
- Landry's G61.0
- Larrey-Weil (leptospiral jaundice) A27.0
- larynx J38.7
- legionnaires' A48.1
  - nonpneumonic A48.2
- Lenegre's I44.2
- lens H27.9
  - specified NEC H27.8
- Lev's (acquired complete heart block) I44.2
- Lewy body (dementia) G31.83 [*F02.80*]
  - with behavioral disturbance G31.83 [*F02.81*]
- Lichtheim's (subacute combined sclerosis with pernicious anemia) D51.0
- Lightwood's (renal tubular acidosis) N25.89
- Lignac's (cystinosis) E72.04
- lip K13.0
- lipid-storage E75.6
  - specified NEC E75.5
- Lipschütz's N76.6
- liver (chronic) (organic) K76.9
  - alcoholic (chronic) K70.9
    - acute — *see* Disease, liver, alcoholic, hepatitis
    - cirrhosis K70.30
      - with ascites K70.31
    - failure K70.40
      - with coma K70.41
    - fatty liver K70.0
    - fibrosis K70.2
    - hepatitis K70.10
      - with ascites K70.11
    - sclerosis K70.2
  - cystic, congenital Q44.6
  - drug-induced (idiosyncratic) (toxic) (predictable) (unpredictable) — *see* Disease, liver, toxic
  - end stage K72.90
    - due to hepatitis — *see* Hepatitis
  - fatty, nonalcoholic (NAFLD) K76.0
    - alcoholic K70.0
  - fibrocystic (congenital) Q44.6
  - fluke
    - Chinese B66.1
    - oriental B66.1
    - sheep B66.3
  - gestational alloimmune (GALD) P78.84
  - glycogen storage E74.09 [*K77*]
  - in (due to)
    - schistosomiasis (bilharziasis) B65.9 [*K77*]
  - inflammatory K75.9
    - alcoholic K70.1 ☑
    - specified NEC K75.89
  - polycystic (congenital) Q44.6
  - toxic K71.9
    - with
      - cholestasis K71.0
      - cirrhosis (liver) K71.7
      - fibrosis (liver) K71.7
      - focal nodular hyperplasia K71.8
      - hepatic granuloma K71.8
      - hepatic necrosis K71.10
        - with coma K71.11
      - hepatitis NEC K71.6
        - acute K71.2
        - chronic
          - active K71.50
            - with ascites K71.51
          - lobular K71.4
          - persistent K71.3
        - lupoid K71.50
          - with ascites K71.51
      - peliosis hepatis K71.8
      - veno-occlusive disease (VOD) of liver K71.8
    - veno-occlusive K76.5
- Lobo's (keloid blastomycosis) B48.0
- Lobstein's (brittle bones and blue sclera) Q78.0
- Ludwig's (submaxillary cellulitis) K12.2
- lumbosacral region M53.87

Disease — *continued*
- lung J98.4
  - black J60
  - congenital Q33.9
  - cystic J98.4
    - congenital Q33.0
  - fibroid (chronic) — *see* Fibrosis, lung
  - fluke B66.4
    - oriental B66.4
  - in
    - amyloidosis E85.4 [*J99*]
    - sarcoidosis D86.0
    - Sjögren's syndrome M35.02
    - systemic
      - lupus erythematosus M32.13
      - sclerosis M34.81
  - interstitial J84.9
    - of childhood, specified NEC J84.848
    - respiratory bronchiolitis J84.115
    - specified NEC J84.89
  - obstructive (chronic) J43.9
    - with
      - acute
        - bronchitis J44.0
        - exacerbation NEC J44.1
        - lower respiratory infection J44.0
      - alveolitis, allergic J67.9
      - asthma J44.9
      - bronchiectasis J47.9
        - with
          - exacerbation (acute) J47.1
          - lower respiratory infection J47.0
      - bronchitis J44.9
        - with
          - exacerbation (acute) J44.1
          - lower respiratory infection J44.0
      - emphysema J43.9
      - hypersensitivity pneumonitis J67.9
    - decompensated J44.1
      - with
        - exacerbation (acute) J44.1
  - polycystic J98.4
    - congenital Q33.0
  - rheumatoid (diffuse) (interstitial) — *see* Rheumatoid, lung
- Lutembacher's (atrial septal defect with mitral stenosis) Q21.1
- Lyme A69.20
- lymphatic (gland) (system) (channel) (vessel) I89.9
- lymphoproliferative D47.9
  - specified NEC D47.Z9
  - T-gamma D47.Z9
  - X-linked D82.3
- Magitot's M27.2
- malarial — *see* Malaria
- malignant (*see also* Neoplasm, malignant, by site)
- Manson's B65.1
- maple bark J67.6
- maple-syrup-urine E71.0
- Marburg (virus) A98.3
- Marion's (bladder neck obstruction) N32.0
- Marsh's (exophthalmic goiter) — *see* Hyperthyroidism, with, goiter (diffuse)
- mastoid (process) — *see* Disorder, ear, middle
- Mathieu's (leptospiral jaundice) A27.0
- Maxcy's A75.2
- McArdle (-Schmid-Pearson) (glycogenosis V) E74.04
- mediastinum J98.59
- medullary center (idiopathic) (respiratory) G93.89
- Meige's (chronic hereditary edema) Q82.0
- meningococcal — *see* Infection, meningococcal
- mental F99
  - organic F09
- mesenchymal M35.9
- mesenteric embolic (*see also* Ischemia, intestine, acute) K55.039
- metabolic, metabolism E88.9
  - bilirubin E80.7
- metal-polisher's J62.8
- metastatic (*see also* Neoplasm, secondary, by site) C79.9
- microvascular - code to condition
- microvillus
  - atrophy Q43.8
  - inclusion (MVD) Q43.8
- middle ear — *see* Disorder, ear, middle
- Mikulicz' (dryness of mouth, absent or decreased lacrimation) K11.8
- Milroy's (chronic hereditary edema) Q82.0
- Minamata — *see* Poisoning, mercury
- minicore G71.2
- Minor's G95.19

Disease

Disease — *continued*

Minot's (hemorrhagic disease, newborn) P53
Minot-von Willebrand-Jürgens (angiohemophilia) D68.0
Mitchell's (erythromelalgia) I73.81
mitral (valve) I05.9
  nonrheumatic I34.9
mixed connective tissue M35.1
moldy hay J67.0 ☑
Monge's T70.29 ☑
Morgagni-Adams-Stokes (syncope with heart block) I45.9
Morgagni's (syndrome) (hyperostosis frontalis interna) M85.2
Morton's (with metatarsalgia) — *see* Lesion, nerve, plantar
Morvan's G60.8
motor neuron (bulbar) (mixed type) (spinal) G12.20
  amyotrophic lateral sclerosis G12.21
  familial G12.24
  progressive bulbar palsy G12.22
  specified NEC G12.29
moyamoya I67.5
mu heavy chain disease C88.2
multicore G71.2
muscle (*see also* Disorder, muscle)
  inflammatory — *see* Myositis
  ocular (external) — *see* Strabismus
musculoskeletal system, soft tissue (*see also* Disorder, soft tissue)
  specified NEC — *see* Disorder, soft tissue, specified type NEC
mushroom workers' J67.5
mycotic B49
myelodysplastic, not classified C94.6
myeloproliferative, not classified C94.6
  chronic D47.1
myocardium, myocardial (*see also* Degeneration, myocardial) I51.5
  primary (idiopathic) I42.9
myoneural G70.9
Naegeli's D69.1
nails L60.9
  specified NEC L60.8
Nairobi (sheep virus) A93.8
nasal J34.9
nemaline body G71.2
nerve — *see* Disorder, nerve
nervous system G98.8
  autonomic G90.9
  central G96.9
    specified NEC G96.8
  congenital Q07.9
  parasympathetic G90.9
  specified NEC G98.8
  sympathetic G90.9
  vegetative G90.9
neuromuscular system G70.9
Newcastle B30.8
Nicolas (-Durand)-Favre (climatic bubo) A55
nipple N64.9
  Paget's C50.01 ☑
    female C50.01 ☑
    male C50.02 ☑
Nishimoto (-Takeuchi) I67.5
nonarthropod-borne NOS (viral) B34.9
  enterovirus NEC B34.1
nonautoimmune hemolytic D59.4
  drug-induced D59.2
Nonne-Milroy-Meige (chronic hereditary edema) Q82.0
nose J34.9
nucleus pulposus — *see* Disorder, disc
nutritional E63.9
oast-house-urine E72.19
  ocular
    herpesviral B00.50
    zoster B02.30
obliterative vascular I77.1
Ohara's — *see* Tularemia
Opitz's (congestive splenomegaly) D73.2
Oppenheim-Urbach (necrobiosis lipoidica diabeticorum) — *see* E08-E13 with .620
optic nerve NEC — *see* Disorder, nerve, optic
orbit — *see* Disorder, orbit
Oriental liver fluke B66.1
Oriental lung fluke B66.4
Ormond's N13.5
Oropouche virus A93.0
Osler-Rendu (familial hemorrhagic telangiectasia) I78.0
osteofibrocystic E21.0

Disease — *continued*

Otto's M24.7
outer ear — *see* Disorder, ear, external
ovary (noninflammatory) N83.9
  cystic N83.20 ☑
  inflammatory — *see* Salpingo-oophoritis
  polycystic E28.2
  specified NEC N83.8
Owren's (congenital) — *see* Defect, coagulation
pancreas K86.9
  cystic K86.2
  fibrocystic E84.9
  specified NEC K86.89
panvalvular I08.9
  specified NEC I08.8
parametrium (noninflammatory) N83.9
parasitic B89
  cerebral NEC B71.9 *[G94]*
  intestinal NOS B82.9
  mouth B37.0
  skin NOS B88.9
  specified type — *see* Infestation
  tongue B37.0
parathyroid (gland) E21.5
  specified NEC E21.4
Parkinson's G20
parodontal K05.6
Parrot's (syphilitic osteochondritis) A50.02
Parry's (exophthalmic goiter) — *see* Hyperthyroidism, with, goiter (diffuse)
Parson's (exophthalmic goiter) — *see* Hyperthyroidism, with, goiter (diffuse)
Paxton's (white piedra) B36.2
pearl-worker's — *see* Osteomyelitis, specified type NEC
Pellegrini-Stieda (calcification, knee joint) — *see* Bursitis, tibial collateral
pelvis, pelvic
  female NOS N94.9
    specified NEC N94.89
  gonococcal (acute) (chronic) A54.24
  inflammatory (female) N73.9
    acute N73.0
    chlamydial A56.11
    chronic N73.1
    specified NEC N73.8
    syphilitic (secondary) A51.42
      late A52.76
    tuberculous A18.17
  organ, female N94.9
  peritoneum, female NEC N94.89
penis N48.9
  inflammatory N48.29
    abscess N48.21
    cellulitis N48.22
  specified NEC N48.89
periapical tissues NOS K04.90
periodontal K05.6
  specified NEC K05.5
periosteum — *see* Disorder, bone, specified type NEC
peripheral
  arterial I73.9
  autonomic nervous system G90.9
  nerves — *see* Polyneuropathy
  vascular NOS I73.9
peritoneum K66.9
  pelvic, female NEC N94.89
  specified NEC K66.8
persistent mucosal (middle ear) H66.20
  left H66.22
    with right H66.23
  right H66.21
    with left H66.23
Petit's — *see* Hernia, abdomen, specified site NEC
pharynx J39.2
  specified NEC J39.2
Phocas' — *see* Mastopathy, cystic
photochromogenic (acid-fast bacilli) (pulmonary) A31.0
  nonpulmonary A31.9
Pick's G31.01 *[F02.80]*
  with behavioral disturbance G31.01 *[F02.81]*
  brain G31.01 *[F02.80]*
    with behavioral disturbance G31.01 *[F02.81]*
  of pericardium (pericardial pseudocirrhosis of liver) I31.1
pigeon fancier's J67.2
pineal gland E34.8
pink — *see* Poisoning, mercury
Pinkus' (lichen nitidus) L44.1
pinworm B80

Disease — *continued*

Piry virus A93.8
pituitary (gland) E23.7
pituitary-snuff-taker's J67.8
pleura (cavity) J94.9
  specified NEC J94.8
pneumatic drill (hammer) T75.21 ☑
Pollitzer's (hidradenitis suppurativa) L73.2
polycystic
  kidney or renal Q61.3
    adult type Q61.2
    childhood type NEC Q61.19
      collecting duct dilatation Q61.11
  liver or hepatic Q44.6
  lung or pulmonary J98.4
    congenital Q33.0
  ovary, ovaries E28.2
  spleen Q89.09
polyethylene T84.05 ☑
Pompe's (glycogenosis II) E74.02
Posadas-Wernicke B38.9
Potain's (pulmonary edema) — *see* Edema, lung
prepuce N47.8
  inflammatory N47.7
    balanoposthitis N47.6
Pringle's (tuberous sclerosis) Q85.1
prion, central nervous system A81.9
  specified NEC A81.89
prostate N42.9
  specified NEC N42.89
protozoal B64
  acanthamebiasis — *see* Acanthamebiasis
  African trypanosomiasis — *see* African trypanosomiasis
  babesiosis B60.0
  Chagas disease — *see* Chagas disease
  intestine, intestinal A07.9
  leishmaniasis — *see* Leishmaniasis
  malaria — *see* Malaria
  naegleriasis B60.2
  pneumocystosis B59
  specified organism NEC B60.8
  toxoplasmosis — *see* Toxoplasmosis
pseudo-Hurler's E77.0
psychiatric F99
psychotic — *see* Psychosis
Puente's (simple glandular cheilitis) K13.0
puerperal (*see also* Puerperal) O90.89
pulmonary (*see also* Disease, lung)
  artery I28.9
  chronic obstructive J44.9
    with
      acute bronchitis J44.0
      exacerbation (acute) J44.1
      lower respiratory infection (acute) J44.0
    decompensated J44.1
      with
        exacerbation (acute) J44.1
  heart I27.9
    specified NEC I27.89
  hypertensive (vascular) (*see also* Hypertension, pulmonary) I27.20
    primary (idiopathic) I27.0
  valve I37.9
    rheumatic I09.89
pulp (dental) NOS K04.90
pulseless M31.4
Putnam's (subacute combined sclerosis with pernicious anemia) D51.0
Pyle (-Cohn) (metaphyseal dysplasia) Q78.5
ragpicker's or ragsorter's A22.1
Raynaud's — *see* Raynaud's disease
reactive airway — *see* Asthma
Reclus' (cystic) — *see* Mastopathy, cystic
rectum K62.9
  specified NEC K62.89
Refsum's (heredopathia atactica polyneuritiformis) G60.1
renal (functional) (pelvis) (*see also* Disease, kidney) N28.9
  with
    edema — *see* Nephrosis
    glomerular lesion — *see* Glomerulonephritis
      with edema — *see* Nephrosis
    interstitial nephritis N12
  acute N28.9
  chronic (*see also* Disease, kidney, chronic) N18.9
  cystic, congenital Q61.9
  diabetic — *see* E08-E13 with .22
  end-stage (failure) N18.6
    due to hypertension I12.0
  fibrocystic (congenital) Q61.8

Disease — *continued*
renal — *continued*
hypertensive — *see* Hypertension, kidney
lupus M32.14
phosphate-losing (tubular) N25.0
polycystic (congenital) Q61.3
adult type Q61.2
childhood type NEC Q61.19
collecting duct dilatation Q61.11
rapidly progressive N01.9
subacute N01.9
Rendu-Osler-Weber (familial hemorrhagic
telangiectasia) I78.0
renovascular (arteriosclerotic) — *see* Hypertension,
kidney
respiratory (tract) J98.9
acute or subacute NOS J06.9
due to
chemicals, gases, fumes or vapors (inhalation)
J68.3
external agent J70.9
specified NEC J70.8
radiation J70.0
smoke inhalation J70.5
noninfectious J39.8
chronic NOS J98.9
due to
chemicals, gases, fumes or vapors J68.4
external agent J70.9
specified NEC J70.8
radiation J70.1
newborn P27.9
specified NEC P27.8
due to
chemicals, gases, fumes or vapors J68.9
acute or subacute NEC J68.3
chronic J68.4
external agent J70.9
specified NEC J70.8
newborn P28.9
specified type NEC P28.89
upper J39.9
acute or subacute J06.9
noninfectious NEC J39.8
specified NEC J39.8
streptococcal J06.9
retina, retinal H35.9
Batten's or Batten-Mayou E75.4 *[H36]*
specified NEC H35.89
rheumatoid — *see* Arthritis, rheumatoid
rickettsial NOS A79.9
specified type NEC A79.89
Riga (-Fede) (cachectic aphthae) K14.0
Riggs' (compound periodontitis) — *see*
Periodontitis
Ritter's L00
Rivalta's (cervicofacial actinomycosis) A42.2
Robles' (onchocerciasis) B73.01
Roger's (congenital interventricular septal defect)
Q21.0
Rosenthal's (factor XI deficiency) D68.1
Rossbach's (hyperchlorhydria) K31.89
psychogenic F45.8
Ross River B33.1
Rotes Quérol — *see* Hyperostosis, ankylosing
Roth (-Bernhardt) — *see* Mononeuropathy, lower
limb, meralgia paresthetica
Runeberg's (progressive pernicious anemia) D51.0
sacroiliac NEC M53.3
salivary gland or duct K11.9
inclusion B25.9
specified NEC K11.8
virus B25.9
sandworm B76.9
Schimmelbusch's — *see* Mastopathy, cystic
Schmorl's — *see* Schmorl's disease or nodes
Schönlein (-Henoch) (purpura rheumatica) D69.0
Schottmüller's — *see* Fever, paratyphoid
Schultz's (agranulocytosis) — *see* Agranulocytosis
Schwalbe-Ziehen-Oppenheim G24.1
Schwartz-Jampel G71.13
sclera H15.9
specified NEC H15.89
scrofulous (tuberculous) A18.2
scrotum N50.9
sebaceous glands L73.9
semilunar cartilage, cystic (*see also* Derangement,
knee, meniscus, cystic)
seminal vesicle N50.9
serum NEC (*see also* Reaction, serum) T80.69 ☑
sexually transmitted A64
anogenital

sexually transmitted — *continued*
herpesviral infection — *see* Herpes, anogenital
warts A63.0
chancroid A57
chlamydial infection — *see* Chlamydia
gonorrhea — *see* Gonorrhea
granuloma inguinale A58
specified organism NEC A63.8
syphilis — *see* Syphilis
trichomoniasis — *see* Trichomoniasis
Sézary C84.1 ☑
shimamushi (scrub typhus) A75.3
shipyard B30.0
sickle-cell D57.1
with crisis (vasoocclusive pain) D57.00
with
acute chest syndrome D57.01
splenic sequestration D57.02
elliptocytosis D57.8 ☑
Hb-C D57.20
with crisis (vasoocclusive pain) D57.219
with
acute chest syndrome D57.211
splenic sequestration D57.212
without crisis D57.20
Hb-SD D57.80
with crisis D57.819
with
acute chest syndrome D57.811
splenic sequestration D57.812
Hb-SE D57.80
with crisis D57.819
with
acute chest syndrome D57.811
splenic sequestration D57.812
specified NEC D57.80
with crisis D57.819
with
acute chest syndrome D57.811
splenic sequestration D57.812
spherocytosis D57.80
with crisis D57.819
with
acute chest syndrome D57.811
splenic sequestration D57.812
thalassemia D57.40
with crisis (vasoocclusive pain) D57.419
with
acute chest syndrome D57.411
splenic sequestration D57.412
without crisis D57.40
silo-filler's J68.8
bronchitis J68.0
pneumonitis J68.0
pulmonary edema J68.1
simian B B00.4
Simons' (progressive lipodystrophy) E88.1
sin nombre virus B33.4
sinus — *see* Sinusitis
Sirkari's B55.0
sixth B08.20
due to human herpesvirus 6 B08.21
due to human herpesvirus 7 B08.22
skin L98.9
due to metabolic disorder NEC E88.9 *[L99]*
specified NEC L98.8
slim (HIV) B20
small vessel I73.9
Sneddon-Wilkinson (subcorneal pustular
dermatosis) L13.1
South African creeping B88.0
spinal (cord) G95.9
congenital Q06.9
specified NEC G95.89
spine (*see also* Spondylopathy)
joint — *see* Dorsopathy
tuberculous A18.01
spinocerebellar (hereditary) G11.9
specified NEC G11.8
spleen D73.9
amyloid E85.4 *[D77]*
organic D73.9
polycystic Q89.09
postinfectional D73.89
sponge-diver's — *see* Toxicity, venom, marine
animal, sea anemone
Startle Q89.8
Steinert's G71.11
Sticker's (erythema infectiosum) B08.3
Stieda's (calcification, knee joint) — *see* Bursitis,
tibial collateral

Disease — *continued*
Stokes' (exophthalmic goiter) — *see*
Hyperthyroidism, with, goiter (diffuse)
Stokes-Adams (syncope with heart block) I45.9
stomach K31.9
functional, psychogenic F45.8
specified NEC K31.89
stonemason's J62.8
storage
glycogen — *see* Disease, glycogen storage
mucopolysaccharide — *see*
Mucopolysaccharidosis
striatopallidal system NEC G25.89
Stuart-Prower (congenital factor X deficiency) D68.2
Stuart's (congenital factor X deficiency) D68.2
subcutaneous tissue — *see* Disease, skin
supporting structures of teeth K08.9
specified NEC K08.89
suprarenal (capsule) (gland) E27.9
hyperfunction E27.0
specified NEC E27.8
sweat glands L74.9
specified NEC L74.8
Sweeley-Klionsky E75.21
Swift (-Feer) — *see* Poisoning, mercury
swimming-pool granuloma A31.1
Sylvest's (epidemic pleurodynia) B33.0
sympathetic nervous system G90.9
synovium — *see* Disorder, synovium
syphilitic — *see* Syphilis
systemic tissue mast cell D47.02
tanapox (virus) B08.71
Tangier E78.6
Tarral-Besnier (pityriasis rubra pilaris) L44.0
Tauri's E74.09
tear duct — *see* Disorder, lacrimal system
tendon, tendinous (*see also* Disorder, tendon)
nodular — *see* Trigger finger
terminal vessel I73.9
testis N50.9
thalassemia Hb-S — *see* Disease, sickle-cell,
thalassemia
Thaysen-Gee (nontropical sprue) K90.0
Thomsen G71.12
throat J39.2
septic J02.0
thromboembolic — *see* Embolism
thymus (gland) E32.9
specified NEC E32.8
thyroid (gland) E07.9
heart (*see also* Hyperthyroidism) E05.90 *[I43]*
with thyroid storm E05.91 *[I43]*
specified NEC E07.89
Tietze's M94.0
tongue K14.9
specified NEC K14.8
tonsils, tonsillar (and adenoids) J35.9
tooth, teeth K08.9
hard tissues K03.9
specified NEC K03.89
pulp NEC K04.99
specified NEC K08.89
Tourette's F95.2
trachea NEC J39.8
tricuspid I07.9
nonrheumatic I36.9
triglyceride-storage E75.5
trophoblastic — *see* Mole, hydatidiform
tsutsugamushi A75.3
tube (fallopian) (noninflammatory) N83.9
inflammatory — *see* Salpingitis
specified NEC N83.8
tuberculous NEC — *see* Tuberculosis
tubo-ovarian (noninflammatory) N83.9
inflammatory — *see* Salpingo-oophoritis
specified NEC N83.8
tubotympanic, chronic — *see* Otitis, media,
suppurative, chronic, tubotympanic
tubulo-interstitial N15.9
specified NEC N15.8
tympanum — *see* Disorder, tympanic membrane
Uhl's Q24.8
Underwood's (sclerema neonatorum) P83.0
Unverricht (-Lundborg) — *see* Epilepsy, generalized,
idiopathic
Urbach-Oppenheim (necrobiosis lipoidica
diabeticorum) — *see* E08-E13 with .620
ureter N28.9
in (due to)
schistosomiasis (bilharziasis) B65.0 *[N29]*
urethra N36.9
specified NEC N36.8

Disease - Dislocation

Disease — *continued*
- urinary (tract) N39.9
  - bladder N32.9
    - specified NEC N32.89
  - specified NEC N39.8
- uterus (noninflammatory) N85.9
  - infective — *see* Endometritis
  - inflammatory — *see* Endometritis
  - specified NEC N85.8
- uveal tract (anterior) H21.9
  - posterior H31.9
- vagabond's B85.1
- vagina, vaginal (noninflammatory) N89.9
  - inflammatory NEC N76.89
  - specified NEC N89.8
- valve, valvular I38
  - multiple I08.9
    - specified NEC I08.8
- van Creveld-von Gierke (glycogenosis I) E74.01
- vas deferens N50.9
- vascular I99.9
  - arteriosclerotic — *see* Arteriosclerosis
  - ciliary body NEC — *see* Disorder, iris, vascular
  - hypertensive — *see* Hypertension
  - iris NEC — *see* Disorder, iris, vascular
  - obliterative I77.1
    - peripheral I73.9
  - occlusive I99.8
  - peripheral (occlusive) I73.9
    - in diabetes mellitus — *see* E08-E13 with .51
- vasomotor I73.9
- vasospastic I73.9
- vein I87.9
- venereal (*see also* Disease, sexually transmitted) A64
  - chlamydial NEC A56.8
    - anus A56.3
    - genitourinary NOS A56.2
    - pharynx A56.4
    - rectum A56.3
  - fifth A55
  - sixth A55
  - specified nature or type NEC A63.8
- vertebra, vertebral (*see also* Spondylopathy)
  - disc — *see* Disorder, disc
- vibration — *see* Vibration, adverse effects
- viral, virus (*see also* Disease, by type of virus) B34.9
  - arbovirus NOS A94
  - arthropod-borne NOS A94
  - congenital P35.9
    - specified NEC P35.8
  - Hanta (with renal manifestations) (Dobrava) (Puumala) (Seoul) A98.5
    - with pulmonary manifestations (Andes) (Bayou) (Bermejo) (Black Creek Canal) (Choclo) (Juquitiba) (Laguna negra) (Lechiguanas) (New York) (Oran) (Sin nombre) B33.4
  - Hantaan (Korean hemorrhagic fever) A98.5
  - human immunodeficiency (HIV) B20
  - Kunjin A83.4
  - nonarthropod-borne NOS B34.9
  - Powassan A84.8
  - Rocio (encephalitis) A83.6
  - Sin nombre (Hantavirus) (cardio)-pulmonary syndrome) B33.4
  - Tahyna B33.8
  - vesicular stomatitis A93.8
- vitreous H43.9
  - specified NEC H43.89
- vocal cord J38.3
- Volkmann's, acquired T79.6 ☑
- von Eulenburg's (congenital paramyotonia) G71.19
- von Gierke's (glycogenosis I) E74.01
- von Graefe's — *see* Strabismus, paralytic, ophthalmoplegia, progressive
- von Willebrand (-Jürgens) (angiohemophilia) D68.0
- Vrolik's (osteogenesis imperfecta) Q78.0
- vulva (noninflammatory) N90.9
  - inflammatory NEC N76.89
  - specified NEC N90.89
- Wallgren's (obstruction of splenic vein with collateral circulation) I87.8
- Wassilieff's (leptospiral jaundice) A27.0
- wasting NEC R64
  - due to malnutrition E41
- Waterhouse-Friderichsen A39.1
- Wegner's (syphilitic osteochondritis) A50.02
- Weil's (leptospiral jaundice of lung) A27.0
- Weir Mitchell's (erythromelalgia) I73.81
- Werdnig-Hoffmann G12.0
- Wermer's E31.21
- Werner-His (trench fever) A79.0
- Werner-Schultz (neutropenic splenomegaly) D73.81

Disease — *continued*
- Wernicke-Posadas B38.9
- whipworm B79
- white blood cells D72.9
  - specified NEC D72.89
- white matter R90.82
- white-spot, meaning lichen sclerosus et atrophicus L90.0
  - penis N48.0
  - vulva N90.4
- Wilkie's K55.1
- Wilkinson-Sneddon (subcorneal pustular dermatosis) L13.1
- Willis' — *see* Diabetes
- Wilson's (hepatolenticular degeneration) E83.01
- woolsorter's A22.1
- yaba monkey tumor B08.72
- yaba pox (virus) B08.72
- Zika virus A92.5
  - congenital P35.4
- zoonotic, bacterial A28.9
  - specified type NEC A28.8

Disfigurement (due to scar) L90.5

Disgerminoma — *see* Dysgerminoma

DISH (diffuse idiopathic skeletal hyperostosis) — *see* Hyperostosis, ankylosing

Disinsertion, retina — *see* Detachment, retina

Dislocatable hip, congenital Q65.6

Dislocation (articular)
- with fracture — *see* Fracture
- acromioclavicular (joint) S43.10 ☑
  - with displacement
    - 100%-200% S43.12 ☑
    - more than 200% S43.13 ☑
  - inferior S43.14 ☑
  - posterior S43.15 ☑
- ankle S93.0 ☑
- astragalus — *see* Dislocation, ankle
- atlantoaxial S13.121 ☑
- atlantooccipital S13.111 ☑
- atloidooccipital S13.111 ☑
- breast bone S23.29 ☑
- capsule, joint - code by site under Dislocation
- carpal (bone) — *see* Dislocation, wrist
- carpometacarpal (joint) NEC S63.05 ☑
  - thumb S63.04 ☑
- cartilage (joint) - code by site under Dislocation
- cervical spine (vertebra) — *see* Dislocation, vertebra, cervical
- chronic — *see* Dislocation, recurrent
- clavicle — *see* Dislocation, acromioclavicular joint
- coccyx S33.2 ☑
- congenital NEC Q68.8
- coracoid — *see* Dislocation, shoulder
- costal cartilage S23.29 ☑
- costochondral S23.29 ☑
- cricoarytenoid articulation S13.29 ☑
- cricothyroid articulation S13.29 ☑
- dorsal vertebra — *see* Dislocation, vertebra, thoracic
- ear ossicle — *see* Discontinuity, ossicles, ear
- elbow S53.10 ☑
  - congenital Q68.8
  - pathological — *see* Dislocation, pathological NEC, elbow
  - radial head alone — *see* Dislocation, radial head
  - recurrent — *see* Dislocation, recurrent, elbow
  - traumatic S53.10 ☑
    - anterior S53.11 ☑
    - lateral S53.14 ☑
    - medial S53.13 ☑
    - posterior S53.12 ☑
    - specified type NEC S53.19 ☑
- eye, nontraumatic — *see* Luxation, globe
- eyeball, nontraumatic — *see* Luxation, globe
- femur
  - distal end — *see* Dislocation, knee
  - proximal end — *see* Dislocation, hip
- fibula
  - distal end — *see* Dislocation, ankle
  - proximal end — *see* Dislocation, knee
- finger S63.25 ☑
  - index S63.25 ☑
  - interphalangeal S63.27 ☑
    - distal S63.29 ☑
      - index S63.29 ☑
      - little S63.29 ☑
      - middle S63.29 ☑
      - ring S63.29 ☑
    - index S63.27 ☑
    - little S63.27 ☑
    - middle S63.27 ☑
    - proximal S63.28 ☑

Dislocation — *continued*
- finger — *continued*
  - index S63.28 ☑
  - little S63.28 ☑
  - middle S63.28 ☑
  - ring S63.28 ☑
  - ring S63.27 ☑
  - little S63.25 ☑
  - metacarpophalangeal S63.26 ☑
    - index S63.26 ☑
    - little S63.26 ☑
    - middle S63.26 ☑
    - ring S63.26 ☑
  - middle S63.25 ☑
  - recurrent — *see* Dislocation, recurrent, finger
  - ring S63.25 ☑
  - thumb — *see* Dislocation, thumb
- foot S93.30 ☑
  - recurrent — *see* Dislocation, recurrent, foot
  - specified NEC S93.33 ☑
  - tarsal joint S93.31 ☑
  - tarsometatarsal joint S93.32 ☑
  - toe — *see* Dislocation, toe
- fracture — *see* Fracture
- glenohumeral (joint) — *see* Dislocation, shoulder
- glenoid — *see* Dislocation, shoulder
- habitual — *see* Dislocation, recurrent
- hip S73.00 ☑
  - anterior S73.03 ☑
    - obturator S73.02 ☑
  - central S73.04 ☑
  - congenital (total) Q65.2
    - bilateral Q65.1
    - partial Q65.5
      - bilateral Q65.4
      - unilateral Q65.3 ☑
    - unilateral Q65.0 ☑
  - developmental M24.85 ☑
  - pathological — *see* Dislocation, pathological NEC, hip
  - posterior S73.01 ☑
  - recurrent — *see* Dislocation, recurrent, hip
- humerus, proximal end — *see* Dislocation, shoulder
- incomplete — *see* Subluxation, by site
- incus — *see* Discontinuity, ossicles, ear
- infracoracoid — *see* Dislocation, shoulder
- innominate (pubic junction) (sacral junction) S33.39 ☑
  - acetabulum — *see* Dislocation, hip
- interphalangeal (joint(s))
  - finger S63.279 ☑
    - distal S63.29 ☑
      - index S63.29 ☑
      - little S63.29 ☑
      - middle S63.29 ☑
      - ring S63.29 ☑
    - index S63.27 ☑
    - little S63.27 ☑
    - middle S63.27 ☑
    - proximal S63.28 ☑
      - index S63.28 ☑
      - little S63.28 ☑
      - middle S63.28 ☑
      - ring S63.28 ☑
    - ring S63.27 ☑
  - foot or toe — *see* Dislocation, toe
  - thumb S63.12 ☑
- jaw (cartilage) (meniscus) S03.0 ☑
- joint prosthesis — *see* Complications, joint prosthesis, mechanical, displacement, by site
- knee S83.106 ☑
  - cap — *see* Dislocation, patella
  - congenital Q68.2
  - old M23.8X ☑
  - patella — *see* Dislocation, patella
  - pathological — *see* Dislocation, pathological NEC, knee
  - proximal tibia
    - anteriorly S83.11 ☑
    - laterally S83.14 ☑
    - medially S83.13 ☑
    - posteriorly S83.12 ☑
  - recurrent (*see also* Derangement, knee, specified NEC)
  - specified type NEC S83.19 ☑
- lacrimal gland H04.16 ☑
- lens (complete) H27.10
  - anterior H27.12 ☑
  - congenital Q12.1
  - ocular implant — *see* Complications, intraocular lens
  - partial H27.11 ☑

Dislocation — *continued*
  lens — *continued*
    posterior H27.13 ☑
    traumatic S05.8X ☑
  ligament - code by site under Dislocation
  lumbar (vertebra) — *see* Dislocation, vertebra, lumbar
  lumbosacral (vertebra) (*see also* Dislocation, vertebra, lumbar)
    congenital Q76.49
  mandible S03.0 ☑
  meniscus (knee) — *see* Tear, meniscus
    other sites - code by site under Dislocation
  metacarpal (bone)
    distal end — *see* Dislocation, finger
    proximal end S63.06 ☑
  metacarpophalangeal (joint)
    finger S63.26 ☑
      index S63.26 ☑
      little S63.26 ☑
      middle S63.26 ☑
      ring S63.26 ☑
      thumb S63.11 ☑
  metatarsal (bone) — *see* Dislocation, foot
  metatarsophalangeal (joint(s)) — *see* Dislocation, toe
  midcarpal (joint) S63.03 ☑
  midtarsal (joint) — *see* Dislocation, foot
  neck S13.20 ☑
    specified site NEC S13.29 ☑
    vertebra — *see* Dislocation, vertebra, cervical
  nose (septal cartilage) S03.1 ☑
  occipitoatloid S13.111 ☑
  old — *see* Derangement, joint, specified type NEC
  ossicles, ear — *see* Discontinuity, ossicles, ear
  partial — *see* Subluxation, by site
  patella S83.006 ☑
    congenital Q74.1
    lateral S83.01 ☑
    recurrent (nontraumatic) M22.0 ☑
      incomplete M22.1 ☑
    specified type NEC S83.09 ☑
  pathological NEC M24.30
    ankle M24.37 ☑
    elbow M24.32 ☑
    foot joint M24.37 ☑
    hand joint M24.34 ☑
    hip M24.35 ☑
    knee M24.36 ☑
    lumbosacral joint — *see* subcategory M53.2 ☑
    pelvic region — *see* Dislocation, pathological, hip
    sacroiliac — *see* subcategory M53.2 ☑
    shoulder M24.31 ☑
    wrist M24.33 ☑
  pelvis NEC S33.30 ☑
    specified NEC S33.39 ☑
  phalanx
    finger or hand — *see* Dislocation, finger
    foot or toe — *see* Dislocation, toe
  prosthesis, internal — *see* Complications, prosthetic device, by site, mechanical
  radial head S53.006 ☑
    anterior S53.01 ☑
    posterior S53.02 ☑
    specified type NEC S53.09 ☑
  radiocarpal (joint) S63.02 ☑
  radiohumeral (joint) — *see* Dislocation, radial head
  radioulnar (joint)
    distal S63.01 ☑
    proximal — *see* Dislocation, elbow
  radius
    distal end — *see* Dislocation, wrist
    proximal end — *see* Dislocation, radial head
  recurrent M24.40
    ankle M24.47 ☑
    elbow M24.42 ☑
    finger M24.44 ☑
    foot joint M24.47 ☑
    hand joint M24.44 ☑
    hip M24.45 ☑
    knee M24.46 ☑
      patella — *see* Dislocation, patella, recurrent
    patella — *see* Dislocation, patella, recurrent
    sacroiliac — *see* subcategory M53.2 ☑
    shoulder M24.41 ☑
    toe M24.47 ☑
    vertebra (*see also* subcategory) M43.5 ☑
      atlantoaxial M43.4
        with myelopathy M43.3
    wrist M24.43 ☑
  rib (cartilage) S23.29 ☑
  sacrococcygeal S33.2 ☑

Dislocation — *continued*
  sacroiliac (joint) (ligament) S33.2 ☑
    congenital Q74.2
    recurrent — *see* subcategory M53.2 ☑
  sacrum S33.2 ☑
  scaphoid (bone) (hand) (wrist) — *see* Dislocation, wrist
    foot — *see* Dislocation, foot
  scapula — *see* Dislocation, shoulder, girdle, scapula
  semilunar cartilage, knee — *see* Tear, meniscus
  septal cartilage (nose) S03.1 ☑
  septum (nasal) (old) J34.2
  sesamoid bone - code by site under Dislocation
  shoulder (blade) (ligament) (joint) (traumatic) S43.006 ☑
    acromioclavicular — *see* Dislocation, acromioclavicular
    chronic — *see* Dislocation, recurrent, shoulder
    congenital Q68.8
    girdle S43.30 ☑
      scapula S43.31 ☑
      specified site NEC S43.39 ☑
    humerus S43.00 ☑
      anterior S43.01 ☑
      inferior S43.03 ☑
      posterior S43.02 ☑
    pathological — *see* Dislocation, pathological NEC, shoulder
    recurrent — *see* Dislocation, recurrent, shoulder
    specified type NEC S43.08 ☑
  spine
    cervical — *see* Dislocation, vertebra, cervical
    congenital Q76.49
    due to birth trauma P11.5
    lumbar — *see* Dislocation, vertebra, lumbar
    thoracic — *see* Dislocation, vertebra, thoracic
  spontaneous — *see* Dislocation, pathological
  sternoclavicular (joint) S43.206 ☑
    anterior S43.21 ☑
    posterior S43.22 ☑
  sternum S23.29 ☑
  subglenoid — *see* Dislocation, shoulder
  symphysis pubis S33.4 ☑
  talus — *see* Dislocation, ankle
  tarsal (bone(s)) (joint(s)) — *see* Dislocation, foot
  tarsometatarsal (joint(s)) — *see* Dislocation, foot
  temporomandibular (joint) S03.0 ☑
  thigh, proximal end — *see* Dislocation, hip
  thorax S23.20 ☑
    specified site NEC S23.29 ☑
    vertebra — *see* Dislocation, vertebra
  thumb S63.10 ☑
    interphalangeal joint — *see* Dislocation, interphalangeal (joint), thumb
    metacarpophalangeal joint — *see* Dislocation, metacarpophalangeal (joint), thumb
  thyroid cartilage S13.29 ☑
  tibia
    distal end — *see* Dislocation, ankle
    proximal end — *see* Dislocation, knee
  tibiofibular (joint)
    distal — *see* Dislocation, ankle
    superior — *see* Dislocation, knee
  toe(s) S93.106 ☑
    great S93.10 ☑
      interphalangeal joint S93.11 ☑
      metatarsophalangeal joint S93.12 ☑
    interphalangeal joint S93.119 ☑
    lesser S93.106 ☑
      interphalangeal joint S93.11 ☑
      metatarsophalangeal joint S93.12 ☑
    metatarsophalangeal joint S93.12 ☑
  tooth S03.2 ☑
  trachea S23.29 ☑
  ulna
    distal end S63.07 ☑
    proximal end — *see* Dislocation, elbow
  ulnohumeral (joint) — *see* Dislocation, elbow
  vertebra (articular process) (body) (traumatic)
    cervical S13.101 ☑
      atlantoaxial joint S13.121 ☑
      atlantooccipital joint S13.111 ☑
      atloidooccipital joint S13.111 ☑
      joint between
        C0 and C1 S13.111 ☑
        C1 and C2 S13.121 ☑
        C2 and C3 S13.131 ☑
        C3 and C4 S13.141 ☑
        C4 and C5 S13.151 ☑
        C5 and C6 S13.161 ☑
        C6 and C7 S13.171 ☑
        C7 and T1 S13.181 ☑
      occipitoatloid joint S13.111 ☑

Dislocation — *continued*
  vertebra — *continued*
    congenital Q76.49
    lumbar S33.101 ☑
      joint between
        L1 and L2 S33.111 ☑
        L2 and L3 S33.121 ☑
        L3 and L4 S33.131 ☑
        L4 and L5 S33.141 ☑
      nontraumatic — *see* Displacement, intervertebral disc
      partial — *see* Subluxation, by site
      recurrent NEC — *see* subcategory M43.5 ☑
    thoracic S23.101 ☑
      joint between
        T1 and T2 S23.111 ☑
        T2 and T3 S23.121 ☑
        T3 and T4 S23.123 ☑
        T4 and T5 S23.131 ☑
        T5 and T6 S23.133 ☑
        T6 and T7 S23.141 ☑
        T7 and T8 S23.143 ☑
        T8 and T9 S23.151 ☑
        T9 and T10 S23.153 ☑
        T10 and T11 S23.161 ☑
        T11 and T12 S23.163 ☑
        T12 and L1 S23.171 ☑
  wrist (carpal bone) S63.006 ☑
    carpometacarpal joint — *see* Dislocation, carpometacarpal (joint)
    distal radioulnar joint — *see* Dislocation, radioulnar (joint), distal
    metacarpal bone, proximal — *see* Dislocation, metacarpal (bone), proximal end
    midcarpal — *see* Dislocation, midcarpal (joint)
    radiocarpal joint — *see* Dislocation, radiocarpal (joint)
    recurrent — *see* Dislocation, recurrent, wrist
    specified site NEC S63.09 ☑
    ulna — *see* Dislocation, ulna, distal end
  xiphoid cartilage S23.29 ☑
Disorder (of) (*see also* Disease)
  acantholytic L11.9
    specified NEC L11.8
  acute
    psychotic — *see* Psychosis, acute
    stress F43.0
  adjustment (grief) F43.20
    with
      anxiety F43.22
        with depressed mood F43.23
      conduct disturbance F43.24
        with emotional disturbance F43.25
      depressed mood F43.21
        with anxiety F43.23
      other specified symptom F43.29
  adrenal (capsule) (gland) (medullary) E27.9
    specified NEC E27.8
  adrenogenital E25.9
    drug-induced E25.8
    iatrogenic E25.8
    idiopathic E25.8
  adult personality (and behavior) F69
    specified NEC F68.8
  affective (mood) — *see* Disorder, mood
  aggressive, unsocialized F91.1
  alcohol-related F10.99
    with
      amnestic disorder, persisting F10.96
      anxiety disorder F10.980
      dementia, persisting F10.97
      intoxication F10.929
        with delirium F10.921
        uncomplicated F10.920
      mood disorder F10.94
      other specified F10.988
      psychotic disorder F10.959
        with
          delusions F10.950
          hallucinations F10.951
      sexual dysfunction F10.981
      sleep disorder F10.982
  alcohol use
    mild F10.10
      with
        alcohol-induced
          anxiety disorder F10.180
          bipolar and related disorder F10.14
          depressive disorder F10.14
          psychotic disorder F10.159
          sexual dysfunction F10.181
          sleep disorder F10.182

Disorder

Disorder — *continued*
- alcohol use — *continued*
  - alcohol intoxication F10.129
    - delirium F10.121
  - in remission (early) (sustained) F10.11
  - moderate or severe F10.20
    - with
      - alcohol-induced
        - anxiety disorder F10.280
        - bipolar and related disorder F10.24
        - depressive disorder F10.24
        - major neurocognitive disorder, amnestic-confabulatory type F10.26
        - major neurocognitive disorder, nonamnestic-confabulatory type F10.27
        - mild neurocognitive disorder F10.288
        - psychotic disorder F10.259
        - sexual dysfunction F10.281
        - sleep disorder F10.282
      - alcohol intoxication F10.229
        - delirium F10.221
      - in remission (early) (sustained) F10.21
- allergic — *see* Allergy
- alveolar NEC J84.09
- amino-acid
  - cystathioninuria E72.19
  - cystinosis E72.04
  - cystinuria E72.01
  - glycinuria E72.09
  - homocystinuria E72.11
  - metabolism — *see* Disturbance, metabolism, amino-acid
  - specified NEC E72.89
  - neonatal, transitory P74.8
  - renal transport NEC E72.09
  - transport NEC E72.09
- amnesic, amnestic
  - alcohol-induced F10.96
    - with dependence F10.26
  - due to (secondary to) general medical condition F04
  - psychoactive NEC-induced F19.96
    - with
      - abuse F19.16
      - dependence F19.26
  - sedative, hypnotic or anxiolytic-induced F13.96
    - with dependence F13.26
- amphetamine-type substance use
  - mild F15.10
    - in remission (early) (sustained) F15.11
  - moderate F15.20
    - in remission (early) (sustained) F15.21
  - severe F15.20
    - in remission (early) (sustained) F15.21
- amphetamine (or other stimulant) use
  - mild
    - with
      - amphetamine (or other stimulant)-induced
        - anxiety disorder F15.180
        - bipolar and related disorder F15.14
        - depressive disorder F15.14
        - obsessive-compulsive and related disorder F15.188
        - psychotic disorder F15.159
        - sexual dysfunction F15.181
      - amphetamine, cocaine, or other stimulant intoxication
        - with perceptual disturbances F15.122
        - without perceptual disturbances F15.129
        - intoxication delirium F15.121
  - moderate or severe
    - with
      - amphetamine (or other stimulant)-induced
        - anxiety disorder F15.280
        - obsessive-compulsive and related disorder F15.288
        - sexual dysfunction F15.281
        - bipolar and related disorder F15.24
        - depressive disorder F15.24
        - psychotic disorder F15.259
      - amphetamine, cocaine, or other stimulant intoxication
        - with perceptual disturbances F15.222
        - without perceptual disturbances F15.229
        - intoxication delirium F15.221
- anaerobic glycolysis with anemia D55.2
- anxiety F41.9
  - due to (secondary to)
    - alcohol F10.980
      - in
        - abuse F10.180
        - dependence F10.280

Disorder — *continued*
- anxiety — *continued*
  - amphetamine F15.980
    - in
      - abuse F15.180
      - dependence F15.280
  - anxiolytic F13.980
    - in
      - abuse F13.180
      - dependence F13.280
  - caffeine F15.980
    - in
      - abuse F15.180
      - dependence F15.280
  - cannabis F12.980
    - in
      - abuse F12.180
      - dependence F12.280
  - cocaine F14.980
    - in
      - abuse F14.180
      - dependence F14.180
  - general medical condition F06.4
  - hallucinogen F16.980
    - in
      - abuse F16.180
      - dependence F16.280
  - hypnotic F13.980
    - in
      - abuse F13.180
      - dependence F13.280
  - inhalant F18.980
    - in
      - abuse F18.180
      - dependence F18.280
  - phencyclidine F16.980
    - in
      - abuse F16.180
      - dependence F16.280
  - psychoactive substance NEC F19.980
    - in
      - abuse F19.180
      - dependence F19.280
  - sedative F13.980
    - in
      - abuse F13.180
      - dependence F13.280
  - volatile solvents F18.980
    - in
      - abuse F18.180
      - dependence F18.280
  - generalized F41.1
  - illness F45.21
  - mixed
    - with depression (mild) F41.8
    - specified NEC F41.3
  - organic F06.4
  - phobic F40.9
    - of childhood F40.8
  - specified NEC F41.8
- aortic valve — *see* Endocarditis, aortic
- aromatic amino-acid metabolism E70.9
  - specified NEC E70.8
- arteriole NEC I77.89
- artery NEC I77.89
- articulation — *see* Disorder, joint
- attachment (childhood)
  - disinhibited F94.2
  - reactive F94.1
- attention-deficit hyperactivity (adolescent) (adult) (child) F90.9
  - combined
    - presentation F90.2
    - type F90.2
  - hyperactive
    - impulsive presentation F90.1
    - type F90.1
  - inattentive
    - presentation F90.0
    - type F90.0
  - specified type NEC F90.8
- attention-deficit without hyperactivity (adolescent) (adult) (child) F98.8
- auditory processing (central) H93.25
- autistic F84.0
- autism spectrum F84.0
- autoimmune D89.89
- autonomic nervous system G90.9
  - specified NEC G90.8
- avoidant
  - child or adolescent F40.10
  - restrictive food intake F50.82

Disorder — *continued*
- balance
  - acid-base E87.8
    - mixed E87.4
  - electrolyte E87.8
  - fluid NEC E87.8
- behavioral (disruptive) — *see* Disorder, conduct
- beta-amino-acid metabolism E72.89
- bile acid and cholesterol metabolism E78.70
  - Barth syndrome E78.71
  - other specified E78.79
  - Smith-Lemli-Opitz syndrome E78.72
- bilirubin excretion E80.6
- binge eating F50.81
- binocular
  - movement H51.9
    - convergence
      - excess H51.12
      - insufficiency H51.11
    - internuclear ophthalmoplegia — *see* Ophthalmoplegia, internuclear
    - palsy of conjugate gaze H51.0
    - specified type NEC H51.8
  - vision NEC — *see* Disorder, vision, binocular
- bipolar (I) (type 1) F31.9
  - and related due to a known physiological condition
    - with
      - manic features F06.33
      - manic- or hypomanic-like episodes F06.33
      - mixed features F06.34
  - current (or most recent) episode
    - depressed F31.9
      - with psychotic features F31.5
      - without psychotic features F31.30
        - mild F31.31
        - moderate F31.32
        - severe (without psychotic features) F31.4
          - with psychotic features F31.5
    - hypomanic F31.0
    - manic F31.9
      - with psychotic features F31.2
      - without psychotic features F31.10
        - mild F31.11
        - moderate F31.12
        - severe (without psychotic features) F31.13
          - with psychotic features F31.2
    - mixed F31.60
      - mild F31.61
      - moderate F31.62
      - severe (without psychotic features) F31.63
        - with psychotic features F31.64
    - severe depression (without psychotic features) F31.4
      - with psychotic features F31.5
  - in remission (currently) F31.70
    - in full remission
      - most recent episode
        - depressed F31.76
        - hypomanic F31.72
        - manic F31.74
        - mixed F31.78
    - in partial remission
      - most recent episode
        - depressed F31.75
        - hypomanic F31.71
        - manic F31.73
        - mixed F31.77
  - specified NEC F31.89
  - II (type 2) F31.81
  - organic F06.30
  - single manic episode F30.9
    - mild F30.11
    - moderate F30.12
    - severe (without psychotic symptoms) F30.13
      - with psychotic symptoms F30.2
- bladder N32.9
  - functional NEC N31.9
  - in schistosomiasis B65.0 *[N33]*
  - specified NEC N32.89
- bleeding D68.9
- blood D75.9
  - in congenital early syphilis A50.09 *[D77]*
- body dysmorphic F45.22
- bone M89.9
  - continuity M84.9
    - specified type NEC M84.80
      - ankle M84.87 ☑
      - fibula M84.86 ☑
      - foot M84.87 ☑
      - hand M84.84 ☑
      - humerus M84.82 ☑
      - neck M84.88

☑ **Additional character required**

Disorder — *continued*
- bone — *continued*
  - pelvis M84.859
  - radius M84.83 ☑
  - rib M84.88
  - shoulder M84.81 ☑
  - skull M84.88
  - thigh M84.85 ☑
  - tibia M84.86 ☑
  - ulna M84.83 ☑
  - vertebra M84.88
  - density and structure M85.9
  - cyst (*see also* Cyst, bone, specified type NEC)
    - aneurysmal — *see* Cyst, bone, aneurysmal
    - solitary — *see* Cyst, bone, solitary
  - diffuse idiopathic skeletal hyperostosis — *see* Hyperostosis, ankylosing
  - fibrous dysplasia (monostotic) — *see* Dysplasia, fibrous, bone
  - fluorosis — *see* Fluorosis, skeletal
  - hyperostosis of skull M85.2
  - osteitis condensans — *see* Osteitis, condensans
  - specified type NEC M85.8 ☑
    - ankle M85.87 ☑
    - foot M85.87 ☑
    - forearm M85.83 ☑
    - hand M85.84 ☑
    - lower leg M85.86 ☑
    - multiple sites M85.89
    - neck M85.88
    - rib M85.88
    - shoulder M85.81 ☑
    - skull M85.88
    - thigh M85.85 ☑
    - upper arm M85.82 ☑
    - vertebra M85.88
  - development and growth NEC M89.20
    - carpus M89.24 ☑
    - clavicle M89.21 ☑
    - femur M89.25 ☑
    - fibula M89.26 ☑
    - finger M89.24 ☑
    - humerus M89.22 ☑
    - ilium M89.259
    - ischium M89.259
    - metacarpus M89.24 ☑
    - metatarsus M89.27 ☑
    - multiple sites M89.29
    - neck M89.28
    - radius M89.23 ☑
    - rib M89.28
    - scapula M89.21 ☑
    - skull M89.28
    - tarsus M89.27 ☑
    - tibia M89.26 ☑
    - toe M89.27 ☑
    - ulna M89.23 ☑
    - vertebra M89.28
  - specified type NEC M89.8X ☑
  - brachial plexus G54.0
  - branched-chain amino-acid metabolism E71.2
    - specified NEC E71.19
  - breast N64.9
    - agalactia — *see* Agalactia
    - associated with
      - lactation O92.70
        - specified NEC O92.79
      - pregnancy O92.20
        - specified NEC O92.29
      - puerperium O92.20
        - specified NEC O92.29
    - cracked nipple — *see* Cracked nipple
    - galactorrhea — *see* Galactorrhea
    - hypogalactia O92.4
    - lactation disorder NEC O92.79
    - mastitis — *see* Mastitis
    - nipple infection — *see* Infection, nipple
    - retracted nipple — *see* Retraction, nipple
    - specified type NEC N64.89
  - Briquet's F45.0
  - bullous, in diseases classified elsewhere L14
  - caffeine use
    - mild
      - with
        - caffeine-induced
          - anxiety disorder F15.180
          - sleep disorder F15.182
    - moderate or severe
      - with
        - caffeine-induced
          - anxiety disorder F15.280
          - sleep disorder F15.282

Disorder — *continued*
- cannabis use
  - mild F12.10
    - with
      - cannabis-induced
        - anxiety disorder F12.180
        - psychotic disorder F12.159
        - sleep disorder F12.188
      - cannabis intoxication delirium F12.121
        - with perceptual disturbances F12.122
        - without perceptual disturbances F12.129
    - in remission (early) (sustained) F12.11
  - moderate or severe F12.20
    - with
      - cannabis-induced
        - anxiety disorder F12.280
        - psychotic disorder F12.259
        - sleep disorder F12.288
      - cannabis intoxication
        - with perceptual disturbances F12.222
        - without perceptual disturbances F12.229
      - delirium F12.221
    - in remission (early) (sustained) F12.21
- carbohydrate
  - absorption, intestinal NEC E74.39
  - metabolism (congenital) E74.9
    - specified NEC E74.8
- cardiac, functional I51.89
- carnitine metabolism E71.40
- cartilage M94.9
  - articular NEC — *see* Derangement, joint, articular cartilage
  - chondrocalcinosis — *see* Chondrocalcinosis
  - specified type NEC M94.8X ☑
    - articular — *see* Derangement, joint, articular cartilage
    - multiple sites M94.8X0
- catatonia (due to known physiological condition) (with another mental disorder) F06.1
- catatonic
  - due to (secondary to) known physiological condition F06.1
  - organic F06.1
- central auditory processing H93.25
- cervical
  - region NEC M53.82
  - root (nerve) NEC G54.2
- character NOS F60.9
- childhood disintegrative NEC F84.3
- cholesterol and bile acid metabolism E78.70
  - Barth syndrome E78.71
  - other specified E78.79
  - Smith-Lemli-Opitz syndrome E78.72
- choroid H31.9
  - atrophy — *see* Atrophy, choroid
  - degeneration — *see* Degeneration, choroid
  - detachment — *see* Detachment, choroid
  - dystrophy — *see* Dystrophy, choroid
  - hemorrhage — *see* Hemorrhage, choroid
  - rupture — *see* Rupture, choroid
  - scar — *see* Scar, chorioretinal
  - solar retinopathy — *see* Retinopathy, solar
  - specified type NEC H31.8
- ciliary body — *see* Disorder, iris
  - degeneration — *see* Degeneration, ciliary body
- coagulation (factor) (*see also* Defect, coagulation) D68.9
  - newborn, transient P61.6
- cocaine use
  - mild F14.10
    - with
      - amphetamine, cocaine, or other stimulant intoxication
        - with perceptual disturbances F14.122
        - without perceptual disturbances F14.129
      - cocaine-induced
        - anxiety disorder F14.180
        - bipolar and related disorder F14.14
        - depressive disorder F14.14
        - obsessive-compulsive and related disorder F14.188
        - psychotic disorder F14.159
        - sexual dysfunction F14.181
        - sleep disorder F14.182
      - cocaine intoxication delirium F14.121
    - in remission (early) (sustained) F14.11
  - moderate or severe F14.20
    - with
      - amphetamine, cocaine, or other stimulant intoxication
        - with perceptual disturbances F14.222
        - without perceptual disturbances F14.229

Disorder — *continued*
- cocaine use — *continued*
  - cocaine-induced
    - anxiety disorder F14.280
    - bipolar and related disorder F14.24
    - depressive disorder F14.24
    - obsessive-compulsive and related disorder F14.288
    - psychotic disorder F14.259
    - sexual dysfunction F14.281
    - sleep disorder F14.282
  - cocaine intoxication delirium F14.221
  - in remission (early) (sustained) F14.21
- coccyx NEC M53.3
- cognitive F09
  - due to (secondary to) general medical condition F09
  - persisting R41.89
    - due to
      - alcohol F10.97
        - with dependence F10.27
      - anxiolytics F13.97
        - with dependence F13.27
      - hypnotics F13.97
        - with dependence F13.27
      - sedatives F13.97
        - with dependence F13.27
      - specified substance NEC F19.97
        - with
          - abuse F19.17
          - dependence F19.27
- communication F80.9
  - social pragmatic F80.82
- conduct (childhood) F91.9
  - adjustment reaction — *see* Disorder, adjustment
  - adolescent onset type F91.2
  - childhood onset type F91.1
  - compulsive F63.9
  - confined to family context F91.0
  - depressive F91.8
  - group type F91.2
  - hyperkinetic — *see* Disorder, attention-deficit hyperactivity
  - oppositional defiance F91.3
  - socialized F91.2
  - solitary aggressive type F91.1
  - specified NEC F91.8
  - unsocialized (aggressive) F91.1
- conduction, heart I45.9
- congenital glycosylation (CDG) E74.8
- conjunctiva H11.9
  - infection — *see* Conjunctivitis
- connective tissue, localized L94.9
  - specified NEC L94.8
- conversion (functional neurological symptom disorder)
  - with
    - abnormal movement F44.4
    - anesthesia or sensory loss F44.6
    - attacks or seizures F44.5
    - mixed symptoms F44.7
    - special sensory symptoms F44.6
    - speech symptoms F44.4
    - swallowing symptoms F44.4
    - weakness or paralysis F44.4
- convulsive (secondary) — *see* Convulsions
- cornea H18.9
  - deformity — *see* Deformity, cornea
  - degeneration — *see* Degeneration, cornea
  - deposits — *see* Deposit, cornea
  - due to contact lens H18.82 ☑
    - specified as edema — *see* Edema, cornea
  - edema — *see* Edema, cornea
  - keratitis — *see* Keratitis
  - keratoconjunctivitis — *see* Keratoconjunctivitis
  - membrane change — *see* Change, corneal membrane
  - neovascularization — *see* Neovascularization, cornea
  - scar — *see* Opacity, cornea
  - specified type NEC H18.89 ☑
  - ulcer — *see* Ulcer, cornea
- corpus cavernosum N48.9
- cranial nerve — *see* Disorder, nerve, cranial
- cyclothymic F34.0
- defiant oppositional F91.3
- delusional (persistent) (systematized) F22
  - induced F24
- depersonalization F48.1
- depressive F32.9
  - due to known physiological condition
    - with

Disorder

Disorder — *continued*
  depressive — *continued*
    depressive features F06.31
    major depressive-like episode F06.32
    mixed features F06.34
  major F32.9
    with psychotic symptoms F32.3
    in remission (full) F32.5
      partial F32.4
    recurrent F33.9
      with psychotic features F33.3
    single episode F32.9
      mild F32.0
      moderate F32.1
      severe (without psychotic symptoms) F32.2
        with psychotic symptoms F32.3
  organic F06.31
  persistent F34.1
  recurrent F33.9
    current episode
      mild F33.0
      moderate F33.1
      severe (without psychotic symptoms) F33.2
        with psychotic symptoms F33.3
    in remission F33.40
      full F33.42
      partial F33.41
    specified NEC F33.8
  single episode — *see* Episode, depressive
  specified NEC F32.89
developmental F89
  arithmetical skills F81.2
  coordination (motor) F82
  expressive writing F81.81
  language F80.9
    expressive F80.1
    mixed receptive and expressive F80.2
    receptive type F80.2
    specified NEC F80.89
  learning F81.9
    arithmetical F81.2
    reading F81.0
  mixed F88
  motor coordination or function F82
  pervasive F84.9
    specified NEC F84.8
  phonological F80.0
  reading F81.0
  scholastic skills (*see also* Disorder, learning)
    mixed F81.89
  specified NEC F88
  speech F80.9
    articulation F80.0
    specified NEC F80.89
  written expression F81.81
diaphragm J98.6
digestive (system) K92.9
  newborn P78.9
    specified NEC P78.89
  postprocedural — *see* Complication,
    gastrointestinal
  psychogenic F45.8
disc (intervertebral) M51.9
  with
    myelopathy
      cervical region M50.00
      cervicothoracic region M50.03
      high cervical region M50.01
      lumbar region M51.06
      mid-cervical region M50.020
      sacrococcygeal region M53.3
      thoracic region M51.04
      thoracolumbar region M51.05
    radiculopathy
      cervical region M50.10
      cervicothoracic region M50.13
      high cervical region M50.11
      lumbar region M51.16
      lumbosacral region M51.17
      mid-cervical region M50.120
      sacrococcygeal region M53.3
      thoracic region M51.14
      thoracolumbar region M51.15
  cervical M50.90
    with
      myelopathy M50.00
        C2-C3 M50.01
        C3-C4 M50.01
        C4-C5 M50.021
        C5-C6 M50.022
        C6-C7 M50.023
        C7-T1 M50.03

Disorder — *continued*
  disc — *continued*
      cervicothoracic region M50.03
      high cervical region M50.01
      mid-cervical region M50.020
    neuritis, radiculitis or radiculopathy M50.10
      C2-C3 M50.11
      C3-C4 M50.11
      C4-C5 M50.121
      C5-C6 M50.122
      C6-C7 M50.123
      C7-T1 M50.13
      cervicothoracic region M50.13
      high cervical region M50.11
      mid-cervical region M50.120
    C2-C3 M50.91
    C3-C4 M50.91
    C4-C5 M50.921
    C5-C6 M50.922
    C6-C7 M50.923
    C7-T1 M50.93
    cervicothoracic region M50.93
    degeneration M50.30
      C2-C3 M50.31
      C3-C4 M50.31
      C4-C5 M50.321
      C5-C6 M50.322
      C6-C7 M50.323
      C7-T1 M50.33
      cervicothoracic region M50.33
      high cervical region M50.31
      mid-cervical region M50.320
    displacement M50.20
      C2-C3 M50.21
      C3-C4 M50.21
      C4-C5 M50.221
      C5-C6 M50.222
      C6-C7 M50.223
      C7-T1 M50.23
      cervicothoracic region M50.23
      high cervical region M50.21
      mid-cervical region M50.220
    high cervical region M50.91
    mid-cervical region M50.920
    specified type NEC M50.80
      C2-C3 M50.81
      C3-C4 M50.81
      C4-C5 M50.821
      C5-C6 M50.822
      C6-C7 M50.823
      C7-T1 M50.83
      cervicothoracic region M50.83
      high cervical region M50.81
      mid-cervical region M50.820
  specified NEC
    lumbar region M51.86
    lumbosacral region M51.87
    sacrococcygeal region M53.3
    thoracic region M51.84
    thoracolumbar region M51.85
disinhibited attachment (childhood) F94.2
disintegrative, childhood NEC F84.3
disruptive F91.9
    mood dysregulation F34.81
    specified NEC F91.8
disruptive behavior — *see* Disorder, conduct
dissocial personality F60.2
dissociative F44.9
  affecting
    motor function F44.4
      and sensation F44.7
    sensation F44.6
      and motor function F44.7
  brief reactive F43.0
  due to (secondary to) general medical condition
    F06.8
  mixed F44.7
  organic F06.8
  other specified NEC F44.89
double heterozygous sickling — *see* Disease,
  sickle-cell
dream anxiety F51.5
drug induced hemorrhagic D68.32
drug related F19.99
  abuse — *see* Abuse, drug
  dependence — *see* Dependence, drug
dysmorphic body F45.22
dysthymic F34.1
ear H93.9 ☑
  bleeding — *see* Otorrhagia
  deafness — *see* Deafness
  degenerative H93.09 ☑

Disorder — *continued*
  ear — *continued*
    discharge — *see* Otorrhea
    external H61.9 ☑
      auditory canal stenosis — *see* Stenosis, external
        ear canal
      exostosis — *see* Exostosis, external ear canal
      impacted cerumen — *see* Impaction, cerumen
      otitis — *see* Otitis, externa
      perichondritis — *see* Perichondritis, ear
      pinna — *see* Disorder, pinna
      specified type NEC H61.89 ☑
        in diseases classified elsewhere H62.8X ☑
    inner H83.9 ☑
      vestibular dysfunction — *see* Disorder,
        vestibular function
    middle H74.9 ☑
      adhesive H74.1 ☑
      ossicle — *see* Abnormal, ear ossicles
      polyp — *see* Polyp, ear (middle)
      specified NEC, in diseases classified elsewhere
        H75.8 ☑
    postprocedural — *see* Complications, ear,
      procedure
    specified NEC, in diseases classified elsewhere
      H94.8 ☑
  eating (adult) (psychogenic) F50.9
    anorexia — *see* Anorexia
    binge F50.81
    bulimia F50.2
    child F98.29
      pica F98.3
      rumination disorder F98.21
    pica F50.89
      childhood F98.3
  electrolyte (balance) NEC E87.8
    with
      abortion — *see* Abortion by type complicated
        by specified condition NEC
      ectopic pregnancy O08.5
      molar pregnancy O08.5
    acidosis (metabolic) (respiratory) E87.2
    alkalosis (metabolic) (respiratory) E87.3
  elimination, transepidermal L87.9
    specified NEC L87.8
  emotional (persistent) F34.9
    of childhood F93.9
      specified NEC F93.8
  endocrine E34.9
    postprocedural E89.89
    specified NEC E89.89
  erectile (male) (organic) (*see also* Dysfunction,
    sexual, male, erectile) N52.9
    nonorganic F52.21
  erythematous — *see* Erythema
  esophagus K22.9
    functional K22.4
    psychogenic F45.8
  eustachian tube H69.9 ☑
    infection — *see* Salpingitis, eustachian
    obstruction — *see* Obstruction, eustachian tube
    patulous — *see* Patulous, eustachian tube
    specified NEC H69.8 ☑
  exhibitionistic F65.2
  extrapyramidal G25.9
    in diseases classified elsewhere — *see* category G26
    specified type NEC G25.89
  eye H57.9
    postprocedural — *see* Complication,
      postprocedural, eye
  eyelid H02.9
    cyst — *see* Cyst, eyelid
    degenerative H02.70
      chloasma — *see* Chloasma, eyelid
      madarosis — *see* Madarosis
      specified type NEC H02.79
      vitiligo — *see* Vitiligo, eyelid
      xanthelasma — *see* Xanthelasma
    dermatochalasis — *see* Dermatochalasis
    edema — *see* Edema, eyelid
    elephantiasis — *see* Elephantiasis, eyelid
    foreign body, retained — *see* Foreign body,
      retained, eyelid
    function H02.59
      abnormal innervation syndrome — *see*
        Syndrome, abnormal innervation
      blepharochalasis — *see* Blepharochalasis
      blepharoclonus — *see* Blepharoclonus
      blepharophimosis — *see* Blepharophimosis
      blepharoptosis — *see* Blepharoptosis
      lagophthalmos — *see* Lagophthalmos
      lid retraction — *see* Retraction, lid

☑ **Additional character required**

Disorder — *continued*
  eyelid — *continued*
    hypertrichosis — *see* Hypertrichosis, eyelid
    specified type NEC H02.89
    vascular H02.879
      left H02.876
        lower H02.875
        upper H02.874
      right H02.873
        lower H02.872
        upper H02.871
  factitious
    by proxy F68.A
    imposed on another F68.A
    imposed on self F68.10
      with predominantly
        psychological symptoms F68.11
          with physical symptoms F68.13
        physical symptoms F68.12
          with psychological symptoms F68.13
  factor, coagulation — *see* Defect, coagulation
  fatty acid
    metabolism E71.30
      specified NEC E71.39
    oxidation
      LCAD E71.310
      MCAD E71.311
      SCAD E71.312
      specified deficiency NEC E71.318
  feeding (infant or child) (*see also* Disorder, eating)
      R63.3
    or eating disorder F50.9
    specified NEC F50.9
  feigned (with obvious motivation) Z76.5
    without obvious motivation — *see* Disorder,
        factitious
  female
    hypoactive sexual desire F52.0
    orgasmic F52.31
    sexual interest/arousal F52.22
  fetishistic F65.0
  fibroblastic M72.9
    specified NEC M72.8
  fluency
    adult onset F98.5
    childhood onset F80.81
    following
      cerebral infarction I69.323
      cerebrovascular disease I69.923
        specified disease NEC I69.823
      intracerebral hemorrhage I69.123
      nontraumatic intracranial hemorrhage NEC
          I69.223
      subarachnoid hemorrhage I69.023
    in conditions classified elsewhere R47.82
  fluid balance E87.8
  follicular (skin) L73.9
    specified NEC L73.8
  frotteuristic F65.81
  fructose metabolism E74.10
    essential fructosuria E74.11
    fructokinase deficiency E74.11
    fructose-1, 6-diphosphatase deficiency E74.19
    hereditary fructose intolerance E74.12
    other specified E74.19
  functional polymorphonuclear neutrophils D71
  gallbladder, biliary tract and pancreas in diseases
      classified elsewhere K87
  gambling F63.0
  gamma aminobutyric acid (GABA) metabolism
      E72.81
  gamma-glutamyl cycle E72.89
  gastric (functional) K31.9
    motility K30
    psychogenic F45.8
    secretion K30
  gastrointestinal (functional) NOS K92.9
    newborn P78.9
    psychogenic F45.8
  gender-identity or -role F64.9
    childhood F64.2
    effect on relationship F66
    of adolescence or adulthood F64.0
      nontranssexual F64.8
    specified NEC F64.8
    uncertainty F66
  genito-pelvic pain penetration F52.6
  genitourinary system
    female N94.9
    male N50.9
      psychogenic F45.8

Disorder — *continued*
  globe H44.9
    degenerated condition H44.50
      absolute glaucoma H44.51 ☑
      atrophy H44.52 ☑
      leucocoria H44.53 ☑
    degenerative H44.30
      chalcosis H44.31 ☑
      myopia (*see also* Myopia, degenerative)
          H44.2 ☑
      siderosis H44.32 ☑
      specified type NEC H44.39 ☑
    endophthalmitis — *see* Endophthalmitis
    foreign body, retained — *see* Foreign body,
        intraocular, old, retained
    hemophthalmos — *see* Hemophthalmos
    hypotony H44.40
      due to
        ocular fistula H44.42 ☑
        specified disorder NEC H44.43 ☑
      flat anterior chamber H44.41 ☑
      primary H44.44 ☑
    luxation — *see* Luxation, globe
    specified type NEC H44.89
  glomerular (in) N05.9
    amyloidosis E85.4 *[N08]*
    cryoglobulinemia D89.1 *[N08]*
    disseminated intravascular coagulation
        D65 *[N08]*
    Fabry's disease E75.21 *[N08]*
    familial lecithin cholesterol acyltransferase
        deficiency E78.6 *[N08]*
    Goodpasture's syndrome M31.0
    hemolytic-uremic syndrome D59.3
    Henoch (-Schönlein) purpura D69.0 *[N08]*
    malariae malaria B52.0
    microscopic polyangiitis M31.7 *[N08]*
    multiple myeloma C90.0 ☑ *[N08]*
    mumps B26.83
    schistosomiasis B65.9 *[N08]*
    sepsis NEC A41. ☑ *[N08]*
      streptococcal A40. *[N08]*
    sickle-cell disorders D57. ☑ *[N08]*
    strongyloidiasis B78.9 *[N08]*
    subacute bacterial endocarditis I33.0 *[N08]*
    syphilis A52.75
    systemic lupus erythematosus M32.14
    thrombotic thrombocytopenic purpura M31.1
        [N08]
    Waldenström macroglobulinemia C88.0 *[N08]*
    Wegener's granulomatosis M31.31
  gluconeogenesis E74.4
  glucosaminoglycan metabolism — *see* Disorder,
      metabolism, glucosaminoglycan
  glycine metabolism E72.50
    d-glycericacidemia E72.59
    hyperhydroxyprolinemia E72.59
    hyperoxaluria R82.992
      primary E72.53
    hyperprolinemia E72.59
    non-ketotic hyperglycinemia E72.51
    oxalosis E72.53
    oxaluria E72.53
    sarcosinemia E72.59
    trimethylaminuria E72.52
  glycoprotein metabolism E77.9
    specified NEC E77.8
  habit (and impulse) F63.9
    involving sexual behavior NEC F65.9
    specified NEC F63.89
  hallucinogen use
    mild F16.10
      with
        hallucinogen-induced
          anxiety disorder F16.180
          bipolar and related disorder F16.14
          depressive disorder F16.14
          psychotic disorder F16.159
        hallucinogen intoxication delirium F16.121
        other hallucinogen intoxication F16.129
      in remission (early) (sustained) F16.11
    moderate or severe F16.20
      with
        hallucinogen-induced
          anxiety disorder F16.280
          bipolar and related disorder F16.24
          depressive disorder F16.24
          psychotic disorder F16.259
        hallucinogen intoxication delirium F16.221
        other hallucinogen intoxication F16.229
      in remission (early) (sustained) F16.21
  heart action I49.9

Disorder — *continued*
  hematological D75.9
    newborn (transient) P61.9
      specified NEC P61.8
  hematopoietic organs D75.9
  hemorrhagic D69.9
    drug-induced D68.32
    due to
      extrinsic circulating anticoagulants D68.32
      increase in
        anti-IIa D68.32
        anti-Xa D68.32
      intrinsic
        circulating anticoagulants D68.318
        increase in
          antithrombin D68.318
          anti-VIIIa D68.318
          anti-IXa D68.318
          anti-XIa D68.318
    following childbirth O72.3
  hemostasis — *see* Defect, coagulation
  histidine metabolism E70.40
    histidinemia E70.41
    other specified E70.49
  hoarding F42.3
  hyperkinetic — *see* Disorder, attention-deficit
      hyperactivity
  hyperleucine-isoleucinemia E71.19
  hypervalinemia E71.19
  hypoactive sexual desire F52.0
  hypochondriacal F45.20
    body dysmorphic F45.22
    neurosis F45.21
    other specified F45.29
  identity
    dissociative F44.81
    of childhood F93.8
    illness anxiety F45.21
  immune mechanism (immunity) D89.9
    specified type NEC D89.89
  impaired renal tubular function N25.9
    specified NEC N25.89
  impulse (control) F63.9
  inflammatory
    pelvic, in diseases classified elsewhere — *see*
        category N74
    penis N48.29
      abscess N48.21
      cellulitis N48.22
  inhalant use
    mild F18.10
      with
        inhalant-induced
          anxiety disorder F18.180
          depressive disorder F18.14
          major neurocognitive disorder F18.17
          mild neurocognitive disorder F18.188
          psychotic disorder F18.159
        inhalant intoxication F18.129
        inhalant intoxication delirium F18.121
      in remission (early) (sustained) F18.11
    moderate or severe F18.20
      with
        inhalant-induced
          anxiety disorder F18.280
          depressive disorder F18.24
          major neurocognitive disorder F18.27
          mild neurocognitive disorder F18.288
          psychotic disorder F18.259
        inhalant intoxication F18.229
        inhalant intoxication delirium F18.221
      in remission (early) (sustained) F18.21
  integument, newborn P83.9
    specified NEC P83.88
  intermittent explosive F63.81
  internal secretion pancreas — *see* Increased,
      secretion, pancreas, endocrine
  intestine, intestinal
    carbohydrate absorption NEC E74.39
      postoperative K91.2
    functional NEC K59.9
      postoperative K91.89
    psychogenic F45.8
    vascular K55.9
      chronic K55.1
      specified NEC K55.8
  intraoperative (intraprocedural) — *see*
      Complications, intraoperative
  involuntary emotional expression (IEED) F48.2
  iris H21.9
    adhesions — *see* Adhesions, iris
    atrophy — *see* Atrophy, iris

Disorder

Disorder — *continued*
- iris — *continued*
  - chamber angle recession — *see* Recession,
    - chamber angle
  - cyst — *see* Cyst, iris
  - degeneration — *see* Degeneration, iris
  - in diseases classified elsewhere H22
  - iridodialysis — *see* Iridodialysis
  - iridoschisis — *see* Iridoschisis
  - miotic pupillary cyst — *see* Cyst, pupillary
  - pupillary
    - abnormality — *see* Abnormality, pupillary
    - membrane — *see* Membrane, pupillary
  - specified type NEC H21.89
  - vascular NEC H21.1X ☑
- iron metabolism E83.10
  - specified NEC E83.19
- isovaleric acidemia E71.110
- jaw, developmental M27.0
- temporomandibular (*see also* Anomaly,
  - dentofacial, temporomandibular joint)
    - M26.60 ☑
- joint M25.9
  - derangement — *see* Derangement, joint
  - effusion — *see* Effusion, joint
  - fistula — *see* Fistula, joint
  - hemarthrosis — *see* Hemarthrosis
  - instability — *see* Instability, joint
  - osteophyte — *see* Osteophyte
  - pain — *see* Pain, joint
  - psychogenic F45.8
  - specified type NEC M25.80
    - ankle M25.87 ☑
    - elbow M25.82 ☑
    - foot joint M25.87 ☑
    - hand joint M25.84 ☑
    - hip M25.85 ☑
    - knee M25.86 ☑
    - shoulder M25.81 ☑
    - wrist M25.83 ☑
  - stiffness — *see* Stiffness, joint
- ketone metabolism E71.32
- kidney N28.9
  - functional (tubular) N25.9
  - in
    - schistosomiasis B65.9 *[N29]*
  - tubular function N25.9
  - specified NEC N25.89
- lacrimal system H04.9
  - changes H04.69
    - fistula — *see* Fistula, lacrimal
  - gland H04.19
    - atrophy — *see* Atrophy, lacrimal gland
    - cyst — *see* Cyst, lacrimal, gland
    - dacryops — *see* Dacryops
    - dislocation — *see* Dislocation, lacrimal gland
    - dry eye syndrome — *see* Syndrome, dry eye
    - infection — *see* Dacryoadenitis
    - granuloma — *see* Granuloma, lacrimal
    - inflammation — *see* Inflammation, lacrimal
    - obstruction — *see* Obstruction, lacrimal
  - specified NEC H04.89
- lactation NEC O92.79
- language (developmental) F80.9
  - expressive F80.1
  - mixed receptive and expressive F80.2
  - receptive F80.2
- late luteal phase dysphoric N94.89
- learning (specific) F81.9
  - acalculia R48.8
  - alexia R48.0
  - mathematics F81.2
  - reading F81.0
  - specified
    - with impairment in
      - mathematics F81.2
      - reading F81.0
      - written expression F81.81
  - specified NEC F81.89
  - spelling F81.81
  - written expression F81.81
- lens H27.9
  - aphakia — *see* Aphakia
  - cataract — *see* Cataract
  - dislocation — *see* Dislocation, lens
  - specified type NEC H27.8
- ligament M24.20
  - ankle M24.27 ☑
  - attachment, spine — *see* Enthesopathy, spinal
  - elbow M24.22 ☑
  - foot joint M24.27 ☑
  - hand joint M24.24 ☑

Disorder — *continued*
- ligament — *continued*
  - hip M24.25 ☑
  - knee — *see* Derangement, knee, specified NEC
  - shoulder M24.21 ☑
  - vertebra M24.28
  - wrist M24.23 ☑
- ligamentous attachments (*see also* Enthesopathy)
  - spine — *see* Enthesopathy, spinal
- lipid
  - metabolism, congenital E78.9
  - storage E75.6
    - specified NEC E75.5
- lipoprotein
  - deficiency (familial) E78.6
  - metabolism E78.9
    - specified NEC E78.89
- liver K76.9
  - malarial B54 *[K77]*
- low back (*see also* Dorsopathy, specified NEC)
- lumbosacral
  - plexus G54.1
  - root (nerve) NEC G54.4
- lung, interstitial, drug-induced J70.4
  - acute J70.2
  - chronic J70.3
- lymphoproliferative, post-transplant (PTLD) D47.Z1
- lysine and hydroxylysine metabolism E72.3
- major neurocognitive — *see* Dementia, in (due to)
- male
  - erectile (organic) (*see also* Dysfunction, sexual,
    - male, erectile) N52.9
    - nonorganic F52.21
  - hypoactive sexual desire F52.0
  - orgasmic F52.32
- manic F30.9
  - organic F06.33
- mast cell activation — *see* Activation, mast cell
- mastoid (*see also* Disorder, ear, middle)
  - postprocedural — *see* Complications, ear,
    - procedure
- meniscus — *see* Derangement, knee, meniscus
- menopausal N95.9
  - specified NEC N95.8
- menstrual N92.6
  - psychogenic F45.8
  - specified NEC N92.5
- mental (or behavioral) (nonpsychotic) F99
  - due to (secondary to)
    - amphetamine
      - due to drug abuse — *see* Abuse, drug,
        - stimulant
      - due to drug dependence — *see* Dependence,
        - drug, stimulant
    - brain disease, damage and dysfunction F09
    - caffeine use
      - due to drug abuse — *see* Abuse, drug,
        - stimulant
      - due to drug dependence — *see* Dependence,
        - drug, stimulant
    - cannabis use
      - due to drug abuse — *see* Abuse, drug,
        - cannabis
      - due to drug dependence — *see* Dependence,
        - drug, cannabis
    - general medical condition F09
    - sedative or hypnotic use
      - due to drug abuse — *see* Abuse, drug,
        - sedative
      - due to drug dependence — *see* Dependence,
        - drug, sedative
    - tobacco (nicotine) use — *see* Dependence,
      - drug, nicotine
  - following organic brain damage F07.9
    - frontal lobe syndrome F07.0
    - personality change F07.0
    - postconcussional syndrome F07.81
    - specified NEC F07.89
  - infancy, childhood or adolescence F98.9
  - neurotic — *see* Neurosis
  - organic or symptomatic F09
  - presenile, psychotic F03 ☑
  - problem NEC
  - psychoneurotic — *see* Neurosis
  - psychotic — *see* Psychosis
  - puerperal F53.0
  - senile, psychotic NEC F03 ☑
- metabolic, amino acid, transitory, newborn P74.8
- metabolism NOS E88.9
  - amino-acid E72.9
    - aromatic E70.9
      - albinism — *see* Albinism

Disorder — *continued*
- metabolism NOS — *continued*
  - histidine E70.40
    - histidinemia E70.41
    - other specified E70.49
  - hyperphenylalaninemia E70.1
    - classical phenylketonuria E70.0
  - other specified E70.8
  - tryptophan E70.5
  - tyrosine E70.20
    - hypertyrosinemia E70.21
    - other specified E70.29
  - branched chain E71.2
    - 3-methylglutaconic aciduria E71.111
    - hyperleucine-isoleucinemia E71.19
    - hypervalinemia E71.19
    - isovaleric acidemia E71.110
    - maple syrup urine disease E71.0
    - methylmalonic acidemia E71.120
    - organic aciduria NEC E71.118
    - other specified E71.19
    - proprionate NEC E71.128
    - proprionic acidemia E71.121
  - glycine E72.50
    - d-glycericacidemia E72.59
    - hyperhydroxyprolinemia E72.59
    - hyperoxaluria R82.992
      - primary E72.53
    - hyperprolinemia E72.59
    - non-ketotic hyperglycinemia E72.51
    - other specified E72.59
    - sarcosinemia E72.59
    - trimethylaminuria E72.52
  - hydroxylysine E72.3
  - lysine E72.3
  - ornithine E72.4
  - other specified E72.89
    - beta-amino acid E72.89
    - gamma-glutamyl cycle E72.89
  - straight-chain E72.89
  - sulfur-bearing E72.10
    - homocystinuria E72.11
    - methylenetetrahydrofolate reductase
      - deficiency E72.12
    - other specified E72.19
  - bile acid and cholesterol metabolism E78.70
  - bilirubin E80.7
    - specified NEC E80.6
  - calcium E83.50
    - hypercalcemia E83.52
    - hypocalcemia E83.51
    - other specified E83.59
  - carbohydrate E74.9
    - specified NEC E74.8
  - cholesterol and bile acid metabolism E78.70
  - congenital E88.9
  - copper E83.00
    - Wilson's disease E83.01
    - specified type NEC E83.09
  - cystinuria E72.01
  - fructose E74.10
  - galactose E74.20
  - glucosaminoglycan E76.9
    - mucopolysaccharidosis — *see*
      - Mucopolysaccharidosis
    - specified NEC E76.8
  - glutamine E72.89
  - glycine E72.50
  - glycogen storage (hepatorenal) E74.09
  - glycoprotein E77.9
    - specified NEC E77.8
  - glycosaminoglycan E76.9
    - specified NEC E76.8
  - in labor and delivery O75.89
  - iron E83.10
  - isoleucine E71.19
  - leucine E71.19
  - lipoid E78.9
  - lipoprotein E78.9
    - specified NEC E78.89
  - magnesium E83.40
    - hypermagnesemia E83.41
    - hypomagnesemia E83.42
    - other specified E83.49
  - mineral E83.9
    - specified NEC E83.89
  - mitochondrial E88.40
    - MELAS syndrome E88.41
    - MERRF syndrome (myoclonic epilepsy
      - associated with ragged-red fibers) E88.42
    - other specified E88.49
  - ornithine E72.4

☑ **Additional character required**

Disorder — *continued*
  metabolism NOS — *continued*
    phosphatases E83.30
    phosphorus E83.30
      acid phosphatase deficiency E83.39
      hypophosphatasia E83.39
      hypophosphatemia E83.39
        familial E83.31
      other specified E83.39
      pseudovitamin D deficiency E83.32
    plasma protein NEC E88.09
    porphyrin — *see* Porphyria
    postprocedural E89.89
      specified NEC E89.89
    purine E79.9
      specified NEC E79.8
    pyrimidine E79.9
      specified NEC E79.8
    pyruvate E74.4
    serine E72.89
    sodium E87.8
    specified NEC E88.89
    threonine E72.89
    valine E71.19
    zinc E83.2
  methylmalonic acidemia E71.120
  micturition NEC (*see also* Difficulty, micturition) R39.198
    feeling of incomplete emptying R39.14
    hesitancy R39.11
    poor stream R39.12
    psychogenic F45.8
    split stream R39.13
    straining R39.16
    urgency R39.15
  mild neurocognitive G31.84
  mitochondrial metabolism E88.40
  mitral (valve) — *see* Endocarditis, mitral
  mixed
    anxiety and depressive F41.8
    of scholastic skills (developmental) F81.89
    receptive expressive language F80.2
  mood F39
    bipolar — *see* Disorder, bipolar
    depressive — *see* Disorder, depressive
    due to (secondary to)
      alcohol F10.94
      amphetamine F15.94
        in
          abuse F15.14
          dependence F15.24
      anxiolytic F13.94
        in
          abuse F13.14
          dependence F13.24
      cocaine F14.94
        in
          abuse F14.14
          dependence F14.24
      general medical condition F06.30
      hallucinogen F16.94
        in
          abuse F16.14
          dependence F16.24
      hypnotic F13.94
        in
          abuse F13.14
          dependence F13.24
      inhalant F18.94
        in
          abuse F18.14
          dependence F18.24
      opioid F11.94
        in
          abuse F11.14
          dependence F11.24
      phencyclidine (PCP) F16.94
        in
          abuse F16.14
          dependence F16.24
      physiological condition F06.30
        with
          depressive features F06.31
          major depressive-like episode F06.32
          manic features F06.33
          mixed features F06.34
      psychoactive substance NEC F19.94
        in
          abuse F19.14
          dependence F19.24
      sedative F13.94
        in

Disorder — *continued*
  mood — *continued*
      abuse F13.14
      dependence F13.24
    volatile solvents F18.94
      in
        abuse F18.14
        dependence F18.24
    manic episode F30.9
      with psychotic symptoms F30.2
      in remission (full) F30.4
        partial F30.3
      specified type NEC F30.8
      without psychotic symptoms F30.10
        mild F30.11
        moderate F30.12
        severe F30.13
    organic F06.30
      right hemisphere F07.89
    persistent F34.9
      cyclothymia F34.0
      dysthymia F34.1
      specified type NEC F34.89
    recurrent F39
    right hemisphere organic F07.89
  movement G25.9
    drug-induced G25.70
      akathisia G25.71
      specified NEC G25.79
    hysterical F44.4
    in diseases classified elsewhere — *see* category G26
    periodic limb G47.61
      sleep related G47.61
    specified NEC G25.89
    sleep related NEC G47.69
    stereotyped F98.4
    treatment-induced G25.9
  multiple personality F44.81
  muscle M62.9
    attachment, spine — *see* Enthesopathy, spinal
    in trichinellosis — *see* Trichinellosis, with muscle disorder
    psychogenic F45.8
    specified type NEC M62.89
    tone, newborn P94.9
      specified NEC P94.8
  muscular
    attachments (*see also* Enthesopathy)
      spine — *see* Enthesopathy, spinal
    urethra N36.44
  musculoskeletal system, soft tissue — *see* Disorder, soft tissue
    postprocedural M96.89
    psychogenic F45.8
  myoneural G70.9
    due to lead G70.1
    specified NEC G70.89
    toxic G70.1
  myotonic NEC G71.19
  nail, in diseases classified elsewhere L62
  neck region NEC — *see* Dorsopathy, specified NEC
  neonatal onset multisystemic inflammatory (NOMID) M04.2
  nerve G58.9
    abducent NEC — *see* Strabismus, paralytic, sixth nerve
    accessory G52.8
    acoustic — *see* subcategory H93.3 ☑
    auditory — *see* subcategory H93.3 ☑
    auriculotemporal G50.8
    axillary G54.0
    cerebral — *see* Disorder, nerve, cranial
    cranial G52.9
      eighth — *see* subcategory H93.3 ☑
      eleventh G52.8
      fifth G50.9
      first G52.0
      fourth NEC — *see* Strabismus, paralytic, fourth nerve
      multiple G52.7
      ninth G52.1
      second NEC — *see* Disorder, nerve, optic
      seventh NEC G51.8
      sixth NEC — *see* Strabismus, paralytic, sixth nerve
      specified NEC G52.8
      tenth G52.2
      third NEC — *see* Strabismus, paralytic, third nerve
      twelfth G52.3
    entrapment — *see* Neuropathy, entrapment

Disorder — *continued*
  nerve — *continued*
    facial G51.9
      specified NEC G51.8
    femoral — *see* Lesion, nerve, femoral
    glossopharyngeal NEC G52.1
    hypoglossal G52.3
    intercostal G58.0
    lateral
      cutaneous of thigh — *see* Mononeuropathy, lower limb, meralgia paresthetica
      popliteal — *see* Lesion, nerve, popliteal
    lower limb — *see* Mononeuropathy, lower limb
    medial popliteal — *see* Lesion, nerve, popliteal, medial
    median NEC — *see* Lesion, nerve, median
    multiple G58.7
    oculomotor NEC — *see* Strabismus, paralytic, third nerve
    olfactory G52.0
    optic NEC H47.09 ☑
      hemorrhage into sheath — *see* Hemorrhage, optic nerve
      ischemic H47.01 ☑
    peroneal — *see* Lesion, nerve, popliteal
    phrenic G58.8
    plantar — *see* Lesion, nerve, plantar
    pneumogastric G52.2
    posterior tibial — *see* Syndrome, tarsal tunnel
    radial — *see* Lesion, nerve, radial
    recurrent laryngeal G52.2
    root G54.9
      cervical G54.2
      lumbosacral G54.1
      specified NEC G54.8
      thoracic G54.3
    sciatic NEC — *see* Lesion, nerve, sciatic
    specified NEC G58.8
      lower limb — *see* Mononeuropathy, lower limb, specified NEC
      upper limb — *see* Mononeuropathy, upper limb, specified NEC
    sympathetic G90.9
    tibial — *see* Lesion, nerve, popliteal, medial
    trigeminal G50.9
      specified NEC G50.8
    trochlear NEC — *see* Strabismus, paralytic, fourth nerve
    ulnar — *see* Lesion, nerve, ulnar
    upper limb — *see* Mononeuropathy, upper limb
    vagus G52.2
  nervous system G98.8
    autonomic (peripheral) G90.9
      specified NEC G90.8
    central G96.9
      specified NEC G96.8
    parasympathetic G90.9
    specified NEC G98.8
    sympathetic G90.9
    vegetative G90.9
  neurocognitive R41.9
    major
      with
        aggressive behavior F01.51
        combative behavior F01.51
        violent behavior F01.51
      due to vascular disease, with behavioral disturbance F01.51
      in (due to) (other diseases classified elsewhere) (*see also* Dementia, in (due to)) F02.80
        with
          aggressive behavior F02.81
          combative behavior F02.81
          violent behavior F02.81
      without behavioral disturbance F01.50
    mild G31.84
  neurodevelopmental F89
    specified NEC F88
  neurohypophysis NEC E23.3
  neurological NEC R29.818
  neuromuscular G70.9
    hereditary NEC G71.9
    specified NEC G70.89
    toxic G70.1
  neurotic F48.9
    specified NEC F48.8
  neutrophil, polymorphonuclear D71
  nicotine use — *see* Dependence, drug, nicotine
  nightmare F51.5
  non-rapid eye movement sleep arousal
    sleep terror type F51.4
    sleepwalking type F51.3

Disorder

Disorder — *continued*
- nose J34.9
  - specified NEC J34.89
- obsessive-compulsive F42.9
  - and related disorder due to a known
    - physiological condition F06.8
- odontogenesis NOS K00.9
- opioid use
  - with
    - opioid-induced psychotic disorder F11.959
      - with
        - delusions F11.950
        - hallucinations F11.951
  - due to drug abuse — *see* Abuse, drug, opioid
  - due to drug dependence — *see* Dependence, drug, opioid
  - mild F11.10
    - with
      - opioid-induced
        - anxiety disorder F11.188
        - depressive disorder F11.14
        - sexual dysfunction F11.181
      - opioid intoxication
        - with perceptual disturbances F11.122
        - delirium F11.121
        - without perceptual disturbances F11.129
    - in remission (early) (sustained) F11.11
  - moderate or severe F11.20
    - with
      - opioid-induced
        - anxiety disorder F11.288
        - anxiety disorder F11.988
        - depressive disorder F11.24
        - depressive disorder F11.94
        - sexual dysfunction F11.281
        - sexual dysfunction F11.981
      - opioid intoxication
        - with perceptual disturbances F11.222
        - delirium F11.221
        - without perceptual disturbances F11.229
    - in remission (early) (sustained) F11.21
- oppositional defiant F91.3
- optic
  - chiasm H47.49
    - due to
      - inflammatory disorder H47.41
      - neoplasm H47.42
      - vascular disorder H47.43
  - disc H47.39 ☑
    - coloboma — *see* Coloboma, optic disc
    - drusen — *see* Drusen, optic disc
    - pseudopapilledema — *see* Pseudopapilledema
  - radiations — *see* Disorder, visual, pathway
  - tracts — *see* Disorder, visual, pathway
- orbit H05.9
  - cyst — *see* Cyst, orbit
  - deformity — *see* Deformity, orbit
  - edema — *see* Edema, orbit
  - enophthalmos — *see* Enophthalmos
  - exophthalmos — *see* Exophthalmos
  - hemorrhage — *see* Hemorrhage, orbit
  - inflammation — *see* Inflammation, orbit
  - myopathy — *see* Myopathy, extraocular muscles
  - retained foreign body — *see* Foreign body, orbit, old
  - specified type NEC H05.89
- organic
  - anxiety F06.4
  - catatonic F06.1
  - delusional F06.2
  - dissociative F06.8
  - emotionally labile (asthenic) F06.8
  - mood (affective) F06.30
  - schizophrenia-like F06.2
- orgasmic (female) F52.31
  - male F52.32
- ornithine metabolism E72.4
- overanxious F41.1
  - of childhood F93.8
- pain
  - with related psychological factors F45.42
  - exclusively related to psychological factors F45.41
  - genito-pelvic penetration disorder F52.6
- pancreatic internal secretion E16.9
  - specified NEC E16.8
- panic F41.0
  - with agoraphobia F40.01
- papulosquamous L44.9
  - in diseases classified elsewhere L45
  - specified NEC L44.8
- paranoid F22
  - induced F24
  - shared F24

Disorder — *continued*
- paraphilic F65.9
  - specified NEC F65.89
- parathyroid (gland) E21.5
  - specified NEC E21.4
- parietoalveolar NEC J84.09
- paroxysmal, mixed R56.9
- patella M22.9 ☑
  - chondromalacia — *see* Chondromalacia, patella
  - derangement NEC M22.3X ☑
  - recurrent
    - dislocation — *see* Dislocation, patella, recurrent
    - subluxation — *see* Dislocation, patella, recurrent, incomplete
  - specified NEC M22.8X ☑
- patellofemoral M22.2X ☑
- pedophilic F65.4
- pentose phosphate pathway with anemia D55.1
- perception, due to hallucinogens F16.983
  - in
    - abuse F16.183
    - dependence F16.283
- peripheral nervous system NEC G64
- peroxisomal E71.50
  - biogenesis
    - neonatal adrenoleukodystrophy E71.511
    - specified disorder NEC E71.518
    - Zellweger syndrome E71.510
  - rhizomelic chondrodysplasia punctata E71.540
  - specified form NEC E71.548
    - group 1 E71.518
    - group 2 E71.53
    - group 3 E71.542
  - X-linked adrenoleukodystrophy E71.529
    - adolescent E71.521
    - adrenomyeloneuropathy E71.522
    - childhood E71.520
    - specified form NEC E71.528
  - Zellweger-like syndrome E71.541
- persistent
  - (somatoform) pain F45.41
  - affective (mood) F34.9
- personality (*see also* Personality) F60.9
  - affective F34.0
  - aggressive F60.3
  - amoral F60.2
  - anankastic F60.5
  - antisocial F60.2
  - anxious F60.6
  - asocial F60.2
  - asthenic F60.7
  - avoidant F60.6
  - borderline F60.3
  - change (secondary) due to general medical condition F07.0
  - compulsive F60.5
  - cyclothymic F34.0
  - dependent (passive) F60.7
  - depressive F34.1
  - dissocial F60.2
  - emotional instability F60.3
  - expansive paranoid F60.0
  - explosive F60.3
  - following organic brain damage F07.9
  - histrionic F60.4
  - hyperthymic F34.0
  - hypothymic F34.1
  - hysterical F60.4
  - immature F60.89
  - inadequate F60.7
  - labile F60.3
  - mixed (nonspecific) F60.89
  - moral deficiency F60.2
  - narcissistic F60.81
  - negativistic F60.89
  - obsessional F60.5
  - obsessive (-compulsive) F60.5
  - organic F07.9
  - overconscientious F60.5
  - paranoid F60.0
  - passive (-dependent) F60.7
  - passive-aggressive F60.89
  - pathological NEC F60.9
  - pseudosocial F60.2
  - psychopathic F60.2
  - schizoid F60.1
  - schizotypal F21
  - self-defeating F60.7
  - specified NEC F60.89
  - type A F60.5
  - unstable (emotional) F60.3
- pervasive, developmental F84.9

Disorder — *continued*
- phencyclidine use
  - mild F16.10
    - with
      - phencyclidine-induced
        - anxiety disorder F16.180
        - bipolar and related disorder F16.14
        - depressive disorder F16.14
        - psychotic disorder F16.159
      - phencyclidine intoxication F16.129
      - phencyclidine intoxication delirium F16.121
    - in remission (early) (sustained) F16.11
  - moderate or severe F16.20
    - with
      - phencyclidine-induced
        - anxiety disorder F16.280
        - bipolar and related disorder F16.24
        - depressive disorder F16.24
        - psychotic disorder F16.259
      - phencyclidine intoxication F16.229
      - phencyclidine intoxication delirium F16.221
    - in remission (early) (sustained) F16.21
- phobic anxiety, childhood F40.8
- phosphate-losing tubular N25.0
- pigmentation L81.9
  - choroid, congenital Q14.3
  - diminished melanin formation L81.6
  - iron L81.8
  - specified NEC L81.8
- pinna (noninfective) H61.10 ☑
  - deformity, acquired H61.11 ☑
  - hematoma H61.12 ☑
  - perichondritis — *see* Perichondritis, ear
  - specified type NEC H61.19 ☑
- pituitary gland E23.7
  - iatrogenic (postprocedural) E89.3
  - specified NEC E23.6
- platelets D69.1
- plexus G54.9
  - specified NEC G54.8
- polymorphonuclear neutrophils D71
- porphyrin metabolism — *see* Porphyria
- postconcussional F07.81
- posthallucinogen perception F16.983
  - in
    - abuse F16.183
    - dependence F16.283
- postmenopausal N95.9
  - specified NEC N95.8
- postprocedural (postoperative) — *see* Complications, postprocedural
- post-transplant lymphoproliferative D47.Z1
- post-traumatic stress (PTSD) F43.10
  - acute F43.11
  - chronic F43.12
- premenstrual dysphoric (PMDD) F32.81
- prepuce N47.8
- propionic acidemia E71.121
- prostate N42.9
  - specified NEC N42.89
- psychogenic NOS (*see also* condition) F45.9
  - anxiety F41.8
  - appetite F50.9
  - asthenic F48.8
  - cardiovascular (system) F45.8
  - compulsive F42.8
  - cutaneous F54
  - depressive F32.9
  - digestive (system) F45.8
  - dysmenorrheic F45.8
  - dyspneic F45.8
  - endocrine (system) F54
  - eye NEC F45.8
  - feeding — *see* Disorder, eating
  - functional NEC F45.8
  - gastric F45.8
  - gastrointestinal (system) F45.8
  - genitourinary (system) F45.8
  - heart (function) (rhythm) F45.8
  - hyperventilatory F45.8
  - hypochondriacal — *see* Disorder, hypochondriacal
  - intestinal F45.8
  - joint F45.8
  - learning F81.9
  - limb F45.8
  - lymphatic (system) F45.8
  - menstrual F45.8
  - micturition F45.8
  - monoplegic NEC F44.4
  - motor F44.4
  - muscle F45.8

☑ **Additional character required**

Disorder — *continued*
  psychogenic NOS — *continued*
    musculoskeletal F45.8
    neurocirculatory F45.8
    obsessive F42.8
    occupational F48.8
    organ or part of body NEC F45.8
    paralytic NEC F44.4
    phobic F40.9
    physical NEC F45.8
    rectal F45.8
    respiratory (system) F45.8
    rheumatic F45.8
    sexual (function) F52.9
    skin (allergic) (eczematous) F54
    sleep F51.9
    specified part of body NEC F45.8
    stomach F45.8
  psychological F99
    associated with
      disease classified elsewhere F54
      sexual
        development F66
        relationship F66
      uncertainty about gender identity F64.9
  psychomotor NEC F44.4
    hysterical F44.4
  psychoneurotic (*see also* Neurosis)
    mixed NEC F48.8
  psychophysiologic — *see* Disorder, somatoform
  psychosexual F65.9
    development F66
    identity of childhood F64.2
  psychosomatic NOS — *see* Disorder, somatoform
    multiple F45.0
    undifferentiated F45.1
  psychotic — *see* Psychosis
    transient (acute) F23
  puberty E30.9
    specified NEC E30.8
  pulmonary (valve) — *see* Endocarditis, pulmonary
  purine metabolism E79.9
  pyrimidine metabolism E79.9
  pyruvate metabolism E74.4
  reactive attachment (childhood) F94.1
  reading R48.0
    developmental (specific) F81.0
  receptive language F80.2
  receptor, hormonal, peripheral (*see also* Syndrome, androgen insensitivity) E34.50
  recurrent brief depressive F33.8
  reflex R29.2
  refraction H52.7
    aniseikonia H52.32
    anisometropia H52.31
    astigmatism — *see* Astigmatism
    hypermetropia — *see* Hypermetropia
    myopia — *see* Myopia
    presbyopia H52.4
    specified NEC H52.6
  relationship F68.8
    due to sexual orientation F66
  REM sleep behavior G47.52
  renal function, impaired (tubular) N25.9
  resonance R49.9
    specified NEC R49.8
  respiratory function, impaired (*see also* Failure, respiration)
    postprocedural — *see* Complication, postoperative, respiratory system
    psychogenic F45.8
  retina H35.9
    angioid streaks H35.33
    changes in vascular appearance H35.01 ☑
    degeneration — *see* Degeneration, retina
    dystrophy (hereditary) — *see* Dystrophy, retina
    edema H35.81
    hemorrhage — *see* Hemorrhage, retina
    ischemia H35.82
    macular degeneration — *see* Degeneration, macula
    microaneurysms H35.04 ☑
    microvascular abnormality NEC H35.09
    neovascularization — *see* Neovascularization, retina
    retinopathy — *see* Retinopathy
    separation of layers H35.70
      central serous chorioretinopathy H35.71 ☑
      pigment epithelium detachment (serous) H35.72 ☑
        hemorrhagic H35.73 ☑
    specified type NEC H35.89

Disorder — *continued*
  retina — *continued*
    telangiectasis — *see* Telangiectasis, retina
    vasculitis — *see* Vasculitis, retina
  retroperitoneal K68.9
  right hemisphere organic affective F07.89
  rumination (infant or child) F98.21
  sacrum, sacrococcygeal NEC M53.3
  schizoaffective F25.9
    bipolar type F25.0
    depressive type F25.1
    manic type F25.0
    mixed type F25.0
    specified NEC F25.8
  schizoid of childhood F84.5
  schizophrenia spectrum and other psychotic disorder F29
    specified NEC F28
  schizophreniform F20.81
    brief F23
  schizotypal (personality) F21
  secretion, thyrocalcitonin E07.0
  sedative, hypnotic, or anxiolytic use
    mild F13.10
      with
        sedative, hypnotic, or anxiolytic-induced
          anxiety disorder F13.180
          bipolar and related disorder F13.14
          depressive disorder F13.14
          psychotic disorder F13.159
          sexual dysfunction F13.181
        sedative, hypnotic, or anxiolytic intoxication F13.129
        sedative, hypnotic, or anxiolytic intoxication delirium F13.121
      in remission (early) (sustained) F13.11
    moderate or severe F13.20
      with
        sedative, hypnotic, or anxiolytic-induced
          anxiety disorder F13.280
          bipolar and related disorder F13.24
          depressive disorder F13.24
          major neurocognitive disorder F13.27
          mild neurocognitive disorder F13.288
          psychotic disorder F13.259
          sexual dysfunction F13.281
        sedative, hypnotic, or anxiolytic intoxication F13.229
        sedative, hypnotic, or anxiolytic intoxication delirium F13.221
      in remission (early) (sustained) F13.21
  seizure (*see also* Epilepsy) G40.909
    intractable G40.919
      with status epilepticus G40.911
  semantic pragmatic F80.89
    with autism F84.0
  sense of smell R43.1
    psychogenic F45.8
  separation anxiety, of childhood F93.0
  sexual
    arousal, female F52.22
    aversion F52.1
    function, psychogenic F52.9
    interest/arousal, female F52.22
    masochism F65.51
    maturation F66
    nonorganic F52.9
    preference (*see also* Deviation, sexual) F65.9
      fetishistic transvestism F65.1
    relationship F66
    sadism F65.52
  shyness, of childhood and adolescence F40.10
  sibling rivalry F93.8
  sickle-cell (sickling) (homozygous) — *see* Disease, sickle-cell
    heterozygous D57.3
    specified type NEC D57.8 ☑
    trait D57.3
  sinus (nasal) J34.9
    specified NEC J34.89
  skin L98.9
    atrophic L90.9
      specified NEC L90.8
    granulomatous L92.9
      specified NEC L92.8
    hypertrophic L91.9
      specified NEC L91.8
    infiltrative NEC L98.6
    newborn P83.9
      specified NEC P83.88
    picking F42.4
    psychogenic (allergic) (eczematous) F54

Disorder — *continued*
  sleep G47.9
    breathing-related — *see* Apnea, sleep
    circadian rhythm G47.20
      advance sleep phase type G47.22
      delayed sleep phase type G47.21
      due to
        alcohol
          abuse F10.182
          dependence F10.282
          use F10.982
        amphetamines
          abuse F15.182
          dependence F15.282
          use F15.982
        caffeine
          abuse F15.182
          dependence F15.282
          use F15.982
        cocaine
          abuse F14.182
          dependence F14.282
          use F14.982
        drug NEC
          abuse F19.182
          dependence F19.282
          use F19.982
        opioid
          abuse F11.182
          dependence F11.282
          use F11.982
        psychoactive substance NEC
          abuse F19.182
          dependence F19.282
          use F19.982
        sedative, hypnotic, or anxiolytic
          abuse F13.182
          dependence F13.282
          use F13.982
        stimulant NEC
          abuse F15.182
          dependence F15.282
          use F15.982
      free running type G47.24
      in conditions classified elsewhere G47.27
      irregular sleep wake type G47.23
      jet lag type G47.25
      non-24-hour sleep-wake type G47.24
      shift work type G47.26
      specified NEC G47.29
    due to
      alcohol
        abuse F10.182
        dependence F10.282
        use F10.982
      amphetamine
        abuse F15.182
        dependence F15.282
        use F15.982
      anxiolytic
        abuse F13.182
        dependence F13.282
        use F13.982
      caffeine
        abuse F15.182
        dependence F15.282
        use F15.982
      cocaine
        abuse F14.182
        dependence F14.282
        use F14.982
      drug NEC
        abuse F19.182
        dependence F19.282
        use F19.982
      hypnotic
        abuse F13.182
        dependence F13.282
        use F13.982
      opioid
        abuse F11.182
        dependence F11.282
        use F11.982
      psychoactive substance NEC
        abuse F19.182
        dependence F19.282
        use F19.982
      sedative
        abuse F13.182
        dependence F13.282
        use F13.982
      stimulant NEC

Disorder

Disorder — *continued*
  sleep — *continued*
      abuse F15.182
      dependence F15.282
      use F15.982
    emotional F51.9
    excessive somnolence — *see* Hypersomnia
    hypersomnia type — *see* Hypersomnia
    initiating or maintaining — *see* Insomnia
    nightmares F51.5
    nonorganic F51.9
      specified NEC F51.8
    parasomnia type G47.50
    specified NEC G47.8
    terrors F51.4
    walking F51.3
  sleep-wake pattern or schedule (*see also* Disorder, sleep, circadian rhythm) G47.9
    specified NEC G47.8
  social
    anxiety (of childhood) F40.10
      generalized F40.11
    functioning in childhood F94.9
      specified NEC F94.8
    pragmatic F80.82
  soft tissue M79.9
    ankle M79.9
    due to use, overuse and pressure M70.90
      ankle M70.97 ☑
      bursitis — *see* Bursitis
      foot M70.97 ☑
      forearm M70.93 ☑
      hand M70.94 ☑
      lower leg M70.96 ☑
      multiple sites M70.99
      pelvic region M70.95 ☑
      shoulder region M70.91 ☑
      specified site NEC M70.98
      specified type NEC M70.80
        ankle M70.87 ☑
        foot M70.87 ☑
        forearm M70.83 ☑
        hand M70.84 ☑
        lower leg M70.86 ☑
        multiple sites M70.89
        pelvic region M70.85 ☑
        shoulder region M70.81 ☑
        specified site NEC M70.88
        thigh M70.85 ☑
        upper arm M70.82 ☑
      thigh M70.95 ☑
      upper arm M70.92 ☑
    foot M79.9
    forearm M79.9
    hand M79.9
    lower leg M79.9
    multiple sites M79.9
    occupational — *see* Disorder, soft tissue, due to use, overuse and pressure
    pelvic region M79.9
    shoulder region M79.9
    specified type NEC M79.89
    thigh M79.9
    upper arm M79.9
  somatic symptom F45.1
  somatization F45.0
  somatoform F45.9
    pain (persistent) F45.41
    somatization (multiple) (long-lasting) F45.0
    specified NEC F45.8
    undifferentiated F45.1
  somnolence, excessive — *see* Hypersomnia
  specific
    arithmetical F81.2
    developmental, of motor F82
    reading F81.0
    speech and language F80.9
    spelling F81.81
    written expression F81.81
  speech R47.9
    articulation (functional) (specific) F80.0
    developmental F80.9
    specified NEC R47.89
  speech-sound F80.0
  spelling (specific) F81.81
  spine (*see also* Dorsopathy)
    ligamentous or muscular attachments, peripheral — *see* Enthesopathy, spinal
    specified NEC — *see* Dorsopathy, specified NEC
  stereotyped, habit or movement F98.4
  stimulant use (other) (unspecified)
    mild F15.10

Disorder — *continued*
  stimulant use — *continued*
      in remission (early) (sustained) F15.11
    moderate or severe F15.20
      in remission (early) (sustained) F15.21
  stomach (functional) — *see* Disorder, gastric
  stress F43.9
    acute F43.0
    post-traumatic F43.10
      acute F43.11
      chronic F43.12
  substance use (other) (unknown)
    mild F19.10
      with substance-induced
        anxiety disorder F19.180
        bipolar and related disorder F19.14
        depressive disorder F19.14
        major neurocognitive disorder F19.17
        mild neurocognitive disorder F19.188
        obsessive-compulsive and related disorder F19.188
        sexual dysfunction F19.181
      substance intoxication F19.129
      substance intoxication delirium F19.121
    moderate or severe F19.20
      with substance-induced
        anxiety disorder F19.280
        bipolar and related disorder F19.24
        depressive disorder F19.24
        major neurocognitive disorder F19.27
        mild neurocognitive disorder F19.288
        obsessive-compulsive and related disorder F19.288
        sexual dysfunction F19.281
      in remission (early) (sustained) F19.21
      substance intoxication F19.229
      substance intoxication delirium F19.221
  sulfur-bearing amino-acid metabolism E72.10
  sweat gland (eccrine) L74.9
    apocrine L75.9
      specified NEC L75.8
    specified NEC L74.8
  synovium M67.90
    acromioclavicular M67.91 ☑
    ankle M67.97 ☑
    elbow M67.92 ☑
    foot M67.97 ☑
    forearm M67.93 ☑
    hand M67.94 ☑
    hip M67.95 ☑
    knee M67.96 ☑
    multiple sites M67.99
    rupture — *see* Rupture, synovium
    shoulder M67.91 ☑
    specified type NEC M67.80
      acromioclavicular M67.81 ☑
      ankle M67.87 ☑
      elbow M67.82 ☑
      foot M67.87 ☑
      hand M67.84 ☑
      hip M67.85 ☑
      knee M67.86 ☑
      multiple sites M67.89
      wrist M67.83 ☑
    synovitis — *see* Synovitis
    upper arm M67.92 ☑
    wrist M67.93 ☑
  temperature regulation, newborn P81.9
    specified NEC P81.8
  temporomandibular joint M26.60 ☑
  tendon M67.90
    acromioclavicular M67.91 ☑
    ankle M67.97 ☑
    contracture — *see* Contracture, tendon
    elbow M67.92 ☑
    foot M67.97 ☑
    forearm M67.93 ☑
    hand M67.94 ☑
    hip M67.95 ☑
    knee M67.96 ☑
    multiple sites M67.99
    rupture — *see* Rupture, tendon
    shoulder M67.91 ☑
    specified type NEC M67.80
      acromioclavicular M67.81 ☑
      ankle M67.87 ☑
      elbow M67.82 ☑
      foot M67.87 ☑
      hand M67.84 ☑
      hip M67.85 ☑
      knee M67.86 ☑
      multiple sites M67.89

Disorder — *continued*
  tendon — *continued*
      trunk M67.88
      wrist M67.83 ☑
    synovitis — *see* Synovitis
    tendinitis — *see* Tendinitis
    tenosynovitis — *see* Tenosynovitis
    trunk M67.98
    upper arm M67.92 ☑
    wrist M67.93 ☑
  thoracic root (nerve) NEC G54.3
  thyrocalcitonin hypersecretion E07.0
  thyroid (gland) E07.9
    function NEC, neonatal, transitory P72.2
    iodine-deficiency related E01.8
    specified NEC E07.89
  tic — *see* Tic
  tobacco use
    chewing tobacco (mild) (moderate) (severe)
      in remission (early) (sustained) F17.221
    cigarettes (mild) (moderate) (severe)
      in remission (early) (sustained) F17.211
    mild F17.200
      in remission (early) (sustained) F17.201
    moderate F17.200
      in remission (early) (sustained) F17.201
    severe F17.200
      in remission (early) (sustained) F17.201
    specified product NEC (mild) (moderate) (severe)
      in remission (early) (sustained) F17.291
  tooth K08.9
    development K00.9
      specified NEC K00.8
    eruption K00.6
  Tourette's F95.2
  trance and possession F44.89
  transvestic F65.1
  trauma and stressor-related F43.9
    other specified F43.8
  tricuspid (valve) — *see* Endocarditis, tricuspid
  tryptophan metabolism E70.5
  tubular, phosphate-losing N25.0
  tubulo-interstitial (in)
    brucellosis A23.9 *[N16]*
    cystinosis E72.04
    diphtheria A36.84
    glycogen storage disease E74.00 *[N16]*
    leukemia NEC C95.9 ☑ *[N16]*
    lymphoma NEC C85.9 ☑ *[N16]*
    mixed cryoglobulinemia D89.1 *[N16]*
    multiple myeloma C90.0 ☑ *[N16]*
    Salmonella infection A02.25
    sarcoidosis D86.84
    sepsis A41.9 *[N16]*
      streptococcal A40.9 *[N16]*
    systemic lupus erythematosus M32.15
    toxoplasmosis B58.83
    transplant rejection T86.91 *[N16]*
    Wilson's disease E83.01 *[N16]*
  tubulo-renal function, impaired N25.9
    specified NEC N25.89
  tympanic membrane H73.9 ☑
    atrophy — *see* Atrophy, tympanic membrane
    infection — *see* Myringitis
    perforation — *see* Perforation, tympanum
    specified NEC H73.89 ☑
  unsocialized aggressive F91.1
  urea cycle metabolism E72.20
    argininemia E72.21
    argininosuccinic aciduria E72.22
    citrullinemia E72.23
    ornithine transcarbamylase deficiency E72.4
    other specified E72.29
  ureter (in) N28.9
    schistosomiasis B65.0 *[N29]*
    tuberculosis A18.11
  urethra N36.9
    specified NEC N36.8
  urinary system N39.9
    specified NEC N39.8
  valve, heart
    aortic — *see* Endocarditis, aortic
    mitral — *see* Endocarditis, mitral
    pulmonary — *see* Endocarditis, pulmonary
    rheumatic
      aortic — *see* Endocarditis, aortic, rheumatic
      mitral — *see* Endocarditis, mitral
      pulmonary — *see* Endocarditis, pulmonary, rheumatic
      tricuspid — *see* Endocarditis, tricuspid
    tricuspid — *see* Endocarditis, tricuspid

Disorder — *continued*
  vestibular function H81.9 ☑
    specified NEC — *see* subcategory H81.8 ☑
      in diseases classified elsewhere H82. ☑
    vertigo — *see* Vertigo
  vision, binocular H53.30
    abnormal retinal correspondence H53.31
    diplopia H53.2
    fusion with defective stereopsis H53.32
    simultaneous perception H53.33
    suppression H53.34
  visual
    cortex
      blindness H47.619
        left brain H47.612
        right brain H47.611
        due to
          inflammatory disorder H47.629
            left brain H47.622
            right brain H47.621
          neoplasm H47.639
            left brain H47.632
            right brain H47.631
          vascular disorder H47.649
            left brain H47.642
            right brain H47.641
    pathway H47.9
      due to
        inflammatory disorder H47.51 ☑
        neoplasm H47.52 ☑
        vascular disorder H47.53 ☑
      optic chiasm — *see* Disorder, optic, chiasm
  vitreous body H43.9
    crystalline deposits — *see* Deposit, crystalline
    degeneration — *see* Degeneration, vitreous
    hemorrhage — *see* Hemorrhage, vitreous
    opacities — *see* Opacity, vitreous
    prolapse — *see* Prolapse, vitreous
    specified type NEC H43.89
  voice R49.9
    specified type NEC R49.8
  volatile solvent use
    due to drug abuse — *see* Abuse, drug, inhalant
    due to drug dependence — *see* Dependence, drug, inhalant
  voyeuristic F65.3
  white blood cells D72.9
    specified NEC D72.89
  withdrawing, child or adolescent F40.10
Disorientation R41.0
Displacement, displaced
  acquired traumatic of bone, cartilage, joint, tendon NEC — *see* Dislocation
  adrenal gland (congenital) Q89.1
  appendix, retrocecal (congenital) Q43.8
  auricle (congenital) Q17.4
  bladder (acquired) N32.89
    congenital Q64.19
  brachial plexus (congenital) Q07.8
  brain stem, caudal (congenital) Q04.8
  canaliculus (lacrimalis), congenital Q10.6
  cardia through esophageal hiatus (congenital) Q40.1
  cerebellum, caudal (congenital) Q04.8
  cervix — *see* Malposition, uterus
  colon (congenital) Q43.3
  device, implant or graft (*see also* Complications, by site and type, mechanical) T85.628 ☑
    arterial graft NEC — *see* Complication, cardiovascular device, mechanical, vascular
    breast (implant) T85.42 ☑
    catheter NEC T85.628 ☑
      dialysis (renal) T82.42 ☑
        intraperitoneal T85.621 ☑
      infusion NEC T82.524 ☑
        spinal (epidural) (subdural) T85.620 ☑
      urinary
        cystostomy T83.020 ☑
        Hopkins T83.028 ☑
        ileostomy T83.028 ☑
        indwelling T83.021 ☑
        nephrostomy T83.022 ☑
        specified NEC T83.028 ☑
        urostomy T83.028 ☑
    electronic (electrode) (pulse generator) (stimulator) — *see* Complication, electronic stimulator
    fixation, internal (orthopedic) NEC — *see* Complication, fixation device, mechanical
    gastrointestinal — *see* Complications, prosthetic device, mechanical, gastrointestinal device
    genital NEC T83.428 ☑

Displacement — *continued*
  device — *continued*
    intrauterine contraceptive device (string) T83.32 ☑
    penile prosthesis (cylinder) (implanted) (pump) (reservoir) T83.420 ☑
    testicular prosthesis T83.421 ☑
    heart NEC — *see* Complication, cardiovascular device, mechanical
    joint prosthesis — *see* Complications, joint prosthesis, mechanical
    ocular — *see* Complications, prosthetic device, mechanical, ocular device
    orthopedic NEC — *see* Complication, orthopedic, device or graft, mechanical
    specified NEC T85.628 ☑
    urinary NEC T83.128 ☑
      graft T83.22 ☑
      sphincter, implanted T83.121 ☑
      stent (ileal conduit) (nephroureteral) T83.123 ☑
      ureteral indwelling T83.122 ☑
    vascular NEC — *see* Complication, cardiovascular device, mechanical
    ventricular intracranial shunt T85.02 ☑
  electronic stimulator
    bone T84.320 ☑
    cardiac — *see* Complications, cardiac device, electronic
    nervous system — *see* Complication, prosthetic device, mechanical, electronic nervous system stimulator
    urinary — *see* Complications, electronic stimulator, urinary
  esophageal mucosa into cardia of stomach, congenital Q39.8
  esophagus (acquired) K22.8
    congenital Q39.8
  eyeball (acquired) (lateral) (old) — *see* Displacement, globe
    congenital Q15.8
    current — *see* Avulsion, eye
  fallopian tube (acquired) N83.4 ☑
    congenital Q50.6
    opening (congenital) Q50.6
  gallbladder (congenital) Q44.1
  gastric mucosa (congenital) Q40.2
  globe (acquired) (old) (lateral) H05.21 ☑
    current — *see* Avulsion, eye
  heart (congenital) Q24.8
    acquired I51.89
  hymen (upward) (congenital) Q52.4
  intervertebral disc NEC
    with myelopathy — *see* Disorder, disc, with, myelopathy
    cervical, cervicothoracic (with) M50.20
      myelopathy — *see* Disorder, disc, cervical, with myelopathy
      neuritis, radiculitis or radiculopathy — *see* Disorder, disc, cervical, with neuritis
    due to trauma — *see* Dislocation, vertebra
    lumbar region M51.26
      with
        myelopathy M51.06
        neuritis, radiculitis, radiculopathy or sciatica M51.16
    lumbosacral region M51.27
      with
        neuritis, radiculitis, radiculopathy or sciatica M51.17
    sacrococcygeal region M53.3
    thoracic region M51.24
      with
        myelopathy M51.04
        neuritis, radiculitis, radiculopathy M51.14
    thoracolumbar region M51.25
      with
        myelopathy M51.05
        neuritis, radiculitis, radiculopathy M51.15
  intrauterine device (string) T83.32 ☑
  kidney (acquired) N28.83
    congenital Q63.2
  lachrymal, lacrimal apparatus or duct (congenital) Q10.6
  lens, congenital Q12.1
  macula (congenital) Q14.1
  Meckel's diverticulum Q43.0
    malignant — *see* Table of Neoplasms, small intestine, malignant
  nail (congenital) Q84.6
    acquired L60.8
  opening of Wharton's duct in mouth Q38.4

Displacement — *continued*
  organ or site, congenital NEC — *see* Malposition, congenital
  ovary (acquired) N83.4 ☑
    congenital Q50.39
    free in peritoneal cavity (congenital) Q50.39
    into hernial sac N83.4 ☑
  oviduct (acquired) N83.4 ☑
    congenital Q50.6
  parathyroid (gland) E21.4
  parotid gland (congenital) Q38.4
  punctum lacrimale (congenital) Q10.6
  sacro-iliac (joint) (congenital) Q74.2
    current injury S33.2 ☑
    old — *see* subcategory M53.2 ☑
  salivary gland (any) (congenital) Q38.4
  spleen (congenital) Q89.09
  stomach, congenital Q40.2
  sublingual duct Q38.4
  tongue (downward) (congenital) Q38.3
  tooth, teeth, fully erupted M26.30
    horizontal M26.33
    vertical M26.34
  trachea (congenital) Q32.1
  ureter or ureteric opening or orifice (congenital) Q62.62
  uterine opening of oviducts or fallopian tubes Q50.6
  uterus, uterine — *see* Malposition, uterus
  ventricular septum Q21.0
    with rudimentary ventricle Q20.4
Disproportion
  between native and reconstructed breast N65.1
  fiber-type G71.2
Disruptio uteri — *see* Rupture, uterus
Disruption (of)
  ciliary body NEC H21.89
  closure of
    cornea T81.31 ☑
    craniotomy T81.32 ☑
    fascia (muscular) (superficial) T81.32 ☑
    internal organ or tissue T81.32 ☑
    laceration (external) (internal) T81.33 ☑
    ligament T81.32 ☑
    mucosa T81.31 ☑
    muscle or muscle flap T81.32 ☑
    ribs or rib cage T81.32 ☑
    skin and subcutaneous tissue (full-thickness) (superficial) T81.31 ☑
    skull T81.32 ☑
    sternum (sternotomy) T81.32 ☑
    tendon T81.32 ☑
    traumatic laceration (external) (internal) T81.33 ☑
  family Z63.8
    due to
      absence of family member due to military deployment Z63.31
      absence of family member NEC Z63.32
      alcoholism and drug addiction in family Z63.72
      bereavement Z63.4
      death (assumed) or disappearance of family member Z63.4
      divorce or separation Z63.5
      drug addiction in family Z63.72
      return of family member from military deployment (current or past conflict) Z63.71
      stressful life events NEC Z63.79
  iris NEC H21.89
  ligament(s) (*see also* Sprain)
    knee
      current injury — *see* Dislocation, knee
      old (chronic) — *see* Derangement, knee, ligament, instability, chronic
      spontaneous NEC — *see* Derangement, knee, disruption ligament
  ossicular chain — *see* Discontinuity, ossicles, ear
  pelvic ring (stable) S32.810 ☑
    unstable S32.811 ☑
  wound T81.30 ☑
    episiotomy O90.1
    operation T81.31 ☑
      cesarean O90.0
      external operation wound (superficial) T81.31 ☑
      internal operation wound (deep) T81.32 ☑
    perineal (obstetric) O90.1
    traumatic injury repair T81.33 ☑
  traumatic injury wound repair T81.33 ☑
Dissatisfaction with
  employment Z56.9
  school environment Z55.4

Disorder - Dissatisfaction

ICD-10-CM INDEX TO DISEASES AND INJURIES

Dissecting — see condition
Dissection
  aorta I71.00
    abdominal I71.02
    thoracic I71.01
    thoracoabdominal I71.03
  artery I77.70
    basilar (trunk) I77.75
    carotid I77.71
    cerebral (nonruptured) I67.0
      ruptured — see Hemorrhage, intracranial, subarachnoid
    coronary I25.42
    extremity
      lower I77.77
      upper I77.76
    iliac I77.72
    precerebral
      congenital (nonruptured) Q28.1
      specified site NEC I77.75
    renal I77.73
    specified NEC I77.79
    vertebral I77.74
  precerebral artery, congenital (nonruptured) Q28.1
    Heartland A93.8
  traumatic — see Wound, open, by site
  vascular I99.8
  wound — see Wound, open
Disseminated — see condition
Dissociation
  auriculoventricular or atrioventricular (AV) (any degree) (isorhythmic) I45.89
    with heart block I44.2
  interference I45.89
Dissociative reaction, state F44.9
Dissolution, vertebra — see Osteoporosis
Distension, distention
  abdomen R14.0
  bladder N32.89
  cecum K63.89
  colon K63.89
  gallbladder K82.8
  intestine K63.89
  kidney N28.89
  liver K76.89
  seminal vesicle N50.89
  stomach K31.89
    acute K31.0
    psychogenic F45.8
  ureter — see Dilatation, ureter
  uterus N85.8
Distoma hepaticum infestation B66.3
Distomiasis B66.9
  bile passages B66.3
  hemic B65.9
  hepatic B66.3
    due to Clonorchis sinensis B66.1
  intestinal B66.5
  liver B66.3
    due to Clonorchis sinensis B66.1
  lung B66.4
  pulmonary B66.4
Distomolar (fourth molar) K00.1
Disto-occlusion (Division I) (Division II) M26.212
Distortion(s) (congenital)
  adrenal (gland) Q89.1
  arm NEC Q68.8
  bile duct or passage Q44.5
  bladder Q64.79
  brain Q04.9
  cervix (uteri) Q51.9
  chest (wall) Q67.8
    bones Q76.8
  clavicle Q74.0
  clitoris Q52.6
  coccyx Q76.49
  common duct Q44.5
  coronary Q24.5
  cystic duct Q44.5
  ear (auricle) (external) Q17.3
    inner Q16.5
    middle Q16.4
      ossicles Q16.3
  endocrine NEC Q89.2
  eustachian tube Q17.8
  eye (adnexa) Q15.8
  face bone(s) NEC Q75.8
  fallopian tube Q50.6
  femur NEC Q68.8
  fibula NEC Q68.8
  finger(s) Q68.1
  foot Q66.9 ☑

Distortion(s) — continued
  genitalia, genital organ(s)
    female Q52.8
      external Q52.79
      internal NEC Q52.8
  gyri Q04.8
  hand bone(s) Q68.1
  heart (auricle) (ventricle) Q24.8
    valve (cusp) Q24.8
  hepatic duct Q44.5
  humerus NEC Q68.8
  hymen Q52.4
  intrafamilial communications Z63.8
  jaw NEC M26.89
  labium (majus) (minus) Q52.79
  leg NEC Q68.8
  lens Q12.8
  liver Q44.7
  lumbar spine Q76.49
    with disproportion O33.8
      causing obstructed labor O65.0
  lumbosacral (joint) (region) Q76.49
    kyphosis — see Kyphosis, congenital
    lordosis — see Lordosis, congenital
  nerve Q07.8
  nose Q30.8
  organ
    of Corti Q16.5
    or site not listed — see Anomaly, by site
  ossicles, ear Q16.3
  oviduct Q50.6
  pancreas Q45.3
  parathyroid (gland) Q89.2
  pituitary (gland) Q89.2
  radius NEC Q68.8
  sacroiliac joint Q74.2
  sacrum Q76.49
  scapula Q74.0
  shoulder girdle Q74.0
  skull bone(s) NEC Q75.8
    with
      anencephalus Q00.0
      encephalocele — see Encephalocele
      hydrocephalus Q03.9
        with spina bifida — see Spina bifida, with hydrocephalus
      microcephaly Q02
  spinal cord Q06.8
  spine Q76.49
    kyphosis — see Kyphosis, congenital
    lordosis — see Lordosis, congenital
  spleen Q89.09
  sternum NEC Q76.7
  thorax (wall) Q67.8
    bony Q76.8
  thymus (gland) Q89.2
  thyroid (gland) Q89.2
  tibia NEC Q68.8
  toe(s) Q66.9 ☑
  tongue Q38.3
  trachea (cartilage) Q32.1
  ulna NEC Q68.8
  ureter Q62.8
  urethra Q64.79
    causing obstruction Q64.39
  uterus Q51.9
  vagina Q52.4
  vertebra Q76.49
    kyphosis — see Kyphosis, congenital
    lordosis — see Lordosis, congenital
  visual (see also Disturbance, vision)
    shape and size H53.15
  vulva Q52.79
  wrist (bones) (joint) Q68.8
Distress
  abdomen — see Pain, abdominal
  acute respiratory R06.03
    syndrome (adult) (child) J80
  epigastric R10.13
  fetal P84
    complicating pregnancy — see Stress, fetal
  gastrointestinal (functional) K30
    psychogenic F45.8
  intestinal (functional) NOS K59.9
    psychogenic F45.8
  maternal, during labor and delivery O75.0
  relationship, with spouse or intimate partner Z63.0
  respiratory (adult) (child) R06.03
    newborn P22.9
      specified NEC P22.8
    orthopnea R06.01
    psychogenic F45.8

Distress — continued
  respiratory — continued
    shortness of breath R06.02
    specified type NEC R06.09
Distribution vessel, atypical Q27.9
  coronary artery Q24.5
  precerebral Q28.1
Districhiasis L68.8
Disturbance(s) (see also Disease)
  absorption K90.9
    calcium E58
    carbohydrate K90.49
    fat K90.49
      pancreatic K90.3
    protein K90.49
    starch K90.49
    vitamin — see Deficiency, vitamin
  acid-base equilibrium E87.8
    mixed E87.4
  activity and attention (with hyperkinesis) — see Disorder, attention-deficit hyperactivity
  amino acid transport E72.00
  assimilation, food K90.9
  auditory nerve, except deafness — see subcategory H93.3 ☑
  behavior — see Disorder, conduct
  blood clotting (mechanism) (see also Defect, coagulation) D68.9
  cerebral
    nerve — see Disorder, nerve, cranial
    status, newborn P91.9
      specified NEC P91.88
  circulatory I99.9
  conduct (see also Disorder, conduct) F91.9
    adjustment reaction — see Disorder, adjustment
    compulsive F63.9
    disruptive F91.9
    hyperkinetic — see Disorder, attention-deficit hyperactivity
    socialized F91.2
    specified NEC F91.8
    unsocialized F91.1
  coordination R27.8
  cranial nerve — see Disorder, nerve, cranial
  deep sensibility — see Disturbance, sensation
  digestive K30
    psychogenic F45.8
  electrolyte (see also Imbalance, electrolyte)
    newborn, transitory P74.49
      hyperammonemia P74.6
      hyperchloremia P74.421
      hyperchloremic metabolic acidosis P74.421
      hypochloremia P74.422
      potassium balance
        hyperkalemia P74.31
        hypokalemia P74.32
      sodium balance
        hypernatremia P74.21
        hyponatremia P74.22
      specified type NEC P74.49
  emotions specific to childhood and adolescence F93.9
    with
      anxiety and fearfulness NEC F93.8
      elective mutism F94.0
      oppositional disorder F91.3
      sensitivity (withdrawal) F40.10
      shyness F40.10
      social withdrawal F40.10
    involving relationship problems F93.8
    mixed F93.8
    specified NEC F93.8
  endocrine (gland) E34.9
    neonatal, transitory P72.9
      specified NEC P72.8
  equilibrium R42
  fructose metabolism E74.10
  gait — see Gait
    hysterical F44.4
    psychogenic F44.4
  gastrointestinal (functional) K30
    psychogenic F45.8
  habit, child F98.9
  hearing, except deafness and tinnitus — see Abnormal, auditory perception
  heart, functional (conditions in I44-I50)
    due to presence of (cardiac) prosthesis I97.19 ☑
    postoperative I97.89
      cardiac surgery (see also Infarct, myocardium, associated with revascularization procedure) I97.19 ☑
  hormones E34.9

Disturbance(s) — *continued*
- innervation uterus (parasympathetic) (sympathetic) N85.8
- keratinization NEC
  - gingiva K05.10
    - nonplaque induced K05.11
    - plaque induced K05.10
  - lip K13.0
  - oral (mucosa) (soft tissue) K13.29
  - tongue K13.29
- learning (specific) — *see* Disorder, learning
- memory — *see* Amnesia
  - mild, following organic brain damage F06.8
- mental F99
  - associated with diseases classified elsewhere F54
- metabolism E88.9
  - with
    - abortion — *see* Abortion, by type with other specified complication
    - ectopic pregnancy O08.5
    - molar pregnancy O08.5
  - amino-acid E72.9
    - aromatic E70.9
    - branched-chain E71.2
    - straight-chain E72.89
    - sulfur-bearing E72.10
  - ammonia E72.20
  - arginine E72.21
  - arginosuccinic acid E72.22
  - carbohydrate E74.9
  - cholesterol E78.9
  - citrulline E72.23
  - cystathionine E72.19
  - general E88.9
  - glutamine E72.89
  - histidine E70.40
  - homocystine E72.19
  - hydroxylysine E72.3
  - in labor or delivery O75.89
  - iron E83.10
  - lipoid E78.9
  - lysine E72.3
  - methionine E72.19
  - neonatal, transitory P74.9
    - calcium and magnesium P71.9
      - specified type NEC P71.8
    - carbohydrate metabolism P70.9
      - specified type NEC P70.8
    - specified NEC P74.8
  - ornithine E72.4
  - phosphate E83.39
  - sodium NEC E87.8
  - threonine E72.89
  - tryptophan E70.5
  - tyrosine E70.20
  - urea cycle E72.20
- motor R29.2
- nervous, functional R45.0
- neuromuscular mechanism (eye), due to syphilis A52.15
- nutritional E63.9
  - nail L60.3
- ocular motion H51.9
  - psychogenic F45.8
- oculogyric H51.8
  - psychogenic F45.8
- oculomotor H51.9
  - psychogenic F45.8
- olfactory nerve R43.1
- optic nerve NEC — *see* Disorder, nerve, optic
- oral epithelium, including tongue NEC K13.29
- perceptual due to
  - alcohol withdrawal F10.232
  - amphetamine intoxication F15.922
    - in
      - abuse F15.122
      - dependence F15.222
  - anxiolytic withdrawal F13.232
  - cannabis intoxication (acute) F12.922
    - in
      - abuse F12.122
      - dependence F12.222
  - cocaine intoxication (acute) F14.922
    - in
      - abuse F14.122
      - dependence F14.222
  - hypnotic withdrawal F13.232
  - opioid intoxication (acute) F11.922
    - in
      - abuse F11.122
      - dependence F11.222
  - phencyclidine intoxication (acute) F16.122
  - sedative withdrawal F13.232

Disturbance(s) — *continued*
- personality (pattern) (trait) (*see also* Disorder, personality) F60.9
  - following organic brain damage F07.9
- polyglandular E31.9
  - specified NEC E31.8
- potassium balance, newborn
  - hyperkalemia P74.31
  - hypokalemia P74.32
- psychogenic F45.9
- psychomotor F44.4
- psychophysical visual H53.16
- pupillary — *see* Anomaly, pupil, function
- reflex R29.2
- rhythm, heart I49.9
- salivary secretion K11.7
- sensation (cold) (heat) (localization) (tactile discrimination) (texture) (vibratory) NEC R20.9
  - hysterical F44.6
  - skin R20.9
    - anesthesia R20.0
    - hyperesthesia R20.3
    - hypoesthesia R20.1
    - paresthesia R20.2
    - specified type NEC R20.8
  - smell R43.9
    - and taste (mixed) R43.8
    - anosmia R43.0
    - parosmia R43.1
    - specified NEC R43.8
  - taste R43.9
    - and smell (mixed) R43.8
    - parageusia R43.2
    - specified NEC R43.8
- sensory — *see* Disturbance, sensation
- situational (transient) (*see also* Disorder, adjustment)
  - acute F43.0
- sleep G47.9
  - nonorganic origin F51.9
- smell — *see* Disturbance, sensation, smell
- sociopathic F60.2
- sodium balance, newborn
  - hypernatremia P74.21
  - hyponatremia P74.22
- speech R47.9
  - developmental F80.9
  - specified NEC R47.89
- stomach (functional) K31.9
- sympathetic (nerve) G90.9
- taste — *see* Disturbance, sensation, taste
- temperature
  - regulation, newborn P81.9
    - specified NEC P81.8
  - sense R20.8
    - hysterical F44.6
- tooth
  - eruption K00.6
  - formation K00.4
  - structure, hereditary NEC K00.5
- touch — *see* Disturbance, sensation
- vascular I99.9
  - arteriosclerotic — *see* Arteriosclerosis
- vasomotor I73.9
- vasospastic I73.9
- vision, visual H53.9
  - following
    - cerebral infarction I69.398
    - cerebrovascular disease I69.998
      - specified NEC I69.898
    - intracerebral hemorrhage I69.198
    - nontraumatic intracranial hemorrhage NEC I69.298
    - specified disease NEC I69.898
    - subarachnoid hemorrhage I69.098
  - psychophysical H53.16
  - specified NEC H53.8
  - subjective H53.10
    - day blindness H53.11
    - discomfort H53.14 ☑
    - distortions of shape and size H53.15
    - loss
      - sudden H53.13 ☑
      - transient H53.12 ☑
    - specified type NEC H53.19
- voice R49.9
  - psychogenic F44.4
  - specified NEC R49.8
Diuresis R35.8
Diver's palsy, paralysis or squeeze T70.3 ☑
Diverticulitis (acute) K57.92
- bladder — *see* Cystitis

Diverticulitis — *continued*
- ileum — *see* Diverticulitis, intestine, small
- intestine K57.92
  - with
    - abscess, perforation or peritonitis K57.80
      - with bleeding K57.81
    - bleeding K57.93
  - congenital Q43.8
  - large K57.32
    - with
      - abscess, perforation or peritonitis K57.20
        - with bleeding K57.21
      - bleeding K57.33
    - small intestine K57.52
      - with
        - abscess, perforation or peritonitis K57.40
          - with bleeding K57.41
        - bleeding K57.53
  - small K57.12
    - with
      - abscess, perforation or peritonitis K57.00
        - with bleeding K57.01
      - bleeding K57.13
    - large intestine K57.52
      - with
        - abscess, perforation or peritonitis K57.40
          - with bleeding K57.41
        - bleeding K57.53
Diverticulosis K57.90
- with bleeding K57.91
- large intestine K57.30
  - with
    - bleeding K57.31
    - small intestine K57.50
      - with bleeding K57.51
  - small intestine K57.10
    - with
      - bleeding K57.11
      - large intestine K57.50
        - with bleeding K57.51
Diverticulum, diverticula (multiple) K57.90
- appendix (noninflammatory) K38.2
- bladder (sphincter) N32.3
  - congenital Q64.6
- bronchus (congenital) Q32.4
  - acquired J98.09
- calyx, calyceal (kidney) N28.89
- cardia (stomach) K31.4
- cecum — *see* Diverticulosis, intestine, large
  - congenital Q43.8
- colon — *see* Diverticulosis, intestine, large
  - congenital Q43.8
- duodenum — *see* Diverticulosis, intestine, small
  - congenital Q43.8
- epiphrenic (esophagus) K22.5
- esophagus (congenital) Q39.6
  - acquired (epiphrenic) (pulsion) (traction) K22.5
- eustachian tube — *see* Disorder, eustachian tube, specified NEC
- fallopian tube N83.8
- gastric K31.4
- heart (congenital) Q24.8
- ileum — *see* Diverticulosis, intestine, small
- jejunum — *see* Diverticulosis, intestine, small
- kidney (pelvis) (calyces) N28.89
  - with calculus — *see* Calculus, kidney
- Meckel's (displaced) (hypertrophic) Q43.0
  - malignant — *see* Table of Neoplasms, small intestine, malignant
- midthoracic K22.5
- organ or site, congenital NEC — *see* Distortion
- pericardium (congenital) (cyst) Q24.8
  - acquired I31.8
- pharyngoesophageal (congenital) Q39.6
  - acquired K22.5
- pharynx (congenital) Q38.7
- rectosigmoid — *see* Diverticulosis, intestine, large
  - congenital Q43.8
- rectum — *see* Diverticulosis, intestine, large
- Rokitansky's K22.5
- seminal vesicle N50.89
- sigmoid — *see* Diverticulosis, intestine, large
  - congenital Q43.8
- stomach (acquired) K31.4
  - congenital Q40.2
- trachea (acquired) J39.8
- ureter (acquired) N28.89
  - congenital Q62.8
- ureterovesical orifice N28.89
- urethra (acquired) N36.1
  - congenital Q64.79
- ventricle, left (congenital) Q24.8

Diverticulum - Duplication

Diverticulum — *continued*
  vesical N32.3
    congenital Q64.6
  Zenker's (esophagus) K22.5
Division
  cervix uteri (acquired) N88.8
  glans penis Q55.69
  labia minora (congenital) Q52.79
  ligament (partial or complete) (current) (*see also* Sprain)
    with open wound — *see* Wound, open
  muscle (partial or complete) (current) (*see also* Injury, muscle)
    with open wound — *see* Wound, open
  nerve (traumatic) — *see* Injury, nerve
  spinal cord — *see* Injury, spinal cord, by region
  vein I87.8
Divorce, causing family disruption Z63.5
Dix-Hallpike neurolabyrinthitis — *see* Neuronitis, vestibular
Dizziness R42
  hysterical F44.89
  psychogenic F45.8
DMAC (disseminated mycobacterium avium-intracellulare complex) A31.2
DNR (do not resuscitate) Z66
Doan-Wiseman syndrome (primary splenic neutropenia) — *see* Agranulocytosis
Doehle-Heller aortitis A52.02
Dog bite — *see* Bite
Dohle body panmyelopathic syndrome D72.0
Dolichocephaly Q67.2
Dolichocolon Q43.8
Dolichostenomelia — *see* Syndrome, Marfan's
Donohue's syndrome E34.8
Donor (organ or tissue) Z52.9
  blood (whole) Z52.000
    autologous Z52.010
    specified component (lymphocytes) (platelets) NEC Z52.008
      autologous Z52.018
      specified donor NEC Z52.098
    specified donor NEC Z52.090
    stem cells Z52.001
      autologous Z52.011
      specified donor NEC Z52.091
  bone Z52.20
    autologous Z52.21
    marrow Z52.3
    specified type NEC Z52.29
  cornea Z52.5
  egg (Oocyte) Z52.819
    age 35 and over Z52.812
      anonymous recipient Z52.812
      designated recipient Z52.813
    under age 35 Z52.810
      anonymous recipient Z52.810
      designated recipient Z52.811
  kidney Z52.4
  liver Z52.6
  lung Z52.89
  lymphocyte — *see* Donor, blood, specified components NEC
  Oocyte — *see* Donor, egg
  platelets Z52.008
  potential, examination of Z00.5
  semen Z52.89
  skin Z52.10
    autologous Z52.11
    specified type NEC Z52.19
  specified organ or tissue NEC Z52.89
  sperm Z52.89
Donovanosis A58
Dorsalgia M54.9
  psychogenic F45.41
  specified NEC M54.89
Dorsopathy M53.9
  deforming M43.9
    specified NEC — *see* subcategory M43.8 ☑
  specified NEC M53.80
    cervical region M53.82
    cervicothoracic region M53.83
    lumbar region M53.86
    lumbosacral region M53.87
    occipito-atlanto-axial region M53.81
    sacrococcygeal region M53.88
    thoracic region M53.84
    thoracolumbar region M53.85
Double
  albumin E88.09
  aortic arch Q25.45
  auditory canal Q17.8

Double — *continued*
  auricle (heart) Q20.8
  bladder Q64.79
  cervix Q51.820
    with doubling of uterus (and vagina) Q51.10
      with obstruction Q51.11
  inlet ventricle Q20.4
  kidney with double pelvis (renal) Q63.0
  meatus urinarius Q64.75
  monster Q89.4
  outlet
    left ventricle Q20.2
    right ventricle Q20.1
  pelvis (renal) with double ureter Q62.5
  tongue Q38.3
  ureter (one or both sides) Q62.5
    with double pelvis (renal) Q62.5
  urethra Q64.74
  urinary meatus Q64.75
  uterus Q51.20
    with
      doubling of cervix (and vagina) Q51.10
        with obstruction Q51.11
    complete Q51.21
    in pregnancy or childbirth O34.0 ☑
      causing obstructed labor O65.5
    partial Q51.22
    specified NEC Q51.28
  vagina Q52.10
    with doubling of uterus (and cervix) Q51.10
      with obstruction Q51.11
  vision H53.2
  vulva Q52.79
Douglas' pouch, cul-de-sac — *see* condition
Down syndrome Q90.9
  meiotic nondisjunction Q90.0
  mitotic nondisjunction Q90.1
  mosaicism Q90.1
  translocation Q90.2
DPD (dihydropyrimidine dehydrogenase deficiency) E88.89
Dracontiasis B72
Dracunculiasis, dracunculosis B72
Dream state, hysterical F44.89
Dreschlera (hawaiiensis) (infection) B43.8
Drepanocytic anemia — *see* Disease, sickle-cell
Dresbach's syndrome (elliptocytosis) D58.1
Dressler's syndrome I24.1
Drift, ulnar — *see* Deformity, limb, specified type NEC, forearm
Drinking (alcohol)
  excessive, to excess NEC (without dependence) F10.10
    habitual (continual) (without remission) F10.20
      with remission F10.21
Drip, postnasal (chronic) R09.82
  due to
    allergic rhinitis — *see* Rhinitis, allergic
    common cold J00
    gastroesophageal reflux — *see* Reflux, gastroesophageal
    nasopharyngitis — *see* Nasopharyngitis
    other know condition - code to condition
    sinusitis — *see* Sinusitis
Droop
  facial R29.810
    cerebrovascular disease I69.992
      cerebral infarction I69.392
      intracerebral hemorrhage I69.192
      nontraumatic intracranial hemorrhage NEC I69.292
      specified disease NEC I69.892
      subarachnoid hemorrhage I69.092
Drop (in)
  attack NEC R55
  finger — *see* Deformity, finger
  foot — *see* Deformity, limb, foot, drop
  hematocrit (precipitous) R71.0
  hemoglobin R71.0
  toe — *see* Deformity, toe, specified NEC
  wrist — *see* Deformity, limb, wrist drop
Dropped heart beats I45.9
Dropsy, dropsical (*see also* Hydrops)
  abdomen R18.8
  brain — *see* Hydrocephalus
  cardiac, heart — *see* Failure, heart, congestive
  gangrenous — *see* Gangrene
  heart — *see* Failure, heart, congestive
  kidney — *see* Nephrosis
  lung — *see* Edema, lung
  newborn due to isoimmunization P56.0
  pericardium — *see* Pericarditis

Drowned, drowning (near) T75.1 ☑
Drowsiness R40.0
Drug
  abuse counseling and surveillance Z71.51
  addiction — *see* Dependence
  dependence — *see* Dependence
  habit — *see* Dependence
  harmful use — *see* Abuse, drug
  induced fever R50.2
  overdose — *see* Table of Drugs and Chemicals, by drug, poisoning
  poisoning — *see* Table of Drugs and Chemicals, by drug, poisoning
  resistant organism infection (*see also* Resistant, organism, to, drug) Z16.30
  therapy
    long term (current) (prophylactic) — *see* Therapy, drug long-term (current) (prophylactic)
    short term - omit code
  wrong substance given or taken in error — *see* Table of Drugs and Chemicals, by drug, poisoning
Drunkenness (without dependence) F10.129
  acute in alcoholism F10.229
  chronic (without remission) F10.20
    with remission F10.21
  pathological (without dependence) F10.129
    with dependence F10.229
  sleep F51.9
Drusen
  macula (degenerative) (retina) — *see* Degeneration, macula, drusen
  optic disc H47.32 ☑
Dry, dryness (*see also* condition)
  larynx J38.7
  mouth R68.2
    due to dehydration E86.0
  nose J34.89
  socket (teeth) M27.3
  throat J39.2
DSAP L56.5
Duane's syndrome H50.81 ☑
Dubin-Johnson disease or syndrome E80.6
Dubois' disease (thymus gland) A50.59 *[E35]*
Dubowitz' syndrome Q87.19
Duchenne-Aran muscular atrophy G12.21
Duchenne-Griesinger disease G71.01
Duchenne's
  disease or syndrome
    motor neuron disease G12.22
    muscular dystrophy G71.01
  locomotor ataxia (syphilitic) A52.11
  paralysis
    birth injury P14.0
    due to or associated with
      motor neuron disease G12.22
      muscular dystrophy G71.01
Ducrey's chancre A57
Duct, ductus — *see* condition
Duhring's disease (dermatitis herpetiformis) L13.0
Dullness, cardiac (decreased) (increased) R01.2
Dumb ague — *see* Malaria
Dumbness — *see* Aphasia
Dumdum fever B55.0
Dumping syndrome (postgastrectomy) K91.1
Duodenitis (nonspecific) (peptic) K29.80
  with bleeding K29.81
Duodenocholangitis — *see* Cholangitis
Duodenum, duodenal — *see* condition
Duplay's bursitis or periarthritis — *see* Tendinitis, calcific, shoulder
Duplication, duplex (*see also* Accessory)
  alimentary tract Q45.8
  anus Q43.4
  appendix (and cecum) Q43.4
  biliary duct (any) Q44.5
  bladder Q64.79
  cecum (and appendix) Q43.4
  cervix Q51.820
  chromosome NEC
    with complex rearrangements NEC Q92.5
    seen only at prometaphase Q92.8
  cystic duct Q44.5
  digestive organs Q45.8
  esophagus Q39.8
  frontonasal process Q75.8
  intestine (large) (small) Q43.4
  kidney Q63.0
  liver Q44.7
  pancreas Q45.3
  penis Q55.69
  respiratory organs NEC Q34.8

☑ **Additional character required**

Duplication — *continued*
 salivary duct Q38.4
 spinal cord (incomplete) Q06.2
 stomach Q40.2
Dupré's disease (meningism) R29.1
Dupuytren's contraction or disease M72.0
Durand-Nicolas-Favre disease A55
Durotomy (inadvertent) (incidental) G97.41
Duroziez's disease (congenital mitral stenosis) Q23.2
Dutton's relapsing fever (West African) A68.1
Dwarfism E34.3
 achondroplastic Q77.4
 congenital E34.3
 constitutional E34.3
 hypochondroplastic Q77.4
 hypophyseal E23.0
 infantile E34.3
 Laron-type E34.3
 Lorain (-Levi) type E23.0
 metatropic Q77.8
 nephrotic-glycosuric (with hypophosphatemic
  rickets) E72.09
 nutritional E45
 pancreatic K86.89
 pituitary E23.0
 renal N25.0
 thanatophoric Q77.1
Dyke-Young anemia (secondary) (symptomatic) D59.1
Dysacusis — *see* Abnormal, auditory perception
Dysadrenocortism E27.9
 hyperfunction E27.0
Dysarthria R47.1
 following
  cerebral infarction I69.322
  cerebrovascular disease I69.922
   specified disease NEC I69.822
  intracerebral hemorrhage I69.122
  nontraumatic intracranial hemorrhage NEC I69.222
  subarachnoid hemorrhage I69.022
Dysautonomia (familial) G90.1
Dysbarism T70.3 ☑
Dysbasia R26.2
 angiosclerotica intermittens I73.9
 hysterical F44.4
 lordotica (progressiva) G24.1
 nonorganic origin F44.4
 psychogenic F44.4
Dysbetalipoproteinemia (familial) E78.2
Dyscalculia R48.8
 developmental F81.2
Dyschezia K59.00
Dyschondroplasia (with hemangiomata) Q78.4
Dyschromia (skin) L81.9
Dyscollagenosis M35.9
Dyscranio-pygo-phalangy Q87.0
Dyscrasia
 blood (with) D75.9
  antepartum hemorrhage — *see* Hemorrhage,
   antepartum, with coagulation defect
  newborn P61.9
   specified type NEC P61.8
  intrapartum hemorrhage O67.0
  puerperal, postpartum O72.3
 polyglandular, pluriglandular E31.9
Dysendocrinism E34.9
Dysentery, dysenteric (catarrhal) (diarrhea) (epidemic)
 (hemorrhagic) (infectious) (sporadic) (tropical) A09
 abscess, liver A06.4
 amebic (*see also* Amebiasis) A06.0
  with abscess — *see* Abscess, amebic
  acute A06.0
  chronic A06.1
 arthritis (*see also* category M01 ☑) A09
  bacillary (*see also* category M01 ☑) A03.9
 bacillary A03.9
  arthritis (*see also* category M01 ☑) A03.9
  Boyd A03.2
  Flexner A03.1
  Schmitz (-Stutzer) A03.0
  Shiga (-Kruse) A03.0
  Shigella A03.9
   boydii A03.2
   dysenteriae A03.0
   flexneri A03.1
   group A A03.0
   group B A03.1
   group C A03.2
   group D A03.3
   sonnei A03.3
   specified type NEC A03.8
  Sonne A03.3
  specified type NEC A03.8

Dysentery — *continued*
 balantidial A07.0
 Balantidium coli A07.0
 Boyd's A03.2
 candidal B37.82
 Chilomastix A07.8
 Chinese A03.9
 coccidial A07.3
 Dientamoeba (fragilis) A07.8
 Embadomonas A07.8
 Entamoeba, entamebic — *see* Dysentery, amebic
 Flexner-Boyd A03.2
 Flexner's A03.1
 Giardia lamblia A07.1
 Hiss-Russell A03.1
 Lamblia A07.1
 leishmanial B55.0
 malarial — *see* Malaria
 metazoal B82.0
 monilial B37.82
 protozoal A07.9
 Salmonella A02.0
 schistosomal B65.1
 Schmitz (-Stutzer) A03.0
 Shiga (-Kruse) A03.0
 Shigella NOS — *see* Dysentery, bacillary
 Sonne A03.3
 strongyloidiasis B78.0
 trichomonal A07.8
 viral (*see also* Enteritis, viral) A08.4
Dysequilibrium R42
Dysesthesia R20.8
 hysterical F44.6
Dysfibrinogenemia (congenital) D68.2
Dysfunction
 adrenal E27.9
  hyperfunction E27.0
 autonomic
  due to alcohol G31.2
  somatoform F45.8
 bladder N31.9
  neurogenic NOS — *see* Dysfunction, bladder,
   neuromuscular
  neuromuscular NOS N31.9
   atonic (motor) (sensory) N31.2
   autonomous N31.2
   flaccid N31.2
   nonreflex N31.2
   reflex N31.1
   specified NEC N31.8
   uninhibited N31.0
  bleeding, uterus N93.8
 cerebral G93.89
 colon K59.9
  psychogenic F45.8
 colostomy K94.03
 cystic duct K82.8
 cystostomy (stoma) — *see* Complications,
  cystostomy
 ejaculatory N53.19
  anejaculatory orgasm N53.13
  painful N53.12
  premature F52.4
  retarded N53.11
 endocrine NOS E34.9
 endometrium N85.8
 enterostomy K94.13
 erectile — *see* Dysfunction, sexual, male, erectile
 gallbladder K82.8
 gastrostomy (stoma) K94.23
 gland, glandular NOS E34.9
  meibomian, of eyelid — *see* Dysfunction,
   meibomian gland
 heart I51.89
 hemoglobin D75.89
 hepatic K76.89
 hypophysis E23.7
 hypothalamic NEC E23.3
 ileostomy (stoma) K94.13
 jejunostomy (stoma) K94.13
 kidney — *see* Disease, renal
 labyrinthine — *see* subcategory H83.2 ☑
 left ventricular, following sudden emotional stress
  I51.81
 liver K76.89
 male — *see* Dysfunction, sexual, male
 meibomian gland, of eyelid H02.889
  left H02.886
   lower H02.885
   upper H02.884
   upper and lower eyelids H02.88B
  right H02.883

Dysfunction — *continued*
 meibomian gland — *continued*
  lower H02.882
  upper H02.881
  upper and lower eyelids H02.88A
 orgasmic (female) F52.31
  male F52.32
 ovary E28.9
  specified NEC E28.8
 papillary muscle I51.89
 parathyroid E21.4
 physiological NEC R68.89
  psychogenic F59
 pineal gland E34.8
 pituitary (gland) E23.3
 platelets D69.1
 polyglandular E31.9
  specified NEC E31.8
 psychophysiologic F59
 psychosexual F52.9
  with
   dyspareunia F52.6
   premature ejaculation F52.4
   vaginismus F52.5
 pylorus K31.9
 rectum K59.9
  psychogenic F45.8
 reflex (sympathetic) — *see* Syndrome, pain,
  complex regional I
 segmental — *see* Dysfunction, somatic
 senile R54
 sexual (due to) R37
  alcohol F10.981
  amphetamine F15.981
   in
    abuse F15.181
    dependence F15.281
  anxiolytic F13.981
   in
    abuse F13.181
    dependence F13.281
  cocaine F14.981
   in
    abuse F14.181
    dependence F14.281
  excessive sexual drive F52.8
  failure of genital response (male) F52.21
   female F52.22
  female N94.9
   aversion F52.1
   dyspareunia N94.10
    psychogenic F52.6
   frigidity F52.22
   nymphomania F52.8
   orgasmic F52.31
   psychogenic F52.9
    aversion F52.1
    dyspareunia F52.6
    frigidity F52.22
    nymphomania F52.8
    orgasmic F52.31
    vaginismus F52.5
   vaginismus N94.2
    psychogenic F52.5
  hypnotic F13.981
   in
    abuse F13.181
    dependence F13.281
  inhibited orgasm (female) F52.31
   male F52.32
  lack
   of sexual enjoyment F52.1
   or loss of sexual desire F52.0
  male N53.9
   anejaculatory orgasm N53.13
   ejaculatory N53.19
    painful N53.12
    premature F52.4
    retarded N53.11
   erectile N52.9
    drug induced N52.2
    due to
     disease classified elsewhere N52.1
     drug N52.2
    postoperative (postprocedural) N52.39
     following
      cryotherapy N52.37
      interstitial seed therapy N52.36
      prostate ablative therapy N52.37
      prostatectomy N52.34
       radical N52.31
      radiation therapy N52.35

Dysfunction — *continued*
  sexual — *continued*
        radical cystectomy N52.32
        ultrasound ablative therapy N52.37
        urethral surgery N52.33
     psychogenic F52.21
     specified cause NEC N52.8
     vasculogenic
       arterial insufficiency N52.01
        with corporo-venous occlusive N52.03
       corporo-venous occlusive N52.02
        with arterial insufficiency N52.03
    impotence — *see* Dysfunction, sexual, male, erectile
    psychogenic F52.9
     aversion F52.1
     erectile F52.21
     orgasmic F52.32
     premature ejaculation F52.4
     satyriasis F52.8
     specified type NEC F52.8
    specified type NEC N53.8
   nonorganic F52.9
    specified NEC F52.8
   opioid F11.981
    in
     abuse F11.181
     dependence F11.281
   orgasmic dysfunction (female) F52.31
    male F52.32
   premature ejaculation F52.4
   psychoactive substances NEC F19.981
    in
     abuse F19.181
     dependence F19.281
   psychogenic F52.9
   sedative F13.981
    in
     abuse F13.181
     dependence F13.281
   sexual aversion F52.1
   vaginismus (nonorganic) (psychogenic) F52.5
  sinoatrial node I49.5
  somatic M99.09
   abdomen M99.09
   acromioclavicular M99.07
   cervical region M99.01
   cervicothoracic M99.01
   costochondral M99.08
   costovertebral M99.08
   head region M99.00
   hip M99.05
   lower extremity M99.06
   lumbar region M99.03
   lumbosacral M99.03
   occipitocervical M99.00
   pelvic region M99.05
   pubic M99.05
   rib cage M99.08
   sacral region M99.04
   sacrococcygeal M99.04
   sacroiliac M99.04
   specified NEC M99.09
   sternochondral M99.08
   sternoclavicular M99.07
   thoracic region M99.02
   thoracolumbar M99.02
   upper extremity M99.07
  somatoform autonomic F45.8
  stomach K31.89
   psychogenic F45.8
  suprarenal E27.9
   hyperfunction E27.0
  symbolic R48.9
   specified type NEC R48.8
  temporomandibular (joint) M26.69
   joint-pain syndrome M26.62 ☑
  testicular (endocrine) E29.9
   specified NEC E29.8
  thymus E32.9
  thyroid E07.9
  ureterostomy (stoma) — *see* Complications, stoma, urinary tract
  urethrostomy (stoma) — *see* Complications, stoma, urinary tract
  uterus, complicating delivery O62.9
   hypertonic O62.4
   hypotonic O62.2
    primary O62.0
    secondary O62.1

Dysfunction — *continued*
  ventricular I51.9
   with congestive heart failure (*see also* Failure, heart) I50.9
   left, reversible, following sudden emotional stress I51.81
Dysgenesis
  gonadal (due to chromosomal anomaly) Q96.9
   pure Q99.1
  renal Q60.5
   bilateral Q60.4
   unilateral Q60.3
  reticular D72.0
  tidal platelet D69.3
Dysgerminoma
  specified site — *see* Neoplasm, malignant, by site
  unspecified site
   female C56.9
   male C62.90
Dysgeusia R43.2
Dysgraphia R27.8
Dyshidrosis, dysidrosis L30.1
Dyskaryotic cervical smear R87.619
Dyskeratosis L85.8
  cervix — *see* Dysplasia, cervix
  congenital Q82.8
  uterus NEC N85.8
Dyskinesia G24.9
  biliary (cystic duct or gallbladder) K82.8
  drug induced
   orofacial G24.01
  esophagus K22.4
  hysterical F44.4
  intestinal K59.8
  nonorganic origin F44.4
  orofacial (idiopathic) G24.4
   drug induced G24.01
  psychogenic F44.4
  subacute, drug induced G24.01
  tardive G24.01
   neuroleptic induced G24.01
  trachea J39.8
  tracheobronchial J98.09
Dyslalia (developmental) F80.0
Dyslexia R48.0
  developmental F81.0
Dyslipidemia E78.5
  depressed HDL cholesterol E78.6
  elevated fasting triglycerides E78.1
Dysmaturity (*see also* Light for dates)
  pulmonary (newborn) (Wilson-Mikity) P27.0
Dysmenorrhea (essential) (exfoliative) N94.6
  congestive (syndrome) N94.6
  primary N94.4
  psychogenic F45.8
  secondary N94.5
Dysmetabolic syndrome X E88.81
Dysmetria R27.8
Dysmorphism (due to)
  alcohol Q86.0
  exogenous cause NEC Q86.8
  hydantoin Q86.1
  warfarin Q86.2
Dysmorphophobia (nondelusional) F45.22
  delusional F22
Dysnomia R47.01
Dysorexia R63.0
  psychogenic F50.89
Dysostosis
  cleidocranial, cleidocranialis Q74.0
  craniofacial Q75.1
  Fairbank's (idiopathic familial generalized osteophytosis) Q78.9
  mandibulofacial (incomplete) Q75.4
  multiplex E76.01
  oculomandibular Q75.5
Dyspareunia (female) N94.10
  deep N94.12
  male N53.12
  nonorganic F52.6
  psychogenic F52.6
  secondary N94.19
  specified NEC N94.19
  superficial (introital) N94.11
Dyspepsia R10.13
  atonic K30
  functional (allergic) (congenital) (gastrointestinal) (occupational) (reflex) K30
  intestinal K59.8
  nervous F45.8
  neurotic F45.8
  psychogenic F45.8

Dysphagia R13.10
  cervical R13.19
  following
   cerebral infarction I69.391
   cerebrovascular disease I69.991
    specified NEC I69.891
   intracerebral hemorrhage I69.191
   nontraumatic intracranial hemorrhage NEC I69.291
   specified disease NEC I69.891
   subarachnoid hemorrhage I69.091
  functional (hysterical) F45.8
  hysterical F45.8
  nervous (hysterical) F45.8
  neurogenic R13.19
  oral phase R13.11
  oropharyngeal phase R13.12
  pharyngeal phase R13.13
  pharyngoesophageal phase R13.14
  psychogenic F45.8
  sideropenic D50.1
  spastica K22.4
  specified NEC R13.19
Dysphagocytosis, congenital D71
Dysphasia R47.02
  developmental
   expressive type F80.1
   receptive type F80.2
  following
   cerebrovascular disease I69.921
    cerebral infarction I69.321
   intracerebral hemorrhage I69.121
   nontraumatic intracranial hemorrhage NEC I69.221
   specified disease NEC I69.821
   subarachnoid hemorrhage I69.021
Dysphonia R49.0
  functional F44.4
  hysterical F44.4
  psychogenic F44.4
  spastica J38.3
Dysphoria
  gender F64.9
   in
    adolescence and adulthood F64.0
    children F64.2
   specified NEC F64.8
  postpartal O90.6
Dyspituitarism E23.3
Dysplasia (*see also* Anomaly)
  acetabular, congenital Q65.89
  alveolar capillary, with vein misalignment J84.843
  anus (histologically confirmed) (mild) (moderate) K62.82
   severe D01.3
  arrhythmogenic right ventricular I42.8
  arterial, fibromuscular I77.3
  asphyxiating thoracic (congenital) Q77.2
  brain Q07.9
  bronchopulmonary, perinatal P27.1
  cervix (uteri) N87.9
   mild N87.0
   moderate N87.1
   severe D06.9
  chondroectodermal Q77.6
  colon D12.6
  craniometaphyseal Q78.8
  dentinal K00.5
  diaphyseal, progressive Q78.3
  dystrophic Q77.5
  ectodermal (anhidrotic) (congenital) (hereditary) Q82.4
   hydrotic Q82.8
  epithelial, uterine cervix — *see* Dysplasia, cervix
  eye (congenital) Q11.2
  fibrous
   bone NEC (monostotic) M85.00
    ankle M85.07 ☑
    foot M85.07 ☑
    forearm M85.03 ☑
    hand M85.04 ☑
    lower leg M85.06 ☑
    multiple site M85.09
    neck M85.08
    rib M85.08
    shoulder M85.01 ☑
    skull M85.08
    specified site NEC M85.08
    thigh M85.05 ☑
    toe M85.07 ☑
    upper arm M85.02 ☑
    vertebra M85.08

☑ **Additional character required**

Dysplasia — *continued*
  fibrous — *continued*
    diaphyseal, progressive Q78.3
    jaw M27.8
    polyostotic Q78.1
  florid osseous (*see also* Cyst, calcifying odontogenic)
  high grade, focal D12.6
  hip, congenital Q65.89
  joint, congenital Q74.8
  kidney Q61.4
    multicystic Q61.4
  leg Q74.2
  lung, congenital (not associated with short
    gestation) Q33.6
  mammary (gland) (benign) N60.9 ☑
    cyst (solitary) — *see* Cyst, breast
    cystic — *see* Mastopathy, cystic
    duct ectasia — *see* Ectasia, mammary duct
    fibroadenosis — *see* Fibroadenosis, breast
    fibrosclerosis — *see* Fibrosclerosis, breast
    specified type NEC N60.8 ☑
  metaphyseal Q78.5
  muscle Q79.8
  oculodentodigital Q87.0
  periapical (cemental) (cemento-osseous) — *see*
    Cyst, calcifying odontogenic
  periosteum — *see* Disorder, bone, specified type
    NEC
  polyostotic fibrous Q78.1
  prostate (*see also* Neoplasia, intraepithelial,
    prostate) N42.30
    severe D07.5
    specified NEC N42.39
  renal Q61.4
    multicystic Q61.4
  retinal, congenital Q14.1
  right ventricular, arrhythmogenic I42.8
  septo-optic Q04.4
  skin L98.8
  spinal cord Q06.1
  spondyloepiphyseal Q77.7
  thymic, with immunodeficiency D82.1
  vagina N89.3
    mild N89.0
    moderate N89.1
    severe NEC D07.2
  vulva N90.3
    mild N90.0
    moderate N90.1
    severe NEC D07.1
Dysplasminogenemia E88.02
Dyspnea (nocturnal) (paroxysmal) R06.00
  asthmatic (bronchial) J45.909
    with
      exacerbation (acute) J45.901
      bronchitis J45.909
        with
          exacerbation (acute) J45.901
          status asthmaticus J45.902
        chronic J44.9
      status asthmaticus J45.902
    cardiac — *see* Failure, ventricular, left
  cardiac — *see* Failure, ventricular, left
  functional F45.8
  hyperventilation R06.4
  hysterical F45.8
  newborn P28.89
  orthopnea R06.01
  psychogenic F45.8
  shortness of breath R06.02
  specified type NEC R06.09
Dyspraxia R27.8
  developmental (syndrome) F82
Dysproteinemia E88.09
Dysreflexia, autonomic G90.4
Dysrhythmia
  cardiac I49.9
    newborn
      bradycardia P29.12
      occurring before birth P03.819
        before onset of labor P03.810
        during labor P03.811
      tachycardia P29.11
    postoperative I97.89
  cerebral or cortical — *see* Epilepsy
Dyssomnia — *see* Disorder, sleep
Dyssynergia
  biliary K83.8
  bladder sphincter N36.44
  cerebellaris myoclonica (Hunt's ataxia) G11.1
Dysthymia F34.1
Dysthyroidism E07.9

Dystocia O66.9
  affecting newborn P03.1
  cervical (hypotonic) O62.2
    affecting newborn P03.6
    primary O62.0
    secondary O62.1
  contraction ring O62.4
  fetal O66.9
    abnormality NEC O66.3
    conjoined twins O66.3
    oversize O66.2
  maternal O66.9
  positional O64.9 ☑
  shoulder (girdle) O66.0
    causing obstructed labor O66.0
  uterine NEC O62.4
Dystonia G24.9
  cervical G24.3
  deformans progressiva G24.1
  drug induced NEC G24.09
    acute G24.02
    specified NEC G24.09
  familial G24.1
  idiopathic G24.1
    familial G24.1
    nonfamilial G24.2
    orofacial G24.4
  lenticularis G24.8
  musculorum deformans G24.1
  neuroleptic induced (acute) G24.02
  orofacial (idiopathic) G24.4
  oromandibular G24.4
    due to drug G24.01
  specified NEC G24.8
  torsion (familial) (idiopathic) G24.1
    acquired G24.8
    genetic G24.1
    symptomatic (nonfamilial) G24.2
Dystonic movements R25.8
Dystrophy, dystrophia
  adiposogenital E23.6
  autosomal recessive, childhood type, muscular
    dystrophy resembling Duchenne or Becker
    G71.01
  Becker's type G71.01
  cervical sympathetic G90.2
  choroid (hereditary) H31.20
    central areolar H31.22
    choroideremia H31.21
    gyrate atrophy H31.23
    specified type NEC H31.29
  cornea (hereditary) H18.50
    endothelial H18.51
    epithelial H18.52
    granular H18.53
    lattice H18.54
    macular H18.55
    specified type NEC H18.59
  Duchenne's type G71.01
  due to malnutrition E45
  Erb's G71.02
  Fuchs' H18.51
  Gower's muscular G71.01
  hair L67.8
  infantile neuroaxonal G31.89
  Landouzy-Déjérine G71.02
  Leyden-Möbius G71.09
  muscular G71.00
    autosomal recessive, childhood type, muscular
      dystrophy resembling Duchenne or Becker
      G71.01
    benign (Becker type) G71.01
    scapuloperoneal with early contractures
      [Emery-Dreifuss] G71.09
    congenital (hereditary) (progressive) (with
      specific morphological abnormalities of the
      muscle fiber) G71.09
      myotonic G71.11
    distal G71.09
    Duchenne type G71.01
    Emery-Dreifuss G71.09
    Erb type G71.02
    facioscapulohumeral G71.02
    Gower's G71.01
    hereditary (progressive) G71.09
    Landouzy-Déjérine type G71.02
    limb-girdle G71.09
    myotonic G71.11
    progressive (hereditary) G71.09
      Charcot-Marie (-Tooth) type G60.0
    pseudohypertrophic (infantile) G71.01
    scapulohumeral G71.02

Dystrophy — *continued*
  muscular — *continued*
    scapuloperoneal G71.09
    severe (Duchenne type) G71.01
    specified type NEC G71.09
  myocardium, myocardial — *see* Degeneration,
    myocardial
  myotonic, myotonica G71.11
  nail L60.3
    congenital Q84.6
  nutritional E45
  ocular G71.09
  oculocerebrorenal E72.03
  oculopharyngeal G71.09
  ovarian N83.8
  polyglandular E31.8
  reflex (neuromuscular) (sympathetic) — *see*
    Syndrome, pain, complex regional I
  retinal (hereditary) H35.50
    in
      lipid storage disorders E75.6 *[H36]*
      systemic lipidoses E75.6 *[H36]*
    involving
      pigment epithelium H35.54
      sensory area H35.53
    pigmentary H35.52
    vitreoretinal H35.51
  Salzmann's nodular — *see* Degeneration, cornea,
    nodular
  scapuloperoneal G71.09
  skin NEC L98.8
  sympathetic (reflex) — *see* Syndrome, pain,
    complex regional I
    cervical G90.2
  tapetoretinal H35.54
  thoracic, asphyxiating Q77.2
  unguium L60.3
    congenital Q84.6
  vitreoretinal H35.51
  vulva N90.4
  yellow (liver) — *see* Failure, hepatic
Dysuria R30.0
  psychogenic F45.8

E

Eales' disease H35.06 ☑
Ear (*see also* condition)
  piercing Z41.3
  tropical NEC B36.9 *[H62.40]*
    in
      aspergillosis B44.89
      candidiasis B37.84
      moniliasis B37.84
  wax (impacted) H61.20
    left H61.22
      with right H61.23
    right H61.21
      with left H61.23
Earache — *see* subcategory H92.0 ☑
Early satiety R68.81
Eaton-Lambert syndrome — *see* Syndrome,
  Lambert-Eaton
Eberth's disease (typhoid fever) A01.00
Ebola virus disease A98.4
Ebstein's anomaly or syndrome (heart) Q22.5
Eccentro-osteochondrodysplasia E76.29
Ecchondroma — *see* Neoplasm, bone, benign
Ecchondrosis D48.0
Ecchymosis R58
  conjunctiva — *see* Hemorrhage, conjunctiva
  eye (traumatic) — *see* Contusion, eyeball
  eyelid (traumatic) — *see* Contusion, eyelid
  newborn P54.5
  spontaneous R23.3
  traumatic — *see* Contusion
Echinococciasis — *see* Echinococcus
Echinococcosis — *see* Echinococcus
Echinococcus (infection) B67.90
  granulosus B67.4
    bone B67.2
    liver B67.0
    lung B67.1
    multiple sites B67.32
    specified site NEC B67.39
    thyroid B67.31
  liver NOS B67.8
    granulosus B67.0
    multilocularis B67.5

Echinococcus — *continued*
 lung NEC B67.99
  granulosus B67.1
  multilocularis B67.69
 multilocularis B67.7
  liver B67.5
  multiple sites B67.61
  specified site NEC B67.69
 specified site NEC B67.99
  granulosus B67.39
  multilocularis B67.69
 thyroid NEC B67.99
  granulosus B67.31
  multilocularis B67.69 *[E35]*
Echinorhynchiasis B83.8
Echinostomiasis B66.8
Echolalia R48.8
Echovirus, as cause of disease classified elsewhere
 B97.12
Eclampsia, eclamptic (coma) (convulsions) (delirium)
 (with hypertension) NEC O15.9
 complicating
  labor and delivery O15.1
  postpartum O15.2
  pregnancy O15.0 ☑
  puerperium O15.2
Economic circumstances affecting care Z59.9
Economo's disease A85.8
Ectasia, ectasis
 annuloaortic I35.8
 aorta I77.819
  with aneurysm — *see* Aneurysm, aorta
  abdominal I77.811
  thoracic I77.810
  thoracoabdominal I77.812
 breast — *see* Ectasia, mammary duct
 capillary I78.8
 cornea H18.71 ☑
 gastric antral vascular (GAVE) K31.819
  with hemorrhage K31.811
  without hemorrhage K31.819
 mammary duct N60.4 ☑
 salivary gland (duct) K11.8
 sclera — *see* Sclerectasia
Ecthyma L08.0
 contagiosum B08.02
 gangrenosum L08.0
 infectiosum B08.02
Ectocardia Q24.8
Ectodermal dysplasia (anhidrotic) Q82.4
Ectodermosis erosiva pluriorificialis L51.1
Ectopic, ectopia (congenital)
 abdominal viscera Q45.8
  due to defect in anterior abdominal wall
   Q79.59
 ACTH syndrome E24.3
 adrenal gland Q89.1
 anus Q43.5
 atrial beats I49.1
 beats I49.49
  atrial I49.1
  ventricular I49.3
 bladder Q64.10
 bone and cartilage in lung Q33.5
 brain Q04.8
 breast tissue Q83.8
 cardiac Q24.8
 cerebral Q04.8
 cordis Q24.8
 endometrium — *see* Endometriosis
 gastric mucosa Q40.2
 gestation — *see* Pregnancy, by site
 heart Q24.8
 hormone secretion NEC E34.2
 kidney (crossed) (pelvis) Q63.2
 lens, lentis Q12.1
 mole — *see* Pregnancy, by site
 organ or site NEC — *see* Malposition, congenital
 pancreas Q45.3
 pregnancy — *see* Pregnancy, ectopic
 pupil — *see* Abnormality, pupillary
 renal Q63.2
 sebaceous glands of mouth Q38.6
 spleen Q89.09
 testis Q53.00
  bilateral Q53.02
  unilateral Q53.01
 thyroid Q89.2
 tissue in lung Q33.5
 ureter Q62.63
 ventricular beats I49.3
 vesicae Q64.10

Ectromelia Q73.8
 lower limb — *see* Defect, reduction, limb, lower,
  specified type NEC
 upper limb — *see* Defect, reduction, limb, upper,
  specified type NEC
Ectropion H02.109
 cervix N86
  with cervicitis N72
 congenital Q10.1
 eyelid H02.109
  cicatricial H02.119
   left H02.116
    lower H02.115
    upper H02.114
   right H02.113
    lower H02.112
    upper H02.111
  congenital Q10.1
  left H02.106
   lower H02.105
   upper H02.104
  mechanical H02.129
   left H02.126
    lower H02.125
    upper H02.124
   right H02.123
    lower H02.122
    upper H02.121
  paralytic H02.159
   left H02.156
    lower H02.155
    upper H02.154
   right H02.153
    lower H02.152
    upper H02.151
  right H02.103
   lower H02.102
   upper H02.101
  senile H02.139
   left H02.136
    lower H02.135
    upper H02.134
   right H02.133
    lower H02.132
    upper H02.131
  spastic H02.149
   left H02.146
    lower H02.145
    upper H02.144
   right H02.143
    lower H02.142
    upper H02.141
 iris H21.89
 lip (acquired) K13.0
  congenital Q38.0
 urethra N36.8
 uvea H21.89
Eczema (acute) (chronic) (erythematous) (fissum)
 (rubrum) (squamous) (*see also* Dermatitis) L30.9
 contact — *see* Dermatitis, contact
 dyshydrotic L30.1
 external ear — *see* Otitis, externa, acute, eczematoid
 flexural L20.82
 herpeticum B00.0
 hypertrophicum L28.0
 hypostatic — *see* Varix, leg, with, inflammation
 impetiginous L01.1
 infantile (due to any substance) L20.83
  intertriginous L21.1
  seborrheic L21.1
 intertriginous NEC L30.4
  infantile L21.1
 intrinsic (allergic) L20.84
 lichenified NEC L28.0
 marginatum (hebrae) B35.6
 pustular L30.3
 stasis I87.2
  with varicose veins — *see* Varix, leg, with,
   inflammation
 vaccination, vaccinatum T88.1 ☑
 varicose — *see* Varix, leg, with, inflammation
Eczematid L30.2
Eddowes (-Spurway) syndrome Q78.0
Edema, edematous (infectious) (pitting) (toxic) R60.9
 with nephritis — *see* Nephrosis
 allergic T78.3 ☑
 amputation stump (surgical) (sequelae (late effect))
  T87.89
 angioneurotic (allergic) (any site) (with urticaria)
  T78.3 ☑
  hereditary D84.1
 angiospastic I73.9

Edema — *continued*
 Berlin's (traumatic) S05.8X ☑
 brain (cytotoxic) (vasogenic) G93.6
  due to birth injury P11.0
   newborn (anoxia or hypoxia) P52.4
    birth injury P11.0
  traumatic — *see* Injury, intracranial, cerebral
   edema
 cardiac — *see* Failure, heart, congestive
 cardiovascular — *see* Failure, heart, congestive
 cerebral — *see* Edema, brain
 cerebrospinal — *see* Edema, brain
 cervix (uteri) (acute) N88.8
  puerperal, postpartum O90.89
 chronic hereditary Q82.0
 circumscribed, acute T78.3 ☑
  hereditary D84.1
 conjunctiva H11.42 ☑
 cornea H18.2 ☑
  idiopathic H18.22 ☑
  secondary H18.23 ☑
   due to contact lens H18.21 ☑
 due to
  lymphatic obstruction I89.0
  salt retention E87.0
 epiglottis — *see* Edema, glottis
 essential, acute T78.3 ☑
  hereditary D84.1
 extremities, lower — *see* Edema, legs
 eyelid NEC H02.849
  left H02.846
   lower H02.845
   upper H02.844
  right H02.843
   lower H02.842
   upper H02.841
 familial, hereditary Q82.0
 famine — *see* Malnutrition, severe
 generalized R60.1
 glottis, glottic, glottidis (obstructive) (passive)
  J38.4
  allergic T78.3 ☑
   hereditary D84.1
 heart — *see* Failure, heart, congestive
 heat T67.7 ☑
 hereditary Q82.0
 inanition — *see* Malnutrition, severe
 intracranial G93.6
 iris H21.89
 joint — *see* Effusion, joint
 larynx — *see* Edema, glottis
 legs R60.0
  due to venous obstruction I87.1
  hereditary Q82.0
 localized R60.0
  due to venous obstruction I87.1
 lower limbs — *see* Edema, legs
 lung J81.1
  with heart condition or failure — *see* Failure,
   ventricular, left
  acute J81.0
  chemical (acute) J68.1
   chronic J68.1
  chronic J81.1
   due to
    chemicals, gases, fumes or vapors (inhalation)
     J68.1
    external agent J70.9
     specified NEC J70.8
    radiation J70.1
  due to
   chemicals, fumes or vapors (inhalation) J68.1
   external agent J70.9
    specified NEC J70.8
   high altitude T70.29 ☑
   near drowning T75.1 ☑
   radiation J70.0
  meaning failure, left ventricle I50.1
 lymphatic I89.0
  due to mastectomy I97.2
 macula H35.81
  cystoid, following cataract surgery — *see*
   Complications, postprocedural, following
   cataract surgery
  diabetic — *see* Diabetes, by type, with,
   retinopathy, with macular edema
 malignant — *see* Gangrene, gas
 Milroy's Q82.0
 nasopharynx J39.2
 newborn P83.30
  hydrops fetalis — *see* Hydrops, fetalis
  specified NEC P83.39

Edema — *continued*
nutritional (*see also* Malnutrition, severe)
with dyspigmentation, skin and hair E40
optic disc or nerve — *see* Papilledema
orbit H05.22 ☑
pancreas K86.89
papilla, optic — *see* Papilledema
penis N48.89
periodic T78.3 ☑
hereditary D84.1
pharynx J39.2
pulmonary — *see* Edema, lung
Quincke's T78.3 ☑
hereditary D84.1
renal — *see* Nephrosis
retina H35.81
diabetic — *see* Diabetes, by type, with,
retinopathy, with macular edema
salt E87.0
scrotum N50.89
seminal vesicle N50.89
spermatic cord N50.89
spinal (cord) (vascular) (nontraumatic) G95.19
starvation — *see* Malnutrition, severe
stasis — *see* Hypertension, venous, (chronic)
subglottic — *see* Edema, glottis
supraglottic — *see* Edema, glottis
testis N44.8
tunica vaginalis N50.89
vas deferens N50.89
vulva (acute) N90.89
Edentulism — *see* Absence, teeth, acquired
Edsall's disease T67.2 ☑
Educational handicap Z55.9
specified NEC Z55.8
Edward's syndrome — *see* Trisomy, 18
Effect, adverse
abnormal gravitational (G) forces or states T75.81 ☑
abuse — *see* Maltreatment
air pressure T70.9 ☑
specified NEC T70.8 ☑
altitude (high) — *see* Effect, adverse, high altitude
anesthesia (*see also* Anesthesia) T88.59 ☑
in labor and delivery O74.9
local, toxic
in labor and delivery O74.4
in pregnancy NEC O29.3 ☑
postpartum, puerperal O89.3
postpartum, puerperal O89.9
specified NEC T88.59 ☑
in labor and delivery O74.8
postpartum, puerperal O89.8
spinal and epidural T88.59 ☑
headache T88.59 ☑
in labor and delivery O74.5
postpartum, puerperal O89.4
specified NEC
in labor and delivery O74.6
postpartum, puerperal O89.5
antitoxin — *see* Complications, vaccination
atmospheric pressure T70.9 ☑
due to explosion T70.8 ☑
high T70.3 ☑
low — *see* Effect, adverse, high altitude
specified effect NEC T70.8 ☑
biological, correct substance properly administered
— *see* Effect, adverse, drug
blood (derivatives) (serum) (transfusion) — *see*
Complications, transfusion
chemical substance — *see* Table of Drugs and
Chemicals
cold (temperature) (weather) T69.9 ☑
chilblains T69.1 ☑
frostbite — *see* Frostbite
specified effect NEC T69.8 ☑
drugs and medicaments T88.7 ☑
specified drug — *see* Table of Drugs and
Chemicals, by drug, adverse effect
specified effect - code to condition
electric current, electricity (shock) T75.4 ☑
burn — *see* Burn
exertion (excessive) T73.3 ☑
exposure — *see* Exposure
external cause NEC T75.89 ☑
foodstuffs T78.1 ☑
allergic reaction — *see* Allergy, food
causing anaphylaxis — *see* Shock, anaphylactic,
due to food
noxious — *see* Poisoning, food, noxious
gases, fumes, or vapors T59.9 ☑
specified agent — *see* Table of Drugs and
Chemicals

Effect — *continued*
glue (airplane) sniffing
due to drug abuse — *see* Abuse, drug, inhalant
due to drug dependence — *see* Dependence,
drug, inhalant
heat — *see* Heat
high altitude NEC T70.29 ☑
anoxia T70.29 ☑
on
ears T70.0 ☑
sinuses T70.1 ☑
polycythemia D75.1
high pressure fluids T70.4 ☑
hot weather — *see* Heat
hunger T73.0 ☑
immersion, foot — *see* Immersion
immunization — *see* Complications, vaccination
immunological agents — *see* Complications,
vaccination
infrared (radiation) (rays) NOS T66 ☑
dermatitis or eczema L59.8
infusion — *see* Complications, infusion
lack of care of infants — *see* Maltreatment, child
lightning — *see* Lightning
medical care T88.9 ☑
specified NEC T88.8 ☑
medicinal substance, correct, properly administered
— *see* Effect, adverse, drug
motion T75.3 ☑
noise, on inner ear — *see* subcategory H83.3 ☑
overheated places — *see* Heat
psychosocial, of work environment Z56.5
radiation (diagnostic) (infrared) (natural source)
(therapeutic) (ultraviolet) (X-ray) NOS T66 ☑
dermatitis or eczema — *see* Dermatitis, due to,
radiation
fibrosis of lung J70.1
pneumonitis J70.0
pulmonary manifestations
acute J70.0
chronic J70.1
skin L59.9
radioactive substance NOS
dermatitis or eczema — *see* Radiodermatitis
reduced temperature T69.9 ☑
immersion foot or hand — *see* Immersion
specified effect NEC T69.8 ☑
serum NEC (*see also* Reaction, serum) T80.69 ☑
specified NEC T78.8 ☑
external cause NEC T75.89 ☑
strangulation — *see* Asphyxia, traumatic
submersion T75.1 ☑
thirst T73.1 ☑
toxic — *see* Toxicity
transfusion — *see* Complications, transfusion
ultraviolet (radiation) (rays) NOS T66 ☑
burn — *see* Burn
dermatitis or eczema — *see* Dermatitis, due to,
ultraviolet rays
acute L56.8
vaccine (any) — *see* Complications, vaccination
vibration — *see* Vibration, adverse effects
water pressure NEC T70.9 ☑
specified NEC T70.8 ☑
weightlessness T75.82 ☑
whole blood — *see* Complications, transfusion
work environment Z56.5
Effect(s) (of) (from) — *see* Effect, adverse NEC
Effects, late — *see* Sequelae
Effluvium
anagen L65.1
telogen L65.0
Effort syndrome (psychogenic) F45.8
Effusion
amniotic fluid — *see* Pregnancy, complicated by,
premature rupture of membranes
brain (serous) G93.6
bronchial — *see* Bronchitis
cerebral G93.6
cerebrospinal (*see also* Meningitis)
vessel G93.6
chest — *see* Effusion, pleura
chylous, chyliform (pleura) J94.0
intracranial G93.6
joint M25.40
ankle M25.47 ☑
elbow M25.42 ☑
foot joint M25.47 ☑
hand joint M25.44 ☑
hip M25.45 ☑
knee M25.46 ☑
shoulder M25.41 ☑

Effusion — *continued*
joint — *continued*
specified joint NEC M25.48
wrist M25.43 ☑
malignant pleural J91.0
meninges — *see* Meningitis
pericardium, pericardial (noninflammatory) I31.3
acute — *see* Pericarditis, acute
peritoneal (chronic) R18.8
pleura, pleurisy, pleuritic, pleuropericardial J90
chylous, chyliform J94.0
due to systemic lupus erythematosis M32.13
in conditions classified elsewhere J91.8
influenzal — *see* Influenza, with, respiratory
manifestations NEC
malignant J91.0
newborn P28.89
tuberculous NEC A15.6
primary (progressive) A15.7
spinal — *see* Meningitis
thorax, thoracic — *see* Effusion, pleura
Egg shell nails L60.3
congenital Q84.6
Egyptian splenomegaly B65.1
Ehrlichiosis A77.40
due to
E. chafeensis A77.41
E. sennetsu A79.81
specified organism NEC A77.49
Ehlers-Danlos syndrome (*see also* Syndrome,
Ehlers-Danlos) Q79.60
Eichstedt's disease B36.0
Eisenmenger's
complex or syndrome I27.83
defect Q21.8
Ejaculation
delayed F52.32
painful N53.12
premature F52.4
retarded N53.11
retrograde N53.14
semen, painful N53.12
psychogenic F52.6
Ekbom's syndrome (restless legs) G25.81
Ekman's syndrome (brittle bones and blue sclera) Q78.0
Elastic skin Q82.8
acquired L57.4
Elastofibroma — *see* Neoplasm, connective tissue,
benign
Elastoma (juvenile) Q82.8
Miescher's L87.2
Elastomyofibrosis I42.4
Elastosis
actinic, solar L57.8
atrophicans (senile) L57.4
perforans serpiginosa L87.2
senilis L57.4
Elbow — *see* condition
Electric current, electricity, effects (concussion) (fatal)
(nonfatal) (shock) T75.4 ☑
burn — *see* Burn
Electric feet syndrome E53.8
Electrocution T75.4 ☑
from electroshock gun (taser) T75.4 ☑
Electrolyte imbalance E87.8
with
abortion — *see* Abortion by type, complicated by,
electrolyte imbalance
ectopic pregnancy O08.5
molar pregnancy O08.5
Elephantiasis (nonfilarial) I89.0
arabicum — *see* Infestation, filarial
bancroftian B74.0
congenital (any site) (hereditary) Q82.0
due to
Brugia (malayi) B74.1
timori B74.2
mastectomy I97.2
Wuchereria (bancrofti) B74.0
eyelid H02.859
left H02.856
lower H02.855
upper H02.854
right H02.853
lower H02.852
upper H02.851
filarial, filariensis — *see* Infestation, filarial
glandular I89.0
graecorum A30.9
lymphangiectatic I89.0
lymphatic vessel I89.0
due to mastectomy I97.2

Elephantiasis - Embolism

Elephantiasis — *continued*
  scrotum (nonfilarial) I89.0
  streptococcal I89.0
  surgical I97.89
    postmastectomy I97.2
  telangiectodes I89.0
  vulva (nonfilarial) N90.89
Elevated, elevation
  antibody titer R76.0
  basal metabolic rate R94.8
  blood pressure (*see also* Hypertension)
    reading (incidental) (isolated) (nonspecific), no
      diagnosis of hypertension R03.0
  blood sugar R73.9
  body temperature (of unknown origin) R50.9
  C-reactive protein (CRP) R79.82
  cancer antigen 125 [CA 125] R97.1
  carcinoembryonic antigen [CEA] R97.0
  cholesterol E78.00
    with high triglycerides E78.2
  conjugate, eye H51.0
  diaphragm, congenital Q79.1
  erythrocyte sedimentation rate R70.0
  fasting glucose R73.01
  fasting triglycerides E78.1
  finding on laboratory examination — *see* Findings,
    abnormal, inconclusive, without diagnosis, by
    type of exam
  GFR (glomerular filtration rate) — *see* Findings,
    abnormal, inconclusive, without diagnosis, by
    type of exam
  glucose tolerance (oral) R73.02
  immunoglobulin level R76.8
  indoleacetic acid R82.5
  lactic acid dehydrogenase (LDH) level R74.0
  leukocytes D72.829
  lipoprotein a (Lp(a)) level E78.41
  liver function
    study R94.5
    test R79.89
      alkaline phosphatase R74.8
      aminotransferase R74.0
      bilirubin R17
      hepatic enzyme R74.8
      lactate dehydrogenase R74.0
  Lp(a) (lipoprotein(a)) E78.41
  lymphocytes D72.820
  prostate specific antigen [PSA] R97.20
  Rh titer — *see* Complication(s), transfusion,
    incompatibility reaction, Rh (factor)
  scapula, congenital Q74.0
  sedimentation rate R70.0
  SGOT R74.0
  SGPT R74.0
  transaminase level R74.0
  triglycerides E78.1
    with high cholesterol E78.2
  tumor associated antigens [TAA] NEC R97.8
  tumor specific antigens [TSA] NEC R97.8
  urine level of
    catecholamine R82.5
    indoleacetic acid R82.5
    17-ketosteroids R82.5
    steroids R82.5
    vanillylmandelic acid (VMA) R82.5
  venous pressure I87.8
  white blood cell count D72.829
    specified NEC D72.828
Elliptocytosis (congenital) (hereditary) D58.1
  Hb C (disease) D58.1
  hemoglobin disease D58.1
  sickle-cell (disease) D57.8 ☑
    trait D57.3
Ellison-Zollinger syndrome E16.4
Ellis-van Creveld syndrome (chondroectodermal
  dysplasia) Q77.6
Elongated, elongation (congenital) (*see also* Distortion)
  bone Q79.9
  cervix (uteri) Q51.828
    acquired N88.4
    hypertrophic N88.4
  colon Q43.8
  common bile duct Q44.5
  cystic duct Q44.5
  frenulum, penis Q55.69
  labia minora (acquired) N90.69
  ligamentum patellae Q74.1
  petiolus (epiglottidis) Q31.8
  tooth, teeth K00.2
  uvula Q38.6
Eltor cholera A00.1
Emaciation (due to malnutrition) E41

Embadomoniasis A07.8
Embedded tooth, teeth K01.0
  root only K08.3
Embolic — *see* condition
Embolism (multiple) (paradoxical) I74.9
  air (any site) (traumatic) T79.0 ☑
    following
      abortion — *see* Abortion by type complicated
        by embolism
      ectopic pregnancy O08.2
      infusion, therapeutic injection or transfusion
        T80.0 ☑
      molar pregnancy O08.2
      procedure NEC
        artery T81.719 ☑
          mesenteric T81.710 ☑
          renal T81.711 ☑
          specified NEC T81.718 ☑
        vein T81.72 ☑
    in pregnancy, childbirth or puerperium — *see*
      Embolism, obstetric
  amniotic fluid (pulmonary) (*see also* Embolism,
    obstetric)
    following
      abortion — *see* Abortion by type complicated
        by embolism
      ectopic pregnancy O08.2
      molar pregnancy O08.2
  aorta, aortic I74.10
    abdominal I74.09
      saddle I74.01
    bifurcation I74.09
      saddle I74.01
    thoracic I74.11
  artery I74.9
    auditory, internal I65.8
    basilar — *see* Occlusion, artery, basilar
    carotid (common) (internal) — *see* Occlusion,
      artery, carotid
    cerebellar (anterior inferior) (posterior inferior)
      (superior) I66.3
    cerebral — *see* Occlusion, artery, cerebral
    choroidal (anterior) I65.8
    communicating posterior I65.8
    coronary (*see also* Infarct, myocardium)
      not resulting in infarction I24.0
    extremity I74.4
      lower I74.3
      upper I74.2
    hypophyseal I65.8
    iliac I74.5
    limb I74.4
      lower I74.3
      upper I74.2
    mesenteric (with gangrene) (*see also* Ischemia,
      intestine, acute) K55.059
    ophthalmic — *see* Occlusion, artery, retina
    peripheral I74.4
    pontine I65.8
    precerebral — *see* Occlusion, artery, precerebral
    pulmonary — *see* Embolism, pulmonary
    renal N28.0
    retinal — *see* Occlusion, artery, retina
    septic I76
    specified NEC I74.8
    vertebral — *see* Occlusion, artery, vertebral
  basilar (artery) I65.1
  blood clot
    following
      abortion — *see* Abortion by type complicated
        by embolism
      ectopic or molar pregnancy O08.2
    in pregnancy, childbirth or puerperium — *see*
      Embolism, obstetric
  brain (*see also* Occlusion, artery, cerebral)
    following
      abortion — *see* Abortion by type complicated
        by embolism
      ectopic or molar pregnancy O08.2
    puerperal, postpartum, childbirth — *see*
      Embolism, obstetric
  capillary I78.8
  cardiac (*see also* Infarct, myocardium)
    not resulting in infarction I51.3
  carotid (artery) (common) (internal) — *see*
    Occlusion, artery, carotid
  cavernous sinus (venous) — *see* Embolism,
    intracranial venous sinus
  cerebral — *see* Occlusion, artery, cerebral
  cholesterol — *see* Atheroembolism
  coronary (artery or vein) (systemic) — *see* Occlusion,
    coronary

Embolism — *continued*
  due to device, implant or graft (*see also*
    Complications, by site and type, specified NEC)
    arterial graft NEC T82.818 ☑
    breast (implant) T85.818 ☑
    catheter NEC T85.818 ☑
      dialysis (renal) T82.818 ☑
        intraperitoneal T85.818 ☑
      infusion NEC T82.818 ☑
        spinal (epidural) (subdural) T85.810 ☑
      urinary (indwelling) T83.81 ☑
    electronic (electrode) (pulse generator)
      (stimulator)
      bone T84.81 ☑
      cardiac T82.817 ☑
      nervous system (brain) (peripheral nerve)
        (spinal) T85.810 ☑
      urinary T83.81 ☑
    fixation, internal (orthopedic) NEC T84.81 ☑
    gastrointestinal (bile duct) (esophagus)
      T85.818 ☑
    genital NEC T83.81 ☑
    heart (graft) (valve) T82.817 ☑
    joint prosthesis T84.81 ☑
    ocular (corneal graft) (orbital implant) T85.818 ☑
    orthopedic (bone graft) NEC T86.838
    specified NEC T85.818 ☑
    urinary (graft) NEC T83.81 ☑
    vascular NEC T82.818 ☑
    ventricular intracranial shunt T85.810 ☑
  extremities
    lower — *see* Embolism, vein, lower extremity
      arterial I74.3
    upper I74.2
  eye H34.9
  fat (cerebral) (pulmonary) (systemic) T79.1 ☑
    following
      abortion — *see* Abortion by type complicated
        by embolism
      ectopic or molar pregnancy O08.2
    complicating delivery — *see* Embolism, obstetric
  following
    abortion — *see* Abortion by type complicated by
      embolism
    ectopic or molar pregnancy O08.2
    infusion, therapeutic injection or transfusion
      air T80.0 ☑
  heart (fatty) (*see also* Infarct, myocardium)
    not resulting in infarction I51.3
  hepatic (vein) I82.0
  in pregnancy, childbirth or puerperium — *see*
    Embolism, obstetric
  intestine (artery) (vein) (with gangrene) (*see also*
    Ischemia, intestine, acute) K55.039
  intracranial (*see also* Occlusion, artery, cerebral)
    venous sinus (any) G08
      nonpyogenic I67.6
  intraspinal venous sinuses or veins G08
    nonpyogenic G95.19
  kidney (artery) N28.0
  lateral sinus (venous) — *see* Embolism, intracranial,
    venous sinus
  leg — *see* Embolism, vein, lower extremity
    arterial I74.3
  longitudinal sinus (venous) — *see* Embolism,
    intracranial, venous sinus
  lung (massive) — *see* Embolism, pulmonary
  meninges I66.8
  mesenteric (artery) (vein) (with gangrene) (*see also*
    Ischemia, intestine, acute) K55.059
  obstetric (in) (pulmonary)
    childbirth O88.22
      air O88.02
      amniotic fluid O88.12
      blood clot O88.22
      fat O88.82
      pyemic O88.32
      septic O88.32
      specified type NEC O88.82
    pregnancy O88.21 ☑
      air O88.01 ☑
      amniotic fluid O88.11 ☑
      blood clot O88.21 ☑
      fat O88.81 ☑
      pyemic O88.31 ☑
      septic O88.31 ☑
      specified type NEC O88.81 ☑
    puerperal O88.23
      air O88.03
      amniotic fluid O88.13
      blood clot O88.23
      fat O88.83

☑ **Additional character required**

Embolism — *continued*
  obstetric — *continued*
    pyemic O88.33
    septic O88.33
    specified type NEC O88.83
  ophthalmic — *see* Occlusion, artery, retina
  penis N48.81
  peripheral artery NOS I74.4
  pituitary E23.6
  popliteal (artery) I74.3
  portal (vein) I81
  postoperative, postrpocedural
    artery T81.719 ☑
      mesenteric T81.710 ☑
      renal T81.711 ☑
      specified NEC T81.718 ☑
    vein T81.72 ☑
  precerebral artery — *see* Occlusion, artery, precerebral
  puerperal — *see* Embolism, obstetric
  pulmonary (acute) (artery) (vein) I26.99
    with acute cor pulmonale I26.09
    chronic I27.82
    following
      abortion — *see* Abortion by type complicated by embolism
      ectopic or molar pregnancy O08.2
    healed or old Z86.711
    in pregnancy, childbirth or puerperium — *see* Embolism, obstetric
    multiple subsegmental without acute cor pulmonale I26.94
    personal history of Z86.711
    saddle I26.92
      with acute cor pulmonale I26.02
    septic I26.90
      with acute cor pulmonale I26.01
    single subsegmental without acute cor pulmonale I26.93
    subsegmental NOS I26.93
  pyemic (multiple) I76
    following
      abortion — *see* Abortion by type complicated by embolism
      ectopic or molar pregnancy O08.2
    Hemophilus influenzae A41.3
    pneumococcal A40.3
      with pneumonia J13
    puerperal, postpartum, childbirth (any organism) — *see* Embolism, obstetric
    specified organism NEC A41.89
    staphylococcal A41.2
    streptococcal A40.9
  renal (artery) N28.0
    vein I82.3
  retina, retinal — *see* Occlusion, artery, retina
  saddle
    abdominal aorta I74.01
    pulmonary artery I26.92
      with acute cor pulmonale I26.02
  septic (arterial) I76
    complicating abortion — *see* Abortion, by type, complicated by, embolism
  sinus — *see* Embolism, intracranial, venous sinus
  soap complicating abortion — *see* Abortion, by type, complicated by, embolism
  spinal cord G95.19
    pyogenic origin G06.1
  spleen, splenic (artery) I74.8
  upper extremity I74.2
  vein (acute) I82.90
    antecubital I82.61 ☑
      chronic I82.71 ☑
    axillary I82.A1 ☑
      chronic I82.A2 ☑
    basilic I82.61 ☑
      chronic I82.71 ☑
    brachial I82.62 ☑
      chronic I82.72 ☑
    brachiocephalic (innominate) I82.290
      chronic I82.291
    cephalic I82.61 ☑
      chronic I82.71 ☑
    chronic I82.91
    deep (DVT) I82.40 ☑
      calf I82.4Z ☑
        chronic I82.5Z ☑
      lower leg I82.4Z ☑
        chronic I82.5Z ☑
      thigh I82.4Y ☑
        chronic I82.5Y ☑
      upper leg I82.4Y ☑

Embolism — *continued*
  vein — *continued*
    chronic I82.5Y ☑
    femoral I82.41 ☑
      chronic I82.51 ☑
    iliac (iliofemoral) I82.42 ☑
      chronic I82.52 ☑
    innominate I82.290
      chronic I82.291
    internal jugular I82.C1 ☑
      chronic I82.C2 ☑
    lower extremity
      deep I82.40 ☑
        chronic I82.50 ☑
          specified NEC I82.49 ☑
            chronic NEC I82.59 ☑
        distal
          deep I82.4Z ☑
        proximal
          deep I82.4Y ☑
            chronic I82.5Y ☑
        superficial I82.81 ☑
    popliteal I82.43 ☑
      chronic I82.53 ☑
    radial I82.62 ☑
      chronic I82.72 ☑
    renal I82.3
    saphenous (greater) (lesser) I82.81 ☑
    specified NEC I82.890
      chronic NEC I82.891
    subclavian I82.B1 ☑
      chronic I82.B2 ☑
    thoracic NEC I82.290
      chronic I82.291
    tibial I82.44 ☑
      chronic I82.54 ☑
    ulnar I82.62 ☑
      chronic I82.72 ☑
    upper extremity I82.60 ☑
      chronic I82.70 ☑
      deep I82.62 ☑
        chronic I82.72 ☑
      superficial I82.61 ☑
        chronic I82.71 ☑
    vena cava
      inferior (acute) I82.220
        chronic I82.221
      superior (acute) I82.210
        chronic I82.211
    venous sinus G08
    vessels of brain — *see* Occlusion, artery, cerebral
Embolus — *see* Embolism
Embryoma (*see also* Neoplasm, uncertain behavior, by site)
  benign — *see* Neoplasm, benign, by site
  kidney C64. ☑
  liver C22.0
  malignant (*see also* Neoplasm, malignant, by site)
    kidney C64. ☑
    liver C22.0
    testis C62.9 ☑
      descended (scrotal) C62.1 ☑
      undescended C62.0 ☑
  testis C62.9 ☑
    descended (scrotal) C62.1 ☑
    undescended C62.0 ☑
Embryonic
  circulation Q28.9
  heart Q28.9
  vas deferens Q55.4
Embryopathia NOS Q89.9
Embryotoxon Q13.4
Emesis — *see* Vomiting
Emotional lability R45.86
Emotionality, pathological F60.3
Emotogenic disease — *see* Disorder, psychogenic
Emphysema (atrophic) (bullous) (chronic) (interlobular) (lung) (obstructive) (pulmonary) (senile) (vesicular) J43.9
  cellular tissue (traumatic) T79.7 ☑
    surgical T81.82 ☑
  centrilobular J43.2
  compensatory J98.3
  congenital (interstitial) P25.0
  conjunctiva H11.89
  connective tissue (traumatic) T79.7 ☑
    surgical T81.82 ☑
  due to chemicals, gases, fumes or vapors J68.4
  eyelid(s) — *see* Disorder, eyelid, specified type NEC
    surgical T81.82 ☑
  traumatic T79.7 ☑

Emphysema — *continued*
  interstitial J98.2
    congenital P25.0
    perinatal period P25.0
  laminated tissue T79.7 ☑
    surgical T81.82 ☑
  mediastinal J98.2
    newborn P25.2
  orbit, orbital — *see* Disorder, orbit, specified type NEC
  panacinar J43.1
  panlobular J43.1
  specified NEC J43.8
  subcutaneous (traumatic) T79.7 ☑
    nontraumatic J98.2
    postprocedural T81.82 ☑
    surgical T81.82 ☑
  surgical T81.82 ☑
  thymus (gland) (congenital) E32.8
  traumatic (subcutaneous) T79.7 ☑
  unilateral J43.0
Empty nest syndrome Z60.0
Empyema (acute) (chest) (double) (pleura) (supradiaphragmatic) (thorax) J86.9
  with fistula J86.0
  accessory sinus (chronic) — *see* Sinusitis
  antrum (chronic) — *see* Sinusitis, maxillary
  brain (any part) — *see* Abscess, brain
  ethmoidal (chronic) (sinus) — *see* Sinusitis, ethmoidal
  extradural — *see* Abscess, extradural
  frontal (chronic) (sinus) — *see* Sinusitis, frontal
  gallbladder K81.0
  mastoid (process) (acute) — *see* Mastoiditis, acute
  maxilla, maxillary M27.2
    sinus (chronic) — *see* Sinusitis, maxillary
  nasal sinus (chronic) — *see* Sinusitis
  sinus (accessory) (chronic) (nasal) — *see* Sinusitis
  sphenoidal (sinus) (chronic) — *see* Sinusitis, sphenoidal
  subarachnoid — *see* Abscess, extradural
  subdural — *see* Abscess, subdural
  tuberculous A15.6
  ureter — *see* Ureteritis
  ventricular — *see* Abscess, brain
En coup de sabre lesion L94.1
Enamel pearls K00.2
Enameloma K00.2
Enanthema, viral B09
Encephalitis (chronic) (hemorrhagic) (idiopathic) (nonepidemic) (spurious) (subacute) G04.90
  acute (*see also* Encephalitis, viral) A86
    disseminated G04.00
      infectious G04.01
      noninfectious G04.81
      postimmunization (postvaccination) G04.02
      postinfectious G04.01
    inclusion body A85.8
    necrotizing hemorrhagic G04.30
      postimmunization G04.32
      postinfectious G04.31
      specified NEC G04.39
  arboviral, arbovirus NEC A85.2
  arthropod-borne NEC (viral) A85.2
  Australian A83.4
  California (virus) A83.5
  Central European (tick-borne) A84.1
  Czechoslovakian A84.1
  Dawson's (inclusion body) A81.1
  diffuse sclerosing A81.1
  disseminated, acute G04.00
  due to
    cat scratch disease A28.1
    human immunodeficiency virus (HIV) disease B20 *[G05.3]*
    malaria — *see* Malaria
    rickettsiosis — *see* Rickettsiosis
    smallpox inoculation G04.02
    typhus — *see* Typhus
  Eastern equine A83.2
  endemic (viral) A86
  epidemic NEC (viral) A86
  equine (acute) (infectious) (viral) A83.9
    Eastern A83.2
    Venezuelan A92.2
    Western A83.1
  Far Eastern (tick-borne) A84.0
  following vaccination or other immunization procedure G04.02
  herpes zoster B02.0
  herpesviral B00.4
    due to herpesvirus 6 B10.01

Encephalitis - Encounter

Encephalitis — *continued*
  herpesviral — *continued*
    due to herpesvirus 7 B10.09
    specified NEC B10.09
  Ilheus (virus) A83.8
  inclusion body A81.1
  in (due to)
    actinomycosis A42.82
    adenovirus A85.1
    African trypanosomiasis B56.9 *[G05.3]*
    Chagas' disease (chronic) B57.42
    cytomegalovirus B25.8
    enterovirus A85.0
    herpes (simplex) virus B00.4
      due to herpesvirus 6 B10.01
      due to herpesvirus 7 B10.09
      specified NEC B10.09
    infectious disease NEC B99 ☑ *[G05.3]*
    influenza — *see* Influenza, with, encephalopathy
    listeriosis A32.12
    measles B05.0
    mumps B26.2
    naegleriasis B60.2
    parasitic disease NEC B89 *[G05.3]*
    poliovirus A80.9 *[G05.3]*
    rubella B06.01
    syphilis
      congenital A50.42
      late A52.14
    systemic lupus erythematosus M32.19
    toxoplasmosis (acquired) B58.2
      congenital P37.1
    tuberculosis A17.82
    zoster B02.0
  infectious (acute) (virus) NEC A86
  Japanese (B type) A83.0
  La Crosse A83.5
  lead — *see* Poisoning, lead
  lethargica (acute) (infectious) A85.8
  louping ill A84.8
  lupus erythematosus, systemic M32.19
  lymphatica A87.2
  Mengo A85.8
  meningococcal A39.81
  Murray Valley A83.4
  otitic NEC H66.40 *[G05.3]*
  parasitic NOS B71.9
  periaxial G37.0
  periaxialis (concentrica) (diffuse) G37.5
  postchickenpox B01.11
  postexanthematous NEC B09
  postimmunization G04.02
  postinfectious NEC G04.01
  postmeasles B05.0
  postvaccinal G04.02
  postvaricella B01.11
  postviral NEC A86
  Powassan A84.8
  Rasmussen G04.81
  Rio Bravo A85.8
  Russian
    autumnal A83.0
    spring-summer (taiga) A84.0
  saturnine — *see* Poisoning, lead
  specified NEC G04.81
  St. Louis A83.3
  subacute sclerosing A81.1
  summer A83.0
  suppurative G04.81
  tick-borne A84.9
  Torula, torular (cryptococcal) B45.1
  toxic NEC G92
  trichinosis B75 *[G05.3]*
  type
    B A83.0
    C A83.3
  van Bogaert's A81.1
  Venezuelan equine A92.2
  Vienna A85.8
  viral, virus A86
    arthropod-borne NEC A85.2
      mosquito-borne A83.9
        Australian X disease A83.4
        California virus A83.5
        Eastern equine A83.2
        Japanese (B type) A83.0
        Murray Valley A83.4
        specified NEC A83.8
        St. Louis A83.3
        type B A83.0
        type C A83.3
        Western equine A83.1

Encephalitis — *continued*
  viral, virus — *continued*
    tick-borne A84.9
      biundulant A84.1
      central European A84.1
      Czechoslovakian A84.1
      diphasic meningoencephalitis A84.1
      Far Eastern A84.0
      Russian spring-summer (taiga) A84.0
      specified NEC A84.8
    specified type NEC A85.8
  Western equine A83.1
Encephalocele Q01.9
  frontal Q01.0
  nasofrontal Q01.1
  occipital Q01.2
  specified NEC Q01.8
Encephalocystocele — *see* Encephalocele
Encephaloduroarteriomyosynangiosis (EDAMS) I67.5
Encephalomalacia (brain) (cerebellar) (cerebral) — *see* Softening, brain
Encephalomeningitis — *see* Meningoencephalitis
Encephalomeningocele — *see* Encephalocele
Encephalomeningomyelitis — *see* Meningoencephalitis
Encephalomyelitis (*see also* Encephalitis) G04.90
  acute disseminated G04.00
    infectious G04.01
    noninfectious G04.81
    postimmunization G04.02
    postinfectious G04.01
  acute necrotizing hemorrhagic G04.30
    postimmunization G04.32
    postinfectious G04.31
    specified NEC G04.39
  benign myalgic G93.3
  equine A83.9
    Eastern A83.2
    Venezuelan A92.2
    Western A83.1
  in diseases classified elsewhere G05.3
  myalgic, benign G93.3
  postchickenpox B01.11
  postinfectious NEC G04.01
  postmeasles B05.0
  postvaccinal G04.02
  postvaricella B01.11
  rubella B06.01
  specified NEC G04.81
  Venezuelan equine A92.2
Encephalomyelocele — *see* Encephalocele
Encephalomyelomeningitis — *see* Meningoencephalitis
Encephalomyelopathy G96.9
Encephalomyeloradiculitis (acute) G61.0
Encephalomyeloradiculoneuritis (acute) (Guillain-Barré) G61.0
Encephalomyeloradiculopathy G96.9
Encephalopathia hyperbilirubinemica, newborn P57.9
  due to isoimmunization (conditions in P55 ☑) P57.0
Encephalopathy (acute) G93.40
  acute necrotizing hemorrhagic G04.30
    postimmunization G04.32
    postinfectious G04.31
    specified NEC G04.39
  alcoholic G31.2
  anoxic — *see* Damage, brain, anoxic
  arteriosclerotic I67.2
  centrolobar progressive (Schilder) G37.0
  congenital Q07.9
  degenerative, in specified disease NEC G32.89
  demyelinating callosal G37.1
  due to
    drugs - (*see also* Table of Drugs and Chemicals) G92
  hepatic — *see* Failure, hepatic
  hyperbilirubinemic, newborn P57.9
    due to isoimmunization (conditions in P55 ☑) P57.0
  hypertensive I67.4
  hypoglycemic E16.2
  hypoxic — *see* Damage, brain, anoxic
  hypoxic ischemic P91.60
    mild P91.61
    moderate P91.62
    severe P91.63
  in (due to) (with)
    birth injury P11.1
    hyperinsulinism E16.1 *[G94]*
    influenza — *see* Influenza, with, encephalopathy
    lack of vitamin (*see also* Deficiency, vitamin) E56.9 *[G32.89]*

Encephalopathy — *continued*
  in — *continued*
    neoplastic disease (*see also* Neoplasm) D49.9 *[G13.1]*
    serum (*see also* Reaction, serum) T80.69 ☑
    syphilis A52.17
    trauma (postconcussional) F07.81
      current injury — *see* Injury, intracranial
    vaccination G04.02
  lead — *see* Poisoning, lead
  metabolic G93.41
    drug induced G92
    toxic G92
  myoclonic, early, symptomatic — *see* Epilepsy, generalized, specified NEC
  necrotizing, subacute (Leigh) G31.82
  neonatal P91.819
    in diseases classified elsewhere P91.811
  pellagrous E52 *[G32.89]*
  portosystemic — *see* Failure, hepatic
  postcontusional F07.81
    current injury — *see* Injury, intracranial, diffuse
  posthypoglycemic (coma) E16.1 *[G94]*
  postradiation G93.89
  saturnine — *see* Poisoning, lead
  septic G93.41
  specified NEC G93.49
  spongiform, subacute (viral) A81.09
  toxic G92
    metabolic G92
  traumatic (postconcussional) F07.81
    current injury — *see* Injury, intracranial
  vitamin B deficiency NEC E53.9 *[G32.89]*
    vitamin B1 E51.2
  Wernicke's E51.2
Encephalorrhagia — *see* Hemorrhage, intracranial, intracerebral
Encephalosis, posttraumatic F07.81
Enchondroma (*see also* Neoplasm, bone, benign)
Enchondromatosis (cartilaginous) (multiple) Q78.4
Encopresis R15.9
  functional F98.1
  nonorganic origin F98.1
  psychogenic F98.1
Encounter (with health service) (for) Z76.89
  adjustment and management (of)
    breast implant Z45.81 ☑
    implanted device NEC Z45.89
    myringotomy device (stent) (tube) Z45.82
    neurostimulator (brain) (gastric) (peripheral nerve) (sacral nerve) (spinal cord) (vagus nerve) Z45.42
  administrative purpose only Z02.9
    examination for
      adoption Z02.82
      armed forces Z02.3
      disability determination Z02.71
      driving license Z02.4
      employment Z02.1
      insurance Z02.6
      medical certificate NEC Z02.79
      paternity testing Z02.81
      residential institution admission Z02.2
      school admission Z02.0
      sports Z02.5
    specified reason NEC Z02.89
  aftercare — *see* Aftercare
  antenatal screening Z36.9
    cervical length Z36.86
    chromosomal anomalies Z36.0
    congenital cardiac abnormalities Z36.83
    elevated maternal serum alphafetoprotein level Z36.1
    fetal growth retardation Z36.4
    fetal lung maturity Z36.84
    fetal macrosomia Z36.88
    hydrops fetalis Z36.81
    intrauterine growth restriction (IUGR)/small-for-dates Z36.4
    isoimmunization Z36.5
    large-for-dates Z36.88
    malformations Z36.3
    non-visualized anatomy on a previous scan Z36.2
    nuchal translucency Z36.82
    raised alphafetoprotein level Z36.1
    risk of pre-term labor Z36.86
    specified type NEC Z36.89
    specified follow-up NEC Z36.2
    specified genetic defects NEC Z36.8A
    Streptococcus B Z36.85
    suspected anomaly Z36.3
    uncertain dates Z36.87

Encounter — *continued*
- assisted reproductive fertility procedure cycle Z31.83
- blood typing Z01.83
  - Rh typing Z01.83
- breast augmentation or reduction Z41.1
- breast implant exchange (different material) (different size) Z45.81 ☑
- breast reconstruction following mastectomy Z42.1
- check-up — *see* Examination
- chemotherapy for neoplasm Z51.11
- colonoscopy, screening Z12.11
- counseling — *see* Counseling
- delivery, full-term, uncomplicated O80
  - cesarean, without indication O82
- desensitization to allergens Z51.6
- ear piercing Z41.3
- examination — *see* Examination
- expectant parent(s) (adoptive) pre-birth pediatrician visit Z76.81
- fertility preservation procedure (prior to cancer therapy) (prior to removal of gonads) Z31.84
- fitting (of) — *see* Fitting (and adjustment) (of)
- genetic
  - counseling
    - nonprocreative Z71.83
    - procreative Z31.5
  - testing — *see* Test, genetic
- hearing conservation and treatment Z01.12
- immunotherapy for neoplasm Z51.12
- in vitro fertilization cycle Z31.83
- instruction (in)
  - childbirth Z32.2
  - child care (postpartal) (prenatal) Z32.3
  - natural family planning
    - procreative Z31.61
    - to avoid pregnancy Z30.02
- insulin pump titration Z46.81
- joint prosthesis insertion following prior explantation of joint prosthesis (staged procedure)
  - hip Z47.32
  - knee Z47.33
  - shoulder Z47.31
- laboratory (as part of a general medical examination) Z00.00
  - with abnormal findings Z00.01
- mental health services (for)
  - abuse NEC
    - perpetrator Z69.82
    - victim Z69.81
  - child abuse
    - nonparental
      - perpetrator Z69.021
      - victim Z69.020
    - parental
      - perpetrator Z69.011
      - victim Z69.010
  - child neglect
    - nonparental
      - perpetrator Z69.021
      - victim Z69.020
    - parental
      - perpetrator Z69.011
      - victim Z69.010
  - child psychological abuse
    - nonparental
      - perpetrator Z69.021
      - victim Z69.020
    - parental
      - perpetrator Z69.011
      - victim Z69.010
  - child sexual abuse
    - nonparental
      - perpetrator Z69.021
      - victim Z69.020
    - parental
      - perpetrator Z69.011
      - victim Z69.010
  - non-spousal adult abuse
    - perpetrator Z69.82
    - victim Z69.81
  - spousal or partner
    - abuse
      - perpetrator Z69.12
      - victim Z69.11
    - neglect
      - perpetrator Z69.12
      - victim Z69.11
    - psychological abuse
      - perpetrator Z69.12
      - victim Z69.11

Encounter — *continued*
- mental health services — *continued*
  - violence
    - perpetrator (physical) (sexual) Z69.12
    - victim (physical) Z69.11
      - sexual Z69.81
- observation (for) (ruled out)
  - exposure to (suspected)
    - anthrax Z03.810
    - biological agent NEC Z03.818
- pediatrician visit, by expectant parent(s) (adoptive) Z76.81
- placental sample (taken vaginally) (*see also* Encounter, antenatal screening) Z36.9
- plastic and reconstructive surgery following medical procedure or healed injury NEC Z42.8
- pregnancy
  - supervision of — *see* Pregnancy, supervision of
  - test Z32.00
    - result negative Z32.02
    - result positive Z32.01
- procreative management and counseling for gestational carrier Z31.7
- prophylactic measures Z29.9
  - antivenin Z29.12
  - fluoride administration Z29.3
  - immunotherapy for respiratory syncytial virus (RSV) Z29.11
  - rabies immune globin Z29.14
  - Rho (D) immune globulin Z29.13
  - specified NEC Z29.8
- radiation therapy (antineoplastic) Z51.0
- radiological (as part of a general medical examination) Z00.00
  - with abnormal findings Z00.01
- reconstructive surgery following medical procedure or healed injury NEC Z42.8
- removal (of) (*see also* Removal)
  - artificial
    - arm Z44.00 ☑
      - complete Z44.01 ☑
      - partial Z44.02 ☑
    - eye Z44.2 ☑
    - leg Z44.10 ☑
      - complete Z44.11 ☑
      - partial Z44.12 ☑
  - breast implant Z45.81 ☑
    - tissue expander (with or without synchronous insertion of permanent implant) Z45.81 ☑
  - device Z46.9
    - specified NEC Z46.89
  - external
    - fixation device - code to fracture with seventh character D
    - prosthesis, prosthetic device Z44.9
      - breast Z44.3 ☑
      - specified NEC Z44.8
  - implanted device NEC Z45.89
  - insulin pump Z46.81
  - internal fixation device Z47.2
  - myringotomy device (stent) (tube) Z45.82
  - nervous system device NEC Z46.2
    - brain neuropacemaker Z46.2
    - visual substitution device Z46.2
      - implanted Z45.31
  - non-vascular catheter Z46.82
  - orthodontic device Z46.4
  - stent
    - ureteral Z46.6
  - urinary device Z46.6
- repeat cervical smear to confirm findings of recent normal smear following initial abnormal smear Z01.42
- respirator [ventilator] use during power failure Z99.12
- Rh typing Z01.83
- screening — *see* Screening
- specified NEC Z76.89
- sterilization Z30.2
- suspected condition, ruled out
  - amniotic cavity and membrane Z03.71
  - cervical shortening Z03.75
  - fetal anomaly Z03.73
  - fetal growth Z03.74
  - maternal and fetal conditions NEC Z03.79
  - oligohydramnios Z03.71
  - placental problem Z03.72
  - polyhydramnios Z03.71
- suspected exposure (to), ruled out
  - anthrax Z03.810
  - biological agents NEC Z03.818
- termination of pregnancy, elective Z33.2

Encounter — *continued*
- testing — *see* Test
- therapeutic drug level monitoring Z51.81
- titration, insulin pump Z46.81
- to determine fetal viability of pregnancy O36.80 ☑
- training
  - insulin pump Z46.81
- X-ray of chest (as part of a general medical examination) Z00.00
  - with abnormal findings Z00.01

Encystment — *see* Cyst

Endarteritis (bacterial, subacute) (infective) I77.6
- brain I67.7
- cerebral or cerebrospinal I67.7
- deformans — *see* Arteriosclerosis
- embolic — *see* Embolism
- obliterans (*see also* Arteriosclerosis)
  - pulmonary I28.8
- pulmonary I28.8
- retina — *see* Vasculitis, retina
- senile — *see* Arteriosclerosis
- syphilitic A52.09
  - brain or cerebral A52.04
  - congenital A50.54 [I79.8]
- tuberculous A18.89

Endemic — *see* condition

Endocarditis (chronic) (marantic) (nonbacterial) (thrombotic) (valvular) I38
- with rheumatic fever (conditions in I00)
  - active — *see* Endocarditis, acute, rheumatic
  - inactive or quiescent (with chorea) I09.1
- acute or subacute I33.9
  - infective I33.0
  - rheumatic (aortic) (mitral) (pulmonary) (tricuspid) I01.1
    - with chorea (acute) (rheumatic) (Sydenham's) I02.0
- aortic (heart) (nonrheumatic) (valve) I35.8
  - with
    - mitral disease I08.0
      - with tricuspid (valve) disease I08.3
      - active or acute I01.1
        - with chorea (acute) (rheumatic) (Sydenham's) I02.0
    - rheumatic fever (conditions in I00)
      - active — *see* Endocarditis, acute, rheumatic
      - inactive or quiescent (with chorea) I06.9
    - tricuspid (valve) disease I08.2
      - with mitral (valve) disease I08.3
  - acute or subacute I33.9
  - arteriosclerotic I35.8
  - rheumatic I06.9
    - with mitral disease I08.0
      - with tricuspid (valve) disease I08.3
      - active or acute I01.1
        - with chorea (acute) (rheumatic) (Sydenham's) I02.0
      - active or acute I01.1
        - with chorea (acute) (rheumatic) (Sydenham's) I02.0
    - specified NEC I06.8
  - specified cause NEC I35.8
  - syphilitic A52.03
- arteriosclerotic I38
- atypical verrucous (Libman-Sacks) M32.11
- bacterial (acute) (any valve) (subacute) I33.0
- candidal B37.6
- congenital Q24.8
- constrictive I33.0
- Coxiella burnetii A78 [I39]
- Coxsackie B33.21
- due to
  - prosthetic cardiac valve T82.6 ☑
  - Q fever A78 [I39]
  - Serratia marcescens I33.0
  - typhoid (fever) A01.02
- gonococcal A54.83
- infectious or infective (acute) (any valve) (subacute) I33.0
- lenta (acute) (any valve) (subacute) I33.0
- Libman-Sacks M32.11
- listerial A32.82
- Löffler's I42.3
- malignant (acute) (any valve) (subacute) I33.0
- meningococcal A39.51
- mitral (chronic) (double) (fibroid) (heart) (inactive) (valve) (with chorea) I05.9
  - with
    - aortic (valve) disease I08.0
      - with tricuspid (valve) disease I08.3
      - active or acute I01.1

Endocarditis — *continued*
  mitral — *continued*
        with chorea (acute) (rheumatic)
          (Sydenham's) I02.0
      rheumatic fever (conditions in I00)
        active — *see* Endocarditis, acute, rheumatic
        inactive or quiescent (with chorea) I05.9
      tricuspid (valve) disease I08.1
        with aortic (valve) disease I08.3
      active or acute I01.1
        with chorea (acute) (rheumatic) (Sydenham's)
          I02.0
      bacterial I33.0
    arteriosclerotic I34.8
    nonrheumatic I34.8
      acute or subacute I33.9
    specified NEC I05.8
  monilial B37.6
  multiple valves I08.9
    specified disorders I08.8
  mycotic (acute) (any valve) (subacute) I33.0
  pneumococcal (acute) (any valve) (subacute) I33.0
  pulmonary (chronic) (heart) (valve) I37.8
    with rheumatic fever (conditions in I00)
      active — *see* Endocarditis, acute, rheumatic
      inactive or quiescent (with chorea) I09.89
        with aortic, mitral or tricuspid disease I08.8
    acute or subacute I33.9
      rheumatic I01.1
        with chorea (acute) (rheumatic) (Sydenham's)
          I02.0
    arteriosclerotic I37.8
    congenital Q22.2
    rheumatic (chronic) (inactive) (with chorea) I09.89
      active or acute I01.1
        with chorea (acute) (rheumatic) (Sydenham's)
          I02.0
    syphilitic A52.03
  purulent (acute) (any valve) (subacute) I33.0
  Q fever A78 *[I39]*
  rheumatic (chronic) (inactive) (with chorea) I09.1
    active or acute (aortic) (mitral) (pulmonary)
      (tricuspid) I01.1
      with chorea (acute) (rheumatic) (Sydenham's)
        I02.0
  rheumatoid — *see* Rheumatoid, carditis
  septic (acute) (any valve) (subacute) I33.0
  streptococcal (acute) (any valve) (subacute) I33.0
  subacute — *see* Endocarditis, acute
  suppurative (acute) (any valve) (subacute) I33.0
  syphilitic A52.03
  toxic I33.9
  tricuspid (chronic) (heart) (inactive) (rheumatic)
    (valve) (with chorea) I07.9
    with
      aortic (valve) disease I08.2
        mitral (valve) disease I08.3
      mitral (valve) disease I08.1
        aortic (valve) disease I08.3
      rheumatic fever (conditions in I00)
        active — *see* Endocarditis, acute, rheumatic
        inactive or quiescent (with chorea) I07.8
    active or acute I01.1
      with chorea (acute) (rheumatic) (Sydenham's)
        I02.0
    arteriosclerotic I36.8
    nonrheumatic I36.8
      acute or subacute I33.9
    specified cause, except rheumatic I36.8
  tuberculous — *see* Tuberculosis, endocarditis
  typhoid A01.02
  ulcerative (acute) (any valve) (subacute) I33.0
  vegetative (acute) (any valve) (subacute) I33.0
  verrucous (atypical) (nonbacterial) (nonrheumatic)
    M32.11
Endocardium, endocardial (*see also* condition)
  cushion defect Q21.2
Endocervicitis (*see also* Cervicitis)
  due to intrauterine (contraceptive) device T83.69 ☑
  hyperplastic N72
Endocrine — *see* condition
Endocrinopathy, pluriglandular E31.9
Endodontic
  overfill M27.52
  underfill M27.53
Endodontitis K04.01
  irreversible K04.02
  reversible K04.01
Endomastoiditis — *see* Mastoiditis
Endometrioma N80.9
Endometriosis N80.9
  appendix N80.5

Endometriosis — *continued*
  bladder N80.8
  bowel N80.5
  broad ligament N80.3
  cervix N80.0
  colon N80.5
  cul-de-sac (Douglas') N80.3
  exocervix N80.0
  fallopian tube N80.2
  female genital organ NEC N80.8
  gallbladder N80.8
  in scar of skin N80.6
  internal N80.0
  intestine N80.5
  lung N80.8
  myometrium N80.0
  ovary N80.1
  parametrium N80.3
  pelvic peritoneum N80.3
  peritoneal (pelvic) N80.3
  rectovaginal septum N80.4
  rectum N80.5
  round ligament N80.3
  skin (scar) N80.6
  specified site NEC N80.8
  stromal D39.0
  thorax N80.8
  umbilicus N80.8
  uterus (internal) N80.0
  vagina N80.4
  vulva N80.8
Endometritis (decidual) (nonspecific) (purulent)
  (senile) (atrophic) (suppurative) N71.9
  with ectopic pregnancy O08.0
  acute N71.0
  blenorrhagic (gonococcal) (acute) (chronic) A54.24
  cervix, cervical (with erosion or ectropion) (*see also*
    Cervicitis)
    hyperplastic N72
  chlamydial A56.11
  chronic N71.1
  following
    abortion — *see* Abortion by type complicated by
      genital infection
    ectopic or molar pregnancy O08.0
  gonococcal, gonorrheal (acute) (chronic) A54.24
  hyperplastic (*see also* Hyperplasia, endometrial)
    N85.00
    cervix N72
  puerperal, postpartum, childbirth O86.12
  subacute N71.0
  tuberculous A18.17
Endometrium — *see* condition
Endomyocardiopathy, South African I42.3
Endomyocarditis — *see* Endocarditis
Endomyofibrosis I42.3
Endomyometritis — *see* Endometritis
Endopericarditis — *see* Endocarditis
Endoperineuritis — *see* Disorder, nerve
Endophlebitis — *see* Phlebitis
Endophthalmia — *see* Endophthalmitis, purulent
Endophthalmitis (acute) (infective) (metastatic)
  (subacute) H44.009
  bleb associated H59.4 ☑ (*see also* Bleb, inflamed
    (infected), postprocedural)
  gonorrheal A54.39
  in (due to)
    cysticercosis B69.1
    onchocerciasis B73.01
    toxocariasis B83.0
  panuveitis — *see* Panuveitis
  parasitic H44.12 ☑
  purulent H44.00 ☑
    panophthalmitis — *see* Panophthalmitis
    vitreous abscess H44.02 ☑
  specified NEC H44.19
  sympathetic — *see* Uveitis, sympathetic
Endosalpingioma D28.2
Endosalpingiosis N94.89
Endosteitis — *see* Osteomyelitis
Endothelioma, bone — *see* Neoplasm, bone,
  malignant
Endotheliosis (hemorrhagic infectional) D69.8
Endotoxemia - code to condition
Endotrachelitis — *see* Cervicitis
Engelmann (-Camurati) syndrome Q78.3
English disease — *see* Rickets
Engman's disease L30.3
Engorgement
  breast N64.59
    newborn P83.4
    puerperal, postpartum O92.79

Engorgement — *continued*
  lung (passive) — *see* Edema, lung
  pulmonary (passive) — *see* Edema, lung
  stomach K31.89
  venous, retina — *see* Occlusion, retina, vein,
    engorgement
Enlargement, enlarged (*see also* Hypertrophy)
  adenoids J35.2
    with tonsils J35.3
  alveolar ridge K08.89
    congenital — *see* Anomaly, alveolar
  apertures of diaphragm (congenital) Q79.1
  gingival K06.1
  heart, cardiac — *see* Hypertrophy, cardiac
  labium majus, childhood asymmetric (CALME)
    N90.61
  lacrimal gland, chronic H04.03 ☑
  liver — *see* Hypertrophy, liver
  lymph gland or node R59.9
    generalized R59.1
    localized R59.0
  orbit H05.34 ☑
  organ or site, congenital NEC — *see* Anomaly, by
    site
  parathyroid (gland) E21.0
  pituitary fossa R93.0
  prostate N40.0
    with lower urinary tract symptoms (LUTS) N40.1
    without lower urinary tract symptoms (LUTS)
      N40.0
  sella turcica R93.0
  spleen — *see* Splenomegaly
  thymus (gland) (congenital) E32.0
  thyroid (gland) — *see* Goiter
  tongue K14.8
  tonsils J35.1
    with adenoids J35.3
  uterus N85.2
  vestibular aqueduct Q16.5
Enophthalmos H05.40 ☑
  due to
    orbital tissue atrophy H05.41 ☑
    trauma or surgery H05.42 ☑
Enostosis M27.8
Entamebic, entamebiasis — *see* Amebiasis
Entanglement
  umbilical cord(s) O69.82 ☑
    with compression O69.2 ☑
    around neck (with compression) O69.81 ☑
      with compression O69.1 ☑
      without compression O69.81 ☑
    of twins in monoamniotic sac O69.2 ☑
    without compression O69.82 ☑
Enteralgia — *see* Pain, abdominal
Enteric — *see* condition
Enteritis (acute) (diarrheal) (hemorrhagic)
  (noninfective) K52.9
  adenovirus A08.2
  aertrycke infection A02.0
  allergic K52.29
    with
      eosinophilic gastritis or gastroenteritis K52.81
      food protein-induced enterocolitis syndrome
        K52.21
      food protein-induced enteropathy K52.22
      FPIES K52.21
  amebic (acute) A06.0
    with abscess — *see* Abscess, amebic
    chronic A06.1
      with abscess — *see* Abscess, amebic
      nondysenteric A06.2
    nondysenteric A06.2
  astrovirus A08.32
  bacillary NOS A03.9
  bacterial A04.9
    specified NEC A04.8
  calicivirus A08.31
  candidal B37.82
  Chilomastix A07.8
  choleriformis A00.1
  chronic (noninfectious) K52.9
    ulcerative — *see* Colitis, ulcerative
  cicatrizing (chronic) — *see* Enteritis, regional, small
    intestine
  Clostridium
    botulinum (food poisoning) A05.1
    difficile
      not specified as recurrent A04.72
      recurrent A04.71
  coccidial A07.3
  coxsackie virus A08.39
  dietetic (*see also* Enteritis, allergic) K52.29

☑ **Additional character required**

Enteritis — *continued*
  drug-induced K52.1
  due to
    astrovirus A08.32
    calicivirus A08.31
    coxsackie virus A08.39
    drugs K52.1
    echovirus A08.39
    enterovirus NEC A08.39
    food hypersensitivity (*see also* Enteritis, allergic)
      K52.29
    infectious organism (bacterial) (viral) — *see*
      Enteritis, infectious
    torovirus A08.39
    Yersinia enterocolitica A04.6
  echovirus A08.39
  eltor A00.1
  enterovirus NEC A08.39
  eosinophilic K52.81
  epidemic (infectious) A09
  fulminant (*see also* Ischemia, intestine, acute)
    K55.019
  gangrenous — *see* Enteritis, infectious
  giardial A07.1
  infectious NOS A09
    due to
      adenovirus A08.2
      Aerobacter aerogenes A04.8
      Arizona (bacillus) A02.0
      bacteria NOS A04.9
        specified NEC A04.8
      Campylobacter A04.5
      Clostridium difficile
        not specified as recurrent A04.72
        recurrent A04.71
      Clostridium perfringens A04.8
      Enterobacter aerogenes A04.8
      enterovirus A08.39
      Escherichia coli A04.4
        enteroaggregative A04.4
        enterohemorrhagic A04.3
        enteroinvasive A04.2
        enteropathogenic A04.0
        enterotoxigenic A04.1
        specified NEC A04.4
      specified
        bacteria NEC A04.8
        virus NEC A08.39
      Staphylococcus A04.8
      virus NEC A08.4
        specified type NEC A08.39
      Yersinia enterocolitica A04.6
    specified organism NEC A08.8
  influenzal — *see* Influenza, with, digestive
    manifestations
  ischemic K55.9
    acute (*see also* Ischemia, intestine, acute) K55.019
    chronic K55.1
  microsporidial A07.8
  mucomembranous, myxomembranous — *see*
    Syndrome, irritable bowel
  mucous — *see* Syndrome, irritable bowel
  necroticans A05.2
  necrotizing of newborn — *see* Enterocolitis,
    necrotizing, in newborn
  neurogenic — *see* Syndrome, irritable bowel
  newborn necrotizing — *see* Enterocolitis,
    necrotizing, in newborn
  noninfectious K52.9
  norovirus A08.11
  parasitic NEC B82.9
  paratyphoid (fever) — *see* Fever, paratyphoid
  protozoal A07.9
    specified NEC A07.8
  radiation K52.0
  regional (of) K50.90
    with
      complication K50.919
        abscess K50.914
        fistula K50.913
        intestinal obstruction K50.912
        rectal bleeding K50.911
        specified complication NEC K50.918
    colon — *see* Enteritis, regional, large intestine
    duodenum — *see* Enteritis, regional, small
      intestine
    ileum — *see* Enteritis, regional, small intestine
    jejunum — *see* Enteritis, regional, small intestine
    large bowel — *see* Enteritis, regional, large
      intestine
    large intestine (colon) (rectum) K50.10
      with

Enteritis — *continued*
  regional — *continued*
    complication K50.119
      abscess K50.114
      fistula K50.113
      intestinal obstruction K50.112
      rectal bleeding K50.111
      small intestine (duodenum) (ileum)
        (jejunum) involvement K50.80
        with
          complication K50.819
            abscess K50.814
            fistula K50.813
            intestinal obstruction K50.812
            rectal bleeding K50.811
            specified complication NEC K50.818
      specified complication NEC K50.118
    rectum — *see* Enteritis, regional, large intestine
    small intestine (duodenum) (ileum) (jejunum)
      K50.00
      with
        complication K50.019
          abscess K50.014
          fistula K50.013
          intestinal obstruction K50.012
          large intestine (colon) (rectum)
            involvement K50.80
            with
              complication K50.819
                abscess K50.814
                fistula K50.813
                intestinal obstruction K50.812
                rectal bleeding K50.811
                specified complication NEC K50.818
          rectal bleeding K50.011
          specified complication NEC K50.018
    rotaviral A08.0
    Salmonella, salmonellosis (arizonae) (cholerae-suis)
      (enteritidis) (typhimurium) A02.0
    segmental — *see* Enteritis, regional
    septic A09
    Shigella — *see* Infection, Shigella
    small round structured NEC A08.19
    spasmodic, spastic — *see* Syndrome, irritable bowel
    staphylococcal A04.8
      due to food A05.0
    torovirus A08.39
    toxic NEC K52.1
      due to Clostridium difficile
        not specified as recurrent A04.72
        recurrent A04.71
    trichomonal A07.8
    tuberculous A18.32
    typhosa A01.00
    ulcerative (chronic) — *see* Colitis, ulcerative
    viral A08.4
      adenovirus A08.2
      enterovirus A08.39
      Rotavirus A08.0
      small round structured NEC A08.19
      specified NEC A08.39
      virus specified NEC A08.39
Enterobiasis B80
Enterobius vermicularis (infection) (infestation) B80
Enterocele (*see also* Hernia, abdomen)
  pelvic, pelvis (acquired) (congenital) N81.5
  vagina, vaginal (acquired) (congenital) NEC N81.5
Enterocolitis (*see also* Enteritis) K52.9
  due to Clostridium difficile
    not specified as recurrent A04.72
    recurrent A04.71
  fulminant ischemic (*see also* Ischemia, intestine,
    acute) K55.059
  granulomatous — *see* Enteritis, regional
  hemorrhagic (acute) (*see also* Ischemia, intestine,
    acute) K55.059
    chronic K55.1
  infectious NEC A09
  ischemic K55.9
  necrotizing K55.30
    with
      perforation K55.33
      pneumatosis K55.32
        and perforation K55.33
    due to Clostridium difficile
      not specified as recurrent A04.72
      recurrent A04.71
    in non-newborn K55.30
      stage 1 (without pneumatosis, without
        perforation) K55.31
      stage 2 (with pneumatosis, without
        perforation) K55.32

Enterocolitis — *continued*
  necrotizing — *continued*
    stage 3 (with pneumatosis, with perforation)
      K55.33
    in newborn P77.9
      stage 1 (without pneumatosis, without
        perforation) P77.1
      stage 2 (with pneumatosis, without
        perforation) P77.2
      stage 3 (with pneumatosis, with perforation)
        P77.3
    without pneumatosis or perforation K55.31
  noninfectious K52.9
    newborn — *see* Enterocolitis, necrotizing, in
      newborn
  pseudomembranous (newborn)
    not specified as recurrent A04.72
    recurrent A04.71
  radiation K52.0
    newborn — *see* Enterocolitis, necrotizing, in
      newborn
  ulcerative (chronic) — *see* Pancolitis, ulcerative
    (chronic)
Enterogastritis — *see* Enteritis
Enteropathy K63.9
  food protein-induced K52.22
  celiac-gluten-sensitive K90.0
    non-celiac K90.41
  hemorrhagic, terminal (*see also* Ischemia, intestine,
    acute) K55.059
  protein-losing K90.49
Enteroperitonitis — *see* Peritonitis
Enteroptosis K63.4
Enterorrhagia K92.2
Enterospasm (*see also* Syndrome, irritable, bowel)
  psychogenic F45.8
Enterostenosis (*see also* Obstruction, intestine,
  specified NEC) K56.699
Enterostomy
  complication — *see* Complication, enterostomy
  status Z93.4
Enterovirus, as cause of disease classified elsewhere
  B97.10
    coxsackievirus B97.11
    echovirus B97.12
    other specified B97.19
Enthesopathy (peripheral) M77.9
  Achilles tendinitis — *see* Tendinitis, Achilles
  ankle and tarsus M77.5 ☑
    specified type NEC — *see* Enthesopathy, foot,
      specified type NEC
  anterior tibial syndrome M76.81 ☑
  calcaneal spur — *see* Spur, bone, calcaneal
  elbow region M77.8
    lateral epicondylitis — *see* Epicondylitis, lateral
    medial epicondylitis — *see* Epicondylitis, medial
  foot NEC M77.9
    metatarsalgia — *see* Metatarsalgia
    specified type NEC M77.5 ☑
  forearm M77.9
  gluteal tendinitis — *see* Tendinitis, gluteal
  hand M77.9
  hip — *see* Enthesopathy, lower limb, specified type
    NEC
  iliac crest spur — *see* Spur, bone, iliac crest
  iliotibial band syndrome — *see* Syndrome, iliotibial
    band
  knee — *see* Enthesopathy, lower limb, lower leg,
    specified type NEC
  lateral epicondylitis — *see* Epicondylitis, lateral
  lower limb (excluding foot) M76.9
    Achilles tendinitis — *see* Tendinitis, Achilles
    ankle and tarsus M77.5 ☑
      specified type NEC — *see* Enthesopathy, foot,
        specified type NEC
    anterior tibial syndrome M76.81 ☑
    gluteal tendinitis — *see* Tendinitis, gluteal
    iliac crest spur — *see* Spur, bone, iliac crest
    iliotibial band syndrome — *see* Syndrome,
      iliotibial band
    patellar tendinitis — *see* Tendinitis, patellar
    pelvic region — *see* Enthesopathy, lower limb,
      specified type NEC
    peroneal tendinitis — *see* Tendinitis, peroneal
    posterior tibial syndrome M76.82 ☑
    psoas tendinitis — *see* Tendinitis, psoas
    specified type NEC M76.89 ☑
    tibial collateral bursitis — *see* Bursitis, tibial
      collateral
  medial epicondylitis — *see* Epicondylitis, medial
  metatarsalgia — *see* Metatarsalgia
  multiple sites M77.9

Enthesopathy - Epilepsy

Enthesopathy — *continued*
  patellar tendinitis — *see* Tendinitis, patellar
  pelvis M77.9
  periarthritis of wrist — *see* Periarthritis, wrist
  peroneal tendinitis — *see* Tendinitis, peroneal
  posterior tibial syndrome M76.82 ☑
  psoas tendinitis — *see* Tendinitis, psoas
  shoulder M77.9
  shoulder region — *see* Lesion, shoulder
  specified site NEC M77.9
  specified type NEC M77.8
  spinal M46.00
    cervical region M46.02
    cervicothoracic region M46.03
    lumbar region M46.06
    lumbosacral region M46.07
    multiple sites M46.09
    occipito-atlanto-axial region M46.01
    sacrococcygeal region M46.08
    thoracic region M46.04
    thoracolumbar region M46.05
  tibial collateral bursitis — *see* Bursitis, tibial
    collateral
  upper arm M77.9
  wrist and carpus NEC M77.8
    calcaneal spur — *see* Spur, bone, calcaneal
    periarthritis of wrist — *see* Periarthritis, wrist
Entomophobia F40.218
Entomophthoromycosis B46.8
Entrance, air into vein — *see* Embolism, air
Entrapment, nerve — *see* Neuropathy, entrapment
Entropion (eyelid) (paralytic) H02.009
  cicatricial H02.019
    left H02.016
      lower H02.015
      upper H02.014
    right H02.013
      lower H02.012
      upper H02.011
  congenital Q10.2
  left H02.006
    lower H02.005
    upper H02.004
  mechanical H02.029
    left H02.026
      lower H02.025
      upper H02.024
    right H02.023
      lower H02.022
      upper H02.021
  right H02.003
    lower H02.002
    upper H02.001
  senile H02.039
    left H02.036
      lower H02.035
      upper H02.034
    right H02.033
      lower H02.032
      upper H02.031
  spastic H02.049
    left H02.046
      lower H02.045
      upper H02.044
    right H02.043
      lower H02.042
      upper H02.041
Enucleated eye (traumatic, current) S05.7 ☑
Enuresis R32
  functional F98.0
  habit disturbance F98.0
  nocturnal N39.44
    psychogenic F98.0
  nonorganic origin F98.0
  psychogenic F98.0
Eosinopenia — *see* Agranulocytosis
Eosinophilia (allergic) (hereditary) (idiopathic)
  (secondary) D72.1
  with
    angiolymphoid hyperplasia (ALHE) D18.01
  infiltrative J82
  Löffler's J82
  peritoneal — *see* Peritonitis, eosinophilic
  pulmonary NEC J82
  tropical (pulmonary) J82
Eosinophilia-myalgia syndrome M35.8
Ependymitis (acute) (cerebral) (chronic) (granular) —
  see Encephalomyelitis
Ependymoblastoma
  specified site — *see* Neoplasm, malignant, by site
  unspecified site C71.9

Ependymoma (epithelial) (malignant)
  anaplastic
    specified site — *see* Neoplasm, malignant, by site
    unspecified site C71.9
  benign
    specified site — *see* Neoplasm, benign, by site
    unspecified site D33.2
  myxopapillary D43.2
    specified site — *see* Neoplasm, uncertain
      behavior, by site
    unspecified site D43.2
  papillary D43.2
    specified site — *see* Neoplasm, uncertain
      behavior, by site
    unspecified site D43.2
  specified site — *see* Neoplasm, malignant, by site
  unspecified site C71.9
Ependymopathy G93.89
Ephelis, ephelides L81.2
Epiblepharon (congenital) Q10.3
Epicanthus, epicanthic fold (eyelid) (congenital) Q10.3
Epicondylitis (elbow)
  lateral M77.1 ☑
  medial M77.0 ☑
Epicystitis — *see* Cystitis
Epidemic — *see* condition
Epidermidalization, cervix — *see* Dysplasia, cervix
Epidermis, epidermal — *see* condition
Epidermodysplasia verruciformis B07.8
Epidermolysis
  bullosa (congenital) Q81.9
    acquired L12.30
      drug-induced L12.31
      specified cause NEC L12.35
    dystrophica Q81.2
    letalis Q81.1
    simplex Q81.0
    specified NEC Q81.8
  necroticans combustiformis L51.2
    due to drug — *see* Table of Drugs and Chemicals,
      by drug
Epidermophytid — *see* Dermatophytosis
Epidermophytosis (infected) — *see* Dermatophytosis
Epididymis — *see* condition
Epididymitis (acute) (nonvenereal) (recurrent)
  (residual) N45.1
  with orchitis N45.3
  blennorrhagic (gonococcal) A54.23
  caseous (tuberculous) A18.15
  chlamydial A56.19
  filarial (*see also* Infestation, filarial) B74.9 *[N51]*
  gonococcal A54.23
  syphilitic A52.76
  tuberculous A18.15
Epididymo-orchitis (*see also* Epididymitis) N45.3
Epidural — *see* condition
Epigastrium, epigastric — *see* condition
Epigastrocele — *see* Hernia, ventral
Epiglottis — *see* condition
Epiglottitis, epiglottiditis (acute) J05.10
  with obstruction J05.11
  chronic J37.0
Epignathus Q89.4
Epilepsia partialis continua (*see also* Kozhevnikof's
  epilepsy) G40.1 ☑
Epilepsy, epileptic, epilepsia (attack) (cerebral)
  (convulsion) (fit) (seizure) G40.909
  Note: the following terms are to be considered
    equivalent to intractable: pharmacoresistant
    (pharmacologically resistant), treatment
    resistant, refractory (medically) and poorly
    controlled
  with
    complex partial seizures — *see* Epilepsy,
      localization-related, symptomatic, with
      complex partial seizures
    grand mal seizures on awakening — *see* Epilepsy,
      generalized, specified NEC
    myoclonic absences — *see* Epilepsy, generalized,
      specified NEC
    myoclonic-astatic seizures — *see* Epilepsy,
      generalized, specified NEC
    simple partial seizures — *see* Epilepsy,
      localization-related, symptomatic, with
      simple partial seizures
  akinetic — *see* Epilepsy, generalized, specified NEC
  benign childhood with centrotemporal EEG spikes
    — *see* Epilepsy, localization-related, idiopathic
  benign myoclonic in infancy G40.80 ☑
  Bravais-jacksonian — *see* Epilepsy, localization-
    related, symptomatic, with simple partial
    seizures

Epilepsy — *continued*
  childhood
    with occipital EEG paroxysms — *see* Epilepsy,
      localization-related, idiopathic
    absence G40.A09
      intractable G40.A19
        with status epilepticus G40.A11
        without status epilepticus G40.A19
      not intractable G40.A09
        with status epilepticus G40.A01
        without status epilepticus G40.A09
  climacteric — *see* Epilepsy, specified NEC
  cysticercosis B69.0
  deterioration (mental) F06.8
  due to syphilis A52.19
  focal — *see* Epilepsy, localization-related,
    symptomatic, with simple partial seizures
  generalized
    idiopathic G40.309
      intractable G40.319
        with status epilepticus G40.311
        without status epilepticus G40.319
      not intractable G40.309
        with status epilepticus G40.301
        without status epilepticus G40.309
    specified NEC G40.409
      intractable G40.419
        with status epilepticus G40.411
        without status epilepticus G40.419
      not intractable G40.409
        with status epilepticus G40.401
        without status epilepticus G40.409
  impulsive petit mal — *see* Epilepsy, juvenile
    myoclonic
  intractable G40.919
    with status epilepticus G40.911
    without status epilepticus G40.919
  juvenile absence G40.A09
    intractable G40.A19
      with status epilepticus G40.A11
      without status epilepticus G40.A19
    not intractable G40.A09
      with status epilepticus G40.A01
      without status epilepticus G40.A09
  juvenile myoclonic G40.B09
    intractable G40.B19
      with status epilepticus G40.B11
      without status epilepticus G40.B19
    not intractable G40.B09
      with status epilepticus G40.B01
      without status epilepticus G40.B09
  localization-related (focal) (partial)
    idiopathic G40.009
      with seizures of localized onset G40.009
        intractable G40.019
          with status epilepticus G40.011
          without status epilepticus G40.019
        not intractable G40.009
          with status epilepticus G40.001
          without status epilepticus G40.009
    symptomatic
      with complex partial seizures G40.209
        intractable G40.219
          with status epilepticus G40.211
          without status epilepticus G40.219
        not intractable G40.209
          with status epilepticus G40.201
          without status epilepticus G40.209
      with simple partial seizures G40.109
        intractable G40.119
          with status epilepticus G40.111
          without status epilepticus G40.119
        not intractable G40.109
          with status epilepticus G40.101
          without status epilepticus G40.109
  myoclonus, myoclonic — *see* Epilepsy, generalized,
    specified NEC
  progressive — *see* Epilepsy, generalized,
    idiopathic
  not intractable G40.909
    with status epilepticus G40.901
    without status epilepticus G40.909
  on awakening — *see* Epilepsy, generalized,
    specified NEC
  parasitic NOS B71.9 *[G94]*
  partialis continua (*see also* Kozhevnikof's epilepsy)
    G40.1 ☑
  peripheral — *see* Epilepsy, specified NEC
  procursiva — *see* Epilepsy, localization-related,
    symptomatic, with simple partial seizures
  progressive (familial) myoclonic — *see* Epilepsy,
    generalized, idiopathic

☑ **Additional character required**

Epilepsy — continued
reflex — see Epilepsy, specified NEC
related to
  alcohol G40.509
    not intractable G40.509
      with status epilepticus G40.501
      without status epilepticus G40.509
  drugs G40.509
    not intractable G40.509
      with status epilepticus G40.501
      without status epilepticus G40.509
  external causes G40.509
    not intractable G40.509
      with status epilepticus G40.501
      without status epilepticus G40.509
  hormonal changes G40.509
    not intractable G40.509
      with status epilepticus G40.501
      without status epilepticus G40.509
  sleep deprivation G40.509
    not intractable G40.509
      with status epilepticus G40.501
      without status epilepticus G40.509
  stress G40.509
    not intractable G40.509
      with status epilepticus G40.501
      without status epilepticus G40.509
somatomotor — see Epilepsy, localization-related, symptomatic, with simple partial seizures
somatosensory — see Epilepsy, localization-related, symptomatic, with simple partial seizures
spasms G40.822
  intractable G40.824
    with status epilepticus G40.823
    without status epilepticus G40.824
  not intractable G40.822
    with status epilepticus G40.821
    without status epilepticus G40.822
  specified NEC G40.802
    intractable G40.804
      with status epilepticus G40.803
      without status epilepticus G40.804
    not intractable G40.802
      with status epilepticus G40.801
      without status epilepticus G40.802
syndromes
  generalized
    idiopathic G40.309
      intractable G40.319
        with status epilepticus G40.311
        without status epilepticus G40.319
      not intractable G40.309
        with status epilepticus G40.301
        without status epilepticus G40.309
    specified NEC G40.409
      intractable G40.419
        with status epilepticus G40.411
        without status epilepticus G40.419
      not intractable G40.409
        with status epilepticus G40.401
        without status epilepticus G40.409
  localization-related (focal) (partial)
    idiopathic G40.009
      with seizures of localized onset G40.009
      intractable G40.019
        with status epilepticus G40.011
        without status epilepticus G40.019
      not intractable G40.009
        with status epilepticus G40.001
        without status epilepticus G40.009
    symptomatic
      with complex partial seizures G40.209
        intractable G40.219
          with status epilepticus G40.211
          without status epilepticus G40.219
        not intractable G40.209
          with status epilepticus G40.201
          without status epilepticus G40.209
      with simple partial seizures G40.109
        intractable G40.119
          with status epilepticus G40.111
          without status epilepticus G40.119
        not intractable G40.109
          with status epilepticus G40.101
          without status epilepticus G40.109
    specified NEC G40.802
      intractable G40.804
        with status epilepticus G40.803
        without status epilepticus G40.804
      not intractable G40.802
        with status epilepticus G40.801
        without status epilepticus G40.802

Epilepsy — continued
tonic (-clonic) — see Epilepsy, generalized, specified NEC
twilight F05
uncinate (gyrus) — see Epilepsy, localization-related, symptomatic, with complex partial seizures
Unverricht (-Lundborg) (familial myoclonic) — see Epilepsy, generalized, idiopathic
visceral — see Epilepsy, specified NEC
visual — see Epilepsy, specified NEC
Epiloia Q85.1
Epimenorrhea N92.0
Epipharyngitis — see Nasopharyngitis
Epiphora H04.20 ☑
  due to
    excess lacrimation H04.21 ☑
    insufficient drainage H04.22 ☑
Epiphyseal arrest — see Arrest, epiphyseal
Epiphyseolysis, epiphysiolysis — see Osteochondropathy
Epiphysitis (see also Osteochondropathy)
  juvenile M92.9
  syphilitic (congenital) A50.02
Epiplocele — see Hernia, abdomen
Epiploitis — see Peritonitis
Epiplosarcomphalocele — see Hernia, umbilicus
Episcleritis (suppurative) H15.10 ☑
  in (due to)
    syphilis A52.71
    tuberculosis A18.51
  nodular H15.12 ☑
  periodica fugax H15.11 ☑
    angioneurotic — see Edema, angioneurotic
  syphilitic (late) A52.71
  tuberculous A18.51
Episode
affective, mixed F39
depersonalization (in neurotic state) F48.1
depressive F32.9
  major F32.9
    mild F32.0
    moderate F32.1
    severe (without psychotic symptoms) F32.2
      with psychotic symptoms F32.3
    recurrent F33.9
      brief F33.8
    specified NEC F32.89
hypomanic F30.8
manic F30.9
  with
    psychotic symptoms F30.2
    remission (full) F30.4
      partial F30.3
  other specified F30.8
  recurrent F31.89
  without psychotic symptoms F30.10
    mild F30.11
    moderate F30.12
    severe (without psychotic symptoms) F30.13
      with psychotic symptoms F30.2
psychotic F23
  organic F06.8
schizophrenic (acute) NEC, brief F23
Epispadias (female) (male) Q64.0
Episplenitis D73.89
Epistaxis (multiple) R04.0
  hereditary I78.0
  vicarious menstruation N94.89
Epithelioma (malignant) (see also Neoplasm, malignant, by site)
  adenoides cysticum — see Neoplasm, skin, benign
  basal cell — see Neoplasm, skin, malignant
  benign — see Neoplasm, benign, by site
  Bowen's — see Neoplasm, skin, in situ
  calcifying, of Malherbe — see Neoplasm, skin, benign
  external site — see Neoplasm, skin, malignant
  intraepidermal, Jadassohn — see Neoplasm, skin, benign
  squamous cell — see Neoplasm, malignant, by site
Epitheliomatosis pigmented Q82.1
Epitheliopathy, multifocal placoid pigment H30.14 ☑
Epithelium, epithelial — see condition
Epituberculosis (with atelectasis) (allergic) A15.7
Eponychia Q84.6
Epstein's
  nephrosis or syndrome — see Nephrosis
  pearl K09.8
Epulis (gingiva) (fibrous) (giant cell) K06.8
Equinia A24.0
Equinovarus (congenital) (talipes) Q66.0 ☑
  acquired — see Deformity, limb, clubfoot

Equivalent
convulsive (abdominal) — see Epilepsy, specified NEC
epileptic (psychic) — see Epilepsy, localization-related, symptomatic, with complex partial seizures
Erb (-Duchenne) paralysis (birth injury) (newborn) P14.0
Erb-Goldflam disease or syndrome G70.00
  with exacerbation (acute) G70.01
  in crisis G70.01
Erb's
  disease G71.02
  palsy, paralysis (brachial) (birth) (newborn) P14.0
    spinal (spastic) syphilitic A52.17
  pseudohypertrophic muscular dystrophy G71.02
Erdheim's syndrome (acromegalic macrospondylitis) E22.0
Erection, painful (persistent) — see Priapism
Ergosterol deficiency (vitamin D) E55.9
  with
    adult osteomalacia M83.8
    rickets — see Rickets
Ergotism (see also Poisoning, food, noxious, plant)
  from ergot used as drug (migraine therapy) — see Table of Drugs and Chemicals
Erosio interdigitalis blastomycetica B37.2
Erosion
artery I77.2
  without rupture I77.89
bone — see Disorder, bone, density and structure, specified NEC
bronchus J98.09
cartilage (joint) — see Disorder, cartilage, specified type NEC
cervix (uteri) (acquired) (chronic) (congenital) N86
  with cervicitis N72
cornea (nontraumatic) — see Ulcer, cornea
  recurrent H18.83 ☑
  traumatic — see Abrasion, cornea
dental (idiopathic) (occupational) (due to diet, drugs or vomiting) K03.2
duodenum, postpyloric — see Ulcer, duodenum
esophagus K22.10
  with bleeding K22.11
gastric — see Ulcer, stomach
gastrojejunal — see Ulcer, gastrojejunal
implanted mesh — see Complications, prosthetic devise or implant, mesh
intestine K63.3
lymphatic vessel I89.8
pylorus, pyloric (ulcer) — see Ulcer, stomach
spine, aneurysmal A52.09
stomach — see Ulcer, stomach
subcutaneous device pocket
  nervous system prosthetic device, implant, or graft T85.890 ☑
  other internal prosthetic device, implant, or graft T85.898 ☑
teeth (idiopathic) (occupational) (due to diet, drugs or vomiting) K03.2
urethra N36.8
uterus N85.8
Erotomania F52.8
Error
metabolism, inborn — see Disorder, metabolism
refractive — see Disorder, refraction
Eructation R14.2
nervous or psychogenic F45.8
Eruption
creeping B76.9
drug (generalized) (taken internally) L27.0
  fixed L27.1
  in contact with skin — see Dermatitis, due to drugs
  localized L27.1
Hutchinson, summer L56.4
Kaposi's varicelliform B00.0
napkin L22
polymorphous light (sun) L56.4
recalcitrant pustular L13.8
ringed R23.8
skin (nonspecific) R21
  creeping (meaning hookworm) B76.9
  due to inoculation/vaccination (generalized) (see also Dermatitis, due to, vaccine) L27.0
    localized L27.1
  erysipeloid A26.0
  feigned L98.1
  Kaposi's varicelliform B00.0
  lichenoid L28.0
  meaning dermatitis — see Dermatitis
  toxic NEC L53.0

☑ **Additional character required**

Eruption - Examination

Eruption — *continued*
tooth, teeth, abnormal (incomplete) (late) (premature) (sequence) K00.6
vesicular R23.8
Erysipelas (gangrenous) (infantile) (newborn) (phlegmonous) (suppurative) A46
external ear A46 *[H62.40]*
puerperal, postpartum O86.89
Erysipeloid A26.9
cutaneous (Rosenbach's) A26.0
disseminated A26.8
sepsis A26.7
specified NEC A26.8
Erythema, erythematous (infectional) (inflammation) L53.9
ab igne L59.0
annulare (centrifugum) (rheumaticum) L53.1
arthriticum epidemicum A25.1
brucellum — *see* Brucellosis
chronic figurate NEC L53.3
chronicum migrans (Borrelia burgdorferi) A69.20
diaper L22
due to
chemical NEC L53.0
in contact with skin L24.5
drug (internal use) — *see* Dermatitis, due to, drugs
elevatum diutinum L95.1
endemic E52
epidemic, arthritic A25.1
figuratum perstans L53.3
gluteal L22
heat - code by site under Burn, first degree
ichthyosiforme congenitum bullous Q80.3
in diseases classified elsewhere L54
induratum (nontuberculous) L52
tuberculous A18.4
infectiosum B08.3
intertrigo L30.4
iris L51.9
marginatum L53.2
in (due to) acute rheumatic fever I00
medicamentosum — *see* Dermatitis, due to, drugs
migrans A26.0
chronicum A69.20
tongue K14.1
multiforme (major) (minor) L51.9
bullous, bullosum L51.1
conjunctiva L51.1
nonbullous L51.0
pemphigoides L12.0
specified NEC L51.8
napkin L22
neonatorum P83.88
toxic P83.1
nodosum L52
tuberculous A18.4
palmar L53.8
pernio T69.1 ☑
rash, newborn P83.88
scarlatiniform (recurrent) (exfoliative) L53.8
solare L55.0
specified NEC L53.8
toxic, toxicum NEC L53.0
newborn P83.1
tuberculous (primary) A18.4
Erythematous, erythematosus — *see* condition
Erythermalgia (primary) I73.81
Erythralgia I73.81
Erythrasma L08.1
Erythredema (polyneuropathy) — *see* Poisoning, mercury
Erythremia (acute) C94.0 ☑
chronic D45
secondary D75.1
Erythroblastopenia (*see also* Aplasia, red cell) D60.9
congenital D61.01
Erythroblastophthisis D61.09
Erythroblastosis (fetalis) (newborn) P55.9
due to
ABO (antibodies) (incompatibility) (isoimmunization) P55.1
Rh (antibodies) (incompatibility) (isoimmunization) P55.0
Erythrocyanosis (crurum) I73.89
Erythrocythemia — *see* Erythremia
Erythrocytosis (megalosplenic) (secondary) D75.0
familial D75.0
oval, hereditary — *see* Elliptocytosis
secondary D75.1
stress D75.1

Erythroderma (secondary) (*see also* Erythema) L53.9
bullous ichthyosiform, congenital Q80.3
desquamativum L21.1
ichthyosiform, congenital (bullous) Q80.3
neonatorum P83.88
psoriaticum L40.8
Erythrodysesthesia, palmar plantar (PPE) L27.1
Erythrogenesis imperfecta D61.09
Erythroleukemia C94.0 ☑
Erythromelalgia I73.81
Erythrophagocytosis D75.89
Erythrophobia F40.298
Erythroplakia, oral epithelium, and tongue K13.29
Erythroplasia (Queyrat) D07.4
specified site — *see* Neoplasm, skin, in situ
unspecified site D07.4
Escherichia coli (E. coli), as cause of disease classified elsewhere B96.20
non-O157 Shiga toxin-producing (with known O group) B96.22
non-Shiga toxin-producing B96.29
O157 with confirmation of Shiga toxin when H antigen is unknown, or is not H7 B96.21
O157:H- (nonmotile) with confirmation of Shiga toxin B96.21
O157:H7 with or without confirmation of Shiga toxin-production B96.21
Shiga toxin-producing (with unspecified O group) (STEC) B96.23
O157 B96.21
O157:H7 with or without confirmation of Shiga toxin-production B96.21
specified NEC B96.22
specified NEC B96.29
Esophagismus K22.4
Esophagitis (acute) (alkaline) (chemical) (chronic) (infectional) (necrotic) (peptic) (postoperative) K20.9
candidal B37.81
due to gastrointestinal reflux disease K21.0
eosinophilic K20.0
reflux K21.0
specified NEC K20.8
tuberculous A18.83
ulcerative K22.10
with bleeding K22.11
Esophagocele K22.5
Esophagomalacia K22.8
Esophagospasm K22.4
Esophagostenosis K22.2
Esophagostomiasis B81.8
Esophagotracheal — *see* condition
Esophagus — *see* condition
Esophoria H50.51
convergence, excess H51.12
divergence, insufficiency H51.8
Esotropia — *see* Strabismus, convergent concomitant
Espundia B55.2
Essential — *see* condition
Esthesioneuroblastoma C30.0
Esthesioneurocytoma C30.0
Esthesioneuroepithelioma C30.0
Esthiomene A55
Estivo-autumnal malaria (fever) B50.9
Estrangement (marital) Z63.5
parent-child NEC Z62.890
Estriasis — *see* Myiasis
Ethanolism — *see* Alcoholism
Etherism — *see* Dependence, drug, inhalant
Ethmoid, ethmoidal — *see* condition
Ethmoiditis (chronic) (nonpurulent) (purulent) (*see also* Sinusitis, ethmoidal)
influenzal — *see* Influenza, with, respiratory manifestations NEC
Woakes' J33.1
Ethylism — *see* Alcoholism
Eulenburg's disease (congenital paramyotonia) G71.19
Eumycetoma B47.0
Eunuchoidism E29.1
hypogonadotropic E23.0
European blastomycosis — *see* Cryptococcosis
Eustachian — *see* condition
Evaluation (for) (of)
development state
adolescent Z00.3
period of
delayed growth in childhood Z00.70
with abnormal findings Z00.71
rapid growth in childhood Z00.2
puberty Z00.3
growth and developmental state (period of rapid growth) Z00.2

Evaluation — *continued*
growth and developmental — *continued*
delayed growth Z00.70
with abnormal findings Z00.71
mental health (status) Z00.8
requested by authority Z04.6
period of
delayed growth in childhood Z00.70
with abnormal findings Z00.71
rapid growth in childhood Z00.2
suspected condition — *see* Observation
Evans syndrome D69.41
Event
apparent life threatening in newborn and infant (ALTE) R68.13
brief resolved unexplained event (BRUE) R68.13
Eventration
colon into chest — *see* Hernia, diaphragm
diaphragm (congenital) Q79.1
Eversion
bladder N32.89
cervix (uteri) N86
with cervicitis N72
foot NEC (*see also* Deformity, valgus, ankle)
congenital Q66.6
punctum lacrimale (postinfectional) (senile) H04.52 ☑
ureter (meatus) N28.89
urethra (meatus) N36.8
uterus N81.4
Evidence
cytologic
of malignancy on anal smear R85.614
of malignancy on cervical smear R87.614
of malignancy on vaginal smear R87.624
Evisceration
birth injury P15.8
traumatic NEC
eye — *see* Enucleated eye
Evulsion — *see* Avulsion
Ewing's sarcoma or tumor — *see* Neoplasm, bone, malignant
Examination (for) (following) (general) (of) (routine) Z00.00
with abnormal findings Z00.01
abuse, physical (alleged), ruled out
adult Z04.71
child Z04.72
adolescent (development state) Z00.3
alleged rape or sexual assault (victim), ruled out
adult Z04.41
child Z04.42
allergy Z01.82
annual (adult) (periodic) (physical) Z00.00
with abnormal findings Z00.01
gynecological Z01.419
with abnormal findings Z01.411
antibody response Z01.84
blood — *see* Examination, laboratory
blood pressure Z01.30
with abnormal findings Z01.31
cancer staging — *see* Neoplasm, malignant, by site
cervical Papanicolaou smear Z12.4
as part of routine gynecological examination Z01.419
with abnormal findings Z01.411
child (over 28 days old) Z00.129
with abnormal findings Z00.121
under 28 days old — *see* Newborn, examination
clinical research control or normal comparison (control) (participant) Z00.6
contraceptive (drug) maintenance (routine) Z30.8
device (intrauterine) Z30.431
dental Z01.20
with abnormal findings Z01.21
developmental — *see* Examination, child
donor (potential) Z00.5
ear Z01.10
with abnormal findings NEC Z01.118
eye Z01.00
with abnormal findings Z01.01
following failed vision screening Z01.020
with abnormal findings Z01.021
following
accident NEC Z04.3
transport Z04.1
work Z04.2
assault, alleged, ruled out
adult Z04.71
child Z04.72
motor vehicle accident Z04.1
treatment (for) Z09

☑ **Additional character required**

Examination — *continued*
  following — *continued*
    combined NEC Z09
      fracture Z09
        malignant neoplasm Z08
      malignant neoplasm Z08
      mental disorder Z09
      specified condition NEC Z09
    follow-up (routine) (following) Z09
      chemotherapy NEC Z09
        malignant neoplasm Z08
      fracture Z09
      malignant neoplasm Z08
      postpartum Z39.2
      psychotherapy Z09
      radiotherapy NEC Z09
        malignant neoplasm Z08
      surgery NEC Z09
        malignant neoplasm Z08
    forced sexual exploitation Z04.81
    forced labor exploitation Z04.82
  gynecological Z01.419
    with abnormal findings Z01.411
    for contraceptive maintenance Z30.8
  health — *see* Examination, medical
  hearing Z01.10
    with abnormal findings NEC Z01.118
    infant or child (over 28 days old) Z00.129
      with abnormal findings Z00.121
    following failed hearing screening Z01.110
  immunity status testing Z01.84
  laboratory (as part of a general medical
    examination) Z00.00
    with abnormal findings Z00.01
    preprocedural Z01.812
  lactating mother Z39.1
  medical (adult) (for) (of) Z00.00
    with abnormal findings Z00.01
    administrative purpose only Z02.9
      specified NEC Z02.89
    admission to
      armed forces Z02.3
      old age home Z02.2
      prison Z02.89
      residential institution Z02.2
      school Z02.0
        following illness or medical treatment Z02.0
      summer camp Z02.89
    adoption Z02.82
    blood alcohol or drug level Z02.83
    camp (summer) Z02.89
    clinical research, normal subject (control)
      (participant) Z00.6
    control subject in clinical research (normal
      comparison) (participant) Z00.6
    donor (potential) Z00.5
    driving license Z02.4
    general (adult) Z00.00
      with abnormal findings Z00.01
    immigration Z02.89
    insurance purposes Z02.6
    marriage Z02.89
    medicolegal reasons NEC Z04.89
    naturalization Z02.89
    participation in sport Z02.5
    paternity testing Z02.81
    population survey Z00.8
    pre-employment Z02.1
    pre-operative — *see* Examination, pre-procedural
    pre-procedural
      cardiovascular Z01.810
      respiratory Z01.811
      specified NEC Z01.818
    preschool children
      for admission to school Z02.0
    prisoners
      for entrance into prison Z02.89
    recruitment for armed forces Z02.3
    specified NEC Z00.8
    sport competition Z02.5
  medicolegal reason NEC Z04.89
    following
      forced sexual exploitation Z04.81
      forced labor exploitation Z04.82
  newborn — *see* Newborn, examination
  pelvic (annual) (periodic) Z01.419
    with abnormal findings Z01.411
  period of rapid growth in childhood Z00.2
  periodic (adult) (annual) (routine) Z00.00
    with abnormal findings Z00.01
  physical (adult) (*see also* Examination, medical Z00.00)
    sports Z02.5

Examination — *continued*
  postpartum
    immediately after delivery Z39.0
    routine follow-up Z39.2
  prenatal (normal pregnancy) (*see also* Pregnancy,
    normal) Z34.9 ☑
  pre-chemotherapy (antineoplastic) Z01.818
  pre-procedural (pre-operative)
    cardiovascular Z01.810
    laboratory Z01.812
    respiratory Z01.811
    specified NEC Z01.818
  prior to chemotherapy (antineoplastic) Z01.818
  psychiatric NEC Z00.8
    follow-up not needing further care Z09
    requested by authority Z04.6
  radiological (as part of a general medical
    examination) Z00.00
    with abnormal findings Z00.01
  repeat cervical smear to confirm findings of recent
    normal smear following initial abnormal smear
    Z01.42
  skin (hypersensitivity) Z01.82
  special (*see also* Examination, by type) Z01.89
    specified type NEC Z01.89
  specified type or reason NEC Z04.89
  teeth Z01.20
    with abnormal findings Z01.21
  urine — *see* Examination, laboratory
  vision Z01.00
    with abnormal findings Z01.01
    following failed vision screening Z01.020
      with abnormal findings Z01.021
    infant or child (over 28 days old) Z00.129
      with abnormal findings Z00.121
Exanthem, exanthema (*see also* Rash)
  with enteroviral vesicular stomatitis B08.4
  Boston A88.0
  epidemic with meningitis A88.0 *[G02]*
  subitum B08.20
    due to human herpesvirus 6 B08.21
    due to human herpesvirus 7 B08.22
  viral, virus B09
    specified type NEC B08.8
Excess, excessive, excessively
  alcohol level in blood R78.0
  androgen (ovarian) E28.1
  attrition, tooth, teeth K03.0
  carotene, carotin (dietary) E67.1
  cold, effects of T69.9 ☑
    specified effect NEC T69.8 ☑
  convergence H51.12
  crying
    in child, adolescent, or adult R45.83
    in infant R68.11
  development, breast N62
  divergence H51.8
  drinking (alcohol) NEC (without dependence)
    F10.10
    habitual (continual) (without remission) F10.20
  eating R63.2
  estrogen E28.0
  fat (*see also* Obesity)
    in heart — *see* Degeneration, myocardial
    localized E65
  foreskin N47.8
  gas R14.0
  glucagon E16.3
  heat — *see* Heat
  intermaxillary vertical dimension of fully erupted
    teeth M26.37
  interocclusal distance of fully erupted teeth M26.37
  kalium E87.5
  large
    colon K59.39
      congenital Q43.8
    infant P08.0
    organ or site, congenital NEC — *see* Anomaly,
      by site
  long
    organ or site, congenital NEC — *see* Anomaly,
      by site
  menstruation (with regular cycle) N92.0
    with irregular cycle N92.1
  napping Z72.821
  natrium E87.0
  number of teeth K00.1
  nutrient (dietary) NEC R63.2
  potassium (K) E87.5
  salivation K11.7
  secretion (*see also* Hypersecretion)
    milk O92.6

Excess — *continued*
  secretion — *continued*
    sputum R09.3
    sweat R61
  sexual drive F52.8
  short
    organ or site, congenital NEC — *see* Anomaly, by site
    umbilical cord in labor or delivery O69.3 ☑
  skin L98.7
    and subcutaneous tissue L98.7
    eyelid (acquired) — *see* Blepharochalasis
      congenital Q10.3
  sodium (Na) E87.0
  spacing of fully erupted teeth M26.32
  sputum R09.3
  sweating R61
  thirst R63.1
    due to deprivation of water T73.1 ☑
  tuberosity of jaw M26.07
  vitamin
    A (dietary) E67.0
      administered as drug (prolonged intake) — *see*
        Table of Drugs and Chemicals, vitamins,
        adverse effect
      overdose or wrong substance given or taken —
        see Table of Drugs and Chemicals, vitamins,
        poisoning
    D (dietary) E67.3
      administered as drug (prolonged intake) — *see*
        Table of Drugs and Chemicals, vitamins,
        adverse effect
      overdose or wrong substance given or taken —
        see Table of Drugs and Chemicals, vitamins,
        poisoning
  weight
    gain R63.5
    loss R63.4
Excitability, abnormal, under minor stress (personality
  disorder) F60.3
Excitation
  anomalous atrioventricular I45.6
  psychogenic F30.8
  reactive (from emotional stress, psychological
    trauma) F30.8
Excitement
  hypomanic F30.8
  manic F30.9
  mental, reactive (from emotional stress,
    psychological trauma) F30.8
  state, reactive (from emotional stress, psychological
    trauma) F30.8
Excoriation (traumatic) (*see also* Abrasion)
  neurotic L98.1
  skin picking disorder F42.4
Exfoliation
  due to erythematous conditions according to
    extent of body surface involved L49.0
    10-19 percent of body surface L49.1
    20-29 percent of body surface L49.2
    30-39 percent of body surface L49.3
    40-49 percent of body surface L49.4
    50-59 percent of body surface L49.5
    60-69 percent of body surface L49.6
    70-79 percent of body surface L49.7
    80-89 percent of body surface L49.8
    90-99 percent of body surface L49.9
    less than 10 percent of body surface L49.0
  teeth, due to systemic causes K08.0
Exfoliative — *see* condition
Exhaustion, exhaustive (physical NEC) R53.83
  battle F43.0
  cardiac — *see* Failure, heart
  delirium F43.0
  due to
    cold T69.8 ☑
    excessive exertion T73.3 ☑
    exposure T73.2 ☑
    neurasthenia F48.8
  heart — *see* Failure, heart
  heat (*see also* Heat, exhaustion) T67.5 ☑
    due to
      salt depletion T67.4 ☑
      water depletion T67.3 ☑
  maternal, complicating delivery O75.81
  mental F48.8
  myocardium, myocardial — *see* Failure, heart
  nervous F48.8
  old age R54
  psychogenic F48.8
  psychosis F43.0
  senile R54
  vital NEC Z73.0

Exhibitionism F65.2
Exocervicitis — *see* Cervicitis
Exomphalos Q79.2
  meaning hernia — *see* Hernia, umbilicus
Exophoria H50.52
  convergence, insufficiency H51.11
  divergence, excess H51.8
Exophthalmos H05.2 ☑
  congenital Q15.8
  constant NEC H05.24 ☑
  displacement, globe — *see* Displacement, globe
  due to thyrotoxicosis (hyperthyroidism) — *see*
    Hyperthyroidism, with, goiter (diffuse)
  dysthyroid — *see* Hyperthyroidism, with, goiter
    (diffuse)
  goiter — *see* Hyperthyroidism, with, goiter (diffuse)
  intermittent NEC H05.25 ☑
  malignant — *see* Hyperthyroidism, with, goiter
    (diffuse)
  orbital
    edema — *see* Edema, orbit
    hemorrhage — *see* Hemorrhage, orbit
  pulsating NEC H05.26 ☑
  thyrotoxic, thyrotropic — *see* Hyperthyroidism,
    with, goiter (diffuse)
Exostosis (*see also* Disorder, bone)
  cartilaginous — *see* Neoplasm, bone, benign
  congenital (multiple) Q78.6
  external ear canal H61.81 ☑
  gonococcal A54.49
  jaw (bone) M27.8
  multiple, congenital Q78.6
  orbit H05.35 ☑
  osteocartilaginous — *see* Neoplasm, bone, benign
  syphilitic A52.77
Exotropia — *see* Strabismus, divergent concomitant
Explanation of
  investigation finding Z71.2
  medication Z71.89
Exposure (to) (*see also* Contact, with) T75.89 ☑
  acariasis Z20.7
  AIDS virus Z20.6
  air pollution Z77.110
  algae and algae toxins Z77.121
  algae bloom Z77.121
  anthrax Z20.810
  aromatic amines Z77.020
  aromatic (hazardous) compounds NEC Z77.028
  aromatic dyes NOS Z77.028
  arsenic Z77.010
  asbestos Z77.090
  bacterial disease NEC Z20.818
  benzene Z77.021
  blue-green algae bloom Z77.121
  body fluids (potentially hazardous) Z77.21
  brown tide Z77.121
  chemicals (chiefly nonmedicinal) (hazardous) NEC
    Z77.098
  cholera Z20.09
  chromium compounds Z77.018
  cold, effects of T69.9 ☑
    specified effect NEC T69.8 ☑
  communicable disease Z20.9
    bacterial NEC Z20.818
    specified NEC Z20.89
    viral NEC Z20.828
    Zika virus Z20.821
  cyanobacteria bloom Z77.121
  disaster Z65.5
  discrimination Z60.5
  dyes Z77.098
  effects of T73.9 ☑
  environmental tobacco smoke (acute) (chronic)
    Z77.22
  Escherichia coli (E. coli) Z20.01
  exhaustion due to T73.2 ☑
  fiberglass — *see* Table of Drugs and Chemicals,
    fiberglass
  German measles Z20.4
  gonorrhea Z20.2
  hazardous metals NEC Z77.018
  hazardous substances NEC Z77.29
  hazards in the physical environment NEC Z77.128
  hazards to health NEC Z77.9
  human immunodeficiency virus (HIV) Z20.6
  human T-lymphotropic virus type-1 (HTLV-1) Z20.89
  implanted
    mesh — *see* Complications, prosthetic devise or
      implant, mesh
    prosthetic materials NEC — *see* Complications,
      prosthetic materials NEC
  infestation (parasitic) NEC Z20.7

Exposure — *continued*
  intestinal infectious disease NEC Z20.09
    Escherichia coli (E. coli) Z20.01
  lead Z77.011
  meningococcus Z20.811
  mold (toxic) Z77.120
  nickel dust Z77.018
  noise Z77.122
  occupational
    air contaminants NEC Z57.39
    dust Z57.2
    environmental tobacco smoke Z57.31
    extreme temperature Z57.6
    noise Z57.0
    radiation Z57.1
    risk factors Z57.9
      specified NEC Z57.8
    toxic agents (gases) (liquids) (solids) (vapors) in
      agriculture Z57.4
    toxic agents (gases) (liquids) (solids) (vapors) in
      industry NEC Z57.5
    vibration Z57.7
  parasitic disease NEC Z20.7
  pediculosis Z20.7
  persecution Z60.5
  pfiesteria piscicida Z77.121
  poliomyelitis Z20.89
  polycyclic aromatic hydrocarbons Z77.028
  pollution
    air Z77.110
    environmental NEC Z77.118
    soil Z77.112
    water Z77.111
  prenatal (drugs) (toxic chemicals) — *see* Newborn,
    affected by, noxious substances transmitted via
    placenta or breast milk
  rabies Z20.3
  radiation, naturally occurring NEC Z77.123
  radon Z77.123
  red tide (Florida) Z77.121
  rubella Z20.4
  second hand tobacco smoke (acute) (chronic) Z77.22
    in the perinatal period P96.81
  sexually-transmitted disease Z20.2
  smallpox (laboratory) Z20.89
  syphilis Z20.2
  terrorism Z65.4
  torture Z65.4
  tuberculosis Z20.1
  uranium Z77.012
  varicella Z20.820
  venereal disease Z20.2
  viral disease NEC Z20.828
  war Z65.5
  water pollution Z77.111
  Zika virus Z20.821
Exsanguination — *see* Hemorrhage
Exstrophy
  abdominal contents Q45.8
  bladder Q64.10
    cloacal Q64.12
    specified type NEC Q64.19
    supravesical fissure Q64.11
Extensive — *see* condition
Extra (*see also* Accessory)
  marker chromosomes (normal individual) Q92.61
    in abnormal individual Q92.62
  rib Q76.6
    cervical Q76.5
Extrasystoles (supraventricular) I49.49
  atrial I49.1
  auricular I49.1
  junctional I49.2
  ventricular I49.3
Extrauterine gestation or pregnancy — *see*
  Pregnancy, by site
Extravasation
  blood R58
  chyle into mesentery I89.8
  pelvicalyceal N13.8
  pyelosinus N13.8
  urine (from ureter) R39.0
  vesicant agent
    antineoplastic chemotherapy T80.810 ☑
    other agent NEC T80.818 ☑
Extremity — *see* condition, limb
Extrophy — *see* Exstrophy
Extroversion
  bladder Q64.19
  uterus N81.4
    complicating delivery O71.2
    postpartal (old) N81.4

Extruded tooth (teeth) M26.34
Extrusion
  breast implant (prosthetic) T85.42 ☑
  eye implant (globe) (ball) T85.328 ☑
  intervertebral disc — *see* Displacement,
    intervertebral disc
  ocular lens implant (prosthetic) — *see*
    Complications, intraocular lens
  vitreous — *see* Prolapse, vitreous
Exudate
  pleural — *see* Effusion, pleura
  retina H35.89
Exudative — *see* condition
Eye, eyeball, eyelid — *see* condition
Eyestrain — *see* Disturbance, vision, subjective
Eyeworm disease of Africa B74.3

F

Faber's syndrome (achlorhydric anemia) D50.9
Fabry (-Anderson) disease E75.21
Faciocephalalgia, autonomic (*see also* Neuropathy,
  peripheral, autonomic) G90.09
Factor(s)
  psychic, associated with diseases classified
    elsewhere F54
  psychological
    affecting physical conditions F54
    or behavioral
      affecting general medical condition F54
      associated with disorders or diseases classified
        elsewhere F54
Fahr disease (of brain) G23.8
Fahr Volhard disease (of kidney) I12. ☑
Failure, failed
  abortion — *see* Abortion, attempted
  aortic (valve) I35.8
    rheumatic I06.8
  attempted abortion — *see* Abortion, attempted
  biventricular I50.82
    due to left heart failure I50.814
  bone marrow — *see* Anemia, aplastic
  cardiac — *see* Failure, heart
  cardiorenal (chronic) (*see also* Failure, renal, and
    Failure, heart) I50.9
    hypertensive I13.2
  cardiorespiratory (*see also* Failure, heart) R09.2
  cardiovascular (chronic) — *see* Failure, heart
  cerebrovascular I67.9
  cervical dilatation in labor O62.0
  circulation, circulatory (peripheral) R57.9
    newborn P29.89
  compensation — *see* Disease, heart
  compliance with medical treatment or regimen —
    see Noncompliance
  congestive — *see* Failure, heart, congestive
  dental implant (endosseous) M27.69
    due to
      failure of dental prosthesis M27.63
      lack of attached gingiva M27.62
      occlusal trauma (poor prosthetic design)
        M27.62
      parafunctional habits M27.62
      periodontal infection (peri-implantitis) M27.62
      poor oral hygiene M27.62
    osseointegration M27.61
      due to
        complications of systemic disease M27.61
        poor bone quality M27.61
      iatrogenic M27.61
    post-osseointegration
      biological M27.62
      due to complications of systemic disease
        M27.62
      iatrogenic M27.62
      mechanical M27.63
    pre-integration M27.61
    pre-osseointegration M27.61
    specified NEC M27.69
  descent of head (at term) of pregnancy (mother)
    O32.4 ☑
  endosseous dental implant — *see* Failure, dental
    implant
  engagement of head (term of pregnancy) (mother)
    O32.4 ☑
  erection (penile) (*see also* Dysfunction, sexual, male,
    erectile) N52.9
    nonorganic F52.21
  examination(s), anxiety concerning Z55.2

☑ **Additional character required**

Failure — *continued*
  expansion terminal respiratory units (newborn) (primary) P28.0
  forceps NOS (with subsequent cesarean delivery) O66.5
  gain weight (child over 28 days old) R62.51
    adult R62.7
    newborn P92.6
  genital response (male) F52.21
    female F52.22
  heart (acute) (senile) (sudden) I50.9
    with
      acute pulmonary edema — *see* Failure, ventricular, left
      decompensation (*see also* Failure, heart, by type as diastolic or systolic, acute and chronic) I50.9
      dilatation — *see* Disease, heart
      hypertension — *see* Hypertension, heart
      normal ejection fraction — *see* Failure, heart, diastolic
      preserved ejection fraction — *see* Failure, heart, diastolic
      reduced ejection fraction — *see* Failure, heart, systolic
    arteriosclerotic I70.90
    biventricular I50.82
      due to left heart failure I50.814
    combined left-right sided I50.82
      due to left heart failure I50.814
    compensated (*see also* Failure, heart, by type as diastolic or systolic, chronic) I50.9
    complicating
      anesthesia (general) (local) or other sedation in labor and delivery O74.2
      in pregnancy O29.12 ☑
      postpartum, puerperal O89.1
      delivery (cesarean) (instrumental) O75.4
    congestive I50.9
      with rheumatic fever (conditions in I00)
        active I01.8
        inactive or quiescent (with chorea) I09.81
      newborn P29.0
      rheumatic (chronic) (inactive) (with chorea) I09.81
        active or acute I01.8
          with chorea I02.0
    decompensated (*see also* Failure, heart, by type as diastolic or systolic, acute and chronic) I50.9
    degenerative — *see* Degeneration, myocardial
    diastolic (congestive) (left ventricular) I50.30
      acute (congestive) I50.31
        and (on) chronic (congestive) I50.33
      chronic (congestive) I50.32
        and (on) acute (congestive) I50.33
      combined with systolic (congestive) I50.40
        acute (congestive) I50.41
          and (on) chronic (congestive) I50.43
        chronic (congestive) I50.42
          and (on) acute (congestive) I50.43
    due to presence of cardiac prosthesis I97.13 ☑
    end stage (*see also* Failure, heart, by type as diastolic or systolic, chronic) I50.84
    following cardiac surgery I97.13 ☑
    high output NOS I50.83
    hypertensive — *see* Hypertension, heart
    left (ventricular) (*see also* Failure, ventricular, left)
      combined diastolic and systolic — *see* Failure, heart, diastolic, combined with systolic
      diastolic — *see* Failure, heart, diastolic
      systolic — *see* Failure, heart, systolic
    low output (syndrome) NOS I50.9
    newborn P29.0
    organic — *see* Disease, heart
    peripartum O90.3
    postprocedural I97.13 ☑
    rheumatic (chronic) (inactive) I09.9
    right (isolated) (ventricular) I50.810
      acute I50.811
        and (on) chronic I50.813
      chronic I50.812
        and acute I50.813
      secondary to left heart failure I50.814
    specified NEC I50.89
    Note: heart failure stages A, B, C, and D are based on the American College of Cardiology and American Heart Association stages of heart failure, which complement and should not be confused with the New York Heart Association Classification of Heart Failure, into Class I, Class II, Class III, and Class IV
    stage A Z91.89

Failure — *continued*
  heart — *continued*
    stage B (*see also* Failure, heart, by type as diastolic or systolic) I50.9
    stage C (*see also* Failure, heart, by type as diastolic or systolic) I50.9
    stage D (*see also* Failure, heart, by type as diastolic or systolic, chronic) I50.84
    systolic (congestive) (left ventricular) I50.20
      acute (congestive) I50.21
        and (on) chronic (congestive) I50.23
      chronic (congestive) I50.22
        and (on) acute (congestive) I50.23
      combined with diastolic (congestive) I50.40
        acute (congestive) I50.41
          and (on) chronic (congestive) I50.43
        chronic (congestive) I50.42
          and (on) acute (congestive) I50.43
    thyrotoxic (*see also* Thyrotoxicosis) E05.90 *[I43]*
      with
        high output (*see also* Thyrotoxicosis) I50.83
        thyroid storm E05.91 *[I43]*
          high output (*see also* Thyrotoxicosis) I50.83
    valvular — *see* Endocarditis
  hepatic K72.90
    with coma K72.91
    acute or subacute K72.00
      with coma K72.01
      due to drugs K71.10
        with coma K71.11
    alcoholic (acute) (chronic) (subacute) K70.40
      with coma K70.41
    chronic K72.10
      with coma K72.11
      due to drugs (acute) (subacute) (chronic) K71.10
        with coma K71.11
    due to drugs (acute) (subacute) (chronic) K71.10
      with coma K71.11
    postprocedural K91.82
  hepatorenal K76.7
  induction (of labor) O61.9
    abortion — *see* Abortion, attempted
    by
      oxytocic drugs O61.0
      prostaglandins O61.0
    instrumental O61.1
    mechanical O61.1
    medical O61.0
    specified NEC O61.8
    surgical O61.1
  intubation during anesthesia T88.4 ☑
    in pregnancy O29.6 ☑
    labor and delivery O74.7
    postpartum, puerperal O89.6
  involution, thymus (gland) E32.0
  kidney (*see also* Disease, kidney, chronic) N19
    acute (*see also* Failure, renal, acute) N17.9
    diabetic — *see* E08-E13 with .22
  lactation (complete) O92.3
    partial O92.4
  Leydig's cell, adult E29.1
  liver — *see* Failure, hepatic
  menstruation at puberty N91.0
  mitral I05.8
  myocardial, myocardium (*see also* Failure, heart) I50.9
    chronic (*see also* Failure, heart, congestive) I50.9
    congestive (*see also* Failure, heart, congestive) I50.9
  orgasm (female) (psychogenic) F52.31
    male F52.32
  ovarian (primary) E28.39
    iatrogenic E89.40
      asymptomatic E89.40
      symptomatic E89.41
    postprocedural (postablative) (postirradiation) (postsurgical) E89.40
      asymptomatic E89.40
      symptomatic E89.41
  ovulation causing infertility N97.0
  polyglandular, autoimmune E31.0
  prosthetic joint implant — *see* Complications, joint prosthesis, mechanical, breakdown, by site
  renal N19
    with
      tubular necrosis (acute) N17.0
    acute N17.9
      with
        cortical necrosis N17.1
        medullary necrosis N17.2
        tubular necrosis N17.0

Failure — *continued*
  renal — *continued*
      specified NEC N17.8
    chronic N18.9
      hypertensive — *see* Hypertension, kidney
    congenital P96.0
    end stage (chronic) N18.6
      due to hypertension I12.0
    following
      abortion — *see* Abortion by type complicated by specified condition NEC
      crushing T79.5 ☑
      ectopic or molar pregnancy O08.4
      labor and delivery (acute) O90.4
    hypertensive — *see* Hypertension, kidney
    postprocedural N99.0
  respiration, respiratory J96.90
    with
      hypercapnia J96.92
      hypercarbia J96.92
      hypoxia J96.91
    acute J96.00
      with
        hypercapnia J96.02
        hypercarbia J96.02
        hypoxia J96.01
    center G93.89
    acute and (on) chronic J96.20
      with
        hypercapnia J96.22
        hypercarbia J96.22
        hypoxia J96.21
    chronic J96.10
      with
        hypercapnia J96.12
        hypercarbia J96.12
        hypoxia J96.11
    newborn P28.5
    postprocedural (acute) J95.821
      acute and chronic J95.822
  rotation
    cecum Q43.3
    colon Q43.3
    intestine Q43.3
    kidney Q63.2
  sedation (conscious) (moderate) during procedure T88.52 ☑
    history of Z92.83
  segmentation (*see also* Fusion)
    fingers — *see* Syndactylism, complex, fingers
    vertebra Q76.49
      with scoliosis Q76.3
  seminiferous tubule, adult E29.1
  senile (general) R54
  sexual arousal (male) F52.21
    female F52.22
  testicular endocrine function E29.1
  to thrive (child over 28 days old) R62.51
    adult R62.7
    newborn P92.6
  transplant T86.92
    bone T86.831
      marrow T86.02
    cornea T86.841
    heart T86.22
      with lung(s) T86.32
    intestine T86.851
    kidney T86.12
    liver T86.42
    lung(s) T86.811
      with heart T86.32
    pancreas T86.891
    skin (allograft) (autograft) T86.821
    specified organ or tissue NEC T86.891
    stem cell (peripheral blood) (umbilical cord) T86.5
  trial of labor (with subsequent cesarean delivery) O66.40
    following previous cesarean delivery O66.41
  tubal ligation N99.89
  urinary — *see* Disease, kidney, chronic
  vacuum extraction NOS (with subsequent cesarean delivery) O66.5
  vasectomy N99.89
  ventouse NOS (with subsequent cesarean delivery) O66.5
  ventricular (*see also* Failure, heart) I50.9
    left (*see also* Failure, heart, left) I50.1
      with rheumatic fever (conditions in I00)
        active I01.8
          with chorea I02.0
        inactive or quiescent (with chorea) I09.81

Failure — *continued*
  ventricular — *continued*
    rheumatic (chronic) (inactive) (with chorea)
      I09.81
      active or acute I01.8
        with chorea I02.0
    right — *see* Failure, heart, right
  vital centers, newborn P91.88
Fainting (fit) R55
Fallen arches — *see* Deformity, limb, flat foot
Falling, falls (repeated) R29.6
  any organ or part — *see* Prolapse
Fallopian
  insufflation Z31.41
  tube — *see* condition
Fallot's
  pentalogy Q21.8
  tetrad or tetralogy Q21.3
  triad or trilogy Q22.3
False (*see also* condition)
  croup J38.5
  joint — *see* Nonunion, fracture
  labor (pains) O47.9
    at or after 37 completed weeks of gestation O47.1
    before 37 completed weeks of gestation O47.0 ☑
  passage, urethra (prostatic) N36.5
  pregnancy F45.8
Family, familial (*see also* condition)
  disruption Z63.8
    involving divorce or separation Z63.5
  Li-Fraumeni (syndrome) Z15.01
  planning advice Z30.09
  problem Z63.9
    specified NEC Z63.8
  retinoblastoma C69.2 ☑
Famine (effects of) T73.0 ☑
  edema — *see* Malnutrition, severe
Fanconi (-de Toni)(-Debré) syndrome E72.09
  with cystinosis E72.04
Fanconi's anemia (congenital pancytopenia) D61.09
Farber's disease or syndrome E75.29
Farcy A24.0
Farmer's
  lung J67.0
  skin L57.8
Farsightedness — *see* Hypermetropia
Fascia — *see* condition
Fasciculation R25.3
Fasciitis M72.9
  diffuse (eosinophilic) M35.4
  infective M72.8
    necrotizing M72.6
  necrotizing M72.6
  nodular M72.4
  perirenal (with ureteral obstruction) N13.5
    with infection N13.6
  plantar M72.2
  specified NEC M72.8
  traumatic (old) M72.8
    current - code by site under Sprain
Fascioliasis B66.3
Fasciolopsis, fasciolopsiasis (intestinal) B66.5
Fascioscapulohumeral myopathy G71.02
Fast pulse R00.0
Fat
  embolism — *see* Embolism, fat
  excessive (*see also* Obesity)
    in heart — *see* Degeneration, myocardial
  in stool R19.5
  localized (pad) E65
    heart — *see* Degeneration, myocardial
    knee M79.4
    retropatellar M79.4
  necrosis
    breast N64.1
    mesentery K65.4
    omentum K65.4
  pad E65
    knee M79.4
Fatigue R53.83
  auditory deafness — *see* Deafness
  chronic R53.82
  combat F43.0
  general R53.83
    psychogenic F48.8
  heat (transient) T67.6 ☑
  muscle M62.89
  myocardium — *see* Failure, heart
  neoplasm-related R53.0
  nervous, neurosis F48.8
  operational F48.8
  psychogenic (general) F48.8

Fatigue — *continued*
  senile R54
  voice R49.8
Fatness — *see* Obesity
Fatty (*see also* condition)
  apron E65
  degeneration — *see* Degeneration, fatty
  heart (enlarged) — *see* Degeneration, myocardial
  liver NEC K76.0
    alcoholic K70.0
    nonalcoholic K76.0
  necrosis — *see* Degeneration, fatty
Fauces — *see* condition
Fauchard's disease (periodontitis) — *see* Periodontitis
Faucitis J02.9
Favism (anemia) D55.0
Favus — *see* Dermatophytosis
Fazio-Londe disease or syndrome G12.1
Fear complex or reaction F40.9
Fear of — *see* Phobia
Feared complaint unfounded Z71.1
Febris, febrile (*see also* Fever)
  flava (*see also* Fever, yellow) A95.9
  melitensis A23.0
  pestis — *see* Plague
  recurrens — *see* Fever, relapsing
  rubra A38.9
Fecal
  incontinence R15.9
  smearing R15.1
  soiling R15.1
  urgency R15.2
Fecalith (impaction) K56.41
  appendix K38.1
  congenital P76.8
Fede's disease K14.0
Feeble rapid pulse due to shock following injury
  T79.4 ☑
Feeble-minded F70
Feeding
  difficulties R63.3
  problem R63.3
    newborn P92.9
      specified NEC P92.8
    nonorganic (adult) — *see* Disorder, eating
Feeling (of)
  foreign body in throat R09.89
Feer's disease — *see* Poisoning, mercury
Feet — *see* condition
Feigned illness Z76.5
Feil-Klippel syndrome (brevicollis) Q76.1
Feinmesser's (hidrotic) ectodermal dysplasia Q82.4
Felinophobia F40.218
Felon (*see also* Cellulitis, digit)
  with lymphangitis — *see* Lymphangitis, acute, digit
Felty's syndrome M05.00
  ankle M05.07 ☑
  elbow M05.02 ☑
  foot joint M05.07 ☑
  hand joint M05.04 ☑
  hip M05.05 ☑
  knee M05.06 ☑
  multiple site M05.09
  shoulder M05.01 ☑
  vertebra — *see* Spondylitis, ankylosing
  wrist M05.03 ☑
Female genital cutting status — *see* Female genital
  mutilation status (FGM)
Female genital mutilation status (FGM) N90.810
  specified NEC N90.818
  type I (clitorectomy status) N90.811
  type II (clitorectomy with excision of labia minora
    status) N90.812
  type III (infibulation status) N90.813
  type IV N90.818
Femur, femoral — *see* condition
Fenestration, fenestrated (*see also* Imperfect, closure)
  aortico-pulmonary Q21.4
  cusps, heart valve NEC Q24.8
    pulmonary Q22.3
  pulmonic cusps Q22.3
Fernell's disease (aortic aneurysm) I71.9
Fertile eunuch syndrome E23.0
Fetid
  breath R19.6
  sweat L75.0
Fetishism F65.0
  transvestic F65.1
Fetus, fetal (*see also* condition)
  alcohol syndrome (dysmorphic) Q86.0
  compressus O31.0 ☑
  hydantoin syndrome Q86.1

Fetus — *continued*
  lung tissue P28.0
  papyraceous O31.0 ☑
Fever (inanition) (of unknown origin) (persistent) (with
  chills) (with rigor) R50.9
  abortus A23.1
  Aden (dengue) A90
  African tick-borne A68.1
  American
    mountain (tick) A93.2
    spotted A77.0
  aphthous B08.8
  arbovirus, arboviral A94
    hemorrhagic A94
    specified NEC A93.8
  Argentinian hemorrhagic A96.0
  Assam B55.0
  Australian Q A78
  Bangkok hemorrhagic A91
  Barmah forest A92.8
  Bartonella A44.0
  bilious, hemoglobinuric B50.8
  blackwater B50.8
  blister B00.1
  Bolivian hemorrhagic A96.1
  Bonvale dam T73.3 ☑
  boutonneuse A77.1
  brain — *see* Encephalitis
  Brazilian purpuric A48.4
  breakbone A90
  Bullis A77.0
  Bunyamwera A92.8
  Burdwan B55.0
  Bwamba A92.8
  Cameroon — *see* Malaria
  Canton A75.9
  catarrhal (acute) J00
    chronic J31.0
  cat-scratch A28.1
  Central Asian hemorrhagic A98.0
  cerebral — *see* Encephalitis
  cerebrospinal meningococcal A39.0
  Chagres B50.9
  Chandipura A92.8
  Changuinola A93.1
  Charcot's (biliary) (hepatic) (intermittent) — *see*
    Calculus, bile duct
  Chikungunya (viral) (hemorrhagic) A92.0
  Chitral A93.1
  Colombo — *see* Fever, paratyphoid
  Colorado tick (virus) A93.2
  congestive (remittent) — *see* Malaria
  Congo virus A98.0
  continued malarial B50.9
  Corsican — *see* Malaria
  Crimean-Congo hemorrhagic A98.0
  Cyprus — *see* Brucellosis
  dandy A90
  deer fly — *see* Tularemia
  dengue (virus) A90
    hemorrhagic A91
    sandfly A93.1
  desert B38.0
  drug induced R50.2
  due to
    conditions classified elsewhere R50.81
    heat T67.01 ☑
  enteric A01.00
  enteroviral exanthematous (Boston exanthem)
    A88.0
  ephemeral (of unknown origin) R50.9
  epidemic hemorrhagic A98.5
  erysipelatous — *see* Erysipelas
  estivo-autumnal (malarial) B50.9
  famine A75.0
  five day A79.0
  following delivery O86.4
  Fort Bragg A27.89
  gastroenteric A01.00
  gastromalarial — *see* Malaria
  Gibraltar — *see* Brucellosis
  glandular — *see* Mononucleosis, infectious
  Guama (viral) A92.8
  Haverhill A25.1
  hay (allergic) J30.1
    with asthma (bronchial) J45.909
      with
        exacerbation (acute) J45.901
        status asthmaticus J45.902
      due to
        allergen other than pollen J30.89
        pollen, any plant or tree J30.1

☑ **Additional character required**

Fever — *continued*
- heat (effects) T67.01 ☑
- hematuric, bilious B50.8
- hemoglobinuric (malarial) (bilious) B50.8
- hemorrhagic (arthropod-borne) NOS A94
  - with renal syndrome A98.5
  - arenaviral A96.9
    - specified NEC A96.8
  - Argentinian A96.0
  - Bangkok A91
  - Bolivian A96.1
  - Central Asian A98.0
  - Chikungunya A92.0
  - Crimean-Congo A98.0
  - dengue (virus) A91
  - epidemic A98.5
  - Junin (virus) A96.0
  - Korean A98.5
  - Kyasanur forest A98.2
  - Machupo (virus) A96.1
  - mite-borne A93.8
  - mosquito-borne A92.8
  - Omsk A98.1
  - Philippine A91
  - Russian A98.5
  - Singapore A91
  - Southeast Asia A91
  - Thailand A91
  - tick-borne NEC A93.8
  - viral A99
    - specified NEC A98.8
- hepatic — *see* Cholecystitis
- herpetic — *see* Herpes
- icterohemorrhagic A27.0
- Indiana A93.8
- infective B99.9
  - specified NEC B99.8
- intermittent (bilious) (*see also* Malaria)
  - of unknown origin R50.9
  - pernicious B50.9
- iodide R50.2
- Japanese river A75.3
- jungle (*see also* Malaria)
  - yellow A95.0
- Junin (virus) hemorrhagic A96.0
- Katayama B65.2
- kedani A75.3
- Kenya (tick) A77.1
- Kew Garden A79.1
- Korean hemorrhagic A98.5
- Lassa A96.2
- Lone Star A77.0
- Machupo (virus) hemorrhagic A96.1
- malaria, malarial — *see* Malaria
- Malta A23.9
- Marseilles A77.1
- marsh — *see* Malaria
- Mayaro (viral) A92.8
- Mediterranean (*see also* Brucellosis) A23.9
  - familial M04.1
  - tick A77.1
- meningeal — *see* Meningitis
- Meuse A79.0
- Mexican A75.2
- mianeh A68.1
- miasmatic — *see* Malaria
- mosquito-borne (viral) A92.9
  - hemorrhagic A92.8
- mountain (*see also* Brucellosis)
  - meaning Rocky Mountain spotted fever A77.0
  - tick (American) (Colorado) (viral) A93.2
- Mucambo (viral) A92.8
- mud A27.9
- Neapolitan — *see* Brucellosis
- neutropenic D70.9
- newborn P81.9
  - environmental P81.0
- Nine-Mile A78
- non-exanthematous tick A93.2
- North Asian tick-borne A77.2
- Omsk hemorrhagic A98.1
- O'nyong-nyong (viral) A92.1
- Oropouche (viral) A93.0
- Oroya A44.0
- paludal — *see* Malaria
- Panama (malarial) B50.9
- Pappataci A93.1
- paratyphoid A01.4
  - A A01.1
  - B A01.2
  - C A01.3
- parrot A70

Fever — *continued*
- periodic (Mediterranean) M04.1
- persistent (of unknown origin) R50.9
- petechial A39.0
- pharyngoconjunctival B30.2
- Philippine hemorrhagic A91
- phlebotomus A93.1
- Piry (virus) A93.8
- Pixuna (viral) A92.8
- Plasmodium ovale B53.0
- polioviral (nonparalytic) A80.4
- Pontiac A48.2
- postimmunization R50.83
- postoperative R50.82
  - due to infection T81.40 ☑
- posttransfusion R50.84
- postvaccination R50.83
- presenting with conditions classified elsewhere R50.81
- pretibial A27.89
- puerperal O86.4
- Q A78
- quadrilateral A78
- quartan (malaria) B52.9
- Queensland (coastal) (tick) A77.3
- quintan A79.0
- rabbit — *see* Tularemia
- rat-bite A25.9
  - due to
    - Spirillum A25.0
    - Streptobacillus moniliformis A25.1
- recurrent — *see* Fever, relapsing
- relapsing (Borrelia) A68.9
  - Carter's (Asiatic) A68.1
  - Dutton's (West African) A68.1
  - Koch's A68.9
  - louse-borne A68.0
  - Novy's
    - louse-borne A68.0
    - tick-borne A68.1
  - Obermeyer's (European) A68.0
  - tick-borne A68.1
- remittent (bilious) (congestive) (gastric) — *see* Malaria
- rheumatic (active) (acute) (chronic) (subacute) I00
  - with central nervous system involvement I02.9
  - active with heart involvement — *see* category I01 ☑
  - inactive or quiescent with
    - cardiac hypertrophy I09.89
    - carditis I09.9
    - endocarditis I09.1
      - aortic (valve) I06.9
        - with mitral (valve) disease I08.0
      - mitral (valve) I05.9
        - with aortic (valve) disease I08.0
      - pulmonary (valve) I09.89
      - tricuspid (valve) I07.8
    - heart disease NEC I09.89
    - heart failure (congestive) (conditions in category I50. ☑) I09.81
    - left ventricular failure (conditions in I50.1- I50.4 ☑) I09.81
    - myocarditis, myocardial degeneration (conditions in I51.4) I09.0
    - pancarditis I09.9
    - pericarditis I09.2
- Rift Valley (viral) A92.4
- Rocky Mountain spotted A77.0
- rose J30.1
- Ross River B33.1
- Russian hemorrhagic A98.5
- San Joaquin (Valley) B38.0
- sandfly A93.1
- Sao Paulo A77.0
- scarlet A38.9
- seven day (leptospirosis) (autumnal) (Japanese) A27.89
  - dengue A90
- shin-bone A79.0
- Singapore hemorrhagic A91
- solar A90
- Songo A98.5
- sore B00.1
- South African tick-bite A68.1
- Southeast Asia hemorrhagic A91
- spinal — *see* Meningitis
- spirillary A25.0
- splenic — *see* Anthrax
- spotted A77.9
  - American A77.0
  - Brazilian A77.0
  - cerebrospinal meningitis A39.0

Fever — *continued*
- spotted — *continued*
  - Colombian A77.0
  - due to Rickettsia
    - australis A77.3
    - conorii A77.1
    - rickettsii A77.0
    - sibirica A77.2
    - specified type NEC A77.8
  - Ehrlichiosis A77.40
    - due to
      - E. chafeensis A77.41
      - specified organism NEC A77.49
  - Rocky Mountain A77.0
- steroid R50.2
- streptobacillary A25.1
- subtertian B50.9
- Sumatran mite A75.3
- sun A90
- swamp A27.9
- swine A02.8
- sylvatic, yellow A95.0
- Tahyna B33.8
- tertian — *see* Malaria, tertian
- Thailand hemorrhagic A91
- thermic T67.01 ☑
- three-day A93.1
- tick
  - American mountain A93.2
  - Colorado A93.2
  - Kemerovo A93.8
  - Mediterranean A77.1
  - mountain A93.2
  - nonexanthematous A93.2
  - Quaranfil A93.8
- tick-bite NEC A93.8
- tick-borne (hemorrhagic) NEC A93.8
- trench A79.0
- tsutsugamushi A75.3
- typhogastric A01.00
- typhoid (abortive) (hemorrhagic) (intermittent) (malignant) A01.00
  - complicated by
    - arthritis A01.04
    - heart involvement A01.02
    - meningitis A01.01
    - osteomyelitis A01.05
    - pneumonia A01.03
    - specified NEC A01.09
- typhomalarial — *see* Malaria
- typhus — *see* Typhus (fever)
- undulant — *see* Brucellosis
- unknown origin R50.9
- uveoparotid D86.89
- valley B38.0
- Venezuelan equine A92.2
- vesicular stomatitis A93.8
- viral hemorrhagic — *see* Fever, hemorrhagic, by type of virus
- Volhynian A79.0
- Wesselsbron (viral) A92.8
- West
  - African B50.8
  - Nile (viral) A92.30
    - with
      - complications NEC A92.39
      - cranial nerve disorders A92.32
      - encephalitis A92.31
      - encephalomyelitis A92.31
      - neurologic manifestation NEC A92.32
      - optic neuritis A92.32
      - polyradiculitis A92.32
- Whitmore's — *see* Melioidosis
- Wolhynian A79.0
- worm B83.9
- yellow A95.9
  - jungle A95.0
  - sylvatic A95.0
  - urban A95.1
- Zika virus A92.5

Fibrillation
- atrial or auricular (established) I48.91
  - chronic I48.20
    - persistent I48.19
  - paroxysmal I48.0
  - permanent I48.21
  - persistent (chronic) (NOS) (other) I48.19
    - longstanding I48.11
- cardiac I49.8
- heart I49.8
- muscular M62.89
- ventricular I49.01

Fibrin - Fibrosis

Fibrin
ball or bodies, pleural (sac) J94.1
chamber, anterior (eye) (gelatinous exudate) — see
Iridocyclitis, acute
Fibrinogenolysis — see Fibrinolysis
Fibrinogenopenia D68.8
acquired D65
congenital D68.2
Fibrinolysis (hemorrhagic) (acquired) D65
antepartum hemorrhage — see Hemorrhage,
antepartum, with coagulation defect
following
abortion — see Abortion by type complicated by
hemorrhage
ectopic or molar pregnancy O08.1
intrapartum O67.0
newborn, transient P60
postpartum O72.3
Fibrinopenia (hereditary) D68.2
acquired D68.4
Fibrinopurulent — see condition
Fibrinous — see condition
Fibroadenoma
cellular intracanalicular D24 ☑
giant D24 ☑
intracanalicular
cellular D24 ☑
giant D24 ☑
specified site — see Neoplasm, benign, by site
unspecified site D24 ☑
juvenile D24 ☑
pericanalicular
specified site — see Neoplasm, benign, by site
unspecified site D24 ☑
phyllodes D24 ☑
prostate D29.1
specified site NEC — see Neoplasm, benign, by site
unspecified site D24 ☑
Fibroadenosis, breast (chronic) (cystic) (diffuse)
(periodic) (segmental) N60.2 ☑
Fibroangioma (see also Neoplasm, benign, by site)
juvenile
specified site — see Neoplasm, benign, by site
unspecified site D10.6
Fibrochondrosarcoma — see Neoplasm, cartilage,
malignant
Fibrocystic
disease (see also Fibrosis, cystic)
breast — see Mastopathy, cystic
jaw M27.49
kidney (congenital) Q61.8
liver Q44.6
pancreas E84.9
kidney (congenital) Q61.8
Fibrodysplasia ossificans progressiva — see Myositis,
ossificans, progressiva
Fibroelastosis (cordis) (endocardial) (endomyocardial)
I42.4
Fibroid (tumor) (see also Neoplasm, connective tissue,
benign)
disease, lung (chronic) — see Fibrosis, lung
heart (disease) — see Myocarditis
in pregnancy or childbirth O34.1 ☑
causing obstructed labor O65.5
induration, lung (chronic) — see Fibrosis, lung
lung — see Fibrosis, lung
pneumonia (chronic) — see Fibrosis, lung
uterus (see also Leiomyoma, uterus) D25.9
Fibrolipoma — see Lipoma
Fibroliposarcoma — see Neoplasm, connective tissue,
malignant
Fibroma (see also Neoplasm, connective tissue, benign)
ameloblastic — see Cyst, calcifying odontogenic
bone (nonossifying) — see Disorder, bone, specified
type NEC
ossifying — see Neoplasm, bone, benign
cementifying — see Neoplasm, bone, benign
chondromyxoid — see Neoplasm, bone, benign
desmoplastic — see Neoplasm, connective tissue,
uncertain behavior
durum — see Neoplasm, connective tissue, benign
fascial — see Neoplasm, connective tissue, benign
invasive — see Neoplasm, connective tissue,
uncertain behavior
molle — see Lipoma
myxoid — see Neoplasm, connective tissue, benign
nasopharynx, nasopharyngeal (juvenile) D10.6
nonosteogenic (nonossifying) — see Dysplasia,
fibrous
odontogenic (central) — see Cyst, calcifying
odontogenic
ossifying — see Neoplasm, bone, benign

Fibroma — continued
periosteal — see Neoplasm, bone, benign
soft — see Lipoma
Fibromatosis M72.9
abdominal — see Neoplasm, connective tissue,
uncertain behavior
aggressive — see Neoplasm, connective tissue,
uncertain behavior
congenital generalized — see Neoplasm,
connective tissue, uncertain behavior
Dupuytren's M72.0
gingival K06.1
palmar (fascial) M72.0
plantar (fascial) M72.2
pseudosarcomatous (proliferative) (subcutaneous)
M72.4
retroperitoneal D48.3
specified NEC M72.8
Fibromyalgia M79.7
Fibromyoma (see also Neoplasm, connective tissue,
benign)
uterus (corpus) (see also Leiomyoma, uterus)
in pregnancy or childbirth — see Fibroid, in
pregnancy or childbirth
causing obstructed labor O65.5
Fibromyositis M79.7
Fibromyxolipoma D17.9
Fibromyxoma — see Neoplasm, connective tissue,
benign
Fibromyxosarcoma — see Neoplasm, connective
tissue, malignant
Fibro-odontoma, ameloblastic — see Cyst, calcifying
odontogenic
Fibro-osteoma — see Neoplasm, bone, benign
Fibroplasia, retrolental H35.17 ☑
Fibropurulent — see condition
Fibrosarcoma (see also Neoplasm, connective tissue,
malignant)
ameloblastic C41.1
upper jaw (bone) C41.0
congenital — see Neoplasm, connective tissue,
malignant
fascial — see Neoplasm, connective tissue,
malignant
infantile — see Neoplasm, connective tissue,
malignant
odontogenic C41.1
upper jaw (bone) C41.0
periosteal — see Neoplasm, bone, malignant
Fibrosclerosis
breast N60.3 ☑
multifocal M35.5
penis (corpora cavernosa) N48.6
Fibrosis, fibrotic
adrenal (gland) E27.8
amnion O41.8X ☑
anal papillae K62.89
arteriocapillary — see Arteriosclerosis
bladder N32.89
interstitial — see Cystitis, chronic, interstitial
localized submucosal — see Cystitis, chronic,
interstitial
panmural — see Cystitis, chronic, interstitial
breast — see Fibrosclerosis, breast
capillary (see also Arteriosclerosis) I70.90
lung (chronic) — see Fibrosis, lung
cardiac — see Myocarditis
cervix N88.8
chorion O41.8X ☑
corpus cavernosum (sclerosing) N48.6
cystic (of pancreas) E84.9
with
distal intestinal obstruction syndrome E84.19
fecal impaction E84.19
intestinal manifestations NEC E84.19
pulmonary manifestations E84.0
specified manifestations NEC E84.8
due to device, implant or graft (see also
Complications, by site and type, specified NEC)
T85.828 ☑
arterial graft NEC T82.828 ☑
breast (implant) T85.828 ☑
catheter NEC T85.828 ☑
dialysis (renal) T82.828 ☑
intraperitoneal T85.828 ☑
infusion NEC T82.828 ☑
spinal (epidural) (subdural) T85.820 ☑
urinary (indwelling) T83.82 ☑
electronic (electrode) (pulse generator)
(stimulator)
bone T84.82 ☑
cardiac T82.827 ☑

Fibrosis — continued
due to device — continued
nervous system (brain) (peripheral nerve)
(spinal) T85.820 ☑
urinary T83.82 ☑
fixation, internal (orthopedic) NEC T84.82 ☑
gastrointestinal (bile duct) (esophagus)
T85.828 ☑
genital NEC T83.82 ☑
heart NEC T82.827 ☑
joint prosthesis T84.82 ☑
ocular (corneal graft) (orbital implant) NEC
T85.828 ☑
orthopedic NEC T84.82 ☑
specified NEC T85.828 ☑
urinary NEC T83.82 ☑
vascular NEC T82.828 ☑
ventricular intracranial shunt T85.820 ☑
ejaculatory duct N50.89
endocardium — see Endocarditis
endomyocardial (tropical) I42.3
epididymis N50.89
eye muscle — see Strabismus, mechanical
heart — see Myocarditis
hepatic — see Fibrosis, liver
hepatolienal (portal hypertension) K76.6
hepatosplenic (portal hypertension) K76.6
infrapatellar fat pad M79.4
intrascrotal N50.89
kidney N26.9
liver K74.0
with sclerosis K74.2
alcoholic K70.2
lung (atrophic) (chronic) (confluent) (massive)
(perialveolar) (peribronchial) J84.10
with
anthracosilicosis J60
anthracosis J60
asbestosis J61
bagassosis J67.1
bauxite J63.1
berylliosis J63.2
byssinosis J66.0
calcicosis J62.8
chalicosis J62.8
dust reticulation J64
farmer's lung J67.0
ganister disease J62.8
graphite J63.3
pneumoconiosis NOS J64
siderosis J63.4
silicosis J62.8
capillary J84.10
congenital P27.8
diffuse (idiopathic) J84.10
chemicals, gases, fumes or vapors (inhalation)
J68.4
interstitial J84.10
acute J84.114
talc J62.0
following radiation J70.1
idiopathic J84.112
postinflammatory J84.10
silicotic J62.8
tuberculous — see Tuberculosis, pulmonary
lymphatic gland I89.8
median bar — see Hyperplasia, prostate
mediastinum (idiopathic) J98.59
meninges G96.19
myocardium, myocardial — see Myocarditis
ovary N83.8
oviduct N83.8
pancreas K86.89
penis NEC N48.6
pericardium I31.0
perineum, in pregnancy or childbirth O34.7 ☑
causing obstructed labor O65.5
pleura J94.1
popliteal fat pad M79.4
prostate (chronic) — see Hyperplasia, prostate
pulmonary (see also Fibrosis, lung) J84.10
congenital P27.8
idiopathic J84.112
rectal sphincter K62.89
retroperitoneal, idiopathic (with ureteral
obstruction) N13.5
with infection N13.6
sclerosing mesenteric (idiopathic) K65.4
scrotum N50.89
seminal vesicle N50.89
senile R54
skin L90.5

☑ **Additional character required**

Fibrosis — *continued*
  spermatic cord N50.89
  spleen D73.89
    in schistosomiasis (bilharziasis) B65.9 *[D77]*
  subepidermal nodular — *see* Neoplasm, skin, benign
  submucous (oral) (tongue) K13.5
  testis N44.8
    chronic, due to syphilis A52.76
  thymus (gland) E32.8
  tongue, submucous K13.5
  tunica vaginalis N50.89
  uterus (non-neoplastic) N85.8
  vagina N89.8
  valve, heart — *see* Endocarditis
  vas deferens N50.89
  vein I87.8
Fibrositis (periarticular) M79.7
  nodular, chronic (Jaccoud's) (rheumatoid) — *see*
    Arthropathy, postrheumatic, chronic
Fibrothorax J94.1
Fibrotic — *see* Fibrosis
Fibrous — *see* condition
Fibroxanthoma (*see also* Neoplasm, connective tissue, benign)
  atypical — *see* Neoplasm, connective tissue, uncertain behavior
  malignant — *see* Neoplasm, connective tissue, malignant
Fibroxanthosarcoma — *see* Neoplasm, connective tissue, malignant
Fiedler's
  disease (icterohemorrhagic leptospirosis) A27.0
  myocarditis (acute) I40.1
Fifth disease B08.3
  venereal A55
Filaria, filarial, filariasis — *see* Infestation, filarial
Filatov's disease — *see* Mononucleosis, infectious
File-cutter's disease — *see* Poisoning, lead
Filling defect
  biliary tract R93.2
  bladder R93.41
  duodenum R93.3
  gallbladder R93.2
  gastrointestinal tract R93.3
  intestine R93.3
  kidney R93.42 ☑
  stomach R93.3
  ureter R93.41
  urinary organs, specified NEC R93.49
Fimbrial cyst Q50.4
Financial problem affecting care NOS Z59.9
  bankruptcy Z59.8
  foreclosure on loan Z59.8
Findings, abnormal, inconclusive, without diagnosis (*see also* Abnormal)
  17-ketosteroids, elevated R82.5
  acetonuria R82.4
  alcohol in blood R78.0
  anisocytosis R71.8
  antenatal screening of mother O28.9
    biochemical O28.1
    chromosomal O28.5
    cytological O28.2
    genetic O28.5
    hematological O28.0
    radiological O28.4
    specified NEC O28.8
    ultrasonic O28.3
  antibody titer, elevated R76.0
  anticardiolipin antibody R76.0
  antiphosphatidylglycerol antibody R76.0
  antiphosphatidylinositol antibody R76.0
  antiphosphatidylserine antibody R76.0
  antiphospholipid antibody R76.0
  bacteriuria R82.71
  bicarbonate E87.8
  bile in urine R82.2
  blood sugar R73.09
    high R73.9
    low (transient) E16.2
  body fluid or substance, specified NEC R88.8
  casts, urine R82.998
  catecholamines R82.5
  cells, urine R82.998
  chloride E87.8
  cholesterol E78.9
    high E78.00
      with high triglycerides E78.2
  chyluria R82.0
  cloudy
    dialysis effluent R88.0
    urine R82.90

Findings — *continued*
  creatinine clearance R94.4
  crystals, urine R82.998
  culture
    blood R78.81
    positive — *see* Positive, culture
  echocardiogram R93.1
  electrolyte level, urinary R82.998
  function study NEC R94.8
    bladder R94.8
    endocrine NEC R94.7
      thyroid R94.6
    kidney R94.4
    liver R94.5
    pancreas R94.8
    placenta R94.8
    pulmonary R94.2
    spleen R94.8
  gallbladder, nonvisualization R93.2
  glucose (tolerance test) (non-fasting) R73.09
  glycosuria R81
  heart
    shadow R93.1
    sounds R01.2
  hematinuria R82.3
  hematocrit drop (precipitous) R71.0
  hemoglobinuria R82.3
  human papillomavirus (HPV) DNA test positive
    cervix
      high risk R87.810
      low risk R87.820
    vagina
      high risk R87.811
      low risk R87.821
  in blood (of substance not normally found in blood) R78.9
    addictive drug NEC R78.4
    alcohol (excessive level) R78.0
    cocaine R78.2
    hallucinogen R78.3
    heavy metals (abnormal level) R78.79
    lead R78.71
    lithium (abnormal level) R78.89
    opiate drug R78.1
    psychotropic drug R78.5
    specified substance NEC R78.89
    steroid agent R78.6
  indoleacetic acid, elevated R82.5
  ketonuria R82.4
  lactic acid dehydrogenase (LDH) R74.0
  liver function test R79.89
  mammogram NEC R92.8
    calcification (calculus) R92.1
    inconclusive result (due to dense breasts) R92.2
    microcalcification R92.0
  mediastinal shift R93.89
  melanin, urine R82.998
  myoglobinuria R82.1
  neonatal screening P09
  nonvisualization of gallbladder R93.2
  odor of urine NOS R82.90
  Papanicolaou cervix R87.619
    non-atypical endometrial cells R87.618
  pneumoencephalogram R93.0
  poikilocytosis R71.8
  potassium (deficiency) E87.6
    excess E87.5
  PPD R76.11
  radiologic (X-ray) R93.89
    abdomen R93.5
    biliary tract R93.2
    breast R92.8
    gastrointestinal tract R93.3
    genitourinary organs R93.89
    head R93.0
    inconclusive due to excess body fat of patient R93.9
    intrathoracic organs NEC R93.1
    musculoskeletal
      limbs R93.6
      other than limb R93.7
    placenta R93.89
    retroperitoneum R93.5
    skin R93.89
    skull R93.0
    subcutaneous tissue R93.89
    testis R93.81 ☑
  red blood cell (count) (morphology) (sickling) (volume) R71.8
  scan NEC R94.8
    bladder R94.8
    bone R94.8
    kidney R94.4

Findings — *continued*
  scan NEC — *continued*
    liver R93.2
    lung R94.2
    pancreas R94.8
    placental R94.8
    spleen R94.8
    thyroid R94.6
  sedimentation rate, elevated R70.0
  SGOT R74.0
  SGPT R74.0
  sodium (deficiency) E87.1
    excess E87.0
  specified body fluid NEC R88.8
  stress test R94.39
  thyroid (function) (metabolic rate) (scan) (uptake) R94.6
  transaminase (level) R74.0
  triglycerides E78.9
    high E78.1
      with high cholesterol E78.2
  tuberculin skin test (without active tuberculosis) R76.11
  urine R82.90
    acetone R82.4
    bacteria R82.71
    bile R82.2
    casts or cells R82.998
    chyle R82.0
    culture positive R82.79
    glucose R81
    hemoglobin R82.3
    ketone R82.4
    sugar R81
  vanillylmandelic acid (VMA), elevated R82.5
  vectorcardiogram (VCG) R94.39
  ventriculogram R93.0
  white blood cell (count) (differential) (morphology) D72.9
  xerography R92.8
Finger — *see* condition
Fire, Saint Anthony's — *see* Erysipelas
Fire-setting
  pathological (compulsive) F63.1
Fish hook stomach K31.89
Fishmeal-worker's lung J67.8
Fissure, fissured
  anus, anal K60.2
    acute K60.0
    chronic K60.1
    congenital Q43.8
  ear, lobule, congenital Q17.8
  epiglottis (congenital) Q31.8
  larynx J38.7
    congenital Q31.8
  lip K13.0
    congenital — *see* Cleft, lip
  nipple N64.0
    associated with
      lactation O92.13
      pregnancy O92.11 ☑
      puerperium O92.12
  nose Q30.2
  palate (congenital) — *see* Cleft, palate
  skin R23.4
  spine (congenital) (*see also* Spina bifida)
    with hydrocephalus — *see* Spina bifida, by site, with hydrocephalus
  tongue (acquired) K14.5
    congenital Q38.3
Fistula (cutaneous) L98.8
  abdomen (wall) K63.2
    bladder N32.2
    intestine NEC K63.2
    ureter N28.89
    uterus N82.5
  abdominorectal K63.2
  abdominosigmoidal K63.2
  abdominothoracic J86.0
  abdominouterine N82.5
    congenital Q51.7
  abdominovesical N32.2
  accessory sinuses — *see* Sinusitis
  actinomycotic — *see* Actinomycosis
  alveolar antrum — *see* Sinusitis, maxillary
  alveolar process K04.6
  anorectal K60.5
  antrobuccal — *see* Sinusitis, maxillary
  antrum — *see* Sinusitis, maxillary
  anus, anal (recurrent) (infectional) K60.3
    congenital Q43.6
      with absence, atresia and stenosis Q42.2
    tuberculous A18.32

Fistula

Fistula — *continued*
  aorta-duodenal I77.2
  appendix, appendicular K38.3
  arteriovenous (acquired) (nonruptured) I77.0
    brain I67.1
      congenital Q28.2
        ruptured — *see* Fistula, arteriovenous, brain,
          ruptured
      ruptured I60.8
        intracerebral I61.8
        intraparenchymal I61.8
        intraventricular I61.5
        subarachnoid I60.8
    cerebral — *see* Fistula, arteriovenous, brain
    congenital (peripheral) (*see also* Malformation,
      arteriovenous)
      brain Q28.2
        ruptured — *see* Fistula, arteriovenous, brain,
          ruptured
      coronary Q24.5
      pulmonary Q25.72
    coronary I25.41
      congenital Q24.5
    pulmonary I28.0
      congenital Q25.72
    surgically created (for dialysis) Z99.2
      complication — *see* Complication,
        arteriovenous, fistula, surgically created
    traumatic — *see* Injury, blood vessel
  artery I77.2
  aural (mastoid) — *see* Mastoiditis, chronic
  auricle (*see also* Disorder, pinna, specified type NEC)
    congenital Q18.1
  Bartholin's gland N82.8
  bile duct (common) (hepatic) K83.3
    with calculus, stones — *see* Calculus, bile duct
  biliary (tract) — *see* Fistula, bile duct
  bladder (sphincter) NEC (*see also* Fistula, vesico-)
    N32.2
    into seminal vesicle N32.2
  bone (*see also* Disorder, bone, specified type NEC)
    with osteomyelitis, chronic — *see* Osteomyelitis,
      chronic, with draining sinus
  brain G93.89
    arteriovenous (acquired) (*see also* Fistula,
      arteriovenous, brain) I67.1
      congenital Q28.2
  branchial (cleft) Q18.0
  branchiogenous Q18.0
  breast N61.0
    puerperal, postpartum or gestational, due to
      mastitis (purulent) — *see* Mastitis, obstetric,
      purulent
  bronchial J86.0
  bronchocutaneous, bronchomediastinal,
    bronchopleural, bronchopleuromediastinal
    (infective) J86.0
    tuberculous NEC A15.5
  bronchoesophageal J86.0
    congenital Q39.2
      with atresia of esophagus Q39.1
  bronchovisceral J86.0
  buccal cavity (infective) K12.2
  cecosigmoidal K63.2
  cecum K63.2
  cerebrospinal (fluid) G96.0
  cervical, lateral Q18.1
  cervicoaural Q18.1
  cervicosigmoidal N82.4
  cervicovesical N82.1
  cervix N82.8
  chest (wall) J86.0
  cholecystenteric — *see* Fistula, gallbladder
  cholecystocolic — *see* Fistula, gallbladder
  cholecystocolonic — *see* Fistula, gallbladder
  cholecystoduodenal — *see* Fistula, gallbladder
  cholecystogastric — *see* Fistula, gallbladder
  cholecystointestinal — *see* Fistula, gallbladder
  choledochoduodenal — *see* Fistula, bile duct
  cholocolic K82.3
  coccyx — *see* Sinus, pilonidal
  colon K63.2
  colostomy K94.09
  colovesical N32.1
  common duct — *see* Fistula, bile duct
  congenital, site not listed — *see* Anomaly, by site
  coronary, arteriovenous I25.41
    congenital Q24.5
  costal region J86.0
  cul-de-sac, Douglas' N82.8
  cystic duct (*see also* Fistula, gallbladder)
    congenital Q44.5

Fistula — *continued*
  dental K04.6
  diaphragm J86.0
  duodenum K31.6
  ear (external) (canal) — *see* Disorder, ear, external,
    specified type NEC
  enterocolic K63.2
  enterocutaneous K63.2
  enterouterine N82.4
    congenital Q51.7
  enterovaginal N82.4
    congenital Q52.2
    large intestine N82.3
    small intestine N82.2
  enterovesical N32.1
  epididymis N50.89
    tuberculous A18.15
  esophagobronchial J86.0
    congenital Q39.2
      with atresia of esophagus Q39.1
  esophagocutaneous K22.8
  esophagopleural-cutaneous J86.0
  esophagotracheal J86.0
    congenital Q39.2
      with atresia of esophagus Q39.1
  esophagus K22.8
    congenital Q39.2
      with atresia of esophagus Q39.1
  ethmoid — *see* Sinusitis, ethmoidal
  eyeball (cornea) (sclera) — *see* Disorder, globe, hypotony
  eyelid H01.8
  fallopian tube, external N82.5
  fecal K63.2
    congenital Q43.6
  from periapical abscess K04.6
  frontal sinus — *see* Sinusitis, frontal
  gallbladder K82.3
    with calculus, cholelithiasis, stones — *see*
      Calculus, gallbladder
  gastric K31.6
  gastrocolic K31.6
    congenital Q40.2
    tuberculous A18.32
  gastroenterocolic K31.6
  gastroesophageal K31.6
  gastrojejunal K31.6
  gastrojejunocolic K31.6
  genital tract (female) N82.9
    specified NEC N82.8
    to intestine NEC N82.4
    to skin N82.5
  hepatic artery-portal vein, congenital Q26.6
  hepatopleural J86.0
  hepatopulmonary J86.0
  ileorectal or ileosigmoidal K63.2
  ileovaginal N82.2
  ileovesical N32.1
  ileum K63.2
  in ano K60.3
    tuberculous A18.32
  inner ear (labyrinth) — *see* subcategory H83.1 ☑
  intestine NEC K63.2
  intestinocolonic (abdominal) K63.2
  intestinoureteral N28.89
  intestinouterine N82.4
  intestinovaginal N82.4
    large intestine N82.3
    small intestine N82.2
  intestinovesical N32.1
  ischiorectal (fossa) K61.39
  jejunum K63.2
  joint M25.10
    ankle M25.17 ☑
    elbow M25.12 ☑
    foot joint M25.17 ☑
    hand joint M25.14 ☑
    hip M25.15 ☑
    knee M25.16 ☑
    shoulder M25.11 ☑
    specified joint NEC M25.18
    tuberculous — *see* Tuberculosis, joint
    vertebrae M25.18
    wrist M25.13 ☑
  kidney N28.89
  labium (majus) (minus) N82.8
  labyrinth — *see* subcategory H83.1 ☑
  lacrimal (gland) (sac) H04.61 ☑
  lacrimonasal duct — *see* Fistula, lacrimal
  laryngotracheal, congenital Q34.8
  larynx J38.7
  lip K13.0
    congenital Q38.0

Fistula — *continued*
  lumbar, tuberculous A18.01
  lung J86.0
  lymphatic I89.8
  mammary (gland) N61.0
  mastoid (process) (region) — *see* Mastoiditis,
    chronic
  maxillary J32.0
  medial, face and neck Q18.8
  mediastinal J86.0
  mediastinobronchial J86.0
  mediastinocutaneous J86.0
  middle ear — *see* subcategory H74.8 ☑
  mouth K12.2
  nasal J34.89
    sinus — *see* Sinusitis
  nasopharynx J39.2
  nipple N64.0
  nose J34.89
  oral (cutaneous) K12.2
    maxillary J32.0
    nasal (with cleft palate) — *see* Cleft, palate
  orbit, orbital — *see* Disorder, orbit, specified type
    NEC
  oroantral J32.0
  oviduct, external N82.5
  palate (hard) M27.8
  pancreatic K86.89
  pancreaticoduodenal K86.89
  parotid (gland) K11.4
    region K12.2
  penis N48.89
  perianal K60.3
  pericardium (pleura) (sac) — *see* Pericarditis
  pericecal K63.2
  perineorectal K60.4
  perineosigmoidal K63.2
  perineum, perineal (with urethral involvement)
    NEC N36.0
    tuberculous A18.13
    ureter N28.89
  perirectal K60.4
    tuberculous A18.32
  peritoneum K65.9
  pharyngoesophageal J39.2
  pharynx J39.2
    branchial cleft (congenital) Q18.0
  pilonidal (infected) (rectum) — *see* Sinus, pilonidal
  pleura, pleural, pleurocutaneous, pleuroperitoneal
    J86.0
    tuberculous NEC A15.6
  pleuropericardial I31.8
  portal vein-hepatic artery, congenital Q26.6
  postauricular H70.81 ☑
  postoperative, persistent T81.83 ☑
    specified site — *see* Fistula, by site
  preauricular (congenital) Q18.1
  prostate N42.89
  pulmonary J86.0
    arteriovenous I28.0
      congenital Q25.72
    tuberculous — *see* Tuberculosis, pulmonary
  pulmonoperitoneal J86.0
  rectolabial N82.4
  rectosigmoid (intercommunicating) K63.2
  rectoureteral N28.89
  rectourethral N36.0
    congenital Q64.73
  rectouterine N82.4
    congenital Q51.7
  rectovaginal N82.3
    congenital Q52.2
    tuberculous A18.18
  rectovesical N32.1
    congenital Q64.79
  rectovesicovaginal N82.3
  rectovulval N82.4
    congenital Q52.79
  rectum (to skin) K60.4
    congenital Q43.6
      with absence, atresia and stenosis Q42.0
    tuberculous A18.32
  renal N28.89
  retroauricular — *see* Fistula, postauricular
  salivary duct or gland (any) K11.4
    congenital Q38.4
  scrotum (urinary) N50.89
    tuberculous A18.15
  semicircular canals — *see* subcategory H83.1 ☑
  sigmoid K63.2
    to bladder N32.1
  sinus — *see* Sinusitis

☑ **Additional character required**

Fistula — *continued*
skin L98.8
to genital tract (female) N82.5
splenocolic D73.89
stercoral K63.2
stomach K31.6
sublingual gland K11.4
submandibular gland K11.4
submaxillary (gland) K11.4
region K12.2
thoracic J86.0
duct I89.8
thoracoabdominal J86.0
thoracogastric J86.0
thoracointestinal J86.0
thorax J86.0
thyroglossal duct Q89.2
thyroid E07.89
trachea, congenital (external) (internal) Q32.1
tracheoesophageal J86.0
congenital Q39.2
with atresia of esophagus Q39.1
following tracheostomy J95.04
traumatic arteriovenous — *see* Injury, blood vessel, by site
tuberculous - code by site under Tuberculosis
typhoid A01.09
umbilicourinary Q64.8
urachus, congenital Q64.4
ureter (persistent) N28.89
ureteroabdominal N28.89
ureterorectal N28.89
ureterosigmoido-abdominal N28.89
ureterovaginal N82.1
ureterovesical N32.2
urethra N36.0
congenital Q64.79
tuberculous A18.13
urethroperineal N36.0
urethroperineovesical N32.2
urethrorectal N36.0
congenital Q64.73
urethroscrotal N50.89
urethrovaginal N82.1
urethrovesical N32.2
urinary (tract) (persistent) (recurrent) N36.0
uteroabdominal N82.5
congenital Q51.7
uteroenteric, uterointestinal N82.4
congenital Q51.7
uterorectal N82.4
congenital Q51.7
uteroureteric N82.1
uterourethral Q51.7
uterovaginal N82.8
uterovesical N82.1
congenital Q51.7
uterus N82.8
vagina (postpartal) (wall) N82.8
vaginocutaneous (postpartal) N82.5
vaginointestinal NEC N82.4
large intestine N82.3
small intestine N82.2
vaginoperineal N82.5
vasocutaneous, congenital Q55.7
vesical NEC N32.2
vesicoabdominal N32.2
vesicocervicovaginal N82.1
vesicocolic N32.1
vesicocutaneous N32.2
vesicoenteric N32.1
vesicointestinal N32.1
vesicometrorectal N82.4
vesicoperineal N32.2
vesicorectal N32.1
congenital Q64.79
vesicosigmoidal N32.1
vesicosigmoidovaginal N82.3
vesicoureteral N32.2
vesicoureterovaginal N82.1
vesicourethral N32.2
vesicourethrorectal N32.1
vesicouterine N82.1
congenital Q51.7
vesicovaginal N82.0
vulvorectal N82.4
congenital Q52.79
Fit R56.9
epileptic — *see* Epilepsy
fainting R55
hysterical F44.5
newborn P90

Fitting (and adjustment) (of)
artificial
arm — *see* Admission, adjustment, artificial, arm
breast Z44.3 ☑
eye Z44.2 ☑
leg — *see* Admission, adjustment, artificial, leg
automatic implantable cardiac defibrillator (with synchronous cardiac pacemaker) Z45.02
brain neuropacemaker Z46.2
implanted Z45.42
cardiac defibrillator — *see* Fitting (and adjustment) (of), automatic implantable cardiac defibrillator
catheter, non-vascular Z46.82
colostomy belt Z46.89
contact lenses Z46.0
CRT-D (resynchronization therapy defibrillator) Z45.02
CRT-P (cardiac resynchronization therapy pacemaker) Z45.018
pulse generator Z45.010
cystostomy device Z46.6
defibrillator, cardiac — *see* Fitting (and adjustment) (of), automatic implantable cardiac defibrillator
dentures Z46.3
device NOS Z46.9
abdominal Z46.89
gastrointestinal NEC Z46.59
implanted NEC Z45.89
nervous system Z46.2
implanted — *see* Admission, adjustment, device, implanted, nervous system
orthodontic Z46.4
orthoptic Z46.0
orthotic Z46.89
prosthetic (external) Z44.9
breast Z44.3 ☑
dental Z46.3
eye Z44.2 ☑
specified NEC Z44.8
specified NEC Z46.89
substitution
auditory Z46.2
implanted — *see* Admission, adjustment, device, implanted, hearing device
nervous system Z46.2
implanted — *see* Admission, adjustment, device, implanted, nervous system
visual Z46.2
implanted Z45.31
urinary Z46.6
gastric lap band Z46.51
gastrointestinal appliance NEC Z46.59
glasses (reading) Z46.0
hearing aid Z46.1
ileostomy device Z46.89
insulin pump Z46.81
intestinal appliance NEC Z46.89
myringotomy device (stent) (tube) Z45.82
neuropacemaker Z46.2
implanted Z45.42
non-vascular catheter Z46.82
orthodontic device Z46.4
orthopedic device (brace) (cast) (corset) (shoes) Z46.89
pacemaker (cardiac) (cardiac resynchronization therapy (CRT-P)) Z45.018
nervous system (brain) (peripheral nerve) (spinal cord) Z46.2
implanted Z45.42
pulse generator Z45.010
portacath (port-a-cath) Z45.2
prosthesis (external) Z44.9
arm — *see* Admission, adjustment, artificial, arm
breast Z44.3 ☑
dental Z46.3
eye Z44.2 ☑
leg — *see* Admission, adjustment, artificial, leg
specified NEC Z44.8
spectacles Z46.0
wheelchair Z46.89
Fitzhugh-Curtis syndrome
due to
Chlamydia trachomatis A74.81
Neisseria gonorrhoea (gonococcal peritonitis) A54.85
Fitz's syndrome (acute hemorrhagic pancreatitis) (*see also* Pancreatitis, acute) K85.80
Fixation
joint — *see* Ankylosis
larynx J38.7
stapes — *see* Ankylosis, ear ossicles
deafness — *see* Deafness, conductive

Fixation — *continued*
uterus (acquired) — *see* Malposition, uterus
vocal cord J38.3
Flabby ridge K06.8
Flaccid (*see also* condition)
palate, congenital Q38.5
Flail
chest S22.5 ☑
newborn (birth injury) P13.8
joint (paralytic) M25.20
ankle M25.27 ☑
elbow M25.22 ☑
foot joint M25.27 ☑
hand joint M25.24 ☑
hip M25.25 ☑
knee M25.26 ☑
shoulder M25.21 ☑
specified joint NEC M25.28
wrist M25.23 ☑
Flajani's disease — *see* Hyperthyroidism, with, goiter (diffuse)
Flap, liver K71.3
Flashbacks (residual to hallucinogen use) F16.283
Flat
chamber (eye) — *see* Disorder, globe, hypotony, flat anterior chamber
chest, congenital Q67.8
foot (acquired) (fixed type) (painful) (postural) (*see also* Deformity, limb, flat foot)
congenital (rigid) (spastic) (everted) Q66.5 ☑
rachitic sequelae (late effect) E64.3
organ or site, congenital NEC — *see* Anomaly, by site
pelvis M95.5
with disproportion (fetopelvic) O33.0
causing obstructed labor O65.0
congenital Q74.2
Flatau-Schilder disease G37.0
Flatback syndrome M40.30
lumbar region M40.36
lumbosacral region M40.37
thoracolumbar region M40.35
Flattening
head, femur M89.8X5
hip — *see* Coxa, plana
lip (congenital) Q18.8
nose (congenital) Q67.4
acquired M95.0
Flatulence R14.3
psychogenic F45.8
Flatus R14.3
vaginalis N89.8
Flax-dresser's disease J66.1
Flea bite — *see* Injury, bite, by site, superficial, insect
Flecks, glaucomatous (subcapsular) — *see* Cataract, complicated
Fleischer (-Kayser) ring (cornea) H18.04 ☑
Fleshy mole O02.0
Flexibilitas cerea — *see* Catalepsy
Flexion
amputation stump (surgical) T87.89
cervix — *see* Malposition, uterus
contracture, joint — *see* Contraction, joint
deformity, joint (*see also* Deformity, limb, flexion) M21.20
hip, congenital Q65.89
uterus (*see also* Malposition, uterus)
lateral — *see* Lateroversion, uterus
Flexner-Boyd dysentery A03.2
Flexner's dysentery A03.1
Flexure — *see* Flexion
Flint murmur (aortic insufficiency) I35.1
Floater, vitreous — *see* Opacity, vitreous
Floating
cartilage (joint) (*see also* Loose, body, joint)
knee — *see* Derangement, knee, loose body
gallbladder, congenital Q44.1
kidney N28.89
congenital Q63.8
spleen D73.89
Flooding N92.0
Floor — *see* condition
Floppy
baby syndrome (nonspecific) P94.2
iris syndrome (intraoperative) (IFIS) H21.81
nonrheumatic mitral valve syndrome I34.1
Flu (*see also* Influenza)
avian (*see also* Influenza, due to, identified novel influenza A virus) J09.X2
bird (*see also* Influenza, due to, identified novel influenza A virus) J09.X2
intestinal NEC A08.4

Flu — continued
swine (viruses that normally cause infections in pigs) (see also Influenza, due to, identified novel influenza A virus) J09.X2
Fluctuating blood pressure I99.8
Fluid
abdomen R18.8
chest J94.8
heart — see Failure, heart, congestive
joint — see Effusion, joint
loss (acute) E86.9
lung — see Edema, lung
overload E87.70
specified NEC E87.79
peritoneal cavity R18.8
pleural cavity J94.8
retention R60.9
Flukes NEC (see also Infestation, fluke)
blood NEC — see Schistosomiasis
liver B66.3
Fluor (vaginalis) N89.8
trichomonal or due to Trichomonas (vaginalis) A59.00
Fluorosis
dental K00.3
skeletal M85.10
ankle M85.17 ☑
foot M85.17 ☑
forearm M85.13 ☑
hand M85.14 ☑
lower leg M85.16 ☑
multiple site M85.19
neck M85.18
rib M85.18
shoulder M85.11 ☑
skull M85.18
specified site NEC M85.18
thigh M85.15 ☑
toe M85.17 ☑
upper arm M85.12 ☑
vertebra M85.18
Flush syndrome E34.0
Flushing R23.2
menopausal N95.1
Flutter
atrial or auricular I48.92
atypical I48.4
type I I48.3
type II I48.4
typical I48.3
heart I49.8
atrial or auricular I48.92
atypical I48.4
type I I48.3
type II I48.4
typical I48.3
ventricular I49.02
ventricular I49.02
FNHTR (febrile nonhemolytic transfusion reaction) R50.84
Fochier's abscess - code by site under Abscess
Focus, Assmann's — see Tuberculosis, pulmonary
Fogo selvagem L10.3
Foix-Alajouanine syndrome G95.19
Fold, folds (anomalous) (see also Anomaly, by site)
Descemet's membrane — see Change, corneal membrane, Descemet's, fold
epicanthic Q10.3
heart Q24.8
Folie à deux F24
Follicle
cervix (nabothian) (ruptured) N88.8
graafian, ruptured, with hemorrhage N83.0 ☑
nabothian N88.8
Follicular — see condition
Folliculitis (superficial) L73.9
abscedens et suffodiens L66.3
cyst N83.0 ☑
decalvans L66.2
deep — see Furuncle, by site
gonococcal (acute) (chronic) A54.01
keloid, keloidalis L73.0
pustular L01.02
ulerythematosa reticulata L66.4
Folliculome lipidique
specified site — see Neoplasm, benign, by site
unspecified site
female D27.9
male D29.20
Følling's disease E70.0
Follow-up — see Examination, follow-up

Fong's syndrome (hereditary osteo-onychodysplasia) Q87.2
Food
allergy L27.2
asphyxia (from aspiration or inhalation) — see Foreign body, by site
choked on — see Foreign body, by site
deprivation T73.0 ☑
specified kind of food NEC E63.8
intoxication — see Poisoning, food
lack of T73.0 ☑
poisoning — see Poisoning, food
rejection NEC — see Disorder, eating
strangulation or suffocation — see Foreign body, by site
toxemia — see Poisoning, food
Foot — see condition
Foramen ovale (nonclosure) (patent) (persistent) Q21.1
Forbes' glycogen storage disease E74.03
Fordyce-Fox disease L75.2
Fordyce's disease (mouth) Q38.6
Forearm — see condition
Foreign body
with
laceration — see Laceration, by site, with foreign body
puncture wound — see Puncture, by site, with foreign body
accidentally left following a procedure T81.509 ☑
aspiration T81.506 ☑
resulting in
adhesions T81.516 ☑
obstruction T81.526 ☑
perforation T81.536 ☑
specified complication NEC T81.596 ☑
cardiac catheterization T81.505 ☑
resulting in
acute reaction T81.60 ☑
aseptic peritonitis T81.61 ☑
specified NEC T81.69 ☑
adhesions T81.515 ☑
obstruction T81.525 ☑
perforation T81.535 ☑
specified complication NEC T81.595 ☑
causing
acute reaction T81.60 ☑
aseptic peritonitis T81.61 ☑
specified complication NEC T81.69 ☑
adhesions T81.519 ☑
aseptic peritonitis T81.61 ☑
obstruction T81.529 ☑
perforation T81.539 ☑
specified complication NEC T81.599 ☑
endoscopy T81.504 ☑
resulting in
adhesions T81.514 ☑
obstruction T81.524 ☑
perforation T81.534 ☑
specified complication NEC T81.594 ☑
immunization T81.503 ☑
resulting in
adhesions T81.513 ☑
obstruction T81.523 ☑
perforation T81.533 ☑
specified complication NEC T81.593 ☑
infusion T81.501 ☑
resulting in
adhesions T81.511 ☑
obstruction T81.521 ☑
perforation T81.531 ☑
specified complication NEC T81.591 ☑
injection T81.503 ☑
resulting in
adhesions T81.513 ☑
obstruction T81.523 ☑
perforation T81.533 ☑
specified complication NEC T81.593 ☑
kidney dialysis T81.502 ☑
resulting in
adhesions T81.512 ☑
obstruction T81.522 ☑
perforation T81.532 ☑
specified complication NEC T81.592 ☑
packing removal T81.507 ☑
resulting in
acute reaction T81.60 ☑
aseptic peritonitis T81.61 ☑
specified NEC T81.69 ☑
adhesions T81.517 ☑
obstruction T81.527 ☑
perforation T81.537 ☑
specified complication NEC T81.597 ☑

Foreign body — continued
accidentally left following a procedure — continued
puncture T81.506 ☑
resulting in
adhesions T81.516 ☑
obstruction T81.526 ☑
perforation T81.536 ☑
specified complication NEC T81.596 ☑
specified procedure NEC T81.508 ☑
resulting in
acute reaction T81.60 ☑
aseptic peritonitis T81.61 ☑
specified NEC T81.69 ☑
adhesions T81.518 ☑
obstruction T81.528 ☑
perforation T81.538 ☑
specified complication NEC T81.598 ☑
surgical operation T81.500 ☑
resulting in
acute reaction T81.60 ☑
aseptic peritonitis T81.61 ☑
specified NEC T81.69 ☑
adhesions T81.510 ☑
obstruction T81.520 ☑
perforation T81.530 ☑
specified complication NEC T81.590 ☑
transfusion T81.501 ☑
resulting in
adhesions T81.511 ☑
obstruction T81.521 ☑
perforation T81.531 ☑
specified complication NEC T81.591 ☑
alimentary tract T18.9 ☑
anus T18.5 ☑
colon T18.4 ☑
esophagus — see Foreign body, esophagus
mouth T18.0 ☑
multiple sites T18.8 ☑
rectosigmoid (junction) T18.5 ☑
rectum T18.5 ☑
small intestine T18.3 ☑
specified site NEC T18.8 ☑
stomach T18.2 ☑
anterior chamber (eye) S05.5 ☑
auditory canal — see Foreign body, entering through orifice, ear
bronchus T17.508 ☑
causing
asphyxiation T17.500 ☑
food (bone) (seed) T17.520 ☑
gastric contents (vomitus) T17.510 ☑
specified type NEC T17.590 ☑
injury NEC T17.508 ☑
food (bone) (seed) T17.528 ☑
gastric contents (vomitus) T17.518 ☑
specified type NEC T17.598 ☑
canthus — see Foreign body, conjunctival sac
ciliary body (eye) S05.5 ☑
conjunctival sac T15.1 ☑
cornea T15.0 ☑
entering through orifice
accessory sinus T17.0 ☑
alimentary canal T18.9 ☑
multiple parts T18.8 ☑
specified part NEC T18.8 ☑
alveolar process T18.0 ☑
antrum (Highmore's) T17.0 ☑
anus T18.5 ☑
appendix T18.4 ☑
auditory canal — see Foreign body, entering through orifice, ear
auricle — see Foreign body, entering through orifice, ear
bladder T19.1 ☑
bronchioles — see Foreign body, respiratory tract, specified site NEC
bronchus (main) — see Foreign body, bronchus
buccal cavity T18.0 ☑
canthus (inner) — see Foreign body, conjunctival sac
cecum T18.4 ☑
cervix (canal) (uteri) T19.3 ☑
colon T18.4 ☑
conjunctival sac — see Foreign body, conjunctival sac
cornea — see Foreign body, cornea
digestive organ or tract NOS T18.9 ☑
multiple parts T18.8 ☑
specified part NEC T18.8 ☑
duodenum T18.3 ☑
ear (external) T16. ☑
esophagus — see Foreign body, esophagus

☑ **Additional character required**

Foreign body — *continued*

entering through orifice — *continued*

eye (external) NOS T15.9 ☑
  conjunctival sac — *see* Foreign body, conjunctival sac
  cornea — *see* Foreign body, cornea
  specified part NEC T15.8 ☑
eyeball (*see also* Foreign body, entering through orifice, eye, specified part NEC)
  with penetrating wound — *see* Puncture, eyeball
eyelid (*see also* Foreign body, conjunctival sac) with
  laceration — *see* Laceration, eyelid, with foreign body
  puncture — *see* Puncture, eyelid, with foreign body
  superficial injury — *see* Foreign body, superficial, eyelid
gastrointestinal tract T18.9 ☑
  multiple parts T18.8 ☑
  specified part NEC T18.8 ☑
genitourinary tract T19.9 ☑
  multiple parts T19.8 ☑
  specified part NEC T19.8 ☑
globe — *see* Foreign body, entering through orifice, eyeball
gum T18.0 ☑
Highmore's antrum T17.0 ☑
hypopharynx — *see* Foreign body, pharynx
ileum T18.3 ☑
intestine (small) T18.3 ☑
  large T18.4 ☑
lacrimal apparatus (punctum) — *see* Foreign body, entering through orifice, eye, specified part NEC
large intestine T18.4 ☑
larynx — *see* Foreign body, larynx
lung — *see* Foreign body, respiratory tract, specified site NEC
maxillary sinus T17.0 ☑
mouth T18.0 ☑
nasal sinus T17.0 ☑
nasopharynx — *see* Foreign body, pharynx
nose (passage) T17.1 ☑
nostril T17.1 ☑
oral cavity T18.0 ☑
palate T18.0 ☑
penis T19.4 ☑
pharynx — *see* Foreign body, pharynx
piriform sinus — *see* Foreign body, pharynx
rectosigmoid (junction) T18.5 ☑
rectum T18.5 ☑
respiratory tract — *see* Foreign body, respiratory tract
sinus (accessory) (frontal) (maxillary) (nasal) T17.0 ☑
  piriform — *see* Foreign body, pharynx
small intestine T18.3 ☑
stomach T18.2 ☑
suffocation by — *see* Foreign body, by site
tear ducts or glands — *see* Foreign body, entering through orifice, eye, specified part NEC
throat — *see* Foreign body, pharynx
tongue T18.0 ☑
tonsil, tonsillar (fossa) — *see* Foreign body, pharynx
trachea — *see* Foreign body, trachea
ureter T19.8 ☑
urethra T19.0 ☑
uterus (any part) T19.3 ☑
vagina T19.2 ☑
vulva T19.2 ☑
esophagus T18.108 ☑
  causing
    injury NEC T18.108 ☑
      food (bone) (seed) T18.128 ☑
      gastric contents (vomitus) T18.118 ☑
      specified type NEC T18.198 ☑
    tracheal compression T18.100 ☑
      food (bone) (seed) T18.120 ☑
      gastric contents (vomitus) T18.110 ☑
      specified type NEC T18.190 ☑
feeling of, in throat R09.89
fragment — *see* Retained, foreign body fragments (type of)
genitourinary tract T19.9 ☑
  bladder T19.1 ☑
  multiple parts T19.8 ☑
  penis T19.4 ☑
  specified site NEC T19.8 ☑
  urethra T19.0 ☑

Foreign body — *continued*

genitourinary tract — *continued*

  uterus T19.3 ☑
    IUD Z97.5
  vagina T19.2 ☑
    contraceptive device Z97.5
  vulva T19.2 ☑
granuloma (old) (soft tissue) (*see also* Granuloma, foreign body)
  skin L92.3
in
  laceration — *see* Laceration, by site, with foreign body
  puncture wound — *see* Puncture, by site, with foreign body
  soft tissue (residual) M79.5
inadvertently left in operation wound — *see* Foreign body, accidentally left during a procedure
ingestion, ingested NOS T18.9 ☑
inhalation or inspiration — *see* Foreign body, by site
internal organ, not entering through a natural orifice - code as specific injury with foreign body
intraocular S05.5 ☑
  old, retained (nonmagnetic) H44.70 ☑
    anterior chamber H44.71 ☑
    ciliary body H44.72 ☑
    iris H44.72 ☑
    lens H44.73 ☑
    magnetic H44.60 ☑
      anterior chamber H44.61 ☑
      ciliary body H44.62 ☑
      iris H44.62 ☑
      lens H44.63 ☑
      posterior wall H44.64 ☑
      specified site NEC H44.69 ☑
      vitreous body H44.65 ☑
    posterior wall H44.74 ☑
    specified site NEC H44.79 ☑
    vitreous body H44.75 ☑
iris — *see* Foreign body, intraocular
lacrimal punctum — *see* Foreign body, entering through orifice, eye, specified part NEC
larynx T17.308 ☑
  causing
    asphyxiation T17.300 ☑
      food (bone) (seed) T17.320 ☑
      gastric contents (vomitus) T17.310 ☑
      specified type NEC T17.390 ☑
    injury NEC T17.308 ☑
      food (bone) (seed) T17.328 ☑
      gastric contents (vomitus) T17.318 ☑
      specified type NEC T17.398 ☑
lens — *see* Foreign body, intraocular
ocular muscle S05.4 ☑
  old, retained — *see* Foreign body, orbit, old
old or residual
  soft tissue (residual) M79.5
operation wound, left accidentally — *see* Foreign body, accidentally left during a procedure
orbit S05.4 ☑
  old, retained H05.5 ☑
pharynx T17.208 ☑
  causing
    asphyxiation T17.200 ☑
      food (bone) (seed) T17.220 ☑
      gastric contents (vomitus) T17.210 ☑
      specified type NEC T17.290 ☑
    injury NEC T17.208 ☑
      food (bone) (seed) T17.228 ☑
      gastric contents (vomitus) T17.218 ☑
      specified type NEC T17.298 ☑
respiratory tract T17.908 ☑
  bronchioles — *see* Foreign body, respiratory tract, specified site NEC
  bronchus — *see* Foreign body, bronchus
  causing
    asphyxiation T17.900 ☑
      food (bone) (seed) T17.920 ☑
      gastric contents (vomitus) T17.910 ☑
      specified type NEC T17.990 ☑
    injury NEC T17.908 ☑
      food (bone) (seed) T17.928 ☑
      gastric contents (vomitus) T17.918 ☑
      specified type NEC T17.998 ☑
  larynx — *see* Foreign body, larynx
  lung — *see* Foreign body, respiratory tract, specified site NEC
  multiple parts — *see* Foreign body, respiratory tract, specified site NEC
  nasal sinus T17.0 ☑

Foreign body — *continued*

respiratory tract — *continued*

  nasopharynx — *see* Foreign body, pharynx
  nose T17.1 ☑
  nostril T17.1 ☑
  pharynx — *see* Foreign body, pharynx
  specified site NEC T17.808 ☑
    causing
      asphyxiation T17.800 ☑
        food (bone) (seed) T17.820 ☑
        gastric contents (vomitus) T17.810 ☑
        specified type NEC T17.890 ☑
      injury NEC T17.808 ☑
        food (bone) (seed) T17.828 ☑
        gastric contents (vomitus) T17.818 ☑
        specified type NEC T17.898 ☑
  throat — *see* Foreign body, pharynx
  trachea — *see* Foreign body, trachea
retained (old) (nonmagnetic) (in)
  anterior chamber (eye) — *see* Foreign body, intraocular, old, retained, anterior chamber
    magnetic — *see* Foreign body, intraocular, old, retained, magnetic, anterior chamber
  ciliary body — *see* Foreign body, intraocular, old, retained, ciliary body
    magnetic — *see* Foreign body, intraocular, old, retained, magnetic, ciliary body
  eyelid H02.819
    left H02.816
      lower H02.815
      upper H02.814
    right H02.813
      lower H02.812
      upper H02.811
  fragments — *see* Retained, foreign body fragments (type of)
  globe — *see* Foreign body, intraocular, old, retained
    magnetic — *see* Foreign body, intraocular, old, retained, magnetic
  intraocular — *see* Foreign body, intraocular, old, retained
    magnetic — *see* Foreign body, intraocular, old, retained, magnetic
  iris — *see* Foreign body, intraocular, old, retained, iris
    magnetic — *see* Foreign body, intraocular, old, retained, magnetic, iris
  lens — *see* Foreign body, intraocular, old, retained, lens
    magnetic — *see* Foreign body, intraocular, old, retained, magnetic, lens
  muscle — *see* Foreign body, retained, soft tissue
  orbit — *see* Foreign body, orbit, old
  posterior wall of globe — *see* Foreign body, intraocular, old, retained, posterior wall
    magnetic — *see* Foreign body, intraocular, old, retained, magnetic, posterior wall
  retrobulbar — *see* Foreign body, orbit, old, retrobulbar
  soft tissue M79.5
  vitreous — *see* Foreign body, intraocular, old, retained, vitreous body
    magnetic — *see* Foreign body, intraocular, old, retained, magnetic, vitreous body
retina S05.5 ☑
superficial, without open wound
  abdomen, abdominal (wall) S30.851 ☑
  alveolar process S00.552 ☑
  ankle S90.55 ☑
  antecubital space — *see* Foreign body, superficial, forearm
  anus S30.857 ☑
  arm (upper) S40.85 ☑
  auditory canal — *see* Foreign body, superficial, ear
  auricle — *see* Foreign body, superficial, ear
  axilla — *see* Foreign body, superficial, arm
  back, lower S30.850 ☑
  breast S20.15 ☑
  brow S00.85 ☑
  buttock S30.850 ☑
  calf — *see* Foreign body, superficial, leg
  canthus — *see* Foreign body, superficial, eyelid
  cheek S00.85 ☑
    internal S00.552 ☑
  chest wall — *see* Foreign body, superficial, thorax
  chin S00.85 ☑
  clitoris S30.854 ☑
  costal region — *see* Foreign body, superficial, thorax
  digit(s)
    hand — *see* Foreign body, superficial, finger
    foot — *see* Foreign body, superficial, toe

Foreign body — *continued*
  superficial — *continued*
    ear S00.45 ☑
    elbow S50.35 ☑
    epididymis S30.853 ☑
    epigastric region S30.851 ☑
    epiglottis S10.15 ☑
    esophagus, cervical S10.15 ☑
    eyebrow — *see* Foreign body, superficial, eyelid
    eyelid S00.25 ☑
    face S00.85 ☑
    finger(s) S60.459 ☑
      index S60.45 ☑
      little S60.45 ☑
      middle S60.45 ☑
      ring S60.45 ☑
    flank S30.851 ☑
    foot (except toe(s) alone) S90.85 ☑
      toe — *see* Foreign body, superficial, toe
    forearm S50.85 ☑
      elbow only — *see* Foreign body, superficial, elbow
    forehead S00.85 ☑
    genital organs, external
      female S30.856 ☑
      male S30.855 ☑
    groin S30.851 ☑
    gum S00.552 ☑
    hand S60.55 ☑
    head S00.95 ☑
      ear — *see* Foreign body, superficial, ear
      eyelid — *see* Foreign body, superficial, eyelid
      lip S00.551 ☑
      nose S00.35 ☑
      oral cavity S00.552 ☑
      scalp S00.05 ☑
      specified site NEC S00.85 ☑
    heel — *see* Foreign body, superficial, foot
    hip S70.25 ☑
    inguinal region S30.851 ☑
    interscapular region S20.459 ☑
    jaw S00.85 ☑
    knee S80.25 ☑
    labium (majus) (minus) S30.854 ☑
    larynx S10.15 ☑
    leg (lower) S80.85 ☑
      knee — *see* Foreign body, superficial, knee
      upper — *see* Foreign body, superficial, thigh
    lip S00.551 ☑
    lower back S30.850 ☑
    lumbar region S30.850 ☑
    malar region S00.85 ☑
    mammary — *see* Foreign body, superficial, breast
    mastoid region S00.85 ☑
    mouth S00.552 ☑
    nail
      finger — *see* Foreign body, superficial, finger
      toe — *see* Foreign body, superficial, toe
    nape S10.85 ☑
    nasal S00.35 ☑
    neck S10.95 ☑
      specified site NEC S10.85 ☑
      throat S10.15 ☑
    nose S00.35 ☑
    occipital region S00.05 ☑
    oral cavity S00.552 ☑
    orbital region — *see* Foreign body, superficial, eyelid
    palate S00.552 ☑
    palm — *see* Foreign body, superficial, hand
    parietal region S00.05 ☑
    pelvis S30.850 ☑
    penis S30.852 ☑
    perineum
      female S30.854 ☑
      male S30.850 ☑
    periocular area — *see* Foreign body, superficial, eyelid
    phalanges
      finger — *see* Foreign body, superficial, finger
      toe — *see* Foreign body, superficial, toe
    pharynx S10.15 ☑
    pinna — *see* Foreign body, superficial, ear
    popliteal space — *see* Foreign body, superficial, knee
    prepuce S30.852 ☑
    pubic region S30.850 ☑
    pudendum
      female S30.856 ☑
      male S30.855 ☑
    sacral region S30.850 ☑
    scalp S00.05 ☑

Foreign body — *continued*
  superficial — *continued*
    scapular region — *see* Foreign body, superficial, shoulder
    scrotum S30.853 ☑
    shin — *see* Foreign body, superficial, leg
    shoulder S40.25 ☑
    sternal region S20.359 ☑
    submaxillary region S00.85 ☑
    submental region S00.85 ☑
    subungual
      finger(s) — *see* Foreign body, superficial, finger
      toe(s) — *see* Foreign body, superficial, toe
    supraclavicular fossa S10.85 ☑
    supraorbital S00.85 ☑
    temple S00.85 ☑
    temporal region S00.85 ☑
    testis S30.853 ☑
    thigh S70.35 ☑
    thorax, thoracic (wall) S20.95 ☑
      back S20.45 ☑
      front S20.35 ☑
    throat S10.15 ☑
    thumb S60.35 ☑
    toe(s) (lesser) S90.456 ☑
      great S90.45 ☑
    tongue S00.552 ☑
    trachea S10.15 ☑
    tunica vaginalis S30.853 ☑
    tympanum, tympanic membrane — *see* Foreign body, superficial, ear
    uvula S00.552 ☑
    vagina S30.854 ☑
    vocal cords S10.15 ☑
    vulva S30.854 ☑
    wrist S60.85 ☑
  swallowed T18.9 ☑
  trachea T17.408 ☑
    causing
      asphyxiation T17.400 ☑
        food (bone) (seed) T17.420 ☑
        gastric contents (vomitus) T17.410 ☑
        specified type NEC T17.490 ☑
      injury NEC T17.408 ☑
        food (bone) (seed) T17.428 ☑
        gastric contents (vomitus) T17.418 ☑
        specified type NEC T17.498 ☑
  type of fragment — *see* Retained, foreign body fragments (type of)
  vitreous (humor) S05.5 ☑

Forestier's disease (rhizomelic pseudopolyarthritis) M35.3
  meaning ankylosing hyperostosis — *see* Hyperostosis, ankylosing
Formation
  hyalin in cornea — *see* Degeneration, cornea
  sequestrum in bone (due to infection) — *see* Osteomyelitis, chronic
  valve
    colon, congenital Q43.8
    ureter (congenital) Q62.39
Formication R20.2
Fort Bragg fever A27.89
Fossa (*see also* condition)
  pyriform — *see* condition
Foster-Kennedy syndrome H47.14 ☑
Fothergill's
  disease (trigeminal neuralgia) (*see also* Neuralgia, trigeminal)
  scarlatina anginosa A38.9
Foul breath R19.6
Foundling Z76.1
Fournier disease or gangrene N49.3
  female N76.89
Fourth
  cranial nerve — *see* condition
  molar K00.1
Foville's (peduncular) disease or syndrome G46.3
Fox (-Fordyce) disease (apocrine miliaria) L75.2
FPIES (food protein-induced enterocolitis syndrome) K52.21
Fracture, burst — *see* Fracture, traumatic, by site
Fracture, chronic — *see* Fracture, pathological, by site
Fracture, insufficiency — *see* Fracture, pathological, by site
Fracture, nontraumatic, NEC
  atypical
    femur M84.750 ☑
      complete
        oblique M84.759 ☑
          left side M84.758 ☑
          right side M84.757 ☑

Fracture, nontraumatic, NEC — *continued*
  atypical — *continued*
        transverse M84.756 ☑
          left side M84.755 ☑
          right side M84.754 ☑
      incomplete M84.753 ☑
        left side M84.752 ☑
        right side M84.751 ☑
Fracture, pathological (pathologic) (*see also* Fracture, traumatic M84.40 ☑)
  ankle M84.47 ☑
  carpus M84.44 ☑
  clavicle M84.41 ☑
  compression (not due to trauma) (*see also* Collapse, vertebra) M48.50 ☑
  dental implant M27.63
  dental restorative material K08.539
    with loss of material K08.531
    without loss of material K08.530
  due to
    neoplastic disease NEC (*see also* Neoplasm) M84.50 ☑
      ankle M84.57 ☑
      carpus M84.54 ☑
      clavicle M84.51 ☑
      femur M84.55 ☑
      fibula M84.56 ☑
      finger M84.54 ☑
      hip M84.559 ☑
      humerus M84.52 ☑
      ilium M84.550 ☑
      ischium M84.550 ☑
      metacarpus M84.54 ☑
      metatarsus M84.57 ☑
      neck M84.58 ☑
      pelvis M84.550 ☑
      radius M84.53 ☑
      rib M84.58 ☑
      scapula M84.51 ☑
      skull M84.58 ☑
      specified site NEC M84.58 ☑
      tarsus M84.57 ☑
      tibia M84.56 ☑
      toe M84.57 ☑
      ulna M84.53 ☑
      vertebra M84.58 ☑
    osteoporosis M80.00 ☑
      disuse — *see* Osteoporosis, specified type NEC, with pathological fracture
      drug-induced — *see* Osteoporosis, drug induced, with pathological fracture
      idiopathic — *see* Osteoporosis, specified type NEC, with pathological fracture
      postmenopausal — *see* Osteoporosis, postmenopausal, with pathological fracture
      postoophorectomy — *see* Osteoporosis, postoophorectomy, with pathological fracture
      postsurgical malabsorption — *see* Osteoporosis, specified type NEC, with pathological fracture
      specified cause NEC — *see* Osteoporosis, specified type NEC, with pathological fracture
    specified disease NEC M84.60 ☑
      ankle M84.67 ☑
      carpus M84.64 ☑
      clavicle M84.61 ☑
      femur M84.65 ☑
      fibula M84.66 ☑
      finger M84.64 ☑
      hip M84.65 ☑
      humerus M84.62 ☑
      ilium M84.650 ☑
      ischium M84.650 ☑
      metacarpus M84.64 ☑
      metatarsus M84.67 ☑
      neck M84.68 ☑
      radius M84.63 ☑
      rib M84.68 ☑
      scapula M84.61 ☑
      skull M84.68 ☑
      tarsus M84.67 ☑
      tibia M84.66 ☑
      toe M84.67 ☑
      ulna M84.63 ☑
      vertebra M84.68 ☑
  femur M84.45 ☑
  fibula M84.46 ☑
  finger M84.44 ☑
  hip M84.459 ☑

☑ **Additional character required**

Fracture, pathological — *continued*
- humerus M84.42 ☑
- ilium M84.454 ☑
- ischium M84.454 ☑
- joint prosthesis — *see* Complications, joint prosthesis, mechanical, breakdown, by site
  - periprosthetic — *see* Fracture, pathological, periprosthetic
- metacarpus M84.44 ☑
- metatarsus M84.47 ☑
- neck M84.48 ☑
- pelvis M84.454 ☑
- periprosthetic M97.9 ☑
  - ankle M97.2 ☑
  - elbow M97.4 ☑
  - finger M97.8 ☑
  - hip M97.0 ☑
  - knee M97.1 ☑
  - other specified joint M97.8 ☑
  - shoulder M97.3 ☑
  - spinal joint M97.8 ☑
  - toe joint M97.8 ☑
  - wrist joint M97.8 ☑
- radius M84.43 ☑
- restorative material (dental) K08.539
  - with loss of material K08.531
  - without loss of material K08.530
- rib M84.48 ☑
- scapula M84.41 ☑
- skull M84.48 ☑
- tarsus M84.47 ☑
- tibia M84.46 ☑
- toe M84.47 ☑
- ulna M84.43 ☑
- vertebra M84.48 ☑

Fracture, traumatic (abduction) (adduction) (separation) (*see also* Fracture, pathological) T14.8 ☑
- acetabulum S32.40 ☑
  - column
    - anterior (displaced) (iliopubic) S32.43 ☑
      - nondisplaced S32.436 ☑
    - posterior (displaced) (ilioischial) S32.443 ☑
      - nondisplaced S32.44 ☑
  - dome (displaced) S32.48 ☑
    - nondisplaced S32.48 ☑
  - specified NEC S32.49 ☑
  - transverse (displaced) S32.45 ☑
    - with associated posterior wall fracture (displaced) S32.46 ☑
      - nondisplaced S32.46 ☑
    - nondisplaced S32.45 ☑
  - wall
    - anterior (displaced) S32.41 ☑
      - nondisplaced S32.41 ☑
    - medial (displaced) S32.47 ☑
      - nondisplaced S32.47 ☑
    - posterior (displaced) S32.42 ☑
      - with associated transverse fracture (displaced) S32.46 ☑
        - nondisplaced S32.46 ☑
      - nondisplaced S32.42 ☑
- acromion — *see* Fracture, scapula, acromial process
- ankle S82.899 ☑
  - bimalleolar (displaced) S82.84 ☑
    - nondisplaced S82.84 ☑
  - lateral malleolus only (displaced) S82.6 ☑
    - nondisplaced S82.6 ☑
  - medial malleolus (displaced) S82.5 ☑
    - associated with Maisonneuve's fracture — *see* Fracture, Maisonneuve's
    - nondisplaced S82.5 ☑
  - talus — *see* Fracture, tarsal, talus
  - trimalleolar (displaced) S82.85 ☑
    - nondisplaced S82.85 ☑
- arm (upper) (*see also* Fracture, humerus, shaft)
  - humerus — *see* Fracture, humerus
  - radius — *see* Fracture, radius
  - ulna — *see* Fracture, ulna
- astragalus — *see* Fracture, tarsal, talus
- atlas — *see* Fracture, neck, cervical vertebra, first
- axis — *see* Fracture, neck, cervical vertebra, second
- back — *see* Fracture, vertebra
- Barton's — *see* Barton's fracture
- base of skull — *see* Fracture, skull, base
- basicervical (basal) (femoral) S72.0 ☑
- Bennett's — *see* Bennett's fracture
- bimalleolar — *see* Fracture, ankle, bimalleolar
- blow-out S02.3 ☑
- bone NEC T14.8 ☑
  - birth injury P13.9
  - following insertion of orthopedic implant, joint prosthesis or bone plate — *see* Fracture,

Fracture, traumatic — *continued*
- bone NEC — *continued*
  - following insertion of orthopedic implant, joint prosthesis or bone plate
  - in (due to) neoplastic disease NEC — *see* Fracture, pathological, due to neoplastic disease
  - pathological (cause unknown) — *see* Fracture, pathological
- breast bone — *see* Fracture, sternum
- bucket handle (semilunar cartilage) — *see* Tear, meniscus
- burst — *see* Fracture, traumatic, by site
- calcaneus — *see* Fracture, tarsal, calcaneus
- carpal bone(s) S62.10 ☑
  - capitate (displaced) S62.13 ☑
    - nondisplaced S62.13 ☑
  - cuneiform — *see* Fracture, carpal bone, triquetrum
  - hamate (body) (displaced) S62.143 ☑
    - hook process (displaced) S62.15 ☑
      - nondisplaced S62.15 ☑
    - nondisplaced S62.14 ☑
  - larger multangular — *see* Fracture, carpal bones, trapezium
  - lunate (displaced) S62.12 ☑
    - nondisplaced S62.12 ☑
  - navicular S62.00 ☑
    - distal pole (displaced) S62.01 ☑
      - nondisplaced S62.01 ☑
    - middle third (displaced) S62.02 ☑
      - nondisplaced S62.02 ☑
    - proximal third (displaced) S62.03 ☑
      - nondisplaced S62.03 ☑
    - volar tuberosity — *see* Fracture, carpal bones, navicular, distal pole
  - os magnum — *see* Fracture, carpal bones, capitate
  - pisiform (displaced) S62.16 ☑
    - nondisplaced S62.16 ☑
  - semilunar — *see* Fracture, carpal bones, lunate
  - smaller multangular — *see* Fracture, carpal bones, trapezoid
  - trapezium (displaced) S62.17 ☑
    - nondisplaced S62.17 ☑
  - trapezoid (displaced) S62.18 ☑
    - nondisplaced S62.18 ☑
  - triquetrum (displaced) S62.11 ☑
    - nondisplaced S62.11 ☑
  - unciform — *see* Fracture, carpal bones, hamate
- cervical — *see* Fracture, vertebra, cervical
- clavicle S42.00 ☑
  - acromial end (displaced) S42.03 ☑
    - nondisplaced S42.03 ☑
  - birth injury P13.4
  - lateral end — *see* Fracture, clavicle, acromial end
  - shaft (displaced) S42.02 ☑
    - nondisplaced S42.02 ☑
  - sternal end (anterior) (displaced) S42.01 ☑
    - nondisplaced S42.01 ☑
    - posterior S42.01 ☑
- coccyx S32.2 ☑
- collapsed — *see* Collapse, vertebra
- collar bone — *see* Fracture, clavicle
- Colles' — *see* Colles' fracture
- coronoid process — *see* Fracture, ulna, upper end, coronoid process
- corpus cavernosum penis S39.840 ☑
- costochondral cartilage S23.41 ☑
- costochondral, costosternal junction — *see* Fracture, rib
- cranium — *see* Fracture, skull
- cricoid cartilage S12.8 ☑
- cuboid (ankle) — *see* Fracture, tarsal, cuboid
- cuneiform
  - foot — *see* Fracture, tarsal, cuneiform
  - wrist — *see* Fracture, carpal, triquetrum
- delayed union — *see* Delay, union, fracture
- dental restorative material K08.539
  - with loss of material K08.531
  - without loss of material K08.530
- due to
  - birth injury — *see* Birth, injury, fracture
  - osteoporosis — *see* Osteoporosis, with fracture
- Dupuytren's — *see* Fracture, ankle, lateral malleolus
- elbow S42.40 ☑
- ethmoid (bone) (sinus) — *see* Fracture, skull, base
- face bone S02.92 ☑
- fatigue (*see also* Fracture, stress)
  - vertebra M48.40 ☑
    - cervical region M48.42 ☑
    - cervicothoracic region M48.43 ☑
    - lumbar region M48.46 ☑

Fracture, traumatic — *continued*
- fatigue — *continued*
  - lumbosacral region M48.47 ☑
  - occipito-atlanto-axial region M48.41 ☑
  - sacrococcygeal region M48.48 ☑
  - thoracic region M48.44 ☑
  - thoracolumbar region M48.45 ☑
- femur, femoral S72.9 ☑
  - basicervical (basal) S72.0 ☑
  - birth injury P13.2
  - capital epiphyseal S79.01 ☑
  - condyles, epicondyles — *see* Fracture, femur, lower end
  - distal end — *see* Fracture, femur, lower end
  - epiphysis
    - head — *see* Fracture, femur, upper end, epiphysis
    - lower — *see* Fracture, femur, lower end, epiphysis
    - upper — *see* Fracture, femur, upper end, epiphysis
  - following insertion of implant, prosthesis or plate M96.66 ☑
  - head — *see* Fracture, femur, upper end, head
  - intertrochanteric — *see* Fracture, femur, trochanteric
  - intratrochanteric — *see* Fracture, femur, trochanteric
  - lower end S72.40 ☑
    - condyle (displaced) S72.41 ☑
      - lateral (displaced) S72.42 ☑
        - nondisplaced S72.42 ☑
      - medial (displaced) S72.43 ☑
        - nondisplaced S72.43 ☑
      - nondisplaced S72.41 ☑
    - epiphysis (displaced) S72.44 ☑
      - nondisplaced S72.44 ☑
    - physeal S79.10 ☑
      - Salter-Harris
        - Type I S79.11 ☑
        - Type II S79.12 ☑
        - Type III S79.13 ☑
        - Type IV S79.14 ☑
      - specified NEC S79.19 ☑
    - specified NEC S72.49 ☑
    - supracondylar (displaced) S72.45 ☑
      - with intracondylar extension (displaced) S72.46 ☑
        - nondisplaced S72.46 ☑
      - nondisplaced S72.45 ☑
    - torus S72.47 ☑
  - neck — *see* Fracture, femur, upper end, neck
  - pertrochanteric — *see* Fracture, femur, trochanteric
  - shaft (lower third) (middle third) (upper third) S72.30 ☑
    - comminuted (displaced) S72.35 ☑
      - nondisplaced S72.35 ☑
    - oblique (displaced) S72.33 ☑
      - nondisplaced S72.33 ☑
    - segmental (displaced) S72.36 ☑
      - nondisplaced S72.36 ☑
    - specified NEC S72.39 ☑
    - spiral (displaced) S72.34 ☑
      - nondisplaced S72.34 ☑
    - transverse (displaced) S72.32 ☑
      - nondisplaced S72.32 ☑
  - specified site NEC — *see* subcategory S72.8 ☑
  - subcapital (displaced) S72.01 ☑
  - subtrochanteric (region) (section) (displaced) S72.2 ☑
    - nondisplaced S72.2 ☑
  - transcervical — *see* Fracture, femur, midcervical
  - transtrochanteric — *see* Fracture, femur, trochanteric
  - trochanteric S72.10 ☑
    - apophyseal (displaced) S72.13 ☑
      - nondisplaced S72.13 ☑
    - greater trochanter (displaced) S72.11 ☑
      - nondisplaced S72.11 ☑
    - intertrochanteric (displaced) S72.14 ☑
      - nondisplaced S72.14 ☑
    - lesser trochanter (displaced) S72.12 ☑
      - nondisplaced S72.12 ☑
  - upper end S72.00 ☑
    - apophyseal (displaced) S72.13 ☑
      - nondisplaced S72.13 ☑
    - cervicotrochanteric — *see* Fracture, femur, upper end, neck, base
    - epiphysis (displaced) S72.02 ☑
      - nondisplaced S72.02 ☑
    - head S72.05 ☑

Fracture, traumatic — *continued*
femur — *continued*
    articular (displaced) S72.06 ☑
      nondisplaced S72.06 ☑
    specified NEC S72.09 ☑
   intertrochanteric (displaced) S72.14 ☑
    nondisplaced S72.14 ☑
   intracapsular S72.01 ☑
   midcervical (displaced) S72.03 ☑
    nondisplaced S72.03 ☑
   neck S72.00 ☑
    base (displaced) S72.04 ☑
      nondisplaced S72.04 ☑
    specified NEC S72.09 ☑
   pertrochanteric — *see* Fracture, femur, upper
    end, trochanteric
   physeal S79.00 ☑
    Salter-Harris type I S79.01 ☑
    specified NEC S79.09 ☑
   subcapital (displaced) S72.01 ☑
   subtrochanteric (displaced) S72.2 ☑
    nondisplaced S72.2 ☑
   transcervical — *see* Fracture, femur, upper end,
    midcervical
   trochanteric S72.10 ☑
    greater (displaced) S72.11 ☑
      nondisplaced S72.11 ☑
    lesser (displaced) S72.12 ☑
      nondisplaced S72.12 ☑
fibula (shaft) (styloid) S82.40 ☑
  comminuted (displaced) S82.45 ☑
    nondisplaced S82.45 ☑
  following insertion of implant, prosthesis or plate
    M96.67 ☑
  involving ankle or malleolus — *see* Fracture,
    fibula, lateral malleolus
  lateral malleolus (displaced) S82.6 ☑
    nondisplaced S82.6 ☑
  lower end
    physeal S89.30 ☑
     Salter-Harris
      Type I S89.31 ☑
      Type II S89.32 ☑
     specified NEC S89.39 ☑
    specified NEC S82.83 ☑
    torus S82.82 ☑
  oblique (displaced) S82.43 ☑
    nondisplaced S82.43 ☑
  segmental (displaced) S82.46 ☑
    nondisplaced S82.46 ☑
  specified NEC S82.49 ☑
  spiral (displaced) S82.44 ☑
    nondisplaced S82.44 ☑
  transverse (displaced) S82.42 ☑
    nondisplaced S82.42 ☑
  upper end
    physeal S89.20 ☑
     Salter-Harris
      Type I S89.21 ☑
      Type II S89.22 ☑
     specified NEC S89.29 ☑
    specified NEC S82.83 ☑
    torus S82.81 ☑
finger (except thumb) S62.60 ☑
  distal phalanx (displaced) S62.63 ☑
    nondisplaced S62.66 ☑
  index S62.60 ☑
    distal phalanx (displaced) S62.63 ☑
     nondisplaced S62.66 ☑
    middle phalanx (displaced) S62.62 ☑
     nondisplaced S62.65 ☑
    proximal phalanx (displaced) S62.61 ☑
     nondisplaced S62.64 ☑
  little S62.60 ☑
    distal phalanx (displaced) S62.63 ☑
     nondisplaced S62.66 ☑
    middle phalanx (displaced) S62.62 ☑
     nondisplaced S62.65 ☑
    proximal phalanx (displaced) S62.61 ☑
     nondisplaced S62.64 ☑
  middle phalanx (displaced) S62.62 ☑
    nondisplaced S62.65 ☑
  middle S62.60 ☑
    distal phalanx (displaced) S62.63 ☑
     nondisplaced S62.66 ☑
    middle phalanx (displaced) S62.62 ☑
     nondisplaced S62.65 ☑
    proximal phalanx (displaced) S62.61 ☑
     nondisplaced S62.64 ☑
  proximal phalanx (displaced) S62.61 ☑
    nondisplaced S62.64 ☑
  ring S62.60 ☑

finger — *continued*
  distal phalanx (displaced) S62.63 ☑
    nondisplaced S62.66 ☑
  middle phalanx (displaced) S62.62 ☑
    nondisplaced S62.65 ☑
  proximal phalanx (displaced) S62.61 ☑
    nondisplaced S62.64 ☑
  thumb — *see* Fracture, thumb
following insertion (intraoperative) (postoperative)
  of orthopedic implant, joint prosthesis or bone
  plate M96.69
  femur M96.66 ☑
  fibula M96.67 ☑
  humerus M96.62 ☑
  pelvis M96.65
  radius M96.63 ☑
  specified bone NEC M96.69
  tibia M96.67 ☑
  ulna M96.63 ☑
foot S92.90 ☑
  astragalus — *see* Fracture, tarsal, talus
  calcaneus — *see* Fracture, tarsal, calcaneus
  cuboid — *see* Fracture, tarsal, cuboid
  cuneiform — *see* Fracture, tarsal, cuneiform
  metatarsal — *see* Fracture, metatarsal
  navicular — *see* Fracture, tarsal, navicular
  sesamoid S92.81 ☑
  specified NEC S92.81 ☑
  talus — *see* Fracture, tarsal, talus
  tarsal — *see* Fracture, tarsal
  toe — *see* Fracture, toe
forearm S52.9 ☑
  radius — *see* Fracture, radius
  ulna — *see* Fracture, ulna
fossa (anterior) (middle) (posterior) S02.19 ☑
fragility — *see* Fracture, pathological, due to
  osteoporosis
frontal (bone) (skull) S02.0 ☑
  sinus S02.19 ☑
glenoid (cavity) (scapula) — *see* Fracture, scapula,
  glenoid cavity
greenstick — *see* Fracture, by site
hallux — *see* Fracture, toe, great
hand S62.9 ☑
  carpal — *see* Fracture, carpal bone
  finger (except thumb) — *see* Fracture, finger
  metacarpal — *see* Fracture, metacarpal
  navicular (scaphoid) (hand) — *see* Fracture, carpal
    bone, navicular
  thumb — *see* Fracture, thumb
healed or old
  with complications - code by Nature of the
    complication
heel bone — *see* Fracture, tarsal, calcaneus
Hill-Sachs S42.29 ☑
hip — *see* Fracture, femur, neck
humerus S42.30 ☑
  anatomical neck — *see* Fracture, humerus, upper
    end
  articular process — *see* Fracture, humerus, lower end
  capitellum — *see* Fracture, humerus, lower end,
    condyle, lateral
  distal end — *see* Fracture, humerus, lower end
  epiphysis
    lower — *see* Fracture, humerus, lower end,
     physeal
    upper — *see* Fracture, humerus, upper end,
     physeal
  external condyle — *see* Fracture, humerus, lower
    end, condyle, lateral
  following insertion of implant, prosthesis or plate
    M96.62 ☑
  great tuberosity — *see* Fracture, humerus, upper
    end, greater tuberosity
  intercondylar — *see* Fracture, humerus, lower end
  internal epicondyle - code as Fracture, humerus,
    lower end, epicondyle, medial
  lesser tuberosity — *see* Fracture, humerus, upper
    end, lesser tuberosity
  lower end S42.40 ☑
    condyle
     lateral (displaced) S42.45 ☑
      nondisplaced S42.45 ☑
     medial (displaced) S42.46 ☑
      nondisplaced S42.46 ☑
    epicondyle
     lateral (displaced) S42.43 ☑
      nondisplaced S42.43 ☑
     medial (displaced) S42.44 ☑
      incarcerated S42.44 ☑
      nondisplaced S42.44 ☑

humerus — *continued*
  physeal S49.10 ☑
    Salter-Harris
     Type I S49.11 ☑
     Type II S49.12 ☑
     Type III S49.13 ☑
     Type IV S49.14 ☑
    specified NEC S49.19 ☑
  specified NEC (displaced) S42.49 ☑
    nondisplaced S42.49 ☑
  supracondylar (simple) (displaced) S42.41 ☑
    with intercondylar fracture — *see* Fracture,
     humerus, lower end
    comminuted (displaced) S42.42 ☑
     nondisplaced S42.42 ☑
    nondisplaced S42.41 ☑
    torus S42.48 ☑
    transcondylar (displaced) S42.47 ☑
     nondisplaced S42.47 ☑
  proximal end — *see* Fracture, humerus, upper end
  shaft S42.30 ☑
    comminuted (displaced) S42.35 ☑
     nondisplaced S42.35 ☑
    greenstick S42.31 ☑
    oblique (displaced) S42.33 ☑
     nondisplaced S42.33 ☑
    segmental (displaced) S42.36 ☑
     nondisplaced S42.36 ☑
    specified NEC S42.39 ☑
    spiral (displaced) S42.34 ☑
     nondisplaced S42.34 ☑
    transverse (displaced) S42.32 ☑
     nondisplaced S42.32 ☑
  supracondylar — *see* Fracture, humerus, lower end
  surgical neck — *see* Fracture, humerus, upper
    end, surgical neck
  trochlea — *see* Fracture, humerus, lower end,
    condyle, medial
  tuberosity — *see* Fracture, humerus, upper end
  upper end S42.20 ☑
    anatomical neck — *see* Fracture, humerus,
     upper end, specified NEC
    articular head — *see* Fracture, humerus, upper
     end, specified NEC
    epiphysis — *see* Fracture, humerus, upper end,
     physeal
    greater tuberosity (displaced) S42.25 ☑
     nondisplaced S42.25 ☑
    lesser tuberosity (displaced) S42.26 ☑
     nondisplaced S42.26 ☑
    physeal S49.00 ☑
     Salter-Harris
      Type I S49.01 ☑
      Type II S49.02 ☑
      Type III S49.03 ☑
      Type IV S49.04 ☑
     specified NEC S49.09 ☑
    specified NEC (displaced) S42.29 ☑
     nondisplaced S42.29 ☑
    surgical neck (displaced) S42.21 ☑
     four-part S42.24 ☑
     nondisplaced S42.21 ☑
     three-part S42.23 ☑
     two-part (displaced) S42.22 ☑
      nondisplaced S42.22 ☑
    torus S42.27 ☑
    transepiphyseal — *see* Fracture, humerus,
     upper end, physeal
hyoid bone S12.8 ☑
ilium S32.30 ☑
  with disruption of pelvic ring — *see* Disruption,
    pelvic ring
  avulsion (displaced) S32.31 ☑
    nondisplaced S32.31 ☑
  specified NEC S32.39 ☑
impaction, impacted - code as Fracture, by site
innominate bone — *see* Fracture, ilium
instep — *see* Fracture, foot
ischium S32.60 ☑
  with disruption of pelvic ring — *see* Disruption,
    pelvic ring
  avulsion (displaced) S32.61 ☑
    nondisplaced S32.61 ☑
  specified NEC S32.69 ☑
jaw (bone) (lower) — *see* Fracture, mandible
  upper — *see* Fracture, maxilla
joint prosthesis — *see* Complications, joint
  prosthesis, mechanical, breakdown, by site
  periprosthetic — *see* Fracture, traumatic,
    periprosthetic
knee cap — *see* Fracture, patella

☑ **Additional character required**

Fracture, traumatic — *continued*
  larynx S12.8 ☑
  late effects — *see* Sequelae, fracture
  leg (lower) S82.9 ☑
    ankle — *see* Fracture, ankle
    femur — *see* Fracture, femur
    fibula — *see* Fracture, fibula
    malleolus — *see* Fracture, ankle
    patella — *see* Fracture, patella
    specified site NEC S82.89 ☑
    tibia — *see* Fracture, tibia
  lumbar spine — *see* Fracture, vertebra, lumbar
  lumbosacral spine S32.9 ☑
  Maisonneuve's (displaced) S82.86 ☑
    nondisplaced S82.86 ☑
  malar bone (*see also* Fracture, maxilla) S02.400 ☑
    left side S02.40B ☑
    right side S02.40A ☑
  malleolus — *see* Fracture, ankle
  malunion — *see* Fracture, by site
  mandible (lower jaw (bone) S02.609 ☑
    alveolus S02.67 ☑
    angle (of jaw) S02.65 ☑
    body, unspecified S02.600 ☑
      left side S02.602 ☑
      right side S02.601 ☑
    condylar process S02.61 ☑
    coronoid process S02.63 ☑
    ramus, unspecified S02.64 ☑
    specified site NEC S02.69 ☑
    subcondylar process S02.62 ☑
    symphysis S02.66 ☑
  manubrium (sterni) S22.21 ☑
    dissociation from sternum S22.23 ☑
  march — *see* Fracture, traumatic, stress, by site
  maxilla, maxillary (bone) (sinus) (superior) (upper jaw) S02.401 ☑
    alveolus S02.42 ☑
    inferior — *see* Fracture, mandible
    LeFort I S02.411 ☑
    LeFort II S02.412 ☑
    LeFort III S02.413 ☑
    left side S02.40D ☑
    right side S02.40C ☑
  metacarpal S62.309 ☑
    base (displaced) S62.319 ☑
      nondisplaced S62.349 ☑
    fifth S62.30 ☑
      base (displaced) S62.31 ☑
        nondisplaced S62.34 ☑
      neck (displaced) S62.33 ☑
        nondisplaced S62.36 ☑
      shaft (displaced) S62.32 ☑
        nondisplaced S62.35 ☑
      specified NEC S62.398 ☑
    first S62.20 ☑
      base NEC (displaced) S62.23 ☑
        nondisplaced S62.23 ☑
      Bennett's — *see* Bennett's fracture
      neck (displaced) S62.25 ☑
        nondisplaced S62.25 ☑
      shaft (displaced) S62.24 ☑
        nondisplaced S62.24 ☑
      specified NEC S62.29 ☑
    fourth S62.30 ☑
      base (displaced) S62.31 ☑
        nondisplaced S62.34 ☑
      neck (displaced) S62.33 ☑
        nondisplaced S62.36 ☑
      shaft (displaced) S62.32 ☑
        nondisplaced S62.35 ☑
      specified NEC S62.39 ☑
    neck (displaced) S62.33 ☑
      nondisplaced S62.36 ☑
    Rolando's — *see* Rolando's fracture
    second S62.30 ☑
      base (displaced) S62.31 ☑
        nondisplaced S62.34 ☑
      neck (displaced) S62.33 ☑
        nondisplaced S62.36 ☑
      shaft (displaced) S62.32 ☑
        nondisplaced S62.35 ☑
      specified NEC S62.39 ☑
    shaft (displaced) S62.32 ☑
      nondisplaced S62.35 ☑
    third S62.30 ☑
      base (displaced) S62.31 ☑
        nondisplaced S62.34 ☑
      neck (displaced) S62.33 ☑
        nondisplaced S62.36 ☑
      shaft (displaced) S62.32 ☑
        nondisplaced S62.35 ☑

Fracture, traumatic — *continued*
  metacarpal — *continued*
    specified NEC S62.39 ☑
    specified NEC S62.399 ☑
  metastatic — *see* Fracture, pathological, due to, neoplastic disease (*see also* Neoplasm)
  metatarsal bone S92.30 ☑
    fifth (displaced) S92.35 ☑
      nondisplaced S92.35 ☑
    first (displaced) S92.31 ☑
      nondisplaced S92.31 ☑
    fourth (displaced) S92.34 ☑
      nondisplaced S92.34 ☑
    physeal S99.10 ☑
      Salter-Harris
        Type I S99.11 ☑
        Type II S99.12 ☑
        Type III S99.13 ☑
        Type IV S99.14 ☑
      specified NEC S99.19 ☑
    second (displaced) S92.32 ☑
      nondisplaced S92.32 ☑
    third (displaced) S92.33 ☑
      nondisplaced S92.33 ☑
  Monteggia's — *see* Monteggia's fracture
  multiple
    hand (and wrist) NEC — *see* Fracture, by site
    ribs — *see* Fracture, rib, multiple
  nasal (bone(s)) S02.2 ☑
  navicular (scaphoid) (foot) (*see also* Fracture, tarsal, navicular)
    hand — *see* Fracture, carpal, navicular
  neck S12.9 ☑
    cervical vertebra S12.9 ☑
      fifth (displaced) S12.400 ☑
        nondisplaced S12.401 ☑
        specified type NEC (displaced) S12.490 ☑
          nondisplaced S12.491 ☑
      first (displaced) S12.000 ☑
        burst (stable) S12.01 ☑
          unstable S12.02 ☑
        lateral mass (displaced) S12.040 ☑
          nondisplaced S12.041 ☑
        nondisplaced S12.001 ☑
        posterior arch (displaced) S12.030 ☑
          nondisplaced S12.031 ☑
        specified type NEC (displaced) S12.090 ☑
          nondisplaced S12.091 ☑
      fourth (displaced) S12.300 ☑
        nondisplaced S12.301 ☑
        specified type NEC (displaced) S12.390 ☑
          nondisplaced S12.391 ☑
      second (displaced) S12.100 ☑
        nondisplaced S12.101 ☑
        dens (anterior) (displaced) (type II) S12.110 ☑
          nondisplaced S12.112 ☑
          posterior S12.111 ☑
        specified type NEC (displaced) S12.120 ☑
          nondisplaced S12.121 ☑
        specified type NEC (displaced) S12.190 ☑
          nondisplaced S12.191 ☑
      seventh (displaced) S12.600 ☑
        nondisplaced S12.601 ☑
        specified type NEC (displaced) S12.690 ☑
          nondisplaced S12.691 ☑
      sixth (displaced) S12.500 ☑
        nondisplaced S12.501 ☑
        specified type NEC (displaced) S12.590 ☑
          nondisplaced S12.591 ☑
      third (displaced) S12.200 ☑
        nondisplaced S12.201 ☑
        specified type NEC (displaced) S12.290 ☑
          nondisplaced S12.291 ☑
    hyoid bone S12.8 ☑
    larynx S12.8 ☑
    specified site NEC S12.8 ☑
    thyroid cartilage S12.8 ☑
    trachea S12.8 ☑
  neoplastic NEC — *see* Fracture, pathological, due to, neoplastic disease
  neural arch — *see* Fracture, vertebra
  newborn — *see* Birth, injury, fracture
  nontraumatic — *see* Fracture, pathological
  nonunion — *see* Nonunion, fracture
  nose, nasal (bone) (septum) S02.2 ☑
  occiput — *see* Fracture, skull, base, occiput
  odontoid process — *see* Fracture, neck, cervical vertebra, second
  olecranon (process) (ulna) — *see* Fracture, ulna, upper end, olecranon process
  orbit, orbital (bone) (region) S02.85 ☑
    floor (blow-out) S02.3 ☑

Fracture, traumatic — *continued*
  orbit — *continued*
    roof S02.12 ☑
    wall S02.85 ☑
      lateral S02.84 ☑
      medial S02.83 ☑
  os
    calcis — *see* Fracture, tarsal, calcaneus
    magnum — *see* Fracture, carpal, capitate
    pubis — *see* Fracture, pubis
  palate S02.8 ☑
  parietal bone (skull) S02.0 ☑
  patella S82.00 ☑
    comminuted (displaced) S82.04 ☑
      nondisplaced S82.04 ☑
    longitudinal (displaced) S82.02 ☑
      nondisplaced S82.02 ☑
    osteochondral (displaced) S82.01 ☑
      nondisplaced S82.01 ☑
    specified NEC S82.09 ☑
    transverse (displaced) S82.03 ☑
      nondisplaced S82.03 ☑
  pedicle (of vertebral arch) — *see* Fracture, vertebra
  pelvis, pelvic (bone) S32.9 ☑
    acetabulum — *see* Fracture, acetabulum
    circle — *see* Disruption, pelvic ring
    following insertion of implant, prosthesis or plate M96.65
    ilium — *see* Fracture, ilium
    ischium — *see* Fracture, ischium
    multiple
      with disruption of pelvic ring (circle) — *see* Disruption, pelvic ring
      without disruption of pelvic ring (circle) S32.82 ☑
    pubis — *see* Fracture, pubis
    specified site NEC S32.89 ☑
    sacrum — *see* Fracture, sacrum
  periprosthetic, around internal prosthetic joint M97.9 ☑
    ankle M97.2 ☑
    elbow M97.4 ☑
    finger M97.8 ☑
    hip M97.0 ☑
    knee M97.1 ☑-
    shoulder M97.3 ☑
    specified joint NEC M97.8 ☑
    spine M97.8 ☑
    toe M97.8 ☑
    wrist M97.8 ☑
  phalanx
    foot — *see* Fracture, toe
    hand — *see* Fracture, finger
  pisiform — *see* Fracture, carpal, pisiform
  pond — *see* Fracture, skull
  prosthetic device, internal — *see* Complications, prosthetic device, by site, mechanical
  pubis S32.50 ☑
    with disruption of pelvic ring — *see* Disruption, pelvic ring
    specified site NEC S32.59 ☑
    superior rim S32.51 ☑
  radius S52.9 ☑
    distal end — *see* Fracture, radius, lower end
    following insertion of implant, prosthesis or plate M96.63 ☑
    head — *see* Fracture, radius, upper end, head
    lower end S52.50 ☑
      Barton's — *see* Barton's fracture
      Colles' — *see* Colles' fracture
      extraarticular NEC S52.55 ☑
      intraarticular NEC S52.57 ☑
      physeal S59.20 ☑
        Salter-Harris
          Type I S59.21 ☑
          Type II S59.22 ☑
          Type III S59.23 ☑
          Type IV S59.24 ☑
        specified NEC S59.29 ☑
      Smith's — *see* Smith's fracture
      specified NEC S52.59 ☑
      styloid process (displaced) S52.51 ☑
        nondisplaced S52.51 ☑
      torus S52.52 ☑
    neck — *see* Fracture, radius, upper end
    proximal end — *see* Fracture, radius, upper end
    shaft S52.30 ☑
      bent bone S52.38 ☑
      comminuted (displaced) S52.35 ☑
        nondisplaced S52.35 ☑
      Galeazzi's — *see* Galeazzi's fracture
      greenstick S52.31 ☑

Fracture, traumatic

Fracture, traumatic — *continued*
  radius — *continued*
    oblique (displaced) S52.33 ☑
      nondisplaced S52.33 ☑
    segmental (displaced) S52.36 ☑
      nondisplaced S52.36 ☑
    specified NEC S52.39 ☑
    spiral (displaced) S52.34 ☑
      nondisplaced S52.34 ☑
    transverse (displaced) S52.32 ☑
      nondisplaced S52.32 ☑
    upper end S52.10 ☑
      head (displaced) S52.12 ☑
        nondisplaced S52.12 ☑
      neck (displaced) S52.13 ☑
        nondisplaced S52.13 ☑
      specified NEC S52.18 ☑
    physeal S59.10 ☑
      Salter-Harris
        Type I S59.11 ☑
        Type II S59.12 ☑
        Type III S59.13 ☑
        Type IV S59.14 ☑
      specified NEC S59.19 ☑
    torus S52.11 ☑
  ramus
    inferior or superior, pubis — *see* Fracture, pubis
    mandible — *see* Fracture, mandible
  restorative material (dental) K08.539
    with loss of material K08.531
    without loss of material K08.530
  rib S22.3 ☑
    with flail chest — *see* Flail, chest
    multiple S22.4 ☑
      with flail chest — *see* Flail, chest
  root, tooth — *see* Fracture, tooth
  sacrum S32.10 ☑
    specified NEC S32.19 ☑
    Type
      1 S32.14 ☑
      2 S32.15 ☑
      3 S32.16 ☑
      4 S32.17 ☑
    Zone
      I S32.119 ☑
        displaced (minimally) S32.111 ☑
          severely S32.112 ☑
        nondisplaced S32.110 ☑
      II S32.129 ☑
        displaced (minimally) S32.121 ☑
          severely S32.122 ☑
        nondisplaced S32.120 ☑
      III S32.139 ☑
        displaced (minimally) S32.131 ☑
          severely S32.132 ☑
        nondisplaced S32.130 ☑
  scaphoid (hand) (*see also* Fracture, carpal, navicular)
    foot — *see* Fracture, tarsal, navicular
  scapula S42.10 ☑
    acromial process (displaced) S42.12 ☑
      nondisplaced S42.12 ☑
    body (displaced) S42.11 ☑
      nondisplaced S42.11 ☑
    coracoid process (displaced) S42.13 ☑
      nondisplaced S42.13 ☑
    glenoid cavity (displaced) S42.14 ☑
      nondisplaced S42.14 ☑
    neck (displaced) S42.15 ☑
      nondisplaced S42.15 ☑
    specified NEC S42.19 ☑
  semilunar bone, wrist — *see* Fracture, carpal, lunate
  sequelae — *see* Sequelae, fracture
  sesamoid bone
    foot S92.81 ☑
    hand — *see* Fracture, carpal
    other — *see* Fracture, traumatic, by site
  shepherd's — *see* Fracture, tarsal, talus
  shoulder (girdle) S42.9 ☑
    blade — *see* Fracture, scapula
  sinus (ethmoid) (frontal) S02.19 ☑
  skull S02.91 ☑
    base S02.10 ☑
      occiput S02.119 ☑
        condyle S02.113 ☑
          type I S02.110 ☑
            left side S02.11B ☑
            right side S02.11A ☑
          type II S02.111 ☑
            left side S02.11D ☑
            right side S02.11C ☑
          type III S02.112 ☑
            left side S02.11F ☑

Fracture, traumatic — *continued*
  skull — *continued*
        right side S02.11E ☑
      specified NEC S02.118 ☑
        left side S02.11H ☑
        right side S02.11G ☑
      specified NEC S02.19 ☑
    birth injury P13.0
    frontal bone S02.0 ☑
    parietal bone S02.0 ☑
    specified site NEC S02.8 ☑
    temporal bone S02.19 ☑
    vault S02.0 ☑
  Smith's — *see* Smith's fracture
  sphenoid (bone) (sinus) S02.19 ☑
  spine — *see* Fracture, vertebra
  spinous process — *see* Fracture, vertebra
  spontaneous (cause unknown) — *see* Fracture, pathological
  stave (of thumb) — *see* Fracture, metacarpal, first
  sternum S22.20 ☑
    with flail chest — *see* Flail, chest
    body S22.22 ☑
    manubrium S22.21 ☑
    xiphoid (process) S22.24 ☑
  stress M84.30 ☑
    ankle M84.37 ☑
    carpus M84.34 ☑
    clavicle M84.31 ☑
    femoral neck M84.359 ☑
    femur M84.35 ☑
    fibula M84.36 ☑
    finger M84.34 ☑
    hip M84.359 ☑
    humerus M84.32 ☑
    ilium M84.350 ☑
    ischium M84.350 ☑
    metacarpus M84.34 ☑
    metatarsus M84.37 ☑
    neck — *see* Fracture, fatigue, vertebra
    pelvis M84.350 ☑
    radius M84.33 ☑
    rib M84.38 ☑
    scapula M84.31 ☑
    skull M84.38 ☑
    tarsus M84.37 ☑
    tibia M84.36 ☑
    toe M84.37 ☑
    ulna M84.33 ☑
  vertebra — *see* Fracture, fatigue, vertebra
  supracondylar, elbow — *see* Fracture, humerus, lower end, supracondylar
  symphysis pubis — *see* Fracture, pubis
  talus (ankle bone) — *see* Fracture, tarsal, talus
  tarsal bone(s) S92.20 ☑
    astragalus — *see* Fracture, tarsal, talus
    calcaneus S92.00 ☑
      anterior process (displaced) S92.02 ☑
        nondisplaced S92.02 ☑
      body (displaced) S92.01 ☑
        nondisplaced S92.01 ☑
      extraarticular NEC (displaced) S92.05 ☑
        nondisplaced S92.05 ☑
      intraarticular (displaced) S92.06 ☑
        nondisplaced S92.06 ☑
      physeal S99.00 ☑
        Salter-Harris
          Type I S99.01 ☑
          Type II S99.02 ☑
          Type III S99.03 ☑
          Type IV S99.04 ☑
        specified NEC S99.09 ☑
      tuberosity (displaced) S92.04 ☑
        avulsion (displaced) S92.03 ☑
          nondisplaced S92.03 ☑
        nondisplaced S92.04 ☑
    cuboid (displaced) S92.21 ☑
      nondisplaced S92.21 ☑
    cuneiform
      intermediate (displaced) S92.23 ☑
        nondisplaced S92.23 ☑
      lateral (displaced) S92.22 ☑
        nondisplaced S92.22 ☑
      medial (displaced) S92.24 ☑
        nondisplaced S92.24 ☑
    navicular (displaced) S92.25 ☑
      nondisplaced S92.25 ☑
    scaphoid — *see* Fracture, tarsal, navicular
    talus S92.10 ☑
      avulsion (displaced) S92.15 ☑
        nondisplaced S92.15 ☑
      body (displaced) S92.12 ☑

Fracture, traumatic — *continued*
  tarsal bone(s) — *continued*
        nondisplaced S92.12 ☑
      dome (displaced) S92.14 ☑
        nondisplaced S92.14 ☑
      head (displaced) S92.12 ☑
        nondisplaced S92.12 ☑
      lateral process (displaced) S92.14 ☑
        nondisplaced S92.14 ☑
      neck (displaced) S92.11 ☑
        nondisplaced S92.11 ☑
      posterior process (displaced) S92.13 ☑
        nondisplaced S92.13 ☑
      specified NEC S92.19 ☑
  temporal bone (styloid) S02.19 ☑
  thorax (bony) S22.9 ☑
    with flail chest — *see* Flail, chest
    rib S22.3 ☑
      multiple S22.4 ☑
        with flail chest — *see* Flail, chest
    sternum S22.20 ☑
      body S22.22 ☑
      manubrium S22.21 ☑
      xiphoid process S22.24 ☑
    vertebra (displaced) S22.009 ☑
      burst (stable) S22.001 ☑
        unstable S22.002 ☑
      eighth S22.069 ☑
        burst (stable) S22.061 ☑
          unstable S22.062 ☑
        specified type NEC S22.068 ☑
        wedge compression S22.060 ☑
      eleventh S22.089 ☑
        burst (stable) S22.081 ☑
          unstable S22.082 ☑
        specified type NEC S22.088 ☑
        wedge compression S22.080 ☑
      fifth S22.059 ☑
        burst (stable) S22.051 ☑
          unstable S22.052 ☑
        specified type NEC S22.058 ☑
        wedge compression S22.050 ☑
      first S22.019 ☑
        burst (stable) S22.011 ☑
          unstable S22.012 ☑
        specified type NEC S22.018 ☑
        wedge compression S22.010 ☑
      fourth S22.049 ☑
        burst (stable) S22.041 ☑
          unstable S22.042 ☑
        specified type NEC S22.048 ☑
        wedge compression S22.040 ☑
      ninth S22.079 ☑
        burst (stable) S22.071 ☑
          unstable S22.072 ☑
        specified type NEC S22.078 ☑
        wedge compression S22.070 ☑
      nondisplaced S22.001 ☑
      second S22.029 ☑
        burst (stable) S22.021 ☑
          unstable S22.022 ☑
        specified type NEC S22.028 ☑
        wedge compression S22.020 ☑
      seventh S22.069 ☑
        burst (stable) S22.061 ☑
          unstable S22.062 ☑
        specified type NEC S22.068 ☑
        wedge compression S22.060 ☑
      sixth S22.059 ☑
        burst (stable) S22.051 ☑
          unstable S22.052 ☑
        specified type NEC S22.058 ☑
        wedge compression S22.050 ☑
      specified type NEC S22.008 ☑
      tenth S22.079 ☑
        burst (stable) S22.071 ☑
          unstable S22.072 ☑
        specified type NEC S22.078 ☑
        wedge compression S22.070 ☑
      third S22.039 ☑
        burst (stable) S22.031 ☑
          unstable S22.032 ☑
        specified type NEC S22.038 ☑
        wedge compression S22.030 ☑
      twelfth S22.089 ☑
        burst (stable) S22.081 ☑
          unstable S22.082 ☑
        specified type NEC S22.088 ☑
        wedge compression S22.080 ☑
      wedge compression S22.000 ☑
  thumb S62.50 ☑
    distal phalanx (displaced) S62.52 ☑

☑ **Additional character required**

Fracture, traumatic — *continued*
  thumb — *continued*
    nondisplaced S62.52 ☑
    proximal phalanx (displaced) S62.51 ☑
      nondisplaced S62.51 ☑
  thyroid cartilage S12.8 ☑
  tibia (shaft) S82.20 ☑
    comminuted (displaced) S82.25 ☑
      nondisplaced S82.25 ☑
    condyles — *see* Fracture, tibia, upper end
    distal end — *see* Fracture, tibia, lower end
    epiphysis
      lower — *see* Fracture, tibia, lower end
      upper — *see* Fracture, tibia, upper end
    following insertion of implant, prosthesis or plate M96.67 ☑
    head (involving knee joint) — *see* Fracture, tibia, upper end
    intercondyloid eminence — *see* Fracture, tibia, upper end
    involving ankle or malleolus — *see* Fracture, ankle, medial malleolus
    lower end S82.30 ☑
      physeal S89.10 ☑
        Salter-Harris
          Type I S89.11 ☑
          Type II S89.12 ☑
          Type III S89.13 ☑
          Type IV S89.14 ☑
        specified NEC S89.19 ☑
      pilon (displaced) S82.87 ☑
        nondisplaced S82.87 ☑
      specified NEC S82.39 ☑
      torus S82.31 ☑
    malleolus — *see* Fracture, ankle, medial malleolus
    oblique (displaced) S82.23 ☑
      nondisplaced S82.23 ☑
    pilon — *see* Fracture, tibia, lower end, pilon
    proximal end — *see* Fracture, tibia, upper end
    segmental (displaced) S82.26 ☑
      nondisplaced S82.26 ☑
    specified NEC S82.29 ☑
    spine — *see* Fracture, tibia, upper end, spine
    spiral (displaced) S82.24 ☑
      nondisplaced S82.24 ☑
    transverse (displaced) S82.22 ☑
      nondisplaced S82.22 ☑
    tuberosity — *see* Fracture, tibia, upper end, tuberosity
    upper end S82.10 ☑
      bicondylar (displaced) S82.14 ☑
        nondisplaced S82.14 ☑
      lateral condyle (displaced) S82.12 ☑
        nondisplaced S82.12 ☑
      medial condyle (displaced) S82.13 ☑
        nondisplaced S82.13 ☑
      physeal S89.00 ☑
        Salter-Harris
          Type I S89.01 ☑
          Type II S89.02 ☑
          Type III S89.03 ☑
          Type IV S89.04 ☑
        specified NEC S89.09 ☑
      plateau — *see* Fracture, tibia, upper end, bicondylar
      spine (displaced) S82.11 ☑
        nondisplaced S82.11 ☑
      torus S82.16 ☑
      specified NEC S82.19 ☑
      tuberosity (displaced) S82.15 ☑
        nondisplaced S82.15 ☑
  toe S92.91 ☑
    great (displaced) S92.40 ☑
      distal phalanx (displaced) S92.42 ☑
        nondisplaced S92.42 ☑
      nondisplaced S92.40 ☑
      proximal phalanx (displaced) S92.41 ☑
        nondisplaced S92.41 ☑
      specified NEC S92.49 ☑
    lesser (displaced) S92.50 ☑
      distal phalanx (displaced) S92.53 ☑
        nondisplaced S92.53 ☑
      middle phalanx (displaced) S92.52 ☑
        nondisplaced S92.52 ☑
      nondisplaced S92.50 ☑
      proximal phalanx (displaced) S92.51 ☑
        nondisplaced S92.51 ☑
      specified NEC S92.59 ☑
    physeal
      phalanx S99.20 ☑
        Salter-Harris
          Type I S99.21 ☑

Fracture, traumatic — *continued*
  toe — *continued*
          Type II S99.22 ☑
          Type III S99.23 ☑
          Type IV S99.24 ☑
        specified NEC S99.29 ☑
  tooth (root) S02.5 ☑
  trachea (cartilage) S12.8 ☑
  transverse process — *see* Fracture, vertebra
  trapezium or trapezoid bone — *see* Fracture, carpal
  trimalleolar — *see* Fracture, ankle, trimalleolar
  triquetrum (cuneiform of carpus) — *see* Fracture, carpal, triquetrum
  trochanter — *see* Fracture, femur, trochanteric
  tuberosity (external) — *see* Fracture, traumatic, by site
  ulna (shaft) S52.20 ☑
    bent bone S52.28 ☑
    coronoid process — *see* Fracture, ulna, upper end, coronoid process
    distal end — *see* Fracture, ulna, lower end
    following insertion of implant, prosthesis or plate M96.63 ☑
    head S52.60 ☑
    lower end S52.60 ☑
      physeal S59.00 ☑
        Salter-Harris
          Type I S59.01 ☑
          Type II S59.02 ☑
          Type III S59.03 ☑
          Type IV S59.04 ☑
        specified NEC S59.09 ☑
      specified NEC S52.69 ☑
      styloid process (displaced) S52.61 ☑
        nondisplaced S52.61 ☑
      torus S52.62 ☑
    proximal end — *see* Fracture, ulna, upper end
    shaft S52.20 ☑
      comminuted (displaced) S52.25 ☑
        nondisplaced S52.25 ☑
      greenstick S52.21 ☑
      Monteggia's — *see* Monteggia's fracture
      oblique (displaced) S52.23 ☑
        nondisplaced S52.23 ☑
      segmental (displaced) S52.26 ☑
        nondisplaced S52.26 ☑
      specified NEC S52.29 ☑
      spiral (displaced) S52.24 ☑
        nondisplaced S52.24 ☑
      transverse (displaced) S52.22 ☑
        nondisplaced S52.22 ☑
    upper end S52.00 ☑
      coronoid process (displaced) S52.04 ☑
        nondisplaced S52.04 ☑
      olecranon process (displaced) S52.02 ☑
        with intraarticular extension S52.03 ☑
        nondisplaced S52.02 ☑
          with intraarticular extension S52.03 ☑
      specified NEC S52.09 ☑
      torus S52.01 ☑
  unciform — *see* Fracture, carpal, hamate
  vault of skull S02.0 ☑
  vertebra, vertebral (arch) (body) (column) (neural arch) (pedicle) (spinous process) (transverse process)
    atlas — *see* Fracture, neck, cervical vertebra, first
    axis — *see* Fracture, neck, cervical vertebra, second
    cervical (teardrop) S12.9 ☑
      axis — *see* Fracture, neck, cervical vertebra, second
      first (atlas) — *see* Fracture, neck, cervical vertebra, first
      second (axis) — *see* Fracture, neck, cervical vertebra, second
    chronic M84.48 ☑
    coccyx S32.2 ☑
    dorsal — *see* Fracture, thorax, vertebra
    lumbar S32.009 ☑
      burst (stable) S32.001 ☑
        unstable S32.002 ☑
      fifth S32.059 ☑
        burst (stable) S32.051 ☑
          unstable S32.052 ☑
        specified type NEC S32.058 ☑
        wedge compression S32.050 ☑
      first S32.019 ☑
        burst (stable) S32.011 ☑
          unstable S32.012 ☑
        specified type NEC S32.018 ☑
        wedge compression S32.010 ☑
      fourth S32.049 ☑
        burst (stable) S32.041 ☑

Fracture, traumatic — *continued*
  vertebra — *continued*
          unstable S32.042 ☑
        specified type NEC S32.048 ☑
        wedge compression S32.040 ☑
      second S32.029 ☑
        burst (stable) S32.021 ☑
          unstable S32.022 ☑
        specified type NEC S32.028 ☑
        wedge compression S32.020 ☑
      specified type NEC S32.008 ☑
      third S32.039 ☑
        burst (stable) S32.031 ☑
          unstable S32.032 ☑
        specified type NEC S32.038 ☑
        wedge compression S32.030 ☑
      wedge compression S32.000 ☑
    metastatic — *see* Collapse, vertebra, in, specified disease NEC (*see also* Neoplasm)
    newborn (birth injury) P11.5
    sacrum S32.10 ☑
      specified NEC S32.19 ☑
      Type
        1 S32.14 ☑
        2 S32.15 ☑
        3 S32.16 ☑
        4 S32.17 ☑
      Zone
        I S32.119 ☑
          displaced (minimally) S32.111 ☑
            severely S32.112 ☑
          nondisplaced S32.110 ☑
        II S32.129 ☑
          displaced (minimally) S32.121 ☑
            severely S32.122 ☑
          nondisplaced S32.120 ☑
        III S32.139 ☑
          displaced (minimally) S32.131 ☑
            severely S32.132 ☑
          nondisplaced S32.130 ☑
    thoracic — *see* Fracture, thorax, vertebra
  vertex S02.0 ☑
  vomer (bone) S02.2 ☑
  wrist S62.10 ☑
    carpal — *see* Fracture, carpal bone
    navicular (scaphoid) (hand) — *see* Fracture, carpal, navicular
  xiphisternum, xiphoid (process) S22.24 ☑
  zygoma S02.402 ☑
    left side S02.40F ☑
    right side S02.40E ☑
Fragile, fragility
  autosomal site Q95.5
  bone, congenital (with blue sclera) Q78.0
  capillary (hereditary) D69.8
  hair L67.8
  nails L60.3
  non-sex chromosome site Q95.5
  X chromosome Q99.2
Fragilitas
  crinium L67.8
  ossium (with blue sclerae) (hereditary) Q78.0
  unguium L60.3
    congenital Q84.6
Fragments, cataract (lens), following cataract surgery H59.02 ☑
  retained foreign body — *see* Retained, foreign body fragments (type of)
Frailty (frail) R54
  mental R41.81
Frambesia, frambesial (tropica) (*see also* Yaws)
  initial lesion or ulcer A66.0
  primary A66.0
Frambeside
  gummatous A66.4
  of early yaws A66.2
Frambesioma A66.1
Franceschetti-Klein (-Wildervanck) disease or syndrome Q75.4
Francis' disease — *see* Tularemia
Franklin disease C88.2
Frank's essential thrombocytopenia D69.3
Fraser's syndrome Q87.0
Freckle(s) L81.2
  malignant melanoma in — *see* Melanoma
  melanotic (Hutchinson's) — *see* Melanoma, in situ
  retinal D49.81
Frederickson's hyperlipoproteinemia, type
  I and V E78.3
  IIA E78.00
  IIB and III E78.2
  IV E78.1

Freeman Sheldon syndrome Q87.0
Freezing (*see also* Effect, adverse, cold) T69.9 ☑
Freiberg's disease (infraction of metatarsal head or osteochondrosis) — *see* Osteochondrosis, juvenile, metatarsus
Frei's disease A55
Fremitus, friction, cardiac R01.2
Frenum, frenulum
   external os Q51.828
   tongue (shortening) (congenital) Q38.1
Frequency micturition (nocturnal) R35.0
   psychogenic F45.8
Frey's syndrome
   auriculotemporal G50.8
   hyperhidrosis L74.52
Friction
   burn — *see* Burn, by site
   fremitus, cardiac R01.2
   precordial R01.2
   sounds, chest R09.89
Friderichsen-Waterhouse syndrome or disease A39.1
Friedländer's B (bacillus) NEC (*see also* condition) A49.8
Friedreich's
   ataxia G11.1
   combined systemic disease G11.1
   facial hemihypertrophy Q67.4
   sclerosis (cerebellum) (spinal cord) G11.1
Frigidity F52.22
Fröhlich's syndrome E23.6
Frontal (*see also* condition)
   lobe syndrome F07.0
Frostbite (superficial) T33.90 ☑
   with
      partial thickness skin loss — *see* Frostbite (superficial), by site
      tissue necrosis T34.90 ☑
   abdominal wall T33.3 ☑
      with tissue necrosis T34.3 ☑
   ankle T33.81 ☑
      with tissue necrosis T34.81 ☑
   arm T33.4 ☑
      with tissue necrosis T34.4 ☑
      finger(s) — *see* Frostbite, finger
      hand — *see* Frostbite, hand
      wrist — *see* Frostbite, wrist
   ear T33.01 ☑
      with tissue necrosis T34.01 ☑
   face T33.09 ☑
      with tissue necrosis T34.09 ☑
   finger T33.53 ☑
      with tissue necrosis T34.53 ☑
   foot T33.82 ☑
      with tissue necrosis T34.82 ☑
   hand T33.52 ☑
      with tissue necrosis T34.52 ☑
   head T33.09 ☑
      with tissue necrosis T34.09 ☑
      ear — *see* Frostbite, ear
      nose — *see* Frostbite, nose
   hip (and thigh) T33.6 ☑
      with tissue necrosis T34.6 ☑
   knee T33.7 ☑
      with tissue necrosis T34.7 ☑
   leg T33.9 ☑
      with tissue necrosis T34.9 ☑
      ankle — *see* Frostbite, ankle
      foot — *see* Frostbite, foot
      knee — *see* Frostbite, knee
      lower T33.7 ☑
         with tissue necrosis T34.7 ☑
      thigh — *see* Frostbite, hip
      toe — *see* Frostbite, toe
   limb
      lower T33.99 ☑
         with tissue necrosis T34.99 ☑
      upper — *see* Frostbite, arm
   neck T33.1 ☑
      with tissue necrosis T34.1 ☑
   nose T33.02 ☑
      with tissue necrosis T34.02 ☑
   pelvis T33.3 ☑
      with tissue necrosis T34.3 ☑
   specified site NEC T33.99 ☑
      with tissue necrosis T34.99 ☑
   thigh — *see* Frostbite, hip
   thorax T33.2 ☑
      with tissue necrosis T34.2 ☑
   toes T33.83 ☑
      with tissue necrosis T34.83 ☑
   trunk T33.99 ☑
      with tissue necrosis T34.99 ☑

Frostbite — *continued*
   wrist T33.51 ☑
      with tissue necrosis T34.51 ☑
Frotteurism F65.81
Frozen (*see also* Effect, adverse, cold) T69.9 ☑
   pelvis (female) N94.89
      male K66.8
   shoulder — *see* Capsulitis, adhesive
Fructokinase deficiency E74.11
Fructose 1,6 diphosphatase deficiency E74.19
Fructosemia (benign) (essential) E74.12
Fructosuria (benign) (essential) E74.11
Fuchs'
   black spot (myopic) (*see also* Myopia, degenerative) H44.2 ☑
   dystrophy (corneal endothelium) H18.51
   heterochromic cyclitis — *see* Cyclitis, Fuchs' heterochromic
Fucosidosis E77.1
Fugue R68.89
   dissociative F44.1
   hysterical (dissociative) F44.1
   postictal in epilepsy — *see* Epilepsy
   reaction to exceptional stress (transient) F43.0
Fulminant, fulminating — *see* condition
Functional (*see also* condition)
   bleeding (uterus) N93.8
Functioning, intellectual, borderline R41.83
Fundus — *see* condition
Fungemia NOS B49
Fungus, fungous
   cerebral G93.89
   disease NOS B49
   infection — *see* Infection, fungus
Funiculitis (acute) (chronic) (endemic) N49.1
   gonococcal (acute) (chronic) A54.23
   tuberculous A18.15
Funnel
   breast (acquired) M95.4
      congenital Q67.6
      sequelae (late effect) of rickets E64.3
   chest (acquired) M95.4
      congenital Q67.6
      sequelae (late effect) of rickets E64.3
   pelvis (acquired) M95.5
      with disproportion (fetopelvic) O33.3 ☑
         causing obstructed labor O65.3
      congenital Q74.2
FUO (fever of unknown origin) R50.9
Furfur L21.0
   microsporon B36.0
Furrier's lung J67.8
Furrowed K14.5
   nail(s) (transverse) L60.4
      congenital Q84.6
   tongue K14.5
      congenital Q38.3
Furuncle L02.92
   abdominal wall L02.221
   ankle — *see* Furuncle, lower limb
   anus K61.0
   antecubital space — *see* Furuncle, upper limb
   arm — *see* Furuncle, upper limb
   auditory canal, external — *see* Abscess, ear, external
   auricle (ear) — *see* Abscess, ear, external
   axilla (region) L02.42 ☑
   back (any part) L02.222
   breast N61.1
   buttock L02.32
   cheek (external) L02.02
   chest wall L02.223
   chin L02.02
   corpus cavernosum N48.21
   ear, external — *see* Abscess, ear, external
   external auditory canal — *see* Abscess, ear, external
   eyelid — *see* Abscess, eyelid
   face L02.02
   femoral (region) — *see* Furuncle, lower limb
   finger — *see* Furuncle, hand
   flank L02.221
   foot L02.62 ☑
   forehead L02.02
   gluteal (region) L02.32
   groin L02.224
   hand L02.52 ☑
   head L02.821
      face L02.02
   hip — *see* Furuncle, lower limb
   kidney — *see* Abscess, kidney
   knee — *see* Furuncle, lower limb
   labium (majus) (minus) N76.4

Furuncle — *continued*
   lacrimal
      gland — *see* Dacryoadenitis
      passages (duct) (sac) — *see* Inflammation, lacrimal, passages, acute
   leg (any part) — *see* Furuncle, lower limb
   lower limb L02.42 ☑
   malignant A22.0
   mouth K12.2
   navel L02.226
   neck L02.12
   nose J34.0
   orbit, orbital — *see* Abscess, orbit
   palmar (space) — *see* Furuncle, hand
   partes posteriores L02.32
   pectoral region L02.223
   penis N48.21
   perineum L02.225
   pinna — *see* Abscess, ear, external
   popliteal — *see* Furuncle, lower limb
   prepatellar — *see* Furuncle, lower limb
   scalp L02.821
   seminal vesicle N49.0
   shoulder — *see* Furuncle, upper limb
   specified site NEC L02.828
   submandibular K12.2
   temple (region) L02.02
   thumb — *see* Furuncle, hand
   toe — *see* Furuncle, foot
   trunk L02.229
      abdominal wall L02.221
      back L02.222
      chest wall L02.223
      groin L02.224
      perineum L02.225
      umbilicus L02.226
   umbilicus L02.226
   upper limb L02.42 ☑
   vulva N76.4
Furunculosis — *see* Furuncle
Fused — *see* Fusion, fused
Fusion, fused (congenital)
   astragaloscaphoid Q74.2
   atria Q21.1
   auditory canal Q16.1
   auricles, heart Q21.1
   binocular with defective stereopsis H53.32
   bone Q79.8
   cervical spine M43.22
   choanal Q30.0
   commissure, mitral valve Q23.2
   cusps, heart valve NEC Q24.8
      mitral Q23.2
      pulmonary Q22.1
      tricuspid Q22.4
   ear ossicles Q16.3
   fingers Q70.0 ☑
   hymen Q52.3
   joint (acquired) (*see also* Ankylosis)
      congenital Q74.8
   kidneys (incomplete) Q63.1
   labium (majus) (minus) Q52.5
   larynx and trachea Q34.8
   limb, congenital Q74.8
      lower Q74.2
      upper Q74.0
   lobes, lung Q33.8
   lumbosacral (acquired) M43.27
      arthrodesis status Z98.1
      congenital Q76.49
      postprocedural status Z98.1
   nares, nose, nasal, nostril(s) Q30.0
   organ or site not listed — *see* Anomaly, by site
   ossicles Q79.9
      auditory Q16.3
   pulmonic cusps Q22.1
   ribs Q76.6
   sacroiliac (joint) (acquired) M43.28
      arthrodesis status Z98.1
      congenital Q74.2
      postprocedural status Z98.1
   spine (acquired) NEC M43.20
      arthrodesis status Z98.1
      cervical region M43.22
      cervicothoracic region M43.23
      congenital Q76.49
      lumbar M43.26
      lumbosacral region M43.27
      occipito-atlanto-axial region M43.21
      postoperative status Z98.1
      sacrococcygeal region M43.28
      thoracic region M43.24

Fusion — *continued*
  spine — *continued*
    thoracolumbar region M43.25
  sublingual duct with submaxillary duct at opening in mouth Q38.4
  testes Q55.1
  toes Q70.2 ☑
  tooth, teeth K00.2
  trachea and esophagus Q39.8
  twins Q89.4
  vagina Q52.4
  ventricles, heart Q21.0
  vertebra (arch) — *see* Fusion, spine
  vulva Q52.5
Fusospirillosis (mouth) (tongue) (tonsil) A69.1
Fussy baby R68.12

G

Gain in weight (abnormal) (excessive) (*see also* Weight, gain)
Gaisböck's disease (polycythemia hypertonica) D75.1
Gait abnormality R26.9
  ataxic R26.0
  falling R29.6
  hysterical (ataxic) (staggering) F44.4
  paralytic R26.1
  spastic R26.1
  specified type NEC R26.89
  staggering R26.0
  unsteadiness R26.81
  walking difficulty NEC R26.2
Galactocele (breast) N64.89
  puerperal, postpartum O92.79
Galactokinase deficiency E74.29
Galactophoritis N61.0
  gestational, puerperal, postpartum O91.2 ☑
Galactorrhea O92.6
  not associated with childbirth N64.3
Galactosemia (classic) (congenital) E74.21
Galactosuria E74.29
Galacturia R82.0
  schistosomiasis (bilharziasis) B65.0
GALD (gestational alloimmune liver disease) P78.84
Galeazzi's fracture S52.37 ☑
Galen's vein — *see* condition
Galeophobia F40.218
Gall duct — *see* condition
Gallbladder (*see also* condition)
  acute K81.0
Gallop rhythm R00.8
Gallstone (colic) (cystic duct) (gallbladder) (impacted) (multiple) (*see also* Calculus, gallbladder)
  with
    cholecystitis — *see* Calculus, gallbladder, with cholecystitis
    bile duct (common) (hepatic) — *see* Calculus, bile duct
  causing intestinal obstruction K56.3
  specified NEC K80.80
    with obstruction K80.81
Gambling Z72.6
  pathological (compulsive) F63.0
Gammopathy (of undetermined significance [MGUS]) D47.2
  associated with lymphoplasmacytic dyscrasia D47.2
  monoclonal D47.2
  polyclonal D89.0
Gamna's disease (siderotic splenomegaly) D73.1
Gamophobia F40.298
Gampsodactylia (congenital) Q66.7 ☑
Gamstorp's disease (adynamia episodica hereditaria) G72.3
Gandy-Nanta disease (siderotic splenomegaly) D73.1
Gang
  membership offenses Z72.810
Gangliocytoma D36.10
Ganglioglioma — *see* Neoplasm, uncertain behavior, by site
Ganglion (compound) (diffuse) (joint) (tendon (sheath)) M67.40
  ankle M67.47 ☑
  foot M67.47 ☑
  forearm M67.43 ☑
  hand M67.44 ☑
  lower leg M67.46 ☑
  multiple sites M67.49
  of yaws (early) (late) A66.6
  pelvic region M67.45 ☑
  periosteal — *see* Periostitis

Ganglion — *continued*
  shoulder region M67.41 ☑
  specified site NEC M67.48
  thigh region M67.45 ☑
  tuberculous A18.09
  upper arm M67.42 ☑
  wrist M67.43 ☑
Ganglioneuroblastoma — *see* Neoplasm, nerve, malignant
Ganglioneuroma D36.10
  malignant — *see* Neoplasm, nerve, malignant
Ganglioneuromatosis D36.10
Ganglionitis
  fifth nerve — *see* Neuralgia, trigeminal
  gasserian (postherpetic) (postzoster) B02.21
  geniculate G51.1
    newborn (birth injury) P11.3
    postherpetic, postzoster B02.21
  herpes zoster B02.21
  postherpetic geniculate B02.21
Gangliosidosis E75.10
  GM1 E75.19
  GM2 E75.00
    other specified E75.09
    Sandhoff disease E75.01
    Tay-Sachs disease E75.02
  GM3 E75.19
  mucolipidosis IV E75.11
Gangosa A66.5
Gangrene, gangrenous (connective tissue) (dropsical) (dry) (moist) (skin) (ulcer) (*see also* Necrosis) I96
  with diabetes (mellitus) — *see* Diabetes, gangrene
  abdomen (wall) I96
  alveolar M27.3
  appendix K35.80
    with
      peritonitis, localized (*see also* Appendicitis) K35.31
  arteriosclerotic (general) (senile) — *see* Arteriosclerosis, extremities, with, gangrene
  auricle I96
  Bacillus welchii A48.0
  bladder (infectious) — *see* Cystitis, specified type NEC
  bowel, cecum, or colon — *see* Gangrene, intestine
  Clostridium perfringens or welchii A48.0
  cornea H18.89 ☑
  corpora cavernosa N48.29
    noninfective N48.89
  cutaneous, spreading I96
  decubital — *see* Ulcer, pressure, by site
  diabetic (any site) — *see* Diabetes, gangrene
  epidemic — *see* Poisoning, food, noxious, plant
  epididymis (infectional) N45.1
  erysipelas — *see* Erysipelas
  emphysematous — *see* Gangrene, gas
  extremity (lower) (upper) I96
  Fournier N49.3
    female N76.89
  fusospirochetal A69.0
  gallbladder — *see* Cholecystitis, acute
  gas (bacillus) A48.0
    following
      abortion — *see* Abortion by type complicated by infection
      ectopic or molar pregnancy O08.0
  glossitis K14.0
  hernia — *see* Hernia, by site, with gangrene
  intestine, intestinal (hemorrhagic) (massive) (*see also* Infarct, intestine) K55.069
    with
      mesenteric embolism (*see also* Infarct, intestine) K55.069
      obstruction — *see* Obstruction, intestine
  laryngitis J04.0
  limb (lower) (upper) I96
  lung J85.0
    spirochetal A69.8
  lymphangitis I89.1
  Meleney's (synergistic) — *see* Ulcer, skin
  mesentery (*see also* Infarct, intestine) K55.069
    with
      embolism (*see also* Infarct, intestine) K55.069
      intestinal obstruction — *see* Obstruction, intestine
  mouth A69.0
  ovary — *see* Oophoritis
  pancreas — *see* Pancreatitis, acute
  penis N48.29
    noninfective N48.89
  perineum I96
  pharynx (*see also* Pharyngitis)
    Vincent's A69.1

Gangrene — *continued*
  presenile I73.1
  progressive synergistic — *see* Ulcer, skin
  pulmonary J85.0
  pulpal (dental) K04.1
  quinsy J36
  Raynaud's (symmetric gangrene) I73.01
  retropharyngeal J39.2
  scrotum N49.3
    noninfective N50.89
  senile (atherosclerotic) — *see* Arteriosclerosis, extremities, with, gangrene
  spermatic cord N49.1
    noninfective N50.89
  spine I96
  spirochetal NEC A69.8
  spreading cutaneous I96
  stomatitis A69.0
  symmetrical I73.01
  testis (infectional) N45.2
    noninfective N44.8
  throat (*see also* Pharyngitis)
    diphtheritic A36.0
    Vincent's A69.1
  thyroid (gland) E07.89
  tooth (pulp) K04.1
  tuberculous NEC — *see* Tuberculosis
  tunica vaginalis N49.1
    noninfective N50.89
  umbilicus I96
  uterus — *see* Endometritis
  uvulitis K12.2
  vas deferens N49.1
    noninfective N50.89
  vulva N76.89
Ganister disease J62.8
Ganser's syndrome (hysterical) F44.89
Gardner-Diamond syndrome (autoerythrocyte sensitization) D69.2
Gargoylism E76.01
Garré's disease, osteitis (sclerosing), osteomyelitis — *see* Osteomyelitis, specified type NEC
Garrod's pad, knuckle M72.1
Gartner's duct
  cyst Q52.4
  persistent Q50.6
Gas R14.3
  asphyxiation, inhalation, poisoning, suffocation NEC — *see* Table of Drugs and Chemicals
  excessive R14.0
  gangrene A48.0
    following
      abortion — *see* Abortion by type complicated by infection
      ectopic or molar pregnancy O08.0
  on stomach R14.0
  pains R14.1
Gastralgia (*see also* Pain, abdominal)
Gastrectasis K31.0
  psychogenic F45.8
Gastric — *see* condition
Gastrinoma
  malignant
    pancreas C25.4
    specified site NEC — *see* Neoplasm, malignant, by site
    unspecified site C25.4
  specified site — *see* Neoplasm, uncertain behavior
  unspecified site D37.9
Gastritis (simple) K29.70
  with bleeding K29.71
  acute (erosive) K29.00
    with bleeding K29.01
  alcoholic K29.20
    with bleeding K29.21
  allergic K29.60
    with bleeding K29.61
  atrophic (chronic) K29.40
    with bleeding K29.41
  chronic (antral) (fundal) K29.50
    with bleeding K29.51
    atrophic K29.40
      with bleeding K29.41
    superficial K29.30
      with bleeding K29.31
  dietary counseling and surveillance Z71.3
  due to diet deficiency E63.9
  eosinophilic K52.81
  giant hypertrophic K29.60
    with bleeding K29.61
  granulomatous K29.60
    with bleeding K29.61

Gastritis - Glaucoma

Gastritis — *continued*
  hypertrophic (mucosa) K29.60
    with bleeding K29.61
  nervous F54
  spastic K29.60
    with bleeding K29.61
  specified NEC K29.60
    with bleeding K29.61
  superficial chronic K29.30
    with bleeding K29.31
  tuberculous A18.83
  viral NEC A08.4
Gastrocarcinoma — *see* Neoplasm, malignant, stomach
Gastrocolic — *see* condition
Gastrodisciasis, gastrodiscoidiasis B66.8
Gastroduodenitis K29.90
  with bleeding K29.91
  virus, viral A08.4
    specified type NEC A08.39
Gastrodynia — *see* Pain, abdominal
Gastroenteritis (acute) (chronic) (noninfectious) (*see also* Enteritis) K52.9
  allergic K52.29
    with
      eosinophilic gastritis or gastroenteritis K52.81
      food protein-induced enterocolitis syndrome K52.21
      food protein-induced enteropathy K52.22
  dietetic (*see also* Gastroenteritis, allergic) K52.29
  drug-induced K52.1
  due to
    Cryptosporidium A07.2
    drugs K52.1
    food poisoning — *see* Intoxication, foodborne
    radiation K52.0
  eosinophilic K52.81
  epidemic (infectious) A09
  food hypersensitivity (*see also* Gastroenteritis, allergic) K52.29
  infectious — *see* Enteritis, infectious
  influenzal — *see* Influenza, with gastroenteritis
  noninfectious K52.9
    specified NEC K52.89
  rotaviral A08.0
  Salmonella A02.0
  toxic K52.1
  viral NEC A08.4
    acute infectious A08.39
      type Norwalk A08.11
    infantile (acute) A08.39
    Norwalk agent A08.11
    rotaviral A08.0
    severe of infants A08.39
    specified type NEC A08.39
Gastroenteropathy (*see also* Gastroenteritis) K52.9
  acute, due to Norwalk agent A08.11
  acute, due to Norovirus A08.11
  infectious A09
Gastroenteroptosis K63.4
Gastroesophageal laceration- hemorrhage syndrome K22.6
Gastrointestinal — *see* condition
Gastrojejunal — *see* condition
Gastrojejunitis (*see also* Enteritis) K52.9
Gastrojejunocolic — *see* condition
Gastroliths K31.89
Gastromalacia K31.89
Gastroparalysis K31.84
  diabetic — *see* Diabetes, gastroparalysis
Gastroparesis K31.84
  diabetic — *see* Diabetes, by type, with gastroparesis
Gastropathy K31.9
  congestive portal K31.89
  erythematous K29.70
  exudative K90.89
  portal hypertensive K31.89
Gastroptosis K31.89
Gastrorrhagia K92.2
  psychogenic F45.8
Gastroschisis (congenital) Q79.3
Gastrospasm (neurogenic) (reflex) K31.89
  neurotic F45.8
  psychogenic F45.8
Gastrostaxis — *see* Gastritis, with bleeding
Gastrostenosis K31.89
Gastrostomy
  attention to Z43.1
  status Z93.1
Gastrosuccorrhea (continuous) (intermittent) K31.89
  neurotic F45.8
  psychogenic F45.8

Gatophobia F40.218
Gaucher's disease or splenomegaly (adult) (infantile) E75.22
Gee (-Herter)(-Thaysen) disease (nontropical sprue) K90.0
Gélineau's syndrome G47.419
  with cataplexy G47.411
Gemination, tooth, teeth K00.2
Gemistocytoma
  specified site — *see* Neoplasm, malignant, by site
  unspecified site C71.9
General, generalized — *see* condition
Genetic
  carrier (status)
    cystic fibrosis Z14.1
    hemophilia A (asymptomatic) Z14.01
      symptomatic Z14.02
    specified NEC Z14.8
  susceptibility to disease NEC Z15.89
    malignant neoplasm Z15.09
      breast Z15.01
      endometrium Z15.04
      ovary Z15.02
      prostate Z15.03
      specified NEC Z15.09
    multiple endocrine neoplasia Z15.81
Genital — *see* condition
Genito-anorectal syndrome A55
Genitourinary system — *see* condition
Genu
  congenital Q74.1
  extrorsum (acquired) (*see also* Deformity, varus, knee)
    congenital Q74.1
    sequelae (late effect) of rickets E64.3
  introrsum (acquired) (*see also* Deformity, valgus, knee)
    congenital Q74.1
    sequelae (late effect) of rickets E64.3
  rachitic (old) E64.3
  recurvatum (acquired) (*see also* Deformity, limb, specified type NEC, lower leg)
    congenital Q68.2
    sequelae (late effect) of rickets E64.3
  valgum (acquired) (knock-knee) M21.06 ☑
    congenital Q74.1
    sequelae (late effect) of rickets E64.3
  varum (acquired) (bowleg) M21.16 ☑
    congenital Q74.1
    sequelae (late effect) of rickets E64.3
Geographic tongue K14.1
Geophagia — *see* Pica
Geotrichosis B48.3
  stomatitis B48.3
Gephyrophobia F40.242
Gerbode defect Q21.0
GERD (gastroesophageal reflux disease) K21.9
Gerhardt's
  disease (erythromelalgia) I73.81
  syndrome (vocal cord paralysis) J38.00
    bilateral J38.02
    unilateral J38.01
German measles (*see also* Rubella)
  exposure to Z20.4
Germinoblastoma (diffuse) C85.9 ☑
  follicular C82.9 ☑
Germinoma — *see* Neoplasm, malignant, by site
Gerontoxon — *see* Degeneration, cornea, senile
Gerstmann-Sträussler-Scheinker syndrome (GSS) A81.82
Gerstmann's syndrome R48.8
  developmental F81.2
Gestation (period) (*see also* Pregnancy)
  ectopic — *see* Pregnancy, by site
  multiple O30.9 ☑
    greater than quadruplets — *see* Pregnancy, multiple (gestation), specified NEC
    specified NEC — *see* Pregnancy, multiple (gestation), specified NEC
Gestational
  mammary abscess O91.11 ☑
  purulent mastitis O91.11 ☑
  subareolar abscess O91.11 ☑
Ghon tubercle, primary infection A15.7
Ghost
  teeth K00.4
  vessels (cornea) H16.41 ☑
Ghoul hand A66.3
Gianotti-Crosti disease L44.4
Giant
  cell
    epulis K06.8
    peripheral granuloma K06.8

Giant — *continued*
  esophagus, congenital Q39.5
  kidney, congenital Q63.3
  urticaria T78.3 ☑
    hereditary D84.1
Giardiasis A07.1
Gibert's disease or pityriasis L42
Giddiness R42
  hysterical F44.89
  psychogenic F45.8
Gierke's disease (glycogenosis I) E74.01
Gigantism (cerebral) (hypophyseal) (pituitary) E22.0
  constitutional E34.4
Gilbert's disease or syndrome E80.4
Gilchrist's disease B40.9
Gilford-Hutchinson disease E34.8
Gilles de la Tourette's disease or syndrome (motor-verbal tic) F95.2
Gingivitis K05.10
  acute (catarrhal) K05.00
    necrotizing A69.1
    nonplaque induced K05.01
    plaque induced K05.00
  chronic (desquamative) (hyperplastic) (simple marginal) (pregnancy associated) (ulcerative) K05.10
    nonplaque induced K05.11
    plaque induced K05.10
  expulsiva — *see* Periodontitis
  necrotizing ulcerative (acute) A69.1
  pellagrous E52
    acute necrotizing A69.1
  Vincent's A69.1
Gingivoglossitis K14.0
Gingivopericementitis — *see* Periodontitis
Gingivosis — *see* Gingivitis, chronic
Gingivostomatitis K05.10
  herpesviral B00.2
  necrotizing ulcerative (acute) A69.1
Gland, glandular — *see* condition
Glanders A24.0
Glanzmann (-Naegeli) disease or thrombasthenia D69.1
Glasgow coma scale
  total score
    3-8 R40.243 ☑
    9-12 R40.242 ☑
    13-15 R40.241 ☑
Glass-blower's disease (cataract) — *see* Cataract, specified NEC
Glaucoma H40.9
  with
    increased episcleral venous pressure H40.81 ☑
    pseudoexfoliation of lens — *see* Glaucoma, open angle, primary, capsular
  absolute H44.51 ☑
  angle-closure (primary) H40.20 ☑
    acute (attack) (crisis) H40.21 ☑
    chronic H40.22 ☑
    intermittent H40.23 ☑
    residual stage H40.24 ☑
  borderline H40.00 ☑
  capsular (with pseudoexfoliation of lens) — *see* Glaucoma, open angle, primary, capsular
  childhood Q15.0
  closed angle — *see* Glaucoma, angle-closure
  congenital Q15.0
  corticosteroid-induced — *see* Glaucoma, secondary, drugs
  hypersecretion H40.82 ☑
  in (due to)
    amyloidosis E85.4 *[H42]*
    aniridia Q13.1 *[H42]*
    concussion of globe — *see* Glaucoma, secondary, trauma
    dislocation of lens — *see* Glaucoma, secondary
    disorder of lens NEC — *see* Glaucoma, secondary
    drugs — *see* Glaucoma, secondary, drugs
    endocrine disease NOS E34.9 *[H42]*
    eye
      inflammation — *see* Glaucoma, secondary, inflammation
      trauma — *see* Glaucoma, secondary, trauma
    hypermature cataract — *see* Glaucoma, secondary
    iridocyclitis — *see* Glaucoma, secondary, inflammation
    lens disorder — *see* Glaucoma, secondary,
    Lowe's syndrome E72.03 *[H42]*
    metabolic disease NOS E88.9 *[H42]*
    ocular disorders NEC — *see* Glaucoma, secondary
    onchocerciasis B73.02

☑ **Additional character required**

Glaucoma — *continued*
  in — *continued*
    pupillary block — *see* Glaucoma, secondary
    retinal vein occlusion — *see* Glaucoma, secondary
    Rieger's anomaly Q13.81 *[H42]*
    rubeosis of iris — *see* Glaucoma, secondary
    tumor of globe — *see* Glaucoma, secondary
  infantile Q15.0
  low tension — *see* Glaucoma, open angle, primary, low-tension
  malignant H40.83 ☑
  narrow angle — *see* Glaucoma, angle-closure
  newborn Q15.0
  noncongestive (chronic) — *see* Glaucoma, open angle
  nonobstructive — *see* Glaucoma, open angle
  obstructive (*see also* Glaucoma, angle-closure)
    due to lens changes — *see* Glaucoma, secondary
  open angle H40.10 ☑
    primary H40.11 ☑
      capsular (with pseudoexfoliation of lens) H40.14 ☑
      low-tension H40.12 ☑
      pigmentary H40.13 ☑
      residual stage H40.15 ☑
  phacolytic — *see* Glaucoma, secondary
  pigmentary — *see* Glaucoma, open angle, primary, pigmentary
  postinfectious — *see* Glaucoma, secondary, inflammation
  secondary (to) H40.5 ☑
    drugs H40.6 ☑
    inflammation H40.4 ☑
    trauma H40.3 ☑
  simple (chronic) H40.11 ☑
  simplex H40.11 ☑
  specified type NEC H40.89
  suspect H40.00 ☑
  syphilitic A52.71
  traumatic (*see also* Glaucoma, secondary, trauma)
    newborn (birth injury) P15.3
  tuberculous A18.59
Glaucomatous flecks (subcapsular) — *see* Cataract, complicated
Glazed tongue K14.4
Gleet (gonococcal) A54.01
Glénard's disease K63.4
Glioblastoma (multiforme)
  with sarcomatous component
    specified site — *see* Neoplasm, malignant, by site
    unspecified site C71.9
  giant cell
    specified site — *see* Neoplasm, malignant, by site
    unspecified site C71.9
  specified site — *see* Neoplasm, malignant, by site
  unspecified site C71.9
Glioma (malignant)
  astrocytic
    specified site — *see* Neoplasm, malignant, by site
    unspecified site C71.9
  mixed
    specified site — *see* Neoplasm, malignant, by site
    unspecified site C71.9
  nose Q30.8
  specified site NEC — *see* Neoplasm, malignant, by site
  subependymal D43.2
    specified site — *see* Neoplasm, uncertain behavior, by site
    unspecified site D43.2
  unspecified site C71.9
Gliomatosis cerebri C71.0
Glioneuroma — *see* Neoplasm, uncertain behavior, by site
Gliosarcoma
  specified site — *see* Neoplasm, malignant, by site
  unspecified site C71.9
Gliosis (cerebral) G93.89
  spinal G95.89
Glisson's disease — *see* Rickets
Globinuria R82.3
Globus (hystericus) F45.8
Glomangioma D18.00
  intra-abdominal D18.03
  intracranial D18.02
  skin D18.01
  specified site NEC D18.09
Glomangiomyoma D18.00
  intra-abdominal D18.03
  intracranial D18.02
  skin D18.01
  specified site NEC D18.09

Glomangiosarcoma — *see* Neoplasm, connective tissue, malignant
Glomerular
  disease in syphilis A52.75
  nephritis — *see* Glomerulonephritis
Glomerulitis — *see* Glomerulonephritis
Glomerulonephritis (*see also* Nephritis) N05.9
  with
    edema — *see* Nephrosis
      minimal change N05.0
      minor glomerular abnormality N05.0
  acute N00.9
  chronic N03.9
  crescentic (diffuse) NEC (*see also* N00-N07 with fourth character .7) N05.7
  dense deposit (*see also* N00-N07 with fourth character .6) N05.6
  diffuse
    crescentic (*see also* N00-N07 with fourth character .7) N05.7
    endocapillary proliferative (*see also* N00-N07 with fourth character .4) N05.4
    membranous (*see also* N00-N07 with fourth character .2) N05.2
    mesangial proliferative (*see also* N00-N07 with fourth character .3) N05.3
    mesangiocapillary (*see also* N00-N07 with fourth character .5) N05.5
    sclerosing N18.9
  endocapillary proliferative (diffuse) NEC (*see also* N00-N07 with fourth character .4) N05.4
  extracapillary NEC (*see also* N00-N07 with fourth character .7) N05.7
  focal (and segmental) (*see also* N00-N07 with fourth character .1) N05.1
  hypocomplementemic — *see* Glomerulonephritis, membranoproliferative
  IgA — *see* Nephropathy, IgA
  immune complex (circulating) NEC N05.8
  in (due to)
    amyloidosis E85.4 *[N08]*
    bilharziasis B65.9 *[N08]*
    cryoglobulinemia D89.1 *[N08]*
    defibrination syndrome D65 *[N08]*
    diabetes mellitus — *see* Diabetes, glomerulosclerosis
    disseminated intravascular coagulation D65 *[N08]*
    Fabry (-Anderson) disease E75.21 *[N08]*
    Goodpasture's syndrome M31.0
    hemolytic-uremic syndrome D59.3
    Henoch (-Schönlein) purpura D69.0 *[N08]*
    lecithin cholesterol acyltransferase deficiency E78.6 *[N08]*
    microscopic polyangiitis M31.7 *[N08]*
    multiple myeloma C90.0 ☑ *[N08]*
    Plasmodium malariae B52.0
    schistosomiasis B65.9 *[N08]*
    sepsis A41.9 *[N08]*
      streptococcal A40 ☑ *[N08]*
    sickle-cell disorders D57. ☑ *[N08]*
    strongyloidiasis B78.9 *[N08]*
    subacute bacterial endocarditis I33.0 *[N08]*
    syphilis (late) congenital A50.59 *[N08]*
    systemic lupus erythematosus M32.14
    thrombotic thrombocytopenic purpura M31.1 *[N08]*
    typhoid fever A01.09
    Waldenström macroglobulinemia C88.0 *[N08]*
    Wegener's granulomatosis M31.31
  latent or quiescent N03.9
  lobular, lobulonodular — *see* Glomerulonephritis, membranoproliferative
  membranoproliferative (diffuse)(type 1 or 3) (*see also* N00-N07 with fourth character .5) N05.5
    dense deposit (type 2) NEC (*see also* N00-N07 with fourth character .6) N05.6
    membranous (diffuse) NEC (*see also* N00-N07 with fourth character .2) N05.2
  mesangial
    IgA/IgG — *see* Nephropathy, IgA
    proliferative (diffuse) NEC (*see also* N00-N07 with fourth character .3) N05.3
  mesangiocapillary (diffuse) NEC (*see also* N00-N07 with fourth character .5) N05.5
  necrotic, necrotizing NEC (*see also* N00-N07 with fourth character .8) N05.8
  nodular — *see* Glomerulonephritis, membranoproliferative
  poststreptococcal NEC N05.9
    acute N00.9
    chronic N03.9
    rapidly progressive N01.9

Glomerulonephritis — *continued*
  proliferative NEC (*see also* N00-N07 with fourth character .8) N05.8
    diffuse (lupus) M32.14
  rapidly progressive N01.9
  sclerosing, diffuse N18.9
  specified pathology NEC (*see also* N00-N07 with fourth character .8) N05.8
  subacute N01.9
Glomerulopathy — *see* Glomerulonephritis
Glomerulosclerosis (*see also* Sclerosis, renal)
  intercapillary (nodular) (with diabetes) — *see* Diabetes, glomerulosclerosis
  intracapillary — *see* Diabetes, glomerulosclerosis
Glossagra K14.6
Glossalgia K14.6
Glossitis (chronic superficial) (gangrenous) (Moeller's) K14.0
  areata exfoliativa K14.1
  atrophic K14.4
  benign migratory K14.1
  cortical superficial, sclerotic K14.0
  Hunter's D51.0
  interstitial, sclerous K14.0
  median rhomboid K14.2
  pellagrous E52
  superficial, chronic K14.0
Glossocele K14.8
Glossodynia K14.6
  exfoliativa K14.4
Glossoncus K14.8
Glossopathy K14.9
Glossophytia K14.3
Glossoplegia K14.8
Glossoptosis K14.8
Glossopyrosis K14.6
Glossotrichia K14.3
Glossy skin L90.8
Glottis — *see* condition
Glottitis (*see also* Laryngitis) J04.0
Glucagonoma
  pancreas
    benign D13.7
    malignant C25.4
    uncertain behavior D37.8
  specified site NEC
    benign — *see* Neoplasm, benign, by site
    malignant — *see* Neoplasm, malignant, by site
    uncertain behavior — *see* Neoplasm, uncertain behavior, by site
  unspecified site
    benign D13.7
    malignant C25.4
    uncertain behavior D37.8
Glucoglycinuria E72.51
Glucose-galactose malabsorption E74.39
Glue
  ear — *see* Otitis, media, nonsuppurative, chronic, mucoid
  sniffing (airplane) — *see* Abuse, drug, inhalant
    dependence — *see* Dependence, drug, inhalant
Glutaric aciduria E72.3
Glycinemia E72.51
Glycinuria (renal) (with ketosis) E72.09
Glycogen
  infiltration — *see* Disease, glycogen storage
  storage disease — *see* Disease, glycogen storage
Glycogenosis (diffuse) (generalized) (*see also* Disease, glycogen storage)
  cardiac E74.02 *[I43]*
  diabetic, secondary — *see* Diabetes, glycogenosis, secondary
  pulmonary interstitial J84.842
Glycopenia E16.2
Glycosuria R81
  renal E74.8
Gnathostoma spinigerum (infection) (infestation), gnathostomiasis (wandering swelling) B83.1
Goiter (plunging) (substernal) E04.9
  with
    hyperthyroidism (recurrent) — *see* Hyperthyroidism, with, goiter
    thyrotoxicosis — *see* Hyperthyroidism, with, goiter
  adenomatous — *see* Goiter, nodular
  cancerous C73
  congenital (nontoxic) E03.0
    diffuse E03.0
    parenchymatous E03.0
    transitory, with normal functioning P72.0
  cystic E04.2
    due to iodine-deficiency E01.1

Goiter — *continued*
  due to
    enzyme defect in synthesis of thyroid hormone
      E07.1
    iodine-deficiency (endemic) E01.2
  dyshormonogenetic (familial) E07.1
  endemic (iodine-deficiency) E01.2
    diffuse E01.0
    multinodular E01.1
  exophthalmic — *see* Hyperthyroidism, with, goiter
  iodine-deficiency (endemic) E01.2
    diffuse E01.0
    multinodular E01.1
    nodular E01.1
  lingual Q89.2
  lymphadenoid E06.3
  malignant C73
  multinodular (cystic) (nontoxic) E04.2
    toxic or with hyperthyroidism E05.20
      with thyroid storm E05.21
  neonatal NEC P72.0
  nodular (nontoxic) (due to) E04.9
    with
      hyperthyroidism E05.20
        with thyroid storm E05.21
      thyrotoxicosis E05.20
        with thyroid storm E05.21
    endemic E01.1
    iodine-deficiency E01.1
    sporadic E04.9
    toxic E05.20
      with thyroid storm E05.21
  nontoxic E04.9
    diffuse (colloid) E04.0
    multinodular E04.2
    simple E04.0
    specified NEC E04.8
    uninodular E04.1
  simple E04.0
  toxic — *see* Hyperthyroidism, with, goiter
  uninodular (nontoxic) E04.1
    toxic or with hyperthyroidism E05.10
      with thyroid storm E05.11
Goiter-deafness syndrome E07.1
Goldberg syndrome Q89.8
Goldberg-Maxwell syndrome E34.51
Goldblatt's hypertension or kidney I70.1
Goldenhar (-Gorlin) syndrome Q87.0
Goldflam-Erb disease or syndrome G70.00
  with exacerbation (acute) G70.01
  in crisis G70.01
Goldscheider's disease Q81.8
Goldstein's disease (familial hemorrhagic
  telangiectasia) I78.0
Golfer's elbow — *see* Epicondylitis, medial
Gonadoblastoma
  specified site — *see* Neoplasm, uncertain behavior,
    by site
  unspecified site
    female D39.10
    male D40.10
Gonecystitis — *see* Vesiculitis
Gongylonemiasis B83.8
Goniosynechiae — *see* Adhesions, iris, goniosynechiae
Gonococcemia A54.86
Gonococcus, gonococcal (disease) (infection) (*see also*
  condition) A54.9
  anus A54.6
  bursa, bursitis A54.49
  conjunctiva, conjunctivitis (neonatorum) A54.31
  endocardium A54.83
  eye A54.30
    conjunctivitis A54.31
    iridocyclitis A54.32
    keratitis A54.33
    newborn A54.31
    other specified A54.39
  fallopian tubes (acute) (chronic) A54.24
  genitourinary (organ) (system) (tract) (acute)
    lower A54.00
      with abscess (accessory gland) (periurethral) A54.1
    upper (*see also* condition) A54.29
  heart A54.83
  iridocyclitis A54.32
  joint A54.42
  lymphatic (gland) (node) A54.89
  meninges, meningitis A54.81
  musculoskeletal A54.40
    arthritis A54.42
    osteomyelitis A54.43
    other specified A54.49
    spondylopathy A54.41

Gonococcus — *continued*
  pelviperitonitis A54.24
  pelvis (acute) (chronic) A54.24
  pharynx A54.5
  proctitis A54.6
  pyosalpinx (acute) (chronic) A54.24
  rectum A54.6
  skin A54.89
  specified site NEC A54.89
  tendon sheath A54.49
  throat A54.5
  urethra (acute) (chronic) A54.01
    with abscess (accessory gland) (periurethral)
      A54.1
  vulva (acute) (chronic) A54.02
Gonocytoma
  specified site — *see* Neoplasm, uncertain behavior,
    by site
  unspecified site
    female D39.10
    male D40.10
Gonorrhea (acute) (chronic) A54.9
  Bartholin's gland (acute) (chronic) (purulent) A54.02
    with abscess (accessory gland) (periurethral)
      A54.1
  bladder A54.01
  cervix A54.03
  conjunctiva, conjunctivitis (neonatorum) A54.31
  contact Z20.2
  Cowper's gland (with abscess) A54.1
  exposure to Z20.2
  fallopian tube (acute) (chronic) A54.24
  kidney (acute) (chronic) A54.21
  lower genitourinary tract A54.00
    with abscess (accessory gland) (periurethral)
      A54.1
  ovary (acute) (chronic) A54.24
  pelvis (acute) (chronic) A54.24
    female pelvic inflammatory disease A54.24
  penis A54.09
  prostate (acute) (chronic) A54.22
  seminal vesicle (acute) (chronic) A54.23
  specified site not listed (*see also* Gonococcus)
    A54.89
  spermatic cord (acute) (chronic) A54.23
  urethra A54.01
    with abscess (accessory gland) (periurethral)
      A54.1
  vagina A54.02
  vas deferens (acute) (chronic) A54.23
  vulva A54.02
Goodall's disease A08.19
Goodpasture's syndrome M31.0
Gopalan's syndrome (burning feet) E53.0
Gorlin-Chaudry-Moss syndrome Q87.0
Gottron's papules L94.4
Gougerot's syndrome (trisymptomatic) L81.7
Gougerot-Blum syndrome (pigmented purpuric
  lichenoid dermatitis) L81.7
Gougerot-Carteaud disease or syndrome (confluent
  reticulate papillomatosis) L83
Gouley's syndrome (constrictive pericarditis) I31.1
Goundou A66.6
Gout, gouty (acute) (attack) (flare) (*see also* Gout,
  chronic) M10.9
  drug-induced M10.20
    ankle M10.27 ☑
    elbow M10.22 ☑
    foot joint M10.27 ☑
    hand joint M10.24 ☑
    hip M10.25 ☑
    knee M10.26 ☑
    multiple site M10.29
    shoulder M10.21 ☑
    vertebrae M10.28
    wrist M10.23 ☑
  idiopathic M10.00
    ankle M10.07 ☑
    elbow M10.02 ☑
    foot joint M10.07 ☑
    hand joint M10.04 ☑
    hip M10.05 ☑
    knee M10.06 ☑
    multiple site M10.09
    shoulder M10.01 ☑
    vertebrae M10.08
    wrist M10.03 ☑
  in (due to) renal impairment M10.30
    ankle M10.37 ☑
    elbow M10.32 ☑
    foot joint M10.37 ☑
    hand joint M10.34 ☑

Gout — *continued*
  in — *continued*
    hip M10.35 ☑
    knee M10.36 ☑
    multiple site M10.39
    shoulder M10.31 ☑
    vertebrae M10.38
    wrist M10.33 ☑
  lead-induced M10.10
    ankle M10.17 ☑
    elbow M10.12 ☑
    foot joint M10.17 ☑
    hand joint M10.14 ☑
    hip M10.15 ☑
    knee M10.16 ☑
    multiple site M10.19
    shoulder M10.11 ☑
    vertebrae M10.18
    wrist M10.13 ☑
  primary — *see* Gout, idiopathic
  saturnine — *see* Gout, lead-induced
  secondary NEC M10.40
    ankle M10.47 ☑
    elbow M10.42 ☑
    foot joint M10.47 ☑
    hand joint M10.44 ☑
    hip M10.45 ☑
    knee M10.46 ☑
    multiple site M10.49
    shoulder M10.41 ☑
    vertebrae M10.48
    wrist M10.43 ☑
  syphilitic (*see also* subcategory M14.8 ☑) A52.77
  tophi — *see* Gout, chronic
Gout, chronic (*see also* Gout, gouty) M1A.9 ☑
  drug-induced M1A.20 ☑
    ankle M1A.27 ☑
    elbow M1A.22 ☑
    foot joint M1A.27 ☑
    hand joint M1A.24 ☑
    hip M1A.25 ☑
    knee M1A.26 ☑
    multiple site M1A.29 ☑
    shoulder M1A.21 ☑
    vertebrae M1A.28 ☑
    wrist M1A.23 ☑
  idiopathic M1A.00 ☑
    ankle M1A.07 ☑
    elbow M1A.02 ☑
    foot joint M1A.07 ☑
    hand joint M1A.04 ☑
    hip M1A.05 ☑
    knee M1A.06 ☑
    multiple site M1A.09 ☑
    shoulder M1A.01 ☑
    vertebrae M1A.08 ☑
    wrist M1A.03 ☑
  in (due to) renal impairment M1A.30 ☑
    ankle M1A.37 ☑
    elbow M1A.32 ☑
    foot joint M1A.37 ☑
    hand joint M1A.34 ☑
    hip M1A.35 ☑
    knee M1A.36 ☑
    multiple site M1A.39 ☑
    shoulder M1A.31 ☑
    vertebrae M1A.38 ☑
    wrist M1A.33 ☑
  lead-induced M1A.10 ☑
    ankle M1A.17 ☑
    elbow M1A.12 ☑
    foot joint M1A.17 ☑
    hand joint M1A.14 ☑
    hip M1A.15 ☑
    knee M1A.16 ☑
    multiple site M1A.19 ☑
    shoulder M1A.11 ☑
    vertebrae M1A.18 ☑
    wrist M1A.13 ☑
  primary — *see* Gout, chronic, idiopathic
  saturnine — *see* Gout, chronic, lead-induced
  secondary NEC M1A.40 ☑
    ankle M1A.47 ☑
    elbow M1A.42 ☑
    foot joint M1A.47 ☑
    hand joint M1A.44 ☑
    hip M1A.45 ☑
    knee M1A.46 ☑
    multiple site M1A.49 ☑
    shoulder M1A.41 ☑
    vertebrae M1A.48 ☑
    wrist M1A.43 ☑

☑ **Additional character required**

Gout, chronic — *continued*
  syphilitic (*see also* subcategory M14.8 ☑) A52.77
  tophi M1A.9 ☑
Gower's
  muscular dystrophy G71.01
  syndrome (vasovagal attack) R55
Gradenigo's syndrome — *see* Otitis, media, suppurative, acute
Graefe's disease — *see* Strabismus, paralytic, ophthalmoplegia, progressive
Graft-versus-host disease D89.813
  acute D89.810
  acute on chronic D89.812
  chronic D89.811
Grainhandler's disease or lung J67.8
Grain mite (itch) B88.0
Grand mal — *see* Epilepsy, generalized, specified NEC
Grand multipara status only (not pregnant) Z64.1
  pregnant — *see* Pregnancy, complicated by, grand multiparity
Granite worker's lung J62.8
Granular (*see also* condition)
  inflammation, pharynx J31.2
  kidney (contracting) — *see* Sclerosis, renal
  liver K74.69
Granulation tissue (abnormal) (excessive) L92.9
  postmastoidectomy cavity — *see* Complications, postmastoidectomy, granulation
Granulocytopenia (primary) (malignant) — *see* Agranulocytosis
Granuloma L92.9
  abdomen K66.8
    from residual foreign body L92.3
    pyogenicum L98.0
  actinic L57.5
  annulare (perforating) L92.0
  apical K04.5
  aural — *see* Otitis, externa, specified NEC
  beryllium (skin) L92.3
  bone
    eosinophilic C96.6
    from residual foreign body — *see* Osteomyelitis, specified type NEC
    lung C96.6
  brain (any site) G06.0
    schistosomiasis B65.9 *[G07]*
  canaliculus lacrimalis — *see* Granuloma, lacrimal
  candidal (cutaneous) B37.2
  cerebral (any site) G06.0
  coccidioidal (primary) (progressive) B38.7
    lung B38.1
    meninges B38.4
  colon K63.89
  conjunctiva H11.22 ☑
  dental K04.5
  ear, middle — *see* Cholesteatoma
  eosinophilic C96.6
    bone C96.6
    lung C96.6
    oral mucosa K13.4
    skin L92.2
  eyelid H01.8
  facial (e) L92.2
  foreign body (in soft tissue) NEC M60.20
    ankle M60.27 ☑
    foot M60.27 ☑
    forearm M60.23 ☑
    hand M60.24 ☑
    in operation wound — *see* Foreign body, accidentally left during a procedure
    lower leg M60.26 ☑
    pelvic region M60.25 ☑
    shoulder region M60.21 ☑
    skin L92.3
    specified site NEC M60.28
    subcutaneous tissue L92.3
    thigh M60.25 ☑
    upper arm M60.22 ☑
  gangraenescens M31.2
  genito-inguinale A58
  giant cell (central) (reparative) (jaw) M27.1
    gingiva (peripheral) K06.8
  gland (lymph) I88.8
  hepatic NEC K75.3
    in (due to)
      berylliosis J63.2 *[K77]*
      sarcoidosis D86.89
  Hodgkin C81.9 ☑
  ileum K63.89
  infectious B99.9
    specified NEC B99.8
  inguinale (Donovan) (venereal) A58

Granuloma — *continued*
  intestine NEC K63.89
  intracranial (any site) G06.0
  intraspinal (any part) G06.1
  iridocyclitis — *see* Iridocyclitis, chronic
  jaw (bone) (central) M27.1
    reparative giant cell M27.1
  kidney (*see also* Infection, kidney) N15.8
  lacrimal H04.81 ☑
  larynx J38.7
  lethal midline (facial) M31.2
  liver NEC — *see* Granuloma, hepatic
  lung (infectious) (*see also* Fibrosis, lung)
    coccidioidal B38.1
    eosinophilic C96.6
  Majocchi's B35.8
  malignant (facial(e)) M31.2
  mandible (central) M27.1
  midline (lethal) M31.2
  monilial (cutaneous) B37.2
  nasal sinus — *see* Sinusitis
  operation wound T81.89 ☑
    foreign body — *see* Foreign body, accidentally left during a procedure
    stitch T81.89 ☑
    talc — *see* Foreign body, accidentally left during a procedure
  oral mucosa K13.4
  orbit, orbital H05.11 ☑
  paracoccidioidal B41.8
  penis, venereal A58
  periapical K04.5
  peritoneum K66.8
    due to ova of helminths NOS (*see also* Helminthiasis) B83.9 *[K67]*
  postmastoidectomy cavity — *see* Complications, postmastoidectomy, recurrent cholesteatoma
  prostate N42.89
  pudendi (ulcerating) A58
  pulp, internal (tooth) K03.3
  pyogenic, pyogenicum (of) (skin) L98.0
    gingiva K06.8
    maxillary alveolar ridge K04.5
    oral mucosa K13.4
  rectum K62.89
  reticulohistiocytic D76.3
  rubrum nasi L74.8
  Schistosoma — *see* Schistosomiasis
  septic (skin) L98.0
  silica (skin) L92.3
  sinus (accessory) (infective) (nasal) — *see* Sinusitis
  skin L92.9
    from residual foreign body L92.3
    pyogenicum L98.0
  spine
    syphilitic (epidural) A52.19
    tuberculous A18.01
  stitch (postoperative) T81.89 ☑
  suppurative (skin) L98.0
  swimming pool A31.1
  talc (*see also* Granuloma, foreign body)
    in operation wound — *see* Foreign body, accidentally left during a procedure
  telangiectaticum (skin) L98.0
  tracheostomy J95.09
  trichophyticum B35.8
  tropicum A66.4
  umbilical P83.81
  umbilicus P83.81
  urethra N36.8
  uveitis — *see* Iridocyclitis, chronic
  vagina A58
  venereum A58
  vocal cord J38.3
Granulomatosis L92.9
  lymphoid C83.8 ☑
  miliary (listerial) A32.89
  necrotizing, respiratory M31.30
  progressive septic D71
  specified NEC L92.8
  Wegener's M31.30
    with renal involvement M31.31
Granulomatous tissue (abnormal) (excessive) L92.9
Granulosis rubra nasi L74.8
Graphite fibrosis (of lung) J63.3
Graphospasm F48.8
  organic G25.89
Grating scapula M89.8X1
Gravel (urinary) — *see* Calculus, urinary
Graves' disease — *see* Hyperthyroidism, with, goiter
Gravis — *see* condition
Grawitz tumor C64. ☑

Gray syndrome (newborn) P93.0
Grayness, hair (premature) L67.1
  congenital Q84.2
Green sickness D50.8
Greenfield's disease
  meaning
    concentric sclerosis (encephalitis periaxialis concentrica) G37.5
    metachromatic leukodystrophy E75.25
Greenstick fracture - code as Fracture, by site
Grey syndrome (newborn) P93.0
Grief F43.21
  prolonged F43.29
  reaction (*see also* Disorder, adjustment) F43.20
Griesinger's disease B76.0
Grinder's lung or pneumoconiosis J62.8
Grinding, teeth
  psychogenic F45.8
  sleep related G47.63
Grip
  Dabney's B33.0
  devil's B33.0
Grippe, grippal (*see also* Influenza)
  Balkan A78
  summer, of Italy A93.1
Grisel's disease M43.6
Groin — *see* condition
Grooved tongue K14.5
Ground itch B76.9
Grover's disease or syndrome L11.1
Growing pains, children R29.898
Growth (fungoid) (neoplastic) (new) (*see also* Neoplasm)
  adenoid (vegetative) J35.8
  benign — *see* Neoplasm, benign, by site
  malignant — *see* Neoplasm, malignant, by site
  rapid, childhood Z00.2
  secondary — *see* Neoplasm, secondary, by site
Gruby's disease B35.0
Gubler-Millard paralysis or syndrome G46.3
Guerin-Stern syndrome Q74.3
Guidance, insufficient anterior (occlusal) M26.54
Guillain-Barré disease or syndrome G61.0
  sequelae G65.0
Guinea worms (infection) (infestation) B72
Guinon's disease (motor-verbal tic) F95.2
Gull's disease E03.4
Gum — *see* condition
Gumboil K04.7
  with sinus K04.6
Gumma (syphilitic) A52.79
  artery A52.09
    cerebral A52.04
  bone A52.77
    of yaws (late) A66.6
  brain A52.19
  cauda equina A52.19
  central nervous system A52.3
  ciliary body A52.71
  congenital A50.59
  eyelid A52.71
  heart A52.06
  intracranial A52.19
  iris A52.71
  kidney A52.75
  larynx A52.73
  leptomeninges A52.19
  liver A52.74
  meninges A52.19
  myocardium A52.06
  nasopharynx A52.73
  neurosyphilitic A52.3
  nose A52.73
  orbit A52.71
  palate (soft) A52.79
  penis A52.76
  pericardium A52.06
  pharynx A52.73
  pituitary A52.79
  scrofulous (tuberculous) A18.4
  skin A52.79
  specified site NEC A52.79
  spinal cord A52.19
  tongue A52.79
  tonsil A52.73
  trachea A52.73
  tuberculous A18.4
  ulcerative due to yaws A66.4
  ureter A52.75
  yaws A66.4
    bone A66.6
Gunn's syndrome Q07.8

Gunshot wound - Hearing examination

Gunshot wound (*see also* Wound, open)
  fracture - code as Fracture, by site
  internal organs — *see* Injury, by site
Gynandrism Q56.0
Gynandroblastoma
  specified site — *see* Neoplasm, uncertain behavior,
    by site
  unspecified site
    female D39.10
    male D40.10
Gynecological examination (periodic) (routine)
  Z01.419
  with abnormal findings Z01.411
Gynecomastia N62
Gynephobia F40.291
Gyrate scalp Q82.8

H

H (Hartnup's) disease E72.02
Haas' disease or osteochondrosis (juvenile) (head of
  humerus) — *see* Osteochondrosis, juvenile, humerus
Habit, habituation
  bad sleep Z72.821
  chorea F95.8
  disturbance, child F98.9
  drug — *see* Dependence, drug
  irregular sleep Z72.821
  laxative F55.2
  spasm — *see* Tic
  tic — *see* Tic
Haemophilus (H.) influenzae, as cause of disease
  classified elsewhere B96.3
Haff disease — *see* Poisoning, mercury
Hageman's factor defect, deficiency or disease D68.2
Haglund's disease or osteochondrosis (juvenile) (os
  tibiale externum) — *see* Osteochondrosis, juvenile,
  tarsus
Hailey-Hailey disease Q82.8
Hair (*see also* condition)
  plucking F63.3
    in stereotyped movement disorder F98.4
  tourniquet syndrome (*see also* Constriction,
    external, by site)
    finger S60.44 ☑
    penis S30.842 ☑
    thumb S60.34 ☑
    toe S90.44 ☑
Hairball in stomach T18.2 ☑
Hair-pulling, pathological (compulsive) F63.3
Hairy black tongue K14.3
Half vertebra Q76.49
Halitosis R19.6
Hallerman-Streiff syndrome Q87.0
Hallervorden-Spatz disease G23.0
Hallopeau's acrodermatitis or disease L40.2
Hallucination R44.3
  auditory R44.0
  gustatory R44.2
  olfactory R44.2
  specified NEC R44.2
  tactile R44.2
  visual R44.1
Hallucinosis (chronic) F28
  alcoholic (acute) F10.951
    in
      abuse F10.151
      dependence F10.251
  drug-induced F19.951
    cannabis F12.951
    cocaine F14.951
    hallucinogen F16.151
    in
      abuse F19.151
        cannabis F12.151
        cocaine F14.151
        hallucinogen F16.151
        inhalant F18.151
        opioid F11.151
        sedative, anxiolytic or hypnotic F13.151
        stimulant NEC F15.151
      dependence F19.251
        cannabis F12.251
        cocaine F14.251
        hallucinogen F16.251
        inhalant F18.251
        opioid F11.251
        sedative, anxiolytic or hypnotic F13.251
        stimulant NEC F15.251
    inhalant F18.951

Hallucinosis — *continued*
  drug-induced — *continued*
    opioid F11.951
    sedative, anxiolytic or hypnotic F13.951
    stimulant NEC F15.951
  organic F06.0
Hallux
  deformity (acquired) NEC M20.5X ☑
  limitus M20.5X ☑
  malleus (acquired) NEC M20.3 ☑
  rigidus (acquired) M20.2 ☑
    congenital Q74.2
    sequelae (late effect) of rickets E64.3
  valgus (acquired) M20.1 ☑
    congenital Q66.6
  varus (acquired) M20.3 ☑
    congenital Q66.3 ☑
Halo, visual H53.19
Hamartoma, hamartoblastoma Q85.9
  epithelial (gingival), odontogenic, central or
    peripheral — *see* Cyst, calcifying odontogenic
Hamartosis Q85.9
Hamman-Rich syndrome J84.114
Hammer toe (acquired) NEC (*see also* Deformity, toe,
  hammer toe)
  congenital Q66.89
  sequelae (late effect) of rickets E64.3
Hand — *see* condition
Hand-foot syndrome L27.1
Handicap, handicapped
  educational Z55.9
    specified NEC Z55.8
Hand-Schüller-Christian disease or syndrome C96.5
Hanging (asphyxia) (strangulation) (suffocation) — *see*
  Asphyxia, traumatic, due to mechanical threat
Hangnail (*see also* Cellulitis, digit)
  with lymphangitis — *see* Lymphangitis, acute, digit
Hangover (alcohol) F10.129
Hanhart's syndrome Q87.0
Hanot-Chauffard (-Troisier) syndrome E83.19
Hanot's cirrhosis or disease K74.3
Hansen's disease — *see* Leprosy
Hantaan virus disease (Korean hemorrhagic fever)
  A98.5
Hantavirus disease (with renal manifestations)
  (Dobrava) (Puumala) (Seoul) A98.5
    with pulmonary manifestations (Andes) (Bayou)
      (Bermejo) (Black Creek Canal) (Choclo)
      (Juquitiba) (Laguna negra) (Lechiguanas) (New
      York) (Oran) (Sin nombre) B33.4
Happy puppet syndrome Q93.51
Harada's disease or syndrome H30.81 ☑
Hardening
  artery — *see* Arteriosclerosis
  brain G93.89
Harelip (complete) (incomplete) — *see* Cleft, lip
Harlequin (newborn) Q80.4
Harley's disease D59.6
Harmful use (of)
  alcohol F10.10
  anxiolytics — *see* Abuse, drug, sedative
  cannabinoids — *see* Abuse, drug, cannabis
  cocaine — *see* Abuse, drug, cocaine
  drug — *see* Abuse, drug
  hallucinogens — *see* Abuse, drug, hallucinogen
  hypnotics — *see* Abuse, drug, sedative
  opioids — *see* Abuse, drug, opioid
  PCP (phencyclidine) — *see* Abuse, drug,
    hallucinogen
  sedatives — *see* Abuse, drug, sedative
  stimulants NEC — *see* Abuse, drug, stimulant
Harris' lines — *see* Arrest, epiphyseal
Hartnup's disease E72.02
Harvester's lung J67.0
Harvesting ovum for in vitro fertilization Z31.83
Hashimoto's disease or thyroiditis E06.3
Hashitoxicosis (transient) E06.3
Hassal-Henle bodies or warts (cornea) H18.49
Haut mal — *see* Epilepsy, generalized, specified NEC
Haverhill fever A25.1
Hay fever (*see also* Fever, hay) J30.1
Hayem-Widal syndrome D59.8
Haygarth's nodes M15.8
Haymaker's lung J67.0
Hb (abnormal)
  Bart's disease D56.0
  disease — *see* Disease, hemoglobin
  trait — *see* Trait
Head — *see* condition
Headache R51
  allergic NEC G44.89
  associated with sexual activity G44.82

Headache — *continued*
  chronic daily R51
  cluster G44.009
    chronic G44.029
      intractable G44.021
      not intractable G44.029
    episodic G44.019
      intractable G44.011
      not intractable G44.019
    intractable G44.001
    not intractable G44.009
  cough (primary) G44.83
  daily chronic R51
  drug-induced NEC G44.40
    intractable G44.41
    not intractable G44.40
  exertional (primary) G44.84
  histamine G44.009
    intractable G44.001
    not intractable G44.009
  hypnic G44.81
  lumbar puncture G97.1
  medication overuse G44.40
    intractable G44.41
    not intractable G44.40
  menstrual — *see* Migraine, menstrual
  migraine (type) (*see also* Migraine) G43.909
  nasal septum R51
  neuralgiform, short lasting unilateral, with
    conjunctival injection and tearing (SUNCT)
    G44.059
    intractable G44.051
    not intractable G44.059
  new daily persistent (NDPH) G44.52
  orgasmic G44.82
  periodic syndromes in adults and children G43.C0
    with refractory migraine G43.C1
      intractable G43.C1
      not intractable G43.C0
    without refractory migraine G43.C0
  postspinal puncture G97.1
  post-traumatic G44.309
    acute G44.319
      intractable G44.311
      not intractable G44.319
    chronic G44.329
      intractable G44.321
      not intractable G44.329
    intractable G44.301
    not intractable G44.309
  pre-menstrual — *see* Migraine, menstrual
  preorgasmic G44.82
  primary
    cough G44.83
    exertional G44.84
    stabbing G44.85
    thunderclap G44.53
  rebound G44.40
    intractable G44.41
    not intractable G44.40
  short lasting unilateral neuralgiform, with
    conjunctival injection and tearing (SUNCT)
    G44.059
    intractable G44.051
    not intractable G44.059
  specified syndrome NEC G44.89
  spinal and epidural anesthesia - induced T88.59 ☑
    in labor and delivery O74.5
    in pregnancy O29.4 ☑
    postpartum, puerperal O89.4
  spinal fluid loss (from puncture) G97.1
  stabbing (primary) G44.85
  tension (-type) G44.209
    chronic G44.229
      intractable G44.221
      not intractable G44.229
    episodic G44.219
      intractable G44.211
      not intractable G44.219
    intractable G44.201
    not intractable G44.209
  thunderclap (primary) G44.53
  vascular NEC G44.1
Healthy
  infant
    accompanying sick mother Z76.3
    receiving care Z76.2
  person accompanying sick person Z76.3
Hearing examination Z01.10
  with abnormal findings NEC Z01.118
  infant or child (over 28 days old) Z00.129
    with abnormal findings Z00.121

☑ **Additional character required**

Hearing examination — *continued*
  following failed hearing screening Z01.110
  for hearing conservation and treatment Z01.12
Heart — *see* condition
Heart beat
  abnormality R00.9
    specified NEC R00.8
  awareness R00.2
  rapid R00.0
  slow R00.1
Heartburn R12
  psychogenic F45.8
Heartland virus disease A93.8
Heat (effects) T67.9 ☑
  apoplexy T67.01 ☑
  burn (*see also* Burn) L55.9
  collapse T67.1 ☑
  cramps T67.2 ☑
  dermatitis or eczema L59.0
  edema T67.7 ☑
  erythema - code by site under Burn, first degree
  excessive T67.9 ☑
    specified effect NEC T67.8 ☑
  exhaustion T67.5 ☑
    anhydrotic T67.3 ☑
    due to
      salt (and water) depletion T67.4 ☑
      water depletion T67.3 ☑
        with salt depletion T67.4 ☑
  fatigue (transient) T67.6 ☑
  fever T67.01 ☑
  hyperpyrexia T67.01 ☑
  prickly L74.0
  prostration — *see* Heat, exhaustion
  pyrexia T67.01 ☑
  rash L74.0
  specified effect NEC T67.8 ☑
  stroke T67.01 ☑
    exertional T67.02 ☑
    specified NEC T67.09 ☑
  sunburn — *see* Sunburn
  syncope T67.1 ☑
Heavy-for-dates NEC (infant) (4000g to 4499g) P08.1
  exceptionally (4500g or more) P08.0
Hebephrenia, hebephrenic (schizophrenia) F20.1
Heberden's disease or nodes (with arthropathy) M15.1
Hebra's
  pityriasis L26
  prurigo L28.2
Heel — *see* condition
Heerfordt's disease D86.89
Hegglin's anomaly or syndrome D72.0
Heilmeyer-Schoner disease D45
Heine-Medin disease A80.9
Heinz body anemia, congenital D58.2
Heliophobia F40.228
Heller's disease or syndrome F84.3
HELLP syndrome (hemolysis, elevated liver enzymes
    and low platelet count) O14.2 ☑
  complicating
    childbirth O14.24
    puerperium O14.25
Helminthiasis (*see also* Infestation, helminth)
  Ancylostoma B76.0
  intestinal B82.0
    mixed types (types classifiable to more than one
      of the titles B65.0-B81.3 and B81.8) B81.4
    specified type NEC B81.8
  mixed types (intestinal) (types classifiable to more
    than one of the titles B65.0-B81.3 and B81.8)
    B81.4
  Necator (americanus) B76.1
  specified type NEC B83.8
Heloma L84
Hemangioblastoma — *see* Neoplasm, connective
  tissue, uncertain behavior
  malignant — *see* Neoplasm, connective tissue,
    malignant
Hemangioendothelioma (*see also* Neoplasm,
    uncertain behavior, by site)
  benign D18.00
    intra-abdominal D18.03
    intracranial D18.02
    skin D18.01
    specified site NEC D18.09
  bone (diffuse) — *see* Neoplasm, bone, malignant
  epithelioid (*see also* Neoplasm, uncertain behavior,
    by site)
    malignant — *see* Neoplasm, malignant, by site
  malignant — *see* Neoplasm, connective tissue,
    malignant
Hemangiofibroma — *see* Neoplasm, benign, by site

Hemangiolipoma — *see* Lipoma
Hemangioma D18.00
  arteriovenous D18.00
    intra-abdominal D18.03
    intracranial D18.02
    skin D18.01
    specified site NEC D18.09
  capillary I78.1
    intra-abdominal D18.03
    intracranial D18.02
    skin D18.01
    specified site NEC D18.09
  cavernous D18.00
    intra-abdominal D18.03
    intracranial D18.02
    skin D18.01
    specified site NEC D18.09
  epithelioid D18.00
    intra-abdominal D18.03
    intracranial D18.02
    skin D18.01
    specified site NEC D18.09
  histiocytoid D18.00
    intra-abdominal D18.03
    intracranial D18.02
    skin D18.01
    specified site NEC D18.09
  infantile D18.00
    intra-abdominal D18.03
    intracranial D18.02
    skin D18.01
    specified site NEC D18.09
  intra-abdominal D18.03
  intracranial D18.02
  intramuscular D18.00
    intra-abdominal D18.03
    intracranial D18.02
    skin D18.01
    specified site NEC D18.09
  intrathoracic structures D18.09
  juvenile D18.00
  malignant — *see* Neoplasm, connective tissue,
    malignant
  plexiform D18.00
    intra-abdominal D18.03
    intracranial D18.02
    skin D18.01
    specified site NEC D18.09
  racemose D18.00
    intra-abdominal D18.03
    intracranial D18.02
    skin D18.01
    specified site NEC D18.09
  sclerosing — *see* Neoplasm, skin, benign
  simplex D18.00
    intra-abdominal D18.03
    intracranial D18.02
    skin D18.01
    specified site NEC D18.09
  skin D18.01
  specified site NEC D18.09
  venous D18.00
    intra-abdominal D18.03
    intracranial D18.02
    skin D18.01
    specified site NEC D18.09
  verrucous keratotic D18.00
    intra-abdominal D18.03
    intracranial D18.02
    skin D18.01
    specified site NEC D18.09
Hemangiomatosis (systemic) I78.8
  involving single site — *see* Hemangioma
Hemangiopericytoma (*see also* Neoplasm, connective
  tissue, uncertain behavior)
  benign — *see* Neoplasm, connective tissue, benign
  malignant — *see* Neoplasm, connective tissue,
    malignant
Hemangiosarcoma — *see* Neoplasm, connective
  tissue, malignant
Hemarthrosis (nontraumatic) M25.00
  ankle M25.07 ☑
  elbow M25.02 ☑
  foot joint M25.07 ☑
  hand joint M25.04 ☑
  hip M25.05 ☑
  in hemophilic arthropathy — *see* Arthropathy,
    hemophilic
  knee M25.06 ☑
  shoulder M25.01 ☑
  specified joint NEC M25.08
  traumatic — *see* Sprain, by site

Hemarthrosis — *continued*
  vertebrae M25.08
  wrist M25.03 ☑
Hematemesis K92.0
  with ulcer - code by site under Ulcer, with
    hemorrhage K27.4
  newborn, neonatal P54.0
    due to swallowed maternal blood P78.2
Hematidrosis L74.8
Hematinuria (*see also* Hemoglobinuria)
  malarial B50.8
Hematobilia K83.8
Hematocele
  female NEC N94.89
    with ectopic pregnancy O00.90
      with intrauterine pregnancy O00.91
    ovary N83.8
  male N50.1
Hematochezia (*see also* Melena) K92.1
Hematochyluria (*see also* Infestation, filarial)
  schistosomiasis (bilharziasis) B65.0
Hematocolpos (with hematometra or hematosalpinx)
  N89.7
Hematocornea — *see* Pigmentation, cornea, stromal
Hematogenous — *see* condition
Hematoma (traumatic) (skin surface intact) (*see also*
  Contusion)
  with
    injury of internal organs — *see* Injury, by site
    open wound — *see* Wound, open
  amputation stump (surgical) (late) T87.89
  aorta, dissecting I71.00
    abdominal I71.02
    thoracic I71.01
    thoracoabdominal I71.03
  aortic intramural — *see* Dissection, aorta
  arterial (complicating trauma) — *see* Injury, blood
    vessel, by site
  auricle — *see* Contusion, ear
    nontraumatic — *see* Disorder, pinna, hematoma
  birth injury NEC P15.8
  brain (traumatic)
    with
      cerebral laceration or contusion (diffuse) — *see*
        Injury, intracranial, diffuse
      focal — *see* Injury, intracranial, focal
    cerebellar, traumatic S06.37 ☑
    newborn NEC P52.4
      birth injury P10.1
    intracerebral, traumatic — *see* Injury, intracranial,
      intracerebral hemorrhage
    nontraumatic — *see* Hemorrhage, intracranial
    subarachnoid, arachnoid, traumatic — *see* Injury,
      intracranial, subarachnoid hemorrhage
    subdural, traumatic — *see* Injury, intracranial,
      subdural hemorrhage
  breast (nontraumatic) N64.89
  broad ligament (nontraumatic) N83.7
    traumatic S37.892 ☑
  cerebellar, traumatic S06.37 ☑
  cerebral — *see* Hematoma, brain
  cerebrum S06.36 ☑
    left S06.35 ☑
    right S06.34 ☑
  cesarean delivery wound O90.2
  complicating delivery (perineal) (pelvic) (vagina)
    (vulva) O71.7
  corpus cavernosum (nontraumatic) N48.89
  epididymis (nontraumatic) N50.1
  epidural (traumatic) — *see* Injury, intracranial,
    epidural hemorrhage
    spinal — *see* Injury, spinal cord, by region
  episiotomy O90.2
  face, birth injury P15.4
  genital organ NEC (nontraumatic)
    female (nonobstetric) N94.89
      traumatic S30.202 ☑
    male N50.1
      traumatic S30.201 ☑
  internal organs — *see* Injury, by site
  intracerebral, traumatic — *see* Injury, intracranial,
    intracerebral hemorrhage
  intraoperative — *see* Complications, intraoperative,
    hemorrhage
  labia (nontraumatic) (nonobstetric) N90.89
  liver (subcapsular) (nontraumatic) K76.89
    birth injury P15.0
  mediastinum — *see* Injury, intrathoracic
  mesosalpinx (nontraumatic) N83.7
    traumatic S37.898 ☑
  muscle - code by site under Contusion

Hematoma - Hemophilia

Hematoma — *continued*
  nontraumatic
    muscle M79.81
    soft tissue M79.81
  obstetrical surgical wound O90.2
  orbit, orbital (nontraumatic) (*see also* Hemorrhage, orbit)
    traumatic — *see* Contusion, orbit
  pelvis (female) (nontraumatic) (nonobstetric) N94.89
    obstetric O71.7
    traumatic — *see* Injury, by site
  penis (nontraumatic) N48.89
    birth injury P15.5
  perianal (nontraumatic) K64.5
  perineal S30.23 ☑
    complicating delivery O71.7
  perirenal — *see* Injury, kidney
  pinna — *see* Contusion, ear
    nontraumatic — *see* Disorder, pinna, hematoma
  placenta O43.89 ☑
  postoperative (postprocedural) — *see* Complication, postprocedural, hematoma
  retroperitoneal (nontraumatic) K66.1
    traumatic S36.892 ☑
  scrotum, superficial S30.22 ☑
    birth injury P15.5
  seminal vesicle (nontraumatic) N50.1
    traumatic S37.892 ☑
  spermatic cord (traumatic) S37.892 ☑
    nontraumatic N50.1
  spinal (cord) (meninges) (*see also* Injury, spinal cord, by region)
    newborn (birth injury) P11.5
  spleen D73.5
    intraoperative — *see* Complications, intraoperative, hemorrhage, spleen
    postprocedural (postoperative) — *see* Complications, postprocedural, hemorrhage, spleen
  sternocleidomastoid, birth injury P15.2
  sternomastoid, birth injury P15.2
  subarachnoid (traumatic) — *see* Injury, intracranial, subarachnoid hemorrhage
    newborn (nontraumatic) P52.5
      due to birth injury P10.3
    nontraumatic — *see* Hemorrhage, intracranial, subarachnoid
  subdural (traumatic) — *see* Injury, intracranial, subdural hemorrhage
    newborn (localized) P52.8
      birth injury P10.0
    nontraumatic — *see* Hemorrhage, intracranial, subdural
  superficial, newborn P54.5
  testis (nontraumatic) N50.1
    birth injury P15.5
  tunica vaginalis (nontraumatic) N50.1
  umbilical cord, complicating delivery O69.5 ☑
  uterine ligament (broad) (nontraumatic) N83.7
    traumatic S37.892 ☑
  vagina (ruptured) (nontraumatic) N89.8
    complicating delivery O71.7
  vas deferens (nontraumatic) N50.1
    traumatic S37.892 ☑
  vitreous — *see* Hemorrhage, vitreous
  vulva (nontraumatic) (nonobstetric) N90.89
    complicating delivery O71.7
    newborn (birth injury) P15.5
Hematometra N85.7
  with hematocolpos N89.7
Hematomyelia (central) G95.19
  newborn (birth injury) P11.5
  traumatic T14.8 ☑
Hematomyelitis G04.90
Hematoperitoneum — *see* Hemoperitoneum
Hematophobia F40.230
Hematopneumothorax (*see* Hemothorax)
Hematopoiesis, cyclic D70.4
Hematoporphyria — *see* Porphyria
Hematorachis, hematorrhachis G95.19
  newborn (birth injury) P11.5
Hematosalpinx N83.6
  with
    hematocolpos N89.7
    hematometra N85.7
      with hematocolpos N89.7
    infectional — *see* Salpingitis
Hematospermia R36.1
Hematothorax (*see* Hemothorax)
Hematuria R31.9
  due to sulphonamide, sulfonamide — *see* Table of Drugs and Chemicals, by drug

Hematuria — *continued*
  benign (familial) (of childhood) (*see also* Hematuria, idiopathic)
    essential microscopic R31.1
  endemic (*see also* Schistosomiasis) B65.0
  gross R31.0
  idiopathic N02.9
    with glomerular lesion
      crescentic (diffuse) glomerulonephritis N02.7
      dense deposit disease N02.6
      endocapillary proliferative glomerulonephritis N02.4
      focal and segmental hyalinosis or sclerosis N02.1
      membranoproliferative (diffuse) N02.5
      membranous (diffuse) N02.2
      mesangial proliferative (diffuse) N02.3
      mesangiocapillary (diffuse) N02.5
      minor abnormality N02.0
      proliferative NEC N02.8
      specified pathology NEC N02.8
    intermittent — *see* Hematuria, idiopathic
  malarial B50.8
  microscopic NEC (with symptoms) R31.29
    asymptomatic R31.21
    benign essential R31.1
  paroxysmal (*see also* Hematuria, idiopathic)
    nocturnal D59.5
  persistent — *see* Hematuria, idiopathic
  recurrent — *see* Hematuria, idiopathic
  tropical (*see also* Schistosomiasis) B65.0
  tuberculous A18.13
Hemeralopia (day blindness) H53.11
  vitamin A deficiency E50.5
Hemi-akinesia R41.4
Hemianalgesia R20.0
Hemianencephaly Q00.0
Hemianesthesia R20.0
Hemianopia, hemianopsia (heteronymous) H53.47
  homonymous H53.46 ☑
  syphilitic A52.71
Hemiathetosis R25.8
Hemiatrophy R68.89
  cerebellar G31.9
  face, facial, progressive (Romberg) G51.8
  tongue K14.8
Hemiballism (us) G25.5
Hemicardia Q24.8
Hemicephalus, hemicephaly Q00.0
Hemichorea G25.5
Hemicolitis, left — *see* Colitis, left sided
Hemicrania
  congenital malformation Q00.0
  continua G44.51
  meaning migraine (*see also* Migraine) G43.909
  paroxysmal G44.039
    chronic G44.049
      intractable G44.041
      not intractable G44.049
    episodic G44.039
      intractable G44.031
      not intractable G44.039
    intractable G44.031
    not intractable G44.039
Hemidystrophy — *see* Hemiatrophy
Hemiectromelia Q73.8
Hemihypalgesia R20.8
Hemihypesthesia R20.1
Hemi-inattention R41.4
Hemimelia Q73.8
  lower limb — *see* Defect, reduction, lower limb, specified type NEC
  upper limb — *see* Defect, reduction, upper limb, specified type NEC
Hemiparalysis — *see* Hemiplegia
Hemiparesis — *see* Hemiplegia
Hemiparesthesia R20.2
Hemiparkinsonism G20
Hemiplegia G81.9 ☑
  alternans facialis G83.89
  ascending NEC G81.90
    spinal G95.89
  congenital (cerebral) G80.8
    spastic G80.2
  embolic (current episode) I63.4 ☑
  flaccid G81.0 ☑
  following
    cerebrovascular disease I69.959
      cerebral infarction I69.35 ☑
      intracerebral hemorrhage I69.15 ☑
      nontraumatic intracranial hemorrhage NEC I69.25 ☑

Hemiplegia — *continued*
  following — *continued*
      specified disease NEC I69.85 ☑
      stroke NOS I69.35 ☑
      subarachnoid hemorrhage I69.05 ☑
  hysterical F44.4
  newborn NEC P91.88
    birth injury P11.9
  spastic G81.1 ☑
    congenital G80.2
  thrombotic (current episode) I63.3 ☑
Hemisection, spinal cord — *see* Injury, spinal cord, by region
Hemispasm (facial) R25.2
Hemisporosis B48.8
Hemitremor R25.1
Hemivertebra Q76.49
  failure of segmentation with scoliosis Q76.3
  fusion with scoliosis Q76.3
Hemochromatosis E83.119
  with refractory anemia D46.1
  due to repeated red blood cell transfusion E83.111
  hereditary (primary) E83.110
  neonatal P78.84
  primary E83.110
  specified NEC E83.118
Hemoglobin (*see also* condition)
  abnormal (disease) — *see* Disease, hemoglobin
  AS genotype D57.3
  Constant Spring D58.2
  E-beta thalassemia D56.5
  fetal, hereditary persistence (HPFH) D56.4
  H Constant Spring D56.0
  low NOS D64.9
  S (Hb S), heterozygous D57.3
Hemoglobinemia D59.9
  due to blood transfusion T80.89 ☑
  paroxysmal D59.6
    nocturnal D59.5
Hemoglobinopathy (mixed) D58.2
  with thalassemia D56.8
  sickle-cell D57.1
    with thalassemia D57.40
      with crisis (vasoocclusive pain) D57.419
        with
          acute chest syndrome D57.411
          splenic sequestration D57.412
      without crisis D57.40
Hemoglobinuria R82.3
  with anemia, hemolytic, acquired (chronic) NEC D59.6
  cold (agglutinin) (paroxysmal) (with Raynaud's syndrome) D59.6
  due to exertion or hemolysis NEC D59.6
  intermittent D59.6
  malarial B50.8
  march D59.6
  nocturnal (paroxysmal) D59.5
  paroxysmal (cold) D59.6
    nocturnal D59.5
Hemolymphangioma D18.1
Hemolysis
  intravascular
    with
      abortion — *see* Abortion, by type, complicated by, hemorrhage
      ectopic or molar pregnancy O08.1
      hemorrhage
        antepartum — *see* Hemorrhage, antepartum, with coagulation defect
        intrapartum (*see also* Hemorrhage, complicating, delivery) O67.0
      postpartum O72.3
  neonatal (excessive) P58.9
  specified NEC P58.8
Hemolytic — *see* condition
Hemopericardium I31.2
  following acute myocardial infarction (current complication) I23.0
  newborn P54.8
  traumatic — *see* Injury, heart, with hemopericardium
Hemoperitoneum K66.1
  infectional K65.9
  traumatic S36.899 ☑
    with open wound — *see* Wound, open, with penetration into peritoneal cavity
Hemophilia (classical) (familial) (hereditary) D66
  A D66
  B D67
  C D68.1
  acquired D68.311

Hemophilia — *continued*
  autoimmune D68.311
  calcipriva (*see also* Defect, coagulation) D68.4
  nonfamilial (*see also* Defect, coagulation) D68.4
  secondary D68.311
  vascular D68.0
Hemophthalmos H44.81 ☑
Hemopneumothorax (*see also* Hemothorax)
  traumatic S27.2 ☑
Hemoptysis R04.2
  newborn P26.9
  tuberculous — *see* Tuberculosis, pulmonary
Hemorrhage, hemorrhagic (concealed) R58
  abdomen R58
  accidental antepartum — *see* Hemorrhage, antepartum
  acute idiopathic pulmonary, in infants R04.81
  adenoid J35.8
  adrenal (capsule) (gland) E27.49
    medulla E27.8
    newborn P54.4
  after delivery — *see* Hemorrhage, postpartum
  alveolar
    lung, newborn P26.8
    process K08.89
  alveolus K08.89
  amputation stump (surgical) T87.89
  anemia (chronic) D50.0
    acute D62
  antepartum (with) O46.90
    with coagulation defect O46.00 ☑
      afibrinogenemia O46.01 ☑
      disseminated intravascular coagulation O46.02 ☑
      hypofibrinogenemia O46.01 ☑
      specified defect NEC O46.09 ☑
    before 20 weeks gestation O20.9
      specified type NEC O20.8
      threatened abortion O20.0
    due to
      abruptio placenta (*see also* Abruptio placentae) O45.9 ☑
      leiomyoma, uterus — *see* Hemorrhage, antepartum, specified cause NEC
      placenta previa O44.1 ☑
    specified cause NEC — *see* subcategory O46.8X ☑
  anus (sphincter) K62.5
  apoplexy (stroke) — *see* Hemorrhage, intracranial, intracerebral
  arachnoid — *see* Hemorrhage, intracranial, subarachnoid
  artery R58
    brain — *see* Hemorrhage, intracranial, intracerebral
  basilar (ganglion) I61.0
  bladder N32.89
  bowel K92.2
    newborn P54.3
  brain (miliary) (nontraumatic) — *see* Hemorrhage, intracranial, intracerebral
    due to
      birth injury P10.1
      syphilis A52.05
    epidural or extradural (traumatic) — *see* Injury, intracranial, epidural hemorrhage
    newborn P52.4
      birth injury P10.1
    subarachnoid — *see* Hemorrhage, intracranial, subarachnoid
    subdural — *see* Hemorrhage, intracranial, subdural
  brainstem (nontraumatic) I61.3
    traumatic S06.38 ☑
  breast N64.59
  bronchial tube — *see* Hemorrhage, lung
  bronchopulmonary — *see* Hemorrhage, lung
  bronchus — *see* Hemorrhage, lung
  bulbar I61.5
  capillary I78.8
    primary D69.8
  cecum K92.2
  cerebellar, cerebellum (nontraumatic) I61.4
    newborn P52.6
    traumatic S06.37 ☑
  cerebral, cerebrum (*see also* Hemorrhage, intracranial, intracerebral)
    newborn (anoxic) P52.4
      birth injury P10.1
    lobe I61.1
  cerebromeningeal I61.8
  cerebrospinal — *see* Hemorrhage, intracranial, intracerebral

Hemorrhage — *continued*
  cervix (uteri) (stump) NEC N88.8
  chamber, anterior (eye) — *see* Hyphema
  childbirth — *see* Hemorrhage, complicating, delivery
  choroid H31.30 ☑
    expulsive H31.31 ☑
  ciliary body — *see* Hyphema
  cochlea — *see* subcategory H83.8 ☑
  colon K92.2
  complicating
    abortion — *see* Abortion, by type, complicated by, hemorrhage
    delivery O67.9
      associated with coagulation defect (afibrinogenemia) (DIC) (hyperfibrinolysis) O67.0
      specified cause NEC O67.8
    surgical procedure — *see* Hemorrhage, intraoperative
  conjunctiva H11.3 ☑
    newborn P54.8
  cord, newborn (stump) P51.9
  corpus luteum (ruptured) cyst N83.1 ☑
  cortical (brain) I61.1
  cranial — *see* Hemorrhage, intracranial
  cutaneous R23.3
    due to autosensitivity, erythrocyte D69.2
    newborn P54.5
  delayed
    following ectopic or molar pregnancy O08.1
    postpartum O72.2
  diathesis (familial) D69.9
  disease D69.9
    newborn P53
    specified type NEC D69.8
  due to or associated with
    afibrinogenemia or other coagulation defect (conditions in categories D65-D69)
      antepartum — *see* Hemorrhage, antepartum, with coagulation defect
      intrapartum O67.0
  dental implant M27.61
  device, implant or graft (*see also* Complications, by site and type, specified NEC) T85.838 ☑
    arterial graft NEC T82.838 ☑
    breast T85.838 ☑
    catheter NEC T85.838 ☑
      dialysis (renal) T82.838 ☑
        intraperitoneal T85.838 ☑
      infusion NEC T82.838 ☑
        spinal (epidural) (subdural) T85.830 ☑
      urinary (indwelling) T83.83 ☑
    electronic (electrode) (pulse generator) (stimulator)
      bone T84.83 ☑
      cardiac T82.837 ☑
      nervous system (brain) (peripheral nerve) (spinal) T85.830 ☑
      urinary T83.83 ☑
    fixation, internal (orthopedic) NEC T84.83 ☑
    gastrointestinal (bile duct) (esophagus) T85.838 ☑
    genital NEC T83.83 ☑
    heart NEC T82.837 ☑
    joint prosthesis T84.83 ☑
    ocular (corneal graft) (orbital implant) NEC T85.838 ☑
    orthopedic NEC T84.83 ☑
      bone graft T86.838 ☑
    specified NEC T85.838 ☑
    urinary NEC T83.83 ☑
    vascular NEC T82.838 ☑
    ventricular intracranial shunt T85.830 ☑
  duodenum, duodenal K92.2
    ulcer — *see* Ulcer, duodenum, with hemorrhage
  dura mater — *see* Hemorrhage, intracranial, subdural
  endotracheal — *see* Hemorrhage, lung
  epicranial subaponeurotic (massive), birth injury P12.2
  epidural (traumatic) (*see also* Injury, intracranial, epidural hemorrhage)
    nontraumatic I62.1
  esophagus K22.8
    varix I85.01
    secondary I85.11
  excessive, following ectopic gestation (subsequent episode) O08.1
  extradural (traumatic) — *see* Injury, intracranial, epidural hemorrhage
    birth injury P10.8

Hemorrhage — *continued*
  extradural — *continued*
    newborn (anoxic) (nontraumatic) P52.8
    nontraumatic I62.1
  eye NEC H57.89
    fundus — *see* Hemorrhage, retina
    lid — *see* Disorder, eyelid, specified type NEC
  fallopian tube N83.6
  fibrinogenolysis — *see* Fibrinolysis
  fibrinolytic (acquired) — *see* Fibrinolysis
  from
    ear (nontraumatic) — *see* Otorrhagia
    tracheostomy stoma J95.01
  fundus, eye — *see* Hemorrhage, retina
  funis — *see* Hemorrhage, umbilicus, cord
  gastric — *see* Hemorrhage, stomach
  gastroenteric K92.2
    newborn P54.3
  gastrointestinal (tract) K92.2
    newborn P54.3
  genital organ, male N50.1
  genitourinary (tract) NOS R31.9
  gingiva K06.8
  globe (eye) — *see* Hemophthalmos
  graafian follicle cyst (ruptured) N83.0 ☑
  gum K06.8
  heart I51.89
  hypopharyngeal (throat) R04.1
  intermenstrual (regular) N92.3
    irregular N92.1
  internal (organs) NEC R58
    capsule I61.0
    ear — *see* subcategory H83.8 ☑
    newborn P54.8
  intestine K92.2
    newborn P54.3
  intra-abdominal R58
  intra-alveolar (lung), newborn P26.8
  intracerebral (nontraumatic) — *see* Hemorrhage, intracranial, intracerebral
  intracranial (nontraumatic) I62.9
    birth injury P10.9
    epidural, nontraumatic I62.1
    extradural, nontraumatic I62.1
    newborn P52.9
      specified NEC P52.8
    intracerebral (nontraumatic) (in) I61.9
      brain stem I61.3
      cerebellum I61.4
      newborn P52.4
        birth injury P10.1
      hemisphere I61.2
        cortical (superficial) I61.1
        subcortical (deep) I61.0
      intraoperative
        during a nervous system procedure G97.31
        during other procedure G97.32
      intraventricular I61.5
      multiple localized I61.6
      postprocedural
        following a nervous system procedure G97.51
        following other procedure G97.52
      specified NEC I61.8
      superficial I61.1
      traumatic (diffuse) — *see* Injury, intracranial, diffuse
        focal — *see* Injury, intracranial, focal
    subarachnoid (nontraumatic) (from) I60.9
      newborn P52.5
        birth injury P10.3
      intracranial (cerebral) artery I60.7
        anterior communicating I60.2
        basilar I60.4
        carotid siphon and bifurcation I60.0 ☑
        communicating I60.7
          anterior I60.2
          posterior I60.3 ☑
        middle cerebral I60.1 ☑
        posterior communicating I60.3 ☑
        specified artery NEC I60.6
        vertebral I60.5 ☑
      specified NEC I60.8
      traumatic S06.6X ☑
    subdural (nontraumatic) I62.00
      acute I62.01
      birth injury P10.0
      chronic I62.03
      newborn (anoxic) (hypoxic) P52.8
        birth injury P10.0
      spinal G95.19
      subacute I62.02

Hemorrhage — *continued*
 intracranial — *continued*
  traumatic — *see* Injury, intracranial, subdural hemorrhage
  traumatic — *see* Injury, intracranial, focal brain injury
 intramedullary NEC G95.19
 intraocular — *see* Hemophthalmos
 intraoperative, intraprocedural — *see* Complication, hemorrhage (hematoma), intraoperative (intraprocedural), by site
 intrapartum — *see* Hemorrhage, complicating, delivery
 intrapelvic
  female N94.89
  male K66.1
 intraperitoneal K66.1
 intrapontine I61.3
 intraprocedural — *see* Complication, hemorrhage (hematoma), intraoperative (intraprocedural), by site
 intrauterine N85.7
  complicating delivery (*see also* Hemorrhage, complicating, delivery) O67.9
  postpartum — *see* Hemorrhage, postpartum
 intraventricular I61.5
  newborn (nontraumatic) (*see also* Newborn, affected by, hemorrhage) P52.3
   due to birth injury P10.2
   grade
    1 P52.0
    2 P52.1
    3 P52.21
    4 P52.22
 intravesical N32.89
 iris (postinfectional) (postinflammatory) (toxic) — *see* Hyphema
 joint (nontraumatic) — *see* Hemarthrosis
 kidney N28.89
 knee (joint) (nontraumatic) — *see* Hemarthrosis, knee
 labyrinth — *see* subcategory H83.8 ☑
 lenticular striate artery I61.0
 ligature, vessel — *see* Hemorrhage, postoperative
 liver K76.89
 lung R04.89
  newborn P26.9
   massive P26.1
   specified NEC P26.8
  tuberculous — *see* Tuberculosis, pulmonary
 massive umbilical, newborn P51.0
 mediastinum — *see* Hemorrhage, lung
 medulla I61.3
 membrane (brain) I60.8
  spinal cord — *see* Hemorrhage, spinal cord
 meninges, meningeal (brain) (middle) I60.8
  spinal cord — *see* Hemorrhage, spinal cord
 mesentery K66.1
 metritis — *see* Endometritis
 mouth K13.79
 mucous membrane NEC R58
  newborn P54.8
 muscle M62.89
 nail (subungual) L60.8
 nasal turbinate R04.0
  newborn P54.8
 navel, newborn P51.9
 newborn P54.9
  specified NEC P54.8
 nipple N64.59
 nose R04.0
  newborn P54.8
 omentum K66.1
 optic nerve (sheath) H47.02 ☑
 orbit, orbital H05.23 ☑
 ovary NEC N83.8
 oviduct N83.6
 pancreas K86.89
 parathyroid (gland) (spontaneous) E21.4
 parturition — *see* Hemorrhage, complicating, delivery
 penis N48.89
 pericardium, pericarditis I31.2
 peritoneum, peritoneal K66.1
 peritonsillar tissue J35.8
  due to infection J36
 petechial R23.3
  due to autosensitivity, erythrocyte D69.2
 pituitary (gland) E23.6
 pleura — *see* Hemorrhage, lung
 polioencephalitis, superior E51.2
 polymyositis — *see* Polymyositis

Hemorrhage — *continued*
 pons, pontine I61.3
 posterior fossa (nontraumatic) I61.8
  newborn P52.6
 postmenopausal N95.0
 postnasal R04.0
 postoperative — *see* Complications, postprocedural, hemorrhage, by site
 postpartum NEC (following delivery of placenta) O72.1
  delayed or secondary O72.2
  retained placenta O72.0
  third stage O72.0
 pregnancy — *see* Hemorrhage, antepartum
 preretinal — *see* Hemorrhage, retina
 prostate N42.1
 puerperal — *see* Hemorrhage, postpartum
  delayed or secondary O72.2
 pulmonary R04.89
  newborn P26.9
   massive P26.1
   specified NEC P26.8
  tuberculous — *see* Tuberculosis, pulmonary
 purpura (primary) D69.3
 rectum (sphincter) K62.5
  newborn P54.2
 recurring, following initial hemorrhage at time of injury T79.2 ☑
 renal N28.89
 respiratory passage or tract R04.9
  specified NEC R04.89
 retina, retinal (vessels) H35.6 ☑
  diabetic — *see* Diabetes, retinal, hemorrhage
 retroperitoneal R58
 scalp R58
 scrotum N50.1
 secondary (nontraumatic) R58
  following initial hemorrhage at time of injury T79.2 ☑
 seminal vesicle N50.1
 skin R23.3
  newborn P54.5
 slipped umbilical ligature P51.8
 spermatic cord N50.1
 spinal (cord) G95.19
  newborn (birth injury) P11.5
 spleen D73.5
  intraoperative — *see* Complications, intraoperative, hemorrhage, spleen
  postprocedural — *see* Complications, postprocedural, hemorrhage, spleen
 stomach K92.2
  newborn P54.3
  ulcer — *see* Ulcer, stomach, with hemorrhage
 subarachnoid (nontraumatic) — *see* Hemorrhage, intracranial, subarachnoid
 subconjunctival (*see also* Hemorrhage, conjunctiva)
  birth injury P15.3
 subcortical (brain) I61.0
 subcutaneous R23.3
 subdiaphragmatic R58
 subdural (acute) (nontraumatic) — *see* Hemorrhage, intracranial, subdural
 subependymal
  newborn P52.0
   with intraventricular extension P52.1
    and intracerebral extension P52.22
 subgaleal P12.2
 subhyaloid — *see* Hemorrhage, retina
 subperiosteal — *see* Disorder, bone, specified type NEC
 subretinal — *see* Hemorrhage, retina
 subtentorial — *see* Hemorrhage, intracranial, subdural
 subungual L60.8
 suprarenal (capsule) (gland) E27.49
  newborn P54.4
 tentorium (traumatic) NEC — *see* Hemorrhage, brain
  newborn (birth injury) P10.4
 testis N50.1
 third stage (postpartum) O72.0
 thorax — *see* Hemorrhage, lung
 throat R04.1
 thymus (gland) E32.8
 thyroid (cyst) (gland) E07.89
 tongue K14.8
 tonsil J35.8
 trachea — *see* Hemorrhage, lung
 tracheobronchial R04.89
  newborn P26.0

Hemorrhage — *continued*
 traumatic - code to specific injury
  cerebellar — *see* Hemorrhage, brain
  intracranial — *see* Hemorrhage, brain
  recurring or secondary (following initial hemorrhage at time of injury) T79.2 ☑
 tuberculous NEC (*see also* Tuberculosis, pulmonary) A15.0
 tunica vaginalis N50.1
 ulcer - code by site under Ulcer, with hemorrhage K27.4
 umbilicus, umbilical
  cord
   after birth, newborn P51.9
   complicating delivery O69.5 ☑
  newborn P51.9
   massive P51.0
   slipped ligature P51.8
  stump P51.9
 urethra (idiopathic) N36.8
 uterus, uterine (abnormal) N93.9
  climacteric N92.4
  complicating delivery — *see* Hemorrhage, complicating, delivery
  dysfunctional or functional N93.8
  intermenstrual (regular) N92.3
   irregular N92.1
  postmenopausal N95.0
  postpartum — *see* Hemorrhage, postpartum
  preclimacteric or premenopausal N92.4
  prepubertal N93.8
  pubertal N92.2
 vagina (abnormal) N93.9
  newborn P54.6
 vas deferens N50.1
 vasa previa O69.4 ☑
 ventricular I61.5
 vesical N32.89
 viscera NEC R58
  newborn P54.8
 vitreous (humor) (intraocular) H43.1 ☑
 vulva N90.89
Hemorrhoids (bleeding) (without mention of degree) K64.9
 1st degree (grade/stage I) (without prolapse outside of anal canal) K64.0
 2nd degree (grade/stage II) (that prolapse with straining but retract spontaneously) K64.1
 3rd degree (grade/stage III) (that prolapse with straining and require manual replacement back inside anal canal) K64.2
 4th degree (grade/stage IV) (with prolapsed tissue that cannot be manually replaced) K64.3
 complicating
  pregnancy O22.4 ☑
  puerperium O87.2
 external K64.4
  with
   thrombosis K64.5
 internal (without mention of degree) K64.8
 prolapsed K64.8
 skin tags
  anus K64.4
  residual K64.4
 specified NEC K64.8
 strangulated (*see also* Hemorrhoids, by degree) K64.8
 thrombosed (*see also* Hemorrhoids, by degree) K64.5
 ulcerated (*see also* Hemorrhoids, by degree) K64.8
Hemosalpinx N83.6
 with
  hematocolpos N89.7
  hematometra N85.7
   with hematocolpos N89.7
Hemosiderosis (dietary) E83.19 ☑
 pulmonary, idiopathic E83.1 ☑ *[J84.03]*
 transfusion T80.89 ☑
Hemothorax (bacterial) (nontuberculous) J94.2
 newborn P54.8
 traumatic S27.1 ☑
  with pneumothorax S27.2 ☑
 tuberculous NEC A15.6
Henoch (-Schönlein) disease or syndrome (purpura) D69.0
Henpue, henpuye A66.6
Hepar lobatum (syphilitic) A52.74
Hepatalgia K76.89
Hepatitis K75.9
 acute B17.9
  with coma K72.01
  with hepatic failure — *see* Failure, hepatic

☑ **Additional character required**

Hepatitis — *continued*
  acute — *continued*
    alcoholic — *see* Hepatitis, alcoholic
    infectious B17.9
    non-viral K72.0 ☑
    viral B17.9
  alcoholic (acute) (chronic) K70.10
    with ascites K70.11
  amebic — *see* Abscess, liver, amebic
  anicteric, (viral) — *see* Hepatitis, viral
  antigen-associated (HAA) — *see* Hepatitis, B
  Australia-antigen (positive) — *see* Hepatitis, B
  autoimmune K75.4
  B B19.10
    with hepatic coma B19.11
    acute B16.9
      with
        delta-agent (coinfection) (without hepatic
          coma) B16.1
          with hepatic coma B16.0
        hepatic coma (without delta-agent
          coinfection) B16.2
    chronic B18.1
      with delta-agent B18.0
  bacterial NEC K75.89
  C (viral) B19.20
    with hepatic coma B19.21
    acute B17.10
      with hepatic coma B17.11
    chronic B18.2
  catarrhal (acute) B15.9
    with hepatic coma B15.0
  cholangiolitic K75.89
  cholestatic K75.89
  chronic K73.9
    active NEC K73.2
    lobular NEC K73.1
    persistent NEC K73.0
    specified NEC K73.8
  cytomegaloviral B25.1
  due to ethanol (acute) (chronic) — *see* Hepatitis,
    alcoholic
  epidemic B15.9
    with hepatic coma B15.0
  fulminant NEC (viral) — *see* Hepatitis, viral
  neonatal giant cell P59.29
  granulomatous NEC K75.3
  herpesviral B00.81
  history of
    B Z86.19
    C Z86.19
  homologous serum — *see* Hepatitis, viral, type B
  in (due to)
    mumps B26.81
    toxoplasmosis (acquired) B58.1
      congenital (active) P37.1 *[K77]*
  infectious, infective B15.9
    acute (subacute) B17.9
    chronic B18.9
  inoculation — *see* Hepatitis, viral, type B
  interstitial (chronic) K74.69
  lupoid NEC K75.4
  malignant NEC (with hepatic failure) K72.90
    with coma K72.91
  neonatal (idiopathic) (toxic) P59.29
  newborn P59.29
  postimmunization — *see* Hepatitis, viral, type B
  post-transfusion — *see* Hepatitis, viral, type B
  reactive, nonspecific K75.2
  serum — *see* Hepatitis, viral, type B
  specified type NEC
    with hepatic failure — *see* Failure, hepatic
  syphilitic (late) A52.74
    congenital (early) A50.08 *[K77]*
      late A50.59 *[K77]*
    secondary A51.45
  toxic (*see also* Disease, liver, toxic) K71.6
  tuberculous A18.83
  viral, virus B19.9
    with hepatic coma B19.0
    acute B17.9
    chronic B18.9
      specified NEC B18.8
      type
        B B18.1
          with delta-agent B18.0
        C B18.2
    congenital P35.3
    coxsackie B33.8 *[K77]*
    cytomegalic inclusion B25.1
    in remission, any type - code to Hepatitis, chronic,
      by type

Hepatitis — *continued*
  viral — *continued*
    non-A, non-B B17.8
    specified type NEC (with or without coma) B17.8
    type
      A B15.9
        with hepatic coma B15.0
      B B19.10
        with hepatic coma B19.11
        acute B16.9
          with
            delta-agent (coinfection) (without
              hepatic coma) B16.1
              with hepatic coma B16.0
            hepatic coma (without delta-agent
              coinfection) B16.2
        chronic B18.1
          with delta-agent B18.0
      C B19.20
        with hepatic coma B19.21
        acute B17.10
          with hepatic coma B17.11
        chronic B18.2
      E B17.2
      non-A, non-B B17.8
Hepatization lung (acute) — *see* Pneumonia, lobar
Hepatoblastoma C22.2
Hepatocarcinoma C22.0
Hepatocholangiocarcinoma C22.0
Hepatocholangioma, benign D13.4
Hepatocholangitis K75.89
Hepatolenticular degeneration E83.01
Hepatoma (malignant) C22.0
  benign D13.4
  embryonal C22.0
Hepatomegaly (*see also* Hypertrophy, liver)
  with splenomegaly R16.2
  congenital Q44.7
  in mononucleosis
    gammaherpesviral B27.09
    infectious specified NEC B27.89
Hepatoptosis K76.89
Hepatorenal syndrome following labor and delivery
  O90.4
Hepatosis K76.89
Hepatosplenomegaly R16.2
  hyperlipemic (Bürger-Grütz type) E78.3 *[K77]*
Hereditary — *see* condition
Heredodegeneration, macular — *see* Dystrophy, retina
Heredopathia atactica polyneuritiformis G60.1
Heredosyphilis — *see* Syphilis, congenital
Herlitz' syndrome Q81.1
Hermansky-Pudlak syndrome E70.331
Hermaphrodite, hermaphroditism (true) Q56.0
  46,XX with streak gonads Q99.1
  46,XX/46,XY Q99.0
  46,XY with streak gonads Q99.1
  chimera 46,XX/46,XY Q99.0
Hernia, hernial (acquired) (recurrent) K46.9
  with
    gangrene — *see* Hernia, by site, with, gangrene
    incarceration — *see* Hernia, by site, with,
      obstruction
    irreducible — *see* Hernia, by site, with,
      obstruction
    obstruction — *see* Hernia, by site, with,
      obstruction
    strangulation — *see* Hernia, by site, with,
      obstruction
  abdomen, abdominal K46.9
    with
      gangrene (and obstruction) K46.1
      obstruction K46.0
    femoral — *see* Hernia, femoral
    incisional — *see* Hernia, incisional
    inguinal — *see* Hernia, inguinal
    specified site NEC K45.8
      with
        gangrene (and obstruction) K45.1
        obstruction K45.0
    umbilical — *see* Hernia, umbilical
    wall — *see* Hernia, ventral
  appendix — *see* Hernia, abdomen
  bladder (mucosa) (sphincter)
    congenital (female) (male) Q79.51
    female — *see* Cystocele
    male N32.89
  brain, congenital — *see* Encephalocele
  cartilage, vertebra — *see* Displacement,
    intervertebral disc
  cerebral, congenital (*see also* Encephalocele)
    endaural Q01.8

Hernia — *continued*
  ciliary body (traumatic) S05.2 ☑
  colon — *see* Hernia, abdomen
  Cooper's — *see* Hernia, abdomen, specified site NEC
  crural — *see* Hernia, femoral
  diaphragm, diaphragmatic K44.9
    with
      gangrene (and obstruction) K44.1
      obstruction K44.0
    congenital Q79.0
  direct (inguinal) — *see* Hernia, inguinal
  diverticulum, intestine — *see* Hernia, abdomen
  double (inguinal) — *see* Hernia, inguinal, bilateral
  due to adhesions (with obstruction) K56.50
  epigastric (*see also* Hernia, ventral) K43.9
  esophageal hiatus — *see* Hernia, hiatal
  external (inguinal) — *see* Hernia, inguinal
  fallopian tube N83.4 ☑
  fascia M62.89
  femoral K41.90
    with
      gangrene (and obstruction) K41.40
        not specified as recurrent K41.40
        recurrent K41.41
      obstruction K41.30
        not specified as recurrent K41.30
        recurrent K41.31
    bilateral K41.20
      with
        gangrene (and obstruction) K41.10
          not specified as recurrent K41.10
          recurrent K41.11
        obstruction K41.00
          not specified as recurrent K41.00
          recurrent K41.01
      not specified as recurrent K41.20
      recurrent K41.21
    unilateral K41.90
      with
        gangrene (and obstruction) K41.40
          not specified as recurrent K41.40
          recurrent K41.41
        obstruction K41.30
          not specified as recurrent K41.30
          recurrent K41.31
      not specified as recurrent K41.90
      recurrent K41.91
    not specified as recurrent K41.90
    recurrent K41.91
  foramen magnum G93.5
    congenital Q01.8
  funicular (umbilical) (*see also* Hernia, umbilicus)
    spermatic (cord) — *see* Hernia, inguinal
  gastrointestinal tract — *see* Hernia, abdomen
  Hesselbach's — *see* Hernia, femoral, specified site
    NEC
  hiatal (esophageal) (sliding) K44.9
    with
      gangrene (and obstruction) K44.1
      obstruction K44.0
    congenital Q40.1
  hypogastric — *see* Hernia, ventral
  incarcerated (*see also* Hernia, by site, with
    obstruction)
    with gangrene — *see* Hernia, by site, with
      gangrene
  incisional K43.2
    with
      gangrene (and obstruction) K43.1
      obstruction K43.0
  indirect (inguinal) — *see* Hernia, inguinal
  inguinal (direct) (external) (funicular) (indirect)
    (internal) (oblique) (scrotal) (sliding) K40.90
    with
      gangrene (and obstruction) K40.40
        not specified as recurrent K40.40
        recurrent K40.41
      obstruction K40.30
        not specified as recurrent K40.30
        recurrent K40.31
    not specified as recurrent K40.90
    recurrent K40.91
    bilateral K40.20
      with
        gangrene (and obstruction) K40.10
          not specified as recurrent K40.10
          recurrent K40.11
        obstruction K40.00
          not specified as recurrent K40.00
          recurrent K40.01
      not specified as recurrent K40.20
      recurrent K40.21

Hernia - Hibernoma

Hernia — *continued*
  inguinal — *continued*
    unilateral K40.90
      with
        gangrene (and obstruction) K40.40
          not specified as recurrent K40.40
          recurrent K40.41
        obstruction K40.30
          not specified as recurrent K40.30
          recurrent K40.31
      not specified as recurrent K40.90
      recurrent K40.91
  internal (*see also* Hernia, abdomen)
    inguinal — *see* Hernia, inguinal
  interstitial — *see* Hernia, abdomen
  intervertebral cartilage or disc — *see* Displacement, intervertebral disc
  intestine, intestinal — *see* Hernia, by site
  intra-abdominal — *see* Hernia, abdomen
  iris (traumatic) S05.2 ☑
  irreducible (*see also* Hernia, by site, with obstruction)
    with gangrene — *see* Hernia, by site, with gangrene
  ischiatic — *see* Hernia, abdomen, specified site NEC
  ischiorectal — *see* Hernia, abdomen, specified site NEC
  lens (traumatic) S05.2 ☑
  linea (alba) (semilunaris) — *see* Hernia, ventral
  Littre's — *see* Hernia, abdomen
  lumbar — *see* Hernia, abdomen, specified site NEC
  lung (subcutaneous) J98.4
  mediastinum J98.59
  mesenteric (internal) — *see* Hernia, abdomen
  midline — *see* Hernia, ventral
  muscle (sheath) M62.89
  nucleus pulposus — *see* Displacement, intervertebral disc
  oblique (inguinal) — *see* Hernia, inguinal
  obstructive (*see also* Hernia, by site, with obstruction)
    with gangrene — *see* Hernia, by site, with gangrene
  obturator — *see* Hernia, abdomen, specified site NEC
  omental — *see* Hernia, abdomen
  ovary N83.4 ☑
  oviduct N83.4 ☑
  paraesophageal (*see also* Hernia, diaphragm)
    congenital Q40.1
  parastomal K43.5
    with
      gangrene (and obstruction) K43.4
      obstruction K43.3
  paraumbilical — *see* Hernia, umbilicus
  perineal — *see* Hernia, abdomen, specified site NEC
  Petit's — *see* Hernia, abdomen, specified site NEC
  postoperative — *see* Hernia, incisional
  pregnant uterus — *see* Abnormal, uterus in pregnancy or childbirth
  prevesical N32.89
  properitoneal — *see* Hernia, abdomen, specified site NEC
  pudendal — *see* Hernia, abdomen, specified site NEC
  rectovaginal N81.6
  retroperitoneal — *see* Hernia, abdomen, specified site NEC
  Richter's — *see* Hernia, abdomen, with obstruction
  Rieux's, Riex's — *see* Hernia, abdomen, specified site NEC
  sac condition (adhesion) (dropsy) (inflammation) (laceration) (suppuration) - code by site under Hernia
  sciatic — *see* Hernia, abdomen, specified site NEC
  scrotum, scrotal — *see* Hernia, inguinal
  sliding (inguinal) (*see also* Hernia, inguinal)
    hiatus — *see* Hernia, hiatal
  spigelian — *see* Hernia, ventral
  spinal — *see* Spina bifida
  strangulated (*see also* Hernia, by site, with obstruction)
    with gangrene — *see* Hernia, by site, with gangrene
  subxiphoid — *see* Hernia, ventral
  supra-umbilicus — *see* Hernia, ventral
  tendon — *see* Disorder, tendon, specified type NEC
  Treitz's (fossa) — *see* Hernia, abdomen, specified site NEC
  tunica vaginalis Q55.29
  umbilicus, umbilical K42.9
    with

Hernia — *continued*
  umbilicus — *continued*
      gangrene (and obstruction) K42.1
      obstruction K42.0
  ureter N28.89
  urethra, congenital Q64.79
  urinary meatus, congenital Q64.79
  uterus N81.4
    pregnant — *see* Abnormal, uterus in pregnancy or childbirth
    vaginal (anterior) (wall) — *see* Cystocele
  Velpeau's — *see* Hernia, femoral
  ventral K43.9
    with
      gangrene (and obstruction) K43.7
      obstruction K43.6
    recurrent — *see* Hernia, incisional
    incisional K43.2
      with
        gangrene (and obstruction) K43.1
        obstruction K43.0
    specified NEC K43.9
      with
        gangrene (and obstruction) K43.7
        obstruction K43.6
  vesical
    congenital (female) (male) Q79.51
    female — *see* Cystocele
    male N32.89
  vitreous (into wound) S05.2 ☑
    into anterior chamber — *see* Prolapse, vitreous
Herniation (*see also* Hernia)
  brain (stem) G93.5
  cerebral G93.5
  mediastinum J98.59
  nucleus pulposus — *see* Displacement, intervertebral disc
Herpangina B08.5
Herpes, herpesvirus, herpetic B00.9
  anogenital A60.9
    perianal skin A60.1
    rectum A60.1
    urogenital tract A60.00
      cervix A60.03
      male genital organ NEC A60.02
      penis A60.01
      specified site NEC A60.09
      vagina A60.04
      vulva A60.04
  blepharitis (zoster) B02.39
    simplex B00.59
  circinatus B35.4
    bullosus L12.0
  conjunctivitis (simplex) B00.53
    zoster B02.31
  cornea B02.33
  encephalitis B00.4
    due to herpesvirus 6 B10.01
    due to herpesvirus 7 B10.09
    specified NEC B10.09
  eye (zoster) B02.30
    simplex B00.50
  eyelid (zoster) B02.39
    simplex B00.59
  facialis B00.1
  febrilis B00.1
  geniculate ganglionitis B02.21
  genital, genitalis A60.00
    female A60.09
    male A60.02
  gestational, gestationis O26.4 ☑
  gingivostomatitis B00.2
  human B00.9
    1 — *see* Herpes, simplex
    2 — *see* Herpes, simplex
    3 — *see* Varicella
    4 — *see* Mononucleosis, Epstein-Barr (virus)
    5 — *see* Disease, cytomegalic inclusion (generalized)
    6
      encephalitis B10.01
      specified NEC B10.81
    7
      encephalitis B10.09
      specified NEC B10.82
    8 B10.89
  infection NEC B10.89
    Kaposi's sarcoma associated B10.89
  iridocyclitis (simplex) B00.51
    zoster B02.32
  iris (vesicular erythema multiforme) L51.9
  iritis (simplex) B00.51

Herpes — *continued*
  Kaposi's sarcoma associated B10.89
  keratitis (simplex) (dendritic) (disciform) (interstitial) B00.52
    zoster (interstitial) B02.33
  keratoconjunctivitis (simplex) B00.52
    zoster B02.33
  labialis B00.1
  lip B00.1
  meningitis (simplex) B00.3
    zoster B02.1
  ophthalmicus (zoster) NEC B02.30
    simplex B00.50
  penis A60.01
  perianal skin A60.1
  pharyngitis, pharyngotonsillitis B00.2
  rectum A60.1
  scrotum A60.02
  sepsis B00.7
  simplex B00.9
    complicated NEC B00.89
    congenital P35.2
    conjunctivitis B00.53
    external ear B00.1
    eyelid B00.59
    hepatitis B00.81
    keratitis (interstitial) B00.52
    myelitis B00.82
    specified complication NEC B00.89
    visceral B00.89
  stomatitis B00.2
  tonsurans B35.0
  visceral B00.89
  vulva A60.04
  whitlow B00.89
  zoster (*see also* condition) B02.9
    auricularis B02.21
    complicated NEC B02.8
    conjunctivitis B02.31
    disseminated B02.7
    encephalitis B02.0
    eye (lid) B02.39
    geniculate ganglionitis B02.21
    keratitis (interstitial) B02.33
    meningitis B02.1
    myelitis B02.24
    neuritis, neuralgia B02.29
    ophthalmicus NEC B02.30
    oticus B02.21
    polyneuropathy B02.23
    specified complication NEC B02.8
    trigeminal neuralgia B02.22
Herpesvirus (human) — *see* Herpes
Herpetophobia F40.218
Herrick's anemia — *see* Disease, sickle-cell
Hers' disease E74.09
Herter-Gee syndrome K90.0
Herxheimer's reaction R68.89
Hesitancy
  of micturition R39.11
  urinary R39.11
Hesselbach's hernia — *see* Hernia, femoral, specified site NEC
Heterochromia (congenital) Q13.2
  cataract — *see* Cataract, complicated
  cyclitis (Fuchs) — *see* Cyclitis, Fuchs' heterochromic
  hair L67.1
  iritis — *see* Cyclitis, Fuchs' heterochromic
  retained metallic foreign body (nonmagnetic) — *see* Foreign body, intraocular, old, retained
    magnetic — *see* Foreign body, intraocular, old, retained, magnetic
  uveitis — *see* Cyclitis, Fuchs' heterochromic
Heterophoria — *see* Strabismus, heterophoria
Heterophyes, heterophyiasis (small intestine) B66.8
Heterotopia, heterotopic (*see also* Malposition, congenital)
  cerebralis Q04.8
Heterotropia — *see* Strabismus
Heubner-Herter disease K90.0
Hexadactylism Q69.9
HGSIL (cytology finding) (high grade squamous intraepithelial lesion on cytologic smear) (Pap smear finding)
  anus R85.613
  cervix R87.613
    biopsy (histology) finding — *see* Neoplasia, intraepithelial, cervix, grade II or grade III
  vagina R87.623
    biopsy (histology) finding — *see* Neoplasia, intraepithelial, vagina, grade II or grade III
Hibernoma — *see* Lipoma

☑ **Additional character required**

Hiccup, hiccough R06.6
   epidemic B33.0
   psychogenic F45.8
Hidden penis (congenital) Q55.64
   acquired N48.83
Hidradenitis (axillaris) (suppurative) L73.2
Hidradenoma (nodular) (*see also* Neoplasm, skin, benign)
   clear cell — *see* Neoplasm, skin, benign
   papillary — *see* Neoplasm, skin, benign
Hidrocystoma — *see* Neoplasm, skin, benign
High
   altitude effects T70.20 ☑
      anoxia T70.29 ☑
      on
         ears T70.0 ☑
         sinuses T70.1 ☑
      polycythemia D75.1
   arch
      foot Q66.7 ☑
      palate, congenital Q38.5
   arterial tension — *see* Hypertension
   basal metabolic rate R94.8
   blood pressure (*see also* Hypertension)
      borderline R03.0
      reading (incidental) (isolated) (nonspecific),
         without diagnosis of hypertension R03.0
   cholesterol E78.00
      with high triglycerides E78.2
   diaphragm (congenital) Q79.1
   expressed emotional level within family Z63.8
   head at term O32.4 ☑
   palate, congenital Q38.5
   risk
      infant NEC Z76.2
      sexual behavior (heterosexual) Z72.51
         bisexual Z72.53
         homosexual Z72.52
   scrotal testis, testes
      bilateral Q53.23
      unilateral Q53.13
   temperature (of unknown origin) R50.9
   thoracic rib Q76.6
   triglycerides E78.1
      with high cholesterol E78.2
Hildenbrand's disease A75.0
Hilum — *see* condition
Hip — *see* condition
Hippel's disease Q85.8
Hippophobia F40.218
Hippus H57.09
Hirschsprung's disease or megacolon Q43.1
Hirsutism, hirsuties L68.0
Hirudiniasis
   external B88.3
   internal B83.4
Hiss-Russell dysentery A03.1
Histidinemia, histidinuria E70.41
Histiocytoma (*see also* Neoplasm, skin, benign)
   fibrous (*see also* Neoplasm, skin, benign)
      atypical — *see* Neoplasm, connective tissue,
         uncertain behavior
      malignant — *see* Neoplasm, connective tissue,
         malignant
Histiocytosis D76.3
   acute differentiated progressive C96.0
   Langerhans' cell NEC C96.6
      multifocal X
         multisystemic (disseminated) C96.0
         unisystemic C96.5
      pulmonary, adult (adult PLCH) J84.82
      unifocal (X) C96.6
   lipid, lipoid D76.3
      essential E75.29
   malignant C96.A
   mononuclear phagocytes NEC D76.1
      Langerhans' cells C96.6
   non-Langerhans cell D76.3
   polyostotic sclerosing D76.3
   sinus, with massive lymphadenopathy D76.3
   syndrome NEC D76.3
   X NEC C96.6
      acute (progressive) C96.0
      chronic C96.6
      multifocal C96.5
      multisystemic C96.0
      unifocal C96.6
Histoplasmosis B39.9
   with pneumonia NEC B39.2
   African B39.5
   American — *see* Histoplasmosis, capsulati

Histoplasmosis — *continued*
   capsulati B39.4
      disseminated B39.3
      generalized B39.3
      pulmonary B39.2
         acute B39.0
         chronic B39.1
   Darling's B39.4
   duboisii B39.5
   lung NEC B39.2
History
   family (of) (*see also* History, personal (of))
      alcohol abuse Z81.1
      allergy NEC Z84.89
      anemia Z83.2
      arthritis Z82.61
      asthma Z82.5
      blindness Z82.1
      cardiac death (sudden) Z82.41
      carrier of genetic disease Z84.81
      chromosomal anomaly Z82.79
      chronic
         disabling disease NEC Z82.8
         lower respiratory disease Z82.5
      colonic polyps Z83.71
      congenital malformations and deformations
         Z82.79
         polycystic kidney Z82.71
      consanguinity Z84.3
      deafness Z82.2
      diabetes mellitus Z83.3
      disability NEC Z82.8
      disease or disorder (of)
         allergic NEC Z84.89
         behavioral NEC Z81.8
         blood and blood-forming organs Z83.2
         cardiovascular NEC Z82.49
         chronic disabling NEC Z82.8
         digestive Z83.79
         ear NEC Z83.52
         endocrine NEC Z83.49
         elevated lipoprotein(a) (Lp(a)) Z83.430
         eye NEC Z83.518
            glaucoma Z83.511
         familial hypercholesterolemia Z83.42
         genitourinary NEC Z84.2
         glaucoma Z83.511
         hematological Z83.2
         immune mechanism Z83.2
         infectious NEC Z83.1
         ischemic heart Z82.49
         kidney Z84.1
         lipoprotein metabolism Z83.438
         mental NEC Z81.8
         metabolic Z83.49
         musculoskeletal NEC Z82.69
         neurological NEC Z82.0
         nutritional Z83.49
         parasitic NEC Z83.1
         psychiatric NEC Z81.8
         respiratory NEC Z83.6
         skin and subcutaneous tissue NEC Z84.0
         specified NEC Z84.89
      drug abuse NEC Z81.3
      elevated lipoprotein(a) (Lp(a)) Z83.430
      epilepsy Z82.0
      familial hypercholesterolemia Z83.42
      genetic disease carrier Z84.81
      glaucoma Z83.511
      hearing loss Z82.2
      human immunodeficiency virus (HIV) infection
         Z83.0
      Huntington's chorea Z82.0
      hyperlipidemia, familial combined Z83.438
      intellectual disability Z81.0
      leukemia Z80.6
      lipidemia NEC Z83.438
      malignant neoplasm (of) NOS Z80.9
         bladder Z80.52
         breast Z80.3
         bronchus Z80.1
         digestive organ Z80.0
         gastrointestinal tract Z80.0
         genital organ Z80.49
            ovary Z80.41
            prostate Z80.42
            specified organ NEC Z80.49
            testis Z80.43
         hematopoietic NEC Z80.7
         intrathoracic organ NEC Z80.2
         kidney Z80.51
         lung Z80.1

History — *continued*
   family — *continued*
         lymphatic NEC Z80.7
         ovary Z80.41
         prostate Z80.42
         respiratory organ NEC Z80.2
         specified site NEC Z80.8
         testis Z80.43
         trachea Z80.1
         urinary organ or tract Z80.59
            bladder Z80.52
            kidney Z80.51
      mental
         disorder NEC Z81.8
      multiple endocrine neoplasia (MEN) syndrome
         Z83.41
      osteoporosis Z82.62
      polycystic kidney Z82.71
      polyps (colon) Z83.71
      psychiatric disorder Z81.8
      psychoactive substance abuse NEC Z81.3
      respiratory condition NEC Z83.6
         asthma and other lower respiratory conditions
            Z82.5
      self-harmful behavior Z81.8
      SIDS (sudden infant death syndrome) Z84.82
      skin condition Z84.0
      specified condition NEC Z84.89
      stroke (cerebrovascular) Z82.3
      substance abuse NEC Z81.4
         alcohol Z81.1
         drug NEC Z81.3
         psychoactive NEC Z81.3
         tobacco Z81.2
      sudden
         cardiac death Z82.41
         infant death syndrome (SIDS) Z84.82
      tobacco abuse Z81.2
      violence, violent behavior Z81.8
      visual loss Z82.1
   personal (of) (*see also* History, family (of))
      abuse
         adult Z91.419
            forced labor or sexual exploitation Z91.42
            physical and sexual Z91.410
            psychological Z91.411
         childhood Z62.819
            forced labor or sexual exploitation in
               childhood Z62.813
            physical Z62.810
            psychological Z62.811
            sexual Z62.810
      alcohol dependence F10.21
      allergy (to) Z88.9
         analgesic agent NEC Z88.6
         anesthetic Z88.4
         antibiotic agent NEC Z88.1
         anti-infective agent NEC Z88.3
         contrast media Z91.041
         drugs, medicaments and biological substances
            Z88.9
            specified NEC Z88.8
         food Z91.018
            additives Z91.02
            eggs Z91.012
            milk products Z91.011
            peanuts Z91.010
            seafood Z91.013
            specified food NEC Z91.018
         insect Z91.038
            bee Z91.030
         latex Z91.040
         medicinal agents Z88.9
            specified NEC Z88.8
         narcotic agent NEC Z88.5
         nonmedicinal agents Z91.048
         penicillin Z88.0
         serum Z88.7
         specified NEC Z91.09
         sulfonamides Z88.2
         vaccine Z88.7
      anaphylactic shock Z87.892
      anaphylaxis Z87.892
      behavioral disorders Z86.59
      benign carcinoid tumor Z86.012
      benign neoplasm Z86.018
         carcinoid Z86.012
         brain Z86.011
         colonic polyps Z86.010
      brain injury (traumatic) Z87.820
      breast implant removal Z98.86
      calculi, renal Z87.442

History

History — *continued*
  personal — *continued*
    cancer — *see* History, personal (of), malignant neoplasm (of)
    cardiac arrest (death), successfully resuscitated Z86.74
    cerebral infarction without residual deficit Z86.73
    cervical dysplasia Z87.410
    chemotherapy for neoplastic condition Z92.21
    childhood abuse — *see* History, personal (of), abuse
    cleft lip (corrected) Z87.730
    cleft palate (corrected) Z87.730
    collapsed vertebra (healed) Z87.311
      due to osteoporosis Z87.310
    combat and operational stress reaction Z86.51
    congenital malformation (corrected) Z87.798
      circulatory system (corrected) Z87.74
      digestive system (corrected) NEC Z87.738
      ear (corrected) Z87.721
      eye (corrected) Z87.720
      face and neck (corrected) Z87.790
      genitourinary system (corrected) NEC Z87.718
      heart (corrected) Z87.74
      integument (corrected) Z87.76
      limb(s) (corrected) Z87.76
      musculoskeletal system (corrected) Z87.76
      neck (corrected) Z87.790
      nervous system (corrected) NEC Z87.728
      respiratory system (corrected) Z87.75
      sense organs (corrected) NEC Z87.728
      specified NEC Z87.798
    contraception Z92.0
    deployment (military) Z91.82
    diabetic foot ulcer Z86.31
    disease or disorder (of) Z87.898
      blood and blood-forming organs Z86.2
      circulatory system Z86.79
        specified condition NEC Z86.79
      connective tissue NEC Z87.39
      digestive system Z87.19
        colonic polyp Z86.010
        peptic ulcer disease Z87.11
        specified condition NEC Z87.19
      ear Z86.69
      endocrine Z86.39
        diabetic foot ulcer Z86.31
        gestational diabetes Z86.32
        specified type NEC Z86.39
      eye Z86.69
      genital (track) system NEC
        female Z87.42
        male Z87.438
      hematological Z86.2
      Hodgkin Z85.71
      immune mechanism Z86.2
      infectious Z86.19
        malaria Z86.13
        Methicillin resistant Staphylococcus aureus (MRSA) Z86.14
        poliomyelitis Z86.12
        specified NEC Z86.19
        tuberculosis Z86.11
      mental NEC Z86.59
      metabolic Z86.39
        diabetic foot ulcer Z86.31
        gestational diabetes Z86.32
        specified type NEC Z86.39
      musculoskeletal NEC Z87.39
      nervous system Z86.69
      nutritional Z86.39
      parasitic Z86.19
      respiratory system NEC Z87.09
      sense organs Z86.69
      skin Z87.2
      specified site or type NEC Z87.898
      subcutaneous tissue Z87.2
      trophoblastic Z87.59
      urinary system NEC Z87.448
    drug dependence — *see* Dependence, drug, by type, in remission
    drug therapy
      antineoplastic chemotherapy Z92.21
      estrogen Z92.23
      immunosuppression Z92.25
      inhaled steroids Z92.240
      monoclonal drug Z92.22
      specified NEC Z92.29
      steroid Z92.241
      systemic steroids Z92.241
    dysplasia
      cervical (mild) (moderate) Z87.410
        severe (grade III) Z86.001

History — *continued*
  personal — *continued*
    prostatic Z87.430
      vaginal (mild) (moderate) Z87.411
        severe (grade III) Z86.002
      vulvar (mild) (moderate) Z87.412
        severe (grade III) Z86.002
    embolism (venous) Z86.718
      pulmonary Z86.711
    encephalitis Z86.61
    estrogen therapy Z92.23
    extracorporeal membrane oxygenation (ECMO) Z92.81
    failed moderate sedation Z92.83
    failed conscious sedation Z92.83
    fall, falling Z91.81
    forced labor or sexual exploitation Z91.42
      in childhood Z62.813
    fracture (healed)
      fatigue Z87.312
      fragility Z87.310
      osteoporosis Z87.310
      pathological NEC Z87.311
      stress Z87.312
      traumatic Z87.81
    gestational diabetes Z86.32
    hepatitis
      B Z86.19
      C Z86.19
    Hodgkin disease Z85.71
    hyperthermia, malignant Z88.4
    hypospadias (corrected) Z87.710
    hysterectomy Z90.710
    immunosuppression therapy Z92.25
    in situ neoplasm
      breast Z86.000
      cervix uteri Z86.001
      digestive organs, specified NEC Z86.004
      esophagus Z86.003
      genital organs, specified NEC Z86.002
      melanoma Z86.006
      middle ear Z86.005
      oral cavity Z86.003
      respiratory system Z86.005
      skin Z86.007
      specified NEC Z86.008
      stomach Z86.003
    infection NEC Z86.19
      central nervous system Z86.61
      latent tuberculosis Z86.15
      Methicillin resistant Staphylococcus aureus (MRSA) Z86.14
      urinary (recurrent) (tract) Z87.440
    injury NEC Z87.828
    in utero procedure during pregnancy Z98.870
    in utero procedure while a fetus Z98.871
    irradiation Z92.3
    kidney stones Z87.442
    latent tuberculosis infection Z86.15
    leukemia Z85.6
    lymphoma (non-Hodgkin) Z85.72
    malignant melanoma (skin) Z85.820
    malignant neoplasm (of) Z85.9
      accessory sinuses Z85.22
      anus NEC Z85.048
        carcinoid Z85.040
      bladder Z85.51
      bone Z85.830
      brain Z85.841
      breast Z85.3
      bronchus NEC Z85.118
        carcinoid Z85.110
      carcinoid — *see* History, personal (of), malignant neoplasm, by site, carcinioid
      cervix Z85.41
      colon NEC Z85.038
        carcinoid Z85.030
      digestive organ Z85.00
        specified NEC Z85.09
      endocrine gland NEC Z85.858
      epididymis Z85.48
      esophagus Z85.01
      eye Z85.840
      gastrointestinal tract — *see* History, malignant neoplasm, digestive organ
      genital organ
        female Z85.40
          specified NEC Z85.44
        male Z85.45
          specified NEC Z85.49
      hematopoietic NEC Z85.79
      intrathoracic organ Z85.20

History — *continued*
  personal — *continued*
      kidney NEC Z85.528
        carcinoid Z85.520
      large intestine NEC Z85.038
        carcinoid Z85.030
      larynx Z85.21
      liver Z85.05
      lung NEC Z85.118
        carcinoid Z85.110
      mediastinum Z85.29
      Merkel cell Z85.821
      middle ear Z85.22
      nasal cavities Z85.22
      nervous system NEC Z85.848
      oral cavity Z85.819
        specified site NEC Z85.818
      ovary Z85.43
      pancreas Z85.07
      pelvis Z85.53
      pharynx Z85.819
        specified site NEC Z85.818
      pelvis Z85.53
      pleura Z85.29
      prostate Z85.46
      rectosigmoid junction NEC Z85.048
        carcinoid Z85.040
      rectum NEC Z85.048
        carcinoid Z85.040
      respiratory organ Z85.20
      sinuses, accessory Z85.22
      skin NEC Z85.828
        melanoma Z85.820
        Merkel cell Z85.821
      small intestine NEC Z85.068
        carcinoid Z85.060
      soft tissue Z85.831
      specified site NEC Z85.89
      stomach NEC Z85.028
        carcinoid Z85.020
      testis Z85.47
      thymus NEC Z85.238
        carcinoid Z85.230
      thyroid Z85.850
      tongue Z85.810
      trachea Z85.12
      ureter Z85.54
      urinary organ or tract Z85.50
        specified NEC Z85.59
      uterus Z85.42
    maltreatment Z91.89
    medical treatment NEC Z92.89
    melanoma Z85.820
      in situ Z86.006
      malignant (skin) Z85.820
    meningitis Z86.61
    mental disorder Z86.59
    Merkel cell carcinoma (skin) Z85.821
    Methicillin resistant Staphylococcus aureus (MRSA) Z86.14
    military deployment Z91.82
    military war, peacekeeping and humanitarian deployment (current or past conflict) Z91.82
    myocardial infarction (old) I25.2
    neglect (in)
      adult Z91.412
      childhood Z62.812
    neoplasia
      anal intraepithelial, III [AIN III] Z86.004
      high-grade prostatic intraepithelial, III [HGPIN III] Z86.002
      vaginal intraepithelial, III [VAIN III] Z86.002
      vulvar intraepithelial, III [VIN III] Z86.002
    neoplasm
      benign Z86.018
        brain Z86.011
        colon polyp Z86.010
      in situ
        breast Z86.000
        cervix uteri Z86.001
        digestive organs, specified NEC Z86.004
        esophagus Z86.003
        genital organs, specified NEC Z86.002
        melanoma Z86.006
        middle ear Z86.005
        oral cavity Z86.003
        respiratory system Z86.005
        skin Z86.007
        specified NEC Z86.008
        stomach Z86.003
      malignant — *see* History of, malignant neoplasm
      uncertain behavior Z86.03

☑ **Additional character required**

History — *continued*
  personal — *continued*
    nephrotic syndrome Z87.441
    nicotine dependence Z87.891
    noncompliance with medical treatment or regimen — *see* Noncompliance
    nutritional deficiency Z86.39
    obstetric complications Z87.59
      childbirth Z87.59
      pregnancy Z87.59
      pre-term labor Z87.51
      puerperium Z87.59
    osteoporosis fractures Z87.31 ☑
    parasuicide (attempt) Z91.5
    physical trauma NEC Z87.828
      self-harm or suicide attempt Z91.5
    poisoning NEC Z91.89
      self-harm or suicide attempt Z91.5
    poor personal hygiene Z91.89
    pneumonia (recurrent) Z87.01
    preterm labor Z87.51
    prolonged reversible ischemic neurologic deficit (PRIND) Z86.73
    procedure during pregnancy Z98.870
    procedure while a fetus Z98.871
    prostatic dysplasia Z87.430
    psychological
      abuse
        adult Z91.411
        child Z62.811
      trauma, specified NEC Z91.49
    radiation therapy Z92.3
    removal
      implant
        breast Z98.86
    renal calculi Z87.442
    respiratory condition NEC Z87.09
    retained foreign body fully removed Z87.821
    risk factors NEC Z91.89
    self-harm Z91.5
    self-poisoning attempt Z91.5
    sex reassignment Z87.890
    sleep-wake cycle problem Z72.821
    specified NEC Z87.898
    steroid therapy (systemic) Z92.241
      inhaled Z92.240
    stroke without residual deficits Z86.73
    substance abuse NEC F10-F19
    sudden cardiac arrest Z86.74
    sudden cardiac death successfully resuscitated Z86.74
    suicide attempt Z91.5
    surgery NEC Z98.890
      with uterine scar Z98.891
      sex reassignment Z87.890
      transplant — *see* Transplant
    thrombophlebitis Z86.72
    thrombosis (venous) Z86.718
      pulmonary Z86.711
    tobacco dependence Z87.891
    transient ischemic attack (TIA) without residual deficits Z86.73
    trauma (physical) NEC Z87.828
      psychological NEC Z91.49
      self-harm Z91.5
    traumatic brain injury Z87.820
    tuberculosis, latent infection Z86.15
    unhealthy sleep-wake cycle Z72.821
    unintended awareness under general anesthesia Z92.84
    urinary calculi Z87.442
    urinary (recurrent) (tract) infection(s) Z87.440
    uterine scar from previous surgery Z98.891
    vaginal dysplasia Z87.411
    venous thrombosis or embolism Z86.718
      pulmonary Z86.711
    vulvar dysplasia Z87.412
His-Werner disease A79.0
HIV (*see also* Human, immunodeficiency virus) B20
  laboratory evidence (nonconclusive) R75
  positive, seropositive Z21
  nonconclusive test (in infants) R75
Hives (bold) — *see* Urticaria
Hoarseness R49.0
Hobo Z59.0
Hodgkin disease — *see* Lymphoma, Hodgkin
Hodgson's disease I71.2
  ruptured I71.1
Hoffa-Kastert disease E88.89
Hoffa's disease E88.89
Hoffmann-Bouveret syndrome I47.9
Hoffmann's syndrome E03.9 *[G73.7]*

Hole (round)
  macula H35.34 ☑
  retina (without detachment) — *see* Break, retina, round hole
    with detachment — *see* Detachment, retina, with retinal, break
Holiday relief care Z75.5
Hollenhorst's plaque — *see* Occlusion, artery, retina
Hollow foot (congenital) Q66.7 ☑
  acquired — *see* Deformity, limb, foot, specified NEC
Holoprosencephaly Q04.2
Holt-Oram syndrome Q87.2
Homelessness Z59.0
Homesickness — *see* Disorder, adjustment
Homocystinemia, homocystinuria E72.11
Homogentisate 1,2-dioxygenase deficiency E70.29
Homologous serum hepatitis (prophylactic) (therapeutic) — *see* Hepatitis, viral, type B
Honeycomb lung J98.4
  congenital Q33.0
Hooded
  clitoris Q52.6
  penis Q55.69
Hookworm (disease) (infection) (infestation) B76.9
  with anemia B76.9 *[D63.8]*
  specified NEC B76.8
Hordeolum (eyelid) (externum) (recurrent) H00.019
  internum H00.029
    left H00.026
      lower H00.025
      upper H00.024
    right H00.023
      lower H00.022
      upper H00.021
    left H00.016
      lower H00.015
      upper H00.014
    right H00.013
      lower H00.012
      upper H00.011
Horn
  cutaneous L85.8
  nail L60.2
    congenital Q84.6
Horner (-Claude Bernard) syndrome G90.2
  traumatic — *see* Injury, nerve, cervical sympathetic
Horseshoe kidney (congenital) Q63.1
Horton's headache or neuralgia G44.099
  intractable G44.091
  not intractable G44.099
Hospital hopper syndrome — *see* Disorder, factitious
Hospitalism in children — *see* Disorder, adjustment
Hostility R45.5
  towards child Z62.3
Hot flashes
  menopausal N95.1
Hourglass (contracture) (*see also* Contraction, hourglass)
  stomach K31.89
    congenital Q40.2
    stricture K31.2
Household, housing circumstance affecting care Z59.9
  specified NEC Z59.8
Housemaid's knee — *see* Bursitis, prepatellar
Hudson (-Stähli) line (cornea) — *see* Pigmentation, cornea, anterior
Human
  bite (open wound) (*see also* Bite)
    intact skin surface — *see* Bite, superficial
  herpesvirus — *see* Herpes
  immunodeficiency virus (HIV) disease (infection) B20
    asymptomatic status Z21
    contact Z20.6
    counseling Z71.7
    dementia B20 *[F02.80]*
      with behavioral disturbance B20 *[F02.81]*
    exposure to Z20.6
    laboratory evidence R75
    type-2 (HIV 2) as cause of disease classified elsewhere B97.35
  papillomavirus (HPV)
    DNA test positive
      high risk
        cervix R87.810
        vagina R87.811
      low risk
        cervix R87.820
        vagina R87.821
    screening for Z11.51
  T-cell lymphotropic virus
    type-1 (HTLV-I) infection B33.3

Human — *continued*
  T-cell lymphotropic virus — *continued*
    as cause of disease classified elsewhere B97.33
    carrier Z22.6
    type-2 (HTLV-II) as cause of disease classified elsewhere B97.34
Humidifier lung or pneumonitis J67.7
Humiliation (experience) in childhood Z62.898
Humpback (acquired) — *see* Kyphosis
Hunchback (acquired) — *see* Kyphosis
Hunger T73.0 ☑
  air, psychogenic F45.8
Hungry bone syndrome E83.81
Hunner's ulcer — *see* Cystitis, chronic, interstitial
Hunter's
  glossitis D51.0
  syndrome E76.1
Huntington's disease or chorea G10
  with dementia G10 *[F02.80]*
    with behavioral disturbance G10 *[F02.81]*
Hunt's
  disease or syndrome (herpetic geniculate ganglionitis) B02.21
  dyssynergia cerebellaris myoclonica G11.1
  neuralgia B02.21
Hurler (-Scheie) disease or syndrome E76.02
Hurst's disease G36.1
Hurthle cell
  adenocarcinoma C73
  adenoma D34
  carcinoma C73
  tumor D34
Hutchinson-Boeck disease or syndrome — *see* Sarcoidosis
Hutchinson-Gilford disease or syndrome E34.8
Hutchinson's
  disease, meaning
    angioma serpiginosum L81.7
    pompholyx (cheiropompholyx) L30.1
    prurigo estivalis L56.4
    summer eruption or summer prurigo L56.4
  melanotic freckle — *see* Melanoma, in situ
    malignant melanoma in — *see* Melanoma
  teeth or incisors (congenital syphilis) A50.52
  triad (congenital syphilis) A50.53
Hyalin plaque, sclera, senile H15.89
Hyaline membrane (disease) (lung) (pulmonary) (newborn) P22.0
Hyalinosis
  cutis (et mucosae) E78.89
  focal and segmental (glomerular) (*see also* N00-N07 with fourth character .1) N05.1
Hyalitis, hyalosis asteroid (*see also* Deposit, crystalline)
  syphilitic (late) A52.71
Hydatid
  cyst or tumor — *see* Echinococcus
  mole — *see* Hydatidiform mole
  Morgagni
    female Q50.5
    male (epididymal) Q55.4
    testicular Q55.29
Hydatidiform mole (benign) (complicating pregnancy) (delivered) (undelivered) O01.9
  classical O01.0
  complete O01.0
  incomplete O01.1
  invasive D39.2
  malignant D39.2
  partial O01.1
Hydatidosis — *see* Echinococcus
Hydradenitis (axillaris) (suppurative) L73.2
Hydradenoma — *see* Hidradenoma
Hydramnios O40. ☑
Hydrancephaly, hydranencephaly Q04.3
  with spina bifida — *see* Spina bifida, with hydrocephalus
Hydrargyrism NEC — *see* Poisoning, mercury
Hydrarthrosis (*see also* Effusion, joint)
  gonococcal A54.42
  intermittent M12.40
    ankle M12.47 ☑
    elbow M12.42 ☑
    foot joint M12.47 ☑
    hand joint M12.44 ☑
    hip M12.45 ☑
    knee M12.46 ☑
    multiple site M12.49
    shoulder M12.41 ☑
    specified joint NEC M12.48
    wrist M12.43 ☑
  of yaws (early) (late) (*see also* subcategory M14.8 ☑) A66.6

Hydrarthrosis - Hypercorticosteronism

Hydrarthrosis — *continued*
  syphilitic (late) A52.77
    congenital A50.55 *[M12.80]*
Hydremia D64.89
Hydrencephalocele (congenital) — *see* Encephalocele
Hydrencephalomeningocele (congenital) — *see*
  Encephalocele
Hydroa R23.8
  aestivale L56.4
  vacciniforme L56.4
Hydroadenitis (axillaris) (suppurative) L73.2
Hydrocalycosis — *see* Hydronephrosis
Hydrocele (spermatic cord) (testis) (tunica vaginalis) N43.3
  canal of Nuck N94.89
  communicating N43.2
    congenital P83.5
  congenital P83.5
  encysted N43.0
  female NEC N94.89
  infected N43.1
  newborn P83.5
  round ligament N94.89
  specified NEC N43.2
  spinalis — *see* Spina bifida
  vulva N90.89
Hydrocephalus (acquired) (external) (internal)
  (malignant) (recurrent) G91.9
  aqueduct Sylvius stricture Q03.0
  causing disproportion O33.6 ☑
    with obstructed labor O66.3
  communicating G91.0
  congenital (external) (internal) Q03.9
    with spina bifida Q05.4
      cervical Q05.0
      dorsal Q05.1
      lumbar Q05.2
      lumbosacral Q05.2
      sacral Q05.3
      thoracic Q05.1
      thoracolumbar Q05.1
    specified NEC Q03.8
  due to toxoplasmosis (congenital) P37.1
  foramen Magendie block (acquired) G91.1
    congenital (*see also* Hydrocephalus, congenital)
      Q03.1
  in (due to)
    infectious disease NEC B89 *[G91.4]*
    neoplastic disease NEC (*see also* Neoplasm) G91.4
    parasitic disease B89 *[G91.4]*
  newborn Q03.9
    with spina bifida — *see* Spina bifida, with
      hydrocephalus
  noncommunicating G91.1
  normal pressure G91.2
    secondary G91.0
  obstructive G91.1
  otitic G93.2
  post-traumatic NEC G91.3
  secondary G91.4
    post-traumatic G91.3
  specified NEC G91.8
  syphilitic, congenital A50.49
Hydrocolpos (congenital) N89.8
Hydrocystoma — *see* Neoplasm, skin, benign
Hydroencephalocele (congenital) — *see*
  Encephalocele
Hydroencephalomeningocele (congenital) — *see*
  Encephalocele
Hydrohematopneumothorax — *see* Hemothorax
Hydromeningitis — *see* Meningitis
Hydromeningocele (spinal) (*see also* Spina bifida)
  cranial — *see* Encephalocele
Hydrometra N85.8
Hydrometrocolpos N89.8
Hydromicrocephaly Q02
Hydromphalos (since birth) Q45.8
Hydromyelia Q06.4
Hydromyelocele — *see* Spina bifida
Hydronephrosis (atrophic) (early) (functionless)
  (intermittent) (primary) (secondary) NEC N13.30
  with
    infection N13.6
    obstruction (by) (of)
      renal calculus N13.2
        with infection N13.6
      ureteral NEC N13.1
        with infection N13.6
        calculus N13.2
          with infection N13.6
      ureteropelvic junction (congenital) Q62.11
        acquired N13.0
          with infection N13.6

Hydronephrosis — *continued*
  with — *continued*
    ureteral stricture NEC N13.1
      with infection N13.6
  congenital Q62.0
    due to acquired occlusion of ureteropelvic
      junction N13.0
  specified type NEC N13.39
  tuberculous A18.11
Hydropericarditis — *see* Pericarditis
Hydropericardium — *see* Pericarditis
Hydroperitoneum R18.8
Hydrophobia — *see* Rabies
Hydrophthalmos Q15.0
Hydropneumohemothorax — *see* Hemothorax
Hydropneumopericarditis — *see* Pericarditis
Hydropneumopericardium — *see* Pericarditis
Hydropneumothorax J94.8
  traumatic — *see* Injury, intrathoracic, lung
  tuberculous NEC A15.6
Hydrops R60.9
  abdominis R18.8
  articulorum intermittens — *see* Hydrarthrosis,
    intermittent
  cardiac — *see* Failure, heart, congestive
  causing obstructed labor (mother) O66.3
  endolymphatic H81.0 ☑
  fetal — *see* Pregnancy, complicated by, hydrops,
    fetalis
  fetalis P83.2
    due to
      ABO isoimmunization P56.0
      alpha thalassemia D56.0
      hemolytic disease P56.90
        specified NEC P56.99
      isoimmunization (ABO) (Rh) P56.0
      other specified nonhemolytic disease NEC
        P83.2
      Rh incompatibility P56.0
    during pregnancy — *see* Pregnancy, complicated
      by, hydrops, fetalis
  gallbladder K82.1
  joint — *see* Effusion, joint
  labyrinth H81.0 ☑
  newborn (idiopathic) P83.2
    due to
      ABO isoimmunization P56.0
      alpha thalassemia D56.0
      hemolytic disease P56.90
        specified NEC P56.99
      isoimmunization (ABO) (Rh) P56.0
      Rh incompatibility P56.0
  nutritional — *see* Malnutrition, severe
  pericardium — *see* Pericarditis
  pleura — *see* Hydrothorax
  spermatic cord — *see* Hydrocele
Hydropyonephrosis N13.6
Hydrorachis Q06.4
Hydrorrhea (nasal) J34.89
  pregnancy — *see* Rupture, membranes, premature
Hydrosadenitis (axillaris) (suppurative) L73.2
Hydrosalpinx (fallopian tube) (follicularis) N70.11
Hydrothorax (double) (pleura) J94.8
  chylous (nonfilarial) I89.8
    filarial (*see also* Infestation, filarial) B74.9 *[J91.8]*
  traumatic — *see* Injury, intrathoracic
  tuberculous NEC (non primary) A15.6
Hydroureter (*see also* Hydronephrosis) N13.4
  with infection N13.6
  congenital Q62.39
Hydroureteronephrosis — *see* Hydronephrosis
Hydrourethra N36.8
Hydroxykynureninuria E70.8
Hydroxylysinemia E72.3
Hydroxyprolinemia E72.59
Hygiene, sleep
  abuse Z72.821
  inadequate Z72.821
  poor Z72.821
Hygroma (congenital) (cystic) D18.1
  praepatellare, prepatellar — *see* Bursitis,
    prepatellar
Hymen — *see* condition
Hymenolepis, hymenolepiasis (diminuta) (infection)
  (infestation) (nana) B71.0
Hypalgesia R20.8
Hyperacidity (gastric) K31.89
  psychogenic F45.8
Hyperactive, hyperactivity F90.9
  basal cell, uterine cervix — *see* Dysplasia, cervix
  bowel sounds R19.12
  cervix epithelial (basal) — *see* Dysplasia, cervix

Hyperactive — *continued*
  child F90.9
    attention deficit — *see* Disorder, attention-deficit
      hyperactivity
  detrusor muscle N32.81
  gastrointestinal K31.89
    psychogenic F45.8
  nasal mucous membrane J34.3
  stomach K31.89
  thyroid (gland) — *see* Hyperthyroidism
Hyperacusis H93.23 ☑
Hyperadrenalism E27.5
Hyperadrenocorticism E24.9
  congenital E25.0
  iatrogenic E24.2
    correct substance properly administered — *see*
      Table of Drugs and Chemicals, by drug,
      adverse effect
    overdose or wrong substance given or taken —
      see Table of Drugs and Chemicals, by drug,
      poisoning
  not associated with Cushing's syndrome E27.0
  pituitary-dependent E24.0
Hyperaldosteronism E26.9
  familial (type I) E26.02
  glucocorticoid-remediable E26.02
  primary (due to (bilateral) adrenal hyperplasia)
    E26.09
  primary NEC E26.09
  secondary E26.1
  specified NEC E26.89
Hyperalgesia R20.8
Hyperalimentation R63.2
  carotene, carotin E67.1
  specified NEC E67.8
  vitamin
    A E67.0
    D E67.3
Hyperaminoaciduria
  arginine E72.21
  cystine E72.01
  lysine E72.3
  ornithine E72.4
Hyperammonemia (congenital) E72.20
Hyperazotemia — *see* Uremia
Hyperbetalipoproteinemia (familial) E78.00
  with prebetalipoproteinemia E78.2
Hyperbicarbonatemia P74.41
Hyperbilirubinemia
  constitutional E80.6
  familial conjugated E80.6
  neonatal (transient) — *see* Jaundice, newborn
Hypercalcemia, hypocalciuric, familial E83.52
Hypercalciuria, idiopathic R82.994
Hypercapnia R06.89
  newborn P84
Hypercarotenemia (dietary) E67.1
Hypercementosis K03.4
Hyperchloremia E87.8
Hyperchlorhydria K31.89
  neurotic F45.8
  psychogenic F45.8
Hypercholesterinemia — *see* Hypercholesterolemia
Hypercholesterolemia (essential) (primary) (pure)
  E78.00
  with hyperglyceridemia, endogenous E78.2
  dietary counseling and surveillance Z71.3
  familial E78.01
  hereditary E78.01
Hyperchylia gastrica, psychogenic F45.8
Hyperchylomicronemia (familial) (primary) E78.3
  with hyperbetalipoproteinemia E78.3
Hypercoagulable (state) D68.59
  activated protein C resistance D68.51
  antithrombin (III) deficiency D68.59
  factor V Leiden mutation D68.51
  primary NEC D68.59
  protein C deficiency D68.59
  protein S deficiency D68.59
  prothrombin gene mutation D68.52
  secondary D68.69
  specified NEC D68.69
Hypercoagulation (state) D68.59
Hypercorticalism, pituitary-dependent E24.0
Hypercorticosolism — *see* Cushing's, syndrome
Hypercorticosteronism E24.2
  correct substance properly administered — *see*
    Table of Drugs and Chemicals, by drug, adverse
    effect
  overdose or wrong substance given or taken —
    see Table of Drugs and Chemicals, by drug,
    poisoning

☑ **Additional character required**

Hypercortisonism E24.2
- correct substance properly administered — *see* Table of Drugs and Chemicals, by drug, adverse effect
- overdose or wrong substance given or taken — *see* Table of Drugs and Chemicals, by drug, poisoning

Hyperekplexia Q89.8

Hyperelectrolytemia E87.8

Hyperemesis R11.10
- with nausea R11.2
- gravidarum (mild) O21.0
  - with
    - carbohydrate depletion O21.1
    - dehydration O21.1
    - electrolyte imbalance O21.1
    - metabolic disturbance O21.1
  - severe (with metabolic disturbance) O21.1
- projectile R11.12
- psychogenic F45.8

Hyperemia (acute) (passive) R68.89
- anal mucosa K62.89
- bladder N32.89
- cerebral I67.89
- conjunctiva H11.43 ☑
- ear internal, acute — *see* subcategory H83.0 ☑
- enteric K59.8
- eye — *see* Hyperemia, conjunctiva
- eyelid (active) (passive) — *see* Disorder, eyelid, specified type NEC
- intestine K59.8
- iris — *see* Disorder, iris, vascular
- kidney N28.89
- labyrinth — *see* subcategory H83.0 ☑
- liver (active) K76.89
- lung (passive) — *see* Edema, lung
- pulmonary (passive) — *see* Edema, lung
- renal N28.89
- retina H35.89
- stomach K31.89

Hyperesthesia (body surface) R20.3
- larynx (reflex) J38.7
  - hysterical F44.89
- pharynx (reflex) J39.2
  - hysterical F44.89

Hyperestrogenism (drug-induced) (iatrogenic) E28.0

Hyperexplexia Q89.8

Hyperfibrinolysis — *see* Fibrinolysis

Hyperfructosemia E74.19

Hyperfunction
- adrenal cortex, not associated with Cushing's syndrome E27.0
  - medulla E27.5
    - adrenomedullary E27.5
  - virilism E25.9
    - congenital E25.0
- ovarian E28.8
- pancreas K86.89
- parathyroid (gland) E21.3
- pituitary (gland) (anterior) E22.9
  - specified NEC E22.8
- polyglandular E31.1
- testicular E29.0

Hypergammaglobulinemia D89.2
- polyclonal D89.0
- Waldenström D89.0

Hypergastrinemia E16.4

Hyperglobulinemia R77.1

Hyperglycemia, hyperglycemic (transient) R73.9
- coma — *see* Diabetes, by type, with coma
- postpancreatectomy E89.1

Hyperglyceridemia (endogenous) (essential) (familial) (hereditary) (pure) E78.1
- mixed E78.3

Hyperglycinemia (non-ketotic) E72.51

Hypergonadism
- ovarian E28.8
- testicular (primary) (infantile) E29.0

Hyperheparinemia D68.32

Hyperhidrosis, hyperidrosis R61
- focal
  - primary L74.519
    - axilla L74.510
    - face L74.511
    - palms L74.512
    - soles L74.513
  - secondary L74.52
- generalized R61
- localized
  - primary L74.519
    - axilla L74.510
    - face L74.511

Hyperhidrosis — *continued*
- localized — *continued*
  - primary — *continued*
    - palms L74.512
    - soles L74.513
  - secondary L74.52
- psychogenic F45.8
- secondary R61
  - focal L74.52

Hyperhistidinemia E70.41

Hyperhomocysteinemia E72.11

Hyperhydroxyprolinemia E72.59

Hyperinsulinism (functional) E16.1
- with
  - coma (hypoglycemic) E15
  - encephalopathy E16.1 *[G94]*
- ectopic E16.1
- therapeutic misadventure (from administration of insulin) — *see* subcategory T38.3 ☑

Hyperkalemia E87.5

Hyperkeratosis (*see also* Keratosis) L85.9
- cervix N88.0
- due to yaws (early) (late) (palmar or plantar) A66.3
- follicularis Q82.8
  - penetrans (in cutem) L87.0
- palmoplantaris climacterica L85.1
- pinta A67.1
- senile (with pruritus) L57.0
- universalis congenita Q80.8
- vocal cord J38.3
- vulva N90.4

Hyperkinesia, hyperkinetic (disease) (reaction) (syndrome) (childhood) (adolescence) (*see also* Disorder, attention-deficit hyperactivity)
- heart I51.89

Hyperleucine-isoleucinemia E71.19

Hyperlipemia, hyperlipidemia E78.5
- combined E78.2
  - familial E78.49
- group
  - A E78.00
  - B E78.1
  - C E78.2
  - D E78.3
- mixed E78.2
- specified NEC E78.49

Hyperlipidosis E75.6
- hereditary NEC E75.5

Hyperlipoproteinemia E78.5
- Fredrickson's type
  - I E78.3
  - IIa E78.00
  - IIb E78.2
  - III E78.2
  - IV E78.1
  - V E78.3
- low-density-lipoprotein-type (LDL) E78.00
- very-low-density-lipoprotein-type (VLDL) E78.1

Hyperlucent lung, unilateral J43.0

Hyperlysinemia E72.3

Hypermagnesemia E83.41
- neonatal P71.8

Hypermenorrhea N92.0

Hypermethioninemia E72.19

Hypermetropia (congenital) H52.0 ☑

Hypermobility, hypermotility
- cecum — *see* Syndrome, irritable bowel
- coccyx — *see* subcategory M53.2 ☑
- colon — *see* Syndrome, irritable bowel
  - psychogenic F45.8
- ileum K58.9
- intestine (*see also* Syndrome, irritable bowel) K58.9
  - psychogenic F45.8
- meniscus (knee) — *see* Derangement, knee, meniscus
- scapula — *see* Instability, joint, shoulder
- stomach K31.89
  - psychogenic F45.8
- syndrome M35.7
- urethra N36.41
  - with intrinsic sphincter deficiency N36.43

Hypernasality R49.21

Hypernatremia E87.0

Hypernephroma C64. ☑

Hyperopia — *see* Hypermetropia

Hyperorexia nervosa F50.2

Hyperornithinemia E72.4

Hyperosmia R43.1

Hyperosmolality E87.0

Hyperostosis (monomelic) (*see also* Disorder, bone, density and structure, specified NEC)
- ankylosing (spine) M48.10
  - cervical region M48.12

Hyperostosis — *continued*
- ankylosing — *continued*
  - cervicothoracic region M48.13
  - lumbar region M48.16
  - lumbosacral region M48.17
  - multiple sites M48.19
  - occipito-atlanto-axial region M48.11
  - sacrococcygeal region M48.18
  - thoracic region M48.14
  - thoracolumbar region M48.15
- cortical (skull) M85.2
  - infantile M89.8X ☑
- frontal, internal of skull M85.2
- interna frontalis M85.2
- skeletal, diffuse idiopathic — *see* Hyperostosis, ankylosing
- skull M85.2
  - congenital Q75.8
- vertebral, ankylosing — *see* Hyperostosis, ankylosing

Hyperovarism E28.8

Hyperoxaluria R82.992
- primary E72.53

Hyperparathyroidism E21.3
- primary E21.0
- secondary (renal) N25.81
  - non-renal E21.1
- specified NEC E21.2
- tertiary E21.2

Hyperpathia R20.8

Hyperperistalsis R19.2
- psychogenic F45.8

Hyperpermeability, capillary I78.8

Hyperphagia R63.2

Hyperphenylalaninemia NEC E70.1

Hyperphoria (alternating) H50.53

Hyperphosphatemia E83.39

Hyperpiesis, hyperpiesia — *see* Hypertension

Hyperpigmentation (*see also* Pigmentation)
- melanin NEC L81.4
- postinflammatory L81.0

Hyperpinealism E34.8

Hyperpituitarism E22.9

Hyperplasia, hyperplastic
- adenoids J35.2
- adrenal (capsule) (cortex) (gland) E27.8
  - with
    - sexual precocity (male) E25.9
      - congenital E25.0
    - virilism, adrenal E25.9
      - congenital E25.0
    - virilization (female) E25.9
      - congenital E25.0
  - congenital E25.0
  - salt-losing E25.0
- adrenomedullary E27.5
- angiolymphoid, eosinophilia (ALHE) D18.01
- appendix (lymphoid) K38.0
- artery, fibromuscular I77.3
- bone (*see also* Hypertrophy, bone)
  - marrow D75.89
- breast (*see also* Hypertrophy, breast)
  - atypical, atypia N60.9 ☑
    - ductal N60.9 ☑
    - lobular N60.9 ☑
- C-cell, thyroid E07.0
- cementation (tooth) (teeth) K03.4
- cervical gland R59.0
- cervix (uteri) (basal cell) (endometrium) (polypoid) (*see also* Dysplasia, cervix)
  - congenital Q51.828
- clitoris, congenital Q52.6
- denture K06.2
- endocervicitis N72
- endometrium, endometrial (adenomatous) (cystic) (glandular) (glandular-cystic) (polypoid) N85.00
  - with atypia N85.02
  - benign N85.01
  - cervix — *see* Dysplasia, cervix
  - complex (without atypia) N85.01
  - simple (without atypia) N85.01
- epithelial L85.9
  - focal, oral, including tongue K13.29
  - nipple N62
  - skin L85.9
  - tongue K13.29
  - vaginal wall N89.3
- erythroid D75.89
- fibromuscular of artery (carotid) (renal) I77.3
- genital
  - female NEC N94.89
  - male N50.89

Hyperplasia - Hypertension

Hyperplasia — *continued*
  gingiva K06.1
  glandularis cystica uteri (interstitialis) (*see also*
    Hyperplasia, endometrial) N85.00
  gum K06.1
  hymen, congenital Q52.4
  irritative, edentulous (alveolar) K06.2
  jaw M26.09
    alveolar M26.79
    lower M26.03
      alveolar M26.72
    upper M26.01
      alveolar M26.71
  kidney (congenital) Q63.3
  labia N90.69
    epithelial N90.3
  liver (congenital) Q44.7
    nodular, focal K76.89
  lymph gland or node R59.9
  mandible, mandibular M26.03
    alveolar M26.72
    unilateral condylar M27.8
  maxilla, maxillary M26.01
    alveolar M26.71
  myometrium, myometrial N85.2
  neuroendocrine cell, of infancy J84.841
  nose
    lymphoid J34.89
    polypoid J33.9
  oral mucosa (irritative) K13.6
  organ or site, congenital NEC — *see* Anomaly, by
    site
  ovary N83.8
  palate, papillary (irritative) K13.6
  pancreatic islet cells E16.9
    alpha E16.8
      with excess
        gastrin E16.4
        glucagon E16.3
    beta E16.1
  parathyroid (gland) E21.0
  pharynx (lymphoid) J39.2
  prostate (adenofibromatous) (nodular) N40.0
    with lower urinary tract symptoms (LUTS) N40.1
    without lower urinary tract symptoms (LUTS)
      N40.0
  renal artery I77.89
  reticulo-endothelial (cell) D75.89
  salivary gland (any) K11.1
  Schimmelbusch's — *see* Mastopathy, cystic
  suprarenal capsule (gland) E27.8
  thymus (gland) (persistent) E32.0
  thyroid (gland) — *see* Goiter
  tonsils (faucial) (infective) (lingual) (lymphoid) J35.1
    with adenoids J35.3
  unilateral condylar M27.8
  uterus, uterine N85.2
    endometrium (glandular) (*see also* Hyperplasia,
      endometrial) N85.00
  vulva N90.69
    epithelial N90.3
Hyperpnea — *see* Hyperventilation
Hyperpotassemia E87.5
Hyperprebetalipoproteinemia (familial) E78.1
Hyperprolactinemia E22.1
Hyperprolinemia (type I) (type II) E72.59
Hyperproteinemia E88.09
Hyperprothrombinemia, causing coagulation factor
  deficiency D68.4
Hyperpyrexia R50.9
  heat (effects) T67.01 ☑
  malignant, due to anesthetic T88.3 ☑
  rheumatic — *see* Fever, rheumatic
  unknown origin R50.9
Hyper-reflexia R29.2
Hypersalivation K11.7
Hypersecretion
  ACTH (not associated with Cushing's syndrome)
    E27.0
    pituitary E24.0
  adrenaline E27.5
  adrenomedullary E27.5
  androgen (testicular) E29.0
    ovarian (drug-induced) (iatrogenic) E28.1
  calcitonin E07.0
  catecholamine E27.5
  corticoadrenal E24.9
  cortisol E24.9
  epinephrine E27.5
  estrogen E28.0
  gastric K31.89
    psychogenic F45.8

Hypersecretion — *continued*
  gastrin E16.4
  glucagon E16.3
  hormone(s)
    ACTH (not associated with Cushing's syndrome)
      E27.0
      pituitary E24.0
    antidiuretic E22.2
    growth E22.0
    intestinal NEC E34.1
    ovarian androgen E28.1
    pituitary E22.9
    testicular E29.0
    thyroid stimulating E05.80
      with thyroid storm E05.81
  insulin — *see* Hyperinsulinism
  lacrimal glands — *see* Epiphora
  medulloadrenal E27.5
  milk O92.6
  ovarian androgens E28.1
  salivary gland (any) K11.7
  thyrocalcitonin E07.0
  upper respiratory J39.8
Hypersegmentation, leukocytic, hereditary D72.0
Hypersensitive, hypersensitiveness, hypersensitivity
  (*see also* Allergy)
  carotid sinus G90.01
  colon — *see* Irritable, colon
  drug T88.7 ☑
  gastrointestinal K52.29
    immediate K52.29
    psychogenic F45.8
  labyrinth — *see* subcategory H83.2 ☑
  pain R20.8
  pneumonitis — *see* Pneumonitis, allergic
  reaction T78.40 ☑
    upper respiratory tract NEC J39.3
Hypersomnia (organic) G47.10
  due to
    alcohol
      abuse F10.182
      dependence F10.282
      use F10.982
    amphetamines
      abuse F15.182
      dependence F15.282
      use F15.982
    caffeine
      abuse F15.182
      dependence F15.282
      use F15.982
    cocaine
      abuse F14.182
      dependence F14.282
      use F14.982
    drug NEC
      abuse F19.182
      dependence F19.282
      use F19.982
    medical condition G47.14
    mental disorder F51.13
    opioid
      abuse F11.182
      dependence F11.282
      use F11.982
    psychoactive substance NEC
      abuse F19.182
      dependence F19.282
      use F19.982
    sedative, hypnotic, or anxiolytic
      abuse F13.182
      dependence F13.282
      use F13.982
    stimulant NEC
      abuse F15.182
      dependence F15.282
      use F15.982
  idiopathic G47.11
    with long sleep time G47.11
    without long sleep time G47.12
  menstrual related G47.13
  nonorganic origin F51.11
    specified NEC F51.19
  not due to a substance or known physiological
    condition F51.11
    specified NEC F51.19
  primary F51.11
  recurrent G47.13
  specified NEC G47.19
Hypersplenia, hypersplenism D73.1
Hyperstimulation, ovaries (associated with induced
  ovulation) N98.1

Hypersusceptibility — *see* Allergy
Hypertelorism (ocular) (orbital) Q75.2
Hypertension, hypertensive (accelerated) (benign)
  (essential) (idiopathic) (malignant) (systemic) I10
  with
    heart failure (congestive) I11.0
    heart involvement (conditions in I50. ☑,
      I51.4- I51.9 due to hypertension) — *see*
      Hypertension, heart
    kidney involvement — *see* Hypertension, kidney
  benign, intracranial G93.2
  borderline R03.0
  cardiorenal (disease) I13.10
    with heart failure I13.0
      with stage 1 through stage 4 chronic kidney
        disease I13.0
      with stage 5 or end stage renal disease I13.2
    without heart failure I13.10
      with stage 1 through stage 4 chronic kidney
        disease I13.10
      with stage 5 or end stage renal disease I13.11
  cardiovascular
    disease (arteriosclerotic) (sclerotic) — *see*
      Hypertension, heart
    renal (disease) — *see* Hypertension, cardiorenal
  chronic venous — *see* Hypertension, venous
    (chronic)
  complicating
    childbirth (labor) O16.4
      pre-existing O10.92
        with
          heart disease O10.12
            with renal disease O10.32
          pre-eclampsia O11.4
          renal disease O10.22
            with heart disease O10.32
          essential O10.02
        secondary O10.42
    pregnancy O16. ☑
      with edema (*see also* Pre-eclampsia) O14.9 ☑
      gestational (pregnancy induced) (without
        proteinuria) O13. ☑
        with proteinuria O14.9 ☑
          mild pre-eclampsia O14.0 ☑
          moderate pre-eclampsia O14.0 ☑
          severe pre-eclampsia O14.1 ☑
            with hemolysis, elevated liver enzymes
              and low platelet count (HELLP)
              O14.2 ☑
      pre-existing O10.91 ☑
        with
          heart disease O10.11 ☑
            with renal disease O10.31 ☑
          pre-eclampsia — *see* category O11 ☑
          renal disease O10.21 ☑
            with heart disease O10.31 ☑
          essential O10.01 ☑
          secondary O10.41 ☑
      transient O13. ☑
    puerperium, pre-existing O16.5
      pre-existing
        with
          heart disease O10.13
            with renal disease O10.33
          pre-eclampsia O11.5
          renal disease O10.23
            with heart disease O10.33
          essential O10.03
      pregnancy-induced O13.9
      secondary O10.43
  crisis I16.9
  due to
    endocrine disorders I15.2
    pheochromocytoma I15.2
    renal disorders NEC I15.1
      arterial I15.0
    renovascular disorders I15.0
    specified disease NEC I15.8
  emergency I16.1
  encephalopathy I67.4
  gestational (without significant proteinuria)
    (pregnancy-induced) (transient) O13. ☑
    with significant proteinuria — *see* Pre-eclampsia
  complicating
    delivery O13.4
    puerperium O13.5
  Goldblatt's I70.1
  heart (disease) (conditions in I51.4-I51.9 due to
    hypertension) I11.9
    with
      heart failure (congestive) I11.0

☑ **Additional character required**

Hypertension — continued
  heart — continued
    kidney disease (chronic) — see Hypertension,
      cardiorenal
  intracranial (benign) G93.2
  kidney I12.9
    with
      heart disease — see Hypertension, cardiorenal
      stage 5 chronic kidney disease (CKD) or end
        stage renal disease (ESRD) I12.0
      stage 1 through stage 4 chronic kidney disease
        I12.9
  lesser circulation I27.0
  maternal O16. ☑
  newborn P29.2
    pulmonary (persistent) P29.30
  ocular H40.05 ☑
  pancreatic duct - code to underlying condition
    with chronic pancreatitis K86.1
  portal (due to chronic liver disease) (idiopathic)
    K76.6
    gastropathy K31.89
    in (due to) schistosomiasis (bilharziasis) B65.9
      [K77]
  postoperative I97.3
  psychogenic F45.8
  pulmonary I27.20
    with
      cor pulmonale (chronic) I27.29
        acute I26.09
      right heart ventricular strain/failure I27.29
        acute I26.09
      right to left shunt related to congenital heart
        disease I27.83
      unclear multifactorial mechanisms I27.29
    arterial (associated) (drug-induced) (toxin-
      induced) I27.21
    chronic thromboembolic I27.24
    due to
      hematologic disorders I27.29
      left heart disease I27.22
      lung diseases and hypoxia I27.23
      metabolic disorders I27.29
      specified systemic disorders NEC I27.29
    group 1 (associated) (drug-induced) (toxin-
      induced) I27.21
    group 2 I27.22
    group 3 I27.23
    group 4 I27.24
    group 5 I27.29
    of newborn (persistent) P29.30
    primary (idiopathic) I27.0
    secondary
      arterial I27.21
      specified NEC I27.29
  renal — see Hypertension, kidney
  renovascular I15.0
  secondary NEC I15.9
    due to
      endocrine disorders I15.2
      pheochromocytoma I15.2
      renal disorders NEC I15.1
        arterial I15.0
      renovascular disorders I15.0
      specified NEC I15.8
  transient R03.0
    of pregnancy O13. ☑
  urgency I16.0
  venous (chronic)
    due to
      deep vein thrombosis — see Syndrome,
        postthrombotic
    idiopathic I87.309
      with
        inflammation I87.32 ☑
          with ulcer I87.33 ☑
        specified complication NEC I87.39 ☑
        ulcer I87.31 ☑
          with inflammation I87.33 ☑
        asymptomatic I87.30 ☑
Hypertensive urgency — see Hypertension
Hyperthecosis ovary E28.8
Hyperthermia (of unknown origin) (see also
  Hyperpyrexia)
  malignant, due to anesthesia T88.3 ☑
  newborn P81.9
    environmental P81.0
Hyperthyroid (recurrent) — see Hyperthyroidism
Hyperthyroidism (latent) (pre-adult) (recurrent) E05.90
  with
    goiter (diffuse) E05.00
      with thyroid storm E05.01

Hyperthyroidism — continued
  with — continued
    nodular (multinodular) E05.20
      with thyroid storm E05.21
      uninodular E05.10
        with thyroid storm E05.11
    storm E05.91
  due to ectopic thyroid tissue E05.30
    with thyroid storm E05.31
  neonatal, transitory P72.1
  specified NEC E05.80
    with thyroid storm E05.81
Hypertony, hypertonia, hypertonicity
  bladder N31.8
  congenital P94.1
  stomach K31.89
    psychogenic F45.8
  uterus, uterine (contractions) (complicating
    delivery) O62.4
Hypertrichosis L68.9
  congenital Q84.2
  eyelid H02.869
    left H02.866
      lower H02.865
      upper H02.864
    right H02.863
      lower H02.862
      upper H02.861
  lanuginosa Q84.2
    acquired L68.1
  localized L68.2
  specified NEC L68.8
Hypertriglyceridemia, essential E78.1
Hypertrophy, hypertrophic
  adenofibromatous, prostate — see Enlargement,
    enlarged, prostate
  adenoids (infective) J35.2
    with tonsils J35.3
  adrenal cortex E27.8
  alveolar process or ridge — see Anomaly, alveolar
  anal papillae K62.89
  artery I77.89
    congenital NEC Q27.8
      digestive system Q27.8
      lower limb Q27.8
      specified site NEC Q27.8
      upper limb Q27.8
  auricular — see Hypertrophy, cardiac
  Bartholin's gland N75.8
  bile duct (common) (hepatic) K83.8
  bladder (sphincter) (trigone) N32.89
  bone M89.30
    carpus M89.34 ☑
    clavicle M89.31 ☑
    femur M89.35 ☑
    fibula M89.36 ☑
    finger M89.34 ☑
    humerus M89.32 ☑
    ilium M89.359
    ischium M89.359
    metacarpus M89.34 ☑
    metatarsus M89.37 ☑
    multiple sites M89.39
    neck M89.38
    radius M89.33 ☑
    rib M89.38
    scapula M89.31 ☑
    skull M89.38
    tarsus M89.37 ☑
    tibia M89.36 ☑
    toe M89.37 ☑
    ulna M89.33 ☑
    vertebra M89.38
  brain G93.89
  breast N62
    cystic — see Mastopathy, cystic
    newborn P83.4
    pubertal, massive N62
    puerperal, postpartum — see Disorder, breast,
      specified type NEC
    senile (parenchymatous) N62
  cardiac (chronic) (idiopathic) I51.7
    with rheumatic fever (conditions in I00)
      active I01.8
      inactive or quiescent (with chorea) I09.89
    congenital NEC Q24.8
    fatty — see Degeneration, myocardial
    hypertensive — see Hypertension, heart
    rheumatic (with chorea) I09.89
      active or acute I01.8
        with chorea I02.0
    valve — see Endocarditis

Hypertrophy — continued
  cartilage — see Disorder, cartilage, specified type
    NEC
  cecum — see Megacolon
  cervix (uteri) N88.8
    congenital Q51.828
    elongation N88.4
  clitoris (cirrhotic) N90.89
    congenital Q52.6
  colon (see also Megacolon)
    congenital Q43.2
  conjunctiva, lymphoid H11.89
  corpora cavernosa N48.89
  cystic duct K82.8
  duodenum K31.89
  endometrium (glandular) (see also Hyperplasia,
    endometrial) N85.00
    cervix N88.8
  epididymis N50.89
  esophageal hiatus (congenital) Q79.1
    with hernia — see Hernia, hiatal
  eyelid — see Disorder, eyelid, specified type NEC
  fat pad E65
    knee (infrapatellar) (popliteal) (prepatellar)
      (retropatellar) M79.4
  foot (congenital) Q74.2
  frenulum, frenum (tongue) K14.8
    lip K13.0
  gallbladder K82.8
  gastric mucosa K29.60
    with bleeding K29.61
  gland, glandular R59.9
    generalized R59.1
    localized R59.0
  gum (mucous membrane) K06.1
  heart (idiopathic) (see also Hypertrophy, cardiac)
    valve (see also Endocarditis) I38
  hemifacial Q67.4
  hepatic — see Hypertrophy, liver
  hiatus (esophageal) Q79.1
  hilus gland R59.0
  hymen, congenital Q52.4
  ileum K63.89
  intestine NEC K63.89
  jejunum K63.89
  kidney (compensatory) N28.81
    congenital Q63.3
  labium (majus) (minus) N90.60
  ligament — see Disorder, ligament
  lingual tonsil (infective) J35.1
    with adenoids J35.3
  lip K13.0
    congenital Q18.6
  liver R16.0
    acute K76.89
    congenital Q44.7
    cirrhotic — see Cirrhosis, liver
    fatty — see Fatty, liver
  lymph, lymphatic gland R59.9
    generalized R59.1
    localized R59.0
    tuberculous — see Tuberculosis, lymph gland
  mammary gland — see Hypertrophy, breast
  Meckel's diverticulum (congenital) Q43.0
    malignant — see Table of Neoplasms, small
      intestine, malignant
  median bar — see Hyperplasia, prostate
  meibomian gland — see Chalazion
  meniscus, knee, congenital Q74.1
  metatarsal head — see Hypertrophy, bone,
    metatarsus
  metatarsus — see Hypertrophy, bone, metatarsus
  mucous membrane
    alveolar ridge K06.2
    gum K06.1
    nose (turbinate) J34.3
  muscle M62.89
  muscular coat, artery I77.89
  myocardium (see also Hypertrophy, cardiac)
    idiopathic I42.2
  myometrium N85.2
  nail L60.2
    congenital Q84.5
  nasal J34.89
    alae J34.89
    bone J34.89
    cartilage J34.89
    mucous membrane (septum) J34.3
    sinus J34.89
    turbinate J34.3
  nasopharynx, lymphoid (infectional) (tissue) (wall)
    J35.2

Hypertrophy - Hypoplasia

Hypertrophy — *continued*
  nipple N62
  organ or site, congenital NEC — *see* Anomaly, by
    site
  ovary N83.8
  palate (hard) M27.8
    soft K13.79
  pancreas, congenital Q45.3
  parathyroid (gland) E21.0
  parotid gland K11.1
  penis N48.89
  pharyngeal tonsil J35.2
  pharynx J39.2
    lymphoid (infectional) (tissue) (wall) J35.2
  pituitary (anterior) (fossa) (gland) E23.6
  prepuce (congenital) N47.8
    female N90.89
  prostate — *see* Enlargement, enlarged, prostate
    congenital Q55.4
  pseudomuscular G71.09
  pylorus (adult) (muscle) (sphincter) K31.1
    congenital or infantile Q40.0
  rectal, rectum (sphincter) K62.89
  rhinitis (turbinate) J31.0
  salivary gland (any) K11.1
    congenital Q38.4
  scaphoid (tarsal) — *see* Hypertrophy, bone, tarsus
  scar L91.0
  scrotum N50.89
  seminal vesicle N50.89
  sigmoid — *see* Megacolon
  skin L91.9
    specified NEC L91.8
  spermatic cord N50.89
  spleen — *see* Splenomegaly
  spondylitis — *see* Spondylosis
  stomach K31.89
  sublingual gland K11.1
  submandibular gland K11.1
  suprarenal cortex (gland) E27.8
  synovial NEC M67.20
    acromioclavicular M67.21 ☑
    ankle M67.27 ☑
    elbow M67.22 ☑
    foot M67.27 ☑
    hand M67.24 ☑
    hip M67.25 ☑
    knee M67.26 ☑
    multiple sites M67.29
    specified site NEC M67.28
    wrist M67.23 ☑
  tendon — *see* Disorder, tendon, specified type
    NEC
  testis N44.8
    congenital Q55.29
  thymic, thymus (gland) (congenital) E32.0
  thyroid (gland) — *see* Goiter
  toe (congenital) Q74.2
    acquired (*see also* Deformity, toe, specified NEC)
  tongue K14.8
    congenital Q38.2
    papillae (foliate) K14.3
  tonsils (faucial) (infective) (lingual) (lymphoid) J35.1
    with adenoids J35.3
  tunica vaginalis N50.89
  ureter N28.89
  urethra N36.8
  uterus N85.2
    neck (with elongation) N88.4
    puerperal O90.89
  uvula K13.79
  vagina N89.8
  vas deferens N50.89
  vein I87.8
  ventricle, ventricular (heart) (*see also* Hypertrophy,
    cardiac)
    congenital Q24.8
    in tetralogy of Fallot Q21.3
  verumontanum N36.8
  vocal cord J38.3
  vulva N90.60
    stasis (nonfilarial) N90.69
Hypertropia H50.2 ☑
Hypertyrosinemia E70.21
Hyperuricemia (asymptomatic) E79.0
Hyperuricosuria R82.993
Hypervalinemia E71.19
Hyperventilation (tetany) R06.4
  hysterical F45.8
  psychogenic F45.8
  syndrome F45.8
Hypervitaminosis (dietary) NEC E67.8

Hypervitaminosis — *continued*
  A E67.0
    administered as drug (prolonged intake) — *see*
      Table of Drugs and Chemicals, vitamins,
      adverse effect
    overdose or wrong substance given or taken —
      see Table of Drugs and Chemicals, vitamins,
      poisoning
  B6 E67.2
  D E67.3
    administered as drug (prolonged intake) — *see*
      Table of Drugs and Chemicals, vitamins,
      adverse effect
    overdose or wrong substance given or taken —
      see Table of Drugs and Chemicals, vitamins,
      poisoning
  K E67.8
    administered as drug (prolonged intake) — *see*
      Table of Drugs and Chemicals, vitamins,
      adverse effect
    overdose or wrong substance given or taken —
      see Table of Drugs and Chemicals, vitamins,
      poisoning
Hypervolemia E87.70
  specified NEC E87.79
Hypesthesia R20.1
  cornea — *see* Anesthesia, cornea
Hyphema H21.0 ☑
  traumatic S05.1 ☑
Hypoacidity, gastric K31.89
  psychogenic F45.8
Hypoadrenalism, hypoadrenia E27.40
  primary E27.1
  tuberculous A18.7
Hypoadrenocorticism E27.40
  pituitary E23.0
  primary E27.1
Hypoalbuminemia E88.09
Hypoaldosteronism E27.40
Hypoalphalipoproteinemia E78.6
Hypobarism T70.29 ☑
Hypobaropathy T70.29 ☑
Hypobetalipoproteinemia (familial) E78.6
Hypocalcemia E83.51
  dietary E58
  neonatal P71.1
    due to cow's milk P71.0
  phosphate-loading (newborn) P71.1
Hypochloremia E87.8
Hypochlorhydria K31.89
  neurotic F45.8
  psychogenic F45.8
Hypochondria, hypochondriac, hypochondriasis
  (reaction) F45.21
  sleep F51.03
Hypochondrogenesis Q77.0
Hypochondroplasia Q77.4
Hypochromasia, blood cells D50.8
Hypocitraturia R82.991
Hypodontia — *see* Anodontia
Hypoeeosinophilia D72.89
Hypoesthesia R20.1
Hypofibrinogenemia D68.8
  acquired D65
  congenital (hereditary) D68.2
Hypofunction
  adrenocortical E27.40
    drug-induced E27.3
    postprocedural E89.6
    primary E27.1
  adrenomedullary, postprocedural E89.6
  cerebral R29.818
  corticoadrenal NEC E27.40
  intestinal K59.8
  labyrinth — *see* subcategory H83.2 ☑
  ovary E28.39
  pituitary (gland) (anterior) E23.0
  testicular E29.1
    postprocedural (postsurgical) (postirradiation)
      (iatrogenic) E89.5
Hypogalactia O92.4
Hypogammaglobulinemia (*see also*
  Agammaglobulinemia) D80.1
  hereditary D80.0
  nonfamilial D80.1
  transient, of infancy D80.7
Hypogenitalism (congenital) — *see* Hypogonadism
Hypoglossia Q38.3
Hypoglycemia (spontaneous) E16.2
  coma E15
    diabetic — *see* Diabetes, by type, with
      hypoglycemia, with coma

Hypoglycemia — *continued*
  diabetic — *see* Diabetes, hypoglycemia
  dietary counseling and surveillance Z71.3
  drug-induced E16.0
    with coma (nondiabetic) E15
  due to insulin E16.0
    with coma (nondiabetic) E15
      therapeutic misadventure — *see* subcategory
        T38.3 ☑
  functional, nonhyperinsulinemic E16.1
  iatrogenic E16.0
    with coma (nondiabetic) E15
  in infant of diabetic mother P70.1
    gestational diabetes P70.0
  infantile E16.1
  leucine-induced E71.19
  neonatal (transitory) P70.4
    iatrogenic P70.3
  reactive (not drug-induced) E16.1
  transitory neonatal P70.4
Hypogonadism
  female E28.39
  hypogonadotropic E23.0
  male E29.1
  ovarian (primary) E28.39
  pituitary E23.0
  testicular (primary) E29.1
Hypohidrosis, hypoidrosis L74.4
Hypoinsulinemia, postprocedural E89.1
Hypokalemia E87.6
Hypoleukocytosis — *see* Agranulocytosis
Hypolipoproteinemia (alpha) (beta) E78.6
Hypomagnesemia E83.42
  neonatal P71.2
Hypomania, hypomanic reaction F30.8
Hypomenorrhea — *see* Oligomenorrhea
Hypometabolism R63.8
Hypomotility
  gastrointestinal (tract) K31.89
    psychogenic F45.8
  intestine K59.8
    psychogenic F45.8
  stomach K31.89
    psychogenic F45.8
Hyponasality R49.22
Hyponatremia E87.1
Hypo-osmolality E87.1
Hypo-ovarianism, hypo-ovarism E28.39
Hypoparathyroidism E20.9
  familial E20.8
  idiopathic E20.0
  neonatal, transitory P71.4
  postprocedural E89.2
  specified NEC E20.8
Hypoperfusion (in)
  newborn P96.89
Hypopharyngitis — *see* Laryngopharyngitis
Hypophoria H50.53
Hypophosphatemia, hypophosphatasia (acquired)
  (congenital) (renal) E83.39
  familial E83.31
Hypophyseal, hypophysis (*see also* condition)
  dwarfism E23.0
  gigantism E22.0
Hypopiesis — *see* Hypotension
Hypopinealism E34.8
Hypopituitarism (juvenile) E23.0
  drug-induced E23.1
  due to
    hypophysectomy E89.3
    radiotherapy E89.3
  iatrogenic NEC E23.1
  postirradiation E89.3
  postpartum O99.285
  postprocedural E89.3
Hypoplasia, hypoplastic
  adrenal (gland), congenital Q89.1
  alimentary tract, congenital Q45.8
    upper Q40.8
  anus, anal (canal) Q42.3
    with fistula Q42.2
  aorta, aortic Q25.42
    ascending, in hypoplastic left heart syndrome
      Q23.4
      valve Q23.1
    in hypoplastic left heart syndrome Q23.4
  areola, congenital Q83.8
  arm (congenital) — *see* Defect, reduction, upper
    limb
  artery (peripheral) Q27.8
    brain (congenital) Q28.3
    coronary Q24.5

☑ **Additional character required**

Hypoplasia — *continued*
  artery — *continued*
    digestive system Q27.8
    lower limb Q27.8
    pulmonary Q25.79
      functional, unilateral J43.0
    retinal (congenital) Q14.1
    specified site NEC Q27.8
    umbilical Q27.0
    upper limb Q27.8
  auditory canal Q17.8
    causing impairment of hearing Q16.9
  biliary duct or passage Q44.5
  bone NOS Q79.9
    face Q75.8
    marrow D61.9
      megakaryocytic D69.49
    skull — *see* Hypoplasia, skull
  brain Q02
    gyri Q04.3
    part of Q04.3
  breast (areola) N64.82
  bronchus Q32.4
  cardiac Q24.8
  carpus — *see* Defect, reduction, upper limb,
      specified type NEC
  cartilage hair Q78.8
  cecum Q42.8
  cementum K00.4
  cephalic Q02
  cerebellum Q04.3
  cervix (uteri), congenital Q51.821
  clavicle (congenital) Q74.0
  coccyx Q76.49
  colon Q42.9
    specified NEC Q42.8
  corpus callosum Q04.0
  cricoid cartilage Q31.2
  digestive organ(s) or tract NEC Q45.8
    upper (congenital) Q40.8
  ear (auricle) (lobe) Q17.2
    middle Q16.4
  enamel of teeth (neonatal) (postnatal) (prenatal)
      K00.4
  endocrine (gland) NEC Q89.2
  endometrium N85.8
  epididymis (congenital) Q55.4
  epiglottis Q31.2
  erythroid, congenital D61.01
  esophagus (congenital) Q39.8
  eustachian tube Q17.8
  eye Q11.2
  eyelid (congenital) Q10.3
  face Q18.8
    bone(s) Q75.8
  femur (congenital) — *see* Defect, reduction, lower
      limb, specified type NEC
  fibula (congenital) — *see* Defect, reduction, lower
      limb, specified type NEC
  finger (congenital) — *see* Defect, reduction, upper
      limb, specified type NEC
  focal dermal Q82.8
  foot — *see* Defect, reduction, lower limb, specified
      type NEC
  gallbladder Q44.0
  genitalia, genital organ(s)
    female, congenital Q52.8
      external Q52.79
      internal NEC Q52.8
    in adiposogenital dystrophy E23.6
  glottis Q31.2
  hair Q84.2
  hand (congenital) — *see* Defect, reduction, upper
      limb, specified type NEC
  heart Q24.8
  humerus (congenital) — *see* Defect, reduction,
      upper limb, specified type NEC
  intestine (small) Q41.9
    large Q42.9
      specified NEC Q42.8
  jaw M26.09
    alveolar M26.79
    lower M26.04
      alveolar M26.74
    upper M26.02
      alveolar M26.73
  kidney(s) Q60.5
    bilateral Q60.4
    unilateral Q60.3
  labium (majus) (minus), congenital Q52.79
  larynx Q31.2
  left heart syndrome Q23.4

Hypoplasia — *continued*
  leg (congenital) — *see* Defect, reduction, lower
      limb
  limb Q73.8
    lower (congenital) — *see* Defect, reduction, lower
        limb
    upper (congenital) — *see* Defect, reduction,
        upper limb
  liver Q44.7
  lung (lobe) (not associated with short gestation)
      Q33.6
    associated with immaturity, low birth weight,
        prematurity, or short gestation P28.0
  mammary (areola), congenital Q83.8
  mandible, mandibular M26.04
    alveolar M26.74
    unilateral condylar M27.8
  maxillary M26.02
    alveolar M26.73
  medullary D61.9
  megakaryocytic D69.49
  metacarpus — *see* Defect, reduction, upper limb,
      specified type NEC
  metatarsus — *see* Defect, reduction, lower limb,
      specified type NEC
  muscle Q79.8
  nail(s) Q84.6
  nose, nasal Q30.1
  optic nerve H47.03 ☑
  osseous meatus (ear) Q17.8
  ovary, congenital Q50.39
  pancreas Q45.0
  parathyroid (gland) Q89.2
  parotid gland Q38.4
  patella Q74.1
  pelvis, pelvic girdle Q74.2
  penis (congenital) Q55.62
  peripheral vascular system Q27.8
    digestive system Q27.8
    lower limb Q27.8
    specified site NEC Q27.8
    upper limb Q27.8
  pituitary (gland) (congenital) Q89.2
  pulmonary (not associated with short gestation)
      Q33.6
    artery, functional J43.0
    associated with short gestation P28.0
  radioulnar — *see* Defect, reduction, upper limb,
      specified type NEC
  radius — *see* Defect, reduction, upper limb
  rectum Q42.1
    with fistula Q42.0
  respiratory system NEC Q34.8
  rib Q76.6
  right heart syndrome Q22.6
  sacrum Q76.49
  scapula Q74.0
  scrotum Q55.1
  shoulder girdle Q74.0
  skin Q82.8
  skull (bone) Q75.8
    with
      anencephaly Q00.0
      encephalocele — *see* Encephalocele
      hydrocephalus Q03.9
        with spina bifida — *see* Spina bifida, by site,
            with hydrocephalus
      microcephaly Q02
  spinal (cord) (ventral horn cell) Q06.1
  spine Q76.49
  sternum Q76.7
  tarsus — *see* Defect, reduction, lower limb, specified
      type NEC
  testis Q55.1
  thymic, with immunodeficiency D82.1
  thymus (gland) Q89.2
    with immunodeficiency D82.1
  thyroid (gland) E03.1
    cartilage Q31.2
  tibiofibular (congenital) — *see* Defect, reduction,
      lower limb, specified type NEC
  toe — *see* Defect, reduction, lower limb, specified
      type NEC
  tongue Q38.3
  Turner's K00.4
  ulna (congenital) — *see* Defect, reduction, upper
      limb
  umbilical artery Q27.0
  unilateral condylar M27.8
  ureter Q62.8
  uterus, congenital Q51.811
  vagina Q52.4

Hypoplasia — *continued*
  vascular NEC peripheral Q27.8
    brain Q28.3
    digestive system Q27.8
    lower limb Q27.8
    specified site NEC Q27.8
    upper limb Q27.8
  vein(s) (peripheral) Q27.8
    brain Q28.3
    digestive system Q27.8
    great Q26.8
    lower limb Q27.8
    specified site NEC Q27.8
    upper limb Q27.8
  vena cava (inferior) (superior) Q26.8
  vertebra Q76.49
  vulva, congenital Q52.79
  zonule (ciliary) Q12.8
Hypoplasminogenemia E88.02
Hypopnea, obstructive sleep apnea G47.33
Hypopotassemia E87.6
Hypoproconvertinemia, congenital (hereditary) D68.2
Hypoproteinemia E77.8
Hypoprothrombinemia (congenital) (hereditary)
    (idiopathic) D68.2
  acquired D68.4
  newborn, transient P61.6
Hypoptyalism K11.7
Hypopyon (eye) (anterior chamber) — *see* Iridocyclitis,
    acute, hypopyon
Hypopyrexia R68.0
Hyporeflexia R29.2
Hyposecretion
  ACTH E23.0
  antidiuretic hormone E23.2
  ovary E28.39
  salivary gland (any) K11.7
  vasopressin E23.2
Hyposegmentation, leukocytic, hereditary D72.0
Hyposiderinemia D50.9
Hypospadias Q54.9
  balanic Q54.0
  coronal Q54.0
  glandular Q54.0
  penile Q54.1
  penoscrotal Q54.2
  perineal Q54.3
  specified NEC Q54.8
Hypospermatogenesis — *see* Oligospermia
Hyposplenism D73.0
Hypostasis pulmonary, passive — *see* Edema, lung
Hypostatic — *see* condition
Hyposthenuria N28.89
Hypotension (arterial) (constitutional) I95.9
  chronic I95.89
  due to (of) hemodialysis I95.3
  drug-induced I95.2
  iatrogenic I95.89
  idiopathic (permanent) I95.0
  intracranial, following ventricular shunting
      (ventriculostomy) G97.2
  intra-dialytic I95.3
  maternal, syndrome (following labor and delivery)
      O26.5 ☑
  neurogenic, orthostatic G90.3
  orthostatic (chronic) I95.1
    due to drugs I95.2
    neurogenic G90.3
  postoperative I95.81
  postural I95.1
  specified NEC I95.89
Hypothermia (accidental) T68 ☑
  due to anesthesia, anesthetic T88.51 ☑
  low environmental temperature T68 ☑
  neonatal P80.9
    environmental (mild) NEC P80.8
    mild P80.8
    severe (chronic) (cold injury syndrome) P80.0
    specified NEC P80.8
  not associated with low environmental
      temperature R68.0
Hypothyroidism (acquired) E03.9
  autoimmune — *see* Thyroiditis, autoimmune
  congenital (without goiter) E03.1
    with goiter (diffuse) E03.0
  due to
    exogenous substance NEC E03.2
    iodine-deficiency, acquired E01.8
      subclinical E02
    irradiation therapy E89.0
    medicament NEC E03.2
    P-aminosalicylic acid (PAS) E03.2

Hypothyroidism - Immunodeficiency

Hypothyroidism — continued
  due to — continued
    phenylbutazone E03.2
    resorcinol E03.2
    sulfonamide E03.2
    surgery E89.0
    thiourea group drugs E03.2
  iatrogenic NEC E03.2
  iodine-deficiency (acquired) E01.8
    congenital — see Syndrome, iodine- deficiency,
      congenital
    subclinical E02
  neonatal, transitory P72.2
  postinfectious E03.3
  postirradiation E89.0
  postprocedural E89.0
  postsurgical E89.0
  specified NEC E03.8
  subclinical, iodine-deficiency related E02
Hypotonia, hypotonicity, hypotony
  bladder N31.2
  congenital (benign) P94.2
  eye — see Disorder, globe, hypotony
Hypotrichosis — see Alopecia
Hypotropia H50.2 ☑
Hypoventilation R06.89
  congenital central alveolar G47.35
  sleep related
    idiopathic nonobstructive alveolar G47.34
    in conditions classified elsewhere G47.36
Hypovitaminosis — see Deficiency, vitamin
Hypovolemia E86.1
  surgical shock T81.19 ☑
  traumatic (shock) T79.4 ☑
Hypoxemia R09.02
  newborn P84
  sleep related, in conditions classified elsewhere
    G47.36
Hypoxia (see also Anoxia) R09.02
  cerebral, during a procedure NEC G97.81
    postprocedural NEC G97.82
  intrauterine P84
  myocardial — see Insufficiency, coronary
  newborn P84
  sleep-related G47.34
Hypsarrhythmia — see Epilepsy, generalized, specified
  NEC
Hysteralgia, pregnant uterus O26.89 ☑
Hysteria, hysterical (conversion) (dissociative state)
  F44.9
  anxiety F41.8
  convulsions F44.5
  psychosis, acute F44.9
Hysteroepilepsy F44.5

I

IBDU (colonic inflammatory bowel disease
  unclassified) K52.3
Ichthyoparasitism due to Vandellia cirrhosa B88.8
Ichthyosis (congenital) Q80.9
  acquired L85.0
  fetalis Q80.4
  hystrix Q80.8
  lamellar Q80.2
  lingual K13.29
  palmaris and plantaris Q82.8
  simplex Q80.0
  vera Q80.8
  vulgaris Q80.0
  X-linked Q80.1
Ichthyotoxism — see Poisoning, fish
  bacterial — see Intoxication, foodborne
Icteroanemia, hemolytic (acquired) D59.9
  congenital — see Spherocytosis
Icterus (see also Jaundice)
  conjunctiva R17
  newborn P59.9
  gravis, newborn P55.0
  hematogenous (acquired) D59.9
  hemolytic (acquired) D59.9
    congenital — see Spherocytosis
  hemorrhagic (acute) (leptospiral) (spirochetal) A27.0
    newborn P53
  infectious B15.9
    with hepatic coma B15.0
    leptospiral A27.0
    spirochetal A27.0
  neonatorum — see Jaundice, newborn
  spirochetal A27.0

Ictus solaris, solis T67.01 ☑
Ideation
  homicidal R45.850
  suicidal R45.851
Identity disorder (child) F64.9
  gender role F64.2
  psychosexual F64.2
Id reaction (due to bacteria) L30.2
Idioglossia F80.0
Idiopathic — see condition
Idiot, idiocy (congenital) F73
  amaurotic (Bielschowsky(-Jansky)) (family) (infantile
    (late)) (juvenile (late)) (Vogt-Spielmeyer) E75.4
  microcephalic Q02
IgE asthma J45.909
IIAC (idiopathic infantile arterial calcification) Q28.8
Ileitis (chronic) (noninfectious) (see also Enteritis) K52.9
  backwash — see Pancolitis, ulcerative (chronic)
  infectious A09
  regional (ulcerative) — see Enteritis, regional, small
    intestine
  segmental — see Enteritis, regional
  terminal (ulcerative) — see Enteritis, regional, small
    intestine
Ileocolitis (see also Enteritis) K52.9
  infectious A09
  regional — see Enteritis, regional
  ulcerative K51.0 ☑
Ileostomy
  attention to Z43.2
  malfunctioning K94.13
  status Z93.2
    with complication — see Complications,
      enterostomy
Ileotyphus — see Typhoid
Ileum — see condition
Ileus (bowel) (colon) (inhibitory) (intestine) K56.7
  adynamic K56.0
  due to gallstone (in intestine) K56.3
  duodenal (chronic) K31.5
  gallstone K56.3
  mechanical NEC (see also Obstruction, intestine,
    specified NEC) K56.699
  meconium P76.0
    in cystic fibrosis E84.11
    meaning meconium plug (without cystic fibrosis)
      P76.0
  myxedema K59.8
  neurogenic K56.0
    Hirschsprung's disease or megacolon Q43.1
  newborn
    due to meconium P76.0
      in cystic fibrosis E84.11
      meaning meconium plug (without cystic
        fibrosis) P76.0
    transitory P76.1
  obstructive (see also Obstruction, intestine,
    specified NEC) K56.699
  paralytic K56.0
  postoperative K91.89
Iliac — see condition
Iliotibial band syndrome M76.3 ☑
Illiteracy Z55.0
Illness (see also Disease) R69
  manic-depressive — see Disorder, bipolar
Imbalance R26.89
  autonomic G90.8
  constituents of food intake E63.1
  electrolyte E87.8
    with
      abortion — see Abortion by type, complicated
        by, electrolyte imbalance
      molar pregnancy O08.5
    due to hyperemesis gravidarum O21.1
    following ectopic or molar pregnancy O08.5
    neonatal, transitory NEC P74.49
      potassium
        hyperkalemia P74.31
        hypokalemia P74.32
      sodium
        hypernatremia P74.21
        hyponatremia P74.22
  endocrine E34.9
  eye muscle NOS H50.9
  hormone E34.9
  hysterical F44.4
  labyrinth — see subcategory H83.2 ☑
  posture R29.3
  protein-energy — see Malnutrition
  sympathetic G90.8
Imbecile, imbecility (I.Q.35-49) F71
Imbedding, intrauterine device T83.39 ☑

Imbibition, cholesterol (gallbladder) K82.4
Imbrication, teeth,, fully erupted M26.30
Imerslund (-Gräsbeck) syndrome D51.1
Immature (see also Immaturity)
  birth (less than 37 completed weeks) — see
    Preterm, newborn
    extremely (less than 28 completed weeks) — see
      Immaturity, extreme
  personality F60.89
Immaturity (less than 37 completed weeks) (see also
  Preterm, newborn)
  extreme of newborn (less than 28 completed weeks
    of gestation) (less than 196 completed days
    of gestation) (unspecified weeks of gestation)
    P07.20
    gestational age
      23 completed weeks (23 weeks, 0 days through
        23 weeks, 6 days) P07.22
      24 completed weeks (24 weeks, 0 days through
        24 weeks, 6 days) P07.23
      25 completed weeks (25 weeks, 0 days through
        25 weeks, 6 days) P07.24
      26 completed weeks (26 weeks, 0 days through
        26 weeks, 6 days) P07.25
      27 completed weeks (27 weeks, 0 days through
        27 weeks, 6 days) P07.26
      less than 23 completed weeks P07.21
  fetus or infant light-for-dates — see Light-for-dates
  lung, newborn P28.0
  organ or site NEC — see Hypoplasia
  pulmonary, newborn P28.0
  reaction F60.89
  sexual (female) (male), after puberty E30.0
Immersion T75.1 ☑
  hand T69.01 ☑
  foot T69.02 ☑
Immobile, immobility
  complete, due to severe physical disability or frailty
    R53.2
  intestine K59.8
  syndrome (paraplegic) M62.3
Immune reconstitution (inflammatory)
  syndrome [IRIS] D89.3
Immunization (see also Vaccination)
  ABO — see Incompatibility, ABO
    in newborn P55.1
  appropriate for age
    child (over 28 days old) Z00.129
      with abnormal findings Z00.121
  complication — see Complications, vaccination
  encounter for Z23
  not done (not carried out) Z28.9
    because (of)
      acute illness of patient Z28.01
      allergy to vaccine (or component) Z28.04
      caregiver refusal Z28.82
      chronic illness of patient Z28.02
      contraindication NEC Z28.09
      delay in delivery of vaccine Z28.83
      group pressure Z28.1
      guardian refusal Z28.82
      immune compromised state of patient Z28.03
      lack of availability of vaccine Z28.83
      manufacturer delay of vaccine Z28.83
      parent refusal Z28.82
      patient's belief Z28.1
      patient had disease being vaccinated against
        Z28.81
      patient refusal Z28.21
      religious beliefs of patient Z28.1
      specified reason NEC Z28.89
        of patient Z28.29
      unavailability of vaccine Z28.83
      unspecified patient reason Z28.20
  Rh factor
    affecting management of pregnancy NEC
      O36.09 ☑
      anti-D antibody O36.01 ☑
    from transfusion — see Complication(s),
      transfusion, incompatibility reaction, Rh
      (factor)
Immunocytoma C83.0 ☑
Immunodeficiency D84.9
  with
    adenosine-deaminase deficiency (see also
      Deficiency, adenosine deaminase) D81.30
    antibody defects D80.9
      specified type NEC D80.8
    hyperimmunoglobulinemia D80.6
    increased immunoglobulin M (IgM) D80.5
    major defect D82.9
      specified type NEC D82.8

Immunodeficiency — *continued*
  with — *continued*
    partial albinism D82.8
    short-limbed stature D82.2
    thrombocytopenia and eczema D82.0
  antibody with
    hyperimmunoglobulinemia D80.6
    near-normal immunoglobulins D80.6
  autosomal recessive, Swiss type D80.0
  combined D81.9
    biotin-dependent carboxylase D81.819
      biotinidase D81.810
      holocarboxylase synthetase D81.818
      specified type NEC D81.818
    severe (SCID) D81.9
      with
        low or normal B-cell numbers D81.2
        low T- and B-cell numbers D81.1
        reticular dysgenesis D81.0
      specified type NEC D81.89
  common variable D83.9
    with
      abnormalities of B-cell numbers and function D83.0
      autoantibodies to B- or T-cells D83.2
      immunoregulatory T-cell disorders D83.1
    specified type NEC D83.8
  following hereditary defective response to Epstein-Barr virus (EBV) D82.3
  selective, immunoglobulin
    A (IgA) D80.2
    G (IgG) (subclasses) D80.3
    M (IgM) D80.4
  severe combined (SCID) D81.9
    due to adenosine deaminase deficiency D81.31
  specified type NEC D84.8
  X-linked, with increased IgM D80.5
Immunotherapy (encounter for)
  antineoplastic Z51.12
Impaction, impacted
  bowel, colon, rectum (*see also* Impaction, fecal) K56.49
    by gallstone K56.3
  calculus — *see* Calculus
  cerumen (ear) (external) H61.2 ☑
  cuspid — *see* Impaction, tooth
  dental (same or adjacent tooth) K01.1
  fecal, feces K56.41
  fracture — *see* Fracture, by site
  gallbladder — *see* Calculus, gallbladder
  gallstone(s) — *see* Calculus, gallbladder
    bile duct (common) (hepatic) — *see* Calculus, bile duct
    cystic duct — *see* Calculus, gallbladder
    in intestine, with obstruction (any part) K56.3
  intestine (calculous) NEC (*see also* Impaction, fecal) K56.49
    gallstone, with ileus K56.3
  intrauterine device (IUD) T83.39 ☑
  molar — *see* Impaction, tooth
  shoulder, causing obstructed labor O66.0
  tooth, teeth K01.1
  turbinate J34.89
Impaired, impairment (function)
  auditory discrimination — *see* Abnormal, auditory perception
  cognitive, mild, so stated G31.84
  dual sensory Z73.82
  fasting glucose R73.01
  glucose tolerance (oral) R73.02
  hearing — *see* Deafness
  heart — *see* Disease, heart
  kidney N28.9
    disorder resulting from N25.9
      specified NEC N25.89
  liver K72.90
    with coma K72.91
  mastication K08.89
  mild cognitive, so stated G31.84
  mobility
    ear ossicles — *see* Ankylosis, ear ossicles
    requiring care provider Z74.09
  myocardium, myocardial — *see* Insufficiency, myocardial
  rectal sphincter R19.8
  renal (acute) (chronic) N28.9
    disorder resulting from N25.9
      specified NEC N25.89
  vision NEC H54.7
    both eyes H54.3
Impediment, speech R47.9
  psychogenic (childhood) F98.8

Impediment — *continued*
  slurring R47.81
  specified NEC R47.89
Impending
  coronary syndrome I20.0
  delirium tremens F10.239
  myocardial infarction I20.0
Imperception auditory (acquired) (*see also* Deafness)
  congenital H93.25
Imperfect
  aeration, lung (newborn) NEC — *see* Atelectasis
  closure (congenital)
    alimentary tract NEC Q45.8
      lower Q43.8
      upper Q40.8
    atrioventricular ostium Q21.2
    atrium (secundum) Q21.1
    branchial cleft NOS Q18.2
      cyst Q18.0
      fistula Q18.0
      sinus Q18.0
    choroid Q14.3
    cricoid cartilage Q31.8
    cusps, heart valve NEC Q24.8
      pulmonary Q22.3
    ductus
      arteriosus Q25.0
      Botalli Q25.0
    ear drum (causing impairment of hearing) Q16.4
    esophagus with communication to bronchus or trachea Q39.1
    eyelid Q10.3
    foramen
      botalli Q21.1
      ovale Q21.1
    genitalia, genital organ(s) or system
      female Q52.8
        external Q52.79
        internal NEC Q52.8
      male Q55.8
    glottis Q31.8
    interatrial ostium or septum Q21.1
    interauricular ostium or septum Q21.1
    interventricular ostium or septum Q21.0
    larynx Q31.8
    lip — *see* Cleft, lip
    nasal septum Q30.3
    nose Q30.2
    omphalomesenteric duct Q43.0
    optic nerve entry Q14.2
    organ or site not listed — *see* Anomaly, by site
    ostium
      interatrial Q21.1
      interauricular Q21.1
      interventricular Q21.0
    palate — *see* Cleft, palate
    preauricular sinus Q18.1
    retina Q14.1
    roof of orbit Q75.8
    sclera Q13.5
    septum
      aorticopulmonary Q21.4
      atrial (secundum) Q21.1
      between aorta and pulmonary artery Q21.4
      heart Q21.9
      interatrial (secundum) Q21.1
      interauricular (secundum) Q21.1
      interventricular Q21.0
        in tetralogy of Fallot Q21.3
      nasal Q30.3
      ventricular Q21.0
        with pulmonary stenosis or atresia, dextraposition of aorta, and hypertrophy of right ventricle Q21.3
        in tetralogy of Fallot Q21.3
    skull Q75.0
      with
        anencephaly Q00.0
        encephalocele — *see* Encephalocele
        hydrocephalus Q03.9
          with spina bifida — *see* Spina bifida, by site, with hydrocephalus
        microcephaly Q02
    spine (with meningocele) — *see* Spina bifida
    trachea Q32.1
    tympanic membrane (causing impairment of hearing) Q16.4
    uterus Q51.818
    vitelline duct Q43.0
  erection — *see* Dysfunction, sexual, male, erectile
  fusion — *see* Imperfect, closure
  inflation, lung (newborn) — *see* Atelectasis

Imperfect — *continued*
  posture R29.3
  rotation, intestine Q43.3
  septum, ventricular Q21.0
Imperfectly descended testis — *see* Cryptorchid
Imperforate (congenital) (*see also* Atresia)
  anus Q42.3
    with fistula Q42.2
  cervix (uteri) Q51.828
  esophagus Q39.0
    with tracheoesophageal fistula Q39.1
  hymen Q52.3
  jejunum Q41.1
  pharynx Q38.8
  rectum Q42.1
    with fistula Q42.0
  urethra Q64.39
  vagina Q52.4
Impervious (congenital) (*see also* Atresia)
  anus Q42.3
    with fistula Q42.2
  bile duct Q44.2
  esophagus Q39.0
    with tracheoesophageal fistula Q39.1
  intestine (small) Q41.9
    large Q42.9
      specified NEC Q42.8
  rectum Q42.1
    with fistula Q42.0
  ureter — *see* Atresia, ureter
  urethra Q64.39
Impetiginization of dermatoses L01.1
Impetigo (any organism) (any site) (circinate) (contagiosa) (simplex) (vulgaris) L01.00
  Bockhart's L01.02
  bullous, bullosa L01.03
  external ear L01.00 *[H62.40]*
  follicularis L01.02
  furfuracea L30.5
  herpetiformis L40.1
    nonobstetrical L40.1
  neonatorum L01.03
  nonbullous L01.01
  specified type NEC L01.09
  ulcerative L01.09
Impingement (on teeth)
  joint — *see* Disorder, joint, specified type NEC
  soft tissue
    anterior M26.81
    posterior M26.82
Implant, endometrial N80.9
Implantation
  anomalous — *see* Anomaly, by site
    ureter Q62.63
  cyst
    external area or site (skin) NEC L72.0
    iris — *see* Cyst, iris, implantation
    vagina N89.8
    vulva N90.7
  dermoid (cyst) — *see* Implantation, cyst
Impotence (sexual) N52.9
  counseling Z70.1
  organic origin (*see also* Dysfunction, sexual, male, erectile) N52.9
  psychogenic F52.21
Impression, basilar Q75.8
Imprisonment, anxiety concerning Z65.1
Improper care (child) (newborn) — *see* Maltreatment
Improperly tied umbilical cord (causing hemorrhage) P51.8
Impulsiveness (impulsive) R45.87
Inability to swallow — *see* Aphagia
Inaccessible, inaccessibility
  health care NEC Z75.3
    due to
      waiting period Z75.2
        for admission to facility elsewhere Z75.1
      other helping agencies Z75.4
Inactive — *see* condition
Inadequate, inadequacy
  aesthetics of dental restoration K08.56
  biologic, constitutional, functional, or social F60.7
  development
    child R62.50
    genitalia
      after puberty NEC E30.0
      congenital
        female Q52.8
          external Q52.79
          internal Q52.8
        male Q55.8
    lungs Q33.6

Inadequate - Inequality

Inadequate — *continued*
  development — *continued*
    associated with short gestation P28.0
    organ or site not listed — *see* Anomaly, by site
  diet (causing nutritional deficiency) E63.9
  eating habits Z72.4
  environment, household Z59.1
  family support Z63.8
  food (supply) NEC Z59.4
    hunger effects T73.0 ☑
  functional F60.7
  household care, due to
    family member
      handicapped or ill Z74.2
      on vacation Z75.5
      temporarily away from home Z74.2
    technical defects in home Z59.1
    temporary absence from home of person
        rendering care Z74.2
  housing (heating) (space) Z59.1
  income (financial) Z59.6
  intrafamilial communication Z63.8
  material resources Z59.9
  mental — *see* Disability, intellectual
  parental supervision or control of child Z62.0
  personality F60.7
  pulmonary
    function R06.89
      newborn P28.5
    ventilation, newborn P28.5
  sample of cytologic smear
    anus R85.615
    cervix R87.615
    vagina R87.625
  social F60.7
    insurance Z59.7
    skills NEC Z73.4
  supervision of child by parent Z62.0
  teaching affecting education Z55.8
  welfare support Z59.7
Inanition R64
  with edema — *see* Malnutrition, severe
  due to
    deprivation of food T73.0 ☑
    malnutrition — *see* Malnutrition
  fever R50.9
Inappropriate
  change in quantitative human chorionic
      gonadotropin (hCG) in early pregnancy O02.81
  diet or eating habits Z72.4
  level of quantitative human chorionic
      gonadotropin (hCG) for gestational age in early
      pregnancy O02.81
  secretion
    antidiuretic hormone (ADH) (excessive) E22.2
      deficiency E23.2
    pituitary (posterior) E22.2
Inattention at or after birth — *see* Neglect
Incarceration, incarcerated
  enterocele K46.0
    gangrenous K46.1
  epiplocele K46.0
    gangrenous K46.1
  exomphalos K42.0
    gangrenous K42.1
  hernia (*see also* Hernia, by site, with obstruction)
    with gangrene — *see* Hernia, by site, with
        gangrene
  iris, in wound — *see* Injury, eye, laceration, with
      prolapse
  lens, in wound — *see* Injury, eye, laceration, with
      prolapse
  omphalocele K42.0
  prison, anxiety concerning Z65.1
  rupture — *see* Hernia, by site
  sarcoepiplocele K46.0
    gangrenous K46.1
  sarcoepiplomphalocele K42.0
    with gangrene K42.1
  uterus N85.8
    gravid O34.51 ☑
      causing obstructed labor O65.5
Incised wound
  external — *see* Laceration
  internal organs — *see* Injury, by site
Incision, incisional
  hernia K43.2
    with
      gangrene (and obstruction) K43.1
      obstruction K43.0
  surgical, complication — *see* Complications, surgical
      procedure

Incision — *continued*
  traumatic
    external — *see* Laceration
    internal organs — *see* Injury, by site
Inclusion
  azurophilic leukocytic D72.0
  blennorrhea (neonatal) (newborn) P39.1
  gallbladder in liver (congenital) Q44.1
Incompatibility
  ABO
    affecting management of pregnancy O36.11 ☑
      anti-A sensitization O36.11 ☑
      anti-B sensitization O36.19 ☑
      specified NEC O36.19 ☑
    infusion or transfusion reaction — *see*
        Complication(s), transfusion, incompatibility
        reaction, ABO
    newborn P55.1
  blood (group) (Duffy) (K) (Kell) (Kidd) (Lewis) (M)(s)
      NEC
    affecting management of pregnancy O36.11 ☑
      anti-A sensitization O36.11 ☑
      anti-B sensitization O36.19 ☑
    infusion or transfusion reaction T80.89 ☑
    newborn P55.8
  divorce or estrangement Z63.5
  Rh (blood group) (factor) Z31.82
    affecting management of pregnancy NEC
        O36.09 ☑
      anti-D antibody O36.01 ☑
    infusion or transfusion reaction — *see*
        Complication(s), transfusion, incompatibility
        reaction, Rh (factor)
    newborn P55.0
  rhesus — *see* Incompatibility, Rh
Incompetency, incompetent, incompetence
  annular
    aortic (valve) — *see* Insufficiency, aortic
    mitral (valve) I34.0
    pulmonary valve (heart) I37.1
  aortic (valve) — *see* Insufficiency, aortic
  cardiac valve — *see* Endocarditis
  cervix, cervical (os) N88.3
    in pregnancy O34.3 ☑
  chronotropic I45.89
    with
      autonomic dysfunction G90.8
      ischemic heart disease I25.89
      left ventricular dysfunction I51.89
      sinus node dysfunction I49.8
  esophagogastric (junction) (sphincter) K22.0
  mitral (valve) — *see* Insufficiency, mitral
  pelvic fundus N81.89
  pubocervical tissue N81.82
  pulmonary valve (heart) I37.1
    congenital Q22.3
  rectovaginal tissue N81.83
  tricuspid (annular) (valve) — *see* Insufficiency,
      tricuspid
  valvular — *see* Endocarditis
    congenital Q24.8
  vein, venous (saphenous) (varicose) — *see* Varix, leg
Incomplete (*see also* condition)
  bladder, emptying R33.9
  defecation R15.0
  expansion lungs (newborn) NEC — *see* Atelectasis
  rotation, intestine Q43.3
Inconclusive
  diagnostic imaging due to excess body fat of
      patient R93.9
  findings on diagnostic imaging of breast NEC R92.8
  mammogram (due to dense breasts) R92.2
Incontinence R32
  anal sphincter R15.9
  coital N39.491
  feces R15.9
    nonorganic origin F98.1
  insensible (urinary) N39.42
  overflow N39.490
  postural (urinary) N39.492
  psychogenic F45.8
  rectal R15.9
  reflex N39.498
  stress (female) (male) N39.3
    and urge N39.46
  urethral sphincter R32
  urge N39.41
    and stress (female) (male) N39.46
  urine (urinary) R32
    continuous N39.45
    due to cognitive impairment, or severe physical
        disability or immobility R39.81

Incontinence — *continued*
  urine — *continued*
    functional R39.81
    insensible N39.42
    mixed (stress and urge) N39.46
    nocturnal N39.44
    nonorganic origin F98.0
    overflow N39.490
    post dribbling N39.43
    postural N39.492
    reflex N39.498
    specified NEC N39.498
    stress (female) (male) N39.3
      and urge N39.46
    total N39.498
    unaware N39.42
    urge N39.41
      and stress (female) (male) N39.46
Incontinentia pigmenti Q82.3
Incoordinate, incoordination
  esophageal-pharyngeal (newborn) — *see*
      Dysphagia
  muscular R27.8
  uterus (action) (contractions) (complicating
      delivery) O62.4
Increase, increased
  abnormal, in development R63.8
  androgens (ovarian) E28.1
  anticoagulants (antithrombin) (anti-VIIIa)
      (anti-IXa) (anti-Xa) (anti-XIa) — *see* Circulating
      anticoagulants
  cold sense R20.8
  estrogen E28.0
  function
    adrenal
      cortex — *see* Cushing's, syndrome
      medulla E27.5
    pituitary (gland) (anterior) (lobe) E22.9
      posterior E22.2
  heat sense R20.8
  intracranial pressure (benign) G93.2
  permeability, capillaries I78.8
  pressure, intracranial G93.2
  secretion
    gastrin E16.4
    glucagon E16.3
    pancreas, endocrine E16.9
      growth hormone-releasing hormone E16.8
      pancreatic polypeptide E16.8
      somatostatin E16.8
      vasoactive-intestinal polypeptide E16.8
  sphericity, lens Q12.4
  splenic activity D73.1
  venous pressure I87.8
    portal K76.6
Increta placenta O43.22 ☑
Incrustation, cornea, foreign body (lead)(zinc) — *see*
    Foreign body, cornea
Incyclophoria H50.54
Incyclotropia — *see* Cyclotropia
Indeterminate sex Q56.4
India rubber skin Q82.8
Indigestion (acid) (bilious) (functional) K30
  catarrhal K31.89
  due to decomposed food NOS A05.9
  nervous F45.8
  psychogenic F45.8
Indirect — *see* condition
Induratio penis plastica N48.6
Induration, indurated
  brain G93.89
  breast (fibrous) N64.51
    puerperal, postpartum O92.29
  broad ligament N83.8
  chancre
    anus A51.1
    congenital A50.07
    extragenital NEC A51.2
  corpora cavernosa (penis) (plastic) N48.6
  liver (chronic) K76.89
  lung (black) (chronic) (fibroid) (*see also* Fibrosis,
      lung) J84.10
    essential brown J84.03
  penile (plastic) N48.6
  phlebitic — *see* Phlebitis
  skin R23.4
Inebriety (without dependence) — *see* Alcohol,
    intoxication
Inefficiency, kidney N28.9
Inelasticity, skin R23.4
Inequality, leg (length) (acquired) (*see also* Deformity,
    limb, unequal length)

☑ **Additional character required**

Inequality — continued
  congenital — see Defect, reduction, lower limb
  lower leg — see Deformity, limb, unequal length
Inertia
  bladder (neurogenic) N31.2
  stomach K31.89
    psychogenic F45.8
  uterus, uterine during labor O62.2
    during latent phase of labor O62.0
    primary O62.0
    secondary O62.1
  vesical (neurogenic) N31.2
Infancy, infantile, infantilism (see also condition)
  celiac K90.0
  genitalia, genitals (after puberty) E30.0
  Herter's (nontropical sprue) K90.0
  intestinal K90.0
  Lorain E23.0
  pancreatic K86.89
  pelvis M95.5
    with disproportion (fetopelvic) O33.1
      causing obstructed labor O65.1
  pituitary E23.0
  renal N25.0
  uterus — see Infantile, genitalia
Infant(s) (see also Infancy)
  excessive crying R68.11
  irritable child R68.12
  lack of care — see Neglect
  liveborn (singleton) Z38.2
    born in hospital Z38.00
      by cesarean Z38.01
    born outside hospital Z38.1
    multiple NEC Z38.8
      born in hospital Z38.68
        by cesarean Z38.69
      born outside hospital Z38.7
    quadruplet Z38.8
      born in hospital Z38.63
        by cesarean Z38.64
      born outside hospital Z38.7
    quintuplet Z38.8
      born in hospital Z38.65
        by cesarean Z38.66
      born outside hospital Z38.7
    triplet Z38.8
      born in hospital Z38.61
        by cesarean Z38.62
      born outside hospital Z38.7
    twin Z38.5
      born in hospital Z38.30
        by cesarean Z38.31
      born outside hospital Z38.4
  of diabetic mother (syndrome of) P70.1
    gestational diabetes P70.0
Infantile (see also condition)
  genitalia, genitals E30.0
  os, uterine E30.0
  penis E30.0
  testis E29.1
  uterus E30.0
Infantilism — see Infancy
Infarct, infarction
  adrenal (capsule) (gland) E27.49
  appendices epiploicae (see also Infarct, intestine) K55.069
  bowel (see also Infarct, intestine) K55.069
  brain (stem) — see Infarct, cerebral
  breast N64.89
  brewer's (kidney) N28.0
  cardiac — see Infarct, myocardium
  cerebellar — see Infarct, cerebral
  cerebral (acute) (chronic) (see also Occlusion, artery cerebral or precerebral, with infarction) I63.9
    aborted I63.9
    cortical I63.9
    due to
      cerebral venous thrombosis, nonpyogenic I63.6
      embolism
        cerebral arteries I63.4 ☑
        precerebral arteries I63.1 ☑
      occlusion NEC
        cerebral arteries I63.5 ☑
        precerebral arteries I63.2 ☑
        small artery I63.81
      stenosis NEC
        cerebral arteries I63.5 ☑
        precerebral arteries I63.2 ☑
        small artery I63.81
      thrombosis
        cerebral artery I63.3 ☑
        precerebral artery I63.0 ☑

Infarct — continued
  cerebral — continued
    intraoperative
      during cardiac surgery I97.810
      during other surgery I97.811
    postprocedural
      following cardiac surgery I97.820
      following other surgery I97.821
    specified NEC I63.89
  colon (acute) (agnogenic) (embolic) (hemorrhagic) (nonocclusive) (nonthrombotic) (occlusive) (segmental) (thrombotic) (with gangrene) (see also Infarct, intestine) K55.049
  coronary artery — see Infarct, myocardium
  embolic — see Embolism
  fallopian tube N83.8
  gallbladder K82.8
  heart — see Infarct, myocardium
  hepatic K76.3
  hypophysis (anterior lobe) E23.6
  impending (myocardium) I20.0
  intestine (acute) (agnogenic) (embolic) (hemorrhagic) (nonocclusive) (nonthrombotic) (occlusive) (thrombotic) (with gangrene) K55.069
    diffuse K55.062
    focal K55.061
    large K55.049
      diffuse K55.042
      focal K55.041
    small K55.029
      diffuse K55.022
      focal K55.021
  kidney N28.0
  lacunar I63.81
  liver K76.3
  lung (embolic) (thrombotic) — see Embolism, pulmonary
  lymph node I89.8
  mesentery, mesenteric (embolic) (thrombotic) (with gangrene) (see also Infarct, intestine) K55.069
  muscle (ischemic) M62.20
    ankle M62.27 ☑
    foot M62.27 ☑
    forearm M62.23 ☑
    hand M62.24 ☑
    lower leg M62.26 ☑
    pelvic region M62.25 ☑
    shoulder region M62.21 ☑
    specified site NEC M62.28
    thigh M62.25 ☑
    upper arm M62.22 ☑
  myocardium, myocardial (acute) (with stated duration of 4 weeks or less) I21.9
    associated with revascularization procedure I21.A9
    diagnosed on ECG, but presenting no symptoms I25.2
    due to
      demand ischemia I21.A1
      ischemic imbalance I21.A1
    healed or old I25.2
    intraoperative (see also Infarct, myocardium, associated with revascularization procedure)
      during cardiac surgery I97.790
      during other surgery I97.791
    non-Q wave I21.4
    non-ST elevation (NSTEMI) I21.4
      subsequent I22.2
    nontransmural I21.4
    past (diagnosed on ECG or other investigation, but currently presenting no symptoms) I25.2
    postprocedural (see also Infarct, myocardium, associated with revascularization procedure)
      following cardiac surgery (see also Infarct, myocardium, type 4 or type 5) I97.190
      following other surgery I97.191
    Q wave (see also, Infarct, myocardium, by site) I21.3
    secondary to
      demand ischemia I21.A1
      ischemic imbalance I21.A1
    ST elevation (STEMI) I21.3
      anterior (anteroapical) (anterolateral) (anteroseptal) (Q wave) (wall) I21.09
        subsequent I22.0
      inferior (diaphragmatic) (inferolateral) (inferoposterior) (wall) NEC I21.19
        subsequent I22.1
      inferoposterior transmural (Q wave) I21.11
    involving

Infarct — continued
  myocardium — continued
    coronary artery of anterior wall NEC I21.09
    coronary artery of inferior wall NEC I21.19
    diagonal coronary artery I21.02
    left anterior descending coronary artery I21.02
    left circumflex coronary artery I21.21
    left main coronary artery I21.01
    oblique marginal coronary artery I21.21
    right coronary artery I21.11
    lateral (apical-lateral) (basal-lateral) (high) I21.29
      subsequent I22.8
    posterior (posterobasal) (posterolateral) (posteroseptal) (true) I21.29
      subsequent I22.8
    septal I21.29
      subsequent I22.8
    specified NEC I21.29
      subsequent I22.8
    subsequent I22.9
    subsequent (recurrent) (reinfarction) I22.9
      anterior (anteroapical) (anterolateral) (anteroseptal) (wall) I22.0
      diaphragmatic (wall) I22.1
      inferior (diaphragmatic) (inferolateral) (inferoposterior) (wall) I22.1
      lateral (apical-lateral) (basal-lateral) (high) I22.8
      non-ST elevation (NSTEMI) I22.2
      posterior (posterobasal) (posterolateral) (posteroseptal) (true) I22.8
      septal I22.8
      specified NEC I22.8
      ST elevation I22.9
        anterior (anteroapical) (anterolateral) (anteroseptal) (wall) I22.0
        inferior (diaphragmatic) (inferolateral) (inferoposterior) (wall) I22.1
        specified NEC I22.8
      subendocardial I22.2
      transmural I22.9
        anterior (anteroapical) (anterolateral) (anteroseptal) (wall) I22.0
        diaphragmatic (wall) I22.1
        inferior (diaphragmatic) (inferolateral) (inferoposterior) (wall) I22.1
        lateral (apical-lateral) (basal-lateral) (high) I22.8
        posterior (posterobasal) (posterolateral) (posteroseptal) (true) I22.8
        specified NEC I22.8
    type 1 (see also Infarction, myocardial, subsequent, by site, or by ST elevation or non-ST elevation) I22.9
    type 2 I21.A1
    type 3 I21.A9
    type 4 I21.A9
    type 5 I21.A9
    syphilitic A52.06
    transmural I21.9
      anterior (anteroapical) (anterolateral) (anteroseptal) (Q wave) (wall) NEC I21.09
      inferior (diaphragmatic) (inferolateral) (inferoposterior) (Q wave) (wall) NEC I21.19
      inferoposterior (Q wave) I21.11
      lateral (apical-lateral) (basal-lateral) (high) NEC I21.29
      posterior (posterobasal) (posterolateral) (posteroseptal) (true) NEC I21.29
      septal NEC I21.29
      specified NEC I21.29
    type 1 (see also Infarction, myocardial, by site, or by ST elevation or non-ST elevation) I21.9
    type 2 I21.A1
    type 3 I21.A9
    type 4 (a) (b) (c) I21.A9
    type 5 I21.A9
  nontransmural I21.4
  omentum (see also Infarct, intestine) K55.069
  ovary N83.8
  pancreas K86.89
  papillary muscle — see Infarct, myocardium
  parathyroid gland E21.4
  pituitary (gland) E23.6
  placenta O43.81 ☑
  prostate N42.89
  pulmonary (artery) (vein) (hemorrhagic) — see Embolism, pulmonary
  renal (embolic) (thrombotic) N28.0
  retina, retinal (artery) — see Occlusion, artery, retina
  spinal (cord) (acute) (embolic) (nonembolic) G95.11

Infarct - Infection

Infarct — *continued*
  spleen D73.5
    embolic or thrombotic I74.8
  subendocardial (acute) (nontransmural) I21.4
  suprarenal (capsule) (gland) E27.49
  testis N50.1
  thrombotic (*see also* Thrombosis)
    artery, arterial — *see* Embolism
  thyroid (gland) E07.89
  ventricle (heart) — *see* Infarct, myocardium
Infecting — *see* condition
Infection, infected, infective (opportunistic) B99.9
  with
    drug resistant organism — *see* Resistance (to),
      drug (*see also* specific organism)
    lymphangitis — *see* Lymphangitis
    organ dysfunction (acute) R65.20
      with septic shock R65.21
  abscess (skin) - code by site under Abscess
  Absidia — *see* Mucormycosis
  Acanthamoeba — *see* Acanthamebiasis
  Acanthocheilonema (perstans) (streptocerca) B74.4
  accessory sinus (chronic) — *see* Sinusitis
  achorion — *see* Dermatophytosis
  Acremonium falciforme B47.0
  acromioclavicular M00.9
  Actinobacillus (actinomycetem-comitans) A28.8
    mallei A24.0
    muris A25.1
  Actinomadura B47.1
  Actinomyces (israelii) (*see also* Actinomycosis) A42.9
  Actinomycetales — *see* Actinomycosis
  actinomycotic NOS — *see* Actinomycosis
  adenoid (and tonsil) J03.90
    chronic J35.02
  adenovirus NEC
    as cause of disease classified elsewhere B97.0
    unspecified nature or site B34.0
  aerogenes capsulatus A48.0
  aertrycke — *see* Infection, salmonella
  alimentary canal NOS — *see* Enteritis, infectious
  Allescheria boydii B48.2
  Alternaria B48.8
  alveolus, alveolar (process) K04.7
  Ameba, amebic (histolytica) — *see* Amebiasis
  amniotic fluid, sac or cavity O41.10 ☑
    chorioamnionitis O41.12 ☑
    placentitis O41.14 ☑
  amputation stump (surgical) — *see* Complication,
    amputation stump, infection
  Ancylostoma (duodenalis) B76.0
  Anisakiasis, Anisakis larvae B81.0
  anthrax — *see* Anthrax
  antrum (chronic) — *see* Sinusitis, maxillary
  anus, anal (papillae) (sphincter) K62.89
  arbovirus (arbor virus) A94
    specified type NEC A93.8
  artificial insemination N98.0
  Ascaris lumbricoides — *see* Ascariasis
  Ascomycetes B47.0
  Aspergillus (flavus) (fumigatus) (terreus) — *see*
    Aspergillosis
  atypical
    acid-fast (bacilli) — *see* Mycobacterium, atypical
    mycobacteria — *see* Mycobacterium, atypical
    virus A81.9
      specified type NEC A81.89
  auditory meatus (external) — *see* Otitis, externa,
    infective
  auricle (ear) — *see* Otitis, externa, infective
  axillary gland (lymph) L04.2
  Bacillus A49.9
    abortus A23.1
    anthracis — *see* Anthrax
    Ducrey's (any location) A57
    Flexner's A03.1
    Friedländer's NEC A49.8
    gas (gangrene) A48.0
    mallei A24.0
    melitensis A23.0
    paratyphoid, paratyphosus A01.4
      A A01.1
      B A01.2
      C A01.3
    Shiga (-Kruse) A03.0
    suipestifer — *see* Infection, salmonella
    swimming pool A31.1
    typhosa A01.00
    welchii — *see* Gangrene, gas
  bacterial NOS A49.9
    as cause of disease classified elsewhere B96.89
      Clostridium perfringens [C. perfringens] B96.7

Infection — *continued*
  bacterial NOS — *continued*
    Bacteroides fragilis [B. fragilis] B96.6
    Enterobacter sakazakii B96.89
    Enterococcus B95.2
    Escherichia coli [E. coli] (*see also* Escherichia
      coli) B96.20
    Helicobacter pylori [H. pylori] B96.81
    Hemophilus influenzae [H. influenzae] B96.3
    Klebsiella pneumoniae [K. pneumoniae] B96.1
    Mycoplasma pneumoniae [M. pneumoniae]
      B96.0
    Proteus (mirabilis) (morganii) B96.4
    Pseudomonas (aeruginosa) (mallei)
      (pseudomallei) B96.5
    Staphylococcus B95.8
      aureus (methicillin susceptible) (MSSA)
        B95.61
      methicillin resistant (MRSA) B95.62
      specified NEC B95.7
    Streptococcus B95.5
      group A B95.0
      group B B95.1
      pneumoniae B95.3
      specified NEC B95.4
    Vibrio vulnificus B96.82
    specified NEC A48.8
  Bacterium
    paratyphosum A01.4
      A A01.1
      B A01.2
      C A01.3
    typhosum A01.00
  Bacteroides NEC A49.8
    fragilis, as cause of disease classified elsewhere
      B96.6
  Balantidium coli A07.0
  Bartholin's gland N75.8
  Basidiobolus B46.8
  bile duct (common) (hepatic) — *see* Cholangitis
  bladder — *see* Cystitis
  Blastomyces, blastomycotic (*see also* Blastomycosis)
    brasiliensis — *see* Paracoccidioidomycosis
    dermatitidis — *see* Blastomycosis
    European — *see* Cryptococcosis
    Loboi B48.0
    North American B40.9
    South American — *see* Paracoccidioidomycosis
  bleb, postprocedure — *see* Blebitis
  bone — *see* Osteomyelitis
  Bordetella — *see* Whooping cough
  Borrelia bergdorfi A69.20
  brain (*see also* Encephalitis) G04.90
    membranes — *see* Meningitis
    septic G06.0
      meninges — *see* Meningitis, bacterial
  branchial cyst Q18.0
  breast — *see* Mastitis
  bronchus — *see* Bronchitis
  Brucella A23.9
    abortus A23.1
    canis A23.3
    melitensis A23.0
    mixed A23.8
    specified NEC A23.8
    suis A23.2
  Brugia (malayi) B74.1
    timori B74.2
  bursa — *see* Bursitis, infective
  buttocks (skin) L08.9
  Campylobacter, intestinal A04.5
    as cause of disease classified elsewhere B96.81
  Candida (albicans) (tropicalis) — *see* Candidiasis
  candiru B88.8
  Capillaria (intestinal) B81.1
    hepatica B83.8
    philippinensis B81.1
  cartilage — *see* Disorder, cartilage, specified type
    NEC
  catheter-related bloodstream (CRBSI) T80.211 ☑
  cat liver fluke B66.0
  cellulitis - code by site under Cellulitis
  central line-associated T80.219 ☑
    bloodstream (CLABSI) T80.211 ☑
    specified NEC T80.218 ☑
  Cephalosporium falciforme B47.0
  cerebrospinal — *see* Meningitis
  cervical gland (lymph) L04.0
  cervix — *see* Cervicitis
  cesarean delivery wound (puerperal) O86.00
  cestodes — *see* Infestation, cestodes
  chest J22

Infection — *continued*
  Chilomastix (intestinal) A07.8
  Chlamydia, chlamydial A74.9
    anus A56.3
    genitourinary tract A56.2
      lower A56.00
      specified NEC A56.19
    lymphogranuloma A55
    pharynx A56.4
    psittaci A70
    rectum A56.3
    sexually transmitted NEC A56.8
  cholera — *see* Cholera
  Cladosporium
    bantianum (brain abscess) B43.1
    carrionii B43.0
    castellanii B36.1
    trichoides (brain abscess) B43.1
    werneckii B36.1
  Clonorchis (sinensis) (liver) B66.1
  Clostridium NEC
    bifermentans A48.0
    botulinum (food poisoning) A05.1
      infant A48.51
      wound A48.52
    difficile
      as cause of disease classified elsewhere B96.89
      foodborne (disease)
        not specified as recurrent A04.72
        recurrent A04.71
      gas gangrene A48.0
      necrotizing enterocolitis
        not specified as recurrent A04.72
        recurrent A04.71
      sepsis A41.4
    gas-forming NEC A48.0
    histolyticum A48.0
    novyi, causing gas gangrene A48.0
    oedematiens A48.0
    perfringens
      as cause of disease classified elsewhere B96.7
      due to food A05.2
      foodborne (disease) A05.2
      gas gangrene A48.0
      sepsis A41.4
    septicum, causing gas gangrene A48.0
    sordellii, causing gas gangrene A48.0
    welchii
      as cause of disease classified elsewhere B96.7
      foodborne (disease) A05.2
      gas gangrene A48.0
      necrotizing enteritis A05.2
      sepsis A41.4
  Coccidioides (immitis) — *see* Coccidioidomycosis
  colon — *see* Enteritis, infectious
  colostomy K94.02
  common duct — *see* Cholangitis
  congenital P39.9
    Candida (albicans) P37.5
    cytomegalovirus P35.1
    hepatitis, viral P35.3
    herpes simplex P35.2
    infectious or parasitic disease P37.9
      specified NEC P37.8
    listeriosis (disseminated) P37.2
    malaria NEC P37.4
      falciparum P37.3
    Plasmodium falciparum P37.3
    poliomyelitis P35.8
    rubella P35.0
    skin P39.4
    toxoplasmosis (acute) (subacute) (chronic) P37.1
    tuberculosis P37.0
    urinary (tract) P39.3
    vaccinia P35.8
    virus P35.9
      specified type NEC P35.8
  Conidiobolus B46.8
  coronavirus NEC B34.2
    as cause of disease classified elsewhere B97.29
    severe acute respiratory syndrome (SARS
      associated) B97.21
  corpus luteum — *see* Salpingo-oophoritis
  Corynebacterium diphtheriae — *see* Diphtheria
  cotia virus B08.8
  Coxiella burnetii A78
  coxsackie — *see* Coxsackie
  Cryptococcus neoformans — *see* Cryptococcosis
  Cryptosporidium A07.2
  Cunninghamella — *see* Mucormycosis
  cyst — *see* Cyst
  cystic duct (*see also* Cholecystitis) K81.9

☑ **Additional character required**

Infection — *continued*
Cysticercus cellulosae — *see* Cysticercosis
cytomegalovirus, cytomegaloviral B25.9
  congenital P35.1
  maternal, maternal care for (suspected) damage
    to fetus O35.3 ☑
  mononucleosis B27.10
    with
      complication NEC B27.19
      meningitis B27.12
      polyneuropathy B27.11
delta-agent (acute), in hepatitis B carrier B17.0
dental (pulpal origin) K04.7
Deuteromycetes B47.0
Dicrocoelium dendriticum B66.2
Dipetalonema (perstans) (streptocerca) B74.4
diphtherial — *see* Diphtheria
Diphyllobothrium (adult) (latum) (pacificum) B70.0
  larval B70.1
Diplogonoporus (grandis) B71.8
Dipylidium caninum B67.4
Dirofilaria B74.8
Dracunculus medinensis B72
Drechslera (hawaiiensis) B43.8
Ducrey Haemophilus (any location) A57
due to or resulting from
  artificial insemination N98.0
  central venous catheter T80.219 ☑
    bloodstream T80.211 ☑
    exit or insertion site T80.212 ☑
    localized T80.212 ☑
    port or reservoir T80.212 ☑
    specified NEC T80.218 ☑
    tunnel T80.212 ☑
  device, implant or graft (*see also* Complications,
    by site and type, infection or inflammation)
    T85.79 ☑
    arterial graft NEC T82.7 ☑
    breast (implant) T85.79 ☑
    catheter NEC T85.79 ☑
      dialysis (renal) T82.7 ☑
        intraperitoneal T85.71 ☑
      infusion NEC T82.7 ☑
        cranial T85.735 ☑
        intrathecal T85.735 ☑
        spinal (epidural) (subdural) T85.735 ☑
        subarachnoid T85.735 ☑
      urinary T83.518 ☑
        cystostomy T83.510 ☑
        Hopkins T83.518 ☑
        ileostomy T83.518 ☑
        nephrostomy T83.512 ☑
        specified NEC T83.518 ☑
        urethral indwelling T83.511 ☑
        urostomy T83.518 ☑
    electronic (electrode) (pulse generator)
      (stimulator)
    bone T84.7 ☑
    cardiac T82.7 ☑
    nervous system T85.738 ☑
      brain T85.731 ☑
      cranial nerve T85.732 ☑
      gastric nerve T85.732 ☑
      generator pocket T85.734 ☑
      neurostimulator generator T85.734 ☑
      peripheral nerve T85.732 ☑
      sacral nerve T85.732 ☑
      spinal cord T85.733 ☑
      vagal nerve T85.732 ☑
    urinary T83.590 ☑
  fixation, internal (orthopedic) NEC — *see*
    Complication, fixation device, infection
  gastrointestinal (bile duct) (esophagus)
    T85.79 ☑
  neurostimulator electrode (lead) T85.732 ☑
  genital NEC T83.69 ☑
  heart NEC T82.7 ☑
    valve (prosthesis) T82.6 ☑
      graft T82.7 ☑
  joint prosthesis — *see* Complication, joint
    prosthesis, infection
  ocular (corneal graft) (orbital implant) NEC
    T85.79 ☑
  orthopedic NEC T84.7 ☑
  penile (cylinder) (pump) (reservoir) T83.61 ☑
  specified NEC T85.79 ☑
  testicular T83.62 ☑
  urinary NEC T83.598 ☑
    ileal conduit stent T83.593 ☑
    implanted neurostimulation T83.590 ☑
    implanted sphincter T83.591 ☑
    indwelling ureteral stent T83.592 ☑

Infection — *continued*
due to or resulting from — *continued*
    nephroureteral stent T83.593 ☑
    specified stent NEC T83.593 ☑
  vascular NEC T82.7 ☑
  ventricular intracranial (communicating) shunt
    T85.730 ☑
  Hickman catheter T80.219 ☑
    bloodstream T80.211 ☑
    localized T80.212 ☑
    specified NEC T80.218 ☑
  immunization or vaccination T88.0 ☑
  infusion, injection or transfusion NEC T80.29 ☑
    acute T80.22 ☑
  injury NEC - code by site under Wound, open
  peripherally inserted central catheter (PICC)
    T80.219 ☑
    bloodstream T80.211 ☑
    localized T80.212 ☑
    specified NEC T80.218 ☑
  portacath (port-a-cath) T80.219 ☑
    bloodstream T80.211 ☑
    localized T80.212 ☑
    specified NEC T80.218 ☑
  pulmonary artery catheter — *see* Infection, due to
    or resulting from, central venous catheter
  surgery T81.40 ☑
  Swan Ganz catheter — *see* Infection, due to or
    resulting from, central venous catheter
  triple lumen catheter T80.219 ☑
    bloodstream T80.211 ☑
    localized T80.212 ☑
    specified NEC T80.218 ☑
  umbilical venous catheter T80.219 ☑
    bloodstream T80.211 ☑
    localized T80.212 ☑
    specified NEC T80.218 ☑
during labor NEC O75.3
ear (middle) (*see also* Otitis media)
  external — *see* Otitis, externa, infective
  inner — *see* subcategory H83.0 ☑
Eberthella typhosa A01.00
Echinococcus — *see* Echinococcus
echovirus
  as cause of disease classified elsewhere B97.12
  unspecified nature or site B34.1
endocardium I33.0
endocervix — *see* Cervicitis
Entamoeba — *see* Amebiasis
enteric — *see* Enteritis, infectious
Enterobacter sakazakii B96.89
Enterobius vermicularis B80
enterostomy K94.12
enterovirus B34.1
  as cause of disease classified elsewhere B97.10
    coxsackievirus B97.11
    echovirus B97.12
    specified NEC B97.19
Entomophthora B46.8
Epidermophyton — *see* Dermatophytosis
epididymis — *see* Epididymitis
episiotomy (puerperal) O86.09
Erysipelothrix (insidiosa) (rhusiopathiae) — *see*
  Erysipeloid
erythema infectiosum B08.3
Escherichia (E.) coli NEC A49.8
  as cause of disease classified elsewhere (*see also*
    Escherichia coli) B96.20
  congenital P39.8
    sepsis P36.4
  generalized A41.51
  intestinal — *see* Enteritis, infectious, due to,
    Escherichia coli
ethmoidal (chronic) (sinus) — *see* Sinusitis,
  ethmoidal
eustachian tube (ear) — *see* Salpingitis,
  eustachian
external auditory canal (meatus) NEC — *see* Otitis,
  externa, infective
eye (purulent) — *see* Endophthalmitis, purulent
eyelid — *see* Inflammation, eyelid
fallopian tube — *see* Salpingo-oophoritis
Fasciola (gigantica) (hepatica) (indica) B66.3
Fasciolopsis (buski) B66.5
filarial — *see* Infestation, filarial
finger (skin) L08.9
  nail L03.01
    fungus B35.1
fish tapeworm B70.0
  larval B70.1
flagellate, intestinal A07.9
fluke — *see* Infestation, fluke

Infection — *continued*
focal
  teeth (pulpal origin) K04.7
  tonsils J35.01
Fonsecaea (compactum) (pedrosoi) B43.0
food — *see* Intoxication, foodborne
foot (skin) L08.9
  dermatophytic fungus B35.3
Francisella tularensis — *see* Tularemia
frontal (sinus) (chronic) — *see* Sinusitis, frontal
fungus NOS B49
  beard B35.0
  dermatophytic — *see* Dermatophytosis
  foot B35.3
  groin B35.6
  hand B35.2
  nail B35.1
  pathogenic to compromised host only B48.8
  perianal (area) B35.6
  scalp B35.0
  skin B36.9
    foot B35.3
    hand B35.2
  toenails B35.1
Fusarium B48.8
gallbladder — *see* Cholecystitis
gas bacillus — *see* Gangrene, gas
gastrointestinal — *see* Enteritis, infectious
generalized NEC — *see* Sepsis
generator pocket, implanted electronic
  neurostimulator T85.734 ☑
genital organ or tract
  female — *see* Disease, pelvis, inflammatory
  male N49.9
    multiple sites N49.8
    specified NEC N49.8
Ghon tubercle, primary A15.7
Giardia lamblia A07.1
gingiva (chronic) K05.10
  acute K05.00
    nonplaque induced K05.01
    plaque induced K05.00
  nonplaque induced K05.11
  plaque induced K05.10
glanders A24.0
glenosporopsis B48.0
Gnathostoma (spinigerum) B83.1
Gongylonema B83.8
gonococcal — *see* Gonococcus
gram-negative bacilli NOS A49.9
guinea worm B72
gum (chronic) K05.10
  acute K05.00
    nonplaque induced K05.01
    plaque induced K05.00
  nonplaque induced K05.11
  plaque induced K05.10
Haemophilus — *see* Infection, Hemophilus
heart — *see* Carditis
Helicobacter pylori A04.8
  as cause of disease classified elsewhere B96.81
helminths B83.9
  intestinal B82.0
    mixed (types classifiable to more than one of
      the titles B65.0-B81.3 and B81.8) B81.4
    specified type NEC B81.8
  specified type NEC B83.8
Hemophilus
  aegyptius, systemic A48.4
  ducrey (any location) A57
  influenzae NEC A49.2
    as cause of disease classified elsewhere B96.3
    generalized A41.3
herpes (simplex) (*see also* Herpes)
  congenital P35.2
  disseminated B00.7
  zoster B02.9
herpesvirus, herpesviral — *see* Herpes
hip (joint) NEC M00.9
  due to internal joint prosthesis
    left T84.52 ☑
    right T84.51 ☑
  skin NEC L08.9
Heterophyes (heterophyes) B66.8
Histoplasma — *see* Histoplasmosis
  American B39.4
  capsulatum B39.4
hookworm B76.9
human
  papilloma virus A63.0
  T-cell lymphotropic virus type-1 (HTLV-1) B33.3
hydrocele N43.0

Infection

Infection — *continued*
- Hymenolepis B71.0
- hypopharynx — *see* Pharyngitis
- inguinal (lymph) glands L04.1
  - due to soft chancre A57
- intervertebral disc, pyogenic M46.30
  - cervical region M46.32
  - cervicothoracic region M46.33
  - lumbar region M46.36
  - lumbosacral region M46.37
  - multiple sites M46.39
  - occipito-atlanto-axial region M46.31
  - sacrococcygeal region M46.38
  - thoracic region M46.34
  - thoracolumbar region M46.35
- intestine, intestinal — *see* Enteritis, infectious
  - specified NEC A08.8
- intra-amniotic affecting newborn NEC P39.2
- Isospora belli or hominis A07.3
- Japanese B encephalitis A83.0
- jaw (bone) (lower) (upper) M27.2
- joint NEC M00.9
  - due to internal joint prosthesis T84.50 ☑
- kidney (cortex) (hematogenous) N15.9
  - with calculus N20.0
    - with hydronephrosis N13.6
  - following ectopic gestation O08.83
  - pelvis and ureter (cystic) N28.85
  - puerperal (postpartum) O86.21
  - specified NEC N15.8
- Klebsiella (K.) pneumoniae NEC A49.8
  - as cause of disease classified elsewhere B96.1
- knee (joint) NEC M00.9
  - joint M00.9
  - due to internal joint prosthesis
    - left T84.54 ☑
    - right T84.53 ☑
  - skin L08.9
- Koch's — *see* Tuberculosis
- labia (majora) (minora) (acute) — *see* Vulvitis
- lacrimal
  - gland — *see* Dacryoadenitis
  - passages (duct) (sac) — *see* Inflammation, lacrimal, passages
- lancet fluke B66.2
- larynx NEC J38.7
- leg (skin) NOS L08.9
- Legionella pneumophila A48.1
  - nonpneumonic A48.2
- Leishmania (*see also* Leishmaniasis)
  - aethiopica B55.1
  - braziliensis B55.2
  - chagasi B55.0
  - donovani B55.0
  - infantum B55.0
  - major B55.1
  - mexicana B55.1
  - tropica B55.1
- lentivirus, as cause of disease classified elsewhere B97.31
- Leptosphaeria senegalensis B47.0
- Leptospira interrogans A27.9
  - autumnalis A27.89
  - canicola A27.89
  - hebdomadis A27.89
  - icterohaemorrhagiae A27.0
  - pomona A27.89
  - specified type NEC A27.89
- leptospirochetal NEC — *see* Leptospirosis
- Listeria monocytogenes (*see also* Listeriosis)
  - congenital P37.2
- Loa loa B74.3
  - with conjunctival infestation B74.3
  - eyelid B74.3
- Loboa loboi B48.0
- local, skin (staphylococcal) (streptococcal) L08.9
  - abscess - code by site under Abscess
  - cellulitis - code by site under Cellulitis
  - specified NEC L08.89
  - ulcer — *see* Ulcer, skin
- Loefflerella mallei A24.0
- lung (*see also* Pneumonia) J18.9
  - atypical Mycobacterium A31.0
  - spirochetal A69.8
  - tuberculous — *see* Tuberculosis, pulmonary
  - virus — *see* Pneumonia, viral
- lymph gland (*see also* Lymphadenitis, acute)
  - mesenteric I88.0
- lymphoid tissue, base of tongue or posterior pharynx, NEC (chronic) J35.03
- Madurella (grisea) (mycetomii) B47.0

Infection — *continued*
- major
  - following ectopic or molar pregnancy O08.0
  - puerperal, postpartum, childbirth O85
- Malassezia furfur B36.0
- Malleomyces
  - mallei A24.0
  - pseudomallei (whitmori) — *see* Melioidosis
- mammary gland N61.0
- Mansonella (ozzardi) (perstans) (streptocerca) B74.4
- mastoid — *see* Mastoiditis
- maxilla, maxillary M27.2
  - sinus (chronic) — *see* Sinusitis, maxillary
- mediastinum J98.51
- Medina (worm) B72
- meibomian cyst or gland — *see* Hordeolum
- meninges — *see* Meningitis, bacterial
- meningococcal (*see also* condition) A39.9
  - adrenals A39.1
  - brain A39.81
  - cerebrospinal A39.0
  - conjunctiva A39.89
  - endocardium A39.51
  - heart A39.50
    - endocardium A39.51
    - myocardium A39.52
    - pericardium A39.53
  - joint A39.83
  - meninges A39.0
  - meningococcemia A39.4
    - acute A39.2
    - chronic A39.3
  - myocardium A39.52
  - pericardium A39.53
  - retrobulbar neuritis A39.82
  - specified site NEC A39.89
- mesenteric lymph nodes or glands NEC I88.0
- Metagonimus B66.8
- metatarsophalangeal M00.9
- methicillin
  - resistant Staphylococcus aureus (MRSA) A49.02
  - susceptible Staphylococcus aureus (MSSA) A49.01
- Microsporum, microsporic — *see* Dermatophytosis
- mixed flora (bacterial) NEC A49.8
- Monilia — *see* Candidiasis
- Monosporium apiospermum B48.2
- mouth, parasitic B37.0
- Mucor — *see* Mucormycosis
- muscle NEC — *see* Myositis, infective
- mycelium NOS B49
- mycetoma B47.9
  - actinomycotic NEC B47.1
  - mycotic NEC B47.0
- Mycobacterium, mycobacterial — *see* Mycobacterium
- Mycoplasma NEC A49.3
  - pneumoniae, as cause of disease classified elsewhere B96.0
- mycotic NOS B49
  - pathogenic to compromised host only B48.8
  - skin NOS B36.9
- myocardium NEC I40.0
- nail (chronic)
  - with lymphangitis — *see* Lymphangitis, acute, digit
  - finger L03.01 ☑
    - fungus B35.1
  - ingrowing L60.0
  - toe L03.03 ☑
    - fungus B35.1
- nasal sinus (chronic) — *see* Sinusitis
- nasopharynx — *see* Nasopharyngitis
- navel L08.82
- Necator americanus B76.1
- Neisseria — *see* Gonococcus
- Neotestudina rosatii B47.0
- newborn P39.9
  - intra-amniotic NEC P39.2
  - skin P39.4
  - specified type NEC P39.8
- nipple N61.0
  - associated with
    - lactation O91.03
    - pregnancy O91.01 ☑
    - puerperium O91.02
- Nocardia — *see* Nocardiosis
- obstetrical surgical wound (puerperal) O86.00
  - incisional site
    - deep O86.02
    - superficial O86.01
  - organ and space site O86.03
  - surgical site specified NEC O86.09

Infection — *continued*
- Oesophagostomum (apiostomum) B81.8
- Oestrus ovis — *see* Myiasis
- Oidium albicans B37.9
- Onchocerca (volvulus) — *see* Onchocerciasis
- oncovirus, as cause of disease classified elsewhere B97.32
- operation wound T81.49 ☑
- Opisthorchis (felineus) (viverrini) B66.0
- orbit, orbital — *see* Inflammation, orbit
- orthopoxvirus NEC B08.09
- ovary — *see* Salpingo-oophoritis
- Oxyuris vermicularis B80
- pancreas (acute) — *see* Pancreatitis, acute
  - abscess — *see* Pancreatitis, acute
  - specified NEC (*see also* Pancreatitis, acute) K85.80
- papillomavirus, as cause of disease classified elsewhere B97.7
- papovavirus NEC B34.4
- Paracoccidioides brasiliensis — *see* Paracoccidioidomycosis
- Paragonimus (westermani) B66.4
- parainfluenza virus B34.8
- parameningococcus NOS A39.9
- parapoxvirus B08.60
  - specified NEC B08.69
- parasitic B89
- Parastrongylus
  - cantonensis B83.2
  - costaricensis B81.3
- paratyphoid A01.4
  - Type A A01.1
  - Type B A01.2
  - Type C A01.3
- paraurethral ducts N34.2
- parotid gland — *see* Sialoadenitis
- parvovirus NEC B34.3
  - as cause of disease classified elsewhere B97.6
- Pasteurella NEC A28.9
  - multocida A28.0
  - pestis — *see* Plague
  - pseudotuberculosis A28.2
  - septica (cat bite) (dog bite) A28.0
  - tularensis — *see* Tularemia
- pelvic, female — *see* Disease, pelvis, inflammatory
- Penicillium (marneffei) B48.4
- penis (glans) (retention) NEC N48.29
- periapical K04.5
- peridental, periodontal K05.20
  - generalized — *see* Periodontitis, aggressive, generalized
  - localized — *see* Periodontitis, aggressive, localized
- perinatal period P39.9
  - specified type NEC P39.8
- perineal repair (puerperal) O86.09
- periorbital — *see* Inflammation, orbit
- perirectal K62.89
- perirenal — *see* Infection, kidney
- peritoneal — *see* Peritonitis
- periureteral N28.89
- Petriellidium boydii B48.2
- pharynx (*see also* Pharyngitis)
  - coxsackievirus B08.5
  - posterior, lymphoid (chronic) J35.03
- Phialophora
  - gougerotii (subcutaneous abscess or cyst) B43.2
  - jeanselmei (subcutaneous abscess or cyst) B43.2
  - verrucosa (skin) B43.0
- Piedraia hortae B36.3
- pinta A67.9
  - intermediate A67.1
  - late A67.2
  - mixed A67.3
  - primary A67.0
- pinworm B80
- pityrosporum furfur B36.0
- pleuro-pneumonia-like organism (PPLO) NEC A49.3
  - as cause of disease classified elsewhere B96.0
- pneumococcus, pneumococcal NEC A49.1
  - as cause of disease classified elsewhere B95.3
  - generalized (purulent) A40.3
    - with pneumonia J13
- Pneumocystis carinii (pneumonia) B59
- Pneumocystis jiroveci (pneumonia) B59
- port or reservoir T80.212 ☑
- postoperative T81.40 ☑
- postoperative wound T81.49 ☑
  - surgical site
    - deep incisional T81.42 ☑
    - organ and space T81.43 ☑
    - specified NEC T81.49 ☑
    - superficial incisional T81.41 ☑

☑ **Additional character required**

Infection — *continued*
  postprocedural T81.40 ☑
  postvaccinal T88.0 ☑
  prepuce NEC N47.7
    with penile inflammation N47.6
  prion — *see* Disease, prion, central nervous system
  prostate (capsule) — *see* Prostatitis
  Proteus (mirabilis) (morganii) (vulgaris) NEC A49.8
    as cause of disease classified elsewhere B96.4
  protozoal NEC B64
    intestinal A07.9
      specified NEC A07.8
    specified NEC B60.8
  Pseudoallescheria boydii B48.2
  Pseudomonas NEC A49.8
    as cause of disease classified elsewhere B96.5
    mallei A24.0
    pneumonia J15.1
    pseudomallei — *see* Melioidosis
  puerperal O86.4
    genitourinary tract NEC O86.89
    major or generalized O85
    minor O86.4
    specified NEC O86.89
  pulmonary — *see* Infection, lung
  purulent — *see* Abscess
  Pyrenochaeta romeroi B47.0
  Q fever A78
  rectum (sphincter) K62.89
  renal (*see also* Infection, kidney)
    pelvis and ureter (cystic) N28.85
  reovirus, as cause of disease classified elsewhere B97.5
  respiratory (tract) NEC J98.8
    acute J22
    chronic J98.8
    influenzal (upper) (acute) — *see* Influenza, with, respiratory manifestations NEC
    lower (acute) J22
      chronic — *see* Bronchitis, chronic
    rhinovirus J00
    syncytial virus (RSV) — *see* Infection, virus, respiratory syncytial (RSV)
    upper (acute) NOS J06.9
      chronic J39.8
      streptococcal J06.9
      viral NOS J06.9
        due to respiratory syncytial virus (RSV) J06.9 [B97.4]
  resulting from
    presence of internal prosthesis, implant, graft — *see* Complications, by site and type, infection
  retortamoniasis A07.8
  retroperitoneal NEC K68.9
  retrovirus B33.3
    as cause of disease classified elsewhere B97.30
      human
        immunodeficiency, type 2 (HIV 2) B97.35
        T-cell lymphotropic
          type I (HTLV-I) B97.33
          type II (HTLV-II) B97.34
      lentivirus B97.31
      oncovirus B97.32
      specified NEC B97.39
  Rhinosporidium (seeberi) B48.1
  rhinovirus
    as cause of disease classified elsewhere B97.89
    unspecified nature or site B34.8
  Rhizopus — *see* Mucormycosis
  rickettsial NOS A79.9
  roundworm (large) NEC B82.0
    Ascariasis (*see also* Ascariasis) B77.9
  rubella — *see* Rubella
  Saccharomyces — *see* Candidiasis
  salivary duct or gland (any) — *see* Sialoadenitis
  Salmonella (aertrycke) (arizonae) (callinarum) (cholerae-suis) (enteritidis) (suipestifer) (typhimurium) A02.9
    with
      (gastro)enteritis A02.0
      sepsis A02.1
      specified manifestation NEC A02.8
    due to food (poisoning) A02.9
    hirschfeldii A01.3
    localized A02.20
      arthritis A02.23
      meningitis A02.21
      osteomyelitis A02.24
      pneumonia A02.22
      pyelonephritis A02.25
      specified NEC A02.29
    paratyphi A01.4

Infection — *continued*
  Salmonella — *continued*
    A A01.1
    B A01.2
    C A01.3
    schottmuelleri A01.2
    typhi, typhosa — *see* Typhoid
  Sarcocystis A07.8
  scabies B86
  Schistosoma — *see* Infestation, Schistosoma
  scrotum (acute) NEC N49.2
  seminal vesicle — *see* Vesiculitis
  septic
    localized, skin — *see* Abscess
  sheep liver fluke B66.3
  Shigella A03.9
    boydii A03.2
    dysenteriae A03.0
    flexneri A03.1
    group
      A A03.0
      B A03.1
      C A03.2
      D A03.3
    Schmitz (-Stutzer) A03.0
    schmitzii A03.0
    shigae A03.0
    sonnei A03.3
    specified NEC A03.8
  shoulder (joint) NEC M00.9
    due to internal joint prosthesis T84.59 ☑
    skin NEC L08.9
  sinus (accessory) (chronic) (nasal) (*see also* Sinusitis)
    pilonidal — *see* Sinus, pilonidal
    skin NEC L08.89
  Skene's duct or gland — *see* Urethritis
  skin (local) (staphylococcal) (streptococcal) L08.9
    abscess - code by site under Abscess
    cellulitis - code by site under Cellulitis
    due to fungus B36.9
      specified type NEC B36.8
    mycotic B36.9
      specified type NEC B36.8
    newborn P39.4
    ulcer — *see* Ulcer, skin
  slow virus A81.9
    specified NEC A81.89
  Sparganum (mansoni) (proliferum) (baxteri) B70.1
  specific (*see also* Syphilis)
    to perinatal period — *see* Infection, congenital
  specified NEC B99.8
  spermatic cord NEC N49.1
  sphenoidal (sinus) — *see* Sinusitis, sphenoidal
  spinal cord NOS (*see also* Myelitis) G04.91
    abscess G06.1
    meninges — *see* Meningitis
    streptococcal G04.89
  Spirillum A25.0
  spirochetal NOS A69.9
    lung A69.8
    specified NEC A69.8
  Spirometra larvae B70.1
  spleen D73.89
  Sporotrichum, Sporothrix (schenckii) — *see* Sporotrichosis
  staphylococcal, unspecified site
    aureus (methicillin susceptible) (MSSA) A49.01
      methicillin resistant (MRSA) A49.02
    as cause of disease classified elsewhere B95.8
      aureus (methicillin susceptible) (MSSA) B95.61
        methicillin resistant (MRSA) B95.62
      specified NEC B95.7
    food poisoning A05.0
    generalized (purulent) A41.2
    pneumonia — *see* Pneumonia, staphylococcal
  Stellantchasmus falcatus B66.8
  streptobacillus moniliformis A25.1
  streptococcal NEC A49.1
    as cause of disease classified elsewhere B95.5
    B genitourinary complicating
      childbirth O98.82
      pregnancy O98.81 ☑
      puerperium O98.83
    congenital
      sepsis P36.10
        group B P36.0
        specified NEC P36.19
    generalized (purulent) A40.9
  Streptomyces B47.1
  Strongyloides (stercoralis) — *see* Strongyloidiasis
  stump (amputation) (surgical) — *see* Complication, amputation stump, infection

Infection — *continued*
  subcutaneous tissue, local L08.9
  suipestifer — *see* Infection, salmonella
  swimming pool bacillus A31.1
  Taenia — *see* Infestation, Taenia
  Taeniarhynchus saginatus B68.1
  tapeworm — *see* Infestation, tapeworm
  tendon (sheath) — *see* Tenosynovitis, infective NEC
  Ternidens diminutus B81.8
  testis — *see* Orchitis
  threadworm B80
  throat — *see* Pharyngitis
  thyroglossal duct K14.8
  toe (skin) L08.9
    cellulitis L03.03 ☑
      fungus B35.1
    nail L03.03 ☑
      fungus B35.1
  tongue NEC K14.0
    parasitic B37.0
  tonsil (and adenoid) (faucial) (lingual) (pharyngeal) — *see* Tonsillitis
  tooth, teeth K04.7
    periapical K04.7
    peridental, periodontal K05.20
      generalized — *see* Periodontitis, aggressive, generalized
      localized — *see* Periodontitis, aggressive, localized
    pulp K04.01
      irreversible K04.02
      reversible K04.01
    socket M27.3
  TORCH — *see* Infection, congenital
    without active infection P00.2
  Torula histolytica — *see* Cryptococcosis
  Toxocara (canis) (cati) (felis) B83.0
  Toxoplasma gondii — *see* Toxoplasma
  trachea, chronic J42
  trematode NEC — *see* Infestation, fluke
  trench fever A79.0
  Treponema pallidum — *see* Syphilis
  Trichinella (spiralis) B75
  Trichomonas A59.9
    cervix A59.09
    intestine A07.8
    prostate A59.02
    specified site NEC A59.8
    urethra A59.03
    urogenitalis A59.00
    vagina A59.01
    vulva A59.01
  Trichophyton, trichophytic — *see* Dermatophytosis
  Trichosporon (beigelii) cutaneum B36.2
  Trichostrongylus B81.2
  Trichuris (trichiura) B79
  Trombicula (irritans) B88.0
  Trypanosoma
    brucei
      gambiense B56.0
      rhodesiense B56.1
    cruzi — *see* Chagas' disease
  tubal — *see* Salpingo-oophoritis
  tuberculous
    latent (LTBI) Z22.7
    NEC — *see* Tuberculosis
  tubo-ovarian — *see* Salpingo-oophoritis
  tunnel T80.212 ☑
  tunica vaginalis N49.1
  tympanic membrane NEC — *see* Myringitis
  typhoid (abortive) (ambulant) (bacillus) — *see* Typhoid
  typhus A75.9
    flea-borne A75.2
    mite-borne A75.3
    recrudescent A75.1
    tick-borne A77.9
      African A77.1
      North Asian A77.2
  umbilicus L08.82
  ureter — *see* Ureteritis
  urethra — *see* Urethritis
  urinary (tract) N39.0
    bladder — *see* Cystitis
    complicating
      pregnancy O23.4 ☑
        specified type NEC O23.3 ☑
    kidney — *see* Infection, kidney
    newborn P39.3
    puerperal (postpartum) O86.20
    tuberculous A18.13
    urethra — *see* Urethritis

Infection - Infestation

Infection — *continued*
uterus, uterine — *see* Endometritis
vaccination T88.0 ☑
vaccinia not from vaccination B08.011
vagina (acute) — *see* Vaginitis
varicella B01.9
varicose veins — *see* Varix
vas deferens NEC N49.1
vesical — *see* Cystitis
Vibrio
  cholerae A00.0
    El Tor A00.1
  parahaemolyticus (food poisoning) A05.3
  vulnificus
    as cause of disease classified elsewhere B96.82
    foodborne intoxication A05.5
Vincent's (gum) (mouth) (tonsil) A69.1
virus, viral NOS B34.9
  adenovirus
    as cause of disease classified elsewhere B97.0
    unspecified nature or site B34.0
  arbovirus, arbovirus arthropod-borne A94
  as cause of disease classified elsewhere B97.89
    adenovirus B97.0
    coronavirus B97.29
      SARS-associated B97.21
    coxsackievirus B97.11
    echovirus B97.12
    enterovirus B97.10
      coxsackievirus B97.11
      echovirus B97.12
      specified NEC B97.19
    human
      immunodeficiency, type 2 (HIV 2) B97.35
      T-cell lymphotropic,
        type I (HTLV-I) B97.33
        type II (HTLV-II) B97.34
      metapneumovirus B97.81
    papillomavirus B97.7
    parvovirus B97.6
    reovirus B97.5
    respiratory syncytial (RSV) — *see* Infection,
      virus, respiratory syncytial (RSV)
    retrovirus B97.30
      human
        immunodeficiency, type 2 (HIV 2) B97.35
        T-cell lymphotropic,
          type I (HTLV-I) B97.33
          type II (HTLV-II) B97.34
      lentivirus B97.31
      oncovirus B97.32
      specified NEC B97.39
    specified NEC B97.89
  central nervous system A89
    atypical A81.9
      specified NEC A81.89
    enterovirus NEC A88.8
      meningitis A87.0
    slow virus A81.9
      specified NEC A81.89
    specified NEC A88.8
  chest J98.8
  cotia B08.8
  coxsackie (*see also* Infection, coxsackie) B34.1
    as cause of disease classified elsewhere B97.11
  ECHO
    as cause of disease classified elsewhere B97.12
    unspecified nature or site B34.1
  encephalitis, tick-borne A84.9
  enterovirus, as cause of disease classified
    elsewhere B97.10
    coxsackievirus B97.11
    echovirus B97.12
    specified NEC B97.19
  exanthem NOS B09
  human papilloma as cause of disease classified
    elsewhere B97.7
  human metapneumovirus as cause of disease
    classified elsewhere B97.81
  intestine — *see* Enteritis, viral
  respiratory syncytial (RSV)
    as cause of disease classified elsewhere B97.4
    bronchiolitis J21.0
    bronchitis J20.5
    bronchopneumonia J12.1
    otitis media H65. ☑ *[B97.4]*
    pneumonia J12.1
    upper respiratory infection J06.9 *[B97.4]*
  rhinovirus
    as cause of disease classified elsewhere B97.89
    unspecified nature or site B34.8
  slow A81.9

Infection — *continued*
virus — *continued*
  specified NEC A81.89
  specified type NEC B33.8
    as cause of disease classified elsewhere B97.89
    unspecified nature or site B34.8
  unspecified nature or site B34.9
  West Nile — *see* Virus, West Nile
vulva (acute) — *see* Vulvitis
West Nile — *see* Virus, West Nile
whipworm B79
worms B83.9
  specified type NEC B83.8
Wuchereria (bancrofti) B74.0
  malayi B74.1
yatapoxvirus B08.70
  specified NEC B08.79
yeast (*see also* Candidiasis) B37.9
yellow fever — *see* Fever, yellow
Yersinia
  enterocolitica (intestinal) A04.6
  pestis — *see* Plague
  pseudotuberculosis A28.2
Zeis' gland — *see* Hordeolum
Zika virus A92.5
  congenital P35.4
zoonotic bacterial NOS A28.9
Zopfia senegalensis B47.0
Infective, infectious — *see* condition
Infertility
female N97.9
  age-related N97.8
  associated with
    anovulation N97.0
    cervical (mucus) disease or anomaly N88.3
    congenital anomaly
      cervix N88.3
      fallopian tube N97.1
      uterus N97.2
      vagina N97.8
    dysmucorrhea N88.3
    fallopian tube disease or anomaly N97.1
    pituitary-hypothalamic origin E23.0
    specified origin NEC N97.8
    Stein-Leventhal syndrome E28.2
    uterine disease or anomaly N97.2
    vaginal disease or anomaly N97.8
  due to
    cervical anomaly N88.3
    fallopian tube anomaly N97.1
    ovarian failure E28.39
    Stein-Leventhal syndrome E28.2
    uterine anomaly N97.2
    vaginal anomaly N97.8
  nonimplantation N97.2
  origin
    cervical N88.3
    tubal (block) (occlusion) (stenosis) N97.1
    uterine N97.2
    vaginal N97.8
male N46.9
  azoospermia N46.01
    extratesticular cause N46.029
      drug therapy N46.021
      efferent duct obstruction N46.023
      infection N46.022
      radiation N46.024
      specified cause NEC N46.029
      systemic disease N46.025
  oligospermia N46.11
    extratesticular cause N46.129
      drug therapy N46.121
      efferent duct obstruction N46.123
      infection N46.122
      radiation N46.124
      specified cause NEC N46.129
      systemic disease N46.125
  specified type NEC N46.8
Infestation B88.9
Acanthocheilonema (perstans) (streptocerca) B74.4
Acariasis B88.0
  demodex folliculorum B88.0
  sarcoptes scabiei B86
  trombiculae B88.0
Agamofilaria streptocerca B74.4
Ancylostoma, ankylostoma (braziliense) (caninum)
  (ceylanicum) (duodenale) B76.0
  americanum B76.1
  new world B76.1
Anisakis larvae, anisakiasis B81.0
arthropod NEC B88.2
Ascaris lumbricoides — *see* Ascariasis

Infestation — *continued*
Balantidium coli A07.0
beef tapeworm B68.1
Bothriocephalus (latus) B70.0
  larval B70.1
broad tapeworm B70.0
  larval B70.1
Brugia (malayi) B74.1
  timori B74.2
candiru B88.8
Capillaria
  hepatica B83.8
  philippinensis B81.1
cat liver fluke B66.0
cestodes B71.9
  diphyllobothrium — *see* Infestation,
    diphyllobothrium
  dipylidiasis B71.1
  hymenolepiasis B71.0
  specified type NEC B71.8
chigger B88.0
chigo, chigoe B88.1
Clonorchis (sinensis) (liver) B66.1
coccidial A07.3
crab-lice B85.3
Cysticercus cellulosae — *see* Cysticercosis
Demodex (folliculorum) B88.0
Dermanyssus gallinae B88.0
Dermatobia (hominis) — *see* Myiasis
Dibothriocephalus (latus) B70.0
  larval B70.1
Dicrocoelium dendriticum B66.2
Diphyllobothrium (adult) (latum) (intestinal)
  (pacificum) B70.0
  larval B70.1
Diplogonoporus (grandis) B71.8
Dipylidium caninum B67.4
Distoma hepaticum B66.3
dog tapeworm B67.4
Dracunculus medinensis B72
dragon worm B72
dwarf tapeworm B71.0
Echinococcus — *see* Echinococcus
Echinostomum ilocanum B66.8
Entamoeba (histolytica) — *see* Infection, Ameba
Enterobius vermicularis B80
eyelid
  in (due to)
    leishmaniasis B55.1
    loiasis B74.3
    onchocerciasis B73.09
    phthiriasis B85.3
    parasitic NOS B89
eyeworm B74.3
Fasciola (gigantica) (hepatica) (indica) B66.3
Fasciolopsis (buski) (intestine) B66.5
filarial B74.9
  bancroftian B74.0
  conjunctiva B74.9
  due to
    Acanthocheilonema (perstans) (streptocerca)
      B74.4
    Brugia (malayi) B74.1
      timori B74.2
    Dracunculus medinensis B72
    guinea worm B72
    loa loa B74.3
    Mansonella (ozzardi) (perstans) (streptocerca)
      B74.4
    Onchocerca volvulus B73.00
      eye B73.00
      eyelid B73.09
    Wuchereria (bancrofti) B74.0
  Malayan B74.1
  ozzardi B74.4
  specified type NEC B74.8
fish tapeworm B70.0
  larval B70.1
fluke B66.9
  blood NOS — *see* Schistosomiasis
  cat liver B66.0
  intestinal B66.5
  liver (sheep) B66.3
    cat B66.0
    Chinese B66.1
    due to clonorchiasis B66.1
    oriental B66.1
  lancet B66.2
  lung (oriental) B66.4
  sheep liver B66.3
  specified type NEC B66.8
fly larvae — *see* Myiasis

☑ **Additional character required**

Infestation — *continued*
Gasterophilus (intestinalis) — *see* Myiasis
Gastrodiscoides hominis B66.8
Giardia lamblia A07.1
Gnathostoma (spinigerum) B83.1
Gongylonema B83.8
guinea worm B72
helminth B83.9
  angiostrongyliasis B83.2
    intestinal B81.3
  gnathostomiasis B83.1
  hirudiniasis, internal B83.4
  intestinal B82.9
    angiostrongyliasis B81.3
    anisakiasis B81.0
    ascariasis — *see* Ascariasis
    capillariasis B81.1
    cysticercosis — *see* Cysticercosis
    diphyllobothriasis — *see* Infestation, diphyllobothriasis
    dracunculiasis B72
    echinococcus — *see* Echinococcosis
    enterobiasis B80
    filariasis — *see* Infestation, filarial
    fluke — *see* Infestation, fluke
    hookworm — *see* Infestation, hookworm
    mixed (types classifiable to more than one of the titles B65.0-B81.3 and B81.8) B81.4
    onchocerciasis — *see* Onchocerciasis
    schistosomiasis — *see* Infestation, schistosoma
    specified
      cestode NEC — *see* Infestation, cestode type NEC B81.8
    strongyloidiasis — *see* Strongyloidiasis
    taenia — *see* Infestation, taenia
    trichinellosis B75
    trichostrongyliasis B81.2
    trichuriasis B79
  specified type NEC B83.8
  syngamiasis B83.3
  visceral larva migrans B83.0
Heterophyes (heterophyes) B66.8
hookworm B76.9
  ancylostomiasis B76.0
  necatoriasis B76.1
  specified type NEC B76.8
Hymenolepis (diminuta) (nana) B71.0
  intestinal NEC B82.9
leeches (aquatic) (land) — *see* Hirudiniasis
Leishmania — *see* Leishmaniasis
lice, louse — *see* Infestation, Pediculus
Linguatula B88.8
Liponyssoides sanguineus B88.0
Loa loa B74.3
  conjunctival B74.3
  eyelid B74.3
louse — *see* Infestation, Pediculus
maggots — *see* Myiasis
Mansonella (ozzardi) (perstans) (streptocerca) B74.4
Medina (worm) B72
Metagonimus (yokogawai) B66.8
microfilaria streptocerca — *see* Onchocerciasis
  eye B73.00
  eyelid B73.09
mites B88.9
  scabic B86
Monilia (albicans) — *see* Candidiasis
mouth B37.0
Necator americanus B76.1
nematode NEC (intestinal) B82.0
  Ancylostoma B76.0
  conjunctiva NEC B83.9
  Enterobius vermicularis B80
  Gnathostoma spinigerum B83.1
  physaloptera B80
  specified NEC B81.8
  trichostrongylus B81.2
  trichuris (trichuria) B79
Oesophagostomum (apiostomum) B81.8
Oestrus ovis (*see also* Myiasis) B87.9
Onchocerca (volvulus) — *see* Onchocerciasis
Opisthorchis (felineus) (viverrini) B66.0
orbit, parasitic NOS B89
Oxyuris vermicularis B80
Paragonimus (westermani) B66.4
parasite, parasitic B89
  eyelid B89
  intestinal NOS B82.9
  mouth B37.0
  skin B88.9
  tongue B37.0

Infestation — *continued*
Parastrongylus
  cantonensis B83.2
  costaricensis B81.3
Pediculus B85.2
  body B85.1
  capitis (humanus) (any site) B85.0
  corporis (humanus) (any site) B85.1
  head B85.0
  mixed (classifiable to more than one of the titles B85.0-B85.3) B85.4
  pubis (any site) B85.3
Pentastoma B88.8
Phthirus (pubis) (any site) B85.3
  with any infestation classifiable to B85.0-B85.2 B85.4
pinworm B80
pork tapeworm (adult) B68.0
protozoal NEC B64
  intestinal A07.9
    specified NEC A07.8
  specified NEC B60.8
pubic, louse B85.3
rat tapeworm B71.0
red bug B88.0
roundworm (large) NEC B82.0
  Ascariasis (*see also* Ascariasis) B77.9
sandflea B88.1
Sarcoptes scabiei B86
scabies B86
Schistosoma B65.9
  bovis B65.8
  cercariae B65.3
  haematobium B65.0
  intercalatum B65.8
  japonicum B65.2
  mansoni B65.1
  mattheei B65.8
  mekongi B65.8
  specified type NEC B65.8
  spindale B65.8
screw worms — *see* Myiasis
skin NOS B88.9
Sparganum (mansoni) (proliferum) (baxteri) B70.1
  larval B70.1
specified type NEC B88.8
Spirometra larvae B70.1
Stellantchasmus falcatus B66.8
Strongyloides stercoralis — *see* Strongyloidiasis
Taenia B68.9
  diminuta B71.0
  echinococcus — *see* Echinococcus
  mediocanellata B68.1
  nana B71.0
  saginata B68.1
  solium (intestinal form) B68.0
    larval form — *see* Cysticercosis
Taeniarhynchus saginatus B68.1
tapeworm B71.9
  beef B68.1
  broad B70.0
    larval B70.1
  dog B67.4
  dwarf B71.0
  fish B70.0
    larval B70.1
  pork B68.0
  rat B71.0
Ternidens diminutus B81.8
Tetranychus molestissimus B88.0
threadworm B80
tongue B37.0
Toxocara (canis) (cati) (felis) B83.0
trematode(s) NEC — *see* Infestation, fluke
Trichinella (spiralis) B75
Trichocephalus B79
Trichomonas — *see* Trichomoniasis
Trichostrongylus B81.2
Trichuris (trichiura) B79
Trombicula (irritans) B88.0
Tunga penetrans B88.1
Uncinaria americana B76.1
Vandellia cirrhosa B88.8
whipworm B79
worms B83.9
  intestinal B82.0
Wuchereria (bancrofti) B74.0
Infiltrate, infiltration
amyloid (generalized) (localized) — *see* Amyloidosis
calcareous NEC R89.7
  localized — *see* Degeneration, by site
calcium salt R89.7

Infiltrate — *continued*
cardiac
  fatty — *see* Degeneration, myocardial
  glycogenic E74.02 *[I43]*
corneal — *see* Edema, cornea
eyelid — *see* Inflammation, eyelid
glycogen, glycogenic — *see* Disease, glycogen storage
heart, cardiac
  fatty — *see* Degeneration, myocardial
  glycogenic E74.02 *[I43]*
inflammatory in vitreous H43.89
kidney N28.89
leukemic — *see* Leukemia
liver K76.89
  fatty — *see* Fatty, liver NEC
  glycogen (*see also* Disease, glycogen storage) E74.03 *[K77]*
lung R91.8
  eosinophilic J82
lymphatic (*see also* Leukemia, lymphatic) C91.9 ☑
  gland I88.9
muscle, fatty M62.89
myocardium, myocardial
  fatty — *see* Degeneration, myocardial
  glycogenic E74.02 *[I43]*
on chest X-ray R91.8
pulmonary R91.8
  with eosinophilia J82
skin (lymphocytic) L98.6
thymus (gland) (fatty) E32.8
urine R39.0
vesicant agent
  antineoplastic chemotherapy T80.810 ☑
  other agent NEC T80.818 ☑
vitreous body H43.89
Infirmity R68.89
senile R54
Inflammation, inflamed, inflammatory (with exudation)
abducent (nerve) — *see* Strabismus, paralytic, sixth nerve
accessory sinus (chronic) — *see* Sinusitis
adrenal (gland) E27.8
alveoli, teeth M27.3
  scorbutic E54
anal canal, anus K62.89
antrum (chronic) — *see* Sinusitis, maxillary
appendix — *see* Appendicitis
arachnoid — *see* Meningitis
areola N61.0
  puerperal, postpartum or gestational — *see* Infection, nipple
areolar tissue NOS L08.9
artery — *see* Arteritis
auditory meatus (external) — *see* Otitis, externa
Bartholin's gland N75.8
bile duct (common) (hepatic) or passage — *see* Cholangitis
bladder — *see* Cystitis
bone — *see* Osteomyelitis
brain (*see also* Encephalitis)
  membrane — *see* Meningitis
breast N61.0
  puerperal, postpartum, gestational — *see* Mastitis, obstetric
broad ligament — *see* Disease, pelvis, inflammatory
bronchi — *see* Bronchitis
catarrhal J00
cecum — *see* Appendicitis
cerebral (*see also* Encephalitis)
  membrane — *see* Meningitis
cerebrospinal
  meningococcal A39.0
cervix (uteri) — *see* Cervicitis
chest J98.8
chorioretinal H30.9 ☑
  cyclitis — *see* Cyclitis
  disseminated H30.10 ☑
    generalized H30.13 ☑
    peripheral H30.12 ☑
    posterior pole H30.11 ☑
  epitheliopathy — *see* Epitheliopathy
  focal H30.00 ☑
    juxtapapillary H30.01 ☑
    macular H30.04 ☑
    paramacular — *see* Inflammation, chorioretinal, focal, macular
    peripheral H30.03 ☑
    posterior pole H30.02 ☑
  specified type NEC H30.89 ☑
choroid — *see* Inflammation, chorioretinal

Inflammation — *continued*
  chronic, postmastoidectomy cavity — *see* Complications, postmastoidectomy, inflammation
  colon — *see* Enteritis
  connective tissue (diffuse) NEC — *see* Disorder, soft tissue, specified type NEC
  cornea — *see* Keratitis
  corpora cavernosa N48.29
  cranial nerve — *see* Disorder, nerve, cranial
  Douglas' cul-de-sac or pouch (chronic) N73.0
  due to device, implant or graft (*see also* Complications, by site and type, infection or inflammation)
    arterial graft T82.7 ☑
    breast (implant) T85.79 ☑
    catheter T85.79 ☑
      dialysis (renal) T82.7 ☑
        intraperitoneal T85.71 ☑
      infusion T82.7 ☑
        cranial T85.735 ☑
        intrathecal T85.735 ☑
        spinal (epidural) (subdural) T85.735 ☑
        subarachnoid T85.735 ☑
      urinary T83.518 ☑
        cystostomy T83.510 ☑
        Hopkins T83.518 ☑
        ileostomy T83.518 ☑
        nephrostomy T83.512 ☑
        specified NEC T83.518 ☑
        urethral indwelling T83.511 ☑
        urostomy T83.518 ☑
    electronic (electrode) (pulse generator) (stimulator)
      bone T84.7 ☑
      cardiac T82.7 ☑
      nervous system T85.738 ☑
        brain T85.731 ☑
        cranial nerve T85.732 ☑
        gastric nerve T85.732 ☑
        neurostimulator generator T85.734 ☑
        peripheral nerve T85.732 ☑
        sacral nerve T85.732 ☑
        spinal cord T85.733 ☑
        vagal nerve T85.732 ☑
      urinary T83.590 ☑
    fixation, internal (orthopedic) NEC — *see* Complication, fixation device, infection
    gastrointestinal (bile duct) (esophagus) T85.79 ☑
      neurostimulator electrode (lead) T85.732 ☑
    genital NEC T83.69 ☑
    heart NEC T82.7 ☑
      valve (prosthesis) T82.6 ☑
        graft T82.7 ☑
    joint prosthesis — *see* Complication, joint prosthesis, infection
    ocular (corneal graft) (orbital implant) NEC T85.79 ☑
    orthopedic NEC T84.7 ☑
    penile (cylinder) (pump) (reservoir) T83.61 ☑
    specified NEC T85.79 ☑
    testicular T83.62 ☑
    urinary NEC T83.598 ☑
      ileal conduit stent T83.593 ☑
      implanted neurostimulation T83.590 ☑
      implanted sphincter T83.591 ☑
      indwelling ureteral stent T83.592 ☑
      nephroureteral stent T83.593 ☑
      specified stent NEC T83.593 ☑
    vascular NEC T82.7 ☑
    ventricular intracranial (communicating) shunt T85.730 ☑
  duodenum K29.80
    with bleeding K29.81
  dura mater — *see* Meningitis
  ear (middle) (*see also* Otitis, media)
    external — *see* Otitis, externa
    inner — *see* subcategory H83.0 ☑
  epididymis — *see* Epididymitis
  esophagus K20.9
  ethmoidal (sinus) (chronic) — *see* Sinusitis, ethmoidal
  eustachian tube (catarrhal) — *see* Salpingitis, eustachian
  eyelid H01.9
    abscess — *see* Abscess, eyelid
    blepharitis — *see* Blepharitis
    chalazion — *see* Chalazion
    dermatosis (noninfectious) — *see* Dermatosis, eyelid
    hordeolum — *see* Hordeolum
    specified NEC H01.8

Inflammation — *continued*
  fallopian tube — *see* Salpingo-oophoritis
  fascia — *see* Myositis
  follicular, pharynx J31.2
  frontal (sinus) (chronic) — *see* Sinusitis, frontal
  gallbladder — *see* Cholecystitis
  gastric — *see* Gastritis
  gastrointestinal — *see* Enteritis
  genital organ (internal) (diffuse)
    female — *see* Disease, pelvis, inflammatory
    male N49.9
      multiple sites N49.8
      specified NEC N49.8
  gland (lymph) — *see* Lymphadenitis
  glottis — *see* Laryngitis
  granular, pharynx J31.2
  gum K05.10
    nonplaque induced K05.11
    plaque induced K05.10
  heart — *see* Carditis
  hepatic duct — *see* Cholangitis
  ileoanal (internal) pouch K91.850
  ileum (*see also* Enteritis)
    regional or terminal — *see* Enteritis, regional
  intestine (any part) — *see* Enteritis
  intestinal pouch K91.850
  jaw (acute) (bone) (chronic) (lower) (suppurative) (upper) M27.2
  joint NEC — *see* Arthritis
    sacroiliac M46.1
  kidney — *see* Nephritis
  knee (joint) M13.169
    tuberculous A18.02
  labium (majus) (minus) — *see* Vulvitis
  lacrimal
    gland — *see* Dacryoadenitis
    passages (duct) (sac) (*see also* Dacryocystitis)
      canaliculitis — *see* Canaliculitis, lacrimal
  larynx — *see* Laryngitis
  leg NOS L08.9
  lip K13.0
  liver (capsule) (*see also* Hepatitis)
    chronic K73.9
    suppurative K75.0
  lung (acute) (*see also* Pneumonia)
    chronic J98.4
  lymph gland or node — *see* Lymphadenitis
  lymphatic vessel — *see* Lymphangitis
  maxilla, maxillary M27.2
    sinus (chronic) — *see* Sinusitis, maxillary
  membranes of brain or spinal cord — *see* Meningitis
  meninges — *see* Meningitis
  mouth K12.1
  muscle — *see* Myositis
  myocardium — *see* Myocarditis
  nasal sinus (chronic) — *see* Sinusitis
  nasopharynx — *see* Nasopharyngitis
  navel L08.82
  nerve NEC — *see* Neuralgia
  nipple N61.0
    puerperal, postpartum or gestational — *see* Infection, nipple
  nose — *see* Rhinitis
  oculomotor (nerve) — *see* Strabismus, paralytic, third nerve
  optic nerve — *see* Neuritis, optic
  orbit (chronic) H05.10
    acute H05.00
      abscess — *see* Abscess, orbit
      cellulitis — *see* Cellulitis, orbit
      osteomyelitis — *see* Osteomyelitis, orbit
      periostitis — *see* Periostitis, orbital
      tenonitis — *see* Tenonitis, eye
    granuloma — *see* Granuloma, orbit
    myositis — *see* Myositis, orbital
  ovary — *see* Salpingo-oophoritis
  oviduct — *see* Salpingo-oophoritis
  pancreas (acute) — *see* Pancreatitis
  parametrium N73.0
  parotid region L08.9
  pelvis, female — *see* Disease, pelvis, inflammatory
  penis (corpora cavernosa) N48.29
  perianal K62.89
  pericardium — *see* Pericarditis
  perineum (female) (male) L08.9
  perirectal K62.89
  peritoneum — *see* Peritonitis
  periuterine — *see* Disease, pelvis, inflammatory
  perivesical — *see* Cystitis
  petrous bone (acute) (chronic) — *see* Petrositis
  pharynx (acute) — *see* Pharyngitis
  pia mater — *see* Meningitis

Inflammation — *continued*
  pleura — *see* Pleurisy
  polyp, colon (*see also* Polyp, colon, inflammatory) K51.40
  prostate (*see also* Prostatitis)
    specified type NEC N41.8
  rectosigmoid — *see* Rectosigmoiditis
  rectum (*see also* Proctitis) K62.89
  respiratory, upper (*see also* Infection, respiratory, upper) J06.9
    acute, due to radiation J70.0
    chronic, due to external agent — *see* condition, respiratory, chronic, due to
    due to
      chemicals, gases, fumes or vapors (inhalation) J68.2
      radiation J70.1
  retina — *see* Chorioretinitis
  retrocecal — *see* Appendicitis
  retroperitoneal — *see* Peritonitis
  salivary duct or gland (any) (suppurative) — *see* Sialoadenitis
  scorbutic, alveoli, teeth E54
  scrotum N49.2
  seminal vesicle — *see* Vesiculitis
  sigmoid — *see* Enteritis
  sinus — *see* Sinusitis
  Skene's duct or gland — *see* Urethritis
  skin L08.9
  spermatic cord N49.1
  sphenoidal (sinus) — *see* Sinusitis, sphenoidal
  spinal
    cord — *see* Encephalitis
    membrane — *see* Meningitis
    nerve — *see* Disorder, nerve
  spine — *see* Spondylopathy, inflammatory
  spleen (capsule) D73.89
  stomach — *see* Gastritis
  subcutaneous tissue L08.9
  suprarenal (gland) E27.8
  synovial — *see* Tenosynovitis
  tendon (sheath) NEC — *see* Tenosynovitis
  testis — *see* Orchitis
  throat (acute) — *see* Pharyngitis
  thymus (gland) E32.8
  thyroid (gland) — *see* Thyroiditis
  tongue K14.0
  tonsil — *see* Tonsillitis
  trachea — *see* Tracheitis
  trochlear (nerve) — *see* Strabismus, paralytic, fourth nerve
  tubal — *see* Salpingo-oophoritis
  tuberculous NEC — *see* Tuberculosis
  tubo-ovarian — *see* Salpingo-oophoritis
  tunica vaginalis N49.1
  tympanic membrane — *see* Tympanitis
  umbilicus, umbilical L08.82
  uterine ligament — *see* Disease, pelvis, inflammatory
  uterus (catarrhal) — *see* Endometritis
  uveal tract (anterior) NOS (*see also* Iridocyclitis)
    posterior — *see* Chorioretinitis
  vagina — *see* Vaginitis
  vas deferens N49.1
  vein (*see also* Phlebitis)
    intracranial or intraspinal (septic) G08
    thrombotic I80.9
      leg — *see* Phlebitis, leg
      lower extremity — *see* Phlebitis, leg
  vocal cord J38.3
  vulva — *see* Vulvitis
  Wharton's duct (suppurative) — *see* Sialoadenitis
Inflation, lung, imperfect (newborn) — *see* Atelectasis
Influenza (bronchial) (epidemic) (respiratory (upper)) (unidentified influenza virus) J11.1
  with
    digestive manifestations J11.2
    encephalopathy J11.81
    enteritis J11.2
    gastroenteritis J11.2
    gastrointestinal manifestations J11.2
    laryngitis J11.1
    myocarditis J11.82
    otitis media J11.83
    pharyngitis J11.1
    pneumonia J11.00
      specified type J11.08
    respiratory manifestations NEC J11.1
    specified manifestation NEC J11.89
  A/H5N1 (*see also* Influenza, due to, identified novel influenza A virus) J09.X2

☑ **Additional character required**

Influenza — continued
avian (see also Influenza, due to, identified novel influenza A virus) J09.X2
bird (see also Influenza, due to, identified novel influenza A virus) J09.X2
novel (2009) H1N1 influenza (see also Influenza, due to, identified influenza virus NEC) J10.1
novel influenza A/H1N1 (see also Influenza, due to, identified influenza virus NEC) J10.1
due to
  avian (see also Influenza, due to, identified novel influenza A virus) J09.X2
  identified influenza virus NEC J10.1
    with
      digestive manifestations J10.2
      encephalopathy J10.81
      enteritis J10.2
      gastroenteritis J10.2
      gastrointestinal manifestations J10.2
      laryngitis J10.1
      myocarditis J10.82
      otitis media J10.83
      pharyngitis J10.1
      pneumonia (unspecified type) J10.00
        with same identified influenza virus J10.01
        specified type NEC J10.08
      respiratory manifestations NEC J10.1
      specified manifestation NEC J10.89
  identified novel influenza A virus J09.X2
    with
      digestive manifestations J09.X3
      encephalopathy J09.X9
      enteritis J09.X3
      gastroenteritis J09.X3
      gastrointestinal manifestations J09.X3
      laryngitis J09.X2
      myocarditis J09.X9
      otitis media J09.X9
      pharyngitis J09.X2
      pneumonia J09.X1
      respiratory manifestations NEC J09.X2
      specified manifestation NEC J09.X9
      upper respiratory symptoms J09.X2
of other animal origin, not bird or swine (see also Influenza, due to, identified novel influenza A virus) J09.X2
swine (viruses that normally cause infections in pigs) (see also Influenza, due to, identified novel influenza A virus) J09.X2
Influenza-like disease — see Influenza
Influenzal — see Influenza
Infraction, Freiberg's (metatarsal head) — see Osteochondrosis, juvenile, metatarsus
Infraeruption of tooth (teeth) M26.34
Infusion complication, misadventure, or reaction — see Complications, infusion
Ingestion
chemical — see Table of Drugs and Chemicals, by substance, poisoning
drug or medicament
  correct substance properly administered — see Table of Drugs and Chemicals, by drug, adverse effect
  overdose or wrong substance given or taken — see Table of Drugs and Chemicals, by drug, poisoning
foreign body — see Foreign body, alimentary tract
multiple drug — see Table of Drugs and Chemicals, multiple
tularemia A21.3
Ingrowing
hair (beard) L73.1
nail (finger) (toe) L60.0
Inguinal (see also condition)
testicle Q53.9
  bilateral Q53.212
  unilateral Q53.112
Inhalant-induced
anxiety disorder F18.980
depressive disorder F18.94
major neurocognitive disorder F18.97
mild neurocognitive disorder F18.988
psychotic disorder F18.959
Inhalation
anthrax A22.1
flame T27.3 ☑
food or foreign body — see Foreign body, by site
gases, fumes, or vapors NEC T59.9 ☑
  specified agent — see Table of Drugs and Chemicals, by substance
liquid or vomitus — see Asphyxia

Inhalation — continued
meconium (newborn) P24.00
  with
    pneumonia (pneumonitis) P24.01
    with respiratory symptoms P24.01
mucus — see Asphyxia, mucus
oil or gasoline (causing suffocation) — see Foreign body, by site
smoke J70.5
  due to chemicals, gases, fumes and vapors J68.9
steam — see Toxicity, vapors
stomach contents or secretions — see Foreign body, by site
  due to anesthesia (general) (local) or other sedation T88.59 ☑
    in labor and delivery O74.0
    in pregnancy O29.01 ☑
    postpartum, puerperal O89.01
Inhibition, orgasm
female F52.31
male F52.32
Inhibitor, systemic lupus erythematosus (presence of) D68.62
Iniencephalus, iniencephaly Q00.2
Injection, traumatic jet (air) (industrial) (water) (paint or dye) T70.4 ☑
Injury (see also specified injury type) T14.90 ☑
abdomen, abdominal S39.91 ☑
  blood vessel — see Injury, blood vessel, abdomen
  cavity — see Injury, intra-abdominal
  contusion S30.1 ☑
  internal — see Injury, intra-abdominal
  intra-abdominal organ — see Injury, intra-abdominal
  nerve — see Injury, nerve, abdomen
  open — see Wound, open, abdomen
  specified NEC S39.81 ☑
  superficial — see Injury, superficial, abdomen
Achilles tendon S86.00 ☑
  laceration S86.02 ☑
  specified type NEC S86.09 ☑
  strain S86.01 ☑
acoustic, resulting in deafness — see Injury, nerve, acoustic
adrenal (gland) S37.819 ☑
  contusion S37.812 ☑
  laceration S37.813 ☑
  specified type NEC S37.818 ☑
alveolar (process) S09.93 ☑
ankle S99.91 ☑
  contusion — see Contusion, ankle
  dislocation — see Dislocation, ankle
  fracture — see Fracture, ankle
  nerve — see Injury, nerve, ankle
  open — see Wound, open, ankle
  specified type NEC S99.81 ☑
  sprain — see Sprain, ankle
  superficial — see Injury, superficial, ankle
anterior chamber, eye — see Injury, eye, specified site NEC
anus — see Injury, abdomen
aorta (thoracic) S25.00 ☑
  abdominal S35.00 ☑
    laceration (minor) (superficial) S35.01 ☑
      major S35.02 ☑
    specified type NEC S35.09 ☑
  laceration (minor) (superficial) S25.01 ☑
    major S25.02 ☑
  specified type NEC S25.09 ☑
arm (upper) S49.9 ☑
  blood vessel — see Injury, blood vessel, arm
  contusion — see Contusion, arm, upper
  fracture — see Fracture, humerus
  lower — see Injury, forearm
  muscle — see Injury, muscle, shoulder
  nerve — see Injury, nerve, arm
  open — see Wound, open, arm
  specified type NEC S49.8 ☑
  superficial — see Injury, superficial, arm
artery (complicating trauma) (see also Injury, blood vessel, by site)
  cerebral or meningeal — see Injury, intracranial
auditory canal (external) (meatus) S09.91 ☑
auricle, auris, ear S09.91 ☑
axilla — see Injury, shoulder
back — see Injury, back, lower
bile duct S36.13 ☑
birth (see also Birth, injury) P15.9
bladder (sphincter) S37.20 ☑
  at delivery O71.5
  contusion S37.22 ☑
  laceration S37.23 ☑

Injury — continued
bladder — continued
  obstetrical trauma O71.5
  specified type NEC S37.29 ☑
blast (air) (hydraulic) (immersion) (underwater) NEC T14.8 ☑
  acoustic nerve trauma — see Injury, nerve, acoustic
  bladder — see Injury, bladder
  brain — see Concussion
  colon — see Injury, intestine, large, blast injury
  ear (primary) S09.31 ☑
    secondary S09.39 ☑
  generalized T70.8 ☑
  lung — see Injury, intrathoracic, lung, blast injury
  multiple body organs T70.8 ☑
  peritoneum S36.81 ☑
  rectum S36.61 ☑
  retroperitoneum S36.898 ☑
  small intestine S36.419 ☑
    duodenum S36.410 ☑
    specified site NEC S36.418 ☑
  specified
    intra-abdominal organ NEC S36.898 ☑
    pelvic organ NEC S37.899 ☑
blood vessel NEC T14.8 ☑
  abdomen S35.9 ☑
    aorta — see Injury, aorta, abdominal
    celiac artery — see Injury, blood vessel, celiac artery
    iliac vessel — see Injury, blood vessel, iliac
    laceration S35.91 ☑
    mesenteric vessel — see Injury, mesenteric
    portal vein — see Injury, blood vessel, portal vein
    renal vessel — see Injury, blood vessel, renal
    specified vessel NEC S35.8X ☑
    splenic vessel — see Injury, blood vessel, splenic
    vena cava — see Injury, vena cava, inferior
  ankle — see Injury, blood vessel, foot
  aorta (abdominal) (thoracic) — see Injury, aorta
  arm (upper) NEC S45.90 ☑
    forearm — see Injury, blood vessel, forearm
    laceration S45.91 ☑
    specified
      site NEC S45.80 ☑
        laceration S45.81 ☑
        specified type NEC S45.89 ☑
      type NEC S45.99 ☑
    superficial vein S45.30 ☑
      laceration S45.31 ☑
      specified type NEC S45.39 ☑
  axillary
    artery S45.00 ☑
      laceration S45.01 ☑
      specified type NEC S45.09 ☑
    vein S45.20 ☑
      laceration S45.21 ☑
      specified type NEC S45.29 ☑
  azygos vein — see Injury, blood vessel, thoracic, specified site NEC
  brachial
    artery S45.10 ☑
      laceration S45.11 ☑
      specified type NEC S45.19 ☑
    vein S45.20 ☑
      laceration S45.219 ☑
      specified type NEC S45.29 ☑
  carotid artery (common) (external) (internal, extracranial) S15.00 ☑
    internal, intracranial S06.8 ☑
    laceration (minor) (superficial) S15.01 ☑
      major S15.02 ☑
    specified type NEC S15.09 ☑
  celiac artery S35.219 ☑
    branch S35.299 ☑
      laceration (minor) (superficial) S35.291 ☑
        major S35.292 ☑
      specified NEC S35.298 ☑
    laceration (minor) (superficial) S35.211 ☑
      major S35.212 ☑
    specified type NEC S35.218 ☑
  cerebral — see Injury, intracranial
  deep plantar — see Injury, blood vessel, plantar artery
  digital (hand) — see Injury, blood vessel, finger
  dorsal
    artery (foot) S95.00 ☑
      laceration S95.01 ☑
      specified type NEC S95.09 ☑
    vein (foot) S95.20 ☑
      laceration S95.21 ☑

Injury

Injury — *continued*
    blood vessel NEC — *continued*
        specified type NEC S95.29 ☑
        due to accidental laceration during procedure
            — *see* Laceration, accidental complicating surgery
        extremity — *see* Injury, blood vessel, limb
        femoral
            artery (common) (superficial) S75.00 ☑
                laceration (minor) (superficial) S75.01 ☑
                    major S75.02 ☑
                specified type NEC S75.09 ☑
            vein (hip level) (thigh level) S75.10 ☑
                laceration (minor) (superficial) S75.11 ☑
                    major S75.12 ☑
                specified type NEC S75.19 ☑
        finger S65.50 ☑
            index S65.50 ☑
                laceration S65.51 ☑
                specified type NEC S65.59 ☑
            laceration S65.51 ☑
            little S65.50 ☑
                laceration S65.51 ☑
                specified type NEC S65.59 ☑
            middle S65.50 ☑
                laceration S65.51 ☑
                specified type NEC S65.59 ☑
            specified type NEC S65.59 ☑
            thumb — *see* Injury, blood vessel, thumb
        foot S95.90 ☑
            dorsal
                artery — *see* Injury, blood vessel, dorsal, artery
                vein — *see* Injury, blood vessel, dorsal, vein
            laceration S95.91 ☑
            plantar artery — *see* Injury, blood vessel, plantar artery
            specified
                site NEC S95.80 ☑
                    laceration S95.81 ☑
                    specified type NEC S95.89 ☑
                specified type NEC S95.99 ☑
        forearm S55.90 ☑
            laceration S55.91 ☑
            radial artery — *see* Injury, blood vessel, radial artery
            specified
                site NEC S55.80 ☑
                    laceration S55.81 ☑
                    specified type NEC S55.89 ☑
                type NEC S55.99 ☑
            ulnar artery — *see* Injury, blood vessel, ulnar artery
            vein S55.20 ☑
                laceration S55.21 ☑
                specified type NEC S55.29 ☑
        gastric
            artery — *see* Injury, mesenteric, artery, branch
            vein — *see* Injury, blood vessel, abdomen
        gastroduodenal artery — *see* Injury, mesenteric, artery, branch
        greater saphenous vein (lower leg level) S85.30 ☑
            hip (and thigh) level S75.20 ☑
                laceration (minor) (superficial) S75.21 ☑
                    major S75.22 ☑
                specified type NEC S75.29 ☑
            laceration S85.31 ☑
            specified type NEC S85.39 ☑
        hand (level) S65.90 ☑
            finger — *see* Injury, blood vessel, finger
            laceration S65.91 ☑
            palmar arch — *see* Injury, blood vessel, palmar arch
            radial artery — *see* Injury, blood vessel, radial artery, hand
            specified
                site NEC S65.80 ☑
                    laceration S65.81 ☑
                    specified type NEC S65.89 ☑
                type NEC S65.99 ☑
            thumb — *see* Injury, blood vessel, thumb
            ulnar artery — *see* Injury, blood vessel, ulnar artery, hand
        head S09.0 ☑
            intracranial — *see* Injury, intracranial
            multiple S09.0 ☑
        hepatic
            artery — *see* Injury, mesenteric, artery
            vein — *see* Injury, vena cava, inferior
        hip S75.90 ☑
            femoral artery — *see* Injury, blood vessel, femoral, artery

Injury — *continued*
    blood vessel NEC — *continued*
        femoral vein — *see* Injury, blood vessel, femoral, vein
        greater saphenous vein — *see* Injury, blood vessel, greater saphenous, hip level
        laceration S75.91 ☑
        specified
            site NEC S75.80 ☑
                laceration S75.81 ☑
                specified type NEC S75.89 ☑
            type NEC S75.99 ☑
        hypogastric (artery) (vein) — *see* Injury, blood vessel, iliac
        iliac S35.5 ☑
            artery S35.51 ☑
            specified vessel NEC S35.5 ☑
            uterine vessel — *see* Injury, blood vessel, uterine
            vein S35.51 ☑
        innominate — *see* Injury, blood vessel, thoracic, innominate
        intercostal (artery) (vein) — *see* Injury, blood vessel, thoracic, intercostal
        jugular vein (external) S15.20 ☑
            internal S15.30 ☑
                laceration (minor) (superficial) S15.31 ☑
                    major S15.32 ☑
                specified type NEC S15.39 ☑
            laceration (minor) (superficial) S15.21 ☑
                major S15.22 ☑
            specified type NEC S15.29 ☑
        leg (level) (lower) S85.90 ☑
            greater saphenous — *see* Injury, blood vessel, greater saphenous
            laceration S85.91 ☑
            lesser saphenous — *see* Injury, blood vessel, lesser saphenous
            peroneal artery — *see* Injury, blood vessel, peroneal artery
            popliteal
                artery — *see* Injury, blood vessel, popliteal, artery
                vein — *see* Injury, blood vessel, popliteal, vein
            specified
                site NEC S85.80 ☑
                    laceration S85.81 ☑
                    specified type NEC S85.89 ☑
                type NEC S85.99 ☑
            thigh — *see* Injury, blood vessel, hip
            tibial artery — *see* Injury, blood vessel, tibial artery
        lesser saphenous vein (lower leg level) S85.40 ☑
            laceration S85.41 ☑
            specified type NEC S85.49 ☑
        limb
            lower — *see* Injury, blood vessel, leg
            upper — *see* Injury, blood vessel, arm
        lower back — *see* Injury, blood vessel, abdomen
            specified NEC — *see* Injury, blood vessel, abdomen, specified, site NEC
        mammary (artery) (vein) — *see* Injury, blood vessel, thoracic, specified site NEC
        mesenteric (inferior) (superior)
            artery — *see* Injury, mesenteric, artery
            vein — *see* Injury, mesenteric, vein
        neck S15.9 ☑
            specified site NEC S15.8 ☑
        ovarian (artery) (vein) — *see* subcategory S35.8 ☑
        palmar arch (superficial) S65.20 ☑
            deep S65.30 ☑
                laceration S65.31 ☑
                specified type NEC S65.39 ☑
            laceration S65.21 ☑
            specified type NEC S65.29 ☑
        pelvis — *see* Injury, blood vessel, abdomen
            specified NEC — *see* Injury, blood vessel, abdomen, specified, site NEC
        peroneal artery S85.20 ☑
            laceration S85.21 ☑
            specified type NEC S85.29 ☑
        plantar artery (deep) (foot) S95.10 ☑
            laceration S95.11 ☑
            specified type NEC S95.19 ☑
        popliteal
            artery S85.00 ☑
                laceration S85.01 ☑
                specified type NEC S85.09 ☑
            vein S85.50 ☑
                laceration S85.51 ☑
                specified type NEC S85.59 ☑
        portal vein S35.319 ☑

Injury — *continued*
    blood vessel NEC — *continued*
        laceration S35.311 ☑
        specified type NEC S35.318 ☑
        precerebral — *see* Injury, blood vessel, neck
        pulmonary (artery) (vein) — *see* Injury, blood vessel, thoracic, pulmonary
        radial artery (forearm level) S55.10 ☑
            hand and wrist (level) S65.10 ☑
                laceration S65.11 ☑
                specified type NEC S65.19 ☑
            laceration S55.11 ☑
            specified type NEC S55.19 ☑
        renal
            artery S35.40 ☑
                laceration S35.41 ☑
                specified NEC S35.49 ☑
            vein S35.40 ☑
                laceration S35.41 ☑
                specified NEC S35.49 ☑
        saphenous vein (greater) (lower leg level) — *see* Injury, blood vessel, greater saphenous
            hip and thigh level — *see* Injury, blood vessel, greater saphenous, hip level
            lesser — *see* Injury, blood vessel, lesser saphenous
        shoulder
            specified NEC — *see* Injury, blood vessel, arm, specified site NEC
            superficial vein — *see* Injury, blood vessel, arm, superficial vein
        specified NEC T14.8 ☑
        splenic
            artery — *see* Injury, blood vessel, celiac artery, branch
            vein S35.329 ☑
                laceration S35.321 ☑
                specified NEC S35.328 ☑
        subclavian — *see* Injury, blood vessel, thoracic, innominate
        thigh — *see* Injury, blood vessel, hip
        thoracic S25.90 ☑
            aorta S25.00 ☑
                laceration (minor) (superficial) S25.01 ☑
                    major S25.02 ☑
                specified type NEC S25.09 ☑
            azygos vein — *see* Injury, blood vessel, thoracic, specified, site NEC
            innominate
                artery S25.10 ☑
                    laceration (minor) (superficial) S25.11 ☑
                        major S25.12 ☑
                    specified type NEC S25.19 ☑
                vein S25.30 ☑
                    laceration (minor) (superficial) S25.31 ☑
                        major S25.32 ☑
                    specified type NEC S25.39 ☑
            intercostal S25.50 ☑
                laceration S25.51 ☑
                specified type NEC S25.59 ☑
            laceration S25.91 ☑
            mammary vessel — *see* Injury, blood vessel, thoracic, specified, site NEC
            pulmonary S25.40 ☑
                laceration (minor) (superficial) S25.41 ☑
                    major S25.42 ☑
                specified type NEC S25.49 ☑
            specified
                site NEC S25.80 ☑
                    laceration S25.81 ☑
                    specified type NEC S25.89 ☑
                type NEC S25.99 ☑
            subclavian — *see* Injury, blood vessel, thoracic, innominate
            vena cava (superior) S25.20 ☑
                laceration (minor) (superficial) S25.21 ☑
                    major S25.22 ☑
                specified type NEC S25.29 ☑
        thumb S65.40 ☑
            laceration S65.41 ☑
            specified type NEC S65.49 ☑
        tibial artery S85.10 ☑
            anterior S85.13 ☑
                laceration S85.14 ☑
                specified injury NEC S85.15 ☑
            laceration S85.11 ☑
            posterior S85.16 ☑
                laceration S85.17 ☑
                specified injury NEC S85.18 ☑
            specified injury NEC S85.12 ☑
        ulnar artery (forearm level) S55.00 ☑
            hand and wrist (level) S65.00 ☑

☑ **Additional character required**

Injury — *continued*
- blood vessel NEC — *continued*
    - laceration S65.01 ☑
    - specified type NEC S65.09 ☑
    - laceration S55.01 ☑
    - specified type NEC S55.09 ☑
    - upper arm (level) — *see* Injury, blood vessel, arm
    - superficial vein — *see* Injury, blood vessel, arm, superficial vein
    - uterine S35.5 ☑
        - artery S35.53 ☑
        - vein S35.53 ☑
    - vena cava — *see* Injury, vena cava
    - vertebral artery S15.10 ☑
        - laceration (minor) (superficial) S15.11 ☑
            - major S15.12 ☑
        - specified type NEC S15.19 ☑
    - wrist (level) — *see* Injury, blood vessel, hand
- brachial plexus S14.3 ☑
    - newborn P14.3
- brain (traumatic) S06.9 ☑
    - diffuse (axonal) S06.2X ☑
    - focal S06.30 ☑
- brainstem S06.38 ☑
- breast NOS S29.9 ☑
- broad ligament — *see* Injury, pelvic organ, specified site NEC
- bronchus, bronchi — *see* Injury, intrathoracic, bronchus
- brow S09.90 ☑
- buttock S39.92 ☑
- canthus, eye S05.90 ☑
- cardiac plexus — *see* Injury, nerve, thorax, sympathetic
- cauda equina S34.3 ☑
- cavernous sinus — *see* Injury, intracranial
- cecum — *see* Injury, colon
- celiac ganglion or plexus — *see* Injury, nerve, lumbosacral, sympathetic
- cerebellum — *see* Injury, intracranial
- cerebral — *see* Injury, intracranial
- cervix (uteri) — *see* Injury, uterus
- cheek (wall) S09.93 ☑
- chest — *see* Injury, thorax
- childbirth (newborn) (*see also* Birth, injury)
    - maternal NEC O71.9
- chin S09.93 ☑
- choroid (eye) — *see* Injury, eye, specified site NEC
- clitoris S39.94 ☑
- coccyx (*see also* Injury, back, lower)
    - complicating delivery O71.6
- colon — *see* Injury, intestine, large
- common bile duct — *see* Injury, liver
- conjunctiva (superficial) — *see* Injury, eye, conjunctiva
- conus medullaris — *see* Injury, spinal, sacral
- cord
    - spermatic (pelvic region) S37.898 ☑
        - scrotal region S39.848 ☑
    - spinal — *see* Injury, spinal cord, by region
- cornea — *see* Injury, eye, specified site NEC
    - abrasion — *see* Injury, eye, cornea, abrasion
- cortex (cerebral) (*see also* Injury, intracranial)
    - visual — *see* Injury, nerve, optic
- costal region NEC S29.9 ☑
- costochondral NEC S29.9 ☑
- cranial
    - cavity — *see* Injury, intracranial
    - nerve — *see* Injury, nerve, cranial
- crushing — *see* Crush
- cutaneous sensory nerve
- cystic duct — *see* Injury, liver
- deep tissue — *see* Contusion, by site
    - meaning pressure ulcer — *see* Ulcer, pressure, unstageable, by site
- delivery (newborn) P15.9
    - maternal NEC O71.9
- Descemet's membrane — *see* Injury, eyeball, penetrating
- diaphragm — *see* Injury, intrathoracic, diaphragm
- duodenum — *see* Injury, intestine, small, duodenum
- ear (auricle) (external) (canal) S09.91 ☑
    - abrasion — *see* Abrasion, ear
    - bite — *see* Bite, ear
    - blister — *see* Blister, ear
    - bruise — *see* Contusion, ear
    - contusion — *see* Contusion, ear
    - external constriction — *see* Constriction, external, ear
    - hematoma — *see* Hematoma, ear
    - inner — *see* Injury, ear, middle

Injury — *continued*
- ear — *continued*
    - laceration — *see* Laceration, ear
    - middle S09.30 ☑
        - blast — *see* Injury, blast, ear
        - specified NEC S09.39 ☑
    - puncture — *see* Puncture, ear
    - superficial — *see* Injury, superficial, ear
- eighth cranial nerve (acoustic or auditory) — *see* Injury, nerve, acoustic
- elbow S59.90 ☑
    - contusion — *see* Contusion, elbow
    - dislocation — *see* Dislocation, elbow
    - fracture — *see* Fracture, ulna, upper end
    - open — *see* Wound, open, elbow
    - specified NEC S59.80 ☑
    - sprain — *see* Sprain, elbow
    - superficial — *see* Injury, superficial, elbow
- eleventh cranial nerve (accessory) — *see* Injury, nerve, accessory
- epididymis S39.94 ☑
- epigastric region S39.91 ☑
- epiglottis NEC S19.89 ☑
- esophageal plexus — *see* Injury, nerve, thorax, sympathetic
- esophagus (thoracic part) (*see also* Injury, intrathoracic, esophagus)
    - cervical NEC S19.85 ☑
- eustachian tube S09.30 ☑
- eye S05.9 ☑
    - avulsion S05.7 ☑
    - ball — *see* Injury, eyeball
    - conjunctiva S05.0 ☑
    - cornea
        - abrasion S05.0 ☑
        - laceration S05.3 ☑
            - with prolapse S05.2 ☑
    - lacrimal apparatus S05.8X ☑
    - orbit penetration S05.4 ☑
    - specified site NEC S05.8X ☑
- eyeball S05.8X ☑
    - contusion S05.1 ☑
    - penetrating S05.6 ☑
        - with
            - foreign body S05.5 ☑
            - prolapse or loss of intraocular tissue S05.2 ☑
            - without prolapse or loss of intraocular tissue S05.3 ☑
    - specified type NEC S05.8 ☑
- eyebrow S09.93 ☑
- eyelid S09.93 ☑
    - abrasion — *see* Abrasion, eyelid
    - contusion — *see* Contusion, eyelid
    - open — *see* Wound, open, eyelid
- face S09.93 ☑
- fallopian tube S37.509 ☑
    - bilateral S37.502 ☑
        - blast injury S37.512 ☑
        - contusion S37.522 ☑
        - laceration S37.532 ☑
        - specified type NEC S37.592 ☑
    - blast injury (primary) S37.519 ☑
        - bilateral S37.512 ☑
        - secondary — *see* Injury, fallopian tube, specified type NEC
        - unilateral S37.511 ☑
    - contusion S37.529 ☑
        - bilateral S37.522 ☑
        - unilateral S37.521 ☑
    - laceration S37.539 ☑
        - bilateral S37.532 ☑
        - unilateral S37.531 ☑
    - specified type NEC S37.599 ☑
        - bilateral S37.592 ☑
        - unilateral S37.591 ☑
    - unilateral S37.501 ☑
        - blast injury S37.511 ☑
        - contusion S37.521 ☑
        - laceration S37.531 ☑
        - specified type NEC S37.591 ☑
- fascia — *see* Injury, muscle
- fifth cranial nerve (trigeminal) — *see* Injury, nerve, trigeminal
- finger (nail) S69.9 ☑
    - blood vessel — *see* Injury, blood vessel, finger
    - contusion — *see* Contusion, finger
    - dislocation — *see* Dislocation, finger
    - fracture — *see* Fracture, finger
    - muscle — *see* Injury, muscle, finger
    - nerve — *see* Injury, nerve, digital, finger
    - open — *see* Wound, open, finger
    - specified NEC S69.8 ☑

Injury — *continued*
- finger — *continued*
    - sprain — *see* Sprain, finger
    - superficial — *see* Injury, superficial, finger
- first cranial nerve (olfactory) — *see* Injury, nerve, olfactory
- flank — *see* Injury, abdomen
- foot S99.92 ☑
    - blood vessel — *see* Injury, blood vessel, foot
    - contusion — *see* Contusion, foot
    - dislocation — *see* Dislocation, foot
    - fracture — *see* Fracture, foot
    - muscle — *see* Injury, muscle, foot
    - open — *see* Wound, open, foot
    - specified type NEC S99.82 ☑
    - sprain — *see* Sprain, foot
    - superficial — *see* Injury, superficial, foot
- forceps NOS P15.9
- forearm S59.91 ☑
    - blood vessel — *see* Injury, blood vessel, forearm
    - contusion — *see* Contusion, forearm
    - fracture — *see* Fracture, forearm
    - muscle — *see* Injury, muscle, forearm
    - nerve — *see* Injury, nerve, forearm
    - open — *see* Wound, open, forearm
    - specified NEC S59.81 ☑
    - superficial — *see* Injury, superficial, forearm
- forehead S09.90 ☑
- fourth cranial nerve (trochlear) — *see* Injury, nerve, trochlear
- gallbladder S36.129 ☑
    - contusion S36.122 ☑
    - laceration S36.123 ☑
    - specified NEC S36.128 ☑
- ganglion
    - celiac, coeliac — *see* Injury, nerve, lumbosacral, sympathetic
    - gasserian — *see* Injury, nerve, trigeminal
    - stellate — *see* Injury, nerve, thorax, sympathetic
    - thoracic sympathetic — *see* Injury, nerve, thorax, sympathetic
- gasserian ganglion — *see* Injury, nerve, trigeminal
- gastric artery — *see* Injury, blood vessel, celiac artery, branch
- gastroduodenal artery — *see* Injury, blood vessel, celiac artery, branch
- gastrointestinal tract — *see* Injury, intra-abdominal
    - with open wound into abdominal cavity — *see* Wound, open, with penetration into peritoneal cavity
    - colon — *see* Injury, intestine, large
    - rectum — *see* Injury, intestine, large, rectum
        - with open wound into abdominal cavity S36.61 ☑
    - specified site NEC — *see* Injury, intra-abdominal, specified, site NEC
    - stomach — *see* Injury, stomach
    - small intestine — *see* Injury, intestine, small
- genital organ(s)
    - external S39.94 ☑
        - specified NEC S39.848 ☑
    - internal S37.90 ☑
        - fallopian tube — *see* Injury, fallopian tube
        - ovary — *see* Injury, ovary
        - prostate — *see* Injury, prostate
        - seminal vesicle — *see* Injury, pelvis, organ, specified site NEC
        - uterus — *see* Injury, uterus
        - vas deferens — *see* Injury, pelvis, organ, specified site NEC
    - obstetrical trauma O71.9
- gland
    - lacrimal laceration — *see* Injury, eye, specified site NEC
    - salivary S09.93 ☑
    - thyroid NEC S19.84 ☑
- globe (eye) S05.90 ☑
    - specified NEC S05.8X ☑
- groin — *see* Injury, abdomen
- gum S09.90 ☑
- hand S69.9 ☑
    - blood vessel — *see* Injury, blood vessel, hand
    - contusion — *see* Contusion, hand
    - fracture — *see* Fracture, hand
    - muscle — *see* Injury, muscle, hand
    - nerve — *see* Injury, nerve, hand
    - open — *see* Wound, open, hand
    - specified NEC S69.8 ☑
    - sprain — *see* Sprain, hand
    - superficial — *see* Injury, superficial, hand
- head S09.90 ☑
    - with loss of consciousness S06.9 ☑
    - specified NEC S09.8 ☑

Injury

Injury — *continued*
- heart S26.90 ☑
  - with hemopericardium S26.00 ☑
    - contusion S26.01 ☑
    - laceration (mild) S26.020 ☑
      - moderate S26.021 ☑
      - major S26.022 ☑
    - specified type NEC S26.09 ☑
  - contusion S26.91 ☑
  - laceration S26.92 ☑
  - specified type NEC S26.99 ☑
  - without hemopericardium S26.10 ☑
    - contusion S26.11 ☑
    - laceration S26.12 ☑
    - specified type NEC S26.19 ☑
- heel — *see* Injury, foot
- hepatic
  - artery — *see* Injury, blood vessel, celiac artery, branch
  - duct — *see* Injury, liver
  - vein — *see* Injury, vena cava, inferior
- hip S79.91 ☑
  - blood vessel — *see* Injury, blood vessel, hip
  - contusion — *see* Contusion, hip
  - dislocation — *see* Dislocation, hip
  - fracture — *see* Fracture, femur, neck
  - muscle — *see* Injury, muscle, hip
  - nerve — *see* Injury, nerve, hip
  - open — *see* Wound, open, hip
  - sprain — *see* Sprain, hip
  - superficial — *see* Injury, superficial, hip
  - specified NEC S79.81 ☑
- hymen S39.94 ☑
- hypogastric
  - blood vessel — *see* Injury, blood vessel, iliac
  - plexus — *see* Injury, nerve, lumbosacral, sympathetic
- ileum — *see* Injury, intestine, small
- iliac region S39.91 ☑
- instrumental (during surgery) — *see* Laceration, accidental complicating surgery
- birth injury — *see* Birth, injury
- nonsurgical — *see* Injury, by site
- obstetrical O71.9
  - bladder O71.5
  - cervix O71.3
  - high vaginal O71.4
  - perineal NOS O70.9
  - urethra O71.5
  - uterus O71.5
    - with rupture or perforation O71.1
- internal T14.8 ☑
  - aorta — *see* Injury, aorta
  - bladder (sphincter) — *see* Injury, bladder
    - with
      - ectopic or molar pregnancy O08.6
      - following ectopic or molar pregnancy O08.6
      - obstetrical trauma O71.5
  - bronchus, bronchi — *see* Injury, intrathoracic, bronchus
  - cecum — *see* Injury, intestine, large
  - cervix (uteri) (*see also* Injury, uterus)
    - with ectopic or molar pregnancy O08.6
    - following ectopic or molar pregnancy O08.6
    - obstetrical trauma O71.3
  - chest — *see* Injury, intrathoracic
  - gastrointestinal tract — *see* Injury, intra-abdominal
  - heart — *see* Injury, heart
  - intestine NEC — *see* Injury, intestine
  - intrauterine — *see* Injury, uterus
  - mesentery — *see* Injury, intra-abdominal, specified, site NEC
  - pelvis, pelvic (organ) S37.90 ☑
    - following ectopic or molar pregnancy (subsequent episode) O08.6
    - obstetrical trauma NEC O71.5
      - rupture or perforation O71.1
    - specified NEC S39.83 ☑
  - rectum — *see* Injury, intestine, large, rectum
  - stomach — *see* Injury, stomach
  - ureter — *see* Injury, ureter
  - urethra (sphincter) following ectopic or molar pregnancy O08.6
  - uterus — *see* Injury, uterus
- interscapular area — *see* Injury, thorax
- intestine
  - large S36.509 ☑
    - ascending (right) S36.500 ☑
      - blast injury (primary) S36.510 ☑
        - secondary S36.590 ☑
      - contusion S36.520 ☑

Injury — *continued*
- intestine — *continued*
  - large — *continued*
    - laceration S36.530 ☑
    - specified type NEC S36.590 ☑
    - blast injury (primary) S36.519 ☑
      - ascending (right) S36.510 ☑
      - descending (left) S36.512 ☑
      - rectum S36.61 ☑
      - sigmoid S36.513 ☑
      - specified site NEC S36.518 ☑
      - transverse S36.511 ☑
    - contusion S36.529 ☑
      - ascending (right) S36.520 ☑
      - descending (left) S36.522 ☑
      - rectum S36.62 ☑
      - sigmoid S36.523 ☑
      - specified site NEC S36.528 ☑
      - transverse S36.521 ☑
    - descending (left) S36.502 ☑
      - blast injury (primary) S36.512 ☑
        - secondary S36.592 ☑
      - contusion S36.522 ☑
      - laceration S36.532 ☑
      - specified type NEC S36.592 ☑
    - laceration S36.539 ☑
      - ascending (right) S36.530 ☑
      - descending (left) S36.532 ☑
      - rectum S36.63 ☑
      - sigmoid S36.533 ☑
      - specified site NEC S36.538 ☑
      - transverse S36.531 ☑
    - rectum S36.60 ☑
      - blast injury (primary) S36.61 ☑
        - secondary S36.69 ☑
      - contusion S36.62 ☑
      - laceration S36.63 ☑
      - specified type NEC S36.69 ☑
    - sigmoid S36.503 ☑
      - blast injury (primary) S36.513 ☑
        - secondary S36.593 ☑
      - contusion S36.523 ☑
      - laceration S36.533 ☑
      - specified type NEC S36.593 ☑
    - specified
      - site NEC S36.508 ☑
        - blast injury (primary) S36.518 ☑
          - secondary S36.598 ☑
        - contusion S36.528 ☑
        - laceration S36.538 ☑
        - specified type NEC S36.598 ☑
      - type NEC S36.599 ☑
        - ascending (right) S36.590 ☑
        - descending (left) S36.592 ☑
        - rectum S36.69 ☑
        - sigmoid S36.593 ☑
        - specified site NEC S36.598 ☑
        - transverse S36.591 ☑
    - transverse S36.501 ☑
      - blast injury (primary) S36.511 ☑
        - secondary S36.591 ☑
      - contusion S36.521 ☑
      - laceration S36.531 ☑
      - specified type NEC S36.591 ☑
  - small S36.409 ☑
    - blast injury (primary) S36.419 ☑
      - duodenum S36.410 ☑
      - secondary S36.499 ☑
        - duodenum S36.490 ☑
        - specified site NEC S36.498 ☑
      - specified site NEC S36.418 ☑
    - contusion S36.429 ☑
      - duodenum S36.420 ☑
      - specified site NEC S36.428 ☑
    - duodenum S36.400 ☑
      - blast injury (primary) S36.410 ☑
        - secondary S36.490 ☑
      - contusion S36.420 ☑
      - laceration S36.430 ☑
      - specified NEC S36.490 ☑
    - laceration S36.439 ☑
      - duodenum S36.430 ☑
      - specified site NEC S36.438 ☑
    - specified
      - type NEC S36.499 ☑
        - duodenum S36.490 ☑
        - specified site NEC S36.498 ☑
      - site NEC S36.408 ☑
- intra-abdominal S36.90 ☑
  - adrenal gland — *see* Injury, adrenal gland
  - bladder — *see* Injury, bladder
  - colon — *see* Injury, intestine, large
  - contusion S36.92 ☑

Injury — *continued*
- intra-abdominal — *continued*
  - fallopian tube — *see* Injury, fallopian tube
  - gallbladder — *see* Injury, gallbladder
  - intestine — *see* Injury, intestine
  - laceration S36.93 ☑
  - liver — *see* Injury, liver
  - kidney — *see* Injury, kidney
  - ovary — *see* Injury, ovary
  - pancreas — *see* Injury, pancreas
  - pelvic NOS S37.90 ☑
  - peritoneum — *see* Injury, intra-abdominal, specified, site NEC
  - prostate — *see* Injury, prostate
  - rectum — *see* Injury, intestine, large, rectum
  - retroperitoneum — *see* Injury, intra-abdominal, specified, site NEC
  - seminal vesicle — *see* Injury, pelvis, organ, specified site NEC
  - small intestine — *see* Injury, intestine, small
  - specified
    - site NEC S36.899 ☑
      - contusion S36.892 ☑
      - laceration S36.893 ☑
      - specified type NEC S36.898 ☑
    - type NEC S36.99 ☑
  - pelvic S37.90 ☑
    - specified
      - site NEC S37.899 ☑
        - specified type NEC S37.898 ☑
      - type NEC S37.99 ☑
  - spleen — *see* Injury, spleen
  - stomach — *see* Injury, stomach
  - ureter — *see* Injury, ureter
  - urethra — *see* Injury, urethra
  - uterus — *see* Injury, uterus
  - vas deferens — *see* Injury, pelvis, organ, specified site NEC
- intracranial (traumatic) S06.9 ☑
  - cerebellar hemorrhage, traumatic — *see* Injury, intracranial, focal
  - cerebral edema, traumatic S06.1X ☑
    - diffuse S06.1X ☑
    - focal S06.1X ☑
  - diffuse (axonal) S06.2X ☑
  - epidural hemorrhage (traumatic) S06.4X ☑
  - focal brain injury S06.30 ☑
    - contusion — *see* Contusion, cerebral
    - laceration — *see* Laceration, cerebral
    - intracerebral hemorrhage, traumatic S06.36 ☑
      - left side S06.35 ☑
      - right side S06.34 ☑
    - subarachnoid hemorrhage, traumatic S06.6X ☑
    - subdural hemorrhage, traumatic S06.5X ☑
  - intraocular — *see* Injury, eyeball, penetrating
- intrathoracic S27.9 ☑
  - bronchus S27.409 ☑
    - bilateral S27.402 ☑
    - blast injury (primary) S27.419 ☑
      - bilateral S27.412 ☑
      - secondary — *see* Injury, intrathoracic, bronchus, specified type NEC
      - unilateral S27.411 ☑
    - contusion S27.429 ☑
      - bilateral S27.422 ☑
      - unilateral S27.421 ☑
    - laceration S27.439 ☑
      - bilateral S27.432 ☑
      - unilateral S27.431 ☑
    - specified type NEC S27.499 ☑
      - bilateral S27.492 ☑
      - unilateral S27.491 ☑
    - unilateral S27.401 ☑
  - diaphragm S27.809 ☑
    - contusion S27.802 ☑
    - laceration S27.803 ☑
    - specified type NEC S27.808 ☑
  - esophagus (thoracic) S27.819 ☑
    - contusion S27.812 ☑
    - laceration S27.813 ☑
    - specified type NEC S27.818 ☑
  - heart — *see* Injury, heart
  - hemopneumothorax S27.2 ☑
  - hemothorax S27.1 ☑
  - lung S27.309 ☑
    - aspiration J69.0
    - bilateral S27.302 ☑
    - blast injury (primary) S27.319 ☑
      - bilateral S27.312 ☑
      - secondary — *see* Injury, intrathoracic, lung, specified type NEC
    - unilateral S27.311 ☑

☑ **Additional character required**

Injury — *continued*
  intrathoracic — *continued*
    contusion S27.329 ☑
      bilateral S27.322 ☑
      unilateral S27.321 ☑
    laceration S27.339 ☑
      bilateral S27.332 ☑
      unilateral S27.331 ☑
    specified type NEC S27.399 ☑
      bilateral S27.392 ☑
      unilateral S27.391 ☑
    unilateral S27.301 ☑
    pleura S27.60 ☑
      laceration S27.63 ☑
      specified type NEC S27.69 ☑
    pneumothorax S27.0 ☑
    specified organ NEC S27.899 ☑
      contusion S27.892 ☑
      laceration S27.893 ☑
      specified type NEC S27.898 ☑
    thoracic duct — *see* Injury, intrathoracic, specified organ NEC
    thymus gland — *see* Injury, intrathoracic, specified organ NEC
    trachea, thoracic S27.50 ☑
      blast (primary) S27.51 ☑
      contusion S27.52 ☑
      laceration S27.53 ☑
      specified type NEC S27.59 ☑
  iris — *see* Injury, eye, specified site NEC
    penetrating — *see* Injury, eyeball, penetrating
  jaw S09.93 ☑
  jejunum — *see* Injury, intestine, small
  joint NOS T14.8 ☑
    old or residual — *see* Disorder, joint, specified type NEC
  kidney S37.00 ☑
    acute (nontraumatic) N17.9
    contusion — *see* Contusion, kidney
    laceration — *see* Laceration, kidney
    specified NEC S37.09 ☑
  knee S89.9 ☑
    contusion — *see* Contusion, knee
    dislocation — *see* Dislocation, knee
    meniscus (lateral) (medial) — *see* Sprain, knee, specified site NEC
      old injury or tear — *see* Derangement, knee, meniscus, due to old injury
    open — *see* Wound, open, knee
    specified NEC S89.8 ☑
    sprain — *see* Sprain, knee
    superficial — *see* Injury, superficial, knee
  labium (majus) (minus) S39.94 ☑
  labyrinth, ear S09.30 ☑
  lacrimal apparatus, duct, gland, or sac — *see* Injury, eye, specified site NEC
  larynx NEC S19.81 ☑
  leg (lower) S89.9 ☑
    blood vessel — *see* Injury, blood vessel, leg
    contusion — *see* Contusion, leg
    fracture — *see* Fracture, leg
    muscle — *see* Injury, muscle, leg
    nerve — *see* Injury, nerve, leg
    open — *see* Wound, open, leg
    specified NEC S89.8 ☑
    superficial — *see* Injury, superficial, leg
  lens, eye — *see* Injury, eye, specified site NEC
    penetrating — *see* Injury, eyeball, penetrating
  limb NEC T14.8 ☑
  lip S09.93 ☑
  liver S36.119 ☑
    contusion S36.112 ☑
    laceration S36.113 ☑
      major (stellate) S36.116 ☑
      minor S36.114 ☑
      moderate S36.115 ☑
      specified NEC S36.118 ☑
  lower back S39.92 ☑
    specified NEC S39.82 ☑
  lumbar, lumbosacral (region) S39.92 ☑
    plexus — *see* Injury, lumbosacral plexus
  lumbosacral plexus S34.4 ☑
  lung (*see also* Injury, intrathoracic, lung)
    aspiration J69.0
    transfusion-related (TRALI) J95.84
  lymphatic thoracic duct — *see* Injury, intrathoracic, specified organ NEC
  malar region S09.93 ☑
  mastoid region S09.90 ☑
  maxilla S09.93 ☑
  mediastinum — *see* Injury, intrathoracic, specified organ NEC

Injury — *continued*
  membrane, brain — *see* Injury, intracranial
  meningeal artery — *see* Injury, intracranial, subdural hemorrhage
  meninges (cerebral) — *see* Injury, intracranial
  mesenteric
    artery
      branch S35.299 ☑
        laceration (minor) (superficial) S35.291 ☑
          major S35.292 ☑
        specified NEC S35.298 ☑
      inferior S35.239 ☑
        laceration (minor) (superficial) S35.231 ☑
          major S35.232 ☑
        specified NEC S35.238 ☑
      superior S35.229 ☑
        laceration (minor) (superficial) S35.221 ☑
          major S35.222 ☑
        specified NEC S35.228 ☑
    plexus (inferior) (superior) — *see* Injury, nerve, lumbosacral, sympathetic
    vein
      inferior S35.349 ☑
        laceration S35.341 ☑
        specified NEC S35.348 ☑
      superior S35.339 ☑
        laceration S35.331 ☑
        specified NEC S35.338 ☑
  mesentery — *see* Injury, intra-abdominal, specified site NEC
  mesosalpinx — *see* Injury, pelvic organ, specified site NEC
  middle ear S09.30 ☑
  midthoracic region NOS S29.9 ☑
  mouth S09.93 ☑
  multiple NOS T07 ☑
  muscle (and fascia) (and tendon)
    abdomen S39.001 ☑
      laceration S39.021 ☑
      specified type NEC S39.091 ☑
      strain S39.011 ☑
    abductor
      thumb, forearm level — *see* Injury, muscle, thumb, abductor
    adductor
      thigh S76.20 ☑
        laceration S76.22 ☑
        specified type NEC S76.29 ☑
        strain S76.21 ☑
    ankle — *see* Injury, muscle, foot
    anterior muscle group, at leg level (lower) S86.20 ☑
      laceration S86.22 ☑
      specified type NEC S86.29 ☑
      strain S86.21 ☑
    arm (upper) — *see* Injury, muscle, shoulder
    biceps (parts NEC) S46.20 ☑
      laceration S46.22 ☑
      long head S46.10 ☑
        laceration S46.12 ☑
        strain S46.11 ☑
      specified type NEC S46.19 ☑
      specified type NEC S46.29 ☑
      strain S46.21 ☑
    extensor
      finger(s) (other than thumb) — *see* Injury, muscle, finger by site, extensor
      forearm level, specified NEC — *see* Injury, muscle, forearm, extensor
      thumb — *see* Injury, muscle, thumb, extensor
      toe (large) (ankle level) (foot level) — *see* Injury, muscle, toe, extensor
    finger
      extensor (forearm level) S56.40 ☑
        hand level S66.309 ☑
          laceration S66.329 ☑
          specified type NEC S66.399 ☑
          strain S66.319 ☑
        laceration S56.429 ☑
        specified type NEC S56.499 ☑
        strain S56.419 ☑
      flexor (forearm level) S56.10 ☑
        hand level S66.109 ☑
          laceration S66.129 ☑
          specified type NEC S66.199 ☑
          strain S66.119 ☑
        laceration S56.129 ☑
        specified type NEC S56.199 ☑
        strain S56.119 ☑
      intrinsic S66.509 ☑
        laceration S66.529 ☑
        specified type NEC S66.599 ☑
        strain S66.519 ☑

Injury — *continued*
  muscle — *continued*
    index
      extensor (forearm level)
        hand level S66.308 ☑
          laceration S66.32 ☑
          specified type NEC S66.39 ☑
          strain S66.31 ☑
        specified type NEC S56.492 ☑
      flexor (forearm level)
        hand level S66.108 ☑
          laceration S66.12 ☑
          specified type NEC S66.19 ☑
          strain S66.11 ☑
        specified type NEC S56.19 ☑
        strain S56.11 ☑
      intrinsic S66.50 ☑
        laceration S66.52 ☑
        specified type NEC S66.59 ☑
        strain S66.51 ☑
    little
      extensor (forearm level)
        hand level S66.30 ☑
          laceration S66.32 ☑
          specified type NEC S66.39 ☑
          strain S66.31 ☑
        laceration S56.42 ☑
        specified type NEC S56.49 ☑
        strain S56.41 ☑
      flexor (forearm level)
        hand level S66.10 ☑
          laceration S66.12 ☑
          specified type NEC S66.19 ☑
          strain S66.11 ☑
        laceration S56.12 ☑
        specified type NEC S56.19 ☑
        strain S56.11 ☑
      intrinsic S66.50 ☑
        laceration S66.52 ☑
        specified type NEC S66.59 ☑
        strain S66.51 ☑
    middle
      extensor (forearm level)
        hand level S66.30 ☑
          laceration S66.32 ☑
          specified type NEC S66.39 ☑
          strain S66.31 ☑
        laceration S56.42 ☑
        specified type NEC S56.49 ☑
        strain S56.41 ☑
      flexor (forearm level)
        hand level S66.10 ☑
          laceration S66.12 ☑
          specified type NEC S66.19 ☑
          strain S66.11 ☑
        laceration S56.12 ☑
        specified type NEC S56.19 ☑
        strain S56.11 ☑
      intrinsic S66.50 ☑
        laceration S66.52 ☑
        specified type NEC S66.59 ☑
        strain S66.51 ☑
    ring
      extensor (forearm level)
        hand level S66.30 ☑
          laceration S66.32 ☑
          specified type NEC S66.39 ☑
          strain S66.31 ☑
        laceration S56.42 ☑
        specified type NEC S56.49 ☑
        strain S56.41 ☑
      flexor (forearm level)
        hand level S66.10 ☑
          laceration S66.12 ☑
          specified type NEC S66.19 ☑
          strain S66.11 ☑
        laceration S56.12 ☑
        specified type NEC S56.19 ☑
        strain S56.11 ☑
      intrinsic S66.50 ☑
        laceration S66.52 ☑
        specified type NEC S66.59 ☑
        strain S66.51 ☑
    flexor
      finger(s) (other than thumb) — *see* Injury, muscle, finger
      forearm level, specified NEC — *see* Injury, muscle, forearm, flexor
      thumb — *see* Injury, muscle, thumb, flexor
      toe (long) (ankle level) (foot level) — *see* Injury, muscle, toe, flexor
    foot S96.90 ☑

Injury

Injury — *continued*
muscle — *continued*
intrinsic S96.20 ☑
laceration S96.22 ☑
specified type NEC S96.29 ☑
strain S96.21 ☑
laceration S96.92 ☑
long extensor, toe — *see* Injury, muscle, toe, extensor
long flexor, toe — *see* Injury, muscle, toe, flexor
specified
site NEC S96.80 ☑
laceration S96.82 ☑
specified type NEC S96.89 ☑
strain S96.81 ☑
type NEC S96.99 ☑
strain S96.91 ☑
forearm (level) S56.90 ☑
extensor S56.50 ☑
laceration S56.52 ☑
specified type NEC S56.59 ☑
strain S56.51 ☑
flexor S56.20 ☑
laceration S56.22 ☑
specified type NEC S56.29 ☑
strain S56.21 ☑
laceration S56.92 ☑
specified S56.99 ☑
site NEC S56.80 ☑
laceration S56.82 ☑
strain S56.81 ☑
type NEC S56.89 ☑
strain S56.91 ☑
hand (level) S66.90 ☑
laceration S66.92 ☑
specified
site NEC S66.80 ☑
laceration S66.82 ☑
specified type NEC S66.89 ☑
strain S66.81 ☑
type NEC S66.99 ☑
strain S66.91 ☑
head S09.10 ☑
laceration S09.12 ☑
specified type NEC S09.19 ☑
strain S09.11 ☑
hip NEC S76.00 ☑
laceration S76.02 ☑
specified type NEC S76.09 ☑
strain S76.01 ☑
intrinsic
ankle and foot level — *see* Injury, muscle, foot, intrinsic
finger (other than thumb) — *see* Injury, muscle, finger by site, intrinsic
foot (level) — *see* Injury, muscle, foot, intrinsic
thumb — *see* Injury, muscle, thumb, intrinsic
leg (level) (lower) S86.90 ☑
Achilles tendon — *see* Injury, Achilles tendon
anterior muscle group — *see* Injury, muscle, anterior muscle group
laceration S86.92 ☑
peroneal muscle group — *see* Injury, muscle, peroneal muscle group
posterior muscle group — *see* Injury, muscle, posterior muscle group, leg level
specified
site NEC S86.80 ☑
laceration S86.82 ☑
specified type NEC S86.89 ☑
strain S86.81 ☑
type NEC S86.99 ☑
strain S86.91 ☑
long
extensor toe, at ankle and foot level — *see* Injury, muscle, toe, extensor
flexor, toe, at ankle and foot level — *see* Injury, muscle, toe, flexor
head, biceps — *see* Injury, muscle, biceps, long head
lower back S39.002 ☑
laceration S39.022 ☑
specified type NEC S39.092 ☑
strain S39.012 ☑
neck (level) S16.9 ☑
laceration S16.2 ☑
specified type NEC S16.8 ☑
strain S16.1 ☑
pelvis S39.003 ☑
laceration S39.023 ☑
specified type NEC S39.093 ☑
strain S39.013 ☑

Injury — *continued*
muscle — *continued*
peroneal muscle group, at leg level (lower) S86.30 ☑
laceration S86.32 ☑
specified type NEC S86.39 ☑
strain S86.31 ☑
posterior muscle (group)
leg level (lower) S86.10 ☑
laceration S86.12 ☑
specified type NEC S86.19 ☑
strain S86.11 ☑
thigh level S76.30 ☑
laceration S76.32 ☑
specified type NEC S76.39 ☑
strain S76.31 ☑
quadriceps (thigh) S76.10 ☑
laceration S76.12 ☑
specified type NEC S76.19 ☑
strain S76.11 ☑
shoulder S46.90 ☑
laceration S46.92 ☑
rotator cuff — *see* Injury, rotator cuff
specified site NEC S46.80 ☑
laceration S46.82 ☑
strain S46.81 ☑
specified type NEC S46.89 ☑
strain S46.91 ☑
specified type NEC S46.99 ☑
thigh NEC (level) S76.90 ☑
adductor — *see* Injury, muscle, adductor, thigh
laceration S76.92 ☑
posterior muscle (group) — *see* Injury, muscle, posterior muscle, thigh level
quadriceps — *see* Injury, muscle, quadriceps
specified
site NEC S76.80 ☑
laceration S76.82 ☑
specified type NEC S76.89 ☑
strain S76.81 ☑
type NEC S76.99 ☑
strain S76.91 ☑
thorax (level) S29.009 ☑
back wall S29.002 ☑
front wall S29.001 ☑
laceration S29.029 ☑
back wall S29.022 ☑
front wall S29.021 ☑
specified type NEC S29.099 ☑
back wall S29.092 ☑
front wall S29.091 ☑
strain S29.019 ☑
back wall S29.012 ☑
front wall S29.011 ☑
thumb
abductor (forearm level) S56.30 ☑
laceration S56.32 ☑
specified type NEC S56.39 ☑
strain S56.31 ☑
extensor (forearm level) S56.30 ☑
hand level S66.20 ☑
laceration S66.22 ☑
specified type NEC S66.29 ☑
strain S66.21 ☑
laceration S56.32 ☑
specified type NEC S56.39 ☑
strain S56.31 ☑
flexor (forearm level) S56.00 ☑
hand level S66.00 ☑
laceration S66.02 ☑
specified type NEC S66.09 ☑
strain S66.01 ☑
laceration S56.02 ☑
specified type NEC S56.09 ☑
strain S56.01 ☑
wrist level — *see* Injury, muscle, thumb, flexor, hand level
intrinsic S66.40 ☑
laceration S66.42 ☑
specified type NEC S66.49 ☑
strain S66.41 ☑
toe (*see also* Injury, muscle, foot)
extensor, long S96.10 ☑
laceration S96.12 ☑
specified type NEC S96.19 ☑
strain S96.11 ☑
flexor, long S96.00 ☑
laceration S96.02 ☑
specified type NEC S96.09 ☑
strain S96.01 ☑
triceps S46.30 ☑
laceration S46.32 ☑

Injury — *continued*
muscle — *continued*
specified type NEC S46.39 ☑
strain S46.31 ☑
wrist (and hand) level — *see* Injury, muscle, hand
musculocutaneous nerve — *see* Injury, nerve, musculocutaneous
myocardium — *see* Injury, heart
nape — *see* Injury, neck
nasal (septum) (sinus) S09.92 ☑
nasopharynx S09.92 ☑
neck S19.9 ☑
specified NEC S19.80 ☑
specified site NEC S19.89 ☑
nerve NEC T14.8 ☑
abdomen S34.9 ☑
peripheral S34.6 ☑
specified site NEC S34.8 ☑
abducens S04.4 ☑
contusion S04.4 ☑
laceration S04.4 ☑
specified type NEC S04.4 ☑
abducent — *see* Injury, nerve, abducens
accessory S04.7 ☑
contusion S04.7 ☑
laceration S04.7 ☑
specified type NEC S04.7 ☑
acoustic S04.6 ☑
contusion S04.6 ☑
laceration S04.6 ☑
specified type NEC S04.6 ☑
ankle S94.9 ☑
cutaneous sensory S94.3 ☑
specified site NEC — *see* subcategory S94.8 ☑
anterior crural, femoral — *see* Injury, nerve, femoral
arm (upper) S44.9 ☑
axillary — *see* Injury, nerve, axillary
cutaneous — *see* Injury, nerve, cutaneous, arm
median — *see* Injury, nerve, median, upper arm
musculocutaneous — *see* Injury, nerve, musculocutaneous
radial — *see* Injury, nerve, radial, upper arm
specified site NEC — *see* subcategory S44.8 ☑
ulnar — *see* Injury, nerve, ulnar, arm
auditory — *see* Injury, nerve, acoustic
axillary S44.3 ☑
brachial plexus — *see* Injury, brachial plexus
cervical sympathetic S14.5 ☑
cranial S04.9 ☑
contusion S04.9 ☑
eighth (acoustic or auditory) — *see* Injury, nerve, acoustic
eleventh (accessory) — *see* Injury, nerve, accessory
fifth (trigeminal) — *see* Injury, nerve, trigeminal
first (olfactory) — *see* Injury, nerve, olfactory
fourth (trochlear) — *see* Injury, nerve, trochlear
laceration S04.9 ☑
ninth (glossopharyngeal) — *see* Injury, nerve, glossopharyngeal
second (optic) — *see* Injury, nerve, optic
seventh (facial) — *see* Injury, nerve, facial
sixth (abducent) — *see* Injury, nerve, abducens
specified
nerve NEC S04.89 ☑
contusion S04.89 ☑
laceration S04.89 ☑
specified type NEC S04.89 ☑
type NEC S04.9 ☑
tenth (pneumogastric or vagus) — *see* Injury, nerve, vagus
third (oculomotor) — *see* Injury, nerve, oculomotor
twelfth (hypoglossal) — *see* Injury, nerve, hypoglossal
cutaneous sensory
ankle (level) S94.3 ☑
arm (upper) (level) S44.5 ☑
foot (level) — *see* Injury, nerve, cutaneous sensory, ankle
forearm (level) S54.3 ☑
hip (level) S74.2 ☑
leg (lower level) S84.2 ☑
shoulder (level) — *see* Injury, nerve, cutaneous sensory, arm
thigh (level) — *see* Injury, nerve, cutaneous sensory, hip
deep peroneal — *see* Injury, nerve, peroneal, foot
digital
finger S64.4 ☑
index S64.49 ☑

☑ **Additional character required**

Injury — *continued*
 muscle — *continued*
  little S64.49 ☑
  middle S64.49 ☑
  ring S64.49 ☑
  thumb S64.3 ☑
  toe — *see* Injury, nerve, ankle, specified site NEC
 eighth cranial (acoustic or auditory) — *see* Injury, nerve, acoustic
 eleventh cranial (accessory) — *see* Injury, nerve, accessory
 facial S04.5 ☑
  contusion S04.5 ☑
  laceration S04.5 ☑
  newborn P11.3
  specified type NEC S04.5 ☑
 femoral (hip level) (thigh level) S74.1 ☑
 fifth cranial (trigeminal) — *see* Injury, nerve, trigeminal
 finger (digital) — *see* Injury, nerve, digital, finger
 first cranial (olfactory) — *see* Injury, nerve, olfactory
 foot S94.9 ☑
  cutaneous sensory S94.3 ☑
  deep peroneal S94.2 ☑
  lateral plantar S94.0 ☑
  medial plantar S94.1 ☑
  specified site NEC — *see* subcategory S94.8 ☑
 forearm (level) S54.9 ☑
  cutaneous sensory — *see* Injury, nerve, cutaneous sensory, forearm
  median — *see* Injury, nerve, median
  radial — *see* Injury, nerve, radial
  specified site NEC — *see* subcategory S54.8 ☑
  ulnar — *see* Injury, nerve, ulnar
 fourth cranial (trochlear) — *see* Injury, nerve, trochlear
 glossopharyngeal S04.89 ☑
  specified type NEC S04.89 ☑
 hand S64.9 ☑
  median — *see* Injury, nerve, median, hand
  radial — *see* Injury, nerve, radial, hand
  specified NEC — *see* subcategory S64.8 ☑
  ulnar — *see* Injury, nerve, ulnar, hand
 hip (level) S74.9 ☑
  cutaneous sensory — *see* Injury, nerve, cutaneous sensory, hip
  femoral — *see* Injury, nerve, femoral
  sciatic — *see* Injury, nerve, sciatic
  specified site NEC — *see* subcategory S74.8 ☑
 hypoglossal S04.89 ☑
  specified type NEC S04.89 ☑
 lateral plantar S94.0 ☑
 leg (lower) S84.9 ☑
  cutaneous sensory — *see* Injury, nerve, cutaneous sensory, leg
  peroneal — *see* Injury, nerve, peroneal
  specified site NEC — *see* subcategory S84.8 ☑
  tibial — *see* Injury, nerve, tibial
  upper — *see* Injury, nerve, thigh
 lower
  back — *see* Injury, nerve, abdomen, specified site NEC
   peripheral — *see* Injury, nerve, abdomen, peripheral
  limb — *see* Injury, nerve, leg
 lumbar spinal — *see* Injury, nerve, spinal, lumbar
 lumbar plexus — *see* Injury, nerve, lumbosacral, sympathetic
 lumbosacral
  plexus — *see* Injury, nerve, lumbosacral, sympathetic
  sympathetic S34.5 ☑
 medial plantar S94.1 ☑
 median (forearm level) S54.1 ☑
  hand (level) S64.1 ☑
  upper arm (level) S44.1 ☑
  wrist (level) — *see* Injury, nerve, median, hand
 musculocutaneous S44.4 ☑
 musculospiral (upper arm level) — *see* Injury, nerve, radial, upper arm
 neck S14.9 ☑
  peripheral S14.4 ☑
  specified site NEC S14.8 ☑
  sympathetic S14.5 ☑
 ninth cranial (glossopharyngeal) — *see* Injury, nerve, glossopharyngeal
 oculomotor S04.1 ☑
  contusion S04.1 ☑
  laceration S04.1 ☑
  specified type NEC S04.1 ☑
 olfactory S04.81 ☑

Injury — *continued*
 muscle — *continued*
  specified type NEC S04.81 ☑
 optic S04.01 ☑
  contusion S04.01 ☑
  laceration S04.01 ☑
  specified type NEC S04.01 ☑
 pelvic girdle — *see* Injury, nerve, hip
 pelvis — *see* Injury, nerve, abdomen, specified site NEC
  peripheral — *see* Injury, nerve, abdomen, peripheral
 peripheral NEC T14.8 ☑
  abdomen — *see* Injury, nerve, abdomen, peripheral
  lower back — *see* Injury, nerve, abdomen, peripheral
  neck — *see* Injury, nerve, neck, peripheral
  pelvis — *see* Injury, nerve, abdomen, peripheral
  specified NEC T14.8 ☑
 peroneal (lower leg level) S84.1 ☑
  foot S94.2 ☑
 plexus
  brachial — *see* Injury, brachial plexus
  celiac, coeliac — *see* Injury, nerve, lumbosacral, sympathetic
  mesenteric, inferior — *see* Injury, nerve, lumbosacral, sympathetic
  sacral — *see* Injury, lumbosacral plexus
  spinal
   brachial — *see* Injury, brachial plexus
   lumbosacral — *see* Injury, lumbosacral plexus
 pneumogastric — *see* Injury, nerve, vagus
 radial (forearm level) S54.2 ☑
  hand (level) S64.2 ☑
  upper arm (level) S44.2 ☑
  wrist (level) — *see* Injury, nerve, radial, hand
 root — *see* Injury, nerve, spinal, root
 sacral plexus — *see* Injury, lumbosacral plexus
 sacral spinal — *see* Injury, nerve, spinal, sacral
 sciatic (hip level) (thigh level) S74.0 ☑
 second cranial (optic) — *see* Injury, nerve, optic
 seventh cranial (facial) — *see* Injury, nerve, facial
 shoulder — *see* Injury, nerve, arm
 sixth cranial (abducent) — *see* Injury, nerve, abducens
 spinal
  plexus — *see* Injury, nerve, plexus, spinal
  root
   cervical S14.2 ☑
   dorsal S24.2 ☑
   lumbar S34.21 ☑
   sacral S34.22 ☑
   thoracic — *see* Injury, nerve, spinal, root, dorsal
 splanchnic — *see* Injury, nerve, lumbosacral, sympathetic
 sympathetic NEC — *see* Injury, nerve, lumbosacral, sympathetic
  cervical — *see* Injury, nerve, cervical sympathetic
 tenth cranial (pneumogastric or vagus) — *see* Injury, nerve, vagus
 thigh (level) — *see* Injury, nerve, hip
  cutaneous sensory — *see* Injury, nerve, cutaneous sensory, hip
  femoral — *see* Injury, nerve, femoral
  sciatic — *see* Injury, nerve, sciatic
  specified NEC — *see* Injury, nerve, hip
 third cranial (oculomotor) — *see* Injury, nerve, oculomotor
 thorax S24.9 ☑
  peripheral S24.3 ☑
  specified site NEC S24.8 ☑
  sympathetic S24.4 ☑
 thumb, digital — *see* Injury, nerve, digital, thumb
 tibial (lower leg level) (posterior) S84.0 ☑
 toe — *see* Injury, nerve, ankle
 trigeminal S04.3 ☑
  contusion S04.3 ☑
  laceration S04.3 ☑
  specified type NEC S04.3 ☑
 trochlear S04.2 ☑
  contusion S04.2 ☑
  laceration S04.2 ☑
  specified type NEC S04.2 ☑
 twelfth cranial (hypoglossal) — *see* Injury, nerve, hypoglossal
 ulnar (forearm level) S54.0 ☑
  arm (upper) (level) S44.0 ☑
  hand (level) S64.0 ☑
  wrist (level) — *see* Injury, nerve, ulnar, hand

Injury — *continued*
 muscle — *continued*
  vagus S04.89 ☑
   specified type NEC S04.89 ☑
  wrist (level) — *see* Injury, nerve, hand
 ninth cranial nerve (glossopharyngeal) — *see* Injury, nerve, glossopharyngeal
 nose (septum) S09.92 ☑
 obstetrical O71.9
  specified NEC O71.89
 occipital (region) (scalp) S09.90 ☑
  lobe — *see* Injury, intracranial
 optic chiasm S04.02 ☑
 optic radiation S04.03 ☑
 optic tract and pathways S04.03 ☑
 orbit, orbital (region) — *see* Injury, eye
  penetrating (with foreign body) — *see* Injury, eye, orbit, penetrating
  specified NEC — *see* Injury, eye, specified site NEC
 ovary, ovarian S37.409 ☑
  bilateral S37.402 ☑
   contusion S37.422 ☑
   laceration S37.432 ☑
   specified type NEC S37.492 ☑
  blood vessel — *see* Injury, blood vessel, ovarian
  contusion S37.429 ☑
   bilateral S37.422 ☑
   unilateral S37.421 ☑
  laceration S37.439 ☑
   bilateral S37.432 ☑
   unilateral S37.431 ☑
  specified type NEC S37.499 ☑
   bilateral S37.492 ☑
   unilateral S37.491 ☑
  unilateral S37.401 ☑
   contusion S37.421 ☑
   laceration S37.431 ☑
   specified type NEC S37.491 ☑
 palate (hard) (soft) S09.93 ☑
 pancreas S36.209 ☑
  body S36.201 ☑
   contusion S36.221 ☑
   laceration S36.231 ☑
    major S36.261 ☑
    minor S36.241 ☑
    moderate S36.251 ☑
   specified type NEC S36.291 ☑
  contusion S36.229 ☑
  head S36.200 ☑
   contusion S36.220 ☑
   laceration S36.230 ☑
    major S36.260 ☑
    minor S36.240 ☑
    moderate S36.250 ☑
   specified type NEC S36.290 ☑
  laceration S36.239 ☑
   major S36.269 ☑
   minor S36.249 ☑
   moderate S36.259 ☑
  specified type NEC S36.299 ☑
  tail S36.202 ☑
   contusion S36.222 ☑
   laceration S36.232 ☑
    major S36.262 ☑
    minor S36.242 ☑
    moderate S36.252 ☑
   specified type NEC S36.292 ☑
 parietal (region) (scalp) S09.90 ☑
  lobe — *see* Injury, intracranial
 patellar ligament (tendon) S76.10 ☑
  laceration S76.12 ☑
  specified NEC S76.19 ☑
  strain S76.11 ☑
 pelvis, pelvic (floor) S39.93 ☑
  complicating delivery O70.1
  joint or ligament, complicating delivery O71.6
  organ S37.90 ☑
   with ectopic or molar pregnancy O08.6
   complication of abortion — *see* Abortion
   contusion S37.92 ☑
   following ectopic or molar pregnancy O08.6
   laceration S37.93 ☑
   obstetrical trauma NEC O71.5
   specified
    site NEC S37.899 ☑
     contusion S37.892 ☑
     laceration S37.893 ☑
     specified type NEC S37.898 ☑
    type NEC S37.99 ☑
  specified NEC S39.83 ☑
 penis S39.94 ☑
 perineum S39.94 ☑

Injury

Injury — *continued*

peritoneum S36.81 ☑
  laceration S36.893 ☑
periurethral tissue — *see* Injury, urethra
  complicating delivery O71.82
phalanges
  foot — *see* Injury, foot
  hand — *see* Injury, hand
pharynx NEC S19.85 ☑
pleura — *see* Injury, intrathoracic, pleura
plexus
  brachial — *see* Injury, brachial plexus
  cardiac — *see* Injury, nerve, thorax, sympathetic
  celiac, coeliac — *see* Injury, nerve, lumbosacral, sympathetic
  esophageal — *see* Injury, nerve, thorax, sympathetic
  hypogastric — *see* Injury, nerve, lumbosacral, sympathetic
  lumbar, lumbosacral — *see* Injury, lumbosacral plexus
  mesenteric — *see* Injury, nerve, lumbosacral, sympathetic
  pulmonary — *see* Injury, nerve, thorax, sympathetic
postcardiac surgery (syndrome) I97.0
prepuce S39.94 ☑
pressure
  injury — *see* Ulcer, pressure, by site
prostate S37.829 ☑
  contusion S37.822 ☑
  laceration S37.823 ☑
  specified type NEC S37.828 ☑
pubic region S39.94 ☑
pudendum S39.94 ☑
pulmonary plexus — *see* Injury, nerve, thorax, sympathetic
rectovaginal septum NEC S39.83 ☑
rectum — *see* Injury, intestine, large, rectum
retina — *see* Injury, eye, specified site NEC
  penetrating — *see* Injury, eyeball, penetrating
retroperitoneal — *see* Injury, intra-abdominal, specified site NEC
rotator cuff (muscle(s)) (tendon(s)) S46.00 ☑
  laceration S46.02 ☑
  specified type NEC S46.09 ☑
  strain S46.01 ☑
round ligament — *see* Injury, pelvic organ, specified site NEC
sacral plexus — *see* Injury, lumbosacral plexus
salivary duct or gland S09.93 ☑
scalp S09.90 ☑
  newborn (birth injury) P12.9
    due to monitoring (electrode) (sampling incision) P12.4
    specified NEC P12.89
      caput succedaneum P12.81
scapular region — *see* Injury, shoulder
sclera — *see* Injury, eye, specified site NEC
  penetrating — *see* Injury, eyeball, penetrating
scrotum S39.94 ☑
second cranial nerve (optic) — *see* Injury, nerve, optic
seminal vesicle — *see* Injury, pelvic organ, specified site NEC
seventh cranial nerve (facial) — *see* Injury, nerve, facial
shoulder S49.9 ☑
  blood vessel — *see* Injury, blood vessel, arm
  contusion — *see* Contusion, shoulder
  dislocation — *see* Dislocation, shoulder
  fracture — *see* Fracture, shoulder
  muscle — *see* Injury, muscle, shoulder
  nerve — *see* Injury, nerve, shoulder
  open — *see* Wound, open, shoulder
  specified type NEC S49.8 ☑
  sprain — *see* Sprain, shoulder girdle
  superficial — *see* Injury, superficial, shoulder
sinus
  cavernous — *see* Injury, intracranial
  nasal S09.92 ☑
sixth cranial nerve (abducent) — *see* Injury, nerve, abducens
skeleton, birth injury P13.9
  specified part NEC P13.8
skin NEC T14.8 ☑
  surface intact — *see* Injury, superficial
skull NEC S09.90 ☑
specified NEC T14.8 ☑
spermatic cord (pelvic region) S37.898 ☑
  scrotal region S39.848 ☑

Injury — *continued*

spinal (cord)
  cervical (neck) S14.109 ☑
    anterior cord syndrome S14.139 ☑
      C1 level S14.131 ☑
      C2 level S14.132 ☑
      C3 level S14.133 ☑
      C4 level S14.134 ☑
      C5 level S14.135 ☑
      C6 level S14.136 ☑
      C7 level S14.137 ☑
      C8 level S14.138 ☑
    Brown-Séquard syndrome S14.149 ☑
      C1 level S14.141 ☑
      C2 level S14.142 ☑
      C3 level S14.143 ☑
      C4 level S14.144 ☑
      C5 level S14.145 ☑
      C6 level S14.146 ☑
      C7 level S14.147 ☑
      C8 level S14.148 ☑
    C1 level S14.101 ☑
    C2 level S14.102 ☑
    C3 level S14.103 ☑
    C4 level S14.104 ☑
    C5 level S14.105 ☑
    C6 level S14.106 ☑
    C7 level S14.107 ☑
    C8 level S14.108 ☑
    central cord syndrome S14.129 ☑
      C1 level S14.121 ☑
      C2 level S14.122 ☑
      C3 level S14.123 ☑
      C4 level S14.124 ☑
      C5 level S14.125 ☑
      C6 level S14.126 ☑
      C7 level S14.127 ☑
      C8 level S14.128 ☑
    complete lesion S14.119 ☑
      C1 level S14.111 ☑
      C2 level S14.112 ☑
      C3 level S14.113 ☑
      C4 level S14.114 ☑
      C5 level S14.115 ☑
      C6 level S14.116 ☑
      C7 level S14.117 ☑
      C8 level S14.118 ☑
    concussion S14.0 ☑
    edema S14.0 ☑
    incomplete lesion specified NEC S14.159 ☑
      C1 level S14.151 ☑
      C2 level S14.152 ☑
      C3 level S14.153 ☑
      C4 level S14.154 ☑
      C5 level S14.155 ☑
      C6 level S14.156 ☑
      C7 level S14.157 ☑
      C8 level S14.158 ☑
    posterior cord syndrome S14.159 ☑
      C1 level S14.151 ☑
      C2 level S14.152 ☑
      C3 level S14.153 ☑
      C4 level S14.154 ☑
      C5 level S14.155 ☑
      C6 level S14.156 ☑
      C7 level S14.157 ☑
      C8 level S14.158 ☑
  dorsal — *see* Injury, spinal, thoracic
  lumbar S34.109 ☑
    complete lesion S34.119 ☑
      L1 level S34.111 ☑
      L2 level S34.112 ☑
      L3 level S34.113 ☑
      L4 level S34.114 ☑
      L5 level S34.115 ☑
    concussion S34.01 ☑
    edema S34.01 ☑
    incomplete lesion S34.129 ☑
      L1 level S34.121 ☑
      L2 level S34.122 ☑
      L3 level S34.123 ☑
      L4 level S34.124 ☑
      L5 level S34.125 ☑
    L1 level S34.101 ☑
    L2 level S34.102 ☑
    L3 level S34.103 ☑
    L4 level S34.104 ☑
    L5 level S34.105 ☑
  nerve root NEC
    cervical — *see* Injury, nerve, spinal, root, cervical
    dorsal — *see* Injury, nerve, spinal, root, dorsal
    lumbar S34.21 ☑

Injury — *continued*

spinal — *continued*
  sacral S34.22 ☑
  thoracic — *see* Injury, nerve, spinal, root, dorsal
  plexus
    brachial — *see* Injury, brachial plexus
    lumbosacral — *see* Injury, lumbosacral plexus
  sacral S34.139 ☑
    complete lesion S34.131 ☑
    incomplete lesion S34.132 ☑
  thoracic S24.109 ☑
    anterior cord syndrome S24.139 ☑
      T1 level S24.131 ☑
      T2-T6 level S24.132 ☑
      T7-T10 level S24.133 ☑
      T11-T12 level S24.134 ☑
    Brown-Séquard syndrome S24.149 ☑
      T1 level S24.141 ☑
      T2-T6 level S24.142 ☑
      T7-T10 level S24.143 ☑
      T11-T12 level S24.144 ☑
    complete lesion S24.119 ☑
      T1 level S24.111 ☑
      T2-T6 level S24.112 ☑
      T7-T10 level S24.113 ☑
      T11-T12 level S24.114 ☑
    concussion S24.0 ☑
    edema S24.0 ☑
    incomplete lesion specified NEC S24.159 ☑
      T1 level S24.151 ☑
      T2-T6 level S24.152 ☑
      T7-T10 level S24.153 ☑
      T11-T12 level S24.154 ☑
    posterior cord syndrome S24.159 ☑
      T1 level S24.151 ☑
      T2-T6 level S24.152 ☑
      T7-T10 level S24.153 ☑
      T11-T12 level S24.154 ☑
    T1 level S24.101 ☑
    T2-T6 level S24.102 ☑
    T7-T10 level S24.103 ☑
    T11-T12 level S24.104 ☑
splanchnic nerve — *see* Injury, nerve, lumbosacral, sympathetic
spleen S36.00 ☑
  contusion S36.029 ☑
    major S36.021 ☑
    minor S36.020 ☑
  laceration S36.039 ☑
    major (massive) (stellate) S36.032 ☑
    moderate S36.031 ☑
    superficial (capsular) (minor) S36.030 ☑
  specified type NEC S36.09 ☑
splenic artery — *see* Injury, blood vessel, celiac artery, branch
stellate ganglion — *see* Injury, nerve, thorax, sympathetic
sternal region S29.9 ☑
stomach S36.30 ☑
  contusion S36.32 ☑
  laceration S36.33 ☑
  specified type NEC S36.39 ☑
subconjunctival — *see* Injury, eye, conjunctiva
subcutaneous NEC T14.8 ☑
submaxillary region S09.93 ☑
submental region S09.93 ☑
subungual
  fingers — *see* Injury, hand
  toes — *see* Injury, foot
superficial NEC T14.8 ☑
  abdomen, abdominal (wall) S30.92 ☑
    abrasion S30.811 ☑
    bite S30.871 ☑
      insect S30.861 ☑
    contusion S30.1 ☑
    external constriction S30.841 ☑
    foreign body S30.851 ☑
  abrasion — *see* Abrasion, by site
  adnexa, eye NEC — *see* Injury, eye, specified site NEC
  alveolar process — *see* Injury, superficial, oral cavity
  ankle S90.91 ☑
    abrasion — *see* Abrasion, ankle
    blister — *see* Blister, ankle
    bite — *see* Bite, ankle
    contusion — *see* Contusion, ankle
    external constriction — *see* Constriction, external, ankle
    foreign body — *see* Foreign body, superficial, ankle
  anus S30.98 ☑

☑ **Additional character required**

Injury — *continued*
 superficial NEC — *continued*
  arm (upper) S40.92 ☑
   abrasion — *see* Abrasion, arm
   bite — *see* Bite, superficial, arm
   blister — *see* Blister, arm (upper)
   contusion — *see* Contusion, arm
   external constriction — *see* Constriction,
    external, arm
   foreign body — *see* Foreign body, superficial,
    arm
  auditory canal (external) (meatus) — *see* Injury,
   superficial, ear
  auricle — *see* Injury, superficial, ear
  axilla — *see* Injury, superficial, arm
  back (*see also* Injury, superficial, thorax, back)
   lower S30.91 ☑
    abrasion S30.810 ☑
    contusion S30.0 ☑
    external constriction S30.840 ☑
    superficial
     bite NEC S30.870 ☑
      insect S30.860 ☑
     foreign body S30.850 ☑
  bite NEC — *see* Bite, superficial NEC, by site
  blister — *see* Blister, by site
  breast S20.10 ☑
   abrasion — *see* Abrasion, breast
   bite — *see* Bite, superficial, breast
   contusion — *see* Contusion, breast
   external constriction — *see* Constriction,
    external, breast
   foreign body — *see* Foreign body, superficial,
    breast
  brow — *see* Injury, superficial, head, specified NEC
  buttock S30.91 ☑
  calf — *see* Injury, superficial, leg
  canthus, eye — *see* Injury, superficial, periocular
   area
  cheek (external) — *see* Injury, superficial, head,
   specified NEC
   internal — *see* Injury, superficial, oral cavity
  chest wall — *see* Injury, superficial, thorax
  chin — *see* Injury, superficial, head NEC
  clitoris S30.95 ☑
  conjunctiva — *see* Injury, eye, conjunctiva
   with foreign body (in conjunctival sac) — *see*
    Foreign body, conjunctival sac
  contusion — *see* Contusion, by site
  costal region — *see* Injury, superficial, thorax
  digit(s)
   hand — *see* Injury, superficial, finger
  ear (auricle) (canal) (external) S00.40 ☑
   abrasion — *see* Abrasion, ear
   bite — *see* Bite, superficial, ear
   contusion — *see* Contusion, ear
   external constriction — *see* Constriction,
    external, ear
   foreign body — *see* Foreign body, superficial,
    ear
  elbow S50.90 ☑
   abrasion — *see* Abrasion, elbow
   bite — *see* Bite, superficial, elbow
   blister — *see* Blister, elbow
   contusion — *see* Contusion, elbow
   external constriction — *see* Constriction,
    external, elbow
   foreign body — *see* Foreign body, superficial,
    elbow
  epididymis S30.94 ☑
  epigastric region S30.92 ☑
  epiglottis — *see* Injury, superficial, throat
  esophagus
   cervical — *see* Injury, superficial, throat
  external constriction — *see* Constriction, external,
   by site
  extremity NEC T14.8 ☑
  eyeball NEC — *see* Injury, eye, specified site NEC
  eyebrow — *see* Injury, superficial, periocular area
  eyelid S00.20 ☑
   abrasion — *see* Abrasion, eyelid
   bite — *see* Bite, superficial, eyelid
   contusion — *see* Contusion, eyelid
   external constriction — *see* Constriction,
    external, eyelid
   foreign body — *see* Foreign body, superficial,
    eyelid
  face NEC — *see* Injury, superficial, head, specified
   NEC
  finger(s) S60.949 ☑
   abrasion — *see* Abrasion, finger
   bite — *see* Bite, superficial, finger

Injury — *continued*
 superficial NEC — *continued*
  blister — *see* Blister, finger
  contusion — *see* Contusion, finger
  external constriction — *see* Constriction,
   external, finger
  foreign body — *see* Foreign body, superficial,
   finger
  insect bite — *see* Bite, by site, superficial, insect
  index S60.94 ☑
  little S60.94 ☑
  middle S60.94 ☑
  ring S60.94 ☑
  flank S30.92 ☑
  foot S90.92 ☑
   abrasion — *see* Abrasion, foot
   bite — *see* Bite, foot
   blister — *see* Blister, foot
   contusion — *see* Contusion, foot
   external constriction — *see* Constriction,
    external, foot
   foreign body — *see* Foreign body, superficial,
    foot
  forearm S50.91 ☑
   abrasion — *see* Abrasion, forearm
   bite — *see* Bite, forearm, superficial
   blister — *see* Blister, forearm
   contusion — *see* Contusion, forearm
   elbow only — *see* Injury, superficial, elbow
   external constriction — *see* Constriction,
    external, forearm
   foreign body — *see* Foreign body, superficial,
    forearm
  forehead — *see* Injury, superficial, head NEC
  foreign body — *see* Foreign body, superficial
  genital organs, external
   female S30.97 ☑
   male S30.96 ☑
  globe (eye) — *see* Injury, eye, specified site NEC
  groin S30.92 ☑
  gum — *see* Injury, superficial, oral cavity
  hand S60.92 ☑
   abrasion — *see* Abrasion, hand
   bite — *see* Bite, superficial, hand
   contusion — *see* Contusion, hand
   external constriction — *see* Constriction,
    external, hand
   foreign body — *see* Foreign body, superficial,
    hand
  head S00.90 ☑
   ear — *see* Injury, superficial, ear
   eyelid — *see* Injury, superficial, eyelid
   nose S00.30 ☑
   oral cavity S00.502 ☑
   scalp S00.00 ☑
   specified site NEC S00.80 ☑
  heel — *see* Injury, superficial, foot
  hip S70.91 ☑
   abrasion — *see* Abrasion, hip
   bite — *see* Bite, superficial, hip
   blister — *see* Blister, hip
   contusion — *see* Contusion, hip
   external constriction — *see* Constriction,
    external, hip
   foreign body — *see* Foreign body, superficial,
    hip
  iliac region — *see* Injury, superficial, abdomen
  inguinal region — *see* Injury, superficial, abdomen
  insect bite — *see* Bite, by site, superficial, insect
  interscapular region — *see* Injury, superficial,
   thorax, back
  jaw — *see* Injury, superficial, head, specified NEC
  knee S80.91 ☑
   abrasion — *see* Abrasion, knee
   bite — *see* Bite, superficial, knee
   blister — *see* Blister, knee
   contusion — *see* Contusion, knee
   external constriction — *see* Constriction,
    external, knee
   foreign body — *see* Foreign body, superficial,
    knee
  labium (majus) (minus) S30.95 ☑
  lacrimal (apparatus) (gland) (sac) — *see* Injury,
   eye, specified site NEC
  larynx — *see* Injury, superficial, throat
  leg (lower) S80.92 ☑
   abrasion — *see* Abrasion, leg
   bite — *see* Bite, superficial, leg
   contusion — *see* Contusion, leg
   external constriction — *see* Constriction,
    external, leg

Injury — *continued*
 superficial NEC — *continued*
  foreign body — *see* Foreign body, superficial,
   leg
  knee — *see* Injury, superficial, knee
  limb NEC T14.8 ☑
  lip S00.501 ☑
  lower back S30.91 ☑
  lumbar region S30.91 ☑
  malar region — *see* Injury, superficial, head,
   specified NEC
  mammary — *see* Injury, superficial, breast
  mastoid region — *see* Injury, superficial, head,
   specified NEC
  mouth — *see* Injury, superficial, oral cavity
  muscle NEC T14.8 ☑
  nail NEC T14.8 ☑
   finger — *see* Injury, superficial, finger
   toe — *see* Injury, superficial, toe
  nasal (septum) — *see* Injury, superficial, nose
  neck S10.90 ☑
   specified site NEC S10.80 ☑
  nose (septum) S00.30 ☑
  occipital region — *see* Injury, superficial, scalp
  oral cavity S00.502 ☑
  orbital region — *see* Injury, superficial, periocular
   area
  palate — *see* Injury, superficial, oral cavity
  palm — *see* Injury, superficial, hand
  parietal region — *see* Injury, superficial, scalp
  pelvis S30.91 ☑
   girdle — *see* Injury, superficial, hip
  penis S30.93 ☑
  perineum
   female S30.95 ☑
   male S30.91 ☑
  periocular area S00.20 ☑
   abrasion — *see* Abrasion, eyelid
   bite — *see* Bite, superficial, eyelid
   contusion — *see* Contusion, eyelid
   external constriction — *see* Constriction,
    external, eyelid
   foreign body — *see* Foreign body, superficial,
    eyelid
  phalanges
   finger — *see* Injury, superficial, finger
   toe — *see* Injury, superficial, toe
  pharynx — *see* Injury, superficial, throat
  pinna — *see* Injury, superficial, ear
  popliteal space — *see* Injury, superficial, knee
  prepuce S30.93 ☑
  pubic region S30.91 ☑
  pudendum
   female S30.97 ☑
   male S30.96 ☑
  sacral region S30.91 ☑
  scalp S00.00 ☑
  scapular region — *see* Injury, superficial, shoulder
  sclera — *see* Injury, eye, specified site NEC
  scrotum S30.94 ☑
  shin — *see* Injury, superficial, leg
  shoulder S40.91 ☑
   abrasion — *see* Abrasion, shoulder
   bite — *see* Bite, superficial, shoulder
   blister — *see* Blister, shoulder
   contusion — *see* Contusion, shoulder
   external constriction — *see* Constriction,
    external, shoulder
   foreign body — *see* Foreign body, superficial,
    shoulder
  skin NEC T14.8 ☑
  sternal region — *see* Injury, superficial, thorax,
   front
  subconjunctival — *see* Injury, eye, specified site
   NEC
  subcutaneous NEC T14.8 ☑
  submaxillary region — *see* Injury, superficial,
   head, specified NEC
  submental region — *see* Injury, superficial, head,
   specified NEC
  subungual
   finger(s) — *see* Injury, superficial, finger
   toe(s) — *see* Injury, superficial, toe
  supraclavicular fossa — *see* Injury, superficial,
   neck
  supraorbital — *see* Injury, superficial, head,
   specified NEC
  temple — *see* Injury, superficial, head, specified
   NEC
  temporal region — *see* Injury, superficial, head,
   specified NEC
  testis S30.94 ☑

Injury - Insomnia

Injury — *continued*
- superficial NEC — *continued*
  - thigh S70.92 ☑
    - abrasion — *see* Abrasion, thigh
    - bite — *see* Bite, superficial, thigh
    - blister — *see* Blister, thigh
    - contusion — *see* Contusion, thigh
    - external constriction — *see* Constriction, external, thigh
    - foreign body — *see* Foreign body, superficial, thigh
  - thorax, thoracic (wall) S20.90 ☑
    - abrasion — *see* Abrasion, thorax
    - back S20.40 ☑
    - bite — *see* Bite, thorax, superficial
    - blister — *see* Blister, thorax
    - contusion — *see* Contusion, thorax
    - external constriction — *see* Constriction, external, thorax
    - foreign body — *see* Foreign body, superficial, thorax
    - front S20.30 ☑
  - throat S10.10 ☑
    - abrasion S10.11 ☑
    - bite S10.17 ☑
      - insect S10.16 ☑
    - blister S10.12 ☑
    - contusion S10.0 ☑
    - external constriction S10.14 ☑
    - foreign body S10.15 ☑
  - thumb S60.93 ☑
    - abrasion — *see* Abrasion, thumb
    - bite — *see* Bite, superficial, thumb
    - blister — *see* Blister, thumb
    - contusion — *see* Contusion, thumb
    - external constriction — *see* Constriction, external, thumb
    - foreign body — *see* Foreign body, superficial, thumb
    - insect bite — *see* Bite, by site, superficial, insect
    - specified type NEC S60.39 ☑
  - toe(s) S90.93 ☑
    - abrasion — *see* Abrasion, toe
    - bite — *see* Bite, toe
    - blister — *see* Blister, toe
    - contusion — *see* Contusion, toe
    - external constriction — *see* Constriction, external, toe
    - foreign body — *see* Foreign body, superficial, toe
    - great S90.93 ☑
  - tongue — *see* Injury, superficial, oral cavity
  - tooth, teeth — *see* Injury, superficial, oral cavity
  - trachea S10.10 ☑
  - tunica vaginalis S30.94 ☑
  - tympanum, tympanic membrane — *see* Injury, superficial, ear
  - uvula — *see* Injury, superficial, oral cavity
  - vagina S30.95 ☑
  - vocal cords — *see* Injury, superficial, throat
  - vulva S30.95 ☑
  - wrist S60.91 ☑
- supraclavicular region — *see* Injury, neck
- supraorbital S09.93 ☑
- suprarenal gland (multiple) — *see* Injury, adrenal
- surgical complication (external or internal site) — *see* Laceration, accidental complicating surgery
- temple S09.90 ☑
- temporal region S09.90 ☑
- tendon (*see also* Injury, muscle, by site)
  - abdomen — *see* Injury, muscle, abdomen
  - Achilles — *see* Injury, Achilles tendon
  - lower back — *see* Injury, muscle, lower back
  - pelvic organs — *see* Injury, muscle, pelvis
- tenth cranial nerve (pneumogastric or vagus) — *see* Injury, nerve, vagus
- testis S39.94 ☑
- thigh S79.92 ☑
  - blood vessel — *see* Injury, blood vessel, hip
  - contusion — *see* Contusion, thigh
  - fracture — *see* Fracture, femur
  - muscle — *see* Injury, muscle, thigh
  - nerve — *see* Injury, nerve, thigh
  - open — *see* Wound, open, thigh
  - specified NEC S79.82 ☑
  - superficial — *see* Injury, superficial, thigh
- third cranial nerve (oculomotor) — *see* Injury, nerve, oculomotor
- thorax, thoracic S29.9 ☑
  - blood vessel — *see* Injury, blood vessel, thorax
  - cavity — *see* Injury, intrathoracic
  - dislocation — *see* Dislocation, thorax

Injury — *continued*
- thorax — *continued*
  - external (wall) S29.9 ☑
    - contusion — *see* Contusion, thorax
    - nerve — *see* Injury, nerve, thorax
    - open — *see* Wound, open, thorax
    - specified NEC S29.8 ☑
    - sprain — *see* Sprain, thorax
    - superficial — *see* Injury, superficial, thorax
  - fracture — *see* Fracture, thorax
  - internal — *see* Injury, intrathoracic
  - intrathoracic organ — *see* Injury, intrathoracic
  - sympathetic ganglion — *see* Injury, nerve, thorax, sympathetic
- throat (*see also* Injury, neck) S19.9 ☑
- thumb S69.9 ☑
  - blood vessel — *see* Injury, blood vessel, thumb
  - contusion — *see* Contusion, thumb
  - dislocation — *see* Dislocation, thumb
  - fracture — *see* Fracture, thumb
  - muscle — *see* Injury, muscle, thumb
  - nerve — *see* Injury, nerve, digital, thumb
  - open — *see* Wound, open, thumb
  - specified NEC S69.8 ☑
  - sprain — *see* Sprain, thumb
  - superficial — *see* Injury, superficial, thumb
- thymus (gland) — *see* Injury, intrathoracic, specified organ NEC
- thyroid (gland) NEC S19.84 ☑
- toe S99.92 ☑
  - contusion — *see* Contusion, toe
  - dislocation — *see* Dislocation, toe
  - fracture — *see* Fracture, toe
  - muscle — *see* Injury, muscle, toe
  - open — *see* Wound, open, toe
  - specified type NEC S99.82 ☑
  - sprain — *see* Sprain, toe
  - superficial — *see* Injury, superficial, toe
- tongue S09.93 ☑
- tonsil S09.93 ☑
- tooth S09.93 ☑
- trachea (cervical) NEC S19.82 ☑
  - thoracic — *see* Injury, intrathoracic, trachea, thoracic
- transfusion-related acute lung (TRALI) J95.84
- tunica vaginalis S39.94 ☑
- twelfth cranial nerve (hypoglossal) — *see* Injury, nerve, hypoglossal
- ureter S37.10 ☑
  - contusion S37.12 ☑
  - laceration S37.13 ☑
  - specified type NEC S37.19 ☑
- urethra (sphincter) S37.30 ☑
  - at delivery O71.5
  - contusion S37.32 ☑
  - laceration S37.33 ☑
  - specified type NEC S37.39 ☑
- urinary organ S37.90 ☑
  - contusion S37.92 ☑
  - laceration S37.93 ☑
  - specified
    - site NEC S37.899 ☑
      - contusion S37.892 ☑
      - laceration S37.893 ☑
      - specified type NEC S37.898 ☑
    - type NEC S37.99 ☑
- uterus, uterine S37.60 ☑
  - with ectopic or molar pregnancy O08.6
  - blood vessel — *see* Injury, blood vessel, iliac
  - contusion S37.62 ☑
  - laceration S37.63 ☑
    - cervix at delivery O71.3
    - rupture associated with obstetrics — *see* Rupture, uterus
  - specified type NEC S37.69 ☑
- uvula S09.93 ☑
- vagina S39.93 ☑
  - abrasion S30.814 ☑
  - bite S31.45 ☑
    - insect S30.864 ☑
    - superficial NEC S30.874 ☑
  - contusion S30.23 ☑
  - crush S38.03 ☑
  - during delivery — *see* Laceration, vagina, during delivery
  - external constriction S30.844 ☑
  - insect bite S30.864 ☑
  - laceration S31.41 ☑
    - with foreign body S31.42 ☑
  - open wound S31.40 ☑
  - puncture S31.43 ☑
    - with foreign body S31.44 ☑

Injury — *continued*
- vagina — *continued*
  - superficial S30.95 ☑
    - foreign body S30.854 ☑
- vas deferens — *see* Injury, pelvic organ, specified site NEC
- vascular NEC T14.8 ☑
- vein — *see* Injury, blood vessel
- vena cava (superior) S25.20 ☑
  - inferior S35.10 ☑
    - laceration (minor) (superficial) S35.11 ☑
      - major S35.12 ☑
    - specified type NEC S35.19 ☑
  - laceration (minor) (superficial) S25.21 ☑
    - major S25.22 ☑
  - specified type NEC S25.29 ☑
- vesical (sphincter) — *see* Injury, bladder
- visual cortex S04.04 ☑
- vitreous (humor) S05.90 ☑
  - specified NEC S05.8X ☑
- vocal cord NEC S19.83 ☑
- vulva S39.94 ☑
  - abrasion S30.814 ☑
  - bite S31.45 ☑
    - insect S30.864 ☑
    - superficial NEC S30.874 ☑
  - contusion S30.23 ☑
  - crush S38.03 ☑
  - during delivery — *see* Laceration, perineum, female, during delivery
  - external constriction S30.844 ☑
  - insect bite S30.864 ☑
  - laceration S31.41 ☑
    - with foreign body S31.42 ☑
  - open wound S31.40 ☑
  - puncture S31.43 ☑
    - with foreign body S31.44 ☑
  - superficial S30.95 ☑
    - foreign body S30.854 ☑
- whiplash (cervical spine) S13.4 ☑
- wrist S69.9 ☑
  - blood vessel — *see* Injury, blood vessel, hand
  - contusion — *see* Contusion, wrist
  - dislocation — *see* Dislocation, wrist
  - fracture — *see* Fracture, wrist
  - muscle — *see* Injury, muscle, hand
  - nerve — *see* Injury, nerve, hand
  - open — *see* Wound, open, wrist
  - specified NEC S69.8 ☑
  - sprain — *see* Sprain, wrist
  - superficial — *see* Injury, superficial, wrist

Inoculation (*see also* Vaccination)
- complication or reaction — *see* Complications, vaccination

Insanity, insane (*see also* Psychosis)
- adolescent — *see* Schizophrenia
- confusional F28
  - acute or subacute F05
- delusional F22
- senile F03 ☑

Insect
- bite — *see* Bite, by site, superficial, insect
- venomous, poisoning NEC (by) — *see* Venom, arthropod

Insensitivity
- adrenocorticotropin hormone (ACTH) E27.49
- androgen E34.50
  - complete E34.51
  - partial E34.52

Insertion
- cord (umbilical) lateral or velamentous O43.12 ☑
- intrauterine contraceptive device (encounter for) — *see* Intrauterine contraceptive device

Insolation (sunstroke) T67.01 ☑

Insomnia (organic) G47.00
- adjustment F51.02
- adjustment disorder F51.02
- behavioral, of childhood Z73.819
  - combined type Z73.812
  - limit setting type Z73.811
  - sleep-onset association type Z73.810
- childhood Z73.819
- chronic F51.04
  - somatized tension F51.04
- conditioned F51.04
- due to
  - alcohol
    - abuse F10.182
    - dependence F10.282
    - use F10.982
  - amphetamines
    - abuse F15.182

☑ **Additional character required**

Insomnia — *continued*
  due to — *continued*
    dependence F15.282
      use F15.982
    anxiety disorder F51.05
    caffeine
      abuse F15.182
      dependence F15.282
      use F15.982
    cocaine
      abuse F14.182
      dependence F14.282
      use F14.982
    depression F51.05
    drug NEC
      abuse F19.182
      dependence F19.282
      use F19.982
    medical condition G47.01
    mental disorder NEC F51.05
    opioid
      abuse F11.182
      dependence F11.282
      use F11.982
    psychoactive substance NEC
      abuse F19.182
      dependence F19.282
      use F19.982
    sedative, hypnotic, or anxiolytic
      abuse F13.182
      dependence F13.282
      use F13.982
    stimulant NEC
      abuse F15.182
      dependence F15.282
      use F15.982
  fatal familial (FFI) A81.83
  idiopathic F51.01
  learned F51.3
  nonorganic origin F51.01
  not due to a substance or known physiological
    condition F51.01
    specified NEC F51.09
  paradoxical F51.03
  primary F51.01
  psychiatric F51.05
  psychophysiologic F51.04
  related to psychopathology F51.05
  short-term F51.02
  specified NEC G47.09
  stress-related F51.02
  transient F51.02
  without objective findings F51.02
Inspiration
  food or foreign body — *see* Foreign body, by site
  mucus — *see* Asphyxia, mucus
Inspissated bile syndrome (newborn) P59.1
Instability
  emotional (excessive) F60.3
  joint (post-traumatic) M25.30
    ankle M25.37 ☑
    due to old ligament injury — *see* Disorder,
      ligament
    elbow M25.32 ☑
    flail — *see* Flail, joint
    foot M25.37 ☑
    hand M25.34 ☑
    hip M25.35 ☑
    knee M25.36 ☑
    lumbosacral — *see* subcategory M53.2 ☑
    prosthesis — *see* Complications, joint prosthesis,
      mechanical, displacement, by site
    sacroiliac — *see* subcategory M53.2 ☑
    secondary to
      old ligament injury — *see* Disorder, ligament
      removal of joint prosthesis M96.89
    shoulder (region) M25.31 ☑
    spine — *see* subcategory M53.2 ☑
    wrist M25.33 ☑
  knee (chronic) M23.5 ☑
  lumbosacral — *see* subcategory M53.2 ☑
  nervous F48.8
  personality (emotional) F60.3
  spine — *see* Instability, joint, spine
  vasomotor R55
Institutional syndrome (childhood) F94.2
Institutionalization, affecting child Z62.22
  disinhibited attachment F94.2
Insufficiency, insufficient
  accommodation, old age H52.4
  adrenal (gland) E27.40
    primary E27.1

Insufficiency — *continued*
  adrenocortical E27.40
    drug-induced E27.3
    iatrogenic E27.3
    primary E27.1
  anatomic crown height K08.89
  anterior (occlusal) guidance M26.54
  anus K62.89
  aortic (valve) I35.1
    with
      mitral (valve) disease I08.0
        with tricuspid (valve) disease I08.3
      stenosis I35.2
      tricuspid (valve) disease I08.2
        with mitral (valve) disease I08.3
    congenital Q23.1
    rheumatic I06.1
      with
        mitral (valve) disease I08.0
          with tricuspid (valve) disease I08.3
        stenosis I06.2
          with mitral (valve) disease I08.0
            with tricuspid (valve) disease I08.3
        tricuspid (valve) disease I08.2
          with mitral (valve) disease I08.3
    specified cause NEC I35.1
    syphilitic A52.03
  arterial I77.1
    basilar G45.0
    carotid (hemispheric) G45.1
    cerebral I67.81
    coronary (acute or subacute) I24.8
    mesenteric K55.1
    peripheral I73.9
    precerebral (multiple) (bilateral) G45.2
    vertebral G45.0
  arteriovenous I99.8
  biliary K83.8
  cardiac (*see also* Insufficiency, myocardial)
    due to presence of (cardiac) prosthesis I97.11 ☑
    postprocedural I97.11 ☑
  cardiorenal, hypertensive I13.2
  cardiovascular — *see* Disease, cardiovascular
  cerebrovascular (acute) I67.81
    with transient focal neurological signs and
      symptoms G45.8
  circulatory NEC I99.8
    newborn P29.89
  clinical crown length K08.89
  convergence H51.11
  coronary (acute or subacute) I24.8
    chronic or with a stated duration of over 4 weeks
      I25.89
  corticoadrenal E27.40
    primary E27.1
  dietary E63.9
  divergence H51.8
  food T73.0 ☑
  gastroesophageal K22.8
  gonadal
    ovary E28.39
    testis E29.1
  heart (*see also* Insufficiency, myocardial)
    newborn P29.0
    valve — *see* Endocarditis
  hepatic — *see* Failure, hepatic
  idiopathic autonomic G90.09
  interocclusal distance of fully erupted teeth (ridge)
    M26.36
  kidney N28.9
    acute N28.9
    chronic N18.9
  lacrimal (secretion) H04.12 ☑
    passages — *see* Stenosis, lacrimal
  liver — *see* Failure, hepatic
  lung — *see* Insufficiency, pulmonary
  mental (congenital) — *see* Disability, intellectual
  mesenteric K55.1
  mitral (valve) I34.0
    with
      aortic valve disease I08.0
        with tricuspid (valve) disease I08.3
      obstruction or stenosis I05.2
        with aortic valve disease I08.0
      tricuspid (valve) disease I08.1
        with aortic (valve) disease I08.3
    congenital Q23.3
    rheumatic I05.1
      with
        aortic valve disease I08.0
          with tricuspid (valve) disease I08.3
        obstruction or stenosis I05.2

Insufficiency — *continued*
  mitral — *continued*
    with aortic valve disease I08.0
      with tricuspid (valve) disease I08.3
      tricuspid (valve) disease I08.1
        with aortic (valve) disease I08.3
    active or acute I01.1
      with chorea, rheumatic (Sydenham's) I02.0
    specified cause, except rheumatic I34.0
  muscle (*see also* Disease, muscle)
    heart — *see* Insufficiency, myocardial
  ocular NEC H50.9
  myocardial, myocardium (with arteriosclerosis)
    (*see also* Failure, heart) I50.9
    with
      rheumatic fever (conditions in I00) I09.0
        active, acute or subacute I01.2
          with chorea I02.0
        inactive or quiescent (with chorea) I09.0
    congenital Q24.8
    hypertensive — *see* Hypertension, heart
    newborn P29.0
    rheumatic I09.0
      active, acute, or subacute I01.2
    syphilitic A52.06
  nourishment T73.0 ☑
  pancreatic K86.89
    exocrine K86.81
  parathyroid (gland) E20.9
  peripheral vascular (arterial) I73.9
  pituitary E23.0
  placental (mother) O36.51 ☑
  platelets D69.6
  prenatal care affecting management of pregnancy
    O09.3 ☑
  progressive pluriglandular E31.0
  pulmonary J98.4
    acute, following surgery (nonthoracic) J95.2
      thoracic J95.1
    chronic, following surgery J95.3
    following
      shock J98.4
      trauma J98.4
    newborn P28.89
    valve I37.1
      with stenosis I37.2
      congenital Q22.2
      rheumatic I09.89
        with aortic, mitral or tricuspid (valve) disease
          I08.8
  pyloric K31.89
  renal (acute) N28.9
    chronic N18.9
  respiratory R06.89
    newborn P28.5
  rotation — *see* Malrotation
  sleep syndrome F51.12
  social insurance Z59.7
  suprarenal E27.40
    primary E27.1
  tarso-orbital fascia, congenital Q10.3
  testis E29.1
  thyroid (gland) (acquired) E03.9
    congenital E03.1
  tricuspid (valve) (rheumatic) I07.1
    with
      aortic (valve) disease I08.2
        with mitral (valve) disease I08.3
      mitral (valve) disease I08.1
        with aortic (valve) disease I08.3
      obstruction or stenosis I07.2
        with aortic (valve) disease I08.2
          with mitral (valve) disease I08.3
    congenital Q22.8
    nonrheumatic I36.1
      with stenosis I36.2
  urethral sphincter R32
  valve, valvular (heart) I38
    aortic — *see* Insufficiency, aortic (valve)
    mitral — *see* Insufficiency, mitral (valve)
    pulmonary — *see* Insufficiency, pulmonary, valve
    tricuspid — *see* Insufficiency, tricuspid (valve)
    congenital Q24.8
  vascular I99.8
    intestine K55.9
      acute (*see also* Ischemia, intestine, acute) K55.059
    mesenteric K55.1
    peripheral I73.9
    renal — *see* Hypertension, kidney
  velopharyngeal
    acquired K13.79
    congenital Q38.8

Insufficiency - Iridocyclitis

Insufficiency — *continued*
  venous (chronic) (peripheral) I87.2
  ventricular — *see* Insufficiency, myocardial
  welfare support Z59.7
Insufflation, fallopian Z31.41
Insular — *see* condition
Insulinoma
  pancreas
    benign D13.7
    malignant C25.4
    uncertain behavior D37.8
  specified site
    benign — *see* Neoplasm, by site, benign
    malignant — *see* Neoplasm, by site, malignant
    uncertain behavior — *see* Neoplasm, by site,
      uncertain behavior
  unspecified site
    benign D13.7
    malignant C25.4
    uncertain behavior D37.8
Insuloma — *see* Insulinoma
Interference
  balancing side M26.56
  non-working side M26.56
Intermenstrual — *see* condition
Intermittent — *see* condition
Internal — *see* condition
Interrogation
  cardiac defibrillator (automatic) (implantable)
    Z45.02
  cardiac pacemaker Z45.018
  cardiac (event) (loop) recorder Z45.09
  infusion pump (implanted) (intrathecal) Z45.1
  neurostimulator Z46.2
Interruption
  aortic arch Q25.21
  bundle of His I44.30
  phase-shift, sleep cycle — *see* Disorder, sleep,
    circadian rhythm
  sleep phase-shift, or 24 hour sleep-wake cycle —
    see Disorder, sleep, circadian rhythm
Interstitial — *see* condition
Intertrigo L30.4
  labialis K13.0
Intervertebral disc — *see* condition
Intestine, intestinal — *see* condition
Intolerance
  carbohydrate K90.49
  disaccharide, hereditary E73.0
  fat NEC K90.49
    pancreatic K90.3
  food K90.49
    dietary counseling and surveillance Z71.3
  fructose E74.10
    hereditary E74.12
  glucose (-galactose) E74.39
  gluten K90.41
  lactose E73.9
    specified NEC E73.8
  lysine E72.3
  milk NEC K90.49
    lactose E73.9
  protein K90.49
  starch NEC K90.49
  sucrose (-isomaltose) E74.31
Intoxicated NEC (without dependence) — *see* Alcohol,
  intoxication
Intoxication
  acid E87.2
  alcoholic (acute) (without dependence) — *see*
    Alcohol, intoxication
  alimentary canal K52.1
  amphetamine (without dependence) (*see also*
    Abuse, drug, stimulant, with intoxication)
    with dependence — *see* Dependence, drug,
      stimulant, with intoxication
    stimulant NEC F15.10
      with
        anxiety disorder F15.180
        intoxication F15.129
          with
            delirium F15.121
            perceptual disturbance F15.122
  anxiolytic (acute) (without dependence) — *see*
    Abuse, drug, sedative, with intoxication
    with dependence — *see* Dependence, drug,
      sedative, with intoxication
  caffeine F15.929
    with dependence — *see* Dependence, drug,
      stimulant, with intoxication
  cannabinoids (acute) (without dependence) — *see*
    Use, cannabis, with intoxication

Intoxication — *continued*
  cannabinoids — *continued*
    with
      abuse — *see* Abuse, drug, cannabis, with
        intoxication
      dependence — *see* Dependence, drug,
        cannabis, with intoxication
  chemical — *see* Table of Drugs and Chemicals
    via placenta or breast milk — *see* - Absorption,
      chemical, through placenta
  cocaine (acute) (without dependence) — *see* Abuse,
    drug, cocaine, with intoxication
    with dependence — *see* Dependence, drug,
      cocaine, with intoxication
  drug
    acute (without dependence) — *see* Abuse, drug,
      by type with intoxication
      with dependence — *see* Dependence, drug, by
        type with intoxication
    addictive
      via placenta or breast milk — *see* Absorption,
        drug, addictive, through placenta
    newborn P93.8
      gray baby syndrome P93.0
    overdose or wrong substance given or taken —
      see Table of Drugs and Chemicals, by drug,
      poisoning
  enteric K52.1
  foodborne A05.9
    bacterial A05.9
    classical (Clostridium botulinum) A05.1
    due to
      Bacillus cereus A05.4
      bacterium A05.9
        specified NEC A05.8
      Clostridium
        botulinum A05.1
        perfringens A05.2
        welchii A05.2
      Salmonella A02.9
        with
          (gastro)enteritis A02.0
          localized infection(s) A02.20
            arthritis A02.23
            meningitis A02.21
            osteomyelitis A02.24
            pneumonia A02.22
            pyelonephritis A02.25
            specified NEC A02.29
          sepsis A02.1
          specified manifestation NEC A02.8
      Staphylococcus A05.0
      Vibrio
        parahaemolyticus A05.3
        vulnificus A05.5
    enterotoxin, staphylococcal A05.0
    noxious — *see* Poisoning, food, noxious
  gastrointestinal K52.1
  hallucinogenic (without dependence) — *see* Abuse,
    drug, hallucinogen, with intoxication
    with dependence — *see* Dependence, drug,
      hallucinogen, with intoxication
  hypnotic (acute) (without dependence) — *see*
    Abuse, drug, sedative, with intoxication
    with dependence — *see* Dependence, drug,
      sedative, with intoxication
  inhalant (acute) (without dependence) — *see*
    Abuse, drug, inhalant, with intoxication
    with dependence — *see* Dependence, drug,
      inhalant, with intoxication
  meaning
    inebriation — *see* category F10 ☑
    poisoning — *see* Table of Drugs and Chemicals
  methyl alcohol (acute) (without dependence) — *see*
    Alcohol, intoxication
  opioid (acute) (without dependence) — *see* Abuse,
    drug, opioid, with intoxication
    with dependence — *see* Dependence, drug,
      opioid, with intoxication
  pathologic NEC (without dependence) — *see*
    Alcohol, intoxication
  phencyclidine (without dependence) — *see* Abuse,
    drug, hallucinogen, with intoxication
    with dependence — *see* Dependence, drug,
      hallucinogen, with intoxication
  potassium (K) E87.5
  psychoactive substance NEC (without dependence)
    — *see* Abuse, drug, psychoactive NEC, with
    intoxication
    with dependence — *see* Dependence, drug,
      psychoactive NEC, with intoxication

Intoxication — *continued*
  sedative (acute) (without dependence) — *see*
    Abuse, drug, sedative, with intoxication
    with dependence — *see* Dependence, drug,
      sedative, with intoxication
  serum (*see also* Reaction, serum) T80.69 ☑
  uremic — *see* Uremia
  volatile solvents (acute) (without dependence) —
    see Abuse, drug, inhalant, with intoxication
    with dependence — *see* Dependence, drug,
      inhalant, with intoxication
  water E87.79
Intraabdominal testis, testes
  bilateral Q53.211
  unilateral Q53.111
Intracranial — *see* condition
Intrahepatic gallbladder Q44.1
Intraligamentous — *see* condition
Intrathoracic (*see also* condition)
  kidney Q63.2
Intrauterine contraceptive device
  checking Z30.431
  insertion Z30.430
    immediately following removal Z30.433
  in situ Z97.5
  management Z30.431
  reinsertion Z30.433
  removal Z30.432
  replacement Z30.433
  retention in pregnancy O26.3 ☑
Intraventricular — *see* condition
Intrinsic deformity — *see* Deformity
Intubation, difficult or failed T88.4 ☑
Intumescence, lens (eye) (cataract) — *see* Cataract
Intussusception (bowel) (colon) (enteric) (ileocecal)
  (ileocolic) (intestine) (rectum) K56.1
    appendix K38.8
    congenital Q43.8
    ureter (with obstruction) N13.5
Invagination (bowel, colon, intestine or rectum) K56.1
Inversion
  albumin-globulin (A-G) ratio E88.09
  bladder N32.89
  cecum — *see* Intussusception
  cervix N88.8
  chromosome in normal individual Q95.1
  circadian rhythm — *see* Disorder, sleep, circadian
    rhythm
  nipple N64.59
    congenital Q83.8
    gestational — *see* Retraction, nipple
    puerperal, postpartum — *see* Retraction, nipple
  nyctohemeral rhythm — *see* Disorder, sleep,
    circadian rhythm
  optic papilla Q14.2
  organ or site, congenital NEC — *see* Anomaly, by
    site
  sleep rhythm — *see* Disorder, sleep, circadian
    rhythm
  testis (congenital) Q55.29
  uterus (chronic) (postinfectional) (postpartal, old)
    N85.5
    postpartum O71.2
  vagina (posthysterectomy) N99.3
  ventricular Q20.5
Investigation (*see also* Examination) Z04.9
  clinical research subject (control) (normal
    comparison) (participant) Z00.6
Involuntary movement, abnormal R25.9
Involution, involutional (*see also* condition)
  breast, cystic — *see* Dysplasia, mammary, specified
    type NEC
  depression (single episode) F32.89
    recurrent episode F33.9
  melancholia (single episode) F32.89
    recurrent episode F33.8
  ovary, senile — *see* Atrophy, ovary
  thymus failure E32.8
I.Q.
  under 20 F73
  20-34 F72
  35-49 F71
  50-69 F70
IRDS (type I) P22.0
  type II P22.1
Irideremia Q13.1
Iridis rubeosis — *see* Disorder, iris, vascular
Iridochoroiditis (panuveitis) — *see* Panuveitis
Iridocyclitis H20.9
  acute H20.0 ☑
    hypopyon H20.05 ☑
    primary H20.01 ☑

☑ **Additional character required**

Iridocyclitis — *continued*
  acute — *continued*
    recurrent H20.02 ☑
    secondary (noninfectious) H20.04 ☑
      infectious H20.03 ☑
  chronic H20.1 ☑
  due to allergy — *see* Iridocyclitis, acute, secondary
  endogenous — *see* Iridocyclitis, acute, primary
  Fuchs' — *see* Cyclitis, Fuchs' heterochromic
  gonococcal A54.32
  granulomatous — *see* Iridocyclitis, chronic
  herpes, herpetic (simplex) B00.51
    zoster B02.32
  hypopyon — *see* Iridocyclitis, acute, hypopyon
  in (due to)
    ankylosing spondylitis M45.9
    gonococcal infection A54.32
    herpes (simplex) virus B00.51
      zoster B02.32
    infectious disease NOS B99 ☑
    parasitic disease NOS B89 *[H22]*
    sarcoidosis D86.83
    syphilis A51.43
    tuberculosis A18.54
    zoster B02.32
  lens-induced H20.2 ☑
  nongranulomatous — *see* Iridocyclitis, acute
  recurrent — *see* Iridocyclitis, acute, recurrent
  rheumatic — *see* Iridocyclitis, chronic
  subacute — *see* Iridocyclitis, acute
  sympathetic — *see* Uveitis, sympathetic
  syphilitic (secondary) A51.43
  tuberculous (chronic) A18.54
  Vogt-Koyanagi H20.82 ☑
Iridocyclochoroiditis (panuveitis) — *see* Panuveitis
Iridodialysis H21.53 ☑
Iridodonesis H21.89
Iridoplegia (complete) (partial) (reflex) H57.09
Iridoschisis H21.25 ☑
Iris (*see also* condition)
  bombé — *see* Membrane, pupillary
Iritis (*see also* Iridocyclitis)
  chronic — *see* Iridocyclitis, chronic
  diabetic — *see* E08-E13 with .39
  due to
    herpes simplex B00.51
    leprosy A30.9 *[H22]*
  gonococcal A54.32
  gouty (*see also* Gout, by type) M10.9 *[H22]*
  granulomatous — *see* Iridocyclitis, chronic
  lens induced — *see* Iridocyclitis, lens-induced
  papulosa (syphilitic) A52.71
  rheumatic — *see* Iridocyclitis, chronic
  syphilitic (secondary) A51.43
    congenital (early) A50.01
    late A52.71
  tuberculous A18.54
Iron — *see* condition
Iron-miner's lung J63.4
Irradiated enamel (tooth, teeth) K03.89
Irradiation effects, adverse T66 ☑
Irreducible, irreducibility — *see* condition
Irregular, irregularity
  action, heart I49.9
  alveolar process K08.89
  bleeding N92.6
  breathing R06.89
  contour of cornea (acquired) — *see* Deformity, cornea
    congenital Q13.4
  contour, reconstructed breast N65.0
  dentin (in pulp) K04.3
  eye movements H55.89
    nystagmus — *see* Nystagmus
    saccadic H55.81
  labor O62.2
  menstruation (cause unknown) N92.6
  periods N92.6
  prostate N42.9
  pupil — *see* Abnormality, pupillary
  reconstructed breast N65.0
  respiratory R06.89
  septum (nasal) J34.2
  shape, organ or site, congenital NEC — *see* Distortion
  sleep-wake pattern (rhythm) G47.23
Irritable, irritability R45.4
  bladder N32.89
  bowel (syndrome) K58.9
    with
      constipation K58.1
      diarrhea K58.0

Irritable — *continued*
  bowel — *continued*
    mixed K58.2
    psychogenic F45.8
    specified NEC K58.8
  bronchial — *see* Bronchitis
  cerebral, in newborn P91.3
  colon (*see also* Irritable, bowel) K58.9
    with diarrhea K58.0
    psychogenic F45.8
  duodenum K59.8
  heart (psychogenic) F45.8
  hip — *see* Derangement, joint, specified type NEC, hip
  ileum K59.8
  infant R68.12
  jejunum K59.8
  rectum K59.8
  stomach K31.89
    psychogenic F45.8
  sympathetic G90.8
  urethra N36.8
Irritation
  anus K62.89
  axillary nerve G54.0
  bladder N32.89
  brachial plexus G54.0
  bronchial — *see* Bronchitis
  cervical plexus G54.2
  cervix — *see* Cervicitis
  choroid, sympathetic — *see* Endophthalmitis
  cranial nerve — *see* Disorder, nerve, cranial
  gastric K31.89
    psychogenic F45.8
  globe, sympathetic — *see* Uveitis, sympathetic
  labyrinth — *see* subcategory H83.2 ☑
  lumbosacral plexus G54.1
  meninges (traumatic) — *see* Injury, intracranial
    nontraumatic — *see* Meningismus
  nerve — *see* Disorder, nerve
  nervous R45.0
  penis N48.89
  perineum NEC L29.3
  peripheral autonomic nervous system G90.8
  peritoneum — *see* Peritonitis
  pharynx J39.2
  plantar nerve — *see* Lesion, nerve, plantar
  spinal (cord) (traumatic) (*see also* Injury, spinal cord, by region)
    nerve G58.9
      root NEC — *see* Radiculopathy
    nontraumatic — *see* Myelopathy
  stomach K31.89
    psychogenic F45.8
  sympathetic nerve NEC G90.8
  ulnar nerve — *see* Lesion, nerve, ulnar
  vagina N89.8
Ischemia, ischemic I99.8
  brain — *see* Ischemia, cerebral
  bowel (transient)
    acute (*see also* Ischemia, intestine, acute) K55.059
    chronic K55.1
    due to mesenteric artery insufficiency K55.1
  cardiac (*see* Disease, heart, ischemic)
  cardiomyopathy I25.5
  cerebral (chronic) (generalized) I67.82
    arteriosclerotic I67.2
    intermittent G45.9
    newborn P91.0
    recurrent focal G45.8
    transient G45.9
  colon chronic (due to mesenteric artery insufficiency) K55.1
  coronary — *see* Disease, heart, ischemic
  demand (coronary) (*see also* Angina) I24.8
    with myocardial infarction I21.A1
    resulting in myocardial infarction I21.A1
  heart (chronic or with a stated duration of over 4 weeks) I25.9
    acute or with a stated duration of 4 weeks or less I24.9
    subacute I24.9
  infarction, muscle — *see* Infarct, muscle
  intestine (large) (small) (transient) K55.9
    acute K55.059
      diffuse K55.052
      focal K55.051
      large K55.039
        diffuse K55.032
        focal K55.031
      small K55.019
        diffuse K55.012
        focal K55.011

Ischemia — *continued*
  intestine — *continued*
    chronic K55.1
    due to mesenteric artery insufficiency K55.1
  kidney N28.0
  mesenteric, acute (*see also* Ischemia, intestine, acute) K55.059
  muscle, traumatic T79.6 ☑
  myocardium, myocardial (chronic or with a stated duration of over 4 weeks) I25.9
    acute, without myocardial infarction I51.3
    silent (asymptomatic) I25.6
    transient of newborn P29.4
  renal N28.0
  retina, retinal — *see* Occlusion, artery, retina
  small bowel
    acute K55.019
      diffuse K55.012
      focal K55.011
    chronic K55.1
    due to mesenteric artery insufficiency K55.1
  spinal cord G95.11
  subendocardial — *see* Insufficiency, coronary
  supply (coronary) (*see also* Angina) I25.9
    due to vasospasm I20.1
Ischial spine — *see* condition
Ischialgia — *see* Sciatica
Ischiopagus Q89.4
Ischium, ischial — *see* condition
Ischuria R34
Iselin's disease or osteochondrosis — *see* Osteochondrosis, juvenile, metatarsus
Islands of
  parotid tissue in
    lymph nodes Q38.6
    neck structures Q38.6
  submaxillary glands in
    fascia Q38.6
    lymph nodes Q38.6
    neck muscles Q38.6
Islet cell tumor, pancreas D13.7
Isoimmunization NEC (*see also* Incompatibility)
  affecting management of pregnancy (ABO) (with hydrops fetalis) O36.11 ☑
    anti-A sensitization O36.11 ☑
    anti-B sensitization O36.19 ☑
    anti-c sensitization O36.09 ☑
    anti-C sensitization O36.09 ☑
    anti-e sensitization O36.09 ☑
    anti-E sensitization O36.09 ☑
    Rh NEC O36.09 ☑
      anti-D antibody O36.01 ☑
    specified NEC O36.19 ☑
  newborn P55.9
    with
      hydrops fetalis P56.0
      kernicterus P57.0
    ABO (blood groups) P55.1
    Rhesus (Rh) factor P55.0
    specified type NEC P55.8
Isolation, isolated
  dwelling Z59.8
  family Z63.79
  social Z60.4
Isoleucinosis E71.19
Isomerism atrial appendages (with asplenia or polysplenia) Q20.6
Isosporiasis, isosporosis A07.3
Isovaleric acidemia E71.110
Issue of
  medical certificate Z02.79
    for disability determination Z02.71
  repeat prescription (appliance) (glasses) (medicinal substance, medicament, medicine) Z76.0
    contraception — *see* Contraception
Itch, itching (*see also* Pruritus)
  baker's L23.6
  barber's B35.0
  bricklayer's L24.5
  cheese B88.0
  clam digger's B65.3
  coolie B76.9
  copra B88.0
  dew B76.9
  dhobi B35.6
  filarial — *see* Infestation, filarial
  grain B88.0
  grocer's B88.0
  ground B76.9
  harvest B88.0
  jock B35.6

Itch - Keratitis

Itch — *continued*
- Malabar B35.5
  - beard B35.0
  - foot B35.3
  - scalp B35.0
- meaning scabies B86
- Norwegian B86
- perianal L29.0
- poultrymen's B88.0
- sarcoptic B86
- scabies B86
- scrub B88.0
- straw B88.0
- swimmer's B65.3
- water B76.9
- winter L29.8

Ivemark's syndrome (asplenia with congenital heart disease) Q89.01
Ivory bones Q78.2
Ixodiasis NEC B88.8

J

Jaccoud's syndrome — *see* Arthropathy, postrheumatic, chronic
Jackson's
- membrane Q43.3
- paralysis or syndrome G83.89
- veil Q43.3

Jacquet's dermatitis (diaper dermatitis) L22
Jadassohn-Pellizari's disease or anetoderma L90.2
Jadassohn's
- blue nevus — *see* Nevus
- intraepidermal epithelioma — *see* Neoplasm, skin, benign

Jaffe-Lichtenstein (-Uehlinger) syndrome — *see* Dysplasia, fibrous, bone NEC
Jakob-Creutzfeldt disease or syndrome — *see* Creutzfeldt-Jakob disease or syndrome
Jaksch-Luzet disease D64.89
Jamaican
- neuropathy G92
- paraplegic tropical ataxic-spastic syndrome G92

Janet's disease F48.8
Janiceps Q89.4
Jansky-Bielschowsky amaurotic idiocy E75.4
Japanese
- B-type encephalitis A83.0
- river fever A75.3

Jaundice (yellow) R17
- acholuric (familial) (splenomegalic) (*see also* Spherocytosis)
  - acquired D59.8
- breast-milk (inhibitor) P59.3
- catarrhal (acute) B15.9
  - with hepatic coma B15.0
- cholestatic (benign) R17
- due to or associated with
  - delayed conjugation P59.8
    - associated with (due to) preterm delivery P59.0
  - preterm delivery P59.0
- epidemic (catarrhal) B15.9
  - with hepatic coma B15.0
  - leptospiral A27.0
  - spirochetal A27.0
- familial nonhemolytic (congenital) (Gilbert) E80.4
  - Crigler-Najjar E80.5
- febrile (acute) B15.9
  - with hepatic coma B15.0
  - leptospiral A27.0
  - spirochetal A27.0
- hematogenous D59.9
- hemolytic (acquired) D59.9
  - congenital — *see* Spherocytosis
- hemorrhagic (acute) (leptospiral) (spirochetal) A27.0
- infectious (acute) (subacute) B15.9
  - with hepatic coma B15.0
  - leptospiral A27.0
  - spirochetal A27.0
- leptospiral (hemorrhagic) A27.0
- malignant (without coma) K72.90
  - with coma K72.91
- newborn P59.9
  - due to or associated with
    - ABO
      - antibodies P55.1
      - incompatibility, maternal/fetal P55.1

Jaundice — *continued*
- newborn — *continued*
  - isoimmunization P55.1
  - absence or deficiency of enzyme system for bilirubin conjugation (congenital) P59.8
  - bleeding P58.1
  - breast milk inhibitors to conjugation P59.3
    - associated with preterm delivery P59.0
  - bruising P58.0
  - Crigler-Najjar syndrome E80.5
  - delayed conjugation P59.8
    - associated with preterm delivery P59.0
  - drugs or toxins
    - given to newborn P58.42
    - transmitted from mother P58.41
  - excessive hemolysis P58.9
    - due to
      - bleeding P58.1
      - bruising P58.0
      - drugs or toxins
        - given to newborn P58.42
        - transmitted from mother P58.41
      - infection P58.2
      - polycythemia P58.3
      - swallowed maternal blood P58.5
    - specified type NEC P58.8
  - galactosemia E74.21
  - Gilbert syndrome E80.4
  - hemolytic disease P55.9
    - ABO isoimmunization P55.1
    - Rh isoimmunization P55.0
    - specified NEC P55.8
  - hepatocellular damage P59.20
    - specified NEC P59.29
  - hereditary hemolytic anemia P58.8
  - hypothyroidism, congenital E03.1
  - incompatibility, maternal/fetal NOS P55.9
  - infection P58.2
  - inspissated bile syndrome P59.1
  - isoimmunization NOS P55.9
  - mucoviscidosis E84.9
  - polycythemia P58.3
  - preterm delivery P59.0
  - Rh
    - antibodies P55.0
    - incompatibility, maternal/fetal P55.0
    - isoimmunization P55.0
  - specified cause NEC P59.8
  - swallowed maternal blood P58.5
- spherocytosis (congenital) D58.0
- neonatal — *see* Jaundice, newborn
- nonhemolytic congenital familial (Gilbert) E80.4
- nuclear, newborn (*see also* Kernicterus of newborn) P57.9
- obstructive (*see also* Obstruction, bile duct) K83.1
- post-immunization — *see* Hepatitis, viral, type, B
- post-transfusion — *see* Hepatitis, viral, type, B
- regurgitation (*see also* Obstruction, bile duct) K83.1
- serum (homologous) (prophylactic) (therapeutic) — *see* Hepatitis, viral, type, B
- spirochetal (hemorrhagic) A27.0
- symptomatic R17
  - newborn P59.9

Jaw — *see* condition
Jaw-winking phenomenon or syndrome Q07.8
Jealousy
- alcoholic F10.988
- childhood F93.8
- sibling F93.8

Jejunitis — *see* Enteritis
Jejunostomy status Z93.4
Jejunum, jejunal — *see* condition
Jensen's disease — *see* Inflammation, chorioretinal, focal, juxtapapillary
Jerks, myoclonic G25.3
Jervell-Lange-Nielsen syndrome I45.81
Jeune's disease Q77.2
Jigger disease B88.1
Job's syndrome (chronic granulomatous disease) D71
Joint (*see also* condition)
- mice — *see* Loose, body, joint
  - knee M23.4 ☑

Jordan's anomaly or syndrome D72.0
Joseph-Diamond-Blackfan anemia (congenital hypoplastic) D61.01
Jungle yellow fever A95.0
Jüngling's disease — *see* Sarcoidosis
Juvenile — *see* condition

K

Kahler's disease C90.0 ☑
Kakke E51.11
Kala-azar B55.0
Kallmann's syndrome E23.0
Kanner's syndrome (autism) — *see* Psychosis, childhood
Kaposi's
- dermatosis (xeroderma pigmentosum) Q82.1
- lichen ruber L44.0
  - acuminatus L44.0
- sarcoma
  - colon C46.4
  - connective tissue C46.1
  - gastrointestinal organ C46.4
  - lung C46.5 ☑
  - lymph node (multiple) C46.3
  - palate (hard) (soft) C46.2
  - rectum C46.4
  - skin (multiple sites) C46.0
  - specified site NEC C46.7
  - stomach C46.4
  - unspecified site C46.9
- varicelliform eruption B00.0
  - vaccinia T88.1 ☑

Kartagener's syndrome or triad (sinusitis, bronchiectasis, situs inversus) Q89.3
Karyotype
- with abnormality except iso (Xq) Q96.2
- 45,X Q96.0
- 46,X
  - iso (Xq) Q96.1
- 46,XX Q98.3
  - with streak gonads Q50.32
  - hermaphrodite (true) Q99.1
  - male Q98.3
- 46,XY
  - with streak gonads Q56.1
  - female Q97.3
  - hermaphrodite (true) Q99.1
- 47,XXX Q97.0
- 47,XXY Q98.0
- 47,XYY Q98.5

Kaschin-Beck disease — *see* Disease, Kaschin-Beck
Katayama's disease or fever B65.2
Kawasaki's syndrome M30.3
Kayser-Fleischer ring (cornea) (pseudosclerosis) H18.04 ☑
Kaznelson's syndrome (congenital hypoplastic anemia) D61.01
Kearns-Sayre syndrome H49.81 ☑
Kedani fever A75.3
Kelis L91.0
Kelly (-Patterson) syndrome (sideropenic dysphagia) D50.1
Keloid, cheloid L91.0
- acne L73.0
- Addison's L94.0
- cornea — *see* Opacity, cornea
- Hawkin's L91.0
- scar L91.0

Keloma L91.0
Kenya fever A77.1
Keratectasia (*see also* Ectasia, cornea)
- congenital Q13.4

Keratinization of alveolar ridge mucosa
- excessive K13.23
- minimal K13.22

Keratinized residual ridge mucosa
- excessive K13.23
- minimal K13.22

Keratitis (nodular) (nonulcerative) (simple) (zonular) H16.9
- with ulceration (central) (marginal) (perforated) (ring) — *see* Ulcer, cornea
- actinic — *see* Photokeratitis
- arborescens (herpes simplex) B00.52
- areolar H16.11 ☑
- bullosa H16.8
- deep H16.309
  - specified type NEC H16.399
- dendritic (a) (herpes simplex) B00.52
- disciform (is) (herpes simplex) B00.52
  - varicella B01.81
- filamentary H16.12 ☑
- gonococcal (congenital or prenatal) A54.33
- herpes, herpetic (simplex) B00.52
  - zoster B02.33
- in (due to)
  - acanthamebiasis B60.13

Keratitis — *continued*
    in — *continued*
        adenovirus B30.0
        exanthema (*see also* Exanthem) B09
        herpes (simplex) virus B00.52
        measles B05.81
        syphilis A50.31
        tuberculosis A18.52
        zoster B02.33
    interstitial (nonsyphilitic) H16.30 ☑
        diffuse H16.32 ☑
        herpes, herpetic (simplex) B00.52
            zoster B02.33
        sclerosing H16.33 ☑
        specified type NEC H16.39 ☑
        syphilitic (congenital) (late) A50.31
        tuberculous A18.52
    macular H16.11 ☑
    nummular H16.11 ☑
    oyster shuckers' H16.8
    parenchymatous — *see* Keratitis, interstitial
    petrificans H16.8
    postmeasles B05.81
    punctata
        leprosa A30.9 [*H16.14* ☑]
        syphilitic (profunda) A50.31
    punctate H16.14 ☑
    purulent H16.8
    rosacea L71.8
    sclerosing H16.33 ☑
    specified type NEC H16.8
    stellate H16.11 ☑
    striate H16.11 ☑
    superficial H16.10 ☑
        with conjunctivitis — *see* Keratoconjunctivitis
        due to light — *see* Photokeratitis
    suppurative H16.8
    syphilitic (congenital) (prenatal) A50.31
    trachomatous A71.1
        sequelae B94.0
    tuberculous A18.52
    vesicular H16.8
    xerotic (*see also* Keratomalacia) H16.8
        vitamin A deficiency E50.4
Keratoacanthoma L85.8
Keratocele — *see* Descemetocele
Keratoconjunctivitis H16.20 ☑
    Acanthamoeba B60.13
    adenoviral B30.0
    epidemic B30.0
    exposure H16.21 ☑
    herpes, herpetic (simplex) B00.52
        zoster B02.33
    in exanthema (*see also* Exanthem) B09
    infectious B30.0
    lagophthalmic — *see* Keratoconjunctivitis, specified
        type NEC
    neurotrophic H16.23 ☑
    phlyctenular H16.25 ☑
    postmeasles B05.81
    shipyard B30.0
    sicca (Sjogren's) M35.0 ☑
        not Sjogren's H16.22 ☑
    specified type NEC H16.29 ☑
    tuberculous (phlyctenular) A18.52
    vernal H16.26 ☑
Keratoconus H18.60 ☑
    congenital Q13.4
    stable H18.61 ☑
    unstable H18.62 ☑
Keratocyst (dental) (odontogenic) — *see* Cyst,
    calcifying odontogenic
Keratoderma, keratodermia (congenital) (palmaris et
    plantaris) (symmetrical) Q82.8
    acquired L85.1
        in diseases classified elsewhere L86
    climactericum L85.1
    gonococcal A54.89
    gonorrheal A54.89
    punctata L85.2
    Reiter's — *see* Reiter's disease
Keratodermatocele — *see* Descemetocele
Keratoglobus H18.79 ☑
    congenital Q15.8
        with glaucoma Q15.0
Keratohemia — *see* Pigmentation, cornea, stromal
Keratoiritis (*see also* Iridocyclitis)
    syphilitic A50.39
    tuberculous A18.54
Keratoma L57.0
    palmaris and plantaris hereditarium Q82.8
    senile L57.0

Keratomalacia H18.44 ☑
    vitamin A deficiency E50.4
Keratomegaly Q13.4
Keratomycosis B49
    nigrans, nigricans (palmaris) B36.1
Keratopathy H18.9
    band H18.42 ☑
    bullous H18.1 ☑
    bullous (aphakic), following cataract surgery
        H59.01 ☑
Keratoscleritis, tuberculous A18.52
Keratosis L57.0
    actinic L57.0
    arsenical L85.8
    congenital, specified NEC Q80.8
    female genital NEC N94.89
    follicularis Q82.8
        acquired L11.0
        congenita Q82.8
        et parafollicularis in cutem penetrans L87.0
        spinulosa (decalvans) Q82.8
        vitamin A deficiency E50.8
    gonococcal A54.89
    male genital (external) N50.89
    nigricans L83
    obturans, external ear (canal) — *see* Cholesteatoma,
        external ear
    palmaris et plantaris (inherited) (symmetrical) Q82.8
        acquired L85.1
    penile N48.89
    pharynx J39.2
    pilaris, acquired L85.8
        punctata (palmaris et plantaris) L85.2
    scrotal N50.89
    seborrheic L82.1
        inflamed L82.0
    senile L57.0
    solar L57.0
    tonsillaris J35.8
    vagina N89.4
    vegetans Q82.8
    vitamin A deficiency E50.8
    vocal cord J38.3
Kerato-uveitis — *see* Iridocyclitis
Kerunoparalysis T75.09 ☑
Kerion (celsi) B35.0
Kernicterus of newborn (not due to isoimmunization)
    P57.9
    due to isoimmunization (conditions in P55.0-P55.9)
        P57.0
    specified type NEC P57.8
Keshan disease E59
Ketoacidosis E87.2
    diabetic — *see* Diabetes, by type, with ketoacidosis
Ketonuria R82.4
Ketosis NEC E88.89
    diabetic — *see* Diabetes, by type, with ketoacidosis
Kew Garden fever A79.1
Kidney — *see* condition
Kienböck's disease (*see also* Osteochondrosis, juvenile,
    hand, carpal lunate)
    adult M93.1
Kimmelstiel (-Wilson) disease — *see* Diabetes,
    Kimmelstiel (-Wilson) disease
Kimura disease D21.9
    specified site (*see* Neoplasm, connective tissue
        benign)
Kink, kinking
    artery I77.1
    hair (acquired) L67.8
    ileum or intestine — *see* Obstruction, intestine
    Lane's — *see* Obstruction, intestine
    organ or site, congenital NEC — *see* Anomaly, by site
    ureter (pelvic junction) N13.5
        with
            hydronephrosis N13.1
                with infection N13.6
            pyelonephritis (chronic) N11.1
        congenital Q62.39
    vein(s) I87.8
        caval I87.1
        peripheral I87.1
Kinnier Wilson's disease (hepatolenticular
    degeneration) E83.01
Kissing spine M48.20
    cervical region M48.22
    cervicothoracic region M48.23
    lumbar region M48.26
    lumbosacral region M48.27
    occipito-atlanto-axial region M48.21
    thoracic region M48.24
    thoracolumbar region M48.25

Klatskin's tumor C24.0
Klauder's disease A26.8
Klebs' disease (*see also* Glomerulonephritis) N05. ☑
Klebsiella (K.) pneumoniae, as cause of disease
    classified elsewhere B96.1
Klein (e)-Levin syndrome G47.13
Kleptomania F63.2
Klinefelter's syndrome Q98.4
    karyotype 47,XXY Q98.0
    male with more than two X chromosomes Q98.1
Klippel-Feil deficiency, disease, or syndrome
    (brevicollis) Q76.1
Klippel's disease I67.2
Klippel-Trenaunay (-Weber) syndrome Q87.2
Klumpke (-Déjerine) palsy, paralysis (birth) (newborn)
    P14.1
Knee — *see* condition
Knock knee (acquired) M21.06 ☑
    congenital Q74.1
Knot(s)
    intestinal, syndrome (volvulus) K56.2
    surfer S89.8 ☑
    umbilical cord (true) O69.2 ☑
Knotting (of)
    hair L67.8
    intestine K56.2
Knuckle pad (Garrod's) M72.1
Koch's
    infection — *see* Tuberculosis
    relapsing fever A68.9
Koch-Weeks' conjunctivitis — *see* Conjunctivitis, acute,
    mucopurulent
Köebner's syndrome Q81.8
Köenig's disease (osteochondritis dissecans) — *see*
    Osteochondritis, dissecans
Köhler-Pellegrini-Steida disease or syndrome
    (calcification, knee joint) — *see* Bursitis, tibial
    collateral
Köhler's disease
    patellar — *see* Osteochondrosis, juvenile, patella
    tarsal navicular — *see* Osteochondrosis, juvenile, tarsus
Koilonychia L60.3
    congenital Q84.6
Kojevnikov's, epilepsy — *see* Kozhevnikof's epilepsy
Koplik's spots B05.9
Kopp's asthma E32.8
Korsakoff's (Wernicke) disease, psychosis or syndrome
    (alcoholic) F10.96
    with dependence F10.26
    drug-induced
        due to drug abuse — *see* Abuse, drug, by type,
            with amnestic disorder
        due to drug dependence — *see* Dependence,
            drug, by type, with amnestic disorder
    nonalcoholic F04
Korsakov's disease, psychosis or syndrome — *see*
    Korsakoff's disease
Korsakow's disease, psychosis or syndrome — *see*
    Korsakoff's disease
Kostmann's disease or syndrome (infantile genetic
    agranulocytosis) — *see* Agranulocytosis
Kozhevnikof's epilepsy G40.109
    intractable G40.119
        with status epilepticus G40.111
        without status epilepticus G40.119
    not intractable G40.109
        with status epilepticus G40.101
        without status epilepticus G40.109
Krabbe's
    disease E75.23
    syndrome, congenital muscle hypoplasia Q79.8
Kraepelin-Morel disease — *see* Schizophrenia
Kraft-Weber-Dimitri disease Q85.8
Kraurosis
    ani K62.89
    penis N48.0
    vagina N89.8
    vulva N90.4
Kreotoxism A05.9
Krukenberg's
    spindle — *see* Pigmentation, cornea, posterior
    tumor C79.6 ☑
Kufs' disease E75.4
Kugelberg-Welander disease G12.1
Kuhnt-Junius degeneration (*see also* Degeneration,
    macula) H35.32 ☑
Kümmell's disease or spondylitis — *see* Spondylopathy,
    traumatic
Kupffer cell sarcoma C22.3
Kuru A81.81
Kussmaul's
    disease M30.0

Kussmaul's — *continued*
  respiration E87.2
    in diabetic acidosis — *see* Diabetes, by type, with
      ketoacidosis
Kwashiorkor E40
  marasmic, marasmus type E42
Kyasanur Forest disease A98.2
Kyphoscoliosis, kyphoscoliotic (acquired) (*see also*
  Scoliosis) M41.9
  congenital Q67.5
  heart (disease) I27.1
  sequelae of rickets E64.3
  tuberculous A18.01
Kyphosis, kyphotic (acquired) M40.209
  cervical region M40.202
  cervicothoracic region M40.203
  congenital Q76.419
    cervical region Q76.412
    cervicothoracic region Q76.413
    occipito-atlanto-axial region Q76.411
    thoracic region Q76.414
    thoracolumbar region Q76.415
  Morquio-Brailsford type (spinal) (*see also*
    subcategory M49.8 🗹) E76.219
  postlaminectomy M96.3
  postradiation therapy M96.2
  postural (adolescent) M40.00
    cervicothoracic region M40.03
    thoracic region M40.04
    thoracolumbar region M40.05
  secondary NEC M40.10
    cervical region M40.12
    cervicothoracic region M40.13
    thoracic region M40.14
    thoracolumbar region M40.15
  sequelae of rickets E64.3
  specified type NEC M40.299
    cervical region M40.292
    cervicothoracic region M40.293
    thoracic region M40.294
    thoracolumbar region M40.295
  syphilitic, congenital A50.56
  thoracic region M40.204
  thoracolumbar region M40.205
  tuberculous A18.01
Kyrle disease L87.0

L

Labia, labium — *see* condition
Labile
  blood pressure R09.89
  vasomotor system I73.9
Labioglossal paralysis G12.29
Labium leporinum — *see* Cleft, lip
Labor — *see* Delivery
Labored breathing — *see* Hyperventilation
Labyrinthitis (circumscribed) (destructive) (diffuse)
  (inner ear) (latent) (purulent) (suppurative) (*see also*
  subcategory) H83.0 🗹
  syphilitic A52.79
Laceration
  with abortion — *see* Abortion, by type, complicated
    by laceration of pelvic organs
  abdomen, abdominal
    wall S31.119 🗹
      with
        foreign body S31.129 🗹
        penetration into peritoneal cavity S31.619 🗹
          with foreign body S31.629 🗹
      epigastric region S31.112 🗹
        with
          foreign body S31.122 🗹
          penetration into peritoneal cavity
            S31.612 🗹
            with foreign body S31.622 🗹
      left
        lower quadrant S31.114 🗹
          with
            foreign body S31.124 🗹
            penetration into peritoneal cavity
              S31.614 🗹
              with foreign body S31.624 🗹
        upper quadrant S31.111 🗹
          with
            foreign body S31.121 🗹
            penetration into peritoneal cavity
              S31.611 🗹
              with foreign body S31.621 🗹
      periumbilic region S31.115 🗹

Laceration — *continued*
  abdomen — *continued*
    with
      foreign body S31.125 🗹
      penetration into peritoneal cavity
        S31.615 🗹
      with foreign body S31.625 🗹
    right
      lower quadrant S31.113 🗹
        with
          foreign body S31.123 🗹
          penetration into peritoneal cavity
            S31.613 🗹
            with foreign body S31.623 🗹
      upper quadrant S31.110 🗹
        with
          foreign body S31.120 🗹
          penetration into peritoneal cavity
            S31.610 🗹
            with foreign body S31.620 🗹
  accidental, complicating surgery — *see*
    Complications, surgical, accidental puncture or
    laceration
  Achilles tendon S86.02 🗹
  adrenal gland S37.813 🗹
  alveolar (process) — *see* Laceration, oral cavity
  ankle S91.01 🗹
    with
      foreign body S91.02 🗹
  antecubital space — *see* Laceration, elbow
  anus (sphincter) S31.831 🗹
    with
      ectopic or molar pregnancy O08.6
      foreign body S31.832 🗹
    complicating delivery — *see* Delivery,
      complicated, by, laceration, anus (sphincter)
    following ectopic or molar pregnancy O08.6
    nontraumatic, nonpuerperal — *see* Fissure, anus
  arm (upper) S41.11 🗹
    with foreign body S41.12 🗹
    lower — *see* Laceration, forearm
  auditory canal (external) (meatus) — *see* Laceration,
    ear
  auricle, ear — *see* Laceration, ear
  axilla — *see* Laceration, arm
  back (*see also* Laceration, thorax, back)
    lower S31.010 🗹
      with
        foreign body S31.020 🗹
          with penetration into retroperitoneal space
            S31.021 🗹
        penetration into retroperitoneal space
          S31.011 🗹
  bile duct S36.13 🗹
  bladder S37.23 🗹
    with ectopic or molar pregnancy O08.6
    following ectopic or molar pregnancy O08.6
    obstetrical trauma O71.5
  blood vessel — *see* Injury, blood vessel
  bowel (*see also* Laceration, intestine)
    with ectopic or molar pregnancy O08.6
    complicating abortion — *see* Abortion, by type,
      complicated by, specified condition NEC
    following ectopic or molar pregnancy O08.6
    obstetrical trauma O71.5
  brain (any part) (cortex) (diffuse) (membrane) (*see*
    also Injury, intracranial, diffuse)
    during birth P10.8
      with hemorrhage P10.1
    focal — *see* Injury, intracranial, focal brain injury
  brainstem S06.38 🗹
  breast S21.01 🗹
    with foreign body S21.02 🗹
  broad ligament S37.893 🗹
    with ectopic or molar pregnancy O08.6
    following ectopic or molar pregnancy O08.6
    laceration syndrome N83.8
    obstetrical trauma O71.6
    syndrome (laceration) N83.8
  buttock S31.801 🗹
    with foreign body S31.802 🗹
    left S31.821 🗹
      with foreign body S31.822 🗹
    right S31.811 🗹
      with foreign body S31.812 🗹
  calf — *see* Laceration, leg
  canaliculus lacrimalis — *see* Laceration, eyelid
  canthus, eye — *see* Laceration, eyelid
  capsule, joint — *see* Sprain
  causing eversion of cervix uteri (old) N86
  central (perineal), complicating delivery O70.9
  cerebellum, traumatic S06.37 🗹

Laceration — *continued*
  cerebral S06.33 🗹
    left side S06.32 🗹
    during birth P10.8
      with hemorrhage P10.1
    right side S06.31 🗹
  cervix (uteri)
    with ectopic or molar pregnancy O08.6
    following ectopic or molar pregnancy O08.6
    nonpuerperal, nontraumatic N88.1
    obstetrical trauma (current) O71.3
    old (postpartal) N88.1
    traumatic S37.63 🗹
  cheek (external) S01.41 🗹
    with foreign body S01.42 🗹
    internal — *see* Laceration, oral cavity
  chest wall — *see* Laceration, thorax
  chin — *see* Laceration, head, specified site NEC
  chordae tendinae NEC I51.1
    concurrent with acute myocardial infarction —
      see Infarct, myocardium
    following acute myocardial infarction (current
      complication) I23.4
  clitoris — *see* Laceration, vulva
  colon — *see* Laceration, intestine, large, colon
  common bile duct S36.13 🗹
  cortex (cerebral) — *see* Injury, intracranial, diffuse
  costal region — *see* Laceration, thorax
  cystic duct S36.13 🗹
  diaphragm S27.803 🗹
  digit(s)
    hand — *see* Laceration, finger
    foot — *see* Laceration, toe
  duodenum S36.430 🗹
  ear (canal) (external) S01.31 🗹
    with foreign body S01.32 🗹
    drum S09.2 🗹
  elbow S51.01 🗹
    with
      foreign body S51.02 🗹
  epididymis — *see* Laceration, testis
  epigastric region — *see* Laceration, abdomen, wall,
    epigastric region
  esophagus K22.8
    traumatic
      cervical S11.21 🗹
        with foreign body S11.22 🗹
      thoracic S27.813 🗹
  eye (ball) S05.3 🗹
    with prolapse or loss of intraocular tissue S05.2 🗹
    penetrating S05.6 🗹
  eyebrow — *see* Laceration, eyelid
  eyelid S01.11 🗹
    with foreign body S01.12 🗹
  face NEC — *see* Laceration, head, specified site NEC
  fallopian tube S37.539 🗹
    bilateral S37.532 🗹
    unilateral S37.531 🗹
  finger(s) S61.219 🗹
    with
      damage to nail S61.319 🗹
        with
          foreign body S61.329 🗹
      foreign body S61.229 🗹
    index S61.218 🗹
      with
        damage to nail S61.318 🗹
          with
            foreign body S61.328 🗹
        foreign body S61.228 🗹
    left S61.211 🗹
      with
        damage to nail S61.311 🗹
          with
            foreign body S61.321 🗹
        foreign body S61.221 🗹
    right S61.210 🗹
      with
        damage to nail S61.310 🗹
          with
            foreign body S61.320 🗹
        foreign body S61.220 🗹
    little S61.218 🗹
      with
        damage to nail S61.318 🗹
          with
            foreign body S61.328 🗹
        foreign body S61.228 🗹
    left S61.217 🗹
      with
        damage to nail S61.317 🗹
          with

🗹 **Additional character required**

Laceration — *continued*
  finger(s) — *continued*
        foreign body S61.327 ☑
      foreign body S61.227 ☑
    right S61.216 ☑
      with
        damage to nail S61.316 ☑
          with
            foreign body S61.326 ☑
        foreign body S61.226 ☑
    middle S61.218 ☑
      with
        damage to nail S61.318 ☑
          with
            foreign body S61.328 ☑
        foreign body S61.228 ☑
      left S61.213 ☑
        with
          damage to nail S61.313 ☑
            with
              foreign body S61.323 ☑
          foreign body S61.223 ☑
      right S61.212 ☑
        with
          damage to nail S61.312 ☑
            with
              foreign body S61.322 ☑
          foreign body S61.222 ☑
    ring S61.218 ☑
      with
        damage to nail S61.318 ☑
          with
            foreign body S61.328 ☑
        foreign body S61.228 ☑
      left S61.215 ☑
        with
          damage to nail S61.315 ☑
            with
              foreign body S61.325 ☑
          foreign body S61.225 ☑
      right S61.214 ☑
        with
          damage to nail S61.314 ☑
            with
              foreign body S61.324 ☑
          foreign body S61.224 ☑
  flank S31.119 ☑
    with foreign body S31.129 ☑
  foot (except toe(s) alone) S91.319 ☑
    with foreign body S91.329 ☑
    left S91.312 ☑
      with foreign body S91.322 ☑
    right S91.311 ☑
      with foreign body S91.321 ☑
    toe — *see* Laceration, toe
  forearm S51.819 ☑
    with
      foreign body S51.829 ☑
    elbow only — *see* Laceration, elbow
    left S51.812 ☑
      with
        foreign body S51.822 ☑
    right S51.811 ☑
      with
        foreign body S51.821 ☑
  forehead S01.81 ☑
    with foreign body S01.82 ☑
  fourchette O70.0
    with ectopic or molar pregnancy O08.6
    complicating delivery O70.0
    following ectopic or molar pregnancy O08.6
  gallbladder S36.123 ☑
  genital organs, external
    female S31.512 ☑
      with foreign body S31.522 ☑
      vagina — *see* Laceration, vagina
      vulva — *see* Laceration, vulva
    male S31.511 ☑
      with foreign body S31.521 ☑
      penis — *see* Laceration, penis
      scrotum — *see* Laceration, scrotum
      testis — *see* Laceration, testis
  groin — *see* Laceration, abdomen, wall
  gum — *see* Laceration, oral cavity
  hand S61.419 ☑
    with
      foreign body S61.429 ☑
    finger — *see* Laceration, finger
    left S61.412 ☑
      with
        foreign body S61.422 ☑
    right S61.411 ☑

Laceration — *continued*
  hand — *continued*
      with
        foreign body S61.421 ☑
    thumb — *see* Laceration, thumb
  head S01.91 ☑
    with foreign body S01.92 ☑
    cheek — *see* Laceration, cheek
    ear — *see* Laceration, ear
    eyelid — *see* Laceration, eyelid
    lip — *see* Laceration, lip
    nose — *see* Laceration, nose
    oral cavity — *see* Laceration, oral cavity
    scalp S01.01 ☑
      with foreign body S01.02 ☑
    specified site NEC S01.81 ☑
      with foreign body S01.82 ☑
    temporomandibular area — *see* Laceration, cheek
  heart — *see* Injury, heart, laceration
  heel — *see* Laceration, foot
  hepatic duct S36.13 ☑
  hip S71.019 ☑
    with foreign body S71.029 ☑
    left S71.012 ☑
      with foreign body S71.022 ☑
    right S71.011 ☑
      with foreign body S71.021 ☑
  hymen — *see* Laceration, vagina
  hypochondrium — *see* Laceration, abdomen, wall
  hypogastric region — *see* Laceration, abdomen, wall
  ileum S36.438 ☑
  inguinal region — *see* Laceration, abdomen, wall
  instep — *see* Laceration, foot
  internal organ — *see* Injury, by site
  interscapular region — *see* Laceration, thorax, back
  intestine
    large
      colon S36.539 ☑
        ascending S36.530 ☑
        descending S36.532 ☑
        sigmoid S36.533 ☑
        specified site NEC S36.538 ☑
      rectum S36.63 ☑
        transverse S36.531 ☑
    small S36.439 ☑
      duodenum S36.430 ☑
      specified site NEC S36.438 ☑
  intra-abdominal organ S36.93 ☑
    intestine — *see* Laceration, intestine
    liver — *see* Laceration, liver
    pancreas — *see* Laceration, pancreas
    peritoneum S36.81 ☑
    specified site NEC S36.893 ☑
    spleen — *see* Laceration, spleen
    stomach — *see* Laceration, stomach
  intracranial NEC (*see also* Injury, intracranial, diffuse)
    birth injury P10.9
  jaw — *see* Laceration, head, specified site NEC
  jejunum S36.438 ☑
  joint capsule — *see* Sprain, by site
  kidney S37.03 ☑
    major (greater than 3 cm) (massive) (stellate) S37.06 ☑
    minor (less than 1 cm) S37.04 ☑
    moderate (1 to 3 cm) S37.05 ☑
      multiple S37.06 ☑
  knee S81.01 ☑
    with foreign body S81.02 ☑
  labium (majus) (minus) — *see* Laceration, vulva
  lacrimal duct — *see* Laceration, eyelid
  large intestine — *see* Laceration, intestine, large
  larynx S11.011 ☑
    with foreign body S11.012 ☑
  leg (lower) S81.819 ☑
    with foreign body S81.829 ☑
    foot — *see* Laceration, foot
    knee — *see* Laceration, knee
    left S81.812 ☑
      with foreign body S81.822 ☑
    right S81.811 ☑
      with foreign body S81.821 ☑
    upper — *see* Laceration, thigh
  ligament — *see* Sprain
  lip S01.511 ☑
    with foreign body S01.521 ☑
  liver S36.113 ☑
    major (stellate) S36.116 ☑
    minor S36.114 ☑
    moderate S36.115 ☑
  loin — *see* Laceration, abdomen, wall
  lower back — *see* Laceration, back, lower

Laceration — *continued*
  lumbar region — *see* Laceration, back, lower
  lung S27.339 ☑
    bilateral S27.332 ☑
    unilateral S27.331 ☑
  malar region — *see* Laceration, head, specified site NEC
  mammary — *see* Laceration, breast
  mastoid region — *see* Laceration, head, specified site NEC
  meninges — *see* Injury, intracranial, diffuse
  meniscus — *see* Tear, meniscus
  mesentery S36.893 ☑
  mesosalpinx S37.893 ☑
  mouth — *see* Laceration, oral cavity
  muscle — *see* Injury, muscle, by site, laceration
  nail
    finger — *see* Laceration, finger, with damage to nail
    toe — *see* Laceration, toe, with damage to nail
  nasal (septum) (sinus) — *see* Laceration, nose
  nasopharynx — *see* Laceration, head, specified site NEC
  neck S11.91 ☑
    with foreign body S11.92 ☑
    involving
      cervical esophagus S11.21 ☑
        with foreign body S11.22 ☑
      larynx — *see* Laceration, larynx
      pharynx — *see* Laceration, pharynx
      thyroid gland — *see* Laceration, thyroid gland
      trachea — *see* Laceration, trachea
    specified site NEC S11.81 ☑
      with foreign body S11.82 ☑
  nerve — *see* Injury, nerve
  nose (septum) (sinus) S01.21 ☑
    with foreign body S01.22 ☑
  ocular NOS S05.3 ☑
    adnexa NOS S01.11 ☑
  oral cavity S01.512 ☑
    with foreign body S01.522 ☑
  orbit (eye) — *see* Wound, open, ocular, orbit
  ovary S37.439 ☑
    bilateral S37.432 ☑
    unilateral S37.431 ☑
  palate — *see* Laceration, oral cavity
  palm — *see* Laceration, hand
  pancreas S36.239 ☑
    body S36.231 ☑
      major S36.261 ☑
      minor S36.241 ☑
      moderate S36.251 ☑
    head S36.230 ☑
      major S36.260 ☑
      minor S36.240 ☑
      moderate S36.250 ☑
    major S36.269 ☑
    minor S36.249 ☑
    moderate S36.259 ☑
    tail S36.232 ☑
      major S36.262 ☑
      minor S36.242 ☑
      moderate S36.252 ☑
  pelvic S31.010 ☑
    with
      foreign body S31.020 ☑
        penetration into retroperitoneal cavity S31.021 ☑
      penetration into retroperitoneal cavity S31.011 ☑
    floor (*see also* Laceration, back, lower)
      with ectopic or molar pregnancy O08.6
      complicating delivery O70.1
      following ectopic or molar pregnancy O08.6
      old (postpartal) N81.89
    organ S37.93 ☑
      with ectopic or molar pregnancy O08.6
      adrenal gland S37.813 ☑
      bladder S37.23 ☑
      fallopian tube — *see* Laceration, fallopian tube
      following ectopic or molar pregnancy O08.6
      kidney — *see* Laceration, kidney
      obstetrical trauma O71.5
      ovary — *see* Laceration, ovary
      prostate S37.823 ☑
      specified site NEC S37.893 ☑
      ureter S37.13 ☑
      urethra S37.33 ☑
      uterus S37.63 ☑
  penis S31.21 ☑
    with foreign body S31.22 ☑

Laceration - Lacrimation

Laceration — *continued*
  perineum
    female S31.41 ☑
      with
        ectopic or molar pregnancy O08.6
        foreign body S31.42 ☑
      during delivery O70.9
        first degree O70.0
        fourth degree O70.3
        second degree O70.1
        third degree (*see also* Delivery, complicated, by, laceration, perineum, third degree) O70.20
      old (postpartal) N81.89
      postpartal N81.89
      secondary (postpartal) O90.1
    male S31.119 ☑
      with foreign body S31.129 ☑
  periocular area (with or without lacrimal passages) — *see* Laceration, eyelid
  peritoneum S36.893 ☑
  periumbilic region — *see* Laceration, abdomen, wall, periumbilic
  periurethral tissue — *see* Laceration, urethra
  phalanges
    finger — *see* Laceration, finger
    toe — *see* Laceration, toe
  pharynx S11.21 ☑
    with foreign body S11.22 ☑
  pinna — *see* Laceration, ear
  popliteal space — *see* Laceration, knee
  prepuce — *see* Laceration, penis
  prostate S37.823 ☑
  pubic region S31.119 ☑
    with foreign body S31.129 ☑
  pudendum — *see* Laceration, genital organs, external
  rectovaginal septum — *see* Laceration, vagina
  rectum S36.63 ☑
  retroperitoneum S36.893 ☑
  round ligament S37.893 ☑
  sacral region — *see* Laceration, back, lower
  sacroiliac region — *see* Laceration, back, lower
  salivary gland — *see* Laceration, oral cavity
  scalp S01.01 ☑
    with foreign body S01.02 ☑
  scapular region — *see* Laceration, shoulder
  scrotum S31.31 ☑
    with foreign body S31.32 ☑
  seminal vesicle S37.893 ☑
  shin — *see* Laceration, leg
  shoulder S41.019 ☑
    with foreign body S41.029 ☑
    left S41.012 ☑
      with foreign body S41.022 ☑
    right S41.011 ☑
      with foreign body S41.021 ☑
  small intestine — *see* Laceration, intestine, small
  spermatic cord — *see* Laceration, testis
  spinal cord (meninges) (*see also* Injury, spinal cord, by region)
    due to injury at birth P11.5
    newborn (birth injury) P11.5
  spleen S36.039 ☑
    major (massive) (stellate) S36.032 ☑
    moderate S36.031 ☑
    superficial (minor) S36.030 ☑
  sternal region — *see* Laceration, thorax, front
  stomach S36.33 ☑
  submaxillary region — *see* Laceration, head, specified site NEC
  submental region — *see* Laceration, head, specified site NEC
  subungual
    finger(s) — *see* Laceration, finger, with damage to nail
    toe(s) — *see* Laceration, toe, with damage to nail
  suprarenal gland — *see* Laceration, adrenal gland
  temple, temporal region — *see* Laceration, head, specified site NEC
  temporomandibular area — *see* Laceration, cheek
  tendon — *see* Injury, muscle, by site, laceration
    Achilles S86.02 ☑
  tentorium cerebelli — *see* Injury, intracranial, diffuse
  testis S31.31 ☑
    with foreign body S31.32 ☑
  thigh S71.11 ☑
    with foreign body S71.12 ☑
  thorax, thoracic (wall) S21.91 ☑
    with foreign body S21.92 ☑
      back S21.22 ☑
        with penetration into thoracic cavity S21.42 ☑

Laceration — *continued*
  thorax — *continued*
    front S21.12 ☑
      with penetration into thoracic cavity S21.32 ☑
    back S21.21 ☑
      with
        foreign body S21.22 ☑
          with penetration into thoracic cavity S21.42 ☑
        penetration into thoracic cavity S21.41 ☑
    breast — *see* Laceration, breast
    front S21.11 ☑
      with
        foreign body S21.12 ☑
          with penetration into thoracic cavity S21.32 ☑
        penetration into thoracic cavity S21.31 ☑
  thumb S61.019 ☑
    with
      damage to nail S61.119 ☑
        with
          foreign body S61.129 ☑
      foreign body S61.029 ☑
    left S61.012 ☑
      with
        damage to nail S61.112 ☑
          with
            foreign body S61.122 ☑
        foreign body S61.022 ☑
    right S61.011 ☑
      with
        damage to nail S61.111 ☑
          with
            foreign body S61.121 ☑
        foreign body S61.021 ☑
  thyroid gland S11.11 ☑
    with foreign body S11.12 ☑
  toe(s) S91.119 ☑
    with
      damage to nail S91.219 ☑
        with
          foreign body S91.229 ☑
      foreign body S91.129 ☑
    great S91.113 ☑
      with
        damage to nail S91.213 ☑
          with
            foreign body S91.223 ☑
        foreign body S91.123 ☑
      left S91.112 ☑
        with
          damage to nail S91.212 ☑
            with
              foreign body S91.222 ☑
          foreign body S91.122 ☑
      right S91.111 ☑
        with
          damage to nail S91.211 ☑
            with
              foreign body S91.221 ☑
          foreign body S91.121 ☑
    lesser S91.116 ☑
      with
        damage to nail S91.216 ☑
          with
            foreign body S91.226 ☑
        foreign body S91.126 ☑
      left S91.115 ☑
        with
          damage to nail S91.215 ☑
            with
              foreign body S91.225 ☑
          foreign body S91.125 ☑
      right S91.114 ☑
        with
          damage to nail S91.214 ☑
            with
              foreign body S91.224 ☑
          foreign body S91.124 ☑
  tongue — *see* Laceration, oral cavity
  trachea S11.021 ☑
    with foreign body S11.022 ☑
  tunica vaginalis — *see* Laceration, testis
  tympanum, tympanic membrane — *see* Laceration, ear, drum
  umbilical region S31.115 ☑
    with foreign body S31.125 ☑
  ureter S37.13 ☑
  urethra S37.33 ☑
    with or following ectopic or molar pregnancy O08.6
    obstetrical trauma O71.5

Laceration — *continued*
  urinary organ NEC S37.893 ☑
  uterus S37.63 ☑
    with ectopic or molar pregnancy O08.6
    following ectopic or molar pregnancy O08.6
    nonpuerperal, nontraumatic N85.8
    obstetrical trauma NEC O71.81
    old (postpartal) N85.8
  uvula — *see* Laceration, oral cavity
  vagina S31.41 ☑
    with
      ectopic or molar pregnancy O08.6
      foreign body S31.42 ☑
    during delivery O71.4
      with perineal laceration — *see* Laceration, perineum, female, during delivery
    following ectopic or molar pregnancy O08.6
    nonpuerperal, nontraumatic N89.8
    old (postpartal) N89.8
  vas deferens S37.893 ☑
  vesical — *see* Laceration, bladder
  vocal cords S11.031 ☑
    with foreign body S11.032 ☑
  vulva S31.41 ☑
    with
      ectopic or molar pregnancy O08.6
      foreign body S31.42 ☑
    complicating delivery O70.0
    following ectopic or molar pregnancy O08.6
    nonpuerperal, nontraumatic N90.89
    old (postpartal) N90.89
  wrist S61.519 ☑
    with
      foreign body S61.529 ☑
    left S61.512 ☑
      with
        foreign body S61.522 ☑
    right S61.511 ☑
      with
        foreign body S61.521 ☑

Lack of
  achievement in school Z55.3
  adequate
    food Z59.4
    intermaxillary vertical dimension of fully erupted teeth M26.36
    sleep Z72.820
  appetite (*see* Anorexia) R63.0
  awareness R41.9
  care
    in home Z74.2
    of infant (at or after birth) T76.02 ☑
      confirmed T74.02 ☑
  cognitive functions R41.9
  coordination R27.9
    ataxia R27.0
    specified type NEC R27.8
  development (physiological) R62.50
    failure to thrive (child over 28 days old) R62.51
      adult R62.7
      newborn P92.6
    short stature R62.52
    specified type NEC R62.59
  energy R53.83
  financial resources Z59.6
  food T73.0 ☑
  growth R62.52
  heating Z59.1
  housing (permanent) (temporary) Z59.0
    adequate Z59.1
  learning experiences in childhood Z62.898
  leisure time (affecting life-style) Z73.2
  material resources Z59.9
  memory (*see also* Amnesia)
    mild, following organic brain damage F06.8
  ovulation N97.0
  parental supervision or control of child Z62.0
  person able to render necessary care Z74.2
  physical exercise Z72.3
  play experience in childhood Z62.898
  posterior occlusal support M26.57
  relaxation (affecting life-style) Z73.2
  sexual
    desire F52.0
    enjoyment F52.1
  shelter Z59.0
  sleep (adequate) Z72.820
  supervision of child by parent Z62.0
  support, posterior occlusal M26.57
  water T73.1 ☑
Lacrimal — *see* condition
Lacrimation, abnormal — *see* Epiphora

☑ **Additional character required**

Lacrimonasal duct — *see* condition
Lactation, lactating (breast) (puerperal, postpartum)
  associated
    cracked nipple O92.13
    retracted nipple O92.03
  defective O92.4
  disorder NEC O92.79
  excessive O92.6
  failed (complete) O92.3
    partial O92.4
  mastitis NEC — *see* Mastitis, obstetric
  mother (care and/or examination) Z39.1
  nonpuerperal N64.3
Lacticemia, excessive E87.2
Lacunar skull Q75.8
Laennec's cirrhosis K70.30
  with ascites K70.31
  nonalcoholic K74.69
Lafora's disease — *see* Epilepsy, generalized, idiopathic
Lag, lid (nervous) — *see* Retraction, lid
Lagophthalmos (eyelid) (nervous) H02.209
  bilateral, upper and lower eyelids H02.20C
  cicatricial H02.219
    bilateral, upper and lower eyelids H02.21C
    left H02.216
      lower H02.215
      upper H02.214
      upper and lower eyelids H02.21B
    right H02.213
      lower H02.212
      upper H02.211
      upper and lower eyelids H02.21A
  keratoconjunctivitis — *see* Keratoconjunctivitis
  left H02.206
    lower H02.205
    upper H02.204
    upper and lower eyelids H02.20B
  mechanical H02.229
    bilateral, upper and lower eyelids H02.22C
    left H02.226
      lower H02.225
      upper H02.224
      upper and lower eyelids H02.22B
    right H02.223
      lower H02.222
      upper H02.221
      upper and lower eyelids H02.22A
  paralytic H02.239
    bilateral, upper and lower eyelids H02.23C
    left H02.236
      lower H02.235
      upper H02.234
      upper and lower eyelids H02.23B
    right H02.233
      lower H02.232
      upper H02.231
      upper and lower eyelids H02.23A
  right H02.203
    lower H02.202
    upper H02.201
    upper and lower eyelids H02.20A
Laki-Lorand factor deficiency — *see* Defect, coagulation, specified type NEC
Lalling F80.0
Lambert-Eaton syndrome — *see* Syndrome, Lambert-Eaton
Lambliasis, lambliosis A07.1
Landau-Kleffner syndrome — *see* Epilepsy, specified NEC
Landouzy-Déjérine dystrophy or facioscapulohumeral atrophy G71.02
Landouzy's disease (icterohemorrhagic leptospirosis) A27.0
Landry-Guillain-Barré, syndrome or paralysis G61.0
Landry's disease or paralysis G61.0
Lane's
  band Q43.3
  kink — *see* Obstruction, intestine
  syndrome K90.2
Langdon Down syndrome — *see* Trisomy, 21
Lapsed immunization schedule status Z28.3
Large
  baby (regardless of gestational age) (4000g to 4499g) P08.1
  ear, congenital Q17.1
  physiological cup Q14.2
  stature R68.89
Large-for-dates NEC (infant) (4000g to 4499g) P08.1
  affecting management of pregnancy O36.6 ☑
  exceptionally (4500g or more) P08.0
Larsen-Johansson disease orosteochondrosis — *see* Osteochondrosis, juvenile, patella

Larsen's syndrome (flattened facies and multiple congenital dislocations) Q74.8
Larva migrans
  cutaneous B76.9
    Ancylostoma B76.0
  visceral B83.0
Laryngeal — *see* condition
Laryngismus (stridulus) J38.5
  congenital P28.89
  diphtheritic A36.2
Laryngitis (acute) (edematous) (fibrinous) (infective) (infiltrative) (malignant) (membranous) (phlegmonous) (pneumococcal) (pseudomembranous) (septic) (subglottic) (suppurative) (ulcerative) J04.0
  with
    influenza, flu, or grippe — *see* Influenza, with, laryngitis
    tracheitis (acute) — *see* Laryngotracheitis
  atrophic J37.0
  catarrhal J37.0
  chronic J37.0
    with tracheitis (chronic) J37.1
  diphtheritic A36.2
  due to external agent — *see* Inflammation, respiratory, upper, due to
  Hemophilus influenzae J04.0
  H. influenzae J04.0
  hypertrophic J37.0
  influenzal — *see* Influenza, with, respiratory manifestations NEC
  obstructive J05.0
  sicca J37.0
  spasmodic J05.0
    acute J04.0
  streptococcal J04.0
  stridulous J05.0
  syphilitic (late) A52.73
    congenital A50.59 *[J99]*
    early A50.03 *[J99]*
  tuberculous A15.5
  Vincent's A69.1
Laryngocele (congenital) (ventricular) Q31.3
Laryngofissure J38.7
  congenital Q31.8
Laryngomalacia (congenital) Q31.5
Laryngopharyngitis (acute) J06.0
  chronic J37.0
  due to external agent — *see* Inflammation, respiratory, upper, due to
Laryngoplegia J38.00
  bilateral J38.02
  unilateral J38.01
Laryngoptosis J38.7
Laryngospasm J38.5
Laryngostenosis J38.6
Laryngotracheitis (acute) (Infectional) (infective) (viral) J04.2
  atrophic J37.1
  catarrhal J37.1
  chronic J37.1
  diphtheritic A36.2
  due to external agent — *see* Inflammation, respiratory, upper, due to
  Hemophilus influenzae J04.2
  hypertrophic J37.1
  influenzal — *see* Influenza, with, respiratory manifestations NEC
  pachydermic J38.7
  sicca J37.1
  spasmodic J38.5
    acute J05.0
  streptococcal J04.2
  stridulous J38.5
  syphilitic (late) A52.73
    congenital A50.59 *[J99]*
    early A50.03 *[J99]*
  tuberculous A15.5
  Vincent's A69.1
Laryngotracheobronchitis — *see* Bronchitis
Larynx, laryngeal — *see* condition
Lassa fever A96.2
Lassitude — *see* Weakness
Late
  talker R62.0
  walker R62.0
Late effect(s) — *see* Sequelae
Latent — *see* condition
Laterocession — *see* Lateroversion
Lateroflexion — *see* Lateroversion
Lateroversion
  cervix — *see* Lateroversion, uterus

Lateroversion — *continued*
  uterus, uterine (cervix) (postinfectional) (postpartal, old) N85.4
    congenital Q51.818
    in pregnancy or childbirth O34.59 ☑
Lathyrism — *see* Poisoning, food, noxious, plant
Launois' syndrome (pituitary gigantism) E22.0
Launois-Bensaude adenolipomatosis E88.89
Laurence-Moon (-Bardet)-Biedl syndrome Q87.89
Lax, laxity (*see also* Relaxation)
  ligament (ous) (*see also* Disorder, ligament)
    familial M35.7
    knee — *see* Derangement, knee
  skin (acquired) L57.4
    congenital Q82.8
Laxative habit F55.2
Lazy leukocyte syndrome D70.8
LTBI (latent tuberculosis infection) Z22.7
Lead miner's lung J63.6
Leak, leakage
  air NEC J93.82
    postprocedural J95.812
  amniotic fluid — *see* Rupture, membranes, premature
  blood (microscopic), fetal, into maternal circulation affecting management of pregnancy — *see* Pregnancy, complicated by
  cerebrospinal fluid G96.0
    from spinal (lumbar) puncture G97.0
  device, implant or graft (*see also* Complications, by site and type, mechanical)
    arterial graft NEC — *see* Complication, cardiovascular device, mechanical, vascular
    breast (implant) T85.43 ☑
    catheter NEC T85.638 ☑
      urinary T83.038 ☑
        cystostomy T83.030 ☑
        Hopkins T83.038 ☑
        ileostomy T83.038 ☑
        indwelling T83.031 ☑
        nephrostomy T83.032 ☑
        specified NEC T83.038 ☑
        urostomy T83.038 ☑
    dialysis (renal) T82.43 ☑
      intraperitoneal T85.631 ☑
    infusion NEC T82.534 ☑
      spinal (epidural) (subdural) T85.630 ☑
    gastrointestinal — *see* Complications, prosthetic device, mechanical, gastrointestinal device
    genital NEC T83.498 ☑
      penile prosthesis (cylinder) (implanted) (pump) (reservoir) T83.490 ☑
      testicular prosthesis T83.491 ☑
    heart NEC — *see* Complication, cardiovascular device, mechanical
    joint prosthesis — *see* Complications, joint prosthesis, mechanical, specified NEC, by site
    ocular NEC — *see* Complications, prosthetic device, mechanical, ocular device
    orthopedic NEC — *see* Complication, orthopedic, device, mechanical
    persistent air J93.82
    specified NEC T85.638 ☑
    urinary NEC (*see also* Complication, genitourinary, device, urinary, mechanical)
      graft T83.23 ☑
    vascular NEC — *see* Complication, cardiovascular device, mechanical
    ventricular intracranial shunt T85.03 ☑
  urine — *see* Incontinence
Leaky heart — *see* Endocarditis
Learning defect (specific) F81.9
Leather bottle stomach C16.9
Leber's
  congenital amaurosis H35.50
  optic atrophy (hereditary) H47.22
Lederer's anemia D59.1
Leeches (external) — *see* Hirudiniasis
Leg — *see* condition
Legg (-Calvé)-Perthes disease, syndrome or osteochondrosis M91.1 ☑
Legionellosis A48.1
  nonpneumonic A48.2
Legionnaires'
  disease A48.1
    nonpneumonic A48.2
  pneumonia A48.1
Leigh's disease G31.82
Leiner's disease L21.1
Leiofibromyoma — *see* Leiomyoma
Leiomyoblastoma — *see* Neoplasm, connective tissue, benign

Leiomyofibroma - Lesion(s)

Leiomyofibroma (*see also* Neoplasm, connective tissue, benign)
  uterus (cervix) (corpus) D25.9
Leiomyoma (*see also* Neoplasm, connective tissue, benign)
  bizarre — *see* Neoplasm, connective tissue, benign
  cellular — *see* Neoplasm, connective tissue, benign
  epithelioid — *see* Neoplasm, connective tissue, benign
  uterus (cervix) (corpus) D25.9
    intramural D25.1
    submucous D25.0
    subserosal D25.2
  vascular — *see* Neoplasm, connective tissue, benign
Leiomyoma, leiomyomatosis (intravascular) — *see* Neoplasm, connective tissue, uncertain behavior
Leiomyosarcoma (*see also* Neoplasm, connective tissue, malignant)
  epithelioid — *see* Neoplasm, connective tissue, malignant
  myxoid — *see* Neoplasm, connective tissue, malignant
Leishmaniasis B55.9
  American (mucocutaneous) B55.2
    cutaneous B55.1
  Asian Desert B55.1
  Brazilian B55.2
  cutaneous (any type) B55.1
  dermal (*see also* Leishmaniasis, cutaneous)
    post-kala-azar B55.0
  eyelid B55.1
  infantile B55.0
  Mediterranean B55.0
  mucocutaneous (American) (New World) B55.2
  naso-oral B55.2
  nasopharyngeal B55.2
  old world B55.1
  tegumentaria diffusa B55.1
  visceral B55.0
Leishmanoid, dermal (*see also* Leishmaniasis, cutaneous)
  post-kala-azar B55.0
Lenegre's disease I44.2
Lengthening, leg — *see* Deformity, limb, unequal length
Lennert's lymphoma — *see* Lymphoma, Lennert's
Lennox-Gastaut syndrome G40.812
  intractable G40.814
    with status epilepticus G40.813
    without status epilepticus G40.814
  not intractable G40.812
    with status epilepticus G40.811
    without status epilepticus G40.812
Lens — *see* condition
Lenticonus (anterior) (posterior) (congenital) Q12.8
Lenticular degeneration, progressive E83.01
Lentiglobus (posterior) (congenital) Q12.8
Lentigo (congenital) L81.4
  maligna (*see also* Melanoma, in situ)
    melanoma — *see* Melanoma
Lentivirus, as cause of disease classified elsewhere B97.31
Leontiasis
  ossium M85.2
  syphilitic (late) A52.78
    congenital A50.59
Lepothrix A48.8
Lepra — *see* Leprosy
Leprechaunism E34.8
Leprosy A30. ☑
  with muscle disorder A30.9 *[M63.80]*
    ankle A30.9 *[M63.87 ☑]*
    foot A30.9 *[M63.87 ☑]*
    forearm A30.9 *[M63.83 ☑]*
    hand A30.9 *[M63.84 ☑]*
    lower leg A30.9 *[M63.86 ☑]*
    multiple sites A30.9 *[M63.89]*
    pelvic region A30.9 *[M63.85 ☑]*
    shoulder region A30.9 *[M63.81 ☑]*
    specified site NEC A30.9 *[M63.88]*
    thigh A30.9 *[M63.85 ☑]*
    upper arm A30.9 *[M63.82 ☑]*
  anesthetic A30.9
  BB A30.3
  BL A30.4
  borderline (infiltrated) (neuritic) A30.3
    lepromatous A30.4
    tuberculoid A30.2
  BT A30.2
  dimorphous (infiltrated) (neuritic) A30.3
  I A30.0
  indeterminate (macular) (neuritic) A30.0

Leprosy — *continued*
  lepromatous (diffuse) (infiltrated) (macular) (neuritic) (nodular) A30.5
    LL A30.5
  macular (early) (neuritic) (simple) A30.9
  maculoanesthetic A30.9
  mixed A30.3
  neural A30.9
  nodular A30.5
  primary neuritic A30.3
  specified type NEC A30.8
  TT A30.1
  tuberculoid (major) (minor) A30.1
Leptocytosis, hereditary D56.9
Leptomeningitis (chronic) (circumscribed) (hemorrhagic) (nonsuppurative) — *see* Meningitis
Leptomeningopathy G96.19
Leptospiral — *see* condition
Leptospirochetal — *see* condition
Leptospirosis A27.9
  canicola A27.89
  due to Leptospira interrogans serovar
    icterohaemorrhagiae A27.0
  icterohemorrhagica A27.0
  pomona A27.89
  Weil's disease A27.0
Leptus dermatitis B88.0
Leriche's syndrome (aortic bifurcation occlusion) I74.09
Leri's pleonosteosis Q78.8
Leri-Weill syndrome Q77.8
Lermoyez' syndrome — *see* Vertigo, peripheral NEC
Lesch-Nyhan syndrome E79.1
Leser-Trélat disease L82.1
  inflamed L82.0
Lesion(s) (nontraumatic)
  abducens nerve — *see* Strabismus, paralytic, sixth nerve
  alveolar process K08.9
  angiocentric immunoproliferative D47.Z9
  anorectal K62.9
  aortic (valve) I35.9
  auditory nerve — *see* subcategory H93.3 ☑
  basal ganglion G25.9
  bile duct — *see* Disease, bile duct
  biomechanical M99.9
    specified type NEC M99.89
      abdomen M99.89
      acromioclavicular M99.87
      cervical region M99.81
      cervicothoracic M99.81
      costochondral M99.88
      costovertebral M99.88
      head region M99.80
      hip M99.85
      lower extremity M99.86
      lumbar region M99.83
      lumbosacral M99.83
      occipitocervical M99.80
      pelvic region M99.85
      pubic M99.85
      rib cage M99.88
      sacral region M99.84
      sacrococcygeal M99.84
      sacroiliac M99.84
      specified NEC M99.89
      sternochondral M99.88
      sternoclavicular M99.87
      thoracic region M99.82
      thoracolumbar M99.82
      upper extremity M99.87
  bladder N32.9
  bone — *see* Disorder, bone
  brachial plexus G54.0
  brain G93.9
    congenital Q04.9
    vascular I67.9
      degenerative I67.9
      hypertensive I67.4
  buccal cavity K13.79
  calcified — *see* Calcification
  canthus — *see* Disorder, eyelid
  carate — *see* Pinta, lesions
  cardia K31.9
  cardiac (*see also* Disease, heart) I51.9
    congenital Q24.9
    valvular — *see* Endocarditis
  cauda equina G83.4
  cecum K63.9
  cerebral — *see* Lesion, brain
  cerebrovascular I67.9
    degenerative I67.9
    hypertensive I67.4

Lesion(s) — *continued*
  cervical (nerve) root NEC G54.2
  chiasmal — *see* Disorder, optic, chiasm
  chorda tympani G51.8
  coin, lung R91.1
  colon K63.9
  combined periodontic - endodontic K05.5
  congenital — *see* Anomaly, by site
  conjunctiva H11.9
  conus medullaris — *see* Injury, conus medullaris
  coronary artery — *see* Ischemia, heart
  cranial nerve G52.9
    eighth — *see* Disorder, ear
    eleventh G52.9
    fifth G50.9
    first G52.0
    fourth — *see* Strabismus, paralytic, fourth nerve
    seventh G51.9
    sixth — *see* Strabismus, paralytic, sixth nerve
    tenth G52.2
    twelfth G52.3
  cystic — *see* Cyst
  degenerative — *see* Degeneration
  duodenum K31.9
  edentulous (alveolar) ridge, associated with trauma, due to traumatic occlusion K06.2
  en coup de sabre L94.1
  eyelid — *see* Disorder, eyelid
  gasserian ganglion G50.8
  gastric K31.9
  gastroduodenal K31.9
  gastrointestinal K63.9
  gingiva, associated with trauma K06.2
  glomerular
    focal and segmental (*see also* N00-N07 with fourth character .1) N05.1
    minimal change (*see also* N00-N07 with fourth character .0) N05.0
  heart (organic) — *see* Disease, heart
  hyperchromic, due to pinta (carate) A67.1
  hyperkeratotic — *see* Hyperkeratosis
  hypothalamic E23.7
  ileocecal K63.9
  ileum K63.9
  iliohypogastric nerve G57.8 ☑
  inflammatory — *see* Inflammation
  intestine K63.9
  intracerebral — *see* Lesion, brain
  intrachiasmal (optic) — *see* Disorder, optic, chiasm
  intracranial, space-occupying R90.0
  joint — *see* Disorder, joint
    sacroiliac (old) M53.3
  keratotic — *see* Keratosis
  kidney — *see* Disease, renal
  laryngeal nerve (recurrent) G52.2
  lip K13.0
  liver K76.9
  lumbosacral
    plexus G54.1
    root (nerve) NEC G54.4
  lung (coin) R91.1
  maxillary sinus J32.0
  mitral I05.9
  Morel-Lavallée — *see* Hematoma, by site
  motor cortex NEC G93.89
  mouth K13.79
  nerve G58.9
    femoral G57.2 ☑
    median G56.1 ☑
      carpal tunnel syndrome — *see* Syndrome, carpal tunnel
    plantar G57.6 ☑
    popliteal (lateral) G57.3 ☑
      medial G57.4 ☑
    radial G56.3 ☑
    sciatic G57.0 ☑
    spinal — *see* Injury, nerve, spinal
    ulnar G56.2 ☑
  nervous system, congenital Q07.9
  nonallopathic — *see* Lesion, biomechanical
  nose (internal) J34.89
  obstructive — *see* Obstruction
  obturator nerve G57.8 ☑
  oral mucosa K13.70
  organ or site NEC — *see* Disease, by site
  osteolytic — *see* Osteolysis
  peptic K27.9
  periodontal, due to traumatic occlusion K05.5
  pharynx J39.2
  pigment, pigmented (skin) L81.9
  pinta — *see* Pinta, lesions
  polypoid — *see* Polyp

☑ **Additional character required**

Lesion(s) — continued
  prechiasmal (optic) — see Disorder, optic, chiasm
  primary (see also Syphilis, primary) A51.0
    carate A67.0
    pinta A67.0
    yaws A66.0
  pulmonary J98.4
    valve I37.9
  pylorus K31.9
  rectosigmoid K63.9
  retina, retinal H35.9
  sacroiliac (joint) (old) M53.3
  salivary gland K11.9
    benign lymphoepithelial K11.8
  saphenous nerve G57.8 ☑
  sciatic nerve G57.0 ☑
  secondary — see Syphilis, secondary
  shoulder (region) M75.9 ☑
    specified NEC M75.8 ☑
  sigmoid K63.9
  sinus (accessory) (nasal) J34.89
  skin L98.9
    suppurative L08.0
  SLAP S43.43 ☑
  spinal cord G95.9
    congenital Q06.9
  spleen D73.89
  stomach K31.9
  superior glenoid labrum S43.43 ☑
  syphilitic — see Syphilis
  tertiary — see Syphilis, tertiary
  thoracic root (nerve) NEC G54.3
  tonsillar fossa J35.9
  tooth, teeth K08.9
    white spot
      chewing surface K02.51
      pit and fissure surface K02.51
      smooth surface K02.61
  traumatic — see specific type of injury by site
  tricuspid (valve) I07.9
    nonrheumatic I36.9
  trigeminal nerve G50.9
  ulcerated or ulcerative — see Ulcer, skin
  uterus N85.9
  vagina N89.8
  vulva N90.89
  vagus nerve G52.2
  valvular — see Endocarditis
  vascular I99.9
    affecting central nervous system I67.9
    following trauma NEC T14.8 ☑
    umbilical cord, complicating delivery O69.5 ☑
  warty — see Verruca
  white spot (tooth)
    chewing surface K02.51
    pit and fissure surface K02.51
    smooth surface K02.61
Lethargic — see condition
Lethargy R53.83
Letterer-Siwe's disease C96.0
Leukemia, leukemic C95.9 ☑
  acute basophilic C94.8 ☑
  acute bilineal C95.0 ☑
  acute erythroid C94.0 ☑
  acute lymphoblastic C91.0 ☑
  acute megakaryoblastic C94.2 ☑
  acute megakaryocytic C94.2 ☑
  acute mixed lineage C95.0 ☑
  acute monoblastic (monoblastic/monocytic)
    C93.0 ☑
  acute monocytic (monoblastic/monocytic) C93.0 ☑
  acute myeloblastic (minimal differentiation) (with
    maturation) C92.0 ☑
  acute myeloid, NOS C92.0 ☑
    with
      11q23-abnormality C92.6 ☑
      dysplasia of remaining hematopoesis and/
        or myelodysplastic disease in its history
        C92.A ☑
      multilineage dysplasia C92.A ☑
      variation of MLL-gene C92.6 ☑
    M6 (a)(b) C94.0 ☑
    M7 C94.2 ☑
  acute myelomonocytic C92.5 ☑
  acute promyelocytic C92.4 ☑
  adult T-cell (HTLV-1-associated) (acute variant)
    (chronic variant) (lymphomatoid variant)
    (smouldering variant) C91.5 ☑
  aggressive NK-cell C94.8 ☑
  AML (1/ETO) (M0) (M1) (M2) (without a FAB
    classification) C92.0 ☑
  AML M3 C92.4 ☑

Leukemia — continued
  AML M4 Eo with inv(16) or t(16;16) C92.5 ☑
  AML M5 C93.0 ☑
  AML M5a C93.0 ☑
  AML M5b C93.0 ☑
  AML Me with t (15;17) and variants C92.4 ☑
  atypical chronic myeloid, BCR/ABL-negative
    C92.2 ☑
  biphenotypic acute C95.0 ☑
  blast cell C95.0 ☑
  Burkitt-type, mature B-cell C91.A ☑
  chronic lymphocytic, of B-cell type C91.1 ☑
  chronic monocytic C93.1 ☑
  chronic myelogenous (Philadelphia chromosome
    (Ph1) positive) (t(9;22)) (q34;q11) (with crisis of
    blast cells) C92.1 ☑
  chronic myeloid, BCR/ABL-positive C92.1 ☑
    atypical, BCR/ABL-negative C92.2 ☑
  chronic myelomonocytic C93.1 ☑
  chronic neutrophilic D47.1
  CMML (-1) (-2) (with eosinophilia) C93.1 ☑
  granulocytic (see also Category) C92 ☑ C92.9 ☑
  hairy cell C91.4 ☑
  juvenile myelomonocytic C93.3 ☑
  lymphoid C91.9 ☑
    specified NEC C91.Z ☑
  mast cell C94.3 ☑
  mature B-cell, Burkitt-type C91.A ☑
  monocytic (subacute) C93.9 ☑
    specified NEC C93.Z ☑
  myelogenous (see also Category) C92 ☑ C92.9 ☑
  myeloid C92.9 ☑
    acute C92.0 ☑
    specified NEC C92.Z ☑
  plasma cell C90.1 ☑
  plasmacytic C90.1 ☑
  prolymphocytic
    of B-cell type C91.3 ☑
    of T-cell type C91.6 ☑
  specified NEC C94.8 ☑
  stem cell, of unclear lineage C95.0 ☑
  subacute lymphocytic C91.9 ☑
  T-cell large granular lymphocytic C91.Z ☑
  unspecified cell type C95.9 ☑
    acute C95.0 ☑
    chronic C95.1 ☑
Leukemoid reaction (see also Reaction, leukemoid)
  D72.823
Leukoaraiosis (hypertensive) I67.81
Leukoariosis — see Leukoaraiosis
Leukocoria — see Disorder, globe, degenerated
  condition, leucocoria
Leukocytopenia D72.819
Leukocytosis D72.829
  eosinophilic D72.1
Leukoderma, leukodermia NEC L81.5
  syphilitic A51.39
    late A52.79
Leukodystrophy E75.29
Leukoedema, oral epithelium K13.29
Leukoencephalitis G04.81
  acute (subacute) hemorrhagic G36.1
    postimmunization or postvaccinal G04.02
  postinfectious G04.01
  subacute sclerosing A81.1
  van Bogaert's (sclerosing) A81.1
Leukoencephalopathy (see also Encephalopathy)
  G93.49
  Binswanger's I67.3
  heroin vapor G92
  metachromatic E75.25
  multifocal (progressive) A81.2
    postimmunization and postvaccinal G04.02
  progressive multifocal A81.2
  reversible, posterior G93.6
  van Bogaert's (sclerosing) A81.1
  vascular, progressive I67.3
Leukoerythroblastosis D75.9
Leukokeratosis (see also Leukoplakia)
  mouth K13.21
  nicotina palati K13.24
  oral mucosa K13.21
  tongue K13.21
  vocal cord J38.3
Leukokraurosis vulva (e) N90.4
Leukoma (cornea) (see also Opacity, cornea)
  adherent H17.0 ☑
  interfering with central vision — see Opacity,
    cornea, central
Leukomalacia, cerebral, newborn P91.2
  periventricular P91.2
Leukomelanopathy, hereditary D72.0

Leukonychia (punctata) (striata) L60.8
  congenital Q84.4
Leukopathia unguium L60.8
  congenital Q84.4
Leukopenia D72.819
  basophilic D72.818
  chemotherapy (cancer) induced D70.1
  congenital D70.0
  cyclic D70.0
  drug induced NEC D70.2
    due to cytoreductive cancer chemotherapy D70.1
  eosinophilic D72.818
  familial D70.0
  infantile genetic D70.0
  malignant D70.9
  periodic D70.0
  transitory neonatal P61.5
Leukopenic — see condition
Leukoplakia
  anus K62.89
  bladder (postinfectional) N32.89
  buccal K13.21
  cervix (uteri) N88.0
  esophagus K22.8
  gingiva K13.21
  hairy (oral mucosa) (tongue) K13.3
  kidney (pelvis) N28.89
  larynx J38.7
  lip K13.21
  mouth K13.21
  oral epithelium, including tongue (mucosa) K13.21
  palate K13.21
  pelvis (kidney) N28.89
  penis (infectional) N48.0
  rectum K62.89
  syphilitic (late) A52.79
  tongue K13.21
  ureter (postinfectional) N28.89
  urethra (postinfectional) N36.8
  uterus N85.8
  vagina N89.4
  vocal cord J38.3
  vulva N90.4
Leukorrhea N89.8
  due to Trichomonas (vaginalis) A59.00
  trichomonal A59.00
Leukosarcoma C85.9 ☑
Levocardia (isolated) Q24.1
  with situs inversus Q89.3
Levotransposition Q20.5
Lev's disease or syndrome (acquired complete heart
  block) I44.2
Levulosuria — see Fructosuria
Levurid L30.2
Lewy body (ies) (dementia) (disease) G31.83
Leyden-Moebius dystrophy G71.09
Leydig cell
  carcinoma
    specified site — see Neoplasm, malignant, by site
    unspecified site
      female C56.9
      male C62.9 ☑
  tumor
    benign
      specified site — see Neoplasm, benign, by site
      unspecified site
        female D27. ☑
        male D29.2 ☑
    malignant
      specified site — see Neoplasm, malignant, by
        site
      unspecified site
        female C56. ☑
        male C62.9 ☑
    specified site — see Neoplasm, uncertain
      behavior, by site
    unspecified site
      female D39.1 ☑
      male D40.1 ☑
Leydig-Sertoli cell tumor
  specified site — see Neoplasm, benign, by site
  unspecified site
    female D27. ☑
    male D29.2 ☑
LGSIL (Low grade squamous intraepithelial lesion on
  cytologic smear of)
  anus R85.612
  cervix R87.612
  vagina R87.622
Liar, pathologic F60.2
Libido
  decreased R68.82

Libman-Sacks - Long-term

ICD-10-CM INDEX TO DISEASES AND INJURIES

Libman-Sacks disease M32.11
Lice (infestation) B85.2
  body (Pediculus corporis) B85.1
  crab B85.3
  head (Pediculus capitis) B85.0
  mixed (classifiable to more than one of the titles
    B85.0-B85.3) B85.4
  pubic (Phthirus pubis) B85.3
Lichen L28.0
  albus L90.0
    penis N48.0
    vulva N90.4
  amyloidosis E85.4 *[L99]*
  atrophicus L90.0
    penis N48.0
    vulva N90.4
  congenital Q82.8
  myxedematosus L98.5
  nitidus L44.1
  pilaris Q82.8
    acquired L85.8
  planopilaris L66.1
  planus (chronicus) L43.9
    annularis L43.8
    bullous L43.1
    follicular L66.1
    hypertrophic L43.0
    moniliformis L44.3
    of Wilson L43.9
    specified NEC L43.8
    subacute (active) L43.3
    tropicus L43.3
  ruber
    acuminatus L44.0
    moniliformis L44.3
    planus L43.9
  sclerosus (et atrophicus) L90.0
    penis N48.0
    vulva N90.4
  scrofulosus (primary) (tuberculous) A18.4
  simplex (chronicus) (circumscriptus) L28.0
  striatus L44.2
  urticatus L28.2
Lichenification L28.0
Lichenoides tuberculosis (primary) A18.4
Lichtheim's disease or syndrome D51.0
Lien migrans D73.89
Ligament — *see* condition
Light
  for gestational age — *see* Light for dates
  headedness R42
Light-for-dates (infant) P05.00
  with weight of
    499 grams or less P05.01
    500-749 grams P05.02
    750-999 grams P05.03
    1000-1249 grams P05.04
    1250-1499 grams P05.05
    1500-1749 grams P05.06
    1750-1999 grams P05.07
    2000-2499 grams P05.08
    2500 grams and over P05.09
  specified NEC P05.09
  and small-for-dates — *see* Small for dates
  affecting management of pregnancy O36.59 ☑
Lightning (effects) (stroke) (struck by) T75.00 ☑
  burn — *see* Burn
  foot E53.8
  shock T75.01 ☑
  specified effect NEC T75.09 ☑
Lightwood-Albright syndrome N25.89
Lightwood's disease or syndrome (renal tubular
  acidosis) N25.89
Lignac (-de Toni) (-Fanconi) (-Debré) disease or
  syndrome E72.09
  with cystinosis E72.04
Ligneous thyroiditis E06.5
Likoff's syndrome I20.8
Limb — *see* condition
Limbic epilepsy personality syndrome F07.0
Limitation, limited
  activities due to disability Z73.6
  cardiac reserve — *see* Disease, heart
  eye muscle duction, traumatic — *see* Strabismus,
    mechanical
  mandibular range of motion M26.52
Lindau (-von Hippel) disease Q85.8
Line(s)
  Beau's L60.4
  Harris' — *see* Arrest, epiphyseal
  Hudson's (cornea) — *see* Pigmentation, cornea,
    anterior

Line(s) — *continued*
  Stähli's (cornea) — *see* Pigmentation, cornea,
    anterior
Linea corneae senilis — *see* Change, cornea, senile
Lingua
  geographica K14.1
  nigra (villosa) K14.3
  plicata K14.5
  tylosis K13.29
Lingual — *see* condition
Linguatulosis B88.8
Linitis (gastric) plastica C16.9
Lip — *see* condition
Lipedema — *see* Edema
Lipemia (*see also* Hyperlipidemia)
  retina, retinalis E78.3
Lipidosis E75.6
  cerebral (infantile) (juvenile) (late) E75.4
  cerebroretinal E75.4
  cerebroside E75.22
  cholesterol (cerebral) E75.5
  glycolipid E75.21
  hepatosplenomegalic E78.3
  sphingomyelin — *see* Niemann-Pick disease or
    syndrome
  sulfatide E75.29
Lipoadenoma — *see* Neoplasm, benign, by site
Lipoblastoma — *see* Lipoma
Lipoblastomatosis — *see* Lipoma
Lipochondrodystrophy E76.01
Lipodermatosclerosis — *see* Varix, leg, with,
  inflammation
  ulcerated — *see* Varix, leg, with, ulcer, with
    inflammation by site
Lipochrome histiocytosis (familial) D71
Lipodystrophia progressiva E88.1
Lipodystrophy (progressive) E88.1
  insulin E88.1
  intestinal K90.81
  mesenteric K65.4
Lipofibroma — *see* Lipoma
Lipofuscinosis, neuronal (with ceroidosis) E75.4
Lipogranuloma, sclerosing L92.8
Lipogranulomatosis E78.89
Lipoid (*see also* condition)
  histiocytosis D76.3
    essential E75.29
  nephrosis N04.9
  proteinosis of Urbach E78.89
Lipoidemia — *see* Hyperlipidemia
Lipoidosis — *see* Lipidosis
Lipoma D17.9
  fetal D17.9
    fat cell D17.9
  infiltrating D17.9
  intramuscular D17.9
  pleomorphic D17.9
  site classification
    arms (skin) (subcutaneous) D17.2 ☑
    connective tissue D17.30
      intra-abdominal D17.5
      intrathoracic D17.4
      peritoneum D17.79
      retroperitoneum D17.79
      specified site NEC D17.39
      spermatic cord D17.6
    face (skin) (subcutaneous) D17.0
    genitourinary organ NEC D17.72
    head (skin) (subcutaneous) D17.0
    intra-abdominal D17.5
    intrathoracic D17.4
    kidney D17.71
    legs (skin) (subcutaneous) D17.2 ☑
    neck (skin) (subcutaneous) D17.0
    peritoneum D17.79
    retroperitoneum D17.79
    skin D17.30
      specified site NEC D17.39
    specified site NEC D17.79
    spermatic cord D17.6
    subcutaneous D17.30
      specified site NEC D17.39
    trunk (skin) (subcutaneous) D17.1
    unspecified D17.9
  spindle cell D17.9
Lipomatosis E88.2
  dolorosa (Dercum) E88.2
  fetal — *see* Lipoma
  Launois-Bensaude E88.89
Lipomyoma — *see* Lipoma
Lipomyxoma — *see* Lipoma

Lipomyxosarcoma — *see* Neoplasm, connective tissue,
  malignant
Lipoprotein metabolism disorder E78.9
Lipoproteinemia E78.5
  broad-beta E78.2
  floating-beta E78.2
  hyper-pre-beta E78.1
Liposarcoma (*see also* Neoplasm, connective tissue,
  malignant)
  dedifferentiated — *see* Neoplasm, connective
    tissue, malignant
  differentiated type — *see* Neoplasm, connective
    tissue, malignant
  embryonal — *see* Neoplasm, connective tissue,
    malignant
  mixed type — *see* Neoplasm, connective tissue,
    malignant
  myxoid — *see* Neoplasm, connective tissue, malignant
  pleomorphic — *see* Neoplasm, connective tissue,
    malignant
  round cell — *see* Neoplasm, connective tissue,
    malignant
  well differentiated type — *see* Neoplasm,
    connective tissue, malignant
Liposynovitis prepatellaris E88.89
Lipping, cervix N86
Lipschütz disease or ulcer N76.6
Lipuria R82.0
  schistosomiasis (bilharziasis) B65.0
Lisping F80.0
Lissauer's paralysis A52.17
Lissencephalia, lissencephaly Q04.3
Listeriosis, listerellosis A32.9
  congenital (disseminated) P37.2
  cutaneous A32.0
  neonatal, newborn (disseminated) P37.2
  oculoglandular A32.81
  specified NEC A32.89
Lithemia E79.0
Lithiasis — *see* Calculus
Lithosis J62.8
Lithuria R82.998
Litigation, anxiety concerning Z65.3
Little leaguer's elbow — *see* Epicondylitis, medial
Little's disease G80.9
Littre's
  gland — *see* condition
  hernia — *see* Hernia, abdomen
Littritis — *see* Urethritis
Livedo (annularis) (racemosa) (reticularis) R23.1
Liver — *see* condition
Living alone (problems with) Z60.2
  with handicapped person Z74.2
Lloyd's syndrome — *see* Adenomatosis, endocrine
Loa loa, loaiasis, loasis B74.3
Lobar — *see* condition
Lobomycosis B48.0
Lobo's disease B48.0
Lobotomy syndrome F07.0
Lobstein (-Ekman) disease or syndrome Q78.0
Lobster-claw hand Q71.6 ☑
Lobulation (congenital) (*see also* Anomaly, by site)
  kidney, Q63.1
  liver, abnormal Q44.7
  spleen Q89.09
Lobule, lobular — *see* condition
Local, localized — *see* condition
Locked-in state G83.5
Locked twins causing obstructed labor O66.1
Locking
  joint — *see* Derangement, joint, specified type NEC
    knee — *see* Derangement, knee
Lockjaw — *see* Tetanus
Löffler's
  endocarditis I42.3
  eosinophilia J82
  pneumonia J82
  syndrome (eosinophilic pneumonitis) J82
Loiasis (with conjunctival infestation) (eyelid) B74.3
Lone Star fever A77.0
Long
  labor O63.9
    first stage O63.0
    second stage O63.1
  QT syndrome I45.81
Long-term (current) (prophylactic) drug therapy
  (use of)
  agents affecting estrogen receptors and estrogen
    levels NEC Z79.818
  anastrozole (Arimidex) Z79.811
  antibiotics Z79.2
    short-term use - omit code

Long-term — *continued*
  anticoagulants Z79.01
  anti-inflammatory, non-steroidal (NSAID) Z79.1
  antiplatelet Z79.02
  antithrombotics Z79.02
  aromatase inhibitors Z79.811
  aspirin Z79.82
  birth control pill or patch Z79.3
  bisphosphonates Z79.83
  contraceptive, oral Z79.3
  drug, specified NEC Z79.899
  estrogen receptor downregulators Z79.818
  Evista Z79.810
  exemestane (Aromasin) Z79.811
  Fareston Z79.810
  fulvestrant (Faslodex) Z79.818
  gonadotropin-releasing hormone (GnRH) agonist
    Z79.818
  goserelin acetate (Zoladex) Z79.818
  hormone replacement Z79.890
  insulin Z79.4
  letrozole (Femara) Z79.811
  leuprolide acetate (leuprorelin) (Lupron) Z79.818
  megestrol acetate (Megace) Z79.818
  methadone for pain management Z79.891
  Nolvadex Z79.810
  non-steroidal anti-inflammatories (NSAID) Z79.1
  opiate analgesic Z79.891
  oral
    antidiabetic Z79.84
    contraceptive Z79.3
    hypoglycemic Z79.84
  raloxifene (Evista) Z79.810
  selective estrogen receptor modulators (SERMs)
    Z79.810
  steroids
    inhaled Z79.51
    systemic Z79.52
  tamoxifen (Nolvadex) Z79.810
  toremifene (Fareston) Z79.810
Longitudinal stripes or grooves, nails L60.8
  congenital Q84.6
Loop
  intestine — *see* Volvulus
  vascular on papilla (optic) Q14.2
Loose (*see also* condition)
  body
    joint M24.00
      ankle M24.07 ☑
      elbow M24.02 ☑
      hand M24.04 ☑
      hip M24.05 ☑
      knee M23.4 ☑
      shoulder (region) M24.01 ☑
      specified site NEC M24.08
      vertebra M24.08
      toe M24.07 ☑
      wrist M24.03 ☑
    knee M23.4 ☑
    sheath, tendon — *see* Disorder, tendon, specified
      type NEC
    cartilage — *see* Loose, body, joint
  skin and subcutaneous tissue (following bariatric
    surgery weight loss) (following dietary weight
    loss) L98.7
  tooth, teeth K08.89
Loosening
  aseptic
    joint prosthesis — *see* Complications, joint
      prosthesis, mechanical, loosening, by site
  epiphysis — *see* Osteochondropathy
  mechanical
    joint prosthesis — *see* Complications, joint
      prosthesis, mechanical, loosening, by site
Looser-Milkman (-Debray) syndrome M83.8
Lop ear (deformity) Q17.3
Lorain (-Levi) short stature syndrome E23.0
Lordosis M40.50
  acquired — *see* Lordosis, specified type NEC
  congenital Q76.429
    lumbar region Q76.426
    lumbosacral region Q76.427
    sacral region Q76.428
    sacrococcygeal region Q76.428
    thoracolumbar region Q76.425
  lumbar region M40.56
  lumbosacral region M40.57
  postsurgical M96.4
  postural — *see* Lordosis, specified type NEC
  rachitic (late effect) (sequelae) E64.3
  sequelae of rickets E64.3

Lordosis — *continued*
  specified type NEC M40.40
    lumbar region M40.46
    lumbosacral region M40.47
    thoracolumbar region M40.45
  thoracolumbar region M40.55
  tuberculous A18.01
Loss (of)
  appetite (*see* Anorexia) R63.0
    hysterical F50.89
    nonorganic origin F50.89
    psychogenic F50.89
  blood — *see* Hemorrhage
  bone — *see* Loss, substance of, bone
  control, sphincter, rectum R15.9
    nonorganic origin F98.1
  consciousness, transient R55
    traumatic — *see* Injury, intracranial
  elasticity, skin R23.4
  family (member) in childhood Z62.898
  fluid (acute) E86.9
  function of labyrinth — *see* subcategory H83.2 ☑
  hair, nonscarring — *see* Alopecia
  hearing (*see also* Deafness)
    central NOS H90.5
    conductive H90.2
      bilateral H90.0
      unilateral
        with
          restricted hearing on the contralateral side
            H90.A1 ☑
          unrestricted hearing on the contralateral
            side H90.1 ☑
    mixed conductive and sensorineural hearing loss
      H90.8
      bilateral H90.6
      unilateral
        with
          restricted hearing on the contralateral side
            H90.A3 ☑
          unrestricted hearing on the contralateral
            side H90.7 ☑
    neural NOS H90.5
    perceptive NOS H90.5
    sensorineural NOS H90.5
      bilateral H90.3
      unilateral
        with
          restricted hearing on the contralateral side
            H90.A2 ☑
          unrestricted hearing on the contralateral
            side H90.4 ☑
    sensory NOS H90.5
  height R29.890
  limb or member, traumatic, current — *see*
    Amputation, traumatic
  love relationship in childhood Z62.898
  memory (*see also* Amnesia)
    mild, following organic brain damage F06.8
  mind — *see* Psychosis
  occlusal vertical dimension of fully erupted teeth
    M26.37
  organ or part — *see* Absence, by site, acquired
  ossicles, ear (partial) H74.32 ☑
  parent in childhood Z63.4
  pregnancy, recurrent N96
    care in current pregnancy O26.2 ☑
    without current pregnancy N96
  recurrent pregnancy — *see* Loss, pregnancy,
    recurrent
  self-esteem, in childhood Z62.898
  sense of
    smell — *see* Disturbance, sensation, smell
    taste — *see* Disturbance, sensation, taste
    touch R20.8
  sensory R44.9
    dissociative F44.6
  sexual desire F52.0
  sight (acquired) (complete) (congenital) — *see*
    Blindness
  substance of
    bone — *see* Disorder, bone, density and structure,
      specified NEC
      horizontal alveolar K06.3
    cartilage — *see* Disorder, cartilage, specified type
      NEC
    auricle (ear) — *see* Disorder, pinna, specified
      type NEC
    vitreous (humor) H15.89
  tooth, teeth — *see* Absence, teeth, acquired
  vision, visual H54.7
    both eyes H54.3

Loss — *continued*
  vision — *continued*
    one eye H54.60
      left (normal vision on right) H54.62
      right (normal vision on left) H54.61
    specified as blindness — *see* Blindness
    subjective
      sudden H53.13 ☑
      transient H53.12 ☑
  vitreous — *see* Prolapse, vitreous
  voice — *see* Aphonia
  weight (abnormal) (cause unknown) R63.4
Louis-Bar syndrome (ataxia-telangiectasia) G11.3
Louping ill (encephalitis) A84.8
Louse, lousiness — *see* Lice
Low
  achiever, school Z55.3
  back syndrome M54.5
  basal metabolic rate R94.8
  birthweight (2499 grams or less) P07.10
    with weight of
      1000-1249 grams P07.14
      1250-1499 grams P07.15
      1500-1749 grams P07.16
      1750-1999 grams P07.17
      2000-2499 grams P07.18
    extreme (999 grams or less) P07.00
      with weight of
        499 grams or less P07.01
        500-749 grams P07.02
        750-999 grams P07.03
    for gestational age — *see* Light for dates
  blood pressure (*see also* Hypotension)
    reading (incidental) (isolated) (nonspecific) R03.1
  cardiac reserve — *see* Disease, heart
  function (*see also* Hypofunction)
    kidney N28.9
  hematocrit D64.9
  hemoglobin D64.9
  income Z59.6
  level of literacy Z55.0
  lying
    kidney N28.89
    organ or site, congenital — *see* Malposition,
      congenital
  output syndrome (cardiac) — *see* Failure, heart
  platelets (blood) — *see* Thrombocytopenia
  reserve, kidney N28.89
  salt syndrome E87.1
  self-esteem R45.81
  set ears Q17.4
  vision H54.2X ☑
    one eye (other eye normal) H54.50
      left (normal vision on right) H54.52A ☑
      other eye blind — *see* Blindness
      right (normal vision on left) H54.511 ☑
Low-density-lipoprotein-type (LDL)
  hyperlipoproteinemia E78.00
Lowe's syndrome E72.03
Lown-Ganong-Levine syndrome I45.6
LSD reaction (acute) (without dependence) F16.90
  with dependence F16.20
L-shaped kidney Q63.8
Ludwig's angina or disease K12.2
Lues (venerea), luetic — *see* Syphilis
Luetscher's syndrome (dehydration) E86.0
Lumbago, lumbalgia M54.5
  with sciatica M54.4 ☑
  due to intervertebral disc disorder M51.17
  due to displacement, intervertebral disc M51.27
    with sciatica M51.17
Lumbar — *see* condition
Lumbarization, vertebra, congenital Q76.49
Lumbermen's itch B88.0
Lump (*see also* Mass)
  breast N63.0
    axillary tail
      left N63.32
      right N63.31
    left
      lower inner quadrant N63.24
      lower outer quadrant N63.23
      overlapping quadrants N63.25
      unspecified quadrant N63.20
      upper inner quadrant N63.22
      upper outer quadrant N63.21
    right
      lower inner quadrant N63.14
      lower outer quadrant N63.13
      overlapping quadrants N63.15
      unspecified quadrant N63.10
      upper inner quadrant N63.12

Lump - Lymphocytic

Lump — continued
   breast — continued
      upper outer quadrant N63.11
      subareolar
         left N63.42
         right N63.41
Lunacy — see Psychosis
Lung — see condition
Lupoid (miliary) of Boeck D86.3
Lupus
   anticoagulant D68.62
      with
         hemorrhagic disorder D68.312
         hypercoagulable state D68.62
         finding without diagnosis R76.0
   discoid (local) L93.0
   erythematosus (discoid) (local) L93.0
      disseminated — see Lupus, erythematosus,
         systemic
      eyelid H01.129
         left H01.126
            lower H01.125
            upper H01.124
         right H01.123
            lower H01.122
            upper H01.121
      profundus L93.2
      specified NEC L93.2
      subacute cutaneous L93.1
      systemic M32.9
         with organ or system involvement M32.10
            endocarditis M32.11
            lung M32.13
            pericarditis M32.12
            renal (glomerular) M32.14
               tubulo-interstitial M32.15
            specified organ or system NEC M32.19
         drug-induced M32.0
         inhibitor (presence of) D68.62
            with
               hemorrhagic disorder D68.312
               hypercoagulable state D68.62
               finding without diagnosis R76.0
         specified NEC M32.8
   exedens A18.4
   hydralazine M32.0
      correct substance properly administered — see
         Table of Drugs and Chemicals, by drug,
         adverse effect
      overdose or wrong substance given or taken —
         see Table of Drugs and Chemicals, by drug,
         poisoning
   nephritis (chronic) M32.14
   nontuberculous, not disseminated L93.0
   panniculitis L93.2
   pernio (Besnier) D86.3
   systemic — see Lupus, erythematosus, systemic
   tuberculous A18.4
      eyelid A18.4
   vulgaris A18.4
      eyelid A18.4
Luteinoma D27. ☑
Lutembacher's disease or syndrome (atrial septal
   defect with mitral stenosis) Q21.1
Luteoma D27. ☑
Lutz (-Splendore-de Almeida) disease — see
   Paracoccidioidomycosis
Luxation (see also Dislocation)
   eyeball (nontraumatic) — see Luxation, globe
      birth injury P15.3
   globe, nontraumatic H44.82 ☑
   lacrimal gland — see Dislocation, lacrimal gland
   lens (old) (partial) (spontaneous)
      congenital Q12.1
      syphilitic A50.39
Lycanthropy F22
Lyell's syndrome L51.2
   due to drug L51.2
      correct substance properly administered — see
         Table of Drugs and Chemicals, by drug,
         adverse effect
      overdose or wrong substance given or taken —
         see Table of Drugs and Chemicals, by drug,
         poisoning
Lyme disease A69.20
Lymph
   gland or node — see condition
   scrotum — see Infestation, filarial
Lymphadenitis I88.9
   with ectopic or molar pregnancy O08.0
   acute L04.9
      axilla L04.2

Lymphadenitis — continued
   acute — continued
      face L04.0
      head L04.0
      hip L04.3
      limb
         lower L04.3
         upper L04.2
      neck L04.0
      shoulder L04.2
      specified site NEC L04.8
      trunk L04.1
   anthracosis (occupational) J60
   any site, except mesenteric I88.9
      chronic I88.1
      subacute I88.1
   breast
      gestational — see Mastitis, obstetric
      puerperal, postpartum (nonpurulent) O91.22
   chancroidal (congenital) A57
   chronic I88.1
      mesenteric I88.0
   due to
      Brugia (malayi) B74.1
         timori B74.2
      chlamydial lymphogranuloma A55
      diphtheria (toxin) A36.89
      lymphogranuloma venereum A55
      Wuchereria bancrofti B74.0
   following ectopic or molar pregnancy O08.0
   gonorrheal A54.89
   infective — see Lymphadenitis, acute
   mesenteric (acute) (chronic) (nonspecific)
      (subacute) I88.0
      due to Salmonella typhi A01.09
      tuberculous A18.39
   mycobacterial A31.8
   purulent — see Lymphadenitis, acute
   pyogenic — see Lymphadenitis, acute
   regional, nonbacterial I88.8
   septic — see Lymphadenitis, acute
   subacute, unspecified site I88.1
   suppurative — see Lymphadenitis, acute
   syphilitic (early) (secondary) A51.49
      late A52.79
   tuberculous — see Tuberculosis, lymph gland
   venereal (chlamydial) A55
Lymphadenoid goiter E06.3
Lymphadenopathy (generalized) R59.1
   angioimmunoblastic, with dysproteinemia (AILD)
      C86.5
   due to toxoplasmosis (acquired) B58.89
      congenital (acute) (subacute) (chronic) P37.1
   localized R59.0
   syphilitic (early) (secondary) A51.49
Lymphadenosis R59.1
Lymphangiectasis I89.0
   conjunctiva H11.89
   postinfectional I89.0
   scrotum I89.0
Lymphangiectatic elephantiasis, nonfilarial I89.0
Lymphangioendothelioma D18.1
   malignant — see Neoplasm, connective tissue,
      malignant
Lymphangioleiomyomatosis J84.81
Lymphangioma D18.1
   capillary D18.1
   cavernous D18.1
   cystic D18.1
   malignant — see Neoplasm, connective tissue,
      malignant
Lymphangiomyoma D18.1
Lymphangiomyomatosis J84.81
Lymphangiosarcoma — see Neoplasm, connective
   tissue, malignant
Lymphangitis I89.1
   with
      abscess - code by site under Abscess
      cellulitis - code by site under Cellulitis
      ectopic or molar pregnancy O08.0
   acute L03.91
      abdominal wall L03.321
      ankle — see Lymphangitis, acute, lower limb
      arm — see Lymphangitis, acute, upper limb
      auricle (ear) — see Lymphangitis, acute, ear
      axilla L03.12 ☑
      back (any part) L03.322
      buttock L03.327
      cervical (meaning neck) L03.222
      cheek (external) L03.212
      chest wall L03.323
      digit

Lymphangitis — continued
   acute — continued
      finger — see Lymphangitis, acute, finger
      toe — see Lymphangitis, acute, toe
      ear (external) H60.1 ☑
      external auditory canal — see Lymphangitis,
         acute, ear
      eyelid — see Abscess, eyelid
      face NEC L03.212
      finger (intrathecal) (periosteal) (subcutaneous)
         (subcuticular) L03.02 ☑
      foot — see Lymphangitis, acute, lower limb
      gluteal (region) L03.327
      groin L03.324
      hand — see Lymphangitis, acute, upper limb
      head NEC L03.891
         face (any part, except ear, eye and nose)
            L03.212
      heel — see Lymphangitis, acute, lower limb
      hip — see Lymphangitis, acute, lower limb
      jaw (region) L03.212
      knee — see Lymphangitis, acute, lower limb
      leg — see Lymphangitis, acute, lower limb
      lower limb L03.12 ☑
         toe — see Lymphangitis, acute, toe
      navel L03.326
      neck (region) L03.222
      orbit, orbital — see Cellulitis, orbit
      pectoral (region) L03.323
      perineal, perineum L03.325
      scalp (any part) L03.891
      shoulder — see Lymphangitis, acute, upper limb
      specified site NEC L03.898
      thigh — see Lymphangitis, acute, lower limb
      thumb (intrathecal) (periosteal) (subcutaneous)
         (subcuticular) — see Lymphangitis, acute,
         finger
      toe (intrathecal) (periosteal) (subcutaneous)
         (subcuticular) L03.04 ☑
      trunk L03.329
         abdominal wall L03.321
         back (any part) L03.322
         buttock L03.327
         chest wall L03.323
         groin L03.324
         perineal, perineum L03.325
         umbilicus L03.326
      umbilicus L03.326
      upper limb L03.12 ☑
         axilla — see Lymphangitis, acute, axilla
         finger — see Lymphangitis, acute, finger
         thumb — see Lymphangitis, acute, finger
         wrist — see Lymphangitis, acute, upper limb
   breast
      gestational — see Mastitis, obstetric
   chancroidal A57
   chronic (any site) I89.1
   due to
      Brugia (malayi) B74.1
         timori B74.2
      Wuchereria bancrofti B74.0
   following ectopic or molar pregnancy O08.89
   penis
      acute N48.29
      gonococcal (acute) (chronic) A54.09
   puerperal, postpartum, childbirth O86.89
   strumous, tuberculous A18.2
   subacute (any site) I89.1
   tuberculous — see Tuberculosis, lymph gland
Lymphatic (vessel) — see condition
Lymphatism E32.8
Lymphectasia I89.0
Lymphedema (acquired) (see also Elephantiasis)
   congenital Q82.0
   hereditary (chronic) (idiopathic) Q82.0
   postmastectomy I97.2
   praecox I89.0
   secondary I89.0
   surgical NEC I97.89
      postmastectomy (syndrome) I97.2
Lymphoblastic — see condition
Lymphoblastoma (diffuse) — see Lymphoma,
   lymphoblastic (diffuse)
   giant follicular — see Lymphoma, lymphoblastic
      (diffuse)
   macrofollicular — see Lymphoma, lymphoblastic
      (diffuse)
Lymphocele I89.8
Lymphocytic
   chorioencephalitis (acute) (serous) A87.2
   choriomeningitis (acute) (serous) A87.2
   meningoencephalitis A87.2

Lymphocytoma, benign cutis L98.8
Lymphocytopenia D72.810
Lymphocytosis (symptomatic) D72.820
   infectious (acute) B33.8
Lymphoepithelioma — *see* Neoplasm, malignant, by
   site
Lymphogranuloma (malignant) (*see also* Lymphoma,
   Hodgkin)
   chlamydial A55
   inguinale A55
   venereum (any site) (chlamydial) (with stricture of
     rectum) A55
Lymphogranulomatosis (malignant) (*see also*
   Lymphoma, Hodgkin)
   benign (Boeck's sarcoid) (Schaumann's) D86.1
Lymphohistiocytosis, hemophagocytic (familial) D76.1
Lymphoid — *see* condition
Lymphoma (of) (malignant) C85.90
   adult T-cell (HTLV-1-associated) (acute variant)
     (chronic variant) (lymphomatoid variant)
     (smouldering variant) C91.5 ☑
   anaplastic large cell
     ALK-negative C84.7 ☑
     ALK-positive C84.6 ☑
     CD30 ☑ positive C84.6 ☑
     primary cutaneous C86.6
   angioimmunoblastic T-cell C86.5
   BALT C88.4
   B-cell C85.1 ☑
   B-precursor C83.5 ☑
   blastic NK-cell C84.6
   blastic plasmacytoid dendritic cell neoplasm
     (BPDCN) C86.4
   bronchial-associated lymphoid tissue
     [BALT-lymphoma] C88.4
   Burkitt (atypical) C83.7 ☑
   Burkitt-like C83.7 ☑
   centrocytic C83.1 ☑
   cutaneous follicle center C82.6 ☑
   cutaneous T-cell C84.A ☑
   diffuse follicle center C82.5 ☑
   diffuse large cell C83.3 ☑
     anaplastic C83.3 ☑
     B-cell C83.3 ☑
     CD30 ☑ positive C83.3 ☑
     centroblastic C83.3 ☑
     immunoblastic C83.3 ☑
     plasmablastic C83.3 ☑
     subtype not specified C83.3 ☑
     T-cell rich C83.3 ☑
   enteropathy-type (associated) (intestinal) T-cell C86.2
   extranodal NK/T-cell, nasal type C86.0
   extranodal marginal zone B-cell lymphoma
     of mucosa-associated lymphoid tissue
     [MALT-lymphoma] C88.4
   follicular C82.9 ☑
     grade
       I C82.0 ☑
       II C82.1 ☑
       III C82.2 ☑
       IIIa C82.3 ☑
       IIIb C82.4 ☑
     specified NEC C82.8 ☑
   hepatosplenic T-cell (alpha-beta) (gamma-delta)
     C86.1
   histiocytic C85.9 ☑
     true C96.A
   Hodgkin C81.9 ☑
     lymphocyte-rich (classical) C81.4 ☑
     lymphocyte depleted (classical) C81.3 ☑
     mixed cellularity (classical) C81.2 ☑
     nodular sclerosis (classical) C81.1 ☑
     specified NEC (classical) C81.7 ☑
     lymphocyte-rich classical C81.4 ☑
     lymphocyte depleted classical C81.3 ☑
     mixed cellularity classical C81.2 ☑
     nodular
       lymphocyte predominant C81.0 ☑
       sclerosis (classical) C81.1 ☑
   intravascular large B-cell C83.8 ☑
   Lennert's C84.4 ☑
   lymphoblastic B-cell C83.5 ☑
   lymphoblastic (diffuse) C83.5 ☑
   lymphoblastic T-cell C83.5 ☑
   lymphoepithelioid C84.4 ☑
   lymphoplasmacytic C83.0 ☑
     with IgM-production C88.0
   MALT C88.4
   mantle cell C83.1 ☑
   mature T-cell NEC C84.4 ☑
   mature T/NK-cell C84.9 ☑
     specified NEC C84.Z ☑

Lymphoma — *continued*
   mediastinal (thymic) large B-cell C85.2 ☑
   Mediterranean C88.3
   mucosa-associated lymphoid tissue
     [MALT-lymphoma] C88.4
   NK/T cell C84.9 ☑
   nodal marginal zone C83.0 ☑
   non-follicular (diffuse) C83.9 ☑
     specified NEC C83.8 ☑
   non-Hodgkin (*see also* Lymphoma, by type) C85.9 ☑
     specified NEC C85.8 ☑
   non-leukemic variant of B-CLL C83.0 ☑
   peripheral T-cell, not classified C84.4 ☑
   primary cutaneous
     anaplastic large cell C86.6
     CD30 ☑ positive large T-cell C86.6
   primary effusion B-cell C83.8 ☑
   SALT C88.4
   skin-associated lymphoid tissue [SALT-lymphoma]
     C88.4
   small cell B-cell C83.0 ☑
   splenic marginal zone C83.0 ☑
   subcutaneous panniculitis-like T-cell C86.3
   T-precursor C83.5 ☑
   true histiocytic C96.A
Lymphomatosis — *see* Lymphoma
Lymphopathia venereum, veneris A55
Lymphopenia D72.810
Lymphoplasmacytic leukemia — *see* Leukemia,
   chronic lymphocytic, B-cell type
Lymphoproliferation, X-linked disease D82.3
Lymphoreticulosis, benign (of inoculation) A28.1
Lymphorrhea I89.8
Lymphosarcoma (diffuse) (*see also* Lymphoma) C85.9 ☑
Lymphostasis I89.8
Lypemania — *see* Melancholia
Lysine and hydroxylysine metabolism disorder E72.3
Lyssa — *see* Rabies

M

Macacus ear Q17.3
Maceration, wet feet, tropical (syndrome) T69.02 ☑
MacLeod's syndrome J43.0
Macrocephalia, macrocephaly Q75.3
Macrocheilia, macrochilia (congenital) Q18.6
Macrocolon (*see also* Megacolon) Q43.1
Macrocornea Q15.8
   with glaucoma Q15.0
Macrocytic — *see* condition
Macrocytosis D75.89
Macrodactylia, macrodactylism (fingers) (thumbs)
   Q74.0
   toes Q74.2
Macrodontia K00.2
Macrogenia M26.05
Macrogenitosomia (adrenal) (male) (praecox) E25.9
   congenital E25.0
Macroglobulinemia (idiopathic) (primary) C88.0
   monoclonal (essential) D47.2
   Waldenström C88.0
Macroglossia (congenital) Q38.2
   acquired K14.8
Macrognathia, macrognathism (congenital)
   (mandibular) (maxillary) M26.09
Macrogyria (congenital) Q04.8
Macrohydrocephalus — *see* Hydrocephalus
Macromastia — *see* Hypertrophy, breast
Macrophthalmos Q11.3
   in congenital glaucoma Q15.0
Macropsia H53.15
Macrosigmoid K59.39
   congenital Q43.2
Macrospondylitis , acromegalic E22.0
Macrostomia (congenital) Q18.4
Macrotia (external ear) (congenital) Q17.1
Macula
   cornea, corneal — *see* Opacity, cornea
   degeneration (atrophic) (exudative) (senile)
     (*see also* Degeneration, macula)
     hereditary — *see* Dystrophy, retina
Maculae ceruleae B85.1
Maculopathy, toxic — *see* Degeneration, macula, toxic
Madarosis (eyelid) H02.729
   left H02.726
     lower H02.725
     upper H02.724
   right H02.723
     lower H02.722
     upper H02.721

Madelung's
   deformity (radius) Q74.0
   disease
     radial deformity Q74.0
     symmetrical lipomas, neck E88.89
Madness — *see* Psychosis
Madura
   foot B47.9
     actinomycotic B47.1
     mycotic B47.0
Maduromycosis B47.0
Maffucci's syndrome Q78.4
Magnesium metabolism disorder — *see* Disorder,
   metabolism, magnesium
Main en griffe (acquired) (*see also* Deformity, limb,
   clawhand)
   congenital Q74.0
Maintenance (encounter for)
   antineoplastic chemotherapy Z51.11
   antineoplastic radiation therapy Z51.0
   methadone F11.20
Majocchi's
   disease L81.7
   granuloma B35.8
Major — *see* condition
Malabar itch (any site) B35.5
Malabsorption K90.9
   calcium K90.89
   carbohydrate K90.49
   disaccharide E73.9
   fat K90.49
   galactose E74.20
   glucose (-galactose) E74.39
   intestinal K90.9
     specified NEC K90.89
   isomaltose E74.31
   lactose E73.9
   methionine E72.19
   monosaccharide E74.39
   postgastrectomy K91.2
   postsurgical K91.2
   protein K90.49
   starch K90.49
   sucrose E74.39
   syndrome K90.9
     postsurgical K91.2
Malacia, bone (adult) M83.9
   juvenile — *see* Rickets
Malacoplakia
   bladder N32.89
   pelvis (kidney) N28.89
   ureter N28.89
   urethra N36.8
Malacosteon, juvenile — *see* Rickets
Maladaptation — *see* Maladjustment
Maladie de Roger Q21.0
Maladjustment
   conjugal Z63.0
     involving divorce or estrangement Z63.5
   educational Z55.4
   family Z63.9
   marital Z63.0
     involving divorce or estrangement Z63.5
   occupational NEC Z56.89
   simple, adult — *see* Disorder, adjustment
   situational — *see* Disorder, adjustment
   social Z60.9
     due to
       acculturation difficulty Z60.3
       discrimination and persecution (perceived)
         Z60.5
       exclusion and isolation Z60.4
       life-cycle (phase of life) transition Z60.0
       rejection Z60.4
       specified reason NEC Z60.8
Malaise R53.81
Malakoplakia — *see* Malacoplakia
Malaria, malarial (fever) B54
   with
     blackwater fever B50.8
       hemoglobinuric (bilious) B50.8
       hemoglobinuria B50.8
   accidentally induced (therapeutically) - code by
     type under Malaria
   algid B50.9
   cerebral B50.0 *[G94]*
   clinically diagnosed (without parasitological
     confirmation) B54
   congenital NEC P37.4
     falciparum P37.3
   congestion, congestive B54
   continued (fever) B50.9

Malaria - Malformation

Malaria — *continued*
- estivo-autumnal B50.9
- falciparum B50.9
  - with complications NEC B50.8
    - cerebral B50.0 *[G94]*
  - severe B50.8
- hemorrhagic B54
- malariae B52.9
  - with
    - complications NEC B52.8
    - glomerular disorder B52.0
- malignant (tertian) — *see* Malaria, falciparum
- mixed infections - code to first listed type in B50-B53
- ovale B53.0
- parasitologically confirmed NEC B53.8
- pernicious, acute — *see* Malaria, falciparum
- Plasmodium (P.)
  - falciparum NEC — *see* Malaria, falciparum
  - malariae NEC B52.9
    - with Plasmodium
      - falciparum (and or vivax) — *see* Malaria, falciparum
      - vivax (*see also* Malaria, vivax)
        - and falciparum — *see* Malaria, falciparum
  - ovale B53.0
    - with Plasmodium malariae (*see also* Malaria, malariae)
      - and vivax (*see also* Malaria, vivax)
        - and falciparum — *see* Malaria, falciparum
  - simian B53.1
    - with Plasmodium malariae (*see also* Malaria, malariae)
      - and vivax (*see also* Malaria, vivax)
        - and falciparum — *see* Malaria, falciparum
  - vivax NEC B51.9
    - with Plasmodium falciparum — *see* Malaria, falciparum
- quartan — *see* Malaria, malariae
- quotidian — *see* Malaria, falciparum
- recurrent B54
- remittent B54
- specified type NEC (parasitologically confirmed) B53.8
- spleen B54
- subtertian (fever) — *see* Malaria, falciparum
- tertian (benign) (*see also* Malaria, vivax)
  - malignant B50.9
- tropical B50.9
- typhoid B54
- vivax B51.9
  - with
    - complications NEC B51.8
    - ruptured spleen B51.0
Malassimilation K90.9
Malassez's disease (cystic) N50.89
Mal de los pintos — *see* Pinta
Mal de mer T75.3 ☑
Maldescent, testis Q53.9
- bilateral Q53.20
  - abdominal Q53.211
  - perineal Q53.22
- unilateral Q53.10
  - abdominal Q53.111
  - perineal Q53.12
Maldevelopment (*see also* Anomaly)
- brain Q07.9
- colon Q43.9
- hip Q74.2
  - congenital dislocation Q65.2
    - bilateral Q65.1
    - unilateral Q65.0 ☑
- mastoid process Q75.8
- middle ear Q16.4
  - except ossicles Q16.4
  - ossicles Q16.3
- ossicles Q16.3
- spine Q76.49
- toe Q74.2
Male type pelvis Q74.2
- with disproportion (fetopelvic) O33.3 ☑
  - causing obstructed labor O65.3
Malformation (congenital) (*see also* Anomaly)
- adrenal gland Q89.1
- affecting multiple systems with skeletal changes NEC Q87.5
- alimentary tract Q45.9
  - specified type NEC Q45.8
  - upper Q40.9
    - specified type NEC Q40.8
- aorta Q25.40
  - absence Q25.41

Malformation — *continued*
- aorta — *continued*
  - aneurysm, congenital Q25.43
  - aplasia Q25.41
  - atresia Q25.29
    - aortic arch Q25.21
  - coarctation (preductal) (postductal) Q25.1
  - dilatation, congenital Q25.44
  - hypoplasia Q25.42
  - patent ductus arteriosus Q25.0
  - specified type NEC Q25.49
  - stenosis Q25.1
    - supravalvular Q25.3
- aortic valve Q23.9
  - specified NEC Q23.8
- arteriovenous, aneurysmatic (congenital) Q27.30
  - brain Q28.2
    - ruptured I60.8
      - intracerebral I61.8
      - intraparenchymal I61.8
      - intraventricular I61.5
      - subarachnoid I60.8
  - cerebral (*see also* Malformation, arteriovenous, brain) Q28.2
  - peripheral Q27.30
    - digestive system — *see* Angiodysplasia
      - congenital Q27.33
    - lower limb Q27.32
    - other specified site Q27.39
    - renal vessel Q27.34
    - upper limb Q27.31
  - precerebral vessels (nonruptured) Q28.0
- auricle
  - ear (congenital) Q17.3
    - acquired H61.119
      - left H61.112
        - with right H61.113
      - right H61.111
        - with left H61.113
- bile duct Q44.5
- bladder Q64.79
  - aplasia Q64.5
  - diverticulum Q64.6
  - exstrophy — *see* Exstrophy, bladder
  - neck obstruction Q64.31
- bone Q79.9
  - face Q75.9
    - specified type NEC Q75.8
  - skull Q75.9
    - specified type NEC Q75.8
- brain (multiple) Q04.9
  - arteriovenous Q28.2
  - specified type NEC Q04.8
- branchial cleft Q18.2
- breast Q83.9
  - specified type NEC Q83.8
- broad ligament Q50.6
- bronchus Q32.4
- bursa Q79.9
- cardiac
  - chambers Q20.9
    - specified type NEC Q20.8
  - septum Q21.9
    - specified type NEC Q21.8
- cerebral Q04.9
  - vessels Q28.3
- cervix uteri Q51.9
  - specified type NEC Q51.828
- Chiari
  - Type I G93.5
  - Type II Q07.01
- choroid (congenital) Q14.3
  - plexus Q07.8
- circulatory system Q28.9
- cochlea Q16.5
- cornea Q13.4
- coronary vessels Q24.5
- corpus callosum (congenital) Q04.0
- diaphragm Q79.1
- digestive system NEC, specified type NEC Q45.8
- dura Q07.9
  - brain Q04.9
  - spinal Q06.9
- ear Q17.9
  - causing impairment of hearing Q16.9
  - external Q17.9
    - accessory auricle Q17.0
    - causing impairment of hearing Q16.9
    - absence of
      - auditory canal Q16.1
      - auricle Q16.0
  - macrotia Q17.1

Malformation — *continued*
- ear — *continued*
  - microtia Q17.2
  - misplacement Q17.4
  - misshapen NEC Q17.3
  - prominence Q17.5
  - specified type NEC Q17.8
  - inner Q16.5
  - middle Q16.4
    - absence of eustachian tube Q16.2
    - ossicles (fusion) Q16.3
  - ossicles Q16.3
  - specified type NEC Q17.8
- epididymis Q55.4
- esophagus Q39.9
  - specified type NEC Q39.8
- eye Q15.9
  - lid Q10.3
  - specified NEC Q15.8
- fallopian tube Q50.6
- genital organ — *see* Anomaly, genitalia
- great
  - artery Q25.9
    - aorta — *see* Malformation, aorta
    - pulmonary artery — *see* Malformation, pulmonary, artery
    - specified type NEC Q25.8
  - vein Q26.9
    - anomalous
      - portal venous connection Q26.5
      - pulmonary venous connection Q26.4
        - partial Q26.3
        - total Q26.2
    - persistent left superior vena cava Q26.1
    - portal vein-hepatic artery fistula Q26.6
    - specified type NEC Q26.8
    - vena cava stenosis, congenital Q26.0
- gum Q38.6
- hair Q84.2
- heart Q24.9
  - specified type NEC Q24.8
- integument Q84.9
  - specified type NEC Q84.8
- internal ear Q16.5
- intestine Q43.9
  - specified type NEC Q43.8
- iris Q13.2
- joint Q74.9
  - ankle Q74.2
  - lumbosacral Q76.49
  - sacroiliac Q74.2
  - specified type NEC Q74.8
- kidney Q63.9
  - accessory Q63.0
  - giant Q63.3
  - horseshoe Q63.1
  - hydronephrosis Q62.0
  - malposition Q63.2
  - specified type NEC Q63.8
- lacrimal apparatus Q10.6
- lip Q38.0
- lingual Q38.3
- liver Q44.7
- lung Q33.9
- meninges or membrane (congenital) Q07.9
  - cerebral Q04.8
  - spinal (cord) Q06.9
- middle ear Q16.4
  - ossicles Q16.3
- mitral valve Q23.9
  - specified NEC Q23.8
- Mondini's (congenital) (malformation, cochlea) Q16.5
- mouth (congenital) Q38.6
- multiple types NEC Q89.7
- musculoskeletal system Q79.9
- myocardium Q24.8
- nail Q84.6
- nervous system (central) Q07.9
- nose Q30.9
  - specified type NEC Q30.8
- optic disc Q14.2
- orbit Q10.7
- ovary Q50.39
- palate Q38.5
- parathyroid gland Q89.2
- pelvic organs or tissues NEC
  - in pregnancy or childbirth O34.8 ☑
    - causing obstructed labor O65.5
- penis Q55.69
  - aplasia Q55.5
  - curvature (lateral) Q55.61
  - hypoplasia Q55.62

☑ **Additional character required**

Malformation — *continued*
pericardium Q24.8
peripheral vascular system Q27.9
specified type NEC Q27.8
pharynx Q38.8
precerebral vessels Q28.1
prostate Q55.4
pulmonary
arteriovenous Q25.72
artery Q25.9
atresia Q25.5
specified type NEC Q25.79
stenosis Q25.6
valve Q22.3
renal artery Q27.2
respiratory system Q34.9
retina Q14.1
scrotum — *see* Malformation, testis and scrotum
seminal vesicles Q55.4
sense organs NEC Q07.9
skin Q82.9
specified NEC Q89.8
spinal
cord Q06.9
nerve root Q07.8
spine Q76.49
kyphosis — *see* Kyphosis, congenital
lordosis — *see* Lordosis, congenital
spleen Q89.09
stomach Q40.3
specified type NEC Q40.2
teeth, tooth K00.9
tendon Q79.9
testis and scrotum Q55.20
aplasia Q55.0
hypoplasia Q55.1
polyorchism Q55.21
retractile testis Q55.22
scrotal transposition Q55.23
specified NEC Q55.29
throat Q38.8
thorax, bony Q76.9
thyroid gland Q89.2
tongue (congenital) Q38.3
hypertrophy Q38.2
tie Q38.1
trachea Q32.1
tricuspid valve Q22.9
specified type NEC Q22.8
umbilical cord NEC (complicating delivery) O69.89 ☑
umbilicus Q89.9
ureter Q62.8
agenesis Q62.4
duplication Q62.5
malposition — *see* Malposition, congenital, ureter
obstructive defect — *see* Defect, obstructive, ureter
vesico-uretero-renal reflux Q62.7
urethra Q64.79
aplasia Q64.5
duplication Q64.74
posterior valves Q64.2
prolapse Q64.71
stricture Q64.32
urinary system Q64.9
uterus Q51.9
specified type NEC Q51.818
vagina Q52.4
vascular system, peripheral Q27.9
vas deferens Q55.4
atresia Q55.3
venous — *see* Anomaly, vein(s)
vulva Q52.70
Malfunction (*see also* Dysfunction)
cardiac electronic device T82.119 ☑
electrode T82.110 ☑
pulse generator T82.111 ☑
specified type NEC T82.118 ☑
catheter device NEC T85.618 ☑
cystostomy T83.010 ☑
dialysis (renal) (vascular) T82.41 ☑
intraperitoneal T85.611 ☑
infusion NEC T82.514 ☑
cranial T85.610 ☑
epidural T85.610 ☑
intrathecal T85.610 ☑
spinal T85.610 ☑
subarachnoid T85.610 ☑
subdural T85.610 ☑
urinary (*see also* Breakdown, device, catheter) T83.018 ☑

Malfunction — *continued*
colostomy K94.03
valve K94.03
cystostomy (stoma) N99.512
catheter T83.010 ☑
enteric stoma K94.13
enterostomy K94.13
esophagostomy K94.33
gastroenteric K31.89
gastrostomy K94.23
ileostomy K94.13
valve K94.13
intrathecal infusion pump T85.615 ☑
jejunostomy K94.13
nervous system device, implant or graft, specified NEC T85.615 ☑
pacemaker — *see* Malfunction, cardiac electronic device
prosthetic device, internal — *see* Complications, prosthetic device, by site, mechanical
tracheostomy J95.03
urinary device NEC — *see* Complication, genitourinary, device, urinary, mechanical
valve
colostomy K94.03
heart T82.09 ☑
ileostomy K94.13
vascular graft or shunt NEC — *see* Complication, cardiovascular device, mechanical, vascular
ventricular (communicating shunt) T85.01 ☑
Malherbe's tumor — *see* Neoplasm, skin, benign
Malibu disease L98.8
Malignancy (*see also* Neoplasm, malignant, by site)
unspecified site (primary) C80.1
Malignant — *see* condition
Malingerer, malingering Z76.5
Mallet finger (acquired) — *see* Deformity, finger, mallet finger
congenital Q74.0
sequelae of rickets E64.3
Malleus A24.0
Mallory's bodies R89.7
Mallory-Weiss syndrome K22.6
Malnutrition E46
degree
first E44.1
mild (protein) E44.1
moderate (protein) E44.0
second E44.0
severe (protein-energy) E43
intermediate form E42
with
kwashiorkor (and marasmus) E42
marasmus E41
third E43
following gastrointestinal surgery K91.2
intrauterine
light-for-dates — *see* Light for dates
small-for-dates — *see* Small for dates
lack of care, or neglect (child) (infant) T76.02 ☑
confirmed T74.02 ☑
malignant E40
protein E46
calorie E46
mild E44.1
moderate E44.0
severe E43
intermediate form E42
with
kwashiorkor (and marasmus) E42
marasmus E41
energy E46
mild E44.1
moderate E44.0
severe E43
intermediate form E42
with
kwashiorkor (and marasmus) E42
marasmus E41
severe (protein-energy) E43
with
kwashiorkor (and marasmus) E42
marasmus E41
Malocclusion (teeth) M26.4
Angle's M26.219
class I M26.211
class II M26.212
class III M26.213
due to
abnormal swallowing M26.59
mouth breathing M26.59
tongue, lip or finger habits M26.59
temporomandibular (joint) M26.69

Malposition
cervix — *see* Malposition, uterus
congenital
adrenal (gland) Q89.1
alimentary tract Q45.8
lower Q43.8
upper Q40.8
aorta Q25.49
appendix Q43.8
arterial trunk Q20.0
artery (peripheral) Q27.8
coronary Q24.5
digestive system Q27.8
lower limb Q27.8
pulmonary Q25.79
specified site NEC Q27.8
upper limb Q27.8
auditory canal Q17.8
causing impairment of hearing Q16.9
auricle (ear) Q17.4
causing impairment of hearing Q16.9
cervical Q18.2
biliary duct or passage Q44.5
bladder (mucosa) — *see* Exstrophy, bladder
brachial plexus Q07.8
brain tissue Q04.8
breast Q83.8
bronchus Q32.4
cecum Q43.8
clavicle Q74.0
colon Q43.8
digestive organ or tract NEC Q45.8
lower Q43.8
upper Q40.8
ear (auricle) (external) Q17.4
ossicles Q16.3
endocrine (gland) NEC Q89.2
epiglottis Q31.8
eustachian tube Q17.8
eye Q15.8
facial features Q18.8
fallopian tube Q50.6
finger(s) Q68.1
supernumerary Q69.0
foot Q66.9 ☑
gallbladder Q44.1
gastrointestinal tract Q45.8
genitalia, genital organ(s) or tract
female Q52.8
external Q52.79
internal NEC Q52.8
male Q55.8
glottis Q31.8
hand Q68.1
heart Q24.8
dextrocardia Q24.0
with complete transposition of viscera Q89.3
hepatic duct Q44.5
hip (joint) Q65.89
intestine (large) (small) Q43.8
with anomalous adhesions, fixation or malrotation Q43.3
joint NEC Q68.8
kidney Q63.2
larynx Q31.8
limb Q68.8
lower Q68.8
upper Q68.8
liver Q44.7
lung (lobe) Q33.8
nail(s) Q84.6
nerve Q07.8
nervous system NEC Q07.8
nose, nasal (septum) Q30.8
organ or site not listed — *see* Anomaly, by site
ovary Q50.39
pancreas Q45.3
parathyroid (gland) Q89.2
patella Q74.1
peripheral vascular system Q27.8
pituitary (gland) Q89.2
respiratory organ or system NEC Q34.8
rib (cage) Q76.6
supernumerary in cervical region Q76.5
scapula Q74.0
shoulder Q74.0
spinal cord Q06.8
spleen Q89.09
sternum NEC Q76.7
stomach Q40.2
symphysis pubis Q74.2
thymus (gland) Q89.2

Malposition - Mass

Malposition — *continued*
  congenital — *continued*
    thyroid (gland) (tissue) Q89.2
      cartilage Q31.8
    toe(s) Q66.9 ☑
      supernumerary Q69.2
    tongue Q38.3
    trachea Q32.1
    ureter Q62.60
      deviation Q62.61
      displacement Q62.62
      ectopia Q62.63
      specified type NEC Q62.69
    uterus Q51.818
    vein(s) (peripheral) Q27.8
      great Q26.8
    vena cava (inferior) (superior) Q26.8
  device, implant or graft (*see also* Complications, by
      site and type, mechanical) T85.628 ☑
    arterial graft NEC — *see* Complication,
        cardiovascular device, mechanical, vascular
    breast (implant) T85.42 ☑
    catheter NEC T85.628 ☑
      cystostomy T83.020 ☑
      dialysis (renal) T82.42 ☑
        intraperitoneal T85.621 ☑
      infusion NEC T82.524 ☑
        spinal (epidural) (subdural) T85.620 ☑
      urinary (*see also* Displacement, device, catheter,
          urinary) T83.028 ☑
    electronic (electrode) (pulse generator)
        (stimulator)
      bone T84.320 ☑
      cardiac T82.129 ☑
        electrode T82.120 ☑
        pulse generator T82.121 ☑
        specified type NEC T82.128 ☑
      nervous system — *see* Complication, prosthetic
          device, mechanical, electronic nervous
          system stimulator
      urinary — *see* Complication, genitourinary,
          device, urinary, mechanical
    fixation, internal (orthopedic) NEC — *see*
        Complication, fixation device, mechanical
    gastrointestinal — *see* Complications,
        prosthetic device, mechanical,
        gastrointestinal device
    genital NEC T83.428 ☑
      intrauterine contraceptive device (string)
          T83.32 ☑
      penile prosthesis (cylinder) (implanted) (pump)
          (reservoir) T83.420 ☑
      testicular prosthesis T83.421 ☑
    heart NEC — *see* Complication, cardiovascular
        device, mechanical
    joint prosthesis — *see* Complication, joint
        prosthesis, mechanical
    ocular NEC — *see* Complications, prosthetic
        device, mechanical, ocular device
    orthopedic NEC — *see* Complication, orthopedic,
        device, mechanical
    specified NEC T85.628 ☑
    urinary NEC (*see also* Complication, genitourinary,
        device, urinary, mechanical)
      graft T83.22 ☑
    vascular NEC — *see* Complication, cardiovascular
        device, mechanical
    ventricular intracranial shunt T85.02 ☑
  fetus — *see* Pregnancy, complicated by
      (management affected by), presentation, fetal
  gallbladder K82.8
  gastrointestinal tract, congenital Q45.8
  heart, congenital NEC Q24.8
  joint prosthesis — *see* Complications, joint
      prosthesis, mechanical, displacement, by site
  stomach K31.89
    congenital Q40.2
  tooth, teeth, fully erupted M26.30
  uterus (acute) (acquired) (adherent) (asymptomatic)
      (postinfectional) (postpartal, old) N85.4
    anteflexion or anteversion N85.4
      congenital Q51.818
    flexion N85.4
      lateral — *see* Lateroversion, uterus
    inversion N85.5
    lateral (flexion) (version) — *see* Lateroversion,
        uterus
    in pregnancy or childbirth — *see* subcategory
        O34.5 ☑
    retroflexion or retroversion — *see* Retroversion,
        uterus
Malposture R29.3

Malrotation
  cecum Q43.3
  colon Q43.3
  intestine Q43.3
  kidney Q63.2
Maltreatment
  adult
    abandonment
      confirmed T74.01 ☑
      suspected T76.01 ☑
    bullying
      confirmed T74.31 ☑
      suspected T76.31 ☑
    confirmed T74.91 ☑
    history of Z91.419
    intimidation (through social media)
      confirmed T74.31 ☑
      suspected T76.31 ☑
    neglect
      confirmed T74.01 ☑
      suspected T76.01 ☑
    physical abuse
      confirmed T74.11 ☑
      suspected T76.11 ☑
    psychological abuse
      confirmed T74.31 ☑
      suspected T76.31 ☑
      history of Z91.411
    sexual abuse
      confirmed T74.21 ☑
      suspected T76.21 ☑
    suspected T76.91 ☑
  child
    abandonment
      confirmed T74.02 ☑
      suspected T76.02 ☑
    bullying
      confirmed T74.32 ☑
      suspected T76.32 ☑
    confirmed T74.92 ☑
    history of — *see* History, personal (of), abuse
    intimidation (through social media)
      confirmed T74.32 ☑
      suspected T76.32 ☑
    neglect
      confirmed T74.02 ☑
      history of — *see* History, personal (of), abuse
      suspected T76.02 ☑
    physical abuse
      confirmed T74.12 ☑
      history of — *see* History, personal (of), abuse
      suspected T76.12 ☑
    psychological abuse
      confirmed T74.32 ☑
      history of — *see* History, personal (of), abuse
      suspected T76.32 ☑
    sexual abuse
      confirmed T74.22 ☑
      history of — *see* History, personal (of), abuse
      suspected T76.22 ☑
    suspected T76.92 ☑
  personal history of Z91.89
Malta fever — *see* Brucellosis
Maltworker's lung J67.4
Malunion, fracture — *see* Fracture, by site
Mammillitis N61.0
  puerperal, postpartum O91.02
Mammitis — *see* Mastitis
Mammogram (examination) Z12.39
  routine Z12.31
Mammoplasia N62
Management (of)
  bone conduction hearing device (implanted)
      Z45.320
  cardiac pacemaker NEC Z45.018
  cerebrospinal fluid drainage device Z45.41
  cochlear device (implanted) Z45.321
  contraceptive Z30.9
    specified NEC Z30.8
  implanted device Z45.9
    specified NEC Z45.89
  infusion pump Z45.1
  procreative Z31.9
    male factor infertility in female Z31.81
    specified NEC Z31.89
  prosthesis (external) (*see also* Fitting) Z44.9
    implanted Z45.9
      specified NEC Z45.89
  renal dialysis catheter Z49.01
  vascular access device Z45.2
Mangled — *see* specified injury by site

Mania (monopolar) (*see also* Disorder, mood, manic
    episode)
  with psychotic symptoms F30.2
  without psychotic symptoms F30.10
    mild F30.11
    moderate F30.12
    severe F30.13
  Bell's F30.8
  chronic (recurrent) F31.89
  hysterical F44.89
  puerperal F30.8
  recurrent F31.89
Manic depression F31.9
Manic-depressive insanity, psychosis, or syndrome —
    see Disorder, bipolar
Mannosidosis E77.1
Mansonelliasis, mansonellosis B74.4
Manson's
  disease B65.1
  schistosomiasis B65.1
Manual — *see* condition
Maple-bark-stripper's lung (disease) J67.6
Maple-syrup-urine disease E71.0
Marable's syndrome (celiac artery compression) I77.4
Marasmus E41
  due to malnutrition E41
  intestinal E41
  nutritional E41
  senile R54
  tuberculous NEC — *see* Tuberculosis
Marble
  bones Q78.2
  skin R23.8
Marburg virus disease A98.3
March
  fracture — *see* Fracture, traumatic, stress, by site
  hemoglobinuria D59.6
Marchesani (-Weill) syndrome Q87.0
Marchiafava (-Bignami) syndrome or disease G37.1
Marchiafava-Micheli syndrome D59.5
Marcus Gunn's syndrome Q07.8
Marfan's syndrome — *see* Syndrome, Marfan's
Marie-Bamberger disease — *see* Osteoarthropathy,
    hypertrophic, specified NEC
Marie-Charcot-Tooth neuropathic muscular atrophy
    G60.0
Marie's
  cerebellar ataxia (late-onset) G11.2
  disease or syndrome (acromegaly) E22.0
Marie-Strümpell arthritis, disease or spondylitis — *see*
    Spondylitis, ankylosing
Marion's disease (bladder neck obstruction) N32.0
Marital conflict Z63.0
Mark
  port wine Q82.5
  raspberry Q82.5
  strawberry Q82.5
  stretch L90.6
  tattoo L81.8
Marker heterochromatin — *see* Extra, marker
    chromosomes
Maroteaux-Lamy syndrome (mild) (severe) E76.29
Marrow (bone)
  arrest D61.9
  poor function D75.89
Marseilles fever A77.1
Marsh fever — *see* Malaria
Marshall's (hidrotic) ectodermal dysplasia Q82.4
Marsh's disease (exophthalmic goiter) E05.00
  with storm E05.01
Masculinization (female) with adrenal hyperplasia
    E25.9
  congenital E25.0
Masculinovoblastoma D27. ☑
Masochism (sexual) F65.51
Mason's lung J62.8
Mass
  abdominal R19.00
    epigastric R19.06
    generalized R19.07
    left lower quadrant R19.04
    left upper quadrant R19.02
    periumbilic R19.05
    right lower quadrant R19.03
    right upper quadrant R19.01
    specified site NEC R19.09
  breast (*see also* Lump, breast) N63.0
  chest R22.2
  cystic — *see* Cyst
  ear H93.8 ☑
  head R22.0

Mass — *continued*
intra-abdominal (diffuse) (generalized) — *see* Mass, abdominal
kidney N28.89
liver R16.0
localized (skin) R22.9
chest R22.2
head R22.0
limb
lower R22.4 ☑
upper R22.3 ☑
neck R22.1
trunk R22.2
lung R91.8
malignant — *see* Neoplasm, malignant, by site
neck R22.1
pelvic (diffuse) (generalized) — *see* Mass, abdominal
specified organ NEC — *see* Disease, by site
splenic R16.1
substernal thyroid — *see* Goiter
superficial (localized) R22.9
umbilical (diffuse) (generalized) R19.09
Massive — *see* condition
Mast cell
disease, systemic tissue D47.02
leukemia C94.3 ☑
neoplasm
malignant C96.20
specified type NEC C96.29
of uncertain behavior NEC D47.09
sarcoma C96.22
tumor D47.09
Mastalgia N64.4
Masters-Allen syndrome N83.8
Mastitis (acute) (diffuse) (nonpuerperal) (subacute) N61.0
with abscess N61.1
chronic (cystic) — *see* Mastopathy, cystic
cystic (Schimmelbusch's type) — *see* Mastopathy, cystic
fibrocystic — *see* Mastopathy, cystic
infective N61.0
newborn P39.0
interstitial, gestational or puerperal — *see* Mastitis, obstetric
neonatal (noninfective) P83.4
infective P39.0
obstetric (interstitial) (nonpurulent)
associated with
lactation O91.23
pregnancy O91.21 ☑
puerperium O91.22
purulent
associated with
lactation O91.13
pregnancy O91.11 ☑
puerperium O91.12
periductal — *see* Ectasia, mammary duct
phlegmonous — *see* Mastopathy, cystic
plasma cell — *see* Ectasia, mammary duct
without abscess N61.0
Mastocytoma (extracutaneous) D47.09
malignant C96.29
solitary D47.01
Mastocytosis D47.09
aggressive systemic C96.21
cutaneous (diffuse) (maculopapular) D47.01
congenital Q82.2
of neonatal onset Q82.2
of newborn onset Q82.2
indolent systemic D47.02
isolated bone marrow D47.02
malignant C96.29
systemic (indolent) (smoldering)
with an associated hematological non-mast cell lineage disease (SM-AHNMD) D47.02
Mastodynia N64.4
Mastoid — *see* condition
Mastoidalgia — *see* subcategory H92.0 ☑
Mastoiditis (coalescent) (hemorrhagic) (suppurative) H70.9 ☑
acute, subacute H70.00 ☑
complicated NEC H70.09 ☑
subperiosteal H70.01 ☑
chronic (necrotic) (recurrent) H70.1 ☑
in (due to)
infectious disease NEC B99 ☑ *[H75.0 ☑]*
parasitic disease NEC B89 *[H75.0 ☑]*
tuberculosis A18.03
petrositis — *see* Petrositis
postauricular fistula — *see* Fistula, postauricular
specified NEC H70.89 ☑
tuberculous A18.03

Mastopathy, mastopathia N64.9
chronica cystica — *see* Mastopathy, cystic
cystic (chronic) (diffuse) N60.1 ☑
with epithelial proliferation N60.3 ☑
diffuse cystic — *see* Mastopathy, cystic
estrogenic, oestrogenica N64.89
ovarian origin N64.89
Mastoplasia, mastoplastia N62
Masturbation (excessive) F98.8
Maternal care (for) — *see* Pregnancy (complicated by) (management affected by)
Mathieu's disease (leptospiral jaundice) A27.0
Mauclaire's disease or osteochondrosis — *see* Osteochondrosis, juvenile, hand, metacarpal
Maxcy's disease A75.2
Maxilla, maxillary — *see* condition
May (-Hegglin) anomaly or syndrome D72.0
McArdle (-Schmid)(-Pearson) disease (glycogen storage) E74.04
McCune-Albright syndrome Q78.1
McQuarrie's syndrome (idiopathic familial hypoglycemia) E16.2
Meadow's syndrome Q86.1
Measles (black) (hemorrhagic) (suppressed) B05.9
with
complications NEC B05.89
encephalitis B05.0
intestinal complications B05.4
keratitis (keratoconjunctivitis) B05.81
meningitis B05.1
otitis media B05.3
pneumonia B05.2
French — *see* Rubella
German — *see* Rubella
Liberty — *see* Rubella
Meatitis, urethral — *see* Urethritis
Meatus, meatal — *see* condition
Meat-wrappers' asthma J68.8
Meckel-Gruber syndrome Q61.9
Meckel's diverticulitis, diverticulum (displaced) (hypertrophic) Q43.0
malignant — *see* Table of Neoplasms, small intestine, malignant
Meconium
ileus, newborn P76.0
in cystic fibrosis E84.11
meaning meconium plug (without cystic fibrosis) P76.0
obstruction, newborn P76.0
due to fecaliths P76.0
in mucoviscidosis E84.11
peritonitis P78.0
plug syndrome (newborn) NEC P76.0
Median (*see also* condition)
arcuate ligament syndrome I77.4
bar (prostate) (vesical orifice) — *see* Hyperplasia, prostate
rhomboid glossitis K14.2
Mediastinal shift R93.89
Mediastinitis (acute) (chronic) J98.51
syphilitic A52.73
tuberculous A15.8
Mediastinopericarditis (*see also* Pericarditis)
acute I30.9
adhesive I31.0
chronic I31.8
rheumatic I09.2
Mediastinum, mediastinal — *see* condition
Medicine poisoning — *see* Table of Drugs and Chemicals, by drug, poisoning
Mediterranean
fever — *see* Brucellosis
familial M04.1
tick A77.1
kala-azar B55.0
leishmaniasis B55.0
tick fever A77.1
Medulla — *see* condition
Medullary cystic kidney Q61.5
Medullated fibers
optic (nerve) Q14.8
retina Q14.1
Medulloblastoma
desmoplastic C71.6
specified site — *see* Neoplasm, malignant, by site
unspecified site C71.6
Medulloepithelioma (*see also* Neoplasm, malignant, by site)
teratoid — *see* Neoplasm, malignant, by site
Medullomyoblastoma
specified site — *see* Neoplasm, malignant, by site
unspecified site C71.6

Meekeren-Ehlers-Danlos syndrome (*see also* Syndrome, Ehlers-Danlos) Q79.69
Megacolon (acquired) (functional) (not Hirschsprung's disease) (in) K59.39
Chagas' disease B57.32
congenital, congenitum (aganglionic) Q43.1
Hirschsprung's (disease) Q43.1
toxic NEC K59.31
due to Clostridium difficile
not specified as recurrent A04.72
recurrent A04.71
Megaesophagus (functional) K22.0
congenital Q39.5
in (due to) Chagas' disease B57.31
Megalencephaly Q04.5
Megalerythema (epidemic) B08.3
Megaloappendix Q43.8
Megalocephalus, megalocephaly NEC Q75.3
Megalocornea Q15.8
with glaucoma Q15.0
Megalocytic anemia D53.1
Megalodactylia (fingers) (thumbs) (congenital) Q74.0
toes Q74.2
Megaloduodenum Q43.8
Megaloesophagus (functional) K22.0
congenital Q39.5
Megalogastria (acquired) K31.89
congenital Q40.2
Megalophthalmos Q11.3
Megalopia H53.15
Megalosplenia — *see* Splenomegaly
Megaloureter N28.82
congenital Q62.2
Megarectum K62.89
Megasigmoid K59.39
congenital Q43.2
Megaureter N28.82
congenital Q62.2
Megavitamin-B6 syndrome E67.2
Megrim — *see* Migraine
Meibomian
cyst, infected — *see* Hordeolum
gland — *see* condition
sty, stye — *see* Hordeolum
Meibomitis — *see* Hordeolum
Meige-Milroy disease (chronic hereditary edema) Q82.0
Meige's syndrome Q82.0
Melalgia, nutritional E53.8
Melancholia F32.9
climacteric (single episode) F32.89
recurrent episode F33.8
hypochondriac F45.29
intermittent (single episode) F32.89
recurrent episode F33.8
involutional (single episode) F32.89
recurrent episode F33.8
menopausal (single episode) F32.89
recurrent episode F33.8
puerperal F32.89
reactive (emotional stress or trauma) F32.3
recurrent F33.9
senile F03 ☑
stuporous (single episode) F32.89
recurrent episode F33.8
Melanemia R79.89
Melanoameloblastoma — *see* Neoplasm, bone, benign
Melanoblastoma — *see* Melanoma
Melanocarcinoma — *see* Melanoma
Melanocytoma, eyeball D31.9 ☑
Melanocytosis, neurocutaneous Q82.8
Melanoderma, melanodermia L81.4
Melanodontia, infantile K03.89
Melanodontoclasia K03.89
Melanoepithelioma — *see* Melanoma
Melanoma (malignant) C43.9
acral lentiginous, malignant — *see* Melanoma, skin, by site
amelanotic — *see* Melanoma, skin, by site
balloon cell — *see* Melanoma, skin, by site
benign — *see* Nevus
desmoplastic, malignant — *see* Melanoma, skin, by site
epithelioid cell — *see* Melanoma, skin, by site
with spindle cell, mixed — *see* Melanoma, skin, by site
in
giant pigmented nevus — *see* Melanoma, skin, by site
Hutchinson's melanotic freckle — *see* Melanoma, skin, by site
junctional nevus — *see* Melanoma, skin, by site

Melanoma - Meningioma

Melanoma — *continued*
  in — *continued*
    precancerous melanosis — *see* Melanoma, skin,
      by site
  in situ D03.9
    abdominal wall D03.59
    ala nasi D03.39
    ankle D03.7 ☑
    anus, anal (margin) (skin) D03.51
    arm D03.6 ☑
    auditory canal D03.2 ☑
    auricle (ear) D03.2 ☑
    auricular canal (external) D03.2 ☑
    axilla, axillary fold D03.59
    back D03.59
    breast D03.52
    brow D03.39
    buttock D03.59
    canthus (eye) D03.1 ☑
    cheek (external) D03.39
    chest wall D03.59
    chin D03.39
    choroid D03.8
    conjunctiva D03.8
    ear (external) D03.2 ☑
    external meatus (ear) D03.2 ☑
    eye D03.8
    eyebrow D03.39
    eyelid (lower) (upper) D03.1 ☑
    face D03.30
      specified NEC D03.39
    female genital organ (external) NEC D03.8
    finger D03.6 ☑
    flank D03.59
    foot D03.7 ☑
    forearm D03.6 ☑
    forehead D03.39
    foreskin D03.8
    gluteal region D03.59
    groin D03.59
    hand D03.6 ☑
    heel D03.7 ☑
    helix D03.2 ☑
    hip D03.7 ☑
    interscapular region D03.59
    iris D03.8
    jaw D03.39
    knee D03.7 ☑
    labium (majus) (minus) D03.8
    lacrimal gland D03.8
    leg D03.7 ☑
    lip (lower) (upper) D03.0
    lower limb NEC D03.7 ☑
    male genital organ (external) NEC D03.8
    nail D03.9
      finger D03.6 ☑
      toe D03.7 ☑
    neck D03.4
    nose (external) D03.39
    orbit D03.8
    penis D03.8
    perianal skin D03.51
    perineum D03.51
    pinna D03.2 ☑
    popliteal fossa or space D03.7 ☑
    prepuce D03.8
    pudendum D03.8
    retina D03.8
    retrobulbar D03.8
    scalp D03.4
    scrotum D03.8
    shoulder D03.6 ☑
    specified site NEC D03.8
    submammary fold D03.52
    temple D03.39
    thigh D03.7 ☑
    toe D03.7 ☑
    trunk NEC D03.59
    umbilicus D03.59
    upper limb NEC D03.6 ☑
    vulva D03.8
  juvenile — *see* Nevus
  malignant, of soft parts except skin — *see*
    Neoplasm, connective tissue, malignant
  metastatic
    breast C79.81
    genital organ C79.82
    specified site NEC C79.89
  neurotropic, malignant — *see* Melanoma, skin, by
    site
  nodular — *see* Melanoma, skin, by site
  regressing, malignant — *see* Melanoma, skin, by site

Melanoma — *continued*
  skin C43.9
    abdominal wall C43.59
    ala nasi C43.31
    ankle C43.7 ☑
    anus, anal (skin) C43.51
    arm C43.6 ☑
    auditory canal (external) C43.2 ☑
    auricle (ear) C43.2 ☑
    auricular canal (external) C43.2 ☑
    axilla, axillary fold C43.59
    back C43.59
    breast (female) (male) C43.52
    brow C43.39
    buttock C43.59
    canthus (eye) C43.1 ☑
    cheek (external) C43.39
    chest wall C43.59
    chin C43.39
    ear (external) C43.2 ☑
    elbow C43.6 ☑
    external meatus (ear) C43.2 ☑
    eyebrow C43.39
    eyelid (lower) (upper) C43.1 ☑
    face C43.30
      specified NEC C43.39
    female genital organ (external) NEC C51.9
    finger C43.6 ☑
    flank C43.59
    foot C43.7 ☑
    forearm C43.6 ☑
    forehead C43.39
    foreskin C60.0
    glabella C43.39
    gluteal region C43.59
    groin C43.59
    hand C43.6 ☑
    heel C43.7 ☑
    helix C43.2 ☑
    hip C43.7 ☑
    interscapular region C43.59
    jaw (external) C43.39
    knee C43.7 ☑
    labium C51.9
      majus C51.0
      minus C51.1
    leg C43.7 ☑
    lip (lower) (upper) C43.0
    lower limb NEC C43.7 ☑
    male genital organ (external) NEC C63.9
    nail
      finger C43.6 ☑
      toe C43.7 ☑
    nasolabial groove C43.39
    nates C43.59
    neck C43.4
    nose (external) C43.31
    overlapping site C43.8
    palpebra C43.1 ☑
    penis C60.9
    perianal skin C43.51
    perineum C43.51
    pinna C43.2 ☑
    popliteal fossa or space C43.7 ☑
    prepuce C60.0
    pudendum C51.9
    scalp C43.4
    scrotum C63.2
    shoulder C43.6 ☑
    skin NEC C43.9
    submammary fold C43.52
    temple C43.39
    thigh C43.7 ☑
    toe C43.7 ☑
    trunk NEC C43.59
    umbilicus C43.59
    upper limb NEC C43.6 ☑
    vulva C51.9
      overlapping sites C51.8
  spindle cell
    with epithelioid, mixed — *see* Melanoma, skin,
      by site
    type A C69.4 ☑
    type B C69.4 ☑
  superficial spreading — *see* Melanoma, skin, by site
Melanosarcoma (*see also* Melanoma)
  epithelioid cell — *see* Melanoma
Melanosis L81.4
  addisonian E27.1
    tuberculous A18.7
  adrenal E27.1
  colon K63.89

Melanosis — *continued*
  conjunctiva — *see* Pigmentation, conjunctiva
    congenital Q13.89
  cornea (presenile) (senile) (*see also* Pigmentation,
    cornea)
    congenital Q13.4
  eye NEC H57.89
    congenital Q15.8
  lenticularis progressiva Q82.1
  liver K76.89
  precancerous (*see also* Melanoma, in situ)
    malignant melanoma in — *see* Melanoma
  Riehl's L81.4
  sclera H15.89
    congenital Q13.89
  suprarenal E27.1
  tar L81.4
  toxic L81.4
Melanuria R82.998
MELAS syndrome E88.41
Melasma L81.1
  adrenal (gland) E27.1
  suprarenal (gland) E27.1
Melena K92.1
  with ulcer - code by site under Ulcer, with
    hemorrhage K27.4
  due to swallowed maternal blood P78.2
  newborn, neonatal P54.1
    due to swallowed maternal blood P78.2
Meleney's
  gangrene (cutaneous) — *see* Ulcer, skin
  ulcer (chronic undermining) — *see* Ulcer, skin
Melioidosis A24.9
  acute A24.1
  chronic A24.2
  fulminating A24.1
  pneumonia A24.1
  pulmonary (chronic) A24.2
    acute A24.1
    subacute A24.2
  sepsis A24.1
  specified NEC A24.3
  subacute A24.2
Melitensis, febris A23.0
Melkersson (-Rosenthal) syndrome G51.2
Mellitus, diabetes — *see* Diabetes
Melorheostosis (bone) — *see* Disorder, bone, density
  and structure, specified NEC
Meloschisis Q18.4
Melotia Q17.4
Membrana
  capsularis lentis posterior Q13.89
  epipapillaris Q14.2
Membranacea placenta O43.19 ☑
Membranaceous uterus N85.8
Membrane(s), membranous (*see also* condition)
  cyclitic — *see* Membrane, pupillary
  folds, congenital — *see* Web
  Jackson's Q43.3
  over face of newborn P28.9
  premature rupture — *see* Rupture, membranes,
    premature
  pupillary H21.4 ☑
    persistent Q13.89
  retained (with hemorrhage) (complicating delivery)
    O72.2
    without hemorrhage O73.1
  secondary cataract — *see* Cataract, secondary
  unruptured (causing asphyxia) — *see* Asphyxia,
    newborn
  vitreous — *see* Opacity, vitreous, membranes and
    strands
Membranitis — *see* Chorioamnionitis
Memory disturbance, lack or loss (*see also* Amnesia)
  mild, following organic brain damage F06.8
Menadione deficiency E56.1
Menarche
  delayed E30.0
  precocious E30.1
Mendacity, pathologic F60.2
Mendelson's syndrome (due to anesthesia) J95.4
  in labor and delivery O74.0
  in pregnancy O29.01 ☑
  obstetric O74.0
  postpartum, puerperal O89.01
Ménétrier's disease or syndrome K29.60
  with bleeding K29.61
Ménière's disease, syndrome or vertigo H81.0 ☑
Meninges, meningeal — *see* condition
Meningioma (*see also* Neoplasm, meninges, benign)
  angioblastic — *see* Neoplasm, meninges, benign
  angiomatous — *see* Neoplasm, meninges, benign

☑ **Additional character required**

Meningioma — *continued*
  endotheliomatous — *see* Neoplasm, meninges, benign
  fibroblastic — *see* Neoplasm, meninges, benign
  fibrous — *see* Neoplasm, meninges, benign
  hemangioblastic — *see* Neoplasm, meninges, benign
  hemangiopericytic — *see* Neoplasm, meninges, benign
  malignant — *see* Neoplasm, meninges, malignant
  meningiothelial — *see* Neoplasm, meninges, benign
  meningotheliomatous — *see* Neoplasm, meninges, benign
  mixed — *see* Neoplasm, meninges, benign
  multiple — *see* Neoplasm, meninges, uncertain behavior
  papillary — *see* Neoplasm, meninges, uncertain behavior
  psammomatous — *see* Neoplasm, meninges, benign
  syncytial — *see* Neoplasm, meninges, benign
  transitional — *see* Neoplasm, meninges, benign
Meningiomatosis (diffuse) — *see* Neoplasm, meninges, uncertain behavior
Meningism — *see* Meningismus
Meningismus (infectional) (pneumococcal) R29.1
  due to serum or vaccine R29.1
  influenzal — *see* Influenza, with, manifestations NEC
Meningitis (basal) (basic) (brain) (cerebral) (cervical) (congestive) (diffuse) (hemorrhagic) (infantile) (membranous) (metastatic) (nonspecific) (pontine) (progressive) (simple) (spinal) (subacute) (sympathetic) (toxic) G03.9
  abacterial G03.0
  actinomycotic A42.81
  adenoviral A87.1
  arbovirus A87.8
  aseptic (acute) G03.0
  bacterial G00.9
    Escherichia coli (E. coli) G00.8
    Friedländer (bacillus) G00.8
    gram-negative G00.9
    H. influenzae G00.0
    Klebsiella G00.8
    pneumococcal G00.1
    specified organism NEC G00.8
    staphylococcal G00.3
    streptococcal (acute) G00.2
  benign recurrent (Mollaret) G03.2
  candidal B37.5
  caseous (tuberculous) A17.0
  cerebrospinal A39.0
  chronic NEC G03.1
  clear cerebrospinal fluid NEC G03.0
  coxsackievirus A87.0
  cryptococcal B45.1
  diplococcal (gram positive) A39.0
  echovirus A87.0
  enteroviral A87.0
  eosinophilic B83.2
  epidemic NEC A39.0
  Escherichia coli (E. coli) G00.8
  fibrinopurulent G00.9
    specified organism NEC G00.8
  Friedländer (bacillus) G00.8
  gonococcal A54.81
  gram-negative cocci G00.9
  gram-positive cocci G00.9
  Haemophilus (influenzae) G00.0
  H. influenzae G00.0
  in (due to)
    adenovirus A87.1
    African trypanosomiasis B56.9 *[G02]*
    anthrax A22.8
    bacterial disease NEC A48.8 *[G01]*
    Chagas' disease (chronic) B57.41
    chickenpox B01.0
    coccidioidomycosis B38.4
    Diplococcus pneumoniae G00.1
    enterovirus A87.0
    herpes (simplex) virus B00.3
      zoster B02.1
    infectious mononucleosis B27.92
    leptospirosis A27.81
    Listeria monocytogenes A32.11
    Lyme disease A69.21
    measles B05.1
    mumps (virus) B26.1
    neurosyphilis (late) A52.13
    parasitic disease NEC B89 *[G02]*
    poliovirus A80.9 *[G02]*

Meningitis — *continued*
  in — *continued*
    preventive immunization, inoculation or vaccination G03.8
    rubella B06.02
    Salmonella infection A02.21
    specified cause NEC G03.8
    Streptococcal pneumoniae G00.1
    typhoid fever A01.01
    varicella B01.0
    viral disease NEC A87.8
    whooping cough A37.90
    zoster B02.1
  infectious G00.9
  influenzal (H. influenzae) G00.0
  Klebsiella G00.8
  leptospiral (aseptic) A27.81
  lymphocytic (acute) (benign) (serous) A87.2
  meningococcal A39.0
  Mima polymorpha G00.8
  Mollaret (benign recurrent) G03.2
  monilial B37.5
  mycotic NEC B49 *[G02]*
  Neisseria A39.0
  nonbacterial G03.0
  nonpyogenic NEC G03.0
  ossificans G96.19
  pneumococcal streptococcus pneumoniae G00.1
  poliovirus A80.9 *[G02]*
  postmeasles B05.1
  purulent G00.9
    specified organism NEC G00.8
  pyogenic G00.9
    specified organism NEC G00.8
  Salmonella (arizonae) (Cholerae-Suis) (enteritidis) (typhimurium) A02.21
  septic G00.9
    specified organism NEC G00.8
  serosa circumscripta NEC G03.0
  serous NEC G93.2
  specified organism NEC G00.8
  sporotrichosis B42.81
  staphylococcal G00.3
  sterile G03.0
  Streptococcal (acute) G00.2
    pneumoniae G00.1
  suppurative G00.9
    specified organism NEC G00.8
  syphilitic (late) (tertiary) A52.13
    acute A51.41
    congenital A50.41
    secondary A51.41
  Torula histolytica (cryptococcal) B45.1
  traumatic (complication of injury) T79.8 ☑
  tuberculous A17.0
  typhoid A01.01
  viral NEC A87.9
  Yersinia pestis A20.3
Meningocele (spinal) (*see also* Spina bifida)
  with hydrocephalus — *see* Spina bifida, by site, with hydrocephalus
  acquired (traumatic) G96.19
  cerebral — *see* Encephalocele
Meningocerebritis — *see* Meningoencephalitis
Meningococcemia A39.4
  acute A39.2
  chronic A39.3
Meningococcus, meningococcal (*see also* condition) A39.9
  adrenalitis, hemorrhagic A39.1
  carrier (suspected) of Z22.31
  meningitis (cerebrospinal) A39.0
Meningoencephalitis (*see also* Encephalitis) G04.90
  acute NEC (*see also* Encephalitis, viral) A86
  bacterial NEC G04.2
  California A83.5
  diphasic A84.1
  eosinophilic B83.2
  epidemic A39.81
  herpesviral, herpetic B00.4
    due to herpesvirus 6 B10.01
    due to herpesvirus 7 B10.09
    specified NEC B10.09
  in (due to)
    blastomycosis NEC B40.81
    diseases classified elsewhere G05.3
    free-living amebae B60.2
    Hemophilus influenzae (H .influenzae) G00.0
    herpes B00.4
      due to herpesvirus 6 B10.01
      due to herpesvirus 7 B10.09
      specified NEC B10.09

Meningoencephalitis — *continued*
  in — *continued*
    H. influenzae G00.0
    Lyme disease A69.22
    mercury — *see* subcategory T56.1 ☑
    mumps B26.2
    Naegleria (amebae) (organisms) (fowleri) B60.2
    Parastrongylus cantonensis B83.2
    toxoplasmosis (acquired) B58.2
      congenital P37.1
  infectious (acute) (viral) A86
  influenzal (H. influenzae) G00.0
  Listeria monocytogenes A32.12
  lymphocytic (serous) A87.2
  mumps B26.2
  parasitic NEC B89 *[G05.3]*
  pneumococcal G04.2
  primary amebic B60.2
  specific (syphilitic) A52.14
  specified organism NEC G04.81
  staphylococcal G04.2
  streptococcal G04.2
  syphilitic A52.14
  toxic NEC G92
    due to mercury — *see* subcategory T56.1 ☑
  tuberculous A17.82
  virus NEC A86
Meningoencephalocele (*see also* Encephalocele)
  syphilitic A52.19
    congenital A50.49
Meningoencephalomyelitis (*see also* Meningoencephalitis)
  acute NEC (viral) A86
    disseminated G04.00
      postimmunization or postvaccination G04.02
      postinfectious G04.01
    due to
      actinomycosis A42.82
      Torula B45.1
      Toxoplasma or toxoplasmosis (acquired) B58.2
        congenital P37.1
    postimmunization or postvaccination G04.02
Meningoencephalomyelopathy G96.9
Meningoencephalopathy G96.9
Meningomyelitis (*see also* Meningoencephalitis)
  bacterial NEC G04.2
  blastomycotic NEC B40.81
  cryptococcal B45.1
  in diseases classified elsewhere G05.4
  meningococcal A39.81
  syphilitic A52.14
  tuberculous A17.82
Meningomyelocele (*see also* Spina bifida)
  syphilitic A52.19
Meningomyeloneuritis — *see* Meningoencephalitis
Meningoradiculitis — *see* Meningitis
Meningovascular — *see* condition
Menkes' disease or syndrome E83.09
  meaning maple-syrup-urine disease E71.0
Menometrorrhagia N92.1
Menopause, menopausal (asymptomatic) (state) Z78.0
  arthritis (any site) NEC — *see* Arthritis, specified form NEC
  bleeding N92.4
  depression (single episode) F32.89
    agitated (single episode) F32.2
      recurrent episode F33.9
    psychotic (single episode) F32.89
      recurrent episode F33.9
    recurrent episode F33.8
  melancholia (single episode) F32.89
    recurrent episode F33.8
  paranoid state F22
  premature E28.319
    asymptomatic E28.319
      postirradiation E89.40
      postsurgical E89.40
    symptomatic E28.310
      postirradiation E89.41
      postsurgical E89.41
  psychosis NEC F28
  symptomatic N95.1
  toxic polyarthritis NEC — *see* Arthritis, specified form NEC
Menorrhagia (primary) N92.0
  climacteric N92.4
    menopausal N92.4
  menopausal N92.4
  perimenopausal N92.4
  postclimacteric N95.0
  postmenopausal N95.0

Menorrhagia - Micturition

Menorrhagia — *continued*
  preclimacteric or premenopausal N92.4
  pubertal (menses retained) N92.2
Menostaxis N92.0
Menses, retention N94.89
Menstrual — *see* Menstruation
Menstruation
  absent — *see* Amenorrhea
  anovulatory N97.0
  cycle, irregular N92.6
  delayed N91.0
  disorder N93.9
    psychogenic F45.8
  during pregnancy O20.8
  excessive (with regular cycle) N92.0
    with irregular cycle N92.1
    at puberty N92.2
  frequent N92.0
  infrequent — *see* Oligomenorrhea
  irregular N92.6
    specified NEC N92.5
  latent N92.5
  membranous N92.5
  painful (*see also* Dysmenorrhea) N94.6
    primary N94.4
    psychogenic F45.8
    secondary N94.5
  passage of clots N92.0
  precocious E30.1
  protracted N92.5
  rare — *see* Oligomenorrhea
  retained N94.89
  retrograde N92.5
  scanty — *see* Oligomenorrhea
  suppression N94.89
  vicarious (nasal) N94.89
Mental (*see also* condition)
  deficiency — *see* Disability, intellectual
  deterioration — *see* Psychosis
  disorder — *see* Disorder, mental
  exhaustion F48.8
  insufficiency (congenital) — *see* Disability,
    intellectual
  observation without need for further medical care
    Z03.89
  retardation — *see* Disability, intellectual
  subnormality — *see* Disability, intellectual
  upset — *see* Disorder, mental
Meralgia paresthetica G57.1 ☑
Mercurial — *see* condition
Mercurialism — *see* subcategory T56.1 ☑
MERRF syndrome (myoclonic epilepsy associated with
  ragged-red fiber) E88.42
Merkel cell tumor — *see* Carcinoma, Merkel cell
Merocele — *see* Hernia, femoral
Meromelia
  lower limb — *see* Defect, reduction, lower limb
  intercalary
    femur — *see* Defect, reduction, lower limb,
      specified type NEC
      tibiofibular (complete) (incomplete) — *see*
        Defect, reduction, lower limb
  upper limb — *see* Defect, reduction, upper limb
    intercalary, humeral, radioulnar — *see* Agenesis,
      arm, with hand present
Merzbacher-Pelizaeus disease E75.29
Mesaortitis — *see* Aortitis
Mesarteritis — *see* Arteritis
Mesencephalitis — *see* Encephalitis
Mesenchymoma (*see also* Neoplasm, connective tissue,
  uncertain behavior)
  benign — *see* Neoplasm, connective tissue, benign
  malignant — *see* Neoplasm, connective tissue,
    malignant
Mesenteritis
  retractile K65.4
  sclerosing K65.4
Mesentery, mesenteric — *see* condition
Mesiodens, mesiodentes K00.1
Mesio-occlusion M26.213
Mesocolon — *see* condition
Mesonephroma (malignant) — *see* Neoplasm,
  malignant, by site
  benign — *see* Neoplasm, benign, by site
Mesophlebitis — *see* Phlebitis
Mesostromal dysgenesia Q13.89
Mesothelioma (malignant) C45.9
  benign
    mesentery D19.1
    mesocolon D19.1
    omentum D19.1
    peritoneum D19.1

Mesothelioma — *continued*
  benign — *continued*
    pleura D19.0
    specified site NEC D19.7
    unspecified site D19.9
  biphasic C45.9
    benign
      mesentery D19.1
      mesocolon D19.1
      omentum D19.1
      peritoneum D19.1
      pleura D19.0
      specified site NEC D19.7
      unspecified site D19.9
  cystic D48.4
  epithelioid C45.9
    benign
      mesentery D19.1
      mesocolon D19.1
      omentum D19.1
      peritoneum D19.1
      pleura D19.0
      specified site NEC D19.7
      unspecified site D19.9
  fibrous C45.9
    benign
      mesentery D19.1
      mesocolon D19.1
      omentum D19.1
      peritoneum D19.1
      pleura D19.0
      specified site NEC D19.7
      unspecified site D19.9
  site classification
    liver C45.7
    lung C45.7
    mediastinum C45.7
    mesentery C45.1
    mesocolon C45.1
    omentum C45.1
    pericardium C45.2
    peritoneum C45.1
    pleura C45.0
      parietal C45.0
    retroperitoneum C45.7
    specified site NEC C45.7
    unspecified C45.9
Metabolic syndrome E88.81
Metagonimiasis B66.8
Metagonimus infestation (intestine) B66.8
Metal
  pigmentation L81.8
  polisher's disease J62.8
Metamorphopsia H53.15
Metaplasia
  apocrine (breast) — *see* Dysplasia, mammary,
    specified type NEC
  cervix (squamous) — *see* Dysplasia, cervix
  endometrium (squamous) (uterus) N85.8
  esophagus K22.7 ☑
  kidney (pelvis) (squamous) N28.89
  myelogenous D73.1
  myeloid (agnogenic) (megakaryocytic) D73.1
  spleen D73.1
  squamous cell, bladder N32.89
Metastasis, metastatic
  abscess — *see* Abscess
  calcification E83.59
  cancer
    from specified site — *see* Neoplasm, malignant,
      by site
    to specified site — *see* Neoplasm, secondary, by
      site
  deposits (in) — *see* Neoplasm, secondary, by site
  disease (*see also* Neoplasm, secondary, by site)
    C79.9
  spread (to) — *see* Neoplasm, secondary, by site
Metastrongyliasis B83.8
Metatarsalgia M77.4 ☑
  anterior G57.6 ☑
  Morton's G57.6 ☑
Metatarsus, metatarsal (*see also* condition)
  adductus, congenital Q66.22 ☑
  valgus (abductus), congenital Q66.6
  varus (congenital) Q66.22 ☑
    primus Q66.21 ☑
Methadone use — *see* Use, opioid
Methemoglobinemia D74.9
  acquired (with sulfhemoglobinemia) D74.8
  congenital D74.0
    enzymatic (congenital) D74.0
  Hb M disease D74.0

Methemoglobinemia — *continued*
  hereditary D74.0
  toxic D74.8
Methemoglobinuria — *see* Hemoglobinuria
Methioninemia E72.19
Methylmalonic acidemia E71.120
Metritis (catarrhal) (hemorrhagic) (septic) (suppurative)
  (*see also* Endometritis)
  cervical — *see* Cervicitis
Metropathia hemorrhagica N93.8
Metroperitonitis — *see* Peritonitis, pelvic, female
Metrorrhagia N92.1
  climacteric N92.4
  menopausal N92.4
  perimenopausal N92.4
  postpartum NEC (atonic) (following delivery of
    placenta) O72.1
    delayed or secondary O72.2
  preclimacteric or premenopausal N92.4
  psychogenic F45.8
Metrorrhexis — *see* Rupture, uterus
Metrosalpingitis N70.91
Metrostaxis N93.8
Metrovaginitis — *see* Endometritis
Meyer-Schwickerath and Weyers syndrome Q87.0
Meynert's amentia (nonalcoholic) F04
  alcoholic F10.96
    with dependence F10.26
Mibelli's disease (porokeratosis) Q82.8
Mice, joint — *see* Loose, body, joint
  knee M23.4 ☑
Micrencephalon, micrencephaly Q02
Microalbuminuria R80.9
Microaneurysm, retinal (*see also* Disorder, retina,
  microaneurysms)
  diabetic — *see* E08-E13 with .31
Microangiopathy (peripheral) I73.9
  thrombotic M31.1
Microcalcifications, breast R92.0
Microcephalus, microcephalic, microcephaly Q02
  due to toxoplasmosis (congenital) P37.1
Microcheilia Q18.7
Microcolon (congenital) Q43.8
Microcornea (congenital) Q13.4
Microcytic — *see* condition
Microdeletions NEC Q93.88
Microdontia K00.2
Microdrepanocytosis D57.40
  with crisis (vasoocclusive pain) D57.419
    with
      acute chest syndrome D57.411
      splenic sequestration D57.412
Microembolism
  atherothrombotic — *see* Atheroembolism
  retinal — *see* Occlusion, artery, retina
Microencephalon Q02
Microfilaria streptocerca infestation — *see*
  Onchocerciasis
Microgastria (congenital) Q40.2
Microgenia M26.06
Microgenitalia, congenital
  female Q52.8
  male Q55.8
Microglioma — *see* Lymphoma, non-Hodgkin,
  specified NEC
Microglossia (congenital) Q38.3
Micrognathia, micrognathism (congenital)
  (mandibular) (maxillary) M26.09
Microgyria (congenital) Q04.3
Microinfarct of heart — *see* Insufficiency, coronary
Microlentia (congenital) Q12.8
Microlithiasis, alveolar, pulmonary J84.02
Micromastia N64.82
Micromyelia (congenital) Q06.8
Micropenis Q55.62
Microphakia (congenital) Q12.8
Microphthalmos, microphthalmia (congenital) Q11.2
  due to toxoplasmosis P37.1
Micropsia H53.15
Microscopic polyangiitis (polyarteritis) M31.7
Microsporidiosis B60.8
  intestinal A07.8
Microsporon furfur infestation B36.0
Microsporosis (*see also* Dermatophytosis)
  nigra B36.1
Microstomia (congenital) Q18.5
Microtia (congenital) (external ear) Q17.2
Microtropia H50.40
Microvillus inclusion disease (MVD) (MVID) Q43.8
Micturition
  disorder NEC (*see also* Difficulty, micturition) R39.198
    psychogenic F45.8

☑ **Additional character required**

Micturition — *continued*
 frequency R35.0
  psychogenic F45.8
 hesitancy R39.11
 incomplete emptying R39.14
 nocturnal R35.1
 painful R30.9
  dysuria R30.0
  psychogenic F45.8
  tenesmus R30.1
 poor stream R39.12
 position dependent R39.192
 split stream R39.13
 straining R39.16
 urgency R39.15
Mid plane — *see* condition
Middle
 ear — *see* condition
 lobe (right) syndrome J98.19
Miescher's elastoma L87.2
Mietens' syndrome Q87.2
Migraine (idiopathic) G43.909
 with refractory migraine G43.919
  with status migrainosus G43.911
  without status migrainosus G43.919
 with aura (acute-onset) (prolonged) (typical)
  (without headache) G43.109
  with refractory migraine G43.119
   with status migrainosus G43.111
   without status migrainosus G43.119
  intractable G43.119
   with status migrainosus G43.111
   without status migrainosus G43.119
  not intractable G43.109
   with status migrainosus G43.101
   without status migrainosus G43.109
  persistent G43.509
   with cerebral infarction G43.609
    with refractory migraine G43.619
     with status migrainosus G43.611
     without status migrainosus G43.619
    intractable G43.619
     with status migrainosus G43.611
     without status migrainosus G43.619
    not intractable G43.609
     with status migrainosus G43.601
     without status migrainosus G43.609
    without refractory migraine G43.609
     with status migrainosus G43.601
     without status migrainosus G43.609
   without cerebral infarction G43.509
    with refractory migraine G43.519
     with status migrainosus G43.511
     without status migrainosus G43.519
    intractable G43.519
     with status migrainosus G43.511
     without status migrainosus G43.519
    not intractable G43.509
     with status migrainosus G43.501
     without status migrainosus G43.509
    without refractory migraine G43.509
     with status migrainosus G43.501
     without status migrainosus G43.509
  without mention of refractory migraine G43.109
   with status migrainosus G43.101
   without status migrainosus G43.109
 abdominal G43.D0
  with refractory migraine G43.D1
  intractable G43.D1
  not intractable G43.D0
  without refractory migraine G43.D0
 basilar — *see* Migraine, with aura
 classical — *see* Migraine, with aura
 common — *see* Migraine, without aura
 complicated G43.109
 equivalents — *see* Migraine, with aura
 familiar — *see* Migraine, hemiplegic
 hemiplegic G43.409
  with refractory migraine G43.419
   with status migrainosus G43.411
   without status migrainosus G43.419
  intractable G43.419
   with status migrainosus G43.411
   without status migrainosus G43.419
  not intractable G43.409
   with status migrainosus G43.401
   without status migrainosus G43.409
  without refractory migraine G43.409
   with status migrainosus G43.401
   without status migrainosus G43.409
 intractable G43.919
  with status migrainosus G43.911

Migraine — *continued*
 intractable — *continued*
  without status migrainosus G43.919
 menstrual G43.829
  with refractory migraine G43.839
   with status migrainosus G43.831
   without status migrainosus G43.839
  intractable G43.839
   with status migrainosus G43.831
   without status migrainosus G43.839
  not intractable 4G43.829
   with status migrainosus G43.821
   without status migrainosus G43.829
  without refractory migraine G43.829
   with status migrainosus G43.821
   without status migrainosus G43.829
 menstrually related — *see* Migraine, menstrual
 not intractable G43.909
  with status migrainosus G43.901
  without status migrainosus G43.919
 ophthalmoplegic G43.B0
  with refractory migraine G43.B1
  intractable G43.B1
  not intractable G43.B0
  without refractory migraine G43.B0
 persistent aura (with, without) cerebral infarction —
  see Migraine, with aura, persistent
 preceded or accompanied by transient focal
  neurological phenomena — *see* Migraine, with
  aura
 pre-menstrual — *see* Migraine, menstrual
 pure menstrual — *see* Migraine, menstrual
 retinal — *see* Migraine, with aura
 specified NEC G43.809
  intractable G43.819
   with status migrainosus G43.811
   without status migrainosus G43.819
  not intractable G43.809
   with status migrainosus G43.801
   without status migrainosus G43.809
 sporadic — *see* Migraine, hemiplegic
 transformed — *see* Migraine, without aura, chronic
 triggered seizures — *see* Migraine, with aura
 without aura G43.009
  with refractory migraine G43.019
   with status migrainosus G43.011
   without status migrainosus G43.019
  chronic G43.709
   with refractory migraine G43.719
    with status migrainosus G43.711
    without status migrainosus G43.719
   intractable
    with status migrainosus G43.711
    without status migrainosus G43.719
   not intractable
    with status migrainosus G43.701
    without status migrainosus G43.709
   without refractory migraine G43.709
    with status migrainosus G43.701
    without status migrainosus G43.709
  intractable
   with status migrainosus G43.011
   without status migrainosus G43.019
  not intractable
   with status migrainosus G43.001
   without status migrainosus G43.009
  without mention of refractory migraine G43.009
   with status migrainosus G43.001
   without status migrainosus G43.009
  without refractory migraineG43.909
   with status migrainosus G43.901
   without status migrainosus G43.919
Migrant, social Z59.0
Migration, anxiety concerning Z60.3
Migratory, migrating (*see also* condition)
 person Z59.0
 testis Q55.29
Mikity-Wilson disease or syndrome P27.0
Mikulicz' disease or syndrome K11.8
Miliaria L74.3
 alba L74.1
 apocrine L75.2
 crystallina L74.1
 profunda L74.2
 rubra L74.0
 tropicalis L74.2
Miliary — *see* condition
Milium L72.0
 colloid L57.8
Milk
 crust L21.0
 excessive secretion O92.6

Milk — *continued*
 poisoning — *see* Poisoning, food, noxious
 retention O92.79
 sickness — *see* Poisoning, food, noxious
 spots I31.0
Milk-alkali disease or syndrome E83.52
Milk-leg (deep vessels) (nonpuerperal) — *see*
 Embolism, vein, lower extremity
 complicating pregnancy O22.3 ☑
 puerperal, postpartum, childbirth O87.1
Milkman's disease or syndrome M83.8
Milky urine — *see* Chyluria
Millard-Gubler (-Foville) paralysis or syndrome G46.3
Millar's asthma J38.5
Miller Fisher syndrome G61.0
Mills' disease — *see* Hemiplegia
Millstone maker's pneumoconiosis J62.8
Milroy's disease (chronic hereditary edema) Q82.0
Minamata disease T56.1 ☑
Miners' asthma or lung J60
Minkowski-Chauffard syndrome — *see* Spherocytosis
Minor — *see* condition
Minor's disease (hematomyelia) G95.19
Minot's disease (hemorrhagic disease), newborn P53
Minot-von Willebrand-Jurgens disease or syndrome
 (angiohemophilia) D68.0
Minus (and plus) hand (intrinsic) — *see* Deformity,
 limb, specified type NEC, forearm
Miosis (pupil) H57.03
Mirizzi's syndrome (hepatic duct stenosis) K83.1
Mirror writing F81.0
Misadventure (of) (prophylactic) (therapeutic) (*see also*
 Complications) T88.9 ☑
 administration of insulin (by accident) — *see*
  subcategory T38.3 ☑
 infusion — *see* Complications, infusion
 local applications (of fomentations, plasters, etc.)
  T88.9 ☑
  burn or scald — *see* Burn
  specified NEC T88.8 ☑
 medical care (early) (late) T88.9 ☑
  adverse effect of drugs or chemicals — *see* Table
   of Drugs and Chemicals
 medical care (early) (late)
  burn or scald — *see* Burn
  specified NEC T88.8 ☑
 specified NEC T88.8 ☑
 surgical procedure (early) (late) — *see*
  Complications, surgical procedure
 transfusion — *see* Complications, transfusion
 vaccination or other immunological procedure —
  see Complications, vaccination
Miscarriage O03.9
Misdirection, aqueous H40.83 ☑
Misperception, sleep state F51.02
Misplaced, misplacement
 ear Q17.4
 kidney (acquired) N28.89
  congenital Q63.2
 organ or site, congenital NEC — *see* Malposition,
  congenital
Missed
 abortion O02.1
 delivery O36.4 ☑
Missing (*see also* Absence)
 string of intrauterine contraceptive device
  T83.32 ☑
Misuse of drugs F19.99
Mitchell's disease (erythromelalgia) I73.81
Mite(s) (infestation) B88.9
 diarrhea B88.0
 grain (itch) B88.0
 hair follicle (itch) B88.0
 in sputum B88.0
Mitral — *see* condition
Mittelschmerz N94.0
Mixed — *see* condition
MMN (multifocal motor neuropathy) G61.82
MNGIE (Mitochondrial Neurogastrointestinal
 Encephalopathy) syndrome E88.49
Mobile, mobility
 cecum Q43.3
 excessive — *see* Hypermobility
 gallbladder, congenital Q44.1
 kidney N28.89
 organ or site, congenital NEC — *see* Malposition,
  congenital
Mobitz heart block (atrioventricular) I44.1
Moebius, Möbius
 disease (ophthalmoplegic migraine) — *see*
  Migraine, ophthalmoplegic

Moebius — *continued*
  syndrome Q87.0
    congenital oculofacial paralysis (with other anomalies) Q87.0
    ophthalmoplegic migraine — *see* Migraine, ophthalmoplegic
Moeller's glossitis K14.0
Mohr's syndrome (Types I and II) Q87.0
Mola destruens D39.2
Molar pregnancy O02.0
Molarization of premolars K00.2
Molding, head (during birth) - omit code
Mole (pigmented) (*see also* Nevus)
  blood O02.0
  Breus' O02.0
  cancerous — *see* Melanoma
  carneous O02.0
  destructive D39.2
  fleshy O02.0
  hydatid, hydatidiform (benign) (complicating pregnancy) (delivered) (undelivered) O01.9
    classical O01.0
    complete O01.0
    incomplete O01.1
    invasive D39.2
    malignant D39.2
    partial O01.1
  intrauterine O02.0
  invasive (hydatidiform) D39.2
  malignant
    meaning
      malignant hydatidiform mole D39.2
      melanoma — *see* Melanoma
  nonhydatidiform O02.0
  nonpigmented — *see* Nevus
  pregnancy NEC O02.0
  skin — *see* Nevus
  tubal O00.10 ☑
    with intrauterine pregnancy O00.11 ☑
  vesicular — *see* Mole, hydatidiform
Molimen, molimina (menstrual) N94.3
Molluscum contagiosum (epitheliale) B08.1
Mönckeberg's arteriosclerosis, disease, or sclerosis — *see* Arteriosclerosis, extremities
Mondini's malformation (cochlea) Q16.5
Mondor's disease I80.8
Monge's disease T70.29 ☑
Monilethrix (congenital) Q84.1
Moniliasis (*see also* Candidiasis) B37.9
  neonatal P37.5
Monitoring (encounter for)
  therapeutic drug level Z51.81
Monkey malaria B53.1
Monkeypox B04
Monoarthritis M13.10
  ankle M13.17 ☑
  elbow M13.12 ☑
  foot joint M13.17 ☑
  hand joint M13.14 ☑
  hip M13.15 ☑
  knee M13.16 ☑
  shoulder M13.11 ☑
  wrist M13.13 ☑
Monoblastic — *see* condition
Monochromat (ism), monochromatopsia (acquired) (congenital) H53.51
Monocytic — *see* condition
Monocytopenia D72.818
Monocytosis (symptomatic) D72.821
Monomania — *see* Psychosis
Mononeuritis G58.9
  cranial nerve — *see* Disorder, nerve, cranial
  femoral nerve G57.2 ☑
  lateral
    cutaneous nerve of thigh G57.1 ☑
    popliteal nerve G57.3 ☑
  lower limb G57.9 ☑
    specified nerve NEC G57.8 ☑
  medial popliteal nerve G57.4 ☑
  median nerve G56.1 ☑
  multiplex G58.7
  plantar nerve G57.6 ☑
  posterior tibial nerve G57.5 ☑
  radial nerve G56.3 ☑
  sciatic nerve G57.0 ☑
  specified NEC G58.8
  tibial nerve G57.4 ☑
  ulnar nerve G56.2 ☑
  upper limb G56.9 ☑
    specified nerve NEC G56.8 ☑
  vestibular — *see* subcategory H93.3 ☑

Mononeuropathy G58.9
  carpal tunnel syndrome — *see* Syndrome, carpal tunnel
  diabetic NEC — *see* E08-E13 with .41
  femoral nerve — *see* Lesion, nerve, femoral
  ilioinguinal nerve G57.8 ☑
  in diseases classified elsewhere — *see* category G59
  intercostal G58.0
  lower limb G57.9 ☑
    causalgia — *see* Causalgia, lower limb
    femoral nerve — *see* Lesion, nerve, femoral
    meralgia paresthetica G57.1 ☑
    plantar nerve — *see* Lesion, nerve, plantar
    popliteal nerve — *see* Lesion, nerve, popliteal
    sciatic nerve — *see* Lesion, nerve, sciatic
    specified NEC G57.8 ☑
    tarsal tunnel syndrome — *see* Syndrome, tarsal tunnel
  median nerve — *see* Lesion, nerve, median
  multiplex G58.7
  obturator nerve G57.8 ☑
  popliteal nerve — *see* Lesion, nerve, popliteal
  radial nerve — *see* Lesion, nerve, radial
  saphenous nerve G57.8 ☑
  specified NEC G58.8
  tarsal tunnel syndrome — *see* Syndrome, tarsal tunnel
  tuberculous A17.83
  ulnar nerve — *see* Lesion, nerve, ulnar
  upper limb G56.9 ☑
    carpal tunnel syndrome — *see* Syndrome, carpal tunnel
    causalgia — *see* Causalgia
    median nerve — *see* Lesion, nerve, median
    radial nerve — *see* Lesion, nerve, radial
    specified site NEC G56.8 ☑
    ulnar nerve — *see* Lesion, nerve, ulnar
Mononucleosis, infectious B27.90
  with
    complication NEC B27.99
    meningitis B27.92
    polyneuropathy B27.91
  cytomegaloviral B27.10
    with
      complication NEC B27.19
      meningitis B27.12
      polyneuropathy B27.11
  Epstein-Barr (virus) B27.00
    with
      complication NEC B27.09
      meningitis B27.02
      polyneuropathy B27.01
  gammaherpesviral B27.00
    with
      complication NEC B27.09
      meningitis B27.02
      polyneuropathy B27.01
  specified NEC B27.80
    with
      complication NEC B27.89
      meningitis B27.82
      polyneuropathy B27.81
Monoplegia G83.3 ☑
  congenital (cerebral) G80.8
    spastic G80.1
  embolic (current episode) I63.4 ☑
  following
    cerebrovascular disease
      cerebral infarction
        lower limb I69.34 ☑
        upper limb I69.33 ☑
      intracerebral hemorrhage
        lower limb I69.14 ☑
        upper limb I69.13 ☑
      lower limb I69.94 ☑
      nontraumatic intracranial hemorrhage NEC
        lower limb I69.24 ☑
        upper limb I69.23 ☑
      specified disease NEC
        lower limb I69.84 ☑
        upper limb I69.83 ☑
      stroke NOS
        lower limb I69.34 ☑
        upper limb I69.33 ☑
      subarachnoid hemorrhage
        lower limb I69.04 ☑
        upper limb I69.03 ☑
      upper limb I69.93 ☑
  hysterical (transient) F44.4
  lower limb G83.1 ☑
  psychogenic (conversion reaction) F44.4
  thrombotic (current episode) I63.3 ☑

Monoplegia — *continued*
  transient R29.818
  upper limb G83.2 ☑
Monorchism, monorchidism Q55.0
Monosomy (*see also* Deletion, chromosome) Q93.9
  specified NEC Q93.89
  whole chromosome
    meiotic nondisjunction Q93.0
    mitotic nondisjunction Q93.1
    mosaicism Q93.1
  X Q96.9
Monster, monstrosity (single) Q89.7
  acephalic Q00.0
  twin Q89.4
Monteggia's fracture (-dislocation) S52.27 ☑
Mooren's ulcer (cornea) — *see* Ulcer, cornea, Mooren's
Moore's syndrome — *see* Epilepsy, specified NEC
Mooser-Neill reaction A75.2
Mooser's bodies A75.2
Morbidity not stated or unknown R69
Morbilli — *see* Measles
Morbus (*see also* Disease)
  angelicus, anglorum E55.0
  Beigel B36.2
  caducus — *see* Epilepsy
  celiacus K90.0
  comitialis — *see* Epilepsy
  cordis (*see also* Disease, heart) I51.9
    valvulorum — *see* Endocarditis
  coxae senilis M16.9
    tuberculous A18.02
  hemorrhagicus neonatorum P53
  maculosus neonatorum P54.5
Morel (-Stewart)(-Morgagni) syndrome M85.2
Morel-Kraepelin disease — *see* Schizophrenia
Morel-Moore syndrome M85.2
Morgagni's
  cyst, organ, hydatid, or appendage
    female Q50.5
    male (epididymal) Q55.4
      testicular Q55.29
  syndrome M85.2
Morgagni-Stokes-Adams syndrome I45.9
Morgagni-Stewart-Morel syndrome M85.2
Morgagni-Turner (-Albright) syndrome Q96.9
Moria F07.0
Moron (I.Q.50-69) F70
Morphea L94.0
Morphinism (without remission) F11.20
  with remission F11.21
Morphinomania (without remission) F11.20
  with remission F11.21
Morquio (-Ullrich)(-Brailsford) disease or syndrome — *see* Mucopolysaccharidosis
Mortification (dry) (moist) — *see* Gangrene
Morton's metatarsalgia (neuralgia)(neuroma) (syndrome) G57.6 ☑
Morvan's disease or syndrome G60.8
Mosaicism, mosaic (autosomal) (chromosomal)
  45,X/other cell lines NEC with abnormal sex chromosome Q96.4
  45,X/46,XX Q96.3
  sex chromosome
    female Q97.8
    lines with various numbers of X chromosomes Q97.2
    male Q98.7
  XY Q96.3
Moschowitz' disease M31.1
Mother yaw A66.0
Motion sickness (from travel, any vehicle) (from roundabouts or swings) T75.3 ☑
Mottled, mottling, teeth (enamel) (endemic) (nonendemic) K00.3
Mounier-Kuhn syndrome Q32.4
  with bronchiectasis J47.9
    exacerbation (acute) J47.1
    lower respiratory infection J47.0
  acquired J98.09
    with bronchiectasis J47.9
      with
        exacerbation (acute) J47.1
        lower respiratory infection J47.0
Mountain
  sickness T70.29 ☑
    with polycythemia , acquired (acute) D75.1
  tick fever A93.2
Mouse, joint — *see* Loose, body, joint
  knee M23.4 ☑
Mouth — *see* condition
Movable
  coccyx — *see* subcategory M53.2 ☑

Movable — *continued*
kidney N28.89
congenital Q63.8
spleen D73.89
Movements, dystonic R25.8
Moyamoya disease I67.5
MRSA (Methicillin resistant Staphylococcus aureus)
infection A49.02
as the cause of diseases classified elsewhere
B95.62
sepsis A41.02
MSD (multiple sulfatase deficiency) E75.26
MSSA (Methicillin susceptible Staphylococcus
aureus)
infection A49.01
as the cause of diseases classified elsewhere
B95.61
sepsis A41.01
Mucha-Habermann disease L41.0
Mucinosis (cutaneous) (focal) (papular) (reticular
erythematous) (skin) L98.5
oral K13.79
Mucocele
appendix K38.8
buccal cavity K13.79
gallbladder K82.1
lacrimal sac, chronic H04.43 ☑
nasal sinus J34.1
nose J34.1
salivary gland (any) K11.6
sinus (accessory) (nasal) J34.1
turbinate (bone) (middle) (nasal) J34.1
uterus N85.8
Mucolipidosis
I E77.1
II, III E77.0
IV E75.11
Mucopolysaccharidosis E76.3
beta-gluduronidase deficiency E76.29
cardiopathy E76.3 *[I52]*
Hunter's syndrome E76.1
Hurler's syndrome E76.01
Hurler-Scheie syndrome E76.02
Maroteaux-Lamy syndrome E76.29
Morquio syndrome E76.219
A E76.210
B E76.211
classic E76.210
Sanfilippo syndrome E76.22
Scheie's syndrome E76.03
specified NEC E76.29
type
I
Hurler's syndrome E76.01
Hurler-Scheie syndrome E76.02
Scheie's syndrome E76.03
II E76.1
III E76.22
IV E76.219
IVA E76.210
IVB E76.211
VI E76.29
VII E76.29
Mucormycosis B46.5
cutaneous B46.3
disseminated B46.4
gastrointestinal B46.2
generalized B46.4
pulmonary B46.0
rhinocerebral B46.1
skin B46.3
subcutaneous B46.3
Mucositis (ulcerative) K12.30
due to drugs NEC K12.32
gastrointestinal K92.81
mouth (oral) (oropharyngeal) K12.30
due to antineoplastic therapy K12.31
due to drugs NEC K12.32
due to radiation K12.33
specified NEC K12.39
viral K12.39
nasal J34.81
oral cavity — *see* Mucositis, mouth
oral soft tissues — *see* Mucositis, mouth
vagina and vulva N76.81
Mucositis necroticans agranulocytica — *see*
Agranulocytosis
Mucous (*see also* condition)
patches (syphilitic) A51.39
congenital A50.07
Mucoviscidosis E84.9
with meconium obstruction E84.11

Mucus
asphyxia or suffocation — *see* Asphyxia, mucus
in stool R19.5
plug — *see* Asphyxia, mucus
Muguet B37.0
Mulberry molars (congenital syphilis) A50.52
Müllerian mixed tumor
specified site — *see* Neoplasm, malignant, by site
unspecified site C54.9
Multicystic kidney (development) Q61.4
Multiparity (grand) Z64.1
affecting management of pregnancy, labor and
delivery (supervision only) O09.4 ☑
requiring contraceptive management — *see*
Contraception
Multipartita placenta O43.19 ☑
Multiple, multiplex (*see also* condition)
digits (congenital) Q69.9
endocrine neoplasia — *see* Neoplasia, endocrine,
multiple (MEN)
personality F44.81
Mumps B26.9
arthritis B26.85
complication NEC B26.89
encephalitis B26.2
hepatitis B26.81
meningitis (aseptic) B26.1
meningoencephalitis B26.2
myocarditis B26.82
oophoritis B26.89
orchitis B26.0
pancreatitis B26.3
polyneuropathy B26.84
Mumu (*see also* Infestation, filarial) B74.9 *[N51]*
Münchhausen's syndrome — *see* Disorder, factitious
Münchmeyer's syndrome — *see* Myositis, ossificans,
progressiva
Mural — *see* condition
Murmur (cardiac) (heart) (organic) R01.1
abdominal R19.15
aortic (valve) — *see* Endocarditis, aortic
benign R01.0
diastolic — *see* Endocarditis
Flint I35.1
functional R01.0
Graham Steell I37.1
innocent R01.0
mitral (valve) — *see* Insufficiency, mitral
nonorganic R01.0
presystolic, mitral — *see* Insufficiency, mitral
pulmonic (valve) I37.8
systolic R01.1
tricuspid (valve) I07.9
valvular — *see* Endocarditis
Murri's disease (intermittent hemoglobinuria) D59.6
Muscle, muscular (*see also* condition)
carnitine (palmityltransferase) deficiency E71.314
Musculoneuralgia — *see* Neuralgia
Mushroom-workers' (pickers') disease or lung J67.5
Mushrooming hip — *see* Derangement, joint, specified
NEC, hip
Mutation(s)
factor V Leiden D68.51
surfactant, of lung J84.83
prothrombin gene D68.52
Mutism (*see also* Aphasia)
deaf (acquired) (congenital) NEC H91.3
elective (adjustment reaction) (childhood) F94.0
hysterical F44.4
selective (childhood) F94.0
MVD (microvillus inclusion disease) Q43.8
MVID (microvillus inclusion disease) Q43.8
Myalgia M79.10
auxiliary muscles, head and neck M79.12
epidemic (cervical) B33.0
mastication muscle M79.11
site specified NEC M79.18
traumatic NEC T14.8 ☑
Myasthenia G70.9
congenital G70.2
cordis — *see* Failure, heart
developmental G70.2
gravis G70.00
with exacerbation (acute) G70.01
in crisis G70.01
neonatal, transient P94.0
pseudoparalytica G70.00
with exacerbation (acute) G70.01
in crisis G70.01
stomach, psychogenic F45.8
syndrome
in

Myasthenia — *continued*
syndrome — *continued*
diabetes mellitus — *see* E08-E13 with .44
neoplastic disease (*see also* Neoplasm)
D49.9 *[G73.3]*
pernicious anemia D51.0 *[G73.3]*
thyrotoxicosis E05.90 *[G73.3]*
with thyroid storm E05.91 *[G73.3]*
Myasthenic M62.81
Mycelium infection B49
Mycetismus — *see* Poisoning, food, noxious,
mushroom
Mycetoma B47.9
actinomycotic B47.1
bone (mycotic) B47.9 *[M90.80]*
eumycotic B47.0
foot B47.9
actinomycotic B47.1
mycotic B47.0
madurae NEC B47.9
mycotic B47.0
maduromycotic B47.0
mycotic B47.0
nocardial B47.1
Mycobacteriosis — *see* Mycobacterium
Mycobacterium, mycobacterial (infection) A31.9
anonymous A31.9
atypical A31.9
cutaneous A31.1
pulmonary A31.0
tuberculous — *see* Tuberculosis, pulmonary
specified site NEC A31.8
avium (intracellulare complex) A31.0
balnei A31.1
battey A31.0
chelonei A31.8
cutaneous A31.1
extrapulmonary systemic A31.8
fortuitum A31.8
intracellulare (Battey bacillus) A31.0
kansasii (yellow bacillus) A31.0
kakaferifu A31.8
kasongo A31.8
leprae (*see also* Leprosy) A30.9
luciflavum A31.1
marinum (M. balnei) A31.1
nonspecific — *see* Mycobacterium, atypical
pulmonary (atypical) A31.0
tuberculous — *see* Tuberculosis, pulmonary
scrofulaceum A31.8
simiae A31.8
systemic, extrapulmonary A31.8
szulgai A31.8
terrae A31.8
triviale A31.8
tuberculosis (human, bovine) — *see* Tuberculosis
ulcerans A31.1
xenopi A31.8
Mycoplasma (M.) pneumoniae, as cause of disease
classified elsewhere B96.0
Mycosis, mycotic B49
cutaneous NEC B36.9
ear B36.9
in
aspergillosis B44.89
candidiasis B37.84
moniliasis B37.84
fungoides (extranodal) (solid organ) C84.0 ☑
mouth B37.0
nails B35.1
opportunistic B48.8
skin NEC B36.9
specified NEC B48.8
stomatitis B37.0
vagina, vaginitis (candidal) B37.3
Mydriasis (pupil) H57.04
Myelatelia Q06.1
Myelinolysis, pontine, central G37.2
Myelitis (acute) (ascending) (childhood) (chronic)
(descending) (diffuse) (disseminated) (idiopathic)
(pressure) (progressive) (spinal cord) (subacute)
(*see also* Encephalitis) G04.91
herpes simplex B00.82
herpes zoster B02.24
in diseases classified elsewhere G05.4
necrotizing, subacute G37.4
optic neuritis in G36.0
postchickenpox B01.12
postherpetic B02.24
postimmunization G04.02
postinfectious NEC G04.89
postvaccinal G04.02

Myelitis - Myopathy

Myelitis — *continued*
    specified NEC G04.89
    syphilitic (transverse) A52.14
    toxic G92
    transverse (in demyelinating diseases of central
        nervous system) G37.3
    tuberculous A17.82
    varicella B01.12
Myeloblastic — *see* condition
Myeloblastoma
    granular cell (*see also* Neoplasm, connective tissue)
        malignant — *see* Neoplasm, connective tissue,
            malignant
        tongue D10.1
Myelocele — *see* Spina bifida
Myelocystocele — *see* Spina bifida
Myelocytic — *see* condition
Myelodysplasia D46.9
    specified NEC D46.Z
    spinal cord (congenital) Q06.1
Myelodysplastic syndrome D46.9
    with
        5q deletion D46.C
        isolated del (5q) chromosomal abnormality D46.C
    specified NEC D46.Z
Myeloencephalitis — *see* Encephalitis
Myelofibrosis D75.81
    with myeloid metaplasia D47.4
    acute C94.4 ☑
    idiopathic (chronic) D47.4
    primary D47.1
    secondary D75.81
        in myeloproliferative disease D47.4
Myelogenous — *see* condition
Myeloid — *see* condition
Myelokathexis D70.9
Myeloleukodystrophy E75.29
Myelolipoma — *see* Lipoma
Myeloma (multiple) C90.0 ☑
    monostotic C90.3 ☑
        plasma cell C90.0 ☑
    plasma cell C90.0 ☑
    solitary (*see also* Plasmacytoma, solitary) C90.3 ☑
Myelomalacia G95.89
Myelomatosis C90.0 ☑
Myelomeningitis — *see* Meningoencephalitis
Myelomeningocele (spinal cord) — *see* Spina bifida
Myelo-osteo-musculodysplasia hereditaria Q79.8
Myelopathic
    anemia D64.89
    muscle atrophy — *see* Atrophy, muscle, spinal
    pain syndrome G89.0
Myelopathy (spinal cord) G95.9
    drug-induced G95.89
    in (due to)
        degeneration or displacement, intervertebral disc
            NEC — *see* Disorder, disc, with, myelopathy
        infection — *see* Encephalitis
        intervertebral disc disorder (*see also* Disorder,
            disc, with, myelopathy)
        mercury — *see* subcategory T56.1 ☑
        neoplastic disease (*see also* Neoplasm) D49.9
            [G99.2]
        pernicious anemia D51.0 *[G99.2]*
        spondylosis — *see* Spondylosis, with myelopathy
            NEC
    necrotic (subacute) (vascular) G95.19
    radiation-induced G95.89
    spondylogenic NEC — *see* Spondylosis, with
        myelopathy NEC
    toxic G95.89
    transverse, acute G37.3
    vascular G95.19
    vitamin B12 E53.8 *[G32.0]*
Myelophthisis D61.82
Myeloradiculitis G04.91
Myeloradiculodysplasia (spinal) Q06.1
Myelosarcoma C92.3 ☑
Myelosclerosis D75.89
    with myeloid metaplasia D47.4
    disseminated, of nervous system G35
    megakaryocytic D47.4
        with myeloid metaplasia D47.4
Myelosis
    acute C92.0 ☑
    aleukemic C92.9 ☑
    chronic D47.1
    erythremic (acute) C94.0 ☑
    megakaryocytic C94.2 ☑
    nonleukemic D72.828
    subacute C92.9 ☑
Myiasis (cavernous) B87.9

Myiasis — *continued*
    aural B87.4
    creeping B87.0
    cutaneous B87.0
    dermal B87.0
    ear (external) (middle) B87.4
    eye B87.2
    genitourinary B87.81
    intestinal B87.82
    laryngeal B87.3
    nasopharyngeal B87.3
    ocular B87.2
    orbit B87.2
    skin B87.0
    specified site NEC B87.89
    traumatic B87.1
    wound B87.1
Myoadenoma, prostate — *see* Hyperplasia, prostate
Myoblastoma
    granular cell (*see also* Neoplasm, connective tissue,
        benign)
        malignant — *see* Neoplasm, connective tissue,
            malignant
    tongue D10.1
Myocardial — *see* condition
Myocardiopathy (congestive) (constrictive) (familial)
    (hypertrophic nonobstructive) (idiopathic)
    (infiltrative) (obstructive) (primary) (restrictive)
    (sporadic) (*see also* Cardiomyopathy) I42.9
    alcoholic I42.6
    cobalt-beer I42.6
    glycogen storage E74.02 *[I43]*
    hypertrophic obstructive I42.1
    in (due to)
        beriberi E51.12
        cardiac glycogenosis E74.02 *[I43]*
        Friedreich's ataxia G11.1 *[I43]*
        myotonia atrophica G71.11 *[I43]*
        progressive muscular dystrophy G71.09 *[I43]*
    obscure (African) I42.8
    secondary I42.9
    thyrotoxic E05.90 *[I43]*
        with storm E05.91 *[I43]*
    toxic NEC I42.7
Myocarditis (with arteriosclerosis)(chronic)(fibroid)
    (interstitial) (old) (progressive) (senile) I51.4
    with
        rheumatic fever (conditions in I00) I09.0
            active — *see* Myocarditis, acute, rheumatic
            inactive or quiescent (with chorea) I09.0
    active I40.9
        rheumatic I01.2
            with chorea (acute) (rheumatic) (Sydenham's)
                I02.0
    acute or subacute (interstitial) I40.9
        due to
            streptococcus (beta-hemolytic) I01.2
        idiopathic I40.1
        rheumatic I01.2
            with chorea (acute) (rheumatic) (Sydenham's)
                I02.0
        specified NEC I40.8
    aseptic of newborn B33.22
    bacterial (acute) I40.0
    Coxsackie (virus) B33.22
    diphtheritic A36.81
    eosinophilic I40.1
    epidemic of newborn (Coxsackie) B33.22
    Fiedler's (acute) (isolated) I40.1
    giant cell (acute) (subacute) I40.1
    gonococcal A54.83
    granulomatous (idiopathic) (isolated) (nonspecific)
        I40.1
    hypertensive — *see* Hypertension, heart
    idiopathic (granulomatous) I40.1
    in (due to)
        diphtheria A36.81
        epidemic louse-borne typhus A75.0 *[I41]*
        Lyme disease A69.29
        sarcoidosis D86.85
        scarlet fever A38.1
        toxoplasmosis (acquired) B58.81
        typhoid A01.02
        typhus NEC A75.9 *[I41]*
    infective I40.0
    influenzal — *see* Influenza, with, myocarditis
    isolated (acute) I40.1
    meningococcal A39.52
    mumps B26.82
    nonrheumatic, active I40.9
    parenchymatous I40.9
    pneumococcal I40.0

Myocarditis — *continued*
    rheumatic (chronic) (inactive) (with chorea) I09.0
        active or acute I01.2
            with chorea (acute) (rheumatic) (Sydenham's)
                I02.0
    rheumatoid — *see* Rheumatoid, carditis
    septic I40.0
    staphylococcal I40.0
    suppurative I40.0
    syphilitic (chronic) A52.06
    toxic I40.8
        rheumatic — *see* Myocarditis, acute, rheumatic
    tuberculous A18.84
    typhoid A01.02
    valvular — *see* Endocarditis
    virus, viral I40.0
        of newborn (Coxsackie) B33.22
Myocardium, myocardial — *see* condition
Myocardosis — *see* Cardiomyopathy
Myoclonus, myoclonic, myoclonia (familial) (essential)
    (multifocal) (simplex) G25.3
    drug-induced G25.3
    epilepsy (*see also* Epilepsy, generalized, specified
        NEC) G40.4 ☑
        familial (progressive) G25.3
    epileptica G40.409
        with status epilepticus G40.401
    facial G51.3 ☑
    familial progressive G25.3
    Friedreich's G25.3
    jerks G25.3
    massive G25.3
    palatal G25.3
    pharyngeal G25.3
Myocytolysis I51.5
Myodiastasis — *see* Diastasis, muscle
Myoendocarditis — *see* Endocarditis
Myoepithelioma — *see* Neoplasm, benign, by site
Myofasciitis (acute) — *see* Myositis
Myofibroma (*see also* Neoplasm, connective tissue,
    benign)
    uterus (cervix) (corpus) — *see* Leiomyoma
Myofibromatosis D48.1
    infantile Q89.8
Myofibrosis M62.89
    heart — *see* Myocarditis
    scapulohumeral — *see* Lesion, shoulder, specified
        NEC
Myofibrositis M79.7
    scapulohumeral — *see* Lesion, shoulder, specified
        NEC
Myoglobulinuria, myoglobinuria (primary) R82.1
Myokymia, facial G51.4
Myolipoma — *see* Lipoma
Myoma (*see also* Neoplasm, connective tissue, benign)
    malignant — *see* Neoplasm, connective tissue,
        malignant
    prostate D29.1
    uterus (cervix) (corpus) — *see* Leiomyoma
Myomalacia M62.89
Myometritis — *see* Endometritis
Myometrium — *see* condition
Myonecrosis, clostridial A48.0
Myopathy G72.9
    acute
        necrotizing G72.81
        quadriplegic G72.81
    alcoholic G72.1
    benign congenital G71.2
    central core G71.2
    centronuclear G71.2
    congenital (benign) G71.2
    critical illness G72.81
    distal G71.09
    drug-induced G72.0
    endocrine NEC E34.9 *[G73.7]*
    extraocular muscles H05.82 ☑
    facioscapulohumeral G71.02
    hereditary G71.9
        specified NEC G71.8
    immune NEC G72.49
    in (due to)
        Addison's disease E27.1 *[G73.7]*
        alcohol G72.1
        amyloidosis E85.9 *[G73.7]*
        cretinism E00.9 *[G73.7]*
        Cushing's syndrome E24.9 *[G73.7]*
        drugs G72.0
        endocrine disease NEC E34.9 *[G73.7]*
        giant cell arteritis M31.6 *[G73.7]*
        glycogen storage disease E74.00 *[G73.7]*
        hyperadrenocorticism E24.9 *[G73.7]*

☑ **Additional character required**

Myopathy — *continued*
in — *continued*
hyperparathyroidism NEC E21.3 *[G73.7]*
hypoparathyroidism E20.9 *[G73.7]*
hypopituitarism E23.0 *[G73.7]*
hypothyroidism E03.9 *[G73.7]*
infectious disease NEC B99 ☑ *[G73.7]*
lipid storage disease E75.6 *[G73.7]*
metabolic disease NEC E88.9 *[G73.7]*
myxedema E03.9 *[G73.7]*
parasitic disease NEC B89 *[G73.7]*
polyarteritis nodosa M30.0 *[G73.7]*
rheumatoid arthritis — *see* Rheumatoid, myopathy
sarcoidosis D86.87
scleroderma M34.82
sicca syndrome M35.03
Sjögren's syndrome M35.03
systemic lupus erythematosus M32.19
thyrotoxicosis (hyperthyroidism) E05.90 *[G73.7]*
with thyroid storm E05.91 *[G73.7]*
toxic agent NEC G72.2
inflammatory NEC G72.49
intensive care (ICU) G72.81
limb-girdle G71.09
mitochondrial NEC G71.3
mytonic, proximal (PROMM) G71.11
myotubular G71.2
nemaline G71.2
ocular G71.09
oculopharyngeal G71.09
of critical illness G72.81
primary G71.9
specified NEC G71.8
progressive NEC G72.89
proximal myotonic (PROMM) G71.11
rod G71.2
scapulohumeral G71.02
specified NEC G72.89
toxic G72.2
Myopericarditis (*see also* Pericarditis)
chronic rheumatic I09.2
Myopia (axial) (congenital) H52.1 ☑
degenerative (malignant) H44.20
with
choroidal neovascularization H44.2A ☑
foveoschisis H44.2D ☑
macular hole H44.2B ☑
retinal detachment H44.2C ☑
specified maculopathy NEC H44.2E ☑
bilateral H44.23
left eye H44.22
right eye H44.21
malignant (*see also* Myopia, degenerative) H44.2 ☑
pernicious (*see also* Myopia, degenerative) H44.2 ☑
progressive high (degenerative) (*see also* Myopia, degenerative) H44.2 ☑
Myosarcoma — *see* Neoplasm, connective tissue, malignant
Myosis (pupil) H57.03
stromal (endolymphatic) D39.0
Myositis M60.9
clostridial A48.0
due to posture — *see* Myositis, specified type NEC
epidemic B33.0
fibrosa or fibrous (chronic), Volkmann's T79.6 ☑
foreign body granuloma — *see* Granuloma, foreign body
in (due to)
bilharziasis B65.9 *[M63.8 ☑]*
cysticercosis B69.81
leprosy A30.9 *[M63.8 ☑]*
mycosis B49 *[M63.8 ☑]*
sarcoidosis D86.87
schistosomiasis B65.9 *[M63.8 ☑]*
syphilis
late A52.78
secondary A51.49
toxoplasmosis (acquired) B58.82
trichinellosis B75 *[M63.8 ☑]*
tuberculosis A18.09
inclusion body [IBM] G72.41
infective M60.009
arm M60.002
left M60.001
right M60.000
leg M60.005
left M60.004
right M60.003
lower limb M60.005
ankle M60.07 ☑
foot M60.07 ☑

Myositis — *continued*
infective — *continued*
lower leg M60.06 ☑
thigh M60.05 ☑
toe M60.07 ☑
multiple sites M60.09
specified site NEC M60.08
upper limb M60.002
finger M60.04 ☑
forearm M60.03 ☑
hand M60.04 ☑
shoulder region M60.01 ☑
upper arm M60.02 ☑
interstitial M60.10
ankle M60.17 ☑
foot M60.17 ☑
forearm M60.13 ☑
hand M60.14 ☑
lower leg M60.16 ☑
multiple sites M60.19
shoulder region M60.11 ☑
specified site NEC M60.18
thigh M60.15 ☑
upper arm M60.12 ☑
mycotic B49 *[M63.8 ☑]*
orbital, chronic H05.12 ☑
ossificans or ossifying (circumscripta) (*see also* Ossification, muscle, specified NEC)
in (due to)
burns M61.30
ankle M61.37 ☑
foot M61.37 ☑
forearm M61.33 ☑
hand M61.34 ☑
lower leg M61.36 ☑
multiple sites M61.39
pelvic region M61.35 ☑
shoulder region M61.31 ☑
specified site NEC M61.38
thigh M61.35 ☑
upper arm M61.32 ☑
quadriplegia or paraplegia M61.20
ankle M61.27 ☑
foot M61.27 ☑
forearm M61.23 ☑
hand M61.24 ☑
lower leg M61.26 ☑
multiple sites M61.29
pelvic region M61.25 ☑
shoulder region M61.21 ☑
specified site NEC M61.28
thigh M61.25 ☑
upper arm M61.22 ☑
progressiva M61.10
ankle M61.17 ☑
finger M61.14 ☑
foot M61.17 ☑
forearm M61.13 ☑
hand M61.14 ☑
lower leg M61.16 ☑
multiple sites M61.19
pelvic region M61.15 ☑
shoulder region M61.11 ☑
specified site NEC M61.18
thigh M61.15 ☑
toe M61.17 ☑
upper arm M61.12 ☑
traumatica M61.00
ankle M61.07 ☑
foot M61.07 ☑
forearm M61.03 ☑
hand M61.04 ☑
lower leg M61.06 ☑
multiple sites M61.09
pelvic region M61.05 ☑
shoulder region M61.01 ☑
specified site NEC M61.08
thigh M61.05 ☑
upper arm M61.02 ☑
purulent — *see* Myositis, infective
specified type NEC M60.80
ankle M60.87 ☑
foot M60.87 ☑
forearm M60.83 ☑
hand M60.84 ☑
lower leg M60.86 ☑
multiple sites M60.89
pelvic region M60.85 ☑
shoulder region M60.81 ☑
specified site NEC M60.88
thigh M60.85 ☑
upper arm M60.82 ☑

Myositis — *continued*
suppurative — *see* Myositis, infective
traumatic (old) — *see* Myositis, specified type NEC
Myospasia impulsiva F95.2
Myotonia (acquisita) (intermittens) M62.89
atrophica G71.11
chondrodystrophic G71.13
congenita (acetazolamide responsive) (dominant) (recessive) G71.12
drug-induced G71.14
dystrophica G71.11
fluctuans G71.19
levior G71.12
permanens G71.19
symptomatic G71.19
Myotonic pupil — *see* Anomaly, pupil, function, tonic pupil
Myriapodiasis B88.2
Myringitis H73.2 ☑
with otitis media — *see* Otitis, media
acute H73.00 ☑
bullous H73.01 ☑
specified NEC H73.09 ☑
bullous — *see* Myringitis, acute, bullous
chronic H73.1 ☑
Mysophobia F40.228
Mytilotoxism — *see* Poisoning, fish
Myxadenitis labialis K13.0
Myxedema (adult) (idiocy) (infantile) (*see also* Hypothyroidism) E03.9
circumscribed E05.90
with storm E05.91
coma E03.5
congenital E00.1
cutis L98.5
localized (pretibial) E05.90
with storm E05.91
papular L98.5
Myxochondrosarcoma — *see* Neoplasm, cartilage, malignant
Myxofibroma — *see* Neoplasm, connective tissue, benign
odontogenic — *see* Cyst, calcifying odontogenic
Myxofibrosarcoma — *see* Neoplasm, connective tissue, malignant
Myxolipoma D17.9
Myxoliposarcoma — *see* Neoplasm, connective tissue, malignant
Myxoma (*see also* Neoplasm, connective tissue, benign)
nerve sheath — *see* Neoplasm, nerve, benign
odontogenic — *see* Cyst, calcifying odontogenic
Myxosarcoma — *see* Neoplasm, connective tissue, malignant

N

Naegeli's
disease Q82.8
leukemia, monocytic C93.1 ☑
Naegleriasis (with meningoencephalitis) B60.2
Naffziger's syndrome G54.0
Naga sore — *see* Ulcer, skin
Nägele's pelvis M95.5
with disproportion (fetopelvic) O33.0
causing obstructed labor O65.0
Nail (*see also* condition)
biting F98.8
patella syndrome Q87.2
Nanism, nanosomia — *see* Dwarfism
Nanophyetiasis B66.8
Nanukayami A27.89
Napkin rash L22
Narcolepsy G47.419
with cataplexy G47.411
in conditions classified elsewhere G47.429
with cataplexy G47.421
Narcosis R06.89
Narcotism — *see* Dependence
NARP (Neuropathy, Ataxia and Retinitis pigmentosa) syndrome E88.49
Narrow
anterior chamber angle H40.03 ☑
gingival width (of periodontal soft tissue) K05.5
pelvis — *see* Contraction, pelvis
Narrowing (*see also* Stenosis)
artery I77.1
auditory, internal I65.8
basilar — *see* Occlusion, artery, basilar
carotid — *see* Occlusion, artery, carotid

Narrowing — *continued*
  artery — *continued*
    cerebellar — *see* Occlusion, artery, cerebellar
    cerebral — *see* Occlusion artery, cerebral
    choroidal — *see* Occlusion, artery, precerebral,
      specified NEC
    communicating posterior — *see* Occlusion, artery,
      precerebral, specified NEC
    coronary (*see also* Disease, heart, ischemic,
      atherosclerotic)
      congenital Q24.5
        syphilitic A50.54 *[I52]*
      due to syphilis NEC A52.06
    hypophyseal — *see* Occlusion, artery, precerebral,
      specified NEC
    pontine — *see* Occlusion, artery, precerebral,
      specified NEC
    precerebral — *see* Occlusion, artery, precerebral
    vertebral — *see* Occlusion, artery, vertebral
  auditory canal (external) — *see* Stenosis, external
    ear canal
  eustachian tube — *see* Obstruction, eustachian
    tube
  eyelid — *see* Disorder, eyelid function
  larynx J38.6
  mesenteric artery (*see also* Ischemia, intestine,
    acute) K55.059
  palate M26.89
  palpebral fissure — *see* Disorder, eyelid function
  ureter N13.5
    with infection N13.6
  urethra — *see* Stricture, urethra
Narrowness, abnormal, eyelid Q10.3
Nasal — *see* condition
Nasolachrymal, nasolacrimal — *see* condition
Nasopharyngeal (*see also* condition)
  pituitary gland Q89.2
  torticollis M43.6
Nasopharyngitis (acute) (infective) (streptococcal)
  (subacute) J00
  chronic (suppurative) (ulcerative) J31.1
Nasopharynx, nasopharyngeal — *see* condition
Natal tooth, teeth K00.6
Nausea (without vomiting) R11.0
  with vomiting R11.2
  gravidarum — *see* Hyperemesis, gravidarum
  marina T75.3 ☑
  navalis T75.3 ☑
Navel — *see* condition
Neapolitan fever — *see* Brucellosis
Near drowning T75.1 ☑
Nearsightedness — *see* Myopia
Near-syncope R55
Nebula, cornea — *see* Opacity, cornea
Necator americanus infestation B76.1
Necatoriasis B76.1
Neck — *see* condition
Necrobiosis R68.89
  lipoidica NEC L92.1
    with diabetes — *see* E08-E13 with .620
Necrolysis, toxic epidermal L51.2
  due to drug
    correct substance properly administered — *see*
      Table of Drugs and Chemicals, by drug,
      adverse effect
    overdose or wrong substance given or taken —
      see Table of Drugs and Chemicals, by drug,
      poisoning
Necrophilia F65.89
Necrosis, necrotic (ischemic) (*see also* Gangrene)
  adrenal (capsule) (gland) E27.49
  amputation stump (surgical) (late) T87.50
    arm T87.5 ☑
    leg T87.5 ☑
  antrum J32.0
  aorta (hyaline) (*see also* Aneurysm, aorta)
    cystic medial — *see* Dissection, aorta
  artery I77.5
  bladder (aseptic) (sphincter) N32.89
  bone (*see also* Osteonecrosis) M87.9
    aseptic or avascular — *see* Osteonecrosis
      idiopathic M87.00
    ethmoid J32.2
    jaw M27.2
    tuberculous — *see* Tuberculosis, bone
  brain I67.89
  breast (aseptic) (fat) (segmental) N64.1
  bronchus J98.09
  central nervous system NEC I67.89
  cerebellar I67.89
  cerebral I67.89
  colon (*see also* Infarct, intestine) K55.049

Necrosis — *continued*
  cornea H18.89 ☑
  cortical (acute) (renal) N17.1
  cystic medial (aorta) — *see* Dissection, aorta
  dental pulp K04.1
  esophagus K22.8
  ethmoid (bone) J32.2
  eyelid — *see* Disorder, eyelid, degenerative
  fat, fatty (generalized) (*see also* Disorder, soft tissue,
    specified type NEC)
    abdominal wall K65.4
    breast (aseptic) (segmental) N64.1
    localized — *see* Degeneration, by site, fatty
    mesentery K65.4
    omentum K65.4
    pancreas K86.89
    peritoneum K65.4
    skin (subcutaneous), newborn P83.0
    subcutaneous, due to birth injury P15.6
  gallbladder — *see* Cholecystitis, acute
  heart — *see* Infarct, myocardium
  hip, aseptic or avascular — *see* Osteonecrosis, by
    type, femur
  intestine (acute) (hemorrhagic) (massive) (*see also*
    Infarct, intestine) K55.069
  jaw M27.2
  kidney (bilateral) N28.0
    acute N17.9
    cortical (acute) (bilateral) N17.1
      with ectopic or molar pregnancy O08.4
    medullary (bilateral) (in acute renal failure)
      (papillary) N17.2
    papillary (bilateral) (in acute renal failure) N17.2
    tubular N17.0
      with ectopic or molar pregnancy O08.4
      complicating
        abortion — *see* Abortion, by type,
          complicated by, tubular necrosis
        ectopic or molar pregnancy O08.4
        pregnancy — *see* Pregnancy, complicated by,
          diseases of, specified type or system NEC
      following ectopic or molar pregnancy O08.4
      traumatic T79.5 ☑
  larynx J38.7
  liver (with hepatic failure) (cell) — *see* Failure,
    hepatic
    hemorrhagic, central K76.2
  lung J85.0
  lymphatic gland — *see* Lymphadenitis, acute
  mammary gland (fat) (segmental) N64.1
  mastoid (chronic) — *see* Mastoiditis, chronic
  medullary (acute) (renal) N17.2
  mesentery (*see also* Infarct, intestine) K55.069
    fat K65.4
  mitral valve — *see* Insufficiency, mitral
  myocardium, myocardial — *see* Infarct, myocardium
  nose J34.0
  omentum (with mesenteric infarction) (*see also*
    Infarct, intestine) K55.069
    fat K65.4
  orbit, orbital — *see* Osteomyelitis, orbit
  ossicles, ear — *see* Abnormal, ear ossicles
  ovary N70.92
  pancreas (aseptic) (duct) (fat) K86.89
    acute (infective) — *see* Pancreatitis, acute
    infective — *see* Pancreatitis, acute
  papillary (acute) (renal) N17.2
  perineum N90.89
  peritoneum (with mesenteric infarction) (*see also*
    Infarct, intestine) K55.069
    fat K65.4
  pharynx J02.9
    in granulocytopenia — *see* Neutropenia
    Vincent's A69.1
  phosphorus — *see* subcategory T54.2 ☑
  pituitary (gland) E23.0
    postpartum O99.285
    Sheehan O99.285
  pressure — *see* Ulcer, pressure, by site
  pulmonary J85.0
  pulp (dental) K04.1
  radiation — *see* Necrosis, by site
  radium — *see* Necrosis, by site
  renal — *see* Necrosis, kidney
  sclera H15.89
  scrotum N50.89
  skin or subcutaneous tissue NEC I96
  spine, spinal (column) (*see also* Osteonecrosis, by
    type, vertebra)
    cord G95.19
  spleen D73.5
  stomach K31.89

Necrosis — *continued*
  stomatitis (ulcerative) A69.0
  subcutaneous fat, newborn P83.88
  subendocardial (acute) I21.4
    chronic I25.89
  suprarenal (capsule) (gland) E27.49
  testis N50.89
  thymus (gland) E32.8
  tonsil J35.8
  trachea J39.8
  tuberculous NEC — *see* Tuberculosis
  tubular (acute) (anoxic) (renal) (toxic) N17.0
    postprocedural N99.0
  vagina N89.8
  vertebra (*see also* Osteonecrosis, by type, vertebra)
    tuberculous A18.01
  vulva N90.89
  X-ray — *see* Necrosis, by site
Necrospermia — *see* Infertility, male
Need (for)
  care provider because (of)
    assistance with personal care Z74.1
    continuous supervision required Z74.3
    impaired mobility Z74.09
    no other household member able to render care
      Z74.2
    specified reason NEC Z74.8
  immunization — *see* Vaccination
  vaccination — *see* Vaccination
Neglect
  adult
    confirmed T74.01 ☑
    history of Z91.412
    suspected T76.01 ☑
  child (childhood)
    confirmed T74.02 ☑
    history of Z62.812
    suspected T76.02 ☑
  emotional, in childhood Z62.898
  hemispatial R41.4
  left-sided R41.4
  sensory R41.4
  visuospatial R41.4
Neisserian infection NEC — *see* Gonococcus
Nelaton's syndrome G60.8
Nelson's syndrome E24.1
Nematodiasis (intestinal) B82.0
  Ancylostoma B76.0
Neonatal (*see also* Newborn)
  acne L70.4
  bradycardia P29.12
  tachycardia P29.11
  screening, abnormal findings on P09
  tooth, teeth K00.6
Neonatorum — *see* condition
Neoplasia
  endocrine, multiple (MEN) E31.20
    type I E31.21
    type IIA E31.22
    type IIB E31.23
  intraepithelial (histologically confirmed)
    anal (AIN) (histologically confirmed) K62.82
      grade I K62.82
      grade II K62.82
      severe D01.3
    cervical glandular (histologically confirmed)
      D06.9
    cervix (uteri) (CIN) (histologically confirmed)
      N87.9
      glandular D06.9
      grade I N87.0
      grade II N87.1
      grade III (severe dysplasia) (*see also* Carcinoma,
        cervix uteri, in situ) D06.9
    prostate (histologically confirmed) (PIN)
      N42.31
      grade I N42.31
      grade II N42.31
      grade III (severe dysplasia) D07.5
    vagina (histologically confirmed) (VAIN) N89.3
      grade I N89.0
      grade II N89.1
      grade III (severe dysplasia) D07.2
    vulva (histologically confirmed) (VIN) N90.3
      grade I N90.0
      grade II N90.1
      grade III (severe dysplasia) D07.1
Neoplasm, neoplastic (*see also* Table of Neoplasms)
  lipomatous, benign — *see* Lipoma
  malignant mast cell C96.20
    specified type NEC C96.29
  mast cell, of uncertain behavior NEC D47.09

☑ **Additional character required**

Neovascularization
  ciliary body — *see* Disorder, iris, vascular
  cornea H16.40 ☑
    deep H16.44 ☑
    ghost vessels — *see* Ghost, vessels
    localized H16.43 ☑
    pannus — *see* Pannus
  iris — *see* Disorder, iris, vascular
  retina H35.05 ☑
Nephralgia N23
Nephritis, nephritic (albuminuric) (azotemic)
  (congenital) (disseminated) (epithelial) (familial)
  (focal) (granulomatous) (hemorrhagic) (infantile)
  (nonsuppurative, excretory) (uremic) N05.9
  with
    dense deposit disease N05.6
    diffuse
      crescentic glomerulonephritis N05.7
      endocapillary proliferative glomerulonephritis
        N05.4
      membranous glomerulonephritis N05.2
      mesangial proliferative glomerulonephritis N05.3
      mesangiocapillary glomerulonephritis N05.5
    edema — *see* Nephrosis
    focal and segmental glomerular lesions N05.1
    foot process disease N04.9
    glomerular lesion
      diffuse sclerosing N05.8
      hypocomplementemic — *see* Nephritis,
        membranoproliferative
      IgA — *see* Nephropathy, IgA
      lobular, lobulonodular — *see* Nephritis,
        membranoproliferative
      nodular — *see* Nephritis,
        membranoproliferative
    lesion of
      glomerulonephritis, proliferative N05.8
      renal necrosis N05.9
    minor glomerular abnormality N05.0
    specified morphological changes NEC N05.8
  acute N00.9
    with
      dense deposit disease N00.6
      diffuse
        crescentic glomerulonephritis N00.7
        endocapillary proliferative
          glomerulonephritis N00.4
        membranous glomerulonephritis N00.2
        mesangial proliferative glomerulonephritis
          N00.3
        mesangiocapillary glomerulonephritis N00.5
      focal and segmental glomerular lesions N00.1
      minor glomerular abnormality N00.0
      specified morphological changes NEC N00.8
  amyloid E85.4 *[N08]*
  antiglomerular basement membrane (anti-GBM)
    antibody NEC
    in Goodpasture's syndrome M31.0
  antitubular basement membrane (tubulo-
    interstitial) NEC N12
  toxic — *see* Nephropathy, toxic
  arteriolar — *see* Hypertension, kidney
  arteriosclerotic — *see* Hypertension, kidney
  ascending — *see* Nephritis, tubulo-interstitial
  atrophic N03.9
  Balkan (endemic) N15.0
  calculous, calculus — *see* Calculus, kidney
  cardiac — *see* Hypertension, kidney
  cardiovascular — *see* Hypertension, kidney
  chronic N03.9
    with
      dense deposit disease N03.6
      diffuse
        crescentic glomerulonephritis N03.7
        endocapillary proliferative
          glomerulonephritis N03.4
        membranous glomerulonephritis N03.2
        mesangial proliferative glomerulonephritis
          N03.3
        mesangiocapillary glomerulonephritis N03.5
      focal and segmental glomerular lesions N03.1
      minor glomerular abnormality N03.0
      specified morphological changes NEC N03.8
    arteriosclerotic — *see* Hypertension, kidney
  cirrhotic N26.9
  complicating pregnancy O26.83 ☑
  croupous N00.9
  degenerative — *see* Nephrosis
  diffuse sclerosing N05.8
  due to
    diabetes mellitus — *see* E08-E13 with .21
    subacute bacterial endocarditis I33.0

Nephritis — *continued*
  due to — *continued*
    systemic lupus erythematosus (chronic) M32.14
    typhoid fever A01.09
  gonococcal (acute) (chronic) A54.21
  hypocomplementemic — *see* Nephritis,
    membranoproliferative
  IgA — *see* Nephropathy, IgA
  immune complex (circulating) NEC N05.8
  infective — *see* Nephritis, tubulo-interstitial
  interstitial — *see* Nephritis, tubulo-interstitial
  lead N14.3
  membranoproliferative (diffuse) (type 1 or 3) (*see also*
    N00-N07 with fourth character .5) N05.5
    type 2 (*see also* N00-N07 with fourth character .6)
      N05.6
  minimal change N05.0
  necrotic, necrotizing NEC (*see also* N00-N07 with
    fourth character .8) N05.8
  nephrotic — *see* Nephrosis
  nodular — *see* Nephritis, membranoproliferative
  polycystic Q61.3
    adult type Q61.2
    autosomal
      dominant Q61.2
      recessive NEC Q61.19
    childhood type NEC Q61.19
    infantile type NEC Q61.19
  poststreptococcal N05.9
    acute N00.9
    chronic N03.9
    rapidly progressive N01.9
  proliferative NEC (*see also* N00-N07 with fourth
    character .8) N05.8
  purulent — *see* Nephritis, tubulo-interstitial
  rapidly progressive N01.9
    with
      dense deposit disease N01.6
      diffuse
        crescentic glomerulonephritis N01.7
        endocapillary proliferative
          glomerulonephritis N01.4
        membranous glomerulonephritis N01.2
        mesangial proliferative glomerulonephritis
          N01.3
        mesangiocapillary glomerulonephritis N01.5
      focal and segmental glomerular lesions N01.1
      minor glomerular abnormality N01.0
      specified morphological changes NEC N01.8
  salt losing or wasting NEC N28.89
  saturnine N14.3
  sclerosing, diffuse N05.8
  septic — *see* Nephritis, tubulo-interstitial
  specified pathology NEC (*see also* N00-N07 with
    fourth character .8) N05.8
  subacute N01.9
  suppurative — *see* Nephritis, tubulo-interstitial
  syphilitic (late) A52.75
    congenital A50.59 *[N08]*
    early (secondary) A51.44
  toxic — *see* Nephropathy, toxic
  tubal, tubular — *see* Nephritis, tubulo-interstitial
  tuberculous A18.11
  tubulo-interstitial (in) N12
    acute (infectious) N10
    chronic (infectious) N11.9
      nonobstructive N11.8
        reflux-associated N11.0
      obstructive N11.1
      specified NEC N11.8
    due to
      brucellosis A23.9 *[N16]*
      cryoglobulinemia D89.1 *[N16]*
      glycogen storage disease E74.00 *[N16]*
    Sjögren's syndrome M35.04
  vascular — *see* Hypertension, kidney
  war N00.9
Nephroblastoma (epithelial) (mesenchymal) C64 ☑
Nephrocalcinosis E83.59 *[N29]*
Nephrocystitis, pustular — *see* Nephritis, tubulo-
  interstitial
Nephrolithiasis (congenital) (pelvis) (recurrent)
  (*see also* Calculus, kidney)
Nephroma C64 ☑
  mesoblastic D41.0 ☑
Nephronephritis — *see* Nephrosis
Nephronophthisis Q61.5
Nephropathia epidemica A98.5
Nephropathy (*see also* Nephritis) N28.9
  with
    edema — *see* Nephrosis
    glomerular lesion — *see* Glomerulonephritis

Nephropathy — *continued*
  amyloid, hereditary E85.0
  analgesic N14.0
    with medullary necrosis, acute N17.2
  Balkan (endemic) N15.0
  chemical — *see* Nephropathy, toxic
  diabetic — *see* E08-E13 with .21
  drug-induced N14.2
    specified NEC N14.1
  focal and segmental hyalinosis or sclerosis N02.1
  heavy metal-induced N14.3
  hereditary NEC N07.9
    with
      dense deposit disease N07.6
      diffuse
        crescentic glomerulonephritis N07.7
        endocapillary proliferative
          glomerulonephritis N07.4
        membranous glomerulonephritis N07.2
        mesangial proliferative glomerulonephritis
          N07.3
        mesangiocapillary glomerulonephritis N07.5
      focal and segmental glomerular lesions N07.1
      minor glomerular abnormality N07.0
      specified morphological changes NEC N07.8
  hypercalcemic N25.89
  hypertensive — *see* Hypertension, kidney
  hypokalemic (vacuolar) N25.89
  IgA N02.8
    with glomerular lesion N02.9
      focal and segmental hyalinosis or sclerosis
        N02.1
      membranoproliferative (diffuse) N02.5
      membranous (diffuse) N02.2
      mesangial proliferative (diffuse) N02.3
      mesangiocapillary (diffuse) N02.5
      proliferative NEC N02.8
      specified pathology NEC N02.8
  lead N14.3
  membranoproliferative (diffuse) N02.5
  membranous (diffuse) N02.2
  mesangial (IgA/IgG) — *see* Nephropathy, IgA
    proliferative (diffuse) N02.3
  mesangiocapillary (diffuse) N02.5
  obstructive N13.8
  phenacetin N17.2
  phosphate-losing N25.0
  potassium depletion N25.89
  pregnancy-related O26.83 ☑
  proliferative NEC (*see also* N00-N07 with fourth
    character .8) N05.8
  protein-losing N25.89
  saturnine N14.3
  sickle-cell D57. ☑ *[N08]*
  toxic NEC N14.4
    due to
      drugs N14.2
        analgesic N14.0
        specified NEC N14.1
      heavy metals N14.3
  vasomotor N17.0
  water-losing N25.89
Nephroptosis N28.83
Nephropyosis — *see* Abscess, kidney
Nephrorrhagia N28.89
Nephrosclerosis (arteriolar)(arteriosclerotic) (chronic)
  (hyaline) (*see also* Hypertension, kidney)
  hyperplastic — *see* Hypertension, kidney
  senile N26.9
Nephrosis, nephrotic (Epstein's) (syndrome)
  (congenital) N04.9
  with
    foot process disease N04.9
    glomerular lesion N04.1
    hypocomplementemic N04.5
  acute N04.9
  anoxic — *see* Nephrosis, tubular
  chemical — *see* Nephrosis, tubular
  cholemic K76.7
  diabetic — *see* E08-E13 with .21
  Finnish type (congenital) Q89.8
  hemoglobin N10
  hemoglobinuric — *see* Nephrosis, tubular
  in
    amyloidosis E85.4 *[N08]*
    diabetes mellitus — *see* E08-E13 with .21
    epidemic hemorrhagic fever A98.5
    malaria (malariae) B52.0
  ischemic — *see* Nephrosis, tubular
  lipoid N04.9
  lower nephron — *see* Nephrosis, tubular
  malarial (malariae) B52.0

Nephrosis - Neuropathy

Nephrosis — *continued*
  minimal change N04.0
  myoglobin N10
  necrotizing — *see* Nephrosis, tubular
  osmotic (sucrose) N25.89
  radiation N04.9
  syphilitic (late) A52.75
  toxic — *see* Nephrosis, tubular
  tubular (acute) N17.0
    postprocedural N99.0
    radiation N04.9
Nephrosonephritis, hemorrhagic (endemic) A98.5
Nephrostomy
  attention to Z43.6
  status Z93.6
Nerve (*see also* condition)
  injury — *see* Injury, nerve, by body site
Nerves R45.0
Nervous (*see also* condition) R45.0
  heart F45.8
  stomach F45.8
  tension R45.0
Nervousness R45.0
Nesidioblastoma
  pancreas D13.7
  specified site NEC — *see* Neoplasm, benign, by site
  unspecified site D13.7
Nettleship's syndrome — *see* Urticaria pigmentosa
Neumann's disease or syndrome L10.1
Neuralgia, neuralgic (acute) M79.2
  accessory (nerve) G52.8
  acoustic (nerve) — *see* subcategory H93.3 ☑
  auditory (nerve) — *see* subcategory H93.3 ☑
  ciliary G44.009
    intractable G44.001
    not intractable G44.009
  cranial
    nerve (*see also* Disorder, nerve, cranial)
      fifth or trigeminal — *see* Neuralgia, trigeminal
    postherpetic, postzoster B02.29
  ear — *see* subcategory H92.0 ☑
  facialis vera G51.1
  Fothergill's — *see* Neuralgia, trigeminal
  glossopharyngeal (nerve) G52.1
  Horton's G44.099
    intractable G44.091
    not intractable G44.099
  Hunt's B02.21
  hypoglossal (nerve) G52.3
  infraorbital — *see* Neuralgia, trigeminal
  malarial — *see* Malaria
  migrainous G44.009
    intractable G44.001
    not intractable G44.009
  Morton's G57.6 ☑
  nerve, cranial — *see* Disorder, nerve, cranial
  nose G52.0
  occipital M54.81
  olfactory G52.0
  penis N48.9
  perineum R10.2
  postherpetic NEC B02.29
    trigeminal B02.22
  pubic region R10.2
  scrotum R10.2
  Sluder's G44.89
  specified nerve NEC G58.8
  spermatic cord R10.2
  sphenopalatine (ganglion) G90.09
  trifacial — *see* Neuralgia, trigeminal
  trigeminal G50.0
    postherpetic, postzoster B02.22
  vagus (nerve) G52.2
  writer's F48.8
    organic G25.89
Neurapraxia — *see* Injury, nerve
Neurasthenia F48.8
  cardiac F45.8
  gastric F45.8
  heart F45.8
Neurilemmoma (*see also* Neoplasm, nerve, benign)
  acoustic (nerve) D33.3
  malignant (*see also* Neoplasm, nerve, malignant)
    acoustic (nerve) C72.4 ☑
Neurilemmosarcoma — *see* Neoplasm, nerve, malignant
Neurinoma — *see* Neoplasm, nerve, benign
Neurinomatosis — *see* Neoplasm, nerve, uncertain behavior
Neuritis (rheumatoid) M79.2
  abducens (nerve) — *see* Strabismus, paralytic, sixth nerve

Neuritis — *continued*
  accessory (nerve) G52.8
  acoustic (nerve) (*see also* subcategory) H93.3 ☑
    in (due to)
      infectious disease NEC B99 ☑ *[H94.0 ☑]*
      parasitic disease NEC B89 *[H94.0 ☑]*
    syphilitic A52.15
  alcoholic G62.1
    with psychosis — *see* Psychosis, alcoholic
  amyloid, any site E85.4 *[G63]*
  auditory (nerve) — *see* subcategory H93.3 ☑
  brachial — *see* Radiculopathy
    due to displacement, intervertebral disc — *see* Disorder, disc, cervical, with neuritis
  cranial nerve
    due to Lyme disease A69.22
    eighth or acoustic or auditory — *see* subcategory H93.3 ☑
    eleventh or accessory G52.8
    fifth or trigeminal G51.0
    first or olfactory G52.0
    fourth or trochlear — *see* Strabismus, paralytic, fourth nerve
    second or optic — *see* Neuritis, optic
    seventh or facial G51.8
      newborn (birth injury) P11.3
    sixth or abducent — *see* Strabismus, paralytic, sixth nerve
    tenth or vagus G52.2
    third or oculomotor — *see* Strabismus, paralytic, third nerve
    twelfth or hypoglossal G52.3
  Déjérine-Sottas G60.0
  diabetic (mononeuropathy) — *see* E08-E13 with .41
    polyneuropathy — *see* E08-E13 with .42
  due to
    beriberi E51.11
    displacement, prolapse or rupture, intervertebral disc — *see* Disorder, disc, with, radiculopathy
    herniation, nucleus pulposus M51.9 *[G55]*
  endemic E51.11
  facial G51.8
    newborn (birth injury) P11.3
  general — *see* Polyneuropathy
  geniculate ganglion G51.1
    due to herpes (zoster) B02.21
  gouty (*see also* Gout, by type) M10.9 *[G63]*
  hypoglossal (nerve) G52.3
  ilioinguinal (nerve) G57.9 ☑
  infectious (multiple) NEC G61.0
  interstitial hypertrophic progressive G60.0
  lumbar M54.16
  lumbosacral M54.17
  multiple (*see also* Polyneuropathy)
    endemic E51.11
    infective, acute G61.0
  multiplex endemica E51.11
  nerve root — *see* Radiculopathy
  oculomotor (nerve) — *see* Strabismus, paralytic, third nerve
  olfactory nerve G52.0
  optic (nerve) (hereditary) (sympathetic) H46.9
    with demyelination G36.0
    in myelitis G36.0
    nutritional H46.2
    papillitis — *see* Papillitis, optic
    retrobulbar H46.1 ☑
    specified type NEC H46.8
    toxic H46.3
  peripheral (nerve) G62.9
    multiple — *see* Polyneuropathy
    single — *see* Mononeuritis
  pneumogastric (nerve) G52.2
  postherpetic, postzoster B02.29
  progressive hypertrophic interstitial G60.0
  retrobulbar (*see also* Neuritis, optic, retrobulbar)
    in (due to)
      late syphilis A52.15
      meningococcal infection A39.82
    meningococcal A39.82
    syphilitic A52.15
  sciatic (nerve) (*see also* Sciatica)
    due to displacement of intervertebral disc — *see* Disorder, disc, with, radiculopathy
  serum (*see also* Reaction, serum) T80.69 ☑
  shoulder-girdle G54.5
  specified nerve NEC G58.8
  spinal (nerve) root — *see* Radiculopathy
  syphilitic A52.15
  thenar (median) G56.1 ☑
  thoracic M54.14
  toxic NEC G62.2

Neuritis — *continued*
  trochlear (nerve) — *see* Strabismus, paralytic, fourth nerve
  vagus (nerve) G52.2
Neuroastrocytoma — *see* Neoplasm, uncertain behavior, by site
Neuroavitaminosis E56.9 *[G99.8]*
Neuroblastoma
  olfactory C30.0
  specified site — *see* Neoplasm, malignant, by site
  unspecified site C74.90
Neurochorioretinitis — *see* Chorioretinitis
Neurocirculatory asthenia F45.8
Neurocysticercosis B69.0
Neurocytoma — *see* Neoplasm, benign, by site
Neurodermatitis (circumscribed) (circumscripta) (local) L28.0
  atopic L20.81
  diffuse (Brocq) L20.81
  disseminated L20.81
Neuroencephalomyelopathy, optic G36.0
Neuroepithelioma (*see also* Neoplasm, malignant, by site)
  olfactory C30.0
Neurofibroma (*see also* Neoplasm, nerve, benign)
  melanotic — *see* Neoplasm, nerve, benign
  multiple — *see* Neurofibromatosis
  plexiform — *see* Neoplasm, nerve, benign
Neurofibromatosis (multiple) (nonmalignant) Q85.00
  acoustic Q85.02
  malignant — *see* Neoplasm, nerve, malignant
  specified NEC Q85.09
  type 1 (von Recklinghausen) Q85.01
  type 2 Q85.02
Neurofibrosarcoma — *see* Neoplasm, nerve, malignant
Neurogenic (*see also* condition)
  bladder (*see also* Dysfunction, bladder, neuromuscular) N31.9
    cauda equina syndrome G83.4
  bowel NEC K59.2
  heart F45.8
Neuroglioma — *see* Neoplasm, uncertain behavior, by site
Neurolabyrinthitis (of Dix and Hallpike) — *see* Neuronitis, vestibular
Neurolathyrism — *see* Poisoning, food, noxious, plant
Neuroleprosy A30.9
Neuroma (*see also* Neoplasm, nerve, benign)
  acoustic (nerve) D33.3
  amputation (stump) (traumatic) (surgical complication) (late) T87.3 ☑
    arm T87.3 ☑
    leg T87.3 ☑
  digital (toe) G57.6 ☑
  interdigital G58.8
    lower limb (toe) G57.8 ☑
    upper limb G56.8 ☑
  intermetatarsal G57.8 ☑
  Morton's G57.6 ☑
  nonneoplastic
    arm G56.9 ☑
    leg G57.9 ☑
    lower extremity G57.9 ☑
    upper extremity G56.9 ☑
  optic (nerve) D33.3
  plantar G57.6 ☑
  plexiform — *see* Neoplasm, nerve, benign
  surgical (nonneoplastic)
    arm G56.9 ☑
    leg G57.9 ☑
    lower extremity G57.9 ☑
    upper extremity G56.9 ☑
Neuromyalgia — *see* Neuralgia
Neuromyasthenia (epidemic) (postinfectious) G93.3
Neuromyelitis G36.9
  ascending G61.0
  optica G36.0
Neuromyopathy G70.9
  paraneoplastic D49.9 *[G13.0]*
Neuromyotonia (Isaacs) G71.19
Neuronevus — *see* Nevus
Neuronitis G58.9
  ascending (acute) G57.2 ☑
  vestibular H81.2 ☑
Neuroparalytic — *see* condition
Neuropathy, neuropathic G62.9
  acute motor G62.81
  alcoholic G62.1
    with psychosis — *see* Psychosis, alcoholic
  arm G56.9 ☑
  autonomic, peripheral — *see* Neuropathy, peripheral, autonomic

☑ **Additional character required**

Neuropathy — *continued*
  axillary G56.9 ☑
  bladder N31.9
    atonic (motor) (sensory) N31.2
    autonomous N31.2
    flaccid N31.2
    nonreflex N31.2
    reflex N31.1
    uninhibited N31.0
  brachial plexus G54.0
  cervical plexus G54.2
  chronic
    progressive segmentally demyelinating G62.89
    relapsing demyelinating G62.89
  Déjérine-Sottas G60.0
  diabetic — *see* E08-E13 with .40
    mononeuropathy — *see* E08-E13 with .41
    polyneuropathy — *see* E08-E13 with .42
  entrapment G58.9
    iliohypogastric nerve G57.8 ☑
    ilioinguinal nerve G57.8 ☑
    lateral cutaneous nerve of thigh G57.1 ☑
    median nerve G56.0 ☑
    obturator nerve G57.8 ☑
    peroneal nerve G57.3 ☑
    posterior tibial nerve G57.5 ☑
    saphenous nerve G57.8 ☑
    ulnar nerve G56.2 ☑
  facial nerve G51.9
  hereditary G60.9
    motor and sensory (types I-IV) G60.0
    sensory G60.8
    specified NEC G60.8
  hypertrophic G60.0
    Charcot-Marie-Tooth G60.0
    Déjérine-Sottas G60.0
    interstitial progressive G60.0
    of infancy G60.0
    Refsum G60.1
  idiopathic G60.9
    progressive G60.3
    specified NEC G60.8
  in association with hereditary ataxia G60.2
  intercostal G58.0
  ischemic — *see* Disorder, nerve
  Jamaica (ginger) G62.2
  leg NEC G57.9 ☑
  lower extremity G57.9 ☑
  lumbar plexus G54.1
  median nerve G56.1 ☑
  motor and sensory (*see also* Polyneuropathy)
    hereditary (types I-IV) G60.0
  multifocal motor (MMN) G61.82
  multiple (acute) (chronic) — *see* Polyneuropathy
  optic (nerve) (*see also* Neuritis, optic)
    ischemic H47.01 ☑
  paraneoplastic (sensorial) (Denny Brown) D49.9 *[G13.0]*
  peripheral (nerve) (*see also* Polyneuropathy) G62.9
    autonomic G90.9
      idiopathic G90.09
      in (due to)
        amyloidosis E85.4 *[G99.0]*
        diabetes mellitus — *see* E08-E13 with .43
        endocrine disease NEC E34.9 *[G99.0]*
        gout M10.00 *[G99.0]*
        hyperthyroidism E05.90 *[G99.0]*
          with thyroid storm E05.91 *[G99.0]*
        metabolic disease NEC E88.9 *[G99.0]*
    idiopathic G60.9
      progressive G60.3
    in (due to)
      antitetanus serum G62.0
      arsenic G62.2
      drugs NEC G62.0
      lead G62.2
      organophosphate compounds G62.2
      toxic agent NEC G62.2
  plantar nerves G57.6 ☑
  progressive
    hypertrophic interstitial G60.0
    inflammatory G62.81
  radicular NEC — *see* Radiculopathy
  sacral plexus G54.1
  sciatic G57.0 ☑
  serum G61.1
  toxic NEC G62.2
  trigeminal sensory G50.8
  ulnar nerve G56.2 ☑
  uremic N18.9 *[G63]*
  vitamin B12 E53.8 *[G63]*
    with anemia (pernicious) D51.0 *[G63]*
      due to dietary deficiency D51.3 *[G63]*

Neurophthisis (*see also* Disorder, nerve)
  peripheral, diabetic — *see* E08-E13 with .42
Neuroretinitis — *see* Chorioretinitis
Neuroretinopathy, hereditary optic H47.22
Neurosarcoma — *see* Neoplasm, nerve, malignant
Neurosclerosis — *see* Disorder, nerve
Neurosis, neurotic F48.9
  anankastic F42.8
  anxiety (state) F41.1
    panic type F41.0
  asthenic F48.8
  bladder F45.8
  cardiac (reflex) F45.8
  cardiovascular F45.8
  character F60.9
  colon F45.8
  compensation F68.10
  compulsive, compulsion F42.8
  conversion F44.9
  craft F48.8
  cutaneous F45.8
  depersonalization F48.1
  depressive (reaction) (type) F34.1
  environmental F48.8
  excoriation L98.1
  fatigue F48.8
  functional — *see* Disorder, somatoform
  gastric F45.8
  gastrointestinal F45.8
  heart F45.8
  hypochondriacal F45.21
  hysterical F44.9
  incoordination F45.8
    larynx F45.8
    vocal cord F45.8
  intestine F45.8
  larynx (sensory) F45.8
    hysterical F44.4
  mixed NEC F48.8
  musculoskeletal F45.8
  obsessional F42.8
  obsessive-compulsive F42.8
  occupational F48.8
  ocular NEC F45.8
  organ — *see* Disorder, somatoform
  pharynx F45.8
  phobic F40.9
  posttraumatic (situational) F43.10
    acute F43.11
    chronic F43.12
  psychasthenic (type) F48.8
  railroad F48.8
  rectum F45.8
  respiratory F45.8
  rumination F45.8
  sexual F65.9
  situational F48.8
  social F40.10
    generalized F40.11
  specified type NEC F48.8
  state F48.9
    with depersonalization episode F48.1
  stomach F45.8
  traumatic F43.10
    acute F43.11
    chronic F43.12
  vasomotor F45.8
  visceral F45.8
  war F48.8
Neurospongioblastosis diffusa Q85.1
Neurosyphilis (arrested) (early) (gumma) (late) (latent) (recurrent) (relapse) A52.3
  with ataxia (cerebellar) (locomotor) (spastic) (spinal) A52.19
  aneurysm (cerebral) A52.05
  arachnoid (adhesive) A52.13
  arteritis (any artery) (cerebral) A52.04
  asymptomatic A52.2
  congenital A50.40
  dura (mater) A52.13
  general paresis A52.17
  hemorrhagic A52.05
  juvenile (asymptomatic) (meningeal) A50.40
  leptomeninges (aseptic) A52.13
  meningeal, meninges (adhesive) A52.13
  meningitis A52.13
  meningovascular (diffuse) A52.13
  optic atrophy A52.15
  parenchymatous (degenerative) A52.19
  paresis, paretic A52.17
    juvenile A50.45
  remission in (sustained) A52.3

Neurosyphilis — *continued*
  serological (without symptoms) A52.2
  specified nature or site NEC A52.19
  tabes, tabetic (dorsalis) A52.11
    juvenile A50.45
  taboparesis A52.17
    juvenile A50.45
  thrombosis (cerebral) A52.05
  vascular (cerebral) NEC A52.05
Neurothekeoma — *see* Neoplasm, nerve, benign
Neurotic — *see* Neurosis
Neurotoxemia — *see* Toxemia
Neutroclusion M26.211
Neutropenia, neutropenic (chronic) (genetic) (idiopathic) (immune) (infantile) (malignant) (pernicious) (splenic) D70.9
  congenital (primary) D70.0
  cyclic D70.4
  cytoreductive cancer chemotherapy sequela D70.1
  drug-induced D70.2
    due to cytoreductive cancer chemotherapy D70.1
  due to infection D70.3
  fever D70.9
  neonatal, transitory (isoimmune) (maternal transfer) P61.5
  periodic D70.4
  secondary (cyclic) (periodic) (splenic) D70.4
    drug-induced D70.2
      due to cytoreductive cancer chemotherapy D70.1
  toxic D70.8
Neutrophilia, hereditary giant D72.0
Nevocarcinoma — *see* Melanoma
Nevus D22.9
  achromic — *see* Neoplasm, skin, benign
  amelanotic — *see* Neoplasm, skin, benign
  angiomatous D18.00
    intra-abdominal D18.03
    intracranial D18.02
    skin D18.01
    specified site NEC D18.09
  araneus I78.1
  balloon cell — *see* Neoplasm, skin, benign
  bathing trunk D48.5
  blue — *see* Neoplasm, skin, benign
    cellular — *see* Neoplasm, skin, benign
    giant — *see* Neoplasm, skin, benign
    Jadassohn's — *see* Neoplasm, skin, benign
    malignant — *see* Melanoma
  capillary D18.00
    intra-abdominal D18.03
    intracranial D18.02
    skin D18.01
    specified site NEC D18.09
  cavernous D18.00
    intra-abdominal D18.03
    intracranial D18.02
    skin D18.01
    specified site NEC D18.09
  cellular — *see* Neoplasm, skin, benign
    blue — *see* Neoplasm, skin, benign
  choroid D31.3 ☑
  comedonicus Q82.5
  conjunctiva D31.0 ☑
  dermal — *see* Neoplasm, skin, benign
    with epidermal nevus — *see* Neoplasm, skin, benign
  dysplastic — *see* Neoplasm, skin, benign
  eye D31.9 ☑
  flammeus Q82.5
  hemangiomatous D18.00
    intra-abdominal D18.03
    intracranial D18.02
    skin D18.01
    specified site NEC D18.09
  iris D31.4 ☑
  lacrimal gland D31.5 ☑
  lymphatic D18.1
  magnocellular
    specified site — *see* Neoplasm, benign, by site
    unspecified site D31.40
  malignant — *see* Melanoma
  meaning hemangioma D18.00
    intra-abdominal D18.03
    intracranial D18.02
    skin D18.01
    specified site NEC D18.09
  mouth (mucosa) D10.30
    specified site NEC D10.39
    white sponge Q38.6
  multiplex Q85.1
  non-neoplastic I78.1

Nevus — *continued*
- oral mucosa D10.30
  - specified site NEC D10.39
  - white sponge Q38.6
- orbit D31.6 ☑
- pigmented
  - giant (*see also* Neoplasm, skin, uncertain behavior) D48.5
    - malignant melanoma in — *see* Melanoma
- portwine Q82.5
- retina D31.2 ☑
- retrobulbar D31.6 ☑
- sanguineous Q82.5
- senile I78.1
- skin D22.9
  - abdominal wall D22.5
  - ala nasi D22.39
  - ankle D22.7 ☑
  - anus, anal D22.5
  - arm D22.6 ☑
  - auditory canal (external) D22.2 ☑
  - auricle (ear) D22.2 ☑
  - auricular canal (external) D22.2 ☑
  - axilla, axillary fold D22.5
  - back D22.5
  - breast D22.5
  - brow D22.39
  - buttock D22.5
  - canthus (eye) D22.1 ☑
  - cheek (external) D22.39
  - chest wall D22.5
  - chin D22.39
  - ear (external) D22.2 ☑
  - external meatus (ear) D22.2 ☑
  - eyebrow D22.39
  - eyelid (lower) (upper) D22.1 ☑
  - face D22.30
    - specified NEC D22.39
  - female genital organ (external) NEC D28.0
  - finger D22.6 ☑
  - flank D22.5
  - foot D22.7 ☑
  - forearm D22.6 ☑
  - forehead D22.39
  - foreskin D29.0
  - genital organ (external) NEC
    - female D28.0
    - male D29.9
  - gluteal region D22.5
  - groin D22.5
  - hand D22.6 ☑
  - heel D22.7 ☑
  - helix D22.2 ☑
  - hip D22.7 ☑
  - interscapular region D22.5
  - jaw D22.39
  - knee D22.7 ☑
  - labium (majus) (minus) D28.0
  - leg D22.7 ☑
  - lip (lower) (upper) D22.0
  - lower limb D22.7 ☑
  - male genital organ (external) D29.9
  - nail D22.9
    - finger D22.6 ☑
    - toe D22.7 ☑
  - nasolabial groove D22.39
  - nates D22.5
  - neck D22.4
  - nose (external) D22.39
  - palpebra D22.1 ☑
  - penis D29.0
  - perianal skin D22.5
  - perineum D22.5
  - pinna D22.2 ☑
  - popliteal fossa or space D22.7 ☑
  - prepuce D29.0
  - pudendum D28.0
  - scalp D22.4
  - scrotum D29.4
  - shoulder D22.6 ☑
  - submammary fold D22.5
  - temple D22.39
  - thigh D22.7 ☑
  - toe D22.7 ☑
  - trunk NEC D22.5
  - umbilicus D22.5
  - upper limb D22.6 ☑
  - vulva D28.0
- specified site NEC — *see* Neoplasm, by site, benign
- spider I78.1
- stellar I78.1
- strawberry Q82.5

Nevus — *continued*
- Sutton's benign D22.9
- unius lateris Q82.5
- Unna's Q82.5
- vascular Q82.5
- verrucous Q82.5

Newborn (infant) (liveborn) (singleton) Z38.2
- acne L70.4
- abstinence syndrome P96.1
- affected by
  - abnormalities of membranes P02.9
    - specified NEC P02.8
  - abruptio placenta P02.1
  - amino-acid metabolic disorder, transitory P74.8
  - amniocentesis (while in utero) P00.6
  - amnionitis P02.78
  - apparent life threatening event (ALTE) R68.13
  - bleeding (into)
    - cerebral cortex P52.22
    - germinal matrix P52.0
    - ventricles P52.1
  - breech delivery P03.0
  - cardiac arrest P29.81
  - cardiomyopathy I42.8
    - congenital I42.4
  - cerebral ischemia P91.0
  - Cesarean delivery P03.4
  - chemotherapy agents P04.11
  - chorioamnionitis P02.78
  - cocaine (crack) P04.41
  - complications of labor and delivery P03.9
    - specified NEC P03.89
  - compression of umbilical cord NEC P02.5
  - contracted pelvis P03.1
  - cyanosis P28.2
  - delivery P03.9
    - Cesarean P03.4
    - forceps P03.2
    - vacuum extractor P03.3
  - drugs of addiction P04.40
    - cocaine P04.41
    - hallucinogens P04.42
    - specified drug NEC P04.49
  - environmental chemicals P04.6
  - entanglement (knot) in umbilical cord P02.5
  - fetal (intrauterine)
    - growth retardation P05.9
    - inflammatory response syndrome (FIRS) P02.70
    - malnutrition not light or small for gestational age P05.2
  - FIRS (fetal inflammatory response syndrome) P02.70
  - forceps delivery P03.2
  - heart rate abnormalities
    - bradycardia P29.12
    - intrauterine P03.819
      - before onset of labor P03.810
      - during labor P03.811
    - tachycardia P29.11
  - hemorrhage (antepartum) P02.1
    - cerebellar (nontraumatic) P52.6
    - intracerebral (nontraumatic) P52.4
    - intracranial (nontraumatic) P52.9
      - specified NEC P52.8
    - intraventricular (nontraumatic) P52.3
      - grade 1 P52.0
      - grade 2 P52.1
      - grade 3 P52.21
      - grade 4 P52.22
    - posterior fossa (nontraumatic) P52.6
    - subarachnoid (nontraumatic) P52.5
    - subependymal P52.0
      - with intracerebral extension P52.22
      - with intraventricular extension P52.1
        - with enlargement of ventricles P52.21
      - without intraventricular extension P52.0
  - hypoxic ischemic encephalopathy [HIE] P91.60
    - mild P91.61
    - moderate P91.62
    - severe P91.63
  - induction of labor P03.89
  - intestinal perforation P78.0
  - intrauterine (fetal) blood loss P50.9
    - due to (from)
      - cut end of co-twin cord P50.5
      - hemorrhage into
        - co-twin P50.3
        - maternal circulation P50.4
      - placenta P50.2
      - ruptured cord blood P50.1
      - vasa previa P50.0
    - specified NEC P50.8

Newborn — *continued*
- affected by — *continued*
  - intrauterine (fetal) hemorrhage P50.9
  - intrauterine (in utero) procedure P96.5
  - malpresentation (malposition) NEC P03.1
  - maternal (complication of) (use of)
    - alcohol P04.3
    - amphetamines P04.16
    - analgesia (maternal) P04.0
    - anesthesia (maternal) P04.0
    - anticonvulsants P04.13
    - antidepressants P04.15
    - antineoplastic chemotherapy P04.11
    - anxiolytics P04.1A
    - blood loss P02.1
    - cannabis P04.81
    - circulatory disease P00.3
    - condition P00.9
      - specified NEC P00.89
    - cytotoxic drugs P04.12
    - delivery P03.9
      - Cesarean P03.4
      - forceps P03.2
      - vacuum extractor P03.3
    - diabetes mellitus (pre-existing) P70.1
    - disorder P00.9
      - specified NEC P00.89
    - drugs (addictive) (illegal) NEC P04.49
    - ectopic pregnancy P01.4
    - gestational diabetes P70.0
    - hemorrhage P02.1
    - hypertensive disorder P00.0
    - incompetent cervix P01.0
    - infectious disease P00.2
    - injury P00.5
    - labor and delivery P03.9
    - malpresentation before labor P01.7
    - maternal death P01.6
    - medical procedure P00.7
    - medication P04.19
      - specified type NEC P04.18
    - multiple pregnancy P01.5
    - nutritional disorder P00.4
    - oligohydramnios P01.2
    - opiates P04.14
      - administered for procedures during pregnancy or labor and delivery P04.0
    - parasitic disease P00.2
    - periodontal disease P00.81
    - placenta previa P02.0
    - polyhydramnios P01.3
    - precipitate delivery P03.5
    - pregnancy P01.9
      - specified P01.8
    - premature rupture of membranes P01.1
    - renal disease P00.1
    - respiratory disease P00.3
    - sedative-hypnotics P04.17
    - surgical procedure P00.6
    - tranquilizers administered for procedures during pregnancy or labor and delivery P04.0
    - urinary tract disease P00.1
    - uterine contraction (abnormal) P03.6
  - meconium peritonitis P78.0
  - medication (legal) (maternal use) (prescribed) P04.19
  - membrane abnormalities P02.9
    - specified NEC P02.8
  - membranitis P02.78
  - methamphetamine(s) P04.49
  - mixed metabolic and respiratory acidosis P84
  - neonatal abstinence syndrome P96.1
  - noxious substances transmitted via placenta or breast milk P04.9
    - cannabis P04.81
    - specified NEC P04.89
  - nutritional supplements P04.5
  - placenta previa P02.0
  - placental
    - abnormality (functional) (morphological) P02.20
      - specified NEC P02.29
    - dysfunction P02.29
    - infarction P02.29
    - insufficiency P02.29
    - separation NEC P02.1
    - transfusion syndromes P02.3
  - placentitis P02.78
  - precipitate delivery P03.5
  - prolapsed cord P02.4
  - respiratory arrest P28.81
  - slow intrauterine growth P05.9

☑ **Additional character required**

Newborn — *continued*
  affected by — *continued*
    tobacco P04.2
    twin to twin transplacental transfusion P02.3
    umbilical cord (tightly) around neck P02.5
    umbilical cord condition P02.60
      short cord P02.69
      specified NEC P02.69
    uterine contractions (abnormal) P03.6
    vasa previa P02.69
      from intrauterine blood loss P50.0
  apnea P28.4
    primary P28.3
    obstructive P28.4
    sleep (central) (obstructive) (primary) P28.3
  born in hospital Z38.00
    by cesarean Z38.01
  born outside hospital Z38.1
  breast buds P96.89
  breast engorgement P83.4
  check-up — *see* Newborn, examination
  convulsion P90
  dehydration P74.1
  examination
    8 to 28 days old Z00.111
    under 8 days old Z00.110
  fever P81.9
    environmentally-induced P81.0
  hyperbilirubinemia P59.9
    of prematurity P59.0
  hypernatremia P74.21
  hyponatremia P74.22
  infection P39.9
    candidal P37.5
    specified NEC P39.8
    urinary tract P39.3
  jaundice P59.9
    due to
      breast milk inhibitor P59.3
      hepatocellular damage P59.20
        specified NEC P59.29
      preterm delivery P59.0
    of prematurity P59.0
    specified NEC P59.8
  late metabolic acidosis P74.0
  mastitis P39.0
    infective P39.0
    noninfective P83.4
  multiple born NEC Z38.8
    born in hospital Z38.68
      by cesarean Z38.69
    born outside hospital Z38.7
  omphalitis P38.9
    with mild hemorrhage P38.1
    without hemorrhage P38.9
  post-term P08.21
  prolonged gestation (over 42 completed weeks)
    P08.22
  quadruplet Z38.8
    born in hospital Z38.63
      by cesarean Z38.64
    born outside hospital Z38.7
  quintuplet Z38.8
    born in hospital Z38.65
      by cesarean Z38.66
    born outside hospital Z38.7
  seizure P90
  sepsis (congenital) P36.9
    due to
      anaerobes NEC P36.5
      Escherichia coli P36.4
      Staphylococcus P36.30
        aureus P36.2
        specified NEC P36.39
      Streptococcus P36.10
        group B P36.0
        specified NEC P36.19
      specified NEC P36.8
  triplet Z38.8
    born in hospital Z38.61
      by cesarean Z38.62
    born outside hospital Z38.7
  twin Z38.5
    born in hospital Z38.30
      by cesarean Z38.31
    born outside hospital Z38.4
  vomiting P92.09
    bilious P92.01
  weight check Z00.111
Newcastle conjunctivitis or disease B30.8
Nezelof's syndrome (pure alymphocytosis) D81.4
Niacin (amide) deficiency E52

Nicolas (-Durand)-Favre disease A55
Nicotine — *see* Tobacco
Nicotinic acid deficiency E52
Niemann-Pick disease or syndrome E75.249
  specified NEC E75.248
  type
    A E75.240
    B E75.241
    C E75.242
    D E75.243
Night
  blindness — *see* Blindness, night
  sweats R61
  terrors (child) F51.4
Nightmares (REM sleep type) F51.5
NIHSS (National Institutes of Health Stroke Scale)
  score R29.7 ☑
Nipple — *see* condition
Nisbet's chancre A57
Nishimoto (-Takeuchi) disease I67.5
Nitritoid crisis or reaction — *see* Crisis, nitritoid
Nitrosohemoglobinemia D74.8
Njovera A65
Nocardiosis, nocardiasis A43.9
  cutaneous A43.1
  lung A43.0
  pneumonia A43.0
  pulmonary A43.0
  specified site NEC A43.8
Nocturia R35.1
  psychogenic F45.8
Nocturnal — *see* condition
Nodal rhythm I49.8
Node(s) (*see also* Nodule)
  Bouchard's (with arthropathy) M15.2
  Haygarth's M15.8
  Heberden's (with arthropathy) M15.1
  larynx J38.7
  lymph — *see* condition
  milker's B08.03
  Osler's I33.0
  Schmorl's — *see* Schmorl's disease
  singer's J38.2
  teacher's J38.2
  tuberculous — *see* Tuberculosis, lymph gland
  vocal cord J38.2
Nodule(s), nodular
  actinomycotic — *see* Actinomycosis
  breast NEC (*see also* Lump, breast) N63.0
  colloid (cystic), thyroid E04.1
  cutaneous — *see* Swelling, localized
  endometrial (stromal) D26.1
  Haygarth's M15.8
  inflammatory — *see* Inflammation
  juxta-articular
    syphilitic A52.77
    yaws A66.7
  larynx J38.7
  lung, solitary (subsegmental branch of the
    bronchial tree) R91.1
    multiple R91.8
  milker's B08.03
  prostate N40.2
    with lower urinary tract symptoms (LUTS) N40.3
    without lower urinary tract symptoms (LUTS) N40.2
  pulmonary, solitary (subsegmental branch of the
    bronchial tree) R91.1
  retrocardiac R09.89
  rheumatoid M06.30
    ankle M06.37 ☑
    elbow M06.32 ☑
    foot joint M06.37 ☑
    hand joint M06.34 ☑
    hip M06.35 ☑
    knee M06.36 ☑
    multiple site M06.39
    shoulder M06.31 ☑
    vertebra M06.38
    wrist M06.33 ☑
  scrotum (inflammatory) N49.2
  singer's J38.2
  solitary, lung (subsegmental branch of the
    bronchial tree) R91.1
    multiple R91.8
  subcutaneous — *see* Swelling, localized
  teacher's J38.2
  thyroid (cold) (gland) (nontoxic) E04.1
    with thyrotoxicosis E05.20
      with thyroid storm E05.21
    toxic or with hyperthyroidism E05.20
      with thyroid storm E05.21
  vocal cord J38.2

Noma (gangrenous) (hospital) (infective) A69.0
  auricle I96
  mouth A69.0
  pudendi N76.89
  vulvae N76.89
Nomad, nomadism Z59.0
NOMID (neonatal onset multisystemic inflammatory
  disorder) M04.2
Nonadherence to medical treatment Z91.19
Nonautoimmune hemolytic anemia D59.4
  drug-induced D59.2
Nonclosure (*see also* Imperfect, closure)
  ductus arteriosus (Botallo's) Q25.0
  foramen
    botalli Q21.1
    ovale Q21.1
Noncompliance Z91.19
  with
    dietary regimen Z91.11
    dialysis Z91.15
    medical treatment Z91.19
    medication regimen NEC Z91.14
      underdosing (*see also* Table of Drugs and
        Chemicals, categories T36-T50, with final
        character 6) Z91.14
      intentional NEC Z91.128
        due to financial hardship of patient Z91.120
      unintentional NEC Z91.138
        due to patient's age related debility
          Z91.130
    renal dialysis Z91.15
Nondescent (congenital) (*see also* Malposition,
  congenital)
  cecum Q43.3
  colon Q43.3
  testicle Q53.9
    bilateral Q53.20
      abdominal Q53.211
      perineal Q53.22
    unilateral Q53.10
      abdominal Q53.111
      perineal Q53.12
Nondevelopment
  brain Q02
    part of Q04.3
  heart Q24.8
  organ or site, congenital NEC — *see* Hypoplasia
Nonengagement
  head NEC O32.4 ☑
    in labor, causing obstructed labor O64.8 ☑
Nonexanthematous tick fever A93.2
Nonexpansion, lung (newborn) P28.0
Nonfunctioning
  cystic duct (*see also* Disease, gallbladder) K82.8
  gallbladder (*see also* Disease, gallbladder) K82.8
  kidney N28.9
  labyrinth — *see* subcategory H83.2 ☑
Non-Hodgkin lymphoma NEC — *see* Lymphoma,
  non-Hodgkin
Non-working side interference M26.56
Nonimplantation, ovum N97.2
Noninsufflation, fallopian tube N97.1
Non-ketotic hyperglycinemia E72.51
Nonne-Milroy syndrome Q82.0
Nonovulation N97.0
Non-palpable testicle(s)
  bilateral R39.84
  unilateral R39.83
Nonpatent fallopian tube N97.1
Nonpneumatization, lung NEC P28.0
Nonrotation — *see* Malrotation
Nonsecretion, urine — *see* Anuria
Nonunion
  fracture — *see* Fracture, by site
  joint, following fusion or arthrodesis M96.0
  organ or site, congenital NEC — *see* Imperfect,
    closure
  symphysis pubis, congenital Q74.2
Nonvisualization, gallbladder R93.2
Nonvital, nonvitalized tooth K04.99
Noonan's syndrome Q87.19
Normocytic anemia (infectional) due to blood loss
  (chronic) D50.0
  acute D62
Norrie's disease (congenital) Q15.8
North American blastomycosis B40.9
Norwegian itch B86
Nose, nasal — *see* condition
Nosebleed R04.0
Nose-picking F98.8
Nosomania F45.21
Nosophobia F45.22

Nostalgia - Obstruction

Nostalgia F43.20
Notch of iris Q13.2
Notching nose, congenital (tip) Q30.2
Nothnagel's
  syndrome — *see* Strabismus, paralytic, third nerve
  vasomotor acroparesthesia I73.89
Novy's relapsing fever A68.9
  louse-borne A68.0
  tick-borne A68.1
Noxious
  foodstuffs, poisoning by — *see* Poisoning, food,
    noxious, plant
  substances transmitted through placenta or breast
    milk P04.9
Nucleus pulposus — *see* condition
Numbness R20.0
Nuns' knee — *see* Bursitis, prepatellar
Nursemaid's elbow S53.03 ☑
Nutcracker esophagus K22.4
Nutmeg liver K76.1
Nutrient element deficiency E61.9
  specified NEC E61.8
Nutrition deficient or insufficient (*see also*
  Malnutrition) E46
  due to
    insufficient food T73.0 ☑
    lack of
      care (child) T76.02 ☑
        adult T76.01 ☑
      food T73.0 ☑
Nutritional stunting E45
Nyctalopia (night blindness) — *see* Blindness, night
Nycturia R35.1
  psychogenic F45.8
Nymphomania F52.8
Nystagmus H55.00
  benign paroxysmal — *see* Vertigo, benign
    paroxysmal
  central positional H81.4
  congenital H55.01
  dissociated H55.04
  latent H55.02
  miners' H55.09
  positional
    benign paroxysmal H81.4
    central H81.4
  specified form NEC H55.09
  visual deprivation H55.03

O

Obermeyer's relapsing fever (European) A68.0
Obesity E66.9
  with alveolar hypoventilation E66.2
  adrenal E27.8
  complicating
    childbirth O99.214
    pregnancy O99.21 ☑
    puerperium O99.215
  constitutional E66.9
  dietary counseling and surveillance Z71.3
  drug-induced E66.1
  due to
    drug E66.1
    excess calories E66.09
      morbid E66.01
      severe E66.01
  endocrine E66.8
  endogenous E66.8
  exogenous E66.09
  familial E66.8
  glandular E66.8
  hypothyroid — *see* Hypothyroidism
  hypoventilation syndrome (OHS) E66.2
  morbid E66.01
    with
      alveolar hypoventilation E66.2
      obesity hypoventilation syndrome (OHS) E66.2
    due to excess calories E66.01
  nutritional E66.09
  pituitary E23.6
  severe E66.01
  specified type NEC E66.8
Oblique — *see* condition
Obliteration
  appendix (lumen) K38.8
  artery I77.1
  bile duct (noncalculous) K83.1
  common duct (noncalculous) K83.1
  cystic duct — *see* Obstruction, gallbladder

Obliteration — *continued*
  disease, arteriolar I77.1
  endometrium N85.8
  eye, anterior chamber — *see* Disorder, globe,
    hypotony
  fallopian tube N97.1
  lymphatic vessel I89.0
    due to mastectomy I97.2
  organ or site, congenital NEC — *see* Atresia, by site
  ureter N13.5
    with infection N13.6
  urethra — *see* Stricture, urethra
  vein I87.8
  vestibule (oral) K08.89
Observation (following) (for) (without need for further
  medical care) Z04.9
  accident NEC Z04.3
    at work Z04.2
    transport Z04.1
  adverse effect of drug Z03.6
  alleged rape or sexual assault (victim), ruled out
    adult Z04.41
    child Z04.42
  criminal assault Z04.89
  development state
    adolescent Z00.3
    period of rapid growth in childhood Z00.2
    puberty Z00.3
  disease, specified NEC Z03.89
  following work accident Z04.2
  forced sexual exploitation Z04.81
  forced labor exploitation Z04.82
  growth and development state — *see* Observation,
    development state
  injuries (accidental) NEC (*see also* Observation,
    accident)
  newborn (for)
    suspected condition, related to exposure from
      the mother or birth process — *see* - Newborn,
      affected by, maternal
    ruled out Z05.9
      cardiac Z05.0
      connective tissue Z05.73
      gastrointestinal Z05.5
      genetic Z05.41
      genitourinary Z05.6
      immunologic Z05.43
      infectious Z05.1
      metabolic Z05.42
      musculoskeletal Z05.72
      neurological Z05.2
      respiratory Z05.3
      skin and subcutaneous tissue Z05.71
      specified condition NEC Z05.8
  postpartum
    immediately after delivery Z39.0
    routine follow-up Z39.2
  pregnancy (normal) (without complication)
    Z34.9 ☑
    high risk O09.9 ☑
  suicide attempt, alleged NEC Z03.89
    self-poisoning Z03.6
  suspected, ruled out (*see also* Suspected condition,
    ruled out)
    abuse, physical
      adult Z04.71
      child Z04.72
    accident at work Z04.2
    adult battering victim Z04.71
    child battering victim Z04.72
    condition NEC Z03.89
      newborn (*see also* Observation, newborn (for),
        suspected condition, ruled out) Z05.9
    drug poisoning or adverse effect Z03.6
    exposure (to)
      anthrax Z03.810
      biological agent NEC Z03.818
    inflicted injury NEC Z04.89
    suicide attempt, alleged Z03.89
      self-poisoning Z03.6
    toxic effects from ingested substance (drug)
      (poison) Z03.6
    toxic effects from ingested substance (drug)
      (poison) Z03.6
Obsession, obsessional state F42.8
  mixed thoughts and acts F42.2
Obsessive-compulsive neurosis or reaction F42.8
Obstetric embolism, septic — *see* Embolism, obstetric,
  septic
Obstetrical trauma (complicating delivery) O71.9
  with or following ectopic or molar pregnancy O08.6
  specified type NEC O71.89

Obstipation — *see* Constipation
Obstruction, obstructed, obstructive
  airway J98.8
    with
      allergic alveolitis J67.9
      asthma J45.909
        with
          exacerbation (acute) J45.901
          status asthmaticus J45.902
      bronchiectasis J47.9
        with
          exacerbation (acute) J47.1
          lower respiratory infection J47.0
      bronchitis (chronic) J44.9
      emphysema J43.9
    chronic J44.9
      with
        allergic alveolitis — *see* Pneumonitis,
          hypersensitivity
        bronchiectasis J47.9
          with
            exacerbation (acute) J47.1
            lower respiratory infection J47.0
    due to
      foreign body — *see* Foreign body, by site,
        causing asphyxia
      inhalation of fumes or vapors J68.9
      laryngospasm J38.5
  ampulla of Vater K83.1
  aortic (heart) (valve) — *see* Stenosis, aortic
  aortoiliac I74.09
  aqueduct of Sylvius G91.1
    congenital Q03.0
      with spina bifida — *see* Spina bifida, by site,
        with hydrocephalus
  Arnold-Chiari — *see* Arnold-Chiari disease
  artery (*see also* Atherosclerosis, artery) I70.9 ☑
    stent — *see* Restenosis, stent
    basilar (complete) (partial) — *see* Occlusion,
      artery, basilar
    carotid (complete) (partial) — *see* Occlusion,
      artery, carotid
    cerebellar — *see* Occlusion, artery, cerebellar
    cerebral (anterior) (middle) (posterior) — *see*
      Occlusion, artery, cerebral
    precerebral — *see* Occlusion, artery, precerebral
    renal N28.0
    retinal NEC — *see* Occlusion, artery, retina
    vertebral (complete) (partial) — *see* Occlusion,
      artery, vertebral
  band (intestinal) (*see also* Obstruction, intestine,
    specified NEC) K56.699
  bile duct or passage (common) (hepatic)
    (noncalculous) K83.1
    with calculus K80.51
    congenital (causing jaundice) Q44.3
  biliary (duct) (tract) K83.1
    gallbladder K82.0
  bladder-neck (acquired) N32.0
    congenital Q64.31
    due to hyperplasia (hypertrophy) of prostate —
      see Hyperplasia, prostate
  bowel — *see* Obstruction, intestine
  bronchus J98.09
  canal, ear — *see* Stenosis, external ear canal
  cardia K22.2
  caval veins (inferior) (superior) I87.1
  cecum — *see* Obstruction, intestine
  circulatory I99.8
  colon — *see* Obstruction, intestine
  common duct (noncalculous) K83.1
  coronary (artery) — *see* Occlusion, coronary
  cystic duct (*see also* Obstruction, gallbladder)
    with calculus K80.21
  device, implant or graft (*see also* Complications, by
    site and type, mechanical) T85.698 ☑
    arterial graft NEC — *see* Complication,
      cardiovascular device, mechanical, vascular
    catheter NEC T85.628 ☑
      cystostomy T83.090 ☑
      dialysis (renal) T82.49 ☑
        intraperitoneal T85.691 ☑
      Hopkins T83.098 ☑
      ileostomy T83.098 ☑
      infusion NEC T82.594 ☑
        spinal (epidural) (subdural) T85.690 ☑
      nephrostomy T83.092 ☑
      urethral indwelling T83.091 ☑
      urinary T83.098 ☑
      urostomy T83.098 ☑
    due to infection T85.79 ☑

Obstruction — *continued*
  device — *continued*
    gastrointestinal — *see* Complications, prosthetic device, mechanical, gastrointestinal device
    genital NEC T83.498 ☑
      intrauterine contraceptive device T83.39 ☑
      penile prosthesis (cylinder) (implanted) (pump) (reservoir) T83.490 ☑
      testicular prosthesis T83.491 ☑
    heart NEC — *see* Complication, cardiovascular device, mechanical
    joint prosthesis — *see* Complications, joint prosthesis, mechanical, specified NEC, by site
    orthopedic NEC — *see* Complication, orthopedic, device, mechanical
    specified NEC T85.628 ☑
    urinary NEC (*see also* Complication, genitourinary, device, urinary, mechanical)
      graft T83.29 ☑
    vascular NEC — *see* Complication, cardiovascular device, mechanical
    ventricular intracranial shunt T85.09 ☑
  due to foreign body accidentally left in operative wound T81.529 ☑
  duodenum K31.5
  ejaculatory duct N50.89
  esophagus K22.2
  eustachian tube (complete) (partial) H68.10 ☑
    cartilagenous (extrinsic) H68.13 ☑
      intrinsic H68.12 ☑
    osseous H68.11 ☑
  fallopian tube (bilateral) N97.1
  fecal K56.41
    with hernia — *see* Hernia, by site, with obstruction
  foramen of Monro (congenital) Q03.8
    with spina bifida — *see* Spina bifida, by site, with hydrocephalus
  foreign body — *see* Foreign body
  gallbladder K82.0
    with calculus, stones K80.21
    congenital Q44.1
  gastric outlet K31.1
  gastrointestinal — *see* Obstruction, intestine
  hepatic K76.89
    duct (noncalculous) K83.1
  hepatobiliary K83.1
  ileum — *see* Obstruction, intestine
  iliofemoral (artery) I74.5
  intestine K56.609
    complete K56.601
    incomplete K56.600
    partial K56.600
    with
      adhesions (intestinal) (peritoneal) K56.50
        complete K56.52
        incomplete K56.51
        partial K56.51
    adynamic K56.0
    by gallstone K56.3
    congenital (small) Q41.9
      large Q42.9
        specified part NEC Q42.8
    neurogenic K56.0
      Hirschsprung's disease or megacolon Q43.1
    newborn P76.9
      due to
        fecaliths P76.8
        inspissated milk P76.2
        meconium (plug) P76.0
          in mucoviscidosis E84.11
      specified NEC P76.8
    postoperative K91.30
      complete K91.32
      incomplete K91.31
      partial K91.31
    reflex K56.0
    specified NEC K56.699
      complete K56.691
      incomplete K56.690
      partial K56.690
    volvulus K56.2
  intracardiac ball valve prosthesis T82.09 ☑
  jejunum — *see* Obstruction, intestine
  joint prosthesis — *see* Complications, joint prosthesis, mechanical, specified NEC, by site
  kidney (calices) N28.89
  labor — *see* Delivery
  lacrimal (passages) (duct)
    by
      dacryolith — *see* Dacryolith
      stenosis — *see* Stenosis, lacrimal

Obstruction — *continued*
  lacrimal — *continued*
    congenital Q10.5
    neonatal H04.53 ☑
  lacrimonasal duct — *see* Obstruction, lacrimal
  lacteal, with steatorrhea K90.2
  laryngitis — *see* Laryngitis
  larynx NEC J38.6
    congenital Q31.8
  lung J98.4
    disease, chronic J44.9
  lymphatic I89.0
  meconium (plug)
    newborn P76.0
      due to fecaliths P76.0
      in mucoviscidosis E84.11
  mitral — *see* Stenosis, mitral
  nasal J34.89
  nasolacrimal duct (*see also* Obstruction, lacrimal)
    congenital Q10.5
  nasopharynx J39.2
  nose J34.89
  organ or site, congenital NEC — *see* Atresia, by site
  pancreatic duct K86.89
  parotid duct or gland K11.8
  pelviureteral junction N13.5
    with hydronephrosis N13.0
    congenital Q62.39
  pharynx J39.2
  portal (circulation) (vein) I81
  prostate (*see also* Hyperplasia, prostate)
    valve (urinary) N32.0
  pulmonary valve (heart) I37.0
  pyelonephritis (chronic) N11.1
  pylorus
    adult K31.1
    congenital or infantile Q40.0
  rectosigmoid — *see* Obstruction, intestine
  rectum K62.4
  renal N28.89
    outflow N13.8
    pelvis, congenital Q62.39
  respiratory J98.8
    chronic J44.9
  retinal (vessels) H34.9
  salivary duct (any) K11.8
    with calculus K11.5
  sigmoid — *see* Obstruction, intestine
  sinus (accessory) (nasal) J34.89
  Stensen's duct K11.8
  stomach NEC K31.89
    acute K31.0
    congenital Q40.2
    due to pylorospasm K31.3
  submandibular duct K11.8
  submaxillary gland K11.8
    with calculus K11.5
  thoracic duct I89.0
  thrombotic — *see* Thrombosis
  trachea J39.8
  tracheostomy airway J95.03
  tricuspid (valve) — *see* Stenosis, tricuspid
  upper respiratory, congenital Q34.8
  ureter (functional) (pelvic junction) NEC N13.5
    with
      hydronephrosis N13.1
        with infection N13.6
      pyelonephritis (chronic) N11.1
    congenital Q62.39
    due to calculus — *see* Calculus, ureter
  urethra NEC N36.8
    congenital Q64.39
  urinary (moderate) N13.9
    due to hyperplasia (hypertrophy) of prostate — *see* Hyperplasia, prostate
    organ or tract (lower) N13.9
    prostatic valve N32.0
    specified NEC N13.8
  uropathy N13.9
  uterus N85.8
  vagina N89.5
  valvular — *see* Endocarditis
  vein, venous I87.1
    caval (inferior) (superior) I87.1
    thrombotic — *see* Thrombosis
  vena cava (inferior) (superior) I87.1
  vesical NEC N32.0
  vesicourethral orifice N32.0
    congenital Q64.31
  vessel NEC I99.8
    stent — *see* Restenosis, stent
Obturator — *see* condition

Occlusal wear, teeth K03.0
Occlusio pupillae — *see* Membrane, pupillary
Occlusion, occluded
  anus K62.4
    congenital Q42.3
      with fistula Q42.2
  aortoiliac (chronic) I74.09
  aqueduct of Sylvius G91.1
    congenital Q03.0
      with spina bifida — *see* Spina bifida, by site, with hydrocephalus
  artery (*see also* Atherosclerosis, artery) I70.9 ☑
    auditory, internal I65.8
    basilar I65.1
      with
        infarction I63.22
        due to
          embolism I63.12
          thrombosis I63.02
    brain or cerebral I66.9
      with infarction (due to) I63.5 ☑
        embolism I63.4 ☑
        thrombosis I63.3 ☑
    carotid I65.2 ☑
      with
        infarction I63.23 ☑
        due to
          embolism I63.13 ☑
          thrombosis I63.03 ☑
    cerebellar (anterior inferior) (posterior inferior) (superior) I66.3
      with infarction I63.54 ☑
        due to
          embolism I63.44 ☑
          thrombosis I63.34 ☑
    cerebral I66.9
      with infarction I63.50
        due to
          embolism I63.40
            specified NEC I63.49
          thrombosis I63.30
            specified NEC I63.39
      anterior I66.1 ☑
        with infarction I63.52 ☑
          due to
            embolism I63.42 ☑
            thrombosis I63.32 ☑
      middle I66.0 ☑
        with infarction I63.51 ☑
          due to
            embolism I63.41 ☑
            thrombosis I63.31 ☑
      posterior I66.2 ☑
        with infarction I63.53 ☑
          due to
            embolism I63.43 ☑
            thrombosis I63.33 ☑
      specified NEC I66.8
        with infarction I63.59
          due to
            embolism I63.4 ☑
            thrombosis I63.3 ☑
    choroidal (anterior) — *see* Occlusion, artery, precerebral, specified NEC
    communicating posterior — *see* Occlusion, artery, precerebral, specified NEC
    complete
      coronary I25.82
      extremities I70.92
    coronary (acute) (thrombotic) (without myocardial infarction) I24.0
      with myocardial infarction — *see* Infarction, myocardium
      chronic total I25.82
      complete I25.82
      healed or old I25.2
      total (chronic) I25.82
    hypophyseal — *see* Occlusion, artery, precerebral, specified NEC
    iliac I74.5
    lower extremities due to stenosis or stricture I77.1
    mesenteric (embolic) (thrombotic) (*see also* Infarct, intestine) K55.069
    perforating — *see* Occlusion, artery, cerebral, specified NEC
    peripheral I77.9
      thrombotic or embolic I74.4
    pontine — *see* Occlusion, artery, precerebral, specified NEC
    precerebral I65.9
      with infarction I63.20
        specified NEC I63.29

Occlusion — *continued*
  artery — *continued*
    due to
      embolism I63.10
        specified NEC I63.19
      thrombosis I63.00
        specified NEC I63.09
    basilar — *see* Occlusion, artery, basilar
    carotid — *see* Occlusion, artery, carotid
    puerperal O88.23
    specified NEC I65.8
      with infarction I63.29
        due to
          embolism I63.19
          thrombosis I63.09
    vertebral — *see* Occlusion, artery, vertebral
    renal N28.0
    retinal
      central H34.1 ☑
      partial H34.21 ☑
      branch H34.23 ☑
      transient H34.0 ☑
    spinal — *see* Occlusion, artery, precerebral, vertebral
    total (chronic)
      coronary I25.82
      extremities I70.92
    vertebral I65.0 ☑
      with
        infarction I63.21 ☑
          due to
            embolism I63.11 ☑
            thrombosis I63.01 ☑
  basilar artery — *see* Occlusion, artery, basilar
  bile duct (common) (hepatic) (noncalculous) K83.1
  bowel — *see* Obstruction, intestine
  carotid (artery) (common) (internal) — *see* Occlusion, artery, carotid
  centric (of teeth) M26.59
    maximum intercuspation discrepancy M26.55
  cerebellar (artery) — *see* Occlusion, artery, cerebellar
  cerebral (artery) — *see* Occlusion, artery, cerebral
  cerebrovascular (*see also* Occlusion, artery, cerebral)
    with infarction I63.5 ☑
  cervical canal — *see* Stricture, cervix
  cervix (uteri) — *see* Stricture, cervix
  choanal Q30.0
  choroidal (artery) — *see* Occlusion, artery, precerebral, specified NEC
  colon — *see* Obstruction, intestine
  communicating posterior artery — *see* Occlusion, artery, precerebral, specified NEC
  coronary (artery) (vein) (thrombotic) (*see also* Infarct, myocardium)
    chronic total I25.82
    healed or old I25.2
    not resulting in infarction I24.0
    total (chronic) I25.82
  cystic duct — *see* Obstruction, gallbladder
  embolic — *see* Embolism
  fallopian tube N97.1
    congenital Q50.6
  gallbladder (*see also* Obstruction, gallbladder)
    congenital (causing jaundice) Q44.1
  gingiva, traumatic K06.2
  hymen N89.6
    congenital Q52.3
  hypophyseal (artery) — *see* Occlusion, artery, precerebral, specified NEC
  iliac artery I74.5
  intestine — *see* Obstruction, intestine
  lacrimal passages — *see* Obstruction, lacrimal
  lung J98.4
  lymph or lymphatic channel I89.0
  mammary duct N64.89
  mesenteric artery (embolic) (thrombotic) (*see also* Infarct, intestine) K55.069
  nose J34.89
    congenital Q30.0
  organ or site, congenital NEC — *see* Atresia, by site
  oviduct N97.1
    congenital Q50.6
  peripheral arteries
    due to stricture or stenosis I77.1
    upper extremity I74.2
  pontine (artery) — *see* Occlusion, artery, precerebral, specified NEC
  posterior lingual, of mandibular teeth M26.29
  precerebral artery — *see* Occlusion, artery, precerebral
  punctum lacrimale — *see* Obstruction, lacrimal

Occlusion — *continued*
  pupil — *see* Membrane, pupillary
  pylorus, adult (*see also* Stricture, pylorus) K31.1
  renal artery N28.0
  retina, retinal
    artery — *see* Occlusion, artery, retinal
    vein (central) H34.81 ☑
      engorgement H34.82 ☑
      tributary H34.83 ☑
    vessels H34.9
  spinal artery — *see* Occlusion, artery, precerebral, vertebral
  teeth (mandibular) (posterior lingual) M26.29
  thoracic duct I89.0
  thrombotic — *see* Thrombosis, artery
  traumatic
    edentulous (alveolar) ridge K06.2
    gingiva K06.2
    periodontal K05.5
  tubal N97.1
  ureter (complete) (partial) N13.5
    congenital Q62.10
  ureteropelvic junction N13.5
    congenital Q62.11
  ureterovesical orifice N13.5
    congenital Q62.12
  urethra — *see* Stricture, urethra
  uterus N85.8
  vagina N89.5
  vascular NEC I99.8
  vein — *see* Thrombosis
    retinal — *see* Occlusion, retinal, vein
  vena cava (inferior) (superior) — *see* Embolism, vena cava
  ventricle (brain) NEC G91.1
  vertebral (artery) — *see* Occlusion, artery, vertebral
  vessel (blood) I99.8
  vulva N90.5
Occult
  blood in feces (stools) R19.5
Occupational
  problems NEC Z56.89
Ochlophobia — *see* Agoraphobia
Ochronosis (endogenous) E70.29
Ocular muscle — *see* condition
Oculogyric crisis or disturbance H51.8
  psychogenic F45.8
Oculomotor syndrome H51.9
Oculopathy
  syphilitic NEC A52.71
    congenital
      early A50.01
      late A50.30
    early (secondary) A51.43
    late A52.71
Oddi's sphincter spasm K83.4
Odontalgia K08.89
Odontoameloblastoma — *see* Cyst, calcifying odontogenic
Odontoclasia K03.89
Odontodysplasia, regional K00.4
Odontogenesis imperfecta K00.5
Odontoma (ameloblastic) (complex) (compound) (fibroameloblastic) — *see* Cyst, calcifying odontogenic
Odontomyelitis (closed) (open) K04.01
  irreversible K04.02
  reversible K04.01
Odontorrhagia K08.89
Odontosarcoma, ameloblastic C41.1
  upper jaw (bone) C41.0
Oestriasis — *see* Myiasis
Oguchi's disease H53.63
Ohara's disease — *see* Tularemia
OHS (obesity hypoventilation syndrome) E66.2
Oidiomycosis — *see* Candidiasis
Oidium albicans infection — *see* Candidiasis
Old age (without mention of debility) R54
  dementia F03 ☑
Old (previous) myocardial infarction I25.2
Olfactory — *see* condition
Oligemia — *see* Anemia
Oligoastrocytoma
  specified site — *see* Neoplasm, malignant, by site
  unspecified site C71.9
Oligocythemia D64.9
Oligodendroblastoma
  specified site — *see* Neoplasm, malignant
  unspecified site C71.9
Oligodendroglioma
  anaplastic type
    specified site — *see* Neoplasm, malignant, by site
    unspecified site C71.9

Oligodendroglioma — *continued*
  specified site — *see* Neoplasm, malignant, by site
  unspecified site C71.9
Oligodontia — *see* Anodontia
Oligoencephalon Q02
Oligohidrosis L74.4
Oligohydramnios O41.0 ☑
Oligohydrosis L74.4
Oligomenorrhea N91.5
  primary N91.3
  secondary N91.4
Oligophrenia (*see also* Disability, intellectual)
  phenylpyruvic E70.0
Oligospermia N46.11
  due to
    drug therapy N46.121
    efferent duct obstruction N46.123
    infection N46.122
    radiation N46.124
    specified cause NEC N46.129
    systemic disease N46.125
Oligotrichia — *see* Alopecia
Oliguria R34
  with, complicating or following ectopic or molar pregnancy O08.4
  postprocedural N99.0
Ollier's disease Q78.4
Omentitis — *see* Peritonitis
Omenotocele — *see* Hernia, abdomen, specified site NEC
Omentum, omental — *see* condition
Omphalitis (congenital) (newborn) P38.9
  with mild hemorrhage P38.1
  without hemorrhage P38.9
  not of newborn L08.82
  tetanus A33
Omphalocele Q79.2
Omphalomesenteric duct, persistent Q43.0
Omphalorrhagia, newborn P51.9
Omsk hemorrhagic fever A98.1
Onanism (excessive) F98.8
Onchocerciasis, onchocercosis B73.1
  with
    eye disease B73.00
      endophthalmitis B73.01
      eyelid B73.09
      glaucoma B73.02
      specified NEC B73.09
    eye NEC B73.00
    eyelid B73.09
Oncocytoma — *see* Neoplasm, benign, by site
Oncovirus, as cause of disease classified elsewhere B97.32
Ondine's curse — *see* Apnea, sleep
Oneirophrenia F23
Onychauxis L60.2
  congenital Q84.5
Onychia (*see also* Cellulitis, digit)
  with lymphangitis — *see* Lymphangitis, acute, digit
  candidal B37.2
  dermatophytic B35.1
Onychitis (*see also* Cellulitis, digit)
  with lymphangitis — *see* Lymphangitis, acute, digit
Onychocryptosis L60.0
Onychodystrophy L60.3
  congenital Q84.6
Onychogryphosis, onychogryposis L60.2
Onycholysis L60.1
Onychomadesis L60.8
Onychomalacia L60.3
Onychomycosis (finger) (toe) B35.1
Onycho-osteodysplasia Q87.2
Onychophagia F98.8
Onychophosis L60.8
Onychoptosis L60.8
Onychorrhexis L60.3
  congenital Q84.6
Onychoschizia L60.3
Onyxis (finger) (toe) L60.0
Onyxitis (*see also* Cellulitis, digit)
  with lymphangitis — *see* Lymphangitis, acute, digit
Oophoritis (cystic) (infectional) (interstitial) N70.92
  with salpingitis N70.93
  acute N70.02
    with salpingitis N70.03
  chronic N70.12
    with salpingitis N70.13
  complicating abortion — *see* Abortion, by type, complicated by, oophoritis
Oophorocele N83.4 ☑
Opacity, opacities
  cornea H17. ☑

☑ **Additional character required**

Opacity — *continued*
  cornea — *continued*
    central H17.1 ☑
    congenital Q13.3
    degenerative — *see* Degeneration, cornea
    hereditary — *see* Dystrophy, cornea
    inflammatory — *see* Keratitis
    minor H17.81 ☑
    peripheral H17.82 ☑
    sequelae of trachoma (healed) B94.0
    specified NEC H17.89
  enamel (teeth) (fluoride) (nonfluoride) K00.3
  lens — *see* Cataract
  snowball — *see* Deposit, crystalline
  vitreous (humor) NEC H43.39 ☑
    congenital Q14.0
    membranes and strands H43.31 ☑
Opalescent dentin (hereditary) K00.5
Open, opening
  abnormal, organ or site, congenital — *see*
      Imperfect, closure
  angle with
    borderline
      findings
        high risk H40.02 ☑
        low risk H40.01 ☑
      intraocular pressure H40.00 ☑
    cupping of discs H40.01 ☑
    glaucoma (primary) — *see* Glaucoma, open angle
  bite
    anterior M26.220
    posterior M26.221
  false — *see* Imperfect, closure
  margin on tooth restoration K08.51
  restoration margins of tooth K08.51
  wound — *see* Wound, open
Operational fatigue F48.8
Operative — *see* condition
Operculitis — *see* Periodontitis
Operculum — *see* Break, retina
Ophiasis L63.2
Ophthalmia (*see also* Conjunctivitis) H10.9
  actinic rays — *see* Photokeratitis
  allergic (acute) — *see* Conjunctivitis, acute, atopic
  blennorrhagic (gonococcal) (neonatorum) A54.31
  diphtheritic A36.86
  Egyptian A71.1
  electrica — *see* Photokeratitis
  gonococcal (neonatorum) A54.31
  metastatic — *see* Endophthalmitis, purulent
  migraine — *see* Migraine, ophthalmoplegic
  neonatorum, newborn P39.1
    gonococcal A54.31
  nodosa H16.24 ☑
  purulent — *see* Conjunctivitis, acute, mucopurulent
  spring — *see* Conjunctivitis, acute, atopic
  sympathetic — *see* Uveitis, sympathetic
Ophthalmitis — *see* Ophthalmia
Ophthalmocele (congenital) Q15.8
Ophthalmoneuromyelitis G36.0
Ophthalmoplegia (*see also* Strabismus, paralytic)
  anterior internuclear — *see* Ophthalmoplegia,
      internuclear
  ataxia-areflexia G61.0
  diabetic — *see* E08-E13 with .39
  exophthalmic E05.00
    with thyroid storm E05.01
  external H49.88 ☑
    progressive H49.4 ☑
      with pigmentary retinopathy — *see* Kearns-
          Sayre syndrome
    total H49.3 ☑
  internal (complete) (total) H52.51 ☑
  internuclear H51.2 ☑
  migraine — *see* Migraine, ophthalmoplegic
  Parinaud's H49.88 ☑
  progressive external — *see* Ophthalmoplegia,
      external, progressive
  supranuclear, progressive G23.1
  total (external) — *see* Ophthalmoplegia, external,
      total
Opioid(s)
  abuse — *see* Abuse, drug, opioids
  dependence — *see* Dependence, drug, opioids
  induced, without use disorder
    anxiety disorder F11.988
    delirium F11.921
    depressive disorder F11.94
    sexual dysfunction F11.981
    sleep disorder F11.982
Opisthognathism M26.09
Opisthorchiasis (felineus) (viverrini) B66.0

Opitz' disease D73.2
Opiumism — *see* Dependence, drug, opioid
Oppenheim's disease G70.2
Oppenheim-Urbach disease (necrobiosis lipoidica
    diabeticorum) — *see* E08-E13 with .620
Optic nerve — *see* condition
Orbit — *see* condition
Orchioblastoma C62.9 ☑
Orchitis (gangrenous) (nonspecific) (septic)
    (suppurative) N45.2
  blennorrhagic (gonococcal) (acute) (chronic) A54.23
  chlamydial A56.19
  filarial (*see also* Infestation, filarial) B74.9 *[N51]*
  gonococcal (acute) (chronic) A54.23
  mumps B26.0
  syphilitic A52.76
  tuberculous A18.15
Orf (virus disease) B08.02
Organic (*see also* condition)
  brain syndrome F09
  heart — *see* Disease, heart
  mental disorder F09
  psychosis F09
Orgasm
  anejaculatory N53.13
Oriental
  bilharziasis B65.2
  schistosomiasis B65.2
Orifice — *see* condition
Origin of both great vessels from right ventricle Q20.1
Ormond's disease (with ureteral obstruction) N13.5
  with infection N13.6
Ornithine metabolism disorder E72.4
Ornithinemia (Type I) (Type II) E72.4
Ornithosis A70
Orotaciduria, oroticaciduria (congenital) (hereditary)
    (pyrimidine deficiency) E79.8
  anemia D53.0
Orthodontics
  adjustment Z46.4
  fitting Z46.4
Orthopnea R06.01
Orthopoxvirus B08.09
Os, uterus — *see* condition
Osgood-Schlatter disease or osteochondrosis — *see*
    Osteochondrosis, juvenile, tibia
Osler (-Weber)-Rendu disease I78.0
Osler's nodes I33.0
Osmidrosis L75.0
Osseous — *see* condition
Ossification
  artery — *see* Arteriosclerosis
  auricle (ear) — *see* Disorder, pinna, specified type
      NEC
  bronchial J98.09
  cardiac — *see* Degeneration, myocardial
  cartilage (senile) — *see* Disorder, cartilage, specified
      type NEC
  coronary (artery) — *see* Disease, heart, ischemic,
      atherosclerotic
  diaphragm J98.6
  ear, middle — *see* Otosclerosis
  falx cerebri G96.19
  fontanel, premature Q75.0
  heart (*see also* Degeneration, myocardial)
    valve — *see* Endocarditis
  larynx J38.7
  ligament — *see* Disorder, tendon, specified type
      NEC
    posterior longitudinal — *see* Spondylopathy,
        specified NEC
  meninges (cerebral) (spinal) G96.19
  multiple, eccentric centers — *see* Disorder, bone,
      development or growth
  muscle (*see also* Calcification, muscle)
    due to burns — *see* Myositis, ossificans, in, burns
    paralytic — *see* Myositis, ossificans, in,
        quadriplegia
    progressive — *see* Myositis, ossificans, progressiva
    specified NEC M61.50
      ankle M61.57 ☑
      foot M61.57 ☑
      forearm M61.53 ☑
      hand M61.54 ☑
      lower leg M61.56 ☑
      multiple sites M61.59
      pelvic region M61.55 ☑
      shoulder region M61.51 ☑
      specified site NEC M61.58
      thigh M61.55 ☑
      upper arm M61.52 ☑
    traumatic — *see* Myositis, ossificans, traumatica

Ossification — *continued*
  myocardium, myocardial — *see* Degeneration,
      myocardial
  penis N48.89
  periarticular — *see* Disorder, joint, specified type
      NEC
  pinna — *see* Disorder, pinna, specified type NEC
  rider's bone — *see* Ossification, muscle, specified
      NEC
  sclera H15.89
  subperiosteal, post-traumatic M89.8X ☑
  tendon — *see* Disorder, tendon, specified type NEC
  trachea J39.8
  tympanic membrane — *see* Disorder, tympanic
      membrane, specified NEC
  vitreous (humor) — *see* Deposit, crystalline
Osteitis (*see also* Osteomyelitis)
  alveolar M27.3
  condensans M85.30
    ankle M85.37 ☑
    foot M85.37 ☑
    forearm M85.33 ☑
    hand M85.34 ☑
    lower leg M85.36 ☑
    multiple site M85.39
    neck M85.38
    rib M85.38
    shoulder M85.31 ☑
    skull M85.38
    specified site NEC M85.38
    thigh M85.35 ☑
    toe M85.37 ☑
    upper arm M85.32 ☑
    vertebra M85.38
  deformans M88.9
    in (due to)
      malignant neoplasm of bone C41.9 *[M90.60]*
      neoplastic disease (*see also* Neoplasm) D49.9
          [M90.60]
        carpus D49.9 *[M90.64 ☑]*
        clavicle D49.9 *[M90.61 ☑]*
        femur D49.9 *[M90.65 ☑]*
        fibula D49.9 *[M90.66 ☑]*
        finger D49.9 *[M90.64 ☑]*
        humerus D49.9 *[M90.62 ☑]*
        ilium D49.9 *[M90.65 ☑]*
        ischium D49.9 *[M90.65 ☑]*
        metacarpus D49.9 *[M90.64 ☑]*
        metatarsus D49.9 *[M90.67 ☑]*
        multiple sites D49.9 *[M90.69]*
        neck D49.9 *[M90.68]*
        radius D49.9 *[M90.63 ☑]*
        rib D49.9 *[M90.68]*
        scapula D49.9 *[M90.61 ☑]*
        skull D49.9 *[M90.68]*
        tarsus D49.9 *[M90.67 ☑]*
        tibia D49.9 *[M90.66 ☑]*
        toe D49.9 *[M90.67 ☑]*
        ulna D49.9 *[M90.63 ☑]*
        vertebra D49.9 *[M90.68]*
    skull M88.0
    specified NEC — *see* Paget's disease, bone, by site
    vertebra M88.1
  due to yaws A66.6
  fibrosa NEC — *see* Cyst, bone, by site
    circumscripta — *see* Dysplasia, fibrous, bone NEC
    cystica (generalisata) E21.0
    disseminata Q78.1
    osteoplastica E21.0
  fragilitans Q78.0
  Garr's (sclerosing) — *see* Osteomyelitis, specified
      type NEC
  jaw (acute) (chronic) (lower) (suppurative) (upper)
      M27.2
  parathyroid E21.0
  petrous bone (acute) (chronic) — *see* Petrositis
  sclerotic, nonsuppurative — *see* Osteomyelitis,
      specified type NEC
  tuberculosa A18.09
    cystica D86.89
    multiplex cystoides D86.89
Osteoarthritis M19.90
  ankle M19.07 ☑
  elbow M19.02 ☑
  foot joint M19.07 ☑
  generalized M15.9
    erosive M15.4
    primary M15.0
    specified NEC M15.8
  hand joint M19.04 ☑
    first carpometacarpal joint M18.9
  hip M16.1 ☑

Osteoarthritis — *continued*
  hip — *continued*
    bilateral M16.0
    due to hip dysplasia (unilateral) M16.3 ☑
      bilateral M16.2
    interphalangeal
      distal (Heberden) M15.1
      proximal (Bouchard) M15.2
    knee M17.1 ☑
      bilateral M17.0
    shoulder M19.01 ☑
    spine — *see* Spondylosis
    wrist M19.03 ☑
  post-traumatic NEC M19.92
    ankle M19.17 ☑
    elbow M19.12 ☑
    foot joint M19.17 ☑
    hand joint M19.14 ☑
      first carpometacarpal joint M18.3 ☑
        bilateral M18.2
    hip M16.5 ☑
      bilateral M16.4
    knee M17.3 ☑
      bilateral M17.2
    shoulder M19.11 ☑
    wrist M19.13 ☑
  primary M19.91
    ankle M19.07 ☑
    elbow M19.02 ☑
    foot joint M19.07 ☑
    hand joint M19.04 ☑
      first carpometacarpal joint M18.1 ☑
        bilateral M18.0
    hip M16.1 ☑
      bilateral M16.0
    knee M17.1 ☑
      bilateral M17.0
    multiple sites M89.49
    shoulder M19.01 ☑
    spine — *see* Spondylosis
    wrist M19.03 ☑
  secondary M19.93
    ankle M19.27 ☑
    elbow M19.22 ☑
    foot joint M19.27 ☑
    hand joint M19.24 ☑
      first carpometacarpal joint M18.5 ☑
        bilateral M18.4
    hip M16.7 ☑
      bilateral M16.6
    knee M17.5 ☑
      bilateral M17.4
    multiple M15.3
    shoulder M19.21 ☑
    spine — *see* Spondylosis
    wrist M19.23 ☑
Osteoarthropathy (hypertrophic) M19.90
  ankle — *see* Osteoarthritis, primary, ankle
  elbow — *see* Osteoarthritis, primary, elbow
  foot joint — *see* Osteoarthritis, primary, foot
  hand joint — *see* Osteoarthritis, primary, hand joint
  knee joint — *see* Osteoarthritis, primary, knee
  multiple site — *see* Osteoarthritis, primary, multiple joint
  pulmonary (*see also* Osteoarthropathy, specified type NEC)
    hypertrophic — *see* Osteoarthropathy, hypertrophic, specified type NEC
    secondary hypertrophic — *see* Osteoarthropathy, specified type NEC
  shoulder — *see* Osteoarthritis, primary, shoulder
  specified joint NEC — *see* Osteoarthritis, primary, specified joint NEC
  specified type NEC M89.40
    carpus M89.44 ☑
    clavicle M89.41 ☑
    femur M89.45 ☑
    fibula M89.46 ☑
    finger M89.44 ☑
    humerus M89.42 ☑
    ilium M89.459
    ischium M89.459
    metacarpus M89.44 ☑
    metatarsus M89.47 ☑
    multiple sites M89.49
    neck M89.48
    radius M89.43 ☑
    rib M89.48
    scapula M89.41 ☑
    skull M89.48
    tarsus M89.47 ☑
    tibia M89.46 ☑

Osteoarthropathy — *continued*
  specified type NEC — *continued*
    toe M89.47 ☑
    ulna M89.43 ☑
    vertebra M89.48
  secondary — *see* Osteoarthropathy, specified type NEC
  spine — *see* Spondylosis
  wrist — *see* Osteoarthritis, primary, wrist
Osteoarthrosis (degenerative) (hypertrophic) (joint) (*see also* Osteoarthritis)
  deformans alkaptonurica E70.29 *[M36.8]*
  erosive M15.4
  generalized M15.9
    primary M15.0
  polyarticular M15.9
  spine — *see* Spondylosis
Osteoblastoma — *see* Neoplasm, bone, benign
  aggressive — *see* Neoplasm, bone, uncertain behavior
Osteochondroarthrosis deformans endemica — *see* Disease, Kaschin-Beck
Osteochondritis (*see also* Osteochondropathy, by site)
  Brailsford's — *see* Osteochondrosis, juvenile, radius
  dissecans M93.20
    ankle M93.27 ☑
    elbow M93.22 ☑
    foot M93.27 ☑
    hand M93.24 ☑
    hip M93.25 ☑
    knee M93.26 ☑
    multiple sites M93.29
    shoulder joint M93.21 ☑
    specified site NEC M93.28
    wrist M93.23 ☑
  juvenile M92.9
    patellar — *see* Osteochondrosis, juvenile, patella
  syphilitic (congenital) (early) A50.02 *[M90.80]*
    ankle A50.02 *[M90.87 ☑]*
    elbow A50.02 *[M90.82 ☑]*
    foot A50.02 *[M90.87 ☑]*
    forearm A50.02 *[M90.83 ☑]*
    hand A50.02 *[M90.84 ☑]*
    hip A50.02 *[M90.85 ☑]*
    knee A50.02 *[M90.86 ☑]*
    multiple sites A50.02 *[M90.89]*
    shoulder joint A50.02 *[M90.81 ☑]*
    specified site NEC A50.02 *[M90.88]*
Osteochondrodysplasia Q78.9
  with defects of growth of tubular bones and spine Q77.9
    specified NEC Q77.8
  specified NEC Q78.8
Osteochondrodystrophy E78.9
Osteochondrolysis — *see* Osteochondritis, dissecans
Osteochondroma — *see* Neoplasm, bone, benign
Osteochondromatosis D48.0
  syndrome Q78.4
Osteochondromyxosarcoma — *see* Neoplasm, bone, malignant
Osteochondropathy M93.90
  ankle M93.97 ☑
  elbow M93.92 ☑
  foot M93.97 ☑
  hand M93.94 ☑
  hip M93.95 ☑
  Kienböck's disease of adults M93.1
  knee M93.96 ☑
  multiple joints M93.99
  osteochondritis dissecans — *see* Osteochondritis, dissecans
  osteochondrosis — *see* Osteochondrosis
  shoulder region M93.91 ☑
  slipped upper femoral epiphysis — *see* Slipped, epiphysis, upper femoral
  specified joint NEC M93.98
  specified type NEC M93.80
    ankle M93.87 ☑
    elbow M93.82 ☑
    foot M93.87 ☑
    hand M93.84 ☑
    hip M93.85 ☑
    knee M93.86 ☑
    multiple joints M93.89
    shoulder region M93.81 ☑
    specified joint NEC M93.88
    wrist M93.83 ☑
  syphilitic, congenital
    early A50.02 *[M90.80]*
    late A50.56 *[M90.80]*
  wrist M93.93 ☑

Osteochondrosarcoma — *see* Neoplasm, bone, malignant
Osteochondrosis (*see also* Osteochondropathy, by site)
  acetabulum (juvenile) M91.0
  adult — *see* Osteochondropathy, specified type NEC, by site
  astragalus (juvenile) — *see* Osteochondrosis, juvenile, tarsus
  Blount's — *see* Osteochondrosis, juvenile, tibia
  Buchanan's M91.0
  Burns' — *see* Osteochondrosis, juvenile, ulna
  calcaneus (juvenile) — *see* Osteochondrosis, juvenile, tarsus
  capitular epiphysis (femur) (juvenile) — *see* Legg-Calvé-Perthes disease
  carpal (juvenile) (lunate) (scaphoid) — *see* Osteochondrosis, juvenile, hand, carpal lunate
    adult M93.1
  coxae juvenilis — *see* Legg-Calvé-Perthes disease
  deformans juvenilis, coxae — *see* Legg-Calvé-Perthes disease
  Diaz's — *see* Osteochondrosis, juvenile, tarsus
  dissecans (knee) (shoulder) — *see* Osteochondritis, dissecans
  femoral capital epiphysis (juvenile) — *see* Legg-Calvé-Perthes disease
  femur (head), juvenile — *see* Legg-Calvé-Perthes disease
  fibula (juvenile) — *see* Osteochondrosis, juvenile, fibula
  foot NEC (juvenile) M92.8
  Freiberg's — *see* Osteochondrosis, juvenile, metatarsus
  Haas' (juvenile) — *see* Osteochondrosis, juvenile, humerus
  Haglund's — *see* Osteochondrosis, juvenile, tarsus
  hip (juvenile) — *see* Legg-Calvé-Perthes disease
  humerus (capitulum) (head) (juvenile) — *see* Osteochondrosis, juvenile, humerus
  ilium, iliac crest (juvenile) M91.0
  ischiopubic synchondrosis M91.0
  Iselin's — *see* Osteochondrosis, juvenile, metatarsus
  juvenile, juvenilis M92.9
    after congenital dislocation of hip reduction — *see* Osteochondrosis, juvenile, hip, specified NEC
    arm — *see* Osteochondrosis, juvenile, upper limb NEC
    capitular epiphysis (femur) — *see* Legg-Calvé-Perthes disease
    clavicle, sternal epiphysis — *see* Osteochondrosis, juvenile, upper limb NEC
    coxae — *see* Legg-Calvé-Perthes disease
    deformans M92.9
    fibula M92.5 ☑
    foot NEC M92.8
    hand M92.20 ☑
      carpal lunate M92.21 ☑
      metacarpal head M92.22 ☑
      specified site NEC M92.29 ☑
    head of femur — *see* Legg-Calvé-Perthes disease
    hip and pelvis M91.9 ☑
      coxa plana — *see* Coxa, plana
      femoral head — *see* Legg-Calvé-Perthes disease
      pelvis M91.0
      pseudocoxalgia — *see* Pseudocoxalgia
      specified NEC M91.8 ☑
    humerus M92.0 ☑
    limb
      lower NEC M92.8
      upper NEC — *see* Osteochondrosis, juvenile, upper limb NEC
    medial cuneiform bone — *see* Osteochondrosis, juvenile, tarsus
    metatarsus M92.7 ☑
    patella M92.4 ☑
    radius M92.1 ☑
    specified site NEC M92.8
    spine M42.00
      cervical region M42.02
      cervicothoracic region M42.03
      lumbar region M42.06
      lumbosacral region M42.07
      multiple sites M42.09
      occipito-atlanto-axial region M42.01
      sacrococcygeal region M42.08
      thoracic region M42.04
      thoracolumbar region M42.05
    tarsus M92.6 ☑
    tibia M92.5 ☑
    ulna M92.1 ☑
    upper limb NEC M92.3 ☑

Osteochondrosis — continued
  juvenile — continued
    vertebra (body) (epiphyseal plates) (Calvé's) (Scheuermann's) — see Osteochondrosis, juvenile, spine
    Kienböck's — see Osteochondrosis, juvenile, hand, carpal lunate
      adult M93.1
    Köhler's
      patellar — see Osteochondrosis, juvenile, patella
      tarsal navicular — see Osteochondrosis, juvenile, tarsus
    Legg-Perthes (-Calvé)(-Waldenström) — see Legg-Calvé-Perthes disease
    limb
      lower NEC (juvenile) M92.8
      upper NEC (juvenile) — see Osteochondrosis, juvenile, upper limb NEC
    lunate bone (carpal) (juvenile) (see also Osteochondrosis, juvenile, hand, carpal lunate)
      adult M93.1
    Mauclaire's — see Osteochondrosis, juvenile, hand, metacarpal
    metacarpal (head) (juvenile) — see Osteochondrosis, juvenile, hand, metacarpal
    metatarsus (fifth) (head) (juvenile) (second) — see Osteochondrosis, juvenile, metatarsus
    navicular (juvenile) — see Osteochondrosis, juvenile, tarsus
    os
      calcis (juvenile) — see Osteochondrosis, juvenile, tarsus
      tibiale externum (juvenile) — see Osteochondrosis, juvenile, tarsus
    Osgood-Schlatter — see Osteochondrosis, juvenile, tibia
    Panner's — see Osteochondrosis, juvenile, humerus
    patellar center (juvenile) (primary) (secondary) — see Osteochondrosis, juvenile, patella
    pelvis (juvenile) M91.0
    Pierson's M91.0
    radius (head) (juvenile) — see Osteochondrosis, juvenile, radius
    Scheuermann's — see Osteochondrosis, juvenile, spine
    Sever's — see Osteochondrosis, juvenile, tarsus
    Sinding-Larsen — see Osteochondrosis, juvenile, patella
    spine M42.9
      adult M42.10
        cervical region M42.12
        cervicothoracic region M42.13
        lumbar region M42.16
        lumbosacral region M42.17
        multiple sites M42.19
        occipito-atlanto-axial region M42.11
        sacrococcygeal region M42.18
        thoracic region M42.14
        thoracolumbar region M42.15
      juvenile — see Osteochondrosis, juvenile, spine
    symphysis pubis (juvenile) M91.0
    syphilitic (congenital) A50.02
    talus (juvenile) — see Osteochondrosis, juvenile, tarsus
    tarsus (navicular) (juvenile) — see Osteochondrosis, juvenile, tarsus
    tibia (proximal) (tubercle) (juvenile) — see Osteochondrosis, juvenile, tibia
    tuberculous — see Tuberculosis, bone
    ulna (lower) (juvenile) — see Osteochondrosis, juvenile, ulna
    van Neck's M91.0
    vertebral — see Osteochondrosis, spine
Osteoclastoma D48.0
  malignant — see Neoplasm, bone, malignant
Osteodynia — see Disorder, bone, specified type NEC
Osteodystrophy Q78.9
  azotemic N25.0
  congenital Q78.9
  parathyroid, secondary E21.1
  renal N25.0
Osteofibroma — see Neoplasm, bone, benign
Osteofibrosarcoma — see Neoplasm, bone, malignant
Osteogenesis imperfecta Q78.0
Osteogenic — see condition
Osteolysis M89.50
  carpus M89.54 ☑
  clavicle M89.51 ☑
  femur M89.55 ☑
  fibula M89.56 ☑
  finger M89.54 ☑
  humerus M89.52 ☑

Osteolysis — continued
  ilium M89.559
  ischium M89.559
  joint prosthesis (periprosthetic) — see Complications, joint prosthesis, mechanical, periprosthetic, osteolysis, by site
  metacarpus M89.54 ☑
  metatarsus M89.57 ☑
  multiple sites M89.59
  neck M89.58
  periprosthetic — see Complications, joint prosthesis, mechanical, periprosthetic, osteolysis, by site
  radius M89.53 ☑
  rib M89.58
  scapula M89.51 ☑
  skull M89.58
  tarsus M89.57 ☑
  tibia M89.56 ☑
  toe M89.57 ☑
  ulna M89.53 ☑
  vertebra M89.58
Osteoma (see also Neoplasm, bone, benign)
  osteoid (see also Neoplasm, bone, benign)
    giant — see Neoplasm, bone, benign
Osteomalacia M83.9
  adult M83.9
    drug-induced NEC M83.5
    due to
      malabsorption (postsurgical) M83.2
      malnutrition M83.3
    specified NEC M83.8
  aluminium-induced M83.4
  infantile — see Rickets
  juvenile — see Rickets
  oncogenic E83.89
  pelvis M83.8
  puerperal M83.0
  senile M83.1
  vitamin-D-resistant in adults E83.31 [M90.8 ☑]
    carpus E83.31 [M90.84 ☑]
    clavicle E83.31 [M90.81 ☑]
    femur E83.31 [M90.85 ☑]
    fibula E83.31 [M90.86 ☑]
    finger E83.31 [M90.84 ☑]
    humerus E83.31 [M90.82 ☑]
    ilium E83.31 [M90.859]
    ischium E83.31 [M90.859]
    metacarpus E83.31 [M90.84 ☑]
    metatarsus E83.31 [M90.87 ☑]
    multiple sites E83.31 [M90.89]
    neck E83.31 [M90.88]
    radius E83.31 [M90.83 ☑]
    rib E83.31 [M90.88]
    scapula E83.31 [M90.819]
    skull E83.31 [M90.88]
    tarsus E83.31 [M90.879]
    tibia E83.31 [M90.869]
    toe E83.31 [M90.879]
    ulna E83.31 [M90.839]
    vertebra E83.31 [M90.88]
Osteomyelitis (general) (infective) (localized) (neonatal) (purulent) (septic) (staphylococcal) (streptococcal) (suppurative) (with periostitis) M86.9
  acute M86.10
    carpus M86.14 ☑
    clavicle M86.11 ☑
    femur M86.15 ☑
    fibula M86.16 ☑
    finger M86.14 ☑
    hematogenous M86.00
      carpus M86.04 ☑
      clavicle M86.01 ☑
      femur M86.05 ☑
      fibula M86.06 ☑
      finger M86.04 ☑
      humerus M86.02 ☑
      ilium M86.059
      ischium M86.059
      mandible M27.2
      metacarpus M86.04 ☑
      metatarsus M86.07 ☑
      multiple sites M86.09
      neck M86.08
      orbit H05.02 ☑
      petrous bone — see Petrositis
      radius M86.03 ☑
      rib M86.08
      scapula M86.01 ☑
      skull M86.08
      tarsus M86.07 ☑
      tibia M86.06 ☑

Osteomyelitis — continued
  acute — continued
    toe M86.07 ☑
    ulna M86.03 ☑
    vertebra — see Osteomyelitis, vertebra
    humerus M86.12 ☑
    ilium M86.18
    ischium M86.18
    mandible M27.2
    metacarpus M86.14 ☑
    metatarsus M86.17 ☑
    multiple sites M86.19
    neck M86.18
    orbit H05.02 ☑
    petrous bone — see Petrositis
    radius M86.13 ☑
    rib M86.18
    scapula M86.11 ☑
    skull M86.18
    tarsus M86.17 ☑
    tibia M86.16 ☑
    toe M86.17 ☑
    ulna M86.13 ☑
    vertebra — see Osteomyelitis, vertebra
  chronic (or old) M86.60
    with draining sinus M86.40
      carpus M86.44 ☑
      clavicle M86.41 ☑
      femur M86.45 ☑
      fibula M86.46 ☑
      finger M86.44 ☑
      humerus M86.42 ☑
      ilium M86.459
      ischium M86.459
      mandible M27.2
      metacarpus M86.44 ☑
      metatarsus M86.47 ☑
      multiple sites M86.49
      neck M86.48
      orbit H05.02 ☑
      petrous bone — see Petrositis
      radius M86.43 ☑
      rib M86.48
      scapula M86.41 ☑
      skull M86.48
      tarsus M86.47 ☑
      tibia M86.46 ☑
      toe M86.47 ☑
      ulna M86.43 ☑
      vertebra — see Osteomyelitis, vertebra
    carpus M86.64 ☑
    clavicle M86.61 ☑
    femur M86.65 ☑
    fibula M86.66 ☑
    finger M86.64 ☑
    hematogenous NEC M86.50
      carpus M86.54 ☑
      clavicle M86.51 ☑
      femur M86.55 ☑
      fibula M86.56 ☑
      finger M86.54 ☑
      humerus M86.52 ☑
      ilium M86.559
      ischium M86.559
      mandible M27.2
      metacarpus M86.54 ☑
      metatarsus M86.57 ☑
      multifocal M86.30
        carpus M86.34 ☑
        clavicle M86.31 ☑
        femur M86.35 ☑
        fibula M86.36 ☑
        finger M86.34 ☑
        humerus M86.32 ☑
        ilium M86.359
        ischium M86.359
        metacarpus M86.34 ☑
        metatarsus M86.37 ☑
        multiple sites M86.39
        neck M86.38
        radius M86.33 ☑
        rib M86.38
        scapula M86.31 ☑
        skull M86.38
        tarsus M86.37 ☑
        tibia M86.36 ☑
        toe M86.37 ☑
        ulna M86.33 ☑
        vertebra — see Osteomyelitis, vertebra
      multiple sites M86.59
      neck M86.58
      orbit H05.02 ☑

Osteomyelitis - Osteopathy

Osteomyelitis — *continued*
  chronic — *continued*
    petrous bone — *see* Petrositis
    radius M86.53 ☑
    rib M86.58
    scapula M86.51 ☑
    skull M86.58
    tarsus M86.57 ☑
    tibia M86.56 ☑
    toe M86.57 ☑
    ulna M86.53 ☑
    vertebra — *see* Osteomyelitis, vertebra
    humerus M86.62 ☑
    ilium M86.659
    ischium M86.659
    mandible M27.2
    metacarpus M86.64 ☑
    metatarsus M86.67 ☑
    multifocal — *see* Osteomyelitis, chronic,
      hematogenous, multifocal
    multiple sites M86.69
    neck M86.68
    orbit H05.02 ☑
    petrous bone — *see* Petrositis
    radius M86.63 ☑
    rib M86.68
    scapula M86.61 ☑
    skull M86.68
    tarsus M86.67 ☑
    tibia M86.66 ☑
    toe M86.67 ☑
    ulna M86.63 ☑
    vertebra — *see* Osteomyelitis, vertebra
  echinococcal B67.2
  Garr's — *see* Osteomyelitis, specified type NEC
  in diabetes mellitus — *see* E08-E13 with .69
  jaw (acute) (chronic) (lower) (neonatal)
    (suppurative) (upper) M27.2
  nonsuppurating — *see* Osteomyelitis, specified
    type NEC
  orbit H05.02 ☑
  petrous bone — *see* Petrositis
  Salmonella (arizonae) (cholerae-suis) (enteritidis)
    (typhimurium) A02.24
  sclerosing, nonsuppurative — *see* Osteomyelitis,
    specified type NEC
  specified type NEC (*see also* subcategory) M86.8X ☑
    mandible M27.2
    orbit H05.02 ☑
    petrous bone — *see* Petrositis
    vertebra — *see* Osteomyelitis, vertebra
  subacute M86.20
    carpus M86.24 ☑
    clavicle M86.21 ☑
    femur M86.25 ☑
    fibula M86.26 ☑
    finger M86.24 ☑
    humerus M86.22 ☑
    mandible M27.2
    metacarpus M86.24 ☑
    metatarsus M86.27 ☑
    multiple sites M86.29
    neck M86.28
    orbit H05.02 ☑
    petrous bone — *see* Petrositis
    radius M86.23 ☑
    rib M86.28
    scapula M86.21 ☑
    skull M86.28
    tarsus M86.27 ☑
    tibia M86.26 ☑
    toe M86.27 ☑
    ulna M86.23 ☑
    vertebra — *see* Osteomyelitis, vertebra
  syphilitic A52.77
    congenital (early) A50.02 *[M90.80]*
  tuberculous — *see* Tuberculosis, bone
  typhoid A01.05
  vertebra M46.20
    cervical region M46.22
    cervicothoracic region M46.23
    lumbar region M46.26
    lumbosacral region M46.27
    occipito-atlanto-axial region M46.21
    sacrococcygeal region M46.28
    thoracic region M46.24
    thoracolumbar region M46.25
Osteomyelofibrosis D47.4
Osteomyelosclerosis D75.89
Osteonecrosis M87.9
  due to
    drugs — *see* Osteonecrosis, secondary, due to, drugs

Osteonecrosis — *continued*
  due to — *continued*
    trauma — *see* Osteonecrosis, secondary, due to,
      trauma
  idiopathic aseptic M87.00
    ankle M87.07 ☑
    carpus M87.03 ☑
    clavicle M87.01 ☑
    femur M87.05 ☑
    fibula M87.06 ☑
    finger M87.04 ☑
    humerus M87.02 ☑
    ilium M87.050
    ischium M87.050
    metacarpus M87.04 ☑
    metatarsus M87.07 ☑
    multiple sites M87.09
    neck M87.08
    pelvis M87.050
    radius M87.03 ☑
    rib M87.08
    scapula M87.01 ☑
    skull M87.08
    tarsus M87.07 ☑
    tibia M87.06 ☑
    toe M87.07 ☑
    ulna M87.03 ☑
    vertebra M87.08
  secondary NEC M87.30
    carpus M87.33 ☑
    clavicle M87.31 ☑
    due to
      drugs M87.10
        carpus M87.13 ☑
        clavicle M87.11 ☑
        femur M87.15 ☑
        fibula M87.16 ☑
        finger M87.14 ☑
        humerus M87.12 ☑
        ilium M87.159
        ischium M87.159
        jaw M87.180
        metacarpus M87.14 ☑
        metatarsus M87.17 ☑
        multiple sites M87.19
        neck M87.18 ☑
        radius M87.13 ☑
        rib M87.18 ☑
        scapula M87.11 ☑
        skull M87.18 ☑
        tarsus M87.17 ☑
        tibia M87.16 ☑
        toe M87.17 ☑
        ulna M87.13 ☑
        vertebra M87.18 ☑
      hemoglobinopathy NEC D58.2 *[M90.50]*
        carpus D58.2 *[M90.54 ☑]*
        clavicle D58.2 *[M90.51 ☑]*
        femur D58.2 *[M90.55 ☑]*
        fibula D58.2 *[M90.56 ☑]*
        finger D58.2 *[M90.54 ☑]*
        humerus D58.2 *[M90.52 ☑]*
        ilium D58.2 *[M90.55 ☑]*
        ischium D58.2 *[M90.55 ☑]*
        metacarpus D58.2 *[M90.54 ☑]*
        metatarsus D58.2 *[M90.57 ☑]*
        multiple sites D58.2 *[M90.58]*
        neck D58.2 *[M90.58]*
        radius D58.2 *[M90.53 ☑]*
        rib D58.2 *[M90.58]*
        scapula D58.2 *[M90.51 ☑]*
        skull D58.2 *[M90.58]*
        tarsus D58.2 *[M90.57 ☑]*
        tibia D58.2 *[M90.56 ☑]*
        toe D58.2 *[M90.57 ☑]*
        ulna D58.2 *[M90.53 ☑]*
        vertebra D58.2 *[M90.58]*
      trauma (previous) M87.20
        carpus M87.23 ☑
        clavicle M87.21 ☑
        femur M87.25 ☑
        fibula M87.26 ☑
        finger M87.24 ☑
        humerus M87.22 ☑
        ilium M87.25 ☑
        ischium M87.25 ☑
        metacarpus M87.24 ☑
        metatarsus M87.27 ☑
        multiple sites M87.29
        neck M87.28
        radius M87.23 ☑
        rib M87.28

Osteonecrosis — *continued*
  secondary NEC — *continued*
    scapula M87.21 ☑
    skull M87.28
    tarsus M87.27 ☑
    tibia M87.26 ☑
    toe M87.27 ☑
    ulna M87.23 ☑
    vertebra M87.28
    femur M87.35 ☑
    fibula M87.36 ☑
    finger M87.34 ☑
    humerus M87.32 ☑
    ilium M87.350
    in
      caisson disease T70.3 ☑ *[M90.50]*
        carpus T70.3 ☑ *[M90.54]*
        clavicle T70.3 ☑ *[M90.51 ☑]*
        femur T70.3 ☑ *[M90.55 ☑]*
        fibula T70.3 ☑ *[M90.56 ☑]*
        finger T70.3 ☑ *[M90.54 ☑]*
        humerus T70.3 ☑ *[M90.52 ☑]*
        ilium T70.3 ☑ *[M90.55 ☑]*
        ischium T70.3 ☑ *[M90.55 ☑]*
        metacarpus T70.3 ☑ *[M90.54 ☑]*
        metatarsus T70.3 ☑ *[M90.57 ☑]*
        multiple sites T70.3 ☑ *[M90.59]*
        neck T70.3 ☑ *[M90.58]*
        radius T70.3 ☑ *[M90.53 ☑]*
        rib T70.3 ☑ *[M90.58]*
        scapula T70.3 ☑ *[M90.51 ☑]*
        skull T70.3 ☑ *[M90.58]*
        tarsus T70.3 ☑ *[M90.57 ☑]*
        tibia T70.3 ☑ *[M90.56 ☑]*
        toe T70.3 ☑ *[M90.57 ☑]*
        ulna T70.3 ☑ *[M90.53 ☑]*
        vertebra T70.3 ☑ *[M90.58]*
    ischium M87.350
    metacarpus M87.34 ☑
    metatarsus M87.37 ☑
    multiple site M87.39
    neck M87.38
    radius M87.33 ☑
    rib M87.38
    scapula M87.319
    skull M87.38
    tarsus M87.379
    tibia M87.366
    toe M87.379
    ulna M87.33 ☑
    vertebra M87.38
  specified type NEC M87.80
    carpus M87.83 ☑
    clavicle M87.81 ☑
    femur M87.85 ☑
    fibula M87.86 ☑
    finger M87.84 ☑
    humerus M87.82 ☑
    ilium M87.85 ☑
    ischium M87.85 ☑
    metacarpus M87.84 ☑
    metatarsus M87.87 ☑
    multiple sites M87.89
    neck M87.88
    radius M87.83 ☑
    rib M87.88
    scapula M87.81 ☑
    skull M87.88
    tarsus M87.87 ☑
    tibia M87.86 ☑
    toe M87.87 ☑
    ulna M87.83 ☑
    vertebra M87.88
Osteo-onycho-arthro-dysplasia Q87.2
Osteo-onychodysplasia, hereditary Q87.2
Osteopathia condensans disseminata Q78.8
Osteopathy (*see also* Osteomyelitis, Osteonecrosis,
  Osteoporosis)
  after poliomyelitis M89.60
    carpus M89.64 ☑
    clavicle M89.61 ☑
    femur M89.65 ☑
    fibula M89.66 ☑
    finger M89.64 ☑
    humerus M89.62 ☑
    ilium M89.659
    ischium M89.659
    metacarpus M89.64 ☑
    metatarsus M89.67 ☑
    multiple sites M89.69
    neck M89.68
    radius M89.63 ☑

☑ **Additional character required**

Osteopathy — *continued*
  after poliomyelitis — *continued*
    rib M89.68
    scapula M89.61 ☑
    skull M89.68
    tarsus M89.67 ☑
    tibia M89.66 ☑
    toe M89.67 ☑
    ulna M89.63 ☑
    vertebra M89.68
  in (due to)
    renal osteodystrophy N25.0
    specified diseases classified elsewhere — *see* subcategory M90.8 ☑
Osteopenia M85.8 ☑
  borderline M85.8 ☑
Osteoperiostitis — *see* Osteomyelitis, specified type NEC
Osteopetrosis (familial) Q78.2
Osteophyte M25.70
  ankle M25.77 ☑
  elbow M25.72 ☑
  foot joint M25.77 ☑
  hand joint M25.74 ☑
  hip M25.75 ☑
  knee M25.76 ☑
  shoulder M25.71 ☑
  spine M25.78
  vertebrae M25.78
  wrist M25.73 ☑
Osteopoikilosis Q78.8
Osteoporosis (female) (male) M81.0
  with current pathological fracture M80.00 ☑
  age-related M81.0
    with current pathologic fracture M80.00 ☑
      carpus M80.04 ☑
      clavicle M80.01 ☑
      fibula M80.06 ☑
      finger M80.04 ☑
      humerus M80.02 ☑
      ilium M80.05 ☑
      ischium M80.05 ☑
      metacarpus M80.04 ☑
      metatarsus M80.07 ☑
      pelvis M80.05 ☑
      radius M80.03 ☑
      scapula M80.01 ☑
      tarsus M80.07 ☑
      tibia M80.06 ☑
      toe M80.07 ☑
      ulna M80.03 ☑
      vertebra M80.08 ☑
  disuse M81.8
    with current pathological fracture M80.80 ☑
      carpus M80.84 ☑
      clavicle M80.81 ☑
      fibula M80.86 ☑
      finger M80.84 ☑
      humerus M80.82 ☑
      ilium M80.85 ☑
      ischium M80.85 ☑
      metacarpus M80.84 ☑
      metatarsus M80.87 ☑
      pelvis M80.85 ☑
      radius M80.83 ☑
      scapula M80.81 ☑
      tarsus M80.87 ☑
      tibia M80.86 ☑
      toe M80.87 ☑
      ulna M80.83 ☑
      vertebra M80.88 ☑
  drug-induced — *see* Osteoporosis, specified type NEC
  idiopathic — *see* Osteoporosis, specified type NEC
  involutional — *see* Osteoporosis, age-related
  Lequesne M81.6
  localized M81.6
  postmenopausal M81.0
    with pathological fracture M80.00 ☑
      carpus M80.04 ☑
      clavicle M80.01 ☑
      fibula M80.06 ☑
      finger M80.04 ☑
      humerus M80.02 ☑
      ilium M80.05 ☑
      ischium M80.05 ☑
      metacarpus M80.04 ☑
      metatarsus M80.07 ☑
      pelvis M80.05 ☑
      radius M80.03 ☑
      scapula M80.01 ☑
      tarsus M80.07 ☑

Osteoporosis — *continued*
  postmenopausal — *continued*
    tibia M80.06 ☑
    toe M80.07 ☑
    ulna M80.03 ☑
    vertebra M80.08 ☑
  postoophorectomy — *see* Osteoporosis, specified type NEC
  postsurgical malabsorption — *see* Osteoporosis, specified type NEC
  post-traumatic — *see* Osteoporosis, specified type NEC
  senile — *see* Osteoporosis, age-related
  specified type NEC M81.8
    with pathological fracture M80.80 ☑
      carpus M80.84 ☑
      clavicle M80.81 ☑
      fibula M80.86 ☑
      finger M80.84 ☑
      humerus M80.82 ☑
      ilium M80.85 ☑
      ischium M80.85 ☑
      metacarpus M80.84 ☑
      metatarsus M80.87 ☑
      pelvis M80.85 ☑
      radius M80.83 ☑
      scapula M80.81 ☑
      tarsus M80.87 ☑
      tibia M80.86 ☑
      toe M80.87 ☑
      ulna M80.83 ☑
      vertebra M80.88 ☑
Osteopsathyrosis (idiopathica) Q78.0
Osteoradionecrosis, jaw (acute) (chronic) (lower) (suppurative) (upper) M27.2
Osteosarcoma (any form) — *see* Neoplasm, bone, malignant
Osteosclerosis Q78.2
  acquired M85.8 ☑
  congenita Q77.4
  fragilitas (generalisata) Q78.2
  myelofibrosis D75.81
Osteosclerotic anemia D64.89
Osteosis
  cutis L94.2
  renal fibrocystic N25.0
Österreicher-Turner syndrome Q87.2
Ostium
  atrioventriculare commune Q21.2
  primum (arteriosum) (defect) (persistent) Q21.2
  secundum (arteriosum) (defect) (patent) (persistent) Q21.1
Ostrum-Furst syndrome Q75.8
Otalgia — *see* subcategory H92.0 ☑
Otitis (acute) H66.90
  with effusion (*see also* Otitis, media, nonsuppurative)
    purulent — *see* Otitis, media, suppurative
  adhesive — *see* subcategory H74.1 ☑
  chronic (*see also* Otitis, media, chronic)
    with effusion (*see also* Otitis, media, nonsuppurative, chronic)
  externa H60.9 ☑
    abscess — *see* Abscess, ear, external
    acute (noninfective) H60.50 ☑
      actinic H60.51 ☑
      chemical H60.52 ☑
      contact H60.53 ☑
      eczematoid H60.54 ☑
      infective — *see* Otitis, externa, infective
      reactive H60.55 ☑
      specified NEC H60.59 ☑
    cellulitis — *see* Cellulitis, ear
    chronic H60.6 ☑
    diffuse — *see* Otitis, externa, infective, diffuse
    hemorrhagic — *see* Otitis, externa, infective, hemorrhagic
    in (due to)
      aspergillosis B44.89
      candidiasis B37.84
      erysipelas A46 *[H62.40]*
      herpes (simplex) virus infection B00.1
        zoster B02.8
      impetigo L01.00 *[H62.40]*
      infectious disease NEC B99 ☑ *[H62.4 ☑]*
      mycosis NEC B36.9 *[H62.40]*
      parasitic disease NEC B89 *[H62.40]*
      viral disease NEC B34.9 *[H62.40]*
      zoster B02.8
    infective NEC H60.39 ☑
      abscess — *see* Abscess, ear, external
      cellulitis — *see* Cellulitis, ear

Otitis — *continued*
  externa — *continued*
    diffuse H60.31 ☑
    hemorrhagic H60.32 ☑
    swimmer's ear — *see* Swimmer's, ear
    malignant H60.2 ☑
    mycotic NEC B36.9 *[H62.40]*
      in
        aspergillosis B44.89
        candidiasis B37.84
        moniliasis B37.84
    necrotizing — *see* Otitis, externa, malignant
    Pseudomonas aeruginosa — *see* Otitis, externa, malignant
    reactive — *see* Otitis, externa, acute, reactive
    specified NEC — *see* subcategory H60.8 ☑
    tropical NEC B36.9 *[H62.40]*
      in
        aspergillosis B44.89
        candidiasis B37.84
        moniliasis B37.84
  insidiosa — *see* Otosclerosis
  interna — *see* subcategory H83.0 ☑
  media (hemorrhagic) (staphylococcal) (streptococcal) H66.9 ☑
    with effusion (nonpurulent) — *see* Otitis, media, nonsuppurative
    acute, subacute H66.90
      allergic — *see* Otitis, media, nonsuppurative, acute, allergic
      exudative — *see* Otitis, media, suppurative, acute
      mucoid — *see* Otitis, media, nonsuppurative, acute
      necrotizing (*see also* Otitis, media, suppurative, acute)
        in
          measles B05.3
          scarlet fever A38.0
      nonsuppurative NEC — *see* Otitis, media, nonsuppurative, acute
      purulent — *see* Otitis, media, suppurative, acute
      sanguinous — *see* Otitis, media, nonsuppurative, acute
      secretory — *see* Otitis, media, nonsuppurative, acute, serous
      seromucinous — *see* Otitis, media, nonsuppurative, acute
      serous — *see* Otitis, media, nonsuppurative, acute, serous
      suppurative — *see* Otitis, media, suppurative, acute
    allergic — *see* Otitis, media, nonsuppurative
    catarrhal — *see* Otitis, media, nonsuppurative
    chronic H66.90
      with effusion (nonpurulent) — *see* Otitis, media, nonsuppurative, chronic
      allergic — *see* Otitis, media, nonsuppurative, chronic, allergic
      benign suppurative — *see* Otitis, media, suppurative, chronic, tubotympanic
      catarrhal — *see* Otitis, media, nonsuppurative, chronic, serous
      exudative — *see* Otitis, media, nonsuppurative, chronic
      mucinous — *see* Otitis, media, nonsuppurative, chronic, mucoid
      mucoid — *see* Otitis, media, nonsuppurative, chronic, mucoid
      nonsuppurative NEC — *see* Otitis, media, nonsuppurative, chronic
      purulent — *see* Otitis, media, suppurative, chronic
      secretory — *see* Otitis, media, nonsuppurative, chronic, mucoid
      seromucinous — *see* Otitis, media, nonsuppurative, chronic
      serous — *see* Otitis, media, nonsuppurative, chronic, serous
      suppurative — *see* Otitis, media, suppurative, chronic
      transudative — *see* Otitis, media, nonsuppurative, chronic, mucoid
    exudative — *see* Otitis, media, suppurative
    in (due to) (with)
      influenza — *see* Influenza, with, otitis media
      measles B05.3
      scarlet fever A38.0
      tuberculosis A18.6
      viral disease NEC B34. ☑ *[H67. ☑]*
    mucoid — *see* Otitis, media, nonsuppurative
    nonsuppurative H65.9 ☑

Otitis — *continued*
  media — *continued*
    acute or subacute NEC H65.19 ☑
      allergic H65.11 ☑
        recurrent H65.11 ☑
      recurrent H65.19 ☑
      secretory — *see* Otitis, media,
        nonsuppurative, serous
      serous H65.0 ☑
        recurrent H65.0 ☑
    chronic H65.49 ☑
      allergic H65.41 ☑
      mucoid H65.3 ☑
      serous H65.2 ☑
    postmeasles B05.3
    purulent — *see* Otitis, media, suppurative
    secretory — *see* Otitis, media, nonsuppurative
    seromucinous — *see* Otitis, media, nonsuppurative
    serous — *see* Otitis, media, nonsuppurative
    suppurative H66.4 ☑
      acute H66.00 ☑
        with rupture of ear drum H66.01 ☑
        recurrent H66.00 ☑
          with rupture of ear drum H66.01 ☑
      chronic (*see also* subcategory) H66.3 ☑
        atticoantral H66.2 ☑
        benign — *see* Otitis, media, suppurative,
          chronic, tubotympanic
        tubotympanic H66.1 ☑
    transudative — *see* Otitis, media, nonsuppurative
    tuberculous A18.6
Otocephaly Q18.2
Otolith syndrome — *see* subcategory H81.8 ☑
Otomycosis (diffuse) NEC B36.9 *[H62.40]*
  in
    aspergillosis B44.89
    candidiasis B37.84
    moniliasis B37.84
Otoporosis — *see* Otosclerosis
Otorrhagia (nontraumatic) H92.2 ☑
  traumatic - code by Type of injury
Otorrhea H92.1 ☑
  cerebrospinal G96.0
Otosclerosis (general) H80.9 ☑
  cochlear (endosteal) H80.2 ☑
  involving
    otic capsule — *see* Otosclerosis, cochlear
    oval window
      nonobliterative H80.0 ☑
      obliterative H80.1 ☑
    round window — *see* Otosclerosis, cochlear
  nonobliterative — *see* Otosclerosis, involving, oval
    window, nonobliterative
  obliterative — *see* Otosclerosis, involving, oval
    window, obliterative
  specified NEC H80.8 ☑
Otospongiosis — *see* Otosclerosis
Otto's disease or pelvis M24.7
Outcome of delivery Z37.9
  multiple births Z37.9
    all liveborn Z37.50
      quadruplets Z37.52
      quintuplets Z37.53
      sextuplets Z37.54
      specified number NEC Z37.59
      triplets Z37.51
    all stillborn Z37.7
    some liveborn Z37.60
      quadruplets Z37.62
      quintuplets Z37.63
      sextuplets Z37.64
      specified number NEC Z37.69
      triplets Z37.61
  single NEC Z37.9
    liveborn Z37.0
    stillborn Z37.1
  twins NEC Z37.9
    both liveborn Z37.2
    both stillborn Z37.4
    one liveborn, one stillborn Z37.3
Outlet — *see* condition
Ovalocytosis (congenital) (hereditary) — *see* Elliptocytosis
Ovarian — *see* Condition
Ovaritis (cystic) — *see* Oophoritis
Ovary, ovarian (*see also* condition)
  resistant syndrome E28.39
  vein syndrome N13.8
Overactive (*see also* Hyperfunction)
  adrenal cortex NEC E27.0
  bladder N32.81
  hypothalamus E23.3

Overactive — *continued*
  thyroid — *see* Hyperthyroidism
Overactivity R46.3
  child — *see* Disorder, attention-deficit hyperactivity
Overbite (deep) (excessive) (horizontal) (vertical)
  M26.29
Overbreathing — *see* Hyperventilation
Overconscientious personality F60.5
Overdevelopment — *see* Hypertrophy
Overdistension — *see* Distension
Overdose, overdosage (drug) — *see* Table of Drugs and
  Chemicals, by drug, poisoning
Overeating R63.2
  nonorganic origin F50.89
  psychogenic F50.89
Overexertion (effects) (exhaustion) T73.3 ☑
Overexposure (effects) T73.9 ☑
  exhaustion T73.2 ☑
Overfeeding — *see* Overeating
  newborn P92.4
Overfill, endodontic M27.52
Overgrowth, bone — *see* Hypertrophy, bone
Overhanging of dental restorative material
  (unrepairable) K08.52
Overheated (places) (effects) — *see* Heat
Overjet (excessive horizontal) M26.23
Overlaid, overlying (suffocation) — *see* Asphyxia,
  traumatic, due to mechanical threat
Overlap, excessive horizontal (teeth) M26.23
Overlapping toe (acquired) (*see also* Deformity, toe,
  specified NEC)
  congenital (fifth toe) Q66.89
Overload
  circulatory, due to transfusion (blood) (blood
    components) (TACO) E87.71
  fluid E87.70
    due to transfusion (blood) (blood components)
      E87.71
    specified NEC E87.79
  iron, due to repeated red blood cell transfusions
    E83.111
  potassium (K) E87.5
  sodium (Na) E87.0
Overnutrition — *see* Hyperalimentation
Overproduction (*see also* Hypersecretion)
  ACTH E27.0
  catecholamine E27.5
  growth hormone E22.0
Overprotection, child by parent Z62.1
Overriding
  aorta Q25.49
  finger (acquired) — *see* Deformity, finger
    congenital Q68.1
  toe (acquired) (*see also* Deformity, toe, specified
    NEC)
    congenital Q66.89
Overstrained R53.83
  heart — *see* Hypertrophy, cardiac
Overuse, muscle NEC M70.8 ☑
Overweight E66.3
Overworked R53.83
Oviduct — *see* condition
Ovotestis Q56.0
Ovulation (cycle)
  failure or lack of N97.0
  pain N94.0
Ovum — *see* condition
Owren's disease or syndrome (parahemophilia) D68.2
Ox heart — *see* Hypertrophy, cardiac
Oxalosis E72.53
Oxaluria E72.53
Oxycephaly, oxycephalic Q75.0
  syphilitic, congenital A50.02
Oxyuriasis B80
Oxyuris vermicularis (infestation) B80
Ozena J31.0

P

Pachyderma, pachydermia L85.9
  larynx (verrucosa) J38.7
Pachydermatocele (congenital) Q82.8
Pachydermoperiostosis (*see also* Osteoarthropathy,
  hypertrophic, specified type NEC)
  clubbed nail M89.40 *[L62]*
Pachygyria Q04.3
Pachymeningitis (adhesive) (basal) (brain) (cervical)
  (chronic)(circumscribed) (external) (fibrous)
  (hemorrhagic) (hypertrophic) (internal) (purulent)
  (spinal) (suppurative) — *see* Meningitis

Pachyonychia (congenital) Q84.5
Pacinian tumor — *see* Neoplasm, skin, benign
Pad, knuckle or Garrod's M72.1
Paget-Schroetter syndrome I82.890
Paget's disease
  with infiltrating duct carcinoma — *see* Neoplasm,
    breast, malignant
  bone M88.9
    carpus M88.84 ☑
    clavicle M88.81 ☑
    femur M88.85 ☑
    fibula M88.86 ☑
    finger M88.84 ☑
    humerus M88.82 ☑
    ilium M88.85 ☑
    in neoplastic disease — *see* Osteitis, deformans, in
      neoplastic disease
    ischium M88.85 ☑
    metacarpus M88.84 ☑
    metatarsus M88.87 ☑
    multiple sites M88.89
    neck M88.88
    radius M88.83 ☑
    rib M88.88
    scapula M88.81 ☑
    skull M88.0
    specified NEC M88.88
    tarsus M88.87 ☑
    tibia M88.86 ☑
    toe M88.87 ☑
    ulna M88.83 ☑
    vertebra M88.1
  breast (female) C50.01 ☑
    male C50.02 ☑
  extramammary (*see also* Neoplasm, skin, malignant)
    anus C21.0
      margin C44.590
      skin C44.590
  intraductal carcinoma — *see* Neoplasm, breast,
    malignant
  malignant — *see* Neoplasm, skin, malignant
    breast (female) C50.01 ☑
      male C50.02 ☑
    unspecified site (female) C50.01 ☑
      male C50.02 ☑
  mammary — *see* Paget's disease, breast
  nipple — *see* Paget's disease, breast
  osteitis deformans — *see* Paget's disease, bone
Pain(s) (*see also* Painful) R52
  abdominal R10.9
    colic R10.83
    generalized R10.84
      with acute abdomen R10.0
    lower R10.30
      left quadrant R10.32
      pelvic or perineal R10.2
      periumbilical R10.33
      right quadrant R10.31
    rebound — *see* Tenderness, abdominal, rebound
    severe with abdominal rigidity R10.0
    tenderness — *see* Tenderness, abdominal
    upper R10.10
      epigastric R10.13
      left quadrant R10.12
      right quadrant R10.11
  acute R52
    due to trauma G89.11
    neoplasm related G89.3
    postprocedural NEC G89.18
    post-thoracotomy G89.12
    specified by site - code to Pain, by site
  adnexa (uteri) R10.2
  anginoid — *see* Pain, precordial
  anus K62.89
  arm — *see* Pain, limb, upper
  axillary (axilla) M79.62 ☑
  back (postural) M54.9
  bladder R39.89
    associated with micturition — *see* Micturition,
      painful
    chronic R39.82
  bone — *see* Disorder, bone, specified type NEC
  breast N64.4
  broad ligament R10.2
  cancer associated (acute) (chronic) G89.3
  cecum — *see* Pain, abdominal
  cervicobrachial M53.1
  chest (central) R07.9
    anterior wall R07.89
    atypical R07.89
    ischemic I20.9
    musculoskeletal R07.89

☑ **Additional character required**

Pain(s) — *continued*
  chest — *continued*
    non-cardiac R07.89
    on breathing R07.1
    pleurodynia R07.81
    precordial R07.2
    wall (anterior) R07.89
  chronic G89.29
    associated with significant psychosocial
      dysfunction G89.4
    due to trauma G89.21
    neoplasm related G89.3
    postoperative NEC G89.28
    postprocedural NEC G89.28
    post-thoracotomy G89.22
    specified NEC G89.29
  coccyx M53.3
  colon — *see* Pain, abdominal
  coronary — *see* Angina
  costochondral R07.1
  diaphragm R07.1
  due to cancer G89.3
  due to device, implant or graft (*see also* Complications,
    by site and type, specified NEC) T85.848 ☑
    arterial graft NEC T82.848 ☑
    breast (implant) T85.848 ☑
    catheter NEC T85.848 ☑
      dialysis (renal) T82.848 ☑
        intraperitoneal T85.848 ☑
      infusion NEC T82.848 ☑
        spinal (epidural) (subdural) T85.840 ☑
      urinary (indwelling) T83.84 ☑
    electronic (electrode) (pulse generator)
      (stimulator)
      bone T84.84 ☑
      cardiac T82.847 ☑
      nervous system (brain) (peripheral nerve)
        (spinal) T85.840 ☑
      urinary T83.84 ☑
    fixation, internal (orthopedic) NEC T84.84 ☑
    gastrointestinal (bile duct) (esophagus)
      T85.848 ☑
    genital NEC T83.84 ☑
    heart NEC T82.847 ☑
    infusion NEC T85.848 ☑
    joint prosthesis T84.84 ☑
    ocular (corneal graft) (orbital implant) NEC
      T85.848 ☑
    orthopedic NEC T84.84 ☑
    specified NEC T85.848 ☑
    urinary NEC T83.84 ☑
    vascular NEC T82.848 ☑
    ventricular intracranial shunt T85.840 ☑
  due to malignancy (primary) (secondary) G89.3
  ear — *see* subcategory H92.0 ☑
  epigastric, epigastrium R10.13
  eye — *see* Pain, ocular
  face, facial R51
    atypical G50.1
  female genital organs NEC N94.89
  finger — *see* Pain, limb, upper
  flank — *see* Pain, abdominal
  foot — *see* Pain, limb, lower
  gallbladder K82.9
  gas (intestinal) R14.1
  gastric — *see* Pain, abdominal
  generalized NOS R52
  genital organ
    female N94.89
    male N50.89
  groin — *see* Pain, abdominal, lower
  hand — *see* Pain, limb, upper
  head — *see* Headache
  heart — *see* Pain, precordial
  infra-orbital — *see* Neuralgia, trigeminal
  intercostal R07.82
  intermenstrual N94.0
  jaw R68.84
  joint M25.50
    ankle M25.57 ☑
    elbow M25.52 ☑
    finger M25.54 ☑
    foot M25.57 ☑
    hand M25.54 ☑
    hip M25.55 ☑
    knee M25.56 ☑
    shoulder M25.51 ☑
    toe M25.57 ☑
    wrist M25.53 ☑
  kidney N23
  laryngeal R07.0
  leg — *see* Pain, limb, lower

Pain(s) — *continued*
  limb M79.609
    lower M79.60 ☑
      foot M79.67 ☑
      lower leg M79.66 ☑
      thigh M79.65 ☑
      toe M79.67 ☑
    upper M79.60 ☑
      axilla M79.62 ☑
      finger M79.64 ☑
      forearm M79.63 ☑
      hand M79.64 ☑
      upper arm M79.62 ☑
  loin M54.5
  low back M54.5
  lumbar region M54.5
  mandibular R68.84
  mastoid — *see* subcategory H92.0 ☑
  maxilla R68.84
  menstrual (*see also* Dysmenorrhea) N94.6
  metacarpophalangeal (joint) — *see* Pain, joint, hand
  metatarsophalangeal (joint) — *see* Pain, joint, foot
  mouth K13.79
  muscle — *see* Myalgia
  musculoskeletal (*see also* Pain, by site) M79.18
  myofascial M79.18
  nasal J34.89
  nasopharynx J39.2
  neck NEC M54.2
  nerve NEC — *see* Neuralgia
  neuromuscular — *see* Neuralgia
  nose J34.89
  ocular H57.1 ☑
  ophthalmic — *see* Pain, ocular
  orbital region — *see* Pain, ocular
  ovary N94.89
  over heart — *see* Pain, precordial
  ovulation N94.0
  pelvic (female) R10.2
  penis N48.89
  pericardial — *see* Pain, precordial
  perineal, perineum R10.2
  pharynx J39.2
  pleura, pleural, pleuritic R07.81
  postoperative NOS G89.18
  postprocedural NOS G89.18
  post-thoracotomy G89.12
  precordial (region) R07.2
  premenstrual N94.3
  psychogenic (persistent) (any site) F45.41
  radicular (spinal) — *see* Radiculopathy
  rectum K62.89
  respiration R07.1
  retrosternal R07.2
  rheumatoid, muscular — *see* Myalgia
  rib R07.81
  root (spinal) — *see* Radiculopathy
  round ligament (stretch) R10.2
  sacroiliac M53.3
  sciatic — *see* Sciatica
  scrotum N50.82
  seminal vesicle N50.89
  shoulder M25.51 ☑
  spermatic cord N50.89
  spinal root — *see* Radiculopathy
  spine M54.9
    cervical M54.2
    low back M54.5
      with sciatica M54.4 ☑
    thoracic M54.6
  stomach — *see* Pain, abdominal
  substernal R07.2
  temporomandibular (joint) M26.62 ☑
  testis N50.81 ☑
  thoracic spine M54.6
    with radicular and visceral pain M54.14
  throat R07.0
  tibia — *see* Pain, limb, lower
  toe — *see* Pain, limb, lower
  tongue K14.6
  tooth K08.89
  trigeminal — *see* Neuralgia, trigeminal
  tumor associated G89.3
  ureter N23
  urinary (organ) (system) N23
  uterus NEC N94.89
  vagina R10.2
  vertebrogenic (syndrome) M54.89
  vesical R39.89
    associated with micturition — *see* Micturition,
      painful
  vulva R10.2

Painful (*see also* Pain)
  coitus
    female N94.10
    male N53.12
    psychogenic F52.6
  ejaculation (semen) N53.12
    psychogenic F52.6
  erection — *see* Priapism
  feet syndrome E53.8
  joint replacement (hip) (knee) T84.84 ☑
  menstruation — *see* Dysmenorrhea
    psychogenic F45.8
  micturition — *see* Micturition, painful
  respiration R07.1
  scar NEC L90.5
  wire sutures T81.89 ☑
Painter's colic — *see* subcategory T56.0 ☑
Palate — *see* condition
Palatoplegia K13.79
Palatoschisis — *see* Cleft, palate
Palilalia R48.8
Palliative care Z51.5
Pallor R23.1
  optic disc, temporal — *see* Atrophy, optic
Palmar (*see also* condition)
  fascia — *see* condition
Palpable
  cecum K63.89
  kidney N28.89
  ovary N83.8
  prostate N42.9
  spleen — *see* Splenomegaly
Palpitations (heart) R00.2
  psychogenic F45.8
Palsy (*see also* Paralysis) G83.9
  atrophic diffuse (progressive) G12.22
  Bell's (*see also* Palsy, facial)
    newborn P11.3
  brachial plexus NEC G54.0
    newborn (birth injury) P14.3
  brain — *see* Palsy, cerebral
  bulbar (progressive) (chronic) G12.22
    of childhood (Fazio-Londe) G12.1
    pseudo NEC G12.29
    supranuclear (progressive) G23.1
  cerebral (congenital) G80.9
    ataxic G80.4
    athetoid G80.3
    choreathetoid G80.3
    diplegic G80.8
      spastic G80.1
    dyskinetic G80.3
      athetoid G80.3
      choreathetoid G80.3
      distonic G80.3
    dystonic G80.3
    hemiplegic G80.8
      spastic G80.2
    mixed G80.8
    monoplegic G80.8
      spastic G80.1
    paraplegic G80.8
      spastic G80.1
    quadriplegic G80.8
      spastic G80.0
    spastic G80.1
      diplegic G80.1
      hemiplegic G80.2
      monoplegic G80.1
      quadriplegic G80.0
      specified NEC G80.1
      tetraplegic G80.0
    specified NEC G80.8
    syphilitic A52.12
      congenital A50.49
    tetraplegic G80.8
      spastic G80.0
  cranial nerve (*see also* Disorder, nerve, cranial)
    multiple G52.7
      in
        infectious disease B99 ☑ *[G53]*
        neoplastic disease (*see also* Neoplasm) D49.9
          [G53]
        parasitic disease B89 *[G53]*
        sarcoidosis D86.82
  creeping G12.22
  diver's T70.3 ☑
  Erb's P14.0
  facial G51.0
    newborn (birth injury) P11.3
  glossopharyngeal G52.1
  Klumpke (-Déjérine) P14.1

Palsy - Paraganglioma

Palsy — continued
- lead — see subcategory T56.0 ☑
- median nerve (tardy) G56.1 ☑
- nerve G58.9
  - specified NEC G58.8
- peroneal nerve (acute) (tardy) G57.3 ☑
- progressive supranuclear G23.1
- pseudobulbar NEC G12.29
- radial nerve (acute) G56.3 ☑
- seventh nerve (see also Palsy, facial)
  - newborn P11.3
- shaking — see Parkinsonism
- spastic (cerebral) (spinal) G80.1
- ulnar nerve (tardy) G56.2 ☑
- wasting G12.29

Paludism — see Malaria
Panangiitis M30.0
Panaris, panaritium (see also Cellulitis, digit)
- with lymphangitis — see Lymphangitis, acute, digit

Panarteritis nodosa M30.0
- brain or cerebral I67.7

Pancake heart R93.1
- with cor pulmonale (chronic) I27.81

Pancarditis (acute) (chronic) I51.89
- rheumatic I09.89
  - active or acute I01.8

Pancoast's syndrome or tumor C34.1 ☑
Pancolitis, ulcerative (chronic) K51.00
- with
  - complication K51.019
    - abscess K51.014
    - fistula K51.013
    - obstruction K51.012
    - rectal bleeding K51.011
    - specified complication NEC K51.018

Pancreas, pancreatic — see condition
Pancreatitis (annular) (apoplectic) (calcareous)
(edematous) (hemorrhagic) (malignant) (recurrent)
(subacute) (suppurative) K85.90
- with necrosis (uninfected) K85.91
  - infected K85.92
- acute (without necrosis or infection) K85.90
  - with necrosis (uninfected) K85.91
    - infected K85.92
  - alcohol induced (without necrosis or infection) K85.20
    - with necrosis (uninfected) K85.21
      - infected K85.22
  - biliary (without necrosis or infection) K85.10
    - with necrosis (uninfected) K85.11
      - infected K85.12
  - drug induced (without necrosis or infection) K85.30
    - with necrosis (uninfected) K85.31
      - infected K85.32
  - gallstone (without necrosis or infection) K85.10
    - with necrosis (uninfected) K85.11
      - infected K85.12
  - idiopathic (without necrosis or infection) K85.00
    - with necrosis (uninfected) K85.01
      - infected K85.02
  - specified NEC (without necrosis or infection) K85.80
    - with necrosis (uninfected) K85.81
      - infected K85.82
- chronic (infectious) K86.1
  - alcohol-induced K86.0
  - recurrent K86.1
  - relapsing K86.1
- cystic (chronic) K86.1
- cytomegaloviral B25.2
- fibrous (chronic) K86.1
- gangrenous — see Pancreatitis, acute
- gallstone (without necrosis or infection) K85.10
  - with necrosis (uninfected) K85.11
    - infected K85.12
- interstitial (chronic) K86.1
  - acute (see also Pancreatitis, acute) K85.80
- mumps B26.3
- recurrent (chronic) K86.1
- relapsing, chronic K86.1
- syphilitic A52.74

Pancreatoblastoma — see Neoplasm, pancreas, malignant
Pancreolithiasis K86.89
Pancytolysis D75.89
Pancytopenia (acquired) D61.818
- with
  - malformations D61.09
  - myelodysplastic syndrome — see Syndrome, myelodysplastic
  - antineoplastic chemotherapy induced D61.810

Pancytopenia — continued
- congenital D61.09
- drug-induced NEC D61.811

PANDAS (pediatric autoimmune neuropsychiatric disorders associated with streptococcal infections syndrome) D89.89
Panencephalitis, subacute, sclerosing A81.1
Panhematopenia D61.9
- congenital D61.09
- constitutional D61.09
- splenic, primary D73.1

Panhemocytopenia D61.9
- congenital D61.09
- constitutional D61.09

Panhypogonadism E29.1
Panhypopituitarism E23.0
- prepubertal E23.0

Panic (attack) (state) F41.0
- reaction to exceptional stress (transient) F43.0

Panmyelopathy, familial, constitutional D61.09
Panmyelophthisis D61.82
- congenital D61.09

Panmyelosis (acute) (with myelofibrosis) C94.4 ☑
Panner's disease — see Osteochondrosis, juvenile, humerus
Panneuritis endemica E51.11
Panniculitis (nodular) (nonsuppurative) M79.3
- back M54.00
  - cervical region M54.02
  - cervicothoracic region M54.03
  - lumbar region M54.06
  - lumbosacral region M54.07
  - multiple sites M54.09
  - occipito-atlanto-axial region M54.01
  - sacrococcygeal region M54.08
  - thoracic region M54.04
  - thoracolumbar region M54.05
- lupus L93.2
- mesenteric K65.4
- neck M54.02
  - cervicothoracic region M54.03
  - occipito-atlanto-axial region M54.01
- relapsing M35.6

Panniculus adiposus (abdominal) E65
Pannus (allergic) (cornea) (degenerativus) (keratic) H16.42 ☑
- abdominal (symptomatic) E65
- trachomatosus, trachomatous (active) A71.1

Panophthalmitis H44.01 ☑
Pansinusitis (chronic) (hyperplastic) (nonpurulent) (purulent) J32.4
- acute J01.40
  - recurrent J01.41
- tuberculous A15.8

Panuveitis (sympathetic) H44.11 ☑
Panvalvular disease I08.9
- specified NEC I08.8

PAPA (pyogenic arthritis, pyoderma gangrenosum, and acne syndrome) M04.8
Papanicolaou smear, cervix Z12.4
- as part of routine gynecological examination Z01.419
  - with abnormal findings Z01.411
- for suspected neoplasm Z12.4
- nonspecific abnormal finding R87.619
- routine Z01.419
  - with abnormal findings Z01.411

Papilledema (choked disc) H47.10
- associated with
  - decreased ocular pressure H47.12
  - increased intracranial pressure H47.11
  - retinal disorder H47.13
- Foster-Kennedy syndrome H47.14 ☑

Papillitis H46.00
- anus K62.89
- chronic lingual K14.4
- necrotizing, kidney N17.2
- optic H46.0 ☑
- rectum K62.89
- renal, necrotizing N17.2
- tongue K14.0

Papilloma (see also Neoplasm, benign, by site)
- acuminatum (female) (male) (anogenital) A63.0
- basal cell L82.1
  - inflamed L82.0
- benign pinta (primary) A67.0
- bladder (urinary) (transitional cell) D41.4
- choroid plexus (lateral ventricle) (third ventricle) D33.0
  - anaplastic C71.5
  - fourth ventricle D33.1
  - malignant C71.5

Papilloma — continued
- renal pelvis (transitional cell) D41.1 ☑
  - benign D30.1 ☑
- Schneiderian
  - specified site — see Neoplasm, benign, by site
  - unspecified site D14.0
- serous surface
  - borderline malignancy
    - specified site — see Neoplasm, uncertain behavior, by site
    - unspecified site D39.10
  - specified site — see Neoplasm, benign, by site
  - unspecified site D27.9
- transitional (cell)
  - bladder (urinary) D41.4
  - inverted type — see Neoplasm, uncertain behavior, by site
  - renal pelvis D41.1 ☑
  - ureter D41.2 ☑
- ureter (transitional cell) D41.2 ☑
  - benign D30.2 ☑
- urothelial — see Neoplasm, uncertain behavior, by site
- villous — see Neoplasm, uncertain behavior, by site
  - adenocarcinoma in — see Neoplasm, malignant, by site
  - in situ — see Neoplasm, in situ
- yaws, plantar or palmar A66.1

Papillomata, multiple, of yaws A66.1
Papillomatosis (see also Neoplasm, benign, by site)
- confluent and reticulated L83
- cystic, breast — see Mastopathy, cystic
- ductal, breast — see Mastopathy, cystic
- intraductal (diffuse) — see Neoplasm, benign, by site
- subareolar duct D24 ☑

Papillomavirus, as cause of disease classified elsewhere B97.7
Papillon-Léage and Psaume syndrome Q87.0
Papule(s) R23.8
- carate (primary) A67.0
- fibrous, of nose D22.39
- Gottron's L94.4
- pinta (primary) A67.0

Papulosis
- lymphomatoid C86.6
- malignant I77.89

Papyraceous fetus O31.0 ☑
Para-albuminemia E88.09
Paracephalus Q89.7
Parachute mitral valve Q23.2
Paracoccidioidomycosis B41.9
- disseminated B41.7
- generalized B41.7
- mucocutaneous-lymphangitic B41.8
- pulmonary B41.0
- specified NEC B41.8
- visceral B41.8

Paradentosis K05.4
Paraffinoma T88.8 ☑
Paraganglioma D44.7
- adrenal D35.0 ☑
  - malignant C74.1 ☑
- aortic body D44.7
  - malignant C75.5
- carotid body D44.6
  - malignant C75.4
- chromaffin (see also Neoplasm, benign, by site)
  - malignant — see Neoplasm, malignant, by site
- extra-adrenal D44.7
  - malignant C75.5
    - specified site — see Neoplasm, malignant, by site
    - unspecified site C75.5
  - specified site — see Neoplasm, uncertain behavior, by site
  - unspecified site D44.7
- gangliocytic D13.2
  - specified site — see Neoplasm, benign, by site
  - unspecified site D13.2
- glomus jugulare D44.7
  - malignant C75.5
- jugular D44.7
- malignant C75.5
  - specified site — see Neoplasm, malignant, by site
  - unspecified site C75.5
- nonchromaffin D44.7
  - malignant C75.5
    - specified site — see Neoplasm, malignant, by site
    - unspecified site C75.5

☑ **Additional character required**

Paraganglioma — *continued*
  nonchromaffin — *continued*
    specified site — *see* Neoplasm, uncertain
      behavior, by site
    unspecified site D44.7
    parasympathetic D44.7
      specified site — *see* Neoplasm, uncertain
        behavior, by site
      unspecified site D44.7
    specified site — *see* Neoplasm, uncertain behavior,
      by site
    sympathetic D44.7
      specified site — *see* Neoplasm, uncertain
        behavior, by site
      unspecified site D44.7
  unspecified site D44.7
Parageusia R43.2
  psychogenic F45.8
Paragonimiasis B66.4
Paragranuloma, Hodgkin — *see* Lymphoma, Hodgkin,
  specified NEC
Parahemophilia (*see also* Defect, coagulation) D68.2
Parakeratosis R23.4
  variegata L41.0
Paralysis, paralytic (complete) (incomplete) G83.9
  with
    syphilis A52.17
  abducens, abducent (nerve) — *see* Strabismus,
    paralytic, sixth nerve
  abductor, lower extremity G57.9 ☑
  accessory nerve G52.8
  accommodation (*see also* Paresis, of accommodation)
    hysterical F44.89
  acoustic nerve (except Deafness) — *see*
    subcategory H93.3 ☑
  agitans (*see also* Parkinsonism) G20
    arteriosclerotic G21.4
  alternating (oculomotor) G83.89
  amyotrophic G12.21
  ankle G57.9 ☑
  anus (sphincter) K62.89
  arm — *see* Monoplegia, upper limb
  ascending (spinal), acute G61.0
  association G12.29
  asthenic bulbar G70.00
    with exacerbation (acute) G70.01
    in crisis G70.01
  ataxic (hereditary) G11.9
    general (syphilitic) A52.17
  atrophic G58.9
    infantile, acute — *see* Poliomyelitis, paralytic
    progressive G12.22
    spinal (acute) — *see* Poliomyelitis, paralytic
  axillary G54.0
  Babinski-Nageotte's G83.89
  Bell's G51.0
    newborn P11.3
  Benedikt's G46.3
  birth injury P14.9
    spinal cord P11.5
  bladder (neurogenic) (sphincter) N31.2
  bowel, colon or intestine K56.0
  brachial plexus G54.0
    birth injury P14.3
    newborn (birth injury) P14.3
  brain G83.9
    diplegia G83.0
    triplegia G83.89
  bronchial J98.09
  Brown-Séquard G83.81
  bulbar (chronic) (progressive) G12.22
    infantile — *see* Poliomyelitis, paralytic
    poliomyelitic — *see* Poliomyelitis, paralytic
    pseudo G12.29
  bulbospinal G70.00
    with exacerbation (acute) G70.01
    in crisis G70.01
  cardiac (*see also* Failure, heart) I50.9
  cerebrocerebellar, diplegic G80.1
  cervical
    plexus G54.2
    sympathetic G90.09
  Céstan-Chenais G46.3
  Charcot-Marie-Tooth type G60.0
  Clark's G80.9
  colon K56.0
  compressed air T70.3 ☑
  compression
    arm G56.9 ☑
    leg G57.9 ☑
    lower extremity G57.9 ☑
    upper extremity G56.9 ☑

Paralysis — *continued*
  congenital (cerebral) — *see* Palsy, cerebral
  conjugate movement (gaze) (of eye) H51.0
    cortical (nuclear) (supranuclear) H51.0
  cordis — *see* Failure, heart
  cranial or cerebral nerve G52.9
  creeping G12.22
  crossed leg G83.89
  crutch — *see* Injury, brachial plexus
  deglutition R13.0
    hysterical F44.4
  dementia A52.17
  descending (spinal) NEC G12.29
  diaphragm (flaccid) J98.6
    due to accidental dissection of phrenic nerve
      during procedure — *see* Puncture, accidental
      complicating surgery
  digestive organs NEC K59.8
  diplegic — *see* Diplegia
  divergence (nuclear) H51.8
  diver's T70.3 ☑
  Duchenne's
    birth injury P14.0
    due to or associated with
      motor neuron disease G12.22
      muscular dystrophy G71.01
    due to intracranial or spinal birth injury — *see* Palsy,
      cerebral
  embolic (current episode) I63.4 ☑
  Erb (-Duchenne) (birth) (newborn) P14.0
  Erb's syphilitic spastic spinal A52.17
  esophagus K22.8
  eye muscle (extrinsic) H49.9
    intrinsic (*see also* Paresis, of accommodation)
  facial (nerve) G51.0
    birth injury P11.3
    congenital P11.3
    following operation NEC — *see* Puncture,
      accidental complicating surgery
    newborn (birth injury) P11.3
  familial (recurrent) (periodic) G72.3
    spastic G11.4
  fauces J39.2
  finger G56.9 ☑
  gait R26.1
  gastric nerve (nondiabetic) G52.2
  gaze, conjugate H51.0
  general (progressive) (syphilitic) A52.17
    juvenile A50.45
  glottis J38.00
    bilateral J38.02
    unilateral J38.01
  gluteal G54.1
  Gubler (-Millard) G46.3
  hand — *see* Monoplegia, upper limb
  heart — *see* Arrest, cardiac
  hemiplegic — *see* Hemiplegia
  hyperkalemic periodic (familial) G72.3
  hypoglossal (nerve) G52.3
  hypokalemic periodic G72.3
  hysterical F44.4
  ileus K56.0
  infantile (*see also* Poliomyelitis, paralytic) A80.30
    bulbar — *see* Poliomyelitis, paralytic
    cerebral — *see* Palsy, cerebral
    spastic — *see* Palsy, cerebral, spastic
  infective — *see* Poliomyelitis, paralytic
  inferior nuclear G83.9
  internuclear — *see* Ophthalmoplegia, internuclear
  intestine K56.0
  iris H57.09
    due to diphtheria (toxin) A36.89
  ischemic, Volkmann's (complicating trauma)
    T79.6 ☑
  Jackson's G83.89
  jake — *see* Poisoning, food, noxious, plant
  Jamaica ginger (jake) G62.2
  juvenile general A50.45
  Klumpke (-Déjérine) (birth) (newborn) P14.1
  labioglossal (laryngeal) (pharyngeal) G12.29
  Landry's G61.0
  laryngeal nerve (recurrent) (superior) (unilateral)
    J38.00
    bilateral J38.02
    unilateral J38.01
  larynx J38.00
    bilateral J38.02
    due to diphtheria (toxin) A36.2
    unilateral J38.01
  lateral G12.23
  lead — *see* subcategory T56.0 ☑
  left side — *see* Hemiplegia

Paralysis — *continued*
  leg G83.1 ☑
    both — *see* Paraplegia
    crossed G83.89
    hysterical F44.4
    psychogenic F44.4
    transient or transitory R29.818
      traumatic NEC — *see* Injury, nerve, leg
  levator palpebrae superioris — *see* Blepharoptosis,
    paralytic
  limb — *see* Monoplegia
  lip K13.0
  Lissauer's A52.17
  lower limb — *see* Monoplegia, lower limb
    both — *see* Paraplegia
  lung J98.4
  median nerve G56.1 ☑
  medullary (tegmental) G83.89
  mesencephalic NEC G83.89
    tegmental G83.89
  middle alternating G83.89
  Millard-Gubler-Foville G46.3
  monoplegic — *see* Monoplegia
  motor G83.9
  muscle, muscular NEC G72.89
    due to nerve lesion G58.9
    eye (extrinsic) H49.9
      intrinsic — *see* Paresis, of accommodation
      oblique — *see* Strabismus, paralytic, fourth
        nerve
    iris sphincter H21.9
    ischemic (Volkmann's) (complicating trauma)
      T79.6 ☑
    progressive G12.21
    progressive, spinal G12.25
    spinal progressive G12.25
    pseudohypertrophic G71.02
  musculocutaneous nerve G56.9 ☑
  musculospiral G56.9 ☑
  nerve (*see also* Disorder, nerve)
    abducent — *see* Strabismus, paralytic, sixth nerve
    accessory G52.8
    auditory (except Deafness) — *see* subcategory
      H93.3 ☑
    birth injury P14.9
    cranial or cerebral G52.9
    facial G51.0
      birth injury P11.3
      congenital P11.3
      newborn (birth injury) P11.3
    fourth or trochlear — *see* Strabismus, paralytic,
      fourth nerve
    newborn (birth injury) P14.9
    oculomotor — *see* Strabismus, paralytic, third
      nerve
    phrenic (birth injury) P14.2
    radial G56.3 ☑
    seventh or facial G51.0
      newborn (birth injury) P11.3
    sixth or abducent — *see* Strabismus, paralytic,
      sixth nerve
    syphilitic A52.15
    third or oculomotor — *see* Strabismus, paralytic,
      third nerve
    trigeminal G50.9
    trochlear — *see* Strabismus, paralytic, fourth nerve
    ulnar G56.2 ☑
  normokalemic periodic G72.3
  ocular H49.9
    alternating G83.89
  oculofacial, congenital (Moebius) Q87.0
  oculomotor (external bilateral) (nerve) — *see*
    Strabismus, paralytic, third nerve
  palate (soft) K13.79
  paratrigeminal G50.9
  periodic (familial) (hyperkalemic) (hypokalemic)
    (myotonic) (normokalemic) (potassium
    sensitive) (secondary) G72.3
  peripheral autonomic nervous system — *see*
    Neuropathy, peripheral, autonomic
  peroneal (nerve) G57.3 ☑
  pharynx J39.2
  phrenic nerve G56.8 ☑
  plantar nerve(s) G57.6 ☑
  pneumogastric nerve G52.2
  poliomyelitis (current) — *see* Poliomyelitis, paralytic
  popliteal nerve G57.3 ☑
  postepileptic transitory G83.84
  progressive (atrophic) (bulbar) (spinal) G12.22
    general A52.17
    infantile acute — *see* Poliomyelitis, paralytic
    supranuclear G23.1

Paralysis - Parkinsonism

Paralysis — *continued*
  pseudobulbar G12.29
  pseudohypertrophic (muscle) G71.09
  psychogenic F44.4
  quadriceps G57.9 ☑
  quadriplegic — *see* Tetraplegia
  radial nerve G56.3 ☑
  rectus muscle (eye) H49.9
  recurrent isolated sleep G47.53
  respiratory (muscle) (system) (tract) R06.81
    center NEC G93.89
    congenital P28.89
    newborn P28.89
  right side — *see* Hemiplegia
  saturnine — *see* subcategory T56.0 ☑
  sciatic nerve G57.0 ☑
  senile G83.9
  shaking — *see* Parkinsonism
  shoulder G56.9 ☑
  sleep, recurrent isolated G47.53
  spastic G83.9
    cerebral — *see* Palsy, cerebral, spastic
    congenital (cerebral) — *see* Palsy, cerebral, spastic
    familial G11.4
    hereditary G11.4
    quadriplegic G80.0
    syphilitic (spinal) A52.17
  sphincter, bladder — *see* Paralysis, bladder
  spinal (cord) G83.9
    accessory nerve G52.8
    acute — *see* Poliomyelitis, paralytic
    ascending acute G61.0
    atrophic (acute) (*see also* Poliomyelitis, paralytic)
      spastic, syphilitic A52.17
    congenital NEC — *see* Palsy, cerebral
    infantile — *see* Poliomyelitis, paralytic
    hereditary G95.89
    progressive G12.21
      muscle G12.25
    sequelae NEC G83.89
  sternomastoid G52.8
  stomach K31.84
    diabetic — *see* Diabetes, by type, with gastroparesis
    nerve G52.2
      diabetic — *see* Diabetes, by type, with gastroparesis
  stroke — *see* Infarct, brain
  subcapsularis G56.8 ☑
  supranuclear (progressive) G23.1
  sympathetic G90.8
    cervical G90.09
    nervous system — *see* Neuropathy, peripheral, autonomic
  syndrome G83.9
    specified NEC G83.89
  syphilitic spastic spinal (Erb's) A52.17
  thigh G57.9 ☑
  throat J39.2
    diphtheritic A36.0
    muscle J39.2
  thrombotic (current episode) I63.3 ☑
  thumb G56.9 ☑
  tick — *see* Toxicity, venom, arthropod, specified NEC
  Todd's (postepileptic transitory paralysis) G83.84
  toe G57.6 ☑
  tongue K14.8
  transient R29.5
    arm or leg NEC R29.818
    traumatic NEC — *see* Injury, nerve
  trapezius G52.8
  traumatic, transient NEC — *see* Injury, nerve
  trembling — *see* Parkinsonism
  triceps brachii G56.9 ☑
  trigeminal nerve G50.9
  trochlear (nerve) — *see* Strabismus, paralytic, fourth nerve
  ulnar nerve G56.2 ☑
  upper limb — *see* Monoplegia, upper limb
  uremic N18.9 *[G99.8]*
  uveoparotitic D86.89
  uvula K13.79
    postdiphtheritic A36.0
  vagus nerve G52.2
  vasomotor NEC G90.8
  velum palati K13.79
  vesical — *see* Paralysis, bladder
  vestibular nerve (except Vertigo) — *see* subcategory H93.3 ☑
  vocal cords J38.00
    bilateral J38.02
    unilateral J38.01

Paralysis — *continued*
  Volkmann's (complicating trauma) T79.6 ☑
  wasting G12.29
  Weber's G46.3
  wrist G56.9 ☑
Paramedial urethrovesical orifice Q64.79
Paramenia N92.6
Parametritis (*see also* Disease, pelvis, inflammatory) N73.2
  acute N73.0
  complicating abortion — *see* Abortion, by type, complicated by, parametritis
Parametrium, parametric — *see* condition
Paramnesia — *see* Amnesia
Paramolar K00.1
Paramyloidosis E85.89
Paramyoclonus multiplex G25.3
Paramyotonia (congenita) G71.19
Parangi — *see* Yaws
Paranoia (querulans) F22
  senile F03 ☑
Paranoid
  dementia (senile) F03 ☑
    praecox — *see* Schizophrenia
  personality F60.0
  psychosis (climacteric) (involutional) (menopausal) F22
    psychogenic (acute) F23
    senile F03 ☑
  reaction (acute) F23
    chronic F22
  schizophrenia F20.0
  state (climacteric) (involutional) (menopausal) (simple) F22
    senile F03 ☑
  tendencies F60.0
  traits F60.0
  trends F60.0
  type, psychopathic personality F60.0
Paraparesis — *see* Paraplegia
Paraphasia R47.02
Paraphilia F65.9
Paraphimosis (congenital) N47.2
  chancroidal A57
Paraphrenia, paraphrenic (late) F22
  schizophrenia F20.0
Paraplegia (lower) G82.20
  ataxic — *see* Degeneration, combined, spinal cord
  complete G82.21
  congenital (cerebral) G80.8
    spastic G80.1
  familial spastic G11.4
  functional (hysterical) F44.4
  hereditary, spastic G11.4
  hysterical F44.4
  incomplete G82.22
  Pott's A18.01
  psychogenic F44.4
  spastic
    Erb's spinal, syphilitic A52.17
    hereditary G11.4
    tropical G04.1
  syphilitic (spastic) A52.17
  traumatic
    current injury - code to injury with seventh character A
    sequela of previous injury - code to injury with seventh character S
  tropical spastic G04.1
Parapoxvirus B08.60
  specified NEC B08.69
Paraproteinemia D89.2
  benign (familial) D89.2
  monoclonal D47.2
  secondary to malignant disease D47.2
Parapsoriasis L41.9
  en plaques L41.4
  guttata L41.1
  large plaque L41.4
  retiform, retiformis L41.5
  small plaque L41.3
  specified NEC L41.8
  varioliformis (acuta) L41.0
Parasitic (*see also* condition)
  disease NEC B89
  stomatitis B37.0
  sycosis (beard) (scalp) B35.0
  twin Q89.4
Parasitism B89
  intestinal B82.9
  skin B88.9
  specified — *see* Infestation

Parasitophobia F40.218
Parasomnia G47.50
  due to
    alcohol
      abuse F10.182
      dependence F10.282
      use F10.982
    amphetamines
      abuse F15.182
      dependence F15.282
      use F15.982
    caffeine
      abuse F15.182
      dependence F15.282
      use F15.982
    cocaine
      abuse F14.182
      dependence F14.282
      use F14.982
    drug NEC
      abuse F19.182
      dependence F19.282
      use F19.982
    opioid
      abuse F11.182
      dependence F11.282
      use F11.982
    psychoactive substance NEC
      abuse F19.182
      dependence F19.282
      use F19.982
    sedative, hypnotic, or anxiolytic
      abuse F13.182
      dependence F13.282
      use F13.982
    stimulant NEC
      abuse F15.182
      dependence F15.282
      use F15.982
  in conditions classified elsewhere G47.54
  nonorganic origin F51.8
  organic G47.50
  specified NEC G47.59
Paraspadias Q54.9
Paraspasmus facialis G51.8
Parasuicide (attempt)
  history of (personal) Z91.5
    in family Z81.8
Parathyroid gland — *see* condition
Parathyroid tetany E20.9
Paratrachoma A74.0
Paratyphilitis — *see* Appendicitis
Paratyphoid (fever) — *see* Fever, paratyphoid
Paratyphus — *see* Fever, paratyphoid
Paraurethral duct Q64.79
Paraurethritis (*see also* Urethritis)
  gonococcal (acute) (chronic) (with abscess) A54.1
Paravaccinia NEC B08.04
Paravaginitis — *see* Vaginitis
Parencephalitis (*see also* Encephalitis)
  sequelae G09
Parent-child conflict — *see* Conflict, parent-child
  estrangement NEC Z62.890
Paresis (*see also* Paralysis)
  accommodation — *see* Paresis, of accommodation
  Bernhardt's G57.1 ☑
  bladder (sphincter) (*see also* Paralysis, bladder)
    tabetic A52.17
  bowel, colon or intestine K56.0
  extrinsic muscle, eye H49.9
  general (progressive) (syphilitic) A52.17
    juvenile A50.45
  heart — *see* Failure, heart
  insane (syphilitic) A52.17
  juvenile (general) A50.45
  of accommodation H52.52 ☑
  peripheral progressive (idiopathic) G60.3
  pseudohypertrophic G71.09
  senile G83.9
  syphilitic (general) A52.17
    congenital A50.45
  vesical NEC N31.2
Paresthesia (*see also* Disturbance, sensation, skin) R20.2
  Bernhardt G57.1 ☑
Paretic — *see* condition
Parinaud's
  conjunctivitis H10.89
  oculoglandular syndrome H10.89
  ophthalmoplegia H49.88 ☑
Parkinsonism (idiopathic) (primary) G20

Parkinsonism — *continued*
    with neurogenic orthostatic hypotension
        (symptomatic) G90.3
    arteriosclerotic G21.4
    dementia G31.83 *[F02.80]*
        with behavioral disturbance G31.83 *[F02.81]*
    due to
        drugs NEC G21.19
            neuroleptic G21.11
    medication-induced NEC G21.19
    neuroleptic induced G21.11
    postencephalitic G21.3
    secondary G21.9
        due to
            arteriosclerosis G21.4
            drugs NEC G21.19
                neuroleptic G21.11
            encephalitis G21.3
            external agents NEC G21.2
            syphilis A52.19
        specified NEC G21.8
    syphilitic A52.19
    treatment-induced NEC G21.19
    vascular G21.4
Parkinson's disease, syndrome or tremor — *see*
    Parkinsonism
Parodontitis — *see* Periodontitis
Parodontosis K05.4
Paronychia (*see also* Cellulitis, digit)
    with lymphangitis — *see* Lymphangitis, acute, digit
    candidal (chronic) B37.2
    tuberculous (primary) A18.4
Parorexia (psychogenic) F50.89
Parosmia R43.1
    psychogenic F45.8
Parotid gland — *see* condition
Parotitis, parotiditis (allergic)(nonspecific toxic)
    (purulent) (septic) (suppurative) (*see also*
    Sialoadenitis)
    epidemic — *see* Mumps
    infectious — *see* Mumps
    postoperative K91.89
    surgical K91.89
Parrot fever A70
Parrot's disease (early congenital syphilitic
    pseudoparalysis) A50.02
Parry-Romberg syndrome G51.8
Parry's disease or syndrome E05.00
    with thyroid storm E05.01
Pars planitis — *see* Cyclitis
Parsonage (-Aldren)-Turner syndrome G54.5
Parson's disease (exophthalmic goiter) E05.00
    with thyroid storm E05.01
Particolored infant Q82.8
Parturition — *see* Delivery
Parulis K04.7
    with sinus K04.6
Parvovirus, as cause of disease classified elsewhere B97.6
Pasini and Pierini's atrophoderma L90.3
Passage
    false, urethra N36.5
    meconium (newborn) during delivery P03.82
    of sounds or bougies — *see* Attention to, artificial,
        opening
Passive — *see* condition
    smoking Z77.22
Pasteurella septica A28.0
Pasteurellosis — *see* Infection, Pasteurella
PAT (paroxysmal atrial tachycardia) I47.1
Patau's syndrome — *see* Trisomy, 13
Patches
    mucous (syphilitic) A51.39
        congenital A50.07
    smokers' (mouth) K13.24
Patellar — *see* condition
Patent (*see also* Imperfect, closure)
    canal of Nuck Q52.4
    cervix N88.3
    ductus arteriosus or Botallo's Q25.0
    foramen
        botalli Q21.1
        ovale Q21.1
    interauricular septum Q21.1
    interventricular septum Q21.0
    omphalomesenteric duct Q43.0
    os (uteri) — *see* Patent, cervix
    ostium secundum Q21.1
    urachus Q64.4
    vitelline duct Q43.0
Paterson (-Brown)(-Kelly) syndrome or web D50.1
Pathologic, pathological (*see also* condition)
    asphyxia R09.01

Pathologic — *continued*
    fire-setting F63.1
    gambling F63.0
    ovum O02.0
    resorption, tooth K03.3
    stealing F63.2
Pathology (of) — *see* Disease
    periradicular, associated with previous endodontic
        treatment NEC M27.59
Pattern, sleep-wake, irregular G47.23
Patulous (*see also* Imperfect, closure (congenital))
    alimentary tract Q45.8
        lower Q43.8
        upper Q40.8
    eustachian tube H69.0 ☑
Pause, sinoatrial I49.5
Paxton's disease B36.2
Pearl(s)
    enamel K00.2
    Epstein's K09.8
Pearl-worker's disease — *see* Osteomyelitis, specified
    type NEC
Pectenosis K62.4
Pectoral — *see* condition
Pectus
    carinatum (congenital) Q67.7
        acquired M95.4
        rachitic sequelae (late effect) E64.3
    excavatum (congenital) Q67.6
        acquired M95.4
        rachitic sequelae (late effect) E64.3
    recurvatum (congenital) Q67.6
Pedatrophia E41
Pederosis F65.4
Pediculosis (infestation) B85.2
    capitis (head-louse) (any site) B85.0
    corporis (body-louse) (any site) B85.1
    eyelid B85.0
    mixed (classifiable to more than one of the titles
        B85.0-B85.3) B85.4
    pubis (pubic louse) (any site) B85.3
    vestimenti B85.1
    vulvae B85.3
Pediculus (infestation) — *see* Pediculosis
Pedophilia F65.4
Peg-shaped teeth K00.2
Pelade — *see* Alopecia, areata
Pelger-Huët anomaly or syndrome D72.0
Peliosis (rheumatica) D69.0
    hepatis K76.4
        with toxic liver disease K71.8
Pelizaeus-Merzbacher disease E75.29
Pellagra (alcoholic) (with polyneuropathy) E52
Pellagra-cerebellar-ataxia-renal aminoaciduria
    syndrome E72.02
Pellegrini (-Stieda) disease or syndrome — *see* Bursitis,
    tibial collateral
Pellizzi's syndrome E34.8
Pel's crisis A52.11
Pelvic (*see also* condition)
    examination (periodic) (routine) Z01.419
        with abnormal findings Z01.411
    kidney, congenital Q63.2
Pelviolithiasis — *see* Calculus, kidney
Pelviperitonitis (*see also* Peritonitis, pelvic)
    gonococcal A54.24
    puerperal O85
Pelvis — *see* condition or type
Pemphigoid L12.9
    benign, mucous membrane L12.1
    bullous L12.0
    cicatricial L12.1
    juvenile L12.2
    ocular L12.1
    specified NEC L12.8
Pemphigus L10.9
    benign familial (chronic) Q82.8
    Brazilian L10.3
    circinatus L13.0
    conjunctiva L12.1
    drug-induced L10.5
    erythematosus L10.4
    foliaceus L10.2
    gangrenous — *see* Gangrene
    neonatorum L01.03
    ocular L12.1
    paraneoplastic L10.81
    specified NEC L10.89
    syphilitic (congenital) A50.06
    vegetans L10.1
    vulgaris L10.0
    wildfire L10.3

Pendred's syndrome E07.1
Pendulous
    abdomen, in pregnancy — *see* Pregnancy,
        complicated by, abnormal, pelvic organs or
        tissues NEC
    breast N64.89
Penetrating wound (*see also* Puncture)
    with internal injury — *see* Injury, by site
    eyeball — *see* Puncture, eyeball
    orbit (with or without foreign body) — *see*
        Puncture, orbit
    uterus by instrument with or following ectopic or
        molar pregnancy O08.6
Penicillosis B48.4
Penis — *see* condition
Penitis N48.29
Pentalogy of Fallot Q21.8
Pentasomy X syndrome Q97.1
Pentosuria (essential) E74.8
Percreta placenta O43.23 ☑
Peregrinating patient — *see* Disorder, factitious
Perforation, perforated (nontraumatic) (of)
    accidental during procedure (blood vessel) (nerve)
        (organ) — *see* Complication, accidental
        puncture or laceration
    antrum — *see* Sinusitis, maxillary
    appendix K35.32
        with localized peritonitis K35.32
    atrial septum, multiple Q21.1
    attic, ear — *see* Perforation, tympanum, attic
    bile duct (common) (hepatic) K83.2
        cystic K82.2
    bladder (urinary)
        with or following ectopic or molar pregnancy
            O08.6
        obstetrical trauma O71.5
        traumatic S37.29 ☑
            at delivery O71.5
    bowel K63.1
        with or following ectopic or molar pregnancy
            O08.6
        newborn P78.0
        obstetrical trauma O71.5
        traumatic — *see* Laceration, intestine
    broad ligament N83.8
        with or following ectopic or molar pregnancy
            O08.6
        obstetrical trauma O71.6
    by
        device, implant or graft (*see also* Complications,
            by site and type, mechanical) T85.628 ☑
            arterial graft NEC — *see* Complication,
                cardiovascular device, mechanical, vascular
            breast (implant) T85.49 ☑
            catheter NEC T85.698 ☑
                cystostomy T83.090 ☑
                dialysis (renal) T82.49 ☑
                    intraperitoneal T85.691 ☑
                infusion NEC T82.594 ☑
                    spinal (epidural) (subdural) T85.690 ☑
                urinary (*see also* Complications, catheter,
                    urinary) T83.098 ☑
            electronic (electrode) (pulse generator)
                (stimulator)
                bone T84.390 ☑
                cardiac T82.199 ☑
                    electrode T82.190 ☑
                    pulse generator T82.191 ☑
                    specified type NEC T82.198 ☑
                nervous system — *see* Complication,
                    prosthetic device, mechanical, electronic
                    nervous system stimulator
                urinary — *see* Complication, genitourinary,
                    device, urinary, mechanical
            fixation, internal (orthopedic) NEC — *see*
                Complication, fixation device, mechanical
            gastrointestinal — *see* Complications,
                prosthetic device, mechanical,
                gastrointestinal device
            genital NEC T83.498 ☑
                intrauterine contraceptive device T83.39 ☑
                penile prosthesis T83.490 ☑
            heart NEC — *see* Complication, cardiovascular
                device, mechanical
            joint prosthesis — *see* Complications, joint
                prosthesis, mechanical, specified NEC, by
                site
            ocular NEC — *see* Complications, prosthetic
                device, mechanical, ocular device
            orthopedic NEC — *see* Complication,
                orthopedic, device, mechanical
            specified NEC T85.628 ☑

Perforation - Periepididymitis

Perforation — *continued*
  by — *continued*
    urinary NEC (*see also* Complication,
        genitourinary, device, urinary, mechanical)
      graft T83.29 ☑
    vascular NEC — *see* Complication,
        cardiovascular device, mechanical
    ventricular intracranial shunt T85.09 ☑
    foreign body left accidentally in operative wound
        T81.539 ☑
    instrument (any) during a procedure, accidental
        — *see* Puncture, accidental complicating
        surgery
  cecum K35.32
    with localized peritonitis K35.32
  cervix (uteri) N88.8
    with or following ectopic or molar pregnancy
        O08.6
    obstetrical trauma O71.3
  colon K63.1
    newborn P78.0
    obstetrical trauma O71.5
    traumatic — *see* Laceration, intestine, large
  common duct (bile) K83.2
  cornea (due to ulceration) — *see* Ulcer, cornea,
      perforated
  cystic duct K82.2
  diverticulum (intestine) K57.80
    with bleeding K57.81
    large intestine K57.20
      with
        bleeding K57.21
        small intestine K57.40
          with bleeding K57.41
    small intestine K57.00
      with
        bleeding K57.01
        large intestine K57.40
          with bleeding K57.41
  ear drum — *see* Perforation, tympanum
  esophagus K22.3
  ethmoidal sinus — *see* Sinusitis, ethmoidal
  frontal sinus — *see* Sinusitis, frontal
  gallbladder K82.2
  heart valve — *see* Endocarditis
  ileum K63.1
    newborn P78.0
    obstetrical trauma O71.5
    traumatic — *see* Laceration, intestine, small
  instrumental, surgical (accidental) (blood vessel)
      (nerve) (organ) — *see* Puncture, accidental
      complicating surgery
  intestine NEC K63.1
    with ectopic or molar pregnancy O08.6
    newborn P78.0
    obstetrical trauma O71.5
    traumatic — *see* Laceration, intestine
    ulcerative NEC K63.1
      newborn P78.0
  jejunum, jejunal K63.1
    obstetrical trauma O71.5
    traumatic — *see* Laceration, intestine, small
    ulcer — *see* Ulcer, gastrojejunal, with perforation
  joint prosthesis — *see* Complications, joint
      prosthesis, mechanical, specified NEC, by site
  mastoid (antrum) (cell) — *see* Disorder, mastoid,
      specified NEC
  maxillary sinus — *see* Sinusitis, maxillary
  membrana tympani — *see* Perforation, tympanum
  nasal
    septum J34.89
      congenital Q30.3
      syphilitic A52.73
    sinus J34.89
      congenital Q30.8
      due to sinusitis — *see* Sinusitis
  palate (*see also* Cleft, palate) Q35.9
    syphilitic A52.79
  palatine vault (*see also* Cleft, palate, hard) Q35.1
    syphilitic A52.79
    congenital A50.59
  pars flaccida (ear drum) — *see* Perforation,
      tympanum, attic
  pelvic
    floor S31.030 ☑
      with
        ectopic or molar pregnancy O08.6
        penetration into retroperitoneal space
            S31.031 ☑
        retained foreign body S31.040 ☑
          with penetration into retroperitoneal space
              S31.041 ☑

Perforation — *continued*
  pelvic — *continued*
    following ectopic or molar pregnancy O08.6
    obstetrical trauma O70.1
  organ S37.99 ☑
    adrenal gland S37.818 ☑
    bladder — *see* Perforation, bladder
    fallopian tube S37.599 ☑
      bilateral S37.592 ☑
      unilateral S37.591 ☑
    kidney S37.09 ☑
    obstetrical trauma O71.5
    ovary S37.499 ☑
      bilateral S37.492 ☑
      unilateral S37.491 ☑
    prostate S37.828 ☑
    specified organ NEC S37.898 ☑
    ureter — *see* Perforation, ureter
    urethra — *see* Perforation, urethra
    uterus — *see* Perforation, uterus
  perineum — *see* Laceration, perineum
  pharynx J39.2
  rectum K63.1
    newborn P78.0
    obstetrical trauma O71.5
    traumatic S36.63 ☑
  root canal space due to endodontic treatment
      M27.51
  sigmoid K63.1
    newborn P78.0
    obstetrical trauma O71.5
    traumatic S36.533 ☑
  sinus (accessory) (chronic) (nasal) J34.89
  sphenoidal sinus — *see* Sinusitis, sphenoidal
  surgical (accidental) (by instrument) (blood vessel)
      (nerve) (organ) — *see* Puncture, accidental
      complicating surgery
  traumatic
    external — *see* Puncture
    eye — *see* Puncture, eyeball
    internal organ — *see* Injury, by site
  tympanum, tympanic (membrane) (persistent post-
      traumatic) (postinflammatory) H72.9 ☑
    attic H72.1 ☑
      multiple — *see* Perforation, tympanum,
          multiple
      total — *see* Perforation, tympanum, total
    central H72.0 ☑
      multiple — *see* Perforation, tympanum,
          multiple
      total — *see* Perforation, tympanum, total
    marginal NEC — *see* subcategory H72.2 ☑
    multiple H72.81 ☑
    pars flaccida — *see* Perforation, tympanum, attic
    total H72.82 ☑
    traumatic, current episode S09.2 ☑
  typhoid, gastrointestinal — *see* Typhoid
  ulcer — *see* Ulcer, by site, with perforation
  ureter N28.89
    traumatic S37.19 ☑
  urethra N36.8
    with ectopic or molar pregnancy O08.6
    following ectopic or molar pregnancy O08.6
    obstetrical trauma O71.5
    traumatic S37.39 ☑
      at delivery O71.5
  uterus
    with ectopic or molar pregnancy O08.6
    by intrauterine contraceptive device T83.39 ☑
    following ectopic or molar pregnancy O08.6
    obstetrical trauma O71.1
    traumatic S37.69 ☑
      obstetric O71.1
  uvula K13.79
    syphilitic A52.79
  vagina
    obstetrical trauma O71.4
    other trauma — *see* Puncture, vagina
Periadenitis mucosa necrotica recurrens K12.0
Periappendicitis (acute) — *see* Appendicitis
Periarteritis nodosa (disseminated) (infectious)
    (necrotizing) M30.0
Periarthritis (joint) (*see also* Enthesopathy)
    Duplay's M75.0
    gonococcal A54.42
    humeroscapularis — *see* Capsulitis, adhesive
    scapulohumeral — *see* Capsulitis, adhesive
    shoulder — *see* Capsulitis, adhesive
    wrist M77.2 ☑
Periarthrosis (angioneural) — *see* Enthesopathy
Pericapsulitis, adhesive (shoulder) — *see* Capsulitis,
    adhesive

Pericarditis (with decompensation) (with effusion)
    I31.9
  with rheumatic fever (conditions in I00)
    active — *see* Pericarditis, rheumatic
    inactive or quiescent I09.2
  acute (hemorrhagic) (nonrheumatic) (Sicca) I30.9
    with chorea (acute) (rheumatic) (Sydenham's)
        I02.0
    benign I30.8
    nonspecific I30.0
    rheumatic I01.0
      with chorea (acute) (Sydenham's) I02.0
  adhesive or adherent (chronic) (external) (internal)
      I31.0
    acute — *see* Pericarditis, acute
    rheumatic I09.2
  bacterial (acute) (subacute) (with serous or
      seropurulent effusion) I30.1
  calcareous I31.1
  cholesterol (chronic) I31.8
    acute I30.9
  chronic (nonrheumatic) I31.9
    rheumatic I09.2
  constrictive (chronic) I31.1
  coxsackie B33.23
  fibrinocaseous (tuberculous) A18.84
  fibrinopurulent I30.1
  fibrinous I30.8
  fibrous I31.0
  gonococcal A54.83
  idiopathic I30.0
  in systemic lupus erythematosus M32.12
  infective I30.1
  meningococcal A39.53
  neoplastic (chronic) I31.8
    acute I30.9
  obliterans, obliterating I31.0
  plastic I31.0
  pneumococcal I30.1
  postinfarction I24.1
  purulent I30.1
  rheumatic (active) (acute) (with effusion) (with
      pneumonia) I01.0
    with chorea (acute) (rheumatic) (Sydenham's)
        I02.0
    chronic or inactive (with chorea) I09.2
  rheumatoid — *see* Rheumatoid, carditis
  septic I30.1
  serofibrinous I30.8
  staphylococcal I30.1
  streptococcal I30.1
  suppurative I30.1
  syphilitic A52.06
  tuberculous A18.84
  uremic N18.9 *[I32]*
  viral I30.1
Pericardium, pericardial — *see* condition
Pericellulitis — *see* Cellulitis
Pericementitis (chronic) (suppurative) (*see also*
    Periodontitis)
  acute K05.20
    generalized — *see* Periodontitis, aggressive,
        generalized
    localized — *see* Periodontitis, aggressive, localized
Perichondritis
  auricle — *see* Perichondritis, ear
  bronchus J98.09
  ear (external) H61.00 ☑
    acute H61.01 ☑
    chronic H61.02 ☑
  external auditory canal — *see* Perichondritis, ear
  larynx J38.7
    syphilitic A52.73
    typhoid A01.09
  nose J34.89
  pinna — *see* Perichondritis, ear
  trachea J39.8
Periclasia K05.4
Pericoronitis — *see* Periodontitis
Pericystitis N30.90
  with hematuria N30.91
Peridiverticulitis (intestine) K57.92
  cecum — *see* Diverticulitis, intestine, large
  colon — *see* Diverticulitis, intestine, large
  duodenum — *see* Diverticulitis, intestine, small
  intestine — *see* Diverticulitis, intestine
  jejunum — *see* Diverticulitis, intestine, small
  rectosigmoid — *see* Diverticulitis, intestine, large
  rectum — *see* Diverticulitis, intestine, large
  sigmoid — *see* Diverticulitis, intestine, large
Periendocarditis — *see* Endocarditis
Periepididymitis N45.1

☑ **Additional character required**

Perifolliculitis L01.02
  abscedens, caput, scalp L66.3
  capitis, abscedens (et suffodiens) L66.3
  superficial pustular L01.02
Perihepatitis K65.8
Perilabyrinthitis (acute) — see subcategory H83.0 ☑
Perimeningitis — see Meningitis
Perimetritis — see Endometritis
Perimetrosalpingitis — see Salpingo-oophoritis
Perineocele N81.81
Perinephric, perinephritic — see condition
Perinephritis (see also Infection, kidney)
  purulent — see Abscess, kidney
Perineum, perineal — see condition
Perineuritis NEC — see Neuralgia
Periodic — see condition
Periodontitis (chronic) (complex) (compound) (local)
    (simplex) K05.30
  acute K05.20
    generalized K05.229
      moderate K05.222
      severe K05.223
      slight K05.221
    localized K05.219
      moderate K05.212
      severe K05.213
      slight K05.211
  apical K04.5
    acute (pulpal origin) K04.4
  generalized K05.329
    moderate K05.322
    severe K05.323
    slight K05.321
  localized K05.319
    moderate K05.312
    severe K05.313
    slight K05.311
Periodontoclasia K05.4
Periodontosis (juvenile) K05.4
Periods (see also Menstruation)
  heavy N92.0
  irregular N92.6
  shortened intervals (irregular) N92.1
Perionychia (see also Cellulitis, digit)
  with lymphangitis — see Lymphangitis, acute,
    digit
Periodophoritis — see Salpingo-oophoritis
Periorchitis N45.2
Periosteum, periosteal — see condition
Periostitis (albuminosa) (circumscribed) (diffuse)
    (infective) (monomelic) (see also Osteomyelitis)
  alveolar M27.3
  alveolodental M27.3
  dental M27.3
  gonorrheal A54.43
  jaw (lower) (upper) M27.2
  orbit H05.03 ☑
  syphilitic A52.77
    congenital (early) A50.02 [M90.80]
    secondary A51.46
  tuberculous — see Tuberculosis, bone
  yaws (hypertrophic) (early) (late) A66.6 [M90.80]
Periostosis (hyperplastic) (see also Disorder, bone,
    specified type NEC)
  with osteomyelitis — see Osteomyelitis, specified
    type NEC
Peripartum
  cardiomyopathy O90.3
Periphlebitis — see Phlebitis
Periproctitis K62.89
Periprostatitis — see Prostatitis
Perirectal — see condition
Perirenal — see condition
Perisalpingitis — see Salpingo-oophoritis
Perisplenitis (infectional) D73.89
Peristalsis, visible or reversed R19.2
Peritendinitis — see Enthesopathy
Peritoneum, peritoneal — see condition
Peritonitis (adhesive) (bacterial) (fibrinous)
    (hemorrhagic) (idiopathic) (localized) (perforative)
    (primary) (with adhesions) (with effusion) K65.9
  with or following
    abscess K65.1
    appendicitis
      with perforation or rupture K35.32
      generalized (see also Appendicitis) K35.20
      localized (see also Appendicitis) K35.30
    diverticular disease (intestine) K57.80
      with bleeding K57.81
      large intestine K57.20
        with
          bleeding K57.21

Peritonitis — continued
  with or following — continued
    small intestine K57.40
      with bleeding K57.41
    small intestine K57.00
      with
        bleeding K57.01
        large intestine K57.40
          with bleeding K57.41
    ectopic or molar pregnancy O08.0
  acute (generalized) K65.0
  aseptic T81.61 ☑
  bile, biliary K65.3
  chemical T81.61 ☑
  chlamydial A74.81
  complicating abortion — see Abortion, by type,
    complicated by, pelvic peritonitis
  congenital P78.1
  chronic proliferative K65.8
  diaphragmatic K65.0
  diffuse K65.0
  diphtheritic A36.89
  disseminated K65.0
  due to
    bile K65.3
    foreign
      body or object accidentally left during a
        procedure (instrument) (sponge) (swab)
        T81.599 ☑
      substance accidentally left during a procedure
        (chemical) (powder) (talc) T81.61 ☑
    talc T81.61 ☑
    urine K65.8
  eosinophilic K65.8
    acute K65.0
  fibrocaseous (tuberculous) A18.31
  fibropurulent K65.0
  following ectopic or molar pregnancy O08.0
  general (ized) K65.0
  gonococcal A54.85
  meconium (newborn) P78.0
  neonatal P78.1
    meconium P78.0
  pancreatic K65.0
  paroxysmal, familial E85.0
    benign E85.0
  pelvic
    female N73.5
      acute N73.3
      chronic N73.4
        with adhesions N73.6
    male K65.0
  periodic, familial E85.0
  proliferative, chronic K65.8
  puerperal, postpartum, childbirth O85
  purulent K65.0
  septic K65.0
  specified NEC K65.8
  spontaneous bacterial K65.2
  subdiaphragmatic K65.0
  subphrenic K65.0
  suppurative K65.0
  syphilitic A52.74
    congenital (early) A50.08 [K67]
  talc T81.61 ☑
  tuberculous A18.31
  urine K65.8
Peritonsillar — see condition
Peritonsillitis J36
Perityphlitis K37
Periureteritis N28.89
Periurethral — see condition
Periurethritis (gangrenous) — see Urethritis
Periuterine — see condition
Perivaginitis — see Vaginitis
Perivasculitis, retinal H35.06 ☑
Perivasitis (chronic) N49.1
Perivesiculitis (seminal) — see Vesiculitis
Perlèche NEC K13.0
  due to
    candidiasis B37.83
    moniliasis B37.83
    riboflavin deficiency E53.0
    vitamin B2 (riboflavin) deficiency E53.0
Pernicious — see condition
Pernio, perniosis T69.1 ☑
Perpetrator (of abuse) — see Index to External Causes
  of Injury, Perpetrator
Persecution
  delusion F22
  social Z60.5
Perseveration (tonic) R48.8

Persistence, persistent (congenital)
  anal membrane Q42.3
    with fistula Q42.2
  arteria stapedia Q16.3
  atrioventricular canal Q21.2
  branchial cleft NOS Q18.2
    cyst Q18.0
    fistula Q18.0
    sinus Q18.0
  bulbus cordis in left ventricle Q21.8
  canal of Cloquet Q14.0
  capsule (opaque) Q12.8
  cilioretinal artery or vein Q14.8
  cloaca Q43.7
  communication — see Fistula, congenital
  convolutions
    aortic arch Q25.46
    fallopian tube Q50.6
    oviduct Q50.6
    uterine tube Q50.6
  double aortic arch Q25.45
  ductus arteriosus (Botalli) Q25.0
  fetal
    circulation P29.38
    form of cervix (uteri) Q51.828
    hemoglobin, hereditary (HPFH) D56.4
  foramen
    Botalli Q21.1
    ovale Q21.1
  Gartner's duct Q52.4
  hemoglobin, fetal (hereditary) (HPFH) D56.4
  hyaloid
    artery (generally incomplete) Q14.0
    system Q14.8
  hymen, in pregnancy or childbirth — see
    Pregnancy, complicated by, abnormal, vulva
  lanugo Q84.2
  left
    posterior cardinal vein Q26.8
    root with right arch of aorta Q25.49
    superior vena cava Q26.1
  Meckel's diverticulum Q43.0
    malignant — see Table of Neoplasms, small
      intestine, malignant
  mucosal disease (middle ear) — see Otitis, media,
    suppurative, chronic, tubotympanic
  nail(s), anomalous Q84.6
  omphalomesenteric duct Q43.0
  organ or site not listed — see Anomaly, by site
  ostium
    atrioventriculare commune Q21.2
    primum Q21.2
    secundum Q21.1
  ovarian rests in fallopian tube Q50.6
  pancreatic tissue in intestinal tract Q43.8
  primary (deciduous)
    teeth K00.6
    vitreous hyperplasia Q14.0
  pupillary membrane Q13.89
  right aortic arch Q25.47
  rhesus (Rh) titer — see Complication(s), transfusion,
    incompatibility reaction, Rh (factor)
  sinus
    urogenitalis
      female Q52.8
      male Q55.8
    venosus with imperfect incorporation in right
      auricle Q26.8
  thymus (gland) (hyperplasia) E32.0
  thyroglossal duct Q89.2
  thyrolingual duct Q89.2
  truncus arteriosus or communis Q20.0
  tunica vasculosa lentis Q12.2
  umbilical sinus Q64.4
  urachus Q64.4
  vitelline duct Q43.0
Person (with)
  admitted for clinical research, as a control subject
    (normal comparison) (participant) Z00.6
  awaiting admission to adequate facility elsewhere
    Z75.1
  concern (normal) about sick person in family
    Z63.6
  consulting on behalf of another Z71.0
  feigning illness Z76.5
  living (in)
    alone Z60.2
    boarding school Z59.3
    residential institution Z59.3
    without
      adequate housing (heating) (space) Z59.1
      housing (permanent) (temporary) Z59.0

Person — *continued*
  living — *continued*
    person able to render necessary care Z74.2
    shelter Z59.0
  on waiting list Z75.1
  sick or handicapped in family Z63.6
Personality (disorder) F60.9
  accentuation of traits (type A pattern) Z73.1
  affective F34.0
  aggressive F60.3
  amoral F60.2
  anacastic, anankastic F60.5
  antisocial F60.2
  anxious F60.6
  asocial F60.2
  asthenic F60.7
  avoidant F60.6
  borderline F60.3
  change due to organic condition (enduring) F07.0
  compulsive F60.5
  cycloid F34.0
  cyclothymic F34.0
  dependent F60.7
  depressive F34.1
  dissocial F60.2
  dual F44.81
  eccentric F60.89
  emotionally unstable F60.3
  expansive paranoid F60.0
  explosive F60.3
  fanatic F60.0
  haltose type F60.89
  histrionic F60.4
  hyperthymic F34.0
  hypothymic F34.1
  hysterical F60.4
  immature F60.89
  inadequate F60.7
  labile (emotional) F60.3
  mixed (nonspecific) F60.89
  morally defective F60.2
  multiple F44.81
  narcissistic F60.81
  obsessional F60.5
  obsessive (-compulsive) F60.5
  organic F07.0
  overconscientious F60.5
  paranoid F60.0
  passive (-dependent) F60.7
  passive-aggressive F60.89
  pathologic F60.9
  pattern defect or disturbance F60.9
  pseudopsychopathic (organic) F07.0
  pseudoretarded (organic) F07.0
  psychoinfantile F60.4
  psychoneurotic NEC F60.89
  psychopathic F60.2
  querulant F60.0
  sadistic F60.89
  schizoid F60.1
  self-defeating F60.89
  sensitive paranoid F60.0
  sociopathic (amoral) (antisocial) (asocial) (dissocial)
    F60.2
  specified NEC F60.89
  type A Z73.1
  unstable (emotional) F60.3
Perthes' disease — *see* Legg-Calvé-Perthes disease
Pertussis (*see also* Whooping cough) A37.90
Perversion, perverted
  appetite F50.89
    psychogenic F50.89
  function
    pituitary gland E23.2
      posterior lobe E22.2
  sense of smell and taste R43.8
    psychogenic F45.8
  sexual — *see* Deviation, sexual
Pervious, congenital (*see also* Imperfect, closure)
  ductus arteriosus Q25.0
Pes (congenital) (*see also* Talipes)
  acquired (*see also* Deformity, limb, foot, specified
    NEC)
  planus — *see* Deformity, limb, flat foot
  adductus Q66.89
  cavus Q66.7 ☑
  deformity NEC, acquired — *see* Deformity, limb,
    foot, specified NEC
  planus (acquired) (any degree) (*see also* Deformity,
    limb, flat foot)
    rachitic sequelae (late effect) E64.3
  valgus Q66.6

Pest, pestis — *see* Plague
Petechia, petechiae R23.3
  newborn P54.5
Petechial typhus A75.9
Peter's anomaly Q13.4
Petit mal seizure — *see* Epilepsy, childhood, absence
Petit's hernia — *see* Hernia, abdomen, specified site
  NEC
Petrellidosis B48.2
Petrositis H70.20 ☑
  acute H70.21 ☑
  chronic H70.22 ☑
Peutz-Jeghers disease or syndrome Q85.8
Peyronie's disease N48.6
PFAPA (periodic fever, aphthous stomatitis, pharyngitis,
  and adenopathy syndrome) M04.8
Pfeiffer's disease — *see* Mononucleosis, infectious
Phagedena (dry) (moist) (sloughing) (*see also*
  Gangrene)
  geometric L88
  penis N48.29
  tropical — *see* Ulcer, skin
  vulva N76.6
Phagedenic — *see* condition
Phakoma H35.89
Phakomatosis (*see also* specific eponymous
  syndromes) Q85.9
  Bourneville's Q85.1
  specified NEC Q85.8
Phantom limb syndrome (without pain) G54.7
  with pain G54.6
Pharyngeal pouch syndrome D82.1
Pharyngitis (acute) (catarrhal)(gangrenous) (infective)
  (malignant) (membranous) (phlegmonous)
  (pseudomembranous) (simple) (subacute)
  (suppurative) (ulcerative) (viral) J02.9
  with influenza, flu, or grippe — *see* Influenza, with,
    pharyngitis
  aphthous B08.5
  atrophic J31.2
  chlamydial A56.4
  chronic (atrophic) (granular) (hypertrophic) J31.2
  coxsackievirus B08.5
  diphtheritic A36.0
  enteroviral vesicular B08.5
  follicular (chronic) J31.2
  fusospirochetal A69.1
  gonococcal A54.5
  granular (chronic) J31.2
  herpesviral B00.2
  hypertrophic J31.2
  infectional, chronic J31.2
  influenzal — *see* Influenza, with, respiratory
    manifestations NEC
  lymphonodular, acute (enteroviral) B08.8
  pneumococcal J02.8
  purulent J02.9
  putrid J02.9
  septic J02.0
  sicca J31.2
  specified organism NEC J02.8
  staphylococcal J02.8
  streptococcal J02.0
  syphilitic, congenital (early) A50.03
  tuberculous A15.8
  vesicular, enteroviral B08.5
  viral NEC J02.8
Pharyngoconjunctivitis, viral B30.2
Pharyngolaryngitis (acute) J06.0
  chronic J37.0
Pharyngoplegia J39.2
Pharyngotonsillitis, herpesviral B00.2
Pharyngotracheitis, chronic J42
Pharynx, pharyngeal — *see* condition
Phencyclidine-induced
  anxiety disorder F16.980
  bipolar and related disorder F16.94
  depressive disorder F16.94
  psychotic disorder F16.959
Phenomenon
  Arthus' — *see* Arthus' phenomenon
  jaw-winking Q07.8
  lupus erythematosus (LE) cell M32.9
  Raynaud's (secondary) I73.00
    with gangrene I73.01
  vasomotor R55
  vasospastic I73.9
  vasovagal R55
  Wenckebach's I44.1
Phenylketonuria E70.1
  classical E70.0
  maternal E70.1

Pheochromoblastoma
  specified site — *see* Neoplasm, malignant, by site
  unspecified site C74.10
Pheochromocytoma
  malignant
    specified site — *see* Neoplasm, malignant, by site
    unspecified site C74.10
  specified site — *see* Neoplasm, benign, by site
  unspecified site D35.00
Pheohyphomycosis — *see* Chromomycosis
Pheomycosis — *see* Chromomycosis
Phimosis (congenital) (due to infection) N47.1
  chancroidal A57
Phlebectasia (*see also* Varix)
  congenital Q27.4
Phlebitis (infective) (pyemic) (septic) (suppurative)
  I80.9
  antepartum — *see* Thrombophlebitis, antepartum
  blue — *see* Phlebitis, leg, deep
  breast, superficial I80.8
  cavernous (venous) sinus — *see* Phlebitis,
    intracranial (venous) sinus
  calf muscular vein (NOS) I80.25 ☑
  cerebral (venous) sinus — *see* Phlebitis, intracranial
    (venous) sinus
  chest wall, superficial I80.8
  cranial (venous) sinus — *see* Phlebitis, intracranial
    (venous) sinus
  deep (vessels) — *see* Phlebitis, leg, deep
  due to implanted device — *see* Complications, by
    site and type, specified NEC
  during or resulting from a procedure T81.72 ☑
  femoral vein (superficial) I80.1 ☑
  femoropopliteal vein I80.0 ☑
  gastrocnemial vein I80.25 ☑
  gestational — *see* Phlebopathy, gestational
  hepatic veins I80.8
  iliac vein (common) (external) (internal) I80.21 ☑
  iliofemoral — *see* Phlebitis, femoral vein
  intracranial (venous) sinus (any) G08
    nonpyogenic I67.6
  intraspinal venous sinuses and veins G08
    nonpyogenic G95.19
  lateral (venous) sinus — *see* Phlebitis, intracranial
    (venous) sinus
  leg I80.3
    antepartum — *see* Thrombophlebitis, antepartum
    deep (vessels) NEC I80.20 ☑
      iliac I80.21 ☑
      popliteal vein I80.22 ☑
      specified vessel NEC I80.29 ☑
      tibial vein (anterior) (posterior) I80.23 ☑
    femoral vein (superficial) I80.1 ☑
    superficial (vessels) I80.0 ☑
  longitudinal sinus — *see* Phlebitis, intracranial
    (venous) sinus
  lower limb — *see* Phlebitis, leg
  migrans, migrating (superficial) I82.1
  pelvic
    with ectopic or molar pregnancy O08.0
    following ectopic or molar pregnancy O08.0
    puerperal, postpartum O87.1
  peroneal vein I80.24 ☑
  popliteal vein — *see* Phlebitis, leg, deep, popliteal
  portal (vein) K75.1
  postoperative T81.72 ☑
  pregnancy — *see* Thrombophlebitis, antepartum
  puerperal, postpartum, childbirth O87.0
    deep O87.1
    pelvic O87.1
    superficial O87.0
  retina — *see* Vasculitis, retina
  saphenous (accessory) (great) (long) (small) — *see*
    Phlebitis, leg, superficial
  sinus (meninges) — *see* Phlebitis, intracranial
    (venous) sinus
  soleal vein I80.25 ☑
  specified site NEC I80.8
  syphilitic A52.09
  tibial vein — *see* Phlebitis, leg, deep, tibial
  ulcerative I80.9
    leg — *see* Phlebitis, leg
  umbilicus I80.8
  uterus (septic) — *see* Endometritis
  varicose (leg) (lower limb) — *see* Varix, leg, with,
    inflammation
Phlebofibrosis I87.8
Phleboliths I87.8
Phlebopathy,
  gestational O22.9 ☑
  puerperal O87.9
Phlebosclerosis I87.8

☑ **Additional character required**

Phlebothrombosis (*see also* Thrombosis)
  antepartum — *see* Thrombophlebitis, antepartum
  pregnancy — *see* Thrombophlebitis, antepartum
  puerperal — *see* Thrombophlebitis, puerperal
Phlebotomus fever A93.1
Phlegmasia
  alba dolens O87.1
    nonpuerperal — *see* Phlebitis, femoral vein
  cerulea dolens — *see* Phlebitis, leg, deep
Phlegmon — *see* Abscess
Phlegmonous — *see* condition
Phlyctenulosis (allergic) (keratoconjunctivitis)
  (nontuberculous) (*see also* Keratoconjunctivitis)
  cornea — *see* Keratoconjunctivitis
  tuberculous A18.52
Phobia, phobic F40.9
  animal F40.218
    spiders F40.210
  examination F40.298
  reaction F40.9
  simple F40.298
  social F40.10
    generalized F40.11
  specific (isolated) F40.298
    animal F40.218
      spiders F40.210
    blood F40.230
    injection F40.231
    injury F40.233
    men F40.290
    natural environment F40.228
      thunderstorms F40.220
    situational F40.248
      bridges F40.242
      closed in spaces F40.240
      flying F40.243
      heights F40.241
    specified focus NEC F40.298
    transfusion F40.231
    women F40.291
  specified NEC F40.8
    medical care NEC F40.232
  state F40.9
Phocas' disease — *see* Mastopathy, cystic
Phocomelia Q73.1
  lower limb — *see* Agenesis, leg, with foot present
  upper limb — *see* Agenesis, arm, with hand present
Phoria H50.50
Phosphate-losing tubular disorder N25.0
Phosphatemia E83.39
Phosphaturia E83.39
Photodermatitis (sun) L56.8
  chronic L57.8
  due to drug L56.8
  light other than sun L59.8
Photokeratitis H16.13 ☑
Photophobia H53.14 ☑
Photophthalmia — *see* Photokeratitis
Photopsia H53.19
Photoretinitis — *see* Retinopathy, solar
Photosensitivity, photosensitization (sun) skin L56.8
  light other than sun L59.8
Phrenitis — *see* Encephalitis
Phrynoderma (vitamin A deficiency) E50.8
Phthiriasis (pubis) B85.3
  with any infestation classifiable to B85.0-B85.2
    B85.4
Phthirus infestation — *see* Phthiriasis
Phthisis (*see also* Tuberculosis)
  bulbi (infectional) — *see* Disorder, globe,
    degenerated condition, atrophy
  eyeball (due to infection) — *see* Disorder, globe,
    degenerated condition, atrophy
Phycomycosis — *see* Zygomycosis
Physalopteriasis B81.8
Physical restraint status Z78.1
Phytobezoar T18.9 ☑
  intestine T18.3 ☑
  stomach T18.2 ☑
Pian — *see* Yaws
Pianoma A66.1
Pica F50.89
  in adults F50.89
  infant or child F98.3
Picking, nose F98.8
Pick-Niemann disease — *see* Niemann-Pick disease or
  syndrome
Pick's
  cerebral atrophy G31.01 *[F02.80]*
    with behavioral disturbance G31.01 *[F02.81]*
  disease or syndrome (brain) G31.01 *[F02.80]*
    with behavioral disturbance G31.01 *[F02.81]*

Pick's — *continued*
  disease or syndrome — *continued*
    brain G31.01 *[F02.80]*
      with behavioral disturbance G31.01 *[F02.81]*
    pericardium (pericardial pseudocirrhosis of liver)
      I31.1
    syndrome
      brain G31.01 *[F02.80]*
        with behavioral disturbance G31.01 *[F02.81]*
      of heart (pericardial pseudocirrhosis of liver)
        I31.1
Pickwickian syndrome E66.2
Piebaldism E70.39
Piedra (beard) (scalp) B36.8
  black B36.3
  white B36.2
Pierre Robin deformity or syndrome Q87.0
Pierson's disease or osteochondrosis M91.0
Pig-bel A05.2
Pigeon
  breast or chest (acquired) M95.4
    congenital Q67.7
      rachitic sequelae (late effect) E64.3
  breeder's disease or lung J67.2
  fancier's disease or lung J67.2
  toe — *see* Deformity, toe, specified NEC
Pigmentation (abnormal) (anomaly) L81.9
  conjunctiva H11.13 ☑
  cornea (anterior) H18.01 ☑
    posterior H18.05 ☑
    stromal H18.06 ☑
  diminished melanin formation NEC L81.6
  iron L81.8
  lids, congenital Q82.8
  limbus corneae — *see* Pigmentation, cornea
  metals L81.8
  optic papilla, congenital Q14.2
  retina, congenital (grouped) (nevoid) Q14.1
  scrotum, congenital Q82.8
  tattoo L81.8
Piles (*see also* Hemorrhoids) K64.9
Pili
  annulati or torti (congenital) Q84.1
  incarnati L73.1
Pill roller hand (intrinsic) — *see* Parkinsonism
Pilomatrixoma — *see* Neoplasm, skin, benign
  malignant — *see* Neoplasm, skin, malignant
Pilonidal — *see* condition
Pimple R23.8
PIN — *see* Neoplasia, intraepithelial, prostate
Pinched nerve — *see* Neuropathy, entrapment
Pindborg tumor — *see* Cyst, calcifying odontogenic
Pineal body or gland — *see* condition
Pinealoblastoma C75.3
Pinealoma D44.5
  malignant C75.3
Pineoblastoma C75.3
Pineocytoma D44.5
Pinguecula H11.15 ☑
Pingueculitis H10.81 ☑
Pinhole meatus (*see also* Stricture, urethra) N35.919
Pink
  disease — *see* subcategory T56.1 ☑
  eye — *see* Conjunctivitis, acute, mucopurulent
Pinkus' disease (lichen nitidus) L44.1
Pinpoint
  meatus — *see* Stricture, urethra
  os (uteri) — *see* Stricture, cervix
Pins and needles R20.2
Pinta A67.9
  cardiovascular lesions A67.2
  chancre (primary) A67.0
  erythematous plaques A67.1
  hyperchromic lesions A67.1
  hyperkeratosis A67.1
  lesions A67.9
    cardiovascular A67.2
    hyperchromic A67.1
    intermediate A67.1
    late A67.2
    mixed A67.3
    primary A67.0
    skin (achromic) (cicatricial) (dyschromic) A67.2
      hyperchromic A67.1
      mixed (achromic and hyperchromic) A67.3
  papule (primary) A67.0
  skin lesions (achromic) (cicatricial) (dyschromic)
    A67.2
    hyperchromic A67.1
    mixed (achromic and hyperchromic) A67.3
  vitiligo A67.2
Pintids A67.1

Pinworm (disease) (infection) (infestation) B80
Piroplasmosis B60.0
Pistol wound — *see* Gunshot wound
Pitchers' elbow — *see* Derangement, joint, specified
  type NEC, elbow
Pithecoid pelvis Q74.2
  with disproportion (fetopelvic) O33.0
    causing obstructed labor O65.0
Pithiatism F48.8
Pitted — *see* Pitting
Pitting (*see also* Edema) R60.9
  lip R60.0
  nail L60.8
  teeth K00.4
Pituitary gland — *see* condition
Pituitary-snuff-taker's disease J67.0
Pityriasis (capitis) L21.0
  alba L30.5
  circinata (et maculata) L42
  furfuracea L21.0
  Hebra's L26
  lichenoides L41.0
    chronica L41.1
    et varioliformis (acuta) L41.0
  maculata (et circinata) L30.5
  nigra B36.1
  pilaris, Hebra's L44.0
  rosea L42
  rotunda L44.8
  rubra (Hebra) pilaris L44.0
  simplex L30.5
  specified type NEC L30.5
  streptogenes L30.5
  versicolor (scrotal) B36.0
Placenta, placental — *see* Pregnancy, complicated
  by (care of) (management affected by), specified
  condition
Placentitis O41.14 ☑
Plagiocephaly Q67.3
Plague A20.9
  abortive A20.8
  ambulatory A20.8
  asymptomatic A20.8
  bubonic A20.0
  cellulocutaneous A20.1
  cutaneobubonic A20.1
  lymphatic gland A20.0
  meningitis A20.3
  pharyngeal A20.8
  pneumonic (primary) (secondary) A20.2
  pulmonary, pulmonic A20.2
  septicemic A20.7
  tonsillar A20.8
    septicemic A20.7
Planning, family
  contraception Z30.9
  procreation Z31.69
Plaque(s)
  artery, arterial — *see* Arteriosclerosis
  calcareous — *see* Calcification
  coronary, lipid rich I25.83
  epicardial I31.8
  erythematous, of pinta A67.1
  Hollenhorst's — *see* Occlusion, artery, retina
  lipid rich, coronary I25.83
  pleural (without asbestos) J92.9
    with asbestos J92.0
  tongue K13.29
Plasmacytoma C90.3 ☑
  extramedullary C90.2 ☑
  medullary C90.0 ☑
  solitary C90.3 ☑
Plasmacytopenia D72.818
Plasmacytosis D72.822
Plaster ulcer — *see* Ulcer, pressure, by site
Plateau iris syndrome (post-iridectomy)
  (postprocedural) (without glaucoma) H21.82
  with glaucoma H40.22 ☑
Platybasia Q75.8
Platyonychia (congenital) Q84.6
  acquired L60.8
Platypelloid pelvis M95.5
  with disproportion (fetopelvic) O33.0
    causing obstructed labor O65.0
  congenital Q74.2
Platyspondylisis Q76.49
Plaut (-Vincent) disease (*see also* Vincent's) A69.1
Plethora R23.2
  newborn P61.1
Pleura, pleural — *see* condition
Pleuralgia R07.81

Pleurisy - Pneumonia

Pleurisy (acute) (adhesive) (chronic) (costal)
  (diaphragmatic) (double) (dry) (fibrinous) (fibrous)
  (interlobar) (latent) (plastic) (primary) (residual)
  (sicca) (sterile) (subacute) (unresolved) R09.1
    with
      adherent pleura J86.0
      effusion J90
        chylous, chyliform J94.0
        tuberculous (non primary) A15.6
          primary (progressive) A15.7
        tuberculosis — see Pleurisy, tuberculous (non
          primary)
    encysted — see Pleurisy, with effusion
    exudative — see Pleurisy, with effusion
    fibrinopurulent, fibropurulent — see Pyothorax
    hemorrhagic — see Hemothorax
    pneumococcal J90
    purulent — see Pyothorax
    septic — see Pyothorax
    serofibrinous — see Pleurisy, with effusion
    seropurulent — see Pyothorax
    serous — see Pleurisy, with effusion
    staphylococcal J86.9
    streptococcal J90
    suppurative — see Pyothorax
    traumatic (post) (current) — see Injury, intrathoracic,
      pleura
    tuberculous (with effusion) (non primary) A15.6
      primary (progressive) A15.7
Pleuritis sicca — see Pleurisy
Pleurobronchopneumonia — see Pneumonia,
  broncho-
Pleurodynia R07.81
    epidemic B33.0
    viral B33.0
Pleuropericarditis (see also Pericarditis)
    acute I30.9
Pleuropneumonia (acute) (bilateral) (double) (septic)
  (see also Pneumonia) J18.8
    chronic — see Fibrosis, lung
Pleuro-pneumonia-like-organism (PPLO), as cause of
  disease classified elsewhere B96.0
Pleurorrhea — see Pleurisy, with effusion
Plexitis, brachial G54.0
Plica
    polonica B85.0
    syndrome, knee M67.5 ☑
    tonsil J35.8
Plicated tongue K14.5
Plug
    bronchus NEC J98.09
    meconium (newborn) NEC syndrome P76.0
    mucus — see Asphyxia, mucus
Plumbism — see subcategory T56.0 ☑
Plummer's disease E05.20
    with thyroid storm E05.21
Plummer-Vinson syndrome D50.1
Pluricarential syndrome of infancy E40
Plus (and minus) hand (intrinsic) — see Deformity,
  limb, specified type NEC, forearm
Pneumathemia — see Air, embolism
Pneumatic hammer (drill) syndrome T75.21 ☑
Pneumatocele (lung) J98.4
    intracranial G93.89
    tension J44.9
Pneumatosis
    cystoides intestinalis K63.89
    intestinalis K63.89
    peritonei K66.8
Pneumaturia R39.89
Pneumoblastoma — see Neoplasm, lung, malignant
Pneumocephalus G93.89
Pneumococcemia A40.3
Pneumococcus, pneumococcal — see condition
Pneumoconiosis (due to) (inhalation of) J64
    with tuberculosis (any type in A15 ☑) J65
    aluminum J63.0
    asbestos J61
    bagasse, bagassosis J67.1
    bauxite J63.1
    beryllium J63.2
    coal miners' (simple) J60
    coalworkers' (simple) J60
    collier's J60
    cotton dust J66.0
    diatomite (diatomaceous earth) J62.8
    dust
      inorganic NEC J63.6
      lime J62.8
      marble J62.8
      organic NEC J66.8
    fumes or vapors (from silo) J68.9

Pneumoconiosis — continued
    graphite J63.3
    grinder's J62.8
    kaolin J62.8
    mica J62.8
    millstone maker's J62.8
    mineral fibers NEC J61
    miner's J60
    moldy hay J67.0
    potter's J62.8
    rheumatoid — see Rheumatoid, lung
    sandblaster's J62.8
    silica, silicate NEC J62.8
      with carbon J60
    stonemason's J62.8
    talc (dust) J62.0
Pneumocystis carinii pneumonia B59
Pneumocystis jiroveci (pneumonia) B59
Pneumocystosis (with pneumonia) B59
Pneumohemopericardium I31.2
Pneumohemothorax J94.2
    traumatic S27.2 ☑
Pneumohydropericardium — see Pericarditis
Pneumohydrothorax — see Hydrothorax
Pneumomediastinum J98.2
    congenital or perinatal P25.2
Pneumomycosis B49 [J99]
Pneumonia (acute) (double) (migratory) (purulent)
  (septic) (unresolved) J18.9
    with
      lung abscess J85.1
        due to specified organism — see Pneumonia,
          in (due to)
      influenza — see Influenza, with, pneumonia
    adenoviral J12.0
    adynamic J18.2
    alba J50.04
    allergic (eosinophilic) J82
    alveolar — see Pneumonia, lobar
    anaerobes J15.8
    anthrax A22.1
    apex, apical — see Pneumonia, lobar
    Ascaris B77.81
    aspiration J69.0
      due to
        aspiration of microorganisms
          bacterial J15.9
          viral J12.9
        food (regurgitated) J69.0
        gastric secretions J69.0
        milk (regurgitated) J69.0
        oils, essences J69.1
        solids, liquids NEC J69.8
        vomitus J69.0
      newborn P24.81
        amniotic fluid (clear) P24.11
        blood P24.21
        liquor (amnii) P24.11
        meconium P24.01
        milk P24.31
        mucus P24.11
        food (regurgitated) P24.31
        specified NEC P24.81
        stomach contents P24.31
      postprocedural J95.4
    atypical NEC J18.9
    bacillus J15.9
      specified NEC J15.8
    bacterial J15.9
      specified NEC J15.8
    Bacteroides (fragilis) (oralis) (melaninogenicus)
      J15.8
    basal, basic, basilar — see Pneumonia, by type
    bronchiolitis obliterans organized (BOOP) J84.89
    broncho-, bronchial (confluent) (croupous) (diffuse)
      (disseminated) (hemorrhagic) (involving lobes)
      (lobar) (terminal) J18.0
      allergic (eosinophilic) J82
      aspiration — see Pneumonia, aspiration
      bacterial J15.9
        specified NEC J15.8
      chronic — see Fibrosis, lung
      diplococcal J13
      Eaton's agent J15.7
      Escherichia coli (E. coli) J15.5
      Friedländer's bacillus J15.0
      Hemophilus influenzae J14
      hypostatic J18.2
      inhalation (see also Pneumonia, aspiration)
        due to fumes or vapors (chemical) J68.0
        of oils or essences J69.1
      Klebsiella (pneumoniae) J15.0

Pneumonia — continued
    broncho-, bronchial — continued
      lipid, lipoid J69.1
        endogenous J84.89
      Mycoplasma (pneumoniae) J15.7
      pleuro-pneumonia-like-organisms (PPLO) J15.7
      pneumococcal J13
      Proteus J15.6
      Pseudomonas J15.1
      Serratia marcescens J15.6
      specified organism NEC J16.8
      staphylococcal — see Pneumonia, staphylococcal
      streptococcal NEC J15.4
        group B J15.3
        pneumoniae J13
      viral, virus — see Pneumonia, viral
    Butyrivibrio (fibriosolvens) J15.8
    Candida B37.1
    caseous — see Tuberculosis, pulmonary
    catarrhal — see Pneumonia, broncho
    chlamydial J16.0
      congenital P23.1
    cholesterol J84.89
    cirrhotic (chronic) — see Fibrosis, lung
    Clostridium (haemolyticum) (novyi) J15.8
    confluent — see Pneumonia, broncho
    congenital (infective) P23.9
      due to
        bacterium NEC P23.6
        Chlamydia P23.1
        Escherichia coli P23.4
        Haemophilus influenzae P23.6
        infective organism NEC P23.8
        Klebsiella pneumoniae P23.6
        Mycoplasma P23.6
        Pseudomonas P23.5
        Staphylococcus P23.2
        Streptococcus (except group B) P23.6
          group B P23.3
        viral agent P23.0
      specified NEC P23.8
    croupous — see Pneumonia, lobar
    cryptogenic organizing J84.116
    cytomegalic inclusion B25.0
    cytomegaloviral B25.0
    deglutition — see Pneumonia, aspiration
    desquamative interstitial J84.117
    diffuse — see Pneumonia, broncho
    diplococcal, diplococcus (broncho-) (lobar) J13
    disseminated (focal) — see Pneumonia, broncho
    Eaton's agent J15.7
    embolic, embolism — see Embolism, pulmonary
    Enterobacter J15.6
    eosinophilic J82
    Escherichia coli (E. coli) J15.5
    Eubacterium J15.8
    fibrinous — see Pneumonia, lobar
    fibroid, fibrous (chronic) — see Fibrosis, lung
    Friedländer's bacillus J15.0
    Fusobacterium (nucleatum) J15.8
    gangrenous J85.0
    giant cell (measles) B05.2
    gonococcal A54.84
    gram-negative bacteria NEC J15.6
      anaerobic J15.8
    Hemophilus influenzae (broncho) (lobar) J14
    human metapneumovirus J12.3
    hypostatic (broncho) (lobar) J18.2
    in (due to)
      actinomycosis A42.0
      adenovirus J12.0
      anthrax A22.1
      ascariasis B77.81
      aspergillosis B44.9
      Bacillus anthracis A22.1
      Bacterium anitratum J15.6
      candidiasis B37.1
      chickenpox B01.2
      Chlamydia J16.0
        neonatal P23.1
      coccidioidomycosis B38.2
        acute B38.0
        chronic B38.1
      cytomegalovirus disease B25.0
      Diplococcus (pneumoniae) J13
      Eaton's agent J15.7
      Enterobacter J15.6
      Escherichia coli (E. coli) J15.5
      Friedländer's bacillus J15.0
      fumes and vapors (chemical) (inhalation) J68.0
      gonorrhea A54.84
      Hemophilus influenzae (H. influenzae) J14

Pneumonia — *continued*
  in — *continued*
    Herellea J15.6
    histoplasmosis B39.2
      acute B39.0
      chronic B39.1
    human metapneumovirus J12.3
    Klebsiella (pneumoniae) J15.0
    measles B05.2
    Mycoplasma (pneumoniae) J15.7
    nocardiosis, nocardiasis A43.0
    ornithosis A70
    parainfluenza virus J12.2
    pleuro-pneumonia-like-organism (PPLO) J15.7
    pneumococcus J13
    pneumocystosis (Pneumocystis carinii)
      (Pneumocystis jiroveci) B59
    Proteus J15.6
    Pseudomonas NEC J15.1
      pseudomallei A24.1
    psittacosis A70
    Q fever A78
    respiratory syncytial virus (RSV) J12.1
    rheumatic fever I00 *[J17]*
    rubella B06.81
    Salmonella (infection) A02.22
      typhi A01.03
    schistosomiasis B65.9 *[J17]*
    Serratia marcescens J15.6
    specified
      bacterium NEC J15.8
      organism NEC J16.8
    spirochetal NEC A69.8
    Staphylococcus J15.20
      aureus (methicillin susceptible) (MSSA) J15.211
        methicillin resistant (MRSA) J15.212
      specified NEC J15.29
    Streptococcus J15.4
      group B J15.3
      pneumoniae J13
      specified NEC J15.4
    toxoplasmosis B58.3
    tularemia A21.2
    typhoid (fever) A01.03
    varicella B01.2
    virus — *see* Pneumonia, viral
    whooping cough A37.91
      due to
        Bordetella parapertussis A37.11
        Bordetella pertussis A37.01
        specified NEC A37.81
    Yersinia pestis A20.2
  inhalation of food or vomit — *see* Pneumonia,
    aspiration
  interstitial J84.9
    chronic J84.111
    desquamative J84.117
    due to
      collagen vascular disease J84.17
      known underlying cause J84.17
    idiopathic NOS J84.111
    in disease classified elsewhere J84.17
    lymphocytic (due to collagen vascular disease) (in
      diseases classified elsewhere) J84.17
    lymphoid J84.2
    non-specific J84.89
      due to
        collagen vascular disease J84.17
        known underlying cause J84.17
      idiopathic J84.113
      in diseases classified elsewhere J84.17
    plasma cell B59
    pseudomonas J15.1
    usual J84.112
      due to collagen vascular disease J84.17
      idiopathic J84.112
      in diseases classified elsewhere J84.17
  Klebsiella (pneumoniae) J15.0
  lipid, lipoid (exogenous) J69.1
    endogenous J84.89
  lobar (disseminated) (double) (interstitial) J18.1
    bacterial J15.9
      specified NEC J15.8
    chronic — *see* Fibrosis, lung
    Escherichia coli (E. coli) J15.5
    Friedländer's bacillus J15.0
    Hemophilus influenzae J14
    hypostatic J18.2
    Klebsiella (pneumoniae) J15.0
    pneumococcal J13
    Proteus J15.6
    Pseudomonas J15.1

Pneumonia — *continued*
  lobar — *continued*
    specified organism NEC J16.8
    staphylococcal — *see* Pneumonia, staphylococcal
    streptococcal NEC J15.4
    Streptococcus pneumoniae J13
    viral, virus — *see* Pneumonia, viral
  lobular — *see* Pneumonia, broncho
  Löffler's J82
  lymphoid interstitial J84.2
  massive — *see* Pneumonia, lobar
  meconium P24.01
  MRSA (Methicillin resistant Staphylococcus aureus)
    J15.212
  MSSA (methicillin susceptible Staphylococcus
    aureus) J15.211
  multilobar — *see* Pneumonia, by type
  Mycoplasma (pneumoniae) J15.7
  necrotic J85.0
  neonatal P23.9
    aspiration — *see* Aspiration, by substance, with
      pneumonia
  nitrogen dioxide J68.0
  organizing J84.89
    due to
      collagen vascular disease J84.17
      known underlying cause J84.17
    in diseases classified elsewhere J84.17
  orthostatic J18.2
  parainfluenza virus J12.2
  parenchymatous — *see* Fibrosis, lung
  passive J18.2
  patchy — *see* Pneumonia, broncho
  Peptococcus J15.8
  Peptostreptococcus J15.8
  plasma cell (of infants) B59
  pleurolobar — *see* Pneumonia, lobar
  pleuro-pneumonia-like organism (PPLO) J15.7
  pneumococcal (broncho) (lobar) J13
  Pneumocystis (carinii) (jiroveci) B59
  postinfectional NEC B99 ☑ *[J17]*
  postmeasles B05.2
  Proteus J15.6
  Pseudomonas J15.1
  psittacosis A70
  radiation J70.0
  respiratory syncytial virus (RSV) J12.1
  resulting from a procedure J95.89
  rheumatic I00 *[J17]*
  Salmonella (arizonae) (cholerae-suis) (enteritidis)
    (typhimurium) A02.22
    typhi A01.03
    typhoid fever A01.03
  SARS-associated coronavirus J12.81
  segmented, segmental — *see* Pneumonia, broncho-
  Serratia marcescens J15.6
  specified NEC J18.8
    bacterium NEC J15.8
    organism NEC J16.8
    virus NEC J12.89
  spirochetal NEC A69.8
  staphylococcal (broncho) (lobar) J15.20
    aureus (methicillin susceptible) (MSSA) J15.211
      methicillin resistant (MRSA) J15.212
    specified NEC J15.29
  static, stasis J18.2
  streptococcal NEC (broncho) (lobar) J15.4
    group
      A J15.4
      B J15.3
      specified NEC J15.4
  Streptococcus pneumoniae J13
  syphilitic, congenital (early) A50.04
  traumatic (complication) (early) (secondary)
    T79.8 ☑
  tuberculous (any) — *see* Tuberculosis, pulmonary
  tularemic A21.2
  varicella B01.2
  Veillonella J15.8
  ventilator associated J95.851
  viral, virus (broncho) (interstitial) (lobar) J12.9
    adenoviral J12.0
    congenital P23.0
    human metapneumovirus J12.3
    parainfluenza J12.2
    respiratory syncytial (RSV) J12.1
    SARS-associated coronavirus J12.81
    specified NEC J12.89
  white (congenital) A50.04
Pneumonic — *see* condition
Pneumonitis (acute) (primary) (*see also* Pneumonia)
  air-conditioner J67.7

Pneumonitis — *continued*
  allergic (due to) J67.9
    organic dust NEC J67.8
    red cedar dust J67.8
    sequoiosis J67.8
    wood dust J67.8
  aspiration J69.0
    due to
      anesthesia J95.4
        during
          labor and delivery O74.0
          pregnancy O29.01 ☑
          puerperium O89.01
      fumes or gases J68.0
    obstetric O74.0
  chemical (due to gases, fumes or vapors)
    (inhalation) J68.0
    due to anesthesia J95.4
  cholesterol J84.89
  crack (cocaine) J68.0
  chronic — *see* Fibrosis, lung
  congenital rubella P35.0
  due to
    beryllium J68.0
    cadmium J68.0
    crack (cocaine) J68.0
    detergent J69.8
    fluorocarbon-polymer J68.0
    food, vomit (aspiration) J69.0
    fumes or vapors J68.0
    gases, fumes or vapors (inhalation) J68.0
    inhalation
      blood J69.8
      essences J69.1
      food (regurgitated), milk, vomit J69.0
      oils, essences J69.1
      saliva J69.0
      solids, liquids NEC J69.8
    manganese J68.0
    nitrogen dioxide J68.0
    oils, essences J69.1
    solids, liquids NEC J69.8
    toxoplasmosis (acquired) B58.3
      congenital P37.1
    vanadium J68.0
    ventilator J95.851
  eosinophilic J82
  hypersensitivity J67.9
    air conditioner lung J67.7
    bagassosis J67.1
    bird fancier's lung J67.2
    farmer's lung J67.0
    maltworker's lung J67.4
    maple bark-stripper's lung J67.6
    mushroom worker's lung J67.5
    specified organic dust NEC J67.8
    suberosis J67.3
  interstitial (chronic) J84.89
    acute J84.114
    lymphoid J84.2
    non-specific J84.89
      idiopathic J84.113
  lymphoid, interstitial J84.2
  meconium P24.01
  postanesthetic J95.4
    correct substance properly administered — *see*
      Table of Drugs and Chemicals, by drug,
      adverse effect
    in labor and delivery O74.0
    in pregnancy O29.01 ☑
    obstetric O74.0
    overdose or wrong substance given or taken
      (by accident) — *see* Table of Drugs and
      Chemicals, by drug, poisoning
    postpartum, puerperal O89.01
  postoperative J95.4
    obstetric O74.0
  radiation J70.0
  rubella, congenital P35.0
  ventilation (air-conditioning) J67.7
  ventilator associated J95.851
  wood-dust J67.8
Pneumonoconiosis — *see* Pneumoconiosis
Pneumoparotid K11.8
Pneumopathy NEC J98.4
  alveolar J84.09
  due to organic dust NEC J66.8
  parietoalveolar J84.09
Pneumopericarditis (*see also* Pericarditis)
  acute I30.9
Pneumopericardium (*see also* Pericarditis)
  congenital P25.3

Pneumopericardium - Polyneuropathy

Pneumopericardium — *continued*
  newborn P25.3
  traumatic (post) — *see* Injury, heart
Pneumophagia (psychogenic) F45.8
Pneumopleurisy, pneumopleuritis (*see also*
  Pneumonia) J18.8
Pneumopyopericardium I30.1
Pneumopyothorax — *see* Pyopneumothorax
  with fistula J86.0
Pneumorrhagia (*see also* Hemorrhage, lung)
  tuberculous — *see* Tuberculosis, pulmonary
Pneumothorax NOS J93.9
  acute J93.83
  chronic J93.81
  congenital P25.1
  perinatal period P25.1
  postprocedural J95.811
  specified NEC J93.83
  spontaneous NOS J93.83
    newborn P25.1
    primary J93.11
    secondary J93.12
    tension J93.0
  tense valvular, infectional J93.0
  tension (spontaneous) J93.0
  traumatic S27.0 ☑
    with hemothorax S27.2 ☑
  tuberculous — *see* Tuberculosis, pulmonary
Podagra (*see also* Gout) M10.9
Podencephalus Q01.9
Poikilocytosis R71.8
Poikiloderma L81.6
  Civatte's L57.3
  congenital Q82.8
  vasculare atrophicans L94.5
Poikilodermatomyositis M33.10
  with
    myopathy M33.12
    respiratory involvement M33.11
    specified organ involvement NEC M33.19
Pointed ear (congenital) Q17.3
Poison ivy, oak, sumac or other plant dermatitis
  (allergic) (contact) L23.7
Poisoning (acute) (*see also* Table of Drugs and
  Chemicals)
  algae and toxins T65.82 ☑
  Bacillus B (aertrycke) (cholerae (suis))
    (paratyphosus) (suipestifer) A02.9
    botulinus A05.1
  bacterial toxins A05.9
  berries, noxious — *see* Poisoning, food, noxious,
    berries
  botulism A05.1
  ciguatera fish T61.0 ☑
  Clostridium botulinum A05.1
  death-cap (Amanita phalloides) (Amanita verna) —
    see Poisoning, food, noxious, mushrooms
  drug — *see* Table of Drugs and Chemicals, by drug,
    poisoning
  epidemic, fish (noxious) — *see* Poisoning, seafood
    bacterial A05.9
  fava bean D55.0
  fish (noxious) T61.9 ☑
    bacterial — *see* Intoxication, foodborne, by agent
    ciguatera fish — *see* Poisoning, ciguatera fish
    scombroid fish — *see* Poisoning, scombroid fish
    specified type NEC T61.77 ☑
  food NEC A05.9
    bacterial — *see* Intoxication, foodborne, by agent
    due to
      Bacillus (aertrycke) (choleraesuis)
        (paratyphosus) (suipestifer) A02.9
        botulinus A05.1
      Clostridium (perfringens) (Welchii) A05.2
      salmonella (aertrycke) (callinarum)
        (choleraesuis) (enteritidis) (paratyphi)
        (suipestifer) A02.9
        with
          gastroenteritis A02.0
          sepsis A02.1
      staphylococcus A05.0
      Vibrio
        parahaemolyticus A05.3
        vulnificus A05.5
    noxious or naturally toxic T62.9 ☑
      berries — *see* subcategory T62.1 ☑
      fish — *see* Poisoning, fish
      mushrooms — *see* subcategory T62.0X ☑
      plants NEC — *see* subcategory T62.2X ☑
      seafood — *see* Poisoning, seafood
      specified NEC — *see* subcategory T62.8X ☑
    ichthyotoxism — *see* Poisoning, seafood

Poisoning — *continued*
  kreotoxism, food A05.9
  latex T65.81 ☑
  lead T56.0 ☑
  mushroom — *see* Poisoning, food, noxious,
    mushroom
  mussels (*see also* Poisoning, shellfish)
    bacterial — *see* Intoxication, foodborne, by agent
  nicotine (tobacco) T65.2 ☑
  noxious foodstuffs — *see* Poisoning, food, noxious
  plants, noxious — *see* Poisoning, food, noxious,
    plants NEC
  ptomaine — *see* Poisoning, food
  radiation J70.0
  Salmonella (arizonae) (cholerae-suis) (enteritidis)
    (typhimurium) A02.9
  scombroid fish T61.1 ☑
  seafood (noxious) T61.9 ☑
    bacterial — *see* Intoxication, foodborne, by agent
    fish — *see* Poisoning, fish
    shellfish — *see* Poisoning, shellfish
    specified NEC — *see* subcategory T61.8X ☑
  shellfish (amnesic) (azaspiracid) (diarrheic)
    (neurotoxic) (noxious) (paralytic) T61.78 ☑
    bacterial — *see* Intoxication, foodborne, by agent
    ciguatera mollusk — *see* Poisoning, ciguatera fish
  specified substance NEC T65.891 ☑
  Staphylococcus, food A05.0
  tobacco (nicotine) T65.2 ☑
  water E87.79
Poker spine — *see* Spondylitis, ankylosing
Poland syndrome Q79.8
Polioencephalitis (acute) (bulbar) A80.9
  inferior G12.22
  influenzal — *see* Influenza, with, encephalopathy
  superior hemorrhagic (acute) (Wernicke's) E51.2
  Wernicke's E51.2
Polioencephalomyelitis (acute) (anterior) A80.9
  with beriberi E51.2
Polioencephalopathy, superior hemorrhagic E51.2
  with
    beriberi E51.11
    pellagra E52
Poliomeningoencephalitis — *see* Meningoencephalitis
Poliomyelitis (acute) (anterior) (epidemic) A80.9
  with paralysis (bulbar) — *see* Poliomyelitis, paralytic
  abortive A80.4
  ascending (progressive) — *see* Poliomyelitis,
    paralytic
  bulbar (paralytic) — *see* Poliomyelitis, paralytic
  congenital P35.8
  nonepidemic A80.9
  nonparalytic A80.4
  paralytic A80.30
    specified NEC A80.39
    vaccine-associated A80.0
      wild virus
        imported A80.1
        indigenous A80.2
  spinal, acute A80.9
Poliosis (eyebrow) (eyelashes) L67.1
  circumscripta, acquired L67.1
Pollakiuria R35.0
  psychogenic F45.8
Pollinosis J30.1
Pollitzer's disease L73.2
Polyadenitis (*see also* Lymphadenitis)
  malignant A20.0
Polyalgia M79.89
Polyangiitis M30.0
  microscopic M31.7
  overlap syndrome M30.8
Polyarteritis
  microscopic M31.7
  nodosa M30.0
    with lung involvement M30.1
    juvenile M30.2
    related condition NEC M30.8
Polyarthralgia — *see* Pain, joint
Polyarthritis, polyarthropathy (*see also* Arthritis) M13.0
  due to or associated with other specified conditions
    — *see* Arthritis
  epidemic (Australian) (with exanthema) B33.1
  infective — *see* Arthritis, pyogenic or pyemic
  inflammatory M06.4
  juvenile (chronic) (seronegative) M08.3
  migratory M13.8 ☑
  rheumatic, acute — *see* Fever, rheumatic
Polyarthrosis M15.9
  post-traumatic M15.3
  primary M15.0
  specified NEC M15.8

Polycarential syndrome of infancy E40
Polychondritis (atrophic) (chronic) (*see also* Disorder,
  cartilage, specified type NEC)
  relapsing M94.1
Polycoria Q13.2
Polycystic (disease)
  degeneration, kidney Q61.3
    autosomal dominant (adult type) Q61.2
    autosomal recessive (infantile type) NEC Q61.19
  kidney Q61.3
    autosomal
      dominant Q61.2
      recessive NEC Q61.19
    autosomal dominant (adult type) Q61.2
    autosomal recessive (childhood type) NEC Q61.19
    infantile type NEC Q61.19
  liver Q44.6
  lung J98.4
    congenital Q33.0
  ovary, ovaries E28.2
  spleen Q89.09
Polycythemia (secondary) D75.1
  acquired D75.1
  benign (familial) D75.0
  due to
    donor twin P61.1
    erythropoietin D75.1
    fall in plasma volume D75.1
    high altitude D75.1
    maternal-fetal transfusion P61.1
    stress D75.1
  emotional D75.1
  erythropoietin D75.1
  familial (benign) D75.0
  Gaisböck's (hypertonica) D75.1
  high altitude D75.1
  hypertonica D75.1
  hypoxemic D75.1
  neonatorum P61.1
  nephrogenous D75.1
  relative D75.1
  secondary D75.1
  spurious D75.1
  stress D75.1
  vera D45
Polycytosis cryptogenica D75.1
Polydactylism, polydactyly Q69.9
  toes Q69.2
Polydipsia R63.1
Polydystrophy, pseudo-Hurler E77.0
Polyembryoma — *see* Neoplasm, malignant, by site
Polyglandular
  deficiency E31.0
  dyscrasia E31.9
  dysfunction E31.9
  syndrome E31.8
Polyhydramnios O40. ☑
Polymastia Q83.1
Polymenorrhea N92.0
Polymyalgia M35.3
  arteritica, giant cell M31.5
  rheumatica M35.3
    with giant cell arteritis M31.5
Polymyositis (acute) (chronic) (hemorrhagic) M33.20
  with
    myopathy M33.22
    respiratory involvement M33.21
    skin involvement — *see* Dermatopolymyositis
    specified organ involvement NEC M33.29
  ossificans (generalisata) (progressiva) — *see*
    Myositis, ossificans, progressiva
Polyneuritis, polyneuritic (*see also* Polyneuropathy)
  acute (post-)infective G61.0
  alcoholic G62.1
  cranialis G52.7
  demyelinating, chronic inflammatory (CIDP)
    G61.81
  diabetic — *see* Diabetes, polyneuropathy
  diphtheritic A36.83
  due to lack of vitamin NEC E56.9 *[G63]*
  endemic E51.11
  erythredema — *see* subcategory T56.1 ☑
  febrile G61.0
  hereditary ataxic G60.1
  idiopathic, acute G61.0
  infective (acute) G61.0
  inflammatory, chronic demyelinating (CIDP) G61.81
  nutritional E63.9 *[G63]*
  postinfective (acute) G61.0
  specified NEC G62.89
Polyneuropathy (peripheral) G62.9
  alcoholic G62.1

☑ **Additional character required**

Polyneuropathy — continued
  amyloid (Portuguese) E85.1 *[G63]*
    transthyretin-related (ATTR) familial E85.1 *[G63]*
  arsenical G62.2
  critical illness G62.81
  demyelinating, chronic inflammatory (CIDP) G61.81
  diabetic — *see* Diabetes, polyneuropathy
  drug-induced G62.0
  hereditary G60.9
    specified NEC G60.8
  idiopathic G60.9
    progressive G60.3
  in (due to)
    alcohol G62.1
      sequelae G65.2
    amyloidosis, familial (Portuguese) E85.1 *[G63]*
    antitetanus serum G61.1
    arsenic G62.2
      sequelae G65.2
    avitaminosis NEC E56.9 *[G63]*
    beriberi E51.11
    collagen vascular disease NEC M35.9 *[G63]*
    deficiency (of)
      B (-complex) vitamins E53.9 *[G63]*
      vitamin B6 E53.1 *[G63]*
    diabetes — *see* Diabetes, polyneuropathy
    diphtheria A36.83
    drug or medicament G62.0
      correct substance properly administered — *see* Table of Drugs and Chemicals, by drug, adverse effect
      overdose or wrong substance given or taken — *see* Table of Drugs and Chemicals, by drug, poisoning
    endocrine disease NEC E34.9 *[G63]*
    herpes zoster B02.23
    hypoglycemia E16.2 *[G63]*
    infectious
      disease NEC B99 ☑ *[G63]*
      mononucleosis B27.91
    lack of vitamin NEC E56.9 *[G63]*
    lead G62.2
      sequelae G65.2
    leprosy A30.9 *[G63]*
    Lyme disease A69.22
    metabolic disease NEC E88.9 *[G63]*
    microscopic polyangiitis M31.7 *[G63]*
    mumps B26.84
    neoplastic disease (*see also* Neoplasm) D49.9 *[G63]*
    nutritional deficiency NEC E63.9 *[G63]*
    organophosphate compounds G62.2
      sequelae G65.2
    parasitic disease NEC B89 *[G63]*
    pellagra E52 *[G63]*
    polyarteritis nodosa M30.0
    porphyria E80.20 *[G63]*
    radiation G62.82
    rheumatoid arthritis — *see* Rheumatoid, polyneuropathy
    sarcoidosis D86.89
    serum G61.1
    syphilis (late) A52.15
      congenital A50.43
    systemic
      connective tissue disorder M35.9 *[G63]*
      lupus erythematosus M32.19
    toxic agent NEC G62.2
      sequelae G65.2
    transthyretin-related (ATTR) familial amyloid E85.1
    triorthocresyl phosphate G62.2
      sequelae G65.2
    tuberculosis A17.89
    uremia N18.9 *[G63]*
    vitamin B12 deficiency E53.8 *[G63]*
      with anemia (pernicious) D51.0 *[G63]*
        due to dietary deficiency D51.3 *[G63]*
    zoster B02.23
  inflammatory G61.9
    chronic demyelinating (CIDP) G61.81
    sequelae G65.1
    specified NEC G61.89
  lead G62.2
    sequelae G65.2
  nutritional NEC E63.9 *[G63]*
  postherpetic (zoster) B02.23
  progressive G60.3
  radiation-induced G62.82
  sensory (hereditary) (idiopathic) G60.8
  specified NEC G62.89
  syphilitic (late) A52.15
    congenital A50.43

Polyopia H53.8
Polyorchism, polyorchidism Q55.21
Polyosteoarthritis (*see also* Osteoarthritis, generalized) M15.9
  post-traumatic M15.3
  specified NEC M15.8
Polyostotic fibrous dysplasia Q78.1
Polyotia Q17.0
Polyp, polypus
  accessory sinus J33.8
  adenocarcinoma in — *see* Neoplasm, malignant, by site
  adenocarcinoma in situ in — *see* Neoplasm, in situ, by site
  adenoid tissue J33.0
  adenomatous (*see also* Neoplasm, benign, by site)
    adenocarcinoma in — *see* Neoplasm, malignant, by site
    adenocarcinoma in situ in — *see* Neoplasm, in situ, by site
    carcinoma in — *see* Neoplasm, malignant, by site
    carcinoma in situ in — *see* Neoplasm, in situ, by site
    multiple — *see* Neoplasm, benign
      adenocarcinoma in — *see* Neoplasm, malignant, by site
      adenocarcinoma in situ in — *see* Neoplasm, in situ, by site
  antrum J33.8
  anus, anal (canal) K62.0
  Bartholin's gland N84.3
  bladder D41.4
  carcinoma in — *see* Neoplasm, malignant, by site
  carcinoma in situ in — *see* Neoplasm, in situ, by site
  cecum D12.0
  cervix (uteri) N84.1
    in pregnancy or childbirth — *see* Pregnancy, complicated by, abnormal, cervix
    mucous N84.1
    nonneoplastic N84.1
  choanal J33.0
  cholesterol K82.4
  clitoris N84.3
  colon K63.5
    adenomatous D12.6
      ascending D12.2
      cecum D12.0
      descending D12.4
    hyperplastic, (any site) K63.5
    inflammatory K51.40
      with
        abscess K51.414
        complication K51.419
          specified NEC K51.418
        fistula K51.413
        intestinal obstruction K51.412
        rectal bleeding K51.411
    sigmoid D12.5
    transverse D12.3
  corpus uteri N84.0
  dental K04.01
    irreversible K04.02
    reversible K04.01
  duodenum K31.7
  ear (middle) H74.4 ☑
  endometrium N84.0
  ethmoidal (sinus) J33.8
  fallopian tube N84.8
  female genital tract N84.9
    specified NEC N84.8
  frontal (sinus) J33.8
  gallbladder K82.4
  gingiva, gum K06.8
  labia, labium (majus) (minus) N84.3
  larynx (mucous) J38.1
    adenomatous D14.1
  malignant — *see* Neoplasm, malignant, by site
  maxillary (sinus) J33.8
  middle ear — *see* Polyp, ear (middle)
  myometrium N84.0
  nares
    anterior J33.9
    posterior J33.0
  nasal (mucous) J33.9
    cavity J33.0
    septum J33.0
  nasopharyngeal J33.0
  nose (mucous) J33.9
  oviduct N84.8
  pharynx J39.2
  placenta O90.89
  prostate — *see* Enlargement, enlarged, prostate

Polyp — continued
  pudenda, pudendum N84.3
  pulpal (dental) K04.01
    irreversible K04.02
    reversible K04.01
  rectum (nonadenomatous) K62.1
    adenomatous — *see* Polyp, adenomatous
  septum (nasal) J33.0
  sinus (accessory) (ethmoidal) (frontal) (maxillary) (sphenoidal) J33.8
  sphenoidal (sinus) J33.8
  stomach K31.7
    adenomatous D13.1
  tube, fallopian N84.8
  turbinate, mucous membrane J33.8
  umbilical, newborn P83.6
  ureter N28.89
  urethra N36.2
  uterus (body) (corpus) (mucous) N84.0
    cervix N84.1
    in pregnancy or childbirth — *see* Pregnancy, complicated by, tumor, uterus
  vagina N84.2
  vocal cord (mucous) J38.1
  vulva N84.3
Polyphagia R63.2
Polyploidy Q92.7
Polypoid — *see* condition
Polyposis (*see also* Polyp)
  coli (adenomatous) D12.6
    adenocarcinoma in C18.9
    adenocarcinoma in situ in — *see* Neoplasm, in situ, by site
    carcinoma in C18.9
  colon (adenomatous) D12.6
  familial D12.6
    adenocarcinoma in situ in — *see* Neoplasm, in situ, by site
  intestinal (adenomatous) D12.6
  malignant lymphomatous C83.1 ☑
  multiple, adenomatous (*see also* Neoplasm, benign) D36.9
Polyradiculitis — *see* Polyneuropathy
Polyradiculoneuropathy (acute) (postinfective) (segmentally demyelinating) G61.0
Polyserositis
  due to pericarditis I31.1
  pericardial I31.1
  periodic, familial E85.0
  tuberculous A19.9
    acute A19.1
    chronic A19.8
Polysplenia syndrome Q89.09
Polysyndactyly (*see also* Syndactylism, syndactyly) Q70.4
Polytrichia L68.3
Polyunguia Q84.6
Polyuria R35.8
  nocturnal R35.1
  psychogenic F45.8
Pompe's disease (glycogen storage) E74.02
Pompholyx L30.1
Poncet's disease (tuberculous rheumatism) A18.09
Pond fracture — *see* Fracture, skull
Ponos B55.0
Pons, pontine — *see* condition
Poor
  aesthetic of existing restoration of tooth K08.56
  contractions, labor O62.2
  gingival margin to tooth restoration K08.51
  personal hygiene R46.0
  prenatal care, affecting management of pregnancy — *see* Pregnancy, complicated by, insufficient, prenatal care
  sucking reflex (newborn) R29.2
  urinary stream R39.12
  vision NEC H54.7
Poradenitis, nostras inguinalis or venerea A55
Porencephaly (congenital) (developmental) (true) Q04.6
  acquired G93.0
  nondevelopmental G93.0
  traumatic (post) F07.89
Porocephaliasis B88.8
Porokeratosis Q82.8
Poroma, eccrine — *see* Neoplasm, skin, benign
Porphyria (South African) E80.20
  acquired E80.20
  acute intermittent (hepatic) (Swedish) E80.21
  cutanea tarda (hereditary) (symptomatic) E80.1

Porphyria - Pregnancy

Porphyria — *continued*
  due to drugs E80.20
    correct substance properly administered — *see*
      Table of Drugs and Chemicals, by drug,
      adverse effect
    overdose or wrong substance given or taken —
      see Table of Drugs and Chemicals, by drug,
      poisoning
  erythropoietic (congenital) (hereditary) E80.0
  hepatocutaneous type E80.1
  secondary E80.20
  toxic NEC E80.20
  variegata E80.20
Porphyrinuria — *see* Porphyria
Porphyruria — *see* Porphyria
Portal — *see* condition
Port wine nevus, mark, or stain Q82.5
Posadas-Wernicke disease B38.9
Positive
  culture (nonspecific)
    blood R78.81
    bronchial washings R84.5
    cerebrospinal fluid R83.5
    cervix uteri R87.5
    nasal secretions R84.5
    nipple discharge R89.5
    nose R84.5
      staphylococcus (Methicillin susceptible) Z22.321
        Methicillin resistant Z22.322
    peritoneal fluid R85.5
    pleural fluid R84.5
    prostatic secretions R86.5
    saliva R85.5
    seminal fluid R86.5
    sputum R84.5
    synovial fluid R89.5
    throat scrapings R84.5
    urine R82.79
    vagina R87.5
    vulva R87.5
    wound secretions R89.5
  PPD (skin test) R76.11
  serology for syphilis A53.0
    false R76.8
    with signs or symptoms - code as Syphilis, by site
      and stage
  skin test, tuberculin (without active tuberculosis)
    R76.11
  test, human immunodeficiency virus (HIV) R75
  VDRL A53.0
    with signs or symptoms - code by site and stage
      under Syphilis A53.9
  Wassermann reaction A53.0
Postcardiotomy syndrome I97.0
Postcaval ureter Q62.62
Postcholecystectomy syndrome K91.5
Postclimacteric bleeding N95.0
Postcommissurotomy syndrome I97.0
Postconcussional syndrome F07.81
Postcontusional syndrome F07.81
Postcricoid region — *see* condition
Post-dates (40-42 weeks) (pregnancy) (mother) O48.0
  more than 42 weeks gestation O48.1
Postencephalitic syndrome F07.89
Posterior — *see* condition
Posterolateral sclerosis (spinal cord) — *see*
  Degeneration, combined
Postexanthematous — *see* condition
Postfebrile — *see* condition
Postgastrectomy dumping syndrome K91.1
Posthemiplegic chorea — *see* Monoplegia
Posthemorrhagic anemia (chronic) D50.0
  acute D62
  newborn P61.3
Postherpetic neuralgia (zoster) B02.29
  trigeminal B02.22
Posthitis N47.7
Postimmunization complication or reaction — *see*
  Complications, vaccination
Postinfectious — *see* condition
Postlaminectomy syndrome NEC M96.1
Postleukotomy syndrome F07.0
Postmastectomy lymphedema (syndrome) I97.2
Postmaturity, postmature (over 42 weeks)
  maternal (over 42 weeks gestation) O48.1
  newborn P08.22
Postmeasles complication NEC (*see also* condition)
  B05.89
Postmenopausal
  endometrium (atrophic) N95.8
    suppurative (*see also* Endometritis) N71.9
  osteoporosis — *see* Osteoporosis, postmenopausal

Postnasal drip R09.82
  due to
    allergic rhinitis — *see* Rhinitis, allergic
    common cold J00
    gastroesophageal reflux — *see* Reflux,
      gastroesophageal
    nasopharyngitis — *see* Nasopharyngitis
    other know condition - code to condition
    sinusitis — *see* Sinusitis
Postnatal — *see* condition
Postoperative (postprocedural) — *see* Complication,
  postoperative
  pneumothorax, therapeutic Z98.3
  state NEC Z98.890
Postpancreatectomy hyperglycemia E89.1
Postpartum — *see* Puerperal
Postphlebitic syndrome — *see* Syndrome,
  postthrombotic
Postpoliomyelitic (*see also* condition)
  osteopathy — *see* Osteopathy, after poliomyelitis
Postpolio (myelitic) syndrome G14
Postprocedural (*see also* Postoperative)
  hypoinsulinemia E89.1
Postschizophrenic depression F32.89
Postsurgery status (*see also* Status (post))
  pneumothorax, therapeutic Z98.3
Post-term (40-42 weeks) (pregnancy) (mother) O48.0
  infant P08.21
  more than 42 weeks gestation (mother) O48.1
Post-traumatic brain syndrome, nonpsychotic F07.81
Post-typhoid abscess A01.09
Postures, hysterical F44.2
Postvaccinal reaction or complication — *see*
  Complications, vaccination
Postvalvulotomy syndrome I97.0
Potain's
  disease (pulmonary edema) — *see* Edema, lung
  syndrome (gastrectasis with dyspepsia) K31.0
Potter's
  asthma J62.8
  facies Q60.6
  lung J62.8
  syndrome (with renal agenesis) Q60.6
Pott's
  curvature (spinal) A18.01
  disease or paraplegia A18.01
  spinal curvature A18.01
  tumor, puffy — *see* Osteomyelitis, specified type
    NEC
Pouch
  bronchus Q32.4
  Douglas' — *see* condition
  esophagus, esophageal, congenital Q39.6
    acquired K22.5
  gastric K31.4
  Hartmann's K82.8
  pharynx, pharyngeal (congenital) Q38.7
Pouchitis K91.850
Poultrymen's itch B88.0
Poverty NEC Z59.6
  extreme Z59.5
Poxvirus NEC B08.8
Prader-Willi syndrome Q87.11
Prader-Willi-like syndrome Q87.19
Preauricular appendage or tag Q17.0
Prebetalipoproteinemia (acquired) (essential)
  (familial) (hereditary) (primary) (secondary) E78.1
  with chylomicronemia E78.3
Precipitate labor or delivery O62.3
Preclimacteric bleeding (menorrhagia) N92.4
Precocious
  adrenarche E30.1
  menarche E30.1
  menstruation E30.1
  pubarche E30.1
  puberty E30.1
    central E22.8
  sexual development NEC E30.1
  thelarche E30.8
Precocity, sexual (constitutional) (cryptogenic) (female)
  (idiopathic) (male) E30.1
  with adrenal hyperplasia E25.9
    congenital E25.0
Precordial pain R07.2
Predeciduous teeth K00.2
Prediabetes, prediabetic R73.03
  complicating
    pregnancy — *see* Pregnancy, complicated by,
      diseases of, specified type or system NEC
    puerperium O99.89
Predislocation status of hip at birth Q65.6
Pre-eclampsia O14.9 ☑

Pre-eclampsia — *continued*
  with pre-existing hypertension — *see* Hypertension,
    complicating pregnancy, pre-existing, with,
    pre-eclampsia
  complicating
    childbirth O14.94
    puerperium O14.95
  mild O14.0 ☑
    complicating
      childbirth O14.04
      puerperium O14.05
  moderate O14.0 ☑
    complicating
      childbirth O14.04
      puerperium O14.05
  severe O14.1 ☑
    with hemolysis, elevated liver enzymes and low
      platelet count (HELLP) O14.2 ☑
    complicating
      childbirth O14.24
      puerperium O14.25
    complicating
      childbirth O14.14
      puerperium O14.15
Pre-eruptive color change, teeth, tooth K00.8
Pre-excitation atrioventricular conduction I45.6
Preglaucoma H40.00 ☑
Pregnancy (single) (uterine) (*see also* Delivery and
  Puerperal)
  Note: The Tabular must be reviewed for assignment
    of the appropriate character indicating the
    trimester of the pregnancy
  Note: The Tabular must be reviewed for assignment
    of appropriate seventh character for multiple
    gestation codes in Chapter 15
  abdominal (ectopic) O00.00
    with intrauterine pregnancy O00.01
    with viable fetus O36.7 ☑
  ampullar O00.10 ☑
    with intrauterine pregnancy O00.11 ☑
  biochemical O02.81
  broad ligament O00.80
    with intrauterine pregnancy O00.81
  cervical O00.80
    with intrauterine pregnancy O00.81
  chemical O02.81
  complicated NOS O26.9 ☑
  complicated by (care of) (management affected by)
    abnormal, abnormality
      cervix O34.4 ☑
        causing obstructed labor O65.5
      cord (umbilical) O69.9 ☑
      fetal heart rate or rhythm O36.83 ☑
      findings on antenatal screening of mother
        O28.9
        biochemical O28.1
        cytological O28.2
        chromosomal O28.5
        genetic O28.5
        hematological O28.0
        radiological O28.4
        specified NEC O28.8
        ultrasonic O28.3
      glucose (tolerance) NEC O99.810
      pelvic organs O34.9 ☑
        specified NEC O34.8 ☑
          causing obstructed labor O65.5
      pelvis (bony) (major) NEC O33.0
      perineum O34.7 ☑
      position
        placenta O44.0 ☑
          with hemorrhage O44.1 ☑
        uterus O34.59 ☑
      uterus O34.59 ☑
        causing obstructed labor O65.5
        congenital O34.0 ☑
      vagina O34.6 ☑
        causing obstructed labor O65.5
      vulva O34.7 ☑
        causing obstructed labor O65.5
    abruptio placentae — *see* Abruptio placentae
    abscess or cellulitis
      bladder O23.1 ☑
      breast O91.11 ☑
      genital organ or tract O23.9 ☑
    abuse
      physical O9A.31 ☑
      psychological O9A.51 ☑
      sexual O9A.41 ☑
    adverse effect anesthesia O29.9 ☑
      aspiration pneumonitis O29.01 ☑
      cardiac arrest O29.11 ☑

Pregnancy — *continued*
  complicated by — *continued*
    cardiac complication NEC O29.19 ☑
    cardiac failure O29.12 ☑
    central nervous system complication NEC O29.29 ☑
    cerebral anoxia O29.21 ☑
    failed or difficult intubation O29.6 ☑
    inhalation of stomach contents or secretions NOS O29.01 ☑
    local, toxic reaction O29.3X ☑
    Mendelson's syndrome O29.01 ☑
    pressure collapse of lung O29.02 ☑
    pulmonary complications NEC O29.09 ☑
    specified NEC O29.8X ☑
    spinal and epidural type NEC O29.5X ☑
      induced headache O29.4 ☑
  albuminuria (*see also* Proteinuria, gestational) O12.1 ☑
  alcohol use O99.31 ☑
  amnionitis O41.12 ☑
  anaphylactoid syndrome of pregnancy O88.01 ☑
  anemia (conditions in D50-D64) (pre-existing) O99.01 ☑
    complicating the puerperium O99.03
  antepartum hemorrhage O46.9 ☑
    with coagulation defect — *see* Hemorrhage, antepartum, with coagulation defect
    specified NEC O46.8X ☑
  appendicitis O99.61 ☑
  atrophy (yellow) (acute) liver (subacute) O26.61 ☑
  bariatric surgery status O99.84 ☑
  bicornis or bicornuate uterus O34.0 ☑
  biliary tract problems O26.61 ☑
  breech presentation O32.1 ☑
  cardiovascular diseases (conditions in I00-I09, I00-I09, I00-I09) O99.41 ☑
  cerebrovascular disorders (conditions in I60-I69) O99.41 ☑
  cervical shortening O26.87 ☑
  cervicitis O23.51 ☑
  chloasma (gravidarum) O26.89 ☑
  cholestasis (intrahepatic) O26.61 ☑
  cholecystitis O99.61 ☑
  chorioamnionitis O41.12 ☑
  circulatory system disorder (conditions in I00-I09, I00-I09, O99.41 ☑)
  compound presentation O32.6 ☑
  conjoined twins O30.02 ☑
  connective system disorders (conditions in M00-M99) O99.89
  contracted pelvis (general) O33.1
    inlet O33.2
    outlet O33.3 ☑
  convulsions (eclamptic) (uremic) (*see also* Eclampsia) O15.9
  cracked nipple O92.11 ☑
  cystitis O23.1 ☑
  cystocele O34.8 ☑
  death of fetus (near term) O36.4 ☑
    early pregnancy O02.1
    of one fetus or more in multiple gestation O31.2 ☑
  deciduitis O41.14 ☑
  decreased fetal movement O36.81 ☑
  dental problems O99.61 ☑
  diabetes (mellitus) O24.91 ☑
    gestational (pregnancy induced) — *see* Diabetes, gestational
    pre-existing O24.31 ☑
      specified NEC O24.81 ☑
      type 1 O24.01 ☑
      type 2 O24.11 ☑
  digestive system disorders (conditions in K00-K93) O99.61 ☑
  diseases of — *see* Pregnancy, complicated by, specified body system disease
    biliary tract O26.61 ☑
    blood NEC (conditions in D65-D77) O99.11 ☑
    liver O26.61 ☑
    specified NEC O99.89
  disorders of — *see* Pregnancy, complicated by, specified body system disorder
    amniotic fluid and membranes O41.9 ☑
      specified NEC O41.8X ☑
    biliary tract O26.61 ☑
    ear and mastoid process (conditions in H60-H95) O99.89
    eye and adnexa (conditions in H00-H59) O99.89
    liver O26.61 ☑
    skin (conditions in L00-L99) O99.71 ☑
    specified NEC O99.89

Pregnancy — *continued*
  complicated by — *continued*
    displacement, uterus NEC O34.59 ☑
      causing obstructed labor O65.5
    disproportion (due to) O33.9
      fetal (ascites) (hydrops) (meningomyelocele) (sacral teratoma) (tumor) deformities NEC O33.7 ☑
      generally contracted pelvis O33.1
      hydrocephalus fetus O33.6 ☑
      inlet contraction of pelvis O33.2
      mixed maternal and fetal origin O33.4 ☑
      specified NEC O33.8
    double uterus O34.0 ☑
      causing obstructed labor O65.5
    drug use (conditions in F11-F19) O99.32 ☑
    eclampsia, eclamptic (coma) (convulsions) (delirium) (nephritis) (uremia) (*see also* Eclampsia) O15. ☑
    ectopic pregnancy — *see* Pregnancy, ectopic
    edema O12.0 ☑
      with
        gestational hypertension, mild (*see also* Pre-eclampsia) O14.0 ☑
        proteinuria O12.2 ☑
    effusion, amniotic fluid — *see* Pregnancy, complicated by, premature rupture of membranes
    elderly
      multigravida O09.52 ☑
      primigravida O09.51 ☑
    embolism (*see also* Embolism, obstetric, pregnancy) O88. ☑
    endocrine diseases NEC O99.28 ☑
    endometritis O86.12
    excessive weight gain O26.0 ☑
    exhaustion O26.81 ☑
      during labor and delivery O75.81
    face presentation O32.3 ☑
    failed induction of labor O61.9
      instrumental O61.1
      mechanical O61.1
      medical O61.0
      specified NEC O61.8
      surgical O61.1
    failed or difficult intubation for anesthesia O29.6 ☑
    false labor (pains) O47.9
      at or after 37 completed weeks of pregnancy O47.1
      before 37 completed weeks of pregnancy O47.0 ☑
    fatigue O26.81 ☑
      during labor and delivery O75.81
    fatty metamorphosis of liver O26.61 ☑
    female genital mutilation O34.8 ☑ *[N90.81 ☑]*
    fetal (maternal care for)
      abnormality or damage O35.9 ☑
        acid-base balance O68
        specified type NEC O35.8 ☑
      acidemia O68
      acidosis O68
      alkalosis O68
      anemia and thrombocytopenia O36.82 ☑
      anencephaly O35.0 ☑
      bradycardia O36.83 ☑
      chromosomal abnormality (conditions in Q90-Q99) O35.1 ☑
      conjoined twins O30.02 ☑
      damage from
        amniocentesis O35.7 ☑
        biopsy procedures O35.7 ☑
        drug addiction O35.5 ☑
        hematological investigation O35.7 ☑
        intrauterine contraceptive device O35.7 ☑
        maternal
          alcohol addiction O35.4 ☑
          cytomegalovirus infection O35.3 ☑
          disease NEC O35.8 ☑
          drug addiction O35.5 ☑
          listeriosis O35.8 ☑
          rubella O35.3 ☑
          toxoplasmosis O35.8 ☑
          viral infection O35.3 ☑
        medical procedure NEC O35.7 ☑
        radiation O35.6 ☑
      death (near term) O36.4 ☑
        early pregnancy O02.1
      decreased movement O36.81 ☑
      depressed heart rate tones O36.83 ☑
      disproportion due to deformity (fetal) O33.7 ☑
      excessive growth (large for dates) O36.6 ☑

Pregnancy — *continued*
  complicated by — *continued*
    growth retardation O36.59 ☑
      light for dates O36.59 ☑
      small for dates O36.59 ☑
    heart rate irregularity (abnormal variability) (bradycardia) (decelerations) (tachycardia) O36.83 ☑
    hereditary disease O35.2 ☑
    hydrocephalus O35.0 ☑
    intrauterine death O36.4 ☑
    non-reassuring heart rate or rhythm O36.83 ☑
    poor growth O36.59 ☑
      light for dates O36.59 ☑
      small for dates O36.59 ☑
    problem O36.9 ☑
      specified NEC O36.89 ☑
    reduction (elective) O31.3 ☑
    selective termination O31.3 ☑
    spina bifida O35.0 ☑
    thrombocytopenia O36.82 ☑
  fibroid (tumor) (uterus) O34.1 ☑
  fissure of nipple O92.11 ☑
  gallstones O99.61 ☑
  gastric banding status O99.84 ☑
  gastric bypass status O99.84 ☑
  genital herpes (asymptomatic) (history of) (inactive) O98.3 ☑
  genital tract infection O23.9 ☑
  glomerular diseases (conditions in N00-N07) O26.83 ☑
    with hypertension, pre-existing — *see* Hypertension, complicating, pregnancy, pre-existing, with, renal disease
  gonorrhea O98.21 ☑
  grand multiparity O09.4 ☑
  habitual aborter — *see* Pregnancy, complicated by, recurrent pregnancy loss
  HELLP syndrome (hemolysis, elevated liver enzymes and low platelet count) O14.2 ☑
  hemorrhage
    antepartum — *see* Hemorrhage, antepartum
    before 20 completed weeks gestation O20.9
      specified NEC O20.8
    due to premature separation, placenta (*see also* Abruptio placentae) O45.9 ☑
    early O20.9
      specified NEC O20.8
    threatened abortion O20.0
  hemorrhoids O22.4 ☑
  hepatitis (viral) O98.41 ☑
  herniation of uterus O34.59 ☑
  high
    head at term O32.4 ☑
    risk — *see* Supervision (of) (for), high-risk
    history of in utero procedure during previous pregnancy O09.82 ☑
  HIV O98.71 ☑
  human immunodeficiency virus (HIV) disease O98.71 ☑
  hydatidiform mole (*see also* Mole, hydatidiform) O01.9
  hydramnios O40. ☑
  hydrocephalic fetus (disproportion) O33.6 ☑
  hydrops
    amnii O40. ☑
    fetalis O36.2 ☑
      associated with isoimmunization (*see also* Pregnancy, complicated by, isoimmunization) O36.11 ☑
  hydrorrhea O42.90
  hyperemesis (gravidarum) (mild) (*see also* Hyperemesis, gravidarum) O21.0
  hypertension — *see* Hypertension, complicating pregnancy
  hypertensive
    heart and renal disease, pre-existing — *see* Hypertension, complicating, pregnancy, pre-existing, with, heart disease, with renal disease
    heart disease, pre-existing — *see* Hypertension, complicating, pregnancy, pre-existing, with, heart disease
    renal disease, pre-existing — *see* Hypertension, complicating, pregnancy, pre-existing, with, renal disease
  hypotension O26.5 ☑
  immune disorders NEC (conditions in D80-D89) O99.11 ☑
  incarceration, uterus O34.51 ☑
  incompetent cervix O34.3 ☑
  inconclusive fetal viability O36.80 ☑

Pregnancy

Pregnancy — *continued*
  complicated by — *continued*
    infection(s) O98.91 ☑
      amniotic fluid or sac O41.10 ☑
      bladder O23.1 ☑
      carrier state NEC O99.830
        streptococcus B O99.820
      genital organ or tract O23.9 ☑
        specified NEC O23.59 ☑
      genitourinary tract O23.9 ☑
      gonorrhea O98.21 ☑
      hepatitis (viral) O98.41 ☑
      HIV O98.71 ☑
      human immunodeficiency virus (HIV) O98.71 ☑
      kidney O23.0 ☑
      nipple O91.01 ☑
      parasitic disease O98.91 ☑
        specified NEC O98.81 ☑
      protozoal disease O98.61 ☑
      sexually transmitted NEC O98.31 ☑
      specified type NEC O98.81 ☑
      syphilis O98.11 ☑
      tuberculosis O98.01 ☑
      urethra O23.2 ☑
      urinary (tract) O23.4 ☑
        specified NEC O23.3 ☑
      viral disease O98.51 ☑
    injury or poisoning (conditions in S00-T88) O9A.21 ☑
      due to abuse
        physical O9A.31 ☑
        psychological O9A.51 ☑
        sexual O9A.41 ☑
    insufficient
      prenatal care O09.3 ☑
      weight gain O26.1 ☑
    insulin resistance O26.89 ☑
    intrauterine fetal death (near term) O36.4 ☑
      early pregnancy O02.1
      multiple gestation (one fetus or more) O31.2 ☑
    isoimmunization O36.11 ☑
      anti-A sensitization O36.11 ☑
      anti-B sensitization O36.19 ☑
      Rh O36.09 ☑
        anti-D antibody O36.01 ☑
      specified NEC O36.19 ☑
    laceration of uterus NEC O71.81
    malformation
      placenta, placental (vessel) O43.10 ☑
        specified NEC O43.19 ☑
      uterus (congenital) O34.0 ☑
    malnutrition (conditions in E40-E46) O25.1 ☑
    maternal hypotension syndrome O26.5 ☑
    mental disorders (conditions in F01-F09, F01-F09) O99.34 ☑
      alcohol use O99.31 ☑
      drug use O99.32 ☑
      smoking O99.33 ☑
    mentum presentation O32.3 ☑
    metabolic disorders O99.28 ☑
    missed
      abortion O02.1
      delivery O36.4 ☑
    multiple gestations O30.9 ☑
      conjoined twins O30.02 ☑
      specified number of multiples NEC — *see* Pregnancy, multiple (gestation), specified NEC
      quadruplet — *see* Pregnancy, quadruplet
      specified complication NEC O31.8X ☑
      triplet — *see* Pregnancy, triplet
      twin — *see* Pregnancy, twin
    musculoskeletal condition (conditions is M00-M99) O99.89
    necrosis, liver (conditions in K72 ☑) O26.61 ☑
    neoplasm
      benign
        cervix O34.4 ☑
        corpus uteri O34.1 ☑
        uterus O34.1 ☑
      malignant O9A.11 ☑
    nephropathy NEC O26.83 ☑
    nervous system condition (conditions in G00-G99) O99.35 ☑
    nutritional diseases NEC O99.28 ☑
    obesity (pre-existing) O99.21 ☑
    obesity surgery status O99.84 ☑
    oblique lie or presentation O32.2 ☑
    older mother — *see* Pregnancy, complicated by, elderly
    oligohydramnios O41.0 ☑

Pregnancy — *continued*
  complicated by — *continued*
    with premature rupture of membranes (*see also* Pregnancy, complicated by, premature rupture of membranes) O42. ☑
    onset (spontaneous) of labor after 37 completed weeks of gestation but before 39 completed weeks gestation, with delivery by (planned) cesarean section O75.82
    oophoritis O23.52 ☑
    overdose, drug (*see also* Table of Drugs and Chemicals, by drug, poisoning) O9A.21 ☑
    oversize fetus O33.5 ☑
    papyraceous fetus O31.0 ☑
    pelvic inflammatory disease O99.89
    periodontal disease O99.61 ☑
    peripheral neuritis O26.82 ☑
    peritoneal (pelvic) adhesions O99.89
    phlebitis O22.9 ☑
    phlebopathy O22.9 ☑
    phlebothrombosis (superficial) O22.2 ☑
      deep O22.3 ☑
    placenta accreta O43.21 ☑
    placenta increta O43.22 ☑
    placenta percreta O43.23 ☑
    placenta previa O44.0 ☑
      complete O44.0 ☑
        with hemorrhage O44.1 ☑
      marginal O44.2 ☑
        with hemorrhage O44.3 ☑
      partial O44.2 ☑
        with hemorrhage O44.3 ☑
    placental disorder O43.9 ☑
      specified NEC O43.89 ☑
    placental dysfunction O43.89 ☑
    placental infarction O43.81 ☑
    placental insufficiency O36.51 ☑
    placental transfusion syndromes
      fetomaternal O43.01 ☑
      fetus to fetus O43.02 ☑
      maternofetal O43.01 ☑
    placentitis O41.14 ☑
    pneumonia O99.51 ☑
    poisoning (*see also* Table of Drugs and Chemicals) O9A.21 ☑
    polyhydramnios O40 ☑
    polymorphic eruption of pregnancy O26.86
    poor obstetric history NEC O09.29 ☑
    postmaturity (post-term) (40 to 42 weeks) O48.0
      more than 42 completed weeks gestation (prolonged) O48.1
    pre-eclampsia O14.9 ☑
      mild O14.0 ☑
      moderate O14.0 ☑
      severe O14.1 ☑
        with hemolysis, elevated liver enzymes and low platelet count (HELLP) O14.2 ☑
    premature labor — *see* Pregnancy, complicated by, preterm labor
    premature rupture of membranes O42.90
      full-term, unspecified as to length of time between rupture and onset of labor O42.92
      with onset of labor
        within 24 hours O42.00
          at or after 37 weeks gestation, onset of labor within 24 hours of rupture O42.02
          pre-term (before 37 completed weeks of gestation) O42.01 ☑
        after 24 hours O42.10
          at or after 37 weeks gestation, onset of labor more than 24 hours following rupture O42.12
          pre-term (before 37 completed weeks of gestation) O42.11 ☑
        at or after 37 weeks gestation, unspecified as to length of time between rupture and onset of labor O42.92
        pre-term (before 37 completed weeks of gestation) O42.91 ☑
    premature separation of placenta (*see also* Abruptio placentae) O45.9 ☑
    presentation, fetal — *see* Delivery, complicated by, malposition
    preterm delivery O60.10 ☑
    preterm labor
      with delivery O60.10 ☑
        preterm O60.10 ☑
        term O60.20 ☑
      second trimester
        with term delivery O60.22 ☑
        without delivery O60.02

Pregnancy — *continued*
  complicated by — *continued*
    with preterm delivery
      second trimester O60.12 ☑
      third trimester O60.13 ☑
    third trimester
      with term delivery O60.23 ☑
      without delivery O60.03
      with third trimester preterm delivery O60.14 ☑
      without delivery O60.00
        second trimester O60.02
        third trimester O60.03
    previous history of — *see* Pregnancy, supervision of, high-risk
    prolapse, uterus O34.52 ☑
    proteinuria (gestational) (*see also* Proteinuria, gestational) O12.1 ☑
      with edema O12.2 ☑
    pruritic urticarial papules and plaques of pregnancy (PUPPP) O26.86
    pruritus (neurogenic) O26.89 ☑
    psychosis or psychoneurosis (puerperal) F53.1
    ptyalism O26.89 ☑
    PUPPP (pruritic urticarial papules and plaques of pregnancy) O26.86
    pyelitis O23.0 ☑
    recurrent pregnancy loss O26.2 ☑
    renal disease or failure NEC O26.83 ☑
      with secondary hypertension, pre-existing — *see* Hypertension, complicating, pregnancy, pre-existing, secondary
      hypertensive, pre-existing — *see* Hypertension, complicating, pregnancy, pre-existing, with, renal disease
    respiratory condition (conditions in J00-J99) O99.51 ☑
    retained, retention
      dead ovum O02.0
      intrauterine contraceptive device O26.3 ☑
    retroversion, uterus O34.53 ☑
    Rh immunization, incompatibility or sensitization NEC O36.09 ☑
      anti-D antibody O36.01 ☑
    rupture
      amnion (premature) (*see also* Pregnancy, complicated by, premature rupture of membranes) O42 ☑
      membranes (premature) (*see also* Pregnancy, complicated by, premature rupture of membranes) O42 ☑
      uterus (during labor) O71.1
        before onset of labor O71.0 ☑
    salivation (excessive) O26.89 ☑
    salpingitis O23.52 ☑
    salpingo-oophoritis O23.52 ☑
    sepsis (conditions in A40 ☑, A41 ☑) O98.81 ☑
    size date discrepancy (uterine) O26.84 ☑
    skin condition (conditions in L00-L99) O99.71 ☑
    smoking (tobacco) O99.33 ☑
    social problem O09.7 ☑
    specified condition NEC O26.89 ☑
    spotting O26.85 ☑
    streptococcus group B (GBS) carrier state O99.820
    subluxation of symphysis (pubis) O26.71 ☑
    syphilis (conditions in A50-A53) O98.11 ☑
    threatened
      abortion O20.0
      labor O47.9
        at or after 37 weeks of gestation O47.1
        before 37 completed weeks of gestation O47.0 ☑
    thrombophlebitis (superficial) O22.2 ☑
    thrombosis O22.9 ☑
      cerebral venous O22.5 ☑
      cerebrovenous sinus O22.5 ☑
      deep O22.3 ☑
    tobacco use disorder (smoking) O99.33 ☑
    torsion of uterus O34.59 ☑
    toxemia O14.9 ☑
    transverse lie or presentation O32.2 ☑
    tuberculosis (conditions in A15-A19) O98.01 ☑
    tumor (benign)
      cervix O34.4 ☑
      malignant O9A.11 ☑
      uterus O34.1 ☑
    unstable lie O32.0 ☑
    upper respiratory infection O99.51 ☑
    urethritis O23.2 ☑
    uterine size date discrepancy O26.84 ☑
    vaginitis or vulvitis O23.59 ☑

☑ **Additional character required**

Pregnancy — *continued*
  complicated by — *continued*
    varicose veins (lower extremities) O22.0 ☑
      genitals O22.1 ☑
      legs O22.0 ☑
      perineal O22.1 ☑
      vaginal or vulval O22.1 ☑
    venereal disease NEC (conditions in A63.8)
      O98.31 ☑
    venous disorders O22.9 ☑
      specified NEC O22.8X ☑
    viral diseases (conditions in A80-B09, A80-B09)
      O98.51 ☑
    very young mother — *see* Pregnancy,
      complicated by, young mother
    vomiting O21.9
      due to diseases classified elsewhere O21.8
      hyperemesis gravidarum (mild) (*see also*
        Hyperemesis, gravidarum) O21.0
      late (occurring after 20 weeks of gestation)
        O21.2
    young mother
      multigravida O09.62 ☑
      primigravida O09.61 ☑
  concealed O09.3 ☑
  continuing following
    elective fetal reduction of one or more fetus
      O31.3 ☑
    intrauterine death of one or more fetus O31.2 ☑
    spontaneous abortion of one or more fetus
      O31.1 ☑
  cornual O00.80
    with intrauterine pregnancy O00.81
  ectopic (ruptured) O00.90
    with intrauterine pregnancy O00.91
    abdominal O00.00
      with
        intrauterine pregnancy O00.01
          viable fetus O36.7 ☑
    cervical O00.80
      with intrauterine pregnancy O00.81
    complicated (by) O08.9
      afibrinogenemia O08.1
      cardiac arrest O08.81
      chemical damage of pelvic organ(s) O08.6
      circulatory collapse O08.3
      defibrination syndrome O08.1
      electrolyte imbalance O08.5
      embolism (amniotic fluid) (blood clot)
        (pulmonary) (septic) O08.2
      endometritis O08.0
      genital tract and pelvic infection O08.0
      hemorrhage (delayed) (excessive) O08.1
      infection
        genital tract or pelvic O08.0
          kidney O08.83
          urinary tract O08.83
      intravascular coagulation O08.1
      laceration of pelvic organ(s) O08.6
      metabolic disorder O08.5
      oliguria O08.4
      oophoritis O08.0
      parametritis O08.0
      pelvic peritonitis O08.0
      perforation of pelvic organ(s) O08.6
      renal failure or shutdown O08.4
      salpingitis or salpingo-oophoritis O08.0
      sepsis O08.82
      shock O08.83
        septic O08.82
      specified condition NEC O08.89
      tubular necrosis (renal) O08.4
      uremia O08.4
      urinary infection O08.83
      venous complication NEC O08.7
        embolism O08.2
    cornual O00.80
      with intrauterine pregnancy O00.81
    intraligamentous O00.80
      with intrauterine pregnancy O00.81
    mural O00.80
      with intrauterine pregnancy O00.81
    ovarian O00.20 ☑
      with intrauterine pregnancy O00.21 ☑
    specified site NEC O00.80
      with intrauterine pregnancy O00.81
    tubal (ruptured) O00.10 ☑
      with intrauterine pregnancy O00.11 ☑
  examination (normal) Z34.9 ☑
    high-risk — *see* Pregnancy, supervision of, high-risk
    first Z34.0 ☑
    specified Z34.8 ☑

Pregnancy — *continued*
  extrauterine — *see* Pregnancy, ectopic
  fallopian O00.10 ☑
    with intrauterine pregnancy O00.11 ☑
  false F45.8
  gestational carrier Z33.3
  heptachorionic, hepta-amniotic (septuplets)
    O30.83 ☑
  hexachorionic, hexa-amniotic (sextuplets)
    O30.83 ☑
  hidden O09.3 ☑
  high-risk — *see* Pregnancy, supervision of, high-risk
  incidental finding Z33.1
  interstitial O00.80
    with intrauterine pregnancy O00.81
  intraligamentous O00.80
    with intrauterine pregnancy O00.81
  intramural O00.80
    with intrauterine pregnancy O00.81
  intraperitoneal O00.00
    with intrauterine pregnancy O00.01
  isthmian O00.10 ☑
    with intrauterine pregnancy O00.11 ☑
  mesometric (mural) O00.80
    with intrauterine pregnancy O00.81
  molar NEC O02.0
    complicated (by) O08.9
      afibrinogenemia O08.1
      cardiac arrest O08.81
      chemical damage of pelvic organ(s) O08.6
      circulatory collapse O08.3
      defibrination syndrome O08.1
      electrolyte imbalance O08.5
      embolism (amniotic fluid) (blood clot)
        (pulmonary) (septic) O08.2
      endometritis O08.0
      genital tract and pelvic infection O08.0
      hemorrhage (delayed) (excessive) O08.1
      infection
        genital tract or pelvic O08.0
          kidney O08.83
          urinary tract O08.83
      intravascular coagulation O08.1
      laceration of pelvic organ(s) O08.6
      metabolic disorder O08.5
      oliguria O08.4
      oophoritis O08.0
      parametritis O08.0
      pelvic peritonitis O08.0
      perforation of pelvic organ(s) O08.6
      renal failure or shutdown O08.4
      salpingitis or salpingo-oophoritis O08.0
      sepsis O08.82
      shock O08.3
        septic O08.82
      specified condition NEC O08.89
      tubular necrosis (renal) O08.4
      uremia O08.4
      urinary infection O08.83
      venous complication NEC O08.7
        embolism O08.2
    hydatidiform (*see also* Mole, hydatidiform) O01.9
  multiple (gestation) O30.9 ☑
    greater than quadruplets — *see* Pregnancy,
      multiple (gestation), specified NEC
    specified NEC O30.80 ☑
      with
        two or more monoamniotic fetuses O30.82 ☑
        two or more monochorionic fetuses
          O30.81 ☑
      number of chorions and amnions are both
        equal to the number of fetuses O30.83 ☑
      two or more monoamniotic fetuses O30.82 ☑
      two or more monochorionic fetuses O30.81 ☑
      unable to determine number of placenta and
        number of amniotic sacs O30.89 ☑
      unspecified number of placenta and
        unspecified number of amniotic sacs
        O30.80 ☑
  mural O00.80
    with intrauterine pregnancy O00.81
  normal (supervision of) Z34.9 ☑
    high-risk — *see* Pregnancy, supervision of,
      high-risk
    first Z34.0 ☑
    specified Z34.8 ☑
  ovarian O00.20 ☑
    with intrauterine pregnancy O00.21 ☑
  pentachorionic, penta-amniotic (quintuplets)
    O30.83 ☑
  postmature (40 to 42 weeks) O48.0
    more than 42 weeks gestation O48.1

Pregnancy — *continued*
  post-term (40 to 42 weeks) O48.0
  prenatal care only Z34.9 ☑
    high-risk — *see* Pregnancy, supervision of,
      high-risk
    first Z34.0 ☑
    specified Z34.8 ☑
  prolonged (more than 42 weeks gestation) O48.1
  quadruplet O30.20 ☑
    with
      two or more monoamniotic fetuses O30.22 ☑
      two or more monochorionic fetuses O30.21 ☑
    quadrachorionic/quadra-amniotic O30.23 ☑
    two or more monoamniotic fetuses O30.22 ☑
    two or more monochorionic fetuses O30.21 ☑
    unable to determine number of placenta and
      number of amniotic sacs O30.29 ☑
    unspecified number of placenta and unspecified
      number of amniotic sacs O30.20 ☑
  quintuplet — *see* Pregnancy, multiple (gestation),
    specified NEC
  sextuplet — *see* Pregnancy, multiple (gestation),
    specified NEC
  supervision of
    concealed pregnancy O09.3 ☑
    elderly mother
      multigravida O09.52 ☑
      primigravida O09.51 ☑
    hidden pregnancy O09.3 ☑
    high-risk O09.9 ☑
      due to (history of)
        ectopic pregnancy O09.1 ☑
        elderly — *see* Pregnancy, supervision, elderly
          mother
        grand multiparity O09.4 ☑
        infertility O09.0 ☑
        insufficient prenatal care O09.3 ☑
        in utero procedure during previous
          pregnancy O09.82 ☑
        in vitro fertilization O09.81 ☑
        molar pregnancy O09.A ☑
        multiple previous pregnancies O09.4 ☑
        older mother — *see* Pregnancy, supervision
          of, elderly mother
        poor reproductive or obstetric history NEC
          O09.29 ☑
        pre-term labor O09.21 ☑
        previous
          neonatal death O09.29 ☑
        social problems O09.7 ☑
        specified NEC O09.89 ☑
        very young mother — *see* Pregnancy,
          supervision, young mother
      resulting from in vitro fertilization O09.81 ☑
    normal Z34.9 ☑
      first Z34.0 ☑
      specified NEC Z34.8 ☑
    young mother
      multigravida O09.62 ☑
      primigravida O09.61 ☑
  triplet O30.10 ☑
    with
      two or more monoamniotic fetuses O30.12 ☑
      two or more monochorionic fetuses O30.11 ☑
    trichorionic/triamniotic O30.13 ☑
    two or more monoamniotic fetuses O30.12 ☑
    two or more monochorionic fetuses O30.11 ☑
    unable to determine number of placenta and
      number of amniotic sacs O30.19 ☑
    unspecified number of placenta and unspecified
      number of amniotic sacs O30.10 ☑
  tubal (with abortion) (with rupture) O00.10 ☑
    with intrauterine pregnancy O00.11 ☑
  twin O30.00 ☑
    conjoined O30.02 ☑
    dichorionic/diamniotic (two placenta, two
      amniotic sacs) O30.04 ☑
    monochorionic/diamniotic (one placenta, two
      amniotic sacs) O30.03 ☑
    monochorionic/monoamniotic (one placenta,
      one amniotic sac) O30.01 ☑
    unable to determine number of placenta and
      number of amniotic sacs O30.09 ☑
    unspecified number of placenta and unspecified
      number of amniotic sacs O30.00 ☑
  unwanted Z64.0
  weeks of gestation
    8 weeks Z3A.08
    9 weeks Z3A.09
    10 weeks Z3A.10
    11 weeks Z3A.11
    12 weeks Z3A.12

☑ **Additional character required**

Pregnancy - Presence

Pregnancy — *continued*
  weeks of gestation — *continued*
    13 weeks Z3A.13
    14 weeks Z3A.14
    15 weeks Z3A.15
    16 weeks Z3A.16
    17 weeks Z3A.17
    18 weeks Z3A.18
    19 weeks Z3A.19
    20 weeks Z3A.20
    21 weeks Z3A.21
    22 weeks Z3A.22
    23 weeks Z3A.23
    24 weeks Z3A.24
    25 weeks Z3A.25
    26 weeks Z3A.26
    27 weeks Z3A.27
    28 weeks Z3A.28
    29 weeks Z3A.29
    30 weeks Z3A.30
    31 weeks Z3A.31
    32 weeks Z3A.32
    33 weeks Z3A.33
    34 weeks Z3A.34
    35 weeks Z3A.35
    36 weeks Z3A.36
    37 weeks Z3A.37
    38 weeks Z3A.38
    39 weeks Z3A.39
    40 weeks Z3A.40
    41 weeks Z3A.41
    42 weeks Z3A.42
    greater than 42 weeks Z3A.49
    less than 8 weeks Z3A.01
    not specified Z3A.00
Preiser's disease — *see* Osteonecrosis, secondary, due to, trauma, metacarpus
Pre-kwashiorkor — *see* Malnutrition, severe
Preleukemia (syndrome) D46.9
Preluxation, hip, congenital Q65.6
Premature (*see also* condition)
  adrenarche E27.0
  aging E34.8
  beats I49.40
    atrial I49.1
    auricular I49.1
    supraventricular I49.1
  birth NEC — *see* Preterm, newborn
  closure, foramen ovale Q21.8
  contraction
    atrial I49.1
    atrioventricular I49.2
    auricular I49.1
    auriculoventricular I49.49
    heart (extrasystole) I49.49
    junctional I49.2
    ventricular I49.3
  delivery (*see also* Pregnancy, complicated by, preterm labor) O60.10 ☑
  ejaculation F52.4
  infant NEC — *see* Preterm, newborn
    light-for-dates — *see* Light for dates
  labor — *see* Pregnancy, complicated by, preterm labor
  lungs P28.0
  menopause E28.319
    asymptomatic E28.319
    symptomatic E28.310
  newborn
    extreme (less than 28 completed weeks) — *see* Immaturity, extreme
    less than 37 completed weeks — *see* Preterm, newborn
  puberty E30.1
  rupture membranes or amnion — *see* Pregnancy, complicated by, premature rupture of membranes
  senility E34.8
  thelarche E30.8
  ventricular systole I49.3
Prematurity NEC (less than 37 completed weeks) — *see* Preterm, newborn
  extreme (less than 28 completed weeks) — *see* Immaturity, extreme
Premenstrual
  dysphoric disorder (PMDD) F32.81
  tension (syndrome) N94.3
Premolarization, cuspids K00.2
Prenatal
  care, normal pregnancy — *see* Pregnancy, normal
  screening of mother (*see also* Encounter, antenatal screening) Z36.9
  teeth K00.6

Preparatory care for subsequent treatment NEC
  for dialysis Z49.01
    peritoneal Z49.02
Prepartum — *see* condition
Preponderance, left or right ventricular I51.7
Prepuce — *see* condition
PRES (posterior reversible encephalopathy syndrome) I67.83
Presbycardia R54
Presbycusis, presbyacusia H91.1 ☑
Presbyesophagus K22.8
Presbyophrenia F03 ☑
Presbyopia H52.4
Prescription of contraceptives (initial) Z30.019
  barrier Z30.018
  diaphragm Z30.018
  emergency (postcoital) Z30.012
  implantable subdermal Z30.017
  injectable Z30.013
  intrauterine contraceptive device Z30.014
  pills Z30.011
  postcoital (emergency) Z30.012
  repeat Z30.40
    barrier Z30.49
    diaphragm Z30.49
    implantable subdermal Z30.46
    injectable Z30.42
    pills Z30.41
    specified type NEC Z30.49
    transdermal patch hormonal Z30.45
    vaginal ring hormonal Z30.44
  specified type NEC Z30.018
    transdermal patch hormonal Z30.016
    vaginal ring hormonal Z30.015
Presence (of)
  ankle-joint implant (functional) (prosthesis) Z96.66 ☑
  aortocoronary (bypass) graft Z95.1
  arterial-venous shunt (dialysis) Z99.2
  artificial
    eye (globe) Z97.0
    heart (fully implantable) (mechanical) Z95.812
      valve Z95.2
    larynx Z96.3
    lens (intraocular) Z96.1
    limb (complete) (partial) Z97.1 ☑
      arm Z97.1 ☑
        bilateral Z97.15
      leg Z97.1 ☑
        bilateral Z97.16
  audiological implant (functional) Z96.29
  bladder implant (functional) Z96.0
  bone
    conduction hearing device Z96.29
    implant (functional) NEC Z96.7
    joint (prosthesis) — *see* Presence, joint implant
  cardiac
    defibrillator (functional) (with synchronous cardiac pacemaker) Z95.810
    implant or graft Z95.9
      specified type NEC Z95.818
    pacemaker Z95.0
    resynchronization therapy
      defibrillator Z95.810
      pacemaker Z95.0
  cerebrospinal fluid drainage device Z98.2
  cochlear implant (functional) Z96.21
  contact lens (es) Z97.3
  coronary artery graft or prosthesis Z95.5
  CRT-D (cardiac resynchronization therapy defibrillator) Z95.810
  CRT-P (cardiac resynchronization therapy pacemaker) Z95.0
  cardioverter-defibrillator (ICD) Z95.810
  CSF shunt Z98.2
  dental prosthesis device Z97.2
  dentures Z97.2
  device (external) NEC Z97.8
    cardiac NEC Z95.818
    heart assist Z95.811
    implanted (functional) Z96.9
      specified NEC Z96.89
    prosthetic Z97.8
  ear implant Z96.20
    cochlear implant Z96.21
    myringotomy tube Z96.22
    specified type NEC Z96.29
  elbow-joint implant (functional) (prosthesis) Z96.62 ☑
  endocrine implant (functional) NEC Z96.49
  eustachian tube stent or device (functional) Z96.29
  external hearing-aid or device Z97.4

Presence — *continued*
  finger-joint implant (functional) (prosthetic) Z96.69 ☑
  functional implant Z96.9
    specified NEC Z96.89
  graft
    cardiac NEC Z95.818
    vascular NEC Z95.828
  hearing-aid or device (external) Z97.4
    implant (bone) (cochlear) (functional) Z96.21
  heart assist device Z95.811
  heart valve implant (functional) Z95.2
    prosthetic Z95.2
    specified type NEC Z95.4
    xenogenic Z95.3
  hip-joint implant (functional) (prosthesis) Z96.64 ☑
  ICD (cardioverter-defibrillator) Z95.810
  implanted device (artificial) (functional) (prosthetic) Z96.9
    automatic cardiac defibrillator (with synchronous cardiac pacemaker) Z95.810
    cardiac pacemaker Z95.0
    cochlear Z96.21
    dental Z96.5
    heart Z95.812
    heart valve Z95.2
      prosthetic Z95.2
      specified NEC Z95.4
      xenogenic Z95.3
    insulin pump Z96.41
    intraocular lens Z96.1
    joint Z96.60
      ankle Z96.66 ☑
      elbow Z96.62 ☑
      finger Z96.69 ☑
      hip Z96.64 ☑
      knee Z96.65 ☑
      shoulder Z96.61 ☑
      specified NEC Z96.698
      wrist Z96.63 ☑
    larynx Z96.3
    myringotomy tube Z96.22
    otological Z96.20
      cochlear Z96.21
      eustachian stent Z96.29
      myringotomy Z96.22
      specified NEC Z96.29
      stapes Z96.29
    skin Z96.81
    skull plate Z96.7
    specified NEC Z96.89
    urogenital Z96.0
  insulin pump (functional) Z96.41
  intestinal bypass or anastomosis Z98.0
  intraocular lens (functional) Z96.1
  intrauterine contraceptive device (IUD) Z97.5
  intravascular implant (functional) (prosthetic) NEC Z95.9
    coronary artery Z95.5
    defibrillator (with synchronous cardiac pacemaker) Z95.810
    peripheral vessel (with angioplasty) Z95.820
  joint implant (prosthetic) (any) Z96.60
    ankle — *see* Presence, ankle joint implant
    elbow — *see* Presence, elbow joint implant
    finger — *see* Presence, finger joint implant
    hip — *see* Presence, hip joint implant
    knee — *see* Presence, knee joint implant
    shoulder — *see* Presence, shoulder joint implant
    specified joint NEC Z96.698
    wrist — *see* Presence, wrist joint implant
  knee-joint implant (functional) (prosthesis) Z96.65 ☑
  laryngeal implant (functional) Z96.3
  mandibular implant (dental) Z96.5
  myringotomy tube(s) Z96.22
  neurostimulator (brain) (gastric) (peripheral nerve) (sacral nerve) (spinal cord) (vagus nerve) Z96.82
  orthopedic-joint implant (prosthetic) (any) — *see* Presence, joint implant
  otological implant (functional) Z96.29
  shoulder-joint implant (functional) (prosthesis) Z96.61 ☑
  skull-plate implant Z96.7
  spectacles Z97.3
  stapes implant (functional) Z96.29
  systemic lupus erythematosus [SLE] inhibitor D68.62
  tendon implant (functional) (graft) Z96.7
  tooth root(s) implant Z96.5
  ureteral stent Z96.0
  urethral stent Z96.0

☑ **Additional character required**

Presence — *continued*
    urogenital implant (functional) Z96.0
    vascular implant or device Z95.9
        access port device Z95.828
        specified type NEC Z95.828
    wrist-joint implant (functional) (prosthesis)
        Z96.63 ☑
Presenile (*see also* condition)
    dementia F03 ☑
    premature aging E34.8
Presentation, fetal — *see* Delivery , complicated by, malposition
Prespondylolisthesis (congenital) Q76.2
Pressure
    area, skin — *see* Ulcer, pressure, by site
    brachial plexus G54.0
    brain G93.5
        injury at birth NEC P11.1
    cerebral — *see* Pressure, brain
    chest R07.89
    cone, tentorial G93.5
    hyposystolic (*see also* Hypotension)
        incidental reading, without diagnosis of hypotension R03.1
    increased
        intracranial (benign) G93.2
            injury at birth P11.0
        intraocular H40.05 ☑
    injury — *see* Ulcer, pressure, by site
    lumbosacral plexus G54.1
    mediastinum J98.59
    necrosis (chronic) — *see* Ulcer, pressure, by site
    parental, inappropriate (excessive) Z62.6
    sore (chronic) — *see* Ulcer, pressure, by site
    spinal cord G95.20
    ulcer (chronic) — *see* Ulcer, pressure, by site
    venous, increased I87.8
Pre-syncope R55
Preterm
    delivery (*see also* Pregnancy, complicated by, preterm labor) O60.10 ☑
    labor — *see* Pregnancy, complicated by, preterm labor
    newborn (infant) P07.30
        gestational age
            28 completed weeks (28 weeks, 0 days through 28 weeks, 6 days) P07.31
            29 completed weeks (29 weeks, 0 days through 29 weeks, 6 days) P07.32
            30 completed weeks (30 weeks, 0 days through 30 weeks, 6 days) P07.33
            31 completed weeks (31 weeks, 0 days through 31 weeks, 6 days) P07.34
            32 completed weeks (32 weeks, 0 days through 32 weeks, 6 days) P07.35
            33 completed weeks (33 weeks, 0 days through 33 weeks, 6 days) P07.36
            34 completed weeks (34 weeks, 0 days through 34 weeks, 6 days) P07.37
            35 completed weeks (35 weeks, 0 days through 35 weeks, 6 days) P07.38
            36 completed weeks (36 weeks, 0 days through 36 weeks, 6 days) P07.39
Previa
    placenta (total) (without hemorrhage) O44.0 ☑
        with hemorrhage O44.1 ☑
        complete O44.0 ☑
            with hemorrhage O44.1 ☑
        low (*see also* Delivery, complicated, by, placenta, low) O44.4 ☑
            with hemorrhage O44.5 ☑
        marginal O44.2 ☑
            with hemorrhage O44.3 ☑
        partial O44.2 ☑
            with hemorrhage O44.3 ☑
    vasa O69.4 ☑
Priapism N48.30
    due to
        disease classified elsewhere N48.32
        drug N48.33
        specified cause NEC N48.39
        trauma N48.31
Prickling sensation (skin) R20.2
Prickly heat L74.0
Primary — *see* condition
Primigravida
    elderly, affecting management of pregnancy, labor and delivery (supervision only) — *see* Pregnancy, complicated by, elderly, primigravida
    older, affecting management of pregnancy, labor and delivery (supervision only) —

Primigravida — *continued*
    older — *continued*
        see Pregnancy, complicated by, elderly, primigravida
    very young, affecting management of pregnancy, labor and delivery (supervision only) — *see* Pregnancy, complicated by, young mother, primigravida
Primipara
    elderly, affecting management of pregnancy, labor and delivery (supervision only) — *see* Pregnancy, complicated by, elderly, primigravida
    older, affecting management of pregnancy, labor and delivery (supervision only) — *see* Pregnancy, complicated by, elderly, primigravida
    very young, affecting management of pregnancy, labor and delivery (supervision only) — *see* Pregnancy, complicated by, young mother, primigravida
Primus varus Q66.21 ☑
PRIND (Prolonged reversible ischemic neurologic deficit) I63.9
Pringle's disease (tuberous sclerosis) Q85.1
Prinzmetal angina I20.1
Prizefighter ear — *see* Cauliflower ear
Problem (with) (related to)
    academic Z55.8
    acculturation Z60.3
    adjustment (to)
        change of job Z56.1
        life-cycle transition Z60.0
        pension Z60.0
        retirement Z60.0
    adopted child Z62.821
    alcoholism in family Z63.72
    atypical parenting situation Z62.9
    bankruptcy Z59.8
    behavioral (adult) F69
        drug seeking Z76.5
    birth of sibling affecting child Z62.898
    care (of)
        provider dependency Z74.9
            specified NEC Z74.8
        sick or handicapped person in family or household Z63.6
    child
        abuse (affecting the child) — *see* Maltreatment, child
        custody or support proceedings Z65.3
        in welfare custody Z62.21
        in care of non-parental family member Z62.21
        in foster care Z62.21
        living in orphanage or group home Z62.22
    child-rearing Z62.9
        specified NEC Z62.898
    communication (developmental) F80.9
    conflict or discord (with)
        boss Z56.4
        classmates Z55.4
        counselor Z64.4
        employer Z56.4
        family Z63.9
            specified NEC Z63.8
        probation officer Z64.4
        social worker Z64.4
        teachers Z55.4
        workmates Z56.4
    conviction in legal proceedings Z65.0
        with imprisonment Z65.1
    counselor Z64.4
    creditors Z59.8
    digestive K92.9
    drug addict in family Z63.72
    ear — *see* Disorder, ear
    economic Z59.9
        affecting care Z59.9
        specified NEC Z59.8
    education Z55.9
        specified NEC Z55.8
    employment Z56.9
        change of job Z56.1
        discord Z56.4
        environment Z56.5
        sexual harassment Z56.81
        specified NEC Z56.89
        stress NEC Z56.6
        stressful schedule Z56.3
        threat of job loss Z56.2
        unemployment Z56.0
    enuresis, child F98.0

Problem — *continued*
    eye H57.9
    failed examinations (school) Z55.2
    falling Z91.81
    family (*see also* Disruption, family) Z63.9
        specified NEC Z63.8
    feeding (elderly) (infant) R63.3
        newborn P92.9
            breast P92.5
            overfeeding P92.4
            slow P92.2
            specified NEC P92.8
            underfeeding P92.3
        nonorganic F50.89
    finance Z59.9
        specified NEC Z59.8
    foreclosure on loan Z59.8
    foster child Z62.822
    frightening experience(s) in childhood Z62.898
    genital NEC
        female N94.9
        male N50.9
    health care Z75.9
        specified NEC Z75.8
    hearing — *see* Deafness
    homelessness Z59.0
    housing Z59.9
        inadequate Z59.1
        isolated Z59.8
        specified NEC Z59.8
    identity (of childhood) F93.8
    illegitimate pregnancy (unwanted) Z64.0
    illiteracy Z55.0
    impaired mobility Z74.09
    imprisonment or incarceration Z65.1
    inadequate teaching affecting education Z55.8
    inappropriate (excessive) parental pressure Z62.6
    influencing health status NEC Z78.9
    in-law Z63.1
    institutionalization, affecting child Z62.22
    intrafamilial communication Z63.8
    jealousy, child F93.8
    landlord Z59.2
    language (developmental) F80.9
    learning (developmental) F81.9
    legal Z65.3
        conviction without imprisonment Z65.0
        imprisonment Z65.1
        release from prison Z65.2
    life-management Z73.9
        specified NEC Z73.89
    life-style Z72.9
        gambling Z72.6
        high-risk sexual behavior (heterosexual) Z72.51
            bisexual Z72.53
            homosexual Z72.52
        inappropriate eating habits Z72.4
        self-damaging behavior NEC Z72.89
        specified NEC Z72.89
        tobacco use Z72.0
    literacy Z55.9
        low level Z55.0
        specified NEC Z55.8
    living alone Z60.2
    lodgers Z59.2
    loss of love relationship in childhood Z62.898
    marital Z63.0
        involving
            divorce Z63.5
            estrangement Z63.5
            gender identity F66
    mastication K08.89
    medical
        care, within family Z63.6
        facilities Z75.9
            specified NEC Z75.8
    mental F48.9
    multiparity Z64.1
    negative life events in childhood Z62.9
        altered pattern of family relationships Z62.898
        frightening experience Z62.898
        loss of
            love relationship Z62.898
            self-esteem Z62.898
        physical abuse (alleged) — *see* Maltreatment, child
        removal from home Z62.29
        specified event NEC Z62.898
    neighbor Z59.2
    neurological NEC R29.818
    new step-parent affecting child Z62.898
    none (feared complaint unfounded) Z71.1

Problem — *continued*
occupational NEC Z56.89
parent-child — *see* Conflict, parent-child
personal hygiene Z91.89
personality F69
phase-of-life transition, adjustment Z60.0
presence of sick or disabled person in family or
household Z63.79
needing care Z63.6
primary support group (family) Z63.9
specified NEC Z63.8
probation officer Z64.4
psychiatric F99
psychosexual (development) F66
psychosocial Z65.9
religious or spiritual Z65.8
specified NEC Z65.8
relationship Z63.9
childhood F93.8
release from prison Z65.2
religious or spiritual Z65.8
removal from home affecting child Z62.29
seeking and accepting known hazardous and
harmful
behavioral or psychological interventions Z65.8
chemical, nutritional or physical interventions
Z65.8
sexual function (nonorganic) F52.9
sight H54.7
sleep disorder, child F51.9
smell — *see* Disturbance, sensation, smell
social
environment Z60.9
specified NEC Z60.8
exclusion and rejection Z60.4
worker Z64.4
speech R47.9
developmental F80.9
specified NEC R47.89
swallowing — *see* Dysphagia
taste — *see* Disturbance, sensation, taste
tic, child F95.0
underachievement in school Z55.3
unemployment Z56.0
threatened Z56.2
unwanted pregnancy Z64.0
upbringing Z62.9
specified NEC Z62.898
urinary N39.9
voice production R47.89
work schedule (stressful) Z56.3
Procedure (surgical)
converted
arthroscopic to open Z53.33
laparoscopic to open Z53.31
specified procedure NEC to open Z53.39
thoracoscopic to open Z53.32
for purpose other than remedying health state
Z41.9
specified NEC Z41.8
not done Z53.9
because of
administrative reasons Z53.8
contraindication Z53.09
smoking Z53.01
patient's decision Z53.20
for reasons of belief or group pressure
Z53.1
left against medical advice (AMA) Z53.21
specified reason NEC Z53.29
specified reason NEC Z53.8
Procidentia (uteri) N81.3
Proctalgia K62.89
fugax K59.4
spasmodic K59.4
Proctitis K62.89
amebic (acute) A06.0
chlamydial A56.3
gonococcal A54.6
granulomatous — *see* Enteritis, regional, large
intestine
herpetic A60.1
radiation K62.7
tuberculous A18.32
ulcerative (chronic) K51.20
with
complication K51.219
abscess K51.214
fistula K51.213
obstruction K51.212
rectal bleeding K51.211
specified NEC K51.218

Proctocele
female (without uterine prolapse) N81.6
with uterine prolapse N81.2
complete N81.3
male K62.3
Proctocolitis
food-induced eosinophilic K52.82
food protein-induced K52.82
milk protein-induced K52.82
mucosal — *see* Rectosigmoiditis, ulcerative
Proctoptosis K62.3
Proctorrhagia K62.5
Proctosigmoiditis K63.89
ulcerative (chronic) — *see* Rectosigmoiditis,
ulcerative
Proctospasm K59.4
psychogenic F45.8
Profichet's disease — *see* Disorder, soft tissue, specified
type NEC
Progeria E34.8
Prognathism (mandibular) (maxillary) M26.19
Progonoma (melanotic) — *see* Neoplasm, benign, by
site
Progressive — *see* condition
Prolactinoma
specified site — *see* Neoplasm, benign, by site
unspecified site D35.2
Prolapse, prolapsed
anus, anal (canal) (sphincter) K62.2
arm or hand O32.2 ☑
causing obstructed labor O64.4 ☑
bladder (mucosa) (sphincter) (acquired)
congenital Q79.4
female — *see* Cystocele
male N32.89
breast implant (prosthetic) T85.49 ☑
cecostomy K94.09
cecum K63.4
cervix, cervical (hypertrophied) N81.2
anterior lip, obstructing labor O65.5
congenital Q51.828
postpartal, old N81.2
stump N81.85
ciliary body (traumatic) — *see* Laceration, eye(ball),
with prolapse or loss of interocular tissue
colon (pedunculated) K63.4
colostomy K94.09
disc (intervertebral) — *see* Displacement,
intervertebral disc
eye implant (orbital) T85.398 ☑
lens (ocular) — *see* Complications, intraocular
lens
fallopian tube N83.4 ☑
gastric (mucosa) K31.89
genital, female N81.9
specified NEC N81.89
globe, nontraumatic — *see* Luxation, globe
ileostomy bud K94.19
intervertebral disc — *see* Displacement,
intervertebral disc
intestine (small) K63.4
iris (traumatic) — *see* Laceration, eye(ball), with
prolapse or loss of interocular tissue
nontraumatic H21.89
kidney N28.83
congenital Q63.2
laryngeal muscles or ventricle J38.7
liver K76.89
meatus urinarius N36.8
mitral (valve) I34.1
ocular lens implant — *see* Complications,
intraocular lens
organ or site, congenital NEC — *see* Malposition,
congenital
ovary N83.4 ☑
pelvic floor, female N81.89
perineum, female N81.89
rectum (mucosa) (sphincter) K62.3
due to trichuris trichuria B79
spleen D73.89
stomach K31.89
umbilical cord
complicating delivery O69.0 ☑
urachus, congenital Q64.4
ureter N28.89
with obstruction N13.5
with infection N13.6
ureterovesical orifice N28.89
urethra (acquired) (infected) (mucosa) N36.8
congenital Q64.71
urinary meatus N36.8
congenital Q64.72

Prolapse — *continued*
uterovaginal N81.4
complete N81.3
incomplete N81.2
uterus (with prolapse of vagina) N81.4
complete N81.3
congenital Q51.818
first degree N81.2
in pregnancy or childbirth — *see* Pregnancy,
complicated by, abnormal, uterus
incomplete N81.2
postpartal (old) N81.4
second degree N81.2
third degree N81.3
uveal (traumatic) — *see* Laceration, eye(ball), with
prolapse or loss of interocular tissue
vagina (anterior) (wall) — *see* Cystocele
with prolapse of uterus N81.4
complete N81.3
incomplete N81.2
posterior wall N81.6
posthysterectomy N99.3
vitreous (humor) H43.0 ☑
in wound — *see* Laceration, eye(ball), with
prolapse or loss of interocular tissue
womb — *see* Prolapse, uterus
Prolapsus, female N81.9
specified NEC N81.89
Proliferation(s)
prostate, atypical small acinar N42.32
primary cutaneous CD30 ☑ positive large T-cell
C86.6
Proliferative — *see* condition
Prolonged, prolongation (of)
bleeding (time) (idiopathic) R79.1
coagulation (time) R79.1
gestation (over 42 completed weeks)
mother O48.1
newborn P08.22
interval I44.0
labor O63.9
first stage O63.0
second stage O63.1
partial thromboplastin time (PTT) R79.1
pregnancy (more than 42 weeks gestation) O48.1
prothrombin time R79.1
QT interval R94.31
uterine contractions in labor O62.4
Prominence, prominent
auricle (congenital) (ear) Q17.5
ischial spine or sacral promontory
with disproportion (fetopelvic) O33.0
causing obstructed labor O65.0
nose (congenital) acquired M95.0
Promiscuity — *see* High, risk, sexual behavior
Pronation
ankle — *see* Deformity, limb, foot, specified NEC
foot (*see also* Deformity, limb, foot, specified NEC)
congenital Q74.2
Prophylactic
administration of
antibiotics, long-term Z79.2
short-term use - omit code
drug (*see also* Long-term (current) drug therapy
(use of)) Z79.899
medication Z79.899
organ removal (for neoplasia management) Z40.00
breast Z40.01
fallopian tube(s) Z40.03
with ovary(s) Z40.02
ovary(s) Z40.02
specified site NEC Z40.09
surgery Z40.9
for risk factors related to malignant neoplasm —
see Prophylactic, organ removal
specified NEC Z40.8
vaccination Z23
Propionic acidemia E71.121
Proptosis (ocular) (*see also* Exophthalmos)
thyroid — *see* Hyperthyroidism, with goiter
Prosecution, anxiety concerning Z65.3
Prosopagnosia R48.3
Prostadynia N42.81
Prostate, prostatic — *see* condition
Prostatism — *see* Hyperplasia, prostate
Prostatitis (congestive) (suppurative) (with cystitis)
N41.9
acute N41.0
cavitary N41.8
chronic N41.1
diverticular N41.8
due to Trichomonas (vaginalis) A59.02

Prostatitis — *continued*
   fibrous N41.1
   gonococcal (acute) (chronic) A54.22
   granulomatous N41.4
   hypertrophic N41.1
   subacute N41.1
   trichomonal A59.02
   tuberculous A18.14
Prostatocystitis N41.3
Prostatorrhea N42.89
Prostatosis N42.82
Prostration R53.83
   heat (*see also* Heat, exhaustion)
      anhydrotic T67.3 ☑
      due to
         salt (and water) depletion T67.4 ☑
         water depletion T67.3 ☑
   nervous F48.8
   senile R54
Protanomaly (anomalous trichromat) H53.54
Protanopia (complete) (incomplete) H53.54
Protection (against) (from) — *see* Prophylactic
Protein
   deficiency NEC — *see* Malnutrition
   malnutrition — *see* Malnutrition
   sickness (*see also* Reaction, serum) T80.69 ☑
Proteinemia R77.9
Proteinosis
   alveolar (pulmonary) J84.01
   lipid or lipoid (of Urbach) E78.89
Proteinuria R80.9
   Bence Jones R80.3
   complicating pregnancy — *see* Proteinuria,
      gestational
   gestational
      complicating
         childbirth O12.14
         pregnancy O12.1 ☑
            with edema O12.2 ☑
         puerperium O12.15
   idiopathic R80.0
   isolated R80.0
      with glomerular lesion N06.9
         dense deposit disease N06.6
         diffuse
            crescentic glomerulonephritis N06.7
            endocapillary proliferative
               glomerulonephritis N06.4
            mesangiocapillary glomerulonephritis N06.5
         focal and segmental hyalinosis or sclerosis
            N06.1
         membranous (diffuse) N06.2
         mesangial proliferative (diffuse) N06.3
         minimal change N06.0
         specified pathology NEC N06.8
   orthostatic R80.2
      with glomerular lesion — *see* Proteinuria, isolated,
         with glomerular lesion
   persistent R80.1
      with glomerular lesion — *see* Proteinuria, isolated,
         with glomerular lesion
   postural R80.2
      with glomerular lesion — *see* Proteinuria, isolated,
         with glomerular lesion
   pre-eclamptic — *see* Pre-eclampsia
   puerperal O12.15
   specified type NEC R80.8
Proteolysis, pathologic D65
Proteus (mirabilis) (morganii), as cause of disease
   classified elsewhere B96.4
Prothrombin gene mutation D68.52
Protoporphyria, erythropoietic E80.0
Protozoal (*see also* condition)
   disease B64
      specified NEC B60.8
Protrusion, protrusio
   acetabuli M24.7
   acetabulum (into pelvis) M24.7
   device, implant or graft (*see also* Complications, by
      site and type, mechanical) T85.698 ☑
      arterial graft NEC — *see* Complication,
         cardiovascular device, mechanical, vascular
      breast (implant) T85.49 ☑
      catheter NEC T85.698 ☑
         cystostomy T83.090 ☑
         dialysis (renal) T82.49 ☑
            intraperitoneal T85.691 ☑
         infusion NEC T82.594 ☑
            spinal (epidural) (subdural) T85.690 ☑
         urinary (*see also* Complications, catheter,
            urinary) T83.098 ☑

Protrusion — *continued*
   device — *continued*
      electronic (electrode) (pulse generator)
         (stimulator)
         bone T84.390 ☑
         nervous system — *see* Complication, prosthetic
            device, mechanical, electronic nervous
            system stimulator
      fixation, internal (orthopedic) NEC — *see*
         Complication, fixation device, mechanical
      gastrointestinal — *see* Complications, prosthetic
         device, mechanical, gastrointestinal device
      genital NEC T83.498 ☑
         intrauterine contraceptive device T83.39 ☑
         penile prosthesis (cylinder) (implanted) (pump)
            (reservoir) T83.490 ☑
         testicular prosthesis T83.491 ☑
      heart NEC — *see* Complication, cardiovascular
         device, mechanical
      joint prosthesis — *see* Complications, joint
         prosthesis, mechanical, specified NEC, by site
      ocular NEC — *see* Complications, prosthetic
         device, mechanical, ocular device
      orthopedic NEC — *see* Complication, orthopedic,
         device, mechanical
      specified NEC T85.628 ☑
      urinary NEC (*see also* Complication, genitourinary,
         device, urinary, mechanical)
         graft T83.29 ☑
      vascular NEC — *see* Complication, cardiovascular
         device, mechanical
      ventricular intracranial shunt T85.09 ☑
   intervertebral disc — *see* Displacement,
      intervertebral disc
   joint prosthesis — *see* Complications, joint
      prosthesis, mechanical, specified NEC, by site
   nucleus pulposus — *see* Displacement,
      intervertebral disc
Prune belly (syndrome) Q79.4
Prurigo (ferox) (gravis) (Hebrae) (Hebra's) (mitis)
   (simplex) L28.2
   Besnier's L20.0
   estivalis L56.4
   nodularis L28.1
   psychogenic F45.8
Pruritus, pruritic (essential) L29.9
   ani, anus L29.0
      psychogenic F45.8
   anogenital L29.3
      psychogenic F45.8
   due to onchocerca volvulus B73.1
   gravidarum — *see* Pregnancy, complicated by,
      specified pregnancy-related condition NEC
   hiemalis L29.8
   neurogenic (any site) F45.8
   perianal L29.0
   psychogenic (any site) F45.8
   scroti, scrotum L29.1
      psychogenic F45.8
   senile, senilis L29.8
   specified NEC L29.8
      psychogenic F45.8
   Trichomonas A59.9
   vulva, vulvae L29.2
      psychogenic F45.8
Pseudarthrosis, pseudoarthrosis (bone) — *see*
   Nonunion, fracture
   clavicle, congenital Q74.0
   joint, following fusion or arthrodesis M96.0
Pseudoaneurysm — *see* Aneurysm
Pseudoangioma I81
Pseudoangina (pectoris) — *see* Angina
Pseudoarteriosus Q28.8
Pseudoarthrosis — *see* Pseudarthrosis
Pseudobulbar affect (PBA) F48.2
Pseudochromhidrosis L67.8
Pseudocirrhosis, liver, pericardial I31.1
Pseudocowpox B08.03
Pseudocoxalgia M91.3 ☑
Pseudocroup J38.5
Pseudo-Cushing's syndrome, alcohol-induced E24.4
Pseudocyesis F45.8
Pseudocyst
   lung J98.4
   pancreas K86.3
   retina — *see* Cyst, retina
Pseudoelephantiasis neuroarthritica Q82.0
Pseudoexfoliation, capsule (lens) — *see* Cataract,
   specified NEC
Pseudofolliculitis barbae L73.1
Pseudoglioma H44.89

Pseudohemophilia (Bernuth's) (hereditary) (type B)
   D68.0
   Type A D69.8
   vascular D69.8
Pseudohermaphroditism Q56.3
   adrenal E25.8
   female Q56.2
      with adrenocortical disorder E25.8
      without adrenocortical disorder Q56.2
      adrenal (congenital) E25.0
      unspecified E25.9
   male Q56.1
      with
         adrenocortical disorder E25.8
         androgen resistance E34.51
         cleft scrotum Q56.1
         feminizing testis E34.51
         5-alpha-reductase deficiency E29.1
      without gonadal disorder Q56.1
      adrenal E25.8
      unspecified E25.9
Pseudo-Hurler's polydystrophy E77.0
Pseudohydrocephalus G93.2
Pseudohypertrophic muscular dystrophy (Erb's)
   G71.02
Pseudohypertrophy, muscle G71.09
Pseudohypoparathyroidism E20.1
Pseudoinsomnia F51.03
Pseudoleukemia, infantile D64.89
Pseudomembranous — *see* condition
Pseudomenses (newborn) P54.6
Pseudomenstruation (newborn) P54.6
Pseudomeningocele (cerebral) (infective) (post-
   traumatic) G96.19
   postprocedural (spinal) G97.82
Pseudomonas
   aeruginosa, as cause of disease classified elsewhere
      B96.5
   mallei infection A24.0
      as cause of disease classified elsewhere B96.5
      pseudomallei, as cause of disease classified
         elsewhere B96.5
Pseudomyotonia G71.19
Pseudomyxoma peritonei C78.6
Pseudoneuritis, optic (nerve) (disc) (papilla),
   congenital Q14.2
Pseudo-obstruction intestine (acute) (chronic)
   (idiopathic) (intermittent secondary) (primary) K59.8
Pseudopapilledema H47.33 ☑
   congenital Q14.2
Pseudoparalysis
   arm or leg R29.818
   atonic, congenital P94.2
Pseudopelade L66.0
Pseudophakia Z96.1
Pseudopolyarthritis, rhizomelic M35.3
Pseudopolycythemia D75.1
Pseudopseudohypoparathyroidism E20.1
Pseudopterygium H11.81 ☑
Pseudoptosis (eyelid) — *see* Blepharochalasis
Pseudopuberty, precocious
   female heterosexual E25.8
   male isosexual E25.8
Pseudorickets (renal) N25.0
Pseudorubella B08.20
Pseudosclerema, newborn P83.88
Pseudosclerosis (brain)
   of Westphal (Strümpell) E83.01
   Jakob's — *see* Creutzfeldt-Jakob disease or
      syndrome
   spastic — *see* Creutzfeldt-Jakob disease or
      syndrome
Pseudotetanus — *see* Convulsions
Pseudotetany R29.0
   hysterical F44.5
Pseudotruncus arteriosus Q25.49
Pseudotuberculosis A28.2
   enterocolitis A04.8
   pasteurella (infection) A28.0
Pseudotumor
   cerebri G93.2
   orbital H05.11 ☑
Pseudoxanthoma elasticum Q82.8
Psilosis (sprue) (tropical) K90.1
   nontropical K90.0
Psittacosis A70
Psoitis M60.88
Psoriasis L40.9
   arthropathic L40.50
      arthritis mutilans L40.52
      distal interphalangeal L40.51
      juvenile L40.54

Psoriasis — *continued*
  arthropathic — *continued*
    other specified L40.59
    spondylitis L40.53
  buccal K13.29
  flexural L40.8
  guttate L40.4
  mouth K13.29
  nummular L40.0
  plaque L40.0
  psychogenic F54
  pustular (generalized) L40.1
    palmaris et plantaris L40.3
  specified NEC L40.8
  vulgaris L40.0
Psychasthenia F48.8
Psychiatric disorder or problem F99
Psychogenic (*see also* condition)
  factors associated with physical conditions F54
Psychological and behavioral factors affecting
  medical condition F59
Psychoneurosis, psychoneurotic (*see also* Neurosis)
  anxiety (state) F41.1
  depersonalization F48.1
  hypochondriacal F45.21
  hysteria F44.9
  neurasthenic F48.8
  personality NEC F60.89
Psychopathy, psychopathic
  affectionless F94.2
  autistic F84.5
  constitution, post-traumatic F07.81
  personality — *see* Disorder, personality
  sexual — *see* Deviation, sexual
  state F60.2
Psychosexual identity disorder of childhood F64.2
Psychosis, psychotic F29
  acute (transient) F23
    hysterical F44.9
  affective — *see* Disorder, mood
  alcoholic F10.959
    with
      abuse F10.159
      anxiety disorder F10.980
        with
          abuse F10.180
          dependence F10.280
      delirium tremens F10.231
      delusions F10.950
        with
          abuse F10.150
          dependence F10.250
      dementia F10.97
        with dependence F10.27
      dependence F10.259
      hallucinosis F10.951
        with
          abuse F10.151
          dependence F10.251
      mood disorder F10.94
        with
          abuse F10.14
          dependence F10.24
      paranoia F10.950
        with
          abuse F10.150
          dependence F10.250
      persisting amnesia F10.96
        with dependence F10.26
    amnestic confabulatory F10.96
      with dependence F10.26
    delirium tremens F10.231
    Korsakoff's, Korsakov's, Korsakow's F10.26
    paranoid type F10.950
      with
        abuse F10.150
        dependence F10.250
  anergastic — *see* Psychosis, organic
  arteriosclerotic (simple type) (uncomplicated)
    F01.50
    with behavioral disturbance F01.51
  childhood F84.0
    atypical F84.8
  climacteric — *see* Psychosis, involutional
  confusional F29
    acute or subacute F05
    reactive F23
  cycloid F23
  depressive — *see* Disorder, depressive
  disintegrative (childhood) F84.3

Psychosis — *continued*
  drug-induced — *see* F11-F19 with .x59
    paranoid and hallucinatory states — *see* F11-F19
      with .x50 or .x51
  due to or associated with
    addiction, drug — *see* F11-F19 with .x59
    dependence
      alcohol F10.259
      drug — *see* F11-F19 with .x59
    epilepsy F06.8
    Huntington's chorea F06.8
    ischemia, cerebrovascular (generalized) F06.8
    multiple sclerosis F06.8
    physical disease F06.8
    presenile dementia F03 ☑
    senile dementia F03 ☑
    vascular disease (arteriosclerotic) (cerebral)
      F01.50
      with behavioral disturbance F01.51
  epileptic F06.8
  episode F23
    due to or associated with physical condition F06.8
  exhaustive F43.0
  hallucinatory, chronic F28
  hypomanic F30.8
  hysterical (acute) F44.9
  induced F24
  infantile F84.0
    atypical F84.8
  infective (acute) (subacute) F05
  involutional F28
    depressive — *see* Disorder, depressive
    melancholic — *see* Disorder, depressive
    paranoid (state) F22
  Korsakoff's, Korsakov's, Korsakow's (nonalcoholic)
    F04
    alcoholic F10.96
      in dependence F10.26
    induced by other psychoactive substance — *see*
      categories F11-F19 with .x5x
  mania, manic (single episode) F30.2
    recurrent type F31.89
  manic-depressive — *see* Disorder, bipolar
  menopausal — *see* Psychosis, involutional
  mixed schizophrenic and affective F25.8
  multi-infarct (cerebrovascular) F01.50
    with behavioral disturbance F01.51
  nonorganic F29
    specified NEC F28
  organic F09
    due to or associated with
      arteriosclerosis (cerebral) — *see* Psychosis,
        arteriosclerotic
      cerebrovascular disease, arteriosclerotic — *see*
        Psychosis, arteriosclerotic
      childbirth — *see* Psychosis, puerperal
      Creutzfeldt-Jakob disease or syndrome — *see*
        Creutzfeldt-Jakob disease or syndrome
      dependence, alcohol F10.259
      disease
        alcoholic liver F10.259
        brain, arteriosclerotic — *see* Psychosis,
          arteriosclerotic
        cerebrovascular F01.50
          with behavioral disturbance F01.51
        Creutzfeldt-Jakob — *see* Creutzfeldt-Jakob
          disease or syndrome
      endocrine or metabolic F06.8
        acute or subacute F05
        liver, alcoholic F10.259
      epilepsy transient (acute) F05
      infection
        brain (intracranial) F06.8
          acute or subacute F05
      intoxication
        alcoholic (acute) F10.259
        drug F11-F19 with .x59
      ischemia, cerebrovascular (generalized) — *see*
        Psychosis, arteriosclerotic
      puerperium — *see* Psychosis, puerperal
      trauma, brain (birth) (from electric current)
        (surgical) F06.8
        acute or subacute F05
    infective F06.8
      acute or subacute F05
    post-traumatic F06.8
      acute or subacute F05
  paranoiac F22
  paranoid (climacteric) (involutional) (menopausal) F22
    psychogenic (acute) F23
    schizophrenic F20.0
  senile F03 ☑

Psychosis — *continued*
  postpartum (NOS) F53.1
  presbyophrenic (type) F03 ☑
  presenile F03 ☑
  psychogenic (paranoid) F23
    depressive F32.3
  puerperal (NOS) F53.1
    specified type — *see* Psychosis, by type
  reactive (brief) (transient) (emotional stress)
    (psychological trauma) F23
    depressive F32.3
      recurrent F33.3
    excitative type F30.8
  schizoaffective F25.9
    depressive type F25.1
    manic type F25.0
  schizophrenia, schizophrenic — *see* Schizophrenia
  schizophrenia-like, in epilepsy F06.2
  schizophreniform F20.81
    affective type F25.9
    brief F23
    confusional type F23
    mixed type F25.0
  senile NEC F03 ☑
    depressed or paranoid type F03 ☑
    simple deterioration F03 ☑
    specified type - code to condition
  shared F24
  situational (reactive) F23
  symbiotic (childhood) F84.3
  symptomatic F09
Psychosomatic — *see* Disorder, psychosomatic
Psychosyndrome, organic F07.9
Psychotic episode due to or associated with physical
  condition F06.8
Pterygium (eye) H11.00 ☑
  amyloid H11.01 ☑
  central H11.02 ☑
  colli Q18.3
  double H11.03 ☑
  peripheral
    progressive H11.05 ☑
    stationary H11.04 ☑
  recurrent H11.06 ☑
Ptilosis (eyelid) — *see* Madarosis
Ptomaine (poisoning) — *see* Poisoning, food
Ptosis (*see also* Blepharoptosis)
  adiposa (false) — *see* Blepharoptosis
  breast N64.81
  brow H57.81 ☑
  cecum K63.4
  colon K63.4
  congenital (eyelid) Q10.0
    specified site NEC — *see* Anomaly, by site
  eyebrow H57.81 ☑
  eyelid — *see* Blepharoptosis
    congenital Q10.0
  gastric K31.89
  intestine K63.4
  kidney N28.83
  liver K76.89
  renal N28.83
  splanchnic K63.4
  spleen D73.89
  stomach K31.89
  viscera K63.4
PTP D69.51
Ptyalism (periodic) K11.7
  hysterical F45.8
  pregnancy — *see* Pregnancy, complicated by,
    specified pregnancy-related condition NEC
  psychogenic F45.8
Ptyalolithiasis K11.5
Pubarche, precocious E30.1
Pubertas praecox E30.1
Puberty (development state) Z00.3
  bleeding (excessive) N92.2
  delayed E30.0
  precocious (constitutional) (cryptogenic)
    (idiopathic) E30.1
    central E22.8
    due to
      ovarian hyperfunction E28.1
        estrogen E28.0
      testicular hyperfunction E29.0
  premature E30.1
    due to
      adrenal cortical hyperfunction E25.8
      pineal tumor E34.8
      pituitary (anterior) hyperfunction E22.8
Puckering, macula — *see* Degeneration, macula,
  puckering

☑ **Additional character required**

Pudenda, pudendum — *see* condition
Puente's disease (simple glandular cheilitis) K13.0
Puerperal, puerperium (complicated by, complications)
  abnormal glucose (tolerance test) O99.815
  abscess
    areola O91.02
      associated with lactation O91.03
    Bartholin's gland O86.19
    breast O91.12
      associated with lactation O91.13
    cervix (uteri) O86.11
    genital organ NEC O86.19
    kidney O86.21
    mammary O91.12
      associated with lactation O91.13
    nipple O91.02
      associated with lactation O91.03
    peritoneum O85
    subareolar O91.12
      associated with lactation O91.13
    urinary tract — *see* Puerperal, infection, urinary
    uterus O86.12
    vagina (wall) O86.13
    vaginorectal O86.13
    vulvovaginal gland O86.13
  adnexitis O86.19
  afibrinogenemia, or other coagulation defect O72.3
  albuminuria (acute) (subacute) — *see* Proteinuria, gestational
  alcohol use O99.315
  anemia O90.81
    pre-existing (pre-pregnancy) O99.03
  anesthetic death O89.8
  apoplexy O99.43
  bariatric surgery status O99.845
  blood disorder NEC O99.13
  blood dyscrasia O72.3
  cardiomyopathy O90.3
  cerebrovascular disorder (conditions in I60-I69) O99.43
  cervicitis O86.11
  circulatory system disorder O99.43
  coagulopathy (any) O99.13
    with hemorrhage O72.3
  complications O90.9
    specified NEC O90.89
  convulsions — *see* Eclampsia
  cystitis O86.22
  cystopyelitis O86.29
  delirium NEC F05
  diabetes O24.93
    gestational — *see* Puerperal, gestational diabetes
    pre-existing O24.33
      specified NEC O24.83
      type 1 O24.03
      type 2 O24.13
  digestive system disorder O99.63
  disease O90.9
    breast NEC O92.29
    cerebrovascular (acute) O99.43
    nonobstetric NEC O99.89
    tubo-ovarian O86.19
    Valsuani's O99.03
  disorder O90.9
    biliary tract O26.63
    lactation O92.70
    liver O26.63
    nonobstetric NEC O99.89
  disruption
    cesarean wound O90.0
    episiotomy wound O90.1
    perineal laceration wound O90.1
  drug use O99.325
  eclampsia (with pre-existing hypertension) O15.2
  embolism (pulmonary) (blood clot) — *see* Embolism, obstetric, puerperal
  endocrine, nutritional or metabolic disease NEC O99.285
  endophlebitis — *see* Puerperal, phlebitis
  endotrachelitis O86.11
  failure
    lactation (complete) O92.3
      partial O92.4
    renal, acute O90.4
  fever (of unknown origin) O86.4
    septic O85
  fissure, nipple O92.12
    associated with lactation O92.13
  fistula
    breast (due to mastitis) O91.12
      associated with lactation O91.13

Puerperal — *continued*
  fistula — *continued*
    nipple O91.02
      associated with lactation O91.03
  galactophoritis O91.22
    associated with lactation O91.23
  galactorrhea O92.6
  gastric banding status O99.845
  gastric bypass status O99.845
  gastrointestinal disease NEC O99.63
  gestational
    diabetes O24.439
      diet controlled O24.430
      insulin (and diet) controlled O24.434
      oral drug controlled (antidiabetic) (hypoglycemic) O24.435
    edema O12.05
      with proteinuria O12.25
    proteinuria O12.15
  gonorrhea O98.23
  hematoma, subdural O99.43
  hemiplegia, cerebral O99.355
    due to cerebrovascular disorder O99.43
  hemorrhage O72.1
    brain O99.43
    bulbar O99.43
    cerebellar O99.43
    cerebral O99.43
    cortical O99.43
    delayed or secondary O72.2
    extradural O99.43
    internal capsule O99.43
    intracranial O99.43
    intrapontine O99.43
    meningeal O99.43
    pontine O99.43
    retained placenta O72.0
    subarachnoid O99.43
    subcortical O99.43
    subdural O99.43
    third stage O72.0
    uterine, delayed O72.2
    ventricular O99.43
  hemorrhoids O87.2
  hepatorenal syndrome O90.4
  hypertension — *see* Hypertension, complicating, puerperium
  hypertrophy, breast O92.29
  induration breast (fibrous) O92.29
  infection O86.4
    cervix O86.11
    generalized O85
    genital tract NEC O86.19
      obstetric surgical wound O86.09
    kidney (bacillus coli) O86.21
    maternal O98.93
      carrier state NEC O99.835
      gonorrhea O98.23
      human immunodeficiency virus (HIV) O98.73
      protozoal O98.63
      sexually transmitted NEC O98.33
      specified NEC O98.83
      streptococcus group B (GBS) carrier state O99.825
      syphilis O98.13
      tuberculosis O98.03
      viral hepatitis O98.43
      viral NEC O98.53
    nipple O91.02
      associated with lactation O91.03
    peritoneum O85
    renal O86.21
    specified NEC O86.89
    urinary (asymptomatic) (tract) NEC O86.20
      bladder O86.22
      kidney O86.21
      specified site NEC O86.29
      urethra O86.22
    vagina O86.13
    vein — *see* Puerperal, phlebitis
  ischemia, cerebral O99.43
  lymphangitis O86.89
    breast O91.22
      associated with lactation O91.23
  malignancy O9A.13
  malnutrition O25.3
  mammillitis O91.02
    associated with lactation O91.03
  mammitis O91.22
    associated with lactation O91.23
  mania F30.8

Puerperal — *continued*
  mastitis O91.22
    associated with lactation O91.23
    purulent O91.12
      associated with lactation O91.13
  melancholia — *see* Disorder, depressive
  mental disorder NEC O99.345
  metroperitonitis O85
  metrorrhagia — *see* Hemorrhage, postpartum
  metrosalpingitis O86.19
  metrovaginitis O86.13
  milk leg O87.1
  monoplegia, cerebral O99.43
  mood disturbance O90.6
  necrosis, liver (acute) (subacute) (conditions in subcategory K72.0 ☑) O26.63
    with renal failure O90.4
  nervous system disorder O99.355
  neuritis O90.89
  obesity (pre-existing prior to pregnancy) O99.215
  obesity surgery status O99.845
  occlusion, precerebral artery O99.43
  paralysis
    bladder (sphincter) O90.89
    cerebral O99.43
  paralytic stroke O99.43
  parametritis O85
  paravaginitis O86.13
  pelviperitonitis O85
  perimetritis O86.12
  perimetrosalpingitis O86.19
  perinephritis O86.21
  periphlebitis — *see* Puerperal phlebitis
  peritoneal infection O85
  peritonitis (pelvic) O85
  perivaginitis O86.13
  phlebitis O87.0
    deep O87.1
    pelvic O87.1
    superficial O87.0
  phlebothrombosis, deep O87.1
  phlegmasia alba dolens O87.1
  placental polyp O90.89
  pneumonia, embolic — *see* Embolism, obstetric, puerperal
  pre-eclampsia — *see* Pre-eclampsia
  psychosis (NOS) F53.1
  pyelitis O86.21
  pyelocystitis O86.29
  pyelonephritis O86.21
  pyelonephrosis O86.21
  pyemia O85
  pyocystitis O86.29
  pyohemia O85
  pyometra O86.12
  pyonephritis O86.21
  pyosalpingitis O86.19
  pyrexia (of unknown origin) O86.4
  renal
    disease NEC O90.89
    failure O90.4
  respiratory disease NEC O99.53
  retention
    decidua — *see* Retention, decidua
    placenta O72.0
    secundines — *see* Retention, secundines
  retracted nipple O92.02
  salpingo-ovaritis O86.19
  salpingoperitonitis O85
  secondary perineal tear O90.1
  sepsis (pelvic) O85
  sepsis O85
  septic thrombophlebitis O86.81
  skin disorder NEC O99.73
  specified condition NEC O99.89
  stroke O99.43
  subinvolution (uterus) O90.89
  subluxation of symphysis (pubis) O26.73
  suppuration — *see* Puerperal, abscess
  tetanus A34
  thelitis O91.02
    associated with lactation O91.03
  thrombocytopenia O72.3
  thrombophlebitis (superficial) O87.0
    deep O87.1
    pelvic O87.1
    septic O86.81
  thrombosis (venous) — *see* Thrombosis, puerperal
  thyroiditis O90.5
  toxemia (eclamptic) (pre-eclamptic) (with convulsions) O15.2

Puerperal - Puncture

Puerperal — *continued*
  trauma, non-obstetric O9A.23
    caused by abuse (physical) (suspected) O9A.33
      confirmed O9A.33
      psychological (suspected) O9A.53
        confirmed O9A.53
      sexual (suspected) O9A.43
        confirmed O9A.43
  uremia (due to renal failure) O90.4
  urethritis O86.22
  vaginitis O86.13
  varicose veins (legs) O87.4
    vulva or perineum O87.8
  venous O87.9
  vulvitis O86.19
  vulvovaginitis O86.13
  white leg O87.1
Puerperium — *see* Puerperal
Pulmolithiasis J98.4
Pulmonary — *see* condition
Pulpitis (acute) (anachoretic) (chronic) (hyperplastic) (putrescent) (suppurative) (ulcerative) K04.01
  irreversible K04.02
  reversible K04.01
Pulpless tooth K04.99
Pulse
  alternating R00.8
  bigeminal R00.8
  fast R00.0
  feeble, rapid due to shock following injury T79.4 ☑
  rapid R00.0
  weak R09.89
Pulsus alternans or trigeminus R00.8
Punch drunk F07.81
Punctum lacrimale occlusion — *see* Obstruction, lacrimal
Puncture
  abdomen, abdominal
    wall S31.139 ☑
      with
        foreign body S31.149 ☑
        penetration into peritoneal cavity S31.639 ☑
          with foreign body S31.649 ☑
      epigastric region S31.132 ☑
        with
          foreign body S31.142 ☑
          penetration into peritoneal cavity S31.632 ☑
            with foreign body S31.642 ☑
      left
        lower quadrant S31.134 ☑
          with
            foreign body S31.144 ☑
            penetration into peritoneal cavity S31.634 ☑
              with foreign body S31.644 ☑
        upper quadrant S31.131 ☑
          with
            foreign body S31.141 ☑
            penetration into peritoneal cavity S31.631 ☑
              with foreign body S31.641 ☑
      periumbilic region S31.135 ☑
        with
          foreign body S31.145 ☑
          penetration into peritoneal cavity S31.635 ☑
            with foreign body S31.645 ☑
      right
        lower quadrant S31.133 ☑
          with
            foreign body S31.143 ☑
            penetration into peritoneal cavity S31.633 ☑
              with foreign body S31.643 ☑
        upper quadrant S31.130 ☑
          with
            foreign body S31.140 ☑
            penetration into peritoneal cavity S31.630 ☑
              with foreign body S31.640 ☑
  accidental, complicating surgery — *see* Complication, accidental puncture or laceration
  alveolar (process) — *see* Puncture, oral cavity
  ankle S91.039 ☑
    with
      foreign body S91.049 ☑
    left S91.032 ☑
      with
        foreign body S91.042 ☑
    right S91.031 ☑
      with
        foreign body S91.041 ☑

Puncture — *continued*
  anus S31.833 ☑
    with foreign body S31.834 ☑
  arm (upper) S41.139 ☑
    with foreign body S41.149 ☑
    left S41.132 ☑
      with foreign body S41.142 ☑
    lower — *see* Puncture, forearm
    right S41.131 ☑
      with foreign body S41.141 ☑
  auditory canal (external) (meatus) — *see* Puncture, ear
  auricle, ear — *see* Puncture, ear
  axilla — *see* Puncture, arm
  back (*see also* Puncture, thorax, back)
    lower S31.030 ☑
      with
        foreign body S31.040 ☑
        with penetration into retroperitoneal space S31.041 ☑
        penetration into retroperitoneal space S31.031 ☑
  bladder (traumatic) S37.29 ☑
    nontraumatic N32.89
  breast S21.039 ☑
    with foreign body S21.049 ☑
    left S21.032 ☑
      with foreign body S21.042 ☑
    right S21.031 ☑
      with foreign body S21.041 ☑
  buttock S31.803 ☑
    with foreign body S31.804 ☑
    left S31.823 ☑
      with foreign body S31.824 ☑
    right S31.813 ☑
      with foreign body S31.814 ☑
  by
    device, implant or graft — *see* Complications, by site and type, mechanical
    foreign body left accidentally in operative wound T81.539 ☑
    instrument (any) during a procedure, accidental — *see* Puncture, accidental complicating surgery
  calf — *see* Puncture, leg
  canaliculus lacrimalis — *see* Puncture, eyelid
  canthus, eye — *see* Puncture, eyelid
  cervical esophagus S11.23 ☑
    with foreign body S11.24 ☑
  cheek (external) S01.439 ☑
    with foreign body S01.449 ☑
    left S01.432 ☑
      with foreign body S01.442 ☑
    right S01.431 ☑
      with foreign body S01.441 ☑
    internal — *see* Puncture, oral cavity
  chest wall — *see* Puncture, thorax
  chin — *see* Puncture, head, specified site NEC
  clitoris — *see* Puncture, vulva
  costal region — *see* Puncture, thorax
  digit(s)
    hand — *see* Puncture, finger
    foot — *see* Puncture, toe
  ear (canal) (external) S01.339 ☑
    with foreign body S01.349 ☑
    left S01.332 ☑
      with foreign body S01.342 ☑
    right S01.331 ☑
      with foreign body S01.341 ☑
    drum S09.2 ☑
  elbow S51.039 ☑
    with
      foreign body S51.049 ☑
    left S51.032 ☑
      with
        foreign body S51.042 ☑
    right S51.031 ☑
      with
        foreign body S51.041 ☑
  epididymis — *see* Puncture, testis
  epigastric region — *see* Puncture, abdomen, wall, epigastric
  epiglottis S11.83 ☑
    with foreign body S11.84 ☑
  esophagus
    cervical S11.23 ☑
      with foreign body S11.24 ☑
    thoracic S27.818 ☑
  eyeball S05.6 ☑
    with foreign body S05.5 ☑
  eyebrow — *see* Puncture, eyelid

Puncture — *continued*
  eyelid S01.13 ☑
    with foreign body S01.14 ☑
    left S01.132 ☑
      with foreign body S01.142 ☑
    right S01.131 ☑
      with foreign body S01.141 ☑
  face NEC — *see* Puncture, head, specified site NEC
  finger(s) S61.239 ☑
    with
      damage to nail S61.339 ☑
        with
          foreign body S61.349 ☑
      foreign body S61.249 ☑
    index S61.238 ☑
      with
        damage to nail S61.338 ☑
          with
            foreign body S61.348 ☑
        foreign body S61.248 ☑
      left S61.231 ☑
        with
          damage to nail S61.331 ☑
            with
              foreign body S61.341 ☑
          foreign body S61.241 ☑
      right S61.230 ☑
        with
          damage to nail S61.330 ☑
            with
              foreign body S61.340 ☑
          foreign body S61.240 ☑
    little S61.238 ☑
      with
        damage to nail S61.338 ☑
          with
            foreign body S61.348 ☑
        foreign body S61.248 ☑
      left S61.237 ☑
        with
          damage to nail S61.337 ☑
            with
              foreign body S61.347 ☑
          foreign body S61.247 ☑
      right S61.236 ☑
        with
          damage to nail S61.336 ☑
            with
              foreign body S61.346 ☑
          foreign body S61.246 ☑
    middle S61.238 ☑
      with
        damage to nail S61.338 ☑
          with
            foreign body S61.348 ☑
        foreign body S61.248 ☑
      left S61.233 ☑
        with
          damage to nail S61.333 ☑
            with
              foreign body S61.343 ☑
          foreign body S61.243 ☑
      right S61.232 ☑
        with
          damage to nail S61.332 ☑
            with
              foreign body S61.342 ☑
          foreign body S61.242 ☑
    ring S61.238 ☑
      with
        damage to nail S61.338 ☑
          with
            foreign body S61.348 ☑
        foreign body S61.248 ☑
      left S61.235 ☑
        with
          damage to nail S61.335 ☑
            with
              foreign body S61.345 ☑
          foreign body S61.245 ☑
      right S61.234 ☑
        with
          damage to nail S61.334 ☑
            with
              foreign body S61.344 ☑
          foreign body S61.244 ☑
  flank S31.139 ☑
    with foreign body S31.149 ☑
  foot (except toe(s) alone) S91.339 ☑
    with foreign body S91.349 ☑
    left S91.332 ☑
      with foreign body S91.342 ☑

☑ **Additional character required**

Puncture — *continued*
  foot — *continued*
    right S91.331 ☑
      with foreign body S91.341 ☑
    toe — *see* Puncture, toe
  forearm S51.839 ☑
    with
      foreign body S51.849 ☑
    elbow only — *see* Puncture, elbow
    left S51.832 ☑
      with
        foreign body S51.842 ☑
    right S51.831 ☑
      with
        foreign body S51.841 ☑
  forehead — *see* Puncture, head, specified site NEC
  genital organs, external
    female S31.532 ☑
      with foreign body S31.542 ☑
      vagina — *see* Puncture, vagina
      vulva — *see* Puncture, vulva
    male S31.531 ☑
      with foreign body S31.541 ☑
      penis — *see* Puncture, penis
      scrotum — *see* Puncture, scrotum
      testis — *see* Puncture, testis
  groin — *see* Puncture, abdomen, wall
  gum — *see* Puncture, oral cavity
  hand S61.439 ☑
    with
      foreign body S61.449 ☑
    finger — *see* Puncture, finger
    left S61.432 ☑
      with
        foreign body S61.442 ☑
    right S61.431 ☑
      with
        foreign body S61.441 ☑
    thumb — *see* Puncture, thumb
  head S01.93 ☑
    with foreign body S01.94 ☑
    cheek — *see* Puncture, cheek
    ear — *see* Puncture, ear
    eyelid — *see* Puncture, eyelid
    lip — *see* Puncture, oral cavity
    nose — *see* Puncture, nose
    oral cavity — *see* Puncture, oral cavity
    scalp S01.03 ☑
      with foreign body S01.04 ☑
    specified site NEC S01.83 ☑
      with foreign body S01.84 ☑
    temporomandibular area — *see* Puncture, cheek
  heart S26.99 ☑
    with hemopericardium S26.09 ☑
    without hemopericardium S26.19 ☑
  heel — *see* Puncture, foot
  hip S71.039 ☑
    with foreign body S71.049 ☑
    left S71.032 ☑
      with foreign body S71.042 ☑
    right S71.031 ☑
      with foreign body S71.041 ☑
  hymen — *see* Puncture, vagina
  hypochondrium — *see* Puncture, abdomen, wall
  hypogastric region — *see* Puncture, abdomen, wall
  inguinal region — *see* Puncture, abdomen, wall
  instep — *see* Puncture, foot
  internal organs — *see* Injury, by site
  interscapular region — *see* Puncture, thorax, back
  intestine
    large
      colon S36.599 ☑
        ascending S36.590 ☑
        descending S36.592 ☑
        sigmoid S36.593 ☑
        specified site NEC S36.598 ☑
        transverse S36.591 ☑
      rectum S36.69 ☑
    small S36.499 ☑
      duodenum S36.490 ☑
      specified site NEC S36.498 ☑
  intra-abdominal organ S36.99 ☑
    gallbladder S36.128 ☑
    intestine — *see* Puncture, intestine
    liver S36.118 ☑
    pancreas — *see* Puncture, pancreas
    peritoneum S36.81 ☑
    specified site NEC S36.898 ☑
    spleen S36.09 ☑
    stomach S36.39 ☑
  jaw — *see* Puncture, head, specified site NEC

Puncture — *continued*
  knee S81.039 ☑
    with foreign body S81.049 ☑
    left S81.032 ☑
      with foreign body S81.042 ☑
    right S81.031 ☑
      with foreign body S81.041 ☑
  labium (majus) (minus) — *see* Puncture, vulva
  lacrimal duct — *see* Puncture, eyelid
  larynx S11.013 ☑
    with foreign body S11.014 ☑
  leg (lower) S81.839 ☑
    with foreign body S81.849 ☑
    foot — *see* Puncture, foot
    knee — *see* Puncture, knee
    left S81.832 ☑
      with foreign body S81.842 ☑
    right S81.831 ☑
      with foreign body S81.841 ☑
    upper — *see* Puncture, thigh
  lip S01.531 ☑
    with foreign body S01.541 ☑
  loin — *see* Puncture, abdomen, wall
  lower back — *see* Puncture, back, lower
  lumbar region — *see* Puncture, back, lower
  malar region — *see* Puncture, head, specified site NEC
  mammary — *see* Puncture, breast
  mastoid region — *see* Puncture, head, specified site NEC
  mouth — *see* Puncture, oral cavity
  nail
    finger — *see* Puncture, finger, with damage to nail
    toe — *see* Puncture, toe, with damage to nail
  nasal (septum) (sinus) — *see* Puncture, nose
  nasopharynx — *see* Puncture, head, specified site NEC
  neck S11.93 ☑
    with foreign body S11.94 ☑
    involving
      cervical esophagus — *see* Puncture, cervical esophagus
      larynx — *see* Puncture, larynx
      pharynx — *see* Puncture, pharynx
      thyroid gland — *see* Puncture, thyroid gland
      trachea — *see* Puncture, trachea
    specified site NEC S11.83 ☑
      with foreign body S11.84 ☑
  nose (septum) (sinus) S01.23 ☑
    with foreign body S01.24 ☑
  ocular — *see* Puncture, eyeball
  oral cavity S01.532 ☑
    with foreign body S01.542 ☑
  orbit S05.4 ☑
  palate — *see* Puncture, oral cavity
  palm — *see* Puncture, hand
  pancreas S36.299 ☑
    body S36.291 ☑
    head S36.290 ☑
    tail S36.292 ☑
  pelvis — *see* Puncture, back, lower
  penis S31.23 ☑
    with foreign body S31.24 ☑
  perineum
    female S31.43 ☑
      with foreign body S31.44 ☑
    male S31.139 ☑
      with foreign body S31.149 ☑
  periocular area (with or without lacrimal passages) — *see* Puncture, eyelid
  phalanges
    finger — *see* Puncture, finger
    toe — *see* Puncture, toe
  pharynx S11.23 ☑
    with foreign body S11.24 ☑
  pinna — *see* Puncture, ear
  popliteal space — *see* Puncture, knee
  prepuce — *see* Puncture, penis
  pubic region S31.139 ☑
    with foreign body S31.149 ☑
  pudendum — *see* Puncture, genital organs, external
  rectovaginal septum — *see* Puncture, vagina
  sacral region — *see* Puncture, back, lower
  sacroiliac region — *see* Puncture, back, lower
  salivary gland — *see* Puncture, oral cavity
  scalp S01.03 ☑
    with foreign body S01.04 ☑
  scapular region — *see* Puncture, shoulder
  scrotum S31.33 ☑
    with foreign body S31.34 ☑
  shin — *see* Puncture, leg

Puncture — *continued*
  shoulder S41.039 ☑
    with foreign body S41.049 ☑
    left S41.032 ☑
      with foreign body S41.042 ☑
    right S41.031 ☑
      with foreign body S41.041 ☑
  spermatic cord — *see* Puncture, testis
  sternal region — *see* Puncture, thorax, front
  submaxillary region — *see* Puncture, head, specified site NEC
  submental region — *see* Puncture, head, specified site NEC
  subungual
    finger(s) — *see* Puncture, finger, with damage to nail
    toe — *see* Puncture, toe, with damage to nail
  supraclavicular fossa — *see* Puncture, neck, specified site NEC
  temple, temporal region — *see* Puncture, head, specified site NEC
  temporomandibular area — *see* Puncture, cheek
  testis S31.33 ☑
    with foreign body S31.34 ☑
  thigh S71.139 ☑
    with foreign body S71.149 ☑
    left S71.132 ☑
      with foreign body S71.142 ☑
    right S71.131 ☑
      with foreign body S71.141 ☑
  thorax, thoracic (wall) S21.93 ☑
    with foreign body S21.94 ☑
    back S21.23 ☑
      with
        foreign body S21.24 ☑
          with penetration S21.44 ☑
        penetration S21.43 ☑
    breast — *see* Puncture, breast
    front S21.13 ☑
      with
        foreign body S21.14 ☑
          with penetration S21.34 ☑
        penetration S21.33 ☑
  throat — *see* Puncture, neck
  thumb S61.039 ☑
    with
      damage to nail S61.139 ☑
        with
          foreign body S61.149 ☑
      foreign body S61.049 ☑
    left S61.032 ☑
      with
        damage to nail S61.132 ☑
          with
            foreign body S61.142 ☑
        foreign body S61.042 ☑
    right S61.031 ☑
      with
        damage to nail S61.131 ☑
          with
            foreign body S61.141 ☑
        foreign body S61.041 ☑
  thyroid gland S11.13 ☑
    with foreign body S11.14 ☑
  toe(s) S91.139 ☑
    with
      damage to nail S91.239 ☑
        with
          foreign body S91.249 ☑
      foreign body S91.149 ☑
    great S91.133 ☑
      with
        damage to nail S91.233 ☑
          with
            foreign body S91.243 ☑
        foreign body S91.143 ☑
      left S91.132 ☑
        with
          damage to nail S91.232 ☑
            with
              foreign body S91.242 ☑
          foreign body S91.142 ☑
      right S91.131 ☑
        with
          damage to nail S91.231 ☑
            with
              foreign body S91.241 ☑
          foreign body S91.141 ☑
    lesser S91.136 ☑
      with
        damage to nail S91.236 ☑
          with

Puncture — *continued*
  toe(s) — *continued*
          foreign body S91.246 ☑
        foreign body S91.146 ☑
      left S91.135 ☑
        with
          damage to nail S91.235 ☑
            with
              foreign body S91.245 ☑
          foreign body S91.145 ☑
      right S91.134 ☑
        with
          damage to nail S91.234 ☑
            with
              foreign body S91.244 ☑
          foreign body S91.144 ☑
  tongue — *see* Puncture, oral cavity
  trachea S11.023 ☑
    with foreign body S11.024 ☑
  tunica vaginalis — *see* Puncture, testis
  tympanum, tympanic membrane S09.2 ☑
  umbilical region S31.135 ☑
    with foreign body S31.145 ☑
  uvula — *see* Puncture, oral cavity
  vagina S31.43 ☑
    with foreign body S31.44 ☑
  vocal cords S11.033 ☑
    with foreign body S11.034 ☑
  vulva S31.43 ☑
    with foreign body S31.44 ☑
  wrist S61.539 ☑
    with
      foreign body S61.549 ☑
    left S61.532 ☑
      with
        foreign body S61.542 ☑
    right S61.531 ☑
      with
        foreign body S61.541 ☑
PUO (pyrexia of unknown origin) R50.9
Pupillary membrane (persistent) Q13.89
Pupillotonia — *see* Anomaly, pupil, function, tonic pupil
Purpura D69.2
  abdominal D69.0
  allergic D69.0
  anaphylactoid D69.0
  annularis telangiectodes L81.7
  arthritic D69.0
  autoerythrocyte sensitization D69.2
  autoimmune D69.0
  bacterial D69.0
  Bateman's (senile) D69.2
  capillary fragility (hereditary) (idiopathic) D69.8
  cryoglobulinemic D89.1
  Devil's pinches D69.2
  fibrinolytic — *see* Fibrinolysis
  fulminans, fulminous D65
  gangrenous D65
  hemorrhagic, hemorrhagica D69.3
    not due to thrombocytopenia D69.0
  Henoch (-Schönlein) (allergic) D69.0
  hypergammaglobulinemic (benign) (Waldenström)
      D89.0
  idiopathic (thrombocytopenic) D69.3
    nonthrombocytopenic D69.0
  immune thrombocytopenic D69.3
  infectious D69.0
  malignant D69.0
  neonatorum P54.5
  nervosa D69.0
  newborn P54.5
  nonthrombocytopenic D69.2
    hemorrhagic D69.0
    idiopathic D69.0
  nonthrombopenic D69.2
  peliosis rheumatica D69.0
  posttransfusion (post-transfusion) (from (fresh)
      whole blood or blood products) D69.51
  primary D69.49
  red cell membrane sensitivity D69.2
  rheumatica D69.2
  Schönlein (-Henoch) (allergic) D69.0
  scorbutic E54 *[D77]*
  senile D69.2
  simplex D69.2
  symptomatica D69.0
  telangiectasia annularis L81.7
  thrombocytopenic D69.49
    congenital D69.42
    hemorrhagic D69.3
    hereditary D69.42
    idiopathic D69.3

Purpura — *continued*
  thrombocytopenic — *continued*
    immune D69.3
    neonatal, transitory P61.0
    thrombotic M31.1
  thrombohemolytic — *see* Fibrinolysis
  thrombolytic — *see* Fibrinolysis
  thrombopenic D69.49
  thrombotic, thrombocytopenic M31.1
  toxic D69.0
  vascular D69.0
  visceral symptoms D69.0
Purpuric spots R23.3
Purulent — *see* condition
Pus
  in
    stool R19.5
    urine N39.0
  tube (rupture) — *see* Salpingo-oophoritis
Pustular rash L08.0
Pustule (nonmalignant) L08.9
  malignant A22.0
Pustulosis palmaris et plantaris L40.3
Putnam (-Dana) disease or syndrome — *see*
  Degeneration, combined
Putrescent pulp (dental) K04.1
Pyarthritis, pyarthrosis — *see* Arthritis, pyogenic or
  pyemic
  tuberculous — *see* Tuberculosis, joint
Pyelectasis — *see* Hydronephrosis
Pyelitis (congenital) (uremic) (*see also* Pyelonephritis)
  with
    calculus — *see* category N20 ☑
      with hydronephrosis N13.6
    contracted kidney N11.9
  acute N10
  chronic N11.9
    with calculus — *see* category N20 ☑
      with hydronephrosis N13.6
  cystica N28.84
  puerperal (postpartum) O86.21
  tuberculous A18.11
Pyelocystitis — *see* Pyelonephritis
Pyelonephritis (*see also* Nephritis, tubulo-interstitial)
  with
    calculus — *see* category N20 ☑
      with hydronephrosis N13.6
    contracted kidney N11.9
  acute N10
  calculous — *see* category N20 ☑
    with hydronephrosis N13.6
  chronic N11.9
    with calculus — *see* category N20 ☑
      with hydronephrosis N13.6
    associated with ureteral obstruction or stricture
      N11.1
    nonobstructive N11.8
      with reflux (vesicoureteral) N11.0
    obstructive N11.1
    specified NEC N11.8
  in (due to)
    brucellosis A23.9 *[N16]*
    cryoglobulinemia (mixed) D89.1 *[N16]*
    cystinosis E72.04
    diphtheria A36.84
    glycogen storage disease E74.09 *[N16]*
    leukemia NEC C95.9 ☑ *[N16]*
    lymphoma NEC C85.90 *[N16]*
    multiple myeloma C90.0 ☑ *[N16]*
    obstruction N11.1
    Salmonella infection A02.25
    sarcoidosis D86.84
    sepsis A41.9 *[N16]*
    Sjögren's disease M35.04
    toxoplasmosis B58.83
    transplant rejection T86.91 *[N16]*
    Wilson's disease E83.01 *[N16]*
  nonobstructive N12
    with reflux (vesicoureteral) N11.0
    chronic N11.8
  syphilitic A52.75
Pyelonephrosis (obstructive) N11.1
  chronic N11.9
Pyelophlebitis I80.8
Pyeloureteritis cystica N28.85
Pyemia, pyemic (fever) (infection) (purulent) (*see also*
  Sepsis)
  joint — *see* Arthritis, pyogenic or pyemic
  liver K75.1
  pneumococcal A40.3
  portal K75.1
  postvaccinal T88.0 ☑

Pyemia — *continued*
  puerperal, postpartum, childbirth O85
  specified organism NEC A41.89
  tuberculous — *see* Tuberculosis, miliary
Pygopagus Q89.4
Pyknoepilepsy (idiopathic) — *see* Pyknolepsy
Pyknolepsy G40.A09
  intractable G40.A19
    with status epilepticus G40.A11
    without status epilepticus G40.A19
  not intractable G40.A09
    with status epilepticus G40.A01
    without status epilepticus G40.A09
Pylephlebitis K75.1
Pyle's syndrome Q78.5
Pylethrombophlebitis K75.1
Pylethrombosis K75.1
Pyloritis K29.90
  with bleeding K29.91
Pylorospasm (reflex) NEC K31.3
  congenital or infantile Q40.0
  newborn Q40.0
  neurotic F45.8
  psychogenic F45.8
Pylorus, pyloric — *see* condition
Pyoarthrosis — *see* Arthritis, pyogenic or pyemic
Pyocele
  mastoid — *see* Mastoiditis, acute
  sinus (accessory) — *see* Sinusitis
  turbinate (bone) J32.9
  urethra (*see also* Urethritis) N34.0
Pyocolpos — *see* Vaginitis
Pyocystitis N30.80
  with hematuria N30.81
Pyoderma, pyodermia L08.0
  gangrenosum L88
  newborn P39.4
  phagedenic L88
  vegetans L08.81
Pyodermatitis L08.0
  vegetans L08.81
Pyogenic — *see* condition
Pyohydronephrosis N13.6
Pyometra, pyometrium, pyometritis — *see*
  Endometritis
Pyomyositis (tropical) — *see* Myositis, infective
Pyonephritis N12
Pyonephrosis N13.6
  tuberculous A18.11
Pyo-oophoritis — *see* Salpingo-oophoritis
Pyo-ovarium — *see* Salpingo-oophoritis
Pyopericarditis, pyopericardium I30.1
Pyophlebitis — *see* Phlebitis
Pyopneumopericardium I30.1
Pyopneumothorax (infective) J86.9
  with fistula J86.0
  tuberculous NEC A15.6
Pyosalpinx, pyosalpingitis (*see also* Salpingo-
  oophoritis)
Pyothorax J86.9
  with fistula J86.0
  tuberculous NEC A15.6
Pyoureter N28.89
  tuberculous A18.11
Pyramidopallidonigral syndrome G20
Pyrexia (of unknown origin) R50.9
  atmospheric T67.01 ☑
  during labor NEC O75.2
  heat T67.01 ☑
  newborn P81.9
    environmentally-induced P81.0
  persistent R50.9
  puerperal O86.4
Pyroglobulinemia NEC E88.09
Pyromania F63.1
Pyrosis R12
Pyuria (bacterial) (sterile) R82.81

Q

Q fever A78
  with pneumonia A78
Quadricuspid aortic valve Q23.8
Quadrilateral fever A78
Quadriparesis — *see* Quadriplegia
  meaning muscle weakness M62.81
Quadriplegia G82.50
  complete
    C1-C4 level G82.51
    C5-C7 level G82.53

☑ **Additional character required**

Quadriplegia — *continued*
  congenital (cerebral) (spinal) G80.8
    spastic G80.0
  embolic (current episode) I63.4 ☑
  functional R53.2
  incomplete
    C1-C4 level G82.52
    C5-C7 level G82.54
  thrombotic (current episode) I63.3 ☑
  traumatic - code to injury with seventh character S
    current episode — *see* Injury, spinal (cord),
      cervical
Quadruplet, pregnancy — *see* Pregnancy, quadruplet
Quarrelsomeness F60.3
Queensland fever A77.3
Quervain's disease M65.4
  thyroid E06.1
Queyrat's erythroplasia D07.4
  penis D07.4
  specified site — *see* Neoplasm, skin, in situ
  unspecified site D07.4
Quincke's disease or edema T78.3 ☑
  hereditary D84.1
Quinsy (gangrenous) J36
Quintan fever A79.0
Quintuplet, pregnancy — *see* Pregnancy, quintuplet

R

Rabbit fever — *see* Tularemia
Rabies A82.9
  contact Z20.3
  exposure to Z20.3
  inoculation reaction — *see* Complications,
    vaccination
  sylvatic A82.0
  urban A82.1
Rachischisis — *see* Spina bifida
Rachitic (*see also* condition)
  deformities of spine (late effect) (sequelae) E64.3
  pelvis (late effect) (sequelae) E64.3
    with disproportion (fetopelvic) O33.0
      causing obstructed labor O65.0
Rachitis, rachitism (acute) (tarda) (*see also* Rickets)
  renalis N25.0
  sequelae E64.3
Radial nerve — *see* condition
Radiation
  burn — *see* Burn
  effects NOS T66 ☑
  sickness NOS T66 ☑
  therapy, encounter for Z51.0
Radiculitis (pressure) (vertebrogenic) — *see*
  Radiculopathy
Radiculomyelitis (*see also* Encephalitis)
  toxic, due to
    Clostridium tetani A35
    Corynebacterium diphtheriae A36.82
Radiculopathy M54.10
  cervical region M54.12
  cervicothoracic region M54.13
  due to
    disc disorder
      C3 M50.11
      C4 M50.11
      C5 M50.121
      C6 M50.122
      C7 M50.123
      C8 M50.13
    displacement of intervertebral disc — *see*
      Disorder, disc, with, radiculopathy
  leg M54.1 ☑
  lumbar region M54.16
  lumbosacral region M54.17
  occipito-atlanto-axial region M54.11
  postherpetic B02.29
  sacrococcygeal region M54.18
  syphilitic A52.11
  thoracic region (with visceral pain) M54.14
  thoracolumbar region M54.15
Radiodermal burns (acute, chronic, or occupational)
  — *see* Burn
Radiodermatitis L58.9
  acute L58.0
  chronic L58.1
Radiotherapy session Z51.0
RAEB (refractory anemia with excess blasts) D46.2 ☑
Rage, meaning rabies — *see* Rabies
Ragpicker's disease A22.1
Ragsorter's disease A22.1

Raillietiniasis B71.8
Railroad neurosis F48.8
Railway spine F48.8
Raised (*see also* Elevated)
  antibody titer R76.0
Rake teeth, tooth M26.39
Rales R09.89
Ramifying renal pelvis Q63.8
Ramsay-Hunt disease or syndrome (*see also* Hunt's
  disease) B02.21
  meaning dyssynergia cerebellaris myoclonica G11.1
Ranula K11.6
  congenital Q38.4
Rape
  adult
    confirmed T74.21 ☑
    suspected T76.21 ☑
  alleged, observation or examination, ruled out
    adult Z04.41
    child Z04.42
  child
    confirmed T74.22 ☑
    suspected T76.22 ☑
Rapid
  feeble pulse, due to shock, following injury T79.4 ☑
  heart (beat) R00.0
    psychogenic F45.8
  second stage (delivery) O62.3
  time-zone change syndrome G47.25
Rarefaction, bone — *see* Disorder, bone, density and
  structure, specified NEC
Rash (toxic) R21
  canker A38.9
  diaper L22
  drug (internal use) L27.0
    contact (*see also* Dermatitis, due to, drugs,
      external) L25.1
  following immunization T88.1 ☑
  food — *see* Dermatitis, due to, food
  heat L74.0
  napkin (psoriasiform) L22
  nettle — *see* Urticaria
  pustular L08.0
  rose R21
    epidemic B06.9
  scarlet A38.9
  serum (*see also* Reaction, serum) T80.69 ☑
  wandering tongue K14.1
Rasmussen aneurysm — *see* Tuberculosis, pulmonary
Rasmussen encephalitis G04.81
Rat-bite fever A25.9
  due to Streptobacillus moniliformis A25.1
  spirochetal (morsus muris) A25.0
Rathke's pouch tumor D44.3
Raymond (-Céstan) syndrome I65.8
Raynaud's disease, phenomenon or syndrome
  (secondary) I73.00
  with gangrene (symmetric) I73.01
RDS (newborn) (type I) P22.0
  type II P22.1
Reaction (*see also* Disorder)
  adaptation — *see* Disorder, adjustment
  adjustment (anxiety) (conduct disorder)
    (depressiveness) (distress) — *see* Disorder,
      adjustment
    with
      mutism, elective (child) (adolescent) F94.0
  adverse
    food (any) (ingested) NEC T78.1 ☑
      anaphylactic — *see* Shock, anaphylactic, due
        to food
  affective — *see* Disorder, mood
  allergic — *see* Allergy
  anaphylactic — *see* Shock, anaphylactic
  anaphylactoid — *see* Shock, anaphylactic
  anesthesia — *see* Anesthesia, complication
  antitoxin (prophylactic) (therapeutic) — *see*
    Complications, vaccination
  anxiety F41.1
  Arthus — *see* Arthus' phenomenon
  asthenic F48.8
  combat and operational stress F43.0
  compulsive F42.8
  conversion F44.9
  crisis, acute F43.0
  deoxyribonuclease (DNA) (DNase) hypersensitivity
    D69.2
  depressive (single episode) F32.9
    affective (single episode) F31.4
      recurrent episode F33.9
    neurotic F34.1
    psychoneurotic F34.1

Reaction — *continued*
  depressive — *continued*
    psychotic F32.3
    recurrent — *see* Disorder, depressive, recurrent
  dissociative F44.9
  drug NEC T88.7 ☑
    addictive — *see* Dependence, drug
      transmitted via placenta or breast milk — *see*
        Absorption, drug, addictive, through
          placenta
    allergic — *see* Allergy, drug
    lichenoid L43.2
    newborn P93.8
      gray baby syndrome P93.0
    overdose or poisoning (by accident) — *see* Table
      of Drugs and Chemicals, by drug, poisoning
    photoallergic L56.1
    phototoxic L56.0
    withdrawal — *see* Dependence, by drug, with,
      withdrawal
      infant of dependent mother P96.1
      newborn P96.1
    wrong substance given or taken (by accident) —
      see Table of Drugs and Chemicals, by drug,
        poisoning
  fear F40.9
    child (abnormal) F93.8
  febrile nonhemolytic transfusion (FNHTR) R50.84
  fluid loss, cerebrospinal G97.1
  foreign
    body NEC — *see* Granuloma, foreign body
      in operative wound (inadvertently left) — *see*
        Foreign body, accidentally left during a
          procedure
    substance accidentally left during a procedure
      (chemical) (powder) (talc) T81.60 ☑
      aseptic peritonitis T81.61 ☑
      body or object (instrument) (sponge) (swab) —
        see Foreign body, accidentally left during a
          procedure
      specified reaction NEC T81.69 ☑
  grief — *see* Disorder, adjustment
  Herxheimer's R68.89
  hyperkinetic — *see* Hyperkinesia
  hypochondriacal F45.20
  hypoglycemic, due to insulin E16.0
    with coma (diabetic) — *see* Diabetes, coma
      nondiabetic E15
    therapeutic misadventure — *see* subcategory
      T38.3 ☑
  hypomanic F30.8
  hysterical F44.9
  immunization — *see* Complications, vaccination
  incompatibility
    ABO blood group (infusion) (transfusion) — *see*
      Complication(s), transfusion, incompatibility
        reaction, ABO
      delayed serologic T80.39 ☑
    minor blood group (Duffy) (E) (K) (Kell) (Kidd)
      (Lewis) (M) (N) (P)(s) T80.89 ☑
    Rh (factor) (infusion) (transfusion) — *see*
      Complication(s), transfusion, incompatibility
        reaction, Rh (factor)
  inflammatory — *see* Infection
  infusion — *see* Complications, infusion
  inoculation (immune serum) — *see* Complications,
    vaccination
  insulin T38.3 ☑
  involutional psychotic — *see* Disorder, depressive
  leukemoid D72.823
    basophilic D72.823
    lymphocytic D72.823
    monocytic D72.823
    myelocytic D72.823
    neutrophilic D72.823
  LSD (acute)
    due to drug abuse — *see* Abuse, drug,
      hallucinogen
    due to drug dependence — *see* Dependence,
      drug, hallucinogen
  lumbar puncture G97.1
  manic-depressive — *see* Disorder, bipolar
  neurasthenic F48.8
  neurogenic — *see* Neurosis
  neurotic F48.9
  neurotic-depressive F34.1
  nitritoid — *see* Crisis, nitritoid
  nonspecific
    to
      cell mediated immunity measurement of
        gamma interferon antigen response
          without active tuberculosis R76.12

Reaction — *continued*
  nonspecific — *continued*
    QuantiFERON-TB test (QFT) without active
      tuberculosis R76.12
    tuberculin test (*see also* Reaction, tuberculin
      skin test) R76.11
  obsessive-compulsive F42.8
  organic, acute or subacute — *see* Delirium
  paranoid (acute) F23
    chronic F22
    senile F03 ☑
  passive dependency F60.7
  phobic F40.9
  post-traumatic stress, uncomplicated Z73.3
  psychogenic F99
  psychoneurotic (*see also* Neurosis)
    compulsive F42.8
    depersonalization F48.1
    depressive F34.1
    hypochondriacal F45.20
    neurasthenic F48.8
    obsessive F42.8
  psychophysiologic — *see* Disorder, somatoform
  psychosomatic — *see* Disorder, somatoform
  psychotic — *see* Psychosis
  scarlet fever toxin — *see* Complications, vaccination
  schizophrenic F23
    acute (brief) (undifferentiated) F23
    latent F21
    undifferentiated (acute) (brief) F23
  serological for syphilis — *see* Serology for syphilis
  serum T80.69 ☑
    anaphylactic (immediate) (*see also* Shock,
      anaphylactic) T80.59 ☑
    specified reaction NEC
      due to
        administration of blood and blood products
          T80.61 ☑
        immunization T80.62 ☑
        serum specified NEC T80.69 ☑
        vaccination T80.62 ☑
  situational — *see* Disorder, adjustment
  somatization — *see* Disorder, somatoform
  spinal puncture G97.1
  stress (severe) F43.9
    acute (agitation) ("daze") (disorientation)
      (disturbance of consciousness) (flight
      reaction) (fugue) F43.0
    specified NEC F43.8
  surgical procedure — *see* Complications, surgical
    procedure
  tetanus antitoxin — *see* Complications, vaccination
  toxic, to local anesthesia T88.59 ☑
    in labor and delivery O74.4
    in pregnancy O29.3X ☑
    postpartum, puerperal O89.3
  toxin-antitoxin — *see* Complications, vaccination
  transfusion (blood) (bone marrow) (lymphocytes)
    (allergic) — *see* Complications, transfusion
  tuberculin skin test, abnormal R76.11
  vaccination (any) — *see* Complications, vaccination
  withdrawing, child or adolescent F93.8
Reactive airway disease — *see* Asthma
Reactive depression — *see* Reaction, depressive
Rearrangement
  chromosomal
    balanced (in) Q95.9
      abnormal individual (autosomal) Q95.2
      non-sex (autosomal) chromosomes Q95.2
      sex/non-sex chromosomes Q95.3
      specified NEC Q95.8
Recalcitrant patient — *see* Noncompliance
Recanalization, thrombus — *see* Thrombosis
Recession, receding
  chamber angle (eye) H21.55 ☑
  chin M26.09
  gingival (postinfective) (postoperative)
    generalized K06.020
      minimal K06.021
      moderate K06.022
      severe K06.023
    localized K06.010
      minimal K06.011
      moderate K06.012
      severe K06.013
Recklinghausen disease Q85.01
  bones E21.0
Reclus' disease (cystic) — *see* Mastopathy, cystic
Recrudescent typhus (fever) A75.1
Recruitment, auditory H93.21 ☑
Rectalgia K62.89
Rectitis K62.89

Rectocele
  female (without uterine prolapse) N81.6
    with uterine prolapse N81.4
      incomplete N81.2
  in pregnancy — *see* Pregnancy, complicated by,
    abnormal, pelvic organs or tissues NEC
  male K62.3
Rectosigmoid junction — *see* condition
Rectosigmoiditis K63.89
  ulcerative (chronic) K51.30
    with
      complication K51.319
        abscess K51.314
        fistula K51.313
        obstruction K51.312
        rectal bleeding K51.311
        specified NEC K51.318
Rectourethral — *see* condition
Rectovaginal — *see* condition
Rectovesical — *see* condition
Rectum, rectal — *see* condition
Recurrent — *see* condition
  pregnancy loss — *see* Loss (of), pregnancy,
    recurrent
Red bugs B88.0
Red-cedar lung or pneumonitis J67.8
Red tide (*see also* Table of Drugs and Chemicals)
  T65.82 ☑
Reduced
  mobility Z74.09
  ventilatory or vital capacity R94.2
Redundant, redundancy
  anus (congenital) Q43.8
  clitoris N90.89
  colon (congenital) Q43.8
  foreskin (congenital) N47.8
  intestine (congenital) Q43.8
  labia N90.69
  organ or site, congenital NEC — *see* Accessory
  panniculus (abdominal) E65
  prepuce (congenital) N47.8
  pylorus K31.89
  rectum (congenital) Q43.8
  scrotum N50.89
  sigmoid (congenital) Q43.8
  skin L98.7
    and subcutaneous tissue L98.7
    of face L57.4
      eyelids — *see* Blepharochalasis
  stomach K31.89
Reduplication — *see* Duplication
Reflex R29.2
  hyperactive gag J39.2
  pupillary, abnormal — *see* Anomaly, pupil, function
  vasoconstriction I73.9
  vasovagal R55
Reflux K21.9
  acid K21.9
  esophageal K21.9
    with esophagitis K21.0
    newborn P78.83
  gastroesophageal K21.9
    with esophagitis K21.0
  mitral — *see* Insufficiency, mitral
  ureteral — *see* Reflux, vesicoureteral
  vesicoureteral (with scarring) N13.70
    with
      nephropathy N13.729
        with hydroureter N13.739
          bilateral N13.732
          unilateral N13.731
        bilateral N13.722
        unilateral N13.721
      without hydroureter N13.729
        bilateral N13.722
        unilateral N13.721
      pyelonephritis (chronic) N11.0
    congenital Q62.7
    without nephropathy N13.71
Reforming, artificial openings — *see* Attention to,
  artificial, opening
Refractive error — *see* Disorder, refraction
Refsum's disease or syndrome G60.1
Refusal of
  food, psychogenic F50.89
  treatment (because of) Z53.20
    left against medical advice (AMA) Z53.21
    patient's decision NEC Z53.29
    reasons of belief or group pressure Z53.1
Regional — *see* condition
Regurgitation R11.10
  aortic (valve) — *see* Insufficiency, aortic

Regurgitation — *continued*
  food (*see also* Vomiting)
    with reswallowing — *see* Rumination
    newborn P92.1
  gastric contents — *see* Vomiting
  heart — *see* Endocarditis
  mitral (valve) — *see* Insufficiency, mitral
    congenital Q23.3
  myocardial — *see* Endocarditis
  pulmonary (valve) (heart) I37.1
    congenital Q22.2
    syphilitic A52.03
  tricuspid — *see* Insufficiency, tricuspid
  valve, valvular — *see* Endocarditis
    congenital Q24.8
  vesicoureteral — *see* Reflux, vesicoureteral
Reifenstein syndrome E34.52
Reinsertion
  implantable subdermal contraceptive Z30.46
  intrauterine contraceptive device Z30.433
Reiter's disease, syndrome, or urethritis M02.30
  ankle M02.37 ☑
  elbow M02.32 ☑
  foot joint M02.37 ☑
  hand joint M02.34 ☑
  hip M02.35 ☑
  knee M02.36 ☑
  multiple site M02.39
  shoulder M02.31 ☑
  vertebra M02.38
  wrist M02.33 ☑
Reichmann's disease or syndrome K31.89
Rejection
  food, psychogenic F50.89
  transplant T86.91
    bone T86.830
      marrow T86.01
    cornea T86.840
    heart T86.21
      with lung(s) T86.31
    intestine T86.850
    kidney T86.11
    liver T86.41
    lung(s) T86.810
      with heart T86.31
    organ (immune or nonimmune cause) T86.91
    pancreas T86.890
    skin (allograft) (autograft) T86.820
    specified NEC T86.890
    stem cell (peripheral blood) (umbilical cord) T86.5
Relapsing fever A68.9
  Carter's (Asiatic) A68.1
  Dutton's (West African) A68.1
  Koch's A68.9
  louse-borne (epidemic) A68.0
  Novy's (American) A68.1
  Obermeyers's (European) A68.0
  Spirillum A68.9
  tick-borne (endemic) A68.1
Relationship
  occlusal
    open anterior M26.220
    open posterior M26.221
Relaxation
  anus (sphincter) K62.89
    psychogenic F45.8
  arch (foot) (*see also* Deformity, limb, flat foot)
  back ligaments — *see* Instability, joint, spine
  bladder (sphincter) N31.2
  cardioesophageal K21.9
  cervix — *see* Incompetency, cervix
  diaphragm J98.6
  joint (capsule) (ligament) (paralytic) — *see* Flail, joint
    congenital NEC Q74.8
  lumbosacral (joint) — *see* subcategory M53.2 ☑
  pelvic floor N81.89
  perineum N81.89
  posture R29.3
  rectum (sphincter) K62.89
  sacroiliac (joint) — *see* subcategory M53.2 ☑
  scrotum N50.89
  urethra (sphincter) N36.44
  vesical N31.2
Release from prison, anxiety concerning Z65.2
Remains
  canal of Cloquet Q14.0
  capsule (opaque) Q14.8
Remittent fever (malarial) B54
Remnant
  canal of Cloquet Q14.0
  capsule (opaque) Q14.8
  cervix, cervical stump (acquired) (postoperative) N88.8

☑ **Additional character required**

Remnant — *continued*
cystic duct, postcholecystectomy K91.5
fingernail L60.8
congenital Q84.6
meniscus, knee — *see* Derangement, knee, meniscus, specified NEC
thyroglossal duct Q89.2
tonsil J35.8
infected (chronic) J35.01
urachus Q64.4
Removal (from) (of)
artificial
arm Z44.00 ☑
complete Z44.01 ☑
partial Z44.02 ☑
eye Z44.2 ☑
leg Z44.10 ☑
complete Z44.11 ☑
partial Z44.12 ☑
breast implant Z45.81 ☑
cardiac pulse generator (battery) (end-of-life) Z45.010
catheter (urinary) (indwelling) Z46.6
from artificial opening — *see* Attention to, artificial, opening
non-vascular Z46.82
vascular NEC Z45.2
drains Z48.03
device Z46.9
contraceptive Z30.432
implantable subdermal Z30.46
implanted NEC Z45.89
specified NEC Z46.89
dressing (nonsurgical) Z48.00
surgical Z48.01
external
fixation device - code to fracture with seventh character D
prosthesis, prosthetic device Z44.9
breast Z44.3 ☑
specified NEC Z44.8
home in childhood (to foster home or institution) Z62.29
ileostomy Z43.2
insulin pump Z46.81
myringotomy device (stent) (tube) Z45.82
nervous system device NEC Z46.2
brain neuropacemaker Z46.2
visual substitution device Z46.2
implanted Z45.31
non-vascular catheter Z46.82
orthodontic device Z46.4
organ, prophylactic (for neoplasia management) — *see* Prophylactic, organ removal
staples Z48.02
stent
ureteral Z46.6
suture Z48.02
urinary device Z46.6
vascular access device or catheter Z45.2
Ren
arcuatus Q63.1
mobile, mobilis N28.89
congenital Q63.8
unguliformis Q63.1
Renal — *see* condition
Rendu-Osler-Weber disease or syndrome I78.0
Reninoma D41.0 ☑
Renon-Delille syndrome E23.3
Reovirus, as cause of disease classified elsewhere B97.5
Repeated falls NEC R29.6
Replaced chromosome by dicentric ring Q93.2
Replacement by artificial or mechanical device or prosthesis of
bladder Z96.0
blood vessel NEC Z95.828
bone NEC Z96.7
cochlea Z96.21
coronary artery Z95.5
eustachian tube Z96.29
eye globe Z97.0
heart Z95.812
valve Z95.2
prosthetic Z95.2
specified NEC Z95.4
xenogenic Z95.3
intestine Z96.89
joint Z96.60
hip — *see* Presence, hip joint implant
knee — *see* Presence, knee joint implant
specified site NEC Z96.698
larynx Z96.3

Replacement — *continued*
lens Z96.1
limb(s) — *see* Presence, artificial, limb
mandible NEC (for tooth root implant(s)) Z96.5
organ NEC Z96.89
peripheral vessel NEC Z95.828
stapes Z96.29
teeth Z97.2
tendon Z96.7
tissue NEC Z96.89
tooth root(s) Z96.5
vessel NEC Z95.828
coronary (artery) Z95.5
Request for expert evidence Z04.89
Reserve, decreased or low
cardiac — *see* Disease, heart
kidney N28.89
Residual (*see also* condition)
ovary syndrome N99.83
state, schizophrenic F20.5
urine R39.198
Resistance, resistant (to)
activated protein C D68.51
complicating pregnancy O26.89 ☑
insulin E88.81
organism(s)
to
drug Z16.30
aminoglycosides Z16.29
amoxicillin Z16.11
ampicillin Z16.11
antibiotic(s) Z16.20
multiple Z16.24
specified NEC Z16.29
antifungal Z16.32
antimicrobial (single) Z16.30
multiple Z16.35
specified NEC Z16.39
antimycobacterial (single) Z16.341
multiple Z16.342
antiparasitic Z16.31
antiviral Z16.33
beta lactam antibiotics Z16.10
specified NEC Z16.19
cephalosporins Z16.19
extended beta lactamase (ESBL) Z16.12
fluoroquinolones Z16.23
macrolides Z16.29
methicillin — *see* MRSA
multiple drugs (MDRO)
antibiotics Z16.24
antimicrobial Z16.35
antimycobacterials Z16.342
penicillins Z16.11
quinine (and related compounds) Z16.31
quinolones Z16.23
sulfonamides Z16.29
tetracyclines Z16.29
tuberculostatics (single) Z16.341
multiple Z16.342
vancomycin Z16.21
related antibiotics Z16.22
thyroid hormone E07.89
Resorption
dental (roots) K03.3
alveoli M26.79
teeth (external) (internal) (pathological) (roots) K03.3
Respiration
Cheyne-Stokes R06.3
decreased due to shock, following injury T79.4 ☑
disorder of, psychogenic F45.8
insufficient, or poor R06.89
newborn P28.5
painful R07.1
sighing, psychogenic F45.8
Respiratory (*see also* condition)
distress syndrome (newborn) (type I) P22.0
type II P22.1
syncytial virus, as cause of disease classified elsewhere (*see also* Virus, respiratory syncytial (RSV)) B97.4
Respite care Z75.5
Response (drug)
photoallergic L56.1
phototoxic L56.0
Restenosis
stent
vascular
end stent
adjacent to stent — *see* Arteriosclerosis
within the stent

Restenosis — *continued*
stent — *continued*
coronary T82.855 ☑
peripheral T82.856 ☑
in stent
coronary vessel T82.855 ☑
peripheral vessel T82.856 ☑
Restless legs (syndrome) G25.81
Restlessness R45.1
Restriction of housing space Z59.1
Restoration (of)
dental
aesthetically inadequate or displeasing K08.56
defective K08.50
specified NEC K08.59
failure of marginal integrity K08.51
failure of periodontal anatomical integrity K08.54
organ continuity from previous sterilization (tuboplasty) (vasoplasty) Z31.0
aftercare Z31.42
tooth (existing)
contours biologically incompatible with oral health K08.54
open margins K08.51
overhanging K08.52
poor aesthetic K08.56
poor gingival margins K08.51
unsatisfactory, of tooth K08.50
specified NEC K08.59
Restorative material (dental)
allergy to K08.55
fractured K08.539
with loss of material K08.531
without loss of material K08.530
unrepairable overhanging of K08.52
Rests, ovarian, in fallopian tube Q50.6
Restzustand (schizophrenic) F20.5
Retained (*see also* Retention)
cholelithiasis following cholecystectomy K91.86
foreign body fragments (type of) Z18.9
acrylics Z18.2
animal quill(s) or spines Z18.31
cement Z18.83
concrete Z18.83
crystalline Z18.83
depleted isotope Z18.09
depleted uranium Z18.01
diethylhexyl phthalates Z18.2
glass Z18.81
isocyanate Z18.2
magnetic metal Z18.11
metal Z18.10
nonmagnetic metal Z18.12
nontherapeutic radioactive Z18.09
organic NEC Z18.39
plastic Z18.2
quill(s) (animal) Z18.31
radioactive (nontherapeutic) NEC Z18.09
specified NEC Z18.89
spine(s) (animal) Z18.31
stone Z18.83
tooth (teeth) Z18.32
wood Z18.33
fragments (type of) Z18.9
acrylics Z18.2
animal quill(s) or spines Z18.31
cement Z18.83
concrete Z18.83
crystalline Z18.83
depleted isotope Z18.09
depleted uranium Z18.01
diethylhexyl phthalates Z18.2
glass Z18.81
isocyanate Z18.2
magnetic metal Z18.11
metal Z18.10
nonmagnetic metal Z18.12
nontherapeutic radioactive Z18.09
organic NEC Z18.39
plastic Z18.2
quill(s) (animal) Z18.31
radioactive (nontherapeutic) NEC Z18.09
specified NEC Z18.89
spine(s) (animal) Z18.31
stone Z18.83
tooth (teeth) Z18.32
wood Z18.33
gallstones, following cholecystectomy K91.86
Retardation
development, developmental, specific — *see* Disorder, developmental

Remnant - Retardation

ICD-10-CM INDEX TO DISEASES AND INJURIES

Retardation — *continued*
endochondral bone growth — *see* Disorder, bone, development or growth
growth R62.50
due to malnutrition E45
mental — *see* Disability, intellectual
motor function, specific F82
physical (child) R62.52
due to malnutrition E45
reading (specific) F81.0
spelling (specific) (without reading disorder) F81.81
Retching — *see* Vomiting
Retention (*see also* Retained)
bladder — *see* Retention, urine
carbon dioxide E87.2
cholelithiasis following cholecystectomy K91.86
cyst — *see* Cyst
dead
fetus (at or near term) (mother) O36.4 ☑
early fetal death O02.1
ovum O02.0
decidua (fragments) (following delivery) (with hemorrhage) O72.2
without hemorrhage O73.1
deciduous tooth K00.6
dental root K08.3
fecal — *see* Constipation
fetus
dead O36.4 ☑
early O02.1
fluid R60.9
foreign body (*see also* Foreign body, retained)
current trauma - code as Foreign body, by site or type
gallstones, following cholecystectomy K91.86
gastric K31.89
intrauterine contraceptive device, in pregnancy — *see* Pregnancy, complicated by, retention, intrauterine device
membranes (complicating delivery) (with hemorrhage) O72.2
with abortion — *see* Abortion, by type
without hemorrhage O73.1
meniscus — *see* Derangement, meniscus
menses N94.89
milk (puerperal, postpartum) O92.79
nitrogen, extrarenal R39.2
ovary syndrome N99.83
placenta (total) (with hemorrhage) O72.0
without hemorrhage O73.0
portions or fragments (with hemorrhage) O72.2
without hemorrhage O73.1
products of conception
early pregnancy (dead fetus) O02.1
following
delivery (with hemorrhage) O72.2
without hemorrhage O73.1
secundines (following delivery) (with hemorrhage) O72.0
without hemorrhage O73.0
complicating puerperium (delayed hemorrhage) O72.2
partial O72.2
without hemorrhage O73.1
smegma, clitoris N90.89
urine R33.9
due to hyperplasia (hypertrophy) of prostate — *see* Hyperplasia, prostate
drug-induced R33.0
organic R33.8
drug-induced R33.0
psychogenic F45.8
specified NEC R33.8
water (in tissues) — *see* Edema
Reticular erythematous mucinosis L98.5
Reticulation, dust — *see* Pneumoconiosis
Reticulocytosis R70.1
Reticuloendotheliosis
acute infantile C96.0
leukemic C91.4 ☑
nonlipid C96.0
Reticulohistiocytoma (giant-cell) D76.3
Reticuloid, actinic L57.1
Reticulosis (skin)
acute of infancy C96.0
hemophagocytic, familial D76.1
histiocytic medullary C96.A
lipomelanotic I89.8
malignant (midline) C86.0
polymorphic C86.0
Sézary — *see* Sézary disease

Retina, retinal (*see also* condition)
dark area D49.81
Retinitis (*see also* Inflammation, chorioretinal)
albuminurica N18.9 *[H32]*
diabetic — *see* Diabetes, retinitis
disciformis — *see* Degeneration, macula
focal — *see* Inflammation, chorioretinal, focal
gravidarum — *see* Pregnancy, complicated by, specified pregnancy-related condition NEC
juxtapapillaris — *see* Inflammation, chorioretinal, focal, juxtapapillary
luetic — *see* Retinitis, syphilitic
pigmentosa H35.52
proliferans — *see* Disorder, globe, degenerative, specified type NEC
proliferating — *see* Disorder, globe, degenerative, specified type NEC
renal N18.9 *[H32]*
syphilitic (early) (secondary) A51.43
central, recurrent A52.71
congenital (early) A50.01 *[H32]*
late A52.71
tuberculous A18.53
Retinoblastoma C69.2 ☑
differentiated C69.2 ☑
undifferentiated C69.2 ☑
Retinochoroiditis (*see also* Inflammation, chorioretinal)
disseminated — *see* Inflammation, chorioretinal, disseminated
syphilitic A52.71
focal — *see* Inflammation, chorioretinal
juxtapapillaris — *see* Inflammation, chorioretinal, focal, juxtapapillary
Retinopathy (background) H35.00
arteriosclerotic I70.8 *[H35.0 ☑]*
atherosclerotic I70.8 *[H35.0 ☑]*
central serous — *see* Chorioretinopathy, central serous
Coats H35.02 ☑
diabetic — *see* Diabetes, retinopathy
exudative H35.02 ☑
hypertensive H35.03 ☑
in (due to)
diabetes — *see* Diabetes, retinopathy
sickle-cell disorders D57. ☑ *[H36]*
of prematurity H35.10 ☑
stage 0 H35.11 ☑
stage 1 H35.12 ☑
stage 2 H35.13 ☑
stage 3 H35.14 ☑
stage 4 H35.15 ☑
stage 5 H35.16 ☑
pigmentary, congenital — *see* Dystrophy, retina
proliferative NEC H35.2 ☑
diabetic — *see* Diabetes, retinopathy, proliferative
sickle-cell D57. ☑ *[H36]*
solar H31.02 ☑
Retinoschisis H33.10 ☑
congenital Q14.1
specified type NEC H33.19 ☑
Retortamoniasis A07.8
Retractile testis Q55.22
Retraction
cervix — *see* Retroversion, uterus
drum (membrane) — *see* Disorder, tympanic membrane, specified NEC
finger — *see* Deformity, finger
lid H02.539
left H02.536
lower H02.535
upper H02.534
right H02.533
lower H02.532
upper H02.531
lung J98.4
mediastinum J98.59
nipple N64.53
associated with
lactation O92.03
pregnancy O92.01 ☑
puerperium O92.02
congenital Q83.8
palmar fascia M72.0
pleura — *see* Pleurisy
ring, uterus (Bandl's) (pathological) O62.4
sternum (congenital) Q76.7
acquired M95.4
uterus — *see* Retroversion, uterus
valve (heart) — *see* Endocarditis
Retrobulbar — *see* condition
Retrocecal — *see* condition
Retrocession — *see* Retroversion

Retrodisplacement — *see* Retroversion
Retroflection, retroflexion — *see* Retroversion
Retrognathia, retrognathism (mandibular) (maxillary) M26.19
Retrograde menstruation N92.5
Retroperineal — *see* condition
Retroperitoneal — *see* condition
Retroperitonitis K68.9
Retropharyngeal — *see* condition
Retroplacental — *see* condition
Retroposition — *see* Retroversion
Retroprosthetic membrane T85.398 ☑
Retrosternal thyroid (congenital) Q89.2
Retroversion, retroverted
cervix — *see* Retroversion, uterus
female NEC — *see* Retroversion, uterus
iris H21.89
testis (congenital) Q55.29
uterus (acquired) (acute) (any degree) (asymptomatic) (cervix) (postinfectional) (postpartal, old) N85.4
congenital Q51.818
in pregnancy O34.53 ☑
Retrovirus, as cause of disease classified elsewhere B97.30
human
immunodeficiency, type 2 (HIV 2) B97.35
T-cell lymphotropic
type I (HTLV-I) B97.33
type II (HTLV-II) B97.34
lentivirus B97.31
oncovirus B97.32
specified NEC B97.39
Retrusion, premaxilla (developmental) M26.09
Rett's disease or syndrome F84.2
Reverse peristalsis R19.2
Reye's syndrome G93.7
Rh (factor)
hemolytic disease (newborn) P55.0
incompatibility, immunization or sensitization
affecting management of pregnancy NEC O36.09 ☑
anti-D antibody O36.01 ☑
newborn P55.0
transfusion reaction — *see* Complication(s), transfusion, incompatibility reaction, Rh (factor)
negative mother affecting newborn P55.0
titer elevated — *see* Complication(s), transfusion, incompatibility reaction, Rh (factor)
transfusion reaction — *see* Complication(s), transfusion, incompatibility reaction, Rh (factor)
Rhabdomyolysis (idiopathic) NEC M62.82
traumatic T79.6 ☑
Rhabdomyoma (*see also* Neoplasm, connective tissue, benign)
adult — *see* Neoplasm, connective tissue, benign
fetal — *see* Neoplasm, connective tissue, benign
glycogenic — *see* Neoplasm, connective tissue, benign
Rhabdomyosarcoma (any type) — *see* Neoplasm, connective tissue, malignant
Rhabdosarcoma — *see* Rhabdomyosarcoma
Rhesus (factor) incompatibility — *see* Rh, incompatibility
Rheumatic (acute) (subacute)
adherent pericardium I09.2
chronic I09.89
coronary arteritis I01.8
degeneration, myocardium I09.0
fever (acute) — *see* Fever, rheumatic
heart — *see* Disease, heart, rheumatic
myocardial degeneration — *see* Degeneration, myocardium
myocarditis (chronic) (inactive) (with chorea) I09.0
active or acute I01.2
with chorea (acute) (rheumatic) (Sydenham's) I02.0
pancarditis, acute I01.8
with chorea (acute (rheumatic) Sydenham's) I02.0
pericarditis (active) (acute) (with effusion) (with pneumonia) I01.0
with chorea (acute) (rheumatic) (Sydenham's) I02.0
chronic or inactive I09.2
pneumonia I00 *[J17]*
torticollis M43.6
typhoid fever A01.09
Rheumatism (articular) (neuralgic) (nonarticular) M79.0
gout — *see* Arthritis, rheumatoid

Rheumatism — *continued*
  intercostal, meaning Tietze's disease M94.0
  palindromic (any site) M12.30
    ankle M12.37 ☑
    elbow M12.32 ☑
    foot joint M12.37 ☑
    hand joint M12.34 ☑
    hip M12.35 ☑
    knee M12.36 ☑
    multiple site M12.39
    shoulder M12.31 ☑
    specified joint NEC M12.38
    vertebrae M12.38
    wrist M12.33 ☑
  sciatic M54.4 ☑
Rheumatoid (*see also* condition)
  arthritis (*see also* Arthritis, rheumatoid)
    with involvement of organs NEC M05.60
      ankle M05.67 ☑
      elbow M05.62 ☑
      foot joint M05.67 ☑
      hand joint M05.64 ☑
      hip M05.65 ☑
      knee M05.66 ☑
      multiple site M05.69
      shoulder M05.61 ☑
      vertebra — *see* Spondylitis, ankylosing
      wrist M05.63 ☑
    seronegative — *see* Arthritis, rheumatoid, seronegative
    seropositive — *see* Arthritis, rheumatoid, seropositive
  carditis M05.30
    ankle M05.37 ☑
    elbow M05.32 ☑
    foot joint M05.37 ☑
    hand joint M05.34 ☑
    hip M05.35 ☑
    knee M05.36 ☑
    multiple site M05.39
    shoulder M05.31 ☑
    vertebra — *see* Spondylitis, ankylosing
    wrist M05.33 ☑
  endocarditis — *see* Rheumatoid, carditis
  lung (disease) M05.10
    ankle M05.17 ☑
    elbow M05.12 ☑
    foot joint M05.17 ☑
    hand joint M05.14 ☑
    hip M05.15 ☑
    knee M05.16 ☑
    multiple site M05.19
    shoulder M05.11 ☑
    vertebra — *see* Spondylitis, ankylosing
    wrist M05.13 ☑
  myocarditis — *see* Rheumatoid, carditis
  myopathy M05.40
    ankle M05.47 ☑
    elbow M05.42 ☑
    foot joint M05.47 ☑
    hand joint M05.44 ☑
    hip M05.45 ☑
    knee M05.46 ☑
    multiple site M05.49
    shoulder M05.41 ☑
    vertebra — *see* Spondylitis, ankylosing
    wrist M05.43 ☑
  pericarditis — *see* Rheumatoid, carditis
  polyarthritis — *see* Arthritis, rheumatoid
  polyneuropathy M05.50
    ankle M05.57 ☑
    elbow M05.52 ☑
    foot joint M05.57 ☑
    hand joint M05.54 ☑
    hip M05.55 ☑
    knee M05.56 ☑
    multiple site M05.59
    shoulder M05.51 ☑
    vertebra — *see* Spondylitis, ankylosing
    wrist M05.53 ☑
  vasculitis M05.20
    ankle M05.27 ☑
    elbow M05.22 ☑
    foot joint M05.27 ☑
    hand joint M05.24 ☑
    hip M05.25 ☑
    knee M05.26 ☑
    multiple site M05.29
    shoulder M05.21 ☑
    vertebra — *see* Spondylitis, ankylosing
    wrist M05.23 ☑

Rhinitis (atrophic) (catarrhal) (chronic) (croupous) (fibrinous) (granulomatous) (hyperplastic) (hypertrophic) (membranous) (obstructive) (purulent) (suppurative) (ulcerative) J31.0
  with
    sore throat — *see* Nasopharyngitis
  acute J00
  allergic J30.9
    with asthma J45.909
      with
        exacerbation (acute) J45.901
        status asthmaticus J45.902
    due to
      food J30.5
      pollen J30.1
    nonseasonal J30.89
    perennial J30.89
    seasonal NEC J30.2
    specified NEC J30.89
  infective J00
  pneumococcal J00
  syphilitic A52.73
    congenital A50.05 *[J99]*
  tuberculous A15.8
  vasomotor J30.0
Rhinoantritis (chronic) — *see* Sinusitis, maxillary
Rhinodacryolith — *see* Dacryolith
Rhinolith (nasal sinus) J34.89
Rhinomegaly J34.89
Rhinopharyngitis (acute) (subacute) (*see also* Nasopharyngitis)
  chronic J31.1
  destructive ulcerating A66.5
  mutilans A66.5
Rhinophyma L71.1
Rhinorrhea J34.89
  cerebrospinal (fluid) G96.0
  paroxysmal — *see* Rhinitis, allergic
  spasmodic — *see* Rhinitis, allergic
Rhinosalpingitis — *see* Salpingitis, eustachian
Rhinoscleroma A48.8
Rhinosporidiosis B48.1
Rhinovirus infection NEC B34.8
Rhizomelic chondrodysplasia punctata E71.540
Rhythm
  atrioventricular nodal I49.8
  disorder I49.9
    coronary sinus I49.8
    ectopic I49.8
    nodal I49.8
  escape I49.9
  heart, abnormal I49.9
  idioventricular I44.2
  nodal I49.8
  sleep, inversion G47.2 ☑
    nonorganic origin — *see* Disorder, sleep, circadian rhythm, psychogenic
Rhytidosis facialis L98.8
Rib (*see also* condition)
  cervical Q76.5
Riboflavin deficiency E53.0
Rice bodies (*see also* Loose, body, joint)
  knee M23.4 ☑
Richter syndrome — *see* Leukemia, chronic lymphocytic, B-cell type
Richter's hernia — *see* Hernia, abdomen, with obstruction
Ricinism — *see* Poisoning, food, noxious, plant
Rickets (active) (acute) (adolescent) (chest wall) (congenital) (current) (infantile) (intestinal) E55.0
  adult — *see* Osteomalacia
  celiac K90.0
  hypophosphatemic with nephrotic-glycosuric dwarfism E72.09
  inactive E64.3
  kidney N25.0
  renal N25.0
  sequelae, any E64.3
  vitamin-D-resistant E83.31 *[M90.80]*
Rickettsial disease A79.9
  specified type NEC A79.89
Rickettsialpox (Rickettsia akari) A79.1
Rickettsiosis A79.9
  due to
    Ehrlichia sennetsu A79.81
    Rickettsia akari (rickettsialpox) A79.1
  specified type NEC A79.89
  tick-borne A77.9
  vesicular A79.1
Rider's bone — *see* Ossification, muscle, specified NEC
Ridge, alveolus (*see also* condition)
  flabby K06.8

Ridged ear, congenital Q17.3
Riedel's
  lobe, liver Q44.7
  struma, thyroiditis or disease E06.5
Rieger's anomaly or syndrome Q13.81
Riehl's melanosis L81.4
Rietti-Greppi-Micheli anemia D56.9
Rieux's hernia — *see* Hernia, abdomen, specified site NEC
Riga (-Fede) disease K14.0
Riggs' disease — *see* Periodontitis
Right aortic arch Q25.47
Right middle lobe syndrome J98.11
Rigid, rigidity (*see also* condition)
  abdominal R19.30
    with severe abdominal pain R10.0
    epigastric R19.36
    generalized R19.37
    left lower quadrant R19.34
    left upper quadrant R19.32
    periumbilic R19.35
    right lower quadrant R19.33
    right upper quadrant R19.31
  articular, multiple, congenital Q68.8
  cervix (uteri) in pregnancy — *see* Pregnancy, complicated by, abnormal, cervix
  hymen (acquired) (congenital) N89.6
  nuchal R29.1
  pelvic floor in pregnancy — *see* Pregnancy, complicated by, abnormal, pelvic organs or tissues NEC
  perineum or vulva in pregnancy — *see* Pregnancy, complicated by, abnormal, vulva
  spine — *see* Dorsopathy, specified NEC
  vagina in pregnancy — *see* Pregnancy, complicated by, abnormal, vagina
Rigors R68.89
  with fever R50.9
Riley-Day syndrome G90.1
RIND (reversible ischemic neurologic deficit) I63.9
Ring(s)
  aorta (vascular) Q25.45
  Bandl's O62.4
  contraction, complicating delivery O62.4
  esophageal, lower (muscular) K22.2
  Fleischer's (cornea) H18.04 ☑
  hymenal, tight (acquired) (congenital) N89.6
  Kayser-Fleischer (cornea) H18.04 ☑
  retraction, uterus, pathological O62.4
  Schatzki's (esophagus) (lower) K22.2
    congenital Q39.3
  Soemmerring's — *see* Cataract, secondary
  vascular (congenital) Q25.8
    aorta Q25.45
Ringed hair (congenital) Q84.1
Ringworm B35.9
  beard B35.0
  black dot B35.0
  body B35.4
  Burmese B35.5
  corporeal B35.4
  foot B35.3
  groin B35.6
  hand B35.2
  honeycomb B35.0
  nails B35.1
  perianal (area) B35.6
  scalp B35.0
  specified NEC B35.8
  Tokelau B35.5
Rise, venous pressure I87.8
Rising, PSA following treatment for malignant neoplasm of prostate R97.21
Risk
  for
    dental caries Z91.849
      high Z91.843
      low Z91.841
      moderate Z91.842
  suicidal
    meaning personal history of attempted suicide Z91.5
    meaning suicidal ideation — *see* Ideation, suicidal
Ritter's disease L00
Rivalry, sibling Z62.891
Rivalta's disease A42.2
River blindness B73.01
Robert's pelvis Q74.2
  with disproportion (fetopelvic) O33.0
    causing obstructed labor O65.0
Robin (-Pierre) syndrome Q87.0
Robinow-Silvermann-Smith syndrome Q87.19

Robinson's (hidrotic) ectodermal dysplasia or syndrome Q82.4
Robles' disease B73.01
Rocky Mountain (spotted) fever A77.0
Roetheln — *see* Rubella
Roger's disease Q21.0
Rokitansky-Aschoff sinuses (gallbladder) K82.8
Rolando's fracture (displaced) S62.22 ☑
   nondisplaced S62.22 ☑
Romano-Ward (prolonged QT interval) syndrome I45.81
Romberg's disease or syndrome G51.8
Roof, mouth — *see* condition
Rosacea L71.9
   acne L71.9
   keratitis L71.8
   specified NEC L71.8
Rosary, rachitic E55.0
Rose
   cold J30.1
   fever J30.1
   rash R21
      epidemic B06.9
Rosenbach's erysipeloid A26.0
Rosenthal's disease or syndrome D68.1
Roseola B09
   infantum B08.20
      due to human herpesvirus 6 B08.21
      due to human herpesvirus 7 B08.22
Rossbach's disease K31.89
   psychogenic F45.8
Ross River disease or fever B33.1
Rostan's asthma (cardiac) — *see* Failure, ventricular, left
Rotation
   anomalous, incomplete or insufficient, intestine Q43.3
   cecum (congenital) Q43.3
   colon (congenital) Q43.3
   spine, incomplete or insufficient — *see* Dorsopathy, deforming, specified NEC
   tooth, teeth, fully erupted M26.35
   vertebra, incomplete or insufficient — *see* Dorsopathy, deforming, specified NEC
Rotes Quérol disease or syndrome — *see* Hyperostosis, ankylosing
Roth (-Bernhardt) disease or syndrome — *see* Meralgia paraesthetica
Rothmund (-Thomson) syndrome Q82.8
Rotor's disease or syndrome E80.6
Round
   back (with wedging of vertebrae) — *see* Kyphosis
      sequelae (late effect) of rickets E64.3
   worms (large) (infestation) NEC B82.0
      Ascariasis (*see also* Ascariasis) B77.9
Roussy-Lévy syndrome G60.0
Rubella (German measles) B06.9
   complication NEC B06.09
      neurological B06.00
   congenital P35.0
   contact Z20.4
   exposure to Z20.4
   maternal
      manifest rubella in infant P35.0
      care for (suspected) damage to fetus O35.3 ☑
      suspected damage to fetus affecting management of pregnancy O35.3 ☑
   specified complications NEC B06.89
Rubeola (meaning measles) — *see* Measles
   meaning rubella — *see* Rubella
Rubeosis, iris — *see* Disorder, iris, vascular
Rubinstein-Taybi syndrome Q87.2
Rudimentary (congenital) (*see also* Agenesis)
   arm — *see* Defect, reduction, upper limb
   bone Q79.9
   cervix uteri Q51.828
   eye Q11.2
   lobule of ear Q17.3
   patella Q74.1
   respiratory organs in thoracopagus Q89.4
   tracheal bronchus Q32.4
   uterus Q51.818
      in male Q56.1
   vagina Q52.0
Ruled out condition — *see* Observation, suspected
Rumination R11.10
   with nausea R11.2
   disorder of infancy F98.21
   neurotic F42.8
   newborn P92.1
   obsessional F42.8
   psychogenic F42.8
Runeberg's disease D51.0

Runny nose R09.89
Rupia (syphilitic) A51.39
   congenital A50.06
   tertiary A52.79
Rupture, ruptured
   abscess (spontaneous) - code by site under Abscess
   aneurysm — *see* Aneurysm
   anus (sphincter) — *see* Laceration, anus
   aorta, aortic I71.8
      abdominal I71.3
      arch I71.1
      ascending I71.1
      descending I71.8
         abdominal I71.3
         thoracic I71.1
      syphilitic A52.01
      thoracoabdominal I71.5
      thorax, thoracic I71.1
      transverse I71.1
      traumatic — *see* Injury, aorta, laceration, major
      valve or cusp (*see also* Endocarditis, aortic) I35.8
   appendix (with peritonitis) (*see also* Appendicitis) K35.32
      with localized peritonitis (*see also* Appendicitis) K35.32
   arteriovenous fistula, brain — *see* Fistula, arteriovenous, brain, ruptured
   artery I77.2
      brain — *see* Hemorrhage, intracranial, intracerebral
      coronary — *see* Infarct, myocardium
      heart — *see* Infarct, myocardium
      pulmonary I28.8
      traumatic (complication) — *see* Injury, blood vessel
   bile duct (common) (hepatic) K83.2
      cystic K82.2
   bladder (sphincter) (nontraumatic) (spontaneous) N32.89
      following ectopic or molar pregnancy O08.6
      obstetrical trauma O71.5
      traumatic S37.29 ☑
   blood vessel (*see also* Hemorrhage)
      brain — *see* Hemorrhage, intracranial, intracerebral
      heart — *see* Infarct, myocardium
      traumatic (complication) — *see* Injury, blood vessel, laceration, major, by site
   bone — *see* Fracture
   bowel (nontraumatic) K63.1
   brain
      aneurysm (congenital) (*see also* Hemorrhage, intracranial, subarachnoid)
         syphilitic A52.05
      hemorrhagic — *see* Hemorrhage, intracranial, intracerebral
   capillaries I78.8
   cardiac (auricle) (ventricle) (wall) I23.3
      with hemopericardium I23.0
      infectional I40.9
      traumatic — *see* Injury, heart
   cartilage (articular) (current) (*see also* Sprain)
      knee S83.3 ☑
      semilunar — *see* Tear, meniscus
   cecum (with peritonitis) K65.0
      with peritoneal abscess K35.33
      traumatic S36.598 ☑
   celiac artery, traumatic — *see* Injury, blood vessel, celiac artery, laceration, major
   cerebral aneurysm (congenital) (*see* Hemorrhage, intracranial, subarachnoid)
   cervix (uteri)
      with ectopic or molar pregnancy O08.6
      following ectopic or molar pregnancy O08.6
      obstetrical trauma O71.3
      traumatic S37.69 ☑
   chordae tendineae NEC I51.1
      concurrent with acute myocardial infarction — *see* Infarct, myocardium
      following acute myocardial infarction (current complication) I23.4
   choroid (direct) (indirect) (traumatic) H31.32 ☑
   circle of Willis I60.6
   colon (nontraumatic) K63.1
      traumatic — *see* Injury, intestine, large
   cornea (traumatic) — *see* Injury, eye, laceration
   coronary (artery) (thrombotic) — *see* Infarct, myocardium
   corpus luteum (infected) (ovary) N83.1 ☑
   cyst — *see* Cyst
   cystic duct K82.2

Rupture — *continued*
   Descemet's membrane — *see* Change, corneal membrane, Descemet's, rupture
      traumatic — *see* Injury, eye, laceration
   diaphragm, traumatic — *see* Injury, intrathoracic, diaphragm
   disc — *see* Rupture, intervertebral disc
   diverticulum (intestine) K57.80
      with bleeding K57.81
      bladder N32.3
      large intestine K57.20
         with
            bleeding K57.21
            small intestine K57.40
               with bleeding K57.41
      small intestine K57.00
         with
            bleeding K57.01
            large intestine K57.40
               with bleeding K57.41
   duodenal stump K31.89
   ear drum (nontraumatic) (*see also* Perforation, tympanum)
      traumatic S09.2 ☑
         due to blast injury — *see* Injury, blast, ear
   esophagus K22.3
   eye (without prolapse or loss of intraocular tissue) — *see* Injury, eye, laceration
   fallopian tube NEC (nonobstetric) (nontraumatic) N83.8
      due to pregnancy O00.10 ☑
         with intrauterine pregnancy O00.11 ☑
   fontanel P13.1
   gallbladder K82.2
      traumatic S36.128 ☑
   gastric (*see also* Rupture, stomach)
      vessel K92.2
   globe (eye) (traumatic) — *see* Injury, eye, laceration
   graafian follicle (hematoma) N83.0 ☑
   heart — *see* Rupture, cardiac
   hymen (nontraumatic) (nonintentional) N89.8
   internal organ, traumatic — *see* Injury, by site
   intervertebral disc — *see* Displacement, intervertebral disc
      traumatic — *see* Rupture, traumatic, intervertebral disc
   intestine NEC (nontraumatic) K63.1
      traumatic — *see* Injury, intestine
   iris (*see also* Abnormality, pupillary)
      traumatic — *see* Injury, eye, laceration
   joint capsule, traumatic — *see* Sprain
   kidney (traumatic) S37.06 ☑
      birth injury P15.8
      nontraumatic N28.89
   lacrimal duct (traumatic) — *see* Injury, eye, specified site NEC
   lens (cataract) (traumatic) — *see* Cataract, traumatic
   ligament, traumatic — *see* Rupture, traumatic, ligament, by site
   liver S36.116 ☑
      birth injury P15.0
   lymphatic vessel I89.8
   marginal sinus (placental) (with hemorrhage) — *see* Hemorrhage, antepartum, specified cause NEC
   membrana tympani (nontraumatic) — *see* Perforation, tympanum
   membranes (spontaneous)
      artificial
         delayed delivery following O75.5
      delayed delivery following — *see* Pregnancy, complicated by, premature rupture of membranes
   meningeal artery I60.8
   meniscus (knee) (*see also* Tear, meniscus)
      old — *see* Derangement, meniscus
      site other than knee - code as Sprain
   mesenteric artery, traumatic — *see* Injury, mesenteric, artery, laceration, major
   mesentery (nontraumatic) K66.8
      traumatic — *see* Injury, intra-abdominal, specified, site NEC
   mitral (valve) I34.8
   muscle (traumatic) (*see also* Strain)
      diastasis — *see* Diastasis, muscle
      nontraumatic M62.10
         ankle M62.17 ☑
         foot M62.17 ☑
         forearm M62.13 ☑
         hand M62.14 ☑
         lower leg M62.16 ☑
         pelvic region M62.15 ☑
         shoulder region M62.11 ☑

☑ **Additional character required**

Rupture — *continued*
  muscle — *continued*
    specified site NEC M62.18
    thigh M62.15 ☑
    upper arm M62.12 ☑
   traumatic — *see* Strain, by site
  musculotendinous junction NEC, nontraumatic — *see* Rupture, tendon, spontaneous
  mycotic aneurysm causing cerebral hemorrhage — *see* Hemorrhage, intracranial, subarachnoid
  myocardium, myocardial — *see* Rupture, cardiac
   traumatic — *see* Injury, heart
  nontraumatic, meaning hernia — *see* Hernia
  obstructed — *see* Hernia, by site, obstructed
  operation wound — *see* Disruption, wound, operation
  ovary, ovarian N83.8
   corpus luteum cyst N83.1 ☑
   follicle (graafian) N83.0 ☑
  oviduct (nonobstetric) (nontraumatic) N83.8
   due to pregnancy O00.10 ☑
    with intrauterine pregnancy O00.11 ☑
  pancreas (nontraumatic) K86.89
   traumatic S36.299 ☑
  papillary muscle NEC I51.2
   following acute myocardial infarction (current complication) I23.5
  pelvic
   floor, complicating delivery O70.1
   organ NEC, obstetrical trauma O71.5
  perineum (nonobstetric) (nontraumatic) N90.89
   complicating delivery — *see* Delivery, complicated, by, laceration, anus (sphincter)
  postoperative wound — *see* Disruption, wound, operation
  prostate (traumatic) S37.828 ☑
  pulmonary
   artery I28.8
   valve (heart) I37.8
   vein I28.8
   vessel I28.8
  pus tube — *see* Salpingitis
  pyosalpinx — *see* Salpingitis
  rectum (nontraumatic) K63.1
   traumatic S36.69 ☑
  retina, retinal (traumatic) (without detachment) (*see also* Break, retina)
   with detachment — *see* Detachment, retina, with retinal, break
  rotator cuff (nontraumatic) M75.10 ☑
   complete M75.12 ☑
   incomplete M75.11 ☑
  sclera — *see* Injury, eye, laceration
  sigmoid (nontraumatic) K63.1
   traumatic S36.593 ☑
  spinal cord (*see also* Injury, spinal cord, by region)
   due to injury at birth P11.5
   newborn (birth injury) P11.5
  spleen (traumatic) S36.09 ☑
   birth injury P15.1
   congenital (birth injury) P15.1
   due to P. vivax malaria B51.0
   nontraumatic D73.5
   spontaneous D73.5
  splenic vein R58
   traumatic — *see* Injury, blood vessel, splenic vein
  stomach (nontraumatic) (spontaneous) K31.89
   traumatic S36.39 ☑
  supraspinatus (complete) (incomplete) (nontraumatic) — *see* Tear, rotator cuff
  symphysis pubis
   obstetric O71.6
   traumatic S33.4 ☑
  synovium (cyst) M66.10
   ankle M66.17 ☑
   elbow M66.12 ☑
   finger M66.14 ☑
   foot M66.17 ☑
   forearm M66.13 ☑
   hand M66.14 ☑
   pelvic region M66.15 ☑
   shoulder region M66.11 ☑
   specified site NEC M66.18
   thigh M66.15 ☑
   toe M66.17 ☑
   upper arm M66.12 ☑
   wrist M66.13 ☑
  tendon (traumatic) — *see* Strain
   nontraumatic (spontaneous) M66.9
    ankle M66.87 ☑
    extensor M66.20
     ankle M66.27 ☑

Rupture — *continued*
  tendon — *continued*
   foot M66.27 ☑
   forearm M66.23 ☑
   hand M66.24 ☑
   lower leg M66.26 ☑
   multiple sites M66.29
   pelvic region M66.25 ☑
   shoulder region M66.21 ☑
   specified site NEC M66.28
   thigh M66.25 ☑
   upper arm M66.22 ☑
   flexor M66.30
    ankle M66.37 ☑
    foot M66.37 ☑
    forearm M66.33 ☑
    hand M66.34 ☑
    lower leg M66.36 ☑
    multiple sites M66.39
    pelvic region M66.35 ☑
    shoulder region M66.31 ☑
    specified site NEC M66.38
    thigh M66.35 ☑
    upper arm M66.32 ☑
   foot M66.87 ☑
   forearm M66.83 ☑
   hand M66.84 ☑
   lower leg M66.86 ☑
   multiple sites M66.89
   pelvic region M66.85 ☑
   shoulder region M66.81 ☑
   specified
    site NEC M66.88
    tendon M66.80
   thigh M66.85 ☑
   upper arm M66.82 ☑
  thoracic duct I89.8
  tonsil J35.8
  traumatic
   aorta — *see* Injury, aorta, laceration, major
   diaphragm — *see* Injury, intrathoracic, diaphragm
   external site — *see* Wound, open, by site
   eye — *see* Injury, eye, laceration
   internal organ — *see* Injury, by site
   intervertebral disc
    cervical S13.0 ☑
    lumbar S33.0 ☑
    thoracic S23.0 ☑
   kidney S37.06 ☑
   ligament (*see also* Sprain)
    ankle — *see* Sprain, ankle
    carpus — *see* Rupture, traumatic, ligament, wrist
    collateral (hand) — *see* Rupture, traumatic, ligament, finger, collateral
    finger (metacarpophalangeal) (interphalangeal) S63.40 ☑
     collateral S63.41 ☑
      index S63.41 ☑
      little S63.41 ☑
      middle S63.41 ☑
      ring S63.41 ☑
     index S63.40 ☑
     little S63.40 ☑
     middle S63.40 ☑
     palmar S63.42 ☑
      index S63.42 ☑
      little S63.42 ☑
      middle S63.42 ☑
      ring S63.42 ☑
     ring S63.40 ☑
     specified site NEC S63.499 ☑
      index S63.49 ☑
      little S63.49 ☑
      middle S63.49 ☑
      ring S63.49 ☑
     volar plate S63.43 ☑
      index S63.43 ☑
      little S63.43 ☑
      middle S63.43 ☑
      ring S63.43 ☑
    foot — *see* Sprain, foot
    radial collateral S53.2 ☑
    radiocarpal — *see* Rupture, traumatic, ligament, wrist, radiocarpal
    ulnar collateral S53.3 ☑
    ulnocarpal — *see* Rupture, traumatic, ligament, wrist, ulnocarpal
    wrist S63.30 ☑
     collateral S63.31 ☑
     radiocarpal S63.32 ☑
     specified site NEC S63.39 ☑
     ulnocarpal (palmar) S63.33 ☑

Rupture — *continued*
  traumatic — *continued*
   liver S36.116 ☑
   membrana tympani — *see* Rupture, ear drum, traumatic
   muscle or tendon — *see* Strain
   myocardium — *see* Injury, heart
   pancreas S36.299 ☑
   rectum S36.69 ☑
   sigmoid S36.593 ☑
   spleen S36.09 ☑
   stomach S36.39 ☑
   symphysis pubis S33.4 ☑
   tympanum, tympanic (membrane) — *see* Rupture, ear drum, traumatic
   ureter S37.19 ☑
   uterus S37.69 ☑
   vagina — *see* Injury, vagina
   vena cava — *see* Injury, vena cava, laceration, major
  tricuspid (heart) (valve) I07.8
  tube, tubal (nonobstetric) (nontraumatic) N83.8
   abscess — *see* Salpingitis
   due to pregnancy O00.10 ☑
    with intrauterine pregnancy O00.11 ☑
  tympanum, tympanic (membrane) (nontraumatic) (*see also* Perforation, tympanic membrane) H72.9 ☑
   traumatic — *see* Rupture, ear drum, traumatic
  umbilical cord, complicating delivery O69.89 ☑
  ureter (traumatic) S37.19 ☑
   nontraumatic N28.89
  urethra (nontraumatic) N36.8
   with ectopic or molar pregnancy O08.6
   following ectopic or molar pregnancy O08.6
   obstetrical trauma O71.5
   traumatic S37.39 ☑
  uterosacral ligament (nonobstetric) (nontraumatic) N83.8
  uterus (traumatic) S37.69 ☑
   before labor O71.0 ☑
   during or after labor O71.1
   nonpuerperal, nontraumatic N85.8
   pregnant (during labor) O71.1
    before labor O71.0 ☑
  vagina — *see* Injury, vagina
  valve, valvular (heart) — *see* Endocarditis
  varicose vein — *see* Varix
  varix — *see* Varix
  vena cava R58
   traumatic — *see* Injury, vena cava, laceration, major
  vesical (urinary) N32.89
  vessel (blood) R58
   pulmonary I28.8
   traumatic — *see* Injury, blood vessel
  viscus R19.8
  vulva complicating delivery O70.0
Russell-Silver syndrome Q87.19
Russian spring-summer type encephalitis A84.0
Rust's disease (tuberculous cervical spondylitis) A18.01
Ruvalcaba-Myhre-Smith syndrome E71.440
Rytand-Lipsitch syndrome I44.2

S

Saber, sabre shin or tibia (syphilitic) A50.56 [M90.8 ☑]
Sac lacrimal — *see* condition
Saccharomyces infection B37.9
Saccharopinuria E72.3
Saccular — *see* condition
Sacculation
  aorta (nonsyphilitic) — *see* Aneurysm, aorta
  bladder N32.3
  intralaryngeal (congenital) (ventricular) Q31.3
  larynx (congenital) (ventricular) Q31.3
  organ or site, congenital — *see* Distortion
  pregnant uterus — *see* Pregnancy, complicated by, abnormal, uterus
  ureter N28.89
  urethra N36.1
  vesical N32.3
Sachs' amaurotic familial idiocy or disease E75.02
Sachs-Tay disease E75.02
Sacks-Libman disease M32.11
Sacralgia M53.3
Sacralization Q76.49
Sacrodynia M53.3
Sacroiliac joint — *see* condition
Sacroiliitis NEC M46.1

Sacrum — *see* condition
Saddle
  back — *see* Lordosis
  embolus
    abdominal aorta I74.01
    pulmonary artery I26.92
      with acute cor pulmonale I26.02
  injury - code to condition
  nose M95.0
    due to syphilis A50.57
Sadism (sexual) F65.52
Sadness, postpartal O90.6
Sadomasochism F65.50
Saemisch's ulcer (cornea) — *see* Ulcer, cornea, central
Sagging
  skin and subcutaneous tissue (following bariatric surgery weight loss) (following dietary weight loss) L98.7
Sahib disease B55.0
Sailors' skin L57.8
Saint
  Anthony's fire — *see* Erysipelas
  triad — *see* Hernia, diaphragm
  Vitus' dance — *see* Chorea, Sydenham's
Salaam
  attack(s) — *see* Epilepsy, spasms
  tic R25.8
Salicylism
  abuse F55.8
  overdose or wrong substance given — *see* Table of Drugs and Chemicals, by drug, poisoning
Salivary duct or gland — *see* condition
Salivation, excessive K11.7
Salmonella — *see* Infection, Salmonella
Salmonellosis A02.0
Salpingitis (catarrhal) (fallopian tube) (nodular) (pseudofollicular) (purulent) (septic) N70.91
  with oophoritis N70.93
  acute N70.01
    with oophoritis N70.03
  chlamydial A56.11
  chronic N70.11
    with oophoritis N70.13
  complicating abortion — *see* Abortion, by type, complicated by, salpingitis
  ear — *see* Salpingitis, eustachian
  eustachian (tube) H68.00 ☑
    acute H68.01 ☑
    chronic H68.02 ☑
  follicularis N70.11
    with oophoritis N70.13
  gonococcal (acute) (chronic) A54.24
  interstitial, chronic N70.11
    with oophoritis N70.13
  isthmica nodosa N70.11
    with oophoritis N70.13
  specific (gonococcal) (acute) (chronic) A54.24
  tuberculous (acute) (chronic) A18.17
  venereal (gonococcal) (acute) (chronic) A54.24
Salpingocele N83.4 ☑
Salpingo-oophoritis (catarrhal) (purulent) (ruptured) (septic) (suppurative) N70.93
  acute N70.03
    with ectopic or molar pregnancy O08.0
    following ectopic or molar pregnancy O08.0
    gonococcal A54.24
  chronic N70.13
  following ectopic or molar pregnancy O08.0
  gonococcal (acute) (chronic) A54.24
  puerperal O86.19
  specific (gonococcal) (acute) (chronic) A54.24
  subacute N70.03
  tuberculous (acute) (chronic) A18.17
  venereal (gonococcal) (acute) (chronic) A54.24
Salpingo-ovaritis — *see* Salpingo-oophoritis
Salpingoperitonitis — *see* Salpingo-oophoritis
Salzmann's nodular dystrophy — *see* Degeneration, cornea, nodular
Sampson's cyst or tumor N80.1
San Joaquin (Valley) fever B38.0
Sandblaster's asthma, lung or pneumoconiosis J62.8
Sander's disease (paranoia) F22
Sandfly fever A93.1
Sandhoff's disease E75.01
Sanfilippo (Type B) (Type C) (Type D) syndrome E76.22
Sanger-Brown ataxia G11.2
Sao Paulo fever or typhus A77.0
Saponification, mesenteric K65.8
Sarcocele (benign)
  syphilitic A52.76
    congenital A50.59
Sarcocystosis A07.8

Sarcoepiplocele — *see* Hernia
Sarcoepiplomphalocele Q79.2
Sarcoid (*see also* Sarcoidosis)
  arthropathy D86.86
  Boeck's D86.9
  Darier-Roussy D86.3
  iridocyclitis D86.83
  meningitis D86.81
  myocarditis D86.85
  myositis D86.87
  pyelonephritis D86.84
  Spiegler-Fendt L08.89
Sarcoidosis D86.9
  with
    cranial nerve palsies D86.82
    hepatic granuloma D86.89
    polyarthritis D86.86
    tubulo-interstitial nephropathy D86.84
  combined sites NEC D86.89
  lung D86.0
    and lymph nodes D86.2
  lymph nodes D86.1
    and lung D86.2
  meninges D86.81
  skin D86.3
  specified type NEC D86.89
Sarcoma (of) (*see also* Neoplasm, connective tissue, malignant)
  alveolar soft part — *see* Neoplasm, connective tissue, malignant
  ameloblastic C41.1
    upper jaw (bone) C41.0
  botryoid — *see* Neoplasm, connective tissue, malignant
  botryoides — *see* Neoplasm, connective tissue, malignant
  cerebellar C71.6
    circumscribed (arachnoidal) C71.6
  circumscribed (arachnoidal) cerebellar C71.6
  clear cell (*see also* Neoplasm, connective tissue, malignant)
    kidney C64. ☑
  dendritic cells (accessory cells) C96.4
  embryonal — *see* Neoplasm, connective tissue, malignant
  endometrial (stromal) C54.1
    isthmus C54.0
  epithelioid (cell) — *see* Neoplasm, connective tissue, malignant
  Ewing's — *see* Neoplasm, bone, malignant
  follicular dendritic cell C96.4
  germinoblastic (diffuse) — *see* Lymphoma, diffuse large cell
    follicular — *see* Lymphoma, follicular, specified NEC
  giant cell (except of bone) (*see also* Neoplasm, connective tissue, malignant)
    bone — *see* Neoplasm, bone, malignant
  glomoid — *see* Neoplasm, connective tissue, malignant
  granulocytic C92.3 ☑
  hemangioendothelial — *see* Neoplasm, connective tissue, malignant
  hemorrhagic, multiple — *see* Sarcoma, Kaposi's
  histiocytic C96.A
  Hodgkin — *see* Lymphoma, Hodgkin
  immunoblastic (diffuse) — *see* Lymphoma, diffuse large cell
  interdigitating dendritic cell C96.4
  Kaposi's
    colon C46.4
    connective tissue C46.1
    gastrointestinal organ C46.4
    lung C46.5 ☑
    lymph node(s) C46.3
    palate (hard) (soft) C46.2
    rectum C46.4
    skin C46.0
    specified site NEC C46.7
    stomach C46.4
    unspecified site C46.9
  Kupffer cell C22.3
  Langerhans cell C96.4
  leptomeningeal — *see* Neoplasm, meninges, malignant
  liver NEC C22.4
  lymphangioendothelial — *see* Neoplasm, connective tissue, malignant
  lymphoblastic — *see* Lymphoma, lymphoblastic (diffuse)
  lymphocytic — *see* Lymphoma, small cell B-cell
  mast cell C96.22

Sarcoma — *continued*
  melanotic — *see* Melanoma
  meningeal — *see* Neoplasm, meninges, malignant
  meningothelial — *see* Neoplasm, meninges, malignant
  mesenchymal (*see also* Neoplasm, connective tissue, malignant)
    mixed — *see* Neoplasm, connective tissue, malignant
  mesothelial — *see* Mesothelioma
  monstrocellular
    specified site — *see* Neoplasm, malignant, by site
    unspecified site C71.9
  myeloid C92.3 ☑
  neurogenic — *see* Neoplasm, nerve, malignant
  odontogenic C41.1
    upper jaw (bone) C41.0
  osteoblastic — *see* Neoplasm, bone, malignant
  osteogenic (*see also* Neoplasm, bone, malignant)
    juxtacortical — *see* Neoplasm, bone, malignant
    periosteal — *see* Neoplasm, bone, malignant
  periosteal (*see also* Neoplasm, bone, malignant)
    osteogenic — *see* Neoplasm, bone, malignant
  pleomorphic cell — *see* Neoplasm, connective tissue, malignant
  reticulum cell (diffuse) — *see* Lymphoma, diffuse large cell
    nodular — *see* Lymphoma, follicular
    pleomorphic cell type — *see* Lymphoma, diffuse large cell
  rhabdoid — *see* Neoplasm, malignant, by site
  round cell — *see* Neoplasm, connective tissue, malignant
  small cell — *see* Neoplasm, connective tissue, malignant
  soft tissue — *see* Neoplasm, connective tissue, malignant
  spindle cell — *see* Neoplasm, connective tissue, malignant
  stromal (endometrial) C54.1
    isthmus C54.0
  synovial (*see also* Neoplasm, connective tissue, malignant)
    biphasic — *see* Neoplasm, connective tissue, malignant
    epithelioid cell — *see* Neoplasm, connective tissue, malignant
    spindle cell — *see* Neoplasm, connective tissue, malignant
Sarcomatosis
  meningeal — *see* Neoplasm, meninges, malignant
  specified site NEC — *see* Neoplasm, connective tissue, malignant
  unspecified site C80.1
Sarcopenia (age-related) M62.84
Sarcosinemia E72.59
Sarcosporidiosis (intestinal) A07.8
Satiety, early R68.81
Saturnine — *see* condition
Saturnism
  overdose or wrong substance given or taken — *see* Table of Drugs and Chemicals, by drug, poisoning
Satyriasis F52.8
Sauriasis — *see* Ichthyosis
SBE (subacute bacterial endocarditis) I33.0
Scabs R23.4
Scabies (any site) B86
Scaglietti-Dagnini syndrome E22.0
Scald — *see* Burn
Scalenus anticus (anterior) syndrome G54.0
Scales R23.4
Scaling, skin R23.4
Scalp — *see* condition
Scapegoating affecting child Z62.3
Scaphocephaly Q75.0
Scapulalgia M89.8X1
Scapulohumeral myopathy G71.02
Scar, scarring (*see also* Cicatrix) L90.5
  adherent L90.5
  atrophic L90.5
  cervix
    in pregnancy or childbirth — *see* Pregnancy, complicated by, abnormal cervix
  cheloid L91.0
  chorioretinal H31.00 ☑
    posterior pole macula H31.01 ☑
    postsurgical H59.81 ☑
    solar retinopathy H31.02 ☑
    specified type NEC H31.09 ☑
  choroid — *see* Scar, chorioretinal
  conjunctiva H11.24 ☑

Scar — *continued*
cornea H17.9
xerophthalmic (*see also* Opacity, cornea)
vitamin A deficiency E50.6
duodenum, obstructive K31.5
hypertrophic L91.0
keloid L91.0
labia N90.89
lung (base) J98.4
macula — *see* Scar, chorioretinal, posterior pole
muscle M62.89
myocardium, myocardial I25.2
painful L90.5
posterior pole (eye) — *see* Scar, chorioretinal,
posterior pole
retina — *see* Scar, chorioretinal
trachea J39.8
transmural uterine, in pregnancy O34.29
uterus N85.8
in pregnancy O34.29
vagina N89.8
postoperative N99.2
vulva N90.89
Scarabiasis B88.2
Scarlatina (anginosa) (maligna) A38.9
myocarditis (acute) A38.1
old — *see* Myocarditis
otitis media A38.0
ulcerosa A38.8
Scarlet fever (albuminuria) (angina) A38.9
Schamberg's disease (progressive pigmentary
dermatosis) L81.7
Schatzki's ring (acquired) (esophagus) (lower) K22.2
congenital Q39.3
Schaufenster krankheit I20.8
Schaumann's
benign lymphogranulomatosis D86.1
disease or syndrome — *see* Sarcoidosis
Scheie's syndrome E76.03
Schenck's disease B42.1
Scheuermann's disease or osteochondrosis — *see*
Osteochondrosis, juvenile, spine
Schilder (-Flatau) disease G37.0
Schilling-type monocytic leukemia C93.0 ☑
Schimmelbusch's disease, cystic mastitis, or
hyperplasia — *see* Mastopathy, cystic
Schistosoma infestation — *see* Infestation,
Schistosoma
Schistosomiasis B65.9
with muscle disorder B65.9 *[M63.80]*
ankle B65.9 *[M63.87* ☑*]*
foot B65.9 *[M63.87* ☑*]*
forearm B65.9 *[M63.83* ☑*]*
hand B65.9 *[M63.84* ☑*]*
lower leg B65.9 *[M63.86* ☑*]*
multiple sites B65.9 *[M63.89]*
pelvic region B65.9 *[M63.85* ☑*]*
shoulder region B65.9 *[M63.81* ☑*]*
specified site NEC B65.9 *[M63.88]*
thigh B65.9 *[M63.85* ☑*]*
upper arm B65.9 *[M63.82* ☑*]*
Asiatic B65.2
bladder B65.0
chestermani B65.8
colon B65.1
cutaneous B65.3
due to
S. haematobium B65.0
S. japonicum B65.2
S. mansoni B65.1
S. mattheii B65.8
Eastern B65.2
genitourinary tract B65.0
intestinal B65.1
lung NEC B65.9 *[J99]*
pneumonia B65.9 *[J17]*
Manson's (intestinal) B65.1
oriental B65.2
pulmonary NEC B65.9 *[J99]*
pneumonia B65.9
Schistosoma
haematobium B65.0
japonicum B65.2
mansoni B65.1
specified type NEC B65.8
urinary B65.0
vesical B65.0
Schizencephaly Q04.6
Schizoaffective psychosis F25.9
Schizodontia K00.2
Schizoid personality F60.1
Schizophrenia, schizophrenic F20.9

Schizophrenia — *continued*
acute (brief) (undifferentiated) F23
atypical (form) F20.3
borderline F21
catalepsy F20.2
catatonic (type) (excited) (withdrawn) F20.2
cenesthopathic, cenesthesiopathic F20.89
childhood type F84.5
chronic undifferentiated F20.5
cyclic F25.0
disorganized (type) F20.1
flexibilitas cerea F20.2
hebephrenic (type) F20.1
incipient F21
latent F21
negative type F20.5
paranoid (type) F20.0
paraphrenic F20.0
post-psychotic depression F32.89
prepsychotic F21
prodromal F21
pseudoneurotic F21
pseudopsychopathic F21
reaction F23
residual (state) (type) F20.5
restzustand F20.5
schizoaffective (type) — *see* Psychosis,
schizoaffective
simple (type) F20.89
simplex F20.89
specified type NEC F20.89
spectrum and other psychotic disorder F29
specified NEC F28
stupor F20.2
syndrome of childhood F84.5
undifferentiated (type) F20.3
chronic F20.5
Schizothymia (persistent) F60.1
Schlatter-Osgood disease or osteochondrosis — *see*
Osteochondrosis, juvenile, tibia
Schlatter's tibia — *see* Osteochondrosis, juvenile,
tibia
Schmidt's syndrome (polyglandular, autoimmune)
E31.0
Schmincke's carcinoma or tumor — *see* Neoplasm,
nasopharynx, malignant
Schmitz (-Stutzer) dysentery A03.0
Schmorl's disease or nodes
lumbar region M51.46
lumbosacral region M51.47
sacrococcygeal region M53.3
thoracic region M51.44
thoracolumbar region M51.45
Schneiderian
papilloma — *see* Neoplasm, nasopharynx, benign
specified site — *see* Neoplasm, benign, by site
unspecified site D14.0
specified site — *see* Neoplasm, malignant, by site
unspecified site C30.0
Scholte's syndrome (malignant carcinoid) E34.0
Scholz (-Bielchowsky-Henneberg) disease or
syndrome E75.25
Schönlein (-Henoch) disease or purpura (primary)
(rheumatic) D69.0
Schottmuller's disease A01.4
Schroeder's syndrome (endocrine hypertensive) E27.0
Schüller-Christian disease or syndrome C96.5
Schultze's type acroparesthesia, simple I73.89
Schultz's disease or syndrome — *see* Agranulocytosis
Schwalbe-Ziehen-Oppenheim disease G24.1
Schwannoma (*see also* Neoplasm, nerve, benign)
malignant (*see also* Neoplasm, nerve, malignant)
with rhabdomyoblastic differentiation — *see*
Neoplasm, nerve, malignant
melanocytic — *see* Neoplasm, nerve, benign
pigmented — *see* Neoplasm, nerve, benign
Schwannomatosis Q85.03
Schwartz (-Jampel) syndrome G71.13
Schwartz-Bartter syndrome E22.2
Schweniger-Buzzi anetoderma L90.1
Sciatic — *see* condition
Sciatica (infective)
with lumbago M54.4 ☑
due to intervertebral disc disorder — *see* Disorder,
disc, with, radiculopathy
due to displacement of intervertebral disc
(with lumbago) — *see* Disorder, disc, with,
radiculopathy
wallet M54.3 ☑
Scimitar syndrome Q26.8
Sclera — *see* condition
Sclerectasia H15.84 ☑

Scleredema
adultorum — *see* Sclerosis, systemic
Buschke's — *see* Sclerosis, systemic
newborn P83.0
Sclerema (adiposum) (edematosum) (neonatorum)
(newborn) P83.0
adultorum — *see* Sclerosis, systemic
Scleriasis — *see* Scleroderma
Scleritis H15.00 ☑
with corneal involvement H15.04 ☑
anterior H15.01 ☑
brawny H15.02 ☑
in (due to) zoster B02.34
posterior H15.03 ☑
specified type NEC H15.09 ☑
syphilitic A52.71
tuberculous (nodular) A18.51
Sclerochoroiditis H31.8
Scleroconjunctivitis — *see* Scleritis
Sclerocystic ovary syndrome E28.2
Sclerodactyly, sclerodactylia L94.3
Scleroderma, sclerodermia (acrosclerotic) (diffuse)
(generalized) (progressive) (pulmonary) (*see also*
Sclerosis, systemic) M34.9
circumscribed L94.0
linear L94.1
localized L94.0
newborn P83.88
systemic M34.9
Sclerokeratitis H16.8
tuberculous A18.52
Scleroma nasi A48.8
Scleromalacia (perforans) H15.05 ☑
Scleromyxedema L98.5
Sclérose en plaques G35
Sclerosis, sclerotic
adrenal (gland) E27.8
Alzheimer's — *see* Disease, Alzheimer's
amyotrophic (lateral) G12.21
aorta, aortic I70.0
valve — *see* Endocarditis, aortic
artery, arterial, arteriolar, arteriovascular — *see*
Arteriosclerosis
ascending multiple G35
brain (generalized) (lobular) G37.9
artery, arterial I67.2
diffuse G37.0
disseminated G35
insular G35
Krabbe's E75.23
miliary G35
multiple G35
presenile (Alzheimer's) — *see* Disease,
Alzheimer's, early onset
senile (arteriosclerotic) I67.2
stem, multiple G35
tuberous Q85.1
bulbar, multiple G35
bundle of His I44.39
cardiac — *see* Disease, heart, ischemic,
atherosclerotic
cardiorenal — *see* Hypertension, cardiorenal
cardiovascular (*see also* Disease, cardiovascular)
renal — *see* Hypertension, cardiorenal
cerebellar — *see* Sclerosis, brain
cerebral — *see* Sclerosis, brain
cerebrospinal (disseminated) (multiple) G35
cerebrovascular I67.2
choroid — *see* Degeneration, choroid
combined (spinal cord) (*see also* Degeneration,
combined)
multiple G35
concentric (Balo) G37.5
cornea — *see* Opacity, cornea
coronary (artery) I25.10
with angina pectoris — *see* Arteriosclerosis,
coronary (artery),
corpus cavernosum
female N90.89
male N48.6
diffuse (brain) (spinal cord) G37.0
disseminated G35
dorsal G35
dorsolateral (spinal cord) — *see* Degeneration,
combined
endometrium N85.5
extrapyramidal G25.9
eye, nuclear (senile) — *see* Cataract, senile, nuclear
focal and segmental (glomerular) (*see also* N00-N07
with fourth character .1) N05.1
Friedreich's (spinal cord) G11.1
funicular (spermatic cord) N50.89

Sclerosis - Screening

Sclerosis — *continued*
- general (vascular) — *see* Arteriosclerosis
- gland (lymphatic) I89.8
- hepatic K74.1
  - alcoholic K70.2
- hereditary
  - cerebellar G11.9
  - spinal (Friedreich's ataxia) G11.1
- hippocampal G93.81
- insular G35
- kidney — *see* Sclerosis, renal
- larynx J38.7
- lateral (amyotrophic) (descending) (spinal) G12.21
  - primary G12.23
- lens, senile nuclear — *see* Cataract, senile, nuclear
- liver K74.1
  - with fibrosis K74.2
    - alcoholic K70.2
  - alcoholic K70.2
  - cardiac K76.1
- lung — *see* Fibrosis, lung
- mastoid — *see* Mastoiditis, chronic
- mesial temporal G93.81
- mitral I05.8
- Mönckeberg's (medial) — *see* Arteriosclerosis, extremities
- multiple (brain stem) (cerebral) (generalized) (spinal cord) G35
- myocardium, myocardial — *see* Disease, heart, ischemic, atherosclerotic
- nuclear (senile), eye — *see* Cataract, senile, nuclear
- ovary N83.8
- pancreas K86.89
- penis N48.6
- peripheral arteries — *see* Arteriosclerosis, extremities
- plaques G35
- pluriglandular E31.8
- polyglandular E31.8
- posterolateral (spinal cord) — *see* Degeneration, combined
- presenile (Alzheimer's) — *see* Disease, Alzheimer's, early onset
- primary, lateral G12.23
- progressive, systemic M34.0
- pulmonary — *see* Fibrosis, lung
  - artery I27.0
  - valve (heart) — *see* Endocarditis, pulmonary
- renal N26.9
  - with
    - cystine storage disease E72.09
    - hypertensive heart disease (conditions in I11 ☑) — *see* Hypertension, cardiorenal
  - arteriolar (hyaline) (hyperplastic) — *see* Hypertension, kidney
- retina (senile) (vascular) H35.00
- senile (vascular) — *see* Arteriosclerosis
- spinal (cord) (progressive) G95.89
  - ascending G61.0
  - combined (*see also* Degeneration, combined)
    - multiple G35
    - syphilitic A52.11
  - disseminated G35
  - dorsolateral — *see* Degeneration, combined
  - hereditary (Friedreich's) (mixed form) G11.1
  - lateral (amyotrophic) G12.21
    - progressive G12.23
  - multiple G35
  - posterior (syphilitic) A52.11
- stomach K31.89
- subendocardial, congenital I42.4
- systemic M34.9
  - with
    - lung involvement M34.81
    - myopathy M34.82
    - polyneuropathy M34.83
  - drug-induced M34.2
  - due to chemicals NEC M34.2
  - progressive M34.0
  - specified NEC M34.89
- temporal (mesial) G93.81
- tricuspid (heart) (valve) I07.8
- tuberous (brain) Q85.1
- tympanic membrane — *see* Disorder, tympanic membrane, specified NEC
- valve, valvular (heart) — *see* Endocarditis
- vascular — *see* Arteriosclerosis
- vein I87.8

Scoliosis (acquired) (postural) M41.9
- adolescent (idiopathic) — *see* Scoliosis, idiopathic, adolescent
- congenital Q67.5

Scoliosis — *continued*
- congenital — *continued*
  - due to bony malformation Q76.3
    - failure of segmentation (hemivertebra) Q76.3
    - hemivertebra fusion Q76.3
  - postural Q67.5
- idiopathic M41.20
  - adolescent M41.129
    - cervical region M41.122
    - cervicothoracic region M41.123
    - lumbar region M41.126
    - lumbosacral region M41.127
    - thoracic region M41.124
    - thoracolumbar region M41.125
  - cervical region M41.22
  - cervicothoracic region M41.23
  - infantile M41.00
    - cervical region M41.02
    - cervicothoracic region M41.03
    - lumbar region M41.06
    - lumbosacral region M41.07
    - sacrococcygeal region M41.08
    - thoracic region M41.04
    - thoracolumbar region M41.05
  - juvenile M41.119
    - cervical region M41.112
    - cervicothoracic region M41.113
    - lumbar region M41.116
    - lumbosacral region M41.117
    - thoracic region M41.114
    - thoracolumbar region M41.115
  - lumbar region M41.26
  - lumbosacral region M41.27
  - thoracic region M41.24
  - thoracolumbar region M41.25
- infantile — *see* Scoliosis, idiopathic, infantile
- neuromuscular M41.40
  - cervical region M41.42
  - cervicothoracic region M41.43
  - lumbar region M41.46
  - lumbosacral region M41.47
  - occipito-atlanto-axial region M41.41
  - thoracic region M41.44
  - thoracolumbar region M41.45
- paralytic — *see* Scoliosis, neuromuscular
- postradiation therapy M96.5
- rachitic (late effect or sequelae) E64.3 *[M49.80]*
  - cervical region E64.3 *[M49.82]*
  - cervicothoracic region E64.3 *[M49.83]*
  - lumbar region E64.3 *[M49.86]*
  - lumbosacral region E64.3 *[M49.87]*
  - multiple sites E64.3 *[M49.89]*
  - occipito-atlanto-axial region E64.3 *[M49.81]*
  - sacrococcygeal region E64.3 *[M49.88]*
  - thoracic region E64.3 *[M49.84]*
  - thoracolumbar region E64.3 *[M49.85]*
- sciatic M54.4 ☑
- secondary (to) NEC M41.50
  - cerebral palsy, Friedreich's ataxia, poliomyelitis, neuromuscular disorders — *see* Scoliosis, neuromuscular
  - cervical region M41.52
  - cervicothoracic region M41.53
  - lumbar region M41.56
  - lumbosacral region M41.57
  - thoracic region M41.54
  - thoracolumbar region M41.55
- specified form NEC M41.80
  - cervical region M41.82
  - cervicothoracic region M41.83
  - lumbar region M41.86
  - lumbosacral region M41.87
  - thoracic region M41.84
  - thoracolumbar region M41.85
- thoracogenic M41.30
  - thoracic region M41.34
  - thoracolumbar region M41.35
- tuberculous A18.01

Scoliotic pelvis
- with disproportion (fetopelvic) O33.0
  - causing obstructed labor O65.0

Scorbutus, scorbutic (*see also* Scurvy)
- anemia D53.2

Score, NIHSS (National Institutes of Health Stroke Scale) R29.7 ☑

Scotoma (arcuate) (Bjerrum) (central) (ring) (*see also* Defect, visual field, localized, scotoma)
- scintillating H53.19

Scratch — *see* Abrasion

Scratchy throat R09.89

Screening (for) Z13.9
- alcoholism Z13.39

Screening — *continued*
- anemia Z13.0
- anomaly, congenital Z13.89
- antenatal, of mother (*see also* Encounter, antenatal screening) Z36.9
- arterial hypertension Z13.6
- arthropod-borne viral disease NEC Z11.59
- autism Z13.41
- bacteriuria, asymptomatic Z13.89
- behavioral disorder Z13.30
  - specified NEC Z13.39
- brain injury, traumatic Z13.850
- bronchitis, chronic Z13.83
- brucellosis Z11.2
- cardiovascular disorder Z13.6
- cataract Z13.5
- chlamydial diseases Z11.8
- cholera Z11.0
- chromosomal abnormalities (nonprocreative) NEC Z13.79
- colonoscopy Z12.11
- congenital
  - dislocation of hip Z13.89
  - eye disorder Z13.5
  - malformation or deformation Z13.89
- contamination NEC Z13.88
- cystic fibrosis Z13.228
- dengue fever Z11.59
- dental disorder Z13.84
- depression (adult) (adolescent) (child) Z13.31
  - maternal Z13.32
  - perinatal Z13.32
- developmental
  - delays Z13.40
    - global (milestones) Z13.42
    - specified NEC Z13.49
  - handicap Z13.42
    - in early childhood Z13.42
- diabetes mellitus Z13.1
- diphtheria Z11.2
- disability, intellectual Z13.39
- disease or disorder Z13.9
  - bacterial NEC Z11.2
    - intestinal infectious Z11.0
    - respiratory tuberculosis Z11.1
  - behavioral Z13.30
    - specified NEC Z13.39
  - blood or blood-forming organ Z13.0
  - cardiovascular Z13.6
  - Chagas' Z11.6
  - chlamydial Z11.8
  - dental Z13.89
  - developmental delays Z13.40
    - global (milestones) Z13.42
    - specified NEC Z13.49
  - digestive tract NEC Z13.818
    - lower GI Z13.811
    - upper GI Z13.810
  - ear Z13.5
  - endocrine Z13.29
  - eye Z13.5
  - genitourinary Z13.89
  - heart Z13.6
  - human immunodeficiency virus (HIV) infection Z11.4
  - immunity Z13.0
  - infection
    - intestinal Z11.0
      - specified NEC Z11.6
    - infectious Z11.9
  - mental health and behavioral Z13.30
    - specified NEC Z13.39
  - metabolic Z13.228
  - neurological Z13.89
  - nutritional Z13.21
    - metabolic Z13.228
      - lipoid disorders Z13.220
  - protozoal Z11.6
    - intestinal Z11.0
  - respiratory Z13.83
  - rheumatic Z13.828
  - rickettsial Z11.8
  - sexually-transmitted NEC Z11.3
    - human immunodeficiency virus (HIV) Z11.4
  - sickle-cell (trait) Z13.0
  - skin Z13.89
  - specified NEC Z13.89
  - spirochetal Z11.8
  - thyroid Z13.29
  - vascular Z13.6
  - venereal Z11.3
  - viral NEC Z11.59

☑ **Additional character required**

Screening — *continued*
disease or disorder — *continued*
human immunodeficiency virus (HIV) Z11.4
intestinal Z11.0
elevated titer Z13.89
emphysema Z13.83
encephalitis, viral (mosquito- or tick-borne) Z11.59
exposure to contaminants (toxic) Z13.88
fever
dengue Z11.59
hemorrhagic Z11.59
yellow Z11.59
filariasis Z11.6
galactosemia Z13.228
gastrointestinal condition Z13.818
genetic (nonprocreative) - for procreative
management — *see* Testing, genetic, for
procreative management
disease carrier status (nonprocreative) Z13.71
specified NEC (nonprocreative) Z13.79
genitourinary condition Z13.89
glaucoma Z13.5
gonorrhea Z11.3
gout Z13.89
helminthiasis (intestinal) Z11.6
hematopoietic malignancy Z12.89
hemoglobinopathies NEC Z13.0
hemorrhagic fever Z11.59
Hodgkin disease Z12.89
human immunodeficiency virus (HIV) Z11.4
human papillomavirus Z11.51
hypertension Z13.6
immunity disorders Z13.0
infant or child (over 28 days old) Z00.129
with abnormal findings Z00.121
infection
mycotic Z11.8
parasitic Z11.8
ingestion of radioactive substance Z13.88
intellectual disability Z13.39
intestinal
helminthiasis Z11.6
infectious disease Z11.0
leishmaniasis Z11.6
leprosy Z11.2
leptospirosis Z11.8
leukemia Z12.89
lymphoma Z12.89
malaria Z11.6
malnutrition Z13.29
metabolic Z13.228
nutritional Z13.21
measles Z11.59
mental health disorder Z13.30
specified NEC Z13.39
metabolic errors, inborn Z13.228
multiphasic Z13.89
musculoskeletal disorder Z13.828
osteoporosis Z13.820
mycoses Z11.8
myocardial infarction (acute) Z13.6
neoplasm (malignant) (of) Z12.9
bladder Z12.6
blood Z12.89
breast Z12.39
routine mammogram Z12.31
cervix Z12.4
colon Z12.11
genitourinary organs NEC Z12.79
bladder Z12.6
cervix Z12.4
ovary Z12.73
prostate Z12.5
testis Z12.71
vagina Z12.72
hematopoietic system Z12.89
intestinal tract Z12.10
colon Z12.11
rectum Z12.12
small intestine Z12.13
lung Z12.2
lymph (glands) Z12.89
nervous system Z12.82
oral cavity Z12.81
prostate Z12.5
rectum Z12.12
respiratory organs Z12.2
skin Z12.83
small intestine Z12.13
specified site NEC Z12.89
stomach Z12.0
nephropathy Z13.89

Screening — *continued*
nervous system disorders NEC Z13.858
neurological condition Z13.89
osteoporosis Z13.820
parasitic infestation Z11.9
specified NEC Z11.8
phenylketonuria Z13.228
plague Z11.2
poisoning (chemical) (heavy metal) Z13.88
poliomyelitis Z11.59
postnatal, chromosomal abnormalities Z13.89
prenatal, of mother (*see also* Encounter, antenatal
screening) Z36.9
protozoal disease Z11.6
intestinal Z11.0
pulmonary tuberculosis Z11.1
radiation exposure Z13.88
respiratory condition Z13.83
respiratory tuberculosis Z11.1
rheumatoid arthritis Z13.828
rubella Z11.59
schistosomiasis Z11.6
sexually-transmitted disease NEC Z11.3
human immunodeficiency virus (HIV) Z11.4
sickle-cell disease or trait Z13.0
skin condition Z13.89
sleeping sickness Z11.6
special Z13.9
specified NEC Z13.89
syphilis Z11.3
tetanus Z11.2
trachoma Z11.8
traumatic brain injury Z13.850
trypanosomiasis Z11.6
tuberculosis, respiratory Z11.1
active Z11.1
latent Z11.7
venereal disease Z11.3
viral encephalitis (mosquito- or tick-borne) Z11.59
whooping cough Z11.2
worms, intestinal Z11.6
yaws Z11.8
yellow fever Z11.59
Scrofula, scrofulosis (tuberculosis of cervical lymph
glands) A18.2
Scrofulide (primary) (tuberculous) A18.4
Scrofuloderma, scrofulodermia (any site) (primary) A18.4
Scrofulosus lichen (primary) (tuberculous) A18.4
Scrofulous — *see* condition
Scrotal tongue K14.5
Scrotum — *see* condition
Scurvy, scorbutic E54
anemia D53.2
gum E54
infantile E54
rickets E55.0 *[M90.80]*
Sealpox B08.62
Seasickness T75.3 ☑
Seatworm (infection) (infestation) B80
Sebaceous (*see also* condition)
cyst — *see* Cyst, sebaceous
Seborrhea, seborrheic L21.9
capillitii R23.8
capitis L21.0
dermatitis L21.9
infantile L21.1
eczema L21.9
infantile L21.1
sicca L21.0
Seckel's syndrome Q87.19
Seclusion, pupil — *see* Membrane, pupillary
Second hand tobacco smoke exposure (acute)
(chronic) Z77.22
in the perinatal period P96.81
Secondary
dentin (in pulp) K04.3
neoplasm, secondaries — *see* Table of Neoplasms,
secondary
Secretion
antidiuretic hormone, inappropriate E22.2
catecholamine, by pheochromocytoma E27.5
hormone
antidiuretic, inappropriate (syndrome) E22.2
by
carcinoid tumor E34.0
pheochromocytoma E27.5
ectopic NEC E34.2
urinary
excessive R35.8
suppression R34
Section
nerve, traumatic — *see* Injury, nerve

Sedative, hypnotic, or anxiolytic-induced
anxiety disorder F13.980
bipolar and related disorder F13.94
delirium F13.921
depressive disorder F13.94
major neurocognitive disorder F13.97
mild neurocognitive disorder F13.988
psychotic disorder F13.959
sexual dysfunction F13.981
sleep disorder F13.982
Segmentation, incomplete (congenital) (*see also*
Fusion)
bone NEC Q78.8
lumbosacral (joint) (vertebra) Q76.49
Seitelberger's syndrome (infantile neuraxonal
dystrophy) G31.89
Seizure(s) (*see also* Convulsions) R56.9
absence G40.A ☑
akinetic — *see* Epilepsy, generalized, specified NEC
atonic — *see* Epilepsy, generalized, specified NEC
autonomic (hysterical) F44.5
convulsive — *see* Convulsions
cortical (focal) (motor) — *see* Epilepsy, localization-
related, symptomatic, with simple partial
seizures
disorder (*see also* Epilepsy) G40.909
due to stroke — *see* Sequelae (of), disease,
cerebrovascular, by type, specified NEC
epileptic — *see* Epilepsy
febrile (simple) R56.00
with status epilepticus G40.901
complex (atypical) (complicated) R56.01
with status epilepticus G40.901
grand mal G40.409
intractable G40.419
with status epilepticus G40.411
without status epilepticus G40.419
not intractable G40.409
with status epilepticus G40.401
without status epilepticus G40.409
heart — *see* Disease, heart
hysterical F44.5
intractable G40.919
with status epilepticus G40.911
Jacksonian (focal) (motor type) (sensory type) — *see*
Epilepsy, localization-related, symptomatic,
with simple partial seizures
newborn P90
nonspecific epileptic
atonic — *see* Epilepsy, generalized, specified NEC
clonic — *see* Epilepsy, generalized, specified NEC
myoclonic — *see* Epilepsy, generalized, specified
NEC
tonic — *see* Epilepsy, generalized, specified NEC
tonic-clonic — *see* Epilepsy, generalized, specified
NEC
partial, developing into secondarily generalized
seizures
complex — *see* Epilepsy, localization-related,
symptomatic, with complex partial seizures
simple — *see* Epilepsy, localization-related,
symptomatic, with simple partial seizures
petit mal G40.A ☑
intractable G40.419
with status epilepticus G40.411
without status epilepticus G40.419
not intractable G40.409
with status epilepticus G40.401
without status epilepticus G40.409
post traumatic R56.1
recurrent G40.909
specified NEC G40.89
uncinate — *see* Epilepsy, localization-related,
symptomatic, with complex partial seizures
Selenium deficiency, dietary E59
Self-damaging behavior (life-style) Z72.89
Self-harm (attempted)
history (personal) Z91.5
in family Z81.8
Self-mutilation (attempted)
history (personal) Z91.5
in family Z81.8
Self-poisoning
history (personal) Z91.5
in family Z81.8
observation following (alleged) attempt Z03.6
Semicoma R40.1
Seminal vesiculitis N49.0
Seminoma C62.9 ☑
specified site — *see* Neoplasm, malignant, by site
Senear-Usher disease or syndrome L10.4
Senectus R54

Senescence - Sequelae

Senescence (without mention of psychosis) R54
Senile, senility (*see also* condition) R41.81
  with
    acute confusional state F05
    mental changes NOS F03 ☑
    psychosis NEC — *see* Psychosis, senile
  asthenia R54
  cervix (atrophic) N88.8
  debility R54
  endometrium (atrophic) N85.8
  fallopian tube (atrophic) — *see* Atrophy, fallopian
    tube
  heart (failure) R54
  ovary (atrophic) — *see* Atrophy, ovary
  premature E34.8
  vagina, vaginitis (atrophic) N95.2
  wart L82.1
Sensation
  burning (skin) R20.8
    tongue K14.6
  loss of R20.8
  prickling (skin) R20.2
  tingling (skin) R20.2
Sense loss
  smell — *see* Disturbance, sensation, smell
  taste — *see* Disturbance, sensation, taste
  touch R20.8
Sensibility disturbance (cortical) (deep) (vibratory)
  R20.9
Sensitive, sensitivity (*see also* Allergy)
  carotid sinus G90.01
  child (excessive) F93.8
  cold, autoimmune D59.1
  dentin K03.89
  gluten (non-celiac) K90.41
  latex Z91.040
  methemoglobin D74.8
  tuberculin, without clinical or radiological
    symptoms R76.11
  visual
    glare H53.71
    impaired contrast H53.72
Sensitiver Beziehungswahn F22
Sensitization, auto-erythrocytic D69.2
Separation
  anxiety, abnormal (of childhood) F93.0
  apophysis, traumatic - code as Fracture, by site
  choroid — *see* Detachment, choroid
  epiphysis, epiphyseal
    nontraumatic (*see also* Osteochondropathy,
      specified type NEC)
      upper femoral — *see* Slipped, epiphysis, upper
        femoral
    traumatic - code as Fracture, by site
  fracture — *see* Fracture
  infundibulum cardiac from right ventricle by a
    partition Q24.3
  joint (traumatic) (current) - code by site under
    Dislocation
  muscle (nontraumatic) — *see* Diastasis, muscle
  pubic bone, obstetrical trauma O71.6
  retina, retinal — *see* Detachment, retina
  symphysis pubis, obstetrical trauma O71.6
  tracheal ring, incomplete, congenital Q32.1
Sepsis (generalized) (unspecified organism) A41.9
  with
    organ dysfunction (acute) (multiple) R65.20
      with septic shock R65.21
  actinomycotic A42.7
  adrenal hemorrhage syndrome (meningococcal) A39.1
  anaerobic A41.4
  Bacillus anthracis A22.7
  Brucella (*see also* Brucellosis) A23.9
  candidal B37.7
  cryptogenic A41.9
  due to device, implant or graft T85.79 ☑
    arterial graft NEC T82.7 ☑
    breast (implant) T85.79 ☑
    catheter NEC T85.79 ☑
      dialysis (renal) T82.7 ☑
        intraperitoneal T85.71 ☑
      infusion NEC T82.7 ☑
        spinal (cranial) (epidural) (intrathecal) (spinal)
          (subarachnoid) (subdural) T85.735 ☑
    urethral indwelling T83.511 ☑
    urinary T83.518 ☑
  ectopic or molar pregnancy O08.82
  electronic (electrode) (pulse generator)
    (stimulator)
    bone T84.7 ☑
    cardiac T82.7 ☑
    nervous system T85.738 ☑

Sepsis — *continued*
  due to device — *continued*
    brain T85.731 ☑
    neurostimulator generator T85.734 ☑
    peripheral nerve T85.732 ☑
    spinal cord T85.733 ☑
    urinary T83.590 ☑
  fixation, internal (orthopedic) — *see*
    Complication, fixation device, infection
  gastrointestinal (bile duct) (esophagus) T85.79 ☑
    neurostimulator electrode (lead) T85.732 ☑
  genital T83.69 ☑
  heart NEC T82.7 ☑
    valve (prosthesis) T82.6 ☑
    graft T82.7 ☑
  joint prosthesis — *see* Complication, joint
    prosthesis, infection
  ocular (corneal graft) (orbital implant) T85.79 ☑
  orthopedic NEC T84.7 ☑
    fixation device, internal — *see* Complication,
      fixation device, infection
  specified NEC T85.79 ☑
  vascular T82.7 ☑
  ventricular intracranial (communicating) shunt
    T85.730 ☑
  during labor O75.3
  Enterococcus A41.81
  Erysipelothrix (rhusiopathiae) (erysipeloid) A26.7
  Escherichia coli (E. coli) A41.5 ☑
  extraintestinal yersiniosis A28.2
  following
    abortion (subsequent episode) O08.0
      current episode — *see* Abortion
    ectopic or molar pregnancy O08.82
    immunization T88.0 ☑
    infusion, therapeutic injection or transfusion NEC
      T80.29 ☑
    obstetrical procedure O86.04
  gangrenous A41.9
  gonococcal A54.86
  Gram-negative (organism) A41.5 ☑
    anaerobic A41.4
  Haemophilus influenzae A41.3
  herpesviral B00.7
  intra-abdominal K65.1
  intraocular — *see* Endophthalmitis, purulent
  Listeria monocytogenes A32.7
  localized - code to specific localized infection
    in operation wound T81.49 ☑
    skin — *see* Abscess
  malleus A24.0
  melioidosis A24.1
  meningeal — *see* Meningitis
  meningococcal A39.4
    acute A39.2
    chronic A39.3
  MSSA (Methicillin susceptible Staphylococcus
    aureus) A41.01
  newborn P36.9
    due to
      anaerobes NEC P36.5
      Escherichia coli P36.4
      Staphylococcus P36.30
        aureus P36.2
        specified NEC P36.39
      Streptococcus P36.10
        group B P36.0
        specified NEC P36.19
      specified NEC P36.8
  Pasteurella multocida A28.0
  pelvic, puerperal, postpartum, childbirth O85
  postprocedural T81.44 ☑
  pneumococcal A40.3
  puerperal, postpartum, childbirth (pelvic) O85
  Salmonella (arizonae) (cholerae-suis) (enteritidis)
    (typhimurium) A02.1
  severe R65.20
    with septic shock R65.21
  skin, localized — *see* Abscess
  Shigella (*see also* Dysentery, bacillary) A03.9
  specified organism NEC A41.89
  Staphylococcus, staphylococcal A41.2
    aureus (methicillin susceptible) (MSSA) A41.01
      methicillin resistant (MRSA) A41.02
    coagulase-negative A41.1
    specified NEC A41.1
  Streptococcus, streptococcal A40.9
    agalactiae A40.1
    group
      A A40.0
      B A40.1
      D A41.81

Sepsis — *continued*
  Streptococcus, streptococcal — *continued*
    neonatal P36.10
      group B P36.0
      specified NEC P36.19
    pneumoniae A40.3
    pyogenes A40.0
    specified NEC A40.8
  tracheostomy stoma J95.02
  tularemic A21.7
  umbilical, umbilical cord (newborn) — *see* Sepsis,
    newborn
  Yersinia pestis A20.7
Septate — *see* Septum
Septic — *see* condition
  arm — *see* Cellulitis, upper limb
    with lymphangitis — *see* Lymphangitis, acute,
      upper limb
  embolus — *see* Embolism
  finger — *see* Cellulitis, digit
    with lymphangitis — *see* Lymphangitis, acute,
      digit
  foot — *see* Cellulitis, lower limb
    with lymphangitis — *see* Lymphangitis, acute,
      lower limb
  gallbladder (acute) K81.0
  hand — *see* Cellulitis, upper limb
    with lymphangitis — *see* Lymphangitis, acute,
      upper limb
  joint — *see* Arthritis, pyogenic or pyemic
  leg — *see* Cellulitis, lower limb
    with lymphangitis — *see* Lymphangitis, acute,
      lower limb
  nail (*see also* Cellulitis, digit)
    with lymphangitis — *see* Lymphangitis, acute,
      digit
  sore (*see also* Abscess)
    throat J02.0
      streptococcal J02.0
  spleen (acute) D73.89
  teeth, tooth (pulpal origin) K04.4
  throat — *see* Pharyngitis
  thrombus — *see* Thrombosis
  toe — *see* Cellulitis, digit
    with lymphangitis — *see* Lymphangitis, acute,
      digit
  tonsils, chronic J35.01
    with adenoiditis J35.03
  uterus — *see* Endometritis
Septicemia A41.9
  meaning sepsis — *see* Sepsis
Septum, septate (congenital) (*see also* Anomaly, by
  site)
  anal Q42.3
    with fistula Q42.2
  aqueduct of Sylvius Q03.0
    with spina bifida — *see* Spina bifida, by site, with
      hydrocephalus
  uterus Q51.20
    complete Q51.21
    partial Q51.22
    specified NEC Q51.28
  vagina Q52.10
    in pregnancy — *see* Pregnancy, complicated by,
      abnormal vagina
      causing obstructed labor O65.5
    longitudinal Q52.129
      microperforate
        left side Q52.124
        right side Q52.123
      nonobstruction Q52.120
      obstructing Q52.129
        left side Q52.122
        right side Q52.121
    transverse Q52.11
Sequelae (of) (*see also* condition)
  abscess, intracranial or intraspinal (conditions in
    G06 ☑) G09
  amputation - code to injury with seventh
    character S
  burn and corrosion - code to injury with seventh
    character S
  calcium deficiency E64.8
  cerebrovascular disease — *see* Sequelae, disease,
    cerebrovascular
  childbirth O94
  contusion - code to injury with seventh character S
  corrosion — *see* Sequelae, burn and corrosion
  crushing injury - code to injury with seventh
    character S
  disease
    cerebrovascular I69.90

☑ **Additional character required**

Sequelae — *continued*
    disease — *continued*
        alteration of sensation I69.998
        aphasia I69.920
        apraxia I69.990
        ataxia I69.993
        cognitive deficits I69.91 ☑
        disturbance of vision I69.998
        dysarthria I69.922
        dysphagia I69.991
        dysphasia I69.921
        facial droop I69.992
        facial weakness I69.992
        fluency disorder I69.923
        hemiplegia I69.95 ☑
        hemorrhage
            intracerebral — *see* Sequelae, hemorrhage,
                intracerebral
            intracranial, nontraumatic NEC — *see*
                Sequelae, hemorrhage, intracranial,
                nontraumatic
            subarachnoid — *see* Sequelae, hemorrhage,
                subarachnoid
        language deficit I69.928
        monoplegia
            lower limb I69.94 ☑
            upper limb I69.93 ☑
        paralytic syndrome I69.96 ☑
        specified effect NEC I69.998
        specified type NEC I69.80
            alteration of sensation I69.898
            aphasia I69.820
            apraxia I69.890
            ataxia I69.893
            cognitive deficits I69.81 ☑
            disturbance of vision I69.898
            dysarthria I69.822
            dysphagia I69.891
            dysphasia I69.821
            facial droop I69.892
            facial weakness I69.892
            fluency disorder I69.823
            hemiplegia I69.85 ☑
            language deficit I69.828
            monoplegia
                lower limb I69.84 ☑
                upper limb I69.83 ☑
            paralytic syndrome I69.86 ☑
            specified effect NEC I69.898
        speech deficit I69.928
            speech deficit I69.828
        stroke NOS — *see* Sequelae, stroke NOS
    dislocation - code to injury with seventh character S
    encephalitis or encephalomyelitis (conditions in
        G04 ☑) G09
        in infectious disease NEC B94.8
        viral B94.1
    external cause - code to injury with seventh
        character S
    foreign body entering natural orifice - code to
        injury with seventh character S
    fracture - code to injury with seventh character S
    frostbite - code to injury with seventh character S
    Hansen's disease B92
    hemorrhage
        intracerebral I69.10
            alteration of sensation I69.198
            aphasia I69.120
            apraxia I69.190
            ataxia I69.193
            cognitive deficits I69.11 ☑
            disturbance of vision I69.198
            dysarthria I69.122
            dysphagia I69.191
            dysphasia I69.121
            facial droop I69.192
            facial weakness I69.192
            fluency disorder I69.123
            hemiplegia I69.15 ☑
            language deficit NEC I69.128
            monoplegia
                lower limb I69.14 ☑
                upper limb I69.13 ☑
            paralytic syndrome I69.16 ☑
            specified effect NEC I69.198
            speech deficit NEC I69.128
        intracranial, nontraumatic NEC I69.20
            alteration of sensation I69.298
            aphasia I69.220
            apraxia I69.290
            ataxia I69.293
            cognitive deficits I69.21 ☑

Sequelae — *continued*
    hemorrhage — *continued*
        disturbance of vision I69.298
        dysarthria I69.222
        dysphagia I69.291
        dysphasia I69.221
        facial droop I69.292
        facial weakness I69.292
        fluency disorder I69.223
        hemiplegia I69.25 ☑
        language deficit NEC I69.228
        monoplegia
            lower limb I69.24 ☑
            upper limb I69.23 ☑
        paralytic syndrome I69.26 ☑
        specified effect NEC I69.298
        speech deficit NEC I69.228
    subarachnoid I69.00
        alteration of sensation I69.098
        aphasia I69.020
        apraxia I69.090
        ataxia I69.093
        cognitive deficits — *see* subcategory I69.01 ☑
        disturbance of vision I69.098
        dysarthria I69.022
        dysphagia I69.091
        dysphasia I69.021
        facial droop I69.092
        facial weakness I69.092
        fluency disorder I69.023
        hemiplegia I69.05 ☑
        language deficit NEC I69.028
        monoplegia
            lower limb I69.04 ☑
            upper limb I69.03 ☑
        paralytic syndrome I69.06 ☑
        specified effect NEC I69.098
        speech deficit NEC I69.028
    hepatitis, viral B94.2
    hyperalimentation E68
    infarction
        cerebral I69.30
            alteration of sensation I69.398
            aphasia I69.320
            apraxia I69.390
            ataxia I69.393
            cognitive deficits I69.31 ☑
            disturbance of vision I69.398
            dysarthria I69.322
            dysphagia I69.391
            dysphasia I69.321
            facial droop I69.392
            facial weakness I69.392
            fluency disorder I69.323
            hemiplegia I69.35 ☑
            language deficit NEC I69.328
            monoplegia
                lower limb I69.34 ☑
                upper limb I69.33 ☑
            paralytic syndrome I69.36 ☑
            specified effect NEC I69.398
            speech deficit NEC I69.328
    infection, pyogenic, intracranial or intraspinal G09
    infectious disease B94.9
        specified NEC B94.8
    injury - code to injury with seventh character S
    leprosy B92
    meningitis
        bacterial (conditions in G00 ☑) G09
        other or unspecified cause (conditions in G03 ☑)
            G09
    muscle (and tendon) injury - code to injury with
        seventh character S
    myelitis — *see* Sequelae, encephalitis
    niacin deficiency E64.8
    nutritional deficiency E64.9
        specified NEC E64.8
    obstetrical condition O94
    parasitic disease B94.9
    phlebitis or thrombophlebitis of intracranial
        or intraspinal venous sinuses and veins
        (conditions in G08) G09
    poisoning - code to poisoning with seventh
        character S
        nonmedicinal substance — *see* Sequelae, toxic
            effect, nonmedicinal substance
    poliomyelitis (acute) B91
    pregnancy O94
    protein-energy malnutrition E64.0
    puerperium O94
    rickets E64.3
    selenium deficiency E64.8

Sequelae — *continued*
    sprain and strain - code to injury with seventh
        character S
    stroke NOS I69.30
        alteration in sensation I69.398
        aphasia I69.320
        apraxia I69.390
        ataxia I69.393
        cognitive deficits I69.31 ☑
        disturbance of vision I69.398
        dysarthria I69.322
        dysphagia I69.391
        dysphasia I69.321
        facial droop I69.392
        facial weakness I69.392
        hemiplegia I69.35 ☑
        language deficit NEC I69.328
        monoplegia
            lower limb I69.34 ☑
            upper limb I69.33 ☑
        paralytic syndrome I69.36 ☑
        specified effect NEC I69.398
        speech deficit NEC I69.328
    tendon and muscle injury - code to injury with
        seventh character S
    thiamine deficiency E64.8
    trachoma B94.0
    tuberculosis B90.9
        bones and joints B90.2
        central nervous system B90.0
        genitourinary B90.1
        pulmonary (respiratory) B90.9
        specified organs NEC B90.8
    viral
        encephalitis B94.1
        hepatitis B94.2
    vitamin deficiency NEC E64.8
        A E64.1
        B E64.8
        C E64.2
    wound, open - code to injury with seventh
        character S
Sequestration (*see also* Sequestrum)
    disk — *see* Displacement, intervertebral disk
    lung, congenital Q33.2
Sequestrum
    bone — *see* Osteomyelitis, chronic
    dental M27.2
    jaw bone M27.2
    orbit — *see* Osteomyelitis, orbit
    sinus (accessory) (nasal) — *see* Sinusitis
Sequoiosis lung or pneumonitis J67.8
Serology for syphilis
    doubtful
        with signs or symptoms - code by site and stage
            under Syphilis
        follow-up of latent syphilis — *see* Syphilis, latent
    negative, with signs or symptoms - code by site and
        stage under Syphilis
    positive A53.0
        with signs or symptoms - code by site and stage
            under Syphilis
    reactivated A53.0
Seroma (*see also* Hematoma)
    postprocedural — *see* Complication,
        postprocedural, seroma
    traumatic, secondary and recurrent T79.2 ☑
Seropurulent — *see* condition
Serositis, multiple K65.8
    pericardial I31.1
    peritoneal K65.8
Serous — *see* condition
Sertoli cell
    adenoma
        specified site — *see* Neoplasm, benign, by site
        unspecified site
            female D27.9
            male D29.20
    carcinoma
        specified site — *see* Neoplasm, malignant, by site
        unspecified site (male) C62.9 ☑
            female C56.9
    tumor
        with lipid storage
            specified site — *see* Neoplasm, benign, by site
            unspecified site
                female D27.9
                male D29.20
        specified site — *see* Neoplasm, benign, by site
        unspecified site
            female D27.9
            male D29.20

Sertoli-Leydig cell tumor - Sialitis

Sertoli-Leydig cell tumor — *see* Neoplasm, benign, by site
  specified site — *see* Neoplasm, benign, by site
  unspecified site
    female D27.9
    male D29.20
Serum
  allergy, allergic reaction (*see also* Reaction, serum) T80.69 ☑
    shock (*see also* Shock, anaphylactic) T80.59 ☑
  arthritis (*see also* Reaction, serum) T80.69 ☑
  complication or reaction NEC (*see also* Reaction, serum) T80.69 ☑
  disease NEC (*see also* Reaction, serum) T80.69 ☑
  hepatitis (*see also* Hepatitis, viral, type B)
    carrier (suspected) of B18.1
  intoxication (*see also* Reaction, serum) T80.69 ☑
  neuritis (*see also* Reaction, serum) T80.69 ☑
  neuropathy G61.1
  poisoning NEC (*see also* Reaction, serum) T80.69 ☑
  rash NEC (*see also* Reaction, serum) T80.69 ☑
  reaction NEC (*see also* Reaction, serum) T80.69 ☑
  sickness NEC (*see also* Reaction, serum) T80.69 ☑
  urticaria (*see also* Reaction, serum) T80.69 ☑
Sesamoiditis M25.8 ☑
Sever's disease or osteochondrosis — *see* Osteochondrosis, juvenile, tarsus
Severe sepsis R65.20
  with septic shock R65.21
Sex
  chromosome mosaics Q97.8
    lines with various numbers of X chromosomes Q97.2
  education Z70.8
  reassignment surgery status Z87.890
Sextuplet pregnancy — *see* Pregnancy, sextuplet
Sexual
  function, disorder of (psychogenic) F52.9
  immaturity (female) (male) E30.0
  impotence (psychogenic) organic origin NEC — *see* Dysfunction, sexual, male
  precocity (constitutional) (cryptogenic)(female) (idiopathic) (male) E30.1
Sexuality, pathologic — *see* Deviation, sexual
Sézary disease C84.1 ☑
Shadow, lung R91.8
Shaking palsy or paralysis — *see* Parkinsonism
Shallowness, acetabulum — *see* Derangement, joint, specified type NEC, hip
Shaver's disease J63.1
Sheath (tendon) — *see* condition
Sheathing, retinal vessels H35.01 ☑
Shedding
  nail L60.8
  premature, primary (deciduous) teeth K00.6
Sheehan's disease or syndrome E23.0
Shelf, rectal K62.89
Shell teeth K00.5
Shellshock (current) F43.0
  lasting state — *see* Disorder, post-traumatic stress
Shield kidney Q63.1
Shift
  auditory threshold (temporary) H93.24 ☑
  mediastinal R93.89
Shifting sleep-work schedule (affecting sleep) G47.26
Shiga (-Kruse) dysentery A03.0
Shiga's bacillus A03.0
Shigella (dysentery) — *see* Dysentery, bacillary
Shigellosis A03.9
  Group A A03.0
  Group B A03.1
  Group C A03.2
  Group D A03.3
Shin splints S86.89 ☑
Shingles — *see* Herpes, zoster
Shipyard disease or eye B30.0
Shirodkar suture, in pregnancy — *see* Pregnancy, complicated by, incompetent cervix
Shock R57.9
  with ectopic or molar pregnancy O08.3
  adrenal (cortical) (Addisonian) E27.2
  adverse food reaction (anaphylactic) — *see* Shock, anaphylactic, due to food
  allergic — *see* Shock, anaphylactic
  anaphylactic T78.2 ☑
    chemical — *see* Table of Drugs and Chemicals
    due to drug or medicinal substance
      correct substance properly administered T88.6 ☑
      overdose or wrong substance given or taken (by accident) — *see* Table of Drugs and Chemicals, by drug, poisoning

Shock — *continued*
  anaphylactic — *continued*
    due to food (nonpoisonous) T78.00 ☑
      additives T78.06 ☑
      dairy products T78.07 ☑
      eggs T78.08 ☑
      fish T78.03 ☑
        shellfish T78.02 ☑
      fruit T78.04 ☑
      milk T78.07 ☑
      nuts T78.05 ☑
        multiple types T78.05 ☑
        peanuts T78.01 ☑
      peanuts T78.01 ☑
      seeds T78.05 ☑
      specified type NEC T78.09 ☑
      vegetable T78.04 ☑
    following sting(s) — *see* Venom
    immunization T80.52 ☑
    serum T80.59 ☑
      blood and blood products T80.51 ☑
      immunization T80.52 ☑
      specified NEC T80.59 ☑
      vaccination T80.52 ☑
  anaphylactoid — *see* Shock, anaphylactic
  anesthetic
    correct substance properly administered T88.2 ☑
    overdose or wrong substance given or taken — *see* Table of Drugs and Chemicals, by drug, poisoning
      specified anesthetic — *see* Table of Drugs and Chemicals, by drug, poisoning
  cardiogenic R57.0
  chemical substance — *see* Table of Drugs and Chemicals
  complicating ectopic or molar pregnancy O08.3
  culture — *see* Disorder, adjustment
  drug
    due to correct substance properly administered T88.6 ☑
    overdose or wrong substance given or taken (by accident) — *see* Table of Drugs and Chemicals, by drug, poisoning
  during or after labor and delivery O75.1
  electric T75.4 ☑
    (taser) T75.4 ☑
  endotoxic R65.21
    postprocedural (resulting from a procedure, not elsewhere classified) T81.12 ☑
  following
    ectopic or molar pregnancy O08.3
    injury (immediate) (delayed) T79.4 ☑
    labor and delivery O75.1
  food (anaphylactic) — *see* Shock, anaphylactic, due to food
  from electroshock gun (taser) T75.4 ☑
  gram-negative R65.21
    postprocedural (resulting from a procedure, not elsewhere classified) T81.12 ☑
  hematologic R57.8
  hemorrhagic R57.8
    surgery (intraoperative) (postoperative) T81.19 ☑
    trauma T79.4 ☑
  hypovolemic R57.1
    surgical T81.19 ☑
    traumatic T79.4 ☑
  insulin E15
    therapeutic misadventure — *see* subcategory T38.3 ☑
  kidney N17.0
    traumatic (following crushing) T79.5 ☑
  liver K72.00
  lightning T75.01 ☑
  lung J80
  obstetric O75.1
    with ectopic or molar pregnancy O08.3
    following ectopic or molar pregnancy O08.3
  pleural (surgical) T81.19 ☑
    due to trauma T79.4 ☑
  postprocedural (postoperative) T81.10 ☑
    with ectopic or molar pregnancy O08.3
    cardiogenic T81.11 ☑
    endotoxic T81.12 ☑
    following ectopic or molar pregnancy O08.3
    gram-negative T81.12 ☑
    hypovolemic T81.19 ☑
    septic T81.12 ☑
    specified type NEC T81.19 ☑
  psychic F43.0
  septic (due to severe sepsis) R65.21
  specified NEC R57.8
  surgical T81.10 ☑

Shock — *continued*
  taser gun (taser) T75.4 ☑
  therapeutic misadventure NEC T81.10 ☑
  thyroxin
    overdose or wrong substance given or taken — *see* Table of Drugs and Chemicals, by drug, poisoning
  toxic, syndrome A48.3
  transfusion — *see* Complications, transfusion
  traumatic (immediate) (delayed) T79.4 ☑
Shoemaker's chest M95.4
Short, shortening, shortness
  arm (acquired) (*see also* Deformity, limb, unequal length)
    congenital Q71.81 ☑
    forearm — *see* Deformity, limb, unequal length
  bowel syndrome K91.2
  breath R06.02
  cervical (complicating pregnancy) O26.87 ☑
    non-gravid uterus N88.3
  common bile duct, congenital Q44.5
  cord (umbilical), complicating delivery O69.3 ☑
  cystic duct, congenital Q44.5
  esophagus (congenital) Q39.8
  femur (acquired) — *see* Deformity, limb, unequal length, femur
    congenital — *see* Defect, reduction, lower limb, longitudinal, femur
  frenum, frenulum, linguae (congenital) Q38.1
  hip (acquired) (*see also* Deformity, limb, unequal length)
    congenital Q65.89
  leg (acquired) (*see also* Deformity, limb, unequal length)
    congenital Q72.81 ☑
    lower leg (*see also* Deformity, limb, unequal length)
  limbed stature, with immunodeficiency D82.2
  lower limb (acquired) (*see also* Deformity, limb, unequal length)
    congenital Q72.81 ☑
  organ or site, congenital NEC — *see* Distortion
  palate, congenital Q38.5
  radius (acquired) (*see also* Deformity, limb, unequal length)
    congenital — *see* Defect, reduction, upper limb, longitudinal, radius
  rib syndrome Q77.2
  stature (child) (hereditary) (idiopathic) NEC R62.52
    constitutional E34.3
    due to endocrine disorder E34.3
    Laron-type E34.3
  tendon (*see also* Contraction, tendon)
    with contracture of joint — *see* Contraction, joint
    Achilles (acquired) M67.0 ☑
      congenital Q66.89
    congenital Q79.8
  thigh (acquired) (*see also* Deformity, limb, unequal length, femur)
    congenital — *see* Defect, reduction, lower limb, longitudinal, femur
  tibialis anterior (tendon) — *see* Contraction, tendon
  umbilical cord
    complicating delivery O69.3 ☑
  upper limb, congenital — *see* Defect, reduction, upper limb, specified type NEC
  urethra N36.8
  uvula, congenital Q38.5
  vagina (congenital) Q52.4
Shortsightedness — *see* Myopia
Shoshin (acute fulminating beriberi) E51.11
Shoulder — *see* condition
Shovel-shaped incisors K00.2
Shower, thromboembolic — *see* Embolism
Shunt
  arterial-venous (dialysis) Z99.2
  arteriovenous, pulmonary (acquired) I28.0
    congenital Q25.72
  cerebral ventricle (communicating) in situ Z98.2
  surgical, prosthetic, with complications — *see* Complications, cardiovascular, device or implant
Shutdown, renal N28.9
Shy-Drager syndrome G90.3
Sialadenitis, sialadenosis (any gland) (chronic) (periodic) (suppurative) — *see* Sialoadenitis
Sialectasia K11.8
Sialidosis E77.1
Sialitis, silitis (any gland) (chronic) (suppurative) — *see* Sialoadenitis

☑ **Additional character required**

Sialoadenitis (any gland) (periodic) (suppurative) K11.20
  acute K11.21
    recurrent K11.22
  chronic K11.23
Sialoadenopathy K11.9
Sialoangitis — *see* Sialoadenitis
Sialodochitis (fibrinosa) — *see* Sialoadenitis
Sialodocholithiasis K11.5
Sialolithiasis K11.5
Sialometaplasia, necrotizing K11.8
Sialorrhea (*see also* Ptyalism)
  periodic — *see* Sialoadenitis
Sialosis K11.7
Siamese twin Q89.4
Sibling rivalry Z62.891
Sicard's syndrome G52.7
Sicca syndrome M35.00
  with
    keratoconjunctivitis M35.01
    lung involvement M35.02
    myopathy M35.03
    renal tubulo-interstitial disorders M35.04
    specified organ involvement NEC M35.09
Sick R69
  or handicapped person in family Z63.79
    needing care at home Z63.6
  sinus (syndrome) I49.5
Sick-euthyroid syndrome E07.81
Sickle-cell
  anemia — *see* Disease, sickle-cell
  trait D57.3
Sicklemia (*see also* Disease, sickle-cell)
  trait D57.3
Sickness
  air (travel) T75.3 ☑
  airplane T75.3 ☑
  alpine T70.29 ☑
  altitude T70.20 ☑
  Andes T70.29 ☑
  aviator's T70.29 ☑
  balloon T70.29 ☑
  car T75.3 ☑
  compressed air T70.3 ☑
  decompression T70.3 ☑
  green D50.8
  milk — *see* Poisoning, food, noxious
  motion T75.3 ☑
  mountain T70.29 ☑
    acute D75.1
  protein (*see also* Reaction, serum) T80.69 ☑
  radiation T66 ☑
  roundabout (motion) T75.3 ☑
  sea T75.3 ☑
  serum NEC (*see also* Reaction, serum) T80.69 ☑
  sleeping (African) B56.9
    by Trypanosoma B56.9
      brucei
        gambiense B56.0
        rhodesiense B56.1
    East African B56.1
    Gambian B56.0
    Rhodesian B56.1
    West African B56.0
  swing (motion) T75.3 ☑
  train (railway) (travel) T75.3 ☑
  travel (any vehicle) T75.3 ☑
Sideropenia — *see* Anemia, iron deficiency
Siderosilicosis J62.8
Siderosis (lung) J63.4
  eye (globe) — *see* Disorder, globe, degenerative, siderosis
Siemens' syndrome (ectodermal dysplasia) Q82.8
Sighing R06.89
  psychogenic F45.8
Sigmoid (*see also* condition)
  flexure — *see* condition
  kidney Q63.1
Sigmoiditis (*see also* Enteritis) K52.9
  infectious A09
  noninfectious K52.9
Silfverskiöld's syndrome Q78.9
Silicosiderosis J62.8
Silicosis, silicotic (simple) (complicated) J62.8
  with tuberculosis J65
Silicotuberculosis J65
Silo-fillers' disease J68.8
  bronchitis J68.0
  pneumonitis J68.0
  pulmonary edema J68.1
Silver's syndrome Q87.19
Simian malaria B53.1

Simmonds' cachexia or disease E23.0
Simons' disease or syndrome (progressive lipodystrophy) E88.1
Simple, simplex — *see* condition
Simulation, conscious (of illness) Z76.5
Simultanagnosia (asimultagnosia) R48.3
Sin Nombre virus disease (Hantavirus) (cardio)-pulmonary syndrome) B33.4
Sinding-Larsen disease or osteochondrosis — *see* Osteochondrosis, juvenile, patella
Singapore hemorrhagic fever A91
Singer's node or nodule J38.2
Single
  atrium Q21.2
  coronary artery Q24.5
  umbilical artery Q27.0
  ventricle Q20.4
Singultus R06.6
  epidemicus B33.0
Sinus (*see also* Fistula)
  abdominal K63.89
  arrest I45.5
  arrhythmia I49.8
  bradycardia R00.1
  branchial cleft (internal) (external) Q18.0
  coccygeal — *see* Sinus, pilonidal
  dental K04.6
  dermal (congenital) Q06.8
    with abscess Q06.8
    coccygeal, pilonidal — *see* Sinus, coccygeal
  infected, skin NEC L08.89
  marginal, ruptured or bleeding — *see* Hemorrhage, antepartum, specified cause NEC
  medial, face and neck Q18.8
  pause I45.5
  pericranii Q01.9
  pilonidal (infected) (rectum) L05.92
    with abscess L05.02
  preauricular Q18.1
  rectovaginal N82.3
  Rokitansky-Aschoff (gallbladder) K82.8
  sacrococcygeal (dermoid) (infected) — *see* Sinus, pilonidal
  tachycardia R00.0
    paroxysmal I47.1
  tarsi syndrome M25.57 ☑
  testis N50.89
  tract (postinfective) — *see* Fistula
  urachus Q64.4
Sinusitis (accessory) (chronic) (hyperplastic) (nasal) (nonpurulent) (purulent) J32.9
  acute J01.90
    ethmoidal J01.20
      recurrent J01.21
    frontal J01.10
      recurrent J01.11
    involving more than one sinus, other than pansinusitis J01.80
      recurrent J01.81
    maxillary J01.00
      recurrent J01.01
    pansinusitis J01.40
      recurrent J01.41
    recurrent J01.91
    specified NEC J01.80
      recurrent J01.81
    sphenoidal J01.30
      recurrent J01.31
  allergic — *see* Rhinitis, allergic
  due to high altitude T70.1 ☑
  ethmoidal J32.2
    acute J01.20
      recurrent J01.21
  frontal J32.1
    acute J01.10
      recurrent J01.11
  influenzal — *see* Influenza, with, respiratory manifestations NEC
  involving more than one sinus but not pansinusitis J32.8
    acute J01.80
      recurrent J01.81
  maxillary J32.0
    acute J01.00
      recurrent J01.01
  sphenoidal J32.3
    acute J01.30
      recurrent J01.31
  tuberculous, any sinus A15.8
Sinusitis-bronchiectasis-situs inversus (syndrome) (triad) Q89.3
Sipple's syndrome E31.22

Sirenomelia (syndrome) Q87.2
Siriasis T67.01 ☑
Sirkari's disease B55.0
Siti A65
Situation, psychiatric F99
Situational
  disturbance (transient) — *see* Disorder, adjustment
    acute F43.0
  maladjustment — *see* Disorder, adjustment
  reaction — *see* Disorder, adjustment
    acute F43.0
Situs inversus or transversus (abdominalis) (thoracis) Q89.3
Sixth disease B08.20
  due to human herpesvirus 6 B08.21
  due to human herpesvirus 7 B08.22
Sjögren-Larsson syndrome Q87.19
Sjögren's syndrome or disease — *see* Sicca syndrome
Skeletal — *see* condition
Skene's gland — *see* condition
Skenitis — *see* Urethritis
Skerljevo A65
Skevas-Zerfus disease — *see* Toxicity, venom, marine animal, sea anemone
Skin (*see also* condition)
  clammy R23.1
  donor — *see* Donor, skin
  hidebound M35.9
Slate-dressers' or slate-miners' lung J62.8
Sleep
  apnea — *see* Apnea, sleep
  deprivation Z72.820
  disorder or disturbance G47.9
    child F51.9
    nonorganic origin F51.9
    specified NEC G47.8
  disturbance G47.9
    nonorganic origin F51.9
  drunkenness F51.9
  rhythm inversion G47.2 ☑
  terrors F51.4
  walking F51.3
    hysterical F44.89
Sleep hygiene
  abuse Z72.821
  inadequate Z72.821
  poor Z72.821
Sleeping sickness — *see* Sickness, sleeping
Sleeplessness — *see* Insomnia
  menopausal N95.1
Sleep-wake schedule disorder G47.20
Slim disease (in HIV infection) B20
Slipped, slipping
  epiphysis (traumatic) (*see also* Osteochondropathy, specified type NEC)
    capital femoral (traumatic)
      acute (on chronic) S79.01 ☑
    current traumatic - code as Fracture, by site
    upper femoral (nontraumatic) M93.00 ☑
      acute M93.01 ☑
        on chronic M93.03 ☑
      chronic M93.02 ☑
  intervertebral disc — *see* Displacement, intervertebral disc
  ligature, umbilical P51.8
  patella — *see* Disorder, patella, derangement NEC
  rib M89.8X8
  sacroiliac joint — *see* subcategory M53.2 ☑
  tendon — *see* Disorder, tendon
  ulnar nerve, nontraumatic — *see* Lesion, nerve, ulnar
  vertebra NEC — *see* Spondylolisthesis
Slocumb's syndrome E27.0
Sloughing (multiple) (phagedena) (skin) (*see also* Gangrene)
  abscess — *see* Abscess
  appendix K38.8
  fascia — *see* Disorder, soft tissue, specified type NEC
  scrotum N50.89
  tendon — *see* Disorder, tendon
  transplanted organ — *see* Rejection, transplant
  ulcer — *see* Ulcer, skin
Slow
  feeding, newborn P92.2
  flow syndrome, coronary I20.8
  heart (beat) R00.1
Slowing, urinary stream R39.198
Sluder's neuralgia (syndrome) G44.89
Slurred, slurring speech R47.81
Small (ness)
  for gestational age — *see* Small for dates
  introitus, vagina N89.6

Small - Spens' syndrome

Small — *continued*
- kidney (unknown cause) N27.9
  - bilateral N27.1
  - unilateral N27.0
- ovary (congenital) Q50.39
- pelvis
  - with disproportion (fetopelvic) O33.1
    - causing obstructed labor O65.1
- uterus N85.8
- white kidney N03.9

Small-and-light-for-dates — *see* Small for dates
Small-for-dates (infant) P05.10
- with weight of
  - 499 grams or less P05.11
  - 500-749 grams P05.12
  - 750-999 grams P05.13
  - 1000-1249 grams P05.14
  - 1250-1499 grams P05.15
  - 1500-1749 grams P05.16
  - 1750-1999 grams P05.17
  - 2000-2499 grams P05.18
  - 2500 grams and over P05.19
- specified NEC P05.19

Smallpox B03
Smearing, fecal R15.1
Smith-Lemli-Opitz syndrome E78.72
Smith's fracture S52.54 ☑
Smoker — *see* Dependence, drug, nicotine
Smoker's
- bronchitis J41.0
- cough J41.0
- palate K13.24
- throat J31.2
- tongue K13.24

Smoking
- passive Z77.22

Smothering spells R06.81
Snaggle teeth, tooth M26.39
Snapping
- finger — *see* Trigger finger
- hip — *see* Derangement, joint, specified type NEC, hip
  - involving the iliotibial band M76.3 ☑
- knee — *see* Derangement, knee
  - involving the iliotibial band M76.3 ☑

Sneddon-Wilkinson disease or syndrome (sub-corneal pustular dermatosis) L13.1
Sneezing (intractable) R06.7
Sniffing
- cocaine
  - abuse — *see* Abuse, drug, cocaine
  - dependence — *see* Dependence, drug, cocaine
- gasoline
  - abuse — *see* Abuse, drug, inhalant
  - dependence — *see* Dependence, drug, inhalant
- glue (airplane)
  - abuse — *see* Abuse, drug, inhalant
  - drug dependence — *see* Dependence, drug, inhalant

Sniffles
- newborn P28.89

Snoring R06.83
Snow blindness — *see* Photokeratitis
Snuffles (non-syphilitic) R06.5
- newborn P28.89
- syphilitic (infant) A50.05 *[J99]*

Social
- exclusion Z60.4
  - due to discrimination or persecution (perceived) Z60.5
- migrant Z59.0
  - acculturation difficulty Z60.3
- rejection Z60.4
  - due to discrimination or persecution Z60.5
- role conflict NEC Z73.5
- skills inadequacy NEC Z73.4
- transplantation Z60.3

Sodoku A25.0
Soemmerring's ring — *see* Cataract, secondary
Soft (*see also* condition)
- nails L60.3

Softening
- bone — *see* Osteomalacia
- brain (necrotic) (progressive) G93.89
  - congenital Q04.8
  - embolic I63.4 ☑
  - hemorrhagic — *see* Hemorrhage, intracranial, intracerebral
  - occlusive I63.5 ☑
  - thrombotic I63.3 ☑
- cartilage M94.2 ☑
  - patella M22.4 ☑
- cerebellar — *see* Softening, brain

Softening — *continued*
- cerebral — *see* Softening, brain
- cerebrospinal — *see* Softening, brain
- myocardial, heart — *see* Degeneration, myocardial
- spinal cord G95.89
- stomach K31.89

Soldier's
- heart F45.8
- patches I31.0

Solitary
- cyst, kidney N28.1
- kidney, congenital Q60.0

Solvent abuse — *see* Abuse, drug, inhalant
- dependence — *see* Dependence, drug, inhalant

Somatization reaction, somatic reaction — *see* Disorder, somatoform
Somnambulism F51.3
- hysterical F44.89

Somnolence R40.0
- nonorganic origin F51.11

Sonne dysentery A03.3
Soor B37.0
Sore
- bed — *see* Ulcer, pressure, by site
- chiclero B55.1
- Delhi B55.1
- desert — *see* Ulcer, skin
- eye H57.1 ☑
- Lahore B55.1
- mouth K13.79
  - canker K12.0
- muscle M79.10
- Naga — *see* Ulcer, skin
- of skin — *see* Ulcer, skin
- oriental B55.1
- pressure — *see* Ulcer, pressure, by site
- skin L98.9
- soft A57
- throat (acute) (*see also* Pharyngitis)
  - with influenza, flu, or grippe — *see* Influenza, with, respiratory manifestations NEC
  - chronic J31.2
  - coxsackie (virus) B08.5
  - diphtheritic A36.0
  - herpesviral B00.2
  - influenzal — *see* Influenza, with, respiratory manifestations NEC
  - septic J02.0
  - streptococcal (ulcerative) J02.0
  - viral NEC J02.8
    - coxsackie B08.5
  - tropical — *see* Ulcer, skin
  - veldt — *see* Ulcer, skin

Soto's syndrome (cerebral gigantism) Q87.3
South African cardiomyopathy syndrome I42.8
Southeast Asian hemorrhagic fever A91
Spacing
- abnormal, tooth, teeth, fully erupted M26.30
- excessive, tooth, fully erupted M26.32

Spade-like hand (congenital) Q68.1
Spading nail L60.8
- congenital Q84.6

Spanish collar N47.1
Sparganosis B70.1
Spasm(s), spastic, spasticity (*see also* condition) R25.2
- accommodation — *see* Spasm, of accommodation
- ampulla of Vater K83.4
- anus, ani (sphincter) (reflex) K59.4
  - psychogenic F45.8
- artery I73.9
  - cerebral G45.9
- Bell's G51.3 ☑
- bladder (sphincter, external or internal) N32.89
  - psychogenic F45.8
- bronchus, bronchiole J98.01
- cardia K22.0
- cardiac I20.1
- carpopedal — *see* Tetany
- cerebral (arteries) (vascular) G45.9
- cervix, complicating delivery O62.4
- ciliary body (of accommodation) — *see* Spasm, of accommodation
- colon (*see also* Irritable, bowel) K58.9
  - with diarrhea K58.0
  - psychogenic F45.8
- common duct K83.8
- compulsive — *see* Tic
- conjugate H51.8
- coronary (artery) I20.1
- diaphragm (reflex) R06.6
  - epidemic B33.0
  - psychogenic F45.8

Spasm(s) — *continued*
- duodenum K59.8
- epidemic diaphragmatic (transient) B33.0
- esophagus (diffuse) K22.4
  - psychogenic F45.8
- facial G51.3 ☑
- fallopian tube N83.8
- gastrointestinal (tract) K31.89
  - psychogenic F45.8
- glottis J38.5
  - hysterical F44.4
  - psychogenic F45.8
    - conversion reaction F44.4
  - reflex through recurrent laryngeal nerve J38.5
- habit — *see* Tic
- heart I20.1
- hemifacial (clonic) G51.3 ☑
- hourglass — *see* Contraction, hourglass
- hysterical F44.4
- infantile — *see* Epilepsy, spasms
- inferior oblique, eye H51.8
- intestinal (*see also* Syndrome, irritable bowel) K58.9
  - psychogenic F45.8
- larynx, laryngeal J38.5
  - hysterical F44.4
  - psychogenic F45.8
    - conversion reaction F44.4
- levator palpebrae superioris — *see* Disorder, eyelid function
- muscle NEC M62.838
  - back M62.830
- nerve, trigeminal G51.0
- nervous F45.8
- nodding F98.4
- occupational F48.8
- oculogyric H51.8
  - psychogenic F45.8
- of accommodation H52.53 ☑
- ophthalmic artery — *see* Occlusion, artery, retina
- perineal, female N94.89
- peroneo-extensor (*see also* Deformity, limb, flat foot)
- pharynx (reflex) J39.2
  - hysterical F45.8
  - psychogenic F45.8
- psychogenic F45.8
- pylorus NEC K31.3
  - adult hypertrophic K31.89
  - congenital or infantile Q40.0
  - psychogenic F45.8
- rectum (sphincter) K59.4
  - psychogenic F45.8
- retinal (artery) — *see* Occlusion, artery, retina
- sigmoid (*see also* Syndrome, irritable bowel) K58.9
  - psychogenic F45.8
- sphincter of Oddi K83.4
- stomach K31.89
  - neurotic F45.8
- throat J39.2
  - hysterical F45.8
  - psychogenic F45.8
- tic F95.9
  - chronic F95.1
  - transient of childhood F95.0
- tongue K14.8
- torsion (progressive) G24.1
- trigeminal nerve — *see* Neuralgia, trigeminal
- ureter N13.5
- urethra (sphincter) N35.919
- uterus N85.8
  - complicating labor O62.4
- vagina N94.2
  - psychogenic F52.5
- vascular I73.9
- vasomotor I73.9
- vein NEC I87.8
- viscera — *see* Pain, abdominal

Spasmodic — *see* condition
Spasmophilia — *see* Tetany
Spasmus nutans F98.4
Spastic, spasticity (*see also* Spasm)
- child (cerebral) (congenital) (paralysis) G80.1

Speaker's throat R49.8
Specific, specified — *see* condition
Speech
- defect, disorder, disturbance, impediment R47.9
  - psychogenic, in childhood and adolescence F98.8
  - slurring R47.81
  - specified NEC R47.89

Spencer's disease A08.19
Spens' syndrome (syncope with heart block) I45.9

☑ **Additional character required**

Sperm counts (fertility testing) Z31.41
    postvasectomy Z30.8
        reversal Z31.42
Spermatic cord — *see* condition
Spermatocele N43.40
    congenital Q55.4
    multiple N43.42
    single N43.41
Spermatocystitis N49.0
Spermatocytoma C62.9 ☑
    specified site — *see* Neoplasm, malignant, by site
Spermatorrhea N50.89
Sphacelus — *see* Gangrene
Sphenoidal — *see* condition
Sphenoiditis (chronic) — *see* Sinusitis, sphenoidal
Sphenopalatine ganglion neuralgia G90.09
Sphericity, increased, lens (congenital) Q12.4
Spherocytosis (congenital) (familial) (hereditary) D58.0
    hemoglobin disease D58.0
    sickle-cell (disease) D57.8 ☑
Spherophakia Q12.4
Sphincter — *see* condition
Sphincteritis, sphincter of Oddi — *see* Cholangitis
Sphingolipidosis E75.3
    specified NEC E75.29
Sphingomyelinosis E75.3
Spicule tooth K00.2
Spider
    bite — *see* Toxicity, venom, spider
    fingers — *see* Syndrome, Marfan's
    nevus I78.1
    toes — *see* Syndrome, Marfan's
    vascular I78.1
Spiegler-Fendt
    benign lymphocytoma L98.8
    sarcoid L08.89
Spielmeyer-Vogt disease E75.4
Spina bifida (aperta) Q05.9
    with hydrocephalus NEC Q05.4
    cervical Q05.5
        with hydrocephalus Q05.0
    dorsal Q05.6
        with hydrocephalus Q05.1
    lumbar Q05.7
        with hydrocephalus Q05.2
    lumbosacral Q05.7
        with hydrocephalus Q05.2
    occulta Q76.0
    sacral Q05.8
        with hydrocephalus Q05.3
    thoracic Q05.6
        with hydrocephalus Q05.1
    thoracolumbar Q05.6
        with hydrocephalus Q05.1
Spindle, Krukenberg's — *see* Pigmentation, cornea, posterior
Spine, spinal — *see* condition
Spiradenoma (eccrine) — *see* Neoplasm, skin, benign
Spirillosis A25.0
Spirillum
    minus A25.0
    obermeieri infection A68.0
Spirochetal — *see* condition
Spirochetosis A69.9
    arthritic, arthritica A69.9
    bronchopulmonary A69.8
    icterohemorrhagic A27.0
    lung A69.8
Spirometrosis B70.1
Spitting blood — *see* Hemoptysis
Splanchnoptosis K63.4
Spleen, splenic — *see* condition
Splenectasis — *see* Splenomegaly
Splenitis (interstitial) (malignant) (nonspecific) D73.89
    malarial (*see also* Malaria) B54 *[D77]*
    tuberculous A18.85
Splenocele D73.89
Splenomegaly, splenomegalia (Bengal) (cryptogenic) (idiopathic) (tropical) R16.1
    with hepatomegaly R16.2
    cirrhotic D73.2
    congenital Q89.09
    congestive, chronic D73.2
    Egyptian B65.1
    Gaucher's E75.22
    malarial (*see also* Malaria) B54 *[D77]*
    neutropenic D73.81
    Niemann-Pick — *see* Niemann-Pick disease or syndrome
    siderotic D73.2
    syphilitic A52.79
        congenital (early) A50.08 *[D77]*

Splenopathy D73.9
Splenoptosis D73.89
Splenosis D73.89
Splinter — *see* Foreign body, superficial, by site
Split, splitting
    foot Q72.7 ☑
    hand Q71.6 ☑
    heart sounds R01.2
    lip, congenital — *see* Cleft, lip
    nails L60.3
    urinary stream R39.13
Spondylarthrosis — *see* Spondylosis
Spondylitis (chronic) (*see also* Spondylopathy, inflammatory)
    ankylopoietica — *see* Spondylitis, ankylosing
    ankylosing (chronic) M45.9
        with lung involvement M45.9 *[J99]*
        cervical region M45.2
        cervicothoracic region M45.3
        juvenile M08.1
        lumbar region M45.6
        lumbosacral region M45.7
        multiple sites M45.0
        occipito-atlanto-axial region M45.1
        sacrococcygeal region M45.8
        thoracic region M45.4
        thoracolumbar region M45.5
    atrophic (ligamentous) — *see* Spondylitis, ankylosing
    deformans (chronic) — *see* Spondylosis
    gonococcal A54.41
    gouty (*see also* Gout, by type, vertebrae) M10.08
    in (due to)
        brucellosis A23.9 *[M49.80]*
            cervical region A23.9 *[M49.82]*
            cervicothoracic region A23.9 *[M49.83]*
            lumbar region A23.9 *[M49.86]*
            lumbosacral region A23.9 *[M49.87]*
            multiple sites A23.9 *[M49.89]*
            occipito-atlanto-axial region A23.9 *[M49.81]*
            sacrococcygeal region A23.9 *[M49.88]*
            thoracic region A23.9 *[M49.84]*
            thoracolumbar region A23.9 *[M49.85]*
        enterobacteria (*see also* subcategory M49.8 ☑) A04.9
        tuberculosis A18.01
    infectious NEC — *see* Spondylopathy, infective
    juvenile ankylosing (chronic) M08.1
    Kümmell's — *see* Spondylopathy, traumatic
    Marie-Strümpell — *see* Spondylitis, ankylosing
    muscularis — *see* Spondylopathy, specified NEC
    psoriatic L40.53
    rheumatoid — *see* Spondylitis, ankylosing
    rhizomelica — *see* Spondylitis, ankylosing
    sacroiliac NEC M46.1
    senescent, senile — *see* Spondylosis
    traumatic (chronic) or post-traumatic — *see* Spondylopathy, traumatic
    tuberculous A18.01
    typhosa A01.05
Spondylolisthesis (acquired) (degenerative) M43.10
    with disproportion (fetopelvic) O33.0
        causing obstructed labor O65.0
    cervical region M43.12
    cervicothoracic region M43.13
    congenital Q76.2
    lumbar region M43.16
    lumbosacral region M43.17
    multiple sites M43.19
    occipito-atlanto-axial region M43.11
    sacrococcygeal region M43.18
    thoracic region M43.14
    thoracolumbar region M43.15
    traumatic (old) M43.10
        acute
            fifth cervical (displaced) S12.430 ☑
                nondisplaced S12.431 ☑
                specified type NEC (displaced) S12.450 ☑
                    nondisplaced S12.451 ☑
                type III S12.44 ☑
            fourth cervical (displaced) S12.330 ☑
                nondisplaced S12.331 ☑
                specified type NEC (displaced) S12.350 ☑
                    nondisplaced S12.351 ☑
                type III S12.34 ☑
            second cervical (displaced) S12.130 ☑
                nondisplaced S12.131 ☑
                specified type NEC (displaced) S12.150 ☑
                    nondisplaced S12.151 ☑
                type III S12.14 ☑
            seventh cervical (displaced) S12.630 ☑
                nondisplaced S12.631 ☑

Spondylolisthesis — *continued*
    traumatic — *continued*
        specified type NEC (displaced) S12.650 ☑
            nondisplaced S12.651 ☑
        type III S12.64 ☑
        sixth cervical (displaced) S12.530 ☑
            nondisplaced S12.531 ☑
            specified type NEC (displaced) S12.550 ☑
                nondisplaced S12.551 ☑
            type III S12.54 ☑
        third cervical (displaced) S12.230 ☑
            nondisplaced S12.231 ☑
            specified type NEC (displaced) S12.250 ☑
                nondisplaced S12.251 ☑
            type III S12.24 ☑
Spondylolysis (acquired) M43.00
    cervical region M43.02
    cervicothoracic region M43.03
    congenital Q76.2
    lumbar region M43.06
    lumbosacral region M43.07
        with disproportion (fetopelvic) O33.0
            causing obstructed labor O65.8
    multiple sites M43.09
    occipito-atlanto-axial region M43.01
    sacrococcygeal region M43.08
    thoracic region M43.04
    thoracolumbar region M43.05
Spondylopathy M48.9
    infective NEC M46.50
        cervical region M46.52
        cervicothoracic region M46.53
        lumbar region M46.56
        lumbosacral region M46.57
        multiple sites M46.59
        occipito-atlanto-axial region M46.51
        sacrococcygeal region M46.58
        thoracic region M46.54
        thoracolumbar region M46.55
    inflammatory M46.90
        cervical region M46.92
        cervicothoracic region M46.93
        lumbar region M46.96
        lumbosacral region M46.97
        multiple sites M46.99
        occipito-atlanto-axial region M46.91
        sacrococcygeal region M46.98
        specified type NEC M46.80
            cervical region M46.82
            cervicothoracic region M46.83
            lumbar region M46.86
            lumbosacral region M46.87
            multiple sites M46.89
            occipito-atlanto-axial region M46.81
            sacrococcygeal region M46.88
            thoracic region M46.84
            thoracolumbar region M46.85
        thoracic region M46.94
        thoracolumbar region M46.95
    neuropathic, in
        syringomyelia and syringobulbia G95.0
        tabes dorsalis A52.11
    specified NEC — *see* subcategory M48.8 ☑
    traumatic M48.30
        cervical region M48.32
        cervicothoracic region M48.33
        lumbar region M48.36
        lumbosacral region M48.37
        occipito-atlanto-axial region M48.31
        sacrococcygeal region M48.38
        thoracic region M48.34
        thoracolumbar region M48.35
Spondylosis M47.9
    with
        disproportion (fetopelvic) O33.0
            causing obstructed labor O65.0
        myelopathy NEC M47.10
            cervical region M47.12
            cervicothoracic region M47.13
            lumbar region M47.16
            occipito-atlanto-axial region M47.11
            thoracic region M47.14
            thoracolumbar region M47.15
        radiculopathy M47.20
            cervical region M47.22
            cervicothoracic region M47.23
            lumbar region M47.26
            lumbosacral region M47.27
            occipito-atlanto-axial region M47.21
            sacrococcygeal region M47.28
            thoracic region M47.24
            thoracolumbar region M47.25

Spondylosis — *continued*
  specified NEC M47.899
    cervical region M47.892
    cervicothoracic region M47.893
    lumbar region M47.896
    lumbosacral region M47.897
    occipito-atlanto-axial region M47.891
    sacrococcygeal region M47.898
    thoracic region M47.894
    thoracolumbar region M47.895
  traumatic — *see* Spondylopathy, traumatic
  without myelopathy or radiculopathy M47.819
    cervical region M47.812
    cervicothoracic region M47.813
    lumbar region M47.816
    lumbosacral region M47.817
    occipito-atlanto-axial region M47.811
    sacrococcygeal region M47.818
    thoracic region M47.814
    thoracolumbar region M47.815
Sponge
  inadvertently left in operation wound — *see*
    Foreign body, accidentally left during a
    procedure
  kidney (medullary) Q61.5
Sponge-diver's disease — *see* Toxicity, venom, marine
  animal, sea anemone
Spongioblastoma (any type) — *see* Neoplasm,
  malignant, by site
  specified site — *see* Neoplasm, malignant, by site
  unspecified site C71.9
Spongioneuroblastoma — *see* Neoplasm, malignant,
  by site
Spontaneous (*see also* condition)
  fracture (cause unknown) — *see* Fracture,
    pathological
Spoon nail L60.3
  congenital Q84.6
Sporadic — *see* condition
Sporothrix schenckii infection — *see* Sporotrichosis
Sporotrichosis B42.9
  arthritis B42.82
  disseminated B42.7
  generalized B42.7
  lymphocutaneous (fixed) (progressive) B42.1
  pulmonary B42.0
  specified NEC B42.89
Spots, spotting (in) (of)
  Bitot's (*see also* Pigmentation, conjunctiva)
    in the young child E50.1
    vitamin A deficiency E50.1
  café, au lait L81.3
  Cayenne pepper I78.1
  cotton wool, retina — *see* Occlusion, artery, retina
  de Morgan's (senile angiomas) I78.1
  Fuchs' black (myopic) (*see also* Myopia,
    degenerative) H44.2 ☑
  intermenstrual (regular) N92.0
    irregular N92.1
  Koplik's B05.9
  liver L81.4
  pregnancy O26.85 ☑
  purpuric R23.3
  ruby I78.1
Spotted fever — *see* Fever, spotted N92.3
Sprain (joint) (ligament)
  acromioclavicular joint or ligament S43.5 ☑
  ankle S93.40 ☑
    calcaneofibular ligament S93.41 ☑
    deltoid ligament S93.42 ☑
    internal collateral ligament — *see* Sprain, ankle,
      specified ligament NEC
    specified ligament NEC S93.49 ☑
    talofibular ligament — *see* Sprain, ankle, specified
      ligament NEC
    tibiofibular ligament S93.43 ☑
  anterior longitudinal, cervical S13.4 ☑
  atlas, atlanto-axial, atlanto-occipital S13.4 ☑
  breast bone — *see* Sprain, sternum
  calcaneofibular — *see* Sprain, ankle
  carpal — *see* Sprain, wrist
  carpometacarpal — *see* Sprain, hand, specified site
    NEC
  cartilage
    costal S23.41 ☑
    semilunar (knee) — *see* Sprain, knee, specified
      site NEC
      with current tear — *see* Tear, meniscus
    thyroid region S13.5 ☑
    xiphoid — *see* Sprain, sternum
  cervical, cervicodorsal, cervicothoracic S13.4 ☑
  chondrosternal S23.421 ☑

Sprain — *continued*
  coracoclavicular S43.8 ☑
  coracohumeral S43.41 ☑
  coronary, knee — *see* Sprain, knee, specified site
    NEC
  costal cartilage S23.41 ☑
  cricoarytenoid articulation or ligament S13.5 ☑
  cricothyroid articulation S13.5 ☑
  cruciate, knee — *see* Sprain, knee, cruciate
  deltoid, ankle — *see* Sprain, ankle
  dorsal (spine) S23.3 ☑
  elbow S53.40 ☑
    radial collateral ligament S53.43 ☑
    radiohumeral S53.41 ☑
    rupture
      radial collateral ligament — *see* Rupture,
        traumatic, ligament, radial collateral
      ulnar collateral ligament — *see* Rupture,
        traumatic, ligament, ulnar collateral
    specified type NEC S53.49 ☑
    ulnar collateral ligament S53.44 ☑
    ulnohumeral S53.42 ☑
  femur, head — *see* Sprain, hip
  fibular collateral, knee — *see* Sprain, knee, collateral
  fibulocalcaneal — *see* Sprain, ankle
  finger(s) S63.61 ☑
    index S63.61 ☑
    interphalangeal (joint) S63.63 ☑
      index S63.63 ☑
      little S63.63 ☑
      middle S63.63 ☑
      ring S63.63 ☑
    little S63.61 ☑
    middle S63.61 ☑
    ring S63.61 ☑
    metacarpophalangeal (joint) S63.65 ☑
    specified site NEC S63.69 ☑
      index S63.69 ☑
      little S63.69 ☑
      middle S63.69 ☑
      ring S63.69 ☑
  foot S93.60 ☑
    specified ligament NEC S93.69 ☑
    tarsal ligament S93.61 ☑
    tarsometatarsal ligament S93.62 ☑
    toe — *see* Sprain, toe
  hand S63.9 ☑
    finger — *see* Sprain, finger
    specified site NEC — *see* subcategory S63.8 ☑
    thumb — *see* Sprain, thumb
  head S03.9 ☑
  hip S73.10 ☑
    iliofemoral ligament S73.11 ☑
    ischiocapsular (ligament) S73.12 ☑
    specified NEC S73.19 ☑
  iliofemoral — *see* Sprain, hip
  innominate
    acetabulum — *see* Sprain, hip
    sacral junction S33.6 ☑
  internal
    collateral, ankle — *see* Sprain, ankle
    semilunar cartilage — *see* Sprain, knee, specified
      site NEC
  interphalangeal
    finger — *see* Sprain, finger, interphalangeal
      (joint)
    toe — *see* Sprain, toe, interphalangeal joint
  ischiocapsular — *see* Sprain, hip
  ischiofemoral — *see* Sprain, hip
  jaw (articular disc) (cartilage) (meniscus) S03.4 ☑
    old M26.69
  knee S83.9 ☑
    collateral ligament S83.40 ☑
      lateral (fibular) S83.42 ☑
      medial (tibial) S83.41 ☑
    cruciate ligament S83.50 ☑
      anterior S83.51 ☑
      posterior S83.52 ☑
    lateral (fibular) collateral ligament S83.42 ☑
    medial (tibial) collateral ligament S83.41 ☑
    patellar ligament S76.11 ☑
    specified site NEC S83.8X ☑
    superior tibiofibular joint (ligament) S83.6 ☑
  lateral collateral, knee — *see* Sprain, knee, collateral
  lumbar (spine) S33.5 ☑
  lumbosacral S33.9 ☑
  mandible (articular disc) S03.4 ☑
    old M26.69
  medial collateral, knee — *see* Sprain, knee, collateral
  meniscus
    jaw S03.4 ☑
      old M26.69

Sprain — *continued*
  meniscus — *continued*
    knee — *see* Sprain, knee, specified site NEC
      with current tear — *see* Tear, meniscus
        old — *see* Derangement, knee, meniscus, due
          to old tear
    mandible S03.4 ☑
      old M26.69
  metacarpal (distal) (proximal) — *see* Sprain, hand,
    specified site NEC
  metacarpophalangeal — *see* Sprain, finger,
    metacarpophalangeal (joint)
  metatarsophalangeal — *see* Sprain, toe,
    metatarsophalangeal joint
  midcarpal — *see* Sprain, hand, specified site NEC
  midtarsal — *see* Sprain, foot, specified site NEC
  neck S13.9 ☑
    anterior longitudinal cervical ligament S13.4 ☑
    atlanto-axial joint S13.4 ☑
    atlanto-occipital joint S13.4 ☑
    cervical spine S13.4 ☑
    cricoarytenoid ligament S13.5 ☑
    cricothyroid ligament S13.5 ☑
    specified site NEC S13.8 ☑
    thyroid region (cartilage) S13.5 ☑
  nose S03.8 ☑
  orbicular, hip — *see* Sprain, hip
  patella — *see* Sprain, knee, specified site NEC
  patellar ligament S76.11 ☑
  pelvis NEC S33.8 ☑
  phalanx
    finger — *see* Sprain, finger
    toe — *see* Sprain, toe
  pubofemoral — *see* Sprain, hip
  radiocarpal — *see* Sprain, wrist
  radiohumeral — *see* Sprain, elbow
  radius, collateral — *see* Rupture, traumatic,
    ligament, radial collateral
  rib (cage) S23.41 ☑
  rotator cuff (capsule) S43.42 ☑
  sacroiliac (region)
    chronic or old — *see* subcategory M53.2 ☑
    joint S33.6 ☑
  scaphoid (hand) — *see* Sprain, hand, specified site
    NEC
  scapula (r) — *see* Sprain, shoulder girdle, specified
    site NEC
  semilunar cartilage (knee) — *see* Sprain, knee,
    specified site NEC
    with current tear — *see* Tear, meniscus
      old — *see* Derangement, knee, meniscus, due
        to old tear
  shoulder joint S43.40 ☑
    acromioclavicular joint (ligament) — *see* Sprain,
      acromioclavicular joint
    blade — *see* Sprain, shoulder, girdle, specified
      site NEC
    coracoclavicular joint (ligament) — *see* Sprain,
      coracoclavicular joint
    coracohumeral ligament — *see* Sprain,
      coracohumeral joint
    girdle S43.9 ☑
      specified site NEC S43.8 ☑
    rotator cuff — *see* Sprain, rotator cuff
    specified site NEC S43.49 ☑
    sternoclavicular joint (ligament) — *see* Sprain,
      sternoclavicular joint
  spine
    cervical S13.4 ☑
    lumbar S33.5 ☑
    thoracic S23.3 ☑
  sternoclavicular joint S43.6 ☑
  sternum S23.429 ☑
    chondrosternal joint S23.421 ☑
    specified site NEC S23.428 ☑
    sternoclavicular (joint) (ligament) S23.420 ☑
  symphysis
    jaw S03.4 ☑
      old M26.69
    mandibular S03.4 ☑
      old M26.69
  talofibular — *see* Sprain, ankle
  tarsal — *see* Sprain, foot, specified site NEC
  tarsometatarsal — *see* Sprain, foot, specified site
    NEC
  temporomandibular S03.4 ☑
    old M26.69
  thorax S23.9 ☑
    ribs S23.41 ☑
    specified site NEC S23.8 ☑
    spine S23.3 ☑
    sternum — *see* Sprain, sternum

☑ **Additional character required**

Sprain — *continued*
  thumb S63.60 ☑
    interphalangeal (joint) S63.62 ☑
    metacarpophalangeal (joint) S63.64 ☑
    specified site NEC S63.68 ☑
  thyroid cartilage or region S13.5 ☑
  tibia (proximal end) — *see* Sprain, knee, specified site NEC
  tibial collateral, knee — *see* Sprain, knee, collateral
  tibiofibular
    distal — *see* Sprain, ankle
    superior — *see* Sprain, knee, specified site NEC
  toe(s) S93.50 ☑
    great S93.50 ☑
    interphalangeal joint S93.51 ☑
      great S93.51 ☑
      lesser S93.51 ☑
    lesser S93.50 ☑
    metatarsophalangeal joint S93.52 ☑
      great S93.52 ☑
      lesser S93.52 ☑
  ulna, collateral — *see* Rupture, traumatic, ligament, ulnar collateral
  ulnohumeral — *see* Sprain, elbow
  wrist S63.50 ☑
    carpal S63.51 ☑
    radiocarpal S63.52 ☑
    specified site NEC S63.59 ☑
  xiphoid cartilage — *see* Sprain, sternum
Sprengel's deformity (congenital) Q74.0
Sprue (tropical) K90.1
  celiac K90.0
  idiopathic K90.49
  meaning thrush B37.0
  nontropical K90.0
Spur, bone (*see also* Enthesopathy)
  calcaneal M77.3 ☑
  iliac crest M76.2 ☑
  nose (septum) J34.89
Spurway's syndrome Q78.0
Sputum
  abnormal (amount) (color) (odor) (purulent) R09.3
  blood-stained R04.2
  excessive (cause unknown) R09.3
Squamous (*see also* condition)
  epithelium in
    cervical canal (congenital) Q51.828
    uterine mucosa (congenital) Q51.818
Squashed nose M95.0
  congenital Q67.4
Squeeze, diver's T70.3 ☑
Squint (*see also* Strabismus)
  accommodative — *see* Strabismus, convergent concomitant
SSADHD (succinic semialdehyde dehydrogenase deficiency) E72.81
St. Hubert's disease A82.9
Stab (*see also* Laceration)
  internal organs — *see* Injury, by site
Stafne's cyst or cavity M27.0
Staggering gait R26.0
  hysterical F44.4
Staghorn calculus — *see* Calculus, kidney
Stähli's line (cornea) (pigment) — *see* Pigmentation, cornea, anterior
Stain, staining
  meconium (newborn) P96.83
  port wine Q82.5
  tooth, teeth (hard tissues) (extrinsic) K03.6
    due to
      accretions K03.6
      deposits (betel) (black) (green) (materia alba) (orange) (soft) (tobacco) K03.6
      metals (copper) (silver) K03.7
      nicotine K03.6
      pulpal bleeding K03.7
      tobacco K03.6
    intrinsic K00.8
Stammering (*see also* Disorder, fluency) F80.81
Standstill
  auricular I45.5
  cardiac — *see* Arrest, cardiac
  sinoatrial I45.5
  ventricular — *see* Arrest, cardiac
Stannosis J63.5
Stanton's disease — *see* Melioidosis
Staphylitis (acute) (catarrhal) (chronic) (gangrenous) (membranous) (suppurative) (ulcerative) K12.2
Staphylococcal scalded skin syndrome L00
Staphylococcemia A41.2
Staphylococcus, staphylococcal (*see also* condition)
  as cause of disease classified elsewhere B95.8

Staphylococcus — *continued*
  as cause of disease — *continued*
    aureus (methicillin susceptible) (MSSA) B95.61
      methicillin resistant (MRSA) B95.62
    specified NEC, as cause of disease classified elsewhere B95.7
Staphyloma (sclera)
  cornea H18.72 ☑
  equatorial H15.81 ☑
  localized (anterior) H15.82 ☑
  posticum H15.83 ☑
  ring H15.85 ☑
Stargardt's disease — *see* Dystrophy, retina
Starvation (inanition) (due to lack of food) T73.0 ☑
  edema — *see* Malnutrition, severe
Stasis
  bile (noncalculous) K83.1
  bronchus J98.09
    with infection — *see* Bronchitis
  cardiac — *see* Failure, heart, congestive
  cecum K59.8
  colon K59.8
  dermatitis I87.2
    with
      varicose ulcer — *see* Varix, leg, with ulcer, with inflammation
      varicose veins — *see* Varix, leg, with, inflammation
    due to postthrombotic syndrome — *see* Syndrome, postthrombotic
  duodenal K31.5
  eczema — *see* Varix, leg, with, inflammation
  edema — *see* Hypertension, venous (chronic), idiopathic
  foot T69.0 ☑
  ileocecal coil K59.8
  ileum K59.8
  intestinal K59.8
  jejunum K59.8
  kidney N19
  liver (cirrhotic) K76.1
  lymphatic I89.8
  pneumonia J18.2
  pulmonary — *see* Edema, lung
  rectal K59.8
  renal N19
    tubular N17.0
  ulcer — *see* Varix, leg, with, ulcer
    without varicose veins I87.2
  urine — *see* Retention, urine
  venous I87.8
State (of)
  affective and paranoid, mixed, organic psychotic F06.8
  agitated R45.1
    acute reaction to stress F43.0
  anxiety (neurotic) F41.1
  apprehension F41.1
  burn-out Z73.0
  climacteric, female Z78.0
    symptomatic N95.1
  compulsive F42.8
    mixed with obsessional thoughts F42.2
  confusional (psychogenic) F44.89
    acute (*see also* Delirium)
      with
        arteriosclerotic dementia F01.50
          with behavioral disturbance F01.51
        senility or dementia F05
      alcoholic F10.231
    epileptic F05
    reactive (from emotional stress, psychological trauma) F44.89
    subacute — *see* Delirium
  convulsive — *see* Convulsions
  crisis F43.0
  depressive F32.9
    neurotic F34.1
  dissociative F44.9
  emotional shock (stress) R45.7
  hypercoagulation — *see* Hypercoagulable
  locked-in G83.5
  menopausal Z78.0
    symptomatic N95.1
  neurotic F48.9
    with depersonalization F48.1
  obsessional F42.8
  oneiroid (schizophrenia-like) F23
  organic
    hallucinatory (nonalcoholic) F06.0
    paranoid (-hallucinatory) F06.2
  panic F41.0

State — *continued*
  paranoid F22
    climacteric F22
    involutional F22
    menopausal F22
    organic F06.2
    senile F03 ☑
    simple F22
  persistent vegetative R40.3
  phobic F40.9
  postleukotomy F07.0
  pregnant
    gestational carrier Z33.3
    incidental Z33.1
  psychogenic, twilight F44.89
  psychopathic (constitutional) F60.2
  psychotic, organic (*see also* Psychosis, organic)
    mixed paranoid and affective F06.8
    senile or presenile F03 ☑
    transient NEC F06.8
      with
        hallucinations F06.0
        depression F06.31
  residual schizophrenic F20.5
  restlessness R45.1
  stress (emotional) R45.7
  tension (mental) F48.9
    specified NEC F48.8
  transient organic psychotic NEC F06.8
    depressive type F06.31
    hallucinatory type F06.0
  twilight
    epileptic F05
    psychogenic F44.89
  vegetative, persistent R40.3
  vital exhaustion Z73.0
  withdrawal, — *see* Withdrawal, state
Status (post) (*see also* Presence (of))
  absence, epileptic — *see* Epilepsy, by type, with status epilepticus
  administration of tPA (rtPA) in a different facility within the last 24 hours prior to admission to current facility Z92.82
  adrenalectomy (unilateral) (bilateral) E89.6
  anastomosis Z98.0
  angioplasty (peripheral) Z98.62
    with implant Z95.820
    coronary artery Z98.61
      with implant Z95.5
  anginosus I20.9
  aortocoronary bypass Z95.1
  arthrodesis Z98.1
  artificial opening (of) Z93.9
    gastrointestinal tract Z93.4
    specified NEC Z93.8
    urinary tract Z93.6
    vagina Z93.8
  asthmaticus — *see* Asthma, by type, with status asthmaticus
  awaiting organ transplant Z76.82
  bariatric surgery Z98.84
  bed confinement Z74.01
  bleb, filtering (vitreous), after glaucoma surgery Z98.83
  breast implant Z98.82
    removal Z98.86
  cataract extraction Z98.4 ☑
  cholecystectomy Z90.49
  clitorectomy N90.811
    with excision of labia minora N90.812
  colectomy (complete) (partial) Z90.49
  colonization — *see* Carrier (suspected) of
  colostomy Z93.3
  convulsivus idiopathicus — *see* Epilepsy, by type, with status epilepticus
  coronary artery angioplasty — *see* Status, angioplasty, coronary artery
  coronary artery bypass graft Z95.1
  cystectomy (urinary bladder) Z90.6
  cystostomy Z93.50
    appendico-vesicostomy Z93.52
    cutaneous Z93.51
    specified NEC Z93.59
  delinquent immunization Z28.3
  dental Z98.818
    crown Z98.811
    fillings Z98.811
    restoration Z98.811
    sealant Z98.810
    specified NEC Z98.818
  deployment (current) (military) Z56.82
  dialysis (hemodialysis) (peritoneal) Z99.2

Status — *continued*
do not resuscitate (DNR) Z66
donor — *see* Donor
embedded fragments — *see* Retained, foreign body
    fragments (type of)
embedded splinter — *see* Retained, foreign body
    fragments (type of)
enterostomy Z93.4
epileptic, epilepticus (*see also* Epilepsy, by type,
    with status epilepticus) G40.901
estrogen receptor
    negative Z17.1
    positive Z17.0
female genital cutting — *see* Female genital
    mutilation status
female genital mutilation — *see* Female genital
    mutilation status
filtering (vitreous) bleb after glaucoma surgery
    Z98.83
gastrectomy (complete) (partial) Z90.3
gastric banding Z98.84
gastric bypass for obesity Z98.84
gastrostomy Z93.1
human immunodeficiency virus (HIV) infection,
    asymptomatic Z21
hysterectomy (complete) (total) Z90.710
    partial (with remaining cervical stump) Z90.711
ileostomy Z93.2
implant
    breast Z98.82
infibulation N90.813
intestinal bypass Z98.0
jejunostomy Z93.4
laryngectomy Z90.02
lapsed immunization schedule Z28.3
lymphaticus E32.8
malignancy
    castrate resistant prostate Z19.2
    hormone resistant Z19.2
    hormone sensitive Z19.1
marmoratus G80.3
mastectomy (unilateral) (bilateral) Z90.1 ☑
military deployment status (current) Z56.82
    in theater or in support of military war,
        peacekeeping and humanitarian operations
        Z56.82
nephrectomy (unilateral) (bilateral) Z90.5
nephrostomy Z93.6
obesity surgery Z98.84
oophorectomy
    bilateral Z90.722
    unilateral Z90.721
organ replacement
    by artificial or mechanical device or prosthesis of
        artery Z95.828
        bladder Z96.0
        blood vessel Z95.828
        breast Z97.8
        eye globe Z97.0
        heart Z95.812
            valve Z95.2
        intestine Z97.8
        joint Z96.60
            hip — *see* Presence, hip joint implant
            knee — *see* Presence, knee joint implant
            specified site NEC Z96.698
        kidney Z97.8
        larynx Z96.3
        lens Z96.1
        limbs — *see* Presence, artificial, limb
        liver Z97.8
        lung Z97.8
        pancreas Z97.8
    by organ transplant (heterologous)(homologous)
        — *see* Transplant
pacemaker
    brain Z96.89
    cardiac Z95.0
    specified NEC Z96.89
pancreatectomy Z90.410
    complete Z90.410
    partial Z90.411
    total Z90.410
physical restraint Z78.1
pneumonectomy (complete) (partial) Z90.2
pneumothorax, therapeutic Z98.3
postcommotio cerebri F07.81
postoperative (postprocedural) NEC Z98.890
    breast implant Z98.82
    dental Z98.818
        crown Z98.811
        fillings Z98.811

Status — *continued*
postoperative — *continued*
    restoration Z98.811
    sealant Z98.810
    specified NEC Z98.818
    uterine scar Z98.891
    pneumothorax, therapeutic Z98.3
postpartum (routine follow-up) Z39.2
    care immediately after delivery Z39.0
postsurgical (postprocedural) NEC Z98.890
    pneumothorax, therapeutic Z98.3
pregnancy, incidental Z33.1
prosthesis coronary angioplasty Z95.5
pseudophakia Z96.1
renal dialysis (hemodialysis) (peritoneal) Z99.2
retained foreign body — *see* Retained, foreign body
    fragments (type of)
reversed jejunal transposition (for bypass) Z98.0
salpingo-oophorectomy
    bilateral Z90.722
    unilateral Z90.721
sex reassignment surgery status Z87.890
shunt
    arteriovenous (for dialysis) Z99.2
    cerebrospinal fluid Z98.2
    ventricular (communicating) (for drainage) Z98.2
splenectomy Z90.81
thymicolymphaticus E32.8
thymicus E32.8
thymolymphaticus E32.8
thyroidectomy (hypothyroidism) E89.0
tooth (teeth) extraction (*see also* Absence, teeth,
    acquired) K08.409
tPA (rtPA) administration in a different facility within
    the last 24 hours prior to admission to current
    facility Z92.82
tracheostomy Z93.0
transplant — *see* Transplant
    organ removed Z98.85
tubal ligation Z98.51
underimmunization Z28.3
ureterostomy Z93.6
urethrostomy Z93.6
vagina, artificial Z93.8
vasectomy Z98.52
wheelchair confinement Z99.3
Stealing
child problem F91.8
    in company with others Z72.810
    pathological (compulsive) F63.2
Steam burn — *see* Burn
Steatocystoma multiplex L72.2
Steatohepatitis (nonalcoholic) (NASH) K75.81
Steatoma L72.3
    eyelid (cystic) — *see* Dermatosis, eyelid
        infected — *see* Hordeolum
Steatorrhea (chronic) K90.9
    with lacteal obstruction K90.2
    idiopathic (adult) (infantile) K90.9
    pancreatic K90.3
    primary K90.0
    tropical K90.1
Steatosis E88.89
    heart — *see* Degeneration, myocardial
    kidney N28.89
    liver NEC K76.0
Steele-Richardson-Olszewski disease or syndrome
    G23.1
Steinbrocker's syndrome G90.8
Steinert's disease G71.11
Stein-Leventhal syndrome E28.2
Stein's syndrome E28.2
STEMI (*see also* - Infarct, myocardium, ST elevation)
    I21.3
Stenocardia I20.8
Stenocephaly Q75.8
Stenosis, stenotic (cicatricial) (*see also* Stricture)
    ampulla of Vater K83.1
    anus, anal (canal) (sphincter) K62.4
        and rectum K62.4
        congenital Q42.3
            with fistula Q42.2
    aorta (ascending) (supraventricular) (congenital)
        Q25.1
        arteriosclerotic I70.0
        calcified I70.0
        supravalvular Q25.3
    aortic (valve) I35.0
        with insufficiency I35.2
        congenital Q23.0
        rheumatic I06.0
            with

Stenosis — *continued*
aortic — *continued*
    incompetency, insufficiency or regurgitation
        I06.2
        with mitral (valve) disease I08.0
            with tricuspid (valve) disease I08.3
        mitral (valve) disease I08.0
            with tricuspid (valve) disease I08.3
        tricuspid (valve) disease I08.2
            with mitral (valve) disease I08.3
    specified cause NEC I35.0
    syphilitic A52.03
aqueduct of Sylvius (congenital) Q03.0
    with spina bifida — *see* Spina bifida, by site, with
        hydrocephalus
    acquired G91.1
artery NEC (*see also* Arteriosclerosis) I77.1
    celiac I77.4
    cerebral — *see* Occlusion, artery, cerebral
    extremities — *see* Arteriosclerosis, extremities
    precerebral — *see* Occlusion, artery, precerebral
    pulmonary (congenital) Q25.6
        acquired I28.8
    renal I70.1
    stent
        coronary T82.855 ☑
        peripheral T82.856 ☑
bile duct (common) (hepatic) K83.1
    congenital Q44.3
bladder-neck (acquired) N32.0
    congenital Q64.31
brain G93.89
bronchus J98.09
    congenital Q32.3
    syphilitic A52.72
cardia (stomach) K22.2
    congenital Q39.3
cardiovascular — *see* Disease, cardiovascular
caudal M48.08
cervix, cervical (canal) N88.2
    congenital Q51.828
    in pregnancy or childbirth — *see* Pregnancy,
        complicated by, abnormal cervix
colon (*see also* Obstruction, intestine)
    congenital Q42.9
    specified NEC Q42.8
colostomy K94.03
common (bile) duct K83.1
    congenital Q44.3
coronary (artery) — *see* Disease, heart, ischemic,
    atherosclerotic
cystic duct — *see* Obstruction, gallbladder
due to presence of device, implant or graft (*see also*
    Complications, by site and type, specified NEC)
    T85.858 ☑
    arterial graft NEC T82.858 ☑
    breast (implant) T85.858 ☑
    catheter T85.858 ☑
        dialysis (renal) T82.858 ☑
            intraperitoneal T85.858 ☑
        infusion NEC T82.858 ☑
            spinal (epidural) (subdural) T85.850 ☑
        urinary (indwelling) T83.85 ☑
    fixation, internal (orthopedic) NEC T84.85 ☑
    gastrointestinal (bile duct) (esophagus)
        T85.858 ☑
    genital NEC T83.85 ☑
    heart NEC T82.857 ☑
    joint prosthesis T84.85 ☑
    ocular (corneal graft) (orbital implant) NEC
        T85.858 ☑
    orthopedic NEC T84.85 ☑
    specified NEC T85.858 ☑
    urinary NEC T83.85 ☑
    vascular NEC T82.858 ☑
    ventricular intracranial shunt T85.850 ☑
duodenum K31.5
    congenital Q41.0
ejaculatory duct NEC N50.89
endocervical os — *see* Stenosis, cervix
enterostomy K94.13
esophagus K22.2
    congenital Q39.3
    syphilitic A52.79
    congenital A50.59 *[K23]*
eustachian tube — *see* Obstruction, eustachian
    tube
external ear canal (acquired) H61.30 ☑
    congenital Q16.1
    due to
        inflammation H61.32 ☑
        trauma H61.31 ☑

☑ **Additional character required**

Stenosis — *continued*
  external ear canal — *continued*
    postprocedural H95.81 ☑
    specified cause NEC H61.39 ☑
  gallbladder — *see* Obstruction, gallbladder
  glottis J38.6
  heart valve (congenital) Q24.8
    aortic Q23.0
    mitral Q23.2
    pulmonary Q22.1
    tricuspid Q22.4
  hepatic duct K83.1
  hymen N89.6
  hypertrophic subaortic (idiopathic) I42.1
  ileum (*see also* Obstruction, intestine, specified
      NEC) K56.699
    congenital Q41.2
  infundibulum cardia Q24.3
  intervertebral foramina (*see also* Lesion,
      biomechanical, specified NEC)
    connective tissue M99.79
      abdomen M99.79
      cervical region M99.71
      cervicothoracic M99.71
      head region M99.70
      lumbar region M99.73
      lumbosacral M99.73
      occipitocervical M99.70
      sacral region M99.74
      sacrococcygeal M99.74
      sacroiliac M99.74
      specified NEC M99.79
      thoracic region M99.72
      thoracolumbar M99.72
    disc M99.79
      abdomen M99.79
      cervical region M99.71
      cervicothoracic M99.71
      head region M99.70
      lower extremity M99.76
      lumbar region M99.73
      lumbosacral M99.73
      occipitocervical M99.70
      pelvic M99.75
      rib cage M99.78
      sacral region M99.74
      sacrococcygeal M99.74
      sacroiliac M99.74
      specified NEC M99.79
      thoracic region M99.72
      thoracolumbar M99.72
      upper extremity M99.77
    osseous M99.69
      abdomen M99.69
      cervical region M99.61
      cervicothoracic M99.61
      head region M99.60
      lower extremity M99.66
      lumbar region M99.63
      lumbosacral M99.63
      occipitocervical M99.60
      pelvic M99.65
      rib cage M99.68
      sacral region M99.64
      sacrococcygeal M99.64
      sacroiliac M99.64
      specified NEC M99.69
      thoracic region M99.62
      thoracolumbar M99.62
      upper extremity M99.67
    subluxation — *see* Stenosis, intervertebral
        foramina, osseous
  intestine (*see also* Obstruction, intestine)
    congenital (small) Q41.9
      large Q42.9
        specified NEC Q42.8
      specified NEC Q41.8
  jejunum (*see also* Obstruction, intestine, specified
      NEC) K56.699
    congenital Q41.1
  lacrimal (passage)
    canaliculi H04.54 ☑
    congenital Q10.5
    duct H04.55 ☑
    punctum H04.56 ☑
    sac H04.57 ☑
  lacrimonasal duct — *see* Stenosis, lacrimal, duct
    congenital Q10.5
  larynx J38.6
    congenital NEC Q31.8
      subglottic Q31.1
    syphilitic A52.73

Stenosis — *continued*
  larynx — *continued*
    congenital A50.59 [*J99*]
  mitral (chronic) (inactive) (valve) I05.0
    with
      aortic valve disease I08.0
      incompetence, insufficiency or regurgitation
          I05.2
    active or acute I01.1
      with rheumatic or Sydenham's chorea I02.0
    congenital Q23.2
    specified cause, except rheumatic I34.2
    syphilitic A52.03
  myocardium, myocardial (*see also* Degeneration,
      myocardial)
    hypertrophic subaortic (idiopathic) I42.1
  nares (anterior) (posterior) J34.89
    congenital Q30.0
  nasal duct (*see also* Stenosis, lacrimal, duct)
    congenital Q10.5
  nasolacrimal duct (*see also* Stenosis, lacrimal, duct)
    congenital Q10.5
  neural canal (*see also* Lesion, biomechanical,
      specified NEC)
    connective tissue M99.49
      abdomen M99.49
      cervical region M99.41
      cervicothoracic M99.41
      head region M99.40
      lower extremity M99.46
      lumbar region M99.43
      lumbosacral M99.43
      occipitocervical M99.40
      pelvic M99.45
      rib cage M99.48
      sacral region M99.44
      sacrococcygeal M99.44
      sacroiliac M99.44
      specified NEC M99.49
      thoracic region M99.42
      thoracolumbar M99.42
      upper extremity M99.47
    intervertebral disc M99.59
      abdomen M99.59
      cervical region M99.51
      cervicothoracic M99.51
      head region M99.50
      lower extremity M99.56
      lumbar region M99.53
      lumbosacral M99.53
      occipitocervical M99.50
      pelvic M99.55
      rib cage M99.58
      sacral region M99.54
      sacrococcygeal M99.54
      sacroiliac M99.54
      specified NEC M99.59
      thoracic region M99.52
      thoracolumbar M99.52
      upper extremity M99.57
    osseous M99.39
      abdomen M99.39
      cervical region M99.31
      cervicothoracic M99.31
      head region M99.30
      lower extremity M99.36
      lumbar region M99.33
      lumbosacral M99.33
      pelvic M99.35
      rib cage M99.38
      occipitocervical M99.30
      sacral region M99.34
      sacrococcygeal M99.34
      sacroiliac M99.34
      specified NEC M99.39
      thoracic region M99.32
      thoracolumbar M99.32
      upper extremity M99.37
    subluxation M99.29
      cervical region M99.21
      cervicothoracic M99.21
      head region M99.20
      lower extremity M99.26
      lumbar region M99.23
      lumbosacral M99.23
      occipitocervical M99.20
      pelvic M99.25
      rib cage M99.28
      sacral region M99.24
      sacrococcygeal M99.24
      sacroiliac M99.24
      specified NEC M99.29

Stenosis — *continued*
  neural canal — *continued*
    thoracic region M99.22
    thoracolumbar M99.22
    upper extremity M99.27
  organ or site, congenital NEC — *see* Atresia, by site
  papilla of Vater K83.1
  pulmonary (artery) (congenital) Q25.6
    with ventricular septal defect, transposition of
        aorta, and hypertrophy of right ventricle
        Q21.3
    acquired I28.8
    in tetralogy of Fallot Q21.3
    infundibular Q24.3
    subvalvular Q24.3
    supravalvular Q25.6
    valve I37.0
      with insufficiency I37.2
      congenital Q22.1
      rheumatic I09.89
        with aortic, mitral or tricuspid (valve) disease
            I08.8
    vein, acquired I28.8
    vessel NEC I28.8
  pulmonic (congenital) Q22.1
    infundibular Q24.3
    subvalvular Q24.3
  pylorus (hypertrophic) (acquired) K31.1
    adult K31.1
    congenital Q40.0
    infantile Q40.0
  rectum (sphincter) — *see* Stricture, rectum
  renal artery I70.1
    congenital Q27.1
  salivary duct (any) K11.8
  sphincter of Oddi K83.1
  spinal M48.00
    cervical region M48.02
    cervicothoracic region M48.03
    lumbar region (NOS) (without neurogenic
        claudication) M48.061
      with neurogenic claudication M48.062
    lumbosacral region M48.07
    occipito-atlanto-axial region M48.01
    sacrococcygeal region M48.08
    thoracic region M48.04
    thoracolumbar region M48.05
  stent
    vascular
      end stent
        adjacent to stent — *see* Arteriosclerosis
        within the stent
          coronary T82.855 ☑
          peripheral T82.856 ☑
      in stent
        coronary vessel T82.855 ☑
        peripheral vessel T82.856 ☑
  stomach, hourglass K31.2
  subaortic (congenital) Q24.4
    hypertrophic (idiopathic) I42.1
  subglottic J38.6
    congenital Q31.1
    postprocedural J95.5
  trachea J39.8
    congenital Q32.1
    syphilitic A52.73
    tuberculous NEC A15.5
  tracheostomy J95.03
  tricuspid (valve) I07.0
    with
      aortic (valve) disease I08.2
      incompetency, insufficiency or regurgitation
          I07.2
        with aortic (valve) disease I08.2
          with mitral (valve) disease I08.3
      mitral (valve) disease I08.1
        with aortic (valve) disease I08.3
    congenital Q22.4
    nonrheumatic I36.0
      with insufficiency I36.2
  tubal N97.1
  ureter — *see* Atresia, ureter
  ureteropelvic junction, congenital Q62.11
  ureterovesical orifice, congenital Q62.12
  urethra (valve) (*see also* Stricture, urethra)
    congenital Q64.32
  urinary meatus, congenital Q64.33
  vagina N89.5
    congenital Q52.4
    in pregnancy — *see* Pregnancy, complicated by,
        abnormal vagina
      causing obstructed labor O65.5

Stenosis - Strangury

Stenosis — *continued*
- valve (cardiac) (heart) (*see also* Endocarditis) I38
  - congenital Q24.8
    - aortic Q23.0
    - mitral Q23.2
    - pulmonary Q22.1
    - tricuspid Q22.4
  - vena cava (inferior) (superior) I87.1
    - congenital Q26.0
  - vesicourethral orifice Q64.31
  - vulva N90.5

Stent jail T82.897 ☑

Stercolith (impaction) K56.41
- appendix K38.1

Stercoraceous, stercoral ulcer K63.3
- anus or rectum K62.6

Stereotypies NEC F98.4

Sterility — *see* Infertility

Sterilization — *see* Encounter (for), sterilization

Sternalgia — *see* Angina

Sternopagus Q89.4

Sternum bifidum Q76.7

Steroid
- effects (adverse) (adrenocortical) (iatrogenic)
  - cushingoid E24.2
    - correct substance properly administered — *see* Table of Drugs and Chemicals, by drug, adverse effect
    - overdose or wrong substance given or taken — *see* Table of Drugs and Chemicals, by drug, poisoning
  - diabetes — *see* category E09 ☑
    - correct substance properly administered — *see* Table of Drugs and Chemicals, by drug, adverse effect
    - overdose or wrong substance given or taken — *see* Table of Drugs and Chemicals, by drug, poisoning
  - fever R50.2
  - insufficiency E27.3
    - correct substance properly administered — *see* Table of Drugs and Chemicals, by drug, adverse effect
    - overdose or wrong substance given or taken — *see* Table of Drugs and Chemicals, by drug, poisoning
  - responder H40.04 ☑

Stevens-Johnson disease or syndrome L51.1
- toxic epidermal necrolysis overlap L51.3

Stewart-Morel syndrome M85.2

Sticker's disease B08.3

Sticky eye — *see* Conjunctivitis, acute, mucopurulent

Stieda's disease — *see* Bursitis, tibial collateral

Stiff neck — *see* Torticollis

Stiff-man syndrome G25.82

Stiffness, joint NEC M25.60
- ankle M25.67 ☑
- ankylosis — *see* Ankylosis, joint
- contracture — *see* Contraction, joint
- elbow M25.62 ☑
- foot M25.67 ☑
- hand M25.64 ☑
- hip M25.65 ☑
- knee M25.66 ☑
- shoulder M25.61 ☑
- wrist M25.63 ☑

Stigmata congenital syphilis A50.59

Stillbirth P95

Still-Felty syndrome — *see* Felty's syndrome

Still's disease or syndrome (juvenile) M08.20
- adult-onset M06.1
- ankle M08.27 ☑
- elbow M08.22 ☑
- foot joint M08.27 ☑
- hand joint M08.24 ☑
- hip M08.25 ☑
- knee M08.26 ☑
- multiple site M08.29
- shoulder M08.21 ☑
- vertebra M08.28
- wrist M08.23 ☑

Stimulation, ovary E28.1

Sting (venomous) (with allergic or anaphylactic shock) — *see* Table of Drugs and Chemicals, by animal or substance, poisoning

Stippled epiphyses Q78.8

Stitch
- abscess T81.41 ☑
- burst (in operation wound) — *see* Disruption, wound, operation

Stokes-Adams disease or syndrome I45.9

Stokes' disease E05.00
- with thyroid storm E05.01

Stokvis (-Talma) disease D74.8

Stoma malfunction
- colostomy K94.03
- enterostomy K94.13
- gastrostomy K94.23
- ileostomy K94.13
- tracheostomy J95.03

Stomach — *see* condition

Stomatitis (denture) (ulcerative) K12.1
- angular K13.0
  - due to dietary or vitamin deficiency E53.0
- aphthous K12.0
- bovine B08.61
- candidal B37.0
- catarrhal K12.1
- diphtheritic A36.89
- due to
  - dietary deficiency E53.0
  - thrush B37.0
  - vitamin deficiency
    - B group NEC E53.9
    - B2 (riboflavin) E53.0
- epidemic B08.8
- epizootic B08.8
- follicular K12.1
- gangrenous A69.0
- Geotrichum B48.3
- herpesviral, herpetic B00.2
- herpetiformis K12.0
- malignant K12.1
- membranous acute K12.1
- monilial B37.0
- mycotic B37.0
- necrotizing ulcerative A69.0
- parasitic B37.0
- septic K12.1
- spirochetal A69.1
- suppurative (acute) K12.2
- ulceromembranous A69.1
- vesicular K12.1
  - with exanthem (enteroviral) B08.4
  - virus disease A93.8
- Vincent's A69.1

Stomatocytosis D58.8

Stomatomycosis B37.0

Stomatorrhagia K13.79

Stone(s) (*see also* Calculus)
- bladder (diverticulum) N21.0
- cystine E72.09
- heart syndrome I50.1
- kidney N20.0
- prostate N42.0
- pulpal (dental) K04.2
- renal N20.0
- salivary gland or duct (any) K11.5
- urethra (impacted) N21.1
- urinary (duct) (impacted) (passage) N20.9
  - bladder (diverticulum) N21.0
  - lower tract N21.9
  - specified NEC N21.8
- xanthine E79.8 *[N22]*

Stonecutter's lung J62.8

Stonemason's asthma, disease, lung or pneumoconiosis J62.8

Stoppage
- heart — *see* Arrest, cardiac
- urine — *see* Retention, urine

Storm, thyroid — *see* Thyrotoxicosis

Strabismus (congenital) (nonparalytic) H50.9
- concomitant H50.40
  - convergent — *see* Strabismus, convergent concomitant
  - divergent — *see* Strabismus, divergent concomitant
- convergent concomitant H50.00
  - accommodative component H50.43
  - alternating H50.05
    - with
      - A pattern H50.06
      - specified nonconcomitances NEC H50.08
      - V pattern H50.07
    - monocular H50.01 ☑
      - with
        - A pattern H50.02 ☑
        - specified nonconcomitances NEC H50.04 ☑
        - V pattern H50.03 ☑
      - intermittent H50.31 ☑
        - alternating H50.32
  - cyclotropia H50.41 ☑

Strabismus — *continued*
- divergent concomitant H50.10
  - alternating H50.15
    - with
      - A pattern H50.16
      - specified nonconcomitances NEC H50.18
      - V pattern H50.17
    - monocular H50.11 ☑
      - with
        - A pattern H50.12 ☑
        - specified nonconcomitances NEC H50.14 ☑
        - V pattern H50.13 ☑
      - intermittent H50.33 ☑
        - alternating H50.34
- Duane's syndrome H50.81 ☑
- due to adhesions, scars H50.69
- heterophoria H50.50
  - alternating H50.55
  - cyclophoria H50.54
  - esophoria H50.51
  - exophoria H50.52
  - vertical H50.53
- heterotropia H50.40
  - intermittent H50.30
- hypertropia H50.2 ☑
- hypotropia — *see* Hypertropia
- latent H50.50
- mechanical H50.60
  - Brown's sheath syndrome H50.61 ☑
  - specified type NEC H50.69
- monofixation syndrome H50.42
- paralytic H49.9
  - abducens nerve H49.2 ☑
  - fourth nerve H49.1 ☑
  - Kearns-Sayre syndrome H49.81 ☑
  - ophthalmoplegia (external)
    - progressive H49.4 ☑
      - with pigmentary retinopathy H49.81 ☑
    - total H49.3 ☑
  - sixth nerve H49.2 ☑
  - specified type NEC H49.88 ☑
  - third nerve H49.0 ☑
  - trochlear nerve H49.1 ☑
- specified type NEC H50.89
- vertical H50.2 ☑

Strain
- back S39.012 ☑
- cervical S16.1 ☑
- eye NEC — *see* Disturbance, vision, subjective
- heart — *see* Disease, heart
- low back S39.012 ☑
- mental NOS Z73.3
- muscle (tendon) — *see* Injury, muscle, by site, strain
- neck S16.1 ☑
- postural (*see also* Disorder, soft tissue, due to use)
- physical NOS Z73.3
  - work-related Z56.6
- psychological NEC Z73.3
- tendon — *see* Injury, muscle, by site, strain

Straining, on urination R39.16

Strand, vitreous — *see* Opacity, vitreous, membranes and strands

Strangulation, strangulated (*see also* Asphyxia, traumatic)
- appendix K38.8
- bladder-neck N32.0
- bowel or colon K56.2
- food or foreign body — *see* Foreign body, by site
- hemorrhoids — *see* Hemorrhoids, with complication
- hernia (*see also* Hernia, by site, with obstruction)
  - with gangrene — *see* Hernia, by site, with gangrene
- intestine (large) (small) K56.2
  - with hernia (*see also* Hernia, by site, with obstruction)
    - with gangrene — *see* Hernia, by site, with gangrene
- mesentery K56.2
- mucus — *see* Asphyxia, mucus
- omentum K56.2
- organ or site, congenital NEC — *see* Atresia, by site
- ovary — *see* Torsion, ovary
- penis N48.89
  - foreign body T19.4 ☑
- rupture — *see* Hernia, by site, with obstruction
- stomach due to hernia (*see also* Hernia, by site, with obstruction)
  - with gangrene — *see* Hernia, by site, with gangrene
- vesicourethral orifice N32.0

Strangury R30.0

☑ **Additional character required**

Straw itch B88.0
Strawberry
  gallbladder K82.4
  mark Q82.5
  tongue (red) (white) K14.3
Streak(s)
  macula, angioid H35.33
  ovarian Q50.32
Strephosymbolia F81.0
  secondary to organic lesion R48.8
Streptobacillary fever A25.1
Streptobacillosis A25.1
Streptobacillus moniliformis A25.1
Streptococcus, streptococcal (*see also* condition)
  as cause of disease classified elsewhere B95.5
  group
    A, as cause of disease classified elsewhere B95.0
    B, as cause of disease classified elsewhere B95.1
    D, as cause of disease classified elsewhere B95.2
  pneumoniae, as cause of disease classified
    elsewhere B95.3
  specified NEC, as cause of disease classified
    elsewhere B95.4
Streptomycosis B47.1
Streptotrichosis A48.8
Stress F43.9
  family — *see* Disruption, family
  fetal P84
    complicating pregnancy O77.9
    due to drug administration O77.1
  mental NEC Z73.3
    work-related Z56.6
  physical NEC Z73.3
    work-related Z56.6
  polycythemia D75.1
  reaction (*see also* Reaction, stress) F43.9
  work schedule Z56.3
Stretching, nerve — *see* Injury, nerve
Striae albicantes, atrophicae or distensae (cutis) L90.6
Stricture (*see also* Stenosis)
  ampulla of Vater K83.1
  anus (sphincter) K62.4
    congenital Q42.3
      with fistula Q42.2
    infantile Q42.3
      with fistula Q42.2
  aorta (ascending) (congenital) Q25.1
    arteriosclerotic I70.0
    calcified I70.0
    supravalvular, congenital Q25.3
  aortic (valve) — *see* Stenosis, aortic
  aqueduct of Sylvius (congenital) Q03.0
    with spina bifida — *see* Spina bifida, by site, with
      hydrocephalus
    acquired G91.1
  artery I77.1
    basilar — *see* Occlusion, artery, basilar
    carotid — *see* Occlusion, artery, carotid
    celiac I77.4
    congenital (peripheral) Q27.8
      cerebral Q28.3
      coronary Q24.5
      digestive system Q27.8
      lower limb Q27.8
      retinal Q14.1
      specified site NEC Q27.8
      umbilical Q27.0
      upper limb Q27.8
    coronary — *see* Disease, heart, ischemic,
      atherosclerotic
      congenital Q24.5
    precerebral — *see* Occlusion, artery, precerebral
    pulmonary (congenital) Q25.6
      acquired I28.8
    renal I70.1
    vertebral — *see* Occlusion, artery, vertebral
  auditory canal (external) (congenital)
    acquired — *see* Stenosis, external ear canal
  bile duct (common) (hepatic) K83.1
    congenital Q44.3
    postoperative K91.89
  bladder N32.89
    neck N32.0
  bowel — *see* Obstruction, intestine
  brain G93.89
  bronchus J98.09
    congenital Q32.3
    syphilitic A52.72
  cardia (stomach) K22.2
    congenital Q39.3
  cardiac (*see also* Disease, heart)
    orifice (stomach) K22.2

Stricture — *continued*
  cecum — *see* Obstruction, intestine
  cervix, cervical (canal) N88.2
    congenital Q51.828
    in pregnancy — *see* Pregnancy, complicated by,
      abnormal cervix
      causing obstructed labor O65.5
  colon (*see also* Obstruction, intestine)
    congenital Q42.9
      specified NEC Q42.8
  colostomy K94.03
  common (bile) duct K83.1
  coronary (artery) — *see* Disease, heart, ischemic,
    atherosclerotic
  cystic duct — *see* Obstruction, gallbladder
  digestive organs NEC, congenital Q45.8
  duodenum K31.5
    congenital Q41.0
  ear canal (external) (congenital) Q16.1
    acquired — *see* Stricture, auditory canal, acquired
  ejaculatory duct N50.89
  enterostomy K94.13
  esophagus K22.2
    congenital Q39.3
    syphilitic A52.79
      congenital A50.59 [K23]
  eustachian tube (*see also* Obstruction, eustachian
    tube)
    congenital Q17.8
  fallopian tube N97.1
    gonococcal A54.24
    tuberculous A18.17
  gallbladder — *see* Obstruction, gallbladder
  glottis J38.6
  heart (*see also* Disease, heart)
    valve (*see also* Endocarditis) I38
      aortic Q23.0
      mitral Q23.2
      pulmonary Q22.1
      tricuspid Q22.4
  hepatic duct K83.1
  hourglass, of stomach K31.2
  hymen N89.6
  hypopharynx J39.2
  ileum (*see also* Obstruction, intestine, specified
    NEC) K56.699
    congenital Q41.2
  intestine (*see also* Obstruction, intestine)
    congenital (small) Q41.9
      large Q42.9
        specified NEC Q42.8
      specified NEC Q41.8
    ischemic K55.1
  jejunum (*see also* Obstruction, intestine, specified
    NEC) K56.699
    congenital Q41.1
  lacrimal passages (*see also* Stenosis, lacrimal)
    congenital Q10.5
  larynx J38.6
    congenital NEC Q31.8
      subglottic Q31.1
    syphilitic A52.73
      congenital A50.59 [J99]
  meatus
    ear (congenital) Q16.1
      acquired — *see* Stricture, auditory canal,
        acquired
    osseous (ear) (congenital) Q16.1
      acquired — *see* Stricture, auditory canal, acquired
    urinarius (*see also* Stricture, urethra)
      congenital Q64.33
  mitral (valve) — *see* Stenosis, mitral
  myocardium, myocardial I51.5
    hypertrophic subaortic (idiopathic) I42.1
  nares (anterior) (posterior) J34.89
    congenital Q30.0
  nasal duct (*see also* Stenosis, lacrimal, duct)
    congenital Q10.5
  nasolacrimal duct (*see also* Stenosis, lacrimal, duct)
    congenital Q10.5
  nasopharynx J39.2
    syphilitic A52.73
  nose J34.89
    congenital Q30.0
  nostril (anterior) (posterior) J34.89
    congenital Q30.0
    syphilitic A52.73
      congenital A50.59 [J99]
  organ or site, congenital NEC — *see* Atresia, by site
  os uteri — *see* Stricture, cervix
  osseous meatus (ear) (congenital) Q16.1
    acquired — *see* Stricture, auditory canal, acquired

Stricture — *continued*
  oviduct — *see* Stricture, fallopian tube
  pelviureteric junction (congenital) Q62.11
    acquired, with hydronephrosis N13.0
  penis, by foreign body T19.4 ☑
  pharynx J39.2
  prostate N42.89
  pulmonary, pulmonic
    artery (congenital) Q25.6
      acquired I28.8
      noncongenital I28.8
    infundibulum (congenital) Q24.3
    valve I37.0
      congenital Q22.1
    vein, acquired I28.8
    vessel NEC I28.8
  punctum lacrimale (*see also* Stenosis, lacrimal,
    punctum)
    congenital Q10.5
  pylorus (hypertrophic) K31.1
    adult K31.1
    congenital Q40.0
    infantile Q40.0
  rectosigmoid (*see also* Obstruction, intestine,
    specified NEC) K56.699
  rectum (sphincter) K62.4
    congenital Q42.1
      with fistula Q42.0
    due to
      chlamydial lymphogranuloma A55
      irradiation K91.89
      lymphogranuloma venereum A55
    gonococcal A54.6
    inflammatory (chlamydial) A55
    syphilitic A52.74
    tuberculous A18.32
  renal artery I70.1
    congenital Q27.1
  salivary duct or gland (any) K11.8
  sigmoid (flexure) — *see* Obstruction, intestine
  spermatic cord N50.89
  stoma (following) (of)
    colostomy K94.03
    enterostomy K94.13
    gastrostomy K94.23
    ileostomy K94.13
    tracheostomy J95.03
  stomach K31.89
    congenital Q40.2
    hourglass K31.2
  subaortic Q24.4
    hypertrophic (acquired) (idiopathic) I42.1
  subglottic J38.6
  syphilitic NEC A52.79
  trachea J39.8
    congenital Q32.1
    syphilitic A52.73
    tuberculous NEC A15.5
  tracheostomy J95.03
  tricuspid (valve) — *see* Stenosis, tricuspid
  tunica vaginalis N50.89
  ureter (postoperative) N13.5
    with
      hydronephrosis N13.1
        with infection N13.6
      pyelonephritis (chronic) N11.1
    congenital — *see* Atresia, ureter
    tuberculous A18.11
  ureteropelvic junction (congenital) Q62.11
    acquired, with hydronephrosis N13.0
  ureterovesical orifice N13.5
    with infection N13.6
  urethra (organic) (spasmodic) (*see also* Stricture,
    urethra, male) N35.919
    associated with schistosomiasis B65.0 [N37]
    congenital Q64.39
      valvular (posterior) Q64.2
    due to
      infection — *see* Stricture, urethra, postinfective
      trauma — *see* Stricture, urethra, post-traumatic
    female N35.92
    gonococcal, gonorrheal A54.01
    infective NEC — *see* Stricture, urethra,
      postinfective
    late effect (sequelae) of injury — *see* Stricture,
      urethra, post-traumatic
    male N35.919
      anterior urethra N35.914
      bulbous urethra N35.912
      meatal N35.911
      membranous urethra N35.913
      overlapping sites N35.916

Stricture - Subluxation

Stricture — *continued*
 urethra — *continued*
  postcatheterization — *see* Stricture, urethra, postprocedural
  postinfective NEC
   female N35.12
   male N35.119
    anterior urethra N35.114
    bulbous urethra N35.112
    meatal N35.111
    membranous urethra N35.113
    overlapping sites N35.116
  postobstetric N35.021
  postoperative — *see* Stricture, urethra, postprocedural
  postprocedural
   female N99.12
   male N99.114
    anterior bulbous urethra N99.113
    bulbous urethra N99.111
    fossa navicularis N99.115
    meatal N99.110
    membranous urethra N99.112
    overlapping sites N99.116
  post-traumatic
   female N35.028
    due to childbirth N35.021
   male N35.014
    anterior urethra N35.013
    bulbous urethra N35.011
    meatal N35.010
    membranous urethra N35.012
    overlapping sites N35.016
  sequela (late effect) of
   childbirth N35.021
   injury — *see* Stricture, urethra, post-traumatic
  specified cause NEC
   female N35.82
   male N35.819
    anterior urethra N35.814
    bulbous urethra N35.812
    meatal N35.811
    membranous urethra N35.813
    overlapping sites N35.816
  syphilitic A52.76
  traumatic — *see* Stricture, urethra, post-traumatic
  valvular (posterior), congenital Q64.2
 urinary meatus — *see* Stricture, urethra
 uterus, uterine (synechiae) N85.6
  os (external) (internal) — *see* Stricture, cervix
 vagina (outlet) — *see* Stenosis, vagina
 valve (cardiac) (heart) (*see also* Endocarditis)
  congenital
   aortic Q23.0
   mitral Q23.2
   pulmonary Q22.1
   tricuspid Q22.4
 vas deferens N50.89
  congenital Q55.4
 vein I87.1
 vena cava (inferior) (superior) NEC I87.1
  congenital Q26.0
 vesicourethral orifice N32.0
  congenital Q64.31
 vulva (acquired) N90.5
Stridor R06.1
 congenital (larynx) P28.89
Stridulous — *see* condition
Stroke (apoplectic) (brain) (embolic) (ischemic) (paralytic) (thrombotic) I63.9
 cryptogenic (*see also* Infarction, cerebral) I63.9
 epileptic — *see* Epilepsy
 heat T67.01 ☑
  exertional T67.02 ☑
  specified NEC T67.09 ☑
 in evolution I63.9
 intraoperative
  during cardiac surgery I97.810
  during other surgery I97.811
 lightning — *see* Lightning
 meaning
  cerebral hemorrhage - code to Hemorrhage, intracranial
  cerebral infarction - code to Infarction, cerebral
 postprocedural
  following cardiac surgery I97.820
  following other surgery I97.821
 sun T67.01 ☑
  specified NEC T67.09 ☑
 unspecified (NOS) I63.9
Stromatosis, endometrial D39.0
Strongyloidiasis, strongyloidosis B78.9

Strongyloidiasis — *continued*
 cutaneous B78.1
 disseminated B78.7
 intestinal B78.0
Strophulus pruriginosus L28.2
Struck by lightning — *see* Lightning
Struma (*see also* Goiter)
 Hashimoto E06.3
 lymphomatosa E06.3
 nodosa (simplex) E04.9
  endemic E01.2
   multinodular E01.1
  multinodular E04.2
   iodine-deficiency related E01.1
  toxic or with hyperthyroidism E05.20
   with thyroid storm E05.21
   multinodular E05.20
    with thyroid storm E05.21
   uninodular E05.10
    with thyroid storm E05.11
  toxicosa E05.20
   with thyroid storm E05.21
   multinodular E05.20
    with thyroid storm E05.21
   uninodular E05.10
    with thyroid storm E05.11
  uninodular E04.1
 ovarii D27. ☑
 Riedel's E06.5
Strumipriva cachexia E03.4
Strümpell-Marie spine — *see* Spondylitis, ankylosing
Strümpell-Westphal pseudosclerosis E83.01
Stuart deficiency disease (factor X) D68.2
Stuart-Prower factor deficiency (factor X) D68.2
Student's elbow — *see* Bursitis, elbow, olecranon
Stump — *see* Amputation
Stunting, nutritional E45
Stupor (catatonic) R40.1
 depressive (single episode) F32.89
  recurrent episode F33.8
 dissociative F44.2
 manic F30.2
 manic-depressive F31.89
 psychogenic (anergic) F44.2
 reaction to exceptional stress (transient) F43.0
Sturge (-Weber) (-Dimitri) (-Kalischer) disease or syndrome Q85.8
Stuttering F80.81
 adult onset F98.5
 childhood onset F80.81
 following cerebrovascular disease — *see* Disorder, fluency. following cerebrovascular disease
 in conditions classified elsewhere R47.82
Sty, stye (external) (internal) (meibomian) (zeisian) — *see* Hordeolum
Subacidity, gastric K31.89
 psychogenic F45.8
Subacute — *see* condition
Subarachnoid — *see* condition
Subcortical — *see* condition
Subcostal syndrome, nerve compression — *see* Mononeuropathy, upper limb, specified site NEC
Subcutaneous, subcuticular — *see* condition
Subdural — *see* condition
Subendocardium — *see* condition
Subependymoma
 specified site — *see* Neoplasm, uncertain behavior, by site
 unspecified site D43.2
Suberosis J67.3
Subglossitis — *see* Glossitis
Subhemophilia D66
Subinvolution
 breast (postlactational) (postpuerperal) N64.89
 puerperal O90.89
 uterus (chronic) (nonpuerperal) N85.3
  puerperal O90.89
Sublingual — *see* condition
Sublinguitis — *see* Sialoadenitis
Subluxatable hip Q65.6
Subluxation (*see also* Dislocation)
 acromioclavicular S43.11 ☑
 ankle S93.0 ☑
 atlantoaxial, recurrent M43.4
  with myelopathy M43.3
 carpometacarpal (joint) NEC S63.05 ☑
  thumb S63.04 ☑
 complex, vertebral — *see* Complex, subluxation
 congenital (*see also* Malposition, congenital)
  hip — *see* Dislocation, hip, congenital, partial
  joint (excluding hip)
   lower limb Q68.8

Subluxation — *continued*
 congenital — *continued*
  shoulder Q68.8
  upper limb Q68.8
 elbow (traumatic) S53.10 ☑
  anterior S53.11 ☑
  lateral S53.14 ☑
  medial S53.13 ☑
  posterior S53.12 ☑
  specified type NEC S53.19 ☑
 finger S63.20 ☑
  index S63.20 ☑
  interphalangeal S63.22 ☑
   distal S63.24 ☑
    index S63.24 ☑
    little S63.24 ☑
    middle S63.24 ☑
    ring S63.24 ☑
   index S63.22 ☑
   little S63.22 ☑
   middle S63.22 ☑
   proximal S63.23 ☑
    index S63.23 ☑
    little S63.23 ☑
    middle S63.23 ☑
    ring S63.23 ☑
   ring S63.22 ☑
  little S63.20 ☑
  metacarpophalangeal S63.21 ☑
   index S63.21 ☑
   little S63.21 ☑
   middle S63.21 ☑
   ring S63.21 ☑
  middle S63.20 ☑
  ring S63.20 ☑
 foot S93.30 ☑
  specified site NEC S93.33 ☑
  tarsal joint S93.31 ☑
  tarsometatarsal joint S93.32 ☑
  toe — *see* Subluxation, toe
 hip S73.00 ☑
  anterior S73.03 ☑
   obturator S73.02 ☑
  central S73.04 ☑
  posterior S73.01 ☑
 interphalangeal (joint)
  finger S63.22 ☑
   distal joint S63.24 ☑
    index S63.24 ☑
    little S63.24 ☑
    middle S63.24 ☑
    ring S63.24 ☑
   index S63.22 ☑
   little S63.22 ☑
   middle S63.22 ☑
   proximal joint S63.23 ☑
    index S63.23 ☑
    little S63.23 ☑
    middle S63.23 ☑
    ring S63.23 ☑
   ring S63.22 ☑
  thumb S63.12 ☑
  toe S93.13 ☑
   great S93.13 ☑
   lesser S93.13 ☑
 joint prosthesis — *see* Complications, joint prosthesis, mechanical, displacement, by site
 knee S83.10 ☑
  cap — *see* Subluxation, patella
  patella — *see* Subluxation, patella
  proximal tibia
   anteriorly S83.11 ☑
   laterally S83.14 ☑
   medially S83.13 ☑
   posteriorly S83.12 ☑
  specified type NEC S83.19 ☑
 lens — *see* Dislocation, lens, partial
 ligament, traumatic — *see* Sprain, by site
 metacarpal (bone)
  proximal end S63.06 ☑
 metacarpophalangeal (joint)
  finger S63.21 ☑
   index S63.21 ☑
   little S63.21 ☑
   middle S63.21 ☑
   ring S63.21 ☑
  thumb S63.11 ☑
 metatarsophalangeal joint S93.14 ☑
  great toe S93.14 ☑
  lesser toe S93.14 ☑
 midcarpal (joint) S63.03 ☑

☑ **Additional character required**

Subluxation — *continued*
  patella S83.00 ☑
    lateral S83.01 ☑
    recurrent (nontraumatic) — *see* Dislocation,
      patella, recurrent, incomplete
    specified type NEC S83.09 ☑
  pathological — *see* Dislocation, pathological
  radial head S53.00 ☑
    anterior S53.01 ☑
    nursemaid's elbow S53.03 ☑
    posterior S53.02 ☑
    specified type NEC S53.09 ☑
  radiocarpal (joint) S63.02 ☑
  radioulnar (joint)
    distal S63.01 ☑
    proximal — *see* Subluxation, elbow
  shoulder
    congenital Q68.8
    girdle S43.30 ☑
      scapula S43.31 ☑
      specified site NEC S43.39 ☑
    traumatic S43.00 ☑
      anterior S43.01 ☑
      inferior S43.03 ☑
      posterior S43.02 ☑
      specified type NEC S43.08 ☑
  sternoclavicular (joint) S43.20 ☑
    anterior S43.21 ☑
    posterior S43.22 ☑
  symphysis (pubis)
  thumb S63.103 ☑
    interphalangeal joint — *see* Subluxation,
      interphalangeal (joint), thumb
    metacarpophalangeal joint — *see* Subluxation,
      metacarpophalangeal (joint), thumb
  toe(s) S93.10 ☑
    great S93.10 ☑
      interphalangeal joint S93.13 ☑
      metatarsophalangeal joint S93.14 ☑
    interphalangeal joint S93.13 ☑
    lesser S93.10 ☑
      interphalangeal joint S93.13 ☑
      metatarsophalangeal joint S93.14 ☑
    metatarsophalangeal joint S93.149 ☑
  ulnohumeral joint — *see* Subluxation, elbow
  vertebral
    recurrent NEC — *see* subcategory M43.5 ☑
    traumatic
      cervical S13.100 ☑
        atlantoaxial joint S13.120 ☑
        atlantooccipital joint S13.110 ☑
        atloidooccipital joint S13.110 ☑
        joint between
          C0 and C1 S13.110 ☑
          C1 and C2 S13.120 ☑
          C2 and C3 S13.130 ☑
          C3 and C4 S13.140 ☑
          C4 and C5 S13.150 ☑
          C5and C6 S13.160 ☑
          C6and C7 S13.170 ☑
          C7and T1 S13.180 ☑
        occipitoatloid joint S13.110 ☑
      lumbar S33.100 ☑
        joint between
          L1and L2 S33.110 ☑
          L2and L3 S33.120 ☑
          L3 and L4 S33.130 ☑
          L4and L5 S33.140 ☑
      thoracic S23.100 ☑
        joint between
          T1and T2 S23.110 ☑
          T2and T3 S23.120 ☑
          T3 and T4 S23.122 ☑
          T4 and T5 S23.130 ☑
          T5 and T6 S23.132 ☑
          T6 and T7 S23.140 ☑
          T7 and T8 S23.142 ☑
          T8 and T9 S23.150 ☑
          T9 and T10 S23.152 ☑
          T10 and T11 S23.160 ☑
          T11 and T12 S23.162 ☑
          T12 and L1 S23.170 ☑
  ulna
    distal end S63.07 ☑
    proximal end — *see* Subluxation, elbow
  wrist (carpal bone) S63.00 ☑
    carpometacarpal joint — *see* Subluxation,
      carpometacarpal (joint)
    distal radioulnar joint — *see* Subluxation,
      radioulnar (joint), distal
    metacarpal bone, proximal — *see* Subluxation,
      metacarpal (bone), proximal end

Subluxation — *continued*
  wrist — *continued*
    midcarpal — *see* Subluxation, midcarpal (joint)
    radiocarpal joint — *see* Subluxation, radiocarpal
      (joint)
    recurrent — *see* Dislocation, recurrent, wrist
    specified site NEC S63.09 ☑
    ulna — *see* Subluxation, ulna, distal end
Submaxillary — *see* condition
Submersion (fatal) (nonfatal) T75.1 ☑
Submucous — *see* condition
Subnormal, subnormality
  accommodation (old age) H52.4
  mental — *see* Disability, intellectual
  temperature (accidental) T68 ☑
Subphrenic — *see* condition
Subscapular nerve — *see* condition
Subseptus uterus Q51.28
Subsiding appendicitis K36
Substance (other psychoactive)-induced
  anxiety disorder F19.980
  bipolar and related disorder F19.94
  delirium F19.921
  depressive disorder F19.94
  major neurocognitive disorder F19.97
  mild neurocognitive disorder F19.988
  obsessive-compulsive and related disorder
    F19.988
  psychotic disorder F19.959
  sexual dysfunction F19.981
  sleep disorder F19.982
Substernal thyroid E04.9
  congenital Q89.2
Substitution disorder F44.9
Subtentorial — *see* condition
Subthyroidism (acquired) (*see also* Hypothyroidism)
  congenital E03.1
Succenturiate placenta O43.19 ☑
Sucking thumb, child (excessive) F98.8
Sudamen, sudamina L74.1
Sudanese kala-azar B55.0
Sudden
  heart failure — *see* Failure, heart
  hearing loss — *see* Deafness, sudden
Sudeck's atrophy, disease, or syndrome — *see*
  Algoneurodystrophy
Suffocation — *see* Asphyxia, traumatic
Sugar
  blood
    high (transient) R73.9
    low (transient) E16.2
  in urine R81
Suicide, suicidal (attempted) T14.91 ☑
  by poisoning — *see* Table of Drugs and Chemicals
  history of (personal) Z91.5
    in family Z81.8
  ideation — *see* Ideation, suicidal
  risk
    meaning personal history of attempted suicide
      Z91.5
    meaning suicidal ideation — *see* Ideation, suicidal
  tendencies
    meaning personal history of attempted suicide
      Z91.5
    meaning suicidal ideation — *see* Ideation, suicidal
  trauma — *see* nature of injury by site
Suipestifer infection — *see* Infection, salmonella
Sulfhemoglobinemia, sulphemoglobinemia (acquired)
  (with methemoglobinemia) D74.8
Sumatran mite fever A75.3
Summer — *see* condition
Sunburn L55.9
  due to
    tanning bed (acute) L56.8
      chronic L57.8
    ultraviolet radiation (acute) L56.8
      chronic L57.8
  first degree L55.0
  second degree L55.1
  third degree L55.2
SUNCT (short lasting unilateral neuralgiform headache
  with conjunctival injection and tearing) G44.059
  intractable G44.051
  not intractable G44.059
Sundowning F05
Sunken acetabulum — *see* Derangement, joint,
  specified type NEC, hip
Sunstroke T67.01 ☑
  specified NEC T67.09 ☑
Superfecundation — *see* Pregnancy, multiple
Superfetation — *see* Pregnancy, multiple
Superinvolution (uterus) N85.8

Supernumerary (congenital)
  aortic cusps Q23.8
  auditory ossicles Q16.3
  bone Q79.8
  breast Q83.1
  carpal bones Q74.0
  cusps, heart valve NEC Q24.8
    aortic Q23.8
    mitral Q23.2
    pulmonary Q22.3
  digit(s) Q69.9
  ear (lobule) Q17.0
  fallopian tube Q50.6
  finger Q69.0
  hymen Q52.4
  kidney Q63.0
  lacrimonasal duct Q10.6
  lobule (ear) Q17.0
  mitral cusps Q23.2
  muscle Q79.8
  nipple(s) Q83.3
  organ or site not listed — *see* Accessory
  ossicles, auditory Q16.3
  ovary Q50.31
  oviduct Q50.6
  pulmonary, pulmonic cusps Q22.3
  rib Q76.6
    cervical or first (syndrome) Q76.5
  roots (of teeth) K00.2
  spleen Q89.09
  tarsal bones Q74.2
  teeth K00.1
  testis Q55.29
  thumb Q69.1
  toe Q69.2
  uterus Q51.28
  vagina Q52.1 ☑
  vertebra Q76.49
Supervision (of)
  contraceptive — *see* Prescription, contraceptives
  dietary (for) Z71.3
    allergy (food) Z71.3
    colitis Z71.3
    diabetes mellitus Z71.3
    food allergy or intolerance Z71.3
    gastritis Z71.3
    hypercholesterolemia Z71.3
    hypoglycemia Z71.3
    intolerance (food) Z71.3
    obesity Z71.3
    specified NEC Z71.3
  healthy infant or child Z76.2
    foundling Z76.1
  high-risk pregnancy — *see* Pregnancy, complicated
    by, high, risk
  lactation Z39.1
  pregnancy — *see* Pregnancy, supervision of
Supplemental teeth K00.1
Suppression
  binocular vision H53.34
  lactation O92.5
  menstruation N94.89
  ovarian secretion E28.39
  renal N28.9
  urine, urinary secretion R34
Suppuration, suppurative (*see also* condition)
  accessory sinus (chronic) — *see* Sinusitis
  adrenal gland
  antrum (chronic) — *see* Sinusitis, maxillary
  bladder — *see* Cystitis
  brain G06.0
    sequelae G09
  breast N61.1
    puerperal, postpartum or gestational — *see*
      Mastitis, obstetric, purulent
  dental periosteum M27.3
  ear (middle) (*see also* Otitis, media)
    external NEC — *see* Otitis, externa, infective
    internal — *see* subcategory H83.0 ☑
  ethmoidal (chronic) (sinus) — *see* Sinusitis,
    ethmoidal
  fallopian tube — *see* Salpingo-oophoritis
  frontal (chronic) (sinus) — *see* Sinusitis, frontal
  gallbladder (acute) K81.0
  gum K05.20
    generalized — *see* Periodontitis, aggressive,
      generalized
    localized — *see* Periodontitis, aggressive, localized
  intracranial G06.0
  joint — *see* Arthritis, pyogenic or pyemic
  labyrinthine — *see* subcategory H83.0 ☑
  lung — *see* Abscess, lung

Suppuration — *continued*
  mammary gland N61.1
    puerperal, postpartum O91.12
      associated with lactation O91.13
  maxilla, maxillary M27.2
    sinus (chronic) — *see* Sinusitis, maxillary
  muscle — *see* Myositis, infective
  nasal sinus (chronic) — *see* Sinusitis
  pancreas, acute (*see also* Pancreatitis, acute) K85.80
  parotid gland — *see* Sialoadenitis
  pelvis, pelvic
    female — *see* Disease, pelvis, inflammatory
    male K65.0
  pericranial — *see* Osteomyelitis
  salivary duct or gland (any) — *see* Sialoadenitis
  sinus (accessory) (chronic) (nasal) — *see* Sinusitis
  sphenoidal sinus (chronic) — *see* Sinusitis, sphenoidal
  thymus (gland) E32.1
  thyroid (gland) E06.0
  tonsil — *see* Tonsillitis
  uterus — *see* Endometritis
Supraeruption of tooth (teeth) M26.34
Supraglottitis J04.30
  with obstruction J04.31
Suprarenal (gland) — *see* condition
Suprascapular nerve — *see* condition
Suprasellar — *see* condition
Surfer's knots or nodules S89.8 ☑
Surgical
  emphysema T81.82 ☑
  procedures, complication or misadventure — *see* Complications, surgical procedures
  shock T81.10 ☑
Surveillance (of) (for) (*see also* Observation)
  alcohol abuse Z71.41
  contraceptive — *see* Prescription, contraceptives
  dietary Z71.3
  drug abuse Z71.51
Susceptibility to disease, genetic Z15.89
  malignant neoplasm Z15.09
    breast Z15.01
    endometrium Z15.04
    ovary Z15.02
    prostate Z15.03
    specified NEC Z15.09
  multiple endocrine neoplasia Z15.81
Suspected condition, ruled out (*see also* Observation, suspected)
  amniotic cavity and membrane Z03.71
  cervical shortening Z03.75
  fetal anomaly Z03.73
  fetal growth Z03.74
  maternal and fetal conditions NEC Z03.79
  newborn (*see also* Observation, newborn, suspected condition ruled out) Z05.9
  oligohydramnios Z03.71
  placental problem Z03.72
  polyhydramnios Z03.71
Suspended uterus
  in pregnancy or childbirth — *see* Pregnancy, complicated by, abnormal uterus
Sutton's nevus D22.9
Suture
  burst (in operation wound) T81.31 ☑
    external operation wound T81.31 ☑
    internal operation wound T81.32 ☑
  inadvertently left in operation wound — *see* Foreign body, accidentally left during a procedure
  removal Z48.02
Swab inadvertently left in operation wound — *see* Foreign body, accidentally left during a procedure
Swallowed, swallowing
  difficulty — *see* Dysphagia
  foreign body — *see* Foreign body, alimentary tract
Swan-neck deformity (finger) — *see* Deformity, finger, swan-neck
Swearing, compulsive F42.8
  in Gilles de la Tourette's syndrome F95.2
Sweat, sweats
  fetid L75.0
  night R61
Sweating, excessive R61
Sweeley-Klionsky disease E75.21
Sweet's disease or dermatosis L98.2
Swelling (of) R60.9
  abdomen, abdominal (not referable to any particular organ) — *see* Mass, abdominal
  ankle — *see* Effusion, joint, ankle
  arm M79.89
    forearm M79.89

Swelling — *continued*
  breast (*see also* Lump, breast) N63.0
  Calabar B74.3
  cervical gland R59.0
  chest, localized R22.2
  ear H93.8 ☑
  extremity (lower) (upper) — *see* Disorder, soft tissue, specified type NEC
  finger M79.89
  foot M79.89
  glands R59.9
    generalized R59.1
    localized R59.0
  hand M79.89
  head (localized) R22.0
  inflammatory — *see* Inflammation
  intra-abdominal — *see* Mass, abdominal
  joint — *see* Effusion, joint
  leg M79.89
    lower M79.89
  limb — *see* Disorder, soft tissue, specified type NEC
  localized (skin) R22.9
    chest R22.2
    head R22.0
    limb
      lower — *see* Mass, localized, limb, lower
      upper — *see* Mass, localized, limb, upper
    neck R22.1
    trunk R22.2
  neck (localized) R22.1
  pelvic — *see* Mass, abdominal
  scrotum N50.89
  splenic — *see* Splenomegaly
  testis N50.89
  toe M79.89
  umbilical R19.09
  wandering, due to Gnathostoma (spinigerum) B83.1
  white — *see* Tuberculosis, arthritis
Swift (-Feer) **disease**
  overdose or wrong substance given or taken — *see* Table of Drugs and Chemicals, by drug, poisoning
Swimmer's
  cramp T75.1 ☑
  ear H60.33 ☑
  itch B65.3
Swimming in the head R42
Swollen — *see* Swelling
Swyer syndrome Q99.1
Sycosis L73.8
  barbae (not parasitic) L73.8
  contagiosa (mycotic) B35.0
  lupoides L73.8
  mycotic B35.0
  parasitic B35.0
  vulgaris L73.8
Sydenham's chorea — *see* Chorea, Sydenham's
Sylvatic yellow fever A95.0
Sylvest's disease B33.0
Symblepharon H11.23 ☑
  congenital Q10.3
Symond's syndrome G93.2
Sympathetic — *see* condition
Sympatheticotonia G90.8
Sympathicoblastoma
  specified site — *see* Neoplasm, malignant, by site
  unspecified site C74.90
Sympathogonioma — *see* Sympathicoblastoma
Symphalangy (fingers) (toes) Q70.9
Symptoms NEC R68.89
  breast NEC N64.59
  cold J00
  development NEC R63.8
  factitious, self-induced — *see* Disorder, factitious
  genital organs, female R10.2
  involving
    abdomen NEC R19.8
    appearance NEC R46.89
    awareness R41.9
      altered mental status R41.82
      amnesia — *see* Amnesia
      borderline intellectual functioning R41.83
      coma — *see* Coma
      disorientation R41.0
      neurologic neglect syndrome R41.4
      senile cognitive decline R41.81
      specified symptom NEC R41.89
    behavior NEC R46.89
    cardiovascular system NEC R09.89
    chest NEC R09.89
    circulatory system NEC R09.89

Symptoms — *continued*
  involving — *continued*
    cognitive functions R41.9
      altered mental status R41.82
      amnesia — *see* Amnesia
      borderline intellectual functioning R41.83
      coma — *see* Coma
      disorientation R41.0
      neurologic neglect syndrome R41.4
      senile cognitive decline R41.81
      specified symptom NEC R41.89
    development NEC R62.50
    digestive system NEC R19.8
    emotional state NEC R45.89
      emotional lability R45.86
    food and fluid intake R63.8
    general perceptions and sensations R44.9
      specified NEC R44.8
    musculoskeletal system R29.91
      specified NEC R29.898
    nervous system R29.90
      specified NEC R29.818
    pelvis NEC R19.8
    respiratory system NEC R09.89
    skin and integument R23.9
    urinary system R39.9
  menopausal N95.1
  metabolism NEC R63.8
  neurotic F48.8
  of infancy R68.19
  pelvis NEC, female R10.2
  skin and integument NEC R23.9
  subcutaneous tissue NEC R23.9
  viral cold J00
Sympus Q74.2
Syncephalus Q89.4
Synchondrosis
  abnormal (congenital) Q78.8
  ischiopubic M91.0
Synchysis (scintillans) (senile) (vitreous body) H43.89
Syncope (near) (pre-) R55
  anginosa I20.8
  bradycardia R00.1
  cardiac R55
  carotid sinus G90.01
  due to spinal (lumbar) puncture G97.1
  heart R55
  heat T67.1 ☑
  laryngeal R05
  psychogenic F48.8
  tussive R05
  vasoconstriction R55
  vasodepressor R55
  vasomotor R55
  vasovagal R55
Syndactylism, syndactyly Q70.9
  complex (with synostosis)
    fingers Q70.0 ☑
    toes Q70.2 ☑
  simple (without synostosis)
    fingers Q70.1 ☑
    toes Q70.3 ☑
Syndrome (*see also* Disease)
  5q minus NOS D46.C
  48,XXXX Q97.1
  49,XXXXX Q97.1
  abdominal
    acute R10.0
    muscle deficiency Q79.4
  abnormal innervation H02.519
    left H02.516
      lower H02.515
      upper H02.514
    right H02.513
      lower H02.512
      upper H02.511
  abstinence, neonatal P96.1
  acid pulmonary aspiration, obstetric O74.0
  acquired immunodeficiency — *see* Human, immunodeficiency virus (HIV) disease
  acute abdominal R10.0
  acute respiratory distress (adult) (child) J80
    idiopathic J84.114
  Adair-Dighton Q78.0
  Adams-Stokes (-Morgagni) I45.9
  adiposogenital E23.6
  adrenal
    hemorrhage (meningococcal) A39.1
    meningococcic A39.1
  adrenocortical — *see* Cushing's, syndrome
  adrenogenital E25.9

☑ **Additional character required**

Syndrome — *continued*
adrenogenital — *continued*
congenital, associated with enzyme deficiency E25.0
afferent loop NEC K91.89
Alagille's Q44.7
alcohol withdrawal (without convulsions) — *see* Dependence, alcohol, with, withdrawal
Alder's D72.0
Aldrich (-Wiskott) D82.0
alien hand R41.4
Alport Q87.81
alveolar hypoventilation E66.2
alveolocapillary block J84.10
amnesic, amnestic (confabulatory) (due to) — *see* Disorder, amnesic
amyostatic (Wilson's disease) E83.01
androgen insensitivity E34.50
complete E34.51
partial E34.52
androgen resistance (*see also* Syndrome, androgen insensitivity) E34.50
Angelman Q93.51
anginal — *see* Angina
ankyloglossia superior Q38.1
anterior
chest wall R07.89
cord G83.82
spinal artery G95.19
compression M47.019
cervical region M47.012
cervicothoracic region M47.013
lumbar region M47.016
occipito-atlanto-axial region M47.011
thoracic region M47.014
thoracolumbar region M47.015
tibial M76.81 ☑
antibody deficiency D80.9
agammaglobulinemic D80.1
hereditary D80.0
congenital D80.0
hypogammaglobulinemic D80.1
hereditary D80.0
anticardiolipin (-antibody) D68.61
antidepressant discontinuation T43.205 ☑
antiphospholipid (-antibody) D68.61
aortic
arch M31.4
bifurcation I74.09
aortomesenteric duodenum occlusion K31.5
apical ballooning (transient left ventricular) I51.81
arcuate ligament I77.4
argentaffin, argentaffinoma E34.0
Arnold-Chiari — *see* Arnold-Chiari disease
Arrillaga-Ayerza I27.0
arterial tortuosity Q87.82
arteriovenous steal T82.898 ☑
Asherman's N85.6
aspiration, of newborn — *see* Aspiration, by substance, with pneumonia
meconium P24.01
ataxia-telangiectasia G11.3
auriculotemporal G50.8
autoerythrocyte sensitization (Gardner-Diamond) D69.2
autoimmune polyglandular E31.0
autoimmune lymphoproliferative [ALPS] D89.82
autoinflammatory M04.9
specified type NEC M04.8
autosomal — *see* Abnormal, autosomes
Avellis' G46.8
Ayerza (-Arrillaga) I27.0
Babinski-Nageotte G83.89
Bakwin-Krida Q78.5
bare lymphocyte D81.6
Barré-Guillain G61.0
Barré-Liéou M53.0
Barrett's — *see* Barrett's, esophagus
Barsony-Polgar K22.4
Barsony-Teschendorf K22.4
Barth E78.71
Bartter's E26.81
basal cell nevus Q87.89
Basedow's E05.00
with thyroid storm E05.01
basilar artery G45.0
Batten-Steinert G71.11
battered
baby or child — *see* Maltreatment, child, physical abuse
spouse — *see* Maltreatment, adult, physical abuse
Beals Q87.40

Syndrome — *continued*
Beau's I51.5
Beck's I65.8
Benedikt's G46.3
Béquez César (-Steinbrinck-Chédiak-Higashi) E70.330
Bernhardt-Roth — *see* Meralgia paresthetica
Bernheim's — *see* Failure, heart, right
big spleen D73.1
bilateral polycystic ovarian E28.2
Bing-Horton's — *see* Horton's headache
Birt-Hogg-Dube syndrome Q87.89
Björck (-Thorsen) E34.0
black
lung J60
widow spider bite — *see* Toxicity, venom, spider, black widow
Blackfan-Diamond D61.01
Blau M04.8
blind loop K90.2
congenital Q43.8
postsurgical K91.2
blue sclera Q78.0
blue toe I75.02 ☑
Boder-Sedgewick G11.3
Boerhaave's K22.3
Borjeson Forssman Lehmann Q89.8
Bouillaud's I01.9
Bourneville (-Pringle) Q85.1
Bouveret (-Hoffman) I47.9
brachial plexus G54.0
bradycardia-tachycardia I49.5
brain (nonpsychotic) F09
with psychosis, psychotic reaction F09
acute or subacute — *see* Delirium
congenital — *see* Disability, intellectual
organic F09
post-traumatic (nonpsychotic) F07.81
psychotic F09
personality change F07.0
postcontusional F07.81
post-traumatic, nonpsychotic F07.81
psycho-organic F09
psychotic F06.8
brain stem stroke G46.3
Brandt's (acrodermatitis enteropathica) E83.2
broad ligament laceration N83.8
Brock's J98.11
bronze baby P83.88
Brown-Sequard G83.81
Brugada I49.8
bubbly lung P27.0
Buchem's M85.2
Budd-Chiari I82.0
bulbar (progressive) G12.22
Bürger-Grütz E78.3
Burke's K86.89
Burnett's (milk-alkali) E83.52
burning feet E53.9
Bywaters' T79.5 ☑
Call-Fleming I67.841
carbohydrate-deficient glycoprotein (CDGS) E77.8
carcinogenic thrombophlebitis I82.1
carcinoid E34.0
cardiac asthma I50.1
cardiacos negros I27.0
cardiofaciocutaneous Q87.89
cardiopulmonary-obesity E66.2
cardiorenal — *see* Hypertension, cardiorenal
cardiorespiratory distress (idiopathic), newborn P22.0
cardiovascular renal — *see* Hypertension, cardiorenal
carotid
artery (hemispheric) (internal) G45.1
body G90.01
sinus G90.01
carpal tunnel G56.0 ☑
Cassidy (-Scholte) E34.0
cat cry Q93.4
cat eye Q92.8
cauda equina G83.4
causalgia — *see* Causalgia
celiac K90.0
artery compression I77.4
axis I77.4
central pain G89.0
cerebellar
hereditary G11.9
stroke G46.4
cerebellomedullary malformation — *see* Spina bifida

Syndrome — *continued*
cerebral
artery
anterior G46.1
middle G46.0
posterior G46.2
gigantism E22.0
cervical (root) M53.1
disc — *see* Disorder, disc, cervical, with neuritis
fusion Q76.1
posterior, sympathicus M53.0
rib Q76.5
sympathetic paralysis G90.2
cervicobrachial (diffuse) M53.1
cervicocranial M53.0
cervicodorsal outlet G54.2
cervicothoracic outlet G54.0
Céstan (-Raymond) I65.8
Charcot's (angina cruris) (intermittent claudication) I73.9
Charcot-Weiss-Baker G90.09
CHARGE Q89.8
Chédiak-Higashi (-Steinbrinck) E70.330
chest wall R07.1
Chiari's (hepatic vein thrombosis) I82.0
Chilaiditi's Q43.3
child maltreatment — *see* Maltreatment, child
chondrocostal junction M94.0
chondroectodermal dysplasia Q77.6
chromosome 4 short arm deletion Q93.3
chromosome 5 short arm deletion Q93.4
chronic
infantile neurological, cutaneous and articular (CINCA) M04.2
pain G89.4
personality F68.8
Churg-Strauss M30.1
Clarke-Hadfield K86.89
Clerambault's automatism G93.89
Clouston's (hidrotic ectodermal dysplasia) Q82.4
clumsiness, clumsy child F82
cluster headache G44.009
intractable G44.001
not intractable G44.009
Coffin-Lowry Q89.8
cold injury (newborn) P80.0
combined immunity deficiency D81.9
compartment (deep) (posterior) (traumatic) T79.A0 ☑
abdomen T79.A3 ☑
lower extremity (hip, buttock, thigh, leg, foot, toes) T79.A2 ☑
nontraumatic
abdomen M79.A3
lower extremity (hip, buttock, thigh, leg, foot, toes) M79.A2 ☑
specified site NEC M79.A9
upper extremity (shoulder, arm, forearm, wrist, hand, fingers) M79.A1 ☑
postprocedural — *see* Syndrome, compartment, nontraumatic
specified site NEC T79.A9 ☑
upper extremity (shoulder, arm, forearm, wrist, hand, fingers) T79.A1 ☑
complex regional pain — *see* Syndrome, pain, complex regional
compression T79.5 ☑
anterior spinal — *see* Syndrome, anterior, spinal artery, compression
cauda equina G83.4
celiac artery I77.4
vertebral artery M47.029
occipito-atlanto-axial region M47.021
cervical region M47.022
concussion F07.81
congenital
affecting multiple systems NEC Q87.89
central alveolar hypoventilation G47.35
facial diplegia Q87.0
muscular hypertrophy-cerebral Q87.89
oculo-auriculovertebral Q87.0
oculofacial diplegia (Moebius) Q87.0
rubella (manifest) P35.0
congestion-fibrosis (pelvic), female N94.89
congestive dysmenorrhea N94.6
Conn's E26.01
connective tissue M35.9
overlap NEC M35.1
conus medullaris G95.81
cord
anterior G83.82
posterior G83.83

Syndrome

Syndrome — *continued*
- coronary
  - acute NEC I24.9
  - insufficiency or intermediate I20.0
  - slow flow I20.8
- Costen's (complex) M26.69
- costochondral junction M94.0
- costoclavicular G54.0
- costovertebral E22.0
- Cowden Q85.8
- craniovertebral M53.0
- Creutzfeldt-Jakob — *see* Creutzfeldt-Jakob disease or syndrome
- cri-du-chat Q93.4
- crib death R99
- cricopharyngeal — *see* Dysphagia
- croup J05.0
- CRPS I — *see* Syndrome, pain, complex regional I
- crush T79.5 ☑
- cubital tunnel — *see* Lesion, nerve, ulnar
- Curschmann (-Batten) (-Steinert) G71.11
- Cushing's E24.9
  - alcohol-induced E24.4
  - due to
    - alcohol
      - drugs E24.2
      - ectopic ACTH E24.3
      - overproduction of pituitary ACTH E24.0
  - drug-induced E24.2
  - overdose or wrong substance given or taken — *see* Table of Drugs and Chemicals, by drug, poisoning
  - pituitary-dependent E24.0
  - specified type NEC E24.8
- cryopyrin-associated periodic M04.2
- cryptophthalmos Q87.0
- cystic duct stump K91.5
- Dana-Putnam D51.0
- Danbolt (-Cross) (acrodermatitis enteropathica) E83.2
- Dandy-Walker Q03.1
  - with spina bifida Q07.01
- Danlos' (*see also* Syndrome, Ehlers-Danlos) Q79.60
- defibrination (*see also* Fibrinolysis)
  - with
    - antepartum hemorrhage — *see* Hemorrhage, antepartum, with coagulation defect
    - intrapartum hemorrhage — *see* Hemorrhage, complicating, delivery
  - newborn P60
  - postpartum O72.3
- Degos' I77.89
- Déjérine-Roussy G89.0
- delayed sleep phase G47.21
- demyelinating G37.9
- dependence — *see* F10-F19 with fourth character .2
- depersonalization (-derealization) F48.1
- De Quervain E34.51
- de Toni-Fanconi (-Debré) E72.09
  - with cystinosis E72.04
- diabetes mellitus-hypertension-nephrosis — *see* Diabetes, nephrosis
- diabetes mellitus in newborn infant P70.2
- diabetes-nephrosis — *see* Diabetes, nephrosis
- diabetic amyotrophy — *see* Diabetes, amyotrophy
- dialysis associated steal T82.898 ☑
- Diamond-Blackfan D61.01
- Diamond-Gardener D69.2
- DIC (diffuse or disseminated intravascular coagulopathy) D65
- di George's D82.1
- Dighton's Q78.0
- disequilibrium E87.8
- Döhle body-panmyelopathic D72.0
- dorsolateral medullary G46.4
- double athetosis G80.3
- Down (*see also* Down syndrome) Q90.9
- Dresbach's (elliptocytosis) D58.1
- Dressler's (postmyocardial infarction) I24.1
  - postcardiotomy I97.0
- drug withdrawal, infant of dependent mother P96.1
- dry eye H04.12 ☑
  - due to abnormality
    - chromosomal Q99.9
      - sex
        - female phenotype Q97.9
        - male phenotype Q98.9
        - specified NEC Q99.8
- dumping (postgastrectomy) K91.1
  - nonsurgical K31.89
- Dupré's (meningism) R29.1
- dysmetabolic X E88.81

Syndrome — *continued*
- dyspraxia, developmental F82
- Eagle-Barrett Q79.4
- Eaton-Lambert — *see* Syndrome, Lambert-Eaton
- Ebstein's Q22.5
- ectopic ACTH E24.3
- eczema-thrombocytopenia D82.0
- Eddowes' Q78.0
- effort (psychogenic) F45.8
- Eisenmenger's I27.83
- Ehlers-Danlos Q79.60
  - classical (cEDS) (classical EDS) Q79.61
  - hypermobile (hEDS) (hypermobile EDS) Q79.62
  - specified NEC Q79.69
  - vascular (vascular EDS) (vEDS) Q79.63
- Ekman's Q78.0
- electric feet E53.8
- Ellis-van Creveld Q77.6
- empty nest Z60.0
- endocrine-hypertensive E27.0
- entrapment — *see* Neuropathy, entrapment
- eosinophilia-myalgia M35.8
- epileptic (*see also* Epilepsy, by type)
  - absence G40.A09
    - intractable G40.A19
      - with status epilepticus G40.A11
      - without status epilepticus G40.A19
    - not intractable G40.A09
      - with status epilepticus G40.A01
      - without status epilepticus G40.A09
- Erdheim-Chester (ECD) E88.89
- Erdheim's E22.0
- erythrocyte fragmentation D59.4
- Evans D69.41
- exhaustion F48.8
- extrapyramidal G25.9
  - specified NEC G25.89
- eye retraction — *see* Strabismus
- eyelid-malar-mandible Q87.0
- Faber's D50.9
- facial pain, paroxysmal G50.0
- Fallot's Q21.3
- familial cold autoinflammatory M04.2
- familial eczema-thrombocytopenia (Wiskott-Aldrich) D82.0
- Fanconi (-de Toni) (-Debré) E72.09
  - with cystinosis E72.04
- Fanconi's (anemia) (congenital pancytopenia) D61.09
- fatigue
  - chronic R53.82
  - psychogenic F48.8
- faulty bowel habit K59.39
- Feil-Klippel (brevicollis) Q76.1
- Felty's — *see* Felty's syndrome
- fertile eunuch E23.0
- fetal
  - alcohol (dysmorphic) Q86.0
  - hydantoin Q86.1
- Fiedler's I40.1
- first arch Q87.0
- fish odor E72.89
- Fisher's G61.0
- Fitzhugh-Curtis
  - due to
    - Chlamydia trachomatis A74.81
    - Neisseria gonorrhoea (gonococcal peritonitis) A54.85
- Fitz's (*see also* Pancreatitis, acute) K85.80
- Flajani (-Basedow) E05.00
  - with thyroid storm E05.01
- flatback — *see* Flatback syndrome
- floppy
  - baby P94.2
  - iris (intraoperative) (IFIS) H21.81
  - mitral valve I34.1
- flush E34.0
- Foix-Alajouanine G95.19
- Fong's Q87.2
- food protein-induced enterocolitis (FPIES) K52.21
- foramen magnum G93.5
- Foster-Kennedy H47.14 ☑
- Foville's (peduncular) G46.3
- fragile X Q99.2
- Franceschetti Q75.4
- Frey's
  - auriculotemporal G50.8
  - hyperhidrosis L74.52
- Friderichsen-Waterhouse A39.1
- Froin's G95.89
- frontal lobe F07.0
- Fukuhara E88.49

Syndrome — *continued*
- functional
  - bowel K59.9
  - prepubertal castrate E29.1
- Gaisböck's D75.1
- ganglion (basal ganglia brain) G25.9
  - geniculi G51.1
- Gardner-Diamond D69.2
- gastroesophageal
  - junction K22.0
  - laceration-hemorrhage K22.6
- gastrojejunal loop obstruction K91.89
- Gee-Herter-Heubner K90.0
- Gelineau's G47.419
  - with cataplexy G47.411
- genito-anorectal A55
- Gerstmann-Sträussler-Scheinker (GSS) A81.82
- Gianotti-Crosti L44.4
- giant platelet (Bernard-Soulier) D69.1
- Gilles de la Tourette's F95.2
- Glass Q87.89
- goiter-deafness E07.1
- Goldberg Q89.8
- Goldberg-Maxwell E34.51
- Good's D83.8
- Gopalan' (burning feet) E53.8
- Gorlin's Q87.89
- Gougerot-Blum L81.7
- Gouley's I31.1
- Gower's R55
- gray or grey (newborn) P93.0
  - platelet D69.1
- Gubler-Millard G46.3
- Guillain-Barré (-Strohl) G61.0
- gustatory sweating G50.8
- Hadfield-Clarke K86.89
- hair tourniquet — *see* Constriction, external, by site
- Hamman's J98.19
- hand-foot L27.1
- hand-shoulder G90.8
- hantavirus (cardio)-pulmonary (HPS) (HCPS) B33.4
- happy puppet Q93.51
- Harada's H30.81 ☑
- Hayem-Faber D50.9
- headache NEC G44.89
  - complicated NEC G44.59
- Heberden's I20.8
- Hedinger's E34.0
- Hegglin's D72.0
- HELLP (hemolysis, elevated liver enzymes and low platelet count) O14.2 ☑
  - complicating
    - childbirth O14.24
    - puerperium O14.25
- hemolytic-uremic D59.3
- hemophagocytic, infection-associated D76.2
- Henoch-Schönlein D69.0
- hepatic flexure K59.8
- hepatopulmonary K76.81
- hepatorenal K76.7
  - following delivery O90.4
  - postoperative or postprocedural K91.83
  - postpartum, puerperal O90.4
- hepatourologic K76.7
- Herter (-Gee) (nontropical sprue) K90.0
- Heubner-Herter K90.0
- Heyd's K76.7
- Hilger's G90.09
- histamine-like (fish poisoning) — *see* Poisoning, fish
- histiocytic D76.3
- histiocytosis NEC D76.3
- HIV infection, acute B20
- Hoffmann-Werdnig G12.0
- Hollander-Simons E88.1
- Hoppe-Goldflam G70.00
  - with exacerbation (acute) G70.01
  - in crisis G70.01
- Horner's G90.2
- hungry bone E83.81
- hunterian glossitis D51.0
- Hutchinson's triad A50.53
- hyperabduction G54.0
- hyperammonemia-hyperornithinemia-homocitrullinemia E72.4
- hypereosinophilic (idiopathic) D72.1
- hyperimmunoglobulin D M04.1
- hyperimmunoglobulin E (IgE) D82.4
- hyperkalemic E87.5
- hyperkinetic — *see* Hyperkinesia
- hypermobility M35.7
- hypernatremia E87.0
- hyperosmolarity E87.0

☑ **Additional character required**

Syndrome — *continued*
- hyperperfusion G97.82
- hypersplenic D73.1
- hypertransfusion, newborn P61.1
- hyperventilation F45.8
- hyperviscosity (of serum)
  - polycythemic D75.1
  - sclerothymic D58.8
- hypoglycemic (familial) (neonatal) E16.2
- hypokalemic E87.6
- hyponatremic E87.1
- hypopituitarism E23.0
- hypoplastic left-heart Q23.4
- hypopotassemia E87.6
- hyposmolality E87.1
- hypotension, maternal O26.5 ☑
- hypothenar hammer I73.89
- hypoventilation, obesity (OHS) E66.2
- ICF (intravascular coagulation-fibrinolysis) D65
- idiopathic
  - cardiorespiratory distress, newborn P22.0
  - nephrotic (infantile) N04.9
- iliotibial band M76.3 ☑
- immobility, immobilization (paraplegic) M62.3
- immune reconstitution D89.3
- immune reconstitution inflammatory [IRIS] D89.3
- immunity deficiency, combined D81.9
- immunodeficiency
  - acquired — *see* Human, immunodeficiency virus (HIV) disease
  - combined D81.9
- impending coronary I20.0
- impingement, shoulder M75.4 ☑
- inappropriate secretion of antidiuretic hormone E22.2
- infant
  - of diabetic mother P70.1
    - gestational diabetes P70.0
- infantilism (pituitary) E23.0
- inferior vena cava I87.1
- inspissated bile (newborn) P59.1
- institutional (childhood) F94.2
- insufficient sleep F51.12
- intermediate coronary (artery) I20.0
- interspinous ligament — *see* Spondylopathy, specified NEC
- intestinal
  - carcinoid E34.0
  - knot K56.2
- intravascular coagulation-fibrinolysis (ICF) D65
- iodine-deficiency, congenital E00.9
  - type
    - mixed E00.2
    - myxedematous E00.1
    - neurological E00.0
- IRDS (idiopathic respiratory distress, newborn) P22.0
- irritable
  - bowel K58.9
    - with
      - constipation K58.1
      - diarrhea K58.0
    - mixed K58.2
    - psychogenic F45.8
    - specified NEC K58.8
  - heart (psychogenic) F45.8
  - weakness F48.8
- ischemic
  - bowel (transient) K55.9
    - chronic K55.1
    - due to mesenteric artery insufficiency K55.1
  - steal T82.898 ☑
- IVC (intravascular coagulopathy) D65
- Ivemark's Q89.01
- Jaccoud's — *see* Arthropathy, postrheumatic, chronic
- Jackson's G83.89
- Jakob-Creutzfeldt — *see* Creutzfeldt-Jakob disease or syndrome
- jaw-winking Q07.8
- Jervell-Lange-Nielsen I45.81
- jet lag G47.25
- Job's D71
- Joseph-Diamond-Blackfan D61.01
- jugular foramen G52.7
- Kabuki Q89.8
- Kanner's (autism) F84.0
- Kartagener's Q89.3
- Kelly's D50.1
- Kimmelstiel-Wilson — *see* Diabetes, specified type, with Kimmelsteil-Wilson disease
- Klein (e)-Levine G47.13

Syndrome — *continued*
- Klippel-Feil (brevicollis) Q76.1
- Köhler-Pellegrini-Steida — *see* Bursitis, tibial collateral
- König's K59.8
- Korsakoff (-Wernicke) (nonalcoholic) F04
  - alcoholic F10.26
- Kostmann's D70.0
- Krabbe's congenital muscle hypoplasia Q79.8
- labyrinthine — *see* subcategory H83.2 ☑
- lacunar NEC G46.7
- Lambert-Eaton G70.80
  - in
    - neoplastic disease G73.1
    - specified disease NEC G70.81
- Landau-Kleffner — *see* Epilepsy, specified NEC
- Larsen's Q74.8
- lateral
  - cutaneous nerve of thigh G57.1 ☑
  - medullary G46.4
- Launois' E22.0
- lazy
  - leukocyte D70.8
  - posture M62.3
- Lemiere I80.8
- Lennox-Gastaut G40.812
  - intractable G40.814
    - with status epilepticus G40.813
    - without status epilepticus G40.814
  - not intractable G40.812
    - with status epilepticus G40.811
    - without status epilepticus G40.812
- lenticular, progressive E83.01
- Leopold-Levi's E05.90
- Lev's I44.2
- Li-Fraumeni Z15.01
- Lichtheim's D51.0
- Lightwood's N25.89
- Lignac (de Toni) (-Fanconi) (-Debré) E72.09
  - with cystinosis E72.04
- Likoff's I20.8
- limbic epilepsy personality F07.0
- liver-kidney K76.7
- lobotomy F07.0
- Loffler's J82
- long arm 18 or 21 deletion Q93.89
- long QT I45.81
- Louis-Barré G11.3
- low
  - atmospheric pressure T70.29 ☑
  - back M54.5
  - output (cardiac) I50.9
- lower radicular, newborn (birth injury) P14.8
- Luetscher's (dehydration) E86.0
- Lupus anticoagulant D68.62
- Lutembacher's Q21.1
- macrophage activation D76.1
  - due to infection D76.2
- magnesium-deficiency R29.0
- Majeed M04.8
- Mal de Debarquement R42
- malabsorption K90.9
  - postsurgical K91.2
- malformation, congenital, due to
  - alcohol Q86.0
  - exogenous cause NEC Q86.8
  - hydantoin Q86.1
  - warfarin Q86.2
- malignant
  - carcinoid E34.0
  - neuroleptic G21.0
- Mallory-Weiss K22.6
- mandibulofacial dysostosis Q75.4
- manic-depressive — *see* Disorder, bipolar
- maple-syrup-urine E71.0
- Marable's I77.4
- Marfan's Q87.40
  - with
    - cardiovascular manifestations Q87.418
      - aortic dilation Q87.410
    - ocular manifestations Q87.42
    - skeletal manifestations Q87.43
- Marie's (acromegaly) E22.0
- mast cell activation — *see* Activation, mast cell
- maternal hypotension — *see* Syndrome, hypotension, maternal
- May (-Hegglin) D72.0
- McArdle (-Schmidt) (-Pearson) E74.04
- McQuarrie's E16.2
- meconium plug (newborn) P76.0
- median arcuate ligament I77.4
- Meekeren-Ehlers-Danlos Q79.6 ☑

Syndrome — *continued*
- megavitamin-B6 E67.2
- Meige G24.4
- MELAS E88.41
- Mendelson's O74.0
- MERRF (myoclonic epilepsy associated with ragged-red fibers) E88.42
- mesenteric
  - artery (superior) K55.1
  - vascular insufficiency K55.1
- metabolic E88.81
- metastatic carcinoid E34.0
- micrognathia-glossoptosis Q87.0
- midbrain NEC G93.89
- middle lobe (lung) J98.19
- middle radicular G54.0
- migraine (*see also* Migraine) G43.909
- Mikulicz' K11.8
- milk-alkali E83.52
- Millard-Gubler G46.3
- Miller-Dieker Q93.88
- Miller-Fisher G61.0
- Minkowski-Chauffard D58.0
- Mirizzi's K83.1
- MNGIE (Mitochondrial Neurogastrointestinal Encephalopathy) E88.49
- Möbius, ophthalmoplegic migraine — *see* Migraine, ophthalmoplegic
- monofixation H50.42
- Morel-Moore M85.2
- Morel-Morgagni M85.2
- Morgagni (-Morel) (-Stewart) M85.2
- Morgagni-Adams-Stokes I45.9
- Muckle-Wells M04.2
- mucocutaneous lymph node (acute febrile) (MCLS) M30.3
- multiple endocrine neoplasia (MEN) — *see* Neoplasia, endocrine, multiple (MEN)
- multiple operations — *see* Disorder, factitious
- Mounier-Kuhn Q32.4
  - with bronchiectasis J47.9
    - with
      - exacerbation (acute) J47.1
      - lower respiratory infection J47.0
  - acquired J98.09
    - with bronchiectasis J47.9
      - with
        - exacerbation (acute) J47.1
        - lower respiratory infection J47.0
- myasthenic G70.9
  - in
    - diabetes mellitus — *see* Diabetes, amyotrophy
    - endocrine disease NEC E34.9 *[G73.3]*
    - neoplastic disease (*see also* Neoplasm) D49.9 *[G73.3]*
    - thyrotoxicosis (hyperthyroidism) E05.90 *[G73.3]*
      - with thyroid storm E05.91 *[G73.3]*
- myelodysplastic D46.9
  - with
    - 5q deletion D46.C
    - isolated del (5q) chromosomal abnormality D46.C
  - lesions, low grade D46.20
  - specified NEC D46.Z
- myelopathic pain G89.0
- myeloproliferative (chronic) D47.1
- myofascial pain M79.18
- Naffziger's G54.0
- nail patella Q87.2
- NARP (Neuropathy, Ataxia and Retinitis pigmentosa) E88.49
- neonatal abstinence P96.1
- nephritic (*see also* Nephritis)
  - with edema — *see* Nephrosis
  - acute N00.9
  - chronic N03.9
  - rapidly progressive N01.9
- nephrotic (congenital) (*see also* Nephrosis) N04.9
  - with
    - dense deposit disease N04.6
    - diffuse
      - crescentic glomerulonephritis N04.7
      - endocapillary proliferative glomerulonephritis N04.4
      - membranous glomerulonephritis N04.2
      - mesangial proliferative glomerulonephritis N04.3
      - mesangiocapillary glomerulonephritis N04.5
    - focal and segmental glomerular lesions N04.1
    - minor glomerular abnormality N04.0
    - specified morphological changes NEC N04.8
  - diabetic — *see* Diabetes, nephrosis

Syndrome — continued
- neurologic neglect R41.4
- Nezelof's D81.4
- Nonne-Milroy-Meige Q82.0
- Nothnagel's vasomotor acroparesthesia I73.89
- obesity hypoventilation (OHS) E66.2
- oculomotor H51.9
- ophthalmoplegia-cerebellar ataxia — see Strabismus, paralytic, third nerve
- oral allergy T78.1 ☑
- oral-facial-digital Q87.0
- organic
  - affective F06.30
  - amnesic (not alcohol- or drug-induced) F04
  - brain F09
  - depressive F06.31
  - hallucinosis F06.0
  - personality F07.0
- Ormond's N13.5
- oro-facial-digital Q87.0
- os trigonum Q68.8
- Osler-Weber-Rendu I78.0
- osteoporosis-osteomalacia M83.8
- Osterreicher-Turner Q87.2
- otolith — see subcategory H81.8 ☑
- oto-palatal-digital Q87.0
- outlet (thoracic) G54.0
- ovary
  - polycystic E28.2
  - resistant E28.39
  - sclerocystic E28.2
- Owren's D68.2
- Paget-Schroetter I82.890
- pain (see also Pain)
  - complex regional I G90.50
    - lower limb G90.52 ☑
    - specified site NEC G90.59
    - upper limb G90.51 ☑
  - complex regional II — see Causalgia
- painful
  - bruising D69.2
  - feet E53.8
  - prostate N42.81
- paralysis agitans — see Parkinsonism
- paralytic G83.9
  - specified NEC G83.89
- Parinaud's H51.0
- parkinsonian — see Parkinsonism
- Parkinson's — see Parkinsonism
- paroxysmal facial pain G50.0
- Parry's E05.00
  - with thyroid storm E05.01
- Parsonage (-Aldren)-Turner G54.5
- patella clunk M25.86 ☑
- Paterson (-Brown) (-Kelly) D50.1
- pectoral girdle I77.89
- pectoralis minor I77.89
- pediatric autoimmune neuropsychiatric disorders associated with streptococcal infections (PANDAS) D89.89
- Pelger-Huet D72.0
- pellagra-cerebellar ataxia-renal aminoaciduria E72.02
- pellagroid E52
- Pellegrini-Stieda — see Bursitis, tibial collateral
- pelvic congestion-fibrosis, female N94.89
- penta X Q97.1
- peptic ulcer — see Ulcer, peptic
- perabduction I77.89
- periodic fever M04.1
- periodic fever, aphthous stomatitis, pharyngitis, and adenopathy [PFAPA] M04.8
- periodic headache, in adults and children — see Headache, periodic syndromes in adults and children
- periurethral fibrosis N13.5
- phantom limb (without pain) G54.7
  - with pain G54.6
- pharyngeal pouch D82.1
- Pick's — see Disease, Pick's
- Pickwickian E66.2
- PIE (pulmonary infiltration with eosinophilia) J82
- pigmentary pallidal degeneration (progressive) G23.0
- pineal E34.8
- pituitary E22.0
- plantar fascia M72.2
- placental transfusion — see Pregnancy, complicated by, placental transfusion syndromes
- plateau iris (post-iridectomy) (postprocedural) H21.82
- Plummer-Vinson D50.1

Syndrome — continued
- pluricarential of infancy E40
- plurideficiency E40
- pluriglandular (compensatory) E31.8
  - autoimmune E31.0
- pneumatic hammer T75.21 ☑
- polyangiitis overlap M30.8
- polycarential of infancy E40
- polyglandular E31.8
  - autoimmune E31.0
- polysplenia Q89.09
- pontine NEC G93.89
- popliteal
  - artery entrapment I77.89
  - web Q87.89
  - post endometrial ablation N99.85
- postcardiac injury
  - postcardiotomy I97.0
  - postmyocardial infarction I24.1
- postcardiotomy I97.0
- post chemoembolization - code to associated conditions
- postcholecystectomy K91.5
- postcommissurotomy I97.0
- postconcussional F07.81
- postcontusional F07.81
- postencephalitic F07.89
- posterior
  - cervical sympathetic M53.0
  - cord G83.83
  - fossa compression G93.5
  - reversible encephalopathy (PRES) I67.83
- postgastrectomy (dumping) K91.1
- postgastric surgery K91.1
- postinfarction I24.1
- postlaminectomy NEC M96.1
- postleukotomy F07.0
- postmastectomy lymphedema I97.2
- postmyocardial infarction I24.1
- postoperative NEC T81.9 ☑
  - blind loop K90.2
- postpartum panhypopituitary (Sheehan) E23.0
- postpolio (myelitic) G14
- postthrombotic I87.009
  - with
    - inflammation I87.02 ☑
      - with ulcer I87.03 ☑
    - specified complication NEC I87.09 ☑
    - ulcer I87.01 ☑
      - with inflammation I87.03 ☑
  - asymptomatic I87.00 ☑
- postvagotomy K91.1
- postvalvulotomy I97.0
- postviral NEC G93.3
  - fatigue G93.3
- Potain's K31.0
- potassium intoxication E87.5
- Prader-Willi Q87.11
- Prader-Willi-like Q87.19
- precerebral artery (multiple) (bilateral) G45.2
- preinfarction I20.0
- preleukemic D46.9
- premature senility E34.8
- premenstrual dysphoric F32.81
- premenstrual tension N94.3
- Prinzmetal-Massumi R07.1
- prune belly Q79.4
- pseudocarpal tunnel (sublimis) — see Syndrome, carpal tunnel
- pseudoparalytica G70.00
  - with exacerbation (acute) G70.01
  - in crisis G70.01
- pseudo -Turner's Q87.19
- psycho-organic (nonpsychotic severity) F07.9
  - acute or subacute F05
  - depressive type F06.31
  - hallucinatory type F06.0
  - nonpsychotic severity F07.0
  - specified NEC F07.89
- pulmonary
  - arteriosclerosis I27.0
  - dysmaturity (Wilson-Mikity) P27.0
  - hypoperfusion (idiopathic) P22.0
  - renal (hemorrhagic) (Goodpasture's) M31.0
- pure
  - motor lacunar G46.5
  - sensory lacunar G46.6
- Putnam-Dana D51.0
- pyogenic arthritis, pyoderma gangrenosum, and acne [PAPA] M04.8
- pyramidopallidonigral G20
- pyriformis — see Lesion, nerve, sciatic

Syndrome — continued
- QT interval prolongation I45.81
- radicular NEC — see Radiculopathy
  - upper limbs, newborn (birth injury) P14.3
- rapid time-zone change G47.25
- Rasmussen G04.81
- Raymond (-Céstan) I65.8
- Raynaud's I73.00
  - with gangrene I73.01
- RDS (respiratory distress syndrome, newborn) P22.0
- reactive airways dysfunction J68.3
- Refsum's G60.1
- Reifenstein E34.52
- renal glomerulohyalinosis-diabetic — see Diabetes, nephrosis
- Rendu-Osler-Weber I78.0
- residual ovary N99.83
- resistant ovary E28.39
- respiratory
  - distress
    - acute J80
      - adult J80
      - child J80
      - idiopathic J84.114
    - newborn (idiopathic) (type I) P22.0
      - type II P22.1
- restless legs G25.81
- retinoblastoma (familial) C69.2 ☑
- retroperitoneal fibrosis N13.5
- retroviral seroconversion (acute) Z21
- Reye's G93.7
- Richter — see Leukemia, chronic lymphocytic, B-cell type
- Ridley's I50.1
- right
  - heart, hypoplastic Q22.6
  - ventricular obstruction — see Failure, heart, right
- Romano-Ward (prolonged QT interval) I45.81
- rotator cuff, shoulder (see also Tear, rotator cuff) M75.10 ☑
- Rotes Quérol — see Hyperostosis, ankylosing
- Roth — see Meralgia paresthetica
- rubella (congenital) P35.0
- Ruvalcaba-Myhre-Smith E71.440
- Rytand-Lipsitch I44.2
- salt
  - depletion E87.1
    - due to heat NEC T67.8 ☑
      - causing heat exhaustion or prostration T67.4 ☑
  - low E87.1
- salt-losing N28.89
- SATB2-associated Q87.89
- Scaglietti-Dagnini E22.0
- scalenus anticus (anterior) G54.0
- scapulocostal — see Mononeuropathy, upper limb, specified site NEC
- scapuloperoneal G71.09
- schizophrenic, of childhood NEC F84.5
- Schnitzler D47.2
- Scholte's E34.0
- Schroeder's E27.0
- Schüller-Christian C96.5
- Schwachman's — see Syndrome, Shwachman's
- Schwartz (-Jampel) G71.13
- Schwartz-Bartter E22.2
- scimitar Q26.8
- sclerocystic ovary E28.2
- Seitelberger's G31.89
- septicemic adrenal hemorrhage A39.1
- seroconversion, retroviral (acute) Z21
- serous meningitis G93.2
- severe acute respiratory (SARS) J12.81
- shaken infant T74.4 ☑
- shock (traumatic) T79.4 ☑
  - kidney N17.0
    - following crush injury T79.5 ☑
  - toxic A48.3
- shock-lung J80
- Shone's - code to specific anomalies
- short
  - bowel K91.2
  - rib Q77.2
- shoulder-hand — see Algoneurodystrophy
- Shwachman's D70.4
- sicca — see Sicca syndrome
- sick
  - cell E87.1
  - sinus I49.5
- sick-euthyroid E07.81
- sideropenic D50.1
- Siemens' ectodermal dysplasia Q82.4

☑ **Additional character required**

Syndrome — *continued*
Silfversköld's Q78.9
Simons' E88.1
sinus tarsi M25.57 ☑
sinusitis-bronchiectasis-situs inversus Q89.3
Sipple's E31.22
sirenomelia Q87.2
Slocumb's E27.0
slow flow, coronary I20.8
Sluder's G44.89
Smith-Magenis Q93.88
Sneddon-Wilkinson L13.1
Soto's Q87.3
South African cardiomyopathy I42.8
spasmodic
　upward movement, eyes H51.8
　winking F95.8
Spen's I45.9
splenic
　agenesis Q89.01
　flexure K59.8
　neutropenia D73.81
Spurway's Q78.0
staphylococcal scalded skin L00
steal
　arteriovenous T82.898 ☑
　ischemic T82.898 ☑
　subclavian G45.8
Stein-Leventhal E28.2
Stein's E28.2
Stevens-Johnson syndrome L51.1
　toxic epidermal necrolysis overlap L51.3
Stewart-Morel M85.2
Stickler Q89.8
stiff baby Q89.8
stiff man G25.82
Still-Felty — *see* Felty's syndrome
Stokes (-Adams) I45.9
stone heart I50.1
straight back, congenital Q76.49
subclavian steal G45.8
subcoracoid-pectoralis minor G54.0
subcostal nerve compression I77.89
subphrenic interposition Q43.3
superior
　cerebellar artery I63.89
　mesenteric artery K55.1
　semi-circular canal dehiscence H83.8X ☑
　vena cava I87.1
supine hypotensive (maternal) — *see* Syndrome, hypotension, maternal
suprarenal cortical E27.0
supraspinatus (*see also* Tear, rotator cuff) M75.10 ☑
Susac G93.49
swallowed blood P78.2
sweat retention L74.0
Swyer Q99.1
Symond's G93.2
sympathetic
　cervical paralysis G90.2
　pelvic, female N94.89
systemic inflammatory response (SIRS), of non-infectious origin (without organ dysfunction) R65.10
　with acute organ dysfunction R65.11
tachycardia-bradycardia I49.5
takotsubo I51.81
TAR (thrombocytopenia with absent radius) Q87.2
tarsal tunnel G57.5 ☑
teething K00.7
tegmental G93.89
telangiectasic-pigmentation-cataract Q82.8
temporal pyramidal apex — *see* Otitis, media, suppurative, acute
temporomandibular joint-pain-dysfunction M26.62 ☑
Terry's (*see also* Myopia, degenerative) H44.2 ☑
testicular feminization (*see also* Syndrome, androgen insensitivity) E34.51
thalamic pain (hyperesthetic) G89.0
thoracic outlet (compression) G54.0
Thorson-Björck E34.0
thrombocytopenia with absent radius (TAR) Q87.2
thyroid-adrenocortical insufficiency E31.0
tibial
　anterior M76.81 ☑
　posterior M76.82 ☑
Tietze's M94.0
time-zone (rapid) G47.25
Toni-Fanconi E72.09
　with cystinosis E72.04
Touraine's Q79.8

Syndrome — *continued*
tourniquet — *see* Constriction, external, by site
toxic shock A48.3
transient left ventricular apical ballooning I51.81
traumatic vasospastic T75.22 ☑
Treacher Collins Q75.4
triple X, female Q97.0
trisomy Q92.9
　13 Q91.7
　　meiotic nondisjunction Q91.4
　　mitotic nondisjunction Q91.5
　　mosaicism Q91.5
　　translocation Q91.6
　18 Q91.3
　　meiotic nondisjunction Q91.0
　　mitotic nondisjunction Q91.1
　　mosaicism Q91.1
　　translocation Q91.2
　20 (q)(p) Q92.8
　21 Q90.9
　　meiotic nondisjunction Q90.0
　　mitotic nondisjunction Q90.1
　　mosaicism Q90.1
　　translocation Q90.2
　22 Q92.8
tropical wet feet T69.0 ☑
Trousseau's I82.1
tumor lysis (following antineoplastic chemotherapy) (spontaneous) NEC E88.3
tumor necrosis factor receptor associated periodic (TRAPS) M04.1
Twiddler's (due to)
　automatic implantable defibrillator T82.198 ☑
　cardiac pacemaker T82.198 ☑
Unverricht (-Lundborg) — *see* Epilepsy, generalized, idiopathic
upward gaze H51.8
uremia, chronic (*see also* Disease, kidney, chronic) N18.9
urethral N34.3
urethro-oculo-articular — *see* Reiter's disease
urohepatic K76.7
vago-hypoglossal G52.7
vascular NEC in cerebrovascular disease G46.8
vasoconstriction, reversible cerebrovascular I67.841
vasomotor I73.9
vasospastic (traumatic) T75.22 ☑
vasovagal R55
van Buchem's M85.2
van der Hoeve's Q78.0
VATER Q87.2
velo-cardio-facial Q93.81
vena cava (inferior) (superior) (obstruction) I87.1
vertebral
　artery G45.0
　　compression — *see* Syndrome, anterior, spinal artery, compression
　steal G45.0
vertebro-basilar artery G45.0
vertebrogenic (pain) M54.89
vertiginous — *see* Disorder, vestibular function
Vinson-Plummer D50.1
virus B34.9
visceral larva migrans B83.0
visual disorientation H53.8
vitamin B6 deficiency E53.1
vitreal corneal H59.01 ☑
vitreous (touch) H59.01 ☑
Vogt-Koyanagi H20.82 ☑
Volkmann's T79.6 ☑
von Schroetter's I82.890
von Willebrand (-Jürgen) D68.0
Waldenström-Kjellberg D50.1
Wallenberg's G46.3
water retention E87.79
Waterhouse (-Friderichsen) A39.1
Weber-Gubler G46.3
Weber-Leyden G46.3
Weber's G46.3
Wegener's M31.30
　with
　　kidney involvement M31.31
　　lung involvement M31.30
　　　with kidney involvement M31.31
Weingarten's (tropical eosinophilia) J82
Weiss-Baker G90.09
Werdnig-Hoffman G12.0
Werner's E31.21
Werner's E34.8
Wernicke-Korsakoff (nonalcoholic) F04
　alcoholic F10.26

Syndrome — *continued*
West's — *see* Epilepsy, spasms
Westphal-Strümpell E83.01
wet
　feet (maceration) (tropical) T69.0 ☑
　lung, newborn P22.1
whiplash S13.4 ☑
whistling face Q87.0
Wilkie's K55.1
Wilkinson-Sneddon L13.1
Williams Q93.82
Willebrand (-Jürgens) D68.0
Wilson's (hepatolenticular degeneration) E83.01
Wiskott-Aldrich D82.0
withdrawal — *see* Withdrawal, state
　drug
　　infant of dependent mother P96.1
　　therapeutic use, newborn P96.2
Woakes' (ethmoiditis) J33.1
Wright's (hyperabduction) G54.0
X I20.9
XXXX Q97.1
XXXXX Q97.1
XXXXY Q98.1
XXY Q98.0
Yao M04.8
yellow nail L60.5
Zahorsky's B08.5
Zellweger syndrome E71.510
Zellweger-like syndrome E71.541
Synechia (anterior) (iris) (posterior) (pupil) (*see also* Adhesions, iris)
　intra-uterine (traumatic) N85.6
Synesthesia R20.8
Syngamiasis, syngamosis B83.3
Synodontia K00.2
Synorchidism, synorchism Q55.1
Synostosis (congenital) Q78.8
　astragalo-scaphoid Q74.2
　radioulnar Q74.0
Synovial sarcoma — *see* Neoplasm, connective tissue, malignant
Synovioma (malignant) (*see also* Neoplasm, connective tissue, malignant)
　benign — *see* Neoplasm, connective tissue, benign
Synoviosarcoma — *see* Neoplasm, connective tissue, malignant
Synovitis (*see also* Tenosynovitis) M65.9
　crepitant
　　hand M70.0 ☑
　　wrist M70.03 ☑
　gonococcal A54.49
　gouty — *see* Gout
　in (due to)
　　crystals M65.8 ☑
　　gonorrhea A54.49
　　syphilis (late) A52.78
　　use, overuse, pressure — *see* Disorder, soft tissue, due to use
　infective NEC — *see* Tenosynovitis, infective NEC
　specified NEC — *see* Tenosynovitis, specified type NEC
　syphilitic A52.78
　　congenital (early) A50.02
　toxic — *see* Synovitis, transient
　transient M67.3 ☑
　　ankle M67.37 ☑
　　elbow M67.32 ☑
　　foot joint M67.37 ☑
　　hand joint M67.34 ☑
　　hip M67.35 ☑
　　knee M67.36 ☑
　　multiple site M67.39
　　pelvic region M67.35 ☑
　　shoulder M67.31 ☑
　　specified joint NEC M67.38
　　wrist M67.33 ☑
　traumatic, current — *see* Sprain
　tuberculous — *see* Tuberculosis, synovitis
　villonodular (pigmented) M12.2 ☑
　　ankle M12.27 ☑
　　elbow M12.22 ☑
　　foot joint M12.27 ☑
　　hand joint M12.24 ☑
　　hip M12.25 ☑
　　knee M12.26 ☑
　　multiple site M12.29
　　pelvic region M12.25 ☑
　　shoulder M12.21 ☑
　　specified joint NEC M12.28
　　vertebrae M12.28
　　wrist M12.23 ☑

Syphilid - Syphilis

Syphilid A51.39
  congenital A50.06
  newborn A50.06
  tubercular (late) A52.79
Syphilis, syphilitic (acquired) A53.9
  abdomen (late) A52.79
  acoustic nerve A52.15
  adenopathy (secondary) A51.49
  adrenal (gland) (with cortical hypofunction) A52.79
  age under 2 years NOS (*see also* Syphilis, congenital, early)
    acquired A51.9
  alopecia (secondary) A51.32
  anemia (late) A52.79 *[D63.8]*
  aneurysm (aorta) (ruptured) A52.01
    central nervous system A52.05
    congenital A50.54 *[I79.0]*
  anus (late) A52.74
    primary A51.1
    secondary A51.39
  aorta (arch) (abdominal) (thoracic) A52.02
    aneurysm A52.01
  aortic (insufficiency) (regurgitation) (stenosis) A52.03
    aneurysm A52.01
  arachnoid (adhesive) (cerebral) (spinal) A52.13
  asymptomatic — *see* Syphilis, latent
  ataxia (locomotor) A52.11
  atrophoderma maculatum A51.39
  auricular fibrillation A52.06
  bladder (late) A52.76
  bone A52.77
    secondary A51.46
  brain A52.17
  breast (late) A52.79
  bronchus (late) A52.72
  bubo (primary) A51.0
  bulbar palsy A52.19
  bursa (late) A52.78
  cardiac decompensation A52.06
  cardiovascular A52.00
  central nervous system (late) (recurrent) (relapse) (tertiary) A52.3
    with
      ataxia A52.11
      general paralysis A52.17
        juvenile A50.45
      paresis (general) A52.17
        juvenile A50.45
      tabes (dorsalis) A52.11
        juvenile A50.45
      taboparesis A52.17
        juvenile A50.45
    aneurysm A52.05
    congenital A50.40
    juvenile A50.40
    remission in (sustained) A52.3
    serology doubtful, negative, or positive A52.3
    specified nature or site NEC A52.19
    vascular A52.05
  cerebral A52.17
    meningovascular A52.13
    nerves (multiple palsies) A52.15
    sclerosis A52.17
    thrombosis A52.05
  cerebrospinal (tabetic type) A52.12
  cerebrovascular A52.05
  cervix (late) A52.76
  chancre (multiple) A51.0
    extragenital A51.2
    Rollet's A51.0
  Charcot's joint A52.16
  chorioretinitis A51.43
    congenital A50.01
    late A52.71
    prenatal A50.01
  choroiditis — *see* Syphilitic chorioretinitis
  choroidoretinitis — *see* Syphilitic chorioretinitis
  ciliary body (secondary) A51.43
    late A52.71
  colon (late) A52.74
  combined spinal sclerosis A52.11
  condyloma (latum) A51.31
  congenital A50.9
    with
      paresis (general) A50.45
      tabes (dorsalis) A50.45
      taboparesis A50.45
    chorioretinitis, choroiditis A50.01 *[H32]*
    early, or less than 2 years after birth NEC A50.2
      with manifestations — *see* Syphilis, congenital, early, symptomatic

Syphilis — *continued*
  congenital — *continued*
    latent (without manifestations) A50.1
      negative spinal fluid test A50.1
      serology positive A50.1
    symptomatic A50.09
      cutaneous A50.06
      mucocutaneous A50.07
      oculopathy A50.01
      osteochondropathy A50.02
      pharyngitis A50.03
      pneumonia A50.04
      rhinitis A50.05
      visceral A50.08
    interstitial keratitis A50.31
    juvenile neurosyphilis A50.45
    late, or 2 years or more after birth NEC A50.7
      chorioretinitis, choroiditis A50.32
      interstitial keratitis A50.31
      juvenile neurosyphilis A50.45
      latent (without manifestations) A50.6
        negative spinal fluid test A50.6
        serology positive A50.6
      symptomatic or with manifestations NEC A50.59
        arthropathy A50.55
        cardiovascular A50.54
        Clutton's joints A50.51
        Hutchinson's teeth A50.52
        Hutchinson's triad A50.53
        osteochondropathy A50.56
        saddle nose A50.57
  conjugal A53.9
    tabes A52.11
  conjunctiva (late) A52.71
  contact Z20.2
  cord bladder A52.19
  cornea, late A52.71
  coronary (artery) (sclerosis) A52.06
  coryza, congenital A50.05
  cranial nerve A52.15
    multiple palsies A52.15
  cutaneous — *see* Syphilis, skin
  dacryocystitis (late) A52.71
  degeneration, spinal cord A52.12
  dementia paralytica A52.17
    juvenilis A50.45
  destruction of bone A52.77
  dilatation, aorta A52.01
  due to blood transfusion A53.9
  dura mater A52.13
  ear A52.79
    inner A52.79
      nerve (eighth) A52.15
      neurorecurrence A52.15
  early A51.9
    cardiovascular A52.00
    central nervous system A52.3
    latent (without manifestations) (less than 2 years after infection) A51.5
      negative spinal fluid test A51.5
      serological relapse after treatment A51.5
      serology positive A51.5
    relapse (treated, untreated) A51.9
    skin A51.39
    symptomatic A51.9
      extragenital chancre A51.2
      primary, except extragenital chancre A51.0
      secondary (*see also* Syphilis, secondary) A51.39
        relapse (treated, untreated) A51.49
    ulcer A51.39
  eighth nerve (neuritis) A52.15
  endemic A65
  endocarditis A52.03
    aortic A52.03
    pulmonary A52.03
  epididymis (late) A52.76
  epiglottis (late) A52.73
  epiphysitis (congenital) (early) A50.02
  episcleritis (late) A52.71
  esophagus A52.79
  eustachian tube A52.73
  exposure to Z20.2
  eye A52.71
  eyelid (late) (with gumma) A52.71
  fallopian tube (late) A52.76
  fracture A52.77
  gallbladder (late) A52.74
  gastric (polyposis) (late) A52.74
  general A53.9
    paralysis A52.17
      juvenile A50.45

Syphilis — *continued*
  genital (primary) A51.0
  glaucoma A52.71
  gumma NEC A52.79
    cardiovascular system A52.00
    central nervous system A52.3
    congenital A50.59
  heart (block) (decompensation) (disease) (failure) A52.06 *[I52]*
    valve NEC A52.03
  hemianesthesia A52.19
  hemianopsia A52.71
  hemiparesis A52.17
  hemiplegia A52.17
  hepatic artery A52.09
  hepatis A52.74
  hepatomegaly, congenital A50.08
  hereditaria tarda — *see* Syphilis, congenital, late
  hereditary — *see* Syphilis, congenital
  Hutchinson's teeth A50.52
  hyalitis A52.71
  inactive — *see* Syphilis, latent
  infantum — *see* Syphilis, congenital
  inherited — *see* Syphilis, congenital
  internal ear A52.79
  intestine (late) A52.74
  iris, iritis (secondary) A51.43
    late A52.71
  joint (late) A52.77
  keratitis (congenital) (interstitial) (late) A50.31
  kidney (late) A52.75
  lacrimal passages (late) A52.71
  larynx (late) A52.73
  late A52.9
    cardiovascular A52.00
    central nervous system A52.3
    kidney A52.75
    latent or 2 years or more after infection (without manifestations) A52.8
      negative spinal fluid test A52.8
      serology positive A52.8
    paresis A52.17
    specified site NEC A52.79
    symptomatic or with manifestations A52.79
    tabes A52.11
  latent A53.0
    with signs or symptoms - code by site and stage under Syphilis
    central nervous system A52.2
    date of infection unspecified A53.0
    early, or less than 2 years after infection A51.5
    follow-up of latent syphilis A53.0
      date of infection unspecified A53.0
      late, or 2 years or more after infection A52.8
    late, or 2 years or more after infection A52.8
    positive serology (only finding) A53.0
      date of infection unspecified A53.0
      early, or less than 2 years after infection A51.5
      late, or 2 years or more after infection A52.8
  lens (late) A52.71
  leukoderma A51.39
    late A52.79
  lienitis A52.79
  lip A51.39
    chancre (primary) A51.2
    late A52.79
  Lissauer's paralysis A52.17
  liver A52.74
  locomotor ataxia A52.11
  lung A52.72
  lymph gland (early) (secondary) A51.49
    late A52.79
  lymphadenitis (secondary) A51.49
  macular atrophy of skin A51.39
    striated A52.79
  mediastinum (late) A52.73
  meninges (adhesive) (brain) (spinal cord) A52.13
  meningitis A52.13
    acute (secondary) A51.41
    congenital A50.41
  meningoencephalitis A52.14
  meningovascular A52.13
    congenital A50.41
  mesarteritis A52.09
    brain A52.04
  middle ear A52.77
  mitral stenosis A52.03
  monoplegia A52.17
  mouth (secondary) A51.39
    late A52.79
  mucocutaneous (secondary) A51.39
    late A52.79

☑ **Additional character required**

Syphilis — *continued*
  mucous
    membrane (secondary) A51.39
      late A52.79
    patches A51.39
      congenital A50.07
  mulberry molars A50.52
  muscle A52.78
  myocardium A52.06
  nasal sinus (late) A52.73
  neonatorum — *see* Syphilis, congenital
  nephrotic syndrome (secondary) A51.44
  nerve palsy (any cranial nerve) A52.15
    multiple A52.15
  nervous system, central A52.3
  neuritis A52.15
    acoustic A52.15
  neurorecidive of retina A52.19
  neuroretinitis A52.19
  newborn — *see* Syphilis, congenital
  nodular superficial (late) A52.79
  nonvenereal A65
  nose (late) A52.73
    saddle back deformity A50.57
  occlusive arterial disease A52.09
  oculopathy A52.71
  ophthalmic (late) A52.71
  optic nerve (atrophy) (neuritis) (papilla) A52.15
  orbit (late) A52.71
  organic A53.9
  osseous (late) A52.77
  osteochondritis (congenital) (early) A50.02 *[M90.80]*
  osteoporosis A52.77
  ovary (late) A52.76
  oviduct (late) A52.76
  palate (late) A52.79
  pancreas (late) A52.74
  paralysis A52.17
    general A52.17
      juvenile A50.45
  paresis (general) A52.17
    juvenile A50.45
  paresthesia A52.19
  Parkinson's disease or syndrome A52.19
  paroxysmal tachycardia A52.06
  pemphigus (congenital) A50.06
  penis (chancre) A51.0
    late A52.76
  pericardium A52.06
  perichondritis, larynx (late) A52.73
  periosteum (late) A52.77
    congenital (early) A50.02 *[M90.80]*
    early (secondary) A51.46
  peripheral nerve A52.79
  petrous bone (late) A52.77
  pharynx (late) A52.73
    secondary A51.39
  pituitary (gland) A52.79
  pleura (late) A52.73
  pneumonia, white A50.04
  pontine lesion A52.17
  portal vein A52.09
  primary A51.0
    anal A51.1
    and secondary — *see* Syphilis, secondary
    central nervous system A52.3
    extragenital chancre NEC A51.2
    fingers A51.2
    genital A51.0
    lip A51.2
    specified site NEC A51.2
    tonsils A51.2
  prostate (late) A52.76
  ptosis (eyelid) A52.71
  pulmonary (late) A52.72
    artery A52.09
  pyelonephritis (late) A52.75
  recently acquired, symptomatic A51.9
  rectum (late) A52.74
  respiratory tract (late) A52.73
  retina, late A52.71
  retrobulbar neuritis A52.15
  salpingitis A52.76
  sclera (late) A52.71
  sclerosis
    cerebral A52.17
    coronary A52.06
    multiple A52.11
  scotoma (central) A52.71
  scrotum (late) A52.76
  secondary (and primary) A51.49
    adenopathy A51.49

Syphilis — *continued*
  secondary — *continued*
    anus A51.39
    bone A51.46
    chorioretinitis, choroiditis A51.43
    hepatitis A51.45
    liver A51.45
    lymphadenitis A51.49
    meningitis (acute) A51.41
    mouth A51.39
    mucous membranes A51.39
    periosteum, periostitis A51.46
    pharynx A51.39
    relapse (treated, untreated) A51.49
    skin A51.39
    specified form NEC A51.49
    tonsil A51.39
    ulcer A51.39
    viscera NEC A51.49
    vulva A51.39
  seminal vesicle (late) A52.76
  seronegative with signs or symptoms - code by site
    and stage under Syphilis
  seropositive
    with signs or symptoms - code by site and stage
      under Syphilis
    follow-up of latent syphilis — *see* Syphilis, latent
    only finding — *see* Syphilis, latent
  seventh nerve (paralysis) A52.15
  sinus, sinusitis (late) A52.73
  skeletal system A52.77
  skin (with ulceration) (early) (secondary) A51.39
    late or tertiary A52.79
  small intestine A52.74
  spastic spinal paralysis A52.17
  spermatic cord (late) A52.76
  spinal (cord) A52.12
  spleen A52.79
  splenomegaly A52.79
  spondylitis A52.77
  staphyloma A52.71
  stigmata (congenital) A50.59
  stomach A52.74
  synovium A52.78
  tabes dorsalis (late) A52.11
    juvenile A50.45
  tabetic type A52.11
    juvenile A50.45
  taboparesis A52.17
    juvenile A50.45
  tachycardia A52.06
  tendon (late) A52.78
  tertiary A52.9
    with symptoms NEC A52.79
    cardiovascular A52.00
    central nervous system A52.3
    multiple NEC A52.79
    specified site NEC A52.79
  testis A52.76
  thorax A52.73
  throat A52.73
  thymus (gland) (late) A52.79
  thyroid (late) A52.79
  tongue (late) A52.79
  tonsil (lingual) (late) A52.73
    primary A51.2
    secondary A51.39
  trachea (late) A52.73
  tunica vaginalis (late) A52.76
  ulcer (any site) (early) (secondary) A51.39
    late A52.79
    perforating A52.79
      foot A52.11
  urethra (late) A52.76
  urogenital (late) A52.76
  uterus (late) A52.76
  uveal tract (secondary) A51.43
    late A52.71
  uveitis (secondary) A51.43
    late A52.71
  uvula (late) (perforated) A52.79
  vagina A51.0
    late A52.76
  valvulitis NEC A52.03
  vascular A52.00
    brain (cerebral) A52.05
  ventriculi A52.74
  vesicae urinariae (late) A52.76
  viscera (abdominal) (late) A52.74
    secondary A51.49
  vitreous (opacities) (late) A52.71
    hemorrhage A52.71

Syphilis — *continued*
  vulva A51.0
    late A52.76
    secondary A51.39
Syphiloma A52.79
  cardiovascular system A52.00
  central nervous system A52.3
  circulatory system A52.00
  congenital A50.59
Syphilophobia F45.29
Syringadenoma (*see also* Neoplasm, skin, benign)
  papillary — *see* Neoplasm, skin, benign
Syringobulbia G95.0
Syringocystadenoma — *see* Neoplasm, skin, benign
  papillary — *see* Neoplasm, skin, benign
Syringoma (*see also* Neoplasm, skin, benign)
  chondroid — *see* Neoplasm, skin, benign
Syringomyelia G95.0
Syringomyelitis — *see* Encephalitis
Syringomyelocele — *see* Spina bifida
Syringopontia G95.0
System, systemic (*see also* condition)
  disease, combined — *see* Degeneration, combined
  inflammatory response syndrome (SIRS) of non-
    infectious origin (without organ dysfunction)
    R65.10
    with acute organ dysfunction R65.11
  lupus erythematosus M32.9
    inhibitor present D68.62

T

Tabacism, tabacosis, tabagism (*see also* Poisoning,
  tobacco)
  meaning dependence (without remission) F17.200
    with
      disorder F17.299
        in remission F17.211
        specified disorder NEC F17.298
      withdrawal F17.203
Tabardillo A75.9
  flea-borne A75.2
  louse-borne A75.0
Tabes, tabetic A52.10
  with
    central nervous system syphilis A52.10
    Charcot's joint A52.16
    cord bladder A52.19
    crisis, viscera (any) A52.19
    paralysis, general A52.17
    paresis (general) A52.17
    perforating ulcer (foot) A52.19
  arthropathy (Charcot) A52.16
  bladder A52.19
  bone A52.11
  cerebrospinal A52.12
  congenital A50.45
  conjugal A52.10
  dorsalis A52.11
    juvenile A50.49
  juvenile A50.49
  latent A52.19
  mesenterica A18.39
  paralysis, insane, general A52.17
  spasmodic A52.17
  syphilis (cerebrospinal) A52.12
Taboparalysis A52.17
Taboparesis (remission) A52.17
  juvenile A50.45
TAC (trigeminal autonomic cephalgia) NEC G44.099
  intractable G44.091
  not intractable G44.099
Tache noir S60.22 ☑
Tachyalimentation K91.2
Tachyarrhythmia, tachyrhythmia — *see* Tachycardia
Tachycardia R00.0
  atrial (paroxysmal) I47.1
  auricular I47.1
  AV nodal re-entry (re-entrant) I47.1
  junctional (paroxysmal) I47.1
  newborn P29.11
  nodal (paroxysmal) I47.1
  non-paroxysmal AV nodal I45.89
  paroxysmal (sustained) (nonsustained) I47.9
    with sinus bradycardia I49.5
    atrial (PAT) I47.1
    atrioventricular (AV) (re-entrant) I47.1
      psychogenic F54
    junctional I47.1
      ectopic I47.1

Tachycardia - Tendinitis

Tachycardia — *continued*
   paroxysmal — *continued*
      nodal I47.1
      psychogenic (atrial) (supraventricular)
         (ventricular) F54
      supraventricular (sustained) I47.1
         psychogenic F54
      ventricular I47.2
         psychogenic F54
   psychogenic F45.8
   sick sinus I49.5
   sinoauricular NOS R00.0
      paroxysmal I47.1
   sinus [sinusal] NOS R00.0
      paroxysmal I47.1
   supraventricular I47.1
   ventricular (paroxysmal) (sustained) I47.2
      psychogenic F54
Tachygastria K31.89
Tachypnea R06.82
   hysterical F45.8
   newborn (idiopathic) (transitory) P22.1
   psychogenic F45.8
   transitory, of newborn P22.1
Taenia (infection) (infestation) B68.9
   diminuta B71.0
   echinococcal infestation B67.90
   mediocanellata B68.1
   nana B71.0
   saginata B68.1
   solium (intestinal form) B68.0
      larval form — *see* Cysticercosis
Taeniasis (intestine) — *see* Taenia
TACO (transfusion associated circulatory overload)
   E87.71
Tag (hypertrophied skin) (infected) L91.8
   adenoid J35.8
   anus K64.4
   hemorrhoidal K64.4
   hymen N89.8
   perineal N90.89
   preauricular Q17.0
   sentinel K64.4
   skin L91.8
      accessory (congenital) Q82.8
      anus K64.4
      congenital Q82.8
      preauricular Q17.0
   tonsil J35.8
   urethra, urethral N36.8
   vulva N90.89
Tahyna fever B33.8
Takahara's disease E80.3
Takayasu's disease or syndrome M31.4
Talcosis (pulmonary) J62.0
Talipes (congenital) Q66.89
   acquired, planus — *see* Deformity, limb, flat foot
   asymmetric Q66.89
   calcaneovalgus Q66.4 ☑
   calcaneovarus Q66.1 ☑
   calcaneus Q66.89
   cavus Q66.7 ☑
   equinovalgus Q66.6
   equinovarus Q66.0 ☑
   equinus Q66.89
   percavus Q66.7 ☑
   planovalgus Q66.6
   planus (acquired) (any degree) (*see also* Deformity,
      limb, flat foot)
      congenital Q66.5 ☑
      due to rickets (sequelae) E64.3
   valgus Q66.6
   varus Q66.3 ☑
Tall stature, constitutional E34.4
Talma's disease M62.89
Talon noir S90.3 ☑
   hand S60.22 ☑
   heel S90.3 ☑
   toe S90.1 ☑
Tamponade, heart I31.4
Tanapox (virus disease) B08.71
Tangier disease E78.6
Tantrum, child problem F91.8
Tapeworm (infection) (infestation) — *see* Infestation,
   tapeworm
Tapia's syndrome G52.7
TAR (thrombocytopenia with absent radius) syndrome
   Q87.2
Tarral-Besnier disease L44.0
Tarsal tunnel syndrome — *see* Syndrome, tarsal
   tunnel
Tarsalgia — *see* Pain, limb, lower

Tarsitis (eyelid) H01.8
   syphilitic A52.71
   tuberculous A18.4
Tartar (teeth) (dental calculus) K03.6
Tattoo (mark) L81.8
Tauri's disease E74.09
Taurodontism K00.2
Taussig-Bing syndrome Q20.1
Taybi's syndrome Q87.2
Tay-Sachs amaurotic familial idiocy or disease E75.02
TBI (traumatic brain injury) S06.9 ☑
Teacher's node or nodule J38.2
Tear, torn (traumatic) (*see also* Laceration)
   with abortion — *see* Abortion
   annular fibrosis M51.35
   anus, anal (sphincter) S31.831 ☑
      complicating delivery
         with third degree perineal laceration (*see also*
            Delivery, complicated, by, laceration,
            perineum, third degree) O70.20
            with mucosa O70.3
         without third degree perineal laceration O70.4
      nontraumatic (healed) (old) K62.81
   articular cartilage, old — *see* Derangement, joint,
      articular cartilage, by site
   bladder
      with ectopic or molar pregnancy O08.6
      following ectopic or molar pregnancy O08.6
      obstetrical O71.5
      traumatic — *see* Injury, bladder
   bowel
      with ectopic or molar pregnancy O08.6
      following ectopic or molar pregnancy O08.6
      obstetrical trauma O71.5
   broad ligament
      with ectopic or molar pregnancy O08.6
      following ectopic or molar pregnancy O08.6
      obstetrical trauma O71.6
   bucket handle (knee) (meniscus) — *see* Tear,
      meniscus
   capsule, joint — *see* Sprain
   cartilage (*see also* Sprain)
      articular, old — *see* Derangement, joint, articular
         cartilage, by site
   cervix
      with ectopic or molar pregnancy O08.6
      following ectopic or molar pregnancy O08.6
      obstetrical trauma (current) O71.3
      old N88.1
      traumatic — *see* Injury, uterus
   dural G97.41
      nontraumatic G96.11
   internal organ — *see* Injury, by site
   knee cartilage
      articular (current) S83.3 ☑
      old — *see* Derangement, knee, meniscus, due to
         old tear
   ligament — *see* Sprain
   meniscus (knee) (current injury) S83.209 ☑
      bucket-handle S83.20 ☑
      lateral
         bucket-handle S83.25 ☑
         complex S83.27 ☑
         peripheral S83.26 ☑
         specified type NEC S83.28 ☑
      medial
         bucket-handle S83.21 ☑
         complex S83.23 ☑
         peripheral S83.22 ☑
         specified type NEC S83.24 ☑
      old — *see* Derangement, knee, meniscus, due to
         old tear
      site other than knee - code as Sprain
      specified type NEC S83.20 ☑
   muscle — *see* Strain
   pelvic
      floor, complicating delivery O70.1
      organ NEC, obstetrical trauma O71.5
         with ectopic or molar pregnancy O08.6
         following ectopic or molar pregnancy O08.6
   perineal, secondary O90.1
   periurethral tissue, obstetrical trauma O71.82
      with ectopic or molar pregnancy O08.6
      following ectopic or molar pregnancy O08.6
   rectovaginal septum — *see* Laceration, vagina
   retina, retinal (without detachment) (horseshoe)
      (*see also* Break, retina, horseshoe)
      with detachment — *see* Detachment, retina, with
         retinal, break
   rotator cuff (nontraumatic) M75.10 ☑
      complete M75.12 ☑
      incomplete M75.11 ☑

Tear — *continued*
   rotator cuff — *continued*
      traumatic S46.01 ☑
         capsule S43.42 ☑
   semilunar cartilage, knee — *see* Tear, meniscus
   supraspinatus (complete) (incomplete)
      (nontraumatic) (*see also* Tear, rotator cuff)
      M75.10 ☑
   tendon — *see* Strain
   tentorial, at birth P10.4
   umbilical cord
      complicating delivery O69.89 ☑
   urethra
      with ectopic or molar pregnancy O08.6
      following ectopic or molar pregnancy O08.6
      obstetrical trauma O71.5
   uterus — *see* Injury, uterus
   vagina — *see* Laceration, vagina
   vessel, from catheter — *see* Puncture, accidental
      complicating surgery
   vulva, complicating delivery O70.0
Tear-stone — *see* Dacryolith
Teeth (*see also* condition)
   grinding
      psychogenic F45.8
      sleep related G47.63
Teething (syndrome) K00.7
Telangiectasia, telangiectasis (verrucous) I78.1
   ataxic (cerebellar) (Louis-Bar) G11.3
   familial I78.0
   hemorrhagic, hereditary (congenital) (senile) I78.0
   hereditary, hemorrhagic (congenital) (senile) I78.0
   juxtafoveal H35.07 ☑
   macular H35.07 ☑
   macularis eruptiva perstans D47.01
   parafoveal H35.07 ☑
   retinal (idiopathic) (juxtafoveal) (macular)
      (parafoveal) H35.07 ☑
   spider I78.1
Telephone scatologia F65.89
Telescoped bowel or intestine K56.1
   congenital Q43.8
Temperature
   body, high (of unknown origin) R50.9
   cold, trauma from T69.9 ☑
      newborn P80.0
      specified effect NEC T69.8 ☑
Temple — *see* condition
Temporal — *see* condition
Temporomandibular joint pain-dysfunction syndrome
   M26.62 ☑
Temporosphenoidal — *see* condition
Tendency
   bleeding — *see* Defect, coagulation
   suicide
      meaning personal history of attempted suicide
         Z91.5
      meaning suicidal ideation — *see* Ideation, suicidal
   to fall R29.6
Tenderness, abdominal R10.819
   epigastric R10.816
   generalized R10.817
   left lower quadrant R10.814
   left upper quadrant R10.812
   periumbilic R10.815
   right lower quadrant R10.813
   right upper quadrant R10.811
   rebound R10.829
      epigastric R10.826
      generalized R10.827
      left lower quadrant R10.824
      left upper quadrant R10.822
      periumbilic R10.825
      right lower quadrant R10.823
      right upper quadrant R10.821
Tendinitis, tendonitis (*see also* Enthesopathy)
   Achilles M76.6 ☑
   adhesive — *see* Tenosynovitis, specified type NEC
      shoulder — *see* Capsulitis, adhesive
   bicipital M75.2 ☑
   calcific M65.2 ☑
      ankle M65.27 ☑
      foot M65.27 ☑
      forearm M65.23 ☑
      hand M65.24 ☑
      lower leg M65.26 ☑
      multiple sites M65.29
      pelvic region M65.25 ☑
      shoulder M75.3 ☑
      specified site NEC M65.28
      thigh M65.25 ☑
      upper arm M65.22 ☑

☑ **Additional character required**

Tendinitis — *continued*
  due to use, overuse, pressure (*see also* Disorder, soft tissue, due to use)
    specified NEC — *see* Disorder, soft tissue, due to use, specified NEC
  gluteal M76.0 ☑
  patellar M76.5 ☑
  peroneal M76.7 ☑
  psoas M76.1 ☑
  tibial (posterior) M76.82 ☑
    anterior M76.81 ☑
  trochanteric — *see* Bursitis, hip, trochanteric
Tendon — *see* condition
Tendosynovitis — *see* Tenosynovitis
Tenesmus (rectal) R19.8
  vesical R30.1
Tennis elbow — *see* Epicondylitis, lateral
Tenonitis (*see also* Tenosynovitis)
  eye (capsule) H05.04 ☑
Tenontosynovitis — *see* Tenosynovitis
Tenontothecitis — *see* Tenosynovitis
Tenophyte — *see* Disorder, synovium, specified type NEC
Tenosynovitis (*see also* Synovitis) M65.9
  adhesive — *see* Tenosynovitis, specified type NEC
    shoulder — *see* Capsulitis, adhesive
  bicipital (calcifying) — *see* Tendinitis, bicipital
  gonococcal A54.49
  in (due to)
    crystals M65.8 ☑
    gonorrhea A54.49
    syphilis (late) A52.78
    use, overuse, pressure (*see also* Disorder, soft tissue, due to use)
      specified NEC — *see* Disorder, soft tissue, due to use, specified NEC
  infective NEC M65.1 ☑
    ankle M65.17 ☑
    foot M65.17 ☑
    forearm M65.13 ☑
    hand M65.14 ☑
    lower leg M65.16 ☑
    multiple sites M65.19
    pelvic region M65.15 ☑
    shoulder region M65.11 ☑
    specified site NEC M65.18
    thigh M65.15 ☑
    upper arm M65.12 ☑
  radial styloid M65.4
  shoulder region M65.81 ☑
    adhesive — *see* Capsulitis, adhesive
  specified type NEC M65.88
    ankle M65.87 ☑
    foot M65.87 ☑
    forearm M65.83 ☑
    hand M65.84 ☑
    lower leg M65.86 ☑
    multiple sites M65.89
    pelvic region M65.85 ☑
    shoulder region M65.81 ☑
    specified site NEC M65.88
    thigh M65.85 ☑
    upper arm M65.82 ☑
  tuberculous — *see* Tuberculosis, tenosynovitis
Tenovaginitis — *see* Tenosynovitis
Tension
  arterial, high (*see also* Hypertension)
    without diagnosis of hypertension R03.0
  headache G44.209
    intractable G44.201
    not intractable G44.209
  nervous R45.0
  pneumothorax J93.0
  premenstrual N94.3
  state (mental) F48.9
Tentorium — *see* condition
Teratencephalus Q89.8
Teratism Q89.7
Teratoblastoma (malignant) — *see* Neoplasm, malignant, by site
Teratocarcinoma (*see also* Neoplasm, malignant, by site)
  liver C22.7
Teratoma (solid) (*see also* Neoplasm, uncertain behavior, by site)
  with embryonal carcinoma, mixed — *see* Neoplasm, malignant, by site
  with malignant transformation — *see* Neoplasm, malignant, by site
  adult (cystic) — *see* Neoplasm, benign, by site
  benign — *see* Neoplasm, benign, by site

Teratoma — *continued*
  combined with choriocarcinoma — *see* Neoplasm, malignant, by site
  cystic (adult) — *see* Neoplasm, benign, by site
  differentiated — *see* Neoplasm, benign, by site
  embryonal (*see also* Neoplasm, malignant, by site)
    liver C22.7
  immature — *see* Neoplasm, malignant, by site
  liver C22.7
    adult, benign, cystic, differentiated type or mature D13.4
  malignant (*see also* Neoplasm, malignant, by site)
    anaplastic — *see* Neoplasm, malignant, by site
    intermediate — *see* Neoplasm, malignant, by site
      specified site — *see* Neoplasm, malignant, by site
      unspecified site C62.90
    undifferentiated — *see* Neoplasm, malignant, by site
  mature — *see* Neoplasm, uncertain behavior, by site
    malignant — *see* Neoplasm, by site, malignant, by site
  ovary D27. ☑
    embryonal, immature or malignant C56 ☑
  solid — *see* Neoplasm, uncertain behavior, by site
  testis C62.9 ☑
    adult, benign, cystic, differentiated type or mature D29.2 ☑
    scrotal C62.1 ☑
    undescended C62.0 ☑
Termination
  anomalous (*see also* Malposition, congenital)
    right pulmonary vein Q26.3
  pregnancy, elective Z33.2
Ternidens diminutus infestation B81.8
Ternidensiasis B81.8
Terror(s) night (child) F51.4
Terrorism, victim of Z65.4
Terry's syndrome (*see also* Myopia, degenerative) H44.2 ☑
Tertiary — *see* condition
Test, tests, testing (for)
  adequacy (for dialysis)
    hemodialysis Z49.31
    peritoneal Z49.32
  blood-alcohol Z04.89
    positive — *see* Findings, abnormal, in blood
  blood-drug Z04.89
    positive — *see* Findings, abnormal, in blood
  blood pressure Z01.30
    abnormal reading — *see* Blood, pressure
  blood typing Z01.83
    Rh typing Z01.83
  cardiac pulse generator (battery) Z45.010
  fertility Z31.41
  genetic
    disease carrier status for procreative management
      female Z31.430
      male Z31.440
    male partner of patient with recurrent pregnancy loss Z31.441
    procreative management NEC
      female Z31.438
      male Z31.448
  hearing Z01.10
    with abnormal findings NEC Z01.118
    infant or child (over 28 days old) Z00.129
      with abnormal findings Z00.121
  HIV (human immunodeficiency virus)
    nonconclusive (in infants) R75
    positive Z21
    seropositive Z21
  immunity status Z01.84
  intelligence NEC Z01.89
  laboratory (as part of a general medical examination) Z00.00
    with abnormal finding Z00.01
    for medicolegal reason NEC Z04.89
  male partner of patient with recurrent pregnancy loss Z31.441
  Mantoux (for tuberculosis) Z11.1
    abnormal result R76.11
  pregnancy, positive first pregnancy — *see* Pregnancy, normal, first
  procreative Z31.49
    fertility Z31.41
  skin, diagnostic
    allergy Z01.82
      special screening examination — *see* Screening, by name of disease
    Mantoux Z11.1
    tuberculin Z11.1

Test — *continued*
  specified NEC Z01.89
  tuberculin Z11.1
    abnormal result R76.11
  vision Z01.00
    with abnormal findings Z01.01
    following failed vision screening Z01.020
      with abnormal findings Z01.021
    infant or child (over 28 days old) Z00.129
      with abnormal findings Z00.121
  Wassermann Z11.3
    positive — *see* Serology for syphilis, positive
Testicle, testicular, testis (*see also* condition)
  feminization syndrome (*see also* Syndrome, androgen insensitivity) E34.51
  migrans Q55.29
Tetanus, tetanic (cephalic) (convulsions) A35
  with
    abortion A34
    ectopic or molar pregnancy O08.0
  following ectopic or molar pregnancy O08.0
  inoculation reaction (due to serum) — *see* Complications, vaccination
  neonatorum A33
  obstetrical A34
  puerperal, postpartum, childbirth A34
Tetany (due to) R29.0
  alkalosis E87.3
  associated with rickets E55.0
  convulsions R29.0
    hysterical F44.5
  functional (hysterical) F44.5
  hyperkinetic R29.0
    hysterical F44.5
  hyperpnea R06.4
    hysterical F44.5
    psychogenic F45.8
  hyperventilation (*see also* Hyperventilation) R06.4
    hysterical F44.5
  neonatal (without calcium or magnesium deficiency) P71.3
  parathyroid (gland) E20.9
  parathyroprival E89.2
  post- (para)thyroidectomy E89.2
  postoperative E89.2
  pseudotetany R29.0
  psychogenic (conversion reaction) F44.5
Tetralogy of Fallot Q21.3
Tetraplegia (chronic) (*see also* Quadriplegia) G82.50
Thailand hemorrhagic fever A91
Thalassanemia — *see* Thalassemia
Thalassemia (anemia) (disease) D56.9
  with other hemoglobinopathy D56.8
  alpha (major) (severe) (triple gene defect) D56.0
    minor D56.3
    silent carrier D56.3
    trait D56.3
  beta (severe) D56.1
    homozygous D56.1
    major D56.1
    minor D56.3
    trait D56.3
  delta-beta (homozygous) D56.2
    minor D56.3
    trait D56.3
  dominant D56.8
  hemoglobin
    C D56.8
    E-beta D56.5
  intermedia D56.1
  major D56.1
  minor D56.3
  mixed D56.8
  sickle-cell — *see* Disease, sickle-cell, thalassemia
  specified type NEC D56.8
  trait D56.3
  variants D56.8
Thanatophoric dwarfism or short stature Q77.1
Thaysen-Gee disease (nontropical sprue) K90.0
Thaysen's disease K90.0
Thecoma D27 ☑
  luteinized D27 ☑
  malignant C56 ☑
Thelarche, premature E30.8
Thelaziasis B83.8
Thelitis N61.0
  puerperal, postpartum or gestational — *see* Infection, nipple
Therapeutic — *see* condition
Therapy
  drug, long-term (current) (prophylactic)

Therapy — *continued*
  drug — *continued*
    agents affecting estrogen receptors and estrogen levels NEC Z79.818
    anastrozole (Arimidex) Z79.811
    antibiotics Z79.2
      short-term use - omit code
    anticoagulants Z79.01
    anti-inflammatory Z79.1
    antiplatelet Z79.02
    antithrombotics Z79.02
    aromatase inhibitors Z79.811
    aspirin Z79.82
    birth control pill or patch Z79.3
    bisphosphonates Z79.83
    contraceptive, oral Z79.3
    drug, specified NEC Z79.899
    estrogen receptor downregulators Z79.818
    Evista Z79.810
    exemestane (Aromasin) Z79.811
    Fareston Z79.810
    fulvestrant (Faslodex) Z79.818
    gonadotropin-releasing hormone (GnRH) agonist Z79.818
    goserelin acetate (Zoladex) Z79.818
    hormone replacement Z79.890
    insulin Z79.4
    letrozole (Femara) Z79.811
    leuprolide acetate (leuprorelin) (Lupron) Z79.818
    megestrol acetate (Megace) Z79.818
    methadone
      for pain management Z79.891
      maintenance therapy F11.20
    Nolvadex Z79.810
    opiate analgesic Z79.891
    oral contraceptive Z79.3
    raloxifene (Evista) Z79.810
    selective estrogen receptor modulators (SERMs) Z79.810
    short term - omit code
    steroids
      inhaled Z79.51
      systemic Z79.52
    tamoxifen (Nolvadex) Z79.810
    toremifene (Fareston) Z79.810
Thermic — *see* condition
Thermography (abnormal) (*see also* Abnormal, diagnostic imaging) R93.89
  breast R92.8
Thermoplegia T67.01 ☑
Thesaurismosis, glycogen — *see* Disease, glycogen storage
Thiamin deficiency E51.9
  specified NEC E51.8
Thiaminic deficiency with beriberi E51.11
Thibierge-Weissenbach syndrome — *see* Sclerosis, systemic
Thickening
  bone — *see* Hypertrophy, bone
  breast N64.59
  endometrium R93.89
  epidermal L85.9
    specified NEC L85.8
  hymen N89.6
  larynx J38.7
  nail L60.2
    congenital Q84.5
  periosteal — *see* Hypertrophy, bone
  pleura J92.9
    with asbestos J92.0
  skin R23.4
  subepiglottic J38.7
  tongue K14.8
  valve, heart — *see* Endocarditis
Thigh — *see* condition
Thinning vertebra — *see* Spondylopathy, specified NEC
Thirst, excessive R63.1
  due to deprivation of water T73.1 ☑
Thomsen disease G71.12
Thoracic (*see also* condition)
  kidney Q63.2
  outlet syndrome G54.0
Thoracogastroschisis (congenital) Q79.8
Thoracopagus Q89.4
Thorax — *see* condition
Thorn's syndrome N28.89
Thorson-Björck syndrome E34.0
Threadworm (infection) (infestation) B80
Threatened
  abortion O20.0
    with subsequent abortion O03.9
  job loss, anxiety concerning Z56.2

Threatened — *continued*
  labor (without delivery) O47.9
    at or after 37 completed weeks of gestation O47.1
    before 37 completed weeks of gestation O47.0 ☑
  loss of job, anxiety concerning Z56.2
  miscarriage O20.0
  unemployment, anxiety concerning Z56.2
Three-day fever A93.1
Threshers' lung J67.0
Thrix annulata (congenital) Q84.1
Throat — *see* condition
Thrombasthenia (Glanzmann) (hemorrhagic) (hereditary) D69.1
Thromboangiitis I73.1
  obliterans (general) I73.1
    cerebral I67.89
    vessels
      brain I67.89
      spinal cord I67.89
Thromboarteritis — *see* Arteritis
Thromboasthenia (Glanzmann) (hemorrhagic) (hereditary) D69.1
Thrombocytasthenia (Glanzmann) D69.1
Thrombocythemia (essential) (hemorrhagic) (idiopathic) (primary) D47.3
Thrombocytopathy (dystrophic) (granulopenic) D69.1
Thrombocytopenia, thrombocytopenic D69.6
  with absent radius (TAR) Q87.2
  congenital D69.42
  dilutional D69.59
  due to
    drugs D69.59
    extracorporeal circulation of blood D69.59
    (massive) blood transfusion D69.59
    platelet alloimmunization D69.59
  essential D69.3
  heparin induced (HIT) D75.82
  hereditary D69.42
  idiopathic D69.3
  neonatal, transitory P61.0
    due to
      exchange transfusion P61.0
      idiopathic maternal thrombocytopenia P61.0
      isoimmunization P61.0
  primary NEC D69.49
    idiopathic D69.3
  puerperal, postpartum O72.3
  secondary D69.59
  transient neonatal P61.0
Thrombocytosis, essential D47.3
  primary D47.3
Thromboembolism — *see* Embolism
Thrombopathy (Bernard-Soulier) D69.1
  constitutional D68.0
  Willebrand-Jurgens D68.0
Thrombopenia — *see* Thrombocytopenia
Thrombophilia D68.59
  primary NEC D68.59
  secondary NEC D68.69
  specified NEC D68.69
Thrombophlebitis I80.9
  antepartum O22.2 ☑
    deep O22.3 ☑
    superficial O22.2 ☑
  calf muscular vein (NOS) I80.25 ☑
  cavernous (venous) sinus G08
    complicating pregnancy O22.5 ☑
    nonpyogenic I67.6
  cerebral (sinus) (vein) G08
    nonpyogenic I67.6
    sequelae G09
  due to implanted device — *see* Complications, by site and type, specified NEC
  during or resulting from a procedure NEC T81.72 ☑
  femoral vein (superficial) I80.1 ☑
  femoropopliteal vein I80.0 ☑
  gastrocnemial vein I80.25 ☑
  hepatic (vein) I80.8
  idiopathic, recurrent I82.1
  iliac vein (common) (external) (internal) I80.21 ☑
  iliofemoral I80.1 ☑
  intracranial venous sinus (any) G08
    nonpyogenic I67.6
    sequelae G09
  intraspinal venous sinuses and veins G08
    nonpyogenic G95.19
  lateral (venous) sinus G08
    nonpyogenic I67.6
  leg I80.3
    superficial I80.0 ☑
  longitudinal (venous) sinus G08
    nonpyogenic I67.6

Thrombophlebitis — *continued*
  lower extremity I80.299
  migrans, migrating I82.1
  pelvic
    with ectopic or molar pregnancy O08.0
    following ectopic or molar pregnancy O08.0
    puerperal O87.1
  peroneal vein I80.24 ☑
  popliteal vein — *see* Phlebitis, leg, deep, popliteal
  portal (vein) K75.1
  postoperative T81.72 ☑
  pregnancy — *see* Thrombophlebitis, antepartum
  puerperal, postpartum, childbirth O87.0
    deep O87.1
    pelvic O87.1
    septic O86.81
    superficial O87.0
  saphenous (greater) (lesser) I80.0 ☑
  sinus (intracranial) G08
    nonpyogenic I67.6
  soleal vein I80.25 ☑
  specified site NEC I80.8
  tibial vein (anterior) (posterior) I80.23 ☑
Thrombosis, thrombotic (bland) (multiple) (progressive) (silent) (vessel) I82.90
  anal K64.5
  antepartum — *see* Thrombophlebitis, antepartum
  aorta, aortic I74.10
    abdominal I74.09
      saddle I74.01
    bifurcation I74.09
    saddle I74.01
    specified site NEC I74.19
    terminal I74.09
    thoracic I74.11
    valve — *see* Endocarditis, aortic
  apoplexy I63.3 ☑
  artery, arteries (postinfectional) I74.9
    auditory, internal — *see* Occlusion, artery, precerebral, specified NEC
    basilar — *see* Occlusion, artery, basilar
    carotid (common) (internal) — *see* Occlusion, artery, carotid
    cerebellar (anterior inferior) (posterior inferior) (superior) — *see* Occlusion, artery, cerebellar
    cerebral — *see* Occlusion, artery, cerebral
    choroidal (anterior) — *see* Occlusion, artery, precerebral, specified NEC
    communicating, posterior — *see* Occlusion, artery, precerebral, specified NEC
    coronary (*see also* Infarct, myocardium)
      not resulting in infarction I24.0
    hepatic I74.8
    hypophyseal — *see* Occlusion, artery, precerebral, specified NEC
    iliac I74.5
    limb I74.4
      lower I74.3
      upper I74.2
    meningeal, anterior or posterior — *see* Occlusion, artery, cerebral, specified NEC
    mesenteric (with gangrene) (*see also* Infarct, intestine) K55.069
    ophthalmic — *see* Occlusion, artery, retina
    pontine — *see* Occlusion, artery, precerebral, specified NEC
    precerebral — *see* Occlusion, artery, precerebral
    pulmonary (iatrogenic) — *see* Embolism, pulmonary
    renal N28.0
    retinal — *see* Occlusion, artery, retina
    spinal, anterior or posterior G95.11
    traumatic NEC T14.8 ☑
    vertebral — *see* Occlusion, artery, vertebral
  atrium, auricular (*see also* Infarct, myocardium)
    following acute myocardial infarction (current complication) I23.6
    not resulting in infarction I51.3
    old I51.3
  basilar (artery) — *see* Occlusion, artery, basilar
  brain (artery) (stem) (*see also* Occlusion, artery, cerebral)
    due to syphilis A52.05
    puerperal O99.43
    sinus — *see* Thrombosis, intracranial venous sinus
  capillary I78.8
  cardiac (*see also* Infarct, myocardium)
    not resulting in infarction I51.3
    old I51.3
    valve — *see* Endocarditis
  carotid (artery) (common) (internal) — *see* Occlusion, artery, carotid

Thrombosis — *continued*
cavernous (venous) sinus — *see* Thrombosis,
intracranial venous sinus
cerebellar artery (anterior inferior) (posterior
inferior) (superior) I66.3
cerebral (artery) — *see* Occlusion, artery, cerebral
cerebrovenous sinus (*see also* Thrombosis,
intracranial venous sinus)
puerperium O87.3
chronic I82.91
coronary (artery) (vein) (*see also* Infarct,
myocardium)
not resulting in infarction I24.0
corpus cavernosum N48.89
cortical I66.9
deep — *see* Embolism, vein, lower extremity
due to device, implant or graft (*see also*
Complications, by site and type, specified NEC)
T85.868 ☑
arterial graft NEC T82.868 ☑
breast (implant) T85.868 ☑
catheter NEC T85.868 ☑
dialysis (renal) T82.868 ☑
intraperitoneal T85.868 ☑
infusion NEC T82.868 ☑
spinal (epidural) (subdural) T85.860 ☑
urinary (indwelling) T83.86 ☑
electronic (electrode) (pulse generator)
(stimulator)
bone T84.86 ☑
cardiac T82.867 ☑
nervous system (brain) (peripheral nerve)
(spinal) T85.860 ☑
urinary T83.86 ☑
fixation, internal (orthopedic) NEC T84.86 ☑
gastrointestinal (bile duct) (esophagus)
T85.868 ☑
genital NEC T83.86 ☑
heart T82.867 ☑
joint prosthesis T84.86 ☑
ocular (corneal graft) (orbital implant) NEC
T85.868 ☑
orthopedic NEC T84.86 ☑
specified NEC T85.868 ☑
urinary NEC T83.86 ☑
vascular NEC T82.868 ☑
ventricular intracranial shunt T85.860 ☑
during the puerperium — *see* Thrombosis,
puerperal
endocardial (*see also* Infarct, myocardium)
not resulting in infarction I51.3
eye — *see* Occlusion, retina
genital organ
female NEC N94.89
pregnancy — *see* Thrombophlebitis,
antepartum
male N50.1
gestational — *see* Phlebopathy, gestational
heart (chamber) (*see also* Infarct, myocardium)
not resulting in infarction I51.3
old I51.3
hepatic (vein) I82.0
artery I74.8
history (of) Z86.718
intestine (with gangrene) (*see also* Infarct, intestine)
K55.069
intracardiac NEC (apical) (atrial) (auricular)
(ventricular) (old) I51.3
intracranial (arterial) I66.9
venous sinus (any) G08
nonpyogenic origin I67.6
puerperium O87.3
intramural (*see also* Infarct, myocardium)
not resulting in infarction I51.3
old I51.3
intraspinal venous sinuses and veins G08
nonpyogenic G95.19
kidney (artery) N28.0
lateral (venous) sinus — *see* Thrombosis, intracranial
venous sinus
leg — *see* Thrombosis, vein, lower extremity
arterial I74.3
liver (venous) I82.0
artery I74.8
portal vein I81
longitudinal (venous) sinus — *see* Thrombosis,
intracranial venous sinus
lower limb — *see* Thrombosis, vein, lower extremity
lung (iatrogenic) (postoperative) — *see* Embolism,
pulmonary
meninges (brain) (arterial) I66.8

Thrombosis — *continued*
mesenteric (artery) (with gangrene) (*see also* Infarct,
intestine) K55.069
vein (inferior) (superior) K55.0 ☑
mitral I34.8
mural (*see also* Infarct, myocardium)
due to syphilis A52.06
not resulting in infarction I51.3
old I51.3
omentum (with gangrene) (*see also* Infarct,
intestine) K55.069
ophthalmic — *see* Occlusion, retina
pampiniform plexus (male) N50.1
parietal (*see also* Infarct, myocardium)
not resulting in infarction I24.0
penis, superficial vein N48.81
perianal venous K64.5
peripheral arteries I74.4
upper I74.2
personal history (of) Z86.718
portal I81
due to syphilis A52.09
precerebral artery — *see* Occlusion, artery,
precerebral
puerperal, postpartum O87.0
brain (artery) O99.43
venous (sinus) O87.3
cardiac O99.43
cerebral (artery) O99.43
venous (sinus) O87.3
superficial O87.0
pulmonary (artery) (iatrogenic) (postoperative)
(vein) — *see* Embolism, pulmonary
renal (artery) N28.0
vein I82.3
resulting from presence of device, implant or graft
— *see* Complications, by site and type, specified
NEC
retina, retinal — *see* Occlusion, retina
scrotum N50.1
seminal vesicle N50.1
sigmoid (venous) sinus — *see* Thrombosis,
intracranial venous sinus
sinus, intracranial (any) — *see* Thrombosis,
intracranial venous sinus
specified site NEC I82.890
chronic I82.891
spermatic cord N50.1
spinal cord (arterial) G95.11
due to syphilis A52.09
pyogenic origin G06.1
spleen, splenic D73.5
artery I74.8
testis N50.1
tumor — *see* Neoplasm, unspecified behavior, by
site
traumatic NEC T14.8 ☑
tricuspid I07.8
tunica vaginalis N50.1
umbilical cord (vessels), complicating delivery
O69.5 ☑
vas deferens N50.1
vein (acute) I82.90
antecubital I82.61 ☑
chronic I82.71 ☑
axillary I82.A1 ☑
chronic I82.A2 ☑
basilic I82.61 ☑
chronic I82.71 ☑
brachial I82.62 ☑
chronic I82.72 ☑
brachiocephalic (innominate) I82.290
chronic I82.291
cerebral, nonpyogenic I67.6
cephalic I82.61 ☑
chronic I82.71 ☑
chronic I82.91
deep (DVT) I82.40 ☑
calf I82.4Z ☑
chronic I82.5Z ☑
lower leg I82.4Z ☑
chronic I82.5Z ☑
thigh I82.4Y ☑
chronic I82.5Y ☑
upper leg I82.4Y ☑
chronic I82.5Y ☑
femoral I82.41 ☑
chronic I82.51 ☑
iliac (iliofemoral) I82.42 ☑
chronic I82.52 ☑
innominate I82.290
chronic I82.291

Thrombosis — *continued*
vein — *continued*
internal jugular I82.C1 ☑
chronic I82.C2 ☑
lower extremity
deep I82.40 ☑
chronic I82.50 ☑
specified NEC I82.49 ☑
chronic NEC I82.59 ☑
distal
deep I82.4Z ☑
proximal
deep I82.4Y ☑
chronic I82.5Y ☑
superficial I82.81 ☑
perianal K64.5
popliteal I82.43 ☑
chronic I82.53 ☑
radial I82.62 ☑
chronic I82.72 ☑
renal I82.3
saphenous (greater) (lesser) I82.81 ☑
specified NEC I82.890
chronic NEC I82.891
subclavian I82.B1 ☑
chronic I82.B2 ☑
thoracic NEC I82.290
chronic I82.291
tibial I82.44 ☑
chronic I82.54 ☑
ulnar I82.62 ☑
chronic I82.72 ☑
upper extremity I82.60 ☑
chronic I82.70 ☑
deep I82.62 ☑
chronic I82.72 ☑
superficial I82.61 ☑
chronic I82.71 ☑
vena cava
inferior I82.220
chronic I82.221
superior I82.210
chronic I82.211
venous, perianal K64.5
ventricle (*see also* Infarct, myocardium)
following acute myocardial infarction (current
complication) I23.6
not resulting in infarction I24.0
old I51.3
Thrombus — *see* Thrombosis
Thrush (*see also* Candidiasis)
oral B37.0
newborn P37.5
vaginal B37.3
Thumb (*see also* condition)
sucking (child problem) F98.8
Thymitis E32.8
Thymoma (benign) D15.0
malignant C37
Thymus, thymic (gland) — *see* condition
Thyrocele — *see* Goiter
Thyroglossal (*see also* condition)
cyst Q89.2
duct, persistent Q89.2
Thyroid (gland) (body) (*see also* condition)
hormone resistance E07.89
lingual Q89.2
nodule (cystic) (nontoxic) (single) E04.1
Thyroiditis E06.9
acute (nonsuppurative) (pyogenic) (suppurative)
E06.0
autoimmune E06.3
chronic (nonspecific) (sclerosing) E06.5
with thyrotoxicosis, transient E06.2
fibrous E06.5
lymphadenoid E06.3
lymphocytic E06.3
lymphoid E06.3
de Quervain's E06.1
drug-induced E06.4
fibrous (chronic) E06.5
giant-cell (follicular) E06.1
granulomatous (de Quervain) (subacute) E06.1
Hashimoto's (struma lymphomatosa) E06.3
iatrogenic E06.4
ligneous E06.5
lymphocytic (chronic) E06.3
lymphoid E06.3
lymphomatous E06.3
nonsuppurative E06.1
postpartum, puerperal O90.5
pseudotuberculous E06.1

Thyroiditis - Torticollis

Thyroiditis — *continued*
  pyogenic E06.0
  radiation E06.4
  Riedel's E06.5
  subacute (granulomatous) E06.1
  suppurative E06.0
  tuberculous A18.81
  viral E06.1
  woody E06.5
Thyrolingual duct, persistent Q89.2
Thyromegaly E01.0
Thyrotoxic
  crisis — *see* Thyrotoxicosis
  heart disease or failure (*see also* Thyrotoxicosis)
    E05.90 *[I43]*
    with thyroid storm E05.91 *[I43]*
  storm — *see* Thyrotoxicosis
Thyrotoxicosis (recurrent) E05.90
  with
    goiter (diffuse) E05.00
      with thyroid storm E05.01
      adenomatous uninodular E05.10
        with thyroid storm E05.11
      multinodular E05.20
        with thyroid storm E05.21
      nodular E05.20
        with thyroid storm E05.21
      uninodular E05.10
        with thyroid storm E05.11
    infiltrative
      dermopathy E05.00
        with thyroid storm E05.01
      ophthalmopathy E05.00
        with thyroid storm E05.01
    single thyroid nodule E05.10
      with thyroid storm E05.11
    thyroid storm E05.91
  due to
    ectopic thyroid nodule or tissue E05.30
      with thyroid storm E05.31
    ingestion of (excessive) thyroid material E05.40
      with thyroid storm E05.41
    overproduction of thyroid-stimulating hormone
      E05.80
      with thyroid storm E05.81
    specified cause NEC E05.80
      with thyroid storm E05.81
  factitia E05.40
    with thyroid storm E05.41
  heart (*see also* Failure, heart, high-output) E05.90 *[I43]*
    with thyroid storm (*see also* Failure, heart, high-output) E05.91 *[I43]*
    failure (*see also* Failure, heart, high-output)
      E05.90 *[I43]*
  neonatal (transient) P72.1
  transient with chronic thyroiditis E06.2
Tibia vara — *see* Osteochondrosis, juvenile, tibia
Tic (disorder) F95.9
  breathing F95.8
  child problem F95.0
  compulsive F95.1
  de la Tourette F95.2
  degenerate (generalized) (localized) G25.69
    facial G25.69
  disorder
    chronic
      motor F95.1
      vocal F95.1
    combined vocal and multiple motor F95.2
    transient F95.0
  douloureux G50.0
    atypical G50.1
    postherpetic, postzoster B02.22
  drug-induced G25.61
  eyelid F95.8
  habit F95.9
    chronic F95.1
    transient of childhood F95.0
  lid, transient of childhood F95.0
  motor-verbal F95.2
  occupational F48.8
  orbicularis F95.8
    transient of childhood F95.0
  organic origin G25.69
  provisional F95.0
  postchoreic G25.69
  psychogenic, compulsive F95.1
  salaam R25.8
  spasm (motor or vocal) F95.9
    chronic F95.1
    transient of childhood F95.0
  specified NEC F95.8

Tick-borne — *see* condition
Tietze's disease or syndrome M94.0
Tight, tightness
  anus K62.89
  chest R07.89
  fascia (lata) M62.89
  foreskin (congenital) N47.1
  hymen, hymenal ring N89.6
  introitus (acquired) (congenital) N89.6
  rectal sphincter K62.89
  tendon — *see* Short, tendon
  urethral sphincter N35.919
Tilting vertebra — *see* Dorsopathy, deforming, specified NEC
Timidity, child F93.8
Tin-miner's lung J63.5
Tinea (intersecta) (tarsi) B35.9
  amiantacea L44.8
  asbestina B35.0
  barbae B35.0
  beard B35.0
  black dot B35.0
  blanca B36.2
  capitis B35.0
  corporis B35.4
  cruris B35.6
  flava B36.0
  foot B35.3
  furfuracea B36.0
  imbricata (Tokelau) B35.5
  kerion B35.0
  manuum B35.2
  microsporic — *see* Dermatophytosis
  nigra B36.1
  nodosa — *see* Piedra
  pedis B35.3
  scalp B35.0
  specified NEC B35.8
  sycosis B35.0
  tonsurans B35.0
  trichophytic — *see* Dermatophytosis
  unguium B35.1
  versicolor B36.0
Tingling sensation (skin) R20.2
Tinnitus NOS H93.1 ☑
  audible H93.1 ☑
  aurium H93.1 ☑
  pulsatile H93.A ☑
  subjective H93.1 ☑
Tipped tooth (teeth) M26.33
Tipping
  pelvis M95.5
    with disproportion (fetopelvic) O33.0
      causing obstructed labor O65.0
  tooth (teeth), fully erupted M26.33
Tiredness R53.83
Tissue — *see* condition
Tobacco (nicotine)
  abuse — *see* Tobacco, use
  dependence — *see* Dependence, drug, nicotine
  harmful use Z72.0
  heart — *see* Tobacco, toxic effect
  maternal use, affecting newborn P04.2
  toxic effect — *see* Table of Drugs and Chemicals, by substance, poisoning
    chewing tobacco — *see* Table of Drugs and Chemicals, by substance, poisoning
    cigarettes — *see* Table of Drugs and Chemicals, by substance, poisoning
  use Z72.0
    complicating
      childbirth O99.334
      pregnancy O99.33 ☑
      puerperium O99.335
    counseling and surveillance Z71.6
    history Z87.891
    withdrawal state (*see also* Dependence, drug, nicotine) F17.203
Tocopherol deficiency E56.0
Todd's
  cirrhosis K74.3
  paralysis (postepileptic) (transitory) G83.84
Toe — *see* condition
Toilet, artificial opening — *see* Attention to, artificial, opening
Tokelau (ringworm) B35.5
Tollwut — *see* Rabies
Tommaselli's disease R31.9
  correct substance properly administered — *see* Table of Drugs and Chemicals, by drug, adverse effect

Tommaselli's — *continued*
  overdose or wrong substance given or taken — *see* Table of Drugs and Chemicals, by drug, poisoning
Tongue (*see also* condition)
  tie Q38.1
Tonic pupil — *see* Anomaly, pupil, function, tonic pupil
Toni-Fanconi syndrome (cystinosis) E72.09
  with cystinosis E72.04
Tonsil — *see* condition
Tonsillitis (acute) (catarrhal) (croupous) (follicular) (gangrenous) (infective) (lacunar) (lingual) (malignant) (membranous) (parenchymatous) (phlegmonous) (pseudomembranous) (purulent) (septic) (subacute) (suppurative) (toxic) (ulcerative) (vesicular) (viral) J03.90
  chronic J35.01
    with adenoiditis J35.03
  diphtheritic A36.0
  hypertrophic J35.01
    with adenoiditis J35.03
  recurrent J03.91
  specified organism NEC J03.80
    recurrent J03.81
  staphylococcal J03.80
    recurrent J03.81
  streptococcal J03.00
    recurrent J03.01
  tuberculous A15.8
  Vincent's A69.1
Tooth, teeth — *see* condition
Toothache K08.89
Topagnosis R20.8
Tophi — *see* Gout, chronic
TORCH infection — *see* Infection, congenital
  without active infection P00.2
Torn — *see* Tear
Tornwaldt's cyst or disease J39.2
Torsion
  accessory tube — *see* Torsion, fallopian tube
  adnexa (female) — *see* Torsion, fallopian tube
  aorta, acquired I77.1
  appendix epididymis N44.04
  appendix testis N44.03
  bile duct (common) (hepatic) K83.8
    congenital Q44.5
  bowel, colon or intestine K56.2
  cervix — *see* Malposition, uterus
  cystic duct K82.8
  dystonia — *see* Dystonia, torsion
  epididymis (appendix) N44.04
  fallopian tube N83.52 ☑
    with ovary N83.53
  gallbladder K82.8
    congenital Q44.1
  hydatid of Morgagni
    female N83.52 ☑
    male N44.03
  kidney (pedicle) (leading to infarction) N28.0
  Meckel's diverticulum (congenital) Q43.0
    malignant — *see* Table of Neoplasms, small intestine, malignant
  mesentery K56.2
  omentum K56.2
  organ or site, congenital NEC — *see* Anomaly, by site
  ovary (pedicle) N83.51 ☑
    with fallopian tube N83.53
    congenital Q50.2
  oviduct — *see* Torsion, fallopian tube
  penis (acquired) N48.82
    congenital Q55.63
  spasm — *see* Dystonia, torsion
  spermatic cord N44.02
    extravaginal N44.01
    intravaginal N44.02
  spleen D73.5
  testis, testicle N44.00
    appendix N44.03
  tibia — *see* Deformity, limb, specified type NEC, lower leg
  uterus — *see* Malposition, uterus
Torticollis (intermittent) (spastic) M43.6
  congenital (sternomastoid) Q68.0
  due to birth injury P15.8
  hysterical F44.4
  ocular R29.891
  psychogenic F45.8
    conversion reaction F44.4
  rheumatic M43.6
  rheumatoid M06.88
  spasmodic G24.3
  traumatic, current S13.4 ☑

☑ **Additional character required**

Tortipelvis G24.1
Tortuous
aortic arch Q25.46
artery I77.1
organ or site, congenital NEC — *see* Distortion
retinal vessel, congenital Q14.1
ureter N13.8
urethra N36.8
vein — *see* Varix
Torture, victim of Z65.4
Torula, torular (histolytica) (infection) — *see* Cryptococcosis
Torulosis — *see* Cryptococcosis
Torus (mandibularis) (palatinus) M27.0
fracture — *see* Fracture, by site, torus
Touraine's syndrome Q79.8
Tourette's syndrome F95.2
Tourniquet syndrome — *see* Constriction, external, by site
Tower skull Q75.0
with exophthalmos Q87.0
Toxemia R68.89
bacterial — *see* Sepsis
burn — *see* Burn
eclamptic (with pre-existing hypertension) — *see* Eclampsia
erysipelatous — *see* Erysipelas
fatigue R68.89
food — *see* Poisoning, food
gastrointestinal K52.1
intestinal K52.1
kidney — *see* Uremia
malarial — *see* Malaria
myocardial — *see* Myocarditis, toxic
of pregnancy — *see* Pre-eclampsia
pre-eclamptic — *see* Pre-eclampsia
small intestine K52.1
staphylococcal, due to food A05.0
stasis R68.89
uremic — *see* Uremia
urinary — *see* Uremia
Toxemica cerebropathia psychica (nonalcoholic) F04
alcoholic — *see* Alcohol, amnestic disorder
Toxic (poisoning) (*see also* condition) T65.91 ☑
effect — *see* Table of Drugs and Chemicals, by substance, poisoning
shock syndrome A48.3
thyroid (gland) — *see* Thyrotoxicosis
Toxicemia — *see* Toxemia
Toxicity — *see* Table of Drugs and Chemicals, by substance, poisoning
fava bean D55.0
food, noxious — *see* Poisoning, food
from drug or nonmedicinal substance — *see* Table of Drugs and Chemicals, by drug
Toxicosis (*see also* Toxemia)
capillary, hemorrhagic D69.0
Toxinfection, gastrointestinal K52.1
Toxocariasis B83.0
Toxoplasma, toxoplasmosis (acquired) B58.9
with
hepatitis B58.1
meningoencephalitis B58.2
ocular involvement B58.00
other organ involvement B58.89
pneumonia, pneumonitis B58.3
congenital (acute) (subacute) (chronic) P37.1
maternal, manifest toxoplasmosis in infant (acute) (subacute) (chronic) P37.1
tPA (rtPA) administration in a different facility within the last 24 hours prior to admission to current facility Z92.82
Trabeculation, bladder N32.89
Trachea — *see* condition
Tracheitis (catarrhal) (infantile) (membranous) (plastic) (septal) (suppurative) (viral) J04.10
with
bronchitis (15 years of age and above) J40
acute or subacute — *see* Bronchitis, acute
chronic J42
tuberculous NEC A15.5
under 15 years of age J20.9
laryngitis (acute) J04.2
chronic J37.1
tuberculous NEC A15.5
acute J04.10
with obstruction J04.11
chronic J42
with
bronchitis (chronic) J42
laryngitis (chronic) J37.1
diphtheritic (membranous) A36.89

Tracheitis — *continued*
due to external agent — *see* Inflammation, respiratory, upper, due to
syphilitic A52.73
tuberculous A15.5
Trachelitis (nonvenereal) — *see* Cervicitis
Tracheobronchial — *see* condition
Tracheobronchitis (15 years of age and above) (*see also* Bronchitis)
due to
Bordetella bronchiseptica A37.80
with pneumonia A37.81
Francisella tularensis A21.8
Tracheobronchomegaly Q32.4
with bronchiectasis J47.9
with
exacerbation (acute) J47.1
lower respiratory infection J47.0
acquired J98.09
with bronchiectasis J47.9
with
exacerbation (acute) J47.1
lower respiratory infection J47.0
Tracheobronchopneumonitis — *see* Pneumonia, broncho-
Tracheocele (external) (internal) J39.8
congenital Q32.1
Tracheomalacia J39.8
congenital Q32.0
Tracheopharyngitis (acute) J06.9
chronic J42
due to external agent — *see* Inflammation, respiratory, upper, due to
Tracheostenosis J39.8
Tracheostomy
complication — *see* Complication, tracheostomy
status Z93.0
attention to Z43.0
malfunctioning J95.03
Trachoma, trachomatous A71.9
active (stage) A71.1
contraction of conjunctiva A71.1
dubium A71.0
initial (stage) A71.0
healed or sequelae B94.0
pannus A71.1
Türck's J37.0
Traction, vitreomacular H43.82 ☑
Train sickness T75.3 ☑
Trait(s)
Hb-S D57.3
hemoglobin
abnormal NEC D58.2
with thalassemia D56.3
C — *see* Disease, hemoglobin C
S (Hb-S) D57.3
Lepore D56.3
personality, accentuated Z73.1
sickle-cell D57.3
with elliptocytosis or spherocytosis D57.3
type A personality Z73.1
Tramp Z59.0
Trance R41.89
hysterical F44.89
Transection
abdomen (partial) S38.3 ☑
aorta (incomplete) (*see also* Injury, aorta)
complete — *see* Injury, aorta, laceration, major
carotid artery (incomplete) (*see also* Injury, blood vessel, carotid, laceration)
complete — *see* Injury, blood vessel, carotid, laceration, major
celiac artery (incomplete) S35.211 ☑
branch (incomplete) S35.291 ☑
complete S35.292 ☑
complete S35.212 ☑
innominate
artery (incomplete) (*see also* Injury, blood vessel, thoracic, innominate, artery, laceration)
complete — *see* Injury, blood vessel, thoracic, innominate, artery, laceration, major
vein (incomplete) (*see also* Injury, blood vessel, thoracic, innominate, vein, laceration)
complete — *see* Injury, blood vessel, thoracic, innominate, vein, laceration, major
jugular vein (external) (incomplete) (*see also* Injury, blood vessel, jugular vein, laceration)
complete — *see* Injury, blood vessel, jugular vein, laceration, major
internal (incomplete) (*see also* Injury, blood vessel, jugular vein, internal, laceration)

Transection — *continued*
jugular vein — *continued*
complete — *see* Injury, blood vessel, jugular vein, internal, laceration, major
mesenteric artery (incomplete) (*see also* Injury, mesenteric, artery, laceration)
complete — *see* Injury, mesenteric artery, laceration, major
pulmonary vessel (incomplete) (*see also* Injury, blood vessel, thoracic, pulmonary, laceration)
complete — *see* Injury, blood vessel, thoracic, pulmonary, laceration, major
subclavian — *see* Transection, innominate
vena cava (incomplete) (*see also* Injury, vena cava)
complete — *see* Injury, vena cava, laceration, major
vertebral artery (incomplete) (*see also* Injury, blood vessel, vertebral, laceration)
complete — *see* Injury, blood vessel, vertebral, laceration, major
Transaminasemia R74.0
Transfusion
associated (red blood cell) hemochromatosis E83.111
blood
ABO incompatible — *see* Complication(s), transfusion, incompatibility reaction, ABO
minor blood group (Duffy) (E) (K) (Kell) (Kidd) (Lewis) (M) (N) (P)(s) T80.89 ☑
reaction or complication — *see* Complications, transfusion
fetomaternal (mother) — *see* Pregnancy, complicated by, placenta, transfusion syndrome
maternofetal (mother) — *see* Pregnancy, complicated by, placenta, transfusion syndrome
placental (syndrome) (mother) — *see* Pregnancy, complicated by, placenta, transfusion syndrome
reaction (adverse) — *see* Complications, transfusion
related acute lung injury (TRALI) J95.84
twin-to-twin — *see* Pregnancy, complicated by, placenta, transfusion syndrome, fetus to fetus
Transient (meaning homeless) (*see also* condition) Z59.0
Translocation
balanced autosomal Q95.9
in normal individual Q95.0
chromosomes NEC Q99.8
balanced and insertion in normal individual Q95.0
Down syndrome Q90.2
trisomy
13 Q91.6
18 Q91.2
21 Q90.2
Translucency, iris — *see* Degeneration, iris
Transmission of chemical substances through the placenta — *see* Absorption, chemical, through placenta
Transparency, lung, unilateral J43.0
Transplant (ed) (status) Z94.9
awaiting organ Z76.82
bone Z94.6
marrow Z94.81
candidate Z76.82
complication — *see* Complication, transplant
cornea Z94.7
heart Z94.1
and lung(s) Z94.3
valve Z95.2
prosthetic Z95.2
specified NEC Z95.4
xenogenic Z95.3
intestine Z94.82
kidney Z94.0
liver Z94.4
lung(s) Z94.2
and heart Z94.3
organ (failure) (infection) (rejection) Z94.9
removal status Z98.85
pancreas Z94.83
skin Z94.5
social Z60.3
specified organ or tissue NEC Z94.89
stem cells Z94.84
tissue Z94.9
Transplants, ovarian, endometrial N80.1
Transposed — *see* Transposition
Transposition (congenital) (*see also* Malposition, congenital)

Transposition - Tuberculosis

Transposition — *continued*
  abdominal viscera Q89.3
  aorta (dextra) Q20.3
  appendix Q43.8
  colon Q43.8
  corrected Q20.5
  great vessels (complete) (partial) Q20.3
  heart Q24.0
    with complete transposition of viscera Q89.3
  intestine (large) (small) Q43.8
  reversed jejunal (for bypass) (status) Z98.0
  scrotum Q55.23
  stomach Q40.2
    with general transposition of viscera Q89.3
  tooth, teeth, fully erupted M26.30
  vessels, great (complete) (partial) Q20.3
  viscera (abdominal) (thoracic) Q89.3
Transsexualism F64.0
Transverse (*see also* condition)
  arrest (deep), in labor O64.0 ☑
  lie (mother) O32.2 ☑
    causing obstructed labor O64.8 ☑
Transvestism, transvestitism (dual-role) F64.1
  fetishistic F65.1
Trapped placenta (with hemorrhage) O72.0
  without hemorrhage O73.0
TRAPS (tumor necrosis factor receptor associated periodic syndrome) M04.1
Trauma, traumatism (*see also* Injury)
  acoustic — *see* subcategory H83.3 ☑
  birth — *see* Birth, injury
  complicating ectopic or molar pregnancy O08.6
  during delivery O71.9
  following ectopic or molar pregnancy O08.6
  obstetric O71.9
    specified NEC O71.89
  occlusal
    primary K08.81
    secondary K08.82
Traumatic (*see also* condition)
  brain injury S06.9 ☑
Treacher Collins syndrome Q75.4
Treitz's hernia — *see* Hernia, abdomen, specified site NEC
Trematode infestation — *see* Infestation, fluke
Trematodiasis — *see* Infestation, fluke
Trembling paralysis — *see* Parkinsonism
Tremor(s) R25.1
  drug induced G25.1
  essential (benign) G25.0
  familial G25.0
  hereditary G25.0
  hysterical F44.4
  intention G25.2
  medication induced postural G25.1
  mercurial — *see* subcategory T56.1 ☑
  Parkinson's — *see* Parkinsonism
  psychogenic (conversion reaction) F44.4
  senilis R54
  specified type NEC G25.2
Trench
  fever A79.0
  foot — *see* Immersion, foot
  mouth A69.1
Treponema pallidum infection — *see* Syphilis
Treponematosis
  due to
    T. pallidum — *see* Syphilis
    T. pertenue — *see* Yaws
Triad
  Hutchinson's (congenital syphilis) A50.53
  Kartagener's Q89.3
  Saint's — *see* Hernia, diaphragm
Trichiasis (eyelid) H02.059
  with entropion — *see* Entropion
  left H02.056
    lower H02.055
    upper H02.054
  right H02.053
    lower H02.052
    upper H02.051
Trichinella spiralis (infection) (infestation) B75
Trichinellosis, trichiniasis, trichinelliasis, trichinosis B75
  with muscle disorder B75 [*M63.80*]
    ankle B75 [*M63.87* ☑]
    foot B75 [*M63.87* ☑]
    forearm B75 [*M63.83* ☑]
    hand B75 [*M63.84* ☑]
    lower leg B75 [*M63.86* ☑]
    multiple sites B75 [*M63.89*]
    pelvic region B75 [*M63.85* ☑]
    shoulder region B75 [*M63.81* ☑]

Trichinellosis — *continued*
  with muscle disorder — *continued*
    specified site NEC B75 [*M63.88*]
    thigh B75 [*M63.85* ☑]
    upper arm B75 [*M63.82* ☑]
Trichobezoar T18.9 ☑
  intestine T18.3 ☑
  stomach T18.2 ☑
Trichocephaliasis, trichocephalosis B79
Trichocephalus infestation B79
Trichoclasis L67.8
Trichoepithelioma (*see also* Neoplasm, skin, benign)
  malignant — *see* Neoplasm, skin, malignant
Trichofolliculoma — *see* Neoplasm, skin, benign
Tricholemmoma — *see* Neoplasm, skin, benign
Trichomoniasis A59.9
  bladder A59.03
  cervix A59.09
  intestinal A07.8
  prostate A59.02
  seminal vesicles A59.09
  specified site NEC A59.8
  urethra A59.03
  urogenitalis A59.00
  vagina A59.01
  vulva A59.01
Trichomycosis
  axillaris A48.8
  nodosa, nodularis B36.8
Trichonodosis L67.8
Trichophytid, trichophyton infection — *see* Dermatophytosis
Trichophytobezoar T18.9 ☑
  intestine T18.3 ☑
  stomach T18.2 ☑
Trichophytosis — *see* Dermatophytosis
Trichoptilosis L67.8
Trichorrhexis (nodosa) (invaginata) L67.0
Trichosis axillaris A48.8
Trichosporosis nodosa B36.2
Trichostasis spinulosa (congenital) Q84.1
Trichostrongyliasis, trichostrongylosis (small intestine) B81.2
Trichostrongylus infection B81.2
Trichotillomania F63.3
Trichromat, trichromatopsia, anomalous (congenital) H53.55
Trichuriasis B79
Trichuris trichiura (infection) (infestation) (any site) B79
Tricuspid (valve) — *see* condition
Trifid (*see also* Accessory)
  kidney (pelvis) Q63.8
  tongue Q38.3
Trigeminal neuralgia — *see* Neuralgia, trigeminal
Trigeminy R00.8
Trigger finger (acquired) M65.30
  congenital Q74.0
  index finger M65.32 ☑
  little finger M65.35 ☑
  middle finger M65.33 ☑
  ring finger M65.34 ☑
  thumb M65.31 ☑
Trigonitis (bladder) (chronic) (pseudomembranous) N30.30
  with hematuria N30.31
Trigonocephaly Q75.0
Trilocular heart — *see* Cor triloculare
Trimethylaminuria E72.52
Tripartite placenta O43.19 ☑
Triphalangeal thumb Q74.0
Triple (*see also* Accessory)
  kidneys Q63.0
  uteri Q51.818
  X, female Q97.0
Triplegia G83.89
  congenital G80.8
Triplet (newborn) (*see also* Newborn, triplet)
  complicating pregnancy — *see* Pregnancy, triplet
Triplication — *see* Accessory
Triploidy Q92.7
Trismus R25.2
  neonatorum A33
  newborn A33
Trisomy (syndrome) Q92.9
  autosomes Q92.9
  chromosome specified NEC Q92.8
    partial Q92.2
      due to unbalanced translocation Q92.5
    whole (nonsex chromosome)
      meiotic nondisjunction Q92.0
      mitotic nondisjunction Q92.0
      mosaicism Q92.1

Trisomy — *continued*
  chromosome specified NEC — *continued*
    specified NEC Q92.8
  due to
    dicentrics — *see* Extra, marker chromosomes
    extra rings — *see* Extra, marker chromosomes
    isochromosomes — *see* Extra, marker chromosomes
  specified NEC Q92.8
  whole chromosome Q92.9
    meiotic nondisjunction Q92.0
    mitotic nondisjunction Q92.1
    mosaicism Q92.1
    partial Q92.9
    specified NEC Q92.8
  13 (partial) Q91.7
    meiotic nondisjunction Q91.4
    mitotic nondisjunction Q91.5
    mosaicism Q91.5
    translocation Q91.6
  18 (partial) Q91.3
    meiotic nondisjunction Q91.0
    mitotic nondisjunction Q91.1
    mosaicism Q91.1
    translocation Q91.2
  20 Q92.8
  21 (partial) Q90.9
    meiotic nondisjunction Q90.0
    mitotic nondisjunction Q90.1
    mosaicism Q90.1
    translocation Q90.2
  22 Q92.8
Tritanomaly, tritanopia H53.55
Trombiculosis, trombiculiasis, trombidiosis B88.0
Trophedema (congenital) (hereditary) Q82.0
Trophoblastic disease (*see also* Mole, hydatidiform) O01.9
Tropholymphedema Q82.0
Trophoneurosis NEC G96.8
  disseminated M34.9
Tropical — *see* condition
Trouble (*see also* Disease)
  heart — *see* Disease, heart
  kidney — *see* Disease, renal
  nervous R45.0
  sinus — *see* Sinusitis
Trousseau's syndrome (thrombophlebitis migrans) I82.1
Truancy, childhood
  from school Z72.810
Truncus
  arteriosus (persistent) Q20.0
  communis Q20.0
Trunk — *see* condition
Trypanosomiasis
  African B56.9
    by Trypanosoma brucei
      gambiense B56.0
      rhodesiense B56.1
  American — *see* Chagas' disease
  Brazilian — *see* Chagas' disease
  by Trypanosoma
    brucei gambiense B56.0
    brucei rhodesiense B56.1
    cruzi — *see* Chagas' disease
  gambiensis, Gambian B56.0
  rhodesiensis, Rhodesian B56.1
  South American — *see* Chagas' disease
  where
    African trypanosomiasis is prevalent B56.9
    Chagas' disease is prevalent B57.2
T-shaped incisors K00.2
Tsutsugamushi (disease) (fever) A75.3
Tube, tubal, tubular — *see* condition
Tubercle (*see also* Tuberculosis)
  brain, solitary A17.81
  Darwin's Q17.8
  Ghon, primary infection A15.7
Tuberculid, tuberculide (indurating, subcutaneous) (lichenoid) (miliary) (papulonecrotic) (primary) (skin) A18.4
Tuberculoma (*see also* Tuberculosis)
  brain A17.81
  meninges (cerebral) (spinal) A17.1
  spinal cord A17.81
Tuberculosis, tubercular, tuberculous (calcification) (calcified) (caseous) (chromogenic acid-fast bacilli) (degeneration) (fibrocaseous) (fistula) (interstitial) (isolated circumscribed lesions) (necrosis) (parenchymatous) (ulcerative) A15.9
  with pneumoconiosis (any condition in J60-J64) J65
  abdomen (lymph gland) A18.39

☑ **Additional character required**

Tuberculosis — *continued*
  abscess (respiratory) A15.9
    bone A18.03
      hip A18.02
      knee A18.02
      sacrum A18.01
      specified site NEC A18.03
      spinal A18.01
      vertebra A18.01
    brain A17.81
    breast A18.89
    Cowper's gland A18.15
    dura (mater) (cerebral) (spinal) A17.81
    epidural (cerebral) (spinal) A17.81
    female pelvis A18.17
    frontal sinus A15.8
    genital organs NEC A18.10
    genitourinary A18.10
    gland (lymphatic) — *see* Tuberculosis, lymph gland
    hip A18.02
    intestine A18.32
    ischiorectal A18.32
    joint NEC A18.02
      hip A18.02
      knee A18.02
      specified NEC A18.02
      vertebral A18.01
    kidney A18.11
    knee A18.02
    latent Z22.7
    lumbar (spine) A18.01
    lung — *see* Tuberculosis, pulmonary
    meninges (cerebral) (spinal) A17.0
    muscle A18.09
    perianal (fistula) A18.32
    perinephritic A18.11
    perirectal A18.32
    rectum A18.32
    retropharyngeal A15.8
    sacrum A18.01
    scrofulous A18.2
    scrotum A18.15
    skin (primary) A18.4
    spinal cord A17.81
    spine or vertebra (column) A18.01
    subdiaphragmatic A18.31
    testis A18.15
    urinary A18.13
    uterus A18.17
  accessory sinus — *see* Tuberculosis, sinus
  Addison's disease A18.7
  adenitis — *see* Tuberculosis, lymph gland
  adenoids A15.8
  adenopathy — *see* Tuberculosis, lymph gland
  adherent pericardium A18.84
  adnexa (uteri) A18.17
  adrenal (capsule) (gland) A18.7
  alimentary canal A18.32
  anemia A18.89
  ankle (joint) (bone) A18.02
  anus A18.32
  apex, apical — *see* Tuberculosis, pulmonary
  appendicitis, appendix A18.32
  arachnoid A17.0
  artery, arteritis A18.89
    cerebral A18.89
  arthritis (chronic) (synovial) A18.02
    spine or vertebra (column) A18.01
  articular — *see* Tuberculosis, joint
  ascites A18.31
  asthma — *see* Tuberculosis, pulmonary
  axilla, axillary (gland) A18.2
  bladder A18.12
  bone A18.03
    hip A18.02
    knee A18.02
    limb NEC A18.03
    sacrum A18.01
    spine or vertebral column A18.01
  bowel (miliary) A18.32
  brain A17.81
  breast A18.89
  broad ligament A18.17
  bronchi, bronchial, bronchus A15.5
    ectasia, ectasis (bronchiectasis) — *see*
      Tuberculosis, pulmonary
    fistula A15.5
      primary (progressive) A15.7
    gland or node A15.4
      primary (progressive) A15.7
    lymph gland or node A15.4
      primary (progressive) A15.7

Tuberculosis — *continued*
  bronchiectasis — *see* Tuberculosis, pulmonary
  bronchitis A15.5
  bronchopleural A15.6
  bronchopneumonia, bronchopneumonic — *see*
    Tuberculosis, pulmonary
  bronchorrhagia A15.5
  bronchotracheal A15.5
  bronze disease A18.7
  buccal cavity A18.83
  bulbourethral gland A18.15
  bursa A18.09
  cachexia A15.9
  cardiomyopathy A18.84
  caries — *see* Tuberculosis, bone
  cartilage A18.02
    intervertebral A18.01
  catarrhal — *see* Tuberculosis, respiratory
  cecum A18.32
  cellulitis (primary) A18.4
  cerebellum A17.81
  cerebral, cerebrum A17.81
  cerebrospinal A17.81
    meninges A17.0
  cervical (lymph gland or node) A18.2
  cervicitis, cervix (uteri) A18.16
  chest — *see* Tuberculosis, respiratory
  chorioretinitis A18.53
  choroid, choroiditis A18.53
  ciliary body A18.54
  colitis A18.32
  collier's J65
  colliquativa (primary) A18.4
  colon A18.32
  complex, primary A15.7
  congenital P37.0
  conjunctiva A18.59
  connective tissue (systemic) A18.89
  contact Z20.1
  cornea (ulcer) A18.52
  Cowper's gland A18.15
  coxae A18.02
  coxalgia A18.02
  cul-de-sac of Douglas A18.17
  curvature, spine A18.01
  cutis (colliquativa) (primary) A18.4
  cyst, ovary A18.18
  cystitis A18.12
  dactylitis A18.03
  diarrhea A18.32
  diffuse — *see* Tuberculosis, miliary
  digestive tract A18.32
  disseminated — *see* Tuberculosis, miliary
  duodenum A18.32
  dura (mater) (cerebral) (spinal) A17.0
    abscess (cerebral) (spinal) A17.81
  dysentery A18.32
  ear (inner) (middle) A18.6
    bone A18.03
    external (primary) A18.4
    skin (primary) A18.4
  elbow A18.02
  emphysema — *see* Tuberculosis, pulmonary
  empyema A15.6
  encephalitis A17.82
  endarteritis A18.89
  endocarditis A18.84
    aortic A18.84
    mitral A18.84
    pulmonary A18.84
    tricuspid A18.84
  endocrine glands NEC A18.82
  endometrium A18.17
  enteric, enterica, enteritis A18.32
  enterocolitis A18.32
  epididymis, epididymitis A18.15
  epidural abscess (cerebral) (spinal) A17.81
  epiglottis A15.5
  episcleritis A18.51
  erythema (induratum) (nodosum) (primary) A18.4
  esophagus A18.83
  eustachian tube A18.6
  exposure (to) Z20.1
  exudative — *see* Tuberculosis, pulmonary
  eye A18.50
  eyelid (primary) (lupus) A18.4
  fallopian tube (acute) (chronic) A18.17
  fascia A18.09
  fauces A15.8
  female pelvic inflammatory disease A18.17
  finger A18.03
  first infection A15.7

Tuberculosis — *continued*
  gallbladder A18.83
  ganglion A18.09
  gastritis A18.83
  gastrocolic fistula A18.32
  gastroenteritis A18.32
  gastrointestinal tract A18.32
  general, generalized — *see* Tuberculosis, miliary
  genital organs A18.10
  genitourinary A18.10
  genu A18.02
  glandula suprarenalis A18.7
  glandular, general A18.2
  glottis A15.5
  grinder's J65
  gum A18.83
  hand A18.03
  heart A18.84
  hematogenous — *see* Tuberculosis, miliary
  hemoptysis — *see* Tuberculosis, pulmonary
  hemorrhage NEC — *see* Tuberculosis, pulmonary
  hemothorax A15.6
  hepatitis A18.83
  hilar lymph nodes A15.4
    primary (progressive) A15.7
  hip (joint) (disease) (bone) A18.02
  hydropneumothorax A15.6
  hydrothorax A15.6
  hypoadrenalism A18.7
  hypopharynx A15.8
  ileocecal (hyperplastic) A18.32
  ileocolitis A18.32
  ileum A18.32
  iliac spine (superior) A18.03
  immunological findings only A15.7
  indurativa (primary) A18.4
  infantile A15.7
  infection A15.9
    without clinical manifestations A15.7
  infraclavicular gland A18.2
  inguinal gland A18.2
  inguinalis A18.2
  intestine (any part) A18.32
  iridocyclitis A18.54
  iris, iritis A18.54
  ischiorectal A18.32
  jaw A18.03
  jejunum A18.32
  joint A18.02
    vertebral A18.01
  keratitis (interstitial) A18.52
  keratoconjunctivitis A18.52
  kidney A18.11
  knee (joint) A18.02
  kyphosis, kyphoscoliosis A18.01
  laryngitis A15.5
  larynx A15.5
  latent Z22.7
  leptomeninges, leptomeningitis (cerebral) (spinal)
    A17.0
  lichenoides (primary) A18.4
  linguae A18.83
  lip A18.83
  liver A18.83
  lordosis A18.01
  lung — *see* Tuberculosis, pulmonary
  lupus vulgaris A18.4
  lymph gland or node (peripheral) A18.2
    abdomen A18.39
    bronchial A15.4
      primary (progressive) A15.7
    cervical A18.2
    hilar A15.4
      primary (progressive) A15.7
    intrathoracic A15.4
      primary (progressive) A15.7
    mediastinal A15.4
      primary (progressive) A15.7
    mesenteric A18.39
    retroperitoneal A18.39
    tracheobronchial A15.4
      primary (progressive) A15.7
  lymphadenitis — *see* Tuberculosis, lymph gland
  lymphangitis — *see* Tuberculosis, lymph gland
  lymphatic (gland) (vessel) — *see* Tuberculosis,
    lymph gland
  mammary gland A18.89
  marasmus A15.9
  mastoiditis A18.03
  mediastinal lymph gland or node A15.4
    primary (progressive) A15.7

Tuberculosis — *continued*
  mediastinitis A15.8
    primary (progressive) A15.7
  mediastinum A15.8
    primary (progressive) A15.7
  medulla A17.81
  melanosis, Addisonian A18.7
  meninges, meningitis (basilar) (cerebral)
      (cerebrospinal) (spinal) A17.0
  meningoencephalitis A17.82
  mesentery, mesenteric (gland or node) A18.39
  miliary A19.9
    acute A19.2
      multiple sites A19.1
      single specified site A19.0
    chronic A19.8
    specified NEC A19.8
  millstone makers' J65
  miner's J65
  molder's J65
  mouth A18.83
  multiple A19.9
    acute A19.1
    chronic A19.8
  muscle A18.09
  myelitis A17.82
  myocardium, myocarditis A18.84
  nasal (passage) (sinus) A15.8
  nasopharynx A15.8
  neck gland A18.2
  nephritis A18.11
  nerve (mononeuropathy) A17.83
  nervous system A17.9
  nose (septum) A15.8
  ocular A18.50
  omentum A18.31
  oophoritis (acute) (chronic) A18.17
  optic (nerve trunk) (papilla) A18.59
  orbit A18.59
  orchitis A18.15
  organ, specified NEC A18.89
  osseous — *see* Tuberculosis, bone
  osteitis — *see* Tuberculosis, bone
  osteomyelitis — *see* Tuberculosis, bone
  otitis media A18.6
  ovary, ovaritis (acute) (chronic) A18.17
  oviduct (acute) (chronic) A18.17
  pachymeningitis A17.0
  palate (soft) A18.83
  pancreas A18.83
  papulonecrotic (a) (primary) A18.4
  parathyroid glands A18.82
  paronychia (primary) A18.4
  parotid gland or region A18.83
  pelvis (bony) A18.03
  penis A18.15
  peribronchitis A15.5
  pericardium, pericarditis A18.84
  perichondritis, larynx A15.5
  periostitis — *see* Tuberculosis, bone
  perirectal fistula A18.32
  peritoneum NEC A18.31
  peritonitis A18.31
  pharynx, pharyngitis A15.8
  phlyctenulosis (keratoconjunctivitis) A18.52
  phthisis NEC — *see* Tuberculosis, pulmonary
  pituitary gland A18.82
  pleura, pleural, pleurisy, pleuritis (fibrinous)
      (obliterative) (purulent) (simple plastic) (with
      effusion) A15.6
    primary (progressive) A15.7
  pneumonia, pneumonic — *see* Tuberculosis,
      pulmonary
  pneumothorax (spontaneous) (tense valvular) —
      see Tuberculosis, pulmonary
  polyneuropathy A17.89
  polyserositis A19.9
    acute A19.1
    chronic A19.8
  potter's J65
  prepuce A18.15
  primary (complex) A15.7
  proctitis A18.32
  prostate, prostatitis A18.14
  pulmonalis — *see* Tuberculosis, pulmonary
  pulmonary (cavitated) (fibrotic) (infiltrative)
      (nodular) A15.0
    childhood type or first infection A15.7
    primary (complex) A15.7
  pyelitis A18.11
  pyelonephritis A18.11
  pyemia — *see* Tuberculosis, miliary

Tuberculosis — *continued*
  pyonephrosis A18.11
  pyopneumothorax A15.6
  pyothorax A15.6
  rectum (fistula) (with abscess) A18.32
  reinfection stage — *see* Tuberculosis, pulmonary
  renal A18.11
  renis A18.11
  respiratory A15.9
    primary A15.7
    specified site NEC A15.8
  retina, retinitis A18.53
  retroperitoneal (lymph gland or node) A18.39
  rheumatism NEC A18.09
  rhinitis A15.8
  sacroiliac (joint) A18.01
  sacrum A18.01
  salivary gland A18.83
  salpingitis (acute) (chronic) A18.17
  sandblaster's J65
  sclera A18.51
  scoliosis A18.01
  scrofulous A18.2
  scrotum A18.15
  seminal tract or vesicle A18.15
  senile A15.9
  septic — *see* Tuberculosis, miliary
  shoulder (joint) A18.02
    blade A18.03
  sigmoid A18.32
  sinus (any nasal) A15.8
    bone A18.03
    epididymis A18.15
  skeletal NEC A18.03
  skin (any site) (primary) A18.4
  small intestine A18.32
  soft palate A18.83
  spermatic cord A18.15
  spine, spinal (column) A18.01
    cord A17.81
    medulla A17.81
    membrane A17.0
    meninges A17.0
  spleen, splenitis A18.85
  spondylitis A18.01
  sternoclavicular joint A18.02
  stomach A18.83
  stonemason's J65
  subcutaneous tissue (cellular) (primary) A18.4
  subcutis (primary) A18.4
  subdeltoid bursa A18.83
  submaxillary (region) A18.83
  supraclavicular gland A18.2
  suprarenal (capsule) (gland) A18.7
  swelling, joint (*see also* category M01 ☑) (*see also*
      Tuberculosis, joint) A18.02
  symphysis pubis A18.02
  synovitis A18.09
    articular A18.02
    spine or vertebra A18.01
  systemic — *see* Tuberculosis, miliary
  tarsitis A18.4
  tendon (sheath) — *see* Tuberculosis, tenosynovitis
  tenosynovitis A18.09
    spine or vertebra A18.01
  testis A18.15
  throat A15.8
  thymus gland A18.82
  thyroid gland A18.81
  tongue A18.83
  tonsil, tonsillitis A15.8
  trachea, tracheal A15.5
    lymph gland or node A15.4
      primary (progressive) A15.7
  tracheobronchial A15.5
    lymph gland or node A15.4
      primary (progressive) A15.7
  tubal (acute) (chronic) A18.17
  tunica vaginalis A18.15
  ulcer (skin) (primary) A18.4
    bowel or intestine A18.32
    specified NEC - code under Tuberculosis, by site
  unspecified site A15.9
  ureter A18.11
  urethra, urethral (gland) A18.13
  urinary organ or tract A18.13
  uterus A18.17
  uveal tract A18.54
  uvula A18.83
  vagina A18.18
  vas deferens A18.15
  verruca, verrucosa (cutis) (primary) A18.4

Tuberculosis — *continued*
  vertebra (column) A18.01
  vesiculitis A18.15
  vulva A18.18
  wrist (joint) A18.02
Tuberculum
  Carabelli — *see* Note at K00.2
  occlusal — *see* Note at K00.2
  paramolare K00.2
Tuberosity, entire maxillary M26.07
Tuberous sclerosis (brain) Q85.1
Tubo-ovarian — *see* condition
Tuboplasty, after previous sterilization Z31.0
  aftercare Z31.42
Tubotympanitis, catarrhal (chronic) — *see* Otitis,
    media, nonsuppurative, chronic, serous
Tularemia A21.9
  with
    conjunctivitis A21.1
    pneumonia A21.2
  abdominal A21.3
  bronchopneumonic A21.2
  conjunctivitis A21.1
  cryptogenic A21.3
  enteric A21.3
  gastrointestinal A21.3
  generalized A21.7
  ingestion A21.3
  intestinal A21.3
  oculoglandular A21.1
  ophthalmic A21.1
  pneumonia (any), pneumonic A21.2
  pulmonary A21.2
  sepsis A21.7
  specified NEC A21.8
  typhoidal A21.7
  ulceroglandular A21.0
Tularensis conjunctivitis A21.1
Tumefaction (*see also* Swelling)
  liver — *see* Hypertrophy, liver
Tumor (*see also* Neoplasm, unspecified behavior, by
    site)
  acinar cell — *see* Neoplasm, uncertain behavior,
      by site
  acinic cell — *see* Neoplasm, uncertain behavior,
      by site
  adenocarcinoid — *see* Neoplasm, malignant, by site
  adenomatoid (*see also* Neoplasm, benign, by site)
    odontogenic — *see* Cyst, calcifying odontogenic
  adnexal (skin) — *see* Neoplasm, skin, benign, by site
  adrenal
    cortical (benign) D35.0 ☑
      malignant C74.0 ☑
    rest — *see* Neoplasm, benign, by site
  alpha-cell
    malignant
      pancreas C25.4
      specified site NEC — *see* Neoplasm, malignant,
          by site
      unspecified site C25.4
    pancreas D13.7
    specified site NEC — *see* Neoplasm, benign, by
        site
    unspecified site D13.7
  aneurysmal — *see* Aneurysm
  aortic body D44.7
    malignant C75.5
  Askin's — *see* Neoplasm, connective tissue,
      malignant
  basal cell (*see also* Neoplasm, skin, uncertain
      behavior) D48.5
  Bednar — *see* Neoplasm, skin, malignant
  benign (unclassified) — *see* Neoplasm, benign, by
      site
  beta-cell
    malignant
      pancreas C25.4
      specified site NEC — *see* Neoplasm, malignant,
          by site
      unspecified site C25.4
    pancreas D13.7
    specified site NEC — *see* Neoplasm, benign, by
        site
    unspecified site D13.7
  Brenner D27.9
    borderline malignancy D39.1 ☑
    malignant C56 ☑
    proliferating D39.1 ☑
  bronchial alveolar, intravascular D38.1
  Brooke's — *see* Neoplasm, skin, benign
  brown fat — *see* Lipoma
  Burkitt — *see* Lymphoma, Burkitt

☑ **Additional character required**

Tumor — *continued*
- calcifying epithelial odontogenic — *see* Cyst, calcifying odontogenic
- carcinoid D3A.00
  - benign D3A.00
    - appendix D3A.020
    - ascending colon D3A.022
    - bronchus (lung) D3A.090
    - cecum D3A.021
    - colon D3A.029
    - descending colon D3A.024
    - duodenum D3A.010
    - foregut NOS D3A.094
    - hindgut NOS D3A.096
    - ileum D3A.012
    - jejunum D3A.011
    - kidney D3A.093
    - large intestine D3A.029
    - lung (bronchus) D3A.090
    - midgut NOS D3A.095
    - rectum D3A.026
    - sigmoid colon D3A.025
    - small intestine D3A.019
    - specified NEC D3A.098
    - stomach D3A.092
    - thymus D3A.091
    - transverse colon D3A.023
  - malignant C7A.00
    - appendix C7A.020
    - ascending colon C7A.022
    - bronchus (lung) C7A.090
    - cecum C7A.021
    - colon C7A.029
    - descending colon C7A.024
    - duodenum C7A.010
    - foregut NOS C7A.094
    - hindgut NOS C7A.096
    - ileum C7A.012
    - jejunum C7A.011
    - kidney C7A.093
    - large intestine C7A.029
    - lung (bronchus) C7A.090
    - midgut NOS C7A.095
    - rectum C7A.026
    - sigmoid colon C7A.025
    - small intestine C7A.019
    - specified NEC C7A.098
    - stomach C7A.092
    - thymus C7A.091
    - transverse colon C7A.023
  - mesentery metastasis C7B.04
  - secondary C7B.00
    - bone C7B.03
    - distant lymph nodes C7B.01
    - liver C7B.02
    - peritoneum C7B.04
    - specified NEC C7B.09
- carotid body D44.6
  - malignant C75.4
- cells (*see also* Neoplasm, unspecified behavior, site)
  - benign — *see* Neoplasm, benign, by site
  - malignant — *see* Neoplasm, malignant, by site
  - uncertain whether benign or malignant — *see* Neoplasm, uncertain behavior, by site
- cervix, in pregnancy or childbirth — *see* Pregnancy, complicated by, tumor, cervix
- chondromatous giant cell — *see* Neoplasm, bone, benign
- chromaffin (*see also* Neoplasm, benign, by site)
  - malignant — *see* Neoplasm, malignant, by site
- Cock's peculiar L72.3
- Codman's — *see* Neoplasm, bone, benign
- dentigerous, mixed — *see* Cyst, calcifying odontogenic
- dermoid — *see* Neoplasm, benign, by site
  - with malignant transformation C56 ☑
- desmoid (extra-abdominal) (*see also* Neoplasm, connective tissue, uncertain behavior)
  - abdominal — *see* Neoplasm, connective tissue, uncertain behavior
- embolus — *see* Neoplasm, secondary, by site
- embryonal (mixed) (*see also* Neoplasm, uncertain behavior, by site)
  - liver C22.7
- endodermal sinus
  - specified site — *see* Neoplasm, malignant, by site
  - unspecified site
    - female C56. ☑
    - male C62.90
- epithelial
  - benign — *see* Neoplasm, benign, by site

Tumor — *continued*
- epithelial — *continued*
  - malignant — *see* Neoplasm, malignant, by site
- Ewing's — *see* Neoplasm, bone, malignant, by site
- fatty — *see* Lipoma
- fibroid — *see* Leiomyoma
- G cell
  - malignant
    - pancreas C25.4
    - specified site NEC — *see* Neoplasm, malignant, by site
    - unspecified site C25.4
  - specified site — *see* Neoplasm, uncertain behavior, by site
  - unspecified site D37.8
- germ cell (*see also* Neoplasm, malignant, by site)
  - mixed — *see* Neoplasm, malignant, by site
- ghost cell, odontogenic — *see* Cyst, calcifying odontogenic
- giant cell (*see also* Neoplasm, uncertain behavior, by site)
  - bone D48.0
    - malignant — *see* Neoplasm, bone, malignant
    - chondromatous — *see* Neoplasm, bone, benign
  - malignant — *see* Neoplasm, malignant, by site
  - soft parts — *see* Neoplasm, connective tissue, uncertain behavior
    - malignant — *see* Neoplasm, connective tissue, malignant
- glomus D18.00
  - intra-abdominal D18.03
  - intracranial D18.02
  - jugulare D44.7
    - malignant C75.5
  - skin D18.01
  - specified site NEC D18.09
- gonadal stromal — *see* Neoplasm, uncertain behavior, by site
- granular cell (*see also* Neoplasm, connective tissue, benign)
  - malignant — *see* Neoplasm, connective tissue, malignant
- granulosa cell D39.1 ☑
  - juvenile D39.1 ☑
  - malignant C56 ☑
- granulosa cell-theca cell D39.1 ☑
  - malignant C56 ☑
- Grawitz's C64 ☑
- hemorrhoidal — *see* Hemorrhoids
- hilar cell D27 ☑
- hilus cell D27 ☑
- Hurthle cell (benign) D34
  - malignant C73
- hydatid — *see* Echinococcus
- hypernephroid (*see also* Neoplasm, uncertain behavior, by site)
- interstitial cell (*see also* Neoplasm, uncertain behavior, by site)
  - benign — *see* Neoplasm, benign, by site
  - malignant — *see* Neoplasm, malignant, by site
- intravascular bronchial alveolar D38.1
- islet cell — *see* Neoplasm, benign, by site
  - malignant — *see* Neoplasm, malignant, by site
    - pancreas C25.4
    - specified site NEC — *see* Neoplasm, malignant, by site
    - unspecified site C25.4
  - pancreas D13.7
  - specified site NEC — *see* Neoplasm, benign, by site
  - unspecified site D13.7
- juxtaglomerular D41.0 ☑
- Klatskin's C24.0
- Krukenberg's C79.6 ☑
- Leydig cell — *see* Neoplasm, uncertain behavior, by site
  - benign — *see* Neoplasm, benign, by site
    - specified site — *see* Neoplasm, benign, by site
    - unspecified site
      - female D27.9
      - male D29.20
  - malignant — *see* Neoplasm, malignant, by site
    - specified site — *see* Neoplasm, malignant, by site
    - unspecified site
      - female C56.9
      - male C62.90
  - specified site — *see* Neoplasm, uncertain behavior, by site
  - unspecified site
    - female D39.10
    - male D40.10

Tumor — *continued*
- lipid cell, ovary D27 ☑
- lipoid cell, ovary D27 ☑
- malignant (*see also* Neoplasm, malignant, by site) C80.1
  - fusiform cell (type) C80.1
  - giant cell (type) C80.1
  - localized, plasma cell — *see* Plasmacytoma, solitary
  - mixed NEC C80.1
  - small cell (type) C80.1
  - spindle cell (type) C80.1
  - unclassified C80.1
- mast cell D47.09
- melanotic, neuroectodermal — *see* Neoplasm, benign, by site
- Merkel cell — *see* Carcinoma, Merkel cell
- mesenchymal
  - malignant — *see* Neoplasm, connective tissue, malignant
  - mixed — *see* Neoplasm, connective tissue, uncertain behavior
- mesodermal, mixed (*see also* Neoplasm, malignant, by site)
  - liver C22.4
- mesonephric (*see also* Neoplasm, uncertain behavior, by site)
  - malignant — *see* Neoplasm, malignant, by site
- metastatic
  - from specified site — *see* Neoplasm, malignant, by site
  - of specified site — *see* Neoplasm, malignant, by site
  - to specified site — *see* Neoplasm, secondary, by site
- mixed NEC (*see also* Neoplasm, benign, by site)
  - malignant — *see* Neoplasm, malignant, by site
- mucinous of low malignant potential
  - specified site — *see* Neoplasm, malignant, by site
  - unspecified site C56.9
- mucocarcinoid
  - specified site — *see* Neoplasm, malignant, by site
  - unspecified site C18.1
- mucoepidermoid — *see* Neoplasm, uncertain behavior, by site
- Müllerian, mixed
  - specified site — *see* Neoplasm, malignant, by site
  - unspecified site C54.9
- myoepithelial — *see* Neoplasm, benign, by site
- neuroectodermal (peripheral) — *see* Neoplasm, malignant, by site
  - primitive
    - specified site — *see* Neoplasm, malignant, by site
    - unspecified site C71.9
- neuroendocrine D3A.8
  - malignant poorly differentiated C7A.1
  - secondary NEC C7B.8
  - specified NEC C7A.8
- neurogenic olfactory C30.0
- nonencapsulated sclerosing C73
- odontogenic (adenomatoid) (benign) (calcifying epithelial) (keratocystic) (squamous) — *see* Cyst, calcifying odontogenic
  - malignant C41.1
  - upper jaw (bone) C41.0
- ovarian stromal D39.1 ☑
- ovary, in pregnancy — *see* Pregnancy, complicated by
- pacinian — *see* Neoplasm, skin, benign
- Pancoast's — *see* Pancoast's syndrome
- papillary (*see also* Papilloma)
  - cystic D37.9
  - mucinous of low malignant potential C56 ☑
    - specified site — *see* Neoplasm, malignant, by site
    - unspecified site C56.9
  - serous of low malignant potential
    - specified site — *see* Neoplasm, malignant, by site
    - unspecified site C56.9
- pelvic, in pregnancy or childbirth — *see* Pregnancy, complicated by
- phantom F45.8
- phyllodes D48.6 ☑
  - benign D24 ☑
  - malignant — *see* Neoplasm, breast, malignant
- Pindborg — *see* Cyst, calcifying odontogenic
- placental site trophoblastic D39.2
- plasma cell (malignant) (localized) — *see* Plasmacytoma, solitary
- polyvesicular vitelline
  - specified site — *see* Neoplasm, malignant, by site

Tumor — *continued*
 polyvesicular vitelline — *continued*
  unspecified site
   female C56.9
   male C62.90
 Pott's puffy — *see* Osteomyelitis, specified NEC
 Rathke's pouch D44.3
 retinal anlage — *see* Neoplasm, benign, by site
 salivary gland type, mixed — *see* Neoplasm, salivary
   gland, benign
  malignant — *see* Neoplasm, salivary gland,
   malignant
 Sampson's N80.1
 Schmincke's — *see* Neoplasm, nasopharynx,
   malignant
 sclerosing stromal D27 ☑
 sebaceous — *see* Cyst, sebaceous
 secondary — *see* Neoplasm, secondary, by site
  carcinoid C7B.00
   bone C7B.03
   distant lymph nodes C7B.01
   liver C7B.02
   peritoneum C7B.04
   specified NEC C7B.09
  neuroendocrine NEC C7B.8
 serous of low malignant potential
  specified site — *see* Neoplasm, malignant, by site
  unspecified site C56.9
 Sertoli cell — *see* Neoplasm, benign, by site
  with lipid storage
   specified site — *see* Neoplasm, benign, by site
   unspecified site
    female D27.9
    male D29.20
  specified site — *see* Neoplasm, benign, by site
  unspecified site
   female D27.9
   male D29.20
 Sertoli-Leydig cell — *see* Neoplasm, benign, by site
  specified site — *see* Neoplasm, benign, by site
  unspecified site
   female D27.9
   male D29.20
 sex cord (-stromal) — *see* Neoplasm, uncertain
   behavior, by site
  with annular tubules D39.1 ☑
 skin appendage — *see* Neoplasm, skin, benign
 smooth muscle — *see* Neoplasm, connective tissue,
   uncertain behavior
 soft tissue
  benign — *see* Neoplasm, connective tissue,
   benign
  malignant — *see* Neoplasm, connective tissue,
   malignant
 sternomastoid (congenital) Q68.0
 stromal
  endometrial D39.0
  gastric D48.1
   benign D21.4
   malignant C16.9
   uncertain behavior D48.1
  gastrointestinal C49.A ☑
   benign D21.4
   esophagus C49.A1
   large intestine C49.A4
   malignant C49.A0
    colon C49.A4
    duodenum C49.A3
    esophagus C49.A1
    ileum C49.A3
    jejunum C49.A3
    large intestine C49.A4
    Meckel diverticulum C49.A3
    omentum C49.A9
    peritoneum C49.A9
    rectum C49.A5
    small intestine C49.A3
    specified site NEC C49.A9
    stomach C49.A2
   rectum C49.A5
   small intestine C49.A3
   specified site NEC C49.A9
   stomach C49.A2
   uncertain behavior D48.1
  intestine
   benign D21.4
   malignant
    large C49.A4
    small C49.A3
   uncertain behavior D48.1
  ovarian D39.1 ☑
  stomach C49.A2

Tumor — *continued*
 stromal — *continued*
  benign D21.4
  malignant C49.A2
  uncertain behavior D48.1
 testicular D40.10
 sweat gland (*see also* Neoplasm, skin, uncertain
   behavior)
  benign — *see* Neoplasm, skin, benign
  malignant — *see* Neoplasm, skin, malignant
 syphilitic, brain A52.17
 testicular stromal D40.1 ☑
 theca cell D27. ☑
 theca cell-granulosa cell D39.1 ☑
 Triton, malignant — *see* Neoplasm, nerve,
   malignant
 trophoblastic, placental site D39.2
 turban D23.4
 uterus (body), in pregnancy or childbirth — *see*
   Pregnancy, complicated by, tumor, uterus
 vagina, in pregnancy or childbirth — *see* Pregnancy,
   complicated by
 varicose — *see* Varix
 von Recklinghausen's — *see* Neurofibromatosis
 vulva or perineum, in pregnancy or childbirth — *see*
   Pregnancy, complicated by
  causing obstructed labor O65.5
 Warthin's — *see* Neoplasm, salivary gland, benign
 Wilms' C64 ☑
 yolk sac — *see* Neoplasm, malignant, by site
  specified site — *see* Neoplasm, malignant, by site
  unspecified site
   female C56.9
   male C62.90
Tumor lysis syndrome (following antineoplastic
  chemotherapy) (spontaneous) NEC E88.3
Tumorlet — *see* Neoplasm, uncertain behavior, by site
Tungiasis B88.1
Tunica vasculosa lentis Q12.2
Turban tumor D23.4
Türck's trachoma J37.0
Turner-Kieser syndrome Q87.2
Turner-like syndrome Q87.19
Turner's
 hypoplasia (tooth) K00.4
 syndrome Q96.9
  specified NEC Q96.8
 tooth K00.4
Turner-Ullrich syndrome Q96.9
Tussis convulsiva — *see* Whooping cough
Twiddler's syndrome (due to)
 automatic implantable defibrillator T82.198 ☑
 cardiac pacemaker T82.198 ☑
Twilight state
 epileptic F05
 psychogenic F44.89
Twin (newborn) (*see also* Newborn, twin)
 conjoined Q89.4
 pregnancy — *see* Pregnancy, twin
Twinning, teeth K00.2
Twist, twisted
 bowel, colon or intestine K56.2
 hair (congenital) Q84.1
 mesentery K56.2
 omentum K56.2
 organ or site, congenital NEC — *see* Anomaly, by site
 ovarian pedicle — *see* Torsion, ovary
Twitching R25.3
Tylosis (acquired) L84
 buccalis K13.29
 linguae K13.29
 palmaris et plantaris (congenital) (inherited) Q82.8
  acquired L85.1
Tympanism R14.0
Tympanites (abdominal) (intestinal) R14.0
Tympanitis — *see* Myringitis
Tympanosclerosis — *see* subcategory H74.0 ☑
Tympanum — *see* condition
Tympany
 abdomen R14.0
 chest R09.89
Type A behavior pattern Z73.1
Typhlitis — *see* Appendicitis
Typhoenteritis — *see* Typhoid
Typhoid (abortive) (ambulant) (any site) (clinical)
  (fever) (hemorrhagic) (infection) (intermittent)
  (malignant) (rheumatic) (Widal negative) A01.00
 with pneumonia A01.03
 abdominal A01.09
 arthritis A01.04
 carrier (suspected) of Z22.0
 cholecystitis (current) A01.09

Typhoid — *continued*
 endocarditis A01.02
 heart involvement A01.02
 inoculation reaction — *see* Complications,
   vaccination
 meningitis A01.01
 mesenteric lymph nodes A01.09
 myocarditis A01.02
 osteomyelitis A01.05
 perichondritis, larynx A01.09
 pneumonia A01.03
 spine A01.05
 specified NEC A01.09
 ulcer (perforating) A01.09
Typhomalaria (fever) — *see* Malaria
Typhomania A01.00
Typhoperitonitis A01.09
Typhus (fever) A75.9
 abdominal, abdominalis — *see* Typhoid
 African tick A77.1
 amarillic A95.9
 brain A75.9 *[G94]*
 cerebral A75.9 *[G94]*
 classical A75.0
 due to Rickettsia
  prowazekii A75.0
   recrudescent A75.1
  tsutsugamushi A75.3
  typhi A75.2
 endemic (flea-borne) A75.2
 epidemic (louse-borne) A75.0
 exanthematic NEC A75.0
 exanthematicus SAI A75.0
  brillii SAI A75.1
  mexicanus SAI A75.2
  typhus murinus A75.2
 flea-borne A75.2
 India tick A77.1
 Kenya (tick) A77.1
 louse-borne A75.0
 Mexican A75.2
 mite-borne A75.3
 murine A75.2
 North Asian tick-borne A77.2
 petechial A75.9
 Queensland tick A77.3
 rat A75.2
 recrudescent A75.1
 recurrens — *see* Fever, relapsing
 Sao Paulo A77.0
 scrub (China) (India) (Malaysia) (New Guinea) A75.3
 shop (of Malaysia) A75.2
 Siberian tick A77.2
 tick-borne A77.9
 tropical (mite-borne) A75.3
Tyrosinemia E70.21
 newborn, transitory P74.5
Tyrosinosis E70.21
Tyrosinuria E70.29

U

Uhl's anomaly or disease Q24.8
Ulcer, ulcerated, ulcerating, ulceration, ulcerative
 alveolar process M27.3
 amebic (intestine) A06.1
  skin A06.7
 anastomotic — *see* Ulcer, gastrojejunal
 anorectal K62.6
 antral — *see* Ulcer, stomach
 anus (sphincter) (solitary) K62.6
 aorta — *see* Aneurysm
 aphthous (oral) (recurrent) K12.0
  genital organ(s)
   female N76.6
   male N50.89
 artery I77.2
 atrophic — *see* Ulcer, skin
  decubitus — *see* Ulcer, pressure, by site
 back L98.429
  with
   bone involvement without evidence of necrosis
    L98.426
   bone necrosis L98.424
   exposed fat layer L98.422
   muscle involvement without evidence of
    necrosis L98.425
   muscle necrosis L98.423
   skin breakdown only L98.421
   specified severity NEC L98.428

Ulcer — *continued*
  Barrett's (esophagus) K22.10
    with bleeding K22.11
  bile duct (common) (hepatic) K83.8
  bladder (solitary) (sphincter) NEC N32.89
    bilharzial B65.9 *[N33]*
    in schistosomiasis (bilharzial) B65.9 *[N33]*
    submucosal — *see* Cystitis, interstitial
    tuberculous A18.12
  bleeding K27.4
  bone — *see* Osteomyelitis, specified type NEC
  bowel — *see* Ulcer, intestine
  breast N61.1
  bronchus J98.09
  buccal (cavity) (traumatic) K12.1
  Buruli A31.1
  buttock L98.419
    with
      bone involvement without evidence of necrosis
        L98.416
      bone necrosis L98.414
      exposed fat layer L98.412
      muscle involvement without evidence of
        necrosis L98.415
      muscle necrosis L98.413
      skin breakdown only L98.411
      specified severity NEC L98.418
  cancerous — *see* Neoplasm, malignant, by site
  cardia K22.10
    with bleeding K22.11
  cardioesophageal (peptic) K22.10
    with bleeding K22.11
  cecum — *see* Ulcer, intestine
  cervix (uteri) (decubitus) (trophic) N86
    with cervicitis N72
  chancroidal A57
  chiclero B55.1
  chronic (cause unknown) — *see* Ulcer, skin
  Cochin-China B55.1
  colon — *see* Ulcer, intestine
  conjunctiva H10.89
  cornea H16.00 ☑
    with hypopyon H16.03 ☑
    central H16.01 ☑
    dendritic (herpes simplex) B00.52
    marginal H16.04 ☑
    Mooren's H16.05 ☑
    mycotic H16.06 ☑
    perforated H16.07 ☑
    ring H16.02 ☑
    tuberculous (phlyctenular) A18.52
  corpus cavernosum (chronic) N48.5
  crural — *see* Ulcer, lower limb
  Curling's — *see* Ulcer, peptic, acute
  Cushing's — *see* Ulcer, peptic, acute
  cystic duct K82.8
  cystitis (interstitial) — *see* Cystitis, interstitial
  decubitus — *see* Ulcer, pressure, by site
  dendritic, cornea (herpes simplex) B00.52
  diabetes, diabetic — *see* Diabetes, ulcer
  Dieulafoy's K25.0
  due to
    infection NEC — *see* Ulcer, skin
    radiation NEC L59.8
    trophic disturbance (any region) — *see* Ulcer, skin
    X-ray L58.1
  duodenum, duodenal (eroded) (peptic) K26.9
    with
      hemorrhage K26.4
        and perforation K26.6
      perforation K26.5
    acute K26.3
      with
        hemorrhage K26.0
          and perforation K26.2
        perforation K26.1
    chronic K26.7
      with
        hemorrhage K26.4
          and perforation K26.6
        perforation K26.5
  dysenteric A09
  elusive — *see* Cystitis, interstitial
  endocarditis (acute) (chronic) (subacute) I28.8
  epiglottis J38.7
  esophagus (peptic) K22.10
    with bleeding K22.11
    due to
      aspirin K22.10
        with bleeding K22.11
      gastrointestinal reflux disease K21.0
      ingestion of chemical or medicament K22.10

Ulcer — *continued*
  esophagus — *continued*
      with bleeding K22.11
    fungal K22.10
      with bleeding K22.11
    infective K22.10
      with bleeding K22.11
    varicose — *see* Varix, esophagus
  eyelid (region) H01.8
  fauces J39.2
  Fenwick (-Hunner) (solitary) — *see* Cystitis,
    interstitial
  fistulous — *see* Ulcer, skin
  foot (indolent) (trophic) — *see* Ulcer, lower limb
  frambesial, initial A66.0
  frenum (tongue) K14.0
  gallbladder or duct K82.8
  gangrenous — *see* Gangrene
  gastric — *see* Ulcer, stomach
  gastrocolic — *see* Ulcer, gastrojejunal
  gastroduodenal — *see* Ulcer, peptic
  gastroesophageal — *see* Ulcer, stomach
  gastrointestinal — *see* Ulcer, gastrojejunal
  gastrojejunal (peptic) K28.9
    with
      hemorrhage K28.4
        and perforation K28.6
      perforation K28.5
    acute K28.3
      with
        hemorrhage K28.0
          and perforation K28.2
        perforation K28.1
    chronic K28.7
      with
        hemorrhage K28.4
          and perforation K28.6
        perforation K28.5
  gastrojejunocolic — *see* Ulcer, gastrojejunal
  gingiva K06.8
  gingivitis K05.10
    nonplaque induced K05.11
    plaque induced K05.10
  glottis J38.7
  granuloma of pudenda A58
  gum K06.8
  gumma, due to yaws A66.4
  heel — *see* Ulcer, lower limb
  hemorrhoid (*see also* Hemorrhoids, by degree)
    K64.8
  Hunner's — *see* Cystitis, interstitial
  hypopharynx J39.2
  hypopyon (chronic) (subacute) — *see* Ulcer, cornea,
    with hypopyon
  hypostaticum — *see* Ulcer, varicose
  ileum — *see* Ulcer, intestine
  intestine, intestinal K63.3
    with perforation K63.1
    amebic A06.1
    duodenal — *see* Ulcer, duodenum
    granulocytopenic (with hemorrhage) — *see*
      Neutropenia
    marginal — *see* Ulcer, gastrojejunal
    perforating K63.1
      newborn P78.0
    primary, small intestine K63.3
    rectum K62.6
    stercoraceous, stercoral K63.3
    tuberculous A18.32
    typhoid (fever) — *see* Typhoid
    varicose I86.8
  jejunum, jejunal — *see* Ulcer, gastrojejunal
  keratitis — *see* Ulcer, cornea
  knee — *see* Ulcer, lower limb
  labium (majus) (minus) N76.6
  laryngitis — *see* Laryngitis
  larynx (aphthous) (contact) J38.7
    diphtheritic A36.2
  leg — *see* Ulcer, lower limb
  lip K13.0
  Lipschütz's N76.6
  lower limb (atrophic) (chronic) (neurogenic)
    (perforating) (pyogenic) (trophic) (tropical)
    L97.909
    with
      bone involvement without evidence of necrosis
        L97.906
      bone necrosis L97.904
      exposed fat layer L97.902
      muscle involvement without evidence of
        necrosis L97.905
      muscle necrosis L97.903

Ulcer — *continued*
  lower limb — *continued*
      skin breakdown only L97.901
      specified severity NEC L97.908
    ankle L97.309
      with
        bone involvement without evidence of
          necrosis L97.306
        bone necrosis L97.304
        exposed fat layer L97.302
        muscle involvement without evidence of
          necrosis L97.305
        muscle necrosis L97.303
        skin breakdown only L97.301
        specified severity NEC L97.308
      left L97.329
        with
          bone involvement without evidence of
            necrosis L97.326
          bone necrosis L97.324
          exposed fat layer L97.322
          muscle involvement without evidence of
            necrosis L97.325
          muscle necrosis L97.323
          skin breakdown only L97.321
          specified severity NEC L97.328
      right L97.319
        with
          bone involvement without evidence of
            necrosis L97.316
          bone necrosis L97.314
          exposed fat layer L97.312
          muscle involvement without evidence of
            necrosis L97.315
          muscle necrosis L97.313
          skin breakdown only L97.311
          specified severity NEC L97.318
    calf L97.209
      with
        bone involvement without evidence of
          necrosis L97.206
        bone necrosis L97.204
        exposed fat layer L97.202
        muscle involvement without evidence of
          necrosis L97.205
        muscle necrosis L97.203
        skin breakdown only L97.201
        specified severity NEC L97.208
      left L97.229
        with
          bone involvement without evidence of
            necrosis L97.226
          bone necrosis L97.224
          exposed fat layer L97.222
          muscle involvement without evidence of
            necrosis L97.225
          muscle necrosis L97.223
          skin breakdown only L97.221
          specified severity NEC L97.228
      right L97.219
        with
          bone involvement without evidence of
            necrosis L97.216
          bone necrosis L97.214
          exposed fat layer L97.212
          muscle involvement without evidence of
            necrosis L97.215
          muscle necrosis L97.213
          skin breakdown only L97.211
          specified severity NEC L97.218
    decubitus — *see* Ulcer, pressure, by site
    foot specified NEC L97.509
      with
        bone involvement without evidence of
          necrosis L97.506
        bone necrosis L97.504
        exposed fat layer L97.502
        muscle involvement without evidence of
          necrosis L97.505
        muscle necrosis L97.503
        skin breakdown only L97.501
        specified severity NEC L97.508
      left L97.529
        with
          bone involvement without evidence of
            necrosis L97.526
          bone necrosis L97.524
          exposed fat layer L97.522
          muscle involvement without evidence of
            necrosis L97.525
          muscle necrosis L97.523
          skin breakdown only L97.521

Ulcer

Ulcer — *continued*
  lower limb — *continued*
    specified severity NEC L97.528
    right L97.519
      with
        bone involvement without evidence of
          necrosis L97.516
        bone necrosis L97.514
        exposed fat layer L97.512
        muscle involvement without evidence of
          necrosis L97.515
        muscle necrosis L97.513
        skin breakdown only L97.511
        specified severity NEC L97.518
    heel L97.409
      with
        bone involvement without evidence of
          necrosis L97.406
        bone necrosis L97.404
        exposed fat layer L97.402
        muscle involvement without evidence of
          necrosis L97.405
        muscle necrosis L97.403
        skin breakdown only L97.401
        specified severity NEC L97.408
    left L97.429
      with
        bone involvement without evidence of
          necrosis L97.426
        bone necrosis L97.424
        exposed fat layer L97.422
        muscle involvement without evidence of
          necrosis L97.425
        muscle necrosis L97.423
        skin breakdown only L97.421
        specified severity NEC L97.428
    right L97.419
      with
        bone involvement without evidence of
          necrosis L97.416
        bone necrosis L97.414
        exposed fat layer L97.412
        muscle involvement without evidence of
          necrosis L97.415
        muscle necrosis L97.413
        skin breakdown only L97.411
        specified severity NEC L97.418
    left L97.929
      with
        bone involvement without evidence of
          necrosis L97.926
        bone necrosis L97.924
        exposed fat layer L97.922
        muscle involvement without evidence of
          necrosis L97.925
        muscle necrosis L97.923
        skin breakdown only L97.921
        specified severity NEC L97.928
    lower leg NOS L97.909
      with
        bone involvement without evidence of
          necrosis L97.906
        bone necrosis L97.904
        exposed fat layer L97.902
        muscle involvement without evidence of
          necrosis L97.905
        muscle necrosis L97.903
        skin breakdown only L97.901
        specified severity NEC L97.908
    left L97.929
      with
        bone involvement without evidence of
          necrosis L97.926
        bone necrosis L97.924
        exposed fat layer L97.922
        muscle involvement without evidence of
          necrosis L97.925
        muscle necrosis L97.923
        skin breakdown only L97.921
        specified severity NEC L97.928
    right L97.919
      with
        bone involvement without evidence of
          necrosis L97.916
        bone necrosis L97.914
        exposed fat layer L97.912
        muscle involvement without evidence of
          necrosis L97.915
        muscle necrosis L97.913
        skin breakdown only L97.911
        specified severity NEC L97.918
    specified site NEC L97.809

Ulcer — *continued*
  lower limb — *continued*
    with
      bone involvement without evidence of
        necrosis L97.806
      bone necrosis L97.804
      exposed fat layer L97.802
      muscle involvement without evidence of
        necrosis L97.805
      muscle necrosis L97.803
      skin breakdown only L97.801
      specified severity NEC L97.808
    left L97.829
      with
        bone involvement without evidence of
          necrosis L97.826
        bone necrosis L97.824
        exposed fat layer L97.822
        muscle involvement without evidence of
          necrosis L97.825
        muscle necrosis L97.823
        skin breakdown only L97.821
        specified severity NEC L97.828
    right L97.819
      with
        bone involvement without evidence of
          necrosis L97.816
        bone necrosis L97.814
        exposed fat layer L97.812
        muscle involvement without evidence of
          necrosis L97.815
        muscle necrosis L97.813
        skin breakdown only L97.811
        specified severity NEC L97.818
  midfoot L97.409
    with
      bone involvement without evidence of
        necrosis L97.406
      bone necrosis L97.404
      exposed fat layer L97.402
      muscle involvement without evidence of
        necrosis L97.405
      muscle necrosis L97.403
      skin breakdown only L97.401
      specified severity NEC L97.408
    left L97.429
      with
        bone involvement without evidence of
          necrosis L97.426
        bone necrosis L97.424
        exposed fat layer L97.422
        muscle involvement without evidence of
          necrosis L97.425
        muscle necrosis L97.423
        skin breakdown only L97.421
        specified severity NEC L97.428
    right L97.419
      with
        bone involvement without evidence of
          necrosis L97.416
        bone necrosis L97.414
        exposed fat layer L97.412
        muscle involvement without evidence of
          necrosis L97.415
        muscle necrosis L97.413
        skin breakdown only L97.411
        specified severity NEC L97.418
  right L97.919
    with
      bone involvement without evidence of
        necrosis L97.916
      bone necrosis L97.914
      exposed fat layer L97.912
      muscle involvement without evidence of
        necrosis L97.915
      muscle necrosis L97.913
      skin breakdown only L97.911
      specified severity NEC L97.918
  thigh L97.109
    with
      bone involvement without evidence of
        necrosis L97.106
      bone necrosis L97.104
      muscle involvement without evidence of
        necrosis L97.105
      exposed fat layer L97.102
      muscle necrosis L97.103
      skin breakdown only L97.101
      specified severity NEC L97.108
    left L97.129
      with

Ulcer — *continued*
  lower limb — *continued*
    bone involvement without evidence of
      necrosis L97.126
    bone necrosis L97.124
    exposed fat layer L97.122
    muscle involvement without evidence of
      necrosis L97.125
    muscle necrosis L97.123
    skin breakdown only L97.121
    specified severity NEC L97.128
  right L97.119
    with
      bone involvement without evidence of
        necrosis L97.116
      bone necrosis L97.114
      exposed fat layer L97.112
      muscle involvement without evidence of
        necrosis L97.115
      muscle necrosis L97.113
      skin breakdown only L97.111
      specified severity NEC L97.118
  toe L97.509
    with
      bone involvement without evidence of
        necrosis L97.506
      bone necrosis L97.504
      exposed fat layer L97.502
      muscle involvement without evidence of
        necrosis L97.505
      muscle necrosis L97.503
      skin breakdown only L97.501
      specified severity NEC L97.508
    left L97.529
      with
        bone involvement without evidence of
          necrosis L97.526
        bone necrosis L97.524
        exposed fat layer L97.522
        muscle involvement without evidence of
          necrosis L97.525
        muscle necrosis L97.523
        skin breakdown only L97.521
        specified severity NEC L97.528
    right L97.519
      with
        bone involvement without evidence of
          necrosis L97.516
        bone necrosis L97.514
        exposed fat layer L97.512
        muscle involvement without evidence of
          necrosis L97.515
        muscle necrosis L97.513
        skin breakdown only L97.511
        specified severity NEC L97.518
  leprous A30.1
  syphilitic A52.19
  varicose — *see* Varix, leg, with, ulcer
  luetic — *see* Ulcer, syphilitic
  lung J98.4
    tuberculous — *see* Tuberculosis, pulmonary
  malignant — *see* Neoplasm, malignant, by site
  marginal NEC — *see* Ulcer, gastrojejunal
  meatus (urinarius) N34.2
  Meckel's diverticulum Q43.0
    malignant — *see* Table of Neoplasms, small
      intestine, malignant
  Meleney's (chronic undermining) — *see* Ulcer, skin
  Mooren's (cornea) — *see* Ulcer, cornea, Mooren's
  mycobacterial (skin) A31.1
  nasopharynx J39.2
  neck, uterus N86
  neurogenic NEC — *see* Ulcer, skin
  nose, nasal (passage) (infective) (septum) J34.0
    skin — *see* Ulcer, skin
    spirochetal A69.8
    varicose (bleeding) I86.8
  oral mucosa (traumatic) K12.1
  palate (soft) K12.1
  penis (chronic) N48.5
  peptic (site unspecified) K27.9
    with
      hemorrhage K27.4
        and perforation K27.6
      perforation K27.5
    acute K27.3
      with
        hemorrhage K27.0
          and perforation K27.2
        perforation K27.1
    chronic K27.7
      with

☑ **Additional character required**

Ulcer — *continued*
  peptic — *continued*
    hemorrhage K27.4
      and perforation K27.6
    perforation K27.5
    esophagus K22.10
      with bleeding K22.11
    newborn P78.82
  perforating K27.5
    skin — *see* Ulcer, skin
  peritonsillar J35.8
  phagedenic (tropical) — *see* Ulcer, skin
  pharynx J39.2
  phlebitis — *see* Phlebitis
  plaster — *see* Ulcer, pressure, by site
  popliteal space — *see* Ulcer, lower limb
  postpyloric — *see* Ulcer, duodenum
  prepuce N47.7
  prepyloric — *see* Ulcer, stomach
  pressure (pressure area) L89.9 ☑
    ankle L89.5 ☑
    back L89.1 ☑
    buttock L89.3 ☑
    coccyx L89.15 ☑
    contiguous site of back, buttock, hip L89.4 ☑
    elbow L89.0 ☑
    face L89.81 ☑
    head L89.81 ☑
    heel L89.6 ☑
    hip L89.2 ☑
    sacral region (tailbone) L89.15 ☑
    specified site NEC L89.89 ☑
    stage 1 (healing) (pre-ulcer skin changes limited to persistent focal edema)
      ankle L89.5 ☑
      back L89.1 ☑
      buttock L89.3 ☑
      coccyx L89.15 ☑
      contiguous site of back, buttock, hip L89.4 ☑
      elbow L89.0 ☑
      face L89.81 ☑
      head L89.81 ☑
      heel L89.6 ☑
      hip L89.2 ☑
      sacral region (tailbone) L89.15 ☑
      specified site NEC L89.89 ☑
    stage 2 (healing) (abrasion, blister, partial thickness skin loss involving epidermis and/or dermis)
      ankle L89.5 ☑
      back L89.1 ☑
      buttock L89.3 ☑
      coccyx L89.15 ☑
      contiguous site of back, buttock, hip L89.4 ☑
      elbow L89.0 ☑
      face L89.81 ☑
      head L89.81 ☑
      heel L89.6 ☑
      hip L89.2 ☑
      sacral region (tailbone) L89.15 ☑
      specified site NEC L89.89 ☑
    stage 3 (healing) (full thickness skin loss involving damage or necrosis of subcutaneous tissue)
      ankle L89.5 ☑
      back L89.1 ☑
      buttock L89.3 ☑
      coccyx L89.15 ☑
      contiguous site of back, buttock, hip L89.4 ☑
      elbow L89.0 ☑
      face L89.81 ☑
      head L89.81 ☑
      heel L89.6 ☑
      hip L89.2 ☑
      sacral region (tailbone) L89.15 ☑
      specified site NEC L89.89 ☑
    stage 4 (healing) (necrosis of soft tissues through to underlying muscle, tendon, or bone)
      ankle L89.5 ☑
      back L89.1 ☑
      buttock L89.3 ☑
      coccyx L89.15 ☑
      contiguous site of back, buttock, hip L89.4 ☑
      elbow L89.0 ☑
      face L89.81 ☑
      head L89.81 ☑
      heel L89.6 ☑
      hip L89.2 ☑
      sacral region (tailbone) L89.15 ☑
      specified site NEC L89.89 ☑
    unspecified stage
      ankle L89.5 ☑
      back L89.1 ☑

Ulcer — *continued*
  pressure — *continued*
    buttock L89.3 ☑
    coccyx L89.15 ☑
    contiguous site of back, buttock, hip L89.4 ☑
    elbow L89.0 ☑
    face L89.81 ☑
    head L89.81 ☑
    heel L89.6 ☑
    hip L89.2 ☑
    sacral region (tailbone) L89.15 ☑
    specified site NEC L89.89 ☑
    unstageable
      ankle L89.5 ☑
      back L89.1 ☑
      buttock L89.3 ☑
      coccyx L89.15 ☑
      contiguous site of back, buttock, hip L89.4 ☑
      elbow L89.0 ☑
      face L89.81 ☑
      head L89.81 ☑
      heel L89.6 ☑
      hip L89.2 ☑
      sacral region (tailbone) L89.15 ☑
      specified site NEC L89.89 ☑
  primary of intestine K63.3
    with perforation K63.1
  prostate N41.9
  pyloric — *see* Ulcer, stomach
  rectosigmoid K63.3
    with perforation K63.1
  rectum (sphincter) (solitary) K62.6
    stercoraceous, stercoral K62.6
  retina — *see* Inflammation, chorioretinal
  rodent (*see also* Neoplasm, skin, malignant)
  sclera — *see* Scleritis
  scrofulous (tuberculous) A18.2
  scrotum N50.89
    tuberculous A18.15
    varicose I86.1
  seminal vesicle N50.89
  sigmoid — *see* Ulcer, intestine
  skin (atrophic) (chronic) (neurogenic) (non-healing) (perforating) (pyogenic) (trophic) (tropical) L98.499
    with gangrene — *see* Gangrene
    amebic A06.7
    back — *see* Ulcer, back
    buttock — *see* Ulcer, buttock
    decubitus — *see* Ulcer, pressure
    lower limb — *see* Ulcer, lower limb
    mycobacterial A31.1
    specified site NEC L98.499
      with
        bone involvement without evidence of necrosis L98.496
        bone necrosis L98.494
        exposed fat layer L98.492
        muscle involvement without evidence of necrosis L98.495
        muscle necrosis L98.493
        skin breakdown only L98.491
        specified severity NEC L98.498
    tuberculous (primary) A18.4
    varicose — *see* Ulcer, varicose
  sloughing — *see* Ulcer, skin
  solitary, anus or rectum (sphincter) K62.6
  sore throat J02.9
    streptococcal J02.0
  spermatic cord N50.89
  spine (tuberculous) A18.01
  stasis (venous) — *see* Varix, leg, with, ulcer
    without varicose veins I87.2
  stercoraceous, stercoral K63.3
    with perforation K63.1
    anus or rectum K62.6
  stoma, stomal — *see* Ulcer, gastrojejunal
  stomach (eroded) (peptic) (round) K25.9
    with
      hemorrhage K25.4
        and perforation K25.6
      perforation K25.5
    acute K25.3
      with
        hemorrhage K25.0
          and perforation K25.2
        perforation K25.1
    chronic K25.7
      with
        hemorrhage K25.4
          and perforation K25.6
        perforation K25.5

Ulcer — *continued*
  stomal — *see* Ulcer, gastrojejunal
  stomatitis K12.1
  stress — *see* Ulcer, peptic
  strumous (tuberculous) A18.2
  submucosal, bladder — *see* Cystitis, interstitial
  syphilitic (any site) (early) (secondary) A51.39
    late A52.79
      perforating A52.79
        foot A52.11
  testis N50.89
  thigh — *see* Ulcer, lower limb
  throat J39.2
    diphtheritic A36.0
  toe — *see* Ulcer, lower limb
  tongue (traumatic) K14.0
  tonsil J35.8
    diphtheritic A36.0
  trachea J39.8
  trophic — *see* Ulcer, skin
  tropical — *see* Ulcer, skin
  tuberculous — *see* Tuberculosis, ulcer
  tunica vaginalis N50.89
  turbinate J34.89
  typhoid (perforating) — *see* Typhoid
  unspecified site — *see* Ulcer, skin
  urethra (meatus) — *see* Urethritis
  uterus N85.8
    cervix N86
      with cervicitis N72
    neck N86
      with cervicitis N72
  vagina N76.5
    in Behçet's disease M35.2 *[N77.0]*
    pessary N89.8
  valve, heart I33.0
  varicose (lower limb, any part) (*see also* Varix, leg, with, ulcer)
    broad ligament I86.2
    esophagus — *see* Varix, esophagus
    inflamed or infected — *see* Varix, leg, with ulcer, with inflammation
    nasal septum I86.8
    perineum I86.3
    scrotum I86.1
    specified site NEC I86.8
    sublingual I86.0
    vulva I86.3
  vas deferens N50.89
  vulva (acute) (infectional) N76.6
    in (due to)
      Behçet's disease M35.2 *[N77.0]*
      herpesviral (herpes simplex) infection A60.04
      tuberculosis A18.18
  vulvobuccal, recurring N76.6
  X-ray L58.1
  yaws A66.4
Ulcerosa scarlatina A38.8
Ulcus (*see also* Ulcer)
  cutis tuberculosum A18.4
  duodeni — *see* Ulcer, duodenum
  durum (syphilitic) A51.0
    extragenital A51.2
  gastrojejunale — *see* Ulcer, gastrojejunal
  hypostaticum — *see* Ulcer, varicose
  molle (cutis) (skin) A57
  serpens corneae — *see* Ulcer, cornea, central
  ventriculi — *see* Ulcer, stomach
Ulegyria Q04.8
Ulerythema
  ophryogenes, congenital Q84.2
  sycosiforme L73.8
Ullrich (-Bonnevie)(-Turner) syndrome (*see also* Turner's syndrome) Q87.19
Ullrich-Feichtiger syndrome Q87.0
Ulnar — *see* condition
Ulorrhagia, ulorrhea K06.8
Umbilicus, umbilical — *see* condition
Unacceptable
  contours of tooth K08.54
  morphology of tooth K08.54
Unavailability (of)
  bed at medical facility Z75.1
  health service-related agencies Z75.4
  medical facilities (at) Z75.3
    due to
      investigation by social service agency Z75.2
      lack of services at home Z75.0
      remoteness from facility Z75.3
      waiting list Z75.1
    home Z75.0
    outpatient clinic Z75.3

Unavailability - Use

Unavailability — *continued*
 schooling Z55.1
 social service agencies Z75.4
Uncinaria americana infestation B76.1
Uncinariasis B76.9
Uncongenial work Z56.5
Unconscious (ness) — *see* Coma
Under observation — *see* Observation
Underachievement in school Z55.3
Underdevelopment (*see also* Undeveloped)
 nose Q30.1
 sexual E30.0
Underdosing (*see also* Table of Drugs and Chemicals,
 categories T36-T50, with final character 6) Z91.14
 intentional NEC Z91.128
  due to financial hardship of patient Z91.120
 unintentional NEC Z91.138
  due to patient's age related debility Z91.130
Underfeeding, newborn P92.3
Underfill, endodontic M27.53
Underimmunization status Z28.3
Undernourishment — *see* Malnutrition
Undernutrition — *see* Malnutrition
Underweight R63.6
 for gestational age — *see* Light for dates
Underwood's disease P83.0
Undescended (*see also* Malposition, congenital)
 cecum Q43.3
 colon Q43.3
 testicle — *see* Cryptorchid
Undeveloped, undevelopment (*see also* Hypoplasia)
 brain (congenital) Q02
 cerebral (congenital) Q02
 heart Q24.8
 lung Q33.6
 testis E29.1
 uterus E30.0
Undiagnosed (disease) R69
Undulant fever — *see* Brucellosis
Unemployment, anxiety concerning Z56.0
 threatened Z56.2
Unequal length (acquired) (limb) (*see also* Deformity,
 limb, unequal length)
 leg (*see also* Deformity, limb, unequal length)
  congenital Q72.9 ☑
Unextracted dental root K08.3
Unguis incarnatus L60.0
Unhappiness R45.2
Unicornate uterus Q51.4
 in pregnancy or childbirth O34.00
Unilateral (*see also* condition)
 development, breast N64.89
 organ or site, congenital NEC — *see* Agenesis, by site
Unilocular heart Q20.8
Union, abnormal (*see also* Fusion)
 larynx and trachea Q34.8
Universal mesentery Q43.3
Unrepairable overhanging of dental restorative
 materials K08.52
Unsatisfactory
 restoration of tooth K08.50
  specified NEC K08.59
 sample of cytologic smear
  anus R85.615
  cervix R87.615
  vagina R87.625
 surroundings Z59.1
  work Z56.5
Unsoundness of mind — *see* Psychosis
Unstable
 back NEC — *see* Instability, joint, spine
 hip (congenital) Q65.6
  acquired — *see* Derangement, joint, specified
   type NEC, hip
 joint — *see* Instability, joint
  secondary to removal of joint prosthesis M96.89
 lie (mother) O32.0 ☑
 lumbosacral joint (congenital) — *see* subcategory
  M53.2 ☑
 sacroiliac — *see* subcategory M53.2 ☑
 spine NEC — *see* Instability, joint, spine
Unsteadiness on feet R26.81
Untruthfulness, child problem F91.8
Unverricht (-Lundborg) disease or epilepsy — *see*
 Epilepsy, generalized, idiopathic
Unwanted pregnancy Z64.0
Upbringing, institutional Z62.22
 away from parents NEC Z62.29
 in care of non-parental family member Z62.21
 in foster care Z62.21
 in orphanage or group home Z62.22
 in welfare custody Z62.21

Upper respiratory — *see* condition
Upset
 gastric K30
 gastrointestinal K30
  psychogenic F45.8
 intestinal (large) (small) K59.9
  psychogenic F45.8
 menstruation N93.9
 mental F48.9
 stomach K30
  psychogenic F45.8
Urachus (*see also* condition)
 patent or persistent Q64.4
Urbach-Oppenheim disease (necrobiosis lipoidica
 diabeticorum) — *see* E08-E13 with .620
Urbach's lipoid proteinosis E78.89
Urbach-Wiethe disease E78.89
Urban yellow fever A95.1
Urea
 blood, high — *see* Uremia
 cycle metabolism disorder — *see* Disorder, urea
  cycle metabolism
Uremia, uremic N19
 with
  ectopic or molar pregnancy O08.4
  polyneuropathy N18.9 *[G63]*
 chronic NOS (*see also* Disease, kidney, chronic)
  N18.9
  due to hypertension — *see* Hypertensive, kidney
 complicating
  ectopic or molar pregnancy O08.4
 congenital P96.0
 extrarenal R39.2
 following ectopic or molar pregnancy O08.4
 newborn P96.0
 prerenal R39.2
Ureter, ureteral — *see* condition
Ureteralgia N23
Ureterectasis — *see* Hydroureter
Ureteritis N28.89
 cystica N28.86
 due to calculus N20.1
  with calculus, kidney N20.2
   with hydronephrosis N13.2
 gonococcal (acute) (chronic) A54.21
 nonspecific N28.89
Ureterocele N28.89
 congenital (orthotopic) Q62.31
 ectopic Q62.32
Ureterolith, ureterolithiasis — *see* Calculus, ureter
Ureterostomy
 attention to Z43.6
 status Z93.6
Urethra, urethral — *see* condition
Urethralgia R39.89
Urethritis (anterior) (posterior) N34.2
 calculous N21.1
 candidal B37.41
 chlamydial A56.01
 diplococcal (gonococcal) A54.01
  with abscess (accessory gland) (periurethral)
   A54.1
 gonococcal A54.01
  with abscess (accessory gland) (periurethral)
   A54.1
 nongonococcal N34.1
  Reiter's — *see* Reiter's disease
 nonspecific N34.1
 nonvenereal N34.1
 postmenopausal N34.2
 puerperal O86.22
 Reiter's — *see* Reiter's disease
 specified NEC N34.2
 trichomonal or due to Trichomonas (vaginalis)
  A59.03
Urethrocele N81.0
 with
  cystocele — *see* Cystocele
  prolapse of uterus — *see* Prolapse, uterus
Urethrolithiasis (with colic or infection) N21.1
Urethrorectal — *see* condition
Urethrorrhagia N36.8
Urethrorrhea R36.9
Urethrostomy
 attention to Z43.6
 status Z93.6
Urethrotrigonitis — *see* Trigonitis
Urethrovaginal — *see* condition
Urgency
 fecal R15.2
 hypertensive — *see* Hypertension
 urinary R39.15

Urhidrosis, uridrosis L74.8
Uric acid in blood (increased) E79.0
Uricacidemia (asymptomatic) E79.0
Uricemia (asymptomatic) E79.0
Uricosuria R82.998
Urinary — *see* condition
Urination
 frequent R35.0
 painful R30.9
Urine
 blood in — *see* Hematuria
 discharge, excessive R35.8
 enuresis, nonorganic origin F98.0
 extravasation R39.0
 frequency R35.0
 incontinence R32
  nonorganic origin F98.0
 intermittent stream R39.198
 pus in N39.0
 retention or stasis R33.9
  organic R33.8
   drug-induced R33.0
  psychogenic F45.8
 secretion
  deficient R34
  excessive R35.8
  frequency R35.0
 stream
  intermittent R39.198
  slowing R39.198
  splitting R39.13
  weak R39.12
Urinemia — *see* Uremia
Urinoma, urethra N36.8
Uroarthritis, infectious (Reiter's) — *see* Reiter's
 disease
Urodialysis R34
Urolithiasis — *see* Calculus, urinary
Uronephrosis — *see* Hydronephrosis
Uropathy N39.9
 obstructive N13.9
  specified NEC N13.8
 reflux N13.9
  specified NEC N13.8
 vesicoureteral reflux-associated — *see* Reflux,
  vesicoureteral
Urosepsis - code to condition
Urticaria L50.9
 with angioneurotic edema T78.3 ☑
  hereditary D84.1
 allergic L50.0
 cholinergic L50.5
 chronic L50.8
 cold, familial L50.2
 contact L50.6
 dermatographic L50.3
 due to
  cold or heat L50.2
  drugs L50.0
  food L50.0
  inhalants L50.0
  plants L50.6
  serum (*see also* Reaction, serum) T80.69 ☑
 factitial L50.3
 familial cold M04.2
 giant T78.3 ☑
  hereditary D84.1
 gigantea T78.3 ☑
 idiopathic L50.1
 larynx T78.3 ☑
  hereditary D84.1
 neonatorum P83.88
 nonallergic L50.1
 papulosa (Hebra) L28.2
 pigmentosa D47.01
  congenital Q82.2
  of neonatal onset Q82.2
  of newborn onset Q82.2
 recurrent periodic L50.8
 serum (*see also* Reaction, serum) T80.69 ☑
 solar L56.3
 specified type NEC L50.8
 thermal (cold) (heat) L50.2
 vibratory L50.4
 xanthelasmoidea — *see* Urticaria pigmentosa
Use (of)
 alcohol Z72.89
  with
   intoxication F10.929
   sleep disorder F10.982
  harmful — *see* Abuse, alcohol
 amphetamines — *see* Use, stimulant NEC

☑ **Additional character required**

Use — *continued*
  caffeine — *see* Use, stimulant NEC
  cannabis F12.90
    with
      anxiety disorder F12.980
      intoxication F12.929
        with
          delirium F12.921
          perceptual disturbance F12.922
        uncomplicated F12.920
      other specified disorder F12.988
      psychosis F12.959
        delusions F12.950
        hallucinations F12.951
      unspecified disorder F12.99
    withdrawal F12.93
  cocaine F14.90
    with
      anxiety disorder F14.980
      intoxication F14.929
        with
          delirium F14.921
          perceptual disturbance F14.922
        uncomplicated F14.920
      other specified disorder F14.988
      psychosis F14.959
        delusions F14.950
        hallucinations F14.951
      sexual dysfunction F14.981
      sleep disorder F14.982
      unspecified disorder F14.99
    harmful — *see* Abuse, drug, cocaine
  drug(s) NEC F19.90
    with sleep disorder F19.982
    harmful — *see* Abuse, drug, by type
  hallucinogen NEC F16.90
    with
      anxiety disorder F16.980
      intoxication F16.929
        with
          delirium F16.921
        uncomplicated F16.920
      mood disorder F16.94
      other specified disorder F16.988
      perception disorder (flashbacks) F16.983
      psychosis F16.959
        delusions F16.950
        hallucinations F16.951
      unspecified disorder F16.99
    harmful — *see* Abuse, drug, hallucinogen NEC
  inhalants F18.90
    with
      anxiety disorder F18.980
      intoxication F18.929
        with delirium F18.921
        uncomplicated F18.920
      mood disorder F18.94
      other specified disorder F18.988
      persisting dementia F18.97
      psychosis F18.959
        delusions F18.950
        hallucinations F18.951
      unspecified disorder F18.99
    harmful — *see* Abuse, drug, inhalant
  methadone — *see* Use, opioid
  nonprescribed drugs F19.90
    harmful — *see* Abuse, non-psychoactive
      substance
  opioid F11.90
    with
      disorder F11.99
        mood F11.94
        sleep F11.982
        specified type NEC F11.988
      intoxication F11.929
        with
          delirium F11.921
          perceptual disturbance F11.922
        uncomplicated F11.920
      withdrawal F11.93
    harmful — *see* Abuse, drug, opioid
  patent medicines F19.90
    harmful — *see* Abuse, non-psychoactive
      substance
  psychoactive drug NEC F19.90
    with
      anxiety disorder F19.980
      intoxication F19.929
        with
          delirium F19.921
          perceptual disturbance F19.922
        uncomplicated F19.920

Use — *continued*
  psychoactive drug NEC — *continued*
      mood disorder F19.94
      other specified disorder F19.988
      persisting
        amnestic disorder F19.96
        dementia F19.97
      psychosis F19.959
        delusions F19.950
        hallucinations F19.951
      sexual dysfunction F19.981
      sleep disorder F19.982
      unspecified disorder F19.99
      withdrawal F19.939
        with
          delirium F19.931
          perceptual disturbance F19.932
        uncomplicated F19.930
    harmful — *see* Abuse, drug NEC, psychoactive
      NEC
  sedative, hypnotic, or anxiolytic F13.90
    with
      anxiety disorder F13.980
      intoxication F13.929
        with
          delirium F13.921
        uncomplicated F13.920
      other specified disorder F13.988
      persisting
        amnestic disorder F13.96
        dementia F13.97
      psychosis F13.959
        delusions F13.950
        hallucinations F13.951
      sexual dysfunction F13.981
      sleep disorder F13.982
      unspecified disorder F13.99
    harmful — *see* Abuse, drug, sedative, hypnotic,
      or anxiolytic
  stimulant NEC F15.90
    with
      anxiety disorder F15.980
      intoxication F15.929
        with
          delirium F15.921
          perceptual disturbance F15.922
        uncomplicated F15.920
      mood disorder F15.94
      other specified disorder F15.988
      psychosis F15.959
        delusions F15.950
        hallucinations F15.951
      sexual dysfunction F15.981
      sleep disorder F15.982
      unspecified disorder F15.99
      withdrawal F15.93
    harmful — *see* Abuse, drug, stimulant NEC
  tobacco Z72.0
    with dependence — *see* Dependence, drug,
      nicotine
  volatile solvents (*see also* Use, inhalant)
    F18.90
    harmful — *see* Abuse, drug, inhalant
Usher-Senear disease or syndrome L10.4
Uta B55.1
Uteromegaly N85.2
Uterovaginal — *see* condition
Uterovesical — *see* condition
Uveal — *see* condition
Uveitis (anterior) (*see also* Iridocyclitis)
  acute — *see* Iridocyclitis, acute
  chronic — *see* Iridocyclitis, chronic
  due to toxoplasmosis (acquired) B58.09
    congenital P37.1
  granulomatous — *see* Iridocyclitis, chronic
  heterochromic — *see* Cyclitis, Fuchs'
      heterochromic
  lens-induced — *see* Iridocyclitis, lens-induced
  posterior — *see* Chorioretinitis
  sympathetic H44.13 ☑
  syphilitic (secondary) A51.43
    congenital (early) A50.01
    late A52.71
  tuberculous A18.54
Uveoencephalitis — *see* Inflammation, chorioretinal
Uveokeratitis — *see* Iridocyclitis
Uveoparotitis D86.89
Uvula — *see* condition
Uvulitis (acute) (catarrhal) (chronic) (membranous)
  (suppurative) (ulcerative) K12.2

V

Vaccination (prophylactic)
  complication or reaction — *see* Complications,
    vaccination
  delayed Z28.9
  encounter for Z23
  not done — *see* Immunization, not done, because
    (of)
Vaccinia (generalized) (localized) T88.1 ☑
  congenital P35.8
  without vaccination B08.011
Vacuum, in sinus (accessory) (nasal) J34.89
Vagabond, vagabondage Z59.0
Vagabond's disease B85.1
Vagina, vaginal — *see* condition
Vaginalitis (tunica) (testis) N49.1
Vaginismus (reflex) N94.2
  functional F52.5
  nonorganic F52.5
  psychogenic F52.5
  secondary N94.2
Vaginitis (acute) (circumscribed) (diffuse)
  (emphysematous) (nonvenereal) (ulcerative) N76.0
  with ectopic or molar pregnancy O08.0
  amebic A06.82
  atrophic, postmenopausal N95.2
  bacterial N76.0
  blennorrhagic (gonococcal) A54.02
  candidal B37.3
  chlamydial A56.02
  chronic N76.1
  due to Trichomonas (vaginalis) A59.01
  following ectopic or molar pregnancy O08.0
  gonococcal A54.02
    with abscess (accessory gland) (periurethral)
      A54.1
  granuloma A58
  in (due to)
    candidiasis B37.3
    herpesviral (herpes simplex) infection A60.04
    pinworm infection B80 *[N77.1]*
  monilial B37.3
  mycotic (candidal) B37.3
  postmenopausal atrophic N95.2
  puerperal (postpartum) O86.13
  senile (atrophic) N95.2
  subacute or chronic N76.1
  syphilitic (early) A51.0
    late A52.76
  trichomonal A59.01
  tuberculous A18.18
Vaginosis — *see* Vaginitis
Vagotonia G52.2
Vagrancy Z59.0
VAIN — *see* Neoplasia, intraepithelial, vagina
Vallecula — *see* condition
Valley fever B38.0
Valsuani's disease — *see* Anemia, obstetric
Valve, valvular (formation) (*see also* condition)
  cerebral ventricle (communicating) in situ Z98.2
  cervix, internal os Q51.828
  congenital NEC — *see* Atresia, by site
  ureter (pelvic junction) (vesical orifice) Q62.39
  urethra (congenital) (posterior) Q64.2
Valvulitis (chronic) — *see* Endocarditis
Valvulopathy — *see* Endocarditis
Van Bogaert's leukoencephalopathy (sclerosing)
  (subacute) A81.1
Van Bogaert-Scherer-Epstein disease or syndrome
  E75.5
Van Buchem's syndrome M85.2
Van Creveld-von Gierke disease E74.01
Van der Hoeve (-de Kleyn) syndrome Q78.0
Van der Woude's syndrome Q38.0
Van Neck's disease or osteochondrosis M91.0
Vanishing lung J44.9
Vapor asphyxia or suffocation T59.9 ☑
  specified agent — *see* Table of Drugs and Chemicals
Variance, lethal ball, prosthetic heart valve T82.09 ☑
Variants, thalassemic D56.8
Variations in hair color L67.1
Varicella B01.9
  with
    complications NEC B01.89
    encephalitis B01.11
    encephalomyelitis B01.11
    meningitis B01.0
    myelitis B01.12
    pneumonia B01.2
  congenital P35.8

Varices - Version

Varices — see Varix
Varicocele (scrotum) (thrombosed) I86.1
  ovary I86.2
  perineum I86.3
  spermatic cord (ulcerated) I86.1
Varicose
  aneurysm (ruptured) I77.0
  dermatitis — see Varix, leg, with, inflammation
  eczema — see Varix, leg, with, inflammation
  phlebitis — see Varix, with, inflammation
  tumor — see Varix
  ulcer (lower limb, any part) (see also Varix, leg, with, ulcer)
    anus (see also Hemorrhoids) K64.8
    esophagus — see Varix, esophagus
    inflamed or infected — see Varix, leg, with ulcer, with inflammation
    nasal septum I86.8
    perineum I86.3
    scrotum I86.1
    specified site NEC I86.8
  vein — see Varix
  vessel — see Varix, leg
Varicosis, varicosities, varicosity — see Varix
Variola (major) (minor) B03
Varioloid B03
Varix (lower limb) I83.90
  with
    bleeding I83.899
    edema I83.899
    inflammation I83.10
      with ulcer (venous) I83.209
    pain I83.819
    rupture I83.899
    specified complication NEC I83.899
    stasis dermatitis I83.10
      with ulcer (venous) I83.209
    swelling I83.899
    ulcer I83.009
      with inflammation I83.209
  aneurysmal I77.0
  asymptomatic I83.9 ☑
  bladder I86.2
  broad ligament I86.2
  complicating
    childbirth (lower extremity) O87.4
      anus or rectum O87.2
      genital (vagina, vulva or perineum) O87.8
    pregnancy (lower extremity) O22.0 ☑
      anus or rectum O22.4 ☑
      genital (vagina, vulva or perineum) O22.1 ☑
    puerperium (lower extremity) O87.4
      anus or rectum O87.2
      genital (vagina, vulva, perineum) O87.8
  congenital (any site) Q27.8
  esophagus (idiopathic) (primary) (ulcerated) I85.00
    bleeding I85.01
    congenital Q27.8
    in (due to)
      alcoholic liver disease I85.10
        bleeding I85.11
      cirrhosis of liver I85.10
        bleeding I85.11
      portal hypertension I85.10
        bleeding I85.11
      schistosomiasis I85.10
        bleeding I85.11
      toxic liver disease I85.10
        bleeding I85.11
    secondary I85.10
      bleeding I85.11
  gastric I86.4
  inflamed or infected I83.10
    ulcerated I83.209
  labia (majora) I86.3
  leg (asymptomatic) I83.90
    with
      edema I83.899
      inflammation I83.10
        with ulcer — see Varix, leg, with, ulcer, with inflammation by site
      pain I83.819
      specified complication NEC I83.899
      swelling I83.899
      ulcer I83.009
        with inflammation I83.209
        ankle I83.003
          with inflammation I83.203
        calf I83.002
          with inflammation I83.202
        foot NEC I83.005
          with inflammation I83.205

Varix — continued
  leg — continued
        heel I83.004
          with inflammation I83.204
        lower leg NEC I83.008
          with inflammation I83.208
        midfoot I83.004
          with inflammation I83.204
        thigh I83.001
          with inflammation I83.201
    bilateral (asymptomatic) I83.93
      with
        edema I83.893
        pain I83.813
        specified complication NEC I83.893
        swelling I83.893
        ulcer I83.0 ☑
          with inflammation I83.209
    left (asymptomatic) I83.92
      with
        edema I83.892
        pain I83.812
        specified complication NEC I83.892
        swelling I83.892
        inflammation I83.12
          with ulcer — see Varix, leg, with, ulcer, with inflammation by site
        ulcer I83.029
          with inflammation I83.229
          ankle I83.023
            with inflammation I83.223
          calf I83.022
            with inflammation I83.222
          foot NEC I83.025
            with inflammation I83.225
          heel I83.024
            with inflammation I83.224
          lower leg NEC I83.028
            with inflammation I83.228
          midfoot I83.024
            with inflammation I83.224
          thigh I83.021
            with inflammation I83.221
    right (asymptomatic) I83.91
      with
        edema I83.891
        pain I83.811
        specified complication NEC I83.891
        swelling I83.891
        inflammation I83.11
          with ulcer — see Varix, leg, with, ulcer, with inflammation by site
        ulcer I83.019
          with inflammation I83.219
          ankle I83.013
            with inflammation I83.213
          calf I83.012
            with inflammation I83.212
          foot NEC I83.015
            with inflammation I83.215
          heel I83.014
            with inflammation I83.214
          lower leg NEC I83.018
            with inflammation I83.218
          midfoot I83.014
            with inflammation I83.214
          thigh I83.011
            with inflammation I83.211
  nasal septum I86.8
  orbit I86.8
    congenital Q27.8
  ovary I86.2
  papillary I78.1
  pelvis I86.2
  perineum I86.3
  pharynx I86.8
  placenta O43.89 ☑
  renal papilla I86.8
  retina H35.09
  scrotum (ulcerated) I86.1
  sigmoid colon I86.8
  specified site NEC I86.8
  spinal (cord) (vessels) I86.8
  spleen, splenic (vein) (with phlebolith) I86.8
  stomach I86.4
  sublingual I86.0
  ulcerated I83.009
    inflamed or infected I83.209
  uterine ligament I86.2
  vagina I86.8
  vocal cord I86.8
  vulva I86.3

Vas deferens — see condition
Vas deferentitis N49.1
Vasa previa O69.4 ☑
  hemorrhage from, affecting newborn P50.0
Vascular (see also condition)
  loop on optic papilla Q14.2
  spasm I73.9
  spider I78.1
Vascularization, cornea — see Neovascularization, cornea
Vasculitis I77.6
  allergic D69.0
  cryoglobulinemic D89.1
  disseminated I77.6
  hypocomplementemic M31.8
  kidney I77.89
  livedoid L95.0
  nodular L95.8
  retina H35.06 ☑
  rheumatic — see Fever, rheumatic
  rheumatoid — see Rheumatoid, vasculitis
  skin (limited to) L95.9
    specified NEC L95.8
  systemic M31.8
Vasculopathy, necrotizing M31.9
  cardiac allograft T86.290
  specified NEC M31.8
Vasitis (nodosa) N49.1
  tuberculous A18.15
Vasodilation I73.9
Vasomotor — see condition
Vasoplasty, after previous sterilization Z31.0
  aftercare Z31.42
Vasospasm (vasoconstriction) I73.9
  cerebral (cerebrovascular) (artery) I67.848
    reversible I67.841
  coronary I20.1
  nerve
    arm — see Mononeuropathy, upper limb
    brachial plexus G54.0
    cervical plexus G54.2
    leg — see Mononeuropathy, lower limb
  peripheral NOS I73.9
  retina (artery) — see Occlusion, artery, retina
Vasospastic — see condition
Vasovagal attack (paroxysmal) R55
  psychogenic F45.8
VATER syndrome Q87.2
Vater's ampulla — see condition
Vegetation, vegetative
  adenoid (nasal fossa) J35.8
  endocarditis (acute) (any valve) (subacute) I33.0
  heart (mycotic) (valve) I33.0
Veil
  Jackson's Q43.3
Vein, venous — see condition
Veldt sore — see Ulcer, skin
Velpeau's hernia — see Hernia, femoral
Venereal
  bubo A55
  disease A64
  granuloma inguinale A58
  lymphogranuloma (Durand-Nicolas-Favre) A55
Venofibrosis I87.8
Venom, venomous — see Table of Drugs and Chemicals, by animal or substance, poisoning
Venous — see condition
Ventilator lung, newborn P27.8
Ventral — see condition
Ventricle, ventricular (see also condition)
  escape I49.3
  inversion Q20.5
Ventriculitis (cerebral) (see also Encephalitis) G04.90
Ventriculostomy status Z98.2
Vernet's syndrome G52.7
Verneuil's disease (syphilitic bursitis) A52.78
Verruca (due to HPV) (filiformis) (simplex) (viral) (vulgaris) B07.9
  acuminata A63.0
  necrogenica (primary) (tuberculosa) A18.4
  plana B07.8
  plantaris B07.0
  seborrheica L82.1
    inflamed L82.0
  senile (seborrheic) L82.1
    inflamed L82.0
  tuberculosa (primary) A18.4
  venereal A63.0
Verrucosities — see Verruca
Verruga peruana, peruviana A44.1
Version
  with extraction

☑ **Additional character required**

Version — *continued*
  cervix — *see* Malposition, uterus
  uterus (postinfectional) (postpartal, old) — *see*
    Malposition, uterus
Vertebra, vertebral — *see* condition
Vertical talus (congenital) Q66.80
  left foot Q66.82
  right foot Q66.81
Vertigo R42
  auditory — *see* Vertigo, aural
  aural H81.31 ☑
  benign paroxysmal (positional) H81.1 ☑
  central (origin) H81.4
  cerebral H81.4
  Dix and Hallpike (epidemic) — *see* Neuronitis,
    vestibular
  due to infrasound T75.23 ☑
  epidemic A88.1
    Dix and Hallpike — *see* Neuronitis, vestibular
    Pedersen's — *see* Neuronitis, vestibular
    vestibular neuronitis — *see* Neuronitis, vestibular
  hysterical F44.89
  infrasound T75.23 ☑
  labyrinthine — *see* subcategory H81.0 ☑
  laryngeal R05
  malignant positional H81.4
  Ménière's — *see* subcategory H81.0 ☑
  menopausal N95.1
  otogenic — *see* Vertigo, aural
  paroxysmal positional, benign — *see* Vertigo,
    benign paroxysmal
  Pedersen's (epidemic) — *see* Neuronitis, vestibular
  peripheral NEC H81.39 ☑
  positional
    benign paroxysmal — *see* Vertigo, benign
      paroxysmal
    malignant H81.4
Very-low-density-lipoprotein-type (VLDL)
  hyperlipoproteinemia E78.1
Vesania — *see* Psychosis
Vesical — *see* condition
Vesicle
  cutaneous R23.8
  seminal — *see* condition
  skin R23.8
Vesicocolic — *see* condition
Vesicoperineal — *see* condition
Vesicorectal — *see* condition
Vesicourethrorectal — *see* condition
Vesicovaginal — *see* condition
Vesicular — *see* condition
Vesiculitis (seminal) N49.0
  amebic A06.82
  gonorrheal (acute) (chronic) A54.23
  trichomonal A59.09
  tuberculous A18.15
Vestibulitis (ear) (*see also* subcategory) H83.0 ☑
  nose (external) J34.89
  vulvar N94.810
Vestibulopathy , acute peripheral (recurrent) — *see*
  Neuronitis, vestibular
Vestige, vestigial (*see also* Persistence)
  branchial Q18.0
  structures in vitreous Q14.0
Vibration
  adverse effects T75.20 ☑
    pneumatic hammer syndrome T75.21 ☑
    specified effect NEC T75.29 ☑
    vasospastic syndrome T75.22 ☑
    vertigo from infrasound T75.23 ☑
  exposure (occupational) Z57.7
  vertigo T75.23 ☑
Vibriosis A28.9
Victim (of)
  crime Z65.4
  disaster Z65.5
  terrorism Z65.4
  torture Z65.4
  war Z65.5
Vidal's disease L28.0
Villaret's syndrome G52.7
Villous — *see* condition
VIN — *see* Neoplasia, intraepithelial, vulva
Vincent's infection (angina) (gingivitis) A69.1
  stomatitis NEC A69.1
Vinson-Plummer syndrome D50.1
Violence, physical R45.6
Viosterol deficiency — *see* Deficiency, calciferol
Vipoma — *see* Neoplasm, malignant, by site
Viremia B34.9
Virilism (adrenal) E25.9
  congenital E25.0

Virilization (female) (suprarenal) E25.9
  congenital E25.0
  isosexual E28.2
Virulent bubo A57
Virus, viral (*see also* condition)
  as cause of disease classified elsewhere B97.89
    respiratory syncytial virus (RSV) — *see* Virus,
      infection, respiratory syncytial (RSV)
  cytomegalovirus B25.9
  human immunodeficiency (HIV) — *see* Human,
    immunodeficiency virus (HIV) disease
  infection — *see* Infection, virus
  respiratory syncytial (RSV)
    as cause of disease classified elsewhere B97.4
    bronchiolitis J21.0
    bronchitis J20.5
    bronchopneumonia J12.1
    otitis media H65. ☑ *[B97.4]*
    pneumonia J12.1
    upper respiratory infection J06.9 *[B97.4]*
  specified NEC B34.8
  swine influenza (viruses that normally cause
    infections in pigs) (*see also* Influenza, due to,
    identified novel influenza A virus) J09.X2
  West Nile (fever) A92.30
    with
      complications NEC A92.39
      cranial nerve disorders A92.32
      encephalitis A92.31
      encephalomyelitis A92.31
      neurologic manifestation NEC A92.32
      optic neuritis A92.32
      polyradiculitis A92.32
Viscera, visceral — *see* condition
Visceroptosis K63.4
Visible peristalsis R19.2
Vision, visual
  binocular, suppression H53.34
  blurred, blurring H53.8
    hysterical F44.6
  defect, defective NEC H54.7
  disorientation (syndrome) H53.8
  disturbance H53.9
    hysterical F44.6
  double H53.2
  examination Z01.00
    with abnormal findings Z01.01
    following failed vision screening Z01.020
      with abnormal findings Z01.021
  field, limitation (defect) — *see* Defect, visual field
  hallucinations R44.1
  halos H53.19
  loss — *see* Loss, vision
    sudden — *see* Disturbance, vision, subjective,
      loss, sudden
  low (both eyes) — *see* Low, vision
  perception, simultaneous without fusion H53.33
Vitality, lack or want of R53.83
  newborn P96.89
Vitamin deficiency — *see* Deficiency, vitamin
Vitelline duct, persistent Q43.0
Vitiligo L80
  eyelid H02.739
    left H02.736
      lower H02.735
      upper H02.734
    right H02.733
      lower H02.732
      upper H02.731
  pinta A67.2
  vulva N90.89
Vitreal corneal syndrome H59.01 ☑
Vitreoretinopathy, proliferative (*see also* Retinopathy,
  proliferative)
  with retinal detachment — *see* Detachment, retina,
    traction
Vitreous (*see also* condition)
  touch syndrome — *see* Complication,
    postprocedural, following cataract surgery
Vocal cord — *see* condition
Vogt-Koyanagi syndrome H20.82 ☑
Vogt's disease or syndrome G80.3
Vogt-Spielmeyer amaurotic idiocy or disease E75.4
Voice
  change R49.9
    specified NEC R49.8
  loss — *see* Aphonia
Volhynian fever A79.0
Volkmann's ischemic contracture or paralysis
  (complicating trauma) T79.6 ☑
Volvulus (bowel) (colon) (intestine) K56.2
  with perforation K56.2

Volvulus — *continued*
  congenital Q43.8
  duodenum K31.5
  fallopian tube — *see* Torsion, fallopian tube
  oviduct — *see* Torsion, fallopian tube
  stomach (due to absence of gastrocolic ligament)
    K31.89
Vomiting R11.10
  with nausea R11.2
  asphyxia — *see* Foreign body, by site, causing
    asphyxia, gastric contents
  bilious (cause unknown) R11.14
    in newborn P92.01
    following gastro-intestinal surgery K91.0
  blood — *see* Hematemesis
  causing asphyxia, choking, or suffocation — *see*
    Foreign body, by site
  cyclical, in migraine, G43.A0
    with refractory migraine G43.A1
    intractable G43.A1
    not intractable G43.A0
    psychogenic F50.89
    without refractory migraine G43.A0
  cyclical syndrome NOS (unrelated to migraine) R11.15
  fecal matter R11.13
  following gastrointestinal surgery K91.0
    psychogenic F50.89
  functional K31.89
  hysterical F50.89
  nervous F50.89
  neurotic F50.89
  newborn NEC P92.09
    bilious P92.01
  periodic R11.10
    psychogenic F50.89
  persistent R11.15
  projectile R11.12
  psychogenic F50.89
  uremic — *see* Uremia
  without nausea R11.11
Vomito negro — *see* Fever, yellow
Von Bezold's abscess — *see* Mastoiditis, acute
Von Economo-Cruchet disease A85.8
Von Eulenburg's disease G71.19
Von Gierke's disease E74.01
Von Hippel (-Lindau) disease or syndrome Q85.8
Von Jaksch's anemia or disease D64.89
Von Recklinghausen
  disease (neurofibromatosis) Q85.01
    bones E21.0
Von Schroetter's syndrome I82.890
Von Willebrand (-Jurgens)(-Minot) disease or
  syndrome D68.0
Von Zumbusch's disease L40.1
Voyeurism F65.3
Vrolik's disease Q78.0
Vulva — *see* condition
Vulvismus N94.2
Vulvitis (acute) (allergic) (atrophic) (hypertrophic)
  (intertriginous) (senile) N76.2
  with ectopic or molar pregnancy O08.0
  adhesive, congenital Q52.79
  blennorrhagic (gonococcal) A54.02
  candidal B37.3
  chlamydial A56.02
  due to Haemophilus ducreyi A57
  following ectopic or molar pregnancy O08.0
  gonococcal A54.02
    with abscess (accessory gland) (periurethral)
      A54.1
  herpesviral A60.04
  leukoplakic N90.4
  monilial B37.3
  puerperal (postpartum) O86.19
  subacute or chronic N76.3
  syphilitic (early) A51.0
    late A52.76
  trichomonal A59.01
  tuberculous A18.18
Vulvodynia N94.819
  specified NEC N94.818
Vulvorectal — *see* condition
Vulvovaginitis (acute) — *see* Vaginitis

W

Waiting list, person on Z75.1
  for organ transplant Z76.82
  undergoing social agency investigation Z75.2
Waldenström-Kjellberg syndrome D50.1

Waldenström - Worn out

Waldenström
  hypergammaglobulinemia D89.0
  syndrome or macroglobulinemia C88.0
Walking
  difficulty R26.2
    psychogenic F44.4
  sleep F51.3
    hysterical F44.89
Wall, abdominal — see condition
Wallenberg's disease or syndrome G46.3
Wallgren's disease I87.8
Wandering
  gallbladder, congenital Q44.1
  in diseases classified elsewhere Z91.83
  kidney, congenital Q63.8
  organ or site, congenital NEC — see Malposition,
    congenital, by site
  pacemaker (heart) I49.8
  spleen D73.89
War neurosis F48.8
Wart (due to HPV) (filiform) (infectious) (viral) B07.9
  anogenital region (venereal) A63.0
  common B07.8
  external genital organs (venereal) A63.0
  flat B07.8
  Hassal-Henle's (of cornea) H18.49
  Peruvian A44.1
  plantar B07.0
  prosector (tuberculous) A18.4
  seborrheic L82.1
    inflamed L82.0
  senile (seborrheic) L82.1
    inflamed L82.0
  tuberculous A18.4
  venereal A63.0
Warthin's tumor — see Neoplasm, salivary gland, benign
Wassilieff's disease A27.0
Wasting
  disease R64
    due to malnutrition E41
  extreme (due to malnutrition) E41
  muscle NEC — see Atrophy, muscle
Water
  clefts (senile cataract) — see Cataract, senile, incipient
  deprivation of T73.1 ☑
  intoxication E87.79
  itch B76.9
  lack of T73.1 ☑
  loading E87.70
  on
    brain — see Hydrocephalus
    chest J94.8
  poisoning E87.79
Waterbrash R12
Waterhouse (-Friderichsen) syndrome or disease
  (meningococcal) A39.1
Water-losing nephritis N25.89
Watermelon stomach K31.819
  with hemorrhage K31.811
  without hemorrhage K31.819
Watsoniasis B66.8
Wax in ear — see Impaction, cerumen
Weak, weakening, weakness (generalized) R53.1
  arches (acquired) (see also Deformity, limb, flat foot)
  bladder (sphincter) R32
  facial R29.810
    following
      cerebrovascular disease I69.992
        cerebral infarction I69.392
        intracerebral hemorrhage I69.192
        nontraumatic intracranial hemorrhage NEC
          I69.292
        specified disease NEC I69.892
        stroke I69.392
        subarachnoid hemorrhage I69.092
  foot (double) (see also Weak, arches)
  heart, cardiac — see Failure, heart
  mind F70
  muscle M62.81
  myocardium — see Failure, heart
  newborn P96.89
  pelvic fundus N81.89
  pubocervical tissue N81.82
  senile R54
  rectovaginal tissue N81.83
  urinary stream R39.12
  valvular — see Endocarditis
Wear, worn (with normal or routine use)
  articular bearing surface of internal joint prosthesis
    — see Complications, joint prosthesis,
    mechanical, wear of articular bearing surfaces,
    by site

Wear — continued
  device, implant or graft — see Complications, by
    site, mechanical complication
  tooth, teeth (approximal) (hard tissues)
    (interproximal) (occlusal) K03.0
Weather, weathered
  effects of
    cold T69.9 ☑
      specified effect NEC T69.8 ☑
    hot — see Heat
    skin L57.8
Weaver's syndrome Q87.3
Web, webbed (congenital)
  duodenal Q43.8
  esophagus Q39.4
  fingers Q70.1 ☑
  larynx (glottic) (subglottic) Q31.0
  neck (pterygium colli) Q18.3
  Paterson-Kelly D50.1
  popliteal syndrome Q87.89
  toes Q70.3 ☑
Weber-Christian disease M35.6
Weber-Cockayne syndrome (epidermolysis bullosa)
  Q81.8
Weber-Gubler syndrome G46.3
Weber-Leyden syndrome G46.3
Weber-Osler syndrome I78.0
Weber's paralysis or syndrome G46.3
Wedge-shaped or wedging vertebra — see Collapse,
  vertebra NEC
Wegener's granulomatosis or syndrome M31.30
  with
    kidney involvement M31.31
    lung involvement M31.30
      with kidney involvement M31.31
Wegner's disease A50.02
Weight
  1000-2499 grams at birth (low) — see Low,
    birthweight
  999 grams or less at birth (extremely low) — see
    Low, birthweight, extreme
  and length below 10th percentile for gestational
    age P05.1 ☑
  below but length above 10th percentile for
    gestational age P05.0 ☑
  gain (abnormal) (excessive) R63.5
    in pregnancy — see Pregnancy, complicated by,
      excessive weight gain
    low — see Pregnancy, complicated by,
      insufficient, weight gain
  loss (abnormal) (cause unknown) R63.4
Weightlessness (effect of) T75.82 ☑
Weil (I)-Marchesani syndrome Q87.19
Weil's disease A27.0
Weingarten's syndrome J82
Weir Mitchell's disease I73.81
Weiss-Baker syndrome G90.09
Wells' disease L98.3
Wen — see Cyst, sebaceous
Wenckebach's block or phenomenon I44.1
Werdnig-Hoffmann syndrome (muscular atrophy)
  G12.0
Werlhof's disease D69.3
Wermer's disease or syndrome E31.21
Werner-His disease A79.0
Werner's disease or syndrome E34.8
Wernicke-Korsakoff's syndrome or psychosis
  (alcoholic) F10.96
  with dependence F10.26
  drug-induced
    due to drug abuse — see Abuse, drug, by type,
      with amnestic disorder
    due to drug dependence — see Dependence,
      drug, by type, with amnestic disorder
  nonalcoholic F04
Wernicke-Posadas disease B38.9
Wernicke's
  developmental aphasia F80.2
  disease or syndrome E51.2
  encephalopathy E51.2
  polioencephalitis, superior E51.2
West African fever B50.8
Westphal-Strümpell syndrome E83.01
West's syndrome — see Epilepsy, spasms
Wet
  feet, tropical (maceration) (syndrome) — see
    Immersion, foot
  lung (syndrome), newborn P22.1
Wharton's duct — see condition
Wheal — see Urticaria
Wheezing R06.2
Whiplash injury S13.4 ☑

Whipple's disease (see also subcategory M14.8 ☑)
  K90.81
Whipworm (disease) (infection) (infestation) B79
Whistling face Q87.0
White (see also condition)
  kidney, small N03.9
  leg, puerperal, postpartum, childbirth O87.1
  mouth B37.0
  patches of mouth K13.29
  spot lesions, teeth
    chewing surface K02.51
    pit and fissure surface K02.51
    smooth surface K02.61
Whitehead L70.0
Whitlow (see also Cellulitis, digit)
  with lymphangitis — see Lymphangitis, acute, digit
  herpesviral B00.89
Whitmore's disease or fever — see Melioidosis
Whooping cough A37.90
  with pneumonia A37.91
    due to Bordetella
      bronchiseptica A37.81
      parapertussis A37.11
      pertussis A37.01
      specified organism NEC A37.81
  due to
    Bordetella
      bronchiseptica A37.80
        with pneumonia A37.81
      parapertussis A37.10
        with pneumonia A37.11
      pertussis A37.00
        with pneumonia A37.01
    specified NEC A37.80
      with pneumonia A37.81
Wichman's asthma J38.5
Wide cranial sutures, newborn P96.3
Widening aorta — see Ectasia, aorta
  with aneurysm — see Aneurysm, aorta
Wilkie's disease or syndrome K55.1
Wilkinson-Sneddon disease or syndrome L13.1
Willebrand (-Jürgens) thrombopathy D68.0
Williams syndrome Q93.82
Willige-Hunt disease or syndrome G23.1
Wilms' tumor C64
Wilson-Mikity syndrome P27.0
Wilson's
  disease or syndrome E83.01
  hepatolenticular degeneration E83.01
  lichen ruber L43.9
Window (see also Imperfect, closure)
  aorticopulmonary Q21.4
Winter — see condition
Wiskott-Aldrich syndrome D82.0
Withdrawal state (see also Dependence, drug by type,
  with withdrawal)
  alcohol
    with perceptual disturbances F10.232
    without perceptual disturbances F10.239
  caffeine F15.93
  cannabis F12.23
  newborn
    correct therapeutic substance properly
      administered P96.2
    infant of dependent mother P96.1
    therapeutic substance, neonatal P96.2
Witts' anemia D50.8
Witzelsucht F07.0
Woakes' ethmoiditis or syndrome J33.1
Wolff-Hirschorn syndrome Q93.3
Wolff-Parkinson-White syndrome I45.6
Wolhynian fever A79.0
Wolman's disease E75.5
Wood lung or pneumonitis J67.8
Woolly, wooly hair (congenital) (nevus) Q84.1
Woolsorter's disease A22.1
Word
  blindness (congenital) (developmental) F81.0
  deafness (congenital) (developmental) H93.25
Worm(s) (infection) (infestation) (see also Infestation,
  helminth)
  guinea B72
  in intestine NEC B82.0
Worm-eaten soles A66.3
Worn out — see Exhaustion
  cardiac
    defibrillator (with synchronous cardiac
      pacemaker) Z45.02
    pacemaker
      battery Z45.010
      lead Z45.018

☑ **Additional character required**

Worn out — *continued*
   device, implant or graft — *see* Complications, by
      site, mechanical
Worried well Z71.1
Worries R45.82
Wound check Z48.0 ☑
   due to injury - code to Injury, by site, using
      appropriate seventh character for subsequent
      encounter
Wound, open T14.8 ☑
   abdomen, abdominal
      wall S31.109 ☑
         with penetration into peritoneal cavity S31.609
            ☑
         bite — *see* Bite, abdomen, wall
         epigastric region S31.102 ☑
            with penetration into peritoneal cavity
               S31.602 ☑
            bite — *see* Bite, abdomen, wall, epigastric
               region
            laceration — *see* Laceration, abdomen, wall,
               epigastric region
            puncture — *see* Puncture, abdomen, wall,
               epigastric region
         laceration — *see* Laceration, abdomen, wall
         left
            lower quadrant S31.104 ☑
               with penetration into peritoneal cavity
                  S31.604 ☑
               bite — *see* Bite, abdomen, wall, left, lower
                  quadrant
               laceration — *see* Laceration, abdomen, wall,
                  left, lower quadrant
               puncture — *see* Puncture, abdomen, wall,
                  left, lower quadrant
            upper quadrant S31.101 ☑
               with penetration into peritoneal cavity
                  S31.601 ☑
               bite — *see* Bite, abdomen, wall, left, upper
                  quadrant
               laceration — *see* Laceration, abdomen, wall,
                  left, upper quadrant
               puncture — *see* Puncture, abdomen, wall,
                  left, upper quadrant
         periumbilic region S31.105 ☑
            with penetration into peritoneal cavity
               S31.605 ☑
            bite — *see* Bite, abdomen, wall, periumbilic
               region
            laceration — *see* Laceration, abdomen, wall,
               periumbilic region
            puncture — *see* Puncture, abdomen, wall,
               periumbilic region
         puncture — *see* Puncture, abdomen, wall
         right
            lower quadrant S31.103 ☑
               with penetration into peritoneal cavity
                  S31.603 ☑
               bite — *see* Bite, abdomen, wall, right, lower
                  quadrant
               laceration — *see* Laceration, abdomen, wall,
                  right, lower quadrant
               puncture — *see* Puncture, abdomen, wall,
                  right, lower quadrant
            upper quadrant S31.100 ☑
               with penetration into peritoneal cavity
                  S31.600 ☑
               bite — *see* Bite, abdomen, wall, right, upper
                  quadrant
               laceration — *see* Laceration, abdomen, wall,
                  right, upper quadrant
               puncture — *see* Puncture, abdomen, wall,
                  right, upper quadrant
      alveolar (process) — *see* Wound, open, oral cavity
      ankle S91.00 ☑
         bite — *see* Bite, ankle
         laceration — *see* Laceration, ankle
         puncture — *see* Puncture, ankle
      antecubital space — *see* Wound, open, elbow
      anterior chamber, eye — *see* Wound, open, ocular
      anus S31.839 ☑
         bite S31.835 ☑
         laceration — *see* Laceration, anus
         puncture — *see* Puncture, anus
      arm (upper) S41.10 ☑
         with amputation — *see* Amputation, traumatic,
            arm
         bite — *see* Bite, arm
         forearm — *see* Wound, open, forearm
         laceration — *see* Laceration, arm
         puncture — *see* Puncture, arm

Wound — *continued*
      auditory canal (external) (meatus) — *see* Wound,
         open, ear
      auricle, ear — *see* Wound, open, ear
      axilla — *see* Wound, open, arm
      back (*see also* Wound, open, thorax, back)
         lower S31.000 ☑
            with penetration into retroperitoneal space
               S31.001 ☑
            bite — *see* Bite, back, lower
            laceration — *see* Laceration, back, lower
            puncture — *see* Puncture, back, lower
      bite — *see* Bite
      blood vessel — *see* Injury, blood vessel
      breast S21.00 ☑
         with amputation — *see* Amputation, traumatic,
            breast
         bite — *see* Bite, breast
         laceration — *see* Laceration, breast
         puncture — *see* Puncture, breast
      buttock S31.809 ☑
         bite — *see* Bite, buttock
         laceration — *see* Laceration, buttock
         left S31.829 ☑
         puncture — *see* Puncture, buttock
         right S31.819 ☑
      calf — *see* Wound, open, leg
      canaliculus lacrimalis — *see* Wound, open, eyelid
      canthus, eye — *see* Wound, open, eyelid
      cervical esophagus S11.20 ☑
         bite S11.25 ☑
         laceration — *see* Laceration, esophagus,
            traumatic, cervical
         puncture — *see* Puncture, cervical esophagus
      cheek (external) S01.40 ☑
         bite — *see* Bite, cheek
         laceration — *see* Laceration, cheek
         puncture — *see* Puncture, cheek
         internal — *see* Wound, open, oral cavity
      chest wall — *see* Wound, open, thorax
      chin — *see* Wound, open, head, specified site NEC
      choroid — *see* Wound, open, ocular
      ciliary body (eye) — *see* Wound, open, ocular
      clitoris S31.40 ☑
         with amputation — *see* Amputation, traumatic,
            clitoris
         bite S31.45 ☑
         laceration — *see* Laceration, vulva
         puncture — *see* Puncture, vulva
      conjunctiva — *see* Wound, open, ocular
      cornea — *see* Wound, open, ocular
      costal region — *see* Wound, open, thorax
      Descemet's membrane — *see* Wound, open, ocular
      digit(s)
         foot — *see* Wound, open, toe
         hand — *see* Wound, open, finger
      ear (canal) (external) S01.30 ☑
         with amputation — *see* Amputation, traumatic,
            ear
         bite — *see* Bite, ear
         laceration — *see* Laceration, ear
         puncture — *see* Puncture, ear
         drum S09.2 ☑
      elbow S51.00 ☑
         bite — *see* Bite, elbow
         laceration — *see* Laceration, elbow
         puncture — *see* Puncture, elbow
      epididymis — *see* Wound, open, testis
      epigastric region S31.102 ☑
         with penetration into peritoneal cavity S31.602 ☑
         bite — *see* Bite, abdomen, wall, epigastric region
         laceration — *see* Laceration, abdomen, wall,
            epigastric region
         puncture — *see* Puncture, abdomen, wall,
            epigastric region
      epiglottis — *see* Wound, open, neck, specified site
         NEC
      esophagus (thoracic) S27.819 ☑
         cervical — *see* Wound, open, cervical esophagus
         laceration S27.813 ☑
         specified type NEC S27.818 ☑
      eye — *see* Wound, open, ocular
      eyeball — *see* Wound, open, ocular
      eyebrow — *see* Wound, open, eyelid
      eyelid S01.10 ☑
         bite — *see* Bite, eyelid
         laceration — *see* Laceration, eyelid
         puncture — *see* Puncture, eyelid
      face NEC — *see* Wound, open, head, specified site
         NEC
      finger(s) S61.209 ☑
         with

Wound — *continued*
      finger(s) — *continued*
         amputation — *see* Amputation, traumatic,
            finger
         damage to nail S61.309 ☑
         bite — *see* Bite, finger
         index S61.208 ☑
            with
               damage to nail S61.308 ☑
            left S61.201 ☑
               with
                  damage to nail S61.301 ☑
            right S61.200 ☑
               with
                  damage to nail S61.300 ☑
         laceration — *see* Laceration, finger
         little S61.208 ☑
            with
               damage to nail S61.308 ☑
            left S61.207 ☑
               with damage to nail S61.307 ☑
            right S61.206 ☑
               with damage to nail S61.306 ☑
         middle S61.208 ☑
            with
               damage to nail S61.308 ☑
            left S61.203 ☑
               with damage to nail S61.303 ☑
            right S61.202 ☑
               with damage to nail S61.302 ☑
         puncture — *see* Puncture, finger
         ring S61.208 ☑
            with
               damage to nail S61.308 ☑
            left S61.205 ☑
               with damage to nail S61.305 ☑
            right S61.204 ☑
               with damage to nail S61.304 ☑
      flank — *see* Wound, open, abdomen, wall
      foot (except toe(s) alone) S91.30 ☑
         with amputation — *see* Amputation, traumatic,
            foot
         bite — *see* Bite, foot
         laceration — *see* Laceration, foot
         puncture — *see* Puncture, foot
         toe — *see* Wound, open, toe
      forearm S51.80 ☑
         with
            amputation — *see* Amputation, traumatic,
               forearm
         bite — *see* Bite, forearm
         elbow only — *see* Wound, open, elbow
         laceration — *see* Laceration, forearm
         puncture — *see* Puncture, forearm
      forehead — *see* Wound, open, head, specified site
         NEC
      genital organs, external
         with amputation — *see* Amputation, traumatic,
            genital organs
         bite — *see* Bite, genital organ
         female S31.502 ☑
            vagina S31.40 ☑
            vulva S31.40 ☑
         laceration — *see* Laceration, genital organ
         male S31.501 ☑
            penis S31.20 ☑
            scrotum S31.30 ☑
            testes S31.30 ☑
         puncture — *see* Puncture, genital organ
      globe (eye) — *see* Wound, open, ocular
      groin — *see* Wound, open, abdomen, wall
      gum — *see* Wound, open, oral cavity
      hand S61.40 ☑
         with
            amputation — *see* Amputation, traumatic, hand
         bite — *see* Bite, hand
         finger(s) — *see* Wound, open, finger
         laceration — *see* Laceration, hand
         puncture — *see* Puncture, hand
         thumb — *see* Wound, open, thumb
      head S01.90 ☑
         bite — *see* Bite, head
         cheek — *see* Wound, open, cheek
         ear — *see* Wound, open, ear
         eyelid — *see* Wound, open, eyelid
         laceration — *see* Laceration, head
         lip — *see* Wound, open, lip
         nose S01.20 ☑
         oral cavity — *see* Wound, open, oral cavity
         puncture — *see* Puncture, head
         scalp — *see* Wound, open, scalp
         specified site NEC S01.80 ☑

Wound

Wound — *continued*
- head — *continued*
  - temporomandibular area — *see* Wound, open, cheek
  - heel — *see* Wound, open, foot
  - hip S71.00 ☑
    - with amputation — *see* Amputation, traumatic, hip
    - bite — *see* Bite, hip
    - laceration — *see* Laceration, hip
    - puncture — *see* Puncture, hip
  - hymen S31.40 ☑
    - bite — *see* Bite, vulva
    - laceration — *see* Laceration, vagina
    - puncture — *see* Puncture, vagina
  - hypochondrium S31.109 ☑
    - bite — *see* Bite, hypochondrium
    - laceration — *see* Laceration, hypochondrium
    - puncture — *see* Puncture, hypochondrium
  - hypogastric region S31.109 ☑
    - bite — *see* Bite, hypogastric region
    - laceration — *see* Laceration, hypogastric region
    - puncture — *see* Puncture, hypogastric region
  - iliac (region) — *see* Wound, open, inguinal region
  - inguinal region S31.109 ☑
    - bite — *see* Bite, abdomen, wall, lower quadrant
    - laceration — *see* Laceration, inguinal region
    - puncture — *see* Puncture, inguinal region
  - instep — *see* Wound, open, foot
  - interscapular region — *see* Wound, open, thorax, back
  - intraocular — *see* Wound, open, ocular
  - iris — *see* Wound, open, ocular
  - jaw — *see* Wound, open, head, specified site NEC
  - knee S81.00 ☑
    - bite — *see* Bite, knee
    - laceration — *see* Laceration, knee
    - puncture — *see* Puncture, knee
  - labium (majus) (minus) — *see* Wound, open, vulva
  - laceration — *see* Laceration, by site
  - lacrimal duct — *see* Wound, open, eyelid
  - larynx S11.019 ☑
    - bite — *see* Bite, larynx
    - laceration — *see* Laceration, larynx
    - puncture — *see* Puncture, larynx
  - left
    - lower quadrant S31.104 ☑
      - with penetration into peritoneal cavity S31.604 ☑
      - bite — *see* Bite, abdomen, wall, left, lower quadrant
      - laceration — *see* Laceration, abdomen, wall, left, lower quadrant
      - puncture — *see* Puncture, abdomen, wall, left, lower quadrant
    - upper quadrant S31.101 ☑
      - with penetration into peritoneal cavity S31.601 ☑
      - bite — *see* Bite, abdomen, wall, left, upper quadrant
      - laceration — *see* Laceration, abdomen, wall, left, upper quadrant
      - puncture — *see* Puncture, abdomen, wall, left, upper quadrant
  - leg (lower) S81.80 ☑
    - with amputation — *see* Amputation, traumatic, leg
    - ankle — *see* Wound, open, ankle
    - bite — *see* Bite, leg
    - foot — *see* Wound, open, foot
    - knee — *see* Wound, open, knee
    - laceration — *see* Laceration, leg
    - puncture — *see* Puncture, leg
    - toe — *see* Wound, open, toe
    - upper — *see* Wound, open, thigh
  - lip S01.501 ☑
    - bite — *see* Bite, lip
    - laceration — *see* Laceration, lip
    - puncture — *see* Puncture, lip
  - loin S31.109 ☑
    - bite — *see* Bite, abdomen, wall
    - laceration — *see* Laceration, loin
    - puncture — *see* Puncture, loin
  - lower back — *see* Wound, open, back, lower
  - lumbar region — *see* Wound, open, back, lower
  - malar region — *see* Wound, open, head, specified site NEC
  - mammary — *see* Wound, open, breast
  - mastoid region — *see* Wound, open, head, specified site NEC
  - mouth — *see* Wound, open, oral cavity
  - nail
    - finger — *see* Wound, open, finger, with damage to nail

Wound — *continued*
- nail — *continued*
  - toe — *see* Wound, open, toe, with damage to nail
- nape (neck) — *see* Wound, open, neck
- nasal (septum) (sinus) — *see* Wound, open, nose
- nasopharynx — *see* Wound, open, head, specified site NEC
- neck S11.90 ☑
  - bite — *see* Bite, neck
  - involving
    - cervical esophagus S11.20 ☑
    - larynx — *see* Wound, open, larynx
    - pharynx S11.20 ☑
    - thyroid S11.10 ☑
    - trachea (cervical) S11.029 ☑
      - bite — *see* Bite, trachea
      - laceration S11.021 ☑
        - with foreign body S11.022 ☑
      - puncture S11.023 ☑
        - with foreign body S11.024 ☑
  - laceration — *see* Laceration, neck
  - puncture — *see* Puncture, neck
  - specified site NEC S11.80 ☑
    - specified type NEC S11.89 ☑
- nose (septum) (sinus) S01.20 ☑
  - with amputation — *see* Amputation, traumatic, nose
  - bite — *see* Bite, nose
  - laceration — *see* Laceration, nose
  - puncture — *see* Puncture, nose
- ocular S05.90 ☑
  - avulsion (traumatic enucleation) S05.7 ☑
  - eyeball S05.6 ☑
    - with foreign body S05.5 ☑
  - eyelid — *see* Wound, open, eyelid
  - laceration and rupture S05.3 ☑
    - with prolapse or loss of intraocular tissue S05.2 ☑
  - orbit (penetrating) (with or without foreign body) S05.4 ☑
  - periocular area — *see* Wound, open, eyelid
  - specified NEC S05.8X ☑
- oral cavity S01.502 ☑
  - bite S01.552 ☑
  - laceration — *see* Laceration, oral cavity
  - puncture — *see* Puncture, oral cavity
- orbit — *see* Wound, open, ocular, orbit
- palate — *see* Wound, open, oral cavity
- palm — *see* Wound, open, hand
- pelvis, pelvic (*see also* Wound, open, back, lower)
  - girdle — *see* Wound, open, hip
- penetrating — *see* Puncture, by site
- penis S31.20 ☑
  - with amputation — *see* Amputation, traumatic, penis
  - bite S31.25 ☑
  - laceration — *see* Laceration, penis
  - puncture — *see* Puncture, penis
- perineum
  - bite — *see* Bite, perineum
  - female S31.502 ☑
  - laceration — *see* Laceration, perineum
  - male S31.501 ☑
  - puncture — *see* Puncture, perineum
- periocular area (with or without lacrimal passages) — *see* Wound, open, eyelid
- periumbilic region S31.105 ☑
  - with penetration into peritoneal cavity S31.605 ☑
  - bite — *see* Bite, abdomen, wall, periumbilic region
  - laceration — *see* Laceration, abdomen, wall, periumbilic region
  - puncture — *see* Puncture, abdomen, wall, periumbilic region
- phalanges
  - finger — *see* Wound, open, finger
  - toe — *see* Wound, open, toe
- pharynx S11.20 ☑
- pinna — *see* Wound, open, ear
- popliteal space — *see* Wound, open, knee
- prepuce — *see* Wound, open, penis
- pubic region — *see* Wound, open, back, lower
- pudendum — *see* Wound, open, genital organs, external
- puncture wound — *see* Puncture
- rectovaginal septum — *see* Wound, open, vagina
- right
  - lower quadrant S31.103 ☑
    - with penetration into peritoneal cavity S31.603 ☑
    - bite — *see* Bite, abdomen, wall, right, lower quadrant

Wound — *continued*
- right — *continued*
  - laceration — *see* Laceration, abdomen, wall, right, lower quadrant
  - puncture — *see* Puncture, abdomen, wall, right, lower quadrant
  - upper quadrant S31.100 ☑
    - with penetration into peritoneal cavity S31.600 ☑
    - bite — *see* Bite, abdomen, wall, right, upper quadrant
    - laceration — *see* Laceration, abdomen, wall, right, upper quadrant
    - puncture — *see* Puncture, abdomen, wall, right, upper quadrant
- sacral region — *see* Wound, open, back, lower
- sacroiliac region — *see* Wound, open, back, lower
- salivary gland — *see* Wound, open, oral cavity
- scalp S01.00 ☑
  - bite S01.05 ☑
  - laceration — *see* Laceration, scalp
  - puncture — *see* Puncture, scalp
- scalpel, newborn (birth injury) P15.8
- scapular region — *see* Wound, open, shoulder
- sclera — *see* Wound, open, ocular
- scrotum S31.30 ☑
  - with amputation — *see* Amputation, traumatic, scrotum
  - bite S31.35 ☑
  - laceration — *see* Laceration, scrotum
  - puncture — *see* Puncture, scrotum
- shin — *see* Wound, open, leg
- shoulder S41.00 ☑
  - with amputation — *see* Amputation, traumatic, arm
  - bite — *see* Bite, shoulder
  - laceration — *see* Laceration, shoulder
  - puncture — *see* Puncture, shoulder
- skin NOS T14.8 ☑
- spermatic cord — *see* Wound, open, testis
- sternal region — *see* Wound, open, thorax, front wall
- submaxillary region — *see* Wound, open, head, specified site NEC
- submental region — *see* Wound, open, head, specified site NEC
- subungual
  - finger(s) — *see* Wound, open, finger
  - toe(s) — *see* Wound, open, toe
- supraclavicular region — *see* Wound, open, neck, specified site NEC
- temple, temporal region — *see* Wound, open, head, specified site NEC
- temporomandibular area — *see* Wound, open, cheek
- testis S31.30 ☑
  - with amputation — *see* Amputation, traumatic, testes
  - bite S31.35 ☑
  - laceration — *see* Laceration, testis
  - puncture — *see* Puncture, testis
- thigh S71.10 ☑
  - with amputation — *see* Amputation, traumatic, hip
  - bite — *see* Bite, thigh
  - laceration — *see* Laceration, thigh
  - puncture — *see* Puncture, thigh
- thorax, thoracic (wall) S21.90 ☑
  - back S21.20 ☑
    - with penetration S21.40 ☑
  - bite — *see* Bite, thorax
  - breast — *see* Wound, open, breast
  - front S21.10 ☑
    - with penetration S21.30 ☑
  - laceration — *see* Laceration, thorax
  - puncture — *see* Puncture, thorax
- throat — *see* Wound, open, neck
- thumb S61.009 ☑
  - with
    - amputation — *see* Amputation, traumatic, thumb
    - damage to nail S61.109 ☑
  - bite — *see* Bite, thumb
  - laceration — *see* Laceration, thumb
  - left S61.002 ☑
    - with
      - damage to nail S61.102 ☑
  - puncture — *see* Puncture, thumb
  - right S61.001 ☑
    - with
      - damage to nail S61.101 ☑
- thyroid (gland) — *see* Wound, open, neck, thyroid

☑ **Additional character required**

Wound — *continued*
   toe(s) S91.109 ☑
      with
         amputation — *see* Amputation, traumatic, toe
         damage to nail S91.209 ☑
      bite — *see* Bite, toe
      great S91.103 ☑
         with
            damage to nail S91.203 ☑
         left S91.102 ☑
            with
               damage to nail S91.202 ☑
         right S91.101 ☑
            with
               damage to nail S91.201 ☑
      laceration — *see* Laceration, toe
      lesser S91.106 ☑
         with
            damage to nail S91.206 ☑
         left S91.105 ☑
            with
               damage to nail S91.205 ☑
         right S91.104 ☑
            with
               damage to nail S91.204 ☑
      puncture — *see* Puncture, toe
   tongue — *see* Wound, open, oral cavity
   trachea (cervical region) — *see* Wound, open, neck, trachea
   tunica vaginalis — *see* Wound, open, testis
   tympanum, tympanic membrane S09.2 ☑
      laceration — *see* Laceration, ear, drum
      puncture — *see* Puncture, tympanum
   umbilical region — *see* Wound, open, abdomen, wall, periumbilic region
   uvula — *see* Wound, open, oral cavity
   vagina S31.40 ☑
      bite S31.45 ☑
      laceration — *see* Laceration, vagina
      puncture — *see* Puncture, vagina
   vocal cord S11.039 ☑
      bite — *see* Bite, vocal cord
      laceration S11.031 ☑
         with foreign body S11.032 ☑
      puncture S11.033 ☑
         with foreign body S11.034 ☑
   vitreous (humor) — *see* Wound, open, ocular
   vulva S31.40 ☑
      with amputation — *see* Amputation, traumatic, vulva
      bite S31.45 ☑
      laceration — *see* Laceration, vulva
      puncture — *see* Puncture, vulva
   wrist S61.50 ☑
      bite — *see* Bite, wrist
      laceration — *see* Laceration, wrist
      puncture — *see* Puncture, wrist
Wound, superficial — *see* Injury (*see also* specified injury type)
Wright's syndrome G54.0
Wrist — *see* condition
Wrong drug (by accident) (given in error) — *see* Table of Drugs and Chemicals, by drug, poisoning
Wry neck — *see* Torticollis
Wuchereria (bancrofti) infestation B74.0
Wuchereriasis B74.0
Wuchernde Struma Langhans C73

X

Xanthelasma (eyelid) (palpebrarum) H02.60
   left H02.66
      lower H02.65
      upper H02.64
   right H02.63
      lower H02.62
      upper H02.61
Xanthelasmatosis (essential) E78.2
Xanthinuria, hereditary E79.8
Xanthoastrocytoma
   specified site — *see* Neoplasm, malignant, by site
   unspecified site C71.9
Xanthofibroma — *see* Neoplasm, connective tissue, benign
Xanthogranuloma D76.3
Xanthoma(s), xanthomatosis (primary) (familial) (hereditary) E75.5
   with
      hyperlipoproteinemia
         Type I E78.3

Xanthoma(s) — *continued*
   with — *continued*
         Type III E78.2
         Type IV E78.1
         Type V E78.3
   bone (generalisata) C96.5
   cerebrotendinous E75.5
   cutaneotendinous E75.5
   disseminatum (skin) E78.2
   eruptive E78.2
   hypercholesterinemic E78.00
   hypercholesterolemic E78.00
   hyperlipidemic E78.5
   joint E75.5
   multiple (skin) E78.2
   tendon (sheath) E75.5
   tubo-eruptive E78.2
   tuberosum E78.2
   tuberous E78.2
   verrucous, oral mucosa K13.4
Xanthosis R23.8
Xenophobia F40.10
Xeroderma (*see also* Ichthyosis)
   acquired L85.0
   eyelid H01.149
      left H01.146
         lower H01.145
         upper H01.144
      right H01.143
         lower H01.142
         upper H01.141
   pigmentosum Q82.1
   vitamin A deficiency E50.8
Xerophthalmia (vitamin A deficiency) E50.7
   unrelated to vitamin A deficiency — *see* Keratoconjunctivitis
Xerosis
   conjunctiva H11.14 ☑
      with Bitot's spots (*see also* Pigmentation, conjunctiva)
         vitamin A deficiency E50.1
      vitamin A deficiency E50.0
   cornea H18.89 ☑
      with ulceration — *see* Ulcer, cornea
         vitamin A deficiency E50.3
      vitamin A deficiency E50.2
   cutis L85.3
   skin L85.3
Xerostomia K11.7
Xiphopagus Q89.4
XO syndrome Q96.9
X-ray (of)
   abnormal findings — *see* Abnormal, diagnostic imaging
   breast (mammogram) (routine) Z12.31
   chest
      routine (as part of a general medical examination) Z00.00
         with abnormal findings Z00.01
   routine (as part of a general medical examination) Z00.00
      with abnormal findings Z00.01
XXXXY syndrome Q98.1
XXY syndrome Q98.0

Y

Yaba pox (virus disease) B08.72
Yatapoxvirus B08.70
   specified NEC B08.79
Yawning R06.89
   psychogenic F45.8
Yaws A66.9
   bone lesions A66.6
   butter A66.1
   chancre A66.0
   cutaneous, less than five years after infection A66.2
   early (cutaneous) (macular) (maculopapular) (micropapular) (papular) A66.2
      frambeside A66.2
      skin lesions NEC A66.2
   eyelid A66.2
   ganglion A66.6
   gangosis, gangosa A66.5
   gumma, gummata A66.4
      bone A66.6
   gummatous
      frambeside A66.4
      osteitis A66.6
      periostitis A66.6

Yaws — *continued*
   hydrarthrosis (*see also* subcategory M14.8 ☑) A66.6
   hyperkeratosis (early) (late) A66.3
   initial lesions A66.0
   joint lesions (*see also* subcategory M14.8 ☑) A66.6
   juxta-articular nodules A66.7
   late nodular (ulcerated) A66.4
   latent (without clinical manifestations) (with positive serology) A66.8
   mother A66.0
   mucosal A66.7
   multiple papillomata A66.1
   nodular, late (ulcerated) A66.4
   osteitis A66.6
   papilloma, plantar or palmar A66.1
   periostitis (hypertrophic) A66.6
   specified NEC A66.7
   ulcers A66.4
   wet crab A66.1
Yeast infection (*see also* Candidiasis) B37.9
Yellow
   atrophy (liver) — *see* Failure, hepatic
   fever — *see* Fever, yellow
   jack — *see* Fever, yellow
   jaundice — *see* Jaundice
   nail syndrome L60.5
Yersiniosis (*see also* Infection, Yersinia)
   extraintestinal A28.2
   intestinal A04.6

Z

Zahorsky's syndrome (herpangina) B08.5
Zellweger's syndrome E71.510
Zenker's diverticulum (esophagus) K22.5
Ziehen-Oppenheim disease G24.1
Zieve's syndrome K70.0
Zika NOS A92.5
   congenital P35.4
Zinc
   deficiency, dietary E60
   metabolism disorder E83.2
Zollinger-Ellison syndrome E16.4
Zona — *see* Herpes, zoster
Zoophobia F40.218
Zoster (herpes) — *see* Herpes, zoster
Zygomycosis B46.9
   specified NEC B46.8
Zymotic — *see* condition

This page intentionally left blank

ICD-10-CM Table of Neoplasms

The list below gives the code numbers for neoplasms by anatomical site. For each site there are six possible code numbers according to whether the neoplasm in question is malignant, benign, in situ, of uncertain behavior, or of unspecified nature. The description of the neoplasm will often indicate which of the six columns is appropriate; e.g., malignant melanoma of skin, benign fibroadenoma of breast, carcinoma in situ of cervix uteri.

Where such descriptors are not present, the remainder of the Index should be consulted where guidance is given to the appropriate column for each morphological (histological) variety listed; e.g., Mesonephroma—see Neoplasm, malignant; Embryoma—see also Neoplasm, uncertain behavior; Disease, Bowen's—see Neoplasm, skin, in situ. However, the guidance in the Index can be overridden if one of the descriptors mentioned above is present; e.g., malignant adenoma of colon is coded to C18.9 and not to D12.6 as the adjective 'malignant' overrides the Index entry 'Adenoma—see also Neoplasm, benign.'

Codes listed with a dash (-) following the code have a required additional character for laterality. The Tabular must be reviewed for the complete code.

Neoplasm	Malignant Primary	Malignant Secondary	Ca in situ	Benign	Uncertain Behavior	Unspecified Behavior
Neoplasm, neoplastic	C80.1	C79.9	D09.9	D36.9	D48.9	D49.9
abdomen, abdominal	C76.2	C79.8-	D09.8	D36.7	D48.7	D49.89
cavity	C76.2	C79.8-	D09.8	D36.7	D48.7	D49.89
organ	C76.2	C79.8-	D09.8	D36.7	D48.7	D49.89
viscera	C76.2	C79.8-	D09.8	D36.7	D48.7	D49.89
wall (see also Neoplasm, abdomen, wall, skin)	C44.509	C79.2-	D04.5	D23.5	D48.5	D49.2
connective tissue	C49.4	C79.8-	-	D21.4	D48.1	D49.2
skin	C44.509	-	-	-	-	-
basal cell carcinoma	C44.519	-	-	-	-	-
specified type NEC	C44.599	-	-	-	-	-
squamous cell carcinoma	C44.529	-	-	-	-	-
abdominopelvic	C76.8	C79.8-	-	D36.7	D48.7	D49.89
accessory sinus — see Neoplasm, sinus						
acoustic nerve	C72.4-	C79.49	-	D33.3	D43.3	D49.7
adenoid (pharynx) (tissue)	C11.1	C79.89	D00.08	D10.6	D37.05	D49.0
adipose tissue (see also Neoplasm, connective tissue)	C49.4	C79.89	-	D21.9	D48.1	D49.2
adnexa (uterine)	C57.4	C79.89	D07.39	D28.7	D39.8	D49.59
adrenal	C74.9-	C79.7-	D09.3	D35.0-	D44.1-	D49.7
capsule	C74.9-	C79.7-	D09.3	D35.0-	D44.1-	D49.7
cortex	C74.0-	C79.7-	D09.3	D35.0-	D44.1-	D49.7
gland	C74.9-	C79.7-	D09.3	D35.0-	D44.1-	D49.7
medulla	C74.1-	C79.7-	D09.3	D35.0-	D44.1-	D49.7
ala nasi (external) (see also Neoplasm, skin, nose)	C44.301	C79.2	D04.39	D23.39	D48.5	D49.2
alimentary canal or tract NEC	C26.9	C78.80	D01.9	D13.9	D37.9	D49.0
alveolar	C03.9	C79.89	D00.03	D10.39	D37.09	D49.0
mucosa	C03.9	C79.89	D00.03	D10.39	D37.09	D49.0
lower	C03.1	C79.89	D00.03	D10.39	D37.09	D49.0
upper	C03.0	C79.89	D00.03	D10.39	D37.09	D49.0
ridge or process	C41.1	C79.51	-	D16.5-	D48.0	D49.2
carcinoma	C03.9	C79.8-	-	-	-	-
lower	C03.1	C79.8-	-	-	-	-
upper	C03.0	C79.8-	-	-	-	-
lower	C41.1	C79.51	-	D16.5-	D48.0	D49.2
mucosa	C03.9	C79.89	D00.03	D10.39	D37.09	D49.0
lower	C03.1	C79.89	D00.03	D10.39	D37.09	D49.0
upper	C03.0	C79.89	D00.03	D10.39	D37.09	D49.0
upper	C41.0	C79.51	-	D16.4-	D48.0	D49.2
sulcus	C06.1	C79.89	D00.02	D10.39	D37.09	D49.0
alveolus	C03.9	C79.89	D00.03	D10.39	D37.09	D49.0
lower	C03.1	C79.89	D00.03	D10.39	D37.09	D49.0
upper	C03.0	C79.89	D00.03	D10.39	D37.09	D49.0
ampulla of Vater	C24.1	C78.89	D01.5	D13.5	D37.6	D49.0
ankle NEC	C76.5-	C79.89	D04.7-	D36.7	D48.7	D49.89
anorectum, anorectal (junction)	C21.8	C78.5	D01.3	D12.9	D37.8	D49.0
antecubital fossa or space	C76.4-	C79.89	D04.6-	D36.7	D48.7	D49.89
antrum (Highmore) (maxillary)	C31.0	C78.39	D02.3	D14.0	D38.5	D49.1
pyloric	C16.3	C78.89	D00.2	D13.1	D37.1	D49.0
tympanicum	C30.1	C78.39	D02.3	D14.0	D38.5	D49.1
anus, anal	C21.0	C78.5	D01.3	D12.9	D37.8	D49.0
canal	C21.1	C78.5	D01.3	D12.9	D37.8	D49.0
cloacogenic zone	C21.2	C78.5	D01.3	D12.9	D37.8	D49.0
margin (see also Neoplasm, anus, skin)	C44.500	C79.2	D04.5	D23.5	D48.5	D49.2
overlapping lesion with rectosigmoid junction or rectum	C21.8	-	-	-	-	-
skin	C44.500	C79.2	D04.5	D23.5	D48.5	D49.2
basal cell carcinoma	C44.510	-	-	-	-	-
specified type NEC	C44.590	-	-	-	-	-
squamous cell carcinoma	C44.520	-	-	-	-	-
sphincter	C21.1	C78.5	D01.3	D12.9	D37.8	D49.0
aorta (thoracic)	C49.3	C79.89	-	D21.3	D48.1	D49.2
abdominal	C49.4	C79.89	-	D21.4	D48.1	D49.2
aortic body	C75.5	C79.89	-	D35.6	D44.7	D49.7

Neoplasm	Malignant Primary	Malignant Secondary	Ca in situ	Benign	Uncertain Behavior	Unspecified Behavior
aponeurosis	C49.9	C79.89	-	D21.9	D48.1	D49.2
palmar	C49.1-	C79.89	-	D21.1-	D48.1	D49.2
plantar	C49.2-	C79.89	-	D21.2-	D48.1	D49.2
appendix	C18.1	C78.5	D01.0	D12.1	D37.3	D49.0
arachnoid	C70.9	C79.49	-	D32.9	D42.9	D49.7
cerebral	C70.0	C79.32	-	D32.0	D42.0	D49.7
spinal	C70.1	C79.49	-	D32.1	D42.1	D49.7
areola	C50.0-	C79.81	D05.-	D24.-	D48.6-	D49.3
arm NEC	C76.4-	C79.89	D04.6-	D36.7	D48.7	D49.89
artery — see Neoplasm, connective tissue						
aryepiglottic fold	C13.1	C79.89	D00.08	D10.7	D37.05	D49.0
hypopharyngeal aspect	C13.1	C79.89	D00.08	D10.7	D37.05	D49.0
laryngeal aspect	C32.1	C78.39	D02.0	D14.1	D38.0	D49.1
marginal zone	C13.1	C79.89	D00.08	D10.7	D37.05	D49.0
arytenoid (cartilage)	C32.3	C78.39	D02.0	D14.1	D38.0	D49.1
fold — see Neoplasm, aryepiglottic						
associated with transplanted organ	C80.2	-	-	-	-	-
atlas	C41.2	C79.51	-	D16.6	D48.0	D49.2
atrium, cardiac	C38.0	C79.89	-	D15.1	D48.7	D49.89
auditory						
canal (external) (skin)	C44.20-	C79.2	D04.2-	D23.2-	D48.5	D49.2
internal	C30.1	C78.39	D02.3	D14.0	D38.5	D49.1
nerve	C72.4-	C79.49	-	D33.3	D43.3	D49.7
tube	C30.1	C78.39	D02.3	D14.0	D38.5	D49.1
opening	C11.2	C79.89	D00.08	D10.6	D37.05	D49.0
auricle, ear (see also Neoplasm, skin, ear)	C44.20-	C79.2	D04.2-	D23.2-	D48.5	D49.2
auricular canal (external) (see also Neoplasm, skin, ear)	C44.20-	C79.2	D04.2-	D23.2-	D48.5	D49.2
internal	C30.1	C78.39	D02.3	D14.0	D38.5	D49.2
autonomic nerve or nervous system NEC (see Neoplasm, nerve, peripheral)						
axilla, axillary	C76.1	C79.89	D09.8	D36.7	D48.7	D49.89
fold (see also Neoplasm, skin, trunk)	C44.509	C79.2	D04.5	D23.5	D48.5	D49.2
back NEC	C76.8	C79.89	D04.5	D36.7	D48.7	D49.89
Bartholin's gland	C51.0	C79.82	D07.1	D28.0	D39.8	D49.59
basal ganglia	C71.0	C79.31	-	D33.0	D43.0	D49.6
basis pedunculi	C71.7	C79.31	-	D33.1	D43.1	D49.6
bile or biliary (tract)	C24.9	C78.89	D01.5	D13.5	D37.6	D49.0
canaliculi (biliferi) (intrahepatic)	C22.1	C78.7	D01.5	D13.4	D37.6	D49.0
canals, interlobular	C22.1	C78.89	D01.5	D13.4	D37.6	D49.0
duct or passage (common) (cystic) (extrahepatic)	C24.0	C78.89	D01.5	D13.5	D37.6	D49.0
interlobular	C22.1	C78.89	D01.5	D13.4	D37.6	D49.0
intrahepatic	C22.1	C78.7	D01.5	D13.4	D37.6	D49.0
and extrahepatic	C24.8	C78.89	D01.5	D13.5	D37.6	D49.0
bladder (urinary)	C67.9	C79.11	D09.0	D30.3	D41.4	D49.4
dome	C67.1	C79.11	D09.0	D30.3	D41.4	D49.4
neck	C67.5	C79.11	D09.0	D30.3	D41.4	D49.4
orifice	C67.9	C79.11	D09.0	D30.3	D41.4	D49.4
ureteric	C67.6	C79.11	D09.0	D30.3	D41.4	D49.4
urethral	C67.5	C79.11	D09.0	D30.3	D41.4	D49.4
overlapping lesion	C67.8					
sphincter	C67.8	C79.11	D09.0	D30.3	D41.4	D49.4
trigone	C67.0	C79.11	D09.0	D30.3	D41.4	D49.4
urachus	C67.7	C79.11	D09.0	D30.3	D41.4	D49.4
wall	C67.9	C79.11	D09.0	D30.3	D41.4	D49.4
anterior	C67.3	C79.11	D09.0	D30.3	D41.4	D49.4
lateral	C67.2	C79.11	D09.0	D30.3	D41.4	D49.4
posterior	C67.4	C79.11	D09.0	D30.3	D41.4	D49.4
blood vessel — see Neoplasm, connective tissue						
bone (periosteum)	C41.9	C79.51	-	D16.9-	D48.0	D49.2
acetabulum	C41.4	C79.51	-	D16.8-	D48.0	D49.2
ankle	C40.3-	C79.51	-	D16.3-	-	-
arm NEC	C40.0-	C79.51	-	D16.0-	-	-
astragalus	C40.3-	C79.51	-	D16.3-	-	-
atlas	C41.2	C79.51	-	D16.6-	D48.0	D49.2
axis	C41.2	C79.51	-	D16.6-	D48.0	D49.2
back NEC	C41.2	C79.51	-	D16.6-	D48.0	D49.2
calcaneus	C40.3-	C79.51	-	D16.3-	-	-
calvarium	C41.0	C79.51	-	D16.4-	D48.0	D49.2
carpus (any)	C40.1-	C79.51	-	D16.1-	-	-
cartilage NEC	C41.9	C79.51	-	D16.9-	D48.0	D49.2
clavicle	C41.3	C79.51	-	D16.7-	D48.0	D49.2
clivus	C41.0	C79.51	-	D16.4-	D48.0	D49.2
coccygeal vertebra	C41.4	C79.51	-	D16.8-	D48.0	D49.2
coccyx	C41.4	C79.51	-	D16.8-	D48.0	D49.2
costal cartilage	C41.3	C79.51	-	D16.7-	D48.0	D49.2
costovertebral joint	C41.3	C79.51	-	D16.7-	D48.0	D49.2
cranial	C41.0	C79.51	-	D16.4-	D48.0	D49.2
cuboid	C40.3-	C79.51	-	D16.3-	-	-
cuneiform	C41.9	C79.51	-	D16.9-	D48.0	D49.2
elbow	C40.0-	C79.51	-	D16.0-	-	-

bone - canthus

Neoplasm	Malignant Primary	Malignant Secondary	Ca in situ	Benign	Uncertain Behavior	Unspecified Behavior
bone — continued						
ethmoid (labyrinth)	C41.0	C79.51	-	D16.4-	D48.0	D49.2
face	C41.0	C79.51	-	D16.4-	D48.0	D49.2
femur (any part)	C40.2-	C79.51	-	D16.2-	-	-
fibula (any part)	C40.2-	C79.51	-	D16.2-	-	-
finger (any)	C40.1-	C79.51	-	D16.1-	-	-
foot	C40.3-	C79.51	-	D16.3-	-	-
forearm	C40.0-	C79.51	-	D16.0-	-	-
frontal	C41.0	C79.51	-	D16.4-	D48.0	D49.2
hand	C40.1-	C79.51	-	D16.1-	-	-
heel	C40.3-	C79.51	-	D16.3-	-	-
hip	C41.4	C79.51	-	D16.8-	D48.0	D49.2
humerus (any part)	C40.0-	C79.51	-	D16.0-	-	-
hyoid	C41.0	C79.51	-	D16.4-	D48.0	D49.2
ilium	C41.4	C79.51	-	D16.8-	D48.0	D49.2
innominate	C41.4	C79.51	-	D16.8-	D48.0	D49.2
intervertebral cartilage or disc	C41.2	C79.51	-	D16.6-	D48.0	D49.2
ischium	C41.4	C79.51	-	D16.8-	D48.0	D49.2
jaw (lower)	C41.1	C79.51	-	D16.5-	D48.0	D49.2
knee	C40.2-	C79.51	-	D16.2-	-	-
leg NEC	C40.2-	C79.51	-	D16.2-	-	-
limb NEC	C40.9-	C79.51	-	D16.9-	-	-
lower (long bones)	C40.2-	C79.51	-	D16.2-	-	-
short bones	C40.3-	C79.51	-	D16.3-	-	-
upper (long bones)	C40.0-	C79.51	-	D16.0-	-	-
short bones	C40.1-	C79.51	-	D16.1-	-	-
malar	C41.0	C79.51	-	D16.4-	D48.0	D49.2
mandible	C41.1	C79.51	-	D16.5-	D48.0	D49.2
marrow NEC (any bone)	C96.9	C79.52	-	-	D47.9	D49.89
mastoid	C41.0	C79.51	-	D16.4-	D48.0	D49.2
maxilla, maxillary (superior)	C41.0	C79.51	-	D16.4-	D48.0	D49.2
inferior	C41.1	C79.51	-	D16.5-	D48.0	D49.2
metacarpus (any)	C40.1-	C79.51	-	D16.1-	-	-
metatarsus (any)	C40.3-	C79.51	-	D16.3-	-	-
overlapping sites	C40.8-	-	-	-	-	-
navicular						
ankle	C40.3-	C79.51	-	-	-	-
hand	C40.1-	C79.51	-	-	-	-
nose, nasal	C41.0	C79.51	-	D16.4-	D48.0	D49.2
occipital	C41.0	C79.51	-	D16.4-	D48.0	D49.2
orbit	C41.0	C79.51	-	D16.4-	D48.0	D49.2
parietal	C41.0	C79.51	-	D16.4-	D48.0	D49.2
patella	C40.2-	C79.51	-	-	-	-
pelvic	C41.4	C79.51	-	D16.8	D48.0	D49.2
phalanges						
foot	C40.3-	C79.51	-	-	-	-
hand	C40.1-	C79.51	-	-	-	-
pubic	C41.4	C79.51	-	D16.8	D48.0	D49.2
radius (any part)	C40.0-	C79.51	-	D16.0-	-	-
rib	C41.3	C79.51	-	D16.7	D48.0	D49.2
sacral vertebra	C41.4	C79.51	-	D16.8	D48.0	D49.2
sacrum	C41.4	C79.51	-	D16.8	D48.0	D49.2
scaphoid						
of ankle	C40.3-	C79.51	-	-	-	-
of hand	C40.1-	C79.51	-	-	-	-
scapula (any part)	C40.0-	C79.51	-	D16.0-	-	-
sella turcica	C41.0	C79.51	-	D16.4-	D48.0	D49.2
shoulder	C40.0-	C79.51	-	D16.0-	-	-
skull	C41.0	C79.51	-	D16.4-	D48.0	D49.2
sphenoid	C41.0	C79.51	-	D16.4-	D48.0	D49.2
spine, spinal (column)	C41.2	C79.51	-	D16.6	D48.0	D49.2
coccyx	C41.4	C79.51	-	D16.8	D48.0	D49.2
sacrum	C41.4	C79.51	-	D16.8	D48.0	D49.2
sternum	C41.3	C79.51	-	D16.7	D48.0	D49.2
tarsus (any)	C40.3-	C79.51	-	-	-	-
temporal	C41.0	C79.51	-	D16.4-	D48.0	D49.2
thumb	C40.1-	C79.51	-	-	-	-
tibia (any part)	C40.2-	C79.51	-	-	-	-
toe (any)	C40.3-	C79.51	-	-	-	-
trapezium	C40.1-	C79.51	-	-	-	-
trapezoid	C40.1-	C79.51	-	-	-	-
turbinate	C41.0	C79.51	-	D16.4-	D48.0	D49.2
ulna (any part)	C40.0-	C79.51	-	D16.0-	-	-
unciform	C40.1-	C79.51	-	-	-	-
vertebra (column)	C41.2	C79.51	-	D16.6	D48.0	D49.2
coccyx	C41.4	C79.51	-	D16.8	D48.0	D49.2
sacrum	C41.4	C79.51	-	D16.8	D48.0	D49.2
vomer	C41.0	C79.51	-	D16.4-	D48.0	D49.2
wrist	C40.1-	C79.51	-	-	-	-
xiphoid process	C41.3	C79.51	-	D16.7	D48.0	D49.2
zygomatic	C41.0	C79.51	-	D16.4-	D48.0	D49.2
book-leaf (mouth) [*ventral surface of tongue and floor of mouth*]	C06.89	C79.89	D00.00	D10.39	D37.09	D49.0
bowel — *see* Neoplasm, intestine						
brachial plexus	C47.1-	C79.89	-	D36.12	D48.2	D49.2
brain NEC	C71.9	C79.31	-	D33.2	D43.2	D49.6
basal ganglia	C71.0	C79.31	-	D33.0	D43.0	D49.6
cerebellopontine angle	C71.6	C79.31	-	D33.1	D43.1	D49.6

Neoplasm	Malignant Primary	Malignant Secondary	Ca in situ	Benign	Uncertain Behavior	Unspecified Behavior
brain NEC — continued						
cerebellum NOS	C71.6	C79.31	-	D33.1	D43.1	D49.6
cerebrum	C71.0	C79.31	-	D33.0	D43.0	D49.6
choroid plexus	C71.7	C79.31	-	D33.1	D43.1	D49.6
corpus callosum	C71.8	C79.31	-	D33.2	D43.2	D49.6
corpus striatum	C71.0	C79.31	-	D33.0	D43.0	D49.6
cortex (cerebral)	C71.0	C79.31	-	D33.0	D43.0	D49.6
frontal lobe	C71.1	C79.31	-	D33.0	D43.0	D49.6
globus pallidus	C71.0	C79.31	-	D33.0	D43.0	D49.6
hippocampus	C71.2	C79.31	-	D33.0	D43.0	D49.6
hypothalamus	C71.0	C79.31	-	D33.0	D43.0	D49.6
internal capsule	C71.0	C79.31	-	D33.0	D43.0	D49.6
medulla oblongata	C71.7	C79.31	-	D33.1	D43.1	D49.6
meninges	C70.0	C79.32	-	D32.0	D42.0	D49.7
midbrain	C71.7	C79.31	-	D33.1	D43.1	D49.6
occipital lobe	C71.4	C79.31	-	D33.0	D43.0	D49.6
overlapping lesion	C71.8	C79.31	-	-	-	-
parietal lobe	C71.3	C79.31	-	D33.0	D43.0	D49.6
peduncle	C71.7	C79.31	-	D33.1	D43.1	D49.6
pons	C71.7	C79.31	-	D33.1	D43.1	D49.6
stem	C71.7	C79.31	-	D33.1	D43.1	D49.6
tapetum	C71.8	C79.31	-	D33.2	D43.2	D49.6
temporal lobe	C71.2	C79.31	-	D33.0	D43.0	D49.6
thalamus	C71.0	C79.31	-	D33.0	D43.0	D49.6
uncus	C71.2	C79.31	-	D33.0	D43.0	D49.6
ventricle (floor)	C71.5	C79.31	-	D33.0	D43.0	D49.6
fourth	C71.7	C79.31	-	D33.1	D43.1	D49.6
branchial (cleft) (cyst) (vestiges)	C10.4	C79.89	D00.08	D10.5	D37.05	D49.0
breast (connective tissue) (glandular tissue) (soft parts)	C50.9-	C79.81	D05.-	D24.-	D48.6-	D49.3
areola	C50.0-	C79.81	D05.-	D24.-	D48.6-	D49.3
axillary tail	C50.6-	C79.81	D05.-	D24.-	D48.6-	D49.3
central portion	C50.1-	C79.81	D05.-	D24.-	D48.6-	D49.3
inner	C50.8-	C79.81	D05.-	D24.-	D48.6-	D49.3
lower	C50.8-	C79.81	D05.-	D24.-	D48.6-	D49.3
lower-inner quadrant	C50.3-	C79.81	D05.-	D24.-	D48.6-	D49.3
lower-outer quadrant	C50.5-	C79.81	D05.-	D24.-	D48.6-	D49.3
mastectomy site (skin) (*see also* Neoplasm, breast, skin)	C44.501	C79.2	-	-	-	-
specified as breast tissue	C50.8-	C79.81	D05.-	D24.-	D48.6-	D49.3
midline	C50.8-	C79.81	D05.-	D24.-	D48.6-	D49.3
nipple	C50.0-	C79.81	D05.-	D24.-	D48.6-	D49.3
outer	C50.8-	C79.81	D05.-	D24.-	D48.6-	D49.3
overlapping lesion	C50.8-	-	-	-	-	-
skin	C44.501	C79.2	D04.5	D23.5	D48.5	D49.2
basal cell carcinoma	C44.511	-	-	-	-	-
specified type NEC	C44.591	-	-	-	-	-
squamous cell carcinoma	C44.521	-	-	-	-	-
tail (axillary)	C50.6-	C79.81	D05.-	D24.-	D48.6-	D49.3
upper	C50.8-	C79.81	D05.-	D24.-	D48.6-	D49.3
upper-inner quadrant	C50.2-	C79.81	D05.-	D24.-	D48.6-	D49.3
upper-outer quadrant	C50.4-	C79.81	D05.-	D24.-	D48.6-	D49.3
broad ligament	C57.1	C79.82	D07.39	D28.2	D39.8	D49.59
bronchiogenic, bronchogenic (lung)	C34.9-	C78.0-	D02.2-	D14.3-	D38.1	D49.1
bronchiole	C34.9-	C78.0-	D02.2-	D14.3-	D38.1	D49.1
bronchus	C34.9-	C78.0-	D02.2-	D14.3-	D38.1	D49.1
carina	C34.0-	C78.0-	D02.2-	D14.3-	D38.1	D49.1
lower lobe of lung	C34.3-	C78.0-	D02.2-	D14.3-	D38.1	D49.1
main	C34.0-	C78.0-	D02.2-	D14.3-	D38.1	D49.1
middle lobe of lung	C34.2	C78.0-	D02.21	D14.31	D38.1	D49.1
overlapping lesion	C34.8-	-	-	-	-	-
upper lobe of lung	C34.1-	C78.0-	D02.2-	D14.3-	D38.1	D49.1
brow	C44.309	C79.2	D04.39	D23.39	D48.5	D49.2
basal cell carcinoma	C44.319	-	-	-	-	-
specified type NEC	C44.399	-	-	-	-	-
squamous cell carcinoma	C44.329	-	-	-	-	-
buccal (cavity)	C06.9	C79.89	D00.00	D10.39	D37.09	D49.0
commissure	C06.0	C79.89	D00.02	D10.39	D37.09	D49.0
groove (lower) (upper)	C06.1	C79.89	D00.02	D10.39	D37.09	D49.0
mucosa	C06.0	C79.89	D00.00	D10.39	D37.09	D49.0
sulcus (lower) (upper)	C06.1	C79.89	D00.02	D10.39	D37.09	D49.0
bulbourethral gland	C68.0	C79.19	D09.19	D30.4	D41.3	D49.59
bursa — *see* Neoplasm, connective tissue						
buttock NEC	C76.3	C79.89	D04.5	D36.7	D48.7	D49.89
calf	C76.5-	C79.89	D04.7-	D36.7	D48.7	D49.89
calvarium	C41.0	C79.51	-	D16.4-	D48.0	D49.2
calyx, renal	C65.-	C79.0-	D09.19	D30.1-	D41.1-	D49.51-
canal						
anal	C21.1	C78.5	D01.3	D12.9	D37.8	D49.0
auditory (external) (*see also* Neoplasm, skin, ear)	C44.20-	C79.2	D04.2-	D23.2-	D48.5	D49.2
auricular (external) (*see also* Neoplasm, skin, ear)	C44.20-	C79.2	D04.2-	D23.2-	D48.5	D49.2
canaliculi, biliary (biliferi) (intrahepatic)	C22.1	C78.7	D01.5	D13.4	D37.6	D49.0
canthus (eye) (inner) (outer)	C44.10-	C79.2	D04.1-	D23.1-	D48.5	D49.2
basal cell carcinoma	C44.11-	-	-	-	-	-
sebaceous cell	C44.13-	-	-	-	-	-
specified type NEC	C44.19-	-	-	-	-	-
squamous cell carcinoma	C44.12-	-	-	-	-	-

Neoplasm	Malignant Primary	Malignant Secondary	Ca in situ	Benign	Uncertain Behavior	Unspecified Behavior
capillary — see Neoplasm, connective tissue						
caput coli	C18.0	C78.5	D01.0	D12.0	D37.4	D49.0
carcinoid — see Tumor, carcinoid						
cardia (gastric)	C16.0	C78.89	D00.2	D13.1	D37.1	D49.0
cardiac orifice (stomach)	C16.0	C78.89	D00.2	D13.1	D37.1	D49.0
cardio-esophageal junction	C16.0	C78.89	D00.2	D13.1	D37.1	D49.0
cardio-esophagus	C16.0	C78.89	D00.2	D13.1	D37.1	D49.0
carina (bronchus)	C34.0-	C78.0-	D02.2-	D14.3-	D38.1	D49.1
carotid (artery)	C49.0	C79.89	-	D21.0	D48.1	D49.2
body	C75.4	C79.89	-	D35.5	D44.6	D49.7
carpus (any bone)	C40.1-	C79.51	-	D16.1-	-	-
cartilage (articular) (joint) NEC (see also Neoplasm, bone)	C41.9	C79.51	-	D16.9-	D48.0	D49.2
arytenoid	C32.3	C78.39	D02.0	D14.1	D38.0	D49.1
auricular	C49.0	C79.89	-	D21.0	D48.1	D49.2
bronchi	C34.0-	C78.39	-	D14.3-	D38.1	D49.1
costal	C41.3	C79.51	-	D16.7	D48.0	D49.2
cricoid	C32.3	C78.39	D02.0	D14.1	D38.0	D49.1
cuneiform	C32.3	C78.39	D02.0	D14.1	D38.0	D49.1
ear (external)	C49.0	C79.89	-	D21.0	D48.1	D49.2
ensiform	C41.3	C79.51	-	D16.7	D48.0	D49.2
epiglottis	C32.1	C78.39	D02.0	D14.1	D38.0	D49.1
anterior surface	C10.1	C79.89	D00.08	D10.5	D37.05	D49.0
eyelid	C49.0	C79.89	-	D21.0	D48.1	D49.2
intervertebral	C41.2	C79.51	-	D16.6	D48.0	D49.2
larynx, laryngeal	C32.3	C78.39	D02.0	D14.1	D38.0	D49.1
nose, nasal	C30.0	C78.39	D02.3	D14.0	D38.5	D49.1
pinna	C49.0	C79.89	-	D21.0	D48.1	D49.2
rib	C41.3	C79.51	-	D16.7	D48.0	D49.2
semilunar (knee)	C40.2-	C79.51	-	D16.2-	D48.0	D49.2
thyroid	C32.3	C78.39	D02.0	D14.1	D38.0	D49.1
trachea	C33	C78.39	D02.1	D14.2	D38.1	D49.1
cauda equina	C72.1	C79.49	-	D33.4	D43.4	D49.7
cavity						
buccal	C06.9	C79.89	D00.00	D10.30	D37.09	D49.0
nasal	C30.0	C78.39	D02.3	D14.0	D38.5	D49.1
oral	C06.9	C79.89	D00.00	D10.30	D37.09	D49.0
peritoneal	C48.2	C78.6	-	D20.1	D48.4	D49.0
tympanic	C30.1	C78.39	D02.3	D14.0	D38.5	D49.1
cecum	C18.0	C78.5	D01.0	D12.0	D37.4	D49.0
central nervous system	C72.9	C79.40	-	-	-	-
cerebellopontine (angle)	C71.6	C79.31	-	D33.1	D43.1	D49.6
cerebellum, cerebellar	C71.6	C79.31	-	D33.1	D43.1	D49.6
cerebrum, cerebra (cortex) (hemisphere) (white matter)	C71.0	C79.31	-	D33.0	D43.0	D49.6
meninges	C70.0	C79.32	-	D32.0	D42.0	D49.7
peduncle	C71.7	C79.31	-	D33.1	D43.1	D49.6
ventricle	C71.5	C79.31	-	D33.0	D43.0	D49.6
fourth	C71.7	C79.31	-	D33.1	D43.1	D49.6
cervical region	C76.0	C79.89	D09.8	D36.7	D48.7	D49.89
cervix (cervical) (uteri) (uterus)	C53.9	C79.82	D06.9	D26.0	D39.0	D49.59
canal	C53.0	C79.82	D06.0	D26.0	D39.0	D49.59
endocervix (canal) (gland)	C53.0	C79.82	D06.0	D26.0	D39.0	D49.59
exocervix	C53.1	C79.82	D06.1	D26.0	D39.0	D49.59
external os	C53.1	C79.82	D06.1	D26.0	D39.0	D49.59
internal os	C53.0	C79.82	D06.0	D26.0	D39.0	D49.59
nabothian gland	C53.0	C79.82	D06.0	D26.0	D39.0	D49.59
overlapping lesion	C53.8	-	-	-	-	-
squamocolumnar junction	C53.8	C79.82	D06.7	D26.0	D39.0	D49.59
stump	C53.8	C79.82	D06.7	D26.0	D39.0	D49.59
cheek	C76.0	C79.89	D09.8	D36.7	D48.7	D49.89
external	C44.309	C79.2	D04.39	D23.39	D48.5	D49.2
basal cell carcinoma	C44.319	-	-	-	-	-
specified type NEC	C44.399	-	-	-	-	-
squamous cell carcinoma	C44.329	-	-	-	-	-
inner aspect	C06.0	C79.89	D00.02	D10.39	D37.09	D49.0
internal	C06.0	C79.89	D00.02	D10.39	D37.09	D49.0
mucosa	C06.0	C79.89	D00.02	D10.39	D37.09	D49.0
chest (wall) NEC	C76.1	C79.89	D09.8	D36.7	D48.7	D49.89
chiasma opticum	C72.3-	C79.49	-	D33.3	D43.3	D49.7
chin	C44.309	C79.2	D04.39	D23.39	D48.5	D49.2
basal cell carcinoma	C44.319	-	-	-	-	-
specified type NEC	C44.399	-	-	-	-	-
squamous cell carcinoma	C44.329	-	-	-	-	-
choana	C11.3	C79.89	D00.08	D10.6	D37.05	D49.0
cholangiole	C22.1	C78.89	D01.5	D13.4	D37.6	D49.0
choledochal duct	C24.0	C78.89	D01.5	D13.5	D37.6	D49.0
choroid	C69.3-	C79.49	D09.2-	D31.3-	D48.7	D49.81
plexus	C71.5	C79.31	-	D33.0	D43.0	D49.6
ciliary body	C69.4-	C79.49	D09.2-	D31.4-	D48.7	D49.89
clavicle	C41.3	C79.51	-	D16.7	D48.0	D49.2
clitoris	C51.2	C79.82	D07.1	D28.0	D39.8	D49.59
clivus	C41.0	C79.51	-	D16.4-	D48.0	D49.2
cloacogenic zone	C21.2	C78.5	D01.3	D12.9	D37.8	D49.0
coccygeal						
body or glomus	C49.5	C79.89	-	D21.5	D48.1	D49.2
vertebra	C41.4	C79.51	-	D16.8	D48.0	D49.2

Neoplasm	Malignant Primary	Malignant Secondary	Ca in situ	Benign	Uncertain Behavior	Unspecified Behavior
coccyx	C41.4	C79.51	-	D16.8	D48.0	D49.2
colon (see also Neoplasm, intestine, large)	C18.9	C78.5	-	-	-	-
with rectum	C19	C78.5	D01.1	D12.7	D37.5	D49.0
column, spinal — see Neoplasm, spine						
columnella (see also Neoplasm, skin, face)	C44.390	C79.2	D04.39	D23.39	D48.5	D49.2
commissure						
labial, lip	C00.6	C79.89	D00.01	D10.39	D37.01	D49.0
laryngeal	C32.0	C78.39	D02.0	D14.1	D38.0	D49.1
common (bile) duct	C24.0	C78.89	D01.5	D13.5	D37.6	D49.0
concha (see also Neoplasm, skin, ear)	C44.20-	C79.2	D04.2-	D23.2-	D48.5	D49.2
nose	C30.0	C78.39	D02.3	D14.0	D38.5	D49.1
conjunctiva	C69.0-	C79.49	D09.2-	D31.0-	D48.7	D49.89
connective tissue NEC	C49.9	C79.89	-	D21.9	D48.1	D49.2

Note: For neoplasms of connective tissue (blood vessel, bursa, fascia, ligament, muscle, peripheral nerves, sympathetic and parasympathetic nerves and ganglia, synovia, tendon, etc.) or of morphological types that indicate connective tissue, code according to the list under "Neoplasm, connective tissue". For sites that do not appear in this list, code to neoplasm of that site; e.g., fibrosarcoma, pancreas (C25.9)

Note: Morphological types that indicate connective tissue appear in their proper place in the Alphabetic Index with the instruction "see Neoplasm, connective tissue ...."

Neoplasm	Malignant Primary	Malignant Secondary	Ca in situ	Benign	Uncertain Behavior	Unspecified Behavior
abdomen	C49.4	C79.89	-	D21.4	D48.1	D49.2
abdominal wall	C49.4	C79.89	-	D21.4	D48.1	D49.2
ankle	C49.2-	C79.89	-	D21.2-	D48.1	D49.2
antecubital fossa or space	C49.1-	C79.89	-	D21.1-	D48.1	D49.2
arm	C49.1-	C79.89	-	D21.1-	D48.1	D49.2
auricle (ear)	C49.0	C79.89	-	D21.0	D48.1	D49.2
axilla	C49.3	C79.89	-	D21.3	D48.1	D49.2
back	C49.6	C79.89	-	D21.6	D48.1	D49.2
breast — see Neoplasm, breast						
buttock	C49.5	C79.89	-	D21.5	D48.1	D49.2
calf	C49.2-	C79.89	-	D21.2-	D48.1	D49.2
cervical region	C49.0	C79.89	-	D21.0	D48.1	D49.2
cheek	C49.0	C79.89	-	D21.0	D48.1	D49.2
chest (wall)	C49.3	C79.89	-	D21.3	D48.1	D49.2
chin	C49.0	C79.89	-	D21.0	D48.1	D49.2
diaphragm	C49.3	C79.89	-	D21.3	D48.1	D49.2
ear (external)	C49.0	C79.89	-	D21.0	D48.1	D49.2
elbow	C49.1-	C79.89	-	D21.1-	D48.1	D49.2
extrarectal	C49.5	C79.89	-	D21.5	D48.1	D49.2
extremity	C49.9	C79.89	-	D21.9	D48.1	D49.2
lower	C49.2-	C79.89	-	D21.2-	D48.1	D49.2
upper	C49.1-	C79.89	-	D21.1-	D48.1	D49.2
eyelid	C49.0	C79.89	-	D21.0	D48.1	D49.2
face	C49.0	C79.89	-	D21.0	D48.1	D49.2
finger	C49.1-	C79.89	-	D21.1-	D48.1	D49.2
flank	C49.6	C79.89	-	D21.6	D48.1	D49.2
foot	C49.2-	C79.89	-	D21.2-	D48.1	D49.2
forearm	C49.1-	C79.89	-	D21.1-	D48.1	D49.2
forehead	C49.0	C79.89	-	D21.0	D48.1	D49.2
gastric	C49.4	C79.89	-	D21.4	D48.1	D49.2
gastrointestinal	C49.4	C79.89	-	D21.4	D48.1	D49.2
gluteal region	C49.5	C79.89	-	D21.5	D48.1	D49.2
great vessels NEC	C49.3	C79.89	-	D21.3	D48.1	D49.2
groin	C49.5	C79.89	-	D21.5	D48.1	D49.2
hand	C49.1-	C79.89	-	D21.1-	D48.1	D49.2
head	C49.0	C79.89	-	D21.0	D48.1	D49.2
heel	C49.2-	C79.89	-	D21.2-	D48.1	D49.2
hip	C49.2-	C79.89	-	D21.2-	D48.1	D49.2
hypochondrium	C49.4	C79.89	-	D21.4	D48.1	D49.2
iliopsoas muscle	C49.5	C79.89	-	D21.5	D48.1	D49.2
infraclavicular region	C49.3	C79.89	-	D21.3	D48.1	D49.2
inguinal (canal) (region)	C49.5	C79.89	-	D21.5	D48.1	D49.2
intestinal	C49.4	C79.89	-	D21.4	D48.1	D49.2
intrathoracic	C49.3	C79.89	-	D21.3	D48.1	D49.2
ischiorectal fossa	C49.5	C79.89	-	D21.5	D48.1	D49.2
jaw	C03.9	C79.89	D00.03	D10.39	D37.09	D49.0
knee	C49.2-	C79.89	-	D21.2-	D48.1	D49.2
leg	C49.2-	C79.89	-	D21.2-	D48.1	D49.2
limb NEC	C49.9	C79.89	-	D21.9	D48.1	D49.2
lower	C49.2-	C79.89	-	D21.2-	D48.1	D49.2
upper	C49.1-	C79.89	-	D21.1-	D48.1	D49.2
nates	C49.5	C79.89	-	D21.5	D48.1	D49.2
neck	C49.0	C79.89	-	D21.0	D48.1	D49.2
orbit	C69.6-	C79.49	D09.2-	D31.6-	D48.1	D49.89
overlapping lesion	C49.8	-	-	-	-	-
pararectal	C49.5	C79.89	-	D21.5	D48.1	D49.2
para-urethral	C49.5	C79.89	-	D21.5	D48.1	D49.2
paravaginal	C49.5	C79.89	-	D21.5	D48.1	D49.2
pelvis (floor)	C49.5	C79.89	-	D21.5	D48.1	D49.2
pelvo-abdominal	C49.8	C79.89	-	D21.6	D48.1	D49.2
perineum	C49.5	C79.89	-	D21.5	D48.1	D49.2
perirectal (tissue)	C49.5	C79.89	-	D21.5	D48.1	D49.2
periurethral (tissue)	C49.5	C79.89	-	D21.5	D48.1	D49.2
popliteal fossa or space	C49.2-	C79.89	-	D21.2-	D48.1	D49.2
presacral	C49.5	C79.89	-	D21.5	D48.1	D49.2

connective - fibula

Neoplasm	Malignant Primary	Malignant Secondary	Ca in situ	Benign	Uncertain Behavior	Unspecified Behavior
connective tissue NEC — *continued*						
psoas muscle	C49.4	C79.89	-	D21.4	D48.1	D49.2
pterygoid fossa	C49.0	C79.89	-	D21.0	D48.1	D49.2
rectovaginal septum or wall	C49.5	C79.89	-	D21.5	D48.1	D49.2
rectovesical	C49.5	C79.89	-	D21.5	D48.1	D49.2
retroperitoneum	C48.0	C78.6	-	D20.0	D48.3	D49.0
sacrococcygeal region	C49.5	C79.89	-	D21.5	D48.1	D49.2
scalp	C49.0	C79.89	-	D21.0	D48.1	D49.2
scapular region	C49.3	C79.89	-	D21.3	D48.1	D49.2
shoulder	C49.1-	C79.89	-	D21.1-	D48.1	D49.2
skin (dermis) NEC (*see also* Neoplasm, skin, by site)	C44.90	C79.2	D04.9	D23.9	D48.5	D49.2
stomach	C49.4	C79.89	-	D21.4	D48.1	D49.2
submental	C49.0	C79.89	-	D21.0	D48.1	D49.2
supraclavicular region	C49.0	C79.89	-	D21.0	D48.1	D49.2
temple	C49.0	C79.89	-	D21.0	D48.1	D49.2
temporal region	C49.0	C79.89	-	D21.0	D48.1	D49.2
thigh	C49.2-	C79.89	-	D21.2-	D48.1	D49.2
thoracic (duct) (wall)	C49.3	C79.89	-	D21.3	D48.1	D49.2
thorax	C49.3	C79.89	-	D21.3	D48.1	D49.2
thumb	C49.1-	C79.89	-	D21.1-	D48.1	D49.2
toe	C49.2-	C79.89	-	D21.2-	D48.1	D49.2
trunk	C49.6	C79.89	-	D21.6	D48.1	D49.2
umbilicus	C49.4	C79.89	-	D21.4	D48.1	D49.2
vesicorectal	C49.5	C79.89	-	D21.5	D48.1	D49.2
wrist	C49.1-	C79.89	-	D21.1-	D48.1	D49.2
conus medullaris	C72.0	C79.49	-	D33.4	D43.4	D49.7
cord (true) (vocal)	C32.0	C78.39	D02.0	D14.1	D38.0	D49.1
false	C32.1	C78.39	D02.0	D14.1	D38.0	D49.1
spermatic	C63.1-	C79.82	D07.69	D29.8	D40.8	D49.59
spinal (cervical) (lumbar) (thoracic)	C72.0	C79.49	-	D33.4	D43.4	D49.7
cornea (limbus)	C69.1-	C79.49	D09.2-	D31.1-	D48.7	D49.89
corpus						
albicans	C56.-	C79.6-	D07.39	D27.-	D39.1-	D49.59
callosum, brain	C71.0	C79.31	-	D33.2	D43.2	D49.6
cavernosum	C60.2	C79.82	D07.4	D29.0	D40.8	D49.59
gastric	C16.2	C78.89	D00.2	D13.1	D37.1	D49.0
overlapping sites	C54.8	-	-	-	-	-
penis	C60.2	C79.82	D07.4	D29.0	D40.8	D49.59
striatum, cerebrum	C71.0	C79.31	-	D33.0	D43.0	D49.6
uteri	C54.9	C79.82	D07.0	D26.1	D39.0	D49.59
isthmus	C54.0	C79.82	D07.0	D26.1	D39.0	D49.59
cortex						
adrenal	C74.0-	C79.7-	D09.3	D35.0-	D44.1-	D49.7
cerebral	C71.0	C79.31	-	D33.0	D43.0	D49.6
costal cartilage	C41.3	C79.51	-	D16.7	D48.0	D49.2
costovertebral joint	C41.3	C79.51	-	D16.7	D48.0	D49.2
Cowper's gland	C68.0	C79.19	D09.19	D30.4	D41.3	D49.59
cranial (fossa, any)	C71.9	C79.31	-	D33.2	D43.2	D49.6
meninges	C70.0	C79.32	-	D32.0	D42.0	D49.7
nerve	C72.50	C79.49	-	D33.3	D43.3	D49.7
specified NEC	C72.59	C79.49	-	D33.3	D43.3	D49.7
craniobuccal pouch	C75.2	C79.89	D09.3	D35.2	D44.3	D49.7
craniopharyngeal (duct) (pouch)	C75.2	C79.89	D09.3	D35.3	D44.4	D49.7
cricoid	C13.0	C79.89	D00.08	D10.7	D37.05	D49.0
cartilage	C32.3	C78.39	D02.0	D14.1	D38.0	D49.1
cricopharynx	C13.0	C79.89	D00.08	D10.7	D37.05	D49.0
crypt of Morgagni	C21.8	C78.5	D01.3	D12.9	D37.8	D49.0
crystalline lens	C69.4-	C79.49	D09.2-	D31.4-	D48.7	D49.89
cul-de-sac (Douglas')	C48.1	C78.6	-	D20.1	D48.4	D49.0
cuneiform cartilage	C32.3	C78.39	D02.0	D14.1	D38.0	D49.1
cutaneous — *see* Neoplasm, skin						
cutis — *see* Neoplasm, skin						
cystic (bile) duct (common)	C24.0	C78.89	D01.5	D13.5	D37.6	D49.0
dermis — *see* Neoplasm, skin						
diaphragm	C49.3	C79.89	-	D21.3	D48.1	D49.2
digestive organs, system, tube, or tract NEC	C26.9	C78.89	D01.9	D13.9	D37.9	D49.0
disc, intervertebral	C41.2	C79.51	-	D16.6	D48.0	D49.2
disease, generalized	C80.0	-	-	-	-	-
disseminated	C80.0	-	-	-	-	-
Douglas' cul-de-sac or pouch	C48.1	C78.6	-	D20.1	D48.4	D49.0
duodenojejunal junction	C17.8	C78.4	D01.49	D13.39	D37.2	D49.0
duodenum	C17.0	C78.4	D01.49	D13.2	D37.2	D49.0
dura (cranial) (mater)	C70.9	C79.49	-	D32.9	D42.9	D49.7
cerebral	C70.0	C79.32	-	D32.0	D42.0	D49.7
spinal	C70.1	C79.49	-	D32.1	D42.1	D49.7
ear (external) (*see also* Neoplasm, skin, ear)	C44.20-	C79.2	D04.2-	D23.2-	D48.5	D49.2
auricle or auris (*see also* Neoplasm, skin, ear)	C44.20-	C79.2	D04.2-	D23.2-	D48.5	D49.2
canal, external (*see also* Neoplasm, skin, ear)	C44.20-	C79.2	D04.2-	D23.2-	D48.5	D49.2
cartilage	C49.0	C79.89	-	D21.0	D48.1	D49.2
external meatus (*see also* Neoplasm, skin, ear)	C44.20-	C79.2	D04.2-	D23.2-	D48.5	D49.2
inner	C30.1	C78.39	D02.3	D14.0	D38.5	D49.1
lobule (*see also* Neoplasm, skin, ear)	C44.20-	C79.2	D04.2-	D23.2-	D48.5	D49.2

Neoplasm	Malignant Primary	Malignant Secondary	Ca in situ	Benign	Uncertain Behavior	Unspecified Behavior
ear — *continued*						
middle	C30.1	C78.39	D02.3	D14.0	D38.5	D49.1
overlapping lesion with accessory sinuses	C31.8	-	-	-	-	-
skin	C44.20-	C79.2	D04.2-	D23.2-	D48.5	D49.2
basal cell carcinoma	C44.21-	-	-	-	-	-
specified type NEC	C44.29-	-	-	-	-	-
squamous cell carcinoma	C44.22-	-	-	-	-	-
earlobe	C44.20-	C79.2	D04.2-	D23.2-	D48.5	D49.2
basal cell carcinoma	C44.21-	-	-	-	-	-
specified type NEC	C44.29-	-	-	-	-	-
squamous cell carcinoma	C44.22-	-	-	-	-	-
ejaculatory duct	C63.7	C79.82	D07.69	D29.8	D40.8	D49.59
elbow NEC	C76.4-	C79.89	D04.6-	D36.7	D48.7	D49.89
endocardium	C38.0	C79.89	-	D15.1	D48.7	D49.89
endocervix (canal) (gland)	C53.0	C79.82	D06.0	D26.0	D39.0	D49.59
endocrine gland NEC	C75.9	C79.89	D09.3	D35.9	D44.9	D49.7
pluriglandular	C75.8	C79.89	D09.3	D35.7	D44.9	D49.7
endometrium (gland) (stroma)	C54.1	C79.82	D07.0	D26.1	D39.0	D49.59
ensiform cartilage	C41.3	C79.51	-	D16.7	D48.0	D49.2
enteric — *see* Neoplasm, intestine						
ependyma (brain)	C71.5	C79.31	-	D33.0	D43.0	D49.6
fourth ventricle	C71.7	C79.31	-	D33.1	D43.1	D49.6
epicardium	C38.0	C79.89	-	D15.1	D48.7	D49.89
epididymis	C63.0-	C79.82	D07.69	D29.3-	D40.8	D49.59
epidural	C72.9	C79.49	-	D33.9	D43.9	D49.7
epiglottis	C32.1	C78.39	D02.0	D14.1	D38.0	D49.1
anterior aspect or surface	C10.1	C79.89	D00.08	D10.5	D37.05	D49.0
cartilage	C32.3	C78.39	D02.0	D14.1	D38.0	D49.1
free border (margin)	C10.1	C79.89	D00.08	D10.5	D37.05	D49.0
junctional region	C10.8	C79.89	D00.08	D10.5	D37.05	D49.0
posterior (laryngeal) surface	C32.1	C78.39	D02.0	D14.1	D38.0	D49.1
suprahyoid portion	C32.1	C78.39	D02.0	D14.1	D38.0	D49.1
esophagogastric junction	C16.0	C78.89	D00.2	D13.1	D37.1	D49.0
esophagus	C15.9	C78.89	D00.1	D13.0	D37.8	D49.0
abdominal	C15.5	C78.89	D00.1	D13.0	D37.8	D49.0
cervical	C15.3	C78.89	D00.1	D13.0	D37.8	D49.0
distal (third)	C15.5	C78.89	D00.1	D13.0	D37.8	D49.0
lower (third)	C15.5	C78.89	D00.1	D13.0	D37.8	D49.0
middle (third)	C15.4	C78.89	D00.1	D13.0	D37.8	D49.0
overlapping lesion	C15.8	-	-	-	-	-
proximal (third)	C15.3	C78.89	D00.1	D13.0	D37.8	D49.0
thoracic	C15.4	C78.89	D00.1	D13.0	D37.8	D49.0
upper (third)	C15.3	C78.89	D00.1	D13.0	D37.8	D49.0
ethmoid (sinus)	C31.1	C78.39	D02.3	D14.0	D38.5	D49.1
bone or labyrinth	C41.0	C79.51	-	D16.4-	D48.0	D49.2
eustachian tube	C30.1	C78.39	D02.3	D14.0	D38.5	D49.1
exocervix	C53.1	C79.82	D06.1	D26.0	D39.0	D49.59
external						
meatus (ear) (*see also* Neoplasm, skin, ear)	C44.20-	C79.2	D04.2-	D23.2-	D48.5	D49.2
os, cervix uteri	C53.1	C79.82	D06.1	D26.0	D39.0	D49.59
extradural	C72.9	C79.49	-	D33.9	D43.9	D49.7
extrahepatic (bile) duct	C24.0	C78.89	D01.5	D13.5	D37.6	D49.0
overlapping lesion with gallbladder	C24.8	-	-	-	-	-
extraocular muscle	C69.6-	C79.49	D09.2-	D31.6-	D48.7	D49.89
extrarectal	C76.3	C79.89	D09.8	D36.7	D48.7	D49.89
extremity	C76.8	C79.89	D04.8	D36.7	D48.7	D49.89
lower	C76.5-	C79.89	D04.7-	D36.7	D48.7	D49.89
upper	C76.4-	C79.89	D04.6-	D36.7	D48.7	D49.89
eye NEC	C69.9-	C79.49	D09.2	D31.9	D48.7	D49.89
overlapping sites	C69.8	-	-	-	-	-
eyeball	C69.9-	C79.49	D09.2-	D31.9-	D48.7	D49.89
eyebrow	C44.309	C79.2	D04.39	D23.39	D48.5	D49.2
basal cell carcinoma	C44.319	-	-	-	-	-
specified type NEC	C44.399	-	-	-	-	-
squamous cell carcinoma	C44.329	-	-	-	-	-
eyelid (lower) (skin) (upper)	C44.10-	-	-	-	-	-
basal cell carcinoma	C44.11-	-	-	-	-	-
sebaceous cell	C44.13-	-	-	-	-	-
specified type NEC	C44.19-	-	-	-	-	-
squamous cell carcinoma	C44.12-	-	-	-	-	-
cartilage	C49.0	C79.89	-	D21.0	D48.1	D49.2
face NEC	C76.0	C79.89	D04.39	D36.7	D48.7	D49.89
fallopian tube (accessory)	C57.0-	C79.82	D07.39	D28.2	D39.8	D49.59
falx (cerebella) (cerebri)	C70.0	C79.32	-	D32.0	D42.0	D49.7
fascia (*see also* Neoplasm, connective tissue)						
palmar	C49.1-	C79.89	-	D21.1-	D48.1	D49.2
plantar	C49.2-	C79.89	-	D21.2-	D48.1	D49.2
fatty tissue — *see* Neoplasm, connective tissue						
fauces, faucial NEC	C10.9	C79.89	D00.08	D10.5	D37.05	D49.0
pillars	C09.1	C79.89	D00.08	D10.5	D37.05	D49.0
tonsil	C09.9	C79.89	D00.08	D10.4	D37.05	D49.0
femur (any part)	C40.2-	-	-	D16.2-	-	-
fetal membrane	C58	C79.82	D07.0	D26.7	D39.2	D49.59
fibrous tissue — *see* Neoplasm, connective tissue						
fibula (any part)	C40.2-	C79.51	-	D16.2-	-	-

Neoplasm	Malignant Primary	Malignant Secondary	Ca in situ	Benign	Uncertain Behavior	Unspecified Behavior
filum terminale	C72.0	C79.49	-	D33.4	D43.4	D49.7
finger NEC	C76.4-	C79.89	D04.6-	D36.7	D48.7	D49.89
flank NEC	C76.8	C79.89	D04.5	D36.7	D48.7	D49.89
follicle, nabothian	C53.0	C79.82	D06.0	D26.0	D39.0	D49.59
foot NEC	C76.5-	C79.89	D04.7-	D36.7	D48.7	D49.89
forearm NEC	C76.4-	C79.89	D04.6-	D36.7	D48.7	D49.89
forehead (skin)	C44.309	C79.2	D04.39	D23.39	D48.5	D49.2
basal cell carcinoma	C44.319	-	-	-	-	-
specified type NEC	C44.399	-	-	-	-	-
squamous cell carcinoma	C44.329	-	-	-	-	-
foreskin	C60.0	C79.82	D07.4	D29.0	D40.8	D49.59
fornix						
pharyngeal	C11.3	C79.89	D00.08	D10.6	D37.05	D49.0
vagina	C52	C79.82	D07.2	D28.1	D39.8	D49.59
fossa (of)						
anterior (cranial)	C71.9	C79.31	-	D33.2	D43.2	D49.6
cranial	C71.9	C79.31	-	D33.2	D43.2	D49.6
ischiorectal	C76.3	C79.89	D09.8	D36.7	D48.7	D49.89
middle (cranial)	C71.9	C79.31	-	D33.2	D43.2	D49.6
piriform	C12	C79.89	D00.08	D10.7	D37.05	D49.0
pituitary	C75.1	C79.89	D09.3	D35.2	D44.3	D49.7
posterior (cranial)	C71.9	C79.31	-	D33.2	D43.2	D49.6
pterygoid	C49.0	C79.89	-	D21.0	D48.1	D49.2
pyriform	C12	C79.89	D00.08	D10.7	D37.05	D49.0
Rosenmuller	C11.2	C79.89	D00.08	D10.6	D37.05	D49.0
tonsillar	C09.0	C79.89	D00.08	D10.5	D37.05	D49.0
fourchette	C51.9	C79.82	D07.1	D28.0	D39.8	D49.59
frenulum						
labii — *see* Neoplasm, lip, internal						
linguae	C02.2	C79.89	D00.07	D10.1	D37.02	D49.0
frontal						
bone	C41.0	C79.51	-	D16.4-	D48.0	D49.2
lobe, brain	C71.1	C79.31	-	D33.0	D43.0	D49.6
pole	C71.1	C79.31	-	D33.0	D43.0	D49.6
sinus	C31.2	C78.39	D02.3	D14.0	D38.5	D49.1
fundus						
stomach	C16.1	C78.89	D00.2	D13.1	D37.1	D49.0
uterus	C54.3	C79.82	D07.0	D26.1	D39.0	D49.59
gall duct (extrahepatic)	C24.0	C78.89	D01.5	D13.5	D37.6	D49.0
intrahepatic	C22.1	C78.7	D01.5	D13.4	D37.6	D49.0
gallbladder	C23	C78.89	D01.5	D13.5	D37.6	D49.0
overlapping lesion with extrahepatic bile ducts	C24.8	-	-	-	-	-
ganglia (*see also* Neoplasm, nerve, peripheral)	C47.9	C79.89	-	D36.10	D48.2	D49.2
basal	C71.0	C79.31	-	D33.0	D43.0	D49.6
cranial nerve	C72.50	C79.49	-	D33.3	D43.3	D49.7
Gartner's duct	C52	C79.82	D07.2	D28.1	D39.8	D49.59
gastric — *see* Neoplasm, stomach						
gastrocolic	C26.9	C78.89	D01.9	D13.9	D37.9	D49.0
gastroesophageal junction	C16.0	C78.89	D00.2	D13.1	D37.1	D49.0
gastrointestinal (tract) NEC	C26.9	C78.89	D01.9	D13.9	D37.9	D49.0
generalized	C80.0	-	-	-	-	-
genital organ or tract						
female NEC	C57.9	C79.82	D07.30	D28.9	D39.9	D49.59
overlapping lesion	C57.8	-	-	-	-	-
specified site NEC	C57.7	C79.82	D07.39	D28.7	D39.8	D49.59
male NEC	C63.9	C79.82	D07.60	D29.9	D40.9	D49.59
overlapping lesion	C63.8	-	-	-	-	-
specified site NEC	C63.7	C79.82	D07.69	D29.8	D40.8	D49.59
genitourinary tract						
female	C57.9	C79.82	D07.30	D28.9	D39.9	D49.59
male	C63.9	C79.82	D07.60	D29.9	D40.9	D49.59
gingiva (alveolar) (marginal)	C03.9	C79.89	D00.03	D10.39	D37.09	D49.0
lower	C03.1	C79.89	D00.03	D10.39	D37.09	D49.0
mandibular	C03.1	C79.89	D00.03	D10.39	D37.09	D49.0
maxillary	C03.0	C79.89	D00.03	D10.39	D37.09	D49.0
upper	C03.0	C79.89	D00.03	D10.39	D37.09	D49.0
gland, glandular (lymphatic) (system) (*see also* Neoplasm, lymph gland)						
endocrine NEC	C75.9	C79.89	D09.3	D35.9	D44.9	D49.7
salivary — *see* Neoplasm, salivary gland						
glans penis	C60.1	C79.82	D07.4	D29.0	D40.8	D49.59
globus pallidus	C71.0	C79.31	-	D33.0	D43.0	D49.6
glomus						
coccygeal	C49.5	C79.89	-	D21.5	D48.1	D49.2
jugularis	C75.5	C79.89	-	D35.6	D44.7	D49.7
glosso-epiglottic fold(s)	C10.1	C79.89	D00.08	D10.5	D37.05	D49.0
glossopalatine fold	C09.1	C79.89	D00.08	D10.5	D37.05	D49.0
glossopharyngeal sulcus	C09.0	C79.89	D00.08	D10.5	D37.05	D49.0
glottis	C32.0	C78.39	D02.0	D14.1	D38.0	D49.1
gluteal region	C76.3	C79.89	D04.5	D36.7	D48.7	D49.89
great vessels NEC	C49.3	C79.89	-	D21.3	D48.1	D49.2
groin NEC	C76.3	C79.89	D04.5	D36.7	D48.7	D49.89
gum	C03.9	C79.89	D00.03	D10.39	D37.09	D49.0
lower	C03.1	C79.89	D00.03	D10.39	D37.09	D49.0
upper	C03.0	C79.89	D00.03	D10.39	D37.09	D49.0
hand NEC	C76.4-	C79.89	D04.6-	D36.7	D48.7	D49.89

Neoplasm	Malignant Primary	Malignant Secondary	Ca in situ	Benign	Uncertain Behavior	Unspecified Behavior
head NEC	C76.0	C79.89	D04.4	D36.7	D48.7	D49.89
heart	C38.0	C79.89	-	D15.1	D48.7	D49.89
heel NEC	C76.5-	C79.89	D04.7-	D36.7	D48.7	D49.89
helix (*see also* Neoplasm, skin, ear)	C44.20-	C79.2	D04.2-	D23.2-	D48.5	D49.2
hematopoietic, hemopoietic tissue NEC	C96.9	-	-	-	-	-
specified NEC	C96.7	-	-	-	-	-
hemisphere, cerebral	C71.0	C79.31	-	D33.0	D43.0	D49.6
hemorrhoidal zone	C21.1	C78.5	D01.3	D12.9	D37.8	D49.0
hepatic (*see also* Index to disease, by histology)	C22.9	C78.7	D01.5	D13.4	D37.6	D49.0
duct (bile)	C24.0	C78.89	D01.5	D13.5	D37.6	D49.0
flexure (colon)	C18.3	C78.5	D01.0	D12.3	D37.4	D49.0
primary	C22.8	C78.7	D01.5	D13.4	D37.6	D49.0
hepatobiliary	C24.9	C78.89	D01.5	D13.5	D37.6	D49.0
hepatoblastoma	C22.2	C78.7	D01.5	D13.4	D37.6	D49.0
hepatoma	C22.0	C78.7	D01.5	D13.4	D37.6	D49.0
hilus of lung	C34.0-	C78.0-	D02.2-	D14.3-	D38.1	D49.1
hip NEC	C76.5-	C79.89	D04.7-	D36.7	D48.7	D49.89
hippocampus, brain	C71.2	C79.31	-	D33.0	D43.0	D49.6
humerus (any part)	C40.0-	C79.51	-	D16.0-	D48.0	D49.2
hymen	C52	C79.82	D07.2	D28.1	D39.8	D49.59
hypopharynx, hypopharyngeal NEC	C13.9	C79.89	D00.08	D10.7	D37.05	D49.0
overlapping lesion	C13.8	-	-	-	-	-
postcricoid region	C13.0	C79.89	D00.08	D10.7	D37.05	D49.0
posterior wall	C13.2	C79.89	D00.08	D10.7	D37.05	D49.0
pyriform fossa (sinus)	C12	C79.89	D00.08	D10.7	D37.05	D49.0
hypophysis	C75.1	C79.89	D09.3	D35.2	D44.3	D49.7
hypothalamus	C71.0	C79.31	-	D33.0	D43.0	D49.6
ileocecum, ileocecal (coil) (junction) (valve)	C18.0	C78.5	D01.0	D12.0	D37.4	D49.0
ileum	C17.2	C78.4	D01.49	D13.39	D37.2	D49.0
ilium	C41.4	C79.51	-	D16.8	D48.0	D49.2
immunoproliferative NEC	C88.9	-	-	-	-	-
infraclavicular (region)	C76.1	C79.89	D04.5	D36.7	D48.7	D49.89
inguinal (region)	C76.3	C79.89	D04.5	D36.7	D48.7	D49.89
insula	C71.0	C79.31	-	D33.0	D43.0	D49.6
insular tissue (pancreas)	C25.4	C78.89	D01.7	D13.7	D37.8	D49.0
brain	C71.0	C79.31	-	D33.0	D43.0	D49.6
interarytenoid fold	C13.1	C79.89	D00.08	D10.7	D37.05	D49.0
hypopharyngeal aspect	C13.1	C79.89	D00.08	D10.7	D37.05	D49.0
laryngeal aspect	C32.1	C78.39	D02.0	D14.1	D38.0	D49.1
marginal zone	C13.1	C79.89	D00.08	D10.7	D37.05	D49.0
interdental papillae	C03.9	C79.89	D00.03	D10.39	D37.09	D49.0
lower	C03.1	C79.89	D00.03	D10.39	D37.09	D49.0
upper	C03.0	C79.89	D00.03	D10.39	D37.09	D49.0
internal						
capsule	C71.0	C79.31	-	D33.0	D43.0	D49.6
os (cervix)	C53.0	C79.82	D06.0	D26.0	D39.0	D49.59
intervertebral cartilage or disc	C41.2	C79.51	-	D16.6	D48.0	D49.2
intestine, intestinal	C26.0	C78.80	D01.40	D13.9	D37.8	D49.0
large	C18.9	C78.5	D01.0	D12.6	D37.4	D49.0
appendix	C18.1	C78.5	D01.0	D12.1	D37.3	D49.0
caput coli	C18.0	C78.5	D01.0	D12.0	D37.4	D49.0
cecum	C18.0	C78.5	D01.0	D12.0	D37.4	D49.0
colon	C18.9	C78.5	D01.0	D12.6	D37.4	D49.0
and rectum	C19	C78.5	D01.1	D12.7	D37.5	D49.0
ascending	C18.2	C78.5	D01.0	D12.2	D37.4	D49.0
caput	C18.0	C78.5	D01.0	D12.0	D37.4	D49.0
descending	C18.6	C78.5	D01.0	D12.4	D37.4	D49.0
distal	C18.6	C78.5	D01.0	D12.4	D37.4	D49.0
left	C18.6	C78.5	D01.0	D12.4	D37.4	D49.0
overlapping lesion	C18.8	-	-	-	-	-
pelvic	C18.7	C78.5	D01.0	D12.5	D37.4	D49.0
right	C18.2	C78.5	D01.0	D12.2	D37.4	D49.0
sigmoid (flexure)	C18.7	C78.5	D01.0	D12.5	D37.4	D49.0
transverse	C18.4	C78.5	D01.0	D12.3	D37.4	D49.0
hepatic flexure	C18.3	C78.5	D01.0	D12.3	D37.4	D49.0
ileocecum, ileocecal (coil) (valve)	C18.0	C78.5	D01.0	D12.0	D37.4	D49.0
overlapping lesion	C18.8	-	-	-	-	-
sigmoid flexure (lower) (upper)	C18.7	C78.5	D01.0	D12.5	D37.4	D49.0
splenic flexure	C18.5	C78.5	D01.0	D12.3	D37.4	D49.0
small	C17.9	C78.4	D01.40	D13.30	D37.2	D49.0
duodenum	C17.0	C78.4	D01.49	D13.2	D37.2	D49.0
ileum	C17.2	C78.4	D01.49	D13.39	D37.2	D49.0
jejunum	C17.1	C78.4	D01.49	D13.39	D37.2	D49.0
overlapping lesion	C17.8	-	-	-	-	-
tract NEC	C26.0	C78.89	D01.40	D13.9	D37.8	D49.0
intra-abdominal	C76.2	C79.89	D09.8	D36.7	D48.7	D49.89
intracranial NEC	C71.9	C79.31	-	D33.2	D43.2	D49.6
intrahepatic (bile) duct	C22.1	C78.7	D01.5	D13.4	D37.6	D49.0
intraocular	C69.9-	C79.49	D09.2-	D31.9-	D48.7	D49.89
intraorbital	C69.6-	C79.49	D09.2-	D31.6-	D48.7	D49.89
intrasellar	C75.1	C79.89	D09.3	D35.2	D44.3	D49.7
intrathoracic (cavity) (organs)	C76.1	C79.89	D09.8	D15.9	D48.7	D49.89
specified NEC	C76.1	C79.89	D09.8	D15.7	-	-
iris	C69.4-	C79.49	D09.2-	D31.4-	D48.7	D49.89
ischiorectal (fossa)	C76.3	C79.89	D09.8	D36.7	D48.7	D49.89
ischium	C41.4	C79.51	-	D16.8	D48.0	D49.2

island - lymph

Neoplasm	Malignant Primary	Malignant Secondary	Ca in situ	Benign	Uncertain Behavior	Unspecified Behavior
island of Reil	C71.0	C79.31	-	D33.0	D43.0	D49.6
islands or islets of Langerhans	C25.4	C78.89	D01.7	D13.7	D37.8	D49.0
isthmus uteri	C54.0	C79.82	D07.0	D26.1	D39.0	D49.59
jaw	C76.0	C79.89	D09.8	D36.7	D48.7	D49.89
bone	C41.1	C79.51	-	D16.5-	D48.0	D49.2
lower	C41.1	C79.51	-	D16.5-	-	-
upper	C41.0	C79.51	-	D16.4-	-	-
carcinoma (any type) (lower) (upper)	C76.0	C79.89				
skin (see also Neoplasm, skin, face)	C44.309	C79.2	D04.39	D23.39	D48.5	D49.2
soft tissues	C03.9	C79.89	D00.03	D10.39	D37.09	D49.0
lower	C03.1	C79.89	D00.03	D10.39	D37.09	D49.0
upper	C03.0	C79.89	D00.03	D10.39	D37.09	D49.0
jejunum	C17.1	C78.4	D01.49	D13.39	D37.2	D49.0
joint NEC (see also Neoplasm, bone)	C41.9	C79.51	-	D16.9-	D48.0	D49.2
acromioclavicular	C40.0-	C79.51	-	D16.0-	-	-
bursa or synovial membrane — see Neoplasm, connective tissue						
costovertebral	C41.3	C79.51	-	D16.7	D48.0	D49.2
sternocostal	C41.3	C79.51	-	D16.7	D48.0	D49.2
temporomandibular	C41.1	C79.51	-	D16.5-	D48.0	D49.2
junction						
anorectal	C21.8	C78.5	D01.3	D12.9	D37.8	D49.0
cardioesophageal	C16.0	C78.89	D00.2	D13.1	D37.1	D49.0
esophagogastric	C16.0	C78.89	D00.2	D13.1	D37.1	D49.0
gastroesophageal	C16.0	C78.89	D00.2	D13.1	D37.1	D49.0
hard and soft palate	C05.9	C79.89	D00.00	D10.39	D37.09	D49.0
ileocecal	C18.0	C78.5	D01.0	D12.0	D37.4	D49.0
pelvirectal	C19	C78.5	D01.1	D12.7	D37.5	D49.0
pelviureteric	C65.-	C79.0-	D09.19	D30.1-	D41.1-	D49.59
rectosigmoid	C19	C78.5	D01.1	D12.7	D37.5	D49.0
squamocolumnar, of cervix	C53.8	C79.82	D06.7	D26.0	D39.0	D49.59
Kaposi's sarcoma — see Kaposi's, sarcoma						
kidney (parenchymal)	C64.-	C79.0-	D09.19	D30.0-	D41.0-	D49.51-
calyx	C65.-	C79.0-	D09.19	D30.1-	D41.1-	D49.51-
hilus	C65.-	C79.0-	D09.19	D30.1-	D41.1-	D49.51-
pelvis	C65.-	C79.0-	D09.19	D30.1-	D41.1-	D49.51-
knee NEC	C76.5-	C79.89	D04.7-	D36.7	D48.7	D49.89
labia (skin)	C51.9	C79.82	D07.1	D28.0	D39.8	D49.59
majora	C51.0	C79.82	D07.1	D28.0	D39.8	D49.59
minora	C51.1	C79.82	D07.1	D28.0	D39.8	D49.59
labial (see also Neoplasm, lip)	C00.9	C79.89	D00.01	D10.0	D37.01	D49.0
sulcus (lower) (upper)	C06.1	C79.89	D00.02	D10.39	D37.09	D49.0
labium (skin)	C51.9	C79.82	D07.1	D28.0	D39.8	D49.59
majus	C51.0	C79.82	D07.1	D28.0	D39.8	D49.59
minus	C51.1	C79.82	D07.1	D28.0	D39.8	D49.59
lacrimal						
canaliculi	C69.5-	C79.49	D09.2-	D31.5-	D48.7	D49.89
duct (nasal)	C69.5-	C79.49	D09.2-	D31.5-	D48.7	D49.89
gland	C69.5-	C79.49	D09.2-	D31.5-	D48.7	D49.89
punctum	C69.5-	C79.49	D09.2-	D31.5-	D48.7	D49.89
sac	C69.5-	C79.49	D09.2-	D31.5-	D48.7	D49.89
Langerhans, islands or islets	C25.4	C78.89	D01.7	D13.7	D37.8	D49.0
laryngopharynx	C13.9	C79.89	D00.08	D10.7	D37.05	D49.0
larynx, laryngeal NEC	C32.9	C78.39	D02.0	D14.1	D38.0	D49.1
aryepiglottic fold	C32.1	C78.39	D02.0	D14.1	D38.0	D49.1
cartilage (arytenoid) (cricoid) (cuneiform) (thyroid)	C32.3	C78.39	D02.0	D14.1	D38.0	D49.1
commissure (anterior) (posterior)	C32.0	C78.39	D02.0	D14.1	D38.0	D49.1
extrinsic NEC	C32.1	C78.39	D02.0	D14.1	D38.0	D49.1
meaning hypopharynx	C13.9	C79.89	D00.08	D10.7	D37.05	D49.0
interarytenoid fold	C32.1	C78.39	D02.0	D14.1	D38.0	D49.1
intrinsic	C32.0	C78.39	D02.0	D14.1	D38.0	D49.1
overlapping lesion	C32.8	-	-	-	-	-
ventricular band	C32.1	C78.39	D02.0	D14.1	D38.0	D49.1
leg NEC	C76.5-	C79.89	D04.7-	D36.7	D48.7	D49.89
lens, crystalline	C69.4-	C79.49	D09.2-	D31.4-	D48.7	D49.89
lid (lower) (upper)	C44.10-	C79.2	D04.1-	D23.1-	D48.5	D49.2
basal cell carcinoma	C44.11-	-	-	-	-	-
sebaceous cell	C44.13-	-	-	-	-	-
specified type NEC	C44.19-	-	-	-	-	-
squamous cell carcinoma	C44.12-	-	-	-	-	-
ligament (see also Neoplasm, connective tissue)						
broad	C57.1	C79.82	D07.39	D28.2	D39.8	D49.59
Mackenrodt's	C57.7	C79.82	D07.39	D28.7	D39.8	D49.59
non-uterine — see Neoplasm, connective tissue						
round	C57.2	C79.82	-	D28.2	D39.8	D49.59
sacro-uterine	C57.3	C79.82	-	D28.2	D39.8	D49.59
uterine	C57.3	C79.82	-	D28.2	D39.8	D49.59
utero-ovarian	C57.7	C79.82	D07.39	D28.2	D39.8	D49.59
uterosacral	C57.3	C79.82	-	D28.2	D39.8	D49.59
limb	C76.8	C79.89	D04.8	D36.7	D48.7	D49.89
lower	C76.5-	C79.89	D04.7-	D36.7	D48.7	D49.89
upper	C76.4-	C79.89	D04.6-	D36.7	D48.7	D49.89
limbus of cornea	C69.1-	C79.49	D09.2-	D31.1-	D48.7	D49.89
lingual NEC (see also Neoplasm, tongue)	C02.9	C79.89	D00.07	D10.1	D37.02	D49.0
lingula, lung	C34.1-	C78.0-	D02.2-	D14.3-	D38.1	D49.1

Neoplasm	Malignant Primary	Malignant Secondary	Ca in situ	Benign	Uncertain Behavior	Unspecified Behavior
lip	C00.9	C79.89	D00.01	D10.0	D37.0	D49.0
buccal aspect — see Neoplasm, lip, internal						
commissure	C00.6	C79.89	D00.01	D10.0	D37.01	D49.0
external	C00.2	C79.89	D00.01	D10.0	D37.01	D49.0
lower	C00.1	C79.89	D00.01	D10.0	D37.01	D49.0
upper	C00.0	C79.89	D00.01	D10.0	D37.01	D49.0
frenulum — see Neoplasm, lip, internal						
inner aspect — see Neoplasm, lip, internal						
internal	C00.5	C79.89	D00.01	D10.0	D37.01	D49.0
lower	C00.4	C79.89	D00.01	D10.0	D37.01	D49.0
upper	C00.3	C79.89	D00.01	D10.0	D37.01	D49.0
lipstick area	C00.2	C79.89	D00.01	D10.0	D37.01	D49.0
lower	C00.1	C79.89	D00.01	D10.0	D37.01	D49.0
upper	C00.0	C79.89	D00.01	D10.0	D37.01	D49.0
lower	C00.1	C79.89	D00.01	D10.0	D37.01	D49.0
internal	C00.4	C79.89	D00.01	D10.0	D37.01	D49.0
mucosa — see Neoplasm, lip, internal						
oral aspect — see Neoplasm, lip, internal						
overlapping lesion	C00.8	-	-	-	-	-
with oral cavity or pharynx	C14.8	-	-	-	-	-
skin (commissure) (lower) (upper)	C44.00	C79.2	D04.0	D23.0	D48.5	D49.2
basal cell carcinoma	C44.01	-	-	-	-	-
specified type NEC	C44.09	-	-	-	-	-
squamous cell carcinoma	C44.02	-	-	-	-	-
upper	C00.0	C79.89	D00.01	D10.0	D37.01	D49.0
internal	C00.3	C79.89	D00.01	D10.0	D37.01	D49.0
vermilion border	C00.2	C79.89	D00.01	D10.0	D37.01	D49.0
lower	C00.1	C79.89	D00.01	D10.0	D37.01	D49.0
upper	C00.0	C79.89	D00.01	D10.0	D37.01	D49.0
lipomatous — see Lipoma, by site						
liver (see also Index to disease, by histology)	C22.9	C78.7	D01.5	D13.4	D37.6	D49.0
primary	C22.8	C78.7	D01.5	D13.4	D37.6	D49.0
lumbosacral plexus	C47.5	C79.89	-	D36.16	D48.2	D49.2
lung	C34.9-	C78.0-	D02.2-	D14.3-	D38.1	D49.1
azygos lobe	C34.1-	C78.0-	D02.2-	D14.3-	D38.1	D49.1
carina	C34.0-	C78.0-	D02.2-	D14.3-	D38.1	D49.1
hilus	C34.0-	C78.0-	D02.2-	D14.3-	D38.1	D49.1
lingula	C34.1-	C78.0-	D02.2-	D14.3-	D38.1	D49.1
lobe NEC	C34.9-	C78.0-	D02.2-	D14.3-	D38.1	D49.1
lower lobe	C34.3-	C78.0-	D02.2-	D14.3-	D38.1	D49.1
main bronchus	C34.0-	C78.0-	D02.2-	D14.3-	D38.1	D49.1
mesothelioma — see Mesothelioma						
middle lobe	C34.2	C78.0-	D02.21	D14.31	D38.1	D49.1
overlapping lesion	C34.8-					
upper lobe	C34.1-	C78.0-	D02.2-	D14.3-	D38.1	D49.1
lymph, lymphatic channel NEC	C49.9	C79.89	-	D21.9	D48.1	D49.2
gland (secondary)	-	C77.9	-	D36.0	D48.7	D49.89
abdominal	-	C77.2	-	D36.0	D48.7	D49.89
aortic	-	C77.2	-	D36.0	D48.7	D49.89
arm	-	C77.3	-	D36.0	D48.7	D49.89
auricular (anterior) (posterior)	-	C77.0	-	D36.0	D48.7	D49.89
axilla, axillary	-	C77.3	-	D36.0	D48.7	D49.89
brachial	-	C77.3	-	D36.0	D48.7	D49.89
bronchial	-	C77.1	-	D36.0	D48.7	D49.89
bronchopulmonary	-	C77.1	-	D36.0	D48.7	D49.89
celiac	-	C77.2	-	D36.0	D48.7	D49.89
cervical	-	C77.0	-	D36.0	D48.7	D49.89
cervicofacial	-	C77.0	-	D36.0	D48.7	D49.89
Cloquet	-	C77.4	-	D36.0	D48.7	D49.89
colic	-	C77.2	-	D36.0	D48.7	D49.89
common duct	-	C77.2	-	D36.0	D48.7	D49.89
cubital	-	C77.3	-	D36.0	D48.7	D49.89
diaphragmatic	-	C77.1	-	D36.0	D48.7	D49.89
epigastric, inferior	-	C77.1	-	D36.0	D48.7	D49.89
epitrochlear	-	C77.3	-	D36.0	D48.7	D49.89
esophageal	-	C77.1	-	D36.0	D48.7	D49.89
face	-	C77.0	-	D36.0	D48.7	D49.89
femoral	-	C77.4	-	D36.0	D48.7	D49.89
gastric	-	C77.2	-	D36.0	D48.7	D49.89
groin	-	C77.4	-	D36.0	D48.7	D49.89
head	-	C77.0	-	D36.0	D48.7	D49.89
hepatic	-	C77.2	-	D36.0	D48.7	D49.89
hilar (pulmonary)	-	C77.1	-	D36.0	D48.7	D49.89
splenic	-	C77.2	-	D36.0	D48.7	D49.89
hypogastric	-	C77.5	-	D36.0	D48.7	D49.89
ileocolic	-	C77.2	-	D36.0	D48.7	D49.89
iliac	-	C77.5	-	D36.0	D48.7	D49.89
infraclavicular	-	C77.3	-	D36.0	D48.7	D49.89
inguina, inguinal	-	C77.4	-	D36.0	D48.7	D49.89
innominate	-	C77.1	-	D36.0	D48.7	D49.89
intercostal	-	C77.1	-	D36.0	D48.7	D49.89
intestinal	-	C77.2	-	D36.0	D48.7	D49.89
intrabdominal	-	C77.2	-	D36.0	D48.7	D49.89
intrapelvic	-	C77.5	-	D36.0	D48.7	D49.89

Neoplasm	Malignant Primary	Malignant Secondary	Ca in situ	Benign	Uncertain Behavior	Unspecified Behavior
lymph, lymphatic channel NEC —continued						
gland — continued						
intrathoracic	-	C77.1	-	D36.0	D48.7	D49.89
jugular	-	C77.0	-	D36.0	D48.7	D49.89
leg	-	C77.4	-	D36.0	D48.7	D49.89
limb						
lower	-	C77.4	-	D36.0	D48.7	D49.89
upper	-	C77.3	-	D36.0	D48.7	D49.89
lower limb	-	C77.4	-	D36.0	D48.7	D49.89
lumbar	-	C77.2	-	D36.0	D48.7	D49.89
mandibular	-	C77.0	-	D36.0	D48.7	D49.89
mediastinal	-	C77.1	-	D36.0	D48.7	D49.89
mesenteric (inferior) (superior)	-	C77.2	-	D36.0	D48.7	D49.89
midcolic	-	C77.2	-	D36.0	D48.7	D49.89
multiple sites in categories C77.0 - C77.5	-	C77.8	-	D36.0	D48.7	D49.89
neck	-	C77.0	-	D36.0	D48.7	D49.89
obturator	-	C77.5	-	D36.0	D48.7	D49.89
occipital	-	C77.0	-	D36.0	D48.7	D49.89
pancreatic	-	C77.2	-	D36.0	D48.7	D49.89
para-aortic	-	C77.2	-	D36.0	D48.7	D49.89
paracervical	-	C77.5	-	D36.0	D48.7	D49.89
parametrial	-	C77.5	-	D36.0	D48.7	D49.89
parasternal	-	C77.1	-	D36.0	D48.7	D49.89
parotid	-	C77.0	-	D36.0	D48.7	D49.89
pectoral	-	C77.3	-	D36.0	D48.7	D49.89
pelvic	-	C77.5	-	D36.0	D48.7	D49.89
peri-aortic	-	C77.2	-	D36.0	D48.7	D49.89
peripancreatic	-	C77.2	-	D36.0	D48.7	D49.89
popliteal	-	C77.4	-	D36.0	D48.7	D49.89
porta hepatis	-	C77.2	-	D36.0	D48.7	D49.89
portal	-	C77.2	-	D36.0	D48.7	D49.89
preauricular	-	C77.0	-	D36.0	D48.7	D49.89
prelaryngeal	-	C77.0	-	D36.0	D48.7	D49.89
presymphysial	-	C77.5	-	D36.0	D48.7	D49.89
pretracheal	-	C77.0	-	D36.0	D48.7	D49.89
primary (any site) NEC	C96.9	-	-	-	-	-
pulmonary (hilar)	-	C77.1	-	D36.0	D48.7	D49.89
pyloric	-	C77.2	-	D36.0	D48.7	D49.89
retroperitoneal	-	C77.2	-	D36.0	D48.7	D49.89
retropharyngeal	-	C77.0	-	D36.0	D48.7	D49.89
Rosenmuller's	-	C77.4	-	D36.0	D48.7	D49.89
sacral	-	C77.5	-	D36.0	D48.7	D49.89
scalene	-	C77.0	-	D36.0	D48.7	D49.89
site NEC	-	C77.9	-	D36.0	D48.7	D49.89
splenic (hilar)	-	C77.2	-	D36.0	D48.7	D49.89
subclavicular	-	C77.3	-	D36.0	D48.7	D49.89
subinguinal	-	C77.4	-	D36.0	D48.7	D49.89
sublingual	-	C77.0	-	D36.0	D48.7	D49.89
submandibular	-	C77.0	-	D36.0	D48.7	D49.89
submaxillary	-	C77.0	-	D36.0	D48.7	D49.89
submental	-	C77.0	-	D36.0	D48.7	D49.89
subscapular	-	C77.3	-	D36.0	D48.7	D49.89
supraclavicular	-	C77.0	-	D36.0	D48.7	D49.89
thoracic	-	C77.1	-	D36.0	D48.7	D49.89
tibial	-	C77.4	-	D36.0	D48.7	D49.89
tracheal	-	C77.1	-	D36.0	D48.7	D49.89
tracheobronchial	-	C77.1	-	D36.0	D48.7	D49.89
upper limb	-	C77.3	-	D36.0	D48.7	D49.89
Virchow's	-	C77.0	-	D36.0	D48.7	D49.89
node (see also Neoplasm, lymph gland)						
primary NEC	C96.9	-	-	-	-	-
vessel (see also Neoplasm, connective tissue)	C49.9	C79.89	-	D21.9	D48.1	D49.2
Mackenrodt's ligament	C57.7	C79.82	D07.39	D28.7	D39.8	D49.59
malar	C41.0	C79.51	-	D16.4-	D48.0	D49.2
region — see Neoplasm, cheek						
mammary gland — see Neoplasm, breast						
mandible	C41.1	C79.51	-	D16.5-	D48.0	D49.2
alveolar						
mucosa (carcinoma)	C03.1	C79.89	D00.03	D10.39	D37.09	D49.0
ridge or process	C41.1	C79.51	-	D16.5-	D48.0	D49.2
marrow (bone) NEC	C96.9	C79.52	-	-	D47.9	D49.89
mastectomy site (skin) (see also Neoplasm, breast, skin)	C44.501	C79.2	-	-	-	-
specified as breast tissue	C50.8-	C79.81	-	-	-	-
mastoid (air cells) (antrum) (cavity)	C30.1	C78.39	D02.3	D14.0	D38.5	D49.1
bone or process	C41.0	C79.51	-	D16.4-	D48.0	D49.2
maxilla, maxillary (superior)	C41.0	C79.51	-	D16.4-	D48.0	D49.2
alveolar						
mucosa	C03.0	C79.89	D00.03	D10.39	D37.09	D49.0
ridge or process (carcinoma)	C41.0	C79.51	-	D16.4-	D48.0	D49.2
antrum	C31.0	C78.39	D02.3	D14.0	D38.5	D49.1
carcinoma	C03.0	C79.51	-	-	-	-
inferior — see Neoplasm, mandible						
sinus	C31.0	C78.39	D02.3	D14.0	D38.5	D49.1
meatus external (ear) (see also Neoplasm, skin, ear)	C44.20-	C79.2	D04.2-	D23.2-	D48.5	D49.2

Neoplasm	Malignant Primary	Malignant Secondary	Ca in situ	Benign	Uncertain Behavior	Unspecified Behavior
Meckel's diverticulum, malignant	C17.3	C78.4	D01.49	D13.39	D37.2	D49.0
mediastinum, mediastinal	C38.3	C78.1	-	D15.2	D38.3	D49.89
anterior	C38.1	C78.1	-	D15.2	D38.3	D49.89
posterior	C38.2	C78.1	-	D15.2	D38.3	D49.89
medulla						
adrenal	C74.1-	C79.7-	D09.3	D35.0-	D44.1-	D49.7
oblongata	C71.7	C79.31	-	D33.1	D43.1	D49.6
meibomian gland	C44.10-	C79.2	D04.1-	D23.1-	D48.5	D49.2
basal cell carcinoma	C44.11-	-	-	-	-	-
sebaceous cell	C44.13-	-	-	-	-	-
specified type NEC	C44.19-	-	-	-	-	-
squamous cell carcinoma	C44.12-	-	-	-	-	-
melanoma — see Melanoma						
meninges	C70.9	C79.49	-	D32.9	D42.9	D49.7
brain	C70.0	C79.32	-	D32.0	D42.0	D49.7
cerebral	C70.0	C79.32	-	D32.0	D42.0	D49.7
cranial	C70.0	C79.32	-	D32.0	D42.0	D49.7
intracranial	C70.0	C79.32	-	D32.0	D42.0	D49.7
spinal (cord)	C70.1	C79.49	-	D32.1	D42.1	D49.7
meniscus, knee joint (lateral) (medial)	C40.2-	C79.51	-	D16.2-	D48.0	D49.2
Merkel cell — see Carcinoma, Merkel cell						
mesentery, mesenteric	C48.1	C78.6	-	D20.1	D48.4	D49.0
mesoappendix	C48.1	C78.6	-	D20.1	D48.4	D49.0
mesocolon	C48.1	C78.6	-	D20.1	D48.4	D49.0
mesopharynx — see Neoplasm, oropharynx						
mesosalpinx	C57.1	C79.82	D07.39	D28.2	D39.8	D49.59
mesothelial tissue — see Mesothelioma						
mesothelioma — see Mesothelioma						
mesovarium	C57.1	C79.82	D07.39	D28.2	D39.8	D49.59
metacarpus (any bone)	C40.1-	C79.51	-	D16.1-	-	-
metastatic NEC (see also Neoplasm, by site, secondary)		C79.9	-	-	-	-
metatarsus (any bone)	C40.3-	C79.51	-	D16.3-	-	-
midbrain	C71.7	C79.31	-	D33.1	D43.1	D49.6
milk duct — see Neoplasm, breast						
mons						
pubis	C51.9	C79.82	D07.1	D28.0	D39.8	D49.59
veneris	C51.9	C79.82	D07.1	D28.0	D39.8	D49.59
motor tract	C72.9	C79.49	-	D33.9	D43.9	D49.7
brain	C71.9	C79.31	-	D33.2	D43.2	D49.6
cauda equina	C72.1	C79.49	-	D33.4	D43.4	D49.7
spinal	C72.0	C79.49	-	D33.4	D43.4	D49.7
mouth	C06.9	C79.89	D00.00	D10.30	D37.09	D49.0
book-leaf	C06.89	C79.89	-	-	-	-
floor	C04.9	C79.89	D00.06	D10.2	D37.09	D49.0
anterior portion	C04.0	C79.89	D00.06	D10.2	D37.09	D49.0
lateral portion	C04.1	C79.89	D00.06	D10.2	D37.09	D49.0
overlapping lesion	C04.8	-	-	-	-	-
overlapping NEC	C06.80	-	-	-	-	-
roof	C05.9	C79.89	D00.00	D10.39	D37.09	D49.0
specified part NEC	C06.89	C79.89	D00.00	D10.39	D37.09	D49.0
vestibule	C06.1	C79.89	D00.00	D10.39	D37.09	D49.0
mucosa						
alveolar (ridge or process)	C03.9	C79.89	D00.03	D10.39	D37.09	D49.0
lower	C03.1	C79.89	D00.03	D10.39	D37.09	D49.0
upper	C03.0	C79.89	D00.03	D10.39	D37.09	D49.0
buccal	C06.0	C79.89	D00.02	D10.39	D37.09	D49.0
cheek	C06.0	C79.89	D00.02	D10.39	D37.09	D49.0
lip — see Neoplasm, lip, internal						
nasal	C30.0	C78.39	D02.3	D14.0	D38.5	D49.1
oral	C06.0	C79.89	D00.02	D10.39	D37.09	D49.0
Mullerian duct						
female	C57.7	C79.82	D07.39	D28.7	D39.8	D49.59
male	C63.7	C79.82	D07.69	D29.8	D40.8	D49.59
muscle (see also Neoplasm, connective tissue)						
extraocular	C69.6-	C79.49	D09.2-	D31.6-	D48.7	D49.89
myocardium	C38.0	C79.89	-	D15.1	D48.7	D49.89
myometrium	C54.2	C79.82	D07.0	D26.1	D39.0	D49.59
myopericardium	C38.0	C79.89	-	D15.1	D48.7	D49.89
nabothian gland (follicle)	C53.0	C79.82	D06.0	D26.0	D39.0	D49.59
nail (see also Neoplasm, skin, limb)	C44.90	C79.2	D04.9	D23.9	D48.5	D49.2
finger (see also Neoplasm, skin, limb, upper)	C44.60-	C79.2	D04.6-	D23.6-	D48.5	D49.2
toe (see also Neoplasm, skin, limb, lower)	C44.70-	C79.2	D04.7-	D23.7-	D48.5	D49.2
nares, naris (anterior) (posterior)	C30.0	C78.39	D02.3	D14.0	D38.5	D49.1
nasal — see Neoplasm, nose						
nasolabial groove (see also Neoplasm, skin, face)	C44.309	C79.2	D04.39	D23.39	D48.5	D49.2
nasolacrimal duct	C69.5-	C79.49	D09.2-	D31.5-	D48.7	D49.89
nasopharynx, nasopharyngeal	C11.9	C79.89	D00.08	D10.6	D37.05	D49.0
floor	C11.3	C79.89	D00.08	D10.6	D37.05	D49.0
overlapping lesion	C11.8					
roof	C11.0	C79.89	D00.08	D10.6	D37.05	D49.0
wall	C11.9	C79.89	D00.08	D10.6	D37.05	D49.0
anterior	C11.3	C79.89	D00.08	D10.6	D37.05	D49.0

Neoplasm	Malignant Primary	Malignant Secondary	Ca in situ	Benign	Uncertain Behavior	Unspecified Behavior
nasopharynx, nasopharyngeal—*continued*						
wall — *continued*						
lateral	C11.2	C79.89	D00.08	D10.6	D37.05	D49.0
posterior	C11.1	C79.89	D00.08	D10.6	D37.05	D49.0
superior	C11.0	C79.89	D00.08	D10.6	D37.05	D49.0
nates (*see also* Neoplasm, skin, trunk)	C44.509	C79.2	D04.5	D23.5	D48.5	D49.2
neck NEC	C76.0	C79.89	D09.8	D36.7	D48.7	D49.89
skin	C44.40	-	-	-	-	-
basal cell carcinoma	C44.41	-	-	-	-	-
specified type NEC	C44.49	-	-	-	-	-
squamous cell carcinoma	C44.42	-	-	-	-	-
nerve (ganglion)	C47.9	C79.89	-	D36.10	D48.2	D49.2
abducens	C72.59	C79.49	-	D33.3	D43.3	D49.7
accessory (spinal)	C72.59	C79.49	-	D33.3	D43.3	D49.7
acoustic	C72.4-	C79.49	-	D33.3	D43.3	D49.7
auditory	C72.4-	C79.49	-	D33.3	D43.3	D49.7
autonomic NEC (*see also* Neoplasm, nerve, peripheral)	C47.9	C79.89	-	D36.10	D48.2	D49.2
brachial	C47.1-	C79.89	-	D36.12	D48.2	D49.2
cranial	C72.50	C79.49	-	D33.3	D43.3	D49.7
specified NEC	C72.59	C79.49	-	D33.3	D43.3	D49.7
facial	C72.59	C79.49	-	D33.3	D43.3	D49.7
femoral	C47.2-	C79.89	-	D36.13	D48.2	D49.2
ganglion NEC (*see also* Neoplasm, nerve, peripheral)	C47.9	C79.89	-	D36.10	D48.2	D49.2
glossopharyngeal	C72.59	C79.49	-	D33.3	D43.3	D49.7
hypoglossal	C72.59	C79.49	-	D33.3	D43.3	D49.7
intercostal	C47.3	C79.89	-	D36.14	D48.2	D49.2
lumbar	C47.6	C79.89	-	D36.17	D48.2	D49.2
median	C47.1-	C79.89	-	D36.12	D48.2	D49.2
obturator	C47.2-	C79.89	-	D36.13	D48.2	D49.2
oculomotor	C72.59	C79.49	-	D33.3	D43.3	D49.7
olfactory	C72.2-	C79.49	-	D33.3	D43.3	D49.7
optic	C72.3-	C79.49	-	D33.3	D43.3	D49.7
parasympathetic NEC	C47.9	C79.89	-	D36.10	D48.2	D49.2
peripheral NEC	C47.9	C79.89	-	D36.10	D48.2	D49.2
abdomen	C47.4	C79.89	-	D36.15	D48.2	D49.2
abdominal wall	C47.4	C79.89	-	D36.15	D48.2	D49.2
ankle	C47.2-	C79.89	-	D36.13	D48.2	D49.2
antecubital fossa or space	C47.1-	C79.89	-	D36.12	D48.2	D49.2
arm	C47.1-	C79.89	-	D36.12	D48.2	D49.2
auricle (ear)	C47.0	C79.89	-	D36.11	D48.2	D49.2
axilla	C47.3	C79.89	-	D36.12	D48.2	D49.2
back	C47.6	C79.89	-	D36.17	D48.2	D49.2
buttock	C47.5	C79.89	-	D36.16	D48.2	D49.2
calf	C47.2-	C79.89	-	D36.13	D48.2	D49.2
cervical region	C47.0	C79.89	-	D36.11	D48.2	D49.2
cheek	C47.0	C79.89	-	D36.11	D48.2	D49.2
chest (wall)	C47.3	C79.89	-	D36.14	D48.2	D49.2
chin	C47.0	C79.89	-	D36.11	D48.2	D49.2
ear (external)	C47.0	C79.89	-	D36.11	D48.2	D49.2
elbow	C47.1-	C79.89	-	D36.12	D48.2	D49.2
extrarectal	C47.5	C79.89	-	D36.16	D48.2	D49.2
extremity	C47.9	C79.89	-	D36.10	D48.2	D49.2
lower	C47.2-	C79.89	-	D36.13	D48.2	D49.2
upper	C47.1-	C79.89	-	D36.12	D48.2	D49.2
eyelid	C47.0	C79.89	-	D36.11	D48.2	D49.2
face	C47.0	C79.89	-	D36.11	D48.2	D49.2
finger	C47.1-	C79.89	-	D36.12	D48.2	D49.2
flank	C47.6	C79.89	-	D36.17	D48.2	D49.2
foot	C47.2-	C79.89	-	D36.13	D48.2	D49.2
forearm	C47.1-	C79.89	-	D36.12	D48.2	D49.2
forehead	C47.0	C79.89	-	D36.11	D48.2	D49.2
gluteal region	C47.5	C79.89	-	D36.16	D48.2	D49.2
groin	C47.5	C79.89	-	D36.16	D48.2	D49.2
hand	C47.1-	C79.89	-	D36.12	D48.2	D49.2
head	C47.0	C79.89	-	D36.11	D48.2	D49.2
heel	C47.2-	C79.89	-	D36.13	D48.2	D49.2
hip	C47.2-	C79.89	-	D36.13	D48.2	D49.2
infraclavicular region	C47.3	C79.89	-	D36.14	D48.2	D49.2
inguinal (canal) (region)	C47.5	C79.89	-	D36.16	D48.2	D49.2
intrathoracic	C47.3	C79.89	-	D36.14	D48.2	D49.2
ischiorectal fossa	C47.5	C79.89	-	D36.16	D48.2	D49.2
knee	C47.2-	C79.89	-	D36.13	D48.2	D49.2
leg	C47.2-	C79.89	-	D36.13	D48.2	D49.2
limb NEC	C47.9	C79.89	-	D36.10	D48.2	D49.2
lower	C47.2-	C79.89	-	D36.13	D48.2	D49.2
upper	C47.1-	C79.89	-	D36.12	D48.2	D49.2
nates	C47.5	C79.89	-	D36.16	D48.2	D49.2
neck	C47.0	C79.89	-	D36.11	D48.2	D49.2
orbit	C69.6-	C79.49	-	D31.6-	D48.7	D49.2
pararectal	C47.5	C79.89	-	D36.16	D48.2	D49.2
paraurethral	C47.5	C79.89	-	D36.16	D48.2	D49.2
paravaginal	C47.5	C79.89	-	D36.16	D48.2	D49.2
pelvis (floor)	C47.5	C79.89	-	D36.16	D48.2	D49.2
pelvo-abdominal	C47.8	C79.89	-	D36.17	D48.2	D49.2
perineum	C47.5	C79.89	-	D36.16	D48.2	D49.2
perirectal (tissue)	C47.5	C79.89	-	D36.16	D48.2	D49.2

Neoplasm	Malignant Primary	Malignant Secondary	Ca in situ	Benign	Uncertain Behavior	Unspecified Behavior
nerve — *continued*						
peripheral NEC — *continued*						
periurethral (tissue)	C47.5	C79.89	-	D36.16	D48.2	D49.2
popliteal fossa or space	C47.2-	C79.89	-	D36.13	D48.2	D49.2
presacral	C47.5	C79.89	-	D36.16	D48.2	D49.2
pterygoid fossa	C47.0	C79.89	-	D36.11	D48.2	D49.2
rectovaginal septum or wall	C47.5	C79.89	-	D36.16	D48.2	D49.2
rectovesical	C47.5	C79.89	-	D36.16	D48.2	D49.2
sacrococcygeal region	C47.5	C79.89	-	D36.16	D48.2	D49.2
scalp	C47.0	C79.89	-	D36.11	D48.2	D49.2
scapular region	C47.3	C79.89	-	D36.14	D48.2	D49.2
shoulder	C47.1-	C79.89	-	D36.12	D48.2	D49.2
submental	C47.0	C79.89	-	D36.11	D48.2	D49.2
supraclavicular region	C47.0	C79.89	-	D36.11	D48.2	D49.2
temple	C47.0	C79.89	-	D36.11	D48.2	D49.2
temporal region	C47.0	C79.89	-	D36.11	D48.2	D49.2
thigh	C47.2-	C79.89	-	D36.13	D48.2	D49.2
thoracic (duct) (wall)	C47.3	C79.89	-	D36.14	D48.2	D49.2
thorax	C47.3	C79.89	-	D36.14	D48.2	D49.2
thumb	C47.1-	C79.89	-	D36.12	D48.2	D49.2
toe	C47.2-	C79.89	-	D36.13	D48.2	D49.2
trunk	C47.6	C79.89	-	D36.17	D48.2	D49.2
umbilicus	C47.4	C79.89	-	D36.15	D48.2	D49.2
vesicorectal	C47.5	C79.89	-	D36.16	D48.2	D49.2
wrist	C47.1-	C79.89	-	D36.12	D48.2	D49.2
radial	C47.1-	C79.89	-	D36.12	D48.2	D49.2
sacral	C47.5	C79.89	-	D36.16	D48.2	D49.2
sciatic	C47.2-	C79.89	-	D36.13	D48.2	D49.2
spinal NEC	C47.9	C79.89	-	D36.10	D48.2	D49.2
accessory	C72.59	C79.49	-	D33.3	D43.3	D49.7
sympathetic NEC (*see also* Neoplasm, nerve, peripheral)	C47.9	C79.89	-	D36.10	D48.2	D49.2
trigeminal	C72.59	C79.49	-	D33.3	D43.3	D49.7
trochlear	C72.59	C79.49	-	D33.3	D43.3	D49.7
ulnar	C47.1-	C79.89	-	D36.12	D48.2	D49.2
vagus	C72.59	C79.49	-	D33.3	D43.3	D49.7
nervous system (central)	C72.9	C79.40	-	D33.9	D43.9	D49.7
autonomic — *see* Neoplasm, nerve, peripheral						
parasympathetic — *see* Neoplasm, nerve, peripheral						
specified site NEC	-	C79.49	-	D33.7	D43.8	-
sympathetic — *see* Neoplasm, nerve, peripheral						
nevus — *see* Nevus						
nipple	C50.0-	C79.81	D05.-	D24.-	-	-
nose, nasal	C76.0	C79.89	D09.8	D36.7	D48.7	D49.89
ala (external) (nasi) (*see also* Neoplasm, nose, skin)	C44.301	C79.2	D04.39	D23.39	D48.5	D49.2
bone	C41.0	C79.51	-	D16.4-	D48.0	D49.2
cartilage	C30.0	C78.39	D02.3	D14.0	D38.5	D49.1
cavity	C30.0	C78.39	D02.3	D14.0	D38.5	D49.1
choana	C11.3	C79.89	D00.08	D10.6	D37.05	D49.0
external (skin) (*see also* Neoplasm, nose, skin)	C44.301	C79.2	D04.39	D23.39	D48.5	D49.2
fossa	C30.0	C78.39	D02.3	D14.0	D38.5	D49.1
internal	C30.0	C78.39	D02.3	D14.0	D38.5	D49.1
mucosa	C30.0	C78.39	D02.3	D14.0	D38.5	D49.1
septum	C30.0	C78.39	D02.3	D14.0	D38.5	D49.1
posterior margin	C11.3	C79.89	D00.08	D10.6	D37.05	D49.0
sinus — *see* Neoplasm, sinus						
skin	C44.301	C79.2	D04.39	D23.39	D48.5	D49.2
basal cell carcinoma	C44.311	-	-	-	-	-
specified type NEC	C44.391	-	-	-	-	-
squamous cell carcinoma	C44.321	-	-	-	-	-
turbinate (mucosa)	C30.0	C78.39	D02.3	D14.0	D38.5	D49.1
bone	C41.0	C79.51	-	D16.4-	D48.0	D49.2
vestibule	C30.0	C78.39	D02.3	D14.0	D38.5	D49.1
nostril	C30.0	C78.39	D02.3	D14.0	D38.5	D49.1
nucleus pulposus	C41.2	C79.51	-	D16.6	D48.0	D49.2
occipital						
bone	C41.0	C79.51	-	D16.4-	D48.0	D49.2
lobe or pole, brain	C71.4	C79.31	-	D33.0	D43.0	D49.6
odontogenic — *see* Neoplasm, jaw bone						
olfactory nerve or bulb	C72.2-	C79.49	-	D33.3	D43.3	D49.7
olive (brain)	C71.7	C79.31	-	D33.1	D43.1	D49.6
omentum	C48.1	C78.6	-	D20.1	D48.4	D49.0
operculum (brain)	C71.0	C79.31	-	D33.0	D43.0	D49.6
optic nerve, chiasm, or tract	C72.3-	C79.49	-	D33.3	D43.3	D49.7
oral (cavity)	C06.9	C79.89	D00.00	D10.30	D37.09	D49.0
ill-defined	C14.8	C79.89	D00.00	D10.30	D37.09	D49.0
mucosa	C06.0	C79.89	D00.02	D10.39	D37.09	D49.0
orbit	C69.6-	C79.49	D09.2-	D31.6-	D48.7	D49.89
autonomic nerve	C69.6-	C79.49	-	D31.6-	D48.7	D49.2
bone	C41.0	C79.51	-	D16.4-	D48.0	D49.2
eye	C69.6-	C79.49	D09.2-	D31.6-	D48.7	D49.89
peripheral nerves	C69.6-	C79.49	-	D31.6-	D48.7	D49.2
soft parts	C69.6-	C79.49	D09.2-	D31.6-	D48.7	D49.89

Neoplasm	Malignant Primary	Malignant Secondary	Ca in situ	Benign	Uncertain Behavior	Unspecified Behavior
organ of Zuckerkandl	C75.5	C79.89	-	D35.6	D44.7	D49.7
oropharynx	C10.9	C79.89	D00.08	D10.5	D37.05	D49.0
branchial cleft (vestige)	C10.4	C79.89	D00.08	D10.5	D37.05	D49.0
junctional region	C10.8	C79.89	D00.08	D10.5	D37.05	D49.0
lateral wall	C10.2	C79.89	D00.08	D10.5	D37.05	D49.0
overlapping lesion	C10.8	-	-	-	-	-
pillars or fauces	C09.1	C79.89	D00.08	D10.5	D37.05	D49.0
posterior wall	C10.3	C79.89	D00.08	D10.5	D37.05	D49.0
vallecula	C10.0	C79.89	D00.08	D10.5	D37.05	D49.0
os						
external	C53.1	C79.82	D06.1	D26.0	D39.0	D49.59
internal	C53.0	C79.82	D06.0	D26.0	D39.0	D49.59
ovary	C56.-	C79.6-	D07.39	D27.-	D39.1-	D49.59
oviduct	C57.0-	C79.82	D07.39	D28.2	D39.8	D49.59
palate	C05.9	C79.89	D00.00	D10.39	D37.09	D49.0
hard	C05.0	C79.89	D00.05	D10.39	D37.09	D49.0
junction of hard and soft palate	C05.9	C79.89	D00.00	D10.39	D37.09	D49.0
overlapping lesions	C05.8	-	-	-	-	-
soft	C05.1	C79.89	D00.04	D10.39	D37.09	D49.0
nasopharyngeal surface	C11.3	C79.89	D00.08	D10.6	D37.05	D49.0
posterior surface	C11.3	C79.89	D00.08	D10.6	D37.05	D49.0
superior surface	C11.3	C79.89	D00.08	D10.6	D37.05	D49.0
palatoglossal arch	C09.1	C79.89	D00.00	D10.5	D37.09	D49.0
palatopharyngeal arch	C09.1	C79.89	D00.00	D10.5	D37.09	D49.0
pallium	C71.0	C79.31	-	D33.0	D43.0	D49.6
palpebra	C44.10-	C79.2	D04.1-	D23.1-	D48.5	D49.2
basal cell carcinoma	C44.11-	-	-	-	-	-
sebaceous cell	C44.13-	-	-	-	-	-
specified type NEC	C44.19-	-	-	-	-	-
squamous cell carcinoma	C44.12-	-	-	-	-	-
pancreas	C25.9	C78.89	D01.7	D13.6	D37.8	D49.0
body	C25.1	C78.89	D01.7	D13.6	D37.8	D49.0
duct (of Santorini) (of Wirsung)	C25.3	C78.89	D01.7	D13.6	D37.8	D49.0
ectopic tissue	C25.7	C78.89	-	D13.6	D37.8	D49.0
head	C25.0	C78.89	D01.7	D13.6	D37.8	D49.0
islet cells	C25.4	C78.89	D01.7	D13.7	D37.8	D49.0
neck	C25.7	C78.89	D01.7	D13.6	D37.8	D49.0
overlapping lesion	C25.8	-	-	-	-	-
tail	C25.2	C78.89	D01.7	D13.6	D37.8	D49.0
para-aortic body	C75.5	C79.89	-	D35.6	D44.7	D49.7
paraganglion NEC	C75.5	C79.89	-	D35.6	D44.7	D49.7
parametrium	C57.3	C79.82	-	D28.2	D39.8	D49.59
paranephric	C48.0	C78.6	-	D20.0	D48.3	D49.0
pararectal	C76.3	C79.89	-	D36.7	D48.7	D49.89
parasagittal (region)	C76.0	C79.89	D09.8	D36.7	D48.7	D49.89
parasellar	C72.9	C79.49	-	D33.9	D43.8	D49.7
parathyroid (gland)	C75.0	C79.89	D09.3	D35.1	D44.2	D49.7
paraurethral	C76.3	C79.89	-	D36.7	D48.7	D49.89
gland	C68.1	C79.19	D09.19	D30.8	D41.8	D49.59
paravaginal	C76.3	C79.89	-	D36.7	D48.7	D49.89
parenchyma, kidney	C64.-	C79.0-	D09.19	D30.0-	D41.0-	D49.51-
parietal						
bone	C41.0	C79.51	-	D16.4-	D48.0	D49.2
lobe, brain	C71.3	C79.31	-	D33.0	D43.0	D49.6
paroophoron	C57.1	C79.82	D07.39	D28.2	D39.8	D49.59
parotid (duct) (gland)	C07	C79.89	D00.00	D11.0	D37.030	D49.0
parovarium	C57.1	C79.82	D07.39	D28.2	D39.8	D49.59
patella	C40.20	C79.51	-	-	-	-
peduncle, cerebral	C71.7	C79.31	-	D33.1	D43.1	D49.6
pelvirectal junction	C19	C78.5	D01.1	D12.7	D37.5	D49.0
pelvis, pelvic	C76.3	C79.89	D09.8	D36.7	D48.7	D49.89
bone	C41.4	C79.51	-	D16.8	D48.0	D49.2
floor	C76.3	C79.89	D09.8	D36.7	D48.7	D49.89
renal	C65.-	C79.0-	D09.19	D30.1-	D41.1-	D49.51-
viscera	C76.3	C79.89	D09.8	D36.7	D48.7	D49.89
wall	C76.3	C79.89	D09.8	D36.7	D48.7	D49.89
pelvo-abdominal	C76.8	C79.89	D09.8	D36.7	D48.7	D49.89
penis	C60.9	C79.82	D07.4	D29.0	D40.8	D49.59
body	C60.2	C79.82	D07.4	D29.0	D40.8	D49.59
corpus (cavernosum)	C60.2	C79.82	D07.4	D29.0	D40.8	D49.59
glans	C60.1	C79.82	D07.4	D29.0	D40.8	D49.59
overlapping sites	C60.8	-	-	-	-	-
skin NEC	C60.9	C79.82	D07.4	D29.0	D40.8	D49.59
periadrenal (tissue)	C48.0	C78.6	-	D20.0	D48.3	D49.0
perianal (skin) (see also Neoplasm, anus, skin)	C44.500	C79.2	D04.5	D23.5	D48.5	D49.2
pericardium	C38.0	C79.89	-	D15.1	D48.7	D49.89
perinephric	C48.0	C78.6	-	D20.0	D48.3	D49.0
perineum	C76.3	C79.89	D09.8	D36.7	D48.7	D49.89
periodontal tissue NEC	C03.9	C79.89	D00.03	D10.39	D37.09	D49.0
periosteum — see Neoplasm, bone						
peripancreatic	C48.0	C78.6	-	D20.0	D48.3	D49.0
peripheral nerve NEC	C47.9	C79.89	-	D36.10	D48.2	D49.2
perirectal (tissue)	C76.3	C79.89	-	D36.7	D48.7	D49.89
perirenal (tissue)	C48.0	C78.6	-	D20.0	D48.3	D49.0
peritoneum, peritoneal (cavity)	C48.2	C78.6	-	D20.1	D48.4	D49.0
benign mesothelial tissue — see Mesothelioma, benign						
overlapping lesion	C48.8	-	-	-	-	-
with digestive organs	C26.9	-	-	-	-	-

Neoplasm	Malignant Primary	Malignant Secondary	Ca in situ	Benign	Uncertain Behavior	Unspecified Behavior
peritoneum, peritoneal — continued						
parietal	C48.1	C78.6	-	D20.1	D48.4	D49.0
pelvic	C48.1	C78.6	-	D20.1	D48.4	D49.0
specified part NEC	C48.1	C78.6	-	D20.1	D48.4	D49.0
peritonsillar (tissue)	C76.0	C79.89	D09.8	D36.7	D48.7	D49.89
periurethral tissue	C76.3	C79.89	-	D36.7	D48.7	D49.89
phalanges						
foot	C40.3-	C79.51	-	D16.3-	-	-
hand	C40.1-	C79.51	-	D16.1-	-	-
pharynx, pharyngeal	C14.0	C79.89	D00.08	D10.9	D37.05	D49.0
bursa	C11.1	C79.89	D00.08	D10.6	D37.05	D49.0
fornix	C11.3	C79.89	D00.08	D10.6	D37.05	D49.0
recess	C11.2	C79.89	D00.08	D10.6	D37.05	D49.0
region	C14.0	C79.89	D00.08	D10.9	D37.05	D49.0
tonsil	C11.1	C79.89	D00.08	D10.6	D37.05	D49.0
wall (lateral) (posterior)	C14.0	C79.89	D00.08	D10.9	D37.05	D49.0
pia mater	C70.9	C79.40	-	D32.9	D42.9	D49.7
cerebral	C70.0	C79.32	-	D32.0	D42.0	D49.7
cranial	C70.0	C79.32	-	D32.0	D42.0	D49.7
spinal	C70.1	C79.49	-	D32.1	D42.1	D49.7
pillars of fauces	C09.1	C79.89	D00.08	D10.5	D37.05	D49.0
pineal (body) (gland)	C75.3	C79.89	D09.3	D35.4	D44.5	D49.7
pinna (ear) NEC (see also Neoplasm, skin, ear)	C44.20-	C79.2	D04.2-	D23.2-	D48.5	D49.2
piriform fossa or sinus	C12	C79.89	D00.08	D10.7	D37.05	D49.0
pituitary (body) (fossa) (gland) (lobe)	C75.1	C79.89	D09.3	D35.2	D44.3	D49.7
placenta	C58	C79.82	D07.0	D26.7	D39.2	D49.59
pleura, pleural (cavity)	C38.4	C78.2	-	D19.0	D38.2	D49.1
overlapping lesion with heart or mediastinum	C38.8	-	-	-	-	-
parietal	C38.4	C78.2	-	D19.0	D38.2	D49.1
visceral	C38.4	C78.2	-	D19.0	D38.2	D49.1
plexus						
brachial	C47.1-	C79.89	-	D36.12	D48.2	D49.2
cervical	C47.0	C79.89	-	D36.11	D48.2	D49.2
choroid	C71.5	C79.31	-	D33.0	D43.0	D49.6
lumbosacral	C47.5	C79.89	-	D36.16	D48.2	D49.2
sacral	C47.5	C79.89	-	D36.16	D48.2	D49.2
pluriendocrine	C75.8	C79.89	D09.3	D35.7	D44.9	D49.7
pole						
frontal	C71.1	C79.31	-	D33.0	D43.0	D49.6
occipital	C71.4	C79.31	-	D33.0	D43.0	D49.6
pons (varolii)	C71.7	C79.31	-	D33.1	D43.1	D49.6
popliteal fossa or space	C76.5-	C79.89	D04.7-	D36.7	D48.7	D49.89
postcricoid (region)	C13.0	C79.89	D00.08	D10.7	D37.05	D49.0
posterior fossa (cranial)	C71.9	C79.31	-	D33.2	D43.2	D49.6
postnasal space	C11.9	C79.89	D00.08	D10.6	D37.05	D49.0
prepuce	C60.0	C79.82	D07.4	D29.0	D40.8	D49.59
prepylorus	C16.4	C78.89	D00.2	D13.1	D37.1	D49.0
presacral (region)	C76.3	C79.89	-	D36.7	D48.7	D49.89
prostate (gland)	C61	C79.82	D07.5	D29.1	D40.0	D49.59
utricle	C68.0	C79.19	D09.19	D30.4	D41.3	D49.59
pterygoid fossa	C49.0	C79.89	-	D21.0	D48.1	D49.2
pubic bone	C41.4	C79.51	-	D16.8	D48.0	D49.2
pudenda, pudendum (female)	C51.9	C79.82	D07.1	D28.0	D39.8	D49.59
pulmonary (see also Neoplasm, lung)	C34.9-	C78.0-	D02.2-	D14.3-	D38.1	D49.1
putamen	C71.0	C79.31	-	D33.0	D43.0	D49.6
pyloric						
antrum	C16.3	C78.89	D00.2	D13.1	D37.1	D49.0
canal	C16.4	C78.89	D00.2	D13.1	D37.1	D49.0
pylorus	C16.4	C78.89	D00.2	D13.1	D37.1	D49.0
pyramid (brain)	C71.7	C79.31	-	D33.1	D43.1	D49.6
pyriform fossa or sinus	C12	C79.89	D00.08	D10.7	D37.05	D49.0
radius (any part)	C40.0-	C79.51	-	D16.0-	-	-
Rathke's pouch	C75.1	C79.89	D09.3	D35.2	D44.3	D49.7
rectosigmoid (junction)	C19	C78.5	D01.1	D12.7	D37.5	D49.0
overlapping lesion with anus or rectum	C21.8	-	-	-	-	-
rectouterine pouch	C48.1	C78.6	-	D20.1	D48.4	D49.0
rectovaginal septum or wall	C76.3	C79.89	D09.8	D36.7	D48.7	D49.89
rectovesical septum	C76.3	C79.89	D09.8	D36.7	D48.7	D49.89
rectum (ampulla)	C20	C78.5	D01.2	D12.8	D37.5	D49.0
and colon	C19	C78.5	D01.1	D12.7	D37.5	D49.0
overlapping lesion with anus or rectosigmoid junction	C21.8	-	-	-	-	-
renal	C64.-	C79.0-	D09.19	D30.0-	D41.0-	D49.51-
calyx	C65.-	C79.0-	D09.19	D30.1-	D41.1-	D49.51-
hilus	C65.-	C79.0-	D09.19	D30.1-	D41.1-	D49.51-
parenchyma	C64.-	C79.0-	D09.19	D30.0-	D41.0-	D49.51-
pelvis	C65.-	C79.0-	D09.19	D30.1-	D41.1-	D49.51-
respiratory						
organs or system NEC	C39.9	C78.30	D02.4	D14.4	D38.6	D49.1
tract NEC	C39.9	C78.30	D02.4	D14.4	D38.5	D49.1
upper	C39.0	C78.30	D02.4	D14.4	D38.5	D49.1
retina	C69.2-	C79.49	D09.2-	D31.2-	D48.7	D49.81
retrobulbar	C69.6-	C79.49	-	D31.6-	D48.7	D49.89
retrocecal	C48.0	C78.6	-	D20.0	D48.3	D49.0
retromolar (area) (triangle) (trigone)	C06.2	C79.89	D00.00	D10.39	D37.09	D49.0
retro-orbital	C76.0	C79.89	D09.8	D36.7	D48.7	D49.89

retroperitoneal - skin

Neoplasm	Malignant Primary	Malignant Secondary	Ca in situ	Benign	Uncertain Behavior	Unspecified Behavior
retroperitoneal (space) (tissue)	C48.0	C78.6	-	D20.0	D48.3	D49.0
retroperitoneum	C48.0	C78.6	-	D20.0	D48.3	D49.0
retropharyngeal	C14.0	C79.89	D00.08	D10.9	D37.05	D49.0
retrovesical (septum)	C76.3	C79.89	D09.8	D36.7	D48.7	D49.89
rhinencephalon	C71.0	C79.31	-	D33.0	D43.0	D49.6
rib	C41.3	C79.51	-	D16.7	D48.0	D49.2
Rosenmuller's fossa	C11.2	C79.89	D00.08	D10.6	D37.05	D49.0
round ligament	C57.2	C79.82	-	D28.2	D39.8	D49.59
sacrococcyx, sacrococcygeal	C41.4	C79.51	-	D16.8	D48.0	D49.2
region	C76.3	C79.89	D09.8	D36.7	D48.7	D49.89
sacrouterine ligament	C57.3	C79.82	-	D28.2	D39.8	D49.59
sacrum, sacral (vertebra)	C41.4	C79.51	-	D16.8	D48.0	D49.2
salivary gland or duct (major)	C08.9	C79.89	D00.00	D11.9	D37.039	D49.0
minor NEC	C06.9	C79.89	D00.00	D10.39	D37.04	D49.0
overlapping lesion	C08.9	-	-	-	-	-
parotid	C07	C79.89	D00.00	D11.0	D37.030	D49.0
pluriglandular	C08.9	C79.89	D00.00	D11.9	D37.039	D49.0
sublingual	C08.1	C79.89	D00.00	D11.7	D37.031	D49.0
submandibular	C08.0	C79.89	D00.00	D11.7	D37.032	D49.0
submaxillary	C08.0	C79.89	D00.00	D11.7	D37.032	D49.0
salpinx (uterine)	C57.0-	C79.82	D07.39	D28.2	D39.8	D49.59
Santorini's duct	C25.3	C78.89	D01.7	D13.6	D37.8	D49.0
scalp	C44.40	C79.2	D04.4	D23.4	D48.5	D49.2
basal cell carcinoma	C44.41	-	-	-	-	-
specified type NEC	C44.49	-	-	-	-	-
squamous cell carcinoma	C44.42	-	-	-	-	-
scapula (any part)	C40.0-	C79.51	-	D16.0-	-	-
scapular region	C76.1	C79.89	D09.8	D36.7	D48.7	D49.89
scar NEC (see also Neoplasm, skin, by site)	C44.90	C79.2	D04.9	D23.9	D48.5	D49.2
sciatic nerve	C47.2-	C79.89	-	D36.13	D48.2	D49.2
sclera	C69.4-	C79.49	D09.2-	D31.4-	D48.7	D49.89
scrotum (skin)	C63.2	C79.82	D07.61	D29.4	D40.8	D49.59
sebaceous gland — see Neoplasm, skin						
sella turcica	C75.1	C79.89	D09.3	D35.2	D44.3	D49.7
bone	C41.0	C79.51	-	D16.4-	D48.0	D49.2
semilunar cartilage (knee)	C40.2-	C79.51	-	D16.2-	D48.0	D49.2
seminal vesicle	C63.7	C79.82	D07.69	D29.8	D40.8	D49.59
septum						
nasal	C30.0	C78.39	D02.3	D14.0	D38.5	D49.1
posterior margin	C11.3	C79.89	D00.08	D10.6	D37.05	D49.0
rectovaginal	C76.3	C79.89	D09.8	D36.7	D48.7	D49.89
rectovesical	C76.3	C79.89	D09.8	D36.7	D48.7	D49.89
urethrovaginal	C57.9	C79.82	D07.30	D28.9	D39.9	D49.59
vesicovaginal	C57.9	C79.82	D07.30	D28.9	D39.9	D49.59
shoulder NEC	C76.4-	C79.89	D04.6-	D36.7	D48.7	D49.89
sigmoid flexure (lower) (upper)	C18.7	C78.5	D01.0	D12.5	D37.4	D49.0
sinus (accessory)	C31.9	C78.39	D02.3	D14.0	D38.5	D49.1
bone (any)	C41.0	C79.51	-	D16.4-	D48.0	D49.2
ethmoidal	C31.1	C78.39	D02.3	D14.0	D38.5	D49.1
frontal	C31.2	C78.39	D02.3	D14.0	D38.5	D49.1
maxillary	C31.0	C78.39	D02.3	D14.0	D38.5	D49.1
nasal, paranasal NEC	C31.9	C78.39	D02.3	D14.0	D38.5	D49.1
overlapping lesion	C31.8	-	-	-	-	-
pyriform	C12	C79.89	D00.08	D10.7	D37.05	D49.0
sphenoid	C31.3	C78.39	D02.3	D14.0	D38.5	D49.1
skeleton, skeletal NEC	C41.9	C79.51	-	D16.9-	D48.0	D49.2
Skene's gland	C68.1	C79.19	D09.19	D30.8	D41.8	D49.59
skin NOS	C44.90	C79.2	D04.9	D23.9	D48.5	D49.2
abdominal wall	C44.509	C79.2	D04.5	D23.5	D48.5	D49.2
basal cell carcinoma	C44.519	-	-	-	-	-
specified type NEC	C44.599	-	-	-	-	-
squamous cell carcinoma	C44.529	-	-	-	-	-
ala nasi (see also Neoplasm, nose, skin)	C44.301	C79.2	D04.39	D23.39	D48.5	D49.2
ankle (see also Neoplasm, skin, limb, lower)	C44.70-	C79.2	D04.7-	D23.7-	D48.5	D49.2
antecubital space (see also Neoplasm, skin, limb, upper)	C44.60-	C79.2	D04.6-	D23.6-	D48.5	D49.2
anus	C44.500	C79.2	D04.5	D23.5	D48.5	D49.2
basal cell carcinoma	C44.510	-	-	-	-	-
specified type NEC	C44.590	-	-	-	-	-
squamous cell carcinoma	C44.520	-	-	-	-	-
arm (see also Neoplasm, skin, limb, upper)	C44.60-	C79.2	D04.6-	D23.6-	D48.5	D49.2
auditory canal (external) (see also Neoplasm, skin, ear)	C44.20-	C79.2	D04.2-	D23.2-	D48.5	D49.2
auricle (ear) (see also Neoplasm, skin, ear)	C44.20-	C79.2	D04.2-	D23.2-	D48.5	D49.2
auricular canal (external) (see also Neoplasm, skin, ear)	C44.20-	C79.2	D04.2-	D23.2-	D48.5	D49.2
axilla, axillary fold (see also Neoplasm, skin, trunk)	C44.509	C79.2	D04.5	D23.5	D48.5	D49.2
back (see also Neoplasm, skin, trunk)	C44.509	C79.2	D04.5	D23.5	D48.5	D49.2
basal cell carcinoma	C44.91					
breast	C44.501	C79.2	D04.5	D23.5	D48.5	D49.2
basal cell carcinoma	C44.511	-	-	-	-	-
specified type NEC	C44.591	-	-	-	-	-
squamous cell carcinoma	C44.521	-	-	-	-	-
brow (see also Neoplasm, skin, face)	C44.309	C79.2	D04.39	D23.39	D48.5	D49.2

Neoplasm	Malignant Primary	Malignant Secondary	Ca in situ	Benign	Uncertain Behavior	Unspecified Behavior
skin NOS — continued						
buttock (see also Neoplasm, skin, trunk)	C44.509	C79.2	D04.5	D23.5	D48.5	D49.2
calf (see also Neoplasm, skin, limb, lower)	C44.70-	C79.2	D04.7-	D23.7-	D48.5	D49.2
canthus (eye) (inner) (outer)	C44.10-	C79.2	D04.1-	D23.1-	D48.5	D49.2
basal cell carcinoma	C44.11-	-	-	-	-	-
sebaceous cell	C44.13-	-	-	-	-	-
specified type NEC	C44.19-	-	-	-	-	-
squamous cell carcinoma	C44.12-	-	-	-	-	-
cervical region (see also Neoplasm, skin, neck)	C44.40	C79.2	D04.4	D23.4	D48.5	D49.2
cheek (external) (see also Neoplasm, skin, face)	C44.309	C79.2	D04.39	D23.39	D48.5	D49.2
chest (wall) (see also Neoplasm, skin, trunk)	C44.509	C79.2	D04.5	D23.5	D48.5	D49.2
chin (see also Neoplasm, skin, face)	C44.309	C79.2	D04.39	D23.39	D48.5	D49.2
clavicular area (see also Neoplasm, skin, trunk)	C44.509	C79.2	D04.5	D23.5	D48.5	D49.2
clitoris	C51.2	C79.82	D07.1	D28.0	D39.8	D49.59
columnella (see also Neoplasm, skin, face)	C44.309	C79.2	D04.39	D23.39	D48.5	D49.2
concha (see also Neoplasm, skin, ear)	C44.20-	C79.2	D04.2-	D23.2-	D48.5	D49.2
ear (external)	C44.20-	C79.2	D04.2-	D23.2-	D48.5	D49.2
basal cell carcinoma	C44.21-	-	-	-	-	-
specified type NEC	C44.29-	-	-	-	-	-
squamous cell carcinoma	C44.22-	-	-	-	-	-
elbow (see also Neoplasm, skin, limb, upper)	C44.60-	C79.2	D04.6-	D23.6-	D48.5	D49.2
eyebrow (see also Neoplasm, skin, face)	C44.309	C79.2	D04.39	D23.39	D48.5	D49.2
eyelid	C44.10-	C79.2	D04.1-	D23.1-	D48.5	D49.2
basal cell carcinoma	C44.11-	-	-	-	-	-
sebaceous cell	C44.13-	-	-	-	-	-
specified type NEC	C44.19-	-	-	-	-	-
squamous cell carcinoma	C44.12-	-	-	-	-	-
face NOS	C44.300	C79.2	D04.30	D23.30	D48.5	D49.2
basal cell carcinoma	C44.310	-	-	-	-	-
specified type NEC	C44.390	-	-	-	-	-
squamous cell carcinoma	C44.320	-	-	-	-	-
female genital organs (external)	C51.9	C79.82	D07.1	D28.0	D39.8	D49.59
clitoris	C51.2	C79.82	D07.1	D28.0	D39.8	D49.59
labium NEC	C51.9	C79.82	D07.1	D28.0	D39.8	D49.59
majus	C51.0	C79.82	D07.1	D28.0	D39.8	D49.59
minus	C51.1	C79.82	D07.1	D28.0	D39.8	D49.59
pudendum	C51.9	C79.82	D07.1	D28.0	D39.8	D49.59
vulva	C51.9	C79.82	D07.1	D28.0	D39.8	D49.59
finger (see also Neoplasm, skin, limb, upper)	C44.60-	C79.2	D04.6-	D23.6-	D48.5	D49.2
flank (see also Neoplasm, skin, trunk)	C44.509	C79.2	D04.5	D23.5	D48.5	D49.2
foot (see also Neoplasm, skin, limb, lower)	C44.70-	C79.2	D04.7-	D23.7-	D48.5	D49.2
forearm (see also Neoplasm, skin, limb, upper)	C44.60-	C79.2	D04.6-	D23.6-	D48.5	D49.2
forehead (see also Neoplasm, skin, face)	C44.309	C79.2	D04.39	D23.39	D48.5	D49.2
glabella (see also Neoplasm, skin, face)	C44.309	C79.2	D04.39	D23.39	D48.5	D49.2
gluteal region (see also Neoplasm, skin, trunk)	C44.509	C79.2	D04.5	D23.5	D48.5	D49.2
groin (see also Neoplasm, skin, trunk)	C44.509	C79.2	D04.5	D23.5	D48.5	D49.2
hand (see also Neoplasm, skin, limb, upper)	C44.60-	C79.2	D04.6-	D23.6-	D48.5	D49.2
head NEC (see also Neoplasm, skin, scalp)	C44.40	C79.2	D04.4	D23.4	D48.5	D49.2
heel (see also Neoplasm, skin, limb, lower)	C44.70-	C79.2	D04.7-	D23.7-	D48.5	D49.2
helix (see also Neoplasm, skin, ear)	C44.20-	C79.2	D04.2-	D23.2-	D48.5	D49.2
hip (see also Neoplasm, skin, limb, lower)	C44.70-	C79.2	D04.7-	D23.7-	D48.5	D49.2
infraclavicular region (see also Neoplasm, skin, trunk)	C44.509	C79.2	D04.5	D23.5	D48.5	D49.2
inguinal region (see also Neoplasm, skin, trunk)	C44.509	C79.2	D04.5	D23.5	D48.5	D49.2
jaw (see also Neoplasm, skin, face)	C44.309	C79.2	D04.39	D23.39	D48.5	D49.2
Kaposi's sarcoma — see Kaposi's, sarcoma, skin						
knee (see also Neoplasm, skin, limb, lower)	C44.70-	C79.2	D04.7-	D23.7-	D48.5	D49.2
labia						
majora	C51.0	C79.82	D07.1	D28.0	D39.8	D49.59
minora	C51.1	C79.82	D07.1	D28.0	D39.8	D49.59
leg (see also Neoplasm, skin, limb, lower)	C44.70-	C79.2	D04.7-	D23.7-	D48.5	D49.2
lid (lower) (upper)	C44.10-	C79.2	D04.1-	D23.1-	D48.5	D49.2
basal cell carcinoma	C44.11-	-	-	-	-	-
sebaceous cell	C44.13-	-	-	-	-	-
specified type NEC	C44.19-	-	-	-	-	-
squamous cell carcinoma	C44.12-	-	-	-	-	-

Neoplasm	Malignant Primary	Malignant Secondary	Ca in situ	Benign	Uncertain Behavior	Unspecified Behavior
skin NOS — continued						
limb NEC	C44.90	C79.2	D04.9	D23.9	D48.5	D49.2
basal cell carcinoma	C44.91	-	-	-	-	-
lower	C44.70-	C79.2	D04.7-	D23.7-	D48.5	D49.2
basal cell carcinoma	C44.71-	-	-	-	-	-
specified type NEC	C44.79-	-	-	-	-	-
squamous cell carcinoma	C44.72-	-	-	-	-	-
upper	C44.60-	C79.2	D04.6-	D23.6-	D48.5	D49.2
basal cell carcinoma	C44.61-	-	-	-	-	-
specified type NEC	C44.69-	-	-	-	-	-
squamous cell carcinoma	C44.62-	-	-	-	-	-
lip (lower) (upper)	C44.00	C79.2	D04.0	D23.0	D48.5	D49.2
basal cell carcinoma	C44.01	-	-	-	-	-
specified type NEC	C44.09	-	-	-	-	-
squamous cell carcinoma	C44.02	-	-	-	-	-
male genital organs	C63.9	C79.82	D07.60	D29.9	D40.8	D49.59
penis	C60.9	C79.82	D07.4	D29.0	D40.8	D49.59
prepuce	C60.0	C79.82	D07.4	D29.0	D40.8	D49.59
scrotum	C63.2	C79.82	D07.61	D29.4	D40.8	D49.59
mastectomy site (skin) (see also Neoplasm, skin, breast)	C44.501	C79.2	-	-	-	-
specified as breast tissue	C50.8-	C79.81	-	-	-	-
meatus, acoustic (external) (see also Neoplasm, skin, ear)	C44.20-	C79.2	D04.2-	D23.2-	D48.5	D49.2
melanotic — see Melanoma						
Merkel cell — see Carcinoma, Merkel cell						
nates (see also Neoplasm, skin, trunk)	C44.509	C79.2	D04.5	D23.5	D48.5	D49.2
neck	C44.40	C79.2	D04.4	D23.4	D48.5	D49.2
basal cell carcinoma	C44.41	-	-	-	-	-
specified type NEC	C44.49	-	-	-	-	-
squamous cell carcinoma	C44.42	-	-	-	-	-
nevus — see Nevus, skin						
nose (external) (see also Neoplasm, nose, skin)	C44.301	C79.2	D04.39	D23.39	D48.5	D49.2
overlapping lesion	C44.80	-	-	-	-	-
basal cell carcinoma	C44.81	-	-	-	-	-
specified type NEC	C44.89	-	-	-	-	-
squamous cell carcinoma	C44.82	-	-	-	-	-
palm (see also Neoplasm, skin, limb, upper)	C44.60-	C79.2	D04.6-	D23.6-	D48.5	D49.2
palpebra	C44.10-	C79.2	D04.1-	D23.1-	D48.5	D49.2
basal cell carcinoma	C44.11-	-	-	-	-	-
sebaceous cell	C44.13-	-	-	-	-	-
specified type NEC	C44.19-	-	-	-	-	-
squamous cell carcinoma	C44.12-	-	-	-	-	-
penis NEC	C60.9	C79.82	D07.4	D29.0	D40.8	D49.59
perianal (see also Neoplasm, skin, anus)	C44.500	C79.2	D04.5	D23.5	D48.5	D49.2
perineum (see also Neoplasm, skin, anus)	C44.500	C79.2	D04.5	D23.5	D48.5	D49.2
pinna (see also Neoplasm, skin, ear)	C44.20-	C79.2	D04.2-	D23.2-	D48.5	D49.2
plantar (see also Neoplasm, skin, limb, lower)	C44.70-	C79.2	D04.7-	D23.7-	D48.5	D49.2
popliteal fossa or space (see also Neoplasm, skin, limb, lower)	C44.70-	C79.2	D04.7-	D23.7-	D48.5	D49.2
prepuce	C60.0	C79.82	D07.4	D29.0	D40.8	D49.59
pubes (see also Neoplasm, skin, trunk)	C44.509	C79.2	D04.5	D23.5	D48.5	D49.2
sacrococcygeal region (see also Neoplasm, skin, trunk)	C44.509	C79.2	D04.5	D23.5	D48.5	D49.2
scalp	C44.40	C79.2	D04.4	D23.4	D48.5	D49.2
basal cell carcinoma	C44.41	-	-	-	-	-
specified type NEC	C44.49	-	-	-	-	-
squamous cell carcinoma	C44.42	-	-	-	-	-
scapular region (see also Neoplasm, skin, trunk)	C44.509	C79.2	D04.5	D23.5	D48.5	D49.2
scrotum	C63.2	C79.82	D07.61	D29.4	D40.8	D49.59
shoulder (see also Neoplasm, skin, limb, upper)	C44.60-	C79.2	D04.6-	D23.6-	D48.5	D49.2
sole (foot) (see also Neoplasm, skin, limb, lower)	C44.70-	C79.2	D04.7-	D23.7-	D48.5	D49.2
specified sites NEC	C44.80	C79.2	D04.8	D23.9	D48.5	D49.2
basal cell carcinoma	C44.81	-	-	-	-	-
specified type NEC	C44.89	-	-	-	-	-
squamous cell carcinoma	C44.82	-	-	-	-	-
specified type NEC	C44.99	-	-	-	-	-
squamous cell carcinoma	C44.92	-	-	-	-	-
submammary fold (see also Neoplasm, skin, trunk)	C44.509	C79.2	D04.5	D23.5	D48.5	D49.2
supraclavicular region (see also Neoplasm, skin, neck)	C44.40	C79.2	D04.4	D23.4	D48.5	D49.2
temple (see also Neoplasm, skin, face)	C44.309	C79.2	D04.39	D23.39	D48.5	D49.2
thigh (see also Neoplasm, skin, limb, lower)	C44.70-	C79.2	D04.7-	D23.7-	D48.5	D49.2
thoracic wall (see also Neoplasm, skin, trunk)	C44.509	C79.2	D04.5	D23.5	D48.5	D49.2
thumb (see also Neoplasm, skin, limb, upper)	C44.60-	C79.2	D04.6-	D23.6-	D48.5	D49.2

Neoplasm	Malignant Primary	Malignant Secondary	Ca in situ	Benign	Uncertain Behavior	Unspecified Behavior
skin NOS — continued						
toe (see also Neoplasm, skin, limb, lower)	C44.70-	C79.2	D04.7-	D23.7-	D48.5	D49.2
tragus (see also Neoplasm, skin, ear)	C44.20-	C79.2	D04.2-	D23.2-	D48.5	D49.2
trunk	C44.509	C79.2	D04.5	D23.5	D48.5	D49.2
basal cell carcinoma	C44.519	-	-	-	-	-
specified type NEC	C44.599	-	-	-	-	-
squamous cell carcinoma	C44.529	-	-	-	-	-
umbilicus (see also Neoplasm, skin, trunk)	C44.509	C79.2	D04.5	D23.5	D48.5	D49.2
vulva	C51.9	C79.82	D07.1	D28.0	D39.8	D49.59
overlapping lesion	C51.8	-	-	-	-	-
wrist (see also Neoplasm, skin, limb, upper)	C44.60-	C79.2	D04.6-	D23.6-	D48.5	D49.2
skull	C41.0	C79.51	-	D16.4-	D48.0	D49.2
soft parts or tissues — see Neoplasm, connective tissue						
specified site NEC	C76.8	C79.89	D09.8	D36.7	D48.7	D49.89
spermatic cord	C63.1-	C79.82	D07.69	D29.8	D40.8	D49.59
sphenoid	C31.3	C78.39	D02.3	D14.0	D38.5	D49.1
bone	C41.0	C79.51	-	D16.4-	D48.0	D49.2
sinus	C31.3	C78.39	D02.3	D14.0	D38.5	D49.1
sphincter						
anal	C21.1	C78.5	D01.3	D12.9	D37.8	D49.0
of Oddi	C24.0	C78.89	D01.5	D13.5	D37.6	D49.0
spine, spinal (column)	C41.2	C79.51	-	D16.6	D48.0	D49.2
bulb	C71.7	C79.31	-	D33.1	D43.1	D49.6
coccyx	C41.4	C79.51	-	D16.8	D48.0	D49.2
cord (cervical) (lumbar) (sacral) (thoracic)	C72.0	C79.49	-	D33.4	D43.4	D49.7
dura mater	C70.1	C79.49	-	D32.1	D42.1	D49.7
lumbosacral	C41.2	C79.51	-	D16.6	D48.0	D49.2
marrow NEC	C96.9	C79.52	-		D47.9	D49.89
membrane	C70.1	C79.49	-	D32.1	D42.1	D49.7
meninges	C70.1	C79.49	-	D32.1	D42.1	D49.7
nerve (root)	C47.9	C79.89	-	D36.10	D48.2	D49.2
pia mater	C70.1	C79.49	-	D32.1	D42.1	D49.7
root	C47.9	C79.89	-	D36.10	D48.2	D49.2
sacrum	C41.4	C79.51	-	D16.8	D48.0	D49.2
spleen, splenic NEC	C26.1	C78.89	D01.7	D13.9	D37.8	D49.0
flexure (colon)	C18.5	C78.5	D01.0	D12.3	D37.4	D49.0
stem, brain	C71.7	C79.31	-	D33.1	D43.1	D49.6
Stensen's duct	C07	C79.89	D00.00	D11.0	D37.030	D49.0
sternum	C41.3	C79.51	-	D16.7	D48.0	D49.2
stomach	C16.9	C78.89	D00.2	D13.1	D37.1	D49.0
antrum (pyloric)	C16.3	C78.89	D00.2	D13.1	D37.1	D49.0
body	C16.2	C78.89	D00.2	D13.1	D37.1	D49.0
cardia	C16.0	C78.89	D00.2	D13.1	D37.1	D49.0
cardiac orifice	C16.0	C78.89	D00.2	D13.1	D37.1	D49.0
corpus	C16.2	C78.89	D00.2	D13.1	D37.1	D49.0
fundus	C16.1	C78.89	D00.2	D13.1	D37.1	D49.0
greater curvature NEC	C16.6	C78.89	D00.2	D13.1	D37.1	D49.0
lesser curvature NEC	C16.5	C78.89	D00.2	D13.1	D37.1	D49.0
overlapping lesion	C16.8	-	-	-	-	-
prepylorus	C16.4	C78.89	D00.2	D13.1	D37.1	D49.0
pylorus	C16.4	C78.89	D00.2	D13.1	D37.1	D49.0
wall NEC	C16.9	C78.89	D00.2	D13.1	D37.1	D49.0
anterior NEC	C16.8	C78.89	D00.2	D13.1	D37.1	D49.0
posterior NEC	C16.8	C78.89	D00.2	D13.1	D37.1	D49.0
stroma, endometrial	C54.1	C79.82	D07.0	D26.1	D39.0	D49.59
stump, cervical	C53.8	C79.82	D06.7	D26.0	D39.0	D49.59
subcutaneous (nodule) (tissue) NEC — see Neoplasm, connective tissue						
subdural	C70.9	C79.32	-	D32.9	D42.9	D49.7
subglottis, subglottic	C32.2	C78.39	D02.0	D14.1	D38.0	D49.1
sublingual	C04.9	C79.89	D00.06	D10.2	D37.09	D49.0
gland or duct	C08.1	C79.89	D00.00	D11.7	D37.031	D49.0
submandibular gland	C08.0	C79.89	D00.00	D11.7	D37.032	D49.0
submaxillary gland or duct	C08.0	C79.89	D00.00	D11.7	D37.032	D49.0
submental	C76.0	C79.89	D09.8	D36.7	D48.7	D49.89
subpleural	C34.9-	C78.0-	D02.2-	D14.3-	D38.1	D49.1
substernal	C38.1	C78.1	-	D15.2	D38.3	D49.89
sudoriferous, sudoriparous gland, site unspecified	C44.90	C79.2	D04.9	D23.9	D48.5	D49.2
specified site — see Neoplasm, skin						
supraclavicular region	C76.0	C79.89	D09.8	D36.7	D48.7	D49.89
supraglottis	C32.1	C78.39	D02.0	D14.1	D38.0	D49.1
suprarenal	C74.9-	C79.7-	D09.3	D35.0-	D44.1-	D49.7
capsule	C74.9-	C79.7-	D09.3	D35.0-	D44.1-	D49.7
cortex	C74.0-	C79.7-	D09.3	D35.0-	D44.1-	D49.7
gland	C74.9-	C79.7-	D09.3	D35.0-	D44.1-	D49.7
medulla	C74.1-	C79.7-	D09.3	D35.0-	D44.1-	D49.7
suprasellar (region)	C71.9	C79.31	-	D33.2	D43.2	D49.6
supratentorial (brain) NEC	C71.0	C79.31	-	D33.0	D43.0	D49.6
sweat gland (apocrine) (eccrine), site unspecified	C44.90	C79.2	D04.9	D23.9	D48.5	D49.2
specified site — see Neoplasm, skin						
sympathetic nerve or nervous system NEC	C47.9	C79.89	-	D36.10	D48.2	D49.2

symphysis - Zuckerkandl

Neoplasm	Malignant Primary	Malignant Secondary	Ca in situ	Benign	Uncertain Behavior	Unspecified Behavior
symphysis pubis	C41.4	C79.51	-	D16.8	D48.0	D49.2
synovial membrane — *see* Neoplasm, connective tissue						
tapetum, brain	C71.8	C79.31	-	D33.2	D43.2	D49.6
tarsus (any bone)	C40.3-	C79.51	-	D16.3-	-	-
temple (skin) (*see also* Neoplasm, skin, face)	C44.309	C79.2	D04.39	D23.39	D48.5	D49.2
temporal						
bone	C41.0	C79.51	-	D16.4-	D48.0	D49.2
lobe or pole	C71.2	C79.31	-	D33.0	D43.0	D49.6
region	C76.0	C79.89	D09.8	D36.7	D48.7	D49.89
skin (*see also* Neoplasm, skin, face)	C44.309	C79.2	D04.39	D23.39	D48.5	D49.2
tendon (sheath) — *see* Neoplasm, connective tissue						
tentorium (cerebelli)	C70.0	C79.32	-	D32.0	D42.0	D49.7
testis, testes	C62.9-	C79.82	D07.69	D29.2-	D40.1-	D49.59
descended	C62.1-	C79.82	D07.69	D29.2-	D40.1-	D49.59
ectopic	C62.0-	C79.82	D07.69	D29.2-	D40.1-	D49.59
retained	C62.0-	C79.82	D07.69	D29.2-	D40.1-	D49.59
scrotal	C62.1-	C79.82	D07.69	D29.2-	D40.1-	D49.59
undescended	C62.0-	C79.82	D07.69	D29.2-	D40.1-	D49.59
unspecified whether descended or undescended	C62.9-	C79.82	D07.69	D29.2-	D40.1-	D49.59
thalamus	C71.0	C79.31	-	D33.0	D43.0	D49.6
thigh NEC	C76.5-	C79.89	D04.7-	D36.7	D48.7	D49.89
thorax, thoracic (cavity) (organs NEC)	C76.1	C79.89	D09.8	D36.7	D48.7	D49.89
duct	C49.3	C79.89	-	D21.3	D48.1	D49.2
wall NEC	C76.1	C79.89	D09.8	D36.7	D48.7	D49.89
throat	C14.0	C79.89	D00.08	D10.9	D37.05	D49.0
thumb NEC	C76.4-	C79.89	D04.6-	D36.7	D48.7	D49.89
thymus (gland)	C37	C79.89	D09.3	D15.0	D38.4	D49.89
thyroglossal duct	C73	C79.89	D09.3	D34	D44.0	D49.7
thyroid (gland)	C73	C79.89	D09.3	D34	D44.0	D49.7
cartilage	C32.3	C78.39	D02.0	D14.1	D38.0	D49.1
tibia (any part)	C40.2-	C79.51	-	D16.2-	-	-
toe NEC	C76.5-	C79.89	D04.7-	D36.7	D48.7	D49.89
tongue	C02.9	C79.89	D00.07	D10.1	D37.02	D49.0
anterior (two-thirds) NEC	C02.3	C79.89	D00.07	D10.1	D37.02	D49.0
dorsal surface	C02.0	C79.89	D00.07	D10.1	D37.02	D49.0
ventral surface	C02.2	C79.89	D00.07	D10.1	D37.02	D49.0
base (dorsal surface)	C01	C79.89	D00.07	D10.1	D37.02	D49.0
border (lateral)	C02.1	C79.89	D00.07	D10.1	D37.02	D49.0
dorsal surface NEC	C02.0	C79.89	D00.07	D10.1	D37.02	D49.0
fixed part NEC	C01	C79.89	D00.07	D10.1	D37.02	D49.0
foramen cecum	C02.0	C79.89	D00.07	D10.1	D37.02	D49.0
frenulum linguae	C02.2	C79.89	D00.07	D10.1	D37.02	D49.0
junctional zone	C02.8	C79.89	D00.07	D10.1	D37.02	D49.0
margin (lateral)	C02.1	C79.89	D00.07	D10.1	D37.02	D49.0
midline NEC	C02.0	C79.89	D00.07	D10.1	D37.02	D49.0
mobile part NEC	C02.3	C79.89	D00.07	D10.1	D37.02	D49.0
overlapping lesion	C02.8	-	-	-	-	-
posterior (third)	C01	C79.89	D00.07	D10.1	D37.02	D49.0
root	C01	C79.89	D00.07	D10.1	D37.02	D49.0
surface (dorsal)	C02.0	C79.89	D00.07	D10.1	D37.02	D49.0
base	C01	C79.89	D00.07	D10.1	D37.02	D49.0
ventral	C02.2	C79.89	D00.07	D10.1	D37.02	D49.0
tip	C02.1	C79.89	D00.07	D10.1	D37.02	D49.0
tonsil	C02.4	C79.89	D00.07	D10.1	D37.02	D49.0
tonsil	C09.9	C79.89	D00.08	D10.4	D37.05	D49.0
fauces, faucial	C09.9	C79.89	D00.08	D10.4	D37.05	D49.0
lingual	C02.4	C79.89	D00.07	D10.1	D37.02	D49.0
overlapping sites	C09.8	-	-	-	-	-
palatine	C09.9	C79.89	D00.08	D10.4	D37.05	D49.0
pharyngeal	C11.1	C79.89	D00.08	D10.6	D37.05	D49.0
pillar (anterior) (posterior)	C09.1	C79.89	D00.08	D10.5	D37.05	D49.0
tonsillar fossa	C09.0	C79.89	D00.08	D10.5	D37.05	D49.0
tooth socket NEC	C03.9	C79.89	D00.03	D10.39	D37.09	D49.0
trachea (cartilage) (mucosa)	C33	C78.39	D02.1	D14.2	D38.1	D49.1
overlapping lesion with bronchus or lung	C34.8-	-	-	-	-	-
tracheobronchial	C34.8-	C78.39	D02.1	D14.2	D38.1	D49.1
overlapping lesion with lung	C34.8-	-	-	-	-	-
tragus (*see also* Neoplasm, skin, ear)	C44.20-	C79.2	D04.2-	D23.2-	D48.5	D49.2
trunk NEC	C76.8	C79.89	D04.5	D36.7	D48.7	D49.89
tubo-ovarian	C57.8	C79.82	D07.39	D28.7	D39.8	D49.59
tunica vaginalis	C63.7	C79.82	D07.69	D29.8	D40.8	D49.59
turbinate (bone)	C41.0	C79.51	-	D16.4-	D48.0	D49.2
nasal	C30.0	C78.39	D02.3	D14.0	D38.5	D49.1
tympanic cavity	C30.1	C78.39	D02.3	D14.0	D38.5	D49.1
ulna (any part)	C40.0-	C79.51	-	D16.0-	-	-
umbilicus, umbilical (*see also* Neoplasm, skin, trunk)	C44.509	C79.2	D04.5	D23.5	D48.5	D49.2
uncus, brain	C71.2	C79.31	-	D33.0	D43.0	D49.6
unknown site or unspecified	C80.1	C79.9	D09.9	D36.9	D48.9	D49.9
urachus	C67.7	C79.11	D09.0	D30.3	D41.4	D49.4
ureter, ureteral	C66.-	C79.19	D09.19	D30.2-	D41.2-	D49.59
orifice (bladder)	C67.6	C79.11	D09.0	D30.3	D41.4	D49.4
ureter-bladder (junction)	C67.6	C79.11	D09.0	D30.3	D41.4	D49.4

Neoplasm	Malignant Primary	Malignant Secondary	Ca in situ	Benign	Uncertain Behavior	Unspecified Behavior
urethra, urethral (gland)	C68.0	C79.19	D09.19	D30.4	D41.3	D49.59
orifice, internal	C67.5	C79.11	D09.0	D30.3	D41.4	D49.4
urethrovaginal (septum)	C57.9	C79.82	D07.30	D28.9	D39.8	D49.59
urinary organ or system	C68.9	C79.10	D09.10	D30.9	D41.9	D49.59
bladder — *see* Neoplasm, bladder						
overlapping lesion	C68.8	-	-	-	-	-
specified sites NEC	C68.8	C79.19	D09.19	D30.8	D41.8	D49.59
utero-ovarian	C57.8	C79.82	D07.39	D28.7	D39.8	D49.59
ligament	C57.1	C79.82	D07.39	D28.2	D39.8	D49.59
uterosacral ligament	C57.3	C79.82	-	D28.2	D39.8	D49.59
uterus, uteri, uterine	C55	C79.82	D07.0	D26.9	D39.0	D49.59
adnexa NEC	C57.4	C79.82	D07.39	D28.7	D39.8	D49.59
body	C54.9	C79.82	D07.0	D26.1	D39.0	D49.59
cervix	C53.9	C79.82	D06.9	D26.0	D39.0	D49.59
cornu	C54.9	C79.82	D07.0	D26.1	D39.0	D49.59
corpus	C54.9	C79.82	D07.0	D26.1	D39.0	D49.59
endocervix (canal) (gland)	C53.0	C79.82	D06.0	D26.0	D39.0	D49.59
endometrium	C54.1	C79.82	D07.0	D26.1	D39.0	D49.59
exocervix	C53.1	C79.82	D06.1	D26.0	D39.0	D49.59
external os	C53.1	C79.82	D06.1	D26.0	D39.0	D49.59
fundus	C54.3	C79.82	D07.0	D26.1	D39.0	D49.59
internal os	C53.0	C79.82	D06.0	D26.0	D39.0	D49.59
isthmus	C54.0	C79.82	D07.0	D26.1	D39.0	D49.59
ligament	C57.3	C79.82	-	D28.2	D39.8	D49.59
broad	C57.1	C79.82	D07.39	D28.2	D39.8	D49.59
round	C57.2	C79.82	-	D28.2	D39.8	D49.59
lower segment	C54.0	C79.82	D07.0	D26.1	D39.0	D49.59
myometrium	C54.2	C79.82	D07.0	D26.1	D39.0	D49.59
overlapping sites	C54.8	-	-	-	-	-
squamocolumnar junction	C53.8	C79.82	D06.7	D26.0	D39.0	D49.59
tube	C57.0-	C79.82	D07.39	D28.2	D39.8	D49.59
utricle, prostatic	C68.0	C79.19	D09.19	D30.4	D41.3	D49.59
uveal tract	C69.4-	C79.49	D09.2-	D31.4-	D48.7	D49.89
uvula	C05.2	C79.89	D00.04	D10.39	D37.09	D49.0
vagina, vaginal (fornix) (vault) (wall)	C52	C79.82	D07.2	D28.1	D39.8	D49.59
vaginovesical	C57.9	C79.82	D07.30	D28.9	D39.9	D49.59
septum	C57.9	C79.82	D07.30	D28.9	D39.9	D49.59
vallecula (epiglottis)	C10.0	C79.89	D00.08	D10.5	D37.05	D49.0
vas deferens	C63.1-	C79.82	D07.69	D29.8	D40.8	D49.59
vascular — *see* Neoplasm, connective tissue						
Vater's ampulla	C24.1	C78.89	D01.5	D13.5	D37.6	D49.0
vein, venous — *see* Neoplasm, connective tissue						
vena cava (abdominal) (inferior)	C49.4	C79.89	-	D21.4	D48.1	D49.2
superior	C49.3	C79.89	-	D21.3	D48.1	D49.2
ventricle (cerebral) (floor) (lateral) (third)	C71.5	C79.31	-	D33.0	D43.0	D49.6
cardiac (left) (right)	C38.0	C79.89	-	D15.1	D48.7	D49.89
fourth	C71.7	C79.31	-	D33.1	D43.1	D49.6
ventricular band of larynx	C32.1	C78.39	D02.0	D14.1	D38.0	D49.1
ventriculus — *see* Neoplasm, stomach						
vermillion border — *see* Neoplasm, lip						
vermis, cerebellum	C71.6	C79.31	-	D33.1	D43.1	D49.6
vertebra (column)	C41.2	C79.51	-	D16.6	D48.0	D49.2
coccyx	C41.4	C79.51	-	D16.8-	D48.0	D49.2
marrow NEC	C96.9	C79.52	-	-	D47.9	D49.89
sacrum	C41.4	C79.51	-	D16.8-	D48.0	D49.2
vesical — *see* Neoplasm, bladder						
vesicle, seminal	C63.7	C79.82	D07.69	D29.8	D40.8	D49.59
vesicocervical tissue	C57.9	C79.82	D07.30	D28.9	D39.9	D49.59
vesicorectal	C76.3	C79.89	D09.8	D36.7	D48.7	D49.89
vesicovaginal	C57.9	C79.82	D07.30	D28.9	D39.9	D49.59
septum	C57.9	C79.82	D07.30	D28.9	D39.8	D49.59
vessel (blood) — *see* Neoplasm, connective tissue						
vestibular gland, greater	C51.0	C79.82	D07.1	D28.0	D39.8	D49.59
vestibule						
mouth	C06.1	C79.89	D00.00	D10.39	D37.09	D49.0
nose	C30.0	C78.39	D02.3	D14.0	D38.5	D49.1
Virchow's gland	C77.0	C77.0	-	D36.0	D48.7	D49.89
viscera NEC	C76.8	C79.89	D09.8	D36.7	D48.7	D49.89
vocal cords (true)	C32.0	C78.39	D02.0	D14.1	D38.0	D49.1
false	C32.1	C78.39	D02.0	D14.1	D38.0	D49.1
vomer	C41.0	C79.51	-	D16.4-	D48.0	D49.2
vulva	C51.9	C79.82	D07.1	D28.0	D39.8	D49.59
vulvovaginal gland	C51.0	C79.82	D07.1	D28.0	D39.8	D49.59
Waldeyer's ring	C14.2	C79.89	D00.08	D10.9	D37.05	D49.0
Wharton's duct	C08.0	C79.89	D00.00	D11.7	D37.032	D49.0
white matter (central) (cerebral)	C71.0	C79.31	-	D33.0	D43.0	D49.6
windpipe	C33	C78.39	D02.1	D14.2	D38.1	D49.1
Wirsung's duct	C25.3	C78.89	D01.7	D13.6	D37.8	D49.0
wolffian (body) (duct)						
female	C57.7	C79.82	D07.39	D28.7	D39.8	D49.59
male	C63.7	C79.82	D07.69	D29.8	D40.8	D49.59
womb — *see* Neoplasm, uterus						
wrist NEC	C76.4-	C79.89	D04.6-	D36.7	D48.7	D49.89
xiphoid process	C41.3	C79.51	-	D16.7	D48.0	D49.2
Zuckerkandl organ	C75.5	C79.89	-	D35.6	D44.7	D49.7

ICD-10-CM Table of Drugs and Chemicals

Substance	Poisoning, Accidental (unintentional)	Poisoning, Intentional self-harm	Poisoning, Assault	Poisoning, Undetermined	Adverse effect	Underdosing
1-propanol	T51.3X1	T51.3X2	T51.3X3	T51.3X4	--	--
2-propanol	T51.2X1	T51.2X2	T51.2X3	T51.2X4	--	--
2,4-D (dichlorophen-oxyacetic acid)	T60.3X1	T60.3X2	T60.3X3	T60.3X4	--	--
2,4-toluene diisocyanate	T65.0X1	T65.0X2	T65.0X3	T65.0X4	--	--
2,4,5-T (trichloro-phenoxyacetic acid)	T60.1X1	T60.1X2	T60.1X3	T60.1X4	--	--
3,4-methylenedioxymethamphetamine	T43.641	T43.642	T43.643	T43.644	--	--
14-hydroxydihydro-morphinone	T40.2X1	T40.2X2	T40.2X3	T40.2X4	T40.2X5	T40.2X6
A						
ABOB	T37.5X1	T37.5X2	T37.5X3	T37.5X4	T37.5X5	T37.5X6
Abrine	T62.2X1	T62.2X2	T62.2X3	T62.2X4	--	--
Abrus (seed)	T62.2X1	T62.2X2	T62.2X3	T62.2X4	--	--
Absinthe	T51.0X1	T51.0X2	T51.0X3	T51.0X4	--	--
beverage	T51.0X1	T51.0X2	T51.0X3	T51.0X4	--	--
Acaricide	T60.8X1	T60.8X2	T60.8X3	T60.8X4	--	--
Acebutolol	T44.7X1	T44.7X2	T44.7X3	T44.7X4	T44.7X5	T44.7X6
Acecarbromal	T42.6X1	T42.6X2	T42.6X3	T42.6X4	T42.6X5	T42.6X6
Aceclidine	T44.1X1	T44.1X2	T44.1X3	T44.1X4	T44.1X5	T44.1X6
Acedapsone	T37.0X1	T37.0X2	T37.0X3	T37.0X4	T37.0X5	T37.0X6
Acefylline piperazine	T48.6X1	T48.6X2	T48.6X3	T48.6X4	T48.6X5	T48.6X6
Acemorphan	T40.2X1	T40.2X2	T40.2X3	T40.2X4	T40.2X5	T40.2X6
Acenocoumarin	T45.511	T45.512	T45.513	T45.514	T45.515	T45.516
Acenocoumarol	T45.511	T45.512	T45.513	T45.514	T45.515	T45.516
Acepifylline	T48.6X1	T48.6X2	T48.6X3	T48.6X4	T48.6X5	T48.6X6
Acepromazine	T43.3X1	T43.3X2	T43.3X3	T43.3X4	T43.3X5	T43.3X6
Acesulfamethoxypyridazine	T37.0X1	T37.0X2	T37.0X3	T37.0X4	T37.0X5	T37.0X6
Acetal	T52.8X1	T52.8X2	T52.8X3	T52.8X4	--	--
Acetaldehyde (vapor)	T52.8X1	T52.8X2	T52.8X3	T52.8X4	--	--
liquid	T65.891	T65.892	T65.893	T65.894	--	--
P-Acetamidophenol	T39.1X1	T39.1X2	T39.1X3	T39.1X4	T39.1X5	T39.1X6
Acetaminophen	T39.1X1	T39.1X2	T39.1X3	T39.1X4	T39.1X5	T39.1X6
Acetaminosalol	T39.1X1	T39.1X2	T39.1X3	T39.1X4	T39.1X5	T39.1X6
Acetanilide	T39.1X1	T39.1X2	T39.1X3	T39.1X4	T39.1X5	T39.1X6
Acetarsol	T37.3X1	T37.3X2	T37.3X3	T37.3X4	T37.3X5	T37.3X6
Acetazolamide	T50.2X1	T50.2X2	T50.2X3	T50.2X4	T50.2X5	T50.2X6
Acetiamine	T45.2X1	T45.2X2	T45.2X3	T45.2X4	T45.2X5	T45.2X6
Acetic						
acid	T54.2X1	T54.2X2	T54.2X3	T54.2X4	--	--
with sodium acetate (ointment)	T49.3X1	T49.3X2	T49.3X3	T49.3X4	T49.3X5	T49.3X6
ester (solvent)(vapor)	T52.8X1	T52.8X2	T52.8X3	T52.8X4	--	--
irrigating solution	T50.3X1	T50.3X2	T50.3X3	T50.3X4	T50.3X5	T50.3X6
medicinal (lotion)	T49.2X1	T49.2X2	T49.2X3	T49.2X4	T49.2X5	T49.2X6
anhydride	T65.891	T65.892	T65.893	T65.894	--	--
ether (vapor)	T52.8X1	T52.8X2	T52.8X3	T52.8X4	--	--
Acetohexamide	T38.3X1	T38.3X2	T38.3X3	T38.3X4	T38.3X5	T38.3X6
Acetohydroxamic acid	T50.991	T50.992	T50.993	T50.994	T50.995	T50.996
Acetomenaphthone	T45.7X1	T45.7X2	T45.7X3	T45.7X4	T45.7X5	T45.7X6
Acetomorphine	T40.1X1	T40.1X2	T40.1X3	T40.1X4	--	--
Acetone (oils)	T52.4X1	T52.4X2	T52.4X3	T52.4X4	--	--
chlorinated	T52.4X1	T52.4X2	T52.4X3	T52.4X4	--	--
vapor	T52.4X1	T52.4X2	T52.4X3	T52.4X4	--	--
Acetonitrile	T52.8X1	T52.8X2	T52.8X3	T52.8X4	--	--
Acetophenazine	T43.3X1	T43.3X2	T43.3X3	T43.3X4	T43.3X5	T43.3X6
Acetophenetedin	T39.1X1	T39.1X2	T39.1X3	T39.1X4	T39.1X5	T39.1X6
Acetophenone	T52.4X1	T52.4X2	T52.4X3	T52.4X4	--	--
Acetorphine	T40.2X1	T40.2X2	T40.2X3	T40.2X4	--	--
Acetosulfone (sodium)	T37.1X1	T37.1X2	T37.1X3	T37.1X4	T37.1X5	T37.1X6
Acetrizoate (sodium)	T50.8X1	T50.8X2	T50.8X3	T50.8X4	T50.8X5	T50.8X6
Acetrizoic acid	T50.8X1	T50.8X2	T50.8X3	T50.8X4	T50.8X5	T50.8X6
Acetyl						
bromide	T53.6X1	T53.6X2	T53.6X3	T53.6X4	--	--
chloride	T53.6X1	T53.6X2	T53.6X3	T53.6X4	--	--
Acetylcarbromal	T42.6X1	T42.6X2	T42.6X3	T42.6X4	T42.6X5	T42.6X6
Acetylcholine						
chloride	T44.1X1	T44.1X2	T44.1X3	T44.1X4	T44.1X5	T44.1X6
derivative	T44.1X1	T44.1X2	T44.1X3	T44.1X4	T44.1X5	T44.1X6
Acetylcysteine	T48.4X1	T48.4X2	T48.4X3	T48.4X4	T48.4X5	T48.4X6
Acetyldigitoxin	T46.0X1	T46.0X2	T46.0X3	T46.0X4	T46.0X5	T46.0X6
Acetyldigoxin	T46.0X1	T46.0X2	T46.0X3	T46.0X4	T46.0X5	T46.0X6
Acetyldihydrocodeine	T40.2X1	T40.2X2	T40.2X3	T40.2X4	--	--
Acetyldihydrocodeinone	T40.2X1	T40.2X2	T40.2X3	T40.2X4	--	--
Acetylene (gas)	T59.891	T59.892	T59.893	T59.894	--	--
dichloride	T53.6X1	T53.6X2	T53.6X3	T53.6X4	--	--
incomplete combustion of	T58.11	T58.12	T58.13	T58.14	--	--
industrial	T59.891	T59.892	T59.893	T59.894	--	--
tetrachloride	T53.6X1	T53.6X2	T53.6X3	T53.6X4	--	--
vapor	T53.6X1	T53.6X2	T53.6X3	T53.6X4	--	--

Substance	Poisoning, Accidental (unintentional)	Poisoning, Intentional self-harm	Poisoning, Assault	Poisoning, Undetermined	Adverse effect	Underdosing
Acetylpheneturide	T42.6X1	T42.6X2	T42.6X3	T42.6X4	T42.6X5	T42.6X6
Acetylphenylhydrazine	T39.8X1	T39.8X2	T39.8X3	T39.8X4	T39.8X5	T39.8X6
Acetylsalicylic acid (salts)	T39.011	T39.012	T39.013	T39.014	T39.015	T39.016
enteric coated	T39.011	T39.012	T39.013	T39.014	T39.015	T39.016
Acetylsulfamethoxypyridazine	T37.0X1	T37.0X2	T37.0X3	T37.0X4	T37.0X5	T37.0X6
Achromycin	T36.4X1	T36.4X2	T36.4X3	T36.4X4	T36.4X5	T36.4X6
ophthalmic preparation	T49.5X1	T49.5X2	T49.5X3	T49.5X4	T49.5X5	T49.5X6
topical NEC	T49.0X1	T49.0X2	T49.0X3	T49.0X4	T49.0X5	T49.0X6
Aciclovir	T37.5X1	T37.5X2	T37.5X3	T37.5X4	T37.5X5	T37.5X6
Acid (corrosive) NEC	T54.2X1	T54.2X2	T54.2X3	T54.2X4	--	--
Acidifying agent NEC	T50.901	T50.902	T50.903	T50.904	T50.905	T50.906
Acipimox	T46.6X1	T46.6X2	T46.6X3	T46.6X4	T46.6X5	T46.6X6
Acitretin	T50.991	T50.992	T50.993	T50.994	T50.995	T50.996
Aclarubicin	T45.1X1	T45.1X2	T45.1X3	T45.1X4	T45.1X5	T45.1X6
Aclatonium napadisilate	T48.1X1	T48.1X2	T48.1X3	T48.1X4	T48.1X5	T48.1X6
Aconite (wild)	T46.991	T46.992	T46.993	T46.994	T46.995	T46.996
Aconitine	T46.991	T46.992	T46.993	T46.994	T46.995	T46.996
Aconitum ferox	T46.991	T46.992	T46.993	T46.994	T46.995	T46.996
Acridine	T65.6X1	T65.6X2	T65.6X3	T65.6X4	--	--
vapor	T59.891	T59.892	T59.893	T59.894	--	--
Acriflavine	T37.91	T37.92	T37.93	T37.94	T37.95	T37.96
Acriflavinium chloride	T49.0X1	T49.0X2	T49.0X3	T49.0X4	T49.0X5	T49.0X6
Acrinol	T49.0X1	T49.0X2	T49.0X3	T49.0X4	T49.0X5	T49.0X6
Acrisorcin	T49.0X1	T49.0X2	T49.0X3	T49.0X4	T49.0X5	T49.0X6
Acrivastine	T45.0X1	T45.0X2	T45.0X3	T45.0X4	T45.0X5	T45.0X6
Acrolein (gas)	T59.891	T59.892	T59.893	T59.894	--	--
liquid	T54.1X1	T54.1X2	T54.1X3	T54.1X4	--	--
Acrylamide	T65.891	T65.892	T65.893	T65.894	--	--
Acrylic resin	T49.3X1	T49.3X2	T49.3X3	T49.3X4	T49.3X5	T49.3X6
Acrylonitrile	T65.891	T65.892	T65.893	T65.894	--	--
Actaea spicata	T62.2X1	T62.2X2	T62.2X3	T62.2X4	--	--
berry	T62.1X1	T62.1X2	T62.1X3	T62.1X4	--	--
Acterol	T37.3X1	T37.3X2	T37.3X3	T37.3X4	T37.3X5	T37.3X6
ACTH	T38.811	T38.812	T38.813	T38.814	T38.815	T38.816
Actinomycin C	T45.1X1	T45.1X2	T45.1X3	T45.1X4	T45.1X5	T45.1X6
Actinomycin D	T45.1X1	T45.1X2	T45.1X3	T45.1X4	T45.1X5	T45.1X6
Activated charcoal (see also Charcoal, medicinal)	T47.6X1	T47.6X2	T47.6X3	T47.6X4	T47.6X5	T47.6X6
Acyclovir	T37.5X1	T37.5X2	T37.5X3	T37.5X4	T37.5X5	T37.5X6
Adenine	T45.2X1	T45.2X2	T45.2X3	T45.2X4	T45.2X5	T45.2X6
arabinoside	T37.5X1	T37.5X2	T37.5X3	T37.5X4	T37.5X5	T37.5X6
Adenosine (phosphate)	T46.2X1	T46.2X2	T46.2X3	T46.2X4	T46.2X5	T46.2X6
ADH	T38.891	T38.892	T38.893	T38.894	T38.895	T38.896
Adhesive NEC	T65.891	T65.892	T65.893	T65.894	--	--
Adicillin	T36.0X1	T36.0X2	T36.0X3	T36.0X4	T36.0X5	T36.0X6
Adiphenine	T44.3X1	T44.3X2	T44.3X3	T44.3X4	T44.3X5	T44.3X6
Adipiodone	T50.8X1	T50.8X2	T50.8X3	T50.8X4	T50.8X5	T50.8X6
Adjunct, pharmaceutical	T50.901	T50.902	T50.903	T50.904	T50.905	T50.906
Adrenal (extract, cortex or medulla)(glucocorticoids) (hormones)(mineral ocorticoids)	T38.0X1	T38.0X2	T38.0X3	T38.0X4	T38.0X5	T38.0X6
ENT agent	T49.6X1	T49.6X2	T49.6X3	T49.6X4	T49.6X5	T49.6X6
ophthalmic preparation	T49.5X1	T49.5X2	T49.5X3	T49.5X4	T49.5X5	T49.5X6
topical NEC	T49.0X1	T49.0X2	T49.0X3	T49.0X4	T49.0X5	T49.0X6
Adrenaline	T44.5X1	T44.5X2	T44.5X3	T44.5X4	T44.5X5	T44.5X6
Adrenalin — see Adrenaline						
Adrenergic NEC	T44.901	T44.902	T44.903	T44.904	T44.905	T44.906
blocking agent NEC	T44.8X1	T44.8X2	T44.8X3	T44.8X4	T44.8X5	T44.8X6
beta, heart	T44.7X1	T44.7X2	T44.7X3	T44.7X4	T44.7X5	T44.7X6
specified NEC	T44.991	T44.992	T44.993	T44.994	T44.995	T44.996
Adrenochrome						
(mono) semicarbazone	T46.991	T46.992	T46.993	T46.994	T46.995	T46.996
derivative	T46.991	T46.992	T46.993	T46.994	T46.995	T46.996
Adrenocorticotrophic hormone	T38.811	T38.812	T38.813	T38.814	T38.815	T38.816
Adrenocorticotrophin	T38.811	T38.812	T38.813	T38.814	T38.815	T38.816
Adriamycin	T45.1X1	T45.1X2	T45.1X3	T45.1X4	T45.1X5	T45.1X6
Aerosol spray NEC	T65.91	T65.92	T65.93	T65.94	--	--
Aerosporin	T36.8X1	T36.8X2	T36.8X3	T36.8X4	T36.8X5	T36.8X6
ENT agent	T49.6X1	T49.6X2	T49.6X3	T49.6X4	T49.6X5	T49.6X6
ophthalmic preparation	T49.5X1	T49.5X2	T49.5X3	T49.5X4	T49.5X5	T49.5X6
topical NEC	T49.0X1	T49.0X2	T49.0X3	T49.0X4	T49.0X5	T49.0X6
Aethusa cynapium	T62.2X1	T62.2X2	T62.2X3	T62.2X4	--	--
Afghanistan black	T40.7X1	T40.7X2	T40.7X3	T40.7X4	T40.7X5	T40.7X6
Aflatoxin	T64.01	T64.02	T64.03	T64.04	--	--
Afloqualone	T42.8X1	T42.8X2	T42.8X3	T42.8X4	T42.8X5	T42.8X6
African boxwood	T62.2X1	T62.2X2	T62.2X3	T62.2X4	--	--

Agar - Ambuphylline

Substance	Poisoning, Accidental (unintentional)	Poisoning, Intentional self-harm	Poisoning, Assault	Poisoning, Undetermined	Adverse effect	Underdosing
Agar	T47.4X1	T47.4X2	T47.4X3	T47.4X4	T47.4X5	T47.4X6
Agonist						
predominantly						
alpha-adrenoreceptor	T44.4X1	T44.4X2	T44.4X3	T44.4X4	T44.4X5	T44.4X6
beta-adrenoreceptor	T44.5X1	T44.5X2	T44.5X3	T44.5X4	T44.5X5	T44.5X6
Agricultural agent NEC	T65.91	T65.92	T65.93	T65.94	--	--
Agrypnal	T42.3X1	T42.3X2	T42.3X3	T42.3X4	T42.3X5	T42.3X6
AHLG	T50.Z11	T50.Z12	T50.Z13	T50.Z14	T50.Z15	T50.Z16
Air contaminant(s), source/type NOS	T65.91	T65.92	T65.93	T65.94	--	--
Ajmaline	T46.2X1	T46.2X2	T46.2X3	T46.2X4	T46.2X5	T46.2X6
Akee	T62.1X1	T62.1X2	T62.1X3	T62.1X4	--	--
Akrinol	T49.0X1	T49.0X2	T49.0X3	T49.0X4	T49.0X5	T49.0X6
Akritoin	T37.8X1	T37.8X2	T37.8X3	T37.8X4	T37.8X5	T37.8X6
Alacepril	T46.4X1	T46.4X2	T46.4X3	T46.4X4	T46.4X5	T46.4X6
Alantolactone	T37.4X1	T37.4X2	T37.4X3	T37.4X4	T37.4X5	T37.4X6
Albamycin	T36.8X1	T36.8X2	T36.8X3	T36.8X4	T36.8X5	T36.8X6
Albendazole	T37.4X1	T37.4X2	T37.4X3	T37.4X4	T37.4X5	T37.4X6
Albumin						
bovine	T45.8X1	T45.8X2	T45.8X3	T45.8X4	T45.8X5	T45.8X6
human serum	T45.8X1	T45.8X2	T45.8X3	T45.8X4	T45.8X5	T45.8X6
salt-poor	T45.8X1	T45.8X2	T45.8X3	T45.8X4	T45.8X5	T45.8X6
normal human serum	T45.8X1	T45.8X2	T45.8X3	T45.8X4	T45.8X5	T45.8X6
Albuterol	T48.6X1	T48.6X2	T48.6X3	T48.6X4	T48.6X5	T48.6X6
Albutoin	T42.0X1	T42.0X2	T42.0X3	T42.0X4	T42.0X5	T42.0X6
Alclometasone	T49.0X1	T49.0X2	T49.0X3	T49.0X4	T49.0X5	T49.0X6
Alcohol	T51.91	T51.92	T51.93	T51.94	--	--
absolute	T51.0X1	T51.0X2	T51.0X3	T51.0X4	--	--
beverage	T51.0X1	T51.0X2	T51.0X3	T51.0X4	--	--
allyl	T51.8X1	T51.8X2	T51.8X3	T51.8X4	--	--
amyl	T51.3X1	T51.3X2	T51.3X3	T51.3X4	--	--
antifreeze	T51.1X1	T51.1X2	T51.1X3	T51.1X4	--	--
beverage	T51.0X1	T51.0X2	T51.0X3	T51.0X4	--	--
butyl	T51.3X1	T51.3X2	T51.3X3	T51.3X4	--	--
dehydrated	T51.0X1	T51.0X2	T51.0X3	T51.0X4	--	--
beverage	T51.0X1	T51.0X2	T51.0X3	T51.0X4	--	--
denatured	T51.0X1	T51.0X2	T51.0X3	T51.0X4	--	--
deterrent NEC	T50.6X1	T50.6X2	T50.6X3	T50.6X4	T50.6X5	T50.6X6
diagnostic (gastric function)	T50.8X1	T50.8X2	T50.8X3	T50.8X4	T50.8X5	T50.8X6
ethyl	T51.0X1	T51.0X2	T51.0X3	T51.0X4	--	--
beverage	T51.0X1	T51.0X2	T51.0X3	T51.0X4	--	--
grain	T51.0X1	T51.0X2	T51.0X3	T51.0X4	--	--
beverage	T51.0X1	T51.0X2	T51.0X3	T51.0X4	--	--
industrial	T51.0X1	T51.0X2	T51.0X3	T51.0X4	--	--
isopropyl	T51.2X1	T51.2X2	T51.2X3	T51.2X4	--	--
methyl	T51.1X1	T51.1X2	T51.1X3	T51.1X4	--	--
preparation for consumption	T51.0X1	T51.0X2	T51.0X3	T51.0X4	--	--
propyl	T51.3X1	T51.3X2	T51.3X3	T51.3X4	--	--
secondary	T51.2X1	T51.2X2	T51.2X3	T51.2X4	--	--
radiator	T51.1X1	T51.1X2	T51.1X3	T51.1X4	--	--
rubbing	T51.2X1	T51.2X2	T51.2X3	T51.2X4	--	--
specified type NEC	T51.8X1	T51.8X2	T51.8X3	T51.8X4	--	--
surgical	T51.0X1	T51.0X2	T51.0X3	T51.0X4	--	--
vapor (from any type of Alcohol)	T59.891	T59.892	T59.893	T59.894	--	--
wood	T51.1X1	T51.1X2	T51.1X3	T51.1X4	--	--
Alcuronium (chloride)	T48.1X1	T48.1X2	T48.1X3	T48.1X4	T48.1X5	T48.1X6
Aldactone	T50.0X1	T50.0X2	T50.0X3	T50.0X4	T50.0X5	T50.0X6
Aldesulfone sodium	T37.1X1	T37.1X2	T37.1X3	T37.1X4	T37.1X5	T37.1X6
Aldicarb	T60.0X1	T60.0X2	T60.0X3	T60.0X4	--	--
Aldomet	T46.5X1	T46.5X2	T46.5X3	T46.5X4	T46.5X5	T46.5X6
Aldosterone	T50.0X1	T50.0X2	T50.0X3	T50.0X4	T50.0X5	T50.0X6
Aldrin (dust)	T60.1X1	T60.1X2	T60.1X3	T60.1X4	--	--
Aleve — see Naproxen						
Alexitol sodium	T47.1X1	T47.1X2	T47.1X3	T47.1X4	T47.1X5	T47.1X6
Alfacalcidol	T45.2X1	T45.2X2	T45.2X3	T45.2X4	T45.2X5	T45.2X6
Alfadolone	T41.1X1	T41.1X2	T41.1X3	T41.1X4	T41.1X5	T41.1X6
Alfaxalone	T41.1X1	T41.1X2	T41.1X3	T41.1X4	T41.1X5	T41.1X6
Alfentanil	T40.4X1	T40.4X2	T40.4X3	T40.4X4	T40.4X5	T40.4X6
Alfuzosin (hydrochloride)	T44.8X1	T44.8X2	T44.8X3	T44.8X4	T44.8X5	T44.8X6
Algae (harmful) (toxin)	T65.821	T65.822	T65.823	T65.824	--	--
Algeldrate	T47.1X1	T47.1X2	T47.1X3	T47.1X4	T47.1X5	T47.1X6
Algin	T47.8X1	T47.8X2	T47.8X3	T47.8X4	T47.8X5	T47.8X6
Alglucerase	T45.3X1	T45.3X2	T45.3X3	T45.3X4	T45.3X5	T45.3X6
Alidase	T45.3X1	T45.3X2	T45.3X3	T45.3X4	T45.3X5	T45.3X6
Alimemazine	T43.3X1	T43.3X2	T43.3X3	T43.3X4	T43.3X5	T43.3X6
Aliphatic thiocyanates	T65.0X1	T65.0X2	T65.0X3	T65.0X4	--	--
Alizapride	T45.0X1	T45.0X2	T45.0X3	T45.0X4	T45.0X5	T45.0X6
Alkali (caustic)	T54.3X1	T54.3X2	T54.3X3	T54.3X4	--	--
Alkaline antiseptic solution (aromatic)	T49.6X1	T49.6X2	T49.6X3	T49.6X4	T49.6X5	T49.6X6
Alkalinizing agents (medicinal)	T50.901	T50.902	T50.903	T50.904	T50.905	T50.906
Alkalizing agent NEC	T50.901	T50.902	T50.903	T50.904	T50.905	T50.906
Alka-seltzer	T39.011	T39.012	T39.013	T39.014	T39.015	T39.016
Alkavervir	T46.5X1	T46.5X2	T46.5X3	T46.5X4	T46.5X5	T46.5X6
Alkonium (bromide)	T49.0X1	T49.0X2	T49.0X3	T49.0X4	T49.0X5	T49.0X6
Alkylating drug NEC	T45.1X1	T45.1X2	T45.1X3	T45.1X4	T45.1X5	T45.1X6
antimyeloproliferative	T45.1X1	T45.1X2	T45.1X3	T45.1X4	T45.1X5	T45.1X6
lymphatic	T45.1X1	T45.1X2	T45.1X3	T45.1X4	T45.1X5	T45.1X6
Alkylisocyanate	T65.0X1	T65.0X2	T65.0X3	T65.0X4	--	--
Allantoin	T49.4X1	T49.4X2	T49.4X3	T49.4X4	T49.4X5	T49.4X6
Allegron	T43.011	T43.012	T43.013	T43.014	T43.015	T43.016
Allethrin	T49.0X1	T49.0X2	T49.0X3	T49.0X4	T49.0X5	T49.0X6
Allobarbital	T42.3X1	T42.3X2	T42.3X3	T42.3X4	T42.3X5	T42.3X6
Allopurinol	T50.4X1	T50.4X2	T50.4X3	T50.4X4	T50.4X5	T50.4X6
Allyl						
alcohol	T51.8X1	T51.8X2	T51.8X3	T51.8X4	--	--
disulfide	T46.6X1	T46.6X2	T46.6X3	T46.6X4	T46.6X5	T46.6X6
Allylestrenol	T38.5X1	T38.5X2	T38.5X3	T38.5X4	T38.5X5	T38.5X6
Allylisopropylacetylurea	T42.6X1	T42.6X2	T42.6X3	T42.6X4	T42.6X5	T42.6X6
Allylisopropylmalonylurea	T42.3X1	T42.3X2	T42.3X3	T42.3X4	T42.3X5	T42.3X6
Allylthiourea	T49.3X1	T49.3X2	T49.3X3	T49.3X4	T49.3X5	T49.3X6
Allyltribromide	T42.6X1	T42.6X2	T42.6X3	T42.6X4	T42.6X5	T42.6X6
Allypropymal	T42.3X1	T42.3X2	T42.3X3	T42.3X4	T42.3X5	T42.3X6
Almagate	T47.1X1	T47.1X2	T47.1X3	T47.1X4	T47.1X5	T47.1X6
Almasilate	T47.1X1	T47.1X2	T47.1X3	T47.1X4	T47.1X5	T47.1X6
Almitrine	T50.7X1	T50.7X2	T50.7X3	T50.7X4	T50.7X5	T50.7X6
Aloes	T47.2X1	T47.2X2	T47.2X3	T47.2X4	T47.2X5	T47.2X6
Aloglutamol	T47.1X1	T47.1X2	T47.1X3	T47.1X4	T47.1X5	T47.1X6
Aloin	T47.2X1	T47.2X2	T47.2X3	T47.2X4	T47.2X5	T47.2X6
Aloxidone	T42.2X1	T42.2X2	T42.2X3	T42.2X4	T42.2X5	T42.2X6
Alpha						
acetyldigoxin	T46.0X1	T46.0X2	T46.0X3	T46.0X4	T46.0X5	T46.0X6
adrenergic blocking drug	T44.6X1	T44.6X2	T44.6X3	T44.6X4	T44.6X5	T44.6X6
amylase	T45.3X1	T45.3X2	T45.3X3	T45.3X4	T45.3X5	T45.3X6
tocoferol (acetate)	T45.2X1	T45.2X2	T45.2X3	T45.2X4	T45.2X5	T45.2X6
tocopherol	T45.2X1	T45.2X2	T45.2X3	T45.2X4	T45.2X5	T45.2X6
Alphadolone	T41.1X1	T41.1X2	T41.1X3	T41.1X4	T41.1X5	T41.1X6
Alphaprodine	T40.4X1	T40.4X2	T40.4X3	T40.4X4	T40.4X5	T40.4X6
Alphaxalone	T41.1X1	T41.1X2	T41.1X3	T41.1X4	T41.1X5	T41.1X6
Alprazolam	T42.4X1	T42.4X2	T42.4X3	T42.4X4	T42.4X5	T42.4X6
Alprenolol	T44.7X1	T44.7X2	T44.7X3	T44.7X4	T44.7X5	T44.7X6
Alprostadil	T46.7X1	T46.7X2	T46.7X3	T46.7X4	T46.7X5	T46.7X6
Alsactide	T38.811	T38.812	T38.813	T38.814	T38.815	T38.816
Alseroxylon	T46.5X1	T46.5X2	T46.5X3	T46.5X4	T46.5X5	T46.5X6
Alteplase	T45.611	T45.612	T45.613	T45.614	T45.615	T45.616
Altizide	T50.2X1	T50.2X2	T50.2X3	T50.2X4	T50.2X5	T50.2X6
Altretamine	T45.1X1	T45.1X2	T45.1X3	T45.1X4	T45.1X5	T45.1X6
Alum (medicinal)	T49.4X1	T49.4X2	T49.4X3	T49.4X4	T49.4X5	T49.4X6
nonmedicinal (ammonium) (potassium)	T56.891	T56.892	T56.893	T56.894	--	--
Aluminium, aluminum						
acetate	T49.2X1	T49.2X2	T49.2X3	T49.2X4	T49.2X5	T49.2X6
solution	T49.0X1	T49.0X2	T49.0X3	T49.0X4	T49.0X5	T49.0X6
aspirin	T39.011	T39.012	T39.013	T39.014	T39.015	T39.016
bis (acetylsalicylate)	T39.011	T39.012	T39.013	T39.014	T39.015	T39.016
carbonate (gel, basic)	T47.1X1	T47.1X2	T47.1X3	T47.1X4	T47.1X5	T47.1X6
chlorhydroxide-complex	T47.1X1	T47.1X2	T47.1X3	T47.1X4	T47.1X5	T47.1X6
chloride	T49.2X1	T49.2X2	T49.2X3	T49.2X4	T49.2X5	T49.2X6
clofibrate	T46.6X1	T46.6X2	T46.6X3	T46.6X4	T46.6X5	T46.6X6
diacetate	T49.2X1	T49.2X2	T49.2X3	T49.2X4	T49.2X5	T49.2X6
glycinate	T47.1X1	T47.1X2	T47.1X3	T47.1X4	T47.1X5	T47.1X6
hydroxide (gel)	T47.1X1	T47.1X2	T47.1X3	T47.1X4	T47.1X5	T47.1X6
hydroxide-magnesium carb. gel	T47.1X1	T47.1X2	T47.1X3	T47.1X4	T47.1X5	T47.1X6
magnesium silicate	T47.1X1	T47.1X2	T47.1X3	T47.1X4	T47.1X5	T47.1X6
nicotinate	T46.7X1	T46.7X2	T46.7X3	T46.7X4	T46.7X5	T46.7X6
ointment (surgical) (topical)	T49.3X1	T49.3X2	T49.3X3	T49.3X4	T49.3X5	T49.3X6
phosphate	T47.1X1	T47.1X2	T47.1X3	T47.1X4	T47.1X5	T47.1X6
salicylate	T39.091	T39.092	T39.093	T39.094	T39.095	T39.096
silicate	T47.1X1	T47.1X2	T47.1X3	T47.1X4	T47.1X5	T47.1X6
sodium silicate	T47.1X1	T47.1X2	T47.1X3	T47.1X4	T47.1X5	T47.1X6
subacetate	T49.2X1	T49.2X2	T49.2X3	T49.2X4	T49.2X5	T49.2X6
sulfate	T49.0X1	T49.0X2	T49.0X3	T49.0X4	T49.0X5	T49.0X6
tannate	T47.6X1	T47.6X2	T47.6X3	T47.6X4	T47.6X5	T47.6X6
topical NEC	T49.3X1	T49.3X2	T49.3X3	T49.3X4	T49.3X5	T49.3X6
Alurate	T42.3X1	T42.3X2	T42.3X3	T42.3X4	T42.3X5	T42.3X6
Alverine	T44.3X1	T44.3X2	T44.3X3	T44.3X4	T44.3X5	T44.3X6
Alvodine	T40.2X1	T40.2X2	T40.2X3	T40.2X4	T40.2X5	T40.2X6
Amanita phalloides	T62.0X1	T62.0X2	T62.0X3	T62.0X4	--	--
Amanitine	T62.0X1	T62.0X2	T62.0X3	T62.0X4	--	--
Amantadine	T42.8X1	T42.8X2	T42.8X3	T42.8X4	T42.8X5	T42.8X6
Ambazone	T49.6X1	T49.6X2	T49.6X3	T49.6X4	T49.6X5	T49.6X6
Ambenonium (chloride)	T44.0X1	T44.0X2	T44.0X3	T44.0X4	T44.0X5	T44.0X6
Ambroxol	T48.4X1	T48.4X2	T48.4X3	T48.4X4	T48.4X5	T48.4X6
Ambuphylline	T48.6X1	T48.6X2	T48.6X3	T48.6X4	T48.6X5	T48.6X6

Substance	Poisoning, Accidental (unintentional)	Poisoning, Intentional self-harm	Poisoning, Assault	Poisoning, Undetermined	Adverse effect	Underdosing
Ambutonium bromide	T44.3X1	T44.3X2	T44.3X3	T44.3X4	T44.3X5	T44.3X6
Amcinonide	T49.0X1	T49.0X2	T49.0X3	T49.0X4	T49.0X5	T49.0X6
Amdinocilline	T36.0X1	T36.0X2	T36.0X3	T36.0X4	T36.0X5	T36.0X6
Ametazole	T50.8X1	T50.8X2	T50.8X3	T50.8X4	T50.8X5	T50.8X6
Amethocaine	T41.3X1	T41.3X2	T41.3X3	T41.3X4	T41.3X5	T41.3X6
- regional	T41.3X1	T41.3X2	T41.3X3	T41.3X4	T41.3X5	T41.3X6
- spinal	T41.3X1	T41.3X2	T41.3X3	T41.3X4	T41.3X5	T41.3X6
Amethopterin	T45.1X1	T45.1X2	T45.1X3	T45.1X4	T45.1X5	T45.1X6
Amezinium metilsulfate	T44.991	T44.992	T44.993	T44.994	T44.995	T44.996
Amfebutamone	T43.291	T43.292	T43.293	T43.294	T43.295	T43.296
Amfepramone	T50.5X1	T50.5X2	T50.5X3	T50.5X4	T50.5X5	T50.5X6
Amfetamine	T43.621	T43.622	T43.623	T43.624	T43.625	T43.626
Amfetaminil	T43.621	T43.622	T43.623	T43.624	T43.625	T43.626
Amfomycin	T36.8X1	T36.8X2	T36.8X3	T36.8X4	T36.8X5	T36.8X6
Amidefrine mesilate	T48.5X1	T48.5X2	T48.5X3	T48.5X4	T48.5X5	T48.5X6
Amidone	T40.3X1	T40.3X2	T40.3X3	T40.3X4	T40.3X5	T40.3X6
Amidopyrine	T39.2X1	T39.2X2	T39.2X3	T39.2X4	T39.2X5	T39.2X6
Amidotrizoate	T50.8X1	T50.8X2	T50.8X3	T50.8X4	T50.8X5	T50.8X6
Amiflamine	T43.1X1	T43.1X2	T43.1X3	T43.1X4	T43.1X5	T43.1X6
Amikacin	T36.5X1	T36.5X2	T36.5X3	T36.5X4	T36.5X5	T36.5X6
Amikhelline	T46.3X1	T46.3X2	T46.3X3	T46.3X4	T46.3X5	T46.3X6
Amiloride	T50.2X1	T50.2X2	T50.2X3	T50.2X4	T50.2X5	T50.2X6
Aminacrine	T49.0X1	T49.0X2	T49.0X3	T49.0X4	T49.0X5	T49.0X6
Amineptine	T43.011	T43.012	T43.013	T43.014	T43.015	T43.016
Aminitrozole	T37.3X1	T37.3X2	T37.3X3	T37.3X4	T37.3X5	T37.3X6
Amino acids	T50.3X1	T50.3X2	T50.3X3	T50.3X4	T50.3X5	T50.3X6
Aminoacetic acid (derivatives)	T50.3X1	T50.3X2	T50.3X3	T50.3X4	T50.3X5	T50.3X6
Aminoacridine	T49.0X1	T49.0X2	T49.0X3	T49.0X4	T49.0X5	T49.0X6
Aminobenzoic acid (-p)	T49.3X1	T49.3X2	T49.3X3	T49.3X4	T49.3X5	T49.3X6
4-Aminobutyric acid	T43.8X1	T43.8X2	T43.8X3	T43.8X4	T43.8X5	T43.8X6
Aminocaproic acid	T45.621	T45.622	T45.623	T45.624	T45.625	T45.626
Aminoethylisothiourium	T45.8X1	T45.8X2	T45.8X3	T45.8X4	T45.8X5	T45.8X6
Aminofenazone	T39.2X1	T39.2X2	T39.2X3	T39.2X4	T39.2X5	T39.2X6
Aminoglutethimide	T45.1X1	T45.1X2	T45.1X3	T45.1X4	T45.1X5	T45.1X6
Aminohippuric acid	T50.8X1	T50.8X2	T50.8X3	T50.8X4	T50.8X5	T50.8X6
Aminomethylbenzoic acid	T45.691	T45.692	T45.693	T45.694	T45.695	T45.696
Aminometradine	T50.2X1	T50.2X2	T50.2X3	T50.2X4	T50.2X5	T50.2X6
Aminopentamide	T44.3X1	T44.3X2	T44.3X3	T44.3X4	T44.3X5	T44.3X6
Aminophenazone	T39.2X1	T39.2X2	T39.2X3	T39.2X4	T39.2X5	T39.2X6
Aminophenol	T54.0X1	T54.0X2	T54.0X3	T54.0X4	--	--
4-Aminophenol derivatives	T39.1X1	T39.1X2	T39.1X3	T39.1X4	T39.1X5	T39.1X6
Aminophenylpyridone	T43.591	T43.592	T43.593	T43.594	T43.595	T43.596
Aminophylline	T48.6X1	T48.6X2	T48.6X3	T48.6X4	T48.6X5	T48.6X6
Aminopterin sodium	T45.1X1	T45.1X2	T45.1X3	T45.1X4	T45.1X5	T45.1X6
Aminopyrine	T39.2X1	T39.2X2	T39.2X3	T39.2X4	T39.2X5	T39.2X6
8-Aminoquinoline drugs	T37.2X1	T37.2X2	T37.2X3	T37.2X4	T37.2X5	T37.2X6
Aminorex	T50.5X1	T50.5X2	T50.5X3	T50.5X4	T50.5X5	T50.5X6
Aminosalicylic acid	T37.1X1	T37.1X2	T37.1X3	T37.1X4	T37.1X5	T37.1X6
Aminosalylum	T37.1X1	T37.1X2	T37.1X3	T37.1X4	T37.1X5	T37.1X6
Amiodarone	T46.2X1	T46.2X2	T46.2X3	T46.2X4	T46.2X5	T46.2X6
Amiphenazole	T50.7X1	T50.7X2	T50.7X3	T50.7X4	T50.7X5	T50.7X6
Amiquinsin	T46.5X1	T46.5X2	T46.5X3	T46.5X4	T46.5X5	T46.5X6
Amisometradine	T50.2X1	T50.2X2	T50.2X3	T50.2X4	T50.2X5	T50.2X6
Amisulpride	T43.591	T43.592	T43.593	T43.594	T43.595	T43.596
Amitriptyline	T43.011	T43.012	T43.013	T43.014	T43.015	T43.016
Amitriptylinoxide	T43.011	T43.012	T43.013	T43.014	T43.015	T43.016
Amlexanox	T48.6X1	T48.6X2	T48.6X3	T48.6X4	T48.6X5	T48.6X6
Ammonia (fumes) (gas) (vapor)	T59.891	T59.892	T59.893	T59.894	--	--
- aromatic spirit	T48.991	T48.992	T48.993	T48.994	T48.995	T48.996
- liquid (household)	T54.3X1	T54.3X2	T54.3X3	T54.3X4	--	--
Ammoniated mercury	T49.0X1	T49.0X2	T49.0X3	T49.0X4	T49.0X5	T49.0X6
Ammonium						
- acid tartrate	T49.5X1	T49.5X2	T49.5X3	T49.5X4	T49.5X5	T49.5X6
- bromide	T42.6X1	T42.6X2	T42.6X3	T42.6X4	T42.6X5	T42.6X6
- carbonate	T54.3X1	T54.3X2	T54.3X3	T54.3X4	--	--
- chloride	T50.991	T50.992	T50.993	T50.994	T50.995	T50.996
- - expectorant	T48.4X1	T48.4X2	T48.4X3	T48.4X4	T48.4X5	T48.4X6
- compounds (household) NEC	T54.3X1	T54.3X2	T54.3X3	T54.3X4	--	--
- - fumes (any usage)	T59.891	T59.892	T59.893	T59.894	--	--
- - industrial	T54.3X1	T54.3X2	T54.3X3	T54.3X4	--	--
- ichthyosulronate	T49.4X1	T49.4X2	T49.4X3	T49.4X4	T49.4X5	T49.4X6
- mandelate	T37.91	T37.92	T37.93	T37.94	T37.95	T37.96
- sulfamate	T60.3X1	T60.3X2	T60.3X3	T60.3X4	--	--
- sulfonate resin	T47.8X1	T47.8X2	T47.8X3	T47.8X4	T47.8X5	T47.8X6
Amobarbital (sodium)	T42.3X1	T42.3X2	T42.3X3	T42.3X4	T42.3X5	T42.3X6
Amodiaquine	T37.2X1	T37.2X2	T37.2X3	T37.2X4	T37.2X5	T37.2X6
Amopyroquin (e)	T37.2X1	T37.2X2	T37.2X3	T37.2X4	T37.2X5	T37.2X6
Amoxapine	T43.011	T43.012	T43.013	T43.014	T43.015	T43.016
Amoxicillin	T36.0X1	T36.0X2	T36.0X3	T36.0X4	T36.0X5	T36.0X6
Amperozide	T43.591	T43.592	T43.593	T43.594	T43.595	T43.596
Amphenidone	T43.591	T43.592	T43.593	T43.594	T43.595	T43.596
Amphetamine NEC	T43.621	T43.622	T43.623	T43.624	T43.625	T43.626
Amphomycin	T36.8X1	T36.8X2	T36.8X3	T36.8X4	T36.8X5	T36.8X6
Amphotalide	T37.4X1	T37.4X2	T37.4X3	T37.4X4	T37.4X5	T37.4X6
Amphotericin B	T36.7X1	T36.7X2	T36.7X3	T36.7X4	T36.7X5	T36.7X6
- topical	T49.0X1	T49.0X2	T49.0X3	T49.0X4	T49.0X5	T49.0X6
Ampicillin	T36.0X1	T36.0X2	T36.0X3	T36.0X4	T36.0X5	T36.0X6
Amprotropine	T44.3X1	T44.3X2	T44.3X3	T44.3X4	T44.3X5	T44.3X6
Amsacrine	T45.1X1	T45.1X2	T45.1X3	T45.1X4	T45.1X5	T45.1X6
Amygdaline	T62.2X1	T62.2X2	T62.2X3	T62.2X4	--	--
Amyl						
- acetate	T52.8X1	T52.8X2	T52.8X3	T52.8X4	--	--
- - vapor	T59.891	T59.892	T59.893	T59.894	--	--
- alcohol	T51.3X1	T51.3X2	T51.3X3	T51.3X4	--	--
- chloride	T53.6X1	T53.6X2	T53.6X3	T53.6X4	--	--
- formate	T52.8X1	T52.8X2	T52.8X3	T52.8X4	--	--
- nitrite	T46.3X1	T46.3X2	T46.3X3	T46.3X4	T46.3X5	T46.3X6
- propionate	T65.891	T65.892	T65.893	T65.894	--	--
Amylase	T47.5X1	T47.5X2	T47.5X3	T47.5X4	T47.5X5	T47.5X6
Amyleine, regional	T41.3X1	T41.3X2	T41.3X3	T41.3X4	T41.3X5	T41.3X6
Amylene						
- dichloride	T53.6X1	T53.6X2	T53.6X3	T53.6X4	--	--
- hydrate	T51.3X1	T51.3X2	T51.3X3	T51.3X4	--	--
Amylmetacresol	T49.6X1	T49.6X2	T49.6X3	T49.6X4	T49.6X5	T49.6X6
Amylobarbitone	T42.3X1	T42.3X2	T42.3X3	T42.3X4	T42.3X5	T42.3X6
Amylocaine, regional	T41.3X1	T41.3X2	T41.3X3	T41.3X4	T41.3X5	T41.3X6
- infiltration (subcutaneous)	T41.3X1	T41.3X2	T41.3X3	T41.3X4	T41.3X5	T41.3X6
- nerve block (peripheral) (plexus)	T41.3X1	T41.3X2	T41.3X3	T41.3X4	T41.3X5	T41.3X6
- spinal	T41.3X1	T41.3X2	T41.3X3	T41.3X4	T41.3X5	T41.3X6
- topical (surface)	T41.3X1	T41.3X2	T41.3X3	T41.3X4	T41.3X5	T41.3X6
Amylopectin	T47.6X1	T47.6X2	T47.6X3	T47.6X4	T47.6X5	T47.6X6
Amytal (sodium)	T42.3X1	T42.3X2	T42.3X3	T42.3X4	T42.3X5	T42.3X6
Anabolic steroid	T38.7X1	T38.7X2	T38.7X3	T38.7X4	T38.7X5	T38.7X6
Analeptic NEC	T50.7X1	T50.7X2	T50.7X3	T50.7X4	T50.7X5	T50.7X6
Analgesic	T39.91	T39.92	T39.93	T39.94	T39.95	T39.96
- anti-inflammatory NEC	T39.91	T39.92	T39.93	T39.94	T39.95	T39.96
- - propionic acid derivative	T39.311	T39.312	T39.313	T39.314	T39.315	T39.316
- antirheumatic NEC	T39.4X1	T39.4X2	T39.4X3	T39.4X4	T39.4X5	T39.4X6
- aromatic NEC	T39.1X1	T39.1X2	T39.1X3	T39.1X4	T39.1X5	T39.1X6
- narcotic NEC	T40.601	T40.602	T40.603	T40.604	T40.605	T40.606
- - combination	T40.601	T40.602	T40.603	T40.604	T40.605	T40.606
- - obstetric	T40.601	T40.602	T40.603	T40.604	T40.605	T40.606
- non-narcotic NEC	T39.91	T39.92	T39.93	T39.94	T39.95	T39.96
- - combination	T39.91	T39.92	T39.93	T39.94	T39.95	T39.96
- pyrazole	T39.2X1	T39.2X2	T39.2X3	T39.2X4	T39.2X5	T39.2X6
- specified NEC	T39.8X1	T39.8X2	T39.8X3	T39.8X4	T39.8X5	T39.8X6
Analgin	T39.2X1	T39.2X2	T39.2X3	T39.2X4	T39.2X5	T39.2X6
Anamirta cocculus	T62.1X1	T62.1X2	T62.1X3	T62.1X4	--	--
Ancillin	T36.0X1	T36.0X2	T36.0X3	T36.0X4	T36.0X5	T36.0X6
Ancrod	T45.691	T45.692	T45.693	T45.694	T45.695	T45.696
Androgen	T38.7X1	T38.7X2	T38.7X3	T38.7X4	T38.7X5	T38.7X6
Androgen-estrogen mixture	T38.7X1	T38.7X2	T38.7X3	T38.7X4	T38.7X5	T38.7X6
Androstalone	T38.7X1	T38.7X2	T38.7X3	T38.7X4	T38.7X5	T38.7X6
Androstanolone	T38.7X1	T38.7X2	T38.7X3	T38.7X4	T38.7X5	T38.7X6
Androsterone	T38.7X1	T38.7X2	T38.7X3	T38.7X4	T38.7X5	T38.7X6
Anemone pulsatilla	T62.2X1	T62.2X2	T62.2X3	T62.2X4	--	--
Anesthesia						
- caudal	T41.3X1	T41.3X2	T41.3X3	T41.3X4	T41.3X5	T41.3X6
- endotracheal	T41.0X1	T41.0X2	T41.0X3	T41.0X4	T41.0X5	T41.0X6
- epidural	T41.3X1	T41.3X2	T41.3X3	T41.3X4	T41.3X5	T41.3X6
- inhalation	T41.0X1	T41.0X2	T41.0X3	T41.0X4	T41.0X5	T41.0X6
- local	T41.3X1	T41.3X2	T41.3X3	T41.3X4	T41.3X5	T41.3X6
- mucosal	T41.3X1	T41.3X2	T41.3X3	T41.3X4	T41.3X5	T41.3X6
- muscle relaxation	T48.1X1	T48.1X2	T48.1X3	T48.1X4	T48.1X5	T48.1X6
- nerve blocking	T41.3X1	T41.3X2	T41.3X3	T41.3X4	T41.3X5	T41.3X6
- plexus blocking	T41.3X1	T41.3X2	T41.3X3	T41.3X4	T41.3X5	T41.3X6
- potentiated	T41.201	T41.202	T41.203	T41.204	T41.205	T41.206
- rectal	T41.201	T41.202	T41.203	T41.204	T41.205	T41.206
- - general	T41.201	T41.202	T41.203	T41.204	T41.205	T41.206
- - local	T41.3X1	T41.3X2	T41.3X3	T41.3X4	T41.3X5	T41.3X6
- regional	T41.3X1	T41.3X2	T41.3X3	T41.3X4	T41.3X5	T41.3X6
- surface	T41.3X1	T41.3X2	T41.3X3	T41.3X4	T41.3X5	T41.3X6
Anesthetic NEC (*see also* Anesthesia)	T41.41	T41.42	T41.43	T41.44	T41.45	T41.46
- with muscle relaxant	T41.201	T41.202	T41.203	T41.204	T41.205	T41.206
- - general	T41.201	T41.202	T41.203	T41.204	T41.205	T41.206
- - local	T41.3X1	T41.3X2	T41.3X3	T41.3X4	T41.3X5	T41.3X6
- gaseous NEC	T41.0X1	T41.0X2	T41.0X3	T41.0X4	T41.0X5	T41.0X6
- general NEC	T41.201	T41.202	T41.203	T41.204	T41.205	T41.206
- halogenated hydrocarbon derivatives NEC	T41.0X1	T41.0X2	T41.0X3	T41.0X4	T41.0X5	T41.0X6
- infiltration NEC	T41.3X1	T41.3X2	T41.3X3	T41.3X4	T41.3X5	T41.3X6
- intravenous NEC	T41.1X1	T41.1X2	T41.1X3	T41.1X4	T41.1X5	T41.1X6

Substance	Poisoning, Accidental (unintentional)	Poisoning, Intentional self-harm	Poisoning, Assault	Poisoning, Undetermined	Adverse effect	Underdosing
Anesthetic NEC — *continued*						
local NEC	T41.3X1	T41.3X2	T41.3X3	T41.3X4	T41.3X5	T41.3X6
rectal	T41.201	T41.202	T41.203	T41.204	T41.205	T41.206
general	T41.201	T41.202	T41.203	T41.204	T41.205	T41.206
local	T41.3X1	T41.3X2	T41.3X3	T41.3X4	T41.3X5	T41.3X6
regional NEC	T41.3X1	T41.3X2	T41.3X3	T41.3X4	T41.3X5	T41.3X6
spinal NEC	T41.3X1	T41.3X2	T41.3X3	T41.3X4	T41.3X5	T41.3X6
thiobarbiturate	T41.1X1	T41.1X2	T41.1X3	T41.1X4	T41.1X5	T41.1X6
topical	T41.3X1	T41.3X2	T41.3X3	T41.3X4	T41.3X5	T41.3X6
Aneurine	T45.2X1	T45.2X2	T45.2X3	T45.2X4	T45.2X5	T45.2X6
Angio-Conray	T50.8X1	T50.8X2	T50.8X3	T50.8X4	T50.8X5	T50.8X6
Angiotensin	T44.5X1	T44.5X2	T44.5X3	T44.5X4	T44.5X5	T44.5X6
Angiotensinamide	T44.991	T44.992	T44.993	T44.994	T44.995	T44.996
Anhydrohydroxy-progesterone	T38.5X1	T38.5X2	T38.5X3	T38.5X4	T38.5X5	T38.5X6
Anhydron	T50.2X1	T50.2X2	T50.2X3	T50.2X4	T50.2X5	T50.2X6
Anileridine	T40.4X1	T40.4X2	T40.4X3	T40.4X4	T40.4X5	T40.4X6
Aniline (dye) (liquid)	T65.3X1	T65.3X2	T65.3X3	T65.3X4	--	--
analgesic	T39.1X1	T39.1X2	T39.1X3	T39.1X4	T39.1X5	T39.1X6
derivatives, therapeutic NEC	T39.1X1	T39.1X2	T39.1X3	T39.1X4	T39.1X5	T39.1X6
vapor	T65.3X1	T65.3X2	T65.3X3	T65.3X4	--	--
Aniscoropine	T44.3X1	T44.3X2	T44.3X3	T44.3X4	T44.3X5	T44.3X6
Anise oil	T47.5X1	T47.5X2	T47.5X3	T47.5X4	T47.5X5	T47.5X6
Anisidine	T65.3X1	T65.3X2	T65.3X3	T65.3X4	--	--
Anisindione	T45.511	T45.512	T45.513	T45.514	T45.515	T45.516
Anisotropine methyl-bromide	T44.3X1	T44.3X2	T44.3X3	T44.3X4	T44.3X5	T44.3X6
Anistreplase	T45.611	T45.612	T45.613	T45.614	T45.615	T45.616
Anorexiant (central)	T50.5X1	T50.5X2	T50.5X3	T50.5X4	T50.5X5	T50.5X6
Anorexic agents	T50.5X1	T50.5X2	T50.5X3	T50.5X4	T50.5X5	T50.5X6
Ansamycin	T36.6X1	T36.6X2	T36.6X3	T36.6X4	T36.6X5	T36.6X6
Ant (bite) (sting)	T63.421	T63.422	T63.423	T63.424	--	--
Ant poison — *see* Insecticide						
Antabuse	T50.6X1	T50.6X2	T50.6X3	T50.6X4	T50.6X5	T50.6X6
Antacid NEC	T47.1X1	T47.1X2	T47.1X3	T47.1X4	T47.1X5	T47.1X6
Antagonist						
aldosterone	T50.0X1	T50.0X2	T50.0X3	T50.0X4	T50.0X5	T50.0X6
alpha-adrenoreceptor	T44.6X1	T44.6X2	T44.6X3	T44.6X4	T44.6X5	T44.6X6
anticoagulant	T45.7X1	T45.7X2	T45.7X3	T45.7X4	T45.7X5	T45.7X6
beta-adrenoreceptor	T44.7X1	T44.7X2	T44.7X3	T44.7X4	T44.7X5	T44.7X6
extrapyramidal NEC	T44.3X1	T44.3X2	T44.3X3	T44.3X4	T44.3X5	T44.3X6
folic acid	T45.1X1	T45.1X2	T45.1X3	T45.1X4	T45.1X5	T45.1X6
H2 receptor	T47.0X1	T47.0X2	T47.0X3	T47.0X4	T47.0X5	T47.0X6
heavy metal	T45.8X1	T45.8X2	T45.8X3	T45.8X4	T45.8X5	T45.8X6
narcotic analgesic	T50.7X1	T50.7X2	T50.7X3	T50.7X4	T50.7X5	T50.7X6
opiate	T50.7X1	T50.7X2	T50.7X3	T50.7X4	T50.7X5	T50.7X6
pyrimidine	T45.1X1	T45.1X2	T45.1X3	T45.1X4	T45.1X5	T45.1X6
serotonin	T46.5X1	T46.5X2	T46.5X3	T46.5X4	T46.5X5	T46.5X6
Antazolin (e)	T45.0X1	T45.0X2	T45.0X3	T45.0X4	T45.0X5	T45.0X6
Anterior pituitary hormone NEC	T38.811	T38.812	T38.813	T38.814	T38.815	T38.816
Anthelmintic NEC	T37.4X1	T37.4X2	T37.4X3	T37.4X4	T37.4X5	T37.4X6
Anthiolimine	T37.4X1	T37.4X2	T37.4X3	T37.4X4	T37.4X5	T37.4X6
Anthralin	T49.4X1	T49.4X2	T49.4X3	T49.4X4	T49.4X5	T49.4X6
Anthramycin	T45.1X1	T45.1X2	T45.1X3	T45.1X4	T45.1X5	T45.1X6
Antiadrenergic NEC	T44.8X1	T44.8X2	T44.8X3	T44.8X4	T44.8X5	T44.8X6
Antiallergic NEC	T45.0X1	T45.0X2	T45.0X3	T45.0X4	T45.0X5	T45.0X6
Anti-anemic (drug) (preparation)	T45.8X1	T45.8X2	T45.8X3	T45.8X4	T45.8X5	T45.8X6
Antiandrogen NEC	T38.6X1	T38.6X2	T38.6X3	T38.6X4	T38.6X5	T38.6X6
Antianxiety drug NEC	T43.501	T43.502	T43.503	T43.504	T43.505	T43.506
Antiaris toxicaria	T65.891	T65.892	T65.893	T65.894	--	--
Antiarteriosclerotic drug	T46.6X1	T46.6X2	T46.6X3	T46.6X4	T46.6X5	T46.6X6
Antiasthmatic drug NEC	T48.6X1	T48.6X2	T48.6X3	T48.6X4	T48.6X5	T48.6X6
Antibiotic NEC	T36.91	T36.92	T36.93	T36.94	T36.95	T36.96
aminoglycoside	T36.5X1	T36.5X2	T36.5X3	T36.5X4	T36.5X5	T36.5X6
anticancer	T45.1X1	T45.1X2	T45.1X3	T45.1X4	T45.1X5	T45.1X6
antifungal	T36.7X1	T36.7X2	T36.7X3	T36.7X4	T36.7X5	T36.7X6
antimycobacterial	T36.5X1	T36.5X2	T36.5X3	T36.5X4	T36.5X5	T36.5X6
antineoplastic	T45.1X1	T45.1X2	T45.1X3	T45.1X4	T45.1X5	T45.1X6
cephalosporin (group)	T36.1X1	T36.1X2	T36.1X3	T36.1X4	T36.1X5	T36.1X6
chloramphenicol (group)	T36.2X1	T36.2X2	T36.2X3	T36.2X4	T36.2X5	T36.2X6
ENT	T49.6X1	T49.6X2	T49.6X3	T49.6X4	T49.6X5	T49.6X6
eye	T49.5X1	T49.5X2	T49.5X3	T49.5X4	T49.5X5	T49.5X6
fungicidal (local)	T49.0X1	T49.0X2	T49.0X3	T49.0X4	T49.0X5	T49.0X6
intestinal	T36.8X1	T36.8X2	T36.8X3	T36.8X4	T36.8X5	T36.8X6
b-lactam NEC	T36.1X1	T36.1X2	T36.1X3	T36.1X4	T36.1X5	T36.1X6
local	T49.0X1	T49.0X2	T49.0X3	T49.0X4	T49.0X5	T49.0X6
macrolides	T36.3X1	T36.3X2	T36.3X3	T36.3X4	T36.3X5	T36.3X6
polypeptide	T36.8X1	T36.8X2	T36.8X3	T36.8X4	T36.8X5	T36.8X6
specified NEC	T36.8X1	T36.8X2	T36.8X3	T36.8X4	T36.8X5	T36.8X6
tetracycline (group)	T36.4X1	T36.4X2	T36.4X3	T36.4X4	T36.4X5	T36.4X6
throat	T49.6X1	T49.6X2	T49.6X3	T49.6X4	T49.6X5	T49.6X6
Anticancer agents NEC	T45.1X1	T45.1X2	T45.1X3	T45.1X4	T45.1X5	T45.1X6
Anticholesterolemic drug NEC	T46.6X1	T46.6X2	T46.6X3	T46.6X4	T46.6X5	T46.6X6

Substance	Poisoning, Accidental (unintentional)	Poisoning, Intentional self-harm	Poisoning, Assault	Poisoning, Undetermined	Adverse effect	Underdosing
Anticholinergic NEC	T44.3X1	T44.3X2	T44.3X3	T44.3X4	T44.3X5	T44.3X6
Anticholinesterase	T44.0X1	T44.0X2	T44.0X3	T44.0X4	T44.0X5	T44.0X6
organophosphorus	T44.0X1	T44.0X2	T44.0X3	T44.0X4	T44.0X5	T44.0X6
insecticide	T60.0X1	T60.0X2	T60.0X3	T60.0X4	--	--
nerve gas	T59.891	T59.892	T59.893	T59.894	--	--
reversible	T44.0X1	T44.0X2	T44.0X3	T44.0X4	T44.0X5	T44.0X6
ophthalmological	T49.5X1	T49.5X2	T49.5X3	T49.5X4	T49.5X5	T49.5X6
Anticoagulant NEC	T45.511	T45.512	T45.513	T45.514	T45.515	T45.516
antagonist	T45.7X1	T45.7X2	T45.7X3	T45.7X4	T45.7X5	T45.7X6
Anti-common-cold drug NEC	T48.5X1	T48.5X2	T48.5X3	T48.5X4	T48.5X5	T48.5X6
Anticonvulsant	T42.71	T42.72	T42.73	T42.74	T42.75	T42.76
barbiturate	T42.3X1	T42.3X2	T42.3X3	T42.3X4	T42.3X5	T42.3X6
combination (with barbiturate)	T42.3X1	T42.3X2	T42.3X3	T42.3X4	T42.3X5	T42.3X6
hydantoin	T42.0X1	T42.0X2	T42.0X3	T42.0X4	T42.0X5	T42.0X6
hypnotic NEC	T42.6X1	T42.6X2	T42.6X3	T42.6X4	T42.6X5	T42.6X6
oxazolidinedione	T42.2X1	T42.2X2	T42.2X3	T42.2X4	T42.2X5	T42.2X6
pyrimidinedione	T42.6X1	T42.6X2	T42.6X3	T42.6X4	T42.6X5	T42.6X6
specified NEC	T42.6X1	T42.6X2	T42.6X3	T42.6X4	T42.6X5	T42.6X6
succinimide	T42.2X1	T42.2X2	T42.2X3	T42.2X4	T42.2X5	T42.2X6
Anti-D immunoglobulin (human)	T50.Z11	T50.Z12	T50.Z13	T50.Z14	T50.Z15	T50.Z16
Antidepressant	T43.201	T43.202	T43.203	T43.204	T43.205	T43.206
monoamine oxidase inhibitor	T43.1X1	T43.1X2	T43.1X3	T43.1X4	T43.1X5	T43.1X6
selective serotonin norepinephrine reuptake inhibitor	T43.211	T43.212	T43.213	T43.214	T43.215	T43.216
selective serotonin reuptake inhibitor	T43.221	T43.222	T43.223	T43.224	T43.225	T43.226
specified NEC	T43.291	T43.292	T43.293	T43.294	T43.295	T43.296
tetracyclic	T43.021	T43.022	T43.023	T43.024	T43.025	T43.026
triazolopyridine	T43.211	T43.212	T43.213	T43.214	T43.215	T43.216
tricyclic	T43.011	T43.012	T43.013	T43.014	T43.015	T43.016
Antidiabetic NEC	T38.3X1	T38.3X2	T38.3X3	T38.3X4	T38.3X5	T38.3X6
biguanide	T38.3X1	T38.3X2	T38.3X3	T38.3X4	T38.3X5	T38.3X6
and sulfonyl combined	T38.3X1	T38.3X2	T38.3X3	T38.3X4	T38.3X5	T38.3X6
combined	T38.3X1	T38.3X2	T38.3X3	T38.3X4	T38.3X5	T38.3X6
sulfonylurea	T38.3X1	T38.3X2	T38.3X3	T38.3X4	T38.3X5	T38.3X6
Antidiarrheal drug NEC	T47.6X1	T47.6X2	T47.6X3	T47.6X4	T47.6X5	T47.6X6
absorbent	T47.6X1	T47.6X2	T47.6X3	T47.6X4	T47.6X5	T47.6X6
Antidiphtheria serum	T50.Z11	T50.Z12	T50.Z13	T50.Z14	T50.Z15	T50.Z16
Antidiuretic hormone	T38.891	T38.892	T38.893	T38.894	T38.895	T38.896
Antidote NEC	T50.6X1	T50.6X2	T50.6X3	T50.6X4	T50.6X5	T50.6X6
heavy metal	T45.8X1	T45.8X2	T45.8X3	T45.8X4	T45.8X5	T45.8X6
Antidysrhythmic NEC	T46.2X1	T46.2X2	T46.2X3	T46.2X4	T46.2X5	T46.2X6
Antiemetic drug	T45.0X1	T45.0X2	T45.0X3	T45.0X4	T45.0X5	T45.0X6
Antiepilepsy agent	T42.71	T42.72	T42.73	T42.74	T42.75	T42.76
combination	T42.5X1	T42.5X2	T42.5X3	T42.5X4	T42.5X5	T42.5X6
mixed	T42.5X1	T42.5X2	T42.5X3	T42.5X4	T42.5X5	T42.5X6
specified, NEC	T42.6X1	T42.6X2	T42.6X3	T42.6X4	T42.6X5	T42.6X6
Antiestrogen NEC	T38.6X1	T38.6X2	T38.6X3	T38.6X4	T38.6X5	T38.6X6
Antifertility pill	T38.4X1	T38.4X2	T38.4X3	T38.4X4	T38.4X5	T38.4X6
Antifibrinolytic drug	T45.621	T45.622	T45.623	T45.624	T45.625	T45.626
Antifilarial drug	T37.4X1	T37.4X2	T37.4X3	T37.4X4	T37.4X5	T37.4X6
Antiflatulent	T47.5X1	T47.5X2	T47.5X3	T47.5X4	T47.5X5	T47.5X6
Antifreeze	T65.91	T65.92	T65.93	T65.94	--	--
alcohol	T51.1X1	T51.1X2	T51.1X3	T51.1X4	--	--
ethylene glycol	T51.8X1	T51.8X2	T51.8X3	T51.8X4	--	--
Antifungal						
antibiotic (systemic)	T36.7X1	T36.7X2	T36.7X3	T36.7X4	T36.7X5	T36.7X6
anti-infective NEC	T37.91	T37.92	T37.93	T37.94	T37.95	T37.96
disinfectant, local	T49.0X1	T49.0X2	T49.0X3	T49.0X4	T49.0X5	T49.0X6
nonmedicinal (spray)	T60.3X1	T60.3X2	T60.3X3	T60.3X4	--	--
topical	T49.0X1	T49.0X2	T49.0X3	T49.0X4	T49.0X5	T49.0X6
Anti-gastric-secretion drug NEC	T47.1X1	T47.1X2	T47.1X3	T47.1X4	T47.1X5	T47.1X6
Antigonadotrophin NEC	T38.6X1	T38.6X2	T38.6X3	T38.6X4	T38.6X5	T38.6X6
Antihallucinogen	T43.501	T43.502	T43.503	T43.504	T43.505	T43.506
Antihelmintics	T37.4X1	T37.4X2	T37.4X3	T37.4X4	T37.4X5	T37.4X6
Antihemophilic						
factor	T45.8X1	T45.8X2	T45.8X3	T45.8X4	T45.8X5	T45.8X6
fraction	T45.8X1	T45.8X2	T45.8X3	T45.8X4	T45.8X5	T45.8X6
globulin concentrate	T45.7X1	T45.7X2	T45.7X3	T45.7X4	T45.7X5	T45.7X6
human plasma	T45.8X1	T45.8X2	T45.8X3	T45.8X4	T45.8X5	T45.8X6
plasma, dried	T45.7X1	T45.7X2	T45.7X3	T45.7X4	T45.7X5	T45.7X6
Antihemorrhoidal preparation	T49.2X1	T49.2X2	T49.2X3	T49.2X4	T49.2X5	T49.2X6
Antiheparin drug	T45.7X1	T45.7X2	T45.7X3	T45.7X4	T45.7X5	T45.7X6
Antihistamine	T45.0X1	T45.0X2	T45.0X3	T45.0X4	T45.0X5	T45.0X6
Antihookworm drug	T37.4X1	T37.4X2	T37.4X3	T37.4X4	T37.4X5	T37.4X6

Substance	Poisoning, Accidental (unintentional)	Poisoning, Intentional self-harm	Poisoning, Assault	Poisoning, Undetermined	Adverse effect	Underdosing
Anti-human lymphocytic globulin	T50.Z11	T50.Z12	T50.Z13	T50.Z14	T50.Z15	T50.Z16
Antihyperlipidemic drug	T46.6X1	T46.6X2	T46.6X3	T46.6X4	T46.6X5	T46.6X6
Antihypertensive drug NEC	T46.5X1	T46.5X2	T46.5X3	T46.5X4	T46.5X5	T46.5X6
Anti-infective NEC	T37.91	T37.92	T37.93	T37.94	T37.95	T37.96
anthelmintic	T37.4X1	T37.4X2	T37.4X3	T37.4X4	T37.4X5	T37.4X6
antibiotics	T36.91	T36.92	T36.93	T36.94	T36.95	T36.96
specified NEC	T36.8X1	T36.8X2	T36.8X3	T36.8X4	T36.8X5	T36.8X6
antimalarial	T37.2X1	T37.2X2	T37.2X3	T37.2X4	T37.2X5	T37.2X6
antimycobacterial NEC	T37.1X1	T37.1X2	T37.1X3	T37.1X4	T37.1X5	T37.1X6
antibiotics	T36.5X1	T36.5X2	T36.5X3	T36.5X4	T36.5X5	T36.5X6
antiprotozoal NEC	T37.3X1	T37.3X2	T37.3X3	T37.3X4	T37.3X5	T37.3X6
blood	T37.2X1	T37.2X2	T37.2X3	T37.2X4	T37.2X5	T37.2X6
antiviral	T37.5X1	T37.5X2	T37.5X3	T37.5X4	T37.5X5	T37.5X6
arsenical	T37.8X1	T37.8X2	T37.8X3	T37.8X4	T37.8X5	T37.8X6
bismuth, local	T49.0X1	T49.0X2	T49.0X3	T49.0X4	T49.0X5	T49.0X6
ENT	T49.6X1	T49.6X2	T49.6X3	T49.6X4	T49.6X5	T49.6X6
eye NEC	T49.5X1	T49.5X2	T49.5X3	T49.5X4	T49.5X5	T49.5X6
heavy metals NEC	T37.8X1	T37.8X2	T37.8X3	T37.8X4	T37.8X5	T37.8X6
local NEC	T49.0X1	T49.0X2	T49.0X3	T49.0X4	T49.0X5	T49.0X6
specified NEC	T49.0X1	T49.0X2	T49.0X3	T49.0X4	T49.0X5	T49.0X6
mixed	T37.91	T37.92	T37.93	T37.94	T37.95	T37.96
ophthalmic preparation	T49.5X1	T49.5X2	T49.5X3	T49.5X4	T49.5X5	T49.5X6
topical NEC	T49.0X1	T49.0X2	T49.0X3	T49.0X4	T49.0X5	T49.0X6
Anti-inflammatory drug NEC	T39.391	T39.392	T39.393	T39.394	T39.395	T39.396
local	T49.0X1	T49.0X2	T49.0X3	T49.0X4	T49.0X5	T49.0X6
nonsteroidal NEC	T39.391	T39.392	T39.393	T39.394	T39.395	T39.396
propionic acid derivative	T39.311	T39.312	T39.313	T39.314	T39.315	T39.316
specified NEC	T39.391	T39.392	T39.393	T39.394	T39.395	T39.396
Antikaluretic	T50.3X1	T50.3X2	T50.3X3	T50.3X4	T50.3X5	T50.3X6
Antiknock (tetraethyl lead)	T56.0X1	T56.0X2	T56.0X3	T56.0X4	--	--
Antilipemic drug NEC	T46.6X1	T46.6X2	T46.6X3	T46.6X4	T46.6X5	T46.6X6
Antimalarial	T37.2X1	T37.2X2	T37.2X3	T37.2X4	T37.2X5	T37.2X6
prophylactic NEC	T37.2X1	T37.2X2	T37.2X3	T37.2X4	T37.2X5	T37.2X6
pyrimidine derivative	T37.2X1	T37.2X2	T37.2X3	T37.2X4	T37.2X5	T37.2X6
Antimetabolite	T45.1X1	T45.1X2	T45.1X3	T45.1X4	T45.1X5	T45.1X6
Antimitotic agent	T45.1X1	T45.1X2	T45.1X3	T45.1X4	T45.1X5	T45.1X6
Antimony (compounds) (vapor) NEC	T56.891	T56.892	T56.893	T56.894	--	--
anti-infectives	T37.8X1	T37.8X2	T37.8X3	T37.8X4	T37.8X5	T37.8X6
dimercaptosuccinate	T37.3X1	T37.3X2	T37.3X3	T37.3X4	T37.3X5	T37.3X6
hydride	T56.891	T56.892	T56.893	T56.894	--	--
pesticide (vapor)	T60.8X1	T60.8X2	T60.8X3	T60.8X4	--	--
potassium (sodium) tartrate	T37.8X1	T37.8X2	T37.8X3	T37.8X4	T37.8X5	T37.8X6
sodium dimercaptosuccinate	T37.3X1	T37.3X2	T37.3X3	T37.3X4	T37.3X5	T37.3X6
tartrated	T37.8X1	T37.8X2	T37.8X3	T37.8X4	T37.8X5	T37.8X6
Antimuscarinic NEC	T44.3X1	T44.3X2	T44.3X3	T44.3X4	T44.3X5	T44.3X6
Antimycobacterial drug NEC	T37.1X1	T37.1X2	T37.1X3	T37.1X4	T37.1X5	T37.1X6
antibiotics	T36.5X1	T36.5X2	T36.5X3	T36.5X4	T36.5X5	T36.5X6
combination	T37.1X1	T37.1X2	T37.1X3	T37.1X4	T37.1X5	T37.1X6
Antinausea drug	T45.0X1	T45.0X2	T45.0X3	T45.0X4	T45.0X5	T45.0X6
Antinematode drug	T37.4X1	T37.4X2	T37.4X3	T37.4X4	T37.4X5	T37.4X6
Antineoplastic NEC	T45.1X1	T45.1X2	T45.1X3	T45.1X4	T45.1X5	T45.1X6
alkaloidal	T45.1X1	T45.1X2	T45.1X3	T45.1X4	T45.1X5	T45.1X6
antibiotics	T45.1X1	T45.1X2	T45.1X3	T45.1X4	T45.1X5	T45.1X6
combination	T45.1X1	T45.1X2	T45.1X3	T45.1X4	T45.1X5	T45.1X6
estrogen	T38.5X1	T38.5X2	T38.5X3	T38.5X4	T38.5X5	T38.5X6
steroid	T38.7X1	T38.7X2	T38.7X3	T38.7X4	T38.7X5	T38.7X6
Antiparasitic drug (systemic)	T37.91	T37.92	T37.93	T37.94	T37.95	T37.96
local	T49.0X1	T49.0X2	T49.0X3	T49.0X4	T49.0X5	T49.0X6
specified NEC	T37.8X1	T37.8X2	T37.8X3	T37.8X4	T37.8X5	T37.8X6
Antiparkinsonism drug NEC	T42.8X1	T42.8X2	T42.8X3	T42.8X4	T42.8X5	T42.8X6
Antiperspirant NEC	T49.2X1	T49.2X2	T49.2X3	T49.2X4	T49.2X5	T49.2X6
Antiphlogistic NEC	T39.4X1	T39.4X2	T39.4X3	T39.4X4	T39.4X5	T39.4X6
Antiplatyhelmintic drug	T37.4X1	T37.4X2	T37.4X3	T37.4X4	T37.4X5	T37.4X6
Antiprotozoal drug NEC	T37.3X1	T37.3X2	T37.3X3	T37.3X4	T37.3X5	T37.3X6
blood	T37.2X1	T37.2X2	T37.2X3	T37.2X4	T37.2X5	T37.2X6
local	T49.0X1	T49.0X2	T49.0X3	T49.0X4	T49.0X5	T49.0X6
Antipruritic drug NEC	T49.1X1	T49.1X2	T49.1X3	T49.1X4	T49.1X5	T49.1X6
Antipsychotic drug	T43.501	T43.502	T43.503	T43.504	T43.505	T43.506
specified NEC	T43.591	T43.592	T43.593	T43.594	T43.595	T43.596
Antipyretic	T39.91	T39.92	T39.93	T39.94	T39.95	T39.96
specified NEC	T39.8X1	T39.8X2	T39.8X3	T39.8X4	T39.8X5	T39.8X6
Antipyrine	T39.2X1	T39.2X2	T39.2X3	T39.2X4	T39.2X5	T39.2X6
Antirabies hyperimmune serum	T50.Z11	T50.Z12	T50.Z13	T50.Z14	T50.Z15	T50.Z16
Antirheumatic NEC	T39.4X1	T39.4X2	T39.4X3	T39.4X4	T39.4X5	T39.4X6
Antirigidity drug NEC	T42.8X1	T42.8X2	T42.8X3	T42.8X4	T42.8X5	T42.8X6
Antischistosomal drug	T37.4X1	T37.4X2	T37.4X3	T37.4X4	T37.4X5	T37.4X6
Antiscorpion sera	T50.Z11	T50.Z12	T50.Z13	T50.Z14	T50.Z15	T50.Z16
Antiseborrheics	T49.4X1	T49.4X2	T49.4X3	T49.4X4	T49.4X5	T49.4X6
Antiseptics (external) (medicinal)	T49.0X1	T49.0X2	T49.0X3	T49.0X4	T49.0X5	T49.0X6

Substance	Poisoning, Accidental (unintentional)	Poisoning, Intentional self-harm	Poisoning, Assault	Poisoning, Undetermined	Adverse effect	Underdosing
Antistine	T45.0X1	T45.0X2	T45.0X3	T45.0X4	T45.0X5	T45.0X6
Antitapeworm drug	T37.4X1	T37.4X2	T37.4X3	T37.4X4	T37.4X5	T37.4X6
Antitetanus immunoglobulin	T50.Z11	T50.Z12	T50.Z13	T50.Z14	T50.Z15	T50.Z16
Antithrombotic	T45.521	T45.522	T45.523	T45.524	T45.525	T45.526
Antithyroid drug NEC	T38.2X1	T38.2X2	T38.2X3	T38.2X4	T38.2X5	T38.2X6
Antitoxin	T50.Z11	T50.Z12	T50.Z13	T50.Z14	T50.Z15	T50.Z16
diphtheria	T50.Z11	T50.Z12	T50.Z13	T50.Z14	T50.Z15	T50.Z16
gas gangrene	T50.Z11	T50.Z12	T50.Z13	T50.Z14	T50.Z15	T50.Z16
tetanus	T50.Z11	T50.Z12	T50.Z13	T50.Z14	T50.Z15	T50.Z16
Antitrichomonal drug	T37.3X1	T37.3X2	T37.3X3	T37.3X4	T37.3X5	T37.3X6
Antituberculars	T37.1X1	T37.1X2	T37.1X3	T37.1X4	T37.1X5	T37.1X6
antibiotics	T36.5X1	T36.5X2	T36.5X3	T36.5X4	T36.5X5	T36.5X6
Antitussive NEC	T48.3X1	T48.3X2	T48.3X3	T48.3X4	T48.3X5	T48.3X6
codeine mixture	T40.2X1	T40.2X2	T40.2X3	T40.2X4	T40.2X5	T40.2X6
opiate	T40.2X1	T40.2X2	T40.2X3	T40.2X4	T40.2X5	T40.2X6
Antivaricose drug	T46.8X1	T46.8X2	T46.8X3	T46.8X4	T46.8X5	T46.8X6
Antivenin, antivenom (sera)	T50.Z11	T50.Z12	T50.Z13	T50.Z14	T50.Z15	T50.Z16
crotaline	T50.Z11	T50.Z12	T50.Z13	T50.Z14	T50.Z15	T50.Z16
spider bite	T50.Z11	T50.Z12	T50.Z13	T50.Z14	T50.Z15	T50.Z16
Antivertigo drug	T45.0X1	T45.0X2	T45.0X3	T45.0X4	T45.0X5	T45.0X6
Antiviral drug NEC	T37.5X1	T37.5X2	T37.5X3	T37.5X4	T37.5X5	T37.5X6
eye	T49.5X1	T49.5X2	T49.5X3	T49.5X4	T49.5X5	T49.5X6
Antiwhipworm drug	T37.4X1	T37.4X2	T37.4X3	T37.4X4	T37.4X5	T37.4X6
Antrol (*see also* by specific chemical substance)	T60.91	T60.92	T60.93	T60.94	--	--
fungicide	T60.91	T60.92	T60.93	T60.94	--	--
ANTU (alpha naphthylthiourea)	T60.4X1	T60.4X2	T60.4X3	T60.4X4	--	--
Apalcillin	T36.0X1	T36.0X2	T36.0X3	T36.0X4	T36.0X5	T36.0X6
APC	T48.5X1	T48.5X2	T48.5X3	T48.5X4	T48.5X5	T48.5X6
Aplonidine	T44.4X1	T44.4X2	T44.4X3	T44.4X4	T44.4X5	T44.4X6
Apomorphine	T47.7X1	T47.7X2	T47.7X3	T47.7X4	T47.7X5	T47.7X6
Appetite depressants, central	T50.5X1	T50.5X2	T50.5X3	T50.5X4	T50.5X5	T50.5X6
Apraclonidine (hydrochloride)	T44.4X1	T44.4X2	T44.4X3	T44.4X4	T44.4X5	T44.4X6
Apresoline	T46.5X1	T46.5X2	T46.5X3	T46.5X4	T46.5X5	T46.5X6
Aprindine	T46.2X1	T46.2X2	T46.2X3	T46.2X4	T46.2X5	T46.2X6
Aprobarbital	T42.3X1	T42.3X2	T42.3X3	T42.3X4	T42.3X5	T42.3X6
Apronalide	T42.6X1	T42.6X2	T42.6X3	T42.6X4	T42.6X5	T42.6X6
Aprotinin	T45.621	T45.622	T45.623	T45.624	T45.625	T45.626
Aptocaine	T41.3X1	T41.3X2	T41.3X3	T41.3X4	T41.3X5	T41.3X6
Aqua fortis	T54.2X1	T54.2X2	T54.2X3	T54.2X4	--	--
Ara-A	T37.5X1	T37.5X2	T37.5X3	T37.5X4	T37.5X5	T37.5X6
Ara-C	T45.1X1	T45.1X2	T45.1X3	T45.1X4	T45.1X5	T45.1X6
Arachis oil	T49.3X1	T49.3X2	T49.3X3	T49.3X4	T49.3X5	T49.3X6
cathartic	T47.4X1	T47.4X2	T47.4X3	T47.4X4	T47.4X5	T47.4X6
Aralen	T37.2X1	T37.2X2	T37.2X3	T37.2X4	T37.2X5	T37.2X6
Arecoline	T44.1X1	T44.1X2	T44.1X3	T44.1X4	T44.1X5	T44.1X6
Arginine	T50.991	T50.992	T50.993	T50.994	T50.995	T50.996
glutamate	T50.991	T50.992	T50.993	T50.994	T50.995	T50.996
Argyrol	T49.0X1	T49.0X2	T49.0X3	T49.0X4	T49.0X5	T49.0X6
ENT agent	T49.6X1	T49.6X2	T49.6X3	T49.6X4	T49.6X5	T49.6X6
ophthalmic preparation	T49.5X1	T49.5X2	T49.5X3	T49.5X4	T49.5X5	T49.5X6
Aristocort	T38.0X1	T38.0X2	T38.0X3	T38.0X4	T38.0X5	T38.0X6
ENT agent	T49.6X1	T49.6X2	T49.6X3	T49.6X4	T49.6X5	T49.6X6
ophthalmic preparation	T49.5X1	T49.5X2	T49.5X3	T49.5X4	T49.5X5	T49.5X6
topical NEC	T49.0X1	T49.0X2	T49.0X3	T49.0X4	T49.0X5	T49.0X6
Aromatics, corrosive	T54.1X1	T54.1X2	T54.1X3	T54.1X4	--	--
disinfectants	T54.1X1	T54.1X2	T54.1X3	T54.1X4	--	--
Arsenate of lead	T57.0X1	T57.0X2	T57.0X3	T57.0X4	--	--
herbicide	T57.0X1	T57.0X2	T57.0X3	T57.0X4	--	--
Arsenic, arsenicals (compounds) (dust) (vapor) **NEC**	T57.0X1	T57.0X2	T57.0X3	T57.0X4	--	--
anti-infectives	T37.8X1	T37.8X2	T37.8X3	T37.8X4	T37.8X5	T37.8X6
pesticide (dust) (fumes)	T57.0X1	T57.0X2	T57.0X3	T57.0X4	--	--
Arsine (gas)	T57.0X1	T57.0X2	T57.0X3	T57.0X4	--	--
Arsphenamine (silver)	T37.8X1	T37.8X2	T37.8X3	T37.8X4	T37.8X5	T37.8X6
Arsthinol	T37.3X1	T37.3X2	T37.3X3	T37.3X4	T37.3X5	T37.3X6
Artane	T44.3X1	T44.3X2	T44.3X3	T44.3X4	T44.3X5	T44.3X6
Arthropod (venomous) **NEC**	T63.481	T63.482	T63.483	T63.484	--	--
Articaine	T41.3X1	T41.3X2	T41.3X3	T41.3X4	T41.3X5	T41.3X6
Asbestos	T57.8X1	T57.8X2	T57.8X3	T57.8X4	--	--
Ascaridole	T37.4X1	T37.4X2	T37.4X3	T37.4X4	T37.4X5	T37.4X6
Ascorbic acid	T45.2X1	T45.2X2	T45.2X3	T45.2X4	T45.2X5	T45.2X6
Asiaticoside	T49.0X1	T49.0X2	T49.0X3	T49.0X4	T49.0X5	T49.0X6
Asparaginase	T45.1X1	T45.1X2	T45.1X3	T45.1X4	T45.1X5	T45.1X6
Aspidium (oleoresin)	T37.4X1	T37.4X2	T37.4X3	T37.4X4	T37.4X5	T37.4X6
Aspirin (aluminum) (soluble)	T39.011	T39.012	T39.013	T39.014	T39.015	T39.016
Aspoxicillin	T36.0X1	T36.0X2	T36.0X3	T36.0X4	T36.0X5	T36.0X6
Astemizole	T45.0X1	T45.0X2	T45.0X3	T45.0X4	T45.0X5	T45.0X6
Astringent (local)	T49.2X1	T49.2X2	T49.2X3	T49.2X4	T49.2X5	T49.2X6
specified NEC	T49.2X1	T49.2X2	T49.2X3	T49.2X4	T49.2X5	T49.2X6
Astromicin	T36.5X1	T36.5X2	T36.5X3	T36.5X4	T36.5X5	T36.5X6
Ataractic drug NEC	T43.501	T43.502	T43.503	T43.504	T43.505	T43.506
Atenolol	T44.7X1	T44.7X2	T44.7X3	T44.7X4	T44.7X5	T44.7X6
Atonia drug, intestinal	T47.4X1	T47.4X2	T47.4X3	T47.4X4	T47.4X5	T47.4X6

Anti-human lymphocytic globulin - Atonia drug, intestinal

ICD-10-CM TABLE OF DRUGS AND CHEMICALS

Atophan - Benzothiadiazides

Substance	Poisoning, Accidental (unintentional)	Poisoning, Intentional self-harm	Poisoning, Assault	Poisoning, Undetermined	Adverse effect	Underdosing
Atophan	T50.4X1	T50.4X2	T50.4X3	T50.4X4	T50.4X5	T50.4X6
Atracurium besilate	T48.1X1	T48.1X2	T48.1X3	T48.1X4	T48.1X5	T48.1X6
Atropine	T44.3X1	T44.3X2	T44.3X3	T44.3X4	T44.3X5	T44.3X6
derivative	T44.3X1	T44.3X2	T44.3X3	T44.3X4	T44.3X5	T44.3X6
methonitrate	T44.3X1	T44.3X2	T44.3X3	T44.3X4	T44.3X5	T44.3X6
Attapulgite	T47.6X1	T47.6X2	T47.6X3	T47.6X4	T47.6X5	T47.6X6
Auramine	T65.891	T65.892	T65.893	T65.894	--	--
dye	T65.6X1	T65.6X2	T65.6X3	T65.6X4	--	--
fungicide	T60.3X1	T60.3X2	T60.3X3	T60.3X4	--	--
Auranofin	T39.4X1	T39.4X2	T39.4X3	T39.4X4	T39.4X5	T39.4X6
Aurantiin	T46.991	T46.992	T46.993	T46.994	T46.995	T46.996
Aureomycin	T36.4X1	T36.4X2	T36.4X3	T36.4X4	T36.4X5	T36.4X6
ophthalmic preparation	T49.5X1	T49.5X2	T49.5X3	T49.5X4	T49.5X5	T49.5X6
topical NEC	T49.0X1	T49.0X2	T49.0X3	T49.0X4	T49.0X5	T49.0X6
Aurothioglucose	T39.4X1	T39.4X2	T39.4X3	T39.4X4	T39.4X5	T39.4X6
Aurothioglycanide	T39.4X1	T39.4X2	T39.4X3	T39.4X4	T39.4X5	T39.4X6
Aurothiomalate sodium	T39.4X1	T39.4X2	T39.4X3	T39.4X4	T39.4X5	T39.4X6
Aurotioprol	T39.4X1	T39.4X2	T39.4X3	T39.4X4	T39.4X5	T39.4X6
Automobile fuel	T52.0X1	T52.0X2	T52.0X3	T52.0X4	--	--
Autonomic nervous system agent NEC	T44.901	T44.902	T44.903	T44.904	T44.905	T44.906
Avlosulfon	T37.1X1	T37.1X2	T37.1X3	T37.1X4	T37.1X5	T37.1X6
Avomine	T42.6X1	T42.6X2	T42.6X3	T42.6X4	T42.6X5	T42.6X6
Axerophthol	T45.2X1	T45.2X2	T45.2X3	T45.2X4	T45.2X5	T45.2X6
Azacitidine	T45.1X1	T45.1X2	T45.1X3	T45.1X4	T45.1X5	T45.1X6
Azacyclonol	T43.591	T43.592	T43.593	T43.594	T43.595	T43.596
Azadirachta	T60.2X1	T60.2X2	T60.2X3	T60.2X4	--	--
Azanidazole	T37.3X1	T37.3X2	T37.3X3	T37.3X4	T37.3X5	T37.3X6
Azapetine	T46.7X1	T46.7X2	T46.7X3	T46.7X4	T46.7X5	T46.7X6
Azapropazone	T39.2X1	T39.2X2	T39.2X3	T39.2X4	T39.2X5	T39.2X6
Azaribine	T45.1X1	T45.1X2	T45.1X3	T45.1X4	T45.1X5	T45.1X6
Azaserine	T45.1X1	T45.1X2	T45.1X3	T45.1X4	T45.1X5	T45.1X6
Azatadine	T45.0X1	T45.0X2	T45.0X3	T45.0X4	T45.0X5	T45.0X6
Azatepa	T45.1X1	T45.1X2	T45.1X3	T45.1X4	T45.1X5	T45.1X6
Azathioprine	T45.1X1	T45.1X2	T45.1X3	T45.1X4	T45.1X5	T45.1X6
Azelaic acid	T49.0X1	T49.0X2	T49.0X3	T49.0X4	T49.0X5	T49.0X6
Azelastine	T45.0X1	T45.0X2	T45.0X3	T45.0X4	T45.0X5	T45.0X6
Azidocillin	T36.0X1	T36.0X2	T36.0X3	T36.0X4	T36.0X5	T36.0X6
Azidothymidine	T37.5X1	T37.5X2	T37.5X3	T37.5X4	T37.5X5	T37.5X6
Azinphos (ethyl) (methyl)	T60.0X1	T60.0X2	T60.0X3	T60.0X4	--	--
Aziridine (chelating)	T54.1X1	T54.1X2	T54.1X3	T54.1X4	--	--
Azithromycin	T36.3X1	T36.3X2	T36.3X3	T36.3X4	T36.3X5	T36.3X6
Azlocillin	T36.0X1	T36.0X2	T36.0X3	T36.0X4	T36.0X5	T36.0X6
Azobenzene smoke	T65.3X1	T65.3X2	T65.3X3	T65.3X4	--	--
acaricide	T60.8X1	T60.8X2	T60.8X3	T60.8X4	--	--
Azosulfamide	T37.0X1	T37.0X2	T37.0X3	T37.0X4	T37.0X5	T37.0X6
AZT	T37.5X1	T37.5X2	T37.5X3	T37.5X4	T37.5X5	T37.5X6
Aztreonam	T36.1X1	T36.1X2	T36.1X3	T36.1X4	T36.1X5	T36.1X6
Azulfidine	T37.0X1	T37.0X2	T37.0X3	T37.0X4	T37.0X5	T37.0X6
Azuresin	T50.8X1	T50.8X2	T50.8X3	T50.8X4	T50.8X5	T50.8X6
B						
Bacampicillin	T36.0X1	T36.0X2	T36.0X3	T36.0X4	T36.0X5	T36.0X6
Bacillus						
lactobacillus	T47.8X1	T47.8X2	T47.8X3	T47.8X4	T47.8X5	T47.8X6
subtilis	T47.6X1	T47.6X2	T47.6X3	T47.6X4	T47.6X5	T47.6X6
Bacimycin	T49.0X1	T49.0X2	T49.0X3	T49.0X4	T49.0X5	T49.0X6
ophthalmic preparation	T49.5X1	T49.5X2	T49.5X3	T49.5X4	T49.5X5	T49.5X6
Bacitracin zinc	T49.0X1	T49.0X2	T49.0X3	T49.0X4	T49.0X5	T49.0X6
with neomycin	T49.0X1	T49.0X2	T49.0X3	T49.0X4	T49.0X5	T49.0X6
ENT agent	T49.6X1	T49.6X2	T49.6X3	T49.6X4	T49.6X5	T49.6X6
ophthalmic preparation	T49.5X1	T49.5X2	T49.5X3	T49.5X4	T49.5X5	T49.5X6
topical NEC	T49.0X1	T49.0X2	T49.0X3	T49.0X4	T49.0X5	T49.0X6
Baclofen	T42.8X1	T42.8X2	T42.8X3	T42.8X4	T42.8X5	T42.8X6
Baking soda	T50.991	T50.992	T50.993	T50.994	T50.995	T50.996
BAL	T45.8X1	T45.8X2	T45.8X3	T45.8X4	T45.8X5	T45.8X6
Bambuterol	T48.6X1	T48.6X2	T48.6X3	T48.6X4	T48.6X5	T48.6X6
Bamethan (sulfate)	T46.7X1	T46.7X2	T46.7X3	T46.7X4	T46.7X5	T46.7X6
Bamifylline	T48.6X1	T48.6X2	T48.6X3	T48.6X4	T48.6X5	T48.6X6
Bamipine	T45.0X1	T45.0X2	T45.0X3	T45.0X4	T45.0X5	T45.0X6
Baneberry — *see* Actaea spicata						
Banewort — *see* Belladonna						
Barbenyl	T42.3X1	T42.3X2	T42.3X3	T42.3X4	T42.3X5	T42.3X6
Barbexaclone	T42.6X1	T42.6X2	T42.6X3	T42.6X4	T42.6X5	T42.6X6
Barbital	T42.3X1	T42.3X2	T42.3X3	T42.3X4	T42.3X5	T42.3X6
sodium	T42.3X1	T42.3X2	T42.3X3	T42.3X4	T42.3X5	T42.3X6
Barbitone	T42.3X1	T42.3X2	T42.3X3	T42.3X4	T42.3X5	T42.3X6
Barbiturate NEC	T42.3X1	T42.3X2	T42.3X3	T42.3X4	T42.3X5	T42.3X6
with tranquilizer	T42.3X1	T42.3X2	T42.3X3	T42.3X4	T42.3X5	T42.3X6
anesthetic (intravenous)	T41.1X1	T41.1X2	T41.1X3	T41.1X4	T41.1X5	T41.1X6
Barium (carbonate) (chloride) (sulfite)	T57.8X1	T57.8X2	T57.8X3	T57.8X4	--	--
diagnostic agent	T50.8X1	T50.8X2	T50.8X3	T50.8X4	T50.8X5	T50.8X6
pesticide	T60.4X1	T60.4X2	T60.4X3	T60.4X4	--	--
rodenticide	T60.4X1	T60.4X2	T60.4X3	T60.4X4	--	--
sulfate (medicinal)	T50.8X1	T50.8X2	T50.8X3	T50.8X4	T50.8X5	T50.8X6
Barrier cream	T49.3X1	T49.3X2	T49.3X3	T49.3X4	T49.3X5	T49.3X6
Basic fuchsin	T49.0X1	T49.0X2	T49.0X3	T49.0X4	T49.0X5	T49.0X6
Battery acid or fluid	T54.2X1	T54.2X2	T54.2X3	T54.2X4	--	--
Bay rum	T51.8X1	T51.8X2	T51.8X3	T51.8X4	--	--
BCG (vaccine)	T50.A91	T50.A92	T50.A93	T50.A94	T50.A95	T50.A96
BCNU	T45.1X1	T45.1X2	T45.1X3	T45.1X4	T45.1X5	T45.1X6
Bearsfoot	T62.2X1	T62.2X2	T62.2X3	T62.2X4	--	--
Beclamide	T42.6X1	T42.6X2	T42.6X3	T42.6X4	T42.6X5	T42.6X6
Beclomethasone	T44.5X1	T44.5X2	T44.5X3	T44.5X4	T44.5X5	T44.5X6
Bee (sting) (venom)	T63.441	T63.442	T63.443	T63.444	--	--
Befunolol	T49.5X1	T49.5X2	T49.5X3	T49.5X4	T49.5X5	T49.5X6
Bekanamycin	T36.5X1	T36.5X2	T36.5X3	T36.5X4	T36.5X5	T36.5X6
Belladonna (*see also* Nightshade)						
alkaloids	T44.3X1	T44.3X2	T44.3X3	T44.3X4	T44.3X5	T44.3X6
extract	T44.3X1	T44.3X2	T44.3X3	T44.3X4	T44.3X5	T44.3X6
herb	T44.3X1	T44.3X2	T44.3X3	T44.3X4	T44.3X5	T44.3X6
Bemegride	T50.7X1	T50.7X2	T50.7X3	T50.7X4	T50.7X5	T50.7X6
Benactyzine	T44.3X1	T44.3X2	T44.3X3	T44.3X4	T44.3X5	T44.3X6
Benadryl	T45.0X1	T45.0X2	T45.0X3	T45.0X4	T45.0X5	T45.0X6
Benaprizine	T44.3X1	T44.3X2	T44.3X3	T44.3X4	T44.3X5	T44.3X6
Benazepril	T46.4X1	T46.4X2	T46.4X3	T46.4X4	T46.4X5	T46.4X6
Bencyclane	T46.7X1	T46.7X2	T46.7X3	T46.7X4	T46.7X5	T46.7X6
Bendazol	T46.3X1	T46.3X2	T46.3X3	T46.3X4	T46.3X5	T46.3X6
Bendrofluazide	T50.2X1	T50.2X2	T50.2X3	T50.2X4	T50.2X5	T50.2X6
Bendroflumethiazide	T50.2X1	T50.2X2	T50.2X3	T50.2X4	T50.2X5	T50.2X6
Benemid	T50.4X1	T50.4X2	T50.4X3	T50.4X4	T50.4X5	T50.4X6
Benethamine penicillin	T36.0X1	T36.0X2	T36.0X3	T36.0X4	T36.0X5	T36.0X6
Benexate	T47.1X1	T47.1X2	T47.1X3	T47.1X4	T47.1X5	T47.1X6
Benfluorex	T46.6X1	T46.6X2	T46.6X3	T46.6X4	T46.6X5	T46.6X6
Benfotiamine	T45.2X1	T45.2X2	T45.2X3	T45.2X4	T45.2X5	T45.2X6
Benisone	T49.0X1	T49.0X2	T49.0X3	T49.0X4	T49.0X5	T49.0X6
Benomyl	T60.0X1	T60.0X2	T60.0X3	T60.0X4	--	--
Benoquin	T49.8X1	T49.8X2	T49.8X3	T49.8X4	T49.8X5	T49.8X6
Benoxinate	T41.3X1	T41.3X2	T41.3X3	T41.3X4	T41.3X5	T41.3X6
Benperidol	T43.4X1	T43.4X2	T43.4X3	T43.4X4	T43.4X5	T43.4X6
Benproperine	T48.3X1	T48.3X2	T48.3X3	T48.3X4	T48.3X5	T48.3X6
Benserazide	T42.8X1	T42.8X2	T42.8X3	T42.8X4	T42.8X5	T42.8X6
Bentazepam	T42.4X1	T42.4X2	T42.4X3	T42.4X4	T42.4X5	T42.4X6
Bentiromide	T50.8X1	T50.8X2	T50.8X3	T50.8X4	T50.8X5	T50.8X6
Bentonite	T49.3X1	T49.3X2	T49.3X3	T49.3X4	T49.3X5	T49.3X6
Benzalbutyramide	T46.6X1	T46.6X2	T46.6X3	T46.6X4	T46.6X5	T46.6X6
Benzalkonium (chloride)	T49.0X1	T49.0X2	T49.0X3	T49.0X4	T49.0X5	T49.0X6
ophthalmic preparation	T49.5X1	T49.5X2	T49.5X3	T49.5X4	T49.5X5	T49.5X6
Benzamidosalicylate (calcium)	T37.1X1	T37.1X2	T37.1X3	T37.1X4	T37.1X5	T37.1X6
Benzamine	T41.3X1	T41.3X2	T41.3X3	T41.3X4	T41.3X5	T41.3X6
lactate	T49.1X1	T49.1X2	T49.1X3	T49.1X4	T49.1X5	T49.1X6
Benzamphetamine	T50.5X1	T50.5X2	T50.5X3	T50.5X4	T50.5X5	T50.5X6
Benzapril hydrochloride	T46.5X1	T46.5X2	T46.5X3	T46.5X4	T46.5X5	T46.5X6
Benzathine benzylpenicillin	T36.0X1	T36.0X2	T36.0X3	T36.0X4	T36.0X5	T36.0X6
Benzathine penicillin	T36.0X1	T36.0X2	T36.0X3	T36.0X4	T36.0X5	T36.0X6
Benzatropine	T42.8X1	T42.8X2	T42.8X3	T42.8X4	T42.8X5	T42.8X6
Benzbromarone	T50.4X1	T50.4X2	T50.4X3	T50.4X4	T50.4X5	T50.4X6
Benzcarbimine	T45.1X1	T45.1X2	T45.1X3	T45.1X4	T45.1X5	T45.1X6
Benzedrex	T44.991	T44.992	T44.993	T44.994	T44.995	T44.996
Benzedrine (amphetamine)	T43.621	T43.622	T43.623	T43.624	T43.625	T43.626
Benzenamine	T65.3X1	T65.3X2	T65.3X3	T65.3X4	--	--
Benzene	T52.1X1	T52.1X2	T52.1X3	T52.1X4	--	--
homologues (acetyl) (dimethyl)(methyl) (solvent)	T52.2X1	T52.2X2	T52.2X3	T52.2X4	--	--
Benzethonium (chloride)	T49.0X1	T49.0X2	T49.0X3	T49.0X4	T49.0X5	T49.0X6
Benzfetamine	T50.5X1	T50.5X2	T50.5X3	T50.5X4	T50.5X5	T50.5X6
Benzhexol	T44.3X1	T44.3X2	T44.3X3	T44.3X4	T44.3X5	T44.3X6
Benzhydramine (chloride)	T45.0X1	T45.0X2	T45.0X3	T45.0X4	T45.0X5	T45.0X6
Benzidine	T65.891	T65.892	T65.893	T65.894	--	--
Benzilonium bromide	T44.3X1	T44.3X2	T44.3X3	T44.3X4	T44.3X5	T44.3X6
Benzimidazole	T60.3X1	T60.3X2	T60.3X3	T60.3X4	--	--
Benzin (e) — *see* Ligroin						
Benziodarone	T46.3X1	T46.3X2	T46.3X3	T46.3X4	T46.3X5	T46.3X6
Benznidazole	T37.3X1	T37.3X2	T37.3X3	T37.3X4	T37.3X5	T37.3X6
Benzocaine	T41.3X1	T41.3X2	T41.3X3	T41.3X4	T41.3X5	T41.3X6
Benzodiapin	T42.4X1	T42.4X2	T42.4X3	T42.4X4	T42.4X5	T42.4X6
Benzodiazepine NEC	T42.4X1	T42.4X2	T42.4X3	T42.4X4	T42.4X5	T42.4X6
Benzoic acid	T49.0X1	T49.0X2	T49.0X3	T49.0X4	T49.0X5	T49.0X6
with salicylic acid	T49.0X1	T49.0X2	T49.0X3	T49.0X4	T49.0X5	T49.0X6
Benzoin (tincture)	T48.5X1	T48.5X2	T48.5X3	T48.5X4	T48.5X5	T48.5X6
Benzol (benzene)	T52.1X1	T52.1X2	T52.1X3	T52.1X4	--	--
vapor	T52.0X1	T52.0X2	T52.0X3	T52.0X4	--	--
Benzomorphan	T40.2X1	T40.2X2	T40.2X3	T40.2X4	T40.2X5	T40.2X6
Benzonatate	T48.3X1	T48.3X2	T48.3X3	T48.3X4	T48.3X5	T48.3X6
Benzophenones	T49.3X1	T49.3X2	T49.3X3	T49.3X4	T49.3X5	T49.3X6
Benzopyrone	T46.991	T46.992	T46.993	T46.994	T46.995	T46.996
Benzothiadiazides	T50.2X1	T50.2X2	T50.2X3	T50.2X4	T50.2X5	T50.2X6

Substance	Poisoning, Accidental (unintentional)	Poisoning, Intentional self-harm	Poisoning, Assault	Poisoning, Undetermined	Adverse effect	Underdosing
Benzoxonium chloride	T49.0X1	T49.0X2	T49.0X3	T49.0X4	T49.0X5	T49.0X6
Benzoyl peroxide	T49.0X1	T49.0X2	T49.0X3	T49.0X4	T49.0X5	T49.0X6
Benzoylpas calcium	T37.1X1	T37.1X2	T37.1X3	T37.1X4	T37.1X5	T37.1X6
Benzperidin	T43.591	T43.592	T43.593	T43.594	T43.595	T43.596
Benzperidol	T43.591	T43.592	T43.593	T43.594	T43.595	T43.596
Benzphetamine	T50.5X1	T50.5X2	T50.5X3	T50.5X4	T50.5X5	T50.5X6
Benzpyrinium bromide	T44.1X1	T44.1X2	T44.1X3	T44.1X4	T44.1X5	T44.1X6
Benzquinamide	T45.0X1	T45.0X2	T45.0X3	T45.0X4	T45.0X5	T45.0X6
Benzthiazide	T50.2X1	T50.2X2	T50.2X3	T50.2X4	T50.2X5	T50.2X6
Benztropine						
anticholinergic	T44.3X1	T44.3X2	T44.3X3	T44.3X4	T44.3X5	T44.3X6
antiparkinson	T42.8X1	T42.8X2	T42.8X3	T42.8X4	T42.8X5	T42.8X6
Benzydamine	T49.0X1	T49.0X2	T49.0X3	T49.0X4	T49.0X5	T49.0X6
Benzyl						
acetate	T52.8X1	T52.8X2	T52.8X3	T52.8X4	--	--
alcohol	T49.0X1	T49.0X2	T49.0X3	T49.0X4	T49.0X5	T49.0X6
benzoate	T49.0X1	T49.0X2	T49.0X3	T49.0X4	T49.0X5	T49.0X6
benzoic acid	T49.0X1	T49.0X2	T49.0X3	T49.0X4	T49.0X5	T49.0X6
morphine	T40.2X1	T40.2X2	T40.2X3	T40.2X4	--	--
nicotinate	T46.6X1	T46.6X2	T46.6X3	T46.6X4	T46.6X5	T46.6X6
penicillin	T36.0X1	T36.0X2	T36.0X3	T36.0X4	T36.0X5	T36.0X6
Benzylhydrochlorthia-zide	T50.2X1	T50.2X2	T50.2X3	T50.2X4	T50.2X5	T50.2X6
Benzylpenicillin	T36.0X1	T36.0X2	T36.0X3	T36.0X4	T36.0X5	T36.0X6
Benzylthiouracil	T38.2X1	T38.2X2	T38.2X3	T38.2X4	T38.2X5	T38.2X6
Bephenium hydroxy-naphthoate	T37.4X1	T37.4X2	T37.4X3	T37.4X4	T37.4X5	T37.4X6
Bepridil	T46.1X1	T46.1X2	T46.1X3	T46.1X4	T46.1X5	T46.1X6
Bergamot oil	T65.891	T65.892	T65.893	T65.894	--	--
Bergapten	T50.991	T50.992	T50.993	T50.994	T50.995	T50.996
Berries, poisonous	T62.1X1	T62.1X2	T62.1X3	T62.1X4	--	--
Beryllium (compounds)	T56.7X1	T56.7X2	T56.7X3	T56.7X4	--	--
b-acetyldigoxin	T46.0X1	T46.0X2	T46.0X3	T46.0X4	T46.0X5	T46.0X6
beta adrenergic blocking agent, heart	T44.7X1	T44.7X2	T44.7X3	T44.7X4	T44.7X5	T44.7X6
b-benzalbutyramide	T46.6X1	T46.6X2	T46.6X3	T46.6X4	T46.6X5	T46.6X6
Betacarotene	T45.2X1	T45.2X2	T45.2X3	T45.2X4	T45.2X5	T45.2X6
b-eucaine	T49.1X1	T49.1X2	T49.1X3	T49.1X4	T49.1X5	T49.1X6
Beta-Chlor	T42.6X1	T42.6X2	T42.6X3	T42.6X4	T42.6X5	T42.6X6
b-galactosidase	T47.5X1	T47.5X2	T47.5X3	T47.5X4	T47.5X5	T47.5X6
Betahistine	T46.7X1	T46.7X2	T46.7X3	T46.7X4	T46.7X5	T46.7X6
Betaine	T47.5X1	T47.5X2	T47.5X3	T47.5X4	T47.5X5	T47.5X6
Betamethasone	T49.0X1	T49.0X2	T49.0X3	T49.0X4	T49.0X5	T49.0X6
topical	T49.0X1	T49.0X2	T49.0X3	T49.0X4	T49.0X5	T49.0X6
Betamicin	T36.8X1	T36.8X2	T36.8X3	T36.8X4	T36.8X5	T36.8X6
Betanidine	T46.5X1	T46.5X2	T46.5X3	T46.5X4	T46.5X5	T46.5X6
b-sitosterol(s)	T46.6X1	T46.6X2	T46.6X3	T46.6X4	T46.6X5	T46.6X6
Betaxolol	T44.7X1	T44.7X2	T44.7X3	T44.7X4	T44.7X5	T44.7X6
Betazole	T50.8X1	T50.8X2	T50.8X3	T50.8X4	T50.8X5	T50.8X6
Bethanechol	T44.1X1	T44.1X2	T44.1X3	T44.1X4	T44.1X5	T44.1X6
chloride	T44.1X1	T44.1X2	T44.1X3	T44.1X4	T44.1X5	T44.1X6
Bethanidine	T46.5X1	T46.5X2	T46.5X3	T46.5X4	T46.5X5	T46.5X6
Betoxycaine	T41.3X1	T41.3X2	T41.3X3	T41.3X4	T41.3X5	T41.3X6
Betula oil	T49.3X1	T49.3X2	T49.3X3	T49.3X4	T49.3X5	T49.3X6
Bevantolol	T44.7X1	T44.7X2	T44.7X3	T44.7X4	T44.7X5	T44.7X6
Bevonium metilsulfate	T44.3X1	T44.3X2	T44.3X3	T44.3X4	T44.3X5	T44.3X6
Bezafibrate	T46.6X1	T46.6X2	T46.6X3	T46.6X4	T46.6X5	T46.6X6
Bezitramide	T40.4X1	T40.4X2	T40.4X3	T40.4X4	T40.4X5	T40.4X6
BHA	T50.991	T50.992	T50.993	T50.994	T50.995	T50.996
Bhang	T40.7X1	T40.7X2	T40.7X3	T40.7X4	T40.7X5	T40.7X6
BHC (medicinal)	T49.0X1	T49.0X2	T49.0X3	T49.0X4	T49.0X5	T49.0X6
nonmedicinal (vapor)	T53.6X1	T53.6X2	T53.6X3	T53.6X4	--	--
Bialamicol	T37.3X1	T37.3X2	T37.3X3	T37.3X4	T37.3X5	T37.3X6
Bibenzonium bromide	T48.3X1	T48.3X2	T48.3X3	T48.3X4	T48.3X5	T48.3X6
Bibrocathol	T49.5X1	T49.5X2	T49.5X3	T49.5X4	T49.5X5	T49.5X6
Bichloride of mercury — *see* Mercury, chloride						
Bichromates (calcium) (potassium)(sodium) (crystals)	T57.8X1	T57.8X2	T57.8X3	T57.8X4	--	--
fumes	T56.2X1	T56.2X2	T56.2X3	T56.2X4	--	--
Biclotymol	T49.6X1	T49.6X2	T49.6X3	T49.6X4	T49.6X5	T49.6X6
Bicucculine	T50.7X1	T50.7X2	T50.7X3	T50.7X4	T50.7X5	T50.7X6
Bifemelane	T43.291	T43.292	T43.293	T43.294	T43.295	T43.296
Biguanide derivatives, oral	T38.3X1	T38.3X2	T38.3X3	T38.3X4	T38.3X5	T38.3X6
Bile salts	T47.5X1	T47.5X2	T47.5X3	T47.5X4	T47.5X5	T47.5X6
Biligrafin	T50.8X1	T50.8X2	T50.8X3	T50.8X4	T50.8X5	T50.8X6
Bilopaque	T50.8X1	T50.8X2	T50.8X3	T50.8X4	T50.8X5	T50.8X6
Binifibrate	T46.6X1	T46.6X2	T46.6X3	T46.6X4	T46.6X5	T46.6X6
Binitrobenzol	T65.3X1	T65.3X2	T65.3X3	T65.3X4	--	--
Bioflavonoid(s)	T46.991	T46.992	T46.993	T46.994	T46.995	T46.996
Biological substance NEC	T50.901	T50.902	T50.903	T50.904	T50.905	T50.906
Biotin	T45.2X1	T45.2X2	T45.2X3	T45.2X4	T45.2X5	T45.2X6
Biperiden	T44.3X1	T44.3X2	T44.3X3	T44.3X4	T44.3X5	T44.3X6
Bisacodyl	T47.2X1	T47.2X2	T47.2X3	T47.2X4	T47.2X5	T47.2X6
Bisbentiamine	T45.2X1	T45.2X2	T45.2X3	T45.2X4	T45.2X5	T45.2X6
Bisbutiamine	T45.2X1	T45.2X2	T45.2X3	T45.2X4	T45.2X5	T45.2X6
Bisdequalinium (salts) (diacetate)	T49.6X1	T49.6X2	T49.6X3	T49.6X4	T49.6X5	T49.6X6
Bishydroxycoumarin	T45.511	T45.512	T45.513	T45.514	T45.515	T45.516
Bismarsen	T37.8X1	T37.8X2	T37.8X3	T37.8X4	T37.8X5	T37.8X6
Bismuth salts	T47.6X1	T47.6X2	T47.6X3	T47.6X4	T47.6X5	T47.6X6
aluminate	T47.1X1	T47.1X2	T47.1X3	T47.1X4	T47.1X5	T47.1X6
anti-infectives	T37.8X1	T37.8X2	T37.8X3	T37.8X4	T37.8X5	T37.8X6
formic iodide	T49.0X1	T49.0X2	T49.0X3	T49.0X4	T49.0X5	T49.0X6
glycolylarsenate	T49.0X1	T49.0X2	T49.0X3	T49.0X4	T49.0X5	T49.0X6
nonmedicinal (compounds) NEC	T65.91	T65.92	T65.93	T65.94	--	--
subcarbonate	T47.6X1	T47.6X2	T47.6X3	T47.6X4	T47.6X5	T47.6X6
subsalicylate	T37.8X1	T37.8X2	T37.8X3	T37.8X4	T37.8X5	T37.8X6
sulfarsphenamine	T37.8X1	T37.8X2	T37.8X3	T37.8X4	T37.8X5	T37.8X6
Bisoprolol	T44.7X1	T44.7X2	T44.7X3	T44.7X4	T44.7X5	T44.7X6
Bisoxatin	T47.2X1	T47.2X2	T47.2X3	T47.2X4	T47.2X5	T47.2X6
Bisulepin (hydrochloride)	T45.0X1	T45.0X2	T45.0X3	T45.0X4	T45.0X5	T45.0X6
Bithionol	T37.8X1	T37.8X2	T37.8X3	T37.8X4	T37.8X5	T37.8X6
anthelminthic	T37.4X1	T37.4X2	T37.4X3	T37.4X4	T37.4X5	T37.4X6
Bitolterol	T48.6X1	T48.6X2	T48.6X3	T48.6X4	T48.6X5	T48.6X6
Bitoscanate	T37.4X1	T37.4X2	T37.4X3	T37.4X4	T37.4X5	T37.4X6
Bitter almond oil	T62.8X1	T62.8X2	T62.8X3	T62.8X4	--	--
Bittersweet	T62.2X1	T62.2X2	T62.2X3	T62.2X4	--	--
Black						
flag	T60.91	T60.92	T60.93	T60.94	--	--
henbane	T62.2X1	T62.2X2	T62.2X3	T62.2X4	--	--
leaf (40)	T60.91	T60.92	T60.93	T60.94	--	--
widow spider (bite)	T63.311	T63.312	T63.313	T63.314	--	--
antivenin	T50.Z11	T50.Z12	T50.Z13	T50.Z14	T50.Z15	T50.Z16
Blast furnace gas (carbon monoxide from)	T58.8X1	T58.8X2	T58.8X3	T58.8X4	--	--
Bleach	T54.91	T54.92	T54.93	T54.94	--	--
Bleaching agent (medicinal)	T49.4X1	T49.4X2	T49.4X3	T49.4X4	T49.4X5	T49.4X6
Bleomycin	T45.1X1	T45.1X2	T45.1X3	T45.1X4	T45.1X5	T45.1X6
Blockain	T41.3X1	T41.3X2	T41.3X3	T41.3X4	T41.3X5	T41.3X6
infiltration (subcutaneous)	T41.3X1	T41.3X2	T41.3X3	T41.3X4	T41.3X5	T41.3X6
nerve block (peripheral) (plexus)	T41.3X1	T41.3X2	T41.3X3	T41.3X4	T41.3X5	T41.3X6
topical (surface)	T41.3X1	T41.3X2	T41.3X3	T41.3X4	T41.3X5	T41.3X6
Blockers, calcium channel	T46.1X1	T46.1X2	T46.1X3	T46.1X4	T46.1X5	T46.1X6
Blood (derivatives) (natural) (plasma) (whole)	T45.8X1	T45.8X2	T45.8X3	T45.8X4	T45.8X5	T45.8X6
dried	T45.8X1	T45.8X2	T45.8X3	T45.8X4	T45.8X5	T45.8X6
drug affecting NEC	T45.91	T45.92	T45.93	T45.94	T45.95	T45.96
expander NEC	T45.8X1	T45.8X2	T45.8X3	T45.8X4	T45.8X5	T45.8X6
fraction NEC	T45.8X1	T45.8X2	T45.8X3	T45.8X4	T45.8X5	T45.8X6
substitute (macromolecular)	T45.8X1	T45.8X2	T45.8X3	T45.8X4	T45.8X5	T45.8X6
Blue velvet	T40.2X1	T40.2X2	T40.2X3	T40.2X4	--	--
Bone meal	T62.8X1	T62.8X2	T62.8X3	T62.8X4	--	--
Bonine	T45.0X1	T45.0X2	T45.0X3	T45.0X4	T45.0X5	T45.0X6
Bopindolol	T44.7X1	T44.7X2	T44.7X3	T44.7X4	T44.7X5	T44.7X6
Boracic acid	T49.0X1	T49.0X2	T49.0X3	T49.0X4	T49.0X5	T49.0X6
ENT agent	T49.6X1	T49.6X2	T49.6X3	T49.6X4	T49.6X5	T49.6X6
ophthalmic preparation	T49.5X1	T49.5X2	T49.5X3	T49.5X4	T49.5X5	T49.5X6
Borane complex	T57.8X1	T57.8X2	T57.8X3	T57.8X4	--	--
Borate(s)	T57.8X1	T57.8X2	T57.8X3	T57.8X4	--	--
buffer	T50.991	T50.992	T50.993	T50.994	T50.995	T50.996
cleanser	T54.91	T54.92	T54.93	T54.94	--	--
sodium	T57.8X1	T57.8X2	T57.8X3	T57.8X4	--	--
Borax (cleanser)	T54.91	T54.92	T54.93	T54.94	--	--
Bordeaux mixture	T60.3X1	T60.3X2	T60.3X3	T60.3X4	--	--
Boric acid	T49.0X1	T49.0X2	T49.0X3	T49.0X4	T49.0X5	T49.0X6
ENT agent	T49.6X1	T49.6X2	T49.6X3	T49.6X4	T49.6X5	T49.6X6
ophthalmic preparation	T49.5X1	T49.5X2	T49.5X3	T49.5X4	T49.5X5	T49.5X6
Bornaprine	T44.3X1	T44.3X2	T44.3X3	T44.3X4	T44.3X5	T44.3X6
Boron	T57.8X1	T57.8X2	T57.8X3	T57.8X4	--	--
hydride NEC	T57.8X1	T57.8X2	T57.8X3	T57.8X4	--	--
fumes or gas	T57.8X1	T57.8X2	T57.8X3	T57.8X4	--	--
trifluoride	T59.891	T59.892	T59.893	T59.894	--	--
Botox	T48.291	T48.292	T48.293	T48.294	T48.295	T48.296
Botulinus anti-toxin (type A, B)	T50.Z11	T50.Z12	T50.Z13	T50.Z14	T50.Z15	T50.Z16
Brake fluid vapor	T59.891	T59.892	T59.893	T59.894	--	--
Brallobarbital	T42.3X1	T42.3X2	T42.3X3	T42.3X4	T42.3X5	T42.3X6
Bran (wheat)	T47.4X1	T47.4X2	T47.4X3	T47.4X4	T47.4X5	T47.4X6
Brass (fumes)	T56.891	T56.892	T56.893	T56.894	--	--
Brasso	T52.0X1	T52.0X2	T52.0X3	T52.0X4	--	--
Bretylium tosilate	T46.2X1	T46.2X2	T46.2X3	T46.2X4	T46.2X5	T46.2X6
Brevital (sodium)	T41.1X1	T41.1X2	T41.1X3	T41.1X4	T41.1X5	T41.1X6
Brinase	T45.3X1	T45.3X2	T45.3X3	T45.3X4	T45.3X5	T45.3X6
British antilewisite	T45.8X1	T45.8X2	T45.8X3	T45.8X4	T45.8X5	T45.8X6

Substance	Poisoning, Accidental (unintentional)	Poisoning, Intentional self-harm	Poisoning, Assault	Poisoning, Undetermined	Adverse effect	Underdosing
Brodifacoum	T60.4X1	T60.4X2	T60.4X3	T60.4X4	--	--
Bromal (hydrate)	T42.6X1	T42.6X2	T42.6X3	T42.6X4	T42.6X5	T42.6X6
Bromazepam	T42.4X1	T42.4X2	T42.4X3	T42.4X4	T42.4X5	T42.4X6
Bromazine	T45.0X1	T45.0X2	T45.0X3	T45.0X4	T45.0X5	T45.0X6
Brombenzylcyanide	T59.3X1	T59.3X2	T59.3X3	T59.3X4	--	--
Bromelains	T45.3X1	T45.3X2	T45.3X3	T45.3X4	T45.3X5	T45.3X6
Bromethalin	T60.4X1	T60.4X2	T60.4X3	T60.4X4	--	--
Bromhexine	T48.4X1	T48.4X2	T48.4X3	T48.4X4	T48.4X5	T48.4X6
Bromide salts	T42.6X1	T42.6X2	T42.6X3	T42.6X4	T42.6X5	T42.6X6
Bromindione	T45.511	T45.512	T45.513	T45.514	T45.515	T45.516
Bromine						
compounds (medicinal)	T42.6X1	T42.6X2	T42.6X3	T42.6X4	T42.6X5	T42.6X6
sedative	T42.6X1	T42.6X2	T42.6X3	T42.6X4	T42.6X5	T42.6X6
vapor	T59.891	T59.892	T59.893	T59.894	--	--
Bromisoval	T42.6X1	T42.6X2	T42.6X3	T42.6X4	T42.6X5	T42.6X6
Bromisovalum	T42.6X1	T42.6X2	T42.6X3	T42.6X4	T42.6X5	T42.6X6
Bromobenzylcyanide	T59.3X1	T59.3X2	T59.3X3	T59.3X4	--	--
Bromochlorosalicylani-lide	T49.0X1	T49.0X2	T49.0X3	T49.0X4	T49.0X5	T49.0X6
Bromocriptine	T42.8X1	T42.8X2	T42.8X3	T42.8X4	T42.8X5	T42.8X6
Bromodiphenhydramine	T45.0X1	T45.0X2	T45.0X3	T45.0X4	T45.0X5	T45.0X6
Bromoform	T42.6X1	T42.6X2	T42.6X3	T42.6X4	T42.6X5	T42.6X6
Bromophenol blue reagent	T50.991	T50.992	T50.993	T50.994	T50.995	T50.996
Bromopride	T47.8X1	T47.8X2	T47.8X3	T47.8X4	T47.8X5	T47.8X6
Bromosalicylchloranitide	T49.0X1	T49.0X2	T49.0X3	T49.0X4	T49.0X5	T49.0X6
Bromosalicylhydroxamic acid	T37.1X1	T37.1X2	T37.1X3	T37.1X4	T37.1X5	T37.1X6
Bromo-seltzer	T39.1X1	T39.1X2	T39.1X3	T39.1X4	T39.1X5	T39.1X6
Bromoxynil	T60.3X1	T60.3X2	T60.3X3	T60.3X4	--	--
Bromperidol	T43.4X1	T43.4X2	T43.4X3	T43.4X4	T43.4X5	T43.4X6
Brompheniramine	T45.0X1	T45.0X2	T45.0X3	T45.0X4	T45.0X5	T45.0X6
Bromsulfophthalein	T50.8X1	T50.8X2	T50.8X3	T50.8X4	T50.8X5	T50.8X6
Bromural	T42.6X1	T42.6X2	T42.6X3	T42.6X4	T42.6X5	T42.6X6
Bromvaletone	T42.6X1	T42.6X2	T42.6X3	T42.6X4	T42.6X5	T42.6X6
Bronchodilator NEC	T48.6X1	T48.6X2	T48.6X3	T48.6X4	T48.6X5	T48.6X6
Brotizolam	T42.4X1	T42.4X2	T42.4X3	T42.4X4	T42.4X5	T42.4X6
Brovincamine	T46.7X1	T46.7X2	T46.7X3	T46.7X4	T46.7X5	T46.7X6
Brown recluse spider (bite) (venom)	T63.331	T63.332	T63.333	T63.334	--	--
Brown spider (bite) (venom)	T63.391	T63.392	T63.393	T63.394	--	--
Broxaterol	T48.6X1	T48.6X2	T48.6X3	T48.6X4	T48.6X5	T48.6X6
Broxuridine	T45.1X1	T45.1X2	T45.1X3	T45.1X4	T45.1X5	T45.1X6
Broxyquinoline	T37.8X1	T37.8X2	T37.8X3	T37.8X4	T37.8X5	T37.8X6
Bruceine	T48.291	T48.292	T48.293	T48.294	T48.295	T48.296
Brucia	T62.2X1	T62.2X2	T62.2X3	T62.2X4	--	--
Brucine	T65.1X1	T65.1X2	T65.1X3	T65.1X4	--	--
Brunswick green — *see* Copper						
Bruten — *see* Ibuprofen						
Bryonia	T47.2X1	T47.2X2	T47.2X3	T47.2X4	T47.2X5	T47.2X6
Buclizine	T45.0X1	T45.0X2	T45.0X3	T45.0X4	T45.0X5	T45.0X6
Buclosamide	T49.0X1	T49.0X2	T49.0X3	T49.0X4	T49.0X5	T49.0X6
Budesonide	T44.5X1	T44.5X2	T44.5X3	T44.5X4	T44.5X5	T44.5X6
Budralazine	T46.5X1	T46.5X2	T46.5X3	T46.5X4	T46.5X5	T46.5X6
Bufferin	T39.011	T39.012	T39.013	T39.014	T39.015	T39.016
Buflomedil	T46.7X1	T46.7X2	T46.7X3	T46.7X4	T46.7X5	T46.7X6
Buformin	T38.3X1	T38.3X2	T38.3X3	T38.3X4	T38.3X5	T38.3X6
Bufotenine	T40.991	T40.992	T40.993	T40.994	--	--
Bufrolin	T48.6X1	T48.6X2	T48.6X3	T48.6X4	T48.6X5	T48.6X6
Bufylline	T48.6X1	T48.6X2	T48.6X3	T48.6X4	T48.6X5	T48.6X6
Bulk filler	T50.5X1	T50.5X2	T50.5X3	T50.5X4	T50.5X5	T50.5X6
cathartic	T47.4X1	T47.4X2	T47.4X3	T47.4X4	T47.4X5	T47.4X6
Bumetanide	T50.1X1	T50.1X2	T50.1X3	T50.1X4	T50.1X5	T50.1X6
Bunaftine	T46.2X1	T46.2X2	T46.2X3	T46.2X4	T46.2X5	T46.2X6
Bunamiodyl	T50.8X1	T50.8X2	T50.8X3	T50.8X4	T50.8X5	T50.8X6
Bunazosin	T44.6X1	T44.6X2	T44.6X3	T44.6X4	T44.6X5	T44.6X6
Bunitrolol	T44.7X1	T44.7X2	T44.7X3	T44.7X4	T44.7X5	T44.7X6
Buphenine	T46.7X1	T46.7X2	T46.7X3	T46.7X4	T46.7X5	T46.7X6
Bupivacaine	T41.3X1	T41.3X2	T41.3X3	T41.3X4	T41.3X5	T41.3X6
infiltration (subcutaneous)	T41.3X1	T41.3X2	T41.3X3	T41.3X4	T41.3X5	T41.3X6
nerve block (peripheral) (plexus)	T41.3X1	T41.3X2	T41.3X3	T41.3X4	T41.3X5	T41.3X6
spinal	T41.3X1	T41.3X2	T41.3X3	T41.3X4	T41.3X5	T41.3X6
Bupranolol	T44.7X1	T44.7X2	T44.7X3	T44.7X4	T44.7X5	T44.7X6
Buprenorphine	T40.4X1	T40.4X2	T40.4X3	T40.4X4	T40.4X5	T40.4X6
Bupropion	T43.291	T43.292	T43.293	T43.294	T43.295	T43.296
Burimamide	T47.1X1	T47.1X2	T47.1X3	T47.1X4	T47.1X5	T47.1X6
Buserelin	T38.891	T38.892	T38.893	T38.894	T38.895	T38.896
Buspirone	T43.591	T43.592	T43.593	T43.594	T43.595	T43.596
Busulfan, busulphan	T45.1X1	T45.1X2	T45.1X3	T45.1X4	T45.1X5	T45.1X6
Butabarbital (sodium)	T42.3X1	T42.3X2	T42.3X3	T42.3X4	T42.3X5	T42.3X6
Butabarbitone	T42.3X1	T42.3X2	T42.3X3	T42.3X4	T42.3X5	T42.3X6
Butabarpal	T42.3X1	T42.3X2	T42.3X3	T42.3X4	T42.3X5	T42.3X6
Butacaine	T41.3X1	T41.3X2	T41.3X3	T41.3X4	T41.3X5	T41.3X6
Butalamine	T46.7X1	T46.7X2	T46.7X3	T46.7X4	T46.7X5	T46.7X6
Butalbital	T42.3X1	T42.3X2	T42.3X3	T42.3X4	T42.3X5	T42.3X6
Butallylonal	T42.3X1	T42.3X2	T42.3X3	T42.3X4	T42.3X5	T42.3X6
Butamben	T41.3X1	T41.3X2	T41.3X3	T41.3X4	T41.3X5	T41.3X6
Butamirate	T48.3X1	T48.3X2	T48.3X3	T48.3X4	T48.3X5	T48.3X6
Butane (distributed in mobile container)	T59.891	T59.892	T59.893	T59.894	--	--
distributed through pipes	T59.891	T59.892	T59.893	T59.894	--	--
incomplete combustion	T58.11	T58.12	T58.13	T58.14	--	--
Butanilicaine	T41.3X1	T41.3X2	T41.3X3	T41.3X4	T41.3X5	T41.3X6
Butanol	T51.3X1	T51.3X2	T51.3X3	T51.3X4	--	--
Butanone, 2-butanone	T52.4X1	T52.4X2	T52.4X3	T52.4X4	--	--
Butantrone	T49.4X1	T49.4X2	T49.4X3	T49.4X4	T49.4X5	T49.4X6
Butaperazine	T43.3X1	T43.3X2	T43.3X3	T43.3X4	T43.3X5	T43.3X6
Butazolidin	T39.2X1	T39.2X2	T39.2X3	T39.2X4	T39.2X5	T39.2X6
Butetamate	T48.6X1	T48.6X2	T48.6X3	T48.6X4	T48.6X5	T48.6X6
Butethal	T42.3X1	T42.3X2	T42.3X3	T42.3X4	T42.3X5	T42.3X6
Butethamate	T44.3X1	T44.3X2	T44.3X3	T44.3X4	T44.3X5	T44.3X6
Buthalitone (sodium)	T41.1X1	T41.1X2	T41.1X3	T41.1X4	T41.1X5	T41.1X6
Butisol (sodium)	T42.3X1	T42.3X2	T42.3X3	T42.3X4	T42.3X5	T42.3X6
Butizide	T50.2X1	T50.2X2	T50.2X3	T50.2X4	T50.2X5	T50.2X6
Butobarbital	T42.3X1	T42.3X2	T42.3X3	T42.3X4	T42.3X5	T42.3X6
sodium	T42.3X1	T42.3X2	T42.3X3	T42.3X4	T42.3X5	T42.3X6
Butobarbitone	T42.3X1	T42.3X2	T42.3X3	T42.3X4	T42.3X5	T42.3X6
Butoconazole (nitrate)	T49.0X1	T49.0X2	T49.0X3	T49.0X4	T49.0X5	T49.0X6
Butorphanol	T40.4X1	T40.4X2	T40.4X3	T40.4X4	T40.4X5	T40.4X6
Butriptyline	T43.011	T43.012	T43.013	T43.014	T43.015	T43.016
Butropium bromide	T44.3X1	T44.3X2	T44.3X3	T44.3X4	T44.3X5	T44.3X6
Butter of antimony — *see* Antimony						
Buttercups	T62.2X1	T62.2X2	T62.2X3	T62.2X4	--	--
Butyl						
acetate (secondary)	T52.8X1	T52.8X2	T52.8X3	T52.8X4	--	--
alcohol	T51.3X1	T51.3X2	T51.3X3	T51.3X4	--	--
aminobenzoate	T41.3X1	T41.3X2	T41.3X3	T41.3X4	T41.3X5	T41.3X6
butyrate	T52.8X1	T52.8X2	T52.8X3	T52.8X4	--	--
carbinol	T51.3X1	T51.3X2	T51.3X3	T51.3X4	--	--
carbitol	T52.3X1	T52.3X2	T52.3X3	T52.3X4	--	--
cellosolve	T52.3X1	T52.3X2	T52.3X3	T52.3X4	--	--
chloral (hydrate)	T42.6X1	T42.6X2	T42.6X3	T42.6X4	T42.6X5	T42.6X6
formate	T52.8X1	T52.8X2	T52.8X3	T52.8X4	--	--
lactate	T52.8X1	T52.8X2	T52.8X3	T52.8X4	--	--
propionate	T52.8X1	T52.8X2	T52.8X3	T52.8X4	--	--
scopolamine bromide	T44.3X1	T44.3X2	T44.3X3	T44.3X4	T44.3X5	T44.3X6
thiobarbital sodium	T41.1X1	T41.1X2	T41.1X3	T41.1X4	T41.1X5	T41.1X6
Butylated hydroxy-anisole	T50.991	T50.992	T50.993	T50.994	T50.995	T50.996
Butylchloral hydrate	T42.6X1	T42.6X2	T42.6X3	T42.6X4	T42.6X5	T42.6X6
Butyltoluene	T52.2X1	T52.2X2	T52.2X3	T52.2X4	--	--
Butyn	T41.3X1	T41.3X2	T41.3X3	T41.3X4	T41.3X5	T41.3X6
Butyrophenone (-based tranquilizers)	T43.4X1	T43.4X2	T43.4X3	T43.4X4	T43.4X5	T43.4X6
C						
Cabergoline	T42.8X1	T42.8X2	T42.8X3	T42.8X4	T42.8X5	T42.8X6
Cacodyl, cacodylic acid	T57.0X1	T57.0X2	T57.0X3	T57.0X4	--	--
Cactinomycin	T45.1X1	T45.1X2	T45.1X3	T45.1X4	T45.1X5	T45.1X6
Cade oil	T49.4X1	T49.4X2	T49.4X3	T49.4X4	T49.4X5	T49.4X6
Cadexomer iodine	T49.0X1	T49.0X2	T49.0X3	T49.0X4	T49.0X5	T49.0X6
Cadmium (chloride) (fumes) (oxide)	T56.3X1	T56.3X2	T56.3X3	T56.3X4	--	--
sulfide (medicinal) NEC	T49.4X1	T49.4X2	T49.4X3	T49.4X4	T49.4X5	T49.4X6
Cadralazine	T46.5X1	T46.5X2	T46.5X3	T46.5X4	T46.5X5	T46.5X6
Caffeine	T43.611	T43.612	T43.613	T43.614	T43.615	T43.616
Calabar bean	T62.2X1	T62.2X2	T62.2X3	T62.2X4	--	--
Caladium seguinum	T62.2X1	T62.2X2	T62.2X3	T62.2X4	--	--
Calamine (lotion)	T49.3X1	T49.3X2	T49.3X3	T49.3X4	T49.3X5	T49.3X6
Calcifediol	T45.2X1	T45.2X2	T45.2X3	T45.2X4	T45.2X5	T45.2X6
Calciferol	T45.2X1	T45.2X2	T45.2X3	T45.2X4	T45.2X5	T45.2X6
Calcitonin	T50.991	T50.992	T50.993	T50.994	T50.995	T50.996
Calcitriol	T45.2X1	T45.2X2	T45.2X3	T45.2X4	T45.2X5	T45.2X6
Calcium	T50.3X1	T50.3X2	T50.3X3	T50.3X4	T50.3X5	T50.3X6
actylsalicylate	T39.011	T39.012	T39.013	T39.014	T39.015	T39.016
benzamidosalicylate	T37.1X1	T37.1X2	T37.1X3	T37.1X4	T37.1X5	T37.1X6
bromide	T42.6X1	T42.6X2	T42.6X3	T42.6X4	T42.6X5	T42.6X6
bromolactobionate	T42.6X1	T42.6X2	T42.6X3	T42.6X4	T42.6X5	T42.6X6
carbaspirin	T39.011	T39.012	T39.013	T39.014	T39.015	T39.016
carbimide	T50.6X1	T50.6X2	T50.6X3	T50.6X4	T50.6X5	T50.6X6
carbonate	T47.1X1	T47.1X2	T47.1X3	T47.1X4	T47.1X5	T47.1X6
chloride	T50.991	T50.992	T50.993	T50.994	T50.995	T50.996
anhydrous	T50.991	T50.992	T50.993	T50.994	T50.995	T50.996
cyanide	T57.8X1	T57.8X2	T57.8X3	T57.8X4	--	--
dioctyl sulfosuccinate	T47.4X1	T47.4X2	T47.4X3	T47.4X4	T47.4X5	T47.4X6
disodium edathamil	T45.8X1	T45.8X2	T45.8X3	T45.8X4	T45.8X5	T45.8X6
disodium edetate	T45.8X1	T45.8X2	T45.8X3	T45.8X4	T45.8X5	T45.8X6
dobesilate	T46.991	T46.992	T46.993	T46.994	T46.995	T46.996
EDTA	T45.8X1	T45.8X2	T45.8X3	T45.8X4	T45.8X5	T45.8X6
ferrous citrate	T45.4X1	T45.4X2	T45.4X3	T45.4X4	T45.4X5	T45.4X6
folinate	T45.8X1	T45.8X2	T45.8X3	T45.8X4	T45.8X5	T45.8X6

Substance	Poisoning, Accidental (unintentional)	Poisoning, Intentional self-harm	Poisoning, Assault	Poisoning, Undetermined	Adverse effect	Underdosing
Calcium — continued						
glubionate	T50.3X1	T50.3X2	T50.3X3	T50.3X4	T50.3X5	T50.3X6
gluconate	T50.3X1	T50.3X2	T50.3X3	T50.3X4	T50.3X5	T50.3X6
gluconogalactogluc-onate	T50.3X1	T50.3X2	T50.3X3	T50.3X4	T50.3X5	T50.3X6
hydrate, hydroxide	T54.3X1	T54.3X2	T54.3X3	T54.3X4	--	--
hypochlorite	T54.3X1	T54.3X2	T54.3X3	T54.3X4	--	--
iodide	T48.4X1	T48.4X2	T48.4X3	T48.4X4	T48.4X5	T48.4X6
ipodate	T50.8X1	T50.8X2	T50.8X3	T50.8X4	T50.8X5	T50.8X6
lactate	T50.3X1	T50.3X2	T50.3X3	T50.3X4	T50.3X5	T50.3X6
leucovorin	T45.8X1	T45.8X2	T45.8X3	T45.8X4	T45.8X5	T45.8X6
mandelate	T37.91	T37.92	T37.93	T37.94	T37.95	T37.96
oxide	T54.3X1	T54.3X2	T54.3X3	T54.3X4	--	--
pantothenate	T45.2X1	T45.2X2	T45.2X3	T45.2X4	T45.2X5	T45.2X6
phosphate	T50.3X1	T50.3X2	T50.3X3	T50.3X4	T50.3X5	T50.3X6
salicylate	T39.091	T39.092	T39.093	T39.094	T39.095	T39.096
salts	T50.3X1	T50.3X2	T50.3X3	T50.3X4	T50.3X5	T50.3X6
Calculus-dissolving drug	T50.991	T50.992	T50.993	T50.994	T50.995	T50.996
Calomel	T49.0X1	T49.0X2	T49.0X3	T49.0X4	T49.0X5	T49.0X6
Caloric agent	T50.3X1	T50.3X2	T50.3X3	T50.3X4	T50.3X5	T50.3X6
Calusterone	T38.7X1	T38.7X2	T38.7X3	T38.7X4	T38.7X5	T38.7X6
Camazepam	T42.4X1	T42.4X2	T42.4X3	T42.4X4	T42.4X5	T42.4X6
Camomile	T49.0X1	T49.0X2	T49.0X3	T49.0X4	T49.0X5	T49.0X6
Camoquin	T37.2X1	T37.2X2	T37.2X3	T37.2X4	T37.2X5	T37.2X6
Camphor						
insecticide	T60.2X1	T60.2X2	T60.2X3	T60.2X4	--	--
medicinal	T49.8X1	T49.8X2	T49.8X3	T49.8X4	T49.8X5	T49.8X6
Camylofin	T44.3X1	T44.3X2	T44.3X3	T44.3X4	T44.3X5	T44.3X6
Cancer chemotherapy drug regimen	T45.1X1	T45.1X2	T45.1X3	T45.1X4	T45.1X5	T45.1X6
Candeptin	T49.0X1	T49.0X2	T49.0X3	T49.0X4	T49.0X5	T49.0X6
Candicidin	T49.0X1	T49.0X2	T49.0X3	T49.0X4	T49.0X5	T49.0X6
Cannabinol	T40.7X1	T40.7X2	T40.7X3	T40.7X4	T40.7X5	T40.7X6
Cannabis (derivatives)	T40.7X1	T40.7X2	T40.7X3	T40.7X4	T40.7X5	T40.7X6
Canned heat	T51.1X1	T51.1X2	T51.1X3	T51.1X4		
Canrenoic acid	T50.0X1	T50.0X2	T50.0X3	T50.0X4	T50.0X5	T50.0X6
Canrenone	T50.0X1	T50.0X2	T50.0X3	T50.0X4	T50.0X5	T50.0X6
Cantharides, cantharidin, cantharis	T49.8X1	T49.8X2	T49.8X3	T49.8X4	T49.8X5	T49.8X6
Canthaxanthin	T50.991	T50.992	T50.993	T50.994	T50.995	T50.996
Capillary-active drug NEC	T46.901	T46.902	T46.903	T46.904	T46.905	T46.906
Capreomycin	T36.8X1	T36.8X2	T36.8X3	T36.8X4	T36.8X5	T36.8X6
Capsicum	T49.4X1	T49.4X2	T49.4X3	T49.4X4	T49.4X5	T49.4X6
Captafol	T60.3X1	T60.3X2	T60.3X3	T60.3X4	--	--
Captan	T60.3X1	T60.3X2	T60.3X3	T60.3X4	--	--
Captodiame, captodiamine	T43.591	T43.592	T43.593	T43.594	T43.595	T43.596
Captopril	T46.4X1	T46.4X2	T46.4X3	T46.4X4	T46.4X5	T46.4X6
Caramiphen	T44.3X1	T44.3X2	T44.3X3	T44.3X4	T44.3X5	T44.3X6
Carazolol	T44.7X1	T44.7X2	T44.7X3	T44.7X4	T44.7X5	T44.7X6
Carbachol	T44.1X1	T44.1X2	T44.1X3	T44.1X4	T44.1X5	T44.1X6
Carbacrylamine (resin)	T50.3X1	T50.3X2	T50.3X3	T50.3X4	T50.3X5	T50.3X6
Carbamate (insecticide)	T60.0X1	T60.0X2	T60.0X3	T60.0X4	--	--
Carbamate (sedative)	T42.6X1	T42.6X2	T42.6X3	T42.6X4	T42.6X5	T42.6X6
herbicide	T60.0X1	T60.0X2	T60.0X3	T60.0X4	--	--
insecticide	T60.0X1	T60.0X2	T60.0X3	T60.0X4	--	--
Carbamazepine	T42.1X1	T42.1X2	T42.1X3	T42.1X4	T42.1X5	T42.1X6
Carbamide	T47.3X1	T47.3X2	T47.3X3	T47.3X4	T47.3X5	T47.3X6
peroxide	T49.0X1	T49.0X2	T49.0X3	T49.0X4	T49.0X5	T49.0X6
topical	T49.8X1	T49.8X2	T49.8X3	T49.8X4	T49.8X5	T49.8X6
Carbamylcholine chloride	T44.1X1	T44.1X2	T44.1X3	T44.1X4	T44.1X5	T44.1X6
Carbaril	T60.0X1	T60.0X2	T60.0X3	T60.0X4	--	--
Carbarsone	T37.3X1	T37.3X2	T37.3X3	T37.3X4	T37.3X5	T37.3X6
Carbaryl	T60.0X1	T60.0X2	T60.0X3	T60.0X4	--	--
Carbaspirin	T39.011	T39.012	T39.013	T39.014	T39.015	T39.016
Carbazochrome (salicylate) (sodium sulfonate)	T49.4X1	T49.4X2	T49.4X3	T49.4X4	T49.4X5	T49.4X6
Carbenicillin	T36.0X1	T36.0X2	T36.0X3	T36.0X4	T36.0X5	T36.0X6
Carbenoxolone	T47.1X1	T47.1X2	T47.1X3	T47.1X4	T47.1X5	T47.1X6
Carbetapentane	T48.3X1	T48.3X2	T48.3X3	T48.3X4	T48.3X5	T48.3X6
Carbethyl salicylate	T39.091	T39.092	T39.093	T39.094	T39.095	T39.096
Carbidopa (with levodopa)	T42.8X1	T42.8X2	T42.8X3	T42.8X4	T42.8X5	T42.8X6
Carbimazole	T38.2X1	T38.2X2	T38.2X3	T38.2X4	T38.2X5	T38.2X6
Carbinol	T51.1X1	T51.1X2	T51.1X3	T51.1X4	--	--
Carbinoxamine	T45.0X1	T45.0X2	T45.0X3	T45.0X4	T45.0X5	T45.0X6
Carbiphene	T39.8X1	T39.8X2	T39.8X3	T39.8X4	T39.8X5	T39.8X6
Carbitol	T52.3X1	T52.3X2	T52.3X3	T52.3X4	--	--
Carbo medicinalis	T47.6X1	T47.6X2	T47.6X3	T47.6X4	T47.6X5	T47.6X6
Carbocaine	T41.3X1	T41.3X2	T41.3X3	T41.3X4	T41.3X5	T41.3X6
infiltration (subcutaneous)	T41.3X1	T41.3X2	T41.3X3	T41.3X4	T41.3X5	T41.3X6
nerve block (peripheral) (plexus)	T41.3X1	T41.3X2	T41.3X3	T41.3X4	T41.3X5	T41.3X6
topical (surface)	T41.3X1	T41.3X2	T41.3X3	T41.3X4	T41.3X5	T41.3X6
Carbocisteine	T48.4X1	T48.4X2	T48.4X3	T48.4X4	T48.4X5	T48.4X6
Carbocromen	T46.3X1	T46.3X2	T46.3X3	T46.3X4	T46.3X5	T46.3X6
Carbol fuchsin	T49.0X1	T49.0X2	T49.0X3	T49.0X4	T49.0X5	T49.0X6

Substance	Poisoning, Accidental (unintentional)	Poisoning, Intentional self-harm	Poisoning, Assault	Poisoning, Undetermined	Adverse effect	Underdosing
Carbolic acid (see also Phenol)	T54.0X1	T54.0X2	T54.0X3	T54.0X4	--	--
Carbolonium (bromide)	T48.1X1	T48.1X2	T48.1X3	T48.1X4	T48.1X5	T48.1X6
Carbomycin	T36.8X1	T36.8X2	T36.8X3	T36.8X4	T36.8X5	T36.8X6
Carbon						
bisulfide (liquid)	T65.4X1	T65.4X2	T65.4X3	T65.4X4	--	--
vapor	T65.4X1	T65.4X2	T65.4X3	T65.4X4	--	--
dioxide (gas)	T59.7X1	T59.7X2	T59.7X3	T59.7X4	--	--
medicinal	T41.5X1	T41.5X2	T41.5X3	T41.5X4	T41.5X5	T41.5X6
nonmedicinal	T59.7X1	T59.7X2	T59.7X3	T59.7X4	--	--
snow	T49.4X1	T49.4X2	T49.4X3	T49.4X4	T49.4X5	T49.4X6
disulfide (liquid)	T65.4X1	T65.4X2	T65.4X3	T65.4X4	--	--
vapor	T65.4X1	T65.4X2	T65.4X3	T65.4X4	--	--
monoxide (from incomplete combustion)	T58.91	T58.92	T58.93	T58.94		
blast furnace gas	T58.8X1	T58.8X2	T58.8X3	T58.8X4		
butane (distributed in mobile container)	T58.11	T58.12	T58.13	T58.14		
distributed through pipes	T58.11	T58.12	T58.13	T58.14		
charcoal fumes	T58.2X1	T58.2X2	T58.2X3	T58.2X4		
coal	T58.2X1	T58.2X2	T58.2X3	T58.2X4		
coke (in domestic stoves, fireplaces)	T58.2X1	T58.2X2	T58.2X3	T58.2X4		
gas (piped)	T58.11	T58.12	T58.13	T58.14		
solid (in domestic stoves, fireplaces)	T58.2X1	T58.2X2	T58.2X3	T58.2X4		
exhaust gas (motor) not in transit	T58.01	T58.02	T58.03	T58.04		
combustion engine, any not in watercraft	T58.01	T58.02	T58.03	T58.04		
farm tractor, not in transit	T58.01	T58.02	T58.03	T58.04		
gas engine	T58.01	T58.02	T58.03	T58.04		
motor pump	T58.01	T58.02	T58.03	T58.04		
motor vehicle, not in transit	T58.01	T58.02	T58.03	T58.04		
fuel (in domestic use)	T58.2X1	T58.2X2	T58.2X3	T58.2X4		
gas (piped)	T58.11	T58.12	T58.13	T58.14		
in mobile container	T58.11	T58.12	T58.13	T58.14		
piped (natural)	T58.11	T58.12	T58.13	T58.14		
utility	T58.11	T58.12	T58.13	T58.14		
in mobile container	T58.11	T58.12	T58.13	T58.14		
illuminating gas	T58.11	T58.12	T58.13	T58.14		
industrial fuels or gases, any	T58.8X1	T58.8X2	T58.8X3	T58.8X4		
kerosene (in domestic stoves, fireplaces)	T58.2X1	T58.2X2	T58.2X3	T58.2X4		
kiln gas or vapor	T58.8X1	T58.8X2	T58.8X3	T58.8X4		
motor exhaust gas, not in transit	T58.01	T58.02	T58.03	T58.04		
piped gas (manufactured) (natural)	T58.11	T58.12	T58.13	T58.14		
producer gas	T58.8X1	T58.8X2	T58.8X3	T58.8X4		
propane (distributed in mobile container)	T58.11	T58.12	T58.13	T58.14		
distributed through pipes	T58.11	T58.12	T58.13	T58.14		
specified source NEC	T58.8X1	T58.8X2	T58.8X3	T58.8X4		
stove gas	T58.11	T58.12	T58.13	T58.14		
piped	T58.11	T58.12	T58.13	T58.14		
utility gas	T58.11	T58.12	T58.13	T58.14		
piped	T58.11	T58.12	T58.13	T58.14		
water gas	T58.11	T58.12	T58.13	T58.14		
wood (in domestic stoves, fireplaces)	T58.2X1	T58.2X2	T58.2X3	T58.2X4		
tetrachloride (vapor) NEC	T53.0X1	T53.0X2	T53.0X3	T53.0X4	--	--
liquid (cleansing agent) NEC	T53.0X1	T53.0X2	T53.0X3	T53.0X4	--	--
solvent	T53.0X1	T53.0X2	T53.0X3	T53.0X4	--	--
Carbonic acid gas	T59.7X1	T59.7X2	T59.7X3	T59.7X4	--	--
anhydrase inhibitor NEC	T50.2X1	T50.2X2	T50.2X3	T50.2X4	T50.2X5	T50.2X6
Carbophenothion	T60.0X1	T60.0X2	T60.0X3	T60.0X4	--	--
Carboplatin	T45.1X1	T45.1X2	T45.1X3	T45.1X4	T45.1X5	T45.1X6
Carboprost	T48.0X1	T48.0X2	T48.0X3	T48.0X4	T48.0X5	T48.0X6
Carboquone	T45.1X1	T45.1X2	T45.1X3	T45.1X4	T45.1X5	T45.1X6
Carbowax	T49.3X1	T49.3X2	T49.3X3	T49.3X4	T49.3X5	T49.3X6
Carboxymethyl-cellulose	T47.4X1	T47.4X2	T47.4X3	T47.4X4	T47.4X5	T47.4X6
S-Carboxymethyl-cysteine	T48.4X1	T48.4X2	T48.4X3	T48.4X4	T48.4X5	T48.4X6
Carbrital	T42.3X1	T42.3X2	T42.3X3	T42.3X4	T42.3X5	T42.3X6
Carbromal	T42.6X1	T42.6X2	T42.6X3	T42.6X4	T42.6X5	T42.6X6

Substance	Poisoning, Accidental (unintentional)	Poisoning, Intentional self-harm	Poisoning, Assault	Poisoning, Undetermined	Adverse effect	Underdosing
Carbutamide	T38.3X1	T38.3X2	T38.3X3	T38.3X4	T38.3X5	T38.3X6
Carbuterol	T48.6X1	T48.6X2	T48.6X3	T48.6X4	T48.6X5	T48.6X6
Cardiac						
depressants	T46.2X1	T46.2X2	T46.2X3	T46.2X4	T46.2X5	T46.2X6
rhythm regulator	T46.2X1	T46.2X2	T46.2X3	T46.2X4	T46.2X5	T46.2X6
specified NEC	T46.2X1	T46.2X2	T46.2X3	T46.2X4	T46.2X5	T46.2X6
Cardiografin	T50.8X1	T50.8X2	T50.8X3	T50.8X4	T50.8X5	T50.8X6
Cardio-green	T50.8X1	T50.8X2	T50.8X3	T50.8X4	T50.8X5	T50.8X6
Cardiotonic (glycoside) **NEC**	T46.0X1	T46.0X2	T46.0X3	T46.0X4	T46.0X5	T46.0X6
Cardiovascular drug NEC	T46.901	T46.902	T46.903	T46.904	T46.905	T46.906
Cardrase	T50.2X1	T50.2X2	T50.2X3	T50.2X4	T50.2X5	T50.2X6
Carfecillin	T36.0X1	T36.0X2	T36.0X3	T36.0X4	T36.0X5	T36.0X6
Carfenazine	T43.3X1	T43.3X2	T43.3X3	T43.3X4	T43.3X5	T43.3X6
Carfusin	T49.0X1	T49.0X2	T49.0X3	T49.0X4	T49.0X5	T49.0X6
Carindacillin	T36.0X1	T36.0X2	T36.0X3	T36.0X4	T36.0X5	T36.0X6
Carisoprodol	T42.8X1	T42.8X2	T42.8X3	T42.8X4	T42.8X5	T42.8X6
Carmellose	T47.4X1	T47.4X2	T47.4X3	T47.4X4	T47.4X5	T47.4X6
Carminative	T47.5X1	T47.5X2	T47.5X3	T47.5X4	T47.5X5	T47.5X6
Carmofur	T45.1X1	T45.1X2	T45.1X3	T45.1X4	T45.1X5	T45.1X6
Carmustine	T45.1X1	T45.1X2	T45.1X3	T45.1X4	T45.1X5	T45.1X6
Carotene	T45.2X1	T45.2X2	T45.2X3	T45.2X4	T45.2X5	T45.2X6
Carphenazine	T43.3X1	T43.3X2	T43.3X3	T43.3X4	T43.3X5	T43.3X6
Carpipramine	T42.4X1	T42.4X2	T42.4X3	T42.4X4	T42.4X5	T42.4X6
Carprofen	T39.311	T39.312	T39.313	T39.314	T39.315	T39.316
Carpronium chloride	T44.3X1	T44.3X2	T44.3X3	T44.3X4	T44.3X5	T44.3X6
Carrageenan	T47.8X1	T47.8X2	T47.8X3	T47.8X4	T47.8X5	T47.8X6
Carteolol	T44.7X1	T44.7X2	T44.7X3	T44.7X4	T44.7X5	T44.7X6
Carter's Little Pills	T47.2X1	T47.2X2	T47.2X3	T47.2X4	T47.2X5	T47.2X6
Cascara (sagrada)	T47.2X1	T47.2X2	T47.2X3	T47.2X4	T47.2X5	T47.2X6
Cassava	T62.2X1	T62.2X2	T62.2X3	T62.2X4	--	--
Castellani's paint	T49.0X1	T49.0X2	T49.0X3	T49.0X4	T49.0X5	T49.0X6
Castor						
bean	T62.2X1	T62.2X2	T62.2X3	T62.2X4	--	--
oil	T47.2X1	T47.2X2	T47.2X3	T47.2X4	T47.2X5	T47.2X6
Catalase	T45.3X1	T45.3X2	T45.3X3	T45.3X4	T45.3X5	T45.3X6
Caterpillar (sting)	T63.431	T63.432	T63.433	T63.434	--	--
Catha (edulis) (tea)	T43.691	T43.692	T43.693	T43.694	--	--
Cathartic NEC	T47.4X1	T47.4X2	T47.4X3	T47.4X4	T47.4X5	T47.4X6
anthacene derivative	T47.2X1	T47.2X2	T47.2X3	T47.2X4	T47.2X5	T47.2X6
bulk	T47.4X1	T47.4X2	T47.4X3	T47.4X4	T47.4X5	T47.4X6
contact	T47.2X1	T47.2X2	T47.2X3	T47.2X4	T47.2X5	T47.2X6
emollient NEC	T47.4X1	T47.4X2	T47.4X3	T47.4X4	T47.4X5	T47.4X6
irritant NEC	T47.2X1	T47.2X2	T47.2X3	T47.2X4	T47.2X5	T47.2X6
mucilage	T47.4X1	T47.4X2	T47.4X3	T47.4X4	T47.4X5	T47.4X6
saline	T47.3X1	T47.3X2	T47.3X3	T47.3X4	T47.3X5	T47.3X6
vegetable	T47.2X1	T47.2X2	T47.2X3	T47.2X4	T47.2X5	T47.2X6
Cathine	T50.5X1	T50.5X2	T50.5X3	T50.5X4	T50.5X5	T50.5X6
Cathomycin	T36.8X1	T36.8X2	T36.8X3	T36.8X4	T36.8X5	T36.8X6
Cation exchange resin	T50.3X1	T50.3X2	T50.3X3	T50.3X4	T50.3X5	T50.3X6
Caustic(s) NEC	T54.91	T54.92	T54.93	T54.94	--	--
alkali	T54.3X1	T54.3X2	T54.3X3	T54.3X4	--	--
hydroxide	T54.3X1	T54.3X2	T54.3X3	T54.3X4	--	--
potash	T54.3X1	T54.3X2	T54.3X3	T54.3X4	--	--
soda	T54.3X1	T54.3X2	T54.3X3	T54.3X4	--	--
specified NEC	T54.91	T54.92	T54.93	T54.94	--	--
Ceepryn	T49.0X1	T49.0X2	T49.0X3	T49.0X4	T49.0X5	T49.0X6
ENT agent	T49.6X1	T49.6X2	T49.6X3	T49.6X4	T49.6X5	T49.6X6
lozenges	T49.6X1	T49.6X2	T49.6X3	T49.6X4	T49.6X5	T49.6X6
Cefacetrile	T36.1X1	T36.1X2	T36.1X3	T36.1X4	T36.1X5	T36.1X6
Cefaclor	T36.1X1	T36.1X2	T36.1X3	T36.1X4	T36.1X5	T36.1X6
Cefadroxil	T36.1X1	T36.1X2	T36.1X3	T36.1X4	T36.1X5	T36.1X6
Cefalexin	T36.1X1	T36.1X2	T36.1X3	T36.1X4	T36.1X5	T36.1X6
Cefaloglycin	T36.1X1	T36.1X2	T36.1X3	T36.1X4	T36.1X5	T36.1X6
Cefaloridine	T36.1X1	T36.1X2	T36.1X3	T36.1X4	T36.1X5	T36.1X6
Cefalosporins	T36.1X1	T36.1X2	T36.1X3	T36.1X4	T36.1X5	T36.1X6
Cefalotin	T36.1X1	T36.1X2	T36.1X3	T36.1X4	T36.1X5	T36.1X6
Cefamandole	T36.1X1	T36.1X2	T36.1X3	T36.1X4	T36.1X5	T36.1X6
Cefamycin antibiotic	T36.1X1	T36.1X2	T36.1X3	T36.1X4	T36.1X5	T36.1X6
Cefapirin	T36.1X1	T36.1X2	T36.1X3	T36.1X4	T36.1X5	T36.1X6
Cefatrizine	T36.1X1	T36.1X2	T36.1X3	T36.1X4	T36.1X5	T36.1X6
Cefazedone	T36.1X1	T36.1X2	T36.1X3	T36.1X4	T36.1X5	T36.1X6
Cefazolin	T36.1X1	T36.1X2	T36.1X3	T36.1X4	T36.1X5	T36.1X6
Cefbuperazone	T36.1X1	T36.1X2	T36.1X3	T36.1X4	T36.1X5	T36.1X6
Cefetamet	T36.1X1	T36.1X2	T36.1X3	T36.1X4	T36.1X5	T36.1X6
Cefixime	T36.1X1	T36.1X2	T36.1X3	T36.1X4	T36.1X5	T36.1X6
Cefmenoxime	T36.1X1	T36.1X2	T36.1X3	T36.1X4	T36.1X5	T36.1X6
Cefmetazole	T36.1X1	T36.1X2	T36.1X3	T36.1X4	T36.1X5	T36.1X6
Cefminox	T36.1X1	T36.1X2	T36.1X3	T36.1X4	T36.1X5	T36.1X6
Cefonicid	T36.1X1	T36.1X2	T36.1X3	T36.1X4	T36.1X5	T36.1X6
Cefoperazone	T36.1X1	T36.1X2	T36.1X3	T36.1X4	T36.1X5	T36.1X6
Ceforanide	T36.1X1	T36.1X2	T36.1X3	T36.1X4	T36.1X5	T36.1X6
Cefotaxime	T36.1X1	T36.1X2	T36.1X3	T36.1X4	T36.1X5	T36.1X6
Cefotetan	T36.1X1	T36.1X2	T36.1X3	T36.1X4	T36.1X5	T36.1X6
Cefotiam	T36.1X1	T36.1X2	T36.1X3	T36.1X4	T36.1X5	T36.1X6

Substance	Poisoning, Accidental (unintentional)	Poisoning, Intentional self-harm	Poisoning, Assault	Poisoning, Undetermined	Adverse effect	Underdosing
Cefoxitin	T36.1X1	T36.1X2	T36.1X3	T36.1X4	T36.1X5	T36.1X6
Cefpimizole	T36.1X1	T36.1X2	T36.1X3	T36.1X4	T36.1X5	T36.1X6
Cefpiramide	T36.1X1	T36.1X2	T36.1X3	T36.1X4	T36.1X5	T36.1X6
Cefradine	T36.1X1	T36.1X2	T36.1X3	T36.1X4	T36.1X5	T36.1X6
Cefroxadine	T36.1X1	T36.1X2	T36.1X3	T36.1X4	T36.1X5	T36.1X6
Cefsulodin	T36.1X1	T36.1X2	T36.1X3	T36.1X4	T36.1X5	T36.1X6
Ceftazidime	T36.1X1	T36.1X2	T36.1X3	T36.1X4	T36.1X5	T36.1X6
Cefteram	T36.1X1	T36.1X2	T36.1X3	T36.1X4	T36.1X5	T36.1X6
Ceftezole	T36.1X1	T36.1X2	T36.1X3	T36.1X4	T36.1X5	T36.1X6
Ceftizoxime	T36.1X1	T36.1X2	T36.1X3	T36.1X4	T36.1X5	T36.1X6
Ceftriaxone	T36.1X1	T36.1X2	T36.1X3	T36.1X4	T36.1X5	T36.1X6
Cefuroxime	T36.1X1	T36.1X2	T36.1X3	T36.1X4	T36.1X5	T36.1X6
Cefuzonam	T36.1X1	T36.1X2	T36.1X3	T36.1X4	T36.1X5	T36.1X6
Celestone	T38.0X1	T38.0X2	T38.0X3	T38.0X4	T38.0X5	T38.0X6
topical	T49.0X1	T49.0X2	T49.0X3	T49.0X4	T49.0X5	T49.0X6
Celiprolol	T44.7X1	T44.7X2	T44.7X3	T44.7X4	T44.7X5	T44.7X6
Cell stimulants and proliferants	T49.8X1	T49.8X2	T49.8X3	T49.8X4	T49.8X5	T49.8X6
Cellosolve	T52.91	T52.92	T52.93	T52.94	--	--
Cellulose						
cathartic	T47.4X1	T47.4X2	T47.4X3	T47.4X4	T47.4X5	T47.4X6
hydroxyethyl	T47.4X1	T47.4X2	T47.4X3	T47.4X4	T47.4X5	T47.4X6
nitrates (topical)	T49.3X1	T49.3X2	T49.3X3	T49.3X4	T49.3X5	T49.3X6
oxidized	T49.4X1	T49.4X2	T49.4X3	T49.4X4	T49.4X5	T49.4X6
Centipede (bite)	T63.411	T63.412	T63.413	T63.414	--	--
Central nervous system						
depressants	T42.71	T42.72	T42.73	T42.74	T42.75	T42.76
anesthetic (general) NEC	T41.201	T41.202	T41.203	T41.204	T41.205	T41.206
gases NEC	T41.0X1	T41.0X2	T41.0X3	T41.0X4	T41.0X5	T41.0X6
intravenous	T41.1X1	T41.1X2	T41.1X3	T41.1X4	T41.1X5	T41.1X6
barbiturates	T42.3X1	T42.3X2	T42.3X3	T42.3X4	T42.3X5	T42.3X6
benzodiazepines	T42.4X1	T42.4X2	T42.4X3	T42.4X4	T42.4X5	T42.4X6
bromides	T42.6X1	T42.6X2	T42.6X3	T42.6X4	T42.6X5	T42.6X6
cannabis sativa	T40.7X1	T40.7X2	T40.7X3	T40.7X4	T40.7X5	T40.7X6
chloral hydrate	T42.6X1	T42.6X2	T42.6X3	T42.6X4	T42.6X5	T42.6X6
ethanol	T51.0X1	T51.0X2	T51.0X3	T51.0X4	--	--
hallucinogenics	T40.901	T40.902	T40.903	T40.904	T40.905	T40.906
hypnotics	T42.71	T42.72	T42.73	T42.74	T42.75	T42.76
specified NEC	T42.6X1	T42.6X2	T42.6X3	T42.6X4	T42.6X5	T42.6X6
muscle relaxants	T42.8X1	T42.8X2	T42.8X3	T42.8X4	T42.8X5	T42.8X6
paraldehyde	T42.6X1	T42.6X2	T42.6X3	T42.6X4	T42.6X5	T42.6X6
sedatives; sedative-hypnotics	T42.71	T42.72	T42.73	T42.74	T42.75	T42.76
mixed NEC	T42.6X1	T42.6X2	T42.6X3	T42.6X4	T42.6X5	T42.6X6
specified NEC	T42.6X1	T42.6X2	T42.6X3	T42.6X4	T42.6X5	T42.6X6
muscle-tone depressants	T42.8X1	T42.8X2	T42.8X3	T42.8X4	T42.8X5	T42.8X6
stimulants	T43.601	T43.602	T43.603	T43.604	T43.605	T43.606
amphetamines	T43.621	T43.622	T43.623	T43.624	T43.625	T43.626
analeptics	T50.7X1	T50.7X2	T50.7X3	T50.7X4	T50.7X5	T50.7X6
antidepressants	T43.201	T43.202	T43.203	T43.204	T43.205	T43.206
opiate antagonists	T50.7X1	T50.7X2	T50.7X3	T50.7X4	T50.7X5	T50.7X6
specified NEC	T43.691	T43.692	T43.693	T43.694	T43.695	T43.696
Cephalexin	T36.1X1	T36.1X2	T36.1X3	T36.1X4	T36.1X5	T36.1X6
Cephaloglycin	T36.1X1	T36.1X2	T36.1X3	T36.1X4	T36.1X5	T36.1X6
Cephaloridine	T36.1X1	T36.1X2	T36.1X3	T36.1X4	T36.1X5	T36.1X6
Cephalosporins	T36.1X1	T36.1X2	T36.1X3	T36.1X4	T36.1X5	T36.1X6
N (adicillin)	T36.0X1	T36.0X2	T36.0X3	T36.0X4	T36.0X5	T36.0X6
Cephalothin	T36.1X1	T36.1X2	T36.1X3	T36.1X4	T36.1X5	T36.1X6
Cephalotin	T36.1X1	T36.1X2	T36.1X3	T36.1X4	T36.1X5	T36.1X6
Cephradine	T36.1X1	T36.1X2	T36.1X3	T36.1X4	T36.1X5	T36.1X6
Cerbera (odallam)	T62.2X1	T62.2X2	T62.2X3	T62.2X4	--	--
Cerberin	T46.0X1	T46.0X2	T46.0X3	T46.0X4	T46.0X5	T46.0X6
Cerebral stimulants	T43.601	T43.602	T43.603	T43.604	T43.605	T43.606
psychotherapeutic	T43.601	T43.602	T43.603	T43.604	T43.605	T43.606
specified NEC	T43.691	T43.692	T43.693	T43.694	T43.695	T43.696
Cerium oxalate	T45.0X1	T45.0X2	T45.0X3	T45.0X4	T45.0X5	T45.0X6
Cerous oxalate	T45.0X1	T45.0X2	T45.0X3	T45.0X4	T45.0X5	T45.0X6
Ceruletide	T50.8X1	T50.8X2	T50.8X3	T50.8X4	T50.8X5	T50.8X6
Cetalkonium (chloride)	T49.0X1	T49.0X2	T49.0X3	T49.0X4	T49.0X5	T49.0X6
Cethexonium chloride	T49.0X1	T49.0X2	T49.0X3	T49.0X4	T49.0X5	T49.0X6
Cetiedil	T46.7X1	T46.7X2	T46.7X3	T46.7X4	T46.7X5	T46.7X6
Cetirizine	T45.0X1	T45.0X2	T45.0X3	T45.0X4	T45.0X5	T45.0X6
Cetomacrogol	T50.991	T50.992	T50.993	T50.994	T50.995	T50.996
Cetotiamine	T45.2X1	T45.2X2	T45.2X3	T45.2X4	T45.2X5	T45.2X6
Cetoxime	T45.0X1	T45.0X2	T45.0X3	T45.0X4	T45.0X5	T45.0X6
Cetraxate	T47.1X1	T47.1X2	T47.1X3	T47.1X4	T47.1X5	T47.1X6
Cetrimide	T49.0X1	T49.0X2	T49.0X3	T49.0X4	T49.0X5	T49.0X6
Cetrimonium (bromide)	T49.0X1	T49.0X2	T49.0X3	T49.0X4	T49.0X5	T49.0X6
Cetylpyridinium chloride	T49.0X1	T49.0X2	T49.0X3	T49.0X4	T49.0X5	T49.0X6
ENT agent	T49.6X1	T49.6X2	T49.6X3	T49.6X4	T49.6X5	T49.6X6
lozenges	T49.6X1	T49.6X2	T49.6X3	T49.6X4	T49.6X5	T49.6X6
Cevadilla — *see* Sabadilla						
Cevitamic acid	T45.2X1	T45.2X2	T45.2X3	T45.2X4	T45.2X5	T45.2X6
Chalk, precipitated	T47.1X1	T47.1X2	T47.1X3	T47.1X4	T47.1X5	T47.1X6

Substance	Poisoning, Accidental (unintentional)	Poisoning, Intentional self-harm	Poisoning, Assault	Poisoning, Undetermined	Adverse effect	Underdosing
Chamomile	T49.0X1	T49.0X2	T49.0X3	T49.0X4	T49.0X5	T49.0X6
Ch'an su	T46.0X1	T46.0X2	T46.0X3	T46.0X4	T46.0X5	T46.0X6
Charcoal	T47.6X1	T47.6X2	T47.6X3	T47.6X4	T47.6X5	T47.6X6
activated (*see also* Charcoal, medicinal)	T47.6X1	T47.6X2	T47.6X3	T47.6X4	T47.6X5	T47.6X6
fumes (Carbon monoxide)	T58.2X1	T58.2X2	T58.2X3	T58.2X4	--	--
industrial	T58.8X1	T58.8X2	T58.8X3	T58.8X4	--	--
medicinal (activated)	T47.6X1	T47.6X2	T47.6X3	T47.6X4	T47.6X5	T47.6X6
antidiarrheal	T47.6X1	T47.6X2	T47.6X3	T47.6X4	T47.6X5	T47.6X6
poison control	T47.8X1	T47.8X2	T47.8X3	T47.8X4	T47.8X5	T47.8X6
specified use other than for diarrhea	T47.8X1	T47.8X2	T47.8X3	T47.8X4	T47.8X5	T47.8X6
topical	T49.8X1	T49.8X2	T49.8X3	T49.8X4	T49.8X5	T49.8X6
Chaulmosulfone	T37.1X1	T37.1X2	T37.1X3	T37.1X4	T37.1X5	T37.1X6
Chelating agent NEC	T50.6X1	T50.6X2	T50.6X3	T50.6X4	T50.6X5	T50.6X6
Chelidonium majus	T62.2X1	T62.2X2	T62.2X3	T62.2X4	--	--
Chemical substance NEC	T65.91	T65.92	T65.93	T65.94	--	--
Chenodeoxycholic acid	T47.5X1	T47.5X2	T47.5X3	T47.5X4	T47.5X5	T47.5X6
Chenodiol	T47.5X1	T47.5X2	T47.5X3	T47.5X4	T47.5X5	T47.5X6
Chenopodium	T37.4X1	T37.4X2	T37.4X3	T37.4X4	T37.4X5	T37.4X6
Cherry laurel	T62.2X1	T62.2X2	T62.2X3	T62.2X4	--	--
Chinidin (e)	T46.2X1	T46.2X2	T46.2X3	T46.2X4	T46.2X5	T46.2X6
Chiniofon	T37.8X1	T37.8X2	T37.8X3	T37.8X4	T37.8X5	T37.8X6
Chlophedianol	T48.3X1	T48.3X2	T48.3X3	T48.3X4	T48.3X5	T48.3X6
Chloral	T42.6X1	T42.6X2	T42.6X3	T42.6X4	T42.6X5	T42.6X6
derivative	T42.6X1	T42.6X2	T42.6X3	T42.6X4	T42.6X5	T42.6X6
hydrate	T42.6X1	T42.6X2	T42.6X3	T42.6X4	T42.6X5	T42.6X6
Chloralamide	T42.6X1	T42.6X2	T42.6X3	T42.6X4	T42.6X5	T42.6X6
Chloralodol	T42.6X1	T42.6X2	T42.6X3	T42.6X4	T42.6X5	T42.6X6
Chloralose	T60.4X1	T60.4X2	T60.4X3	T60.4X4	--	--
Chlorambucil	T45.1X1	T45.1X2	T45.1X3	T45.1X4	T45.1X5	T45.1X6
Chloramine	T57.8X1	T57.8X2	T57.8X3	T57.8X4	--	--
T	T49.0X1	T49.0X2	T49.0X3	T49.0X4	T49.0X5	T49.0X6
topical	T49.0X1	T49.0X2	T49.0X3	T49.0X4	T49.0X5	T49.0X6
Chloramphenicol	T36.2X1	T36.2X2	T36.2X3	T36.2X4	T36.2X5	T36.2X6
ENT agent	T49.6X1	T49.6X2	T49.6X3	T49.6X4	T49.6X5	T49.6X6
ophthalmic preparation	T49.5X1	T49.5X2	T49.5X3	T49.5X4	T49.5X5	T49.5X6
topical NEC	T49.0X1	T49.0X2	T49.0X3	T49.0X4	T49.0X5	T49.0X6
Chlorate (potassium) (sodium) NEC	T60.3X1	T60.3X2	T60.3X3	T60.3X4	--	--
herbicide	T60.3X1	T60.3X2	T60.3X3	T60.3X4	--	--
Chlorazanil	T50.2X1	T50.2X2	T50.2X3	T50.2X4	T50.2X5	T50.2X6
Chlorbenzene, chlorbenzol	T53.7X1	T53.7X2	T53.7X3	T53.7X4	--	--
Chlorbenzoxamine	T44.3X1	T44.3X2	T44.3X3	T44.3X4	T44.3X5	T44.3X6
Chlorbutol	T42.6X1	T42.6X2	T42.6X3	T42.6X4	T42.6X5	T42.6X6
Chlorcyclizine	T45.0X1	T45.0X2	T45.0X3	T45.0X4	T45.0X5	T45.0X6
Chlordan (e) (dust)	T60.1X1	T60.1X2	T60.1X3	T60.1X4	--	--
Chlordantoin	T49.0X1	T49.0X2	T49.0X3	T49.0X4	T49.0X5	T49.0X6
Chlordiazepoxide	T42.4X1	T42.4X2	T42.4X3	T42.4X4	T42.4X5	T42.4X6
Chlordiethyl benzamide	T49.3X1	T49.3X2	T49.3X3	T49.3X4	T49.3X5	T49.3X6
Chloresium	T49.8X1	T49.8X2	T49.8X3	T49.8X4	T49.8X5	T49.8X6
Chlorethiazol	T42.6X1	T42.6X2	T42.6X3	T42.6X4	T42.6X5	T42.6X6
Chlorethyl — *see* Ethyl chloride						
Chloretone	T42.6X1	T42.6X2	T42.6X3	T42.6X4	T42.6X5	T42.6X6
Chlorex	T53.6X1	T53.6X2	T53.6X3	T53.6X4	--	--
insecticide	T60.1X1	T60.1X2	T60.1X3	T60.1X4	--	--
Chlorfenvinphos	T60.0X1	T60.0X2	T60.0X3	T60.0X4	--	--
Chlorhexadol	T42.6X1	T42.6X2	T42.6X3	T42.6X4	T42.6X5	T42.6X6
Chlorhexamide	T45.1X1	T45.1X2	T45.1X3	T45.1X4	T45.1X5	T45.1X6
Chlorhexidine	T49.0X1	T49.0X2	T49.0X3	T49.0X4	T49.0X5	T49.0X6
Chlorhydroxyquinolin	T49.0X1	T49.0X2	T49.0X3	T49.0X4	T49.0X5	T49.0X6
Chloride of lime (bleach)	T54.3X1	T54.3X2	T54.3X3	T54.3X4	--	--
Chlorimipramine	T43.011	T43.012	T43.013	T43.014	T43.015	T43.016
Chlorinated						
camphene	T53.6X1	T53.6X2	T53.6X3	T53.6X4	--	--
diphenyl	T53.7X1	T53.7X2	T53.7X3	T53.7X4	--	--
hydrocarbons NEC	T53.91	T53.92	T53.93	T53.94	--	--
solvents	T53.91	T53.92	T53.93	T53.94	--	--
lime (bleach)	T54.3X1	T54.3X2	T54.3X3	T54.3X4	--	--
and boric acid solution	T49.0X1	T49.0X2	T49.0X3	T49.0X4	T49.0X5	T49.0X6
naphthalene (insecticide)	T60.1X1	T60.1X2	T60.1X3	T60.1X4	--	--
industrial (non-pesticide)	T53.7X1	T53.7X2	T53.7X3	T53.7X4	--	--
pesticide NEC	T60.8X1	T60.8X2	T60.8X3	T60.8X4	--	--
soda (*see also* sodium hypochlorite)						
solution	T49.0X1	T49.0X2	T49.0X3	T49.0X4	T49.0X5	T49.0X6
Chlorine (fumes) (gas)	T59.4X1	T59.4X2	T59.4X3	T59.4X4	--	--
bleach	T54.3X1	T54.3X2	T54.3X3	T54.3X4	--	--
compound gas NEC	T59.4X1	T59.4X2	T59.4X3	T59.4X4	--	--
disinfectant	T59.4X1	T59.4X2	T59.4X3	T59.4X4	--	--
releasing agents NEC	T59.4X1	T59.4X2	T59.4X3	T59.4X4	--	--
Chlorisondamine chloride	T46.991	T46.992	T46.993	T46.994	T46.995	T46.996
Chlormadinone	T38.5X1	T38.5X2	T38.5X3	T38.5X4	T38.5X5	T38.5X6
Chlormephos	T60.0X1	T60.0X2	T60.0X3	T60.0X4	--	--
Chlormerodrin	T50.2X1	T50.2X2	T50.2X3	T50.2X4	T50.2X5	T50.2X6
Chlormethiazole	T42.6X1	T42.6X2	T42.6X3	T42.6X4	T42.6X5	T42.6X6
Chlormethine	T45.1X1	T45.1X2	T45.1X3	T45.1X4	T45.1X5	T45.1X6
Chlormethylenecycline	T36.4X1	T36.4X2	T36.4X3	T36.4X4	T36.4X5	T36.4X6
Chlormezanone	T42.6X1	T42.6X2	T42.6X3	T42.6X4	T42.6X5	T42.6X6
Chloroacetic acid	T60.3X1	T60.3X2	T60.3X3	T60.3X4	--	--
Chloroacetone	T59.3X1	T59.3X2	T59.3X3	T59.3X4	--	--
Chloroacetophenone	T59.3X1	T59.3X2	T59.3X3	T59.3X4	--	--
Chloroaniline	T53.7X1	T53.7X2	T53.7X3	T53.7X4	--	--
Chlorobenzene, chlorobenzol	T53.7X1	T53.7X2	T53.7X3	T53.7X4	--	--
Chlorobromomethane (fire extinguisher)	T53.6X1	T53.6X2	T53.6X3	T53.6X4	--	--
Chlorobutanol	T49.0X1	T49.0X2	T49.0X3	T49.0X4	T49.0X5	T49.0X6
Chlorocresol	T49.0X1	T49.0X2	T49.0X3	T49.0X4	T49.0X5	T49.0X6
Chlorodehydro-methyltestosterone	T38.7X1	T38.7X2	T38.7X3	T38.7X4	T38.7X5	T38.7X6
Chlorodinitrobenzene	T53.7X1	T53.7X2	T53.7X3	T53.7X4	--	--
dust or vapor	T53.7X1	T53.7X2	T53.7X3	T53.7X4	--	--
Chlorodiphenyl	T53.7X1	T53.7X2	T53.7X3	T53.7X4	--	--
Chloroethane — *see* Ethyl chloride						
Chloroethylene	T53.6X1	T53.6X2	T53.6X3	T53.6X4	--	--
Chlorofluorocarbons	T53.5X1	T53.5X2	T53.5X3	T53.5X4	--	--
Chloroform (fumes) (vapor)	T53.1X1	T53.1X2	T53.1X3	T53.1X4	--	--
anesthetic	T41.0X1	T41.0X2	T41.0X3	T41.0X4	T41.0X5	T41.0X6
solvent	T53.1X1	T53.1X2	T53.1X3	T53.1X4	--	--
water, concentrated	T41.0X1	T41.0X2	T41.0X3	T41.0X4	T41.0X5	T41.0X6
Chloroguanide	T37.2X1	T37.2X2	T37.2X3	T37.2X4	T37.2X5	T37.2X6
Chloromycetin	T36.2X1	T36.2X2	T36.2X3	T36.2X4	T36.2X5	T36.2X6
ENT agent	T49.6X1	T49.6X2	T49.6X3	T49.6X4	T49.6X5	T49.6X6
ophthalmic preparation	T49.5X1	T49.5X2	T49.5X3	T49.5X4	T49.5X5	T49.5X6
otic solution	T49.6X1	T49.6X2	T49.6X3	T49.6X4	T49.6X5	T49.6X6
topical NEC	T49.0X1	T49.0X2	T49.0X3	T49.0X4	T49.0X5	T49.0X6
Chloronitrobenzene	T53.7X1	T53.7X2	T53.7X3	T53.7X4	--	--
dust or vapor	T53.7X1	T53.7X2	T53.7X3	T53.7X4	--	--
Chlorophacinone	T60.4X1	T60.4X2	T60.4X3	T60.4X4	--	--
Chlorophenol	T53.7X1	T53.7X2	T53.7X3	T53.7X4	--	--
Chlorophenothane	T60.1X1	T60.1X2	T60.1X3	T60.1X4	--	--
Chlorophyll	T50.991	T50.992	T50.993	T50.994	T50.995	T50.996
Chloropicrin (fumes)	T53.6X1	T53.6X2	T53.6X3	T53.6X4	--	--
fumigant	T60.8X1	T60.8X2	T60.8X3	T60.8X4	--	--
fungicide	T60.3X1	T60.3X2	T60.3X3	T60.3X4	--	--
pesticide	T60.8X1	T60.8X2	T60.8X3	T60.8X4	--	--
Chloroprocaine	T41.3X1	T41.3X2	T41.3X3	T41.3X4	T41.3X5	T41.3X6
infiltration (subcutaneous)	T41.3X1	T41.3X2	T41.3X3	T41.3X4	T41.3X5	T41.3X6
nerve block (peripheral) (plexus)	T41.3X1	T41.3X2	T41.3X3	T41.3X4	T41.3X5	T41.3X6
spinal	T41.3X1	T41.3X2	T41.3X3	T41.3X4	T41.3X5	T41.3X6
Chloroptic	T49.5X1	T49.5X2	T49.5X3	T49.5X4	T49.5X5	T49.5X6
Chloropurine	T45.1X1	T45.1X2	T45.1X3	T45.1X4	T45.1X5	T45.1X6
Chloropyramine	T45.0X1	T45.0X2	T45.0X3	T45.0X4	T45.0X5	T45.0X6
Chloropyrifos	T60.0X1	T60.0X2	T60.0X3	T60.0X4	--	--
Chloropyrilene	T45.0X1	T45.0X2	T45.0X3	T45.0X4	T45.0X5	T45.0X6
Chloroquine	T37.2X1	T37.2X2	T37.2X3	T37.2X4	T37.2X5	T37.2X6
Chlorothalonil	T60.3X1	T60.3X2	T60.3X3	T60.3X4	--	--
Chlorothen	T45.0X1	T45.0X2	T45.0X3	T45.0X4	T45.0X5	T45.0X6
Chlorothiazide	T50.2X1	T50.2X2	T50.2X3	T50.2X4	T50.2X5	T50.2X6
Chlorothymol	T49.4X1	T49.4X2	T49.4X3	T49.4X4	T49.4X5	T49.4X6
Chlorotrianisene	T38.5X1	T38.5X2	T38.5X3	T38.5X4	T38.5X5	T38.5X6
Chlorovinyldichloro-arsine, not in war	T57.0X1	T57.0X2	T57.0X3	T57.0X4	--	--
Chloroxine	T49.4X1	T49.4X2	T49.4X3	T49.4X4	T49.4X5	T49.4X6
Chloroxylenol	T49.0X1	T49.0X2	T49.0X3	T49.0X4	T49.0X5	T49.0X6
Chlorphenamine	T45.0X1	T45.0X2	T45.0X3	T45.0X4	T45.0X5	T45.0X6
Chlorphenesin	T42.8X1	T42.8X2	T42.8X3	T42.8X4	T42.8X5	T42.8X6
topical (antifungal)	T49.0X1	T49.0X2	T49.0X3	T49.0X4	T49.0X5	T49.0X6
Chlorpheniramine	T45.0X1	T45.0X2	T45.0X3	T45.0X4	T45.0X5	T45.0X6
Chlorphenoxamine	T45.0X1	T45.0X2	T45.0X3	T45.0X4	T45.0X5	T45.0X6
Chlorphentermine	T50.5X1	T50.5X2	T50.5X3	T50.5X4	T50.5X5	T50.5X6
Chlorprocaine — *see* Chloroprocaine						
Chlorproguanil	T37.2X1	T37.2X2	T37.2X3	T37.2X4	T37.2X5	T37.2X6
Chlorpromazine	T43.3X1	T43.3X2	T43.3X3	T43.3X4	T43.3X5	T43.3X6
Chlorpropamide	T38.3X1	T38.3X2	T38.3X3	T38.3X4	T38.3X5	T38.3X6
Chlorprothixene	T43.4X1	T43.4X2	T43.4X3	T43.4X4	T43.4X5	T43.4X6
Chlorquinaldol	T49.0X1	T49.0X2	T49.0X3	T49.0X4	T49.0X5	T49.0X6
Chlorquinol	T49.0X1	T49.0X2	T49.0X3	T49.0X4	T49.0X5	T49.0X6
Chlortalidone	T50.2X1	T50.2X2	T50.2X3	T50.2X4	T50.2X5	T50.2X6
Chlortetracycline	T36.4X1	T36.4X2	T36.4X3	T36.4X4	T36.4X5	T36.4X6
Chlorthalidone	T50.2X1	T50.2X2	T50.2X3	T50.2X4	T50.2X5	T50.2X6
Chlorthiophos	T60.0X1	T60.0X2	T60.0X3	T60.0X4	--	--
Chlortrianisene	T38.5X1	T38.5X2	T38.5X3	T38.5X4	T38.5X5	T38.5X6
Chlor-Trimeton	T45.0X1	T45.0X2	T45.0X3	T45.0X4	T45.0X5	T45.0X6
Chlorthion	T60.0X1	T60.0X2	T60.0X3	T60.0X4	--	--

Substance	Poisoning, Accidental (unintentional)	Poisoning, Intentional self-harm	Poisoning, Assault	Poisoning, Undetermined	Adverse effect	Underdosing
Chlorzoxazone	T42.8X1	T42.8X2	T42.8X3	T42.8X4	T42.8X5	T42.8X6
Choke damp	T59.7X1	T59.7X2	T59.7X3	T59.7X4	--	--
Cholagogues	T47.5X1	T47.5X2	T47.5X3	T47.5X4	T47.5X5	T47.5X6
Cholebrine	T50.8X1	T50.8X2	T50.8X3	T50.8X4	T50.8X5	T50.8X6
Cholecalciferol	T45.2X1	T45.2X2	T45.2X3	T45.2X4	T45.2X5	T45.2X6
Cholecystokinin	T50.8X1	T50.8X2	T50.8X3	T50.8X4	T50.8X5	T50.8X6
Cholera vaccine	T50.A91	T50.A92	T50.A93	T50.A94	T50.A95	T50.A96
Choleretic	T47.5X1	T47.5X2	T47.5X3	T47.5X4	T47.5X5	T47.5X6
Cholesterol-lowering agents	T46.6X1	T46.6X2	T46.6X3	T46.6X4	T46.6X5	T46.6X6
Cholestyramine (resin)	T46.6X1	T46.6X2	T46.6X3	T46.6X4	T46.6X5	T46.6X6
Cholic acid	T47.5X1	T47.5X2	T47.5X3	T47.5X4	T47.5X5	T47.5X6
Choline	T48.6X1	T48.6X2	T48.6X3	T48.6X4	T48.6X5	T48.6X6
chloride	T50.991	T50.992	T50.993	T50.994	T50.995	T50.996
dihydrogen citrate	T50.991	T50.992	T50.993	T50.994	T50.995	T50.996
salicylate	T39.091	T39.092	T39.093	T39.094	T39.095	T39.096
theophyllinate	T48.6X1	T48.6X2	T48.6X3	T48.6X4	T48.6X5	T48.6X6
Cholinergic (drug) **NEC**	T44.1X1	T44.1X2	T44.1X3	T44.1X4	T44.1X5	T44.1X6
muscle tone enhancer	T44.1X1	T44.1X2	T44.1X3	T44.1X4	T44.1X5	T44.1X6
organophosphorus	T44.0X1	T44.0X2	T44.0X3	T44.0X4	T44.0X5	T44.0X6
insecticide	T60.0X1	T60.0X2	T60.0X3	T60.0X4	--	--
nerve gas	T59.891	T59.892	T59.893	T59.894	--	--
trimethyl ammonium propanediol	T44.1X1	T44.1X2	T44.1X3	T44.1X4	T44.1X5	T44.1X6
Cholinesterase reactivator	T50.6X1	T50.6X2	T50.6X3	T50.6X4	T50.6X5	T50.6X6
Cholografin	T50.8X1	T50.8X2	T50.8X3	T50.8X4	T50.8X5	T50.8X6
Chorionic gonadotropin	T38.891	T38.892	T38.893	T38.894	T38.895	T38.896
Chromate	T56.2X1	T56.2X2	T56.2X3	T56.2X4	--	--
dust or mist	T56.2X1	T56.2X2	T56.2X3	T56.2X4	--	--
lead (*see also* lead)	T56.0X1	T56.0X2	T56.0X3	T56.0X4	--	--
paint	T56.0X1	T56.0X2	T56.0X3	T56.0X4	--	--
Chromic						
acid	T56.2X1	T56.2X2	T56.2X3	T56.2X4	--	--
dust or mist	T56.2X1	T56.2X2	T56.2X3	T56.2X4	--	--
phosphate 32P	T45.1X1	T45.1X2	T45.1X3	T45.1X4	T45.1X5	T45.1X6
Chromium	T56.2X1	T56.2X2	T56.2X3	T56.2X4	--	--
compounds — *see* Chromate						
sesquioxide	T50.8X1	T50.8X2	T50.8X3	T50.8X4	T50.8X5	T50.8X6
Chromomycin A3	T45.1X1	T45.1X2	T45.1X3	T45.1X4	T45.1X5	T45.1X6
Chromonar	T46.3X1	T46.3X2	T46.3X3	T46.3X4	T46.3X5	T46.3X6
Chromyl chloride	T56.2X1	T56.2X2	T56.2X3	T56.2X4	--	--
Chrysarobin	T49.4X1	T49.4X2	T49.4X3	T49.4X4	T49.4X5	T49.4X6
Chrysazin	T47.2X1	T47.2X2	T47.2X3	T47.2X4	T47.2X5	T47.2X6
Chymar	T45.3X1	T45.3X2	T45.3X3	T45.3X4	T45.3X5	T45.3X6
ophthalmic preparation	T49.5X1	T49.5X2	T49.5X3	T49.5X4	T49.5X5	T49.5X6
Chymopapain	T45.3X1	T45.3X2	T45.3X3	T45.3X4	T45.3X5	T45.3X6
Chymotrypsin	T45.3X1	T45.3X2	T45.3X3	T45.3X4	T45.3X5	T45.3X6
ophthalmic preparation	T49.5X1	T49.5X2	T49.5X3	T49.5X4	T49.5X5	T49.5X6
Cianidanol	T50.991	T50.992	T50.993	T50.994	T50.995	T50.996
Cianopramine	T43.011	T43.012	T43.013	T43.014	T43.015	T43.016
Cibenzoline	T46.2X1	T46.2X2	T46.2X3	T46.2X4	T46.2X5	T46.2X6
Ciclacillin	T36.0X1	T36.0X2	T36.0X3	T36.0X4	T36.0X5	T36.0X6
Ciclobarbital — *see* Hexobarbital						
Ciclonicate	T46.7X1	T46.7X2	T46.7X3	T46.7X4	T46.7X5	T46.7X6
Ciclopirox (olamine)	T49.0X1	T49.0X2	T49.0X3	T49.0X4	T49.0X5	T49.0X6
Ciclosporin	T45.1X1	T45.1X2	T45.1X3	T45.1X4	T45.1X5	T45.1X6
Cicuta maculata or virosa	T62.2X1	T62.2X2	T62.2X3	T62.2X4	--	--
Cicutoxin	T62.2X1	T62.2X2	T62.2X3	T62.2X4	--	--
Cigarette lighter fluid	T52.0X1	T52.0X2	T52.0X3	T52.0X4	--	--
Cigarettes (tobacco)	T65.221	T65.222	T65.223	T65.224	--	--
Ciguatoxin	T61.01	T61.02	T61.03	T61.04	--	--
Cilazapril	T46.4X1	T46.4X2	T46.4X3	T46.4X4	T46.4X5	T46.4X6
Cimetidine	T47.0X1	T47.0X2	T47.0X3	T47.0X4	T47.0X5	T47.0X6
Cimetropium bromide	T44.3X1	T44.3X2	T44.3X3	T44.3X4	T44.3X5	T44.3X6
Cinchocaine	T41.3X1	T41.3X2	T41.3X3	T41.3X4	T41.3X5	T41.3X6
topical (surface)	T41.3X1	T41.3X2	T41.3X3	T41.3X4	T41.3X5	T41.3X6
Cinchona	T37.2X1	T37.2X2	T37.2X3	T37.2X4	T37.2X5	T37.2X6
Cinchonine alkaloids	T37.2X1	T37.2X2	T37.2X3	T37.2X4	T37.2X5	T37.2X6
Cinchophen	T50.4X1	T50.4X2	T50.4X3	T50.4X4	T50.4X5	T50.4X6
Cinepazide	T46.7X1	T46.7X2	T46.7X3	T46.7X4	T46.7X5	T46.7X6
Cinnamedrine	T48.5X1	T48.5X2	T48.5X3	T48.5X4	T48.5X5	T48.5X6
Cinnarizine	T45.0X1	T45.0X2	T45.0X3	T45.0X4	T45.0X5	T45.0X6
Cinoxacin	T37.8X1	T37.8X2	T37.8X3	T37.8X4	T37.8X5	T37.8X6
Ciprofibrate	T46.6X1	T46.6X2	T46.6X3	T46.6X4	T46.6X5	T46.6X6
Ciprofloxacin	T36.8X1	T36.8X2	T36.8X3	T36.8X4	T36.8X5	T36.8X6
Cisapride	T47.8X1	T47.8X2	T47.8X3	T47.8X4	T47.8X5	T47.8X6
Cisplatin	T45.1X1	T45.1X2	T45.1X3	T45.1X4	T45.1X5	T45.1X6
Citalopram	T43.221	T43.222	T43.223	T43.224	T43.225	T43.226
Citanest	T41.3X1	T41.3X2	T41.3X3	T41.3X4	T41.3X5	T41.3X6
infiltration (subcutaneous)	T41.3X1	T41.3X2	T41.3X3	T41.3X4	T41.3X5	T41.3X6
nerve block (peripheral) (plexus)	T41.3X1	T41.3X2	T41.3X3	T41.3X4	T41.3X5	T41.3X6
Citric acid	T47.5X1	T47.5X2	T47.5X3	T47.5X4	T47.5X5	T47.5X6
Citrovorum (factor)	T45.8X1	T45.8X2	T45.8X3	T45.8X4	T45.8X5	T45.8X6
Claviceps purpurea	T62.2X1	T62.2X2	T62.2X3	T62.2X4	--	--

Substance	Poisoning, Accidental (unintentional)	Poisoning, Intentional self-harm	Poisoning, Assault	Poisoning, Undetermined	Adverse effect	Underdosing
Clavulanic acid	T36.1X1	T36.1X2	T36.1X3	T36.1X4	T36.1X5	T36.1X6
Cleaner, cleansing agent, type not specified	T65.891	T65.892	T65.893	T65.894	--	--
of paint or varnish	T52.91	T52.92	T52.93	T52.94	--	--
specified type NEC	T65.891	T65.892	T65.893	T65.894	--	--
Clebopride	T47.8X1	T47.8X2	T47.8X3	T47.8X4	T47.8X5	T47.8X6
Clefamide	T37.3X1	T37.3X2	T37.3X3	T37.3X4	T37.3X5	T37.3X6
Clemastine	T45.0X1	T45.0X2	T45.0X3	T45.0X4	T45.0X5	T45.0X6
Clematis vitalba	T62.2X1	T62.2X2	T62.2X3	T62.2X4	--	--
Clemizole	T45.0X1	T45.0X2	T45.0X3	T45.0X4	T45.0X5	T45.0X6
penicillin	T36.0X1	T36.0X2	T36.0X3	T36.0X4	T36.0X5	T36.0X6
Clenbuterol	T48.6X1	T48.6X2	T48.6X3	T48.6X4	T48.6X5	T48.6X6
Clidinium bromide	T44.3X1	T44.3X2	T44.3X3	T44.3X4	T44.3X5	T44.3X6
Clindamycin	T36.8X1	T36.8X2	T36.8X3	T36.8X4	T36.8X5	T36.8X6
Clinofibrate	T46.6X1	T46.6X2	T46.6X3	T46.6X4	T46.6X5	T46.6X6
Clioquinol	T37.8X1	T37.8X2	T37.8X3	T37.8X4	T37.8X5	T37.8X6
Cliradon	T40.2X1	T40.2X2	T40.2X3	T40.2X4	--	--
Clobazam	T42.4X1	T42.4X2	T42.4X3	T42.4X4	T42.4X5	T42.4X6
Clobenzorex	T50.5X1	T50.5X2	T50.5X3	T50.5X4	T50.5X5	T50.5X6
Clobetasol	T49.0X1	T49.0X2	T49.0X3	T49.0X4	T49.0X5	T49.0X6
Clobetasone	T49.0X1	T49.0X2	T49.0X3	T49.0X4	T49.0X5	T49.0X6
Clobutinol	T48.3X1	T48.3X2	T48.3X3	T48.3X4	T48.3X5	T48.3X6
Clocortolone	T38.0X1	T38.0X2	T38.0X3	T38.0X4	T38.0X5	T38.0X6
Clodantoin	T49.0X1	T49.0X2	T49.0X3	T49.0X4	T49.0X5	T49.0X6
Clodronic acid	T50.991	T50.992	T50.993	T50.994	T50.995	T50.996
Clofazimine	T37.1X1	T37.1X2	T37.1X3	T37.1X4	T37.1X5	T37.1X6
Clofedanol	T48.3X1	T48.3X2	T48.3X3	T48.3X4	T48.3X5	T48.3X6
Clofenamide	T50.2X1	T50.2X2	T50.2X3	T50.2X4	T50.2X5	T50.2X6
Clofenotane	T49.0X1	T49.0X2	T49.0X3	T49.0X4	T49.0X5	T49.0X6
Clofezone	T39.2X1	T39.2X2	T39.2X3	T39.2X4	T39.2X5	T39.2X6
Clofibrate	T46.6X1	T46.6X2	T46.6X3	T46.6X4	T46.6X5	T46.6X6
Clofibride	T46.6X1	T46.6X2	T46.6X3	T46.6X4	T46.6X5	T46.6X6
Cloforex	T50.5X1	T50.5X2	T50.5X3	T50.5X4	T50.5X5	T50.5X6
Clomethiazole	T42.6X1	T42.6X2	T42.6X3	T42.6X4	T42.6X5	T42.6X6
Clometocillin	T36.0X1	T36.0X2	T36.0X3	T36.0X4	T36.0X5	T36.0X6
Clomifene	T38.5X1	T38.5X2	T38.5X3	T38.5X4	T38.5X5	T38.5X6
Clomiphene	T38.5X1	T38.5X2	T38.5X3	T38.5X4	T38.5X5	T38.5X6
Clomipramine	T43.011	T43.012	T43.013	T43.014	T43.015	T43.016
Clomocycline	T36.4X1	T36.4X2	T36.4X3	T36.4X4	T36.4X5	T36.4X6
Clonazepam	T42.4X1	T42.4X2	T42.4X3	T42.4X4	T42.4X5	T42.4X6
Clonidine	T46.5X1	T46.5X2	T46.5X3	T46.5X4	T46.5X5	T46.5X6
Clonixin	T39.8X1	T39.8X2	T39.8X3	T39.8X4	T39.8X5	T39.8X6
Clopamide	T50.2X1	T50.2X2	T50.2X3	T50.2X4	T50.2X5	T50.2X6
Clopenthixol	T43.4X1	T43.4X2	T43.4X3	T43.4X4	T43.4X5	T43.4X6
Cloperastine	T48.3X1	T48.3X2	T48.3X3	T48.3X4	T48.3X5	T48.3X6
Clophedianol	T48.3X1	T48.3X2	T48.3X3	T48.3X4	T48.3X5	T48.3X6
Cloponone	T36.2X1	T36.2X2	T36.2X3	T36.2X4	T36.2X5	T36.2X6
Cloprednol	T38.0X1	T38.0X2	T38.0X3	T38.0X4	T38.0X5	T38.0X6
Cloral betaine	T42.6X1	T42.6X2	T42.6X3	T42.6X4	T42.6X5	T42.6X6
Cloramfenicol	T36.2X1	T36.2X2	T36.2X3	T36.2X4	T36.2X5	T36.2X6
Clorazepate (dipotassium)	T42.4X1	T42.4X2	T42.4X3	T42.4X4	T42.4X5	T42.4X6
Clorexolone	T50.2X1	T50.2X2	T50.2X3	T50.2X4	T50.2X5	T50.2X6
Clorfenamine	T45.0X1	T45.0X2	T45.0X3	T45.0X4	T45.0X5	T45.0X6
Clorgiline	T43.1X1	T43.1X2	T43.1X3	T43.1X4	T43.1X5	T43.1X6
Clorotepine	T44.3X1	T44.3X2	T44.3X3	T44.3X4	T44.3X5	T44.3X6
Clorox (bleach)	T54.91	T54.92	T54.93	T54.94	--	--
Clorprenaline	T48.6X1	T48.6X2	T48.6X3	T48.6X4	T48.6X5	T48.6X6
Clortermine	T50.5X1	T50.5X2	T50.5X3	T50.5X4	T50.5X5	T50.5X6
Clotiapine	T43.591	T43.592	T43.593	T43.594	T43.595	T43.596
Clotiazepam	T42.4X1	T42.4X2	T42.4X3	T42.4X4	T42.4X5	T42.4X6
Clotibric acid	T46.6X1	T46.6X2	T46.6X3	T46.6X4	T46.6X5	T46.6X6
Clotrimazole	T49.0X1	T49.0X2	T49.0X3	T49.0X4	T49.0X5	T49.0X6
Cloxacillin	T36.0X1	T36.0X2	T36.0X3	T36.0X4	T36.0X5	T36.0X6
Cloxazolam	T42.4X1	T42.4X2	T42.4X3	T42.4X4	T42.4X5	T42.4X6
Cloxiquine	T49.0X1	T49.0X2	T49.0X3	T49.0X4	T49.0X5	T49.0X6
Clozapine	T42.4X1	T42.4X2	T42.4X3	T42.4X4	T42.4X5	T42.4X6
Coagulant NEC	T45.7X1	T45.7X2	T45.7X3	T45.7X4	T45.7X5	T45.7X6
Coal (carbon monoxide from) (*see also* Carbon, monoxide, coal)	T58.2X1	T58.2X2	T58.2X3	T58.2X4	--	--
oil — *see* Kerosene						
tar	T49.1X1	T49.1X2	T49.1X3	T49.1X4	T49.1X5	T49.1X6
fumes	T59.891	T59.892	T59.893	T59.894	--	--
medicinal (ointment)	T49.4X1	T49.4X2	T49.4X3	T49.4X4	T49.4X5	T49.4X6
analgesics NEC	T39.2X1	T39.2X2	T39.2X3	T39.2X4	T39.2X5	T39.2X6
naphtha (solvent)	T52.0X1	T52.0X2	T52.0X3	T52.0X4	--	--
Cobalamine	T45.2X1	T45.2X2	T45.2X3	T45.2X4	T45.2X5	T45.2X6
Cobalt (nonmedicinal) (fumes) (industrial)	T56.891	T56.892	T56.893	T56.894	--	--
medicinal (trace) (chloride)	T45.8X1	T45.8X2	T45.8X3	T45.8X4	T45.8X5	T45.8X6
Cobra (venom)	T63.041	T63.042	T63.043	T63.044	--	--
Coca (leaf)	T40.5X1	T40.5X2	T40.5X3	T40.5X4	T40.5X5	T40.5X6
Cocaine	T40.5X1	T40.5X2	T40.5X3	T40.5X4	T40.5X5	T40.5X6
topical anesthetic	T41.3X1	T41.3X2	T41.3X3	T41.3X4	T41.3X5	T41.3X6

Substance	Poisoning, Accidental (unintentional)	Poisoning, Intentional self-harm	Poisoning, Assault	Poisoning, Undetermined	Adverse effect	Underdosing
Cocarboxylase	T45.3X1	T45.3X2	T45.3X3	T45.3X4	T45.3X5	T45.3X6
Coccidioidin	T50.8X1	T50.8X2	T50.8X3	T50.8X4	T50.8X5	T50.8X6
Cocculus indicus	T62.1X1	T62.1X2	T62.1X3	T62.1X4	--	--
Cochineal	T65.6X1	T65.6X2	T65.6X3	T65.6X4	--	--
medicinal products	T50.991	T50.992	T50.993	T50.994	T50.995	T50.996
Codeine	T40.2X1	T40.2X2	T40.2X3	T40.2X4	T40.2X5	T40.2X6
Cod-liver oil	T45.2X1	T45.2X2	T45.2X3	T45.2X4	T45.2X5	T45.2X6
Coenzyme A	T50.991	T50.992	T50.993	T50.994	T50.995	T50.996
Coffee	T62.8X1	T62.8X2	T62.8X3	T62.8X4	--	--
Cogalactoiso-merase	T50.991	T50.992	T50.993	T50.994	T50.995	T50.996
Cogentin	T44.3X1	T44.3X2	T44.3X3	T44.3X4	T44.3X5	T44.3X6
Coke fumes or gas (carbon monoxide)	T58.2X1	T58.2X2	T58.2X3	T58.2X4	--	--
industrial use	T58.8X1	T58.8X2	T58.8X3	T58.8X4	--	--
Colace	T47.4X1	T47.4X2	T47.4X3	T47.4X4	T47.4X5	T47.4X6
Colaspase	T45.1X1	T45.1X2	T45.1X3	T45.1X4	T45.1X5	T45.1X6
Colchicine	T50.4X1	T50.4X2	T50.4X3	T50.4X4	T50.4X5	T50.4X6
Colchicum	T62.2X1	T62.2X2	T62.2X3	T62.2X4	--	--
Cold cream	T49.3X1	T49.3X2	T49.3X3	T49.3X4	T49.3X5	T49.3X6
Colecalciferol	T45.2X1	T45.2X2	T45.2X3	T45.2X4	T45.2X5	T45.2X6
Colestipol	T46.6X1	T46.6X2	T46.6X3	T46.6X4	T46.6X5	T46.6X6
Colestyramine	T46.6X1	T46.6X2	T46.6X3	T46.6X4	T46.6X5	T46.6X6
Colimycin	T36.8X1	T36.8X2	T36.8X3	T36.8X4	T36.8X5	T36.8X6
Colistimethate	T36.8X1	T36.8X2	T36.8X3	T36.8X4	T36.8X5	T36.8X6
Colistin	T36.8X1	T36.8X2	T36.8X3	T36.8X4	T36.8X5	T36.8X6
sulfate (eye preparation)	T49.5X1	T49.5X2	T49.5X3	T49.5X4	T49.5X5	T49.5X6
Collagen	T50.991	T50.992	T50.993	T50.994	T50.995	T50.996
Collagenase	T49.4X1	T49.4X2	T49.4X3	T49.4X4	T49.4X5	T49.4X6
Collodion	T49.3X1	T49.3X2	T49.3X3	T49.3X4	T49.3X5	T49.3X6
Colocynth	T47.2X1	T47.2X2	T47.2X3	T47.2X4	T47.2X5	T47.2X6
Colophony adhesive	T49.3X1	T49.3X2	T49.3X3	T49.3X4	T49.3X5	T49.3X6
Colorant (see also Dye)	T50.991	T50.992	T50.993	T50.994	T50.995	T50.996
Coloring matter — see Dye(s)						
Combustion gas (after combustion) — see Carbon, monoxide						
prior to combustion	T59.891	T59.892	T59.893	T59.894	--	--
Compazine	T43.3X1	T43.3X2	T43.3X3	T43.3X4	T43.3X5	T43.3X6
Compound						
42 (warfarin)	T60.4X1	T60.4X2	T60.4X3	T60.4X4	--	--
269 (endrin)	T60.1X1	T60.1X2	T60.1X3	T60.1X4	--	--
497 (dieldrin)	T60.1X1	T60.1X2	T60.1X3	T60.1X4	--	--
1080 (sodium fluoroacetate)	T60.4X1	T60.4X2	T60.4X3	T60.4X4	--	--
3422 (parathion)	T60.0X1	T60.0X2	T60.0X3	T60.0X4	--	--
3911 (phorate)	T60.0X1	T60.0X2	T60.0X3	T60.0X4	--	--
3956 (toxaphene)	T60.1X1	T60.1X2	T60.1X3	T60.1X4	--	--
4049 (malathion)	T60.0X1	T60.0X2	T60.0X3	T60.0X4	--	--
4069 (malathion)	T60.0X1	T60.0X2	T60.0X3	T60.0X4	--	--
4124 (dicapthon)	T60.0X1	T60.0X2	T60.0X3	T60.0X4	--	--
E (cortisone)	T38.0X1	T38.0X2	T38.0X3	T38.0X4	T38.0X5	T38.0X6
F (hydrocortisone)	T38.0X1	T38.0X2	T38.0X3	T38.0X4	T38.0X5	T38.0X6
Congener, anabolic	T38.7X1	T38.7X2	T38.7X3	T38.7X4	T38.7X5	T38.7X6
Congo red	T50.8X1	T50.8X2	T50.8X3	T50.8X4	T50.8X5	T50.8X6
Coniine, conine	T62.2X1	T62.2X2	T62.2X3	T62.2X4	--	--
Conium (maculatum)	T62.2X1	T62.2X2	T62.2X3	T62.2X4	--	--
Conjugated estrogenic substances	T38.5X1	T38.5X2	T38.5X3	T38.5X4	T38.5X5	T38.5X6
Contac	T48.5X1	T48.5X2	T48.5X3	T48.5X4	T48.5X5	T48.5X6
Contact lens solution	T49.5X1	T49.5X2	T49.5X3	T49.5X4	T49.5X5	T49.5X6
Contraceptive (oral)	T38.4X1	T38.4X2	T38.4X3	T38.4X4	T38.4X5	T38.4X6
vaginal	T49.8X1	T49.8X2	T49.8X3	T49.8X4	T49.8X5	T49.8X6
Contrast medium, radiography	T50.8X1	T50.8X2	T50.8X3	T50.8X4	T50.8X5	T50.8X6
Convallaria glycosides	T46.0X1	T46.0X2	T46.0X3	T46.0X4	T46.0X5	T46.0X6
Convallaria majalis	T62.2X1	T62.2X2	T62.2X3	T62.2X4	--	--
berry	T62.1X1	T62.1X2	T62.1X3	T62.1X4	--	--
Copper (dust) (fumes) (nonmedicinal) NEC	T56.4X1	T56.4X2	T56.4X3	T56.4X4	--	--
arsenate, arsenite	T57.0X1	T57.0X2	T57.0X3	T57.0X4	--	--
insecticide	T60.2X1	T60.2X2	T60.2X3	T60.2X4	--	--
emetic	T47.7X1	T47.7X2	T47.7X3	T47.7X4	T47.7X5	T47.7X6
fungicide	T60.3X1	T60.3X2	T60.3X3	T60.3X4	--	--
gluconate	T49.0X1	T49.0X2	T49.0X3	T49.0X4	T49.0X5	T49.0X6
insecticide	T60.2X1	T60.2X2	T60.2X3	T60.2X4	--	--
medicinal (trace)	T45.8X1	T45.8X2	T45.8X3	T45.8X4	T45.8X5	T45.8X6
oleate	T49.0X1	T49.0X2	T49.0X3	T49.0X4	T49.0X5	T49.0X6
sulfate	T56.4X1	T56.4X2	T56.4X3	T56.4X4	--	--
cupric	T56.4X1	T56.4X2	T56.4X3	T56.4X4	--	--
fungicide	T60.3X1	T60.3X2	T60.3X3	T60.3X4	--	--
medicinal						
ear	T49.6X1	T49.6X2	T49.6X3	T49.6X4	T49.6X5	T49.6X6

Substance	Poisoning, Accidental (unintentional)	Poisoning, Intentional self-harm	Poisoning, Assault	Poisoning, Undetermined	Adverse effect	Underdosing
Copper — continued						
sulfate — continued						
emetic	T47.7X1	T47.7X2	T47.7X3	T47.7X4	T47.7X5	T47.7X6
eye	T49.5X1	T49.5X2	T49.5X3	T49.5X4	T49.5X5	T49.5X6
cuprous	T56.4X1	T56.4X2	T56.4X3	T56.4X4	--	--
fungicide	T60.3X1	T60.3X2	T60.3X3	T60.3X4	--	--
medicinal						
ear	T49.6X1	T49.6X2	T49.6X3	T49.6X4	T49.6X5	T49.6X6
emetic	T47.7X1	T47.7X2	T47.7X3	T47.7X4	T47.7X5	T47.7X6
eye	T49.5X1	T49.5X2	T49.5X3	T49.5X4	T49.5X5	T49.5X6
Copperhead snake (bite) (venom)	T63.061	T63.062	T63.063	T63.064	--	--
Coral (sting)	T63.691	T63.692	T63.693	T63.694	--	--
snake (bite) (venom)	T63.021	T63.022	T63.023	T63.024	--	--
Corbadrine	T49.6X1	T49.6X2	T49.6X3	T49.6X4	T49.6X5	T49.6X6
Cordite	T65.891	T65.892	T65.893	T65.894	--	--
vapor	T59.891	T59.892	T59.893	T59.894	--	--
Cordran	T49.0X1	T49.0X2	T49.0X3	T49.0X4	T49.0X5	T49.0X6
Corn cures	T49.4X1	T49.4X2	T49.4X3	T49.4X4	T49.4X5	T49.4X6
Corn starch	T49.3X1	T49.3X2	T49.3X3	T49.3X4	T49.3X5	T49.3X6
Cornhusker's lotion	T49.3X1	T49.3X2	T49.3X3	T49.3X4	T49.3X5	T49.3X6
Coronary vasodilator NEC	T46.3X1	T46.3X2	T46.3X3	T46.3X4	T46.3X5	T46.3X6
Corrosive NEC	T54.91	T54.92	T54.93	T54.94	--	--
acid NEC	T54.2X1	T54.2X2	T54.2X3	T54.2X4	--	--
aromatics	T54.1X1	T54.1X2	T54.1X3	T54.1X4	--	--
disinfectant	T54.1X1	T54.1X2	T54.1X3	T54.1X4	--	--
fumes NEC	T54.91	T54.92	T54.93	T54.94	--	--
specified NEC	T54.91	T54.92	T54.93	T54.94	--	--
sublimate	T56.1X1	T56.1X2	T56.1X3	T56.1X4	--	--
Cortate	T38.0X1	T38.0X2	T38.0X3	T38.0X4	T38.0X5	T38.0X6
Cort-Dome	T38.0X1	T38.0X2	T38.0X3	T38.0X4	T38.0X5	T38.0X6
ENT agent	T49.6X1	T49.6X2	T49.6X3	T49.6X4	T49.6X5	T49.6X6
ophthalmic preparation	T49.5X1	T49.5X2	T49.5X3	T49.5X4	T49.5X5	T49.5X6
topical NEC	T49.0X1	T49.0X2	T49.0X3	T49.0X4	T49.0X5	T49.0X6
Cortef	T38.0X1	T38.0X2	T38.0X3	T38.0X4	T38.0X5	T38.0X6
ENT agent	T49.6X1	T49.6X2	T49.6X3	T49.6X4	T49.6X5	T49.6X6
ophthalmic preparation	T49.5X1	T49.5X2	T49.5X3	T49.5X4	T49.5X5	T49.5X6
topical NEC	T49.0X1	T49.0X2	T49.0X3	T49.0X4	T49.0X5	T49.0X6
Corticosteroid	T38.0X1	T38.0X2	T38.0X3	T38.0X4	T38.0X5	T38.0X6
ENT agent	T49.6X1	T49.6X2	T49.6X3	T49.6X4	T49.6X5	T49.6X6
mineral	T50.0X1	T50.0X2	T50.0X3	T50.0X4	T50.0X5	T50.0X6
ophthalmic	T49.5X1	T49.5X2	T49.5X3	T49.5X4	T49.5X5	T49.5X6
topical NEC	T49.0X1	T49.0X2	T49.0X3	T49.0X4	T49.0X5	T49.0X6
Corticotropin	T38.811	T38.812	T38.813	T38.814	T38.815	T38.816
Cortisol	T49.0X1	T49.0X2	T49.0X3	T49.0X4	T49.0X5	T49.0X6
ENT agent	T49.6X1	T49.6X2	T49.6X3	T49.6X4	T49.6X5	T49.6X6
ophthalmic preparation	T49.5X1	T49.5X2	T49.5X3	T49.5X4	T49.5X5	T49.5X6
topical NEC	T49.0X1	T49.0X2	T49.0X3	T49.0X4	T49.0X5	T49.0X6
Cortisone (acetate)	T38.0X1	T38.0X2	T38.0X3	T38.0X4	T38.0X5	T38.0X6
ENT agent	T49.6X1	T49.6X2	T49.6X3	T49.6X4	T49.6X5	T49.6X6
ophthalmic preparation	T49.5X1	T49.5X2	T49.5X3	T49.5X4	T49.5X5	T49.5X6
topical NEC	T49.0X1	T49.0X2	T49.0X3	T49.0X4	T49.0X5	T49.0X6
Cortivazol	T38.0X1	T38.0X2	T38.0X3	T38.0X4	T38.0X5	T38.0X6
Cortogen	T38.0X1	T38.0X2	T38.0X3	T38.0X4	T38.0X5	T38.0X6
ENT agent	T49.6X1	T49.6X2	T49.6X3	T49.6X4	T49.6X5	T49.6X6
ophthalmic preparation	T49.5X1	T49.5X2	T49.5X3	T49.5X4	T49.5X5	T49.5X6
Cortone	T38.0X1	T38.0X2	T38.0X3	T38.0X4	T38.0X5	T38.0X6
ENT agent	T49.6X1	T49.6X2	T49.6X3	T49.6X4	T49.6X5	T49.6X6
ophthalmic preparation	T49.5X1	T49.5X2	T49.5X3	T49.5X4	T49.5X5	T49.5X6
Cortril	T38.0X1	T38.0X2	T38.0X3	T38.0X4	T38.0X5	T38.0X6
ENT agent	T49.6X1	T49.6X2	T49.6X3	T49.6X4	T49.6X5	T49.6X6
ophthalmic preparation	T49.5X1	T49.5X2	T49.5X3	T49.5X4	T49.5X5	T49.5X6
topical NEC	T49.0X1	T49.0X2	T49.0X3	T49.0X4	T49.0X5	T49.0X6
Corynebacterium parvum	T45.1X1	T45.1X2	T45.1X3	T45.1X4	T45.1X5	T45.1X6
Cosmetic preparation	T49.8X1	T49.8X2	T49.8X3	T49.8X4	T49.8X5	T49.8X6
Cosmetics	T49.8X1	T49.8X2	T49.8X3	T49.8X4	T49.8X5	T49.8X6
Cosyntropin	T38.811	T38.812	T38.813	T38.814	T38.815	T38.816
Cotarnine	T45.7X1	T45.7X2	T45.7X3	T45.7X4	T45.7X5	T45.7X6
Co-trimoxazole	T36.8X1	T36.8X2	T36.8X3	T36.8X4	T36.8X5	T36.8X6
Cottonseed oil	T49.3X1	T49.3X2	T49.3X3	T49.3X4	T49.3X5	T49.3X6
Cough mixture (syrup)	T48.4X1	T48.4X2	T48.4X3	T48.4X4	T48.4X5	T48.4X6
containing opiates	T40.2X1	T40.2X2	T40.2X3	T40.2X4	T40.2X5	T40.2X6
expectorants	T48.4X1	T48.4X2	T48.4X3	T48.4X4	T48.4X5	T48.4X6
Coumadin	T45.511	T45.512	T45.513	T45.514	T45.515	T45.516
rodenticide	T60.4X1	T60.4X2	T60.4X3	T60.4X4	--	--
Coumaphos	T60.0X1	T60.0X2	T60.0X3	T60.0X4	--	--
Coumarin	T45.511	T45.512	T45.513	T45.514	T45.515	T45.516
Coumetarol	T45.511	T45.512	T45.513	T45.514	T45.515	T45.516
Cowbane	T62.2X1	T62.2X2	T62.2X3	T62.2X4	--	--
Cozyme	T45.2X1	T45.2X2	T45.2X3	T45.2X4	T45.2X5	T45.2X6
Crack	T40.5X1	T40.5X2	T40.5X3	T40.5X4	--	--
Crataegus extract	T46.0X1	T46.0X2	T46.0X3	T46.0X4	T46.0X5	T46.0X6
Creolin	T54.1X1	T54.1X2	T54.1X3	T54.1X4	--	--
disinfectant	T54.1X1	T54.1X2	T54.1X3	T54.1X4	--	--

Substance	Poisoning, Accidental (unintentional)	Poisoning, Intentional self-harm	Poisoning, Assault	Poisoning, Undetermined	Adverse effect	Underdosing
Creosol (compound)	T49.0X1	T49.0X2	T49.0X3	T49.0X4	T49.0X5	T49.0X6
Creosote (coal tar) (beechwood)	T49.0X1	T49.0X2	T49.0X3	T49.0X4	T49.0X5	T49.0X6
medicinal (expectorant)	T48.4X1	T48.4X2	T48.4X3	T48.4X4	T48.4X5	T48.4X6
syrup	T48.4X1	T48.4X2	T48.4X3	T48.4X4	T48.4X5	T48.4X6
Cresol(s)	T49.0X1	T49.0X2	T49.0X3	T49.0X4	T49.0X5	T49.0X6
and soap solution	T49.0X1	T49.0X2	T49.0X3	T49.0X4	T49.0X5	T49.0X6
Cresyl acetate	T49.0X1	T49.0X2	T49.0X3	T49.0X4	T49.0X5	T49.0X6
Cresylic acid	T49.0X1	T49.0X2	T49.0X3	T49.0X4	T49.0X5	T49.0X6
Crimidine	T60.4X1	T60.4X2	T60.4X3	T60.4X4	--	--
Croconazole	T37.8X1	T37.8X2	T37.8X3	T37.8X4	T37.8X5	T37.8X6
Cromoglicic acid	T48.6X1	T48.6X2	T48.6X3	T48.6X4	T48.6X5	T48.6X6
Cromolyn	T48.6X1	T48.6X2	T48.6X3	T48.6X4	T48.6X5	T48.6X6
Cromonar	T46.3X1	T46.3X2	T46.3X3	T46.3X4	T46.3X5	T46.3X6
Cropropamide	T39.8X1	T39.8X2	T39.8X3	T39.8X4	T39.8X5	T39.8X6
with crotethamide	T50.7X1	T50.7X2	T50.7X3	T50.7X4	T50.7X5	T50.7X6
Crotamiton	T49.0X1	T49.0X2	T49.0X3	T49.0X4	T49.0X5	T49.0X6
Crotethamide	T39.8X1	T39.8X2	T39.8X3	T39.8X4	T39.8X5	T39.8X6
with cropropamide	T50.7X1	T50.7X2	T50.7X3	T50.7X4	T50.7X5	T50.7X6
Croton (oil)	T47.2X1	T47.2X2	T47.2X3	T47.2X4	T47.2X5	T47.2X6
chloral	T42.6X1	T42.6X2	T42.6X3	T42.6X4	T42.6X5	T42.6X6
Crude oil	T52.0X1	T52.0X2	T52.0X3	T52.0X4	--	--
Cryogenine	T39.8X1	T39.8X2	T39.8X3	T39.8X4	T39.8X5	T39.8X6
Cryolite (vapor)	T60.1X1	T60.1X2	T60.1X3	T60.1X4	--	--
insecticide	T60.1X1	T60.1X2	T60.1X3	T60.1X4	--	--
Cryptenamine (tannates)	T46.5X1	T46.5X2	T46.5X3	T46.5X4	T46.5X5	T46.5X6
Crystal violet	T49.0X1	T49.0X2	T49.0X3	T49.0X4	T49.0X5	T49.0X6
Cuckoopint	T62.2X1	T62.2X2	T62.2X3	T62.2X4	--	--
Cumetharol	T45.511	T45.512	T45.513	T45.514	T45.515	T45.516
Cupric						
acetate	T60.3X1	T60.3X2	T60.3X3	T60.3X4	--	--
acetoarsenite	T57.0X1	T57.0X2	T57.0X3	T57.0X4	--	--
arsenate	T57.0X1	T57.0X2	T57.0X3	T57.0X4	--	--
gluconate	T49.0X1	T49.0X2	T49.0X3	T49.0X4	T49.0X5	T49.0X6
oleate	T49.0X1	T49.0X2	T49.0X3	T49.0X4	T49.0X5	T49.0X6
sulfate	T56.4X1	T56.4X2	T56.4X3	T56.4X4	--	--
Cuprous sulfate (*see also* Copper sulfate)	T56.4X1	T56.4X2	T56.4X3	T56.4X4	--	--
Curare, curarine	T48.1X1	T48.1X2	T48.1X3	T48.1X4	T48.1X5	T48.1X6
Cyamemazine	T43.3X1	T43.3X2	T43.3X3	T43.3X4	T43.3X5	T43.3X6
Cyamopsis tetragono-loba	T46.6X1	T46.6X2	T46.6X3	T46.6X4	T46.6X5	T46.6X6
Cyanacetyl hydrazide	T37.1X1	T37.1X2	T37.1X3	T37.1X4	T37.1X5	T37.1X6
Cyanic acid (gas)	T59.891	T59.892	T59.893	T59.894	--	--
Cyanide(s) (compounds) (potassium) (sodium) NEC	T65.0X1	T65.0X2	T65.0X3	T65.0X4	--	--
dust or gas (inhalation) NEC	T57.3X1	T57.3X2	T57.3X3	T57.3X4	--	--
fumigant	T65.0X1	T65.0X2	T65.0X3	T65.0X4	--	--
hydrogen	T57.3X1	T57.3X2	T57.3X3	T57.3X4	--	--
mercuric — *see* Mercury						
pesticide (dust) (fumes)	T65.0X1	T65.0X2	T65.0X3	T65.0X4	--	--
Cyanoacrylate adhesive	T49.3X1	T49.3X2	T49.3X3	T49.3X4	T49.3X5	T49.3X6
Cyanocobalamin	T45.8X1	T45.8X2	T45.8X3	T45.8X4	T45.8X5	T45.8X6
Cyanogen (chloride) (gas) **NEC**	T59.891	T59.892	T59.893	T59.894	--	--
Cyclacillin	T36.0X1	T36.0X2	T36.0X3	T36.0X4	T36.0X5	T36.0X6
Cyclaine	T41.3X1	T41.3X2	T41.3X3	T41.3X4	T41.3X5	T41.3X6
Cyclamate	T50.991	T50.992	T50.993	T50.994	T50.995	T50.996
Cyclamen europaeum	T62.2X1	T62.2X2	T62.2X3	T62.2X4	--	--
Cyclandelate	T46.7X1	T46.7X2	T46.7X3	T46.7X4	T46.7X5	T46.7X6
Cyclazocine	T50.7X1	T50.7X2	T50.7X3	T50.7X4	T50.7X5	T50.7X6
Cyclizine	T45.0X1	T45.0X2	T45.0X3	T45.0X4	T45.0X5	T45.0X6
Cyclobarbital	T42.3X1	T42.3X2	T42.3X3	T42.3X4	T42.3X5	T42.3X6
Cyclobarbitone	T42.3X1	T42.3X2	T42.3X3	T42.3X4	T42.3X5	T42.3X6
Cyclobenzaprine	T48.1X1	T48.1X2	T48.1X3	T48.1X4	T48.1X5	T48.1X6
Cyclodrine	T44.3X1	T44.3X2	T44.3X3	T44.3X4	T44.3X5	T44.3X6
Cycloguanil embonate	T37.2X1	T37.2X2	T37.2X3	T37.2X4	T37.2X5	T37.2X6
Cyclohexane	T52.8X1	T52.8X2	T52.8X3	T52.8X4	--	--
Cyclohexanol	T51.8X1	T51.8X2	T51.8X3	T51.8X4	--	--
Cyclohexanone	T52.4X1	T52.4X2	T52.4X3	T52.4X4	--	--
Cycloheximide	T60.3X1	T60.3X2	T60.3X3	T60.3X4	--	--
Cyclohexyl acetate	T52.8X1	T52.8X2	T52.8X3	T52.8X4	--	--
Cycloleucin	T45.1X1	T45.1X2	T45.1X3	T45.1X4	T45.1X5	T45.1X6
Cyclomethycaine	T41.3X1	T41.3X2	T41.3X3	T41.3X4	T41.3X5	T41.3X6
Cyclopentamine	T44.4X1	T44.4X2	T44.4X3	T44.4X4	T44.4X5	T44.4X6
Cyclopenthiazide	T50.2X1	T50.2X2	T50.2X3	T50.2X4	T50.2X5	T50.2X6
Cyclopentolate	T44.3X1	T44.3X2	T44.3X3	T44.3X4	T44.3X5	T44.3X6
Cyclophosphamide	T45.1X1	T45.1X2	T45.1X3	T45.1X4	T45.1X5	T45.1X6
Cycloplegic drug	T49.5X1	T49.5X2	T49.5X3	T49.5X4	T49.5X5	T49.5X6
Cyclopropane	T41.291	T41.292	T41.293	T41.294	T41.295	T41.296
Cyclopyrabital	T39.8X1	T39.8X2	T39.8X3	T39.8X4	T39.8X5	T39.8X6
Cycloserine	T37.1X1	T37.1X2	T37.1X3	T37.1X4	T37.1X5	T37.1X6
Cyclosporin	T45.1X1	T45.1X2	T45.1X3	T45.1X4	T45.1X5	T45.1X6
Cyclothiazide	T50.2X1	T50.2X2	T50.2X3	T50.2X4	T50.2X5	T50.2X6
Cycrimine	T44.3X1	T44.3X2	T44.3X3	T44.3X4	T44.3X5	T44.3X6
Cyhalothrin	T60.1X1	T60.1X2	T60.1X3	T60.1X4	--	--
Cymarin	T46.0X1	T46.0X2	T46.0X3	T46.0X4	T46.0X5	T46.0X6
Cypermethrin	T60.1X1	T60.1X2	T60.1X3	T60.1X4	--	--
Cyphenothrin	T60.2X1	T60.2X2	T60.2X3	T60.2X4	--	--
Cyproheptadine	T45.0X1	T45.0X2	T45.0X3	T45.0X4	T45.0X5	T45.0X6
Cyproterone	T38.6X1	T38.6X2	T38.6X3	T38.6X4	T38.6X5	T38.6X6
Cysteamine	T50.6X1	T50.6X2	T50.6X3	T50.6X4	T50.6X5	T50.6X6
Cytarabine	T45.1X1	T45.1X2	T45.1X3	T45.1X4	T45.1X5	T45.1X6
Cytisus						
laburnum	T62.2X1	T62.2X2	T62.2X3	T62.2X4	--	--
scoparius	T62.2X1	T62.2X2	T62.2X3	T62.2X4	--	--
Cytochrome C	T47.5X1	T47.5X2	T47.5X3	T47.5X4	T47.5X5	T47.5X6
Cytomel	T38.1X1	T38.1X2	T38.1X3	T38.1X4	T38.1X5	T38.1X6
Cytosine arabinoside	T45.1X1	T45.1X2	T45.1X3	T45.1X4	T45.1X5	T45.1X6
Cytoxan	T45.1X1	T45.1X2	T45.1X3	T45.1X4	T45.1X5	T45.1X6
Cytozyme	T45.7X1	T45.7X2	T45.7X3	T45.7X4	T45.7X5	T45.7X6
D						
2,4-D (dichlorophen-oxyacetic acid)	T60.3X1	T60.3X2	T60.3X3	T60.3X4	--	--
Dacarbazine	T45.1X1	T45.1X2	T45.1X3	T45.1X4	T45.1X5	T45.1X6
Dactinomycin	T45.1X1	T45.1X2	T45.1X3	T45.1X4	T45.1X5	T45.1X6
DADPS	T37.1X1	T37.1X2	T37.1X3	T37.1X4	T37.1X5	T37.1X6
Dakin's solution	T49.0X1	T49.0X2	T49.0X3	T49.0X4	T49.0X5	T49.0X6
Dalapon (sodium)	T60.3X1	T60.3X2	T60.3X3	T60.3X4	--	--
Dalmane	T42.4X1	T42.4X2	T42.4X3	T42.4X4	T42.4X5	T42.4X6
Danazol	T38.6X1	T38.6X2	T38.6X3	T38.6X4	T38.6X5	T38.6X6
Danilone	T45.511	T45.512	T45.513	T45.514	T45.515	T45.516
Danthron	T47.2X1	T47.2X2	T47.2X3	T47.2X4	T47.2X5	T47.2X6
Dantrolene	T42.8X1	T42.8X2	T42.8X3	T42.8X4	T42.8X5	T42.8X6
Dantron	T47.2X1	T47.2X2	T47.2X3	T47.2X4	T47.2X5	T47.2X6
Daphne (gnidium) (mezereum)	T62.2X1	T62.2X2	T62.2X3	T62.2X4	--	--
berry	T62.1X1	T62.1X2	T62.1X3	T62.1X4	--	--
Dapsone	T37.1X1	T37.1X2	T37.1X3	T37.1X4	T37.1X5	T37.1X6
Daraprim	T37.2X1	T37.2X2	T37.2X3	T37.2X4	T37.2X5	T37.2X6
Darnel	T62.2X1	T62.2X2	T62.2X3	T62.2X4	--	--
Darvon	T39.8X1	T39.8X2	T39.8X3	T39.8X4	T39.8X5	T39.8X6
Daunomycin	T45.1X1	T45.1X2	T45.1X3	T45.1X4	T45.1X5	T45.1X6
Daunorubicin	T45.1X1	T45.1X2	T45.1X3	T45.1X4	T45.1X5	T45.1X6
DBI	T38.3X1	T38.3X2	T38.3X3	T38.3X4	T38.3X5	T38.3X6
D-Con	T60.91	T60.92	T60.93	T60.94	--	--
insecticide	T60.2X1	T60.2X2	T60.2X3	T60.2X4	--	--
rodenticide	T60.4X1	T60.4X2	T60.4X3	T60.4X4	--	--
DDAVP	T38.891	T38.892	T38.893	T38.894	T38.895	T38.896
DDE (bis(chlorophenyl)-dichloroethylene)	T60.2X1	T60.2X2	T60.2X3	T60.2X4	--	--
DDS	T37.1X1	T37.1X2	T37.1X3	T37.1X4	T37.1X5	T37.1X6
DDT (dust)	T60.1X1	T60.1X2	T60.1X3	T60.1X4	--	--
Deadly nightshade (*see also* Belladonna)	T62.2X1	T62.2X2	T62.2X3	T62.2X4	--	--
berry	T62.1X1	T62.1X2	T62.1X3	T62.1X4	--	--
Deamino-D-arginine vasopressin	T38.891	T38.892	T38.893	T38.894	T38.895	T38.896
Deanol (aceglumate)	T50.991	T50.992	T50.993	T50.994	T50.995	T50.996
Debrisoquine	T46.5X1	T46.5X2	T46.5X3	T46.5X4	T46.5X5	T46.5X6
Decaborane	T57.8X1	T57.8X2	T57.8X3	T57.8X4	--	--
fumes	T59.891	T59.892	T59.893	T59.894	--	--
Decadron	T38.0X1	T38.0X2	T38.0X3	T38.0X4	T38.0X5	T38.0X6
ENT agent	T49.6X1	T49.6X2	T49.6X3	T49.6X4	T49.6X5	T49.6X6
ophthalmic preparation	T49.5X1	T49.5X2	T49.5X3	T49.5X4	T49.5X5	T49.5X6
topical NEC	T49.0X1	T49.0X2	T49.0X3	T49.0X4	T49.0X5	T49.0X6
Decahydronaphthalene	T52.8X1	T52.8X2	T52.8X3	T52.8X4	--	--
Decalin	T52.8X1	T52.8X2	T52.8X3	T52.8X4	--	--
Decamethonium (bromide)	T48.1X1	T48.1X2	T48.1X3	T48.1X4	T48.1X5	T48.1X6
Decholin	T47.5X1	T47.5X2	T47.5X3	T47.5X4	T47.5X5	T47.5X6
Declomycin	T36.4X1	T36.4X2	T36.4X3	T36.4X4	T36.4X5	T36.4X6
Decongestant, nasal (mucosa)	T48.5X1	T48.5X2	T48.5X3	T48.5X4	T48.5X5	T48.5X6
combination	T48.5X1	T48.5X2	T48.5X3	T48.5X4	T48.5X5	T48.5X6
Deet	T60.8X1	T60.8X2	T60.8X3	T60.8X4	--	--
Deferoxamine	T45.8X1	T45.8X2	T45.8X3	T45.8X4	T45.8X5	T45.8X6
Deflazacort	T38.0X1	T38.0X2	T38.0X3	T38.0X4	T38.0X5	T38.0X6
Deglycyrrhizinized extract of licorice	T48.4X1	T48.4X2	T48.4X3	T48.4X4	T48.4X5	T48.4X6
Dehydrocholic acid	T47.5X1	T47.5X2	T47.5X3	T47.5X4	T47.5X5	T47.5X6
Dehydroemetine	T37.3X1	T37.3X2	T37.3X3	T37.3X4	T37.3X5	T37.3X6
Dekalin	T52.8X1	T52.8X2	T52.8X3	T52.8X4	--	--
Delalutin	T38.5X1	T38.5X2	T38.5X3	T38.5X4	T38.5X5	T38.5X6
Delorazepam	T42.4X1	T42.4X2	T42.4X3	T42.4X4	T42.4X5	T42.4X6
Delphinium	T62.2X1	T62.2X2	T62.2X3	T62.2X4	--	--
Deltamethrin	T60.1X1	T60.1X2	T60.1X3	T60.1X4	--	--
Deltasone	T38.0X1	T38.0X2	T38.0X3	T38.0X4	T38.0X5	T38.0X6
Deltra	T38.0X1	T38.0X2	T38.0X3	T38.0X4	T38.0X5	T38.0X6
Delvinal	T42.3X1	T42.3X2	T42.3X3	T42.3X4	T42.3X5	T42.3X6
Demecarium (bromide)	T49.5X1	T49.5X2	T49.5X3	T49.5X4	T49.5X5	T49.5X6
Demeclocycline	T36.4X1	T36.4X2	T36.4X3	T36.4X4	T36.4X5	T36.4X6
Demecolcine	T45.1X1	T45.1X2	T45.1X3	T45.1X4	T45.1X5	T45.1X6

Substance	Poisoning, Accidental (unintentional)	Poisoning, Intentional self-harm	Poisoning, Assault	Poisoning, Undetermined	Adverse effect	Underdosing
Demegestone	T38.5X1	T38.5X2	T38.5X3	T38.5X4	T38.5X5	T38.5X6
Demelanizing agents	T49.8X1	T49.8X2	T49.8X3	T49.8X4	T49.8X5	T49.8X6
Demephion -O and -S	T60.0X1	T60.0X2	T60.0X3	T60.0X4	--	--
Demerol	T40.2X1	T40.2X2	T40.2X3	T40.2X4	T40.2X5	T40.2X6
Demethylchlortetracycline	T36.4X1	T36.4X2	T36.4X3	T36.4X4	T36.4X5	T36.4X6
Demethyltetracycline	T36.4X1	T36.4X2	T36.4X3	T36.4X4	T36.4X5	T36.4X6
Demeton -O and -S	T60.0X1	T60.0X2	T60.0X3	T60.0X4	--	--
Demulcent (external)	T49.3X1	T49.3X2	T49.3X3	T49.3X4	T49.3X5	T49.3X6
specified NEC	T49.3X1	T49.3X2	T49.3X3	T49.3X4	T49.3X5	T49.3X6
Demulen	T38.4X1	T38.4X2	T38.4X3	T38.4X4	T38.4X5	T38.4X6
Denatured alcohol	T51.0X1	T51.0X2	T51.0X3	T51.0X4	--	--
Dendrid	T49.5X1	T49.5X2	T49.5X3	T49.5X4	T49.5X5	T49.5X6
Dental drug, topical application NEC	T49.7X1	T49.7X2	T49.7X3	T49.7X4	T49.7X5	T49.7X6
Dentifrice	T49.7X1	T49.7X2	T49.7X3	T49.7X4	T49.7X5	T49.7X6
Deodorant spray (feminine hygiene)	T49.8X1	T49.8X2	T49.8X3	T49.8X4	T49.8X5	T49.8X6
Deoxycortone	T50.0X1	T50.0X2	T50.0X3	T50.0X4	T50.0X5	T50.0X6
2-Deoxy-5-fluorouridine	T45.1X1	T45.1X2	T45.1X3	T45.1X4	T45.1X5	T45.1X6
5-Deoxy-5-fluorouridine	T45.1X1	T45.1X2	T45.1X3	T45.1X4	T45.1X5	T45.1X6
Deoxyribonuclease (pancreatic)	T45.3X1	T45.3X2	T45.3X3	T45.3X4	T45.3X5	T45.3X6
Depilatory	T49.4X1	T49.4X2	T49.4X3	T49.4X4	T49.4X5	T49.4X6
Deprenalin	T42.8X1	T42.8X2	T42.8X3	T42.8X4	T42.8X5	T42.8X6
Deprenyl	T42.8X1	T42.8X2	T42.8X3	T42.8X4	T42.8X5	T42.8X6
Depressant, appetite	T50.5X1	T50.5X2	T50.5X3	T50.5X4	T50.5X5	T50.5X6
Depressant						
appetite (central)	T50.5X1	T50.5X2	T50.5X3	T50.5X4	T50.5X5	T50.5X6
cardiac	T46.2X1	T46.2X2	T46.2X3	T46.2X4	T46.2X5	T46.2X6
central nervous system (anesthetic) (*see also* Central nervous system, depressants)	T42.71	T42.72	T42.73	T42.74	T42.75	T42.76
general anesthetic	T41.201	T41.202	T41.203	T41.204	T41.205	T41.206
muscle tone	T42.8X1	T42.8X2	T42.8X3	T42.8X4	T42.8X5	T42.8X6
muscle tone, central	T42.8X1	T42.8X2	T42.8X3	T42.8X4	T42.8X5	T42.8X6
psychotherapeutic	T43.501	T43.502	T43.503	T43.504	T43.505	T43.506
Deptropine	T45.0X1	T45.0X2	T45.0X3	T45.0X4	T45.0X5	T45.0X6
Dequalinium (chloride)	T49.0X1	T49.0X2	T49.0X3	T49.0X4	T49.0X5	T49.0X6
Derris root	T60.2X1	T60.2X2	T60.2X3	T60.2X4	--	--
Deserpidine	T46.5X1	T46.5X2	T46.5X3	T46.5X4	T46.5X5	T46.5X6
Desferrioxamine	T45.8X1	T45.8X2	T45.8X3	T45.8X4	T45.8X5	T45.8X6
Desipramine	T43.011	T43.012	T43.013	T43.014	T43.015	T43.016
Deslanoside	T46.0X1	T46.0X2	T46.0X3	T46.0X4	T46.0X5	T46.0X6
Desloughing agent	T49.4X1	T49.4X2	T49.4X3	T49.4X4	T49.4X5	T49.4X6
Desmethylimipramine	T43.011	T43.012	T43.013	T43.014	T43.015	T43.016
Desmopressin	T38.891	T38.892	T38.893	T38.894	T38.895	T38.896
Desocodeine	T40.2X1	T40.2X2	T40.2X3	T40.2X4	T40.2X5	T40.2X6
Desogestrel	T38.5X1	T38.5X2	T38.5X3	T38.5X4	T38.5X5	T38.5X6
Desomorphine	T40.2X1	T40.2X2	T40.2X3	T40.2X4	--	--
Desonide	T49.0X1	T49.0X2	T49.0X3	T49.0X4	T49.0X5	T49.0X6
Desoximetasone	T49.0X1	T49.0X2	T49.0X3	T49.0X4	T49.0X5	T49.0X6
Desoxycorticosteroid	T50.0X1	T50.0X2	T50.0X3	T50.0X4	T50.0X5	T50.0X6
Desoxycortone	T50.0X1	T50.0X2	T50.0X3	T50.0X4	T50.0X5	T50.0X6
Desoxyephedrine	T43.621	T43.622	T43.623	T43.624	T43.625	T43.626
Detaxtran	T46.6X1	T46.6X2	T46.6X3	T46.6X4	T46.6X5	T46.6X6
Detergent	T49.2X1	T49.2X2	T49.2X3	T49.2X4	T49.2X5	T49.2X6
external medication	T49.2X1	T49.2X2	T49.2X3	T49.2X4	T49.2X5	T49.2X6
local	T49.2X1	T49.2X2	T49.2X3	T49.2X4	T49.2X5	T49.2X6
medicinal	T49.2X1	T49.2X2	T49.2X3	T49.2X4	T49.2X5	T49.2X6
nonmedicinal	T55.1X1	T55.1X2	T55.1X3	T55.1X4	--	--
specified NEC	T55.1X1	T55.1X2	T55.1X3	T55.1X4	--	--
Deterrent, alcohol	T50.6X1	T50.6X2	T50.6X3	T50.6X4	T50.6X5	T50.6X6
Detoxifying agent	T50.6X1	T50.6X2	T50.6X3	T50.6X4	T50.6X5	T50.6X6
Detrothyronine	T38.1X1	T38.1X2	T38.1X3	T38.1X4	T38.1X5	T38.1X6
Dettol (external medication)	T49.0X1	T49.0X2	T49.0X3	T49.0X4	T49.0X5	T49.0X6
Dexamethasone	T38.0X1	T38.0X2	T38.0X3	T38.0X4	T38.0X5	T38.0X6
ENT agent	T49.6X1	T49.6X2	T49.6X3	T49.6X4	T49.6X5	T49.6X6
ophthalmic preparation	T49.5X1	T49.5X2	T49.5X3	T49.5X4	T49.5X5	T49.5X6
topical NEC	T49.0X1	T49.0X2	T49.0X3	T49.0X4	T49.0X5	T49.0X6
Dexamfetamine	T43.621	T43.622	T43.623	T43.624	T43.625	T43.626
Dexamphetamine	T43.621	T43.622	T43.623	T43.624	T43.625	T43.626
Dexbrompheniramine	T45.0X1	T45.0X2	T45.0X3	T45.0X4	T45.0X5	T45.0X6
Dexchlorpheniramine	T45.0X1	T45.0X2	T45.0X3	T45.0X4	T45.0X5	T45.0X6
Dexedrine	T43.621	T43.622	T43.623	T43.624	T43.625	T43.626
Dexetimide	T44.3X1	T44.3X2	T44.3X3	T44.3X4	T44.3X5	T44.3X6
Dexfenfluramine	T50.5X1	T50.5X2	T50.5X3	T50.5X4	T50.5X5	T50.5X6
Dexpanthenol	T45.2X1	T45.2X2	T45.2X3	T45.2X4	T45.2X5	T45.2X6
Dextran (40) (70) (150)	T45.8X1	T45.8X2	T45.8X3	T45.8X4	T45.8X5	T45.8X6
Dextriferron	T45.4X1	T45.4X2	T45.4X3	T45.4X4	T45.4X5	T45.4X6
Dextro calcium pantothenate	T45.2X1	T45.2X2	T45.2X3	T45.2X4	T45.2X5	T45.2X6
Dextro pantothenyl alcohol	T45.2X1	T45.2X2	T45.2X3	T45.2X4	T45.2X5	T45.2X6
Dextroamphetamine	T43.621	T43.622	T43.623	T43.624	T43.625	T43.626
Dextromethorphan	T48.3X1	T48.3X2	T48.3X3	T48.3X4	T48.3X5	T48.3X6
Dextromoramide	T40.4X1	T40.4X2	T40.4X3	T40.4X4	--	--
topical	T49.8X1	T49.8X2	T49.8X3	T49.8X4	T49.8X5	T49.8X6
Dextropropoxyphene	T40.4X1	T40.4X2	T40.4X3	T40.4X4	T40.4X5	T40.4X6
Dextrorphan	T40.2X1	T40.2X2	T40.2X3	T40.2X4	T40.2X5	T40.2X6
Dextrose	T50.3X1	T50.3X2	T50.3X3	T50.3X4	T50.3X5	T50.3X6
concentrated solution, intravenous	T46.8X1	T46.8X2	T46.8X3	T46.8X4	T46.8X5	T46.8X6
Dextrothyroxin	T38.1X1	T38.1X2	T38.1X3	T38.1X4	T38.1X5	T38.1X6
Dextrothyroxine sodium	T38.1X1	T38.1X2	T38.1X3	T38.1X4	T38.1X5	T38.1X6
DFP	T44.0X1	T44.0X2	T44.0X3	T44.0X4	T44.0X5	T44.0X6
DHE	T37.3X1	T37.3X2	T37.3X3	T37.3X4	T37.3X5	T37.3X6
45	T46.5X1	T46.5X2	T46.5X3	T46.5X4	T46.5X5	T46.5X6
Diabinese	T38.3X1	T38.3X2	T38.3X3	T38.3X4	T38.3X5	T38.3X6
Diacetone alcohol	T52.4X1	T52.4X2	T52.4X3	T52.4X4	--	--
Diacetyl monoxime	T50.991	T50.992	T50.993	T50.994	--	--
Diacetylmorphine	T40.1X1	T40.1X2	T40.1X3	T40.1X4	--	--
Diachylon plaster	T49.4X1	T49.4X2	T49.4X3	T49.4X4	T49.4X5	T49.4X6
Diaethylstilboestrolum	T38.5X1	T38.5X2	T38.5X3	T38.5X4	T38.5X5	T38.5X6
Diagnostic agent NEC	T50.8X1	T50.8X2	T50.8X3	T50.8X4	T50.8X5	T50.8X6
Dial (soap)	T49.2X1	T49.2X2	T49.2X3	T49.2X4	T49.2X5	T49.2X6
sedative	T42.3X1	T42.3X2	T42.3X3	T42.3X4	T42.3X5	T42.3X6
Dialkyl carbonate	T52.91	T52.92	T52.93	T52.94	--	--
Diallylbarbituric acid	T42.3X1	T42.3X2	T42.3X3	T42.3X4	T42.3X5	T42.3X6
Diallymal	T42.3X1	T42.3X2	T42.3X3	T42.3X4	T42.3X5	T42.3X6
Dialysis solution (intraperitoneal)	T50.3X1	T50.3X2	T50.3X3	T50.3X4	T50.3X5	T50.3X6
Diaminodiphenylsulfone	T37.1X1	T37.1X2	T37.1X3	T37.1X4	T37.1X5	T37.1X6
Diamorphine	T40.1X1	T40.1X2	T40.1X3	T40.1X4	--	--
Diamox	T50.2X1	T50.2X2	T50.2X3	T50.2X4	T50.2X5	T50.2X6
Diamthazole	T49.0X1	T49.0X2	T49.0X3	T49.0X4	T49.0X5	T49.0X6
Dianthone	T47.2X1	T47.2X2	T47.2X3	T47.2X4	T47.2X5	T47.2X6
Diaphenylsulfone	T37.0X1	T37.0X2	T37.0X3	T37.0X4	T37.0X5	T37.0X6
Diasone (sodium)	T37.1X1	T37.1X2	T37.1X3	T37.1X4	T37.1X5	T37.1X6
Diastase	T47.5X1	T47.5X2	T47.5X3	T47.5X4	T47.5X5	T47.5X6
Diatrizoate	T50.8X1	T50.8X2	T50.8X3	T50.8X4	T50.8X5	T50.8X6
Diazepam	T42.4X1	T42.4X2	T42.4X3	T42.4X4	T42.4X5	T42.4X6
Diazinon	T60.0X1	T60.0X2	T60.0X3	T60.0X4	--	--
Diazomethane (gas)	T59.891	T59.892	T59.893	T59.894	--	--
Diazoxide	T46.5X1	T46.5X2	T46.5X3	T46.5X4	T46.5X5	T46.5X6
Dibekacin	T36.5X1	T36.5X2	T36.5X3	T36.5X4	T36.5X5	T36.5X6
Dibenamine	T44.6X1	T44.6X2	T44.6X3	T44.6X4	T44.6X5	T44.6X6
Dibenzepin	T43.011	T43.012	T43.013	T43.014	T43.015	T43.016
Dibenzheptropine	T45.0X1	T45.0X2	T45.0X3	T45.0X4	T45.0X5	T45.0X6
Dibenzyline	T44.6X1	T44.6X2	T44.6X3	T44.6X4	T44.6X5	T44.6X6
Diborane (gas)	T59.891	T59.892	T59.893	T59.894	--	--
Dibromochloropropane	T60.8X1	T60.8X2	T60.8X3	T60.8X4	--	--
Dibromodulcitol	T45.1X1	T45.1X2	T45.1X3	T45.1X4	T45.1X5	T45.1X6
Dibromoethane	T53.6X1	T53.6X2	T53.6X3	T53.6X4	--	--
Dibromomannitol	T45.1X1	T45.1X2	T45.1X3	T45.1X4	T45.1X5	T45.1X6
Dibromopropamidine isethionate	T49.0X1	T49.0X2	T49.0X3	T49.0X4	T49.0X5	T49.0X6
Dibrompropamidine	T49.0X1	T49.0X2	T49.0X3	T49.0X4	T49.0X5	T49.0X6
Dibucaine	T41.3X1	T41.3X2	T41.3X3	T41.3X4	T41.3X5	T41.3X6
topical (surface)	T41.3X1	T41.3X2	T41.3X3	T41.3X4	T41.3X5	T41.3X6
Dibunate sodium	T48.3X1	T48.3X2	T48.3X3	T48.3X4	T48.3X5	T48.3X6
Dibutoline sulfate	T44.3X1	T44.3X2	T44.3X3	T44.3X4	T44.3X5	T44.3X6
Dicamba	T60.3X1	T60.3X2	T60.3X3	T60.3X4	--	--
Dicapthon	T60.0X1	T60.0X2	T60.0X3	T60.0X4	--	--
Dichlobenil	T60.3X1	T60.3X2	T60.3X3	T60.3X4	--	--
Dichlone	T60.3X1	T60.3X2	T60.3X3	T60.3X4	--	--
Dichloralphenozone	T42.6X1	T42.6X2	T42.6X3	T42.6X4	T42.6X5	T42.6X6
Dichlorbenzidine	T65.3X1	T65.3X2	T65.3X3	T65.3X4	--	--
Dichlorhydrin	T52.8X1	T52.8X2	T52.8X3	T52.8X4	--	--
Dichlorhydroxyquinoline	T37.8X1	T37.8X2	T37.8X3	T37.8X4	T37.8X5	T37.8X6
Dichlorobenzene	T53.7X1	T53.7X2	T53.7X3	T53.7X4	--	--
Dichlorobenzyl alcohol	T49.6X1	T49.6X2	T49.6X3	T49.6X4	T49.6X5	T49.6X6
Dichlorodifluoromethane	T53.5X1	T53.5X2	T53.5X3	T53.5X4	--	--
Dichloroethane	T52.8X1	T52.8X2	T52.8X3	T52.8X4	--	--
Sym-Dichloroethyl ether	T53.6X1	T53.6X2	T53.6X3	T53.6X4	--	--
Dichloroethyl sulfide, not in war	T59.891	T59.892	T59.893	T59.894	--	--
Dichloroethylene	T53.6X1	T53.6X2	T53.6X3	T53.6X4	--	--
Dichloroformoxine, not in war	T59.891	T59.892	T59.893	T59.894	--	--
Dichlorohydrin, alpha-dichlorohydrin	T52.8X1	T52.8X2	T52.8X3	T52.8X4	--	--
Dichloromethane (solvent)	T53.4X1	T53.4X2	T53.4X3	T53.4X4	--	--
vapor	T53.4X1	T53.4X2	T53.4X3	T53.4X4	--	--
Dichloronaphthoquinone	T60.3X1	T60.3X2	T60.3X3	T60.3X4	--	--
Dichlorophen	T37.4X1	T37.4X2	T37.4X3	T37.4X4	T37.4X5	T37.4X6
2,4-Dichlorophenoxyacetic acid	T60.3X1	T60.3X2	T60.3X3	T60.3X4	--	--
Dichloropropene	T60.3X1	T60.3X2	T60.3X3	T60.3X4	--	--
Dichloropropionic acid	T60.3X1	T60.3X2	T60.3X3	T60.3X4	--	--

Dichlorphenamide - Dinoseb

Substance	Poisoning, Accidental (unintentional)	Poisoning, Intentional self-harm	Poisoning, Assault	Poisoning, Undetermined	Adverse effect	Underdosing
Dichlorphenamide	T50.2X1	T50.2X2	T50.2X3	T50.2X4	T50.2X5	T50.2X6
Dichlorvos	T60.0X1	T60.0X2	T60.0X3	T60.0X4	--	--
Diclofenac	T39.391	T39.392	T39.393	T39.394	T39.395	T39.396
Diclofenamide	T50.2X1	T50.2X2	T50.2X3	T50.2X4	T50.2X5	T50.2X6
Diclofensine	T43.291	T43.292	T43.293	T43.294	T43.295	T43.296
Diclonixine	T39.8X1	T39.8X2	T39.8X3	T39.8X4	T39.8X5	T39.8X6
Dicloxacillin	T36.0X1	T36.0X2	T36.0X3	T36.0X4	T36.0X5	T36.0X6
Dicophane	T49.0X1	T49.0X2	T49.0X3	T49.0X4	T49.0X5	T49.0X6
Dicoumarol, dicoumarin, dicumarol	T45.511	T45.512	T45.513	T45.514	T45.515	T45.516
Dicrotophos	T60.0X1	T60.0X2	T60.0X3	T60.0X4	--	--
Dicyanogen (gas)	T65.0X1	T65.0X2	T65.0X3	T65.0X4	--	--
Dicyclomine	T44.3X1	T44.3X2	T44.3X3	T44.3X4	T44.3X5	T44.3X6
Dicycloverine	T44.3X1	T44.3X2	T44.3X3	T44.3X4	T44.3X5	T44.3X6
Dideoxycytidine	T37.5X1	T37.5X2	T37.5X3	T37.5X4	T37.5X5	T37.5X6
Dideoxyinosine	T37.5X1	T37.5X2	T37.5X3	T37.5X4	T37.5X5	T37.5X6
Dieldrin (vapor)	T60.1X1	T60.1X2	T60.1X3	T60.1X4	--	--
Diemal	T42.3X1	T42.3X2	T42.3X3	T42.3X4	T42.3X5	T42.3X6
Dienestrol	T38.5X1	T38.5X2	T38.5X3	T38.5X4	T38.5X5	T38.5X6
Dienoestrol	T38.5X1	T38.5X2	T38.5X3	T38.5X4	T38.5X5	T38.5X6
Dietetic drug NEC	T50.901	T50.902	T50.903	T50.904	T50.905	T50.906
Diethazine	T42.8X1	T42.8X2	T42.8X3	T42.8X4	T42.8X5	T42.8X6
Diethyl						
barbituric acid	T42.3X1	T42.3X2	T42.3X3	T42.3X4	T42.3X5	T42.3X6
carbamazine	T37.4X1	T37.4X2	T37.4X3	T37.4X4	T37.4X5	T37.4X6
carbinol	T51.3X1	T51.3X2	T51.3X3	T51.3X4	--	--
carbonate	T52.8X1	T52.8X2	T52.8X3	T52.8X4	--	--
ether (vapor) (see also ether)	T41.0X1	T41.0X2	T41.0X3	T41.0X4	T41.0X5	T41.0X6
oxide	T52.8X1	T52.8X2	T52.8X3	T52.8X4	--	--
propion	T50.5X1	T50.5X2	T50.5X3	T50.5X4	T50.5X5	T50.5X6
stilbestrol	T38.5X1	T38.5X2	T38.5X3	T38.5X4	T38.5X5	T38.5X6
toluamide (nonmedicinal)	T60.8X1	T60.8X2	T60.8X3	T60.8X4	--	--
medicinal	T49.3X1	T49.3X2	T49.3X3	T49.3X4	T49.3X5	T49.3X6
Diethylcarbamazine	T37.4X1	T37.4X2	T37.4X3	T37.4X4	T37.4X5	T37.4X6
Diethylene						
dioxide	T52.8X1	T52.8X2	T52.8X3	T52.8X4	--	--
glycol (monoacetate) (monobutyl ether) (monoethyl ether)	T52.3X1	T52.3X2	T52.3X3	T52.3X4	--	--
Diethylhexylphthalate	T65.891	T65.892	T65.893	T65.894	--	--
Diethylpropion	T50.5X1	T50.5X2	T50.5X3	T50.5X4	T50.5X5	T50.5X6
Diethylstilbestrol	T38.5X1	T38.5X2	T38.5X3	T38.5X4	T38.5X5	T38.5X6
Diethylstilboestrol	T38.5X1	T38.5X2	T38.5X3	T38.5X4	T38.5X5	T38.5X6
Diethylsulfone-diethylmethane	T42.6X1	T42.6X2	T42.6X3	T42.6X4	T42.6X5	T42.6X6
Diethyltoluamide	T49.0X1	T49.0X2	T49.0X3	T49.0X4	T49.0X5	T49.0X6
Diethyltryptamine (DET)	T40.991	T40.992	T40.993	T40.994	--	
Difebarbamate	T42.3X1	T42.3X2	T42.3X3	T42.3X4	T42.3X5	T42.3X6
Difencloxazine	T40.2X1	T40.2X2	T40.2X3	T40.2X4	T40.2X5	T40.2X6
Difenidol	T45.0X1	T45.0X2	T45.0X3	T45.0X4	T45.0X5	T45.0X6
Difenoxin	T47.6X1	T47.6X2	T47.6X3	T47.6X4	T47.6X5	T47.6X6
Difetarsone	T37.3X1	T37.3X2	T37.3X3	T37.3X4	T37.3X5	T37.3X6
Diffusin	T45.3X1	T45.3X2	T45.3X3	T45.3X4	T45.3X5	T45.3X6
Diflorasone	T49.0X1	T49.0X2	T49.0X3	T49.0X4	T49.0X5	T49.0X6
Diflos	T44.0X1	T44.0X2	T44.0X3	T44.0X4	T44.0X5	T44.0X6
Diflubenzuron	T60.1X1	T60.1X2	T60.1X3	T60.1X4	--	--
Diflucortolone	T49.0X1	T49.0X2	T49.0X3	T49.0X4	T49.0X5	T49.0X6
Diflunisal	T39.091	T39.092	T39.093	T39.094	T39.095	T39.096
Difluoromethyldopa	T42.8X1	T42.8X2	T42.8X3	T42.8X4	T42.8X5	T42.8X6
Difluorophate	T44.0X1	T44.0X2	T44.0X3	T44.0X4	T44.0X5	T44.0X6
Digestant NEC	T47.5X1	T47.5X2	T47.5X3	T47.5X4	T47.5X5	T47.5X6
Digitalin (e)	T46.0X1	T46.0X2	T46.0X3	T46.0X4	T46.0X5	T46.0X6
Digitalis (leaf)(glycoside)	T46.0X1	T46.0X2	T46.0X3	T46.0X4	T46.0X5	T46.0X6
lanata	T46.0X1	T46.0X2	T46.0X3	T46.0X4	T46.0X5	T46.0X6
purpurea	T46.0X1	T46.0X2	T46.0X3	T46.0X4	T46.0X5	T46.0X6
Digitoxin	T46.0X1	T46.0X2	T46.0X3	T46.0X4	T46.0X5	T46.0X6
Digitoxose	T46.0X1	T46.0X2	T46.0X3	T46.0X4	T46.0X5	T46.0X6
Digoxin	T46.0X1	T46.0X2	T46.0X3	T46.0X4	T46.0X5	T46.0X6
Digoxine	T46.0X1	T46.0X2	T46.0X3	T46.0X4	T46.0X5	T46.0X6
Dihydralazine	T46.5X1	T46.5X2	T46.5X3	T46.5X4	T46.5X5	T46.5X6
Dihydrazine	T46.5X1	T46.5X2	T46.5X3	T46.5X4	T46.5X5	T46.5X6
Dihydrocodeine	T40.2X1	T40.2X2	T40.2X3	T40.2X4	T40.2X5	T40.2X6
Dihydrocodeinone	T40.2X1	T40.2X2	T40.2X3	T40.2X4	T40.2X5	T40.2X6
Dihydroergocornine	T46.7X1	T46.7X2	T46.7X3	T46.7X4	T46.7X5	T46.7X6
Dihydroergocristine (mesilate)	T46.7X1	T46.7X2	T46.7X3	T46.7X4	T46.7X5	T46.7X6
Dihydroergokryptine	T46.7X1	T46.7X2	T46.7X3	T46.7X4	T46.7X5	T46.7X6
Dihydroergotamine	T46.5X1	T46.5X2	T46.5X3	T46.5X4	T46.5X5	T46.5X6
Dihydroergotoxine	T46.7X1	T46.7X2	T46.7X3	T46.7X4	T46.7X5	T46.7X6
mesilate	T46.7X1	T46.7X2	T46.7X3	T46.7X4	T46.7X5	T46.7X6
Dihydrohydroxycodeinone	T40.2X1	T40.2X2	T40.2X3	T40.2X4	T40.2X5	T40.2X6
Dihydrohydroxymorphinone	T40.2X1	T40.2X2	T40.2X3	T40.2X4	T40.2X5	T40.2X6
Dihydroisocodeine	T40.2X1	T40.2X2	T40.2X3	T40.2X4	T40.2X5	T40.2X6
Dihydromorphine	T40.2X1	T40.2X2	T40.2X3	T40.2X4	--	--
Dihydromorphinone	T40.2X1	T40.2X2	T40.2X3	T40.2X4	T40.2X5	T40.2X6
Dihydrostreptomycin	T36.5X1	T36.5X2	T36.5X3	T36.5X4	T36.5X5	T36.5X6
Dihydrotachysterol	T45.2X1	T45.2X2	T45.2X3	T45.2X4	T45.2X5	T45.2X6
Dihydroxyaluminum aminoacetate	T47.1X1	T47.1X2	T47.1X3	T47.1X4	T47.1X5	T47.1X6
Dihydroxyaluminum sodium carbonate	T47.1X1	T47.1X2	T47.1X3	T47.1X4	T47.1X5	T47.1X6
Dihydroxyanthraquinone	T47.2X1	T47.2X2	T47.2X3	T47.2X4	T47.2X5	T47.2X6
Dihydroxycodeinone	T40.2X1	T40.2X2	T40.2X3	T40.2X4	T40.2X5	T40.2X6
Dihydroxypropyl theophylline	T50.2X1	T50.2X2	T50.2X3	T50.2X4	T50.2X5	T50.2X6
Diiodohydroxyquin	T37.8X1	T37.8X2	T37.8X3	T37.8X4	T37.8X5	T37.8X6
topical	T49.0X1	T49.0X2	T49.0X3	T49.0X4	T49.0X5	T49.0X6
Diiodohydroxyquinoline	T37.8X1	T37.8X2	T37.8X3	T37.8X4	T37.8X5	T37.8X6
Diiodotyrosine	T38.2X1	T38.2X2	T38.2X3	T38.2X4	T38.2X5	T38.2X6
Diisopromine	T44.3X1	T44.3X2	T44.3X3	T44.3X4	T44.3X5	T44.3X6
Diisopropylamine	T46.3X1	T46.3X2	T46.3X3	T46.3X4	T46.3X5	T46.3X6
Diisopropylfluorophosphonate	T44.0X1	T44.0X2	T44.0X3	T44.0X4	T44.0X5	T44.0X6
Dilantin	T42.0X1	T42.0X2	T42.0X3	T42.0X4	T42.0X5	T42.0X6
Dilaudid	T40.2X1	T40.2X2	T40.2X3	T40.2X4	T40.2X5	T40.2X6
Dilazep	T46.3X1	T46.3X2	T46.3X3	T46.3X4	T46.3X5	T46.3X6
Dill	T47.5X1	T47.5X2	T47.5X3	T47.5X4	T47.5X5	T47.5X6
Diloxanide	T37.3X1	T37.3X2	T37.3X3	T37.3X4	T37.3X5	T37.3X6
Diltiazem	T46.1X1	T46.1X2	T46.1X3	T46.1X4	T46.1X5	T46.1X6
Dimazole	T49.0X1	T49.0X2	T49.0X3	T49.0X4	T49.0X5	T49.0X6
Dimefline	T50.7X1	T50.7X2	T50.7X3	T50.7X4	T50.7X5	T50.7X6
Dimefox	T60.0X1	T60.0X2	T60.0X3	T60.0X4	--	--
Dimemorfan	T48.3X1	T48.3X2	T48.3X3	T48.3X4	T48.3X5	T48.3X6
Dimenhydrinate	T45.0X1	T45.0X2	T45.0X3	T45.0X4	T45.0X5	T45.0X6
Dimercaprol (British anti-lewisite)	T45.8X1	T45.8X2	T45.8X3	T45.8X4	T45.8X5	T45.8X6
Dimercaptopropanol	T45.8X1	T45.8X2	T45.8X3	T45.8X4	T45.8X5	T45.8X6
Dimestrol	T38.5X1	T38.5X2	T38.5X3	T38.5X4	T38.5X5	T38.5X6
Dimetane	T45.0X1	T45.0X2	T45.0X3	T45.0X4	T45.0X5	T45.0X6
Dimethicone	T47.1X1	T47.1X2	T47.1X3	T47.1X4	T47.1X5	T47.1X6
Dimethindene	T45.0X1	T45.0X2	T45.0X3	T45.0X4	T45.0X5	T45.0X6
Dimethisoquin	T49.1X1	T49.1X2	T49.1X3	T49.1X4	T49.1X5	T49.1X6
Dimethisterone	T38.5X1	T38.5X2	T38.5X3	T38.5X4	T38.5X5	T38.5X6
Dimethoate	T60.0X1	T60.0X2	T60.0X3	T60.0X4	--	--
Dimethocaine	T41.3X1	T41.3X2	T41.3X3	T41.3X4	T41.3X5	T41.3X6
Dimethoxanate	T48.3X1	T48.3X2	T48.3X3	T48.3X4	T48.3X5	T48.3X6
Dimethyl						
arsine, arsinic acid	T57.0X1	T57.0X2	T57.0X3	T57.0X4	--	--
carbinol	T51.2X1	T51.2X2	T51.2X3	T51.2X4	--	--
carbonate	T52.8X1	T52.8X2	T52.8X3	T52.8X4	--	--
diguanide	T38.3X1	T38.3X2	T38.3X3	T38.3X4	T38.3X5	T38.3X6
ketone	T52.4X1	T52.4X2	T52.4X3	T52.4X4	--	--
vapor	T52.4X1	T52.4X2	T52.4X3	T52.4X4	--	--
meperidine	T40.2X1	T40.2X2	T40.2X3	T40.2X4	T40.2X5	T40.2X6
parathion	T60.0X1	T60.0X2	T60.0X3	T60.0X4	--	--
phthlate	T49.3X1	T49.3X2	T49.3X3	T49.3X4	T49.3X5	T49.3X6
polysiloxane	T47.8X1	T47.8X2	T47.8X3	T47.8X4	T47.8X5	T47.8X6
sulfate (fumes)	T59.891	T59.892	T59.893	T59.894		
liquid	T65.891	T65.892	T65.893	T65.894		
sulfoxide (nonmedicinal)	T52.8X1	T52.8X2	T52.8X3	T52.8X4		
medicinal	T49.4X1	T49.4X2	T49.4X3	T49.4X4	T49.4X5	T49.4X6
tryptamine	T40.991	T40.992	T40.993	T40.994		
tubocurarine	T48.1X1	T48.1X2	T48.1X3	T48.1X4	T48.1X5	T48.1X6
Dimethylamine sulfate	T49.4X1	T49.4X2	T49.4X3	T49.4X4	T49.4X5	T49.4X6
Dimethylformamide	T52.8X1	T52.8X2	T52.8X3	T52.8X4		
Dimethyltubocurarinium chloride	T48.1X1	T48.1X2	T48.1X3	T48.1X4	T48.1X5	T48.1X6
Dimeticone	T47.1X1	T47.1X2	T47.1X3	T47.1X4	T47.1X5	T47.1X6
Dimetilan	T60.0X1	T60.0X2	T60.0X3	T60.0X4		
Dimetindene	T45.0X1	T45.0X2	T45.0X3	T45.0X4	T45.0X5	T45.0X6
Dimetotiazine	T43.3X1	T43.3X2	T43.3X3	T43.3X4	T43.3X5	T43.3X6
Dimorpholamine	T50.7X1	T50.7X2	T50.7X3	T50.7X4	T50.7X5	T50.7X6
Dimoxyline	T46.3X1	T46.3X2	T46.3X3	T46.3X4	T46.3X5	T46.3X6
Dinitrobenzene	T65.3X1	T65.3X2	T65.3X3	T65.3X4		
vapor	T59.891	T59.892	T59.893	T59.894	--	--
Dinitrobenzol	T65.3X1	T65.3X2	T65.3X3	T65.3X4		
vapor	T59.891	T59.892	T59.893	T59.894		
Dinitrobutylphenol	T65.3X1	T65.3X2	T65.3X3	T65.3X4		
Dinitro (-ortho-)cresol (pesticide) (spray)	T65.3X1	T65.3X2	T65.3X3	T65.3X4		
Dinitrocyclohexylphenol	T65.3X1	T65.3X2	T65.3X3	T65.3X4		
Dinitrophenol	T65.3X1	T65.3X2	T65.3X3	T65.3X4	--	--
Dinoprost	T48.0X1	T48.0X2	T48.0X3	T48.0X4	T48.0X5	T48.0X6
Dinoprostone	T48.0X1	T48.0X2	T48.0X3	T48.0X4	T48.0X5	T48.0X6
Dinoseb	T60.3X1	T60.3X2	T60.3X3	T60.3X4		

Substance	Poisoning, Accidental (unintentional)	Poisoning, Intentional self-harm	Poisoning, Assault	Poisoning, Undetermined	Adverse effect	Underdosing
Dioctyl sulfosuccinate (calcium) (sodium)	T47.4X1	T47.4X2	T47.4X3	T47.4X4	T47.4X5	T47.4X6
Diodone	T50.8X1	T50.8X2	T50.8X3	T50.8X4	T50.8X5	T50.8X6
Diodoquin	T37.8X1	T37.8X2	T37.8X3	T37.8X4	T37.8X5	T37.8X6
Dionin	T40.2X1	T40.2X2	T40.2X3	T40.2X4	T40.2X5	T40.2X6
Diosmin	T46.991	T46.992	T46.993	T46.994	T46.995	T46.996
Dioxane	T52.8X1	T52.8X2	T52.8X3	T52.8X4	--	--
Dioxathion	T60.0X1	T60.0X2	T60.0X3	T60.0X4	--	--
Dioxin	T53.7X1	T53.7X2	T53.7X3	T53.7X4	--	--
Dioxopromethazine	T43.3X1	T43.3X2	T43.3X3	T43.3X4	T43.3X5	T43.3X6
Dioxyline	T46.3X1	T46.3X2	T46.3X3	T46.3X4	T46.3X5	T46.3X6
Dipentene	T52.8X1	T52.8X2	T52.8X3	T52.8X4	--	--
Diperodon	T41.3X1	T41.3X2	T41.3X3	T41.3X4	T41.3X5	T41.3X6
Diphacinone	T60.4X1	T60.4X2	T60.4X3	T60.4X4	--	--
Diphemanil	T44.3X1	T44.3X2	T44.3X3	T44.3X4	T44.3X5	T44.3X6
metilsulfate	T44.3X1	T44.3X2	T44.3X3	T44.3X4	T44.3X5	T44.3X6
Diphenadione	T45.511	T45.512	T45.513	T45.514	T45.515	T45.516
rodenticide	T60.4X1	T60.4X2	T60.4X3	T60.4X4	--	--
Diphenhydramine	T45.0X1	T45.0X2	T45.0X3	T45.0X4	T45.0X5	T45.0X6
Diphenidol	T45.0X1	T45.0X2	T45.0X3	T45.0X4	T45.0X5	T45.0X6
Diphenoxylate	T47.6X1	T47.6X2	T47.6X3	T47.6X4	T47.6X5	T47.6X6
Diphenylamine	T65.3X1	T65.3X2	T65.3X3	T65.3X4	--	--
Diphenylbutazone	T39.2X1	T39.2X2	T39.2X3	T39.2X4	T39.2X5	T39.2X6
Diphenylchloroarsine, not in war	T57.0X1	T57.0X2	T57.0X3	T57.0X4	--	--
Diphenylhydantoin	T42.0X1	T42.0X2	T42.0X3	T42.0X4	T42.0X5	T42.0X6
Diphenylmethane dye	T52.1X1	T52.1X2	T52.1X3	T52.1X4	--	--
Diphenylpyraline	T45.0X1	T45.0X2	T45.0X3	T45.0X4	T45.0X5	T45.0X6
Diphtheria						
antitoxin	T50.Z11	T50.Z12	T50.Z13	T50.Z14	T50.Z15	T50.Z16
toxoid	T50.A91	T50.A92	T50.A93	T50.A94	T50.A95	T50.A96
with tetanus toxoid	T50.A21	T50.A22	T50.A23	T50.A24	T50.A25	T50.A26
with pertussis component	T50.A11	T50.A12	T50.A13	T50.A14	T50.A15	T50.A16
vaccine	T50.A91	T50.A92	T50.A93	T50.A94	T50.A95	T50.A96
combination						
including pertussis	T50.A11	T50.A12	T50.A13	T50.A14	T50.A15	T50.A16
without pertussis	T50.A21	T50.A22	T50.A23	T50.A24	T50.A25	T50.A26
Diphylline	T50.2X1	T50.2X2	T50.2X3	T50.2X4	T50.2X5	T50.2X6
Dipipanone	T40.4X1	T40.4X2	T40.4X3	T40.4X4	--	--
Dipivefrine	T49.5X1	T49.5X2	T49.5X3	T49.5X4	T49.5X5	T49.5X6
Diplovax	T50.B91	T50.B92	T50.B93	T50.B94	T50.B95	T50.B96
Diprophylline	T50.2X1	T50.2X2	T50.2X3	T50.2X4	T50.2X5	T50.2X6
Dipropyline	T48.291	T48.292	T48.293	T48.294	T48.295	T48.296
Dipyridamole	T46.3X1	T46.3X2	T46.3X3	T46.3X4	T46.3X5	T46.3X6
Dipyrone	T39.2X1	T39.2X2	T39.2X3	T39.2X4	T39.2X5	T39.2X6
Diquat (dibromide)	T60.3X1	T60.3X2	T60.3X3	T60.3X4	--	--
Disinfectant	T65.891	T65.892	T65.893	T65.894	--	--
alkaline	T54.3X1	T54.3X2	T54.3X3	T54.3X4	--	--
aromatic	T54.1X1	T54.1X2	T54.1X3	T54.1X4	--	--
intestinal	T37.8X1	T37.8X2	T37.8X3	T37.8X4	T37.8X5	T37.8X6
Disipal	T42.8X1	T42.8X2	T42.8X3	T42.8X4	T42.8X5	T42.8X6
Disodium edetate	T50.6X1	T50.6X2	T50.6X3	T50.6X4	T50.6X5	T50.6X6
Disoprofol	T41.291	T41.292	T41.293	T41.294	T41.295	T41.296
Disopyramide	T46.2X1	T46.2X2	T46.2X3	T46.2X4	T46.2X5	T46.2X6
Distigmine (bromide)	T44.0X1	T44.0X2	T44.0X3	T44.0X4	T44.0X5	T44.0X6
Disulfamide	T50.2X1	T50.2X2	T50.2X3	T50.2X4	T50.2X5	T50.2X6
Disulfanilamide	T37.0X1	T37.0X2	T37.0X3	T37.0X4	T37.0X5	T37.0X6
Disulfiram	T50.6X1	T50.6X2	T50.6X3	T50.6X4	T50.6X5	T50.6X6
Disulfoton	T60.0X1	T60.0X2	T60.0X3	T60.0X4	--	--
Dithiazanine iodide	T37.4X1	T37.4X2	T37.4X3	T37.4X4	T37.4X5	T37.4X6
Dithiocarbamate	T60.0X1	T60.0X2	T60.0X3	T60.0X4	--	--
Dithranol	T49.4X1	T49.4X2	T49.4X3	T49.4X4	T49.4X5	T49.4X6
Diucardin	T50.2X1	T50.2X2	T50.2X3	T50.2X4	T50.2X5	T50.2X6
Diupres	T50.2X1	T50.2X2	T50.2X3	T50.2X4	T50.2X5	T50.2X6
Diuretic NEC	T50.2X1	T50.2X2	T50.2X3	T50.2X4	T50.2X5	T50.2X6
benzothiadiazine	T50.2X1	T50.2X2	T50.2X3	T50.2X4	T50.2X5	T50.2X6
carbonic acid anhydrase inhibitors	T50.2X1	T50.2X2	T50.2X3	T50.2X4	T50.2X5	T50.2X6
furfuryl NEC	T50.2X1	T50.2X2	T50.2X3	T50.2X4	T50.2X5	T50.2X6
loop (high-ceiling)	T50.1X1	T50.1X2	T50.1X3	T50.1X4	T50.1X5	T50.1X6
mercurial NEC	T50.2X1	T50.2X2	T50.2X3	T50.2X4	T50.2X5	T50.2X6
osmotic	T50.2X1	T50.2X2	T50.2X3	T50.2X4	T50.2X5	T50.2X6
purine NEC	T50.2X1	T50.2X2	T50.2X3	T50.2X4	T50.2X5	T50.2X6
saluretic NEC	T50.2X1	T50.2X2	T50.2X3	T50.2X4	T50.2X5	T50.2X6
sulfonamide	T50.2X1	T50.2X2	T50.2X3	T50.2X4	T50.2X5	T50.2X6
thiazide NEC	T50.2X1	T50.2X2	T50.2X3	T50.2X4	T50.2X5	T50.2X6
xanthine	T50.2X1	T50.2X2	T50.2X3	T50.2X4	T50.2X5	T50.2X6
Diurgin	T50.2X1	T50.2X2	T50.2X3	T50.2X4	T50.2X5	T50.2X6
Diuril	T50.2X1	T50.2X2	T50.2X3	T50.2X4	T50.2X5	T50.2X6
Diuron	T60.3X1	T60.3X2	T60.3X3	T60.3X4	--	--
Divalproex	T42.6X1	T42.6X2	T42.6X3	T42.6X4	T42.6X5	T42.6X6
Divinyl ether	T41.0X1	T41.0X2	T41.0X3	T41.0X4	T41.0X5	T41.0X6
Dixanthogen	T49.0X1	T49.0X2	T49.0X3	T49.0X4	T49.0X5	T49.0X6

Substance	Poisoning, Accidental (unintentional)	Poisoning, Intentional self-harm	Poisoning, Assault	Poisoning, Undetermined	Adverse effect	Underdosing
Dixyrazine	T43.3X1	T43.3X2	T43.3X3	T43.3X4	T43.3X5	T43.3X6
D-lysergic acid diethylamide	T40.8X1	T40.8X2	T40.8X3	T40.8X4	--	--
DMCT	T36.4X1	T36.4X2	T36.4X3	T36.4X4	T36.4X5	T36.4X6
DMSO — *see* Dimethyl sulfoxide						
DNBP	T60.3X1	T60.3X2	T60.3X3	T60.3X4	--	--
DNOC	T65.3X1	T65.3X2	T65.3X3	T65.3X4	--	--
Dobutamine	T44.5X1	T44.5X2	T44.5X3	T44.5X4	T44.5X5	T44.5X6
DOCA	T38.0X1	T38.0X2	T38.0X3	T38.0X4	T38.0X5	T38.0X6
Docusate sodium	T47.4X1	T47.4X2	T47.4X3	T47.4X4	T47.4X5	T47.4X6
Dodicin	T49.0X1	T49.0X2	T49.0X3	T49.0X4	T49.0X5	T49.0X6
Dofamium chloride	T49.0X1	T49.0X2	T49.0X3	T49.0X4	T49.0X5	T49.0X6
Dolophine	T40.3X1	T40.3X2	T40.3X3	T40.3X4	T40.3X5	T40.3X6
Doloxene	T39.8X1	T39.8X2	T39.8X3	T39.8X4	T39.8X5	T39.8X6
Domestic gas (after combustion) — *see* Gas, utility						
prior to combustion	T59.891	T59.892	T59.893	T59.894	--	--
Domiodol	T48.4X1	T48.4X2	T48.4X3	T48.4X4	T48.4X5	T48.4X6
Domiphen (bromide)	T49.0X1	T49.0X2	T49.0X3	T49.0X4	T49.0X5	T49.0X6
Domperidone	T45.0X1	T45.0X2	T45.0X3	T45.0X4	T45.0X5	T45.0X6
Dopa	T42.8X1	T42.8X2	T42.8X3	T42.8X4	T42.8X5	T42.8X6
Dopamine	T44.991	T44.992	T44.993	T44.994	T44.995	T44.996
Doriden	T42.6X1	T42.6X2	T42.6X3	T42.6X4	T42.6X5	T42.6X6
Dormiral	T42.3X1	T42.3X2	T42.3X3	T42.3X4	T42.3X5	T42.3X6
Dormison	T42.6X1	T42.6X2	T42.6X3	T42.6X4	T42.6X5	T42.6X6
Dornase	T48.4X1	T48.4X2	T48.4X3	T48.4X4	T48.4X5	T48.4X6
Dorsacaine	T41.3X1	T41.3X2	T41.3X3	T41.3X4	T41.3X5	T41.3X6
Dosulepin	T43.011	T43.012	T43.013	T43.014	T43.015	T43.016
Dothiepin	T43.011	T43.012	T43.013	T43.014	T43.015	T43.016
Doxantrazole	T48.6X1	T48.6X2	T48.6X3	T48.6X4	T48.6X5	T48.6X6
Doxapram	T50.7X1	T50.7X2	T50.7X3	T50.7X4	T50.7X5	T50.7X6
Doxazosin	T44.6X1	T44.6X2	T44.6X3	T44.6X4	T44.6X5	T44.6X6
Doxepin	T43.011	T43.012	T43.013	T43.014	T43.015	T43.016
Doxifluridine	T45.1X1	T45.1X2	T45.1X3	T45.1X4	T45.1X5	T45.1X6
Doxorubicin	T45.1X1	T45.1X2	T45.1X3	T45.1X4	T45.1X5	T45.1X6
Doxycycline	T36.4X1	T36.4X2	T36.4X3	T36.4X4	T36.4X5	T36.4X6
Doxylamine	T45.0X1	T45.0X2	T45.0X3	T45.0X4	T45.0X5	T45.0X6
Dramamine	T45.0X1	T45.0X2	T45.0X3	T45.0X4	T45.0X5	T45.0X6
Drano (drain cleaner)	T54.3X1	T54.3X2	T54.3X3	T54.3X4	--	--
Dressing, live pulp	T49.7X1	T49.7X2	T49.7X3	T49.7X4	T49.7X5	T49.7X6
Drocode	T40.2X1	T40.2X2	T40.2X3	T40.2X4	T40.2X5	T40.2X6
Dromoran	T40.2X1	T40.2X2	T40.2X3	T40.2X4	T40.2X5	T40.2X6
Dromostanolone	T38.7X1	T38.7X2	T38.7X3	T38.7X4	T38.7X5	T38.7X6
Dronabinol	T40.7X1	T40.7X2	T40.7X3	T40.7X4	T40.7X5	T40.7X6
Droperidol	T43.591	T43.592	T43.593	T43.594	T43.595	T43.596
Dropropizine	T48.3X1	T48.3X2	T48.3X3	T48.3X4	T48.3X5	T48.3X6
Drostanolone	T38.7X1	T38.7X2	T38.7X3	T38.7X4	T38.7X5	T38.7X6
Drotaverine	T44.3X1	T44.3X2	T44.3X3	T44.3X4	T44.3X5	T44.3X6
Drotrecogin alfa	T45.511	T45.512	T45.513	T45.514	T45.515	T45.516
Drug NEC	T50.901	T50.902	T50.903	T50.904	T50.905	T50.906
specified NEC	T50.991	T50.992	T50.993	T50.994	T50.995	T50.996
DTIC	T45.1X1	T45.1X2	T45.1X3	T45.1X4	T45.1X5	T45.1X6
Duboisine	T44.3X1	T44.3X2	T44.3X3	T44.3X4	T44.3X5	T44.3X6
Dulcolax	T47.2X1	T47.2X2	T47.2X3	T47.2X4	T47.2X5	T47.2X6
Duponol (C) (EP)	T49.2X1	T49.2X2	T49.2X3	T49.2X4	T49.2X5	T49.2X6
Durabolin	T38.7X1	T38.7X2	T38.7X3	T38.7X4	T38.7X5	T38.7X6
Dyclone	T41.3X1	T41.3X2	T41.3X3	T41.3X4	T41.3X5	T41.3X6
Dyclonine	T41.3X1	T41.3X2	T41.3X3	T41.3X4	T41.3X5	T41.3X6
Dydrogesterone	T38.5X1	T38.5X2	T38.5X3	T38.5X4	T38.5X5	T38.5X6
Dye NEC	T65.6X1	T65.6X2	T65.6X3	T65.6X4	--	--
antiseptic	T49.0X1	T49.0X2	T49.0X3	T49.0X4	T49.0X5	T49.0X6
diagnostic agents	T50.8X1	T50.8X2	T50.8X3	T50.8X4	T50.8X5	T50.8X6
pharmaceutical NEC	T50.901	T50.902	T50.903	T50.904	T50.905	T50.906
Dyflos	T44.0X1	T44.0X2	T44.0X3	T44.0X4	T44.0X5	T44.0X6
Dymelor	T38.3X1	T38.3X2	T38.3X3	T38.3X4	T38.3X5	T38.3X6
Dynamite	T65.3X1	T65.3X2	T65.3X3	T65.3X4	--	--
fumes	T59.891	T59.892	T59.893	T59.894	--	--
Dyphylline	T44.3X1	T44.3X2	T44.3X3	T44.3X4	T44.3X5	T44.3X6
E						
Ear drug NEC	T49.6X1	T49.6X2	T49.6X3	T49.6X4	T49.6X5	T49.6X6
Ear preparations	T49.6X1	T49.6X2	T49.6X3	T49.6X4	T49.6X5	T49.6X6
Echothiophate, echothiopate, ecothiopate	T49.5X1	T49.5X2	T49.5X3	T49.5X4	T49.5X5	T49.5X6
Econazole	T49.0X1	T49.0X2	T49.0X3	T49.0X4	T49.0X5	T49.0X6
Ecothiopate iodide	T49.5X1	T49.5X2	T49.5X3	T49.5X4	T49.5X5	T49.5X6
Ecstasy	T43.641	T43.642	T43.643	T43.644	--	--
Ectylurea	T42.6X1	T42.6X2	T42.6X3	T42.6X4	T42.6X5	T42.6X6
Edathamil disodium	T45.8X1	T45.8X2	T45.8X3	T45.8X4	T45.8X5	T45.8X6
Edecrin	T50.1X1	T50.1X2	T50.1X3	T50.1X4	T50.1X5	T50.1X6
Edetate, disodium (calcium)	T45.8X1	T45.8X2	T45.8X3	T45.8X4	T45.8X5	T45.8X6
Edoxudine	T49.5X1	T49.5X2	T49.5X3	T49.5X4	T49.5X5	T49.5X6
Edrophonium	T44.0X1	T44.0X2	T44.0X3	T44.0X4	T44.0X5	T44.0X6
chloride	T44.0X1	T44.0X2	T44.0X3	T44.0X4	T44.0X5	T44.0X6

Substance	Poisoning, Accidental (unintentional)	Poisoning, Intentional self-harm	Poisoning, Assault	Poisoning, Undetermined	Adverse effect	Underdosing
EDTA	T50.6X1	T50.6X2	T50.6X3	T50.6X4	T50.6X5	T50.6X6
Eflornithine	T37.2X1	T37.2X2	T37.2X3	T37.2X4	T37.2X5	T37.2X6
Efloxate	T46.3X1	T46.3X2	T46.3X3	T46.3X4	T46.3X5	T46.3X6
Elase	T49.8X1	T49.8X2	T49.8X3	T49.8X4	T49.8X5	T49.8X6
Elastase	T47.5X1	T47.5X2	T47.5X3	T47.5X4	T47.5X5	T47.5X6
Elaterium	T47.2X1	T47.2X2	T47.2X3	T47.2X4	T47.2X5	T47.2X6
Elcatonin	T50.991	T50.992	T50.993	T50.994	T50.995	T50.996
Elder	T62.2X1	T62.2X2	T62.2X3	T62.2X4	--	--
berry, (unripe)	T62.1X1	T62.1X2	T62.1X3	T62.1X4	--	--
Electrolyte balance drug	T50.3X1	T50.3X2	T50.3X3	T50.3X4	T50.3X5	T50.3X6
Electrolytes NEC	T50.3X1	T50.3X2	T50.3X3	T50.3X4	T50.3X5	T50.3X6
Electrolytic agent NEC	T50.3X1	T50.3X2	T50.3X3	T50.3X4	T50.3X5	T50.3X6
Elemental diet	T50.901	T50.902	T50.903	T50.904	T50.905	T50.906
Elliptinium acetate	T45.1X1	T45.1X2	T45.1X3	T45.1X4	T45.1X5	T45.1X6
Embramine	T45.0X1	T45.0X2	T45.0X3	T45.0X4	T45.0X5	T45.0X6
Emepronium (salts)	T44.3X1	T44.3X2	T44.3X3	T44.3X4	T44.3X5	T44.3X6
bromide	T44.3X1	T44.3X2	T44.3X3	T44.3X4	T44.3X5	T44.3X6
Emetic NEC	T47.7X1	T47.7X2	T47.7X3	T47.7X4	T47.7X5	T47.7X6
Emetine	T37.3X1	T37.3X2	T37.3X3	T37.3X4	T37.3X5	T37.3X6
Emollient NEC	T49.3X1	T49.3X2	T49.3X3	T49.3X4	T49.3X5	T49.3X6
Emorfazone	T39.8X1	T39.8X2	T39.8X3	T39.8X4	T39.8X5	T39.8X6
Emylcamate	T43.591	T43.592	T43.593	T43.594	T43.595	T43.596
Enalapril	T46.4X1	T46.4X2	T46.4X3	T46.4X4	T46.4X5	T46.4X6
Enalaprilat	T46.4X1	T46.4X2	T46.4X3	T46.4X4	T46.4X5	T46.4X6
Encainide	T46.2X1	T46.2X2	T46.2X3	T46.2X4	T46.2X5	T46.2X6
Endocaine	T41.3X1	T41.3X2	T41.3X3	T41.3X4	T41.3X5	T41.3X6
Endosulfan	T60.2X1	T60.2X2	T60.2X3	T60.2X4	--	--
Endothall	T60.3X1	T60.3X2	T60.3X3	T60.3X4	--	--
Endralazine	T46.5X1	T46.5X2	T46.5X3	T46.5X4	T46.5X5	T46.5X6
Endrin	T60.1X1	T60.1X2	T60.1X3	T60.1X4	--	--
Enflurane	T41.0X1	T41.0X2	T41.0X3	T41.0X4	T41.0X5	T41.0X6
Enhexymal	T42.3X1	T42.3X2	T42.3X3	T42.3X4	T42.3X5	T42.3X6
Enocitabine	T45.1X1	T45.1X2	T45.1X3	T45.1X4	T45.1X5	T45.1X6
Enovid	T38.4X1	T38.4X2	T38.4X3	T38.4X4	T38.4X5	T38.4X6
Enoxacin	T36.8X1	T36.8X2	T36.8X3	T36.8X4	T36.8X5	T36.8X6
Enoxaparin (sodium)	T45.511	T45.512	T45.513	T45.514	T45.515	T45.516
Enpiprazole	T43.591	T43.592	T43.593	T43.594	T43.595	T43.596
Enprofylline	T48.6X1	T48.6X2	T48.6X3	T48.6X4	T48.6X5	T48.6X6
Enprostil	T47.1X1	T47.1X2	T47.1X3	T47.1X4	T47.1X5	T47.1X6
ENT preparations (anti-infectives)	T49.6X1	T49.6X2	T49.6X3	T49.6X4	T49.6X5	T49.6X6
Enterogastrone	T38.891	T38.892	T38.893	T38.894	T38.895	T38.896
Enviomycin	T36.8X1	T36.8X2	T36.8X3	T36.8X4	T36.8X5	T36.8X6
Enzodase	T45.3X1	T45.3X2	T45.3X3	T45.3X4	T45.3X5	T45.3X6
Enzyme NEC	T45.3X1	T45.3X2	T45.3X3	T45.3X4	T45.3X5	T45.3X6
depolymerizing	T49.8X1	T49.8X2	T49.8X3	T49.8X4	T49.8X5	T49.8X6
fibrolytic	T45.3X1	T45.3X2	T45.3X3	T45.3X4	T45.3X5	T45.3X6
gastric	T47.5X1	T47.5X2	T47.5X3	T47.5X4	T47.5X5	T47.5X6
intestinal	T47.5X1	T47.5X2	T47.5X3	T47.5X4	T47.5X5	T47.5X6
local action	T49.4X1	T49.4X2	T49.4X3	T49.4X4	T49.4X5	T49.4X6
proteolytic	T49.4X1	T49.4X2	T49.4X3	T49.4X4	T49.4X5	T49.4X6
thrombolytic	T45.3X1	T45.3X2	T45.3X3	T45.3X4	T45.3X5	T45.3X6
EPAB	T41.3X1	T41.3X2	T41.3X3	T41.3X4	T41.3X5	T41.3X6
Epanutin	T42.0X1	T42.0X2	T42.0X3	T42.0X4	T42.0X5	T42.0X6
Ephedra	T44.991	T44.992	T44.993	T44.994	T44.995	T44.996
Ephedrine	T44.991	T44.992	T44.993	T44.994	T44.995	T44.996
Epichlorhydrin, epichlorohydrin	T52.8X1	T52.8X2	T52.8X3	T52.8X4	--	--
Epicillin	T36.0X1	T36.0X2	T36.0X3	T36.0X4	T36.0X5	T36.0X6
Epiestriol	T38.5X1	T38.5X2	T38.5X3	T38.5X4	T38.5X5	T38.5X6
Epilim — *see* Sodium valproate						
Epimestrol	T38.5X1	T38.5X2	T38.5X3	T38.5X4	T38.5X5	T38.5X6
Epinephrine	T44.5X1	T44.5X2	T44.5X3	T44.5X4	T44.5X5	T44.5X6
Epirubicin	T45.1X1	T45.1X2	T45.1X3	T45.1X4	T45.1X5	T45.1X6
Epitiostanol	T38.7X1	T38.7X2	T38.7X3	T38.7X4	T38.7X5	T38.7X6
Epitizide	T50.2X1	T50.2X2	T50.2X3	T50.2X4	T50.2X5	T50.2X6
EPN	T60.0X1	T60.0X2	T60.0X3	T60.0X4	--	--
EPO	T45.8X1	T45.8X2	T45.8X3	T45.8X4	T45.8X5	T45.8X6
Epoetin alpha	T45.8X1	T45.8X2	T45.8X3	T45.8X4	T45.8X5	T45.8X6
Epomediol	T50.991	T50.992	T50.993	T50.994	T50.995	T50.996
Epoprostenol	T45.521	T45.522	T45.523	T45.524	T45.525	T45.526
Epoxy resin	T65.891	T65.892	T65.893	T65.894	--	--
Eprazinone	T48.4X1	T48.4X2	T48.4X3	T48.4X4	T48.4X5	T48.4X6
Epsilon amino-caproic acid	T45.621	T45.622	T45.623	T45.624	T45.625	T45.626
Epsom salt	T47.3X1	T47.3X2	T47.3X3	T47.3X4	T47.3X5	T47.3X6
Eptazocine	T40.4X1	T40.4X2	T40.4X3	T40.4X4	T40.4X5	T40.4X6
Equanil	T43.591	T43.592	T43.593	T43.594	T43.595	T43.596
Equisetum	T62.2X1	T62.2X2	T62.2X3	T62.2X4	--	--
diuretic	T50.2X1	T50.2X2	T50.2X3	T50.2X4	T50.2X5	T50.2X6
Ergobasine	T48.0X1	T48.0X2	T48.0X3	T48.0X4	T48.0X5	T48.0X6
Ergocalciferol	T45.2X1	T45.2X2	T45.2X3	T45.2X4	T45.2X5	T45.2X6
Ergoloid mesylates	T46.7X1	T46.7X2	T46.7X3	T46.7X4	T46.7X5	T46.7X6
Ergometrine	T48.0X1	T48.0X2	T48.0X3	T48.0X4	T48.0X5	T48.0X6
Ergonovine	T48.0X1	T48.0X2	T48.0X3	T48.0X4	T48.0X5	T48.0X6
Ergot NEC	T64.81	T64.82	T64.83	T64.84	--	--
derivative	T48.0X1	T48.0X2	T48.0X3	T48.0X4	T48.0X5	T48.0X6
medicinal (alkaloids)	T48.0X1	T48.0X2	T48.0X3	T48.0X4	T48.0X5	T48.0X6
prepared	T48.0X1	T48.0X2	T48.0X3	T48.0X4	T48.0X5	T48.0X6
Ergotamine	T46.5X1	T46.5X2	T46.5X3	T46.5X4	T46.5X5	T46.5X6
Ergotocine	T48.0X1	T48.0X2	T48.0X3	T48.0X4	T48.0X5	T48.0X6
Ergotrate	T48.0X1	T48.0X2	T48.0X3	T48.0X4	T48.0X5	T48.0X6
Eritrityl tetranitrate	T46.3X1	T46.3X2	T46.3X3	T46.3X4	T46.3X5	T46.3X6
Erythrityl tetranitrate	T46.3X1	T46.3X2	T46.3X3	T46.3X4	T46.3X5	T46.3X6
Erythrol tetranitrate	T46.3X1	T46.3X2	T46.3X3	T46.3X4	T46.3X5	T46.3X6
Erythromycin (salts)	T36.3X1	T36.3X2	T36.3X3	T36.3X4	T36.3X5	T36.3X6
ophthalmic preparation	T49.5X1	T49.5X2	T49.5X3	T49.5X4	T49.5X5	T49.5X6
topical NEC	T49.0X1	T49.0X2	T49.0X3	T49.0X4	T49.0X5	T49.0X6
Erythropoietin	T45.8X1	T45.8X2	T45.8X3	T45.8X4	T45.8X5	T45.8X6
human	T45.8X1	T45.8X2	T45.8X3	T45.8X4	T45.8X5	T45.8X6
Escin	T46.991	T46.992	T46.993	T46.994	T46.995	T46.996
Esculin	T45.2X1	T45.2X2	T45.2X3	T45.2X4	T45.2X5	T45.2X6
Esculoside	T45.2X1	T45.2X2	T45.2X3	T45.2X4	T45.2X5	T45.2X6
ESDT (ether-soluble tar distillate)	T49.1X1	T49.1X2	T49.1X3	T49.1X4	T49.1X5	T49.1X6
Eserine	T49.5X1	T49.5X2	T49.5X3	T49.5X4	T49.5X5	T49.5X6
Esflurbiprofen	T39.311	T39.312	T39.313	T39.314	T39.315	T39.316
Eskabarb	T42.3X1	T42.3X2	T42.3X3	T42.3X4	T42.3X5	T42.3X6
Eskalith	T43.8X1	T43.8X2	T43.8X3	T43.8X4	T43.8X5	T43.8X6
Esmolol	T44.7X1	T44.7X2	T44.7X3	T44.7X4	T44.7X5	T44.7X6
Estanozolol	T38.7X1	T38.7X2	T38.7X3	T38.7X4	T38.7X5	T38.7X6
Estazolam	T42.4X1	T42.4X2	T42.4X3	T42.4X4	T42.4X5	T42.4X6
Estradiol	T38.5X1	T38.5X2	T38.5X3	T38.5X4	T38.5X5	T38.5X6
with testosterone	T38.7X1	T38.7X2	T38.7X3	T38.7X4	T38.7X5	T38.7X6
benzoate	T38.5X1	T38.5X2	T38.5X3	T38.5X4	T38.5X5	T38.5X6
Estramustine	T45.1X1	T45.1X2	T45.1X3	T45.1X4	T45.1X5	T45.1X6
Estriol	T38.5X1	T38.5X2	T38.5X3	T38.5X4	T38.5X5	T38.5X6
Estrogen	T38.5X1	T38.5X2	T38.5X3	T38.5X4	T38.5X5	T38.5X6
with progesterone	T38.5X1	T38.5X2	T38.5X3	T38.5X4	T38.5X5	T38.5X6
conjugated	T38.5X1	T38.5X2	T38.5X3	T38.5X4	T38.5X5	T38.5X6
Estrone	T38.5X1	T38.5X2	T38.5X3	T38.5X4	T38.5X5	T38.5X6
Estropipate	T38.5X1	T38.5X2	T38.5X3	T38.5X4	T38.5X5	T38.5X6
Etacrynate sodium	T50.1X1	T50.1X2	T50.1X3	T50.1X4	T50.1X5	T50.1X6
Etacrynic acid	T50.1X1	T50.1X2	T50.1X3	T50.1X4	T50.1X5	T50.1X6
Etafedrine	T48.6X1	T48.6X2	T48.6X3	T48.6X4	T48.6X5	T48.6X6
Etafenone	T46.3X1	T46.3X2	T46.3X3	T46.3X4	T46.3X5	T46.3X6
Etambutol	T37.1X1	T37.1X2	T37.1X3	T37.1X4	T37.1X5	T37.1X6
Etamiphyllin	T48.6X1	T48.6X2	T48.6X3	T48.6X4	T48.6X5	T48.6X6
Etamivan	T50.7X1	T50.7X2	T50.7X3	T50.7X4	T50.7X5	T50.7X6
Etamsylate	T45.7X1	T45.7X2	T45.7X3	T45.7X4	T45.7X5	T45.7X6
Etebenecid	T50.4X1	T50.4X2	T50.4X3	T50.4X4	T50.4X5	T50.4X6
Ethacridine	T49.0X1	T49.0X2	T49.0X3	T49.0X4	T49.0X5	T49.0X6
Ethacrynic acid	T50.1X1	T50.1X2	T50.1X3	T50.1X4	T50.1X5	T50.1X6
Ethadione	T42.2X1	T42.2X2	T42.2X3	T42.2X4	T42.2X5	T42.2X6
Ethambutol	T37.1X1	T37.1X2	T37.1X3	T37.1X4	T37.1X5	T37.1X6
Ethamide	T50.2X1	T50.2X2	T50.2X3	T50.2X4	T50.2X5	T50.2X6
Ethamivan	T50.7X1	T50.7X2	T50.7X3	T50.7X4	T50.7X5	T50.7X6
Ethamsylate	T45.7X1	T45.7X2	T45.7X3	T45.7X4	T45.7X5	T45.7X6
Ethanol	T51.0X1	T51.0X2	T51.0X3	T51.0X4	--	--
beverage	T51.0X1	T51.0X2	T51.0X3	T51.0X4	--	--
Ethanolamine oleate	T46.8X1	T46.8X2	T46.8X3	T46.8X4	T46.8X5	T46.8X6
Ethaverine	T44.3X1	T44.3X2	T44.3X3	T44.3X4	T44.3X5	T44.3X6
Ethchlorvynol	T42.6X1	T42.6X2	T42.6X3	T42.6X4	T42.6X5	T42.6X6
Ethebenecid	T50.4X1	T50.4X2	T50.4X3	T50.4X4	T50.4X5	T50.4X6
Ether (vapor)	T41.0X1	T41.0X2	T41.0X3	T41.0X4	T41.0X5	T41.0X6
anesthetic	T41.0X1	T41.0X2	T41.0X3	T41.0X4	T41.0X5	T41.0X6
divinyl	T41.0X1	T41.0X2	T41.0X3	T41.0X4	T41.0X5	T41.0X6
ethyl (medicinal)	T41.0X1	T41.0X2	T41.0X3	T41.0X4	T41.0X5	T41.0X6
nonmedicinal	T52.8X1	T52.8X2	T52.8X3	T52.8X4	--	--
petroleum — *see* Ligroin						
solvent	T52.8X1	T52.8X2	T52.8X3	T52.8X4	--	--
Ethiazide	T50.2X1	T50.2X2	T50.2X3	T50.2X4	T50.2X5	T50.2X6
Ethidium chloride (vapor)	T59.891	T59.892	T59.893	T59.894	--	--
Ethinamate	T42.6X1	T42.6X2	T42.6X3	T42.6X4	T42.6X5	T42.6X6
Ethinylestradiol, ethinyloestradiol	T38.5X1	T38.5X2	T38.5X3	T38.5X4	T38.5X5	T38.5X6
with						
levonorgestrel	T38.4X1	T38.4X2	T38.4X3	T38.4X4	T38.4X5	T38.4X6
norethisterone	T38.4X1	T38.4X2	T38.4X3	T38.4X4	T38.4X5	T38.4X6
Ethiodized oil (131 I)	T50.8X1	T50.8X2	T50.8X3	T50.8X4	T50.8X5	T50.8X6
Ethion	T60.0X1	T60.0X2	T60.0X3	T60.0X4	--	--
Ethionamide	T37.1X1	T37.1X2	T37.1X3	T37.1X4	T37.1X5	T37.1X6
Ethioniamide	T37.1X1	T37.1X2	T37.1X3	T37.1X4	T37.1X5	T37.1X6
Ethisterone	T38.5X1	T38.5X2	T38.5X3	T38.5X4	T38.5X5	T38.5X6
Ethobral	T42.3X1	T42.3X2	T42.3X3	T42.3X4	T42.3X5	T42.3X6
Ethocaine (infiltration) (topical)	T41.3X1	T41.3X2	T41.3X3	T41.3X4	T41.3X5	T41.3X6
nerve block (peripheral) (plexus)	T41.3X1	T41.3X2	T41.3X3	T41.3X4	T41.3X5	T41.3X6
spinal	T41.3X1	T41.3X2	T41.3X3	T41.3X4	T41.3X5	T41.3X6

Substance	Poisoning, Accidental (unintentional)	Poisoning, Intentional self-harm	Poisoning, Assault	Poisoning, Undetermined	Adverse effect	Underdosing
Ethoheptazine	T40.4X1	T40.4X2	T40.4X3	T40.4X4	T40.4X5	T40.4X6
Ethopropazine	T44.3X1	T44.3X2	T44.3X3	T44.3X4	T44.3X5	T44.3X6
Ethosuximide	T42.2X1	T42.2X2	T42.2X3	T42.2X4	T42.2X5	T42.2X6
Ethotoin	T42.0X1	T42.0X2	T42.0X3	T42.0X4	T42.0X5	T42.0X6
Ethoxazene	T37.91	T37.92	T37.93	T37.94	T37.95	T37.96
Ethoxazorutoside	T46.991	T46.992	T46.993	T46.994	T46.995	T46.996
2-Ethoxyethanol	T52.3X1	T52.3X2	T52.3X3	T52.3X4	--	--
Ethoxzolamide	T50.2X1	T50.2X2	T50.2X3	T50.2X4	T50.2X5	T50.2X6
Ethyl						
acetate	T52.8X1	T52.8X2	T52.8X3	T52.8X4	--	--
alcohol	T51.0X1	T51.0X2	T51.0X3	T51.0X4	--	--
beverage	T51.0X1	T51.0X2	T51.0X3	T51.0X4	--	--
aldehyde (vapor)	T59.891	T59.892	T59.893	T59.894	--	--
liquid	T52.8X1	T52.8X2	T52.8X3	T52.8X4	--	--
aminobenzoate	T41.3X1	T41.3X2	T41.3X3	T41.3X4	T41.3X5	T41.3X6
aminophenothiazine	T43.3X1	T43.3X2	T43.3X3	T43.3X4	T43.3X5	T43.3X6
benzoate	T52.8X1	T52.8X2	T52.8X3	T52.8X4	--	--
biscoumacetate	T45.511	T45.512	T45.513	T45.514	T45.515	T45.516
bromide (anesthetic)	T41.0X1	T41.0X2	T41.0X3	T41.0X4	T41.0X5	T41.0X6
carbamate	T45.1X1	T45.1X2	T45.1X3	T45.1X4	T45.1X5	T45.1X6
carbinol	T51.3X1	T51.3X2	T51.3X3	T51.3X4	--	--
carbonate	T52.8X1	T52.8X2	T52.8X3	T52.8X4	--	--
chaulmoograte	T37.1X1	T37.1X2	T37.1X3	T37.1X4	T37.1X5	T37.1X6
chloride (anesthetic)	T41.0X1	T41.0X2	T41.0X3	T41.0X4	T41.0X5	T41.0X6
anesthetic (local)	T41.3X1	T41.3X2	T41.3X3	T41.3X4	T41.3X5	T41.3X6
inhaled	T41.0X1	T41.0X2	T41.0X3	T41.0X4	T41.0X5	T41.0X6
local	T49.4X1	T49.4X2	T49.4X3	T49.4X4	T49.4X5	T49.4X6
solvent	T53.6X1	T53.6X2	T53.6X3	T53.6X4	--	--
dibunate	T48.3X1	T48.3X2	T48.3X3	T48.3X4	T48.3X5	T48.3X6
dichloroarsine (vapor)	T57.0X1	T57.0X2	T57.0X3	T57.0X4	--	--
estranol	T38.7X1	T38.7X2	T38.7X3	T38.7X4	T38.7X5	T38.7X6
ether (see also ether)	T52.8X1	T52.8X2	T52.8X3	T52.8X4	--	--
formate NEC (solvent)	T52.0X1	T52.0X2	T52.0X3	T52.0X4	--	--
fumarate	T49.4X1	T49.4X2	T49.4X3	T49.4X4	T49.4X5	T49.4X6
hydroxyisobutyrate NEC (solvent)	T52.8X1	T52.8X2	T52.8X3	T52.8X4	--	--
iodoacetate	T59.3X1	T59.3X2	T59.3X3	T59.3X4	--	--
lactate NEC (solvent)	T52.8X1	T52.8X2	T52.8X3	T52.8X4	--	--
loflazepate	T42.4X1	T42.4X2	T42.4X3	T42.4X4	T42.4X5	T42.4X6
mercuric chloride	T56.1X1	T56.1X2	T56.1X3	T56.1X4	--	--
methylcarbinol	T51.8X1	T51.8X2	T51.8X3	T51.8X4	--	--
morphine	T40.2X1	T40.2X2	T40.2X3	T40.2X4	T40.2X5	T40.2X6
noradrenaline	T48.6X1	T48.6X2	T48.6X3	T48.6X4	T48.6X5	T48.6X6
oxybutyrate NEC (solvent)	T52.8X1	T52.8X2	T52.8X3	T52.8X4	--	--
Ethylene (gas)	T59.891	T59.892	T59.893	T59.894	--	--
anesthetic (general)	T41.0X1	T41.0X2	T41.0X3	T41.0X4	T41.0X5	T41.0X6
chlorohydrin	T52.8X1	T52.8X2	T52.8X3	T52.8X4	--	--
vapor	T53.6X1	T53.6X2	T53.6X3	T53.6X4	--	--
dichloride	T52.8X1	T52.8X2	T52.8X3	T52.8X4	--	--
vapor	T53.6X1	T53.6X2	T53.6X3	T53.6X4	--	--
dinitrate	T52.3X1	T52.3X2	T52.3X3	T52.3X4	--	--
glycol(s)	T52.8X1	T52.8X2	T52.8X3	T52.8X4	--	--
dinitrate	T52.3X1	T52.3X2	T52.3X3	T52.3X4	--	--
monobutyl ether	T52.3X1	T52.3X2	T52.3X3	T52.3X4	--	--
imine	T54.1X1	T54.1X2	T54.1X3	T54.1X4	--	--
oxide (fumigant) (nonmedicinal)	T59.891	T59.892	T59.893	T59.894	--	--
medicinal	T49.0X1	T49.0X2	T49.0X3	T49.0X4	T49.0X5	T49.0X6
Ethylenediamine theophylline	T48.6X1	T48.6X2	T48.6X3	T48.6X4	T48.6X5	T48.6X6
Ethylenediaminetetra-acetic acid	T50.6X1	T50.6X2	T50.6X3	T50.6X4	T50.6X5	T50.6X6
Ethylenedinitrilotetra-acetate	T50.6X1	T50.6X2	T50.6X3	T50.6X4	T50.6X5	T50.6X6
Ethylestrenol	T38.7X1	T38.7X2	T38.7X3	T38.7X4	T38.7X5	T38.7X6
Ethylhydroxycellulose	T47.4X1	T47.4X2	T47.4X3	T47.4X4	T47.4X5	T47.4X6
Ethylidene						
chloride NEC	T53.6X1	T53.6X2	T53.6X3	T53.6X4	--	--
diacetate	T60.3X1	T60.3X2	T60.3X3	T60.3X4	--	--
dicoumarin	T45.511	T45.512	T45.513	T45.514	T45.515	T45.516
dicoumarol	T45.511	T45.512	T45.513	T45.514	T45.515	T45.516
diethyl ether	T52.0X1	T52.0X2	T52.0X3	T52.0X4	--	--
Ethylmorphine	T40.2X1	T40.2X2	T40.2X3	T40.2X4	T40.2X5	T40.2X6
Ethylnorepinephrine	T48.6X1	T48.6X2	T48.6X3	T48.6X4	T48.6X5	T48.6X6
Ethylparachlorophen-oxyisobutyrate	T46.6X1	T46.6X2	T46.6X3	T46.6X4	T46.6X5	T46.6X6
Ethynodiol	T38.4X1	T38.4X2	T38.4X3	T38.4X4	T38.4X5	T38.4X6
with mestranol diacetate	T38.4X1	T38.4X2	T38.4X3	T38.4X4	T38.4X5	T38.4X6
Etidocaine	T41.3X1	T41.3X2	T41.3X3	T41.3X4	T41.3X5	T41.3X6
infiltration (subcutaneous)	T41.3X1	T41.3X2	T41.3X3	T41.3X4	T41.3X5	T41.3X6
nerve (peripheral) (plexus)	T41.3X1	T41.3X2	T41.3X3	T41.3X4	T41.3X5	T41.3X6
Etidronate	T50.991	T50.992	T50.993	T50.994	T50.995	T50.996
Etidronic acid (disodium salt)	T50.991	T50.992	T50.993	T50.994	T50.995	T50.996
Etifoxine	T42.6X1	T42.6X2	T42.6X3	T42.6X4	T42.6X5	T42.6X6
Etilefrine	T44.4X1	T44.4X2	T44.4X3	T44.4X4	T44.4X5	T44.4X6

Substance	Poisoning, Accidental (unintentional)	Poisoning, Intentional self-harm	Poisoning, Assault	Poisoning, Undetermined	Adverse effect	Underdosing
Etilfen	T42.3X1	T42.3X2	T42.3X3	T42.3X4	T42.3X5	T42.3X6
Etinodiol	T38.4X1	T38.4X2	T38.4X3	T38.4X4	T38.4X5	T38.4X6
Etiroxate	T46.6X1	T46.6X2	T46.6X3	T46.6X4	T46.6X5	T46.6X6
Etizolam	T42.4X1	T42.4X2	T42.4X3	T42.4X4	T42.4X5	T42.4X6
Etodolac	T39.391	T39.392	T39.393	T39.394	T39.395	T39.396
Etofamide	T37.3X1	T37.3X2	T37.3X3	T37.3X4	T37.3X5	T37.3X6
Etofibrate	T46.6X1	T46.6X2	T46.6X3	T46.6X4	T46.6X5	T46.6X6
Etofylline	T46.7X1	T46.7X2	T46.7X3	T46.7X4	T46.7X5	T46.7X6
clofibrate	T46.6X1	T46.6X2	T46.6X3	T46.6X4	T46.6X5	T46.6X6
Etoglucid	T45.1X1	T45.1X2	T45.1X3	T45.1X4	T45.1X5	T45.1X6
Etomidate	T41.1X1	T41.1X2	T41.1X3	T41.1X4	T41.1X5	T41.1X6
Etomide	T39.8X1	T39.8X2	T39.8X3	T39.8X4	T39.8X5	T39.8X6
Etomidoline	T44.3X1	T44.3X2	T44.3X3	T44.3X4	T44.3X5	T44.3X6
Etoposide	T45.1X1	T45.1X2	T45.1X3	T45.1X4	T45.1X5	T45.1X6
Etorphine	T40.2X1	T40.2X2	T40.2X3	T40.2X4	T40.2X5	T40.2X6
Etoval	T42.3X1	T42.3X2	T42.3X3	T42.3X4	T42.3X5	T42.3X6
Etozolin	T50.1X1	T50.1X2	T50.1X3	T50.1X4	T50.1X5	T50.1X6
Etretinate	T50.991	T50.992	T50.993	T50.994	T50.995	T50.996
Etryptamine	T43.691	T43.692	T43.693	T43.694	T43.695	T43.696
Etybenzatropine	T44.3X1	T44.3X2	T44.3X3	T44.3X4	T44.3X5	T44.3X6
Etynodiol	T38.4X1	T38.4X2	T38.4X3	T38.4X4	T38.4X5	T38.4X6
Eucaine	T41.3X1	T41.3X2	T41.3X3	T41.3X4	T41.3X5	T41.3X6
Eucalyptus oil	T49.7X1	T49.7X2	T49.7X3	T49.7X4	T49.7X5	T49.7X6
Eucatropine	T49.5X1	T49.5X2	T49.5X3	T49.5X4	T49.5X5	T49.5X6
Eucodal	T40.2X1	T40.2X2	T40.2X3	T40.2X4	T40.2X5	T40.2X6
Euneryl	T42.3X1	T42.3X2	T42.3X3	T42.3X4	T42.3X5	T42.3X6
Euphthalmine	T44.3X1	T44.3X2	T44.3X3	T44.3X4	T44.3X5	T44.3X6
Eurax	T49.0X1	T49.0X2	T49.0X3	T49.0X4	T49.0X5	T49.0X6
Euresol	T49.4X1	T49.4X2	T49.4X3	T49.4X4	T49.4X5	T49.4X6
Euthroid	T38.1X1	T38.1X2	T38.1X3	T38.1X4	T38.1X5	T38.1X6
Evans blue	T50.8X1	T50.8X2	T50.8X3	T50.8X4	T50.8X5	T50.8X6
Evipal	T42.3X1	T42.3X2	T42.3X3	T42.3X4	T42.3X5	T42.3X6
sodium	T41.1X1	T41.1X2	T41.1X3	T41.1X4	T41.1X5	T41.1X6
Evipan	T42.3X1	T42.3X2	T42.3X3	T42.3X4	T42.3X5	T42.3X6
sodium	T41.1X1	T41.1X2	T41.1X3	T41.1X4	T41.1X5	T41.1X6
Exalamide	T49.0X1	T49.0X2	T49.0X3	T49.0X4	T49.0X5	T49.0X6
Exalgin	T39.1X1	T39.1X2	T39.1X3	T39.1X4	T39.1X5	T39.1X6
Excipients, pharmaceutical	T50.901	T50.902	T50.903	T50.904	T50.905	T50.906
Exhaust gas (engine) (motor vehicle)	T58.01	T58.02	T58.03	T58.04	--	--
Ex-Lax (phenolphthalein)	T47.2X1	T47.2X2	T47.2X3	T47.2X4	T47.2X5	T47.2X6
Expectorant NEC	T48.4X1	T48.4X2	T48.4X3	T48.4X4	T48.4X5	T48.4X6
Extended insulin zinc suspension	T38.3X1	T38.3X2	T38.3X3	T38.3X4	T38.3X5	T38.3X6
External medications (skin) (mucous membrane)	T49.91	T49.92	T49.93	T49.94	T49.95	T49.96
dental agent	T49.7X1	T49.7X2	T49.7X3	T49.7X4	T49.7X5	T49.7X6
ENT agent	T49.6X1	T49.6X2	T49.6X3	T49.6X4	T49.6X5	T49.6X6
ophthalmic preparation	T49.5X1	T49.5X2	T49.5X3	T49.5X4	T49.5X5	T49.5X6
specified NEC	T49.8X1	T49.8X2	T49.8X3	T49.8X4	T49.8X5	T49.8X6
Extrapyramidal antagonist NEC	T44.3X1	T44.3X2	T44.3X3	T44.3X4	T44.3X5	T44.3X6
Eye agents (anti-infective)	T49.5X1	T49.5X2	T49.5X3	T49.5X4	T49.5X5	T49.5X6
Eye drug NEC	T49.5X1	T49.5X2	T49.5X3	T49.5X4	T49.5X5	T49.5X6
F						
FAC (fluorouracil + doxorubicin + cyclophosphamide)	T45.1X1	T45.1X2	T45.1X3	T45.1X4	T45.1X5	T45.1X6
Factor						
I (fibrinogen)	T45.8X1	T45.8X2	T45.8X3	T45.8X4	T45.8X5	T45.8X6
III (thromboplastin)	T45.8X1	T45.8X2	T45.8X3	T45.8X4	T45.8X5	T45.8X6
VIII (antihemophilic Factor) (concentrate)	T45.8X1	T45.8X2	T45.8X3	T45.8X4	T45.8X5	T45.8X6
IX complex	T45.7X1	T45.7X2	T45.7X3	T45.7X4	T45.7X5	T45.7X6
human	T45.8X1	T45.8X2	T45.8X3	T45.8X4	T45.8X5	T45.8X6
Famotidine	T47.0X1	T47.0X2	T47.0X3	T47.0X4	T47.0X5	T47.0X6
Fat suspension, intravenous	T50.991	T50.992	T50.993	T50.994	T50.995	T50.996
Fazadinium bromide	T48.1X1	T48.1X2	T48.1X3	T48.1X4	T48.1X5	T48.1X6
Febarbamate	T42.3X1	T42.3X2	T42.3X3	T42.3X4	T42.3X5	T42.3X6
Fecal softener	T47.4X1	T47.4X2	T47.4X3	T47.4X4	T47.4X5	T47.4X6
Fedrilate	T48.3X1	T48.3X2	T48.3X3	T48.3X4	T48.3X5	T48.3X6
Felodipine	T46.1X1	T46.1X2	T46.1X3	T46.1X4	T46.1X5	T46.1X6
Felypressin	T38.891	T38.892	T38.893	T38.894	T38.895	T38.896
Femoxetine	T43.221	T43.222	T43.223	T43.224	T43.225	T43.226
Fenalcomine	T46.3X1	T46.3X2	T46.3X3	T46.3X4	T46.3X5	T46.3X6
Fenamisal	T37.1X1	T37.1X2	T37.1X3	T37.1X4	T37.1X5	T37.1X6
Fenazone	T39.2X1	T39.2X2	T39.2X3	T39.2X4	T39.2X5	T39.2X6
Fenbendazole	T37.4X1	T37.4X2	T37.4X3	T37.4X4	T37.4X5	T37.4X6
Fenbutrazate	T50.5X1	T50.5X2	T50.5X3	T50.5X4	T50.5X5	T50.5X6
Fencamfamine	T43.691	T43.692	T43.693	T43.694	T43.695	T43.696
Fendiline	T46.1X1	T46.1X2	T46.1X3	T46.1X4	T46.1X5	T46.1X6
Fenetylline	T43.691	T43.692	T43.693	T43.694	T43.695	T43.696
Fenflumizole	T39.391	T39.392	T39.393	T39.394	T39.395	T39.396
Fenfluramine	T50.5X1	T50.5X2	T50.5X3	T50.5X4	T50.5X5	T50.5X6
Fenobarbital	T42.3X1	T42.3X2	T42.3X3	T42.3X4	T42.3X5	T42.3X6

Substance	Poisoning, Accidental (unintentional)	Poisoning, Intentional self-harm	Poisoning, Assault	Poisoning, Undetermined	Adverse effect	Underdosing
Fenofibrate	T46.6X1	T46.6X2	T46.6X3	T46.6X4	T46.6X5	T46.6X6
Fenoprofen	T39.311	T39.312	T39.313	T39.314	T39.315	T39.316
Fenoterol	T48.6X1	T48.6X2	T48.6X3	T48.6X4	T48.6X5	T48.6X6
Fenoverine	T44.3X1	T44.3X2	T44.3X3	T44.3X4	T44.3X5	T44.3X6
Fenoxazoline	T48.5X1	T48.5X2	T48.5X3	T48.5X4	T48.5X5	T48.5X6
Fenproporex	T50.5X1	T50.5X2	T50.5X3	T50.5X4	T50.5X5	T50.5X6
Fenquizone	T50.2X1	T50.2X2	T50.2X3	T50.2X4	T50.2X5	T50.2X6
Fentanyl	T40.4X1	T40.4X2	T40.4X3	T40.4X4	T40.4X5	T40.4X6
Fentazin	T43.3X1	T43.3X2	T43.3X3	T43.3X4	T43.3X5	T43.3X6
Fenthion	T60.0X1	T60.0X2	T60.0X3	T60.0X4	--	--
Fenticlor	T49.0X1	T49.0X2	T49.0X3	T49.0X4	T49.0X5	T49.0X6
Fenylbutazone	T39.2X1	T39.2X2	T39.2X3	T39.2X4	T39.2X5	T39.2X6
Feprazone	T39.2X1	T39.2X2	T39.2X3	T39.2X4	T39.2X5	T39.2X6
Fer de lance (bite) (venom)	T63.061	T63.062	T63.063	T63.064	--	--
Ferric (*see also* Iron)						
chloride	T45.4X1	T45.4X2	T45.4X3	T45.4X4	T45.4X5	T45.4X6
citrate	T45.4X1	T45.4X2	T45.4X3	T45.4X4	T45.4X5	T45.4X6
hydroxide						
colloidal	T45.4X1	T45.4X2	T45.4X3	T45.4X4	T45.4X5	T45.4X6
polymaltose	T45.4X1	T45.4X2	T45.4X3	T45.4X4	T45.4X5	T45.4X6
pyrophosphate	T45.4X1	T45.4X2	T45.4X3	T45.4X4	T45.4X5	T45.4X6
Ferritin	T45.4X1	T45.4X2	T45.4X3	T45.4X4	T45.4X5	T45.4X6
Ferrocholinate	T45.4X1	T45.4X2	T45.4X3	T45.4X4	T45.4X5	T45.4X6
Ferrodextrane	T45.4X1	T45.4X2	T45.4X3	T45.4X4	T45.4X5	T45.4X6
Ferropolimaler	T45.4X1	T45.4X2	T45.4X3	T45.4X4	T45.4X5	T45.4X6
Ferrous (*see also* Iron)						
phosphate	T45.4X1	T45.4X2	T45.4X3	T45.4X4	T45.4X5	T45.4X6
salt	T45.4X1	T45.4X2	T45.4X3	T45.4X4	T45.4X5	T45.4X6
with folic acid	T45.4X1	T45.4X2	T45.4X3	T45.4X4	T45.4X5	T45.4X6
Ferrous fumerate, gluconate, lactate, salt NEC, sulfate (medicinal)	T45.4X1	T45.4X2	T45.4X3	T45.4X4	T45.4X5	T45.4X6
Ferrovanadium (fumes)	T59.891	T59.892	T59.893	T59.894	--	--
Ferrum — *see* Iron						
Fertilizers NEC	T65.891	T65.892	T65.893	T65.894	--	--
with herbicide mixture	T60.3X1	T60.3X2	T60.3X3	T60.3X4	--	--
Fetoxilate	T47.6X1	T47.6X2	T47.6X3	T47.6X4	T47.6X5	T47.6X6
Fiber, dietary	T47.4X1	T47.4X2	T47.4X3	T47.4X4	T47.4X5	T47.4X6
Fiberglass	T65.831	T65.832	T65.833	T65.834	--	--
Fibrinogen (human)	T45.8X1	T45.8X2	T45.8X3	T45.8X4	T45.8X5	T45.8X6
Fibrinolysin (human)	T45.691	T45.692	T45.693	T45.694	T45.695	T45.696
Fibrinolysis						
affecting drug	T45.601	T45.602	T45.603	T45.604	T45.605	T45.606
inhibitor NEC	T45.621	T45.622	T45.623	T45.624	T45.625	T45.626
Fibrinolytic drug	T45.611	T45.612	T45.613	T45.614	T45.615	T45.616
Filix mas	T37.4X1	T37.4X2	T37.4X3	T37.4X4	T37.4X5	T37.4X6
Filtering cream	T49.3X1	T49.3X2	T49.3X3	T49.3X4	T49.3X5	T49.3X6
Fiorinal	T39.011	T39.012	T39.013	T39.014	T39.015	T39.016
Firedamp	T59.891	T59.892	T59.893	T59.894	--	--
Fish, noxious, nonbacterial	T61.91	T61.92	T61.93	T61.94	--	--
ciguatera	T61.01	T61.02	T61.03	T61.04	--	--
scombroid	T61.11	T61.12	T61.13	T61.14	--	--
shell	T61.781	T61.782	T61.783	T61.784	--	--
specified NEC	T61.771	T61.772	T61.773	T61.774	--	--
Flagyl	T37.3X1	T37.3X2	T37.3X3	T37.3X4	T37.3X5	T37.3X6
Flavine adenine dinucleotide	T45.2X1	T45.2X2	T45.2X3	T45.2X4	T45.2X5	T45.2X6
Flavodic acid	T46.991	T46.992	T46.993	T46.994	T46.995	T46.996
Flavoxate	T44.3X1	T44.3X2	T44.3X3	T44.3X4	T44.3X5	T44.3X6
Flaxedil	T48.1X1	T48.1X2	T48.1X3	T48.1X4	T48.1X5	T48.1X6
Flaxseed (medicinal)	T49.3X1	T49.3X2	T49.3X3	T49.3X4	T49.3X5	T49.3X6
Flecainide	T46.2X1	T46.2X2	T46.2X3	T46.2X4	T46.2X5	T46.2X6
Fleroxacin	T36.8X1	T36.8X2	T36.8X3	T36.8X4	T36.8X5	T36.8X6
Floctafenine	T39.8X1	T39.8X2	T39.8X3	T39.8X4	T39.8X5	T39.8X6
Flomax	T44.6X1	T44.6X2	T44.6X3	T44.6X4	T44.6X5	T44.6X6
Flomoxef	T36.1X1	T36.1X2	T36.1X3	T36.1X4	T36.1X5	T36.1X6
Flopropione	T44.3X1	T44.3X2	T44.3X3	T44.3X4	T44.3X5	T44.3X6
Florantyrone	T47.5X1	T47.5X2	T47.5X3	T47.5X4	T47.5X5	T47.5X6
Floraquin	T37.8X1	T37.8X2	T37.8X3	T37.8X4	T37.8X5	T37.8X6
Florinef	T38.0X1	T38.0X2	T38.0X3	T38.0X4	T38.0X5	T38.0X6
ENT agent	T49.6X1	T49.6X2	T49.6X3	T49.6X4	T49.6X5	T49.6X6
ophthalmic preparation	T49.5X1	T49.5X2	T49.5X3	T49.5X4	T49.5X5	T49.5X6
topical NEC	T49.0X1	T49.0X2	T49.0X3	T49.0X4	T49.0X5	T49.0X6
Flowers of sulfur	T49.4X1	T49.4X2	T49.4X3	T49.4X4	T49.4X5	T49.4X6
Floxuridine	T45.1X1	T45.1X2	T45.1X3	T45.1X4	T45.1X5	T45.1X6
Fluanisone	T43.4X1	T43.4X2	T43.4X3	T43.4X4	T43.4X5	T43.4X6
Flubendazole	T37.4X1	T37.4X2	T37.4X3	T37.4X4	T37.4X5	T37.4X6
Fluclorolone acetonide	T49.0X1	T49.0X2	T49.0X3	T49.0X4	T49.0X5	T49.0X6
Flucloxacillin	T36.0X1	T36.0X2	T36.0X3	T36.0X4	T36.0X5	T36.0X6
Fluconazole	T37.8X1	T37.8X2	T37.8X3	T37.8X4	T37.8X5	T37.8X6
Flucytosine	T37.8X1	T37.8X2	T37.8X3	T37.8X4	T37.8X5	T37.8X6
Fludeoxyglucose (18F)	T50.8X1	T50.8X2	T50.8X3	T50.8X4	T50.8X5	T50.8X6
Fludiazepam	T42.4X1	T42.4X2	T42.4X3	T42.4X4	T42.4X5	T42.4X6
Fludrocortisone	T50.0X1	T50.0X2	T50.0X3	T50.0X4	T50.0X5	T50.0X6
ENT agent	T49.6X1	T49.6X2	T49.6X3	T49.6X4	T49.6X5	T49.6X6
ophthalmic preparation	T49.5X1	T49.5X2	T49.5X3	T49.5X4	T49.5X5	T49.5X6
topical NEC	T49.0X1	T49.0X2	T49.0X3	T49.0X4	T49.0X5	T49.0X6
Fludroxycortide	T49.0X1	T49.0X2	T49.0X3	T49.0X4	T49.0X5	T49.0X6
Flufenamic acid	T39.391	T39.392	T39.393	T39.394	T39.395	T39.396
Fluindione	T45.511	T45.512	T45.513	T45.514	T45.515	T45.516
Flumequine	T37.8X1	T37.8X2	T37.8X3	T37.8X4	T37.8X5	T37.8X6
Flumethasone	T49.0X1	T49.0X2	T49.0X3	T49.0X4	T49.0X5	T49.0X6
Flumethiazide	T50.2X1	T50.2X2	T50.2X3	T50.2X4	T50.2X5	T50.2X6
Flumidin	T37.5X1	T37.5X2	T37.5X3	T37.5X4	T37.5X5	T37.5X6
Flunarizine	T46.7X1	T46.7X2	T46.7X3	T46.7X4	T46.7X5	T46.7X6
Flunidazole	T37.8X1	T37.8X2	T37.8X3	T37.8X4	T37.8X5	T37.8X6
Flunisolide	T48.6X1	T48.6X2	T48.6X3	T48.6X4	T48.6X5	T48.6X6
Flunitrazepam	T42.4X1	T42.4X2	T42.4X3	T42.4X4	T42.4X5	T42.4X6
Fluocinolone (acetonide)	T49.0X1	T49.0X2	T49.0X3	T49.0X4	T49.0X5	T49.0X6
Fluocinonide	T49.0X1	T49.0X2	T49.0X3	T49.0X4	T49.0X5	T49.0X6
Fluocortin (butyl)	T49.0X1	T49.0X2	T49.0X3	T49.0X4	T49.0X5	T49.0X6
Fluocortolone	T49.0X1	T49.0X2	T49.0X3	T49.0X4	T49.0X5	T49.0X6
Fluohydrocortisone	T38.0X1	T38.0X2	T38.0X3	T38.0X4	T38.0X5	T38.0X6
ENT agent	T49.6X1	T49.6X2	T49.6X3	T49.6X4	T49.6X5	T49.6X6
ophthalmic preparation	T49.5X1	T49.5X2	T49.5X3	T49.5X4	T49.5X5	T49.5X6
topical NEC	T49.0X1	T49.0X2	T49.0X3	T49.0X4	T49.0X5	T49.0X6
Fluonid	T49.0X1	T49.0X2	T49.0X3	T49.0X4	T49.0X5	T49.0X6
Fluopromazine	T43.3X1	T43.3X2	T43.3X3	T43.3X4	T43.3X5	T43.3X6
Fluoracetate	T60.8X1	T60.8X2	T60.8X3	T60.8X4	--	--
Fluorescein	T50.8X1	T50.8X2	T50.8X3	T50.8X4	T50.8X5	T50.8X6
Fluorhydrocortisone	T50.0X1	T50.0X2	T50.0X3	T50.0X4	T50.0X5	T50.0X6
Fluoride (nonmedicinal) (pesticide) (sodium) NEC	T60.8X1	T60.8X2	T60.8X3	T60.8X4	--	--
hydrogen — *see* Hydrofluoric acid						
medicinal NEC	T50.991	T50.992	T50.993	T50.994	T50.995	T50.996
dental use	T49.7X1	T49.7X2	T49.7X3	T49.7X4	T49.7X5	T49.7X6
not pesticide NEC	T54.91	T54.92	T54.93	T54.94	--	--
stannous	T49.7X1	T49.7X2	T49.7X3	T49.7X4	T49.7X5	T49.7X6
Fluorinated corticosteroids	T38.0X1	T38.0X2	T38.0X3	T38.0X4	T38.0X5	T38.0X6
Fluorine (gas)	T59.5X1	T59.5X2	T59.5X3	T59.5X4	--	--
salt — *see* Fluoride(s)						
Fluoristan	T49.7X1	T49.7X2	T49.7X3	T49.7X4	T49.7X5	T49.7X6
Fluormetholone	T49.0X1	T49.0X2	T49.0X3	T49.0X4	T49.0X5	T49.0X6
Fluoroacetate	T60.8X1	T60.8X2	T60.8X3	T60.8X4	--	--
Fluorocarbon monomer	T53.6X1	T53.6X2	T53.6X3	T53.6X4	--	--
Fluorocytosine	T37.8X1	T37.8X2	T37.8X3	T37.8X4	T37.8X5	T37.8X6
Fluorodeoxyuridine	T45.1X1	T45.1X2	T45.1X3	T45.1X4	T45.1X5	T45.1X6
Fluorometholone	T49.0X1	T49.0X2	T49.0X3	T49.0X4	T49.0X5	T49.0X6
ophthalmic preparation	T49.5X1	T49.5X2	T49.5X3	T49.5X4	T49.5X5	T49.5X6
Fluorophosphate insecticide	T60.0X1	T60.0X2	T60.0X3	T60.0X4	--	--
Fluorosol	T46.3X1	T46.3X2	T46.3X3	T46.3X4	T46.3X5	T46.3X6
Fluorouracil	T45.1X1	T45.1X2	T45.1X3	T45.1X4	T45.1X5	T45.1X6
Fluorphenylalanine	T49.5X1	T49.5X2	T49.5X3	T49.5X4	T49.5X5	T49.5X6
Fluothane	T41.0X1	T41.0X2	T41.0X3	T41.0X4	T41.0X5	T41.0X6
Fluoxetine	T43.221	T43.222	T43.223	T43.224	T43.225	T43.226
Fluoxymesterone	T38.7X1	T38.7X2	T38.7X3	T38.7X4	T38.7X5	T38.7X6
Flupenthixol	T43.4X1	T43.4X2	T43.4X3	T43.4X4	T43.4X5	T43.4X6
Flupentixol	T43.4X1	T43.4X2	T43.4X3	T43.4X4	T43.4X5	T43.4X6
Fluphenazine	T43.3X1	T43.3X2	T43.3X3	T43.3X4	T43.3X5	T43.3X6
Fluprednidene	T49.0X1	T49.0X2	T49.0X3	T49.0X4	T49.0X5	T49.0X6
Fluprednisolone	T38.0X1	T38.0X2	T38.0X3	T38.0X4	T38.0X5	T38.0X6
Fluradoline	T39.8X1	T39.8X2	T39.8X3	T39.8X4	T39.8X5	T39.8X6
Flurandrenolide	T49.0X1	T49.0X2	T49.0X3	T49.0X4	T49.0X5	T49.0X6
Flurandrenolone	T49.0X1	T49.0X2	T49.0X3	T49.0X4	T49.0X5	T49.0X6
Flurazepam	T42.4X1	T42.4X2	T42.4X3	T42.4X4	T42.4X5	T42.4X6
Flurbiprofen	T39.311	T39.312	T39.313	T39.314	T39.315	T39.316
Flurobate	T49.0X1	T49.0X2	T49.0X3	T49.0X4	T49.0X5	T49.0X6
Fluroxene	T41.0X1	T41.0X2	T41.0X3	T41.0X4	T41.0X5	T41.0X6
Fluspirilene	T43.591	T43.592	T43.593	T43.594	T43.595	T43.596
Flutamide	T38.6X1	T38.6X2	T38.6X3	T38.6X4	T38.6X5	T38.6X6
Flutazolam	T42.4X1	T42.4X2	T42.4X3	T42.4X4	T42.4X5	T42.4X6
Fluticasone propionate	T38.0X1	T38.0X2	T38.0X3	T38.0X4	T38.0X5	T38.0X6
Flutoprazepam	T42.4X1	T42.4X2	T42.4X3	T42.4X4	T42.4X5	T42.4X6
Flutropium bromide	T48.6X1	T48.6X2	T48.6X3	T48.6X4	T48.6X5	T48.6X6
Fluvoxamine	T43.221	T43.222	T43.223	T43.224	T43.225	T43.226
Folacin	T45.8X1	T45.8X2	T45.8X3	T45.8X4	T45.8X5	T45.8X6
Folic acid	T45.8X1	T45.8X2	T45.8X3	T45.8X4	T45.8X5	T45.8X6
with ferrous salt	T45.2X1	T45.2X2	T45.2X3	T45.2X4	T45.2X5	T45.2X6
antagonist	T45.1X1	T45.1X2	T45.1X3	T45.1X4	T45.1X5	T45.1X6
Folinic acid	T45.8X1	T45.8X2	T45.8X3	T45.8X4	T45.8X5	T45.8X6
Folium stramoniae	T48.6X1	T48.6X2	T48.6X3	T48.6X4	T48.6X5	T48.6X6
Follicle-stimulating hormone, human	T38.811	T38.812	T38.813	T38.814	T38.815	T38.816
Folpet	T60.3X1	T60.3X2	T60.3X3	T60.3X4	--	--
Fominoben	T48.3X1	T48.3X2	T48.3X3	T48.3X4	T48.3X5	T48.3X6

Food, foodstuffs, noxious, nonbacterial, NEC - Gas NEC

Substance	Poisoning, Accidental (unintentional)	Poisoning, Intentional self-harm	Poisoning, Assault	Poisoning, Undetermined	Adverse effect	Underdosing
Food, foodstuffs, noxious, nonbacterial, NEC	T62.91	T62.92	T62.93	T62.94	--	--
berries	T62.1X1	T62.1X2	T62.1X3	T62.1X4	--	--
fish (*see also* Fish)	T61.91	T61.92	T61.93	T61.94	--	--
mushrooms	T62.0X1	T62.0X2	T62.0X3	T62.0X4	--	--
plants	T62.2X1	T62.2X2	T62.2X3	T62.2X4	--	--
seafood	T61.91	T61.92	T61.93	T61.94	--	--
specified NEC	T61.8X1	T61.8X2	T61.8X3	T61.8X4	--	--
seeds	T62.2X1	T62.2X2	T62.2X3	T62.2X4	--	--
shellfish	T61.781	T61.782	T61.783	T61.784	--	--
specified NEC	T62.8X1	T62.8X2	T62.8X3	T62.8X4	--	--
Fool's parsley	T62.2X1	T62.2X2	T62.2X3	T62.2X4	--	--
Formaldehyde (solution), gas or vapor	T59.2X1	T59.2X2	T59.2X3	T59.2X4	--	--
fungicide	T60.3X1	T60.3X2	T60.3X3	T60.3X4	--	--
Formalin	T59.2X1	T59.2X2	T59.2X3	T59.2X4	--	--
fungicide	T60.3X1	T60.3X2	T60.3X3	T60.3X4	--	--
vapor	T59.2X1	T59.2X2	T59.2X3	T59.2X4	--	--
Formic acid	T54.2X1	T54.2X2	T54.2X3	T54.2X4	--	--
vapor	T59.891	T59.892	T59.893	T59.894	--	--
Foscarnet sodium	T37.5X1	T37.5X2	T37.5X3	T37.5X4	T37.5X5	T37.5X6
Fosfestrol	T38.5X1	T38.5X2	T38.5X3	T38.5X4	T38.5X5	T38.5X6
Fosfomycin	T36.8X1	T36.8X2	T36.8X3	T36.8X4	T36.8X5	T36.8X6
Fosfonet sodium	T37.5X1	T37.5X2	T37.5X3	T37.5X4	T37.5X5	T37.5X6
Fosinopril	T46.4X1	T46.4X2	T46.4X3	T46.4X4	T46.4X5	T46.4X6
sodium	T46.4X1	T46.4X2	T46.4X3	T46.4X4	T46.4X5	T46.4X6
Fowler's solution	T57.0X1	T57.0X2	T57.0X3	T57.0X4	--	--
Foxglove	T62.2X1	T62.2X2	T62.2X3	T62.2X4	--	--
Framycetin	T36.5X1	T36.5X2	T36.5X3	T36.5X4	T36.5X5	T36.5X6
Frangula	T47.2X1	T47.2X2	T47.2X3	T47.2X4	T47.2X5	T47.2X6
extract	T47.2X1	T47.2X2	T47.2X3	T47.2X4	T47.2X5	T47.2X6
Frei antigen	T50.8X1	T50.8X2	T50.8X3	T50.8X4	T50.8X5	T50.8X6
Freon	T53.5X1	T53.5X2	T53.5X3	T53.5X4	--	--
Fructose	T50.3X1	T50.3X2	T50.3X3	T50.3X4	T50.3X5	T50.3X6
Frusemide	T50.1X1	T50.1X2	T50.1X3	T50.1X4	T50.1X5	T50.1X6
FSH	T38.811	T38.812	T38.813	T38.814	T38.815	T38.816
Ftorafur	T45.1X1	T45.1X2	T45.1X3	T45.1X4	T45.1X5	T45.1X6
Fuel						
automobile	T52.0X1	T52.0X2	T52.0X3	T52.0X4	--	--
exhaust gas, not in transit	T58.01	T58.02	T58.03	T58.04	--	--
vapor NEC	T52.0X1	T52.0X2	T52.0X3	T52.0X4	--	--
gas (domestic use) (*see also* Carbon, monoxide, fuel, utility)	T59.891	T59.892	T59.893	T59.894		
utility	T59.891	T59.892	T59.893	T59.894		
in mobile container	T59.891	T59.892	T59.893	T59.894		
incomplete combustion of — *see* Carbon, monoxide, fuel, utility						
piped (natural)	T59.891	T59.892	T59.893	T59.894	--	--
industrial, incomplete combustion	T58.8X1	T58.8X2	T58.8X3	T58.8X4	--	--
Fugillin	T36.8X1	T36.8X2	T36.8X3	T36.8X4	T36.8X5	T36.8X6
Fulminate of mercury	T56.1X1	T56.1X2	T56.1X3	T56.1X4	--	--
Fulvicin	T36.7X1	T36.7X2	T36.7X3	T36.7X4	T36.7X5	T36.7X6
Fumadil	T36.8X1	T36.8X2	T36.8X3	T36.8X4	T36.8X5	T36.8X6
Fumagillin	T36.8X1	T36.8X2	T36.8X3	T36.8X4	T36.8X5	T36.8X6
Fumaric acid	T49.4X1	T49.4X2	T49.4X3	T49.4X4	T49.4X5	T49.4X6
Fumes (from)	T59.91	T59.92	T59.93	T59.94	--	--
carbon monoxide — *see* Carbon, monoxide						
charcoal (domestic use) — *see* Charcoal, fumes						
chloroform — *see* Chloroform						
coke (in domestic stoves, fireplaces) — *see* Coke fumes						
corrosive NEC	T54.91	T54.92	T54.93	T54.94		
ether — *see* ether						
freons	T53.5X1	T53.5X2	T53.5X3	T53.5X4	--	--
hydrocarbons	T59.891	T59.892	T59.893	T59.894	--	--
petroleum (liquefied)	T59.891	T59.892	T59.893	T59.894	--	--
distributed through pipes (pure or mixed with air)	T59.891	T59.892	T59.893	T59.894	--	--
lead — *see* lead						
metal — *see* Metals, or the specified metal						
nitrogen dioxide	T59.0X1	T59.0X2	T59.0X3	T59.0X4		
pesticides — *see* Pesticide						
Fumes — *continued*						
petroleum (liquefied)	T59.891	T59.892	T59.893	T59.894	--	--
distributed through pipes (pure or mixed with air)	T59.891	T59.892	T59.893	T59.894	--	--
polyester	T59.891	T59.892	T59.893	T59.894	--	--
specified source NEC (*see also* substance specified)	T59.891	T59.892	T59.893	T59.894	--	--
sulfur dioxide	T59.1X1	T59.1X2	T59.1X3	T59.1X4	--	--
Fumigant NEC	T60.91	T60.92	T60.93	T60.94	--	--
Fungi, noxious, used as food	T62.0X1	T62.0X2	T62.0X3	T62.0X4	--	--
Fungicide NEC (nonmedicinal)	T60.3X1	T60.3X2	T60.3X3	T60.3X4	--	--
Fungizone	T36.7X1	T36.7X2	T36.7X3	T36.7X4	T36.7X5	T36.7X6
topical	T49.0X1	T49.0X2	T49.0X3	T49.0X4	T49.0X5	T49.0X6
Furacin	T49.0X1	T49.0X2	T49.0X3	T49.0X4	T49.0X5	T49.0X6
Furadantin	T37.91	T37.92	T37.93	T37.94	T37.95	T37.96
Furazolidone	T37.8X1	T37.8X2	T37.8X3	T37.8X4	T37.8X5	T37.8X6
Furazolium chloride	T49.0X1	T49.0X2	T49.0X3	T49.0X4	T49.0X5	T49.0X6
Furfural	T52.8X1	T52.8X2	T52.8X3	T52.8X4	--	--
Furnace (coal burning) (domestic), gas from	T58.2X1	T58.2X2	T58.2X3	T58.2X4		
industrial	T58.8X1	T58.8X2	T58.8X3	T58.8X4	--	--
Furniture polish	T65.891	T65.892	T65.893	T65.894	--	--
Furosemide	T50.1X1	T50.1X2	T50.1X3	T50.1X4	T50.1X5	T50.1X6
Furoxone	T37.91	T37.92	T37.93	T37.94	T37.95	T37.96
Fursultiamine	T45.2X1	T45.2X2	T45.2X3	T45.2X4	T45.2X5	T45.2X6
Fusafungine	T36.8X1	T36.8X2	T36.8X3	T36.8X4	T36.8X5	T36.8X6
Fusel oil (any) (amyl) (butyl) (propyl), vapor	T51.3X1	T51.3X2	T51.3X3	T51.3X4	--	--
Fusidate (ethanolamine) (sodium)	T36.8X1	T36.8X2	T36.8X3	T36.8X4	T36.8X5	T36.8X6
Fusidic acid	T36.8X1	T36.8X2	T36.8X3	T36.8X4	T36.8X5	T36.8X6
Fytic acid, nonasodium	T50.6X1	T50.6X2	T50.6X3	T50.6X4	T50.6X5	T50.6X6
G						
GABA	T43.8X1	T43.8X2	T43.8X3	T43.8X4	T43.8X5	T43.8X6
Gadopentetic acid	T50.8X1	T50.8X2	T50.8X3	T50.8X4	T50.8X5	T50.8X6
Galactose	T50.3X1	T50.3X2	T50.3X3	T50.3X4	T50.3X5	T50.3X6
b-Galactosidase	T47.5X1	T47.5X2	T47.5X3	T47.5X4	T47.5X5	T47.5X6
Galantamine	T44.0X1	T44.0X2	T44.0X3	T44.0X4	T44.0X5	T44.0X6
Gallamine (triethiodide)	T48.1X1	T48.1X2	T48.1X3	T48.1X4	T48.1X5	T48.1X6
Gallium citrate	T50.991	T50.992	T50.993	T50.994	T50.995	T50.996
Gallopamil	T46.1X1	T46.1X2	T46.1X3	T46.1X4	T46.1X5	T46.1X6
Gamboge	T47.2X1	T47.2X2	T47.2X3	T47.2X4	T47.2X5	T47.2X6
Gamimune	T50.Z11	T50.Z12	T50.Z13	T50.Z14	T50.Z15	T50.Z16
Gamma globulin	T50.Z11	T50.Z12	T50.Z13	T50.Z14	T50.Z15	T50.Z16
Gamma-aminobutyric acid	T43.8X1	T43.8X2	T43.8X3	T43.8X4	T43.8X5	T43.8X6
Gamma-benzene hexachloride (medicinal)	T49.0X1	T49.0X2	T49.0X3	T49.0X4	T49.0X5	T49.0X6
nonmedicinal, vapor	T53.6X1	T53.6X2	T53.6X3	T53.6X4	--	--
Gamma-BHC (medicinal) (*see also* Gamma-benzene hexachloride)	T49.0X1	T49.0X2	T49.0X3	T49.0X4	T49.0X5	T49.0X6
Gamulin	T50.Z11	T50.Z12	T50.Z13	T50.Z14	T50.Z15	T50.Z16
Ganciclovir (sodium)	T37.5X1	T37.5X2	T37.5X3	T37.5X4	T37.5X5	T37.5X6
Ganglionic blocking drug NEC	T44.2X1	T44.2X2	T44.2X3	T44.2X4	T44.2X5	T44.2X6
specified NEC	T44.2X1	T44.2X2	T44.2X3	T44.2X4	T44.2X5	T44.2X6
Ganja	T40.7X1	T40.7X2	T40.7X3	T40.7X4	T40.7X5	T40.7X6
Garamycin	T36.5X1	T36.5X2	T36.5X3	T36.5X4	T36.5X5	T36.5X6
ophthalmic preparation	T49.5X1	T49.5X2	T49.5X3	T49.5X4	T49.5X5	T49.5X6
topical NEC	T49.0X1	T49.0X2	T49.0X3	T49.0X4	T49.0X5	T49.0X6
Gardenal	T42.3X1	T42.3X2	T42.3X3	T42.3X4	T42.3X5	T42.3X6
Gardepanyl	T42.3X1	T42.3X2	T42.3X3	T42.3X4	T42.3X5	T42.3X6
Gas NEC	T59.91	T59.92	T59.93	T59.94	--	--
acetylene	T59.891	T59.892	T59.893	T59.894	--	--
incomplete combustion of	T58.11	T58.12	T58.13	T58.14	--	--
air contaminants, source or type not specified	T59.91	T59.92	T59.93	T59.94	--	--
anesthetic	T41.0X1	T41.0X2	T41.0X3	T41.0X4	T41.0X5	T41.0X6
blast furnace	T58.8X1	T58.8X2	T58.8X3	T58.8X4	--	--
butane — *see* butane						
carbon monoxide — *see* Carbon, monoxide						
chlorine	T59.4X1	T59.4X2	T59.4X3	T59.4X4	--	--
coal	T58.2X1	T58.2X2	T58.2X3	T58.2X4	--	--
cyanide	T57.3X1	T57.3X2	T57.3X3	T57.3X4	--	--
dicyanogen	T65.0X1	T65.0X2	T65.0X3	T65.0X4	--	--
domestic — *see* Domestic gas						

Substance	Poisoning, Accidental (unintentional)	Poisoning, Intentional self-harm	Poisoning, Assault	Poisoning, Undetermined	Adverse effect	Underdosing
Gas NEC — *continued*						
exhaust	T58.01	T58.02	T58.03	T58.04	--	--
from utility (for cooking, heating, or lighting) (after combustion) — *see* Carbon, monoxide, fuel, utility						
prior to combustion	T59.891	T59.892	T59.893	T59.894	--	--
from wood or coal-burning stove or fireplace	T58.2X1	T58.2X2	T58.2X3	T58.2X4	--	--
fuel (domestic use) (after combustion) (*see also* Carbon, monoxide, fuel)						
industrial use	T58.8X1	T58.8X2	T58.8X3	T58.8X4	--	--
prior to combustion	T59.891	T59.892	T59.893	T59.894	--	--
utility	T59.891	T59.892	T59.893	T59.894	--	--
in mobile container	T59.891	T59.892	T59.893	T59.894	--	--
incomplete combustion of — *see* Carbon, monoxide, fuel, utility						
piped (natural)	T59.891	T59.892	T59.893	T59.894	--	--
garage	T58.01	T58.02	T58.03	T58.04	--	--
hydrocarbon NEC	T59.891	T59.892	T59.893	T59.894	--	--
incomplete combustion of — *see* Carbon, monoxide, fuel, utility						
liquefied — *see* butane						
piped	T59.891	T59.892	T59.893	T59.894	--	--
hydrocyanic acid	T65.0X1	T65.0X2	T65.0X3	T65.0X4	--	--
illuminating (after combustion)	T58.11	T58.12	T58.13	T58.14	--	--
prior to combustion	T59.891	T59.892	T59.893	T59.894	--	--
incomplete combustion, any — *see* Carbon, monoxide						
kiln	T58.8X1	T58.8X2	T58.8X3	T58.8X4	--	--
lacrimogenic	T59.3X1	T59.3X2	T59.3X3	T59.3X4	--	--
liquefied petroleum — *see* butane						
marsh	T59.891	T59.892	T59.893	T59.894	--	--
motor exhaust, not in transit	T58.01	T58.02	T58.03	T58.04	--	--
mustard, not in war	T59.891	T59.892	T59.893	T59.894	--	--
natural	T59.891	T59.892	T59.893	T59.894	--	--
nerve, not in war	T59.91	T59.92	T59.93	T59.94	--	--
oil	T52.0X1	T52.0X2	T52.0X3	T52.0X4	--	--
petroleum (liquefied) (distributed in mobile containers)	T59.891	T59.892	T59.893	T59.894	--	--
piped (pure or mixed with air)	T59.891	T59.892	T59.893	T59.894	--	--
piped (manufactured) (natural) NEC	T59.891	T59.892	T59.893	T59.894	--	--
producer	T58.8X1	T58.8X2	T58.8X3	T58.8X4	--	--
propane — *see* propane						
refrigerant (chlorofluoro-carbon)	T53.5X1	T53.5X2	T53.5X3	T53.5X4	--	--
not chlorofluoro-carbon	T59.891	T59.892	T59.893	T59.894	--	--
sewer	T59.91	T59.92	T59.93	T59.94	--	--
specified source NEC	T59.91	T59.92	T59.93	T59.94	--	--
stove (after combustion)	T58.11	T58.12	T58.13	T58.14	--	--
prior to combustion	T59.891	T59.892	T59.893	T59.894	--	--
tear	T59.3X1	T59.3X2	T59.3X3	T59.3X4	--	--
therapeutic	T41.5X1	T41.5X2	T41.5X3	T41.5X4	T41.5X5	T41.5X6
utility (for cooking, heating, or lighting) (piped) NEC	T59.891	T59.892	T59.893	T59.894	--	--
in mobile container	T59.891	T59.892	T59.893	T59.894	--	--
incomplete combustion of — *see* Carbon, monoxide, fuel, utilty						
piped (natural)	T59.891	T59.892	T59.893	T59.894	--	--
water	T58.11	T58.12	T58.13	T58.14	--	--
incomplete combustion of — *see* Carbon, monoxide, fuel, utility						
Gaseous substance — *see* Gas						
Gasoline	T52.0X1	T52.0X2	T52.0X3	T52.0X4	--	--
vapor	T52.0X1	T52.0X2	T52.0X3	T52.0X4	--	--
Gastric enzymes	T47.5X1	T47.5X2	T47.5X3	T47.5X4	T47.5X5	T47.5X6
Gastrografin	T50.8X1	T50.8X2	T50.8X3	T50.8X4	T50.8X5	T50.8X6

Substance	Poisoning, Accidental (unintentional)	Poisoning, Intentional self-harm	Poisoning, Assault	Poisoning, Undetermined	Adverse effect	Underdosing
Gastrointestinal drug	T47.91	T47.92	T47.93	T47.94	T47.95	T47.96
biological	T47.8X1	T47.8X2	T47.8X3	T47.8X4	T47.8X5	T47.8X6
specified NEC	T47.8X1	T47.8X2	T47.8X3	T47.8X4	T47.8X5	T47.8X6
Gaultheria procumbens	T62.2X1	T62.2X2	T62.2X3	T62.2X4	--	--
Gefarnate	T44.3X1	T44.3X2	T44.3X3	T44.3X4	T44.3X5	T44.3X6
Gelatin (intravenous)	T45.8X1	T45.8X2	T45.8X3	T45.8X4	T45.8X5	T45.8X6
absorbable (sponge)	T45.7X1	T45.7X2	T45.7X3	T45.7X4	T45.7X5	T45.7X6
Gelfilm	T49.8X1	T49.8X2	T49.8X3	T49.8X4	T49.8X5	T49.8X6
Gelfoam	T45.7X1	T45.7X2	T45.7X3	T45.7X4	T45.7X5	T45.7X6
Gelsemine	T50.991	T50.992	T50.993	T50.994	T50.995	T50.996
Gelsemium (sempervirens)	T62.2X1	T62.2X2	T62.2X3	T62.2X4	--	--
Gemeprost	T48.0X1	T48.0X2	T48.0X3	T48.0X4	T48.0X5	T48.0X6
Gemfibrozil	T46.6X1	T46.6X2	T46.6X3	T46.6X4	T46.6X5	T46.6X6
Gemonil	T42.3X1	T42.3X2	T42.3X3	T42.3X4	T42.3X5	T42.3X6
Gentamicin	T36.5X1	T36.5X2	T36.5X3	T36.5X4	T36.5X5	T36.5X6
ophthalmic preparation	T49.5X1	T49.5X2	T49.5X3	T49.5X4	T49.5X5	T49.5X6
topical NEC	T49.0X1	T49.0X2	T49.0X3	T49.0X4	T49.0X5	T49.0X6
Gentian	T47.5X1	T47.5X2	T47.5X3	T47.5X4	T47.5X5	T47.5X6
violet	T49.0X1	T49.0X2	T49.0X3	T49.0X4	T49.0X5	T49.0X6
Gepefrine	T44.4X1	T44.4X2	T44.4X3	T44.4X4	T44.4X5	T44.4X6
Gestonorone caproate	T38.5X1	T38.5X2	T38.5X3	T38.5X4	T38.5X5	T38.5X6
Gexane	T49.0X1	T49.0X2	T49.0X3	T49.0X4	T49.0X5	T49.0X6
Gila monster (venom)	T63.111	T63.112	T63.113	T63.114	--	--
Ginger	T47.5X1	T47.5X2	T47.5X3	T47.5X4	T47.5X5	T47.5X6
Jamaica — *see* Jamaica, ginger						
Gitalin	T46.0X1	T46.0X2	T46.0X3	T46.0X4	T46.0X5	T46.0X6
amorphous	T46.0X1	T46.0X2	T46.0X3	T46.0X4	T46.0X5	T46.0X6
Gitaloxin	T46.0X1	T46.0X2	T46.0X3	T46.0X4	T46.0X5	T46.0X6
Gitoxin	T46.0X1	T46.0X2	T46.0X3	T46.0X4	T46.0X5	T46.0X6
Glafenine	T39.8X1	T39.8X2	T39.8X3	T39.8X4	T39.8X5	T39.8X6
Glandular extract (medicinal) NEC	T50.Z91	T50.Z92	T50.Z93	T50.Z94	T50.Z95	T50.Z96
Glaucarubin	T37.3X1	T37.3X2	T37.3X3	T37.3X4	T37.3X5	T37.3X6
Glibenclamide	T38.3X1	T38.3X2	T38.3X3	T38.3X4	T38.3X5	T38.3X6
Glibornuride	T38.3X1	T38.3X2	T38.3X3	T38.3X4	T38.3X5	T38.3X6
Gliclazide	T38.3X1	T38.3X2	T38.3X3	T38.3X4	T38.3X5	T38.3X6
Glimidine	T38.3X1	T38.3X2	T38.3X3	T38.3X4	T38.3X5	T38.3X6
Glipizide	T38.3X1	T38.3X2	T38.3X3	T38.3X4	T38.3X5	T38.3X6
Gliquidone	T38.3X1	T38.3X2	T38.3X3	T38.3X4	T38.3X5	T38.3X6
Glisolamide	T38.3X1	T38.3X2	T38.3X3	T38.3X4	T38.3X5	T38.3X6
Glisoxepide	T38.3X1	T38.3X2	T38.3X3	T38.3X4	T38.3X5	T38.3X6
Globin zinc insulin	T38.3X1	T38.3X2	T38.3X3	T38.3X4	T38.3X5	T38.3X6
Globulin						
antilymphocytic	T50.Z11	T50.Z12	T50.Z13	T50.Z14	T50.Z15	T50.Z16
antirhesus	T50.Z11	T50.Z12	T50.Z13	T50.Z14	T50.Z15	T50.Z16
antivenin	T50.Z11	T50.Z12	T50.Z13	T50.Z14	T50.Z15	T50.Z16
antiviral	T50.Z11	T50.Z12	T50.Z13	T50.Z14	T50.Z15	T50.Z16
Glucagon	T38.3X1	T38.3X2	T38.3X3	T38.3X4	T38.3X5	T38.3X6
Glucocorticoids	T38.0X1	T38.0X2	T38.0X3	T38.0X4	T38.0X5	T38.0X6
Glucocorticosteroid	T38.0X1	T38.0X2	T38.0X3	T38.0X4	T38.0X5	T38.0X6
Gluconic acid	T50.991	T50.992	T50.993	T50.994	T50.995	T50.996
Glucosamine sulfate	T39.4X1	T39.4X2	T39.4X3	T39.4X4	T39.4X5	T39.4X6
Glucose	T50.3X1	T50.3X2	T50.3X3	T50.3X4	T50.3X5	T50.3X6
with sodium chloride	T50.3X1	T50.3X2	T50.3X3	T50.3X4	T50.3X5	T50.3X6
Glucosulfone sodium	T37.1X1	T37.1X2	T37.1X3	T37.1X4	T37.1X5	T37.1X6
Glucurolactone	T47.8X1	T47.8X2	T47.8X3	T47.8X4	T47.8X5	T47.8X6
Glue NEC	T52.8X1	T52.8X2	T52.8X3	T52.8X4	--	--
Glutamic acid	T47.5X1	T47.5X2	T47.5X3	T47.5X4	T47.5X5	T47.5X6
Glutaral (medicinal)	T49.0X1	T49.0X2	T49.0X3	T49.0X4	T49.0X5	T49.0X6
nonmedicinal	T65.891	T65.892	T65.893	T65.894	--	--
Glutaraldehyde (nonmedicinal)	T65.891	T65.892	T65.893	T65.894	--	--
medicinal	T49.0X1	T49.0X2	T49.0X3	T49.0X4	T49.0X5	T49.0X6
Glutathione	T50.6X1	T50.6X2	T50.6X3	T50.6X4	T50.6X5	T50.6X6
Glutethimide	T42.6X1	T42.6X2	T42.6X3	T42.6X4	T42.6X5	T42.6X6
Glyburide	T38.3X1	T38.3X2	T38.3X3	T38.3X4	T38.3X5	T38.3X6
Glycerin	T47.4X1	T47.4X2	T47.4X3	T47.4X4	T47.4X5	T47.4X6
Glycerol	T47.4X1	T47.4X2	T47.4X3	T47.4X4	T47.4X5	T47.4X6
borax	T49.6X1	T49.6X2	T49.6X3	T49.6X4	T49.6X5	T49.6X6
intravenous	T50.3X1	T50.3X2	T50.3X3	T50.3X4	T50.3X5	T50.3X6
iodinated	T48.4X1	T48.4X2	T48.4X3	T48.4X4	T48.4X5	T48.4X6
Glycerophosphate	T50.991	T50.992	T50.993	T50.994	T50.995	T50.996
Glyceryl						
gualacolate	T48.4X1	T48.4X2	T48.4X3	T48.4X4	T48.4X5	T48.4X6
nitrate	T46.3X1	T46.3X2	T46.3X3	T46.3X4	T46.3X5	T46.3X6
triacetate (topical)	T49.0X1	T49.0X2	T49.0X3	T49.0X4	T49.0X5	T49.0X6
trinitrate	T46.3X1	T46.3X2	T46.3X3	T46.3X4	T46.3X5	T46.3X6
Glycine	T50.3X1	T50.3X2	T50.3X3	T50.3X4	T50.3X5	T50.3X6
Glyclopyramide	T38.3X1	T38.3X2	T38.3X3	T38.3X4	T38.3X5	T38.3X6
Glycobiarsol	T37.3X1	T37.3X2	T37.3X3	T37.3X4	T37.3X5	T37.3X6
Glycols (ether)	T52.3X1	T52.3X2	T52.3X3	T52.3X4	--	--
Glyconiazide	T37.1X1	T37.1X2	T37.1X3	T37.1X4	T37.1X5	T37.1X6
Glycopyrrolate	T44.3X1	T44.3X2	T44.3X3	T44.3X4	T44.3X5	T44.3X6

Substance	Poisoning, Accidental (unintentional)	Poisoning, Intentional self-harm	Poisoning, Assault	Poisoning, Undetermined	Adverse effect	Underdosing
Glycopyrronium	T44.3X1	T44.3X2	T44.3X3	T44.3X4	T44.3X5	T44.3X6
bromide	T44.3X1	T44.3X2	T44.3X3	T44.3X4	T44.3X5	T44.3X6
Glycoside, cardiac (stimulant)	T46.0X1	T46.0X2	T46.0X3	T46.0X4	T46.0X5	T46.0X6
Glycyclamide	T38.3X1	T38.3X2	T38.3X3	T38.3X4	T38.3X5	T38.3X6
Glycyrrhiza extract	T48.4X1	T48.4X2	T48.4X3	T48.4X4	T48.4X5	T48.4X6
Glycyrrhizic acid	T48.4X1	T48.4X2	T48.4X3	T48.4X4	T48.4X5	T48.4X6
Glycyrrhizinate potassium	T48.4X1	T48.4X2	T48.4X3	T48.4X4	T48.4X5	T48.4X6
Glymidine sodium	T38.3X1	T38.3X2	T38.3X3	T38.3X4	T38.3X5	T38.3X6
Glyphosate	T60.3X1	T60.3X2	T60.3X3	T60.3X4	--	--
Glyphylline	T48.6X1	T48.6X2	T48.6X3	T48.6X4	T48.6X5	T48.6X6
Gold						
colloidal (I98Au)	T45.1X1	T45.1X2	T45.1X3	T45.1X4	T45.1X5	T45.1X6
salts	T39.4X1	T39.4X2	T39.4X3	T39.4X4	T39.4X5	T39.4X6
Golden sulfide of antimony	T56.891	T56.892	T56.893	T56.894	--	--
Goldylocks	T62.2X1	T62.2X2	T62.2X3	T62.2X4	--	--
Gonadal tissue extract	T38.901	T38.902	T38.903	T38.904	T38.905	T38.906
female	T38.5X1	T38.5X2	T38.5X3	T38.5X4	T38.5X5	T38.5X6
male	T38.7X1	T38.7X2	T38.7X3	T38.7X4	T38.7X5	T38.7X6
Gonadorelin	T38.891	T38.892	T38.893	T38.894	T38.895	T38.896
Gonadotropin	T38.891	T38.892	T38.893	T38.894	T38.895	T38.896
chorionic	T38.891	T38.892	T38.893	T38.894	T38.895	T38.896
pituitary	T38.811	T38.812	T38.813	T38.814	T38.815	T38.816
Goserelin	T45.1X1	T45.1X2	T45.1X3	T45.1X4	T45.1X5	T45.1X6
Grain alcohol	T51.0X1	T51.0X2	T51.0X3	T51.0X4	--	--
Gramicidin	T49.0X1	T49.0X2	T49.0X3	T49.0X4	T49.0X5	T49.0X6
Granisetron	T45.0X1	T45.0X2	T45.0X3	T45.0X4	T45.0X5	T45.0X6
Gratiola officinalis	T62.2X1	T62.2X2	T62.2X3	T62.2X4	--	--
Grease	T65.891	T65.892	T65.893	T65.894	--	--
Green hellebore	T62.2X1	T62.2X2	T62.2X3	T62.2X4	--	--
Green soap	T49.2X1	T49.2X2	T49.2X3	T49.2X4	T49.2X5	T49.2X6
Grifulvin	T36.7X1	T36.7X2	T36.7X3	T36.7X4	T36.7X5	T36.7X6
Griseofulvin	T36.7X1	T36.7X2	T36.7X3	T36.7X4	T36.7X5	T36.7X6
Growth hormone	T38.811	T38.812	T38.813	T38.814	T38.815	T38.816
Guaiac reagent	T50.991	T50.992	T50.993	T50.994	T50.995	T50.996
Guaiacol derivatives	T48.4X1	T48.4X2	T48.4X3	T48.4X4	T48.4X5	T48.4X6
Guaifenesin	T48.4X1	T48.4X2	T48.4X3	T48.4X4	T48.4X5	T48.4X6
Guaimesal	T48.4X1	T48.4X2	T48.4X3	T48.4X4	T48.4X5	T48.4X6
Guaiphenesin	T48.4X1	T48.4X2	T48.4X3	T48.4X4	T48.4X5	T48.4X6
Guamecycline	T36.4X1	T36.4X2	T36.4X3	T36.4X4	T36.4X5	T36.4X6
Guanabenz	T46.5X1	T46.5X2	T46.5X3	T46.5X4	T46.5X5	T46.5X6
Guanacline	T46.5X1	T46.5X2	T46.5X3	T46.5X4	T46.5X5	T46.5X6
Guanadrel	T46.5X1	T46.5X2	T46.5X3	T46.5X4	T46.5X5	T46.5X6
Guanatol	T37.2X1	T37.2X2	T37.2X3	T37.2X4	T37.2X5	T37.2X6
Guanethidine	T46.5X1	T46.5X2	T46.5X3	T46.5X4	T46.5X5	T46.5X6
Guanfacine	T46.5X1	T46.5X2	T46.5X3	T46.5X4	T46.5X5	T46.5X6
Guano	T65.891	T65.892	T65.893	T65.894	--	--
Guanochlor	T46.5X1	T46.5X2	T46.5X3	T46.5X4	T46.5X5	T46.5X6
Guanoclor	T46.5X1	T46.5X2	T46.5X3	T46.5X4	T46.5X5	T46.5X6
Guanoctine	T46.5X1	T46.5X2	T46.5X3	T46.5X4	T46.5X5	T46.5X6
Guanoxabenz	T46.5X1	T46.5X2	T46.5X3	T46.5X4	T46.5X5	T46.5X6
Guanoxan	T46.5X1	T46.5X2	T46.5X3	T46.5X4	T46.5X5	T46.5X6
Guar gum (medicinal)	T46.6X1	T46.6X2	T46.6X3	T46.6X4	T46.6X5	T46.6X6
H						
Hachimycin	T36.7X1	T36.7X2	T36.7X3	T36.7X4	T36.7X5	T36.7X6
Hair						
dye	T49.4X1	T49.4X2	T49.4X3	T49.4X4	T49.4X5	T49.4X6
preparation NEC	T49.4X1	T49.4X2	T49.4X3	T49.4X4	T49.4X5	T49.4X6
Halazepam	T42.4X1	T42.4X2	T42.4X3	T42.4X4	T42.4X5	T42.4X6
Halcinolone	T49.0X1	T49.0X2	T49.0X3	T49.0X4	T49.0X5	T49.0X6
Halcinonide	T49.0X1	T49.0X2	T49.0X3	T49.0X4	T49.0X5	T49.0X6
Halethazole	T49.0X1	T49.0X2	T49.0X3	T49.0X4	T49.0X5	T49.0X6
Hallucinogen NOS	T40.901	T40.902	T40.903	T40.904	T40.905	T40.906
specified NEC	T40.991	T40.992	T40.993	T40.994	T40.995	T40.996
Halofantrine	T37.2X1	T37.2X2	T37.2X3	T37.2X4	T37.2X5	T37.2X6
Halofenate	T46.6X1	T46.6X2	T46.6X3	T46.6X4	T46.6X5	T46.6X6
Halometasone	T49.0X1	T49.0X2	T49.0X3	T49.0X4	T49.0X5	T49.0X6
Haloperidol	T43.4X1	T43.4X2	T43.4X3	T43.4X4	T43.4X5	T43.4X6
Haloprogin	T49.0X1	T49.0X2	T49.0X3	T49.0X4	T49.0X5	T49.0X6
Halotex	T49.0X1	T49.0X2	T49.0X3	T49.0X4	T49.0X5	T49.0X6
Halothane	T41.0X1	T41.0X2	T41.0X3	T41.0X4	T41.0X5	T41.0X6
Haloxazolam	T42.4X1	T42.4X2	T42.4X3	T42.4X4	T42.4X5	T42.4X6
Halquinols	T49.0X1	T49.0X2	T49.0X3	T49.0X4	T49.0X5	T49.0X6
Hamamelis	T49.2X1	T49.2X2	T49.2X3	T49.2X4	T49.2X5	T49.2X6
Haptendextran	T45.8X1	T45.8X2	T45.8X3	T45.8X4	T45.8X5	T45.8X6
Harmonyl	T46.5X1	T46.5X2	T46.5X3	T46.5X4	T46.5X5	T46.5X6
Hartmann's solution	T50.3X1	T50.3X2	T50.3X3	T50.3X4	T50.3X5	T50.3X6
Hashish	T40.7X1	T40.7X2	T40.7X3	T40.7X4	T40.7X5	T40.7X6
Hawaiian Woodrose seeds	T40.991	T40.992	T40.993	T40.994	--	--
HCB	T60.3X1	T60.3X2	T60.3X3	T60.3X4	--	--
HCH	T53.6X1	T53.6X2	T53.6X3	T53.6X4	--	--
medicinal	T49.0X1	T49.0X2	T49.0X3	T49.0X4	T49.0X5	T49.0X6
HCN	T57.3X1	T57.3X2	T57.3X3	T57.3X4	--	--
Headache cures, drugs, powders NEC	T50.901	T50.902	T50.903	T50.904	T50.905	T50.906
Heavenly Blue (morning glory)	T40.991	T40.992	T40.993	T40.994	--	--

Substance	Poisoning, Accidental (unintentional)	Poisoning, Intentional self-harm	Poisoning, Assault	Poisoning, Undetermined	Adverse effect	Underdosing
Heavy metal antidote	T45.8X1	T45.8X2	T45.8X3	T45.8X4	T45.8X5	T45.8X6
Hedaquinium	T49.0X1	T49.0X2	T49.0X3	T49.0X4	T49.0X5	T49.0X6
Hedge hyssop	T62.2X1	T62.2X2	T62.2X3	T62.2X4	--	--
Heet	T49.8X1	T49.8X2	T49.8X3	T49.8X4	T49.8X5	T49.8X6
Helenin	T37.4X1	T37.4X2	T37.4X3	T37.4X4	T37.4X5	T37.4X6
Helium (nonmedicinal) NEC	T59.891	T59.892	T59.893	T59.894	--	--
medicinal	T48.991	T48.992	T48.993	T48.994	T48.995	T48.996
Hellebore (black) (green) (white)	T62.2X1	T62.2X2	T62.2X3	T62.2X4	--	--
Hematin	T45.8X1	T45.8X2	T45.8X3	T45.8X4	T45.8X5	T45.8X6
Hematinic preparation	T45.8X1	T45.8X2	T45.8X3	T45.8X4	T45.8X5	T45.8X6
Hematological agent	T45.91	T45.92	T45.93	T45.94	T45.95	T45.96
specified NEC	T45.8X1	T45.8X2	T45.8X3	T45.8X4	T45.8X5	T45.8X6
Hemlock	T62.2X1	T62.2X2	T62.2X3	T62.2X4	--	--
Hemostatic	T45.621	T45.622	T45.623	T45.624	T45.625	T45.626
drug, systemic	T45.621	T45.622	T45.623	T45.624	T45.625	T45.626
Hemostyptic	T49.4X1	T49.4X2	T49.4X3	T49.4X4	T49.4X5	T49.4X6
Henbane	T62.2X1	T62.2X2	T62.2X3	T62.2X4	--	--
Heparin (sodium)	T45.511	T45.512	T45.513	T45.514	T45.515	T45.516
action reverser	T45.7X1	T45.7X2	T45.7X3	T45.7X4	T45.7X5	T45.7X6
Heparin-fraction	T45.511	T45.512	T45.513	T45.514	T45.515	T45.516
Heparinoid (systemic)	T45.511	T45.512	T45.513	T45.514	T45.515	T45.516
Hepatic secretion stimulant	T47.8X1	T47.8X2	T47.8X3	T47.8X4	T47.8X5	T47.8X6
Hepatitis B						
immune globulin	T50.Z11	T50.Z12	T50.Z13	T50.Z14	T50.Z15	T50.Z16
vaccine	T50.B91	T50.B92	T50.B93	T50.B94	T50.B95	T50.B96
Hepronicate	T46.7X1	T46.7X2	T46.7X3	T46.7X4	T46.7X5	T46.7X6
Heptabarb	T42.3X1	T42.3X2	T42.3X3	T42.3X4	T42.3X5	T42.3X6
Heptabarbital	T42.3X1	T42.3X2	T42.3X3	T42.3X4	T42.3X5	T42.3X6
Heptabarbitone	T42.3X1	T42.3X2	T42.3X3	T42.3X4	T42.3X5	T42.3X6
Heptachlor	T60.1X1	T60.1X2	T60.1X3	T60.1X4	--	--
Heptalgin	T40.2X1	T40.2X2	T40.2X3	T40.2X4	T40.2X5	T40.2X6
Heptaminol	T46.3X1	T46.3X2	T46.3X3	T46.3X4	T46.3X5	T46.3X6
Herbicide NEC	T60.3X1	T60.3X2	T60.3X3	T60.3X4	--	--
Heroin	T40.1X1	T40.1X2	T40.1X3	T40.1X4	--	--
Herplex	T49.5X1	T49.5X2	T49.5X3	T49.5X4	T49.5X5	T49.5X6
HES	T45.8X1	T45.8X2	T45.8X3	T45.8X4	T45.8X5	T45.8X6
Hesperidin	T46.991	T46.992	T46.993	T46.994	T46.995	T46.996
Hetacillin	T36.0X1	T36.0X2	T36.0X3	T36.0X4	T36.0X5	T36.0X6
Hetastarch	T45.8X1	T45.8X2	T45.8X3	T45.8X4	T45.8X5	T45.8X6
HETP	T60.0X1	T60.0X2	T60.0X3	T60.0X4	--	--
Hexachlorobenzene (vapor)	T60.3X1	T60.3X2	T60.3X3	T60.3X4	--	--
Hexachlorocyclohexane	T53.6X1	T53.6X2	T53.6X3	T53.6X4	--	--
Hexachlorophene	T49.0X1	T49.0X2	T49.0X3	T49.0X4	T49.0X5	T49.0X6
Hexadiline	T46.3X1	T46.3X2	T46.3X3	T46.3X4	T46.3X5	T46.3X6
Hexadimethrine (bromide)	T45.7X1	T45.7X2	T45.7X3	T45.7X4	T45.7X5	T45.7X6
Hexadylamine	T46.3X1	T46.3X2	T46.3X3	T46.3X4	T46.3X5	T46.3X6
Hexaethyl tetraphos-phate	T60.0X1	T60.0X2	T60.0X3	T60.0X4	--	--
Hexafluorenium bromide	T48.1X1	T48.1X2	T48.1X3	T48.1X4	T48.1X5	T48.1X6
Hexafluronium (bromide)	T48.1X1	T48.1X2	T48.1X3	T48.1X4	T48.1X5	T48.1X6
Hexa-germ	T49.2X1	T49.2X2	T49.2X3	T49.2X4	T49.2X5	T49.2X6
Hexahydrobenzol	T52.8X1	T52.8X2	T52.8X3	T52.8X4	--	--
Hexahydrocresol(s)	T51.8X1	T51.8X2	T51.8X3	T51.8X4	--	--
arsenide	T57.0X1	T57.0X2	T57.0X3	T57.0X4	--	--
arseniurated	T57.0X1	T57.0X2	T57.0X3	T57.0X4	--	--
cyanide	T57.3X1	T57.3X2	T57.3X3	T57.3X4	--	--
gas	T59.891	T59.892	T59.893	T59.894	--	--
fluoride (liquid)	T57.8X1	T57.8X2	T57.8X3	T57.8X4	--	--
vapor	T59.891	T59.892	T59.893	T59.894	--	--
phophorated	T60.0X1	T60.0X2	T60.0X3	T60.0X4	--	--
sulfate	T57.8X1	T57.8X2	T57.8X3	T57.8X4	--	--
sulfide (gas)	T59.6X1	T59.6X2	T59.6X3	T59.6X4	--	--
arseniurated	T57.0X1	T57.0X2	T57.0X3	T57.0X4	--	--
sulfurated	T57.8X1	T57.8X2	T57.8X3	T57.8X4	--	--
Hexahydrophenol	T51.8X1	T51.8X2	T51.8X3	T51.8X4	--	--
Hexalen	T51.8X1	T51.8X2	T51.8X3	T51.8X4	--	--
Hexamethonium bromide	T44.2X1	T44.2X2	T44.2X3	T44.2X4	T44.2X5	T44.2X6
Hexamethylene	T52.8X1	T52.8X2	T52.8X3	T52.8X4	--	--
Hexamethylmelamine	T45.1X1	T45.1X2	T45.1X3	T45.1X4	T45.1X5	T45.1X6
Hexamidine	T49.0X1	T49.0X2	T49.0X3	T49.0X4	T49.0X5	T49.0X6
Hexamine (mandelate)	T37.8X1	T37.8X2	T37.8X3	T37.8X4	T37.8X5	T37.8X6
Hexanone, 2-hexanone	T52.4X1	T52.4X2	T52.4X3	T52.4X4	--	--
Hexanuorenium	T48.1X1	T48.1X2	T48.1X3	T48.1X4	T48.1X5	T48.1X6
Hexapropymate	T42.6X1	T42.6X2	T42.6X3	T42.6X4	T42.6X5	T42.6X6
Hexasonium iodide	T44.3X1	T44.3X2	T44.3X3	T44.3X4	T44.3X5	T44.3X6
Hexcarbacholine bromide	T48.1X1	T48.1X2	T48.1X3	T48.1X4	T48.1X5	T48.1X6
Hexemal	T42.3X1	T42.3X2	T42.3X3	T42.3X4	T42.3X5	T42.3X6
Hexestrol	T38.5X1	T38.5X2	T38.5X3	T38.5X4	T38.5X5	T38.5X6
Hexethal (sodium)	T42.3X1	T42.3X2	T42.3X3	T42.3X4	T42.3X5	T42.3X6
Hexetidine	T37.8X1	T37.8X2	T37.8X3	T37.8X4	T37.8X5	T37.8X6
Hexobarbital	T42.3X1	T42.3X2	T42.3X3	T42.3X4	T42.3X5	T42.3X6
rectal	T41.291	T41.292	T41.293	T41.294	T41.295	T41.296
sodium	T41.1X1	T41.1X2	T41.1X3	T41.1X4	T41.1X5	T41.1X6
Hexobendine	T46.3X1	T46.3X2	T46.3X3	T46.3X4	T46.3X5	T46.3X6

Hexocyclium - Iloprost

Substance	Poisoning, Accidental (unintentional)	Poisoning, Intentional self-harm	Poisoning, Assault	Poisoning, Undetermined	Adverse effect	Underdosing
Hexocyclium	T44.3X1	T44.3X2	T44.3X3	T44.3X4	T44.3X5	T44.3X6
metilsulfate	T44.3X1	T44.3X2	T44.3X3	T44.3X4	T44.3X5	T44.3X6
Hexoestrol	T38.5X1	T38.5X2	T38.5X3	T38.5X4	T38.5X5	T38.5X6
Hexone	T52.4X1	T52.4X2	T52.4X3	T52.4X4	--	--
Hexoprenaline	T48.6X1	T48.6X2	T48.6X3	T48.6X4	T48.6X5	T48.6X6
Hexylcaine	T41.3X1	T41.3X2	T41.3X3	T41.3X4	T41.3X5	T41.3X6
Hexylresorcinol	T52.2X1	T52.2X2	T52.2X3	T52.2X4	--	--
HGH (human growth hormone)	T38.811	T38.812	T38.813	T38.814	T38.815	T38.816
Hinkle's pills	T47.2X1	T47.2X2	T47.2X3	T47.2X4	T47.2X5	T47.2X6
Histalog	T50.8X1	T50.8X2	T50.8X3	T50.8X4	T50.8X5	T50.8X6
Histamine (phosphate)	T50.8X1	T50.8X2	T50.8X3	T50.8X4	T50.8X5	T50.8X6
Histoplasmin	T50.8X1	T50.8X2	T50.8X3	T50.8X4	T50.8X5	T50.8X6
Holly berries	T62.2X1	T62.2X2	T62.2X3	T62.2X4	--	--
Homatropine	T44.3X1	T44.3X2	T44.3X3	T44.3X4	T44.3X5	T44.3X6
methylbromide	T44.3X1	T44.3X2	T44.3X3	T44.3X4	T44.3X5	T44.3X6
Homochlorcyclizine	T45.0X1	T45.0X2	T45.0X3	T45.0X4	T45.0X5	T45.0X6
Homosalate	T49.3X1	T49.3X2	T49.3X3	T49.3X4	T49.3X5	T49.3X6
Homo-tet	T50.Z11	T50.Z12	T50.Z13	T50.Z14	T50.Z15	T50.Z16
Hormone	T38.801	T38.802	T38.803	T38.804	T38.805	T38.806
adrenal cortical steroids	T38.0X1	T38.0X2	T38.0X3	T38.0X4	T38.0X5	T38.0X6
androgenic	T38.7X1	T38.7X2	T38.7X3	T38.7X4	T38.7X5	T38.7X6
anterior pituitary NEC	T38.811	T38.812	T38.813	T38.814	T38.815	T38.816
antidiabetic agents	T38.3X1	T38.3X2	T38.3X3	T38.3X4	T38.3X5	T38.3X6
antidiuretic	T38.891	T38.892	T38.893	T38.894	T38.895	T38.896
cancer therapy	T45.1X1	T45.1X2	T45.1X3	T45.1X4	T45.1X5	T45.1X6
follicle stimulating	T38.811	T38.812	T38.813	T38.814	T38.815	T38.816
gonadotropic	T38.891	T38.892	T38.893	T38.894	T38.895	T38.896
pituitary	T38.811	T38.812	T38.813	T38.814	T38.815	T38.816
growth	T38.811	T38.812	T38.813	T38.814	T38.815	T38.816
luteinizing	T38.811	T38.812	T38.813	T38.814	T38.815	T38.816
ovarian	T38.5X1	T38.5X2	T38.5X3	T38.5X4	T38.5X5	T38.5X6
oxytocic	T48.0X1	T48.0X2	T48.0X3	T48.0X4	T48.0X5	T48.0X6
parathyroid (derivatives)	T50.991	T50.992	T50.993	T50.994	T50.995	T50.996
pituitary (posterior) NEC	T38.891	T38.892	T38.893	T38.894	T38.895	T38.896
anterior	T38.811	T38.812	T38.813	T38.814	T38.815	T38.816
specified, NEC	T38.891	T38.892	T38.893	T38.894	T38.895	T38.896
thyroid	T38.1X1	T38.1X2	T38.1X3	T38.1X4	T38.1X5	T38.1X6
Hornet (sting)	T63.451	T63.452	T63.453	T63.454	--	--
Horse anti-human lymphocytic serum	T50.Z11	T50.Z12	T50.Z13	T50.Z14	T50.Z15	T50.Z16
Horticulture agent NEC	T65.91	T65.92	T65.93	T65.94	--	--
with pesticide	T60.91	T60.92	T60.93	T60.94	--	--
Human						
albumin	T45.8X1	T45.8X2	T45.8X3	T45.8X4	T45.8X5	T45.8X6
growth hormone (HGH)	T38.811	T38.812	T38.813	T38.814	T38.815	T38.816
immune serum	T50.Z11	T50.Z12	T50.Z13	T50.Z14	T50.Z15	T50.Z16
Hyaluronidase	T45.3X1	T45.3X2	T45.3X3	T45.3X4	T45.3X5	T45.3X6
Hyazyme	T45.3X1	T45.3X2	T45.3X3	T45.3X4	T45.3X5	T45.3X6
Hycodan	T40.2X1	T40.2X2	T40.2X3	T40.2X4	T40.2X5	T40.2X6
Hydantoin derivative NEC	T42.0X1	T42.0X2	T42.0X3	T42.0X4	T42.0X5	T42.0X6
Hydeltra	T38.0X1	T38.0X2	T38.0X3	T38.0X4	T38.0X5	T38.0X6
Hydergine	T44.6X1	T44.6X2	T44.6X3	T44.6X4	T44.6X5	T44.6X6
Hydrabamine penicillin	T36.0X1	T36.0X2	T36.0X3	T36.0X4	T36.0X5	T36.0X6
Hydralazine	T46.5X1	T46.5X2	T46.5X3	T46.5X4	T46.5X5	T46.5X6
Hydrargaphen	T49.0X1	T49.0X2	T49.0X3	T49.0X4	T49.0X5	T49.0X6
Hydrargyri amino-chloridum	T49.0X1	T49.0X2	T49.0X3	T49.0X4	T49.0X5	T49.0X6
Hydrastine	T48.291	T48.292	T48.293	T48.294	T48.295	T48.296
Hydrazine	T54.1X1	T54.1X2	T54.1X3	T54.1X4	--	--
monoamine oxidase inhibitors	T43.1X1	T43.1X2	T43.1X3	T43.1X4	T43.1X5	T43.1X6
Hydrazoic acid, azides	T54.2X1	T54.2X2	T54.2X3	T54.2X4	--	--
Hydriodic acid	T48.4X1	T48.4X2	T48.4X3	T48.4X4	T48.4X5	T48.4X6
Hydrocarbon gas	T59.891	T59.892	T59.893	T59.894	--	--
incomplete combustion of — see Carbon, monoxide, fuel, utility						
liquefied (mobile container)	T59.891	T59.892	T59.893	T59.894	--	--
piped (natural)	T59.891	T59.892	T59.893	T59.894	--	--
Hydrochloric acid (liquid)	T54.2X1	T54.2X2	T54.2X3	T54.2X4	--	--
medicinal (digestant)	T47.5X1	T47.5X2	T47.5X3	T47.5X4	T47.5X5	T47.5X6
vapor	T59.891	T59.892	T59.893	T59.894	--	--
Hydrochlorothiazide	T50.2X1	T50.2X2	T50.2X3	T50.2X4	T50.2X5	T50.2X6
Hydrocodone	T40.2X1	T40.2X2	T40.2X3	T40.2X4	T40.2X5	T40.2X6
Hydrocortisone (derivatives)	T38.0X1	T38.0X2	T38.0X3	T38.0X4	T38.0X5	T38.0X6
aceponate	T49.0X1	T49.0X2	T49.0X3	T49.0X4	T49.0X5	T49.0X6
ENT agent	T49.6X1	T49.6X2	T49.6X3	T49.6X4	T49.6X5	T49.6X6
ophthalmic preparation	T49.5X1	T49.5X2	T49.5X3	T49.5X4	T49.5X5	T49.5X6
topical NEC	T49.0X1	T49.0X2	T49.0X3	T49.0X4	T49.0X5	T49.0X6
Hydrocortone	T38.0X1	T38.0X2	T38.0X3	T38.0X4	T38.0X5	T38.0X6
ENT agent	T49.6X1	T49.6X2	T49.6X3	T49.6X4	T49.6X5	T49.6X6
ophthalmic preparation	T49.5X1	T49.5X2	T49.5X3	T49.5X4	T49.5X5	T49.5X6
topical NEC	T49.0X1	T49.0X2	T49.0X3	T49.0X4	T49.0X5	T49.0X6

Substance	Poisoning, Accidental (unintentional)	Poisoning, Intentional self-harm	Poisoning, Assault	Poisoning, Undetermined	Adverse effect	Underdosing
Hydrocyanic acid (liquid)	T57.3X1	T57.3X2	T57.3X3	T57.3X4	--	--
gas	T65.0X1	T65.0X2	T65.0X3	T65.0X4	--	--
Hydroflumethiazide	T50.2X1	T50.2X2	T50.2X3	T50.2X4	T50.2X5	T50.2X6
Hydrofluoric acid (liquid)	T54.2X1	T54.2X2	T54.2X3	T54.2X4	--	--
vapor	T59.891	T59.892	T59.893	T59.894	--	--
Hydrogen	T59.891	T59.892	T59.893	T59.894	--	--
arsenide	T57.0X1	T57.0X2	T57.0X3	T57.0X4	--	--
arseniureted	T57.0X1	T57.0X2	T57.0X3	T57.0X4	--	--
chloride	T57.8X1	T57.8X2	T57.8X3	T57.8X4	--	--
cyanide (salts)	T57.3X1	T57.3X2	T57.3X3	T57.3X4	--	--
gas	T57.3X1	T57.3X2	T57.3X3	T57.3X4	--	--
fluoride	T59.5X1	T59.5X2	T59.5X3	T59.5X4	--	--
vapor	T59.5X1	T59.5X2	T59.5X3	T59.5X4	--	--
peroxide	T49.0X1	T49.0X2	T49.0X3	T49.0X4	T49.0X5	T49.0X6
phosphureted	T57.1X1	T57.1X2	T57.1X3	T57.1X4	--	--
sulfide	T59.6X1	T59.6X2	T59.6X3	T59.6X4	--	--
arseniureted	T57.0X1	T57.0X2	T57.0X3	T57.0X4	--	--
sulfureted	T59.6X1	T59.6X2	T59.6X3	T59.6X4	--	--
Hydromethylpyridine	T46.7X1	T46.7X2	T46.7X3	T46.7X4	T46.7X5	T46.7X6
Hydromorphinol	T40.2X1	T40.2X2	T40.2X3	T40.2X4	--	--
Hydromorphinone	T40.2X1	T40.2X2	T40.2X3	T40.2X4	T40.2X5	T40.2X6
Hydromorphone	T40.2X1	T40.2X2	T40.2X3	T40.2X4	T40.2X5	T40.2X6
Hydromox	T50.2X1	T50.2X2	T50.2X3	T50.2X4	T50.2X5	T50.2X6
Hydrophilic lotion	T49.3X1	T49.3X2	T49.3X3	T49.3X4	T49.3X5	T49.3X6
Hydroquinidine	T46.2X1	T46.2X2	T46.2X3	T46.2X4	T46.2X5	T46.2X6
Hydroquinone	T52.2X1	T52.2X2	T52.2X3	T52.2X4	--	--
vapor	T59.891	T59.892	T59.893	T59.894	--	--
Hydrosulfuric acid (gas)	T59.6X1	T59.6X2	T59.6X3	T59.6X4	--	--
Hydrotalcite	T47.1X1	T47.1X2	T47.1X3	T47.1X4	T47.1X5	T47.1X6
Hydrous wool fat	T49.3X1	T49.3X2	T49.3X3	T49.3X4	T49.3X5	T49.3X6
Hydroxide, caustic	T54.3X1	T54.3X2	T54.3X3	T54.3X4	--	--
Hydroxocobalamin	T45.8X1	T45.8X2	T45.8X3	T45.8X4	T45.8X5	T45.8X6
Hydroxyamphetamine	T49.5X1	T49.5X2	T49.5X3	T49.5X4	T49.5X5	T49.5X6
Hydroxycarbamide	T45.1X1	T45.1X2	T45.1X3	T45.1X4	T45.1X5	T45.1X6
Hydroxychloroquine	T37.8X1	T37.8X2	T37.8X3	T37.8X4	T37.8X5	T37.8X6
Hydroxydihydrocodeinone	T40.2X1	T40.2X2	T40.2X3	T40.2X4	T40.2X5	T40.2X6
Hydroxyestrone	T38.5X1	T38.5X2	T38.5X3	T38.5X4	T38.5X5	T38.5X6
Hydroxyethyl starch	T45.8X1	T45.8X2	T45.8X3	T45.8X4	T45.8X5	T45.8X6
Hydroxymethylpenta-none	T52.4X1	T52.4X2	T52.4X3	T52.4X4	--	--
Hydroxyphenamate	T43.591	T43.592	T43.593	T43.594	T43.595	T43.596
Hydroxyphenylbutazone	T39.2X1	T39.2X2	T39.2X3	T39.2X4	T39.2X5	T39.2X6
Hydroxyprogesterone	T38.5X1	T38.5X2	T38.5X3	T38.5X4	T38.5X5	T38.5X6
caproate	T38.5X1	T38.5X2	T38.5X3	T38.5X4	T38.5X5	T38.5X6
Hydroxyquinoline (derivatives) NEC	T37.8X1	T37.8X2	T37.8X3	T37.8X4	T37.8X5	T37.8X6
Hydroxystilbamidine	T37.3X1	T37.3X2	T37.3X3	T37.3X4	T37.3X5	T37.3X6
Hydroxytoluene (nonmedicinal)	T54.0X1	T54.0X2	T54.0X3	T54.0X4	--	--
medicinal	T49.0X1	T49.0X2	T49.0X3	T49.0X4	T49.0X5	T49.0X6
Hydroxyurea	T45.1X1	T45.1X2	T45.1X3	T45.1X4	T45.1X5	T45.1X6
Hydroxyzine	T43.591	T43.592	T43.593	T43.594	T43.595	T43.596
Hyoscine	T44.3X1	T44.3X2	T44.3X3	T44.3X4	T44.3X5	T44.3X6
Hyoscyamine	T44.3X1	T44.3X2	T44.3X3	T44.3X4	T44.3X5	T44.3X6
Hyoscyamus	T44.3X1	T44.3X2	T44.3X3	T44.3X4	T44.3X5	T44.3X6
dry extract	T44.3X1	T44.3X2	T44.3X3	T44.3X4	T44.3X5	T44.3X6
Hypaque	T50.8X1	T50.8X2	T50.8X3	T50.8X4	T50.8X5	T50.8X6
Hypertussis	T50.Z11	T50.Z12	T50.Z13	T50.Z14	T50.Z15	T50.Z16
Hypnotic	T42.71	T42.72	T42.73	T42.74	T42.75	T42.76
anticonvulsant	T42.71	T42.72	T42.73	T42.74	T42.75	T42.76
specified NEC	T42.6X1	T42.6X2	T42.6X3	T42.6X4	T42.6X5	T42.6X6
Hypochlorite	T49.0X1	T49.0X2	T49.0X3	T49.0X4	T49.0X5	T49.0X6
Hypophysis, posterior	T38.891	T38.892	T38.893	T38.894	T38.895	T38.896
Hypotensive NEC	T46.5X1	T46.5X2	T46.5X3	T46.5X4	T46.5X5	T46.5X6
Hypromellose	T49.5X1	T49.5X2	T49.5X3	T49.5X4	T49.5X5	T49.5X6
I						
Ibacitabine	T37.5X1	T37.5X2	T37.5X3	T37.5X4	T37.5X5	T37.5X6
Ibopamine	T44.991	T44.992	T44.993	T44.994	T44.995	T44.996
Ibufenac	T39.311	T39.312	T39.313	T39.314	T39.315	T39.316
Ibuprofen	T39.311	T39.312	T39.313	T39.314	T39.315	T39.316
Ibuproxam	T39.311	T39.312	T39.313	T39.314	T39.315	T39.316
Ibuterol	T48.6X1	T48.6X2	T48.6X3	T48.6X4	T48.6X5	T48.6X6
Ichthammol	T49.0X1	T49.0X2	T49.0X3	T49.0X4	T49.0X5	T49.0X6
Ichthyol	T49.4X1	T49.4X2	T49.4X3	T49.4X4	T49.4X5	T49.4X6
Idarubicin	T45.1X1	T45.1X2	T45.1X3	T45.1X4	T45.1X5	T45.1X6
Idrocilamide	T42.8X1	T42.8X2	T42.8X3	T42.8X4	T42.8X5	T42.8X6
Ifenprodil	T46.7X1	T46.7X2	T46.7X3	T46.7X4	T46.7X5	T46.7X6
Ifosfamide	T45.1X1	T45.1X2	T45.1X3	T45.1X4	T45.1X5	T45.1X6
Iletin	T38.3X1	T38.3X2	T38.3X3	T38.3X4	T38.3X5	T38.3X6
Ilex	T62.2X1	T62.2X2	T62.2X3	T62.2X4	--	--
Illuminating gas (after combustion)	T58.11	T58.12	T58.13	T58.14	--	--
prior to combustion	T59.891	T59.892	T59.893	T59.894	--	--
Ilopan	T45.2X1	T45.2X2	T45.2X3	T45.2X4	T45.2X5	T45.2X6
Iloprost	T46.7X1	T46.7X2	T46.7X3	T46.7X4	T46.7X5	T46.7X6

Substance	Poisoning, Accidental (unintentional)	Poisoning, Intentional self-harm	Poisoning, Assault	Poisoning, Undetermined	Adverse effect	Underdosing
Ilotycin	T36.3X1	T36.3X2	T36.3X3	T36.3X4	T36.3X5	T36.3X6
ophthalmic preparation	T49.5X1	T49.5X2	T49.5X3	T49.5X4	T49.5X5	T49.5X6
topical NEC	T49.0X1	T49.0X2	T49.0X3	T49.0X4	T49.0X5	T49.0X6
Imidazole-4-carboxamide	T45.1X1	T45.1X2	T45.1X3	T45.1X4	T45.1X5	T45.1X6
Imipenem	T36.0X1	T36.0X2	T36.0X3	T36.0X4	T36.0X5	T36.0X6
Imipramine	T43.011	T43.012	T43.013	T43.014	T43.015	T43.016
Iminostilbene	T42.1X1	T42.1X2	T42.1X3	T42.1X4	T42.1X5	T42.1X6
Immu-G	T50.Z11	T50.Z12	T50.Z13	T50.Z14	T50.Z15	T50.Z16
Immuglobin	T50.Z11	T50.Z12	T50.Z13	T50.Z14	T50.Z15	T50.Z16
Immune						
globulin	T50.Z11	T50.Z12	T50.Z13	T50.Z14	T50.Z15	T50.Z16
serum globulin	T50.Z11	T50.Z12	T50.Z13	T50.Z14	T50.Z15	T50.Z16
Immunoglobin human (intravenous) (normal)	T50.Z11	T50.Z12	T50.Z13	T50.Z14	T50.Z15	T50.Z16
unmodified	T50.Z11	T50.Z12	T50.Z13	T50.Z14	T50.Z15	T50.Z16
Immunosuppressive drug	T45.1X1	T45.1X2	T45.1X3	T45.1X4	T45.1X5	T45.1X6
Immu-tetanus	T50.Z11	T50.Z12	T50.Z13	T50.Z14	T50.Z15	T50.Z16
Indalpine	T43.221	T43.222	T43.223	T43.224	T43.225	T43.226
Indanazoline	T48.5X1	T48.5X2	T48.5X3	T48.5X4	T48.5X5	T48.5X6
Indandione (derivatives)	T45.511	T45.512	T45.513	T45.514	T45.515	T45.516
Indapamide	T46.5X1	T46.5X2	T46.5X3	T46.5X4	T46.5X5	T46.5X6
Indendione (derivatives)	T45.511	T45.512	T45.513	T45.514	T45.515	T45.516
Indenolol	T44.7X1	T44.7X2	T44.7X3	T44.7X4	T44.7X5	T44.7X6
Inderal	T44.7X1	T44.7X2	T44.7X3	T44.7X4	T44.7X5	T44.7X6
Indian						
hemp	T40.7X1	T40.7X2	T40.7X3	T40.7X4	T40.7X5	T40.7X6
tobacco	T62.2X1	T62.2X2	T62.2X3	T62.2X4	--	--
Indigo carmine	T50.8X1	T50.8X2	T50.8X3	T50.8X4	T50.8X5	T50.8X6
Indobufen	T45.521	T45.522	T45.523	T45.524	T45.525	T45.526
Indocin	T39.2X1	T39.2X2	T39.2X3	T39.2X4	T39.2X5	T39.2X6
Indocyanine green	T50.8X1	T50.8X2	T50.8X3	T50.8X4	T50.8X5	T50.8X6
Indometacin	T39.391	T39.392	T39.393	T39.394	T39.395	T39.396
Indomethacin	T39.391	T39.392	T39.393	T39.394	T39.395	T39.396
farnesil	T39.4X1	T39.4X2	T39.4X3	T39.4X4	T39.4X5	T39.4X6
Indoramin	T44.6X1	T44.6X2	T44.6X3	T44.6X4	T44.6X5	T44.6X6
Industrial						
alcohol	T51.0X1	T51.0X2	T51.0X3	T51.0X4	--	--
fumes	T59.891	T59.892	T59.893	T59.894	--	--
solvents (fumes) (vapors)	T52.91	T52.92	T52.93	T52.94	--	--
Influenza vaccine	T50.B91	T50.B92	T50.B93	T50.B94	T50.B95	T50.B96
Ingested substance NEC	T65.91	T65.92	T65.93	T65.94	--	--
INH	T37.1X1	T37.1X2	T37.1X3	T37.1X4	T37.1X5	T37.1X6
Inhalation, gas (noxious) — see Gas						
Inhibitor						
angiotensin-converting enzyme	T46.4X1	T46.4X2	T46.4X3	T46.4X4	T46.4X5	T46.4X6
carbonic anhydrase	T50.2X1	T50.2X2	T50.2X3	T50.2X4	T50.2X5	T50.2X6
fibrinolysis	T45.621	T45.622	T45.623	T45.624	T45.625	T45.626
monoamine oxidase NEC	T43.1X1	T43.1X2	T43.1X3	T43.1X4	T43.1X5	T43.1X6
hydrazine	T43.1X1	T43.1X2	T43.1X3	T43.1X4	T43.1X5	T43.1X6
postsynaptic	T43.8X1	T43.8X2	T43.8X3	T43.8X4	T43.8X5	T43.8X6
prothrombin synthesis	T45.511	T45.512	T45.513	T45.514	T45.515	T45.516
Ink	T65.891	T65.892	T65.893	T65.894	--	--
Inorganic substance NEC	T57.91	T57.92	T57.93	T57.94	--	--
Inosine pranobex	T37.5X1	T37.5X2	T37.5X3	T37.5X4	T37.5X5	T37.5X6
Inositol	T50.991	T50.992	T50.993	T50.994	T50.995	T50.996
nicotinate	T46.7X1	T46.7X2	T46.7X3	T46.7X4	T46.7X5	T46.7X6
Inproquone	T45.1X1	T45.1X2	T45.1X3	T45.1X4	T45.1X5	T45.1X6
Insect (sting), venomous	T63.481	T63.482	T63.483	T63.484	--	--
ant	T63.421	T63.422	T63.423	T63.424	--	--
bee	T63.441	T63.442	T63.443	T63.444	--	--
caterpillar	T63.431	T63.432	T63.433	T63.434	--	--
hornet	T63.451	T63.452	T63.453	T63.454	--	--
wasp	T63.461	T63.462	T63.463	T63.464	--	--
Insecticide NEC	T60.91	T60.92	T60.93	T60.94	--	--
carbamate	T60.0X1	T60.0X2	T60.0X3	T60.0X4	--	--
chlorinated	T60.1X1	T60.1X2	T60.1X3	T60.1X4	--	--
mixed	T60.91	T60.92	T60.93	T60.94	--	--
organochlorine	T60.1X1	T60.1X2	T60.1X3	T60.1X4	--	--
organophosphorus	T60.0X1	T60.0X2	T60.0X3	T60.0X4	--	--
Insular tissue extract	T38.3X1	T38.3X2	T38.3X3	T38.3X4	T38.3X5	T38.3X6
Insulin (amorphous) (globin) (isophane) (Lente) (NPH) (Semilente) (Ultralente)	T38.3X1	T38.3X2	T38.3X3	T38.3X4	T38.3X5	T38.3X6
defalan	T38.3X1	T38.3X2	T38.3X3	T38.3X4	T38.3X5	T38.3X6
human	T38.3X1	T38.3X2	T38.3X3	T38.3X4	T38.3X5	T38.3X6
injection, soluble	T38.3X1	T38.3X2	T38.3X3	T38.3X4	T38.3X5	T38.3X6
biphasic	T38.3X1	T38.3X2	T38.3X3	T38.3X4	T38.3X5	T38.3X6
intermediate acting	T38.3X1	T38.3X2	T38.3X3	T38.3X4	T38.3X5	T38.3X6
protamine zinc	T38.3X1	T38.3X2	T38.3X3	T38.3X4	T38.3X5	T38.3X6
slow acting	T38.3X1	T38.3X2	T38.3X3	T38.3X4	T38.3X5	T38.3X6
zinc						
protamine injection	T38.3X1	T38.3X2	T38.3X3	T38.3X4	T38.3X5	T38.3X6
suspension (amorphous) (crystalline)	T38.3X1	T38.3X2	T38.3X3	T38.3X4	T38.3X5	T38.3X6

Substance	Poisoning, Accidental (unintentional)	Poisoning, Intentional self-harm	Poisoning, Assault	Poisoning, Undetermined	Adverse effect	Underdosing
Interferon (alpha) (beta) (gamma)	T37.5X1	T37.5X2	T37.5X3	T37.5X4	T37.5X5	T37.5X6
Intestinal motility control drug	T47.6X1	T47.6X2	T47.6X3	T47.6X4	T47.6X5	T47.6X6
biological	T47.8X1	T47.8X2	T47.8X3	T47.8X4	T47.8X5	T47.8X6
Intranarcon	T41.1X1	T41.1X2	T41.1X3	T41.1X4	T41.1X5	T41.1X6
Intravenous						
amino acids	T50.991	T50.992	T50.993	T50.994	T50.995	T50.996
fat suspension	T50.991	T50.992	T50.993	T50.994	T50.995	T50.996
Inulin	T50.8X1	T50.8X2	T50.8X3	T50.8X4	T50.8X5	T50.8X6
Invert sugar	T50.3X1	T50.3X2	T50.3X3	T50.3X4	T50.3X5	T50.3X6
Inza — see Naproxen						
Iobenzamic acid	T50.8X1	T50.8X2	T50.8X3	T50.8X4	T50.8X5	T50.8X6
Iocarmic acid	T50.8X1	T50.8X2	T50.8X3	T50.8X4	T50.8X5	T50.8X6
Iocetamic acid	T50.8X1	T50.8X2	T50.8X3	T50.8X4	T50.8X5	T50.8X6
Iodamide	T50.8X1	T50.8X2	T50.8X3	T50.8X4	T50.8X5	T50.8X6
Iodide NEC (see also Iodine)	T49.0X1	T49.0X2	T49.0X3	T49.0X4	T49.0X5	T49.0X6
mercury (ointment)	T49.0X1	T49.0X2	T49.0X3	T49.0X4	T49.0X5	T49.0X6
methylate	T49.0X1	T49.0X2	T49.0X3	T49.0X4	T49.0X5	T49.0X6
potassium (expectorant) NEC	T48.4X1	T48.4X2	T48.4X3	T48.4X4	T48.4X5	T48.4X6
Iodinated						
contrast medium	T50.8X1	T50.8X2	T50.8X3	T50.8X4	T50.8X5	T50.8X6
glycerol	T48.4X1	T48.4X2	T48.4X3	T48.4X4	T48.4X5	T48.4X6
human serum albumin (131I)	T50.8X1	T50.8X2	T50.8X3	T50.8X4	T50.8X5	T50.8X6
Iodine (antiseptic, external) (tincture) NEC	T49.0X1	T49.0X2	T49.0X3	T49.0X4	T49.0X5	T49.0X6
125 (see also Radiation sickness, and Exposure to radioactive isotopes)	T50.8X1	T50.8X2	T50.8X3	T50.8X4	T50.8X5	T50.8X6
therapeutic	T50.991	T50.992	T50.993	T50.994	T50.995	T50.996
131 (see also Radiation sickness, and Exposure to radioactive isotopes)	T50.8X1	T50.8X2	T50.8X3	T50.8X4	T50.8X5	T50.8X6
therapeutic	T38.2X1	T38.2X2	T38.2X3	T38.2X4	T38.2X5	T38.2X6
diagnostic	T50.8X1	T50.8X2	T50.8X3	T50.8X4	T50.8X5	T50.8X6
for thyroid conditions (antithyroid)	T38.2X1	T38.2X2	T38.2X3	T38.2X4	T38.2X5	T38.2X6
solution	T49.0X1	T49.0X2	T49.0X3	T49.0X4	T49.0X5	T49.0X6
vapor	T59.891	T59.892	T59.893	T59.894	--	--
Iodipamide	T50.8X1	T50.8X2	T50.8X3	T50.8X4	T50.8X5	T50.8X6
Iodized (poppy seed) oil	T50.8X1	T50.8X2	T50.8X3	T50.8X4	T50.8X5	T50.8X6
Iodobismitol	T37.8X1	T37.8X2	T37.8X3	T37.8X4	T37.8X5	T37.8X6
Iodochlorhydroxyquin	T37.8X1	T37.8X2	T37.8X3	T37.8X4	T37.8X5	T37.8X6
topical	T49.0X1	T49.0X2	T49.0X3	T49.0X4	T49.0X5	T49.0X6
Iodochlorhydroxyquinoline	T37.8X1	T37.8X2	T37.8X3	T37.8X4	T37.8X5	T37.8X6
Iodocholesterol (131I)	T50.8X1	T50.8X2	T50.8X3	T50.8X4	T50.8X5	T50.8X6
Iodoform	T49.0X1	T49.0X2	T49.0X3	T49.0X4	T49.0X5	T49.0X6
Iodohippuric acid	T50.8X1	T50.8X2	T50.8X3	T50.8X4	T50.8X5	T50.8X6
Iodopanoic acid	T50.8X1	T50.8X2	T50.8X3	T50.8X4	T50.8X5	T50.8X6
Iodophthalein (sodium)	T50.8X1	T50.8X2	T50.8X3	T50.8X4	T50.8X5	T50.8X6
Iodopyracet	T50.8X1	T50.8X2	T50.8X3	T50.8X4	T50.8X5	T50.8X6
Iodoquinol	T37.8X1	T37.8X2	T37.8X3	T37.8X4	T37.8X5	T37.8X6
Iodoxamic acid	T50.8X1	T50.8X2	T50.8X3	T50.8X4	T50.8X5	T50.8X6
Iofendylate	T50.8X1	T50.8X2	T50.8X3	T50.8X4	T50.8X5	T50.8X6
Ioglycamic acid	T50.8X1	T50.8X2	T50.8X3	T50.8X4	T50.8X5	T50.8X6
Iohexol	T50.8X1	T50.8X2	T50.8X3	T50.8X4	T50.8X5	T50.8X6
Ion exchange resin						
anion	T47.8X1	T47.8X2	T47.8X3	T47.8X4	T47.8X5	T47.8X6
cation	T50.3X1	T50.3X2	T50.3X3	T50.3X4	T50.3X5	T50.3X6
cholestyramine	T46.6X1	T46.6X2	T46.6X3	T46.6X4	T46.6X5	T46.6X6
intestinal	T47.8X1	T47.8X2	T47.8X3	T47.8X4	T47.8X5	T47.8X6
Iopamidol	T50.8X1	T50.8X2	T50.8X3	T50.8X4	T50.8X5	T50.8X6
Iopanoic acid	T50.8X1	T50.8X2	T50.8X3	T50.8X4	T50.8X5	T50.8X6
Iophenoic acid	T50.8X1	T50.8X2	T50.8X3	T50.8X4	T50.8X5	T50.8X6
Iopodate, sodium	T50.8X1	T50.8X2	T50.8X3	T50.8X4	T50.8X5	T50.8X6
Iopodic acid	T50.8X1	T50.8X2	T50.8X3	T50.8X4	T50.8X5	T50.8X6
Iopromide	T50.8X1	T50.8X2	T50.8X3	T50.8X4	T50.8X5	T50.8X6
Iopydol	T50.8X1	T50.8X2	T50.8X3	T50.8X4	T50.8X5	T50.8X6
Iotalamic acid	T50.8X1	T50.8X2	T50.8X3	T50.8X4	T50.8X5	T50.8X6
Iothalamate	T50.8X1	T50.8X2	T50.8X3	T50.8X4	T50.8X5	T50.8X6
Iothiouracil	T38.2X1	T38.2X2	T38.2X3	T38.2X4	T38.2X5	T38.2X6
Iotrol	T50.8X1	T50.8X2	T50.8X3	T50.8X4	T50.8X5	T50.8X6
Iotrolan	T50.8X1	T50.8X2	T50.8X3	T50.8X4	T50.8X5	T50.8X6
Iotroxate	T50.8X1	T50.8X2	T50.8X3	T50.8X4	T50.8X5	T50.8X6
Iotroxic acid	T50.8X1	T50.8X2	T50.8X3	T50.8X4	T50.8X5	T50.8X6
Ioversol	T50.8X1	T50.8X2	T50.8X3	T50.8X4	T50.8X5	T50.8X6
Ioxaglate	T50.8X1	T50.8X2	T50.8X3	T50.8X4	T50.8X5	T50.8X6
Ioxaglic acid	T50.8X1	T50.8X2	T50.8X3	T50.8X4	T50.8X5	T50.8X6
Ioxitalamic acid	T50.8X1	T50.8X2	T50.8X3	T50.8X4	T50.8X5	T50.8X6
Ipecac	T47.7X1	T47.7X2	T47.7X3	T47.7X4	T47.7X5	T47.7X6
Ipecacuanha	T48.4X1	T48.4X2	T48.4X3	T48.4X4	T48.4X5	T48.4X6

Substance	Poisoning, Accidental (unintentional)	Poisoning, Intentional self-harm	Poisoning, Assault	Poisoning, Undetermined	Adverse effect	Underdosing
Ipodate, calcium	T50.8X1	T50.8X2	T50.8X3	T50.8X4	T50.8X5	T50.8X6
Ipral	T42.3X1	T42.3X2	T42.3X3	T42.3X4	T42.3X5	T42.3X6
Ipratropium (bromide)	T48.6X1	T48.6X2	T48.6X3	T48.6X4	T48.6X5	T48.6X6
Ipriflavone	T46.3X1	T46.3X2	T46.3X3	T46.3X4	T46.3X5	T46.3X6
Iprindole	T43.011	T43.012	T43.013	T43.014	T43.015	T43.016
Iproclozide	T43.1X1	T43.1X2	T43.1X3	T43.1X4	T43.1X5	T43.1X6
Iprofenin	T50.8X1	T50.8X2	T50.8X3	T50.8X4	T50.8X5	T50.8X6
Iproheptine	T49.2X1	T49.2X2	T49.2X3	T49.2X4	T49.2X5	T49.2X6
Iproniazid	T43.1X1	T43.1X2	T43.1X3	T43.1X4	T43.1X5	T43.1X6
Iproplatin	T45.1X1	T45.1X2	T45.1X3	T45.1X4	T45.1X5	T45.1X6
Iproveratril	T46.1X1	T46.1X2	T46.1X3	T46.1X4	T46.1X5	T46.1X6
Iron (compounds) (medicinal) **NEC**	T45.4X1	T45.4X2	T45.4X3	T45.4X4	T45.4X5	T45.4X6
ammonium	T45.4X1	T45.4X2	T45.4X3	T45.4X4	T45.4X5	T45.4X6
dextran injection	T45.4X1	T45.4X2	T45.4X3	T45.4X4	T45.4X5	T45.4X6
nonmedicinal	T56.891	T56.892	T56.893	T56.894	--	--
salts	T45.4X1	T45.4X2	T45.4X3	T45.4X4	T45.4X5	T45.4X6
sorbitex	T45.4X1	T45.4X2	T45.4X3	T45.4X4	T45.4X5	T45.4X6
sorbitol citric acid complex	T45.4X1	T45.4X2	T45.4X3	T45.4X4	T45.4X5	T45.4X6
Irrigating fluid (vaginal)	T49.8X1	T49.8X2	T49.8X3	T49.8X4	T49.8X5	T49.8X6
eye	T49.5X1	T49.5X2	T49.5X3	T49.5X4	T49.5X5	T49.5X6
Isepamicin	T36.5X1	T36.5X2	T36.5X3	T36.5X4	T36.5X5	T36.5X6
Isoaminile (citrate)	T48.3X1	T48.3X2	T48.3X3	T48.3X4	T48.3X5	T48.3X6
Isoamyl nitrite	T46.3X1	T46.3X2	T46.3X3	T46.3X4	T46.3X5	T46.3X6
Isobenzan	T60.1X1	T60.1X2	T60.1X3	T60.1X4	--	--
Isobutyl acetate	T52.8X1	T52.8X2	T52.8X3	T52.8X4	--	--
Isocarboxazid	T43.1X1	T43.1X2	T43.1X3	T43.1X4	T43.1X5	T43.1X6
Isoconazole	T49.0X1	T49.0X2	T49.0X3	T49.0X4	T49.0X5	T49.0X6
Isocyanate	T65.0X1	T65.0X2	T65.0X3	T65.0X4	--	--
Isoephedrine	T44.991	T44.992	T44.993	T44.994	T44.995	T44.996
Isoetarine	T48.6X1	T48.6X2	T48.6X3	T48.6X4	T48.6X5	T48.6X6
Isoethadione	T42.2X1	T42.2X2	T42.2X3	T42.2X4	T42.2X5	T42.2X6
Isoetharine	T44.5X1	T44.5X2	T44.5X3	T44.5X4	T44.5X5	T44.5X6
Isoflurane	T41.0X1	T41.0X2	T41.0X3	T41.0X4	T41.0X5	T41.0X6
Isoflurophate	T44.0X1	T44.0X2	T44.0X3	T44.0X4	T44.0X5	T44.0X6
Isomaltose, ferric complex	T45.4X1	T45.4X2	T45.4X3	T45.4X4	T45.4X5	T45.4X6
Isometheptene	T44.3X1	T44.3X2	T44.3X3	T44.3X4	T44.3X5	T44.3X6
Isoniazid	T37.1X1	T37.1X2	T37.1X3	T37.1X4	T37.1X5	T37.1X6
with						
rifampicin	T36.6X1	T36.6X2	T36.6X3	T36.6X4	T36.6X5	T36.6X6
thioacetazone	T37.1X1	T37.1X2	T37.1X3	T37.1X4	T37.1X5	T37.1X6
Isonicotinic acid hydrazide	T37.1X1	T37.1X2	T37.1X3	T37.1X4	T37.1X5	T37.1X6
Isonipecaine	T40.4X1	T40.4X2	T40.4X3	T40.4X4	T40.4X5	T40.4X6
Isopentaquine	T37.2X1	T37.2X2	T37.2X3	T37.2X4	T37.2X5	T37.2X6
Isophane insulin	T38.3X1	T38.3X2	T38.3X3	T38.3X4	T38.3X5	T38.3X6
Isophorone	T65.891	T65.892	T65.893	T65.894	--	--
Isophosphamide	T45.1X1	T45.1X2	T45.1X3	T45.1X4	T45.1X5	T45.1X6
Isopregnenone	T38.5X1	T38.5X2	T38.5X3	T38.5X4	T38.5X5	T38.5X6
Isoprenaline	T48.6X1	T48.6X2	T48.6X3	T48.6X4	T48.6X5	T48.6X6
Isopromethazine	T43.3X1	T43.3X2	T43.3X3	T43.3X4	T43.3X5	T43.3X6
Isopropamide	T44.3X1	T44.3X2	T44.3X3	T44.3X4	T44.3X5	T44.3X6
iodide	T44.3X1	T44.3X2	T44.3X3	T44.3X4	T44.3X5	T44.3X6
Isopropanol	T51.2X1	T51.2X2	T51.2X3	T51.2X4	--	--
Isopropyl						
acetate	T52.8X1	T52.8X2	T52.8X3	T52.8X4	--	--
alcohol	T51.2X1	T51.2X2	T51.2X3	T51.2X4	--	--
medicinal	T49.4X1	T49.4X2	T49.4X3	T49.4X4	T49.4X5	T49.4X6
ether	T52.8X1	T52.8X2	T52.8X3	T52.8X4	--	--
Isopropylaminophenazone	T39.2X1	T39.2X2	T39.2X3	T39.2X4	T39.2X5	T39.2X6
Isoproterenol	T48.6X1	T48.6X2	T48.6X3	T48.6X4	T48.6X5	T48.6X6
Isosorbide dinitrate	T46.3X1	T46.3X2	T46.3X3	T46.3X4	T46.3X5	T46.3X6
Isothipendyl	T45.0X1	T45.0X2	T45.0X3	T45.0X4	T45.0X5	T45.0X6
Isotretinoin	T50.991	T50.992	T50.993	T50.994	T50.995	T50.996
Isoxazolyl penicillin	T36.0X1	T36.0X2	T36.0X3	T36.0X4	T36.0X5	T36.0X6
Isoxicam	T39.391	T39.392	T39.393	T39.394	T39.395	T39.396
Isoxsuprine	T46.7X1	T46.7X2	T46.7X3	T46.7X4	T46.7X5	T46.7X6
Ispagula	T47.4X1	T47.4X2	T47.4X3	T47.4X4	T47.4X5	T47.4X6
husk	T47.4X1	T47.4X2	T47.4X3	T47.4X4	T47.4X5	T47.4X6
Isradipine	T46.1X1	T46.1X2	T46.1X3	T46.1X4	T46.1X5	T46.1X6
I-thyroxine sodium	T38.1X1	T38.1X2	T38.1X3	T38.1X4	T38.1X5	T38.1X6
Itraconazole	T37.8X1	T37.8X2	T37.8X3	T37.8X4	T37.8X5	T37.8X6
Itramin tosilate	T46.3X1	T46.3X2	T46.3X3	T46.3X4	T46.3X5	T46.3X6
Ivermectin	T37.4X1	T37.4X2	T37.4X3	T37.4X4	T37.4X5	T37.4X6
Izoniazid	T37.1X1	T37.1X2	T37.1X3	T37.1X4	T37.1X5	T37.1X6
with thioacetazone	T37.1X1	T37.1X2	T37.1X3	T37.1X4	T37.1X5	T37.1X6
J						
Jalap	T47.2X1	T47.2X2	T47.2X3	T47.2X4	T47.2X5	T47.2X6
Jamaica						
dogwood (bark)	T39.8X1	T39.8X2	T39.8X3	T39.8X4	T39.8X5	T39.8X6
ginger	T65.891	T65.892	T65.893	T65.894	--	--
root	T62.2X1	T62.2X2	T62.2X3	T62.2X4	--	--
Jatropha	T62.2X1	T62.2X2	T62.2X3	T62.2X4	--	--
curcas	T62.2X1	T62.2X2	T62.2X3	T62.2X4	--	--
Jectofer	T45.4X1	T45.4X2	T45.4X3	T45.4X4	T45.4X5	T45.4X6

Substance	Poisoning, Accidental (unintentional)	Poisoning, Intentional self-harm	Poisoning, Assault	Poisoning, Undetermined	Adverse effect	Underdosing
Jellyfish (sting)	T63.621	T63.622	T63.623	T63.624	--	--
Jequirity (bean)	T62.2X1	T62.2X2	T62.2X3	T62.2X4	--	--
Jimson weed (stramonium)	T62.2X1	T62.2X2	T62.2X3	T62.2X4	--	--
seeds	T62.2X1	T62.2X2	T62.2X3	T62.2X4	--	--
Josamycin	T36.3X1	T36.3X2	T36.3X3	T36.3X4	T36.3X5	T36.3X6
Juniper tar	T49.1X1	T49.1X2	T49.1X3	T49.1X4	T49.1X5	T49.1X6
K						
Kallidinogenase	T46.7X1	T46.7X2	T46.7X3	T46.7X4	T46.7X5	T46.7X6
Kallikrein	T46.7X1	T46.7X2	T46.7X3	T46.7X4	T46.7X5	T46.7X6
Kanamycin	T36.5X1	T36.5X2	T36.5X3	T36.5X4	T36.5X5	T36.5X6
Kantrex	T36.5X1	T36.5X2	T36.5X3	T36.5X4	T36.5X5	T36.5X6
Kaolin	T47.6X1	T47.6X2	T47.6X3	T47.6X4	T47.6X5	T47.6X6
light	T47.6X1	T47.6X2	T47.6X3	T47.6X4	T47.6X5	T47.6X6
Karaya (gum)	T47.4X1	T47.4X2	T47.4X3	T47.4X4	T47.4X5	T47.4X6
Kebuzone	T39.2X1	T39.2X2	T39.2X3	T39.2X4	T39.2X5	T39.2X6
Kelevan	T60.1X1	T60.1X2	T60.1X3	T60.1X4	--	--
Kemithal	T41.1X1	T41.1X2	T41.1X3	T41.1X4	T41.1X5	T41.1X6
Kenacort	T38.0X1	T38.0X2	T38.0X3	T38.0X4	T38.0X5	T38.0X6
Keratolytic drug NEC	T49.4X1	T49.4X2	T49.4X3	T49.4X4	T49.4X5	T49.4X6
anthracene	T49.4X1	T49.4X2	T49.4X3	T49.4X4	T49.4X5	T49.4X6
Keratoplastic NEC	T49.4X1	T49.4X2	T49.4X3	T49.4X4	T49.4X5	T49.4X6
Kerosene, kerosine (fuel) (solvent) **NEC**	T52.0X1	T52.0X2	T52.0X3	T52.0X4	--	--
insecticide	T52.0X1	T52.0X2	T52.0X3	T52.0X4	--	--
vapor	T52.0X1	T52.0X2	T52.0X3	T52.0X4	--	--
Ketamine	T41.291	T41.292	T41.293	T41.294	T41.295	T41.296
Ketazolam	T42.4X1	T42.4X2	T42.4X3	T42.4X4	T42.4X5	T42.4X6
Ketazon	T39.2X1	T39.2X2	T39.2X3	T39.2X4	T39.2X5	T39.2X6
Ketobemidone	T40.4X1	T40.4X2	T40.4X3	T40.4X4	--	--
Ketoconazole	T49.0X1	T49.0X2	T49.0X3	T49.0X4	T49.0X5	T49.0X6
Ketols	T52.4X1	T52.4X2	T52.4X3	T52.4X4	--	--
Ketone oils	T52.4X1	T52.4X2	T52.4X3	T52.4X4	--	--
Ketoprofen	T39.311	T39.312	T39.313	T39.314	T39.315	T39.316
Ketorolac	T39.8X1	T39.8X2	T39.8X3	T39.8X4	T39.8X5	T39.8X6
Ketotifen	T45.0X1	T45.0X2	T45.0X3	T45.0X4	T45.0X5	T45.0X6
Khat	T43.691	T43.692	T43.693	T43.694	--	--
Khellin	T46.3X1	T46.3X2	T46.3X3	T46.3X4	T46.3X5	T46.3X6
Khelloside	T46.3X1	T46.3X2	T46.3X3	T46.3X4	T46.3X5	T46.3X6
Kiln gas or vapor (carbon monoxide)	T58.8X1	T58.8X2	T58.8X3	T58.8X4	--	--
Kitasamycin	T36.3X1	T36.3X2	T36.3X3	T36.3X4	T36.3X5	T36.3X6
Konsyl	T47.4X1	T47.4X2	T47.4X3	T47.4X4	T47.4X5	T47.4X6
Kosam seed	T62.2X1	T62.2X2	T62.2X3	T62.2X4	--	--
Krait (venom)	T63.091	T63.092	T63.093	T63.094	--	--
Kwell (insecticide)	T60.1X1	T60.1X2	T60.1X3	T60.1X4	--	--
anti-infective (topical)	T49.0X1	T49.0X2	T49.0X3	T49.0X4	T49.0X5	T49.0X6
L						
Labetalol	T44.8X1	T44.8X2	T44.8X3	T44.8X4	T44.8X5	T44.8X6
Laburnum (seeds)	T62.2X1	T62.2X2	T62.2X3	T62.2X4	--	--
leaves	T62.2X1	T62.2X2	T62.2X3	T62.2X4	--	--
Lachesine	T49.5X1	T49.5X2	T49.5X3	T49.5X4	T49.5X5	T49.5X6
Lacidipine	T46.5X1	T46.5X2	T46.5X3	T46.5X4	T46.5X5	T46.5X6
Lacquer	T65.6X1	T65.6X2	T65.6X3	T65.6X4	--	--
Lacrimogenic gas	T59.3X1	T59.3X2	T59.3X3	T59.3X4	--	--
Lactated potassic saline	T50.3X1	T50.3X2	T50.3X3	T50.3X4	T50.3X5	T50.3X6
Lactic acid	T49.8X1	T49.8X2	T49.8X3	T49.8X4	T49.8X5	T49.8X6
Lactobacillus						
acidophilus	T47.6X1	T47.6X2	T47.6X3	T47.6X4	T47.6X5	T47.6X6
compound	T47.6X1	T47.6X2	T47.6X3	T47.6X4	T47.6X5	T47.6X6
bifidus, lyophilized	T47.6X1	T47.6X2	T47.6X3	T47.6X4	T47.6X5	T47.6X6
bulgaricus	T47.6X1	T47.6X2	T47.6X3	T47.6X4	T47.6X5	T47.6X6
sporogenes	T47.6X1	T47.6X2	T47.6X3	T47.6X4	T47.6X5	T47.6X6
Lactoflavin	T45.2X1	T45.2X2	T45.2X3	T45.2X4	T45.2X5	T45.2X6
Lactose (as excipient)	T50.901	T50.902	T50.903	T50.904	T50.905	T50.906
Lactuca (virosa) (extract)	T42.6X1	T42.6X2	T42.6X3	T42.6X4	T42.6X5	T42.6X6
Lactucarium	T42.6X1	T42.6X2	T42.6X3	T42.6X4	T42.6X5	T42.6X6
Lactulose	T47.3X1	T47.3X2	T47.3X3	T47.3X4	T47.3X5	T47.3X6
Laevo — *see* Levo-						
Lanatosides	T46.0X1	T46.0X2	T46.0X3	T46.0X4	T46.0X5	T46.0X6
Lanolin	T49.3X1	T49.3X2	T49.3X3	T49.3X4	T49.3X5	T49.3X6
Largactil	T43.3X1	T43.3X2	T43.3X3	T43.3X4	T43.3X5	T43.3X6
Larkspur	T62.2X1	T62.2X2	T62.2X3	T62.2X4	--	--
Laroxyl	T43.011	T43.012	T43.013	T43.014	T43.015	T43.016
Lasix	T50.1X1	T50.1X2	T50.1X3	T50.1X4	T50.1X5	T50.1X6
Lassar's paste	T49.4X1	T49.4X2	T49.4X3	T49.4X4	T49.4X5	T49.4X6
Latamoxef	T36.1X1	T36.1X2	T36.1X3	T36.1X4	T36.1X5	T36.1X6
Latex	T65.811	T65.812	T65.813	T65.814	--	--
Lathyrus (seed)	T62.2X1	T62.2X2	T62.2X3	T62.2X4	--	--
Laudanum	T40.0X1	T40.0X2	T40.0X3	T40.0X4	T40.0X5	T40.0X6
Laudexium	T48.1X1	T48.1X2	T48.1X3	T48.1X4	T48.1X5	T48.1X6
Laughing gas	T41.0X1	T41.0X2	T41.0X3	T41.0X4	T41.0X5	T41.0X6
Laurel, black or cherry	T62.2X1	T62.2X2	T62.2X3	T62.2X4	--	--
Laurolinium	T49.0X1	T49.0X2	T49.0X3	T49.0X4	T49.0X5	T49.0X6
Lauryl sulfoacetate	T49.2X1	T49.2X2	T49.2X3	T49.2X4	T49.2X5	T49.2X6

Substance	Poisoning, Accidental (unintentional)	Poisoning, Intentional self-harm	Poisoning, Assault	Poisoning, Undetermined	Adverse effect	Underdosing
Laxative NEC	T47.4X1	T47.4X2	T47.4X3	T47.4X4	T47.4X5	T47.4X6
osmotic	T47.3X1	T47.3X2	T47.3X3	T47.3X4	T47.3X5	T47.3X6
saline	T47.3X1	T47.3X2	T47.3X3	T47.3X4	T47.3X5	T47.3X6
stimulant	T47.2X1	T47.2X2	T47.2X3	T47.2X4	T47.2X5	T47.2X6
L-dopa	T42.8X1	T42.8X2	T42.8X3	T42.8X4	T42.8X5	T42.8X6
Lead (dust) (fumes) (vapor) NEC	T56.0X1	T56.0X2	T56.0X3	T56.0X4	--	--
acetate	T49.2X1	T49.2X2	T49.2X3	T49.2X4	T49.2X5	T49.2X6
alkyl (fuel additive)	T56.0X1	T56.0X2	T56.0X3	T56.0X4	--	--
anti-infectives	T37.8X1	T37.8X2	T37.8X3	T37.8X4	T37.8X5	T37.8X6
antiknock compound (tetraethyl)	T56.0X1	T56.0X2	T56.0X3	T56.0X4	--	--
arsenate, arsenite (dust) (herbicide) (insecticide) (vapor)	T57.0X1	T57.0X2	T57.0X3	T57.0X4	--	--
carbonate	T56.0X1	T56.0X2	T56.0X3	T56.0X4	--	--
paint	T56.0X1	T56.0X2	T56.0X3	T56.0X4	--	--
chromate	T56.0X1	T56.0X2	T56.0X3	T56.0X4	--	--
paint	T56.0X1	T56.0X2	T56.0X3	T56.0X4	--	--
dioxide	T56.0X1	T56.0X2	T56.0X3	T56.0X4	--	--
inorganic	T56.0X1	T56.0X2	T56.0X3	T56.0X4	--	--
iodide	T56.0X1	T56.0X2	T56.0X3	T56.0X4	--	--
pigment (paint)	T56.0X1	T56.0X2	T56.0X3	T56.0X4	--	--
monoxide (dust)	T56.0X1	T56.0X2	T56.0X3	T56.0X4	--	--
paint	T56.0X1	T56.0X2	T56.0X3	T56.0X4	--	--
organic	T56.0X1	T56.0X2	T56.0X3	T56.0X4	--	--
oxide	T56.0X1	T56.0X2	T56.0X3	T56.0X4	--	--
paint	T56.0X1	T56.0X2	T56.0X3	T56.0X4	--	--
paint	T56.0X1	T56.0X2	T56.0X3	T56.0X4	--	--
salts	T56.0X1	T56.0X2	T56.0X3	T56.0X4	--	--
specified compound NEC	T56.0X1	T56.0X2	T56.0X3	T56.0X4	--	--
tetra-ethyl	T56.0X1	T56.0X2	T56.0X3	T56.0X4	--	--
Lebanese red	T40.7X1	T40.7X2	T40.7X3	T40.7X4	T40.7X5	T40.7X6
Lefetamine	T39.8X1	T39.8X2	T39.8X3	T39.8X4	T39.8X5	T39.8X6
Lenperone	T43.4X1	T43.4X2	T43.4X3	T43.4X4	T43.4X5	T43.4X6
Lente lietin (insulin)	T38.3X1	T38.3X2	T38.3X3	T38.3X4	T38.3X5	T38.3X6
Leptazol	T50.7X1	T50.7X2	T50.7X3	T50.7X4	T50.7X5	T50.7X6
Leptophos	T60.0X1	T60.0X2	T60.0X3	T60.0X4	--	--
Leritine	T40.2X1	T40.2X2	T40.2X3	T40.2X4	T40.2X5	T40.2X6
Letosteine	T48.4X1	T48.4X2	T48.4X3	T48.4X4	T48.4X5	T48.4X6
Letter	T38.1X1	T38.1X2	T38.1X3	T38.1X4	T38.1X5	T38.1X6
Lettuce opium	T42.6X1	T42.6X2	T42.6X3	T42.6X4	T42.6X5	T42.6X6
Leucinocaine	T41.3X1	T41.3X2	T41.3X3	T41.3X4	T41.3X5	T41.3X6
Leucocianidol	T46.991	T46.992	T46.993	T46.994	T46.995	T46.996
Leucovorin (factor)	T45.8X1	T45.8X2	T45.8X3	T45.8X4	T45.8X5	T45.8X6
Leukeran	T45.1X1	T45.1X2	T45.1X3	T45.1X4	T45.1X5	T45.1X6
Leuprolide	T38.891	T38.892	T38.893	T38.894	T38.895	T38.896
Levalbuterol	T48.6X1	T48.6X2	T48.6X3	T48.6X4	T48.6X5	T48.6X6
Levallorphan	T50.7X1	T50.7X2	T50.7X3	T50.7X4	T50.7X5	T50.7X6
Levamisole	T37.4X1	T37.4X2	T37.4X3	T37.4X4	T37.4X5	T37.4X6
Levanil	T42.6X1	T42.6X2	T42.6X3	T42.6X4	T42.6X5	T42.6X6
Levarterenol	T44.4X1	T44.4X2	T44.4X3	T44.4X4	T44.4X5	T44.4X6
Levdropropizine	T48.3X1	T48.3X2	T48.3X3	T48.3X4	T48.3X5	T48.3X6
Levobunolol	T49.5X1	T49.5X2	T49.5X3	T49.5X4	T49.5X5	T49.5X6
Levocabastine (hydrochloride)	T45.0X1	T45.0X2	T45.0X3	T45.0X4	T45.0X5	T45.0X6
Levocarnitine	T50.991	T50.992	T50.993	T50.994	T50.995	T50.996
Levodopa	T42.8X1	T42.8X2	T42.8X3	T42.8X4	T42.8X5	T42.8X6
with carbidopa	T42.8X1	T42.8X2	T42.8X3	T42.8X4	T42.8X5	T42.8X6
Levo-dromoran	T40.2X1	T40.2X2	T40.2X3	T40.2X4	T40.2X5	T40.2X6
Levoglutamide	T50.991	T50.992	T50.993	T50.994	T50.995	T50.996
Levoid	T38.1X1	T38.1X2	T38.1X3	T38.1X4	T38.1X5	T38.1X6
Levo-iso-methadone	T40.3X1	T40.3X2	T40.3X3	T40.3X4	T40.3X5	T40.3X6
Levomepromazine	T43.3X1	T43.3X2	T43.3X3	T43.3X4	T43.3X5	T43.3X6
Levonordefrin	T49.6X1	T49.6X2	T49.6X3	T49.6X4	T49.6X5	T49.6X6
Levonorgestrel	T38.4X1	T38.4X2	T38.4X3	T38.4X4	T38.4X5	T38.4X6
with ethinylestradiol	T38.5X1	T38.5X2	T38.5X3	T38.5X4	T38.5X5	T38.5X6
Levopromazine	T43.3X1	T43.3X2	T43.3X3	T43.3X4	T43.3X5	T43.3X6
Levoprome	T42.6X1	T42.6X2	T42.6X3	T42.6X4	T42.6X5	T42.6X6
Levopropoxyphene	T40.4X1	T40.4X2	T40.4X3	T40.4X4	T40.4X5	T40.4X6
Levopropylhexedrine	T50.5X1	T50.5X2	T50.5X3	T50.5X4	T50.5X5	T50.5X6
Levoproxyphylline	T48.6X1	T48.6X2	T48.6X3	T48.6X4	T48.6X5	T48.6X6
Levorphanol	T40.4X1	T40.4X2	T40.4X3	T40.4X4	T40.4X5	T40.4X6
Levothyroxine	T38.1X1	T38.1X2	T38.1X3	T38.1X4	T38.1X5	T38.1X6
sodium	T38.1X1	T38.1X2	T38.1X3	T38.1X4	T38.1X5	T38.1X6
Levsin	T44.3X1	T44.3X2	T44.3X3	T44.3X4	T44.3X5	T44.3X6
Levulose	T50.3X1	T50.3X2	T50.3X3	T50.3X4	T50.3X5	T50.3X6
Lewisite (gas), **not in war**	T57.0X1	T57.0X2	T57.0X3	T57.0X4	--	--
Librium	T42.4X1	T42.4X2	T42.4X3	T42.4X4	T42.4X5	T42.4X6
Lidex	T49.0X1	T49.0X2	T49.0X3	T49.0X4	T49.0X5	T49.0X6
Lidocaine	T41.3X1	T41.3X2	T41.3X3	T41.3X4	T41.3X5	T41.3X6
regional	T41.3X1	T41.3X2	T41.3X3	T41.3X4	T41.3X5	T41.3X6
spinal	T41.3X1	T41.3X2	T41.3X3	T41.3X4	T41.3X5	T41.3X6
Lidofenin	T50.8X1	T50.8X2	T50.8X3	T50.8X4	T50.8X5	T50.8X6
Lidoflazine	T46.1X1	T46.1X2	T46.1X3	T46.1X4	T46.1X5	T46.1X6
Lighter fluid	T52.0X1	T52.0X2	T52.0X3	T52.0X4	--	--
Lignin hemicellulose	T47.6X1	T47.6X2	T47.6X3	T47.6X4	T47.6X5	T47.6X6
Lignocaine	T41.3X1	T41.3X2	T41.3X3	T41.3X4	T41.3X5	T41.3X6
regional	T41.3X1	T41.3X2	T41.3X3	T41.3X4	T41.3X5	T41.3X6
spinal	T41.3X1	T41.3X2	T41.3X3	T41.3X4	T41.3X5	T41.3X6
Ligroin (e) (solvent)	T52.0X1	T52.0X2	T52.0X3	T52.0X4	--	--
vapor	T59.891	T59.892	T59.893	T59.894	--	--
Ligustrum vulgare	T62.2X1	T62.2X2	T62.2X3	T62.2X4	--	--
Lily of the valley	T62.2X1	T62.2X2	T62.2X3	T62.2X4	--	--
Lime (chloride)	T54.3X1	T54.3X2	T54.3X3	T54.3X4	--	--
Limonene	T52.8X1	T52.8X2	T52.8X3	T52.8X4	--	--
Lincomycin	T36.8X1	T36.8X2	T36.8X3	T36.8X4	T36.8X5	T36.8X6
Lindane (insecticide) (nonmedicinal) (vapor)	T53.6X1	T53.6X2	T53.6X3	T53.6X4	--	--
medicinal	T49.0X1	T49.0X2	T49.0X3	T49.0X4	T49.0X5	T49.0X6
Liniments NEC	T49.91	T49.92	T49.93	T49.94	T49.95	T49.96
Linoleic acid	T46.6X1	T46.6X2	T46.6X3	T46.6X4	T46.6X5	T46.6X6
Linolenic acid	T46.6X1	T46.6X2	T46.6X3	T46.6X4	T46.6X5	T46.6X6
Linseed	T47.4X1	T47.4X2	T47.4X3	T47.4X4	T47.4X5	T47.4X6
Liothyronine	T38.1X1	T38.1X2	T38.1X3	T38.1X4	T38.1X5	T38.1X6
Liotrix	T38.1X1	T38.1X2	T38.1X3	T38.1X4	T38.1X5	T38.1X6
Lipancreatin	T47.5X1	T47.5X2	T47.5X3	T47.5X4	T47.5X5	T47.5X6
Lipo-alprostadil	T46.7X1	T46.7X2	T46.7X3	T46.7X4	T46.7X5	T46.7X6
Lipo-Lutin	T38.5X1	T38.5X2	T38.5X3	T38.5X4	T38.5X5	T38.5X6
Lipotropic drug NEC	T50.901	T50.902	T50.903	T50.904	T50.905	T50.906
Liquefied petroleum gases	T59.891	T59.892	T59.893	T59.894	--	--
piped (pure or mixed with air)	T59.891	T59.892	T59.893	T59.894	--	--
Liquid						
paraffin	T47.4X1	T47.4X2	T47.4X3	T47.4X4	T47.4X5	T47.4X6
petrolatum	T47.4X1	T47.4X2	T47.4X3	T47.4X4	T47.4X5	T47.4X6
topical	T49.3X1	T49.3X2	T49.3X3	T49.3X4	T49.3X5	T49.3X6
specified NEC	T65.891	T65.892	T65.893	T65.894	--	--
substance	T65.91	T65.92	T65.93	T65.94	--	--
Liquor creosolis compositus	T65.891	T65.892	T65.893	T65.894	--	--
Liquorice	T48.4X1	T48.4X2	T48.4X3	T48.4X4	T48.4X5	T48.4X6
extract	T47.8X1	T47.8X2	T47.8X3	T47.8X4	T47.8X5	T47.8X6
Lisinopril	T46.4X1	T46.4X2	T46.4X3	T46.4X4	T46.4X5	T46.4X6
Lisuride	T42.8X1	T42.8X2	T42.8X3	T42.8X4	T42.8X5	T42.8X6
Lithane	T43.8X1	T43.8X2	T43.8X3	T43.8X4	T43.8X5	T43.8X6
Lithium	T56.891	T56.892	T56.893	T56.894	--	--
gluconate	T43.591	T43.592	T43.593	T43.594	T43.595	T43.596
salts (carbonate)	T43.591	T43.592	T43.593	T43.594	T43.595	T43.596
Lithonate	T43.8X1	T43.8X2	T43.8X3	T43.8X4	T43.8X5	T43.8X6
Liver						
extract	T45.8X1	T45.8X2	T45.8X3	T45.8X4	T45.8X5	T45.8X6
for parenteral use	T45.8X1	T45.8X2	T45.8X3	T45.8X4	T45.8X5	T45.8X6
fraction 1	T45.8X1	T45.8X2	T45.8X3	T45.8X4	T45.8X5	T45.8X6
hydrolysate	T45.8X1	T45.8X2	T45.8X3	T45.8X4	T45.8X5	T45.8X6
Lizard (bite) (venom)	T63.121	T63.122	T63.123	T63.124	--	--
LMD	T45.8X1	T45.8X2	T45.8X3	T45.8X4	T45.8X5	T45.8X6
Lobelia	T62.2X1	T62.2X2	T62.2X3	T62.2X4	--	--
Lobeline	T50.7X1	T50.7X2	T50.7X3	T50.7X4	T50.7X5	T50.7X6
Local action drug NEC	T49.8X1	T49.8X2	T49.8X3	T49.8X4	T49.8X5	T49.8X6
Locorten	T49.0X1	T49.0X2	T49.0X3	T49.0X4	T49.0X5	T49.0X6
Lofepramine	T43.011	T43.012	T43.013	T43.014	T43.015	T43.016
Lolium temulentum	T62.2X1	T62.2X2	T62.2X3	T62.2X4	--	--
Lomotil	T47.6X1	T47.6X2	T47.6X3	T47.6X4	T47.6X5	T47.6X6
Lomustine	T45.1X1	T45.1X2	T45.1X3	T45.1X4	T45.1X5	T45.1X6
Lonidamine	T45.1X1	T45.1X2	T45.1X3	T45.1X4	T45.1X5	T45.1X6
Loperamide	T47.6X1	T47.6X2	T47.6X3	T47.6X4	T47.6X5	T47.6X6
Loprazolam	T42.4X1	T42.4X2	T42.4X3	T42.4X4	T42.4X5	T42.4X6
Lorajmine	T46.2X1	T46.2X2	T46.2X3	T46.2X4	T46.2X5	T46.2X6
Loratidine	T45.0X1	T45.0X2	T45.0X3	T45.0X4	T45.0X5	T45.0X6
Lorazepam	T42.4X1	T42.4X2	T42.4X3	T42.4X4	T42.4X5	T42.4X6
Lorcainide	T46.2X1	T46.2X2	T46.2X3	T46.2X4	T46.2X5	T46.2X6
Lormetazepam	T42.4X1	T42.4X2	T42.4X3	T42.4X4	T42.4X5	T42.4X6
Lotions NEC	T49.91	T49.92	T49.93	T49.94	T49.95	T49.96
Lotusate	T42.3X1	T42.3X2	T42.3X3	T42.3X4	T42.3X5	T42.3X6
Lovastatin	T46.6X1	T46.6X2	T46.6X3	T46.6X4	T46.6X5	T46.6X6
Lowila	T49.2X1	T49.2X2	T49.2X3	T49.2X4	T49.2X5	T49.2X6
Loxapine	T43.591	T43.592	T43.593	T43.594	T43.595	T43.596
Lozenges (throat)	T49.6X1	T49.6X2	T49.6X3	T49.6X4	T49.6X5	T49.6X6
LSD	T40.8X1	T40.8X2	T40.8X3	T40.8X4	--	--
L-Tryptophan — *see* amino acid						
Lubricant, eye	T49.5X1	T49.5X2	T49.5X3	T49.5X4	T49.5X5	T49.5X6
Lubricating oil NEC	T52.0X1	T52.0X2	T52.0X3	T52.0X4	--	--
Lucanthone	T37.4X1	T37.4X2	T37.4X3	T37.4X4	T37.4X5	T37.4X6
Luminal	T42.3X1	T42.3X2	T42.3X3	T42.3X4	T42.3X5	T42.3X6
Lung irritant (gas) NEC	T59.91	T59.92	T59.93	T59.94	--	--
Luteinizing hormone	T38.811	T38.812	T38.813	T38.814	T38.815	T38.816
Lutocylol	T38.5X1	T38.5X2	T38.5X3	T38.5X4	T38.5X5	T38.5X6

Lutromone - Meprylcaine

Substance	Poisoning, Accidental (unintentional)	Poisoning, Intentional self-harm	Poisoning, Assault	Poisoning, Undetermined	Adverse effect	Underdosing
Lutromone	T38.5X1	T38.5X2	T38.5X3	T38.5X4	T38.5X5	T38.5X6
Lututrin	T48.291	T48.292	T48.293	T48.294	T48.295	T48.296
Lye (concentrated)	T54.3X1	T54.3X2	T54.3X3	T54.3X4	--	--
Lygranum (skin test)	T50.8X1	T50.8X2	T50.8X3	T50.8X4	T50.8X5	T50.8X6
Lymecycline	T36.4X1	T36.4X2	T36.4X3	T36.4X4	T36.4X5	T36.4X6
Lymphogranuloma venereum antigen	T50.8X1	T50.8X2	T50.8X3	T50.8X4	T50.8X5	T50.8X6
Lynestrenol	T38.4X1	T38.4X2	T38.4X3	T38.4X4	T38.4X5	T38.4X6
Lyovac Sodium Edecrin	T50.1X1	T50.1X2	T50.1X3	T50.1X4	T50.1X5	T50.1X6
Lypressin	T38.891	T38.892	T38.893	T38.894	T38.895	T38.896
Lysergic acid diethylamide	T40.8X1	T40.8X2	T40.8X3	T40.8X4	--	--
Lysergide	T40.8X1	T40.8X2	T40.8X3	T40.8X4	--	--
Lysine vasopressin	T38.891	T38.892	T38.893	T38.894	T38.895	T38.896
Lysol	T54.1X1	T54.1X2	T54.1X3	T54.1X4	--	--
Lysozyme	T49.0X1	T49.0X2	T49.0X3	T49.0X4	T49.0X5	T49.0X6
Lytta (vitatta)	T49.8X1	T49.8X2	T49.8X3	T49.8X4	T49.8X5	T49.8X6
M						
Mace	T59.3X1	T59.3X2	T59.3X3	T59.3X4	--	--
Macrogol	T50.991	T50.992	T50.993	T50.994	T50.995	T50.996
Macrolide						
anabolic drug	T38.7X1	T38.7X2	T38.7X3	T38.7X4	T38.7X5	T38.7X6
antibiotic	T36.3X1	T36.3X2	T36.3X3	T36.3X4	T36.3X5	T36.3X6
Mafenide	T49.0X1	T49.0X2	T49.0X3	T49.0X4	T49.0X5	T49.0X6
Magaldrate	T47.1X1	T47.1X2	T47.1X3	T47.1X4	T47.1X5	T47.1X6
Magic mushroom	T40.991	T40.992	T40.993	T40.994	--	--
Magnamycin	T36.8X1	T36.8X2	T36.8X3	T36.8X4	T36.8X5	T36.8X6
Magnesia magma	T47.1X1	T47.1X2	T47.1X3	T47.1X4	T47.1X5	T47.1X6
Magnesium NEC	T56.891	T56.892	T56.893	T56.894	--	--
carbonate	T47.1X1	T47.1X2	T47.1X3	T47.1X4	T47.1X5	T47.1X6
citrate	T47.4X1	T47.4X2	T47.4X3	T47.4X4	T47.4X5	T47.4X6
hydroxide	T47.1X1	T47.1X2	T47.1X3	T47.1X4	T47.1X5	T47.1X6
oxide	T47.1X1	T47.1X2	T47.1X3	T47.1X4	T47.1X5	T47.1X6
peroxide	T49.0X1	T49.0X2	T49.0X3	T49.0X4	T49.0X5	T49.0X6
salicylate	T39.091	T39.092	T39.093	T39.094	T39.095	T39.096
silicofluoride	T50.3X1	T50.3X2	T50.3X3	T50.3X4	T50.3X5	T50.3X6
sulfate	T47.4X1	T47.4X2	T47.4X3	T47.4X4	T47.4X5	T47.4X6
thiosulfate	T45.0X1	T45.0X2	T45.0X3	T45.0X4	T45.0X5	T45.0X6
trisilicate	T47.1X1	T47.1X2	T47.1X3	T47.1X4	T47.1X5	T47.1X6
Malathion (medicinal)	T49.0X1	T49.0X2	T49.0X3	T49.0X4	T49.0X5	T49.0X6
insecticide	T60.0X1	T60.0X2	T60.0X3	T60.0X4	--	--
Male fern extract	T37.4X1	T37.4X2	T37.4X3	T37.4X4	T37.4X5	T37.4X6
M-AMSA	T45.1X1	T45.1X2	T45.1X3	T45.1X4	T45.1X5	T45.1X6
Mandelic acid	T37.8X1	T37.8X2	T37.8X3	T37.8X4	T37.8X5	T37.8X6
Manganese (dioxide) (salts)	T57.2X1	T57.2X2	T57.2X3	T57.2X4	--	--
medicinal	T50.991	T50.992	T50.993	T50.994	T50.995	T50.996
Mannitol	T47.3X1	T47.3X2	T47.3X3	T47.3X4	T47.3X5	T47.3X6
hexanitrate	T46.3X1	T46.3X2	T46.3X3	T46.3X4	T46.3X5	T46.3X6
Mannomustine	T45.1X1	T45.1X2	T45.1X3	T45.1X4	T45.1X5	T45.1X6
MAO inhibitors	T43.1X1	T43.1X2	T43.1X3	T43.1X4	T43.1X5	T43.1X6
Mapharsen	T37.8X1	T37.8X2	T37.8X3	T37.8X4	T37.8X5	T37.8X6
Maphenide	T49.0X1	T49.0X2	T49.0X3	T49.0X4	T49.0X5	T49.0X6
Maprotiline	T43.021	T43.022	T43.023	T43.024	T43.025	T43.026
Marcaine	T41.3X1	T41.3X2	T41.3X3	T41.3X4	T41.3X5	T41.3X6
infiltration (subcutaneous)	T41.3X1	T41.3X2	T41.3X3	T41.3X4	T41.3X5	T41.3X6
nerve block (peripheral) (plexus)	T41.3X1	T41.3X2	T41.3X3	T41.3X4	T41.3X5	T41.3X6
Marezine	T45.0X1	T45.0X2	T45.0X3	T45.0X4	T45.0X5	T45.0X6
Marihuana	T40.7X1	T40.7X2	T40.7X3	T40.7X4	T40.7X5	T40.7X6
Marijuana	T40.7X1	T40.7X2	T40.7X3	T40.7X4	T40.7X5	T40.7X6
Marine (sting)	T63.691	T63.692	T63.693	T63.694	--	--
animals (sting)	T63.691	T63.692	T63.693	T63.694	--	--
plants (sting)	T63.711	T63.712	T63.713	T63.714	--	--
Marplan	T43.1X1	T43.1X2	T43.1X3	T43.1X4	T43.1X5	T43.1X6
Marsh gas	T59.891	T59.892	T59.893	T59.894	--	--
Marsilid	T43.1X1	T43.1X2	T43.1X3	T43.1X4	T43.1X5	T43.1X6
Matulane	T45.1X1	T45.1X2	T45.1X3	T45.1X4	T45.1X5	T45.1X6
Mazindol	T50.5X1	T50.5X2	T50.5X3	T50.5X4	T50.5X5	T50.5X6
MCPA	T60.3X1	T60.3X2	T60.3X3	T60.3X4	--	--
MDMA	T43.641	T43.642	T43.643	T43.644	--	--
Meadow saffron	T62.2X1	T62.2X2	T62.2X3	T62.2X4	--	--
Measles virus vaccine (attenuated)	T50.B91	T50.B92	T50.B93	T50.B94	T50.B95	T50.B96
Meat, noxious	T62.8X1	T62.8X2	T62.8X3	T62.8X4	--	--
Meballymal	T42.3X1	T42.3X2	T42.3X3	T42.3X4	T42.3X5	T42.3X6
Mebanazine	T43.1X1	T43.1X2	T43.1X3	T43.1X4	T43.1X5	T43.1X6
Mebaral	T42.3X1	T42.3X2	T42.3X3	T42.3X4	T42.3X5	T42.3X6
Mebendazole	T37.4X1	T37.4X2	T37.4X3	T37.4X4	T37.4X5	T37.4X6
Mebeverine	T44.3X1	T44.3X2	T44.3X3	T44.3X4	T44.3X5	T44.3X6
Mebhydrolin	T45.0X1	T45.0X2	T45.0X3	T45.0X4	T45.0X5	T45.0X6
Mebumal	T42.3X1	T42.3X2	T42.3X3	T42.3X4	T42.3X5	T42.3X6
Mebutamate	T43.591	T43.592	T43.593	T43.594	T43.595	T43.596
Mecamylamine	T44.2X1	T44.2X2	T44.2X3	T44.2X4	T44.2X5	T44.2X6
Mechlorethamine	T45.1X1	T45.1X2	T45.1X3	T45.1X4	T45.1X5	T45.1X6
Mecillinam	T36.0X1	T36.0X2	T36.0X3	T36.0X4	T36.0X5	T36.0X6
Meclizine (hydrochloride)	T45.0X1	T45.0X2	T45.0X3	T45.0X4	T45.0X5	T45.0X6
Meclocycline	T36.4X1	T36.4X2	T36.4X3	T36.4X4	T36.4X5	T36.4X6
Meclofenamate	T39.391	T39.392	T39.393	T39.394	T39.395	T39.396
Meclofenamic acid	T39.391	T39.392	T39.393	T39.394	T39.395	T39.396
Meclofenoxate	T43.691	T43.692	T43.693	T43.694	T43.695	T43.696
Meclozine	T45.0X1	T45.0X2	T45.0X3	T45.0X4	T45.0X5	T45.0X6
Mecobalamin	T45.8X1	T45.8X2	T45.8X3	T45.8X4	T45.8X5	T45.8X6
Mecoprop	T60.3X1	T60.3X2	T60.3X3	T60.3X4	--	--
Mecrilate	T49.3X1	T49.3X2	T49.3X3	T49.3X4	T49.3X5	T49.3X6
Mecysteine	T48.4X1	T48.4X2	T48.4X3	T48.4X4	T48.4X5	T48.4X6
Medazepam	T42.4X1	T42.4X2	T42.4X3	T42.4X4	T42.4X5	T42.4X6
Medicament NEC	T50.901	T50.902	T50.903	T50.904	T50.905	T50.906
Medinal	T42.3X1	T42.3X2	T42.3X3	T42.3X4	T42.3X5	T42.3X6
Medomin	T42.3X1	T42.3X2	T42.3X3	T42.3X4	T42.3X5	T42.3X6
Medrogestone	T38.5X1	T38.5X2	T38.5X3	T38.5X4	T38.5X5	T38.5X6
Medroxalol	T44.8X1	T44.8X2	T44.8X3	T44.8X4	T44.8X5	T44.8X6
Medroxyprogesterone acetate (depot)	T38.5X1	T38.5X2	T38.5X3	T38.5X4	T38.5X5	T38.5X6
Medrysone	T49.0X1	T49.0X2	T49.0X3	T49.0X4	T49.0X5	T49.0X6
Mefenamic acid	T39.391	T39.392	T39.393	T39.394	T39.395	T39.396
Mefenorex	T50.5X1	T50.5X2	T50.5X3	T50.5X4	T50.5X5	T50.5X6
Mefloquine	T37.2X1	T37.2X2	T37.2X3	T37.2X4	T37.2X5	T37.2X6
Mefruside	T50.2X1	T50.2X2	T50.2X3	T50.2X4	T50.2X5	T50.2X6
Megahallucinogen	T40.901	T40.902	T40.903	T40.904	T40.905	T40.906
Megestrol	T38.5X1	T38.5X2	T38.5X3	T38.5X4	T38.5X5	T38.5X6
Meglumine						
antimoniate	T37.8X1	T37.8X2	T37.8X3	T37.8X4	T37.8X5	T37.8X6
diatrizoate	T50.8X1	T50.8X2	T50.8X3	T50.8X4	T50.8X5	T50.8X6
iodipamide	T50.8X1	T50.8X2	T50.8X3	T50.8X4	T50.8X5	T50.8X6
iotroxate	T50.8X1	T50.8X2	T50.8X3	T50.8X4	T50.8X5	T50.8X6
MEK (methyl ethyl ketone)	T52.4X1	T52.4X2	T52.4X3	T52.4X4	--	--
Meladinin	T49.3X1	T49.3X2	T49.3X3	T49.3X4	T49.3X5	T49.3X6
Meladrazine	T44.3X1	T44.3X2	T44.3X3	T44.3X4	T44.3X5	T44.3X6
Melaleuca alternifolia oil	T49.0X1	T49.0X2	T49.0X3	T49.0X4	T49.0X5	T49.0X6
Melanizing agents	T49.3X1	T49.3X2	T49.3X3	T49.3X4	T49.3X5	T49.3X6
Melanocyte-stimulating hormone	T38.891	T38.892	T38.893	T38.894	T38.895	T38.896
Melarsonyl potassium	T37.3X1	T37.3X2	T37.3X3	T37.3X4	T37.3X5	T37.3X6
Melarsoprol	T37.3X1	T37.3X2	T37.3X3	T37.3X4	T37.3X5	T37.3X6
Melia azedarach	T62.2X1	T62.2X2	T62.2X3	T62.2X4	--	--
Melitracen	T43.011	T43.012	T43.013	T43.014	T43.015	T43.016
Mellaril	T43.3X1	T43.3X2	T43.3X3	T43.3X4	T43.3X5	T43.3X6
Meloxine	T49.3X1	T49.3X2	T49.3X3	T49.3X4	T49.3X5	T49.3X6
Melperone	T43.4X1	T43.4X2	T43.4X3	T43.4X4	T43.4X5	T43.4X6
Melphalan	T45.1X1	T45.1X2	T45.1X3	T45.1X4	T45.1X5	T45.1X6
Memantine	T43.8X1	T43.8X2	T43.8X3	T43.8X4	T43.8X5	T43.8X6
Menadiol	T45.7X1	T45.7X2	T45.7X3	T45.7X4	T45.7X5	T45.7X6
sodium sulfate	T45.7X1	T45.7X2	T45.7X3	T45.7X4	T45.7X5	T45.7X6
Menadione	T45.7X1	T45.7X2	T45.7X3	T45.7X4	T45.7X5	T45.7X6
sodium bisulfite	T45.7X1	T45.7X2	T45.7X3	T45.7X4	T45.7X5	T45.7X6
Menaphthone	T45.7X1	T45.7X2	T45.7X3	T45.7X4	T45.7X5	T45.7X6
Menaquinone	T45.7X1	T45.7X2	T45.7X3	T45.7X4	T45.7X5	T45.7X6
Menatetrenone	T45.7X1	T45.7X2	T45.7X3	T45.7X4	T45.7X5	T45.7X6
Meningococcal vaccine	T50.A91	T50.A92	T50.A93	T50.A94	T50.A95	T50.A96
Menningovax (-AC) (-C)	T50.A91	T50.A92	T50.A93	T50.A94	T50.A95	T50.A96
Menotropins	T38.811	T38.812	T38.813	T38.814	T38.815	T38.816
Menthol	T48.5X1	T48.5X2	T48.5X3	T48.5X4	T48.5X5	T48.5X6
Mepacrine	T37.2X1	T37.2X2	T37.2X3	T37.2X4	T37.2X5	T37.2X6
Meparfynol	T42.6X1	T42.6X2	T42.6X3	T42.6X4	T42.6X5	T42.6X6
Mepartricin	T36.7X1	T36.7X2	T36.7X3	T36.7X4	T36.7X5	T36.7X6
Mepazine	T43.3X1	T43.3X2	T43.3X3	T43.3X4	T43.3X5	T43.3X6
Mepenzolate	T44.3X1	T44.3X2	T44.3X3	T44.3X4	T44.3X5	T44.3X6
bromide	T44.3X1	T44.3X2	T44.3X3	T44.3X4	T44.3X5	T44.3X6
Meperidine	T40.4X1	T40.4X2	T40.4X3	T40.4X4	T40.4X5	T40.4X6
Mephebarbital	T42.3X1	T42.3X2	T42.3X3	T42.3X4	T42.3X5	T42.3X6
Mephenamin (e)	T42.8X1	T42.8X2	T42.8X3	T42.8X4	T42.8X5	T42.8X6
Mephenesin	T42.8X1	T42.8X2	T42.8X3	T42.8X4	T42.8X5	T42.8X6
Mephenhydramine	T45.0X1	T45.0X2	T45.0X3	T45.0X4	T45.0X5	T45.0X6
Mephenoxalone	T42.8X1	T42.8X2	T42.8X3	T42.8X4	T42.8X5	T42.8X6
Mephentermine	T44.991	T44.992	T44.993	T44.994	T44.995	T44.996
Mephenytoin	T42.0X1	T42.0X2	T42.0X3	T42.0X4	T42.0X5	T42.0X6
with phenobarbital	T42.3X1	T42.3X2	T42.3X3	T42.3X4	T42.3X5	T42.3X6
Mephobarbital	T42.3X1	T42.3X2	T42.3X3	T42.3X4	T42.3X5	T42.3X6
Mephosfolan	T60.0X1	T60.0X2	T60.0X3	T60.0X4	--	--
Mepindolol	T44.7X1	T44.7X2	T44.7X3	T44.7X4	T44.7X5	T44.7X6
Mepiperphenidol	T44.3X1	T44.3X2	T44.3X3	T44.3X4	T44.3X5	T44.3X6
Mepitiostane	T38.7X1	T38.7X2	T38.7X3	T38.7X4	T38.7X5	T38.7X6
Mepivacaine	T41.3X1	T41.3X2	T41.3X3	T41.3X4	T41.3X5	T41.3X6
epidural	T41.3X1	T41.3X2	T41.3X3	T41.3X4	T41.3X5	T41.3X6
Meprednisone	T38.0X1	T38.0X2	T38.0X3	T38.0X4	T38.0X5	T38.0X6
Meprobam	T43.591	T43.592	T43.593	T43.594	T43.595	T43.596
Meprobamate	T43.591	T43.592	T43.593	T43.594	T43.595	T43.596
Meproscillarin	T46.0X1	T46.0X2	T46.0X3	T46.0X4	T46.0X5	T46.0X6
Meprylcaine	T41.3X1	T41.3X2	T41.3X3	T41.3X4	T41.3X5	T41.3X6

Substance	Poisoning, Accidental (unintentional)	Poisoning, Intentional self-harm	Poisoning, Assault	Poisoning, Undetermined	Adverse effect	Underdosing
Meptazinol	T39.8X1	T39.8X2	T39.8X3	T39.8X4	T39.8X5	T39.8X6
Mepyramine	T45.0X1	T45.0X2	T45.0X3	T45.0X4	T45.0X5	T45.0X6
Mequitazine	T43.3X1	T43.3X2	T43.3X3	T43.3X4	T43.3X5	T43.3X6
Meralluride	T50.2X1	T50.2X2	T50.2X3	T50.2X4	T50.2X5	T50.2X6
Merbaphen	T50.2X1	T50.2X2	T50.2X3	T50.2X4	T50.2X5	T50.2X6
Merbromin	T49.0X1	T49.0X2	T49.0X3	T49.0X4	T49.0X5	T49.0X6
Mercaptobenzothiazole salts	T49.0X1	T49.0X2	T49.0X3	T49.0X4	T49.0X5	T49.0X6
Mercaptomerin	T50.2X1	T50.2X2	T50.2X3	T50.2X4	T50.2X5	T50.2X6
Mercaptopurine	T45.1X1	T45.1X2	T45.1X3	T45.1X4	T45.1X5	T45.1X6
Mercumatilin	T50.2X1	T50.2X2	T50.2X3	T50.2X4	T50.2X5	T50.2X6
Mercuramide	T50.2X1	T50.2X2	T50.2X3	T50.2X4	T50.2X5	T50.2X6
Mercurochrome	T49.0X1	T49.0X2	T49.0X3	T49.0X4	T49.0X5	T49.0X6
Mercurophylline	T50.2X1	T50.2X2	T50.2X3	T50.2X4	T50.2X5	T50.2X6
Mercury, mercurial, mercuric, mercurous (compounds) (cyanide) (fumes) (nonmedicinal) (vapor) **NEC**	T56.1X1	T56.1X2	T56.1X3	T56.1X4	--	--
ammoniated	T49.0X1	T49.0X2	T49.0X3	T49.0X4	T49.0X5	T49.0X6
anti-infective						
local	T49.0X1	T49.0X2	T49.0X3	T49.0X4	T49.0X5	T49.0X6
systemic	T37.8X1	T37.8X2	T37.8X3	T37.8X4	T37.8X5	T37.8X6
topical	T49.0X1	T49.0X2	T49.0X3	T49.0X4	T49.0X5	T49.0X6
chloride (ammoniated)	T49.0X1	T49.0X2	T49.0X3	T49.0X4	T49.0X5	T49.0X6
fungicide	T56.1X1	T56.1X2	T56.1X3	T56.1X4	--	--
diuretic NEC	T50.2X1	T50.2X2	T50.2X3	T50.2X4	T50.2X5	T50.2X6
fungicide	T56.1X1	T56.1X2	T56.1X3	T56.1X4	--	--
organic (fungicide)	T56.1X1	T56.1X2	T56.1X3	T56.1X4	--	--
oxide, yellow	T49.0X1	T49.0X2	T49.0X3	T49.0X4	T49.0X5	T49.0X6
Mersalyl	T50.2X1	T50.2X2	T50.2X3	T50.2X4	T50.2X5	T50.2X6
Merthiolate	T49.0X1	T49.0X2	T49.0X3	T49.0X4	T49.0X5	T49.0X6
ophthalmic preparation	T49.5X1	T49.5X2	T49.5X3	T49.5X4	T49.5X5	T49.5X6
Meruvax	T50.B91	T50.B92	T50.B93	T50.B94	T50.B95	T50.B96
Mesalazine	T47.8X1	T47.8X2	T47.8X3	T47.8X4	T47.8X5	T47.8X6
Mescal buttons	T40.991	T40.992	T40.993	T40.994	--	--
Mescaline	T40.991	T40.992	T40.993	T40.994	--	--
Mesna	T48.4X1	T48.4X2	T48.4X3	T48.4X4	T48.4X5	T48.4X6
Mesoglycan	T46.6X1	T46.6X2	T46.6X3	T46.6X4	T46.6X5	T46.6X6
Mesoridazine	T43.3X1	T43.3X2	T43.3X3	T43.3X4	T43.3X5	T43.3X6
Mestanolone	T38.7X1	T38.7X2	T38.7X3	T38.7X4	T38.7X5	T38.7X6
Mesterolone	T38.7X1	T38.7X2	T38.7X3	T38.7X4	T38.7X5	T38.7X6
Mestranol	T38.5X1	T38.5X2	T38.5X3	T38.5X4	T38.5X5	T38.5X6
Mesulergine	T42.8X1	T42.8X2	T42.8X3	T42.8X4	T42.8X5	T42.8X6
Mesulfen	T49.0X1	T49.0X2	T49.0X3	T49.0X4	T49.0X5	T49.0X6
Mesuximide	T42.2X1	T42.2X2	T42.2X3	T42.2X4	T42.2X5	T42.2X6
Metabutethamine	T41.3X1	T41.3X2	T41.3X3	T41.3X4	T41.3X5	T41.3X6
Metactesylacetate	T49.0X1	T49.0X2	T49.0X3	T49.0X4	T49.0X5	T49.0X6
Metacycline	T36.4X1	T36.4X2	T36.4X3	T36.4X4	T36.4X5	T36.4X6
Metaldehyde (snail killer) **NEC**	T60.8X1	T60.8X2	T60.8X3	T60.8X4	--	--
Metals (heavy) (nonmedicinal)	T56.91	T56.92	T56.93	T56.94	--	--
dust, fumes, or vapor NEC	T56.91	T56.92	T56.93	T56.94	--	--
light NEC	T56.91	T56.92	T56.93	T56.94	--	--
dust, fumes, or vapor NEC	T56.91	T56.92	T56.93	T56.94	--	--
specified NEC	T56.891	T56.892	T56.893	T56.894	--	--
thallium	T56.811	T56.812	T56.813	T56.814	--	--
Metamfetamine	T43.621	T43.622	T43.623	T43.624	T43.625	T43.626
Metamizole sodium	T39.2X1	T39.2X2	T39.2X3	T39.2X4	T39.2X5	T39.2X6
Metampicillin	T36.0X1	T36.0X2	T36.0X3	T36.0X4	T36.0X5	T36.0X6
Metamucil	T47.4X1	T47.4X2	T47.4X3	T47.4X4	T47.4X5	T47.4X6
Metandienone	T38.7X1	T38.7X2	T38.7X3	T38.7X4	T38.7X5	T38.7X6
Metandrostenolone	T38.7X1	T38.7X2	T38.7X3	T38.7X4	T38.7X5	T38.7X6
Metaphen	T49.0X1	T49.0X2	T49.0X3	T49.0X4	T49.0X5	T49.0X6
Metaphos	T60.0X1	T60.0X2	T60.0X3	T60.0X4	--	--
Metapramine	T43.011	T43.012	T43.013	T43.014	T43.015	T43.016
Metaproterenol	T48.291	T48.292	T48.293	T48.294	T48.295	T48.296
Metaraminol	T44.4X1	T44.4X2	T44.4X3	T44.4X4	T44.4X5	T44.4X6
Metaxalone	T42.8X1	T42.8X2	T42.8X3	T42.8X4	T42.8X5	T42.8X6
Metenolone	T38.7X1	T38.7X2	T38.7X3	T38.7X4	T38.7X5	T38.7X6
Metergoline	T42.8X1	T42.8X2	T42.8X3	T42.8X4	T42.8X5	T42.8X6
Metescufylline	T46.991	T46.992	T46.993	T46.994	T46.995	T46.996
Metetoin	T42.0X1	T42.0X2	T42.0X3	T42.0X4	T42.0X5	T42.0X6
Metformin	T38.3X1	T38.3X2	T38.3X3	T38.3X4	T38.3X5	T38.3X6
Methacholine	T44.1X1	T44.1X2	T44.1X3	T44.1X4	T44.1X5	T44.1X6
Methacycline	T36.4X1	T36.4X2	T36.4X3	T36.4X4	T36.4X5	T36.4X6
Methadone	T40.3X1	T40.3X2	T40.3X3	T40.3X4	T40.3X5	T40.3X6
Methallenestril	T38.5X1	T38.5X2	T38.5X3	T38.5X4	T38.5X5	T38.5X6
Methallenoestril	T38.5X1	T38.5X2	T38.5X3	T38.5X4	T38.5X5	T38.5X6
Methamphetamine	T43.621	T43.622	T43.623	T43.624	T43.625	T43.626
Methampyrone	T39.2X1	T39.2X2	T39.2X3	T39.2X4	T39.2X5	T39.2X6
Methandienone	T38.7X1	T38.7X2	T38.7X3	T38.7X4	T38.7X5	T38.7X6
Methandriol	T38.7X1	T38.7X2	T38.7X3	T38.7X4	T38.7X5	T38.7X6
Methandrostenolone	T38.7X1	T38.7X2	T38.7X3	T38.7X4	T38.7X5	T38.7X6
Methane	T59.891	T59.892	T59.893	T59.894	--	--
Methanethiol	T59.891	T59.892	T59.893	T59.894	--	--
Methaniazide	T37.1X1	T37.1X2	T37.1X3	T37.1X4	T37.1X5	T37.1X6
Methanol (vapor)	T51.1X1	T51.1X2	T51.1X3	T51.1X4	--	--
Methantheline	T44.3X1	T44.3X2	T44.3X3	T44.3X4	T44.3X5	T44.3X6
Methanthelinium bromide	T44.3X1	T44.3X2	T44.3X3	T44.3X4	T44.3X5	T44.3X6
Methaphenilene	T45.0X1	T45.0X2	T45.0X3	T45.0X4	T45.0X5	T45.0X6
Methapyrilene	T45.0X1	T45.0X2	T45.0X3	T45.0X4	T45.0X5	T45.0X6
Methaqualone (compound)	T42.6X1	T42.6X2	T42.6X3	T42.6X4	T42.6X5	T42.6X6
Metharbital	T42.3X1	T42.3X2	T42.3X3	T42.3X4	T42.3X5	T42.3X6
Methazolamide	T50.2X1	T50.2X2	T50.2X3	T50.2X4	T50.2X5	T50.2X6
Methdilazine	T43.3X1	T43.3X2	T43.3X3	T43.3X4	T43.3X5	T43.3X6
Methedrine	T43.621	T43.622	T43.623	T43.624	T43.625	T43.626
Methenamine (mandelate)	T37.8X1	T37.8X2	T37.8X3	T37.8X4	T37.8X5	T37.8X6
Methenolone	T38.7X1	T38.7X2	T38.7X3	T38.7X4	T38.7X5	T38.7X6
Methergine	T48.0X1	T48.0X2	T48.0X3	T48.0X4	T48.0X5	T48.0X6
Methetoin	T42.0X1	T42.0X2	T42.0X3	T42.0X4	T42.0X5	T42.0X6
Methiacil	T38.2X1	T38.2X2	T38.2X3	T38.2X4	T38.2X5	T38.2X6
Methicillin	T36.0X1	T36.0X2	T36.0X3	T36.0X4	T36.0X5	T36.0X6
Methimazole	T38.2X1	T38.2X2	T38.2X3	T38.2X4	T38.2X5	T38.2X6
Methiodal sodium	T50.8X1	T50.8X2	T50.8X3	T50.8X4	T50.8X5	T50.8X6
Methionine	T50.991	T50.992	T50.993	T50.994	T50.995	T50.996
Methisazone	T37.5X1	T37.5X2	T37.5X3	T37.5X4	T37.5X5	T37.5X6
Methisoprinol	T37.5X1	T37.5X2	T37.5X3	T37.5X4	T37.5X5	T37.5X6
Methitural	T42.3X1	T42.3X2	T42.3X3	T42.3X4	T42.3X5	T42.3X6
Methixene	T44.3X1	T44.3X2	T44.3X3	T44.3X4	T44.3X5	T44.3X6
Methobarbital, methobarbitone	T42.3X1	T42.3X2	T42.3X3	T42.3X4	T42.3X5	T42.3X6
Methocarbamol	T42.8X1	T42.8X2	T42.8X3	T42.8X4	T42.8X5	T42.8X6
skeletal muscle relaxant	T48.1X1	T48.1X2	T48.1X3	T48.1X4	T48.1X5	T48.1X6
Methohexital	T41.1X1	T41.1X2	T41.1X3	T41.1X4	T41.1X5	T41.1X6
Methohexitone	T41.1X1	T41.1X2	T41.1X3	T41.1X4	T41.1X5	T41.1X6
Methoin	T42.0X1	T42.0X2	T42.0X3	T42.0X4	T42.0X5	T42.0X6
Methopholine	T39.8X1	T39.8X2	T39.8X3	T39.8X4	T39.8X5	T39.8X6
Methopromazine	T43.3X1	T43.3X2	T43.3X3	T43.3X4	T43.3X5	T43.3X6
Methorate	T48.3X1	T48.3X2	T48.3X3	T48.3X4	T48.3X5	T48.3X6
Methoserpidine	T46.5X1	T46.5X2	T46.5X3	T46.5X4	T46.5X5	T46.5X6
Methotrexate	T45.1X1	T45.1X2	T45.1X3	T45.1X4	T45.1X5	T45.1X6
Methotrimeprazine	T43.3X1	T43.3X2	T43.3X3	T43.3X4	T43.3X5	T43.3X6
Methoxa-Dome	T49.3X1	T49.3X2	T49.3X3	T49.3X4	T49.3X5	T49.3X6
Methoxamine	T44.4X1	T44.4X2	T44.4X3	T44.4X4	T44.4X5	T44.4X6
Methoxsalen	T50.991	T50.992	T50.993	T50.994	T50.995	T50.996
Methoxyaniline	T65.3X1	T65.3X2	T65.3X3	T65.3X4	--	--
Methoxybenzyl penicillin	T36.0X1	T36.0X2	T36.0X3	T36.0X4	T36.0X5	T36.0X6
Methoxychlor	T53.7X1	T53.7X2	T53.7X3	T53.7X4	--	--
Methoxy-DDT	T53.7X1	T53.7X2	T53.7X3	T53.7X4	--	--
2-Methoxyethanol	T52.3X1	T52.3X2	T52.3X3	T52.3X4	--	--
Methoxyflurane	T41.0X1	T41.0X2	T41.0X3	T41.0X4	T41.0X5	T41.0X6
Methoxyphenamine	T48.6X1	T48.6X2	T48.6X3	T48.6X4	T48.6X5	T48.6X6
Methoxypromazine	T43.3X1	T43.3X2	T43.3X3	T43.3X4	T43.3X5	T43.3X6
5-Methoxypsoralen (5-MOP)	T50.991	T50.992	T50.993	T50.994	T50.995	T50.996
8-Methoxypsoralen (8-MOP)	T50.991	T50.992	T50.993	T50.994	T50.995	T50.996
Methscopolamine bromide	T44.3X1	T44.3X2	T44.3X3	T44.3X4	T44.3X5	T44.3X6
Methsuximide	T42.2X1	T42.2X2	T42.2X3	T42.2X4	T42.2X5	T42.2X6
Methyclothiazide	T50.2X1	T50.2X2	T50.2X3	T50.2X4	T50.2X5	T50.2X6
Methyl						
acetate	T52.4X1	T52.4X2	T52.4X3	T52.4X4	--	--
acetone	T52.4X1	T52.4X2	T52.4X3	T52.4X4	--	--
acrylate	T65.891	T65.892	T65.893	T65.894	--	--
alcohol	T51.1X1	T51.1X2	T51.1X3	T51.1X4	--	--
aminophenol	T65.3X1	T65.3X2	T65.3X3	T65.3X4	--	--
amphetamine	T43.621	T43.622	T43.623	T43.624	T43.625	T43.626
androstanolone	T38.7X1	T38.7X2	T38.7X3	T38.7X4	T38.7X5	T38.7X6
atropine	T44.3X1	T44.3X2	T44.3X3	T44.3X4	T44.3X5	T44.3X6
benzene	T52.2X1	T52.2X2	T52.2X3	T52.2X4	--	--
benzoate	T52.8X1	T52.8X2	T52.8X3	T52.8X4	--	--
benzol	T52.2X1	T52.2X2	T52.2X3	T52.2X4	--	--
bromide (gas)	T59.891	T59.892	T59.893	T59.894	--	--
fumigant	T60.8X1	T60.8X2	T60.8X3	T60.8X4	--	--
butanol	T51.3X1	T51.3X2	T51.3X3	T51.3X4	--	--
carbinol	T51.1X1	T51.1X2	T51.1X3	T51.1X4	--	--
carbonate	T52.8X1	T52.8X2	T52.8X3	T52.8X4	--	--
CCNU	T45.1X1	T45.1X2	T45.1X3	T45.1X4	T45.1X5	T45.1X6
cellosolve	T52.91	T52.92	T52.93	T52.94	--	--
cellulose	T47.4X1	T47.4X2	T47.4X3	T47.4X4	T47.4X5	T47.4X6
chloride (gas)	T59.891	T59.892	T59.893	T59.894	--	--
chloroformate	T59.3X1	T59.3X2	T59.3X3	T59.3X4	--	--
cyclohexane	T52.8X1	T52.8X2	T52.8X3	T52.8X4	--	--
cyclohexanol	T51.8X1	T51.8X2	T51.8X3	T51.8X4	--	--
cyclohexanone	T52.8X1	T52.8X2	T52.8X3	T52.8X4	--	--
cyclohexyl acetate	T52.8X1	T52.8X2	T52.8X3	T52.8X4	--	--
demeton	T60.0X1	T60.0X2	T60.0X3	T60.0X4	--	--
dihydromorphinone	T40.2X1	T40.2X2	T40.2X3	T40.2X4	T40.2X5	T40.2X6
ergometrine	T48.0X1	T48.0X2	T48.0X3	T48.0X4	T48.0X5	T48.0X6
ergonovine	T48.0X1	T48.0X2	T48.0X3	T48.0X4	T48.0X5	T48.0X6
ethyl ketone	T52.4X1	T52.4X2	T52.4X3	T52.4X4	--	--

Methyl - Monoxidine hydrochloride

Substance	Poisoning, Accidental (unintentional)	Poisoning, Intentional self-harm	Poisoning, Assault	Poisoning, Undetermined	Adverse effect	Underdosing
Methyl — *continued*						
glucamine antimonate	T37.8X1	T37.8X2	T37.8X3	T37.8X4	T37.8X5	T37.8X6
hydrazine	T65.891	T65.892	T65.893	T65.894	--	--
iodide	T65.891	T65.892	T65.893	T65.894	--	--
isobutyl ketone	T52.4X1	T52.4X2	T52.4X3	T52.4X4	--	--
isothiocyanate	T60.3X1	T60.3X2	T60.3X3	T60.3X4	--	--
mercaptan	T59.891	T59.892	T59.893	T59.894	--	--
morphine NEC	T40.2X1	T40.2X2	T40.2X3	T40.2X4	T40.2X5	T40.2X6
nicotinate	T49.4X1	T49.4X2	T49.4X3	T49.4X4	T49.4X5	T49.4X6
paraben	T49.0X1	T49.0X2	T49.0X3	T49.0X4	T49.0X5	T49.0X6
parafynol	T42.6X1	T42.6X2	T42.6X3	T42.6X4	T42.6X5	T42.6X6
parathion	T60.0X1	T60.0X2	T60.0X3	T60.0X4	--	--
peridol	T43.4X1	T43.4X2	T43.4X3	T43.4X4	T43.4X5	T43.4X6
phenidate	T43.631	T43.632	T43.633	T43.634	T43.635	T43.636
prednisolone	T38.0X1	T38.0X2	T38.0X3	T38.0X4	T38.0X5	T38.0X6
ENT agent	T49.6X1	T49.6X2	T49.6X3	T49.6X4	T49.6X5	T49.6X6
ophthalmic preparation	T49.5X1	T49.5X2	T49.5X3	T49.5X4	T49.5X5	T49.5X6
topical NEC	T49.0X1	T49.0X2	T49.0X3	T49.0X4	T49.0X5	T49.0X6
propylcarbinol	T51.3X1	T51.3X2	T51.3X3	T51.3X4	--	--
rosaniline NEC	T49.0X1	T49.0X2	T49.0X3	T49.0X4	T49.0X5	T49.0X6
salicylate	T49.2X1	T49.2X2	T49.2X3	T49.2X4	T49.2X5	T49.2X6
sulfate (fumes)	T59.891	T59.892	T59.893	T59.894	--	--
liquid	T52.8X1	T52.8X2	T52.8X3	T52.8X4	--	--
sulfonal	T42.6X1	T42.6X2	T42.6X3	T42.6X4	T42.6X5	T42.6X6
testosterone	T38.7X1	T38.7X2	T38.7X3	T38.7X4	T38.7X5	T38.7X6
thiouracil	T38.2X1	T38.2X2	T38.2X3	T38.2X4	T38.2X5	T38.2X6
Methylamphetamine	T43.621	T43.622	T43.623	T43.624	T43.625	T43.626
Methylated spirit	T51.1X1	T51.1X2	T51.1X3	T51.1X4	--	--
Methylatropine nitrate	T44.3X1	T44.3X2	T44.3X3	T44.3X4	T44.3X5	T44.3X6
Methylbenactyzium bromide	T44.3X1	T44.3X2	T44.3X3	T44.3X4	T44.3X5	T44.3X6
Methylbenzethonium chloride	T49.0X1	T49.0X2	T49.0X3	T49.0X4	T49.0X5	T49.0X6
Methylcellulose	T47.4X1	T47.4X2	T47.4X3	T47.4X4	T47.4X5	T47.4X6
laxative	T47.4X1	T47.4X2	T47.4X3	T47.4X4	T47.4X5	T47.4X6
Methylchlorophenoxy-acetic acid	T60.3X1	T60.3X2	T60.3X3	T60.3X4	--	--
Methyldopa	T46.5X1	T46.5X2	T46.5X3	T46.5X4	T46.5X5	T46.5X6
Methyldopate	T46.5X1	T46.5X2	T46.5X3	T46.5X4	T46.5X5	T46.5X6
Methylene						
blue	T50.6X1	T50.6X2	T50.6X3	T50.6X4	T50.6X5	T50.6X6
chloride or dichloride (solvent) NEC	T53.4X1	T53.4X2	T53.4X3	T53.4X4	--	--
Methylenedioxyamphet-amine	T43.621	T43.622	T43.623	T43.624	T43.625	T43.626
Methylenedioxymetham-phetamine	T43.641	T43.642	T43.643	T43.644	--	--
Methylergometrine	T48.0X1	T48.0X2	T48.0X3	T48.0X4	T48.0X5	T48.0X6
Methylergonovine	T48.0X1	T48.0X2	T48.0X3	T48.0X4	T48.0X5	T48.0X6
Methylestrenolone	T38.5X1	T38.5X2	T38.5X3	T38.5X4	T38.5X5	T38.5X6
Methylethyl cellulose	T50.991	T50.992	T50.993	T50.994	T50.995	T50.996
Methylhexabital	T42.3X1	T42.3X2	T42.3X3	T42.3X4	T42.3X5	T42.3X6
Methylmorphine	T40.2X1	T40.2X2	T40.2X3	T40.2X4	T40.2X5	T40.2X6
Methylparaben (ophthalmic)	T49.5X1	T49.5X2	T49.5X3	T49.5X4	T49.5X5	T49.5X6
Methylparafynol	T42.6X1	T42.6X2	T42.6X3	T42.6X4	T42.6X5	T42.6X6
Methylpentynol, methylpenthynol	T42.6X1	T42.6X2	T42.6X3	T42.6X4	T42.6X5	T42.6X6
Methylphenidate	T43.631	T43.632	T43.633	T43.634	T43.635	T43.636
Methylphenobarbital	T42.3X1	T42.3X2	T42.3X3	T42.3X4	T42.3X5	T42.3X6
Methylpolysiloxane	T47.1X1	T47.1X2	T47.1X3	T47.1X4	T47.1X5	T47.1X6
Methylprednisolone — *see* Methyl, prednisolone						
Methylrosaniline	T49.0X1	T49.0X2	T49.0X3	T49.0X4	T49.0X5	T49.0X6
Methylrosanilinium chloride	T49.0X1	T49.0X2	T49.0X3	T49.0X4	T49.0X5	T49.0X6
Methyltestosterone	T38.7X1	T38.7X2	T38.7X3	T38.7X4	T38.7X5	T38.7X6
Methylthionine chloride	T50.6X1	T50.6X2	T50.6X3	T50.6X4	T50.6X5	T50.6X6
Methylthioninium chloride	T50.6X1	T50.6X2	T50.6X3	T50.6X4	T50.6X5	T50.6X6
Methylthiouracil	T38.2X1	T38.2X2	T38.2X3	T38.2X4	T38.2X5	T38.2X6
Methyprylon	T42.6X1	T42.6X2	T42.6X3	T42.6X4	T42.6X5	T42.6X6
Methysergide	T46.5X1	T46.5X2	T46.5X3	T46.5X4	T46.5X5	T46.5X6
Metiamide	T47.1X1	T47.1X2	T47.1X3	T47.1X4	T47.1X5	T47.1X6
Meticillin	T36.0X1	T36.0X2	T36.0X3	T36.0X4	T36.0X5	T36.0X6
Meticrane	T50.2X1	T50.2X2	T50.2X3	T50.2X4	T50.2X5	T50.2X6
Metildigoxin	T46.0X1	T46.0X2	T46.0X3	T46.0X4	T46.0X5	T46.0X6
Metipranolol	T49.5X1	T49.5X2	T49.5X3	T49.5X4	T49.5X5	T49.5X6
Metirosine	T46.5X1	T46.5X2	T46.5X3	T46.5X4	T46.5X5	T46.5X6
Metisazone	T37.5X1	T37.5X2	T37.5X3	T37.5X4	T37.5X5	T37.5X6
Metixene	T44.3X1	T44.3X2	T44.3X3	T44.3X4	T44.3X5	T44.3X6
Metizoline	T48.5X1	T48.5X2	T48.5X3	T48.5X4	T48.5X5	T48.5X6
Metoclopramide	T45.0X1	T45.0X2	T45.0X3	T45.0X4	T45.0X5	T45.0X6
Metofenazate	T43.3X1	T43.3X2	T43.3X3	T43.3X4	T43.3X5	T43.3X6
Metofoline	T39.8X1	T39.8X2	T39.8X3	T39.8X4	T39.8X5	T39.8X6
Metolazone	T50.2X1	T50.2X2	T50.2X3	T50.2X4	T50.2X5	T50.2X6
Metopon	T40.2X1	T40.2X2	T40.2X3	T40.2X4	T40.2X5	T40.2X6
Metoprine	T45.1X1	T45.1X2	T45.1X3	T45.1X4	T45.1X5	T45.1X6
Metoprolol	T44.7X1	T44.7X2	T44.7X3	T44.7X4	T44.7X5	T44.7X6
Metrifonate	T60.0X1	T60.0X2	T60.0X3	T60.0X4	--	--
Metrizamide	T50.8X1	T50.8X2	T50.8X3	T50.8X4	T50.8X5	T50.8X6
Metrizoic acid	T50.8X1	T50.8X2	T50.8X3	T50.8X4	T50.8X5	T50.8X6
Metronidazole	T37.8X1	T37.8X2	T37.8X3	T37.8X4	T37.8X5	T37.8X6
Metycaine	T41.3X1	T41.3X2	T41.3X3	T41.3X4	T41.3X5	T41.3X6
infiltration (subcutaneous)	T41.3X1	T41.3X2	T41.3X3	T41.3X4	T41.3X5	T41.3X6
nerve block (peripheral) (plexus)	T41.3X1	T41.3X2	T41.3X3	T41.3X4	T41.3X5	T41.3X6
topical (surface)	T41.3X1	T41.3X2	T41.3X3	T41.3X4	T41.3X5	T41.3X6
Metyrapone	T50.8X1	T50.8X2	T50.8X3	T50.8X4	T50.8X5	T50.8X6
Mevinphos	T60.0X1	T60.0X2	T60.0X3	T60.0X4	--	--
Mexazolam	T42.4X1	T42.4X2	T42.4X3	T42.4X4	T42.4X5	T42.4X6
Mexenone	T49.3X1	T49.3X2	T49.3X3	T49.3X4	T49.3X5	T49.3X6
Mexiletine	T46.2X1	T46.2X2	T46.2X3	T46.2X4	T46.2X5	T46.2X6
Mezereon	T62.2X1	T62.2X2	T62.2X3	T62.2X4	--	--
berries	T62.1X1	T62.1X2	T62.1X3	T62.1X4	--	--
Mezlocillin	T36.0X1	T36.0X2	T36.0X3	T36.0X4	T36.0X5	T36.0X6
Mianserin	T43.021	T43.022	T43.023	T43.024	T43.025	T43.026
Micatin	T49.0X1	T49.0X2	T49.0X3	T49.0X4	T49.0X5	T49.0X6
Miconazole	T49.0X1	T49.0X2	T49.0X3	T49.0X4	T49.0X5	T49.0X6
Micronomicin	T36.5X1	T36.5X2	T36.5X3	T36.5X4	T36.5X5	T36.5X6
Midazolam	T42.4X1	T42.4X2	T42.4X3	T42.4X4	T42.4X5	T42.4X6
Midecamycin	T36.3X1	T36.3X2	T36.3X3	T36.3X4	T36.3X5	T36.3X6
Mifepristone	T38.6X1	T38.6X2	T38.6X3	T38.6X4	T38.6X5	T38.6X6
Milk of magnesia	T47.1X1	T47.1X2	T47.1X3	T47.1X4	T47.1X5	T47.1X6
Millipede (tropical) (venomous)	T63.411	T63.412	T63.413	T63.414	--	--
Miltown	T43.591	T43.592	T43.593	T43.594	T43.595	T43.596
Milverine	T44.3X1	T44.3X2	T44.3X3	T44.3X4	T44.3X5	T44.3X6
Minaprine	T43.291	T43.292	T43.293	T43.294	T43.295	T43.296
Minaxolone	T41.291	T41.292	T41.293	T41.294	T41.295	T41.296
Mineral						
acids	T54.2X1	T54.2X2	T54.2X3	T54.2X4	--	--
oil (laxative)(medicinal)	T47.4X1	T47.4X2	T47.4X3	T47.4X4	T47.4X5	T47.4X6
emulsion	T47.2X1	T47.2X2	T47.2X3	T47.2X4	T47.2X5	T47.2X6
nonmedicinal	T52.0X1	T52.0X2	T52.0X3	T52.0X4	--	--
topical	T49.3X1	T49.3X2	T49.3X3	T49.3X4	T49.3X5	T49.3X6
salt NEC	T50.3X1	T50.3X2	T50.3X3	T50.3X4	T50.3X5	T50.3X6
spirits	T52.0X1	T52.0X2	T52.0X3	T52.0X4	--	--
Mineralocorticosteroid	T50.0X1	T50.0X2	T50.0X3	T50.0X4	T50.0X5	T50.0X6
Minocycline	T36.4X1	T36.4X2	T36.4X3	T36.4X4	T36.4X5	T36.4X6
Minoxidil	T46.7X1	T46.7X2	T46.7X3	T46.7X4	T46.7X5	T46.7X6
Miokamycin	T36.3X1	T36.3X2	T36.3X3	T36.3X4	T36.3X5	T36.3X6
Miotic drug	T49.5X1	T49.5X2	T49.5X3	T49.5X4	T49.5X5	T49.5X6
Mipafox	T60.0X1	T60.0X2	T60.0X3	T60.0X4	--	--
Mirex	T60.1X1	T60.1X2	T60.1X3	T60.1X4	--	--
Mirtazapine	T43.021	T43.022	T43.023	T43.024	T43.025	T43.026
Misonidazole	T37.3X1	T37.3X2	T37.3X3	T37.3X4	T37.3X5	T37.3X6
Misoprostol	T47.1X1	T47.1X2	T47.1X3	T47.1X4	T47.1X5	T47.1X6
Mithramycin	T45.1X1	T45.1X2	T45.1X3	T45.1X4	T45.1X5	T45.1X6
Mitobronitol	T45.1X1	T45.1X2	T45.1X3	T45.1X4	T45.1X5	T45.1X6
Mitoguazone	T45.1X1	T45.1X2	T45.1X3	T45.1X4	T45.1X5	T45.1X6
Mitolactol	T45.1X1	T45.1X2	T45.1X3	T45.1X4	T45.1X5	T45.1X6
Mitomycin	T45.1X1	T45.1X2	T45.1X3	T45.1X4	T45.1X5	T45.1X6
Mitopodozide	T45.1X1	T45.1X2	T45.1X3	T45.1X4	T45.1X5	T45.1X6
Mitotane	T45.1X1	T45.1X2	T45.1X3	T45.1X4	T45.1X5	T45.1X6
Mitoxantrone	T45.1X1	T45.1X2	T45.1X3	T45.1X4	T45.1X5	T45.1X6
Mivacurium chloride	T48.1X1	T48.1X2	T48.1X3	T48.1X4	T48.1X5	T48.1X6
Miyari bacteria	T47.6X1	T47.6X2	T47.6X3	T47.6X4	T47.6X5	T47.6X6
Moclobemide	T43.1X1	T43.1X2	T43.1X3	T43.1X4	T43.1X5	T43.1X6
Moderil	T46.5X1	T46.5X2	T46.5X3	T46.5X4	T46.5X5	T46.5X6
Mofebutazone	T39.2X1	T39.2X2	T39.2X3	T39.2X4	T39.2X5	T39.2X6
Mogadon — *see* Nitrazepam						
Molindone	T43.591	T43.592	T43.593	T43.594	T43.595	T43.596
Molsidomine	T46.3X1	T46.3X2	T46.3X3	T46.3X4	T46.3X5	T46.3X6
Mometasone	T49.0X1	T49.0X2	T49.0X3	T49.0X4	T49.0X5	T49.0X6
Monistat	T49.0X1	T49.0X2	T49.0X3	T49.0X4	T49.0X5	T49.0X6
Monkshood	T62.2X1	T62.2X2	T62.2X3	T62.2X4	--	--
Monoamine oxidase inhibitor NEC	T43.1X1	T43.1X2	T43.1X3	T43.1X4	T43.1X5	T43.1X6
hydrazine	T43.1X1	T43.1X2	T43.1X3	T43.1X4	T43.1X5	T43.1X6
Monobenzone	T49.4X1	T49.4X2	T49.4X3	T49.4X4	T49.4X5	T49.4X6
Monochloroacetic acid	T60.3X1	T60.3X2	T60.3X3	T60.3X4	--	--
Monochlorobenzene	T53.7X1	T53.7X2	T53.7X3	T53.7X4	--	--
Monoethanolamine	T46.8X1	T46.8X2	T46.8X3	T46.8X4	T46.8X5	T46.8X6
oleate	T46.8X1	T46.8X2	T46.8X3	T46.8X4	T46.8X5	T46.8X6
Monooctanoin	T50.991	T50.992	T50.993	T50.994	T50.995	T50.996
Monophenylbutazone	T39.2X1	T39.2X2	T39.2X3	T39.2X4	T39.2X5	T39.2X6
Monosodium glutamate	T65.891	T65.892	T65.893	T65.894	--	--
Monosulfiram	T49.0X1	T49.0X2	T49.0X3	T49.0X4	T49.0X5	T49.0X6
Monoxide, carbon — *see* Carbon, monoxide						
Monoxidine hydrochloride	T46.1X1	T46.1X2	T46.1X3	T46.1X4	T46.1X5	T46.1X6

Substance	Poisoning, Accidental (unintentional)	Poisoning, Intentional self-harm	Poisoning, Assault	Poisoning, Undetermined	Adverse effect	Underdosing
Monuron	T60.3X1	T60.3X2	T60.3X3	T60.3X4	--	--
Moperone	T43.4X1	T43.4X2	T43.4X3	T43.4X4	T43.4X5	T43.4X6
Mopidamol	T45.1X1	T45.1X2	T45.1X3	T45.1X4	T45.1X5	T45.1X6
MOPP (mechloreth-amine + vincristine + prednisone + procarba-zine)	T45.1X1	T45.1X2	T45.1X3	T45.1X4	T45.1X5	T45.1X6
Morfin	T40.2X1	T40.2X2	T40.2X3	T40.2X4	T40.2X5	T40.2X6
Morinamide	T37.1X1	T37.1X2	T37.1X3	T37.1X4	T37.1X5	T37.1X6
Morning glory seeds	T40.991	T40.992	T40.993	T40.994	--	--
Moroxydine	T37.5X1	T37.5X2	T37.5X3	T37.5X4	T37.5X5	T37.5X6
Morphazinamide	T37.1X1	T37.1X2	T37.1X3	T37.1X4	T37.1X5	T37.1X6
Morphine	T40.2X1	T40.2X2	T40.2X3	T40.2X4	T40.2X5	T40.2X6
antagonist	T50.7X1	T50.7X2	T50.7X3	T50.7X4	T50.7X5	T50.7X6
Morpholinylethylmorphine	T40.2X1	T40.2X2	T40.2X3	T40.2X4	--	--
Morsuximide	T42.2X1	T42.2X2	T42.2X3	T42.2X4	T42.2X5	T42.2X6
Mosapramine	T43.591	T43.592	T43.593	T43.594	T43.595	T43.596
Moth balls (see also Pesticide)	T60.2X1	T60.2X2	T60.2X3	T60.2X4	--	--
naphthalene	T60.2X1	T60.2X2	T60.2X3	T60.2X4	--	--
paradichlorobenzene	T60.1X1	T60.1X2	T60.1X3	T60.1X4	--	--
Motor exhaust gas	T58.01	T58.02	T58.03	T58.04	--	--
Mouthwash (antiseptic) (zinc chloride)	T49.6X1	T49.6X2	T49.6X3	T49.6X4	T49.6X5	T49.6X6
Moxastine	T45.0X1	T45.0X2	T45.0X3	T45.0X4	T45.0X5	T45.0X6
Moxaverine	T44.3X1	T44.3X2	T44.3X3	T44.3X4	T44.3X5	T44.3X6
Moxisylyte	T46.7X1	T46.7X2	T46.7X3	T46.7X4	T46.7X5	T46.7X6
Mucilage, plant	T47.4X1	T47.4X2	T47.4X3	T47.4X4	T47.4X5	T47.4X6
Mucolytic drug	T48.4X1	T48.4X2	T48.4X3	T48.4X4	T48.4X5	T48.4X6
Mucomyst	T48.4X1	T48.4X2	T48.4X3	T48.4X4	T48.4X5	T48.4X6
Mucous membrane agents (external)	T49.91	T49.92	T49.93	T49.94	T49.95	T49.96
specified NEC	T49.8X1	T49.8X2	T49.8X3	T49.8X4	T49.8X5	T49.8X6
Multiple unspecified drugs, medicaments and biological substances	T50.911	T50.912	T50.913	T50.914	T50.915	T50.916
Mumps						
immune globulin (human)	T50.Z11	T50.Z12	T50.Z13	T50.Z14	T50.Z15	T50.Z16
skin test antigen	T50.8X1	T50.8X2	T50.8X3	T50.8X4	T50.8X5	T50.8X6
vaccine	T50.B91	T50.B92	T50.B93	T50.B94	T50.B95	T50.B96
Mumpsvax	T50.B91	T50.B92	T50.B93	T50.B94	T50.B95	T50.B96
Mupirocin	T49.0X1	T49.0X2	T49.0X3	T49.0X4	T49.0X5	T49.0X6
Muriatic acid — see Hydrochloric acid						
Muromonab-CD3	T45.1X1	T45.1X2	T45.1X3	T45.1X4	T45.1X5	T45.1X6
Muscle-action drug NEC	T48.201	T48.202	T48.203	T48.204	T48.205	T48.206
Muscle affecting agents NEC	T48.201	T48.202	T48.203	T48.204	T48.205	T48.206
oxytocic	T48.0X1	T48.0X2	T48.0X3	T48.0X4	T48.0X5	T48.0X6
relaxants	T48.201	T48.202	T48.203	T48.204	T48.205	T48.206
central nervous system	T42.8X1	T42.8X2	T42.8X3	T42.8X4	T42.8X5	T42.8X6
skeletal	T48.1X1	T48.1X2	T48.1X3	T48.1X4	T48.1X5	T48.1X6
smooth	T44.3X1	T44.3X2	T44.3X3	T44.3X4	T44.3X5	T44.3X6
Muscle relaxant — see Relaxant, muscle						
Muscle-tone depressant, central NEC	T42.8X1	T42.8X2	T42.8X3	T42.8X4	T42.8X5	T42.8X6
specified NEC	T42.8X1	T42.8X2	T42.8X3	T42.8X4	T42.8X5	T42.8X6
Mushroom, noxious	T62.0X1	T62.0X2	T62.0X3	T62.0X4	--	--
Mussel, noxious	T61.781	T61.782	T61.783	T61.784	--	--
Mustard (emetic)	T47.7X1	T47.7X2	T47.7X3	T47.7X4	T47.7X5	T47.7X6
black	T47.7X1	T47.7X2	T47.7X3	T47.7X4	T47.7X5	T47.7X6
gas, not in war	T59.91	T59.92	T59.93	T59.94	--	--
nitrogen	T45.1X1	T45.1X2	T45.1X3	T45.1X4	T45.1X5	T45.1X6
Mustine	T45.1X1	T45.1X2	T45.1X3	T45.1X4	T45.1X5	T45.1X6
M-vac	T45.1X1	T45.1X2	T45.1X3	T45.1X4	T45.1X5	T45.1X6
Mycifradin	T36.5X1	T36.5X2	T36.5X3	T36.5X4	T36.5X5	T36.5X6
topical	T49.0X1	T49.0X2	T49.0X3	T49.0X4	T49.0X5	T49.0X6
Mycitracin	T36.8X1	T36.8X2	T36.8X3	T36.8X4	T36.8X5	T36.8X6
ophthalmic preparation	T49.5X1	T49.5X2	T49.5X3	T49.5X4	T49.5X5	T49.5X6
Mycostatin	T36.7X1	T36.7X2	T36.7X3	T36.7X4	T36.7X5	T36.7X6
topical	T49.0X1	T49.0X2	T49.0X3	T49.0X4	T49.0X5	T49.0X6
Mycotoxins	T64.81	T64.82	T64.83	T64.84	--	--
aflatoxin	T64.01	T64.02	T64.03	T64.04	--	--
specified NEC	T64.81	T64.82	T64.83	T64.84	--	--
Mydriacyl	T44.3X1	T44.3X2	T44.3X3	T44.3X4	T44.3X5	T44.3X6
Mydriatic drug	T49.5X1	T49.5X2	T49.5X3	T49.5X4	T49.5X5	T49.5X6
Myelobromal	T45.1X1	T45.1X2	T45.1X3	T45.1X4	T45.1X5	T45.1X6
Myleran	T45.1X1	T45.1X2	T45.1X3	T45.1X4	T45.1X5	T45.1X6
Myochrysin (e)	T39.2X1	T39.2X2	T39.2X3	T39.2X4	T39.2X5	T39.2X6
Myoneural blocking agents	T48.1X1	T48.1X2	T48.1X3	T48.1X4	T48.1X5	T48.1X6
Myralact	T49.0X1	T49.0X2	T49.0X3	T49.0X4	T49.0X5	T49.0X6
Myristica fragrans	T62.2X1	T62.2X2	T62.2X3	T62.2X4	--	--
Myristicin	T65.891	T65.892	T65.893	T65.894	--	--
Mysoline	T42.3X1	T42.3X2	T42.3X3	T42.3X4	T42.3X5	T42.3X6

Substance	Poisoning, Accidental (unintentional)	Poisoning, Intentional self-harm	Poisoning, Assault	Poisoning, Undetermined	Adverse effect	Underdosing
N						
Nabilone	T40.7X1	T40.7X2	T40.7X3	T40.7X4	T40.7X5	T40.7X6
Nabumetone	T39.391	T39.392	T39.393	T39.394	T39.395	T39.396
Nadolol	T44.7X1	T44.7X2	T44.7X3	T44.7X4	T44.7X5	T44.7X6
Nafcillin	T36.0X1	T36.0X2	T36.0X3	T36.0X4	T36.0X5	T36.0X6
Nafoxidine	T38.6X1	T38.6X2	T38.6X3	T38.6X4	T38.6X5	T38.6X6
Naftazone	T46.991	T46.992	T46.993	T46.994	T46.995	T46.996
Naftidrofuryl (oxalate)	T46.7X1	T46.7X2	T46.7X3	T46.7X4	T46.7X5	T46.7X6
Naftifine	T49.0X1	T49.0X2	T49.0X3	T49.0X4	T49.0X5	T49.0X6
Nail polish remover	T52.91	T52.92	T52.93	T52.94	--	--
Nalbuphine	T40.4X1	T40.4X2	T40.4X3	T40.4X4	T40.4X5	T40.4X6
Naled	T60.0X1	T60.0X2	T60.0X3	T60.0X4	--	--
Nalidixic acid	T37.8X1	T37.8X2	T37.8X3	T37.8X4	T37.8X5	T37.8X6
Nalorphine	T50.7X1	T50.7X2	T50.7X3	T50.7X4	T50.7X5	T50.7X6
Naloxone	T50.7X1	T50.7X2	T50.7X3	T50.7X4	T50.7X5	T50.7X6
Naltrexone	T50.7X1	T50.7X2	T50.7X3	T50.7X4	T50.7X5	T50.7X6
Namenda	T43.8X1	T43.8X2	T43.8X3	T43.8X4	T43.8X5	T43.8X6
Nandrolone	T38.7X1	T38.7X2	T38.7X3	T38.7X4	T38.7X5	T38.7X6
Naphazoline	T48.5X1	T48.5X2	T48.5X3	T48.5X4	T48.5X5	T48.5X6
Naphtha (painters') (petroleum)	T52.0X1	T52.0X2	T52.0X3	T52.0X4	--	--
solvent	T52.0X1	T52.0X2	T52.0X3	T52.0X4	--	--
vapor	T52.0X1	T52.0X2	T52.0X3	T52.0X4	--	--
Naphthalene (non-chlorinated)	T60.2X1	T60.2X2	T60.2X3	T60.2X4	--	--
chlorinated	T60.1X1	T60.1X2	T60.1X3	T60.1X4	--	--
vapor	T60.1X1	T60.1X2	T60.1X3	T60.1X4	--	--
insecticide or moth repellent	T60.2X1	T60.2X2	T60.2X3	T60.2X4	--	--
chlorinated	T60.1X1	T60.1X2	T60.1X3	T60.1X4	--	--
vapor	T60.2X1	T60.2X2	T60.2X3	T60.2X4	--	--
chlorinated	T60.1X1	T60.1X2	T60.1X3	T60.1X4	--	--
Naphthol	T65.891	T65.892	T65.893	T65.894	--	--
Naphthylamine	T65.891	T65.892	T65.893	T65.894	--	--
Naphthylthiourea (ANTU)	T60.4X1	T60.4X2	T60.4X3	T60.4X4	--	--
Naprosyn — see Naproxen						
Naproxen	T39.311	T39.312	T39.313	T39.314	T39.315	T39.316
Narcotic (drug)	T40.601	T40.602	T40.603	T40.604	T40.605	T40.606
analgesic NEC	T40.601	T40.602	T40.603	T40.604	T40.605	T40.606
antagonist	T50.7X1	T50.7X2	T50.7X3	T50.7X4	T50.7X5	T50.7X6
specified NEC	T40.691	T40.692	T40.693	T40.694	T40.695	T40.696
synthetic	T40.4X1	T40.4X2	T40.4X3	T40.4X4	T40.4X5	T40.4X6
Narcotine	T48.3X1	T48.3X2	T48.3X3	T48.3X4	T48.3X5	T48.3X6
Nardil	T43.1X1	T43.1X2	T43.1X3	T43.1X4	T43.1X5	T43.1X6
Nasal drug NEC	T49.6X1	T49.6X2	T49.6X3	T49.6X4	T49.6X5	T49.6X6
Natamycin	T49.0X1	T49.0X2	T49.0X3	T49.0X4	T49.0X5	T49.0X6
Natrium cyanide — see Cyanide(s)						
Natural						
blood (product)	T45.8X1	T45.8X2	T45.8X3	T45.8X4	T45.8X5	T45.8X6
gas (piped)	T59.891	T59.892	T59.893	T59.894	--	--
incomplete combustion	T58.11	T58.12	T58.13	T58.14	--	--
Nealbarbital	T42.3X1	T42.3X2	T42.3X3	T42.3X4	T42.3X5	T42.3X6
Nectadon	T48.3X1	T48.3X2	T48.3X3	T48.3X4	T48.3X5	T48.3X6
Nedocromil	T48.6X1	T48.6X2	T48.6X3	T48.6X4	T48.6X5	T48.6X6
Nefopam	T39.8X1	T39.8X2	T39.8X3	T39.8X4	T39.8X5	T39.8X6
Nematocyst (sting)	T63.691	T63.692	T63.693	T63.694	--	--
Nembutal	T42.3X1	T42.3X2	T42.3X3	T42.3X4	T42.3X5	T42.3X6
Nemonapride	T43.591	T43.592	T43.593	T43.594	T43.595	T43.596
Neoarsphenamine	T37.8X1	T37.8X2	T37.8X3	T37.8X4	T37.8X5	T37.8X6
Neocinchophen	T50.4X1	T50.4X2	T50.4X3	T50.4X4	T50.4X5	T50.4X6
Neomycin (derivatives)	T36.5X1	T36.5X2	T36.5X3	T36.5X4	T36.5X5	T36.5X6
with						
bacitracin	T49.0X1	T49.0X2	T49.0X3	T49.0X4	T49.0X5	T49.0X6
neostigmine	T44.0X1	T44.0X2	T44.0X3	T44.0X4	T44.0X5	T44.0X6
ENT agent	T49.6X1	T49.6X2	T49.6X3	T49.6X4	T49.6X5	T49.6X6
ophthalmic preparation	T49.5X1	T49.5X2	T49.5X3	T49.5X4	T49.5X5	T49.5X6
topical NEC	T49.0X1	T49.0X2	T49.0X3	T49.0X4	T49.0X5	T49.0X6
Neonal	T42.3X1	T42.3X2	T42.3X3	T42.3X4	T42.3X5	T42.3X6
Neoprontosil	T37.0X1	T37.0X2	T37.0X3	T37.0X4	T37.0X5	T37.0X6
Neosalvarsan	T37.8X1	T37.8X2	T37.8X3	T37.8X4	T37.8X5	T37.8X6
Neosilversalvarsan	T37.8X1	T37.8X2	T37.8X3	T37.8X4	T37.8X5	T37.8X6
Neosporin	T36.8X1	T36.8X2	T36.8X3	T36.8X4	T36.8X5	T36.8X6
ENT agent	T49.6X1	T49.6X2	T49.6X3	T49.6X4	T49.6X5	T49.6X6
ophthalmic preparation	T49.5X1	T49.5X2	T49.5X3	T49.5X4	T49.5X5	T49.5X6
topical NEC	T49.0X1	T49.0X2	T49.0X3	T49.0X4	T49.0X5	T49.0X6
Neostigmine bromide	T44.0X1	T44.0X2	T44.0X3	T44.0X4	T44.0X5	T44.0X6
Neraval	T42.3X1	T42.3X2	T42.3X3	T42.3X4	T42.3X5	T42.3X6
Neravan	T42.3X1	T42.3X2	T42.3X3	T42.3X4	T42.3X5	T42.3X6
Nerium oleander	T62.2X1	T62.2X2	T62.2X3	T62.2X4	--	--
Nerve gas, not in war	T59.91	T59.92	T59.93	T59.94	--	--
Nesacaine	T41.3X1	T41.3X2	T41.3X3	T41.3X4	T41.3X5	T41.3X6
infiltration (subcutaneous)	T41.3X1	T41.3X2	T41.3X3	T41.3X4	T41.3X5	T41.3X6
nerve block (peripheral) (plexus)	T41.3X1	T41.3X2	T41.3X3	T41.3X4	T41.3X5	T41.3X6
Netilmicin	T36.5X1	T36.5X2	T36.5X3	T36.5X4	T36.5X5	T36.5X6

Neurobarb - Octotiamine

Substance	Poisoning, Accidental (unintentional)	Poisoning, Intentional self-harm	Poisoning, Assault	Poisoning, Undetermined	Adverse effect	Underdosing
Neurobarb	T42.3X1	T42.3X2	T42.3X3	T42.3X4	T42.3X5	T42.3X6
Neuroleptic drug NEC	T43.501	T43.502	T43.503	T43.504	T43.505	T43.506
Neuromuscular blocking drug	T48.1X1	T48.1X2	T48.1X3	T48.1X4	T48.1X5	T48.1X6
Neutral insulin injection	T38.3X1	T38.3X2	T38.3X3	T38.3X4	T38.3X5	T38.3X6
Neutral spirits	T51.0X1	T51.0X2	T51.0X3	T51.0X4	--	--
beverage	T51.0X1	T51.0X2	T51.0X3	T51.0X4	--	--
Niacin	T46.7X1	T46.7X2	T46.7X3	T46.7X4	T46.7X5	T46.7X6
Niacinamide	T45.2X1	T45.2X2	T45.2X3	T45.2X4	T45.2X5	T45.2X6
Nialamide	T43.1X1	T43.1X2	T43.1X3	T43.1X4	T43.1X5	T43.1X6
Niaprazine	T42.6X1	T42.6X2	T42.6X3	T42.6X4	T42.6X5	T42.6X6
Nicametate	T46.7X1	T46.7X2	T46.7X3	T46.7X4	T46.7X5	T46.7X6
Nicardipine	T46.1X1	T46.1X2	T46.1X3	T46.1X4	T46.1X5	T46.1X6
Nicergoline	T46.7X1	T46.7X2	T46.7X3	T46.7X4	T46.7X5	T46.7X6
Nickel (carbonyl) (tetra-carbonyl)(fumes) (vapor)	T56.891	T56.892	T56.893	T56.894	--	--
Nickelocene	T56.891	T56.892	T56.893	T56.894	--	--
Niclosamide	T37.4X1	T37.4X2	T37.4X3	T37.4X4	T37.4X5	T37.4X6
Nicofuranose	T46.7X1	T46.7X2	T46.7X3	T46.7X4	T46.7X5	T46.7X6
Nicomorphine	T40.2X1	T40.2X2	T40.2X3	T40.2X4	--	--
Nicorandil	T46.3X1	T46.3X2	T46.3X3	T46.3X4	T46.3X5	T46.3X6
Nicotiana (plant)	T62.2X1	T62.2X2	T62.2X3	T62.2X4	--	--
Nicotinamide	T45.2X1	T45.2X2	T45.2X3	T45.2X4	T45.2X5	T45.2X6
Nicotine (insecticide) (spray) (sulfate) NEC	T60.2X1	T60.2X2	T60.2X3	T60.2X4	--	--
from tobacco	T65.291	T65.292	T65.293	T65.294	--	--
cigarettes	T65.221	T65.222	T65.223	T65.224	--	--
not insecticide	T65.291	T65.292	T65.293	T65.294	--	--
Nicotinic acid	T46.7X1	T46.7X2	T46.7X3	T46.7X4	T46.7X5	T46.7X6
Nicotinyl alcohol	T46.7X1	T46.7X2	T46.7X3	T46.7X4	T46.7X5	T46.7X6
Nicoumalone	T45.511	T45.512	T45.513	T45.514	T45.515	T45.516
Nifedipine	T46.1X1	T46.1X2	T46.1X3	T46.1X4	T46.1X5	T46.1X6
Nifenazone	T39.2X1	T39.2X2	T39.2X3	T39.2X4	T39.2X5	T39.2X6
Nifuraldezone	T37.91	T37.92	T37.93	T37.94	T37.95	T37.96
Nifuratel	T37.8X1	T37.8X2	T37.8X3	T37.8X4	T37.8X5	T37.8X6
Nifurtimox	T37.3X1	T37.3X2	T37.3X3	T37.3X4	T37.3X5	T37.3X6
Nifurtoinol	T37.8X1	T37.8X2	T37.8X3	T37.8X4	T37.8X5	T37.8X6
Nightshade, deadly (solanum) (see also Belladonna)	T62.2X1	T62.2X2	T62.2X3	T62.2X4	--	--
berry	T62.1X1	T62.1X2	T62.1X3	T62.1X4	--	--
Nikethamide	T50.7X1	T50.7X2	T50.7X3	T50.7X4	T50.7X5	T50.7X6
Nilstat	T36.7X1	T36.7X2	T36.7X3	T36.7X4	T36.7X5	T36.7X6
topical	T49.0X1	T49.0X2	T49.0X3	T49.0X4	T49.0X5	T49.0X6
Nilutamide	T38.6X1	T38.6X2	T38.6X3	T38.6X4	T38.6X5	T38.6X6
Nimesulide	T39.391	T39.392	T39.393	T39.394	T39.395	T39.396
Nimetazepam	T42.4X1	T42.4X2	T42.4X3	T42.4X4	T42.4X5	T42.4X6
Nimodipine	T46.1X1	T46.1X2	T46.1X3	T46.1X4	T46.1X5	T46.1X6
Nimorazole	T37.3X1	T37.3X2	T37.3X3	T37.3X4	T37.3X5	T37.3X6
Nimustine	T45.1X1	T45.1X2	T45.1X3	T45.1X4	T45.1X5	T45.1X6
Niridazole	T37.4X1	T37.4X2	T37.4X3	T37.4X4	T37.4X5	T37.4X6
Nisentil	T40.2X1	T40.2X2	T40.2X3	T40.2X4	T40.2X5	T40.2X6
Nisoldipine	T46.1X1	T46.1X2	T46.1X3	T46.1X4	T46.1X5	T46.1X6
Nitramine	T65.3X1	T65.3X2	T65.3X3	T65.3X4	--	--
Nitrate, organic	T46.3X1	T46.3X2	T46.3X3	T46.3X4	T46.3X5	T46.3X6
Nitrazepam	T42.4X1	T42.4X2	T42.4X3	T42.4X4	T42.4X5	T42.4X6
Nitrefazole	T50.6X1	T50.6X2	T50.6X3	T50.6X4	T50.6X5	T50.6X6
Nitrendipine	T46.1X1	T46.1X2	T46.1X3	T46.1X4	T46.1X5	T46.1X6
Nitric						
acid (liquid)	T54.2X1	T54.2X2	T54.2X3	T54.2X4	--	--
vapor	T59.891	T59.892	T59.893	T59.894	--	--
oxide (gas)	T59.0X1	T59.0X2	T59.0X3	T59.0X4	--	--
Nitrimidazine	T37.3X1	T37.3X2	T37.3X3	T37.3X4	T37.3X5	T37.3X6
Nitrite, amyl (medicinal) (vapor)	T46.3X1	T46.3X2	T46.3X3	T46.3X4	T46.3X5	T46.3X6
Nitroaniline	T65.3X1	T65.3X2	T65.3X3	T65.3X4	--	--
vapor	T59.891	T59.892	T59.893	T59.894	--	--
Nitrobenzene, nitrobenzol	T65.3X1	T65.3X2	T65.3X3	T65.3X4	--	--
vapor	T65.3X1	T65.3X2	T65.3X3	T65.3X4	--	--
Nitrocellulose	T65.891	T65.892	T65.893	T65.894	--	--
lacquer	T65.891	T65.892	T65.893	T65.894	--	--
Nitrodiphenyl	T65.3X1	T65.3X2	T65.3X3	T65.3X4	--	--
Nitrofural	T49.0X1	T49.0X2	T49.0X3	T49.0X4	T49.0X5	T49.0X6
Nitrofurantoin	T37.8X1	T37.8X2	T37.8X3	T37.8X4	T37.8X5	T37.8X6
Nitrofurazone	T49.0X1	T49.0X2	T49.0X3	T49.0X4	T49.0X5	T49.0X6
Nitrogen	T59.0X1	T59.0X2	T59.0X3	T59.0X4	--	--
mustard	T45.1X1	T45.1X2	T45.1X3	T45.1X4	T45.1X5	T45.1X6
Nitroglycerin, nitro-glycerol (medicinal)	T46.3X1	T46.3X2	T46.3X3	T46.3X4	T46.3X5	T46.3X6
nonmedicinal	T65.5X1	T65.5X2	T65.5X3	T65.5X4	--	--
fumes	T65.5X1	T65.5X2	T65.5X3	T65.5X4	--	--
Nitroglycol	T52.3X1	T52.3X2	T52.3X3	T52.3X4	--	--
Nitrohydrochloric acid	T54.2X1	T54.2X2	T54.2X3	T54.2X4	--	--
Nitromersol	T49.0X1	T49.0X2	T49.0X3	T49.0X4	T49.0X5	T49.0X6
Nitronaphthalene	T65.891	T65.892	T65.893	T65.894	--	--
Nitrophenol	T54.0X1	T54.0X2	T54.0X3	T54.0X4	--	--
Nitropropane	T52.8X1	T52.8X2	T52.8X3	T52.8X4	--	--
Nitroprusside	T46.5X1	T46.5X2	T46.5X3	T46.5X4	T46.5X5	T46.5X6
Nitrosodimethylamine	T65.3X1	T65.3X2	T65.3X3	T65.3X4	--	--
Nitrothiazol	T37.4X1	T37.4X2	T37.4X3	T37.4X4	T37.4X5	T37.4X6
Nitrotoluene, nitrotoluol	T65.3X1	T65.3X2	T65.3X3	T65.3X4	--	--
vapor	T65.3X1	T65.3X2	T65.3X3	T65.3X4	--	--
Nitrous						
acid (liquid)	T54.2X1	T54.2X2	T54.2X3	T54.2X4	--	--
fumes	T59.891	T59.892	T59.893	T59.894	--	--
ether spirit	T46.3X1	T46.3X2	T46.3X3	T46.3X4	T46.3X5	T46.3X6
oxide	T41.0X1	T41.0X2	T41.0X3	T41.0X4	T41.0X5	T41.0X6
Nitroxoline	T37.8X1	T37.8X2	T37.8X3	T37.8X4	T37.8X5	T37.8X6
Nitrozone	T49.0X1	T49.0X2	T49.0X3	T49.0X4	T49.0X5	T49.0X6
Nizatidine	T47.0X1	T47.0X2	T47.0X3	T47.0X4	T47.0X5	T47.0X6
Nizofenone	T43.8X1	T43.8X2	T43.8X3	T43.8X4	T43.8X5	T43.8X6
Noctec	T42.6X1	T42.6X2	T42.6X3	T42.6X4	T42.6X5	T42.6X6
Noludar	T42.6X1	T42.6X2	T42.6X3	T42.6X4	T42.6X5	T42.6X6
Nomegestrol	T38.5X1	T38.5X2	T38.5X3	T38.5X4	T38.5X5	T38.5X6
Nomifensine	T43.291	T43.292	T43.293	T43.294	T43.295	T43.296
Nonoxinol	T49.8X1	T49.8X2	T49.8X3	T49.8X4	T49.8X5	T49.8X6
Nonylphenoxy (polyethoxy-ethanol)	T49.8X1	T49.8X2	T49.8X3	T49.8X4	T49.8X5	T49.8X6
Noptil	T42.3X1	T42.3X2	T42.3X3	T42.3X4	T42.3X5	T42.3X6
Noradrenaline	T44.4X1	T44.4X2	T44.4X3	T44.4X4	T44.4X5	T44.4X6
Noramidopyrine	T39.2X1	T39.2X2	T39.2X3	T39.2X4	T39.2X5	T39.2X6
methanesulfonate sodium	T39.2X1	T39.2X2	T39.2X3	T39.2X4	T39.2X5	T39.2X6
Norbormide	T60.4X1	T60.4X2	T60.4X3	T60.4X4	--	--
Nordazepam	T42.4X1	T42.4X2	T42.4X3	T42.4X4	T42.4X5	T42.4X6
Norepinephrine	T44.4X1	T44.4X2	T44.4X3	T44.4X4	T44.4X5	T44.4X6
Norethandrolone	T38.7X1	T38.7X2	T38.7X3	T38.7X4	T38.7X5	T38.7X6
Norethindrone	T38.4X1	T38.4X2	T38.4X3	T38.4X4	T38.4X5	T38.4X6
Norethisterone (acetate) (enantate)	T38.4X1	T38.4X2	T38.4X3	T38.4X4	T38.4X5	T38.4X6
with ethinylestradiol	T38.5X1	T38.5X2	T38.5X3	T38.5X4	T38.5X5	T38.5X6
Noretynodrel	T38.5X1	T38.5X2	T38.5X3	T38.5X4	T38.5X5	T38.5X6
Norfenefrine	T44.4X1	T44.4X2	T44.4X3	T44.4X4	T44.4X5	T44.4X6
Norfloxacin	T36.8X1	T36.8X2	T36.8X3	T36.8X4	T36.8X5	T36.8X6
Norgestrel	T38.4X1	T38.4X2	T38.4X3	T38.4X4	T38.4X5	T38.4X6
Norgestrienone	T38.4X1	T38.4X2	T38.4X3	T38.4X4	T38.4X5	T38.4X6
Norlestrin	T38.4X1	T38.4X2	T38.4X3	T38.4X4	T38.4X5	T38.4X6
Norlutin	T38.4X1	T38.4X2	T38.4X3	T38.4X4	T38.4X5	T38.4X6
Normal serum albumin (human), salt-poor	T45.8X1	T45.8X2	T45.8X3	T45.8X4	T45.8X5	T45.8X6
Normethandrone	T38.5X1	T38.5X2	T38.5X3	T38.5X4	T38.5X5	T38.5X6
Normison — see Benzodiazepine						
Normorphine	T40.2X1	T40.2X2	T40.2X3	T40.2X4	--	--
Norpseudoephedrine	T50.5X1	T50.5X2	T50.5X3	T50.5X4	T50.5X5	T50.5X6
Nortestosterone (furanpropionate)	T38.7X1	T38.7X2	T38.7X3	T38.7X4	T38.7X5	T38.7X6
Nortriptyline	T43.011	T43.012	T43.013	T43.014	T43.015	T43.016
Noscapine	T48.3X1	T48.3X2	T48.3X3	T48.3X4	T48.3X5	T48.3X6
Nose preparations	T49.6X1	T49.6X2	T49.6X3	T49.6X4	T49.6X5	T49.6X6
Novobiocin	T36.5X1	T36.5X2	T36.5X3	T36.5X4	T36.5X5	T36.5X6
Novocain (infiltration) (topical)	T41.3X1	T41.3X2	T41.3X3	T41.3X4	T41.3X5	T41.3X6
nerve block (peripheral) (plexus)	T41.3X1	T41.3X2	T41.3X3	T41.3X4	T41.3X5	T41.3X6
spinal	T41.3X1	T41.3X2	T41.3X3	T41.3X4	T41.3X5	T41.3X6
Noxious foodstuff	T62.91	T62.92	T62.93	T62.94	--	--
specified NEC	T62.8X1	T62.8X2	T62.8X3	T62.8X4	--	--
Noxiptiline	T43.011	T43.012	T43.013	T43.014	T43.015	T43.016
Noxytiolin	T49.0X1	T49.0X2	T49.0X3	T49.0X4	T49.0X5	T49.0X6
NPH Iletin (insulin)	T38.3X1	T38.3X2	T38.3X3	T38.3X4	T38.3X5	T38.3X6
Numorphan	T40.2X1	T40.2X2	T40.2X3	T40.2X4	--	--
Nunol	T42.3X1	T42.3X2	T42.3X3	T42.3X4	T42.3X5	T42.3X6
Nupercaine (spinal anesthetic)	T41.3X1	T41.3X2	T41.3X3	T41.3X4	T41.3X5	T41.3X6
topical (surface)	T41.3X1	T41.3X2	T41.3X3	T41.3X4	T41.3X5	T41.3X6
Nutmeg oil (liniment)	T49.3X1	T49.3X2	T49.3X3	T49.3X4	T49.3X5	T49.3X6
Nutritional supplement	T50.901	T50.902	T50.903	T50.904	T50.905	T50.906
Nux vomica	T65.1X1	T65.1X2	T65.1X3	T65.1X4	--	--
Nydrazid	T37.1X1	T37.1X2	T37.1X3	T37.1X4	T37.1X5	T37.1X6
Nylidrin	T46.7X1	T46.7X2	T46.7X3	T46.7X4	T46.7X5	T46.7X6
Nystatin	T36.7X1	T36.7X2	T36.7X3	T36.7X4	T36.7X5	T36.7X6
topical	T49.0X1	T49.0X2	T49.0X3	T49.0X4	T49.0X5	T49.0X6
Nytol	T45.0X1	T45.0X2	T45.0X3	T45.0X4	T45.0X5	T45.0X6
O						
Obidoxime chloride	T50.6X1	T50.6X2	T50.6X3	T50.6X4	T50.6X5	T50.6X6
Octafonium (chloride)	T49.3X1	T49.3X2	T49.3X3	T49.3X4	T49.3X5	T49.3X6
Octamethyl pyrophos-phoramide	T60.0X1	T60.0X2	T60.0X3	T60.0X4	--	--
Octanoin	T50.991	T50.992	T50.993	T50.994	T50.995	T50.996
Octatropine methyl-bromide	T44.3X1	T44.3X2	T44.3X3	T44.3X4	T44.3X5	T44.3X6
Octotiamine	T45.2X1	T45.2X2	T45.2X3	T45.2X4	T45.2X5	T45.2X6

Substance	Poisoning, Accidental (unintentional)	Poisoning, Intentional self-harm	Poisoning, Assault	Poisoning, Undetermined	Adverse effect	Underdosing
Octoxinol (9)	T49.8X1	T49.8X2	T49.8X3	T49.8X4	T49.8X5	T49.8X6
Octreotide	T38.991	T38.992	T38.993	T38.994	T38.995	T38.996
Octyl nitrite	T46.3X1	T46.3X2	T46.3X3	T46.3X4	T46.3X5	T46.3X6
Oestradiol	T38.5X1	T38.5X2	T38.5X3	T38.5X4	T38.5X5	T38.5X6
Oestriol	T38.5X1	T38.5X2	T38.5X3	T38.5X4	T38.5X5	T38.5X6
Oestrogen	T38.5X1	T38.5X2	T38.5X3	T38.5X4	T38.5X5	T38.5X6
Oestrone	T38.5X1	T38.5X2	T38.5X3	T38.5X4	T38.5X5	T38.5X6
Ofloxacin	T36.8X1	T36.8X2	T36.8X3	T36.8X4	T36.8X5	T36.8X6
Oil (of)	T65.891	T65.892	T65.893	T65.894	--	--
bitter almond	T62.8X1	T62.8X2	T62.8X3	T62.8X4	--	--
cloves	T49.7X1	T49.7X2	T49.7X3	T49.7X4	T49.7X5	T49.7X6
colors	T65.6X1	T65.6X2	T65.6X3	T65.6X4	--	--
fumes	T59.891	T59.892	T59.893	T59.894	--	--
lubricating	T52.0X1	T52.0X2	T52.0X3	T52.0X4	--	--
niobe	T52.8X1	T52.8X2	T52.8X3	T52.8X4	--	--
vitriol (liquid)	T54.2X1	T54.2X2	T54.2X3	T54.2X4	--	--
fumes	T54.2X1	T54.2X2	T54.2X3	T54.2X4	--	--
wintergreen (bitter) NEC	T49.3X1	T49.3X2	T49.3X3	T49.3X4	T49.3X5	T49.3X6
Oily preparation (for skin)	T49.3X1	T49.3X2	T49.3X3	T49.3X4	T49.3X5	T49.3X6
Ointment NEC	T49.3X1	T49.3X2	T49.3X3	T49.3X4	T49.3X5	T49.3X6
Olanzapine	T43.591	T43.592	T43.593	T43.594	T43.595	T43.596
Oleander	T62.2X1	T62.2X2	T62.2X3	T62.2X4	--	--
Oleandomycin	T36.3X1	T36.3X2	T36.3X3	T36.3X4	T36.3X5	T36.3X6
Oleandrin	T46.0X1	T46.0X2	T46.0X3	T46.0X4	T46.0X5	T46.0X6
Oleic acid	T46.6X1	T46.6X2	T46.6X3	T46.6X4	T46.6X5	T46.6X6
Oleovitamin A	T45.2X1	T45.2X2	T45.2X3	T45.2X4	T45.2X5	T45.2X6
Oleum ricini	T47.2X1	T47.2X2	T47.2X3	T47.2X4	T47.2X5	T47.2X6
Olive oil (medicinal) **NEC**	T47.4X1	T47.4X2	T47.4X3	T47.4X4	T47.4X5	T47.4X6
Olivomycin	T45.1X1	T45.1X2	T45.1X3	T45.1X4	T45.1X5	T45.1X6
Olsalazine	T47.8X1	T47.8X2	T47.8X3	T47.8X4	T47.8X5	T47.8X6
Omeprazole	T47.1X1	T47.1X2	T47.1X3	T47.1X4	T47.1X5	T47.1X6
OMPA	T60.0X1	T60.0X2	T60.0X3	T60.0X4	--	--
Oncovin	T45.1X1	T45.1X2	T45.1X3	T45.1X4	T45.1X5	T45.1X6
Ondansetron	T45.0X1	T45.0X2	T45.0X3	T45.0X4	T45.0X5	T45.0X6
Ophthaine	T41.3X1	T41.3X2	T41.3X3	T41.3X4	T41.3X5	T41.3X6
Ophthetic	T41.3X1	T41.3X2	T41.3X3	T41.3X4	T41.3X5	T41.3X6
Opiate NEC	T40.601	T40.602	T40.603	T40.604	T40.605	T40.606
antagonists	T50.7X1	T50.7X2	T50.7X3	T50.7X4	T50.7X5	T50.7X6
Opioid NEC	T40.2X1	T40.2X2	T40.2X3	T40.2X4	T40.2X5	T40.2X6
Opipramol	T43.011	T43.012	T43.013	T43.014	T43.015	T43.016
Opium alkaloids (total)	T40.0X1	T40.0X2	T40.0X3	T40.0X4	T40.0X5	T40.0X6
standardized powdered	T40.0X1	T40.0X2	T40.0X3	T40.0X4	T40.0X5	T40.0X6
tincture (camphorated)	T40.0X1	T40.0X2	T40.0X3	T40.0X4	T40.0X5	T40.0X6
Oracon	T38.4X1	T38.4X2	T38.4X3	T38.4X4	T38.4X5	T38.4X6
Oragrafin	T50.8X1	T50.8X2	T50.8X3	T50.8X4	T50.8X5	T50.8X6
Oral contraceptives	T38.4X1	T38.4X2	T38.4X3	T38.4X4	T38.4X5	T38.4X6
Oral rehydration salts	T50.3X1	T50.3X2	T50.3X3	T50.3X4	T50.3X5	T50.3X6
Orazamide	T50.991	T50.992	T50.993	T50.994	T50.995	T50.996
Orciprenaline	T48.291	T48.292	T48.293	T48.294	T48.295	T48.296
Organidin	T48.4X1	T48.4X2	T48.4X3	T48.4X4	T48.4X5	T48.4X6
Organonitrate NEC	T46.3X1	T46.3X2	T46.3X3	T46.3X4	T46.3X5	T46.3X6
Organophosphates	T60.0X1	T60.0X2	T60.0X3	T60.0X4	--	--
Orimune	T50.B91	T50.B92	T50.B93	T50.B94	T50.B95	T50.B96
Orinase	T38.3X1	T38.3X2	T38.3X3	T38.3X4	T38.3X5	T38.3X6
Ormeloxifene	T38.6X1	T38.6X2	T38.6X3	T38.6X4	T38.6X5	T38.6X6
Ornidazole	T37.3X1	T37.3X2	T37.3X3	T37.3X4	T37.3X5	T37.3X6
Ornithine aspartate	T50.991	T50.992	T50.993	T50.994	T50.995	T50.996
Ornoprostil	T47.1X1	T47.1X2	T47.1X3	T47.1X4	T47.1X5	T47.1X6
Orphenadrine (hydrochloride)	T42.8X1	T42.8X2	T42.8X3	T42.8X4	T42.8X5	T42.8X6
Ortal (sodium)	T42.3X1	T42.3X2	T42.3X3	T42.3X4	T42.3X5	T42.3X6
Orthoboric acid	T49.0X1	T49.0X2	T49.0X3	T49.0X4	T49.0X5	T49.0X6
ENT agent	T49.6X1	T49.6X2	T49.6X3	T49.6X4	T49.6X5	T49.6X6
ophthalmic preparation	T49.5X1	T49.5X2	T49.5X3	T49.5X4	T49.5X5	T49.5X6
Orthocaine	T41.3X1	T41.3X2	T41.3X3	T41.3X4	T41.3X5	T41.3X6
Orthodichlorobenzene	T53.7X1	T53.7X2	T53.7X3	T53.7X4	--	--
Ortho-Novum	T38.4X1	T38.4X2	T38.4X3	T38.4X4	T38.4X5	T38.4X6
Orthotolidine (reagent)	T54.2X1	T54.2X2	T54.2X3	T54.2X4	--	--
Osmic acid (liquid)	T54.2X1	T54.2X2	T54.2X3	T54.2X4	--	--
fumes	T54.2X1	T54.2X2	T54.2X3	T54.2X4	--	--
Osmotic diuretics	T50.2X1	T50.2X2	T50.2X3	T50.2X4	T50.2X5	T50.2X6
Otilonium bromide	T44.3X1	T44.3X2	T44.3X3	T44.3X4	T44.3X5	T44.3X6
Otorhinolaryngological drug NEC	T49.6X1	T49.6X2	T49.6X3	T49.6X4	T49.6X5	T49.6X6
Ouabain (e)	T46.0X1	T46.0X2	T46.0X3	T46.0X4	T46.0X5	T46.0X6
Ovarian						
hormone	T38.5X1	T38.5X2	T38.5X3	T38.5X4	T38.5X5	T38.5X6
stimulant	T38.5X1	T38.5X2	T38.5X3	T38.5X4	T38.5X5	T38.5X6
Ovral	T38.4X1	T38.4X2	T38.4X3	T38.4X4	T38.4X5	T38.4X6
Ovulen	T38.4X1	T38.4X2	T38.4X3	T38.4X4	T38.4X5	T38.4X6
Oxacillin	T36.0X1	T36.0X2	T36.0X3	T36.0X4	T36.0X5	T36.0X6
Oxalic acid	T54.2X1	T54.2X2	T54.2X3	T54.2X4	--	--
ammonium salt	T50.991	T50.992	T50.993	T50.994	T50.995	T50.996
Oxamniquine	T37.4X1	T37.4X2	T37.4X3	T37.4X4	T37.4X5	T37.4X6
Oxanamide	T43.591	T43.592	T43.593	T43.594	T43.595	T43.596
Oxandrolone	T38.7X1	T38.7X2	T38.7X3	T38.7X4	T38.7X5	T38.7X6
Oxantel	T37.4X1	T37.4X2	T37.4X3	T37.4X4	T37.4X5	T37.4X6
Oxapium iodide	T44.3X1	T44.3X2	T44.3X3	T44.3X4	T44.3X5	T44.3X6
Oxaprotiline	T43.021	T43.022	T43.023	T43.024	T43.025	T43.026
Oxaprozin	T39.311	T39.312	T39.313	T39.314	T39.315	T39.316
Oxatomide	T45.0X1	T45.0X2	T45.0X3	T45.0X4	T45.0X5	T45.0X6
Oxazepam	T42.4X1	T42.4X2	T42.4X3	T42.4X4	T42.4X5	T42.4X6
Oxazimedrine	T50.5X1	T50.5X2	T50.5X3	T50.5X4	T50.5X5	T50.5X6
Oxazolam	T42.4X1	T42.4X2	T42.4X3	T42.4X4	T42.4X5	T42.4X6
Oxazolidine derivatives	T42.2X1	T42.2X2	T42.2X3	T42.2X4	T42.2X5	T42.2X6
Oxazolidinedione (derivative)	T42.2X1	T42.2X2	T42.2X3	T42.2X4	T42.2X5	T42.2X6
Ox bile extract	T47.5X1	T47.5X2	T47.5X3	T47.5X4	T47.5X5	T47.5X6
Oxcarbazepine	T42.1X1	T42.1X2	T42.1X3	T42.1X4	T42.1X5	T42.1X6
Oxedrine	T44.4X1	T44.4X2	T44.4X3	T44.4X4	T44.4X5	T44.4X6
Oxeladin (citrate)	T48.3X1	T48.3X2	T48.3X3	T48.3X4	T48.3X5	T48.3X6
Oxendolone	T38.5X1	T38.5X2	T38.5X3	T38.5X4	T38.5X5	T38.5X6
Oxetacaine	T41.3X1	T41.3X2	T41.3X3	T41.3X4	T41.3X5	T41.3X6
Oxethazine	T41.3X1	T41.3X2	T41.3X3	T41.3X4	T41.3X5	T41.3X6
Oxetorone	T39.8X1	T39.8X2	T39.8X3	T39.8X4	T39.8X5	T39.8X6
Oxiconazole	T49.0X1	T49.0X2	T49.0X3	T49.0X4	T49.0X5	T49.0X6
Oxidizing agent NEC	T54.91	T54.92	T54.93	T54.94	--	--
Oxipurinol	T50.4X1	T50.4X2	T50.4X3	T50.4X4	T50.4X5	T50.4X6
Oxitriptan	T43.291	T43.292	T43.293	T43.294	T43.295	T43.296
Oxitropium bromide	T48.6X1	T48.6X2	T48.6X3	T48.6X4	T48.6X5	T48.6X6
Oxodipine	T46.1X1	T46.1X2	T46.1X3	T46.1X4	T46.1X5	T46.1X6
Oxolamine	T48.3X1	T48.3X2	T48.3X3	T48.3X4	T48.3X5	T48.3X6
Oxolinic acid	T37.8X1	T37.8X2	T37.8X3	T37.8X4	T37.8X5	T37.8X6
Oxomemazine	T43.3X1	T43.3X2	T43.3X3	T43.3X4	T43.3X5	T43.3X6
Oxophenarsine	T37.3X1	T37.3X2	T37.3X3	T37.3X4	T37.3X5	T37.3X6
Oxprenolol	T44.7X1	T44.7X2	T44.7X3	T44.7X4	T44.7X5	T44.7X6
Oxsoralen	T49.3X1	T49.3X2	T49.3X3	T49.3X4	T49.3X5	T49.3X6
Oxtriphylline	T48.6X1	T48.6X2	T48.6X3	T48.6X4	T48.6X5	T48.6X6
Oxybate sodium	T41.291	T41.292	T41.293	T41.294	T41.295	T41.296
Oxybuprocaine	T41.3X1	T41.3X2	T41.3X3	T41.3X4	T41.3X5	T41.3X6
Oxybutynin	T44.3X1	T44.3X2	T44.3X3	T44.3X4	T44.3X5	T44.3X6
Oxychlorosene	T49.0X1	T49.0X2	T49.0X3	T49.0X4	T49.0X5	T49.0X6
Oxycodone	T40.2X1	T40.2X2	T40.2X3	T40.2X4	T40.2X5	T40.2X6
Oxyfedrine	T46.3X1	T46.3X2	T46.3X3	T46.3X4	T46.3X5	T46.3X6
Oxygen	T41.5X1	T41.5X2	T41.5X3	T41.5X4	T41.5X5	T41.5X6
Oxylone	T49.0X1	T49.0X2	T49.0X3	T49.0X4	T49.0X5	T49.0X6
ophthalmic preparation	T49.5X1	T49.5X2	T49.5X3	T49.5X4	T49.5X5	T49.5X6
Oxymesterone	T38.7X1	T38.7X2	T38.7X3	T38.7X4	T38.7X5	T38.7X6
Oxymetazoline	T48.5X1	T48.5X2	T48.5X3	T48.5X4	T48.5X5	T48.5X6
Oxymetholone	T38.7X1	T38.7X2	T38.7X3	T38.7X4	T38.7X5	T38.7X6
Oxymorphone	T40.2X1	T40.2X2	T40.2X3	T40.2X4	T40.2X5	T40.2X6
Oxypertine	T43.591	T43.592	T43.593	T43.594	T43.595	T43.596
Oxyphenbutazone	T39.2X1	T39.2X2	T39.2X3	T39.2X4	T39.2X5	T39.2X6
Oxyphencyclimine	T44.3X1	T44.3X2	T44.3X3	T44.3X4	T44.3X5	T44.3X6
Oxyphenisatine	T47.2X1	T47.2X2	T47.2X3	T47.2X4	T47.2X5	T47.2X6
Oxyphenonium bromide	T44.3X1	T44.3X2	T44.3X3	T44.3X4	T44.3X5	T44.3X6
Oxypolygelatin	T45.8X1	T45.8X2	T45.8X3	T45.8X4	T45.8X5	T45.8X6
Oxyquinoline (derivatives)	T37.8X1	T37.8X2	T37.8X3	T37.8X4	T37.8X5	T37.8X6
Oxytetracycline	T36.4X1	T36.4X2	T36.4X3	T36.4X4	T36.4X5	T36.4X6
Oxytocic drug NEC	T48.0X1	T48.0X2	T48.0X3	T48.0X4	T48.0X5	T48.0X6
Oxytocin (synthetic)	T48.0X1	T48.0X2	T48.0X3	T48.0X4	T48.0X5	T48.0X6
Ozone	T59.891	T59.892	T59.893	T59.894	--	--
P						
PABA	T49.3X1	T49.3X2	T49.3X3	T49.3X4	T49.3X5	T49.3X6
Packed red cells	T45.8X1	T45.8X2	T45.8X3	T45.8X4	T45.8X5	T45.8X6
Padimate	T49.3X1	T49.3X2	T49.3X3	T49.3X4	T49.3X5	T49.3X6
Paint NEC	T65.6X1	T65.6X2	T65.6X3	T65.6X4	--	--
cleaner	T52.91	T52.92	T52.93	T52.94	--	--
fumes NEC	T59.891	T59.892	T59.893	T59.894	--	--
lead (fumes)	T56.0X1	T56.0X2	T56.0X3	T56.0X4	--	--
solvent NEC	T52.8X1	T52.8X2	T52.8X3	T52.8X4	--	--
stripper	T52.8X1	T52.8X2	T52.8X3	T52.8X4	--	--
Palfium	T40.2X1	T40.2X2	T40.2X3	T40.2X4	--	--
Palm kernel oil	T50.991	T50.992	T50.993	T50.994	T50.995	T50.996
Paludrine	T37.2X1	T37.2X2	T37.2X3	T37.2X4	T37.2X5	T37.2X6
PAM (pralidoxime)	T50.6X1	T50.6X2	T50.6X3	T50.6X4	T50.6X5	T50.6X6
Pamaquine (naphthoute)	T37.2X1	T37.2X2	T37.2X3	T37.2X4	T37.2X5	T37.2X6
Panadol	T39.1X1	T39.1X2	T39.1X3	T39.1X4	T39.1X5	T39.1X6
Pancreatic						
digestive secretion stimulant	T47.8X1	T47.8X2	T47.8X3	T47.8X4	T47.8X5	T47.8X6
dornase	T45.3X1	T45.3X2	T45.3X3	T45.3X4	T45.3X5	T45.3X6
Pancreatin	T47.5X1	T47.5X2	T47.5X3	T47.5X4	T47.5X5	T47.5X6
Pancrelipase	T47.5X1	T47.5X2	T47.5X3	T47.5X4	T47.5X5	T47.5X6
Pancuronium (bromide)	T48.1X1	T48.1X2	T48.1X3	T48.1X4	T48.1X5	T48.1X6
Pangamic acid	T45.2X1	T45.2X2	T45.2X3	T45.2X4	T45.2X5	T45.2X6
Panthenol	T45.2X1	T45.2X2	T45.2X3	T45.2X4	T45.2X5	T45.2X6
topical	T49.8X1	T49.8X2	T49.8X3	T49.8X4	T49.8X5	T49.8X6
Pantopon	T40.0X1	T40.0X2	T40.0X3	T40.0X4	T40.0X5	T40.0X6
Pantothenic acid	T45.2X1	T45.2X2	T45.2X3	T45.2X4	T45.2X5	T45.2X6

Substance	Poisoning, Accidental (unintentional)	Poisoning, Intentional self-harm	Poisoning, Assault	Poisoning, Undetermined	Adverse effect	Underdosing
Panwarfin	T45.511	T45.512	T45.513	T45.514	T45.515	T45.516
Papain	T47.5X1	T47.5X2	T47.5X3	T47.5X4	T47.5X5	T47.5X6
digestant	T47.5X1	T47.5X2	T47.5X3	T47.5X4	T47.5X5	T47.5X6
Papaveretum	T40.0X1	T40.0X2	T40.0X3	T40.0X4	T40.0X5	T40.0X6
Papaverine	T44.3X1	T44.3X2	T44.3X3	T44.3X4	T44.3X5	T44.3X6
Para-acetamidophenol	T39.1X1	T39.1X2	T39.1X3	T39.1X4	T39.1X5	T39.1X6
Para-aminobenzoic acid	T49.3X1	T49.3X2	T49.3X3	T49.3X4	T49.3X5	T49.3X6
Para-aminophenol derivatives	T39.1X1	T39.1X2	T39.1X3	T39.1X4	T39.1X5	T39.1X6
Para-aminosalicylic acid	T37.1X1	T37.1X2	T37.1X3	T37.1X4	T37.1X5	T37.1X6
Paracetaldehyde	T42.6X1	T42.6X2	T42.6X3	T42.6X4	T42.6X5	T42.6X6
Paracetamol	T39.1X1	T39.1X2	T39.1X3	T39.1X4	T39.1X5	T39.1X6
Parachlorophenol (camphorated)	T49.0X1	T49.0X2	T49.0X3	T49.0X4	T49.0X5	T49.0X6
Paracodin	T40.2X1	T40.2X2	T40.2X3	T40.2X4	T40.2X5	T40.2X6
Paradione	T42.2X1	T42.2X2	T42.2X3	T42.2X4	T42.2X5	T42.2X6
Paraffin(s) (wax)	T52.0X1	T52.0X2	T52.0X3	T52.0X4	--	--
liquid (medicinal)	T47.4X1	T47.4X2	T47.4X3	T47.4X4	T47.4X5	T47.4X6
nonmedicinal	T52.0X1	T52.0X2	T52.0X3	T52.0X4	--	--
Paraformaldehyde	T60.3X1	T60.3X2	T60.3X3	T60.3X4	--	--
Paraldehyde	T42.6X1	T42.6X2	T42.6X3	T42.6X4	T42.6X5	T42.6X6
Paramethadione	T42.2X1	T42.2X2	T42.2X3	T42.2X4	T42.2X5	T42.2X6
Paramethasone	T38.0X1	T38.0X2	T38.0X3	T38.0X4	T38.0X5	T38.0X6
acetate	T49.0X1	T49.0X2	T49.0X3	T49.0X4	T49.0X5	T49.0X6
Paraoxon	T60.0X1	T60.0X2	T60.0X3	T60.0X4	--	--
Paraquat	T60.3X1	T60.3X2	T60.3X3	T60.3X4	--	--
Parasympatholytic NEC	T44.3X1	T44.3X2	T44.3X3	T44.3X4	T44.3X5	T44.3X6
Parasympathomimetic drug NEC	T44.1X1	T44.1X2	T44.1X3	T44.1X4	T44.1X5	T44.1X6
Parathion	T60.0X1	T60.0X2	T60.0X3	T60.0X4	--	--
Parathormone	T50.991	T50.992	T50.993	T50.994	T50.995	T50.996
Parathyroid extract	T50.991	T50.992	T50.993	T50.994	T50.995	T50.996
Paratyphoid vaccine	T50.A91	T50.A92	T50.A93	T50.A94	T50.A95	T50.A96
Paredrine	T44.4X1	T44.4X2	T44.4X3	T44.4X4	T44.4X5	T44.4X6
Paregoric	T40.0X1	T40.0X2	T40.0X3	T40.0X4	T40.0X5	T40.0X6
Pargyline	T46.5X1	T46.5X2	T46.5X3	T46.5X4	T46.5X5	T46.5X6
Paris green	T57.0X1	T57.0X2	T57.0X3	T57.0X4	--	--
insecticide	T57.0X1	T57.0X2	T57.0X3	T57.0X4	--	--
Parnate	T43.1X1	T43.1X2	T43.1X3	T43.1X4	T43.1X5	T43.1X6
Paromomycin	T36.5X1	T36.5X2	T36.5X3	T36.5X4	T36.5X5	T36.5X6
Paroxypropione	T45.1X1	T45.1X2	T45.1X3	T45.1X4	T45.1X5	T45.1X6
Parzone	T40.2X1	T40.2X2	T40.2X3	T40.2X4	T40.2X5	T40.2X6
PAS	T37.1X1	T37.1X2	T37.1X3	T37.1X4	T37.1X5	T37.1X6
Pasiniazid	T37.1X1	T37.1X2	T37.1X3	T37.1X4	T37.1X5	T37.1X6
PBB (polybrominated biphenyls)	T65.891	T65.892	T65.893	T65.894	--	--
PCB	T65.891	T65.892	T65.893	T65.894	--	--
PCP						
meaning pentachlorophenol	T60.1X1	T60.1X2	T60.1X3	T60.1X4	--	--
fungicide	T60.3X1	T60.3X2	T60.3X3	T60.3X4	--	--
herbicide	T60.3X1	T60.3X2	T60.3X3	T60.3X4	--	--
insecticide	T60.1X1	T60.1X2	T60.1X3	T60.1X4	--	--
meaning phencyclidine	T40.991	T40.992	T40.993	T40.994	--	--
Peach kernel oil (emulsion)	T47.4X1	T47.4X2	T47.4X3	T47.4X4	T47.4X5	T47.4X6
Peanut oil (emulsion) **NEC**	T47.4X1	T47.4X2	T47.4X3	T47.4X4	T47.4X5	T47.4X6
topical	T49.3X1	T49.3X2	T49.3X3	T49.3X4	T49.3X5	T49.3X6
Pearly Gates (morning glory seeds)	T40.991	T40.992	T40.993	T40.994	--	--
Pecazine	T43.3X1	T43.3X2	T43.3X3	T43.3X4	T43.3X5	T43.3X6
Pectin	T47.6X1	T47.6X2	T47.6X3	T47.6X4	T47.6X5	T47.6X6
Pefloxacin	T37.8X1	T37.8X2	T37.8X3	T37.8X4	T37.8X5	T37.8X6
Pegademase, bovine	T50.Z91	T50.Z92	T50.Z93	T50.Z94	T50.Z95	T50.Z96
Pelletierine tannate	T37.4X1	T37.4X2	T37.4X3	T37.4X4	T37.4X5	T37.4X6
Pemirolast (potassium)	T48.6X1	T48.6X2	T48.6X3	T48.6X4	T48.6X5	T48.6X6
Pemoline	T50.7X1	T50.7X2	T50.7X3	T50.7X4	T50.7X5	T50.7X6
Pempidine	T44.2X1	T44.2X2	T44.2X3	T44.2X4	T44.2X5	T44.2X6
Penamecillin	T36.0X1	T36.0X2	T36.0X3	T36.0X4	T36.0X5	T36.0X6
Penbutolol	T44.7X1	T44.7X2	T44.7X3	T44.7X4	T44.7X5	T44.7X6
Penethamate	T36.0X1	T36.0X2	T36.0X3	T36.0X4	T36.0X5	T36.0X6
Penfluridol	T43.591	T43.592	T43.593	T43.594	T43.595	T43.596
Penflutizide	T50.2X1	T50.2X2	T50.2X3	T50.2X4	T50.2X5	T50.2X6
Pengitoxin	T46.0X1	T46.0X2	T46.0X3	T46.0X4	T46.0X5	T46.0X6
Penicillamine	T50.6X1	T50.6X2	T50.6X3	T50.6X4	T50.6X5	T50.6X6
Penicillin (any)	T36.0X1	T36.0X2	T36.0X3	T36.0X4	T36.0X5	T36.0X6
Penicillinase	T45.3X1	T45.3X2	T45.3X3	T45.3X4	T45.3X5	T45.3X6
Penicilloyl polylysine	T50.8X1	T50.8X2	T50.8X3	T50.8X4	T50.8X5	T50.8X6
Penimepicycline	T36.4X1	T36.4X2	T36.4X3	T36.4X4	T36.4X5	T36.4X6
Pentachloroethane	T53.6X1	T53.6X2	T53.6X3	T53.6X4	--	--
Pentachloronaphthalene	T53.7X1	T53.7X2	T53.7X3	T53.7X4	--	--
Pentachlorophenol (pesticide)	T60.1X1	T60.1X2	T60.1X3	T60.1X4	--	--
fungicide	T60.3X1	T60.3X2	T60.3X3	T60.3X4	--	--
herbicide	T60.3X1	T60.3X2	T60.3X3	T60.3X4	--	--
insecticide	T60.1X1	T60.1X2	T60.1X3	T60.1X4	--	--
Pentaerythritol	T46.3X1	T46.3X2	T46.3X3	T46.3X4	T46.3X5	T46.3X6
chloral	T42.6X1	T42.6X2	T42.6X3	T42.6X4	T42.6X5	T42.6X6
tetranitrate NEC	T46.3X1	T46.3X2	T46.3X3	T46.3X4	T46.3X5	T46.3X6
Pentaerythrityl tetranitrate	T46.3X1	T46.3X2	T46.3X3	T46.3X4	T46.3X5	T46.3X6
Pentagastrin	T50.8X1	T50.8X2	T50.8X3	T50.8X4	T50.8X5	T50.8X6
Pentalin	T53.6X1	T53.6X2	T53.6X3	T53.6X4	--	--
Pentamethonium bromide	T44.2X1	T44.2X2	T44.2X3	T44.2X4	T44.2X5	T44.2X6
Pentamidine	T37.3X1	T37.3X2	T37.3X3	T37.3X4	T37.3X5	T37.3X6
Pentanol	T51.3X1	T51.3X2	T51.3X3	T51.3X4	--	--
Pentapyrrolinium (bitartrate)	T44.2X1	T44.2X2	T44.2X3	T44.2X4	T44.2X5	T44.2X6
Pentaquine	T37.2X1	T37.2X2	T37.2X3	T37.2X4	T37.2X5	T37.2X6
Pentazocine	T40.4X1	T40.4X2	T40.4X3	T40.4X4	T40.4X5	T40.4X6
Pentetrazole	T50.7X1	T50.7X2	T50.7X3	T50.7X4	T50.7X5	T50.7X6
Penthienate bromide	T44.3X1	T44.3X2	T44.3X3	T44.3X4	T44.3X5	T44.3X6
Pentifylline	T46.7X1	T46.7X2	T46.7X3	T46.7X4	T46.7X5	T46.7X6
Pentobarbital	T42.3X1	T42.3X2	T42.3X3	T42.3X4	T42.3X5	T42.3X6
sodium	T42.3X1	T42.3X2	T42.3X3	T42.3X4	T42.3X5	T42.3X6
Pentobarbitone	T42.3X1	T42.3X2	T42.3X3	T42.3X4	T42.3X5	T42.3X6
Pentolonium tartrate	T44.2X1	T44.2X2	T44.2X3	T44.2X4	T44.2X5	T44.2X6
Pentosan polysulfate (sodium)	T39.8X1	T39.8X2	T39.8X3	T39.8X4	T39.8X5	T39.8X6
Pentostatin	T45.1X1	T45.1X2	T45.1X3	T45.1X4	T45.1X5	T45.1X6
Pentothal	T41.1X1	T41.1X2	T41.1X3	T41.1X4	T41.1X5	T41.1X6
Pentoxifylline	T46.7X1	T46.7X2	T46.7X3	T46.7X4	T46.7X5	T46.7X6
Pentoxyverine	T48.3X1	T48.3X2	T48.3X3	T48.3X4	T48.3X5	T48.3X6
Pentrinat	T46.3X1	T46.3X2	T46.3X3	T46.3X4	T46.3X5	T46.3X6
Pentylenetetrazole	T50.7X1	T50.7X2	T50.7X3	T50.7X4	T50.7X5	T50.7X6
Pentylsalicylamide	T37.1X1	T37.1X2	T37.1X3	T37.1X4	T37.1X5	T37.1X6
Pentymal	T42.3X1	T42.3X2	T42.3X3	T42.3X4	T42.3X5	T42.3X6
Peplomycin	T45.1X1	T45.1X2	T45.1X3	T45.1X4	T45.1X5	T45.1X6
Peppermint (oil)	T47.5X1	T47.5X2	T47.5X3	T47.5X4	T47.5X5	T47.5X6
Pepsin	T47.5X1	T47.5X2	T47.5X3	T47.5X4	T47.5X5	T47.5X6
digestant	T47.5X1	T47.5X2	T47.5X3	T47.5X4	T47.5X5	T47.5X6
Pepstatin	T47.1X1	T47.1X2	T47.1X3	T47.1X4	T47.1X5	T47.1X6
Peptavlon	T50.8X1	T50.8X2	T50.8X3	T50.8X4	T50.8X5	T50.8X6
Perazine	T43.3X1	T43.3X2	T43.3X3	T43.3X4	T43.3X5	T43.3X6
Percaine (spinal)	T41.3X1	T41.3X2	T41.3X3	T41.3X4	T41.3X5	T41.3X6
topical (surface)	T41.3X1	T41.3X2	T41.3X3	T41.3X4	T41.3X5	T41.3X6
Perchloroethylene	T53.3X1	T53.3X2	T53.3X3	T53.3X4	--	--
medicinal	T37.4X1	T37.4X2	T37.4X3	T37.4X4	T37.4X5	T37.4X6
vapor	T53.3X1	T53.3X2	T53.3X3	T53.3X4	--	--
Percodan	T40.2X1	T40.2X2	T40.2X3	T40.2X4	T40.2X5	T40.2X6
Percogesic (*see also* acetaminophen)	T45.0X1	T45.0X2	T45.0X3	T45.0X4	T45.0X5	T45.0X6
Percorten	T38.0X1	T38.0X2	T38.0X3	T38.0X4	T38.0X5	T38.0X6
Pergolide	T42.8X1	T42.8X2	T42.8X3	T42.8X4	T42.8X5	T42.8X6
Pergonal	T38.811	T38.812	T38.813	T38.814	T38.815	T38.816
Perhexilene	T46.3X1	T46.3X2	T46.3X3	T46.3X4	T46.3X5	T46.3X6
Perhexiline (maleate)	T46.3X1	T46.3X2	T46.3X3	T46.3X4	T46.3X5	T46.3X6
Periactin	T45.0X1	T45.0X2	T45.0X3	T45.0X4	T45.0X5	T45.0X6
Periciazine	T43.3X1	T43.3X2	T43.3X3	T43.3X4	T43.3X5	T43.3X6
Periclor	T42.6X1	T42.6X2	T42.6X3	T42.6X4	T42.6X5	T42.6X6
Perindopril	T46.4X1	T46.4X2	T46.4X3	T46.4X4	T46.4X5	T46.4X6
Perisoxal	T39.8X1	T39.8X2	T39.8X3	T39.8X4	T39.8X5	T39.8X6
Peritoneal dialysis solution	T50.3X1	T50.3X2	T50.3X3	T50.3X4	T50.3X5	T50.3X6
Peritrate	T46.3X1	T46.3X2	T46.3X3	T46.3X4	T46.3X5	T46.3X6
Perlapine	T42.4X1	T42.4X2	T42.4X3	T42.4X4	T42.4X5	T42.4X6
Permanganate	T65.891	T65.892	T65.893	T65.894	--	--
Permethrin	T60.1X1	T60.1X2	T60.1X3	T60.1X4	--	--
Pernocton	T42.3X1	T42.3X2	T42.3X3	T42.3X4	T42.3X5	T42.3X6
Pernoston	T42.3X1	T42.3X2	T42.3X3	T42.3X4	T42.3X5	T42.3X6
Peronine	T40.2X1	T40.2X2	T40.2X3	T40.2X4	--	--
Perphenazine	T43.3X1	T43.3X2	T43.3X3	T43.3X4	T43.3X5	T43.3X6
Pertofrane	T43.011	T43.012	T43.013	T43.014	T43.015	T43.016
Pertussis						
immune serum (human)	T50.Z11	T50.Z12	T50.Z13	T50.Z14	T50.Z15	T50.Z16
vaccine (with diphtheria toxoid) (with tetanus toxoid)	T50.A11	T50.A12	T50.A13	T50.A14	T50.A15	T50.A16
Peruvian balsam	T49.0X1	T49.0X2	T49.0X3	T49.0X4	T49.0X5	T49.0X6
Peruvoside	T46.0X1	T46.0X2	T46.0X3	T46.0X4	T46.0X5	T46.0X6
Pesticide (dust) (fumes) (vapor) **NEC**	T60.91	T60.92	T60.93	T60.94	--	--
arsenic	T57.0X1	T57.0X2	T57.0X3	T57.0X4	--	--
chlorinated	T60.1X1	T60.1X2	T60.1X3	T60.1X4	--	--
cyanide	T65.0X1	T65.0X2	T65.0X3	T65.0X4	--	--
kerosene	T52.0X1	T52.0X2	T52.0X3	T52.0X4	--	--
mixture (of compounds)	T60.91	T60.92	T60.93	T60.94	--	--
naphthalene	T60.2X1	T60.2X2	T60.2X3	T60.2X4	--	--
organochlorine (compounds)	T60.1X1	T60.1X2	T60.1X3	T60.1X4	--	--
petroleum (distillate) (products) NEC	T60.8X1	T60.8X2	T60.8X3	T60.8X4	--	--
specified ingredient NEC	T60.8X1	T60.8X2	T60.8X3	T60.8X4	--	--
strychnine	T65.1X1	T65.1X2	T65.1X3	T65.1X4	--	--
thallium	T60.4X1	T60.4X2	T60.4X3	T60.4X4	--	--

Substance	Poisoning, Accidental (unintentional)	Poisoning, Intentional self-harm	Poisoning, Assault	Poisoning, Undetermined	Adverse effect	Underdosing
Pethidine	T40.4X1	T40.4X2	T40.4X3	T40.4X4	T40.4X5	T40.4X6
Petrichloral	T42.6X1	T42.6X2	T42.6X3	T42.6X4	T42.6X5	T42.6X6
Petrol	T52.0X1	T52.0X2	T52.0X3	T52.0X4	--	--
vapor	T52.0X1	T52.0X2	T52.0X3	T52.0X4	--	--
Petrolatum	T49.3X1	T49.3X2	T49.3X3	T49.3X4	T49.3X5	T49.3X6
hydrophilic	T49.3X1	T49.3X2	T49.3X3	T49.3X4	T49.3X5	T49.3X6
liquid	T47.4X1	T47.4X2	T47.4X3	T47.4X4	T47.4X5	T47.4X6
topical	T49.3X1	T49.3X2	T49.3X3	T49.3X4	T49.3X5	T49.3X6
nonmedicinal	T52.0X1	T52.0X2	T52.0X3	T52.0X4	--	--
red veterinary	T49.3X1	T49.3X2	T49.3X3	T49.3X4	T49.3X5	T49.3X6
white	T49.3X1	T49.3X2	T49.3X3	T49.3X4	T49.3X5	T49.3X6
Petroleum (products) NEC	T52.0X1	T52.0X2	T52.0X3	T52.0X4	--	--
benzine(s) — see Ligroin						
ether — see Ligroin						
jelly — see Petrolatum						
naphtha — see Ligroin						
pesticide	T60.8X1	T60.8X2	T60.8X3	T60.8X4	--	--
solids	T52.0X1	T52.0X2	T52.0X3	T52.0X4	--	--
solvents	T52.0X1	T52.0X2	T52.0X3	T52.0X4	--	--
vapor	T52.0X1	T52.0X2	T52.0X3	T52.0X4	--	--
Peyote	T40.991	T40.992	T40.993	T40.994	--	--
Phanodorm, phanodorn	T42.3X1	T42.3X2	T42.3X3	T42.3X4	T42.3X5	T42.3X6
Phanquinone	T37.3X1	T37.3X2	T37.3X3	T37.3X4	T37.3X5	T37.3X6
Phanquone	T37.3X1	T37.3X2	T37.3X3	T37.3X4	T37.3X5	T37.3X6
Pharmaceutical						
adjunct NEC	T50.901	T50.902	T50.903	T50.904	T50.905	T50.906
excipient NEC	T50.901	T50.902	T50.903	T50.904	T50.905	T50.906
sweetener	T50.901	T50.902	T50.903	T50.904	T50.905	T50.906
viscous agent	T50.901	T50.902	T50.903	T50.904	T50.905	T50.906
Phemitone	T42.3X1	T42.3X2	T42.3X3	T42.3X4	T42.3X5	T42.3X6
Phenacaine	T41.3X1	T41.3X2	T41.3X3	T41.3X4	T41.3X5	T41.3X6
Phenacemide	T42.6X1	T42.6X2	T42.6X3	T42.6X4	T42.6X5	T42.6X6
Phenacetin	T39.1X1	T39.1X2	T39.1X3	T39.1X4	T39.1X5	T39.1X6
Phenadoxone	T40.2X1	T40.2X2	T40.2X3	T40.2X4	--	--
Phenaglycodol	T43.591	T43.592	T43.593	T43.594	T43.595	T43.596
Phenantoin	T42.0X1	T42.0X2	T42.0X3	T42.0X4	T42.0X5	T42.0X6
Phenaphthazine reagent	T50.991	T50.992	T50.993	T50.994	T50.995	T50.996
Phenazocine	T40.4X1	T40.4X2	T40.4X3	T40.4X4	T40.4X5	T40.4X6
Phenazone	T39.2X1	T39.2X2	T39.2X3	T39.2X4	T39.2X5	T39.2X6
Phenazopyridine	T39.8X1	T39.8X2	T39.8X3	T39.8X4	T39.8X5	T39.8X6
Phenbenicillin	T36.0X1	T36.0X2	T36.0X3	T36.0X4	T36.0X5	T36.0X6
Phenbutrazate	T50.5X1	T50.5X2	T50.5X3	T50.5X4	T50.5X5	T50.5X6
Phencyclidine	T40.991	T40.992	T40.993	T40.994	T40.995	T40.996
Phendimetrazine	T50.5X1	T50.5X2	T50.5X3	T50.5X4	T50.5X5	T50.5X6
Phenelzine	T43.1X1	T43.1X2	T43.1X3	T43.1X4	T43.1X5	T43.1X6
Phenemal	T42.3X1	T42.3X2	T42.3X3	T42.3X4	T42.3X5	T42.3X6
Phenergan	T42.6X1	T42.6X2	T42.6X3	T42.6X4	T42.6X5	T42.6X6
Pheneticillin	T36.0X1	T36.0X2	T36.0X3	T36.0X4	T36.0X5	T36.0X6
Pheneturide	T42.6X1	T42.6X2	T42.6X3	T42.6X4	T42.6X5	T42.6X6
Phenformin	T38.3X1	T38.3X2	T38.3X3	T38.3X4	T38.3X5	T38.3X6
Phenglutarimide	T44.3X1	T44.3X2	T44.3X3	T44.3X4	T44.3X5	T44.3X6
Phenicarbazide	T39.8X1	T39.8X2	T39.8X3	T39.8X4	T39.8X5	T39.8X6
Phenindamine	T45.0X1	T45.0X2	T45.0X3	T45.0X4	T45.0X5	T45.0X6
Phenindione	T45.511	T45.512	T45.513	T45.514	T45.515	T45.516
Pheniprazine	T43.1X1	T43.1X2	T43.1X3	T43.1X4	T43.1X5	T43.1X6
Pheniramine	T45.0X1	T45.0X2	T45.0X3	T45.0X4	T45.0X5	T45.0X6
Phenisatin	T47.2X1	T47.2X2	T47.2X3	T47.2X4	T47.2X5	T47.2X6
Phenmetrazine	T50.5X1	T50.5X2	T50.5X3	T50.5X4	T50.5X5	T50.5X6
Phenobal	T42.3X1	T42.3X2	T42.3X3	T42.3X4	T42.3X5	T42.3X6
Phenobarbital	T42.3X1	T42.3X2	T42.3X3	T42.3X4	T42.3X5	T42.3X6
with						
mephenytoin	T42.3X1	T42.3X2	T42.3X3	T42.3X4	T42.3X5	T42.3X6
phenytoin	T42.3X1	T42.3X2	T42.3X3	T42.3X4	T42.3X5	T42.3X6
sodium	T42.3X1	T42.3X2	T42.3X3	T42.3X4	T42.3X5	T42.3X6
Phenobarbitone	T42.3X1	T42.3X2	T42.3X3	T42.3X4	T42.3X5	T42.3X6
Phenobutiodil	T50.8X1	T50.8X2	T50.8X3	T50.8X4	T50.8X5	T50.8X6
Phenoctide	T49.0X1	T49.0X2	T49.0X3	T49.0X4	T49.0X5	T49.0X6
Phenol	T49.0X1	T49.0X2	T49.0X3	T49.0X4	T49.0X5	T49.0X6
disinfectant	T54.0X1	T54.0X2	T54.0X3	T54.0X4	--	--
in oil injection	T46.8X1	T46.8X2	T46.8X3	T46.8X4	T46.8X5	T46.8X6
medicinal	T49.1X1	T49.1X2	T49.1X3	T49.1X4	T49.1X5	T49.1X6
nonmedicinal NEC	T54.0X1	T54.0X2	T54.0X3	T54.0X4	--	--
pesticide	T60.8X1	T60.8X2	T60.8X3	T60.8X4	--	--
red	T50.8X1	T50.8X2	T50.8X3	T50.8X4	T50.8X5	T50.8X6
Phenolic preparation	T49.1X1	T49.1X2	T49.1X3	T49.1X4	T49.1X5	T49.1X6
Phenolphthalein	T47.2X1	T47.2X2	T47.2X3	T47.2X4	T47.2X5	T47.2X6
Phenolsulfonphthalein	T50.8X1	T50.8X2	T50.8X3	T50.8X4	T50.8X5	T50.8X6
Phenomorphan	T40.2X1	T40.2X2	T40.2X3	T40.2X4	--	--
Phenonyl	T42.3X1	T42.3X2	T42.3X3	T42.3X4	T42.3X5	T42.3X6
Phenoperidine	T40.4X1	T40.4X2	T40.4X3	T40.4X4	--	--
Phenopyrazone	T46.991	T46.992	T46.993	T46.994	T46.995	T46.996
Phenoquin	T50.4X1	T50.4X2	T50.4X3	T50.4X4	T50.4X5	T50.4X6
Phenothiazine (psychotropic) NEC	T43.3X1	T43.3X2	T43.3X3	T43.3X4	T43.3X5	T43.3X6
insecticide	T60.2X1	T60.2X2	T60.2X3	T60.2X4	--	--

Substance	Poisoning, Accidental (unintentional)	Poisoning, Intentional self-harm	Poisoning, Assault	Poisoning, Undetermined	Adverse effect	Underdosing
Phenothrin	T49.0X1	T49.0X2	T49.0X3	T49.0X4	T49.0X5	T49.0X6
Phenoxybenzamine	T46.7X1	T46.7X2	T46.7X3	T46.7X4	T46.7X5	T46.7X6
Phenoxyethanol	T49.0X1	T49.0X2	T49.0X3	T49.0X4	T49.0X5	T49.0X6
Phenoxymethyl penicillin	T36.0X1	T36.0X2	T36.0X3	T36.0X4	T36.0X5	T36.0X6
Phenprobamate	T42.8X1	T42.8X2	T42.8X3	T42.8X4	T42.8X5	T42.8X6
Phenprocoumon	T45.511	T45.512	T45.513	T45.514	T45.515	T45.516
Phensuximide	T42.2X1	T42.2X2	T42.2X3	T42.2X4	T42.2X5	T42.2X6
Phentermine	T50.5X1	T50.5X2	T50.5X3	T50.5X4	T50.5X5	T50.5X6
Phenthicillin	T36.0X1	T36.0X2	T36.0X3	T36.0X4	T36.0X5	T36.0X6
Phentolamine	T46.7X1	T46.7X2	T46.7X3	T46.7X4	T46.7X5	T46.7X6
Phenyl						
butazone	T39.2X1	T39.2X2	T39.2X3	T39.2X4	T39.2X5	T39.2X6
enediamine	T65.3X1	T65.3X2	T65.3X3	T65.3X4	--	--
hydrazine	T65.3X1	T65.3X2	T65.3X3	T65.3X4	--	--
antineoplastic	T45.1X1	T45.1X2	T45.1X3	T45.1X4	T45.1X5	T45.1X6
mercuric compounds — see Mercury						
salicylate	T49.3X1	T49.3X2	T49.3X3	T49.3X4	T49.3X5	T49.3X6
Phenylalanine mustard	T45.1X1	T45.1X2	T45.1X3	T45.1X4	T45.1X5	T45.1X6
Phenylbutazone	T39.2X1	T39.2X2	T39.2X3	T39.2X4	T39.2X5	T39.2X6
Phenylenediamine	T65.3X1	T65.3X2	T65.3X3	T65.3X4	--	--
Phenylephrine	T44.4X1	T44.4X2	T44.4X3	T44.4X4	T44.4X5	T44.4X6
Phenylethylbiguanide	T38.3X1	T38.3X2	T38.3X3	T38.3X4	T38.3X5	T38.3X6
Phenylmercuric						
acetate	T49.0X1	T49.0X2	T49.0X3	T49.0X4	T49.0X5	T49.0X6
borate	T49.0X1	T49.0X2	T49.0X3	T49.0X4	T49.0X5	T49.0X6
nitrate	T49.0X1	T49.0X2	T49.0X3	T49.0X4	T49.0X5	T49.0X6
Phenylmethylbarbitone	T42.3X1	T42.3X2	T42.3X3	T42.3X4	T42.3X5	T42.3X6
Phenylpropanol	T47.5X1	T47.5X2	T47.5X3	T47.5X4	T47.5X5	T47.5X6
Phenylpropanolamine	T44.991	T44.992	T44.993	T44.994	T44.995	T44.996
Phenylsulfthion	T60.0X1	T60.0X2	T60.0X3	T60.0X4	--	--
Phenyltoloxamine	T45.0X1	T45.0X2	T45.0X3	T45.0X4	T45.0X5	T45.0X6
Phenyramidol, phenyramidon	T39.8X1	T39.8X2	T39.8X3	T39.8X4	T39.8X5	T39.8X6
Phenytoin	T42.0X1	T42.0X2	T42.0X3	T42.0X4	T42.0X5	T42.0X6
with Phenobarbital	T42.3X1	T42.3X2	T42.3X3	T42.3X4	T42.3X5	T42.3X6
pHisoHex	T49.2X1	T49.2X2	T49.2X3	T49.2X4	T49.2X5	T49.2X6
Pholcodine	T48.3X1	T48.3X2	T48.3X3	T48.3X4	T48.3X5	T48.3X6
Pholedrine	T46.991	T46.992	T46.993	T46.994	T46.995	T46.996
Phorate	T60.0X1	T60.0X2	T60.0X3	T60.0X4	--	--
Phosdrin	T60.0X1	T60.0X2	T60.0X3	T60.0X4	--	--
Phosfolan	T60.0X1	T60.0X2	T60.0X3	T60.0X4	--	--
Phosgene (gas)	T59.891	T59.892	T59.893	T59.894	--	--
Phosphamidon	T60.0X1	T60.0X2	T60.0X3	T60.0X4	--	--
Phosphate	T65.891	T65.892	T65.893	T65.894	--	--
laxative	T47.4X1	T47.4X2	T47.4X3	T47.4X4	T47.4X5	T47.4X6
organic	T60.0X1	T60.0X2	T60.0X3	T60.0X4	--	--
solvent	T52.91	T52.92	T52.93	T52.94	--	--
tricresyl	T65.891	T65.892	T65.893	T65.894	--	--
Phosphine	T57.1X1	T57.1X2	T57.1X3	T57.1X4	--	--
fumigant	T57.1X1	T57.1X2	T57.1X3	T57.1X4	--	--
Phospholine	T49.5X1	T49.5X2	T49.5X3	T49.5X4	T49.5X5	T49.5X6
Phosphoric acid	T54.2X1	T54.2X2	T54.2X3	T54.2X4	--	--
Phosphorus (compound) NEC	T57.1X1	T57.1X2	T57.1X3	T57.1X4	--	--
pesticide	T60.0X1	T60.0X2	T60.0X3	T60.0X4	--	--
Phthalates	T65.891	T65.892	T65.893	T65.894	--	--
Phthalic anhydride	T65.891	T65.892	T65.893	T65.894	--	--
Phthalimidoglutarimide	T42.6X1	T42.6X2	T42.6X3	T42.6X4	T42.6X5	T42.6X6
Phthalylsulfathiazole	T37.0X1	T37.0X2	T37.0X3	T37.0X4	T37.0X5	T37.0X6
Phylloquinone	T45.7X1	T45.7X2	T45.7X3	T45.7X4	T45.7X5	T45.7X6
Physeptone	T40.3X1	T40.3X2	T40.3X3	T40.3X4	T40.3X5	T40.3X6
Physostigma venenosum	T62.2X1	T62.2X2	T62.2X3	T62.2X4	--	--
Physostigmine	T49.5X1	T49.5X2	T49.5X3	T49.5X4	T49.5X5	T49.5X6
Phytolacca decandra	T62.2X1	T62.2X2	T62.2X3	T62.2X4	--	--
berries	T62.1X1	T62.1X2	T62.1X3	T62.1X4	--	--
Phytomenadione	T45.7X1	T45.7X2	T45.7X3	T45.7X4	T45.7X5	T45.7X6
Phytonadione	T45.7X1	T45.7X2	T45.7X3	T45.7X4	T45.7X5	T45.7X6
Picoperine	T48.3X1	T48.3X2	T48.3X3	T48.3X4	T48.3X5	T48.3X6
Picosulfate (sodium)	T47.2X1	T47.2X2	T47.2X3	T47.2X4	T47.2X5	T47.2X6
Picric (acid)	T54.2X1	T54.2X2	T54.2X3	T54.2X4	--	--
Picrotoxin	T50.7X1	T50.7X2	T50.7X3	T50.7X4	T50.7X5	T50.7X6
Piketoprofen	T49.0X1	T49.0X2	T49.0X3	T49.0X4	T49.0X5	T49.0X6
Pilocarpine	T44.1X1	T44.1X2	T44.1X3	T44.1X4	T44.1X5	T44.1X6
Pilocarpus (jaborandi) extract	T44.1X1	T44.1X2	T44.1X3	T44.1X4	T44.1X5	T44.1X6
Pilsicainide (hydrochloride)	T46.2X1	T46.2X2	T46.2X3	T46.2X4	T46.2X5	T46.2X6
Pimaricin	T36.7X1	T36.7X2	T36.7X3	T36.7X4	T36.7X5	T36.7X6
Pimeclone	T50.7X1	T50.7X2	T50.7X3	T50.7X4	T50.7X5	T50.7X6
Pimelic ketone	T52.8X1	T52.8X2	T52.8X3	T52.8X4	--	--
Pimethixene	T45.0X1	T45.0X2	T45.0X3	T45.0X4	T45.0X5	T45.0X6
Piminodine	T40.2X1	T40.2X2	T40.2X3	T40.2X4	T40.2X5	T40.2X6
Pimozide	T43.591	T43.592	T43.593	T43.594	T43.595	T43.596
Pinacidil	T46.5X1	T46.5X2	T46.5X3	T46.5X4	T46.5X5	T46.5X6
Pinaverium bromide	T44.3X1	T44.3X2	T44.3X3	T44.3X4	T44.3X5	T44.3X6
Pinazepam	T42.4X1	T42.4X2	T42.4X3	T42.4X4	T42.4X5	T42.4X6
Pindolol	T44.7X1	T44.7X2	T44.7X3	T44.7X4	T44.7X5	T44.7X6

Pindone - Pramoxine

Substance	Poisoning, Accidental (unintentional)	Poisoning, Intentional self-harm	Poisoning, Assault	Poisoning, Undetermined	Adverse effect	Underdosing
Pindone	T60.4X1	T60.4X2	T60.4X3	T60.4X4	--	--
Pine oil (disinfectant)	T65.891	T65.892	T65.893	T65.894	--	--
Pinkroot	T37.4X1	T37.4X2	T37.4X3	T37.4X4	T37.4X5	T37.4X6
Pipadone	T40.2X1	T40.2X2	T40.2X3	T40.2X4	--	--
Pipamazine	T45.0X1	T45.0X2	T45.0X3	T45.0X4	T45.0X5	T45.0X6
Pipamperone	T43.4X1	T43.4X2	T43.4X3	T43.4X4	T43.4X5	T43.4X6
Pipazetate	T48.3X1	T48.3X2	T48.3X3	T48.3X4	T48.3X5	T48.3X6
Pipemidic acid	T37.8X1	T37.8X2	T37.8X3	T37.8X4	T37.8X5	T37.8X6
Pipenzolate bromide	T44.3X1	T44.3X2	T44.3X3	T44.3X4	T44.3X5	T44.3X6
Piperacetazine	T43.3X1	T43.3X2	T43.3X3	T43.3X4	T43.3X5	T43.3X6
Piperacillin	T36.0X1	T36.0X2	T36.0X3	T36.0X4	T36.0X5	T36.0X6
Piperazine	T37.4X1	T37.4X2	T37.4X3	T37.4X4	T37.4X5	T37.4X6
estrone sulfate	T38.5X1	T38.5X2	T38.5X3	T38.5X4	T38.5X5	T38.5X6
Piper cubeba	T62.2X1	T62.2X2	T62.2X3	T62.2X4	--	--
Piperidione	T48.3X1	T48.3X2	T48.3X3	T48.3X4	T48.3X5	T48.3X6
Piperidolate	T44.3X1	T44.3X2	T44.3X3	T44.3X4	T44.3X5	T44.3X6
Piperocaine	T41.3X1	T41.3X2	T41.3X3	T41.3X4	T41.3X5	T41.3X6
infiltration (subcutaneous)	T41.3X1	T41.3X2	T41.3X3	T41.3X4	T41.3X5	T41.3X6
nerve block (peripheral) (plexus)	T41.3X1	T41.3X2	T41.3X3	T41.3X4	T41.3X5	T41.3X6
topical (surface)	T41.3X1	T41.3X2	T41.3X3	T41.3X4	T41.3X5	T41.3X6
Piperonyl butoxide	T60.8X1	T60.8X2	T60.8X3	T60.8X4	--	--
Pipethanate	T44.3X1	T44.3X2	T44.3X3	T44.3X4	T44.3X5	T44.3X6
Pipobroman	T45.1X1	T45.1X2	T45.1X3	T45.1X4	T45.1X5	T45.1X6
Pipotiazine	T43.3X1	T43.3X2	T43.3X3	T43.3X4	T43.3X5	T43.3X6
Pipoxizine	T45.0X1	T45.0X2	T45.0X3	T45.0X4	T45.0X5	T45.0X6
Pipradrol	T43.691	T43.692	T43.693	T43.694	T43.695	T43.696
Piprinhydrinate	T45.0X1	T45.0X2	T45.0X3	T45.0X4	T45.0X5	T45.0X6
Pirarubicin	T45.1X1	T45.1X2	T45.1X3	T45.1X4	T45.1X5	T45.1X6
Pirazinamide	T37.1X1	T37.1X2	T37.1X3	T37.1X4	T37.1X5	T37.1X6
Pirbuterol	T48.6X1	T48.6X2	T48.6X3	T48.6X4	T48.6X5	T48.6X6
Pirenzepine	T47.1X1	T47.1X2	T47.1X3	T47.1X4	T47.1X5	T47.1X6
Piretanide	T50.1X1	T50.1X2	T50.1X3	T50.1X4	T50.1X5	T50.1X6
Piribedil	T42.8X1	T42.8X2	T42.8X3	T42.8X4	T42.8X5	T42.8X6
Piridoxilate	T46.3X1	T46.3X2	T46.3X3	T46.3X4	T46.3X5	T46.3X6
Piritramide	T40.4X1	T40.4X2	T40.4X3	T40.4X4	--	--
Piromidic acid	T37.8X1	T37.8X2	T37.8X3	T37.8X4	T37.8X5	T37.8X6
Piroxicam	T39.391	T39.392	T39.393	T39.394	T39.395	T39.396
beta-cyclodextrin complex	T39.8X1	T39.8X2	T39.8X3	T39.8X4	T39.8X5	T39.8X6
Pirozadil	T46.6X1	T46.6X2	T46.6X3	T46.6X4	T46.6X5	T46.6X6
Piscidia (bark) (erythrina)	T39.8X1	T39.8X2	T39.8X3	T39.8X4	T39.8X5	T39.8X6
Pitch	T65.891	T65.892	T65.893	T65.894	--	--
Pitkin's solution	T41.3X1	T41.3X2	T41.3X3	T41.3X4	T41.3X5	T41.3X6
Pitocin	T48.0X1	T48.0X2	T48.0X3	T48.0X4	T48.0X5	T48.0X6
Pitressin (tannate)	T38.891	T38.892	T38.893	T38.894	T38.895	T38.896
Pituitary extracts (posterior)	T38.891	T38.892	T38.893	T38.894	T38.895	T38.896
anterior	T38.811	T38.812	T38.813	T38.814	T38.815	T38.816
Pituitrin	T38.891	T38.892	T38.893	T38.894	T38.895	T38.896
Pivampicillin	T36.0X1	T36.0X2	T36.0X3	T36.0X4	T36.0X5	T36.0X6
Pivmecillinam	T36.0X1	T36.0X2	T36.0X3	T36.0X4	T36.0X5	T36.0X6
Placental hormone	T38.891	T38.892	T38.893	T38.894	T38.895	T38.896
Placidyl	T42.6X1	T42.6X2	T42.6X3	T42.6X4	T42.6X5	T42.6X6
Plague vaccine	T50.A91	T50.A92	T50.A93	T50.A94	T50.A95	T50.A96
Plant						
food or fertilizer NEC	T65.891	T65.892	T65.893	T65.894	--	--
containing herbicide	T60.3X1	T60.3X2	T60.3X3	T60.3X4	--	--
noxious, used as food	T62.2X1	T62.2X2	T62.2X3	T62.2X4	--	--
berries	T62.1X1	T62.1X2	T62.1X3	T62.1X4	--	--
seeds	T62.2X1	T62.2X2	T62.2X3	T62.2X4	--	--
specified type NEC	T62.2X1	T62.2X2	T62.2X3	T62.2X4	--	--
Plasma	T45.8X1	T45.8X2	T45.8X3	T45.8X4	T45.8X5	T45.8X6
expander NEC	T45.8X1	T45.8X2	T45.8X3	T45.8X4	T45.8X5	T45.8X6
protein fraction (human)	T45.8X1	T45.8X2	T45.8X3	T45.8X4	T45.8X5	T45.8X6
Plasmanate	T45.8X1	T45.8X2	T45.8X3	T45.8X4	T45.8X5	T45.8X6
Plasminogen (tissue) activator	T45.611	T45.612	T45.613	T45.614	T45.615	T45.616
Plaster dressing	T49.3X1	T49.3X2	T49.3X3	T49.3X4	T49.3X5	T49.3X6
Plastic dressing	T49.3X1	T49.3X2	T49.3X3	T49.3X4	T49.3X5	T49.3X6
Plegicil	T43.3X1	T43.3X2	T43.3X3	T43.3X4	T43.3X5	T43.3X6
Plicamycin	T45.1X1	T45.1X2	T45.1X3	T45.1X4	T45.1X5	T45.1X6
Podophyllotoxin	T49.8X1	T49.8X2	T49.8X3	T49.8X4	T49.8X5	T49.8X6
Podophyllum (resin)	T49.4X1	T49.4X2	T49.4X3	T49.4X4	T49.4X5	T49.4X6
Poison NEC	T65.91	T65.92	T65.93	T65.94	--	--
Poisonous berries	T62.1X1	T62.1X2	T62.1X3	T62.1X4	--	--
Pokeweed (any part)	T62.2X1	T62.2X2	T62.2X3	T62.2X4	--	--
Poldine metilsulfate	T44.3X1	T44.3X2	T44.3X3	T44.3X4	T44.3X5	T44.3X6
Polidexide (sulfate)	T46.6X1	T46.6X2	T46.6X3	T46.6X4	T46.6X5	T46.6X6
Polidocanol	T46.8X1	T46.8X2	T46.8X3	T46.8X4	T46.8X5	T46.8X6
Poliomyelitis vaccine	T50.B91	T50.B92	T50.B93	T50.B94	T50.B95	T50.B96
Polish (car) (floor) (furni-ture) (metal) (porcelain) (silver)	T65.891	T65.892	T65.893	T65.894	--	--
abrasive	T65.891	T65.892	T65.893	T65.894	--	--
porcelain	T65.891	T65.892	T65.893	T65.894	--	--
Poloxalkol	T47.4X1	T47.4X2	T47.4X3	T47.4X4	T47.4X5	T47.4X6
Poloxamer	T47.4X1	T47.4X2	T47.4X3	T47.4X4	T47.4X5	T47.4X6

Substance	Poisoning, Accidental (unintentional)	Poisoning, Intentional self-harm	Poisoning, Assault	Poisoning, Undetermined	Adverse effect	Underdosing
Polyaminostyrene resins	T50.3X1	T50.3X2	T50.3X3	T50.3X4	T50.3X5	T50.3X6
Polycarbophil	T47.4X1	T47.4X2	T47.4X3	T47.4X4	T47.4X5	T47.4X6
Polychlorinated biphenyl	T65.891	T65.892	T65.893	T65.894	--	--
Polycycline	T36.4X1	T36.4X2	T36.4X3	T36.4X4	T36.4X5	T36.4X6
Polyester fumes	T59.891	T59.892	T59.893	T59.894	--	--
Polyester resin hardener	T52.91	T52.92	T52.93	T52.94	--	--
fumes	T59.891	T59.892	T59.893	T59.894	--	--
Polyestradiol phosphate	T38.5X1	T38.5X2	T38.5X3	T38.5X4	T38.5X5	T38.5X6
Polyethanolamine alkyl sulfate	T49.2X1	T49.2X2	T49.2X3	T49.2X4	T49.2X5	T49.2X6
Polyethylene adhesive	T49.3X1	T49.3X2	T49.3X3	T49.3X4	T49.3X5	T49.3X6
Polyferose	T45.4X1	T45.4X2	T45.4X3	T45.4X4	T45.4X5	T45.4X6
Polygeline	T45.8X1	T45.8X2	T45.8X3	T45.8X4	T45.8X5	T45.8X6
Polymyxin	T36.8X1	T36.8X2	T36.8X3	T36.8X4	T36.8X5	T36.8X6
B	T36.8X1	T36.8X2	T36.8X3	T36.8X4	T36.8X5	T36.8X6
ENT agent	T49.6X1	T49.6X2	T49.6X3	T49.6X4	T49.6X5	T49.6X6
ophthalmic preparation	T49.5X1	T49.5X2	T49.5X3	T49.5X4	T49.5X5	T49.5X6
topical NEC	T49.0X1	T49.0X2	T49.0X3	T49.0X4	T49.0X5	T49.0X6
E sulfate (eye preparation)	T49.5X1	T49.5X2	T49.5X3	T49.5X4	T49.5X5	T49.5X6
Polynoxylin	T49.0X1	T49.0X2	T49.0X3	T49.0X4	T49.0X5	T49.0X6
Polyoestradiol phosphate	T38.5X1	T38.5X2	T38.5X3	T38.5X4	T38.5X5	T38.5X6
Polyoxymethyleneurea	T49.0X1	T49.0X2	T49.0X3	T49.0X4	T49.0X5	T49.0X6
Polysilane	T47.8X1	T47.8X2	T47.8X3	T47.8X4	T47.8X5	T47.8X6
Polytetrafluoroethylene (inhaled)	T59.891	T59.892	T59.893	T59.894	--	--
Polythiazide	T50.2X1	T50.2X2	T50.2X3	T50.2X4	T50.2X5	T50.2X6
Polyvidone	T45.8X1	T45.8X2	T45.8X3	T45.8X4	T45.8X5	T45.8X6
Polyvinylpyrrolidone	T45.8X1	T45.8X2	T45.8X3	T45.8X4	T45.8X5	T45.8X6
Pontocaine (hydrochloride) (infiltration) (topical)	T41.3X1	T41.3X2	T41.3X3	T41.3X4	T41.3X5	T41.3X6
nerve block (peripheral) (plexus)	T41.3X1	T41.3X2	T41.3X3	T41.3X4	T41.3X5	T41.3X6
spinal	T41.3X1	T41.3X2	T41.3X3	T41.3X4	T41.3X5	T41.3X6
Porfiromycin	T45.1X1	T45.1X2	T45.1X3	T45.1X4	T45.1X5	T45.1X6
Posterior pituitary hormone NEC	T38.891	T38.892	T38.893	T38.894	T38.895	T38.896
Pot	T40.7X1	T40.7X2	T40.7X3	T40.7X4	T40.7X5	T40.7X6
Potash (caustic)	T54.3X1	T54.3X2	T54.3X3	T54.3X4	--	--
Potassic saline injection (lactated)	T50.3X1	T50.3X2	T50.3X3	T50.3X4	T50.3X5	T50.3X6
Potassium (salts) NEC	T50.3X1	T50.3X2	T50.3X3	T50.3X4	T50.3X5	T50.3X6
aminobenzoate	T45.8X1	T45.8X2	T45.8X3	T45.8X4	T45.8X5	T45.8X6
aminosalicylate	T37.1X1	T37.1X2	T37.1X3	T37.1X4	T37.1X5	T37.1X6
antimony 'tartrate'	T37.8X1	T37.8X2	T37.8X3	T37.8X4	T37.8X5	T37.8X6
arsenite (solution)	T57.0X1	T57.0X2	T57.0X3	T57.0X4	--	--
bichromate	T56.2X1	T56.2X2	T56.2X3	T56.2X4	--	--
bisulfate	T47.3X1	T47.3X2	T47.3X3	T47.3X4	T47.3X5	T47.3X6
bromide	T42.6X1	T42.6X2	T42.6X3	T42.6X4	T42.6X5	T42.6X6
canrenoate	T50.0X1	T50.0X2	T50.0X3	T50.0X4	T50.0X5	T50.0X6
carbonate	T54.3X1	T54.3X2	T54.3X3	T54.3X4	--	--
chlorate NEC	T65.891	T65.892	T65.893	T65.894	--	--
chloride	T50.3X1	T50.3X2	T50.3X3	T50.3X4	T50.3X5	T50.3X6
citrate	T50.991	T50.992	T50.993	T50.994	T50.995	T50.996
cyanide	T65.0X1	T65.0X2	T65.0X3	T65.0X4	--	--
ferric hexacyanoferrate (medicinal)	T50.6X1	T50.6X2	T50.6X3	T50.6X4	T50.6X5	T50.6X6
nonmedicinal	T65.891	T65.892	T65.893	T65.894	--	--
fluoride	T57.8X1	T57.8X2	T57.8X3	T57.8X4	--	--
glucaldrate	T47.1X1	T47.1X2	T47.1X3	T47.1X4	T47.1X5	T47.1X6
hydroxide	T54.3X1	T54.3X2	T54.3X3	T54.3X4	--	--
iodate	T49.0X1	T49.0X2	T49.0X3	T49.0X4	T49.0X5	T49.0X6
iodide	T48.4X1	T48.4X2	T48.4X3	T48.4X4	T48.4X5	T48.4X6
nitrate	T57.8X1	T57.8X2	T57.8X3	T57.8X4	--	--
oxalate	T65.891	T65.892	T65.893	T65.894	--	--
perchlorate (nonmedicinal) NEC	T65.891	T65.892	T65.893	T65.894	--	--
antithyroid	T38.2X1	T38.2X2	T38.2X3	T38.2X4	T38.2X5	T38.2X6
medicinal	T38.2X1	T38.2X2	T38.2X3	T38.2X4	T38.2X5	T38.2X6
permanganate (nonmedicinal)	T65.891	T65.892	T65.893	T65.894	--	--
medicinal	T49.0X1	T49.0X2	T49.0X3	T49.0X4	T49.0X5	T49.0X6
sulfate	T47.2X1	T47.2X2	T47.2X3	T47.2X4	T47.2X5	T47.2X6
Potassium-removing resin	T50.3X1	T50.3X2	T50.3X3	T50.3X4	T50.3X5	T50.3X6
Potassium-retaining drug	T50.3X1	T50.3X2	T50.3X3	T50.3X4	T50.3X5	T50.3X6
Povidone	T45.8X1	T45.8X2	T45.8X3	T45.8X4	T45.8X5	T45.8X6
iodine	T49.0X1	T49.0X2	T49.0X3	T49.0X4	T49.0X5	T49.0X6
Practolol	T44.7X1	T44.7X2	T44.7X3	T44.7X4	T44.7X5	T44.7X6
Prajmalium bitartrate	T46.2X1	T46.2X2	T46.2X3	T46.2X4	T46.2X5	T46.2X6
Pralidoxime (iodide)	T50.6X1	T50.6X2	T50.6X3	T50.6X4	T50.6X5	T50.6X6
chloride	T50.6X1	T50.6X2	T50.6X3	T50.6X4	T50.6X5	T50.6X6
Pramiverine	T44.3X1	T44.3X2	T44.3X3	T44.3X4	T44.3X5	T44.3X6
Pramocaine	T49.1X1	T49.1X2	T49.1X3	T49.1X4	T49.1X5	T49.1X6
Pramoxine	T49.1X1	T49.1X2	T49.1X3	T49.1X4	T49.1X5	T49.1X6

Substance	Poisoning, Accidental (unintentional)	Poisoning, Intentional self-harm	Poisoning, Assault	Poisoning, Undetermined	Adverse effect	Underdosing
Prasterone	T38.7X1	T38.7X2	T38.7X3	T38.7X4	T38.7X5	T38.7X6
Pravastatin	T46.6X1	T46.6X2	T46.6X3	T46.6X4	T46.6X5	T46.6X6
Prazepam	T42.4X1	T42.4X2	T42.4X3	T42.4X4	T42.4X5	T42.4X6
Praziquantel	T37.4X1	T37.4X2	T37.4X3	T37.4X4	T37.4X5	T37.4X6
Prazitone	T43.291	T43.292	T43.293	T43.294	T43.295	T43.296
Prazosin	T44.6X1	T44.6X2	T44.6X3	T44.6X4	T44.6X5	T44.6X6
Prednicarbate	T49.0X1	T49.0X2	T49.0X3	T49.0X4	T49.0X5	T49.0X6
Prednimustine	T45.1X1	T45.1X2	T45.1X3	T45.1X4	T45.1X5	T45.1X6
Prednisolone	T38.0X1	T38.0X2	T38.0X3	T38.0X4	T38.0X5	T38.0X6
ENT agent	T49.6X1	T49.6X2	T49.6X3	T49.6X4	T49.6X5	T49.6X6
ophthalmic preparation	T49.5X1	T49.5X2	T49.5X3	T49.5X4	T49.5X5	T49.5X6
steaglate	T49.0X1	T49.0X2	T49.0X3	T49.0X4	T49.0X5	T49.0X6
topical NEC	T49.0X1	T49.0X2	T49.0X3	T49.0X4	T49.0X5	T49.0X6
Prednisone	T38.0X1	T38.0X2	T38.0X3	T38.0X4	T38.0X5	T38.0X6
Prednylidene	T38.0X1	T38.0X2	T38.0X3	T38.0X4	T38.0X5	T38.0X6
Pregnandiol	T38.5X1	T38.5X2	T38.5X3	T38.5X4	T38.5X5	T38.5X6
Pregneninolone	T38.5X1	T38.5X2	T38.5X3	T38.5X4	T38.5X5	T38.5X6
Preludin	T43.691	T43.692	T43.693	T43.694	T43.695	T43.696
Premarin	T38.5X1	T38.5X2	T38.5X3	T38.5X4	T38.5X5	T38.5X6
Premedication anesthetic	T41.201	T41.202	T41.203	T41.204	T41.205	T41.206
Prenalterol	T44.5X1	T44.5X2	T44.5X3	T44.5X4	T44.5X5	T44.5X6
Prenoxdiazine	T48.3X1	T48.3X2	T48.3X3	T48.3X4	T48.3X5	T48.3X6
Prenylamine	T46.3X1	T46.3X2	T46.3X3	T46.3X4	T46.3X5	T46.3X6
Preparation H	T49.8X1	T49.8X2	T49.8X3	T49.8X4	T49.8X5	T49.8X6
Preparation, local	T49.4X1	T49.4X2	T49.4X3	T49.4X4	T49.4X5	T49.4X6
Preservative (nonmedicinal)	T65.891	T65.892	T65.893	T65.894	--	--
medicinal	T50.901	T50.902	T50.903	T50.904	T50.905	T50.906
wood	T60.91	T60.92	T60.93	T60.94	--	--
Prethcamide	T50.7X1	T50.7X2	T50.7X3	T50.7X4	T50.7X5	T50.7X6
Pride of China	T62.2X1	T62.2X2	T62.2X3	T62.2X4	--	--
Pridinol	T44.3X1	T44.3X2	T44.3X3	T44.3X4	T44.3X5	T44.3X6
Prifinium bromide	T44.3X1	T44.3X2	T44.3X3	T44.3X4	T44.3X5	T44.3X6
Prilocaine	T41.3X1	T41.3X2	T41.3X3	T41.3X4	T41.3X5	T41.3X6
infiltration (subcutaneous)	T41.3X1	T41.3X2	T41.3X3	T41.3X4	T41.3X5	T41.3X6
nerve block (peripheral) (plexus)	T41.3X1	T41.3X2	T41.3X3	T41.3X4	T41.3X5	T41.3X6
regional	T41.3X1	T41.3X2	T41.3X3	T41.3X4	T41.3X5	T41.3X6
Primaquine	T37.2X1	T37.2X2	T37.2X3	T37.2X4	T37.2X5	T37.2X6
Primidone	T42.6X1	T42.6X2	T42.6X3	T42.6X4	T42.6X5	T42.6X6
Primula (veris)	T62.2X1	T62.2X2	T62.2X3	T62.2X4	--	--
Prinadol	T40.2X1	T40.2X2	T40.2X3	T40.2X4	T40.2X5	T40.2X6
Priscol, Priscoline	T44.6X1	T44.6X2	T44.6X3	T44.6X4	T44.6X5	T44.6X6
Pristinamycin	T36.3X1	T36.3X2	T36.3X3	T36.3X4	T36.3X5	T36.3X6
Privet	T62.2X1	T62.2X2	T62.2X3	T62.2X4	--	--
berries	T62.1X1	T62.1X2	T62.1X3	T62.1X4	--	--
Privine	T44.4X1	T44.4X2	T44.4X3	T44.4X4	T44.4X5	T44.4X6
Pro-Banthine	T44.3X1	T44.3X2	T44.3X3	T44.3X4	T44.3X5	T44.3X6
Probarbital	T42.3X1	T42.3X2	T42.3X3	T42.3X4	T42.3X5	T42.3X6
Probenecid	T50.4X1	T50.4X2	T50.4X3	T50.4X4	T50.4X5	T50.4X6
Probucol	T46.6X1	T46.6X2	T46.6X3	T46.6X4	T46.6X5	T46.6X6
Procainamide	T46.2X1	T46.2X2	T46.2X3	T46.2X4	T46.2X5	T46.2X6
Procaine	T41.3X1	T41.3X2	T41.3X3	T41.3X4	T41.3X5	T41.3X6
benzylpenicillin	T36.0X1	T36.0X2	T36.0X3	T36.0X4	T36.0X5	T36.0X6
nerve block (periphreal) (plexus)	T41.3X1	T41.3X2	T41.3X3	T41.3X4	T41.3X5	T41.3X6
penicillin G	T36.0X1	T36.0X2	T36.0X3	T36.0X4	T36.0X5	T36.0X6
regional	T41.3X1	T41.3X2	T41.3X3	T41.3X4	T41.3X5	T41.3X6
spinal	T41.3X1	T41.3X2	T41.3X3	T41.3X4	T41.3X5	T41.3X6
Procalmidol	T43.591	T43.592	T43.593	T43.594	T43.595	T43.596
Procarbazine	T45.1X1	T45.1X2	T45.1X3	T45.1X4	T45.1X5	T45.1X6
Procaterol	T44.5X1	T44.5X2	T44.5X3	T44.5X4	T44.5X5	T44.5X6
Prochlorperazine	T43.3X1	T43.3X2	T43.3X3	T43.3X4	T43.3X5	T43.3X6
Procyclidine	T44.3X1	T44.3X2	T44.3X3	T44.3X4	T44.3X5	T44.3X6
Producer gas	T58.8X1	T58.8X2	T58.8X3	T58.8X4	--	--
Profadol	T40.4X1	T40.4X2	T40.4X3	T40.4X4	T40.4X5	T40.4X6
Profenamine	T44.3X1	T44.3X2	T44.3X3	T44.3X4	T44.3X5	T44.3X6
Profenil	T44.3X1	T44.3X2	T44.3X3	T44.3X4	T44.3X5	T44.3X6
Proflavine	T49.0X1	T49.0X2	T49.0X3	T49.0X4	T49.0X5	T49.0X6
Progabide	T42.6X1	T42.6X2	T42.6X3	T42.6X4	T42.6X5	T42.6X6
Progesterone	T38.5X1	T38.5X2	T38.5X3	T38.5X4	T38.5X5	T38.5X6
Progestin	T38.5X1	T38.5X2	T38.5X3	T38.5X4	T38.5X5	T38.5X6
oral contraceptive	T38.4X1	T38.4X2	T38.4X3	T38.4X4	T38.4X5	T38.4X6
Progestogen NEC	T38.5X1	T38.5X2	T38.5X3	T38.5X4	T38.5X5	T38.5X6
Progestone	T38.5X1	T38.5X2	T38.5X3	T38.5X4	T38.5X5	T38.5X6
Proglumide	T47.1X1	T47.1X2	T47.1X3	T47.1X4	T47.1X5	T47.1X6
Proguanil	T37.2X1	T37.2X2	T37.2X3	T37.2X4	T37.2X5	T37.2X6
Prolactin	T38.811	T38.812	T38.813	T38.814	T38.815	T38.816
Prolintane	T43.691	T43.692	T43.693	T43.694	T43.695	T43.696
Proloid	T38.1X1	T38.1X2	T38.1X3	T38.1X4	T38.1X5	T38.1X6
Proluton	T38.5X1	T38.5X2	T38.5X3	T38.5X4	T38.5X5	T38.5X6
Promacetin	T37.1X1	T37.1X2	T37.1X3	T37.1X4	T37.1X5	T37.1X6
Promazine	T43.3X1	T43.3X2	T43.3X3	T43.3X4	T43.3X5	T43.3X6
Promedol	T40.2X1	T40.2X2	T40.2X3	T40.2X4	--	--
Promegestone	T38.5X1	T38.5X2	T38.5X3	T38.5X4	T38.5X5	T38.5X6

Substance	Poisoning, Accidental (unintentional)	Poisoning, Intentional self-harm	Poisoning, Assault	Poisoning, Undetermined	Adverse effect	Underdosing
Promethazine (teoclate)	T43.3X1	T43.3X2	T43.3X3	T43.3X4	T43.3X5	T43.3X6
Promin	T37.1X1	T37.1X2	T37.1X3	T37.1X4	T37.1X5	T37.1X6
Pronase	T45.3X1	T45.3X2	T45.3X3	T45.3X4	T45.3X5	T45.3X6
Pronestyl (hydrochloride)	T46.2X1	T46.2X2	T46.2X3	T46.2X4	T46.2X5	T46.2X6
Pronetalol	T44.7X1	T44.7X2	T44.7X3	T44.7X4	T44.7X5	T44.7X6
Prontosil	T37.0X1	T37.0X2	T37.0X3	T37.0X4	T37.0X5	T37.0X6
Propachlor	T60.3X1	T60.3X2	T60.3X3	T60.3X4	--	--
Propafenone	T46.2X1	T46.2X2	T46.2X3	T46.2X4	T46.2X5	T46.2X6
Propallylonal	T42.3X1	T42.3X2	T42.3X3	T42.3X4	T42.3X5	T42.3X6
Propamidine	T49.0X1	T49.0X2	T49.0X3	T49.0X4	T49.0X5	T49.0X6
Propane (distributed in mobile container)	T59.891	T59.892	T59.893	T59.894	--	--
distributed through pipes	T59.891	T59.892	T59.893	T59.894	--	--
incomplete combustion	T58.11	T58.12	T58.13	T58.14	--	--
Propanidid	T41.291	T41.292	T41.293	T41.294	T41.295	T41.296
Propanil	T60.3X1	T60.3X2	T60.3X3	T60.3X4	--	--
1-Propanol	T51.3X1	T51.3X2	T51.3X3	T51.3X4	--	--
2-Propanol	T51.2X1	T51.2X2	T51.2X3	T51.2X4	--	--
Propantheline	T44.3X1	T44.3X2	T44.3X3	T44.3X4	T44.3X5	T44.3X6
bromide	T44.3X1	T44.3X2	T44.3X3	T44.3X4	T44.3X5	T44.3X6
Proparacaine	T41.3X1	T41.3X2	T41.3X3	T41.3X4	T41.3X5	T41.3X6
Propatylnitrate	T46.3X1	T46.3X2	T46.3X3	T46.3X4	T46.3X5	T46.3X6
Propicillin	T36.0X1	T36.0X2	T36.0X3	T36.0X4	T36.0X5	T36.0X6
Propiolactone	T49.0X1	T49.0X2	T49.0X3	T49.0X4	T49.0X5	T49.0X6
Propiomazine	T45.0X1	T45.0X2	T45.0X3	T45.0X4	T45.0X5	T45.0X6
Propionaldehyde (medicinal)	T42.6X1	T42.6X2	T42.6X3	T42.6X4	T42.6X5	T42.6X6
Propionate (calcium) (sodium)	T49.0X1	T49.0X2	T49.0X3	T49.0X4	T49.0X5	T49.0X6
Propion gel	T49.0X1	T49.0X2	T49.0X3	T49.0X4	T49.0X5	T49.0X6
Propitocaine	T41.3X1	T41.3X2	T41.3X3	T41.3X4	T41.3X5	T41.3X6
infiltration (subcutaneous)	T41.3X1	T41.3X2	T41.3X3	T41.3X4	T41.3X5	T41.3X6
nerve block (peripheral) (plexus)	T41.3X1	T41.3X2	T41.3X3	T41.3X4	T41.3X5	T41.3X6
Propofol	T41.291	T41.292	T41.293	T41.294	T41.295	T41.296
Propoxur	T60.0X1	T60.0X2	T60.0X3	T60.0X4	--	--
Propoxycaine	T41.3X1	T41.3X2	T41.3X3	T41.3X4	T41.3X5	T41.3X6
infiltration (subcutaneous)	T41.3X1	T41.3X2	T41.3X3	T41.3X4	T41.3X5	T41.3X6
nerve block (peripheral) (plexus)	T41.3X1	T41.3X2	T41.3X3	T41.3X4	T41.3X5	T41.3X6
topical (surface)	T41.3X1	T41.3X2	T41.3X3	T41.3X4	T41.3X5	T41.3X6
Propoxyphene	T40.4X1	T40.4X2	T40.4X3	T40.4X4	T40.4X5	T40.4X6
Propranolol	T44.7X1	T44.7X2	T44.7X3	T44.7X4	T44.7X5	T44.7X6
Propyl						
alcohol	T51.3X1	T51.3X2	T51.3X3	T51.3X4	--	--
carbinol	T51.3X1	T51.3X2	T51.3X3	T51.3X4	--	--
hexadrine	T44.4X1	T44.4X2	T44.4X3	T44.4X4	T44.4X5	T44.4X6
iodone	T50.8X1	T50.8X2	T50.8X3	T50.8X4	T50.8X5	T50.8X6
thiouracil	T38.2X1	T38.2X2	T38.2X3	T38.2X4	T38.2X5	T38.2X6
Propylaminopheno-thiazine	T43.3X1	T43.3X2	T43.3X3	T43.3X4	T43.3X5	T43.3X6
Propylene	T59.891	T59.892	T59.893	T59.894	--	--
Propylhexedrine	T48.5X1	T48.5X2	T48.5X3	T48.5X4	T48.5X5	T48.5X6
Propyliodone	T50.8X1	T50.8X2	T50.8X3	T50.8X4	T50.8X5	T50.8X6
Propylparaben (ophthalmic)	T49.5X1	T49.5X2	T49.5X3	T49.5X4	T49.5X5	T49.5X6
Propylthiouracil	T38.2X1	T38.2X2	T38.2X3	T38.2X4	T38.2X5	T38.2X6
Propyphenazone	T39.2X1	T39.2X2	T39.2X3	T39.2X4	T39.2X5	T39.2X6
Proquazone	T39.391	T39.392	T39.393	T39.394	T39.395	T39.396
Proscillaridin	T46.0X1	T46.0X2	T46.0X3	T46.0X4	T46.0X5	T46.0X6
Prostacyclin	T45.521	T45.522	T45.523	T45.524	T45.525	T45.526
Prostaglandin (I2)	T45.521	T45.522	T45.523	T45.524	T45.525	T45.526
E1	T46.7X1	T46.7X2	T46.7X3	T46.7X4	T46.7X5	T46.7X6
E2	T48.0X1	T48.0X2	T48.0X3	T48.0X4	T48.0X5	T48.0X6
F2 alpha	T48.0X1	T48.0X2	T48.0X3	T48.0X4	T48.0X5	T48.0X6
Prostigmin	T44.0X1	T44.0X2	T44.0X3	T44.0X4	T44.0X5	T44.0X6
Prosultiamine	T45.2X1	T45.2X2	T45.2X3	T45.2X4	T45.2X5	T45.2X6
Protamine sulfate	T45.7X1	T45.7X2	T45.7X3	T45.7X4	T45.7X5	T45.7X6
zinc insulin	T38.3X1	T38.3X2	T38.3X3	T38.3X4	T38.3X5	T38.3X6
Protease	T47.5X1	T47.5X2	T47.5X3	T47.5X4	T47.5X5	T47.5X6
Protectant, skin NEC	T49.3X1	T49.3X2	T49.3X3	T49.3X4	T49.3X5	T49.3X6
Protein hydrolysate	T50.991	T50.992	T50.993	T50.994	T50.995	T50.996
Prothiaden — see Dothiepin hydrochloride						
Prothionamide	T37.1X1	T37.1X2	T37.1X3	T37.1X4	T37.1X5	T37.1X6
Prothipendyl	T43.591	T43.592	T43.593	T43.594	T43.595	T43.596
Prothoate	T60.0X1	T60.0X2	T60.0X3	T60.0X4	--	--
Prothrombin						
activator	T45.7X1	T45.7X2	T45.7X3	T45.7X4	T45.7X5	T45.7X6
synthesis inhibitor	T45.511	T45.512	T45.513	T45.514	T45.515	T45.516
Protionamide	T37.1X1	T37.1X2	T37.1X3	T37.1X4	T37.1X5	T37.1X6
Protirelin	T38.891	T38.892	T38.893	T38.894	T38.895	T38.896
Protokylol	T48.6X1	T48.6X2	T48.6X3	T48.6X4	T48.6X5	T48.6X6
Protopam	T50.6X1	T50.6X2	T50.6X3	T50.6X4	T50.6X5	T50.6X6
Protoveratrine(s) (A) (B)	T46.5X1	T46.5X2	T46.5X3	T46.5X4	T46.5X5	T46.5X6
Protriptyline	T43.011	T43.012	T43.013	T43.014	T43.015	T43.016
Provera	T38.5X1	T38.5X2	T38.5X3	T38.5X4	T38.5X5	T38.5X6
Provitamin A	T45.2X1	T45.2X2	T45.2X3	T45.2X4	T45.2X5	T45.2X6

Proxibarbal - Reserpin

Substance	Poisoning, Accidental (unintentional)	Poisoning, Intentional self-harm	Poisoning, Assault	Poisoning, Undetermined	Adverse effect	Underdosing
Proxibarbal	T42.3X1	T42.3X2	T42.3X3	T42.3X4	T42.3X5	T42.3X6
Proxymetacaine	T41.3X1	T41.3X2	T41.3X3	T41.3X4	T41.3X5	T41.3X6
Proxyphylline	T48.6X1	T48.6X2	T48.6X3	T48.6X4	T48.6X5	T48.6X6
Prozac — see Fluoxetine hydrochloride						
Prunus						
laurocerasus	T62.2X1	T62.2X2	T62.2X3	T62.2X4	--	--
virginiana	T62.2X1	T62.2X2	T62.2X3	T62.2X4	--	--
Prussian blue						
commercial	T65.891	T65.892	T65.893	T65.894		
therapeutic	T50.6X1	T50.6X2	T50.6X3	T50.6X4	T50.6X5	T50.6X6
Prussic acid	T65.0X1	T65.0X2	T65.0X3	T65.0X4		
vapor	T57.3X1	T57.3X2	T57.3X3	T57.3X4		
Pseudoephedrine	T44.991	T44.992	T44.993	T44.994	T44.995	T44.996
Psilocin	T40.991	T40.992	T40.993	T40.994	--	--
Psilocybin	T40.991	T40.992	T40.993	T40.994	--	--
Psilocybine	T40.991	T40.992	T40.993	T40.994	--	--
Psoralene (nonmedicinal)	T65.891	T65.892	T65.893	T65.894		
Psoralens (medicinal)	T50.991	T50.992	T50.993	T50.994	T50.995	T50.996
PSP (phenolsulfonphthalein)	T50.8X1	T50.8X2	T50.8X3	T50.8X4	T50.8X5	T50.8X6
Psychodysleptic drug NOS	T40.901	T40.902	T40.903	T40.904	T40.905	T40.906
specified NEC	T40.991	T40.992	T40.993	T40.994	T40.995	T40.996
Psychostimulant	T43.601	T43.602	T43.603	T43.604	T43.605	T43.606
amphetamine	T43.621	T43.622	T43.623	T43.624	T43.625	T43.626
caffeine	T43.611	T43.612	T43.613	T43.614	T43.615	T43.616
methylphenidate	T43.631	T43.632	T43.633	T43.634	T43.635	T43.636
specified NEC	T43.691	T43.692	T43.693	T43.694	T43.695	T43.696
Psychotherapeutic drug NEC	T43.91	T43.92	T43.93	T43.94	T43.95	T43.96
antidepressants (see also Antidepressant)	T43.201	T43.202	T43.203	T43.204	T43.205	T43.206
specified NEC	T43.8X1	T43.8X2	T43.8X3	T43.8X4	T43.8X5	T43.8X6
tranquilizers NEC	T43.501	T43.502	T43.503	T43.504	T43.505	T43.506
Psychotomimetic agents	T40.901	T40.902	T40.903	T40.904	T40.905	T40.906
Psychotropic drug NEC	T43.91	T43.92	T43.93	T43.94	T43.95	T43.96
specified NEC	T43.8X1	T43.8X2	T43.8X3	T43.8X4	T43.8X5	T43.8X6
Psyllium hydrophilic mucilloid	T47.4X1	T47.4X2	T47.4X3	T47.4X4	T47.4X5	T47.4X6
Pteroylglutamic acid	T45.8X1	T45.8X2	T45.8X3	T45.8X4	T45.8X5	T45.8X6
Pteroyltriglutamate	T45.1X1	T45.1X2	T45.1X3	T45.1X4	T45.1X5	T45.1X6
PTFE — see Polytetrafluoroethylene						
Pulp						
devitalizing paste	T49.7X1	T49.7X2	T49.7X3	T49.7X4	T49.7X5	T49.7X6
dressing	T49.7X1	T49.7X2	T49.7X3	T49.7X4	T49.7X5	T49.7X6
Pulsatilla	T62.2X1	T62.2X2	T62.2X3	T62.2X4	--	--
Pumpkin seed extract	T37.4X1	T37.4X2	T37.4X3	T37.4X4	T37.4X5	T37.4X6
Purex (bleach)	T54.91	T54.92	T54.93	T54.94	--	--
Purgative NEC (see also Cathartic)	T47.4X1	T47.4X2	T47.4X3	T47.4X4	T47.4X5	T47.4X6
Purine analogue (antineoplastic)	T45.1X1	T45.1X2	T45.1X3	T45.1X4	T45.1X5	T45.1X6
Purine diuretics	T50.2X1	T50.2X2	T50.2X3	T50.2X4	T50.2X5	T50.2X6
Purinethol	T45.1X1	T45.1X2	T45.1X3	T45.1X4	T45.1X5	T45.1X6
PVP	T45.8X1	T45.8X2	T45.8X3	T45.8X4	T45.8X5	T45.8X6
Pyrabital	T39.8X1	T39.8X2	T39.8X3	T39.8X4	T39.8X5	T39.8X6
Pyramidon	T39.2X1	T39.2X2	T39.2X3	T39.2X4	T39.2X5	T39.2X6
Pyrantel	T37.4X1	T37.4X2	T37.4X3	T37.4X4	T37.4X5	T37.4X6
Pyrathiazine	T45.0X1	T45.0X2	T45.0X3	T45.0X4	T45.0X5	T45.0X6
Pyrazinamide	T37.1X1	T37.1X2	T37.1X3	T37.1X4	T37.1X5	T37.1X6
Pyrazinoic acid (amide)	T37.1X1	T37.1X2	T37.1X3	T37.1X4	T37.1X5	T37.1X6
Pyrazole (derivatives)	T39.2X1	T39.2X2	T39.2X3	T39.2X4	T39.2X5	T39.2X6
Pyrazolone analgesic NEC	T39.2X1	T39.2X2	T39.2X3	T39.2X4	T39.2X5	T39.2X6
Pyrethrin, pyrethrum (nonmedicinal)	T60.2X1	T60.2X2	T60.2X3	T60.2X4	--	--
Pyrethrum extract	T49.0X1	T49.0X2	T49.0X3	T49.0X4	T49.0X5	T49.0X6
Pyribenzamine	T45.0X1	T45.0X2	T45.0X3	T45.0X4	T45.0X5	T45.0X6
Pyridine	T52.8X1	T52.8X2	T52.8X3	T52.8X4	--	--
aldoxime methiodide	T50.6X1	T50.6X2	T50.6X3	T50.6X4	T50.6X5	T50.6X6
aldoxime methyl chloride	T50.6X1	T50.6X2	T50.6X3	T50.6X4	T50.6X5	T50.6X6
vapor	T59.891	T59.892	T59.893	T59.894		
Pyridium	T39.8X1	T39.8X2	T39.8X3	T39.8X4	T39.8X5	T39.8X6
Pyridostigmine bromide	T44.0X1	T44.0X2	T44.0X3	T44.0X4	T44.0X5	T44.0X6
Pyridoxal phosphate	T45.2X1	T45.2X2	T45.2X3	T45.2X4	T45.2X5	T45.2X6
Pyridoxine	T45.2X1	T45.2X2	T45.2X3	T45.2X4	T45.2X5	T45.2X6
Pyrilamine	T45.0X1	T45.0X2	T45.0X3	T45.0X4	T45.0X5	T45.0X6
Pyrimethamine	T37.2X1	T37.2X2	T37.2X3	T37.2X4	T37.2X5	T37.2X6
with sulfadoxine	T37.2X1	T37.2X2	T37.2X3	T37.2X4	T37.2X5	T37.2X6
Pyrimidine antagonist	T45.1X1	T45.1X2	T45.1X3	T45.1X4	T45.1X5	T45.1X6
Pyriminil	T60.4X1	T60.4X2	T60.4X3	T60.4X4		
Pyrithione zinc	T49.4X1	T49.4X2	T49.4X3	T49.4X4	T49.4X5	T49.4X6
Pyrithyldione	T42.6X1	T42.6X2	T42.6X3	T42.6X4	T42.6X5	T42.6X6
Pyrogallic acid	T49.0X1	T49.0X2	T49.0X3	T49.0X4	T49.0X5	T49.0X6
Pyrogallol	T49.0X1	T49.0X2	T49.0X3	T49.0X4	T49.0X5	T49.0X6
Pyroxylin	T49.3X1	T49.3X2	T49.3X3	T49.3X4	T49.3X5	T49.3X6

Substance	Poisoning, Accidental (unintentional)	Poisoning, Intentional self-harm	Poisoning, Assault	Poisoning, Undetermined	Adverse effect	Underdosing
Pyrrobutamine	T45.0X1	T45.0X2	T45.0X3	T45.0X4	T45.0X5	T45.0X6
Pyrrolizidine alkaloids	T62.8X1	T62.8X2	T62.8X3	T62.8X4		
Pyrvinium chloride	T37.4X1	T37.4X2	T37.4X3	T37.4X4	T37.4X5	T37.4X6
PZI	T38.3X1	T38.3X2	T38.3X3	T38.3X4	T38.3X5	T38.3X6
Q						
Quaalude	T42.6X1	T42.6X2	T42.6X3	T42.6X4	T42.6X5	T42.6X6
Quarternary ammonium						
anti-infective	T49.0X1	T49.0X2	T49.0X3	T49.0X4	T49.0X5	T49.0X6
ganglion blocking	T44.2X1	T44.2X2	T44.2X3	T44.2X4	T44.2X5	T44.2X6
parasympatholytic	T44.3X1	T44.3X2	T44.3X3	T44.3X4	T44.3X5	T44.3X6
Quazepam	T42.4X1	T42.4X2	T42.4X3	T42.4X4	T42.4X5	T42.4X6
Quicklime	T54.3X1	T54.3X2	T54.3X3	T54.3X4		
Quillaja extract	T48.4X1	T48.4X2	T48.4X3	T48.4X4	T48.4X5	T48.4X6
Quinacrine	T37.2X1	T37.2X2	T37.2X3	T37.2X4	T37.2X5	T37.2X6
Quinaglute	T46.2X1	T46.2X2	T46.2X3	T46.2X4	T46.2X5	T46.2X6
Quinalbarbital	T42.3X1	T42.3X2	T42.3X3	T42.3X4	T42.3X5	T42.3X6
Quinalbarbitone sodium	T42.3X1	T42.3X2	T42.3X3	T42.3X4	T42.3X5	T42.3X6
Quinalphos	T60.0X1	T60.0X2	T60.0X3	T60.0X4		
Quinapril	T46.4X1	T46.4X2	T46.4X3	T46.4X4	T46.4X5	T46.4X6
Quinestradiol	T38.5X1	T38.5X2	T38.5X3	T38.5X4	T38.5X5	T38.5X6
Quinestradol	T38.5X1	T38.5X2	T38.5X3	T38.5X4	T38.5X5	T38.5X6
Quinestrol	T38.5X1	T38.5X2	T38.5X3	T38.5X4	T38.5X5	T38.5X6
Quinethazone	T50.2X1	T50.2X2	T50.2X3	T50.2X4	T50.2X5	T50.2X6
Quingestanol	T38.4X1	T38.4X2	T38.4X3	T38.4X4	T38.4X5	T38.4X6
Quinidine	T46.2X1	T46.2X2	T46.2X3	T46.2X4	T46.2X5	T46.2X6
Quinine	T37.2X1	T37.2X2	T37.2X3	T37.2X4	T37.2X5	T37.2X6
Quiniobine	T37.8X1	T37.8X2	T37.8X3	T37.8X4	T37.8X5	T37.8X6
Quinisocaine	T49.1X1	T49.1X2	T49.1X3	T49.1X4	T49.1X5	T49.1X6
Quinocide	T37.2X1	T37.2X2	T37.2X3	T37.2X4	T37.2X5	T37.2X6
Quinoline (derivatives) NEC	T37.8X1	T37.8X2	T37.8X3	T37.8X4	T37.8X5	T37.8X6
Quinupramine	T43.011	T43.012	T43.013	T43.014	T43.015	T43.016
Quotane	T41.3X1	T41.3X2	T41.3X3	T41.3X4	T41.3X5	T41.3X6
R						
Rabies						
immune globulin (human)	T50.Z11	T50.Z12	T50.Z13	T50.Z14	T50.Z15	T50.Z16
vaccine	T50.B91	T50.B92	T50.B93	T50.B94	T50.B95	T50.B96
Racemoramide	T40.2X1	T40.2X2	T40.2X3	T40.2X4		
Racemorphan	T40.2X1	T40.2X2	T40.2X3	T40.2X4	T40.2X5	T40.2X6
Racepinefrin	T44.5X1	T44.5X2	T44.5X3	T44.5X4	T44.5X5	T44.5X6
Raclopride	T43.591	T43.592	T43.593	T43.594	T43.595	T43.596
Radiator alcohol	T51.1X1	T51.1X2	T51.1X3	T51.1X4		
Radioactive drug NEC	T50.8X1	T50.8X2	T50.8X3	T50.8X4	T50.8X5	T50.8X6
Radio-opaque (drugs) (materials)	T50.8X1	T50.8X2	T50.8X3	T50.8X4	T50.8X5	T50.8X6
Ramifenazone	T39.2X1	T39.2X2	T39.2X3	T39.2X4	T39.2X5	T39.2X6
Ramipril	T46.4X1	T46.4X2	T46.4X3	T46.4X4	T46.4X5	T46.4X6
Ranitidine	T47.0X1	T47.0X2	T47.0X3	T47.0X4	T47.0X5	T47.0X6
Ranunculus	T62.2X1	T62.2X2	T62.2X3	T62.2X4		
Rat poison NEC	T60.4X1	T60.4X2	T60.4X3	T60.4X4	--	--
Rattlesnake (venom)	T63.011	T63.012	T63.013	T63.014		
Raubasine	T46.7X1	T46.7X2	T46.7X3	T46.7X4	T46.7X5	T46.7X6
Raudixin	T46.5X1	T46.5X2	T46.5X3	T46.5X4	T46.5X5	T46.5X6
Rautensin	T46.5X1	T46.5X2	T46.5X3	T46.5X4	T46.5X5	T46.5X6
Rautina	T46.5X1	T46.5X2	T46.5X3	T46.5X4	T46.5X5	T46.5X6
Rautotal	T46.5X1	T46.5X2	T46.5X3	T46.5X4	T46.5X5	T46.5X6
Rauwiloid	T46.5X1	T46.5X2	T46.5X3	T46.5X4	T46.5X5	T46.5X6
Rauwoldin	T46.5X1	T46.5X2	T46.5X3	T46.5X4	T46.5X5	T46.5X6
Rauwolfia (alkaloids)	T46.5X1	T46.5X2	T46.5X3	T46.5X4	T46.5X5	T46.5X6
Razoxane	T45.1X1	T45.1X2	T45.1X3	T45.1X4	T45.1X5	T45.1X6
Realgar	T57.0X1	T57.0X2	T57.0X3	T57.0X4	--	--
Recombinant (R) — see specific protein						
Red blood cells, packed	T45.8X1	T45.8X2	T45.8X3	T45.8X4	T45.8X5	T45.8X6
Red squill (scilliroside)	T60.4X1	T60.4X2	T60.4X3	T60.4X4	--	--
Reducing agent, industrial NEC	T65.891	T65.892	T65.893	T65.894	--	--
Refrigerant gas (chlorofluoro-carbon)	T53.5X1	T53.5X2	T53.5X3	T53.5X4	--	--
not chlorofluoro-carbon	T59.891	T59.892	T59.893	T59.894	--	--
Regroton	T50.2X1	T50.2X2	T50.2X3	T50.2X4	T50.2X5	T50.2X6
Rehydration salts (oral)	T50.3X1	T50.3X2	T50.3X3	T50.3X4	T50.3X5	T50.3X6
Rela	T42.8X1	T42.8X2	T42.8X3	T42.8X4	T42.8X5	T42.8X6
Relaxant, muscle						
anesthetic	T48.1X1	T48.1X2	T48.1X3	T48.1X4	T48.1X5	T48.1X6
central nervous system	T42.8X1	T42.8X2	T42.8X3	T42.8X4	T42.8X5	T42.8X6
skeletal NEC	T48.1X1	T48.1X2	T48.1X3	T48.1X4	T48.1X5	T48.1X6
smooth NEC	T44.3X1	T44.3X2	T44.3X3	T44.3X4	T44.3X5	T44.3X6
Remoxipride	T43.591	T43.592	T43.593	T43.594	T43.595	T43.596
Renese	T50.2X1	T50.2X2	T50.2X3	T50.2X4	T50.2X5	T50.2X6
Renografin	T50.8X1	T50.8X2	T50.8X3	T50.8X4	T50.8X5	T50.8X6
Replacement solution	T50.3X1	T50.3X2	T50.3X3	T50.3X4	T50.3X5	T50.3X6
Reproterol	T48.6X1	T48.6X2	T48.6X3	T48.6X4	T48.6X5	T48.6X6
Rescinnamine	T46.5X1	T46.5X2	T46.5X3	T46.5X4	T46.5X5	T46.5X6
Reserpin (e)	T46.5X1	T46.5X2	T46.5X3	T46.5X4	T46.5X5	T46.5X6

Substance	Poisoning, Accidental (unintentional)	Poisoning, Intentional self-harm	Poisoning, Assault	Poisoning, Undetermined	Adverse effect	Underdosing
Resorcin, resorcinol (nonmedicinal)	T65.891	T65.892	T65.893	T65.894	--	--
medicinal	T49.4X1	T49.4X2	T49.4X3	T49.4X4	T49.4X5	T49.4X6
Respaire	T48.4X1	T48.4X2	T48.4X3	T48.4X4	T48.4X5	T48.4X6
Respiratory drug NEC	T48.901	T48.902	T48.903	T48.904	T48.905	T48.906
antiasthmatic NEC	T48.6X1	T48.6X2	T48.6X3	T48.6X4	T48.6X5	T48.6X6
anti-common-cold NEC	T48.5X1	T48.5X2	T48.5X3	T48.5X4	T48.5X5	T48.5X6
expectorant NEC	T48.4X1	T48.4X2	T48.4X3	T48.4X4	T48.4X5	T48.4X6
stimulant	T48.901	T48.902	T48.903	T48.904	T48.905	T48.906
Retinoic acid	T49.0X1	T49.0X2	T49.0X3	T49.0X4	T49.0X5	T49.0X6
Retinol	T45.2X1	T45.2X2	T45.2X3	T45.2X4	T45.2X5	T45.2X6
Rh (D) immune globulin (human)	T50.Z11	T50.Z12	T50.Z13	T50.Z14	T50.Z15	T50.Z16
Rhodine	T39.011	T39.012	T39.013	T39.014	T39.015	T39.016
RhoGAM	T50.Z11	T50.Z12	T50.Z13	T50.Z14	T50.Z15	T50.Z16
Rhubarb						
dry extract	T47.2X1	T47.2X2	T47.2X3	T47.2X4	T47.2X5	T47.2X6
tincture, compound	T47.2X1	T47.2X2	T47.2X3	T47.2X4	T47.2X5	T47.2X6
Ribavirin	T37.5X1	T37.5X2	T37.5X3	T37.5X4	T37.5X5	T37.5X6
Riboflavin	T45.2X1	T45.2X2	T45.2X3	T45.2X4	T45.2X5	T45.2X6
Ribostamycin	T36.5X1	T36.5X2	T36.5X3	T36.5X4	T36.5X5	T36.5X6
Ricin	T62.2X1	T62.2X2	T62.2X3	T62.2X4	--	--
Ricinus communis	T62.2X1	T62.2X2	T62.2X3	T62.2X4	--	--
Rickettsial vaccine NEC	T50.A91	T50.A92	T50.A93	T50.A94	T50.A95	T50.A96
Rifabutin	T36.6X1	T36.6X2	T36.6X3	T36.6X4	T36.6X5	T36.6X6
Rifamide	T36.6X1	T36.6X2	T36.6X3	T36.6X4	T36.6X5	T36.6X6
Rifampicin	T36.6X1	T36.6X2	T36.6X3	T36.6X4	T36.6X5	T36.6X6
with isoniazid	T37.1X1	T37.1X2	T37.1X3	T37.1X4	T37.1X5	T37.1X6
Rifampin	T36.6X1	T36.6X2	T36.6X3	T36.6X4	T36.6X5	T36.6X6
Rifamycin	T36.6X1	T36.6X2	T36.6X3	T36.6X4	T36.6X5	T36.6X6
Rifaximin	T36.6X1	T36.6X2	T36.6X3	T36.6X4	T36.6X5	T36.6X6
Rimantadine	T37.5X1	T37.5X2	T37.5X3	T37.5X4	T37.5X5	T37.5X6
Rimazolium metilsulfate	T39.8X1	T39.8X2	T39.8X3	T39.8X4	T39.8X5	T39.8X6
Rimifon	T37.1X1	T37.1X2	T37.1X3	T37.1X4	T37.1X5	T37.1X6
Rimiterol	T48.6X1	T48.6X2	T48.6X3	T48.6X4	T48.6X5	T48.6X6
Ringer (lactate) solution	T50.3X1	T50.3X2	T50.3X3	T50.3X4	T50.3X5	T50.3X6
Ristocetin	T36.8X1	T36.8X2	T36.8X3	T36.8X4	T36.8X5	T36.8X6
Ritalin	T43.631	T43.632	T43.633	T43.634	T43.635	T43.636
Ritodrine	T44.5X1	T44.5X2	T44.5X3	T44.5X4	T44.5X5	T44.5X6
Roach killer — *see* Insecticide						
Rociverine	T44.3X1	T44.3X2	T44.3X3	T44.3X4	T44.3X5	T44.3X6
Rocky Mountain spotted fever vaccine	T50.A91	T50.A92	T50.A93	T50.A94	T50.A95	T50.A96
Rodenticide NEC	T60.4X1	T60.4X2	T60.4X3	T60.4X4	--	--
Rohypnol	T42.4X1	T42.4X2	T42.4X3	T42.4X4	T42.4X5	T42.4X6
Rokitamycin	T36.3X1	T36.3X2	T36.3X3	T36.3X4	T36.3X5	T36.3X6
Rolaids	T47.1X1	T47.1X2	T47.1X3	T47.1X4	T47.1X5	T47.1X6
Rolitetracycline	T36.4X1	T36.4X2	T36.4X3	T36.4X4	T36.4X5	T36.4X6
Romilar	T48.3X1	T48.3X2	T48.3X3	T48.3X4	T48.3X5	T48.3X6
Ronifibrate	T46.6X1	T46.6X2	T46.6X3	T46.6X4	T46.6X5	T46.6X6
Rosaprostol	T47.1X1	T47.1X2	T47.1X3	T47.1X4	T47.1X5	T47.1X6
Rose bengal sodium (131I)	T50.8X1	T50.8X2	T50.8X3	T50.8X4	T50.8X5	T50.8X6
Rose water ointment	T49.3X1	T49.3X2	T49.3X3	T49.3X4	T49.3X5	T49.3X6
Rosoxacin	T37.8X1	T37.8X2	T37.8X3	T37.8X4	T37.8X5	T37.8X6
Rotenone	T60.2X1	T60.2X2	T60.2X3	T60.2X4	--	--
Rotoxamine	T45.0X1	T45.0X2	T45.0X3	T45.0X4	T45.0X5	T45.0X6
Rough-on-rats	T60.4X1	T60.4X2	T60.4X3	T60.4X4	--	--
Roxatidine	T47.0X1	T47.0X2	T47.0X3	T47.0X4	T47.0X5	T47.0X6
Roxithromycin	T36.3X1	T36.3X2	T36.3X3	T36.3X4	T36.3X5	T36.3X6
Rt-PA	T45.611	T45.612	T45.613	T45.614	T45.615	T45.616
Rubbing alcohol	T51.2X1	T51.2X2	T51.2X3	T51.2X4	--	--
Rubefacient	T49.4X1	T49.4X2	T49.4X3	T49.4X4	T49.4X5	T49.4X6
Rubella vaccine	T50.B91	T50.B92	T50.B93	T50.B94	T50.B95	T50.B96
Rubeola vaccine	T50.B91	T50.B92	T50.B93	T50.B94	T50.B95	T50.B96
Rubidium chloride Rb82	T50.8X1	T50.8X2	T50.8X3	T50.8X4	T50.8X5	T50.8X6
Rubidomycin	T45.1X1	T45.1X2	T45.1X3	T45.1X4	T45.1X5	T45.1X6
Rue	T62.2X1	T62.2X2	T62.2X3	T62.2X4	--	--
Rufocromomycin	T45.1X1	T45.1X2	T45.1X3	T45.1X4	T45.1X5	T45.1X6
Russel's viper venin	T45.7X1	T45.7X2	T45.7X3	T45.7X4	T45.7X5	T45.7X6
Ruta (graveolens)	T62.2X1	T62.2X2	T62.2X3	T62.2X4	--	--
Rutinum	T46.991	T46.992	T46.993	T46.994	T46.995	T46.996
Rutoside	T46.991	T46.992	T46.993	T46.994	T46.995	T46.996
S						
Sabadilla (plant)	T62.2X1	T62.2X2	T62.2X3	T62.2X4	--	--
pesticide	T60.2X1	T60.2X2	T60.2X3	T60.2X4	--	--
Saccharated iron oxide	T45.8X1	T45.8X2	T45.8X3	T45.8X4	T45.8X5	T45.8X6
Saccharin	T50.901	T50.902	T50.903	T50.904	T50.905	T50.906
Saccharomyces boulardii	T47.6X1	T47.6X2	T47.6X3	T47.6X4	T47.6X5	T47.6X6
Safflower oil	T46.6X1	T46.6X2	T46.6X3	T46.6X4	T46.6X5	T46.6X6
Safrazine	T43.1X1	T43.1X2	T43.1X3	T43.1X4	T43.1X5	T43.1X6
Salazosulfapyridine	T37.0X1	T37.0X2	T37.0X3	T37.0X4	T37.0X5	T37.0X6
Salbutamol	T48.6X1	T48.6X2	T48.6X3	T48.6X4	T48.6X5	T48.6X6
Salicylamide	T39.091	T39.092	T39.093	T39.094	T39.095	T39.096
Salicylate NEC	T39.091	T39.092	T39.093	T39.094	T39.095	T39.096
methyl	T49.3X1	T49.3X2	T49.3X3	T49.3X4	T49.3X5	T49.3X6
theobromine calcium	T50.2X1	T50.2X2	T50.2X3	T50.2X4	T50.2X5	T50.2X6
Salicylazosulfapyridine	T37.0X1	T37.0X2	T37.0X3	T37.0X4	T37.0X5	T37.0X6
Salicylhydroxamic acid	T49.0X1	T49.0X2	T49.0X3	T49.0X4	T49.0X5	T49.0X6
Salicylic acid	T49.4X1	T49.4X2	T49.4X3	T49.4X4	T49.4X5	T49.4X6
with benzoic acid	T49.4X1	T49.4X2	T49.4X3	T49.4X4	T49.4X5	T49.4X6
congeners	T39.091	T39.092	T39.093	T39.094	T39.095	T39.096
derivative	T39.091	T39.092	T39.093	T39.094	T39.095	T39.096
salts	T39.091	T39.092	T39.093	T39.094	T39.095	T39.096
Salinazid	T37.1X1	T37.1X2	T37.1X3	T37.1X4	T37.1X5	T37.1X6
Salmeterol	T48.6X1	T48.6X2	T48.6X3	T48.6X4	T48.6X5	T48.6X6
Salol	T49.3X1	T49.3X2	T49.3X3	T49.3X4	T49.3X5	T49.3X6
Salsalate	T39.091	T39.092	T39.093	T39.094	T39.095	T39.096
Salt substitute	T50.901	T50.902	T50.903	T50.904	T50.905	T50.906
Salt-replacing drug	T50.901	T50.902	T50.903	T50.904	T50.905	T50.906
Salt-retaining mineralocorticoid	T50.0X1	T50.0X2	T50.0X3	T50.0X4	T50.0X5	T50.0X6
Saluretic NEC	T50.2X1	T50.2X2	T50.2X3	T50.2X4	T50.2X5	T50.2X6
Saluron	T50.2X1	T50.2X2	T50.2X3	T50.2X4	T50.2X5	T50.2X6
Salvarsan 606 (neosilver) (silver)	T37.8X1	T37.8X2	T37.8X3	T37.8X4	T37.8X5	T37.8X6
Sambucus canadensis	T62.2X1	T62.2X2	T62.2X3	T62.2X4	--	--
berry	T62.1X1	T62.1X2	T62.1X3	T62.1X4	--	--
Sandril	T46.5X1	T46.5X2	T46.5X3	T46.5X4	T46.5X5	T46.5X6
Sanguinaria canadensis	T62.2X1	T62.2X2	T62.2X3	T62.2X4	--	--
Saniflush (cleaner)	T54.2X1	T54.2X2	T54.2X3	T54.2X4	--	--
Santonin	T37.4X1	T37.4X2	T37.4X3	T37.4X4	T37.4X5	T37.4X6
Santyl	T49.8X1	T49.8X2	T49.8X3	T49.8X4	T49.8X5	T49.8X6
Saralasin	T46.5X1	T46.5X2	T46.5X3	T46.5X4	T46.5X5	T46.5X6
Sarcolysin	T45.1X1	T45.1X2	T45.1X3	T45.1X4	T45.1X5	T45.1X6
Sarkomycin	T45.1X1	T45.1X2	T45.1X3	T45.1X4	T45.1X5	T45.1X6
Saroten	T43.011	T43.012	T43.013	T43.014	T43.015	T43.016
Saturnine — *see* Lead						
Savin (oil)	T49.4X1	T49.4X2	T49.4X3	T49.4X4	T49.4X5	T49.4X6
Scammony	T47.2X1	T47.2X2	T47.2X3	T47.2X4	T47.2X5	T47.2X6
Scarlet red	T49.8X1	T49.8X2	T49.8X3	T49.8X4	T49.8X5	T49.8X6
Scheele's green	T57.0X1	T57.0X2	T57.0X3	T57.0X4	--	--
insecticide	T57.0X1	T57.0X2	T57.0X3	T57.0X4	--	--
Schizontozide (blood) (tissue)	T37.2X1	T37.2X2	T37.2X3	T37.2X4	T37.2X5	T37.2X6
Schradan	T60.0X1	T60.0X2	T60.0X3	T60.0X4	--	--
Schweinfurth green	T57.0X1	T57.0X2	T57.0X3	T57.0X4	--	--
insecticide	T57.0X1	T57.0X2	T57.0X3	T57.0X4	--	--
Scilla, rat poison	T60.4X1	T60.4X2	T60.4X3	T60.4X4	--	--
Scillaren	T60.4X1	T60.4X2	T60.4X3	T60.4X4	--	--
Sclerosing agent	T46.8X1	T46.8X2	T46.8X3	T46.8X4	T46.8X5	T46.8X6
Scombrotoxin	T61.11	T61.12	T61.13	T61.14	--	--
Scopolamine	T44.3X1	T44.3X2	T44.3X3	T44.3X4	T44.3X5	T44.3X6
Scopolia extract	T44.3X1	T44.3X2	T44.3X3	T44.3X4	T44.3X5	T44.3X6
Scouring powder	T65.891	T65.892	T65.893	T65.894	--	--
Sea						
anemone (sting)	T63.631	T63.632	T63.633	T63.634	--	--
cucumber (sting)	T63.691	T63.692	T63.693	T63.694	--	--
snake (bite) (venom)	T63.091	T63.092	T63.093	T63.094	--	--
urchin spine (puncture)	T63.691	T63.692	T63.693	T63.694	--	--
Seafood	T61.91	T61.92	T61.93	T61.94	--	--
specified NEC	T61.8X1	T61.8X2	T61.8X3	T61.8X4	--	--
Secbutabarbital	T42.3X1	T42.3X2	T42.3X3	T42.3X4	T42.3X5	T42.3X6
Secbutabarbitone	T42.3X1	T42.3X2	T42.3X3	T42.3X4	T42.3X5	T42.3X6
Secnidazole	T37.3X1	T37.3X2	T37.3X3	T37.3X4	T37.3X5	T37.3X6
Secobarbital	T42.3X1	T42.3X2	T42.3X3	T42.3X4	T42.3X5	T42.3X6
Seconal	T42.3X1	T42.3X2	T42.3X3	T42.3X4	T42.3X5	T42.3X6
Secretin	T50.8X1	T50.8X2	T50.8X3	T50.8X4	T50.8X5	T50.8X6
Sedative NEC	T42.71	T42.72	T42.73	T42.74	T42.75	T42.76
mixed NEC	T42.6X1	T42.6X2	T42.6X3	T42.6X4	T42.6X5	T42.6X6
Sedormid	T42.6X1	T42.6X2	T42.6X3	T42.6X4	T42.6X5	T42.6X6
Seed disinfectant or dressing	T60.8X1	T60.8X2	T60.8X3	T60.8X4	--	--
Seeds (poisonous)	T62.2X1	T62.2X2	T62.2X3	T62.2X4	--	--
Selegiline	T42.8X1	T42.8X2	T42.8X3	T42.8X4	T42.8X5	T42.8X6
Selenium NEC	T56.891	T56.892	T56.893	T56.894	--	--
disulfide or sulfide	T49.4X1	T49.4X2	T49.4X3	T49.4X4	T49.4X5	T49.4X6
fumes	T59.891	T59.892	T59.893	T59.894	--	--
sulfide	T49.4X1	T49.4X2	T49.4X3	T49.4X4	T49.4X5	T49.4X6
Selenomethionine (75Se)	T50.8X1	T50.8X2	T50.8X3	T50.8X4	T50.8X5	T50.8X6
Selsun	T49.4X1	T49.4X2	T49.4X3	T49.4X4	T49.4X5	T49.4X6
Semustine	T45.1X1	T45.1X2	T45.1X3	T45.1X4	T45.1X5	T45.1X6
Senega syrup	T48.4X1	T48.4X2	T48.4X3	T48.4X4	T48.4X5	T48.4X6
Senna	T47.2X1	T47.2X2	T47.2X3	T47.2X4	T47.2X5	T47.2X6
Sennoside A+B	T47.2X1	T47.2X2	T47.2X3	T47.2X4	T47.2X5	T47.2X6
Septisol	T49.2X1	T49.2X2	T49.2X3	T49.2X4	T49.2X5	T49.2X6
Seractide	T38.811	T38.812	T38.813	T38.814	T38.815	T38.816
Serax	T42.4X1	T42.4X2	T42.4X3	T42.4X4	T42.4X5	T42.4X6
Serenesil	T42.6X1	T42.6X2	T42.6X3	T42.6X4	T42.6X5	T42.6X6
Serenium (hydrochloride)	T37.91	T37.92	T37.93	T37.94	T37.95	T37.96
Serepax — *see* Oxazepam						
Sermorelin	T38.891	T38.892	T38.893	T38.894	T38.895	T38.896
Sernyl	T41.1X1	T41.1X2	T41.1X3	T41.1X4	T41.1X5	T41.1X6

Serotonin - Sodium

Substance	Poisoning, Accidental (unintentional)	Poisoning, Intentional self-harm	Poisoning, Assault	Poisoning, Undetermined	Adverse effect	Underdosing
Serotonin	T50.991	T50.992	T50.993	T50.994	T50.995	T50.996
Serpasil	T46.5X1	T46.5X2	T46.5X3	T46.5X4	T46.5X5	T46.5X6
Serrapeptase	T45.3X1	T45.3X2	T45.3X3	T45.3X4	T45.3X5	T45.3X6
Serum						
antibotulinus	T50.Z11	T50.Z12	T50.Z13	T50.Z14	T50.Z15	T50.Z16
anticytotoxic	T50.Z11	T50.Z12	T50.Z13	T50.Z14	T50.Z15	T50.Z16
antidiphtheria	T50.Z11	T50.Z12	T50.Z13	T50.Z14	T50.Z15	T50.Z16
antimeningococcus	T50.Z11	T50.Z12	T50.Z13	T50.Z14	T50.Z15	T50.Z16
anti-Rh	T50.Z11	T50.Z12	T50.Z13	T50.Z14	T50.Z15	T50.Z16
anti-snake-bite	T50.Z11	T50.Z12	T50.Z13	T50.Z14	T50.Z15	T50.Z16
antitetanic	T50.Z11	T50.Z12	T50.Z13	T50.Z14	T50.Z15	T50.Z16
antitoxic	T50.Z11	T50.Z12	T50.Z13	T50.Z14	T50.Z15	T50.Z16
complement (inhibitor)	T45.8X1	T45.8X2	T45.8X3	T45.8X4	T45.8X5	T45.8X6
convalescent	T50.Z11	T50.Z12	T50.Z13	T50.Z14	T50.Z15	T50.Z16
hemolytic complement	T45.8X1	T45.8X2	T45.8X3	T45.8X4	T45.8X5	T45.8X6
immune (human)	T50.Z11	T50.Z12	T50.Z13	T50.Z14	T50.Z15	T50.Z16
protective NEC	T50.Z11	T50.Z12	T50.Z13	T50.Z14	T50.Z15	T50.Z16
Setastine	T45.0X1	T45.0X2	T45.0X3	T45.0X4	T45.0X5	T45.0X6
Setoperone	T43.591	T43.592	T43.593	T43.594	T43.595	T43.596
Sewer gas	T59.91	T59.92	T59.93	T59.94	--	--
Shampoo	T55.0X1	T55.0X2	T55.0X3	T55.0X4	--	--
Shellfish, noxious, nonbacterial	T61.781	T61.782	T61.783	T61.784	--	--
Sildenafil	T46.7X1	T46.7X2	T46.7X3	T46.7X4	T46.7X5	T46.7X6
Silibinin	T50.991	T50.992	T50.993	T50.994	T50.995	T50.996
Silicone NEC	T65.891	T65.892	T65.893	T65.894	--	--
medicinal	T49.3X1	T49.3X2	T49.3X3	T49.3X4	T49.3X5	T49.3X6
Silvadene	T49.0X1	T49.0X2	T49.0X3	T49.0X4	T49.0X5	T49.0X6
Silver	T49.0X1	T49.0X2	T49.0X3	T49.0X4	T49.0X5	T49.0X6
anti-infectives	T49.0X1	T49.0X2	T49.0X3	T49.0X4	T49.0X5	T49.0X6
arsphenamine	T37.8X1	T37.8X2	T37.8X3	T37.8X4	T37.8X5	T37.8X6
colloidal	T49.0X1	T49.0X2	T49.0X3	T49.0X4	T49.0X5	T49.0X6
nitrate	T49.0X1	T49.0X2	T49.0X3	T49.0X4	T49.0X5	T49.0X6
ophthalmic preparation	T49.5X1	T49.5X2	T49.5X3	T49.5X4	T49.5X5	T49.5X6
toughened (keratolytic)	T49.4X1	T49.4X2	T49.4X3	T49.4X4	T49.4X5	T49.4X6
nonmedicinal (dust)	T56.891	T56.892	T56.893	T56.894	--	--
protein	T49.5X1	T49.5X2	T49.5X3	T49.5X4	T49.5X5	T49.5X6
salvarsan	T37.8X1	T37.8X2	T37.8X3	T37.8X4	T37.8X5	T37.8X6
sulfadiazine	T49.4X1	T49.4X2	T49.4X3	T49.4X4	T49.4X5	T49.4X6
Silymarin	T50.991	T50.992	T50.993	T50.994	T50.995	T50.996
Simaldrate	T47.1X1	T47.1X2	T47.1X3	T47.1X4	T47.1X5	T47.1X6
Simazine	T60.3X1	T60.3X2	T60.3X3	T60.3X4	--	--
Simethicone	T47.1X1	T47.1X2	T47.1X3	T47.1X4	T47.1X5	T47.1X6
Simfibrate	T46.6X1	T46.6X2	T46.6X3	T46.6X4	T46.6X5	T46.6X6
Simvastatin	T46.6X1	T46.6X2	T46.6X3	T46.6X4	T46.6X5	T46.6X6
Sincalide	T50.8X1	T50.8X2	T50.8X3	T50.8X4	T50.8X5	T50.8X6
Sinequan	T43.011	T43.012	T43.013	T43.014	T43.015	T43.016
Singoserp	T46.5X1	T46.5X2	T46.5X3	T46.5X4	T46.5X5	T46.5X6
Sintrom	T45.511	T45.512	T45.513	T45.514	T45.515	T45.516
Sisomicin	T36.5X1	T36.5X2	T36.5X3	T36.5X4	T36.5X5	T36.5X6
Sitosterols	T46.6X1	T46.6X2	T46.6X3	T46.6X4	T46.6X5	T46.6X6
Skeletal muscle relaxants	T48.1X1	T48.1X2	T48.1X3	T48.1X4	T48.1X5	T48.1X6
Skin						
agents (external)	T49.91	T49.92	T49.93	T49.94	T49.95	T49.96
specified NEC	T49.8X1	T49.8X2	T49.8X3	T49.8X4	T49.8X5	T49.8X6
test antigen	T50.8X1	T50.8X2	T50.8X3	T50.8X4	T50.8X5	T50.8X6
Sleep-eze	T45.0X1	T45.0X2	T45.0X3	T45.0X4	T45.0X5	T45.0X6
Sleeping draught, pill	T42.71	T42.72	T42.73	T42.74	T42.75	T42.76
Smallpox vaccine	T50.B11	T50.B12	T50.B13	T50.B14	T50.B15	T50.B16
Smelter fumes NEC	T56.91	T56.92	T56.93	T56.94	--	--
Smog	T59.1X1	T59.1X2	T59.1X3	T59.1X4	--	--
Smoke NEC	T59.811	T59.812	T59.813	T59.814	--	--
Smooth muscle relaxant	T44.3X1	T44.3X2	T44.3X3	T44.3X4	T44.3X5	T44.3X6
Snail killer NEC	T60.8X1	T60.8X2	T60.8X3	T60.8X4	--	--
Snake venom or bite	T63.001	T63.002	T63.003	T63.004	--	--
hemocoagulase	T45.7X1	T45.7X2	T45.7X3	T45.7X4	T45.7X5	T45.7X6
Snuff	T65.211	T65.212	T65.213	T65.214	--	--
Soap (powder) (product)	T55.0X1	T55.0X2	T55.0X3	T55.0X4	--	--
enema	T47.4X1	T47.4X2	T47.4X3	T47.4X4	T47.4X5	T47.4X6
medicinal, soft	T49.2X1	T49.2X2	T49.2X3	T49.2X4	T49.2X5	T49.2X6
superfatted	T49.2X1	T49.2X2	T49.2X3	T49.2X4	T49.2X5	T49.2X6
Sobrerol	T48.4X1	T48.4X2	T48.4X3	T48.4X4	T48.4X5	T48.4X6
Soda (caustic)	T54.3X1	T54.3X2	T54.3X3	T54.3X4	--	--
bicarb	T47.1X1	T47.1X2	T47.1X3	T47.1X4	T47.1X5	T47.1X6
chlorinated — *see* Sodium, hypochlorite						
Sodium						
acetosulfone	T37.1X1	T37.1X2	T37.1X3	T37.1X4	T37.1X5	T37.1X6
acetrizoate	T50.8X1	T50.8X2	T50.8X3	T50.8X4	T50.8X5	T50.8X6
acid phosphate	T50.3X1	T50.3X2	T50.3X3	T50.3X4	T50.3X5	T50.3X6
alginate	T47.8X1	T47.8X2	T47.8X3	T47.8X4	T47.8X5	T47.8X6
amidotrizoate	T50.8X1	T50.8X2	T50.8X3	T50.8X4	T50.8X5	T50.8X6
aminopterin	T45.1X1	T45.1X2	T45.1X3	T45.1X4	T45.1X5	T45.1X6
amylosulfate	T47.8X1	T47.8X2	T47.8X3	T47.8X4	T47.8X5	T47.8X6
Sodium — *continued*						
amytal	T42.3X1	T42.3X2	T42.3X3	T42.3X4	T42.3X5	T42.3X6
antimony gluconate	T37.3X1	T37.3X2	T37.3X3	T37.3X4	T37.3X5	T37.3X6
arsenate	T57.0X1	T57.0X2	T57.0X3	T57.0X4	--	--
aurothiomalate	T39.4X1	T39.4X2	T39.4X3	T39.4X4	T39.4X5	T39.4X6
aurothiosulfate	T39.4X1	T39.4X2	T39.4X3	T39.4X4	T39.4X5	T39.4X6
barbiturate	T42.3X1	T42.3X2	T42.3X3	T42.3X4	T42.3X5	T42.3X6
basic phosphate	T47.4X1	T47.4X2	T47.4X3	T47.4X4	T47.4X5	T47.4X6
bicarbonate	T47.1X1	T47.1X2	T47.1X3	T47.1X4	T47.1X5	T47.1X6
bichromate	T57.8X1	T57.8X2	T57.8X3	T57.8X4	--	--
biphosphate	T50.3X1	T50.3X2	T50.3X3	T50.3X4	T50.3X5	T50.3X6
bisulfate	T65.891	T65.892	T65.893	T65.894	--	--
borate						
cleanser	T57.8X1	T57.8X2	T57.8X3	T57.8X4	--	--
eye	T49.5X1	T49.5X2	T49.5X3	T49.5X4	T49.5X5	T49.5X6
therapeutic	T49.8X1	T49.8X2	T49.8X3	T49.8X4	T49.8X5	T49.8X6
bromide	T42.6X1	T42.6X2	T42.6X3	T42.6X4	T42.6X5	T42.6X6
cacodylate (nonmedicinal) NEC	T50.8X1	T50.8X2	T50.8X3	T50.8X4	T50.8X5	T50.8X6
anti-infective	T37.8X1	T37.8X2	T37.8X3	T37.8X4	T37.8X5	T37.8X6
herbicide	T60.3X1	T60.3X2	T60.3X3	T60.3X4	--	--
calcium edetate	T45.8X1	T45.8X2	T45.8X3	T45.8X4	T45.8X5	T45.8X6
carbonate NEC	T54.3X1	T54.3X2	T54.3X3	T54.3X4	--	--
chlorate NEC	T65.891	T65.892	T65.893	T65.894	--	--
herbicide	T54.91	T54.92	T54.93	T54.94	--	--
chloride	T50.3X1	T50.3X2	T50.3X3	T50.3X4	T50.3X5	T50.3X6
with glucose	T50.3X1	T50.3X2	T50.3X3	T50.3X4	T50.3X5	T50.3X6
chromate	T65.891	T65.892	T65.893	T65.894	--	--
citrate	T50.991	T50.992	T50.993	T50.994	T50.995	T50.996
cromoglicate	T48.6X1	T48.6X2	T48.6X3	T48.6X4	T48.6X5	T48.6X6
cyanide	T65.0X1	T65.0X2	T65.0X3	T65.0X4	--	--
cyclamate	T50.3X1	T50.3X2	T50.3X3	T50.3X4	T50.3X5	T50.3X6
dehydrocholate	T45.8X1	T45.8X2	T45.8X3	T45.8X4	T45.8X5	T45.8X6
diatrizoate	T50.8X1	T50.8X2	T50.8X3	T50.8X4	T50.8X5	T50.8X6
dibunate	T48.4X1	T48.4X2	T48.4X3	T48.4X4	T48.4X5	T48.4X6
dioctyl sulfosuccinate	T47.4X1	T47.4X2	T47.4X3	T47.4X4	T47.4X5	T47.4X6
dipantoyl ferrate	T45.8X1	T45.8X2	T45.8X3	T45.8X4	T45.8X5	T45.8X6
edetate	T45.8X1	T45.8X2	T45.8X3	T45.8X4	T45.8X5	T45.8X6
ethacrynate	T50.1X1	T50.1X2	T50.1X3	T50.1X4	T50.1X5	T50.1X6
feredetate	T45.8X1	T45.8X2	T45.8X3	T45.8X4	T45.8X5	T45.8X6
fluoride — *see* Fluoride						
fluoroacetate (dust) (pesticide)	T60.4X1	T60.4X2	T60.4X3	T60.4X4	--	--
free salt	T50.3X1	T50.3X2	T50.3X3	T50.3X4	T50.3X5	T50.3X6
fusidate	T36.8X1	T36.8X2	T36.8X3	T36.8X4	T36.8X5	T36.8X6
glucaldrate	T47.1X1	T47.1X2	T47.1X3	T47.1X4	T47.1X5	T47.1X6
glucosulfone	T37.1X1	T37.1X2	T37.1X3	T37.1X4	T37.1X5	T37.1X6
glutamate	T45.8X1	T45.8X2	T45.8X3	T45.8X4	T45.8X5	T45.8X6
hydrogen carbonate	T50.3X1	T50.3X2	T50.3X3	T50.3X4	T50.3X5	T50.3X6
hydroxide	T54.3X1	T54.3X2	T54.3X3	T54.3X4	--	--
hypochlorite (bleach) NEC	T54.3X1	T54.3X2	T54.3X3	T54.3X4	--	--
disinfectant	T54.3X1	T54.3X2	T54.3X3	T54.3X4	--	--
medicinal (anti-infective) (external)	T49.0X1	T49.0X2	T49.0X3	T49.0X4	T49.0X5	T49.0X6
vapor	T54.3X1	T54.3X2	T54.3X3	T54.3X4	--	--
hyposulfite	T49.0X1	T49.0X2	T49.0X3	T49.0X4	T49.0X5	T49.0X6
indigotin disulfonate	T50.8X1	T50.8X2	T50.8X3	T50.8X4	T50.8X5	T50.8X6
iodide	T50.991	T50.992	T50.993	T50.994	T50.995	T50.996
I-131	T50.8X1	T50.8X2	T50.8X3	T50.8X4	T50.8X5	T50.8X6
therapeutic	T38.2X1	T38.2X2	T38.2X3	T38.2X4	T38.2X5	T38.2X6
iodohippurate (131I)	T50.8X1	T50.8X2	T50.8X3	T50.8X4	T50.8X5	T50.8X6
iopodate	T50.8X1	T50.8X2	T50.8X3	T50.8X4	T50.8X5	T50.8X6
iothalamate	T50.8X1	T50.8X2	T50.8X3	T50.8X4	T50.8X5	T50.8X6
iron edetate	T45.4X1	T45.4X2	T45.4X3	T45.4X4	T45.4X5	T45.4X6
lactate (compound solution)	T45.8X1	T45.8X2	T45.8X3	T45.8X4	T45.8X5	T45.8X6
lauryl (sulfate)	T49.2X1	T49.2X2	T49.2X3	T49.2X4	T49.2X5	T49.2X6
L-triiodothyronine	T38.1X1	T38.1X2	T38.1X3	T38.1X4	T38.1X5	T38.1X6
magnesium citrate	T50.991	T50.992	T50.993	T50.994	T50.995	T50.996
mersalate	T50.2X1	T50.2X2	T50.2X3	T50.2X4	T50.2X5	T50.2X6
metasilicate	T65.891	T65.892	T65.893	T65.894	--	--
metrizoate	T50.8X1	T50.8X2	T50.8X3	T50.8X4	T50.8X5	T50.8X6
monofluoroacetate (pesticide)	T60.1X1	T60.1X2	T60.1X3	T60.1X4	--	--
morrhuate	T46.8X1	T46.8X2	T46.8X3	T46.8X4	T46.8X5	T46.8X6
nafcillin	T36.0X1	T36.0X2	T36.0X3	T36.0X4	T36.0X5	T36.0X6
nitrate (oxidizing agent)	T65.891	T65.892	T65.893	T65.894	--	--
nitrite	T50.6X1	T50.6X2	T50.6X3	T50.6X4	T50.6X5	T50.6X6
nitroferricyanide	T46.5X1	T46.5X2	T46.5X3	T46.5X4	T46.5X5	T46.5X6
nitroprusside	T46.5X1	T46.5X2	T46.5X3	T46.5X4	T46.5X5	T46.5X6
oxalate	T65.891	T65.892	T65.893	T65.894	--	--
oxide/peroxide	T65.891	T65.892	T65.893	T65.894	--	--
oxybate	T41.291	T41.292	T41.293	T41.294	T41.295	T41.296
para-aminohippurate	T50.8X1	T50.8X2	T50.8X3	T50.8X4	T50.8X5	T50.8X6

Substance	Poisoning, Accidental (unintentional)	Poisoning, Intentional self-harm	Poisoning, Assault	Poisoning, Undetermined	Adverse effect	Underdosing
Sodium — *continued*						
perborate (nonmedicinal) NEC	T65.891	T65.892	T65.893	T65.894	--	--
medicinal	T49.0X1	T49.0X2	T49.0X3	T49.0X4	T49.0X5	T49.0X6
soap	T55.0X1	T55.0X2	T55.0X3	T55.0X4	--	--
percarbonate — *see* Sodium, perborate						
pertechnetate Tc99m	T50.8X1	T50.8X2	T50.8X3	T50.8X4	T50.8X5	T50.8X6
phosphate						
cellulose	T45.8X1	T45.8X2	T45.8X3	T45.8X4	T45.8X5	T45.8X6
dibasic	T47.2X1	T47.2X2	T47.2X3	T47.2X4	T47.2X5	T47.2X6
monobasic	T47.2X1	T47.2X2	T47.2X3	T47.2X4	T47.2X5	T47.2X6
phytate	T50.6X1	T50.6X2	T50.6X3	T50.6X4	T50.6X5	T50.6X6
picosulfate	T47.2X1	T47.2X2	T47.2X3	T47.2X4	T47.2X5	T47.2X6
polyhydroxyaluminium monocarbonate	T47.1X1	T47.1X2	T47.1X3	T47.1X4	T47.1X5	T47.1X6
polystyrene sulfonate	T50.3X1	T50.3X2	T50.3X3	T50.3X4	T50.3X5	T50.3X6
propionate	T49.0X1	T49.0X2	T49.0X3	T49.0X4	T49.0X5	T49.0X6
propyl hydroxybenzoate	T50.991	T50.992	T50.993	T50.994	T50.995	T50.996
psylliate	T46.8X1	T46.8X2	T46.8X3	T46.8X4	T46.8X5	T46.8X6
removing resins	T50.3X1	T50.3X2	T50.3X3	T50.3X4	T50.3X5	T50.3X6
salicylate	T39.091	T39.092	T39.093	T39.094	T39.095	T39.096
salt NEC	T50.3X1	T50.3X2	T50.3X3	T50.3X4	T50.3X5	T50.3X6
selenate	T60.2X1	T60.2X2	T60.2X3	T60.2X4	--	--
stibogluconate	T37.3X1	T37.3X2	T37.3X3	T37.3X4	T37.3X5	T37.3X6
sulfate	T47.4X1	T47.4X2	T47.4X3	T47.4X4	T47.4X5	T47.4X6
sulfoxone	T37.1X1	T37.1X2	T37.1X3	T37.1X4	T37.1X5	T37.1X6
tetradecyl sulfate	T46.8X1	T46.8X2	T46.8X3	T46.8X4	T46.8X5	T46.8X6
thiopental	T41.1X1	T41.1X2	T41.1X3	T41.1X4	T41.1X5	T41.1X6
thiosalicylate	T39.091	T39.092	T39.093	T39.094	T39.095	T39.096
thiosulfate	T50.6X1	T50.6X2	T50.6X3	T50.6X4	T50.6X5	T50.6X6
tolbutamide	T38.3X1	T38.3X2	T38.3X3	T38.3X4	T38.3X5	T38.3X6
(L) -triiodothyronine	T38.1X1	T38.1X2	T38.1X3	T38.1X4	T38.1X5	T38.1X6
tyropanoate	T50.8X1	T50.8X2	T50.8X3	T50.8X4	T50.8X5	T50.8X6
valproate	T42.6X1	T42.6X2	T42.6X3	T42.6X4	T42.6X5	T42.6X6
versenate	T50.6X1	T50.6X2	T50.6X3	T50.6X4	T50.6X5	T50.6X6
Sodium-free salt	T50.901	T50.902	T50.903	T50.904	T50.905	T50.906
Sodium-removing resin	T50.3X1	T50.3X2	T50.3X3	T50.3X4	T50.3X5	T50.3X6
Soft soap	T55.0X1	T55.0X2	T55.0X3	T55.0X4	--	--
Solanine	T62.2X1	T62.2X2	T62.2X3	T62.2X4	--	--
berries	T62.1X1	T62.1X2	T62.1X3	T62.1X4	--	--
Solanum dulcamara	T62.2X1	T62.2X2	T62.2X3	T62.2X4	--	--
berries	T62.1X1	T62.1X2	T62.1X3	T62.1X4	--	--
Solapsone	T37.1X1	T37.1X2	T37.1X3	T37.1X4	T37.1X5	T37.1X6
Solar lotion	T49.3X1	T49.3X2	T49.3X3	T49.3X4	T49.3X5	T49.3X6
Solasulfone	T37.1X1	T37.1X2	T37.1X3	T37.1X4	T37.1X5	T37.1X6
Soldering fluid	T65.891	T65.892	T65.893	T65.894		
Solid substance	T65.91	T65.92	T65.93	T65.94	--	--
specified NEC	T65.891	T65.892	T65.893	T65.894	--	--
Solvent, industrial NEC	T52.91	T52.92	T52.93	T52.94	--	--
naphtha	T52.0X1	T52.0X2	T52.0X3	T52.0X4	--	--
petroleum	T52.0X1	T52.0X2	T52.0X3	T52.0X4	--	--
specified NEC	T52.8X1	T52.8X2	T52.8X3	T52.8X4	--	--
Soma	T42.8X1	T42.8X2	T42.8X3	T42.8X4	T42.8X5	T42.8X6
Somatorelin	T38.891	T38.892	T38.893	T38.894	T38.895	T38.896
Somatostatin	T38.991	T38.992	T38.993	T38.994	T38.995	T38.996
Somatotropin	T38.811	T38.812	T38.813	T38.814	T38.815	T38.816
Somatrem	T38.811	T38.812	T38.813	T38.814	T38.815	T38.816
Somatropin	T38.811	T38.812	T38.813	T38.814	T38.815	T38.816
Sominex	T45.0X1	T45.0X2	T45.0X3	T45.0X4	T45.0X5	T45.0X6
Somnos	T42.6X1	T42.6X2	T42.6X3	T42.6X4	T42.6X5	T42.6X6
Somonal	T42.3X1	T42.3X2	T42.3X3	T42.3X4	T42.3X5	T42.3X6
Soneryl	T42.3X1	T42.3X2	T42.3X3	T42.3X4	T42.3X5	T42.3X6
Soothing syrup	T50.901	T50.902	T50.903	T50.904	T50.905	T50.906
Sopor	T42.6X1	T42.6X2	T42.6X3	T42.6X4	T42.6X5	T42.6X6
Soporific	T42.71	T42.72	T42.73	T42.74	T42.75	T42.76
Soporific drug	T42.71	T42.72	T42.73	T42.74	T42.75	T42.76
specified type NEC	T42.6X1	T42.6X2	T42.6X3	T42.6X4	T42.6X5	T42.6X6
Sorbide nitrate	T46.3X1	T46.3X2	T46.3X3	T46.3X4	T46.3X5	T46.3X6
Sorbitol	T47.4X1	T47.4X2	T47.4X3	T47.4X4	T47.4X5	T47.4X6
Sotalol	T44.7X1	T44.7X2	T44.7X3	T44.7X4	T44.7X5	T44.7X6
Sotradecol	T46.8X1	T46.8X2	T46.8X3	T46.8X4	T46.8X5	T46.8X6
Soysterol	T46.6X1	T46.6X2	T46.6X3	T46.6X4	T46.6X5	T46.6X6
Spacoline	T44.3X1	T44.3X2	T44.3X3	T44.3X4	T44.3X5	T44.3X6
Spanish fly	T49.8X1	T49.8X2	T49.8X3	T49.8X4	T49.8X5	T49.8X6
Sparine	T43.3X1	T43.3X2	T43.3X3	T43.3X4	T43.3X5	T43.3X6
Sparteine	T48.0X1	T48.0X2	T48.0X3	T48.0X4	T48.0X5	T48.0X6
Spasmolytic						
anticholinergics	T44.3X1	T44.3X2	T44.3X3	T44.3X4	T44.3X5	T44.3X6
autonomic	T44.3X1	T44.3X2	T44.3X3	T44.3X4	T44.3X5	T44.3X6
bronchial NEC	T48.6X1	T48.6X2	T48.6X3	T48.6X4	T48.6X5	T48.6X6
quaternary ammonium	T44.3X1	T44.3X2	T44.3X3	T44.3X4	T44.3X5	T44.3X6
skeletal muscle NEC	T48.1X1	T48.1X2	T48.1X3	T48.1X4	T48.1X5	T48.1X6
Spectinomycin	T36.5X1	T36.5X2	T36.5X3	T36.5X4	T36.5X5	T36.5X6

Substance	Poisoning, Accidental (unintentional)	Poisoning, Intentional self-harm	Poisoning, Assault	Poisoning, Undetermined	Adverse effect	Underdosing
Speed	T43.621	T43.622	T43.623	T43.624	T43.625	T43.626
Spermicide	T49.8X1	T49.8X2	T49.8X3	T49.8X4	T49.8X5	T49.8X6
Spider (bite) (venom)	T63.391	T63.392	T63.393	T63.394		
antivenin	T50.Z11	T50.Z12	T50.Z13	T50.Z14	T50.Z15	T50.Z16
Spigelia (root)	T37.4X1	T37.4X2	T37.4X3	T37.4X4	T37.4X5	T37.4X6
Spindle inactivator	T50.4X1	T50.4X2	T50.4X3	T50.4X4	T50.4X5	T50.4X6
Spiperone	T43.4X1	T43.4X2	T43.4X3	T43.4X4	T43.4X5	T43.4X6
Spiramycin	T36.3X1	T36.3X2	T36.3X3	T36.3X4	T36.3X5	T36.3X6
Spirapril	T46.4X1	T46.4X2	T46.4X3	T46.4X4	T46.4X5	T46.4X6
Spirilene	T43.591	T43.592	T43.593	T43.594	T43.595	T43.596
Spirit(s) (neutral) NEC	T51.0X1	T51.0X2	T51.0X3	T51.0X4	--	--
beverage	T51.0X1	T51.0X2	T51.0X3	T51.0X4	--	--
industrial	T51.0X1	T51.0X2	T51.0X3	T51.0X4	--	--
mineral	T52.0X1	T52.0X2	T52.0X3	T52.0X4	--	--
of salt — *see* Hydrochloric acid						
surgical	T51.0X1	T51.0X2	T51.0X3	T51.0X4	--	--
Spironolactone	T50.0X1	T50.0X2	T50.0X3	T50.0X4	T50.0X5	T50.0X6
Spiroperidol	T43.4X1	T43.4X2	T43.4X3	T43.4X4	T43.4X5	T43.4X6
Sponge, absorbable (gelatin)	T45.7X1	T45.7X2	T45.7X3	T45.7X4	T45.7X5	T45.7X6
Sporostacin	T49.0X1	T49.0X2	T49.0X3	T49.0X4	T49.0X5	T49.0X6
Spray (aerosol)	T65.91	T65.92	T65.93	T65.94	--	--
cosmetic	T65.891	T65.892	T65.893	T65.894	--	--
medicinal NEC	T50.901	T50.902	T50.903	T50.904	T50.905	T50.906
pesticides — *see* Pesticide						
specified content — *see* specific substance						
Spurge flax	T62.2X1	T62.2X2	T62.2X3	T62.2X4	--	--
Spurges	T62.2X1	T62.2X2	T62.2X3	T62.2X4	--	--
Sputum viscosity-lowering drug	T48.4X1	T48.4X2	T48.4X3	T48.4X4	T48.4X5	T48.4X6
Squill	T46.0X1	T46.0X2	T46.0X3	T46.0X4	T46.0X5	T46.0X6
rat poison	T60.4X1	T60.4X2	T60.4X3	T60.4X4	--	--
Squirting cucumber (cathartic)	T47.2X1	T47.2X2	T47.2X3	T47.2X4	T47.2X5	T47.2X6
Stains	T65.6X1	T65.6X2	T65.6X3	T65.6X4	--	--
Stannous fluoride	T49.7X1	T49.7X2	T49.7X3	T49.7X4	T49.7X5	T49.7X6
Stanolone	T38.7X1	T38.7X2	T38.7X3	T38.7X4	T38.7X5	T38.7X6
Stanozolol	T38.7X1	T38.7X2	T38.7X3	T38.7X4	T38.7X5	T38.7X6
Staphisagria or stavesacre (pediculicide)	T49.0X1	T49.0X2	T49.0X3	T49.0X4	T49.0X5	T49.0X6
Starch	T50.901	T50.902	T50.903	T50.904	T50.905	T50.906
Stelazine	T43.3X1	T43.3X2	T43.3X3	T43.3X4	T43.3X5	T43.3X6
Stemetil	T43.3X1	T43.3X2	T43.3X3	T43.3X4	T43.3X5	T43.3X6
Stepronin	T48.4X1	T48.4X2	T48.4X3	T48.4X4	T48.4X5	T48.4X6
Sterculia	T47.4X1	T47.4X2	T47.4X3	T47.4X4	T47.4X5	T47.4X6
Sternutator gas	T59.891	T59.892	T59.893	T59.894	--	--
Steroid	T38.0X1	T38.0X2	T38.0X3	T38.0X4	T38.0X5	T38.0X6
anabolic	T38.7X1	T38.7X2	T38.7X3	T38.7X4	T38.7X5	T38.7X6
androgenic	T38.7X1	T38.7X2	T38.7X3	T38.7X4	T38.7X5	T38.7X6
antineoplastic, hormone	T38.7X1	T38.7X2	T38.7X3	T38.7X4	T38.7X5	T38.7X6
estrogen	T38.5X1	T38.5X2	T38.5X3	T38.5X4	T38.5X5	T38.5X6
ENT agent	T49.6X1	T49.6X2	T49.6X3	T49.6X4	T49.6X5	T49.6X6
ophthalmic preparation	T49.5X1	T49.5X2	T49.5X3	T49.5X4	T49.5X5	T49.5X6
topical NEC	T49.0X1	T49.0X2	T49.0X3	T49.0X4	T49.0X5	T49.0X6
Stibine	T56.891	T56.892	T56.893	T56.894	--	--
Stibogluconate	T37.3X1	T37.3X2	T37.3X3	T37.3X4	T37.3X5	T37.3X6
Stibophen	T37.4X1	T37.4X2	T37.4X3	T37.4X4	T37.4X5	T37.4X6
Stilbamidine (isetionate)	T37.3X1	T37.3X2	T37.3X3	T37.3X4	T37.3X5	T37.3X6
Stilbestrol	T38.5X1	T38.5X2	T38.5X3	T38.5X4	T38.5X5	T38.5X6
Stilboestrol	T38.5X1	T38.5X2	T38.5X3	T38.5X4	T38.5X5	T38.5X6
Stimulant						
central nervous system (*see also* Psychostimulant)	T43.601	T43.602	T43.603	T43.604	T43.605	T43.606
analeptics	T50.7X1	T50.7X2	T50.7X3	T50.7X4	T50.7X5	T50.7X6
opiate antagonist	T50.7X1	T50.7X2	T50.7X3	T50.7X4	T50.7X5	T50.7X6
psychotherapeutic NEC (*see also* Psychotherapeutic drug)	T43.601	T43.602	T43.603	T43.604	T43.605	T43.606
specified NEC	T43.691	T43.692	T43.693	T43.694	T43.695	T43.696
respiratory	T48.901	T48.902	T48.903	T48.904	T48.905	T48.906
Stone-dissolving drug	T50.901	T50.902	T50.903	T50.904	T50.905	T50.906
Storage battery (cells) (acid)	T54.2X1	T54.2X2	T54.2X3	T54.2X4	--	--
Stovaine	T41.3X1	T41.3X2	T41.3X3	T41.3X4	T41.3X5	T41.3X6
infiltration (subcutaneous)	T41.3X1	T41.3X2	T41.3X3	T41.3X4	T41.3X5	T41.3X6
nerve block (peripheral) (plexus)	T41.3X1	T41.3X2	T41.3X3	T41.3X4	T41.3X5	T41.3X6
spinal	T41.3X1	T41.3X2	T41.3X3	T41.3X4	T41.3X5	T41.3X6
topical (surface)	T41.3X1	T41.3X2	T41.3X3	T41.3X4	T41.3X5	T41.3X6
Stovarsal	T37.8X1	T37.8X2	T37.8X3	T37.8X4	T37.8X5	T37.8X6
Stove gas — *see* Gas, stove						
Stoxil	T49.5X1	T49.5X2	T49.5X3	T49.5X4	T49.5X5	T49.5X6

Stramonium - Syrosingopine

Substance	Poisoning, Accidental (unintentional)	Poisoning, Intentional self-harm	Poisoning, Assault	Poisoning, Undetermined	Adverse effect	Underdosing
Stramonium	T48.6X1	T48.6X2	T48.6X3	T48.6X4	T48.6X5	T48.6X6
natural state	T62.2X1	T62.2X2	T62.2X3	T62.2X4	--	--
Streptodornase	T45.3X1	T45.3X2	T45.3X3	T45.3X4	T45.3X5	T45.3X6
Streptoduocin	T36.5X1	T36.5X2	T36.5X3	T36.5X4	T36.5X5	T36.5X6
Streptokinase	T45.611	T45.612	T45.613	T45.614	T45.615	T45.616
Streptomycin (derivative)	T36.5X1	T36.5X2	T36.5X3	T36.5X4	T36.5X5	T36.5X6
Streptonivicin	T36.5X1	T36.5X2	T36.5X3	T36.5X4	T36.5X5	T36.5X6
Streptovarycin	T36.5X1	T36.5X2	T36.5X3	T36.5X4	T36.5X5	T36.5X6
Streptozocin	T45.1X1	T45.1X2	T45.1X3	T45.1X4	T45.1X5	T45.1X6
Streptozotocin	T45.1X1	T45.1X2	T45.1X3	T45.1X4	T45.1X5	T45.1X6
Stripper (paint) (solvent)	T52.8X1	T52.8X2	T52.8X3	T52.8X4	--	--
Strobane	T60.1X1	T60.1X2	T60.1X3	T60.1X4	--	--
Strofantina	T46.0X1	T46.0X2	T46.0X3	T46.0X4	T46.0X5	T46.0X6
Strophanthin (g) (k)	T46.0X1	T46.0X2	T46.0X3	T46.0X4	T46.0X5	T46.0X6
Strophanthus	T46.0X1	T46.0X2	T46.0X3	T46.0X4	T46.0X5	T46.0X6
Strophantin	T46.0X1	T46.0X2	T46.0X3	T46.0X4	T46.0X5	T46.0X6
Strophantin-g	T46.0X1	T46.0X2	T46.0X3	T46.0X4	T46.0X5	T46.0X6
Strychnine (nonmedicinal) (pesticide) (salts)	T65.1X1	T65.1X2	T65.1X3	T65.1X4	--	--
medicinal	T48.291	T48.292	T48.293	T48.294	T48.295	T48.296
Strychnos (ignatii) — see Strychnine						
Styramate	T42.8X1	T42.8X2	T42.8X3	T42.8X4	T42.8X5	T42.8X6
Styrene	T65.891	T65.892	T65.893	T65.894	--	--
Succinimide, antiepileptic or anticonvulsant	T42.2X1	T42.2X2	T42.2X3	T42.2X4	T42.2X5	T42.2X6
mercuric — see Mercury						
Succinylcholine	T48.1X1	T48.1X2	T48.1X3	T48.1X4	T48.1X5	T48.1X6
Succinylsulfathiazole	T37.0X1	T37.0X2	T37.0X3	T37.0X4	T37.0X5	T37.0X6
Sucralfate	T47.1X1	T47.1X2	T47.1X3	T47.1X4	T47.1X5	T47.1X6
Sucrose	T50.3X1	T50.3X2	T50.3X3	T50.3X4	T50.3X5	T50.3X6
Sufentanil	T40.4X1	T40.4X2	T40.4X3	T40.4X4	T40.4X5	T40.4X6
Sulbactam	T36.0X1	T36.0X2	T36.0X3	T36.0X4	T36.0X5	T36.0X6
Sulbenicillin	T36.0X1	T36.0X2	T36.0X3	T36.0X4	T36.0X5	T36.0X6
Sulbentine	T49.0X1	T49.0X2	T49.0X3	T49.0X4	T49.0X5	T49.0X6
Sulfacetamide	T49.0X1	T49.0X2	T49.0X3	T49.0X4	T49.0X5	T49.0X6
ophthalmic preparation	T49.5X1	T49.5X2	T49.5X3	T49.5X4	T49.5X5	T49.5X6
Sulfachlorpyridazine	T37.0X1	T37.0X2	T37.0X3	T37.0X4	T37.0X5	T37.0X6
Sulfacitine	T37.0X1	T37.0X2	T37.0X3	T37.0X4	T37.0X5	T37.0X6
Sulfadiasulfone sodium	T37.0X1	T37.0X2	T37.0X3	T37.0X4	T37.0X5	T37.0X6
Sulfadiazine	T37.0X1	T37.0X2	T37.0X3	T37.0X4	T37.0X5	T37.0X6
silver (topical)	T49.0X1	T49.0X2	T49.0X3	T49.0X4	T49.0X5	T49.0X6
Sulfadimethoxine	T37.0X1	T37.0X2	T37.0X3	T37.0X4	T37.0X5	T37.0X6
Sulfadimidine	T37.0X1	T37.0X2	T37.0X3	T37.0X4	T37.0X5	T37.0X6
Sulfadoxine	T37.0X1	T37.0X2	T37.0X3	T37.0X4	T37.0X5	T37.0X6
with pyrimethamine	T37.2X1	T37.2X2	T37.2X3	T37.2X4	T37.2X5	T37.2X6
Sulfaethidole	T37.0X1	T37.0X2	T37.0X3	T37.0X4	T37.0X5	T37.0X6
Sulfafurazole	T37.0X1	T37.0X2	T37.0X3	T37.0X4	T37.0X5	T37.0X6
Sulfaguanidine	T37.0X1	T37.0X2	T37.0X3	T37.0X4	T37.0X5	T37.0X6
Sulfalene	T37.0X1	T37.0X2	T37.0X3	T37.0X4	T37.0X5	T37.0X6
Sulfaloxate	T37.0X1	T37.0X2	T37.0X3	T37.0X4	T37.0X5	T37.0X6
Sulfaloxic acid	T37.0X1	T37.0X2	T37.0X3	T37.0X4	T37.0X5	T37.0X6
Sulfamazone	T39.2X1	T39.2X2	T39.2X3	T39.2X4	T39.2X5	T39.2X6
Sulfamerazine	T37.0X1	T37.0X2	T37.0X3	T37.0X4	T37.0X5	T37.0X6
Sulfameter	T37.0X1	T37.0X2	T37.0X3	T37.0X4	T37.0X5	T37.0X6
Sulfamethazine	T37.0X1	T37.0X2	T37.0X3	T37.0X4	T37.0X5	T37.0X6
Sulfamethizole	T37.0X1	T37.0X2	T37.0X3	T37.0X4	T37.0X5	T37.0X6
Sulfamethoxazole	T37.0X1	T37.0X2	T37.0X3	T37.0X4	T37.0X5	T37.0X6
with trimethoprim	T36.8X1	T36.8X2	T36.8X3	T36.8X4	T36.8X5	T36.8X6
Sulfamethoxydiazine	T37.0X1	T37.0X2	T37.0X3	T37.0X4	T37.0X5	T37.0X6
Sulfamethoxypyridazine	T37.0X1	T37.0X2	T37.0X3	T37.0X4	T37.0X5	T37.0X6
Sulfamethylthiazole	T37.0X1	T37.0X2	T37.0X3	T37.0X4	T37.0X5	T37.0X6
Sulfametoxydiazine	T37.0X1	T37.0X2	T37.0X3	T37.0X4	T37.0X5	T37.0X6
Sulfamidopyrine	T39.2X1	T39.2X2	T39.2X3	T39.2X4	T39.2X5	T39.2X6
Sulfamonomethoxine	T37.0X1	T37.0X2	T37.0X3	T37.0X4	T37.0X5	T37.0X6
Sulfamoxole	T37.0X1	T37.0X2	T37.0X3	T37.0X4	T37.0X5	T37.0X6
Sulfamylon	T49.0X1	T49.0X2	T49.0X3	T49.0X4	T49.0X5	T49.0X6
Sulfan blue (diagnostic dye)	T50.8X1	T50.8X2	T50.8X3	T50.8X4	T50.8X5	T50.8X6
Sulfanilamide	T37.0X1	T37.0X2	T37.0X3	T37.0X4	T37.0X5	T37.0X6
Sulfanilylguanidine	T37.0X1	T37.0X2	T37.0X3	T37.0X4	T37.0X5	T37.0X6
Sulfaperin	T37.0X1	T37.0X2	T37.0X3	T37.0X4	T37.0X5	T37.0X6
Sulfaphenazole	T37.0X1	T37.0X2	T37.0X3	T37.0X4	T37.0X5	T37.0X6
Sulfaphenylthiazole	T37.0X1	T37.0X2	T37.0X3	T37.0X4	T37.0X5	T37.0X6
Sulfaproxyline	T37.0X1	T37.0X2	T37.0X3	T37.0X4	T37.0X5	T37.0X6
Sulfapyridine	T37.0X1	T37.0X2	T37.0X3	T37.0X4	T37.0X5	T37.0X6
Sulfapyrimidine	T37.0X1	T37.0X2	T37.0X3	T37.0X4	T37.0X5	T37.0X6
Sulfarsphenamine	T37.8X1	T37.8X2	T37.8X3	T37.8X4	T37.8X5	T37.8X6
Sulfasalazine	T37.0X1	T37.0X2	T37.0X3	T37.0X4	T37.0X5	T37.0X6
Sulfasuxidine	T37.0X1	T37.0X2	T37.0X3	T37.0X4	T37.0X5	T37.0X6
Sulfasymazine	T37.0X1	T37.0X2	T37.0X3	T37.0X4	T37.0X5	T37.0X6
Sulfated amylopectin	T47.8X1	T47.8X2	T47.8X3	T47.8X4	T47.8X5	T47.8X6
Sulfathiazole	T37.0X1	T37.0X2	T37.0X3	T37.0X4	T37.0X5	T37.0X6
Sulfatostearate	T49.2X1	T49.2X2	T49.2X3	T49.2X4	T49.2X5	T49.2X6
Sulfinpyrazone	T50.4X1	T50.4X2	T50.4X3	T50.4X4	T50.4X5	T50.4X6
Sulfiram	T49.0X1	T49.0X2	T49.0X3	T49.0X4	T49.0X5	T49.0X6
Sulfisomidine	T37.0X1	T37.0X2	T37.0X3	T37.0X4	T37.0X5	T37.0X6
Sulfisoxazole	T37.0X1	T37.0X2	T37.0X3	T37.0X4	T37.0X5	T37.0X6
ophthalmic preparation	T49.5X1	T49.5X2	T49.5X3	T49.5X4	T49.5X5	T49.5X6
Sulfobromophthalein (sodium)	T50.8X1	T50.8X2	T50.8X3	T50.8X4	T50.8X5	T50.8X6
Sulfobromphthalein	T50.8X1	T50.8X2	T50.8X3	T50.8X4	T50.8X5	T50.8X6
Sulfogaiacol	T48.4X1	T48.4X2	T48.4X3	T48.4X4	T48.4X5	T48.4X6
Sulfomyxin	T36.8X1	T36.8X2	T36.8X3	T36.8X4	T36.8X5	T36.8X6
Sulfonal	T42.6X1	T42.6X2	T42.6X3	T42.6X4	T42.6X5	T42.6X6
Sulfonamide NEC	T37.0X1	T37.0X2	T37.0X3	T37.0X4	T37.0X5	T37.0X6
eye	T49.5X1	T49.5X2	T49.5X3	T49.5X4	T49.5X5	T49.5X6
Sulfonazide	T37.1X1	T37.1X2	T37.1X3	T37.1X4	T37.1X5	T37.1X6
Sulfones	T37.1X1	T37.1X2	T37.1X3	T37.1X4	T37.1X5	T37.1X6
Sulfonethylmethane	T42.6X1	T42.6X2	T42.6X3	T42.6X4	T42.6X5	T42.6X6
Sulfonmethane	T42.6X1	T42.6X2	T42.6X3	T42.6X4	T42.6X5	T42.6X6
Sulfonphthal, sulfonphthol	T50.8X1	T50.8X2	T50.8X3	T50.8X4	T50.8X5	T50.8X6
Sulfonylurea derivatives, oral	T38.3X1	T38.3X2	T38.3X3	T38.3X4	T38.3X5	T38.3X6
Sulforidazine	T43.3X1	T43.3X2	T43.3X3	T43.3X4	T43.3X5	T43.3X6
Sulfoxone	T37.1X1	T37.1X2	T37.1X3	T37.1X4	T37.1X5	T37.1X6
Sulfur, sulfurated, sulfuric, sulfurous, sulfuryl (compounds NEC) (medicinal)	T49.4X1	T49.4X2	T49.4X3	T49.4X4	T49.4X5	T49.4X6
acid	T54.2X1	T54.2X2	T54.2X3	T54.2X4	--	--
dioxide (gas)	T59.1X1	T59.1X2	T59.1X3	T59.1X4	--	--
ether — see Ether(s)						
hydrogen	T59.6X1	T59.6X2	T59.6X3	T59.6X4	--	--
medicinal (keratolytic) (ointment) NEC	T49.4X1	T49.4X2	T49.4X3	T49.4X4	T49.4X5	T49.4X6
ointment	T49.0X1	T49.0X2	T49.0X3	T49.0X4	T49.0X5	T49.0X6
pesticide (vapor)	T60.91	T60.92	T60.93	T60.94	--	--
vapor NEC	T59.891	T59.892	T59.893	T59.894	--	--
Sulfuric acid	T54.2X1	T54.2X2	T54.2X3	T54.2X4	--	--
Sulglicotide	T47.1X1	T47.1X2	T47.1X3	T47.1X4	T47.1X5	T47.1X6
Sulindac	T39.391	T39.392	T39.393	T39.394	T39.395	T39.396
Sulisatin	T47.2X1	T47.2X2	T47.2X3	T47.2X4	T47.2X5	T47.2X6
Sulisobenzone	T49.3X1	T49.3X2	T49.3X3	T49.3X4	T49.3X5	T49.3X6
Sulkowitch's reagent	T50.8X1	T50.8X2	T50.8X3	T50.8X4	T50.8X5	T50.8X6
Sulmetozine	T44.3X1	T44.3X2	T44.3X3	T44.3X4	T44.3X5	T44.3X6
Suloctidil	T46.7X1	T46.7X2	T46.7X3	T46.7X4	T46.7X5	T46.7X6
Sulph- (see also Sulf-)						
Sulphadiazine	T37.0X1	T37.0X2	T37.0X3	T37.0X4	T37.0X5	T37.0X6
Sulphadimethoxine	T37.0X1	T37.0X2	T37.0X3	T37.0X4	T37.0X5	T37.0X6
Sulphadimidine	T37.0X1	T37.0X2	T37.0X3	T37.0X4	T37.0X5	T37.0X6
Sulphadione	T37.1X1	T37.1X2	T37.1X3	T37.1X4	T37.1X5	T37.1X6
Sulphafurazole	T37.0X1	T37.0X2	T37.0X3	T37.0X4	T37.0X5	T37.0X6
Sulphamethizole	T37.0X1	T37.0X2	T37.0X3	T37.0X4	T37.0X5	T37.0X6
Sulphamethoxazole	T37.0X1	T37.0X2	T37.0X3	T37.0X4	T37.0X5	T37.0X6
Sulphan blue	T50.8X1	T50.8X2	T50.8X3	T50.8X4	T50.8X5	T50.8X6
Sulphaphenazole	T37.0X1	T37.0X2	T37.0X3	T37.0X4	T37.0X5	T37.0X6
Sulphapyridine	T37.0X1	T37.0X2	T37.0X3	T37.0X4	T37.0X5	T37.0X6
Sulphasalazine	T37.0X1	T37.0X2	T37.0X3	T37.0X4	T37.0X5	T37.0X6
Sulphinpyrazone	T50.4X1	T50.4X2	T50.4X3	T50.4X4	T50.4X5	T50.4X6
Sulpiride	T43.591	T43.592	T43.593	T43.594	T43.595	T43.596
Sulprostone	T48.0X1	T48.0X2	T48.0X3	T48.0X4	T48.0X5	T48.0X6
Sulpyrine	T39.2X1	T39.2X2	T39.2X3	T39.2X4	T39.2X5	T39.2X6
Sultamicillin	T36.0X1	T36.0X2	T36.0X3	T36.0X4	T36.0X5	T36.0X6
Sulthiame	T42.6X1	T42.6X2	T42.6X3	T42.6X4	T42.6X5	T42.6X6
Sultiame	T42.6X1	T42.6X2	T42.6X3	T42.6X4	T42.6X5	T42.6X6
Sultopride	T43.591	T43.592	T43.593	T43.594	T43.595	T43.596
Sumatriptan	T39.8X1	T39.8X2	T39.8X3	T39.8X4	T39.8X5	T39.8X6
Sunflower seed oil	T46.6X1	T46.6X2	T46.6X3	T46.6X4	T46.6X5	T46.6X6
Superinone	T48.4X1	T48.4X2	T48.4X3	T48.4X4	T48.4X5	T48.4X6
Suprofen	T39.311	T39.312	T39.313	T39.314	T39.315	T39.316
Suramin (sodium)	T37.4X1	T37.4X2	T37.4X3	T37.4X4	T37.4X5	T37.4X6
Surfacaine	T41.3X1	T41.3X2	T41.3X3	T41.3X4	T41.3X5	T41.3X6
Surital	T41.1X1	T41.1X2	T41.1X3	T41.1X4	T41.1X5	T41.1X6
Sutilains	T45.3X1	T45.3X2	T45.3X3	T45.3X4	T45.3X5	T45.3X6
Suxamethonium (chloride)	T48.1X1	T48.1X2	T48.1X3	T48.1X4	T48.1X5	T48.1X6
Suxethonium (chloride)	T48.1X1	T48.1X2	T48.1X3	T48.1X4	T48.1X5	T48.1X6
Suxibuzone	T39.2X1	T39.2X2	T39.2X3	T39.2X4	T39.2X5	T39.2X6
Sweet niter spirit	T46.3X1	T46.3X2	T46.3X3	T46.3X4	T46.3X5	T46.3X6
Sweet oil (birch)	T49.3X1	T49.3X2	T49.3X3	T49.3X4	T49.3X5	T49.3X6
Sweetener	T50.901	T50.902	T50.903	T50.904	T50.905	T50.906
Sym-dichloroethyl ether	T53.6X1	T53.6X2	T53.6X3	T53.6X4	--	--
Sympatholytic NEC	T44.8X1	T44.8X2	T44.8X3	T44.8X4	T44.8X5	T44.8X6
haloalkylamine	T44.8X1	T44.8X2	T44.8X3	T44.8X4	T44.8X5	T44.8X6
Sympathomimetic NEC	T44.901	T44.902	T44.903	T44.904	T44.905	T44.906
anti-common-cold	T48.5X1	T48.5X2	T48.5X3	T48.5X4	T48.5X5	T48.5X6
bronchodilator	T48.6X1	T48.6X2	T48.6X3	T48.6X4	T48.6X5	T48.6X6
specified NEC	T44.991	T44.992	T44.993	T44.994	T44.995	T44.996
Synagis	T50.B91	T50.B92	T50.B93	T50.B94	T50.B95	T50.B96
Synalar	T49.0X1	T49.0X2	T49.0X3	T49.0X4	T49.0X5	T49.0X6
Synthroid	T38.1X1	T38.1X2	T38.1X3	T38.1X4	T38.1X5	T38.1X6
Syntocinon	T48.0X1	T48.0X2	T48.0X3	T48.0X4	T48.0X5	T48.0X6
Syrosingopine	T46.5X1	T46.5X2	T46.5X3	T46.5X4	T46.5X5	T46.5X6

Substance	Poisoning, Accidental (unintentional)	Poisoning, Intentional self-harm	Poisoning, Assault	Poisoning, Undetermined	Adverse effect	Underdosing
Systemic drug	T45.91	T45.92	T45.93	T45.94	T45.95	T45.96
specified NEC	T45.8X1	T45.8X2	T45.8X3	T45.8X4	T45.8X5	T45.8X6
T						
2,4,5-T (trichloro-phenoxyacetic acid)	T60.3X1	T60.3X2	T60.3X3	T60.3X4	--	--
Tablets (see also specified substance)	T50.901	T50.902	T50.903	T50.904	T50.905	T50.906
Tace	T38.5X1	T38.5X2	T38.5X3	T38.5X4	T38.5X5	T38.5X6
Tacrine	T44.0X1	T44.0X2	T44.0X3	T44.0X4	T44.0X5	T44.0X6
Tadalafil	T46.7X1	T46.7X2	T46.7X3	T46.7X4	T46.7X5	T46.7X6
Talampicillin	T36.0X1	T36.0X2	T36.0X3	T36.0X4	T36.0X5	T36.0X6
Talbutal	T42.3X1	T42.3X2	T42.3X3	T42.3X4	T42.3X5	T42.3X6
Talc powder	T49.3X1	T49.3X2	T49.3X3	T49.3X4	T49.3X5	T49.3X6
Talcum	T49.3X1	T49.3X2	T49.3X3	T49.3X4	T49.3X5	T49.3X6
Taleranol	T38.6X1	T38.6X2	T38.6X3	T38.6X4	T38.6X5	T38.6X6
Tamoxifen	T38.6X1	T38.6X2	T38.6X3	T38.6X4	T38.6X5	T38.6X6
Tamsulosin	T44.6X1	T44.6X2	T44.6X3	T44.6X4	T44.6X5	T44.6X6
Tandearil, tanderil	T39.2X1	T39.2X2	T39.2X3	T39.2X4	T39.2X5	T39.2X6
Tannic acid	T49.2X1	T49.2X2	T49.2X3	T49.2X4	T49.2X5	T49.2X6
medicinal (astringent)	T49.2X1	T49.2X2	T49.2X3	T49.2X4	T49.2X5	T49.2X6
Tannin — see Tannic acid						
Tansy	T62.2X1	T62.2X2	T62.2X3	T62.2X4	--	--
TAO	T36.3X1	T36.3X2	T36.3X3	T36.3X4	T36.3X5	T36.3X6
Tapazole	T38.2X1	T38.2X2	T38.2X3	T38.2X4	T38.2X5	T38.2X6
Tar NEC	T52.0X1	T52.0X2	T52.0X3	T52.0X4	--	--
camphor	T60.1X1	T60.1X2	T60.1X3	T60.1X4	--	--
distillate	T49.1X1	T49.1X2	T49.1X3	T49.1X4	T49.1X5	T49.1X6
fumes	T59.891	T59.892	T59.893	T59.894	--	--
medicinal	T49.1X1	T49.1X2	T49.1X3	T49.1X4	T49.1X5	T49.1X6
ointment	T49.1X1	T49.1X2	T49.1X3	T49.1X4	T49.1X5	T49.1X6
Taractan	T43.591	T43.592	T43.593	T43.594	T43.595	T43.596
Tarantula (venomous)	T63.321	T63.322	T63.323	T63.324	--	--
Tartar emetic	T37.8X1	T37.8X2	T37.8X3	T37.8X4	T37.8X5	T37.8X6
Tartaric acid	T65.891	T65.892	T65.893	T65.894	--	--
Tartrate, laxative	T47.4X1	T47.4X2	T47.4X3	T47.4X4	T47.4X5	T47.4X6
Tartrated antimony (anti-infective)	T37.8X1	T37.8X2	T37.8X3	T37.8X4	T37.8X5	T37.8X6
Tauromustine	T45.1X1	T45.1X2	T45.1X3	T45.1X4	T45.1X5	T45.1X6
TCA — see Trichloroacetic acid						
TCDD	T53.7X1	T53.7X2	T53.7X3	T53.7X4	--	--
TDI (vapor)	T65.0X1	T65.0X2	T65.0X3	T65.0X4	--	--
Tear						
gas	T59.3X1	T59.3X2	T59.3X3	T59.3X4	--	--
solution	T49.5X1	T49.5X2	T49.5X3	T49.5X4	T49.5X5	T49.5X6
Teclothiazide	T50.2X1	T50.2X2	T50.2X3	T50.2X4	T50.2X5	T50.2X6
Teclozan	T37.3X1	T37.3X2	T37.3X3	T37.3X4	T37.3X5	T37.3X6
Tegafur	T45.1X1	T45.1X2	T45.1X3	T45.1X4	T45.1X5	T45.1X6
Tegretol	T42.1X1	T42.1X2	T42.1X3	T42.1X4	T42.1X5	T42.1X6
Teicoplanin	T36.8X1	T36.8X2	T36.8X3	T36.8X4	T36.8X5	T36.8X6
Telepaque	T50.8X1	T50.8X2	T50.8X3	T50.8X4	T50.8X5	T50.8X6
Tellurium	T56.891	T56.892	T56.893	T56.894	--	--
fumes	T56.891	T56.892	T56.893	T56.894	--	--
TEM	T45.1X1	T45.1X2	T45.1X3	T45.1X4	T45.1X5	T45.1X6
Temazepam	T42.4X1	T42.4X2	T42.4X3	T42.4X4	T42.4X5	T42.4X6
Temocillin	T36.0X1	T36.0X2	T36.0X3	T36.0X4	T36.0X5	T36.0X6
Tenamfetamine	T43.621	T43.622	T43.623	T43.624	T43.625	T43.626
Teniposide	T45.1X1	T45.1X2	T45.1X3	T45.1X4	T45.1X5	T45.1X6
Tenitramine	T46.3X1	T46.3X2	T46.3X3	T46.3X4	T46.3X5	T46.3X6
Tenoglicin	T48.4X1	T48.4X2	T48.4X3	T48.4X4	T48.4X5	T48.4X6
Tenonitrozole	T37.3X1	T37.3X2	T37.3X3	T37.3X4	T37.3X5	T37.3X6
Tenoxicam	T39.391	T39.392	T39.393	T39.394	T39.395	T39.396
TEPA	T45.1X1	T45.1X2	T45.1X3	T45.1X4	T45.1X5	T45.1X6
TEPP	T60.0X1	T60.0X2	T60.0X3	T60.0X4	--	--
Teprotide	T46.5X1	T46.5X2	T46.5X3	T46.5X4	T46.5X5	T46.5X6
Terazosin	T44.6X1	T44.6X2	T44.6X3	T44.6X4	T44.6X5	T44.6X6
Terbufos	T60.0X1	T60.0X2	T60.0X3	T60.0X4	--	--
Terbutaline	T48.6X1	T48.6X2	T48.6X3	T48.6X4	T48.6X5	T48.6X6
Terconazole	T49.0X1	T49.0X2	T49.0X3	T49.0X4	T49.0X5	T49.0X6
Terfenadine	T45.0X1	T45.0X2	T45.0X3	T45.0X4	T45.0X5	T45.0X6
Teriparatide (acetate)	T50.991	T50.992	T50.993	T50.994	T50.995	T50.996
Terizidone	T37.1X1	T37.1X2	T37.1X3	T37.1X4	T37.1X5	T37.1X6
Terlipressin	T38.891	T38.892	T38.893	T38.894	T38.895	T38.896
Terodiline	T46.3X1	T46.3X2	T46.3X3	T46.3X4	T46.3X5	T46.3X6
Teroxalene	T37.4X1	T37.4X2	T37.4X3	T37.4X4	T37.4X5	T37.4X6
Terpin (cis) hydrate	T48.4X1	T48.4X2	T48.4X3	T48.4X4	T48.4X5	T48.4X6
Terramycin	T36.4X1	T36.4X2	T36.4X3	T36.4X4	T36.4X5	T36.4X6
Tertatolol	T44.7X1	T44.7X2	T44.7X3	T44.7X4	T44.7X5	T44.7X6
Tessalon	T48.3X1	T48.3X2	T48.3X3	T48.3X4	T48.3X5	T48.3X6
Testolactone	T38.7X1	T38.7X2	T38.7X3	T38.7X4	T38.7X5	T38.7X6
Testosterone	T38.7X1	T38.7X2	T38.7X3	T38.7X4	T38.7X5	T38.7X6
Tetanus toxoid or vaccine	T50.A91	T50.A92	T50.A93	T50.A94	T50.A95	T50.A96
antitoxin	T50.Z11	T50.Z12	T50.Z13	T50.Z14	T50.Z15	T50.Z16
immune globulin (human)	T50.Z11	T50.Z12	T50.Z13	T50.Z14	T50.Z15	T50.Z16
toxoid	T50.A91	T50.A92	T50.A93	T50.A94	T50.A95	T50.A96
with diphtheria toxoid	T50.A21	T50.A22	T50.A23	T50.A24	T50.A25	T50.A26
with pertussis	T50.A11	T50.A12	T50.A13	T50.A14	T50.A15	T50.A16

Substance	Poisoning, Accidental (unintentional)	Poisoning, Intentional self-harm	Poisoning, Assault	Poisoning, Undetermined	Adverse effect	Underdosing
Tetrabenazine	T43.591	T43.592	T43.593	T43.594	T43.595	T43.596
Tetracaine	T41.3X1	T41.3X2	T41.3X3	T41.3X4	T41.3X5	T41.3X6
nerve block (peripheral) (plexus)	T41.3X1	T41.3X2	T41.3X3	T41.3X4	T41.3X5	T41.3X6
regional	T41.3X1	T41.3X2	T41.3X3	T41.3X4	T41.3X5	T41.3X6
spinal	T41.3X1	T41.3X2	T41.3X3	T41.3X4	T41.3X5	T41.3X6
Tetrachlorethylene — see Tetrachloroethylene						
Tetrachlormethiazide	T50.2X1	T50.2X2	T50.2X3	T50.2X4	T50.2X5	T50.2X6
2,3,7,8-Tetrachlorodibenzo-p-dioxin	T53.7X1	T53.7X2	T53.7X3	T53.7X4	--	--
Tetrachloroethane	T53.6X1	T53.6X2	T53.6X3	T53.6X4	--	--
vapor	T53.6X1	T53.6X2	T53.6X3	T53.6X4	--	--
paint or varnish	T53.6X1	T53.6X2	T53.6X3	T53.6X4	--	--
Tetrachloroethylene (liquid)	T53.3X1	T53.3X2	T53.3X3	T53.3X4	--	--
medicinal	T37.4X1	T37.4X2	T37.4X3	T37.4X4	T37.4X5	T37.4X6
vapor	T53.3X1	T53.3X2	T53.3X3	T53.3X4	--	--
Tetrachloromethane — see Carbon tetrachloride						
Tetracosactide	T38.811	T38.812	T38.813	T38.814	T38.815	T38.816
Tetracosactrin	T38.811	T38.812	T38.813	T38.814	T38.815	T38.816
Tetracycline	T36.4X1	T36.4X2	T36.4X3	T36.4X4	T36.4X5	T36.4X6
ophthalmic preparation	T49.5X1	T49.5X2	T49.5X3	T49.5X4	T49.5X5	T49.5X6
topical NEC	T49.0X1	T49.0X2	T49.0X3	T49.0X4	T49.0X5	T49.0X6
Tetradifon	T60.8X1	T60.8X2	T60.8X3	T60.8X4	--	--
Tetradotoxin	T61.771	T61.772	T61.773	T61.774	--	--
Tetraethyl						
lead	T56.0X1	T56.0X2	T56.0X3	T56.0X4	--	--
pyrophosphate	T60.0X1	T60.0X2	T60.0X3	T60.0X4	--	--
Tetraethylammonium chloride	T44.2X1	T44.2X2	T44.2X3	T44.2X4	T44.2X5	T44.2X6
Tetraethylthiuram disulfide	T50.6X1	T50.6X2	T50.6X3	T50.6X4	T50.6X5	T50.6X6
Tetrahydroaminoacridine	T44.0X1	T44.0X2	T44.0X3	T44.0X4	T44.0X5	T44.0X6
Tetrahydrocannabinol	T40.7X1	T40.7X2	T40.7X3	T40.7X4	T40.7X5	T40.7X6
Tetrahydrofuran	T52.8X1	T52.8X2	T52.8X3	T52.8X4	--	--
Tetrahydronaphthalene	T52.8X1	T52.8X2	T52.8X3	T52.8X4	--	--
Tetrahydrozoline	T49.5X1	T49.5X2	T49.5X3	T49.5X4	T49.5X5	T49.5X6
Tetralin	T52.8X1	T52.8X2	T52.8X3	T52.8X4	--	--
Tetramethrin	T60.2X1	T60.2X2	T60.2X3	T60.2X4	--	--
Tetramethylthiuram (disulfide) NEC	T60.3X1	T60.3X2	T60.3X3	T60.3X4	--	--
medicinal	T49.0X1	T49.0X2	T49.0X3	T49.0X4	T49.0X5	T49.0X6
Tetramisole	T37.4X1	T37.4X2	T37.4X3	T37.4X4	T37.4X5	T37.4X6
Tetranicotinoyl fructose	T46.7X1	T46.7X2	T46.7X3	T46.7X4	T46.7X5	T46.7X6
Tetrazepam	T42.4X1	T42.4X2	T42.4X3	T42.4X4	T42.4X5	T42.4X6
Tetronal	T42.6X1	T42.6X2	T42.6X3	T42.6X4	T42.6X5	T42.6X6
Tetryl	T65.3X1	T65.3X2	T65.3X3	T65.3X4	--	--
Tetrylammonium chloride	T44.2X1	T44.2X2	T44.2X3	T44.2X4	T44.2X5	T44.2X6
Tetryzoline	T49.5X1	T49.5X2	T49.5X3	T49.5X4	T49.5X5	T49.5X6
Thalidomide	T45.1X1	T45.1X2	T45.1X3	T45.1X4	T45.1X5	T45.1X6
Thallium (compounds) (dust) NEC	T56.811	T56.812	T56.813	T56.814	--	--
pesticide	T60.4X1	T60.4X2	T60.4X3	T60.4X4	--	--
THC	T40.7X1	T40.7X2	T40.7X3	T40.7X4	T40.7X5	T40.7X6
Thebacon	T48.3X1	T48.3X2	T48.3X3	T48.3X4	T48.3X5	T48.3X6
Thebaine	T40.2X1	T40.2X2	T40.2X3	T40.2X4	T40.2X5	T40.2X6
Thenoic acid	T49.6X1	T49.6X2	T49.6X3	T49.6X4	T49.6X5	T49.6X6
Thenyldiamine	T45.0X1	T45.0X2	T45.0X3	T45.0X4	T45.0X5	T45.0X6
Theobromine (calcium salicylate)	T48.6X1	T48.6X2	T48.6X3	T48.6X4	T48.6X5	T48.6X6
sodium salicylate	T48.6X1	T48.6X2	T48.6X3	T48.6X4	T48.6X5	T48.6X6
Theophyllamine	T48.6X1	T48.6X2	T48.6X3	T48.6X4	T48.6X5	T48.6X6
Theophylline	T48.6X1	T48.6X2	T48.6X3	T48.6X4	T48.6X5	T48.6X6
aminobenzoic acid	T48.6X1	T48.6X2	T48.6X3	T48.6X4	T48.6X5	T48.6X6
ethylenediamine	T48.6X1	T48.6X2	T48.6X3	T48.6X4	T48.6X5	T48.6X6
piperazine p-amino-benzoate	T48.6X1	T48.6X2	T48.6X3	T48.6X4	T48.6X5	T48.6X6
Thiabendazole	T37.4X1	T37.4X2	T37.4X3	T37.4X4	T37.4X5	T37.4X6
Thialbarbital	T41.1X1	T41.1X2	T41.1X3	T41.1X4	T41.1X5	T41.1X6
Thiamazole	T38.2X1	T38.2X2	T38.2X3	T38.2X4	T38.2X5	T38.2X6
Thiambutosine	T37.1X1	T37.1X2	T37.1X3	T37.1X4	T37.1X5	T37.1X6
Thiamine	T45.2X1	T45.2X2	T45.2X3	T45.2X4	T45.2X5	T45.2X6
Thiamphenicol	T36.2X1	T36.2X2	T36.2X3	T36.2X4	T36.2X5	T36.2X6
Thiamylal	T41.1X1	T41.1X2	T41.1X3	T41.1X4	T41.1X5	T41.1X6
sodium	T41.1X1	T41.1X2	T41.1X3	T41.1X4	T41.1X5	T41.1X6
Thiazesim	T43.291	T43.292	T43.293	T43.294	T43.295	T43.296
Thiazides (diuretics)	T50.2X1	T50.2X2	T50.2X3	T50.2X4	T50.2X5	T50.2X6
Thiazinamium metilsulfate	T43.3X1	T43.3X2	T43.3X3	T43.3X4	T43.3X5	T43.3X6
Thiethylperazine	T43.3X1	T43.3X2	T43.3X3	T43.3X4	T43.3X5	T43.3X6
Thimerosal	T49.0X1	T49.0X2	T49.0X3	T49.0X4	T49.0X5	T49.0X6
ophthalmic preparation	T49.5X1	T49.5X2	T49.5X3	T49.5X4	T49.5X5	T49.5X6
Thioacetazone	T37.1X1	T37.1X2	T37.1X3	T37.1X4	T37.1X5	T37.1X6
with isoniazid	T37.1X1	T37.1X2	T37.1X3	T37.1X4	T37.1X5	T37.1X6

Thiobarbital sodium - Tranquilizer NEC

Substance	Poisoning, Accidental (unintentional)	Poisoning, Intentional self-harm	Poisoning, Assault	Poisoning, Undetermined	Adverse effect	Underdosing
Thiobarbital sodium	T41.1X1	T41.1X2	T41.1X3	T41.1X4	T41.1X5	T41.1X6
Thiobarbiturate anesthetic	T41.1X1	T41.1X2	T41.1X3	T41.1X4	T41.1X5	T41.1X6
Thiobismol	T37.8X1	T37.8X2	T37.8X3	T37.8X4	T37.8X5	T37.8X6
Thiobutabarbital sodium	T41.1X1	T41.1X2	T41.1X3	T41.1X4	T41.1X5	T41.1X6
Thiocarbamate (insecticide)	T60.0X1	T60.0X2	T60.0X3	T60.0X4	--	--
Thiocarbamide	T38.2X1	T38.2X2	T38.2X3	T38.2X4	T38.2X5	T38.2X6
Thiocarbarsone	T37.8X1	T37.8X2	T37.8X3	T37.8X4	T37.8X5	T37.8X6
Thiocarlide	T37.1X1	T37.1X2	T37.1X3	T37.1X4	T37.1X5	T37.1X6
Thioctamide	T50.991	T50.992	T50.993	T50.994	T50.995	T50.996
Thioctic acid	T50.991	T50.992	T50.993	T50.994	T50.995	T50.996
Thiofos	T60.0X1	T60.0X2	T60.0X3	T60.0X4	--	--
Thioglycolate	T49.4X1	T49.4X2	T49.4X3	T49.4X4	T49.4X5	T49.4X6
Thioglycolic acid	T65.891	T65.892	T65.893	T65.894	--	--
Thioguanine	T45.1X1	T45.1X2	T45.1X3	T45.1X4	T45.1X5	T45.1X6
Thiomercaptomerin	T50.2X1	T50.2X2	T50.2X3	T50.2X4	T50.2X5	T50.2X6
Thiomerin	T50.2X1	T50.2X2	T50.2X3	T50.2X4	T50.2X5	T50.2X6
Thiomersal	T49.0X1	T49.0X2	T49.0X3	T49.0X4	T49.0X5	T49.0X6
Thionazin	T60.0X1	T60.0X2	T60.0X3	T60.0X4	--	--
Thiopental (sodium)	T41.1X1	T41.1X2	T41.1X3	T41.1X4	T41.1X5	T41.1X6
Thiopentone (sodium)	T41.1X1	T41.1X2	T41.1X3	T41.1X4	T41.1X5	T41.1X6
Thiopropazate	T43.3X1	T43.3X2	T43.3X3	T43.3X4	T43.3X5	T43.3X6
Thioproperazine	T43.3X1	T43.3X2	T43.3X3	T43.3X4	T43.3X5	T43.3X6
Thioridazine	T43.3X1	T43.3X2	T43.3X3	T43.3X4	T43.3X5	T43.3X6
Thiosinamine	T49.3X1	T49.3X2	T49.3X3	T49.3X4	T49.3X5	T49.3X6
Thiotepa	T45.1X1	T45.1X2	T45.1X3	T45.1X4	T45.1X5	T45.1X6
Thiothixene	T43.4X1	T43.4X2	T43.4X3	T43.4X4	T43.4X5	T43.4X6
Thiouracil (benzyl) (methyl) (propyl)	T38.2X1	T38.2X2	T38.2X3	T38.2X4	T38.2X5	T38.2X6
Thiourea	T38.2X1	T38.2X2	T38.2X3	T38.2X4	T38.2X5	T38.2X6
Thiphenamil	T44.3X1	T44.3X2	T44.3X3	T44.3X4	T44.3X5	T44.3X6
Thiram	T60.3X1	T60.3X2	T60.3X3	T60.3X4	--	--
medicinal	T49.2X1	T49.2X2	T49.2X3	T49.2X4	T49.2X5	T49.2X6
Thonzylamine (systemic)	T45.0X1	T45.0X2	T45.0X3	T45.0X4	T45.0X5	T45.0X6
mucosal decongestant	T48.5X1	T48.5X2	T48.5X3	T48.5X4	T48.5X5	T48.5X6
Thorazine	T43.3X1	T43.3X2	T43.3X3	T43.3X4	T43.3X5	T43.3X6
Thorium dioxide suspension	T50.8X1	T50.8X2	T50.8X3	T50.8X4	T50.8X5	T50.8X6
Thornapple	T62.2X1	T62.2X2	T62.2X3	T62.2X4	--	--
Throat drug NEC	T49.6X1	T49.6X2	T49.6X3	T49.6X4	T49.6X5	T49.6X6
Thrombin	T45.7X1	T45.7X2	T45.7X3	T45.7X4	T45.7X5	T45.7X6
Thrombolysin	T45.611	T45.612	T45.613	T45.614	T45.615	T45.616
Thromboplastin	T45.7X1	T45.7X2	T45.7X3	T45.7X4	T45.7X5	T45.7X6
Thurfyl nicotinate	T46.7X1	T46.7X2	T46.7X3	T46.7X4	T46.7X5	T46.7X6
Thymol	T49.0X1	T49.0X2	T49.0X3	T49.0X4	T49.0X5	T49.0X6
Thymopentin	T37.5X1	T37.5X2	T37.5X3	T37.5X4	T37.5X5	T37.5X6
Thymoxamine	T46.7X1	T46.7X2	T46.7X3	T46.7X4	T46.7X5	T46.7X6
Thymus extract	T38.891	T38.892	T38.893	T38.894	T38.895	T38.896
Thyreotrophic hormone	T38.811	T38.812	T38.813	T38.814	T38.815	T38.816
Thyroglobulin	T38.1X1	T38.1X2	T38.1X3	T38.1X4	T38.1X5	T38.1X6
Thyroid (hormone)	T38.1X1	T38.1X2	T38.1X3	T38.1X4	T38.1X5	T38.1X6
Thyrolar	T38.1X1	T38.1X2	T38.1X3	T38.1X4	T38.1X5	T38.1X6
Thyrotrophin	T38.811	T38.812	T38.813	T38.814	T38.815	T38.816
Thyrotropic hormone	T38.811	T38.812	T38.813	T38.814	T38.815	T38.816
Thyroxine	T38.1X1	T38.1X2	T38.1X3	T38.1X4	T38.1X5	T38.1X6
Tiabendazole	T37.4X1	T37.4X2	T37.4X3	T37.4X4	T37.4X5	T37.4X6
Tiamizide	T50.2X1	T50.2X2	T50.2X3	T50.2X4	T50.2X5	T50.2X6
Tianeptine	T43.291	T43.292	T43.293	T43.294	T43.295	T43.296
Tiapamil	T46.1X1	T46.1X2	T46.1X3	T46.1X4	T46.1X5	T46.1X6
Tiapride	T43.591	T43.592	T43.593	T43.594	T43.595	T43.596
Tiaprofenic acid	T39.311	T39.312	T39.313	T39.314	T39.315	T39.316
Tiaramide	T39.8X1	T39.8X2	T39.8X3	T39.8X4	T39.8X5	T39.8X6
Ticarcillin	T36.0X1	T36.0X2	T36.0X3	T36.0X4	T36.0X5	T36.0X6
Ticlatone	T49.0X1	T49.0X2	T49.0X3	T49.0X4	T49.0X5	T49.0X6
Ticlopidine	T45.521	T45.522	T45.523	T45.524	T45.525	T45.526
Ticrynafen	T50.1X1	T50.1X2	T50.1X3	T50.1X4	T50.1X5	T50.1X6
Tidiacic	T50.991	T50.992	T50.993	T50.994	T50.995	T50.996
Tiemonium	T44.3X1	T44.3X2	T44.3X3	T44.3X4	T44.3X5	T44.3X6
iodide	T44.3X1	T44.3X2	T44.3X3	T44.3X4	T44.3X5	T44.3X6
Tienilic acid	T50.1X1	T50.1X2	T50.1X3	T50.1X4	T50.1X5	T50.1X6
Tifenamil	T44.3X1	T44.3X2	T44.3X3	T44.3X4	T44.3X5	T44.3X6
Tigan	T45.0X1	T45.0X2	T45.0X3	T45.0X4	T45.0X5	T45.0X6
Tigloidine	T44.3X1	T44.3X2	T44.3X3	T44.3X4	T44.3X5	T44.3X6
Tilactase	T47.5X1	T47.5X2	T47.5X3	T47.5X4	T47.5X5	T47.5X6
Tiletamine	T41.291	T41.292	T41.293	T41.294	T41.295	T41.296
Tilidine	T40.4X1	T40.4X2	T40.4X3	T40.4X4	--	--
Timepidium bromide	T44.3X1	T44.3X2	T44.3X3	T44.3X4	T44.3X5	T44.3X6
Timiperone	T43.4X1	T43.4X2	T43.4X3	T43.4X4	T43.4X5	T43.4X6
Timolol	T44.7X1	T44.7X2	T44.7X3	T44.7X4	T44.7X5	T44.7X6
Tin (chloride) (dust) (oxide) NEC	T56.6X1	T56.6X2	T56.6X3	T56.6X4	--	--
anti-infectives	T37.8X1	T37.8X2	T37.8X3	T37.8X4	T37.8X5	T37.8X6
Tincture, iodine — *see* Iodine						
Tindal	T43.3X1	T43.3X2	T43.3X3	T43.3X4	T43.3X5	T43.3X6
Tinidazole	T37.3X1	T37.3X2	T37.3X3	T37.3X4	T37.3X5	T37.3X6
Tinoridine	T39.8X1	T39.8X2	T39.8X3	T39.8X4	T39.8X5	T39.8X6
Tiocarlide	T37.1X1	T37.1X2	T37.1X3	T37.1X4	T37.1X5	T37.1X6
Tioclomarol	T45.511	T45.512	T45.513	T45.514	T45.515	T45.516
Tioconazole	T49.0X1	T49.0X2	T49.0X3	T49.0X4	T49.0X5	T49.0X6
Tioguanine	T45.1X1	T45.1X2	T45.1X3	T45.1X4	T45.1X5	T45.1X6
Tiopronin	T50.991	T50.992	T50.993	T50.994	T50.995	T50.996
Tiotixene	T43.4X1	T43.4X2	T43.4X3	T43.4X4	T43.4X5	T43.4X6
Tioxolone	T49.4X1	T49.4X2	T49.4X3	T49.4X4	T49.4X5	T49.4X6
Tipepidine	T48.3X1	T48.3X2	T48.3X3	T48.3X4	T48.3X5	T48.3X6
Tiquizium bromide	T44.3X1	T44.3X2	T44.3X3	T44.3X4	T44.3X5	T44.3X6
Tiratricol	T38.1X1	T38.1X2	T38.1X3	T38.1X4	T38.1X5	T38.1X6
Tisopurine	T50.4X1	T50.4X2	T50.4X3	T50.4X4	T50.4X5	T50.4X6
Titanium (compounds) (vapor)	T56.891	T56.892	T56.893	T56.894	--	--
dioxide	T49.3X1	T49.3X2	T49.3X3	T49.3X4	T49.3X5	T49.3X6
ointment	T49.3X1	T49.3X2	T49.3X3	T49.3X4	T49.3X5	T49.3X6
oxide	T49.3X1	T49.3X2	T49.3X3	T49.3X4	T49.3X5	T49.3X6
tetrachloride	T56.891	T56.892	T56.893	T56.894	--	--
Titanocene	T56.891	T56.892	T56.893	T56.894	--	--
Titroid	T38.1X1	T38.1X2	T38.1X3	T38.1X4	T38.1X5	T38.1X6
Tizanidine	T42.8X1	T42.8X2	T42.8X3	T42.8X4	T42.8X5	T42.8X6
TMTD	T60.3X1	T60.3X2	T60.3X3	T60.3X4	--	--
TNT (fumes)	T65.3X1	T65.3X2	T65.3X3	T65.3X4	--	--
Toadstool	T62.0X1	T62.0X2	T62.0X3	T62.0X4	--	--
Tobacco NEC	T65.291	T65.292	T65.293	T65.294	--	--
cigarettes	T65.221	T65.222	T65.223	T65.224	--	--
indian	T62.2X1	T62.2X2	T62.2X3	T62.2X4	--	--
smoke, second-hand	T65.221	T65.222	T65.223	T65.224	--	--
Tobramycin	T36.5X1	T36.5X2	T36.5X3	T36.5X4	T36.5X5	T36.5X6
Tocainide	T46.2X1	T46.2X2	T46.2X3	T46.2X4	T46.2X5	T46.2X6
Tocoferol	T45.2X1	T45.2X2	T45.2X3	T45.2X4	T45.2X5	T45.2X6
Tocopherol	T45.2X1	T45.2X2	T45.2X3	T45.2X4	T45.2X5	T45.2X6
acetate	T45.2X1	T45.2X2	T45.2X3	T45.2X4	T45.2X5	T45.2X6
Tocosamine	T48.0X1	T48.0X2	T48.0X3	T48.0X4	T48.0X5	T48.0X6
Todralazine	T46.5X1	T46.5X2	T46.5X3	T46.5X4	T46.5X5	T46.5X6
Tofisopam	T42.4X1	T42.4X2	T42.4X3	T42.4X4	T42.4X5	T42.4X6
Tofranil	T43.011	T43.012	T43.013	T43.014	T43.015	T43.016
Toilet deodorizer	T65.891	T65.892	T65.893	T65.894	--	--
Tolamolol	T44.7X1	T44.7X2	T44.7X3	T44.7X4	T44.7X5	T44.7X6
Tolazamide	T38.3X1	T38.3X2	T38.3X3	T38.3X4	T38.3X5	T38.3X6
Tolazoline	T46.7X1	T46.7X2	T46.7X3	T46.7X4	T46.7X5	T46.7X6
Tolbutamide (sodium)	T38.3X1	T38.3X2	T38.3X3	T38.3X4	T38.3X5	T38.3X6
Tolciclate	T49.0X1	T49.0X2	T49.0X3	T49.0X4	T49.0X5	T49.0X6
Tolmetin	T39.391	T39.392	T39.393	T39.394	T39.395	T39.396
Tolnaftate	T49.0X1	T49.0X2	T49.0X3	T49.0X4	T49.0X5	T49.0X6
Tolonidine	T46.5X1	T46.5X2	T46.5X3	T46.5X4	T46.5X5	T46.5X6
Toloxatone	T42.6X1	T42.6X2	T42.6X3	T42.6X4	T42.6X5	T42.6X6
Tolperisone	T44.3X1	T44.3X2	T44.3X3	T44.3X4	T44.3X5	T44.3X6
Tolserol	T42.8X1	T42.8X2	T42.8X3	T42.8X4	T42.8X5	T42.8X6
Toluene (liquid)	T52.2X1	T52.2X2	T52.2X3	T52.2X4	--	--
diisocyanate	T65.0X1	T65.0X2	T65.0X3	T65.0X4	--	--
Toluidine	T65.891	T65.892	T65.893	T65.894	--	--
vapor	T59.891	T59.892	T59.893	T59.894	--	--
Toluol (liquid)	T52.2X1	T52.2X2	T52.2X3	T52.2X4	--	--
vapor	T52.2X1	T52.2X2	T52.2X3	T52.2X4	--	--
Toluylenediamine	T65.3X1	T65.3X2	T65.3X3	T65.3X4	--	--
Tolylene-2,4-diisocyanate	T65.0X1	T65.0X2	T65.0X3	T65.0X4	--	--
Tonic NEC	T50.901	T50.902	T50.903	T50.904	T50.905	T50.906
Topical action drug NEC	T49.91	T49.92	T49.93	T49.94	T49.95	T49.96
ear, nose or throat	T49.6X1	T49.6X2	T49.6X3	T49.6X4	T49.6X5	T49.6X6
eye	T49.5X1	T49.5X2	T49.5X3	T49.5X4	T49.5X5	T49.5X6
skin	T49.91	T49.92	T49.93	T49.94	T49.95	T49.96
specified NEC	T49.8X1	T49.8X2	T49.8X3	T49.8X4	T49.8X5	T49.8X6
Toquizine	T44.3X1	T44.3X2	T44.3X3	T44.3X4	T44.3X5	T44.3X6
Toremifene	T38.6X1	T38.6X2	T38.6X3	T38.6X4	T38.6X5	T38.6X6
Tosylchloramide sodium	T49.8X1	T49.8X2	T49.8X3	T49.8X4	T49.8X5	T49.8X6
Toxaphene (dust) (spray)	T60.1X1	T60.1X2	T60.1X3	T60.1X4	--	--
Toxin, diphtheria (Schick Test)	T50.8X1	T50.8X2	T50.8X3	T50.8X4	T50.8X5	T50.8X6
Toxoid						
combined	T50.A21	T50.A22	T50.A23	T50.A24	T50.A25	T50.A26
diphtheria	T50.A91	T50.A92	T50.A93	T50.A94	T50.A95	T50.A96
tetanus	T50.A91	T50.A92	T50.A93	T50.A94	T50.A95	T50.A96
Trace element NEC	T45.8X1	T45.8X2	T45.8X3	T45.8X4	T45.8X5	T45.8X6
Tractor fuel NEC	T52.0X1	T52.0X2	T52.0X3	T52.0X4	--	--
Tragacanth	T50.991	T50.992	T50.993	T50.994	T50.995	T50.996
Tramadol	T40.4X1	T40.4X2	T40.4X3	T40.4X4	T40.4X5	T40.4X6
Tramazoline	T48.5X1	T48.5X2	T48.5X3	T48.5X4	T48.5X5	T48.5X6
Tranexamic acid	T45.621	T45.622	T45.623	T45.624	T45.625	T45.626
Tranilast	T45.0X1	T45.0X2	T45.0X3	T45.0X4	T45.0X5	T45.0X6
Tranquilizer NEC	T43.501	T43.502	T43.503	T43.504	T43.505	T43.506
with hypnotic or sedative	T42.6X1	T42.6X2	T42.6X3	T42.6X4	T42.6X5	T42.6X6
benzodiazepine NEC	T42.4X1	T42.4X2	T42.4X3	T42.4X4	T42.4X5	T42.4X6
butyrophenone NEC	T43.4X1	T43.4X2	T43.4X3	T43.4X4	T43.4X5	T43.4X6
carbamate	T43.591	T43.592	T43.593	T43.594	T43.595	T43.596
dimethylamine	T43.3X1	T43.3X2	T43.3X3	T43.3X4	T43.3X5	T43.3X6
ethylamine	T43.3X1	T43.3X2	T43.3X3	T43.3X4	T43.3X5	T43.3X6

Substance	Poisoning, Accidental (unintentional)	Poisoning, Intentional self-harm	Poisoning, Assault	Poisoning, Undetermined	Adverse effect	Underdosing
Tranquilizer NEC — *continued*						
hydroxyzine	T43.591	T43.592	T43.593	T43.594	T43.595	T43.596
major NEC	T43.501	T43.502	T43.503	T43.504	T43.505	T43.506
penothiazine NEC	T43.3X1	T43.3X2	T43.3X3	T43.3X4	T43.3X5	T43.3X6
phenothiazine-based	T43.3X1	T43.3X2	T43.3X3	T43.3X4	T43.3X5	T43.3X6
piperazine NEC	T43.3X1	T43.3X2	T43.3X3	T43.3X4	T43.3X5	T43.3X6
piperidine	T43.3X1	T43.3X2	T43.3X3	T43.3X4	T43.3X5	T43.3X6
propylamine	T43.3X1	T43.3X2	T43.3X3	T43.3X4	T43.3X5	T43.3X6
specified NEC	T43.591	T43.592	T43.593	T43.594	T43.595	T43.596
thioxanthene NEC	T43.591	T43.592	T43.593	T43.594	T43.595	T43.596
Tranxene	T42.4X1	T42.4X2	T42.4X3	T42.4X4	T42.4X5	T42.4X6
Tranylcypromine	T43.1X1	T43.1X2	T43.1X3	T43.1X4	T43.1X5	T43.1X6
Trapidil	T46.3X1	T46.3X2	T46.3X3	T46.3X4	T46.3X5	T46.3X6
Trasentine	T44.3X1	T44.3X2	T44.3X3	T44.3X4	T44.3X5	T44.3X6
Travert	T50.3X1	T50.3X2	T50.3X3	T50.3X4	T50.3X5	T50.3X6
Trazodone	T43.211	T43.212	T43.213	T43.214	T43.215	T43.216
Trecator	T37.1X1	T37.1X2	T37.1X3	T37.1X4	T37.1X5	T37.1X6
Treosulfan	T45.1X1	T45.1X2	T45.1X3	T45.1X4	T45.1X5	T45.1X6
Tretamine	T45.1X1	T45.1X2	T45.1X3	T45.1X4	T45.1X5	T45.1X6
Tretinoin	T49.0X1	T49.0X2	T49.0X3	T49.0X4	T49.0X5	T49.0X6
Tretoquinol	T48.6X1	T48.6X2	T48.6X3	T48.6X4	T48.6X5	T48.6X6
Triacetin	T49.0X1	T49.0X2	T49.0X3	T49.0X4	T49.0X5	T49.0X6
Triacetoxyanthracene	T49.4X1	T49.4X2	T49.4X3	T49.4X4	T49.4X5	T49.4X6
Triacetyloleandomycin	T36.3X1	T36.3X2	T36.3X3	T36.3X4	T36.3X5	T36.3X6
Triamcinolone	T38.0X1	T38.0X2	T38.0X3	T38.0X4	T38.0X5	T38.0X6
ENT agent	T49.6X1	T49.6X2	T49.6X3	T49.6X4	T49.6X5	T49.6X6
hexacetonide	T49.0X1	T49.0X2	T49.0X3	T49.0X4	T49.0X5	T49.0X6
ophthalmic preparation	T49.5X1	T49.5X2	T49.5X3	T49.5X4	T49.5X5	T49.5X6
topical NEC	T49.0X1	T49.0X2	T49.0X3	T49.0X4	T49.0X5	T49.0X6
Triampyzine	T44.3X1	T44.3X2	T44.3X3	T44.3X4	T44.3X5	T44.3X6
Triamterene	T50.2X1	T50.2X2	T50.2X3	T50.2X4	T50.2X5	T50.2X6
Triazine (herbicide)	T60.3X1	T60.3X2	T60.3X3	T60.3X4	--	--
Triaziquone	T45.1X1	T45.1X2	T45.1X3	T45.1X4	T45.1X5	T45.1X6
Triazolam	T42.4X1	T42.4X2	T42.4X3	T42.4X4	T42.4X5	T42.4X6
Triazole (herbicide)	T60.3X1	T60.3X2	T60.3X3	T60.3X4	--	--
Tribenoside	T46.991	T46.992	T46.993	T46.994	T46.995	T46.996
Tribromacetaldehyde	T42.6X1	T42.6X2	T42.6X3	T42.6X4	T42.6X5	T42.6X6
Tribromoethanol, rectal	T41.291	T41.292	T41.293	T41.294	T41.295	T41.296
Tribromomethane	T42.6X1	T42.6X2	T42.6X3	T42.6X4	T42.6X5	T42.6X6
Trichlorethane	T53.2X1	T53.2X2	T53.2X3	T53.2X4	--	--
Trichlorethylene	T53.2X1	T53.2X2	T53.2X3	T53.2X4	--	--
Trichlorfon	T60.0X1	T60.0X2	T60.0X3	T60.0X4	--	--
Trichlormethiazide	T50.2X1	T50.2X2	T50.2X3	T50.2X4	T50.2X5	T50.2X6
Trichlormethine	T45.1X1	T45.1X2	T45.1X3	T45.1X4	T45.1X5	T45.1X6
Trichloroacetic acid, Trichloracetic acid	T54.2X1	T54.2X2	T54.2X3	T54.2X4	--	--
medicinal	T49.4X1	T49.4X2	T49.4X3	T49.4X4	T49.4X5	T49.4X6
Trichloroethane	T53.2X1	T53.2X2	T53.2X3	T53.2X4	--	--
Trichloroethanol	T42.6X1	T42.6X2	T42.6X3	T42.6X4	T42.6X5	T42.6X6
Trichloroethyl phosphate	T42.6X1	T42.6X2	T42.6X3	T42.6X4	T42.6X5	T42.6X6
Trichloroethylene (liquid) (vapor)	T53.2X1	T53.2X2	T53.2X3	T53.2X4	--	--
anesthetic (gas)	T41.0X1	T41.0X2	T41.0X3	T41.0X4	T41.0X5	T41.0X6
vapor NEC	T53.2X1	T53.2X2	T53.2X3	T53.2X4	--	--
Trichlorofluoromethane NEC	T53.5X1	T53.5X2	T53.5X3	T53.5X4	--	--
Trichloronate	T60.0X1	T60.0X2	T60.0X3	T60.0X4	--	--
2,4,5-Trichlorophen-oxyacetic acid	T60.3X1	T60.3X2	T60.3X3	T60.3X4	--	--
Trichloropropane	T53.6X1	T53.6X2	T53.6X3	T53.6X4	--	--
Trichlorotriethylamine	T45.1X1	T45.1X2	T45.1X3	T45.1X4	T45.1X5	T45.1X6
Trichomonacides NEC	T37.3X1	T37.3X2	T37.3X3	T37.3X4	T37.3X5	T37.3X6
Trichomycin	T36.7X1	T36.7X2	T36.7X3	T36.7X4	T36.7X5	T36.7X6
Triclobisonium chloride	T49.0X1	T49.0X2	T49.0X3	T49.0X4	T49.0X5	T49.0X6
Triclocarban	T49.0X1	T49.0X2	T49.0X3	T49.0X4	T49.0X5	T49.0X6
Triclofos	T42.6X1	T42.6X2	T42.6X3	T42.6X4	T42.6X5	T42.6X6
Triclosan	T49.0X1	T49.0X2	T49.0X3	T49.0X4	T49.0X5	T49.0X6
Tricresyl phosphate	T65.891	T65.892	T65.893	T65.894	--	--
solvent	T52.91	T52.92	T52.93	T52.94	--	--
Tricyclamol chloride	T44.3X1	T44.3X2	T44.3X3	T44.3X4	T44.3X5	T44.3X6
Tridesilon	T49.0X1	T49.0X2	T49.0X3	T49.0X4	T49.0X5	T49.0X6
Tridihexethyl iodide	T44.3X1	T44.3X2	T44.3X3	T44.3X4	T44.3X5	T44.3X6
Tridione	T42.2X1	T42.2X2	T42.2X3	T42.2X4	T42.2X5	T42.2X6
Trientine	T45.8X1	T45.8X2	T45.8X3	T45.8X4	T45.8X5	T45.8X6
Triethanolamine NEC	T54.3X1	T54.3X2	T54.3X3	T54.3X4	--	--
detergent	T54.3X1	T54.3X2	T54.3X3	T54.3X4	--	--
trinitrate (biphosphate)	T46.3X1	T46.3X2	T46.3X3	T46.3X4	T46.3X5	T46.3X6
Triethanomelamine	T45.1X1	T45.1X2	T45.1X3	T45.1X4	T45.1X5	T45.1X6
Triethylenemelamine	T45.1X1	T45.1X2	T45.1X3	T45.1X4	T45.1X5	T45.1X6
Triethylenephosphoramide	T45.1X1	T45.1X2	T45.1X3	T45.1X4	T45.1X5	T45.1X6
Triethylenethiophosphoramide	T45.1X1	T45.1X2	T45.1X3	T45.1X4	T45.1X5	T45.1X6
Trifluoperazine	T43.3X1	T43.3X2	T43.3X3	T43.3X4	T43.3X5	T43.3X6
Trifluoroethyl vinyl ether	T41.0X1	T41.0X2	T41.0X3	T41.0X4	T41.0X5	T41.0X6
Trifluperidol	T43.4X1	T43.4X2	T43.4X3	T43.4X4	T43.4X5	T43.4X6
Triflupromazine	T43.3X1	T43.3X2	T43.3X3	T43.3X4	T43.3X5	T43.3X6
Trifluridine	T37.5X1	T37.5X2	T37.5X3	T37.5X4	T37.5X5	T37.5X6
Triflusal	T45.521	T45.522	T45.523	T45.524	T45.525	T45.526
Trihexyphenidyl	T44.3X1	T44.3X2	T44.3X3	T44.3X4	T44.3X5	T44.3X6
Triiodothyronine	T38.1X1	T38.1X2	T38.1X3	T38.1X4	T38.1X5	T38.1X6
Trilene	T41.0X1	T41.0X2	T41.0X3	T41.0X4	T41.0X5	T41.0X6
Trilostane	T38.991	T38.992	T38.993	T38.994	T38.995	T38.996
Trimebutine	T44.3X1	T44.3X2	T44.3X3	T44.3X4	T44.3X5	T44.3X6
Trimecaine	T41.3X1	T41.3X2	T41.3X3	T41.3X4	T41.3X5	T41.3X6
Trimeprazine (tartrate)	T44.3X1	T44.3X2	T44.3X3	T44.3X4	T44.3X5	T44.3X6
Trimetaphan camsilate	T44.2X1	T44.2X2	T44.2X3	T44.2X4	T44.2X5	T44.2X6
Trimetazidine	T46.7X1	T46.7X2	T46.7X3	T46.7X4	T46.7X5	T46.7X6
Trimethadione	T42.2X1	T42.2X2	T42.2X3	T42.2X4	T42.2X5	T42.2X6
Trimethaphan	T44.2X1	T44.2X2	T44.2X3	T44.2X4	T44.2X5	T44.2X6
Trimethidinium	T44.2X1	T44.2X2	T44.2X3	T44.2X4	T44.2X5	T44.2X6
Trimethobenzamide	T45.0X1	T45.0X2	T45.0X3	T45.0X4	T45.0X5	T45.0X6
Trimethoprim	T37.8X1	T37.8X2	T37.8X3	T37.8X4	T37.8X5	T37.8X6
with sulfamethoxazole	T36.8X1	T36.8X2	T36.8X3	T36.8X4	T36.8X5	T36.8X6
Trimethylcarbinol	T51.3X1	T51.3X2	T51.3X3	T51.3X4	--	--
Trimethylpsoralen	T49.3X1	T49.3X2	T49.3X3	T49.3X4	T49.3X5	T49.3X6
Trimeton	T45.0X1	T45.0X2	T45.0X3	T45.0X4	T45.0X5	T45.0X6
Trimetrexate	T45.1X1	T45.1X2	T45.1X3	T45.1X4	T45.1X5	T45.1X6
Trimipramine	T43.011	T43.012	T43.013	T43.014	T43.015	T43.016
Trimustine	T45.1X1	T45.1X2	T45.1X3	T45.1X4	T45.1X5	T45.1X6
Trinitrine	T46.3X1	T46.3X2	T46.3X3	T46.3X4	T46.3X5	T46.3X6
Trinitrobenzol	T65.3X1	T65.3X2	T65.3X3	T65.3X4	--	--
Trinitrophenol	T65.3X1	T65.3X2	T65.3X3	T65.3X4	--	--
Trinitrotoluene (fumes)	T65.3X1	T65.3X2	T65.3X3	T65.3X4	--	--
Trional	T42.6X1	T42.6X2	T42.6X3	T42.6X4	T42.6X5	T42.6X6
Triorthocresyl phosphate	T65.891	T65.892	T65.893	T65.894	--	--
Trioxide of arsenic	T57.0X1	T57.0X2	T57.0X3	T57.0X4	--	--
Trioxysalen	T49.4X1	T49.4X2	T49.4X3	T49.4X4	T49.4X5	T49.4X6
Tripamide	T50.2X1	T50.2X2	T50.2X3	T50.2X4	T50.2X5	T50.2X6
Triparanol	T46.6X1	T46.6X2	T46.6X3	T46.6X4	T46.6X5	T46.6X6
Tripelennamine	T45.0X1	T45.0X2	T45.0X3	T45.0X4	T45.0X5	T45.0X6
Triperiden	T44.3X1	T44.3X2	T44.3X3	T44.3X4	T44.3X5	T44.3X6
Triperidol	T43.4X1	T43.4X2	T43.4X3	T43.4X4	T43.4X5	T43.4X6
Triphenylphosphate	T65.891	T65.892	T65.893	T65.894	--	--
Triple						
bromides	T42.6X1	T42.6X2	T42.6X3	T42.6X4	T42.6X5	T42.6X6
carbonate	T47.1X1	T47.1X2	T47.1X3	T47.1X4	T47.1X5	T47.1X6
vaccine						
DPT	T50.A11	T50.A12	T50.A13	T50.A14	T50.A15	T50.A16
including pertussis	T50.A11	T50.A12	T50.A13	T50.A14	T50.A15	T50.A16
MMR	T50.B91	T50.B92	T50.B93	T50.B94	T50.B95	T50.B96
Triprolidine	T45.0X1	T45.0X2	T45.0X3	T45.0X4	T45.0X5	T45.0X6
Trisodium hydrogen edetate	T50.6X1	T50.6X2	T50.6X3	T50.6X4	T50.6X5	T50.6X6
Trisoralen	T49.3X1	T49.3X2	T49.3X3	T49.3X4	T49.3X5	T49.3X6
Trisulfapyrimidines	T37.0X1	T37.0X2	T37.0X3	T37.0X4	T37.0X5	T37.0X6
Trithiozine	T44.3X1	T44.3X2	T44.3X3	T44.3X4	T44.3X5	T44.3X6
Tritiozine	T44.3X1	T44.3X2	T44.3X3	T44.3X4	T44.3X5	T44.3X6
Tritoqualine	T45.0X1	T45.0X2	T45.0X3	T45.0X4	T45.0X5	T45.0X6
Trofosfamide	T45.1X1	T45.1X2	T45.1X3	T45.1X4	T45.1X5	T45.1X6
Troleandomycin	T36.3X1	T36.3X2	T36.3X3	T36.3X4	T36.3X5	T36.3X6
Trolnitrate (phosphate)	T46.3X1	T46.3X2	T46.3X3	T46.3X4	T46.3X5	T46.3X6
Tromantadine	T37.5X1	T37.5X2	T37.5X3	T37.5X4	T37.5X5	T37.5X6
Trometamol	T50.2X1	T50.2X2	T50.2X3	T50.2X4	T50.2X5	T50.2X6
Tromethamine	T50.2X1	T50.2X2	T50.2X3	T50.2X4	T50.2X5	T50.2X6
Tronothane	T41.3X1	T41.3X2	T41.3X3	T41.3X4	T41.3X5	T41.3X6
Tropacine	T44.3X1	T44.3X2	T44.3X3	T44.3X4	T44.3X5	T44.3X6
Tropatepine	T44.3X1	T44.3X2	T44.3X3	T44.3X4	T44.3X5	T44.3X6
Tropicamide	T44.3X1	T44.3X2	T44.3X3	T44.3X4	T44.3X5	T44.3X6
Trospium chloride	T44.3X1	T44.3X2	T44.3X3	T44.3X4	T44.3X5	T44.3X6
Troxerutin	T46.991	T46.992	T46.993	T46.994	T46.995	T46.996
Troxidone	T42.2X1	T42.2X2	T42.2X3	T42.2X4	T42.2X5	T42.2X6
Tryparsamide	T37.3X1	T37.3X2	T37.3X3	T37.3X4	T37.3X5	T37.3X6
Trypsin	T45.3X1	T45.3X2	T45.3X3	T45.3X4	T45.3X5	T45.3X6
Tryptizol	T43.011	T43.012	T43.013	T43.014	T43.015	T43.016
TSH	T38.811	T38.812	T38.813	T38.814	T38.815	T38.816
Tuaminoheptane	T48.5X1	T48.5X2	T48.5X3	T48.5X4	T48.5X5	T48.5X6
Tuberculin, purified protein derivative (PPD)	T50.8X1	T50.8X2	T50.8X3	T50.8X4	T50.8X5	T50.8X6
Tubocurare	T48.1X1	T48.1X2	T48.1X3	T48.1X4	T48.1X5	T48.1X6
Tubocurarine (chloride)	T48.1X1	T48.1X2	T48.1X3	T48.1X4	T48.1X5	T48.1X6
Tulobuterol	T48.6X1	T48.6X2	T48.6X3	T48.6X4	T48.6X5	T48.6X6
Turpentine (spirits of)	T52.8X1	T52.8X2	T52.8X3	T52.8X4	--	--
vapor	T52.8X1	T52.8X2	T52.8X3	T52.8X4	--	--
Tybamate	T43.591	T43.592	T43.593	T43.594	T43.595	T43.596
Tyloxapol	T48.4X1	T48.4X2	T48.4X3	T48.4X4	T48.4X5	T48.4X6
Tymazoline	T48.5X1	T48.5X2	T48.5X3	T48.5X4	T48.5X5	T48.5X6
Typhoid-paratyphoid vaccine	T50.A91	T50.A92	T50.A93	T50.A94	T50.A95	T50.A96
Typhus vaccine	T50.A91	T50.A92	T50.A93	T50.A94	T50.A95	T50.A96
Tyropanoate	T50.8X1	T50.8X2	T50.8X3	T50.8X4	T50.8X5	T50.8X6
Tyrothricin	T49.6X1	T49.6X2	T49.6X3	T49.6X4	T49.6X5	T49.6X6
ENT agent	T49.6X1	T49.6X2	T49.6X3	T49.6X4	T49.6X5	T49.6X6
ophthalmic preparation	T49.5X1	T49.5X2	T49.5X3	T49.5X4	T49.5X5	T49.5X6

Ufenamate - Veratrum

Substance	Poisoning, Accidental (unintentional)	Poisoning, Intentional self-harm	Poisoning, Assault	Poisoning, Undetermined	Adverse effect	Underdosing
U						
Ufenamate	T39.391	T39.392	T39.393	T39.394	T39.395	T39.396
Ultraviolet light protectant	T49.3X1	T49.3X2	T49.3X3	T49.3X4	T49.3X5	T49.3X6
Undecenoic acid	T49.0X1	T49.0X2	T49.0X3	T49.0X4	T49.0X5	T49.0X6
Undecoylium	T49.0X1	T49.0X2	T49.0X3	T49.0X4	T49.0X5	T49.0X6
Undecylenic acid (derivatives)	T49.0X1	T49.0X2	T49.0X3	T49.0X4	T49.0X5	T49.0X6
Unna's boot	T49.3X1	T49.3X2	T49.3X3	T49.3X4	T49.3X5	T49.3X6
Unsaturated fatty acid	T46.6X1	T46.6X2	T46.6X3	T46.6X4	T46.6X5	T46.6X6
Uracil mustard	T45.1X1	T45.1X2	T45.1X3	T45.1X4	T45.1X5	T45.1X6
Uramustine	T45.1X1	T45.1X2	T45.1X3	T45.1X4	T45.1X5	T45.1X6
Urapidil	T46.5X1	T46.5X2	T46.5X3	T46.5X4	T46.5X5	T46.5X6
Urari	T48.1X1	T48.1X2	T48.1X3	T48.1X4	T48.1X5	T48.1X6
Urate oxidase	T50.4X1	T50.4X2	T50.4X3	T50.4X4	T50.4X5	T50.4X6
Urea	T47.3X1	T47.3X2	T47.3X3	T47.3X4	T47.3X5	T47.3X6
peroxide	T49.0X1	T49.0X2	T49.0X3	T49.0X4	T49.0X5	T49.0X6
stibamine	T37.4X1	T37.4X2	T37.4X3	T37.4X4	T37.4X5	T37.4X6
topical	T49.8X1	T49.8X2	T49.8X3	T49.8X4	T49.8X5	T49.8X6
Urethane	T45.1X1	T45.1X2	T45.1X3	T45.1X4	T45.1X5	T45.1X6
Urginea (maritima) (scilla) — *see* Squill						
Uric acid metabolism drug NEC	T50.4X1	T50.4X2	T50.4X3	T50.4X4	T50.4X5	T50.4X6
Uricosuric agent	T50.4X1	T50.4X2	T50.4X3	T50.4X4	T50.4X5	T50.4X6
Urinary anti-infective	T37.8X1	T37.8X2	T37.8X3	T37.8X4	T37.8X5	T37.8X6
Urofollitropin	T38.812	T38.812	T38.813	T38.814	T38.815	T38.816
Urokinase	T45.611	T45.612	T45.613	T45.614	T45.615	T45.616
Urokon	T50.8X1	T50.8X2	T50.8X3	T50.8X4	T50.8X5	T50.8X6
Ursodeoxycholic acid	T50.991	T50.992	T50.993	T50.994	T50.995	T50.996
Ursodiol	T50.991	T50.992	T50.993	T50.994	T50.995	T50.996
Urtica	T62.2X1	T62.2X2	T62.2X3	T62.2X4	--	--
Utility gas — *see* Gas, utility						
V						
Vaccine NEC	T50.Z91	T50.Z92	T50.Z93	T50.Z94	T50.Z95	T50.Z96
antineoplastic	T50.Z91	T50.Z92	T50.Z93	T50.Z94	T50.Z95	T50.Z96
bacterial NEC	T50.A91	T50.A92	T50.A93	T50.A94	T50.A95	T50.A96
with						
other bacterial component	T50.A21	T50.A22	T50.A23	T50.A24	T50.A25	T50.A26
pertussis component	T50.A11	T50.A12	T50.A13	T50.A14	T50.A15	T50.A16
viral-rickettsial component	T50.A21	T50.A22	T50.A23	T50.A24	T50.A25	T50.A26
mixed NEC	T50.A21	T50.A22	T50.A23	T50.A24	T50.A25	T50.A26
BCG	T50.A91	T50.A92	T50.A93	T50.A94	T50.A95	T50.A96
cholera	T50.A91	T50.A92	T50.A93	T50.A94	T50.A95	T50.A96
diphtheria	T50.A91	T50.A92	T50.A93	T50.A94	T50.A95	T50.A96
with tetanus	T50.A21	T50.A22	T50.A23	T50.A24	T50.A25	T50.A26
and pertussis	T50.A11	T50.A12	T50.A13	T50.A14	T50.A15	T50.A16
influenza	T50.B91	T50.B92	T50.B93	T50.B94	T50.B95	T50.B96
measles	T50.B91	T50.B92	T50.B93	T50.B94	T50.B95	T50.B96
with mumps and rubella	T50.B91	T50.B92	T50.B93	T50.B94	T50.B95	T50.B96
meningococcal	T50.A91	T50.A92	T50.A93	T50.A94	T50.A95	T50.A96
mumps	T50.B91	T50.B92	T50.B93	T50.B94	T50.B95	T50.B96
paratyphoid	T50.A91	T50.A92	T50.A93	T50.A94	T50.A95	T50.A96
pertussis	T50.A11	T50.A12	T50.A13	T50.A14	T50.A15	T50.A16
with diphtheria	T50.A11	T50.A12	T50.A13	T50.A14	T50.A15	T50.A16
and tetanus	T50.A11	T50.A12	T50.A13	T50.A14	T50.A15	T50.A16
with other component	T50.A11	T50.A12	T50.A13	T50.A14	T50.A15	T50.A16
plague	T50.A91	T50.A92	T50.A93	T50.A94	T50.A95	T50.A96
poliomyelitis	T50.B91	T50.B92	T50.B93	T50.B94	T50.B95	T50.B96
poliovirus	T50.B91	T50.B92	T50.B93	T50.B94	T50.B95	T50.B96
rabies	T50.B91	T50.B92	T50.B93	T50.B94	T50.B95	T50.B96
respiratory syncytial virus	T50.B91	T50.B92	T50.B93	T50.B94	T50.B95	T50.B96
rickettsial NEC	T50.A91	T50.A92	T50.A93	T50.A94	T50.A95	T50.A96
with						
bacterial component	T50.A21	T50.A22	T50.A23	T50.A24	T50.A25	T50.A26
Rocky Mountain spotted fever	T50.A91	T50.A92	T50.A93	T50.A94	T50.A95	T50.A96
rubella	T50.B91	T50.B92	T50.B93	T50.B94	T50.B95	T50.B96
sabin oral	T50.B91	T50.B92	T50.B93	T50.B94	T50.B95	T50.B96
smallpox	T50.B11	T50.B12	T50.B13	T50.B14	T50.B15	T50.B16
TAB	T50.A91	T50.A92	T50.A93	T50.A94	T50.A95	T50.A96
tetanus	T50.A91	T50.A92	T50.A93	T50.A94	T50.A95	T50.A96
typhoid	T50.A91	T50.A92	T50.A93	T50.A94	T50.A95	T50.A96
typhus	T50.A91	T50.A92	T50.A93	T50.A94	T50.A95	T50.A96
viral NEC	T50.B91	T50.B92	T50.B93	T50.B94	T50.B95	T50.B96
yellow fever	T50.B91	T50.B92	T50.B93	T50.B94	T50.B95	T50.B96
Vaccinia immune globulin	T50.Z11	T50.Z12	T50.Z13	T50.Z14	T50.Z15	T50.Z16
Vaginal contraceptives	T49.8X1	T49.8X2	T49.8X3	T49.8X4	T49.8X5	T49.8X6
Valerian						
root	T42.6X1	T42.6X2	T42.6X3	T42.6X4	T42.6X5	T42.6X6
tincture	T42.6X1	T42.6X2	T42.6X3	T42.6X4	T42.6X5	T42.6X6
Valethamate bromide	T44.3X1	T44.3X2	T44.3X3	T44.3X4	T44.3X5	T44.3X6
Valisone	T49.0X1	T49.0X2	T49.0X3	T49.0X4	T49.0X5	T49.0X6
Valium	T42.4X1	T42.4X2	T42.4X3	T42.4X4	T42.4X5	T42.4X6

Substance	Poisoning, Accidental (unintentional)	Poisoning, Intentional self-harm	Poisoning, Assault	Poisoning, Undetermined	Adverse effect	Underdosing
Valmid	T42.6X1	T42.6X2	T42.6X3	T42.6X4	T42.6X5	T42.6X6
Valnoctamide	T42.6X1	T42.6X2	T42.6X3	T42.6X4	T42.6X5	T42.6X6
Valproate (sodium)	T42.6X1	T42.6X2	T42.6X3	T42.6X4	T42.6X5	T42.6X6
Valproic acid	T42.6X1	T42.6X2	T42.6X3	T42.6X4	T42.6X5	T42.6X6
Valpromide	T42.6X1	T42.6X2	T42.6X3	T42.6X4	T42.6X5	T42.6X6
Vanadium	T56.891	T56.892	T56.893	T56.894		
Vancomycin	T36.8X1	T36.8X2	T36.8X3	T36.8X4	T36.8X5	T36.8X6
Vapor (*see also* Gas)	T59.91	T59.92	T59.93	T59.94		
kiln (carbon monoxide)	T58.8X1	T58.8X2	T58.8X3	T58.8X4	--	--
lead — *see* lead						
specified source NEC	T59.891	T59.892	T59.893	T59.894		
Vardenafil	T46.7X1	T46.7X2	T46.7X3	T46.7X4	T46.7X5	T46.7X6
Varicose reduction drug	T46.8X1	T46.8X2	T46.8X3	T46.8X4	T46.8X5	T46.8X6
Varnish	T65.4X1	T65.4X2	T65.4X3	T65.4X4		
cleaner	T52.91	T52.92	T52.93	T52.94		
Vaseline	T49.3X1	T49.3X2	T49.3X3	T49.3X4	T49.3X5	T49.3X6
Vasodilan	T46.7X1	T46.7X2	T46.7X3	T46.7X4	T46.7X5	T46.7X6
Vasodilator						
coronary NEC	T46.3X1	T46.3X2	T46.3X3	T46.3X4	T46.3X5	T46.3X6
peripheral NEC	T46.7X1	T46.7X2	T46.7X3	T46.7X4	T46.7X5	T46.7X6
Vasopressin	T38.891	T38.892	T38.893	T38.894	T38.895	T38.896
Vasopressor drugs	T38.891	T38.892	T38.893	T38.894	T38.895	T38.896
Vecuronium bromide	T48.1X1	T48.1X2	T48.1X3	T48.1X4	T48.1X5	T48.1X6
Vegetable extract, astringent	T49.2X1	T49.2X2	T49.2X3	T49.2X4	T49.2X5	T49.2X6
Venlafaxine	T43.211	T43.212	T43.213	T43.214	T43.215	T43.216
Venom, venomous (bite) (sting)	T63.91	T63.92	T63.93	T63.94		
amphibian NEC	T63.831	T63.832	T63.833	T63.834	--	--
animal NEC	T63.891	T63.892	T63.893	T63.894	--	--
ant	T63.421	T63.422	T63.423	T63.424	--	--
arthropod NEC	T63.481	T63.482	T63.483	T63.484	--	--
bee	T63.441	T63.442	T63.443	T63.444	--	--
centipede	T63.411	T63.412	T63.413	T63.414	--	--
fish	T63.591	T63.592	T63.593	T63.594	--	--
frog	T63.811	T63.812	T63.813	T63.814	--	--
hornet	T63.451	T63.452	T63.453	T63.454	--	--
insect NEC	T63.481	T63.482	T63.483	T63.484	--	--
lizard	T63.121	T63.122	T63.123	T63.124	--	--
marine						
animals	T63.691	T63.692	T63.693	T63.694	--	--
bluebottle	T63.611	T63.612	T63.613	T63.614	--	--
jellyfish NEC	T63.621	T63.622	T63.623	T63.624	--	--
Portugese Man-o-war	T63.611	T63.612	T63.613	T63.614	--	--
sea anemone	T63.631	T63.632	T63.633	T63.634	--	--
specified NEC	T63.691	T63.692	T63.693	T63.694	--	--
fish	T63.591	T63.592	T63.593	T63.594	--	--
plants	T63.711	T63.712	T63.713	T63.714	--	--
sting ray	T63.511	T63.512	T63.513	T63.514	--	--
millipede (tropical)	T63.411	T63.412	T63.413	T63.414	--	--
plant NEC	T63.791	T63.792	T63.793	T63.794	--	--
marine	T63.711	T63.712	T63.713	T63.714	--	--
reptile	T63.191	T63.192	T63.193	T63.194	--	--
gila monster	T63.111	T63.112	T63.113	T63.114	--	--
lizard NEC	T63.121	T63.122	T63.123	T63.124	--	--
scorpion	T63.2X1	T63.2X2	T63.2X3	T63.2X4	--	--
snake	T63.001	T63.002	T63.003	T63.004	--	--
African NEC	T63.081	T63.082	T63.083	T63.084	--	--
American (North) (South) NEC	T63.061	T63.062	T63.063	T63.064	--	--
Asian	T63.081	T63.082	T63.083	T63.084	--	--
Australian	T63.071	T63.072	T63.073	T63.074	--	--
cobra	T63.041	T63.042	T63.043	T63.044	--	--
coral snake	T63.021	T63.022	T63.023	T63.024	--	--
rattlesnake	T63.011	T63.012	T63.013	T63.014	--	--
specified NEC	T63.091	T63.092	T63.093	T63.094	--	--
taipan	T63.031	T63.032	T63.033	T63.034	--	--
specified NEC	T63.891	T63.892	T63.893	T63.894	--	--
spider	T63.301	T63.302	T63.303	T63.304	--	--
black widow	T63.311	T63.312	T63.313	T63.314	--	--
brown recluse	T63.331	T63.332	T63.333	T63.334	--	--
specified NEC	T63.391	T63.392	T63.393	T63.394	--	--
tarantula	T63.321	T63.322	T63.323	T63.324	--	--
sting ray	T63.511	T63.512	T63.513	T63.514	--	--
toad	T63.821	T63.822	T63.823	T63.824	--	--
wasp	T63.461	T63.462	T63.463	T63.464	--	--
Venous sclerosing drug NEC	T46.8X1	T46.8X2	T46.8X3	T46.8X4	T46.8X5	T46.8X6
Ventolin — *see* Albuterol						
Veramon	T42.3X1	T42.3X2	T42.3X3	T42.3X4	T42.3X5	T42.3X6
Verapamil	T46.1X1	T46.1X2	T46.1X3	T46.1X4	T46.1X5	T46.1X6
Veratrine	T46.5X1	T46.5X2	T46.5X3	T46.5X4	T46.5X5	T46.5X6
Veratrum						
album	T62.2X1	T62.2X2	T62.2X3	T62.2X4	--	--
alkaloids	T46.5X1	T46.5X2	T46.5X3	T46.5X4	T46.5X5	T46.5X6
viride	T62.2X1	T62.2X2	T62.2X3	T62.2X4	--	--

Substance	Poisoning, Accidental (unintentional)	Poisoning, Intentional self-harm	Poisoning, Assault	Poisoning, Undetermined	Adverse effect	Underdosing
Verdigris	T60.3X1	T60.3X2	T60.3X3	T60.3X4	--	--
Veronal	T42.3X1	T42.3X2	T42.3X3	T42.3X4	T42.3X5	T42.3X6
Veroxil	T37.4X1	T37.4X2	T37.4X3	T37.4X4	T37.4X5	T37.4X6
Versenate	T50.6X1	T50.6X2	T50.6X3	T50.6X4	T50.6X5	T50.6X6
Versidyne	T39.8X1	T39.8X2	T39.8X3	T39.8X4	T39.8X5	T39.8X6
Vetrabutine	T48.0X1	T48.0X2	T48.0X3	T48.0X4	T48.0X5	T48.0X6
Vidarabine	T37.5X1	T37.5X2	T37.5X3	T37.5X4	T37.5X5	T37.5X6
Vienna						
green	T57.0X1	T57.0X2	T57.0X3	T57.0X4	--	--
insecticide	T60.2X1	T60.2X2	T60.2X3	T60.2X4	--	--
red	T57.0X1	T57.0X2	T57.0X3	T57.0X4	--	--
pharmaceutical dye	T50.991	T50.992	T50.993	T50.994	T50.995	T50.996
Vigabatrin	T42.6X1	T42.6X2	T42.6X3	T42.6X4	T42.6X5	T42.6X6
Viloxazine	T43.291	T43.292	T43.293	T43.294	T43.295	T43.296
Viminol	T39.8X1	T39.8X2	T39.8X3	T39.8X4	T39.8X5	T39.8X6
Vinbarbital, vinbarbitone	T42.3X1	T42.3X2	T42.3X3	T42.3X4	T42.3X5	T42.3X6
Vinblastine	T45.1X1	T45.1X2	T45.1X3	T45.1X4	T45.1X5	T45.1X6
Vinburnine	T46.7X1	T46.7X2	T46.7X3	T46.7X4	T46.7X5	T46.7X6
Vincamine	T45.1X1	T45.1X2	T45.1X3	T45.1X4	T45.1X5	T45.1X6
Vincristine	T45.1X1	T45.1X2	T45.1X3	T45.1X4	T45.1X5	T45.1X6
Vindesine	T45.1X1	T45.1X2	T45.1X3	T45.1X4	T45.1X5	T45.1X6
Vinesthene, vinethene	T41.0X1	T41.0X2	T41.0X3	T41.0X4	T41.0X5	T41.0X6
Vinorelbine tartrate	T45.1X1	T45.1X2	T45.1X3	T45.1X4	T45.1X5	T45.1X6
Vinpocetine	T46.7X1	T46.7X2	T46.7X3	T46.7X4	T46.7X5	T46.7X6
Vinyl						
acetate	T65.891	T65.892	T65.893	T65.894	--	--
bital	T42.3X1	T42.3X2	T42.3X3	T42.3X4	T42.3X5	T42.3X6
bromide	T65.891	T65.892	T65.893	T65.894	--	--
chloride	T59.891	T59.892	T59.893	T59.894	--	--
ether	T41.0X1	T41.0X2	T41.0X3	T41.0X4	T41.0X5	T41.0X6
Vinylbital	T42.3X1	T42.3X2	T42.3X3	T42.3X4	T42.3X5	T42.3X6
Vinylidene chloride	T65.891	T65.892	T65.893	T65.894	--	--
Vioform	T37.8X1	T37.8X2	T37.8X3	T37.8X4	T37.8X5	T37.8X6
topical	T49.0X1	T49.0X2	T49.0X3	T49.0X4	T49.0X5	T49.0X6
Viomycin	T36.8X1	T36.8X2	T36.8X3	T36.8X4	T36.8X5	T36.8X6
Viosterol	T45.2X1	T45.2X2	T45.2X3	T45.2X4	T45.2X5	T45.2X6
Viper (venom)	T63.091	T63.092	T63.093	T63.094	--	--
Viprynium	T37.4X1	T37.4X2	T37.4X3	T37.4X4	T37.4X5	T37.4X6
Viquidil	T46.7X1	T46.7X2	T46.7X3	T46.7X4	T46.7X5	T46.7X6
Viral vaccine NEC	T50.B91	T50.B92	T50.B93	T50.B94	T50.B95	T50.B96
Virginiamycin	T36.8X1	T36.8X2	T36.8X3	T36.8X4	T36.8X5	T36.8X6
Virugon	T37.5X1	T37.5X2	T37.5X3	T37.5X4	T37.5X5	T37.5X6
Viscous agent	T50.901	T50.902	T50.903	T50.904	T50.905	T50.906
Visine	T49.5X1	T49.5X2	T49.5X3	T49.5X4	T49.5X5	T49.5X6
Visnadine	T46.3X1	T46.3X2	T46.3X3	T46.3X4	T46.3X5	T46.3X6
Vitamin NEC	T45.2X1	T45.2X2	T45.2X3	T45.2X4	T45.2X5	T45.2X6
A	T45.2X1	T45.2X2	T45.2X3	T45.2X4	T45.2X5	T45.2X6
B NEC	T45.2X1	T45.2X2	T45.2X3	T45.2X4	T45.2X5	T45.2X6
nicotinic acid	T46.7X1	T46.7X2	T46.7X3	T46.7X4	T46.7X5	T46.7X6
B1	T45.2X1	T45.2X2	T45.2X3	T45.2X4	T45.2X5	T45.2X6
B2	T45.2X1	T45.2X2	T45.2X3	T45.2X4	T45.2X5	T45.2X6
B6	T45.2X1	T45.2X2	T45.2X3	T45.2X4	T45.2X5	T45.2X6
B12	T45.2X1	T45.2X2	T45.2X3	T45.2X4	T45.2X5	T45.2X6
B15	T45.2X1	T45.2X2	T45.2X3	T45.2X4	T45.2X5	T45.2X6
C	T45.2X1	T45.2X2	T45.2X3	T45.2X4	T45.2X5	T45.2X6
D	T45.2X1	T45.2X2	T45.2X3	T45.2X4	T45.2X5	T45.2X6
D2	T45.2X1	T45.2X2	T45.2X3	T45.2X4	T45.2X5	T45.2X6
D3	T45.2X1	T45.2X2	T45.2X3	T45.2X4	T45.2X5	T45.2X6
E	T45.2X1	T45.2X2	T45.2X3	T45.2X4	T45.2X5	T45.2X6
E acetate	T45.2X1	T45.2X2	T45.2X3	T45.2X4	T45.2X5	T45.2X6
hematopoietic	T45.8X1	T45.8X2	T45.8X3	T45.8X4	T45.8X5	T45.8X6
K NEC	T45.7X1	T45.7X2	T45.7X3	T45.7X4	T45.7X5	T45.7X6
K1	T45.7X1	T45.7X2	T45.7X3	T45.7X4	T45.7X5	T45.7X6
K2	T45.7X1	T45.7X2	T45.7X3	T45.7X4	T45.7X5	T45.7X6
PP	T45.2X1	T45.2X2	T45.2X3	T45.2X4	T45.2X5	T45.2X6
ulceroprotectant	T47.1X1	T47.1X2	T47.1X3	T47.1X4	T47.1X5	T47.1X6
Vleminckx's solution	T49.4X1	T49.4X2	T49.4X3	T49.4X4	T49.4X5	T49.4X6
Voltaren — *see* Diclofenac sodium						
W						
Warfarin	T45.511	T45.512	T45.513	T45.514	T45.515	T45.516
rodenticide	T60.4X1	T60.4X2	T60.4X3	T60.4X4	--	--
sodium	T45.511	T45.512	T45.513	T45.514	T45.515	T45.516
Wasp (sting)	T63.461	T63.462	T63.463	T63.464	--	--
Water						
balance drug	T50.3X1	T50.3X2	T50.3X3	T50.3X4	T50.3X5	T50.3X6
distilled	T50.3X1	T50.3X2	T50.3X3	T50.3X4	T50.3X5	T50.3X6
gas — *see* Gas, water incomplete combustion of — *see* Carbon, monoxide, fuel, utility						
hemlock	T62.2X1	T62.2X2	T62.2X3	T62.2X4	--	--
moccasin (venom)	T63.061	T63.062	T63.063	T63.064	--	--
purified	T50.3X1	T50.3X2	T50.3X3	T50.3X4	T50.3X5	T50.3X6
Wax (paraffin) (petroleum)	T52.0X1	T52.0X2	T52.0X3	T52.0X4	--	--
automobile	T65.891	T65.892	T65.893	T65.894	--	--
floor	T52.0X1	T52.0X2	T52.0X3	T52.0X4	--	--
Weed killers NEC	T60.3X1	T60.3X2	T60.3X3	T60.3X4	--	--
Welldorm	T42.6X1	T42.6X2	T42.6X3	T42.6X4	T42.6X5	T42.6X6
White						
arsenic	T57.0X1	T57.0X2	T57.0X3	T57.0X4	--	--
hellebore	T62.2X1	T62.2X2	T62.2X3	T62.2X4	--	--
lotion (keratolytic)	T49.4X1	T49.4X2	T49.4X3	T49.4X4	T49.4X5	T49.4X6
spirit	T52.0X1	T52.0X2	T52.0X3	T52.0X4	--	--
Whitewash	T65.891	T65.892	T65.893	T65.894	--	--
Whole blood (human)	T45.8X1	T45.8X2	T45.8X3	T45.8X4	T45.8X5	T45.8X6
Wild						
black cherry	T62.2X1	T62.2X2	T62.2X3	T62.2X4	--	--
poisonous plants NEC	T62.2X1	T62.2X2	T62.2X3	T62.2X4	--	--
Window cleaning fluid	T65.891	T65.892	T65.893	T65.894	--	--
Wintergreen (oil)	T49.3X1	T49.3X2	T49.3X3	T49.3X4	T49.3X5	T49.3X6
Wisterine	T62.2X1	T62.2X2	T62.2X3	T62.2X4	--	--
Witch hazel	T49.2X1	T49.2X2	T49.2X3	T49.2X4	T49.2X5	T49.2X6
Wood alcohol or spirit	T51.1X1	T51.1X2	T51.1X3	T51.1X4	--	--
Wool fat (hydrous)	T49.3X1	T49.3X2	T49.3X3	T49.3X4	T49.3X5	T49.3X6
Woorali	T48.1X1	T48.1X2	T48.1X3	T48.1X4	T48.1X5	T48.1X6
Wormseed, American	T37.4X1	T37.4X2	T37.4X3	T37.4X4	T37.4X5	T37.4X6
X						
Xamoterol	T44.5X1	T44.5X2	T44.5X3	T44.5X4	T44.5X5	T44.5X6
Xanthine diuretics	T50.2X1	T50.2X2	T50.2X3	T50.2X4	T50.2X5	T50.2X6
Xanthinol nicotinate	T46.7X1	T46.7X2	T46.7X3	T46.7X4	T46.7X5	T46.7X6
Xanthotoxin	T49.3X1	T49.3X2	T49.3X3	T49.3X4	T49.3X5	T49.3X6
Xantinol nicotinate	T46.7X1	T46.7X2	T46.7X3	T46.7X4	T46.7X5	T46.7X6
Xantocillin	T36.0X1	T36.0X2	T36.0X3	T36.0X4	T36.0X5	T36.0X6
Xenon (127Xe) (133Xe)	T50.8X1	T50.8X2	T50.8X3	T50.8X4	T50.8X5	T50.8X6
Xenysalate	T49.4X1	T49.4X2	T49.4X3	T49.4X4	T49.4X5	T49.4X6
Xibornol	T37.8X1	T37.8X2	T37.8X3	T37.8X4	T37.8X5	T37.8X6
Xigris	T45.511	T45.512	T45.513	T45.514	T45.515	T45.516
Xipamide	T50.2X1	T50.2X2	T50.2X3	T50.2X4	T50.2X5	T50.2X6
Xylene (vapor)	T52.2X1	T52.2X2	T52.2X3	T52.2X4	--	--
Xylocaine (infiltration) (topical)	T41.3X1	T41.3X2	T41.3X3	T41.3X4	T41.3X5	T41.3X6
nerve block (peripheral) (plexus)	T41.3X1	T41.3X2	T41.3X3	T41.3X4	T41.3X5	T41.3X6
spinal	T41.3X1	T41.3X2	T41.3X3	T41.3X4	T41.3X5	T41.3X6
Xylol (vapor)	T52.2X1	T52.2X2	T52.2X3	T52.2X4	--	--
Xylometazoline	T48.5X1	T48.5X2	T48.5X3	T48.5X4	T48.5X5	T48.5X6
Y						
Yeast	T45.2X1	T45.2X2	T45.2X3	T45.2X4	T45.2X5	T45.2X6
dried	T45.2X1	T45.2X2	T45.2X3	T45.2X4	T45.2X5	T45.2X6
Yellow						
fever vaccine	T50.B91	T50.B92	T50.B93	T50.B94	T50.B95	T50.B96
jasmine	T62.2X1	T62.2X2	T62.2X3	T62.2X4	--	--
phenolphthalein	T47.2X1	T47.2X2	T47.2X3	T47.2X4	T47.2X5	T47.2X6
Yew	T62.2X1	T62.2X2	T62.2X3	T62.2X4	--	--
Yohimbic acid	T40.991	T40.992	T40.993	T40.994	T40.995	T40.996
Z						
Zactane	T39.8X1	T39.8X2	T39.8X3	T39.8X4	T39.8X5	T39.8X6
Zalcitabine	T37.5X1	T37.5X2	T37.5X3	T37.5X4	T37.5X5	T37.5X6
Zaroxolyn	T50.2X1	T50.2X2	T50.2X3	T50.2X4	T50.2X5	T50.2X6
Zephiran (topical)	T49.0X1	T49.0X2	T49.0X3	T49.0X4	T49.0X5	T49.0X6
ophthalmic preparation	T49.5X1	T49.5X2	T49.5X3	T49.5X4	T49.5X5	T49.5X6
Zeranol	T38.7X1	T38.7X2	T38.7X3	T38.7X4	T38.7X5	T38.7X6
Zerone	T51.1X1	T51.1X2	T51.1X3	T51.1X4	--	--
Zidovudine	T37.5X1	T37.5X2	T37.5X3	T37.5X4	T37.5X5	T37.5X6
Zimeldine	T43.221	T43.222	T43.223	T43.224	T43.225	T43.226
Zinc (compounds) (fumes) (vapor) NEC	T56.5X1	T56.5X2	T56.5X3	T56.5X4	--	--
anti-infectives	T49.0X1	T49.0X2	T49.0X3	T49.0X4	T49.0X5	T49.0X6
antivaricose	T46.8X1	T46.8X2	T46.8X3	T46.8X4	T46.8X5	T46.8X6
bacitracin	T49.0X1	T49.0X2	T49.0X3	T49.0X4	T49.0X5	T49.0X6
chloride (mouthwash)	T49.6X1	T49.6X2	T49.6X3	T49.6X4	T49.6X5	T49.6X6
chromate	T56.5X1	T56.5X2	T56.5X3	T56.5X4	--	--
gelatin	T49.3X1	T49.3X2	T49.3X3	T49.3X4	T49.3X5	T49.3X6
oxide	T49.3X1	T49.3X2	T49.3X3	T49.3X4	T49.3X5	T49.3X6
plaster	T49.3X1	T49.3X2	T49.3X3	T49.3X4	T49.3X5	T49.3X6
peroxide	T49.0X1	T49.0X2	T49.0X3	T49.0X4	T49.0X5	T49.0X6
pesticides	T56.5X1	T56.5X2	T56.5X3	T56.5X4	--	--
phosphide	T60.4X1	T60.4X2	T60.4X3	T60.4X4	--	--
pyrithionate	T49.4X1	T49.4X2	T49.4X3	T49.4X4	T49.4X5	T49.4X6
stearate	T49.3X1	T49.3X2	T49.3X3	T49.3X4	T49.3X5	T49.3X6
sulfate	T49.5X1	T49.5X2	T49.5X3	T49.5X4	T49.5X5	T49.5X6
ENT agent	T49.6X1	T49.6X2	T49.6X3	T49.6X4	T49.6X5	T49.6X6
ophthalmic solution	T49.5X1	T49.5X2	T49.5X3	T49.5X4	T49.5X5	T49.5X6
topical NEC	T49.0X1	T49.0X2	T49.0X3	T49.0X4	T49.0X5	T49.0X6
undecylenate	T49.0X1	T49.0X2	T49.0X3	T49.0X4	T49.0X5	T49.0X6
Zineb	T60.0X1	T60.0X2	T60.0X3	T60.0X4	--	--
Zinostatin	T45.1X1	T45.1X2	T45.1X3	T45.1X4	T45.1X5	T45.1X6

Zipeprol - Zyprexa

Substance	Poisoning, Accidental (unintentional)	Poisoning, Intentional self-harm	Poisoning, Assault	Poisoning, Undetermined	Adverse effect	Underdosing
Zipeprol	T48.3X1	T48.3X2	T48.3X3	T48.3X4	T48.3X5	T48.3X6
Zofenopril	T46.4X1	T46.4X2	T46.4X3	T46.4X4	T46.4X5	T46.4X6
Zolpidem	T42.6X1	T42.6X2	T42.6X3	T42.6X4	T42.6X5	T42.6X6
Zomepirac	T39.391	T39.392	T39.393	T39.394	T39.395	T39.396
Zopiclone	T42.6X1	T42.6X2	T42.6X3	T42.6X4	T42.6X5	T42.6X6
Zorubicin	T45.1X1	T45.1X2	T45.1X3	T45.1X4	T45.1X5	T45.1X6

Substance	Poisoning, Accidental (unintentional)	Poisoning, Intentional self-harm	Poisoning, Assault	Poisoning, Undetermined	Adverse effect	Underdosing
Zotepine	T43.591	T43.592	T43.593	T43.594	T43.595	T43.596
Zovant	T45.511	T45.512	T45.513	T45.514	T45.515	T45.516
Zoxazolamine	T42.8X1	T42.8X2	T42.8X3	T42.8X4	T42.8X5	T42.8X6
Zuclopenthixol	T43.4X1	T43.4X2	T43.4X3	T43.4X4	T43.4X5	T43.4X6
Zygadenus (venenosus)	T62.2X1	T62.2X2	T62.2X3	T62.2X4	--	--
Zyprexa	T43.591	T43.592	T43.593	T43.594	T43.595	T43.596

ICD-10-CM Index to External Causes of Injuries

The vertical yellow line appears at the 2nd and 4th indentations throughout the index.

A

Abandonment (causing exposure to weather conditions) (with intent to injure or kill) NEC X58 ☑
Abuse (adult) (child) (mental) (physical) (sexual) X58 ☑
Accident (to) X58 ☑
  aircraft (in transit) (powered) (*see also* Accident, transport, aircraft)
    due to, caused by cataclysm — *see* Forces of nature, by type
  animal-rider — *see* Accident, transport, animal-rider
  animal-drawn vehicle — *see* Accident, transport, animal-drawn vehicle occupant
  automobile — *see* Accident, transport, car occupant
  bare foot water skiier V94.4 ☑
  boat, boating (*see also* Accident, watercraft)
    striking swimmer
      powered V94.11 ☑
      unpowered V94.12 ☑
  bus — *see* Accident, transport, bus occupant
  cable car, not on rails V98.0 ☑
    on rails — *see* Accident, transport, streetcar occupant
  car — *see* Accident, transport, car occupant
  caused by, due to
    animal NEC W64 ☑
    chain hoist W24.0 ☑
    cold (excessive) — *see* Exposure, cold
    corrosive liquid, substance — *see* Table of Drugs and Chemicals
    cutting or piercing instrument — *see* Contact, with, by type of instrument
    drive belt W24.0 ☑
    electric
      current — *see* Exposure, electric current
      motor (*see also* Contact, with, by type of machine) W31.3 ☑
      current (of) W86.8 ☑
    environmental factor NEC X58 ☑
    explosive material — *see* Explosion
    fire, flames — *see* Exposure, fire
    firearm missile — *see* Discharge, firearm by type
    heat (excessive) — *see* Heat
    hot — *see* Contact, with, hot
    ignition — *see* Ignition
    lifting device W24.0 ☑
    lightning — *see* subcategory T75.0 ☑
      causing fire — *see* Exposure, fire
    machine, machinery — *see* Contact, with, by type of machine
    natural factor NEC X58 ☑
    pulley (block) W24.0 ☑
    radiation — *see* Radiation
    steam X13.1 ☑
      inhalation X13.0 ☑
      pipe X16 ☑
    thunderbolt — *see* subcategory T75.0 ☑
      causing fire — *see* Exposure, fire
    transmission device W24.1 ☑
  coach — *see* Accident, transport, bus occupant
  coal car — *see* Accident, transport, industrial vehicle occupant
  diving (*see also* Fall, into, water)
    with
      drowning or submersion — *see* Drowning
  forklift — *see* Accident, transport, industrial vehicle occupant
  heavy transport vehicle NOS — *see* Accident, transport, truck occupant
  ice yacht V98.2 ☑
  in
    medical, surgical procedure
      as, or due to misadventure — *see* Misadventure
      causing an abnormal reaction or later complication without mention of misadventure (*see also* Complication of or following, by type of procedure) Y84.9
  land yacht V98.1 ☑
  late effect of — *see* W00-X58 with 7th character S
  logging car — *see* Accident, transport, industrial vehicle occupant
  machine, machinery (*see also* Contact, with, by type of machine)
    on board watercraft V93.69 ☑
      explosion — *see* Explosion, in, watercraft

Accident — *continued*
  machine — *continued*
    fire — *see* Burn, on board watercraft
    powered craft V93.63 ☑
      ferry boat V93.61 ☑
      fishing boat V93.62 ☑
      jetskis V93.63 ☑
      liner V93.61 ☑
      merchant ship V93.60 ☑
      passenger ship V93.61 ☑
      sailboat V93.64 ☑
  mine tram — *see* Accident, transport, industrial vehicle occupant
  mobility scooter (motorized) — *see* Accident, transport, pedestrian, conveyance, specified type NEC
  motor scooter — *see* Accident, transport, motorcyclist
  motor vehicle NOS (traffic) (*see also* Accident, transport) V89.2 ☑
    nontraffic V89.0 ☑
    three-wheeled NOS — *see* Accident, transport, three-wheeled motor vehicle occupant
  motorcycle NOS — *see* Accident, transport, motorcyclist
  nonmotor vehicle NOS (nontraffic) (*see also* Accident, transport) V89.1 ☑
    traffic NOS V89.3 ☑
  nontraffic (victim's mode of transport NOS) V88.9 ☑
    collision (between) V88.7 ☑
      bus and truck V88.5 ☑
      car and:
        bus V88.3 ☑
        pickup V88.2 ☑
        three-wheeled motor vehicle V88.0 ☑
        train V88.6 ☑
        truck V88.4 ☑
        two-wheeled motor vehicle V88.0 ☑
        van V88.2 ☑
      specified vehicle NEC and:
        three-wheeled motor vehicle V88.1 ☑
        two-wheeled motor vehicle V88.1 ☑
    known mode of transport — *see* Accident, transport, by type of vehicle
    noncollision V88.8 ☑
  on board watercraft V93.89 ☑
    powered craft V93.83 ☑
      ferry boat V93.81 ☑
      fishing boat V93.82 ☑
      jetskis V93.83 ☑
      liner V93.81 ☑
      merchant ship V93.80 ☑
      passenger ship V93.81 ☑
    unpowered craft V93.88 ☑
      canoe V93.85 ☑
      inflatable V93.86 ☑
        in tow
          recreational V94.31 ☑
          specified NEC V94.32 ☑
      kayak V93.85 ☑
      sailboat V93.84 ☑
      surf-board V93.88 ☑
      water skis V93.87 ☑
      windsurfer V93.88 ☑
  parachutist V97.29 ☑
    entangled in object V97.21 ☑
    injured on landing V97.22 ☑
  pedal cycle — *see* Accident, transport, pedal cyclist
  pedestrian (on foot)
    with
      another pedestrian W51 ☑
        with fall W03 ☑
          due to ice or snow W00.0 ☑
      on pedestrian conveyance NEC V00.09 ☑
      roller skater (in-line) V00.01 ☑
      skate boarder V00.02 ☑
      transport vehicle — *see* Accident, transport
    on pedestrian conveyance — *see* Accident, transport, pedestrian, conveyance
  pick-up truck or van — *see* Accident, transport, pickup truck occupant
  quarry truck — *see* Accident, transport, industrial vehicle occupant
  railway vehicle (any) (in motion) — *see* Accident, transport, railway vehicle occupant
    due to cataclysm — *see* Forces of nature, by type

Accident — *continued*
  scooter (non-motorized) — *see* Accident, transport, pedestrian, conveyance, scooter
  sequelae of — *see* W00-X58 with 7th character S
  skateboard — *see* Accident, transport, pedestrian, conveyance, skateboard
  ski (ing) — *see* Accident, transport, pedestrian, conveyance
    lift V98.3 ☑
  specified cause NEC X58 ☑
  streetcar — *see* Accident, transport, streetcar occupant
  traffic (victim's mode of transport NOS) V87.9 ☑
    collision (between) V87.7 ☑
      bus and truck V87.5 ☑
      car and:
        bus V87.3 ☑
        pickup V87.2 ☑
        three-wheeled motor vehicle V87.0 ☑
        train V87.6 ☑
        truck V87.4 ☑
        two-wheeled motor vehicle V87.0 ☑
        van V87.2 ☑
      specified vehicle NEC V86.39 ☑
        and
          three-wheeled motor vehicle V87.1 ☑
          two-wheeled motor vehicle V87.1 ☑
        driver V86.09 ☑
        person on outside V86.29 ☑
        passenger V86.19 ☑
        while boarding or alighting V86.49 ☑
    known mode of transport — *see* Accident, transport, by type of vehicle
    noncollision V87.8 ☑
  transport (involving injury to) V99 ☑
    18 wheeler — *see* Accident, transport, truck occupant
    agricultural vehicle occupant (nontraffic) V84.9 ☑
      driver V84.5 ☑
      hanger-on V84.7 ☑
      passenger V84.6 ☑
      traffic V84.3 ☑
        driver V84.0 ☑
        hanger-on V84.2 ☑
        passenger V84.1 ☑
      while boarding or alighting V84.4 ☑
    aircraft NEC V97.89 ☑
      military NEC V97.818 ☑
        with civilian aircraft V97.810 ☑
        civilian injured by V97.811 ☑
      occupant injured (in)
        nonpowered craft accident V96.9 ☑
          balloon V96.00 ☑
            collision V96.03 ☑
            crash V96.01 ☑
            explosion V96.05 ☑
            fire V96.04 ☑
            forced landing V96.02 ☑
            specified type NEC V96.09 ☑
          glider V96.20 ☑
            collision V96.23 ☑
            crash V96.21 ☑
            explosion V96.25 ☑
            fire V96.24 ☑
            forced landing V96.22 ☑
            specified type NEC V96.29 ☑
          hang glider V96.10 ☑
            collision V96.13 ☑
            crash V96.11 ☑
            explosion V96.15 ☑
            fire V96.14 ☑
            forced landing V96.12 ☑
            specified type NEC V96.19 ☑
          specified craft NEC V96.8 ☑
        powered craft accident V95.9 ☑
          fixed wing NEC
            commercial V95.30 ☑
              collision V95.33 ☑
              crash V95.31 ☑
              explosion V95.35 ☑
              fire V95.34 ☑
              forced landing V95.32 ☑
              specified type NEC V95.39 ☑
            private V95.20 ☑
              collision V95.23 ☑
              crash V95.21 ☑

Accident

Accident — *continued*
  transport — *continued*
        explosion V95.25 ☑
        fire V95.24 ☑
        forced landing V95.22 ☑
        specified type NEC V95.29 ☑
     glider V95.10 ☑
      collision V95.13 ☑
      crash V95.11 ☑
      explosion V95.15 ☑
      fire V95.14 ☑
      forced landing V95.12 ☑
      specified type NEC V95.19 ☑
     helicopter V95.00 ☑
      collision V95.03 ☑
      crash V95.01 ☑
      explosion V95.05 ☑
      fire V95.04 ☑
      forced landing V95.02 ☑
      specified type NEC V95.09 ☑
     spacecraft V95.40 ☑
      collision V95.43 ☑
      crash V95.41 ☑
      explosion V95.45 ☑
      fire V95.44 ☑
      forced landing V95.42 ☑
      specified type NEC V95.49 ☑
     specified craft NEC V95.8 ☑
     ultralight V95.10 ☑
      collision V95.13 ☑
      crash V95.11 ☑
      explosion V95.15 ☑
      fire V95.14 ☑
      forced landing V95.12 ☑
      specified type NEC V95.19 ☑
    specified accident NEC V97.0 ☑
    while boarding or alighting V97.1 ☑
   person (injured by)
    falling from, in or on aircraft V97.0 ☑
    machinery on aircraft V97.89 ☑
    on ground with aircraft involvement V97.39 ☑
    rotating propeller V97.32 ☑
    struck by object falling from aircraft V97.31 ☑
    sucked into aircraft jet V97.33 ☑
    while boarding or alighting aircraft V97.1 ☑
  airport (battery-powered) passenger vehicle — *see* Accident, transport, industrial vehicle occupant
  all-terrain vehicle occupant (nontraffic) V86.95 ☑
    driver V86.55 ☑
    dune buggy — *see* Accident, transport, dune buggy occupant
    hanger-on V86.75 ☑
    passenger V86.65 ☑
    snowmobile — *see* Accident, transport, snowmobile occupant
    specified type NEC V86.99 ☑
     driver V86.59 ☑
     passenger V86.69 ☑
     person on outside V86.79 ☑
    traffic V86.35 ☑
     driver V86.05 ☑
     hanger-on V86.25 ☑
     passenger V86.15 ☑
    while boarding or alighting V86.45 ☑
  ambulance occupant (traffic) V86.31 ☑
    driver V86.01 ☑
    hanger-on V86.21 ☑
    nontraffic V86.91 ☑
     driver V86.51 ☑
     hanger-on V86.71 ☑
     passenger V86.61 ☑
    passenger V86.11 ☑
    while boarding or alighting V86.41 ☑
  animal-drawn vehicle occupant (in) V80.929 ☑
    collision (with)
     animal V80.12 ☑
      being ridden V80.711 ☑
     animal-drawn vehicle V80.721 ☑
     bus V80.42 ☑
     car V80.42 ☑
     fixed or stationary object V80.82 ☑
     military vehicle V80.920 ☑
     nonmotor vehicle V80.791 ☑
     pedal cycle V80.22 ☑
     pedestrian V80.12 ☑
     pickup V80.42 ☑
     railway train or vehicle V80.62 ☑
     specified motor vehicle NEC V80.52 ☑
     streetcar V80.731 ☑
     truck V80.42 ☑

Accident — *continued*
  transport — *continued*
      two- or three-wheeled motor vehicle V80.32 ☑
      van V80.42 ☑
    noncollision V80.02 ☑
    specified circumstance NEC V80.928 ☑
  animal-rider V80.919 ☑
    collision (with)
     animal V80.11 ☑
      being ridden V80.710 ☑
     animal-drawn vehicle V80.720 ☑
     bus V80.41 ☑
     car V80.41 ☑
     fixed or stationary object V80.81 ☑
     military vehicle V80.910 ☑
     nonmotor vehicle V80.790 ☑
     pedal cycle V80.21 ☑
     pedestrian V80.11 ☑
     pickup V80.41 ☑
     railway train or vehicle V80.61 ☑
     specified motor vehicle NEC V80.51 ☑
     streetcar V80.730 ☑
     truck V80.41 ☑
     two- or three-wheeled motor vehicle V80.31 ☑
     van V80.41 ☑
    noncollision V80.018 ☑
     specified as horse rider V80.010 ☑
    specified circumstance NEC V80.918 ☑
  armored car — *see* Accident, transport, truck occupant
  battery-powered truck (baggage) (mail) — *see* Accident, transport, industrial vehicle occupant
  bus occupant V79.9 ☑
    collision (with)
     animal (traffic) V70.9 ☑
      being ridden (traffic) V76.9 ☑
       nontraffic V76.3 ☑
       while boarding or alighting V76.4 ☑
      nontraffic V70.3 ☑
      while boarding or alighting V70.4 ☑
     animal-drawn vehicle (traffic) V76.9 ☑
      nontraffic V76.3 ☑
      while boarding or alighting V76.4 ☑
     bus (traffic) V74.9 ☑
      nontraffic V74.3 ☑
      while boarding or alighting V74.4 ☑
     car (traffic) V73.9 ☑
      nontraffic V73.3 ☑
      while boarding or alighting V73.4 ☑
     motor vehicle NOS (traffic) V79.60 ☑
      nontraffic V79.20 ☑
      specified type NEC (traffic) V79.69 ☑
       nontraffic V79.29 ☑
     pedal cycle (traffic) V71.9 ☑
      nontraffic V71.3 ☑
      while boarding or alighting V71.4 ☑
     pickup truck (traffic) V73.9 ☑
      nontraffic V73.3 ☑
      while boarding or alighting V73.4 ☑
     railway vehicle (traffic) V75.9 ☑
      nontraffic V75.3 ☑
      while boarding or alighting V75.4 ☑
     specified vehicle NEC (traffic) V76.9 ☑
      nontraffic V76.3 ☑
      while boarding or alighting V76.4 ☑
     stationary object (traffic) V77.9 ☑
      nontraffic V77.3 ☑
      while boarding or alighting V77.4 ☑
     streetcar (traffic) V76.9 ☑
      nontraffic V76.3 ☑
      while boarding or alighting V76.4 ☑
     three wheeled motor vehicle (traffic) V72.9 ☑
      nontraffic V72.3 ☑
      while boarding or alighting V72.4 ☑
     truck (traffic) V74.9 ☑
      nontraffic V74.3 ☑
      while boarding or alighting V74.4 ☑
     two wheeled motor vehicle (traffic) V72.9 ☑
      nontraffic V72.3 ☑
      while boarding or alighting V72.4 ☑
     van (traffic) V73.9 ☑
      nontraffic V73.3 ☑
      while boarding or alighting V73.4 ☑
    driver
     collision (with)
      animal (traffic) V70.5 ☑
       being ridden (traffic) V76.5 ☑
        nontraffic V76.0 ☑
       nontraffic V70.0 ☑

Accident — *continued*
  transport — *continued*
      animal-drawn vehicle (traffic) V76.5 ☑
       nontraffic V76.0 ☑
      bus (traffic) V74.5 ☑
       nontraffic V74.0 ☑
      car (traffic) V73.5 ☑
       nontraffic V73.0 ☑
      motor vehicle NOS (traffic) V79.40 ☑
       nontraffic V79.00 ☑
      specified type NEC (traffic) V79.49 ☑
       nontraffic V79.09 ☑
      pedal cycle (traffic) V71.5 ☑
       nontraffic V71.0 ☑
      pickup truck (traffic) V73.5 ☑
       nontraffic V73.0 ☑
      railway vehicle (traffic) V75.5 ☑
       nontraffic V75.0 ☑
      specified vehicle NEC (traffic) V76.5 ☑
       nontraffic V76.0 ☑
      stationary object (traffic) V77.5 ☑
       nontraffic V77.0 ☑
      streetcar (traffic) V76.5 ☑
       nontraffic V76.0 ☑
      three wheeled motor vehicle (traffic) V72.5 ☑
       nontraffic V72.0 ☑
      truck (traffic) V74.5 ☑
       nontraffic V74.0 ☑
      two wheeled motor vehicle (traffic) V72.5 ☑
       nontraffic V72.0 ☑
      van (traffic) V73.5 ☑
       nontraffic V73.0 ☑
     noncollision accident (traffic) V78.5 ☑
      nontraffic V78.0 ☑
    noncollision accident (traffic) V78.9 ☑
     nontraffic V78.3 ☑
     while boarding or alighting V78.4 ☑
    nontraffic V79.3 ☑
    hanger-on
     collision (with)
      animal (traffic) V70.7 ☑
       being ridden (traffic) V76.7 ☑
        nontraffic V76.2 ☑
       nontraffic V70.2 ☑
      animal-drawn vehicle (traffic) V76.7 ☑
       nontraffic V76.2 ☑
      bus (traffic) V74.7 ☑
       nontraffic V74.2 ☑
      car (traffic) V73.7 ☑
       nontraffic V73.2 ☑
      pedal cycle (traffic) V71.7 ☑
       nontraffic V71.2 ☑
      pickup truck (traffic) V73.7 ☑
       nontraffic V73.2 ☑
      railway vehicle (traffic) V75.7 ☑
       nontraffic V75.2 ☑
      specified vehicle NEC (traffic) V76.7 ☑
       nontraffic V76.2 ☑
      stationary object (traffic) V77.7 ☑
       nontraffic V77.2 ☑
      streetcar (traffic) V76.7 ☑
       nontraffic V76.2 ☑
      three wheeled motor vehicle (traffic) V72.7 ☑
       nontraffic V72.2 ☑
      truck (traffic) V74.7 ☑
       nontraffic V74.2 ☑
      two wheeled motor vehicle (traffic) V72.7 ☑
       nontraffic V72.2 ☑
      van (traffic) V73.7 ☑
       nontraffic V73.2 ☑
     noncollision accident (traffic) V78.7 ☑
      nontraffic V78.2 ☑
    passenger
     collision (with)
      animal (traffic) V70.6 ☑
       being ridden (traffic) V76.6 ☑
        nontraffic V76.1 ☑
       nontraffic V70.1 ☑
      animal-drawn vehicle (traffic) V76.6 ☑
       nontraffic V76.1 ☑
      bus (traffic) V74.6 ☑
       nontraffic V74.1 ☑
      car (traffic) V73.6 ☑
       nontraffic V73.1 ☑
      motor vehicle NOS (traffic) V79.50 ☑
       nontraffic V79.10 ☑
      specified type NEC (traffic) V79.59 ☑
       nontraffic V79.19 ☑

Accident — *continued*
  transport — *continued*
    pedal cycle (traffic) V71.6 ☑
      nontraffic V71.1 ☑
    pickup truck (traffic) V73.6 ☑
      nontraffic V73.1 ☑
    railway vehicle (traffic) V75.6 ☑
      nontraffic V75.1 ☑
    specified vehicle NEC (traffic) V76.6 ☑
      nontraffic V76.1 ☑
    stationary object (traffic) V77.6 ☑
      nontraffic V77.1 ☑
    streetcar (traffic) V76.6 ☑
      nontraffic V76.1 ☑
    three wheeled motor vehicle (traffic)
      V72.6 ☑
      nontraffic V72.1 ☑
    truck (traffic) V74.6 ☑
      nontraffic V74.1 ☑
    two wheeled motor vehicle (traffic)
      V72.6 ☑
      nontraffic V72.1 ☑
    van (traffic) V73.6 ☑
      nontraffic V73.1 ☑
   noncollision accident (traffic) V78.6 ☑
    nontraffic V78.1 ☑
  specified type NEC V79.88 ☑
   military vehicle V79.81 ☑
 cable car, not on rails V98.0 ☑
  on rails — *see* Accident, transport, streetcar
   occupant
 car occupant V49.9 ☑
  ambulance occupant — *see* Accident, transport,
   ambulance occupant
  collision (with)
   animal (traffic) V40.9 ☑
    being ridden (traffic) V46.9 ☑
     nontraffic V46.3 ☑
      while boarding or alighting V46.4 ☑
    nontraffic V40.3 ☑
    while boarding or alighting V40.4 ☑
   animal-drawn vehicle (traffic) V46.9 ☑
    nontraffic V46.3 ☑
    while boarding or alighting V46.4 ☑
   bus (traffic) V44.9 ☑
    nontraffic V44.3 ☑
    while boarding or alighting V44.4 ☑
   car (traffic) V43.92 ☑
    nontraffic V43.32 ☑
    while boarding or alighting V43.42 ☑
   motor vehicle NOS (traffic) V49.60 ☑
    nontraffic V49.20 ☑
    specified type NEC (traffic) V49.69 ☑
     nontraffic V49.29 ☑
   pedal cycle (traffic) V41.9 ☑
    nontraffic V41.3 ☑
    while boarding or alighting V41.4 ☑
   pickup truck (traffic) V43.93 ☑
    nontraffic V43.33 ☑
    while boarding or alighting V43.43 ☑
   railway vehicle (traffic) V45.9 ☑
    nontraffic V45.3 ☑
    while boarding or alighting V45.4 ☑
   specified vehicle NEC (traffic) V46.9 ☑
    nontraffic V46.3 ☑
    while boarding or alighting V46.4 ☑
   sport utility vehicle (traffic) V43.91 ☑
    nontraffic V43.31 ☑
    while boarding or alighting V43.41 ☑
   stationary object (traffic) V47.9 ☑
    nontraffic V47.3 ☑
    while boarding or alighting V47.4 ☑
   streetcar (traffic) V46.9 ☑
    nontraffic V46.3 ☑
    while boarding or alighting V46.4 ☑
   three wheeled motor vehicle (traffic) V42.9 ☑
    nontraffic V42.3 ☑
    while boarding or alighting V42.4 ☑
   truck (traffic) V44.9 ☑
    nontraffic V44.3 ☑
    while boarding or alighting V44.4 ☑
   two wheeled motor vehicle (traffic) V42.9 ☑
    nontraffic V42.3 ☑
    while boarding or alighting V42.4 ☑
   van (traffic) V43.94 ☑
    nontraffic V43.34 ☑
    while boarding or alighting V43.44 ☑
  driver
   collision (with)
    animal (traffic) V40.5 ☑
     being ridden (traffic) V46.5 ☑
      nontraffic V46.0 ☑

Accident — *continued*
  transport — *continued*
    nontraffic V40.0 ☑
   animal-drawn vehicle (traffic) V46.5 ☑
    nontraffic V46.0 ☑
   bus (traffic) V44.5 ☑
    nontraffic V44.0 ☑
   car (traffic) V43.52 ☑
    nontraffic V43.02 ☑
   motor vehicle NOS (traffic) V49.40 ☑
    nontraffic V49.00 ☑
    specified type NEC (traffic) V49.49 ☑
     nontraffic V49.09 ☑
   pedal cycle (traffic) V41.5 ☑
    nontraffic V41.0 ☑
   pickup truck (traffic) V43.53 ☑
    nontraffic V43.03 ☑
   railway vehicle (traffic) V45.5 ☑
    nontraffic V45.0 ☑
   specified vehicle NEC (traffic) V46.5 ☑
    nontraffic V46.0 ☑
   sport utility vehicle (traffic) V43.51 ☑
    nontraffic V43.01 ☑
   stationary object (traffic) V47.5 ☑
    nontraffic V47.0 ☑
   streetcar (traffic) V46.5 ☑
    nontraffic V46.0 ☑
   three wheeled motor vehicle (traffic)
    V42.5 ☑
    nontraffic V42.0 ☑
   truck (traffic) V44.5 ☑
    nontraffic V44.0 ☑
   two wheeled motor vehicle (traffic)
    V42.5 ☑
    nontraffic V42.0 ☑
   van (traffic) V43.54 ☑
    nontraffic V43.04 ☑
   noncollision accident (traffic) V48.5 ☑
    nontraffic V48.0 ☑
  noncollision accident (traffic) V48.9 ☑
   nontraffic V48.3 ☑
   while boarding or alighting V48.4 ☑
  nontraffic V49.3 ☑
  hanger-on
   collision (with)
    animal (traffic) V40.7 ☑
     being ridden (traffic) V46.7 ☑
      nontraffic V46.2 ☑
     nontraffic V40.2 ☑
   animal-drawn vehicle (traffic) V46.7 ☑
    nontraffic V46.2 ☑
   bus (traffic) V44.7 ☑
    nontraffic V44.2 ☑
   car (traffic) V43.72 ☑
    nontraffic V43.22 ☑
   pedal cycle (traffic) V41.7 ☑
    nontraffic V41.2 ☑
   pickup truck (traffic) V43.73 ☑
    nontraffic V43.23 ☑
   railway vehicle (traffic) V45.7 ☑
    nontraffic V45.2 ☑
   specified vehicle NEC (traffic) V46.7 ☑
    nontraffic V46.2 ☑
   sport utility vehicle (traffic) V43.71 ☑
    nontraffic V43.21 ☑
   stationary object (traffic) V47.7 ☑
    nontraffic V47.2 ☑
   streetcar (traffic) V46.7 ☑
    nontraffic V46.2 ☑
   three wheeled motor vehicle (traffic)
    V42.7 ☑
    nontraffic V42.2 ☑
   truck (traffic) V44.7 ☑
    nontraffic V44.2 ☑
   two wheeled motor vehicle (traffic)
    V42.7 ☑
    nontraffic V42.2 ☑
   van (traffic) V43.74 ☑
    nontraffic V43.24 ☑
   noncollision accident (traffic) V48.7 ☑
    nontraffic V48.2 ☑
  passenger
   collision (with)
    animal (traffic) V40.6 ☑
     being ridden (traffic) V46.6 ☑
      nontraffic V46.1 ☑
     nontraffic V40.1 ☑
   animal-drawn vehicle (traffic) V46.6 ☑
    nontraffic V46.1 ☑
   bus (traffic) V44.6 ☑
    nontraffic V44.1 ☑
   car (traffic) V43.62 ☑

Accident — *continued*
  transport — *continued*
    nontraffic V43.12 ☑
   motor vehicle NOS (traffic) V49.50 ☑
    nontraffic V49.10 ☑
    specified type NEC (traffic) V49.59 ☑
     nontraffic V49.19 ☑
   pedal cycle (traffic) V41.6 ☑
    nontraffic V41.1 ☑
   pickup truck (traffic) V43.63 ☑
    nontraffic V43.13 ☑
   railway vehicle (traffic) V45.6 ☑
    nontraffic V45.1 ☑
   specified vehicle NEC (traffic) V46.6 ☑
    nontraffic V46.1 ☑
   sport utility vehicle (traffic) V43.61 ☑
    nontraffic V43.11 ☑
   stationary object (traffic) V47.6 ☑
    nontraffic V47.1 ☑
   streetcar (traffic) V46.6 ☑
    nontraffic V46.1 ☑
   three wheeled motor vehicle (traffic)
    V42.6 ☑
    nontraffic V42.1 ☑
   truck (traffic) V44.6 ☑
    nontraffic V44.1 ☑
   two wheeled motor vehicle (traffic)
    V42.6 ☑
    nontraffic V42.1 ☑
   van (traffic) V43.64 ☑
    nontraffic V43.14 ☑
   noncollision accident (traffic) V48.6 ☑
    nontraffic V48.1 ☑
   specified type NEC V49.88 ☑
    military vehicle V49.81 ☑
 coal car — *see* Accident, transport, industrial
  vehicle occupant
 construction vehicle occupant (nontraffic)
  V85.9 ☑
  driver V85.5 ☑
  hanger-on V85.7 ☑
  passenger V85.6 ☑
  traffic V85.3 ☑
   driver V85.0 ☑
   hanger-on V85.2 ☑
   passenger V85.1 ☑
  while boarding or alighting V85.4 ☑
 dirt bike rider (nontraffic) V86.96 ☑
  driver V86.56 ☑
  hanger-on V86.76 ☑
  passenger V86.66 ☑
  traffic V86.36 ☑
   driver V86.06 ☑
   hanger-on V86.26 ☑
   passenger V86.16 ☑
  while boarding or alighting V86.46 ☑
 due to cataclysm — *see* Forces of nature, by type
 dune buggy occupant (nontraffic) V86.93 ☑
  driver V86.53 ☑
  hanger-on V86.73 ☑
  passenger V86.63 ☑
  traffic V86.33 ☑
   driver V86.03 ☑
   hanger-on V86.23 ☑
   passenger V86.13 ☑
  while boarding or alighting V86.43 ☑
 forklift — *see* Accident, transport, industrial
  vehicle occupant
 go cart — *see* Accident, transport, all-terrain
  vehicle occupant
 golf cart — *see* Accident, transport, all-terrain
  vehicle occupant
 heavy transport vehicle occupant — *see* Accident,
  transport, truck occupant
 ice yacht V98.2 ☑
 industrial vehicle occupant (nontraffic) V83.9 ☑
  driver V83.5 ☑
  hanger-on V83.7 ☑
  passenger V83.6 ☑
  traffic V83.3 ☑
   driver V83.0 ☑
   hanger-on V83.2 ☑
   passenger V83.1 ☑
  while boarding or alighting V83.4 ☑
 interurban electric car — *see* Accident, transport,
  streetcar
 land yacht V98.1 ☑
 logging car — *see* Accident, transport, industrial
  vehicle occupant
 military vehicle occupant (traffic) V86.34 ☑
  driver V86.04 ☑
  hanger-on V86.24 ☑

Accident

Accident

ICD-10-CM INDEX TO EXTERNAL CAUSES OF INJURIES

Accident — *continued*
  transport — *continued*
    nontraffic V86.94 ☑
      driver V86.54 ☑
      hanger-on V86.74 ☑
      passenger V86.64 ☑
      passenger V86.14 ☑
      while boarding or alighting V86.44 ☑
    mine tram — *see* Accident, transport, industrial vehicle occupant
    motorcoach — *see* Accident, transport, bus occupant
    motor/cross bike rider (*see also* Accident, transport, dirt bike rider) V86.96 ☑
    motorcyclist V29.9 ☑
      collision (with)
        animal (traffic) V20.9 ☑
          being ridden (traffic) V26.9 ☑
            nontraffic V26.2 ☑
            while boarding or alighting V26.3 ☑
          nontraffic V20.2 ☑
          while boarding or alighting V20.3 ☑
        animal-drawn vehicle (traffic) V26.9 ☑
          nontraffic V26.2 ☑
          while boarding or alighting V26.3 ☑
        bus (traffic) V24.9 ☑
          nontraffic V24.2 ☑
          while boarding or alighting V24.3 ☑
        car (traffic) V23.9 ☑
          nontraffic V23.2 ☑
          while boarding or alighting V23.3 ☑
        motor vehicle NOS (traffic) V29.60 ☑
          nontraffic V29.20 ☑
          specified type NEC (traffic) V29.69 ☑
            nontraffic V29.29 ☑
        pedal cycle (traffic) V21.9 ☑
          nontraffic V21.2 ☑
          while boarding or alighting V21.3 ☑
        pickup truck (traffic) V23.9 ☑
          nontraffic V23.2 ☑
          while boarding or alighting V23.3 ☑
        railway vehicle (traffic) V25.9 ☑
          nontraffic V25.2 ☑
          while boarding or alighting V25.3 ☑
        specified vehicle NEC (traffic) V26.9 ☑
          nontraffic V26.2 ☑
          while boarding or alighting V26.3 ☑
        stationary object (traffic) V27.9 ☑
          nontraffic V27.2 ☑
          while boarding or alighting V27.3 ☑
        streetcar (traffic) V26.9 ☑
          nontraffic V26.2 ☑
          while boarding or alighting V26.3 ☑
        three wheeled motor vehicle (traffic) V22.9 ☑
          nontraffic V22.2 ☑
          while boarding or alighting V22.3 ☑
        truck (traffic) V24.9 ☑
          nontraffic V24.2 ☑
          while boarding or alighting V24.3 ☑
        two wheeled motor vehicle (traffic) V22.9 ☑
          nontraffic V22.2 ☑
          while boarding or alighting V22.3 ☑
        van (traffic) V23.9 ☑
          nontraffic V23.2 ☑
          while boarding or alighting V23.3 ☑
      driver
        collision (with)
          animal (traffic) V20.4 ☑
            being ridden (traffic) V26.4 ☑
              nontraffic V26.0 ☑
            nontraffic V20.0 ☑
          animal-drawn vehicle (traffic) V26.4 ☑
            nontraffic V26.0 ☑
          bus (traffic) V24.4 ☑
            nontraffic V24.0 ☑
          car (traffic) V23.4 ☑
            nontraffic V23.0 ☑
          motor vehicle NOS (traffic) V29.40 ☑
            nontraffic V29.00 ☑
          specified type NEC (traffic) V29.49 ☑
            nontraffic V29.09 ☑
          pedal cycle (traffic) V21.4 ☑
            nontraffic V21.0 ☑
          pickup truck (traffic) V23.4 ☑
            nontraffic V23.0 ☑
          railway vehicle (traffic) V25.4 ☑
            nontraffic V25.0 ☑
          specified vehicle NEC (traffic) V26.4 ☑
            nontraffic V26.0 ☑
          stationary object (traffic) V27.4 ☑
            nontraffic V27.0 ☑
          streetcar (traffic) V26.4 ☑

Accident — *continued*
  transport — *continued*
          nontraffic V26.0 ☑
        three wheeled motor vehicle (traffic) V22.4 ☑
          nontraffic V22.0 ☑
        truck (traffic) V24.4 ☑
          nontraffic V24.0 ☑
        two wheeled motor vehicle (traffic) V22.4 ☑
          nontraffic V22.0 ☑
        van (traffic) V23.4 ☑
          nontraffic V23.0 ☑
      noncollision accident (traffic) V28.4 ☑
        nontraffic V28.0 ☑
      noncollision accident (traffic) V28.9 ☑
        nontraffic V28.2 ☑
        while boarding or alighting V28.3 ☑
      nontraffic V29.3 ☑
      passenger
        collision (with)
          animal (traffic) V20.5 ☑
            being ridden (traffic) V26.5 ☑
              nontraffic V26.1 ☑
            nontraffic V20.1 ☑
          animal-drawn vehicle (traffic) V26.5 ☑
            nontraffic V26.1 ☑
          bus (traffic) V24.5 ☑
            nontraffic V24.1 ☑
          car (traffic) V23.5 ☑
            nontraffic V23.1 ☑
          motor vehicle NOS (traffic) V29.50 ☑
            nontraffic V29.10 ☑
          specified type NEC (traffic) V29.59 ☑
            nontraffic V29.19 ☑
          pedal cycle (traffic) V21.5 ☑
            nontraffic V21.1 ☑
          pickup truck (traffic) V23.5 ☑
            nontraffic V23.1 ☑
          railway vehicle (traffic) V25.5 ☑
            nontraffic V25.1 ☑
          specified vehicle NEC (traffic) V26.5 ☑
            nontraffic V26.1 ☑
          stationary object (traffic) V27.5 ☑
            nontraffic V27.1 ☑
          streetcar (traffic) V26.5 ☑
            nontraffic V26.1 ☑
          three wheeled motor vehicle (traffic) V22.5 ☑
            nontraffic V22.1 ☑
          truck (traffic) V24.5 ☑
            nontraffic V24.1 ☑
          two wheeled motor vehicle (traffic) V22.5 ☑
            nontraffic V22.1 ☑
          van (traffic) V23.5 ☑
            nontraffic V23.1 ☑
        noncollision accident (traffic) V28.5 ☑
          nontraffic V28.1 ☑
      specified type NEC V29.88 ☑
      military vehicle V29.81 ☑
    motor vehicle NEC occupant (traffic) V89.2 ☑
    occupant (of)
      aircraft (powered) V95.9 ☑
        fixed wing
          commercial — *see* Accident, transport, aircraft, occupant, powered, fixed wing, commercial
          private — *see* Accident, transport, aircraft, occupant, powered, fixed wing, private
        nonpowered V96.9 ☑
        specified NEC V95.8 ☑
      airport battery-powered vehicle — *see* Accident, transport, industrial vehicle occupant
      all-terrain vehicle (ATV) — *see* Accident, transport, all-terrain vehicle occupant
      animal-drawn vehicle — *see* Accident, transport, animal-drawn vehicle occupant
      automobile — *see* Accident, transport, car occupant
      balloon V96.00 ☑
      battery-powered vehicle — *see* Accident, transport, industrial vehicle occupant
      bicycle — *see* Accident, transport, pedal cyclist
        motorized — *see* Accident, transport, motorcycle rider
      boat NEC — *see* Accident, watercraft
      bulldozer — *see* Accident, transport, construction vehicle occupant
      bus — *see* Accident, transport, bus occupant

Accident — *continued*
  transport — *continued*
      cable car (on rails) (*see also* Accident, transport, streetcar occupant)
        not on rails V98.0 ☑
      car (*see also* Accident, transport, car occupant)
        cable (on rails) (*see also* Accident, transport, streetcar occupant)
          not on rails V98.0 ☑
      coach — *see* Accident, transport, bus occupant
      coal-car — *see* Accident, transport, industrial vehicle occupant
      digger — *see* Accident, transport, construction vehicle occupant
      dump truck — *see* Accident, transport, construction vehicle occupant
      earth-leveler — *see* Accident, transport, construction vehicle occupant
      farm machinery (self-propelled) — *see* Accident, transport, agricultural vehicle occupant
      forklift — *see* Accident, transport, industrial vehicle occupant
      glider (unpowered) V96.20 ☑
        hang V96.10 ☑
        powered (microlight) (ultralight) — *see* Accident, transport, aircraft, occupant, powered, glider
      glider (unpowered) NEC V96.20 ☑
      hang-glider V96.10 ☑
      harvester — *see* Accident, transport, agricultural vehicle occupant
      heavy (transport) vehicle — *see* Accident, transport, truck occupant
      helicopter — *see* Accident, transport, aircraft, occupant, helicopter
      ice-yacht V98.2 ☑
      kite (carrying person) V96.8 ☑
      land-yacht V98.1 ☑
      logging car — *see* Accident, transport, industrial vehicle occupant
      mechanical shovel — *see* Accident, transport, construction vehicle occupant
      microlight — *see* Accident, transport, aircraft, occupant, powered, glider
      minibus — *see* Accident, transport, pickup truck occupant
      minivan — *see* Accident, transport, pickup truck occupant
      moped — *see* Accident, transport, motorcycle
      motor scooter — *see* Accident, transport, motorcycle
      motorcycle (with sidecar) — *see* Accident, transport, motorcycle
      off-road motor-vehicle (*see also* Accident, transport, all-terrain vehicle occupant) V86.99 ☑
      pedal cycle (*see also* Accident, transport, pedal cyclist)
      pick-up (truck) — *see* Accident, transport, pickup truck occupant
      railway (train) (vehicle) (subterranean) (elevated) — *see* Accident, transport, railway vehicle occupant
      rickshaw — *see* Accident, transport, pedal cycle
        motorized — *see* Accident, transport, three-wheeled motor vehicle
        pedal driven — *see* Accident, transport, pedal cyclist
      road-roller — *see* Accident, transport, construction vehicle occupant
      ship NOS V94.9 ☑
      ski-lift (chair) (gondola) V98.3 ☑
      snowmobile — *see* Accident, transport, snowmobile occupant
      spacecraft, spaceship — *see* Accident, transport, aircraft, occupant, spacecraft
      sport utility vehicle — *see* Accident, transport, pickup truck occupant
      streetcar (interurban) (operating on public street or highway) — *see* Accident, transport, streetcar occupant
      SUV — *see* Accident, transport, pickup truck occupant
      téléférique V98.0 ☑
      three-wheeled vehicle (motorized) (*see also* Accident, transport, three-wheeled motor vehicle occupant)
        nonmotorized — *see* Accident, transport, pedal cycle
      tractor (farm) (and trailer) — *see* Accident, transport, agricultural vehicle occupant

☑ **Additional character required**

Accident — continued
  transport — continued
    train — see Accident, transport, railway vehicle occupant
    tram — see Accident, transport, streetcar occupant
      in mine or quarry — see Accident, transport, industrial vehicle occupant
    tricycle — see Accident, transport, pedal cycle
      motorized — see Accident, transport, three-wheeled motor vehicle
    trolley — see Accident, transport, streetcar occupant
      in mine or quarry — see Accident, transport, industrial vehicle occupant
    tub, in mine or quarry — see Accident, transport, industrial vehicle occupant
    ultralight — see Accident, transport, aircraft, occupant, powered, glider
    van — see Accident, transport, van occupant
    vehicle NEC V89.9 ☑
      heavy transport — see Accident, transport, truck occupant
      motor (traffic) NEC V89.2 ☑
        nontraffic NEC V89.0 ☑
    watercraft NOS V94.9 ☑
      causing drowning — see Drowning, resulting from accident to boat
  off-road motor-vehicle (see also Accident, transport, all-terrain vehicle occupant) V86.99 ☑
  parachutist V97.29 ☑
    after accident to aircraft — see Accident, transport, aircraft
    entangled in object V97.21 ☑
    injured on landing V97.22 ☑
  pedal cyclist V19.9 ☑
    collision (with)
      animal (traffic) V10.9 ☑
        being ridden (traffic) V16.9 ☑
          nontraffic V16.2 ☑
            while boarding or alighting V16.3 ☑
        nontraffic V10.2 ☑
          while boarding or alighting V10.3 ☑
      animal-drawn vehicle (traffic) V16.9 ☑
        nontraffic V16.2 ☑
          while boarding or alighting V16.3 ☑
      bus (traffic) V14.9 ☑
        nontraffic V14.2 ☑
          while boarding or alighting V14.3 ☑
      car (traffic) V13.9 ☑
        nontraffic V13.2 ☑
          while boarding or alighting V13.3 ☑
      motor vehicle NOS (traffic) V19.60 ☑
        nontraffic V19.20 ☑
        specified type NEC (traffic) V19.69 ☑
          nontraffic V19.29 ☑
      pedal cycle (traffic) V11.9 ☑
        nontraffic V11.2 ☑
          while boarding or alighting V11.3 ☑
      pickup truck (traffic) V13.9 ☑
        nontraffic V13.2 ☑
          while boarding or alighting V13.3 ☑
      railway vehicle (traffic) V15.9 ☑
        nontraffic V15.2 ☑
          while boarding or alighting V15.3 ☑
      specified vehicle NEC (traffic) V16.9 ☑
        nontraffic V16.2 ☑
          while boarding or alighting V16.3 ☑
      stationary object (traffic) V17.9 ☑
        nontraffic V17.2 ☑
          while boarding or alighting V17.3 ☑
      streetcar (traffic) V16.9 ☑
        nontraffic V16.2 ☑
          while boarding or alighting V16.3 ☑
      three wheeled motor vehicle (traffic) V12.9 ☑
        nontraffic V12.2 ☑
          while boarding or alighting V12.3 ☑
      truck (traffic) V14.9 ☑
        nontraffic V14.2 ☑
          while boarding or alighting V14.3 ☑
      two wheeled motor vehicle (traffic) V12.9 ☑
        nontraffic V12.2 ☑
          while boarding or alighting V12.3 ☑
      van (traffic) V13.9 ☑
        nontraffic V13.2 ☑
          while boarding or alighting V13.3 ☑
    driver
      collision (with)
        animal (traffic) V10.4 ☑
          being ridden (traffic) V16.4 ☑

Accident — continued
  transport — continued
          nontraffic V16.0 ☑
        nontraffic V10.0 ☑
        animal-drawn vehicle (traffic) V16.4 ☑
          nontraffic V16.0 ☑
        bus (traffic) V14.4 ☑
          nontraffic V14.0 ☑
        car (traffic) V13.4 ☑
          nontraffic V13.0 ☑
        motor vehicle NOS (traffic) V19.40 ☑
          nontraffic V19.00 ☑
          specified type NEC (traffic) V19.49 ☑
            nontraffic V19.09 ☑
        pedal cycle (traffic) V11.4 ☑
          nontraffic V11.0 ☑
        pickup truck (traffic) V13.4 ☑
          nontraffic V13.0 ☑
        railway vehicle (traffic) V15.4 ☑
          nontraffic V15.0 ☑
        specified vehicle NEC (traffic) V16.4 ☑
          nontraffic V16.0 ☑
        stationary object (traffic) V17.4 ☑
          nontraffic V17.0 ☑
        streetcar (traffic) V16.4 ☑
          nontraffic V16.0 ☑
        three wheeled motor vehicle (traffic) V12.4 ☑
          nontraffic V12.0 ☑
        truck (traffic) V14.4 ☑
          nontraffic V14.0 ☑
        two wheeled motor vehicle (traffic) V12.4 ☑
          nontraffic V12.0 ☑
        van (traffic) V13.4 ☑
          nontraffic V13.0 ☑
      noncollision accident (traffic) V18.4 ☑
        nontraffic V18.0 ☑
    noncollision accident (traffic) V18.9 ☑
      nontraffic V18.2 ☑
      while boarding or alighting V18.3 ☑
    nontraffic V19.3 ☑
    passenger
      collision (with)
        animal (traffic) V10.5 ☑
          being ridden (traffic) V16.5 ☑
            nontraffic V16.1 ☑
          nontraffic V10.1 ☑
        animal-drawn vehicle (traffic) V16.5 ☑
          nontraffic V16.1 ☑
        bus (traffic) V14.5 ☑
          nontraffic V14.1 ☑
        car (traffic) V13.5 ☑
          nontraffic V13.1 ☑
        motor vehicle NOS (traffic) V19.50 ☑
          nontraffic V19.10 ☑
          specified type NEC (traffic) V19.59 ☑
            nontraffic V19.19 ☑
        pedal cycle (traffic) V11.5 ☑
          nontraffic V11.1 ☑
        pickup truck (traffic) V13.5 ☑
          nontraffic V13.1 ☑
        railway vehicle (traffic) V15.5 ☑
          nontraffic V15.1 ☑
        specified vehicle NEC (traffic) V16.5 ☑
          nontraffic V16.1 ☑
        stationary object (traffic) V17.5 ☑
          nontraffic V17.1 ☑
        streetcar (traffic) V16.5 ☑
          nontraffic V16.1 ☑
        three wheeled motor vehicle (traffic) V12.5 ☑
          nontraffic V12.1 ☑
        truck (traffic) V14.5 ☑
          nontraffic V14.1 ☑
        two wheeled motor vehicle (traffic) V12.5 ☑
          nontraffic V12.1 ☑
        van (traffic) V13.5 ☑
          nontraffic V13.1 ☑
      noncollision accident (traffic) V18.5 ☑
        nontraffic V18.1 ☑
    specified type NEC V19.88 ☑
    military vehicle V19.81 ☑
  pedestrian
    conveyance (occupant) V09.9 ☑
      baby stroller V00.828 ☑
        collision (with) V09.9 ☑
          animal being ridden or animal drawn vehicle V06.99 ☑
            nontraffic V06.09 ☑
            traffic V06.19 ☑

Accident — continued
  transport — continued
        bus or heavy transport V04.99 ☑
          nontraffic V04.09 ☑
          traffic V04.19 ☑
        car V03.99 ☑
          nontraffic V03.09 ☑
          traffic V03.19 ☑
        pedal cycle V01.99 ☑
          nontraffic V01.09 ☑
          traffic V01.19 ☑
        pick-up truck or van V03.99 ☑
          nontraffic V03.09 ☑
          traffic V03.19 ☑
        railway (train) (vehicle) V05.99 ☑
          nontraffic V05.09 ☑
          traffic V05.19 ☑
        streetcar V06.99 ☑
          nontraffic V06.09 ☑
          traffic V06.19 ☑
        stationary object V00.822 ☑
        two- or three-wheeled motor vehicle V02.99 ☑
          nontraffic V02.09 ☑
          traffic V02.19 ☑
        vehicle V09.9 ☑
          animal-drawn V06.99 ☑
            nontraffic V06.09 ☑
            traffic V06.19 ☑
          motor
            nontraffic V09.00 ☑
            traffic V09.20 ☑
      fall V00.821 ☑
      nontraffic V09.1 ☑
        involving motor vehicle NEC V09.00 ☑
      traffic V09.3 ☑
        involving motor vehicle NEC V09.20 ☑
    flat-bottomed NEC V00.388 ☑
      collision (with) V09.9 ☑
        animal being ridden or animal drawn vehicle V06.99 ☑
          nontraffic V06.09 ☑
          traffic V06.19 ☑
        bus or heavy transport V04.99 ☑
          nontraffic V04.09 ☑
          traffic V04.19 ☑
        car V03.99 ☑
          nontraffic V03.09 ☑
          traffic V03.19 ☑
        pedal cycle V01.99 ☑
          nontraffic V01.09 ☑
          traffic V01.19 ☑
        pick-up truck or van V03.99 ☑
          nontraffic V03.09 ☑
          traffic V03.19 ☑
        railway (train) (vehicle) V05.99 ☑
          nontraffic V05.09 ☑
          traffic V05.19 ☑
        stationary object V00.382 ☑
        streetcar V06.99 ☑
          nontraffic V06.09 ☑
          traffic V06.19 ☑
        two- or three-wheeled motor vehicle V02.99 ☑
          nontraffic V02.09 ☑
          traffic V02.19 ☑
        vehicle V09.9 ☑
          animal-drawn V06.99 ☑
            nontraffic V06.09 ☑
            traffic V06.19 ☑
          motor
            nontraffic V09.00 ☑
            traffic V09.20 ☑
      fall V00.381 ☑
      nontraffic V09.1 ☑
        involving motor vehicle NEC V09.00 ☑
      snow
        board — see Accident, transport, pedestrian, conveyance, snow board
        ski — see Accident, transport, pedestrian, conveyance, skis (snow)
      traffic V09.3 ☑
        involving motor vehicle NEC V09.20 ☑
    gliding type NEC V00.288 ☑
      collision (with) V09.9 ☑
        animal being ridden or animal drawn vehicle V06.99 ☑
          nontraffic V06.09 ☑
          traffic V06.19 ☑
        bus or heavy transport V04.99 ☑
          nontraffic V04.09 ☑

Accident

Accident — *continued*
  transport — *continued*
    traffic V04.19 ☑
    car V03.99 ☑
      nontraffic V03.09 ☑
      traffic V03.19 ☑
    pedal cycle V01.99 ☑
      nontraffic V01.09 ☑
      traffic V01.19 ☑
    pick-up truck or van V03.99 ☑
      nontraffic V03.09 ☑
      traffic V03.19 ☑
    railway (train) (vehicle) V05.99 ☑
      nontraffic V05.09 ☑
      traffic V05.19 ☑
    stationary object V00.282 ☑
    streetcar V06.99 ☑
      nontraffic V06.09 ☑
      traffic V06.19 ☑
    two- or three-wheeled motor vehicle
      V02.99 ☑
      nontraffic V02.09 ☑
      traffic V02.19 ☑
    vehicle V09.9 ☑
      animal-drawn V06.99 ☑
        nontraffic V06.09 ☑
        traffic V06.19 ☑
      motor
        nontraffic V09.00 ☑
        traffic V09.20 ☑
    fall V00.281 ☑
    heelies — *see* Accident, transport,
      pedestrian, conveyance, heelies
    ice skate — *see* Accident, transport,
      pedestrian, conveyance, ice skate
    nontraffic V09.1 ☑
      involving motor vehicle NEC V09.00 ☑
    sled — *see* Accident, transport, pedestrian,
      conveyance, sled
    traffic V09.3 ☑
      involving motor vehicle NEC V09.20 ☑
      wheelies — *see* Accident, transport,
        pedestrian, conveyance, heelies
  heelies V00.158 ☑
    colliding with stationary object V00.152 ☑
    fall V00.151 ☑
  ice skates V00.218 ☑
    collision (with) V09.9 ☑
      animal being ridden or animal drawn
        vehicle V06.99 ☑
        nontraffic V06.09 ☑
        traffic V06.19 ☑
      bus or heavy transport V04.99 ☑
        nontraffic V04.09 ☑
        traffic V04.19 ☑
      car V03.99 ☑
        nontraffic V03.09 ☑
        traffic V03.19 ☑
      pedal cycle V01.99 ☑
        nontraffic V01.09 ☑
        traffic V01.19 ☑
      pick-up truck or van V03.99 ☑
        nontraffic V03.09 ☑
        traffic V03.19 ☑
      railway (train) (vehicle) V05.99 ☑
        nontraffic V05.09 ☑
        traffic V05.19 ☑
      streetcar V06.99 ☑
        nontraffic V06.09 ☑
        traffic V06.19 ☑
      stationary object V00.212 ☑
      two- or three-wheeled motor vehicle
        V02.99 ☑
        nontraffic V02.09 ☑
        traffic V02.19 ☑
      vehicle V09.9 ☑
        animal-drawn V06.99 ☑
          nontraffic V06.09 ☑
          traffic V06.19 ☑
        motor
          nontraffic V09.00 ☑
          traffic V09.20 ☑
    fall V00.211 ☑
    nontraffic V09.1 ☑
      involving motor vehicle NEC V09.00 ☑
    traffic V09.3 ☑
      involving motor vehicle NEC V09.20 ☑
  motorized mobility scooter V00.838 ☑
    collision with stationary object V00.832 ☑
    fall from V00.831 ☑
  nontraffic V09.1 ☑
    involving motor vehicle V09.00 ☑

Accident — *continued*
  transport — *continued*
    military V09.01 ☑
    specified type NEC V09.09 ☑
  roller skates (non in-line) V00.128 ☑
    collision (with) V09.9 ☑
      animal being ridden or animal drawn
        vehicle V06.91 ☑
        nontraffic V06.01 ☑
        traffic V06.11 ☑
      bus or heavy transport V04.91 ☑
        nontraffic V04.01 ☑
        traffic V04.11 ☑
      car V03.91 ☑
        nontraffic V03.01 ☑
        traffic V03.11 ☑
      pedal cycle V01.91 ☑
        nontraffic V01.01 ☑
        traffic V01.11 ☑
      pick-up truck or van V03.91 ☑
        nontraffic V03.01 ☑
        traffic V03.11 ☑
      railway (train) (vehicle) V05.91 ☑
        nontraffic V05.01 ☑
        traffic V05.11 ☑
      streetcar V06.91 ☑
        nontraffic V06.01 ☑
        traffic V06.11 ☑
      stationary object V00.122 ☑
      two- or three-wheeled motor vehicle
        V02.91 ☑
        nontraffic V02.01 ☑
        traffic V02.11 ☑
      vehicle V09.9 ☑
        animal-drawn V06.91 ☑
          nontraffic V06.01 ☑
          traffic V06.11 ☑
        motor
          nontraffic V09.00 ☑
          traffic V09.20 ☑
    fall V00.121 ☑
    in-line V00.118 ☑
      collision — *see also* Accident, transport,
        pedestrian, conveyance occupant,
        roller skates, collision
        with stationary object V00.112 ☑
      fall V00.111 ☑
    nontraffic V09.1 ☑
      involving motor vehicle NEC V09.00 ☑
    traffic V09.3 ☑
      involving motor vehicle NEC V09.20 ☑
  rolling shoes V00.158 ☑
    colliding with stationary object V00.152 ☑
    fall V00.151 ☑
  rolling type NEC V00.188 ☑
    collision (with) V09.9 ☑
      animal being ridden or animal drawn
        vehicle V06.99 ☑
        nontraffic V06.09 ☑
        traffic V06.19 ☑
      bus or heavy transport V04.99 ☑
        nontraffic V04.09 ☑
        traffic V04.19 ☑
      car V03.99 ☑
        nontraffic V03.09 ☑
        traffic V03.19 ☑
      pedal cycle V01.99 ☑
        nontraffic V01.09 ☑
        traffic V01.19 ☑
      pick-up truck or van V03.99 ☑
        nontraffic V03.09 ☑
        traffic V03.19 ☑
      railway (train) (vehicle) V05.99 ☑
        nontraffic V05.09 ☑
        traffic V05.19 ☑
      stationary object V00.182 ☑
      streetcar V06.99 ☑
        nontraffic V06.09 ☑
        traffic V06.19 ☑
      two- or three-wheeled motor vehicle
        V02.99 ☑
        nontraffic V02.09 ☑
        traffic V02.19 ☑
      vehicle V09.9 ☑
        animal-drawn V06.99 ☑
          nontraffic V06.09 ☑
          traffic V06.19 ☑
        motor
          nontraffic V09.00 ☑
          traffic V09.20 ☑
    fall V00.181 ☑

Accident — *continued*
  transport — *continued*
    in-line roller skate — *see* Accident,
      transport, pedestrian, conveyance,
      roller skate, in-line
    nontraffic V09.1 ☑
      involving motor vehicle NEC V09.00 ☑
    roller skate — *see* Accident, transport,
      pedestrian, conveyance, roller skate
    scooter (non-motorized) — *see* Accident,
      transport, pedestrian, conveyance,
      scooter
    skateboard — *see* Accident, transport,
      pedestrian, conveyance, skateboard
    traffic V09.3 ☑
      involving motor vehicle NEC V09.20 ☑
  scooter (non-motorized) V00.148 ☑
    collision (with) V09.9 ☑
      animal being ridden or animal drawn
        vehicle V06.99 ☑
        nontraffic V06.09 ☑
        traffic V06.19 ☑
      bus or heavy transport V04.99 ☑
        nontraffic V04.09 ☑
        traffic V04.19 ☑
      car V03.99 ☑
        nontraffic V03.09 ☑
        traffic V03.19 ☑
      pedal cycle V01.99 ☑
        nontraffic V01.09 ☑
        traffic V01.19 ☑
      pick-up truck or van V03.99 ☑
        nontraffic V03.09 ☑
        traffic V03.19 ☑
      railway (train) (vehicle) V05.99 ☑
        nontraffic V05.09 ☑
        traffic V05.19 ☑
      streetcar V06.99 ☑
        nontraffic V06.09 ☑
        traffic V06.19 ☑
      stationary object V00.142 ☑
      two- or three-wheeled motor vehicle
        V02.99 ☑
        nontraffic V02.09 ☑
        traffic V02.19 ☑
      vehicle V09.9 ☑
        animal-drawn V06.99 ☑
          nontraffic V06.09 ☑
          traffic V06.19 ☑
        motor
          nontraffic V09.00 ☑
          traffic V09.20 ☑
    fall V00.141 ☑
    nontraffic V09.1 ☑
      involving motor vehicle NEC V09.00 ☑
    traffic V09.3 ☑
      involving motor vehicle NEC V09.20 ☑
  skate board V00.138 ☑
    collision (with) V09.9 ☑
      animal being ridden or animal drawn
        vehicle V06.92 ☑
        nontraffic V06.02 ☑
        traffic V06.12 ☑
      bus or heavy transport V04.92 ☑
        nontraffic V04.02 ☑
        traffic V04.12 ☑
      car V03.92 ☑
        nontraffic V03.02 ☑
        traffic V03.12 ☑
      pedal cycle V01.92 ☑
        nontraffic V01.02 ☑
        traffic V01.12 ☑
      pick-up truck or van V03.92 ☑
        nontraffic V03.02 ☑
        traffic V03.12 ☑
      railway (train) (vehicle) V05.92 ☑
        nontraffic V05.02 ☑
        traffic V05.12 ☑
      streetcar V06.92 ☑
        nontraffic V06.02 ☑
        traffic V06.12 ☑
      stationary object V00.132 ☑
      two- or three-wheeled motor vehicle
        V02.92 ☑
        nontraffic V02.02 ☑
        traffic V02.12 ☑
      vehicle V09.9 ☑
        animal-drawn V06.92 ☑
          nontraffic V06.02 ☑
          traffic V06.12 ☑
        motor
          nontraffic V09.00 ☑

☑ **Additional character required**

Accident — *continued*
  transport — *continued*
        traffic V09.20 ☑
      fall V00.131 ☑
      nontraffic V09.1 ☑
        involving motor vehicle NEC V09.00 ☑
      traffic V09.3 ☑
        involving motor vehicle NEC V09.20 ☑
    sled V00.228 ☑
      collision (with) V09.9 ☑
        animal being ridden or animal drawn
          vehicle V06.99 ☑
          nontraffic V06.09 ☑
          traffic V06.19 ☑
        bus or heavy transport V04.99 ☑
          nontraffic V04.09 ☑
          traffic V04.19 ☑
        car V03.99 ☑
          nontraffic V03.09 ☑
          traffic V03.19 ☑
        pedal cycle V01.99 ☑
          nontraffic V01.09 ☑
          traffic V01.19 ☑
        pick-up truck or van V03.99 ☑
          nontraffic V03.09 ☑
          traffic V03.19 ☑
        railway (train) (vehicle) V05.99 ☑
          nontraffic V05.09 ☑
          traffic V05.19 ☑
        streetcar V06.99 ☑
          nontraffic V06.09 ☑
          traffic V06.19 ☑
        stationary object V00.222 ☑
        two- or three-wheeled motor vehicle
          V02.99 ☑
          nontraffic V02.09 ☑
          traffic V02.19 ☑
        vehicle V09.9 ☑
          animal-drawn V06.99 ☑
            nontraffic V06.09 ☑
            traffic V06.19 ☑
          motor
            nontraffic V09.00 ☑
            traffic V09.20 ☑
      fall V00.221 ☑
      nontraffic V09.1 ☑
        involving motor vehicle NEC V09.00 ☑
      traffic V09.3 ☑
        involving motor vehicle NEC V09.20 ☑
    skis (snow) V00.328 ☑
      collision (with) V09.9 ☑
        animal being ridden or animal drawn
          vehicle V06.99 ☑
          nontraffic V06.09 ☑
          traffic V06.19 ☑
        bus or heavy transport V04.99 ☑
          nontraffic V04.09 ☑
          traffic V04.19 ☑
        car V03.99 ☑
          nontraffic V03.09 ☑
          traffic V03.19 ☑
        pedal cycle V01.99 ☑
          nontraffic V01.09 ☑
          traffic V01.19 ☑
        pick-up truck or van V03.99 ☑
          nontraffic V03.09 ☑
          traffic V03.19 ☑
        railway (train) (vehicle) V05.99 ☑
          nontraffic V05.09 ☑
          traffic V05.19 ☑
        streetcar V06.99 ☑
          nontraffic V06.09 ☑
          traffic V06.19 ☑
        stationary object V00.322 ☑
        two- or three-wheeled motor vehicle
          V02.99 ☑
          nontraffic V02.09 ☑
          traffic V02.19 ☑
        vehicle V09.9 ☑
          animal-drawn V06.99 ☑
            nontraffic V06.09 ☑
            traffic V06.19 ☑
          motor
            nontraffic V09.00 ☑
            traffic V09.20 ☑
      fall V00.321 ☑
      nontraffic V09.1 ☑
        involving motor vehicle NEC V09.00 ☑
      traffic V09.3 ☑
        involving motor vehicle NEC V09.20 ☑
    snow board V00.318 ☑
      collision (with) V09.9 ☑

        animal being ridden or animal drawn
          vehicle V06.99 ☑
          nontraffic V06.09 ☑
          traffic V06.19 ☑
        bus or heavy transport V04.99 ☑
          nontraffic V04.09 ☑
          traffic V04.19 ☑
        car V03.99 ☑
          nontraffic V03.09 ☑
          traffic V03.19 ☑
        pedal cycle V01.99 ☑
          nontraffic V01.09 ☑
          traffic V01.19 ☑
        pick-up truck or van V03.99 ☑
          nontraffic V03.09 ☑
          traffic V03.19 ☑
        railway (train) (vehicle) V05.99 ☑
          nontraffic V05.09 ☑
          traffic V05.19 ☑
        streetcar V06.99 ☑
          nontraffic V06.09 ☑
          traffic V06.19 ☑
        stationary object V00.312 ☑
        two- or three-wheeled motor vehicle
          V02.99 ☑
          nontraffic V02.09 ☑
          traffic V02.19 ☑
        vehicle V09.9 ☑
          animal-drawn V06.99 ☑
            nontraffic V06.09 ☑
            traffic V06.19 ☑
          motor
            nontraffic V09.00 ☑
            traffic V09.20 ☑
      fall V00.311 ☑
      nontraffic V09.1 ☑
        involving motor vehicle NEC V09.00 ☑
      traffic V09.3 ☑
        involving motor vehicle NEC V09.20 ☑
    specified type NEC V00.898 ☑
      collision (with) V09.9 ☑
        animal being ridden or animal drawn
          vehicle V06.99 ☑
          nontraffic V06.09 ☑
          traffic V06.19 ☑
        bus or heavy transport V04.99 ☑
          nontraffic V04.09 ☑
          traffic V04.19 ☑
        car V03.99 ☑
          nontraffic V03.09 ☑
          traffic V03.19 ☑
        pedal cycle V01.99 ☑
          nontraffic V01.09 ☑
          traffic V01.19 ☑
        pick-up truck or van V03.99 ☑
          nontraffic V03.09 ☑
          traffic V03.19 ☑
        railway (train) (vehicle) V05.99 ☑
          nontraffic V05.09 ☑
          traffic V05.19 ☑
        streetcar V06.99 ☑
          nontraffic V06.09 ☑
          traffic V06.19 ☑
        stationary object V00.892 ☑
        two- or three-wheeled motor vehicle
          V02.99 ☑
          nontraffic V02.09 ☑
          traffic V02.19 ☑
        vehicle V09.9 ☑
          animal-drawn V06.99 ☑
            nontraffic V06.09 ☑
            traffic V06.19 ☑
          motor
            nontraffic V09.00 ☑
            traffic V09.20 ☑
      fall V00.891 ☑
      nontraffic V09.1 ☑
        involving motor vehicle NEC V09.00 ☑
      traffic V09.3 ☑
        involving motor vehicle NEC V09.20 ☑
    traffic V09.3 ☑
      involving motor vehicle V09.20 ☑
        military V09.21 ☑
        specified type NEC V09.29 ☑
    wheelchair (powered) V00.818 ☑
      collision (with) V09.9 ☑
        animal being ridden or animal drawn
          vehicle V06.99 ☑
          nontraffic V06.09 ☑
          traffic V06.19 ☑

        bus or heavy transport V04.99 ☑
          nontraffic V04.09 ☑
          traffic V04.19 ☑
        car V03.99 ☑
          nontraffic V03.09 ☑
          traffic V03.19 ☑
        pedal cycle V01.99 ☑
          nontraffic V01.09 ☑
          traffic V01.19 ☑
        pick-up truck or van V03.99 ☑
          nontraffic V03.09 ☑
          traffic V03.19 ☑
        railway (train) (vehicle) V05.99 ☑
          nontraffic V05.09 ☑
          traffic V05.19 ☑
        streetcar V06.99 ☑
          nontraffic V06.09 ☑
          traffic V06.19 ☑
        stationary object V00.812 ☑
        two- or three-wheeled motor vehicle
          V02.99 ☑
          nontraffic V02.09 ☑
          traffic V02.19 ☑
        vehicle V09.9 ☑
          animal-drawn V06.99 ☑
            nontraffic V06.09 ☑
            traffic V06.19 ☑
          motor
            nontraffic V09.00 ☑
            traffic V09.20 ☑
      fall V00.811 ☑
      nontraffic V09.1 ☑
        involving motor vehicle NEC V09.00 ☑
      traffic V09.3 ☑
        involving motor vehicle NEC V09.20 ☑
    wheeled shoe V00.158 ☑
      colliding with stationary object V00.152 ☑
      fall V00.151 ☑
  on foot (*see also* Accident, pedestrian)
    collision (with)
      animal being ridden or animal drawn
        vehicle V06.90 ☑
        nontraffic V06.00 ☑
        traffic V06.10 ☑
      bus or heavy transport V04.90 ☑
        nontraffic V04.00 ☑
        traffic V04.10 ☑
      car V03.90 ☑
        nontraffic V03.00 ☑
        traffic V03.10 ☑
      pedal cycle V01.90 ☑
        nontraffic V01.00 ☑
        traffic V01.10 ☑
      pick-up truck or van V03.90 ☑
        nontraffic V03.00 ☑
        traffic V03.10 ☑
      railway (train) (vehicle) V05.90 ☑
        nontraffic V05.00 ☑
        traffic V05.10 ☑
      streetcar V06.90 ☑
        nontraffic V06.00 ☑
        traffic V06.10 ☑
      two- or three-wheeled motor vehicle
        V02.90 ☑
        nontraffic V02.00 ☑
        traffic V02.10 ☑
      vehicle V09.9 ☑
        animal-drawn V06.90 ☑
          nontraffic V06.00 ☑
          traffic V06.10 ☑
        motor
          nontraffic V09.00 ☑
          traffic V09.20 ☑
    nontraffic V09.1 ☑
      involving motor vehicle V09.00 ☑
        military V09.01 ☑
        specified type NEC V09.09 ☑
    traffic V09.3 ☑
      involving motor vehicle V09.20 ☑
        military V09.21 ☑
        specified type NEC V09.29 ☑
  person NEC (unknown way or transportation)
    V99 ☑
    collision (between)
      bus (with)
        heavy transport vehicle (traffic) V87.5 ☑
          nontraffic V88.5 ☑
      car (with)
        nontraffic V88.5 ☑
        bus (traffic) V87.3 ☑

Accident

Accident — *continued*
  transport — *continued*
        nontraffic V88.3 ☑
      heavy transport vehicle (traffic) V87.4 ☑
        nontraffic V88.4 ☑
      pick-up truck or van (traffic) V87.2 ☑
        nontraffic V88.2 ☑
      train or railway vehicle (traffic) V87.6 ☑
        nontraffic V88.6 ☑
      two-or three-wheeled motor vehicle
        (traffic) V87.0 ☑
        nontraffic V88.0 ☑
      motor vehicle (traffic) NEC V87.7 ☑
        nontraffic V88.7 ☑
      two-or three-wheeled vehicle (with) (traffic)
        motor vehicle NEC V87.1 ☑
        nontraffic V88.1 ☑
      nonmotor vehicle (collision) (noncollision)
        (traffic) V87.9 ☑
        nontraffic V88.9 ☑
    pickup truck occupant V59.9 ☑
      collision (with)
        animal (traffic) V50.9 ☑
          being ridden (traffic) V56.9 ☑
            nontraffic V56.3 ☑
            while boarding or alighting V56.4 ☑
          nontraffic V50.3 ☑
          while boarding or alighting V50.4 ☑
        animal-drawn vehicle (traffic) V56.9 ☑
          nontraffic V56.3 ☑
          while boarding or alighting V56.4 ☑
        bus (traffic) V54.9 ☑
          nontraffic V54.3 ☑
          while boarding or alighting V54.4 ☑
        car (traffic) V53.9 ☑
          nontraffic V53.3 ☑
          while boarding or alighting V53.4 ☑
        motor vehicle NOS (traffic) V59.60 ☑
          nontraffic V59.20 ☑
          specified type NEC (traffic) V59.69 ☑
            nontraffic V59.29 ☑
        pedal cycle (traffic) V51.9 ☑
          nontraffic V51.3 ☑
          while boarding or alighting V51.4 ☑
        pickup truck (traffic) V53.9 ☑
          nontraffic V53.3 ☑
          while boarding or alighting V53.4 ☑
        railway vehicle (traffic) V55.9 ☑
          nontraffic V55.3 ☑
          while boarding or alighting V55.4 ☑
        specified vehicle NEC (traffic) V56.9 ☑
          nontraffic V56.3 ☑
          while boarding or alighting V56.4 ☑
        stationary object (traffic) V57.9 ☑
          nontraffic V57.3 ☑
          while boarding or alighting V57.4 ☑
        streetcar (traffic) V56.9 ☑
          nontraffic V56.3 ☑
          while boarding or alighting V56.4 ☑
        three wheeled motor vehicle (traffic) V52.9 ☑
          nontraffic V52.3 ☑
          while boarding or alighting V52.4 ☑
        truck (traffic) V54.9 ☑
          nontraffic V54.3 ☑
          while boarding or alighting V54.4 ☑
        two wheeled motor vehicle (traffic) V52.9 ☑
          nontraffic V52.3 ☑
          while boarding or alighting V52.4 ☑
        van (traffic) V53.9 ☑
          nontraffic V53.3 ☑
          while boarding or alighting V53.4 ☑
      driver
        collision (with)
          animal (traffic) V50.5 ☑
            being ridden (traffic) V56.5 ☑
              nontraffic V56.0 ☑
            nontraffic V50.0 ☑
          animal-drawn vehicle (traffic) V56.5 ☑
            nontraffic V56.0 ☑
          bus (traffic) V54.5 ☑
            nontraffic V54.0 ☑
          car (traffic) V53.5 ☑
            nontraffic V53.0 ☑
          motor vehicle NOS (traffic) V59.40 ☑
            nontraffic V59.00 ☑
            specified type NEC (traffic) V59.49 ☑
              nontraffic V59.09 ☑
          pedal cycle (traffic) V51.5 ☑
            nontraffic V51.0 ☑
          pickup truck (traffic) V53.5 ☑
            nontraffic V53.0 ☑
          railway vehicle (traffic) V55.5 ☑

Accident — *continued*
  transport — *continued*
        nontraffic V55.0 ☑
        specified vehicle NEC (traffic) V56.5 ☑
          nontraffic V56.0 ☑
        stationary object (traffic) V57.5 ☑
          nontraffic V57.0 ☑
        streetcar (traffic) V56.5 ☑
          nontraffic V56.0 ☑
        three wheeled motor vehicle (traffic)
          V52.5 ☑
          nontraffic V52.0 ☑
        truck (traffic) V54.5 ☑
          nontraffic V54.0 ☑
        two wheeled motor vehicle (traffic)
          V52.5 ☑
          nontraffic V52.0 ☑
        van (traffic) V53.5 ☑
          nontraffic V53.0 ☑
      noncollision accident (traffic) V58.5 ☑
        nontraffic V58.0 ☑
      noncollision accident (traffic) V58.9 ☑
        nontraffic V58.3 ☑
        while boarding or alighting V58.4 ☑
      nontraffic V59.3 ☑
      hanger-on
        collision (with)
          animal (traffic) V50.7 ☑
            being ridden (traffic) V56.7 ☑
              nontraffic V56.2 ☑
            nontraffic V50.2 ☑
          animal-drawn vehicle (traffic) V56.7 ☑
            nontraffic V56.2 ☑
          bus (traffic) V54.7 ☑
            nontraffic V54.2 ☑
          car (traffic) V53.7 ☑
            nontraffic V53.2 ☑
          pedal cycle (traffic) V51.7 ☑
            nontraffic V51.2 ☑
          pickup truck (traffic) V53.7 ☑
            nontraffic V53.2 ☑
          railway vehicle (traffic) V55.7 ☑
            nontraffic V55.2 ☑
          specified vehicle NEC (traffic) V56.7 ☑
            nontraffic V56.2 ☑
          stationary object (traffic) V57.7 ☑
            nontraffic V57.2 ☑
          streetcar (traffic) V56.7 ☑
            nontraffic V56.2 ☑
          three wheeled motor vehicle (traffic)
            V52.7 ☑
            nontraffic V52.2 ☑
          truck (traffic) V54.7 ☑
            nontraffic V54.2 ☑
          two wheeled motor vehicle (traffic)
            V52.7 ☑
            nontraffic V52.2 ☑
          van (traffic) V53.7 ☑
            nontraffic V53.2 ☑
        noncollision accident (traffic) V58.7 ☑
          nontraffic V58.2 ☑
      passenger
        collision (with)
          animal (traffic) V50.6 ☑
            being ridden (traffic) V56.6 ☑
              nontraffic V56.1 ☑
            nontraffic V50.1 ☑
          animal-drawn vehicle (traffic) V56.6 ☑
            nontraffic V56.1 ☑
          bus (traffic) V54.6 ☑
            nontraffic V54.1 ☑
          car (traffic) V53.6 ☑
            nontraffic V53.1 ☑
          motor vehicle NOS (traffic) V59.50 ☑
            nontraffic V59.10 ☑
            specified type NEC (traffic) V59.59 ☑
              nontraffic V59.19 ☑
          pedal cycle (traffic) V51.6 ☑
            nontraffic V51.1 ☑
          pickup truck (traffic) V53.6 ☑
            nontraffic V53.1 ☑
          railway vehicle (traffic) V55.6 ☑
            nontraffic V55.1 ☑
          specified vehicle NEC (traffic) V56.6 ☑
            nontraffic V56.1 ☑
          stationary object (traffic) V57.6 ☑
            nontraffic V57.1 ☑
          streetcar (traffic) V56.6 ☑
            nontraffic V56.1 ☑
          three wheeled motor vehicle (traffic)
            V52.6 ☑
            nontraffic V52.1 ☑

Accident — *continued*
  transport — *continued*
        truck (traffic) V54.6 ☑
          nontraffic V54.1 ☑
        two wheeled motor vehicle (traffic)
          V52.6 ☑
          nontraffic V52.1 ☑
        van (traffic) V53.6 ☑
          nontraffic V53.1 ☑
      noncollision accident (traffic) V58.6 ☑
        nontraffic V58.1 ☑
      specified type NEC V59.88 ☑
      military vehicle V59.81 ☑
    quarry truck — *see* Accident, transport, industrial
      vehicle occupant
    race car — *see* Accident, transport, motor vehicle
      NEC occupant
    railway vehicle occupant V81.9 ☑
      collision (with) V81.3 ☑
        motor vehicle (non-military) (traffic) V81.1 ☑
          military V81.83 ☑
          nontraffic V81.0 ☑
        rolling stock V81.2 ☑
        specified object NEC V81.3 ☑
      during derailment V81.7 ☑
        with antecedent collision — *see* Accident,
          transport, railway vehicle occupant,
          collision
      explosion V81.81 ☑
      fall (in railway vehicle) V81.5 ☑
        during derailment V81.7 ☑
          with antecedent collision — *see* Accident,
            transport, railway vehicle occupant,
            collision
        from railway vehicle V81.6 ☑
          during derailment V81.7 ☑
            with antecedent collision — *see* Accident,
              transport, railway vehicle occupant,
              collision
        while boarding or alighting V81.4 ☑
      fire V81.81 ☑
      object falling onto train V81.82 ☑
      specified type NEC V81.89 ☑
      while boarding or alighting V81.4 ☑
    ski lift V98.3 ☑
    snowmobile occupant (nontraffic) V86.92 ☑
      driver V86.52 ☑
      hanger-on V86.72 ☑
      passenger V86.62 ☑
      traffic V86.32 ☑
        driver V86.02 ☑
        hanger-on V86.22 ☑
        passenger V86.12 ☑
      while boarding or alighting V86.42 ☑
    specified NEC V98.8 ☑
    sport utility vehicle occupant (*see also* Accident,
      transport, pickup truck occupant)
    streetcar occupant V82.9 ☑
      collision (with) V82.3 ☑
        motor vehicle (traffic) V82.1 ☑
          nontraffic V82.0 ☑
        rolling stock V82.2 ☑
      during derailment V82.7 ☑
        with antecedent collision — *see* Accident,
          transport, streetcar occupant, collision
      fall (in streetcar) V82.5 ☑
        during derailment V82.7 ☑
          with antecedent collision — *see* Accident,
            transport, streetcar occupant, collision
        from streetcar V82.6 ☑
          during derailment V82.7 ☑
            with antecedent collision — *see* Accident,
              transport, streetcar occupant,
              collision
        while boarding or alighting V82.4 ☑
      while boarding or alighting V82.4 ☑
      specified type NEC V82.8 ☑
      while boarding or alighting V82.4 ☑
    three-wheeled motor vehicle occupant V39.9 ☑
      collision (with)
        animal (traffic) V30.9 ☑
          being ridden (traffic) V36.9 ☑
            nontraffic V36.3 ☑
            while boarding or alighting V36.4 ☑
          nontraffic V30.3 ☑
          while boarding or alighting V30.4 ☑
        animal-drawn vehicle (traffic) V36.9 ☑
          nontraffic V36.3 ☑
          while boarding or alighting V36.4 ☑
        bus (traffic) V34.9 ☑
          nontraffic V34.3 ☑
          while boarding or alighting V34.4 ☑

Accident — *continued*
  transport — *continued*
    car (traffic) V33.9 ☑
      nontraffic V33.3 ☑
      while boarding or alighting V33.4 ☑
    motor vehicle NOS (traffic) V39.60 ☑
      nontraffic V39.20 ☑
      specified type NEC (traffic) V39.69 ☑
        nontraffic V39.29 ☑
    pedal cycle (traffic) V31.9 ☑
      nontraffic V31.3 ☑
      while boarding or alighting V31.4 ☑
    pickup truck (traffic) V33.9 ☑
      nontraffic V33.3 ☑
      while boarding or alighting V33.4 ☑
    railway vehicle (traffic) V35.9 ☑
      nontraffic V35.3 ☑
      while boarding or alighting V35.4 ☑
    specified vehicle NEC (traffic) V36.9 ☑
      nontraffic V36.3 ☑
      while boarding or alighting V36.4 ☑
    stationary object (traffic) V37.9 ☑
      nontraffic V37.3 ☑
      while boarding or alighting V37.4 ☑
    streetcar (traffic) V36.9 ☑
      nontraffic V36.3 ☑
      while boarding or alighting V36.4 ☑
    three wheeled motor vehicle (traffic) V32.9 ☑
      nontraffic V32.3 ☑
      while boarding or alighting V32.4 ☑
    truck (traffic) V34.9 ☑
      nontraffic V34.3 ☑
      while boarding or alighting V34.4 ☑
    two wheeled motor vehicle (traffic) V32.9 ☑
      nontraffic V32.3 ☑
      while boarding or alighting V32.4 ☑
    van (traffic) V33.9 ☑
      nontraffic V33.3 ☑
      while boarding or alighting V33.4 ☑
  driver
    collision (with)
      animal (traffic) V30.5 ☑
        being ridden (traffic) V36.5 ☑
          nontraffic V36.0 ☑
        nontraffic V30.0 ☑
      animal-drawn vehicle (traffic) V36.5 ☑
        nontraffic V36.0 ☑
      bus (traffic) V34.5 ☑
        nontraffic V34.0 ☑
      car (traffic) V33.5 ☑
        nontraffic V33.0 ☑
      motor vehicle NOS (traffic) V39.40 ☑
        nontraffic V39.00 ☑
        specified type NEC (traffic) V39.49 ☑
          nontraffic V39.09 ☑
      pedal cycle (traffic) V31.5 ☑
        nontraffic V31.0 ☑
      pickup truck (traffic) V33.5 ☑
        nontraffic V33.0 ☑
      railway vehicle (traffic) V35.5 ☑
        nontraffic V35.0 ☑
      specified vehicle NEC (traffic) V36.5 ☑
        nontraffic V36.0 ☑
      stationary object (traffic) V37.5 ☑
        nontraffic V37.0 ☑
      streetcar (traffic) V36.5 ☑
        nontraffic V36.0 ☑
      three wheeled motor vehicle (traffic) V32.5 ☑
        nontraffic V32.0 ☑
      truck (traffic) V34.5 ☑
        nontraffic V34.0 ☑
      two wheeled motor vehicle (traffic) V32.5 ☑
        nontraffic V32.0 ☑
      van (traffic) V33.5 ☑
        nontraffic V33.0 ☑
    noncollision accident (traffic) V38.5 ☑
      nontraffic V38.0 ☑
  noncollision accident (traffic) V38.9 ☑
    nontraffic V38.3 ☑
    while boarding or alighting V38.4 ☑
  nontraffic V39.3 ☑
  hanger-on
    collision (with)
      animal (traffic) V30.7 ☑
        being ridden (traffic) V36.7 ☑
          nontraffic V36.2 ☑
        nontraffic V30.2 ☑
      animal-drawn vehicle (traffic) V36.7 ☑
        nontraffic V36.2 ☑
      bus (traffic) V34.7 ☑
        nontraffic V34.2 ☑

Accident — *continued*
  transport — *continued*
      car (traffic) V33.7 ☑
        nontraffic V33.2 ☑
      pedal cycle (traffic) V31.7 ☑
        nontraffic V31.2 ☑
      pickup truck (traffic) V33.7 ☑
        nontraffic V33.2 ☑
      railway vehicle (traffic) V35.7 ☑
        nontraffic V35.2 ☑
      specified vehicle NEC (traffic) V36.7 ☑
        nontraffic V36.2 ☑
      stationary object (traffic) V37.7 ☑
        nontraffic V37.2 ☑
      streetcar (traffic) V36.7 ☑
        nontraffic V36.2 ☑
      three wheeled motor vehicle (traffic) V32.7 ☑
        nontraffic V32.2 ☑
      truck (traffic) V34.7 ☑
        nontraffic V34.2 ☑
      two wheeled motor vehicle (traffic) V32.7 ☑
        nontraffic V32.2 ☑
      van (traffic) V33.7 ☑
        nontraffic V33.2 ☑
    noncollision accident (traffic) V38.7 ☑
      nontraffic V38.2 ☑
  passenger
    collision (with)
      animal (traffic) V30.6 ☑
        being ridden (traffic) V36.6 ☑
          nontraffic V36.1 ☑
        nontraffic V30.1 ☑
      animal-drawn vehicle (traffic) V36.6 ☑
        nontraffic V36.1 ☑
      bus (traffic) V34.6 ☑
        nontraffic V34.1 ☑
      car (traffic) V33.6 ☑
        nontraffic V33.1 ☑
      motor vehicle NOS (traffic) V39.50 ☑
        nontraffic V39.10 ☑
        specified type NEC (traffic) V39.59 ☑
          nontraffic V39.19 ☑
      pedal cycle (traffic) V31.6 ☑
        nontraffic V31.1 ☑
      pickup truck (traffic) V33.6 ☑
        nontraffic V33.1 ☑
      railway vehicle (traffic) V35.6 ☑
        nontraffic V35.1 ☑
      specified vehicle NEC (traffic) V36.6 ☑
        nontraffic V36.1 ☑
      stationary object (traffic) V37.6 ☑
        nontraffic V37.1 ☑
      streetcar (traffic) V36.6 ☑
        nontraffic V36.1 ☑
      three wheeled motor vehicle (traffic) V32.6 ☑
        nontraffic V32.1 ☑
      truck (traffic) V34.6 ☑
        nontraffic V34.1 ☑
      two wheeled motor vehicle (traffic) V32.6 ☑
        nontraffic V32.1 ☑
      van (traffic) V33.6 ☑
        nontraffic V33.1 ☑
    noncollision accident (traffic) V38.6 ☑
      nontraffic V38.1 ☑
  specified type NEC V39.89 ☑
    military vehicle V39.81 ☑
  tractor (farm) (and trailer) — *see* Accident, transport, agricultural vehicle occupant
  tram — *see* Accident, transport, streetcar
    in mine or quarry — *see* Accident, transport, industrial vehicle occupant
  trolley — *see* Accident, transport, streetcar
    in mine or quarry — *see* Accident, transport, industrial vehicle occupant
  truck (heavy) occupant V69.9 ☑
    collision (with)
      animal (traffic) V60.9 ☑
        being ridden (traffic) V66.9 ☑
          nontraffic V66.3 ☑
          while boarding or alighting V66.4 ☑
        nontraffic V60.3 ☑
        while boarding or alighting V60.4 ☑
      animal-drawn vehicle (traffic) V66.9 ☑
        nontraffic V66.3 ☑
        while boarding or alighting V66.4 ☑
      bus (traffic) V64.9 ☑
        nontraffic V64.3 ☑
        while boarding or alighting V64.4 ☑

Accident — *continued*
  transport — *continued*
      car (traffic) V63.9 ☑
        nontraffic V63.3 ☑
        while boarding or alighting V63.4 ☑
      motor vehicle NOS (traffic) V69.60 ☑
        nontraffic V69.20 ☑
        specified type NEC (traffic) V69.69 ☑
          nontraffic V69.29 ☑
      pedal cycle (traffic) V61.9 ☑
        nontraffic V61.3 ☑
        while boarding or alighting V61.4 ☑
      pickup truck (traffic) V63.9 ☑
        nontraffic V63.3 ☑
        while boarding or alighting V63.4 ☑
      railway vehicle (traffic) V65.9 ☑
        nontraffic V65.3 ☑
        while boarding or alighting V65.4 ☑
      specified vehicle NEC (traffic) V66.9 ☑
        nontraffic V66.3 ☑
        while boarding or alighting V66.4 ☑
      stationary object (traffic) V67.9 ☑
        nontraffic V67.3 ☑
        while boarding or alighting V67.4 ☑
      streetcar (traffic) V66.9 ☑
        nontraffic V66.3 ☑
        while boarding or alighting V66.4 ☑
      three wheeled motor vehicle (traffic) V62.9 ☑
        nontraffic V62.3 ☑
        while boarding or alighting V62.4 ☑
      truck (traffic) V64.9 ☑
        nontraffic V64.3 ☑
        while boarding or alighting V64.4 ☑
      two wheeled motor vehicle (traffic) V62.9 ☑
        nontraffic V62.3 ☑
        while boarding or alighting V62.4 ☑
      van (traffic) V63.9 ☑
        nontraffic V63.3 ☑
        while boarding or alighting V63.4 ☑
    driver
      collision (with)
        animal (traffic) V60.5 ☑
          being ridden (traffic) V66.5 ☑
            nontraffic V66.0 ☑
          nontraffic V60.0 ☑
        animal-drawn vehicle (traffic) V66.5 ☑
          nontraffic V66.0 ☑
        bus (traffic) V64.5 ☑
          nontraffic V64.0 ☑
        car (traffic) V63.5 ☑
          nontraffic V63.0 ☑
        motor vehicle NOS (traffic) V69.40 ☑
          nontraffic V69.00 ☑
          specified type NEC (traffic) V69.49 ☑
            nontraffic V69.09 ☑
        pedal cycle (traffic) V61.5 ☑
          nontraffic V61.0 ☑
        pickup truck (traffic) V63.5 ☑
          nontraffic V63.0 ☑
        railway vehicle (traffic) V65.5 ☑
          nontraffic V65.0 ☑
        specified vehicle NEC (traffic) V66.5 ☑
          nontraffic V66.0 ☑
        stationary object (traffic) V67.5 ☑
          nontraffic V67.0 ☑
        streetcar (traffic) V66.5 ☑
          nontraffic V66.0 ☑
        three wheeled motor vehicle (traffic) V62.5 ☑
          nontraffic V62.0 ☑
        truck (traffic) V64.5 ☑
          nontraffic V64.0 ☑
        two wheeled motor vehicle (traffic) V62.5 ☑
          nontraffic V62.0 ☑
        van (traffic) V63.5 ☑
          nontraffic V63.0 ☑
      noncollision accident (traffic) V68.5 ☑
        nontraffic V68.0 ☑
    dump — *see* Accident, transport, construction vehicle occupant
    hanger-on
      collision (with)
        animal (traffic) V60.7 ☑
          being ridden (traffic) V66.7 ☑
            nontraffic V66.2 ☑
          nontraffic V60.2 ☑
        animal-drawn vehicle (traffic) V66.7 ☑
          nontraffic V66.2 ☑
        bus (traffic) V64.7 ☑
          nontraffic V64.2 ☑
        car (traffic) V63.7 ☑

☑ **Additional character required**

Accident

Accident — *continued*
  transport — *continued*
      nontraffic V63.2 ☑
      pedal cycle (traffic) V61.7 ☑
        nontraffic V61.2 ☑
      pickup truck (traffic) V63.7 ☑
        nontraffic V63.2 ☑
      railway vehicle (traffic) V65.7 ☑
        nontraffic V65.2 ☑
      specified vehicle NEC (traffic) V66.7 ☑
        nontraffic V66.2 ☑
      stationary object (traffic) V67.7 ☑
        nontraffic V67.2 ☑
      streetcar (traffic) V66.7 ☑
        nontraffic V66.2 ☑
      three wheeled motor vehicle (traffic) V62.7 ☑
        nontraffic V62.2 ☑
      truck (traffic) V64.7 ☑
        nontraffic V64.2 ☑
      two wheeled motor vehicle (traffic) V62.7 ☑
        nontraffic V62.2 ☑
      van (traffic) V63.7 ☑
        nontraffic V63.2 ☑
    noncollision accident (traffic) V68.7 ☑
      nontraffic V68.2 ☑
    noncollision accident (traffic) V68.9 ☑
      nontraffic V68.3 ☑
      while boarding or alighting V68.4 ☑
    nontraffic V69.3 ☑
    passenger
      collision (with)
        animal (traffic) V60.6 ☑
          being ridden (traffic) V66.6 ☑
            nontraffic V66.1 ☑
          nontraffic V60.1 ☑
        animal-drawn vehicle (traffic) V66.6 ☑
          nontraffic V66.1 ☑
        bus (traffic) V64.6 ☑
          nontraffic V64.1 ☑
        car (traffic) V63.6 ☑
          nontraffic V63.1 ☑
        motor vehicle NOS (traffic) V69.50 ☑
          nontraffic V69.10 ☑
          specified type NEC (traffic) V69.59 ☑
            nontraffic V69.19 ☑
        pedal cycle (traffic) V61.6 ☑
          nontraffic V61.1 ☑
        pickup truck (traffic) V63.6 ☑
          nontraffic V63.1 ☑
        railway vehicle (traffic) V65.6 ☑
          nontraffic V65.1 ☑
        specified vehicle NEC (traffic) V66.6 ☑
          nontraffic V66.1 ☑
        stationary object (traffic) V67.6 ☑
          nontraffic V67.1 ☑
        streetcar (traffic) V66.6 ☑
          nontraffic V66.1 ☑
        three wheeled motor vehicle (traffic) V62.6 ☑
          nontraffic V62.1 ☑
        truck (traffic) V64.6 ☑
          nontraffic V64.1 ☑
        two wheeled motor vehicle (traffic) V62.6 ☑
          nontraffic V62.1 ☑
        van (traffic) V63.6 ☑
          nontraffic V63.1 ☑
      noncollision accident (traffic) V68.6 ☑
        nontraffic V68.1 ☑
    pickup — *see* Accident, transport, pickup truck occupant
    specified type NEC V69.88 ☑
      military vehicle V69.81 ☑
  van occupant V59.9 ☑
    collision (with)
      animal (traffic) V50.9 ☑
        being ridden (traffic) V56.9 ☑
          nontraffic V56.3 ☑
          while boarding or alighting V56.4 ☑
        nontraffic V50.3 ☑
        while boarding or alighting V50.4 ☑
      animal-drawn vehicle (traffic) V56.9 ☑
        nontraffic V56.3 ☑
        while boarding or alighting V56.4 ☑
      bus (traffic) V54.9 ☑
        nontraffic V54.3 ☑
        while boarding or alighting V54.4 ☑
      car (traffic) V53.9 ☑
        nontraffic V53.3 ☑
        while boarding or alighting V53.4 ☑

Accident — *continued*
  transport — *continued*
      motor vehicle NOS (traffic) V59.60 ☑
        nontraffic V59.20 ☑
        specified type NEC (traffic) V59.69 ☑
          nontraffic V59.29 ☑
      pedal cycle (traffic) V51.9 ☑
        nontraffic V51.3 ☑
        while boarding or alighting V51.4 ☑
      pickup truck (traffic) V53.9 ☑
        nontraffic V53.3 ☑
        while boarding or alighting V53.4 ☑
      railway vehicle (traffic) V55.9 ☑
        nontraffic V55.3 ☑
        while boarding or alighting V55.4 ☑
      specified vehicle NEC (traffic) V56.9 ☑
        nontraffic V56.3 ☑
        while boarding or alighting V56.4 ☑
      stationary object (traffic) V57.9 ☑
        nontraffic V57.3 ☑
        while boarding or alighting V57.4 ☑
      streetcar (traffic) V56.9 ☑
        nontraffic V56.3 ☑
        while boarding or alighting V56.4 ☑
      three wheeled motor vehicle (traffic) V52.9 ☑
        nontraffic V52.3 ☑
        while boarding or alighting V52.4 ☑
      truck (traffic) V54.9 ☑
        nontraffic V54.3 ☑
        while boarding or alighting V54.4 ☑
      two wheeled motor vehicle (traffic) V52.9 ☑
        nontraffic V52.3 ☑
        while boarding or alighting V52.4 ☑
      van (traffic) V53.9 ☑
        nontraffic V53.3 ☑
        while boarding or alighting V53.4 ☑
    driver
      collision (with)
        animal (traffic) V50.5 ☑
          being ridden (traffic) V56.5 ☑
            nontraffic V56.0 ☑
          nontraffic V50.0 ☑
        animal-drawn vehicle (traffic) V56.5 ☑
          nontraffic V56.0 ☑
        bus (traffic) V54.5 ☑
          nontraffic V54.0 ☑
        car (traffic) V53.5 ☑
          nontraffic V53.0 ☑
        motor vehicle NOS (traffic) V59.40 ☑
          nontraffic V59.00 ☑
          specified type NEC (traffic) V59.49 ☑
            nontraffic V59.09 ☑
        pedal cycle (traffic) V51.5 ☑
          nontraffic V51.0 ☑
        pickup truck (traffic) V53.5 ☑
          nontraffic V53.0 ☑
        railway vehicle (traffic) V55.5 ☑
          nontraffic V55.0 ☑
        specified vehicle NEC (traffic) V56.5 ☑
          nontraffic V56.0 ☑
        stationary object (traffic) V57.5 ☑
          nontraffic V57.0 ☑
        streetcar (traffic) V56.5 ☑
          nontraffic V56.0 ☑
        three wheeled motor vehicle (traffic) V52.5 ☑
          nontraffic V52.0 ☑
        truck (traffic) V54.5 ☑
          nontraffic V54.0 ☑
        two wheeled motor vehicle (traffic) V52.5 ☑
          nontraffic V52.0 ☑
        van (traffic) V53.5 ☑
          nontraffic V53.0 ☑
      noncollision accident (traffic) V58.5 ☑
        nontraffic V58.0 ☑
    noncollision accident (traffic) V58.9 ☑
      nontraffic V58.3 ☑
      while boarding or alighting V58.4 ☑
    nontraffic V59.3 ☑
    hanger-on
      collision (with)
        animal (traffic) V50.7 ☑
          being ridden (traffic) V56.7 ☑
            nontraffic V56.2 ☑
          nontraffic V50.2 ☑
        animal-drawn vehicle (traffic) V56.7 ☑
          nontraffic V56.2 ☑
        bus (traffic) V54.7 ☑
          nontraffic V54.2 ☑
        car (traffic) V53.7 ☑
          nontraffic V53.2 ☑

Accident — *continued*
  transport — *continued*
      pedal cycle (traffic) V51.7 ☑
        nontraffic V51.2 ☑
      pickup truck (traffic) V53.7 ☑
        nontraffic V53.2 ☑
      railway vehicle (traffic) V55.7 ☑
        nontraffic V55.2 ☑
      specified vehicle NEC (traffic) V56.7 ☑
        nontraffic V56.2 ☑
      stationary object (traffic) V57.7 ☑
        nontraffic V57.2 ☑
      streetcar (traffic) V56.7 ☑
        nontraffic V56.2 ☑
      three wheeled motor vehicle (traffic) V52.7 ☑
        nontraffic V52.2 ☑
      truck (traffic) V54.7 ☑
        nontraffic V54.2 ☑
      two wheeled motor vehicle (traffic) V52.7 ☑
        nontraffic V52.2 ☑
      van (traffic) V53.7 ☑
        nontraffic V53.2 ☑
    noncollision accident (traffic) V58.7 ☑
      nontraffic V58.2 ☑
    passenger
      collision (with)
        animal (traffic) V50.6 ☑
          being ridden (traffic) V56.6 ☑
            nontraffic V56.1 ☑
          nontraffic V50.1 ☑
        animal-drawn vehicle (traffic) V56.6 ☑
          nontraffic V56.1 ☑
        bus (traffic) V54.6 ☑
          nontraffic V54.1 ☑
        car (traffic) V53.6 ☑
          nontraffic V53.1 ☑
        motor vehicle NOS (traffic) V59.50 ☑
          nontraffic V59.10 ☑
          specified type NEC (traffic) V59.59 ☑
            nontraffic V59.19 ☑
        pedal cycle (traffic) V51.6 ☑
          nontraffic V51.1 ☑
        pickup truck (traffic) V53.6 ☑
          nontraffic V53.1 ☑
        railway vehicle (traffic) V55.6 ☑
          nontraffic V55.1 ☑
        specified vehicle NEC (traffic) V56.6 ☑
          nontraffic V56.1 ☑
        stationary object (traffic) V57.6 ☑
          nontraffic V57.1 ☑
        streetcar (traffic) V56.6 ☑
          nontraffic V56.1 ☑
        three wheeled motor vehicle (traffic) V52.6 ☑
          nontraffic V52.1 ☑
        truck (traffic) V54.6 ☑
          nontraffic V54.1 ☑
        two wheeled motor vehicle (traffic) V52.6 ☑
          nontraffic V52.1 ☑
        van (traffic) V53.6 ☑
          nontraffic V53.1 ☑
      noncollision accident (traffic) V58.6 ☑
        nontraffic V58.1 ☑
    specified type NEC V59.88 ☑
      military vehicle V59.81 ☑
  watercraft occupant — *see* Accident, watercraft
  vehicle NEC V89.9 ☑
    animal-drawn NEC — *see* Accident, transport, animal-drawn vehicle occupant
    special
      agricultural — *see* Accident, transport, agricultural vehicle occupant
      construction — *see* Accident, transport, construction vehicle occupant
      industrial — *see* Accident, transport, industrial vehicle occupant
    three-wheeled NEC (motorized) — *see* Accident, transport, three-wheeled motor vehicle occupant
  watercraft V94.9 ☑
    causing
      drowning — *see* Drowning, due to, accident to, watercraft
      injury NEC V91.89 ☑
        crushed between craft and object V91.19 ☑
          powered craft V91.13 ☑
            ferry boat V91.11 ☑
            fishing boat V91.12 ☑
            jetskis V91.13 ☑

☑ **Additional character required**

Accident — continued
  watercraft — continued
        liner V91.11 ☑
        merchant ship V91.10 ☑
        passenger ship V91.11 ☑
      unpowered craft V91.18 ☑
        canoe V91.15 ☑
        inflatable V91.16 ☑
        kayak V91.15 ☑
        sailboat V91.14 ☑
        surf-board V91.18 ☑
        windsurfer V91.18 ☑
      fall on board V91.29 ☑
        powered craft V91.23 ☑
        ferry boat V91.21 ☑
        fishing boat V91.22 ☑
        jetskis V91.23 ☑
        liner V91.21 ☑
        merchant ship V91.20 ☑
        passenger ship V91.21 ☑
      unpowered craft
        canoe V91.25 ☑
        inflatable V91.26 ☑
        kayak V91.25 ☑
        sailboat V91.24 ☑
      fire on board causing burn V91.09 ☑
        powered craft V91.03 ☑
        ferry boat V91.01 ☑
        fishing boat V91.02 ☑
        jetskis V91.03 ☑
        liner V91.01 ☑
        merchant ship V91.00 ☑
        passenger ship V91.01 ☑
      unpowered craft V91.08 ☑
        canoe V91.05 ☑
        inflatable V91.06 ☑
        kayak V91.05 ☑
        sailboat V91.04 ☑
        surf-board V91.08 ☑
        water skis V91.07 ☑
        windsurfer V91.08 ☑
      hit by falling object V91.39 ☑
        powered craft V91.33 ☑
        ferry boat V91.31 ☑
        fishing boat V91.32 ☑
        jetskis V91.33 ☑
        liner V91.31 ☑
        merchant ship V91.30 ☑
        passenger ship V91.31 ☑
      unpowered craft V91.38 ☑
        canoe V91.35 ☑
        inflatable V91.36 ☑
        kayak V91.35 ☑
        sailboat V91.34 ☑
        surf-board V91.38 ☑
        water skis V91.37 ☑
        windsurfer V91.38 ☑
      specified type NEC V91.89 ☑
        powered craft V91.83 ☑
        ferry boat V91.81 ☑
        fishing boat V91.82 ☑
        jetskis V91.83 ☑
        liner V91.81 ☑
        merchant ship V91.80 ☑
        passenger ship V91.81 ☑
      unpowered craft V91.88 ☑
        canoe V91.85 ☑
        inflatable V91.86 ☑
        kayak V91.85 ☑
        sailboat V91.84 ☑
        surf-board V91.88 ☑
        water skis V91.87 ☑
        windsurfer V91.88 ☑
    due to, caused by cataclysm — *see* Forces of nature, by type
    military NEC V94.818 ☑
      with civilian watercraft V94.810 ☑
      civilian in water injured by V94.811 ☑
    nonpowered, struck by
      nonpowered vessel V94.22 ☑
      powered vessel V94.21 ☑
    specified type NEC V94.89 ☑
    striking swimmer
      powered V94.11 ☑
      unpowered V94.12 ☑
Acid throwing (assault) Y08.89 ☑
Activity (involving) (of victim at time of event) Y93.9
  aerobic and step exercise (class) Y93.A3
  alpine skiing Y93.23
  animal care NEC Y93.K9
  arts and handcrafts NEC Y93.D9
  athletics NEC Y93.79

Activity — continued
  athletics played as a team or group NEC Y93.69
  athletics played individually NEC Y93.59
  baking Y93.G3
  ballet Y93.41
  barbells Y93.B3
  BASE (Building, Antenna, Span, Earth) jumping Y93.33
  baseball Y93.64
  basketball Y93.67
  bathing (personal) Y93.E1
  beach volleyball Y93.68
  bike riding Y93.55
  blackout game Y93.85
  boogie boarding Y93.18
  bowling Y93.54
  boxing Y93.71
  brass instrument playing Y93.J4
  building construction Y93.H3
  bungee jumping Y93.34
  calisthenics Y93.A2
  canoeing (in calm and turbulent water) Y93.16
  capture the flag Y93.6A
  cardiorespiratory exercise NEC Y93.A9
  caregiving (providing) NEC Y93.F9
    bathing Y93.F1
    lifting Y93.F2
  cellular
    communication device Y93.C2
    telephone Y93.C2
  challenge course Y93.A5
  cheerleading Y93.45
  choking game Y93.85
  circuit training Y93.A4
  cleaning
    floor Y93.E5
  climbing NEC Y93.39
    mountain Y93.31
    rock Y93.31
    wall Y93.31
  clothing care and maintenance NEC Y93.E9
  combatives Y93.75
  computer
    keyboarding Y93.C1
    technology NEC Y93.C9
  confidence course Y93.A5
  construction (building) Y93.H3
  cooking and baking Y93.G3
  cool down exercises Y93.A2
  cricket Y93.69
  crocheting Y93.D1
  cross country skiing Y93.24
  dancing (all types) Y93.41
  digging
    dirt Y93.H1
  dirt digging Y93.H1
  dishwashing Y93.G1
  diving (platform) (springboard) Y93.12
    underwater Y93.15
  dodge ball Y93.6A
  downhill skiing Y93.23
  drum playing Y93.J2
  dumbbells Y93.B3
  electronic
    devices NEC Y93.C9
      hand held interactive Y93.C2
    game playing (using) (with)
      interactive device Y93.C2
      keyboard or other stationary device Y93.C1
  elliptical machine Y93.A1
  exercise(s)
    machines ((primarily) for)
      cardiorespiratory conditioning Y93.A1
      muscle strengthening Y93.B1
    muscle strengthening (non-machine) NEC Y93.B9
  external motion NEC Y93.I9
    rollercoaster Y93.I1
  fainting game Y93.85
  field hockey Y93.65
  figure skating (pairs) (singles) Y93.21
  flag football Y93.62
  floor mopping and cleaning Y93.E5
  food preparation and clean up Y93.G1
  football (American) NOS Y93.61
    flag Y93.62
    tackle Y93.61
    touch Y93.62
  four square Y93.6A
  free weights Y93.B3
  frisbee (ultimate) Y93.74
  furniture
    building Y93.D3

Activity — continued
  furniture — continued
    finishing Y93.D3
    repair Y93.D3
  game playing (electronic)
    using keyboard or other stationary device Y93.C1
    using interactive device Y93.C2
  gardening Y93.H2
  golf Y93.53
  grass drills Y93.A6
  grilling and smoking food Y93.G2
  grooming and shearing an animal Y93.K3
  guerilla drills Y93.A6
  gymnastics (rhythmic) Y93.43
  handball Y93.73
  hand held interactive electronic device Y93.C2
  hang gliding Y93.35
  hiking (on level or elevated terrain) Y93.01
  hockey (ice) Y93.22
    field Y93.65
  horseback riding Y93.52
  household (interior) maintenance NEC Y93.E9
  ice NEC Y93.29
    dancing Y93.21
    hockey Y93.22
    skating Y93.21
  inline roller skating Y93.51
  ironing Y93.E4
  judo Y93.75
  jumping (off) NEC Y93.39
    BASE (Building, Antenna, Span, Earth) Y93.33
    bungee Y93.34
    jacks Y93.A2
    rope Y93.56
  jumping jacks Y93.A2
  jumping rope Y93.56
  karate Y93.75
  kayaking (in calm and turbulent water) Y93.16
  keyboarding (computer) Y93.C1
  kickball Y93.6A
  knitting Y93.D1
  lacrosse Y93.65
  land maintenance NEC Y93.H9
  landscaping Y93.H2
  laundry Y93.E2
  machines (exercise)
    primarily for cardiorespiratory conditioning Y93.A1
    primarily for muscle strengthening Y93.B1
  maintenance
    exterior building NEC Y93.H9
    household (interior) NEC Y93.E9
    land Y93.H9
    property Y93.H9
  marching (on level or elevated terrain) Y93.01
  martial arts Y93.75
  microwave oven Y93.G3
  milking an animal Y93.K2
  mopping (floor) Y93.E5
  mountain climbing Y93.31
  muscle strengthening
    exercises (non-machine) NEC Y93.B9
    machines Y93.B1
  musical keyboard (electronic) playing Y93.J1
  nordic skiing Y93.24
  obstacle course Y93.A5
  oven (microwave) Y93.G3
  packing up and unpacking in moving to a new residence Y93.E6
  parasailing Y93.19
  pass out game Y93.85
  percussion instrument playing NEC Y93.J2
  personal
    bathing and showering Y93.E1
    hygiene NEC Y93.E8
    showering Y93.E1
  physical games generally associated with school recess, summer camp and children Y93.6A
  physical training NEC Y93.A9
  piano playing Y93.J1
  pilates Y93.B4
  platform diving Y93.12
  playing musical instrument
    brass instrument Y93.J4
    drum Y93.J2
    musical keyboard (electronic) Y93.J1
    percussion instrument NEC Y93.J2
    piano Y93.J1
    string instrument Y93.J3
    winds instrument Y93.J4

Activity - Assault

Activity — *continued*
property maintenance
  exterior NEC Y93.H9
  interior NEC Y93.E9
pruning (garden and lawn) Y93.H2
pull-ups Y93.B2
push-ups Y93.B2
racquetball Y93.73
rafting (in calm and turbulent water) Y93.16
raking (leaves) Y93.H1
rappelling Y93.32
refereeing a sports activity Y93.81
residential relocation Y93.E6
rhythmic gymnastics Y93.43
rhythmic movement NEC Y93.49
riding
  horseback Y93.52
  rollercoaster Y93.I1
rock climbing Y93.31
rollercoaster riding Y93.I1
roller skating (inline) Y93.51
rough housing and horseplay Y93.83
rowing (in calm and turbulent water) Y93.16
rugby Y93.63
running Y93.02
SCUBA diving Y93.15
sewing Y93.D2
shoveling Y93.H1
  dirt Y93.H1
  snow Y93.H1
showering (personal) Y93.E1
sit-ups Y93.B2
skateboarding Y93.51
skating (ice) Y93.21
  roller Y93.51
skiing (alpine) (downhill) Y93.23
  cross country Y93.24
  nordic Y93.24
  water Y93.17
sledding (snow) Y93.23
sleeping (sleep) Y93.84
smoking and grilling food Y93.G2
snorkeling Y93.15
snow NEC Y93.29
  boarding Y93.23
  shoveling Y93.H1
  sledding Y93.23
  tubing Y93.23
soccer Y93.66
softball Y93.64
specified NEC Y93.89
spectator at an event Y93.82
sports NEC Y93.79
  sports played as a team or group NEC Y93.69
  sports played individually NEC Y93.59
springboard diving Y93.12
squash Y93.73
stationary bike Y93.A1
step (stepping) exercise (class) Y93.A3
stepper machine Y93.A1
stove Y93.G3
string instrument playing Y93.J3
surfing Y93.18
  wind Y93.18
swimming Y93.11
tackle football Y93.61
tap dancing Y93.41
tennis Y93.73
tobogganing Y93.23
touch football Y93.62
track and field events (non-running) Y93.57
  running Y93.02
trampoline Y93.44
treadmill Y93.A1
trimming shrubs Y93.H2
tubing (in calm and turbulent water) Y93.16
  snow Y93.23
ultimate frisbee Y93.74
underwater diving Y93.15
unpacking in moving to a new residence Y93.E6
use of stove, oven and microwave oven Y93.G3
vacuuming Y93.E3
volleyball (beach) (court) Y93.68
wake boarding Y93.17
walking an animal Y93.K1
walking (on level or elevated terrain) Y93.01
  an animal Y93.K1
wall climbing Y93.31
warm up and cool down exercises Y93.A2
water NEC Y93.19
  aerobics Y93.14
  craft NEC Y93.19

Activity — *continued*
water NEC — *continued*
  exercise Y93.14
  polo Y93.13
  skiing Y93.17
  sliding Y93.18
  survival training and testing Y93.19
weeding (garden and lawn) Y93.H2
wind instrument playing Y93.J4
windsurfing Y93.18
wrestling Y93.72
yoga Y93.42
Adverse effect of drugs — *see* Table of Drugs and Chemicals
Aerosinusitis — *see* Air, pressure
After-effect, late — *see* Sequelae
Air
blast in war operations — *see* War operations, air blast
pressure
  change, rapid
    during
      ascent W94.29 ☑
        while (in) (surfacing from)
          aircraft W94.23 ☑
          deep water diving W94.21 ☑
          underground W94.22 ☑
      descent W94.39 ☑
        in
          aircraft W94.31 ☑
          water W94.32 ☑
  high, prolonged W94.0 ☑
  low, prolonged W94.12 ☑
    due to residence or long visit at high altitude W94.11 ☑
Alpine sickness W94.11 ☑
Altitude sickness W94.11 ☑
Anaphylactic shock, anaphylaxis — *see* Table of Drugs and Chemicals
Andes disease W94.11 ☑
Arachnidism, arachnoidism X58 ☑
Arson (with intent to injure or kill) X97 ☑
Asphyxia, asphyxiation
by
  food (bone) (seed) — *see* categories T17 ☑ and T18 ☑
  gas (*see also* Table of Drugs and Chemicals)
    legal
      execution — *see* Legal, intervention, gas
      intervention — *see* Legal, intervention, gas
from
  fire (*see also* Exposure, fire)
    in war operations — *see* War operations, fire
  ignition — *see* Ignition
  vomitus T17.81 ☑
in war operations — *see* War operations, restriction of airway
Aspiration
food (any type) (into respiratory tract) (with asphyxia, obstruction respiratory tract, suffocation) — *see* categories T17 ☑ and T18 ☑
foreign body — *see* Foreign body, aspiration
vomitus (with asphyxia, obstruction respiratory tract, suffocation) T17.81 ☑
Assassination (attempt) — *see* Assault
Assault (homicidal) (by) (in) Y09
arson X97 ☑
bite (of human being) Y04.1 ☑
bodily force Y04.8 ☑
  bite Y04.1 ☑
  bumping into Y04.2 ☑
  sexual — *see* subcategories T74.0 ☑, T76.0 ☑
  unarmed fight Y04.0 ☑
bomb X96.9 ☑
  antipersonnel X96.0 ☑
  fertilizer X96.3 ☑
  gasoline X96.1 ☑
  letter X96.2 ☑
  petrol X96.1 ☑
  pipe X96.3 ☑
  specified NEC X96.8 ☑
brawl (hand) (fists) (foot) (unarmed) Y04.0 ☑
burning, burns (by fire) NEC X97 ☑
  acid Y08.89 ☑
  caustic, corrosive substance Y08.89 ☑
  chemical from swallowing caustic, corrosive substance — *see* Table of Drugs and Chemicals
  cigarette(s) X97 ☑
  hot object X98.9 ☑
    fluid NEC X98.2 ☑
    household appliance X98.3 ☑

Assault — *continued*
burning, burns — *continued*
  specified NEC X98.8 ☑
  steam X98.0 ☑
  tap water X98.1 ☑
  vapors X98.0 ☑
scalding — *see* Assault, burning
  steam X98.0 ☑
  vitriol Y08.89 ☑
caustic, corrosive substance (gas) Y08.89 ☑
crashing of
  aircraft Y08.81 ☑
  motor vehicle Y03.8 ☑
    pushed in front of Y02.0 ☑
    run over Y03.0 ☑
    specified NEC Y03.8 ☑
cutting or piercing instrument X99.9 ☑
  dagger X99.2 ☑
  glass X99.0 ☑
  knife X99.1 ☑
  specified NEC X99.8 ☑
  sword X99.2 ☑
dagger X99.2 ☑
drowning (in) X92.9 ☑
  bathtub X92.0 ☑
  natural water X92.3 ☑
  specified NEC X92.8 ☑
  swimming pool X92.1 ☑
    following fall X92.2 ☑
dynamite X96.8 ☑
explosive(s) (material) X96.9 ☑
fight (hand) (fists) (foot) (unarmed) Y04.0 ☑
  with weapon — *see* Assault, by type of weapon
fire X97 ☑
firearm X95.9 ☑
  airgun X95.01 ☑
  handgun X93 ☑
  hunting rifle X94.1 ☑
  larger X94.9 ☑
    specified NEC X94.8 ☑
  machine gun X94.2 ☑
  shotgun X94.0 ☑
  specified NEC X95.8 ☑
gunshot (wound) NEC — *see* Assault, firearm, by type
incendiary device X97 ☑
injury Y09
  to child due to criminal abortion attempt NEC Y08.89 ☑
knife X99.1 ☑
late effect of — *see* X92-Y08 with 7th character S
placing before moving object NEC Y02.8 ☑
  motor vehicle Y02.0 ☑
poisoning — *see* categories T36-T65 with 7th character S
puncture, any part of body — *see* Assault, cutting or piercing instrument
pushing
  before moving object NEC Y02.8 ☑
    motor vehicle Y02.0 ☑
    subway train Y02.1 ☑
    train Y02.1 ☑
from high place Y01 ☑
rape T74.2 ☑
scalding — *see* Assault, burning
sequelae of — *see* X92-Y08 with 7th character S
sexual (by bodily force) T74.2 ☑
shooting — *see* Assault, firearm
specified means NEC Y08.89 ☑
stab, any part of body — *see* Assault, cutting or piercing instrument
steam X98.0 ☑
striking against
  other person Y04.2 ☑
  sports equipment Y08.09 ☑
    baseball bat Y08.02 ☑
    hockey stick Y08.01 ☑
struck by
  sports equipment Y08.09 ☑
    baseball bat Y08.02 ☑
    hockey stick Y08.01 ☑
submersion — *see* Assault, drowning
violence Y09
weapon Y09
  blunt Y00 ☑
  cutting or piercing — *see* Assault, cutting or piercing instrument
  firearm — *see* Assault, firearm
wound Y09
  cutting — *see* Assault, cutting or piercing instrument
  gunshot — *see* Assault, firearm

☑ **Additional character required**

Assault — *continued*
  wound — *continued*
    knife X99.1 ☑
    piercing — *see* Assault, cutting or piercing instrument
    puncture — *see* Assault, cutting or piercing instrument
    stab — *see* Assault, cutting or piercing instrument
Attack by mammals NEC W55.89 ☑
Avalanche — *see* Landslide
Aviator's disease — *see* Air, pressure

B

Barotitis, barodontalgia, barosinusitis, barotrauma (otitic) (sinus) — *see* Air, pressure
Battered (baby) (child) (person) (syndrome) X58 ☑
Bayonet wound W26.1 ☑
  in
    legal intervention — *see* Legal, intervention, sharp object, bayonet
    war operations — *see* War operations, combat
    stated as undetermined whether accidental or intentional Y28.8 ☑
    suicide (attempt) X78.2 ☑
Bean in nose — *see* categories T17 and T18 ☑
Bed set on fire NEC — *see* Exposure, fire, uncontrolled, building, bed
Beheading (by guillotine)
    homicide X99.9 ☑
    legal execution — *see* Legal, intervention
Bending, injury in (prolonged) (static) X50.1 ☑
Bends — *see* Air, pressure, change
Bite, bitten by
    alligator W58.01 ☑
    arthropod (nonvenomous) NEC W57 ☑
    bull W55.21 ☑
    cat W55.01 ☑
    cow W55.21 ☑
    crocodile W58.11 ☑
    dog W54.0 ☑
    goat W55.31 ☑
    hoof stock NEC W55.31 ☑
    horse W55.11 ☑
    human being (accidentally) W50.3 ☑
      with intent to injure or kill Y04.1 ☑
      as, or caused by, a crowd or human stampede (with fall) W52 ☑
      assault Y04.1 ☑
      homicide (attempt) Y04.1 ☑
      in
        fight Y04.1 ☑
    insect (nonvenomous) W57 ☑
    lizard (nonvenomous) W59.01 ☑
    mammal NEC W55.81 ☑
      marine W56.31 ☑
    marine animal (nonvenomous) W56.81 ☑
    millipede W57 ☑
    moray eel W56.51 ☑
    mouse W53.01 ☑
    person(s) (accidentally) W50.3 ☑
      with intent to injure or kill Y04.1 ☑
      as, or caused by, a crowd or human stampede (with fall) W52 ☑
      assault Y04.1 ☑
      homicide (attempt) Y04.1 ☑
      in
        fight Y04.1 ☑
    pig W55.41 ☑
    raccoon W55.51 ☑
    rat W53.11 ☑
    reptile W59.81 ☑
      lizard W59.01 ☑
      snake W59.11 ☑
      turtle W59.21 ☑
      terrestrial W59.81 ☑
    rodent W53.81 ☑
      mouse W53.01 ☑
      rat W53.11 ☑
      specified NEC W53.81 ☑
      squirrel W53.21 ☑
    shark W56.41 ☑
    sheep W55.31 ☑
    snake (nonvenomous) W59.11 ☑
    spider (nonvenomous) W57 ☑
    squirrel W53.21 ☑
Blast (air) in war operations — *see* War operations, blast
Blizzard X37.2 ☑

Blood alcohol level Y90.9
    less than 20mg/100ml Y90.0
    presence in blood, level not specified Y90.9
    20-39mg/100ml Y90.1
    40-59mg/100ml Y90.2
    60-79mg/100ml Y90.3
    80-99mg/100ml Y90.4
    100-119mg/100ml Y90.5
    120-199mg/100ml Y90.6
    200-239mg/100ml Y90.7
Blow X58 ☑
    by law-enforcing agent, police (on duty) — *see* Legal, intervention, manhandling
      blunt object — *see* Legal, intervention, blunt object
Blowing up — *see* Explosion
Brawl (hand) (fists) (foot) Y04.0 ☑
Breakage (accidental) (part of)
    ladder (causing fall) W11 ☑
    scaffolding (causing fall) W12 ☑
Broken
    glass, contact with — *see* Contact, with, glass
    power line (causing electric shock) W85 ☑
Bumping against, into (accidentally)
    object NEC W22.8 ☑
      with fall — *see* Fall, due to, bumping against, object
      caused by crowd or human stampede (with fall) W52 ☑
      sports equipment W21.9 ☑
    person(s) W51 ☑
      with fall W03 ☑
        due to ice or snow W00.0 ☑
      assault Y04.2 ☑
      caused by, a crowd or human stampede (with fall) W52 ☑
      homicide (attempt) Y04.2 ☑
      sports equipment W21.9 ☑
Burn, burned, burning (accidental) (by) (from) (on)
    acid NEC — *see* Table of Drugs and Chemicals
    bed linen — *see* Exposure, fire, uncontrolled, in building, bed
    blowtorch X08.8 ☑
      with ignition of clothing NEC X06.2 ☑
        nightwear X05 ☑
    bonfire, campfire (controlled) (*see also* Exposure, fire, controlled, not in building)
      uncontrolled — *see* Exposure, fire, uncontrolled, not in building
    candle X08.8 ☑
      with ignition of clothing NEC X06.2 ☑
        nightwear X05 ☑
    caustic liquid, substance (external) (internal) NEC — *see* Table of Drugs and Chemicals
    chemical (external) (internal) (*see also* Table of Drugs and Chemicals)
      in war operations — *see* War operations. fire
    cigar(s) or cigarette(s) X08.8 ☑
      with ignition of clothing NEC X06.2 ☑
        nightwear X05 ☑
    clothes, clothing NEC (from controlled fire) X06.2 ☑
      with conflagration — *see* Exposure, fire, uncontrolled, building
      not in building or structure — *see* Exposure, fire, uncontrolled, not in building
    cooker (hot) X15.8 ☑
      stated as undetermined whether accidental or intentional Y27.3 ☑
      suicide (attempt) X77.3 ☑
    electric blanket X16 ☑
    engine (hot) X17 ☑
    fire, flames — *see* Exposure, fire
    flare, Very pistol — *see* Discharge, firearm NEC
    heat
      from appliance (electrical) (household) X15.8 ☑
        cooker X15.8 ☑
        hotplate X15.2 ☑
        kettle X15.8 ☑
        light bulb X15.8 ☑
        saucepan X15.3 ☑
        skillet X15.3 ☑
        stove X15.0 ☑
        stated as undetermined whether accidental or intentional Y27.3 ☑
        suicide (attempt) X77.3 ☑
        toaster X15.1 ☑
      in local application or packing during medical or surgical procedure Y63.5
    heating
      appliance, radiator or pipe X16 ☑
    homicide (attempt) — *see* Assault, burning

Burn — *continued*
  hot
    air X14.1 ☑
    cooker X15.8 ☑
    drink X10.0 ☑
    engine X17 ☑
    fat X10.2 ☑
    fluid NEC X12 ☑
    food X10.1 ☑
    gases X14.1 ☑
    heating appliance X16 ☑
    household appliance NEC X15.8 ☑
    kettle X15.8 ☑
    liquid NEC X12 ☑
    machinery X17 ☑
    metal (molten) (liquid) NEC X18 ☑
    object (not producing fire or flames) NEC X19 ☑
    oil (cooking) X10.2 ☑
    pipe(s) X16 ☑
    radiator X16 ☑
    saucepan (glass) (metal) X15.3 ☑
    stove (kitchen) X15.0 ☑
    substance NEC X19 ☑
      caustic or corrosive NEC — *see* Table of Drugs and Chemicals
    toaster X15.1 ☑
    tool X17 ☑
    vapor X13.1 ☑
    water (tap) — *see* Contact, with, hot, tap water
  hotplate X15.2 ☑
    suicide (attempt) X77.3 ☑
  ignition — *see* Ignition
  in war operations — *see* War operations, fire
  inflicted by other person X97 ☑
    by hot objects, hot vapor, and steam — *see* Assault, burning, hot object
  internal, from swallowed caustic, corrosive liquid, substance — *see* Table of Drugs and Chemicals
  iron (hot) X15.8 ☑
    stated as undetermined whether accidental or intentional Y27.3 ☑
    suicide (attempt) X77.3 ☑
  kettle (hot) X15.8 ☑
    stated as undetermined whether accidental or intentional Y27.3 ☑
    suicide (attempt) X77.3 ☑
  lamp (flame) X08.8 ☑
    with ignition of clothing NEC X06.2 ☑
      nightwear X05 ☑
  lighter (cigar) (cigarette) X08.8 ☑
    with ignition of clothing NEC X06.2 ☑
      nightwear X05 ☑
  lightning — *see* subcategory T75.0 ☑
    causing fire — *see* Exposure, fire
  liquid (boiling) (hot) NEC X12 ☑
    stated as undetermined whether accidental or intentional Y27.2 ☑
    suicide (attempt) X77.2 ☑
  local application of externally applied substance in medical or surgical care Y63.5
  on board watercraft
    due to
      accident to watercraft V91.09 ☑
        powered craft V91.03 ☑
          ferry boat V91.01 ☑
          fishing boat V91.02 ☑
          jetskis V91.03 ☑
          liner V91.01 ☑
          merchant ship V91.00 ☑
          passenger ship V91.01 ☑
        unpowered craft V91.08 ☑
          canoe V91.05 ☑
          inflatable V91.06 ☑
          kayak V91.05 ☑
          sailboat V91.04 ☑
          surf-board V91.08 ☑
          water skis V91.07 ☑
          windsurfer V91.08 ☑
      fire on board V93.09 ☑
        ferry boat V93.01 ☑
        fishing boat V93.02 ☑
        jetskis V93.03 ☑
        liner V93.01 ☑
        merchant ship V93.00 ☑
        passenger ship V93.01 ☑
        powered craft NEC V93.03 ☑

Burn — *continued*
- on board watercraft — *continued*
  - sailboat V93.04 ☑
  - specified heat source NEC on board V93.19 ☑
    - ferry boat V93.11 ☑
    - fishing boat V93.12 ☑
    - jetskis V93.13 ☑
    - liner V93.11 ☑
    - merchant ship V93.10 ☑
    - passenger ship V93.11 ☑
    - powered craft NEC V93.13 ☑
    - sailboat V93.14 ☑
- machinery (hot) X17 ☑
- matches X08.8 ☑
  - with ignition of clothing NEC X06.2 ☑
    - nightwear X05 ☑
- mattress — *see* Exposure, fire, uncontrolled, building, bed
- medicament, externally applied Y63.5
- metal (hot) (liquid) (molten) NEC X18 ☑
- nightwear (nightclothes, nightdress, gown, pajamas, robe) X05 ☑
- object (hot) NEC X19 ☑
- pipe (hot) X16 ☑
  - smoking X08.8 ☑
    - with ignition of clothing NEC X06.2 ☑
      - nightwear X05 ☑
- powder — *see* Powder burn
- radiator (hot) X16 ☑
- saucepan (hot) (glass) (metal) X15.3 ☑
  - stated as undetermined whether accidental or intentional Y27.3 ☑
  - suicide (attempt) X77.3 ☑
- self-inflicted X76 ☑
  - stated as undetermined whether accidental or intentional Y26 ☑
- steam X13.1 ☑
  - pipe X16 ☑
    - stated as undetermined whether accidental or intentional Y27.8 ☑
  - stated as undetermined whether accidental or intentional Y27.0 ☑
  - suicide (attempt) X77.0 ☑
- stove (hot) (kitchen) X15.0 ☑
  - stated as undetermined whether accidental or intentional Y27.3 ☑
  - suicide (attempt) X77.3 ☑
- substance (hot) NEC X19 ☑
  - boiling X12 ☑
    - stated as undetermined whether accidental or intentional Y27.2 ☑
    - suicide (attempt) X77.2 ☑
  - molten (metal) X18 ☑
- suicide (attempt) NEC X76 ☑
  - hot
    - household appliance X77.3 ☑
    - object X77.9 ☑
- stated as undetermined whether accidental or intentional Y27.0 ☑
- therapeutic misadventure
  - heat in local application or packing during medical or surgical procedure Y63.5
  - overdose of radiation Y63.2
- toaster (hot) X15.1 ☑
  - stated as undetermined whether accidental or intentional Y27.3 ☑
  - suicide (attempt) X77.3 ☑
- tool (hot) X17 ☑
- torch, welding X08.8 ☑
  - with ignition of clothing NEC X06.2 ☑
    - nightwear X05 ☑
- trash fire (controlled) — *see* Exposure, fire, controlled, not in building
  - uncontrolled — *see* Exposure, fire, uncontrolled, not in building
- vapor (hot) X13.1 ☑
  - stated as undetermined whether accidental or intentional Y27.0 ☑
  - suicide (attempt) X77.0 ☑
- Very pistol — *see* Discharge, firearm NEC
Butted by animal W55.82 ☑
- bull W55.22 ☑
- cow W55.22 ☑
- goat W55.32 ☑
- horse W55.12 ☑
- pig W55.42 ☑
- sheep W55.32 ☑

C

Caisson disease — *see* Air, pressure, change
Campfire (exposure to) (controlled) (*see also* Exposure, fire, controlled, not in building)
- uncontrolled — *see* Exposure, fire, uncontrolled, not in building
Capital punishment (any means) — *see* Legal, intervention
Car sickness T75.3 ☑
Casualty (not due to war) NEC X58 ☑
- war — *see* War operations
Cat
- bite W55.01 ☑
- scratch W55.03 ☑
Cataclysm, cataclysmic (any injury) NEC — *see* Forces of nature
Catching fire — *see* Exposure, fire
Caught
- between
  - folding object W23.0 ☑
  - objects (moving) (stationary and moving) W23.0 ☑
    - and machinery — *see* Contact, with, by type of machine
    - stationary W23.1 ☑
  - sliding door and door frame W23.0 ☑
- by, in
  - machinery (moving parts of) — *see* Contact, with, by type of machine
  - washing-machine wringer W23.0 ☑
- under packing crate (due to losing grip) W23.1 ☑
Cave-in caused by cataclysmic earth surface movement or eruption — *see* Landslide
Change(s) in air pressure — *see* Air, pressure, change
Choked, choking (on) (any object except food or vomitus)
- food (bone) (seed) — *see* categories T17 ☑ and T18 ☑
- vomitus T17.81 ☑
Civil insurrection — *see* War operations
Cloudburst (any injury) X37.8 ☑
Cold, exposure to (accidental) (excessive) (extreme) (natural) (place) NEC — *see* Exposure, cold
Collapse
- building W20.1 ☑
  - burning (uncontrolled fire) X00.2 ☑
- dam or man-made structure (causing earth movement) X36.0 ☑
- machinery — *see* Contact, with, by type of machine
- structure W20.1 ☑
  - burning (uncontrolled fire) X00.2 ☑
Collision (accidental) NEC (*see also* Accident, transport) V89.9 ☑
- pedestrian W51 ☑
  - with fall W03 ☑
    - due to ice or snow W00.0 ☑
    - involving pedestrian conveyance — *see* Accident, transport, pedestrian, conveyance
  - and
    - crowd or human stampede (with fall) W52 ☑
    - object W22.8 ☑
      - with fall — *see* Fall, due to, bumping against, object
  - person(s) — *see* Collision, pedestrian
- transport vehicle NEC V89.9 ☑
  - and
    - avalanche, fallen or not moving — *see* Accident, transport
      - falling or moving — *see* Landslide
    - landslide, fallen or not moving — *see* Accident, transport
      - falling or moving — *see* Landslide
    - due to cataclysm — *see* Forces of nature, by type
    - intentional, purposeful suicide (attempt) — *see* Suicide, collision
Combustion, spontaneous — *see* Ignition
Complication (delayed) of or following (medical or surgical procedure) Y84.9
- with misadventure — *see* Misadventure
- amputation of limb(s) Y83.5
- anastomosis (arteriovenous) (blood vessel) (gastrojejunal) (tendon) (natural or artificial material) Y83.2
- aspiration (of fluid) Y84.4
  - tissue Y84.8
- biopsy Y84.8
- blood
  - sampling Y84.7
  - transfusion
    - procedure Y84.8
- bypass Y83.2

Complication — *continued*
- catheterization (urinary) Y84.6
  - cardiac Y84.0
- colostomy Y83.3
- cystostomy Y83.3
- dialysis (kidney) Y84.1
- drug — *see* Table of Drugs and Chemicals
- due to misadventure — *see* Misadventure
- duodenostomy Y83.3
- electroshock therapy Y84.3
- external stoma, creation of Y83.3
- formation of external stoma Y83.3
- gastrostomy Y83.3
- graft Y83.2
- hypothermia (medically-induced) Y84.8
- implant, implantation (of)
  - artificial
    - internal device (cardiac pacemaker) (electrodes in brain) (heart valve prosthesis) (orthopedic) Y83.1
    - material or tissue (for anastomosis or bypass) Y83.2
      - with creation of external stoma Y83.3
  - natural tissues (for anastomosis or bypass) Y83.2
    - with creation of external stoma Y83.3
- infusion
  - procedure Y84.8
- injection — *see* Table of Drugs and Chemicals
  - procedure Y84.8
- insertion of gastric or duodenal sound Y84.5
- insulin-shock therapy Y84.3
- paracentesis (abdominal) (thoracic) (aspirative) Y84.4
- procedures other than surgical operation — *see* Complication of or following, by type of procedure
- radiological procedure or therapy Y84.2
- removal of organ (partial) (total) NEC Y83.6
- sampling
  - blood Y84.7
  - fluid NEC Y84.4
  - tissue Y84.8
- shock therapy Y84.3
- surgical operation NEC (*see also* Complication of or following, by type of operation) Y83.9
  - reconstructive NEC Y83.4
    - with
      - anastomosis, bypass or graft Y83.2
      - formation of external stoma Y83.3
  - specified NEC Y83.8
- transfusion (*see also* Table of Drugs and Chemicals)
  - procedure Y84.8
- transplant, transplantation (heart) (kidney) (liver) (whole organ, any) Y83.0
  - partial organ Y83.4
- ureterostomy Y83.3
- vaccination (*see also* Table of Drugs and Chemicals)
  - procedure Y84.8
Compression
- divers' squeeze — *see* Air, pressure, change
- trachea by
  - food (lodged in esophagus) — *see* categories T17 ☑ and T18 ☑
  - vomitus (lodged in esophagus) T17.81 ☑
Conflagration — *see* Exposure, fire, uncontrolled
Constriction (external)
- hair W49.01 ☑
- jewelry W49.04 ☑
- ring W49.04 ☑
- rubber band W49.03 ☑
- specified item NEC W49.09 ☑
- string W49.02 ☑
- thread W49.02 ☑
Contact (accidental)
- with
  - abrasive wheel (metalworking) W31.1 ☑
  - alligator W58.09 ☑
    - bite W58.01 ☑
    - crushing W58.03 ☑
    - strike W58.02 ☑
  - amphibian W62.9 ☑
    - frog W62.0 ☑
    - toad W62.1 ☑
  - animal (nonvenomous) NEC W64 ☑
    - marine W56.89 ☑
      - bite W56.81 ☑
      - dolphin — *see* Contact, with, dolphin
      - fish NEC — *see* Contact, with, fish
      - mammal — *see* Contact, with, mammal, marine
      - orca — *see* Contact, with, orca
      - sea lion — *see* Contact, with, sea lion

☑ **Additional character required**

Contact — *continued*
  with — *continued*
      shark — *see* Contact, with, shark
      strike W56.82 ☑
    animate mechanical force NEC W64 ☑
    arrow W21.89 ☑
      not thrown, projected or falling W45.8 ☑
    arthropods (nonvenomous) W57 ☑
    axe W27.0 ☑
    band-saw (industrial) W31.2 ☑
    bayonet — *see* Bayonet wound
    bee(s) X58 ☑
    bench-saw (industrial) W31.2 ☑
    bird W61.99 ☑
      bite W61.91 ☑
      chicken — *see* Contact, with, chicken
      duck — *see* Contact, with, duck
      goose — *see* Contact, with, goose
      macaw — *see* Contact, with, macaw
      parrot — *see* Contact, with, parrot
      psittacine — *see* Contact, with, psittacine
      strike W61.92 ☑
      turkey — *see* Contact, with, turkey
    blender W29.0 ☑
    boiling water X12 ☑
      stated as undetermined whether accidental or
        intentional Y27.2 ☑
      suicide (attempt) X77.2 ☑
    bore, earth-drilling or mining (land) (seabed)
      W31.0 ☑
    buffalo — *see* Contact, with, hoof stock NEC
    bull W55.29 ☑
      bite W55.21 ☑
      gored W55.22 ☑
      strike W55.22 ☑
    bumper cars W31.81 ☑
    camel — *see* Contact, with, hoof stock NEC
    can
      lid W26.8 ☑
      opener W27.4 ☑
        powered W29.0 ☑
    cat W55.09 ☑
      bite W55.01 ☑
      scratch W55.03 ☑
    caterpillar (venomous) X58 ☑
    centipede (venomous) X58 ☑
    chain
      hoist W24.0 ☑
        agricultural operations W30.89 ☑
      saw W29.3 ☑
    chicken W61.39 ☑
      peck W61.33 ☑
      strike W61.32 ☑
    chisel W27.0 ☑
    circular saw W31.2 ☑
    cobra X58 ☑
    combine (harvester) W30.0 ☑
    conveyer belt W24.1 ☑
    cooker (hot) X15.8 ☑
      stated as undetermined whether accidental or
        intentional Y27.3 ☑
      suicide (attempt) X77.3 ☑
    coral X58 ☑
    cotton gin W31.82 ☑
    cow W55.29 ☑
      bite W55.21 ☑
      strike W55.22 ☑
    crane W24.0 ☑
      agricultural operations W30.89 ☑
    crocodile W58.19 ☑
      bite W58.11 ☑
      crushing W58.13 ☑
      strike W58.12 ☑
    dagger W26.1 ☑
      stated as undetermined whether accidental or
        intentional Y28.2 ☑
      suicide (attempt) X78.2 ☑
    dairy equipment W31.82 ☑
    dart W21.89 ☑
      not thrown, projected or falling W45.8 ☑
    deer — *see* Contact, with, hoof stock NEC
    derrick W24.0 ☑
      agricultural operations W30.89 ☑
        hay W30.2 ☑
    dog W54.8 ☑
      bite W54.0 ☑
      strike W54.1 ☑
    dolphin W56.09 ☑
      bite W56.01 ☑
      strike W56.02 ☑
    donkey — *see* Contact, with, hoof stock NEC
    drill (powered) W29.8 ☑

Contact — *continued*
  with — *continued*
      earth (land) (seabed) W31.0 ☑
      nonpowered W27.8 ☑
    drive belt W24.0 ☑
      agricultural operations W30.89 ☑
    dry ice — *see* Exposure, cold, man-made
    dryer (clothes) (powered) (spin) W29.2 ☑
    duck W61.69 ☑
      bite W61.61 ☑
      strike W61.62 ☑
    earth (-)
      drilling machine (industrial) W31.0 ☑
      scraping machine in stationary use W31.83 ☑
    edge of stiff paper W26.2 ☑
    electric
      beater W29.0 ☑
      blanket X16 ☑
      fan W29.2 ☑
        commercial W31.82 ☑
      knife W29.1 ☑
      mixer W29.0 ☑
    elevator (building) W24.0 ☑
      agricultural operations W30.89 ☑
      grain W30.3 ☑
    engine(s), hot NEC X17 ☑
    excavating machine W31.0 ☑
    farm machine W30.9 ☑
    feces — *see* Contact, with, by type of animal
    fer de lance X58 ☑
    fish W56.59 ☑
      bite W56.51 ☑
      shark — *see* Contact, with, shark
      strike W56.52 ☑
    flying horses W31.81 ☑
    forging (metalworking) machine W31.1 ☑
    fork W27.4 ☑
    forklift (truck) W24.0 ☑
      agricultural operations W30.89 ☑
    frog W62.0 ☑
    garden
      cultivator (powered) W29.3 ☑
        riding W30.89 ☑
      fork W27.1 ☑
    gas turbine W31.3 ☑
    Gila monster X58 ☑
    giraffe — *see* Contact, with, hoof stock NEC
    glass (sharp) (broken) W25 ☑
      with subsequent fall W18.02 ☑
      assault X99.0 ☑
      due to fall — *see* Fall, by type
      stated as undetermined whether accidental or
        intentional Y28.0 ☑
      suicide (attempt) X78.0 ☑
    goat W55.39 ☑
      bite W55.31 ☑
      strike W55.32 ☑
    goose W61.59 ☑
      bite W61.51 ☑
      strike W61.52 ☑
    hand
      saw W27.0 ☑
      tool (not powered) NEC W27.8 ☑
        powered W29.8 ☑
    harvester W30.0 ☑
    hay-derrick W30.2 ☑
    heat NEC X19 ☑
      from appliance (electrical) (household) — *see*
        Contact, with, hot, household appliance
        heating appliance X16 ☑
    heating
      appliance (hot) X16 ☑
      pad (electric) X16 ☑
    hedge-trimmer (powered) W29.3 ☑
    hoe W27.1 ☑
    hoist (chain) (shaft) NEC W24.0 ☑
      agricultural W30.89 ☑
    hoof stock NEC W55.39 ☑
      bite W55.31 ☑
      strike W55.32 ☑
    hornet(s) X58 ☑
    horse W55.19 ☑
      bite W55.11 ☑
      strike W55.12 ☑
    hot
      air X14.1 ☑
        inhalation X14.0 ☑
      cooker X15.8 ☑
      drinks X10.0 ☑
      engine X17 ☑
      fats X10.2 ☑
      fluids NEC X12 ☑

Contact — *continued*
  with — *continued*
      assault X98.2 ☑
      suicide (attempt) X77.2 ☑
      undetermined whether accidental or
        intentional Y27.2 ☑
      food X10.1 ☑
      gases X14.1 ☑
        inhalation X14.0 ☑
      heating appliance X16 ☑
      household appliance X15.8 ☑
        assault X98.3 ☑
        cooker X15.8 ☑
        hotplate X15.2 ☑
        kettle X15.8 ☑
        light bulb X15.8 ☑
        object NEC X19 ☑
          assault X98.8 ☑
          stated as undetermined whether accidental
            or intentional Y27.9 ☑
          suicide (attempt) X77.8 ☑
        saucepan X15.3 ☑
        skillet X15.3 ☑
        stove X15.0 ☑
        stated as undetermined whether accidental
          or intentional Y27.3 ☑
        suicide (attempt) X77.3 ☑
        toaster X15.1 ☑
      kettle X15.8 ☑
      light bulb X15.8 ☑
      liquid NEC (*see also* Burn) X12 ☑
        drinks X10.0 ☑
        stated as undetermined whether accidental
          or intentional Y27.2 ☑
        suicide (attempt) X77.2 ☑
        tap water X11.8 ☑
          stated as undetermined whether accidental
            or intentional Y27.1 ☑
          suicide (attempt) X77.1 ☑
      machinery X17 ☑
      metal (molten) (liquid) NEC X18 ☑
      object (not producing fire or flames) NEC
        X19 ☑
      oil (cooking) X10.2 ☑
      pipe X16 ☑
      plate X15.2 ☑
      radiator X16 ☑
      saucepan (glass) (metal) X15.3 ☑
      skillet X15.3 ☑
      stove (kitchen) X15.0 ☑
      substance NEC X19 ☑
      tap-water X11.8 ☑
        assault X98.1 ☑
        heated on stove X12 ☑
          stated as undetermined whether accidental
            or intentional Y27.2 ☑
          suicide (attempt) X77.2 ☑
        in bathtub X11.0 ☑
        running X11.1 ☑
        stated as undetermined whether accidental
          or intentional Y27.1 ☑
        suicide (attempt) X77.1 ☑
      toaster X15.1 ☑
      tool X17 ☑
      vapors X13.1 ☑
        inhalation X13.0 ☑
      water (tap) X11.8 ☑
        boiling X12 ☑
          stated as undetermined whether accidental
            or intentional Y27.2 ☑
          suicide (attempt) X77.2 ☑
        heated on stove X12 ☑
          stated as undetermined whether accidental
            or intentional Y27.2 ☑
          suicide (attempt) X77.2 ☑
        in bathtub X11.0 ☑
        running X11.1 ☑
        stated as undetermined whether accidental
          or intentional Y27.1 ☑
        suicide (attempt) X77.1 ☑
      hotplate X15.2 ☑
    ice-pick W27.4 ☑
    insect (nonvenomous) NEC W57 ☑
    kettle (hot) X15.8 ☑
    knife W26.0 ☑
      assault X99.1 ☑
      electric W29.1 ☑
      stated as undetermined whether accidental or
        intentional Y28.1 ☑
      suicide (attempt) X78.1 ☑
    lathe (metalworking) W31.1 ☑
      turnings W45.8 ☑

ICD-10-CM INDEX TO EXTERNAL CAUSES OF INJURIES

Contact

Contact — *continued*
  with — *continued*
    woodworking W31.2 ☑
  lawnmower (powered) (ridden) W28 ☑
    causing electrocution W86.8 ☑
      suicide (attempt) X83.1 ☑
    unpowered W27.1 ☑
  lift, lifting (devices) W24.0 ☑
    agricultural operations W30.89 ☑
    shaft W24.0 ☑
  liquefied gas — *see* Exposure, cold, man-made
  liquid air, hydrogen, nitrogen — *see* Exposure,
      cold, man-made
  lizard (nonvenomous) W59.09 ☑
    bite W59.01 ☑
    strike W59.02 ☑
  llama — *see* Contact, with, hoof stock NEC
  macaw W61.19 ☑
    bite W61.11 ☑
    strike W61.12 ☑
  machine, machinery W31.9 ☑
    abrasive wheel W31.1 ☑
    agricultural including animal-powered W30.9 ☑
      combine harvester W30.0 ☑
      grain storage elevator W30.3 ☑
      hay derrick W30.2 ☑
      power take-off device W30.1 ☑
      reaper W30.0 ☑
      specified NEC W30.89 ☑
      thresher W30.0 ☑
      transport vehicle, stationary W30.81 ☑
    band saw W31.2 ☑
    bench saw W31.2 ☑
    circular saw W31.2 ☑
    commercial NEC W31.82 ☑
    drilling, metal (industrial) W31.1 ☑
    earth-drilling W31.0 ☑
    earthmoving or scraping W31.89 ☑
    excavating W31.89 ☑
    forging machine W31.1 ☑
    gas turbine W31.3 ☑
    hot X17 ☑
    internal combustion engine W31.3 ☑
    land drill W31.0 ☑
    lathe W31.1 ☑
    lifting (devices) W24.0 ☑
    metal drill W31.1 ☑
    metalworking (industrial) W31.1 ☑
    milling, metal W31.1 ☑
    mining W31.0 ☑
    molding W31.2 ☑
    overhead plane W31.2 ☑
    power press, metal W31.1 ☑
    prime mover W31.3 ☑
    printing W31.89 ☑
    radial saw W31.2 ☑
    recreational W31.81 ☑
    roller-coaster W31.81 ☑
    rolling mill, metal W31.1 ☑
    sander W31.2 ☑
    seabed drill W31.0 ☑
    shaft
      hoist W31.0 ☑
      lift W31.0 ☑
    specified NEC W31.89 ☑
    spinning W31.89 ☑
    steam engine W31.3 ☑
    transmission W24.1 ☑
    undercutter W31.0 ☑
    water driven turbine W31.3 ☑
    weaving W31.89 ☑
    woodworking or forming (industrial) W31.2 ☑
  mammal (feces) (urine) W55.89 ☑
    bull — *see* Contact, with, bull
    cat — *see* Contact, with, cat
    cow — *see* Contact, with, cow
    goat — *see* Contact, with, goat
    hoof stock — *see* Contact, with, hoof stock
    horse — *see* Contact, with, horse
    marine W56.39 ☑
      dolphin — *see* Contact, with, dolphin
      orca — *see* Contact, with, orca
      sea lion — *see* Contact, with, sea lion
      specified NEC W56.39 ☑
        bite W56.31 ☑
        strike W56.32 ☑
    pig — *see* Contact, with, pig
    raccoon — *see* Contact, with, raccoon
    rodent — *see* Contact, with, rodent
    sheep — *see* Contact, with, sheep
    specified NEC W55.89 ☑
      bite W55.81 ☑

Contact — *continued*
  with — *continued*
    strike W55.82 ☑
  marine
    animal W56.89 ☑
      bite W56.81 ☑
      dolphin — *see* Contact, with, dolphin
      fish NEC — *see* Contact, with, fish
      mammal — *see* Contact, with, mammal,
          marine
      orca — *see* Contact, with, orca
      sea lion — *see* Contact, with, sea lion
      shark — *see* Contact, with, shark
      strike W56.82 ☑
  meat
    grinder (domestic) W29.0 ☑
      industrial W31.82 ☑
      nonpowered W27.4 ☑
    slicer (domestic) W29.0 ☑
      industrial W31.82 ☑
  merry go round W31.81 ☑
  metal, hot (liquid) (molten) NEC X18 ☑
  millipede W57 ☑
  nail W45.0 ☑
    gun W29.4 ☑
  needle (sewing) W27.3 ☑
    hypodermic W46.0 ☑
      contaminated W46.1 ☑
  object (blunt) NEC
    hot NEC X19 ☑
    legal intervention — *see* Legal, intervention,
        blunt object
    sharp NEC W45.8 ☑
      inflicted by other person NEC W45.8 ☑
        stated as
          intentional homicide (attempt) —
              see Assault, cutting or piercing
              instrument
      legal intervention — *see* Legal, intervention,
          sharp object
      self-inflicted X78.9 ☑
  orca W56.29 ☑
    bite W56.21 ☑
    strike W56.22 ☑
  overhead plane W31.2 ☑
  paper (as sharp object) W26.2 ☑
  paper-cutter W27.5 ☑
  parrot W61.09 ☑
    bite W61.01 ☑
    strike W61.02 ☑
  pig W55.49 ☑
    bite W55.41 ☑
    strike W55.42 ☑
  pipe, hot X16 ☑
  pitchfork W27.1 ☑
  plane (metal) (wood) W27.0 ☑
    overhead W31.2 ☑
  plant thorns, spines, sharp leaves or other
      mechanisms W60 ☑
  powered
    garden cultivator W29.3 ☑
    household appliance, implement, or machine
        W29.8 ☑
    saw (industrial) W31.2 ☑
      hand W29.8 ☑
  printing machine W31.89 ☑
  psittacine bird W61.29 ☑
    bite W61.21 ☑
    macaw — *see* Contact, with, macaw
    parrot — *see* Contact, with, parrot
    strike W61.22 ☑
  pulley (block) (transmission) W24.0 ☑
    agricultural operations W30.89 ☑
  raccoon W55.59 ☑
    bite W55.51 ☑
    strike W55.52 ☑
  radial-saw (industrial) W31.2 ☑
  radiator (hot) X16 ☑
  rake W27.1 ☑
  rattlesnake X58 ☑
  reaper W30.0 ☑
  reptile W59.89 ☑
    lizard — *see* Contact, with, lizard
    snake — *see* Contact, with, snake
    specified NEC W59.89 ☑
      bite W59.81 ☑
      crushing W59.83 ☑
      strike W59.82 ☑
    turtle — *see* Contact, with, turtle
  rivet gun (powered) W29.4 ☑
  road scraper — *see* Accident, transport,
      construction vehicle

Contact — *continued*
  with — *continued*
    rodent (feces) (urine) W53.89 ☑
      bite W53.81 ☑
      mouse W53.09 ☑
        bite W53.01 ☑
      rat W53.19 ☑
        bite W53.11 ☑
      specified NEC W53.89 ☑
        bite W53.81 ☑
      squirrel W53.29 ☑
        bite W53.21 ☑
  roller coaster W31.81 ☑
  rope NEC W24.0 ☑
    agricultural operations W30.89 ☑
  saliva — *see* Contact, with, by type of animal
  sander W29.8 ☑
    industrial W31.2 ☑
  saucepan (hot) (glass) (metal) X15.3 ☑
  saw W27.0 ☑
    band (industrial) W31.2 ☑
    bench (industrial) W31.2 ☑
    chain W29.3 ☑
    hand W27.0 ☑
  sawing machine, metal W31.1 ☑
  scissors W27.2 ☑
  scorpion X58 ☑
  screwdriver W27.0 ☑
    powered W29.8 ☑
  sea
    anemone, cucumber or urchin (spine) X58 ☑
    lion W56.19 ☑
      bite W56.11 ☑
      strike W56.12 ☑
  serpent — *see* Contact, with, snake, by type
  sewing-machine (electric) (powered) W29.2 ☑
    not powered W27.8 ☑
  shaft (hoist) (lift) (transmission) NEC W24.0 ☑
    agricultural W30.89 ☑
  shark W56.49 ☑
    bite W56.41 ☑
    strike W56.42 ☑
  sharp object(s) W26.9 ☑
    specified NEC W26.8 ☑
  shears (hand) W27.2 ☑
    powered (industrial) W31.1 ☑
    domestic W29.2 ☑
  sheep W55.39 ☑
    bite W55.31 ☑
    strike W55.32 ☑
  shovel W27.8 ☑
    steam — *see* Accident, transport, construction
        vehicle
  snake (nonvenomous) W59.19 ☑
    bite W59.11 ☑
    crushing W59.13 ☑
    strike W59.12 ☑
  spade W27.1 ☑
  spider (venomous) X58 ☑
  spin-drier W29.2 ☑
  spinning machine W31.89 ☑
  splinter W45.8 ☑
  sports equipment W21.9 ☑
  staple gun (powered) W29.8 ☑
  steam X13.1 ☑
    engine W31.3 ☑
    inhalation X13.0 ☑
    pipe X16 ☑
    shovel W31.89 ☑
  stove (hot) (kitchen) X15.0 ☑
  substance, hot NEC X19 ☑
    molten (metal) X18 ☑
  sword W26.1 ☑
    assault X99.2 ☑
    stated as undetermined whether accidental or
        intentional Y28.2 ☑
    suicide (attempt) X78.2 ☑
  tarantula X58 ☑
  thresher W30.0 ☑
  tin can lid W26.8 ☑
  toad W62.1 ☑
  toaster (hot) X15.1 ☑
  tool W27.8 ☑
    hand (not powered) W27.8 ☑
      auger W27.0 ☑
      axe W27.0 ☑
      can opener W27.4 ☑
      chisel W27.0 ☑
      fork W27.4 ☑
      garden W27.1 ☑
      handsaw W27.0 ☑
      hoe W27.1 ☑

Contact — *continued*
  with — *continued*
    ice-pick W27.4 ☑
    kitchen utensil W27.4 ☑
    manual
      lawn mower W27.1 ☑
      sewing machine W27.8 ☑
    meat grinder W27.4 ☑
    needle (sewing) W27.3 ☑
      hypodermic W46.0 ☑
        contaminated W46.1 ☑
    paper cutter W27.5 ☑
    pitchfork W27.1 ☑
    rake W27.1 ☑
    scissors W27.2 ☑
    screwdriver W27.0 ☑
    specified NEC W27.8 ☑
    workbench W27.0 ☑
   hot X17 ☑
   powered W29.8 ☑
    blender W29.0 ☑
      commercial W31.82 ☑
    can opener W29.0 ☑
      commercial W31.82 ☑
    chainsaw W29.3 ☑
    clothes dryer W29.2 ☑
      commercial W31.82 ☑
    dishwasher W29.2 ☑
      commercial W31.82 ☑
    edger W29.3 ☑
    electric fan W29.2 ☑
      commercial W31.82 ☑
    electric knife W29.1 ☑
    food processor W29.0 ☑
      commercial W31.82 ☑
    garbage disposal W29.0 ☑
      commercial W31.82 ☑
    garden tool W29.3 ☑
    hedge trimmer W29.3 ☑
    ice maker W29.0 ☑
      commercial W31.82 ☑
    kitchen appliance W29.0 ☑
      commercial W31.82 ☑
    lawn mower W28 ☑
    meat grinder W29.0 ☑
      commercial W31.82 ☑
    mixer W29.0 ☑
      commercial W31.82 ☑
    rototiller W29.3 ☑
    sewing machine W29.2 ☑
      commercial W31.82 ☑
    washing machine W29.2 ☑
      commercial W31.82 ☑
   transmission device (belt, cable, chain, gear, pinion, shaft) W24.1 ☑
    agricultural operations W30.89 ☑
   turbine (gas) (water-driven) W31.3 ☑
   turkey W61.49 ☑
    peck W61.43 ☑
    strike W61.42 ☑
   turtle (nonvenomous) W59.29 ☑
    bite W59.21 ☑
    strike W59.22 ☑
    terrestrial W59.89 ☑
      bite W59.81 ☑
      crushing W59.83 ☑
      strike W59.82 ☑
   under-cutter W31.0 ☑
   urine — *see* Contact, with, by type of animal
   vehicle
    agricultural use (transport) — *see* Accident, transport, agricultural vehicle
      not on public highway W30.81 ☑
    industrial use (transport) — *see* Accident, transport, industrial vehicle
      not on public highway W31.83 ☑
    off-road use (transport) — *see* Accident, transport, all-terrain or off-road vehicle
      not on public highway W31.83 ☑
    special construction use (transport) — *see* Accident, transport, construction vehicle
      not on public highway W31.83 ☑
   venomous
    animal X58 ☑
    arthropods X58 ☑
    lizard X58 ☑
    marine animal NEC X58 ☑
    marine plant NEC X58 ☑
    millipedes (tropical) X58 ☑
    plant(s) X58 ☑
    snake X58 ☑
    spider X58 ☑

Contact — *continued*
  with — *continued*
   viper X58 ☑
   washing-machine (powered) W29.2 ☑
   wasp X58 ☑
   weaving-machine W31.89 ☑
   winch W24.0 ☑
    agricultural operations W30.89 ☑
   wire NEC W24.0 ☑
    agricultural operations W30.89 ☑
   wood slivers W45.8 ☑
   yellow jacket X58 ☑
   zebra — *see* Contact, with, hoof stock NEC
  pressure X50.9 ☑
  stress X50.9 ☑
Coup de soleil X32 ☑
Crash
  aircraft (in transit) (powered) V95.9 ☑
   balloon V96.01 ☑
   fixed wing NEC (private) V95.21 ☑
    commercial V95.31 ☑
   glider V96.21 ☑
    hang V96.11 ☑
    powered V95.11 ☑
   helicopter V95.01 ☑
   in war operations — *see* War operations, destruction of aircraft
   microlight V95.11 ☑
   nonpowered V96.9 ☑
    specified NEC V96.8 ☑
   powered NEC V95.8 ☑
   stated as
    homicide (attempt) Y08.81 ☑
    suicide (attempt) X83.0 ☑
   ultralight V95.11 ☑
  spacecraft V95.41 ☑
  transport vehicle NEC (*see also* Accident, transport) V89.9 ☑
   homicide (attempt) Y03.8 ☑
   motor NEC (traffic) V89.2 ☑
    homicide (attempt) Y03.8 ☑
    suicide (attempt) — *see* Suicide, collision
Cruelty (mental) (physical) (sexual) X58 ☑
Crushed (accidentally) X58 ☑
  between objects (moving) (stationary and moving) W23.0 ☑
   stationary W23.1 ☑
  by
   alligator W58.03 ☑
   avalanche NEC — *see* Landslide
   cave-in W20.0 ☑
    caused by cataclysmic earth surface movement — *see* Landslide
   crocodile W58.13 ☑
   crowd or human stampede W52 ☑
   falling
    aircraft V97.39 ☑
      in war operations — *see* War operations, destruction of aircraft
    earth, material W20.0 ☑
      caused by cataclysmic earth surface movement — *see* Landslide
    object NEC W20.8 ☑
   landslide NEC — *see* Landslide
   lizard (nonvenomous) W59.09 ☑
   machinery — *see* Contact, with, by type of machine
   reptile NEC W59.89 ☑
   snake (nonvenomous) W59.13 ☑
  in
   machinery — *see* Contact, with, by type of machine
Cut, cutting (any part of body) (accidental) (*see also* Contact, with, by object or machine)
  during medical or surgical treatment as misadventure — *see* Index to Diseases and Injuries, Complications
  homicide (attempt) — *see* Assault, cutting or piercing instrument
  inflicted by other person — *see* Assault, cutting or piercing instrument
  legal
   execution — *see* Legal, intervention
   intervention — *see* Legal, intervention, sharp object
  machine NEC (*see also* Contact, with, by type of machine) W31.9 ☑
  self-inflicted — *see* Suicide, cutting or piercing instrument
  suicide (attempt) — *see* Suicide, cutting or piercing instrument
Cyclone (any injury) X37.1 ☑

D

Decapitation (accidental circumstances) NEC X58 ☑
  homicide X99.9 ☑
  legal execution — *see* Legal, intervention
Dehydration from lack of water X58 ☑
Deprivation X58 ☑
Derailment (accidental)
  railway (rolling stock) (train) (vehicle) (without antecedent collision) V81.7 ☑
   with antecedent collision — *see* Accident, transport, railway vehicle occupant
  streetcar (without antecedent collision) V82.7 ☑
   with antecedent collision — *see* Accident, transport, streetcar occupant
Descent
  parachute (voluntary) (without accident to aircraft) V97.29 ☑
  due to accident to aircraft — *see* Accident, transport, aircraft
Desertion X58 ☑
Destitution X58 ☑
Disability, late effect or sequela of injury — *see* Sequelae
Discharge (accidental)
  airgun W34.010 ☑
   assault X95.01 ☑
   homicide (attempt) X95.01 ☑
   stated as undetermined whether accidental or intentional Y24.0 ☑
   suicide (attempt) X74.01 ☑
  BB gun — *see* Discharge, airgun
  firearm (accidental) W34.00 ☑
   assault X95.9 ☑
   handgun (pistol) (revolver) W32.0 ☑
    assault X93 ☑
    homicide (attempt) X93 ☑
    legal intervention — *see* Legal, intervention, firearm, handgun
    stated as undetermined whether accidental or intentional Y22 ☑
    suicide (attempt) X72 ☑
   homicide (attempt) X95.9 ☑
   hunting rifle W33.02 ☑
    assault X94.1 ☑
    homicide (attempt) X94.1 ☑
    legal intervention
      injuring
        bystander Y35.032 ☑
        law enforcement personnel Y35.031 ☑
        suspect Y35.033 ☑
        unspecified person Y35.039 ☑
    stated as undetermined whether accidental or intentional Y23.1 ☑
    suicide (attempt) X73.1 ☑
   larger W33.00 ☑
    assault X94.9 ☑
    homicide (attempt) X94.9 ☑
    hunting rifle — *see* Discharge, firearm, hunting rifle
    legal intervention — *see* Legal, intervention, firearm by type of firearm
    machine gun — *see* Discharge, firearm, machine gun
    shotgun — *see* Discharge, firearm, shotgun
    specified NEC W33.09 ☑
      assault X94.8 ☑
      homicide (attempt) X94.8 ☑
      legal intervention
        injuring
          bystander Y35.092 ☑
          law enforcement personnel Y35.091 ☑
          suspect Y35.093 ☑
          unspecified person Y35.099 ☑
      stated as undetermined whether accidental or intentional Y23.8 ☑
      suicide (attempt) X73.8 ☑
    stated as undetermined whether accidental or intentional Y23.9 ☑
    suicide (attempt) X73.9 ☑
   legal intervention
    injuring
      bystander Y35.002 ☑
      law enforcement personnel Y35.001 ☑
      suspect Y35.03 ☑
      unspecified person Y35.009 ☑
    using rubber bullet
      injuring
        bystander Y35.042 ☑
        law enforcement personnel Y35.041 ☑
        suspect Y35.043 ☑
        unspecified person Y35.049 ☑

Discharge — *continued*
  firearm — *continued*
    machine gun W33.03 ☑
      assault X94.2 ☑
      homicide (attempt) X94.2 ☑
      legal intervention — *see* Legal, intervention, firearm, machine gun
      stated as undetermined whether accidental or intentional Y23.3 ☑
      suicide (attempt) X73.2 ☑
    pellet gun — *see* Discharge, airgun
    shotgun W33.01 ☑
      assault X94.0 ☑
      homicide (attempt) X94.0 ☑
      legal intervention — *see* Legal, intervention, firearm, specified NEC
      stated as undetermined whether accidental or intentional Y23.0 ☑
      suicide (attempt) X73.0 ☑
    specified NEC W34.09 ☑
      assault X95.8 ☑
      homicide (attempt) X95.8 ☑
      legal intervention — *see* Legal, intervention, firearm, specified NEC
      stated as undetermined whether accidental or intentional Y24.8 ☑
      suicide (attempt) X74.8 ☑
    stated as undetermined whether accidental or intentional Y24.9 ☑
    suicide (attempt) X74.9 ☑
    Very pistol W34.09 ☑
      assault X95.8 ☑
      homicide (attempt) X95.8 ☑
      stated as undetermined whether accidental or intentional Y24.8 ☑
      suicide (attempt) X74.8 ☑
  firework(s) W39 ☑
    stated as undetermined whether accidental or intentional Y25 ☑
  gas-operated gun NEC W34.018 ☑
    airgun — *see* Discharge, airgun
    assault X95.09 ☑
    homicide (attempt) X95.09 ☑
    paintball gun — *see* Discharge, paintball gun
    stated as undetermined whether accidental or intentional Y24.8 ☑
    suicide (attempt) X74.09 ☑
  gun NEC (*see also* Discharge, firearm NEC)
    air — *see* Discharge, airgun
    BB — *see* Discharge, airgun
    for single hand use — *see* Discharge, firearm, handgun
    hand — *see* Discharge, firearm, handgun
    machine — *see* Discharge, firearm, machine gun
    other specified — *see* Discharge, firearm NEC
    paintball — *see* Discharge, paintball gun
    pellet — *see* Discharge, airgun
  handgun — *see* Discharge, firearm, handgun
  machine gun — *see* Discharge, firearm, machine gun
  paintball gun W34.011 ☑
    assault X95.02 ☑
    homicide (attempt) X95.02 ☑
    stated as undetermined whether accidental or intentional Y24.8 ☑
    suicide (attempt) X74.02 ☑
  pistol — *see* Discharge, firearm, handgun
    flare — *see* Discharge, firearm, Very pistol
    pellet — *see* Discharge, airgun
    Very — *see* Discharge, firearm, Very pistol
  revolver — *see* Discharge, firearm, handgun
  rifle (hunting) — *see* Discharge, firearm, hunting rifle
  shotgun — *see* Discharge, firearm, shotgun
  spring-operated gun NEC W34.018 ☑
    assault X95.09 ☑
    homicide (attempt) X95.09 ☑
    stated as undetermined whether accidental or intentional Y24.8 ☑
    suicide (attempt) X74.09 ☑
Disease
  Andes W94.11 ☑
  aviator's — *see* Air, pressure
  range W94.11 ☑
Diver's disease, palsy, paralysis, squeeze — *see* Air, pressure
Diving (into water) — *see* Accident, diving
Dog bite W54.0 ☑
Dragged by transport vehicle NEC (*see also* Accident, transport) V09.9 ☑
Drinking poison (accidental) — *see* Table of Drugs and Chemicals
Dropped (accidentally) while being carried or supported by other person W04 ☑

Drowning (accidental) W74 ☑
  assault X92.9 ☑
  due to
    accident (to)
      machinery — *see* Contact, with, by type of machine
      watercraft V90.89 ☑
        burning V90.29 ☑
          powered V90.23 ☑
            merchant ship V90.20 ☑
            passenger ship V90.21 ☑
            fishing boat V90.22 ☑
            jetskis V90.23 ☑
          unpowered V90.28 ☑
            canoe V90.25 ☑
            inflatable V90.26 ☑
            kayak V90.25 ☑
            sailboat V90.24 ☑
            water skis V90.27 ☑
        crushed V90.39 ☑
          powered V90.33 ☑
            merchant ship V90.30 ☑
            passenger ship V90.31 ☑
            fishing boat V90.32 ☑
            jetskis V90.33 ☑
          unpowered V90.38 ☑
            canoe V90.35 ☑
            inflatable V90.36 ☑
            kayak V90.35 ☑
            sailboat V90.34 ☑
            water skis V90.37 ☑
        overturning V90.09 ☑
          powered V90.03 ☑
            merchant ship V90.00 ☑
            passenger ship V90.01 ☑
            fishing boat V90.02 ☑
            jetskis V90.03 ☑
          unpowered V90.08 ☑
            canoe V90.05 ☑
            inflatable V90.06 ☑
            kayak V90.05 ☑
            sailboat V90.04 ☑
        sinking V90.19 ☑
          powered V90.13 ☑
            merchant ship V90.10 ☑
            passenger ship V90.11 ☑
            fishing boat V90.12 ☑
            jetskis V90.13 ☑
          unpowered V90.18 ☑
            canoe V90.15 ☑
            inflatable V90.16 ☑
            kayak V90.15 ☑
            sailboat V90.14 ☑
        specified type NEC V90.89 ☑
          powered V90.83 ☑
            merchant ship V90.80 ☑
            passenger ship V90.81 ☑
            fishing boat V90.82 ☑
            jetskis V90.83 ☑
          unpowered V90.88 ☑
            canoe V90.85 ☑
            inflatable V90.86 ☑
            kayak V90.85 ☑
            sailboat V90.84 ☑
            water skis V90.87 ☑
  avalanche — *see* Landslide
  cataclysmic
    earth surface movement NEC — *see* Forces of nature, earth movement
    storm — *see* Forces of nature, cataclysmic storm
  cloudburst X37.8 ☑
  cyclone X37.1 ☑
  fall overboard (from) V92.09 ☑
    powered craft V92.03 ☑
      ferry boat V92.01 ☑
      liner V92.01 ☑
      merchant ship V92.00 ☑
      passenger ship V92.01 ☑
      fishing boat V92.02 ☑
      jetskis V92.03 ☑
    unpowered craft V92.08 ☑
      canoe V92.05 ☑
      inflatable V92.06 ☑
      kayak V92.05 ☑
      sailboat V92.04 ☑
      surf-board V92.08 ☑
      water skis V92.07 ☑
      windsurfer V92.08 ☑
  resulting from
    accident to watercraft — *see* Drowning, due to, accident to, watercraft
    being washed overboard (from) V92.29 ☑

Drowning — *continued*
  due to — *continued*
    powered craft V92.23 ☑
      ferry boat V92.21 ☑
      liner V92.21 ☑
      merchant ship V92.20 ☑
      passenger ship V92.21 ☑
      fishing boat V92.22 ☑
      jetskis V92.23 ☑
    unpowered craft V92.28 ☑
      canoe V92.25 ☑
      inflatable V92.26 ☑
      kayak V92.25 ☑
      sailboat V92.24 ☑
      surf-board V92.28 ☑
      water skis V92.27 ☑
      windsurfer V92.28 ☑
    motion of watercraft V92.19 ☑
      powered craft V92.13 ☑
        ferry boat V92.11 ☑
        liner V92.11 ☑
        merchant ship V92.10 ☑
        passenger ship V92.11 ☑
        fishing boat V92.12 ☑
        jetskis V92.13 ☑
      unpowered craft
        canoe V92.15 ☑
        inflatable V92.16 ☑
        kayak V92.15 ☑
        sailboat V92.14 ☑
    hurricane X37.0 ☑
    jumping into water from watercraft (involved in accident) (*see also* Drowning, due to, accident to, watercraft)
      without accident to or on watercraft W16.711 ☑
    tidal wave NEC — *see* Forces of nature, tidal wave
    torrential rain X37.8 ☑
  following
    fall
      into
        bathtub W16.211 ☑
        bucket W16.221 ☑
        fountain — *see* Drowning, following, fall, into, water, specified NEC
        quarry — *see* Drowning, following, fall, into, water, specified NEC
        reservoir — *see* Drowning, following, fall, into, water, specified NEC
        swimming-pool W16.011 ☑
          striking
            bottom W16.021 ☑
            wall W16.031 ☑
          stated as undetermined whether accidental or intentional Y21.3 ☑
          suicide (attempt) X71.2 ☑
        water NOS W16.41 ☑
          natural (lake) (open sea) (river) (stream) (pond) W16.111 ☑
            striking
              bottom W16.121 ☑
              side W16.131 ☑
          specified NEC W16.311 ☑
            striking
              bottom W16.321 ☑
              wall W16.331 ☑
    overboard NEC — *see* Drowning, due to, fall overboard
  jump or dive
    from boat W16.711 ☑
      striking bottom W16.721 ☑
    into
      fountain — *see* Drowning, following, jump or dive, into, water, specified NEC
      quarry — *see* Drowning, following, jump or dive, into, water, specified NEC
      reservoir — *see* Drowning, following, jump or dive, into, water, specified NEC
      swimming-pool W16.511 ☑
        striking
          bottom W16.521 ☑
          wall W16.531 ☑
        suicide (attempt) X71.2 ☑
      water NOS W16.91 ☑
        natural (lake) (open sea) (river) (stream) (pond) W16.611 ☑
        specified NEC W16.811 ☑
          striking
            bottom W16.821 ☑
            wall W16.831 ☑
        striking bottom W16.621 ☑
  homicide (attempt) X92.9 ☑

Drowning — *continued*
in
bathtub (accidental) W65 ☑
assault X92.0 ☑
following fall W16.211 ☑
stated as undetermined whether accidental
or intentional Y21.1 ☑
stated as undetermined whether accidental or
intentional Y21.0 ☑
suicide (attempt) X71.0 ☑
lake — *see* Drowning, in, natural water
natural water (lake) (open sea) (river) (stream)
(pond) W69 ☑
assault X92.3 ☑
following
dive or jump W16.611 ☑
striking bottom W16.621 ☑
fall W16.111 ☑
striking
bottom W16.121 ☑
side W16.131 ☑
stated as undetermined whether accidental or
intentional Y21.4 ☑
suicide (attempt) X71.3 ☑
quarry — *see* Drowning, in, specified place NEC
quenching tank — *see* Drowning, in, specified
place NEC
reservoir — *see* Drowning, in, specified place NEC
river — *see* Drowning, in, natural water
sea — *see* Drowning, in, natural water
specified place NEC W73 ☑
assault X92.8 ☑
following
dive or jump W16.811 ☑
striking
bottom W16.821 ☑
wall W16.831 ☑
fall W16.311 ☑
striking
bottom W16.321 ☑
wall W16.331 ☑
stated as undetermined whether accidental or
intentional Y21.8 ☑
suicide (attempt) X71.8 ☑
stream — *see* Drowning, in, natural water
swimming-pool W67 ☑
assault X92.1 ☑
following fall X92.2 ☑
following
dive or jump W16.511 ☑
striking
bottom W16.521 ☑
wall W16.531 ☑
fall W16.011 ☑
striking
bottom W16.021 ☑
wall W16.031 ☑
stated as undetermined whether accidental or
intentional Y21.2 ☑
following fall Y21.3 ☑
suicide (attempt) X71.1 ☑
following fall X71.2 ☑
war operations — *see* War operations, restriction
of airway
resulting from accident to watercraft— *see*
Drowning, due to, accident, watercraft
self-inflicted X71.9 ☑
stated as undetermined whether accidental or
intentional Y21.9 ☑
suicide (attempt) X71.9 ☑

E

Earth (surface) movement NEC — *see* Forces of nature,
earth movement
Earth falling (on) W20.0 ☑
caused by cataclysmic earth surface movement or
eruption — *see* Landslide
Earthquake (any injury) X34 ☑
Effect(s) (adverse) of
air pressure (any) — *see* Air, pressure
cold, excessive (exposure to) — *see* Exposure, cold
heat (excessive) — *see* Heat
hot place (weather) — *see* Heat
insolation X30 ☑
late — *see* Sequelae
motion — *see* Motion
nuclear explosion or weapon in war operations —
see War operations, nuclear weapon
radiation — *see* Radiation
travel — *see* Travel

Electric shock (accidental) (by) (in) — *see* Exposure,
electric current
Electrocution (accidental) — *see* Exposure, electric
current
Endotracheal tube wrongly placed during anesthetic
procedure
Entanglement
in
bed linen, causing suffocation — *see* category
T71 ☑
wheel of pedal cycle V19.88 ☑
Entry of foreign body or material — *see* Foreign body
Environmental pollution related condition — *see* Z57 ☑
Execution, legal (any method) — *see* Legal,
intervention
Exhaustion
cold — *see* Exposure, cold
due to excessive exertion (*see also* Overexertion)
X50.9 ☑
heat — *see* Heat
Explosion (accidental) (of) (with secondary fire) W40.9 ☑
acetylene W40.1 ☑
aerosol can W36.1 ☑
air tank (compressed) (in machinery) W36.2 ☑
aircraft (in transit) (powered) NEC V95.9 ☑
balloon V96.05 ☑
fixed wing NEC (private) V95.25 ☑
commercial V95.35 ☑
glider V96.25 ☑
hang V96.15 ☑
powered V95.15 ☑
helicopter V95.05 ☑
in war operations — *see* War operations,
destruction of aircraft
microlight V95.15 ☑
nonpowered V96.9 ☑
specified NEC V96.8 ☑
powered NEC V95.8 ☑
stated as
homicide (attempt) Y03.8 ☑
suicide (attempt) X83.0 ☑
ultralight V95.15 ☑
anesthetic gas in operating room W40.1 ☑
antipersonnel bomb W40.8 ☑
assault X96.0 ☑
homicide (attempt) X96.0 ☑
suicide (attempt) X75 ☑
assault X96.9 ☑
bicycle tire W37.0 ☑
blasting (cap) (materials) W40.0 ☑
boiler (machinery), not on transport vehicle W35 ☑
on watercraft — *see* Explosion, in, watercraft
butane W40.1 ☑
caused by other person X96.9 ☑
coal gas W40.1 ☑
detonator W40.0 ☑
dump (munitions) W40.8 ☑
dynamite W40.0 ☑
in
assault X96.8 ☑
homicide (attempt) X96.8 ☑
legal intervention
injuring
bystander Y35.112 ☑
law enforcement personnel Y35.111 ☑
suspect Y35.113 ☑
unspecified person Y35.119 ☑
suicide (attempt) X75 ☑
explosive (material) W40.9 ☑
gas W40.1 ☑
in blasting operation W40.0 ☑
specified NEC W40.8 ☑
in
assault X96.8 ☑
homicide (attempt) X96.8 ☑
legal intervention
injuring
bystander Y35.192 ☑
law enforcement personnel Y35.191 ☑
suspect Y35.193 ☑
unspecified person Y35.199 ☑
suicide (attempt) X75 ☑
factory (munitions) W40.8 ☑
fertilizer bomb W40.8 ☑
assault X96.3 ☑
homicide (attempt) X96.3 ☑
suicide (attempt) X75 ☑
firearm (parts) NEC W34.19 ☑
airgun W34.110 ☑
BB gun W34.110 ☑
gas, air or spring-operated gun NEC W34.118 ☑
hangun W32.1 ☑

Explosion — *continued*
firearm — *continued*
hunting rifle W33.12 ☑
larger firearm W33.10 ☑
specified NEC W33.19 ☑
machine gun W33.13 ☑
paintball gun W34.111 ☑
pellet gun W34.110 ☑
shotgun W33.11 ☑
Very pistol [flare] W34.19 ☑
fire-damp W40.1 ☑
fireworks W39 ☑
gas (coal) (explosive) W40.1 ☑
cylinder W36.9 ☑
aerosol can W36.1 ☑
air tank W36.2 ☑
pressurized W36.3 ☑
specified NEC W36.8 ☑
gasoline (fumes) (tank) not in moving motor vehicle
W40.1 ☑
bomb W40.8 ☑
assault X96.1 ☑
homicide (attempt) X96.1 ☑
suicide (attempt) X75 ☑
in motor vehicle — *see* Accident, transport, by
type of vehicle
grain store W40.8 ☑
grenade W40.8 ☑
in
assault X96.8 ☑
homicide (attempt) X96.8 ☑
legal intervention
injuring
bystander Y35.192 ☑
law enforcement personnel Y35.191 ☑
suspect Y35.193 ☑
unspecified person Y35.199 ☑
suicide (attempt) X75 ☑
handgun (parts) — *see* Explosion, firearm, hangun (parts)
homicide (attempt) X96.9 ☑
antipersonnel bomb — *see* Explosion,
antipersonnel bomb
fertilizer bomb — *see* Explosion, fertilizer bomb
gasoline bomb — *see* Explosion, gasoline bomb
letter bomb — *see* Explosion, letter bomb
pipe bomb — *see* Explosion, pipe bomb
specified NEC X96.8 ☑
hose, pressurized W37.8 ☑
hot water heater, tank (in machinery) W35 ☑
on watercraft — *see* Explosion, in, watercraft
in, on
dump W40.8 ☑
factory W40.8 ☑
mine (of explosive gases) NEC W40.1 ☑
watercraft V93.59 ☑
powered craft V93.53 ☑
ferry boat V93.51 ☑
fishing boat V93.52 ☑
jetskis V93.53 ☑
liner V93.51 ☑
merchant ship V93.50 ☑
passenger ship V93.51 ☑
sailboat V93.54 ☑
letter bomb W40.8 ☑
assault X96.2 ☑
homicide (attempt) X96.2 ☑
suicide (attempt) X75 ☑
machinery (*see also* Contact, with, by type of
machine)
on board watercraft — *see* Explosion, in,
watercraft
pressure vessel — *see* Explosion, by type of vessel
methane W40.1 ☑
mine W40.1 ☑
missile NEC W40.8 ☑
mortar bomb W40.8 ☑
in
assault X96.8 ☑
homicide (attempt) X96.8 ☑
legal intervention
injuring
bystander Y35.192 ☑
law enforcement personnel Y35.191 ☑
suspect Y35.193 ☑
unspecified person Y35.199 ☑
suicide (attempt) X75 ☑
munitions (dump) (factory) W40.8 ☑
pipe, pressurized W37.8 ☑
bomb W40.8 ☑
assault X96.4 ☑
homicide (attempt) X96.4 ☑
suicide (attempt) X75 ☑

Explosion — continued
- pressure, pressurized
  - cooker W38 ☑
  - gas tank (in machinery) W36.3 ☑
  - hose W37.8 ☑
  - pipe W37.8 ☑
  - specified device NEC W38 ☑
  - tire W37.8 ☑
    - bicycle W37.0 ☑
  - vessel (in machinery) W38 ☑
- propane W40.1 ☑
- self-inflicted X75 ☑
- shell (artillery) NEC W40.8 ☑
  - during war operations — see War operations, explosion
  - in
    - legal intervention
      - injuring
        - bystander Y35.122 ☑
        - law enforcement personnel Y35.121 ☑
        - suspect Y35.123 ☑
        - unspecified person Y35.129 ☑
    - war — see War operations, explosion
- spacecraft V95.45 ☑
- steam or water lines (in machinery) W37.8 ☑
- stove W40.9 ☑
- stated as undetermined whether accidental or intentional Y25 ☑
- suicide (attempt) X75 ☑
- tire, pressurized W37.8 ☑
  - bicycle W37.0 ☑
- undetermined whether accidental or intentional Y25 ☑
- vehicle tire NEC W37.8 ☑
  - bicycle W37.0 ☑
- war operations — see War operations, explosion

Exposure (to) X58 ☑
- air pressure change — see Air, pressure
- cold (accidental) (excessive) (extreme) (natural) (place) X31 ☑
  - assault Y08.89 ☑
  - due to
    - man-made conditions W93.8 ☑
      - dry ice (contact) W93.01 ☑
        - inhalation W93.02 ☑
      - liquid air (contact) (hydrogen) (nitrogen) W93.11 ☑
        - inhalation W93.12 ☑
      - refrigeration unit (deep freeze) W93.2 ☑
    - suicide (attempt) X83.2 ☑
    - weather (conditions) X31 ☑
  - homicide (attempt) Y08.89 ☑
  - self-inflicted X83.2 ☑
- due to abandonment or neglect X58 ☑
- electric current W86.8 ☑
  - appliance (faulty) W86.8 ☑
    - domestic W86.0 ☑
  - caused by other person Y08.89 ☑
  - conductor (faulty) W86.1 ☑
  - control apparatus (faulty) W86.1 ☑
  - electric power generating plant, distribution station W86.1 ☑
  - electroshock gun — see Exposure, electric current, taser
  - high-voltage cable W85 ☑
  - homicide (attempt) Y08.89 ☑
  - legal execution (see Legal, intervention, specified means NEC
  - lightning — see subcategory T75.0 ☑
  - live rail W86.8 ☑
  - misadventure in medical or surgical procedure in electroshock therapy Y63.4
  - motor (electric) (faulty) W86.8 ☑
    - domestic W86.0 ☑
  - self-inflicted X83.1 ☑
  - specified NEC W86.8 ☑
    - domestic W86.0 ☑
  - stun gun — see Exposure, electric current, taser
  - suicide (attempt) X83.1 ☑
  - taser W86.8 ☑
    - assault Y08.89 ☑
    - legal intervention — see category Y35 ☑
    - self-harm (intentional) X83.8 ☑
    - undetermined intent Y33 ☑
  - third rail W86.8 ☑
  - transformer (faulty) W86.1 ☑
  - transmission lines W85 ☑
- environmental tobacco smoke X58 ☑
- excessive
  - cold — see Exposure, cold
  - heat (natural) NEC X30 ☑
    - man-made W92 ☑

Exposure — continued
- factor(s) NOS X58 ☑
  - environmental NEC X58 ☑
    - man-made NEC W99 ☑
  - natural NEC — see Forces of nature
  - specified NEC X58 ☑
- fire, flames (accidental) X08.8 ☑
  - assault X97 ☑
  - campfire — see Exposure, fire, controlled, not in building
  - controlled (in)
    - with ignition (of) clothing (see also Ignition, clothes) X06.2 ☑
      - nightwear X05 ☑
    - bonfire — see Exposure, fire, controlled, not in building
    - brazier (in building or structure) (see also Exposure, fire, controlled, building)
      - not in building or structure — see Exposure, fire, controlled, not in building
    - building or structure X02.0 ☑
      - with
        - fall from building X02.3 ☑
        - injury due to building collapse X02.2 ☑
        - from building X02.5 ☑
        - smoke inhalation X02.1 ☑
      - hit by object from building X02.4 ☑
      - specified mode of injury NEC X02.8 ☑
    - fireplace, furnace or stove — see Exposure, fire, controlled, building
    - not in building or structure X03.0 ☑
      - with
        - fall X03.3 ☑
        - smoke inhalation X03.1 ☑
      - hit by object X03.4 ☑
      - specified mode of injury NEC X03.8 ☑
    - trash — see Exposure, fire, controlled, not in building
  - fireplace — see Exposure, fire, controlled, building
  - fittings or furniture (in building or structure) (uncontrolled) — see Exposure, fire, uncontrolled, building
  - forest (uncontrolled) — see Exposure, fire, uncontrolled, not in building
  - grass (uncontrolled) — see Exposure, fire, uncontrolled, not in building
  - hay (uncontrolled) — see Exposure, fire, uncontrolled, not in building
  - homicide (attempt) X97 ☑
  - ignition of highly flammable material X04 ☑
  - in, of, on, starting in
    - machinery — see Contact, with, by type of machine
    - motor vehicle (in motion) (see also Accident, transport, occupant by type of vehicle) V87.8 ☑
      - with collision — see Collision
    - railway rolling stock, train, vehicle V81.81 ☑
      - with collision — see Accident, transport, railway vehicle occupant
    - street car (in motion) V82.8 ☑
      - with collision — see Accident, transport, streetcar occupant
    - transport vehicle NEC (see also Accident, transport)
      - with collision — see Collision
    - war operations (see also War operations, fire)
      - from nuclear explosion — see War operations, nuclear weapons
    - watercraft (in transit) (not in transit) V91.09 ☑
      - localized — see Burn, on board watercraft, due to, fire on board
      - powered craft V91.03 ☑
        - ferry boat V91.01 ☑
        - fishing boat V91.02 ☑
        - jet skis V91.03 ☑
        - liner V91.01 ☑
        - merchant ship V91.00 ☑
        - passenger ship V91.01 ☑
      - unpowered craft V91.08 ☑
        - canoe V91.05 ☑
        - inflatable V91.06 ☑
        - kayak V91.05 ☑
        - sailboat V91.04 ☑
        - surf-board V91.08 ☑
        - waterskis V91.07 ☑
        - windsurfer V91.08 ☑
    - lumber (uncontrolled) — see Exposure, fire, uncontrolled, not in building
    - mine (uncontrolled) — see Exposure, fire, uncontrolled, not in building

Exposure — continued
- fire, flames — continued
  - prairie (uncontrolled) — see Exposure, fire, uncontrolled, not in building
  - resulting from
    - explosion — see Explosion
    - lightning X08.8 ☑
  - self-inflicted X76 ☑
  - specified NEC X08.8 ☑
  - started by other person X97 ☑
  - stove — see Exposure, fire, controlled, building
  - stated as undetermined whether accidental or intentional Y26 ☑
  - suicide (attempt) X76 ☑
  - tunnel (uncontrolled) — see Exposure, fire, uncontrolled, not in building
  - uncontrolled
    - in building or structure X00.0 ☑
      - with
        - fall from building X00.3 ☑
        - injury due to building collapse X00.2 ☑
        - jump from building X00.5 ☑
        - smoke inhalation X00.1 ☑
      - bed X08.00 ☑
        - due to
          - cigarette X08.01 ☑
          - specified material NEC X08.09 ☑
      - furniture NEC X08.20 ☑
        - due to
          - cigarette X08.21 ☑
          - specified material NEC X08.29 ☑
      - hit by object from building X00.4 ☑
      - sofa X08.10 ☑
        - due to
          - cigarette X08.11 ☑
          - specified material NEC X08.19 ☑
      - specified mode of injury NEC X00.8 ☑
    - not in building or structure (any) X01.0 ☑
      - with
        - fall X01.3 ☑
        - smoke inhalation X01.1 ☑
      - hit by object X01.4 ☑
      - specified mode of injury NEC X01.8 ☑
  - undetermined whether accidental or intentional Y26 ☑
- forces of nature NEC — see Forces of nature
- G-forces (abnormal) W49.9 ☑
- gravitational forces (abnormal) W49.9 ☑
- heat (natural) NEC — see Heat
- high-pressure jet (hydraulic) (pneumatic) W49.9 ☑
- hydraulic jet W49.9 ☑
- inanimate mechanical force W49.9 ☑
- jet, high-pressure (hydraulic) (pneumatic) W49.9 ☑
- lightning — see subcategory T75.0 ☑
  - causing fire — see Exposure, fire
- mechanical forces NEC W49.9 ☑
  - animate NEC W64 ☑
  - inanimate NEC W49.9 ☑
- noise W42.9 ☑
  - supersonic W42.0 ☑
- noxious substance — see Table of Drugs and Chemicals
- pneumatic jet W49.9 ☑
- prolonged in deep-freeze unit or refrigerator W93.2 ☑
- radiation — see Radiation
- smoke (see also Exposure, fire)
  - tobacco, second hand Z77.22
- specified factors NEC X58 ☑
- sunlight X32 ☑
  - man-made (sun lamp) W89.8 ☑
    - tanning bed W89.1 ☑
- supersonic waves W42.0 ☑
- transmission line(s), electric W85 ☑
- vibration W49.9 ☑
- waves
  - infrasound W49.9 ☑
  - sound W42.9 ☑
  - supersonic W42.0 ☑
- weather NEC — see Forces of nature

External cause status Y99.9
- child assisting in compensated work for family Y99.8
- civilian activity done for financial or other compensation Y99.0
- civilian activity done for income or pay Y99.0
- family member assisting in compensated work for other family member Y99.8
- hobby not done for income Y99.8
- leisure activity Y99.8
- military activity Y99.1
- off-duty activity of military personnel Y99.8

☑ **Additional character required**

External — *continued*
  recreation or sport not for income or while a
    student Y99.8
  specified NEC Y99.8
  student activity Y99.8
  volunteer activity Y99.2

F

Factors, supplemental
  alcohol
    blood level
      less than 20mg/100ml Y90.0
      presence in blood, level not specified Y90.9
      20-39mg/100ml Y90.1
      40-59mg/100ml Y90.2
      60-79mg/100ml Y90.3
      80-99mg/100ml Y90.4
      100-119mg/100ml Y90.5
      120-199mg/100ml Y90.6
      200-239mg/100ml Y90.7
      240mg/100ml or more Y90.8
      presence in blood, but level not specified Y90.9
  environmental-pollution-related condition — *see*
    Z57 ☑
  nosocomial condition Y95
  work-related condition Y99.0
Failure
  in suture or ligature during surgical procedure
    Y65.2
  mechanical, of instrument or apparatus (any)
    (during any medical or surgical procedure)
    Y65.8
  sterile precautions (during medical and surgical
    care) — *see* Misadventure, failure, sterile
    precautions, by type of procedure
  to
    introduce tube or instrument Y65.4
      endotracheal tube during anesthesia Y65.3
    make curve (transport vehicle) NEC — *see*
      Accident, transport
    remove tube or instrument Y65.4
Fall, falling (accidental) W19 ☑
  building W20.1 ☑
    burning (uncontrolled fire) X00.3 ☑
  down
    embankment W17.81 ☑
    escalator W10.0 ☑
    hill W17.81 ☑
    ladder W11 ☑
    ramp W10.2 ☑
    stairs, steps W10.9 ☑
  due to
    bumping against
      object W18.00 ☑
        sharp glass W18.02 ☑
        specified NEC W18.09 ☑
        sports equipment W18.01 ☑
      person W03 ☑
        due to ice or snow W00.0 ☑
        on pedestrian conveyance — *see* Accident,
          transport, pedestrian, conveyance
    collision with another person W03 ☑
      due to ice or snow W00.0 ☑
      involving pedestrian conveyance — *see*
        Accident, transport, pedestrian,
        conveyance
    grocery cart tipping over W17.82 ☑
    ice or snow W00.9 ☑
      from one level to another W00.2 ☑
      on stairs or steps W00.1 ☑
    involving pedestrian conveyance — *see*
      Accident, transport, pedestrian,
      conveyance
    on same level W00.0 ☑
    slipping (on moving sidewalk) W01.0 ☑
      with subsequent striking against object
        W01.10 ☑
        furniture W01.190 ☑
        sharp object W01.119 ☑
          glass W01.110 ☑
          power tool or machine W01.111 ☑
          specified NEC W01.118 ☑
        specified NEC W01.198 ☑
    striking against
      object W18.00 ☑
        sharp glass W18.02 ☑
        specified NEC W18.09 ☑
        sports equipment W18.01 ☑
      person W03 ☑
        due to ice or snow W00.0 ☑

Fall — *continued*
  due to — *continued*
    on pedestrian conveyance — *see* Accident,
      transport, pedestrian, conveyance
  earth (with asphyxia or suffocation (by pressure))
    — *see* Earth, falling
  from, off, out of
    aircraft NEC (with accident to aircraft NEC) V97.0 ☑
      while boarding or alighting V97.1 ☑
    balcony W13.0 ☑
    bed W06 ☑
    boat, ship, watercraft NEC (with drowning or
      submersion) — *see* Drowning, due to, fall
      overboard
      with hitting bottom or object V94.0 ☑
    bridge W13.1 ☑
    building W13.9 ☑
      burning (uncontrolled fire) X00.3 ☑
    cavity W17.2 ☑
    chair W07 ☑
    cherry picker W17.89 ☑
    cliff W15 ☑
    dock W17.4 ☑
    embankment W17.81 ☑
    escalator W10.0 ☑
    flagpole W13.8 ☑
    furniture NEC W08 ☑
    grocery cart W17.82 ☑
    haystack W17.89 ☑
    high place NEC W17.89 ☑
      stated as undetermined whether accidental or
        intentional Y30 ☑
    hole W17.2 ☑
    incline W10.2 ☑
    ladder W11 ☑
    lifting device W17.89 ☑
    machine, machinery (*see also* Contact, with, by
      type of machine)
      not in operation W17.89 ☑
    manhole W17.1 ☑
    mobile elevated work platform [MEWP] W17.89 ☑
    motorized mobility scooter W05.2 ☑
    one level to another NEC W17.89 ☑
      intentional, purposeful, suicide (attempt) X80 ☑
      stated as undetermined whether accidental or
        intentional Y30 ☑
    pit W17.2 ☑
    playground equipment W09.8 ☑
      jungle gym W09.2 ☑
      slide W09.0 ☑
      swing W09.1 ☑
    quarry W17.89 ☑
    railing W13.9 ☑
    ramp W10.2 ☑
    roof W13.2 ☑
    scaffolding W12 ☑
    scooter (nonmotorized) W05.1 ☑
      motorized mobility W05.2 ☑
    sky lift W17.89 ☑
    stairs, steps W10.9 ☑
      curb W10.1 ☑
      due to ice or snow W00.1 ☑
      escalator W10.0 ☑
      incline W10.2 ☑
      ramp W10.2 ☑
      sidewalk curb W10.1 ☑
      specified NEC W10.8 ☑
    stepladder W11 ☑
    storm drain W17.1 ☑
    streetcar NEC V82.6 ☑
      with antecedent collision — *see* Accident,
        transport, streetcar occupant
      while boarding or alighting V82.4 ☑
    structure NEC W13.8 ☑
      burning (uncontrolled fire) X00.3 ☑
    table W08 ☑
    toilet W18.11 ☑
      with subsequent striking against object
        W18.12 ☑
    train NEC V81.6 ☑
      during derailment (without antecedent
        collision) V81.7 ☑
        with antecedent collision — *see* Accident,
          transport, railway vehicle occupant
      while boarding or alighting V81.4 ☑
    transport vehicle after collision — *see* Accident,
      transport, by type of vehicle, collision
    tree W14 ☑
    vehicle (in motion) NEC (*see also* Accident,
      transport) V89.9 ☑
      motor NEC (*see also* Accident, transport,
        occupant, by type of vehicle) V87.8 ☑

Fall — *continued*
  from — *continued*
    stationary W17.89 ☑
      while boarding or alighting — *see* Accident,
        transport, by type of vehicle, while
        boarding or alighting
    viaduct W13.8 ☑
    wall W13.8 ☑
    watercraft (*see also* Drowning, due to, fall
      overboard)
      with hitting bottom or object V94.0 ☑
    well W17.0 ☑
    wheelchair, non-moving W05.0 ☑
      powered — *see* Accident, transport, pedestrian,
        conveyance occupant, specified type NEC
    window W13.4 ☑
  in, on
    aircraft NEC V97.0 ☑
      with accident to aircraft V97.0 ☑
      while boarding or alighting V97.1 ☑
    bathtub (empty) W18.2 ☑
      filled W16.212 ☑
        causing drowning W16.211 ☑
    escalator W10.0 ☑
    incline W10.2 ☑
    ladder W11 ☑
    machine, machinery — *see* Contact, with, by type
      of machine
    object, edged, pointed or sharp (with cut) — *see*
      Fall, by type
    playground equipment W09.8 ☑
      jungle gym W09.2 ☑
      slide W09.0 ☑
      swing W09.1 ☑
    ramp W10.2 ☑
    scaffolding W12 ☑
    shower W18.2 ☑
      causing drowning W16.211 ☑
    staircase, stairs, steps W10.9 ☑
      curb W10.1 ☑
      due to ice or snow W00.1 ☑
      escalator W10.0 ☑
      incline W10.2 ☑
      specified NEC W10.8 ☑
    streetcar (without antecedent collision) V82.5 ☑
      with antecedent collision — *see* Accident,
        transport, streetcar occupant
      while boarding or alighting V82.4 ☑
    train (without antecedent collision) V81.5 ☑
      with antecedent collision — *see* Accident,
        transport, railway vehicle occupant
      during derailment (without antecedent
        collision) V81.7 ☑
        with antecedent collision — *see* Accident,
          transport, railway vehicle occupant
      while boarding or alighting V81.4 ☑
    transport vehicle after collision — *see* Accident,
      transport, by type of vehicle, collision
    watercraft V93.39 ☑
      due to
        accident to craft V91.29 ☑
          powered craft V91.23 ☑
            ferry boat V91.21 ☑
            fishing boat V91.22 ☑
            jetskis V91.23 ☑
            liner V91.21 ☑
            merchant ship V91.20 ☑
            passenger ship V91.21 ☑
          unpowered craft
            canoe V91.25 ☑
            inflatable V91.26 ☑
            kayak V91.25 ☑
            sailboat V91.24 ☑
        powered craft V93.33 ☑
          ferry boat V93.31 ☑
          fishing boat V93.32 ☑
          jetskis V93.33 ☑
          liner V93.31 ☑
          merchant ship V93.30 ☑
          passenger ship V93.31 ☑
        unpowered craft V93.38 ☑
          canoe V93.35 ☑
          inflatable V93.36 ☑
          kayak V93.35 ☑
          sailboat V93.34 ☑
          surf-board V93.38 ☑
          windsurfer V93.38 ☑
  into
    cavity W17.2 ☑
    dock W17.4 ☑
    fire — *see* Exposure, fire, by type
    haystack W17.89 ☑

Fall — *continued*
  into — *continued*
    hole W17.2 ☑
    lake — *see* Fall, into, water
    manhole W17.1 ☑
    moving part of machinery — *see* Contact, with, by
      type of machine
    ocean — *see* Fall, into, water
    opening in surface NEC W17.89 ☑
    pit W17.2 ☑
    pond — *see* Fall, into, water
    quarry W17.89 ☑
    river — *see* Fall, into, water
    shaft W17.89 ☑
    storm drain W17.1 ☑
    stream — *see* Fall, into, water
    swimming pool (*see also* Fall, into, water, in,
      swimming pool)
      empty W17.3 ☑
    tank W17.89 ☑
    water W16.42 ☑
      causing drowning W16.41 ☑
      from watercraft — *see* Drowning, due to, fall
        overboard
      hitting diving board W21.4 ☑
      in
        bathtub W16.212 ☑
          causing drowning W16.211 ☑
        bucket W16.222 ☑
          causing drowning W16.221 ☑
        natural body of water W16.112 ☑
          causing drowning W16.111 ☑
          striking
            bottom W16.122 ☑
              causing drowning W16.121 ☑
            side W16.132 ☑
              causing drowning W16.131 ☑
        specified water NEC W16.312 ☑
          causing drowning W16.311 ☑
          striking
            bottom W16.322 ☑
              causing drowning W16.321 ☑
            wall W16.332 ☑
              causing drowning W16.331 ☑
        swimming pool W16.012 ☑
          causing drowning W16.011 ☑
          striking
            bottom W16.022 ☑
              causing drowning W16.021 ☑
            wall W16.032 ☑
              causing drowning W16.031 ☑
        utility bucket W16.222 ☑
          causing drowning W16.221 ☑
    well W17.0 ☑
  involving
    bed W06 ☑
    chair W07 ☑
    furniture NEC W08 ☑
    glass — *see* Fall, by type
    playground equipment W09.8 ☑
      jungle gym W09.2 ☑
      slide W09.0 ☑
      swing W09.1 ☑
    roller blades — *see* Accident, transport,
      pedestrian, conveyance
    skateboard(s) — *see* Accident, transport,
      pedestrian, conveyance
    skates (ice) (in line) (roller) — *see* Accident,
      transport, pedestrian, conveyance
    skis — *see* Accident, transport, pedestrian,
      conveyance
    table W08 ☑
    wheelchair, non-moving W05.0 ☑
      powered — *see* Accident, transport, pedestrian,
        conveyance, specified type NEC
  object — *see* Struck by, object, falling
  off
    toilet W18.11 ☑
      with subsequent striking against object
        W18.12 ☑
  on same level W18.30 ☑
    due to
      specified NEC W18.39 ☑
      stepping on an object W18.31 ☑
  out of
    bed W06 ☑
    building NEC W13.8 ☑
    chair W07 ☑
    furniture NEC W08 ☑
    wheelchair, non-moving W05.0 ☑
      powered — *see* Accident, transport, pedestrian,
        conveyance, specified type NEC
    window W13.4 ☑

Fall — *continued*
  over
    animal W01.0 ☑
    cliff W15 ☑
    embankment W17.81 ☑
    small object W01.0 ☑
  rock W20.8 ☑
  same level W18.30 ☑
    from
      being crushed, pushed, or stepped on by a
        crowd or human stampede W52 ☑
      collision, pushing, shoving, by or with other
        person W03 ☑
      slipping, stumbling, tripping W01.0 ☑
    involving ice or snow W00.0 ☑
      involving skates (ice) (roller), skateboard, skis
        — *see* Accident, transport, pedestrian,
        conveyance
  snowslide (avalanche) — *see* Landslide
  stone W20.8 ☑
  structure W20.1 ☑
    burning (uncontrolled fire) X00.3 ☑
  through
    bridge W13.1 ☑
    floor W13.3 ☑
    roof W13.2 ☑
    wall W13.8 ☑
    window W13.4 ☑
  timber W20.8 ☑
  tree (caused by lightning) W20.8 ☑
  while being carried or supported by other person(s)
    W04 ☑
Fallen on by
  animal (not being ridden) NEC W55.89 ☑
Felo-de-se — *see* Suicide
Fight (hand) (fists) (foot) — *see* Assault, fight
Fire (accidental) — *see* Exposure, fire
Firearm discharge — *see* Discharge, firearm
Fireball effects from nuclear explosion in war
  operations — *see* War operations, nuclear weapons
Fireworks (explosion) W39 ☑
Flash burns from explosion — *see* Explosion
Flood (any injury) (caused by) X38 ☑
  collapse of man-made structure causing earth
    movement X36.0 ☑
  tidal wave — *see* Forces of nature, tidal wave
Food (any type) in
  air passages (with asphyxia, obstruction, or
    suffocation) — *see* categories T17 and T18 ☑
  alimentary tract causing asphyxia (due to
    compression of trachea) — *see* categories T17 ☑
    and T18 ☑
Forces of nature X39.8 ☑
  avalanche X36.1 ☑
    causing transport accident — *see* Accident,
      transport, by type of vehicle
  blizzard X37.2 ☑
  cataclysmic storm X37.9 ☑
    with flood X38 ☑
    blizzard X37.2 ☑
    cloudburst X37.8 ☑
    cyclone X37.1 ☑
    dust storm X37.3 ☑
    hurricane X37.0 ☑
    specified storm NEC X37.8 ☑
    storm surge X37.0 ☑
    tornado X37.1 ☑
    twister X37.1 ☑
    typhoon X37.0 ☑
  cloudburst X37.8 ☑
  cold (natural) X31 ☑
  cyclone X37.1 ☑
  dam collapse causing earth movement X36.0 ☑
  dust storm X37.3 ☑
  earth movement X36.1 ☑
    earthquake X34 ☑
    caused by dam or structure collapse X36.0 ☑
  earthquake X34 ☑
  flood (caused by) X38 ☑
    dam collapse X36.0 ☑
    tidal wave — *see* Forces of nature, tidal wave
  heat (natural) X30 ☑
  hurricane X37.0 ☑
  landslide X36.1 ☑
    causing transport accident — *see* Accident,
      transport, by type of vehicle
  lightning — *see* subcategory T75.0 ☑
    causing fire — *see* Exposure, fire
  mudslide X36.1 ☑
    causing transport accident — *see* Accident,
      transport, by type of vehicle
  radiation (natural) X39.08 ☑
    radon X39.01 ☑

Forces — *continued*
    radon X39.01 ☑
    specified force NEC X39.8 ☑
    storm surge X37.0 ☑
  structure collapse causing earth movement
    X36.0 ☑
  sunlight X32 ☑
  tidal wave X37.41 ☑
    due to
      earthquake X37.41 ☑
      landslide X37.43 ☑
      storm X37.42 ☑
      volcanic eruption X37.41 ☑
  tornado X37.1 ☑
  tsunami X37.41 ☑
  twister X37.1 ☑
  typhoon X37.0 ☑
  volcanic eruption X35 ☑
Foreign body
  aspiration — *see* Index to Diseases and Injuries,
    Foreign body, respiratory tract
  embedded in skin W45 ☑
  entering through skin W45.8 ☑
    can lid W26.8 ☑
    nail W45.0 ☑
    paper W26.2 ☑
    specified NEC W45.8 ☑
    splinter W45.8 ☑
Forest fire (exposure to) — *see* Exposure, fire,
  uncontrolled, not in building
Found injured X58 ☑
  from exposure (to) — *see* Exposure
  on
    highway, road (way), street V89.9 ☑
    railway right of way V81.9 ☑
Fracture (circumstances unknown or unspecified)
  X58 ☑
  due to specified cause NEC X58 ☑
Freezing — *see* Exposure, cold
Frostbite X31 ☑
  due to man-made conditions — *see* Exposure, cold,
    man-made
Frozen — *see* Exposure, cold

G

Gored by bull W55.22 ☑
Gunshot wound W34.00 ☑

H

Hailstones, injured by X39.8 ☑
Hanged herself or himself — *see* Hanging, self-inflicted
Hanging (accidental) (*see also* category) T71 ☑
  legal execution — *see* Legal, intervention, specified
    means NEC
Heat (effects of) (excessive) X30 ☑
  due to
    man-made conditions W92 ☑
      on board watercraft V93.29 ☑
        fishing boat V93.22 ☑
        merchant ship V93.20 ☑
        passenger ship V93.21 ☑
        sailboat V93.24 ☑
        specified powered craft NEC V93.23 ☑
    weather (conditions) X30 ☑
  from
    electric heating apparatus causing burning
      X16 ☑
    nuclear explosion in war operations — *see* War
      operations, nuclear weapons
  inappropriate in local application or packing in
    medical or surgical procedure Y63.5
Hemorrhage
  delayed following medical or surgical treatment
    without mention of misadventure — *see* Index
    to Diseases and Injuries, Complication(s)
  during medical or surgical treatment as
    misadventure — *see* Index to Diseases and
    Injuries, Complication(s)
High
  altitude (effects) — *see* Air, pressure, low
  level of radioactivity, effects — *see* Radiation
  pressure (effects) — *see* Air, pressure, high
  temperature, effects — *see* Heat
Hit, hitting (accidental) by — *see* Struck by
Hitting against — *see* Striking against
Homicide (attempt) (justifiable) — *see* Assault

Hot
  place, effects (*see also* Heat)
    weather, effects X30 ☑
House fire (uncontrolled) — *see* Exposure, fire, uncontrolled, building
Humidity, causing problem X39.8 ☑
Hunger X58 ☑
Hurricane (any injury) X37.0 ☑
Hypobarism, hypobaropathy — *see* Air, pressure, low

I

Ictus
  caloris (*see also* Heat)
    solaris X30 ☑
Ignition (accidental) (*see also* Exposure, fire) X08.8 ☑
  anesthetic gas in operating room W40.1 ☑
  apparel X06.2 ☑
    from highly flammable material X04 ☑
    nightwear X05 ☑
  bed linen (sheets) (spreads) (pillows) (mattress)
    — *see* Exposure, fire, uncontrolled, building, bed
  benzine X04 ☑
  clothes, clothing NEC (from controlled fire) X06.2 ☑
    from
      highly flammable material X04 ☑
  ether X04 ☑
    in operating room W40.1 ☑
  explosive material — *see* Explosion
  gasoline X04 ☑
  jewelry (plastic) (any) X06.0 ☑
  kerosene X04 ☑
  material
    explosive — *see* Explosion
    highly flammable with secondary explosion X04 ☑
  nightwear X05 ☑
  paraffin X04 ☑
  petrol X04 ☑
Immersion (accidental) (*see also* Drowning)
  hand or foot due to cold (excessive) X31 ☑
Implantation of quills of porcupine W55.89 ☑
Inanition (from) (hunger) X58 ☑
  thirst X58 ☑
Inappropriate operation performed
  correct operation on wrong side or body part (wrong side) (wrong site) Y65.53
  operation intended for another patient done on wrong patient Y65.52
  wrong operation performed on correct patient Y65.51
Inattention after, at birth (homicide intent) (infanticidal intent) X58 ☑
Incident, adverse
  device
    anesthesiology Y70.8
      accessory Y70.2
      diagnostic Y70.0
      miscellaneous Y70.8
      monitoring Y70.0
      prosthetic Y70.2
      rehabilitative Y70.1
      surgical Y70.3
      therapeutic Y70.1
    cardiovascular Y71.8
      accessory Y71.2
      diagnostic Y71.0
      miscellaneous Y71.8
      monitoring Y71.0
      prosthetic Y71.2
      rehabilitative Y71.1
      surgical Y71.3
      therapeutic Y71.1
    gastroenterology Y73.8
      accessory Y73.2
      diagnostic Y73.0
      miscellaneous Y73.8
      monitoring Y73.0
      prosthetic Y73.2
      rehabilitative Y73.1
      surgical Y73.3
      therapeutic Y73.1
    general
      hospital Y74.8
        accessory Y74.2
        diagnostic Y74.0
        miscellaneous Y74.8
        monitoring Y74.0
        prosthetic Y74.2
        rehabilitative Y74.1
        surgical Y74.3
        therapeutic Y74.1

Incident — *continued*
  device — *continued*
    surgical Y81.8
      accessory Y81.2
      diagnostic Y81.0
      miscellaneous Y81.8
      monitoring Y81.0
      prosthetic Y81.2
      rehabilitative Y81.1
      surgical Y81.3
      therapeutic Y81.1
    gynecological Y76.8
      accessory Y76.2
      diagnostic Y76.0
      miscellaneous Y76.8
      monitoring Y76.0
      prosthetic Y76.2
      rehabilitative Y76.1
      surgical Y76.3
      therapeutic Y76.1
    medical Y82.9
      specified type NEC Y82.8
    neurological Y75.8
      accessory Y75.2
      diagnostic Y75.0
      miscellaneous Y75.8
      monitoring Y75.0
      prosthetic Y75.2
      rehabilitative Y75.1
      surgical Y75.3
      therapeutic Y75.1
    obstetrical Y76.8
      accessory Y76.2
      diagnostic Y76.0
      miscellaneous Y76.8
      monitoring Y76.0
      prosthetic Y76.2
      rehabilitative Y76.1
      surgical Y76.3
      therapeutic Y76.1
    ophthalmic Y77.8
      accessory Y77.2
      diagnostic Y77.0
      miscellaneous Y77.8
      monitoring Y77.0
      prosthetic Y77.2
      rehabilitative Y77.1
      surgical Y77.3
      therapeutic Y77.1
    orthopedic Y79.8
      accessory Y79.2
      diagnostic Y79.0
      miscellaneous Y79.8
      monitoring Y79.0
      prosthetic Y79.2
      rehabilitative Y79.1
      surgical Y79.3
      therapeutic Y79.1
    otorhinolaryngological Y72.8
      accessory Y72.2
      diagnostic Y72.0
      miscellaneous Y72.8
      monitoring Y72.0
      prosthetic Y72.2
      rehabilitative Y72.1
      surgical Y72.3
      therapeutic Y72.1
    personal use Y74.8
      accessory Y74.2
      diagnostic Y74.0
      miscellaneous Y74.8
      monitoring Y74.0
      prosthetic Y74.2
      rehabilitative Y74.1
      surgical Y74.3
      therapeutic Y74.1
    physical medicine Y80.8
      accessory Y80.2
      diagnostic Y80.0
      miscellaneous Y80.8
      monitoring Y80.0
      prosthetic Y80.2
      rehabilitative Y80.1
      surgical Y80.3
      therapeutic Y80.1
    plastic surgical Y81.8
      accessory Y81.2
      diagnostic Y81.0
      miscellaneous Y81.8
      monitoring Y81.0
      prosthetic Y81.2
      rehabilitative Y81.1

Incident — *continued*
  device — *continued*
    surgical Y81.3
    therapeutic Y81.1
    radiological Y78.8
      accessory Y78.2
      diagnostic Y78.0
      miscellaneous Y78.8
      monitoring Y78.0
      prosthetic Y78.2
      rehabilitative Y78.1
      surgical Y78.3
      therapeutic Y78.1
    urology Y73.8
      accessory Y73.2
      diagnostic Y73.0
      miscellaneous Y73.8
      monitoring Y73.0
      prosthetic Y73.2
      rehabilitative Y73.1
      surgical Y73.3
      therapeutic Y73.1
Incineration (accidental) — *see* Exposure, fire
Infanticide — *see* Assault
Infrasound waves (causing injury) W49.9 ☑
Ingestion
  foreign body (causing injury) (with obstruction) — *see* Foreign body, alimentary canal
  poisonous
    plant(s) X58 ☑
    substance NEC — *see* Table of Drugs and Chemicals
Inhalation
  excessively cold substance, man-made — *see* Exposure, cold, man-made
  food (any type) (into respiratory tract) (with asphyxia, obstruction respiratory tract, suffocation) — *see* categories T17 ☑ and T18 ☑
  foreign body — *see* Foreign body, aspiration
  gastric contents (with asphyxia, obstruction respiratory passage, suffocation) T17.81 ☑
  hot air or gases X14.0 ☑
  liquid air, hydrogen, nitrogen W93.12 ☑
    suicide (attempt) X83.2 ☑
  steam X13.0 ☑
    assault X98.0 ☑
    stated as undetermined whether accidental or intentional Y27.0 ☑
    suicide (attempt) X77.0 ☑
  toxic gas — *see* Table of Drugs and Chemicals
  vomitus (with asphyxia, obstruction respiratory passage, suffocation) T17.81 ☑
Injury, injured (accidental(ly)) NOS X58 ☑
  by, caused by, from
    assault — *see* Assault
    law-enforcing agent, police, in course of legal intervention — *see* Legal intervention
    suicide (attempt) X83.8 ☑
  due to, in
    civil insurrection — *see* War operations
    fight (*see also* Assault, fight) Y04.0 ☑
    war operations — *see* War operations
    homicide (*see also* Assault) Y09
    inflicted (by)
      in course of arrest (attempted), suppression of disturbance, maintenance of order, by law-enforcing agents — *see* Legal intervention
      other person
        stated as
          accidental X58 ☑
          intentional, homicide (attempt) — *see* Assault
          undetermined whether accidental or intentional Y33 ☑
    purposely (inflicted) by other person(s) — *see* Assault
    self-inflicted X83.8 ☑
      stated as accidental X58 ☑
    specified cause NEC X58 ☑
    undetermined whether accidental or intentional Y33 ☑
Insolation, effects X30 ☑
Insufficient nourishment X58 ☑
Interruption of respiration (by)
  food (lodged in esophagus) — *see* categories T17 ☑ and T18 ☑
  vomitus (lodged in esophagus) T17.81 ☑
Intervention, legal — *see* Legal intervention
Intoxication
  drug — *see* Table of Drugs and Chemicals
  poison — *see* Table of Drugs and Chemicals

J

Jammed (accidentally)
  between objects (moving) (stationary and moving)
    W23.0 ☑
    stationary W23.1 ☑
Jumped, jumping
  before moving object NEC X81.8 ☑
    motor vehicle X81.0 ☑
    subway train X81.1 ☑
    train X81.1 ☑
    undetermined whether accidental or intentional
      Y31 ☑
  from
    boat (into water) voluntarily, without accident (to
      or on boat) W16.712 ☑
      with
        accident to or on boat — see Accident,
          watercraft
        drowning or submersion W16.711 ☑
          suicide (attempt) X71.3 ☑
        striking bottom W16.722 ☑
          causing drowning W16.721 ☑
    building (see also Jumped, from, high place)
      W13.9 ☑
      burning (uncontrolled fire) X00.5 ☑
    high place NEC W17.89 ☑
      suicide (attempt) X80 ☑
      undetermined whether accidental or
        intentional Y30 ☑
    structure (see also Jumped, from, high place)
      W13.9 ☑
      burning (uncontrolled fire) X00.5 ☑
  into water W16.92 ☑
    causing drowning W16.91 ☑
    from, off watercraft — see Jumped, from, boat
    in
      natural body W16.612 ☑
        causing drowning W16.611 ☑
        striking bottom W16.622 ☑
          causing drowning W16.621 ☑
      specified place NEC W16.812 ☑
        causing drowning W16.811 ☑
        striking
          bottom W16.822 ☑
            causing drowning W16.821 ☑
          wall W16.832 ☑
            causing drowning W16.831 ☑
      swimming pool W16.512 ☑
        causing drowning W16.511 ☑
        striking
          bottom W16.522 ☑
            causing drowning W16.521 ☑
          wall W16.532 ☑
            causing drowning W16.531 ☑
    suicide (attempt) X71.3 ☑

K

Kicked by
  animal NEC W55.82 ☑
  person(s) (accidentally) W50.1 ☑
    with intent to injure or kill Y04.0 ☑
    as, or caused by, a crowd or human stampede
      (with fall) W52 ☑
    assault Y04.0 ☑
    homicide (attempt) Y04.0 ☑
    in
      fight Y04.0 ☑
      legal intervention
        injuring
          bystander Y35.812 ☑
          law enforcement personnel Y35.811 ☑
          suspect Y35.813 ☑
          unspecified person Y35.819 ☑
Kicking
  against
    object W22.8 ☑
      sports equipment W21.9 ☑
      stationary W22.09 ☑
        sports equipment W21.89 ☑
    person — see Striking against, person
  sports equipment W21.9 ☑
  carpet stretcher with knee X50.3 ☑
Killed, killing (accidentally) NOS (see also Injury) X58 ☑
  in
    action — see War operations
    brawl, fight (hand) (fists) (foot) Y04.0 ☑
      by weapon (see also Assault)

Killed — continued
  in — continued
    cutting, piercing — see Assault, cutting or
      piercing instrument
    firearm — see Discharge, firearm, by type,
      homicide
  self
    stated as
      accident NOS X58 ☑
      suicide — see Suicide
    undetermined whether accidental or
      intentional Y33 ☑
Kneeling (prolonged) (static) X50.1 ☑
Knocked down (accidentally) (by) NOS X58 ☑
  animal (not being ridden) NEC (see also Struck by,
    by type of animal)
  crowd or human stampede W52 ☑
  person W51 ☑
    in brawl, fight Y04.0 ☑
  transport vehicle NEC (see also Accident, transport)
    V09.9 ☑

L

Laceration NEC — see Injury
Lack of
  care (helpless person) (infant) (newborn) X58 ☑
  food except as result of abandonment or neglect
    X58 ☑
    due to abandonment or neglect X58 ☑
  water except as result of transport accident X58 ☑
    due to transport accident — see Accident,
      transport, by type
  helpless person, infant, newborn X58 ☑
Landslide (falling on transport vehicle) X36.1 ☑
  caused by collapse of man-made structure X36.0 ☑
Late effect — see Sequelae
Legal
  execution (any method) — see Legal, intervention
  intervention (by)
    baton — see Legal, intervention, blunt object,
      baton
    bayonet — see Legal, intervention, sharp object,
      bayonet
    blow — see Legal, intervention, manhandling
    blunt object
      baton
        injuring
          bystander Y35.312 ☑
          law enforcement personnel Y35.311 ☑
          suspect Y35.313 ☑
          unspecified person Y35.319 ☑
      injuring
        bystander Y35.302 ☑
        law enforcement personnel Y35.301 ☑
        suspect Y35.303 ☑
        unspecified person Y35.309 ☑
      specified NEC
        injuring
          bystander Y35.392 ☑
          law enforcement personnel Y35.391 ☑
          suspect Y35.393 ☑
          unspecified person Y35.399 ☑
      stave
        injuring
          bystander Y35.392 ☑
          law enforcement personnel Y35.391 ☑
          suspect Y35.393 ☑
          unspecified person Y35.399 ☑
    bomb — see Legal, intervention, explosive
    conducted energy device
      injuring
        bystander Y35.832 ☑
        law enforcement personnel Y35.831 ☑
        suspect Y35.833 ☑
        unspecified person Y35.839 ☑
    cutting or piercing instrument — see Legal,
      intervention, sharp object
    dynamite — see Legal, intervention, explosive,
      dynamite
    electroshock device (taser)
      injuring
        bystander Y35.832 ☑
        law enforcement personnel Y35.831 ☑
        suspect Y35.833 ☑
        unspecified person Y35.839 ☑
    explosive(s)
      dynamite
        injuring
          bystander Y35.112 ☑

Legal — continued
  intervention — continued
    law enforcement personnel Y35.111 ☑
    suspect Y35.113 ☑
    unspecified person Y35.119 ☑
  grenade
    injuring
      bystander Y35.192 ☑
      law enforcement personnel Y35.191 ☑
      suspect Y35.193 ☑
      unspecified person Y35.199 ☑
  injuring
    bystander Y35.102 ☑
    law enforcement personnel Y35.101 ☑
    suspect Y35.103 ☑
    unspecified person Y35.109 ☑
  mortar bomb
    injuring
      bystander Y35.192 ☑
      law enforcement personnel Y35.191 ☑
      suspect Y35.193 ☑
      unspecified person Y35.199 ☑
  shell
    injuring
      bystander Y35.122 ☑
      law enforcement personnel Y35.121 ☑
      suspect Y35.123 ☑
      unspecified person Y35.129 ☑
  specified NEC
    injuring
      bystander Y35.192 ☑
      law enforcement personnel Y35.191 ☑
      suspect Y35.193 ☑
      unspecified person Y35.199 ☑
  firearm(s) (discharge)
    handgun
      injuring
        bystander Y35.022 ☑
        law enforcement personnel Y35.021 ☑
        suspect Y35.023 ☑
        unspecified person Y35.029 ☑
    injuring
      bystander Y35.002 ☑
      law enforcement personnel Y35.001 ☑
      suspect Y35.003 ☑
      unspecified person Y35.009 ☑
    machine gun
      injuring
        bystander Y35.012 ☑
        law enforcement personnel Y35.011 ☑
        suspect Y35.013 ☑
        unspecified person Y35.019 ☑
    rifle pellet
      injuring
        bystander Y35.032 ☑
        law enforcement personnel Y35.031 ☑
        suspect Y35.033 ☑
        unspecified person Y35.039 ☑
    rubber bullet
      injuring
        bystander Y35.042 ☑
        law enforcement personnel Y35.041 ☑
        suspect Y35.043 ☑
        unspecified person Y35.049 ☑
    shotgun — see Legal, intervention, firearm,
      specified NEC
    specified NEC
      injuring
        bystander Y35.092 ☑
        law enforcement personnel Y35.091 ☑
        suspect Y35.093 ☑
        unspecified person Y35.099 ☑
  gas (asphyxiation) (poisoning)
    injuring
      bystander Y35.202 ☑
      law enforcement personnel Y35.201 ☑
      suspect Y35.203 ☑
      unspecified person Y35.209 ☑
    specified NEC
      injuring
        bystander Y35.292 ☑
        law enforcement personnel Y35.291 ☑
        suspect Y35.293 ☑
        unspecified person Y35.299 ☑
    tear gas
      injuring
        bystander Y35.212 ☑
        law enforcement personnel Y35.211 ☑
        suspect Y35.213 ☑
        unspecified person Y35.219 ☑
  grenade — see Legal, intervention, explosive,
    grenade

☑ **Additional character required**

Legal — *continued*
  intervention — *continued*
    injuring
      bystander Y35.92 ☑
      law enforcement personnel Y35.91 ☑
      suspect Y35.93 ☑
      unspecified person Y35.99 ☑
    late effect (of) — *see* with 7th character S Y35
    manhandling
      injuring
        bystander Y35.812 ☑
        law enforcement personnel Y35.811 ☑
        suspect Y35.813 ☑
        unspecified person Y35.819 ☑
    sequelae (of) — *see* with 7th character S Y35 ☑
    sharp objects
      bayonet
        injuring
          bystander Y35.412 ☑
          law enforcement personnel Y35.411 ☑
          suspect Y35.413 ☑
          unspecified person Y35.419 ☑
      injuring
        bystander Y35.402 ☑
        law enforcement personnel Y35.401 ☑
        suspect Y35.403 ☑
        unspecified person Y35.409 ☑
      specified NEC
        injuring
          bystander Y35.492 ☑
          law enforcement personnel Y35.491 ☑
          suspect Y35.493 ☑
          unspecified person Y35.499 ☑
    specified means NEC
      injuring
        bystander Y35.892 ☑
        law enforcement personnel Y35.891 ☑
        suspect Y35.893 ☑
    stabbing — *see* Legal, intervention, sharp object
    stave — *see* Legal, intervention, blunt object, stave
    stun gun
      injuring
        bystander Y35.832 ☑
        law enforcement personnel Y35.831 ☑
        suspect Y35.833 ☑
        unspecified person Y35.839 ☑
    taser
      injuring
        bystander Y35.832 ☑
        law enforcement personnel Y35.831 ☑
        suspect Y35.833 ☑
        unspecified person Y35.839 ☑
    tear gas — *see* Legal, intervention, gas, tear gas
    truncheon — *see* Legal, intervention, blunt object, stave
Lifting (*see also* Overexertion)
  heavy objects X50.0 ☑
  weights X50.0 ☑
Lightning (shock) (stroke) (struck by) — *see* subcategory T75.0 ☑
  causing fire — *see* Exposure, fire
Loss of control (transport vehicle) NEC — *see* Accident, transport
Lost at sea NOS — *see* Drowning, due to, fall overboard
Low
  pressure (effects) — *see* Air, pressure, low
  temperature (effects) — *see* Exposure, cold
Lying before train, vehicle or other moving object X81.8 ☑
  subway train X81.1 ☑
  train X81.1 ☑
  undetermined whether accidental or intentional Y31 ☑
Lynching — *see* Assault

M

Malfunction (mechanism or component) (of)
  firearm W34.10 ☑
    airgun W34.110 ☑
    BB gun W34.110 ☑
    gas, air or spring-operated gun NEC W34.118 ☑
    handgun W32.1 ☑
    hunting rifle W33.12 ☑
    larger firearm W33.10 ☑
      specified NEC W33.19 ☑
    machine gun W33.13 ☑
    paintball gun W34.111 ☑
    pellet gun W34.110 ☑

Malfunction — *continued*
  firearm — *continued*
    shotgun W33.11 ☑
    specified NEC W34.19 ☑
    Very pistol [flare] W34.19 ☑
  handgun — *see* Malfunction, firearm, handgun
Maltreatment — *see* Perpetrator
Mangled (accidentally) NOS X58 ☑
Manhandling (in brawl, fight) Y04.0 ☑
  legal intervention — *see* Legal, intervention, manhandling
Manslaughter (nonaccidental) — *see* Assault
Mauled by animal NEC W55.89 ☑
Medical procedure, complication of (delayed or as an abnormal reaction without mention of misadventure) — *see* Complication of or following, by specified type of procedure
  due to or as a result of misadventure — *see* Misadventure
Melting (due to fire) (*see also* Exposure, fire)
  apparel NEC X06.3 ☑
  clothes, clothing NEC X06.3 ☑
    nightwear X05 ☑
  fittings or furniture (burning building) (uncontrolled fire) X00.8 ☑
  nightwear X05 ☑
  plastic jewelry X06.1 ☑
Mental cruelty X58 ☑
Military operations (injuries to military and civilians occurring during peacetime on military property and during routine military exercises and operations) (by) (from) (involving) Y37.90 ☑
  air blast Y37.20 ☑
  aircraft
    destruction — *see* Military operations, destruction of aircraft
    airway restriction — *see* Military operations, restriction of airways
  asphyxiation — *see* Military operations, restriction of airways
  biological weapons Y37.6X ☑
  blast Y37.20 ☑
  blast fragments Y37.20 ☑
  blast wave Y37.20 ☑
  blast wind Y37.20 ☑
  bomb Y37.20 ☑
    dirty Y37.50 ☑
    gasoline Y37.31 ☑
    incendiary Y37.31 ☑
    petrol Y37.31 ☑
  bullet Y37.43 ☑
    incendiary Y37.32 ☑
    rubber Y37.41 ☑
  chemical weapons Y37.7X ☑
  combat
    hand to hand (unarmed) combat Y37.44 ☑
    using blunt or piercing object Y37.45 ☑
  conflagration — *see* Military operations, fire
  conventional warfare NEC Y37.49 ☑
  depth-charge Y37.01 ☑
  destruction of aircraft Y37.10 ☑
    due to
      air to air missile Y37.11 ☑
      collision with other aircraft Y37.12 ☑
      detonation (accidental) of onboard munitions and explosives Y37.14 ☑
      enemy fire or explosives Y37.11 ☑
      explosive placed on aircraft Y37.11 ☑
      onboard fire Y37.13 ☑
      rocket propelled grenade [RPG] Y37.11 ☑
      small arms fire Y37.11 ☑
      surface to air missile Y37.11 ☑
    specified NEC Y37.19 ☑
  detonation (accidental) of
    onboard marine weapons Y37.05 ☑
    own munitions or munitions launch device Y37.24 ☑
  dirty bomb Y37.50 ☑
  explosion (of) Y37.20 ☑
    aerial bomb Y37.21 ☑
    bomb NOS (*see also* Military operations, bomb(s)) Y37.20 ☑
    own munitions or munitions launch device (accidental) Y37.24 ☑
    fragments Y37.20 ☑
    grenade Y37.29 ☑
    guided missile Y37.22 ☑
    improvised explosive device [IED] (person-borne) (roadside) (vehicle-borne) Y37.23 ☑
    land mine Y37.29 ☑
    marine mine (at sea) (in harbor) Y37.02 ☑
    marine weapon Y37.00 ☑

Military — *continued*
  explosion — *continued*
    specified NEC Y37.09 ☑
    sea-based artillery shell Y37.03 ☑
    specified NEC Y37.29 ☑
    torpedo Y37.04 ☑
  fire Y37.30 ☑
    specified NEC Y37.39 ☑
  firearms
    discharge Y37.43 ☑
    pellets Y37.42 ☑
  flamethrower Y37.33 ☑
  fragments (from) (of)
    improvised explosive device [IED] (person-borne) (roadside) (vehicle-borne) Y37.26 ☑
    munitions Y37.25 ☑
    specified NEC Y37.29 ☑
    weapons Y37.27 ☑
  friendly fire Y37.92 ☑
  hand to hand (unarmed) combat Y37.44 ☑
  hot substances — *see* Military operations, fire
  incendiary bullet Y37.32 ☑
  nuclear weapon (effects of) Y37.50 ☑
    acute radiation exposure Y37.54 ☑
    blast pressure Y37.51 ☑
    direct blast Y37.51 ☑
    direct heat Y37.53 ☑
    fallout exposure Y37.54 ☑
    fireball Y37.53 ☑
    indirect blast (struck or crushed by blast debris) (being thrown by blast) Y37.52 ☑
    ionizing radiation (immediate exposure) Y37.54 ☑
    nuclear radiation Y37.54 ☑
    radiation
      ionizing (immediate exposure) Y37.54 ☑
      nuclear Y37.54 ☑
      thermal Y37.53 ☑
    specified NEC Y37.59 ☑
    secondary effects Y37.54 ☑
    thermal radiation Y37.53 ☑
  restriction of air (airway)
    intentional Y37.46 ☑
    unintentional Y37.47 ☑
  rubber bullets Y37.41 ☑
  shrapnel NOS Y37.29 ☑
  suffocation — *see* Military operations, restriction of airways
  unconventional warfare NEC Y37.7X ☑
  underwater blast NOS Y37.00 ☑
  warfare
    conventional NEC Y37.49 ☑
    unconventional NEC Y37.7X ☑
  weapons
    biological weapons Y37.6X ☑
    chemical Y37.7X ☑
    nuclear (effects of) Y37.50 ☑
      acute radiation exposure Y37.54 ☑
      blast pressure Y37.51 ☑
      direct blast Y37.51 ☑
      direct heat Y37.53 ☑
      fallout exposure Y37.54 ☑
      fireball Y37.53 ☑
      indirect blast (struck or crushed by blast debris) (being thrown by blast) Y37.52 ☑
      radiation
        ionizing (immediate exposure) Y37.54 ☑
        nuclear Y37.54 ☑
        thermal Y37.53 ☑
      secondary effects Y37.54 ☑
      specified NEC Y37.59 ☑
    of mass destruction [WMD] Y37.91 ☑
  weapon of mass destruction [WMD] Y37.91 ☑
Misadventure(s) to patient(s) during surgical or medical care Y69
  contaminated medical or biological substance (blood, drug, fluid) Y64.9
    administered (by) NEC Y64.9
      immunization Y64.1
      infusion Y64.0
      injection Y64.1
      specified means NEC Y64.8
      transfusion Y64.0
      vaccination Y64.1
  excessive amount of blood or other fluid during transfusion or infusion Y63.0
  failure
    in dosage Y63.9
      electroshock therapy Y63.4
      inappropriate temperature (too hot or too cold) in local application and packing Y63.5
      infusion

Misadventure(s) — *continued*
  failure — *continued*
      excessive amount of fluid Y63.0
      incorrect dilution of fluid Y63.1
    insulin-shock therapy Y63.4
    nonadministration of necessary drug or
        biological substance Y63.6
    overdose — *see* Table of Drugs and Chemicals
      radiation, in therapy Y63.2
    radiation
      overdose Y63.2
    specified procedure NEC Y63.8
    transfusion
      excessive amount of blood Y63.0
  mechanical, of instrument or apparatus (any)
      (during any procedure) Y65.8
    sterile precautions (during procedure) Y62.9
      aspiration of fluid or tissue (by puncture or
          catheterization, except heart) Y62.6
      biopsy (except needle aspiration) Y62.8
        needle (aspirating) Y62.6
      blood sampling Y62.6
      catheterization Y62.6
        heart Y62.5
      dialysis (kidney) Y62.2
      endoscopic examination Y62.4
      enema Y62.8
      immunization Y62.3
      infusion Y62.1
      injection Y62.3
      needle biopsy Y62.6
      paracentesis (abdominal) (thoracic) Y62.6
      perfusion Y62.2
      puncture (lumbar) Y62.6
      removal of catheter or packing Y62.8
      specified procedure NEC Y62.8
      surgical operation Y62.0
      transfusion Y62.1
      vaccination Y62.3
    suture or ligature during surgical procedure Y65.2
    to introduce or to remove tube or instrument
        — *see* Failure, to
  hemorrhage — *see* Index to Diseases and Injuries,
      Complication(s)
  inadvertent exposure of patient to radiation Y63.3
  inappropriate
    operation performed — *see* Inappropriate
        operation performed
    temperature (too hot or too cold) in local
        application or packing Y63.5
  infusion (*see also* Misadventure, by type, infusion)
      Y69
    excessive amount of fluid Y63.0
    incorrect dilution of fluid Y63.1
    wrong fluid Y65.1
  mismatched blood in transfusion Y65.0
  nonadministration of necessary drug or biological
      substance Y63.6
  overdose — *see* Table of Drugs and Chemicals
      radiation (in therapy) Y63.2
  perforation — *see* Index to Diseases and Injuries,
      Complication(s)
  performance of inappropriate operation — *see*
      Inappropriate operation performed
  puncture — *see* Index to Diseases and Injuries,
      Complication(s)
  specified type NEC Y65.8
    failure
      suture or ligature during surgical operation
          Y65.2
      to introduce or to remove tube or instrument
          — *see* Failure, to
    infusion of wrong fluid Y65.1
    performance of inappropriate operation — *see*
        Inappropriate operation performed
    transfusion of mismatched blood Y65.0
    wrong
      fluid in infusion Y65.1
      placement of endotracheal tube during
          anesthetic procedure Y65.3
  transfusion — *see* Misadventure, by type,
      transfusion
    excessive amount of blood Y63.0
    mismatched blood Y65.0
  wrong
    drug given in error — *see* Table of Drugs and
        Chemicals
    fluid in infusion Y65.1
    placement of endotracheal tube during
        anesthetic procedure Y65.3
Mismatched blood in transfusion Y65.0
Motion sickness T75.3 ☑

Mountain sickness W94.11 ☑
Mudslide (of cataclysmic nature) — *see* Landslide
Murder (attempt) — *see* Assault

N

Nail
  contact with W45.0 ☑
    gun W29.4 ☑
  embedded in skin W45.0 ☑
Neglect (criminal) (homicidal intent) X58 ☑
Noise (causing injury) (pollution) W42.9 ☑
  supersonic W42.0 ☑
Nonadministration (of)
  drug or biological substance (necessary) Y63.6
  surgical and medical care Y66
Nosocomial condition Y95

O

Object
  falling
    from, in, on, hitting
      machinery — *see* Contact, with, by type of
          machine
    set in motion by
      accidental explosion or rupture of pressure vessel
          W38 ☑
      firearm — *see* Discharge, firearm, by type
      machine (ry) — *see* Contact, with, by type of
          machine
Overdose (drug) — *see* Table of Drugs and Chemicals
  radiation Y63.2
Overexertion X50.9 ☑
  from
    prolonged static or awkward postures X50.1 ☑
    repetitive movements X50.3 ☑
    specified strenuous movements or postures NEC
        X50.9 ☑
    strenuous movement or load X50.0 ☑
Overexposure (accidental) (to)
  cold (*see also* Exposure, cold) X31 ☑
    due to man-made conditions — *see* Exposure,
        cold, man-made
  heat (*see also* Heat) X30 ☑
  radiation — *see* Radiation
  radioactivity W88.0 ☑
  sun (sunburn) X32 ☑
  weather NEC — *see* Forces of nature
  wind NEC — *see* Forces of nature
Overheated — *see* Heat
Overturning (accidental)
  machinery — *see* Contact, with, by type of machine
  transport vehicle NEC (*see also* Accident, transport)
      V89.9 ☑
  watercraft (causing drowning, submersion) (*see
      also* Drowning, due to, accident to, watercraft,
      overturning)
    causing injury except drowning or submersion
        — *see* Accident, watercraft, causing, injury NEC

P

Parachute descent (voluntary) (without accident to
    aircraft) V97.29 ☑
  due to accident to aircraft — *see* Accident,
      transport, aircraft
Pecked by bird W61.99 ☑
Perforation during medical or surgical treatment as
    misadventure — *see* Index to Diseases and Injuries,
    Complication(s)
Perpetrator, perpetration, of assault, maltreatment and
    neglect (by) Y07.9
  boyfriend Y07.03
  brother Y07.410
    stepbrother Y07.435
  coach Y07.53
  cousin
    female Y07.491
    male Y07.490
  daycare provider Y07.519
    at-home
      adult care Y07.512
      childcare Y07.510
    care center
      adult care Y07.513
      childcare Y07.511

Perpetrator — *continued*
  family member NEC Y07.499
  father Y07.11
    adoptive Y07.13
    foster Y07.420
    stepfather Y07.430
  foster father Y07.420
  foster mother Y07.421
  girlfriend Y07.04
  healthcare provider Y07.529
    mental health Y07.521
    specified NEC Y07.528
  husband Y07.01
  instructor Y07.53
  mother Y07.12
    adoptive Y07.14
    foster Y07.421
    stepmother Y07.433
  multiple perpetrators Y07.6
  nonfamily member Y07.50
    specified NEC Y07.59
  nurse Y07.528
  occupational therapist Y07.528
  partner of parent
    female Y07.434
    male Y07.432
  physical therapist Y07.528
  sister Y07.411
  speech therapist Y07.528
  stepbrother Y07.435
  stepfather Y07.430
  stepmother Y07.433
  stepsister Y07.436
  teacher Y07.53
  wife Y07.02
Piercing — *see* Contact, with, by type of object or
    machine
Pinched
  between objects (moving) (stationary and moving)
      W23.0 ☑
  stationary W23.1 ☑
Pinned under machine (ry) — *see* Contact, with, by
    type of machine
Place of occurrence Y92.9
  abandoned house Y92.89
  airplane Y92.813
  airport Y92.520
  ambulatory health services establishment NEC
      Y92.538
  ambulatory surgery center Y92.530
  amusement park Y92.831
  apartment (co-op) — *see* Place of occurrence,
      residence, apartment
  assembly hall Y92.29
  bank Y92.510
  barn Y92.71
  baseball field Y92.320
  basketball court Y92.310
  beach Y92.832
  boarding house — *see* Place of occurrence,
      residence, boarding house
  boat Y92.814
  bowling alley Y92.39
  bridge Y92.89
  building under construction Y92.61
  bus Y92.811
    station Y92.521
  cafe Y92.511
  campsite Y92.833
  campus — *see* Place of occurrence, school
  canal Y92.89
  car Y92.810
  casino Y92.59
  children's home — *see* Place of occurrence,
      residence, institutional, orphanage
  church Y92.22
  cinema Y92.26
  clubhouse Y92.29
  coal pit Y92.64
  college (community) Y92.214
  condominium — *see* Place of occurrence, residence,
      apartment
  construction area — *see* Place of occurrence,
      industrial and construction area
  convalescent home — *see* Place of occurrence,
      residence, institutional, nursing home
  court-house Y92.240
  cricket ground Y92.328
  cultural building Y92.258
    art gallery Y92.250
    museum Y92.251
    music hall Y92.252

☑ **Additional character required**

Place — *continued*
cultural building — *continued*
opera house Y92.253
specified NEC Y92.258
theater Y92.254
dancehall Y92.252
day nursery Y92.210
dentist office Y92.531
derelict house Y92.89
desert Y92.820
dock NOS Y92.89
dockyard Y92.62
doctor's office Y92.531
dormitory — *see* Place of occurrence, residence,
institutional, school dormitory
dry dock Y92.62
factory (building) (premises) Y92.63
farm (land under cultivation) (outbuildings) Y92.79
barn Y92.71
chicken coop Y92.72
field Y92.73
hen house Y92.72
house — *see* Place of occurrence, residence,
house
orchard Y92.74
specified NEC Y92.79
football field Y92.321
forest Y92.821
freeway Y92.411
gallery Y92.250
garage (commercial) Y92.59
boarding house Y92.044
military base Y92.135
mobile home Y92.025
nursing home Y92.124
orphanage Y92.114
private house Y92.015
reform school Y92.155
gas station Y92.524
gasworks Y92.69
golf course Y92.39
gravel pit Y92.64
grocery Y92.512
gymnasium Y92.39
handball court Y92.318
harbor Y92.89
harness racing course Y92.39
healthcare provider office Y92.531
highway (interstate) Y92.411
hill Y92.828
hockey rink Y92.330
home — *see* Place of occurrence, residence
hospice — *see* Place of occurrence, residence,
institutional, nursing home
hospital Y92.239
cafeteria Y92.233
corridor Y92.232
operating room Y92.234
patient
bathroom Y92.231
room Y92.230
specified NEC Y92.238
hotel Y92.59
house (*see also* Place of occurrence, residence)
abandoned Y92.89
under construction Y92.61
industrial and construction area (yard) Y92.69
building under construction Y92.61
dock Y92.62
dry dock Y92.62
factory Y92.63
gasworks Y92.69
mine Y92.64
oil rig Y92.65
pit Y92.64
power station Y92.69
shipyard Y92.62
specified NEC Y92.69
tunnel under construction Y92.69
workshop Y92.69
kindergarten Y92.211
lacrosse field Y92.328
lake Y92.828
library Y92.241
mall Y92.59
market Y92.512
marsh Y92.828
military
base — *see* Place of occurrence, residence,
institutional, military base
training ground Y92.84
mine Y92.64

Place — *continued*
mosque Y92.22
motel Y92.59
motorway (interstate) Y92.411
mountain Y92.828
movie-house Y92.26
museum Y92.251
music-hall Y92.252
not applicable Y92.9
nuclear power station Y92.69
nursing home — *see* Place of occurrence, residence,
institutional, nursing home
office building Y92.59
offshore installation Y92.65
oil rig Y92.65
old people's home — *see* Place of occurrence,
residence, institutional, specified NEC
opera-house Y92.253
orphanage — *see* Place of occurrence, residence,
institutional, orphanage
outpatient surgery center Y92.530
park (public) Y92.830
amusement Y92.831
parking garage Y92.89
lot Y92.481
pavement Y92.480
physician office Y92.531
polo field Y92.328
pond Y92.828
post office Y92.242
power station Y92.69
prairie Y92.828
prison — *see* Place of occurrence, residence,
institutional, prison
public
administration building Y92.248
city hall Y92.243
courthouse Y92.240
library Y92.241
post office Y92.242
specified NEC Y92.248
building NEC Y92.29
hall Y92.29
place NOS Y92.89
race course Y92.39
radio station Y92.59
railway line (bridge) Y92.85
ranch (outbuildings) — *see* Place of occurrence,
farm
recreation area Y92.838
amusement park Y92.831
beach Y92.832
campsite Y92.833
park (public) Y92.830
seashore Y92.832
specified NEC Y92.838
religious institution Y92.22
reform school — *see* Place of occurrence, residence,
institutional, reform school
residence (non-institutional) (private) Y92.009
apartment Y92.039
bathroom Y92.031
bedroom Y92.032
kitchen Y92.030
specified NEC Y92.038
bathroom Y92.002
bedroom Y92.003
boarding house Y92.049
bathroom Y92.041
bedroom Y92.042
driveway Y92.043
garage Y92.044
garden Y92.046
kitchen Y92.040
specified NEC Y92.048
swimming pool Y92.045
yard Y92.046
dining room Y92.001
garden Y92.007
home Y92.009
house, single family Y92.019
bathroom Y92.012
bedroom Y92.013
dining room Y92.011
driveway Y92.014
garage Y92.015
garden Y92.017
kitchen Y92.010
specified NEC Y92.018
swimming pool Y92.016
yard Y92.017
institutional Y92.10

Place — *continued*
residence — *continued*
children's home — *see* Place of occurrence,
residence, institutional, orphanage
hospice — *see* Place of occurrence, residence,
institutional, nursing home
military base Y92.139
barracks Y92.133
garage Y92.135
garden Y92.137
kitchen Y92.130
mess hall Y92.131
specified NEC Y92.138
swimming pool Y92.136
yard Y92.137
nursing home Y92.129
bathroom Y92.121
bedroom Y92.122
driveway Y92.123
garage Y92.124
garden Y92.126
kitchen Y92.120
specified NEC Y92.128
swimming pool Y92.125
yard Y92.126
orphanage Y92.119
bathroom Y92.111
bedroom Y92.112
driveway Y92.113
garage Y92.114
garden Y92.116
kitchen Y92.110
specified NEC Y92.118
swimming pool Y92.115
yard Y92.116
prison Y92.149
bathroom Y92.142
cell Y92.143
courtyard Y92.147
dining room Y92.141
kitchen Y92.140
specified NEC Y92.148
swimming pool Y92.146
reform school Y92.159
bathroom Y92.152
bedroom Y92.153
dining room Y92.151
driveway Y92.154
garage Y92.155
garden Y92.157
kitchen Y92.150
specified NEC Y92.158
swimming pool Y92.156
yard Y92.157
school dormitory Y92.169
bathroom Y92.162
bedroom Y92.163
dining room Y92.161
kitchen Y92.160
specified NEC Y92.168
specified NEC Y92.199
bathroom Y92.192
bedroom Y92.193
dining room Y92.191
driveway Y92.194
garage Y92.195
garden Y92.197
kitchen Y92.190
specified NEC Y92.198
swimming pool Y92.196
yard Y92.197
kitchen Y92.000
mobile home Y92.029
bathroom Y92.022
bedroom Y92.023
dining room Y92.021
driveway Y92.024
garage Y92.025
garden Y92.027
kitchen Y92.020
specified NEC Y92.028
swimming pool Y92.026
yard Y92.027
specified place in residence NEC Y92.008
specified residence type NEC Y92.099
bathroom Y92.091
bedroom Y92.092
driveway Y92.093
garage Y92.094
garden Y92.096
kitchen Y92.090
specified NEC Y92.098

Place — *continued*
  residence — *continued*
    swimming pool Y92.095
    yard Y92.096
  restaurant Y92.511
  riding school Y92.39
  river Y92.828
  road Y92.410
  rodeo ring Y92.39
  rugby field Y92.328
  same day surgery center Y92.530
  sand pit Y92.64
  school (private) (public) (state) Y92.219
    college Y92.214
    daycare center Y92.210
    elementary school Y92.211
    high school Y92.213
    kindergarten Y92.211
    middle school Y92.212
    specified NEC Y92.218
    trace school Y92.215
    university Y92.214
    vocational school Y92.215
  sea (shore) Y92.832
  senior citizen center Y92.29
  service area
    airport Y92.520
    bus station Y92.521
    gas station Y92.524
    highway rest stop Y92.523
    railway station Y92.522
  shipyard Y92.62
  shop (commercial) Y92.513
  sidewalk Y92.480
  silo Y92.79
  skating rink (roller) Y92.331
    ice Y92.330
  slaughter house Y92.86
  soccer field Y92.322
  specified place NEC Y92.89
  sports area Y92.39
    athletic
      court Y92.318
        basketball Y92.310
        specified NEC Y92.318
        squash Y92.311
        tennis Y92.312
      field Y92.328
        baseball Y92.320
        cricket ground Y92.328
        football Y92.321
        hockey Y92.328
        soccer Y92.322
        specified NEC Y92.328
    golf course Y92.39
    gymnasium Y92.39
    riding school Y92.39
    skating rink (roller) Y92.331
      ice Y92.330
    stadium Y92.39
    swimming pool Y92.34
  squash court Y92.311
  stadium Y92.39
  steeplechasing course Y92.39
  store Y92.512
  stream Y92.828
  street and highway Y92.410
    bike path Y92.482
    freeway Y92.411
    highway ramp Y92.415
    interstate highway Y92.411
    local residential or business street Y92.414
    motorway Y92.411
    parkway Y92.412
    parking lot Y92.481
    sidewalk Y92.480
    specified NEC Y92.488
    state road Y92.413
  subway car Y92.816
  supermarket Y92.512
  swamp Y92.828
  swimming pool (public) Y92.34
    private (at) Y92.095
      boarding house Y92.045
      military base Y92.136
      mobile home Y92.026
      nursing home Y92.125
      orphanage Y92.115
      prison Y92.146
      reform school Y92.156
      single family residence Y92.016
  synagogue Y92.22

Place — *continued*
  television station Y92.59
  tennis court Y92.312
  theater Y92.254
  trade area Y92.59
    bank Y92.510
    cafe Y92.511
    casino Y92.59
    garage Y92.59
    hotel Y92.59
    market Y92.512
    office building Y92.59
    radio station Y92.59
    restaurant Y92.511
    shop Y92.513
    shopping mall Y92.59
    store Y92.512
    supermarket Y92.512
    television station Y92.59
    warehouse Y92.59
  trailer park, residential — *see* Place of occurrence, residence, mobile home
  trailer site NOS Y92.89
  train Y92.815
    station Y92.522
  truck Y92.812
  tunnel under construction Y92.69
  urgent (health) care center Y92.532
  university Y92.214
  vehicle (transport) Y92.818
    airplane Y92.813
    boat Y92.814
    bus Y92.811
    car Y92.810
    specified NEC Y92.818
    subway car Y92.816
    train Y92.815
    truck Y92.812
  warehouse Y92.59
  water reservoir Y92.89
  wilderness area Y92.828
    desert Y92.820
    forest Y92.821
    marsh Y92.828
    mountain Y92.828
    prairie Y92.828
    specified NEC Y92.828
    swamp Y92.828
  workshop Y92.69
  yard, private Y92.096
    boarding house Y92.046
    single family house Y92.017
    mobile home Y92.027
  youth center Y92.29
  zoo (zoological garden) Y92.834
Plumbism — *see* Table of Drugs and Chemicals, lead
Poisoning (accidental) (by) (*see also* Table of Drugs and Chemicals)
  by plant, thorns, spines, sharp leaves or other mechanisms NEC X58 ☑
  carbon monoxide
    generated by
      motor vehicle — *see* Accident, transport
      watercraft (in transit) (not in transit) V93.89 ☑
        ferry boat V93.81 ☑
        fishing boat V93.82 ☑
        jet skis V93.83 ☑
        liner V93.81 ☑
        merchant ship V93.80 ☑
        passenger ship V93.81 ☑
        powered craft NEC V93.83 ☑
  caused by injection of poisons into skin by plant thorns, spines, sharp leaves X58 ☑
    marine or sea plants (venomous) X58 ☑
  exhaust gas
    generated by
      motor vehicle — *see* Accident, transport
      watercraft (in transit) (not in transit) V93.89 ☑
        ferry boat V93.81 ☑
        fishing boat V93.82 ☑
        jet skis V93.83 ☑
        liner V93.81 ☑
        merchant ship V93.80 ☑
        passenger ship V93.81 ☑
        powered craft NEC V93.83 ☑
  fumes or smoke due to
    explosion (*see also* Explosion) W40.9 ☑
    fire — *see* Exposure, fire
    ignition — *see* Ignition
  gas
    in legal intervention — *see* Legal, intervention, gas
    legal execution — *see* Legal, intervention, gas

Poisoning — *continued*
  in war operations — *see* War operations
  legal
    execution — *see* Legal, intervention, gas
    intervention
      by gas — *see* Legal, intervention, gas
      other specified means — *see* Legal, intervention, specified means NEC
Powder burn (by) (from)
  airgun W34.110 ☑
  BB gun W34.110 ☑
  firearm NEC W34.19 ☑
  gas, air or spring-operated gun NEC W34.118 ☑
  handgun W32.1 ☑
  hunting rifle W33.12 ☑
  larger firearm W33.10 ☑
    specified NEC W33.19 ☑
  machine gun W33.13 ☑
  paintball gun W34.111 ☑
  pellet gun W34.110 ☑
  shotgun W33.11 ☑
  Very pistol [flare] W34.19 ☑
Premature cessation (of) surgical and medical care Y66
Privation (food) (water) X58 ☑
Procedure (operation)
  correct, on wrong side or body part (wrong side) (wrong site) Y65.53
  intended for another patient done on wrong patient Y65.52
  performed on patient not scheduled for surgery Y65.52
  performed on wrong patient Y65.52
  wrong, performed on correct patient Y65.51
Prolonged
  sitting in transport vehicle — *see* Travel, by type of vehicle
  stay in
    high altitude as cause of anoxia, barodontalgia, barotitis or hypoxia W94.11 ☑
    weightless environment X52 ☑
Pulling, excessive (*see also* Overexertion) X50.9 ☑
Puncture, puncturing (*see also* Contact, with, by type of object or machine)
  by
    plant thorns, spines, sharp leaves or other mechanisms NEC W60 ☑
  during medical or surgical treatment as misadventure — *see* Index to Diseases and Injuries, Complication(s)
Pushed, pushing (accidental) (injury in)
  by other person(s) (accidental) W51 ☑
    with fall W03 ☑
      due to ice or snow W00.0 ☑
    as, or caused by, a crowd or human stampede (with fall) W52 ☑
    before moving object NEC Y02.8 ☑
      motor vehicle Y02.0 ☑
      subway train Y02.1 ☑
      train Y02.1 ☑
    from
      high place NEC
        in accidental circumstances W17.89 ☑
        stated as
          intentional, homicide (attempt) Y01 ☑
          undetermined whether accidental or intentional Y30 ☑
      transport vehicle NEC (*see also* Accident, transport) V89.9 ☑
        stated as
          intentional, homicide (attempt) Y08.89 ☑
    overexertion X50.9 ☑

R

Radiation (exposure to)
  arc lamps W89.0 ☑
  atomic power plant (malfunction) NEC W88.1 ☑
  complication of or abnormal reaction to medical radiotherapy Y84.2
  electromagnetic, ionizing W88.0 ☑
  gamma rays W88.1 ☑
  in
    war operations (from or following nuclear explosion) — *see* War operations
  inadvertent exposure of patient (receiving test or therapy) Y63.3
  infrared (heaters and lamps) W90.1 ☑
    excessive heat from W92 ☑
  ionized, ionizing (particles, artificially accelerated)
    radioisotopes W88.1 ☑

☑ **Additional character required**

Radiation — *continued*
  ionized, ionizing — *continued*
    specified NEC W88.8 ☑
    X-rays W88.0 ☑
  isotopes, radioactive — *see* Radiation, radioactive
    isotopes
  laser(s) W90.2 ☑
    in war operations — *see* War operations
    misadventure in medical care Y63.2
  light sources (man-made visible and ultraviolet)
    W89.9 ☑
    natural X32 ☑
    specified NEC W89.8 ☑
    tanning bed W89.1 ☑
    welding light W89.0 ☑
  man-made visible light W89.9 ☑
    specified NEC W89.8 ☑
    tanning bed W89.1 ☑
    welding light W89.0 ☑
  microwave W90.8 ☑
  misadventure in medical or surgical procedure
    Y63.2
  natural NEC X39.08 ☑
    radon X39.01 ☑
  overdose (in medical or surgical procedure) Y63.2
  radar W90.0 ☑
  radioactive isotopes (any) W88.1 ☑
    atomic power plant malfunction W88.1 ☑
    misadventure in medical or surgical treatment
      Y63.2
  radiofrequency W90.0 ☑
  radium NEC W88.1 ☑
  sun X32 ☑
  ultraviolet (light) (man-made) W89.9 ☑
    natural X32 ☑
    specified NEC W89.8 ☑
    tanning bed W89.1 ☑
    welding light W89.0 ☑
  welding arc, torch, or light W89.0 ☑
    excessive heat from W92 ☑
  X-rays (hard) (soft) W88.0 ☑
Range disease W94.11 ☑
Rape (attempted) T74.2 ☑
Rat bite W53.11 ☑
Reaching (prolonged) (static) X50.1 ☑
Reaction, abnormal to medical procedure (*see also*
  Complication of or following, by type of procedure)
  Y84.9
  with misadventure — *see* Misadventure
  biologicals — *see* Table of Drugs and Chemicals
  drugs — *see* Table of Drugs and Chemicals
  vaccine — *see* Table of Drugs and Chemicals
Recoil
  airgun W34.110 ☑
  BB gun W34.110 ☑
  firearm NEC W34.19 ☑
  gas, air or spring-operated gun NEC W34.118 ☑
  handgun W32.1 ☑
  hunting rifle W33.12 ☑
  larger firearm W33.10 ☑
    specified NEC W33.19 ☑
  machine gun W33.13 ☑
  paintball gun W34.111 ☑
  pellet W34.110 ☑
  shotgun W33.11 ☑
  Very pistol [flare] W34.19 ☑
Reduction in
  atmospheric pressure — *see* Air, pressure, change
Rock falling on or hitting (accidentally) (person) W20.8 ☑
  in cave-in W20.0 ☑
Run over (accidentally) (by)
  animal (not being ridden) NEC W55.89 ☑
  machinery — *see* Contact, with, by specified type
    of machine
  transport vehicle NEC (*see also* Accident, transport)
    V09.9 ☑
    intentional homicide (attempt) Y03.0 ☑
    motor NEC V09.20 ☑
      intentional homicide (attempt) Y03.0 ☑
Running
  before moving object X81.8 ☑
    motor vehicle X81.0 ☑
Running off, away
  animal (being ridden) (*see also* Accident, transport)
    V80.918 ☑
    not being ridden W55.89 ☑
  animal-drawn vehicle NEC (*see also* Accident,
    transport) V80.928 ☑
  highway, road (way), street
    transport vehicle NEC (*see also* Accident,
      transport) V89.9 ☑
Rupture pressurized devices — *see* Explosion, by type
  of device

S

Saturnism — *see* Table of Drugs and Chemicals, lead
Scald, scalding (accidental) (by) (from) (in) X19 ☑
  air (hot) X14.1 ☑
  gases (hot) X14.1 ☑
  homicide (attempt) — *see* Assault, burning, hot
    object
  inflicted by other person
    stated as intentional, homicide (attempt) — *see*
      Assault, burning, hot object
  liquid (boiling) (hot) NEC X12 ☑
    stated as undetermined whether accidental or
      intentional Y27.2 ☑
    suicide (attempt) X77.2 ☑
  local application of externally applied substance in
    medical or surgical care Y63.5
  metal (molten) (liquid) (hot) NEC X18 ☑
  self-inflicted X77.9 ☑
    stated as undetermined whether accidental or
      intentional Y27.8 ☑
  steam X13.1 ☑
    assault X98.0 ☑
    stated as undetermined whether accidental or
      intentional Y27.0 ☑
    suicide (attempt) X77.0 ☑
  suicide (attempt) X77.9 ☑
  vapor (hot) X13.1 ☑
    assault X98.0 ☑
    stated as undetermined whether accidental or
      intentional Y27.0 ☑
    suicide (attempt) X77.0 ☑
Scratched by
  cat W55.03 ☑
  person(s) (accidentally) W50.4 ☑
    with intent to injure or kill Y04.0 ☑
    as, or caused by, a crowd or human stampede
      (with fall) W52 ☑
    assault Y04.0 ☑
    homicide (attempt) Y04.0 ☑
    in
      fight Y04.0 ☑
      legal intervention
        injuring
          bystander Y35.892 ☑
          law enforcement personnel Y35.891 ☑
          suspect Y35.893 ☑
Seasickness T75.3 ☑
Self-harm NEC (*see also* External cause by type,
  undetermined whether accidental or intentional)
  intentional — *see* Suicide
  poisoning NEC — *see* Table of drugs and biologicals,
    accident
Self-inflicted (injury) NEC (*see also* External cause
  by type, undetermined whether accidental or
  intentional)
  intentional — *see* Suicide
  poisoning NEC — *see* Table of drugs and biologicals,
    accident
Sequelae (of)
  accident NEC — *see* W00-X58 with 7th character S
  assault (homicidal) (any means) — *see* X92-Y08 with
    7th character S
  homicide, attempt (any means) — *see* X92-Y08 with
    7th character S
  injury undetermined whether accidentally or
    purposely inflicted — *see* Y21-Y33 with 7th
    character S
  intentional self-harm (classifiable to X71-X83) — *see*
    X71-X83 with 7th character S
  legal intervention — *see* with 7th character S Y35 ☑
  motor vehicle accident — *see* V00-V99 with 7th
    character S
  suicide, attempt (any means) — *see* X71-X83 with
    7th character S
  transport accident — *see* V00-V99 with 7th
    character S
  war operations — *see* War operations
Shock
  electric — *see* Exposure, electric current
  from electric appliance (any) (faulty) W86.8 ☑
    domestic W86.0 ☑
    suicide (attempt) X83.1 ☑
Shooting, shot (accidental(ly)) (*see also* Discharge,
  firearm, by type)
  herself or himself — *see* Discharge, firearm by type,
    self-inflicted
  homicide (attempt) — *see* Discharge, firearm by
    type, homicide
  in war operations — *see* War operations

Shooting — *continued*
  inflicted by other person — *see* Discharge, firearm
    by type, homicide
    accidental — *see* Discharge, firearm, by type of
      firearm
  legal
    execution — *see* Legal, intervention, firearm
    intervention — *see* Legal, intervention, firearm
  self-inflicted — *see* Discharge, firearm by type,
    suicide
    accidental — *see* Discharge, firearm, by type of
      firearm
  suicide (attempt) — *see* Discharge, firearm by type,
    suicide
Shoving (accidentally) by other person — *see* Pushed,
  by other person
Sickness
  alpine W94.11 ☑
  motion — *see* Motion
  mountain W94.11 ☑
Sinking (accidental)
  watercraft (causing drowning, submersion) (*see
    also* Drowning, due to, accident to, watercraft,
    sinking)
  causing injury except drowning or submersion
    — *see* Accident, watercraft, causing, injury NEC
Siriasis X32 ☑
Sitting (prolonged) (static) X50.1 ☑
Slashed wrists — *see* Cut, self-inflicted
Slipping (accidental) (on same level) (with fall)
  W01.0 ☑
  on
    ice W00.0 ☑
      with skates — *see* Accident, transport,
        pedestrian, conveyance
    mud W01.0 ☑
    oil W01.0 ☑
    snow W00.0 ☑
      with skis — *see* Accident, transport, pedestrian,
        conveyance
    surface (slippery) (wet) NEC W01.0 ☑
  without fall W18.40 ☑
    due to
      specified NEC W18.49 ☑
      stepping from one level to another W18.43 ☑
      stepping into hole or opening W18.42 ☑
      stepping on object W18.41 ☑
Sliver, wood, contact with W45.8 ☑
Smoldering (due to fire) — *see* Exposure, fire
Sodomy (attempted) by force T74.2 ☑
Sound waves (causing injury) W42.9 ☑
  supersonic W42.0 ☑
Splinter, contact with W45.8 ☑
Stab, stabbing — *see* Cut
Standing (prolonged) (static) X50.1 ☑
Starvation X58 ☑
Status of external cause Y99.9
  child assisting in compensated work for family
    Y99.8
  civilian activity done for financial or other
    compensation Y99.0
  civilian activity done for income or pay Y99.0
  family member assisting in compensated work for
    other family member Y99.8
  hobby not done for income Y99.8
  leisure activity Y99.8
  military activity Y99.1
  off-duty activity of military personnel Y99.8
  recreation or sport not for income or while a
    student Y99.8
  specified NEC Y99.8
  student activity Y99.8
  volunteer activity Y99.2
Stepped on
  by
    animal (not being ridden) NEC W55.89 ☑
    crowd or human stampede W52 ☑
    person W50.0 ☑
Stepping on
  object W22.8 ☑
    with fall W18.31 ☑
    sports equipment W21.9 ☑
    stationary W22.09 ☑
      sports equipment W21.89 ☑
  person W51 ☑
    by crowd or human stampede W52 ☑
  sports equipment W21.9 ☑
Sting
  arthropod, nonvenomous W57 ☑
  insect, nonvenomous W57 ☑
Storm (cataclysmic) — *see* Forces of nature, cataclysmic
  storm

Straining, excessive (see also Overexertion) X50.9 ☑
Strangling — see Strangulation
Strangulation (accidental) — see category T71 ☑
Strenuous movements (see also Overexertion) X50.9 ☑
Striking against
  airbag (automobile) W22.10 ☑
    driver side W22.11 ☑
    front passenger side W22.12 ☑
    specified NEC W22.19 ☑
  bottom when
    diving or jumping into water (in) W16.822 ☑
      causing drowning W16.821 ☑
      from boat W16.722 ☑
        causing drowning W16.721 ☑
      natural body W16.622 ☑
        causing drowning W16.821 ☑
      swimming pool W16.522 ☑
        causing drowning W16.521 ☑
    falling into water (in) W16.322 ☑
      causing drowning W16.321 ☑
      fountain — see Striking against, bottom when, falling into water, specified NEC
      natural body W16.122 ☑
        causing drowning W16.121 ☑
      reservoir — see Striking against, bottom when, falling into water, specified NEC
      specified NEC W16.322 ☑
        causing drowning W16.321 ☑
      swimming pool W16.022 ☑
        causing drowning W16.021 ☑
  diving board (swimming-pool) W21.4 ☑
  object W22.8 ☑
    with
      drowning or submersion — see Drowning
      fall — see Fall, due to, bumping against, object
    caused by crowd or human stampede (with fall) W52 ☑
    furniture W22.03 ☑
    lamppost W22.02 ☑
    sports equipment W21.9 ☑
    stationary W22.09 ☑
      sports equipment W21.89 ☑
    wall W22.01 ☑
  person(s) W51 ☑
    with fall W03 ☑
      due to ice or snow W00.0 ☑
    as, or caused by, a crowd or human stampede (with fall) W52 ☑
    assault Y04.2 ☑
    homicide (attempt) Y04.2 ☑
  sports equipment W21.9 ☑
  wall (when) W22.01 ☑
    diving or jumping into water (in) W16.832 ☑
      causing drowning W16.831 ☑
      swimming pool W16.532 ☑
        causing drowning W16.531 ☑
    falling into water (in) W16.332 ☑
      causing drowning W16.331 ☑
      fountain — see Striking against, wall when, falling into water, specified NEC
      natural body W16.132 ☑
        causing drowning W16.131 ☑
      reservoir — see Striking against, wall when, falling into water, specified NEC
      specified NEC W16.332 ☑
        causing drowning W16.331 ☑
      swimming pool W16.032 ☑
        causing drowning W16.031 ☑
    swimming pool (when) W22.042 ☑
      causing drowning W22.041 ☑
      diving or jumping into water W16.532 ☑
        causing drowning W16.531 ☑
      falling into water W16.032 ☑
        causing drowning W16.031 ☑
Struck (accidentally) by
  airbag (automobile) W22.10 ☑
    driver side W22.11 ☑
    front passenger side W22.12 ☑
    specified NEC W22.19 ☑
  alligator W58.02 ☑
  animal (not being ridden) NEC W55.89 ☑
  avalanche — see Landslide
  ball (hit) (thrown) W21.00 ☑
    assault Y08.09 ☑
    baseball W21.03 ☑
    basketball W21.05 ☑
    golf ball W21.04 ☑
    football W21.01 ☑
    soccer W21.02 ☑
    softball W21.07 ☑
    specified NEC W21.09 ☑
    volleyball W21.06 ☑

Struck — continued
  bat or racquet
    baseball bat W21.11 ☑
      assault Y08.02 ☑
    golf club W21.13 ☑
      assault Y08.09 ☑
    specified NEC W21.19 ☑
      assault Y08.09 ☑
    tennis racquet W21.12 ☑
      assault Y08.09 ☑
  bullet (see also Discharge, firearm by type)
    in war operations — see War operations
  crocodile W58.12 ☑
  dog W54.1 ☑
  flare, Very pistol — see Discharge, firearm NEC
  hailstones X39.8 ☑
  hockey (ice)
    field
      puck W21.221 ☑
      stick W21.211 ☑
    puck W21.220 ☑
    stick W21.210 ☑
    assault Y08.01 ☑
  landslide — see Landslide
  law-enforcement agent (on duty) — see Legal, intervention, manhandling
    with blunt object — see Legal, intervention, blunt object
  lightning — see subcategory T75.0 ☑
    causing fire — see Exposure, fire
  machine — see Contact, with, by type of machine
  mammal NEC W55.89 ☑
    marine W56.32 ☑
  marine animal W56.82 ☑
  missile
    firearm — see Discharge, firearm by type
    in war operations — see War operations, missile
  object W22.8 ☑
    blunt W22.8 ☑
      assault Y00 ☑
      suicide (attempt) X79 ☑
      undetermined whether accidental or intentional Y29 ☑
    falling W20.8 ☑
      from, in, on
        building W20.1 ☑
          burning (uncontrolled fire) X00.4 ☑
        cataclysmic
          earth surface movement NEC — see Landslide
          storm — see Forces of nature, cataclysmic storm
        cave-in W20.0 ☑
        earthquake X34 ☑
        machine (in operation) — see Contact, with, by type of machine
        structure W20.1 ☑
          burning X00.4 ☑
        transport vehicle (in motion) — see Accident, transport, by type of vehicle
        watercraft V93.49 ☑
          due to
            accident to craft V91.39 ☑
              powered craft V91.33 ☑
                ferry boat V91.31 ☑
                fishing boat V91.32 ☑
                jetskis V91.33 ☑
                liner V91.31 ☑
                merchant ship V91.30 ☑
                passenger ship V91.31 ☑
              unpowered craft V91.38 ☑
                canoe V91.35 ☑
                inflatable V91.36 ☑
                kayak V91.35 ☑
                sailboat V91.34 ☑
                surf-board V91.38 ☑
                windsurfer V91.38 ☑
            powered craft V93.43 ☑
              ferry boat V93.41 ☑
              fishing boat V93.42 ☑
              jetskis V93.43 ☑
              liner V93.41 ☑
              merchant ship V93.40 ☑
              passenger ship V93.41 ☑
            unpowered craft V93.48 ☑
              sailboat V93.44 ☑
              surf-board V93.48 ☑
              windsurfer V93.48 ☑
    moving NEC W20.8 ☑
    projected W20.8 ☑
      assault Y00 ☑
      in sports W21.9 ☑

Struck — continued
  object — continued
    assault Y08.09 ☑
    ball W21.00 ☑
      baseball W21.03 ☑
      basketball W21.05 ☑
      football W21.01 ☑
      golf ball W21.04 ☑
      soccer W21.02 ☑
      softball W21.07 ☑
      specified NEC W21.09 ☑
      volleyball W21.06 ☑
    bat or racquet
      baseball bat W21.11 ☑
        assault Y08.02 ☑
      golf club W21.13 ☑
        assault Y08.09 ☑
      specified NEC W21.19 ☑
        assault Y08.09 ☑
      tennis racquet W21.12 ☑
        assault Y08.09 ☑
    hockey (ice)
      field
        puck W21.221 ☑
        stick W21.211 ☑
      puck W21.220 ☑
      stick W21.210 ☑
      assault Y08.01 ☑
    specified NEC W21.89 ☑
  set in motion by explosion — see Explosion
  thrown W20.8 ☑
    assault Y00 ☑
    in sports W21.9 ☑
      assault Y08.09 ☑
      ball W21.00 ☑
        baseball W21.03 ☑
        basketball W21.05 ☑
        football W21.01 ☑
        golf ball W21.04 ☑
        soccer W21.02 ☑
        soft ball W21.07 ☑
        specified NEC W21.09 ☑
        volleyball W21.06 ☑
      bat or racquet
        baseball bat W21.11 ☑
          assault Y08.02 ☑
        golf club W21.13 ☑
          assault Y08.09 ☑
        specified NEC W21.19 ☑
          assault Y08.09 ☑
        tennis racquet W21.12 ☑
          assault Y08.09 ☑
      hockey (ice)
        field
          puck W21.221 ☑
          stick W21.211 ☑
        puck W21.220 ☑
        stick W21.210 ☑
        assault Y08.01 ☑
      specified NEC W21.89 ☑
  other person(s) W50.0 ☑
    with
      blunt object W22.8 ☑
        intentional, homicide (attempt) Y00 ☑
        sports equipment W21.9 ☑
        undetermined whether accidental or intentional Y29 ☑
      fall W03 ☑
        due to ice or snow W00.0 ☑
    as, or caused by, a crowd or human stampede (with fall) W52 ☑
    assault Y04.2 ☑
    homicide (attempt) Y04.2 ☑
    in legal intervention
      injuring
        bystander Y35.812 ☑
        law enforcement personnel Y35.811 ☑
        suspect Y35.813 ☑
        unspecified person Y35.819 ☑
    sports equipment W21.9 ☑
  police (on duty) — see Legal, intervention, manhandling
    with blunt object — see Legal, intervention, blunt object
  sports equipment W21.9 ☑
    assault Y08.09 ☑
    ball W21.00 ☑
      baseball W21.03 ☑
      basketball W21.05 ☑
      football W21.01 ☑
      golf ball W21.04 ☑
      soccer W21.02 ☑

☑ Additional character required

Struck — *continued*
  sports equipment — *continued*
    soft ball W21.07 ☑
    specified NEC W21.09 ☑
    volleyball W21.06 ☑
   bat or racquet
    baseball bat W21.11 ☑
     assault Y08.02 ☑
    golf club W21.13 ☑
     assault Y08.09 ☑
    specified NEC W21.19 ☑
    tennis racquet W21.12 ☑
     assault Y08.09 ☑
   cleats (shoe) W21.31 ☑
   foot wear NEC W21.39 ☑
   football helmet W21.81 ☑
   hockey (ice)
    field
     puck W21.221 ☑
     stick W21.211 ☑
    puck W21.220 ☑
    stick W21.210 ☑
     assault Y08.01 ☑
   skate blades W21.32 ☑
   specified NEC W21.89 ☑
    assault Y08.09 ☑
  thunderbolt — *see* subcategory T75.0 ☑
   causing fire — *see* Exposure, fire
  transport vehicle NEC (*see also* Accident, transport) V09.9 ☑
   intentional, homicide (attempt) Y03.0 ☑
   motor NEC (*see also* Accident, transport) V09.20 ☑
    homicide Y03.0 ☑
  vehicle (transport) NEC — *see* Accident, transport, by type of vehicle
  stationary (falling from jack, hydraulic lift, ramp) W20.8 ☑
Stumbling
  over
   animal NEC W01.0 ☑
    with fall W18.09 ☑
   carpet, rug or (small) object W22.8 ☑
    with fall W18.09 ☑
   person W51 ☑
    with fall W03 ☑
     due to ice or snow W00.0 ☑
  without fall W18.40 ☑
   due to
    specified NEC W18.49 ☑
    stepping from one level to another W18.43 ☑
    stepping into hole or opening W18.42 ☑
    stepping on object W18.41 ☑
Submersion (accidental) — *see* Drowning
Suffocation (accidental) (by external means) (by pressure) (mechanical) (*see also* category) T71 ☑
  due to, by
   avalanche — *see* Landslide
   explosion — *see* Explosion
   fire — *see* Exposure, fire
   food, any type (aspiration) (ingestion) (inhalation) — *see* categories T17 ☑ and T18 ☑
   ignition — *see* Ignition
   landslide — *see* Landslide
   machine (ry) — *see* Contact, with, by type of machine
   vomitus (aspiration) (inhalation) T17.81 ☑
  in
   burning building X00.8 ☑
Suicide, suicidal (attempted) (by) X83.8 ☑
  blunt object X79 ☑
  burning, burns X76 ☑
   hot object X77.9 ☑
    fluid NEC X77.2 ☑
    household appliance X77.3 ☑
    specified NEC X77.8 ☑
    steam X77.0 ☑
    tap water X77.1 ☑
    vapors X77.0 ☑
  caustic substance — *see* Table of Drugs and Chemicals
  cold, extreme X83.2 ☑
  collision of motor vehicle with
   motor vehicle X82.0 ☑
   specified NEC X82.8 ☑
   train X82.1 ☑
   tree X82.2 ☑
  crashing of aircraft X83.0 ☑
  cut (any part of body) X78.9 ☑
  cutting or piercing instrument X78.9 ☑
   dagger X78.2 ☑
   glass X78.0 ☑
   knife X78.1 ☑

Suicide — *continued*
  cutting or piercing instrument — *continued*
   specified NEC X78.8 ☑
   sword X78.2 ☑
  drowning (in) X71.9 ☑
   bathtub X71.0 ☑
   natural water X71.3 ☑
   specified NEC X71.8 ☑
   swimming pool X71.1 ☑
    following fall X71.2 ☑
  electrocution X83.1 ☑
  explosive(s) (material) X75 ☑
  fire, flames X76 ☑
  firearm X74.9 ☑
   airgun X74.01 ☑
   handgun X72 ☑
   hunting rifle X73.1 ☑
   larger X73.9 ☑
    specified NEC X73.8 ☑
   machine gun X73.2 ☑
   shotgun X73.0 ☑
   specified NEC X74.8 ☑
  hanging X83.8 ☑
  hot object — *see* Suicide, burning, hot object
  jumping
   before moving object X81.8 ☑
    motor vehicle X81.0 ☑
    subway train X81.1 ☑
    train X81.1 ☑
   from high place X80 ☑
  late effect of attempt — *see* X71-X83 with 7th character S
  lying before moving object, train, vehicle X81.8 ☑
  poisoning — *see* Table of Drugs and Chemicals
  puncture (any part of body) — *see* Suicide, cutting or piercing instrument
  scald — *see* Suicide, burning, hot object
  sequelae of attempt — *see* X71-X83 with 7th character S
  sharp object (any) — *see* Suicide, cutting or piercing instrument
  shooting — *see* Suicide, firearm
  specified means NEC X83.8 ☑
  stab (any part of body) — *see* Suicide, cutting or piercing instrument
  steam, hot vapors X77.0 ☑
  strangulation X83.8 ☑
  submersion — *see* Suicide, drowning
  suffocation X83.8 ☑
  wound NEC X83.8 ☑
Sunstroke X32 ☑
Supersonic waves (causing injury) W42.0 ☑
Surgical procedure, complication of (delayed or as an abnormal reaction without mention of misadventure) (*see also* Complication of or following, by type of procedure)
  due to or as a result of misadventure — *see* Misadventure
Swallowed, swallowing
  foreign body — *see* Foreign body, alimentary canal
  poison — *see* Table of Drugs and Chemicals
  substance
   caustic or corrosive — *see* Table of Drugs and Chemicals
   poisonous — *see* Table of Drugs and Chemicals

T

Tackle in sport W03 ☑
Terrorism (involving) Y38.80 ☑
  biological weapons Y38.6X ☑
  chemical weapons Y38.7X ☑
  conflagration Y38.3X ☑
  drowning and submersion Y38.89 ☑
  explosion Y38.2X ☑
   destruction of aircraft Y38.1X ☑
   marine weapons Y38.0X ☑
  fire Y38.3X ☑
  firearms Y38.4X ☑
  hot substances Y38.3X ☑
  lasers Y38.89 ☑
  nuclear weapons Y38.5X ☑
  piercing or stabbing instruments Y38.89 ☑
  secondary effects Y38.9X ☑
  specified method NEC Y38.89 ☑
  suicide bomber Y38.81 ☑
Thirst X58 ☑
Threat to breathing
  aspiration — *see* Aspiration
  due to cave-in, falling earth or substance NEC — *see* category T71 ☑

Thrown (accidentally)
  against part (any) of or object in transport vehicle (in motion) NEC (*see also* Accident, transport)
  from
   high place, homicide (attempt) Y01 ☑
   machinery — *see* Contact, with, by type of machine
   transport vehicle NEC (*see also* Accident, transport) V89.9 ☑
  off — *see* Thrown, from
Thunderbolt — *see* subcategory T75.0 ☑
  causing fire — *see* Exposure, fire
Tidal wave (any injury) NEC — *see* Forces of nature, tidal wave
Took
  overdose (drug) — *see* Table of Drugs and Chemicals
  poison — *see* Table of Drugs and Chemicals
Tornado (any injury) X37.1 ☑
Torrential rain (any injury) X37.8 ☑
Torture X58 ☑
Trampled by animal NEC W55.89 ☑
Trapped (accidentally)
  between objects (moving) (stationary and moving) — *see* Caught
  by part (any) of
   motorcycle V29.88 ☑
   pedal cycle V19.88 ☑
   transport vehicle NEC (*see also* Accident, transport) V89.9 ☑
Travel (effects) (sickness) T75.3 ☑
Tree falling on or hitting (accidentally) (person) W20.8 ☑
Tripping
  over
   animal W01.0 ☑
    with fall W01.0 ☑
   carpet, rug or (small) object W22.8 ☑
    with fall W18.09 ☑
   person W51 ☑
    with fall W03 ☑
     due to ice or snow W00.0 ☑
  without fall W18.40 ☑
   due to
    specified NEC W18.49 ☑
    stepping from one level to another W18.43 ☑
    stepping into hole or opening W18.42 ☑
    stepping on object W18.41 ☑
Twisted by person(s) (accidentally) W50.2 ☑
  with intent to injure or kill Y04.0 ☑
  as, or caused by, a crowd or human stampede (with fall) W52 ☑
  assault Y04.0 ☑
  homicide (attempt) Y04.0 ☑
  in
   fight Y04.0 ☑
   legal intervention — *see* Legal, intervention, manhandling
Twisting (prolonged) (static) X50.1 ☑

U

Underdosing of necessary drugs, medicaments or biological substances Y63.6
Undetermined intent (contact) (exposure)
  automobile collision Y32 ☑
  blunt object Y29 ☑
  drowning (submersion) (in) Y21.9 ☑
   bathtub Y21.0 ☑
    after fall Y21.1 ☑
   natural water (lake) (ocean) (pond) (river) (stream) Y21.4 ☑
   specified place NEC Y21.8 ☑
   swimming pool Y21.2 ☑
    after fall Y21.3 ☑
  explosive material Y25 ☑
  fall, jump or push from high place Y30 ☑
  falling, lying or running before moving object Y31 ☑
  fire Y26 ☑
  firearm discharge Y24.9 ☑
   airgun (BB) (pellet) Y24.0 ☑
   handgun (pistol) (revolver) Y22 ☑
   hunting rifle Y23.1 ☑
   larger Y23.9 ☑
    hunting rifle Y23.1 ☑
    machine gun Y23.3 ☑
    military Y23.2 ☑
    shotgun Y23.0 ☑
    specified type NEC Y23.8 ☑

Undetermined — *continued*
firearm discharge — *continued*
machine gun Y23.3 ☑
military Y23.2 ☑
shotgun Y23.0 ☑
specified type NEC Y24.8 ☑
Very pistol Y24.8 ☑
hot object Y27.9 ☑
fluid NEC Y27.2 ☑
household appliance Y27.3 ☑
specified object NEC Y27.8 ☑
steam Y27.0 ☑
tap water Y27.1 ☑
vapor Y27.0 ☑
jump, fall or push from high place Y30 ☑
lying, falling or running before moving object
Y31 ☑
motor vehicle crash Y32 ☑
push, fall or jump from high place Y30 ☑
running, falling or lying before moving object
Y31 ☑
sharp object Y28.9 ☑
dagger Y28.2 ☑
glass Y28.0 ☑
knife Y28.1 ☑
specified object NEC Y28.8 ☑
sword Y28.2 ☑
smoke Y26 ☑
specified event NEC Y33 ☑
Use of hand as hammer X50.3 ☑

V

Vibration (causing injury) W49.9 ☑
Victim (of)
avalanche — *see* Landslide
earth movements NEC — *see* Forces of nature, earth
movement
earthquake X34 ☑
flood — *see* Flood
landslide — *see* Landslide
lightning — *see* subcategory T75.0 ☑
causing fire — *see* Exposure, fire
storm (cataclysmic) NEC — *see* Forces of nature,
cataclysmic storm
volcanic eruption X35 ☑
Volcanic eruption (any injury) X35 ☑
Vomitus, gastric contents in air passages (with
asphyxia, obstruction or suffocation) T17.81 ☑

W

Walked into stationary object (any) W22.09 ☑
furniture W22.03 ☑
lamppost W22.02 ☑
wall W22.01 ☑
War operations (injuries to military personnel
and civilians during war, civil insurrection and
peacekeeping missions) (by) (from) (involving)
Y36.90 ☑
after cessation of hostilities Y36.89 ☑
explosion (of)
bomb placed during war operations Y36.82 ☑
mine placed during war operations Y36.81 ☑
specified NEC Y36.88 ☑
air blast Y36.20 ☑
aircraft
destruction — *see* War operations, destruction
of aircraft
airway restriction — *see* War operations, restriction
of airways
asphyxiation — *see* War operations, restriction of
airways
biological weapons Y36.6X ☑
blast Y36.20 ☑
blast fragments Y36.20 ☑
blast wave Y36.20 ☑
blast wind Y36.20 ☑
bomb Y36.20 ☑
dirty Y36.50 ☑
gasoline Y36.31 ☑
incendiary Y36.31 ☑
petrol Y36.31 ☑
bullet Y36.43 ☑
incendiary Y36.32 ☑
rubber Y36.41 ☑

War — *continued*
chemical weapons Y36.7X ☑
combat
hand to hand (unarmed) combat Y36.44 ☑
using blunt or piercing object Y36.45 ☑
conflagration — *see* War operations, fire
conventional warfare NEC Y36.49 ☑
depth-charge Y36.01 ☑
destruction of aircraft Y36.10 ☑
due to
air to air missile Y36.11 ☑
collision with other aircraft Y36.12 ☑
detonation (accidental) of onboard munitions
and explosives Y36.14 ☑
enemy fire or explosives Y36.11 ☑
explosive placed on aircraft Y36.11 ☑
onboard fire Y36.13 ☑
rocket propelled grenade [RPG] Y36.11 ☑
small arms fire Y36.11 ☑
surface to air missile Y36.11 ☑
specified NEC Y36.19 ☑
detonation (accidental) of
onboard marine weapons Y36.05 ☑
own munitions or munitions launch device
Y36.24 ☑
dirty bomb Y36.50 ☑
explosion (of) Y36.20 ☑
after cessation of hostilities
bomb placed during war operations Y36.82 ☑
mine placed during war operations Y36.81 ☑
aerial bomb Y36.21 ☑
bomb NOS (*see also* War operations, bomb(s))
Y36.20 ☑
own munitions or munitions launch device
(accidental) Y36.24 ☑
fragments Y36.20 ☑
grenade Y36.29 ☑
guided missile Y36.22 ☑
improvised explosive device [IED] (person-borne)
(roadside) (vehicle-borne) Y36.23 ☑
land mine Y36.29 ☑
marine mine (at sea) (in harbor) Y36.02 ☑
marine weapon Y36.00 ☑
specified NEC Y36.09 ☑
sea-based artillery shell Y36.03 ☑
specified NEC Y36.29 ☑
torpedo Y36.04 ☑
fire Y36.30 ☑
specified NEC Y36.39 ☑
firearms
discharge Y36.43 ☑
pellets Y36.42 ☑
flamethrower Y36.33 ☑
fragments (from) (of)
improvised explosive device [IED] (person-borne)
(roadside) (vehicle-borne) Y36.26 ☑
munitions Y36.25 ☑
specified NEC Y36.29 ☑
weapons Y36.27 ☑
friendly fire Y36.92 ☑
hand to hand (unarmed) combat Y36.44 ☑
hot substances — *see* War operations, fire
incendiary bullet Y36.32 ☑
nuclear weapon (effects of) Y36.50 ☑
acute radiation exposure Y36.54 ☑
blast pressure Y36.51 ☑
direct blast Y36.51 ☑
direct heat Y36.53 ☑
fallout exposure Y36.54 ☑
fireball Y36.53 ☑
indirect blast (struck or crushed by blast debris)
(being thrown by blast) Y36.52 ☑
ionizing radiation (immediate exposure)
Y36.54 ☑
nuclear radiation Y36.54 ☑
radiation
ionizing (immediate exposure) Y36.54 ☑
nuclear Y36.54 ☑
thermal Y36.53 ☑
specified NEC Y36.59 ☑
secondary effects Y36.54 ☑
thermal radiation Y36.53 ☑
restriction of air (airway)
intentional Y36.46 ☑
unintentional Y36.47 ☑
rubber bullets Y36.41 ☑

War — *continued*
shrapnel NOS Y36.29 ☑
suffocation — *see* War operations, restriction of
airways
unconventional warfare NEC Y36.7X ☑
underwater blast NOS Y36.00 ☑
warfare
conventional NEC Y36.49 ☑
unconventional NEC Y36.7X ☑
weapons
biological weapons Y36.6X ☑
chemical Y36.7X ☑
nuclear (effects of) Y36.50 ☑
acute radiation exposure Y36.54 ☑
blast pressure Y36.51 ☑
direct blast Y36.51 ☑
direct heat Y36.53 ☑
fallout exposure Y36.54 ☑
fireball Y36.53 ☑
indirect blast (struck or crushed by blast debris)
(being thrown by blast) Y36.52 ☑
radiation
ionizing (immediate exposure) Y36.54 ☑
nuclear Y36.54 ☑
thermal Y36.53 ☑
secondary effects Y36.54 ☑
specified NEC Y36.59 ☑
of mass destruction [WMD] Y36.91 ☑
weapon of mass destruction [WMD] Y36.91 ☑
Washed
away by flood — *see* Flood
off road by storm (transport vehicle) — *see* Forces of
nature, cataclysmic storm
Weather exposure NEC — *see* Forces of nature
Weightlessness (causing injury) (effects of) (in
spacecraft, real or simulated) X52 ☑
Work related condition Y99.0
Wound (accidental) NEC (*see also* Injury) X58 ☑
battle (*see also* War operations) Y36.90 ☑
gunshot — *see* Discharge, firearm by type
Wreck transport vehicle NEC (*see also* Accident,
transport) V89.9 ☑
Wrong
device implanted into correct surgical site Y65.51
fluid in infusion Y65.1
procedure (operation) on correct patient Y65.51
patient, procedure performed on Y65.52

Chapter 1: Certain Infectious and Parasitic Diseases (A00-B99)

Certain infectious and parasitic diseases (A00-B99)

INCLUDES *diseases generally recognized as communicable or transmissible*
Use additional code to identify resistance to antimicrobial drugs (Z16.-)
EXCLUDES1 *certain localized infections - see body system-related chapters*
EXCLUDES2 *carrier or suspected carrier of infectious disease (Z22.-)*

infectious and parasitic diseases complicating pregnancy, childbirth and the puerperium (O98.-)

infectious and parasitic diseases specific to the perinatal period (P35-P39)

influenza and other acute respiratory infections (J00-J22)

This chapter contains the following blocks:

A00-A09   Intestinal infectious diseases
A15-A19   Tuberculosis
A20-A28   Certain zoonotic bacterial diseases
A30-A49   Other bacterial diseases
A50-A64   Infections with a predominantly sexual mode of transmission
A65-A69   Other spirochetal diseases
A70-A74   Other diseases caused by chlamydiae
A75-A79   Rickettsioses
A80-A89   Viral and prion infections of the central nervous system
A90-A99   Arthropod-borne viral fevers and viral hemorrhagic fevers
B00-B09   Viral infections characterized by skin and mucous membrane lesions
B10   Other human herpesviruses
B15-B19   Viral hepatitis
B20   Human immunodeficiency virus [HIV] disease
B25-B34   Other viral diseases
B35-B49   Mycoses
B50-B64   Protozoal diseases
B65-B83   Helminthiases
B85-B89   Pediculosis, acariasis and other infestations
B90-B94   Sequelae of infectious and parasitic diseases
B95-B97   Bacterial and viral infectious agents
B99   Other infectious diseases

Intestinal infectious diseases (A00-A09)

4ᵗʰ **A00 Cholera**

   A00.0 Cholera due to Vibrio cholerae 01, biovar cholerae   cc♡ CC/MCC Exc⊘
   Classical cholera
   A00.1 Cholera due to Vibrio cholerae 01, biovar eltor   cc♡ CC/MCC Exc⊘
   Cholera eltor
   A00.9 Cholera, unspecified   cc♡ CC/MCC Exc⊘

4ᵗʰ **A01 Typhoid and paratyphoid fevers**

   5ᵗʰ **A01.0 Typhoid fever**
   Infection due to Salmonella typhi
      A01.00 Typhoid fever, unspecified   cc♡ CC/MCC Exc⊘
      A01.01 Typhoid meningitis   cc♡ CC/MCC Exc⊘
      A01.02 Typhoid fever with heart involvement   cc♡ CC/MCC Exc⊘
      Typhoid endocarditis
      Typhoid myocarditis
      A01.03 Typhoid pneumonia   cc♡ HCC CC/MCC Exc⊘
      A01.04 Typhoid arthritis   cc♡ HCC CC/MCC Exc⊘
      A01.05 Typhoid osteomyelitis   cc♡ HCC CC/MCC Exc⊘
      A01.09 Typhoid fever with other complications   cc♡ CC/MCC Exc⊘
   A01.1 Paratyphoid fever A   cc♡ CC/MCC Exc⊘
   A01.2 Paratyphoid fever B   cc♡ CC/MCC Exc⊘
   A01.3 Paratyphoid fever C   cc♡ CC/MCC Exc⊘
   A01.4 Paratyphoid fever, unspecified   cc♡ CC/MCC Exc⊘
   Infection due to Salmonella paratyphi NOS

4ᵗʰ **A02 Other salmonella infections**

   INCLUDES *infection or foodborne intoxication due to any Salmonella species other than S. typhi and S. paratyphi*

   A02.0 Salmonella enteritis   cc♡ CC/MCC Exc⊘
   Salmonellosis
   A02.1 Salmonella sepsis   HCC MCC♡ CC/MCC Exc⊘
   5ᵗʰ **A02.2 Localized salmonella infections**
      A02.20 Localized salmonella infection, unspecified
      A02.21 Salmonella meningitis   MCC♡ CC/MCC Exc⊘
      A02.22 Salmonella pneumonia   HCC MCC♡ CC/MCC Exc⊘
      A02.23 Salmonella arthritis   cc♡ HCC CC/MCC Exc⊘
      A02.24 Salmonella osteomyelitis   cc♡ HCC CC/MCC Exc⊘
      A02.25 Salmonella pyelonephritis   cc♡ CC/MCC Exc⊘
      Salmonella tubulo-interstitial nephropathy
      A02.29 Salmonella with other localized infection   cc♡ CC/MCC Exc⊘
   A02.8 Other specified salmonella infections   cc♡ CC/MCC Exc⊘
   A02.9 Salmonella infection, unspecified   cc♡ CC/MCC Exc⊘

4ᵗʰ **A03 Shigellosis**
   DEFINITION: Shigellosis is caused by a group of bacteria called Shigella, leading to diarrhea, fever, and stomach cramps.
   A03.0 Shigellosis due to Shigella dysenteriae   cc♡ CC/MCC Exc⊘
   Group A shigellosis [Shiga-Kruse dysentery]
   A03.1 Shigellosis due to Shigella flexneri
   Group B shigellosis
   A03.2 Shigellosis due to Shigella boydii
   Group C shigellosis
   A03.3 Shigellosis due to Shigella sonnei
   Group D shigellosis
   A03.8 Other shigellosis
   A03.9 Shigellosis, unspecified
   Bacillary dysentery NOS

4ᵗʰ **A04 Other bacterial intestinal infections**
   EXCLUDES1 *bacterial foodborne intoxications, NEC (A05.-)*
   tuberculous enteritis (A18.32)
   A04.0 Enteropathogenic Escherichia coli infection   cc♡ CC/MCC Exc⊘
   A04.1 Enterotoxigenic Escherichia coli infection   cc♡ CC/MCC Exc⊘
   A04.2 Enteroinvasive Escherichia coli infection   cc♡ CC/MCC Exc⊘
   A04.3 Enterohemorrhagic Escherichia coli infection   cc♡ CC/MCC Exc⊘
   A04.4 Other intestinal Escherichia coli infections   cc♡ CC/MCC Exc⊘
   Escherichia coli enteritis NOS
   A04.5 Campylobacter enteritis   cc♡ CC/MCC Exc⊘
   A04.6 Enteritis due to Yersinia enterocolitica   cc♡ CC/MCC Exc⊘
   EXCLUDES1 *extraintestinal yersiniosis (A28.2)*
   5ᵗʰ **A04.7 Enterocolitis due to** Clostridium difficile
   Foodborne intoxication by Clostridium difficile
   Pseudomembranous colitis
      A04.71 Enterocolitis due to Clostridium difficile, **recurrent**   cc♡ CC/MCC Exc⊘
      AHA: Q4 2017
      A04.72 Enterocolitis due to Clostridium difficile, **not specified as recurrent**   cc♡ CC/MCC Exc⊘
      AHA: Q4 2017
   A04.8 Other specified bacterial intestinal infections   cc♡ CC/MCC Exc⊘
   A04.9 Bacterial intestinal infection, unspecified   cc♡ CC/MCC Exc⊘
   Bacterial enteritis NOS

4ᵗʰ **A05 Other bacterial foodborne intoxications, not elsewhere classified**
   EXCLUDES1 *Clostridium difficile foodborne intoxication and infection (A04.7-)*
   Escherichia coli infection (A04.0-A04.4)
   listeriosis (A32.-)
   salmonella foodborne intoxication and infection (A02.-)
   toxic effect of noxious foodstuffs (T61-T62)
   A05.0 Foodborne staphylococcal intoxication   cc♡ CC/MCC Exc⊘
   A05.1 Botulism food poisoning   cc♡ CC/MCC Exc⊘
   Botulism NOS
   Classical foodborne intoxication due to Clostridium botulinum
   EXCLUDES1 *infant botulism (A48.51)*
   wound botulism (A48.52)

Unspecified Code   Other Specified Code   Manifestation Code   Ⓝ Newborn   Ⓟ Pediatric   Ⓜ Maternity   Ⓐ Adult   ♂ Male   ♀ Female
● New Code   ▲ Revised Code Title   ►◄ Revised Text   NOTES   INCLUDES   EXCLUDES1 Not coded here   EXCLUDES2 Not included here
4ᵗʰ 4ᵗʰ character required   5ᵗʰ 5ᵗʰ character required   6ᵗʰ 6ᵗʰ character required   7ᵗʰ 7ᵗʰ character required   Extension 'X' Alert
HAC Hospital-acquired condition (HAC) alert   AHA AHA Coding Clinic©   ☞ Code first alert

A05.2 **Foodborne Clostridium perfringens [Clostridium welchii] intoxication** [CC] [CC/MCC Exc]
Enteritis necroticans
Pig-bel
A05.3 **Foodborne Vibrio parahaemolyticus intoxication** [CC] [CC/MCC Exc]
A05.4 **Foodborne Bacillus cereus intoxication** [CC] [CC/MCC Exc]
A05.5 **Foodborne Vibrio vulnificus intoxication** [CC] [CC/MCC Exc]
A05.8 **Other specified bacterial foodborne intoxications** [CC] [CC/MCC Exc]
A05.9 **Bacterial foodborne intoxication, unspecified**

[4th] A06 **Amebiasis**
[INCLUDES] *infection due to Entamoeba histolytica*
[EXCLUDES1] *other protozoal intestinal diseases (A07.-)*
[EXCLUDES2] *acanthamebiasis (B60.1-)*
Naegleriasis (B60.2)
A06.0 **Acute amebic dysentery** [CC] [CC/MCC Exc]
Acute amebiasis
Intestinal amebiasis NOS
A06.1 **Chronic intestinal amebiasis** [CC] [CC/MCC Exc]
A06.2 **Amebic nondysenteric colitis** [CC] [CC/MCC Exc]
A06.3 **Ameboma of intestine** [CC] [CC/MCC Exc]
Ameboma NOS
A06.4 **Amebic liver abscess** [MCC] [CC/MCC Exc]
Hepatic amebiasis
A06.5 **Amebic lung abscess** [HCC] [MCC] [CC/MCC Exc]
Amebic abscess of lung (and liver)
A06.6 **Amebic brain abscess** [MCC] [CC/MCC Exc]
Amebic abscess of brain (and liver) (and lung)
A06.7 **Cutaneous amebiasis**
[5th] A06.8 **Amebic infection of other sites**
A06.81 **Amebic cystitis** [CC] [CC/MCC Exc]
A06.82 **Other amebic genitourinary infections** [CC] [CC/MCC Exc]
Amebic balanitis
Amebic vesiculitis
Amebic vulvovaginitis
A06.89 **Other amebic infections** [CC] [CC/MCC Exc]
Amebic appendicitis
Amebic splenic abscess
A06.9 **Amebiasis, unspecified**

[4th] A07 **Other protozoal intestinal diseases**
A07.0 **Balantidiasis**
Balantidial dysentery
A07.1 **Giardiasis [lambliasis]** [CC] [CC/MCC Exc]
A07.2 **Cryptosporidiosis** [CC] [HCC] [RxHCC] [CC/MCC Exc]
A07.3 **Isosporiasis** [CC] [CC/MCC Exc]
Infection due to Isospora belli and Isospora hominis
Intestinal coccidiosis
Isosporosis
A07.4 **Cyclosporiasis** [CC] [CC/MCC Exc]
A07.8 **Other specified protozoal intestinal diseases** [CC] [CC/MCC Exc]
Intestinal microsporidiosis
Intestinal trichomoniasis
Sarcocystosis
Sarcosporidiosis
A07.9 **Protozoal intestinal disease, unspecified** [CC] [CC/MCC Exc]
Flagellate diarrhea
Protozoal colitis
Protozoal diarrhea
Protozoal dysentery

[4th] A08 **Viral and other specified intestinal infections**
[EXCLUDES1] *influenza with involvement of gastrointestinal tract (J09.X3, J10.2, J11.2)*
A08.0 **Rotaviral enteritis** [CC] [CC/MCC Exc]
[5th] A08.1 **Acute gastroenteropathy due to Norwalk agent and other small round viruses**
A08.11 **Acute gastroenteropathy due to Norwalk agent** [CC] [CC/MCC Exc]
Acute gastroenteropathy due to Norovirus
Acute gastroenteropathy due to Norwalk-like agent
A08.19 **Acute gastroenteropathy due to other small round viruses** [CC] [CC/MCC Exc]
Acute gastroenteropathy due to small round virus [SRV] NOS
A08.2 **Adenoviral enteritis** [CC] [CC/MCC Exc]
[5th] A08.3 **Other viral enteritis**
A08.31 **Calicivirus enteritis** [CC] [CC/MCC Exc]
A08.32 **Astrovirus enteritis** [CC] [CC/MCC Exc]
A08.39 **Other viral enteritis** [CC] [CC/MCC Exc]
Coxsackie virus enteritis
Echovirus enteritis
Enterovirus enteritis NEC
Torovirus enteritis
A08.4 **Viral intestinal infection, unspecified**
AHA: Q3 2016
Viral enteritis NOS
Viral gastroenteritis NOS
Viral gastroenteropathy NOS
A08.8 **Other specified intestinal infections**

A09 **Infectious gastroenteritis and colitis, unspecified**
Infectious colitis NOS
Infectious enteritis NOS
Infectious gastroenteritis NOS
[EXCLUDES1] *colitis NOS (K52.9)*
diarrhea NOS (R19.7)
enteritis NOS (K52.9)
gastroenteritis NOS (K52.9)
noninfective gastroenteritis and colitis, unspecified (K52.9)

Tuberculosis (A15-A19) (Figure 1.1)

[INCLUDES] *infections due to Mycobacterium tuberculosis and Mycobacterium bovis*
[EXCLUDES1] *congenital tuberculosis (P37.0)*
nonspecific reaction to test for tuberculosis without active tuberculosis (R76.1-)
pneumoconiosis associated with tuberculosis, any type in A15 (J65)
positive PPD (R76.11)
positive tuberculin skin test without active tuberculosis (R76.11)
sequelae of tuberculosis (B90.-)
silicotuberculosis (J65)

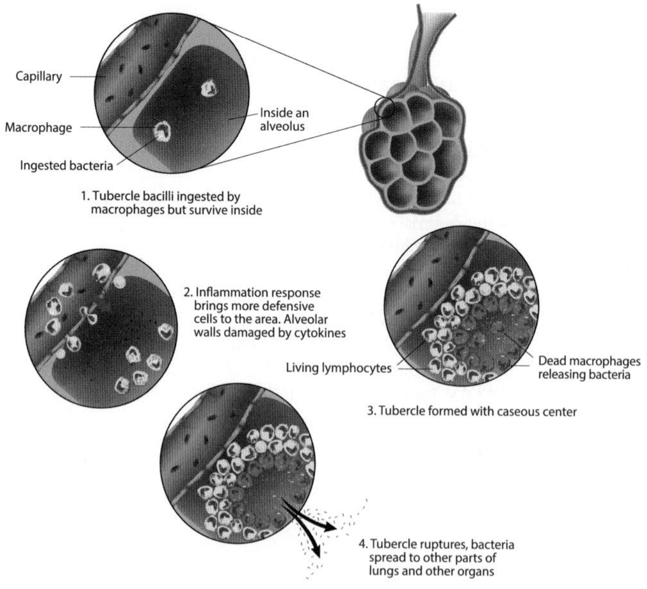
Capillary
Macrophage
Ingested bacteria
Inside an alveolus
1. Tubercle bacilli ingested by macrophages but survive inside
2. Inflammation response brings more defensive cells to the area. Alveolar walls damaged by cytokines
Living lymphocytes
Dead macrophages releasing bacteria
3. Tubercle formed with caseous center
4. Tubercle ruptures, bacteria spread to other parts of lungs and other organs

Figure 1.1 Progression of Tuberculosis

[4th] A15 **Respiratory tuberculosis**
A15.0 **Tuberculosis of lung** [CC] [CC/MCC Exc]
Tuberculous bronchiectasis
Tuberculous fibrosis of lung
Tuberculous pneumonia
Tuberculous pneumothorax

A15.4 **Tuberculosis of** intrathoracic lymph nodes [CC] [CC/MCC Exc]
Tuberculosis of hilar lymph nodes
Tuberculosis of mediastinal lymph nodes
Tuberculosis of tracheobronchial lymph nodes
[EXCLUDES1] *tuberculosis specified as primary (A15.7)*

A15.5 **Tuberculosis of** larynx, trachea **and** bronchus [CC] [CC/MCC Exc]
Tuberculosis of bronchus
Tuberculosis of glottis
Tuberculosis of larynx
Tuberculosis of trachea

A15.6 **Tuberculous pleurisy** [CC] [CC/MCC Exc]
Tuberculosis of pleura Tuberculous empyema
[EXCLUDES1] *primary respiratory tuberculosis (A15.7)*

A15.7 Primary **respiratory tuberculosis** [CC] [CC/MCC Exc]

A15.8 Other **respiratory tuberculosis** [CC] [CC/MCC Exc]
Mediastinal tuberculosis
Nasopharyngeal tuberculosis
Tuberculosis of nose
Tuberculosis of sinus [any nasal]

A15.9 **Respiratory tuberculosis unspecified** [CC] [CC/MCC Exc]

[4th] A17 **Tuberculosis of** nervous system

A17.0 **Tuberculous** meningitis [MCC] [CC/MCC Exc]
Tuberculosis of meninges (cerebral)(spinal)
Tuberculous leptomeningitis
[EXCLUDES1] *tuberculous meningoencephalitis (A17.82)*

A17.1 Meningeal **tuberculoma** [MCC] [CC/MCC Exc]
Tuberculoma of meninges (cerebral) (spinal)
[EXCLUDES2] *tuberculoma of brain and spinal cord (A17.81)*

[5th] A17.8 Other **tuberculosis of** nervous system

A17.81 **Tuberculoma of** brain and spinal cord [MCC] [CC/MCC Exc]
Tuberculous abscess of brain and spinal cord

A17.82 **Tuberculous** meningoencephalitis [MCC] [CC/MCC Exc]
Tuberculous myelitis

A17.83 **Tuberculous** neuritis [MCC]
Tuberculous mononeuropathy

A17.89 Other **tuberculosis of nervous system** [MCC] [CC/MCC Exc]
Tuberculous polyneuropathy

A17.9 **Tuberculosis of nervous system, unspecified** [CC] [CC/MCC Exc]

[4th] A18 **Tuberculosis of** other organs

[5th] A18.0 **Tuberculosis of** bones **and** joints
👁 **See Official Guidelines** "And" I.A.14

A18.01 **Tuberculosis of** spine [CC] [CC/MCC Exc]
Pott's disease or curvature of spine
Tuberculous arthritis
Tuberculous osteomyelitis of spine
Tuberculous spondylitis

A18.02 **Tuberculous** arthritis of other joints [CC] [CC/MCC Exc]
Tuberculosis of hip (joint)
Tuberculosis of knee (joint)

A18.03 **Tuberculosis of** other bones [CC] [CC/MCC Exc]
Tuberculous mastoiditis
Tuberculous osteomyelitis

A18.09 **Other** musculoskeletal **tuberculosis** [CC] [CC/MCC Exc]
Tuberculous myositis
Tuberculous synovitis
Tuberculous tenosynovitis

[5th] A18.1 **Tuberculosis of** genitourinary **system**

A18.10 **Tuberculosis of genitourinary system, unspecified** [CC] [CC/MCC Exc]

A18.11 **Tuberculosis of** kidney and ureter [CC] [CC/MCC Exc]

A18.12 **Tuberculosis of** bladder [CC] [CC/MCC Exc]

A18.13 **Tuberculosis of** other urinary **organs** [CC] [CC/MCC Exc]
Tuberculous urethritis

A18.14 **Tuberculosis of** prostate [A] [CC] ♂ [CC/MCC Exc]

A18.15 **Tuberculosis of** other male genital **organs** [CC] ♂ [CC/MCC Exc]

A18.16 **Tuberculosis of** cervix [CC] ♀ [CC/MCC Exc]

A18.17 **Tuberculous** female pelvic inflammatory disease [CC] ♀ [CC/MCC Exc]
Tuberculous endometritis
Tuberculous oophoritis and salpingitis

A18.18 **Tuberculosis of** other female genital **organs** [CC] ♀ [CC/MCC Exc]
Tuberculous ulceration of vulva

A18.2 **Tuberculous** peripheral lymphadenopathy [CC] [CC/MCC Exc]
Tuberculous adenitis
[EXCLUDES2] *tuberculosis of bronchial and mediastinal lymph nodes (A15.4)*
tuberculosis of mesenteric and retroperitoneal lymph nodes (A18.39)
tuberculous tracheobronchial adenopathy (A15.4)

[5th] A18.3 **Tuberculosis of** intestines, peritoneum and mesenteric glands

A18.31 **Tuberculous** peritonitis [MCC] [CC/MCC Exc]
Tuberculous ascites

A18.32 **Tuberculous** enteritis [CC] [CC/MCC Exc]
Tuberculosis of anus and rectum
Tuberculosis of intestine (large) (small)

A18.39 Retroperitoneal **tuberculosis** [CC] [CC/MCC Exc]
Tuberculosis of mesenteric glands
Tuberculosis of retroperitoneal (lymph glands)

A18.4 **Tuberculosis of** skin and subcutaneous tissue [CC] [CC/MCC Exc]
Erythema induratum, tuberculous
Lupus excedens
Lupus vulgaris NOS
Lupus vulgaris of eyelid
Scrofuloderma
Tuberculosis of external ear
[EXCLUDES2] *lupus erythematosus (L93.-)*
systemic ▶lupus erythematosus◀ (M32.-)

[5th] A18.5 **Tuberculosis of** eye
[EXCLUDES2] *lupus vulgaris of eyelid (A18.4)*

A18.50 **Tuberculosis of eye, unspecified** [CC] [CC/MCC Exc]

A18.51 **Tuberculous** episcleritis [CC] [CC/MCC Exc]

A18.52 **Tuberculous** keratitis [CC] [CC/MCC Exc]
Tuberculous interstitial keratitis
Tuberculous keratoconjunctivitis (interstitial) (phlyctenular)

A18.53 **Tuberculous** chorioretinitis [CC] [CC/MCC Exc]

A18.54 **Tuberculous** iridocyclitis [CC] [CC/MCC Exc]

A18.59 Other **tuberculosis of eye** [CC] [CC/MCC Exc]
Tuberculous conjunctivitis

A18.6 **Tuberculosis of** (inner) (middle) ear [CC] [CC/MCC Exc]
Tuberculous otitis media
[EXCLUDES2] *tuberculosis of external ear (A18.4)*
tuberculous mastoiditis (A18.03)

A18.7 **Tuberculosis of** adrenal glands [CC] [CC/MCC Exc]
Tuberculous Addison's disease

[5th] A18.8 **Tuberculosis of** other specified organs

A18.81 **Tuberculosis of** thyroid gland [CC] [CC/MCC Exc]

A18.82 **Tuberculosis of** other endocrine glands [CC] [CC/MCC Exc]
Tuberculosis of pituitary gland
Tuberculosis of thymus gland

A18.83 **Tuberculosis of** digestive tract organs, **not elsewhere classified** [CC] [CC/MCC Exc]
[EXCLUDES1] *tuberculosis of intestine (A18.32)*

A18.84 **Tuberculosis of** heart [CC] [CC/MCC Exc]
Tuberculous cardiomyopathy
Tuberculous endocarditis
Tuberculous myocarditis
Tuberculous pericarditis

A18.85 **Tuberculosis of** spleen [CC] [CC/MCC Exc]

A18.89 **Tuberculosis of** other sites [CC] [CC/MCC Exc]
Tuberculosis of muscle
Tuberculous cerebral arteritis

[4th] A19 Miliary **tuberculosis**
[INCLUDES] *disseminated tuberculosis*
generalized tuberculosis
tuberculous polyserositis

A19.0 **Acute miliary tuberculosis of a** single specified site [MCC] [CC/MCC Exc]

A19.1 **Acute miliary tuberculosis of** multiple sites [MCC] [CC/MCC Exc]

A19.2 **Acute miliary tuberculosis, unspecified** [MCC] [CC/MCC Exc]

A19.8 Other **miliary tuberculosis** [MCC] [CC/MCC Exc]

A19.9 **Miliary tuberculosis, unspecified** [MCC] [CC/MCC Exc]

Unspecified Code | Other Specified Code | Manifestation Code | [N] Newborn | [P] Pediatric | [M] Maternity | [A] Adult | ♂ Male | ♀ Female
● New Code | ▲ Revised Code Title | ▶◀ Revised Text | [NOTES] | [INCLUDES] | [EXCLUDES1] Not coded here | [EXCLUDES2] Not included here
[4th] 4th character required | [5th] 5th character required | [6th] 6th character required | [7th] 7th character required | Extension 'X' Alert
[HAC] Hospital-acquired condition (HAC) alert | AHA AHA Coding Clinic© | Code first alert

When symbols appear on a code that requires a 7th character extension, refer to Appendix B to identify applicable 7th character codes.

Certain zoonotic bacterial diseases (A20-A28)

A20 Plague
INCLUDES *infection due to Yersinia pestis*
- A20.0 Bubonic **plague**   MCC CC/MCC Exc
- A20.1 Cellulocutaneous **plague**   MCC CC/MCC Exc
- A20.2 Pneumonic **plague**   HCC MCC CC/MCC Exc
- A20.3 **Plague** meningitis   MCC CC/MCC Exc
- A20.7 Septicemic **plague**   HCC MCC CC/MCC Exc
- A20.8 Other **forms of plague**   MCC CC/MCC Exc
  - Abortive plague
  - Asymptomatic plague
  - Pestis minor
- A20.9 **Plague,** unspecified   MCC CC/MCC Exc

A21 Tularemia
INCLUDES *deer-fly fever*
infection due to Francisella tularensis
rabbit fever
- A21.0 Ulceroglandular **tularemia**   CC CC/MCC Exc
- A21.1 Oculoglandular **tularemia**   CC CC/MCC Exc
  - Ophthalmic tularemia
- A21.2 Pulmonary **tularemia**   CC HCC CC/MCC Exc
- A21.3 Gastrointestinal **tularemia**   CC CC/MCC Exc
  - Abdominal tularemia
- A21.7 Generalized **tularemia**   CC CC/MCC Exc
- A21.8 Other **forms of tularemia**   CC CC/MCC Exc
- A21.9 **Tularemia,** unspecified   CC CC/MCC Exc

A22 Anthrax
INCLUDES *infection due to Bacillus anthracis*
- A22.0 Cutaneous **anthrax**   CC CC/MCC Exc
  - Malignant carbuncle
  - Malignant pustule
- A22.1 Pulmonary **anthrax**   HCC MCC CC/MCC Exc
  - Inhalation anthrax
  - Ragpicker's disease
  - Woolsorter's disease
- A22.2 Gastrointestinal **anthrax**   CC CC/MCC Exc
- A22.7 **Anthrax** sepsis   HCC MCC CC/MCC Exc
- A22.8 Other **forms of anthrax**   CC CC/MCC Exc
  - Anthrax meningitis
- A22.9 **Anthrax,** unspecified   CC CC/MCC Exc

A23 Brucellosis
INCLUDES *Malta fever*
Mediterranean fever
undulant fever
- A23.0 **Brucellosis due to Brucella** melitensis
- A23.1 **Brucellosis due to Brucella** abortus
- A23.2 **Brucellosis due to Brucella** suis
- A23.3 **Brucellosis due to Brucella** canis
- A23.8 Other **brucellosis**   CC CC/MCC Exc
- A23.9 **Brucellosis,** unspecified   CC CC/MCC Exc

A24 Glanders and melioidosis
- A24.0 **Glanders**   CC CC/MCC Exc
  - Infection due to Pseudomonas mallei
  - Malleus
- A24.1 Acute and fulminating **melioidosis**   CC CC/MCC Exc
  - Melioidosis pneumonia
  - Melioidosis sepsis
- A24.2 Subacute and chronic **melioidosis**   CC CC/MCC Exc
- A24.3 Other **melioidosis**   CC CC/MCC Exc
- A24.9 **Melioidosis,** unspecified   CC CC/MCC Exc
  - Infection due to Pseudomonas pseudomallei NOS
  - Whitmore's disease

A25 Rat-bite fevers
- A25.0 **Spirillosis**   CC CC/MCC Exc
  - Sodoku
- A25.1 **Streptobacillosis**   CC CC/MCC Exc
  - Epidemic arthritic erythema
  - Haverhill fever
  - Streptobacillary rat-bite fever

- A25.9 **Rat-bite fever,** unspecified   CC CC/MCC Exc

A26 Erysipeloid
- A26.0 Cutaneous **erysipeloid**
  - Erythema migrans
- A26.7 **Erysipelothrix** sepsis   HCC MCC CC/MCC Exc
- A26.8 Other **forms of erysipeloid**
- A26.9 **Erysipeloid,** unspecified

A27 Leptospirosis
- A27.0 **Leptospirosis** icterohemorrhagica   CC CC/MCC Exc
  - Leptospiral or spirochetal jaundice (hemorrhagic)
  - Weil's disease
- A27.8 Other **forms of leptospirosis**
  - A27.81 Aseptic meningitis **in leptospirosis**   MCC CC/MCC Exc
  - A27.89 Other **forms of leptospirosis**   CC CC/MCC Exc
- A27.9 **Leptospirosis,** unspecified   CC CC/MCC Exc

A28 Other zoonotic bacterial diseases, not elsewhere classified
- A28.0 **Pasteurellosis**   CC CC/MCC Exc
- A28.1 **Cat-scratch disease**   CC CC/MCC Exc
  - Cat-scratch fever
- A28.2 Extraintestinal **yersiniosis**   CC CC/MCC Exc
  - *EXCLUDES1* *enteritis due to Yersinia enterocolitica (A04.6)*
  - *plague (A20.-)*
- A28.8 **Other specified zoonotic bacterial diseases, not elsewhere classified**   CC CC/MCC Exc
- A28.9 **Zoonotic bacterial disease,** unspecified   CC CC/MCC Exc

Other bacterial diseases (A30-A49)

A30 Leprosy [Hansen's disease]
INCLUDES *infection due to Mycobacterium leprae*
EXCLUDES1 *sequelae of leprosy (B92)*
- A30.0 Indeterminate **leprosy**   CC CC/MCC Exc
  - **AHA:** Q3 2016
  - I leprosy
- A30.1 Tuberculoid **leprosy**   CC CC/MCC Exc
  - **AHA:** Q3 2016
  - TT leprosy
- A30.2 Borderline tuberculoid **leprosy**   CC CC/MCC Exc
  - **AHA:** Q3 2016
  - BT leprosy
- A30.3 Borderline **leprosy**   CC CC/MCC Exc
  - **AHA:** Q3 2016
  - BB leprosy
- A30.4 Borderline lepromatous **leprosy**   CC CC/MCC Exc
  - **AHA:** Q3 2016
  - BL leprosy
- A30.5 Lepromatous **leprosy**   CC CC/MCC Exc
  - **AHA:** Q3 2016
  - LL leprosy
- A30.8 Other **forms of leprosy**   CC CC/MCC Exc
  - **AHA:** Q3 2016
- A30.9 **Leprosy,** unspecified   CC CC/MCC Exc
  - **AHA:** Q3 2016

A31 Infection due to other mycobacteria
EXCLUDES2 *leprosy (A30.-)*
tuberculosis (A15-A19)
- A31.0 Pulmonary **mycobacterial infection**   CC HCC RxHCC CC/MCC Exc
  - **AHA:** Q3 2016
  - Infection due to Mycobacterium avium
  - Infection due to Mycobacterium intracellulare [Battey bacillus]
  - Infection due to Mycobacterium kansasii
- A31.1 Cutaneous **mycobacterial infection**   CC CC/MCC Exc
  - **AHA:** Q3 2016
  - Buruli ulcer
  - Infection due to Mycobacterium marinum
  - Infection due to Mycobacterium ulcerans
- A31.2 Disseminated **mycobacterium avium-intracellulare complex (DMAC)**   CC HCC RxHCC CC/MCC Exc
  - **AHA:** Q3 2016
  - MAC sepsis

PD*in* Unacceptable principal diagnosis symbol per Medicare code edits   *POA* Code exempt from diagnosis present on admission requirement
❓ Questionable admission   CC Complication or comorbidity   MCC Major complication or comorbidity   CC/MCC Exc CC/MCC exclusion
HCC HCC diagnosis code   RxHCC RxHCC diagnosis code   MACRA MACRA code   **DEFINITION** Describes condition/terminology
TIP Coding guidance   👁 Official Guideline Reference   Z1 Z code as first-listed diagnosis

A31.8 Other **mycobacterial infections** CC꜀ CC/MCC Exc
>>AHA: Q3 2016

A31.9 **Mycobacterial infection, unspecified** CC꜀ CC/MCC Exc
>>AHA: Q3 2016
>>Atypical mycobacterial infection NOS
>>Mycobacteriosis NOS

4ᵀᴴ **A32 Listeriosis**
>>INCLUDES listerial foodborne infection
>>EXCLUDES1 neonatal (disseminated) listeriosis (P37.2)

>A32.0 Cutaneous **listeriosis** CC꜀ CC/MCC Exc
>>AHA: Q3 2016

5ᵀᴴ A32.1 **Listerial meningitis and meningoencephalitis**
>>A32.11 **Listerial** meningitis CC꜀ CC/MCC Exc
>>>AHA: Q3 2016
>>A32.12 **Listerial** meningoencephalitis CC꜀ CC/MCC Exc
>>>AHA: Q3 2016

>A32.7 **Listerial** sepsis HCC MCC꜀ CC/MCC Exc
>>AHA: Q3 2016

5ᵀᴴ A32.8 Other **forms of listeriosis**
>>A32.81 Oculoglandular **listeriosis** CC꜀ CC/MCC Exc
>>>AHA: Q3 2016
>>A32.82 **Listerial** endocarditis CC꜀ CC/MCC Exc
>>>AHA: Q3 2016
>>A32.89 Other **forms of listeriosis** CC꜀ CC/MCC Exc
>>>AHA: Q3 2016
>>>Listerial cerebral arteritis

>A32.9 **Listeriosis, unspecified** CC꜀ CC/MCC Exc
>>AHA: Q3 2016

A33 **Tetanus neonatorum** N MCC꜀ CC/MCC Exc
>>AHA: Q3 2016

A34 **Obstetrical tetanus** M CC꜀ ♀ CC/MCC Exc
>>AHA: Q3 2016

A35 **Other tetanus** MCC꜀ CC/MCC Exc
>>AHA: Q3 2016
>>Tetanus NOS
>>EXCLUDES1 obstetrical tetanus (A34)
>>>>tetanus neonatorum (A33)

4ᵀᴴ **A36 Diphtheria**
>A36.0 Pharyngeal **diphtheria** CC꜀ CC/MCC Exc
>>AHA: Q3 2016
>>Diphtheritic membranous angina
>>Tonsillar diphtheria

>A36.1 Nasopharyngeal **diphtheria** CC꜀ CC/MCC Exc
>>AHA: Q3 2016

>A36.2 Laryngeal **diphtheria** CC꜀ CC/MCC Exc
>>AHA: Q3 2016
>>Diphtheritic laryngotracheitis

>A36.3 Cutaneous **diphtheria** CC꜀ CC/MCC Exc
>>AHA: Q3 2016
>>EXCLUDES2 erythrasma (L08.1)

5ᵀᴴ A36.8 Other **diphtheria**
>>A36.81 **Diphtheritic** cardiomyopathy CC꜀ HCC RxHCC CC/MCC Exc
>>>AHA: Q3 2016
>>>Diphtheritic myocarditis
>>A36.82 **Diphtheritic** radiculomyelitis CC꜀ CC/MCC Exc
>>>AHA: Q3 2016
>>A36.83 **Diphtheritic** polyneuritis CC꜀ CC/MCC Exc
>>>AHA: Q3 2016
>>A36.84 **Diphtheritic** tubulo-interstitial nephropathy CC꜀ CC/MCC Exc
>>>AHA: Q3 2016
>>A36.85 **Diphtheritic** cystitis CC꜀ CC/MCC Exc
>>>AHA: Q3 2016
>>A36.86 **Diphtheritic** conjunctivitis CC꜀ CC/MCC Exc
>>>AHA: Q3 2016
>>A36.89 Other **diphtheritic complications** CC꜀ CC/MCC Exc
>>>AHA: Q3 2016
>>>Diphtheritic peritonitis

>A36.9 **Diphtheria, unspecified** CC꜀ CC/MCC Exc
>>AHA: Q3 2016

4ᵀᴴ A37 Whooping **cough**

5ᵀᴴ A37.0 Whooping cough due to Bordetella pertussis
>>A37.00 Whooping cough due to Bordetella pertussis without pneumonia CC꜀ CC/MCC Exc
>>>AHA: Q3 2016
>>A37.01 Whooping cough due to Bordetella pertussis with pneumonia MCC꜀ CC/MCC Exc
>>>AHA: Q3 2016

5ᵀᴴ A37.1 Whooping cough due to Bordetella parapertussis
>>A37.10 Whooping cough due to Bordetella parapertussis without pneumonia CC꜀ CC/MCC Exc
>>>AHA: Q3 2016
>>A37.11 Whooping cough due to Bordetella parapertussis with pneumonia MCC꜀ CC/MCC Exc
>>>AHA: Q3 2016

5ᵀᴴ A37.8 Whooping cough due to other Bordetella species
>>A37.80 Whooping cough due to other Bordetella species without pneumonia CC꜀ CC/MCC Exc
>>>AHA: Q3 2016
>>A37.81 Whooping cough due to other Bordetella species with pneumonia MCC꜀ CC/MCC Exc
>>>AHA: Q3 2016

5ᵀᴴ A37.9 Whooping cough, unspecified species
>>A37.90 Whooping cough, unspecified species without pneumonia CC꜀ CC/MCC Exc
>>>AHA: Q3 2016
>>A37.91 Whooping cough, unspecified species with pneumonia MCC꜀ CC/MCC Exc
>>>AHA: Q3 2016

4ᵀᴴ **A38 Scarlet fever**
>>INCLUDES scarlatina
>>EXCLUDES2 streptococcal sore throat (J02.0)

>A38.0 **Scarlet fever** with otitis media CC꜀ CC/MCC Exc
>>AHA: Q3 2016

>A38.1 **Scarlet fever** with myocarditis CC꜀ CC/MCC Exc
>>AHA: Q3 2016

>A38.8 **Scarlet fever** with other complications CC꜀ CC/MCC Exc
>>AHA: Q3 2016

>A38.9 **Scarlet fever,** uncomplicated CC꜀ CC/MCC Exc
>>AHA: Q3 2016
>>Scarlet fever, NOS

4ᵀᴴ A39 Meningococcal **infection**
>A39.0 Meningococcal **meningitis** MCC꜀ CC/MCC Exc
>>AHA: Q3 2016

>A39.1 Waterhouse-Friderichsen **syndrome** HCC MCC꜀ RxHCC CC/MCC Exc
>>AHA: Q3 2016
>>Meningococcal hemorrhagic adrenalitis
>>Meningococcic adrenal syndrome

>A39.2 Acute **meningococcemia** HCC MCC꜀ CC/MCC Exc
>>AHA: Q3 2016

>A39.3 Chronic **meningococcemia** HCC MCC꜀ CC/MCC Exc
>>AHA: Q3 2016

>A39.4 **Meningococcemia, unspecified** HCC MCC꜀ CC/MCC Exc
>>AHA: Q3 2016

5ᵀᴴ A39.5 **Meningococcal** heart disease
>>A39.50 **Meningococcal carditis, unspecified** MCC꜀ CC/MCC Exc
>>>AHA: Q3 2016
>>A39.51 **Meningococcal** endocarditis MCC꜀ CC/MCC Exc
>>>AHA: Q3 2016
>>A39.52 **Meningococcal** myocarditis MCC꜀ CC/MCC Exc
>>>AHA: Q3 2016
>>A39.53 **Meningococcal** pericarditis MCC꜀ CC/MCC Exc
>>>AHA: Q3 2016

5ᵀᴴ A39.8 Other **meningococcal infections**
>>A39.81 **Meningococcal** encephalitis MCC꜀ CC/MCC Exc
>>>AHA: Q3 2016
>>A39.82 **Meningococcal** retrobulbar neuritis CC꜀ CC/MCC Exc
>>>AHA: Q3 2016
>>A39.83 **Meningococcal** arthritis CC꜀ HCC CC/MCC Exc
>>>AHA: Q3 2016
>>A39.84 Postmeningococcal **arthritis** CC꜀ HCC CC/MCC Exc
>>>AHA: Q3 2016

Unspecified Code   Other Specified Code   Manifestation Code   N Newborn   P Pediatric   M Maternity   A Adult   ♂ Male   ♀ Female
● New Code   ▲ Revised Code Title   ▶◀ Revised Text   NOTES   INCLUDES   EXCLUDES1 Not coded here   EXCLUDES2 Not included here
4ᵀᴴ 4ᵗʰ character required   5ᵀᴴ 5ᵗʰ character required   6ᵀᴴ 6ᵗʰ character required   7ᵀᴴ 7ᵗʰ character required   Extension 'X' Alert
HAC Hospital-acquired condition (HAC) alert   AHA AHA Coding Clinic©   ☞ Code first alert

A39.89 Other meningococcal infections   CC CC/MCC Exc
> **AHA:** Q3 2016
> Meningococcal conjunctivitis

A39.9 **Meningococcal infection, unspecified**   CC CC/MCC Exc
> **AHA:** Q3 2016
> Meningococcal disease NOS

A40 Streptococcal sepsis
> 👁 **See Official Guidelines** "Puerperal sepsis" I.C.15.k
> ☞ **Code first** postprocedural streptococcal sepsis (T81.4-)
> streptococcal sepsis during labor (O75.3)
> streptococcal sepsis following abortion or ectopic or molar pregnancy (O03-O07, O08.0)
> streptococcal sepsis following immunization (T88.0)
> streptococcal sepsis following infusion, transfusion or therapeutic injection (T80.2-)
> EXCLUDES1   neonatal (P36.0-P36.1)
> > puerperal sepsis (O85)
> > sepsis due to Streptococcus, group D (A41.81)

A40.0 **Sepsis due to streptococcus,** group A   HCC MCC CC/MCC Exc
> **AHA:** Q3 2016

A40.1 **Sepsis due to streptococcus,** group B   HCC MCC CC/MCC Exc
> **AHA:** Q1 2019, Q4 2018, Q3 2016

A40.3 **Sepsis due to Streptococcus** pneumoniae   HCC MCC
> **AHA:** Q3 2016
> Pneumococcal sepsis

A40.8 Other streptococcal sepsis   HCC MCC CC/MCC Exc
> **AHA:** Q3 2016

A40.9 **Streptococcal sepsis, unspecified**   HCC MCC CC/MCC Exc
> **AHA:** Q3 2016

A41 Other sepsis
> 👁 **See Official Guidelines** "Puerperal sepsis" I.C.15.k
> ☞ **Code first** postprocedural sepsis (T81.4-)
> sepsis during labor (O75.3)
> sepsis following abortion, ectopic or molar pregnancy (O03-O07, O08.0)
> sepsis following immunization (T88.0)
> sepsis following infusion, transfusion or therapeutic injection (T80.2-)
> EXCLUDES1   bacteremia NOS (R78.81)
> > neonatal (P36.-)
> > puerperal sepsis (O85)
> > streptococcal sepsis (A40.-)
> EXCLUDES2   sepsis (due to) (in) actinomycotic (A42.7)
> > sepsis (due to) (in) anthrax (A22.7)
> > sepsis (due to) (in) candidal (B37.7)
> > sepsis (due to) (in) Erysipelothrix (A26.7)
> > sepsis (due to) (in) extraintestinal yersiniosis (A28.2)
> > sepsis (due to) (in) gonococcal (A54.86)
> > sepsis (due to) (in) herpesviral (B00.7)
> > sepsis (due to) (in) listerial (A32.7)
> > sepsis (due to) (in) melioidosis (A24.1)
> > sepsis (due to) (in) meningococcal (A39.2-A39.4)
> > sepsis (due to) (in) plague (A20.7)
> > sepsis (due to) (in) tularemia (A21.7)
> > toxic shock syndrome (A48.3)

A41.0 **Sepsis** due to Staphylococcus aureus
> **A41.01** **Sepsis due to** Methicillin susceptible **Staphylococcus aureus**   HCC MCC CC/MCC Exc
> > **AHA:** Q3 2016
> > MSSA sepsis
> > Staphylococcus aureus sepsis NOS
> **A41.02** **Sepsis due to** Methicillin resistant **Staphylococcus aureus**   HCC MCC CC/MCC Exc
> > 👁 **See Official Guidelines** "Combination codes for MRSA infections" I.C.1.e.1.a
> > **AHA:** Q3 2016

A41.1 **Sepsis due to other specified staphylococcus**   HCC MCC CC/MCC Exc
> **AHA:** Q3 2016
> Coagulase negative staphylococcus sepsis

A41.2 **Sepsis due to unspecified staphylococcus**   HCC MCC CC/MCC Exc
> **AHA:** Q3 2016

A41.3 **Sepsis due to** Hemophilus influenzae   HCC MCC CC/MCC Exc
> **AHA:** Q3 2016

A41.4 **Sepsis due to** anaerobes   HCC MCC CC/MCC Exc
> **AHA:** Q3 2016
> EXCLUDES1   gas gangrene (A48.0)

A41.5 **Sepsis due to** other Gram-negative organisms
> **A41.50** **Gram-negative sepsis, unspecified**   HCC MCC CC/MCC Exc
> > **AHA:** Q3 2016
> > Gram-negative sepsis NOS
> **A41.51** **Sepsis due to** Escherichia coli [E. coli]   HCC MCC CC/MCC Exc
> > **AHA:** Q1 2018, Q3 2016
> **A41.52** **Sepsis due to** Pseudomonas   HCC MCC CC/MCC Exc
> > **AHA:** Q3 2016
> > Pseudomonas aeruginosa
> **A41.53** **Sepsis due to** Serratia   HCC MCC CC/MCC Exc
> > **AHA:** Q3 2016
> **A41.59** Other **Gram-negative sepsis**   HCC MCC CC/MCC Exc
> > **AHA:** Q1 2019, Q3 2016

A41.8 Other specified sepsis
> **A41.81** **Sepsis due to** Enterococcus   HCC MCC CC/MCC Exc
> > **AHA:** Q3 2016
> **A41.89** Other specified sepsis   HCC MCC CC/MCC Exc
> > **AHA:** Q3 2016

A41.9 **Sepsis, unspecified organism**   HCC MCC CC/MCC Exc
> 👁 **See Official Guidelines** "Sepsis" I.C.1.d.1.a, "Severe sepsis" I.C.1.d.1.b
> **AHA:** Q4 2018, Q3 2016
> Septicemia NOS

A42 Actinomycosis
> EXCLUDES1   actinomycetoma (B47.1)

A42.0 Pulmonary **actinomycosis**   CC HCC CC/MCC Exc
> **AHA:** Q3 2016

A42.1 Abdominal **actinomycosis**   CC CC/MCC Exc

A42.2 Cervicofacial **actinomycosis**   CC CC/MCC Exc
> **AHA:** Q3 2016

A42.7 **Actinomycotic** sepsis   HCC MCC CC/MCC Exc
> **AHA:** Q3 2016

A42.8 Other forms of actinomycosis
> **A42.81** **Actinomycotic** meningitis   CC CC/MCC Exc
> > **AHA:** Q3 2016
> **A42.82** **Actinomycotic** encephalitis   CC CC/MCC Exc
> > **AHA:** Q3 2016
> **A42.89** Other **forms of actinomycosis**   CC CC/MCC Exc
> > **AHA:** Q3 2016

A42.9 **Actinomycosis, unspecified**   CC CC/MCC Exc
> **AHA:** Q3 2016

A43 Nocardiosis
> **A43.0** Pulmonary **nocardiosis**   CC HCC CC/MCC Exc
> > **AHA:** Q3 2016
> **A43.1** Cutaneous **nocardiosis**   CC CC/MCC Exc
> > **AHA:** Q3 2016
> **A43.8** Other forms **of nocardiosis**   CC CC/MCC Exc
> > **AHA:** Q3 2016
> **A43.9** **Nocardiosis, unspecified**   CC CC/MCC Exc
> > **AHA:** Q3 2016

A44 Bartonellosis
> **A44.0** Systemic **bartonellosis**   CC CC/MCC Exc
> > **AHA:** Q3 2016
> > Oroya fever
> **A44.1** Cutaneous and mucocutaneous **bartonellosis**   CC CC/MCC Exc
> > **AHA:** Q3 2016
> > Verruga peruana
> **A44.8** Other **forms of bartonellosis**   CC CC/MCC Exc
> > **AHA:** Q3 2016
> **A44.9** **Bartonellosis, unspecified**   CC CC/MCC Exc
> > **AHA:** Q3 2016

A46 Erysipelas
> **AHA:** Q3 2016
> EXCLUDES1   postpartum or puerperal erysipelas (O86.89)

A48 Other bacterial diseases, **not elsewhere classified**
> EXCLUDES1   actinomycetoma (B47.1)

A48.0 **Gas gangrene** HCC MCC CC/MCC Exc
AHA: Q4 2017, Q3 2016
Clostridial cellulitis
Clostridial myonecrosis

A48.1 **Legionnaires' disease** HCC MCC CC/MCC Exc
AHA: Q3 2016

A48.2 **Nonpneumonic Legionnaires' disease [Pontiac fever]**
AHA: Q3 2016

A48.3 **Toxic shock syndrome** HCC MCC CC/MCC Exc
AHA: Q3 2016
Use additional code to identify the organism (B95, B96)
EXCLUDES1 *endotoxic shock NOS (R57.8)*
sepsis NOS (A41.9)

A48.4 **Brazilian purpuric fever**
AHA: Q3 2016
Systemic Hemophilus aegyptius infection

5ᵗʰ A48.5 **Other specified botulism**
Non-foodborne intoxication due to toxins of Clostridium botulinum [C. botulinum]
EXCLUDES1 *food poisoning due to toxins of Clostridium botulinum (A05.1)*

A48.51 **Infant botulism** P CC/MCC Exc
AHA: Q3 2016

A48.52 **Wound botulism** CC/MCC Exc
AHA: Q3 2016
Non-foodborne botulism NOS
Use additional code for associated wound

A48.8 **Other specified bacterial diseases**
AHA: Q3 2016

4ᵗʰ A49 Bacterial infection **of unspecified site**
EXCLUDES1 *bacterial agents as the cause of diseases classified elsewhere (B95-B96)*
chlamydial infection NOS (A74.9)
meningococcal infection NOS (A39.9)
rickettsial infection NOS (A79.9)
spirochetal infection NOS (A69.9)

5ᵗʰ A49.0 Staphylococcal infection, **unspecified site**
A49.01 Methicillin susceptible **Staphylococcus aureus infection, unspecified site**
AHA: Q3 2016
Methicillin susceptible Staphylococcus aureus (MSSA) infection
Staphylococcus aureus infection NOS
A49.02 Methicillin resistant **Staphylococcus aureus infection, unspecified site**
AHA: Q3 2016
Methicillin resistant Staphylococcus aureus (MRSA) infection

A49.1 Streptococcal **infection, unspecified site**
AHA: Q3 2016

A49.2 Hemophilus influenzae **infection, unspecified site**
AHA: Q3 2016

A49.3 Mycoplasma **infection, unspecified site**
AHA: Q3 2016

A49.8 Other bacterial **infections of unspecified site**
AHA: Q3 2016

A49.9 Bacterial infection, **unspecified**
AHA: Q3 2016
EXCLUDES1 *bacteremia NOS (R78.81)*

Infections with a predominantly sexual mode of transmission (A50-A64)

EXCLUDES1 *human immunodeficiency virus [HIV] disease (B20)*
nonspecific and nongonococcal urethritis (N34.1)
Reiter's disease (M02.3-)

4ᵗʰ A50 Congenital **syphilis**
5ᵗʰ A50.0 Early **congenital syphilis,** symptomatic
Any congenital syphilitic condition specified as early or manifest less than two years after birth.
A50.01 **Early congenital** syphilitic oculopathy CC/MCC Exc

A50.02 **Early congenital** syphilitic osteochondropathy CC CC/MCC Exc

A50.03 **Early congenital** syphilitic pharyngitis CC CC/MCC Exc
Early congenital syphilitic laryngitis

A50.04 **Early congenital** syphilitic pneumonia CC CC/MCC Exc

A50.05 **Early congenital** syphilitic rhinitis CC CC/MCC Exc

A50.06 **Early** cutaneous **congenital syphilis** CC CC/MCC Exc

A50.07 **Early** mucocutaneous **congenital syphilis** CC CC/MCC Exc

A50.08 **Early** visceral **congenital syphilis** CC CC/MCC Exc

A50.09 Other **early congenital syphilis, symptomatic** CC CC/MCC Exc

A50.1 Early **congenital syphilis,** latent
Congenital syphilis without clinical manifestations, with positive serological reaction and negative spinal fluid test, less than two years after birth.

A50.2 **Early congenital syphilis, unspecified** CC CC/MCC Exc
Congenital syphilis NOS less than two years after birth.

5ᵗʰ A50.3 Late **congenital syphilitic** oculopathy
EXCLUDES1 *Hutchinson's triad (A50.53)*
A50.30 **Late congenital syphilitic oculopathy, unspecified** CC CC/MCC Exc
A50.31 **Late congenital syphilitic interstitial keratitis** CC CC/MCC Exc
A50.32 **Late congenital** syphilitic chorioretinitis CC CC/MCC Exc
A50.39 Other **late congenital syphilitic oculopathy** CC CC/MCC Exc

5ᵗʰ A50.4 Late **congenital** neurosyphilis [**juvenile** neurosyphilis]
Use additional code to identify any associated mental disorder
EXCLUDES1 *Hutchinson's triad (A50.53)*
A50.40 **Late congenital neurosyphilis, unspecified** CC CC/MCC Exc
Juvenile neurosyphilis NOS
A50.41 **Late congenital syphilitic** meningitis MCC CC/MCC Exc
A50.42 **Late congenital syphilitic** encephalitis MCC CC/MCC Exc
A50.43 **Late congenital syphilitic** polyneuropathy CC CC/MCC Exc
A50.44 **Late congenital syphilitic** optic nerve atrophy CC CC/MCC Exc
A50.45 **Juvenile general paresis** CC CC/MCC Exc
Dementia paralytica juvenilis
Juvenile tabetoparetic neurosyphilis
A50.49 **Other late congenital neurosyphilis** CC CC/MCC Exc
Juvenile tabes dorsalis

5ᵗʰ A50.5 Other late **congenital syphilis,** symptomatic
Any congenital syphilitic condition specified as late or manifest two years or more after birth.
A50.51 Clutton's joints CC CC/MCC Exc
A50.52 Hutchinson's teeth CC CC/MCC Exc
A50.53 Hutchinson's triad CC CC/MCC Exc
A50.54 **Late congenital** cardiovascular syphilis CC CC/MCC Exc
A50.55 **Late congenital** syphilitic arthropathy CC HCC CC/MCC Exc
A50.56 **Late congenital syphilitic osteochondropathy** CC CC/MCC Exc
A50.57 **Syphilitic** saddle nose CC CC/MCC Exc
A50.59 Other **late congenital syphilis, symptomatic** CC CC/MCC Exc

A50.6 Late **congenital syphilis,** latent
Congenital syphilis without clinical manifestations, with positive serological reaction and negative spinal fluid test, two years or more after birth.

A50.7 **Late congenital syphilis, unspecified**
Congenital syphilis NOS two years or more after birth.

A50.9 **Congenital syphilis, unspecified**

4ᵗʰ A51 Early **syphilis**
A51.0 Primary genital **syphilis**
Syphilitic chancre NOS
A51.1 Primary anal **syphilis**
A51.2 **Primary syphilis of other sites**
5ᵗʰ A51.3 Secondary **syphilis of** skin and mucous membranes
A51.31 Condyloma latum CC CC/MCC Exc
A51.32 Syphilitic alopecia CC CC/MCC Exc
A51.39 Other secondary syphilis of skin CC CC/MCC Exc
Syphilitic leukoderma
Syphilitic mucous patch
EXCLUDES1 *late syphilitic leukoderma (A52.79)*

Unspecified Code Other Specified Code Manifestation Code N Newborn P Pediatric M Maternity A Adult ♂ Male ♀ Female
● New Code ▲ Revised Code Title ►◄ Revised Text **NOTES** *INCLUDES* EXCLUDES1 Not coded here EXCLUDES2 Not included here
4ᵗʰ 4ᵗʰ character required 5ᵗʰ 5ᵗʰ character required 6ᵗʰ 6ᵗʰ character required 7ᵗʰ 7ᵗʰ character required 7ᵗʰ Extension 'X' Alert
HAC Hospital-acquired condition (HAC) alert AHA AHA Coding Clinic© ☞ Code first alert

A51.4 Other secondary **syphilis** 5ᵗʰ

    A51.41 **Secondary syphilitic** meningitis MCC꜀ CC/MCC Exc⊘

    A51.42 **Secondary syphilitic female pelvic disease** cc꜀ ♀ CC/MCC Exc⊘

    A51.43 **Secondary syphilitic** oculopathy cc꜀ CC/MCC Exc⊘
        Secondary syphilitic chorioretinitis
        Secondary syphilitic iridocyclitis, iritis
        Secondary syphilitic uveitis

    A51.44 **Secondary syphilitic** nephritis cc꜀ CC/MCC Exc⊘

    A51.45 **Secondary syphilitic** hepatitis cc꜀ CC/MCC Exc⊘

    A51.46 **Secondary syphilitic** osteopathy cc꜀ CC/MCC Exc⊘

    A51.49 **Other secondary syphilitic conditions** cc꜀
        Secondary syphilitic lymphadenopathy
        Secondary syphilitic myositis

A51.5 Early **syphilis,** latent
    Syphilis (acquired) without clinical manifestations, with positive serological reaction and negative spinal fluid test, less than two years after infection.

A51.9 **Early syphilis, unspecified**

A52 Late **syphilis** 4ᵗʰ

  A52.0 Cardiovascular **and** cerebrovascular **syphilis** 5ᵗʰ

    A52.00 **Cardiovascular syphilis, unspecified** cc꜀ CC/MCC Exc⊘

    A52.01 **Syphilitic** aneurysm of aorta cc꜀ CC/MCC Exc⊘

    A52.02 **Syphilitic** aortitis cc꜀ CC/MCC Exc⊘

    A52.03 **Syphilitic** endocarditis cc꜀ CC/MCC Exc⊘
        Syphilitic aortic valve incompetence or stenosis
        Syphilitic mitral valve stenosis
        Syphilitic pulmonary valve regurgitation

    A52.04 **Syphilitic** cerebral arteritis cc꜀ RxHCC CC/MCC Exc⊘

    A52.05 **Other cerebrovascular syphilis** cc꜀ CC/MCC Exc⊘
        Syphilitic cerebral aneurysm (ruptured) (non-ruptured)
        Syphilitic cerebral thrombosis

    A52.06 Other **syphilitic** heart involvement cc꜀ CC/MCC Exc⊘
        Syphilitic coronary artery disease
        Syphilitic myocarditis
        Syphilitic pericarditis

    A52.09 Other cardiovascular **syphilis** cc꜀ CC/MCC Exc⊘

  A52.1 Symptomatic **neurosyphilis** 5ᵗʰ

    A52.10 **Symptomatic neurosyphilis, unspecified** cc꜀ CC/MCC Exc⊘

    A52.11 **Tabes dorsalis** cc꜀ CC/MCC Exc⊘
        Locomotor ataxia (progressive)
        Tabetic neurosyphilis

    A52.12 Other cerebrospinal **syphilis** cc꜀ CC/MCC Exc⊘

    A52.13 **Late syphilitic** meningitis MCC꜀ CC/MCC Exc⊘

    A52.14 **Late syphilitic** encephalitis MCC꜀ CC/MCC Exc⊘

    A52.15 **Late syphilitic** neuropathy cc꜀ CC/MCC Exc⊘
        Late syphilitic acoustic neuritis
        Late syphilitic optic (nerve) atrophy
        Late syphilitic polyneuropathy
        Late syphilitic retrobulbar neuritis

    A52.16 **Charcôt's arthropathy (tabetic)** cc꜀ CC/MCC Exc⊘

    A52.17 **General paresis** cc꜀ CC/MCC Exc⊘
        Dementia paralytica

    A52.19 Other symptomatic **neurosyphilis** cc꜀ CC/MCC Exc⊘
        Syphilitic parkinsonism

  A52.2 Asymptomatic **neurosyphilis** cc꜀ CC/MCC Exc⊘

  A52.3 **Neurosyphilis, unspecified** cc꜀ CC/MCC Exc⊘
    Gumma (syphilitic)
    Syphilis (late)
    Syphiloma

  A52.7 Other symptomatic **late syphilis** 5ᵗʰ

    A52.71 **Late syphilitic** oculopathy cc꜀ CC/MCC Exc⊘
        Late syphilitic chorioretinitis
        Late syphilitic episcleritis

    A52.72 **Syphilis of** lung and bronchus cc꜀ CC/MCC Exc⊘

    A52.73 **Symptomatic late syphilis of** other respiratory organs cc꜀ CC/MCC Exc⊘

    A52.74 **Syphilis of** liver **and** other viscera cc꜀ CC/MCC Exc⊘
        Late syphilitic peritonitis

    A52.75 **Syphilis of** kidney **and** ureter cc꜀ CC/MCC Exc⊘
        Syphilitic glomerular disease

    A52.76 Other genitourinary **symptomatic late syphilis** cc꜀ CC/MCC Exc⊘
        Late syphilitic female pelvic inflammatory disease

    A52.77 **Syphilis of** bone and joint cc꜀ CC/MCC Exc⊘

    A52.78 **Syphilis of** other musculoskeletal tissue cc꜀ CC/MCC Exc⊘
        Late syphilitic bursitis
        Syphilis [stage unspecified] of bursa
        Syphilis [stage unspecified] of muscle
        Syphilis [stage unspecified] of synovium
        Syphilis [stage unspecified] of tendon

    A52.79 Other symptomatic late **syphilis** cc꜀ CC/MCC Exc⊘
        Late syphilitic leukoderma
        Syphilis of adrenal gland
        Syphilis of pituitary gland
        Syphilis of thyroid gland
        Syphilitic splenomegaly
        EXCLUDES1 *syphilitic leukoderma (secondary) (A51.39)*

  A52.8 Late **syphilis,** latent
    Syphilis (acquired) without clinical manifestations, with positive serological reaction and negative spinal fluid test, two years or more after infection

  A52.9 **Late syphilis, unspecified**

A53 Other and unspecified syphilis 4ᵗʰ

  A53.0 **Latent syphilis, unspecified as early or late**
    Latent syphilis NOS
    Positive serological reaction for syphilis

  A53.9 **Syphilis, unspecified**
    Infection due to Treponema pallidum NOS
    Syphilis (acquired) NOS
    EXCLUDES1 *syphilis NOS under two years of age (A50.2)*

A54 Gonococcal **infection** 4ᵗʰ

  A54.0 **Gonococcal infection of** lower genitourinary tract without periurethral or accessory gland abscess 5ᵗʰ
    EXCLUDES1 *gonococcal infection with genitourinary gland abscess (A54.1)*
         gonococcal infection with periurethral abscess (A54.1)

    A54.00 **Gonococcal infection of** lower genitourinary tract, **unspecified** cc꜀ CC/MCC Exc⊘

    A54.01 **Gonococcal** cystitis **and** urethritis, **unspecified** cc꜀ CC/MCC Exc⊘

    A54.02 **Gonococcal** vulvovaginitis, **unspecified** cc꜀ ♀ CC/MCC Exc⊘

    A54.03 **Gonococcal** cervicitis, **unspecified** cc꜀ ♀ CC/MCC Exc⊘

    A54.09 Other **gonococcal infection of lower genitourinary tract** cc꜀ CC/MCC Exc⊘

  A54.1 **Gonococcal infection of** lower genitourinary tract with **periurethral and accessory gland abscess** cc꜀ CC/MCC Exc⊘
    Gonococcal Bartholin's gland abscess

  A54.2 **Gonococcal** pelviperitonitis **and** other gonococcal genitourinary **infection** 5ᵗʰ

    A54.21 **Gonococcal infection of** kidney **and** ureter cc꜀ CC/MCC Exc⊘

    A54.22 **Gonococcal** prostatitis cc꜀ ♂ CC/MCC Exc⊘

    A54.23 **Gonococcal infection of other male genital organs** cc꜀ ♂ CC/MCC Exc⊘
        Gonococcal epididymitis
        Gonococcal orchitis

    A54.24 **Gonococcal female pelvic inflammatory disease** cc꜀ ♀ CC/MCC Exc⊘
        Gonococcal pelviperitonitis
        EXCLUDES1 *gonococcal peritonitis (A54.85)*

    A54.29 Other **gonococcal genitourinary infections** cc꜀ CC/MCC Exc⊘

  A54.3 **Gonococcal infection of** eye 5ᵗʰ

    A54.30 **Gonococcal infection of eye, unspecified** cc꜀ CC/MCC Exc⊘

    A54.31 **Gonococcal** conjunctivitis cc꜀ CC/MCC Exc⊘
        Ophthalmia neonatorum due to gonococcus

    A54.32 **Gonococcal** iridocyclitis cc꜀ CC/MCC Exc⊘

    A54.33 **Gonococcal** keratitis cc꜀ CC/MCC Exc⊘

    A54.39 Other **gonococcal eye infection** cc꜀ CC/MCC Exc⊘
        Gonococcal endophthalmia

  A54.4 **Gonococcal infection of** musculoskeletal system 5ᵗʰ

    A54.40 **Gonococcal infection of musculoskeletal system, unspecified** cc꜀ HCC CC/MCC Exc⊘

PDxₐ Unacceptable principal diagnosis symbol per Medicare code edits PoA Code exempt from diagnosis present on admission requirement
⁇ Questionable admission cc꜀ Complication or comorbidity MCC꜀ Major complication or comorbidity CC/MCC Exc⊘ CC/MCC exclusion
HCC HCC diagnosis code RxHCC RxHCC diagnosis code MACRA code **DEFINITION** Describes condition/terminology
TIP Coding guidance 👁 Official Guideline Reference Z1 Z code as first-listed diagnosis

456 When symbols appear on a code that requires a 7th character extension, refer to Appendix B to identify applicable 7th character codes. **2020 ICD-10-CM**

A54.41 **Gonococcal** spondylopathy   ♂ HCC CC/MCC Exc

A54.42 **Gonococcal** arthritis   ♂ HCC CC/MCC Exc

EXCLUDES2 *gonococcal infection of spine (A54.41)*

A54.43 **Gonococcal** osteomyelitis   ♂ HCC CC/MCC Exc

EXCLUDES2 *gonococcal infection of spine (A54.41)*

A54.49 **Gonococcal infection of** other musculoskeletal tissue   ♂ HCC CC/MCC Exc
Gonococcal bursitis
Gonococcal myositis
Gonococcal synovitis
Gonococcal tenosynovitis

A54.5 **Gonococcal** pharyngitis

A54.6 **Gonococcal infection of** anus **and** rectum

A54.8 **Other gonococcal infections**

A54.81 **Gonococcal** meningitis   MCC CC/MCC Exc

A54.82 **Gonococcal** brain abscess   ♂ CC/MCC Exc

A54.83 **Gonococcal** heart infection   ♂ CC/MCC Exc
Gonococcal endocarditis
Gonococcal myocarditis
Gonococcal pericarditis

A54.84 **Gonococcal** pneumonia   ♂ HCC CC/MCC Exc

A54.85 **Gonococcal** peritonitis   ♂ HCC CC/MCC Exc

EXCLUDES1 *gonococcal pelviperitonitis (A54.24)*

A54.86 **Gonococcal sepsis**   HCC MCC CC/MCC Exc

A54.89 **Other gonococcal infections**   ♂ CC/MCC Exc
Gonococcal keratoderma
Gonococcal lymphadenitis

A54.9 **Gonococcal infection, unspecified**   ♂ CC/MCC Exc

A55 Chlamydial **lymphogranuloma (venereum)**
Climatic or tropical bubo
Durand-Nicolas-Favre disease
Esthiomene
Lymphogranuloma inguinale

A56 Other **sexually transmitted chlamydial diseases**

INCLUDES *sexually transmitted diseases due to Chlamydia trachomatis*

EXCLUDES1 *neonatal chlamydial conjunctivitis (P39.1)*
neonatal chlamydial pneumonia (P23.1)

EXCLUDES2 *chlamydial lymphogranuloma (A55)*
conditions classified to A74.-

A56.0 **Chlamydial infection of** lower genitourinary tract

A56.00 **Chlamydial infection of lower genitourinary tract, unspecified**

A56.01 **Chlamydial** cystitis **and** urethritis

A56.02 **Chlamydial** vulvovaginitis   ♀

A56.09 Other **chlamydial infection of lower genitourinary tract**
Chlamydial cervicitis

A56.1 **Chlamydial infection of** pelviperitoneum **and** other genitourinary organs

A56.11 **Chlamydial** female pelvic inflammatory disease   ♀

A56.19 Other **chlamydial genitourinary infection**
Chlamydial epididymitis
Chlamydial orchitis

A56.2 **Chlamydial infection of genitourinary tract, unspecified**

A56.3 **Chlamydial infection of** anus **and** rectum

A56.4 **Chlamydial infection of** pharynx

A56.8 **Sexually transmitted chlamydial infection of** other sites

A57 **Chancroid**
Ulcus molle

A58 **Granuloma inguinale**
Donovanosis

A59 **Trichomoniasis**

EXCLUDES2 *intestinal trichomoniasis (A07.8)*

A59.0 Urogenital **trichomoniasis**

A59.00 **Urogenital trichomoniasis, unspecified**
Fluor (vaginalis) due to Trichomonas
Leukorrhea (vaginalis) due to Trichomonas

A59.01 **Trichomonal** vulvovaginitis   ♀

A59.02 **Trichomonal** prostatitis   ♂

A59.03 **Trichomonal** cystitis **and** urethritis

A59.09 Other **urogenital trichomoniasis**
Trichomonas cervicitis

A59.8 **Trichomoniasis of** other sites

A59.9 **Trichomoniasis, unspecified**

A60 Anogenital herpesviral **[herpes simplex] infections**

A60.0 **Herpesviral infection of** genitalia **and** urogenital tract

A60.00 **Herpesviral infection of urogenital system, unspecified**

A60.01 **Herpesviral infection of** penis   ♂

A60.02 **Herpesviral infection of** other male genital organs   ♂

A60.03 **Herpesviral** cervicitis   ♀

A60.04 **Herpesviral** vulvovaginitis   ♀
Herpesviral [herpes simplex] ulceration
Herpesviral [herpes simplex] vaginitis
Herpesviral [herpes simplex] vulvitis

A60.09 **Herpesviral infection of** other urogenital tract

A60.1 **Herpesviral infection of** perianal skin **and** rectum

A60.9 **Anogenital herpesviral infection, unspecified**

A63 Other **predominantly** sexually transmitted diseases, **not elsewhere classified**

EXCLUDES2 *molluscum contagiosum (B08.1)*
papilloma of cervix (D26.0)

A63.0 **Anogenital (venereal) warts**
Anogenital warts due to (human) papillomavirus [HPV]
Condyloma acuminatum

A63.8 **Other specified predominantly sexually transmitted diseases**

A64 **Unspecified sexually transmitted disease**

Other spirochetal diseases (A65-A69)

EXCLUDES2 *leptospirosis (A27.-)*
syphilis (A50-A53)

A65 **Nonvenereal syphilis**
Bejel
Endemic syphilis
Njovera

A66 **Yaws**

INCLUDES *bouba*
frambesia (tropica)
pian

A66.0 Initial lesions **of yaws**
Chancre of yaws
Frambesia, initial or primary
Initial frambesial ulcer
Mother yaw

A66.1 **Multiple** papillomata **and** wet crab **yaws**
Frambesioma
Pianoma
Plantar or palmar papilloma of yaws

A66.2 Other **early** skin lesions **of yaws**
Cutaneous yaws, less than five years after infection
Early yaws (cutaneous)(macular)(maculopapular) (micropapular)(papular)
Frambeside of early yaws

A66.3 Hyperkeratosis **of yaws**
Ghoul hand
Hyperkeratosis, palmar or plantar (early) (late) due to yaws
Worm-eaten soles

A66.4 Gummata and ulcers **of yaws**
Gummatous frambeside
Nodular late yaws (ulcerated)

A66.5 **Gangosa**
Rhinopharyngitis mutilans

A66.6 Bone **and** joint lesions **of yaws**   HCC
Yaws ganglion
Yaws goundou
Yaws gumma, bone
Yaws gummatous osteitis or periostitis
Yaws hydrarthrosis
Yaws osteitis
Yaws periostitis (hypertrophic)

Unspecified Code   Other Specified Code   Manifestation Code   N Newborn   P Pediatric   M Maternity   A Adult   ♂ Male   ♀ Female
● New Code   ▲ Revised Code Title   ▶◀ Revised Text   NOTES   INCLUDES   EXCLUDES1 Not coded here   EXCLUDES2 Not included here
4th character required   5th character required   6th character required   7th character required   Extension 'X' Alert
HAC Hospital-acquired condition (HAC) alert   AHA AHA Coding Clinic©   ☛ Code first alert

2020 ICD-10-CM   When symbols appear on a code that requires a 7th character extension, refer to Appendix B to identify applicable 7th character codes.   **457**

A66.7 **Other manifestations of yaws**
    Juxta-articular nodules of yaws
    Mucosal yaws

A66.8 **Latent yaws**
    Yaws without clinical manifestations, with positive serology

A66.9 **Yaws, unspecified**

A67 **Pinta [carate]**

A67.0 **Primary lesions of pinta**
    Chancre (primary) of pinta
    Papule (primary) of pinta

A67.1 **Intermediate lesions of pinta**
    Erythematous plaques of pinta
    Hyperchromic lesions of pinta
    Hyperkeratosis of pinta
    Pintids

A67.2 **Late lesions of pinta**
    Achromic skin lesions of pinta
    Cicatricial skin lesions of pinta
    Dyschromic skin lesions of pinta

A67.3 **Mixed lesions of pinta**
    Achromic with hyperchromic skin lesions of pinta [carate]

A67.9 **Pinta, unspecified**

A68 **Relapsing fevers**
    INCLUDES   recurrent fever
    EXCLUDES2 Lyme disease (A69.2-)

A68.0 **Louse-borne relapsing fever**   CC CC/MCC Exc
    Relapsing fever due to Borrelia recurrentis

A68.1 **Tick-borne relapsing fever**   CC CC/MCC Exc
    Relapsing fever due to any Borrelia species other than
    Borrelia recurrentis

A68.9 **Relapsing fever, unspecified**   CC CC/MCC Exc

A69 **Other spirochetal infections**

A69.0 **Necrotizing ulcerative stomatitis**
    Cancrum oris
    Fusospirochetal gangrene
    Noma
    Stomatitis gangrenosa

A69.1 **Other Vincent's infections**   CC CC/MCC Exc
    Fusospirochetal pharyngitis
    Necrotizing ulcerative (acute) gingivitis
    Necrotizing ulcerative (acute) gingivostomatitis
    Spirochetal stomatitis
    Trench mouth
    Vincent's angina
    Vincent's gingivitis

A69.2 **Lyme disease**
    Erythema chronicum migrans due to Borrelia burgdorferi

A69.20 **Lyme disease, unspecified**

A69.21 **Meningitis due to Lyme disease**   CC CC/MCC Exc

A69.22 **Other neurologic disorders in Lyme disease**   CC CC/MCC Exc
    Cranial neuritis
    Meningoencephalitis
    Polyneuropathy

A69.23 **Arthritis due to Lyme disease**   CC HCC CC/MCC Exc

A69.29 **Other conditions associated with Lyme disease**   CC CC/MCC Exc
    AHA: Q3 2016
    Myopericarditis due to Lyme disease

A69.8 **Other specified spirochetal infections**

A69.9 **Spirochetal infection, unspecified**

Other diseases caused by chlamydiae (A70-A74)

    EXCLUDES1 sexually transmitted chlamydial diseases (A55-A56)

A70 **Chlamydia psittaci infections**   CC CC/MCC Exc
    Ornithosis
    Parrot fever
    Psittacosis

A71 **Trachoma**
    EXCLUDES1 sequelae of trachoma (B94.0)

A71.0 **Initial stage of trachoma**
    Trachoma dubium

A71.1 **Active stage of trachoma**
    Granular conjunctivitis (trachomatous)
    Trachomatous follicular conjunctivitis
    Trachomatous pannus

A71.9 **Trachoma, unspecified**

A74 **Other diseases caused by chlamydiae**
    EXCLUDES1 neonatal chlamydial conjunctivitis (P39.1)
                 neonatal chlamydial pneumonia (P23.1)
                  Reiter's disease (M02.3-)
                  sexually transmitted chlamydial diseases (A55-A56)
    EXCLUDES2 chlamydial pneumonia (J16.0)

A74.0 **Chlamydial conjunctivitis**
    Paratrachoma

A74.8 **Other chlamydial diseases**

A74.81 **Chlamydial peritonitis**

A74.89 **Other chlamydial diseases**

A74.9 **Chlamydial infection, unspecified**
    Chlamydiosis NOS

Rickettsioses (A75-A79)

A75 **Typhus fever**
    EXCLUDES1 rickettsiosis due to Ehrlichia sennetsu (A79.81)

A75.0 **Epidemic louse-borne typhus fever due to Rickettsia prowazekii**   CC CC/MCC Exc
    Classical typhus (fever)
    Epidemic (louse-borne) typhus

A75.1 **Recrudescent typhus [Brill's disease]**   CC CC/MCC Exc
    Brill-Zinsser disease

A75.2 **Typhus fever due to Rickettsia typhi**   CC CC/MCC Exc
    Murine (flea-borne) typhus

A75.3 **Typhus fever due to Rickettsia tsutsugamushi**   CC CC/MCC Exc
    Scrub (mite-borne) typhus
    Tsutsugamushi fever

A75.9 **Typhus fever, unspecified**   CC CC/MCC Exc
    Typhus (fever) NOS

A77 **Spotted fever [tick-borne rickettsioses]**

A77.0 **Spotted fever due to Rickettsia rickettsii**   CC CC/MCC Exc
    Rocky Mountain spotted fever
    Sao Paulo fever

A77.1 **Spotted fever due to Rickettsia conorii**   CC CC/MCC Exc
    African tick typhus
    Boutonneuse fever
    India tick typhus
    Kenya tick typhus
    Marseilles fever
    Mediterranean tick fever

A77.2 **Spotted fever due to Rickettsia sibirica**   CC CC/MCC Exc
    North Asian tick fever
    Siberian tick typhus

A77.3 **Spotted fever due to Rickettsia australis**   CC CC/MCC Exc
    Queensland tick typhus

A77.4 **Ehrlichiosis**
    EXCLUDES1 Rickettsiosis due to Ehrlichia sennetsu (A79.81)

A77.40 **Ehrlichiosis, unspecified**   CC CC/MCC Exc

A77.41 **Ehrlichiosis chafeensis [E. chafeensis]**   CC CC/MCC Exc

A77.49 **Other ehrlichiosis**   CC CC/MCC Exc

A77.8 **Other spotted fevers**   CC CC/MCC Exc

A77.9 **Spotted fever, unspecified**   CC CC/MCC Exc
    Tick-borne typhus NOS

A78 **Q fever**   CC CC/MCC Exc
    Infection due to Coxiella burnetii
    Nine Mile fever
    Quadrilateral fever

A79 **Other rickettsioses**

A79.0 **Trench fever**   CC CC/MCC Exc
    Quintan fever
    Wolhynian fever

A79.1 **Rickettsialpox due to Rickettsia akari**   CC CC/MCC Exc
    Kew Garden fever
    Vesicular rickettsiosis

PDx Unacceptable principal diagnosis symbol per Medicare code edits   PDx Code exempt from diagnosis present on admission requirement
? Questionable admission   CC Complication or comorbidity   MCC Major complication or comorbidity   CC/MCC Exc CC/MCC exclusion
HCC HCC diagnosis code   RxHCC RxHCC diagnosis code   MACRA MACRA code   DEFINITION Describes condition/terminology
TIP Coding guidance   👁 Official Guideline Reference   Z1 Z code as first-listed diagnosis

458   When symbols appear on a code that requires a 7th character extension, refer to Appendix B to identify applicable 7th character codes.   **2020 ICD-10-CM**

A79.8 Other **specified rickettsioses**
- **A79.81** **Rickettsiosis due to** Ehrlichia sennetsu   cc CC/MCC Exc
- **A79.89** Other specified rickettsioses   cc CC/MCC Exc

A79.9 **Rickettsiosis, unspecified**   cc CC/MCC Exc
  Rickettsial infection NOS

Viral and prion infections of the central nervous system (A80-A89)

EXCLUDES1 postpolio syndrome (G14)
  sequelae of poliomyelitis (B91)
  sequelae of viral encephalitis (B94.1)

A80 **Acute** poliomyelitis
- **A80.0** **Acute paralytic poliomyelitis,** vaccine-associated   MCC CC/MCC Exc
- **A80.1** **Acute paralytic poliomyelitis,** wild virus, imported   MCC CC/MCC Exc
- **A80.2** **Acute paralytic poliomyelitis,** wild virus, indigenous   MCC CC/MCC Exc
- **A80.3** **Acute paralytic poliomyelitis,** other and unspecified
  - **A80.30** **Acute paralytic poliomyelitis, unspecified**   MCC CC/MCC Exc
  - **A80.39** Other **acute paralytic poliomyelitis**   MCC CC/MCC Exc
- **A80.4** **Acute** nonparalytic **poliomyelitis**
- **A80.9** **Acute poliomyelitis, unspecified**

A81 **Atypical virus infections of central nervous system**
  INCLUDES diseases of the central nervous system caused by prions
  Use additional code to identify:
  dementia with behavioral disturbance (F02.81)
  dementia without behavioral disturbance (F02.80)
- **A81.0** **Creutzfeldt-Jakob disease**
  - **A81.00** **Creutzfeldt-Jakob disease, unspecified**   cc HCC RxHCC CC/MCC Exc
    Jakob-Creutzfeldt disease, unspecified
  - **A81.01** Variant **Creutzfeldt-Jakob disease**   cc HCC RxHCC CC/MCC Exc
    vCJD
  - **A81.09** Other **Creutzfeldt-Jakob disease**   cc HCC RxHCC CC/MCC Exc
    CJD
    Familial Creutzfeldt-Jakob disease
    Iatrogenic Creutzfeldt-Jakob disease
    Sporadic Creutzfeldt-Jakob disease
    Subacute spongiform encephalopathy (with dementia)
- **A81.1** **Subacute sclerosing panencephalitis**   cc HCC RxHCC CC/MCC Exc
    Dawson's inclusion body encephalitis
    Van Bogaert's sclerosing leukoencephalopathy
- **A81.2** **Progressive multifocal leukoencephalopathy**   cc HCC RxHCC CC/MCC Exc
    Multifocal leukoencephalopathy NOS
- **A81.8** **Other atypical virus infections of central nervous system**
  - **A81.81** **Kuru**   cc HCC RxHCC CC/MCC Exc
  - **A81.82** **Gerstmann-Sträussler-Scheinker syndrome**   cc HCC RxHCC CC/MCC Exc
    GSS syndrome
  - **A81.83** **Fatal familial insomnia**   cc HCC RxHCC CC/MCC Exc
    FFI
  - **A81.89** **Other atypical virus infections of central nervous system**   cc HCC RxHCC CC/MCC Exc
- **A81.9** **Atypical virus infection of central nervous system, unspecified**   cc HCC RxHCC CC/MCC Exc
    Prion diseases of the central nervous system NOS

A82 **Rabies**
- **A82.0** Sylvatic **rabies**   cc CC/MCC Exc
- **A82.1** Urban **rabies**   cc CC/MCC Exc
- **A82.9** **Rabies, unspecified**   cc CC/MCC Exc

A83 **Mosquito-borne viral encephalitis**
  INCLUDES mosquito-borne viral meningoencephalitis
  EXCLUDES2 Venezuelan equine encephalitis (A92.2)
    West Nile fever (A92.3-)
    West Nile virus (A92.3-)
- **A83.0** Japanese **encephalitis**   MCC CC/MCC Exc
- **A83.1** Western equine **encephalitis**   MCC CC/MCC Exc
- **A83.2** Eastern equine **encephalitis**   MCC CC/MCC Exc
- **A83.3** St Louis **encephalitis**   MCC CC/MCC Exc
- **A83.4** Australian **encephalitis**   MCC CC/MCC Exc
    Kunjin virus disease

- **A83.5** California **encephalitis**   MCC CC/MCC Exc
    California meningoencephalitis
    La Crosse encephalitis
- **A83.6** **Rocio virus disease**   MCC CC/MCC Exc
- **A83.8** Other **mosquito-borne viral encephalitis**   MCC CC/MCC Exc
- **A83.9** **Mosquito-borne viral encephalitis, unspecified**   MCC CC/MCC Exc

A84 **Tick-borne viral encephalitis**
  INCLUDES tick-borne viral meningoencephalitis
- **A84.0** Far Eastern **tick-borne encephalitis [Russian spring-summer encephalitis]**   MCC CC/MCC Exc
- **A84.1** Central European **tick-borne encephalitis**   MCC CC/MCC Exc
- **A84.8** Other **tick-borne viral encephalitis**   MCC CC/MCC Exc
    Louping ill
    Powassan virus disease
- **A84.9** **Tick-borne viral encephalitis, unspecified**   MCC CC/MCC Exc

A85 **Other viral encephalitis, not elsewhere classified**
  INCLUDES specified viral encephalomyelitis NEC
    specified viral meningoencephalitis NEC
  EXCLUDES1 benign myalgic encephalomyelitis (G93.3)
    encephalitis due to cytomegalovirus (B25.8)
    encephalitis due to herpesvirus NEC (B10.0-)
    encephalitis due to herpesvirus [herpes simplex] (B00.4)
    encephalitis due to measles virus (B05.0)
    encephalitis due to mumps virus (B26.2)
    encephalitis due to poliomyelitis virus (A80.-)
    encephalitis due to zoster (B02.0)
    lymphocytic choriomeningitis (A87.2)
- **A85.0** Enteroviral **encephalitis**   cc CC/MCC Exc
    Enteroviral encephalomyelitis
- **A85.1** Adenoviral **encephalitis**   cc CC/MCC Exc
    Adenoviral meningoencephalitis
- **A85.2** **Arthropod-borne viral encephalitis, unspecified**   MCC CC/MCC Exc
    EXCLUDES1 West nile virus with encephalitis (A92.31)
- **A85.8** **Other specified viral encephalitis**   cc CC/MCC Exc
    Encephalitis lethargica
    Von Economo-Cruchet disease

A86 **Unspecified viral encephalitis**   cc CC/MCC Exc
    Viral encephalomyelitis NOS
    Viral meningoencephalitis NOS

A87 Viral **meningitis**
    EXCLUDES1 meningitis due to herpesvirus [herpes simplex] (B00.3)
      meningitis due to herpesvirus [herpes simplex] (B00.3)
      meningitis due to measles virus (B05.1)
      meningitis due to mumps virus (B26.1)
      meningitis due to poliomyelitis virus (A80.-)
      meningitis due to zoster (B02.1)
- **A87.0** Enteroviral **meningitis**   cc CC/MCC Exc
    Coxsackievirus meningitis
    Echovirus meningitis
- **A87.1** Adenoviral **meningitis**   cc CC/MCC Exc
- **A87.2** **Lymphocytic choriomeningitis**   cc CC/MCC Exc
    Lymphocytic meningoencephalitis
- **A87.8** Other **viral meningitis**   cc CC/MCC Exc
- **A87.9** **Viral meningitis, unspecified**   cc CC/MCC Exc

A88 **Other viral infections of central nervous system, not elsewhere classified**
    EXCLUDES1 viral encephalitis NOS (A86)
      viral meningitis NOS (A87.9)
- **A88.0** **Enteroviral exanthematous fever [Boston exanthem]**   cc CC/MCC Exc
- **A88.1** **Epidemic vertigo**
- **A88.8** **Other specified viral infections of central nervous system**   cc CC/MCC Exc

A89 **Unspecified viral infection of central nervous system**   cc CC/MCC Exc

Arthropod-borne viral fevers and viral hemorrhagic fevers (A90-A99)

A90 **Dengue fever [classical dengue]**   cc CC/MCC Exc
  AHA: Q3 2016
  EXCLUDES1 dengue hemorrhagic fever (A91)

Unspecified Code   Other Specified Code   Manifestation Code   N Newborn   P Pediatric   M Maternity   A Adult   ♂ Male   ♀ Female
● New Code   ▲ Revised Code Title   ▶◀ Revised Text   NOTES   INCLUDES   EXCLUDES1 Not coded here   EXCLUDES2 Not included here
4ᵗʰ 4ᵗʰ character required   5ᵗʰ 5ᵗʰ character required   6ᵗʰ 6ᵗʰ character required   7ᵗʰ 7ᵗʰ character required   Extension 'X' Alert
HAC Hospital-acquired condition (HAC) alert   AHA AHA Coding Clinic©   ☞ Code first alert

A91 Dengue hemorrhagic fever   CC CC/MCC Exc

4ᵗʰ A92 Other mosquito-borne viral fevers
     EXCLUDES1 *Ross River disease (B33.1)*
     A92.0 Chikungunya virus disease   CC CC/MCC Exc
         Chikungunya (hemorrhagic) fever
     A92.1 O'nyong-nyong fever   CC CC/MCC Exc
     A92.2 Venezuelan equine fever   CC CC/MCC Exc
         Venezuelan equine encephalitis
         Venezuelan equine encephalomyelitis virus disease
    5ᵗʰ A92.3 West Nile virus infection
         West Nile fever
       A92.30 West Nile virus infection, unspecified   MCC CC/MCC Exc
           West Nile fever NOS
           West Nile fever without complications
           West Nile virus NOS
       A92.31 West Nile virus infection with encephalitis   MCC CC/MCC Exc
           AHA: Q3 2016
           West Nile encephalitis
           West Nile encephalomyelitis
       A92.32 West Nile virus infection with other neurologic manifestation   MCC CC/MCC Exc
           Use additional code to specify the neurologic manifestation
       A92.39 West Nile virus infection with other complications   MCC CC/MCC Exc
           Use additional code to specify the other conditions
     A92.4 Rift Valley fever   CC CC/MCC Exc
     A92.5 Zika virus disease   CC CC/MCC Exc
         👁 See Official Guidelines "Zika virus infections" I.C.1.f.1
         AHA: Q4 2018, Q4 2016
         Zika virus fever
         Zika virus infection
         Zika NOS
         EXCLUDES1 *congenital Zika virus disease (P35.4)*
     A92.8 Other specified mosquito-borne viral fevers   CC CC/MCC Exc
     A92.9 Mosquito-borne viral fever, unspecified   CC CC/MCC Exc

4ᵗʰ A93 Other arthropod-borne viral fevers, not elsewhere classified
     A93.0 Oropouche virus disease   CC CC/MCC Exc
         Oropouche fever
     A93.1 Sandfly fever   CC CC/MCC Exc
         Pappataci fever
         Phlebotomus fever
     A93.2 Colorado tick fever   CC CC/MCC Exc
     A93.8 Other specified arthropod-borne viral fevers   CC CC/MCC Exc
         Piry virus disease
         Vesicular stomatitis virus disease [Indiana fever]

A94 Unspecified arthropod-borne viral fever   CC CC/MCC Exc
     Arboviral fever NOS
     Arbovirus infection NOS

4ᵗʰ A95 Yellow fever
     A95.0 Sylvatic yellow fever   CC CC/MCC Exc
         Jungle yellow fever
     A95.1 Urban yellow fever   CC CC/MCC Exc
     A95.9 Yellow fever, unspecified   CC CC/MCC Exc

4ᵗʰ A96 Arenaviral hemorrhagic fever
     A96.0 Junin hemorrhagic fever   CC CC/MCC Exc
         Argentinian hemorrhagic fever
     A96.1 Machupo hemorrhagic fever   CC CC/MCC Exc
         Bolivian hemorrhagic fever
     A96.2 Lassa fever
     A96.8 Other arenaviral hemorrhagic fevers   CC CC/MCC Exc
     A96.9 Arenaviral hemorrhagic fever, unspecified   CC CC/MCC Exc

4ᵗʰ A98 Other viral hemorrhagic fevers, not elsewhere classified
     EXCLUDES1 *chikungunya hemorrhagic fever (A92.0)*
                 dengue hemorrhagic fever (A91)
     A98.0 Crimean-Congo hemorrhagic fever   CC CC/MCC Exc
         Central Asian hemorrhagic fever
     A98.1 Omsk hemorrhagic fever   CC CC/MCC Exc
     A98.2 Kyasanur Forest disease
     A98.3 Marburg virus disease
     A98.4 Ebola virus disease

A98.5 Hemorrhagic fever with renal syndrome   CC CC/MCC Exc
     Epidemic hemorrhagic fever
     Korean hemorrhagic fever
     Russian hemorrhagic fever
     Hantaan virus disease
     Hantavirus disease with renal manifestations
     Nephropathia epidemica
     Songo fever
     EXCLUDES1 *hantavirus (cardio)-pulmonary syndrome (B33.4)*
A98.8 Other specified viral hemorrhagic fevers   CC CC/MCC Exc
A99 Unspecified viral hemorrhagic fever   CC CC/MCC Exc

Viral infections characterized by skin and mucous membrane lesions (B00-B09)

4ᵗʰ B00 Herpesviral [herpes simplex] infections
     EXCLUDES1 *congenital herpesviral infections (P35.2)*
     EXCLUDES2 *anogenital herpesviral infection (A60.-)*
                 gammaherpesviral mononucleosis (B27.0-)
                 herpangina (B08.5)
     B00.0 Eczema herpeticum
         Kaposi's varicelliform eruption
     B00.1 Herpesviral vesicular dermatitis (Figure 1.2)
         Herpes simplex facialis
         Herpes simplex labialis
         Herpes simplex otitis externa
         Vesicular dermatitis of ear
         Vesicular dermatitis of lip

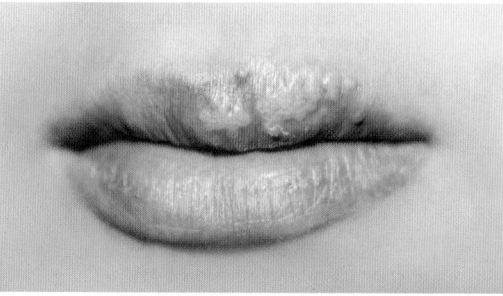

Figure 1.2 Oral Herpes

     B00.2 Herpesviral gingivostomatitis and pharyngotonsillitis   CC CC/MCC Exc
         Herpesviral pharyngitis
     B00.3 Herpesviral meningitis   MCC CC/MCC Exc
     B00.4 Herpesviral encephalitis   MCC CC/MCC Exc
         Herpesviral meningoencephalitis
         Simian B disease
         EXCLUDES1 *herpesviral encephalitis due to herpesvirus 6 and 7 (B10.01, B10.09)*
                 non-simplex herpesviral encephalitis (B10.0-)
    5ᵗʰ B00.5 Herpesviral ocular disease
       B00.50 Herpesviral ocular disease, unspecified   CC CC/MCC Exc
       B00.51 Herpesviral iridocyclitis   CC CC/MCC Exc
           Herpesviral iritis
           Herpesviral uveitis, anterior
       B00.52 Herpesviral keratitis   CC CC/MCC Exc
           Herpesviral keratoconjunctivitis
       B00.53 Herpesviral conjunctivitis   CC CC/MCC Exc
       B00.59 Other herpesviral disease of eye   CC CC/MCC Exc
           Herpesviral dermatitis of eyelid
     B00.7 Disseminated herpesviral disease   HCC MCC CC/MCC Exc
         Herpesviral sepsis
    5ᵗʰ B00.8 Other forms of herpesviral infections
       B00.81 Herpesviral hepatitis   CC CC/MCC Exc
       B00.82 Herpes simplex myelitis   HCC MCC RxHCC CC/MCC Exc
       B00.89 Other herpesviral infection   CC CC/MCC Exc
           Herpesviral whitlow
     B00.9 Herpesviral infection, unspecified
         Herpes simplex infection NOS

PDxᴺ Unacceptable principal diagnosis symbol per Medicare code edits   🔒 Code exempt from diagnosis present on admission requirement
   ❓ Questionable admission   CC Complication or comorbidity   MCC Major complication or comorbidity   CC/MCC Exc CC/MCC exclusion
   HCC HCC diagnosis code   RxHCC RxHCC diagnosis code   MACRA code   **DEFINITION** Describes condition/terminology
   TIP Coding guidance   👁 Official Guideline Reference   Z1 Z code as first-listed diagnosis

B01 Varicella [chickenpox]
  B01.0 Varicella meningitis   cc CC/MCC Exc
  B01.1 Varicella encephalitis, myelitis and encephalomyelitis
    Postchickenpox encephalitis, myelitis and encephalomyelitis
    B01.11 Varicella encephalitis and encephalomyelitis   MCC CC/MCC Exc
      Postchickenpox encephalitis and encephalomyelitis
    B01.12 Varicella myelitis   HCC MCC RxHCC CC/MCC Exc
      Postchickenpox myelitis
  B01.2 Varicella pneumonia   MCC CC/MCC Exc
  B01.8 Varicella with other complications
    B01.81 Varicella keratitis   cc CC/MCC Exc
    B01.89 Other varicella complications   cc CC/MCC Exc
  B01.9 Varicella without complication   cc CC/MCC Exc
    Varicella NOS
B02 Zoster [herpes zoster]
  INCLUDES shingles
    zona
  B02.0 Zoster encephalitis   cc CC/MCC Exc
    Zoster meningoencephalitis
  B02.1 Zoster meningitis   MCC CC/MCC Exc
    AHA: Q1 2019
  B02.2 Zoster with other nervous system involvement
    B02.21 Postherpetic geniculate ganglionitis   cc RxHCC CC/MCC Exc
    B02.22 Postherpetic trigeminal neuralgia   cc RxHCC CC/MCC Exc
    B02.23 Postherpetic polyneuropathy   cc RxHCC CC/MCC Exc
    B02.24 Postherpetic myelitis   HCC MCC RxHCC CC/MCC Exc
      Herpes zoster myelitis
    B02.29 Other postherpetic nervous system involvement   cc RxHCC CC/MCC Exc
      Postherpetic radiculopathy
  B02.3 Zoster ocular disease
    B02.30 Zoster ocular disease, unspecified   cc CC/MCC Exc
    B02.31 Zoster conjunctivitis   cc CC/MCC Exc
    B02.32 Zoster iridocyclitis   cc CC/MCC Exc
    B02.33 Zoster keratitis   cc CC/MCC Exc
      Herpes zoster keratoconjunctivitis
    B02.34 Zoster scleritis   cc CC/MCC Exc
    B02.39 Other herpes zoster eye disease   cc CC/MCC Exc
      Zoster blepharitis
  B02.7 Disseminated zoster   cc CC/MCC Exc
  B02.8 Zoster with other complications   cc CC/MCC Exc
    Herpes zoster otitis externa
  B02.9 Zoster without complications
    Zoster NOS
B03 Smallpox   cc CC/MCC Exc
  NOTES In 1980 the 33rd World Health Assembly declared that smallpox had been eradicated. The classification is maintained for surveillance purposes.
B04 Monkeypox   cc CC/MCC Exc
B05 Measles
  INCLUDES morbilli
  EXCLUDES1 subacute sclerosing panencephalitis (A81.1)
  B05.0 Measles complicated by encephalitis   MCC CC/MCC Exc
    Postmeasles encephalitis
  B05.1 Measles complicated by meningitis   cc CC/MCC Exc
    Postmeasles meningitis
  B05.2 Measles complicated by pneumonia   MCC CC/MCC Exc
    Postmeasles pneumonia
  B05.3 Measles complicated by otitis media
    Postmeasles otitis media
  B05.4 Measles with intestinal complications   cc CC/MCC Exc
  B05.8 Measles with other complications
    B05.81 Measles keratitis and keratoconjunctivitis   cc CC/MCC Exc
    B05.89 Other measles complications   cc CC/MCC Exc
  B05.9 Measles without complication
    Measles NOS
B06 Rubella [German measles]
  EXCLUDES1 congenital rubella (P35.0)

B06.0 Rubella with neurological complications
  B06.00 Rubella with neurological complication, unspecified   cc CC/MCC Exc
  B06.01 Rubella encephalitis   MCC CC/MCC Exc
    Rubella meningoencephalitis
  B06.02 Rubella meningitis   cc CC/MCC Exc
  B06.09 Other neurological complications of rubella   cc CC/MCC Exc
B06.8 Rubella with other complications
  B06.81 Rubella pneumonia   cc CC/MCC Exc
  B06.82 Rubella arthritis   cc HCC CC/MCC Exc
  B06.89 Other rubella complications   cc CC/MCC Exc
B06.9 Rubella without complication
  Rubella NOS
B07 Viral warts
  INCLUDES verruca simplex
    verruca vulgaris
    viral warts due to human papillomavirus
  EXCLUDES2 anogenital (venereal) warts (A63.0)
    papilloma of bladder (D41.4)
    papilloma of cervix (D26.0)
    papilloma larynx (D14.1)
  B07.0 Plantar wart
    Verruca plantaris
  B07.8 Other viral warts
    Common wart
    Flat wart
    Verruca plana
  B07.9 Viral wart, unspecified
B08 Other viral infections characterized by skin and mucous membrane lesions, not elsewhere classified
  EXCLUDES1 vesicular stomatitis virus disease (A93.8)
  B08.0 Other orthopoxvirus infections
    EXCLUDES2 monkeypox (B04)
    B08.01 Cowpox and vaccinia not from vaccine
      B08.010 Cowpox
      B08.011 Vaccinia not from vaccine
        EXCLUDES1 vaccinia (from vaccination) (generalized) (T88.1)
    B08.02 Orf virus disease
      Contagious pustular dermatitis
      Ecthyma contagiosum
    B08.03 Pseudocowpox [milker's node]
    B08.04 Paravaccinia, unspecified
    B08.09 Other orthopoxvirus infections
      Orthopoxvirus infection NOS
  B08.1 Molluscum contagiosum
  B08.2 Exanthema subitum [sixth disease]
    Roseola infantum
    B08.20 Exanthema subitum [sixth disease], unspecified   P
      Roseola infantum, unspecified
    B08.21 Exanthema subitum [sixth disease] due to human herpesvirus 6   P
      Roseola infantum due to human herpesvirus 6
    B08.22 Exanthema subitum [sixth disease] due to human herpesvirus 7   P
      Roseola infantum due to human herpesvirus 7
  B08.3 Erythema infectiosum [fifth disease]   cc CC/MCC Exc
  B08.4 Enteroviral vesicular stomatitis with exanthem
    Hand, foot and mouth disease
  B08.5 Enteroviral vesicular pharyngitis
    Herpangina
  B08.6 Parapoxvirus infections
    B08.60 Parapoxvirus infection, unspecified
    B08.61 Bovine stomatitis
    B08.62 Sealpox
    B08.69 Other parapoxvirus infections
  B08.7 Yatapoxvirus infections
    B08.70 Yatapoxvirus infection, unspecified
    B08.71 Tanapox virus disease   cc CC/MCC Exc

Unspecified Code   Other Specified Code   Manifestation Code   N Newborn   P Pediatric   M Maternity   A Adult   ♂ Male   ♀ Female
● New Code   ▲ Revised Code Title   ►◄ Revised Text   NOTES   INCLUDES   EXCLUDES1 Not coded here   EXCLUDES2 Not included here
4th character required   5th character required   6th character required   7th character required   Extension 'X' Alert
HAC Hospital-acquired condition (HAC) alert   AHA AHA Coding Clinic©   📕 Code first alert

B08.72 **Yaba pox virus disease**
Yaba monkey tumor disease

B08.79 Other **yatapoxvirus infections**

B08.8 **Other specified viral infections characterized by skin and mucous membrane lesions**
Enteroviral lymphonodular pharyngitis
Foot-and-mouth disease
Poxvirus NEC

B09 **Unspecified viral infection characterized by skin and mucous membrane lesions**
Viral enanthema NOS
Viral exanthema NOS

Other human herpesviruses (B10)

B10 **Other human herpesviruses**
EXCLUDES2 *cytomegalovirus (B25.9)*
Epstein-Barr virus (B27.0-)
herpes NOS (B00.9)
herpes simplex (B00.-)
herpes zoster (B02.-)
human herpesvirus NOS (B00.-)
human herpesvirus 1 and 2 (B00.-)
human herpesvirus 3 (B01.-, B02.-)
human herpesvirus 4 (B27.0-)
human herpesvirus 5 (B25.-)
varicella (B01.-)
zoster (B02.-)

B10.0 **Other human herpesvirus** encephalitis
EXCLUDES2 *herpes encephalitis NOS (B00.4)*
herpes simplex encephalitis (B00.4)
human herpesvirus encephalitis (B00.4)
simian B herpes virus encephalitis (B00.4)

B10.01 **Human** herpesvirus 6 **encephalitis** MCC CC/MCC Exc

B10.09 Other **human herpesvirus encephalitis** MCC CC/MCC Exc
Human herpesvirus 7 encephalitis

B10.8 **Other human herpesvirus** infection

B10.81 **Human** herpesvirus 6 **infection**

B10.82 **Human** herpesvirus 7 **infection**

B10.89 Other **human herpesvirus infection**
Human herpesvirus 8 infection
Kaposi's sarcoma-associated herpesvirus infection

Viral hepatitis (B15-B19)

EXCLUDES1 *sequelae of viral hepatitis (B94.2)*
EXCLUDES2 *cytomegaloviral hepatitis (B25.1)*
herpesviral [herpes simplex] hepatitis (B00.81)

B15 **Acute** hepatitis A

B15.0 **Hepatitis A** with hepatic coma MCC CC/MCC Exc

B15.9 **Hepatitis A** without hepatic coma CC CC/MCC Exc
Hepatitis A (acute)(viral) NOS

B16 **Acute** hepatitis B **(Figure 1.3)**

B16.0 **Acute hepatitis B** with delta-agent with hepatic coma MCC CC/MCC Exc

B16.1 **Acute hepatitis B** with delta-agent without hepatic coma CC CC/MCC Exc

B16.2 **Acute hepatitis B** without delta-agent with hepatic coma MCC CC/MCC Exc

B16.9 **Acute hepatitis B** without delta-agent and without hepatic coma CC CC/MCC Exc
AHA: Q3 2016
Hepatitis B (acute) (viral) NOS

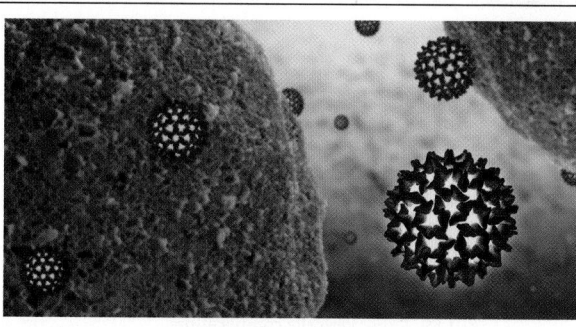

Figure 1.3 Hepatitis B Virus

B17 **Other acute viral hepatitis**

B17.0 Acute delta -(super) infection of hepatitis B carrier CC CC/MCC Exc

B17.1 **Acute** hepatitis C

B17.10 **Acute hepatitis C** without hepatic coma CC CC/MCC Exc
Acute hepatitis C NOS

B17.11 **Acute hepatitis C** with hepatic coma MCC CC/MCC Exc

B17.2 **Acute** hepatitis E CC CC/MCC Exc

B17.8 **Other specified acute viral hepatitis** CC CC/MCC Exc
Hepatitis non-A non-B (acute) (viral) NEC

B17.9 **Acute viral hepatitis, unspecified** CC CC/MCC Exc
Acute hepatitis NOS
Acute infectious hepatitis NOS

B18 Chronic viral hepatitis
INCLUDES *Carrier of viral hepatitis*

B18.0 **Chronic viral** hepatitis B with delta-agent CC HCC RxHCC CC/MCC Exc

B18.1 **Chronic** viral hepatitis B without delta-agent CC HCC RxHCC CC/MCC Exc
Carrier of viral hepatitis B
Chronic (viral) hepatitis B

B18.2 **Chronic viral** hepatitis C HCC RxHCC
AHA: Q1 2018, Q1 2017
Carrier of viral hepatitis C

B18.8 Other **chronic viral hepatitis** CC HCC RxHCC CC/MCC Exc
Carrier of other viral hepatitis

B18.9 **Chronic viral hepatitis, unspecified** CC HCC RxHCC CC/MCC Exc
Carrier of unspecified viral hepatitis

B19 **Unspecified viral hepatitis**

B19.0 **Unspecified viral hepatitis with hepatic coma** MCC CC/MCC Exc

B19.1 **Unspecified viral** hepatitis B

B19.10 **Unspecified viral hepatitis B without hepatic coma** CC CC/MCC Exc
Unspecified viral hepatitis B NOS

B19.11 **Unspecified viral hepatitis B with hepatic coma** MCC CC/MCC Exc

B19.2 **Unspecified viral** hepatitis C

B19.20 **Unspecified viral hepatitis C without hepatic coma**
Viral hepatitis C NOS

B19.21 **Unspecified viral hepatitis C with hepatic coma** MCC CC/MCC Exc

B19.9 **Unspecified viral hepatitis without hepatic coma** CC CC/MCC Exc
Viral hepatitis NOS

Human immunodeficiency virus [HIV] disease (B20)

B20 **Human immunodeficiency virus [HIV] disease** CC HCC RxHCC CC/MCC Exc
See Official Guidelines "Patient admitted for HIV-related condition" I.C.1.a.2.a, "Patient with HIV disease admitted for unrelated condition" I.C.1.a.2.b, "Asymptomatic human immunodeficiency virus" I.C.1.a.2.d, "Previously diagnosed HIV-related illness" I.C.1.a.2.f, "HIV Infection in Pregnancy, Childbirth and the Puerperium" I.C.1.a.2.g

TIP: (1) If the patient is treated for an HIV-related condition, code first B20 followed by the condition being treated. (2) If the patient is treated for a non-HIV-related condition, such as an injury, code first the unrelated condition, followed by B20.

AHA: Q1 2019

INCLUDES *acquired immune deficiency syndrome [AIDS]*
AIDS-related complex [ARC]
HIV infection, symptomatic

PDxⁿ Unacceptable principal diagnosis symbol per Medicare code edits   POA Code exempt from diagnosis present on admission requirement
❓ Questionable admission   CC Complication or comorbidity   MCC Major complication or comorbidity   CC/MCC Exc CC/MCC exclusion
HCC HCC diagnosis code   RxHCC RxHCC diagnosis code   MACRA code   **DEFINITION** Describes condition/terminology
TIP Coding guidance   👁 Official Guideline Reference   Z1 Z code as first-listed diagnosis

☞ **Code first** Human immunodeficiency virus [HIV] disease complicating pregnancy, childbirth and the puerperium, if applicable (O98.7-)
Use additional code(s) to identify all manifestations of HIV infection
EXCLUDES1 asymptomatic human immunodeficiency virus [HIV] infection status (Z21)
exposure to HIV virus (Z20.6)
inconclusive serologic evidence of HIV (R75)

Other viral diseases (B25-B34)

4ᵗʰ **B25 Cytomegaloviral disease**
EXCLUDES1 congenital cytomegalovirus infection (P35.1)
cytomegaloviral mononucleosis (B27.1-)
B25.0 **Cytomegaloviral** pneumonitis HCC MCC RxHCC CC/MCC Exc
B25.1 **Cytomegaloviral** hepatitis CC HCC RxHCC
B25.2 **Cytomegaloviral** pancreatitis HCC MCC RxHCC CC/MCC Exc
B25.8 Other **cytomegaloviral diseases** CC HCC RxHCC CC/MCC Exc
Cytomegaloviral encephalitis
B25.9 **Cytomegaloviral disease, unspecified** CC HCC RxHCC CC/MCC Exc

4ᵗʰ **B26 Mumps**
DEFINITION: Mumps is a highly contagious viral disease that causes swelling and pain in the salivary glands.
INCLUDES epidemic parotitis
infectious parotitis
B26.0 **Mumps** orchitis CC ♂ CC/MCC Exc
B26.1 **Mumps** meningitis MCC CC/MCC Exc
B26.2 **Mumps** encephalitis MCC CC/MCC Exc
B26.3 **Mumps** pancreatitis CC CC/MCC Exc
5ᵗʰ B26.8 **Mumps with other complications**
B26.81 **Mumps** hepatitis CC CC/MCC Exc
B26.82 **Mumps** myocarditis CC CC/MCC Exc
B26.83 **Mumps** nephritis CC CC/MCC Exc
B26.84 **Mumps** polyneuropathy CC CC/MCC Exc
B26.85 **Mumps** arthritis CC HCC CC/MCC Exc
B26.89 **Other mumps complications** CC CC/MCC Exc
B26.9 **Mumps** without complication
Mumps NOS
Mumps parotitis NOS

4ᵗʰ **B27 Infectious** mononucleosis
INCLUDES glandular fever
monocytic angina
Pfeiffer's disease
5ᵗʰ B27.0 Gammaherpesviral **mononucleosis (Figure 1.4)**
Mononucleosis due to Epstein-Barr virus
B27.00 **Gammaherpesviral mononucleosis** without complication
B27.01 **Gammaherpesviral mononucleosis** with polyneuropathy
B27.02 **Gammaherpesviral mononucleosis** with meningitis
B27.09 **Gammaherpesviral mononucleosis with other complications**
Hepatomegaly in gammaherpesviral mononucleosis

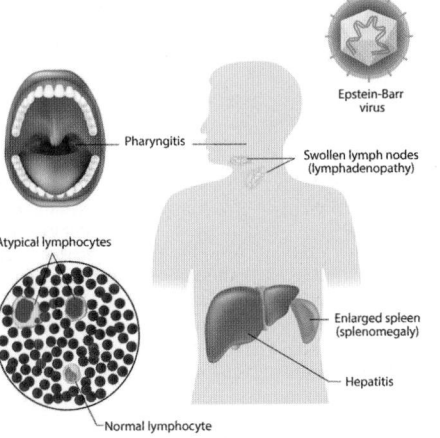

Figure 1.4 Symptoms of Mononucleosis Due to Epstein-Barr Virus

5ᵗʰ B27.1 Cytomegaloviral **mononucleosis**
B27.10 **Cytomegaloviral mononucleosis** without complications
B27.11 **Cytomegaloviral mononucleosis** with polyneuropathy
B27.12 **Cytomegaloviral mononucleosis** with meningitis
B27.19 **Cytomegaloviral mononucleosis with other complication**
Hepatomegaly in cytomegaloviral mononucleosis
5ᵗʰ B27.8 Other **infectious mononucleosis**
B27.80 **Other infectious mononucleosis** without complication
B27.81 **Other infectious mononucleosis** with polyneuropathy
B27.82 **Other infectious mononucleosis** with meningitis
B27.89 **Other infectious mononucleosis with other complication**
Hepatomegaly in other infectious mononucleosis
5ᵗʰ B27.9 **Infectious mononucleosis,** unspecified
B27.90 **Infectious mononucleosis, unspecified** without complication
B27.91 **Infectious mononucleosis, unspecified** with polyneuropathy
B27.92 **Infectious mononucleosis, unspecified** with meningitis
B27.99 **Infectious mononucleosis, unspecified** with other complication
Hepatomegaly in unspecified infectious mononucleosis

4ᵗʰ **B30 Viral conjunctivitis**
EXCLUDES1 herpesviral [herpes simplex] ocular disease (B00.5)
ocular zoster (B02.3)
B30.0 Keratoconjunctivitis **due to adenovirus**
Epidemic keratoconjunctivitis
Shipyard eye
B30.1 Conjunctivitis **due to adenovirus**
Acute adenoviral follicular conjunctivitis
Swimming-pool conjunctivitis
B30.2 **Viral** pharyngoconjunctivitis
B30.3 **Acute epidemic** hemorrhagic conjunctivitis **(enteroviral)**
Conjunctivitis due to coxsackievirus 24
Conjunctivitis due to enterovirus 70
Hemorrhagic conjunctivitis (acute)(epidemic)
B30.8 Other **viral conjunctivitis**
Newcastle conjunctivitis
B30.9 **Viral conjunctivitis, unspecified**

4ᵗʰ **B33 Other viral diseases, not elsewhere classified**
B33.0 **Epidemic myalgia**
Bornholm disease
B33.1 **Ross River disease** CC CC/MCC Exc
Epidemic polyarthritis and exanthema
Ross River fever
5ᵗʰ B33.2 **Viral carditis**
Coxsackie (virus) carditis
B33.20 **Viral carditis, unspecified** CC CC/MCC Exc
B33.21 **Viral** endocarditis CC CC/MCC Exc
B33.22 **Viral** myocarditis CC CC/MCC Exc
B33.23 **Viral** pericarditis CC CC/MCC Exc
B33.24 **Viral** cardiomyopathy HCC RxHCC
B33.3 **Retrovirus infections, not elsewhere classified**
Retrovirus infection NOS
B33.4 **Hantavirus (cardio)-pulmonary syndrome [HPS] [HCPS]** CC CC/MCC Exc
Hantavirus disease with pulmonary manifestations
Sin nombre virus disease
Use additional code to identify any associated acute kidney failure (N17.9)
EXCLUDES1 hantavirus disease with renal manifestations (A98.5)
hemorrhagic fever with renal manifestations (A98.5)

Unspecified Code   Other Specified Code   Manifestation Code   N Newborn   P Pediatric   M Maternity   A Adult   ♂ Male   ♀ Female
● New Code   ▲ Revised Code Title   ►◄ Revised Text   NOTES   INCLUDES   EXCLUDES1 Not coded here   EXCLUDES2 Not included here
4ᵗʰ 4ᵗʰ character required   5ᵗʰ 5ᵗʰ character required   6ᵗʰ 6ᵗʰ character required   7ᵗʰ 7ᵗʰ character required   7ᵗʰ Extension 'X' Alert
HAC Hospital-acquired condition (HAC) alert   AHA AHA Coding Clinic©   ☞ Code first alert

2020 ICD-10-CM   When symbols appear on a code that requires a 7th character extension, refer to Appendix B to identify applicable 7th character codes.   **463**

B33.8 **Other specified viral diseases**
      EXCLUDES1 *anogenital human papillomavirus infection (A63.0)*
                viral warts due to human papillomavirus infection (B07)

🔵 B34 **Viral infection of** unspecified site
      EXCLUDES1 *anogenital human papillomavirus infection (A63.0)*
                cytomegaloviral disease NOS (B25.9)
                herpesvirus [herpes simplex] infection NOS (B00.9)
                retrovirus infection NOS (B33.3)
                viral agents as the cause of diseases classified elsewhere (B97.-)
                viral warts due to human papillomavirus infection (B07)

      B34.0 Adenovirus **infection, unspecified**
      B34.1 Enterovirus **infection, unspecified**
            Coxsackievirus infection NOS
            Echovirus infection NOS
      B34.2 Coronavirus **infection, unspecified**
            EXCLUDES1 *pneumonia due to SARS-associated coronavirus (J12.81)*
      B34.3 Parvovirus **infection, unspecified**   cc⊘ CC/MCC Exc
      B34.4 Papovavirus **infection, unspecified**
      B34.8 Other viral **infections of unspecified site**
      B34.9 Viral **infection, unspecified**
            AHA: Q3 2016
            Viremia NOS

Mycoses (B35-B49)

      EXCLUDES2 *hypersensitivity pneumonitis due to organic dust (J67.-)*
                mycosis fungoides (C84.0-)

🔵 B35 **Dermatophytosis**
      INCLUDES *favus*
               infections due to species of Epidermophyton, Micro-sporum and Trichophyton
               tinea, any type except those in B36.-

      B35.0 **Tinea** barbae **and tinea** capitis
            Beard ringworm
            Kerion
            Scalp ringworm
            Sycosis, mycotic
      B35.1 **Tinea** unguium
            Dermatophytic onychia
            Dermatophytosis of nail
            Onychomycosis
            Ringworm of nails
      B35.2 **Tinea** manuum
            Dermatophytosis of hand
            Hand ringworm
      B35.3 **Tinea** pedis
            Athlete's foot
            Dermatophytosis of foot
            Foot ringworm
      B35.4 **Tinea** corporis
            Ringworm of the body
      B35.5 **Tinea** imbricata
            Tokelau
      B35.6 **Tinea** cruris
            Dhobi itch
            Groin ringworm
            Jock itch
      B35.8 Other **dermatophytoses**
            Disseminated dermatophytosis
            Granulomatous dermatophytosis
      B35.9 **Dermatophytosis, unspecified**
            Ringworm NOS
🔵 B36 **Other superficial mycoses**
      B36.0 **Pityriasis versicolor**
            Tinea flava
            Tinea versicolor
      B36.1 **Tinea nigra**
            Keratomycosis nigricans palmaris
            Microsporosis nigra
            Pityriasis nigra

      B36.2 **White piedra**
            Tinea blanca
      B36.3 **Black piedra**
      B36.8 **Other specified superficial mycoses**
      B36.9 **Superficial mycosis, unspecified**
🔵 B37 **Candidiasis**
      INCLUDES *candidosis*
               moniliasis
      EXCLUDES1 *neonatal candidiasis (P37.5)*
      B37.0 **Candidal** stomatitis   cc⊘ CC/MCC Exc
            Oral thrush
      B37.1 Pulmonary **candidiasis**   HCC MCC⊘ RxHCC CC/MCC Exc
            Candidal bronchitis
            Candidal pneumonia
      B37.2 **Candidiasis of** skin **and** nail
            Candidal onychia
            Candidal paronychia
            EXCLUDES2 *diaper dermatitis (L22)*
      B37.3 **Candidiasis of** vulva **and** vagina   ♀
            Candidal vulvovaginitis
            Monilial vulvovaginitis
            Vaginal thrush
   5️⃣ B37.4 **Candidiasis of** other urogenital sites
            B37.41 **Candidal** cystitis **and** urethritis   cc⊘ HAC CC/MCC Exc
            B37.42 **Candidal** balanitis   ♂
            B37.49 **Other urogenital candidiasis**   cc⊘ HAC CC/MCC Exc
                   Candidal pyelonephritis
      B37.5 **Candidal** meningitis   MCC⊘ CC/MCC Exc
      B37.6 **Candidal** endocarditis   MCC⊘ CC/MCC Exc
      B37.7 **Candidal** sepsis   HCC MCC⊘ RxHCC CC/MCC Exc
            Disseminated candidiasis
            Systemic candidiasis
   5️⃣ B37.8 **Candidiasis of** other sites
            B37.81 **Candidal** esophagitis   HCC MCC⊘ RxHCC CC/MCC Exc
            B37.82 **Candidal** enteritis   MCC⊘ CC/MCC Exc
                   Candidal proctitis
            B37.83 **Candidal** cheilitis   cc⊘ CC/MCC Exc
            B37.84 **Candidal** otitis externa   cc⊘ CC/MCC Exc
            B37.89 Other **sites of candidiasis**   cc⊘ CC/MCC Exc
                   Candidal osteomyelitis
      B37.9 **Candidiasis, unspecified**
            Thrush NOS
🔵 B38 **Coccidioidomycosis**
      B38.0 Acute pulmonary **coccidioidomycosis**   cc⊘ HCC CC/MCC Exc
      B38.1 Chronic pulmonary **coccidioidomycosis**   cc⊘ HCC CC/MCC Exc
      B38.2 Pulmonary **coccidioidomycosis, unspecified** cc⊘ HCC CC/MCC Exc
      B38.3 Cutaneous **coccidioidomycosis**   cc⊘ CC/MCC Exc
      B38.4 Coccidioidomycosis **meningitis**   MCC⊘ CC/MCC Exc
      B38.7 Disseminated **coccidioidomycosis**   cc⊘ CC/MCC Exc
            Generalized coccidioidomycosis
   5️⃣ B38.8 Other forms **of coccidioidomycosis**
            B38.81 Prostatic **coccidioidomycosis**   cc⊘ ♂ CC/MCC Exc
            B38.89 Other forms **of coccidioidomycosis**   cc⊘ CC/MCC Exc
      B38.9 **Coccidioidomycosis, unspecified**   cc⊘ CC/MCC Exc
🔵 B39 **Histoplasmosis**
      📖 **Code first** associated AIDS (B20)
      Use additional code for any associated manifestations, such as:
            endocarditis (I39)
            meningitis (G02)
            pericarditis (I32)
            retinitis (H32)
      B39.0 Acute pulmonary **histoplasmosis capsulati**   HCC MCC⊘ CC/MCC Exc
      B39.1 Chronic pulmonary **histoplasmosis capsulati** HCC MCC⊘ CC/MCC Exc
      B39.2 Pulmonary **histoplasmosis capsulati, unspecified** HCC MCC⊘ CC/MCC Exc
      B39.3 Disseminated **histoplasmosis capsulati**   cc⊘ CC/MCC Exc
            Generalized histoplasmosis capsulati
      B39.4 **Histoplasmosis capsulati, unspecified**
            American histoplasmosis
      B39.5 **Histoplasmosis** duboisii
            African histoplasmosis
      B39.9 **Histoplasmosis, unspecified**

PDx🔒 Unacceptable principal diagnosis symbol per Medicare code edits   🔒 Code exempt from diagnosis present on admission requirement
❓ Questionable admission   cc⊘ Complication or comorbidity   MCC⊘ Major complication or comorbidity   CC/MCC Exc CC/MCC exclusion
HCC HCC diagnosis code   RxHCC RxHCC diagnosis code   MACRA MACRA code   **DEFINITION** Describes condition/terminology
TIP Coding guidance   👁 Official Guideline Reference   📋 Z code as first-listed diagnosis

464   When symbols appear on a code that requires a 7th character extension, refer to Appendix B to identify applicable 7th character codes.   **2020 ICD-10-CM**

4ᵗʰ **B40 Blastomycosis**

> EXCLUDES1 Brazilian blastomycosis (B41.-)
>
> keloidal blastomycosis (B48.0)

B40.0 Acute pulmonary **blastomycosis** cc⊘ HCC CC/MCC Exc

B40.1 Chronic pulmonary **blastomycosis** cc⊘ HCC CC/MCC Exc

B40.2 Pulmonary **blastomycosis, unspecified** cc⊘ HCC CC/MCC Exc

B40.3 Cutaneous **blastomycosis** cc⊘ CC/MCC Exc

B40.7 Disseminated **blastomycosis** cc⊘ CC/MCC Exc

Generalized blastomycosis

5ᵗʰ **B40.8** Other forms **of blastomycosis**

B40.81 **Blastomycotic meningoencephalitis** cc⊘ CC/MCC Exc

Meningomyelitis due to blastomycosis

B40.89 Other forms **of blastomycosis** cc⊘ CC/MCC Exc

B40.9 **Blastomycosis, unspecified** cc⊘ CC/MCC Exc

4ᵗʰ **B41 Paracoccidioidomycosis**

> INCLUDES Brazilian blastomycosis
>
> Lutz' disease

B41.0 Pulmonary **paracoccidioidomycosis** cc⊘ HCC CC/MCC Exc

B41.7 Disseminated **paracoccidioidomycosis** cc⊘ CC/MCC Exc

Generalized paracoccidioidomycosis

B41.8 Other forms **of paracoccidioidomycosis** cc⊘ CC/MCC Exc

B41.9 **Paracoccidioidomycosis, unspecified** cc⊘ CC/MCC Exc

4ᵗʰ **B42 Sporotrichosis**

B42.0 Pulmonary **sporotrichosis**

B42.1 Lymphocutaneous **sporotrichosis**

B42.7 Disseminated **sporotrichosis**

Generalized sporotrichosis

5ᵗʰ **B42.8** Other forms **of sporotrichosis**

B42.81 Cerebral **sporotrichosis**

Meningitis due to sporotrichosis

B42.82 **Sporotrichosis** arthritis HCC

B42.89 Other forms **of sporotrichosis**

B42.9 **Sporotrichosis, unspecified**

4ᵗʰ **B43 Chromomycosis and pheomycotic abscess**

B43.0 Cutaneous **chromomycosis**

Dermatitis verrucosa

B43.1 **Pheomycotic** brain abscess

Cerebral chromomycosis

B43.2 Subcutaneous **pheomycotic abscess and cyst**

B43.8 Other forms **of chromomycosis**

B43.9 **Chromomycosis, unspecified**

4ᵗʰ **B44 Aspergillosis**

> INCLUDES aspergilloma

B44.0 Invasive pulmonary **aspergillosis** HCC MCC⊘ RxHCC CC/MCC Exc

B44.1 Other pulmonary **aspergillosis** cc⊘ HCC RxHCC CC/MCC Exc

B44.2 Tonsillar **aspergillosis** cc⊘ HCC RxHCC CC/MCC Exc

B44.7 Disseminated **aspergillosis** cc⊘ HCC RxHCC CC/MCC Exc

Generalized aspergillosis

5ᵗʰ **B44.8** Other forms **of aspergillosis**

B44.81 Allergic bronchopulmonary **aspergillosis** cc⊘ HCC RxHCC CC/MCC Exc

B44.89 Other forms **of aspergillosis** cc⊘ HCC RxHCC CC/MCC Exc

B44.9 **Aspergillosis, unspecified** cc⊘ HCC RxHCC CC/MCC Exc

4ᵗʰ **B45 Cryptococcosis**

B45.0 Pulmonary **cryptococcosis** cc⊘ HCC RxHCC CC/MCC Exc

B45.1 Cerebral **cryptococcosis** HCC MCC⊘ RxHCC CC/MCC Exc

Cryptococcal meningitis

Cryptococcosis meningocerebralis

B45.2 Cutaneous **cryptococcosis** cc⊘ HCC RxHCC CC/MCC Exc

B45.3 Osseous **cryptococcosis** cc⊘ HCC RxHCC CC/MCC Exc

B45.7 Disseminated **cryptococcosis** cc⊘ HCC RxHCC CC/MCC Exc

Generalized cryptococcosis

B45.8 Other forms **of cryptococcosis** cc⊘ HCC RxHCC CC/MCC Exc

B45.9 **Cryptococcosis, unspecified** cc⊘ HCC RxHCC CC/MCC Exc

4ᵗʰ **B46 Zygomycosis**

B46.0 Pulmonary **mucormycosis** HCC MCC⊘ RxHCC CC/MCC Exc

B46.1 Rhinocerebral **mucormycosis** HCC MCC⊘ RxHCC CC/MCC Exc

B46.2 Gastrointestinal **mucormycosis** HCC MCC⊘ RxHCC CC/MCC Exc

B46.3 Cutaneous **mucormycosis** HCC MCC⊘ RxHCC CC/MCC Exc

Subcutaneous mucormycosis

B46.4 Disseminated **mucormycosis** HCC MCC⊘ RxHCC CC/MCC Exc

Generalized mucormycosis

B46.5 **Mucormycosis, unspecified** HCC MCC⊘ RxHCC CC/MCC Exc

B46.8 Other **zygomycoses** HCC MCC⊘ RxHCC CC/MCC Exc

Entomophthoromycosis

B46.9 **Zygomycosis, unspecified** HCC MCC⊘ RxHCC CC/MCC Exc

Phycomycosis NOS

4ᵗʰ **B47 Mycetoma**

B47.0 **Eumycetoma** cc⊘ CC/MCC Exc

Madura foot, mycotic

Maduromycosis

B47.1 **Actinomycetoma** cc⊘ CC/MCC Exc

B47.9 **Mycetoma, unspecified** cc⊘ CC/MCC Exc

Madura foot NOS

4ᵗʰ **B48 Other mycoses, not elsewhere classified**

B48.0 **Lobomycosis**

Keloidal blastomycosis

Lobo's disease

B48.1 **Rhinosporidiosis**

B48.2 **Allescheriasis** cc⊘ CC/MCC Exc

Infection due to Pseudallescheria boydii

> EXCLUDES1 eumycetoma (B47.0)

B48.3 **Geotrichosis** cc⊘ CC/MCC Exc

Geotrichum stomatitis

B48.4 **Penicillosis** cc⊘ HCC RxHCC CC/MCC Exc

B48.8 Other specified mycoses cc⊘ HCC RxHCC CC/MCC Exc

Adiaspiromycosis

Infection of tissue and organs by Alternaria

Infection of tissue and organs by Drechslera

Infection of tissue and organs by Fusarium

Infection of tissue and organs by saprophytic fungi NEC

B49 Unspecified mycosis cc⊘ CC/MCC Exc

Fungemia NOS

Protozoal diseases (B50-B64)

> EXCLUDES1 amebiasis (A06.-)
>
> other protozoal intestinal diseases (A07.-)

4ᵗʰ **B50 Plasmodium** falciparum **malaria**

> INCLUDES mixed infections of Plasmodium falciparum with any other Plasmodium species

B50.0 **Plasmodium falciparum malaria** with cerebral complications cc⊘ CC/MCC Exc

Cerebral malaria NOS

B50.8 Other severe and complicated **Plasmodium falciparum malaria** cc⊘ CC/MCC Exc

Severe or complicated Plasmodium falciparum malaria NOS

B50.9 **Plasmodium falciparum malaria, unspecified** MCC⊘ CC/MCC Exc

4ᵗʰ **B51 Plasmodium** vivax **malaria**

> INCLUDES mixed infections of Plasmodium vivax with other Plasmodium species, except Plasmodium falciparum

> EXCLUDES1 plasmodium vivax with Plasmodium falciparum (B50.-)

B51.0 **Plasmodium vivax malaria** with rupture of spleen cc⊘ CC/MCC Exc

B51.8 **Plasmodium vivax malaria** with other complications cc⊘ CC/MCC Exc

B51.9 **Plasmodium vivax malaria** without complication cc⊘ CC/MCC Exc

Plasmodium vivax malaria NOS

4ᵗʰ **B52 Plasmodium** malariae **malaria**

> INCLUDES mixed infections of Plasmodium malariae with other Plasmodium species, except Plasmodium falciparum and Plasmodium vivax

> EXCLUDES1 Plasmodium falciparum (B50.-)
>
> Plasmodium vivax (B51.-)

B52.0 **Plasmodium malariae malaria** with nephropathy cc⊘ CC/MCC Exc

B52.8 **Plasmodium malariae malaria** with other complications cc⊘ CC/MCC Exc

B52.9 **Plasmodium malariae malaria** without complication cc⊘ CC/MCC Exc

Plasmodium malariae malaria NOS

| Unspecified Code | Other Specified Code | Manifestation Code | Ⓝ Newborn | Ⓟ Pediatric | Ⓜ Maternity | Ⓐ Adult | ♂ Male | ♀ Female |

● New Code ▲ Revised Code Title ▶◀ Revised Text **NOTES** INCLUDES EXCLUDES1 Not coded here EXCLUDES2 Not included here

4ᵗʰ 4ᵗʰ character required 5ᵗʰ 5ᵗʰ character required 6ᵗʰ 6ᵗʰ character required 7ᵗʰ 7ᵗʰ character required 7ᵗʰ Extension 'X' Alert

HAC Hospital-acquired condition (HAC) alert AHA AHA Coding Clinic© 📖 Code first alert

B53 Other specified **malaria**

    B53.0 Plasmodium ovale **malaria** `cc` `cc/mcc Exc`

        EXCLUDES1 *Plasmodium ovale with Plasmodium falciparum (B50.-)*

            Plasmodium ovale with Plasmodium malariae (B52.-)

            Plasmodium ovale with Plasmodium vivax (B51.-)

    B53.1 **Malaria due to** simian plasmodia `cc` `cc/mcc Exc`

        EXCLUDES1 *Malaria due to simian plasmodia with Plasmodium falciparum (B50.-)*

            Malaria due to simian plasmodia with Plasmodium malariae (B52.-)

            Malaria due to simian plasmodia with Plasmodium ovale (B53.0)

            Malaria due to simian plasmodia with Plasmodium vivax (B51.-)

    B53.8 Other **malaria, not elsewhere classified** `cc` `cc/mcc Exc`

B54 **Unspecified malaria** `cc` `cc/mcc Exc`

B55 **Leishmaniasis**

    B55.0 Visceral **leishmaniasis** `cc` `cc/mcc Exc`

        Kala-azar

        Post-kala-azar dermal leishmaniasis

    B55.1 Cutaneous **leishmaniasis** `cc` `cc/mcc Exc`

    B55.2 Mucocutaneous **leishmaniasis** `cc` `cc/mcc Exc`

    B55.9 **Leishmaniasis, unspecified** `cc` `cc/mcc Exc`

B56 **African trypanosomiasis**

    B56.0 Gambiense **trypanosomiasis** `cc` `cc/mcc Exc`

        Infection due to Trypanosoma brucei gambiense

        West African sleeping sickness

    B56.1 Rhodesiense **trypanosomiasis** `cc` `cc/mcc Exc`

        East African sleeping sickness

        Infection due to Trypanosoma brucei rhodesiense

    B56.9 **African trypanosomiasis, unspecified** `cc` `cc/mcc Exc`

        Sleeping sickness NOS

B57 **Chagas' disease**

    INCLUDES *American trypanosomiasis*

           infection due to Trypanosoma cruzi

    B57.0 Acute **Chagas' disease** with heart involvement `cc` `cc/mcc Exc`

        Acute Chagas' disease with myocarditis

    B57.1 Acute **Chagas' disease** without heart involvement `cc` `cc/mcc Exc`

        Acute Chagas' disease NOS

    B57.2 **Chagas' disease** (chronic) **with heart involvement** `cc` `cc/mcc Exc`

        American trypanosomiasis NOS

        Chagas' disease (chronic) NOS

        Chagas' disease (chronic) with myocarditis

        Trypanosomiasis NOS

    B57.3 **Chagas' disease** (chronic) **with digestive system involvement**

        B57.30 **Chagas' disease with digestive system involvement, unspecified** `cc` `cc/mcc Exc`

        B57.31 Megaesophagus **in Chagas' disease** `cc` `cc/mcc Exc`

        B57.32 Megacolon **in Chagas' disease** `cc` `cc/mcc Exc`

        B57.39 Other digestive system involvement **in Chagas' disease** `cc` `cc/mcc Exc`

    B57.4 **Chagas' disease (chronic)** with nervous system involvement

        B57.40 **Chagas' disease with nervous system involvement, unspecified** `cc` `cc/mcc Exc`

        B57.41 Meningitis **in Chagas' disease** `cc` `cc/mcc Exc`

        B57.42 Meningoencephalitis **in Chagas' disease** `cc` `cc/mcc Exc`

        B57.49 Other nervous system involvement **in Chagas' disease** `cc` `cc/mcc Exc`

    B57.5 **Chagas' disease (chronic)** with other organ involvement `cc` `cc/mcc Exc`

B58 **Toxoplasmosis**

    INCLUDES *infection due to Toxoplasma gondii*

    EXCLUDES1 *congenital toxoplasmosis (P37.1)*

    B58.0 **Toxoplasma** oculopathy

        B58.00 **Toxoplasma oculopathy, unspecified** `cc` `cc/mcc Exc`

        B58.01 **Toxoplasma** chorioretinitis `cc` `cc/mcc Exc`

        B58.09 Other **toxoplasma oculopathy** `cc` `cc/mcc Exc`

           Toxoplasma uveitis

    B58.1 **Toxoplasma** hepatitis `cc` `cc/mcc Exc`

    B58.2 **Toxoplasma** meningoencephalitis `HCC` `MCC` `RxHCC` `cc/mcc Exc`

    B58.3 Pulmonary **toxoplasmosis** `HCC` `MCC` `RxHCC` `cc/mcc Exc`

    B58.8 **Toxoplasmosis** with other organ involvement

        B58.81 **Toxoplasma** myocarditis `MCC` `cc/mcc Exc`

        B58.82 **Toxoplasma** myositis `cc` `cc/mcc Exc`

        B58.83 **Toxoplasma** tubulo-interstitial nephropathy `cc` `cc/mcc Exc`

           Toxoplasma pyelonephritis

        B58.89 **Toxoplasmosis** with other organ involvement `cc` `cc/mcc Exc`

    B58.9 **Toxoplasmosis, unspecified** `cc` `cc/mcc Exc`

B59 **Pneumocystosis** `HCC` `MCC` `RxHCC` `cc/mcc Exc`

    Pneumonia due to Pneumocystis carinii

    Pneumonia due to Pneumocystis jiroveci

B60 Other protozoal diseases, not elsewhere classified

    EXCLUDES1 *cryptosporidiosis (A07.2)*

           intestinal microsporidiosis (A07.8)

           isosporiasis (A07.3)

    B60.0 **Babesiosis** `cc` `cc/mcc Exc`

        Piroplasmosis

    B60.1 **Acanthamebiasis**

        B60.10 **Acanthamebiasis, unspecified** `cc` `cc/mcc Exc`

        B60.11 Meningoencephalitis **due to Acanthamoeba (culbertsoni)**

        B60.12 Conjunctivitis **due to Acanthamoeba**

        B60.13 Keratoconjunctivitis **due to Acanthamoeba** `PDxIn`

        B60.19 Other **acanthamebic disease** `cc` `cc/mcc Exc`

    B60.2 **Naegleriasis** `cc` `cc/mcc Exc`

        Primary amebic meningoencephalitis

    B60.8 **Other specified protozoal diseases**

        Microsporidiosis

B64 **Unspecified protozoal disease**

Helminthiases (B65-B83)

B65 **Schistosomiasis [bilharziasis]**

    INCLUDES *snail fever*

    B65.0 **Schistosomiasis due to Schistosoma** haematobium **[urinary schistosomiasis]** `cc` `cc/mcc Exc`

    B65.1 **Schistosomiasis due to Schistosoma** mansoni **[intestinal schistosomiasis]** `cc` `cc/mcc Exc`

    B65.2 **Schistosomiasis due to Schistosoma** japonicum `cc` `cc/mcc Exc`

        Asiatic schistosomiasis

    B65.3 **Cercarial dermatitis** `cc` `cc/mcc Exc`

        Swimmer's itch

    B65.8 Other **schistosomiasis** `cc` `cc/mcc Exc`

        Infection due to Schistosoma intercalatum

        Infection due to Schistosoma mattheei

        Infection due to Schistosoma mekongi

    B65.9 **Schistosomiasis, unspecified** `cc` `cc/mcc Exc`

B66 **Other fluke infections**

    B66.0 **Opisthorchiasis** `cc` `cc/mcc Exc`

        Infection due to cat liver fluke

        Infection due to Opisthorchis (felineus)(viverrini)

    B66.1 **Clonorchiasis** `cc` `cc/mcc Exc`

        Chinese liver fluke disease

        Infection due to Clonorchis sinensis

        Oriental liver fluke disease

    B66.2 **Dicroceliasis** `cc` `cc/mcc Exc`

        Infection due to Dicrocoelium dendriticum

        Lancet fluke infection

    B66.3 **Fascioliasis** `cc` `cc/mcc Exc`

        Infection due to Fasciola gigantica

        Infection due to Fasciola hepatica

        Infection due to Fasciola indica

        Sheep liver fluke disease

    B66.4 **Paragonimiasis** `cc` `HCC` `cc/mcc Exc`

        Infection due to Paragonimus species

        Lung fluke disease

        Pulmonary distomiasis

B66.5 Fasciolopsiasis CC CC/MCC Exc
Infection due to Fasciolopsis buski
Intestinal distomiasis

B66.8 Other specified fluke infections CC CC/MCC Exc
Echinostomiasis
Heterophyiasis
Metagonimiasis
Nanophyetiasis
Watsoniasis

B66.9 Fluke infection, unspecified

B67 Echinococcosis

INCLUDES hydatidosis

B67.0 Echinococcus granulosus infection of liver CC CC/MCC Exc
B67.1 Echinococcus granulosus infection of lung CC HCC CC/MCC Exc
B67.2 Echinococcus granulosus infection of bone CC CC/MCC Exc
B67.3 Echinococcus granulosus infection, other and multiple sites
　B67.31 Echinococcus granulosus infection, thyroid gland CC CC/MCC Exc
　B67.32 Echinococcus granulosus infection, multiple sites CC CC/MCC Exc
　B67.39 Echinococcus granulosus infection, other sites CC CC/MCC Exc
B67.4 Echinococcus granulosus infection, unspecified CC CC/MCC Exc
Dog tapeworm (infection)
B67.5 Echinococcus multilocularis infection of liver CC CC/MCC Exc
B67.6 Echinococcus multilocularis infection, other and multiple sites
　B67.61 Echinococcus multilocularis infection, multiple sites CC CC/MCC Exc
　B67.69 Echinococcus multilocularis infection, other sites CC CC/MCC Exc
B67.7 Echinococcus multilocularis infection, unspecified CC CC/MCC Exc
B67.8 Echinococcosis, unspecified, of liver CC CC/MCC Exc
B67.9 Echinococcosis, other and unspecified
　B67.90 Echinococcosis, unspecified CC CC/MCC Exc
Echinococcosis NOS
　B67.99 Other echinococcosis CC CC/MCC Exc

B68 Taeniasis (Figure 1.5)

EXCLUDES1 cysticercosis (B69.-)

B68.0 Taenia solium taeniasis CC CC/MCC Exc
Pork tapeworm (infection)
B68.1 Taenia saginata taeniasis CC CC/MCC Exc
Beef tapeworm (infection)
Infection due to adult tapeworm Taenia saginata
B68.9 Taeniasis, unspecified CC CC/MCC Exc

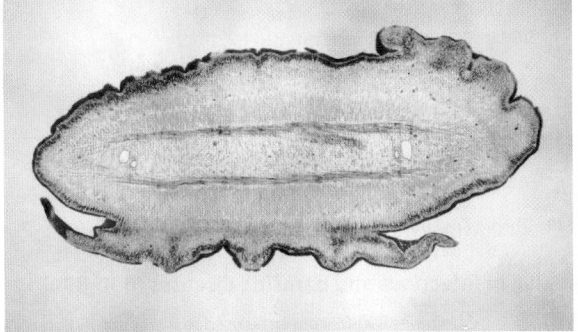

Figure 1.5 Taeniasis

B69 Cysticercosis

INCLUDES cysticerciasis infection due to larval form of Taenia solium

B69.0 Cysticercosis of central nervous system CC CC/MCC Exc
B69.1 Cysticercosis of eye CC CC/MCC Exc
B69.8 Cysticercosis of other sites
　B69.81 Myositis in cysticercosis CC CC/MCC Exc
　B69.89 Cysticercosis of other sites CC CC/MCC Exc
B69.9 Cysticercosis, unspecified CC CC/MCC Exc

B70 Diphyllobothriasis and sparganosis
B70.0 Diphyllobothriasis CC CC/MCC Exc
Diphyllobothrium (adult) (latum) (pacificum) infection
Fish tapeworm (infection)
EXCLUDES2 larval diphyllobothriasis (B70.1)
B70.1 Sparganosis CC CC/MCC Exc
Infection due to Sparganum (mansoni) (proliferum)
Infection due to Spirometra larva
Larval diphyllobothriasis
Spirometrosis

B71 Other cestode infections
B71.0 Hymenolepiasis CC CC/MCC Exc
Dwarf tapeworm infection
Rat tapeworm (infection)
B71.1 Dipylidiasis CC CC/MCC Exc
B71.8 Other specified cestode infections
Coenurosis
B71.9 Cestode infection, unspecified
Tapeworm (infection) NOS

B72 Dracunculiasis CC CC/MCC Exc

INCLUDES guinea worm infection
infection due to Dracunculus medinensis

B73 Onchocerciasis

INCLUDES onchocerca volvulus infection
onchocercosis
river blindness

B73.0 Onchocerciasis with eye disease
　B73.00 Onchocerciasis with eye involvement, unspecified CC CC/MCC Exc
　B73.01 Onchocerciasis with endophthalmitis CC CC/MCC Exc
　B73.02 Onchocerciasis with glaucoma CC CC/MCC Exc
　B73.09 Onchocerciasis with other eye involvement CC CC/MCC Exc
Infestation of eyelid due to onchocerciasis
B73.1 Onchocerciasis without eye disease

B74 Filariasis

EXCLUDES2 onchocerciasis (B73)
tropical (pulmonary) eosinophilia NOS (J82)

B74.0 Filariasis due to Wuchereria bancrofti CC CC/MCC Exc
Bancroftian elephantiasis
Bancroftian filariasis
B74.1 Filariasis due to Brugia malayi CC CC/MCC Exc
B74.2 Filariasis due to Brugia timori CC CC/MCC Exc
B74.3 Loiasis
Calabar swelling
Eyeworm disease of Africa
Loa loa infection
B74.4 Mansonelliasis CC CC/MCC Exc
Infection due to Mansonella ozzardi
Infection due to Mansonella perstans
Infection due to Mansonella streptocerca
B74.8 Other filariases CC CC/MCC Exc
Dirofilariasis
B74.9 Filariasis, unspecified CC CC/MCC Exc

B75 Trichinellosis

INCLUDES infection due to Trichinella species
trichiniasis

B76 Hookworm diseases

INCLUDES uncinariasis

B76.0 Ancylostomiasis CC CC/MCC Exc
Infection due to Ancylostoma species
B76.1 Necatoriasis CC CC/MCC Exc
Infection due to Necator americanus
B76.8 Other hookworm diseases CC CC/MCC Exc
B76.9 Hookworm disease, unspecified CC CC/MCC Exc
Cutaneous larva migrans NOS

B77 Ascariasis

INCLUDES ascaridiasis
roundworm infection

B77.0 Ascariasis with intestinal complications CC CC/MCC Exc

Unspecified Code　Other Specified Code　Manifestation Code　N Newborn　P Pediatric　M Maternity　A Adult　♂ Male　♀ Female
● New Code　▲ Revised Code Title　▶◀ Revised Text　NOTES　*INCLUDES*　*EXCLUDES1* Not coded here　*EXCLUDES2* Not included here
4th character required　5th character required　6th character required　7th character required　Extension 'X' Alert
HAC Hospital-acquired condition (HAC) alert　AHA AHA Coding Clinic©　☛ Code first alert

[5th] **B77.8 Ascariasis** with other complications
- **B77.81 Ascariasis** pneumonia MCC CC/MCC Excl
- **B77.89 Ascariasis** with other complications CC CC/MCC Excl

B77.9 Ascariasis, unspecified CC CC/MCC Excl

[4th] **B78 Strongyloidiasis**

EXCLUDES1 *trichostrongyliasis (B81.2)*

- **B78.0** Intestinal **strongyloidiasis** CC CC/MCC Excl
- **B78.1** Cutaneous **strongyloidiasis**
- **B78.7** Disseminated **strongyloidiasis** CC CC/MCC Excl
- **B78.9 Strongyloidiasis, unspecified** CC CC/MCC Excl

B79 Trichuriasis CC CC/MCC Excl

INCLUDES *trichocephaliasis*
whipworm (disease)(infection)

B80 Enterobiasis CC CC/MCC Excl

INCLUDES *oxyuriasis*
pinworm infection
threadworm infection

[4th] **B81 Other intestinal helminthiases, not elsewhere classified**

EXCLUDES1 *angiostrongyliasis due to:*
Angiostrongylus cantonensis (B83.2)
Parastrongylus cantonensis (B83.2)

B81.0 Anisakiasis CC CC/MCC Excl
Infection due to Anisakis larva

B81.1 Intestinal capillariasis CC CC/MCC Excl
Capillariasis NOS
Infection due to Capillaria philippinensis
EXCLUDES2 *hepatic capillariasis (B83.8)*

B81.2 Trichostrongyliasis CC CC/MCC Excl

B81.3 Intestinal angiostrongyliasis CC CC/MCC Excl
Angiostrongyliasis due to:
Angiostrongylus costaricensis
Parastrongylus costaricensis

B81.4 Mixed intestinal helminthiases CC CC/MCC Excl
Infection due to intestinal helminths classified to more than one of the categories B65.0-B81.3 and B81.8
Mixed helminthiasis NOS

B81.8 Other specified intestinal helminthiases CC CC/MCC Excl
Infection due to Oesophagostomum species [esophagostomiasis]
Infection due to Ternidens diminutus [ternidensiasis]

[4th] **B82 Unspecified intestinal parasitism**
- **B82.0 Intestinal** helminthiasis**, unspecified** CC CC/MCC Excl
- **B82.9 Intestinal** parasitism**, unspecified**

[4th] **B83 Other helminthiases**

EXCLUDES1 *capillariasis NOS (B81.1)*
EXCLUDES2 *intestinal capillariasis (B81.1)*

B83.0 Visceral larva migrans
Toxocariasis

B83.1 Gnathostomiasis
Wandering swelling

B83.2 Angiostrongyliasis due to Parastrongylus cantonensis
Eosinophilic meningoencephalitis due to Parastrongylus cantonensis
EXCLUDES2 *intestinal angiostrongyliasis (B81.3)*

B83.3 Syngamiasis
Syngamosis

B83.4 Internal hirudiniasis
EXCLUDES2 *external hirudiniasis (B88.3)*

B83.8 Other specified helminthiases
Acanthocephaliasis
Gongylonemiasis
Hepatic capillariasis
Metastrongyliasis
Thelaziasis

B83.9 Helminthiasis, unspecified
Worms NOS
EXCLUDES1 *intestinal helminthiasis NOS (B82.0)*

Pediculosis, acariasis and other infestations (B85-B89)

[4th] **B85 Pediculosis and phthiriasis**

DEFINITION: Pediculosis and phthiriasis are infestation of lice, which are small, parasitic insects.

B85.0 Pediculosis due to Pediculus humanus capitis
Head-louse infestation

B85.1 Pediculosis due to Pediculus humanus corporis
Body-louse infestation

B85.2 Pediculosis, unspecified

B85.3 Phthiriasis
Infestation by crab-louse
Infestation by Phthirus pubis

B85.4 Mixed **pediculosis and phthiriasis**
Infestation classifiable to more than one of the categories B85.0-B85.3

B86 Scabies
Sarcoptic itch

[4th] **B87 Myiasis**

INCLUDES *infestation by larva of flies*

B87.0 Cutaneous **myiasis**
Creeping myiasis

B87.1 Wound **myiasis**
Traumatic myiasis

B87.2 Ocular **myiasis**

B87.3 Nasopharyngeal **myiasis**
Laryngeal myiasis

B87.4 Aural **myiasis**

[5th] **B87.8 Myiasis of other sites**
- **B87.81** Genitourinary **myiasis**
- **B87.82** Intestinal **myiasis**
- **B87.89 Myiasis of** other sites

B87.9 Myiasis, unspecified

[4th] **B88 Other infestations**

B88.0 Other acariasis
Acarine dermatitis
Dermatitis due to Demodex species
Dermatitis due to Dermanyssus gallinae
Dermatitis due to Liponyssoides sanguineus
Trombiculosis
EXCLUDES2 *scabies (B86)*

B88.1 Tungiasis [sandflea infestation]

B88.2 Other arthropod infestations
Scarabiasis

B88.3 External hirudiniasis
Leech infestation NOS
EXCLUDES2 *internal hirudiniasis (B83.4)*

B88.8 Other specified infestations
Ichthyoparasitism due to Vandellia cirrhosa
Linguatulosis
Porocephaliasis

B88.9 Infestation, unspecified
Infestation (skin) NOS
Infestation by mites NOS
Skin parasites NOS

B89 Unspecified parasitic disease

Sequelae of infectious and parasitic diseases (B90-B94)

NOTES Categories B90-B94 are to be used to indicate conditions in categories A00-B89 as the cause of sequelae, which are themselves classified elsewhere. The 'sequelae' include conditions specified as such; they also include residuals of diseases classifiable to the above categories if there is evidence that the disease itself is no longer present. Codes from these categories are not to be used for chronic infections. Code chronic current infections to active infectious disease as appropriate.

☞ **Code first** condition resulting from (sequela) the infectious or parasitic disease

[4th] **B90 Sequelae of tuberculosis**
- **B90.0 Sequelae of** central nervous system **tuberculosis** POA
- **B90.1 Sequelae of** genitourinary **tuberculosis** POA

PDx Unacceptable principal diagnosis symbol per Medicare code edits | POA Code exempt from diagnosis present on admission requirement
? Questionable admission | CC Complication or comorbidity | MCC Major complication or comorbidity | CC/MCC Excl CC/MCC exclusion
HCC HCC diagnosis code | RxHCC RxHCC diagnosis code | MACRA code | **DEFINITION** Describes condition/terminology
TIP Coding guidance | 👁 Official Guideline Reference | Z1 Z code as first-listed diagnosis

B90.2 Sequelae of tuberculosis of bones and joints `POA`

B90.8 Sequelae of tuberculosis of other organs `POA`

EXCLUDES2 sequelae of respiratory tuberculosis (B90.9)

B90.9 Sequelae of respiratory and unspecified tuberculosis `POA`

Sequelae of tuberculosis NOS

B91 Sequelae of poliomyelitis `POA`

EXCLUDES1 postpolio syndrome (G14)

B92 Sequelae of leprosy `POA`

🔵 B94 Sequelae of other and unspecified infectious and parasitic diseases

B94.0 Sequelae of trachoma `POA`

B94.1 Sequelae of viral encephalitis `POA`

B94.2 Sequelae of viral hepatitis `POA`

B94.8 Sequelae of other specified infectious and parasitic diseases `POA`

B94.9 Sequelae of unspecified infectious and parasitic disease `POA`

Bacterial and viral infectious agents (B95-B97)

NOTES These categories are provided for use as supplementary or additional codes to identify the infectious agent(s) in diseases classified elsewhere.

🔵 B95 Streptococcus, Staphylococcus, and Enterococcus as the cause of diseases classified elsewhere

👁 **See Official Guidelines** "Multiple coding for a single condition" I.B.7, "Infectious agents as the cause of diseases classified to other chapters" I.C.1.b, "Puerperal sepsis" I.C.15.k

TIP: Code first the type of infection from elsewhere in the book.

B95.0 **Streptococcus,** group A, **as the cause of diseases classified elsewhere** `PDxIn`

AHA: Q1 2018

B95.1 **Streptococcus,** group B, **as the cause of diseases classified elsewhere** `PDxIn`

AHA: Q2 2019, Q1 2018, Q4 2018

B95.2 **Enterococcus as the cause of diseases classified elsewhere** `PDxIn`

AHA: Q1 2018

B95.3 **Streptococcus** pneumoniae **as the cause of diseases classified elsewhere** `PDxIn`

AHA: Q1 2018

B95.4 Other **streptococcus as the cause of diseases classified elsewhere** `PDxIn`

AHA: Q1 2018

B95.5 **Unspecified streptococcus as the cause of diseases classified elsewhere** `PDxIn`

AHA: Q1 2018

🔵 B95.6 **Staphylococcus** aureus **as the cause of diseases classified elsewhere**

B95.61 **Methicillin** susceptible **Staphylococcus aureus infection as the cause of diseases classified elsewhere** `PDxIn`

AHA: Q1 2018

Methicillin susceptible Staphylococcus aureus (MSSA) infection as the cause of diseases classified elsewhere

Staphylococcus aureus infection NOS as the cause of diseases classified elsewhere

B95.62 **Methicillin** resistant **Staphylococcus aureus infection as the cause of diseases classified elsewhere** `PDxIn`

👁 **See Official Guidelines** "Combination codes for MRSA infections" I.C.1.e.1.a, "Other codes for MRSA infection" I.C.1.e.1.b

AHA: Q1 2018, Q1 2016

Methicillin resistant staphylococcus aureus (MRSA) infection as the cause of diseases classified elsewhere

B95.7 **Other staphylococcus as the cause of diseases classified elsewhere** `PDxIn`

AHA: Q1 2018

B95.8 **Unspecified staphylococcus as the cause of diseases classified elsewhere** `PDxIn`

AHA: Q1 2018

🔵 B96 Other bacterial agents **as the cause of diseases classified elsewhere**

👁 **See Official Guidelines** "Multiple coding for a single condition" I.B.7, "Infectious agents as the cause of diseases classified to other chapters" I.C.1.b, "Puerperal sepsis" I.C.15.k

TIP: Code first the type of infection from elsewhere in the book.

B96.0 Mycoplasma pneumoniae [M. pneumoniae] **as the cause of diseases classified elsewhere** `PDxIn`

AHA: Q1 2018

Pleuro-pneumonia-like-organism [PPLO]

B96.1 Klebsiella pneumoniae [K. pneumoniae] **as the cause of diseases classified elsewhere** `PDxIn`

AHA: Q1 2018

🔵 B96.2 Escherichia coli [E. coli] **as the cause of diseases classified elsewhere**

B96.20 **Unspecified Escherichia coli [E. coli] as the cause of diseases classified elsewhere** `PDxIn`

AHA: Q1 2018, Q4 2018

Escherichia coli [E. coli] NOS

▲ B96.21 **Shiga toxin-producing Escherichia coli [E. coli] ▶[STEC]◀ O157 as the cause of diseases classified elsewhere** `PDxIn`

AHA: Q1 2018

E. coli O157:H- (nonmotile) with confirmation of Shiga toxin

E. coli O157 with confirmation of Shiga toxin when H antigen is unknown, or is not H7

O157:H7 Escherichia coli [E.coli] with or without confirmation of Shiga toxin-production

Shiga toxin-producing Escherichia coli [E.coli] O157:H7 with or without confirmation of Shiga toxin-production

STEC O157:H7 with or without confirmation of Shiga toxin-production

▲ B96.22 **Other specified Shiga toxin-producing Escherichia coli [E. coli] ▶[STEC]◀ as the cause of diseases classified elsewhere** `PDxIn`

AHA: Q1 2018

Non-O157 Shiga toxin-producing Escherichia coli [E.coli]

Non-O157 Shiga toxin-producing Escherichia coli [E.coli] with known O group

▲ B96.23 **Unspecified Shiga toxin-producing Escherichia coli [E. coli] ▶[STEC]◀ as the cause of diseases classified elsewhere** `PDxIn`

AHA: Q1 2018

Shiga toxin-producing Escherichia coli [E. coli] with unspecified O group

STEC NOS

B96.29 Other **Escherichia coli [E. coli] as the cause of diseases classified elsewhere** `PDxIn`

AHA: Q1 2018

Non-Shiga toxin-producing E. coli

B96.3 Hemophilus influenzae [H. influenzae] **as the cause of diseases classified elsewhere** `PDxIn`

AHA: Q1 2018

B96.4 Proteus (mirabilis) (morganii) **as the cause of diseases classified elsewhere** `PDxIn`

AHA: Q1 2018

B96.5 Pseudomonas (aeruginosa) (mallei) (pseudomallei) **as the cause of diseases classified elsewhere** `PDxIn`

AHA: Q1 2018, Q1 2015

B96.6 Bacteroides fragilis [B. fragilis] **as the cause of diseases classified elsewhere** `PDxIn`

AHA: Q1 2018

B96.7 Clostridium perfringens [C. perfringens] **as the cause of diseases classified elsewhere** `PDxIn`

AHA: Q1 2018

🔵 B96.8 Other specified bacterial agents **as the cause of diseases classified elsewhere**

B96.81 Helicobacter pylori [H. pylori] **as the cause of diseases classified elsewhere** `PDxIn`

AHA: Q1 2018

Unspecified Code Other Specified Code Manifestation Code Ⓝ Newborn Ⓟ Pediatric Ⓜ Maternity Ⓐ Adult ♂ Male ♀ Female
● New Code ▲ Revised Code Title ▶◀ Revised Text **NOTES** *INCLUDES* *EXCLUDES1* Not coded here *EXCLUDES2* Not included here
🔵 4th character required 🔵 5th character required 🔵 6th character required 🔵 7th character required 🔵 Extension 'X' Alert
HAC Hospital-acquired condition (HAC) alert **AHA** AHA Coding Clinic© 📢 Code first alert

B96.82 Vibrio vulnificus as the cause of diseases classified elsewhere   PDxIn
    AHA: Q1 2018

B96.89 Other specified bacterial agents as the cause of diseases classified elsewhere   PDxIn
    AHA: Q1 2018

B97 Viral agents as the cause of diseases classified elsewhere
    👁 **See Official Guidelines** "Infectious agents as the cause of diseases classified to other chapters" I.C.1.b
    TIP: Code first the type of infection from elsewhere in the book.

B97.0 Adenovirus as the cause of diseases classified elsewhere   PDxIn
    AHA: Q1 2018

B97.1 Enterovirus as the cause of diseases classified elsewhere

    B97.10 Unspecified enterovirus as the cause of diseases classified elsewhere   PDxIn
        AHA: Q1 2018

    B97.11 Coxsackievirus as the cause of diseases classified elsewhere   PDxIn
        AHA: Q1 2018

    B97.12 Echovirus as the cause of diseases classified elsewhere   PDxIn
        AHA: Q1 2018

    B97.19 Other enterovirus as the cause of diseases classified elsewhere   PDxIn
        AHA: Q1 2018

B97.2 Coronavirus as the cause of diseases classified elsewhere

    B97.21 SARS-associated coronavirus as the cause of diseases classified elsewhere   CC PDxIn CC/MCC Exc
        AHA: Q1 2018
        EXCLUDES1 pneumonia due to SARS-associated coronavirus (J12.81)

    B97.29 Other coronavirus as the cause of diseases classified elsewhere   PDxIn
        AHA: Q1 2018

B97.3 Retrovirus as the cause of diseases classified elsewhere
    EXCLUDES1 Human immunodeficiency virus [HIV] disease (B20)

    B97.30 Unspecified retrovirus as the cause of diseases classified elsewhere   PDxIn
        AHA: Q1 2018

    B97.31 Lentivirus as the cause of diseases classified elsewhere   PDxIn
        AHA: Q1 2018

    B97.32 Oncovirus as the cause of diseases classified elsewhere   PDxIn
        AHA: Q1 2018

    B97.33 Human T-cell lymphotrophic virus, type I [HTLV-I] as the cause of diseases classified elsewhere   CC PDxIn CC/MCC Exc
        AHA: Q1 2018

    B97.34 Human T-cell lymphotrophic virus, type II [HTLV-II] as the cause of diseases classified elsewhere   CC PDxIn CC/MCC Exc
        AHA: Q1 2018

    B97.35 Human immunodeficiency virus, type 2 [HIV 2] as the cause of diseases classified elsewhere   CC HCC RxHCC PDxIn CC/MCC Exc
        AHA: Q1 2018

    B97.39 Other retrovirus as the cause of diseases classified elsewhere   PDxIn
        AHA: Q1 2018

B97.4 Respiratory syncytial virus as the cause of diseases classified elsewhere   PDxIn
    AHA: Q1 2018
    RSV as the cause of diseases classified elsewhere
    ☛ **Code first** related disorders, such as:
        otitis media (H65.-)
        upper respiratory infection (J06.9)
    EXCLUDES2 acute bronchiolitis due to respiratory syncytial virus (RSV) (J21.0)
        acute bronchitis due to respiratory syncytial virus (RSV) (J20.5)
        respiratory syncytial virus (RSV) pneumonia (J12.1)

B97.5 Reovirus as the cause of diseases classified elsewhere   PDxIn
    AHA: Q1 2018

B97.6 Parvovirus as the cause of diseases classified elsewhere   PDxIn
    AHA: Q1 2018

B97.7 Papillomavirus as the cause of diseases classified elsewhere   PDxIn
    AHA: Q1 2018

B97.8 Other viral agents as the cause of diseases classified elsewhere

    B97.81 Human metapneumovirus as the cause of diseases classified elsewhere   PDxIn
        AHA: Q1 2018

    B97.89 Other viral agents as the cause of diseases classified elsewhere   PDxIn
        AHA: Q1 2018, Q3 2016

Other infectious diseases (B99)

B99 Other and unspecified infectious diseases
    B99.8 Other infectious disease
    B99.9 Unspecified infectious disease

PDxIn Unacceptable principal diagnosis symbol per Medicare code edits   PDxIn Code exempt from diagnosis present on admission requirement
❓ Questionable admission   CC Complication or comorbidity   MCC Major complication or comorbidity   CC/MCC Exc CC/MCC exclusion
HCC HCC diagnosis code   RxHCC RxHCC diagnosis code   MACRA code   **DEFINITION** Describes condition/terminology
TIP Coding guidance   👁 Official Guideline Reference   Z1 Z code as first-listed diagnosis

Chapter 2: Neoplasms (C00-D49)

Neoplasms (C00-D49)

This chapter contains the following blocks:

C00-C14	Malignant neoplasms of lip, oral cavity and pharynx
C15-C26	Malignant neoplasms of digestive organs
C30-C39	Malignant neoplasms of respiratory and intrathoracic organs
C40-C41	Malignant neoplasms of bone and articular cartilage
C43-C44	Melanoma and other malignant neoplasms of skin
C45-C49	Malignant neoplasms of mesothelial and soft tissue
C50	Malignant neoplasms of breast
C51-C58	Malignant neoplasms of female genital organs
C60-C63	Malignant neoplasms of male genital organs
C64-C68	Malignant neoplasms of urinary tract
C69-C72	Malignant neoplasms of eye, brain and other parts of central nervous system
C73-C75	Malignant neoplasms of thyroid and other endocrine glands
C7A	Malignant neuroendocrine tumors
C7B	Secondary neuroendocrine tumors
C76-C80	Malignant neoplasms of ill-defined, other secondary and unspecified sites
C81-C96	Malignant neoplasms of lymphoid, hematopoietic and related tissue
D00-D09	In situ neoplasms
D10-D36	Benign neoplasms, except benign neuroendocrine tumors
D3A	Benign neuroendocrine tumors
D37-D48	Neoplasms of uncertain behavior, polycythemia vera and myelodysplastic syndromes
D49	Neoplasms of unspecified behavior

[NOTES] Functional activity

All neoplasms are classified in this chapter, whether they are functionally active or not. An additional code from Chapter 4 may be used, to identify functional activity associated with any neoplasm.

Morphology [Histology]

Chapter 2 classifies neoplasms primarily by site (topography), with broad groupings for behavior, malignant, in situ, benign, etc. The Table of Neoplasms should be used to identify the correct topography code. In a few cases, such as for malignant melanoma and certain neuroendocrine tumors, the morphology (histologic type) is included in the category and codes.

Primary malignant neoplasms overlapping site boundaries

A primary malignant neoplasm that overlaps two or more contiguous (next to each other) sites should be classified to the subcategory/code .8 ('overlapping lesion'), unless the combination is specifically indexed elsewhere. For multiple neoplasms of the same site that are not contiguous, such as tumors in different quadrants of the same breast, codes for each site should be assigned.

Malignant neoplasm of ectopic tissue

Malignant neoplasms of ectopic tissue are to be coded to the site mentioned, e.g., ectopic pancreatic malignant neoplasms are coded to pancreas, unspecified (C25.9).

Malignant neoplasms (C00-C96)

Malignant neoplasms, stated or presumed to be primary (of specified sites), and certain specified histologies, except neuroendocrine, and of lymphoid, hematopoietic and related tissue (C00-C75)

Malignant neoplasms of lip, oral cavity and pharynx (C00-C14)

[4th] **C00 Malignant neoplasm of lip**

Use additional code to identify:
- alcohol abuse and dependence (F10.-)
- history of tobacco dependence (Z87.891)
- tobacco dependence (F17.-)
- tobacco use (Z72.0)

[EXCLUDES1] *malignant melanoma of lip (C43.0)*
Merkel cell carcinoma of lip (C4A.0)
other and unspecified malignant neoplasm of skin of lip (C44.0-)

C00.0 Malignant neoplasm of external upper lip
Malignant neoplasm of lipstick area of upper lip
Malignant neoplasm of upper lip NOS
Malignant neoplasm of vermilion border of upper lip

C00.1 Malignant neoplasm of external lower lip
Malignant neoplasm of lower lip NOS
Malignant neoplasm of lipstick area of lower lip
Malignant neoplasm of vermilion border of lower lip

C00.2 Malignant neoplasm of external lip, unspecified
Malignant neoplasm of vermilion border of lip NOS

C00.3 Malignant neoplasm of upper lip, inner aspect
Malignant neoplasm of buccal aspect of upper lip
Malignant neoplasm of frenulum of upper lip
Malignant neoplasm of mucosa of upper lip
Malignant neoplasm of oral aspect of upper lip

C00.4 Malignant neoplasm of lower lip, inner aspect
Malignant neoplasm of buccal aspect of lower lip
Malignant neoplasm of frenulum of lower lip
Malignant neoplasm of mucosa of lower lip
Malignant neoplasm of oral aspect of lower lip

C00.5 Malignant neoplasm of lip, unspecified, inner aspect
Malignant neoplasm of buccal aspect of lip, unspecified
Malignant neoplasm of frenulum of lip, unspecified
Malignant neoplasm of mucosa of lip, unspecified
Malignant neoplasm of oral aspect of lip, unspecified

C00.6 Malignant neoplasm of commissure of lip, unspecified

C00.8 Malignant neoplasm of overlapping sites of lip

C00.9 Malignant neoplasm of lip, unspecified

C01 Malignant neoplasm of base of tongue [HCC]
Malignant neoplasm of dorsal surface of base of tongue
Malignant neoplasm of fixed part of tongue NOS
Malignant neoplasm of posterior third of tongue

Use additional code to identify:
- alcohol abuse and dependence (F10.-)
- history of tobacco dependence (Z87.891)
- tobacco dependence (F17.-)
- tobacco use (Z72.0)

[4th] **C02 Malignant neoplasm of other and unspecified parts of tongue**

Use additional code to identify:
- alcohol abuse and dependence (F10.-)
- history of tobacco dependence (Z87.891)
- tobacco dependence (F17.-)
- tobacco use (Z72.0)

C02.0 Malignant neoplasm of dorsal surface of tongue [HCC]
Malignant neoplasm of anterior two-thirds of tongue, dorsal surface
[EXCLUDES2] *malignant neoplasm of dorsal surface of base of tongue (C01)*

C02.1 Malignant neoplasm of border of tongue [HCC]
Malignant neoplasm of tip of tongue

C02.2 Malignant neoplasm of ventral surface of tongue [HCC]
Malignant neoplasm of anterior two-thirds of tongue, ventral surface
Malignant neoplasm of frenulum linguae

C02.3 Malignant neoplasm of anterior two-thirds of tongue, part unspecified [HCC]
Malignant neoplasm of middle third of tongue NOS
Malignant neoplasm of mobile part of tongue NOS

C02.4 Malignant neoplasm of lingual tonsil [HCC]
[EXCLUDES2] *malignant neoplasm of tonsil NOS (C09.9)*

C02.8 Malignant neoplasm of overlapping sites of tongue [HCC]
Malignant neoplasm of two or more contiguous sites of tongue

C02.9 Malignant neoplasm of tongue, unspecified [HCC]

Unspecified Code | Other Specified Code | Manifestation Code | [N] Newborn | [P] Pediatric | [M] Maternity | [A] Adult | ♂ Male | ♀ Female
● New Code | ▲ Revised Code Title | ►◄ Revised Text | [NOTES] | *INCLUDES* | [EXCLUDES1] Not coded here | [EXCLUDES2] Not included here
[4th] 4th character required | [5th] 5th character required | [6th] 6th character required | [7th] 7th character required | [X] Extension 'X' Alert
[HAC] Hospital-acquired condition (HAC) alert | AHA AHA Coding Clinic© | ☞ Code first alert

When symbols appear on a code that requires a 7th character extension, refer to Appendix B to identify applicable 7th character codes.

C03 **Malignant neoplasm of** gum
  INCLUDES   malignant neoplasm of alveolar (ridge) mucosa
          malignant neoplasm of gingiva
  Use additional code to identify:
    alcohol abuse and dependence (F10.-)
    history of tobacco dependence (Z87.891)
    tobacco dependence (F17.-)
    tobacco use (Z72.0)
  EXCLUDES2 malignant odontogenic neoplasms (C41.0-C41.1)
  C03.0 **Malignant neoplasm of** upper **gum**   HCC
  C03.1 **Malignant neoplasm of** lower **gum**   HCC
  C03.9 **Malignant neoplasm of gum, unspecified**   HCC
C04 **Malignant neoplasm of** floor of mouth
  Use additional code to identify:
    alcohol abuse and dependence (F10.-)
    history of tobacco dependence (Z87.891)
    tobacco dependence (F17.-)
    tobacco use (Z72.0)
  C04.0 **Malignant neoplasm of** anterior **floor of mouth**   HCC
      Malignant neoplasm of anterior to the premolar-canine junction
  C04.1 **Malignant neoplasm of** lateral **floor of mouth**   HCC
  C04.8 **Malignant neoplasm of** overlapping sites **of floor of mouth**   HCC
  C04.9 **Malignant neoplasm of floor of mouth, unspecified**   HCC
C05 **Malignant neoplasm of** palate
  Use additional code to identify:
    alcohol abuse and dependence (F10.-)
    history of tobacco dependence (Z87.891)
    tobacco dependence (F17.-)
    tobacco use (Z72.0)
  EXCLUDES1 Kaposi's sarcoma of palate (C46.2)
  C05.0 **Malignant neoplasm of** hard **palate**   HCC
  C05.1 **Malignant neoplasm of** soft **palate**   HCC
      EXCLUDES2 malignant neoplasm of nasopharyngeal surface of soft palate (C11.3)
  C05.2 **Malignant neoplasm of** uvula   HCC
  C05.8 **Malignant neoplasm of** overlapping sites **of palate**   HCC
  C05.9 **Malignant neoplasm of palate, unspecified**   HCC
      Malignant neoplasm of roof of mouth
C06 **Malignant neoplasm of** other **and** unspecified parts of mouth
  Use additional code to identify:
    alcohol abuse and dependence (F10.-)
    history of tobacco dependence (Z87.891)
    tobacco dependence (F17.-)
    tobacco use (Z72.0)
  C06.0 **Malignant neoplasm of** cheek mucosa   HCC
      Malignant neoplasm of buccal mucosa NOS
      Malignant neoplasm of internal cheek
  C06.1 **Malignant neoplasm of** vestibule **of mouth**   HCC
      Malignant neoplasm of buccal sulcus (upper) (lower)
      Malignant neoplasm of labial sulcus (upper) (lower)
  C06.2 **Malignant neoplasm of** retromolar area   HCC
  C06.8 **Malignant neoplasm of** overlapping sites **of other and unspecified parts of mouth**
      C06.80 **Malignant neoplasm of overlapping sites of unspecified parts of mouth**   HCC
      C06.89 **Malignant neoplasm of overlapping sites of** other **parts of mouth**   HCC
          'book leaf' neoplasm [ventral surface of tongue and floor of mouth]
  C06.9 **Malignant neoplasm of mouth, unspecified**   HCC
      Malignant neoplasm of minor salivary gland, unspecified site
      Malignant neoplasm of oral cavity NOS
C07 **Malignant neoplasm of** parotid gland   HCC
  Use additional code to identify:
    alcohol abuse and dependence (F10.-)
    exposure to environmental tobacco smoke (Z77.22)
    exposure to tobacco smoke in the perinatal period (P96.81)
    history of tobacco dependence (Z87.891)

occupational exposure to environmental tobacco smoke (Z57.31)
tobacco dependence (F17.-)
tobacco use (Z72.0)
C08 **Malignant neoplasm of** other **and** unspecified major salivary glands
  INCLUDES   malignant neoplasm of salivary ducts
  Use additional code to identify:
    alcohol abuse and dependence (F10.-)
    exposure to environmental tobacco smoke (Z77.22)
    exposure to tobacco smoke in the perinatal period (P96.81)
    history of tobacco dependence (Z87.891)
    occupational exposure to environmental tobacco smoke (Z57.31)
    tobacco dependence (F17.-)
    tobacco use (Z72.0)
  EXCLUDES1 malignant neoplasms of specified minor salivary glands which are classified according to their anatomical location
  EXCLUDES2 malignant neoplasms of minor salivary glands NOS (C06.9)
          malignant neoplasm of parotid gland (C07)
  C08.0 **Malignant neoplasm of** submandibular gland   HCC
      Malignant neoplasm of submaxillary gland
  C08.1 **Malignant neoplasm of** sublingual gland   HCC
  C08.9 **Malignant neoplasm of major salivary gland, unspecified**   HCC
      Malignant neoplasm of salivary gland (major) NOS
C09 **Malignant neoplasm of** tonsil
  Use additional code to identify:
    alcohol abuse and dependence (F10.-)
    exposure to environmental tobacco smoke (Z77.22)
    exposure to tobacco smoke in the perinatal period (P96.81)
    history of tobacco dependence (Z87.891)
    occupational exposure to environmental tobacco smoke (Z57.31)
    tobacco dependence (F17.-)
    tobacco use (Z72.0)
  EXCLUDES2 malignant neoplasm of lingual tonsil (C02.4)
          malignant neoplasm of pharyngeal tonsil (C11.1)
  C09.0 **Malignant neoplasm of** tonsillar fossa   HCC
  C09.1 **Malignant neoplasm of** tonsillar pillar (anterior) (posterior)   HCC
  C09.8 **Malignant neoplasm of** overlapping sites **of tonsil**   HCC
  C09.9 **Malignant neoplasm of tonsil, unspecified**   HCC
      Malignant neoplasm of tonsil NOS
      Malignant neoplasm of faucial tonsils
      Malignant neoplasm of palatine tonsils
C10 **Malignant neoplasm of** oropharynx
  Use additional code to identify:
    alcohol abuse and dependence (F10.-)
    exposure to environmental tobacco smoke (Z77.22)
    exposure to tobacco smoke in the perinatal period (P96.81)
    history of tobacco dependence (Z87.891)
    occupational exposure to environmental tobacco smoke (Z57.31)
    tobacco dependence (F17.-)
    tobacco use (Z72.0)
  EXCLUDES2 malignant neoplasm of tonsil (C09.-)
  C10.0 **Malignant neoplasm of** vallecula   HCC
  C10.1 **Malignant neoplasm of** anterior surface of epiglottis   HCC
      Malignant neoplasm of epiglottis, free border [margin]
      Malignant neoplasm of glossoepiglottic fold(s)
      EXCLUDES2 malignant neoplasm of epiglottis (suprahyoid portion) NOS (C32.1)
  C10.2 **Malignant neoplasm of** lateral wall **of oropharynx**   HCC
  C10.3 **Malignant neoplasm of** posterior wall **of oropharynx**   HCC
  C10.4 **Malignant neoplasm of** branchial cleft   HCC
      Malignant neoplasm of branchial cyst [site of neoplasm]
  C10.8 **Malignant neoplasm of** overlapping sites **of oropharynx**   HCC
      Malignant neoplasm of junctional region of oropharynx
  C10.9 **Malignant neoplasm of oropharynx, unspecified**   HCC
C11 **Malignant neoplasm of** nasopharynx
  Use additional code to identify:
    exposure to environmental tobacco smoke (Z77.22)
    exposure to tobacco smoke in the perinatal period (P96.81)
    history of tobacco dependence (Z87.891)

PDₓ Unacceptable principal diagnosis symbol per Medicare code edits   POA Code exempt from diagnosis present on admission requirement
? Questionable admission   cc Complication or comorbidity   MCC Major complication or comorbidity   CC/MCC Excl CC/MCC exclusion
HCC HCC diagnosis code   RxHCC RxHCC diagnosis code   MACRA code   **DEFINITION** Describes condition/terminology
TIP Coding guidance   ◉ Official Guideline Reference   Z1 Z code as first-listed diagnosis

occupational exposure to environmental tobacco smoke (Z57.31)
tobacco dependence (F17.-)
tobacco use (Z72.0)

C11.0 **Malignant neoplasm of** superior wall **of nasopharynx** `HCC`
Malignant neoplasm of roof of nasopharynx

C11.1 **Malignant neoplasm of** posterior wall **of nasopharynx** `HCC`
Malignant neoplasm of adenoid
Malignant neoplasm of pharyngeal tonsil

C11.2 **Malignant neoplasm of** lateral wall **of nasopharynx** `HCC`
Malignant neoplasm of fossa of Rosenmüller
Malignant neoplasm of opening of auditory tube
Malignant neoplasm of pharyngeal recess

C11.3 **Malignant neoplasm of** anterior wall **of nasopharynx** `HCC`
Malignant neoplasm of floor of nasopharynx
Malignant neoplasm of nasopharyngeal (anterior) (posterior)
  surface of soft palate
Malignant neoplasm of posterior margin of nasal choana
Malignant neoplasm of posterior margin of nasal septum

C11.8 **Malignant neoplasm of** overlapping sites **of nasopharynx** `HCC`

C11.9 **Malignant neoplasm of nasopharynx, unspecified** `HCC`
Malignant neoplasm of nasopharyngeal wall NOS

C12 **Malignant neoplasm of** pyriform sinus `HCC`
AHA: Q2 2002, Q4 2002
Malignant neoplasm of pyriform fossa
Use additional code to identify:
  exposure to environmental tobacco smoke (Z77.22)
  exposure to tobacco smoke in the perinatal period (P96.81)
  history of tobacco dependence (Z87.891)
  occupational exposure to environmental tobacco smoke (Z57.31)
  tobacco dependence (F17.-)
  tobacco use (Z72.0)

C13 **Malignant neoplasm of** hypopharynx
Use additional code to identify:
  exposure to environmental tobacco smoke (Z77.22)
  exposure to tobacco smoke in the perinatal period (P96.81)
  history of tobacco dependence (Z87.891)
  occupational exposure to environmental tobacco smoke (Z57.31)
  tobacco dependence (F17.-)
  tobacco use (Z72.0)
  EXCLUDES2 malignant neoplasm of pyriform sinus (C12)

C13.0 **Malignant neoplasm of** postcricoid region `HCC`

C13.1 **Malignant neoplasm of** aryepiglottic fold, hypopharyngeal aspect `HCC`
Malignant neoplasm of aryepiglottic fold, marginal zone
Malignant neoplasm of aryepiglottic fold NOS
Malignant neoplasm of interarytenoid fold, marginal zone
Malignant neoplasm of interarytenoid fold NOS
  EXCLUDES2 malignant neoplasm of aryepiglottic fold or
    interarytenoid fold, laryngeal aspect (C32.1)

C13.2 **Malignant neoplasm of** posterior wall **of hypopharynx** `HCC`

C13.8 **Malignant neoplasm of** overlapping sites **of hypopharynx** `HCC`

C13.9 **Malignant neoplasm of hypopharynx, unspecified** `HCC`
Malignant neoplasm of hypopharyngeal wall NOS

C14 **Malignant neoplasm of other and ill-defined sites in the** lip, oral cavity and pharynx
Use additional code to identify:
  alcohol abuse and dependence (F10.-)
  exposure to environmental tobacco smoke (Z77.22)
  exposure to tobacco smoke in the perinatal period (P96.81)
  history of tobacco dependence (Z87.891)
  occupational exposure to environmental tobacco smoke (Z57.31)
  tobacco dependence (F17.-)
  tobacco use (Z72.0)
  EXCLUDES1 malignant neoplasm of oral cavity NOS (C06.9)

C14.0 **Malignant neoplasm of pharynx, unspecified** `HCC`

C14.2 **Malignant neoplasm of** Waldeyer's ring `HCC`

C14.8 **Malignant neoplasm of** overlapping sites of lip, oral cavity and pharynx `HCC`
Primary malignant neoplasm of two or more contiguous sites
  of lip, oral cavity and pharynx

EXCLUDES1 'book leaf' neoplasm [ventral surface of tongue and
  floor of mouth] (C06.89)

Malignant neoplasms of digestive organs (C15-C26)

EXCLUDES1 Kaposi's sarcoma of gastrointestinal sites (C46.4)
EXCLUDES2 gastrointestinal stromal tumors (C49.A-)

C15 **Malignant neoplasm of** esophagus
Use additional code to identify:
  alcohol abuse and dependence (F10.-)

C15.3 **Malignant neoplasm of** upper third **of esophagus** `HCC`

C15.4 **Malignant neoplasm of** middle third **of esophagus** `HCC`

C15.5 **Malignant neoplasm of** lower third **of esophagus** `HCC`
  EXCLUDES1 malignant neoplasm of cardio-esophageal junction
    (C16.0)

C15.8 **Malignant neoplasm of** overlapping sites **of esophagus** `HCC`

C15.9 **Malignant neoplasm of esophagus, unspecified** `HCC`

C16 **Malignant neoplasm of** stomach
Use additional code to identify:
  alcohol abuse and dependence (F10.-)
  EXCLUDES2 malignant carcinoid tumor of the stomach (C7A.092)

C16.0 **Malignant neoplasm of** cardia `HCC` `RxHCC`
Malignant neoplasm of cardiac orifice
Malignant neoplasm of cardio-esophageal junction
Malignant neoplasm of esophagus and stomach
Malignant neoplasm of gastro-esophageal junction

C16.1 **Malignant neoplasm of** fundus **of stomach** `HCC` `RxHCC`

C16.2 **Malignant neoplasm of** body **of stomach** `HCC` `RxHCC`

C16.3 **Malignant neoplasm of** pyloric antrum `HCC` `RxHCC`
Malignant neoplasm of gastric antrum

C16.4 **Malignant neoplasm of** pylorus `HCC` `RxHCC`
Malignant neoplasm of prepylorus
Malignant neoplasm of pyloric canal

C16.5 **Malignant neoplasm of** lesser curvature **of stomach, unspecified** `HCC` `RxHCC`
Malignant neoplasm of lesser curvature of stomach, not
  classifiable to C16.1-C16.4

C16.6 **Malignant neoplasm of** greater curvature **of stomach, unspecified** `HCC` `RxHCC`
Malignant neoplasm of greater curvature of stomach, not
  classifiable to C16.0-C16.4

C16.8 **Malignant neoplasm of** overlapping sites **of stomach** `HCC` `RxHCC`

C16.9 **Malignant neoplasm of stomach, unspecified** `HCC` `RxHCC`
Gastric cancer NOS

C17 **Malignant neoplasm of** small intestine
  EXCLUDES1 malignant carcinoid tumors of the small intestine (C7A.01)

C17.0 **Malignant neoplasm of** duodenum `HCC` `RxHCC`

C17.1 **Malignant neoplasm of** jejunum `HCC` `RxHCC`

C17.2 **Malignant neoplasm of** ileum `HCC` `RxHCC`
  EXCLUDES1 malignant neoplasm of ileocecal valve (C18.0)

C17.3 Meckel's diverticulum, **malignant** `HCC` `RxHCC`
  EXCLUDES1 Meckel's diverticulum, congenital (Q43.0)

C17.8 **Malignant neoplasm of** overlapping sites **of small intestine** `HCC` `RxHCC`

C17.9 **Malignant neoplasm of small intestine, unspecified** `HCC` `RxHCC`

C18 **Malignant neoplasm of** colon
  EXCLUDES1 malignant carcinoid tumors of the colon (C7A.02-)

C18.0 **Malignant neoplasm of** cecum `HCC`
Malignant neoplasm of ileocecal valve

C18.1 **Malignant neoplasm of** appendix `HCC`

C18.2 **Malignant neoplasm of** ascending colon `HCC`

C18.3 **Malignant neoplasm of** hepatic flexure `HCC`

C18.4 **Malignant neoplasm of** transverse colon `HCC`

C18.5 **Malignant neoplasm of** splenic flexure `HCC`

C18.6 **Malignant neoplasm of** descending colon `HCC`

C18.7 **Malignant neoplasm of** sigmoid colon `HCC`
Malignant neoplasm of sigmoid (flexure)
  EXCLUDES1 malignant neoplasm of rectosigmoid junction (C19)

C18.8 **Malignant neoplasm of** overlapping sites **of colon** `HCC`

Unspecified Code	Other Specified Code	Manifestation Code	N Newborn	P Pediatric	M Maternity	A Adult	♂ Male	♀ Female	

● New Code ▲ Revised Code Title ◄ Revised Text **NOTES** *INCLUDES* *EXCLUDES1* Not coded here *EXCLUDES2* Not included here
④ᵗʰ 4th character required ⑤ᵗʰ 5th character required ⑥ᵗʰ 6th character required ⑦ᵗʰ 7th character required ⑦ˣ Extension 'X' Alert
HAC Hospital-acquired condition (HAC) alert **AHA** AHA Coding Clinic© ☛ **Code first alert**

C18.9 **Malignant neoplasm of colon, unspecified** `HCC`
Malignant neoplasm of large intestine NOS

C19 **Malignant neoplasm of** rectosigmoid junction `HCC`
AHA: Q2 2002, Q4 2002
Malignant neoplasm of colon with rectum
Malignant neoplasm of rectosigmoid (colon)
EXCLUDES1 *malignant carcinoid tumors of the colon (C7A.02-)*

C20 **Malignant neoplasm of** rectum `HCC`
Malignant neoplasm of rectal ampulla
EXCLUDES1 *malignant carcinoid tumor of the rectum (C7A.026)*

C21 **Malignant neoplasm of** anus and anal canal
EXCLUDES2 *malignant carcinoid tumors of the colon (C7A.02-)*
malignant melanoma of anal margin (C43.51)
malignant melanoma of anal skin (C43.51)
malignant melanoma of perianal skin (C43.51)
other and unspecified malignant neoplasm of anal margin (C44.500, C44.510, C44.520, C44.590)
other and unspecified malignant neoplasm of anal skin (C44.500, C44.510, C44.520, C44.590)
other and unspecified malignant neoplasm of perianal skin (C44.500, C44.510, C44.520, C44.590)

C21.0 **Malignant neoplasm of** anus, unspecified `HCC`
C21.1 **Malignant neoplasm of** anal canal `HCC`
Malignant neoplasm of anal sphincter
C21.2 **Malignant neoplasm of** cloacogenic zone `HCC`
C21.8 **Malignant neoplasm of** overlapping sites **of rectum, anus and anal canal** `HCC`
Malignant neoplasm of anorectal junction
Malignant neoplasm of anorectum
Primary malignant neoplasm of two or more contiguous sites of rectum, anus and anal canal

C22 **Malignant neoplasm of** liver and intrahepatic bile ducts
EXCLUDES1 *malignant neoplasm of biliary tract NOS (C24.9)*
secondary malignant neoplasm of liver and intrahepatic bile duct (C78.7)
Use additional code to identify:
alcohol abuse and dependence (F10.-)
hepatitis B (B16.-, B18.0-B18.1)
hepatitis C (B17.1-, B18.2)

C22.0 **Liver cell** carcinoma `HCC` `RxHCC`
AHA: Q1 2016
Hepatocellular carcinoma
Hepatoma
C22.1 Intrahepatic bile duct **carcinoma** `HCC` `RxHCC`
Cholangiocarcinoma
EXCLUDES1 *malignant neoplasm of hepatic duct (C24.0)*
C22.2 **Hepatoblastoma** `HCC` `RxHCC`
C22.3 Angiosarcoma **of liver** `HCC` `RxHCC`
Kupffer cell sarcoma
C22.4 Other **sarcomas of liver** `HCC` `RxHCC`
C22.7 Other specified carcinomas of liver `HCC` `RxHCC`
C22.8 **Malignant neoplasm of liver,** primary, **unspecified** as to type `HCC` `RxHCC`
C22.9 **Malignant neoplasm of liver,** not specified as primary or secondary `HCC` `RxHCC`

C23 **Malignant neoplasm of** gallbladder `HCC` `RxHCC`
C24 **Malignant neoplasm of other and unspecified parts of** biliary tract
EXCLUDES1 *malignant neoplasm of intrahepatic bile duct (C22.1)*
C24.0 **Malignant neoplasm of** extrahepatic bile duct `HCC` `RxHCC`
Malignant neoplasm of biliary duct or passage NOS
Malignant neoplasm of common bile duct
Malignant neoplasm of cystic duct
Malignant neoplasm of hepatic duct
C24.1 **Malignant neoplasm of** ampulla of Vater `HCC` `RxHCC`
C24.8 **Malignant neoplasm of** overlapping sites **of biliary tract** `HCC` `RxHCC`
Malignant neoplasm involving both intrahepatic and extrahepatic bile ducts
Primary malignant neoplasm of two or more contiguous sites of biliary tract
C24.9 **Malignant neoplasm of biliary tract, unspecified** `HCC` `RxHCC`

C25 **Malignant neoplasm of** pancreas
Code also exocrine pancreatic insufficiency (K86.81)
Use additional code to identify:
alcohol abuse and dependence (F10.-)
C25.0 **Malignant neoplasm of** head of pancreas `HCC` `RxHCC`
C25.1 **Malignant neoplasm of** body of pancreas `HCC` `RxHCC`
AHA: Q4 2018
C25.2 **Malignant neoplasm of** tail of pancreas `HCC` `RxHCC`
C25.3 **Malignant neoplasm of** pancreatic duct `HCC` `RxHCC`
C25.4 **Malignant neoplasm of** endocrine pancreas `HCC` `RxHCC`
Malignant neoplasm of islets of Langerhans
Use additional code to identify any functional activity.
C25.7 **Malignant neoplasm of** other parts of pancreas `HCC` `RxHCC`
Malignant neoplasm of neck of pancreas
C25.8 **Malignant neoplasm of** overlapping sites of pancreas `HCC` `RxHCC`
C25.9 **Malignant neoplasm of pancreas, unspecified** `HCC` `RxHCC`
AHA: Q4 2017

C26 **Malignant neoplasm of other and ill-defined** digestive organs
EXCLUDES1 *malignant neoplasm of peritoneum and retroperitoneum (C48.-)*
C26.0 **Malignant neoplasm of** intestinal tract**, part unspecified** `HCC`
Malignant neoplasm of intestine NOS
C26.1 **Malignant neoplasm of** spleen `HCC`
EXCLUDES1 *Hodgkin lymphoma (C81.-)*
non-Hodgkin lymphoma (C82-C85)
C26.9 **Malignant neoplasm of** ill-defined sites **within the digestive system** `HCC`
Malignant neoplasm of alimentary canal or tract NOS
Malignant neoplasm of gastrointestinal tract NOS
EXCLUDES1 *malignant neoplasm of abdominal NOS (C76.2)*
malignant neoplasm of intra-abdominal NOS (C76.2)

Malignant neoplasms of respiratory and intrathoracic organs (C30-C39)

INCLUDES *malignant neoplasm of middle ear*
EXCLUDES1 *mesothelioma (C45.-)*

C30 **Malignant neoplasm of** nasal cavity and middle ear
C30.0 **Malignant neoplasm of** nasal cavity `HCC`
Malignant neoplasm of cartilage of nose
Malignant neoplasm of nasal concha
Malignant neoplasm of internal nose
Malignant neoplasm of septum of nose
Malignant neoplasm of vestibule of nose
EXCLUDES1 *malignant neoplasm of nasal bone (C41.0)*
malignant neoplasm of nose NOS (C76.0)
malignant neoplasm of olfactory bulb (C72.2-)
malignant neoplasm of posterior margin of nasal septum and choana (C11.3)
malignant melanoma of skin of nose (C43.31)
malignant neoplasm of turbinates (C41.0)
other and unspecified malignant neoplasm of skin of nose C44.301, C44.311, C44.321, C44.391)
C30.1 **Malignant neoplasm of** middle ear `HCC`
Malignant neoplasm of antrum tympanicum
Malignant neoplasm of auditory tube
Malignant neoplasm of eustachian tube
Malignant neoplasm of inner ear
Malignant neoplasm of mastoid air cells
Malignant neoplasm of tympanic cavity
EXCLUDES1 *malignant neoplasm of auricular canal (external) (C43.2-,C44.2-)*
malignant neoplasm of bone of ear (meatus) (C41.0)
malignant neoplasm of cartilage of ear (C49.0)
malignant melanoma of skin of (external) ear (C43.2-)
other and unspecified malignant neoplasm of skin of (external) ear (C44.2-)

`PDx` Unacceptable principal diagnosis symbol per Medicare code edits `POA` Code exempt from diagnosis present on admission requirement
? Questionable admission `CC` Complication or comorbidity `MCC` Major complication or comorbidity `CC/MCC Excl` CC/MCC exclusion
`HCC` HCC diagnosis code `RxHCC` RxHCC diagnosis code MACRA code **DEFINITION** Describes condition/terminology
TIP Coding guidance 👁 Official Guideline Reference `Z1` Z code as first-listed diagnosis

C31 - C40

⁴ᵗʰ **C31** Malignant neoplasm of accessory sinuses

    C31.0 **Malignant neoplasm of** maxillary **sinus** `HCC`
        Malignant neoplasm of antrum (Highmore) (maxillary)

    C31.1 **Malignant neoplasm of** ethmoidal **sinus** `HCC`

    C31.2 **Malignant neoplasm of** frontal **sinus** `HCC`

    C31.3 **Malignant neoplasm of** sphenoid **sinus** `HCC`

    C31.8 **Malignant neoplasm of** overlapping sites **of accessory sinuses** `HCC`

    C31.9 **Malignant neoplasm of accessory sinus, unspecified** `HCC`

⁴ᵗʰ **C32** Malignant neoplasm of larynx

    Use additional code to identify:
      alcohol abuse and dependence (F10.-)
      exposure to environmental tobacco smoke (Z77.22)
      exposure to tobacco smoke in the perinatal period (P96.81)
      history of tobacco dependence (Z87.891)
      occupational exposure to environmental tobacco smoke (Z57.31)
      tobacco dependence (F17.-)
      tobacco use (Z72.0)

    C32.0 **Malignant neoplasm of** glottis `HCC`
        Malignant neoplasm of intrinsic larynx
        Malignant neoplasm of laryngeal commissure (anterior) (posterior)
        Malignant neoplasm of vocal cord (true) NOS

    C32.1 **Malignant neoplasm of** supraglottis `HCC`
        Malignant neoplasm of aryepiglottic fold or interarytenoid fold, laryngeal aspect
        Malignant neoplasm of epiglottis (suprahyoid portion) NOS
        Malignant neoplasm of extrinsic larynx
        Malignant neoplasm of false vocal cord
        Malignant neoplasm of posterior (laryngeal) surface of epiglottis
        Malignant neoplasm of ventricular bands

        `EXCLUDES2` *malignant neoplasm of anterior surface of epiglottis (C10.1)*
          malignant neoplasm of aryepiglottic fold or interarytenoid fold, hypopharyngeal aspect (C13.1)
          malignant neoplasm of aryepiglottic fold or interarytenoid fold, marginal zone (C13.1)
          malignant neoplasm of aryepiglottic fold or interarytenoid fold NOS (C13.1)

    C32.2 **Malignant neoplasm of** subglottis `HCC`

    C32.3 **Malignant neoplasm of** laryngeal cartilage `HCC`

    C32.8 **Malignant neoplasm of** overlapping sites **of larynx** `HCC`

    C32.9 **Malignant neoplasm of larynx, unspecified** `HCC`

C33 **Malignant neoplasm of** trachea `HCC` `RxHCC`

    Use additional code to identify:
      exposure to environmental tobacco smoke (Z77.22)
      exposure to tobacco smoke in the perinatal period (P96.81)
      history of tobacco dependence (Z87.891)
      occupational exposure to environmental tobacco smoke (Z57.31)
      tobacco dependence (F17.-)
      tobacco use (Z72.0)

⁴ᵗʰ **C34** Malignant neoplasm of bronchus and lung

    Use additional code to identify:
      exposure to environmental tobacco smoke (Z77.22)
      exposure to tobacco smoke in the perinatal period (P96.81)
      history of tobacco dependence (Z87.891)
      occupational exposure to environmental tobacco smoke (Z57.31)
      tobacco dependence (F17.-)
      tobacco use (Z72.0)

    `EXCLUDES1` *Kaposi's sarcoma of lung (C46.5-)*
      malignant carcinoid tumor of the bronchus and lung (C7A.090)

    ⁵ᵗʰ **C34.0** **Malignant neoplasm of** main bronchus
        Malignant neoplasm of carina
        Malignant neoplasm of hilus (of lung)

        C34.00 **Malignant neoplasm of unspecified main bronchus** `HCC` `RxHCC`

        C34.01 **Malignant neoplasm of** right **main bronchus** `HCC` `RxHCC`

        C34.02 **Malignant neoplasm of** left **main bronchus** `HCC` `RxHCC`

---

    ⁵ᵗʰ **C34.1** **Malignant neoplasm of** upper lobe, **bronchus or lung**

        C34.10 **Malignant neoplasm of upper lobe, unspecified bronchus or lung** `HCC` `RxHCC`

        C34.11 **Malignant neoplasm of upper lobe,** right **bronchus or lung** `HCC` `RxHCC`

        C34.12 **Malignant neoplasm of upper lobe,** left **bronchus or lung** `HCC` `RxHCC`

    C34.2 **Malignant neoplasm of** middle lobe, **bronchus or lung** `HCC` `RxHCC`

    ⁵ᵗʰ **C34.3** **Malignant neoplasm of** lower lobe, **bronchus or lung**

        C34.30 **Malignant neoplasm of lower lobe, unspecified bronchus or lung** `HCC` `RxHCC`

        C34.31 **Malignant neoplasm of lower lobe,** right **bronchus or lung** `HCC` `RxHCC`

        C34.32 **Malignant neoplasm of lower lobe,** left **bronchus or lung** `HCC` `RxHCC`

    ⁵ᵗʰ **C34.8** **Malignant neoplasm of** overlapping sites **of bronchus and lung**

        C34.80 **Malignant neoplasm of overlapping sites of unspecified bronchus and lung** `HCC` `RxHCC`

        C34.81 **Malignant neoplasm of overlapping sites of** right **bronchus and lung** `HCC` `RxHCC`

        C34.82 **Malignant neoplasm of overlapping sites of** left **bronchus and lung** `HCC` `RxHCC`

    ⁵ᵗʰ **C34.9** **Malignant neoplasm of** unspecified part **of bronchus or lung**

        C34.90 **Malignant neoplasm of unspecified part of unspecified bronchus or lung** `HCC` `RxHCC`
          Lung cancer NOS

        C34.91 **Malignant neoplasm of unspecified part of** right **bronchus or lung** `HCC` `RxHCC`

        C34.92 **Malignant neoplasm of unspecified part of** left **bronchus or lung** `HCC` `RxHCC`

C37 **Malignant neoplasm of** thymus `HCC`

    `EXCLUDES1` *malignant carcinoid tumor of the thymus (C7A.091)*

⁴ᵗʰ **C38** Malignant neoplasm of heart, mediastinum and pleura

    `EXCLUDES1` *mesothelioma (C45.-)*

    C38.0 **Malignant neoplasm of** heart `HCC`
        Malignant neoplasm of pericardium
        `EXCLUDES1` *malignant neoplasm of great vessels (C49.3)*

    C38.1 **Malignant neoplasm of** anterior mediastinum `HCC`

    C38.2 **Malignant neoplasm of** posterior mediastinum `HCC`

    C38.3 **Malignant neoplasm of** mediastinum, **part unspecified** `HCC`

    C38.4 **Malignant neoplasm of** pleura `HCC` `RxHCC`

    C38.8 **Malignant neoplasm of** overlapping sites **of heart, mediastinum and pleura** `HCC`

⁴ᵗʰ **C39** Malignant neoplasm of other and ill-defined sites in the respiratory system and intrathoracic organs

    Use additional code to identify:
      exposure to environmental tobacco smoke (Z77.22)
      exposure to tobacco smoke in the perinatal period (P96.81)
      history of tobacco dependence (Z87.891)
      occupational exposure to environmental tobacco smoke (Z57.31)
      tobacco dependence (F17.-)
      tobacco use (Z72.0)

    `EXCLUDES1` *intrathoracic malignant neoplasm NOS (C76.1)*
      thoracic malignant neoplasm NOS (C76.1)

    C39.0 **Malignant neoplasm of** upper **respiratory tract, part unspecified** `HCC`

    C39.9 **Malignant neoplasm of** lower **respiratory tract, part unspecified** `HCC`
        Malignant neoplasm of respiratory tract NOS

Malignant neoplasms of bone and articular cartilage (C40-C41)

    `INCLUDES` *malignant neoplasm of cartilage (articular) (joint)*
      malignant neoplasm of periosteum
    `EXCLUDES1` *malignant neoplasm of bone marrow NOS (C96.9)*
      malignant neoplasm of synovia (C49.-)

⁴ᵗʰ **C40** Malignant neoplasm of bone and articular cartilage of limbs
    Use additional code to identify major osseous defect, if applicable (M89.7-)

🔟 C40.0 **Malignant neoplasm of** scapula and long bones of upper limb
    C40.00 **Malignant neoplasm of scapula and long bones of unspecified upper limb** `HCC` `RxHCC`
    C40.01 **Malignant neoplasm of scapula and long bones of** right **upper limb** `HCC` `RxHCC`
    C40.02 **Malignant neoplasm of scapula and long bones of** left **upper limb** `HCC` `RxHCC`

🔟 C40.1 **Malignant neoplasm of** short bones of upper limb
    C40.10 **Malignant neoplasm of short bones of unspecified upper limb** `HCC` `RxHCC`
    C40.11 **Malignant neoplasm of short bones of** right **upper limb** `HCC` `RxHCC`
    C40.12 **Malignant neoplasm of short bones of** left **upper limb** `HCC` `RxHCC`

🔟 C40.2 **Malignant neoplasm of** long bones of lower limb
    C40.20 **Malignant neoplasm of long bones of unspecified lower limb** `HCC` `RxHCC`
    C40.21 **Malignant neoplasm of long bones of** right **lower limb** `HCC` `RxHCC`
    C40.22 **Malignant neoplasm of long bones of** left **lower limb** `HCC` `RxHCC`

🔟 C40.3 **Malignant neoplasm of** short bones of lower limb
    C40.30 **Malignant neoplasm of short bones of unspecified lower limb** `HCC` `RxHCC`
    C40.31 **Malignant neoplasm of short bones of** right **lower limb** `HCC` `RxHCC`
    C40.32 **Malignant neoplasm of short bones of** left **lower limb** `HCC` `RxHCC`

🔟 C40.8 **Malignant neoplasm of** overlapping sites **of bone and articular cartilage of limb**
    C40.80 **Malignant neoplasm of overlapping sites of bone and articular cartilage of unspecified limb** `HCC` `RxHCC`
    C40.81 **Malignant neoplasm of overlapping sites of bone and articular cartilage of** right **limb** `CC` `HCC` `RxHCC` `CC/MCC Exc`
    C40.82 **Malignant neoplasm of overlapping sites of bone and articular cartilage of** left **limb** `HCC` `RxHCC`

🔟 C40.9 **Malignant neoplasm of** unspecified bones **and articular cartilage of limb**
    C40.90 **Malignant neoplasm of unspecified bones and articular cartilage of unspecified limb** `HCC` `RxHCC`
    C40.91 **Malignant neoplasm of unspecified bones and articular cartilage of** right **limb** `HCC` `RxHCC`
    C40.92 **Malignant neoplasm of unspecified bones and articular cartilage of** left **limb** `HCC` `RxHCC`

4️⃣ C41 **Malignant neoplasm of bone and articular cartilage of** other and unspecified sites
    EXCLUDES1 *malignant neoplasm of bones of limbs (C40.-)*
          malignant neoplasm of cartilage of ear (C49.0)
          malignant neoplasm of cartilage of eyelid (C49.0)
          malignant neoplasm of cartilage of larynx (C32.3)
          malignant neoplasm of cartilage of limbs (C40.-)
          malignant neoplasm of cartilage of nose (C30.0)

    C41.0 **Malignant neoplasm of bones of** skull and face `HCC` `RxHCC`
        Malignant neoplasm of maxilla (superior)
        Malignant neoplasm of orbital bone
        EXCLUDES2 *carcinoma, any type except intraosseous or odontogenic of:*
            maxillary sinus (C31.0)
            upper jaw (C03.0)
            malignant neoplasm of jaw bone (lower) (C41.1)

    C41.1 **Malignant neoplasm of** mandible `HCC` `RxHCC`
        Malignant neoplasm of inferior maxilla
        Malignant neoplasm of lower jaw bone
        EXCLUDES2 *carcinoma, any type except intraosseous or odontogenic of:*
            jaw NOS (C03.9)
            lower (C03.1)
            malignant neoplasm of upper jaw bone (C41.0)

    C41.2 **Malignant neoplasm of** vertebral column `HCC` `RxHCC`
        EXCLUDES1 *malignant neoplasm of sacrum and coccyx (C41.4)*

    C41.3 **Malignant neoplasm of** ribs, sternum and clavicle `HCC` `RxHCC`
    C41.4 **Malignant neoplasm of** pelvic bones, sacrum and coccyx `HCC` `RxHCC`
    C41.9 **Malignant neoplasm of** bone and articular cartilage, **unspecified** `HCC` `RxHCC`

Melanoma and other malignant neoplasms of skin (C43-C44)

4️⃣ C43 **Malignant melanoma of** skin
    EXCLUDES1 *melanoma in situ (D03.-)*
    EXCLUDES2 *malignant melanoma of skin of genital organs (C51-C52, C60.-, C63.-)*
            Merkel cell carcinoma (C4A.-)
            sites other than skin-code to malignant neoplasm of the site

    C43.0 **Malignant melanoma of** lip `HCC`
        EXCLUDES1 *malignant neoplasm of vermilion border of lip (C00.0-C00.2)*

🔟 C43.1 **Malignant melanoma of** eyelid, including canthus
    C43.10 **Malignant melanoma of unspecified eyelid, including canthus** `HCC`
   6️⃣ C43.11 **Malignant melanoma of** right **eyelid, including canthus**
        C43.111 **Malignant melanoma of right** upper **eyelid, including canthus** `HCC`
            AHA: Q4 2018
        C43.112 **Malignant melanoma of right** lower **eyelid, including canthus** `HCC`
            AHA: Q4 2018
   6️⃣ C43.12 **Malignant melanoma of** left **eyelid, including canthus**
        C43.121 **Malignant melanoma of left** upper **eyelid, including canthus** `HCC`
            AHA: Q4 2018
        C43.122 **Malignant melanoma of left** lower **eyelid, including canthus** `HCC`
            AHA: Q4 2018

🔟 C43.2 **Malignant melanoma of** ear and external auricular canal
    C43.20 **Malignant melanoma of unspecified ear and external auricular canal** `HCC`
    C43.21 **Malignant melanoma of** right **ear and external auricular canal** `HCC`
    C43.22 **Malignant melanoma of** left **ear and external auricular canal** `HCC`

🔟 C43.3 **Malignant melanoma of** other and unspecified parts of face
    C43.30 **Malignant melanoma of unspecified part of face** `HCC`
    C43.31 **Malignant melanoma of** nose `HCC`
    C43.39 **Malignant melanoma of** other parts of face `HCC`
    C43.4 **Malignant melanoma of** scalp and neck `HCC`

🔟 C43.5 **Malignant melanoma of** trunk
    EXCLUDES2 *malignant neoplasm of anus NOS (C21.0)*
            malignant neoplasm of scrotum (C63.2)
    C43.51 **Malignant melanoma of** anal skin `HCC`
        Malignant melanoma of anal margin
        Malignant melanoma of perianal skin
    C43.52 **Malignant melanoma of** skin of breast `HCC`
    C43.59 **Malignant melanoma of** other part of trunk `HCC`

🔟 C43.6 **Malignant melanoma of** upper limb, including shoulder
    C43.60 **Malignant melanoma of unspecified upper limb, including shoulder** `HCC`
    C43.61 **Malignant melanoma of** right **upper limb, including shoulder** `HCC`
    C43.62 **Malignant melanoma of** left **upper limb, including shoulder** `HCC`

🔟 C43.7 **Malignant melanoma of** lower limb, including hip
    C43.70 **Malignant melanoma of unspecified lower limb, including hip** `HCC`
    C43.71 **Malignant melanoma of** right **lower limb, including hip** `HCC`
    C43.72 **Malignant melanoma of** left **lower limb, including hip** `HCC`
    C43.8 **Malignant melanoma of** overlapping sites **of skin** `HCC`

PDx🚫 Unacceptable principal diagnosis symbol per Medicare code edits   POA Code exempt from diagnosis present on admission requirement
❓ Questionable admission   CC Complication or comorbidity   MCC Major complication or comorbidity   CC/MCC Exc CC/MCC exclusion
`HCC` HCC diagnosis code   `RxHCC` RxHCC diagnosis code   MACRA MACRA code   **DEFINITION** Describes condition/terminology
TIP Coding guidance   👁 Official Guideline Reference   Z1 Z code as first-listed diagnosis

When symbols appear on a code that requires a 7th character extension, refer to Appendix B to identify applicable 7th character codes.   **2020 ICD-10-CM**

C43.9 **Malignant melanoma of skin, unspecified** [HCC]
Malignant melanoma of unspecified site of skin
Melanoma (malignant) NOS

[4th] C4A **Merkel cell carcinoma**

C4A.0 **Merkel cell carcinoma of lip** [HCC] [RxHCC]
[EXCLUDES1] *malignant neoplasm of vermilion border of lip (C00.0-C00.2)*

[5th] C4A.1 **Merkel cell carcinoma of eyelid, including canthus**
C4A.10 **Merkel cell carcinoma of unspecified eyelid, including canthus** [HCC] [RxHCC]
[6th] C4A.11 **Merkel cell carcinoma of right eyelid, including canthus**
C4A.111 **Merkel cell carcinoma of right upper eyelid, including canthus** [HCC] [RxHCC]
AHA: Q4 2018
C4A.112 **Merkel cell carcinoma of right lower eyelid, including canthus** [HCC] [RxHCC]
AHA: Q4 2018
[6th] C4A.12 **Merkel cell carcinoma of left eyelid, including canthus**
C4A.121 **Merkel cell carcinoma of left upper eyelid, including canthus** [HCC] [RxHCC]
AHA: Q4 2018
C4A.122 **Merkel cell carcinoma of left lower eyelid, including canthus** [HCC] [RxHCC]
AHA: Q4 2018

[5th] C4A.2 **Merkel cell carcinoma of ear and external auricular canal**
C4A.20 **Merkel cell carcinoma of unspecified ear and external auricular canal** [HCC] [RxHCC]
C4A.21 **Merkel cell carcinoma of right ear and external auricular canal** [HCC] [RxHCC]
C4A.22 **Merkel cell carcinoma of left ear and external auricular canal** [HCC] [RxHCC]

[5th] C4A.3 **Merkel cell carcinoma of other and unspecified parts of face**
C4A.30 **Merkel cell carcinoma of unspecified part of face** [HCC] [RxHCC]
C4A.31 **Merkel cell carcinoma of nose** [HCC] [RxHCC]
C4A.39 **Merkel cell carcinoma of other parts of face** [HCC] [RxHCC]

C4A.4 **Merkel cell carcinoma of scalp and neck** [HCC] [RxHCC]

[5th] C4A.5 **Merkel cell carcinoma of trunk**
[EXCLUDES2] *malignant neoplasm of anus NOS (C21.0)*
malignant neoplasm of scrotum (C63.2)
C4A.51 **Merkel cell carcinoma of anal skin** [HCC] [RxHCC]
Merkel cell carcinoma of anal margin
Merkel cell carcinoma of perianal skin
C4A.52 **Merkel cell carcinoma of skin of breast** [HCC] [RxHCC]
C4A.59 **Merkel cell carcinoma of other part of trunk** [HCC] [RxHCC]

[5th] C4A.6 **Merkel cell carcinoma of upper limb, including shoulder**
C4A.60 **Merkel cell carcinoma of unspecified upper limb, including shoulder** [HCC] [RxHCC]
C4A.61 **Merkel cell carcinoma of right upper limb, including shoulder** [HCC] [RxHCC]
C4A.62 **Merkel cell carcinoma of left upper limb, including shoulder** [HCC] [RxHCC]

[5th] C4A.7 **Merkel cell carcinoma of lower limb, including hip**
C4A.70 **Merkel cell carcinoma of unspecified lower limb, including hip** [HCC] [RxHCC]
C4A.71 **Merkel cell carcinoma of right lower limb, including hip** [HCC] [RxHCC]
C4A.72 **Merkel cell carcinoma of left lower limb, including hip** [HCC] [RxHCC]

C4A.8 **Merkel cell carcinoma of overlapping sites** [HCC] [RxHCC]
C4A.9 **Merkel cell carcinoma, unspecified** [HCC] [RxHCC]
Merkel cell carcinoma of unspecified site
Merkel cell carcinoma NOS

[4th] C44 **Other and unspecified malignant neoplasm of skin (Figure 2.1)**
[INCLUDES] *malignant neoplasm of sebaceous glands*
malignant neoplasm of sweat glands
[EXCLUDES1] *Kaposi's sarcoma of skin (C46.0)*
malignant melanoma of skin (C43.-)
malignant neoplasm of skin of genital organs (C51-C52, C60.-, C63.2)
Merkel cell carcinoma (C4A.-)

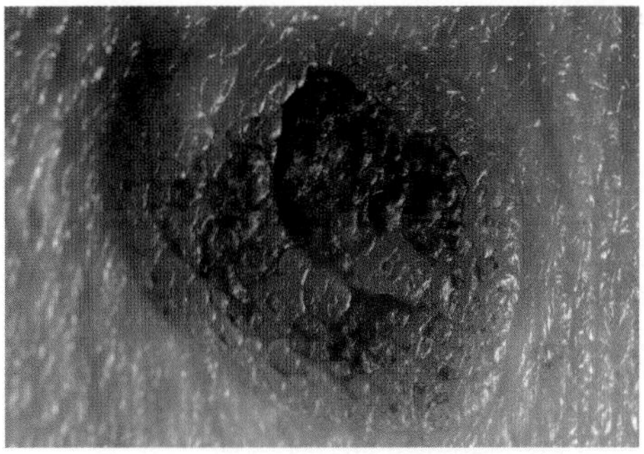

Figure 2.1 Malignant Neoplasm of Skin

[5th] C44.0 **Other and unspecified malignant neoplasm of skin of lip**
[EXCLUDES1] *malignant neoplasm of lip (C00.-)*
C44.00 **Unspecified malignant neoplasm of skin of lip**
C44.01 **Basal cell carcinoma of skin of lip**
C44.02 **Squamous cell carcinoma of skin of lip**
C44.09 **Other specified malignant neoplasm of skin of lip**

[5th] C44.1 **Other and unspecified malignant neoplasm of skin of eyelid, including canthus**
[EXCLUDES1] *connective tissue of eyelid (C49.0)*
The appropriate 7th character is to be added to each code that specifies laterality from subcategory C44.1*:
1 – upper eyelid
2 – lower eyelid

[6th] C44.10 **Unspecified malignant neoplasm of skin of eyelid, including canthus**
C44.101 **Unspecified malignant neoplasm of skin of unspecified eyelid, including canthus**
[7th] C44.102 **Unspecified malignant neoplasm of skin of right eyelid, including canthus**
AHA: Q4 2018
[7th] C44.109 **Unspecified malignant neoplasm of skin of left eyelid, including canthus**
AHA: Q4 2018

[6th] C44.11 **Basal cell carcinoma of skin of eyelid, including canthus**
C44.111 **Basal cell carcinoma of skin of unspecified eyelid, including canthus**
[7th] C44.112 **Basal cell carcinoma of skin of right eyelid, including canthus**
AHA: Q4 2018
[7th] C44.119 **Basal cell carcinoma of skin of left eyelid, including canthus**
AHA: Q4 2018

[6th] C44.12 **Squamous cell carcinoma of skin of eyelid, including canthus**
C44.121 **Squamous cell carcinoma of skin of unspecified eyelid, including canthus**
[7th] C44.122 **Squamous cell carcinoma of skin of right eyelid, including canthus**
AHA: Q4 2018
[7th] C44.129 **Squamous cell carcinoma of skin of left eyelid, including canthus**
AHA: Q4 2018

[6th] C44.13 **Sebaceous cell carcinoma of skin of eyelid, including canthus**
C44.131 **Sebaceous cell carcinoma of skin of unspecified eyelid, including canthus**
AHA: Q4 2018
[7th] C44.132 **Sebaceous cell carcinoma of skin of right eyelid, including canthus**
AHA: Q4 2018
[7th] C44.139 **Sebaceous cell carcinoma of skin of left eyelid, including canthus**
AHA: Q4 2018

[6th] C44.19 **Other specified malignant neoplasm of skin of eyelid, including canthus**

Unspecified Code Other Specified Code Manifestation Code [N] Newborn [P] Pediatric [M] Maternity [A] Adult ♂ Male ♀ Female
● New Code ▲ Revised Code Title ►◄ Revised Text [NOTES] [INCLUDES] [EXCLUDES1] Not coded here [EXCLUDES2] Not included here
[4th] 4th character required [5th] 5th character required [6th] 6th character required [7th] 7th character required [x7th] Extension 'X' Alert
[HAC] Hospital-acquired condition (HAC) alert **AHA** AHA Coding Clinic© ☞ Code first alert

 When symbols appear on a code that requires a 7th character extension, refer to Appendix B to identify applicable 7th character codes.

*CMS does not include 7th character options for several codes under category C44. The publisher added the 7th character options. At press time, CMS did not issue an errata to correct these errors.

C44.191 Other specified malignant neoplasm of skin of unspecified eyelid, including canthus

[7th] C44.192 Other specified malignant neoplasm of skin of right eyelid, including canthus
AHA: Q4 2018

[7th] C44.199 Other specified malignant neoplasm of skin of left eyelid, including canthus
AHA: Q4 2018

[5th] **C44.2 Other and unspecified malignant neoplasm of skin of ear and external auricular canal**

EXCLUDES1 *connective tissue of ear (C49.0)*

[6th] **C44.20 Unspecified malignant neoplasm of skin of ear and external auricular canal**

C44.201 Unspecified malignant neoplasm of skin of unspecified ear and external auricular canal

C44.202 Unspecified malignant neoplasm of skin of right ear and external auricular canal

C44.209 Unspecified malignant neoplasm of skin of left ear and external auricular canal

[6th] **C44.21 Basal cell carcinoma of skin of ear and external auricular canal**

C44.211 Basal cell carcinoma of skin of unspecified ear and external auricular canal

C44.212 Basal cell carcinoma of skin of right ear and external auricular canal

C44.219 Basal cell carcinoma of skin of left ear and external auricular canal

[6th] **C44.22 Squamous cell carcinoma of skin of ear and external auricular canal**

C44.221 Squamous cell carcinoma of skin of unspecified ear and external auricular canal

C44.222 Squamous cell carcinoma of skin of right ear and external auricular canal

C44.229 Squamous cell carcinoma of skin of left ear and external auricular canal

[6th] **C44.29 Other specified malignant neoplasm of skin of ear and external auricular canal**

C44.291 Other specified malignant neoplasm of skin of unspecified ear and external auricular canal

C44.292 Other specified malignant neoplasm of skin of right ear and external auricular canal

C44.299 Other specified malignant neoplasm of skin of left ear and external auricular canal

[5th] **C44.3 Other and unspecified malignant neoplasm of skin of other and unspecified parts of face**

[6th] **C44.30 Unspecified malignant neoplasm of skin of other and unspecified parts of face**

C44.300 Unspecified malignant neoplasm of skin of unspecified part of face

C44.301 Unspecified malignant neoplasm of skin of nose

C44.309 Unspecified malignant neoplasm of skin of other parts of face

[6th] **C44.31 Basal cell carcinoma of skin of other and unspecified parts of face**

C44.310 Basal cell carcinoma of skin of unspecified parts of face

C44.311 Basal cell carcinoma of skin of nose

C44.319 Basal cell carcinoma of skin of other parts of face

[6th] **C44.32 Squamous cell carcinoma of skin of other and unspecified parts of face**

C44.320 Squamous cell carcinoma of skin of unspecified parts of face

C44.321 Squamous cell carcinoma of skin of nose

C44.329 Squamous cell carcinoma of skin of other parts of face

[6th] **C44.39 Other specified malignant neoplasm of skin of other and unspecified parts of face**

C44.390 Other specified malignant neoplasm of skin of unspecified parts of face

C44.391 Other specified malignant neoplasm of skin of nose

C44.399 Other specified malignant neoplasm of skin of other parts of face

[5th] **C44.4 Other and unspecified malignant neoplasm of skin of scalp and neck**

C44.40 Unspecified malignant neoplasm of skin of scalp and neck

C44.41 Basal cell carcinoma of skin of scalp and neck

C44.42 Squamous cell carcinoma of skin of scalp and neck

C44.49 Other specified malignant neoplasm of skin of scalp and neck

[5th] **C44.5 Other and unspecified malignant neoplasm of skin of trunk**

EXCLUDES1 *anus NOS (C21.0)*
scrotum (C63.2)

[6th] **C44.50 Unspecified malignant neoplasm of skin of trunk**

C44.500 Unspecified malignant neoplasm of anal skin
Unspecified malignant neoplasm of anal margin
Unspecified malignant neoplasm of perianal skin

C44.501 Unspecified malignant neoplasm of skin of breast

C44.509 Unspecified malignant neoplasm of skin of other part of trunk

[6th] **C44.51 Basal cell carcinoma of skin of trunk**

C44.510 Basal cell carcinoma of anal skin
Basal cell carcinoma of anal margin
Basal cell carcinoma of perianal skin

C44.511 Basal cell carcinoma of skin of breast

C44.519 Basal cell carcinoma of skin of other part of trunk

[6th] **C44.52 Squamous cell carcinoma of skin of trunk**

C44.520 Squamous cell carcinoma of anal skin
Squamous cell carcinoma of anal margin
Squamous cell carcinoma of perianal skin

C44.521 Squamous cell carcinoma of skin of breast

C44.529 Squamous cell carcinoma of skin of other part of trunk

[6th] **C44.59 Other specified malignant neoplasm of skin of trunk**

C44.590 Other specified malignant neoplasm of anal skin
Other specified malignant neoplasm of anal margin
Other specified malignant neoplasm of perianal skin

C44.591 Other specified malignant neoplasm of skin of breast

C44.599 Other specified malignant neoplasm of skin of other part of trunk

[5th] **C44.6 Other and unspecified malignant neoplasm of skin of upper limb, including shoulder**

[6th] **C44.60 Unspecified malignant neoplasm of skin of upper limb, including shoulder**

C44.601 Unspecified malignant neoplasm of skin of unspecified upper limb, including shoulder

C44.602 Unspecified malignant neoplasm of skin of right upper limb, including shoulder

C44.609 Unspecified malignant neoplasm of skin of left upper limb, including shoulder

[6th] **C44.61 Basal cell carcinoma of skin of upper limb, including shoulder**

C44.611 Basal cell carcinoma of skin of unspecified upper limb, including shoulder

C44.612 Basal cell carcinoma of skin of right upper limb, including shoulder

C44.619 Basal cell carcinoma of skin of left upper limb, including shoulder

[6th] C44.62 Squamous cell carcinoma of skin of upper limb, including shoulder
- C44.621 Squamous cell carcinoma of skin of unspecified upper limb, including shoulder
- C44.622 Squamous cell carcinoma of skin of right upper limb, including shoulder
- C44.629 Squamous cell carcinoma of skin of left upper limb, including shoulder

[6th] C44.69 Other specified malignant neoplasm of skin of upper limb, including shoulder
- C44.691 Other specified malignant neoplasm of skin of unspecified upper limb, including shoulder
- C44.692 Other specified malignant neoplasm of skin of right upper limb, including shoulder
- C44.699 Other specified malignant neoplasm of skin of left upper limb, including shoulder

[5th] C44.7 Other and unspecified malignant neoplasm of skin of lower limb, including hip

[6th] C44.70 Unspecified malignant neoplasm of skin of lower limb, including hip
- C44.701 Unspecified malignant neoplasm of skin of unspecified lower limb, including hip
- C44.702 Unspecified malignant neoplasm of skin of right lower limb, including hip
- C44.709 Unspecified malignant neoplasm of skin of left lower limb, including hip

[6th] C44.71 Basal cell carcinoma of skin of lower limb, including hip
- C44.711 Basal cell carcinoma of skin of unspecified lower limb, including hip
- C44.712 Basal cell carcinoma of skin of right lower limb, including hip
- C44.719 Basal cell carcinoma of skin of left lower limb, including hip

[6th] C44.72 Squamous cell carcinoma of skin of lower limb, including hip
- C44.721 Squamous cell carcinoma of skin of unspecified lower limb, including hip
- C44.722 Squamous cell carcinoma of skin of right lower limb, including hip
- C44.729 Squamous cell carcinoma of skin of left lower limb, including hip

[6th] C44.79 Other specified malignant neoplasm of skin of lower limb, including hip
- C44.791 Other specified malignant neoplasm of skin of unspecified lower limb, including hip
- C44.792 Other specified malignant neoplasm of skin of right lower limb, including hip
- C44.799 Other specified malignant neoplasm of skin of left lower limb, including hip

[5th] C44.8 Other and unspecified malignant neoplasm of overlapping sites of skin
- C44.80 Unspecified malignant neoplasm of overlapping sites of skin
- C44.81 Basal cell carcinoma of overlapping sites of skin
- C44.82 Squamous cell carcinoma of overlapping sites of skin
- C44.89 Other specified malignant neoplasm of overlapping sites of skin

[5th] C44.9 Other and unspecified malignant neoplasm of skin, unspecified
- C44.90 Unspecified malignant neoplasm of skin, unspecified
  Malignant neoplasm of unspecified site of skin
- C44.91 Basal cell carcinoma of skin, unspecified
- C44.92 Squamous cell carcinoma of skin, unspecified
- C44.99 Other specified malignant neoplasm of skin, unspecified

Malignant neoplasms of mesothelial and soft tissue (C45-C49)

[4th] C45 Mesothelioma
- C45.0 Mesothelioma of pleura [HCC] [RxHCC]
  AHA: Q2 2017
  [EXCLUDES1] *other malignant neoplasm of pleura (C38.4)*
- C45.1 Mesothelioma of peritoneum [HCC] [RxHCC]
  Mesothelioma of cul-de-sac
  Mesothelioma of mesentery
  Mesothelioma of mesocolon
  Mesothelioma of omentum
  Mesothelioma of peritoneum (parietal) (pelvic)
  [EXCLUDES1] *other malignant neoplasm of soft tissue of peritoneum (C48.-)*
- C45.2 Mesothelioma of pericardium [HCC] [RxHCC]
  [EXCLUDES1] *other malignant neoplasm of pericardium (C38.0)*
- C45.7 Mesothelioma of other sites [HCC] [RxHCC]
- C45.9 Mesothelioma, unspecified [HCC] [RxHCC]

[4th] C46 Kaposi's sarcoma
☞ Code first any human immunodeficiency virus [HIV] disease (B20)
- C46.0 Kaposi's sarcoma of skin [HCC] [RxHCC]
- C46.1 Kaposi's sarcoma of soft tissue [HCC] [RxHCC]
  Kaposi's sarcoma of blood vessel
  Kaposi's sarcoma of connective tissue
  Kaposi's sarcoma of fascia
  Kaposi's sarcoma of ligament
  Kaposi's sarcoma of lymphatic(s) NEC
  Kaposi's sarcoma of muscle
  [EXCLUDES2] *Kaposi's sarcoma of lymph glands and nodes (C46.3)*
- C46.2 Kaposi's sarcoma of palate [HCC] [RxHCC]
- C46.3 Kaposi's sarcoma of lymph nodes [HCC] [RxHCC]
- C46.4 Kaposi's sarcoma of gastrointestinal sites [HCC] [RxHCC]

[5th] C46.5 Kaposi's sarcoma of lung
- C46.50 Kaposi's sarcoma of unspecified lung [HCC] [RxHCC]
- C46.51 Kaposi's sarcoma of right lung [HCC] [RxHCC]
- C46.52 Kaposi's sarcoma of left lung [HCC] [RxHCC]
- C46.7 Kaposi's sarcoma of other sites [HCC] [RxHCC]
- C46.9 Kaposi's sarcoma, unspecified [HCC] [RxHCC]
  Kaposi's sarcoma of unspecified site

[4th] C47 Malignant neoplasm of peripheral nerves and autonomic nervous system
[INCLUDES] *malignant neoplasm of sympathetic and parasympathetic nerves and ganglia*
[EXCLUDES1] *Kaposi's sarcoma of soft tissue (C46.1)*
- C47.0 Malignant neoplasm of peripheral nerves of head, face and neck [HCC] [RxHCC]
  [EXCLUDES1] *malignant neoplasm of peripheral nerves of orbit (C69.6-)*

[5th] C47.1 Malignant neoplasm of peripheral nerves of upper limb, including shoulder
- C47.10 Malignant neoplasm of peripheral nerves of unspecified upper limb, including shoulder [HCC] [RxHCC]
- C47.11 Malignant neoplasm of peripheral nerves of right upper limb, including shoulder [HCC] [RxHCC]
- C47.12 Malignant neoplasm of peripheral nerves of left upper limb, including shoulder [HCC] [RxHCC]

[5th] C47.2 Malignant neoplasm of peripheral nerves of lower limb, including hip
- C47.20 Malignant neoplasm of peripheral nerves of unspecified lower limb, including hip [HCC] [RxHCC]
- C47.21 Malignant neoplasm of peripheral nerves of right lower limb, including hip [HCC] [RxHCC]
- C47.22 Malignant neoplasm of peripheral nerves of left lower limb, including hip [HCC] [RxHCC]
- C47.3 Malignant neoplasm of peripheral nerves of thorax [HCC] [RxHCC]
- C47.4 Malignant neoplasm of peripheral nerves of abdomen [HCC] [RxHCC]
- C47.5 Malignant neoplasm of peripheral nerves of pelvis [HCC] [RxHCC]
- C47.6 Malignant neoplasm of peripheral nerves of trunk, unspecified [HCC] [RxHCC]
  Malignant neoplasm of peripheral nerves of unspecified part of trunk

Unspecified Code · Other Specified Code · Manifestation Code · [N] Newborn · [P] Pediatric · [M] Maternity · [A] Adult · ♂ Male · ♀ Female
● New Code · ▲ Revised Code Title · ►◄ Revised Text · [NOTES] · [INCLUDES] · [EXCLUDES1] Not coded here · [EXCLUDES2] Not included here
[4th] 4th character required · [5th] 5th character required · [6th] 6th character required · [7th] 7th character required · [X] Extension 'X' Alert
[HAC] Hospital-acquired condition (HAC) alert · AHA AHA Coding Clinic© · ☞ Code first alert

When symbols appear on a code that requires a 7th character extension, refer to Appendix B to identify applicable 7th character codes.

C47.8   **Malignant neoplasm of** overlapping sites **of peripheral nerves and autonomic nervous system** `HCC` `RxHCC`

C47.9   **Malignant neoplasm of peripheral nerves and autonomic nervous system, unspecified** `HCC` `RxHCC`
Malignant neoplasm of unspecified site of peripheral nerves and autonomic nervous system

C48   **Malignant neoplasm of** retroperitoneum and peritoneum

EXCLUDES1   Kaposi's sarcoma of connective tissue (C46.1)
mesothelioma (C45.-)

C48.0   **Malignant neoplasm of** retroperitoneum   `HCC` `RxHCC`

C48.1   **Malignant neoplasm of specified parts of** peritoneum   `HCC` `RxHCC`
Malignant neoplasm of cul-de-sac
Malignant neoplasm of mesentery
Malignant neoplasm of mesocolon
Malignant neoplasm of omentum
Malignant neoplasm of parietal peritoneum
Malignant neoplasm of pelvic peritoneum

C48.2   **Malignant neoplasm of** peritoneum, **unspecified**   `HCC` `RxHCC`

C48.8   **Malignant neoplasm of** overlapping sites **of retroperitoneum and peritoneum**   `HCC` `RxHCC`

C49   **Malignant neoplasm of** other connective and soft tissue

INCLUDES   malignant neoplasm of blood vessel
malignant neoplasm of bursa
malignant neoplasm of cartilage
malignant neoplasm of fascia
malignant neoplasm of fat
malignant neoplasm of ligament, except uterine
malignant neoplasm of lymphatic vessel
malignant neoplasm of muscle
malignant neoplasm of synovia
malignant neoplasm of tendon (sheath)

EXCLUDES1   malignant neoplasm of cartilage (of):
articular (C40-C41)
larynx (C32.3)
nose (C30.0)
malignant neoplasm of connective tissue of breast (C50.-)

EXCLUDES2   Kaposi's sarcoma of soft tissue (C46.1)
malignant neoplasm of heart (C38.0)
malignant neoplasm of peripheral nerves and autonomic nervous system (C47.-)
malignant neoplasm of peritoneum (C48.2)
malignant neoplasm of retroperitoneum (C48.0)
malignant neoplasm of uterine ligament (C57.3)
mesothelioma (C45.-)

C49.0   **Malignant neoplasm of connective and soft tissue of** head, face and neck   `HCC` `RxHCC`
Malignant neoplasm of connective tissue of ear
Malignant neoplasm of connective tissue of eyelid
EXCLUDES1   connective tissue of orbit (C69.6-)

C49.1   **Malignant neoplasm of connective and soft tissue of** upper limb, including shoulder

C49.10   **Malignant neoplasm of connective and soft tissue of** unspecified upper limb, including shoulder   `HCC` `RxHCC`

C49.11   **Malignant neoplasm of connective and soft tissue of** right **upper limb, including shoulder**   `HCC` `RxHCC`

C49.12   **Malignant neoplasm of connective and soft tissue of** left **upper limb, including shoulder**   `HCC` `RxHCC`

C49.2   **Malignant neoplasm of connective and soft tissue of** lower limb, including hip

C49.20   **Malignant neoplasm of connective and soft tissue of** unspecified lower limb, including hip   `HCC` `RxHCC`

C49.21   **Malignant neoplasm of connective and soft tissue of** right **lower limb, including hip**   `HCC` `RxHCC`

C49.22   **Malignant neoplasm of connective and soft tissue of** left **lower limb, including hip**   `HCC` `RxHCC`

C49.3   **Malignant neoplasm of connective and soft tissue of** thorax   `HCC` `RxHCC`
AHA: Q3 2015

Malignant neoplasm of axilla
Malignant neoplasm of diaphragm
Malignant neoplasm of great vessels
EXCLUDES1   malignant neoplasm of breast (C50.-)
malignant neoplasm of heart (C38.0)
malignant neoplasm of mediastinum (C38.1-C38.3)
malignant neoplasm of thymus (C37)

C49.4   **Malignant neoplasm of connective and soft tissue of** abdomen   `HCC` `RxHCC`
Malignant neoplasm of abdominal wall
Malignant neoplasm of hypochondrium

C49.5   **Malignant neoplasm of connective and soft tissue of** pelvis   `HCC` `RxHCC`
Malignant neoplasm of buttock
Malignant neoplasm of groin
Malignant neoplasm of perineum

C49.6   **Malignant neoplasm of connective and soft tissue of** trunk, **unspecified**   `HCC` `RxHCC`
Malignant neoplasm of back NOS

C49.8   **Malignant neoplasm of** overlapping sites **of connective and soft tissue**   `HCC` `RxHCC`
Primary malignant neoplasm of two or more contiguous sites of connective and soft tissue

C49.9   **Malignant neoplasm of connective and soft tissue, unspecified**   `HCC` `RxHCC`

C49.A   Gastrointestinal stromal tumor

C49.A0   **Gastrointestinal stromal tumor, unspecified site**   `HCC` `RxHCC`
AHA: Q4 2016

C49.A1   **Gastrointestinal stromal tumor of** esophagus   `HCC` `RxHCC`
AHA: Q4 2016

C49.A2   **Gastrointestinal stromal tumor of** stomach   `HCC` `RxHCC`
AHA: Q4 2016

C49.A3   **Gastrointestinal stromal tumor** of small intestine   `HCC` `RxHCC`
AHA: Q4 2016

C49.A4   **Gastrointestinal stromal tumor** of large intestine   `HCC` `RxHCC`
AHA: Q4 2016

C49.A5   **Gastrointestinal stromal tumor** of rectum   `HCC` `RxHCC`
AHA: Q4 2016

C49.A9   **Gastrointestinal stromal tumor of** other sites   `HCC` `RxHCC`
AHA: Q4 2016

Malignant neoplasms of breast (C50)

C50   **Malignant neoplasm of** breast **(Figure 2.2)**

INCLUDES   connective tissue of breast
Paget's disease of breast
Paget's disease of nipple

Use additional code to identify estrogen receptor status (Z17.0, Z17.1)

EXCLUDES1   skin of breast (C44.501, C44.511, C44.521, C44.591)

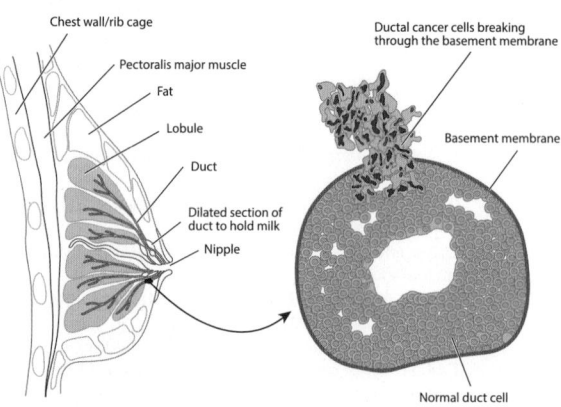

Figure 2.2 Malignant Neoplasm of the Breast

[5th] C50.0 Malignant neoplasm of nipple and areola
[6th] C50.01 Malignant neoplasm of nipple and areola, female
C50.011 Malignant neoplasm of nipple and areola, right female breast [HCC] [RxHCC] ♀
C50.012 Malignant neoplasm of nipple and areola, left female breast [HCC] [RxHCC] ♀
C50.019 Malignant neoplasm of nipple and areola, unspecified female breast [HCC] [RxHCC] ♀
[6th] C50.02 Malignant neoplasm of nipple and areola, male
C50.021 Malignant neoplasm of nipple and areola, right male breast [HCC] [RxHCC] ♂
C50.022 Malignant neoplasm of nipple and areola, left male breast [HCC] [RxHCC] ♂
C50.029 Malignant neoplasm of nipple and areola, unspecified male breast [HCC] [RxHCC] ♂

[5th] C50.1 Malignant neoplasm of central portion of breast
[6th] C50.11 Malignant neoplasm of central portion of breast, female
C50.111 Malignant neoplasm of central portion of right female breast [HCC] [RxHCC] ♀
C50.112 Malignant neoplasm of central portion of left female breast [HCC] [RxHCC] ♀
C50.119 Malignant neoplasm of central portion of unspecified female breast [HCC] [RxHCC] ♀
[6th] C50.12 Malignant neoplasm of central portion of breast, male
C50.121 Malignant neoplasm of central portion of right male breast [HCC] [RxHCC] ♂
C50.122 Malignant neoplasm of central portion of left male breast [HCC] [RxHCC] ♂
C50.129 Malignant neoplasm of central portion of unspecified male breast [HCC] [RxHCC] ♂

[5th] C50.2 Malignant neoplasm of upper-inner quadrant of breast
[6th] C50.21 Malignant neoplasm of upper-inner quadrant of breast, female
C50.211 Malignant neoplasm of upper-inner quadrant of right female breast [HCC] [RxHCC] ♀
C50.212 Malignant neoplasm of upper-inner quadrant of left female breast [HCC] [RxHCC] ♀
C50.219 Malignant neoplasm of upper-inner quadrant of unspecified female breast [HCC] [RxHCC] ♀
[6th] C50.22 Malignant neoplasm of upper-inner quadrant of breast, male
C50.221 Malignant neoplasm of upper-inner quadrant of right male breast [HCC] [RxHCC] ♂
C50.222 Malignant neoplasm of upper-inner quadrant of left male breast [HCC] [RxHCC] ♂
C50.229 Malignant neoplasm of upper-inner quadrant of unspecified male breast [HCC] [RxHCC] ♂

[5th] C50.3 Malignant neoplasm of lower-inner quadrant of breast
[6th] C50.31 Malignant neoplasm of lower-inner quadrant of breast, female
C50.311 Malignant neoplasm of lower-inner quadrant of right female breast [HCC] [RxHCC] ♀
C50.312 Malignant neoplasm of lower-inner quadrant of left female breast [HCC] [RxHCC] ♀
C50.319 Malignant neoplasm of lower-inner quadrant of unspecified female breast [HCC] [RxHCC] ♀
[6th] C50.32 Malignant neoplasm of lower-inner quadrant of breast, male
C50.321 Malignant neoplasm of lower-inner quadrant of right male breast [HCC] [RxHCC] ♂
C50.322 Malignant neoplasm of lower-inner quadrant of left male breast [HCC] [RxHCC] ♂
C50.329 Malignant neoplasm of lower-inner quadrant of unspecified male breast [HCC] [RxHCC] ♂

[5th] C50.4 Malignant neoplasm of upper-outer quadrant of breast
[6th] C50.41 Malignant neoplasm of upper-outer quadrant of breast, female
C50.411 Malignant neoplasm of upper-outer quadrant of right female breast [HCC] [RxHCC] ♀
C50.412 Malignant neoplasm of upper-outer quadrant of left female breast [HCC] [RxHCC] ♀
C50.419 Malignant neoplasm of upper-outer quadrant of unspecified female breast [HCC] [RxHCC] ♀
[6th] C50.42 Malignant neoplasm of upper-outer quadrant of breast, male
C50.421 Malignant neoplasm of upper-outer quadrant of right male breast [HCC] [RxHCC] ♂
C50.422 Malignant neoplasm of upper-outer quadrant of left male breast [HCC] [RxHCC] ♂
C50.429 Malignant neoplasm of upper-outer quadrant of unspecified male breast [HCC] [RxHCC] ♂

[5th] C50.5 Malignant neoplasm of lower-outer quadrant of breast
[6th] C50.51 Malignant neoplasm of lower-outer quadrant of breast, female
C50.511 Malignant neoplasm of lower-outer quadrant of right female breast [HCC] [RxHCC] ♀
C50.512 Malignant neoplasm of lower-outer quadrant of left female breast [HCC] [RxHCC] ♀
C50.519 Malignant neoplasm of lower-outer quadrant of unspecified female breast [HCC] [RxHCC] ♀
[6th] C50.52 Malignant neoplasm of lower-outer quadrant of breast, male
C50.521 Malignant neoplasm of lower-outer quadrant of right male breast [HCC] [RxHCC] ♂
C50.522 Malignant neoplasm of lower-outer quadrant of left male breast [HCC] [RxHCC] ♂
C50.529 Malignant neoplasm of lower-outer quadrant of unspecified male breast [HCC] [RxHCC] ♂

[5th] C50.6 Malignant neoplasm of axillary tail of breast
[6th] C50.61 Malignant neoplasm of axillary tail of breast, female
C50.611 Malignant neoplasm of axillary tail of right female breast [HCC] [RxHCC] ♀
C50.612 Malignant neoplasm of axillary tail of left female breast [HCC] [RxHCC] ♀
C50.619 Malignant neoplasm of axillary tail of unspecified female breast [HCC] [RxHCC] ♀
[6th] C50.62 Malignant neoplasm of axillary tail of breast, male
C50.621 Malignant neoplasm of axillary tail of right male breast [HCC] [RxHCC] ♂
C50.622 Malignant neoplasm of axillary tail of left male breast [HCC] [RxHCC] ♂
C50.629 Malignant neoplasm of axillary tail of unspecified male breast [HCC] [RxHCC] ♂

[5th] C50.8 Malignant neoplasm of overlapping sites of breast
[6th] C50.81 Malignant neoplasm of overlapping sites of breast, female
C50.811 Malignant neoplasm of overlapping sites of right female breast [HCC] [RxHCC] ♀
C50.812 Malignant neoplasm of overlapping sites of left female breast [HCC] [RxHCC] ♀
C50.819 Malignant neoplasm of overlapping sites of unspecified female breast [HCC] [RxHCC] ♀
[6th] C50.82 Malignant neoplasm of overlapping sites of breast, male
C50.821 Malignant neoplasm of overlapping sites of right male breast [HCC] [RxHCC] ♂
C50.822 Malignant neoplasm of overlapping sites of left male breast [HCC] [RxHCC] ♂
C50.829 Malignant neoplasm of overlapping sites of unspecified male breast [HCC] [RxHCC] ♂

[5th] C50.9 Malignant neoplasm of breast of unspecified site
- [6th] C50.91 Malignant neoplasm of breast of unspecified site, female
  - C50.911 **Malignant neoplasm of unspecified site of right female breast** [HCC] [RxHCC] ♀
  - C50.912 **Malignant neoplasm of unspecified site of left female breast** [HCC] [RxHCC] ♀
  - C50.919 **Malignant neoplasm of unspecified site of unspecified female breast** [HCC] [RxHCC] ♀
- [6th] C50.92 Malignant neoplasm of breast of unspecified site, male
  - C50.921 **Malignant neoplasm of unspecified site of right male breast** [HCC] [RxHCC] ♂
  - C50.922 **Malignant neoplasm of unspecified site of left male breast** [HCC] [RxHCC] ♂
  - C50.929 **Malignant neoplasm of unspecified site of unspecified male breast** [HCC] [RxHCC] ♂

Malignant neoplasms of female genital organs (C51-C58)

[INCLUDES] *malignant neoplasm of skin of female genital organs*

[4th] C51 Malignant neoplasm of vulva

[EXCLUDES1] *carcinoma in situ of vulva (D07.1)*

- C51.0 **Malignant neoplasm of labium majus** [HCC] ♀
  Malignant neoplasm of Bartholin's [greater vestibular] gland
- C51.1 **Malignant neoplasm of labium minus** [HCC] ♀
- C51.2 **Malignant neoplasm of clitoris** [HCC] ♀
- C51.8 **Malignant neoplasm of overlapping sites of vulva** [HCC] ♀
- C51.9 **Malignant neoplasm of vulva, unspecified** [HCC] ♀
  Malignant neoplasm of external female genitalia NOS
  Malignant neoplasm of pudendum

C52 **Malignant neoplasm of vagina** [HCC] ♀

[EXCLUDES1] *carcinoma in situ of vagina (D07.2)*

[4th] C53 Malignant neoplasm of cervix uteri

[EXCLUDES1] *carcinoma in situ of cervix uteri (D06.-)*

- C53.0 **Malignant neoplasm of endocervix** [HCC] ♀
- C53.1 **Malignant neoplasm of exocervix** [HCC] ♀
- C53.8 **Malignant neoplasm of overlapping sites of cervix uteri** [HCC] ♀
- C53.9 **Malignant neoplasm of cervix uteri, unspecified** [HCC] ♀
  AHA: Q4 2017

[4th] C54 Malignant neoplasm of corpus uteri
- C54.0 **Malignant neoplasm of isthmus uteri** [HCC] ♀
  Malignant neoplasm of lower uterine segment
- C54.1 **Malignant neoplasm of endometrium** [HCC] ♀
- C54.2 **Malignant neoplasm of myometrium** [HCC] ♀
- C54.3 **Malignant neoplasm of fundus uteri** [HCC] ♀
- C54.8 **Malignant neoplasm of overlapping sites of corpus uteri** [HCC] ♀
- C54.9 **Malignant neoplasm of corpus uteri, unspecified** [HCC] ♀

C55 **Malignant neoplasm of uterus, part unspecified** [HCC] ♀

[4th] C56 Malignant neoplasm of ovary

Use additional code to identify any functional activity
- C56.1 **Malignant neoplasm of right ovary** [HCC] ♀
- C56.2 **Malignant neoplasm of left ovary** [HCC] ♀
- C56.9 **Malignant neoplasm of unspecified ovary** [HCC] ♀

[4th] C57 Malignant neoplasm of other and unspecified female genital organs
- [5th] C57.0 Malignant neoplasm of fallopian tube
  Malignant neoplasm of oviduct
  Malignant neoplasm of uterine tube
  - C57.00 **Malignant neoplasm of unspecified fallopian tube** [HCC] ♀
  - C57.01 **Malignant neoplasm of right fallopian tube** [HCC] ♀
  - C57.02 **Malignant neoplasm of left fallopian tube** [HCC] ♀
- [5th] C57.1 Malignant neoplasm of broad ligament
  - C57.10 **Malignant neoplasm of unspecified broad ligament** [HCC] ♀
  - C57.11 **Malignant neoplasm of right broad ligament** [HCC] ♀
  - C57.12 **Malignant neoplasm of left broad ligament** [HCC] ♀
- [5th] C57.2 Malignant neoplasm of round ligament
  - C57.20 **Malignant neoplasm of unspecified round ligament** [HCC] ♀
  - C57.21 **Malignant neoplasm of right round ligament** [HCC] ♀
  - C57.22 **Malignant neoplasm of left round ligament** [HCC] ♀
- C57.3 **Malignant neoplasm of parametrium** [HCC] ♀
  Malignant neoplasm of uterine ligament NOS
- C57.4 **Malignant neoplasm of uterine adnexa, unspecified** [HCC] ♀
- C57.7 **Malignant neoplasm of other specified female genital organs** [HCC] ♀
  Malignant neoplasm of wolffian body or duct
- C57.8 **Malignant neoplasm of overlapping sites of female genital organs** [HCC] ♀
  Primary malignant neoplasm of two or more contiguous sites of the female genital organs whose point of origin cannot be determined
  Primary tubo-ovarian malignant neoplasm whose point of origin cannot be determined
  Primary utero-ovarian malignant neoplasm whose point of origin cannot be determined
- C57.9 **Malignant neoplasm of female genital organ, unspecified** [HCC] ♀
  Malignant neoplasm of female genitourinary tract NOS

C58 **Malignant neoplasm of placenta** [M] [HCC] ♀

[INCLUDES] *choriocarcinoma NOS*
chorionepithelioma NOS

[EXCLUDES1] *chorioadenoma (destruens) (D39.2)*
hydatidiform mole NOS (O01.9)
invasive hydatidiform mole (D39.2)
male choriocarcinoma NOS (C62.9-)
malignant hydatidiform mole (D39.2)

Malignant neoplasms of male genital organs (C60-C63)(Figure 2.3)

[INCLUDES] *malignant neoplasm of skin of male genital organs*

[4th] C60 Malignant neoplasm of penis
- C60.0 **Malignant neoplasm of prepuce** [HCC] ♂
  Malignant neoplasm of foreskin
- C60.1 **Malignant neoplasm of glans penis** [HCC] ♂
- C60.2 **Malignant neoplasm of body of penis** [HCC] ♂
  Malignant neoplasm of corpus cavernosum
- C60.8 **Malignant neoplasm of overlapping sites of penis** [HCC] ♂
- C60.9 **Malignant neoplasm of penis, unspecified** [HCC] ♂
  Malignant neoplasm of skin of penis NOS

C61 **Malignant neoplasm of prostate** [HCC] ♂

AHA: Q1 2017

Use additional code to identify:
hormone sensitivity status (Z19.1-Z19.2)
rising PSA following treatment for malignant neoplasm of prostate (R97.21)

[EXCLUDES1] *malignant neoplasm of seminal vesicle (C63.7)*

[4th] C62 Malignant neoplasm of testis

Use additional code to identify any functional activity
- [5th] C62.0 Malignant neoplasm of undescended testis
  Malignant neoplasm of ectopic testis
  Malignant neoplasm of retained testis
  - C62.00 **Malignant neoplasm of unspecified undescended testis** [HCC] ♂
  - C62.01 **Malignant neoplasm of undescended right testis** [HCC] ♂
  - C62.02 **Malignant neoplasm of undescended left testis** [HCC] ♂
- [5th] C62.1 Malignant neoplasm of descended testis
  Malignant neoplasm of scrotal testis
  - C62.10 **Malignant neoplasm of unspecified descended testis** [HCC] ♂
  - C62.11 **Malignant neoplasm of descended right testis** [HCC] ♂
  - C62.12 **Malignant neoplasm of descended left testis** [HCC] ♂
- [5th] C62.9 Malignant neoplasm of testis, unspecified whether descended or undescended
  - C62.90 **Malignant neoplasm of unspecified testis, unspecified whether descended or undescended** [HCC] ♂
    Malignant neoplasm of testis NOS

[PDx] Unacceptable principal diagnosis symbol per Medicare code edits [POA] Code exempt from diagnosis present on admission requirement
[?] Questionable admission [CC] Complication or comorbidity [MCC] Major complication or comorbidity [CC/MCC Exc] CC/MCC exclusion
[HCC] HCC diagnosis code [RxHCC] RxHCC diagnosis code MACRA code **DEFINITION** Describes condition/terminology
TIP Coding guidance 👁 Official Guideline Reference [Z1] Z code as first-listed diagnosis

C62.91   Malignant neoplasm of right testis, unspecified whether descended or undescended   HCC ♂

C62.92   Malignant neoplasm of left testis, unspecified whether descended or undescended   HCC ♂

🔄 C63   Malignant neoplasm of other and unspecified male genital organs

   🔵 C63.0   Malignant neoplasm of epididymis

     C63.00   Malignant neoplasm of unspecified epididymis   HCC ♂

     C63.01   Malignant neoplasm of right epididymis   HCC ♂

     C63.02   Malignant neoplasm of left epididymis   HCC ♂

   🔵 C63.1   Malignant neoplasm of spermatic cord

     C63.10   Malignant neoplasm of unspecified spermatic cord   HCC ♂

     C63.11   Malignant neoplasm of right spermatic cord   HCC ♂

     C63.12   Malignant neoplasm of left spermatic cord   HCC ♂

   C63.2   Malignant neoplasm of scrotum   HCC ♂
     Malignant neoplasm of skin of scrotum

   C63.7   **Malignant neoplasm of other specified male genital organs**   HCC ♂
     Malignant neoplasm of seminal vesicle
     Malignant neoplasm of tunica vaginalis

   C63.8   Malignant neoplasm of overlapping sites of male genital organs   HCC ♂
     Primary malignant neoplasm of two or more contiguous sites of male genital organs whose point of origin cannot be determined

   C63.9   Malignant neoplasm of male genital organ, unspecified   HCC ♂
     Malignant neoplasm of male genitourinary tract NOS

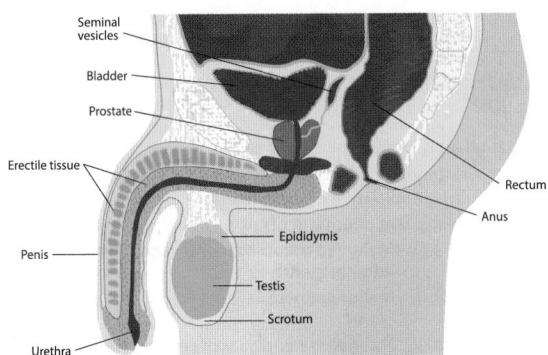

Seminal vesicles — Bladder — Prostate — Erectile tissue — Penis — Urethra — Rectum — Anus — Epididymis — Testis — Scrotum

Figure 2.3 Male Reproductive Tract

Malignant neoplasms of urinary tract (C64-C68)

🔄 C64   Malignant neoplasm of kidney, except renal pelvis
   EXCLUDES1   malignant carcinoid tumor of the kidney (C7A.093)
       malignant neoplasm of renal calyces (C65.-)
       malignant neoplasm of renal pelvis (C65.-)

   C64.1   Malignant neoplasm of right kidney, except renal pelvis   HCC RxHCC

   C64.2   Malignant neoplasm of left kidney, except renal pelvis   HCC RxHCC

   C64.9   Malignant neoplasm of unspecified kidney, except renal pelvis   HCC RxHCC

🔄 C65   Malignant neoplasm of renal pelvis
   INCLUDES   malignant neoplasm of pelviureteric junction
       malignant neoplasm of renal calyces

   C65.1   Malignant neoplasm of right renal pelvis   HCC RxHCC

   C65.2   Malignant neoplasm of left renal pelvis   HCC RxHCC

   C65.9   Malignant neoplasm of unspecified renal pelvis   HCC RxHCC

🔄 C66   Malignant neoplasm of ureter
   EXCLUDES1   malignant neoplasm of ureteric orifice of bladder (C67.6)

   C66.1   Malignant neoplasm of right ureter   HCC

   C66.2   Malignant neoplasm of left ureter   HCC

   C66.9   Malignant neoplasm of unspecified ureter   HCC

🔄 C67   Malignant neoplasm of bladder (Figure 2.4)

   C67.0   Malignant neoplasm of trigone of bladder   HCC

   C67.1   Malignant neoplasm of dome of bladder   HCC

C67.2   Malignant neoplasm of lateral wall of bladder   HCC

C67.3   Malignant neoplasm of anterior wall of bladder   HCC

C67.4   Malignant neoplasm of posterior wall of bladder   HCC

C67.5   Malignant neoplasm of bladder neck   HCC
   Malignant neoplasm of internal urethral orifice

C67.6   Malignant neoplasm of ureteric orifice   HCC

C67.7   Malignant neoplasm of urachus   HCC

C67.8   Malignant neoplasm of overlapping sites of bladder   HCC

C67.9   Malignant neoplasm of bladder, unspecified   HCC
   AHA: Q1 2016

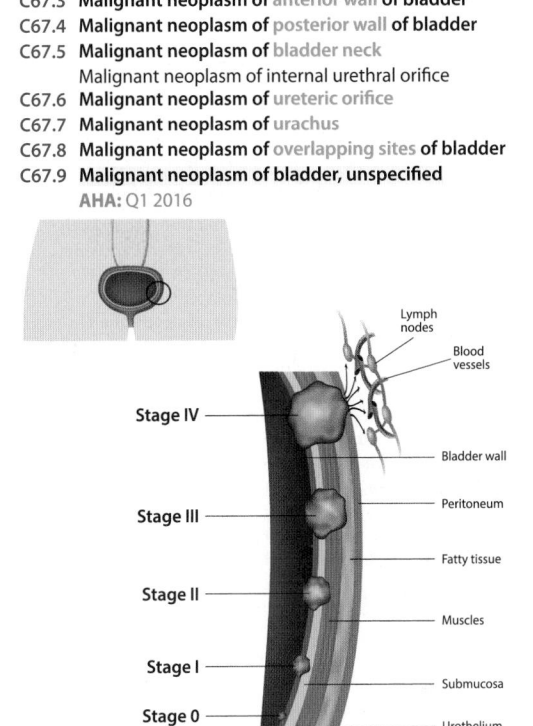

Lymph nodes — Blood vessels — Stage IV — Bladder wall — Stage III — Peritoneum — Fatty tissue — Stage II — Muscles — Stage I — Submucosa — Stage 0 — Urothelium

Figure 2.4 Malignant Neoplasm of Bladder

🔄 C68   Malignant neoplasm of other and unspecified urinary organs
   EXCLUDES1   malignant neoplasm of female genitourinary tract NOS (C57.9)
       malignant neoplasm of male genitourinary tract NOS (C63.9)

   C68.0   Malignant neoplasm of urethra   HCC
     EXCLUDES1   malignant neoplasm of urethral orifice of bladder (C67.5)

   C68.1   Malignant neoplasm of paraurethral glands   CC HCC CC/MCC EXC

   C68.8   Malignant neoplasm of overlapping sites of urinary organs   HCC
     Primary malignant neoplasm of two or more contiguous sites of urinary organs whose point of origin cannot be determined

   C68.9   Malignant neoplasm of urinary organ, unspecified   HCC
     Malignant neoplasm of urinary system NOS

Malignant neoplasms of eye, brain and other parts of central nervous system (C69-C72)

🔄 C69   Malignant neoplasm of eye and adnexa
   EXCLUDES1   malignant neoplasm of connective tissue of eyelid (C49.0)
       malignant neoplasm of eyelid (skin) (C43.1-, C44.1-)
       malignant neoplasm of optic nerve (C72.3-)

   🔵 C69.0   Malignant neoplasm of conjunctiva

     C69.00   Malignant neoplasm of unspecified conjunctiva   HCC

     C69.01   Malignant neoplasm of right conjunctiva   HCC

     C69.02   Malignant neoplasm of left conjunctiva   HCC

   🔵 C69.1   Malignant neoplasm of cornea

     C69.10   Malignant neoplasm of unspecified cornea   HCC

     C69.11   Malignant neoplasm of right cornea   HCC

     C69.12   Malignant neoplasm of left cornea   HCC

   🔵 C69.2   Malignant neoplasm of retina
     EXCLUDES1   dark area on retina (D49.81)
       neoplasm of unspecified behavior of retina and choroid (D49.81)
       retinal freckle (D49.81)

Unspecified Code   Other Specified Code   Manifestation Code   N Newborn   P Pediatric   M Maternity   A Adult   ♂ Male   ♀ Female
● New Code   ▲ Revised Code Title   ▶◀ Revised Text   NOTES   INCLUDES   EXCLUDES1 Not coded here   EXCLUDES2 Not included here
🔄 4th character required   🔵 5th character required   6th character required   7th character required   Extension 'X' Alert
HAC Hospital-acquired condition (HAC) alert   AHA AHA Coding Clinic©   ☞ Code first alert

C69.20 **Malignant neoplasm of unspecified retina** [HCC]
C69.21 **Malignant neoplasm of right retina** [HCC]
C69.22 **Malignant neoplasm of left retina** [HCC]

[5th] **C69.3 Malignant neoplasm of choroid**
C69.30 **Malignant neoplasm of unspecified choroid** [HCC]
C69.31 **Malignant neoplasm of right choroid** [HCC]
C69.32 **Malignant neoplasm of left choroid** [HCC]

[5th] **C69.4 Malignant neoplasm of ciliary body**
C69.40 **Malignant neoplasm of unspecified ciliary body** [HCC]
C69.41 **Malignant neoplasm of right ciliary body** [HCC]
C69.42 **Malignant neoplasm of left ciliary body** [HCC]

[5th] **C69.5 Malignant neoplasm of lacrimal gland and duct**
Malignant neoplasm of lacrimal sac
Malignant neoplasm of nasolacrimal duct
C69.50 **Malignant neoplasm of unspecified lacrimal gland and duct** [HCC]
C69.51 **Malignant neoplasm of right lacrimal gland and duct** [HCC]
C69.52 **Malignant neoplasm of left lacrimal gland and duct** [HCC]

[5th] **C69.6 Malignant neoplasm of orbit**
Malignant neoplasm of connective tissue of orbit
Malignant neoplasm of extraocular muscle
Malignant neoplasm of peripheral nerves of orbit
Malignant neoplasm of retrobulbar tissue
Malignant neoplasm of retro-ocular tissue
[EXCLUDES1] *malignant neoplasm of orbital bone (C41.0)*
C69.60 **Malignant neoplasm of unspecified orbit** [HCC]
C69.61 **Malignant neoplasm of right orbit** [HCC]
C69.62 **Malignant neoplasm of left orbit** [HCC]

[5th] **C69.8 Malignant neoplasm of overlapping sites of eye and adnexa**
C69.80 **Malignant neoplasm of overlapping sites of unspecified eye and adnexa** [HCC]
C69.81 **Malignant neoplasm of overlapping sites of right eye and adnexa** [HCC]
C69.82 **Malignant neoplasm of overlapping sites of left eye and adnexa** [HCC]

[5th] **C69.9 Malignant neoplasm of unspecified site of eye**
Malignant neoplasm of eyeball
C69.90 **Malignant neoplasm of unspecified site of unspecified eye** [HCC]
C69.91 **Malignant neoplasm of unspecified site of right eye** [HCC]
C69.92 **Malignant neoplasm of unspecified site of left eye** [HCC]

[4th] **C70 Malignant neoplasm of meninges**
C70.0 **Malignant neoplasm of cerebral meninges** [HCC]
C70.1 **Malignant neoplasm of spinal meninges** [HCC]
C70.9 **Malignant neoplasm of meninges, unspecified** [HCC]

[4th] **C71 Malignant neoplasm of brain**
[EXCLUDES1] *malignant neoplasm of cranial nerves (C72.2-C72.5)*
retrobulbar malignant neoplasm (C69.6-)
C71.0 **Malignant neoplasm of cerebrum, except lobes and ventricles** [HCC]
Malignant neoplasm of supratentorial NOS
C71.1 **Malignant neoplasm of frontal lobe** [HCC]
C71.2 **Malignant neoplasm of temporal lobe** [HCC]
C71.3 **Malignant neoplasm of parietal lobe** [HCC]
C71.4 **Malignant neoplasm of occipital lobe** [HCC]
C71.5 **Malignant neoplasm of cerebral ventricle** [HCC]
[EXCLUDES1] *malignant neoplasm of fourth cerebral ventricle (C71.7)*
C71.6 **Malignant neoplasm of cerebellum** [HCC]
C71.7 **Malignant neoplasm of brain stem** [HCC]
Malignant neoplasm of fourth cerebral ventricle
Infratentorial malignant neoplasm NOS
C71.8 **Malignant neoplasm of overlapping sites of brain** [HCC]
C71.9 **Malignant neoplasm of brain, unspecified** [HCC]

[4th] **C72 Malignant neoplasm of spinal cord, cranial nerves and other parts of central nervous system**
[EXCLUDES1] *malignant neoplasm of meninges (C70.-)*
malignant neoplasm of peripheral nerves and autonomic nervous system (C47.-)
C72.0 **Malignant neoplasm of spinal cord** [HCC]
C72.1 **Malignant neoplasm of cauda equina** [HCC]

[5th] **C72.2 Malignant neoplasm of olfactory nerve**
Malignant neoplasm of olfactory bulb
C72.20 **Malignant neoplasm of unspecified olfactory nerve** [HCC]
C72.21 **Malignant neoplasm of right olfactory nerve** [HCC]
C72.22 **Malignant neoplasm of left olfactory nerve** [HCC]

[5th] **C72.3 Malignant neoplasm of optic nerve**
C72.30 **Malignant neoplasm of unspecified optic nerve** [HCC]
C72.31 **Malignant neoplasm of right optic nerve** [HCC]
C72.32 **Malignant neoplasm of left optic nerve** [HCC]

[5th] **C72.4 Malignant neoplasm of acoustic nerve**
C72.40 **Malignant neoplasm of unspecified acoustic nerve** [HCC]
C72.41 **Malignant neoplasm of right acoustic nerve** [HCC]
C72.42 **Malignant neoplasm of left acoustic nerve** [HCC]

[5th] **C72.5 Malignant neoplasm of other and unspecified cranial nerves**
C72.50 **Malignant neoplasm of unspecified cranial nerve** [HCC]
Malignant neoplasm of cranial nerve NOS
C72.59 **Malignant neoplasm of other cranial nerves** [HCC]
C72.9 **Malignant neoplasm of central nervous system, unspecified** [HCC]
Malignant neoplasm of unspecified site of central nervous system
Malignant neoplasm of nervous system NOS

Malignant neoplasms of thyroid and other endocrine glands (C73-C75)

C73 Malignant neoplasm of thyroid gland [HCC] [RxHCC]
Use additional code to identify any functional activity

[4th] **C74 Malignant neoplasm of adrenal gland**
[5th] **C74.0 Malignant neoplasm of cortex of adrenal gland**
C74.00 **Malignant neoplasm of cortex of unspecified adrenal gland** [HCC] [RxHCC]
C74.01 **Malignant neoplasm of cortex of right adrenal gland** [HCC] [RxHCC]
C74.02 **Malignant neoplasm of cortex of left adrenal gland** [HCC] [RxHCC]

[5th] **C74.1 Malignant neoplasm of medulla of adrenal gland**
C74.10 **Malignant neoplasm of medulla of unspecified adrenal gland** [HCC] [RxHCC]
C74.11 **Malignant neoplasm of medulla of right adrenal gland** [HCC] [RxHCC]
C74.12 **Malignant neoplasm of medulla of left adrenal gland** [HCC] [RxHCC]

[5th] **C74.9 Malignant neoplasm of unspecified part of adrenal gland**
C74.90 **Malignant neoplasm of unspecified part of unspecified adrenal gland** [HCC] [RxHCC]
C74.91 **Malignant neoplasm of unspecified part of right adrenal gland** [HCC] [RxHCC]
C74.92 **Malignant neoplasm of unspecified part of left adrenal gland** [HCC] [RxHCC]

[4th] **C75 Malignant neoplasm of other endocrine glands and related structures**
[EXCLUDES1] *malignant carcinoid tumors (C7A.0-)*
malignant neoplasm of adrenal gland (C74.-)
malignant neoplasm of endocrine pancreas (C25.4)
malignant neoplasm of islets of Langerhans (C25.4)
malignant neoplasm of ovary (C56.-)
malignant neoplasm of testis (C62.-)
malignant neoplasm of thymus (C37)
malignant neoplasm of thyroid gland (C73)
malignant neuroendocrine tumors (C7A.-)
C75.0 **Malignant neoplasm of parathyroid gland** [HCC] [RxHCC]
C75.1 **Malignant neoplasm of pituitary gland** [HCC]

[PDx] Unacceptable principal diagnosis symbol per Medicare code edits [POA] Code exempt from diagnosis present on admission requirement
[?] Questionable admission [CC] Complication or comorbidity [MCC] Major complication or comorbidity [CC/MCC Exc] CC/MCC exclusion
[HCC] HCC diagnosis code [RxHCC] RxHCC diagnosis code MACRA code **DEFINITION** Describes condition/terminology
TIP Coding guidance 👁 Official Guideline Reference [Z1] Z code as first-listed diagnosis

C75.2 Malignant neoplasm of craniopharyngeal duct `HCC`
C75.3 Malignant neoplasm of pineal gland `HCC`
C75.4 Malignant neoplasm of carotid body `HCC` `RxHCC`
C75.5 Malignant neoplasm of aortic body and other paraganglia `HCC` `RxHCC`
C75.8 Malignant neoplasm with pluriglandular involvement, unspecified `HCC` `RxHCC`
C75.9 Malignant neoplasm of endocrine gland, unspecified `HCC` `RxHCC`

Malignant neuroendocrine tumors (C7A)

C7A Malignant neuroendocrine tumors
　　Code also any associated multiple endocrine neoplasia [MEN] syndromes (E31.2-)
　　Use additional code to identify any associated endocrine syndrome, such as:
　　carcinoid syndrome (E34.0)
　　EXCLUDES2 malignant pancreatic islet cell tumors (C25.4)
　　　　Merkel cell carcinoma (C4A.-)

C7A.0 Malignant carcinoid tumors
　　C7A.00 Malignant carcinoid tumor of unspecified site `HCC` `RxHCC`
　　C7A.01 Malignant carcinoid tumors of the small intestine
　　　　C7A.010 Malignant carcinoid tumor of the duodenum `HCC` `RxHCC`
　　　　C7A.011 Malignant carcinoid tumor of the jejunum `HCC` `RxHCC`
　　　　C7A.012 Malignant carcinoid tumor of the ileum `HCC` `RxHCC`
　　　　C7A.019 Malignant carcinoid tumor of the small intestine, unspecified portion `HCC` `RxHCC`
　　C7A.02 Malignant carcinoid tumors of the appendix, large intestine, and rectum
　　　　C7A.020 Malignant carcinoid tumor of the appendix `HCC` `RxHCC`
　　　　C7A.021 Malignant carcinoid tumor of the cecum `HCC` `RxHCC`
　　　　C7A.022 Malignant carcinoid tumor of the ascending colon `HCC` `RxHCC`
　　　　C7A.023 Malignant carcinoid tumor of the transverse colon `HCC` `RxHCC`
　　　　C7A.024 Malignant carcinoid tumor of the descending colon `HCC` `RxHCC`
　　　　C7A.025 Malignant carcinoid tumor of the sigmoid colon `HCC` `RxHCC`
　　　　C7A.026 Malignant carcinoid tumor of the rectum `HCC` `RxHCC`
　　　　C7A.029 Malignant carcinoid tumor of the large intestine, unspecified portion `HCC` `RxHCC`
　　　　　　Malignant carcinoid tumor of the colon NOS
　　C7A.09 Malignant carcinoid tumors of other sites
　　　　C7A.090 Malignant carcinoid tumor of the bronchus and lung `HCC` `RxHCC`
　　　　C7A.091 Malignant carcinoid tumor of the thymus `HCC` `RxHCC`
　　　　C7A.092 Malignant carcinoid tumor of the stomach `HCC` `RxHCC`
　　　　C7A.093 Malignant carcinoid tumor of the kidney `HCC` `RxHCC`
　　　　C7A.094 Malignant carcinoid tumor of the foregut, unspecified `HCC` `RxHCC`
　　　　C7A.095 Malignant carcinoid tumor of the midgut, unspecified `HCC` `RxHCC`
　　　　C7A.096 Malignant carcinoid tumor of the hindgut, unspecified `HCC` `RxHCC`
　　　　C7A.098 Malignant carcinoid tumors of other sites `HCC` `RxHCC`

C7A.1 Malignant poorly differentiated neuroendocrine tumors `HCC` `RxHCC`
　　Malignant poorly differentiated neuroendocrine tumor NOS
　　Malignant poorly differentiated neuroendocrine carcinoma, any site
　　High grade neuroendocrine carcinoma, any site

C7A.8 Other malignant neuroendocrine tumors `HCC` `RxHCC`

Secondary neuroendocrine tumors (C7B)

C7B Secondary neuroendocrine tumors
　　Use additional code to identify any functional activity
　　C7B.0 Secondary carcinoid tumors
　　　　C7B.00 Secondary carcinoid tumors, unspecified site `HCC` `RxHCC`
　　　　C7B.01 Secondary carcinoid tumors of distant lymph nodes `HCC` `RxHCC`
　　　　C7B.02 Secondary carcinoid tumors of liver `HCC` `RxHCC`
　　　　C7B.03 Secondary carcinoid tumors of bone `HCC` `RxHCC`
　　　　C7B.04 Secondary carcinoid tumors of peritoneum `HCC` `RxHCC`
　　　　　　Mesentery metastasis of carcinoid tumor
　　　　C7B.09 Secondary carcinoid tumors of other sites `HCC` `RxHCC`
　　C7B.1 Secondary Merkel cell carcinoma `HCC` `RxHCC`
　　　　Merkel cell carcinoma nodal presentation
　　　　Merkel cell carcinoma visceral metastatic presentation
　　C7B.8 Other secondary neuroendocrine tumors `HCC` `RxHCC`

Malignant neoplasms of ill-defined, other secondary and unspecified sites (C76-C80)

C76 Malignant neoplasm of other and ill-defined sites
　　EXCLUDES1 malignant neoplasm of female genitourinary tract NOS (C57.9)
　　　　malignant neoplasm of male genitourinary tract NOS (C63.9)
　　　　malignant neoplasm of lymphoid, hematopoietic and related tissue (C81-C96)
　　　　malignant neoplasm of skin (C44.-)
　　　　malignant neoplasm of unspecified site NOS (C80.1)
　　C76.0 Malignant neoplasm of head, face and neck `HCC`
　　　　Malignant neoplasm of cheek NOS
　　　　Malignant neoplasm of nose NOS
　　C76.1 Malignant neoplasm of thorax `HCC`
　　　　Intrathoracic malignant neoplasm NOS
　　　　Malignant neoplasm of axilla NOS
　　　　Thoracic malignant neoplasm NOS
　　C76.2 Malignant neoplasm of abdomen `HCC`
　　C76.3 Malignant neoplasm of pelvis `HCC`
　　　　Malignant neoplasm of groin NOS
　　　　Malignant neoplasm of sites overlapping systems within the pelvis
　　　　Rectovaginal (septum) malignant neoplasm
　　　　Rectovesical (septum) malignant neoplasm
　　C76.4 Malignant neoplasm of upper limb
　　　　C76.40 Malignant neoplasm of unspecified upper limb `HCC`
　　　　C76.41 Malignant neoplasm of right upper limb `HCC`
　　　　C76.42 Malignant neoplasm of left upper limb `HCC`
　　C76.5 Malignant neoplasm of lower limb
　　　　C76.50 Malignant neoplasm of unspecified lower limb `HCC`
　　　　C76.51 Malignant neoplasm of right lower limb `HCC`
　　　　C76.52 Malignant neoplasm of left lower limb `HCC`
　　C76.8 Malignant neoplasm of other specified ill-defined sites `HCC`
　　　　Malignant neoplasm of overlapping ill-defined sites

C77 Secondary and unspecified malignant neoplasm of lymph nodes
　　EXCLUDES1 malignant neoplasm of lymph nodes, specified as primary (C81-C86, C88, C96.-)
　　　　mesentery metastasis of carcinoid tumor (C7B.04)
　　　　secondary carcinoid tumors of distant lymph nodes (C7B.01)
　　C77.0 Secondary and unspecified malignant neoplasm of lymph nodes of head, face and neck `HCC` `RxHCC`
　　　　Secondary and unspecified malignant neoplasm of supraclavicular lymph nodes
　　C77.1 Secondary and unspecified malignant neoplasm of intrathoracic lymph nodes `HCC` `RxHCC`
　　C77.2 Secondary and unspecified malignant neoplasm of intra-abdominal lymph nodes `HCC` `RxHCC`
　　C77.3 Secondary and unspecified malignant neoplasm of axilla and upper limb lymph nodes `HCC` `RxHCC`
　　　　Secondary and unspecified malignant neoplasm of pectoral lymph nodes

---

Unspecified Code　Other Specified Code　Manifestation Code　N Newborn　P Pediatric　M Maternity　A Adult　♂ Male　♀ Female
● New Code　▲ Revised Code Title　►◄ Revised Text　NOTES　INCLUDES　EXCLUDES1 Not coded here　EXCLUDES2 Not included here
4th character required　5th character required　6th character required　7th character required　Extension 'X' Alert
HAC Hospital-acquired condition (HAC) alert　AHA AHA Coding Clinic©　📖 Code first alert

C77.4 **Secondary and unspecified malignant neoplasm of** inguinal and lower limb **lymph nodes** `HCC` `RxHCC`

C77.5 **Secondary and unspecified malignant neoplasm of** intrapelvic **lymph nodes** `HCC` `RxHCC`

C77.8 **Secondary and unspecified malignant neoplasm of lymph nodes of** multiple regions `HCC` `RxHCC`

C77.9 **Secondary and unspecified malignant neoplasm of lymph node, unspecified** `HCC` `RxHCC`

4ᵗʰ **C78 Secondary malignant neoplasm of** respiratory and digestive organs

EXCLUDES1 secondary carcinoid tumors of liver (C7B.02)

secondary carcinoid tumors of peritoneum (C7B.04)

EXCLUDES2 lymph node metastases (C77.0)

5ᵗʰ C78.0 **Secondary malignant neoplasm of** lung

C78.00 **Secondary malignant neoplasm of unspecified lung** `HCC` `RxHCC`

C78.01 **Secondary malignant neoplasm of** right **lung** `HCC` `RxHCC`

C78.02 **Secondary malignant neoplasm of** left **lung** `HCC` `RxHCC`

C78.1 **Secondary malignant neoplasm of** mediastinum `HCC` `RxHCC`

C78.2 **Secondary malignant neoplasm of** pleura `HCC` `RxHCC`

5ᵗʰ C78.3 **Secondary malignant neoplasm of** other and unspecified respiratory organs

C78.30 **Secondary malignant neoplasm of unspecified respiratory organ** `HCC` `RxHCC`

C78.39 **Secondary malignant neoplasm of** other **respiratory organs** `HCC` `RxHCC`

C78.4 **Secondary malignant neoplasm of** small intestine `HCC` `RxHCC`

C78.5 **Secondary malignant neoplasm of** large intestine and rectum `HCC` `RxHCC`

C78.6 **Secondary malignant neoplasm of** retroperitoneum and peritoneum `HCC` `RxHCC`
AHA: Q2 2017

C78.7 **Secondary malignant neoplasm of** liver and intrahepatic bile duct `HCC` `RxHCC`

5ᵗʰ C78.8 **Secondary malignant neoplasm of** other and unspecified digestive organs

C78.80 **Secondary malignant neoplasm of unspecified digestive organ** `HCC` `RxHCC`

C78.89 **Secondary malignant neoplasm of** other **digestive organs** `HCC` `RxHCC`
Code also exocrine pancreatic insufficiency (K86.81)

4ᵗʰ **C79 Secondary malignant neoplasm of** other and unspecified sites

EXCLUDES1 secondary carcinoid tumors (C7B.-)

secondary neuroendocrine tumors (C7B.-)

5ᵗʰ C79.0 **Secondary malignant neoplasm of** kidney and renal pelvis

C79.00 **Secondary malignant neoplasm of unspecified kidney and renal pelvis** `HCC` `RxHCC`

C79.01 **Secondary malignant neoplasm of** right **kidney and renal pelvis** `HCC` `RxHCC`

C79.02 **Secondary malignant neoplasm of** left **kidney and renal pelvis** `HCC` `RxHCC`

5ᵗʰ C79.1 **Secondary malignant neoplasm of** bladder and other and unspecified urinary organs

C79.10 **Secondary malignant neoplasm of unspecified urinary organs** `HCC` `RxHCC`

C79.11 **Secondary malignant neoplasm of** bladder `HCC` `RxHCC`
EXCLUDES2 lymph node metastases (C77.0)

C79.19 **Secondary malignant neoplasm of** other **urinary organs** `HCC` `RxHCC`

C79.2 **Secondary malignant neoplasm of** skin `HCC` `RxHCC`
EXCLUDES1 secondary Merkel cell carcinoma (C7B.1)

5ᵗʰ C79.3 **Secondary malignant neoplasm of** brain and cerebral meninges

C79.31 **Secondary malignant neoplasm of** brain `HCC` `RxHCC`

C79.32 **Secondary malignant neoplasm of** cerebral meninges `HCC` `RxHCC`

5ᵗʰ C79.4 **Secondary malignant neoplasm of** other and unspecified parts of nervous system

C79.40 **Secondary malignant neoplasm of unspecified part of nervous system** `HCC` `RxHCC`

C79.49 **Secondary malignant neoplasm of** other parts of nervous system `HCC` `RxHCC`

5ᵗʰ C79.5 **Secondary malignant neoplasm of** bone and bone marrow
EXCLUDES1 secondary carcinoid tumors of bone (C7B.03)

C79.51 **Secondary malignant neoplasm of** bone `HCC` `RxHCC`

C79.52 **Secondary malignant neoplasm of** bone marrow `HCC` `RxHCC`

5ᵗʰ C79.6 **Secondary malignant neoplasm of** ovary

C79.60 **Secondary malignant neoplasm of unspecified ovary** `HCC` `RxHCC` ♀

C79.61 **Secondary malignant neoplasm of** right **ovary** `HCC` `RxHCC` ♀

C79.62 **Secondary malignant neoplasm of** left **ovary** `HCC` `RxHCC` ♀

5ᵗʰ C79.7 **Secondary malignant neoplasm of** adrenal gland

C79.70 **Secondary malignant neoplasm of unspecified adrenal gland** `HCC` `RxHCC`

C79.71 **Secondary malignant neoplasm of** right **adrenal gland** `HCC` `RxHCC`

C79.72 **Secondary malignant neoplasm of** left **adrenal gland** `HCC` `RxHCC`

5ᵗʰ C79.8 **Secondary malignant neoplasm of** other specified sites

C79.81 **Secondary malignant neoplasm of** breast `HCC` `RxHCC`

C79.82 **Secondary malignant neoplasm of** genital organs `HCC` `RxHCC`

C79.89 **Secondary malignant neoplasm of other specified sites** `HCC` `RxHCC`
AHA: Q2 2017

C79.9 **Secondary malignant neoplasm of unspecified site** `HCC` `RxHCC`
Metastatic cancer NOS
Metastatic disease NOS
EXCLUDES1 carcinomatosis NOS (C80.0)

generalized cancer NOS (C80.0)

malignant (primary) neoplasm of unspecified site (C80.1)

4ᵗʰ **C80 Malignant neoplasm** without specification of site

EXCLUDES1 malignant carcinoid tumor of unspecified site (C7A.00)

malignant neoplasm of specified multiple sites- code to each site

C80.0 **Disseminated malignant neoplasm, unspecified** `HCC` `RxHCC`
Carcinomatosis NOS
Generalized cancer, unspecified site (primary) (secondary)
Generalized malignancy, unspecified site (primary) (secondary)

C80.1 **Malignant (primary) neoplasm, unspecified** `HCC`
Cancer NOS
Cancer unspecified site (primary)
Carcinoma unspecified site (primary)
Malignancy unspecified site (primary)
EXCLUDES1 secondary malignant neoplasm of unspecified site (C79.9)

C80.2 **Malignant neoplasm associated with** transplanted organ `HCC` `PDx`
☞ **Code first** complication of transplanted organ (T86.-)
Use additional code to identify the specific malignancy

Malignant neoplasms of lymphoid, hematopoietic and related tissue (C81-C96)

EXCLUDES2 Kaposi's sarcoma of lymph nodes (C46.3)

secondary and unspecified neoplasm of lymph nodes (C77.-)

secondary neoplasm of bone marrow (C79.52)

secondary neoplasm of spleen (C78.89)

4ᵗʰ **C81** Hodgkin **lymphoma**

EXCLUDES1 personal history of Hodgkin lymphoma (Z85.71)

5ᵗʰ C81.0 Nodular lymphocyte predominant Hodgkin lymphoma

C81.00 **Nodular lymphocyte predominant Hodgkin lymphoma, unspecified site** `HCC`

C81.01 **Nodular lymphocyte predominant Hodgkin lymphoma, lymph nodes of** head, face, and neck `HCC`

C81.02 **Nodular lymphocyte predominant Hodgkin lymphoma,** intrathoracic **lymph nodes** `HCC`

`PDx` Unacceptable principal diagnosis symbol per Medicare code edits   `POA` Code exempt from diagnosis present on admission requirement
? Questionable admission   `✧` Complication or comorbidity   `MCC` Major complication or comorbidity   `CC/MCC` CC/MCC exclusion
`HCC` HCC diagnosis code   `RxHCC` RxHCC diagnosis code   MACRA code   **DEFINITION** Describes condition/terminology
TIP Coding guidance   ✎ Official Guideline Reference   `Z` Z code as first-listed diagnosis

486

When symbols appear on a code that requires a 7th character extension, refer to Appendix B to identify applicable 7th character codes.

2020 ICD-10-CM

C81.03 **Nodular lymphocyte predominant Hodgkin lymphoma,** intra-abdominal **lymph nodes** `HCC`

C81.04 **Nodular lymphocyte predominant Hodgkin lymphoma, lymph nodes of** axilla and upper limb `HCC`

C81.05 **Nodular lymphocyte predominant Hodgkin lymphoma, lymph nodes of** inguinal region and lower limb `HCC`

C81.06 **Nodular lymphocyte predominant Hodgkin lymphoma,** intrapelvic **lymph nodes** `HCC`

C81.07 **Nodular lymphocyte predominant Hodgkin lymphoma,** spleen `HCC`

C81.08 **Nodular lymphocyte predominant Hodgkin lymphoma, lymph nodes of** multiple sites `HCC`

C81.09 **Nodular lymphocyte predominant Hodgkin lymphoma,** extranodal and solid organ sites `HCC`

5ᵗʰ C81.1 Nodular sclerosis **Hodgkin lymphoma**
Nodular sclerosis classical Hodgkin lymphoma

C81.10 **Nodular sclerosis Hodgkin lymphoma, unspecified site** `HCC`

C81.11 **Nodular sclerosis Hodgkin lymphoma, lymph nodes of** head, face, and neck `HCC`

C81.12 **Nodular sclerosis Hodgkin lymphoma,** intrathoracic **lymph nodes** `HCC`

C81.13 **Nodular sclerosis Hodgkin lymphoma,** intra-abdominal **lymph nodes** `HCC`

C81.14 **Nodular sclerosis Hodgkin lymphoma, lymph nodes of** axilla and upper limb `HCC`

C81.15 **Nodular sclerosis Hodgkin lymphoma, lymph nodes of** inguinal region and lower limb `HCC`

C81.16 **Nodular sclerosis Hodgkin lymphoma,** intrapelvic **lymph nodes** `HCC`

C81.17 **Nodular sclerosis Hodgkin lymphoma,** spleen `HCC`

C81.18 **Nodular sclerosis Hodgkin lymphoma, lymph nodes of** multiple sites `HCC`

C81.19 **Nodular sclerosis Hodgkin lymphoma,** extranodal and solid organ sites `HCC`

5ᵗʰ C81.2 Mixed cellularity **Hodgkin lymphoma**
Mixed cellularity classical Hodgkin lymphoma

C81.20 **Mixed cellularity Hodgkin lymphoma, unspecified site** `HCC`

C81.21 **Mixed cellularity Hodgkin lymphoma, lymph nodes of** head, face, and neck `HCC`

C81.22 **Mixed cellularity Hodgkin lymphoma,** intrathoracic **lymph nodes** `HCC`

C81.23 **Mixed cellularity Hodgkin lymphoma,** intra-abdominal **lymph nodes** `HCC`

C81.24 **Mixed cellularity Hodgkin lymphoma, lymph nodes of** axilla and upper limb `HCC`

C81.25 **Mixed cellularity Hodgkin lymphoma, lymph nodes of** inguinal region and lower limb `HCC`

C81.26 **Mixed cellularity Hodgkin lymphoma,** intrapelvic **lymph nodes** `HCC`

C81.27 **Mixed cellularity Hodgkin lymphoma,** spleen `HCC`

C81.28 **Mixed cellularity Hodgkin lymphoma, lymph nodes of** multiple sites `HCC`

C81.29 **Mixed cellularity Hodgkin lymphoma,** extranodal and solid organ sites `HCC`

5ᵗʰ C81.3 Lymphocyte depleted **Hodgkin lymphoma**
Lymphocyte depleted classical Hodgkin lymphoma

C81.30 **Lymphocyte depleted Hodgkin lymphoma, unspecified site** `HCC`

C81.31 **Lymphocyte depleted Hodgkin lymphoma, lymph nodes of** head, face, and neck `HCC`

C81.32 **Lymphocyte depleted Hodgkin lymphoma,** intrathoracic **lymph nodes** `HCC`

C81.33 **Lymphocyte depleted Hodgkin lymphoma,** intra-abdominal **lymph nodes** `HCC`

C81.34 **Lymphocyte depleted Hodgkin lymphoma, lymph nodes of** axilla and upper limb `HCC`

C81.35 **Lymphocyte depleted Hodgkin lymphoma, lymph nodes of** inguinal region and lower limb `HCC`

C81.36 **Lymphocyte depleted Hodgkin lymphoma,** intrapelvic **lymph nodes** `HCC`

C81.37 **Lymphocyte depleted Hodgkin lymphoma,** spleen `HCC`

C81.38 **Lymphocyte depleted Hodgkin lymphoma, lymph nodes of** multiple sites `HCC`

C81.39 **Lymphocyte depleted Hodgkin lymphoma,** extranodal and solid organ sites `HCC`

5ᵗʰ C81.4 Lymphocyte-rich **Hodgkin lymphoma**
Lymphocyte-rich classical Hodgkin lymphoma
EXCLUDES1 nodular lymphocyte predominant Hodgkin lymphoma (C81.0-)

C81.40 **Lymphocyte-rich Hodgkin lymphoma, unspecified site** `HCC`

C81.41 **Lymphocyte-rich Hodgkin lymphoma, lymph nodes of** head, face, and neck `HCC`

C81.42 **Lymphocyte-rich Hodgkin lymphoma,** intrathoracic **lymph nodes** `HCC`

C81.43 **Lymphocyte-rich Hodgkin lymphoma,** intra-abdominal **lymph nodes** `HCC`

C81.44 **Lymphocyte-rich Hodgkin lymphoma, lymph nodes of** axilla and upper limb `HCC`

C81.45 **Lymphocyte-rich Hodgkin lymphoma, lymph nodes of** inguinal region and lower limb `HCC`

C81.46 **Lymphocyte-rich Hodgkin lymphoma,** intrapelvic **lymph nodes** `HCC`

C81.47 **Lymphocyte-rich Hodgkin lymphoma,** spleen `HCC`

C81.48 **Lymphocyte-rich Hodgkin lymphoma, lymph nodes of** multiple sites `HCC`

C81.49 **Lymphocyte-rich Hodgkin lymphoma,** extranodal and solid organ sites `HCC`

5ᵗʰ C81.7 Other **Hodgkin lymphoma**
Classical Hodgkin lymphoma NOS
Other classical Hodgkin lymphoma

C81.70 **Other Hodgkin lymphoma, unspecified site** `HCC`

C81.71 **Other Hodgkin lymphoma, lymph nodes of** head, face, and neck `HCC`

C81.72 **Other Hodgkin lymphoma,** intrathoracic **lymph nodes** `HCC`

C81.73 **Other Hodgkin lymphoma,** intra-abdominal **lymph nodes** `HCC`

C81.74 **Other Hodgkin lymphoma, lymph nodes of** axilla and upper limb `HCC`

C81.75 **Other Hodgkin lymphoma, lymph nodes of** inguinal region and lower limb `HCC`

C81.76 **Other Hodgkin lymphoma,** intrapelvic **lymph nodes** `HCC`

C81.77 **Other Hodgkin lymphoma,** spleen `HCC`

C81.78 **Other Hodgkin lymphoma, lymph nodes of** multiple sites `HCC`

C81.79 **Other Hodgkin lymphoma,** extranodal and solid organ sites `HCC`

5ᵗʰ C81.9 Hodgkin lymphoma, unspecified

C81.90 **Hodgkin lymphoma, unspecified, unspecified site** `HCC`

C81.91 **Hodgkin lymphoma, unspecified, lymph nodes of** head, face, and neck `HCC`

C81.92 **Hodgkin lymphoma, unspecified,** intrathoracic **lymph nodes** `HCC`

C81.93 **Hodgkin lymphoma, unspecified,** intra-abdominal **lymph nodes** `HCC`

C81.94 **Hodgkin lymphoma, unspecified, lymph nodes of** axilla and upper limb `HCC`

C81.95 **Hodgkin lymphoma, unspecified, lymph nodes of** inguinal region and lower limb `HCC`

C81.96 **Hodgkin lymphoma, unspecified,** intrapelvic **lymph nodes** `HCC`

C81.97 **Hodgkin lymphoma, unspecified,** spleen `HCC`

C81.98 **Hodgkin lymphoma, unspecified, lymph nodes of** multiple sites `HCC`

C81.99 **Hodgkin lymphoma, unspecified,** extranodal and solid organ sites `HCC`

[4th] **C82 Follicular lymphoma**
[INCLUDES] *follicular lymphoma with or without diffuse areas*
[EXCLUDES1] *mature T/NK-cell lymphomas (C84.-)*
personal history of non-Hodgkin lymphoma (Z85.72)

[5th] **C82.0 Follicular lymphoma grade I**
- C82.00 **Follicular lymphoma grade I, unspecified site** [HCC]
- C82.01 **Follicular lymphoma grade I, lymph nodes of head, face, and neck** [HCC]
- C82.02 **Follicular lymphoma grade I, intrathoracic lymph nodes** [HCC]
- C82.03 **Follicular lymphoma grade I, intra-abdominal lymph nodes** [HCC]
- C82.04 **Follicular lymphoma grade I, lymph nodes of axilla and upper limb** [HCC]
- C82.05 **Follicular lymphoma grade I, lymph nodes of inguinal region and lower limb** [HCC]
- C82.06 **Follicular lymphoma grade I, intrapelvic lymph nodes** [HCC]
- C82.07 **Follicular lymphoma grade I, spleen** [HCC]
- C82.08 **Follicular lymphoma grade I, lymph nodes of multiple sites** [HCC]
- C82.09 **Follicular lymphoma grade I, extranodal and solid organ sites** [HCC]

[5th] **C82.1 Follicular lymphoma grade II**
- C82.10 **Follicular lymphoma grade II, unspecified site** [HCC]
- C82.11 **Follicular lymphoma grade II, lymph nodes of head, face, and neck** [HCC]
- C82.12 **Follicular lymphoma grade II, intrathoracic lymph nodes** [HCC]
- C82.13 **Follicular lymphoma grade II, intra-abdominal lymph nodes** [HCC]
- C82.14 **Follicular lymphoma grade II, lymph nodes of axilla and upper limb** [HCC]
- C82.15 **Follicular lymphoma grade II, lymph nodes of inguinal region and lower limb** [HCC]
- C82.16 **Follicular lymphoma grade II, intrapelvic lymph nodes** [HCC]
- C82.17 **Follicular lymphoma grade II, spleen** [CC] [HCC] [CC/MCC Exc]
- C82.18 **Follicular lymphoma grade II, lymph nodes of multiple sites** [HCC]
- C82.19 **Follicular lymphoma grade II, extranodal and solid organ sites** [HCC]

[5th] **C82.2 Follicular lymphoma grade III, unspecified**
- C82.20 **Follicular lymphoma grade III, unspecified, unspecified site** [HCC]
- C82.21 **Follicular lymphoma grade III, unspecified, lymph nodes of head, face, and neck** [HCC]
- C82.22 **Follicular lymphoma grade III, unspecified, intrathoracic lymph nodes** [HCC]
- C82.23 **Follicular lymphoma grade III, unspecified, intra-abdominal lymph nodes** [HCC]
- C82.24 **Follicular lymphoma grade III, unspecified, lymph nodes of axilla and upper limb** [HCC]
- C82.25 **Follicular lymphoma grade III, unspecified, lymph nodes of inguinal region and lower limb** [HCC]
- C82.26 **Follicular lymphoma grade III, unspecified, intrapelvic lymph nodes** [HCC]
- C82.27 **Follicular lymphoma grade III, unspecified, spleen** [HCC]
- C82.28 **Follicular lymphoma grade III, unspecified, lymph nodes of multiple sites** [HCC]
- C82.29 **Follicular lymphoma grade III, unspecified, extranodal and solid organ sites** [HCC]

[5th] **C82.3 Follicular lymphoma grade IIIa**
- C82.30 **Follicular lymphoma grade IIIa, unspecified site** [HCC]
- C82.31 **Follicular lymphoma grade IIIa, lymph nodes of head, face, and neck** [HCC]
- C82.32 **Follicular lymphoma grade IIIa, intrathoracic lymph nodes** [HCC]
- C82.33 **Follicular lymphoma grade IIIa, intra-abdominal lymph nodes** [HCC]
- C82.34 **Follicular lymphoma grade IIIa, lymph nodes of axilla and upper limb** [HCC]
- C82.35 **Follicular lymphoma grade IIIa, lymph nodes of inguinal region and lower limb** [HCC]
- C82.36 **Follicular lymphoma grade IIIa, intrapelvic lymph nodes** [HCC]
- C82.37 **Follicular lymphoma grade IIIa, spleen** [HCC]
- C82.38 **Follicular lymphoma grade IIIa, lymph nodes of multiple sites** [HCC]
- C82.39 **Follicular lymphoma grade IIIa, extranodal and solid organ sites** [HCC]

[5th] **C82.4 Follicular lymphoma grade IIIb**
- C82.40 **Follicular lymphoma grade IIIb, unspecified site** [HCC]
- C82.41 **Follicular lymphoma grade IIIb, lymph nodes of head, face, and neck** [HCC]
- C82.42 **Follicular lymphoma grade IIIb, intrathoracic lymph nodes** [HCC]
- C82.43 **Follicular lymphoma grade IIIb, intra-abdominal lymph nodes** [HCC]
- C82.44 **Follicular lymphoma grade IIIb, lymph nodes of axilla and upper limb** [HCC]
- C82.45 **Follicular lymphoma grade IIIb, lymph nodes of inguinal region and lower limb** [HCC]
- C82.46 **Follicular lymphoma grade IIIb, intrapelvic lymph nodes** [HCC]
- C82.47 **Follicular lymphoma grade IIIb, spleen** [HCC]
- C82.48 **Follicular lymphoma grade IIIb, lymph nodes of multiple sites** [HCC]
- C82.49 **Follicular lymphoma grade IIIb, extranodal and solid organ sites** [HCC]

[5th] **C82.5 Diffuse follicle center lymphoma**
- C82.50 **Diffuse follicle center lymphoma, unspecified site** [HCC]
- C82.51 **Diffuse follicle center lymphoma, lymph nodes of head, face, and neck** [HCC]
- C82.52 **Diffuse follicle center lymphoma, intrathoracic lymph nodes** [HCC]
- C82.53 **Diffuse follicle center lymphoma, intra-abdominal lymph nodes** [HCC]
- C82.54 **Diffuse follicle center lymphoma, lymph nodes of axilla and upper limb** [HCC]
- C82.55 **Diffuse follicle center lymphoma, lymph nodes of inguinal region and lower limb** [HCC]
- C82.56 **Diffuse follicle center lymphoma, intrapelvic lymph nodes** [HCC]
- C82.57 **Diffuse follicle center lymphoma, spleen** [HCC]
- C82.58 **Diffuse follicle center lymphoma, lymph nodes of multiple sites** [HCC]
- C82.59 **Diffuse follicle center lymphoma, extranodal and solid organ sites** [HCC]

[5th] **C82.6 Cutaneous follicle center lymphoma**
- C82.60 **Cutaneous follicle center lymphoma, unspecified site** [HCC]
- C82.61 **Cutaneous follicle center lymphoma, lymph nodes of head, face, and neck** [HCC]
- C82.62 **Cutaneous follicle center lymphoma, intrathoracic lymph nodes** [HCC]
- C82.63 **Cutaneous follicle center lymphoma, intra-abdominal lymph nodes** [HCC]
- C82.64 **Cutaneous follicle center lymphoma, lymph nodes of axilla and upper limb** [HCC]
- C82.65 **Cutaneous follicle center lymphoma, lymph nodes of inguinal region and lower limb** [HCC]
- C82.66 **Cutaneous follicle center lymphoma, intrapelvic lymph nodes** [HCC]
- C82.67 **Cutaneous follicle center lymphoma, spleen** [HCC]
- C82.68 **Cutaneous follicle center lymphoma, lymph nodes of multiple sites** [HCC]
- C82.69 **Cutaneous follicle center lymphoma, extranodal and solid organ sites** [HCC]

[5th] **C82.8 Other types of follicular lymphoma**

C82.80 Other types of follicular lymphoma, unspecified site `HCC`

C82.81 Other types of follicular lymphoma, lymph nodes of head, face, and neck `HCC`

C82.82 Other types of follicular lymphoma, intrathoracic lymph nodes `HCC`

C82.83 Other types of follicular lymphoma, intra-abdominal lymph nodes `HCC`

C82.84 Other types of follicular lymphoma, lymph nodes of axilla and upper limb `HCC`

C82.85 Other types of follicular lymphoma, lymph nodes of inguinal region and lower limb `HCC`

C82.86 Other types of follicular lymphoma, intrapelvic lymph nodes `HCC`

C82.87 Other types of follicular lymphoma, spleen `HCC`

C82.88 Other types of follicular lymphoma, lymph nodes of multiple sites `HCC`

C82.89 Other types of follicular lymphoma, extranodal and solid organ sites `HCC`

⑤ C82.9 Follicular lymphoma, unspecified

C82.90 Follicular lymphoma, unspecified, unspecified site `HCC`

C82.91 Follicular lymphoma, unspecified, lymph nodes of head, face, and neck `HCC`

C82.92 Follicular lymphoma, unspecified, intrathoracic lymph nodes `HCC`

C82.93 Follicular lymphoma, unspecified, intra-abdominal lymph nodes `HCC`

C82.94 Follicular lymphoma, unspecified, lymph nodes of axilla and upper limb `HCC`

C82.95 Follicular lymphoma, unspecified, lymph nodes of inguinal region and lower limb `HCC`

C82.96 Follicular lymphoma, unspecified, intrapelvic lymph nodes `HCC`

C82.97 Follicular lymphoma, unspecified, spleen `HCC`

C82.98 Follicular lymphoma, unspecified, lymph nodes of multiple sites `HCC`

C82.99 Follicular lymphoma, unspecified, extranodal and solid organ sites `HCC`

④ C83 Non-follicular lymphoma

EXCLUDES1 personal history of non-Hodgkin lymphoma (Z85.72)

⑤ C83.0 Small cell B-cell lymphoma

Lymphoplasmacytic lymphoma
Nodal marginal zone lymphoma
Non-leukemic variant of B-CLL
Splenic marginal zone lymphoma

EXCLUDES1 chronic lymphocytic leukemia (C91.1)
mature T/NK-cell lymphomas (C84.-)
Waldenström macroglobulinemia (C88.0)

C83.00 Small cell B-cell lymphoma, unspecified site `cc` `HCC` `CC/MCC Exc`

C83.01 Small cell B-cell lymphoma, lymph nodes of head, face, and neck `cc` `HCC` `CC/MCC Exc`

C83.02 Small cell B-cell lymphoma, intrathoracic lymph nodes `HCC`

C83.03 Small cell B-cell lymphoma, intra-abdominal lymph nodes `HCC`

C83.04 Small cell B-cell lymphoma, lymph nodes of axilla and upper limb `HCC`

C83.05 Small cell B-cell lymphoma, lymph nodes of inguinal region and lower limb `HCC`

C83.06 Small cell B-cell lymphoma, intrapelvic lymph nodes `HCC`

C83.07 Small cell B-cell lymphoma, spleen `HCC`

C83.08 Small cell B-cell lymphoma, lymph nodes of multiple sites `HCC`

C83.09 Small cell B-cell lymphoma, extranodal and solid organ sites `HCC`

⑤ C83.1 Mantle cell lymphoma

Centrocytic lymphoma
Malignant lymphomatous polyposis

C83.10 Mantle cell lymphoma, unspecified site `HCC`

C83.11 Mantle cell lymphoma, lymph nodes of head, face, and neck `HCC`

C83.12 Mantle cell lymphoma, intrathoracic lymph nodes `HCC`

C83.13 Mantle cell lymphoma, intra-abdominal lymph nodes `HCC`

C83.14 Mantle cell lymphoma, lymph nodes of axilla and upper limb `HCC`

C83.15 Mantle cell lymphoma, lymph nodes of inguinal region and lower limb `HCC`

C83.16 Mantle cell lymphoma, intrapelvic lymph nodes `HCC`

C83.17 Mantle cell lymphoma, spleen `HCC`

C83.18 Mantle cell lymphoma, lymph nodes of multiple sites `HCC`

C83.19 Mantle cell lymphoma, extranodal and solid organ sites `HCC`

⑤ C83.3 Diffuse large B-cell lymphoma

Anaplastic diffuse large B-cell lymphoma
CD30-positive diffuse large B-cell lymphoma
Centroblastic diffuse large B-cell lymphoma
Diffuse large B-cell lymphoma, subtype not specified
Immunoblastic diffuse large B-cell lymphoma
Plasmablastic diffuse large B-cell lymphoma
Diffuse large B-cell lymphoma, subtype not specified
T-cell rich diffuse large B-cell lymphoma

EXCLUDES1 mediastinal (thymic) large B-cell lymphoma (C85.2-)
mature T/NK-cell lymphomas (C84.-)

C83.30 Diffuse large B-cell lymphoma, unspecified site `HCC`

C83.31 Diffuse large B-cell lymphoma, lymph nodes of head, face, and neck `HCC`

C83.32 Diffuse large B-cell lymphoma, intrathoracic lymph nodes `HCC`

C83.33 Diffuse large B-cell lymphoma, intra-abdominal lymph nodes `HCC`

C83.34 Diffuse large B-cell lymphoma, lymph nodes of axilla and upper limb `HCC`

C83.35 Diffuse large B-cell lymphoma, lymph nodes of inguinal region and lower limb `HCC`

C83.36 Diffuse large B-cell lymphoma, intrapelvic lymph nodes `HCC`

C83.37 Diffuse large B-cell lymphoma, spleen `HCC`

C83.38 Diffuse large B-cell lymphoma, lymph nodes of multiple sites `HCC`

C83.39 Diffuse large B-cell lymphoma, extranodal and solid organ sites `HCC`

⑤ C83.5 Lymphoblastic (diffuse) lymphoma

B-precursor lymphoma
Lymphoblastic B-cell lymphoma
Lymphoblastic lymphoma NOS
Lymphoblastic T-cell lymphoma
T-precursor lymphoma

C83.50 Lymphoblastic (diffuse) lymphoma, unspecified site `HCC`

C83.51 Lymphoblastic (diffuse) lymphoma, lymph nodes of head, face, and neck `HCC`

C83.52 Lymphoblastic (diffuse) lymphoma, intrathoracic lymph nodes `HCC`

C83.53 Lymphoblastic (diffuse) lymphoma, intra-abdominal lymph nodes `HCC`

C83.54 Lymphoblastic (diffuse) lymphoma, lymph nodes of axilla and upper limb `HCC`

C83.55 Lymphoblastic (diffuse) lymphoma, lymph nodes of inguinal region and lower limb `HCC`

C83.56 Lymphoblastic (diffuse) lymphoma, intrapelvic lymph nodes `HCC`

C83.57 Lymphoblastic (diffuse) lymphoma, spleen `HCC`

C83.58 Lymphoblastic (diffuse) lymphoma, lymph nodes of multiple sites `HCC`

C83.59 Lymphoblastic (diffuse) lymphoma, extranodal and solid organ sites `HCC`

C83.7 **Burkitt** lymphoma
Atypical Burkitt lymphoma
Burkitt-like lymphoma
EXCLUDES1 mature B-cell leukemia Burkitt type (C91.A-)

C83.70 **Burkitt lymphoma, unspecified site** HCC

C83.71 **Burkitt lymphoma, lymph nodes of** head, face, and neck HCC

C83.72 **Burkitt lymphoma, intrathoracic lymph nodes** HCC

C83.73 **Burkitt lymphoma, intra-abdominal lymph nodes** HCC

C83.74 **Burkitt lymphoma, lymph nodes of** axilla and upper limb HCC

C83.75 **Burkitt lymphoma, lymph nodes of** inguinal region and lower limb HCC

C83.76 **Burkitt lymphoma, intrapelvic lymph nodes** HCC

C83.77 **Burkitt lymphoma, spleen** HCC

C83.78 **Burkitt lymphoma, lymph nodes of** multiple sites HCC

C83.79 **Burkitt lymphoma, extranodal and solid organ sites** HCC

C83.8 Other non-follicular lymphoma
Intravascular large B-cell lymphoma
Lymphoid granulomatosis
Primary effusion B-cell lymphoma
EXCLUDES1 mediastinal (thymic) large B-cell lymphoma (C85.2-)
T-cell rich B-cell lymphoma (C83.3-)

C83.80 **Other non-follicular lymphoma, unspecified site** HCC

C83.81 **Other non-follicular lymphoma, lymph nodes of** head, face, and neck HCC

C83.82 **Other non-follicular lymphoma, intrathoracic lymph nodes** HCC

C83.83 **Other non-follicular lymphoma, intra-abdominal lymph nodes** HCC

C83.84 **Other non-follicular lymphoma, lymph nodes of** axilla and upper limb HCC

C83.85 **Other non-follicular lymphoma, lymph nodes of** inguinal region and lower limb HCC

C83.86 **Other non-follicular lymphoma, intrapelvic lymph nodes** HCC

C83.87 **Other non-follicular lymphoma, spleen** HCC

C83.88 **Other non-follicular lymphoma, lymph nodes of** multiple sites HCC

C83.89 **Other non-follicular lymphoma, extranodal and solid organ sites** HCC

C83.9 Non-follicular (diffuse) lymphoma, unspecified

C83.90 **Non-follicular (diffuse) lymphoma, unspecified, unspecified site** HCC

C83.91 **Non-follicular (diffuse) lymphoma, unspecified, lymph nodes of** head, face, and neck HCC

C83.92 **Non-follicular (diffuse) lymphoma, unspecified, intrathoracic lymph nodes** HCC

C83.93 **Non-follicular (diffuse) lymphoma, unspecified, intra-abdominal lymph nodes** HCC

C83.94 **Non-follicular (diffuse) lymphoma, unspecified, lymph nodes of** axilla and upper limb HCC

C83.95 **Non-follicular (diffuse) lymphoma, unspecified, lymph nodes of** inguinal region and lower limb HCC

C83.96 **Non-follicular (diffuse) lymphoma, unspecified, intrapelvic lymph nodes** HCC

C83.97 **Non-follicular (diffuse) lymphoma, unspecified, spleen** HCC

C83.98 **Non-follicular (diffuse) lymphoma, unspecified, lymph nodes of** multiple sites HCC

C83.99 **Non-follicular (diffuse) lymphoma, unspecified, extranodal and solid organ sites** HCC

C84 Mature T/NK-cell lymphomas
EXCLUDES1 personal history of non-Hodgkin lymphoma (Z85.72)

C84.0 **Mycosis fungoides**
EXCLUDES1 peripheral T-cell lymphoma, not classified (C84.4-)

C84.00 **Mycosis fungoides, unspecified site** HCC RxHCC

C84.01 **Mycosis fungoides, lymph nodes of** head, face, and neck HCC RxHCC

C84.02 **Mycosis fungoides, intrathoracic lymph nodes** HCC RxHCC

C84.03 **Mycosis fungoides, intra-abdominal lymph nodes** HCC RxHCC

C84.04 **Mycosis fungoides, lymph nodes of** axilla and upper limb HCC RxHCC

C84.05 **Mycosis fungoides, lymph nodes of** inguinal region and lower limb HCC RxHCC

C84.06 **Mycosis fungoides, intrapelvic lymph nodes** HCC RxHCC

C84.07 **Mycosis fungoides, spleen** HCC RxHCC

C84.08 **Mycosis fungoides, lymph nodes of** multiple sites HCC RxHCC

C84.09 **Mycosis fungoides, extranodal and solid organ sites** HCC RxHCC

C84.1 Sézary disease

C84.10 **Sézary disease, unspecified site** HCC RxHCC

C84.11 **Sézary disease, lymph nodes of** head, face, and neck HCC RxHCC

C84.12 **Sézary disease, intrathoracic lymph nodes** HCC RxHCC

C84.13 **Sézary disease, intra-abdominal lymph nodes** HCC RxHCC

C84.14 **Sézary disease, lymph nodes of** axilla and upper limb HCC RxHCC

C84.15 **Sézary disease, lymph nodes of** inguinal region and lower limb HCC RxHCC

C84.16 **Sézary disease, intrapelvic lymph nodes** HCC RxHCC

C84.17 **Sézary disease, spleen** HCC RxHCC

C84.18 **Sézary disease, lymph nodes of** multiple sites HCC RxHCC

C84.19 **Sézary disease, extranodal and solid organ sites** HCC RxHCC

C84.4 Peripheral T-cell lymphoma, not classified
Lennert's lymphoma
Lymphoepithelioid lymphoma
Mature T-cell lymphoma, not elsewhere classified

C84.40 **Peripheral T-cell lymphoma, not classified, unspecified site** HCC

C84.41 **Peripheral T-cell lymphoma, not classified, lymph nodes of** head, face, and neck HCC

C84.42 **Peripheral T-cell lymphoma, not classified, intrathoracic lymph nodes** HCC

C84.43 **Peripheral T-cell lymphoma, not classified, intra-abdominal lymph nodes** HCC

C84.44 **Peripheral T-cell lymphoma, not classified, lymph nodes of** axilla and upper limb HCC

C84.45 **Peripheral T-cell lymphoma, not classified, lymph nodes of** inguinal region and lower limb HCC

C84.46 **Peripheral T-cell lymphoma, not classified, intrapelvic lymph nodes** HCC

C84.47 **Peripheral T-cell lymphoma, not classified, spleen** HCC

C84.48 **Peripheral T-cell lymphoma, not classified, lymph nodes of** multiple sites HCC

C84.49 **Peripheral T-cell lymphoma, not classified, extranodal and solid organ sites** HCC

C84.6 Anaplastic large cell lymphoma, ALK-positive
Anaplastic large cell lymphoma, CD30-positive

C84.60 **Anaplastic large cell lymphoma, ALK-positive, unspecified site** HCC

C84.61 **Anaplastic large cell lymphoma, ALK-positive, lymph nodes of** head, face, and neck HCC

C84.62 **Anaplastic large cell lymphoma, ALK-positive, intrathoracic lymph nodes** HCC

C84.63 **Anaplastic large cell lymphoma, ALK-positive, intra-abdominal lymph nodes** HCC

C84.64 **Anaplastic large cell lymphoma, ALK-positive, lymph nodes of** axilla and upper limb HCC

C84.65 **Anaplastic large cell lymphoma, ALK-positive, lymph nodes of** inguinal region and lower limb HCC

C84.66 **Anaplastic large cell lymphoma, ALK-positive, intrapelvic lymph nodes** HCC

C84.67 **Anaplastic large cell lymphoma, ALK-positive, spleen** HCC

C84.68 **Anaplastic large cell lymphoma, ALK-positive, lymph nodes of** multiple sites HCC

Unacceptable principal diagnosis symbol per Medicare code edits — Code exempt from diagnosis present on admission requirement — Questionable admission — Complication or comorbidity — Major complication or comorbidity — CC/MCC exclusion — HCC diagnosis code — RxHCC diagnosis code — MACRA code — **DEFINITION** Describes condition/terminology — **TIP** Coding guidance — Official Guideline Reference — Z code as first-listed diagnosis

490

When symbols appear on a code that requires a 7th character extension, refer to Appendix B to identify applicable 7th character codes.

2020 ICD-10-CM

C84.69 **Anaplastic large cell lymphoma, ALK-positive,** extranodal and solid organ sites `HCC`

🔟 C84.7 **Anaplastic large cell lymphoma,** ALK-negative

EXCLUDES1 *primary cutaneous CD30-positive T-cell proliferations (C86.6-)*

C84.70 **Anaplastic large cell lymphoma, ALK-negative, unspecified site** `HCC`

C84.71 **Anaplastic large cell lymphoma, ALK-negative, lymph nodes of** head, face, and neck `HCC`

C84.72 **Anaplastic large cell lymphoma, ALK-negative,** intrathoracic **lymph nodes** `HCC`

C84.73 **Anaplastic large cell lymphoma, ALK-negative,** intra-abdominal **lymph nodes** `HCC`

C84.74 **Anaplastic large cell lymphoma, ALK-negative, lymph nodes of** axilla and upper limb `HCC`

C84.75 **Anaplastic large cell lymphoma, ALK-negative, lymph nodes of** inguinal region and lower limb `HCC`

C84.76 **Anaplastic large cell lymphoma, ALK-negative,** intrapelvic **lymph nodes** `HCC`

C84.77 **Anaplastic large cell lymphoma, ALK-negative,** spleen `HCC`

C84.78 **Anaplastic large cell lymphoma, ALK-negative, lymph nodes of** multiple sites `HCC`

C84.79 **Anaplastic large cell lymphoma, ALK-negative,** extranodal and solid organ sites `HCC`

🔟 C84.A **Cutaneous T-cell lymphoma,** unspecified

C84.A0 **Cutaneous T-cell lymphoma, unspecified, unspecified site** `HCC`

C84.A1 **Cutaneous T-cell lymphoma, unspecified lymph nodes of** head, face, and neck `HCC`

C84.A2 **Cutaneous T-cell lymphoma, unspecified,** intrathoracic **lymph nodes** `HCC`

C84.A3 **Cutaneous T-cell lymphoma, unspecified,** intra-abdominal **lymph nodes** `HCC`

C84.A4 **Cutaneous T-cell lymphoma, unspecified, lymph nodes of** axilla and upper limb `HCC`

C84.A5 **Cutaneous T-cell lymphoma, unspecified, lymph nodes of** inguinal region and lower limb `HCC`

C84.A6 **Cutaneous T-cell lymphoma, unspecified,** intrapelvic **lymph nodes** `HCC`

C84.A7 **Cutaneous T-cell lymphoma, unspecified,** spleen `HCC`

C84.A8 **Cutaneous T-cell lymphoma, unspecified, lymph nodes of** multiple sites `HCC`

C84.A9 **Cutaneous T-cell lymphoma, unspecified,** extranodal and solid organ sites `HCC`

🔟 C84.Z Other mature **T/NK-cell lymphomas**

NOTES If T-cell lineage or involvement is mentioned in conjunction with a specific lymphoma, code to the more specific description.

EXCLUDES1 *angioimmunoblastic T-cell lymphoma (C86.5)*

blastic NK-cell lymphoma (C86.4)

enteropathy-type T-cell lymphoma (C86.2)

extranodal NK-cell lymphoma, nasal type (C86.0)

hepatosplenic T-cell lymphoma (C86.1)

primary cutaneous CD30-positive T-cell proliferations (C86.6)

subcutaneous panniculitis-like T-cell lymphoma (C86.3)

T-cell leukemia (C91.1-)

C84.Z0 **Other mature T/NK-cell lymphomas, unspecified site** `HCC`

C84.Z1 **Other mature T/NK-cell lymphomas, lymph nodes of** head, face, and neck `HCC`

C84.Z2 **Other mature T/NK-cell lymphomas,** intrathoracic **lymph nodes** `HCC`

C84.Z3 **Other mature T/NK-cell lymphomas,** intra-abdominal **lymph nodes** `HCC`

C84.Z4 **Other mature T/NK-cell lymphomas, lymph nodes of** axilla and upper limb `HCC`

C84.Z5 **Other mature T/NK-cell lymphomas, lymph nodes of** inguinal region and lower limb `HCC`

C84.Z6 **Other mature T/NK-cell lymphomas,** intrapelvic **lymph nodes** `HCC`

C84.Z7 **Other mature T/NK-cell lymphomas,** spleen `HCC`

C84.Z8 **Other mature T/NK-cell lymphomas, lymph nodes of** multiple sites `HCC`

C84.Z9 **Other mature T/NK-cell lymphomas,** extranodal and solid organ sites `HCC`

🔟 C84.9 **Mature T/NK-cell lymphomas,** unspecified

NK/T cell lymphoma NOS

EXCLUDES1 *mature T-cell lymphoma, not elsewhere classified (C84.4-)*

C84.90 **Mature T/NK-cell lymphomas, unspecified, unspecified site** `HCC`

C84.91 **Mature T/NK-cell lymphomas, unspecified, lymph nodes of** head, face, and neck `HCC`

C84.92 **Mature T/NK-cell lymphomas, unspecified,** intrathoracic **lymph nodes** `HCC`

C84.93 **Mature T/NK-cell lymphomas, unspecified,** intra-abdominal **lymph nodes** `HCC`

C84.94 **Mature T/NK-cell lymphomas, unspecified, lymph nodes of** axilla and upper limb `HCC`

C84.95 **Mature T/NK-cell lymphomas, unspecified, lymph nodes of** inguinal region and lower limb `HCC`

C84.96 **Mature T/NK-cell lymphomas, unspecified,** intrapelvic **lymph nodes** `HCC`

C84.97 **Mature T/NK-cell lymphomas, unspecified,** spleen `HCC`

C84.98 **Mature T/NK-cell lymphomas, unspecified, lymph nodes of** multiple sites `HCC`

C84.99 **Mature T/NK-cell lymphomas, unspecified,** extranodal and solid organ sites `HCC`

4️⃣ C85 Other specified **and** unspecified **types of** non-Hodgkin **lymphoma**

EXCLUDES1 *other specified types of T/NK-cell lymphoma (C86.-)*

personal history of non-Hodgkin lymphoma (Z85.72)

🔟 C85.1 Unspecified **B-cell lymphoma**

NOTES If B-cell lineage or involvement is mentioned in conjunction with a specific lymphoma, code to the more specific description.

C85.10 **Unspecified B-cell lymphoma, unspecified site** `HCC`

C85.11 **Unspecified B-cell lymphoma, lymph nodes of** head, face, and neck `HCC`

C85.12 **Unspecified B-cell lymphoma,** intrathoracic **lymph nodes** `HCC`

C85.13 **Unspecified B-cell lymphoma,** intra-abdominal **lymph nodes** `HCC`

C85.14 **Unspecified B-cell lymphoma, lymph nodes of** axilla and upper limb `HCC`

C85.15 **Unspecified B-cell lymphoma, lymph nodes of** inguinal region and lower limb `HCC`

C85.16 **Unspecified B-cell lymphoma,** intrapelvic **lymph nodes** `HCC`

C85.17 **Unspecified B-cell lymphoma,** spleen `HCC`

C85.18 **Unspecified B-cell lymphoma, lymph nodes of** multiple sites `HCC`

C85.19 **Unspecified B-cell lymphoma,** extranodal and solid organ sites `HCC`

🔟 C85.2 Mediastinal (thymic) **large B-cell lymphoma**

C85.20 **Mediastinal (thymic) large B-cell lymphoma, unspecified site** `HCC`

C85.21 **Mediastinal (thymic) large B-cell lymphoma, lymph nodes of** head, face, and neck `HCC`

C85.22 **Mediastinal (thymic) large B-cell lymphoma,** intrathoracic **lymph nodes** `HCC`

C85.23 **Mediastinal (thymic) large B-cell lymphoma,** intra-abdominal **lymph nodes** `HCC`

C85.24 **Mediastinal (thymic) large B-cell lymphoma, lymph nodes of** axilla and upper limb `HCC`

C85.25 **Mediastinal (thymic) large B-cell lymphoma, lymph nodes of** inguinal region and lower limb `HCC`

C85.26 **Mediastinal (thymic) large B-cell lymphoma,** intrapelvic **lymph nodes** `HCC`

Unspecified Code Other Specified Code Manifestation Code N Newborn P Pediatric M Maternity A Adult ♂ Male ♀ Female
● New Code ▲ Revised Code Title ►◄ Revised Text **NOTES** *INCLUDES* *EXCLUDES1* Not coded here *EXCLUDES2* Not included here
4️⃣ 4th character required 5️⃣ 5th character required 6️⃣ 6th character required 7️⃣ 7th character required 🅧 Extension 'X' Alert
HAC Hospital-acquired condition (HAC) alert **AHA** AHA Coding Clinic© ☛ Code first alert

2020 ICD-10-CM   When symbols appear on a code that requires a 7th character extension, refer to Appendix B to identify applicable 7th character codes.   **491**

CHAPTER 2: NEOPLASMS (C00-D49)

C84.69 - C85.26

C85.27 **Mediastinal (thymic) large B-cell lymphoma,** spleen `HCC`

C85.28 **Mediastinal (thymic) large B-cell lymphoma, lymph nodes of** multiple sites `HCC`

C85.29 **Mediastinal (thymic) large B-cell lymphoma,** extranodal and solid organ sites `HCC`

C85.8 Other specified **types of** non-Hodgkin **lymphoma**

C85.80 **Other specified types of non-Hodgkin lymphoma, unspecified site** `HCC`

C85.81 **Other specified types of non-Hodgkin lymphoma, lymph nodes of** head, face, and neck `HCC`

C85.82 **Other specified types of non-Hodgkin lymphoma,** intrathoracic **lymph nodes** `HCC`

C85.83 **Other specified types of non-Hodgkin lymphoma,** intra-abdominal **lymph nodes** `HCC`

C85.84 **Other specified types of non-Hodgkin lymphoma, lymph nodes of** axilla and upper limb `HCC`

C85.85 **Other specified types of non-Hodgkin lymphoma, lymph nodes of** inguinal region and lower limb `HCC`

C85.86 **Other specified types of non-Hodgkin lymphoma,** intrapelvic **lymph nodes** `HCC`

C85.87 **Other specified types of non-Hodgkin lymphoma,** spleen `HCC`

C85.88 **Other specified types of non-Hodgkin lymphoma, lymph nodes of** multiple sites `HCC`

C85.89 **Other specified types of non-Hodgkin lymphoma,** extranodal and solid organ sites `HCC`

C85.9 Non-Hodgkin **lymphoma,** unspecified

Lymphoma NOS
Malignant lymphoma NOS
Non-Hodgkin lymphoma NOS

C85.90 **Non-Hodgkin lymphoma, unspecified, unspecified site** `HCC`

C85.91 **Non-Hodgkin lymphoma, unspecified, lymph nodes of** head, face, and neck `HCC`

C85.92 **Non-Hodgkin lymphoma, unspecified,** intrathoracic **lymph nodes** `HCC`

C85.93 **Non-Hodgkin lymphoma, unspecified,** intra-abdominal **lymph nodes** `HCC`

C85.94 **Non-Hodgkin lymphoma, unspecified, lymph nodes of** axilla and upper limb `HCC`

C85.95 **Non-Hodgkin lymphoma, unspecified, lymph nodes of** inguinal region and lower limb `HCC`

C85.96 **Non-Hodgkin lymphoma, unspecified,** intrapelvic **lymph nodes** `HCC`

C85.97 **Non-Hodgkin lymphoma, unspecified,** spleen `HCC`

C85.98 **Non-Hodgkin lymphoma, unspecified, lymph nodes of** multiple sites `HCC`

C85.99 **Non-Hodgkin lymphoma, unspecified,** extranodal and solid organ sites `HCC`

C86 Other specified **types of T/NK-cell lymphoma**

EXCLUDES1 *anaplastic large cell lymphoma, ALK negative (C84.7-)*
anaplastic large cell lymphoma, ALK positive (C84.6-)
mature T/NK-cell lymphomas (C84.-)
other specified types of non-Hodgkin lymphoma (C85.8-)

C86.0 Extranodal **NK/T-cell lymphoma,** nasal type `HCC`

C86.1 Hepatosplenic **T-cell lymphoma** `HCC`
Alpha-beta and gamma delta types

C86.2 Enteropathy-type (intestinal) **T-cell lymphoma** `HCC`
Enteropathy associated T-cell lymphoma

C86.3 Subcutaneous panniculitis-like **T-cell lymphoma** `HCC`

C86.4 Blastic **NK-cell lymphoma** `HCC`
Blastic plasmacytoid dendritic cell neoplasm (BPDCN)

C86.5 Angioimmunoblastic **T-cell lymphoma** `HCC`
Angioimmunoblastic lymphadenopathy with dysproteinemia (AILD)

C86.6 Primary cutaneous CD30-positive **T-cell proliferations** `HCC`
Lymphomatoid papulosis
Primary cutaneous anaplastic large cell lymphoma
Primary cutaneous CD30-positive large T-cell lymphoma

C88 **Malignant** immunoproliferative **diseases and certain** other B-cell lymphomas

EXCLUDES1 *B-cell lymphoma, unspecified (C85.1-)*
personal history of other malignant neoplasms of lymphoid, hematopoietic and related tissues (Z85.79)

C88.0 Waldenström **macroglobulinemia** `HCC`
Lymphoplasmacytic lymphoma with IgM-production
Macroglobulinemia (idiopathic) (primary)
EXCLUDES1 *small cell B-cell lymphoma (C83.0)*

C88.2 Heavy chain **disease** `HCC`
Franklin disease
Gamma heavy chain disease
Mu heavy chain disease

C88.3 **Immunoproliferative** small intestinal **disease** `HCC`
Alpha heavy chain disease
Mediterranean lymphoma

C88.4 **Extranodal marginal zone B-cell lymphoma of mucosa-associated lymphoid tissue** [MALT-lymphoma] `HCC`
Lymphoma of skin-associated lymphoid tissue [SALT-lymphoma]
Lymphoma of bronchial-associated lymphoid tissue [BALT-lymphoma]
EXCLUDES1 *high malignant (diffuse large B-cell) lymphoma (C83.3-)*

C88.8 Other **malignant immunoproliferative diseases** `HCC`

C88.9 **Malignant immunoproliferative disease, unspecified** `HCC`
Immunoproliferative disease NOS

C90 Multiple myeloma **and malignant plasma cell neoplasms**

See Official Guidelines "Leukemia, Multiple Myeloma, and Malignant Plasma Cell Neoplasms in remission vs. personal history" I.C.2.n

EXCLUDES1 *personal history of other malignant neoplasms of lymphoid, hematopoietic and related tissues (Z85.79)*

C90.0 **Multiple myeloma**
Kahler's disease
Medullary plasmacytoma
Myelomatosis
Plasma cell myeloma
EXCLUDES1 *solitary myeloma (C90.3-)*
solitary plasmacytoma (C90.3-)

C90.00 **Multiple myeloma** not having achieved remission `HCC` `RxHCC`
Multiple myeloma with failed remission
Multiple myeloma NOS

C90.01 **Multiple myeloma** in remission `HCC` `RxHCC`

C90.02 **Multiple myeloma** in relapse `HCC` `RxHCC`

C90.1 **Plasma cell** leukemia
Plasmacytic leukemia

C90.10 **Plasma cell leukemia** not having achieved remission `HCC` `RxHCC`
AHA: Q2 2019
Plasma cell leukemia with failed remission
Plasma cell leukemia NOS

C90.11 **Plasma cell leukemia** in remission `HCC` `RxHCC`

C90.12 **Plasma cell leukemia** in relapse `HCC` `RxHCC`

C90.2 Extramedullary **plasmacytoma**

C90.20 **Extramedullary plasmacytoma** not having achieved remission `HCC` `RxHCC`
Extramedullary plasmacytoma with failed remission
Extramedullary plasmacytoma NOS

C90.21 **Extramedullary plasmacytoma** in remission `HCC` `RxHCC`

C90.22 **Extramedullary plasmacytoma** in relapse `HCC` `RxHCC`

C90.3 Solitary **plasmacytoma**
Localized malignant plasma cell tumor NOS
Plasmacytoma NOS
Solitary myeloma

C90.30 **Solitary plasmacytoma** not having achieved remission `HCC` `RxHCC`
Solitary plasmacytoma with failed remission
Solitary plasmacytoma NOS

C90.31 **Solitary plasmacytoma** in remission `HCC` `RxHCC`

C90.32 **Solitary plasmacytoma** in relapse `HCC` `RxHCC`

Unacceptable principal diagnosis symbol per Medicare code edits   Code exempt from diagnosis present on admission requirement
Questionable admission   Complication or comorbidity   Major complication or comorbidity   CC/MCC exclusion
`HCC` HCC diagnosis code   `RxHCC` RxHCC diagnosis code   MACRA code   **DEFINITION** Describes condition/terminology
TIP Coding guidance   Official Guideline Reference   Z code as first-listed diagnosis

C91 **Lymphoid** leukemia
   EXCLUDES1 *personal history of leukemia (Z85.6)*
  C91.0 Acute lymphoblastic **leukemia [ALL]**
    NOTES   Codes ▶ in subcategory ◀ C91.0- should only be used for T-cell and B-cell precursor leukemia
    C91.00 **Acute lymphoblastic leukemia** not having achieved remission HCC
     Acute lymphoblastic leukemia with failed remission
     Acute lymphoblastic leukemia NOS
    C91.01 **Acute lymphoblastic leukemia,** in remission HCC
    C91.02 **Acute lymphoblastic leukemia,** in relapse HCC
  C91.1 Chronic lymphocytic **leukemia of** B-cell type
   Lymphoplasmacytic leukemia
   Richter syndrome
   EXCLUDES1 *lymphoplasmacytic lymphoma (C83.0-)*
    C91.10 **Chronic lymphocytic leukemia of B-cell type** not having achieved remission HCC
     Chronic lymphocytic leukemia of B-cell type with failed remission
     Chronic lymphocytic leukemia of B-cell type NOS
    C91.11 **Chronic lymphocytic leukemia of B-cell type** in remission HCC
    C91.12 **Chronic lymphocytic leukemia of B-cell type** in relapse HCC
  C91.3 Prolymphocytic **leukemia of** B-cell type
    C91.30 **Prolymphocytic leukemia of B-cell type** not having achieved remission HCC
     Prolymphocytic leukemia of B-cell type with failed remission
     Prolymphocytic leukemia of B-cell type NOS
    C91.31 **Prolymphocytic leukemia of B-cell type,** in remission HCC
    C91.32 **Prolymphocytic leukemia of B-cell type,** in relapse HCC
  C91.4 Hairy cell **leukemia**
   Leukemic reticuloendotheliosis
    C91.40 **Hairy cell leukemia** not having achieved remission HCC
     Hairy cell leukemia with failed remission
     Hairy cell leukemia NOS
    C91.41 **Hairy cell leukemia,** in remission HCC
    C91.42 **Hairy cell leukemia,** in relapse HCC
  C91.5 Adult T-cell **lymphoma/leukemia (HTLV-1-associated)**
   Acute variant of adult T-cell lymphoma/leukemia (HTLV-1-associated)
   Chronic variant of adult T-cell lymphoma/leukemia (HTLV-1-associated)
   Lymphomatoid variant of adult T-cell lymphoma/leukemia (HTLV-1-associated)
   Smouldering variant of adult T-cell lymphoma/leukemia (HTLV-1-associated)
    C91.50 **Adult T-cell lymphoma/leukemia (HTLV-1-associated)** not having achieved remission A HCC
     Adult T-cell lymphoma/leukemia (HTLV-1-associated) with failed remission
     Adult T-cell lymphoma/leukemia (HTLV-1-associated) NOS
    C91.51 **Adult T-cell lymphoma/leukemia (HTLV-1-associated),** in remission A HCC
    C91.52 **Adult T-cell lymphoma/leukemia (HTLV-1-associated),** in relapse A HCC
  C91.6 Prolymphocytic **leukemia of** T-cell type
    C91.60 **Prolymphocytic leukemia of T-cell type** not having achieved remission HCC
     Prolymphocytic leukemia of T-cell type with failed remission
     Prolymphocytic leukemia of T-cell type NOS
    C91.61 **Prolymphocytic leukemia of T-cell type,** in remission HCC
    C91.62 **Prolymphocytic leukemia of T-cell type,** in relapse HCC
  C91.A Mature B-cell **leukemia** Burkitt-type
   EXCLUDES1 *Burkitt lymphoma (C83.7-)*

    C91.A0 **Mature B-cell leukemia Burkitt-type** not having achieved remission HCC
     Mature B-cell leukemia Burkitt-type with failed remission
     Mature B-cell leukemia Burkitt-type NOS
    C91.A1 **Mature B-cell leukemia Burkitt-type,** in remission HCC
    C91.A2 **Mature B-cell leukemia Burkitt-type,** in relapse HCC
  C91.Z Other **lymphoid leukemia**
   T-cell large granular lymphocytic leukemia (associated with rheumatoid arthritis)
    C91.Z0 Other **lymphoid leukemia** not having achieved remission HCC
     AHA: Q2 2019
     Other lymphoid leukemia with failed remission
     Other lymphoid leukemia NOS
    C91.Z1 Other **lymphoid leukemia,** in remission HCC
    C91.Z2 Other **lymphoid leukemia,** in relapse HCC
  C91.9 **Lymphoid leukemia,** unspecified
    C91.90 **Lymphoid leukemia, unspecified** not having achieved remission HCC
     Lymphoid leukemia with failed remission
     Lymphoid leukemia NOS
    C91.91 **Lymphoid leukemia, unspecified,** in remission HCC
    C91.92 **Lymphoid leukemia, unspecified,** in relapse HCC

C92 Myeloid **leukemia**
  INCLUDES *granulocytic leukemia*
         myelogenous leukemia
  EXCLUDES1 *personal history of leukemia (Z85.6)*
  C92.0 Acute myeloblastic **leukemia**
   Acute myeloblastic leukemia, minimal differentiation
   Acute myeloblastic leukemia (with maturation)
   Acute myeloblastic leukemia 1/ETO
   Acute myeloblastic leukemia M0
   Acute myeloblastic leukemia M1
   Acute myeloblastic leukemia M2
   Acute myeloblastic leukemia with t(8;21)
   Acute myeloblastic leukemia (without a FAB classification) NOS
   Refractory anemia with excess blasts in transformation [RAEB T]
   EXCLUDES1 *acute exacerbation of chronic myeloid leukemia (C92.10)*
       refractory anemia with excess of blasts not in transformation (D46.2-)
    C92.00 **Acute myeloblastic leukemia,** not having achieved remission HCC
     Acute myeloblastic leukemia with failed remission
     Acute myeloblastic leukemia NOS
    C92.01 **Acute myeloblastic leukemia,** in remission HCC
    C92.02 **Acute myeloblastic leukemia,** in relapse HCC
  C92.1 Chronic myeloid **leukemia,** BCR/ABL-positive
   Chronic myelogenous leukemia, Philadelphia chromosome (Ph1) positive
   Chronic myelogenous leukemia, t(9;22) (q34;q11)
   Chronic myelogenous leukemia with crisis of blast cells
   EXCLUDES1 *atypical chronic myeloid leukemia BCR/ABL-negative (C92.2-)*
       chronic myelomonocytic leukemia (C93.1-)
       chronic myeloproliferative disease (D47.1)
    C92.10 **Chronic myeloid leukemia, BCR/ABL-positive,** not having achieved remission HCC RxHCC
     Chronic myeloid leukemia, BCR/ABL-positive with failed remission
     Chronic myeloid leukemia, BCR/ABL-positive NOS
    C92.11 **Chronic myeloid leukemia, BCR/ABL-positive,** in remission HCC RxHCC
    C92.12 **Chronic myeloid leukemia, BCR/ABL-positive,** in relapse HCC RxHCC
  C92.2 Atypical chronic **myeloid leukemia,** BCR/ABL-negative
    C92.20 **Atypical chronic myeloid leukemia, BCR/ABL-negative,** not having achieved remission HCC RxHCC
     Atypical chronic myeloid leukemia, BCR/ABL-negative with failed remission
     Atypical chronic myeloid leukemia, BCR/ABL-negative NOS

C92.21 **Atypical chronic myeloid leukemia, BCR/ABL-negative,** in remission [HCC] [RxHCC]

C92.22 **Atypical chronic myeloid leukemia, BCR/ABL-negative,** in relapse [HCC] [RxHCC]

[5th] C92.3 Myeloid sarcoma
A malignant tumor of immature myeloid cells
Chloroma
Granulocytic sarcoma

C92.30 **Myeloid sarcoma,** not having achieved remission [HCC] [RxHCC]
Myeloid sarcoma with failed remission
Myeloid sarcoma NOS

C92.31 **Myeloid sarcoma,** in remission [HCC] [RxHCC]

C92.32 **Myeloid sarcoma,** in relapse [HCC] [RxHCC]

[5th] C92.4 Acute promyelocytic **leukemia**
AML M3
AML Me with t(15;17) and variants

C92.40 **Acute promyelocytic leukemia, not having achieved remission** [HCC]
Acute promyelocytic leukemia with failed remission
Acute promyelocytic leukemia NOS

C92.41 **Acute promyelocytic leukemia,** in remission [HCC]

C92.42 **Acute promyelocytic leukemia,** in relapse [HCC]

[5th] C92.5 Acute myelomonocytic **leukemia**
AML M4
AML M4 Eo with inv(16) or t(16;16)

C92.50 **Acute myelomonocytic leukemia,** not having achieved remission [HCC]
Acute myelomonocytic leukemia with failed remission
Acute myelomonocytic leukemia NOS

C92.51 **Acute myelomonocytic leukemia, in remission** [HCC]

C92.52 **Acute myelomonocytic leukemia, in relapse** [HCC]

[5th] C92.6 Acute myeloid **leukemia with** 11q23-abnormality
Acute myeloid leukemia with variation of MLL-gene

C92.60 **Acute myeloid leukemia with 11q23-abnormality** not having achieved remission [HCC]
Acute myeloid leukemia with 11q23-abnormality with failed remission
Acute myeloid leukemia with 11q23-abnormality NOS

C92.61 **Acute myeloid leukemia with 11q23-abnormality** in remission [HCC]

C92.62 **Acute myeloid leukemia with 11q23-abnormality** in relapse [HCC]

[5th] C92.A Acute myeloid **leukemia with** multilineage dysplasia
Acute myeloid leukemia with dysplasia of remaining hematopoesis and/or myelodysplastic disease in its history

C92.A0 **Acute myeloid leukemia with multilineage dysplasia,** not having achieved remission [HCC]
Acute myeloid leukemia with multilineage dysplasia with failed remission
Acute myeloid leukemia with multilineage dysplasia NOS

C92.A1 **Acute myeloid leukemia with multilineage dysplasia,** in remission [HCC]

C92.A2 **Acute myeloid leukemia with multilineage dysplasia,** in relapse [HCC]

[5th] C92.Z Other **myeloid leukemia**

C92.Z0 Other **myeloid leukemia** not having achieved remission [HCC] [RxHCC]
Myeloid leukemia NEC with failed remission
Myeloid leukemia NEC

C92.Z1 Other **myeloid leukemia,** in remission [HCC] [RxHCC]

C92.Z2 Other **myeloid leukemia,** in relapse [HCC] [RxHCC]

[5th] C92.9 **Myeloid leukemia,** unspecified

C92.90 **Myeloid leukemia, unspecified,** not having achieved remission [HCC] [RxHCC]
Myeloid leukemia, unspecified with failed remission
Myeloid leukemia, unspecified NOS

C92.91 **Myeloid leukemia, unspecified** in remission [HCC] [RxHCC]

C92.92 **Myeloid leukemia, unspecified** in relapse [HCC] [RxHCC]

[4th] C93 Monocytic **leukemia**
[INCLUDES] *monocytoid leukemia*
[EXCLUDES1] *personal history of leukemia (Z85.6)*

[5th] C93.0 Acute **monoblastic/monocytic leukemia**
AML M5
AML M5a
AML M5b

C93.00 **Acute monoblastic/monocytic leukemia,** not having achieved remission [HCC]
Acute monoblastic/monocytic leukemia with failed remission
Acute monoblastic/monocytic leukemia NOS

C93.01 **Acute monoblastic/monocytic leukemia,** in remission [HCC]

C93.02 **Acute monoblastic/monocytic leukemia,** in relapse [HCC]

[5th] C93.1 Chronic **myelomonocytic leukemia**
Chronic monocytic leukemia
CMML-1
CMML-2
CMML with eosinophilia

C93.10 **Chronic myelomonocytic leukemia** not having achieved remission [HCC] [RxHCC]
Chronic myelomonocytic leukemia with failed remission
Chronic myelomonocytic leukemia NOS

C93.11 **Chronic myelomonocytic leukemia,** in remission [HCC] [RxHCC]

C93.12 **Chronic myelomonocytic leukemia,** in relapse [HCC] [RxHCC]

[5th] C93.3 Juvenile **myelomonocytic leukemia**

C93.30 **Juvenile myelomonocytic leukemia,** not having achieved remission [P] [HCC] [RxHCC]
Juvenile myelomonocytic leukemia with failed remission
Juvenile myelomonocytic leukemia NOS

C93.31 **Juvenile myelomonocytic leukemia,** in remission [P] [HCC] [RxHCC]

C93.32 **Juvenile myelomonocytic leukemia,** in relapse [P] [HCC] [RxHCC]

[5th] C93.Z Other **monocytic leukemia**

C93.Z0 **Other monocytic leukemia,** not having achieved remission [HCC] [RxHCC]
Other monocytic leukemia NOS

C93.Z1 **Other monocytic leukemia,** in remission [HCC] [RxHCC]

C93.Z2 **Other monocytic leukemia,** in relapse [HCC] [RxHCC]

[5th] C93.9 **Monocytic leukemia,** unspecified

C93.90 **Monocytic leukemia, unspecified,** not having achieved remission [HCC] [RxHCC]
Monocytic leukemia, unspecified with failed remission
Monocytic leukemia, unspecified NOS

C93.91 **Monocytic leukemia, unspecified** in remission [HCC] [RxHCC]

C93.92 **Monocytic leukemia, unspecified** in relapse [HCC] [RxHCC]

[4th] C94 Other **leukemias of** specified cell type
[EXCLUDES1] *leukemic reticuloendotheliosis (C91.4-)*
myelodysplastic syndromes (D46.-)
personal history of leukemia (Z85.6)
plasma cell leukemia (C90.1-)

[5th] C94.0 Acute erythroid **leukemia**
Acute myeloid leukemia M6(a)(b)
Erythroleukemia

C94.00 **Acute erythroid leukemia, not having achieved remission** [HCC]
Acute erythroid leukemia with failed remission
Acute erythroid leukemia NOS

C94.01 **Acute erythroid leukemia,** in remission [HCC]

C94.02 **Acute erythroid leukemia,** in relapse [HCC]

[5th] C94.2 Acute megakaryoblastic **leukemia**
Acute myeloid leukemia M7
Acute megakaryocytic leukemia

C94.20 **Acute megakaryoblastic leukemia** not having achieved remission [HCC]
Acute megakaryoblastic leukemia with failed remission
Acute megakaryoblastic leukemia NOS

C94.21 **Acute megakaryoblastic leukemia,** in remission [HCC]

C94.22 **Acute megakaryoblastic leukemia,** in relapse [HCC]

[PDx] Unacceptable principal diagnosis symbol per Medicare code edits [POA] Code exempt from diagnosis present on admission requirement
[?] Questionable admission [CC] Complication or comorbidity [MCC] Major complication or comorbidity [CC/MCC Exc] CC/MCC exclusion
[HCC] HCC diagnosis code [RxHCC] RxHCC diagnosis code MACRA code **DEFINITION** Describes condition/terminology
TIP Coding guidance 👁 Official Guideline Reference [Z-1] Z code as first-listed diagnosis

5ᵗʰ	**C94.3**	Mast cell leukemia	
	C94.30	**Mast cell leukemia** not having achieved remission	HCC RxHCC
		Mast cell leukemia with failed remission	
		Mast cell leukemia NOS	
	C94.31	**Mast cell leukemia,** in remission	HCC RxHCC
	C94.32	**Mast cell leukemia,** in relapse	HCC RxHCC

5ᵗʰ **C94.4** Acute panmyelosis with myelofibrosis
    Acute myelofibrosis
    EXCLUDES1   *myelofibrosis NOS (D75.81)*
           secondary myelofibrosis NOS (D75.81)

    C94.40 **Acute panmyelosis with myelofibrosis** not having achieved remission   HCC
         Acute myelofibrosis NOS
         Acute panmyelosis with myelofibrosis with failed remission
         Acute panmyelosis NOS
    C94.41 **Acute panmyelosis with myelofibrosis,** in remission   HCC
    C94.42 **Acute panmyelosis with myelofibrosis,** in relapse   HCC

C94.6 Myelodysplastic disease, not classified   HCC
    Myeloproliferative disease, not classified

5ᵗʰ **C94.8** Other specified leukemias
    Aggressive NK-cell leukemia
    Acute basophilic leukemia
    C94.80 **Other specified leukemias** not having achieved remission   HCC RxHCC
         Other specified leukemia with failed remission
         Other specified leukemias NOS
    C94.81 **Other specified leukemias,** in remission   HCC RxHCC
    C94.82 **Other specified leukemias,** in relapse   HCC RxHCC

4ᵗʰ **C95** Leukemia of unspecified cell type
    EXCLUDES1   *personal history of leukemia (Z85.6)*

5ᵗʰ **C95.0** Acute leukemia of unspecified cell type
    Acute bilineal leukemia
    Acute mixed lineage leukemia
    Biphenotypic acute leukemia
    Stem cell leukemia of unclear lineage
    EXCLUDES1   *acute exacerbation of unspecified chronic leukemia (C95.10)*
    C95.00 **Acute leukemia of unspecified cell type** not having achieved remission   HCC
         Acute leukemia of unspecified cell type with failed remission
         Acute leukemia NOS
    C95.01 **Acute leukemia of unspecified cell type,** in remission   HCC
    C95.02 **Acute leukemia of unspecified cell type,** in relapse   HCC

5ᵗʰ **C95.1** Chronic leukemia of unspecified cell type
    C95.10 **Chronic leukemia of unspecified cell type** not having achieved remission   HCC
         Chronic leukemia of unspecified cell type with failed remission
         Chronic leukemia NOS
    C95.11 **Chronic leukemia of unspecified cell type,** in remission   HCC
    C95.12 **Chronic leukemia of unspecified cell type,** in relapse   HCC

5ᵗʰ **C95.9** Leukemia, unspecified
    C95.90 **Leukemia, unspecified** not having achieved remission   HCC
         Leukemia, unspecified with failed remission
         Leukemia NOS
    C95.91 **Leukemia, unspecified,** in remission   HCC
    C95.92 **Leukemia, unspecified,** in relapse   HCC

4ᵗʰ **C96** Other and unspecified malignant neoplasms of lymphoid, hematopoietic and related tissue
    EXCLUDES1   *personal history of other malignant neoplasms of lymphoid, hematopoietic and related tissues (Z85.79)*

C96.0 Multifocal and multisystemic (disseminated) Langerhans-cell histiocytosis   HCC
    Histiocytosis X, multisystemic
    Letterer-Siwe disease
    EXCLUDES1   *adult pulmonary Langerhans cell histiocytosis (J84.82)*
           multifocal and unisystemic Langerhans-cell histiocytosis (C96.5)
           unifocal Langerhans-cell histiocytosis (C96.6)

5ᵗʰ **C96.2** Malignant mast cell neoplasm
    EXCLUDES1   *indolent mastocytosis (D47.02)*
           mast cell leukemia (C94.30)
           mastocytosis (congenital) (cutaneous) (Q82.2)
    C96.20 **Malignant mast cell neoplasm, unspecified**   HCC RxHCC
         AHA: Q4 2017
    C96.21 **Aggressive systemic** mastocytosis   HCC RxHCC
         AHA: Q4 2017
    C96.22 **Mast cell** sarcoma   HCC RxHCC
         AHA: Q4 2017
    C96.29 **Other** malignant mast cell neoplasm   HCC RxHCC
         AHA: Q4 2017

C96.4 Sarcoma of dendritic cells (accessory cells)   HCC
    Follicular dendritic cell sarcoma
    Interdigitating dendritic cell sarcoma
    Langerhans cell sarcoma

C96.5 Multifocal and unisystemic Langerhans-cell histiocytosis   HCC
    Hand-Schüller-Christian disease
    Histiocytosis X, multifocal
    EXCLUDES1   *multifocal and multisystemic (disseminated) Langerhans-cell histiocytosis (C96.0)*
           unifocal Langerhans-cell histiocytosis (C96.6)

C96.6 Unifocal Langerhans-cell histiocytosis   HCC
    Eosinophilic granuloma
    Histiocytosis X, unifocal
    Histiocytosis X NOS
    Langerhans-cell histiocytosis NOS
    EXCLUDES1   *multifocal and multisystemic (disseminated) Langerhans-cell histiocytosis (C96.0)*
           multifocal and unisystemic Langerhans-cell histiocytosis (C96.5)

C96.A Histiocytic sarcoma   HCC
    Malignant histiocytosis
C96.Z Other specified malignant neoplasms of lymphoid, hematopoietic and related tissue   HCC
C96.9 Malignant neoplasm of lymphoid, hematopoietic and related tissue, unspecified   HCC

In situ neoplasms (D00-D09)

INCLUDES   *Bowen's disease*
             erythroplasia
             grade III intraepithelial neoplasia
             Queyrat's erythroplasia

4ᵗʰ **D00** Carcinoma in situ of oral cavity, esophagus and stomach
    EXCLUDES1   *melanoma in situ (D03.-)*

5ᵗʰ **D00.0** Carcinoma in situ of lip, oral cavity and pharynx
    Use additional code to identify:
         exposure to environmental tobacco smoke (Z77.22)
         exposure to tobacco smoke in the perinatal period (P96.81)
         history of tobacco dependence (Z87.891)
         occupational exposure to environmental tobacco smoke (Z57.31)
         tobacco dependence (F17.-)
         tobacco use (Z72.0)
    EXCLUDES1   *carcinoma in situ of aryepiglottic fold or interarytenoid fold, laryngeal aspect (D02.0)*
           carcinoma in situ of epiglottis NOS (D02.0)
           carcinoma in situ of epiglottis suprahyoid portion (D02.0)
           carcinoma in situ of skin of lip (D03.0, D04.0)

Unspecified Code   Other Specified Code   Manifestation Code   N Newborn   P Pediatric   M Maternity   A Adult   ♂ Male   ♀ Female
● New Code   ▲ Revised Code Title   ►◄ Revised Text   **NOTES**   *INCLUDES*   *EXCLUDES1* Not coded here   *EXCLUDES2* Not included here
4ᵗʰ 4ᵗʰ character required   5ᵗʰ 5ᵗʰ character required   6ᵗʰ 6ᵗʰ character required   7ᵗʰ 7ᵗʰ character required   7ᵗʰ Extension 'X' Alert
HAC Hospital-acquired condition (HAC) alert   **AHA** AHA Coding Clinic©   📌 Code first alert

D00.00 **Carcinoma in situ of** oral cavity, **unspecified site**

D00.01 **Carcinoma in situ of** labial mucosa and vermilion border

D00.02 **Carcinoma in situ of** buccal mucosa

D00.03 **Carcinoma in situ of** gingiva and edentulous alveolar ridge

D00.04 **Carcinoma in situ of** soft palate

D00.05 **Carcinoma in situ of** hard palate

D00.06 **Carcinoma in situ of** floor of mouth

D00.07 **Carcinoma in situ of** tongue

D00.08 **Carcinoma in situ of** pharynx

Carcinoma in situ of aryepiglottic fold NOS

Carcinoma in situ of hypopharyngeal aspect of aryepiglottic fold

Carcinoma in situ of marginal zone of aryepiglottic fold

D00.1 **Carcinoma in situ of** esophagus

D00.2 **Carcinoma in situ of** stomach

🔵 D01 **Carcinoma in situ of** other and unspecified digestive organs

EXCLUDES1 *melanoma in situ (D03.-)*

D01.0 **Carcinoma in situ of** colon

EXCLUDES1 *carcinoma in situ of rectosigmoid junction (D01.1)*

D01.1 **Carcinoma in situ of** rectosigmoid junction

D01.2 **Carcinoma in situ of** rectum

D01.3 **Carcinoma in situ of** anus and anal canal

Anal intraepithelial neoplasia III [AIN III]

Severe dysplasia of anus

EXCLUDES1 *anal intraepithelial neoplasia I and II [AIN I and AIN II] (K62.82)*

carcinoma in situ of anal margin (D04.5)

carcinoma in situ of anal skin (D04.5)

carcinoma in situ of perianal skin (D04.5)

🔵 D01.4 **Carcinoma in situ of** other and unspecified **parts of** intestine

EXCLUDES1 *carcinoma in situ of ampulla of Vater (D01.5)*

D01.40 **Carcinoma in situ of unspecified part of intestine**

D01.49 **Carcinoma in situ of** other **parts of intestine**

D01.5 **Carcinoma in situ of** liver, gallbladder and bile ducts

Carcinoma in situ of ampulla of Vater

D01.7 **Carcinoma in situ of other specified** digestive organs

Carcinoma in situ of pancreas

D01.9 **Carcinoma in situ of** digestive organ, **unspecified**

🔵 D02 **Carcinoma in situ of** middle ear and respiratory system

Use additional code to identify:

exposure to environmental tobacco smoke (Z77.22)

exposure to tobacco smoke in the perinatal period (P96.81)

history of tobacco dependence (Z87.891)

occupational exposure to environmental tobacco smoke (Z57.31)

tobacco dependence (F17.-)

tobacco use (Z72.0)

EXCLUDES1 *melanoma in situ (D03.-)*

D02.0 **Carcinoma in situ of** larynx

Carcinoma in situ of aryepiglottic fold or interarytenoid fold, laryngeal aspect

Carcinoma in situ of epiglottis (suprahyoid portion)

EXCLUDES1 *carcinoma in situ of aryepiglottic fold or interarytenoid fold NOS (D00.08)*

carcinoma in situ of hypopharyngeal aspect (D00.08)

carcinoma in situ of marginal zone (D00.08)

D02.1 **Carcinoma in situ of** trachea

🔵 D02.2 **Carcinoma in situ of** bronchus and lung

D02.20 **Carcinoma in situ of unspecified bronchus and lung**

D02.21 **Carcinoma in situ of** right **bronchus and lung**

D02.22 **Carcinoma in situ of** left **bronchus and lung**

D02.3 **Carcinoma in situ of** other parts **of respiratory system**

Carcinoma in situ of accessory sinuses

Carcinoma in situ of middle ear

Carcinoma in situ of nasal cavities

EXCLUDES1 *carcinoma in situ of ear (external) (skin) (D04.2-)*

carcinoma in situ of nose NOS D09.8

carcinoma in situ of skin of nose (D04.3)

D02.4 **Carcinoma in situ of respiratory system, unspecified**

🔵 D03 Melanoma in situ

D03.0 **Melanoma in situ of** lip   HCC

🔵 D03.1 **Melanoma in situ of** eyelid, including canthus

D03.10 **Melanoma in situ of unspecified eyelid, including canthus**   HCC

🔵 D03.11 **Melanoma in situ of** right **eyelid, including canthus**

D03.111 **Melanoma in situ of right** upper **eyelid, including canthus**   HCC

AHA: Q4 2018

D03.112 **Melanoma in situ of right** lower **eyelid, including canthus**   HCC

AHA: Q4 2018

🔵 D03.12 **Melanoma in situ of** left **eyelid, including canthus**

D03.121 **Melanoma in situ of left** upper **eyelid, including canthus**   HCC

AHA: Q4 2018

D03.122 **Melanoma in situ of left** lower **eyelid, including canthus**   HCC

AHA: Q4 2018

🔵 D03.2 **Melanoma in situ of** ear and external auricular canal

D03.20 **Melanoma in situ of unspecified ear and external auricular canal**   HCC

D03.21 **Melanoma in situ of** right **ear and external auricular canal**   HCC

D03.22 **Melanoma in situ of** left **ear and external auricular canal**   HCC

🔵 D03.3 **Melanoma in situ of** other and unspecified parts of face

D03.30 **Melanoma in situ of unspecified part of face**   HCC

D03.39 **Melanoma in situ of** other **parts of face**   HCC

D03.4 **Melanoma in situ of** scalp and neck   HCC

🔵 D03.5 **Melanoma in situ of** trunk

D03.51 **Melanoma in situ of** anal skin   HCC

Melanoma in situ of anal margin

Melanoma in situ of perianal skin

D03.52 **Melanoma in situ of** breast (skin) (soft tissue)   HCC

D03.59 **Melanoma in situ of** other **part of trunk**   HCC

🔵 D03.6 **Melanoma in situ of** upper limb, including shoulder

D03.60 **Melanoma in situ of unspecified upper limb, including shoulder**   HCC

D03.61 **Melanoma in situ of** right **upper limb, including shoulder**   HCC

D03.62 **Melanoma in situ of** left **upper limb, including shoulder**   HCC

🔵 D03.7 **Melanoma in situ of** lower limb, including hip

D03.70 **Melanoma in situ of unspecified lower limb, including hip**   HCC

D03.71 **Melanoma in situ of** right **lower limb, including hip**   HCC

D03.72 **Melanoma in situ of** left **lower limb, including hip** HCC

D03.8 **Melanoma in situ of** other **sites**   HCC

Melanoma in situ of scrotum

EXCLUDES1 *carcinoma in situ of scrotum (D07.61)*

D03.9 **Melanoma in situ, unspecified**   HCC

🔵 D04 **Carcinoma in situ of** skin

EXCLUDES1 *erythroplasia of Queyrat (penis) NOS (D07.4)*

melanoma in situ (D03.-)

D04.0 **Carcinoma in situ of skin of lip**

EXCLUDES2 *carcinoma in situ of vermilion border of lip (D00.01)*

🔵 D04.1 **Carcinoma in situ of skin of** eyelid, including canthus

D04.10 **Carcinoma in situ of skin of unspecified eyelid, including canthus**

🔵 D04.11 **Carcinoma in situ of skin of** right **eyelid, including canthus**

D04.111 **Carcinoma in situ of skin of right** upper **eyelid, including canthus**

AHA: Q4 2018

D04.112 **Carcinoma in situ of skin of right** lower **eyelid, including canthus**

AHA: Q4 2018

When symbols appear on a code that requires a 7th character extension, refer to Appendix B to identify applicable 7th character codes.   **2020 ICD-10-CM**

[6th] D04.12 Carcinoma in situ of skin of left eyelid, including canthus
D04.121 Carcinoma in situ of skin of left upper eyelid, including canthus
AHA: Q4 2018
D04.122 Carcinoma in situ of skin of left lower eyelid, including canthus
AHA: Q4 2018
[5th] D04.2 Carcinoma in situ of skin of ear and external auricular canal
D04.20 Carcinoma in situ of skin of unspecified ear and external auricular canal
D04.21 Carcinoma in situ of skin of right ear and external auricular canal
D04.22 Carcinoma in situ of skin of left ear and external auricular canal
[5th] D04.3 Carcinoma in situ of skin of other and unspecified parts of face
D04.30 Carcinoma in situ of skin of unspecified part of face
D04.39 Carcinoma in situ of skin of other parts of face
D04.4 Carcinoma in situ of skin of scalp and neck
D04.5 Carcinoma in situ of skin of trunk
Carcinoma in situ of anal margin
Carcinoma in situ of anal skin
Carcinoma in situ of perianal skin
Carcinoma in situ of skin of breast
EXCLUDES1 *carcinoma in situ of anus NOS (D01.3)*
carcinoma in situ of scrotum (D07.61)
carcinoma in situ of skin of genital organs (D07.-)
[5th] D04.6 Carcinoma in situ of skin of upper limb, including shoulder
D04.60 Carcinoma in situ of skin of unspecified upper limb, including shoulder
D04.61 Carcinoma in situ of skin of right upper limb, including shoulder
D04.62 Carcinoma in situ of skin of left upper limb, including shoulder
[5th] D04.7 Carcinoma in situ of skin of lower limb, including hip
D04.70 Carcinoma in situ of skin of unspecified lower limb, including hip
D04.71 Carcinoma in situ of skin of right lower limb, including hip
D04.72 Carcinoma in situ of skin of left lower limb, including hip
D04.8 Carcinoma in situ of skin of other sites
D04.9 Carcinoma in situ of skin, unspecified
[4th] D05 Carcinoma in situ of breast
EXCLUDES1 *carcinoma in situ of skin of breast (D04.5)*
melanoma in situ of breast (skin) (D03.5)
Paget's disease of breast or nipple (C50.-)
[5th] D05.0 Lobular carcinoma in situ of breast
D05.00 Lobular carcinoma in situ of unspecified breast
D05.01 Lobular carcinoma in situ of right breast
D05.02 Lobular carcinoma in situ of left breast
[5th] D05.1 Intraductal carcinoma in situ of breast
D05.10 Intraductal carcinoma in situ of unspecified breast
D05.11 Intraductal carcinoma in situ of right breast
D05.12 Intraductal carcinoma in situ of left breast
[5th] D05.8 Other specified type of carcinoma in situ of breast
D05.80 Other specified type of carcinoma in situ of unspecified breast
D05.81 Other specified type of carcinoma in situ of right breast
D05.82 Other specified type of carcinoma in situ of left breast
[5th] D05.9 Unspecified type of carcinoma in situ of breast
D05.90 Unspecified type of carcinoma in situ of unspecified breast
D05.91 Unspecified type of carcinoma in situ of right breast
D05.92 Unspecified type of carcinoma in situ of left breast

[4th] D06 Carcinoma in situ of cervix uteri
INCLUDES *cervical adenocarcinoma in situ*
cervical intraepithelial glandular neoplasia
cervical intraepithelial neoplasia III [CIN III]
severe dysplasia of cervix uteri
EXCLUDES1 *cervical intraepithelial neoplasia II [CIN II] (N87.1)*
cytologic evidence of malignancy of cervix without histologic confirmation (R87.614)
high grade squamous intraepithelial lesion (HGSIL) of cervix (R87.613)
melanoma in situ of cervix (D03.5)
moderate cervical dysplasia (N87.1)
D06.0 Carcinoma in situ of endocervix ♀
D06.1 Carcinoma in situ of exocervix ♀
D06.7 Carcinoma in situ of other parts of cervix ♀
D06.9 Carcinoma in situ of cervix, unspecified ♀
[4th] D07 Carcinoma in situ of other and unspecified genital organs
EXCLUDES1 *melanoma in situ of trunk (D03.5)*
D07.0 Carcinoma in situ of endometrium ♀
D07.1 Carcinoma in situ of vulva ♀
Severe dysplasia of vulva
Vulvar intraepithelial neoplasia III [VIN III]
EXCLUDES1 *moderate dysplasia of vulva (N90.1)*
vulvar intraepithelial neoplasia II [VIN II] (N90.1)
D07.2 Carcinoma in situ of vagina ♀
Severe dysplasia of vagina
Vaginal intraepithelial neoplasia III [VAIN III]
EXCLUDES1 *moderate dysplasia of vagina (N89.1)*
vaginal intraepithelial neoplasia II [VIN II] (N89.1)
[5th] D07.3 Carcinoma in situ of other and unspecified female genital organs
D07.30 Carcinoma in situ of unspecified female genital organs ♀
D07.39 Carcinoma in situ of other female genital organs ♀
D07.4 Carcinoma in situ of penis ♂
Erythroplasia of Queyrat NOS
D07.5 Carcinoma in situ of prostate ♂
Prostatic intraepithelial neoplasia III (PIN III)
Severe dysplasia of prostate
EXCLUDES1 *dysplasia (mild) (moderate) of prostate (N42.3-)*
prostatic intraepithelial neoplasia II [PIN II] (N42.3-)
[5th] D07.6 Carcinoma in situ of other and unspecified male genital organs
D07.60 Carcinoma in situ of unspecified male genital organs ♂
D07.61 Carcinoma in situ of scrotum ♂
D07.69 Carcinoma in situ of other male genital organs ♂
[4th] D09 Carcinoma in situ of other and unspecified sites
EXCLUDES1 *melanoma in situ (D03.-)*
D09.0 Carcinoma in situ of bladder
[5th] D09.1 Carcinoma in situ of other and unspecified urinary organs
D09.10 Carcinoma in situ of unspecified urinary organ
D09.19 Carcinoma in situ of other urinary organs
[5th] D09.2 Carcinoma in situ of eye
EXCLUDES1 *carcinoma in situ of skin of eyelid (D04.1-)*
D09.20 Carcinoma in situ of unspecified eye
D09.21 Carcinoma in situ of right eye
D09.22 Carcinoma in situ of left eye
D09.3 Carcinoma in situ of thyroid and other endocrine glands
EXCLUDES1 *carcinoma in situ of endocrine pancreas (D01.7)*
carcinoma in situ of ovary (D07.39)
carcinoma in situ of testis (D07.69)
D09.8 Carcinoma in situ of other specified sites
D09.9 Carcinoma in situ, unspecified

Unspecified Code Other Specified Code Manifestation Code [N] Newborn [P] Pediatric [M] Maternity [A] Adult ♂ Male ♀ Female
● New Code ▲ Revised Code Title ►◄ Revised Text NOTES INCLUDES EXCLUDES1 Not coded here EXCLUDES2 Not included here
[4th] 4th character required [5th] 5th character required [6th] 6th character required [7th] 7th character required [X] Extension 'X' Alert
[HAC] Hospital-acquired condition (HAC) alert AHA AHA Coding Clinic© ☞ Code first alert

Benign neoplasms, except benign neuroendocrine tumors (D10-D36)

🔹 **D10 Benign neoplasm of** mouth and pharynx

D10.0 Benign neoplasm of lip

Benign neoplasm of lip (frenulum) (inner aspect) (mucosa) (vermilion border)

EXCLUDES1 benign neoplasm of skin of lip (D22.0, D23.0)

D10.1 Benign neoplasm of tongue

Benign neoplasm of lingual tonsil

D10.2 Benign neoplasm of floor of mouth

🔹 **D10.3 Benign neoplasm of** other **and** unspecified **parts of mouth**

D10.30 Benign neoplasm of unspecified part of mouth

D10.39 Benign neoplasm of other **parts of mouth**

Benign neoplasm of minor salivary gland NOS

EXCLUDES1 benign odontogenic neoplasms (D16.4-D16.5)

benign neoplasm of mucosa of lip (D10.0)

benign neoplasm of nasopharyngeal surface of soft palate (D10.6)

D10.4 Benign neoplasm of tonsil

Benign neoplasm of tonsil (faucial) (palatine)

EXCLUDES1 benign neoplasm of lingual tonsil (D10.1)

benign neoplasm of pharyngeal tonsil (D10.6)

benign neoplasm of tonsillar fossa (D10.5)

benign neoplasm of tonsillar pillars (D10.5)

D10.5 Benign neoplasm of other parts of oropharynx

Benign neoplasm of epiglottis, anterior aspect

Benign neoplasm of tonsillar fossa

Benign neoplasm of tonsillar pillars

Benign neoplasm of vallecula

EXCLUDES1 benign neoplasm of epiglottis NOS (D14.1)

benign neoplasm of epiglottis, suprahyoid portion (D14.1)

D10.6 Benign neoplasm of nasopharynx

Benign neoplasm of pharyngeal tonsil

Benign neoplasm of posterior margin of septum and choanae

D10.7 Benign neoplasm of hypopharynx

D10.9 Benign neoplasm of pharynx, unspecified

🔹 **D11 Benign neoplasm of** major salivary glands

EXCLUDES1 benign neoplasms of specified minor salivary glands which are classified according to their anatomical location

benign neoplasms of minor salivary glands NOS (D10.39)

D11.0 Benign neoplasm of parotid gland

D11.7 Benign neoplasm of other **major salivary glands**

Benign neoplasm of sublingual salivary gland

Benign neoplasm of submandibular salivary gland

D11.9 Benign neoplasm of major salivary gland, unspecified

🔹 **D12 Benign neoplasm of** colon, rectum, anus and anal canal

EXCLUDES1 benign carcinoid tumors of the large intestine, and rectum (D3A.02-)

polyp of colon NOS (K63.5)

D12.0 Benign neoplasm of cecum

AHA: Q3 2018

Benign neoplasm of ileocecal valve

D12.1 Benign neoplasm of appendix

EXCLUDES1 benign carcinoid tumor of the appendix (D3A.020)

D12.2 Benign neoplasm of ascending colon

AHA: Q2 2018, Q1 2017

D12.3 Benign neoplasm of transverse colon

AHA: Q1 2017

Benign neoplasm of hepatic flexure

Benign neoplasm of splenic flexure

D12.4 Benign neoplasm of descending colon

AHA: Q2 2015

D12.5 Benign neoplasm of sigmoid colon

D12.6 Benign neoplasm of colon, unspecified

AHA: Q1 2017

Adenomatosis of colon

Benign neoplasm of large intestine NOS

Polyposis (hereditary) of colon

EXCLUDES1 inflammatory polyp of colon (K51.4-)

D12.7 Benign neoplasm of rectosigmoid junction

D12.8 Benign neoplasm of rectum

AHA: Q1 2018

EXCLUDES1 benign carcinoid tumor of the rectum (D3A.026)

D12.9 Benign neoplasm of anus and anal canal

Benign neoplasm of anus NOS

EXCLUDES1 benign neoplasm of anal margin (D22.5, D23.5)

benign neoplasm of anal skin (D22.5, D23.5)

benign neoplasm of perianal skin (D22.5, D23.5)

🔹 **D13 Benign neoplasm of** other and ill-defined parts of digestive system

EXCLUDES1 benign stromal tumors of digestive system (D21.4)

D13.0 Benign neoplasm of esophagus

D13.1 Benign neoplasm of stomach

EXCLUDES1 benign carcinoid tumor of the stomach (D3A.092)

D13.2 Benign neoplasm of duodenum

EXCLUDES1 benign carcinoid tumor of the duodenum (D3A.010)

🔹 **D13.3 Benign neoplasm of** other **and** unspecified **parts of** small intestine

EXCLUDES1 benign carcinoid tumors of the small intestine (D3A.01-)

benign neoplasm of ileocecal valve (D12.0)

D13.30 Benign neoplasm of unspecified part of small intestine

D13.39 Benign neoplasm of other **parts of small intestine**

D13.4 Benign neoplasm of liver

Benign neoplasm of intrahepatic bile ducts

D13.5 Benign neoplasm of extrahepatic bile ducts

D13.6 Benign neoplasm of pancreas

EXCLUDES1 benign neoplasm of endocrine pancreas (D13.7)

D13.7 Benign neoplasm of endocrine pancreas

Islet cell tumor

Benign neoplasm of islets of Langerhans

Use additional code to identify any functional activity.

D13.9 Benign neoplasm of ill-defined sites **within the digestive system**

Benign neoplasm of digestive system NOS

Benign neoplasm of intestine NOS

Benign neoplasm of spleen

🔹 **D14 Benign neoplasm of** middle ear and respiratory system

D14.0 Benign neoplasm of middle ear, nasal cavity and accessory sinuses

Benign neoplasm of cartilage of nose

EXCLUDES1 benign neoplasm of auricular canal (external) (D22.2-, D23.2-)

benign neoplasm of bone of ear (D16.4)

benign neoplasm of bone of nose (D16.4)

benign neoplasm of cartilage of ear (D21.0)

benign neoplasm of ear (external)(skin) (D22.2-, D23.2-)

benign neoplasm of nose NOS (D36.7)

benign neoplasm of skin of nose (D22.39, D23.39)

benign neoplasm of olfactory bulb (D33.3)

benign neoplasm of posterior margin of septum and choanae (D10.6)

polyp of accessory sinus (J33.8)

polyp of ear (middle) (H74.4)

polyp of nasal (cavity) (J33.-)

D14.1 Benign neoplasm of larynx

Adenomatous polyp of larynx

Benign neoplasm of epiglottis (suprahyoid portion)

EXCLUDES1 benign neoplasm of epiglottis, anterior aspect (D10.5)

polyp (nonadenomatous) of vocal cord or larynx (J38.1)

D14.2 Benign neoplasm of trachea

🔹 **D14.3 Benign neoplasm of** bronchus and lung

EXCLUDES1 benign carcinoid tumor of the bronchus and lung (D3A.090)

🔲 Unacceptable principal diagnosis symbol per Medicare code edits   🔲 Code exempt from diagnosis present on admission requirement

❓ Questionable admission   🔲 Complication or comorbidity   🔲 Major complication or comorbidity   🔲 CC/MCC exclusion

🔲 HCC diagnosis code   🔲 RxHCC diagnosis code   MACRA code   **DEFINITION** Describes condition/terminology

TIP Coding guidance   ◉ Official Guideline Reference   🔲 Z code as first-listed diagnosis

498

When symbols appear on a code that requires a 7th character extension, refer to Appendix B to identify applicable 7th character codes.

2020 ICD-10-CM

D14.30 Benign neoplasm of unspecified bronchus and lung
D14.31 Benign neoplasm of right bronchus and lung
D14.32 Benign neoplasm of left bronchus and lung
D14.4 Benign neoplasm of respiratory system, unspecified

[4th] D15 Benign neoplasm of other and unspecified intrathoracic organs
[EXCLUDES1] *benign neoplasm of mesothelial tissue (D19.-)*
D15.0 Benign neoplasm of thymus
[EXCLUDES1] *benign carcinoid tumor of the thymus (D3A.091)*
D15.1 Benign neoplasm of heart
[EXCLUDES1] *benign neoplasm of great vessels (D21.3)*
D15.2 Benign neoplasm of mediastinum
D15.7 Benign neoplasm of other specified intrathoracic organs
D15.9 Benign neoplasm of intrathoracic organ, unspecified

[4th] D16 Benign neoplasm of bone and articular cartilage
[EXCLUDES1] *benign neoplasm of connective tissue of ear (D21.0)*
benign neoplasm of connective tissue of eyelid (D21.0)
benign neoplasm of connective tissue of larynx (D14.1)
benign neoplasm of connective tissue of nose (D14.0)
benign neoplasm of synovia (D21.-)
[5th] D16.0 Benign neoplasm of scapula and long bones of upper limb
D16.00 Benign neoplasm of scapula and long bones of unspecified upper limb
D16.01 Benign neoplasm of scapula and long bones of right upper limb
D16.02 Benign neoplasm of scapula and long bones of left upper limb
[5th] D16.1 Benign neoplasm of short bones of upper limb
D16.10 Benign neoplasm of short bones of unspecified upper limb
D16.11 Benign neoplasm of short bones of right upper limb
D16.12 Benign neoplasm of short bones of left upper limb
[5th] D16.2 Benign neoplasm of long bones of lower limb
D16.20 Benign neoplasm of long bones of unspecified lower limb
D16.21 Benign neoplasm of long bones of right lower limb
D16.22 Benign neoplasm of long bones of left lower limb
[5th] D16.3 Benign neoplasm of short bones of lower limb
D16.30 Benign neoplasm of short bones of unspecified lower limb
D16.31 Benign neoplasm of short bones of right lower limb
D16.32 Benign neoplasm of short bones of left lower limb
D16.4 Benign neoplasm of bones of skull and face
Benign neoplasm of maxilla (superior)
Benign neoplasm of orbital bone
Keratocyst of maxilla
Keratocystic odontogenic tumor of maxilla
[EXCLUDES2] *benign neoplasm of lower jaw bone (D16.5)*
D16.5 Benign neoplasm of lower jaw bone
Keratocyst of mandible
Keratocystic odontogenic tumor of mandible
D16.6 Benign neoplasm of vertebral column
[EXCLUDES1] *benign neoplasm of sacrum and coccyx (D16.8)*
D16.7 Benign neoplasm of ribs, sternum and clavicle
D16.8 Benign neoplasm of pelvic bones, sacrum and coccyx
D16.9 Benign neoplasm of bone and articular cartilage, unspecified

[4th] D17 Benign lipomatous neoplasm
D17.0 Benign lipomatous neoplasm of skin and subcutaneous tissue of head, face and neck
D17.1 Benign lipomatous neoplasm of skin and subcutaneous tissue of trunk
[5th] D17.2 Benign lipomatous neoplasm of skin and subcutaneous tissue of limb
D17.20 Benign lipomatous neoplasm of skin and subcutaneous tissue of unspecified limb
D17.21 Benign lipomatous neoplasm of skin and subcutaneous tissue of right arm
D17.22 Benign lipomatous neoplasm of skin and subcutaneous tissue of left arm
D17.23 Benign lipomatous neoplasm of skin and subcutaneous tissue of right leg
D17.24 Benign lipomatous neoplasm of skin and subcutaneous tissue of left leg
[5th] D17.3 Benign lipomatous neoplasm of skin and subcutaneous tissue of other and unspecified sites
D17.30 Benign lipomatous neoplasm of skin and subcutaneous tissue of unspecified sites
D17.39 Benign lipomatous neoplasm of skin and subcutaneous tissue of other sites
D17.4 Benign lipomatous neoplasm of intrathoracic organs
D17.5 Benign lipomatous neoplasm of intra-abdominal organs
[EXCLUDES1] *benign lipomatous neoplasm of peritoneum and retroperitoneum (D17.79)*
D17.6 Benign lipomatous neoplasm of spermatic cord ♂
[5th] D17.7 Benign lipomatous neoplasm of other sites
D17.71 Benign lipomatous neoplasm of kidney
D17.72 Benign lipomatous neoplasm of other genitourinary organ
D17.79 Benign lipomatous neoplasm of other sites
Benign lipomatous neoplasm of peritoneum
Benign lipomatous neoplasm of retroperitoneum
D17.9 Benign lipomatous neoplasm, unspecified
Lipoma NOS

[4th] D18 Hemangioma and lymphangioma, any site
[EXCLUDES1] *benign neoplasm of glomus jugulare (D35.6)*
blue or pigmented nevus (D22.-)
nevus NOS (D22.-)
vascular nevus (Q82.5)
[5th] D18.0 Hemangioma
Angioma NOS
Cavernous nevus
D18.00 Hemangioma unspecified site
D18.01 Hemangioma of skin and subcutaneous tissue
D18.02 Hemangioma of intracranial structures [HCC]
D18.03 Hemangioma of intra-abdominal structures
D18.09 Hemangioma of other sites
D18.1 Lymphangioma, any site
AHA: Q2 2018, Q3 2018

[4th] D19 Benign neoplasm of mesothelial tissue
D19.0 Benign neoplasm of mesothelial tissue of pleura
D19.1 Benign neoplasm of mesothelial tissue of peritoneum
D19.7 Benign neoplasm of mesothelial tissue of other sites
D19.9 Benign neoplasm of mesothelial tissue, unspecified
Benign mesothelioma NOS

[4th] D20 Benign neoplasm of soft tissue of retroperitoneum and peritoneum
[EXCLUDES1] *benign lipomatous neoplasm of peritoneum and retroperitoneum (D17.79)*
benign neoplasm of mesothelial tissue (D19.-)
D20.0 Benign neoplasm of soft tissue of retroperitoneum
D20.1 Benign neoplasm of soft tissue of peritoneum

[4th] D21 Other benign neoplasms of connective and other soft tissue
[INCLUDES] *benign neoplasm of blood vessel*
benign neoplasm of bursa
benign neoplasm of cartilage
benign neoplasm of fascia
benign neoplasm of fat
benign neoplasm of ligament, except uterine
benign neoplasm of lymphatic channel
benign neoplasm of muscle
benign neoplasm of synovia
benign neoplasm of tendon (sheath)
benign stromal tumors
[EXCLUDES1] *benign neoplasm of articular cartilage (D16.-)*
benign neoplasm of cartilage of larynx (D14.1)
benign neoplasm of cartilage of nose (D14.0)
benign neoplasm of connective tissue of breast (D24.-)

Unspecified Code | Other Specified Code | Manifestation Code | [N] Newborn | [P] Pediatric | [M] Maternity | [A] Adult | ♂ Male | ♀ Female
● New Code ▲ Revised Code Title ►◄ Revised Text [NOTES] [INCLUDES] [EXCLUDES1] Not coded here [EXCLUDES2] Not included here
[4th] 4th character required [5th] 5th character required [6th] 6th character required [7th] 7th character required [7th] Extension 'X' Alert
[HAC] Hospital-acquired condition (HAC) alert AHA AHA Coding Clinic© ☞ Code first alert

When symbols appear on a code that requires a 7th character extension, refer to Appendix B to identify applicable 7th character codes.

benign neoplasm of peripheral nerves and autonomic nervous system (D36.1-)

benign neoplasm of peritoneum (D20.1)

benign neoplasm of retroperitoneum (D20.0)

benign neoplasm of uterine ligament, any (D28.2)

benign neoplasm of vascular tissue (D18.-)

hemangioma (D18.0-)

lipomatous neoplasm (D17.-)

lymphangioma (D18.1)

uterine leiomyoma (D25.-)

D21.0 Benign neoplasm of connective and other soft tissue of head, face and neck

Benign neoplasm of connective tissue of ear

Benign neoplasm of connective tissue of eyelid

EXCLUDES1 benign neoplasm of connective tissue of orbit (D31.6-)

D21.1 Benign neoplasm of connective and other soft tissue of upper limb, including shoulder

D21.10 Benign neoplasm of connective and other soft tissue of unspecified upper limb, including shoulder

D21.11 Benign neoplasm of connective and other soft tissue of right upper limb, including shoulder

D21.12 Benign neoplasm of connective and other soft tissue of left upper limb, including shoulder

D21.2 Benign neoplasm of connective and other soft tissue of lower limb, including hip

D21.20 Benign neoplasm of connective and other soft tissue of unspecified lower limb, including hip

D21.21 Benign neoplasm of connective and other soft tissue of right lower limb, including hip

D21.22 Benign neoplasm of connective and other soft tissue of left lower limb, including hip

D21.3 Benign neoplasm of connective and other soft tissue of thorax

Benign neoplasm of axilla

Benign neoplasm of diaphragm

Benign neoplasm of great vessels

EXCLUDES1 benign neoplasm of heart (D15.1)

benign neoplasm of mediastinum (D15.2)

benign neoplasm of thymus (D15.0)

D21.4 Benign neoplasm of connective and other soft tissue of abdomen

Benign stromal tumors of abdomen

D21.5 Benign neoplasm of connective and other soft tissue of pelvis

EXCLUDES1 benign neoplasm of any uterine ligament (D28.2)

uterine leiomyoma (D25.-)

D21.6 Benign neoplasm of connective and other soft tissue of trunk, unspecified

Benign neoplasm of ►connective and other soft tissue◄ back NOS

D21.9 Benign neoplasm of connective and other soft tissue, unspecified

D22 Melanocytic nevi

INCLUDES atypical nevus

blue hairy pigmented nevus

nevus NOS

D22.0 Melanocytic nevi of lip

D22.1 Melanocytic nevi of eyelid, including canthus

D22.10 Melanocytic nevi of unspecified eyelid, including canthus

D22.11 Melanocytic nevi of right eyelid, including canthus

D22.111 Melanocytic nevi of right upper eyelid, including canthus

AHA: Q4 2018

D22.112 Melanocytic nevi of right lower eyelid, including canthus

AHA: Q4 2018

D22.12 Melanocytic nevi of left eyelid, including canthus

D22.121 Melanocytic nevi of left upper eyelid, including canthus

AHA: Q4 2018

D22.122 Melanocytic nevi of left lower eyelid, including canthus

AHA: Q4 2018

D22.2 Melanocytic nevi of ear and external auricular canal

D22.20 Melanocytic nevi of unspecified ear and external auricular canal

D22.21 Melanocytic nevi of right ear and external auricular canal

D22.22 Melanocytic nevi of left ear and external auricular canal

D22.3 Melanocytic nevi of other and unspecified parts of face

D22.30 Melanocytic nevi of unspecified part of face

D22.39 Melanocytic nevi of other parts of face

D22.4 Melanocytic nevi of scalp and neck

D22.5 Melanocytic nevi of trunk

Melanocytic nevi of anal margin

Melanocytic nevi of anal skin

Melanocytic nevi of perianal skin

Melanocytic nevi of skin of breast

D22.6 Melanocytic nevi of upper limb, including shoulder

D22.60 Melanocytic nevi of unspecified upper limb, including shoulder

D22.61 Melanocytic nevi of right upper limb, including shoulder

D22.62 Melanocytic nevi of left upper limb, including shoulder

D22.7 Melanocytic nevi of lower limb, including hip

D22.70 Melanocytic nevi of unspecified lower limb, including hip

D22.71 Melanocytic nevi of right lower limb, including hip

D22.72 Melanocytic nevi of left lower limb, including hip

D22.9 Melanocytic nevi, unspecified

D23 Other benign neoplasms of skin

INCLUDES benign neoplasm of hair follicles

benign neoplasm of sebaceous glands

benign neoplasm of sweat glands

EXCLUDES1 benign lipomatous neoplasms of skin (D17.0-D17.3)

EXCLUDES2 melanocytic nevi (D22.-)

D23.0 Other benign neoplasm of skin of lip

EXCLUDES1 benign neoplasm of vermilion border of lip (D10.0)

D23.1 Other benign neoplasm of skin of eyelid, including canthus

D23.10 Other benign neoplasm of skin of unspecified eyelid, including canthus

D23.11 Other benign neoplasm of skin of right eyelid, including canthus

D23.111 Other benign neoplasm of skin of right upper eyelid, including canthus

AHA: Q4 2018

D23.112 Other benign neoplasm of skin of right lower eyelid, including canthus

AHA: Q4 2018

D23.12 Other benign neoplasm of skin of left eyelid, including canthus

D23.121 Other benign neoplasm of skin of left upper eyelid, including canthus

AHA: Q4 2018

D23.122 Other benign neoplasm of skin of left lower eyelid, including canthus

AHA: Q4 2018

D23.2 Other benign neoplasm of skin of ear and external auricular canal

D23.20 Other benign neoplasm of skin of unspecified ear and external auricular canal

D23.21 Other benign neoplasm of skin of right ear and external auricular canal

D23.22 Other benign neoplasm of skin of left ear and external auricular canal

---

PDx Unacceptable principal diagnosis symbol per Medicare code edits   Code exempt from diagnosis present on admission requirement   Questionable admission   Complication or comorbidity   MCC Major complication or comorbidity   CC/MCC CC/MCC exclusion   HCC HCC diagnosis code   RxHCC RxHCC diagnosis code   MACRA code   DEFINITION Describes condition/terminology   TIP Coding guidance   Official Guideline Reference   Z code as first-listed diagnosis

[5th] D23.3 Other benign neoplasm of skin of other and unspecified parts of face
D23.30 Other benign neoplasm of skin of unspecified part of face
D23.39 Other benign neoplasm of skin of other parts of face
D23.4 Other benign neoplasm of skin of scalp and neck
D23.5 Other benign neoplasm of skin of trunk
Other benign neoplasm of anal margin
Other benign neoplasm of anal skin
Other benign neoplasm of perianal skin
Other benign neoplasm of skin of breast
EXCLUDES1 *benign neoplasm of anus NOS (D12.9)*
[5th] D23.6 Other benign neoplasm of skin of upper limb, including shoulder
D23.60 Other benign neoplasm of skin of unspecified upper limb, including shoulder
D23.61 Other benign neoplasm of skin of right upper limb, including shoulder
D23.62 Other benign neoplasm of skin of left upper limb, including shoulder
[5th] D23.7 Other benign neoplasm of skin of lower limb, including hip
D23.70 Other benign neoplasm of skin of unspecified lower limb, including hip
D23.71 Other benign neoplasm of skin of right lower limb, including hip
D23.72 Other benign neoplasm of skin of left lower limb, including hip
D23.9 Other benign neoplasm of skin, unspecified
[4th] D24 Benign neoplasm of breast
INCLUDES *benign neoplasm of connective tissue of breast*
benign neoplasm of soft parts of breast
fibroadenoma of breast
EXCLUDES2 *adenofibrosis of breast (N60.2)*
benign cyst of breast (N60.-)
benign mammary dysplasia (N60.-)
benign neoplasm of skin of breast (D22.5, D23.5)
fibrocystic disease of breast (N60.-)
D24.1 Benign neoplasm of right breast
D24.2 Benign neoplasm of left breast
D24.9 Benign neoplasm of unspecified breast
[4th] D25 Leiomyoma of uterus (Figure 2.5)
INCLUDES *uterine fibroid*
uterine fibromyoma
uterine myoma
D25.0 Submucous leiomyoma of uterus ♀
D25.1 Intramural leiomyoma of uterus ♀
Interstitial leiomyoma of uterus
D25.2 Subserosal leiomyoma of uterus ♀
Subperitoneal leiomyoma of uterus
D25.9 Leiomyoma of uterus, unspecified ♀

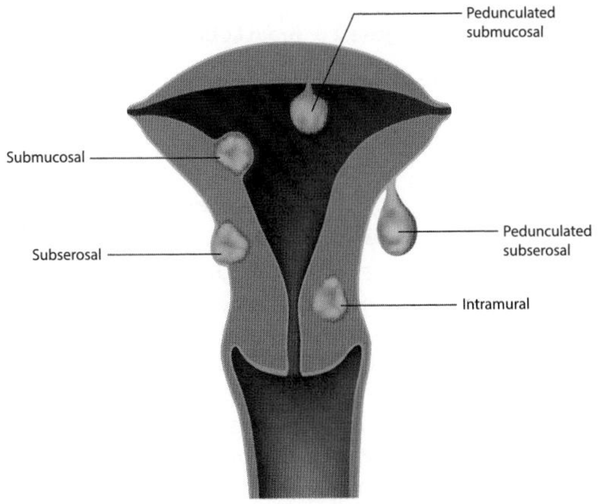

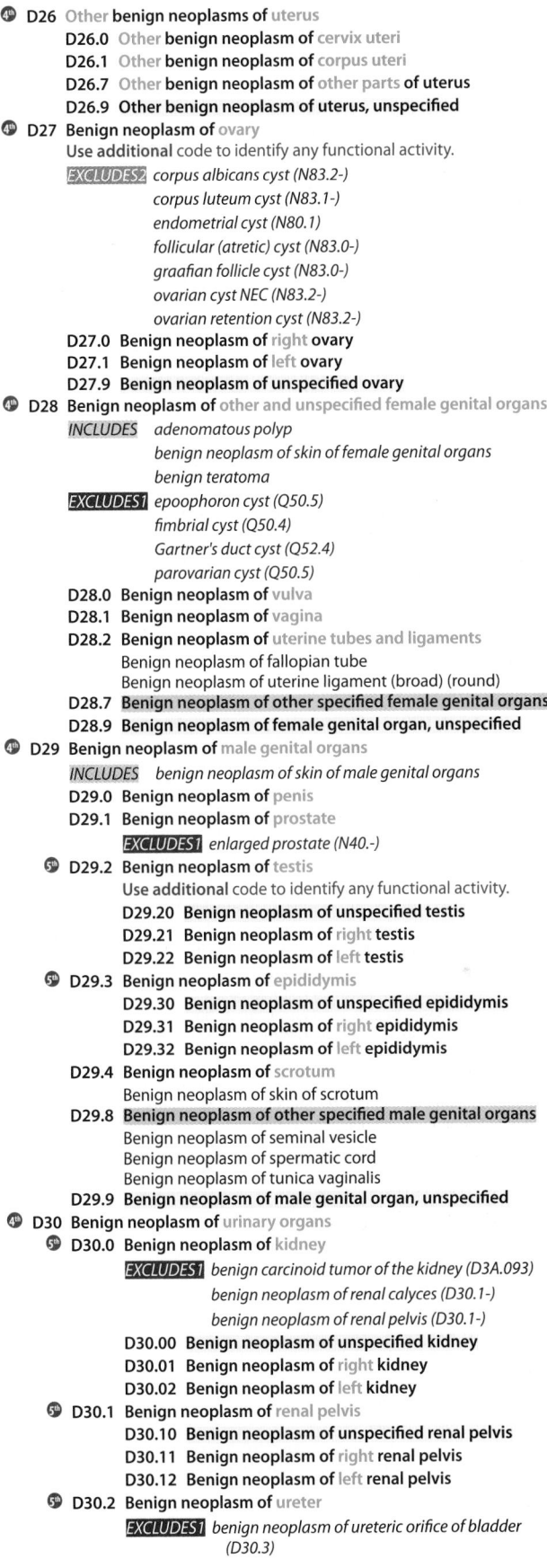

Figure 2.5 Uterine Fibroids

[4th] D26 Other benign neoplasms of uterus
D26.0 Other benign neoplasm of cervix uteri ♀
D26.1 Other benign neoplasm of corpus uteri ♀
D26.7 Other benign neoplasm of other parts of uterus ♀
D26.9 Other benign neoplasm of uterus, unspecified ♀
[4th] D27 Benign neoplasm of ovary
Use additional code to identify any functional activity.
EXCLUDES2 *corpus albicans cyst (N83.2-)*
corpus luteum cyst (N83.1-)
endometrial cyst (N80.1)
follicular (atretic) cyst (N83.0-)
graafian follicle cyst (N83.0-)
ovarian cyst NEC (N83.2-)
ovarian retention cyst (N83.2-)
D27.0 Benign neoplasm of right ovary ♀
D27.1 Benign neoplasm of left ovary ♀
D27.9 Benign neoplasm of unspecified ovary ♀
[4th] D28 Benign neoplasm of other and unspecified female genital organs
INCLUDES *adenomatous polyp*
benign neoplasm of skin of female genital organs
benign teratoma
EXCLUDES1 *epoophoron cyst (Q50.5)*
fimbrial cyst (Q50.4)
Gartner's duct cyst (Q52.4)
parovarian cyst (Q50.5)
D28.0 Benign neoplasm of vulva ♀
D28.1 Benign neoplasm of vagina ♀
D28.2 Benign neoplasm of uterine tubes and ligaments ♀
Benign neoplasm of fallopian tube
Benign neoplasm of uterine ligament (broad) (round)
D28.7 Benign neoplasm of other specified female genital organs ♀
D28.9 Benign neoplasm of female genital organ, unspecified ♀
[4th] D29 Benign neoplasm of male genital organs
INCLUDES *benign neoplasm of skin of male genital organs*
D29.0 Benign neoplasm of penis ♂
D29.1 Benign neoplasm of prostate ♂
EXCLUDES1 *enlarged prostate (N40.-)*
[5th] D29.2 Benign neoplasm of testis
Use additional code to identify any functional activity.
D29.20 Benign neoplasm of unspecified testis ♂
D29.21 Benign neoplasm of right testis ♂
D29.22 Benign neoplasm of left testis ♂
[5th] D29.3 Benign neoplasm of epididymis
D29.30 Benign neoplasm of unspecified epididymis ♂
D29.31 Benign neoplasm of right epididymis ♂
D29.32 Benign neoplasm of left epididymis ♂
D29.4 Benign neoplasm of scrotum ♂
Benign neoplasm of skin of scrotum
D29.8 Benign neoplasm of other specified male genital organs ♂
Benign neoplasm of seminal vesicle
Benign neoplasm of spermatic cord
Benign neoplasm of tunica vaginalis
D29.9 Benign neoplasm of male genital organ, unspecified ♂
[4th] D30 Benign neoplasm of urinary organs
[5th] D30.0 Benign neoplasm of kidney
EXCLUDES1 *benign carcinoid tumor of the kidney (D3A.093)*
benign neoplasm of renal calyces (D30.1-)
benign neoplasm of renal pelvis (D30.1-)
D30.00 Benign neoplasm of unspecified kidney
D30.01 Benign neoplasm of right kidney
D30.02 Benign neoplasm of left kidney
[5th] D30.1 Benign neoplasm of renal pelvis
D30.10 Benign neoplasm of unspecified renal pelvis
D30.11 Benign neoplasm of right renal pelvis
D30.12 Benign neoplasm of left renal pelvis
[5th] D30.2 Benign neoplasm of ureter
EXCLUDES1 *benign neoplasm of ureteric orifice of bladder (D30.3)*

Unspecified Code Other Specified Code Manifestation Code [N] Newborn [P] Pediatric [M] Maternity [A] Adult ♂ Male ♀ Female
● New Code ▲ Revised Code Title ►◄ Revised Text NOTES INCLUDES EXCLUDES1 Not coded here EXCLUDES2 Not included here
[4th] 4th character required [5th] 5th character required [6th] 6th character required [7th] 7th character required [X] Extension 'X' Alert
[HAC] Hospital-acquired condition (HAC) alert AHA AHA Coding Clinic© ☞ Code first alert

D30.20 **Benign neoplasm of unspecified ureter**
D30.21 **Benign neoplasm of** right **ureter**
D30.22 **Benign neoplasm of** left **ureter**
D30.3 **Benign neoplasm of** bladder
Benign neoplasm of ureteric orifice of bladder
Benign neoplasm of urethral orifice of bladder
D30.4 **Benign neoplasm of** urethra
EXCLUDES1 *benign neoplasm of urethral orifice of bladder (D30.3)*
D30.8 **Benign neoplasm of other specified urinary organs**
Benign neoplasm of paraurethral glands
D30.9 **Benign neoplasm of urinary organ, unspecified**
Benign neoplasm of urinary system NOS
D31 **Benign neoplasm of** eye and adnexa
EXCLUDES1 *benign neoplasm of connective tissue of eyelid (D21.0)*
benign neoplasm of optic nerve (D33.3)
benign neoplasm of skin of eyelid (D22.1-, D23.1-)
D31.0 **Benign neoplasm of** conjunctiva
D31.00 **Benign neoplasm of unspecified conjunctiva**
D31.01 **Benign neoplasm of** right **conjunctiva**
D31.02 **Benign neoplasm of** left **conjunctiva**
D31.1 **Benign neoplasm of** cornea
D31.10 **Benign neoplasm of unspecified cornea**
D31.11 **Benign neoplasm of** right **cornea**
D31.12 **Benign neoplasm of** left **cornea**
D31.2 **Benign neoplasm of** retina
EXCLUDES1 *dark area on retina (D49.81)*
hemangioma of retina (D49.81)
neoplasm of unspecified behavior of retina and choroid (D49.81)
retinal freckle (D49.81)
D31.20 **Benign neoplasm of unspecified retina**
D31.21 **Benign neoplasm of** right **retina**
D31.22 **Benign neoplasm of** left **retina**
D31.3 **Benign neoplasm of** choroid
D31.30 **Benign neoplasm of unspecified choroid**
D31.31 **Benign neoplasm of** right **choroid**
D31.32 **Benign neoplasm of** left **choroid**
D31.4 **Benign neoplasm of** ciliary body
D31.40 **Benign neoplasm of unspecified ciliary body**
D31.41 **Benign neoplasm of** right **ciliary body**
D31.42 **Benign neoplasm of** left **ciliary body**
D31.5 **Benign neoplasm of** lacrimal gland and duct
Benign neoplasm of lacrimal sac
Benign neoplasm of nasolacrimal duct
D31.50 **Benign neoplasm of unspecified lacrimal gland and duct**
D31.51 **Benign neoplasm of** right **lacrimal gland and duct**
D31.52 **Benign neoplasm of** left **lacrimal gland and duct**
D31.6 **Benign neoplasm of** unspecified site of orbit
Benign neoplasm of connective tissue of orbit
Benign neoplasm of extraocular muscle
Benign neoplasm of peripheral nerves of orbit
Benign neoplasm of retrobulbar tissue
Benign neoplasm of retro-ocular tissue
EXCLUDES1 *benign neoplasm of orbital bone (D16.4)*
D31.60 **Benign neoplasm of unspecified site of unspecified orbit**
D31.61 **Benign neoplasm of unspecified site of** right **orbit**
D31.62 **Benign neoplasm of unspecified site of** left **orbit**
D31.9 **Benign neoplasm of unspecified part of** eye
Benign neoplasm of eyeball
D31.90 **Benign neoplasm of unspecified part of unspecified eye**
D31.91 **Benign neoplasm of unspecified part of** right **eye**
D31.92 **Benign neoplasm of unspecified part of** left **eye**
D32 **Benign neoplasm of** meninges
D32.0 **Benign neoplasm of** cerebral **meninges**   HCC
D32.1 **Benign neoplasm of** spinal **meninges**   HCC

D32.9 **Benign neoplasm of meninges, unspecified**   HCC
Meningioma NOS
D33 **Benign neoplasm of** brain and other parts of central nervous system (Figure 2.6)
EXCLUDES1 *angioma (D18.0-)*
benign neoplasm of meninges (D32.-)
benign neoplasm of peripheral nerves and autonomic nervous system (D36.1-)
hemangioma (D18.0-)
neurofibromatosis (Q85.0-)
retro-ocular benign neoplasm (D31.6-)
D33.0 **Benign neoplasm of brain,** supratentorial   HCC
Benign neoplasm of cerebral ventricle
Benign neoplasm of cerebrum
Benign neoplasm of frontal lobe
Benign neoplasm of occipital lobe
Benign neoplasm of parietal lobe
Benign neoplasm of temporal lobe
EXCLUDES1 *benign neoplasm of fourth ventricle (D33.1)*
D33.1 **Benign neoplasm of brain,** infratentorial   HCC
Benign neoplasm of brain stem
Benign neoplasm of cerebellum
Benign neoplasm of fourth ventricle
D33.2 **Benign neoplasm of brain, unspecified**   HCC
D33.3 **Benign neoplasm of** cranial nerves   HCC
Benign neoplasm of olfactory bulb
D33.4 **Benign neoplasm of** spinal cord   HCC
D33.7 **Benign neoplasm of other specified** parts of central nervous system   HCC
D33.9 **Benign neoplasm of central nervous system, unspecified**   HCC
Benign neoplasm of nervous system (central) NOS

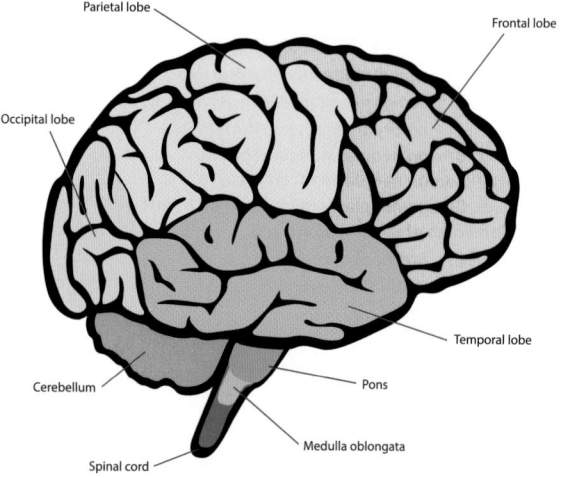

Figure 2.6 Brain Lobes

D34 **Benign neoplasm of** thyroid gland
Use additional code to identify any functional activity
D35 **Benign neoplasm of** other and unspecified endocrine glands
Use additional code to identify any functional activity
EXCLUDES1 *benign neoplasm of endocrine pancreas (D13.7)*
benign neoplasm of ovary (D27.-)
benign neoplasm of testis (D29.2.-)
benign neoplasm of thymus (D15.0)
D35.0 **Benign neoplasm of** adrenal gland
D35.00 **Benign neoplasm of unspecified adrenal gland**
D35.01 **Benign neoplasm of** right **adrenal gland**
D35.02 **Benign neoplasm of** left **adrenal gland**
D35.1 **Benign neoplasm of** parathyroid **gland**
D35.2 **Benign neoplasm of** pituitary **gland**   HCC
D35.3 **Benign neoplasm of** craniopharyngeal duct   HCC
D35.4 **Benign neoplasm of** pineal **gland**   HCC

PDxₐ Unacceptable principal diagnosis symbol per Medicare code edits   ₚₒₓ Code exempt from diagnosis present on admission requirement
? Questionable admission   ℀ Complication or comorbidity   MCC Major complication or comorbidity   CC/MCC CC/MCC exclusion
HCC HCC diagnosis code   RxHCC RxHCC diagnosis code   MACRA code   **DEFINITION** Describes condition/terminology
TIP Coding guidance   ◉ Official Guideline Reference   Z1 Z code as first-listed diagnosis

502

When symbols appear on a code that requires a 7th character extension, refer to Appendix B to identify applicable 7th character codes.

2020 ICD-10-CM

D35.5 **Benign neoplasm of** carotid body

D35.6 **Benign neoplasm of** aortic body and other paraganglia
Benign tumor of glomus jugulare

D35.7 **Benign neoplasm of other specified endocrine glands**

D35.9 **Benign neoplasm of endocrine gland, unspecified**
Benign neoplasm of unspecified endocrine gland

4ᵗʰ **D36 Benign neoplasm of** other and unspecified sites

D36.0 **Benign neoplasm of** lymph nodes
EXCLUDES1 lymphangioma (D18.1)

5ᵗʰ **D36.1 Benign neoplasm of** peripheral nerves and autonomic nervous system
EXCLUDES1 benign neoplasm of peripheral nerves of orbit (D31.6-)
neurofibromatosis (Q85.0-)

D36.10 **Benign neoplasm of peripheral nerves and autonomic nervous system, unspecified**

D36.11 **Benign neoplasm of peripheral nerves and autonomic nervous system of** face, head, and neck

D36.12 **Benign neoplasm of peripheral nerves and autonomic nervous system,** upper limb, including shoulder

D36.13 **Benign neoplasm of peripheral nerves and autonomic nervous system of** lower limb, including hip

D36.14 **Benign neoplasm of peripheral nerves and autonomic nervous system of** thorax

D36.15 **Benign neoplasm of peripheral nerves and autonomic nervous system of** abdomen

D36.16 **Benign neoplasm of peripheral nerves and autonomic nervous system of** pelvis

D36.17 **Benign neoplasm of peripheral nerves and autonomic nervous system of** trunk, **unspecified**

D36.7 **Benign neoplasm of other specified** sites
Benign neoplasm of back NOS
Benign neoplasm of nose NOS

D36.9 **Benign neoplasm, unspecified site**

Benign neuroendocrine tumors (D3A)

4ᵗʰ **D3A Benign neuroendocrine tumors**
Code also any associated multiple endocrine neoplasia [MEN] syndromes (E31.2-)
Use additional code to identify any associated endocrine syndrome, such as:
carcinoid syndrome (E34.0)
EXCLUDES2 benign pancreatic islet cell tumors (D13.7)

5ᵗʰ **D3A.0** Benign carcinoid tumors

D3A.00 **Benign carcinoid tumor of unspecified site**
Carcinoid tumor NOS

6ᵗʰ **D3A.01 Benign carcinoid tumors of the** small intestine

D3A.010 **Benign carcinoid tumor of the** duodenum

D3A.011 **Benign carcinoid tumor of the** jejunum

D3A.012 **Benign carcinoid tumor of the** ileum

D3A.019 **Benign carcinoid tumor of the small intestine, unspecified portion**

6ᵗʰ **D3A.02 Benign carcinoid tumors of the** appendix, large intestine, and rectum

D3A.020 **Benign carcinoid tumor of the** appendix

D3A.021 **Benign carcinoid tumor of the** cecum

D3A.022 **Benign carcinoid tumor of the** ascending colon

D3A.023 **Benign carcinoid tumor of the** transverse colon

D3A.024 **Benign carcinoid tumor of the** descending colon

D3A.025 **Benign carcinoid tumor of the** sigmoid colon

D3A.026 **Benign carcinoid tumor of the** rectum

D3A.029 **Benign carcinoid tumor of the large intestine, unspecified portion**
Benign carcinoid tumor of the colon NOS

6ᵗʰ D3A.09 **Benign carcinoid tumors of** other sites

D3A.090 **Benign carcinoid tumor of the** bronchus and lung

D3A.091 **Benign carcinoid tumor of the** thymus

D3A.092 **Benign carcinoid tumor of the** stomach

D3A.093 **Benign carcinoid tumor of the** kidney

D3A.094 **Benign carcinoid tumor of the** foregut, **unspecified**

D3A.095 **Benign carcinoid tumor of the** midgut, **unspecified**

D3A.096 **Benign carcinoid tumor of the** hindgut, **unspecified**

D3A.098 **Benign carcinoid tumors of** other sites

D3A.8 Other **benign neuroendocrine tumors**
Neuroendocrine tumor NOS

Neoplasms of uncertain behavior, polycythemia vera and myelodysplastic syndromes (D37-D48)

NOTES Categories D37-D44, and D48 classify by site neoplasms of uncertain behavior, i.e., histologic confirmation whether the neoplasm is malignant or benign cannot be made.
EXCLUDES1 neoplasms of unspecified behavior (D49.-)

4ᵗʰ **D37 Neoplasm of uncertain behavior of** oral cavity and digestive organs
EXCLUDES1 stromal tumors of uncertain behavior of digestive system (D48.1)

5ᵗʰ **D37.0 Neoplasm of uncertain behavior of** lip, oral cavity and pharynx
EXCLUDES1 neoplasm of uncertain behavior of aryepiglottic fold or interarytenoid fold, laryngeal aspect (D38.0)
neoplasm of uncertain behavior of epiglottis NOS (D38.0)
neoplasm of uncertain behavior of skin of lip (D48.5)
neoplasm of uncertain behavior of suprahyoid portion of epiglottis (D38.0)

D37.01 **Neoplasm of uncertain behavior of** lip
Neoplasm of uncertain behavior of vermilion border of lip

D37.02 **Neoplasm of uncertain behavior of** tongue

6ᵗʰ **D37.03 Neoplasm of uncertain behavior of the** major salivary glands

D37.030 **Neoplasm of uncertain behavior of the** parotid **salivary glands**

D37.031 **Neoplasm of uncertain behavior of the** sublingual **salivary glands**

D37.032 **Neoplasm of uncertain behavior of the** submandibular **salivary glands**

D37.039 **Neoplasm of uncertain behavior of the major salivary glands, unspecified**

D37.04 **Neoplasm of uncertain behavior of the** minor salivary glands
Neoplasm of uncertain behavior of submucosal salivary glands of lip
Neoplasm of uncertain behavior of submucosal salivary glands of cheek
Neoplasm of uncertain behavior of submucosal salivary glands of hard palate
Neoplasm of uncertain behavior of submucosal salivary glands of soft palate

D37.05 **Neoplasm of uncertain behavior of** pharynx
Neoplasm of uncertain behavior of aryepiglottic fold of pharynx NOS
Neoplasm of uncertain behavior of hypopharyngeal aspect of aryepiglottic fold of pharynx
Neoplasm of uncertain behavior of marginal zone of aryepiglottic fold of pharynx

D37.09 **Neoplasm of uncertain behavior of other specified sites of the oral cavity**

D37.1 **Neoplasm of uncertain behavior of** stomach

D37.2 **Neoplasm of uncertain behavior of** small intestine

D37.3 **Neoplasm of uncertain behavior of** appendix

Unspecified Code | Other Specified Code | Manifestation Code | N Newborn | P Pediatric | M Maternity | A Adult | ♂ Male | ♀ Female
● New Code | ▲ Revised Code Title | ▶◀ Revised Text | NOTES | INCLUDES | EXCLUDES1 Not coded here | EXCLUDES2 Not included here
4ᵗʰ 4ᵗʰ character required | 5ᵗʰ 5ᵗʰ character required | 6ᵗʰ 6ᵗʰ character required | 7ᵗʰ 7ᵗʰ character required | 7ˣ Extension 'X' Alert
HAC Hospital-acquired condition (HAC) alert | AHA AHA Coding Clinic© | ☛ Code first alert

D37.4 **Neoplasm of uncertain behavior of** colon

D37.5 **Neoplasm of uncertain behavior of** rectum

Neoplasm of uncertain behavior of rectosigmoid junction

D37.6 **Neoplasm of uncertain behavior of** liver, gallbladder and bile ducts

Neoplasm of uncertain behavior of ampulla of Vater

D37.8 Neoplasm of uncertain behavior of other specified digestive organs

Neoplasm of uncertain behavior of anal canal
Neoplasm of uncertain behavior of anal sphincter
Neoplasm of uncertain behavior of anus NOS
Neoplasm of uncertain behavior of esophagus
Neoplasm of uncertain behavior of intestine NOS
Neoplasm of uncertain behavior of pancreas

EXCLUDES1 neoplasm of uncertain behavior of anal margin (D48.5)

neoplasm of uncertain behavior of anal skin (D48.5)

neoplasm of uncertain behavior of perianal skin (D48.5)

D37.9 **Neoplasm of uncertain behavior of digestive organ, unspecified**

D38 **Neoplasm of uncertain behavior of** middle ear and respiratory and intrathoracic organs

EXCLUDES1 neoplasm of uncertain behavior of heart (D48.7)

D38.0 **Neoplasm of uncertain behavior of** larynx

Neoplasm of uncertain behavior of aryepiglottic fold or interarytenoid fold, laryngeal aspect
Neoplasm of uncertain behavior of epiglottis (suprahyoid portion)

EXCLUDES1 neoplasm of uncertain behavior of aryepiglottic fold or interarytenoid fold NOS (D37.05)

neoplasm of uncertain behavior of hypopharyngeal aspect of aryepiglottic fold (D37.05)

neoplasm of uncertain behavior of marginal zone of aryepiglottic fold (D37.05)

D38.1 **Neoplasm of uncertain behavior of** trachea, bronchus and lung

D38.2 **Neoplasm of uncertain behavior of** pleura

D38.3 **Neoplasm of uncertain behavior of** mediastinum

D38.4 **Neoplasm of uncertain behavior of** thymus

D38.5 **Neoplasm of uncertain behavior of** other respiratory organs

Neoplasm of uncertain behavior of accessory sinuses
Neoplasm of uncertain behavior of cartilage of nose
Neoplasm of uncertain behavior of middle ear
Neoplasm of uncertain behavior of nasal cavities

EXCLUDES1 neoplasm of uncertain behavior of ear (external) (skin) (D48.5)

neoplasm of uncertain behavior of nose NOS (D48.7)

neoplasm of uncertain behavior of skin of nose (D48.5)

D38.6 **Neoplasm of uncertain behavior of respiratory organ, unspecified**

D39 **Neoplasm of uncertain behavior of** female genital organs

D39.0 **Neoplasm of uncertain behavior of** uterus ♀

D39.1 **Neoplasm of uncertain behavior of** ovary

Use additional code to identify any functional activity.

D39.10 **Neoplasm of uncertain behavior of unspecified ovary** ♀

D39.11 **Neoplasm of uncertain behavior of** right ovary ♀

D39.12 **Neoplasm of uncertain behavior of** left ovary ♀

D39.2 **Neoplasm of uncertain behavior of** placenta M ♀

Chorioadenoma destruens
Invasive hydatidiform mole
Malignant hydatidiform mole

EXCLUDES1 hydatidiform mole NOS (O01.9)

D39.8 Neoplasm of uncertain behavior of other specified female genital organs ♀

Neoplasm of uncertain behavior of skin of female genital organs

D39.9 **Neoplasm of uncertain behavior of female genital organ, unspecified** ♀

D40 **Neoplasm of uncertain behavior of** male genital organs

D40.0 **Neoplasm of uncertain behavior of** prostate ♂

D40.1 **Neoplasm of uncertain behavior of** testis

D40.10 **Neoplasm of uncertain behavior of unspecified testis** ♂

D40.11 **Neoplasm of uncertain behavior of** right testis ♂

D40.12 **Neoplasm of uncertain behavior of** left testis ♂

D40.8 Neoplasm of uncertain behavior of other specified male genital organs ♂

Neoplasm of uncertain behavior of skin of male genital organs

D40.9 **Neoplasm of uncertain behavior of male genital organ, unspecified** ♂

D41 **Neoplasm of uncertain behavior of** urinary organs

D41.0 **Neoplasm of uncertain behavior of** kidney

EXCLUDES1 neoplasm of uncertain behavior of renal pelvis (D41.1-)

D41.00 **Neoplasm of uncertain behavior of unspecified kidney**

D41.01 **Neoplasm of uncertain behavior of** right kidney

D41.02 **Neoplasm of uncertain behavior of** left kidney

D41.1 **Neoplasm of uncertain behavior of** renal pelvis

D41.10 **Neoplasm of uncertain behavior of unspecified renal pelvis**

D41.11 **Neoplasm of uncertain behavior of** right renal pelvis

D41.12 **Neoplasm of uncertain behavior of** left renal pelvis

D41.2 **Neoplasm of uncertain behavior of** ureter

D41.20 **Neoplasm of uncertain behavior of unspecified ureter**

D41.21 **Neoplasm of uncertain behavior of** right ureter

D41.22 **Neoplasm of uncertain behavior of** left ureter

D41.3 **Neoplasm of uncertain behavior of** urethra

D41.4 **Neoplasm of uncertain behavior of** bladder

D41.8 Neoplasm of uncertain behavior of other specified urinary organs

D41.9 **Neoplasm of uncertain behavior of unspecified urinary organ**

D42 **Neoplasm of uncertain behavior of** meninges

D42.0 **Neoplasm of uncertain behavior of** cerebral meninges HCC

D42.1 **Neoplasm of uncertain behavior of** spinal meninges HCC

D42.9 **Neoplasm of uncertain behavior of meninges, unspecified** HCC

D43 **Neoplasm of uncertain behavior of** brain and central nervous system

EXCLUDES1 neoplasm of uncertain behavior of peripheral nerves and autonomic nervous system (D48.2)

D43.0 **Neoplasm of uncertain behavior of brain,** supratentorial HCC

Neoplasm of uncertain behavior of cerebral ventricle
Neoplasm of uncertain behavior of cerebrum
Neoplasm of uncertain behavior of frontal lobe
Neoplasm of uncertain behavior of occipital lobe
Neoplasm of uncertain behavior of parietal lobe
Neoplasm of uncertain behavior of temporal lobe

EXCLUDES1 neoplasm of uncertain behavior of fourth ventricle (D43.1)

D43.1 **Neoplasm of uncertain behavior of brain,** infratentorial HCC

Neoplasm of uncertain behavior of brain stem
Neoplasm of uncertain behavior of cerebellum
Neoplasm of uncertain behavior of fourth ventricle

D43.2 **Neoplasm of uncertain behavior of brain, unspecified** HCC

D43.3 **Neoplasm of uncertain behavior of** cranial nerves HCC

D43.4 **Neoplasm of uncertain behavior of** spinal cord HCC

D43.8 Neoplasm of uncertain behavior of other specified parts of central nervous system HCC

D43.9 **Neoplasm of uncertain behavior of central nervous system, unspecified** HCC

Neoplasm of uncertain behavior of nervous system (central) NOS

D44 **Neoplasm of uncertain behavior of** endocrine glands

EXCLUDES1 multiple endocrine adenomatosis (E31.2-)

multiple endocrine neoplasia (E31.2-)

neoplasm of uncertain behavior of endocrine pancreas (D37.8)

neoplasm of uncertain behavior of ovary (D39.1-)

neoplasm of uncertain behavior of testis (D40.1-)

neoplasm of uncertain behavior of thymus (D38.4)

PDX Unacceptable principal diagnosis symbol per Medicare code edits   PDX Code exempt from diagnosis present on admission requirement
❓ Questionable admission   CC Complication or comorbidity   MCC Major complication or comorbidity   CC/MCC CC/MCC exclusion
HCC HCC diagnosis code   RxHCC RxHCC diagnosis code   MACRA code   **DEFINITION** Describes condition/terminology
TIP Coding guidance   ◉ Official Guideline Reference   Z1 Z code as first-listed diagnosis

When symbols appear on a code that requires a 7th character extension, refer to Appendix B to identify applicable 7th character codes.   **2020 ICD-10-CM**

D44.0 Neoplasm of uncertain behavior of thyroid gland

5ᵗʰ D44.1 Neoplasm of uncertain behavior of adrenal gland
Use additional code to identify any functional activity.

D44.10 Neoplasm of uncertain behavior of unspecified adrenal gland

D44.11 Neoplasm of uncertain behavior of right adrenal gland

D44.12 Neoplasm of uncertain behavior of left adrenal gland

D44.2 Neoplasm of uncertain behavior of parathyroid gland

D44.3 Neoplasm of uncertain behavior of pituitary gland   HCC
Use additional code to identify any functional activity.

D44.4 Neoplasm of uncertain behavior of craniopharyngeal duct   HCC

D44.5 Neoplasm of uncertain behavior of pineal gland   HCC

D44.6 Neoplasm of uncertain behavior of carotid body   HCC

D44.7 Neoplasm of uncertain behavior of aortic body and other paraganglia   HCC
AHA: Q4 2016

D44.9 Neoplasm of uncertain behavior of unspecified endocrine gland

D45 Polycythemia vera   HCC
DEFINITION: Polycythemia vera (PV) is a rare blood cancer, in which the bone marrow makes too many red blood cells.
EXCLUDES1 familial polycythemia (D75.0)
secondary polycythemia (D75.1)

4ᵗʰ D46 Myelodysplastic syndromes
Use additional code for adverse effect, if applicable, to identify drug (T36-T50 with fifth or sixth character 5)
EXCLUDES2 drug-induced aplastic anemia (D61.1)

D46.0 Refractory anemia without ring sideroblasts, so stated   HCC RxHCC
Refractory anemia without sideroblasts, without excess of blasts

D46.1 Refractory anemia with ring sideroblasts   HCC RxHCC
RARS

5ᵗʰ D46.2 Refractory anemia with excess of blasts [RAEB]

D46.20 Refractory anemia with excess of blasts, unspecified   HCC RxHCC
RAEB NOS

D46.21 Refractory anemia with excess of blasts 1   HCC RxHCC
RAEB 1

D46.22 Refractory anemia with excess of blasts 2   HCC RxHCC
RAEB 2

D46.A Refractory cytopenia with multilineage dysplasia   HCC RxHCC

D46.B Refractory cytopenia with multilineage dysplasia and ring sideroblasts   HCC RxHCC
RCMD RS

D46.C Myelodysplastic syndrome with isolated del(5q) chromosomal abnormality   HCC RxHCC
Myelodysplastic syndrome with 5q deletion
5q minus syndrome NOS

D46.4 Refractory anemia, unspecified   HCC RxHCC

D46.Z Other myelodysplastic syndromes   HCC RxHCC
EXCLUDES1 chronic myelomonocytic leukemia (C93.1-)

D46.9 Myelodysplastic syndrome, unspecified   HCC RxHCC
Myelodysplasia NOS

4ᵗʰ D47 Other neoplasms of uncertain behavior of lymphoid, hematopoietic and related tissue

5ᵗʰ D47.0 Mast cell neoplasms of uncertain behavior
EXCLUDES1 congenital cutaneous mastocytosis (Q82.2)
histiocytic neoplasms of uncertain behavior (D47.Z9)
malignant mast cell neoplasm (C96.2-)

D47.01 Cutaneous mastocytosis
AHA: Q4 2017
Diffuse cutaneous mastocytosis
Maculopapular cutaneous mastocytosis
Solitary mastocytoma
Telangiectasia macularis eruptiva perstans
Urticaria pigmentosa
EXCLUDES1 congenital (diffuse) (maculopapular) cutaneous mastocytosis (Q82.2)
congenital urticaria pigmentosa (Q82.2)
extracutaneous mastocytoma (D47.09)

D47.02 Systemic mastocytosis
AHA: Q4 2017
Indolent systemic mastocytosis
Isolated bone marrow mastocytosis
Smoldering systemic mastocytosis
Systemic mastocytosis, with an associated hematological non-mast cell lineage disease (SM-AHNMD)
Code also, if applicable, any associated hematological non-mast cell lineage disease, such as:
acute myeloid leukemia (C92.6-, C92.A-)
chronic myelomonocytic leukemia (C93.1-)
essential thrombocytosis (D47.3)
hypereosinophilic syndrome (D72.1)
myelodysplastic syndrome (D46.9)
myeloproliferative syndrome (D47.1)
non-Hodgkin lymphoma (C82-C85)
plasma cell myeloma (C90.0-)
polycythemia vera (D45)
EXCLUDES1 aggressive systemic mastocytosis (C96.21)
mast cell leukemia (C94.3-)

D47.09 Other mast cell neoplasms of uncertain behavior
AHA: Q4 2017
Extracutaneous mastocytoma
Mast cell tumor NOS
Mastocytoma NOS
Mastocytosis NOS

D47.1 Chronic myeloproliferative disease   HCC
Chronic neutrophilic leukemia
Myeloproliferative disease, unspecified
EXCLUDES1 atypical chronic myeloid leukemia BCR/ABL-negative (C92.2-)
chronic myeloid leukemia BCR/ABL-positive (C92.1-)
myelofibrosis NOS (D75.81)
myelophthisic anemia (D61.82)
myelophthisis (D61.82)
secondary myelofibrosis NOS (D75.81)

D47.2 Monoclonal gammopathy
Monoclonal gammopathy of undetermined significance [MGUS]

D47.3 Essential (hemorrhagic) thrombocythemia   HCC
Essential thrombocytosis
Idiopathic hemorrhagic thrombocythemia

D47.4 Osteomyelofibrosis   HCC RxHCC
Chronic idiopathic myelofibrosis
Myelofibrosis (idiopathic) (with myeloid metaplasia)
Myelosclerosis (megakaryocytic) with myeloid metaplasia
Secondary myelofibrosis in myeloproliferative disease
EXCLUDES1 acute myelofibrosis (C94.4-)

5ᵗʰ D47.Z Other specified neoplasms of uncertain behavior of lymphoid, hematopoietic and related tissue

D47.Z1 Post-transplant lymphoproliferative disorder (PTLD)   HCC PDxn.
☛ Code first complications of transplanted organs and tissue (T86.-)

D47.Z2 Castleman disease   HCC
AHA: Q4 2016
Code also if applicable human herpesvirus 8 infection (B10.89)
EXCLUDES2 Kaposi's sarcoma (C46-)

D47.Z9 Other specified neoplasms of uncertain behavior of lymphoid, hematopoietic and related tissue   HCC
Histiocytic tumors of uncertain behavior

D47.9 Neoplasm of uncertain behavior of lymphoid, hematopoietic and related tissue, unspecified   HCC
Lymphoproliferative disease NOS

4ᵗʰ D48 Neoplasm of uncertain behavior of other and unspecified sites
EXCLUDES1 neurofibromatosis (nonmalignant) (Q85.0-)

D48.0 Neoplasm of uncertain behavior of bone and articular cartilage

---

Unspecified Code   Other Specified Code   Manifestation Code   N Newborn   P Pediatric   M Maternity   A Adult   ♂ Male   ♀ Female
● New Code   ▲ Revised Code Title   ▶◀ Revised Text   NOTES   INCLUDES   EXCLUDES1 Not coded here   EXCLUDES2 Not included here
4ᵗʰ 4ᵗʰ character required   5ᵗʰ 5ᵗʰ character required   6ᵗʰ 6ᵗʰ character required   7ᵗʰ 7ᵗʰ character required   ⑦ Extension 'X' Alert
HAC Hospital-acquired condition (HAC) alert   AHA AHA Coding Clinic©   ☛ Code first alert

2020 ICD-10-CM   When symbols appear on a code that requires a 7th character extension, refer to Appendix B to identify applicable 7th character codes.   505

EXCLUDES1 *neoplasm of uncertain behavior of cartilage of ear (D48.1)*

neoplasm of uncertain behavior of cartilage of larynx (D38.0)

neoplasm of uncertain behavior of cartilage of nose (D38.5)

neoplasm of uncertain behavior of connective tissue of eyelid (D48.1)

neoplasm of uncertain behavior of synovia (D48.1)

D48.1 Neoplasm of uncertain behavior of connective and other soft tissue

Neoplasm of uncertain behavior of connective tissue of ear

Neoplasm of uncertain behavior of connective tissue of eyelid

Stromal tumors of uncertain behavior of digestive system

EXCLUDES1 *neoplasm of uncertain behavior of articular cartilage (D48.0)*

neoplasm of uncertain behavior of cartilage of larynx (D38.0)

neoplasm of uncertain behavior of cartilage of nose (D38.5)

neoplasm of uncertain behavior of connective tissue of breast (D48.6-)

D48.2 Neoplasm of uncertain behavior of peripheral nerves and autonomic nervous system

EXCLUDES1 *neoplasm of uncertain behavior of peripheral nerves of orbit (D48.7)*

D48.3 Neoplasm of uncertain behavior of retroperitoneum

D48.4 Neoplasm of uncertain behavior of peritoneum

D48.5 Neoplasm of uncertain behavior of skin

Neoplasm of uncertain behavior of anal margin

Neoplasm of uncertain behavior of anal skin

Neoplasm of uncertain behavior of perianal skin

Neoplasm of uncertain behavior of skin of breast

EXCLUDES1 *neoplasm of uncertain behavior of anus NOS (D37.8)*

neoplasm of uncertain behavior of skin of genital organs (D39.8, D40.8)

neoplasm of uncertain behavior of vermilion border of lip (D37.0)

5ᵗʰ **D48.6 Neoplasm of uncertain behavior of** breast

Neoplasm of uncertain behavior of connective tissue of breast

Cystosarcoma phyllodes

EXCLUDES1 *neoplasm of uncertain behavior of skin of breast (D48.5)*

D48.60 Neoplasm of uncertain behavior of unspecified breast

D48.61 Neoplasm of uncertain behavior of right **breast**

D48.62 Neoplasm of uncertain behavior of left **breast**

D48.7 Neoplasm of uncertain behavior of other specified sites

Neoplasm of uncertain behavior of eye

Neoplasm of uncertain behavior of heart

Neoplasm of uncertain behavior of peripheral nerves of orbit

EXCLUDES1 *neoplasm of uncertain behavior of connective tissue (D48.1)*

neoplasm of uncertain behavior of skin of eyelid (D48.5)

D48.9 Neoplasm of uncertain behavior, unspecified

Neoplasms of unspecified behavior (D49)

4ᵗʰ **D49 Neoplasms of** unspecified **behavior**

NOTES Category D49 classifies by site neoplasms of unspecified morphology and behavior. The term 'mass', unless otherwise stated, is not to be regarded as a neoplastic growth.

INCLUDES *'growth' NOS*

neoplasm NOS

new growth NOS

tumor NOS

EXCLUDES1 *neoplasms of uncertain behavior (D37-D44, D48)*

D49.0 Neoplasm of unspecified behavior of digestive system

EXCLUDES1 *neoplasm of unspecified behavior of margin of anus (D49.2)*

neoplasm of unspecified behavior of perianal skin (D49.2)

neoplasm of unspecified behavior of skin of anus (D49.2)

D49.1 Neoplasm of unspecified behavior of respiratory system

D49.2 Neoplasm of unspecified behavior of bone, soft tissue, and skin

EXCLUDES1 *neoplasm of unspecified behavior of anal canal (D49.0)*

neoplasm of unspecified behavior of anus NOS (D49.0)

neoplasm of unspecified behavior of bone marrow (D49.89)

neoplasm of unspecified behavior of cartilage of larynx (D49.1)

neoplasm of unspecified behavior of cartilage of nose (D49.1)

neoplasm of unspecified behavior of connective tissue of breast (D49.3)

neoplasm of unspecified behavior of skin of genital organs (D49.59)

neoplasm of unspecified behavior of vermilion border of lip (D49.0)

D49.3 Neoplasm of unspecified behavior of breast

EXCLUDES1 *neoplasm of unspecified behavior of skin of breast (D49.2)*

D49.4 Neoplasm of unspecified behavior of bladder

5ᵗʰ **D49.5 Neoplasm of unspecified behavior of** other genitourinary organs

6ᵗʰ **D49.51 Neoplasm** of unspecified behavior of **kidney**

D49.511 Neoplasm of unspecified behavior of right **kidney**

AHA: Q4 2016

D49.512 Neoplasm of unspecified behavior of left **kidney**

AHA: Q4 2016

D49.519 Neoplasm of unspecified behavior of unspecified kidney

AHA: Q4 2016

D49.59 Neoplasm of unspecified behavior of other genitourinary organ

AHA: Q4 2016

D49.6 Neoplasm of unspecified behavior of brain   HCC

EXCLUDES1 *neoplasm of unspecified behavior of cerebral meninges (D49.7)*

neoplasm of unspecified behavior of cranial nerves (D49.7)

D49.7 Neoplasm of unspecified behavior of endocrine glands and other parts of nervous system

EXCLUDES1 *neoplasm of unspecified behavior of peripheral, sympathetic, and parasympathetic nerves and ganglia (D49.2)*

5ᵗʰ **D49.8 Neoplasm of unspecified behavior of** other specified sites

EXCLUDES1 *neoplasm of unspecified behavior of eyelid (skin) (D49.2)*

neoplasm of unspecified behavior of eyelid cartilage (D49.2)

neoplasm of unspecified behavior of great vessels (D49.2)

neoplasm of unspecified behavior of optic nerve (D49.7)

D49.81 Neoplasm of unspecified behavior of retina and choroid

Dark area on retina

Retinal freckle

D49.89 Neoplasm of unspecified behavior of other specified sites

D49.9 Neoplasm of unspecified behavior of unspecified site

PDx Unacceptable principal diagnosis symbol per Medicare code edits   POA Code exempt from diagnosis present on admission requirement

? Questionable admission   CC Complication or comorbidity   MCC Major complication or comorbidity   CC/MCC CC/MCC exclusion

HCC HCC diagnosis code   RxHCC RxHCC diagnosis code   MACRA code   **DEFINITION** Describes condition/terminology

TIP Coding guidance   👁 Official Guideline Reference   Z1 Z code as first-listed diagnosis

When symbols appear on a code that requires a 7th character extension, refer to Appendix B to identify applicable 7th character codes.

2020 ICD-10-CM

Chapter 3: Diseases of Blood/Blood-Forming Organs & Disorders Involving Immune Mechanism (D50-D89)

Diseases of the blood and blood-forming organs and certain disorders involving the immune mechanism (D50-D89)

EXCLUDES2 autoimmune disease (systemic) NOS (M35.9)

certain conditions originating in the perinatal period (P00-P96)

complications of pregnancy, childbirth and the puerperium (O00-O9A)

congenital malformations, deformations and chromosomal abnormalities (Q00-Q99)

endocrine, nutritional and metabolic diseases (E00-E88)

human immunodeficiency virus [HIV] disease (B20)

injury, poisoning and certain other consequences of external causes (S00-T88)

neoplasms (C00-D49)

symptoms, signs and abnormal clinical and laboratory findings, not elsewhere classified (R00-R94)

This chapter contains the following blocks:

D50-D53   Nutritional anemias
D55-D59   Hemolytic anemias
D60-D64   Aplastic and other anemias and other bone marrow failure syndromes
D65-D69   Coagulation defects, purpura and other hemorrhagic conditions
D70-D77   Other disorders of blood and blood-forming organs
D78   Intraoperative and postprocedural complications of the spleen
D80-D89   Certain disorders involving the immune mechanism

Nutritional anemias (D50-D53)

D50 Iron deficiency anemia

INCLUDES   asiderotic anemia
           hypochromic anemia

D50.0 Iron deficiency anemia secondary to blood loss (chronic)
Posthemorrhagic anemia (chronic)
EXCLUDES1 acute posthemorrhagic anemia (D62)
          congenital anemia from fetal blood loss (P61.3)

D50.1 Sideropenic dysphagia
Kelly-Paterson syndrome
Plummer-Vinson syndrome

D50.8 Other iron deficiency anemias
Iron deficiency anemia due to inadequate dietary iron intake

D50.9 Iron deficiency anemia, unspecified

D51 Vitamin B12 deficiency anemia

EXCLUDES1 vitamin B12 deficiency (E53.8)

D51.0 Vitamin B12 deficiency anemia due to intrinsic factor deficiency
Addison anemia
Biermer anemia
Pernicious (congenital) anemia
Congenital intrinsic factor deficiency

D51.1 Vitamin B12 deficiency anemia due to selective vitamin B12 malabsorption with proteinuria
Imerslund (Gräsbeck) syndrome
Megaloblastic hereditary anemia

D51.2 Transcobalamin II deficiency

D51.3 Other dietary vitamin B12 deficiency anemia
Vegan anemia

D51.8 Other vitamin B12 deficiency anemias

D51.9 Vitamin B12 deficiency anemia, unspecified

D52 Folate deficiency anemia

EXCLUDES1 folate deficiency without anemia (E53.8)

D52.0 Dietary folate deficiency anemia
Nutritional megaloblastic anemia

D52.1 Drug-induced folate deficiency anemia
Use additional code for adverse effect, if applicable, to identify drug (T36-T50 with fifth or sixth character 5)

D52.8 Other folate deficiency anemias

D52.9 Folate deficiency anemia, unspecified
Folic acid deficiency anemia NOS

D53 Other nutritional anemias

INCLUDES   megaloblastic anemia unresponsive to vitamin B12 or folate therapy

D53.0 Protein deficiency anemia
Amino-acid deficiency anemia
Orotaciduric anemia
EXCLUDES1 Lesch-Nyhan syndrome (E79.1)

D53.1 Other megaloblastic anemias, not elsewhere classified
Megaloblastic anemia NOS
EXCLUDES1 Di Guglielmo's disease (C94.0)

D53.2 Scorbutic anemia
EXCLUDES1 scurvy (E54)

D53.8 Other specified nutritional anemias
Anemia associated with deficiency of copper
Anemia associated with deficiency of molybdenum
Anemia associated with deficiency of zinc
EXCLUDES1 nutritional deficiencies without anemia, such as:
          copper deficiency NOS (E61.0)
          molybdenum deficiency NOS (E61.5)
          zinc deficiency NOS (E60)

D53.9 Nutritional anemia, unspecified
AHA: Q4 2018
Simple chronic anemia
EXCLUDES1 anemia NOS (D64.9)

Hemolytic anemias (D55-D59)

D55 Anemia due to enzyme disorders

EXCLUDES1 drug-induced enzyme deficiency anemia (D59.2)

D55.0 Anemia due to glucose-6-phosphate dehydrogenase [G6PD] deficiency   HCC
Favism
G6PD deficiency anemia
EXCLUDES1 glucose-6-phosphate dehydrogenase (G6PD) deficiency without anemia (D75.A)

D55.1 Anemia due to other disorders of glutathione metabolism   HCC
Anemia (due to) enzyme deficiencies, except G6PD, related to the hexose monophosphate [HMP] shunt pathway
Anemia (due to) hemolytic nonspherocytic (hereditary), type I

D55.2 Anemia due to disorders of glycolytic enzymes   HCC
Hemolytic nonspherocytic (hereditary) anemia, type II
Hexokinase deficiency anemia
Pyruvate kinase [PK] deficiency anemia
Triose-phosphate isomerase deficiency anemia
EXCLUDES1 disorders of glycolysis not associated with anemia (E74.8)

D55.3 Anemia due to disorders of nucleotide metabolism   HCC

D55.8 Other anemias due to enzyme disorders   HCC

D55.9 Anemia due to enzyme disorder, unspecified   HCC

D56 Thalassemia

EXCLUDES1 sickle-cell thalassemia (D57.4-)

D56.0 Alpha thalassemia   HCC RxHCC
Alpha thalassemia major
Hemoglobin H Constant Spring
Hemoglobin H disease
Hydrops fetalis due to alpha thalassemia
Severe alpha thalassemia
Triple gene defect alpha thalassemia

Unspecified Code   Other Specified Code   Manifestation Code   N Newborn   P Pediatric   M Maternity   A Adult   ♂ Male   ♀ Female
● New Code   ▲ Revised Code Title   ▶◀ Revised Text   NOTES   INCLUDES   EXCLUDES1 Not coded here   EXCLUDES2 Not included here
4ᵗʰ character required   5ᵗʰ character required   6ᵗʰ character required   7ᵗʰ character required   Extension 'X' Alert
HAC Hospital-acquired condition (HAC) alert   AHA AHA Coding Clinic©   📌 Code first alert

Use additional code, if applicable, for hydrops fetalis due to alpha thalassemia (P56.99)

[EXCLUDES1] *alpha thalassemia trait or minor (D56.3)*
asymptomatic alpha thalassemia (D56.3)
hydrops fetalis due to isoimmunization (P56.0)
hydrops fetalis not due to immune hemolysis (P83.2)

D56.1 Beta thalassemia [HCC] [RxHCC]
Beta thalassemia major
Cooley's anemia
Homozygous beta thalassemia
Severe beta thalassemia
Thalassemia intermedia
Thalassemia major
[EXCLUDES1] *beta thalassemia minor (D56.3)*
beta thalassemia trait (D56.3)
delta-beta thalassemia (D56.2)
hemoglobin E-beta thalassemia (D56.5)
sickle-cell beta thalassemia (D57.4-)

D56.2 Delta-beta thalassemia [HCC]
Homozygous delta-beta thalassemia
[EXCLUDES1] *delta-beta thalassemia minor (D56.3)*
delta-beta thalassemia trait (D56.3)

D56.3 Thalassemia minor
Alpha thalassemia minor
Alpha thalassemia silent carrier
Alpha thalassemia trait
Beta thalassemia minor
Beta thalassemia trait
Delta-beta thalassemia minor
Delta-beta thalassemia trait
Thalassemia trait NOS
[EXCLUDES1] *alpha thalassemia (D56.0)*
beta thalassemia (D56.1)
delta-beta thalassemia (D56.2)
hemoglobin E-beta thalassemia (D56.5)
sickle-cell trait (D57.3)

D56.4 Hereditary persistence of fetal hemoglobin [HPFH] [HCC]

D56.5 Hemoglobin E-beta thalassemia [HCC] [RxHCC]
[EXCLUDES1] *beta thalassemia (D56.1)*
beta thalassemia minor (D56.3)
beta thalassemia trait (D56.3)
delta-beta thalassemia (D56.2)
delta-beta thalassemia trait (D56.3)
hemoglobin E disease (D58.2)
other hemoglobinopathies (D58.2)
sickle-cell beta thalassemia (D57.4-)

D56.8 Other thalassemias [HCC]
Dominant thalassemia
Hemoglobin C thalassemia
Mixed thalassemia
Thalassemia with other hemoglobinopathy
[EXCLUDES1] *hemoglobin C disease (D58.2)*
hemoglobin E disease (D58.2)
other hemoglobinopathies (D58.2)
sickle-cell anemia (D57.-)
sickle-cell thalassemia (D57.4)

D56.9 Thalassemia, unspecified
Mediterranean anemia (with other hemoglobinopathy)

[4th] **D57 Sickle-cell disorders**
Use additional code for any associated fever (R50.81)
[EXCLUDES1] *other hemoglobinopathies (D58.-)*

[5th] **D57.0 Hb-SS disease with crisis**
Sickle-cell disease NOS with crisis
Hb-SS disease with vasoocclusive pain
D57.00 Hb-SS disease with crisis, unspecified [HCC] [RxHCC]
D57.01 Hb-SS disease with acute chest syndrome [HCC] [RxHCC]
D57.02 Hb-SS disease with splenic sequestration [HCC] [RxHCC]

D57.1 Sickle-cell disease without crisis [HCC] [RxHCC]
Hb-SS disease without crisis
Sickle-cell anemia NOS
Sickle-cell disease NOS
Sickle-cell disorder NOS

[5th] **D57.2 Sickle-cell/Hb-C disease**
Hb-SC disease
Hb-S/Hb-C disease
D57.20 Sickle-cell/Hb-C disease without crisis [HCC] [RxHCC]
[6th] **D57.21 Sickle-cell/Hb-C disease with crisis**
D57.211 Sickle-cell/Hb-C disease with acute chest syndrome [HCC] [RxHCC]
D57.212 Sickle-cell/Hb-C disease with splenic sequestration [HCC] [MCC] [RxHCC] [CC/MCC Exc]
D57.219 Sickle-cell/Hb-C disease with crisis, unspecified [HCC] [RxHCC]
Sickle-cell/Hb-C disease with crisis NOS

D57.3 Sickle-cell trait [HCC]
Hb-S trait
Heterozygous hemoglobin S

[5th] **D57.4 Sickle-cell thalassemia**
Sickle-cell beta thalassemia
Thalassemia Hb-S disease
D57.40 Sickle-cell thalassemia without crisis [HCC] [RxHCC]
Microdrepanocytosis
Sickle-cell thalassemia NOS
[6th] **D57.41 Sickle-cell thalassemia with crisis**
Sickle-cell thalassemia with vasoocclusive pain
D57.411 Sickle-cell thalassemia with acute chest syndrome [HCC] [RxHCC]
D57.412 Sickle-cell thalassemia with splenic sequestration [HCC] [MCC] [RxHCC] [CC/MCC Exc]
D57.419 Sickle-cell thalassemia with crisis, unspecified [HCC] [RxHCC]
Sickle-cell thalassemia with crisis NOS

[5th] **D57.8 Other sickle-cell disorders**
Hb-SD disease
Hb-SE disease
D57.80 Other sickle-cell disorders without crisis [HCC] [RxHCC]
[6th] **D57.81 Other sickle-cell disorders with crisis**
D57.811 Other sickle-cell disorders with acute chest syndrome [HCC] [RxHCC]
D57.812 Other sickle-cell disorders with splenic sequestration [HCC] [RxHCC]
D57.819 Other sickle-cell disorders with crisis, unspecified [HCC] [RxHCC]
Other sickle-cell disorders with crisis NOS

[4th] **D58 Other hereditary hemolytic anemias**
[EXCLUDES1] *hemolytic anemia of the newborn (P55.-)*

D58.0 Hereditary spherocytosis [HCC]
Acholuric (familial) jaundice
Congenital (spherocytic) hemolytic icterus
Minkowski-Chauffard syndrome

D58.1 Hereditary elliptocytosis [HCC]
Elliptocytosis (congenital)
Ovalocytosis (congenital) (hereditary)

D58.2 Other hemoglobinopathies [HCC]
Abnormal hemoglobin NOS
Congenital Heinz body anemia
Hb-C disease
Hb-D disease
Hb-E disease
Hemoglobinopathy NOS
Unstable hemoglobin hemolytic disease
[EXCLUDES1] *familial polycythemia (D75.0)*
Hb-M disease (D74.0)
hemoglobin E-beta thalassemia (D56.5)
hereditary persistence of fetal hemoglobin [HPFH] (D56.4)
high-altitude polycythemia (D75.1)
methemoglobinemia (D74.-)
other hemoglobinopathies with thalassemia (D56.8)

[PDx] Unacceptable principal diagnosis symbol per Medicare code edits [POA] Code exempt from diagnosis present on admission requirement
[?] Questionable admission [CC] Complication or comorbidity [MCC] Major complication or comorbidity [CC/MCC Exc] CC/MCC exclusion
[HCC] HCC diagnosis code [RxHCC] RxHCC diagnosis code MACRA code **DEFINITION** Describes condition/terminology
TIP Coding guidance 👁 Official Guideline Reference [Z-1] Z code as first-listed diagnosis

When symbols appear on a code that requires a 7th character extension, refer to Appendix B to identify applicable 7th character codes.

D58.8 Other specified hereditary hemolytic anemias   `HCC`
Stomatocytosis

D58.9 Hereditary hemolytic anemia, unspecified   `HCC`

4ᵗʰ **D59** Acquired hemolytic anemia

D59.0 Drug-induced autoimmune hemolytic anemia   `HCC` `RxHCC`
Use additional code for adverse effect, if applicable, to identify drug (T36-T50 with fifth or sixth character 5)

D59.1 Other autoimmune hemolytic anemias   `HCC` `RxHCC`
Autoimmune hemolytic disease (cold type) (warm type)
Chronic cold hemagglutinin disease
Cold agglutinin disease
Cold agglutinin hemoglobinuria
Cold type (secondary) (symptomatic) hemolytic anemia
Warm type (secondary) (symptomatic) hemolytic anemia
EXCLUDES1 Evans syndrome (D69.41)

hemolytic disease of newborn (P55.-)

paroxysmal cold hemoglobinuria (D59.6)

D59.2 Drug-induced nonautoimmune hemolytic anemia   `HCC` `RxHCC`
Drug-induced enzyme deficiency anemia
Use additional code for adverse effect, if applicable, to identify drug (T36-T50 with fifth or sixth character 5)

D59.3 Hemolytic-uremic syndrome   `HCC` `MCC` `RxHCC` `CC/MCC Exc`
Use additional code to identify associated:
E. coli infection (B96.2-)
Pneumococcal pneumonia (J13)
Shigella dysenteriae (A03.9)

D59.4 Other nonautoimmune hemolytic anemias   `CC` `HCC` `RxHCC` `CC/MCC Exc`
Mechanical hemolytic anemia
Microangiopathic hemolytic anemia
Toxic hemolytic anemia

D59.5 Paroxysmal nocturnal hemoglobinuria
[Marchiafava-Micheli]   `HCC` `RxHCC`
EXCLUDES1 hemoglobinuria NOS (R82.3)

D59.6 Hemoglobinuria due to hemolysis from other external causes   `HCC` `RxHCC`
Hemoglobinuria from exertion
March hemoglobinuria
Paroxysmal cold hemoglobinuria
Use additional code (Chapter 20) to identify external cause
EXCLUDES1 hemoglobinuria NOS (R82.3)

D59.8 Other acquired hemolytic anemias   `HCC` `RxHCC`

D59.9 Acquired hemolytic anemia, unspecified   `CC` `HCC` `RxHCC` `CC/MCC Exc`
Idiopathic hemolytic anemia, chronic

Aplastic and other anemias and other bone marrow failure syndromes (D60-D64)

4ᵗʰ **D60** Acquired pure red cell aplasia [erythroblastopenia]
INCLUDES red cell aplasia (acquired) (adult) (with thymoma)
EXCLUDES1 congenital red cell aplasia (D61.01)

D60.0 Chronic acquired pure red cell aplasia   `HCC` `MCC` `RxHCC` `CC/MCC Exc`

D60.1 Transient acquired pure red cell aplasia   `HCC` `MCC` `RxHCC` `CC/MCC Exc`

D60.8 Other acquired pure red cell aplasias   `HCC` `MCC` `RxHCC` `CC/MCC Exc`

D60.9 Acquired pure red cell aplasia, unspecified   `HCC` `MCC` `RxHCC` `CC/MCC Exc`

4ᵗʰ **D61** Other aplastic anemias and other bone marrow failure syndromes
EXCLUDES1 neutropenia (D70.-)

5ᵗʰ **D61.0** Constitutional aplastic anemia

D61.01 Constitutional (pure) red blood cell aplasia   `CC` `HCC` `RxHCC` `CC/MCC Exc`
Blackfan-Diamond syndrome
Congenital (pure) red cell aplasia
Familial hypoplastic anemia
Primary (pure) red cell aplasia
Red cell (pure) aplasia of infants
EXCLUDES1 acquired red cell aplasia (D60.9)

D61.09 Other constitutional aplastic anemia   `CC` `HCC` `RxHCC` `CC/MCC Exc`
Fanconi's anemia
Pancytopenia with malformations

D61.1 Drug-induced aplastic anemia   `HCC` `MCC` `RxHCC` `CC/MCC Exc`
Use additional code for adverse effect, if applicable, to identify drug (T36-T50 with fifth or sixth character 5)

D61.2 Aplastic anemia due to other external agents   `HCC` `MCC` `RxHCC` `CC/MCC Exc`
☞ Code first, if applicable, toxic effects of substances chiefly nonmedicinal as to source (T51-T65)

D61.3 Idiopathic aplastic anemia   `HCC` `MCC` `RxHCC` `CC/MCC Exc`

5ᵗʰ **D61.8** Other specified aplastic anemias and other bone marrow failure syndromes

6ᵗʰ **D61.81** Pancytopenia
EXCLUDES1 pancytopenia (due to) (with) aplastic anemia (D61.9)

pancytopenia (due to) (with) bone marrow infiltration (D61.82)

pancytopenia (due to) (with) congenital (pure) red cell aplasia (D61.01)

pancytopenia (due to) (with) hairy cell leukemia (C91.4-)

pancytopenia (due to) (with) human immunodeficiency virus disease (B20.-)

pancytopenia (due to) (with) leukoerythroblastic anemia (D61.82)

pancytopenia (due to) (with) myeloproliferative disease (D47.1)

EXCLUDES2 pancytopenia (due to) (with) myelodysplastic syndromes (D46.-)

D61.810 Antineoplastic chemotherapy induced pancytopenia   `CC` `HCC` `CC/MCC Exc`
EXCLUDES2 aplastic anemia due to antineoplastic chemotherapy (D61.1)

D61.811 Other drug-induced pancytopenia   `CC` `HCC` `CC/MCC Exc`
EXCLUDES2 aplastic anemia due to drugs (D61.1)

D61.818 Other pancytopenia   `CC` `HCC` `CC/MCC Exc`
AHA: Q1 2019

D61.82 Myelophthisis   `CC` `HCC` `RxHCC` `CC/MCC Exc`
Leukoerythroblastic anemia
Myelophthisic anemia
Panmyelophthisis
Code also the underlying disorder, such as:
malignant neoplasm of breast (C50.-)
tuberculosis (A15.-)
EXCLUDES1 idiopathic myelofibrosis (D47.1)

myelofibrosis NOS (D75.81)

myelofibrosis with myeloid metaplasia (D47.4)

primary myelofibrosis (D47.1)

secondary myelofibrosis (D75.81)

D61.89 Other specified aplastic anemias and other bone marrow failure syndromes   `HCC` `MCC` `RxHCC` `CC/MCC Exc`

D61.9 Aplastic anemia, unspecified   `HCC` `RxHCC`
Hypoplastic anemia NOS
Medullary hypoplasia

D62 Acute posthemorrhagic anemia
EXCLUDES1 anemia due to chronic blood loss (D50.0)

blood loss anemia NOS (D50.0)

congenital anemia from fetal blood loss (P61.3)

4ᵗʰ **D63** Anemia in chronic diseases classified elsewhere

D63.0 Anemia in neoplastic disease
⬭ See Official Guidelines "Anemia associated with malignancy" I.C.2. c.1, "Encounter for complication associated with a neoplasm" I.C.2.I.4
☞ Code first neoplasm (C00-D49)
EXCLUDES1 aplastic anemia due to antineoplastic chemotherapy (D61.1)

EXCLUDES2 anemia due to antineoplastic chemotherapy (D64.81)

Unspecified Code   Other Specified Code   Manifestation Code   Ⓝ Newborn   Ⓟ Pediatric   Ⓜ Maternity   Ⓐ Adult   ♂ Male   ♀ Female
● New Code   ▲ Revised Code Title   ▶◀ Revised Text   **NOTES**   *INCLUDES*   *EXCLUDES1* Not coded here   *EXCLUDES2* Not included here
4ᵗʰ 4ᵗʰ character required   5ᵗʰ 5ᵗʰ character required   6ᵗʰ 6ᵗʰ character required   7ᵗʰ 7ᵗʰ character required   7ᵗʰ Extension 'X' Alert
`HAC` Hospital-acquired condition (HAC) alert   **AHA** AHA Coding Clinic®   ☞ Code first alert

D63.1 **Anemia in chronic kidney disease**
Erythropoietin resistant anemia (EPO resistant anemia)
Code first underlying chronic kidney disease (CKD) (N18.-)

D63.8 **Anemia in other chronic diseases classified elsewhere**
Code first underlying disease, such as:
diphyllobothriasis (B70.0)
hookworm disease (B76.0-B76.9)
hypothyroidism (E00.0-E03.9)
malaria (B50.0-B54)
symptomatic late syphilis (A52.79)
tuberculosis (A18.89)

[4th] **D64 Other anemias**
[EXCLUDES1] *refractory anemia (D46.-)*
refractory anemia with excess blasts in transformation [RAEB T] (C92.0-)

D64.0 **Hereditary sideroblastic anemia** [HCC] [RxHCC]
Sex-linked hypochromic sideroblastic anemia

D64.1 **Secondary sideroblastic anemia due to disease** [HCC] [RxHCC]
Code first underlying disease

D64.2 **Secondary sideroblastic anemia due to drugs and toxins** [HCC] [RxHCC]
Code first poisoning due to drug or toxin, if applicable (T36-T65 with fifth or sixth character 1-4 or 6)
Use additional code for adverse effect, if applicable, to identify drug (T36-T50 with fifth or sixth character 5)

D64.3 **Other sideroblastic anemias** [HCC] [RxHCC]
Sideroblastic anemia NOS
Pyridoxine-responsive sideroblastic anemia NEC

D64.4 **Congenital dyserythropoietic anemia**
Dyshematopoietic anemia (congenital)
[EXCLUDES1] *Blackfan-Diamond syndrome (D61.01)*
Di Guglielmo's disease (C94.0)

[5th] D64.8 **Other specified anemias**

D64.81 **Anemia due to antineoplastic chemotherapy**
Antineoplastic chemotherapy induced anemia
[EXCLUDES1] *aplastic anemia due to antineoplastic chemotherapy (D61.1)*
[EXCLUDES2] *anemia in neoplastic disease (D63.0)*

D64.89 **Other specified anemias**
Infantile pseudoleukemia

D64.9 **Anemia, unspecified**
AHA: Q4 2018

Coagulation defects, purpura and other hemorrhagic conditions (D65-D69)

D65 Disseminated intravascular coagulation [defibrination syndrome] [HCC] [MCC] [CC/MCC Exc]
AHA: Q2 2019
Afibrinogenemia, acquired
Consumption coagulopathy
Diffuse or disseminated intravascular coagulation [DIC]
Fibrinolytic hemorrhage, acquired
Fibrinolytic purpura
Purpura fulminans
[EXCLUDES1] *disseminated intravascular coagulation (complicating):*
abortion or ectopic or molar pregnancy (O00-O07, O08.1)
in newborn (P60)
pregnancy, childbirth and the puerperium (O45.0, O46.0, O67.0, O72.3)

D66 Hereditary factor VIII deficiency [HCC] [MCC] [CC/MCC Exc]
Classical hemophilia
Deficiency factor VIII (with functional defect)
Hemophilia NOS
Hemophilia A
[EXCLUDES1] *factor VIII deficiency with vascular defect (D68.0)*

D67 Hereditary factor IX deficiency [HCC] [MCC] [CC/MCC Exc]
Christmas disease
Factor IX deficiency (with functional defect)
Hemophilia B
Plasma thromboplastin component [PTC] deficiency

[4th] **D68 Other coagulation defects**
[EXCLUDES1] *abnormal coagulation profile (R79.1)*
coagulation defects complicating abortion or ectopic or molar pregnancy (O00-O07, O08.1)
coagulation defects complicating pregnancy, childbirth and the puerperium (O45.0, O46.0, O67.0, O72.3)

D68.0 **Von Willebrand's disease** [CC] [HCC] [CC/MCC Exc]
Angiohemophilia
Factor VIII deficiency with vascular defect
Vascular hemophilia
[EXCLUDES1] *capillary fragility (hereditary) (D69.8)*
factor VIII deficiency NOS (D66)
factor VIII deficiency with functional defect (D66)

D68.1 **Hereditary factor XI deficiency** [CC] [HCC] [CC/MCC Exc]
Hemophilia C
Plasma thromboplastin antecedent [PTA] deficiency
Rosenthal's disease

D68.2 **Hereditary deficiency of other clotting factors** [CC] [HCC] [CC/MCC Exc]
AC globulin deficiency
Congenital afibrinogenemia
Deficiency of factor I [fibrinogen]
Deficiency of factor II [prothrombin]
Deficiency of factor V [labile]
Deficiency of factor VII [stable]
Deficiency of factor X [Stuart-Prower]
Deficiency of factor XII [Hageman]
Deficiency of factor XIII [fibrin stabilizing]
Dysfibrinogenemia (congenital)
Hypoproconvertinemia
Owren's disease
Proaccelerin deficiency

[5th] D68.3 **Hemorrhagic disorder due to circulating anticoagulants**

[6th] D68.31 **Hemorrhagic disorder due to intrinsic circulating anticoagulants, antibodies, or inhibitors**

D68.311 **Acquired hemophilia** [CC] [HCC] [CC/MCC Exc]
Autoimmune hemophilia
Autoimmune inhibitors to clotting factors
Secondary hemophilia

D68.312 **Antiphospholipid antibody with hemorrhagic disorder** [CC] [HCC] [CC/MCC Exc]
Lupus anticoagulant (LAC) with hemorrhagic disorder
Systemic lupus erythematosus [SLE] inhibitor with hemorrhagic disorder
[EXCLUDES1] *antiphospholipid antibody, finding without diagnosis (R76.0)*
antiphospholipid antibody syndrome (D68.61)
antiphospholipid antibody with hypercoagulable state (D68.61)
lupus anticoagulant (LAC) finding without diagnosis (R76.0)
lupus anticoagulant (LAC) with hypercoagulable state (D68.62)
systemic lupus erythematosus [SLE] inhibitor finding without diagnosis (R76.0)
systemic lupus erythematosus [SLE] inhibitor with hypercoagulable state (D68.62)

D68.318 **Other hemorrhagic disorder due to intrinsic circulating anticoagulants, antibodies, or inhibitors** [CC] [HCC] [CC/MCC Exc]
Antithromboplastinemia
Antithromboplastinogenemia
Hemorrhagic disorder due to intrinsic increase in antithrombin

[PDx] Unacceptable principal diagnosis symbol per Medicare code edits [POA] Code exempt from diagnosis present on admission requirement
[?] Questionable admission [CC] Complication or comorbidity [MCC] Major complication or comorbidity [CC/MCC Exc] CC/MCC exclusion
[HCC] HCC diagnosis code [RxHCC] RxHCC diagnosis code MACRA code **DEFINITION** Describes condition/terminology
TIP Coding guidance 👁 Official Guideline Reference [Z-1] Z code as first-listed diagnosis

Hemorrhagic disorder due to intrinsic
increase in anti-VIIIa
Hemorrhagic disorder due to intrinsic
increase in anti-IXa
Hemorrhagic disorder due to intrinsic
increase in anti-XIa

**D68.32 Hemorrhagic disorder due to extrinsic circulating
anticoagulants** `CC` `HCC` `CC/MCC Exc`
AHA: Q1 2016
Drug-induced hemorrhagic disorder
Hemorrhagic disorder due to increase in anti-IIa
Hemorrhagic disorder due to increase in anti-Xa
Hyperheparinemia
Use additional code for adverse effect, if applicable,
to identify drug (T45.515, T45.525)

D68.4 Acquired coagulation factor deficiency `CC` `HCC` `CC/MCC Exc`
Deficiency of coagulation factor due to liver disease
Deficiency of coagulation factor due to vitamin K deficiency
EXCLUDES1 *vitamin K deficiency of newborn (P53)*

5ᵗʰ **D68.5 Primary thrombophilia**
Primary hypercoagulable states
EXCLUDES1 *antiphospholipid syndrome (D68.61)*
lupus anticoagulant (D68.62)
secondary activated protein C resistance (D68.69)
*secondary antiphospholipid antibody syndrome
(D68.69)*
*secondary lupus anticoagulant with
hypercoagulable state (D68.69)*
*secondary systemic lupus erythematosus [SLE]
inhibitor with hypercoagulable state (D68.69)*
*systemic lupus erythematosus [SLE] inhibitor finding
without diagnosis (R76.0)*
*systemic lupus erythematosus [SLE] inhibitor with
hemorrhagic disorder (D68.312)*
thrombotic thrombocytopenic purpura (M31.1)

D68.51 Activated protein C resistance `HCC` `RxHCC`
Factor V Leiden mutation
D68.52 Prothrombin gene mutation `HCC` `RxHCC`
D68.59 Other primary thrombophilia `HCC` `RxHCC`
Antithrombin III deficiency
Hypercoagulable state NOS
Primary hypercoagulable state NEC
Primary thrombophilia NEC
Protein C deficiency
Protein S deficiency
Thrombophilia NOS

5ᵗʰ **D68.6 Other thrombophilia**
Other hypercoagulable states
EXCLUDES1 *diffuse or disseminated intravascular coagulation
[DIC] (D65)*
heparin induced thrombocytopenia (HIT) (D75.82)
hyperhomocysteinemia (E72.11)

D68.61 Antiphospholipid syndrome `HCC` `RxHCC`
Anticardiolipin syndrome
Antiphospholipid antibody syndrome
EXCLUDES1 *anti-phospholipid antibody, finding without
diagnosis (R76.0)*
*anti-phospholipid antibody with
hemorrhagic disorder (D68.312)*
lupus anticoagulant syndrome (D68.62)
D68.62 Lupus anticoagulant syndrome `HCC` `RxHCC`
Lupus anticoagulant
Presence of systemic lupus erythematosus [SLE]
inhibitor
EXCLUDES1 *anticardiolipin syndrome (D68.61)*
antiphospholipid syndrome (D68.61)
*lupus anticoagulant (LAC) finding without
diagnosis (R76.0)*
*lupus anticoagulant (LAC) with
hemorrhagic disorder (D68.312)*

D68.69 Other thrombophilia `HCC` `RxHCC`
Hypercoagulable states NEC
Secondary hypercoagulable state NOS
D68.8 Other specified coagulation defects `CC` `HCC` `CC/MCC Exc`
EXCLUDES1 *hemorrhagic disease of newborn (P53)*
D68.9 Coagulation defect, unspecified `CC` `HCC` `CC/MCC Exc`
4ᵗʰ **D69 Purpura and other hemorrhagic conditions**
EXCLUDES1 *benign hypergammaglobulinemic purpura (D89.0)*
cryoglobulinemic purpura (D89.1)
essential (hemorrhagic) thrombocythemia (D47.3)
hemorrhagic thrombocythemia (D47.3)
purpura fulminans (D65)
thrombotic thrombocytopenic purpura (M31.1)
Waldenström hypergammaglobulinemic purpura (D89.0)

D69.0 Allergic purpura `CC` `HCC` `CC/MCC Exc`
Allergic vasculitis
Nonthrombocytopenic hemorrhagic purpura
Nonthrombocytopenic idiopathic purpura
Purpura anaphylactoid
Purpura Henoch(-Schönlein)
Purpura rheumatica
Vascular purpura
EXCLUDES1 *thrombocytopenic hemorrhagic purpura (D69.3)*
D69.1 Qualitative platelet defects `CC` `HCC` `CC/MCC Exc`
Bernard-Soulier [giant platelet] syndrome
Glanzmann's disease
Grey platelet syndrome
Thromboasthenia (hemorrhagic) (hereditary)
Thrombocytopathy
EXCLUDES1 *von Willebrand's disease (D68.0)*
D69.2 Other nonthrombocytopenic purpura `HCC`
Purpura NOS
Purpura simplex
Senile purpura
D69.3 Immune thrombocytopenic purpura `CC` `HCC` `CC/MCC Exc`
Hemorrhagic (thrombocytopenic) purpura
Idiopathic thrombocytopenic purpura
Tidal platelet dysgenesis
5ᵗʰ **D69.4 Other primary thrombocytopenia**
EXCLUDES1 *transient neonatal thrombocytopenia (P61.0)*
Wiskott-Aldrich syndrome (D82.0)
D69.41 Evans syndrome `CC` `HCC` `CC/MCC Exc`
**D69.42 Congenital and hereditary thrombocytopenia
purpura** `CC` `HCC` `CC/MCC Exc`
Congenital thrombocytopenia
Hereditary thrombocytopenia
☞ **Code first** congenital or hereditary disorder, such as:
thrombocytopenia with absent radius (TAR
syndrome) (Q87.2)
D69.49 Other primary thrombocytopenia `HCC`
Megakaryocytic hypoplasia
Primary thrombocytopenia NOS
5ᵗʰ **D69.5 Secondary thrombocytopenia**
EXCLUDES1 *heparin induced thrombocytopenia (HIT) (D75.82)*
transient thrombocytopenia of newborn (P61.0)
D69.51 Posttransfusion purpura
Posttransfusion purpura from whole blood (fresh) or
blood products
PTP
D69.59 Other secondary thrombocytopenia
D69.6 Thrombocytopenia, unspecified `HCC`
D69.8 Other specified hemorrhagic conditions `HCC`
Capillary fragility (hereditary)
Vascular pseudohemophilia
D69.9 Hemorrhagic condition, unspecified `HCC`

Unspecified Code   Other Specified Code   Manifestation Code   **N** Newborn   **P** Pediatric   **M** Maternity   **A** Adult   ♂ Male   ♀ Female
● New Code   ▲ Revised Code Title   ►◄ Revised Text   **NOTES**   *INCLUDES*   *EXCLUDES1* Not coded here   *EXCLUDES2* Not included here
4ᵗʰ 4ᵗʰ character required   **5ᵗʰ** 5ᵗʰ character required   **6ᵗʰ** 6ᵗʰ character required   **7ᵗʰ** 7ᵗʰ character required   **⊗** Extension 'X' Alert
HAC Hospital-acquired condition (HAC) alert   **AHA** AHA Coding Clinic®   ☞ Code first alert

Other disorders of blood and blood-forming organs (D70-D77)

D70 Neutropenia

DEFINITION: Neutropenia is an abnormally low level of neutrophils, which are a common type of white blood cell important to fight infections.

INCLUDES agranulocytosis

decreased absolute neutrophil count (ANC)

Use additional code for any associated:

fever (R50.81)

mucositis (J34.81, K12.3-, K92.81, N76.81)

EXCLUDES1 neutropenic splenomegaly (D73.81)

transient neonatal neutropenia (P61.5)

D70.0 Congenital agranulocytosis cc⊘ HCC CC/MCC Exc⊘

Congenital neutropenia

Infantile genetic agranulocytosis

Kostmann's disease

D70.1 Agranulocytosis secondary to cancer chemotherapy cc⊘ HCC CC/MCC Exc⊘

Code also underlying neoplasm

Use additional code for adverse effect, if applicable, to identify drug (T45.1X5)

D70.2 Other drug-induced agranulocytosis cc⊘ HCC CC/MCC Exc⊘

Use additional code for adverse effect, if applicable, to identify drug (T36-T50 with fifth or sixth character 5)

D70.3 Neutropenia due to infection cc⊘ HCC CC/MCC Exc⊘

D70.4 Cyclic neutropenia cc⊘ HCC CC/MCC Exc⊘

Cyclic hematopoiesis

Periodic neutropenia

D70.8 Other neutropenia cc⊘ HCC CC/MCC Exc⊘

D70.9 Neutropenia, unspecified cc⊘ HCC CC/MCC Exc⊘

AHA: Q2 2019

D71 Functional disorders of polymorphonuclear neutrophils cc⊘ HCC CC/MCC Exc⊘

Cell membrane receptor complex [CR3] defect

Chronic (childhood) granulomatous disease

Congenital dysphagocytosis

Progressive septic granulomatosis

D72 Other disorders of white blood cells

EXCLUDES1 basophilia (D72.824)

immunity disorders (D80-D89)

neutropenia (D70)

preleukemia (syndrome) (D46.9)

D72.0 Genetic anomalies of leukocytes HCC

Alder (granulation) (granulocyte) anomaly

Alder syndrome

Hereditary leukocytic hypersegmentation

Hereditary leukocytic hyposegmentation

Hereditary leukomelanopathy

May-Hegglin (granulation) (granulocyte) anomaly

May-Hegglin syndrome

Pelger-Huët (granulation) (granulocyte) anomaly

Pelger-Huët syndrome

EXCLUDES1 Chédiak (-Steinbrinck)-Higashi syndrome (E70.330)

D72.1 Eosinophilia

Allergic eosinophilia

Hereditary eosinophilia

EXCLUDES1 Löffler's syndrome (J82)

pulmonary eosinophilia (J82)

D72.8 Other specified disorders of white blood cells

EXCLUDES1 leukemia (C91-C95)

D72.81 Decreased white blood cell count

EXCLUDES1 neutropenia (D70.-)

D72.810 Lymphocytopenia

Decreased lymphocytes

D72.818 Other decreased white blood cell count

Basophilic leukopenia

Eosinophilic leukopenia

Monocytopenia

Other decreased leukocytes

Plasmacytopenia

D72.819 Decreased white blood cell count, unspecified

Decreased leukocytes, unspecified

Leukocytopenia, unspecified

Leukopenia

EXCLUDES1 malignant leukopenia (D70.9)

D72.82 Elevated white blood cell count

EXCLUDES1 eosinophilia (D72.1)

D72.820 Lymphocytosis (symptomatic)

Elevated lymphocytes

D72.821 Monocytosis (symptomatic)

EXCLUDES1 infectious mononucleosis (B27.-)

D72.822 Plasmacytosis

D72.823 Leukemoid reaction

Basophilic leukemoid reaction

Leukemoid reaction NOS

Lymphocytic leukemoid reaction

Monocytic leukemoid reaction

Myelocytic leukemoid reaction

Neutrophilic leukemoid reaction

D72.824 Basophilia

D72.825 Bandemia

Bandemia without diagnosis of specific infection

EXCLUDES1 confirmed infection - code to infection

leukemia (C91.-, C92.-, C93.-, C94.-, C95.-)

D72.828 Other elevated white blood cell count

D72.829 Elevated white blood cell count, unspecified

Elevated leukocytes, unspecified

Leukocytosis, unspecified

D72.89 Other specified disorders of white blood cells

Abnormality of white blood cells NEC

D72.9 Disorder of white blood cells, unspecified

Abnormal leukocyte differential NOS

D73 Diseases of spleen

D73.0 Hyposplenism

Atrophy of spleen

EXCLUDES1 asplenia (congenital) (Q89.01)

postsurgical absence of spleen (Z90.81)

D73.1 Hypersplenism

EXCLUDES1 neutropenic splenomegaly (D73.81)

primary splenic neutropenia (D73.81)

splenitis, splenomegaly in late syphilis (A52.79)

splenitis, splenomegaly in tuberculosis (A18.85)

splenomegaly NOS (R16.1)

splenomegaly congenital (Q89.0)

D73.2 Chronic congestive splenomegaly

D73.3 Abscess of spleen

D73.4 Cyst of spleen

D73.5 Infarction of spleen

Splenic rupture, nontraumatic

Torsion of spleen

EXCLUDES1 rupture of spleen due to Plasmodium vivax malaria (B51.0)

traumatic rupture of spleen (S36.03-)

D73.8 Other diseases of spleen

D73.81 Neutropenic splenomegaly

Werner-Schultz disease

D73.89 Other diseases of spleen

Fibrosis of spleen NOS

Perisplenitis

Splenitis NOS

D73.9 Disease of spleen, unspecified

D74 Methemoglobinemia

DEFINITION: Methemoglobinemia is caused by elevated levels of methemoglobin, a protein in red blood cells (RBCs) that carries and distributes oxygen to the body

---

PDx⊘ Unacceptable principal diagnosis symbol per Medicare code edits   POA⊘ Code exempt from diagnosis present on admission requirement   ❓ Questionable admission   cc⊘ Complication or comorbidity   MCC⊘ Major complication or comorbidity   CC/MCC Exc⊘ CC/MCC exclusion   HCC HCC diagnosis code   RxHCC RxHCC diagnosis code   MACRA MACRA code   **DEFINITION** Describes condition/terminology   👁 Official Guideline Reference   Z1 Z code as first-listed diagnosis   **TIP** Coding guidance

D74.0 Congenital methemoglobinemia [CC] [CC/MCC Exc]
Congenital NADH-methemoglobin reductase deficiency
Hemoglobin-M [Hb-M] disease
Methemoglobinemia, hereditary

D74.8 Other methemoglobinemias [CC] [CC/MCC Exc]
Acquired methemoglobinemia (with sulfhemoglobinemia)
Toxic methemoglobinemia

D74.9 Methemoglobinemia, unspecified [CC] [CC/MCC Exc]

[4th] **D75 Other and unspecified diseases of blood and blood-forming organs**
[EXCLUDES2] *acute lymphadenitis (L04.-)*
chronic lymphadenitis (I88.1)
enlarged lymph nodes (R59.-)
hypergammaglobulinemia NOS (D89.2)
lymphadenitis NOS (I88.9)
mesenteric lymphadenitis (acute) (chronic) (I88.0)

D75.0 Familial erythrocytosis
Benign polycythemia
Familial polycythemia
[EXCLUDES1] *hereditary ovalocytosis (D58.1)*

D75.1 Secondary polycythemia
Acquired polycythemia
Emotional polycythemia
Erythrocytosis NOS
Hypoxemic polycythemia
Nephrogenous polycythemia
Polycythemia due to erythropoietin
Polycythemia due to fall in plasma volume
Polycythemia due to high altitude
Polycythemia due to stress
Polycythemia NOS
Relative polycythemia
[EXCLUDES1] *polycythemia neonatorum (P61.1)*
polycythemia vera (D45)

[5th] D75.8 Other specified diseases of blood and blood-forming organs

D75.81 Myelofibrosis [CC] [HCC] [RxHCC] [CC/MCC Exc]
Myelofibrosis NOS
Secondary myelofibrosis NOS
☛ **Code first** the underlying disorder, such as:
malignant neoplasm of breast (C50.-)
Use additional code, if applicable, for associated therapy-related myelodysplastic syndrome (D46.-)
Use additional code for adverse effect, if applicable, to identify drug (T45.1X5)
[EXCLUDES1] *acute myelofibrosis (C94.4-)*
idiopathic myelofibrosis (D47.1)
leukoerythroblastic anemia (D61.82)
myelofibrosis with myeloid metaplasia (D47.4)
myelophthisic anemia (D61.82)
myelophthisis (D61.82)
primary myelofibrosis (D47.1)

D75.82 Heparin induced thrombocytopenia (HIT) [CC] [HCC] [CC/MCC Exc]

D75.89 Other specified diseases of blood and blood-forming organs

D75.9 Disease of blood and blood-forming organs, unspecified

● D75.A Glucose-6-phosphate dehydrogenase (G6PD) deficiency without anemia
[EXCLUDES1] *glucose-6-phosphate dehydrogenase (G6PD) deficiency with anemia (D55.0)*

[4th] **D76 Other specified diseases with participation of lymphoreticular and reticulohistiocytic tissue**
[EXCLUDES1] *(Abt-) Letterer-Siwe disease (C96.0)*
eosinophilic granuloma (C96.6)
Hand-Schüller-Christian disease (C96.5)
histiocytic medullary reticulosis (C96.9)
histiocytic sarcoma (C96.A)
histiocytosis X, multifocal (C96.5)
histiocytosis X, unifocal (C96.6)
Langerhans-cell histiocytosis, multifocal (C96.5)
Langerhans-cell histiocytosis NOS (C96.6)
Langerhans-cell histiocytosis, unifocal (C96.6)
leukemic reticuloendotheliosis (C91.4-)
lipomelanotic reticulosis (I89.8)
malignant histiocytosis (C96.A)
malignant reticulosis (C86.0)
nonlipid reticuloendotheliosis (C96.0)

D76.1 Hemophagocytic lymphohistiocytosis [CC] [HCC] [CC/MCC Exc]
Familial hemophagocytic reticulosis
Histiocytoses of mononuclear phagocytes

D76.2 Hemophagocytic syndrome, infection-associated [CC] [HCC] [CC/MCC Exc]
Use additional code to identify infectious agent or disease.

D76.3 Other histiocytosis syndromes [CC] [HCC] [CC/MCC Exc]
Reticulohistiocytoma (giant-cell)
Sinus histiocytosis with massive lymphadenopathy
Xanthogranuloma

D77 Other disorders of blood and blood-forming organs in diseases classified elsewhere
☛ **Code first** underlying disease, such as:
amyloidosis (E85.-)
congenital early syphilis (A50.0)
echinococcosis (B67.0-B67.9)
malaria (B50.0-B54)
schistosomiasis [bilharziasis] (B65.0-B65.9)
vitamin C deficiency (E54)
[EXCLUDES1] *rupture of spleen due to Plasmodium vivax malaria (B51.0)*
splenitis, splenomegaly in late syphilis (A52.79)
splenitis, splenomegaly in tuberculosis (A18.85)

Intraoperative and postprocedural complications of the spleen (D78)

[4th] **D78 Intraoperative and postprocedural complications of the spleen**

[5th] D78.0 Intraoperative hemorrhage and hematoma of the spleen complicating a procedure
[EXCLUDES1] *intraoperative hemorrhage and hematoma of the spleen due to accidental puncture or laceration during a procedure (D78.1-)*

D78.01 Intraoperative hemorrhage and hematoma of the spleen complicating a procedure on the spleen [CC] [CC/MCC Exc]

D78.02 Intraoperative hemorrhage and hematoma of the spleen complicating other procedure [CC] [CC/MCC Exc]

[5th] D78.1 Accidental puncture and laceration of the spleen during a procedure

D78.11 Accidental puncture and laceration of the spleen during a procedure on the spleen [CC] [CC/MCC Exc]

D78.12 Accidental puncture and laceration of the spleen during other procedure [CC] [CC/MCC Exc]

[5th] D78.2 Postprocedural hemorrhage of the spleen following a procedure

D78.21 Postprocedural hemorrhage of the spleen following a procedure on the spleen [CC] [CC/MCC Exc]

D78.22 Postprocedural hemorrhage of the spleen following other procedure [CC] [CC/MCC Exc]

[5th] D78.3 Postprocedural hematoma and seroma of the spleen following a procedure

D78.31 Postprocedural hematoma of the spleen following a procedure on the spleen [CC] [CC/MCC Exc]

D78.32 Postprocedural hematoma of the spleen following other procedure [CC] [CC/MCC Exc]

D78.33 Postprocedural seroma of the spleen following a procedure on the spleen [CC] [CC/MCC Exc]

D78.34 Postprocedural seroma of the spleen following other procedure [CC] [CC/MCC Exc]

Unspecified Code | Other Specified Code | Manifestation Code | [N] Newborn | [P] Pediatric | [M] Maternity | [A] Adult | ♂ Male | ♀ Female
● New Code | ▲ Revised Code Title | ►◄ Revised Text | [NOTES] | INCLUDES | [EXCLUDES1] Not coded here | [EXCLUDES2] Not included here
[4th] 4th character required | [5th] 5th character required | [6th] 6th character required | [7th] 7th character required | [x7th] Extension 'X' Alert
[HAC] Hospital-acquired condition (HAC) alert | AHA AHA Coding Clinic© | ☛ Code first alert

D74.0 - D78.34
CHAPTER 3: DISEASES OF BLOOD/BLOOD-FORMING ORGANS & DISORDERS INVOLVING IMMUNE MECHANISM (D50-D89)

5ᵗʰ **D78.8 Other intraoperative and postprocedural complications of the spleen**
Use additional code, if applicable, to further specify disorder

D78.81 Other intraoperative complications of the spleen CC CC/MCC Exc

D78.89 Other postprocedural complications of the spleen CC CC/MCC Exc

Certain disorders involving the immune mechanism (D80-D89)

INCLUDES *defects in the complement system*

immunodeficiency disorders, except human immunodeficiency virus [HIV] disease

sarcoidosis

EXCLUDES1 *autoimmune disease (systemic) NOS (M35.9)*

functional disorders of polymorphonuclear neutrophils (D71)

human immunodeficiency virus [HIV] disease (B20)

4ᵗʰ **D80 Immunodeficiency with predominantly antibody defects**

D80.0 Hereditary hypogammaglobulinemia CC HCC RxHCC CC/MCC Exc
Autosomal recessive agammaglobulinemia (Swiss type)
X-linked agammaglobulinemia [Bruton] (with growth hormone deficiency)

D80.1 Nonfamilial hypogammaglobulinemia CC HCC RxHCC CC/MCC Exc
Agammaglobulinemia with immunoglobulin-bearing B-lymphocytes
Common variable agammaglobulinemia [CVAgamma]
Hypogammaglobulinemia NOS

D80.2 Selective deficiency of immunoglobulin A [IgA] CC HCC RxHCC CC/MCC Exc

D80.3 Selective deficiency of immunoglobulin G [IgG] subclasses CC HCC RxHCC CC/MCC Exc

D80.4 Selective deficiency of immunoglobulin M [IgM] CC HCC RxHCC CC/MCC Exc

D80.5 Immunodeficiency with increased immunoglobulin M [IgM] CC HCC RxHCC CC/MCC Exc

D80.6 Antibody deficiency with near-normal immunoglobulins or with hyperimmunoglobulinemia CC HCC RxHCC CC/MCC Exc

D80.7 Transient hypogammaglobulinemia of infancy CC HCC RxHCC CC/MCC Exc

D80.8 Other immunodeficiencies with predominantly antibody defects CC HCC RxHCC CC/MCC Exc
Kappa light chain deficiency

D80.9 Immunodeficiency with predominantly antibody defects, unspecified CC HCC RxHCC CC/MCC Exc

4ᵗʰ **D81 Combined immunodeficiencies**

EXCLUDES1 *autosomal recessive agammaglobulinemia (Swiss type) (D80.0)*

D81.0 Severe combined immunodeficiency [SCID] with reticular dysgenesis CC HCC RxHCC CC/MCC Exc

D81.1 Severe combined immunodeficiency [SCID] with low T- and B-cell numbers CC HCC RxHCC CC/MCC Exc

D81.2 Severe combined immunodeficiency [SCID] with low or normal B-cell numbers CC HCC RxHCC CC/MCC Exc

5ᵗʰ **D81.3 Adenosine deaminase [ADA] deficiency**

● **D81.30 Adenosine deaminase deficiency, unspecified** CC CC/MCC Exc
ADA deficiency NOS

● **D81.31 Severe combined immunodeficiency due to adenosine deaminase deficiency** CC CC/MCC Exc
ADA deficiency with SCID
Adenosine deaminase [ADA] deficiency with severe combined immunodeficiency

● **D81.32 Adenosine deaminase 2 deficiency** CC CC/MCC Exc
ADA2 deficiency
Adenosine deaminase deficiency type 2
Code also, if applicable, any associated manifestations, such as:
polyarteritis nodosa (M30.0)
stroke (I63.-)

● **D81.39 Other adenosine deaminase deficiency** CC CC/MCC Exc
Adenosine deaminase [ADA] deficiency type 1, NOS
Adenosine deaminase [ADA] deficiency type 1, without SCID
Adenosine deaminase [ADA] deficiency type 1, without severe combined immunodeficiency
Partial ADA deficiency (type 1)
Partial adenosine deaminase deficiency (type 1)

D81.4 Nezelof's syndrome CC HCC RxHCC CC/MCC Exc

D81.5 Purine nucleoside phosphorylase [PNP] deficiency CC HCC RxHCC

D81.6 Major histocompatibility complex class I deficiency CC HCC RxHCC CC/MCC Exc
Bare lymphocyte syndrome

D81.7 Major histocompatibility complex class II deficiency CC HCC RxHCC CC/MCC Exc

5ᵗʰ **D81.8 Other combined immunodeficiencies**

6ᵗʰ **D81.81 Biotin-dependent carboxylase deficiency**
Multiple carboxylase deficiency
EXCLUDES1 *biotin-dependent carboxylase deficiency due to dietary deficiency of biotin (E53.8)*

D81.810 Biotinidase deficiency

D81.818 Other biotin-dependent carboxylase deficiency
Holocarboxylase synthetase deficiency
Other multiple carboxylase deficiency

D81.819 Biotin-dependent carboxylase deficiency, unspecified
Multiple carboxylase deficiency, unspecified

D81.89 Other combined immunodeficiencies CC HCC RxHCC CC/MCC Exc

D81.9 Combined immunodeficiency, unspecified CC HCC RxHCC CC/MCC Exc
Severe combined immunodeficiency disorder [SCID] NOS

4ᵗʰ **D82 Immunodeficiency associated with other major defects**

EXCLUDES1 *ataxia telangiectasia [Louis-Bar] (G11.3)*

D82.0 Wiskott-Aldrich syndrome CC HCC RxHCC CC/MCC Exc
Immunodeficiency with thrombocytopenia and eczema

D82.1 Di George's syndrome CC HCC RxHCC CC/MCC Exc
Pharyngeal pouch syndrome
Thymic alymphoplasia
Thymic aplasia or hypoplasia with immunodeficiency

D82.2 Immunodeficiency with short-limbed stature HCC RxHCC

D82.3 Immunodeficiency following hereditary defective response to Epstein-Barr virus HCC RxHCC
X-linked lymphoproliferative disease

D82.4 Hyperimmunoglobulin E [IgE] syndrome HCC RxHCC

D82.8 Immunodeficiency associated with other specified major defects HCC RxHCC

D82.9 Immunodeficiency associated with major defect, unspecified HCC RxHCC

4ᵗʰ **D83 Common variable immunodeficiency**

D83.0 Common variable immunodeficiency with predominant abnormalities of B-cell numbers and function CC HCC RxHCC CC/MCC Exc

D83.1 Common variable immunodeficiency with predominant immunoregulatory T-cell disorders CC HCC RxHCC CC/MCC Exc

D83.2 Common variable immunodeficiency with autoantibodies to B- or T-cells CC HCC RxHCC CC/MCC Exc

D83.8 Other common variable immunodeficiencies CC HCC RxHCC CC/MCC Exc

D83.9 Common variable immunodeficiency, unspecified CC HCC RxHCC CC/MCC Exc

4ᵗʰ **D84 Other immunodeficiencies**

D84.0 Lymphocyte function antigen-1 [LFA-1] defect HCC RxHCC

D84.1 Defects in the complement system HCC RxHCC
C1 esterase inhibitor [C1-INH] deficiency

D84.8 Other specified immunodeficiencies CC HCC RxHCC CC/MCC Exc

D84.9 Immunodeficiency, unspecified CC HCC RxHCC CC/MCC Exc

4ᵗʰ **D86 Sarcoidosis**

DEFINITION: Sarcoidosis is a rare condition in which immune cells form granulomas (lumps) in the bodies organs, but most often in the lungs and lymph nodes of the chest.

D86.0 Sarcoidosis of lung HCC

D86.1 Sarcoidosis of lymph nodes

D86.2 Sarcoidosis of lung with sarcoidosis of lymph nodes HCC

POꜞ Unacceptable principal diagnosis symbol per Medicare code edits   POꜞ Code exempt from diagnosis present on admission requirement
❓ Questionable admission   CC Complication or comorbidity   MCC Major complication or comorbidity   CC/MCC Exc CC/MCC exclusion
HCC HCC diagnosis code   RxHCC RxHCC diagnosis code   MACRA code   **DEFINITION** Describes condition/terminology
TIP Coding guidance   👁 Official Guideline Reference   Z1 Z code as first-listed diagnosis

D86.3 **Sarcoidosis of** skin
🔵 D86.8 **Sarcoidosis of** other sites
    D86.81 **Sarcoid** meningitis
    D86.82 Multiple cranial nerve palsies **in sarcoidosis**   `HCC` `RxHCC`
    D86.83 **Sarcoid** iridocyclitis
    D86.84 **Sarcoid** pyelonephritis
        Tubulo-interstitial nephropathy in sarcoidosis
    D86.85 **Sarcoid** myocarditis
    D86.86 **Sarcoid** arthropathy
        Polyarthritis in sarcoidosis
    D86.87 **Sarcoid** myositis
    D86.89 **Sarcoidosis of other sites**
        Hepatic granuloma
        Uveoparotid fever [Heerfordt]
D86.9 **Sarcoidosis, unspecified**
🔵 D89 **Other disorders involving the immune mechanism, not elsewhere classified**
    EXCLUDES1   *hyperglobulinemia NOS (R77.1)*
              monoclonal gammopathy (of undetermined significance) (D47.2)
    EXCLUDES2   *transplant failure and rejection (T86.-)*
D89.0 **Polyclonal hypergammaglobulinemia**
    Benign hypergammaglobulinemic purpura
    Polyclonal gammopathy NOS
D89.1 **Cryoglobulinemia**   `HCC`
    Cryoglobulinemic purpura
    Cryoglobulinemic vasculitis
    Essential cryoglobulinemia
    Idiopathic cryoglobulinemia
    Mixed cryoglobulinemia
    Primary cryoglobulinemia
    Secondary cryoglobulinemia
D89.2 **Hypergammaglobulinemia, unspecified**
D89.3 **Immune reconstitution syndrome**   `HCC` `RxHCC`
    Immune reconstitution inflammatory syndrome [IRIS]
    Use additional code for adverse effect, if applicable, to identify drug (T36-T50 with fifth or sixth character 5)
🔵 D89.4 **Mast cell activation syndrome and related disorders**
    EXCLUDES1   *aggressive systemic mastocytosis (C96.21)*
              congenital cutaneous mastocytosis (Q82.2)
              (non-congenital) cutaneous mastocytosis (D47.01)
              (indolent) systemic mastocytosis (D47.02)
              malignant mast cell neoplasm (C96.2-)
              malignant mastocytoma (C96.29)
              mast cell leukemia (C94.3-)
              mast cell sarcoma (C96.22)
              mastocytoma NOS (D47.09)
              other mast cell neoplasms of uncertain behavior (D47.09)
              systemic mastocytosis associated with a clonal hematologic non-mast cell lineage disease (SM-AHNMD) (D47.02)
    D89.40 **Mast cell activation, unspecified**   `HCC` `RxHCC`
        AHA: Q4 2016
        Mast cell activation disorder, unspecified
        Mast cell activation syndrome, NOS
    D89.41 Monoclonal **mast cell activation syndrome**   `HCC` `RxHCC`
        AHA: Q4 2016
    D89.42 Idiopathic **mast cell activation syndrome**   `HCC` `RxHCC`
        AHA: Q4 2016
    D89.43 Secondary **mast cell activation**   `HCC` `RxHCC`
        AHA: Q4 2016
        Secondary mast cell activation syndrome
        Code also underlying etiology, if known
    D89.49 Other **mast cell activation disorder**   `HCC` `RxHCC`
        AHA: Q4 2016
        Other mast cell activation syndrome

🔵 D89.8 **Other specified disorders involving the immune mechanism, not elsewhere classified**
    🔵 D89.81 **Graft-versus-host disease**
        ☞ **Code first** underlying cause, such as:
            complications of transplanted organs and tissue (T86.-)
            complications of blood transfusion (T80.89)
        Use additional code to identify associated manifestations, such as:
            desquamative dermatitis (L30.8)
            diarrhea (R19.7)
            elevated bilirubin (R17)
            hair loss (L65.9)
        D89.810 Acute **graft-versus-host disease**   `cc` `HCC` `RxHCC` `PDxn` `CC/MCC Exc`
        D89.811 Chronic **graft-versus-host disease**   `cc` `HCC` `RxHCC` `PDxn` `CC/MCC Exc`
        D89.812 Acute on chronic **graft-versus-host disease**   `cc` `HCC` `RxHCC` `PDxn` `CC/MCC Exc`
        D89.813 **Graft-versus-host disease, unspecified**   `cc` `HCC` `RxHCC` `PDxn` `CC/MCC Exc`
    D89.82 **Autoimmune lymphoproliferative syndrome [ALPS]**   `HCC` `RxHCC`
    D89.89 **Other specified disorders involving the immune mechanism, not elsewhere classified**   `HCC` `RxHCC`
        EXCLUDES1   *human immunodeficiency virus disease (B20)*
D89.9 **Disorder involving the immune mechanism, unspecified**   `HCC` `RxHCC`
    AHA: Q3 2015
    Immune disease NOS

Unspecified Code   Other Specified Code   Manifestation Code   ℕ Newborn   ℙ Pediatric   𝕄 Maternity   𝔸 Adult   ♂ Male   ♀ Female

● New Code   ▲ Revised Code Title   ►◄ Revised Text   **NOTES**   *INCLUDES*   *EXCLUDES1* Not coded here   *EXCLUDES2* Not included here

🔵 4th character required   🔵 5th character required   🔵 6th character required   🔵 7th character required   🔵 Extension 'X' Alert

`HAC` Hospital-acquired condition (HAC) alert   **AHA** AHA Coding Clinic©   ☞ Code first alert

2020 ICD-10-CM   When symbols appear on a code that requires a 7th character extension, refer to Appendix B to identify applicable 7th character codes.   **515**

NOTES

Chapter 4: Endocrine, Nutritional and Metabolic Diseases (E00-E89)

Anatomy of the Endocrine System

Introduction

The endocrine system is a series of ductless glands that secrete hormones directly into the blood. These hormones target specific organs and help the body to maintain homeostasis.

1. An Outline of the Endocrine System

a) The endocrine system (Figure 4.a) is primarily responsible for maintaining the body's homeostasis through various hormones.

b) The endocrine system is based on the ductless endocrine glands that secrete their hormones directly into the blood stream. These hormones are further carried to the target organs through the blood stream.

c) The pituitary gland (or hypophysis) is regarded as the master gland of the endocrine system. This gland is monitored and controlled by the hypothalamus of the brain.

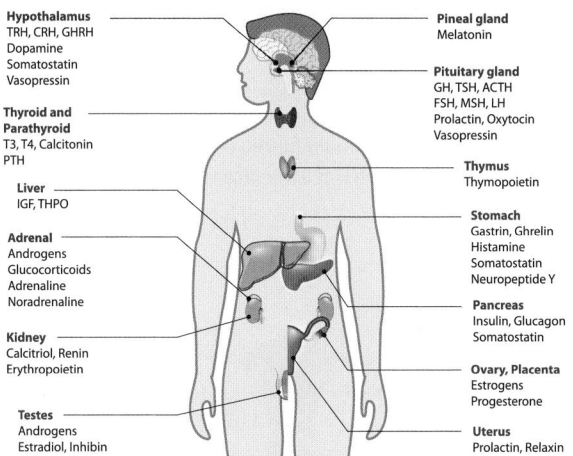

Figure 4.a Endocrine System Anatomy and Hormones

2. The Endocrine Hormones

a) The names of various endocrine hormones of the body are as follows:

   i) epinephrine
   ii) norepinephrine
   iii) oxytocin
   iv) vasopressin
   v) insulin
   vi) growth hormone
   vii) cortisol
   viii) estrogen
   ix) testosterone

b) The hormones monitor and control the processes of cellular respiration, growth, reproduction and electrolyte balances of the body. They also regulate the reproductive cycles, growth and the secretion of other hormones.

3. The Hypothalamus (of the Brain)

a) The hypothalamus controls the secretions of the pituitary gland.

b) The hypothalamus controls and monitors the secretions of the endocrine system.

c) The endocrine system can influence the functions of the hypothalamus via negative feedback mechanisms.

4. The Major Endocrine Glands

a) The names of the major endocrine glands are as follows:

   i) anterior pituitary gland
   ii) posterior pituitary gland
   iii) pineal gland
   iv) thyroid gland
   v) parathyroid gland
   vi) thymus

   vii) adrenal gland
   viii) pancreatic islets
   ix) ovaries
   x) testes

5. The Anatomy of the Anterior Pituitary Gland

The anterior pituitary gland is constituted by the glandular epithelium and generates the following hormones, which are listed below:

a) **Growth Hormone**

   The growth hormone stimulates cell metabolism and growth of bones and muscles.

b) **Thyroid Stimulating Hormone (TSH)**

   The TSH stimulates the thyroid gland for the production of T3, T4 and calcitonin hormones.

c) **Adrenocorticotropic Hormone (ACTH)**

   The ACTH stimulates the adrenal cortex for the secretion of the hormone cortisol.

d) **Melanocyte Stimulating Hormone (MSH)**

   The MSH stimulates melanocytes for the production of melanin, which causes darkening of the skin.

e) **Luteinizing Hormone (LH)**

   The LH stimulates the production of testosterone in males and progesterone in females.

f) **Prolactin**

   The Prolactin provides stimulation for milk production in the mammary glands of female after child birth.

6. The Anatomy of the Posterior Pituitary Gland

The posterior pituitary gland is also known as neurohypophysis. It is made up of the posterior lobe of the pituitary gland. The hormones of the posterior pituitary gland are listed below:

a) **Antidiuretic Hormone (ADH)/Vasopressin**

   Function of vasopressin is to enhance water re-absorption in the kidney tubules. Deficiency of vasopressin can cause Diabetes insipidus.

b) **Oxytocin**

   Oxytocin facilitates childbirth by causing the contraction of uterine smooth muscles. It also facilitates lactation by causing constriction of the mammary glands during breastfeeding.

7. The Anatomy of the Thyroid Gland

a) The thyroid gland is located below the thyroid cartilage in the neck region. It is one of the largest endocrine glands in the body.

b) The overactive thyroid gland causes excessive secretion of thyroid hormone or hyperthyroidism.

c) The underactive thyroid gland causes a condition of lack of thyroid hormone, which is known as the hypothyroidism.

d) The hormone calcitonin is secreted by the extrafollicular cells of the thyroid gland. It causes an increased excretion of the calcium and phosphate ions via the kidneys.

8. The Anatomy of the Parathyroid Glands

a) The parathyroid glands are four in number and remain embedded in the posterior surface of the thyroid gland in the neck region. These glands secrete parathyroid hormone or parathormone (PTH).

b) PTH stimulates the bone cells to release calcium and phosphate into the blood stream.

c) A deficiency of PTH causes hypoparathyroidism.

d) The high levels of PTH can result in the condition of hyperparathyroidism.

9. The Anatomy of Adrenal Glands

a) The adrenal (or suprarenal) glands are located on top of each kidney.

b) The adrenal gland is divided into the following components:

   i) adrenal medulla (or the inner portion)
   ii) adrenal cortex (or the outer portion)

c) The hormones epinephrine (or adrenalin) and norepinephrine (or noradrenalin) are produced by the adrenal medulla.

d) The adrenal cortex is divided into the following three layers:

   i) outer layer of adrenal cortex secretes aldosterone, which is a mineralocorticoid hormone and regulates sodium reabsorption and potassium excretion by the kidney.

   ii) hormone cortisol (or hydrocortisone) is secreted by the middle layer of adrenal cortex. It stimulates the liver to manufacture glucose from the circulating amino acids. The cortisol also possesses anti-inflammatory properties.

   iii) adrenal male sex hormones (or androgens) are produced by the inner layer of the adrenal cortex. These hormones enhance the male sex characteristics. The androgens are also the precursors of all estrogens (or the female sex hormones) and stimulate the female sex drive. Testosterone is the primary and most well-known androgen.

e) A deficit of adrenal cortex hormones causes Addison's disease.

f) An increased secretion of adrenal cortex causes Cushing's syndrome.

10. The Anatomy of the Pancreas

a) The pancreas is a glandular organ of both digestive and endocrine systems.

b) The islets of Langerhans of pancreas constitute its endocrine portion, and produce insulin and glucagon hormones for the regulation of blood glucose levels.

c) The blood glucose concentration is regulated by the negative feedback mechanism.

d) The clinical abnormality of diabetes mellitus is caused by the insufficient production of insulin.

11. The Anatomy of the Testes and Ovaries

a) Each of the two testes is the component of the reproductive and endocrine systems and produces the male sex hormone, testosterone.

b) Testosterone is responsible for the development of secondary male sex characteristics, which include facial and chest hairs, narrow hips, broad shoulders and deep voice.

c) Each of the two ovaries is an ovum-producing reproductive organ and secretes estrogen and progesterone, which are the female sex hormones.

d) Estrogen and progesterone are responsible for the development of the female reproductive organs and the development of secondary female sex characteristics, which include the fat deposition on thighs, hips and legs, high-pitched voice, broad hips and breast enlargement.

12. The Anatomy of the Thymus Gland

a) The thymus gland is regarded as a specialized organ of the immune system that produces the hormone thymosin.

b) Thymosin stimulates the production of the T-lymphocyte white blood cells (or T cells) that are critical cells of the adaptive immune system and protect the body against the invasion of foreign microbes.

13. The Anatomy of the Pineal Gland

a) The pineal gland is also known as the pineal body, epiphysis cerebri or epiphysis. It is a small endocrine gland located near the thalamus inside the human brain.

b) The pineal gland secretes the following hormones:

   i) melatonin, which regulates the body rhythms (wake and sleep patterns) and inhibits the functions of the reproductive system.

   ii) serotonin, which acts as a neurotransmitter and vasoconstrictor.

Common Pathologies

Adrenal Insufficiency
This is a condition in which the production of steroid hormones such as cortisol and aldosterone becomes low. Symptoms include fatigue, stomach upset, dehydration, and skin changes. Addison's disease is a type of adrenal insufficiency.

Cushing's Syndrome
This is a condition in which overproduction of a pituitary gland hormone (ACTH) leads to an overactive adrenal gland. A similar condition called Cushing's disease may occur in people, particularly children, who take high doses of corticosteroid medications.

Gigantism (acromegaly) and other growth hormone problems
This is a condition in which, if the pituitary gland produces too much growth hormone, a child's bones and body parts may grow abnormally fast. If growth hormone levels are too low, a child can stop growing in height.

Hyperthyroidism
This is a condition in which the thyroid gland produces too much thyroid hormone, leading to weight loss, fast heart rate, sweating, and nervousness. The most common cause for an overactive thyroid is an autoimmune disorder called Grave's disease.

Hypothyroidism
This is a condition in which, the thyroid gland does not produce enough thyroid hormone, leading to fatigue, constipation, dry skin, and depression. The underactive gland can cause slowed development in children. Some types of hypothyroidism are present at birth.

Hypopituitarism
This is a condition in which the pituitary gland releases little or no hormones. It may be caused by a number of different diseases. Women with this condition may stop getting their periods.

Polycystic Ovary Syndrome (PCOS) (Figure 4.b)
This is a condition in which overproduction of androgens interfere with the development of eggs and their release from the female ovaries. PCOS is a leading cause of infertility.

Precocious Puberty
This is a condition in which abnormally early puberty occurs when glands tell the body to release sex hormones too soon in life.

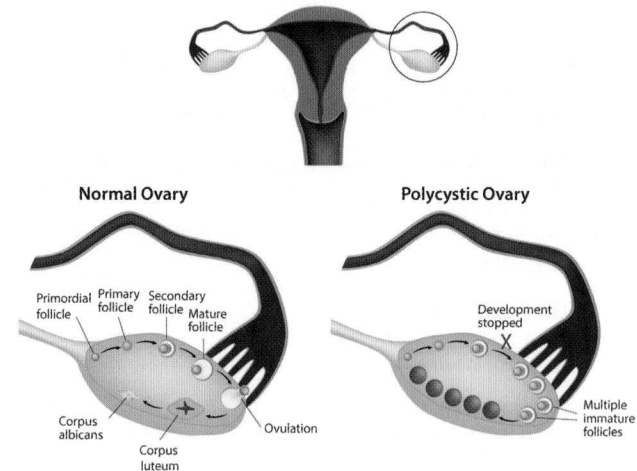

Figure 4.b Polycystic Ovary Syndrome (PCOS)

Endocrine, nutritional and metabolic diseases (E00-E89)

NOTES All neoplasms, whether functionally active or not, are classified in Chapter 2. Appropriate codes in this chapter (i.e. E05.8, E07.0, E16-E31, E34.-) may be used as additional codes to indicate either functional activity by neoplasms and ectopic endocrine tissue or hyperfunction and hypofunction of endocrine glands associated with neoplasms and other conditions classified elsewhere.

EXCLUDES1 transitory endocrine and metabolic disorders specific to newborn (P70-P74)

This chapter contains the following blocks:

E00-E07   Disorders of thyroid gland
E08-E13   Diabetes mellitus
E15-E16   Other disorders of glucose regulation and pancreatic internal secretion
E20-E35   Disorders of other endocrine glands
E36   Intraoperative complications of endocrine system
E40-E46   Malnutrition
E50-E64   Other nutritional deficiencies
E65-E68   Overweight, obesity and other hyperalimentation
E70-E88   Metabolic disorders
E89   Postprocedural endocrine and metabolic complications and disorders, not elsewhere classified

Disorders of thyroid gland (E00-E07)

④ E00 Congenital iodine-deficiency syndrome
   Use additional code (F70-F79) to identify associated intellectual disabilities.
   EXCLUDES1 subclinical iodine-deficiency hypothyroidism (E02)
   E00.0 **Congenital iodine-deficiency syndrome, neurological type** `RxHCC`
         Endemic cretinism, neurological type
   E00.1 **Congenital iodine-deficiency syndrome, myxedematous type** `RxHCC`
         Endemic hypothyroid cretinism
         Endemic cretinism, myxedematous type
   E00.2 **Congenital iodine-deficiency syndrome, mixed type** `RxHCC`
         Endemic cretinism, mixed type
   E00.9 **Congenital iodine-deficiency syndrome, unspecified** `RxHCC`
         Congenital iodine-deficiency hypothyroidism NOS
         Endemic cretinism NOS

④ E01 Iodine-deficiency related thyroid disorders and allied conditions
   EXCLUDES1 congenital iodine-deficiency syndrome (E00.-)
               subclinical iodine-deficiency hypothyroidism (E02)
   E01.0 **Iodine-deficiency related diffuse (endemic) goiter** `RxHCC`
   E01.1 **Iodine-deficiency related multinodular (endemic) goiter** `RxHCC`
         Iodine-deficiency related nodular goiter
   E01.2 **Iodine-deficiency related (endemic) goiter, unspecified** `RxHCC`
         Endemic goiter NOS
   E01.8 **Other iodine-deficiency related thyroid disorders and allied conditions** `RxHCC`
         Acquired iodine-deficiency hypothyroidism NOS
   E02   **Subclinical iodine-deficiency hypothyroidism** `RxHCC`

④ E03 Other hypothyroidism
   EXCLUDES1 iodine-deficiency related hypothyroidism (E00-E02)
               postprocedural hypothyroidism (E89.0)
   E03.0 **Congenital hypothyroidism with diffuse goiter** `RxHCC`
         Congenital parenchymatous goiter (nontoxic)
         Congenital goiter (nontoxic) NOS
         EXCLUDES1 transitory congenital goiter with normal function (P72.0)
   E03.1 **Congenital hypothyroidism without goiter** `RxHCC`
         Aplasia of thyroid (with myxedema)
         Congenital atrophy of thyroid
         Congenital hypothyroidism NOS
   E03.2 **Hypothyroidism due to medicaments and other exogenous substances** `RxHCC`
         ☛ **Code first** poisoning due to drug or toxin, if applicable (T36-T65 with fifth or sixth character 1-4 or 6)

Use additional code for adverse effect, if applicable, to identify drug (T36-T50 with fifth or sixth character 5)
   E03.3 **Postinfectious hypothyroidism** `RxHCC`
   E03.4 **Atrophy of thyroid (acquired)** `RxHCC`
         EXCLUDES1 congenital atrophy of thyroid (E03.1)
   E03.5 **Myxedema coma** `HCC` `MCC` `RxHCC` `CC/MCC Exc`
   E03.8 **Other specified hypothyroidism** `RxHCC`
   E03.9 **Hypothyroidism, unspecified** `RxHCC`
         Myxedema NOS

④ E04 Other nontoxic goiter
   EXCLUDES1 congenital goiter (NOS) (diffuse) (parenchymatous) (E03.0)
               iodine-deficiency related goiter (E00-E02)
   E04.0 **Nontoxic diffuse goiter** `RxHCC`
         Diffuse (colloid) nontoxic goiter
         Simple nontoxic goiter
   E04.1 **Nontoxic single thyroid nodule** `RxHCC`
         Colloid nodule (cystic) (thyroid)
         Nontoxic uninodular goiter
         Thyroid (cystic) nodule NOS
   E04.2 **Nontoxic multinodular goiter** `RxHCC`
         Cystic goiter NOS
         Multinodular (cystic) goiter NOS
   E04.8 **Other specified nontoxic goiter** `RxHCC`
   E04.9 **Nontoxic goiter, unspecified** `RxHCC`
         Goiter NOS
         Nodular goiter (nontoxic) NOS

④ E05 Thyrotoxicosis [hyperthyroidism]
   EXCLUDES1 chronic thyroiditis with transient thyrotoxicosis (E06.2)
               neonatal thyrotoxicosis (P72.1)
   ⑤ E05.0 Thyrotoxicosis with diffuse goiter
         Exophthalmic or toxic goiter NOS
         Graves' disease
         Toxic diffuse goiter
         E05.00 **Thyrotoxicosis with diffuse goiter without thyrotoxic crisis or storm** `RxHCC`
         E05.01 **Thyrotoxicosis with diffuse goiter with thyrotoxic crisis or storm** `MCC` `RxHCC` `CC/MCC Exc`
   ⑤ E05.1 Thyrotoxicosis with toxic single thyroid nodule
         Thyrotoxicosis with toxic uninodular goiter
         E05.10 **Thyrotoxicosis with toxic single thyroid nodule without thyrotoxic crisis or storm** `RxHCC`
         E05.11 **Thyrotoxicosis with toxic single thyroid nodule with thyrotoxic crisis or storm** `MCC` `RxHCC` `CC/MCC Exc`
   ⑤ E05.2 Thyrotoxicosis with toxic multinodular goiter
         Toxic nodular goiter NOS
         E05.20 **Thyrotoxicosis with toxic multinodular goiter without thyrotoxic crisis or storm** `RxHCC`
         E05.21 **Thyrotoxicosis with toxic multinodular goiter with thyrotoxic crisis or storm** `MCC` `RxHCC` `CC/MCC Exc`
   ⑤ E05.3 Thyrotoxicosis from ectopic thyroid tissue
         E05.30 **Thyrotoxicosis from ectopic thyroid tissue without thyrotoxic crisis or storm** `RxHCC`
         E05.31 **Thyrotoxicosis from ectopic thyroid tissue with thyrotoxic crisis or storm** `MCC` `RxHCC` `CC/MCC Exc`
   ⑤ E05.4 Thyrotoxicosis factitia
         E05.40 **Thyrotoxicosis factitia without thyrotoxic crisis or storm** `RxHCC`
         E05.41 **Thyrotoxicosis factitia with thyrotoxic crisis or storm** `MCC` `RxHCC` `CC/MCC Exc`
   ⑤ E05.8 Other thyrotoxicosis
         Overproduction of thyroid-stimulating hormone
         E05.80 **Other thyrotoxicosis without thyrotoxic crisis or storm** `RxHCC`
         E05.81 **Other thyrotoxicosis with thyrotoxic crisis or storm** `MCC` `RxHCC` `CC/MCC Exc`
   ⑤ E05.9 Thyrotoxicosis, unspecified
         Hyperthyroidism NOS
         E05.90 **Thyrotoxicosis, unspecified without thyrotoxic crisis or storm** `RxHCC`
         E05.91 **Thyrotoxicosis, unspecified with thyrotoxic crisis or storm** `MCC` `RxHCC` `CC/MCC Exc`

Unspecified Code   Other Specified Code   Manifestation Code   Ⓝ Newborn   Ⓟ Pediatric   Ⓜ Maternity   Ⓐ Adult   ♂ Male   ♀ Female
● New Code   ▲ Revised Code Title   ►◄ Revised Text   **NOTES**   *INCLUDES*   *EXCLUDES1* Not coded here   *EXCLUDES2* Not included here
④ 4th character required   ⑤ 5th character required   ⑥ 6th character required   ⑦ 7th character required   Ⓧ Extension 'X' Alert
HAC Hospital-acquired condition (HAC) alert   **AHA** AHA Coding Clinic©   ☛ Code first alert

E06   **Thyroiditis**
> *EXCLUDES1*   *postpartum thyroiditis (O90.5)*

   E06.0   Acute **thyroiditis**   `CC` `RxHCC` `CC/MCC Exc`
     Abscess of thyroid
     Pyogenic thyroiditis
     Suppurative thyroiditis
     Use additional code (B95-B97) to identify infectious agent.

   E06.1   Subacute **thyroiditis**   `RxHCC`
     de Quervain thyroiditis
     Giant-cell thyroiditis
     Granulomatous thyroiditis
     Nonsuppurative thyroiditis
     Viral thyroiditis
> *EXCLUDES1*   *autoimmune thyroiditis (E06.3)*

   E06.2   Chronic **thyroiditis** with transient thyrotoxicosis   `RxHCC`
> *EXCLUDES1*   *autoimmune thyroiditis (E06.3)*

   E06.3   Autoimmune **thyroiditis**   `RxHCC`
     Hashimoto's thyroiditis
     Hashitoxicosis (transient)
     Lymphadenoid goiter
     Lymphocytic thyroiditis
     Struma lymphomatosa

   E06.4   Drug-induced **thyroiditis**   `RxHCC`
     Use additional code for adverse effect, if applicable, to identify
       drug (T36-T50 with fifth or sixth character 5)

   E06.5   **Other chronic thyroiditis**   `RxHCC`
     Chronic fibrous thyroiditis
     Chronic thyroiditis NOS
     Ligneous thyroiditis
     Riedel thyroiditis

   E06.9   **Thyroiditis, unspecified**   `RxHCC`

E07   **Other disorders of thyroid**

   E07.0   **Hypersecretion of calcitonin**   `RxHCC`
     C-cell hyperplasia of thyroid
     Hypersecretion of thyrocalcitonin

   E07.1   **Dyshormonogenetic goiter**   `RxHCC`
     Familial dyshormogenetic goiter
     Pendred's syndrome
> *EXCLUDES1*   *transitory congenital goiter with normal function*
>   *(P72.0)*

   E07.8   **Other specified disorders of thyroid**
     E07.81   **Sick-euthyroid syndrome**   `CC` `CC/MCC Exc`
       Euthyroid sick-syndrome
     E07.89   Other specified disorders of thyroid   `RxHCC`
       Abnormality of thyroid-binding globulin
       Hemorrhage of thyroid
       Infarction of thyroid

   E07.9   **Disorder of thyroid, unspecified**   `RxHCC`

Diabetes mellitus (E08-E13)

E08   **Diabetes mellitus** due to underlying condition
   👁 **See Official Guidelines** "Assigning and sequencing secondary
     diabetes codes and its causes" I.C.4.a.6.b
   ☞ **Code first** the underlying condition, such as:
     congenital rubella (P35.0)
     Cushing's syndrome (E24.-)
     cystic fibrosis (E84.-)
     malignant neoplasm (C00-C96)
     malnutrition (E40-E46)
     pancreatitis and other diseases of the pancreas (K85-K86.-)
   Use additional code to identify control using:
     insulin (Z79.4)
     oral antidiabetic drugs (Z79.84)
     oral hypoglycemic drugs (Z79.84)
> *EXCLUDES1*   *drug or chemical induced diabetes mellitus (E09.-)*
>   *gestational diabetes (O24.4-)*
>   *neonatal diabetes mellitus (P70.2)*
>   *postpancreatectomy diabetes mellitus (E13.-)*
>   *postprocedural diabetes mellitus (E13.-)*
>   *secondary diabetes mellitus NEC (E13.-)*

      type 1 diabetes mellitus (E10.-)
      type 2 diabetes mellitus (E11.-)

   E08.0   **Diabetes mellitus due to underlying condition with** hyperosmolarity
     E08.00   **Diabetes mellitus due to underlying condition with hyperosmolarity** without nonketotic hyperglycemic-hyperosmolar coma (NKHHC)   `HAC` `HCC` `MCC` `RxHCC` `CC/MCC Exc`
     E08.01   **Diabetes mellitus due to underlying condition with hyperosmolarity** with coma   `HAC` `HCC` `MCC` `RxHCC` `CC/MCC Exc`

   E08.1   **Diabetes mellitus due to underlying condition with** ketoacidosis
     E08.10   **Diabetes mellitus due to underlying condition with ketoacidosis** without coma   `HAC` `HCC` `MCC` `RxHCC` `CC/MCC Exc`
     E08.11   **Diabetes mellitus due to underlying condition with ketoacidosis** with coma   `HCC` `MCC` `RxHCC` `CC/MCC Exc`

   E08.2   **Diabetes mellitus due to underlying condition with** kidney complications
     E08.21   **Diabetes mellitus due to underlying condition with diabetic** nephropathy   `HCC` `RxHCC`
       Diabetes mellitus due to underlying condition with
         intercapillary glomerulosclerosis
       Diabetes mellitus due to underlying condition with
         intracapillary glomerulonephrosis
       Diabetes mellitus due to underlying condition with
         Kimmelstiel-Wilson disease
     E08.22   **Diabetes mellitus due to underlying condition with diabetic** chronic kidney disease   `HCC` `RxHCC`
       Use additional code to identify stage of chronic
         kidney disease (N18.1-N18.6)
     E08.29   **Diabetes mellitus due to underlying condition with other diabetic kidney complication**   `HCC` `RxHCC`
       Renal tubular degeneration in diabetes mellitus due
         to underlying condition

   E08.3   **Diabetes mellitus due to underlying condition with** ophthalmic complications
     E08.31   **Diabetes mellitus due to underlying condition with** unspecified diabetic retinopathy **(Figure 4.1)**
       E08.311   **Diabetes mellitus due to underlying condition with unspecified diabetic retinopathy with macular edema**   `HCC` `RxHCC`
       E08.319   **Diabetes mellitus due to underlying condition with unspecified diabetic retinopathy without macular edema**   `HCC` `RxHCC`

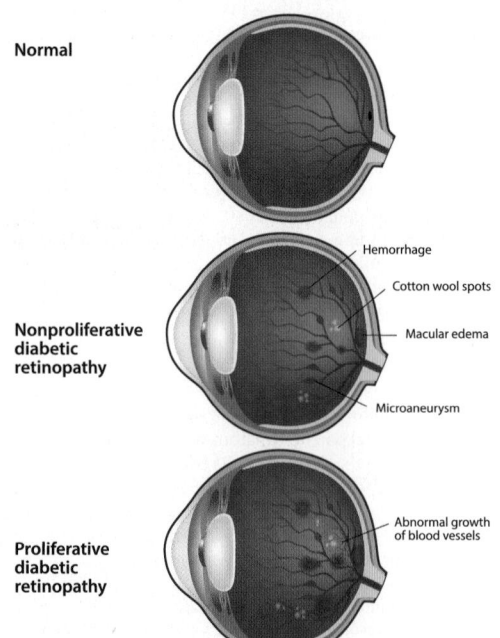

Normal

Nonproliferative diabetic retinopathy

Hemorrhage
Cotton wool spots
Macular edema
Microaneurysm

Proliferative diabetic retinopathy

Abnormal growth of blood vessels

Figure 4.1   Diabetic Retinopathy

6ᵗʰ **E08.32** **Diabetes mellitus due to underlying condition** with mild nonproliferative diabetic retinopathy

Diabetes mellitus due to underlying condition with nonproliferative diabetic retinopathy NOS

One of the following 7th characters is to be assigned to codes in subcategory E08.32 to designate laterality of the disease:
- 1 = right eye
- 2 = left eye
- 3 = bilateral
- 9 = unspecified eye

7ᵗʰ **E08.321** **Diabetes mellitus due to underlying condition with mild nonproliferative diabetic retinopathy** with macular edema HCC RxHCC

7ᵗʰ **E08.329** **Diabetes mellitus due to underlying condition with mild nonproliferative diabetic retinopathy** without macular edema HCC RxHCC

6ᵗʰ **E08.33** **Diabetes mellitus due to underlying condition with** moderate nonproliferative diabetic retinopathy

One of the following 7th characters is to be assigned to codes in subcategory E08.33 to designate laterality of the disease:
- 1 = right eye
- 2 = left eye
- 3 = bilateral
- 9 = unspecified eye

7ᵗʰ **E08.331** **Diabetes mellitus due to underlying condition with moderate nonproliferative diabetic retinopathy** with macular edema HCC RxHCC

7ᵗʰ **E08.339** **Diabetes mellitus due to underlying condition with moderate nonproliferative diabetic retinopathy** without macular edema HCC RxHCC

6ᵗʰ **E08.34** **Diabetes mellitus due to underlying condition with** severe nonproliferative diabetic retinopathy

One of the following 7th characters is to be assigned to codes in subcategory E08.34 to designate laterality of the disease:
- 1 = right eye
- 2 = left eye
- 3 = bilateral
- 9 = unspecified eye

7ᵗʰ **E08.341** **Diabetes mellitus due to underlying condition with severe nonproliferative diabetic retinopathy** with macular edema HCC RxHCC

7ᵗʰ **E08.349** **Diabetes mellitus due to underlying condition with severe nonproliferative diabetic retinopathy** without macular edema HCC RxHCC

6ᵗʰ **E08.35** **Diabetes mellitus due to underlying condition with** proliferative diabetic retinopathy

One of the following 7th characters is to be assigned to codes in subcategory E08.35 to designate laterality of the disease:
- 1 = right eye
- 2 = left eye
- 3 = bilateral
- 9 = unspecified eye

7ᵗʰ **E08.351** **Diabetes mellitus due to underlying condition with proliferative diabetic retinopathy** with macular edema HCC RxHCC

7ᵗʰ **E08.352** **Diabetes mellitus due to underlying condition with proliferative diabetic retinopathy** with traction retinal detachment involving the macula HCC RxHCC

7ᵗʰ **E08.353** **Diabetes mellitus due to underlying condition with proliferative diabetic retinopathy** with traction retinal detachment not involving the macula HCC RxHCC

7ᵗʰ **E08.354** **Diabetes mellitus due to underlying condition with proliferative diabetic retinopathy** with combined traction retinal detachment and rhegmatogenous retinal detachment HCC RxHCC

7ᵗʰ **E08.355** **Diabetes mellitus due to underlying condition with** stable **proliferative diabetic retinopathy** HCC RxHCC

7ᵗʰ **E08.359** **Diabetes mellitus due to underlying condition with proliferative diabetic retinopathy** without macular edema HCC RxHCC

7ᵗʰ **E08.36** **Diabetes mellitus due to underlying condition with diabetic** cataract HCC RxHCC

7ᵗʰ **E08.37** **Diabetes mellitus due to underlying condition with diabetic** macular edema, resolved following treatment HCC RxHCC

One of the following 7th characters is to be assigned to code E08.37 to designate laterality of the disease:
- 1 = right eye
- 2 = left eye
- 3 = bilateral
- 9 = unspecified eye

E08.39 **Diabetes mellitus due to underlying condition with other diabetic ophthalmic complication** HCC RxHCC

Use additional code to identify manifestation, such as: diabetic glaucoma (H40-H42)

5ᵗʰ **E08.4** **Diabetes mellitus due to underlying condition with** neurological complications

E08.40 **Diabetes mellitus due to underlying condition with diabetic** neuropathy, **unspecified** HCC RxHCC

E08.41 **Diabetes mellitus due to underlying condition with diabetic** mononeuropathy HCC RxHCC

E08.42 **Diabetes mellitus due to underlying condition with diabetic** polyneuropathy HCC RxHCC

Diabetes mellitus due to underlying condition with diabetic neuralgia

E08.43 **Diabetes mellitus due to underlying condition with diabetic** autonomic (poly)neuropathy HCC RxHCC

AHA: Q4 2013

Diabetes mellitus due to underlying condition with diabetic gastroparesis

E08.44 **Diabetes mellitus due to underlying condition with diabetic** amyotrophy HCC RxHCC

E08.49 **Diabetes mellitus due to underlying condition with other diabetic neurological complication** HCC RxHCC

5ᵗʰ **E08.5** **Diabetes mellitus due to underlying condition with** circulatory complications

E08.51 **Diabetes mellitus due to underlying condition with diabetic** peripheral angiopathy without gangrene HCC RxHCC

E08.52 **Diabetes mellitus due to underlying condition with diabetic** peripheral angiopathy with gangrene CC HCC RxHCC CC/MCC Exc

Diabetes mellitus due to underlying condition with diabetic gangrene

E08.59 **Diabetes mellitus due to underlying condition with other circulatory complications** HCC RxHCC

5ᵗʰ **E08.6** **Diabetes mellitus due to underlying condition with** other specified complications

6ᵗʰ **E08.61** **Diabetes mellitus due to underlying condition with** diabetic arthropathy

E08.610 **Diabetes mellitus due to underlying condition with diabetic** neuropathic arthropathy HCC RxHCC

Diabetes mellitus due to underlying condition with Charcôt's joints

E08.618 **Diabetes mellitus due to underlying condition with other diabetic arthropathy** HCC RxHCC

6ᵗʰ **E08.62** **Diabetes mellitus due to underlying condition with** skin complications

---

Unspecified Code   Other Specified Code   Manifestation Code   Ⓝ Newborn   Ⓟ Pediatric   Ⓜ Maternity   Ⓐ Adult   ♂ Male   ♀ Female
● New Code   ▲ Revised Code Title   ▶◀ Revised Text   **NOTES**   *INCLUDES*   *EXCLUDES1* Not coded here   *EXCLUDES2* Not included here
4ᵗʰ 4th character required   5ᵗʰ 5th character required   6ᵗʰ 6th character required   7ᵗʰ 7th character required   Ⓧ Extension 'X' Alert
HAC Hospital-acquired condition (HAC) alert   **AHA** AHA Coding Clinic©   ☞ Code first alert

E08.620 **Diabetes mellitus due to underlying condition with diabetic dermatitis** [HCC] [RxHCC]
Diabetes mellitus due to underlying condition with diabetic necrobiosis lipoidica

E08.621 **Diabetes mellitus due to underlying condition with foot ulcer** [HCC] [RxHCC]
Use additional code to identify site of ulcer (L97.4-, L97.5-)

E08.622 **Diabetes mellitus due to underlying condition with other skin ulcer** [HCC] [RxHCC]
Use additional code to identify site of ulcer (L97.1-L97.9, L98.41-L98.49)

E08.628 **Diabetes mellitus due to underlying condition with other skin complications** [HCC] [RxHCC]

[6th] E08.63 **Diabetes mellitus due to underlying condition with oral complications**

E08.630 **Diabetes mellitus due to underlying condition with periodontal disease** [HCC] [RxHCC]

E08.638 **Diabetes mellitus due to underlying condition with other oral complications** [HCC] [RxHCC]

[6th] E08.64 **Diabetes mellitus due to underlying condition with hypoglycemia**

E08.641 **Diabetes mellitus due to underlying condition with hypoglycemia with coma** [HCC] MCC [RxHCC] CC/MCC Exc

E08.649 **Diabetes mellitus due to underlying condition with hypoglycemia without coma** [HCC] [RxHCC]

E08.65 **Diabetes mellitus due to underlying condition with hyperglycemia** [HCC] [RxHCC]

E08.69 **Diabetes mellitus due to underlying condition with other specified complication** [HCC] [RxHCC]
AHA: Q4 2016
Use additional code to identify complication

E08.8 **Diabetes mellitus due to underlying condition with unspecified complications** [HCC] [RxHCC]

E08.9 **Diabetes mellitus due to underlying condition without complications** [HCC] [RxHCC]

[4th] E09 **Drug or chemical induced diabetes mellitus**

👁 **See Official Guidelines** "Secondary diabetes mellitus" I.C.4.a.6, "Assigning and sequencing secondary diabetes codes and its causes" I.C.4.a.6.b

☞ **Code first** poisoning due to drug or toxin, if applicable (T36-T65 with fifth or sixth character 1-4 or 6)

Use additional code for adverse effect, if applicable, to identify drug (T36-T50 with fifth or sixth character 5)

Use additional code to identify control using:
- insulin (Z79.4)
- oral antidiabetic drugs (Z79.84)
- oral hypoglycemic drugs (Z79.84)

[EXCLUDES1] *diabetes mellitus due to underlying condition (E08.-)*
gestational diabetes (O24.4-)
neonatal diabetes mellitus (P70.2)
postpancreatectomy diabetes mellitus (E13.-)
postprocedural diabetes mellitus (E13.-)
secondary diabetes mellitus NEC (E13.-)
type 1 diabetes mellitus (E10.-)
type 2 diabetes mellitus (E11.-)

[5th] E09.0 **Drug or chemical induced diabetes mellitus with hyperosmolarity**

E09.00 **Drug or chemical induced diabetes mellitus with hyperosmolarity without nonketotic hyperglycemic-hyperosmolar coma (NKHHC)** [HAC] [HCC] MCC [RxHCC] CC/MCC Exc

E09.01 **Drug or chemical induced diabetes mellitus with hyperosmolarity with coma** [HAC] [HCC] MCC [RxHCC] CC/MCC Exc

[5th] E09.1 **Drug or chemical induced diabetes mellitus with ketoacidosis**

E09.10 **Drug or chemical induced diabetes mellitus with ketoacidosis without coma** [HAC] [HCC] MCC [RxHCC] CC/MCC Exc

E09.11 **Drug or chemical induced diabetes mellitus with ketoacidosis with coma** [HCC] MCC [RxHCC] CC/MCC Exc

[5th] E09.2 **Drug or chemical induced diabetes mellitus with kidney complications**

E09.21 **Drug or chemical induced diabetes mellitus with diabetic nephropathy** [HCC] [RxHCC]
Drug or chemical induced diabetes mellitus with intercapillary glomerulosclerosis
Drug or chemical induced diabetes mellitus with intracapillary glomerulonephrosis
Drug or chemical induced diabetes mellitus with Kimmelstiel-Wilson disease

E09.22 **Drug or chemical induced diabetes mellitus with diabetic chronic kidney disease** [HCC] [RxHCC]
Use additional code to identify stage of chronic kidney disease (N18.1-N18.6)

E09.29 **Drug or chemical induced diabetes mellitus with other diabetic kidney complication** [HCC] [RxHCC]
Drug or chemical induced diabetes mellitus with renal tubular degeneration

[5th] E09.3 **Drug or chemical induced diabetes mellitus with ophthalmic complications**

[6th] E09.31 **Drug or chemical induced diabetes mellitus with unspecified diabetic retinopathy**

E09.311 **Drug or chemical induced diabetes mellitus with unspecified diabetic retinopathy with macular edema** [HCC] [RxHCC]

E09.319 **Drug or chemical induced diabetes mellitus with unspecified diabetic retinopathy without macular edema** [HCC] [RxHCC]

[6th] E09.32 **Drug or chemical induced diabetes mellitus with mild nonproliferative diabetic retinopathy**
Drug or chemical induced diabetes mellitus with nonproliferative diabetic retinopathy NOS
One of the following 7th characters is to be assigned to codes in subcategory E09.32 to designate laterality of the disease:
- **1 = right eye**
- **2 = left eye**
- **3 = bilateral**
- **9 = unspecified eye**

[7th] E09.321 **Drug or chemical induced diabetes mellitus with mild nonproliferative diabetic retinopathy with macular edema** [HCC] [RxHCC]

[7th] E09.329 **Drug or chemical induced diabetes mellitus with mild nonproliferative diabetic retinopathy without macular edema** [HCC] [RxHCC]

[6th] E09.33 **Drug or chemical induced diabetes mellitus with moderate nonproliferative diabetic retinopathy**
One of the following 7th characters is to be assigned to codes in subcategory E09.33 to designate laterality of the disease:
- **1 = right eye**
- **2 = left eye**
- **3 = bilateral**
- **9 = unspecified eye**

[7th] E09.331 **Drug or chemical induced diabetes mellitus with moderate nonproliferative diabetic retinopathy with macular edema** [HCC] [RxHCC]

[7th] E09.339 **Drug or chemical induced diabetes mellitus with moderate nonproliferative diabetic retinopathy without macular edema** [HCC] [RxHCC]

[6th] E09.34 **Drug or chemical induced diabetes mellitus with severe nonproliferative diabetic retinopathy**
One of the following 7th characters is to be assigned to codes in subcategory E09.34 to designate laterality of the disease:
- **1 = right eye**
- **2 = left eye**
- **3 = bilateral**
- **9 = unspecified eye**

PDx Unacceptable principal diagnosis symbol per Medicare code edits; POA Code exempt from diagnosis present on admission requirement
[?] Questionable admission; CC Complication or comorbidity; MCC Major complication or comorbidity; CC/MCC Exc CC/MCC exclusion
[HCC] HCC diagnosis code; [RxHCC] RxHCC diagnosis code; MACRA code; **DEFINITION** Describes condition/terminology
TIP Coding guidance; 👁 Official Guideline Reference; [Z1] Z code as first-listed diagnosis

◐7ᵗʰ E09.341 **Drug or chemical induced diabetes mellitus with severe nonproliferative diabetic retinopathy** with macular edema **HCC** **RxHCC**

◐7ᵗʰ E09.349 **Drug or chemical induced diabetes mellitus with severe nonproliferative diabetic retinopathy** without macular edema **HCC** **RxHCC**

◐6ᵗʰ E09.35 **Drug or chemical induced diabetes mellitus with** proliferative **diabetic retinopathy**

One of the following 7th characters is to be assigned to codes in subcategory E09.35 to designate laterality of the disease:
- **1 = right eye**
- **2 = left eye**
- **3 = bilateral**
- **9 = unspecified eye**

◐7ᵗʰ E09.351 **Drug or chemical induced diabetes mellitus with proliferative diabetic retinopathy** with macular edema **HCC** **RxHCC**

◐7ᵗʰ E09.352 **Drug or chemical induced diabetes mellitus with proliferative diabetic retinopathy** with traction retinal detachment involving the macula **HCC** **RxHCC**

◐7ᵗʰ E09.353 **Drug or chemical induced diabetes mellitus with proliferative diabetic retinopathy** with traction retinal detachment not involving the macula **HCC** **RxHCC**

◐7ᵗʰ E09.354 **Drug or chemical induced diabetes mellitus with proliferative diabetic retinopathy with** combined traction retinal detachment and rhegmatogenous retinal detachment **HCC** **RxHCC**

◐7ᵗʰ E09.355 **Drug or chemical induced diabetes mellitus with** stable **proliferative diabetic retinopathy** **HCC** **RxHCC**

◐7ᵗʰ E09.359 **Drug or chemical induced diabetes mellitus with proliferative diabetic retinopathy** without macular edema **HCC** **RxHCC**

E09.36 **Drug or chemical induced diabetes mellitus with diabetic** cataract **HCC** **RxHCC**

◐7ᵗʰ E09.37 **Drug or chemical induced diabetes mellitus with** diabetic macular edema, resolved following treatment **HCC** **RxHCC**

One of the following 7th characters is to be assigned to code E09.37 to designate laterality of the disease:
- **1 = right eye**
- **2 = left eye**
- **3 = bilateral**
- **9 = unspecified eye**

E09.39 **Drug or chemical induced diabetes mellitus with other diabetic ophthalmic complication** **HCC** **RxHCC**

Use additional code to identify manifestation, such as: diabetic glaucoma (H40-H42)

◐5ᵗʰ E09.4 **Drug or chemical induced diabetes mellitus with** neurological complications

E09.40 **Drug or chemical induced diabetes mellitus with neurological complications with diabetic** neuropathy, **unspecified** **HCC** **RxHCC**

E09.41 **Drug or chemical induced diabetes mellitus with neurological complications with diabetic** mononeuropathy **HCC** **RxHCC**

E09.42 **Drug or chemical induced diabetes mellitus with neurological complications with diabetic** polyneuropathy **HCC** **RxHCC**

Drug or chemical induced diabetes mellitus with diabetic neuralgia

E09.43 **Drug or chemical induced diabetes mellitus with neurological complications with diabetic** autonomic (poly)neuropathy **HCC** **RxHCC**

AHA: Q4 2013

Drug or chemical induced diabetes mellitus with diabetic gastroparesis

E09.44 **Drug or chemical induced diabetes mellitus with neurological complications with diabetic** amyotrophy **HCC** **RxHCC**

E09.49 **Drug or chemical induced diabetes mellitus with neurological complications with other diabetic neurological complication** **HCC** **RxHCC**

◐5ᵗʰ E09.5 **Drug or chemical induced diabetes mellitus with** circulatory complications

E09.51 **Drug or chemical induced diabetes mellitus with diabetic peripheral angiopathy** without gangrene **HCC** **RxHCC**

E09.52 **Drug or chemical induced diabetes mellitus with diabetic peripheral angiopathy** with gangrene cc° **HCC** **RxHCC** CC/MCC Exc

Drug or chemical induced diabetes mellitus with diabetic gangrene

E09.59 **Drug or chemical induced diabetes mellitus with other circulatory complications** **HCC** **RxHCC**

◐5ᵗʰ E09.6 **Drug or chemical induced diabetes mellitus with other specified complications**

◐6ᵗʰ E09.61 **Drug or chemical induced diabetes mellitus with diabetic** arthropathy

E09.610 **Drug or chemical induced diabetes mellitus with diabetic** neuropathic **arthropathy** **HCC** **RxHCC**

Drug or chemical induced diabetes mellitus with Charcôt's joints

E09.618 **Drug or chemical induced diabetes mellitus with other diabetic arthropathy** **HCC** **RxHCC**

◐6ᵗʰ E09.62 **Drug or chemical induced diabetes mellitus with** skin complications

E09.620 **Drug or chemical induced diabetes mellitus with** diabetic dermatitis **HCC** **RxHCC**

Drug or chemical induced diabetes mellitus with diabetic necrobiosis lipoidica

E09.621 **Drug or chemical induced diabetes mellitus with** foot ulcer **HCC** **RxHCC**

Use additional code to identify site of ulcer (L97.4-, L97.5-)

E09.622 **Drug or chemical induced diabetes mellitus with** other skin ulcer **HCC** **RxHCC**

Use additional code to identify site of ulcer (L97.1-L97.9, L98.41-L98.49)

E09.628 **Drug or chemical induced diabetes mellitus with other skin complications** **HCC** **RxHCC**

◐6ᵗʰ E09.63 **Drug or chemical induced diabetes mellitus with** oral complications

E09.630 **Drug or chemical induced diabetes mellitus with** periodontal disease **HCC** **RxHCC**

E09.638 **Drug or chemical induced diabetes mellitus with other oral complications** **HCC** **RxHCC**

◐6ᵗʰ E09.64 **Drug or chemical induced diabetes mellitus with** hypoglycemia

E09.641 **Drug or chemical induced diabetes mellitus with hypoglycemia** with coma **HCC** **MCC** **RxHCC** CC/MCC Exc

E09.649 **Drug or chemical induced diabetes mellitus with hypoglycemia** without coma **HCC** **RxHCC**

E09.65 **Drug or chemical induced diabetes mellitus with** hyperglycemia cc° **HCC** **RxHCC** CC/MCC Exc

E09.69 **Drug or chemical induced diabetes mellitus with other specified complication** cc° **HCC** **RxHCC** CC/MCC Exc

Use additional code to identify complication

E09.8 **Drug or chemical induced diabetes mellitus with unspecified complications** cc° **HCC** **RxHCC** CC/MCC Exc

E09.9 **Drug or chemical induced diabetes mellitus without complications** cc° **HCC** **RxHCC** CC/MCC Exc

◐4ᵗʰ E10 Type 1 **diabetes mellitus**

INCLUDES brittle diabetes (mellitus)

diabetes (mellitus) due to autoimmune process

diabetes (mellitus) due to immune mediated pancreatic islet beta-cell destruction

idiopathic diabetes (mellitus)

juvenile onset diabetes (mellitus)

ketosis-prone diabetes (mellitus)

Unspecified Code   Other Specified Code   Manifestation Code   N Newborn   P Pediatric   M Maternity   A Adult   ♂ Male   ♀ Female
● New Code   ▲ Revised Code Title   ►◄ Revised Text   **NOTES**   *INCLUDES*   *EXCLUDES1* Not coded here   *EXCLUDES2* Not included here
④ 4ᵗʰ character required   ⑤ 5ᵗʰ character required   ⑥ 6ᵗʰ character required   ⑦ 7ᵗʰ character required   ⑦ Extension 'X' Alert
HAC Hospital-acquired condition (HAC) alert   **AHA** AHA Coding Clinic©   📋 Code first alert

EXCLUDES1 *diabetes mellitus due to underlying condition (E08.-)*
drug or chemical induced diabetes mellitus (E09.-)
gestational diabetes (O24.4-)
hyperglycemia NOS (R73.9)
neonatal diabetes mellitus (P70.2)
postpancreatectomy diabetes mellitus (E13.-)
postprocedural diabetes mellitus (E13.-)
secondary diabetes mellitus NEC (E13.-)
type 2 diabetes mellitus (E11.-)

⑤ **E10.1 Type 1 diabetes mellitus with** ketoacidosis

E10.10 Type 1 diabetes mellitus with ketoacidosis without coma `HAC` `HCC` `MCC` `RxHCC` `CC/MCC Excl.`
AHA: Q3 2013

E10.11 Type 1 diabetes mellitus with ketoacidosis with coma `HCC` `MCC` `RxHCC` `CC/MCC Excl.`

⑤ **E10.2 Type 1 diabetes mellitus with** kidney complications

E10.21 Type 1 diabetes mellitus with diabetic nephropathy `HCC` `RxHCC`
Type 1 diabetes mellitus with intercapillary glomerulosclerosis
Type 1 diabetes mellitus with intracapillary glomerulonephrosis
Type 1 diabetes mellitus with Kimmelstiel-Wilson disease

E10.22 Type 1 diabetes mellitus with diabetic chronic kidney disease `HCC` `RxHCC`
Use additional code to identify stage of chronic kidney disease (N18.1-N18.6)

E10.29 Type 1 diabetes mellitus with other diabetic kidney complication `HCC` `RxHCC`
AHA: Q1 2016
Type 1 diabetes mellitus with renal tubular degeneration

⑤ **E10.3 Type 1 diabetes mellitus with** ophthalmic complications

⑥ **E10.31 Type 1 diabetes mellitus with unspecified diabetic retinopathy**

E10.311 Type 1 diabetes mellitus with unspecified diabetic retinopathy with macular edema `HCC` `RxHCC`

E10.319 Type 1 diabetes mellitus with unspecified diabetic retinopathy without macular edema `HCC` `RxHCC`

⑥ **E10.32 Type 1 diabetes mellitus with** mild nonproliferative diabetic retinopathy
Type 1 diabetes mellitus with nonproliferative diabetic retinopathy NOS
One of the following 7th characters is to be assigned to codes in subcategory E10.32 to designate laterality of the disease:
1 = right eye
2 = left eye
3 = bilateral
9 = unspecified eye

⑦ **E10.321 Type 1 diabetes mellitus with mild nonproliferative diabetic retinopathy with macular edema** `HCC` `RxHCC`

⑦ **E10.329 Type 1 diabetes mellitus with mild nonproliferative diabetic retinopathy without macular edema** `HCC` `RxHCC`

⑥ **E10.33 Type 1 diabetes mellitus with** moderate nonproliferative **diabetic retinopathy**
One of the following 7th characters is to be assigned to codes in subcategory E10.33 to designate laterality of the disease:
1 = right eye
2 = left eye
3 = bilateral
9 = unspecified eye

⑦ **E10.331 Type 1 diabetes mellitus with moderate nonproliferative diabetic retinopathy with macular edema** `HCC` `RxHCC`

⑦ **E10.339 Type 1 diabetes mellitus with moderate nonproliferative diabetic retinopathy** without macular edema `HCC` `RxHCC`

⑥ **E10.34 Type 1 diabetes mellitus with** severe nonproliferative **diabetic retinopathy**
One of the following 7th characters is to be assigned to codes in subcategory E10.34 to designate laterality of the disease:
1 = right eye
2 = left eye
3 = bilateral
9 = unspecified eye

⑦ **E10.341 Type 1 diabetes mellitus with severe nonproliferative diabetic retinopathy with macular edema** `HCC` `RxHCC`

⑦ **E10.349 Type 1 diabetes mellitus with severe nonproliferative diabetic retinopathy** without macular edema `HCC` `RxHCC`

⑥ **E10.35 Type 1 diabetes mellitus with** proliferative **diabetic retinopathy**
One of the following 7th characters is to be assigned to codes in subcategory E10.35 to designate laterality of the disease:
1 = right eye
2 = left eye
3 = bilateral
9 = unspecified eye

⑦ **E10.351 Type 1 diabetes mellitus with proliferative diabetic retinopathy** with macular edema `HCC` `RxHCC`

⑦ **E10.352 Type 1 diabetes mellitus with proliferative diabetic retinopathy** with traction retinal detachment involving the macula `HCC` `RxHCC`

⑦ **E10.353 Type 1 diabetes mellitus with proliferative diabetic retinopathy** with traction retinal detachment not involving the macula `HCC` `RxHCC`

⑦ **E10.354 Type 1 diabetes mellitus with proliferative diabetic retinopathy** with combined traction retinal detachment and rhegmatogenous retinal detachment `HCC` `RxHCC`

⑦ **E10.355 Type 1 diabetes mellitus with** stable proliferative diabetic retinopathy `HCC` `RxHCC`

⑦ **E10.359 Type 1 diabetes mellitus with proliferative diabetic retinopathy** without macular edema `HCC` `RxHCC`

E10.36 Type 1 diabetes mellitus with diabetic cataract `HCC` `RxHCC`

⑦ **E10.37 Type 1 diabetes mellitus** with diabetic macular edema, resolved following treatment `HCC` `RxHCC`
One of the following 7th characters is to be assigned to code E10.37 to designate laterality of the disease:
1 = right eye
2 = left eye
3 = bilateral
9 = unspecified eye

E10.39 Type 1 diabetes mellitus with other diabetic ophthalmic complication `HCC` `RxHCC`
Use additional code to identify manifestation, such as:
diabetic glaucoma (H40-H42)

⑤ **E10.4 Type 1 diabetes mellitus with** neurological complications

E10.40 Type 1 diabetes mellitus with diabetic neuropathy, unspecified `HCC` `RxHCC`

E10.41 Type 1 diabetes mellitus with diabetic mononeuropathy `HCC` `RxHCC`

E10.42 Type 1 diabetes mellitus with diabetic polyneuropathy `HCC` `RxHCC`
Type 1 diabetes mellitus with diabetic neuralgia

E10.43 Type 1 diabetes mellitus with diabetic autonomic (poly)neuropathy `HCC` `RxHCC`
AHA: Q4 2013
Type 1 diabetes mellitus with diabetic gastroparesis

POA Unacceptable principal diagnosis symbol per Medicare code edits POA Code exempt from diagnosis present on admission requirement
❓ Questionable admission CC Complication or comorbidity MCC Major complication or comorbidity CC/MCC Excl CC/MCC exclusion
`HCC` HCC diagnosis code `RxHCC` RxHCC diagnosis code MACRA code **DEFINITION** Describes condition/terminology
TIP Coding guidance 👁 Official Guideline Reference Z1 Z code as first-listed diagnosis

E10.44 **Type 1 diabetes mellitus with diabetic** amyotrophy `HCC` `RxHCC`

E10.49 **Type 1 diabetes mellitus with other diabetic** neurological complication `HCC` `RxHCC`

5ᵗʰ **E10.5** **Type 1 diabetes mellitus with** circulatory complications

E10.51 **Type 1 diabetes mellitus with diabetic peripheral angiopathy** without gangrene `HCC` `RxHCC`

E10.52 **Type 1 diabetes mellitus with diabetic peripheral angiopathy** with gangrene `CC` `HCC` `CC/MCC Exc`
Type 1 diabetes mellitus with diabetic gangrene

E10.59 **Type 1 diabetes mellitus with other circulatory complications** `HCC` `RxHCC`

5ᵗʰ **E10.6** **Type 1 diabetes mellitus with other specified complications**

6ᵗʰ **E10.61** **Type 1 diabetes mellitus with diabetic** arthropathy

E10.610 **Type 1 diabetes mellitus with diabetic** neuropathic **arthropathy** `HCC` `RxHCC`
Type 1 diabetes mellitus with Charcôt's joints

E10.618 **Type 1 diabetes mellitus with other diabetic arthropathy** `HCC` `RxHCC`

6ᵗʰ **E10.62** **Type 1 diabetes mellitus with** skin complications

E10.620 **Type 1 diabetes mellitus with diabetic** dermatitis `HCC` `RxHCC`
Type 1 diabetes mellitus with diabetic necrobiosis lipoidica

E10.621 **Type 1 diabetes mellitus with** foot ulcer `HCC` `RxHCC`
Use additional code to identify site of ulcer (L97.4-, L97.5-)

E10.622 **Type 1 diabetes mellitus with other skin ulcer** `HCC` `RxHCC`
Use additional code to identify site of ulcer (L97.1-L97.9, L98.41-L98.49)

E10.628 **Type 1 diabetes mellitus with other skin complications** `HCC` `RxHCC`

6ᵗʰ **E10.63** **Type 1 diabetes mellitus with** oral complications

E10.630 **Type 1 diabetes mellitus with** periodontal disease `HCC` `RxHCC`

E10.638 **Type 1 diabetes mellitus with other oral complications** `HCC` `RxHCC`

6ᵗʰ **E10.64** **Type 1 diabetes mellitus with** hypoglycemia

E10.641 **Type 1 diabetes mellitus with hypoglycemia** with coma `HCC` `MCC` `RxHCC` `CC/MCC Exc`

E10.649 **Type 1 diabetes mellitus with hypoglycemia** without coma `HCC` `RxHCC`
AHA: Q1 2016

E10.65 **Type 1 diabetes mellitus with** hyperglycemia `HCC` `RxHCC`
AHA: Q3 2013

E10.69 **Type 1 diabetes mellitus with other specified complication** `HCC` `RxHCC`
Use additional code to identify complication

E10.8 **Type 1 diabetes mellitus with unspecified complications** `HCC` `RxHCC`

E10.9 **Type 1 diabetes mellitus** without complications `HCC` `RxHCC`

4ᵗʰ **E11** **Type 2 diabetes mellitus**

👁 **See Official Guidelines** "Type of diabetes mellitus not documented" I.C.4.a.2, "Diabetes mellitus and the use of insulin and oral hypoglycemics" I.C.4.a.3

TIP: Default to a code from E11.- if the provider does not document the type of diabetes.

INCLUDES diabetes (mellitus) due to insulin secretory defect
diabetes NOS
insulin resistant diabetes (mellitus)

Use additional code to identify control using:
insulin (Z79.4)
oral antidiabetic drugs (Z79.84)
oral hypoglycemic drugs (Z79.84)

EXCLUDES1 diabetes mellitus due to underlying condition (E08.-)
drug or chemical induced diabetes mellitus (E09.-)
gestational diabetes (O24.4-)
neonatal diabetes mellitus (P70.2)
postpancreatectomy diabetes mellitus (E13.-)

postprocedural diabetes mellitus (E13.-)
secondary diabetes mellitus NEC (E13.-)
type 1 diabetes mellitus (E10.-)

5ᵗʰ **E11.0** **Type 2 diabetes mellitus with** hyperosmolarity

E11.00 **Type 2 diabetes mellitus with hyperosmolarity** without nonketotic hyperglycemic-hyperosmolar coma (**NKHHC**) `HAC` `HCC` `RxHCC`

E11.01 **Type 2 diabetes mellitus with hyperosmolarity** with coma `HAC` `HCC` `MCC` `RxHCC` `CC/MCC Exc`

5ᵗʰ **E11.1** **Type 2 diabetes mellitus with** ketoacidosis

E11.10 **Type 2 diabetes mellitus with ketoacidosis** without coma `HCC` `MCC` `RxHCC` `CC/MCC Exc`
AHA: Q4 2017

E11.11 **Type 2 diabetes mellitus with ketoacidosis** with coma `HCC` `MCC` `RxHCC` `CC/MCC Exc`
AHA: Q4 2017

5ᵗʰ **E11.2** **Type 2 diabetes mellitus with** kidney complications

E11.21 **Type 2 diabetes mellitus with diabetic** nephropathy `HCC` `RxHCC`
Type 2 diabetes mellitus with intercapillary glomerulosclerosis
Type 2 diabetes mellitus with intracapillary glomerulonephrosis
Type 2 diabetes mellitus with Kimmelstiel-Wilson disease

E11.22 **Type 2 diabetes mellitus with diabetic** chronic kidney disease `HCC` `RxHCC`
AHA: Q4 2018, Q1 2016, Q2 2016
Use additional code to identify stage of chronic kidney disease (N18.1-N18.6)

E11.29 **Type 2 diabetes mellitus with other diabetic kidney complication** `HCC` `RxHCC`
Type 2 diabetes mellitus with renal tubular degeneration

5ᵗʰ **E11.3** **Type 2 diabetes mellitus with** ophthalmic complications

6ᵗʰ **E11.31** **Type 2 diabetes mellitus with unspecified diabetic retinopathy**

E11.311 **Type 2 diabetes mellitus with unspecified diabetic retinopathy** with macular edema `HCC` `RxHCC`

E11.319 **Type 2 diabetes mellitus with unspecified diabetic retinopathy** without macular edema `HCC` `RxHCC`
AHA: Q3 2013

6ᵗʰ **E11.32** **Type 2 diabetes mellitus with** mild nonproliferative **diabetic retinopathy**
Type 2 diabetes mellitus with nonproliferative diabetic retinopathy NOS
One of the following 7th characters is to be assigned to codes in subcategory E11.32 to designate laterality of the disease:
1 = right eye
2 = left eye
3 = bilateral
9 = unspecified eye

7ᵗʰ **E11.321** **Type 2 diabetes mellitus with mild nonproliferative diabetic retinopathy** with macular edema `HCC` `RxHCC`

7ᵗʰ **E11.329** **Type 2 diabetes mellitus with mild nonproliferative diabetic retinopathy** without macular edema `HCC` `RxHCC`

6ᵗʰ **E11.33** **Type 2 diabetes mellitus with** moderate nonproliferative **diabetic retinopathy**
One of the following 7th characters is to be assigned to codes in subcategory E11.33 to designate laterality of the disease:
1 = right eye
2 = left eye
3 = bilateral
9 = unspecified eye

7ᵗʰ **E11.331** **Type 2 diabetes mellitus with moderate nonproliferative diabetic retinopathy** with macular edema `HCC` `RxHCC`

Unspecified Code   Other Specified Code   Manifestation Code   N Newborn   P Pediatric   M Maternity   A Adult   ♂ Male   ♀ Female
● New Code   ▲ Revised Code Title   ▶◀ Revised Text   NOTES   INCLUDES   EXCLUDES1 Not coded here   EXCLUDES2 Not included here
4ᵗʰ 4ᵗʰ character required   5ᵗʰ 5ᵗʰ character required   6ᵗʰ 6ᵗʰ character required   7ᵗʰ 7ᵗʰ character required   ✗ Extension 'X' Alert
HAC Hospital-acquired condition (HAC) alert   AHA AHA Coding Clinic©   ☛ Code first alert

E11.339 Type 2 diabetes mellitus with moderate nonproliferative diabetic retinopathy without macular edema `HCC` `RxHCC`

E11.34 Type 2 diabetes mellitus with severe nonproliferative diabetic retinopathy

One of the following 7th characters is to be assigned to codes in subcategory E11.34 to designate laterality of the disease:

1 = right eye
2 = left eye
3 = bilateral
9 = unspecified eye

E11.341 Type 2 diabetes mellitus with severe nonproliferative diabetic retinopathy with macular edema `HCC` `RxHCC`

E11.349 Type 2 diabetes mellitus with severe nonproliferative diabetic retinopathy without macular edema `HCC` `RxHCC`

E11.35 Type 2 diabetes mellitus with proliferative diabetic retinopathy

One of the following 7th characters is to be assigned to codes in subcategory E11.35 to designate laterality of the disease:

1 = right eye
2 = left eye
3 = bilateral
9 = unspecified eye

E11.351 Type 2 diabetes mellitus with proliferative diabetic retinopathy with macular edema `HCC` `RxHCC`

E11.352 Type 2 diabetes mellitus with proliferative diabetic retinopathy with traction retinal detachment involving the macula `HCC` `RxHCC`

E11.353 Type 2 diabetes mellitus with proliferative diabetic retinopathy with traction retinal detachment not involving the macula `HCC` `RxHCC`

E11.354 Type 2 diabetes mellitus with proliferative diabetic retinopathy with combined traction retinal detachment and rhegmatogenous retinal detachment `HCC` `RxHCC`

E11.355 Type 2 diabetes mellitus with stable proliferative diabetic retinopathy `HCC` `RxHCC`

E11.359 Type 2 diabetes mellitus with proliferative diabetic retinopathy without macular edema `HCC` `RxHCC`

E11.36 Type 2 diabetes mellitus with diabetic cataract `HCC` `RxHCC`
AHA: Q2 2019, Q2 2016

E11.37 Type 2 diabetes mellitus with diabetic macular edema, resolved following treatment `HCC` `RxHCC`

One of the following 7th characters is to be assigned to code E11.37 to designate laterality of the disease:

1 = right eye
2 = left eye
3 = bilateral
9 = unspecified eye

E11.39 Type 2 diabetes mellitus with other diabetic ophthalmic complication `HCC` `RxHCC`
Use additional code to identify manifestation, such as:
diabetic glaucoma (H40-H42)

E11.4 Type 2 diabetes mellitus with neurological complications

E11.40 Type 2 diabetes mellitus with diabetic neuropathy, unspecified `HCC` `RxHCC`
AHA: Q3 2018

E11.41 Type 2 diabetes mellitus with diabetic mononeuropathy `HCC` `RxHCC`

E11.42 Type 2 diabetes mellitus with diabetic polyneuropathy `HCC` `RxHCC`
AHA: Q1 2016
Type 2 diabetes mellitus with diabetic neuralgia

E11.43 Type 2 diabetes mellitus with diabetic autonomic (poly)neuropathy `HCC` `RxHCC`
AHA: Q2 2016
Type 2 diabetes mellitus with diabetic gastroparesis

E11.44 Type 2 diabetes mellitus with diabetic amyotrophy `HCC` `RxHCC`
AHA: Q2 2016

E11.49 Type 2 diabetes mellitus with other diabetic neurological complication `HCC` `RxHCC`

E11.5 Type 2 diabetes mellitus with circulatory complications

E11.51 Type 2 diabetes mellitus with diabetic peripheral angiopathy without gangrene `HCC` `RxHCC`
AHA: Q3 2018

E11.52 Type 2 diabetes mellitus with diabetic peripheral angiopathy with gangrene `CC` `HCC` `RxHCC` `CC/MCC Exc`
AHA: Q4 2017
Type 2 diabetes mellitus with diabetic gangrene

E11.59 Type 2 diabetes mellitus with other circulatory complications `HCC` `RxHCC`

E11.6 Type 2 diabetes mellitus with other specified complications

E11.61 Type 2 diabetes mellitus with diabetic arthropathy

E11.610 Type 2 diabetes mellitus with diabetic neuropathic arthropathy `HCC` `RxHCC`
AHA: Q2 2016
Type 2 diabetes mellitus with Charcôt's joints

E11.618 Type 2 diabetes mellitus with other diabetic arthropathy `HCC` `RxHCC`
AHA: Q2 2018, Q2 2016

E11.62 Type 2 diabetes mellitus with skin complications

E11.620 Type 2 diabetes mellitus with diabetic dermatitis `HCC` `RxHCC`
Type 2 diabetes mellitus with diabetic necrobiosis lipoidica

E11.621 Type 2 diabetes mellitus with foot ulcer `HCC` `RxHCC`
AHA: Q1 2016
Use additional code to identify site of ulcer (L97.4-, L97.5-)

E11.622 Type 2 diabetes mellitus with other skin ulcer `HCC` `RxHCC`
Use additional code to identify site of ulcer (L97.1-L97.9, L98.41-L98.49)

E11.628 Type 2 diabetes mellitus with other skin complications `HCC` `RxHCC`

E11.63 Type 2 diabetes mellitus with oral complications

E11.630 Type 2 diabetes mellitus with periodontal disease `HCC` `RxHCC`

E11.638 Type 2 diabetes mellitus with other oral complications `HCC` `RxHCC`

E11.64 Type 2 diabetes mellitus with hypoglycemia

E11.641 Type 2 diabetes mellitus with hypoglycemia with coma `HCC` `MCC` `RxHCC` `CC/MCC Exc`

E11.649 Type 2 diabetes mellitus with hypoglycemia without coma `HCC` `RxHCC`
AHA: Q3 2016, Q3 2015

E11.65 Type 2 diabetes mellitus with hyperglycemia `HCC` `RxHCC`
AHA: Q3 2013

E11.69 Type 2 diabetes mellitus with other specified complication `HCC` `RxHCC`
AHA: Q4 2016
Use additional code to identify complication

E11.8 Type 2 diabetes mellitus with unspecified complications `HCC` `RxHCC`

E11.9 Type 2 diabetes mellitus without complications `HCC` `?` `RxHCC`
AHA: Q2 2016, Q4 2016

E13 Other specified diabetes mellitus

See Official Guidelines "Secondary diabetes mellitus" I.C.4.a.6, "Assigning and sequencing secondary diabetes codes and its causes" I.C.4.a.6.b

INCLUDES diabetes mellitus due to genetic defects of beta-cell function
diabetes mellitus due to genetic defects in insulin action
postpancreatectomy diabetes mellitus

PDx Unacceptable principal diagnosis symbol per Medicare code edits   POA Code exempt from diagnosis present on admission requirement
? Questionable admission   CC Complication or comorbidity   MCC Major complication or comorbidity   CC/MCC Exc CC/MCC exclusion
HCC HCC diagnosis code   RxHCC RxHCC diagnosis code   MACRA code   **DEFINITION** Describes condition/terminology
TIP Coding guidance   Official Guideline Reference   Z1 Z code as first-listed diagnosis

526   When symbols appear on a code that requires a 7th character extension, refer to Appendix B to identify applicable 7th character codes.   **2020 ICD-10-CM**

        postprocedural diabetes mellitus
        secondary diabetes mellitus NEC
    Use additional code to identify control using:
        insulin (Z79.4)
        oral antidiabetic drugs (Z79.84)
        oral hypoglycemic drugs (Z79.84)
    EXCLUDES1 diabetes (mellitus) due to autoimmune process (E10.-)
        diabetes (mellitus) due to immune mediated pancreatic islet
            beta-cell destruction (E10.-)
        diabetes mellitus due to underlying condition (E08.-)
        drug or chemical induced diabetes mellitus (E09.-)
        gestational diabetes (O24.4-)
        neonatal diabetes mellitus (P70.2)
        type 1 diabetes mellitus (E10.-)

5th **E13.0** Other specified diabetes mellitus with hyperosmolarity

    E13.00 **Other specified diabetes mellitus with hyperosmolarity without nonketotic hyperglycemic-hyperosmolar coma (NKHHC)** HAC HCC MCC RxHCC CC/MCC Exc.
        EXCLUDES2 type 2 diabetes mellitus (E11.-)

    E13.01 **Other specified diabetes mellitus with hyperosmolarity with coma** HAC HCC MCC RxHCC CC/MCC Exc.

5th **E13.1** Other specified diabetes mellitus with ketoacidosis

    E13.10 **Other specified diabetes mellitus with ketoacidosis without coma** HAC HCC MCC RxHCC CC/MCC Exc.
        AHA: Q2 2016

    E13.11 **Other specified diabetes mellitus with ketoacidosis with coma** HCC MCC RxHCC CC/MCC Exc.

5th **E13.2** Other specified diabetes mellitus with kidney complications

    E13.21 **Other specified diabetes mellitus with diabetic nephropathy** HCC RxHCC
        Other specified diabetes mellitus with intercapillary glomerulosclerosis
        Other specified diabetes mellitus with intracapillary glomerulonephrosis
        Other specified diabetes mellitus with Kimmelstiel-Wilson disease

    E13.22 **Other specified diabetes mellitus with diabetic chronic kidney disease** HCC RxHCC
        Use additional code to identify stage of chronic kidney disease (N18.1-N18.6)

    E13.29 **Other specified diabetes mellitus with other diabetic kidney complication** HCC RxHCC
        Other specified diabetes mellitus with renal tubular degeneration

5th **E13.3** Other specified diabetes mellitus with ophthalmic complications

   6th **E13.31** Other specified diabetes mellitus with unspecified diabetic retinopathy

      E13.311 **Other specified diabetes mellitus with unspecified diabetic retinopathy with macular edema** HCC RxHCC

      E13.319 **Other specified diabetes mellitus with unspecified diabetic retinopathy without macular edema** HCC RxHCC

   6th **E13.32** Other specified diabetes mellitus with mild nonproliferative diabetic retinopathy
      Other specified diabetes mellitus with nonproliferative diabetic retinopathy NOS
      One of the following 7th characters is to be assigned to codes in subcategory E13.32 to designate laterality of the disease:
        1 = right eye
        2 = left eye
        3 = bilateral
        9 = unspecified eye

     7th **E13.321** **Other specified diabetes mellitus with mild nonproliferative diabetic retinopathy with macular edema** HCC RxHCC

     7th **E13.329** **Other specified diabetes mellitus with mild nonproliferative diabetic retinopathy without macular edema** HCC RxHCC

   6th **E13.33** Other specified diabetes mellitus with moderate nonproliferative diabetic retinopathy
      One of the following 7th characters is to be assigned to codes in subcategory E13.33 to designate laterality of the disease:
        1 = right eye
        2 = left eye
        3 = bilateral
        9 = unspecified eye

     7th **E13.331** **Other specified diabetes mellitus with moderate nonproliferative diabetic retinopathy with macular edema** HCC RxHCC

     7th **E13.339** **Other specified diabetes mellitus with moderate nonproliferative diabetic retinopathy without macular edema** HCC RxHCC

   6th **E13.34** Other specified diabetes mellitus with severe nonproliferative diabetic retinopathy
      One of the following 7th characters is to be assigned to codes in subcategory E13.34 to designate laterality of the disease:
        1 = right eye
        2 = left eye
        3 = bilateral
        9 = unspecified eye

     7th **E13.341** **Other specified diabetes mellitus with severe nonproliferative diabetic retinopathy with macular edema** HCC RxHCC

     7th **E13.349** **Other specified diabetes mellitus with severe nonproliferative diabetic retinopathy without macular edema** HCC RxHCC

   6th **E13.35** Other specified diabetes mellitus with proliferative diabetic retinopathy
      One of the following 7th characters is to be assigned to codes in subcategory E13.35 to designate laterality of the disease:
        1 = right eye
        2 = left eye
        3 = bilateral
        9 = unspecified eye

     7th **E13.351** **Other specified diabetes mellitus with proliferative diabetic retinopathy with macular edema** HCC RxHCC

     7th **E13.352** **Other specified diabetes mellitus with proliferative diabetic retinopathy with traction retinal detachment involving the macula** HCC RxHCC

     7th **E13.353** **Other specified diabetes mellitus with proliferative diabetic retinopathy with traction retinal detachment not involving the macula** HCC RxHCC

     7th **E13.354** **Other specified diabetes mellitus with proliferative diabetic retinopathy with combined traction retinal detachment and rhegmatogenous retinal detachment** HCC RxHCC

     7th **E13.355** **Other specified diabetes mellitus with stable proliferative diabetic retinopathy** HCC RxHCC

     7th **E13.359** **Other specified diabetes mellitus with proliferative diabetic retinopathy without macular edema** HCC RxHCC

    E13.36 **Other specified diabetes mellitus with diabetic cataract** HCC RxHCC

   7th **E13.37** **Other specified diabetes mellitus with diabetic macular edema, resolved following treatment** HCC RxHCC
      One of the following 7th characters is to be assigned to code E13.37 to designate laterality of the disease:
        1 = right eye
        2 = left eye
        3 = bilateral
        9 = unspecified eye

Unspecified Code   Other Specified Code   Manifestation Code   N Newborn   P Pediatric   M Maternity   A Adult   ♂ Male   ♀ Female
● New Code   ▲ Revised Code Title   ►◄ Revised Text   NOTES   INCLUDES   EXCLUDES1 Not coded here   EXCLUDES2 Not included here
4th 4th character required   5th 5th character required   6th 6th character required   7th 7th character required   7th Extension 'X' Alert
HAC Hospital-acquired condition (HAC) alert   AHA AHA Coding Clinic©   ☛ Code first alert

E13.39 **Other specified diabetes mellitus with other diabetic ophthalmic complication** HCC RxHCC
Use **additional** code to identify manifestation, such as:
diabetic glaucoma (H40-H42)

5th **E13.4** Other specified diabetes mellitus with neurological complications

E13.40 **Other specified diabetes mellitus with diabetic neuropathy, unspecified** HCC RxHCC

E13.41 **Other specified diabetes mellitus with diabetic mononeuropathy** HCC RxHCC

E13.42 **Other specified diabetes mellitus with diabetic polyneuropathy** HCC RxHCC
Other specified diabetes mellitus with diabetic neuralgia

E13.43 **Other specified diabetes mellitus with diabetic autonomic (poly)neuropathy** HCC RxHCC
AHA: Q4 2013
Other specified diabetes mellitus with diabetic gastroparesis

E13.44 **Other specified diabetes mellitus with diabetic amyotrophy** HCC RxHCC

E13.49 **Other specified diabetes mellitus with other diabetic neurological complication** HCC RxHCC

5th **E13.5** Other specified diabetes mellitus with circulatory complications

E13.51 **Other specified diabetes mellitus with diabetic peripheral angiopathy without gangrene** HCC RxHCC

E13.52 **Other specified diabetes mellitus with diabetic peripheral angiopathy with gangrene** cC HCC RxHCC CC/MCC Exc
Other specified diabetes mellitus with diabetic gangrene

E13.59 **Other specified diabetes mellitus with other circulatory complications** HCC RxHCC

5th **E13.6** Other specified diabetes mellitus with other specified complications

6th E13.61 **Other specified diabetes mellitus with diabetic arthropathy**

E13.610 **Other specified diabetes mellitus with diabetic neuropathic arthropathy** HCC RxHCC
Other specified diabetes mellitus with Charcôt's joints

E13.618 **Other specified diabetes mellitus with other diabetic arthropathy** HCC RxHCC

6th E13.62 **Other specified diabetes mellitus with skin complications**

E13.620 **Other specified diabetes mellitus with diabetic dermatitis** HCC RxHCC
Other specified diabetes mellitus with diabetic necrobiosis lipoidica

E13.621 **Other specified diabetes mellitus with foot ulcer**
Use **additional** code to identify site of ulcer (L97.4-, L97.5-)

E13.622 **Other specified diabetes mellitus with other skin ulcer** HCC RxHCC
Use **additional** code to identify site of ulcer (L97.1-L97.9, L98.41-L98.49)

E13.628 **Other specified diabetes mellitus with other skin complications** HCC RxHCC

6th E13.63 **Other specified diabetes mellitus with oral complications**

E13.630 **Other specified diabetes mellitus with periodontal disease** HCC RxHCC

E13.638 **Other specified diabetes mellitus with other oral complications** HCC RxHCC

6th E13.64 **Other specified diabetes mellitus with hypoglycemia**

E13.641 **Other specified diabetes mellitus with hypoglycemia with coma** HCC MCC RxHCC CC/MCC Exc

E13.649 **Other specified diabetes mellitus with hypoglycemia without coma** HCC RxHCC

E13.65 **Other specified diabetes mellitus with hyperglycemia** HCC RxHCC
AHA: Q3 2018

E13.69 **Other specified diabetes mellitus with other specified complication** HCC RxHCC
AHA: Q4 2016
Use **additional** code to identify complication

E13.8 **Other specified diabetes mellitus with unspecified complications** HCC RxHCC

E13.9 **Other specified diabetes mellitus without complications** HCC ? RxHCC

Other disorders of glucose regulation and pancreatic internal secretion (E15-E16)

E15 Nondiabetic hypoglycemic coma cC HAC HCC CC/MCC Exc
INCLUDES *drug-induced insulin coma in nondiabetic*
hyperinsulinism with hypoglycemic coma
hypoglycemic coma NOS

4th E16 Other disorders of pancreatic internal secretion

E16.0 **Drug-induced hypoglycemia without coma**
EXCLUDES1 *diabetes with hypoglycemia without coma (E09.649)*
Use **additional** code for adverse effect, if applicable, to identify drug (T36-T50 with fifth or sixth character 5)

E16.1 **Other hypoglycemia**
Functional hyperinsulinism
Functional nonhyperinsulinemic hypoglycemia
Hyperinsulinism NOS
Hyperplasia of pancreatic islet beta cells NOS
EXCLUDES1 *diabetes with hypoglycemia (E08.649, E10.649, E11.649, E13.649)*
hypoglycemia in infant of diabetic mother (P70.1)
neonatal hypoglycemia (P70.4)

E16.2 **Hypoglycemia, unspecified**
AHA: Q3 2016
EXCLUDES1 *diabetes with hypoglycemia (E08.649, E10.649, E11.649, E13.649)*

E16.3 **Increased secretion of glucagon** RxHCC
Hyperplasia of pancreatic endocrine cells with glucagon excess

E16.4 **Increased secretion of gastrin** RxHCC
Hypergastrinemia
Hyperplasia of pancreatic endocrine cells with gastrin excess
Zollinger-Ellison syndrome

E16.8 **Other specified disorders of pancreatic internal secretion** RxHCC
Increased secretion from endocrine pancreas of growth hormone-releasing hormone
Increased secretion from endocrine pancreas of pancreatic polypeptide
Increased secretion from endocrine pancreas of somatostatin
Increased secretion from endocrine pancreas of vasoactive-intestinal polypeptide

E16.9 **Disorder of pancreatic internal secretion, unspecified** RxHCC
Islet-cell hyperplasia NOS
Pancreatic endocrine cell hyperplasia NOS

Disorders of other endocrine glands (E20-E35)

EXCLUDES1 *galactorrhea (N64.3)*
gynecomastia (N62)

4th E20 Hypoparathyroidism
EXCLUDES1 *Di George's syndrome (D82.1)*
postprocedural hypoparathyroidism (E89.2)
tetany NOS (R29.0)
transitory neonatal hypoparathyroidism (P71.4)

E20.0 Idiopathic **hypoparathyroidism** HCC RxHCC

E20.1 Pseudohypoparathyroidism

E20.8 **Other hypoparathyroidism** HCC RxHCC

E20.9 **Hypoparathyroidism, unspecified** HCC RxHCC
Parathyroid tetany

PDx **Unacceptable principal diagnosis symbol per Medicare code edits** POA **Code exempt from diagnosis present on admission requirement**
? Questionable admission cC Complication or comorbidity MCC Major complication or comorbidity CC/MCC Exc CC/MCC exclusion
HCC HCC diagnosis code RxHCC RxHCC diagnosis code MACRA MACRA code **DEFINITION** Describes condition/terminology
TIP Coding guidance 👁 Official Guideline Reference Z1 Z code as first-listed diagnosis

E21 Hyperparathyroidism and other disorders of parathyroid gland
  EXCLUDES1 *adult osteomalacia (M83.-)*
        ectopic hyperparathyroidism (E34.2)
        familial hypocalciuric hypercalcemia (E83.52)
        hungry bone syndrome (E83.81)
        infantile and juvenile osteomalacia (E55.0)
  E21.0 Primary **hyperparathyroidism**   `HCC` `RxHCC`
        Hyperplasia of parathyroid
        Osteitis fibrosa cystica generalisata [von Recklinghausen's disease of bone]
  E21.1 Secondary **hyperparathyroidism, not elsewhere classified**   `HCC` `RxHCC`
        EXCLUDES1 *secondary hyperparathyroidism of renal origin (N25.81)*
  E21.2 **Other hyperparathyroidism**   `HCC` `RxHCC`
        Tertiary hyperparathyroidism
        EXCLUDES1 *familial hypocalciuric hypercalcemia (E83.52)*
  E21.3 **Hyperparathyroidism, unspecified**   `HCC` `RxHCC`
  E21.4 Other specified disorders of parathyroid gland   `HCC` `RxHCC`
  E21.5 **Disorder of parathyroid gland, unspecified**   `HCC` `RxHCC`
E22 Hyperfunction of pituitary gland
  EXCLUDES1 *Cushing's syndrome (E24.-)*
        Nelson's syndrome (E24.1)
        overproduction of ACTH not associated with Cushing's disease (E27.0)
        overproduction of pituitary ACTH (E24.0)
        overproduction of thyroid-stimulating hormone (E05.8-)
  E22.0 **Acromegaly and pituitary gigantism**   `HCC` `RxHCC`
        Overproduction of growth hormone
        EXCLUDES1 *constitutional gigantism (E34.4)*
                constitutional tall stature (E34.4)
                increased secretion from endocrine pancreas of growth hormone-releasing hormone (E16.8)
  E22.1 **Hyperprolactinemia**   `cc⊘` `HCC` `RxHCC` `CC/MCC Exc⊘`
        Use additional code for adverse effect, if applicable, to identify drug (T36-T50 with fifth or sixth character 5)
  E22.2 **Syndrome of inappropriate secretion of antidiuretic hormone**   `cc⊘` `HCC` `RxHCC` `CC/MCC Exc⊘`
  E22.8 **Other hyperfunction of pituitary gland**   `cc⊘` `HCC` `RxHCC` `CC/MCC Exc⊘`
        Central precocious puberty
  E22.9 **Hyperfunction of pituitary gland, unspecified**   `cc⊘` `HCC` `RxHCC` `CC/MCC Exc⊘`
E23 Hypofunction and other disorders of the pituitary gland
  INCLUDES *the listed conditions whether the disorder is in the pituitary or the hypothalamus*
  EXCLUDES1 *postprocedural hypopituitarism (E89.3)*
  E23.0 **Hypopituitarism**   `HCC` `RxHCC`
        Fertile eunuch syndrome
        Hypogonadotropic hypogonadism
        Idiopathic growth hormone deficiency
        Isolated deficiency of gonadotropin
        Isolated deficiency of growth hormone
        Isolated deficiency of pituitary hormone
        Kallmann's syndrome
        Lorain-Levi short stature
        Necrosis of pituitary gland (postpartum)
        Panhypopituitarism
        Pituitary cachexia
        Pituitary insufficiency NOS
        Pituitary short stature
        Sheehan's syndrome
        Simmonds' disease
  E23.1 **Drug-induced hypopituitarism**   `HCC` `RxHCC`
        Use additional code for adverse effect, if applicable, to identify drug (T36-T50 with fifth or sixth character 5)
  E23.2 **Diabetes insipidus**   `cc⊘` `HCC` `RxHCC` `CC/MCC Exc⊘`
        EXCLUDES1 *nephrogenic diabetes insipidus (N25.1)*
  E23.3 **Hypothalamic dysfunction, not elsewhere classified**   `HCC` `RxHCC`
        EXCLUDES1 *Prader-Willi syndrome ▶(Q87.11)◀*
                Russell-Silver syndrome ▶(Q87.19)◀

  E23.6 **Other disorders of pituitary gland**   `HCC` `RxHCC`
        Abscess of pituitary
        Adiposogenital dystrophy
  E23.7 **Disorder of pituitary gland, unspecified**   `HCC` `RxHCC`
E24 Cushing's syndrome
  DEFINITION: Cushing syndrome occurs when the body is exposed to high levels of the hormone cortisol for an extended time.
  EXCLUDES1 *congenital adrenal hyperplasia (E25.0)*
  E24.0 Pituitary-dependent **Cushing's disease**   `cc⊘` `HCC` `RxHCC` `CC/MCC Exc⊘`
        Overproduction of pituitary ACTH
        Pituitary-dependent hypercorticalism
  E24.1 Nelson's syndrome   `HCC` `RxHCC`
  E24.2 Drug-induced **Cushing's syndrome**   `cc⊘` `HCC` `RxHCC` `CC/MCC Exc⊘`
        Use additional code for adverse effect, if applicable, to identify drug (T36-T50 with fifth or sixth character 5)
  E24.3 Ectopic ACTH syndrome   `cc⊘` `HCC` `RxHCC` `CC/MCC Exc⊘`
  E24.4 Alcohol-induced pseudo-**Cushing's syndrome**   `cc⊘` `HCC` `RxHCC` `CC/MCC Exc⊘`
  E24.8 **Other Cushing's syndrome**   `cc⊘` `HCC` `RxHCC` `CC/MCC Exc⊘`
  E24.9 **Cushing's syndrome, unspecified** `cc⊘` `HCC` `RxHCC` `CC/MCC Exc⊘`
E25 Adrenogenital disorders
  INCLUDES *adrenogenital syndromes, virilizing or feminizing, whether acquired or due to adrenal hyperplasia consequent on inborn enzyme defects in hormone synthesis*
        Female adrenal pseudohermaphroditism
        Female heterosexual precocious pseudopuberty
        Male isosexual precocious pseudopuberty
        Male macrogenitosomia praecox
        Male sexual precocity with adrenal hyperplasia
        Male virilization (female)
  EXCLUDES1 *indeterminate sex and pseudohermaphroditism (Q56)*
        chromosomal abnormalities (Q90-Q99)
  E25.0 Congenital **adrenogenital disorders** associated with enzyme deficiency   `HCC` `RxHCC`
        Congenital adrenal hyperplasia
        21-Hydroxylase deficiency
        Salt-losing congenital adrenal hyperplasia
  E25.8 **Other adrenogenital disorders**   `HCC` `RxHCC`
        Idiopathic adrenogenital disorder
        Use additional code for adverse effect, if applicable, to identify drug (T36-T50 with fifth or sixth character 5)
  E25.9 **Adrenogenital disorder, unspecified**   `HCC` `RxHCC`
        Adrenogenital syndrome NOS
E26 Hyperaldosteronism
  E26.0 Primary **hyperaldosteronism**
        E26.01 **Conn's syndrome**   `HCC` `RxHCC`
                Code also adrenal adenoma (D35.0-)
        E26.02 **Glucocorticoid-remediable aldosteronism**   `HCC` `RxHCC`
                Familial aldosteronism type I
        E26.09 **Other primary hyperaldosteronism**   `HCC` `RxHCC`
                Primary aldosteronism due to adrenal hyperplasia (bilateral)
  E26.1 Secondary **hyperaldosteronism**   `HCC` `RxHCC`
  E26.8 **Other hyperaldosteronism**
        E26.81 **Bartter's syndrome**   `HCC` `RxHCC`
        E26.89 **Other hyperaldosteronism**   `HCC` `RxHCC`
  E26.9 **Hyperaldosteronism, unspecified**   `HCC` `RxHCC`
        Aldosteronism NOS
        Hyperaldosteronism NOS
E27 Other disorders of adrenal gland
  E27.0 **Other adrenocortical overactivity**   `cc⊘` `HCC` `RxHCC` `CC/MCC Exc⊘`
        Overproduction of ACTH, not associated with Cushing's disease
        Premature adrenarche
        EXCLUDES1 *Cushing's syndrome (E24.-)*
  E27.1 **Primary adrenocortical insufficiency**   `cc⊘` `HCC` `RxHCC` `CC/MCC Exc⊘`
        Addison's disease
        Autoimmune adrenalitis
        EXCLUDES1 *Addison only phenotype adrenoleukodystrophy (E71.528)*
                amyloidosis (E85.-)
                tuberculous Addison's disease (A18.7)
                Waterhouse-Friderichsen syndrome (A39.1)

E27.2 **Addisonian crisis** `CC` `HCC` `RxHCC` `CC/MCC Exc`
Adrenal crisis
Adrenocortical crisis

E27.3 **Drug-induced adrenocortical insufficiency** `CC` `HCC` `RxHCC` `CC/MCC Exc`
Use additional code for adverse effect, if applicable, to identify drug (T36-T50 with fifth or sixth character 5)

5ᵗʰ **E27.4** **Other and unspecified adrenocortical insufficiency**
EXCLUDES1 *adrenoleukodystrophy [Addison-Schilder] (E71.528)*
Waterhouse-Friderichsen syndrome (A39.1)

    E27.40 **Unspecified adrenocortical insufficiency** `CC` `HCC` `RxHCC` `CC/MCC Exc`
Adrenocortical insufficiency NOS
Hypoaldosteronism

    E27.49 **Other adrenocortical insufficiency** `CC` `HCC` `RxHCC` `CC/MCC Exc`
Adrenal hemorrhage
Adrenal infarction

E27.5 **Adrenomedullary hyperfunction** `CC` `HCC` `RxHCC` `CC/MCC Exc`
Adrenomedullary hyperplasia
Catecholamine hypersecretion

E27.8 **Other specified disorders of adrenal gland** `HCC` `RxHCC`
Abnormality of cortisol-binding globulin

E27.9 **Disorder of adrenal gland, unspecified** `HCC` `RxHCC`

4ᵗʰ **E28** **Ovarian dysfunction**
EXCLUDES1 *isolated gonadotropin deficiency (E23.0)*
postprocedural ovarian failure (E89.4-)

    E28.0 **Estrogen excess** ♀
Use additional code for adverse effect, if applicable, to identify drug (T36-T50 with fifth or sixth character 5)

    E28.1 **Androgen excess** ♀
Hypersecretion of ovarian androgens
Use additional code for adverse effect, if applicable, to identify drug (T36-T50 with fifth or sixth character 5)

    E28.2 **Polycystic ovarian syndrome** ♀
Sclerocystic ovary syndrome
Stein-Leventhal syndrome

    5ᵗʰ **E28.3** **Primary ovarian failure**
EXCLUDES1 *pure gonadal dysgenesis (Q99.1)*
Turner's syndrome (Q96.-)

      6ᵗʰ **E28.31** **Premature menopause**
        E28.310 **Symptomatic premature menopause** `A` ♀
Symptoms such as flushing, sleeplessness, headache, lack of concentration, associated with premature menopause
        E28.319 **Asymptomatic premature menopause** `A` ♀
Premature menopause NOS

      E28.39 **Other primary ovarian failure** ♀
Decreased estrogen
Resistant ovary syndrome

    E28.8 **Other ovarian dysfunction** ♀
Ovarian hyperfunction NOS
EXCLUDES1 *postprocedural ovarian failure (E89.4-)*

    E28.9 **Ovarian dysfunction, unspecified** ♀

4ᵗʰ **E29** **Testicular dysfunction**
EXCLUDES1 *androgen insensitivity syndrome (E34.5-)*
azoospermia or oligospermia NOS (N46.0-N46.1)
isolated gonadotropin deficiency (E23.0)
Klinefelter's syndrome (Q98.0-Q98.1, Q98.4)

    E29.0 **Testicular hyperfunction** ♂
Hypersecretion of testicular hormones

    E29.1 **Testicular hypofunction** ♂
Defective biosynthesis of testicular androgen NOS
5-delta-Reductase deficiency (with male pseudohermaphroditism)
Testicular hypogonadism NOS
Use additional code for adverse effect, if applicable, to identify drug (T36-T50 with fifth or sixth character 5)
EXCLUDES1 *postprocedural testicular hypofunction (E89.5)*

    E29.8 **Other testicular dysfunction** ♂

    E29.9 **Testicular dysfunction, unspecified** ♂

4ᵗʰ **E30** **Disorders of puberty, not elsewhere classified**

    E30.0 **Delayed puberty**
Constitutional delay of puberty
Delayed sexual development

    E30.1 **Precocious puberty** `P`
Precocious menstruation
EXCLUDES1 *Albright (-McCune) (-Sternberg) syndrome (Q78.1)*
central precocious puberty (E22.8)
congenital adrenal hyperplasia (E25.0)
female heterosexual precocious pseudopuberty (E25.-)
male isosexual precocious pseudopuberty (E25.-)

    E30.8 **Other disorders of puberty** `P`
Premature thelarche

    E30.9 **Disorder of puberty, unspecified**

4ᵗʰ **E31** **Polyglandular dysfunction**
EXCLUDES1 *ataxia telangiectasia [Louis-Bar] (G11.3)*
dystrophia myotonica [Steinert] (G71.11)
pseudohypoparathyroidism (E20.1)

    E31.0 **Autoimmune polyglandular failure** `HCC` `RxHCC`
Schmidt's syndrome

    E31.1 **Polyglandular hyperfunction** `HCC` `RxHCC`
EXCLUDES1 *multiple endocrine adenomatosis (E31.2-)*
multiple endocrine neoplasia (E31.2-)

    5ᵗʰ **E31.2** **Multiple endocrine neoplasia [MEN] syndromes**
Multiple endocrine adenomatosis
Code also any associated malignancies and other conditions associated with the syndromes

      E31.20 **Multiple endocrine neoplasia [MEN] syndrome, unspecified** `HCC` `RxHCC`
Multiple endocrine adenomatosis NOS
Multiple endocrine neoplasia [MEN] syndrome NOS

      E31.21 **Multiple endocrine neoplasia [MEN] type I** `HCC` `RxHCC`
Wermer's syndrome

      E31.22 **Multiple endocrine neoplasia [MEN] type IIA** `HCC` `RxHCC`
Sipple's syndrome

      E31.23 **Multiple endocrine neoplasia [MEN] type IIB** `HCC` `RxHCC`

    E31.8 **Other polyglandular dysfunction** `HCC` `RxHCC`

    E31.9 **Polyglandular dysfunction, unspecified** `HCC` `RxHCC`

4ᵗʰ **E32** **Diseases of thymus**
EXCLUDES1 *aplasia or hypoplasia of thymus with immunodeficiency (D82.1)*
myasthenia gravis (G70.0)

    E32.0 **Persistent hyperplasia of thymus** `HCC` `RxHCC`
Hypertrophy of thymus

    E32.1 **Abscess of thymus** `CC` `HCC` `RxHCC` `CC/MCC Exc`

    E32.8 **Other diseases of thymus** `HCC` `RxHCC`
EXCLUDES1 *aplasia or hypoplasia with immunodeficiency (D82.1)*
thymoma (D15.0)

    E32.9 **Disease of thymus, unspecified** `HCC` `RxHCC`

4ᵗʰ **E34** **Other endocrine disorders**
EXCLUDES1 *pseudohypoparathyroidism (E20.1)*

    E34.0 **Carcinoid syndrome** `CC` `HCC` `RxHCC` `CC/MCC Exc`
NOTES   May be used as an additional code to identify functional activity associated with a carcinoid tumor.

    E34.1 **Other hypersecretion of intestinal hormones**

    E34.2 **Ectopic hormone secretion, not elsewhere classified**
EXCLUDES1 *ectopic ACTH syndrome (E24.3)*

    E34.3 **Short stature due to endocrine disorder**
Constitutional short stature
Laron-type short stature
EXCLUDES1 *achondroplastic short stature (Q77.4)*
hypochondroplastic short stature (Q77.4)
nutritional short stature (E45)
pituitary short stature (E23.0)
progeria (E34.8)

PDx Unacceptable principal diagnosis symbol per Medicare code edits   PDA Code exempt from diagnosis present on admission requirement
? Questionable admission   `CC` Complication or comorbidity   `MCC` Major complication or comorbidity   `CC/MCC Exc` CC/MCC exclusion
`HCC` HCC diagnosis code   `RxHCC` RxHCC diagnosis code   MACRA code   **DEFINITION** Describes condition/terminology
TIP Coding guidance   👁 Official Guideline Reference   `Z1` Z code as first-listed diagnosis

530   When symbols appear on a code that requires a 7th character extension, refer to Appendix B to identify applicable 7th character codes.   **2020 ICD-10-CM**

short stature in specific dysmorphic syndromes -
    code to syndrome - see Alphabetical Index
short stature NOS (R62.52)

E34.4 Constitutional tall stature HCC RxHCC
Constitutional gigantism

5ᵗʰ **E34.5 Androgen insensitivity syndrome**
E34.50 Androgen insensitivity syndrome, unspecified
Androgen insensitivity NOS
E34.51 Complete androgen insensitivity syndrome
Complete androgen insensitivity
de Quervain syndrome
Goldberg-Maxwell syndrome
E34.52 Partial androgen insensitivity syndrome
Partial androgen insensitivity
Reifenstein syndrome

E34.8 Other specified endocrine disorders
Pineal gland dysfunction
Progeria
EXCLUDES2 pseudohypoparathyroidism (E20.1)

E34.9 Endocrine disorder, unspecified
Endocrine disturbance NOS
Hormone disturbance NOS

E35 Disorders of endocrine glands in diseases classified elsewhere
☞ Code first underlying disease, such as:
late congenital syphilis of thymus gland [Dubois disease] (A50.5)
Use additional code, if applicable, to identify:
sequelae of tuberculosis of other organs (B90.8)
EXCLUDES1 Echinococcus granulosus infection of thyroid gland (B67.3)
meningococcal hemorrhagic adrenalitis (A39.1)
syphilis of endocrine gland (A52.79)
tuberculosis of adrenal gland, except calcification (A18.7)
tuberculosis of endocrine gland NEC (A18.82)
tuberculosis of thyroid gland (A18.81)
Waterhouse-Friderichsen syndrome (A39.1)

Intraoperative complications of endocrine system (E36)

4ᵗʰ **E36 Intraoperative complications of endocrine system**
EXCLUDES2 postprocedural endocrine and metabolic complications and disorders, not elsewhere classified (E89.-)

5ᵗʰ **E36.0 Intraoperative hemorrhage and hematoma of an endocrine system organ or structure complicating a procedure**
EXCLUDES1 intraoperative hemorrhage and hematoma of an endocrine system organ or structure due to accidental puncture or laceration during a procedure (E36.1-)
E36.01 Intraoperative hemorrhage and hematoma of an endocrine system organ or structure complicating an endocrine system procedure CC CC/MCC Exc
E36.02 Intraoperative hemorrhage and hematoma of an endocrine system organ or structure complicating other procedure CC CC/MCC Exc

5ᵗʰ **E36.1 Accidental puncture and laceration of an endocrine system organ or structure during a procedure**
E36.11 Accidental puncture and laceration of an endocrine system organ or structure during an endocrine system procedure CC CC/MCC Exc
E36.12 Accidental puncture and laceration of an endocrine system organ or structure during other procedure CC CC/MCC Exc

E36.8 Other intraoperative complications of endocrine system
Use additional code, if applicable, to further specify disorder

Malnutrition (E40-E46)

EXCLUDES1 intestinal malabsorption (K90.-)
sequelae of protein-calorie malnutrition (E64.0)

---

renal short stature (N25.0)
Russell-Silver syndrome ▶(Q87.19)◀
short-limbed stature with immunodeficiency (D82.2)

EXCLUDES2 nutritional anemias (D50-D53)
starvation (T73.0)

E40 Kwashiorkor HCC MCC CC/MCC Exc
AHA: Q3 2017
Severe malnutrition with nutritional edema with dyspigmentation of skin and hair
EXCLUDES1 marasmic kwashiorkor (E42)

E41 Nutritional marasmus HCC MCC CC/MCC Exc
AHA: Q3 2017
Severe malnutrition with marasmus
EXCLUDES1 marasmic kwashiorkor (E42)

E42 Marasmic kwashiorkor CC HCC CC/MCC Exc
AHA: Q3 2017
Intermediate form severe protein-calorie malnutrition
Severe protein-calorie malnutrition with signs of both kwashiorkor and marasmus

E43 Unspecified severe protein-calorie malnutrition CC HCC CC/MCC Exc
AHA: Q3 2017, Q4 2017
Starvation edema

4ᵗʰ **E44 Protein-calorie malnutrition of moderate and mild degree**
E44.0 Moderate protein-calorie malnutrition HCC MCC CC/MCC Exc
AHA: Q3 2017
E44.1 Mild protein-calorie malnutrition CC HCC CC/MCC Exc
AHA: Q3 2017

E45 Retarded development following protein-calorie malnutrition CC HCC CC/MCC Exc
Nutritional short stature
Nutritional stunting
Physical retardation due to malnutrition

E46 Unspecified protein-calorie malnutrition CC HCC CC/MCC Exc
AHA: Q3 2017
Malnutrition NOS
Protein-calorie imbalance NOS
EXCLUDES1 nutritional deficiency NOS (E63.9)

Other nutritional deficiencies (E50-E64)

EXCLUDES2 nutritional anemias (D50-D53)

4ᵗʰ **E50 Vitamin A deficiency**
EXCLUDES1 sequelae of vitamin A deficiency (E64.1)
E50.0 Vitamin A deficiency with conjunctival xerosis
E50.1 Vitamin A deficiency with Bitot's spot and conjunctival xerosis
Bitot's spot in the young child
E50.2 Vitamin A deficiency with corneal xerosis
E50.3 Vitamin A deficiency with corneal ulceration and xerosis
E50.4 Vitamin A deficiency with keratomalacia
E50.5 Vitamin A deficiency with night blindness
E50.6 Vitamin A deficiency with xerophthalmic scars of cornea
E50.7 Other ocular manifestations of vitamin A deficiency
Xerophthalmia NOS
E50.8 Other manifestations of vitamin A deficiency
Follicular keratosis
Xeroderma
E50.9 Vitamin A deficiency, unspecified
Hypovitaminosis A NOS

4ᵗʰ **E51 Thiamine deficiency**
EXCLUDES1 sequelae of thiamine deficiency (E64.8)
5ᵗʰ **E51.1 Beriberi**
E51.11 Dry beriberi CC CC/MCC Exc
Beriberi NOS
Beriberi with polyneuropathy
E51.12 Wet beriberi CC CC/MCC Exc
Beriberi with cardiovascular manifestations
Cardiovascular beriberi
Shoshin disease
E51.2 Wernicke's encephalopathy MCC CC/MCC Exc
E51.8 Other manifestations of thiamine deficiency CC CC/MCC Exc
E51.9 Thiamine deficiency, unspecified CC CC/MCC Exc

Unspecified Code	Other Specified Code	Manifestation Code	N Newborn	P Pediatric	M Maternity	A Adult	♂ Male	♀ Female

● New Code   ▲ Revised Code Title   ▶◀ Revised Text   NOTES   INCLUDES   EXCLUDES1 Not coded here   EXCLUDES2 Not included here
4ᵗʰ 4ᵗʰ character required   5ᵗʰ 5ᵗʰ character required   6ᵗʰ 6ᵗʰ character required   7ᵗʰ 7ᵗʰ character required   7ₓ Extension 'X' Alert
HAC Hospital-acquired condition (HAC) alert   AHA AHA Coding Clinic©   ☞ Code first alert

E52 Niacin **deficiency [pellagra]**
Niacin (-tryptophan) deficiency
Nicotinamide deficiency
Pellagra (alcoholic)
EXCLUDES1 *sequelae of niacin deficiency (E64.8)*

E53 **Deficiency of** other B group vitamins
EXCLUDES1 *sequelae of vitamin B deficiency (E64.8)*
E53.0 Riboflavin **deficiency**   CC CC/MCC Exc
Ariboflavinosis
Vitamin B2 deficiency
E53.1 Pyridoxine **deficiency**
Vitamin B6 deficiency
EXCLUDES1 *pyridoxine-responsive sideroblastic anemia (D64.3)*
E53.8 **Deficiency of other specified B group vitamins**
Biotin deficiency
Cyanocobalamin deficiency
Folate deficiency
Folic acid deficiency
Pantothenic acid deficiency
Vitamin B12 deficiency
EXCLUDES1 *folate deficiency anemia (D52.-)*
vitamin B12 deficiency anemia (D51.-)
E53.9 **Vitamin B deficiency, unspecified**

E54 Ascorbic acid **deficiency**
Deficiency of vitamin C
Scurvy
EXCLUDES1 *scorbutic anemia (D53.2)*
sequelae of vitamin C deficiency (E64.2)

E55 Vitamin D **deficiency**
EXCLUDES1 *adult osteomalacia (M83.-)*
osteoporosis (M80.-)
sequelae of rickets (E64.3)
E55.0 **Rickets, active**   CC RxHCC CC/MCC Exc
Infantile osteomalacia
Juvenile osteomalacia
EXCLUDES1 *celiac rickets (K90.0)*
Crohn's rickets (K50.-)
hereditary vitamin D-dependent rickets (E83.32)
inactive rickets (E64.3)
renal rickets (N25.0)
sequelae of rickets (E64.3)
vitamin D-resistant rickets (E83.31)
E55.9 **Vitamin D deficiency, unspecified**
Avitaminosis D

E56 **Other vitamin deficiencies**
EXCLUDES1 *sequelae of other vitamin deficiencies (E64.8)*
E56.0 **Deficiency of** vitamin E
E56.1 **Deficiency of** vitamin K
EXCLUDES1 *deficiency of coagulation factor due to vitamin K deficiency (D68.4)*
vitamin K deficiency of newborn (P53)
E56.8 **Deficiency of other vitamins**
E56.9 **Vitamin deficiency, unspecified**

E58 Dietary calcium **deficiency**
EXCLUDES1 *disorders of calcium metabolism (E83.5-)*
sequelae of calcium deficiency (E64.8)

E59 Dietary selenium **deficiency**
Keshan disease
EXCLUDES1 *sequelae of selenium deficiency (E64.8)*

E60 Dietary zinc **deficiency**

E61 **Deficiency of** other nutrient elements
Use additional code for adverse effect, if applicable, to identify drug (T36-T50 with fifth or sixth character 5)
EXCLUDES1 *disorders of mineral metabolism (E83.-)*
iodine deficiency related thyroid disorders (E00-E02)
sequelae of malnutrition and other nutritional deficiencies (E64.-)
E61.0 Copper **deficiency**

E61.1 Iron **deficiency**
EXCLUDES1 *iron deficiency anemia (D50.-)*
E61.2 Magnesium **deficiency**
E61.3 Manganese **deficiency**
E61.4 Chromium **deficiency**
E61.5 Molybdenum **deficiency**
E61.6 Vanadium **deficiency**
E61.7 **Deficiency of** multiple nutrient elements
E61.8 **Deficiency of other specified nutrient elements**
E61.9 **Deficiency of nutrient element, unspecified**

E63 **Other nutritional deficiencies**
EXCLUDES1 *dehydration (E86.0)*
failure to thrive, adult (R62.7)
failure to thrive, child (R62.51)
feeding problems in newborn (P92.-)
sequelae of malnutrition and other nutritional deficiencies (E64.-)
E63.0 Essential fatty acid **[EFA] deficiency**
E63.1 **Imbalance of constituents of food intake**
E63.8 **Other specified nutritional deficiencies**
E63.9 **Nutritional deficiency, unspecified**

E64 **Sequelae of malnutrition and other nutritional deficiencies**
NOTES This category is to be used to indicate conditions in categories E43, E44, E46, E50-E63 as the cause of sequelae, which are themselves classified elsewhere. The 'sequelae' include conditions specified as such; they also include the late effects of diseases classifiable to the above categories if the disease itself is no longer present.
☞ **Code first** condition resulting from (sequela) of malnutrition and other nutritional deficiencies
E64.0 **Sequelae of** protein-calorie **malnutrition**   CC POA HCC CC/MCC Exc
EXCLUDES2 *retarded development following protein-calorie malnutrition (E45)*
E64.1 **Sequelae of** vitamin A **deficiency**   POA
E64.2 **Sequelae of** vitamin C **deficiency**   POA
E64.3 **Sequelae of** rickets   POA
E64.8 **Sequelae of other nutritional deficiencies**   POA
E64.9 **Sequelae of unspecified nutritional deficiency**   POA

Overweight, obesity and other hyperalimentation (E65-E68)

E65 **Localized adiposity**
Fat pad

E66 **Overweight and obesity**
☞ **Code first** obesity complicating pregnancy, childbirth and the puerperium, if applicable (O99.21-)
Use additional code to identify body mass index (BMI), if known (Z68.-)
EXCLUDES1 *adiposogenital dystrophy (E23.6)*
lipomatosis NOS (E88.2)
lipomatosis dolorosa [Dercum] (E88.2)
Prader-Willi syndrome ▶(Q87.11)◀
E66.0 **Obesity** due to excess calories
E66.01 **Morbid (severe) obesity due to excess calories**   HAC HCC RxHCC
AHA: Q4 2018
EXCLUDES1 *morbid (severe) obesity with alveolar hypoventilation (E66.2)*
E66.09 **Other obesity due to excess calories**   ?
E66.1 Drug-induced **obesity**   ?
Use additional code for adverse effect, if applicable, to identify drug (T36-T50 with fifth or sixth character 5)
E66.2 Morbid (severe) **obesity with alveolar hypoventilation**   CC HCC RxHCC CC/MCC Exc
Obesity hypoventilation syndrome (OHS)
Pickwickian syndrome
E66.3 **Overweight**
E66.8 **Other obesity**   ?
E66.9 **Obesity, unspecified**   ?
AHA: Q4 2013
Obesity NOS

POADx Unacceptable principal diagnosis symbol per Medicare code edits   POA Code exempt from diagnosis present on admission requirement
? Questionable admission   CC Complication or comorbidity   MCC Major complication or comorbidity   CC/MCC Exc CC/MCC exclusion
HCC HCC diagnosis code   RxHCC RxHCC diagnosis code   MACRA code   **DEFINITION** Describes condition/terminology
TIP Coding guidance   👁 Official Guideline Reference   Z1 Z code as first-listed diagnosis

E67 Other hyperalimentation

> EXCLUDES1   hyperalimentation NOS (R63.2)
>
> sequelae of hyperalimentation (E68)

E67.0 **Hypervitaminosis A**

E67.1 **Hypercarotenemia**

E67.2 **Megavitamin-B6 syndrome**

E67.3 **Hypervitaminosis D**

E67.8 Other specified hyperalimentation

E68 Sequelae of hyperalimentation

> ☞ **Code first** condition resulting from (sequela) of hyperalimentation

Metabolic disorders (E70-E88)

> EXCLUDES1   androgen insensitivity syndrome (E34.5-)
>
> congenital adrenal hyperplasia (E25.0)
>
> Ehlers-Danlos syndrome ▶(Q79.6-)◀
>
> hemolytic anemias attributable to enzyme disorders (D55.-)
>
> Marfan's syndrome (Q87.4)
>
> 5-alpha-reductase deficiency (E29.1)

E70 Disorders of aromatic amino-acid metabolism

E70.0 **Classical** phenylketonuria

E70.1 **Other** hyperphenylalaninemias

E70.2 **Disorders of** tyrosine metabolism

> EXCLUDES1   transitory tyrosinemia of newborn (P74.5)

E70.20 **Disorder of tyrosine metabolism, unspecified**

E70.21 **Tyrosinemia**

Hypertyrosinemia

E70.29 **Other disorders of tyrosine metabolism**

Alkaptonuria

Ochronosis

E70.3 Albinism

E70.30 **Albinism, unspecified**

E70.31 Ocular albinism

E70.310 X-linked ocular albinism

E70.311 Autosomal recessive ocular albinism

E70.318 **Other ocular albinism**

E70.319 **Ocular albinism, unspecified**

E70.32 Oculocutaneous albinism

> EXCLUDES1   Chediak-Higashi syndrome (E70.330)
>
> Hermansky-Pudlak syndrome (E70.331)

E70.320 Tyrosinase negative oculocutaneous albinism

Albinism I

Oculocutaneous albinism ty-neg

E70.321 Tyrosinase positive oculocutaneous albinism

Albinism II

Oculocutaneous albinism ty-pos

E70.328 **Other oculocutaneous albinism**

Cross syndrome

E70.329 **Oculocutaneous albinism, unspecified**

E70.33 Albinism with hematologic abnormality

E70.330 Chediak-Higashi syndrome

E70.331 Hermansky-Pudlak syndrome

E70.338 **Other albinism with hematologic abnormality**

E70.339 **Albinism with hematologic abnormality, unspecified**

E70.39 Other specified albinism

Piebaldism

E70.4 **Disorders of** histidine metabolism

E70.40 **Disorders of histidine metabolism, unspecified**

E70.41 Histidinemia

E70.49 **Other disorders of histidine metabolism**

E70.5 **Disorders of** tryptophan metabolism

E70.8 **Other disorders of aromatic amino-acid metabolism**

E70.9 **Disorder of aromatic amino-acid metabolism, unspecified**

E71 Disorders of branched-chain amino-acid metabolism and fatty-acid metabolism

E71.0 Maple-syrup-urine disease

E71.1 **Other disorders of** branched-chain **metabolism**

E71.11 **Branched-chain** organic acidurias

E71.110 Isovaleric acidemia

E71.111 3-methylglutaconic aciduria

E71.118 **Other branched-chain organic acidurias**

E71.12 **Disorders of** propionate metabolism

E71.120 Methylmalonic acidemia

E71.121 Propionic acidemia

E71.128 **Other disorders of propionate metabolism**

E71.19 **Other disorders of branched-chain amino-acid metabolism**

Hyperleucine-isoleucinemia

Hypervalinemia

E71.2 **Disorder of branched-chain amino-acid metabolism, unspecified**

E71.3 **Disorders of fatty-acid metabolism**

> EXCLUDES1   peroxisomal disorders (E71.5)
>
> Refsum's disease (G60.1)
>
> Schilder's disease (G37.0)
>
> EXCLUDES2   carnitine deficiency due to inborn error of metabolism (E71.42)

E71.30 **Disorder of fatty-acid metabolism, unspecified**

E71.31 Disorders of fatty-acid oxidation

E71.310 Long chain/very long chain acyl CoA dehydrogenase deficiency

LCAD

VLCAD

E71.311 Medium chain acyl CoA dehydrogenase deficiency

MCAD

E71.312 Short chain acyl CoA dehydrogenase deficiency

SCAD

E71.313 Glutaric aciduria type II

Glutaric aciduria type II A

Glutaric aciduria type II B

Glutaric aciduria type II C

> EXCLUDES1   glutaric aciduria (type 1) NOS (E72.3)

E71.314 Muscle carnitine palmitoyltransferase deficiency

E71.318 **Other disorders of fatty-acid oxidation**

E71.32 **Disorders of** ketone metabolism

E71.39 **Other disorders of fatty-acid metabolism**

E71.4 **Disorders of** carnitine metabolism

> EXCLUDES1   Muscle carnitine palmitoyltransferase deficiency (E71.314)

E71.40 **Disorder of carnitine metabolism, unspecified**

E71.41 Primary carnitine deficiency

E71.42 **Carnitine deficiency due to** inborn errors of metabolism

Code also associated inborn error or metabolism

E71.43 Iatrogenic carnitine deficiency

Carnitine deficiency due to hemodialysis

Carnitine deficiency due to Valproic acid therapy

Unspecified Code   Other Specified Code   Manifestation Code   Ⓝ Newborn   Ⓟ Pediatric   Ⓜ Maternity   Ⓐ Adult   ♂ Male   ♀ Female
● New Code   ▲ Revised Code Title   ▶◀ Revised Text   **NOTES**   *INCLUDES*   EXCLUDES1 Not coded here   EXCLUDES2 Not included here
🕪 4th character required   🕔 5th character required   🕕 6th character required   🕖 7th character required   🕗 Extension 'X' Alert
HAC Hospital-acquired condition (HAC) alert   **AHA** AHA Coding Clinic©   ☞ Code first alert

6ᵗʰ E71.44 Other secondary carnitine deficiency

E71.440 Ruvalcaba-Myhre-Smith syndrome `HCC` `RxHCC`

E71.448 Other secondary carnitine deficiency `HCC` `RxHCC`

5ᵗʰ E71.5 Peroxisomal disorders

EXCLUDES1 Schilder's disease (G37.0)

E71.50 Peroxisomal disorder, unspecified `CC` `HCC` `RxHCC` `CC/MCC Exc`

6ᵗʰ E71.51 Disorders of peroxisome biogenesis

Group 1 peroxisomal disorders

EXCLUDES1 Refsum's disease (G60.1)

E71.510 Zellweger syndrome `CC` `HCC` `RxHCC` `CC/MCC Exc`

E71.511 Neonatal adrenoleukodystrophy `CC` `HCC` `RxHCC` `CC/MCC Exc`

EXCLUDES1 X-linked adrenoleukodystrophy (E71.42-)

E71.518 Other disorders of peroxisome biogenesis `CC` `HCC` `RxHCC` `CC/MCC Exc`

6ᵗʰ E71.52 X-linked adrenoleukodystrophy

E71.520 Childhood cerebral X-linked adrenoleukodystrophy `CC` `HCC` `RxHCC` `CC/MCC Exc`

E71.521 Adolescent X-linked adrenoleukodystrophy `CC` `HCC` `RxHCC` `CC/MCC Exc`

E71.522 Adrenomyeloneuropathy `CC` `HCC` `RxHCC` `CC/MCC Exc`

E71.528 Other X-linked adrenoleukodystrophy `CC` `HCC` `RxHCC` `CC/MCC Exc`

Addison only phenotype adrenoleukodystrophy

Addison-Schilder adrenoleukodystrophy

E71.529 X-linked adrenoleukodystrophy, unspecified type `CC` `HCC` `RxHCC` `CC/MCC Exc`

E71.53 Other group 2 peroxisomal disorders `CC` `HCC` `RxHCC` `CC/MCC Exc`

6ᵗʰ E71.54 Other peroxisomal disorders

E71.540 Rhizomelic chondrodysplasia punctata `CC` `HCC` `RxHCC` `CC/MCC Exc`

EXCLUDES1 chondrodysplasia punctata NOS (Q77.3)

E71.541 Zellweger-like syndrome `CC` `HCC` `RxHCC` `CC/MCC Exc`

E71.542 Other group 3 peroxisomal disorders `CC` `HCC` `RxHCC` `CC/MCC Exc`

E71.548 Other peroxisomal disorders `CC` `HCC` `RxHCC` `CC/MCC Exc`

4ᵗʰ E72 Other disorders of amino-acid metabolism

EXCLUDES1 disorders of:

aromatic amino-acid metabolism (E70.-)

branched-chain amino-acid metabolism (E71.0-E71.2)

fatty-acid metabolism (E71.3)

purine and pyrimidine metabolism (E79.-)

gout (M1A.-, M10.-)

5ᵗʰ E72.0 Disorders of amino-acid transport

EXCLUDES1 disorders of tryptophan metabolism (E70.5)

E72.00 Disorders of amino-acid transport, unspecified `CC` `HCC` `RxHCC` `CC/MCC Exc`

E72.01 Cystinuria `CC` `HCC` `RxHCC` `CC/MCC Exc`

E72.02 Hartnup's disease `CC` `HCC` `RxHCC`

E72.03 Lowe's syndrome `CC` `HCC` `RxHCC`

Use additional code for associated glaucoma (H42)

E72.04 Cystinosis `CC` `HCC` `RxHCC` `CC/MCC Exc`

Fanconi (-de Toni) (-Debré) syndrome with cystinosis

EXCLUDES1 Fanconi (-de Toni) (-Debré) syndrome without cystinosis (E72.09)

E72.09 Other disorders of amino-acid transport `CC` `HCC` `RxHCC` `CC/MCC Exc`

Fanconi (-de Toni) (-Debré) syndrome, unspecified

5ᵗʰ E72.1 Disorders of sulfur-bearing amino-acid metabolism

EXCLUDES1 cystinosis (E72.04)

cystinuria (E72.01)

transcobalamin II deficiency (D51.2)

E72.10 Disorders of sulfur-bearing amino-acid metabolism, unspecified `CC` `HCC` `RxHCC` `CC/MCC Exc`

E72.11 Homocystinuria `CC` `HCC` `RxHCC` `CC/MCC Exc`

Cystathionine synthase deficiency

E72.12 Methylenetetrahydrofolate reductase deficiency `CC` `HCC` `RxHCC` `CC/MCC Exc`

E72.19 Other disorders of sulfur-bearing amino-acid metabolism `CC` `HCC` `RxHCC` `CC/MCC Exc`

Cystathioninuria

Methioninemia

Sulfite oxidase deficiency

5ᵗʰ E72.2 Disorders of urea cycle metabolism

EXCLUDES1 disorders of ornithine metabolism (E72.4)

E72.20 Disorder of urea cycle metabolism, unspecified `CC` `HCC` `RxHCC` `CC/MCC Exc`

Hyperammonemia

EXCLUDES1 hyperammonemia-hyperornithinemia-homocitrullinemia syndrome E72.4

transient hyperammonemia of newborn (P74.6)

E72.21 Argininemia `CC` `HCC` `RxHCC` `CC/MCC Exc`

E72.22 Arginosuccinic aciduria `CC` `HCC` `RxHCC` `CC/MCC Exc`

E72.23 Citrullinemia `CC` `HCC` `RxHCC` `CC/MCC Exc`

E72.29 Other disorders of urea cycle metabolism `CC` `HCC` `RxHCC` `CC/MCC Exc`

E72.3 Disorders of lysine and hydroxylysine metabolism `CC` `HCC` `RxHCC` `CC/MCC Exc`

Glutaric aciduria NOS

Glutaric aciduria (type I)

Hydroxylysinemia

Hyperlysinemia

EXCLUDES1 glutaric aciduria type II (E71.313)

Refsum's disease (G60.1)

Zellweger syndrome (E71.510)

E72.4 Disorders of ornithine metabolism `CC` `HCC` `RxHCC` `CC/MCC Exc`

Hyperammonemia-Hyperornithinemia-Homocitrullinemia syndrome

Ornithinemia (types I, II)

Ornithine transcarbamylase deficiency

EXCLUDES1 hereditary choroidal dystrophy (H31.2-)

5ᵗʰ E72.5 Disorders of glycine metabolism

E72.50 Disorder of glycine metabolism, unspecified `CC` `HCC` `RxHCC` `CC/MCC Exc`

E72.51 Non-ketotic hyperglycinemia `CC` `HCC` `RxHCC` `CC/MCC Exc`

E72.52 Trimethylaminuria `CC` `HCC` `RxHCC` `CC/MCC Exc`

E72.53 Primary hyperoxaluria `CC` `HCC` `RxHCC` `CC/MCC Exc`

AHA: Q4 2018

Oxalosis

Oxaluria

E72.59 Other disorders of glycine metabolism `CC` `HCC` `RxHCC` `CC/MCC Exc`

D-glycericacidemia

Hyperhydroxyprolinemia

Hyperprolinemia (types I, II)

Sarcosinemia

5ᵗʰ E72.8 Other specified disorders of amino-acid metabolism

E72.81 Disorders of gamma aminobutyric acid metabolism `CC` `HCC` `RxHCC` `CC/MCC Exc`

AHA: Q4 2018

4-hydroxybutyric aciduria

Disorders of GABA metabolism

GABA metabolic defect

GABA transaminase deficiency

GABA-T deficiency

Gamma-hydroxybutyric aciduria

SSADHD

Succinic semialdehyde dehydrogenase deficiency

E72.89 Other specified disorders of amino-acid metabolism `CC` `HCC` `RxHCC` `CC/MCC Exc`

AHA: Q4 2018

Disorders of beta-amino-acid metabolism

Disorders of gamma-glutamyl cycle

E72.9 Disorder of amino-acid metabolism, unspecified `CC` `HCC` `RxHCC` `CC/MCC Exc`

PDᵡ Unacceptable principal diagnosis symbol per Medicare code edits   POA Code exempt from diagnosis present on admission requirement

❓ Questionable admission   «CC» Complication or comorbidity   MCC Major complication or comorbidity   CC/MCC Exc CC/MCC exclusion

HCC HCC diagnosis code   RxHCC RxHCC diagnosis code   MACRA code MACRA code   **DEFINITION** Describes condition/terminology

TIP Coding guidance   ◉ Official Guideline Reference   Z1 Z code as first-listed diagnosis

534   When symbols appear on a code that requires a 7th character extension, refer to Appendix B to identify applicable 7th character codes.   **2020 ICD-10-CM**

[4th] **E73 Lactose intolerance**
- **E73.0 Congenital lactase deficiency**
- **E73.1 Secondary lactase deficiency**
- **E73.8 Other lactose intolerance**
- **E73.9 Lactose intolerance, unspecified**

[4th] **E74 Other disorders of carbohydrate metabolism**

[EXCLUDES1] *diabetes mellitus (E08-E13)*
hypoglycemia NOS (E16.2)
increased secretion of glucagon (E16.3)
mucopolysaccharidosis (E76.0-E76.3)

[5th] **E74.0 Glycogen storage disease**
- **E74.00 Glycogen storage disease, unspecified** [CC] [HCC] [RxHCC] [CC/MCC Exc]
- **E74.01 von Gierke disease** [CC] [HCC] [RxHCC] [CC/MCC Exc]
  Type I glycogen storage disease
- **E74.02 Pompe disease** [CC] [HCC] [RxHCC] [CC/MCC Exc]
  Cardiac glycogenosis
  Type II glycogen storage disease
- **E74.03 Cori disease** [CC] [HCC] [RxHCC] [CC/MCC Exc]
  Forbes disease
  Type III glycogen storage disease
- **E74.04 McArdle disease** [CC] [HCC] [RxHCC] [CC/MCC Exc]
  Type V glycogen storage disease
- **E74.09 Other glycogen storage disease** [CC] [HCC] [RxHCC] [CC/MCC Exc]
  Andersen disease
  Hers disease
  Tarui disease
  Glycogen storage disease, types 0, IV, VI-XI
  Liver phosphorylase deficiency
  Muscle phosphofructokinase deficiency

[5th] **E74.1 Disorders of fructose metabolism**

[EXCLUDES1] *muscle phosphofructokinase deficiency (E74.09)*
- **E74.10 Disorder of fructose metabolism, unspecified**
- **E74.11 Essential fructosuria**
  Fructokinase deficiency
- **E74.12 Hereditary fructose intolerance**
  Fructosemia
- **E74.19 Other disorders of fructose metabolism**
  Fructose-1, 6-diphosphatase deficiency

[5th] **E74.2 Disorders of galactose metabolism**
- **E74.20 Disorders of galactose metabolism, unspecified** [CC] [HCC] [RxHCC] [CC/MCC Exc]
- **E74.21 Galactosemia** [CC] [HCC] [RxHCC] [CC/MCC Exc]
- **E74.29 Other disorders of galactose metabolism** [CC] [HCC] [RxHCC] [CC/MCC Exc]
  Galactokinase deficiency

[5th] **E74.3 Other disorders of intestinal carbohydrate absorption**

[EXCLUDES2] *lactose intolerance (E73.-)*
- **E74.31 Sucrase-isomaltase deficiency**
- **E74.39 Other disorders of intestinal carbohydrate absorption**
  Disorder of intestinal carbohydrate absorption NOS
  Glucose-galactose malabsorption
  Sucrase deficiency

E74.4 Disorders of pyruvate metabolism and gluconeogenesis [CC] [HCC] [RxHCC] [CC/MCC Exc]
Deficiency of phosphoenolpyruvate carboxykinase
Deficiency of pyruvate carboxylase
Deficiency of pyruvate dehydrogenase

[EXCLUDES1] *disorders of pyruvate metabolism and gluconeogenesis with anemia (D55.-)*
Leigh's syndrome (G31.82)

E74.8 Other specified disorders of carbohydrate metabolism [CC] [HCC] [RxHCC] [CC/MCC Exc]
Essential pentosuria
Renal glycosuria

E74.9 Disorder of carbohydrate metabolism, unspecified [HCC] [RxHCC]

[4th] **E75 Disorders of sphingolipid metabolism and other lipid storage disorders**

[EXCLUDES1] *mucolipidosis, types I-III (E77.0-E77.1)*
Refsum's disease (G60.1)

[5th] **E75.0 GM2 gangliosidosis**
- **E75.00 GM2 gangliosidosis, unspecified** [CC] [HCC] [RxHCC] [CC/MCC Exc]
- **E75.01 Sandhoff disease** [CC] [HCC] [RxHCC] [CC/MCC Exc]
- **E75.02 Tay-Sachs disease** [CC] [HCC] [RxHCC] [CC/MCC Exc]
- **E75.09 Other GM2 gangliosidosis** [CC] [HCC] [RxHCC] [CC/MCC Exc]
  Adult GM2 gangliosidosis
  Juvenile GM2 gangliosidosis

[5th] **E75.1 Other and unspecified gangliosidosis**
- **E75.10 Unspecified gangliosidosis** [CC] [HCC] [RxHCC] [CC/MCC Exc]
  Gangliosidosis NOS
- **E75.11 Mucolipidosis IV** [CC] [HCC] [RxHCC] [CC/MCC Exc]
- **E75.19 Other gangliosidosis** [CC] [HCC] [RxHCC] [CC/MCC Exc]
  GM1 gangliosidosis
  GM3 gangliosidosis

[5th] **E75.2 Other sphingolipidosis**

[EXCLUDES1] *adrenoleukodystrophy [Addison-Schilder] (E71.528)*
- **E75.21 Fabry (-Anderson) disease** [HCC] [RxHCC]
- **E75.22 Gaucher disease** [HCC] [RxHCC]
- **E75.23 Krabbe disease** [CC] [HCC] [RxHCC] [CC/MCC Exc]
- [6th] **E75.24 Niemann-Pick disease**
  - **E75.240 Niemann-Pick disease type A** [HCC] [RxHCC]
  - **E75.241 Niemann-Pick disease type B** [HCC] [RxHCC]
  - **E75.242 Niemann-Pick disease type C** [HCC] [RxHCC]
  - **E75.243 Niemann-Pick disease type D** [HCC] [RxHCC]
  - **E75.248 Other Niemann-Pick disease** [HCC] [RxHCC]
  - **E75.249 Niemann-Pick disease, unspecified** [HCC] [RxHCC]
- **E75.25 Metachromatic leukodystrophy** [CC] [HCC] [RxHCC] [CC/MCC Exc]
- **E75.26 Sulfatase deficiency** [CC] [HCC] [RxHCC] [CC/MCC Exc]
  Multiple sulfatase deficiency (MSD)
- **E75.29 Other sphingolipidosis** [CC] [HCC] [RxHCC] [CC/MCC Exc]
  Farber's syndrome
  Sulfatide lipidosis

E75.3 Sphingolipidosis, unspecified [HCC] [RxHCC]

E75.4 Neuronal ceroid lipofuscinosis [CC] [HCC] [RxHCC] [CC/MCC Exc]
Batten disease
Bielschowsky-Jansky disease
Kufs disease
Spielmeyer-Vogt disease

E75.5 Other lipid storage disorders [RxHCC]
Cerebrotendinous cholesterosis [van Bogaert-Scherer-Epstein]
Wolman's disease

E75.6 Lipid storage disorder, unspecified [RxHCC]

[4th] **E76 Disorders of glycosaminoglycan metabolism**

[5th] **E76.0 Mucopolysaccharidosis, type I**
- **E76.01 Hurler's syndrome** [CC] [HCC] [RxHCC]
- **E76.02 Hurler-Scheie syndrome** [CC] [HCC] [RxHCC]
- **E76.03 Scheie's syndrome** [CC] [HCC] [RxHCC]

E76.1 Mucopolysaccharidosis, type II [CC] [HCC] [RxHCC]
Hunter's syndrome

[5th] **E76.2 Other mucopolysaccharidoses**
- [6th] **E76.21 Morquio mucopolysaccharidoses**
  - **E76.210 Morquio A mucopolysaccharidoses** [CC] [HCC] [RxHCC]
    Classic Morquio syndrome
    Morquio syndrome A
    Mucopolysaccharidosis, type IVA
  - **E76.211 Morquio B mucopolysaccharidoses** [CC] [HCC] [RxHCC]
    Morquio-like mucopolysaccharidoses
    Morquio-like syndrome
    Morquio syndrome B
    Mucopolysaccharidosis, type IVB
  - **E76.219 Morquio mucopolysaccharidoses, unspecified** [CC] [HCC] [RxHCC]
    Morquio syndrome
    Mucopolysaccharidosis, type IV
- **E76.22 Sanfilippo mucopolysaccharidoses** [CC] [HCC] [RxHCC]
  Mucopolysaccharidosis, type III (A) (B) (C) (D)
  Sanfilippo A syndrome
  Sanfilippo B syndrome
  Sanfilippo C syndrome
  Sanfilippo D syndrome

Unspecified Code | Other Specified Code | Manifestation Code | [N] Newborn | [P] Pediatric | [M] Maternity | [A] Adult | ♂ Male | ♀ Female
● New Code | ▲ Revised Code Title | ►◄ Revised Text | [NOTES] | [INCLUDES] | [EXCLUDES1] Not coded here | [EXCLUDES2] Not included here
[4th] 4th character required | [5th] 5th character required | [6th] 6th character required | [7th] 7th character required | [x] Extension 'X' Alert
[HAC] Hospital-acquired condition (HAC) alert | AHA AHA Coding Clinic© | Code first alert

E76.29 **Other mucopolysaccharidoses** `cc` `HCC` `RxHCC`
beta-Glucuronidase deficiency
Maroteaux-Lamy (mild) (severe) syndrome
Mucopolysaccharidosis, types VI, VII

E76.3 **Mucopolysaccharidosis, unspecified** `cc` `HCC` `RxHCC`

E76.8 **Other disorders of glucosaminoglycan metabolism** `cc` `HCC` `RxHCC`

E76.9 **Glucosaminoglycan metabolism disorder, unspecified** `cc` `HCC` `RxHCC`

4ᵗʰ **E77 Disorders of glycoprotein metabolism**

E77.0 **Defects in post-translational modification of lysosomal enzymes** `HCC` `RxHCC`
Mucolipidosis II [I-cell disease]
Mucolipidosis III [pseudo-Hurler polydystrophy]

E77.1 **Defects in glycoprotein degradation** `HCC` `RxHCC`
Aspartylglucosaminuria
Fucosidosis
Mannosidosis
Sialidosis [mucolipidosis I]

E77.8 **Other disorders of glycoprotein metabolism** `HCC` `RxHCC`

E77.9 **Disorder of glycoprotein metabolism, unspecified** `HCC` `RxHCC`

4ᵗʰ **E78 Disorders of lipoprotein metabolism and other lipidemias**

EXCLUDES1 sphingolipidosis (E75.0-E75.3)

5ᵗʰ **E78.0 Pure hypercholesterolemia**

E78.00 **Pure hypercholesterolemia, unspecified** `RxHCC`
AHA: Q4 2016
Fredrickson's hyperlipoproteinemia, type IIa
Hyperbetalipoproteinemia
Low-density-lipoprotein-type [LDL] hyperlipoproteinemia
(Pure) hypercholesterolemia NOS

E78.01 **Familial hypercholesterolemia** `RxHCC`
AHA: Q4 2016

E78.1 **Pure hyperglyceridemia** `RxHCC`
Elevated fasting triglycerides
Endogenous hyperglyceridemia
Fredrickson's hyperlipoproteinemia, type IV
Hyperlipidemia, group B
Hyperprebetalipoproteinemia
Very-low-density-lipoprotein-type [VLDL] hyperlipoproteinemia

E78.2 **Mixed hyperlipidemia** `RxHCC`
Broad- or floating-betalipoproteinemia
Combined hyperlipidemia NOS
Elevated cholesterol with elevated triglycerides NEC
Fredrickson's hyperlipoproteinemia, type IIb or III
Hyperbetalipoproteinemia with prebetalipoproteinemia
Hypercholesteremia with endogenous hyperglyceridemia
Hyperlipidemia, group C
Tubo-eruptive xanthoma
Xanthoma tuberosum
EXCLUDES1 cerebrotendinous cholesterosis [van Bogaert-Scherer- Epstein] (E75.5)
familial combined hyperlipidemia (E78.49)

E78.3 **Hyperchylomicronemia** `RxHCC`
Chylomicron retention disease
Fredrickson's hyperlipoproteinemia, type I or V
Hyperlipidemia, group D
Mixed hyperglyceridemia

5ᵗʰ **E78.4 Other hyperlipidemia**

E78.41 **Elevated Lipoprotein(a)** `RxHCC`
AHA: Q4 2018
Elevated Lp(a)

E78.49 **Other hyperlipidemia** `RxHCC`
AHA: Q4 2018
Familial combined hyperlipidemia

E78.5 **Hyperlipidemia, unspecified** `RxHCC`

E78.6 **Lipoprotein deficiency** `RxHCC`
Abetalipoproteinemia
Depressed HDL cholesterol
High-density lipoprotein deficiency
Hypoalphalipoproteinemia
Hypobetalipoproteinemia (familial)
Lecithin cholesterol acyltransferase deficiency
Tangier disease

5ᵗʰ **E78.7 Disorders of bile acid and cholesterol metabolism**
EXCLUDES1 Niemann-Pick disease type C (E75.242)

E78.70 **Disorder of bile acid and cholesterol metabolism, unspecified** `RxHCC`

E78.71 **Barth syndrome** `cc`

E78.72 **Smith-Lemli-Opitz syndrome** `cc`

E78.79 **Other disorders of bile acid and cholesterol metabolism** `RxHCC`

5ᵗʰ **E78.8 Other disorders of lipoprotein metabolism**

E78.81 **Lipoid dermatoarthritis** `RxHCC`

E78.89 **Other lipoprotein metabolism disorders** `RxHCC`

E78.9 **Disorder of lipoprotein metabolism, unspecified** `RxHCC`

4ᵗʰ **E79 Disorders of purine and pyrimidine metabolism**

EXCLUDES1 Ataxia-telangiectasia ▶(Q87.19)◀
Bloom's syndrome (Q82.8)
Cockayne's syndrome ▶(Q87.19)◀
calculus of kidney (N20.0)
combined immunodeficiency disorders (D81.-)
Fanconi's anemia (D61.09)
gout (M1A.-, M10.-)
orotaciduric anemia (D53.0)
progeria (E34.8)
Werner's syndrome (E34.8)
xeroderma pigmentosum (Q82.1)

E79.0 **Hyperuricemia without signs of inflammatory arthritis and tophaceous disease**
Asymptomatic hyperuricemia

E79.1 **Lesch-Nyhan syndrome** `cc` `HCC` `RxHCC`
HGPRT deficiency

E79.2 **Myoadenylate deaminase deficiency** `cc` `HCC` `RxHCC`

E79.8 **Other disorders of purine and pyrimidine metabolism** `cc` `HCC` `RxHCC`
Hereditary xanthinuria

E79.9 **Disorder of purine and pyrimidine metabolism, unspecified** `cc` `HCC` `RxHCC`

4ᵗʰ **E80 Disorders of porphyrin and bilirubin metabolism**

INCLUDES defects of catalase and peroxidase

E80.0 **Hereditary erythropoietic porphyria** `cc` `HCC` `RxHCC`
Congenital erythropoietic porphyria
Erythropoietic protoporphyria

E80.1 **Porphyria cutanea tarda** `cc` `HCC` `RxHCC`

5ᵗʰ **E80.2 Other and unspecified porphyria**

E80.20 **Unspecified porphyria** `cc` `HCC` `RxHCC`
Porphyria NOS

E80.21 **Acute intermittent (hepatic) porphyria** `cc` `HCC` `RxHCC`

E80.29 **Other porphyria** `cc` `HCC` `RxHCC`
Hereditary coproporphyria

E80.3 **Defects of catalase and peroxidase** `cc` `HCC` `RxHCC` `CC/MCC Exc`
Acatalasia [Takahara]

E80.4 **Gilbert syndrome**

E80.5 **Crigler-Najjar syndrome**

E80.6 **Other disorders of bilirubin metabolism**
Dubin-Johnson syndrome
Rotor's syndrome

E80.7 **Disorder of bilirubin metabolism, unspecified**

4ᵗʰ **E83 Disorders of mineral metabolism**

EXCLUDES1 dietary mineral deficiency (E58-E61)
parathyroid disorders (E20-E21)
vitamin D deficiency (E55.-)

5ᵗʰ **E83.0 Disorders of copper metabolism**

E83.00 **Disorder of copper metabolism, unspecified** `RxHCC`

E83.01 **Wilson's disease** `RxHCC`
Code also associated Kayser Fleischer ring (H18.04-)

E83.09 **Other disorders of copper metabolism** `RxHCC`
Menkes' (kinky hair) (steely hair) disease

5ᵗʰ **E83.1 Disorders of iron metabolism**

EXCLUDES1 iron deficiency anemia (D50.-)
sideroblastic anemia (D64.0-D64.3)

E83.10 **Disorder of iron metabolism, unspecified** `RxHCC`

PDᵃ Unacceptable principal diagnosis symbol per Medicare code edits   PDᵃ Code exempt from diagnosis present on admission requirement
❓ Questionable admission   `cc` Complication or comorbidity   MCC Major complication or comorbidity   cc/mcc Exc CC/MCC exclusion
`HCC` HCC diagnosis code   `RxHCC` RxHCC diagnosis code   MACRA code   **DEFINITION** Describes condition/terminology
TIP Coding guidance   👁 Official Guideline Reference   Z1 Z code as first-listed diagnosis

[6th] E83.11 **Hemochromatosis**
EXCLUDES1 *GALD (P78.84)*
Gestational alloimmune liver disease (P78.84)
Neonatal hemochromatosis (P78.84)
E83.110 **Hereditary hemochromatosis** [HCC] [RxHCC]
Bronzed diabetes
Pigmentary cirrhosis (of liver)
Primary (hereditary) hemochromatosis
E83.111 **Hemochromatosis due to repeated red blood cell transfusions** [CC] [CC/MCC Exc]
Iron overload due to repeated red blood cell transfusions
Transfusion (red blood cell) associated hemochromatosis
E83.118 **Other hemochromatosis** [RxHCC]
E83.119 **Hemochromatosis, unspecified** [RxHCC]
E83.19 **Other disorders of iron metabolism** [RxHCC]
Use additional code, if applicable, for idiopathic pulmonary hemosiderosis (J84.03)
E83.2 **Disorders of zinc metabolism**
Acrodermatitis enteropathica
[5th] E83.3 **Disorders of phosphorus metabolism and phosphatases**
EXCLUDES1 *adult osteomalacia (M83.-)*
osteoporosis (M80.-)
E83.30 **Disorder of phosphorus metabolism, unspecified** [RxHCC]
E83.31 **Familial hypophosphatemia** [RxHCC]
Vitamin D-resistant osteomalacia
Vitamin D-resistant rickets
EXCLUDES1 *vitamin D-deficiency rickets (E55.0)*
E83.32 **Hereditary vitamin D-dependent rickets (type 1) (type 2)** [RxHCC]
25-hydroxyvitamin D 1-alpha-hydroxylase deficiency
Pseudovitamin D deficiency
Vitamin D receptor defect
E83.39 **Other disorders of phosphorus metabolism** [CC] [RxHCC] [CC/MCC Exc]
Acid phosphatase deficiency
Hypophosphatasia
[5th] E83.4 **Disorders of magnesium metabolism**
E83.40 **Disorders of magnesium metabolism, unspecified**
E83.41 **Hypermagnesemia**
AHA: Q4 2016
E83.42 **Hypomagnesemia**
E83.49 **Other disorders of magnesium metabolism**
[5th] E83.5 **Disorders of calcium metabolism**
EXCLUDES1 *chondrocalcinosis (M11.1-M11.2)*
hungry bone syndrome (E83.81)
hyperparathyroidism (E21.0-E21.3)
E83.50 **Unspecified disorder of calcium metabolism**
E83.51 **Hypocalcemia** [CC] [CC/MCC Exc]
E83.52 **Hypercalcemia**
Familial hypocalciuric hypercalcemia
E83.59 **Other disorders of calcium metabolism**
[5th] E83.8 **Other disorders of mineral metabolism**
E83.81 **Hungry bone syndrome**
E83.89 **Other disorders of mineral metabolism**
E83.9 **Disorder of mineral metabolism, unspecified**
[4th] E84 **Cystic fibrosis**
INCLUDES *mucoviscidosis*
Code also exocrine pancreatic insufficiency (K86.81)
E84.0 **Cystic fibrosis with pulmonary manifestations** [HCC] [MCC] [RxHCC] [CC/MCC Exc]
Use additional code to identify any infectious organism present, such as:
Pseudomonas (B96.5)
[5th] E84.1 **Cystic fibrosis with intestinal manifestations**
E84.11 **Meconium ileus in cystic fibrosis** [N] [HCC] [MCC] [RxHCC] [CC/MCC Exc]
EXCLUDES1 *meconium ileus not due to cystic fibrosis (P76.0)*
E84.19 **Cystic fibrosis with other intestinal manifestations** [CC] [HCC] [RxHCC] [CC/MCC Exc]
Distal intestinal obstruction syndrome
E84.8 **Cystic fibrosis with other manifestations** [CC] [HCC] [RxHCC] [CC/MCC Exc]
E84.9 **Cystic fibrosis, unspecified** [CC] [HCC] [RxHCC] [CC/MCC Exc]
[4th] E85 **Amyloidosis**
DEFINITION: Amyloidosis is a rare disease caused by an abnormal protein (amyloid) that builds up in body tissues and organs.
EXCLUDES2 *Alzheimer's disease (G30.0-)*
E85.0 **Non-neuropathic heredofamilial amyloidosis** [CC] [HCC] [CC/MCC Exc]
Hereditary amyloid nephropathy
Code also associated disorders, such as:
autoinflammatory syndromes (M04.-)
EXCLUDES2 *Transthyretin-related (ATTR) familial amyloid cardiomyopathy (E85.4)*
E85.1 **Neuropathic heredofamilial amyloidosis** [CC] [HCC] [CC/MCC Exc]
AHA: Q4 2013
Amyloid polyneuropathy (Portuguese)
Transthyretin-related (ATTR) familial amyloid polyneuropathy
E85.2 **Heredofamilial amyloidosis, unspecified** [CC] [HCC] [CC/MCC Exc]
E85.3 **Secondary systemic amyloidosis** [CC] [HCC] [CC/MCC Exc]
Hemodialysis-associated amyloidosis
E85.4 **Organ-limited amyloidosis** [CC] [HCC] [CC/MCC Exc]
Localized amyloidosis
Transthyretin-related (ATTR) familial amyloid cardiomyopathy
[5th] E85.8 **Other amyloidosis**
E85.81 **Light chain (AL) amyloidosis** [CC] [HCC] [CC/MCC Exc]
AHA: Q4 2017
E85.82 **Wild-type transthyretin-related (ATTR) amyloidosis** [CC] [HCC] [CC/MCC Exc]
AHA: Q4 2017
Senile systemic amyloidosis (SSA)
E85.89 **Other amyloidosis** [CC] [HCC] [CC/MCC Exc]
AHA: Q4 2017
E85.9 **Amyloidosis, unspecified** [CC] [HCC] [CC/MCC Exc]
[4th] E86 **Volume depletion**
Use additional code(s) for any associated disorders of electrolyte and acid-base balance (E87.-)
EXCLUDES1 *dehydration of newborn (P74.1)*
hypovolemic shock NOS (R57.1)
postprocedural hypovolemic shock (T81.19)
traumatic hypovolemic shock (T79.4)
E86.0 **Dehydration**
AHA: Q2 2019
E86.1 **Hypovolemia**
Depletion of volume of plasma
E86.9 **Volume depletion, unspecified**
AHA: Q2 2019
[4th] E87 **Other disorders of fluid, electrolyte and acid-base balance**
EXCLUDES1 *diabetes insipidus (E23.2)*
electrolyte imbalance associated with hyperemesis gravidarum (O21.1)
electrolyte imbalance following ectopic or molar pregnancy (O08.5)
familial periodic paralysis (G72.3)
E87.0 **Hyperosmolality and hypernatremia** [CC] [CC/MCC Exc]
AHA: Q2 2018
Sodium [Na] excess
Sodium [Na] overload
E87.1 **Hypo-osmolality and hyponatremia** [CC] [CC/MCC Exc]
AHA: Q2 2018
Sodium [Na] deficiency
EXCLUDES1 *syndrome of inappropriate secretion of antidiuretic hormone (E22.2)*
E87.2 **Acidosis** [CC] [CC/MCC Exc]
Acidosis NOS
Lactic acidosis
Metabolic acidosis
Respiratory acidosis
EXCLUDES1 *diabetic acidosis - see categories E08-E10, E13 with ketoacidosis*

Unspecified Code | Other Specified Code | Manifestation Code | [N] Newborn | [P] Pediatric | [M] Maternity | [A] Adult | ♂ Male | ♀ Female
● New Code | ▲ Revised Code Title | ►◄ Revised Text | NOTES | INCLUDES | EXCLUDES1 Not coded here | EXCLUDES2 Not included here
[4th] 4th character required | [5th] 5th character required | [6th] 6th character required | [7th] 7th character required | [x] Extension 'X' Alert
[HAC] Hospital-acquired condition (HAC) alert | AHA AHA Coding Clinic© | ☛ Code first alert

E87.3 **Alkalosis** _CC_ _CC/MCC Exc_
  Alkalosis NOS
  Metabolic alkalosis
  Respiratory alkalosis

E87.4 **Mixed disorder of acid-base balance** _CC_ _CC/MCC Exc_

E87.5 **Hyperkalemia**
  Potassium [K] excess
  Potassium [K] overload

E87.6 **Hypokalemia**
  Potassium [K] deficiency

E87.7 **Fluid overload**
  EXCLUDES1 edema NOS (R60.9)
              fluid retention (R60.9)

  E87.70 **Fluid overload, unspecified**

  E87.71 **Transfusion associated circulatory overload**
    Fluid overload due to transfusion (blood) (blood components)
    TACO

  E87.79 **Other fluid overload**

E87.8 **Other disorders of electrolyte and fluid balance, not elsewhere classified**
  Electrolyte imbalance NOS
  Hyperchloremia
  Hypochloremia

E88 **Other and unspecified metabolic disorders**
  Use additional codes for associated conditions
  EXCLUDES1 histiocytosis X (chronic) (C96.6)

E88.0 **Disorders of plasma-protein metabolism, not elsewhere classified**
  EXCLUDES1 disorder of lipoprotein metabolism (E78.-)
              monoclonal gammopathy (of undetermined significance) (D47.2)
              polyclonal hypergammaglobulinemia (D89.0)
              Waldenström macroglobulinemia (C88.0)

  E88.01 **Alpha-1-antitrypsin deficiency** _HCC_ _RxHCC_
    AAT deficiency

  E88.02 **Plasminogen deficiency** _CC_ _CC/MCC Exc_
    AHA: Q4 2018
    Dysplasminogenemia
    Hypoplasminogenemia
    Type 1 plasminogen deficiency
    Type 2 plasminogen deficiency
    Code also, if applicable, ligneous conjunctivitis (H10.51)
    Use additional code for associated findings, such as:
      hydrocephalus (G91.4)
      otitis media (H67.-)
      respiratory disorder related to plasminogen deficiency (J99)

  E88.09 **Other disorders of plasma-protein metabolism, not elsewhere classified**
    Bisalbuminemia

E88.1 **Lipodystrophy, not elsewhere classified**
  Lipodystrophy NOS
  EXCLUDES1 Whipple's disease (K90.81)

E88.2 **Lipomatosis, not elsewhere classified** _RxHCC_
  Lipomatosis NOS
  Lipomatosis (Check) dolorosa [Dercum]

E88.3 **Tumor lysis syndrome** _MCC_ _CC/MCC Exc_
  AHA: Q2 2019
  Tumor lysis syndrome (spontaneous)
  Tumor lysis syndrome following antineoplastic drug chemotherapy
  Use additional code for adverse effect, if applicable, to identify drug (T45.1X5)

E88.4 **Mitochondrial metabolism disorders**
  EXCLUDES1 disorders of pyruvate metabolism (E74.4)
              Kearns-Sayre syndrome (H49.81)
              Leber's disease (H47.22)
              Leigh's encephalopathy (G31.82)
              Mitochondrial myopathy, NEC (G71.3)
              Reye's syndrome (G93.7)

  E88.40 **Mitochondrial metabolism disorder, unspecified** _CC_ _HCC_ _RxHCC_ _CC/MCC Exc_

  E88.41 **MELAS syndrome** _CC_ _HCC_ _RxHCC_ _CC/MCC Exc_
    Mitochondrial myopathy, encephalopathy, lactic acidosis and stroke-like episodes

  E88.42 **MERRF syndrome** _CC_ _HCC_ _RxHCC_ _CC/MCC Exc_
    Myoclonic epilepsy associated with ragged-red fibers
    Code also progressive myoclonic epilepsy (G40.3-)

  E88.49 **Other mitochondrial metabolism disorders** _CC_ _HCC_ _RxHCC_ _CC/MCC Exc_

E88.8 **Other specified metabolic disorders**

  E88.81 **Metabolic syndrome**
    Dysmetabolic syndrome X
    Use additional codes for associated manifestations, such as:
      obesity (E66.-)

  E88.89 **Other specified metabolic disorders** _HCC_ _RxHCC_
    Launois-Bensaude adenolipomatosis
    EXCLUDES1 adult pulmonary Langerhans cell histiocytosis (J84.82)

E88.9 **Metabolic disorder, unspecified**

Postprocedural endocrine and metabolic complications and disorders, not elsewhere classified (E89)

E89 **Postprocedural endocrine and metabolic complications and disorders, not elsewhere classified**
  EXCLUDES2 intraoperative complications of endocrine system organ or structure (E36.0-, E36.1-, E36.8)

E89.0 **Postprocedural hypothyroidism** _RxHCC_
  Postirradiation hypothyroidism
  Postsurgical hypothyroidism

E89.1 **Postprocedural hypoinsulinemia** _CC_ _CC/MCC Exc_
  See Official Guidelines "Secondary diabetes mellitus due to pancreatectomy" I.C.4.a.6.b.i
  Postpancreatectomy hyperglycemia
  Postsurgical hypoinsulinemia
  Use additional code, if applicable, to identify:
    acquired absence of pancreas (Z90.41-)
    diabetes mellitus (postpancreatectomy) (postprocedural) (E13.-)
    insulin use (Z79.4)
  EXCLUDES1 transient postprocedural hyperglycemia (R73.9)
              transient postprocedural hypoglycemia (E16.2)

E89.2 **Postprocedural hypoparathyroidism** _HCC_ _RxHCC_
  Parathyroprival tetany

E89.3 **Postprocedural hypopituitarism** _HCC_ _RxHCC_
  Postirradiation hypopituitarism

E89.4 **Postprocedural ovarian failure**

  E89.40 **Asymptomatic postprocedural ovarian failure** ♀
    Postprocedural ovarian failure NOS

  E89.41 **Symptomatic postprocedural ovarian failure** ♀
    Symptoms such as flushing, sleeplessness, headache, lack of concentration, associated with postprocedural menopause

E89.5 **Postprocedural testicular hypofunction** ♂

E89.6 **Postprocedural adrenocortical (-medullary) hypofunction** _CC_ _HCC_ _RxHCC_ _CC/MCC Exc_

E89.8 **Other postprocedural endocrine and metabolic complications and disorders**

  E89.81 **Postprocedural hemorrhage of an endocrine system organ or structure following a procedure**

    E89.810 **Postprocedural hemorrhage of an endocrine system organ or structure following an endocrine system procedure** _CC_ _CC/MCC Exc_

    E89.811 **Postprocedural hemorrhage of an endocrine system organ or structure following other procedure** _CC_ _CC/MCC Exc_

PDx Unacceptable principal diagnosis symbol per Medicare code edits   _POA_ Code exempt from diagnosis present on admission requirement
? Questionable admission   _CC_ Complication or comorbidity   _MCC_ Major complication or comorbidity   _CC/MCC Exc_ CC/MCC exclusion
HCC HCC diagnosis code   _RxHCC_ RxHCC diagnosis code   MACRA code   **DEFINITION** Describes condition/terminology
TIP Coding guidance   ◉ Official Guideline Reference   _Z1_ Z code as first-listed diagnosis

E89.82 Postprocedural hematoma and seroma of an endocrine system organ or structure

  E89.820 Postprocedural hematoma of an endocrine system organ or structure following an endocrine system procedure   CC CC/MCC Exc

  E89.821 Postprocedural hematoma of an endocrine system organ or structure following other procedure   CC CC/MCC Exc

  E89.822 Postprocedural seroma of an endocrine system organ or structure following an endocrine system procedure   CC CC/MCC Exc

  E89.823 Postprocedural seroma of an endocrine system organ or structure following other procedure   CC CC/MCC Exc

E89.89 Other postprocedural endocrine and metabolic complications and disorders   CC CC/MCC Exc

  Use additional code, if applicable, to further specify disorder

Unspecified Code Other Specified Code Manifestation Code Ⓝ Newborn Ⓟ Pediatric Ⓜ Maternity Ⓐ Adult ♂ Male ♀ Female
● New Code ▲ Revised Code Title ►◄ Revised Text **NOTES** *INCLUDES* *EXCLUDES1* Not coded here *EXCLUDES2* Not included here
4th character required 5th character required 6th character required 7th character required Extension 'X' Alert
HAC Hospital-acquired condition (HAC) alert AHA AHA Coding Clinic© Code first alert

2020 ICD-10-CM When symbols appear on a code that requires a 7th character extension, refer to Appendix B to identify applicable 7th character codes. **539**

NOTES

Chapter 5: Mental, Behavioral and Neurodevelopmental Disorders (F01-F99)

Mental, Behavioral and Neurodevelopmental disorders (F01-F99)

[INCLUDES] *disorders of psychological development*

[EXCLUDES2] *symptoms, signs and abnormal clinical laboratory findings, not elsewhere classified (R00-R99)*

This chapter contains the following blocks:

F01-F09	Mental disorders due to known physiological conditions
F10-F19	Mental and behavioral disorders due to psychoactive substance use
F20-F29	Schizophrenia, schizotypal, delusional, and other non-mood psychotic disorders
F30-F39	Mood [affective] disorders
F40-F48	Anxiety, dissociative, stress-related, somatoform and other nonpsychotic mental disorders
F50-F59	Behavioral syndromes associated with physiological disturbances and physical factors
F60-F69	Disorders of adult personality and behavior
F70-F79	Intellectual disabilities
F80-F89	Pervasive and specific developmental disorders
F90-F98	Behavioral and emotional disorders with onset usually occurring in childhood and adolescence
F99	Unspecified mental disorder

Mental disorders due to known physiological conditions (F01-F09)

[NOTES] This block comprises a range of mental disorders grouped together on the basis of their having in common a demonstrable etiology in cerebral disease, brain injury, or other insult leading to cerebral dysfunction. The dysfunction may be primary, as in diseases, injuries, and insults that affect the brain directly and selectively; or secondary, as in systemic diseases and disorders that attack the brain only as one of the multiple organs or systems of the body that are involved.

[4th] **F01 Vascular dementia**

Vascular dementia as a result of infarction of the brain due to vascular disease, including hypertensive cerebrovascular disease.

[INCLUDES] *arteriosclerotic dementia*

Code first the underlying physiological condition or sequelae of cerebrovascular disease.

[5th] **F01.5 Vascular dementia**

F01.50 **Vascular dementia** without behavioral disturbance [A] [HCC] [RxHCC]

AHA: Q4 2017

Major neurocognitive disorder without behavioral disturbance

F01.51 **Vascular dementia with behavioral disturbance** [A] [CC] [HCC] [RxHCC] [CC/MCC Exc]

AHA: Q4 2017

Major neurocognitive disorder due to vascular disease, with behavioral disturbance

Major neurocognitive disorder with aggressive behavior

Major neurocognitive disorder with combative behavior

Major neurocognitive disorder with violent behavior

Vascular dementia with aggressive behavior

Vascular dementia with combative behavior

Vascular dementia with violent behavior

Use additional code, if applicable, to identify wandering in vascular dementia (Z91.83)

[4th] **F02** Dementia **in other diseases classified elsewhere**

See Official Guidelines "Etiology/manifestation convention" I.A.13

[INCLUDES] *Major neurocognitive disorder in other diseases classified elsewhere*

Code first the underlying physiological condition, such as:

Alzheimer's (G30.-)
cerebral lipidosis (E75.4)
Creutzfeldt-Jakob disease (A81.0-)
dementia with Lewy bodies (G31.83)
dementia with Parkinsonism (G31.83)
epilepsy and recurrent seizures (G40.-)
frontotemporal dementia (G31.09)
hepatolenticular degeneration (E83.0)
human immunodeficiency virus [HIV] disease (B20)
Huntington's disease (G10)
hypercalcemia (E83.52)
hypothyroidism, acquired (E00-E03.-)
intoxications (T36-T65)
Jakob-Creutzfeldt disease (A81.0-)
multiple sclerosis (G35)
neurosyphilis (A52.17)
niacin deficiency [pellagra] (E52)
Parkinson's disease (G20)
Pick's disease (G31.01)
polyarteritis nodosa (M30.0)
prion disease (A81.9)
systemic lupus erythematosus (M32.-)
traumatic brain injury (S06.-)
trypanosomiasis (B56.-, B57.-)
vitamin B deficiency (E53.8)

[EXCLUDES2] *dementia in alcohol and psychoactive substance disorders (F10-F19, with .17, .27, .97)*

vascular dementia (F01.5-)

[5th] **F02.8 Dementia in other diseases classified elsewhere**

F02.80 **Dementia in other diseases classified elsewhere without behavioral disturbance** [HCC] [RxHCC]

See Official Guidelines "Etiology/manifestation convention" I.A.13

AHA: Q1 2017, Q4 2017, Q2 2016, Q4 2016

Dementia in other diseases classified elsewhere NOS

Major neurocognitive disorder in other diseases classified elsewhere

F02.81 **Dementia in other diseases classified elsewhere with behavioral disturbance** [CC] [HCC] [RxHCC] [CC/MCC Exc]

See Official Guidelines "Etiology/manifestation convention" I.A.13

AHA: Q1 2017, Q2 2017, Q4 2017

Dementia in other diseases classified elsewhere with aggressive behavior

Dementia in other diseases classified elsewhere with combative behavior

Dementia in other diseases classified elsewhere with violent behavior

Major neurocognitive disorder in other diseases classified elsewhere with aggressive behavior

Major neurocognitive disorder in other diseases classified elsewhere with combative behavior

Major neurocognitive disorder in other diseases classified elsewhere with violent behavior

Use additional code, if applicable, to identify wandering in dementia in conditions classified elsewhere (Z91.83)

[4th] **F03 Unspecified dementia**

Presenile dementia NOS

Presenile psychosis NOS

Primary degenerative dementia NOS

Senile dementia NOS

Senile dementia depressed or paranoid type

Senile psychosis NOS

[EXCLUDES1] *senility NOS (R41.81)*

[EXCLUDES2] *mild memory disturbance due to known physiological condition (F06.8)*

senile dementia with delirium or acute confusional state (F05)

Unspecified Code | Other Specified Code | Manifestation Code | [N] Newborn | [P] Pediatric | [M] Maternity | [A] Adult | ♂ Male | ♀ Female
● New Code | ▲ Revised Code Title | ►◄ Revised Text | [NOTES] | [INCLUDES] | [EXCLUDES1] Not coded here | [EXCLUDES2] Not included here
[4th] 4th character required | [5th] 5th character required | [6th] 6th character required | [7th] 7th character required | [X] Extension 'X' Alert
[HAC] Hospital-acquired condition (HAC) alert | AHA AHA Coding Clinic© | Code first alert

🔵 **F03.9 Unspecified dementia**
    F03.90 **Unspecified dementia without behavioral disturbance** A HCC RxHCC
        AHA: Q4 2017
        Dementia NOS
    F03.91 **Unspecified dementia with behavioral disturbance** A cc🔹 HCC RxHCC CC/MCC Exc
        AHA: Q4 2017
        Unspecified dementia with aggressive behavior
        Unspecified dementia with combative behavior
        Unspecified dementia with violent behavior
        Use additional code, if applicable, to identify wandering in unspecified dementia (Z91.83)

F04 Amnestic disorder due to known physiological condition HCC RxHCC
    AHA: Q4 2017
    Korsakov's psychosis or syndrome, nonalcoholic
    ☞ **Code first** the underlying physiological condition
    EXCLUDES1 amnesia NOS (R41.3)
        anterograde amnesia (R41.1)
        dissociative amnesia (F44.0)
        retrograde amnesia (R41.2)
    EXCLUDES2 alcohol-induced or unspecified Korsakov's syndrome (F10.26, F10.96)
        Korsakov's syndrome induced by other psychoactive substances (F13.26, F13.96, F19.16, F19.26, F19.96)

F05 Delirium due to known physiological condition cc🔹 CC/MCC Exc
    AHA: Q2 2019, Q4 2017
    Acute or subacute brain syndrome
    Acute or subacute confusional state (nonalcoholic)
    Acute or subacute infective psychosis
    Acute or subacute organic reaction
    Acute or subacute psycho-organic syndrome
    Delirium of mixed etiology
    Delirium superimposed on dementia
    Sundowning
    ☞ **Code first** the underlying physiological condition
    EXCLUDES1 delirium NOS (R41.0)
    EXCLUDES2 delirium tremens alcohol-induced or unspecified (F10.231, F10.921)

🔵 **F06 Other mental disorders due to known physiological condition**
    INCLUDES mental disorders due to endocrine disorder
        mental disorders due to exogenous hormone
        mental disorders due to exogenous toxic substance
        mental disorders due to primary cerebral disease
        mental disorders due to somatic illness
        mental disorders due to systemic disease affecting the brain
    ☞ **Code first** the underlying physiological condition
    EXCLUDES1 unspecified dementia (F03)
    EXCLUDES2 delirium due to known physiological condition (F05)
        dementia as classified in F01-F02
        other mental disorders associated with alcohol and other psychoactive substances (F10-F19)

    F06.0 **Psychotic disorder with hallucinations due to known physiological condition** cc🔹 CC/MCC Exc
        AHA: Q4 2017
        Organic hallucinatory state (nonalcoholic)
        EXCLUDES2 hallucinations and perceptual disturbance induced by alcohol and other psychoactive substances (F10-F19 with .151, .251, .951)
            schizophrenia (F20.-)

    F06.1 **Catatonic disorder due to known physiological condition**
        AHA: Q4 2017
        Catatonia associated with another mental disorder
        Catatonia NOS
        EXCLUDES1 catatonic stupor (R40.1)
            stupor NOS (R40.1)
        EXCLUDES2 catatonic schizophrenia (F20.2)
            dissociative stupor (F44.2)

    F06.2 **Psychotic disorder with delusions due to known physiological condition** cc🔹 CC/MCC Exc
        AHA: Q4 2017
        Paranoid and paranoid-hallucinatory organic states
        Schizophrenia-like psychosis in epilepsy
        EXCLUDES2 alcohol and drug-induced psychotic disorder (F10-F19 with .150, .250, .950)
            brief psychotic disorder (F23)
            delusional disorder (F22)
            schizophrenia (F20.-)

🔵   F06.3 **Mood disorder due to known physiological condition**
        EXCLUDES2 mood disorders due to alcohol and other psychoactive substances (F10-F19 with .14, .24, .94)
            mood disorders, not due to known physiological condition or unspecified (F30-F39)
    F06.30 **Mood disorder due to known physiological condition, unspecified** cc🔹 CC/MCC Exc
        AHA: Q4 2017
    F06.31 **Mood disorder due to known physiological condition with depressive features** cc🔹 CC/MCC Exc
        AHA: Q4 2017
        Depressive disorder due to known physiological condition, with depressive features
    F06.32 **Mood disorder due to known physiological condition with major depressive-like episode**
        AHA: Q4 2017
        Depressive disorder due to known physiological condition, with major depressive-like episode
    F06.33 **Mood disorder due to known physiological condition with manic features**
        AHA: Q4 2017
        Bipolar and related disorder due to a known physiological condition, with manic features
        Bipolar and related disorder due to known physiological condition, with manic- or hypomanic-like episodes
    F06.34 **Mood disorder due to known physiological condition with mixed features**
        AHA: Q4 2017
        Bipolar and related disorder due to known physiological condition, with mixed features
        Depressive disorder due to known physiological condition, with mixed features

    F06.4 **Anxiety disorder due to known physiological condition** cc🔹 CC/MCC Exc
        AHA: Q4 2017
        EXCLUDES2 anxiety disorders due to alcohol and other psychoactive substances (F10-F19 with .180, .280, .980)
            anxiety disorders, not due to known physiological condition or unspecified (F40.-, F41.-)

    F06.8 **Other specified mental disorders due to known physiological condition**
        AHA: Q4 2017
        Epileptic psychosis NOS
        Obsessive-compulsive and related disorder due to a known physiological condition
        Organic dissociative disorder
        Organic emotionally labile [asthenic] disorder

🔵 **F07 Personality and behavioral disorders due to known physiological condition**
    ☞ **Code first** the underlying physiological condition
    F07.0 **Personality change due to known physiological condition**
        AHA: Q4 2017
        Frontal lobe syndrome
        Limbic epilepsy personality syndrome
        Lobotomy syndrome
        Organic personality disorder
        Organic pseudopsychopathic personality
        Organic pseudoretarded personality
        Postleucotomy syndrome
        ☞ **Code first** underlying physiological condition
        EXCLUDES1 mild cognitive impairment (G31.84)

Pᴅᵪ Unacceptable principal diagnosis symbol per Medicare code edits   Pᴏᵪ Code exempt from diagnosis present on admission requirement
❓ Questionable admission   cc Complication or comorbidity   MCC Major complication or comorbidity   CC/MCC CC/MCC exclusion
HCC HCC diagnosis code   RxHCC RxHCC diagnosis code   MACRA code   **DEFINITION** Describes condition/terminology
TIP Coding guidance   👁 Official Guideline Reference   Z code as first-listed diagnosis

542   When symbols appear on a code that requires a 7th character extension, refer to Appendix B to identify applicable 7th character codes.   **2020 ICD-10-CM**

postconcussional syndrome (F07.81)

postencephalitic syndrome (F07.89)

signs and symptoms involving emotional state (R45.-)

EXCLUDES2 specific personality disorder (F60.-)

5ᵗʰ **F07.8** Other **personality and behavioral disorders due to known physiological condition**

F07.81 **Postconcussional syndrome** cc⊘ CC/MCC Exc

AHA: Q4 2017

Postcontusional syndrome (encephalopathy)

Post-traumatic brain syndrome, nonpsychotic

Use additional code to identify associated post-traumatic headache, if applicable (G44.3-)

EXCLUDES1 current concussion (brain) (S06.0-)

postencephalitic syndrome (F07.89)

F07.89 **Other personality and behavioral disorders due to known physiological condition** PDxIn

AHA: Q4 2017

Postencephalitic syndrome

Right hemispheric organic affective disorder

F07.9 **Unspecified personality and behavioral disorder due to known physiological condition**

AHA: Q4 2017

Organic psychosyndrome

F09 **Unspecified mental disorder due to known physiological condition** cc⊘ CC/MCC Exc

AHA: Q4 2017

Mental disorder NOS due to known physiological condition

Organic brain syndrome NOS

Organic mental disorder NOS

Organic psychosis NOS

Symptomatic psychosis NOS

☛ **Code first** the underlying physiological condition

EXCLUDES1 psychosis NOS (F29)

Mental and behavioral disorders due to psychoactive substance use (F10-F19)

👁 **See Official Guidelines** "Mental and behavioral disorders due to psychoactive substance use" I.C.5.b.1, "Alcohol use during pregnancy, childbirth and the puerperium" I.C.15. l.1

4ᵗʰ **F10** **Alcohol related disorders**

Use additional code for blood alcohol level, if applicable (Y90.-)

5ᵗʰ **F10.1** **Alcohol** abuse

EXCLUDES1 alcohol dependence (F10.2-)

alcohol use, unspecified (F10.9-)

F10.10 **Alcohol abuse, uncomplicated**

AHA: Q4 2017

Alcohol use disorder, mild

F10.11 **Alcohol** abuse, in remission

AHA: Q4 2017

Alcohol use disorder, mild, in early remission

Alcohol use disorder, mild, in sustained remission

6ᵗʰ **F10.12** **Alcohol abuse with** intoxication

F10.120 **Alcohol abuse with intoxication, uncomplicated** HCC

AHA: Q4 2017

F10.121 **Alcohol abuse with intoxication delirium** cc⊘ HCC CC/MCC Exc

AHA: Q4 2017

F10.129 **Alcohol abuse with intoxication, unspecified** HCC

AHA: Q4 2017

F10.14 **Alcohol abuse with alcohol-induced mood disorder** cc⊘ HCC CC/MCC Exc

AHA: Q4 2017

Alcohol use disorder, mild, with alcohol-induced bipolar or related disorder

Alcohol use disorder, mild, with alcohol-induced depressive disorder

6ᵗʰ **F10.15** **Alcohol abuse with** alcohol-induced psychotic disorder

F10.150 **Alcohol abuse with alcohol-induced psychotic disorder with** delusions HCC

AHA: Q4 2017

F10.151 **Alcohol abuse with alcohol-induced psychotic disorder with** hallucinations cc⊘ HCC CC/MCC Exc

AHA: Q4 2017

F10.159 **Alcohol abuse with alcohol-induced psychotic disorder, unspecified** cc⊘ HCC CC/MCC Exc

AHA: Q4 2017

6ᵗʰ **F10.18** **Alcohol abuse with** other alcohol-induced disorders

F10.180 **Alcohol abuse with alcohol-induced anxiety disorder** cc⊘ HCC CC/MCC Exc

AHA: Q4 2017

F10.181 **Alcohol abuse with alcohol-induced sexual dysfunction** cc⊘ HCC CC/MCC Exc

AHA: Q4 2017

F10.182 **Alcohol abuse with alcohol-induced sleep disorder** HCC

AHA: Q4 2017

F10.188 **Alcohol abuse with other alcohol-induced disorder** cc⊘ HCC CC/MCC Exc

AHA: Q4 2017

F10.19 **Alcohol abuse with unspecified alcohol-induced disorder** HCC

AHA: Q4 2017

5ᵗʰ **F10.2** **Alcohol** dependence

EXCLUDES1 alcohol abuse (F10.1-)

alcohol use, unspecified (F10.9-)

EXCLUDES2 toxic effect of alcohol (T51.0-)

F10.20 **Alcohol dependence, uncomplicated** HCC

AHA: Q4 2017

Alcohol use disorder, moderate

Alcohol use disorder, severe

F10.21 **Alcohol dependence, in remission** HCC

AHA: Q4 2017

Alcohol use disorder, moderate, in early remission

Alcohol use disorder, moderate, in sustained remission

Alcohol use disorder, severe, in early remission

Alcohol use disorder, severe, in sustained remission

6ᵗʰ **F10.22** **Alcohol dependence** with intoxication

Acute drunkenness (in alcoholism)

EXCLUDES2 alcohol dependence with withdrawal (F10.23-)

F10.220 **Alcohol dependence with intoxication, uncomplicated** HCC

AHA: Q4 2017

F10.221 **Alcohol dependence with intoxication delirium** cc⊘ HCC CC/MCC Exc

AHA: Q4 2017

F10.229 **Alcohol dependence with intoxication, unspecified** HCC

AHA: Q4 2017

6ᵗʰ **F10.23** **Alcohol dependence with** withdrawal

EXCLUDES2 Alcohol dependence with intoxication (F10.22-)

F10.230 **Alcohol dependence with withdrawal, uncomplicated** cc⊘ HCC CC/MCC Exc

AHA: Q4 2017

F10.231 **Alcohol dependence with withdrawal delirium** cc⊘ HCC CC/MCC Exc

AHA: Q4 2017

F10.232 **Alcohol dependence with withdrawal with perceptual disturbance** cc⊘ HCC CC/MCC Exc

AHA: Q4 2017

F10.239 **Alcohol dependence with withdrawal, unspecified** cc⊘ HCC CC/MCC Exc

AHA: Q4 2017, Q2 2015

F10.24 **Alcohol dependence with alcohol-induced** mood disorder cc⊘ HCC CC/MCC Exc

AHA: Q4 2017

Alcohol use disorder, moderate, with alcohol-induced bipolar or related disorder

---

Unspecified Code	Other Specified Code	Manifestation Code	Ⓝ Newborn	Ⓟ Pediatric	Ⓜ Maternity	Ⓐ Adult	♂ Male	♀ Female

● New Code ▲ Revised Code Title ▶◀ Revised Text **NOTES** *INCLUDES* EXCLUDES1 Not coded here EXCLUDES2 Not included here

4ᵗʰ 4ᵗʰ character required 5ᵗʰ 5ᵗʰ character required 6ᵗʰ 6ᵗʰ character required 7ᵗʰ 7ᵗʰ character required 7ˣ Extension 'X' Alert

HAC Hospital-acquired condition (HAC) alert **AHA** AHA Coding Clinic© ☛ **Code first** alert

Alcohol use disorder, moderate, with alcohol-induced depressive disorder

Alcohol use disorder, severe, with alcohol-induced bipolar or related disorder

Alcohol use disorder, severe, with alcohol-induced depressive disorder

6ᵗʰ **F10.25** **Alcohol dependence with alcohol-induced** psychotic disorder

    F10.250 **Alcohol dependence with alcohol-induced psychotic disorder** with delusions **HCC**
      AHA: Q4 2017

    F10.251 **Alcohol dependence with alcohol-induced psychotic disorder** with hallucinations **cᶜ HCC cc/mcc exc**
      AHA: Q4 2017

    F10.259 **Alcohol dependence with alcohol-induced psychotic disorder, unspecified** **cᶜ HCC cc/mcc exc**
      AHA: Q4 2017

  F10.26 **Alcohol dependence with alcohol-induced** persisting amnestic disorder **HCC**
    AHA: Q4 2017
    Alcohol use disorder, moderate, with alcohol-induced major neurocognitive disorder, amnestic-confabulatory type
    Alcohol use disorder, severe, with alcohol-induced major neurocognitive disorder, amnestic-confabulatory type

  F10.27 **Alcohol dependence with alcohol-induced** persisting dementia **cᶜ HCC cc/mcc exc**
    AHA: Q4 2017
    Alcohol use disorder, moderate, with alcohol-induced major neurocognitive disorder, nonamnestic-confabulatory type
    Alcohol use disorder, severe, with alcohol-induced major neurocognitive disorder, nonamnestic-confabulatory type

6ᵗʰ **F10.28** **Alcohol dependence with** other alcohol-induced disorders

    F10.280 **Alcohol dependence with alcohol-induced** anxiety disorder **cᶜ HCC cc/mcc exc**
      AHA: Q4 2017

    F10.281 **Alcohol dependence with alcohol-induced** sexual dysfunction **cᶜ HCC cc/mcc exc**
      AHA: Q4 2017

    F10.282 **Alcohol dependence with alcohol-induced** sleep disorder **HCC**
      AHA: Q4 2017

    F10.288 **Alcohol dependence with other alcohol-induced disorder** **cᶜ HCC cc/mcc exc**
      AHA: Q4 2017
      Alcohol use disorder, moderate, with alcohol-induced mild neurocognitive disorder
      Alcohol use disorder, severe, with alcohol-induced mild neurocognitive disorder

  F10.29 **Alcohol dependence with unspecified alcohol-induced disorder** **cᶜ HCC cc/mcc exc**
    AHA: Q4 2017

5ᵗʰ **F10.9** **Alcohol** use, unspecified
    👁 **See Official Guidelines** "Psychoactive Substance Use, Unspecified" I.C.5.b.3
    EXCLUDES1 alcohol abuse (F10.1-)
             alcohol dependence (F10.2-)

6ᵗʰ **F10.92** **Alcohol use, unspecified** with intoxication
    F10.920 **Alcohol use, unspecified with intoxication,** uncomplicated **HCC**
      AHA: Q4 2017

    F10.921 **Alcohol use, unspecified with intoxication** delirium **cᶜ HCC cc/mcc exc**
      AHA: Q4 2017

    F10.929 **Alcohol use, unspecified with intoxication, unspecified** **HCC**
      AHA: Q4 2017

F10.94 **Alcohol use, unspecified with alcohol-induced mood disorder** **cᶜ HCC cc/mcc exc**
  AHA: Q4 2017
  Alcohol induced bipolar or related disorder, without use disorder
  Alcohol induced depressive disorder, without use disorder

6ᵗʰ **F10.95** **Alcohol use, unspecified with** alcohol-induced psychotic disorder

    F10.950 **Alcohol use, unspecified with alcohol-induced psychotic disorder** with delusions **HCC**
      AHA: Q4 2017

    F10.951 **Alcohol use, unspecified with alcohol-induced psychotic disorder** with hallucinations **cᶜ HCC cc/mcc exc**
      AHA: Q4 2017

    F10.959 **Alcohol use, unspecified with alcohol-induced psychotic disorder, unspecified** **cᶜ HCC cc/mcc exc**
      AHA: Q4 2017
      Alcohol-induced psychotic disorder without use disorder

  F10.96 **Alcohol use, unspecified with** alcohol-induced persisting amnestic disorder **HCC**
    AHA: Q4 2017
    Alcohol-induced major neurocognitive disorder, amnestic-confabulatory type, without use disorder

  F10.97 **Alcohol use, unspecified** with alcohol-induced persisting dementia **HCC**
    AHA: Q4 2017
    Alcohol-induced major neurocognitive disorder, nonamnestic-confabulatory type, without use disorder

6ᵗʰ **F10.98** **Alcohol use, unspecified with** other alcohol-induced disorders

    F10.980 **Alcohol use, unspecified with alcohol-induced** anxiety disorder **cᶜ HCC cc/mcc exc**
      AHA: Q4 2017
      Alcohol induced anxiety disorder, without use disorder

    F10.981 **Alcohol use, unspecified with alcohol-induced** sexual dysfunction **cᶜ HCC cc/mcc exc**
      AHA: Q4 2017
      Alcohol induced sexual dysfunction, without use disorder

    F10.982 **Alcohol use, unspecified with alcohol-induced** sleep disorder **HCC**
      AHA: Q4 2017
      Alcohol induced sleep disorder, without use disorder

    F10.988 **Alcohol use, unspecified with** other alcohol-induced disorder **cᶜ HCC cc/mcc exc**
      AHA: Q4 2017
      Alcohol induced mild neurocognitive disorder, without use disorder

  F10.99 **Alcohol use, unspecified with unspecified alcohol-induced disorder** **HCC**
    AHA: Q4 2017

4ᵗʰ **F11** Opioid related disorders
  👁 **See Official Guidelines** "Drug use during pregnancy, childbirth, and the puerperium" I.C.15.I.3

5ᵗʰ **F11.1** Opioid abuse
    EXCLUDES1 opioid dependence (F11.2-)
             opioid use, unspecified (F11.9-)

    F11.10 **Opioid abuse,** uncomplicated **HCC**
      AHA: Q4 2017
      Opioid use disorder, mild

    F11.11 **Opioid** abuse, **in remission** **HCC**
      AHA: Q4 2017
      Opioid use disorder, mild, in early remission
      Opioid use disorder, mild, in sustained remission

6ᵗʰ **F11.12** **Opioid abuse** with intoxication
    F11.120 **Opioid abuse with intoxication,** uncomplicated **HCC**
      AHA: Q4 2017

PDₓ Unacceptable principal diagnosis symbol per Medicare code edits POA Code exempt from diagnosis present on admission requirement
❓ Questionable admission cᶜ Complication or comorbidity MCC Major complication or comorbidity cc/mcc exc CC/MCC exclusion
HCC HCC diagnosis code RxHCC RxHCC diagnosis code MACRA code **DEFINITION** Describes condition/terminology
TIP Coding guidance 👁 Official Guideline Reference Zⁱ Z code as first-listed diagnosis

F11.121 Opioid abuse with intoxication
delirium `cc` `HCC` `CC/MCC Exc`
AHA: Q4 2017

F11.122 Opioid abuse with intoxication with
perceptual disturbance `HCC`
AHA: Q4 2017

F11.129 Opioid abuse with intoxication,
unspecified `HCC`
AHA: Q4 2017

F11.14 Opioid abuse with opioid-induced
mood disorder `HCC`
AHA: Q4 2017
Opioid use disorder, mild, with opioid-induced
depressive disorder

6th **F11.15** Opioid abuse with opioid-induced psychotic
disorder

F11.150 Opioid abuse with opioid-induced
psychotic disorder with
delusions `cc` `HCC` `CC/MCC Exc`
AHA: Q4 2017

F11.151 Opioid abuse with opioid-induced
psychotic disorder with
hallucinations `cc` `HCC` `CC/MCC Exc`
AHA: Q4 2017

F11.159 Opioid abuse with opioid-induced
psychotic disorder, unspecified `HCC`
AHA: Q4 2017

6th **F11.18** Opioid abuse with other opioid-induced disorder

F11.181 Opioid abuse with opioid-induced sexual
dysfunction `HCC`
AHA: Q4 2017

F11.182 Opioid abuse with opioid-induced sleep
disorder `HCC`
AHA: Q4 2017

F11.188 Opioid abuse with other opioid-induced
disorder `HCC`
AHA: Q4 2017

F11.19 Opioid abuse with unspecified opioid-induced
disorder `HCC`
AHA: Q4 2017

5th **F11.2** Opioid dependence

EXCLUDES1 opioid abuse (F11.1-)
opioid use, unspecified (F11.9-)
EXCLUDES2 opioid poisoning (T40.0-T40.2-)

F11.20 Opioid dependence, uncomplicated `cc` `HCC`
AHA: Q4 2017
Opioid use disorder, moderate
Opioid use disorder, severe

F11.21 Opioid dependence, in remission `HCC`
AHA: Q4 2017
Opioid use disorder, moderate, in early remission
Opioid use disorder, moderate, in sustained remission
Opioid use disorder, severe, in early remission
Opioid use disorder, severe, in sustained remission

6th **F11.22** Opioid dependence with intoxication

EXCLUDES1 opioid dependence with withdrawal
(F11.23)

F11.220 Opioid dependence with intoxication,
uncomplicated `HCC`
AHA: Q4 2017

F11.221 Opioid dependence with intoxication
delirium `cc` `HCC` `CC/MCC Exc`
AHA: Q4 2017

F11.222 Opioid dependence with intoxication with
perceptual disturbance `cc` `HCC`
AHA: Q4 2017

F11.229 Opioid dependence with intoxication,
unspecified `HCC`
AHA: Q4 2017

F11.23 Opioid dependence with withdrawal `cc` `HCC` `CC/MCC Exc`
AHA: Q4 2017

EXCLUDES1 opioid dependence with intoxication
(F11.22-)

F11.24 Opioid dependence with opioid-induced mood
disorder `HCC`
AHA: Q4 2017
Opioid use disorder, moderate, with opioid induced
depressive disorder

6th **F11.25** Opioid dependence with opioid-induced psychotic
disorder

F11.250 Opioid dependence with opioid-induced
psychotic disorder with
delusions `cc` `HCC` `CC/MCC Exc`
AHA: Q4 2017

F11.251 Opioid dependence with opioid-induced
psychotic disorder with
hallucinations `cc` `HCC` `CC/MCC Exc`
AHA: Q4 2017

F11.259 Opioid dependence with opioid-induced
psychotic disorder, unspecified `cc` `HCC`
AHA: Q4 2017

6th **F11.28** Opioid dependence with other opioid-induced
disorder

F11.281 Opioid dependence with opioid-induced
sexual dysfunction `cc` `HCC`
AHA: Q4 2017

F11.282 Opioid dependence with opioid-induced
sleep disorder `cc` `HCC`
AHA: Q4 2017

F11.288 Opioid dependence with other opioid-
induced disorder `cc` `HCC`
AHA: Q4 2017

F11.29 Opioid dependence with unspecified opioid-
induced disorder `HCC`
AHA: Q4 2017

5th **F11.9** Opioid use, unspecified

👁 See Official Guidelines "Psychoactive Substance Use,
Unspecified" I.C.5.b.3
EXCLUDES1 opioid abuse (F11.1-)
opioid dependence (F11.2-)

F11.90 Opioid use, unspecified, uncomplicated
AHA: Q4 2017

6th **F11.92** Opioid use, unspecified with intoxication

EXCLUDES1 opioid use, unspecified with withdrawal
(F11.93)

F11.920 Opioid use, unspecified with intoxication,
uncomplicated `HCC`
AHA: Q4 2017

F11.921 Opioid use, unspecified with intoxication
delirium `cc` `HCC` `CC/MCC Exc`
AHA: Q4 2017
Opioid-induced delirium

F11.922 Opioid use, unspecified with intoxication
with perceptual disturbance `HCC`
AHA: Q4 2017

F11.929 Opioid use, unspecified with intoxication,
unspecified `HCC`
AHA: Q4 2017

F11.93 Opioid use, unspecified with withdrawal `cc` `HCC` `CC/MCC Exc`
AHA: Q4 2017

EXCLUDES1 opioid use, unspecified with intoxication
(F11.92-)

F11.94 Opioid use, unspecified with opioid-induced mood
disorder `HCC`
AHA: Q4 2017
Opioid induced depressive disorder, without use
disorder

6th **F11.95** Opioid use, unspecified with opioid-induced
psychotic disorder

F11.950 Opioid use, unspecified with opioid-
induced psychotic disorder with
delusions `cc` `HCC` `CC/MCC Exc`
AHA: Q4 2017

Unspecified Code	Other Specified Code	Manifestation Code N Newborn P Pediatric M Maternity A Adult ♂ Male ♀ Female

● New Code ▲ Revised Code Title ▶◀ Revised Text **NOTES** *INCLUDES* *EXCLUDES1* Not coded here *EXCLUDES2* Not included here
4th 4th character required **5th** 5th character required **6th** 6th character required **7th** 7th character required Extension 'X' Alert
HAC Hospital-acquired condition (HAC) alert **AHA** AHA Coding Clinic® 📭 Code first alert

F11.951 **Opioid use, unspecified with opioid-induced psychotic disorder with** hallucinations ㏄ HCC CC/MCC Exc
AHA: Q4 2017

F11.959 **Opioid use, unspecified with opioid-induced psychotic disorder, unspecified** HCC
AHA: Q4 2017

6ᵗʰ **F11.98** **Opioid use, unspecified with** other specified opioid-induced disorder

F11.981 **Opioid use, unspecified with opioid-induced** sexual dysfunction HCC
AHA: Q4 2017
Opioid induced sexual dysfunction, without use disorder

F11.982 **Opioid use, unspecified with opioid-induced** sleep disorder HCC
AHA: Q4 2017
Opioid induced sleep disorder, without use disorder

F11.988 **Opioid use, unspecified with other opioid-induced disorder** HCC
AHA: Q4 2017
Opioid induced anxiety disorder, without use disorder

F11.99 **Opioid use, unspecified with unspecified opioid-induced disorder** HCC
AHA: Q4 2017

4ᵗʰ **F12** Cannabis **related disorders**
👁 **See Official Guidelines** "Alcohol use during pregnancy, childbirth and the puerperium" I.C.15.a.6.l.1
INCLUDES marijuana

5ᵗʰ **F12.1** **Cannabis** abuse
EXCLUDES1 cannabis dependence (F12.2-)
cannabis use, unspecified (F12.9-)

F12.10 **Cannabis abuse,** uncomplicated
AHA: Q4 2017
Cannabis use disorder, mild

F12.11 **Cannabis** abuse, **in remission**
AHA: Q4 2017
Cannabis use disorder, mild, in early remission
Cannabis use disorder, mild, in sustained remission

6ᵗʰ **F12.12** **Cannabis abuse** with intoxication

F12.120 **Cannabis abuse with intoxication,** uncomplicated HCC
AHA: Q4 2017

F12.121 **Cannabis abuse with intoxication** delirium ㏄ HCC CC/MCC Exc
AHA: Q4 2017

F12.122 **Cannabis abuse with intoxication with** perceptual disturbance HCC
AHA: Q4 2017

F12.129 **Cannabis abuse with intoxication,** unspecified HCC
AHA: Q4 2017

6ᵗʰ **F12.15** Cannabis abuse with psychotic disorder

F12.150 **Cannabis abuse with psychotic disorder with** delusions ㏄ HCC CC/MCC Exc
AHA: Q4 2017

F12.151 **Cannabis abuse with psychotic disorder with** hallucinations ㏄ HCC CC/MCC Exc
AHA: Q4 2017

F12.159 **Cannabis abuse with psychotic disorder, unspecified** HCC
AHA: Q4 2017

6ᵗʰ **F12.18** Cannabis abuse with other cannabis-induced disorder

F12.180 **Cannabis abuse with cannabis-induced** anxiety disorder HCC
AHA: Q4 2017

F12.188 **Cannabis abuse with other cannabis-induced disorder** HCC
AHA: Q4 2017
Cannabis use disorder, mild, with cannabis-induced sleep disorder

F12.19 **Cannabis abuse with unspecified cannabis-induced disorder** HCC
AHA: Q4 2017

5ᵗʰ **F12.2** **Cannabis** dependence
EXCLUDES1 cannabis abuse (F12.1-)
cannabis use, unspecified (F12.9-)
EXCLUDES2 cannabis poisoning (T40.7-)

F12.20 **Cannabis dependence,** uncomplicated HCC
AHA: Q4 2017
Cannabis use disorder, moderate
Cannabis use disorder, severe

F12.21 **Cannabis dependence,** in remission HCC
AHA: Q4 2017
Cannabis use disorder, moderate, in early remission
Cannabis use disorder, moderate, in sustained remission
Cannabis use disorder, severe, in early remission
Cannabis use disorder, severe, in sustained remission

6ᵗʰ **F12.22** **Cannabis dependence** with intoxication

F12.220 **Cannabis dependence with intoxication,** uncomplicated HCC

F12.221 **Cannabis dependence with intoxication** delirium ㏄ HCC CC/MCC Exc
AHA: Q4 2017

F12.222 **Cannabis dependence with intoxication with** perceptual disturbance HCC
AHA: Q4 2017

F12.229 **Cannabis dependence with intoxication,** unspecified HCC
AHA: Q4 2017

F12.23 **Cannabis dependence** with withdrawal HCC
AHA: Q4 2018

6ᵗʰ **F12.25** **Cannabis dependence** with psychotic disorder

F12.250 **Cannabis dependence with psychotic disorder with** delusions ㏄ HCC CC/MCC Exc
AHA: Q4 2017

F12.251 **Cannabis dependence with psychotic disorder with** hallucinations ㏄ HCC CC/MCC Exc
AHA: Q4 2017

F12.259 **Cannabis dependence with psychotic disorder, unspecified** HCC
AHA: Q4 2017

6ᵗʰ **F12.28** Cannabis dependence with other cannabis-induced disorder

F12.280 **Cannabis dependence with cannabis-induced** anxiety disorder HCC
AHA: Q4 2017

F12.288 **Cannabis dependence with other cannabis-induced disorder** HCC
AHA: Q4 2017
Cannabis use disorder, moderate, with cannabis-induced sleep disorder
Cannabis use disorder, severe, with cannabis-induced sleep disorder

F12.29 **Cannabis dependence with unspecified cannabis-induced disorder** HCC
AHA: Q4 2017

5ᵗʰ **F12.9** **Cannabis** use, **unspecified**
👁 **See Official Guidelines** "Psychoactive Substance Use, Unspecified" I.C.5.b.3
EXCLUDES1 cannabis abuse (F12.1-)
cannabis dependence (F12.2-)

F12.90 **Cannabis use, unspecified,** uncomplicated
AHA: Q4 2017

6ᵗʰ **F12.92** **Cannabis use, unspecified** with intoxication

F12.920 **Cannabis use, unspecified with intoxication,** uncomplicated HCC
AHA: Q4 2017

F12.921 **Cannabis use, unspecified with intoxication** delirium ㏄ HCC CC/MCC Exc
AHA: Q4 2017

PDxⁿ Unacceptable principal diagnosis symbol per Medicare code edits   ⒫ Code exempt from diagnosis present on admission requirement
? Questionable admission   ㏄ Complication or comorbidity   MCC Major complication or comorbidity   CC/MCC Exc CC/MCC exclusion
HCC HCC diagnosis code   RxHCC RxHCC diagnosis code   MACRA code   **DEFINITION** Describes condition/terminology
TIP Coding guidance   👁 Official Guideline Reference   Z1 Z code as first-listed diagnosis

546   When symbols appear on a code that requires a 7th character extension, refer to Appendix B to identify applicable 7th character codes.   **2020 ICD-10-CM**

F12.922 **Cannabis use, unspecified with intoxication with** perceptual disturbance `HCC`
  AHA: Q4 2017

F12.929 **Cannabis use, unspecified with intoxication, unspecified** `HCC`
  AHA: Q4 2017

F12.93 **Cannabis use, unspecified** with withdrawal `HCC`
  AHA: Q4 2018

6ᵗʰ F12.95 **Cannabis use, unspecified with** psychotic disorder

F12.950 **Cannabis use, unspecified with psychotic disorder with** delusions `cc` `HCC` `CC/MCC Exc`
  AHA: Q4 2017

F12.951 **Cannabis use, unspecified with psychotic disorder with** hallucinations `cc` `HCC` `CC/MCC Exc`
  AHA: Q4 2017

F12.959 **Cannabis use, unspecified with psychotic disorder, unspecified** `HCC`
  AHA: Q4 2017
  Cannabis induced psychotic disorder, without use disorder

6ᵗʰ F12.98 **Cannabis use, unspecified with** other cannabis-induced disorder

F12.980 **Cannabis use, unspecified with** anxiety disorder `HCC`
  AHA: Q4 2017
  Cannabis induced anxiety disorder, without use disorder

F12.988 **Cannabis use, unspecified with other cannabis-induced disorder** `HCC`
  AHA: Q4 2017
  Cannabis induced sleep disorder, without use disorder

F12.99 **Cannabis use, unspecified with unspecified cannabis-induced disorder** `HCC`
  AHA: Q4 2017

4ᵗʰ **F13** Sedative, hypnotic, or anxiolytic related disorders
  👁 **See Official Guidelines** "Alcohol use during pregnancy, childbirth and the puerperium" I.C.15.a.6.l.1

5ᵗʰ F13.1 **Sedative, hypnotic or anxiolytic-related** abuse
  EXCLUDES1 sedative, hypnotic or anxiolytic-related dependence (F13.2-)
        sedative, hypnotic, or anxiolytic use, unspecified (F13.9-)

F13.10 **Sedative, hypnotic or anxiolytic abuse,** uncomplicated `HCC`
  AHA: Q4 2017
  Sedative, hypnotic, or anxiolytic use disorder, mild

F13.11 **Sedative, hypnotic or anxiolytic** abuse, **in remission** `HCC`
  AHA: Q4 2017
  Sedative, hypnotic or anxiolytic use disorder, mild, in early remission
  Sedative, hypnotic or anxiolytic use disorder, mild, in sustained remission

6ᵗʰ F13.12 **Sedative, hypnotic or anxiolytic abuse** with intoxication

F13.120 **Sedative, hypnotic or anxiolytic abuse with intoxication,** uncomplicated `HCC`
  AHA: Q4 2017

F13.121 **Sedative, hypnotic or anxiolytic abuse with intoxication** delirium `cc` `HCC` `CC/MCC Exc`
  AHA: Q4 2017

F13.129 **Sedative, hypnotic or anxiolytic abuse with intoxication, unspecified** `HCC`
  AHA: Q4 2017

F13.14 **Sedative, hypnotic or anxiolytic abuse with sedative, hypnotic or anxiolytic-induced** mood disorder `HCC`
  AHA: Q4 2017
  Sedative, hypnotic, or anxiolytic use disorder, mild, with sedative, hypnotic, or anxiolytic-induced bipolar or related disorder
  Sedative, hypnotic, or anxiolytic use disorder, mild, with sedative, hypnotic, or anxiolytic-induced depressive disorder

6ᵗʰ F13.15 **Sedative, hypnotic or anxiolytic abuse with sedative, hypnotic or anxiolytic-induced** psychotic disorder

F13.150 **Sedative, hypnotic or anxiolytic abuse with sedative, hypnotic or anxiolytic-induced psychotic disorder with** delusions `cc` `HCC` `CC/MCC Exc`
  AHA: Q4 2017

F13.151 **Sedative, hypnotic or anxiolytic abuse with sedative, hypnotic or anxiolytic-induced psychotic disorder with** hallucinations `cc` `HCC` `CC/MCC Exc`
  AHA: Q4 2017

F13.159 **Sedative, hypnotic or anxiolytic abuse with sedative, hypnotic or anxiolytic-induced psychotic disorder, unspecified** `HCC`
  AHA: Q4 2017

6ᵗʰ F13.18 **Sedative, hypnotic or anxiolytic abuse with** other sedative, hypnotic or anxiolytic-induced disorders

F13.180 **Sedative, hypnotic or anxiolytic abuse with sedative, hypnotic or anxiolytic-induced** anxiety disorder `HCC`
  AHA: Q4 2017

F13.181 **Sedative, hypnotic or anxiolytic abuse with sedative, hypnotic or anxiolytic-induced** sexual dysfunction `HCC`
  AHA: Q4 2017

F13.182 **Sedative, hypnotic or anxiolytic abuse with sedative, hypnotic or anxiolytic-induced** sleep disorder `HCC`
  AHA: Q4 2017

F13.188 **Sedative, hypnotic or anxiolytic abuse with other sedative, hypnotic or anxiolytic-induced disorder** `HCC`
  AHA: Q4 2017

F13.19 **Sedative, hypnotic or anxiolytic abuse with unspecified sedative, hypnotic or anxiolytic-induced disorder** `HCC`
  AHA: Q4 2017

5ᵗʰ F13.2 **Sedative, hypnotic or anxiolytic-related** dependence
  EXCLUDES1 sedative, hypnotic or anxiolytic-related abuse (F13.1-)
        sedative, hypnotic, or anxiolytic use, unspecified (F13.9-)
  EXCLUDES2 sedative, hypnotic, or anxiolytic poisoning (T42.-)

F13.20 **Sedative, hypnotic or anxiolytic dependence,** uncomplicated `cc` `HCC`
  AHA: Q4 2017

F13.21 **Sedative, hypnotic or anxiolytic dependence,** in remission `HCC`
  AHA: Q4 2017
  Sedative, hypnotic or anxiolytic use disorder, moderate, in early remission
  Sedative, hypnotic or anxiolytic use disorder, moderate, in sustained remission
  Sedative, hypnotic or anxiolytic use disorder, severe, in early remission
  Sedative, hypnotic or anxiolytic use disorder, severe, in sustained remission

6ᵗʰ F13.22 **Sedative, hypnotic or anxiolytic dependence** with intoxication
  EXCLUDES1 sedative, hypnotic or anxiolytic dependence with withdrawal (F13.23-)

F13.220 **Sedative, hypnotic or anxiolytic dependence with intoxication,** uncomplicated `HCC`
  AHA: Q4 2017

F13.221 **Sedative, hypnotic or anxiolytic dependence with intoxication** delirium `cc` `HCC` `CC/MCC Exc`
  AHA: Q4 2017

F13.229 **Sedative, hypnotic or anxiolytic dependence with intoxication, unspecified** `HCC`
  AHA: Q4 2017

[6th] **F13.23 Sedative, hypnotic or anxiolytic dependence with withdrawal**
Sedative, hypnotic, or anxiolytic use disorder, moderate
Sedative, hypnotic, or anxiolytic use disorder, severe
[EXCLUDES1] *sedative, hypnotic or anxiolytic dependence with intoxication (F13.22-)*

F13.230 Sedative, hypnotic or anxiolytic dependence with withdrawal, uncomplicated [CC] [HCC] [CC/MCC Exc]
AHA: Q4 2017

F13.231 Sedative, hypnotic or anxiolytic dependence with withdrawal delirium [CC] [HCC] [CC/MCC Exc]
AHA: Q4 2017

F13.232 Sedative, hypnotic or anxiolytic dependence with withdrawal with perceptual disturbance [CC] [HCC] [CC/MCC Exc]
AHA: Q4 2017
Sedative, hypnotic, or anxiolytic withdrawal with perceptual disturbances

F13.239 Sedative, hypnotic or anxiolytic dependence with withdrawal, unspecified [CC] [HCC] [CC/MCC Exc]
AHA: Q4 2017
Sedative, hypnotic, or anxiolytic withdrawal without perceptual disturbances

F13.24 Sedative, hypnotic or anxiolytic dependence with sedative, hypnotic or anxiolytic-induced mood disorder [HCC]
AHA: Q4 2017
Sedative, hypnotic, or anxiolytic use disorder, moderate, with sedative, hypnotic, or anxiolytic-induced bipolar or related disorder
Sedative, hypnotic, or anxiolytic use disorder, moderate, with sedative, hypnotic, or anxiolytic-induced depressive disorder
Sedative, hypnotic, or anxiolytic use disorder, severe, with sedative, hypnotic, or anxiolytic-induced bipolar or related disorder
Sedative, hypnotic, or anxiolytic use disorder, severe, with sedative, hypnotic, or anxiolytic-induced depressive disorder

[6th] **F13.25 Sedative, hypnotic or anxiolytic dependence with sedative, hypnotic or anxiolytic-induced psychotic disorder**

F13.250 Sedative, hypnotic or anxiolytic dependence with sedative, hypnotic or anxiolytic-induced psychotic disorder with delusions [CC] [HCC] [CC/MCC Exc]
AHA: Q4 2017

F13.251 Sedative, hypnotic or anxiolytic dependence with sedative, hypnotic or anxiolytic-induced psychotic disorder with hallucinations [CC] [HCC] [CC/MCC Exc]
AHA: Q4 2017

F13.259 Sedative, hypnotic or anxiolytic dependence with sedative, hypnotic or anxiolytic-induced psychotic disorder, unspecified [CC] [HCC]
AHA: Q4 2017

F13.26 Sedative, hypnotic or anxiolytic dependence with sedative, hypnotic or anxiolytic-induced persisting amnestic disorder [CC] [HCC]
AHA: Q4 2017

F13.27 Sedative, hypnotic or anxiolytic dependence with sedative, hypnotic or anxiolytic-induced persisting dementia [CC] [HCC] [CC/MCC Exc]
AHA: Q4 2017
Sedative, hypnotic, or anxiolytic use disorder, moderate, with sedative, hypnotic, or anxiolytic-induced major neurocognitive disorder
Sedative, hypnotic, or anxiolytic use disorder, severe, with sedative, hypnotic, or anxiolytic-induced major neurocognitive disorder

[6th] **F13.28 Sedative, hypnotic or anxiolytic dependence with other sedative, hypnotic or anxiolytic-induced disorders**

F13.280 Sedative, hypnotic or anxiolytic dependence with sedative, hypnotic or anxiolytic-induced anxiety disorder [CC] [HCC]
AHA: Q4 2017

F13.281 Sedative, hypnotic or anxiolytic dependence with sedative, hypnotic or anxiolytic-induced sexual dysfunction [CC] [HCC]
AHA: Q4 2017

F13.282 Sedative, hypnotic or anxiolytic dependence with sedative, hypnotic or anxiolytic-induced sleep disorder [CC] [HCC]
AHA: Q4 2017

F13.288 Sedative, hypnotic or anxiolytic dependence with other sedative, hypnotic or anxiolytic-induced disorder [CC] [HCC]
AHA: Q4 2017
Sedative, hypnotic, or anxiolytic use disorder, moderate, with sedative, hypnotic, or anxiolytic-induced mild neurocognitive disorder
Sedative, hypnotic, or anxiolytic use disorder, severe, with sedative, hypnotic, or anxiolytic-induced mild neurocognitive disorder

F13.29 Sedative, hypnotic or anxiolytic dependence with unspecified sedative, hypnotic or anxiolytic-induced disorder [HCC]
AHA: Q4 2017

[5th] **F13.9 Sedative, hypnotic or anxiolytic-related use, unspecified**
👁 **See Official Guidelines** "Psychoactive Substance Use, Unspecified" I.C.5.b.3
[EXCLUDES1] *sedative, hypnotic or anxiolytic-related abuse (F13.1-)*
sedative, hypnotic or anxiolytic-related dependence (F13.2-)

F13.90 Sedative, hypnotic, or anxiolytic use, unspecified, uncomplicated
AHA: Q4 2017

[6th] **F13.92 Sedative, hypnotic or anxiolytic use, unspecified with intoxication**
[EXCLUDES1] *sedative, hypnotic or anxiolytic use, unspecified with withdrawal (F13.93-)*

F13.920 Sedative, hypnotic or anxiolytic use, unspecified with intoxication, uncomplicated [HCC]
AHA: Q4 2017

F13.921 Sedative, hypnotic or anxiolytic use, unspecified with intoxication delirium [CC] [HCC] [CC/MCC Exc]
AHA: Q4 2017
Sedative, hypnotic, or anxiolytic-induced delirium

F13.929 Sedative, hypnotic or anxiolytic use, unspecified with intoxication, unspecified [HCC]
AHA: Q4 2017

[6th] **F13.93 Sedative, hypnotic or anxiolytic use, unspecified with withdrawal**
[EXCLUDES1] *sedative, hypnotic or anxiolytic use, unspecified with intoxication (F13.92-)*

F13.930 Sedative, hypnotic or anxiolytic use, unspecified with withdrawal, uncomplicated [CC] [HCC] [CC/MCC Exc]
AHA: Q4 2017

F13.931 Sedative, hypnotic or anxiolytic use, unspecified with withdrawal delirium [CC] [HCC] [CC/MCC Exc]
AHA: Q4 2017

F13.932 Sedative, hypnotic or anxiolytic use, unspecified with withdrawal with perceptual disturbances [CC] [HCC] [CC/MCC Exc]
AHA: Q4 2017

[PDx] Unacceptable principal diagnosis symbol per Medicare code edits [POA] Code exempt from diagnosis present on admission requirement
[?] Questionable admission [CC] Complication or comorbidity [MCC] Major complication or comorbidity [CC/MCC Exc] CC/MCC exclusion
[HCC] HCC diagnosis code [RxHCC] RxHCC diagnosis code MACRA code **DEFINITION** Describes condition/terminology
TIP Coding guidance 👁 Official Guideline Reference [Z-1] Z code as first-listed diagnosis

F13.939 **Sedative, hypnotic or anxiolytic use, unspecified with withdrawal, unspecified** [CC] [HCC] [CC/MCC Exc]
AHA: Q4 2017

F13.94 **Sedative, hypnotic or anxiolytic use, unspecified with sedative, hypnotic or anxiolytic-induced mood disorder** [HCC]
AHA: Q4 2017
Sedative, hypnotic, or anxiolytic-induced bipolar or related disorder, without use disorder
Sedative, hypnotic, or anxiolytic-induced depressive disorder, without use disorder

[6th] F13.95 **Sedative, hypnotic or anxiolytic use, unspecified with sedative, hypnotic or anxiolytic-induced psychotic disorder**

F13.950 **Sedative, hypnotic or anxiolytic use, unspecified with sedative, hypnotic or anxiolytic-induced psychotic disorder with delusions** [CC] [HCC] [CC/MCC Exc]
AHA: Q4 2017

F13.951 **Sedative, hypnotic or anxiolytic use, unspecified with sedative, hypnotic or anxiolytic-induced psychotic disorder with hallucinations** [CC] [HCC] [CC/MCC Exc]
AHA: Q4 2017

F13.959 **Sedative, hypnotic or anxiolytic use, unspecified with sedative, hypnotic or anxiolytic-induced psychotic disorder, unspecified** [HCC]
AHA: Q4 2017
Sedative, hypnotic, or anxiolytic-induced psychotic disorder, without use disorder

F13.96 **Sedative, hypnotic or anxiolytic use, unspecified with sedative, hypnotic or anxiolytic-induced persisting amnestic disorder** [HCC]
AHA: Q4 2017

F13.97 **Sedative, hypnotic or anxiolytic use, unspecified with sedative, hypnotic or anxiolytic-induced persisting dementia** [CC] [HCC] [CC/MCC Exc]
AHA: Q4 2017
Sedative, hypnotic, or anxiolytic-induced major neurocognitive disorder, without use disorder

[6th] F13.98 **Sedative, hypnotic or anxiolytic use, unspecified with other sedative, hypnotic or anxiolytic-induced disorders**

F13.980 **Sedative, hypnotic or anxiolytic use, unspecified with sedative, hypnotic or anxiolytic-induced anxiety disorder** [HCC]
AHA: Q4 2017
Sedative, hypnotic, or anxiolytic-induced anxiety disorder, without use disorder

F13.981 **Sedative, hypnotic or anxiolytic use, unspecified with sedative, hypnotic or anxiolytic-induced sexual dysfunction** [HCC]
AHA: Q4 2017
Sedative, hypnotic, or anxiolytic-induced sexual dysfunction disorder, without use disorder

F13.982 **Sedative, hypnotic or anxiolytic use, unspecified with sedative, hypnotic or anxiolytic-induced sleep disorder** [HCC]
AHA: Q4 2017
Sedative, hypnotic, or anxiolytic-induced sleep disorder, without use disorder

F13.988 **Sedative, hypnotic or anxiolytic use, unspecified with other sedative, hypnotic or anxiolytic-induced disorder** [HCC]
AHA: Q4 2017
Sedative, hypnotic, or anxiolytic-induced mild neurocognitive disorder

F13.99 **Sedative, hypnotic or anxiolytic use, unspecified with unspecified sedative, hypnotic or anxiolytic-induced disorder** [HCC]
AHA: Q4 2017

[4th] F14 **Cocaine related disorders**
See Official Guidelines "Alcohol use during pregnancy, childbirth and the puerperium" I.C.15.a.6.l.1
[EXCLUDES2] *other stimulant-related disorders (F15.-)*

[5th] F14.1 **Cocaine abuse**
[EXCLUDES1] *cocaine dependence (F14.2-)*
cocaine use, unspecified (F14.9-)

F14.10 **Cocaine abuse, uncomplicated** [HCC]
AHA: Q4 2017
Cocaine use disorder, mild

F14.11 **Cocaine abuse, in remission** [HCC]
AHA: Q4 2017
Cocaine use disorder, mild, in early remission
Cocaine use disorder, mild, in sustained remission

[6th] F14.12 **Cocaine abuse with intoxication**

F14.120 **Cocaine abuse with intoxication, uncomplicated** [HCC]
AHA: Q4 2017

F14.121 **Cocaine abuse with intoxication with delirium** [CC] [HCC] [CC/MCC Exc]
AHA: Q4 2017

F14.122 **Cocaine abuse with intoxication with perceptual disturbance** [HCC]
AHA: Q4 2017

F14.129 **Cocaine abuse with intoxication, unspecified** [HCC]
AHA: Q4 2017

F14.14 **Cocaine abuse with cocaine-induced mood disorder** [HCC]
AHA: Q4 2017
Cocaine use disorder, mild, with cocaine-induced bipolar or related disorder
Cocaine use disorder, mild, with cocaine-induced depressive disorder

[6th] F14.15 **Cocaine abuse with cocaine-induced psychotic disorder**

F14.150 **Cocaine abuse with cocaine-induced psychotic disorder with delusions** [CC] [HCC] [CC/MCC Exc]
AHA: Q4 2017

F14.151 **Cocaine abuse with cocaine-induced psychotic disorder with hallucinations** [CC] [HCC] [CC/MCC Exc]
AHA: Q4 2017

F14.159 **Cocaine abuse with cocaine-induced psychotic disorder, unspecified** [HCC]
AHA: Q4 2017

[6th] F14.18 **Cocaine abuse with other cocaine-induced disorder**

F14.180 **Cocaine abuse with cocaine-induced anxiety disorder** [HCC]
AHA: Q4 2017

F14.181 **Cocaine abuse with cocaine-induced sexual dysfunction** [HCC]
AHA: Q4 2017

F14.182 **Cocaine abuse with cocaine-induced sleep disorder** [HCC]
AHA: Q4 2017

F14.188 **Cocaine abuse with other cocaine-induced disorder** [HCC]
AHA: Q4 2017
Cocaine use disorder, mild, with cocaine-induced obsessive compulsive or related disorder

F14.19 **Cocaine abuse with unspecified cocaine-induced disorder** [HCC]
AHA: Q4 2017

[5th] F14.2 **Cocaine dependence**
[EXCLUDES1] *cocaine abuse (F14.1-)*
cocaine use, unspecified (F14.9-)
[EXCLUDES2] *cocaine poisoning (T40.5-)*

Unspecified Code Other Specified Code Manifestation Code [N] Newborn [P] Pediatric [M] Maternity [A] Adult ♂ Male ♀ Female
● New Code ▲ Revised Code Title ►◄ Revised Text [NOTES] *INCLUDES* [EXCLUDES1] Not coded here [EXCLUDES2] Not included here
[4th] 4th character required [5th] 5th character required [6th] 6th character required [7th] 7th character required [7th] Extension 'X' Alert
[HAC] Hospital-acquired condition (HAC) alert AHA AHA Coding Clinic© ☛ Code first alert

When symbols appear on a code that requires a 7th character extension, refer to Appendix B to identify applicable 7th character codes.

F14.20 **Cocaine dependence,** uncomplicated HCC
AHA: Q4 2017
Cocaine use disorder, moderate
Cocaine use disorder, severe

F14.21 **Cocaine dependence,** in remission HCC
AHA: Q2 2017, Q4 2017
Cocaine use disorder, moderate, in early remission
Cocaine use disorder, moderate, in sustained remission
Cocaine use disorder, severe, in early remission
Cocaine use disorder, severe, in sustained remission

6ᵗʰ F14.22 **Cocaine dependence with intoxication**
EXCLUDES1 cocaine dependence with withdrawal (F14.23)

F14.220 **Cocaine dependence with intoxication,** uncomplicated HCC
AHA: Q4 2017

F14.221 **Cocaine dependence with intoxication** delirium cc HCC CC/MCC Exc
AHA: Q4 2017

F14.222 **Cocaine dependence with intoxication with** perceptual disturbance cc HCC
AHA: Q4 2017

F14.229 **Cocaine dependence with intoxication,** unspecified cc HCC
AHA: Q4 2017

F14.23 **Cocaine dependence** with withdrawal cc HCC CC/MCC Exc
AHA: Q4 2017
EXCLUDES1 cocaine dependence with intoxication (F14.22-)

F14.24 **Cocaine dependence with cocaine-induced** mood disorder HCC
AHA: Q4 2017
Cocaine use disorder, moderate, with cocaine-induced bipolar or related disorder
Cocaine use disorder, moderate, with cocaine-induced depressive disorder
Cocaine use disorder, severe, with cocaine-induced bipolar or related disorder
Cocaine use disorder, severe, with cocaine-induced depressive disorder

6ᵗʰ F14.25 **Cocaine dependence with cocaine-induced** psychotic disorder

F14.250 **Cocaine dependence with cocaine-induced psychotic disorder with** delusions cc HCC CC/MCC Exc
AHA: Q4 2017

F14.251 **Cocaine dependence with cocaine-induced psychotic disorder with** hallucinations cc HCC CC/MCC Exc
AHA: Q4 2017

F14.259 **Cocaine dependence with cocaine-induced psychotic disorder,** unspecified cc HCC
AHA: Q4 2017

6ᵗʰ F14.28 **Cocaine dependence with other cocaine-induced** disorder

F14.280 **Cocaine dependence with cocaine-induced** anxiety disorder cc HCC
AHA: Q4 2017

F14.281 **Cocaine dependence with cocaine-induced** sexual dysfunction cc HCC
AHA: Q4 2017

F14.282 **Cocaine dependence with cocaine-induced** sleep disorder cc HCC
AHA: Q4 2017

F14.288 **Cocaine dependence with other cocaine-induced disorder** cc HCC
AHA: Q4 2017
Cocaine use disorder, moderate, with cocaine-induced obsessive compulsive or related disorder
Cocaine use disorder, severe, with cocaine-induced obsessive compulsive or related disorder

F14.29 **Cocaine dependence with unspecified cocaine-induced disorder** HCC
AHA: Q4 2017

5ᵗʰ F14.9 **Cocaine** use, unspecified
👁 See Official Guidelines "Psychoactive Substance Use, Unspecified" I.C.5.b.3
EXCLUDES1 cocaine abuse (F14.1-)
cocaine dependence (F14.2-)

F14.90 **Cocaine use, unspecified,** uncomplicated
AHA: Q2 2018, Q4 2017

6ᵗʰ F14.92 **Cocaine use, unspecified** with intoxication

F14.920 **Cocaine use, unspecified with intoxication,** uncomplicated HCC
AHA: Q4 2017

F14.921 **Cocaine use, unspecified with intoxication** delirium cc HCC CC/MCC Exc
AHA: Q4 2017

F14.922 **Cocaine use, unspecified with intoxication with** perceptual disturbance HCC
AHA: Q4 2017

F14.929 **Cocaine use, unspecified with intoxication,** unspecified HCC
AHA: Q4 2017

F14.94 **Cocaine use, unspecified with cocaine-induced** mood disorder HCC
AHA: Q4 2017
Cocaine induced bipolar or related disorder, without use disorder
Cocaine induced depressive disorder, without use disorder

6ᵗʰ F14.95 **Cocaine use, unspecified with cocaine-induced** psychotic disorder

F14.950 **Cocaine use, unspecified with cocaine-induced psychotic disorder with** delusions cc HCC CC/MCC Exc
AHA: Q4 2017

F14.951 **Cocaine use, unspecified with cocaine-induced psychotic disorder with** hallucinations cc HCC CC/MCC Exc
AHA: Q4 2017

F14.959 **Cocaine use, unspecified with cocaine-induced psychotic disorder,** unspecified HCC
AHA: Q4 2017
Cocaine induced psychotic disorder, without use disorder

6ᵗʰ F14.98 **Cocaine use, unspecified with** other specified cocaine-induced disorder

F14.980 **Cocaine use, unspecified with cocaine-induced** anxiety disorder HCC
AHA: Q4 2017
Cocaine induced anxiety disorder, without use disorder

F14.981 **Cocaine use, unspecified with cocaine-induced** sexual dysfunction HCC
AHA: Q4 2017
Cocaine induced sexual dysfunction, without use disorder

F14.982 **Cocaine use, unspecified with cocaine-induced** sleep disorder HCC
AHA: Q4 2017
Cocaine induced sleep disorder, without use disorder

F14.988 **Cocaine use, unspecified with other cocaine-induced disorder** HCC
AHA: Q4 2017
Cocaine induced obsessive compulsive or related disorder

F14.99 **Cocaine use, unspecified with unspecified cocaine-induced disorder** HCC
AHA: Q4 2017

PDxₙ Unacceptable principal diagnosis symbol per Medicare code edits   Pₒₐ Code exempt from diagnosis present on admission requirement
❓ Questionable admission   cc Complication or comorbidity   MCC Major complication or comorbidity   CC/MCC Exc CC/MCC exclusion
HCC HCC diagnosis code   RxHCC RxHCC diagnosis code   MACRA code   DEFINITION Describes condition/terminology
TIP Coding guidance   👁 Official Guideline Reference   Z Z code as first-listed diagnosis

When symbols appear on a code that requires a 7th character extension, refer to Appendix B to identify applicable 7th character codes.
2020 ICD-10-CM

[4th] **F15 Other stimulant related disorders**

See Official Guidelines "Alcohol use during pregnancy, childbirth and the puerperium" I.C.15.a.6.l.1

INCLUDES *amphetamine-related disorders*
caffeine

EXCLUDES2 *cocaine-related disorders (F14.-)*

[5th] **F15.1 Other stimulant abuse**

EXCLUDES1 *other stimulant dependence (F15.2-)*
other stimulant use, unspecified (F15.9-)

F15.10 Other stimulant abuse, uncomplicated HCC
AHA: Q4 2017
Amphetamine type substance use disorder, mild
Other or unspecified stimulant use disorder, mild

F15.11 Other stimulant abuse, in remission HCC
AHA: Q4 2017
Amphetamine type substance use disorder, mild, in early remission
Amphetamine type substance use disorder, mild, in sustained remission
Other or unspecified stimulant use disorder, mild, in early remission
Other or unspecified stimulant use disorder, mild, in sustained remission

[6th] **F15.12 Other stimulant abuse with intoxication**

F15.120 Other stimulant abuse with intoxication, uncomplicated HCC
AHA: Q4 2017

F15.121 Other stimulant abuse with intoxication delirium CC HCC CC/MCC Exc
AHA: Q4 2017

F15.122 Other stimulant abuse with intoxication with perceptual disturbance HCC
AHA: Q4 2017
Amphetamine or other stimulant use disorder, mild, with amphetamine or other stimulant intoxication, with perceptual disturbances

F15.129 Other stimulant abuse with intoxication, unspecified HCC
AHA: Q4 2017
Amphetamine or other stimulant use disorder, mild, with amphetamine or other stimulant intoxication, without perceptual disturbances

F15.14 Other stimulant abuse with stimulant-induced mood disorder HCC
AHA: Q4 2017
Amphetamine or other stimulant use disorder, mild, with amphetamine or other stimulant induced bipolar or related disorder
Amphetamine or other stimulant use disorder, mild, with amphetamine or other stimulant induced depressive disorder

[6th] **F15.15 Other stimulant abuse with stimulant-induced psychotic disorder**

F15.150 Other stimulant abuse with stimulant-induced psychotic disorder with delusions CC HCC CC/MCC Exc
AHA: Q4 2017

F15.151 Other stimulant abuse with stimulant-induced psychotic disorder with hallucinations CC HCC CC/MCC Exc
AHA: Q4 2017

F15.159 Other stimulant abuse with stimulant-induced psychotic disorder, unspecified HCC
AHA: Q4 2017

[6th] **F15.18 Other stimulant abuse with other stimulant-induced disorder**

F15.180 Other stimulant abuse with stimulant-induced anxiety disorder HCC
AHA: Q4 2017

F15.181 Other stimulant abuse with stimulant-induced sexual dysfunction HCC
AHA: Q4 2017

F15.182 Other stimulant abuse with stimulant-induced sleep disorder HCC
AHA: Q4 2017

F15.188 Other stimulant abuse with other stimulant-induced disorder HCC
AHA: Q4 2017
Amphetamine or other stimulant use disorder, mild, with amphetamine or other stimulant induced obsessive-compulsive or related disorder

F15.19 Other stimulant abuse with unspecified stimulant-induced disorder HCC
AHA: Q4 2017

[5th] **F15.2 Other stimulant dependence**

EXCLUDES1 *other stimulant abuse (F15.1-)*
other stimulant use, unspecified (F15.9-)

F15.20 Other stimulant dependence, uncomplicated CC HCC
AHA: Q4 2017
Amphetamine type substance use disorder, moderate
Amphetamine type substance use disorder, severe
Other or unspecified stimulant use disorder, moderate
Other or unspecified stimulant use disorder, severe

F15.21 Other stimulant dependence, in remission HCC
AHA: Q4 2017
Amphetamine type substance use disorder, moderate, in early remission
Amphetamine type substance use disorder, moderate, in sustained remission
Amphetamine type substance use disorder, severe, in early remission
Amphetamine type substance use disorder, severe, in sustained remission
Other or unspecified stimulant use disorder, moderate, in early remission
Other or unspecified stimulant use disorder, moderate, in sustained remission
Other or unspecified stimulant use disorder, severe, in early remission
Other or unspecified stimulant use disorder, severe, in sustained remission

[6th] **F15.22 Other stimulant dependence with intoxication**

EXCLUDES1 *other stimulant dependence with withdrawal (F15.23)*

F15.220 Other stimulant dependence with intoxication, uncomplicated HCC
AHA: Q4 2017

F15.221 Other stimulant dependence with intoxication delirium CC HCC CC/MCC Exc
AHA: Q4 2017

F15.222 Other stimulant dependence with intoxication with perceptual disturbance CC HCC
AHA: Q4 2017
Amphetamine or other stimulant use disorder, moderate, with amphetamine or other stimulant intoxication, with perceptual disturbances
Amphetamine or other stimulant use disorder, severe, with amphetamine or other stimulant intoxication, with perceptual disturbances

F15.229 Other stimulant dependence with intoxication, unspecified HCC
AHA: Q4 2017
Amphetamine or other stimulant use disorder, moderate, with amphetamine or other stimulant intoxication, without perceptual disturbances
Amphetamine or other stimulant use disorder, severe, with amphetamine or other stimulant intoxication, without perceptual disturbances

Unspecified Code Other Specified Code Manifestation Code [N] Newborn [P] Pediatric [M] Maternity [A] Adult ♂ Male ♀ Female
● New Code ▲ Revised Code Title ►◄ Revised Text NOTES INCLUDES EXCLUDES1 Not coded here EXCLUDES2 Not included here
[4th] 4th character required [5th] 5th character required [6th] 6th character required [7th] 7th character required [X] Extension 'X' Alert
HAC Hospital-acquired condition (HAC) alert AHA AHA Coding Clinic© Code first alert

F15.23 Other stimulant dependence with withdrawal `cc` `HCC` `CC/MCC Exc`
AHA: Q4 2017
Amphetamine or other stimulant withdrawal
EXCLUDES1 *other stimulant dependence with intoxication (F15.22-)*

F15.24 Other stimulant dependence with stimulant-induced mood disorder `HCC`
AHA: Q4 2017
Amphetamine or other stimulant use disorder, moderate, with amphetamine or other stimulant-induced bipolar or related disorder
Amphetamine or other stimulant use disorder, moderate, with amphetamine or other stimulant induced depressive disorder
Amphetamine or other stimulant use disorder, severe, with amphetamine or other stimulant-induced bipolar or related disorder
Amphetamine or other stimulant use disorder, severe, with amphetamine or other stimulant-induced depressive disorder

6ᵗʰ F15.25 Other stimulant dependence with stimulant-induced psychotic disorder

   F15.250 Other stimulant dependence with stimulant-induced psychotic disorder with delusions `cc` `HCC` `CC/MCC Exc`
   AHA: Q4 2017

   F15.251 Other stimulant dependence with stimulant-induced psychotic disorder with hallucinations `cc` `HCC` `CC/MCC Exc`
   AHA: Q4 2017

   F15.259 Other stimulant dependence with stimulant-induced psychotic disorder, unspecified `cc` `HCC`
   AHA: Q4 2017

6ᵗʰ F15.28 Other stimulant dependence with other stimulant-induced disorder

   F15.280 Other stimulant dependence with stimulant-induced anxiety disorder `cc` `HCC`
   AHA: Q4 2017

   F15.281 Other stimulant dependence with stimulant-induced sexual dysfunction `cc` `HCC`
   AHA: Q4 2017

   F15.282 Other stimulant dependence with stimulant-induced sleep disorder `cc` `HCC`
   AHA: Q4 2017

   F15.288 Other stimulant dependence with other stimulant-induced disorder `cc` `HCC`
   AHA: Q4 2017
   Amphetamine or other stimulant use disorder, moderate, with amphetamine or other stimulant induced obsessive compulsive or related disorder
   Amphetamine or other stimulant use disorder, severe, with amphetamine or other stimulant induced obsessive compulsive or related disorder

F15.29 Other stimulant dependence with unspecified stimulant-induced disorder `HCC`
AHA: Q4 2017

5ᵗʰ F15.9 Other stimulant use, unspecified
   👁 **See Official Guidelines** "Psychoactive Substance Use, Unspecified" I.C.5.b.3
   EXCLUDES1 *other stimulant abuse (F15.1-)*
   other stimulant dependence (F15.2-)

   F15.90 Other stimulant use, unspecified, uncomplicated
   AHA: Q4 2017

6ᵗʰ F15.92 Other stimulant use, unspecified with intoxication
   EXCLUDES1 *other stimulant use, unspecified with withdrawal (F15.93)*

   F15.920 Other stimulant use, unspecified with intoxication, uncomplicated `HCC`
   AHA: Q4 2017

   F15.921 Other stimulant use, unspecified with intoxication delirium `cc` `HCC` `CC/MCC Exc`
   AHA: Q4 2017
   Amphetamine or other stimulant-induced delirium

   F15.922 Other stimulant use, unspecified with intoxication with perceptual disturbance `HCC`
   AHA: Q4 2017

   F15.929 Other stimulant use, unspecified with intoxication, unspecified `HCC`
   AHA: Q4 2017
   Caffeine intoxication

F15.93 Other stimulant use, unspecified with withdrawal `cc` `HCC` `CC/MCC Exc`
AHA: Q4 2017
Caffeine withdrawal
EXCLUDES1 *other stimulant use, unspecified with intoxication (F15.92-)*

F15.94 Other stimulant use, unspecified with stimulant-induced mood disorder `HCC`
AHA: Q4 2017
Amphetamine or other stimulant-induced bipolar or related disorder, without use disorder
Amphetamine or other stimulant-induced depressive disorder, without use disorder

6ᵗʰ F15.95 Other stimulant use, unspecified with stimulant-induced psychotic disorder

   F15.950 Other stimulant use, unspecified with stimulant-induced psychotic disorder with delusions `cc` `HCC` `CC/MCC Exc`
   AHA: Q4 2017

   F15.951 Other stimulant use, unspecified with stimulant-induced psychotic disorder with hallucinations `cc` `HCC` `CC/MCC Exc`
   AHA: Q4 2017

   F15.959 Other stimulant use, unspecified with stimulant-induced psychotic disorder, unspecified `HCC`
   AHA: Q4 2017
   Amphetamine or other stimulant-induced psychotic disorder, without use disorder

6ᵗʰ F15.98 Other stimulant use, unspecified with other stimulant-induced disorder

   F15.980 Other stimulant use, unspecified with stimulant-induced anxiety disorder `HCC`
   AHA: Q4 2017
   Amphetamine or other stimulant-induced anxiety disorder, without use disorder
   Caffeine induced anxiety disorder, without use disorder

   F15.981 Other stimulant use, unspecified with stimulant-induced sexual dysfunction `HCC`
   AHA: Q4 2017
   Amphetamine or other stimulant-induced sexual dysfunction, without use disorder

   F15.982 Other stimulant use, unspecified with stimulant-induced sleep disorder `HCC`
   AHA: Q4 2017
   Amphetamine or other stimulant-induced sleep disorder, without use disorder
   Caffeine induced sleep disorder, without use disorder

   F15.988 Other stimulant use, unspecified with other stimulant-induced disorder `HCC`
   AHA: Q4 2017
   Amphetamine or other stimulant-induced obsessive compulsive or related disorder, without use disorder

F15.99 Other stimulant use, unspecified with unspecified stimulant-induced disorder `HCC`
AHA: Q4 2017

PDxIn Unacceptable principal diagnosis symbol per Medicare code edits   POA Code exempt from diagnosis present on admission requirement
? Questionable admission   `cc` Complication or comorbidity   `MCC` Major complication or comorbidity   `CC/MCC Exc` CC/MCC exclusion
`HCC` HCC diagnosis code   `RxHCC` RxHCC diagnosis code   MACRA code   **DEFINITION** Describes condition/terminology
TIP Coding guidance   👁 Official Guideline Reference   Z1 Z code as first-listed diagnosis

[4th] **F16 Hallucinogen related disorders**
See Official Guidelines "Alcohol use during pregnancy, childbirth and the puerperium" I.C.15.a.6.l.1
[INCLUDES] *ecstasy*
PCP
phencyclidine

[5th] **F16.1 Hallucinogen abuse**
[EXCLUDES1] *hallucinogen dependence (F16.2-)*
hallucinogen use, unspecified (F16.9-)

F16.10 Hallucinogen abuse, uncomplicated [HCC]
AHA: Q4 2018, Q4 2017
Other hallucinogen use disorder, mild
Phencyclidine use disorder, mild

F16.11 Hallucinogen abuse, in remission [HCC]
AHA: Q4 2017
Other hallucinogen use disorder, mild, in early remission
Other hallucinogen use disorder, mild, in sustained remission
Phencyclidine use disorder, mild, in early remission
Phencyclidine use disorder, mild, in sustained remission

[6th] **F16.12 Hallucinogen abuse with intoxication**

F16.120 Hallucinogen abuse with intoxication, uncomplicated [HCC]
AHA: Q4 2017

F16.121 Hallucinogen abuse with intoxication with delirium [CC] [HCC] [CC/MCC Exc]
AHA: Q4 2017

F16.122 Hallucinogen abuse with intoxication with perceptual disturbance [HCC]
AHA: Q4 2017

F16.129 Hallucinogen abuse with intoxication, unspecified [HCC]
AHA: Q4 2017

F16.14 Hallucinogen abuse with hallucinogen-induced mood disorder [HCC]
AHA: Q4 2017
Other hallucinogen use disorder, mild, with other hallucinogen induced bipolar or related disorder
Other hallucinogen use disorder, mild, with other hallucinogen induced depressive disorder
Phencyclidine use disorder, mild, with phencyclidine induced bipolar or related disorder
Phencyclidine use disorder, mild, with phencyclidine induced depressive disorder

[6th] **F16.15 Hallucinogen abuse with hallucinogen-induced psychotic disorder**

F16.150 Hallucinogen abuse with hallucinogen-induced psychotic disorder with delusions [CC] [HCC] [CC/MCC Exc]
AHA: Q4 2017

F16.151 Hallucinogen abuse with hallucinogen-induced psychotic disorder with hallucinations [CC] [HCC] [CC/MCC Exc]
AHA: Q4 2017

F16.159 Hallucinogen abuse with hallucinogen-induced psychotic disorder, unspecified [HCC]
AHA: Q4 2017

[6th] **F16.18 Hallucinogen abuse with other hallucinogen-induced disorder**

F16.180 Hallucinogen abuse with hallucinogen-induced anxiety disorder [HCC]
AHA: Q4 2017

F16.183 Hallucinogen abuse with hallucinogen persisting perception disorder (flashbacks) [HCC]
AHA: Q4 2017

F16.188 Hallucinogen abuse with other hallucinogen-induced disorder [HCC]
AHA: Q4 2017

F16.19 Hallucinogen abuse with unspecified hallucinogen-induced disorder [HCC]
AHA: Q4 2017

[5th] **F16.2 Hallucinogen dependence**
[EXCLUDES1] *hallucinogen abuse (F16.1-)*
hallucinogen use, unspecified (F16.9-)

F16.20 Hallucinogen dependence, uncomplicated [CC] [HCC]
AHA: Q4 2017
Other hallucinogen use disorder, moderate
Other hallucinogen use disorder, severe
Phencyclidine use disorder, moderate
Phencyclidine use disorder, severe

F16.21 Hallucinogen dependence, in remission [HCC]
AHA: Q4 2017
Other hallucinogen use disorder, moderate, in early remission
Other hallucinogen use disorder, moderate, in sustained remission
Other hallucinogen use disorder, severe, in early remission
Other hallucinogen use disorder, severe, in sustained remission
Phencyclidine use disorder, moderate, in early remission
Phencyclidine use disorder, moderate, in sustained remission
Phencyclidine use disorder, severe, in early remission
Phencyclidine use disorder, severe, in sustained remission

[6th] **F16.22 Hallucinogen dependence with intoxication**

F16.220 Hallucinogen dependence with intoxication, uncomplicated [HCC]
AHA: Q4 2017

F16.221 Hallucinogen dependence with intoxication with delirium [CC] [HCC] [CC/MCC Exc]
AHA: Q4 2017

F16.229 Hallucinogen dependence with intoxication, unspecified [HCC]
AHA: Q4 2017

F16.24 Hallucinogen dependence with hallucinogen-induced mood disorder [HCC]
AHA: Q4 2017
Other hallucinogen use disorder, moderate, with other hallucinogen induced bipolar or related disorder
Other hallucinogen use disorder, moderate, with other hallucinogen induced depressive disorder
Other hallucinogen use disorder, severe, with other hallucinogen-induced bipolar or related disorder
Other hallucinogen use disorder, severe, with other hallucinogen-induced depressive disorder
Phencyclidine use disorder, moderate, with phencyclidine induced bipolar or related disorder
Phencyclidine use disorder, moderate, with phencyclidine induced depressive disorder
Phencyclidine use disorder, severe, with phencyclidine induced bipolar or related disorder
Phencyclidine use disorder, severe, with phencyclidine-induced depressive disorder

[6th] **F16.25 Hallucinogen dependence with hallucinogen-induced psychotic disorder**

F16.250 Hallucinogen dependence with hallucinogen-induced psychotic disorder with delusions [CC] [HCC] [CC/MCC Exc]
AHA: Q4 2017

F16.251 Hallucinogen dependence with hallucinogen-induced psychotic disorder with hallucinations [CC] [HCC] [CC/MCC Exc]
AHA: Q4 2017

F16.259 Hallucinogen dependence with hallucinogen-induced psychotic disorder, unspecified [CC] [HCC]
AHA: Q4 2017

Unspecified Code Other Specified Code Manifestation Code [N] Newborn [P] Pediatric [M] Maternity [A] Adult ♂ Male ♀ Female
● New Code ▲ Revised Code Title ►◄ Revised Text [NOTES] [INCLUDES] [EXCLUDES1] Not coded here [EXCLUDES2] Not included here
[4th] 4th character required [5th] 5th character required [6th] 6th character required [7th] 7th character required [x7] Extension 'X' Alert
[HAC] Hospital-acquired condition (HAC) alert **AHA** AHA Coding Clinic© ☞ **Code first alert**

[6th] **F16.28 Hallucinogen dependence with other hallucinogen-induced disorder**

F16.280 Hallucinogen dependence with hallucinogen-induced anxiety disorder [CC] [HCC]
AHA: Q4 2017

F16.283 Hallucinogen dependence with hallucinogen persisting perception disorder (flashbacks) [CC] [HCC]
AHA: Q4 2017

F16.288 Hallucinogen dependence with other hallucinogen-induced disorder [CC] [HCC]
AHA: Q4 2017

F16.29 Hallucinogen dependence with unspecified hallucinogen-induced disorder [HCC]
AHA: Q4 2017

[5th] **F16.9 Hallucinogen use, unspecified**

👁 **See Official Guidelines** "Psychoactive Substance Use, Unspecified" I.C.5.b.3

[EXCLUDES1] *hallucinogen abuse (F16.1-)*
hallucinogen dependence (F16.2-)

F16.90 Hallucinogen use, unspecified, uncomplicated
AHA: Q4 2017

[6th] **F16.92 Hallucinogen use, unspecified with intoxication**

F16.920 Hallucinogen use, unspecified with intoxication, uncomplicated [HCC]
AHA: Q4 2017

F16.921 Hallucinogen use, unspecified with intoxication with delirium [CC] [HCC] [CC/MCC Exc]
AHA: Q4 2017
Other hallucinogen intoxication delirium

F16.929 Hallucinogen use, unspecified with intoxication, unspecified [HCC]
AHA: Q4 2017

F16.94 Hallucinogen use, unspecified with hallucinogen-induced mood disorder [HCC]
AHA: Q4 2017
Other hallucinogen induced bipolar or related disorder, without use disorder
Other hallucinogen induced depressive disorder, without use disorder
Phencyclidine induced bipolar or related disorder, without use disorder
Phencyclidine induced depressive disorder, without use disorder

[6th] **F16.95 Hallucinogen use, unspecified with hallucinogen-induced psychotic disorder**

F16.950 Hallucinogen use, unspecified with hallucinogen-induced psychotic disorder with delusions [CC] [HCC] [CC/MCC Exc]
AHA: Q4 2017

F16.951 Hallucinogen use, unspecified with hallucinogen-induced psychotic disorder with hallucinations [CC] [HCC] [CC/MCC Exc]
AHA: Q4 2017

F16.959 Hallucinogen use, unspecified with hallucinogen-induced psychotic disorder, unspecified [HCC]
AHA: Q4 2017
Other hallucinogen induced psychotic disorder, without use disorder
Phencyclidine induced psychotic disorder, without use disorder

[6th] **F16.98 Hallucinogen use, unspecified with other specified hallucinogen-induced disorder**

F16.980 Hallucinogen use, unspecified with hallucinogen-induced anxiety disorder [HCC]
AHA: Q4 2017
Other hallucinogen-induced anxiety disorder, without use disorder
Phencyclidine induced anxiety disorder, without use disorder

F16.983 Hallucinogen use, unspecified with hallucinogen persisting perception disorder (flashbacks) [HCC]
AHA: Q4 2017

F16.988 Hallucinogen use, unspecified with other hallucinogen-induced disorder [HCC]
AHA: Q4 2017

F16.99 Hallucinogen use, unspecified with unspecified hallucinogen-induced disorder [HCC]
AHA: Q4 2017

[4th] **F17 Nicotine dependence**

👁 **See Official Guidelines** "Tobacco use during pregnancy, childbirth, and the puerperium" I.C.15.l.2

[EXCLUDES1] *history of tobacco dependence (Z87.891)*
tobacco use NOS (Z72.0)

[EXCLUDES2] *tobacco use (smoking) during pregnancy, childbirth and the puerperium (O99.33-)*
toxic effect of nicotine (T65.2-)

[5th] **F17.2 Nicotine dependence**

[6th] **F17.20 Nicotine dependence, unspecified**

F17.200 Nicotine dependence, unspecified, uncomplicated [PDx]
AHA: Q4 2017, Q1 2016
Tobacco use disorder, mild
Tobacco use disorder, moderate
Tobacco use disorder, severe

F17.201 Nicotine dependence, unspecified, in remission [PDx]
AHA: Q4 2017
Tobacco use disorder, mild, in early remission
Tobacco use disorder, mild, in sustained remission
Tobacco use disorder, moderate, in early remission
Tobacco use disorder, moderate, in sustained remission
Tobacco use disorder, severe, in early remission
Tobacco use disorder, severe, in sustained remission

F17.203 Nicotine dependence unspecified, with withdrawal [CC] [CC/MCC Exc]
AHA: Q4 2017
Tobacco withdrawal

F17.208 Nicotine dependence, unspecified, with other nicotine-induced disorders
AHA: Q4 2017

F17.209 Nicotine dependence, unspecified, with unspecified nicotine-induced disorders
AHA: Q4 2017

[6th] **F17.21 Nicotine dependence, cigarettes**

F17.210 Nicotine dependence, cigarettes, uncomplicated [PDx]
AHA: Q2 2017, Q4 2017

F17.211 Nicotine dependence, cigarettes, in remission [PDx]
AHA: Q4 2017
Tobacco use disorder, cigarettes, mild, in early remission
Tobacco use disorder, cigarettes, mild, in sustained remission
Tobacco use disorder, cigarettes, moderate, in early remission
Tobacco use disorder, cigarettes, moderate, in sustained remission
Tobacco use disorder, cigarettes, severe, in early remission
Tobacco use disorder, cigarettes, severe, in sustained remission

F17.213 Nicotine dependence, cigarettes, with withdrawal [CC] [CC/MCC Exc]
AHA: Q4 2017

[PDx] Unacceptable principal diagnosis symbol per Medicare code edits [POA] Code exempt from diagnosis present on admission requirement
[?] Questionable admission [CC] Complication or comorbidity [MCC] Major complication or comorbidity [CC/MCC Exc] CC/MCC exclusion
[HCC] HCC diagnosis code [RxHCC] RxHCC diagnosis code MACRA code **DEFINITION** Describes condition/terminology
TIP Coding guidance 👁 Official Guideline Reference [Z1] Z code as first-listed diagnosis

F17.218   **Nicotine dependence, cigarettes, with other nicotine-induced disorders**
     AHA: Q4 2017

F17.219   **Nicotine dependence, cigarettes, with unspecified nicotine-induced disorders**
     AHA: Q4 2017

6th F17.22   **Nicotine dependence, chewing tobacco**

F17.220   **Nicotine dependence, chewing tobacco, uncomplicated**   PDxIn
     AHA: Q4 2017

F17.221   **Nicotine dependence, chewing tobacco, in remission**   PDxIn
     AHA: Q4 2017
     Tobacco use disorder, chewing tobacco, mild, in early remission
     Tobacco use disorder, chewing tobacco, mild, in sustained remission
     Tobacco use disorder, chewing tobacco, moderate, in early remission
     Tobacco use disorder, chewing tobacco, moderate, in sustained remission
     Tobacco use disorder, chewing tobacco, severe, in early remission
     Tobacco use disorder, chewing tobacco, severe, in sustained remission

F17.223   **Nicotine dependence, chewing tobacco, with withdrawal**   CC CC/MCC Exc
     AHA: Q4 2017

F17.228   **Nicotine dependence, chewing tobacco, with other nicotine-induced disorders**
     AHA: Q4 2017

F17.229   **Nicotine dependence, chewing tobacco, with unspecified nicotine-induced disorders**
     AHA: Q4 2017

6th F17.29   **Nicotine dependence, other tobacco product**

F17.290   **Nicotine dependence, other tobacco product, uncomplicated**   PDxIn
     AHA: Q2 2017, Q4 2017

F17.291   **Nicotine dependence, other tobacco product, in remission**   PDxIn
     AHA: Q4 2017
     Tobacco use disorder, other tobacco product, mild, in early remission
     Tobacco use disorder, other tobacco product, mild, in sustained remission
     Tobacco use disorder, other tobacco product, moderate, in early remission
     Tobacco use disorder, other tobacco product, moderate, in sustained remission
     Tobacco use disorder, other tobacco product, severe, in early remission
     Tobacco use disorder, other tobacco product, severe, in sustained remission

F17.293   **Nicotine dependence, other tobacco product, with withdrawal**   CC CC/MCC Exc
     AHA: Q4 2017

F17.298   **Nicotine dependence, other tobacco product, with other nicotine-induced disorders**
     AHA: Q4 2017

F17.299   **Nicotine dependence, other tobacco product, with unspecified nicotine-induced disorders**
     AHA: Q4 2017

4th **F18**   **Inhalant related disorders**
     👁 **See Official Guidelines** "Drug use during pregnancy, childbirth and the puerperium" I.C.15.l.3
     INCLUDES   volatile solvents

5th **F18.1**   **Inhalant abuse**
     EXCLUDES1   inhalant dependence (F18.2-)
           inhalant use, unspecified (F18.9-)

F18.10   **Inhalant abuse, uncomplicated**   HCC
     AHA: Q4 2017
     Inhalant use disorder, mild

F18.11   **Inhalant abuse, in remission**   HCC
     AHA: Q4 2017
     Inhalant use disorder, mild, in early remission
     Inhalant use disorder, mild, in sustained remission

6th F18.12   **Inhalant abuse with intoxication**

F18.120   **Inhalant abuse with intoxication, uncomplicated**   HCC
     AHA: Q4 2017

F18.121   **Inhalant abuse with intoxication delirium**   CC HCC CC/MCC Exc
     AHA: Q4 2017

F18.129   **Inhalant abuse with intoxication, unspecified**   HCC
     AHA: Q4 2017

F18.14   **Inhalant abuse with inhalant-induced mood disorder**   HCC
     AHA: Q4 2017
     Inhalant use disorder, mild, with inhalant induced depressive disorder

6th F18.15   **Inhalant abuse with inhalant-induced psychotic disorder**

F18.150   **Inhalant abuse with inhalant-induced psychotic disorder with delusions**   CC HCC CC/MCC Exc
     AHA: Q4 2017

F18.151   **Inhalant abuse with inhalant-induced psychotic disorder with hallucinations**   CC HCC CC/MCC Exc
     AHA: Q4 2017

F18.159   **Inhalant abuse with inhalant-induced psychotic disorder, unspecified**   HCC
     AHA: Q4 2017

F18.17   **Inhalant abuse with inhalant-induced dementia**   CC HCC CC/MCC Exc
     AHA: Q4 2017
     Inhalant use disorder, mild, with inhalant induced major neurocognitive disorder

6th F18.18   **Inhalant abuse with other inhalant-induced disorders**

F18.180   **Inhalant abuse with inhalant-induced anxiety disorder**   HCC
     AHA: Q4 2017

F18.188   **Inhalant abuse with other inhalant-induced disorder**   HCC
     AHA: Q4 2017
     Inhalant use disorder, mild, with inhalant induced mild neurocognitive disorder

F18.19   **Inhalant abuse with unspecified inhalant-induced disorder**   HCC
     AHA: Q4 2017

5th **F18.2**   **Inhalant dependence**
     EXCLUDES1   inhalant abuse (F18.1-)
           inhalant use, unspecified (F18.9-)

F18.20   **Inhalant dependence, uncomplicated**   CC HCC
     AHA: Q4 2017
     Inhalant use disorder, moderate
     Inhalant use disorder, severe

F18.21   **Inhalant dependence, in remission**   HCC
     AHA: Q4 2017
     Inhalant use disorder, moderate, in early remission
     Inhalant use disorder, moderate, in sustained remission
     Inhalant use disorder, severe, in early remission
     Inhalant use disorder, severe, in sustained remission

6th F18.22   **Inhalant dependence with intoxication**

F18.220   **Inhalant dependence with intoxication, uncomplicated**   HCC
     AHA: Q4 2017

F18.221   **Inhalant dependence with intoxication delirium**   CC HCC CC/MCC Exc
     AHA: Q4 2017

F18.229   **Inhalant dependence with intoxication, unspecified**   HCC
     AHA: Q4 2017

Unspecified Code   Other Specified Code   Manifestation Code   N Newborn   P Pediatric   M Maternity   A Adult   ♂ Male   ♀ Female
● New Code   ▲ Revised Code Title   ▶◀ Revised Text   NOTES   INCLUDES   EXCLUDES1 Not coded here   EXCLUDES2 Not included here
4th 4th character required   5th 5th character required   6th 6th character required   7th 7th character required   Extension 'X' Alert
HAC Hospital-acquired condition (HAC) alert   AHA AHA Coding Clinic©   📛 Code first alert

2020 ICD-10-CM   When symbols appear on a code that requires a 7th character extension, refer to Appendix B to identify applicable 7th character codes.   555

F18.24 **Inhalant dependence with inhalant-induced mood disorder** [HCC]
AHA: Q4 2017
Inhalant use disorder, moderate, with inhalant induced depressive disorder
Inhalant use disorder, severe, with inhalant induced depressive disorder

[6th] F18.25 **Inhalant dependence with inhalant-induced psychotic disorder**

F18.250 **Inhalant dependence with inhalant-induced psychotic disorder with delusions** [CC] [HCC] [CC/MCC Exc]
AHA: Q4 2017

F18.251 **Inhalant dependence with inhalant-induced psychotic disorder with hallucinations** [CC] [HCC] [CC/MCC Exc]
AHA: Q4 2017

F18.259 **Inhalant dependence with inhalant-induced psychotic disorder, unspecified** [CC] [HCC]
AHA: Q4 2017

F18.27 **Inhalant dependence with inhalant-induced dementia** [CC] [HCC] [CC/MCC Exc]
AHA: Q4 2017
Inhalant use disorder, moderate, with inhalant induced major neurocognitive disorder
Inhalant use disorder, severe, with inhalant induced major neurocognitive disorder

[6th] F18.28 **Inhalant dependence with other inhalant-induced disorders**

F18.280 **Inhalant dependence with inhalant-induced anxiety disorder** [CC] [HCC]
AHA: Q4 2017

F18.288 **Inhalant dependence with other inhalant-induced disorder** [CC] [HCC]
AHA: Q4 2017
Inhalant use disorder, moderate, with inhalant-induced mild neurocognitive disorder
Inhalant use disorder, severe, with inhalant-induced mild neurocognitive disorder

F18.29 **Inhalant dependence with unspecified inhalant-induced disorder** [HCC]
AHA: Q4 2017

[5th] F18.9 **Inhalant use, unspecified**
👁 **See Official Guidelines** "Psychoactive Substance Use, Unspecified" I.C.5.b.3
[EXCLUDES1] *inhalant abuse (F18.1-)*
inhalant dependence (F18.2-)

F18.90 **Inhalant use, unspecified, uncomplicated**
AHA: Q4 2017

[6th] F18.92 **Inhalant use, unspecified with intoxication**

F18.920 **Inhalant use, unspecified with intoxication, uncomplicated** [HCC]
AHA: Q4 2017

F18.921 **Inhalant use, unspecified with intoxication with delirium** [CC] [HCC] [CC/MCC Exc]
AHA: Q4 2017

F18.929 **Inhalant use, unspecified with intoxication, unspecified** [HCC]
AHA: Q4 2017

F18.94 **Inhalant use, unspecified with inhalant-induced mood disorder** [HCC]
AHA: Q4 2017
Inhalant induced depressive disorder

[6th] F18.95 **Inhalant use, unspecified with inhalant-induced psychotic disorder**

F18.950 **Inhalant use, unspecified with inhalant-induced psychotic disorder with delusions** [CC] [HCC] [CC/MCC Exc]
AHA: Q4 2017

F18.951 **Inhalant use, unspecified with inhalant-induced psychotic disorder with hallucinations** [CC] [HCC] [CC/MCC Exc]
AHA: Q4 2017

F18.959 **Inhalant use, unspecified with inhalant-induced psychotic disorder, unspecified** [HCC]
AHA: Q4 2017

F18.97 **Inhalant use, unspecified with inhalant-induced persisting dementia** [CC] [HCC] [CC/MCC Exc]
AHA: Q4 2017
Inhalant-induced major neurocognitive disorder

[6th] F18.98 **Inhalant use, unspecified with other inhalant-induced disorders**

F18.980 **Inhalant use, unspecified with inhalant-induced anxiety disorder** [HCC]
AHA: Q4 2017

F18.988 **Inhalant use, unspecified with other inhalant-induced disorder** [HCC]
AHA: Q4 2017
Inhalant-induced mild neurocognitive disorder

F18.99 **Inhalant use, unspecified with unspecified inhalant-induced disorder** [HCC]
AHA: Q4 2017

[4th] F19 **Other psychoactive substance related disorders**
👁 **See Official Guidelines** "Alcohol use during pregnancy, childbirth and the puerperium" I.C.15.a.6.l.1
[INCLUDES] *polysubstance drug use (indiscriminate drug use)*

[5th] F19.1 **Other psychoactive substance abuse**
[EXCLUDES1] *other psychoactive substance dependence (F19.2-)*
other psychoactive substance use, unspecified (F19.9-)

F19.10 **Other psychoactive substance abuse, uncomplicated** [HCC]
AHA: Q4 2017
Other (or unknown) substance use disorder, mild

F19.11 **Other psychoactive substance abuse, in remission** [HCC]
AHA: Q4 2017
Other (or unknown) substance use disorder, mild, in early remission
Other (or unknown) substance use disorder, mild, in sustained remission

[6th] F19.12 **Other psychoactive substance abuse with intoxication**

F19.120 **Other psychoactive substance abuse with intoxication, uncomplicated** [HCC]
AHA: Q4 2017

F19.121 **Other psychoactive substance abuse with intoxication delirium** [CC] [HCC] [CC/MCC Exc]
AHA: Q4 2017

F19.122 **Other psychoactive substance abuse with intoxication with perceptual disturbances** [HCC]
AHA: Q4 2017

F19.129 **Other psychoactive substance abuse with intoxication, unspecified** [HCC]
AHA: Q4 2017

F19.14 **Other psychoactive substance abuse with psychoactive substance-induced mood disorder** [HCC]
AHA: Q4 2017
Other (or unknown) substance use disorder, mild, with other (or unknown) substance-induced bipolar or related disorder
Other (or unknown) substance use disorder, mild, with other (or unknown) substance-induced depressive disorder

[6th] F19.15 **Other psychoactive substance abuse with psychoactive substance-induced psychotic disorder**

F19.150 **Other psychoactive substance abuse with psychoactive substance-induced psychotic disorder with delusions** [CC] [HCC] [CC/MCC Exc]
AHA: Q4 2017

[PDx] Unacceptable principal diagnosis symbol per Medicare code edits [POA] Code exempt from diagnosis present on admission requirement
[?] Questionable admission [CC] Complication or comorbidity [MCC] Major complication or comorbidity [CC/MCC Exc] CC/MCC exclusion
[HCC] HCC diagnosis code [RxHCC] RxHCC diagnosis code MACRA code **DEFINITION** Describes condition/terminology
TIP Coding guidance 👁 Official Guideline Reference [Z-1] Z code as first-listed diagnosis

F19.151 **Other psychoactive substance abuse with psychoactive substance-induced psychotic disorder with hallucinations** CC HCC CC/MCC Exc
AHA: Q4 2017

F19.159 **Other psychoactive substance abuse with psychoactive substance-induced psychotic disorder, unspecified** HCC
AHA: Q4 2017

F19.16 **Other psychoactive substance abuse with psychoactive substance-induced persisting amnestic disorder** HCC
AHA: Q4 2017

F19.17 **Other psychoactive substance abuse with psychoactive substance-induced persisting dementia** CC HCC CC/MCC Exc
AHA: Q4 2017
Other (or unknown) substance use disorder, mild, with other (or unknown) substance-induced major neurocognitive disorder

[6th] F19.18 **Other psychoactive substance abuse with other psychoactive substance-induced disorders**

F19.180 **Other psychoactive substance abuse with psychoactive substance-induced anxiety disorder** HCC
AHA: Q4 2017

F19.181 **Other psychoactive substance abuse with psychoactive substance-induced sexual dysfunction** HCC
AHA: Q4 2017

F19.182 **Other psychoactive substance abuse with psychoactive substance-induced sleep disorder** HCC
AHA: Q4 2017

F19.188 **Other psychoactive substance abuse with other psychoactive substance-induced disorder** HCC
AHA: Q4 2017
Other (or unknown) substance use disorder, mild, with other (or unknown) substance induced mild neurocognitive disorder
Other (or unknown) substance use disorder, mild, with other (or unknown) substance induced obsessive-compulsive or related disorder

F19.19 **Other psychoactive substance abuse with unspecified psychoactive substance-induced disorder** HCC
AHA: Q4 2017

[5th] F19.2 **Other psychoactive substance dependence**
EXCLUDES1 *other psychoactive substance abuse (F19.1-)*
other psychoactive substance use, unspecified (F19.9-)

F19.20 **Other psychoactive substance dependence, uncomplicated** CC HCC
AHA: Q4 2017
Other (or unknown) substance use disorder, moderate
Other (or unknown) substance use disorder, severe

F19.21 **Other psychoactive substance dependence, in remission** HCC
AHA: Q4 2017
Other (or unknown) substance use disorder, moderate, in early remission
Other (or unknown) substance use disorder, moderate, in sustained remission
Other (or unknown) substance use disorder, severe, in early remission
Other (or unknown) substance use disorder, severe, in sustained remission

[6th] F19.22 **Other psychoactive substance dependence with intoxication**
EXCLUDES1 *other psychoactive substance dependence with withdrawal (F19.23-)*

F19.220 **Other psychoactive substance dependence with intoxication, uncomplicated** HCC
AHA: Q4 2017

F19.221 **Other psychoactive substance dependence with intoxication delirium** CC HCC CC/MCC Exc
AHA: Q4 2017

F19.222 **Other psychoactive substance dependence with intoxication with perceptual disturbance** CC HCC
AHA: Q4 2017

F19.229 **Other psychoactive substance dependence with intoxication, unspecified** HCC
AHA: Q4 2017

[6th] F19.23 **Other psychoactive substance dependence with withdrawal**
EXCLUDES1 *other psychoactive substance dependence with intoxication (F19.22-)*

F19.230 **Other psychoactive substance dependence with withdrawal, uncomplicated** CC HCC CC/MCC Exc
AHA: Q4 2017

F19.231 **Other psychoactive substance dependence with withdrawal delirium** CC HCC CC/MCC Exc
AHA: Q4 2017

F19.232 **Other psychoactive substance dependence with withdrawal with perceptual disturbance** CC HCC CC/MCC Exc
AHA: Q4 2017

F19.239 **Other psychoactive substance dependence with withdrawal, unspecified** CC HCC CC/MCC Exc
AHA: Q4 2017

F19.24 **Other psychoactive substance dependence with psychoactive substance-induced mood disorder** HCC
AHA: Q4 2017
Other (or unknown) substance use disorder, moderate, with other (or unknown) substance induced bipolar or related disorder
Other (or unknown) substance use disorder, moderate, with other (or unknown) substance induced depressive disorder
Other (or unknown) substance use disorder, severe, with other (or unknown) substance induced bipolar or related disorder
Other (or unknown) substance use disorder, severe, with other (or unknown) substance induced depressive disorder

[6th] F19.25 **Other psychoactive substance dependence with psychoactive substance-induced psychotic disorder**

F19.250 **Other psychoactive substance dependence with psychoactive substance-induced psychotic disorder with delusions** CC HCC CC/MCC Exc
AHA: Q4 2017

F19.251 **Other psychoactive substance dependence with psychoactive substance-induced psychotic disorder with hallucinations** CC HCC CC/MCC Exc
AHA: Q4 2017

F19.259 **Other psychoactive substance dependence with psychoactive substance-induced psychotic disorder, unspecified** CC HCC
AHA: Q4 2017

F19.26 **Other psychoactive substance dependence with psychoactive substance-induced persisting amnestic disorder** CC HCC
AHA: Q4 2017

Unspecified Code | Other Specified Code | Manifestation Code | [N] Newborn | [P] Pediatric | [M] Maternity | [A] Adult | ♂ Male | ♀ Female
● New Code ▲ Revised Code Title ►◄ Revised Text NOTES INCLUDES EXCLUDES1 Not coded here EXCLUDES2 Not included here
[4th] 4th character required [5th] 5th character required [6th] 6th character required [7th] 7th character required [x7th] Extension 'X' Alert
[HAC] Hospital-acquired condition (HAC) alert AHA AHA Coding Clinic© ☞ Code first alert

When symbols appear on a code that requires a 7th character extension, refer to Appendix B to identify applicable 7th character codes.

F19.27 Other psychoactive substance dependence with psychoactive substance-induced persisting dementia cc⊘ HCC CC/MCC Exc
AHA: Q4 2017
Other (or unknown) substance use disorder, moderate, with other (or unknown) substance induced major neurocognitive disorder
Other (or unknown) substance use disorder, severe, with other (or unknown) substance induced major neurocognitive disorder

6ᵗʰ F19.28 Other psychoactive substance dependence with other psychoactive substance-induced disorders

F19.280 Other psychoactive substance dependence with psychoactive substance-induced anxiety disorder cc⊘ HCC
AHA: Q4 2017

F19.281 Other psychoactive substance dependence with psychoactive substance-induced sexual dysfunction cc⊘ HCC
AHA: Q4 2017

F19.282 Other psychoactive substance dependence with psychoactive substance-induced sleep disorder cc⊘ HCC
AHA: Q4 2017

F19.288 Other psychoactive substance dependence with other psychoactive substance-induced disorder cc⊘ HCC
AHA: Q4 2017
Other (or unknown) substance use disorder, moderate, with other (or unknown) substance induced mild neurocognitive disorder
Other (or unknown) substance use disorder, severe, with other (or unknown) substance induced mild neurocognitive disorder
Other (or unknown) substance use disorder, moderate, with other (or unknown) substance induced obsessive compulsive or related disorder
Other (or unknown) substance use disorder, severe, with other (or unknown) substance induced obsessive-compulsive or related disorder

F19.29 Other psychoactive substance dependence with unspecified psychoactive substance-induced disorder HCC
AHA: Q4 2017

5ᵗʰ F19.9 Other psychoactive substance use, unspecified
👁 See Official Guidelines "Psychoactive Substance Use, Unspecified" I.C.5.b.3
EXCLUDES1 other psychoactive substance abuse (F19.1-)
other psychoactive substance dependence (F19.2-)

F19.90 Other psychoactive substance use, unspecified, uncomplicated
AHA: Q4 2017

6ᵗʰ F19.92 Other psychoactive substance use, unspecified with intoxication
EXCLUDES1 other psychoactive substance use, unspecified with withdrawal (F19.93)

F19.920 Other psychoactive substance use, unspecified with intoxication, uncomplicated HCC
AHA: Q4 2017

F19.921 Other psychoactive substance use, unspecified with intoxication with delirium cc⊘ HCC CC/MCC Exc
AHA: Q4 2017
Other (or unknown) substance-induced delirium

F19.922 Other psychoactive substance use, unspecified with intoxication with perceptual disturbance HCC
AHA: Q4 2017

F19.929 Other psychoactive substance use, unspecified with intoxication, unspecified HCC
AHA: Q4 2017

6ᵗʰ F19.93 Other psychoactive substance use, unspecified with withdrawal
EXCLUDES1 other psychoactive substance use, unspecified with intoxication (F19.92-)

F19.930 Other psychoactive substance use, unspecified with withdrawal, uncomplicated cc⊘ HCC CC/MCC Exc
AHA: Q4 2017

F19.931 Other psychoactive substance use, unspecified with withdrawal delirium cc⊘ HCC CC/MCC Exc
AHA: Q4 2017

F19.932 Other psychoactive substance use, unspecified with withdrawal with perceptual disturbance cc⊘ HCC CC/MCC Exc
AHA: Q4 2017

F19.939 Other psychoactive substance use, unspecified with withdrawal, unspecified cc⊘ HCC CC/MCC Exc
AHA: Q4 2017

F19.94 Other psychoactive substance use, unspecified with psychoactive substance-induced mood disorder HCC
AHA: Q4 2017
Other (or unknown) substance-induced bipolar or related disorder, without use disorder
Other (or unknown) substance-induced depressive disorder, without use disorder

5ᵗʰ F19.95 Other psychoactive substance use, unspecified with psychoactive substance-induced psychotic disorder

F19.950 Other psychoactive substance use, unspecified with psychoactive substance-induced psychotic disorder with delusions cc⊘ HCC CC/MCC Exc
AHA: Q4 2017

F19.951 Other psychoactive substance use, unspecified with psychoactive substance-induced psychotic disorder with hallucinations cc⊘ HCC CC/MCC Exc
AHA: Q4 2017

F19.959 Other psychoactive substance use, unspecified with psychoactive substance-induced psychotic disorder, unspecified HCC
AHA: Q4 2017
Other or unknown substance-induced psychotic disorder, without use disorder

F19.96 Other psychoactive substance use, unspecified with psychoactive substance-induced persisting amnestic disorder HCC
AHA: Q4 2017

F19.97 Other psychoactive substance use, unspecified with psychoactive substance-induced persisting dementia cc⊘ HCC CC/MCC Exc
AHA: Q4 2017
Other (or unknown) substance-induced major neurocognitive disorder, without use disorder

6ᵗʰ F19.98 Other psychoactive substance use, unspecified with other psychoactive substance-induced disorders

F19.980 Other psychoactive substance use, unspecified with psychoactive substance-induced anxiety disorder HCC
AHA: Q4 2017
Other (or unknown) substance-induced anxiety disorder, without use disorder

F19.981 Other psychoactive substance use, unspecified with psychoactive substance-induced sexual dysfunction HCC
AHA: Q4 2017
Other (or unknown) substance-induced sexual dysfunction, without use disorder

PDxₐ Unacceptable principal diagnosis symbol per Medicare code edits Pₒₐ Code exempt from diagnosis present on admission requirement
❓ Questionable admission cc⊘ Complication or comorbidity MCC⊘ Major complication or comorbidity CC/MCC Exc CC/MCC exclusion
HCC HCC diagnosis code RxHCC RxHCC diagnosis code MACRA code DEFINITION Describes condition/terminology
TIP Coding guidance 👁 Official Guideline Reference Z1 Z code as first-listed diagnosis

558

When symbols appear on a code that requires a 7th character extension, refer to Appendix B to identify applicable 7th character codes.

2020 ICD-10-CM

F19.982 **Other psychoactive substance use, unspecified with psychoactive substance-induced sleep disorder** [HCC]
AHA: Q4 2017
Other (or unknown) substance-induced sleep disorder, without use disorder

F19.988 **Other psychoactive substance use, unspecified with other psychoactive substance-induced disorder** [HCC]
AHA: Q4 2017
Other (or unknown) substance-induced mild neurocognitive disorder, without use disorder
Other (or unknown) substance-induced obsessive-compulsive or related disorder, without use disorder

F19.99 **Other psychoactive substance use, unspecified with unspecified psychoactive substance-induced disorder** [HCC]
AHA: Q4 2017

Schizophrenia, schizotypal, delusional, and other non-mood psychotic disorders (F20-F29)

[4th] F20 **Schizophrenia**
[EXCLUDES1] *brief psychotic disorder (F23)*
cyclic schizophrenia (F25.0)
mood [affective] disorders with psychotic symptoms (F30.2, F31.2, F31.5, F31.64, F32.3, F33.3)
schizoaffective disorder (F25.-)
schizophrenic reaction NOS (F23)
[EXCLUDES2] *schizophrenic reaction in:*
alcoholism (F10.15-, F10.25-, F10.95-)
brain disease (F06.2)
epilepsy (F06.2)
psychoactive drug use (F11-F19 with .15. .25, .95)
schizotypal disorder (F21)

F20.0 **Paranoid schizophrenia** [CC] [HCC] [RxHCC] [CC/MCC Exc]
AHA: Q4 2017
Paraphrenic schizophrenia
[EXCLUDES1] *involutional paranoid state (F22)*
paranoia (F22)

F20.1 **Disorganized schizophrenia** [CC] [HCC] [RxHCC] [CC/MCC Exc]
AHA: Q4 2017
Hebephrenic schizophrenia
Hebephrenia

F20.2 **Catatonic schizophrenia** [CC] [HCC] [RxHCC] [CC/MCC Exc]
AHA: Q4 2017
Schizophrenic catalepsy
Schizophrenic catatonia
Schizophrenic flexibilitas cerea
[EXCLUDES1] *catatonic stupor (R40.1)*

F20.3 **Undifferentiated schizophrenia** [HCC] [RxHCC]
AHA: Q4 2017
Atypical schizophrenia
[EXCLUDES1] *acute schizophrenia-like psychotic disorder (F23)*
[EXCLUDES2] *post-schizophrenic depression (F32.89)*

F20.5 **Residual schizophrenia** [CC] [HCC] [RxHCC] [CC/MCC Exc]
AHA: Q4 2017
Restzustand (schizophrenic)
Schizophrenic residual state

[5th] F20.8 **Other schizophrenia**

F20.81 **Schizophreniform disorder** [CC] [HCC] [RxHCC] [CC/MCC Exc]
AHA: Q4 2017
Schizophreniform psychosis NOS

F20.89 **Other schizophrenia** [CC] [HCC] [RxHCC] [CC/MCC Exc]
AHA: Q4 2017
Cenesthopathic schizophrenia
Simple schizophrenia

F20.9 **Schizophrenia, unspecified** [HCC] [RxHCC]
AHA: Q2 2019, Q4 2017

F21 **Schizotypal disorder** [HCC]
AHA: Q4 2017
Borderline schizophrenia
Latent schizophrenia
Latent schizophrenic reaction
Prepsychotic schizophrenia
Prodromal schizophrenia
Pseudoneurotic schizophrenia
Pseudopsychopathic schizophrenia
Schizotypal personality disorder
[EXCLUDES2] *Asperger's syndrome (F84.5)*
schizoid personality disorder (F60.1)

F22 **Delusional disorders** [CC] [HCC] [CC/MCC Exc]
AHA: Q4 2017
Delusional dysmorphophobia
Involutional paranoid state
Paranoia
Paranoia querulans
Paranoid psychosis
Paranoid state
Paraphrenia (late)
Sensitiver Beziehungswahn
[EXCLUDES1] *mood [affective] disorders with psychotic symptoms (F30.2, F31.2, F31.5, F31.64, F32.3, F33.3)*
paranoid schizophrenia (F20.0)
[EXCLUDES2] *paranoid personality disorder (F60.0)*
paranoid psychosis, psychogenic (F23)
paranoid reaction (F23)

F23 **Brief psychotic disorder** [CC] [HCC]
AHA: Q2 2019, Q4 2017
Paranoid reaction
Psychogenic paranoid psychosis
[EXCLUDES2] *mood [affective] disorders with psychotic symptoms (F30.2, F31.2, F31.5, F31.64, F32.3, F33.3)*

F24 **Shared psychotic disorder** [HCC]
AHA: Q4 2017
Folie à deux
Induced paranoid disorder
Induced psychotic disorder

[4th] F25 **Schizoaffective disorders**
[EXCLUDES1] *mood [affective] disorders with psychotic symptoms (F30.2, F31.2, F31.5, F31.64, F32.3, F33.3)*
schizophrenia (F20.-)

F25.0 **Schizoaffective disorder, bipolar type** [HCC] [RxHCC]
AHA: Q4 2017
Cyclic schizophrenia
Schizoaffective disorder, manic type
Schizoaffective disorder, mixed type
Schizoaffective psychosis, bipolar type

F25.1 **Schizoaffective disorder, depressive type** [HCC] [RxHCC]
AHA: Q4 2017
Schizoaffective psychosis, depressive type

F25.8 **Other schizoaffective disorders** [HCC] [RxHCC]
AHA: Q4 2017

F25.9 **Schizoaffective disorder, unspecified** [HCC] [RxHCC]
AHA: Q4 2017
Schizoaffective psychosis NOS

F28 **Other psychotic disorder not due to a substance or known physiological condition** [CC] [HCC] [CC/MCC Exc]
AHA: Q4 2017
Chronic hallucinatory psychosis
Other specified schizophrenia spectrum and other psychotic disorder

F29 **Unspecified psychosis not due to a substance or known physiological condition** [CC] [HCC] [CC/MCC Exc]
AHA: Q4 2017
Psychosis NOS
Unspecified schizophrenia spectrum and other psychotic disorder
[EXCLUDES1] *mental disorder NOS (F99)*
unspecified mental disorder due to known physiological condition (F09)

Mood [affective] disorders (F30-F39)

F30 Manic episode

> INCLUDES   bipolar disorder, single manic episode
> mixed affective episode

> EXCLUDES1 bipolar disorder (F31.-)
> major depressive disorder, single episode (F32.-)
> major depressive disorder, recurrent (F33.-)

F30.1 Manic episode without psychotic symptoms

    F30.10 **Manic episode without psychotic symptoms, unspecified** cc⊘ HCC RxHCC CC/MCC Exc⊘
        AHA: Q4 2017

    F30.11 **Manic episode without psychotic symptoms,** mild cc⊘ HCC RxHCC CC/MCC Exc⊘
        AHA: Q4 2017

    F30.12 **Manic episode without psychotic symptoms,** moderate cc⊘ HCC RxHCC CC/MCC Exc⊘
        AHA: Q4 2017

    F30.13 **Manic episode,** severe, **without psychotic symptoms** cc⊘ HCC RxHCC CC/MCC Exc⊘
        AHA: Q4 2017

F30.2 Manic episode, severe with psychotic symptoms cc⊘ HCC RxHCC CC/MCC Exc⊘
    AHA: Q4 2017
    Manic stupor
    Mania with mood-congruent psychotic symptoms
    Mania with mood-incongruent psychotic symptoms

F30.3 Manic episode in partial remission   HCC RxHCC
    AHA: Q4 2017

F30.4 Manic episode in full remission   HCC RxHCC
    AHA: Q4 2017

F30.8 Other manic episodes   HCC RxHCC
    AHA: Q4 2017
    Hypomania

F30.9 Manic episode, unspecified cc⊘ HCC RxHCC CC/MCC Exc⊘
    AHA: Q4 2017
    Mania NOS

F31 Bipolar disorder

> INCLUDES   bipolar I disorder
> bipolar type I disorder
> manic-depressive illness
> manic-depressive psychosis
> manic-depressive reaction

> EXCLUDES1 bipolar disorder, single manic episode (F30.-)
> major depressive disorder, single episode (F32.-)
> major depressive disorder, recurrent (F33.-)

> EXCLUDES2 cyclothymia (F34.0)

F31.0 Bipolar disorder, current episode hypomanic cc⊘ HCC RxHCC CC/MCC Exc⊘
    AHA: Q4 2017

F31.1 Bipolar disorder, current episode manic without psychotic features

    F31.10 **Bipolar disorder, current episode manic without psychotic features, unspecified** cc⊘ HCC RxHCC CC/MCC Exc⊘
        AHA: Q4 2017

    F31.11 **Bipolar disorder, current episode manic without psychotic features,** mild cc⊘ HCC RxHCC CC/MCC Exc⊘
        AHA: Q4 2017

    F31.12 **Bipolar disorder, current episode manic without psychotic features,** moderate cc⊘ HCC RxHCC CC/MCC Exc⊘
        AHA: Q4 2017

    F31.13 **Bipolar disorder, current episode manic without psychotic features,** severe cc⊘ HCC RxHCC CC/MCC Exc⊘
        AHA: Q4 2017

F31.2 Bipolar disorder, current episode manic severe with psychotic features cc⊘ HCC RxHCC CC/MCC Exc⊘
    AHA: Q4 2017
    Bipolar disorder, current episode manic with mood-congruent psychotic symptoms
    Bipolar disorder, current episode manic with mood-incongruent psychotic symptoms
    Bipolar I disorder, current or most recent episode manic with psychotic features

F31.3 Bipolar disorder, current episode depressed, mild or moderate severity

    F31.30 **Bipolar disorder, current episode depressed, mild or moderate severity, unspecified** cc⊘ HCC RxHCC CC/MCC Exc⊘
        AHA: Q4 2017

    F31.31 **Bipolar disorder, current episode depressed,** mild cc⊘ HCC RxHCC CC/MCC Exc⊘
        AHA: Q4 2017

    F31.32 **Bipolar disorder, current episode depressed,** moderate cc⊘ HCC RxHCC CC/MCC Exc⊘
        AHA: Q4 2017

F31.4 Bipolar disorder, current episode depressed, severe, without psychotic features cc⊘ HCC RxHCC CC/MCC Exc⊘
    AHA: Q4 2017

F31.5 Bipolar disorder, current episode depressed, severe, with psychotic features cc⊘ HCC RxHCC CC/MCC Exc⊘
    AHA: Q4 2017
    Bipolar disorder, current episode depressed with mood-incongruent psychotic symptoms
    Bipolar disorder, current episode depressed with mood-congruent psychotic symptoms
    Bipolar I disorder, current or most recent episode depressed, with psychotic features

F31.6 Bipolar disorder, current episode mixed

    F31.60 **Bipolar disorder, current episode mixed, unspecified** cc⊘ HCC RxHCC CC/MCC Exc⊘
        AHA: Q4 2017

    F31.61 **Bipolar disorder, current episode mixed,** mild cc⊘ HCC RxHCC CC/MCC Exc⊘
        AHA: Q4 2017

    F31.62 **Bipolar disorder, current episode mixed,** moderate cc⊘ HCC RxHCC CC/MCC Exc⊘
        AHA: Q4 2017

    F31.63 **Bipolar disorder, current episode mixed, severe,** without psychotic features cc⊘ HCC RxHCC CC/MCC Exc⊘
        AHA: Q4 2017

    F31.64 **Bipolar disorder, current episode mixed, severe,** with psychotic features cc⊘ HCC RxHCC CC/MCC Exc⊘
        AHA: Q4 2017
        Bipolar disorder, current episode mixed with mood-congruent psychotic symptoms
        Bipolar disorder, current episode mixed with mood-incongruent psychotic symptoms

F31.7 Bipolar disorder, currently in remission

    F31.70 **Bipolar disorder, currently in remission, most recent episode unspecified** HCC RxHCC
        AHA: Q4 2017

    F31.71 **Bipolar disorder,** in partial remission, **most recent episode** hypomanic HCC RxHCC
        AHA: Q4 2017

    F31.72 **Bipolar disorder,** in full remission, **most recent episode** hypomanic HCC RxHCC
        AHA: Q4 2017

    F31.73 **Bipolar disorder,** in partial remission, **most recent episode** manic HCC RxHCC
        AHA: Q4 2017

    F31.74 **Bipolar disorder,** in full remission, **most recent episode** manic HCC RxHCC
        AHA: Q4 2017

    F31.75 **Bipolar disorder,** in partial remission, **most recent episode** depressed HCC RxHCC
        AHA: Q4 2017

    F31.76 **Bipolar disorder,** in full remission, **most recent episode** depressed HCC RxHCC
        AHA: Q4 2017

    F31.77 **Bipolar disorder,** in partial remission, **most recent episode** mixed HCC RxHCC
        AHA: Q4 2017

    F31.78 **Bipolar disorder,** in full remission, **most recent episode** mixed HCC RxHCC
        AHA: Q4 2017

PDxⁿ Unacceptable principal diagnosis symbol per Medicare code edits   PDx Code exempt from diagnosis present on admission requirement
❓ Questionable admission   cc Complication or comorbidity   MCC Major complication or comorbidity   CC/MCC CC/MCC exclusion
HCC HCC diagnosis code   RxHCC RxHCC diagnosis code   MACRA code   **DEFINITION** Describes condition/terminology
TIP Coding guidance   ◉ Official Guideline Reference   Z1 Z code as first-listed diagnosis

560   When symbols appear on a code that requires a 7th character extension, refer to Appendix B to identify applicable 7th character codes.   **2020 ICD-10-CM**

[5th] F31.8 Other bipolar disorders
 F31.81 Bipolar II disorder [HCC] [RxHCC]
 AHA: Q4 2017
 Bipolar disorder, type 2
 F31.89 Other bipolar disorder [HCC] [RxHCC]
 AHA: Q4 2017
 Recurrent manic episodes NOS
F31.9 Bipolar disorder, unspecified [HCC] [RxHCC]
 AHA: Q4 2017
 Manic depression

[4th] **F32 Major depressive disorder, single episode**
[INCLUDES] *single episode of agitated depression*
single episode of depressive reaction
single episode of major depression
single episode of psychogenic depression
single episode of reactive depression
single episode of vital depression
[EXCLUDES1] *bipolar disorder (F31.-)*
manic episode (F30.-)
recurrent depressive disorder (F33.-)
[EXCLUDES2] *adjustment disorder (F43.2)*

F32.0 **Major depressive disorder, single episode, mild** [HCC] [RxHCC]
 AHA: Q4 2017
F32.1 **Major depressive disorder, single episode, moderate** [CC] [HCC] [RxHCC] [CC/MCC Exc]
 AHA: Q4 2017
F32.2 **Major depressive disorder, single episode, severe without psychotic features** [CC] [HCC] [RxHCC] [CC/MCC Exc]
 AHA: Q4 2017
F32.3 **Major depressive disorder, single episode, severe with psychotic features** [CC] [HCC] [RxHCC] [CC/MCC Exc]
 AHA: Q4 2017
 Single episode of major depression with mood-congruent psychotic symptoms
 Single episode of major depression with mood-incongruent psychotic symptoms
 Single episode of major depression with psychotic symptoms
 Single episode of psychogenic depressive psychosis
 Single episode of psychotic depression
 Single episode of reactive depressive psychosis
F32.4 **Major depressive disorder, single episode, in partial remission** [HCC] [RxHCC]
 AHA: Q4 2017
F32.5 **Major depressive disorder, single episode, in full remission** [HCC] [RxHCC]
 AHA: Q4 2017
[5th] F32.8 **Other depressive episodes**
 F32.81 Premenstrual dysphoric disorder [RxHCC] ♀
 AHA: Q4 2017, Q4 2016
 [EXCLUDES1] *premenstrual tension syndrome (N94.3)*
 F32.89 **Other specified depressive episodes** [RxHCC]
 AHA: Q4 2017, Q4 2016
 Atypical depression
 Post-schizophrenic depression
 Single episode of 'masked' depression NOS
F32.9 **Major depressive disorder, single episode, unspecified** [RxHCC]
 AHA: Q4 2017
 Depression NOS
 Depressive disorder NOS
 Major depression NOS

[4th] **F33 Major depressive disorder, recurrent**
[INCLUDES] *recurrent episodes of depressive reaction*
recurrent episodes of endogenous depression
recurrent episodes of major depression
recurrent episodes of psychogenic depression
recurrent episodes of reactive depression
recurrent episodes of seasonal depressive disorder
recurrent episodes of vital depression
[EXCLUDES1] *bipolar disorder (F31.-)*
manic episode (F30.-)

F33.0 **Major depressive disorder, recurrent, mild** [HCC] [RxHCC]
 AHA: Q4 2017
F33.1 **Major depressive disorder, recurrent, moderate** [CC] [HCC] [RxHCC] [CC/MCC Exc]
 AHA: Q4 2017
F33.2 **Major depressive disorder, recurrent severe without psychotic features** [CC] [HCC] [RxHCC] [CC/MCC Exc]
 AHA: Q4 2017
F33.3 **Major depressive disorder, recurrent, severe with psychotic symptoms** [CC] [HCC] [RxHCC] [CC/MCC Exc]
 AHA: Q4 2017
 Endogenous depression with psychotic symptoms
 Major depressive disorder, recurrent, with psychotic features
 Recurrent severe episodes of major depression with mood-congruent psychotic symptoms
 Recurrent severe episodes of major depression with mood-incongruent psychotic symptoms
 Recurrent severe episodes of major depression with psychotic symptoms
 Recurrent severe episodes of psychogenic depressive psychosis
 Recurrent severe episodes of psychotic depression
 Recurrent severe episodes of reactive depressive psychosis
[5th] F33.4 **Major depressive disorder, recurrent, in remission**
 F33.40 **Major depressive disorder, recurrent, in remission, unspecified** [CC] [HCC] [RxHCC] [CC/MCC Exc]
 AHA: Q4 2017
 F33.41 **Major depressive disorder, recurrent, in partial remission** [HCC] [RxHCC]
 AHA: Q4 2017
 F33.42 **Major depressive disorder, recurrent, in full remission** [HCC] [RxHCC]
 AHA: Q4 2017
F33.8 **Other recurrent depressive disorders** [CC] [HCC] [RxHCC] [CC/MCC Exc]
 AHA: Q4 2017
 Recurrent brief depressive episodes
F33.9 **Major depressive disorder, recurrent, unspecified** [CC] [HCC] [RxHCC] [CC/MCC Exc]
 AHA: Q4 2017
 Monopolar depression NOS

[4th] **F34 Persistent mood [affective] disorders**
F34.0 **Cyclothymic disorder** [RxHCC]
 AHA: Q4 2017
 Affective personality disorder
 Cycloid personality
 Cyclothymia
 Cyclothymic personality
F34.1 **Dysthymic disorder** [RxHCC]
 AHA: Q4 2017
 Depressive neurosis
 Depressive personality disorder
 Dysthymia
 Neurotic depression
 Persistent anxiety depression
 Persistent depressive disorder
 [EXCLUDES2] *anxiety depression (mild or not persistent) (F41.8)*
[5th] F34.8 **Other persistent mood [affective] disorders**
 F34.81 Disruptive mood dysregulation disorder [CC] [HCC] [RxHCC] [CC/MCC Exc]
 AHA: Q4 2017, Q4 2016
 F34.89 **Other specified persistent mood disorders** [CC] [HCC] [RxHCC] [CC/MCC Exc]
 AHA: Q4 2017, Q4 2016
F34.9 **Persistent mood [affective] disorder, unspecified** [CC] [HCC] [RxHCC] [CC/MCC Exc]
 AHA: Q4 2017

F39 Unspecified mood [affective] disorder [HCC] [RxHCC]
 AHA: Q4 2017
 Affective psychosis NOS

Unspecified Code | Other Specified Code | Manifestation Code | [N] Newborn | [P] Pediatric | [M] Maternity | [A] Adult | ♂ Male | ♀ Female
● New Code | ▲ Revised Code Title | ►◄ Revised Text | [NOTES] | [INCLUDES] | [EXCLUDES1] Not coded here | [EXCLUDES2] Not included here
[4th] 4th character required | [5th] 5th character required | [6th] 6th character required | [7th] 7th character required | [x] Extension 'X' Alert
[HAC] Hospital-acquired condition (HAC) alert | AHA AHA Coding Clinic© | ☞ Code first alert

Anxiety, dissociative, stress-related, somatoform and other nonpsychotic mental disorders (F40-F48)

[4th] **F40 Phobic anxiety disorders**

[5th] **F40.0 Agoraphobia**

F40.00 Agoraphobia, unspecified [RxHCC]
AHA: Q4 2017

F40.01 Agoraphobia with panic disorder [RxHCC]
AHA: Q4 2017
Panic disorder with agoraphobia
[EXCLUDES1] *panic disorder without agoraphobia (F41.0)*

F40.02 Agoraphobia without panic disorder [RxHCC]
AHA: Q4 2017

[5th] **F40.1 Social phobias**
Anthropophobia
Social anxiety disorder
Social anxiety disorder of childhood
Social neurosis

F40.10 Social phobia, unspecified [RxHCC]
AHA: Q4 2017

F40.11 Social phobia, generalized [RxHCC]
AHA: Q4 2017

[5th] **F40.2 Specific (isolated) phobias**
[EXCLUDES2] *dysmorphophobia (nondelusional) (F45.22)*
nosophobia (F45.22)

[6th] **F40.21 Animal type phobia**

F40.210 Arachnophobia [RxHCC]
AHA: Q4 2017
Fear of spiders

F40.218 Other animal type phobia [RxHCC]
AHA: Q4 2017

[6th] **F40.22 Natural environment type phobia**

F40.220 Fear of thunderstorms [RxHCC]
AHA: Q4 2017

F40.228 Other natural environment type phobia [RxHCC]
AHA: Q4 2017

[6th] **F40.23 Blood, injection, injury type phobia**

F40.230 Fear of blood [RxHCC]
AHA: Q4 2017

F40.231 Fear of injections and transfusions [RxHCC]
AHA: Q4 2017

F40.232 Fear of other medical care [RxHCC]
AHA: Q4 2017

F40.233 Fear of injury [RxHCC]
AHA: Q4 2017

[6th] **F40.24 Situational type phobia**

F40.240 Claustrophobia [RxHCC]
AHA: Q4 2017

F40.241 Acrophobia [RxHCC]
AHA: Q4 2017

F40.242 Fear of bridges [RxHCC]
AHA: Q4 2017

F40.243 Fear of flying [RxHCC]
AHA: Q4 2017

F40.248 Other situational type phobia [RxHCC]
AHA: Q4 2017

[6th] **F40.29 Other specified phobia**

F40.290 Androphobia [RxHCC]
AHA: Q4 2017
Fear of men

F40.291 Gynephobia [RxHCC]
AHA: Q4 2017
Fear of women

F40.298 Other specified phobia [RxHCC]
AHA: Q4 2017

F40.8 Other phobic anxiety disorders [RxHCC]
AHA: Q4 2017
Phobic anxiety disorder of childhood

F40.9 Phobic anxiety disorder, unspecified [RxHCC]
AHA: Q4 2017
Phobia NOS
Phobic state NOS

[4th] **F41 Other anxiety disorders**
[EXCLUDES2] *anxiety in:*
acute stress reaction (F43.0)
transient adjustment reaction (F43.2)
neurasthenia (F48.8)
psychophysiologic disorders (F45.-)
separation anxiety (F93.0)

F41.0 Panic disorder [episodic paroxysmal anxiety] [RxHCC]
AHA: Q4 2017
Panic attack
Panic state
[EXCLUDES1] *panic disorder with agoraphobia (F40.01)*

F41.1 Generalized anxiety disorder [RxHCC]
AHA: Q4 2017
Anxiety neurosis
Anxiety reaction
Anxiety state
Overanxious disorder
[EXCLUDES2] *neurasthenia (F48.8)*

F41.3 Other mixed anxiety disorders
AHA: Q4 2017

F41.8 Other specified anxiety disorders
AHA: Q4 2017
Anxiety depression (mild or not persistent)
Anxiety hysteria
Mixed anxiety and depressive disorder

F41.9 Anxiety disorder, unspecified
AHA: Q4 2017
Anxiety NOS

[4th] **F42 Obsessive-compulsive disorder**
[EXCLUDES2] *obsessive-compulsive personality (disorder) (F60.5)*
obsessive-compulsive symptoms occurring in depression (F32-F33)
obsessive-compulsive symptoms occurring in schizophrenia (F20.-)

F42.2 Mixed obsessional thoughts and acts [RxHCC]
AHA: Q4 2017, Q4 2016

F42.3 Hoarding disorder [RxHCC]
AHA: Q4 2017, Q4 2016

F42.4 Excoriation (skin-picking) disorder [RxHCC]
AHA: Q4 2017, Q4 2016
[EXCLUDES1] *factitial dermatitis (L98.1)*
other specified behavioral and emotional disorders with onset usually occurring in early childhood and adolescence (F98.8)

F42.8 Other obsessive-compulsive disorder [RxHCC]
AHA: Q4 2017, Q4 2016
Anancastic neurosis
Obsessive-compulsive neurosis

F42.9 Obsessive-compulsive disorder, unspecified [RxHCC]
AHA: Q4 2017, Q4 2016

[4th] **F43 Reaction to severe stress, and adjustment disorders**

F43.0 Acute stress reaction
AHA: Q4 2017
Acute crisis reaction
Acute reaction to stress
Combat and operational stress reaction
Combat fatigue
Crisis state
Psychic shock

[5th] **F43.1 Post-traumatic stress disorder (PTSD)**
Traumatic neurosis

F43.10 Post-traumatic stress disorder, unspecified [RxHCC]
AHA: Q4 2017

F43.11 Post-traumatic stress disorder, acute [RxHCC]
AHA: Q4 2017

[PDx] Unacceptable principal diagnosis symbol per Medicare code edits [POA] Code exempt from diagnosis present on admission requirement
[Q] Questionable admission [CC] Complication or comorbidity [MCC] Major complication or comorbidity [CC/MCC Exc] CC/MCC exclusion
[HCC] HCC diagnosis code [RxHCC] RxHCC diagnosis code MACRA code **DEFINITION** Describes condition/terminology
TIP Coding guidance 👁 Official Guideline Reference [Z1] Z code as first-listed diagnosis

F43.12 **Post-traumatic stress disorder,** chronic [RxHCC]
AHA: Q4 2017

5ᵗʰ **F43.2** Adjustment **disorders**
Culture shock
Grief reaction
Hospitalism in children
EXCLUDES2 *separation anxiety disorder of childhood (F93.0)*
F43.20 **Adjustment disorder, unspecified**
AHA: Q4 2017
F43.21 **Adjustment disorder** with depressed mood
AHA: Q4 2017
F43.22 **Adjustment disorder** with anxiety
AHA: Q4 2017
F43.23 **Adjustment disorder** with mixed anxiety and depressed mood
AHA: Q4 2017
F43.24 **Adjustment disorder** with disturbance of conduct
AHA: Q4 2017
F43.25 **Adjustment disorder** with mixed disturbance of emotions and conduct
AHA: Q4 2017
F43.29 **Adjustment disorder with other symptoms**
AHA: Q4 2017

F43.8 **Other reactions to severe stress**
AHA: Q4 2017
Other specified trauma and stressor-related disorder
F43.9 **Reaction to severe stress, unspecified**
AHA: Q4 2017
Trauma and stressor-related disorder, NOS

4ᵗʰ **F44** Dissociative **and** conversion **disorders**
INCLUDES conversion hysteria
conversion reaction
hysteria
hysterical psychosis
EXCLUDES2 *malingering [conscious simulation] (Z76.5)*
F44.0 **Dissociative** amnesia [HCC] [RxHCC]
AHA: Q4 2017
EXCLUDES1 *amnesia NOS (R41.3)*
anterograde amnesia (R41.1)
dissociative amnesia with dissociative fugue (F44.1)
retrograde amnesia (R41.2)
EXCLUDES2 *alcohol-or other psychoactive substance-induced amnestic disorder (F10, F13, F19 with .26, .96)*
amnestic disorder due to known physiological condition (F04)
postictal amnesia in epilepsy (G40.-)
F44.1 **Dissociative** fugue [HCC] [RxHCC]
AHA: Q4 2017
Dissociative amnesia with dissociative fugue
EXCLUDES2 *postictal fugue in epilepsy (G40.-)*
F44.2 **Dissociative** stupor [RxHCC]
AHA: Q4 2017
EXCLUDES1 *catatonic stupor (R40.1)*
stupor NOS (R40.1)
EXCLUDES2 *catatonic disorder due to known physiological condition (F06.1)*
depressive stupor (F32, F33)
manic stupor (F30, F31)
F44.4 **Conversion** disorder with motor symptom or deficit [RxHCC]
AHA: Q4 2017
Conversion disorder with abnormal movement
Conversion disorder with speech symptoms
Conversion disorder with swallowing symptoms
Conversion disorder with weakness/paralysis
Dissociative motor disorders
Psychogenic aphonia
Psychogenic dysphonia

F44.5 **Conversion disorder** with seizures or convulsions [RxHCC]
AHA: Q1 2019, Q4 2017
Conversion disorder with attacks or seizures
Dissociative convulsions
F44.6 **Conversion disorder** with sensory symptom or deficit [RxHCC]
AHA: Q4 2017
Conversion disorder with anesthesia or sensory loss
Conversion disorder with special sensory symptoms
Dissociative anesthesia and sensory loss
Psychogenic deafness
F44.7 **Conversion disorder** with mixed symptom presentation [RxHCC]
AHA: Q4 2017
5ᵗʰ **F44.8** Other **dissociative and conversion disorders**
F44.81 **Dissociative** identity **disorder** [HCC] [RxHCC]
AHA: Q4 2017
Multiple personality disorder
F44.89 **Other dissociative and conversion disorders** [RxHCC]
AHA: Q4 2017
Ganser's syndrome
Psychogenic confusion
Psychogenic twilight state
Trance and possession disorders
F44.9 **Dissociative and conversion disorder, unspecified** [RxHCC]
AHA: Q4 2017
Dissociative disorder NOS

4ᵗʰ **F45** Somatoform **disorders**
EXCLUDES2 *dissociative and conversion disorders (F44.-)*
factitious disorders (F68.1-, F68.A)
hair-plucking (F63.3)
lalling (F80.0)
lisping (F80.0)
malingering [conscious simulation] (Z76.5)
nail-biting (F98.8)
psychological or behavioral factors associated with disorders or diseases classified elsewhere (F54)
sexual dysfunction, not due to a substance or known physiological condition (F52.-)
thumb-sucking (F98.8)
tic disorders (in childhood and adolescence) (F95.-)
Tourette's syndrome (F95.2)
trichotillomania (F63.3)
F45.0 **Somatization disorder** [RxHCC]
AHA: Q4 2017
Briquet's disorder
Multiple psychosomatic disorder
F45.1 **Undifferentiated** somatoform **disorder** [RxHCC]
AHA: Q4 2017
Somatic symptom disorder
Undifferentiated psychosomatic disorder
5ᵗʰ **F45.2** Hypochondriacal **disorders**
EXCLUDES2 *delusional dysmorphophobia (F22)*
fixed delusions about bodily functions or shape (F22)
F45.20 **Hypochondriacal disorder, unspecified** [RxHCC]
AHA: Q4 2017
F45.21 **Hypochondriasis** [RxHCC]
AHA: Q4 2017
Hypochondriacal neurosis
Illness anxiety disorder
F45.22 **Body dysmorphic disorder** [RxHCC]
AHA: Q4 2017
Dysmorphophobia (nondelusional)
Nosophobia
F45.29 **Other hypochondriacal disorders** [RxHCC]
AHA: Q4 2017
5ᵗʰ **F45.4** Pain disorders related to psychological factors
EXCLUDES1 *pain NOS (R52)*
F45.41 **Pain disorder exclusively related to psychological factors**
👁 See Official Guidelines "Pain disorders related to psychological factors" I.C.5.a
AHA: Q4 2017
Somatoform pain disorder (persistent)

Unspecified Code   Other Specified Code   Manifestation Code   N Newborn   P Pediatric   M Maternity   A Adult   ♂ Male   ♀ Female
● New Code   ▲ Revised Code Title   ►◄ Revised Text   NOTES   INCLUDES   EXCLUDES1 Not coded here   EXCLUDES2 Not included here
4ᵗʰ 4ᵗʰ character required   5ᵗʰ 5ᵗʰ character required   6ᵗʰ 6ᵗʰ character required   7ᵗʰ 7ᵗʰ character required   Extension 'X' Alert
HAC Hospital-acquired condition (HAC) alert   AHA AHA Coding Clinic©   Code first alert

F45.42 **Pain disorder with related psychological factors**
👁 **See Official Guidelines** "Pain disorders related to psychological factors" I.C.5.a
AHA: Q4 2017
Code also associated acute or chronic pain (G89.-)

F45.8 **Other somatoform disorders** RxHCC
👁 **See Official Guidelines** "Excludes Notes" I.A.12.a
AHA: Q4 2017, Q4 2016
Psychogenic dysmenorrhea
Psychogenic dysphagia, including 'globus hystericus'
Psychogenic pruritus
Psychogenic torticollis
Somatoform autonomic dysfunction
Teeth grinding
EXCLUDES1 sleep related teeth grinding (G47.63)

F45.9 **Somatoform disorder, unspecified** RxHCC
AHA: Q4 2017
Psychosomatic disorder NOS

F48 Other nonpsychotic mental disorders
F48.1 **Depersonalization-derealization syndrome** HCC RxHCC
AHA: Q4 2017

F48.2 **Pseudobulbar affect**
AHA: Q4 2017
Involuntary emotional expression disorder
☞ **Code first** underlying cause, if known, such as:
amyotrophic lateral sclerosis (G12.21)
multiple sclerosis (G35)
sequelae of cerebrovascular disease (I69.-)
sequelae of traumatic intracranial injury (S06.-)

F48.8 **Other specified nonpsychotic mental disorders**
AHA: Q4 2017
Dhat syndrome
Neurasthenia
Occupational neurosis, including writer's cramp
Psychasthenia
Psychasthenic neurosis
Psychogenic syncope

F48.9 **Nonpsychotic mental disorder, unspecified**
AHA: Q4 2017
Neurosis NOS

Behavioral syndromes associated with physiological disturbances and physical factors (F50-F59)

F50 Eating disorders
EXCLUDES1 anorexia NOS (R63.0)
feeding difficulties (R63.3)
feeding problems of newborn (P92.-)
polyphagia (R63.2)
EXCLUDES2 feeding disorder in infancy or childhood (F98.2-)

F50.0 **Anorexia nervosa**
EXCLUDES1 loss of appetite (R63.0)
psychogenic loss of appetite (F50.89)

F50.00 **Anorexia nervosa, unspecified** cc RxHCC CC/MCC Exc
AHA: Q4 2017

F50.01 **Anorexia nervosa, restricting type** cc RxHCC CC/MCC Exc
AHA: Q4 2017

F50.02 **Anorexia nervosa, binge eating/purging type** cc RxHCC CC/MCC Exc
AHA: Q4 2017
EXCLUDES1 bulimia nervosa (F50.2)

F50.2 **Bulimia nervosa** cc RxHCC CC/MCC Exc
AHA: Q4 2017
Bulimia NOS
Hyperorexia nervosa
EXCLUDES1 anorexia nervosa, binge eating/purging type (F50.02)

F50.8 **Other eating disorders**
EXCLUDES2 pica of infancy and childhood (F98.3)

F50.81 **Binge eating disorder**
AHA: Q4 2017, Q4 2016

F50.82 **Avoidant/restrictive food intake disorder**
AHA: Q4 2017

F50.89 **Other specified eating disorder**
AHA: Q4 2017, Q4 2016
Pica in adults
Psychogenic loss of appetite

F50.9 **Eating disorder, unspecified**
AHA: Q4 2017
Atypical anorexia nervosa
Atypical bulimia nervosa
Feeding or eating disorder, unspecified
Other specified feeding disorder

F51 Sleep disorders not due to a substance or known physiological condition
EXCLUDES2 organic sleep disorders (G47.-)

F51.0 **Insomnia not due to a substance or known physiological condition**
EXCLUDES2 alcohol related insomnia (F10.182, F10.282, F10.982)
drug-related insomnia (F11.182, F11.282, F11.982, F13.182, F13.282, F13.982, F14.182, F14.282, F14.982, F15.182, F15.282, F15.982, F19.182, F19.282, F19.982)
insomnia NOS (G47.0-)
insomnia due to known physiological condition (G47.0-)
organic insomnia (G47.0-)
sleep deprivation (Z72.820)

F51.01 **Primary insomnia**
AHA: Q4 2017
Idiopathic insomnia

F51.02 **Adjustment insomnia**
AHA: Q4 2017

F51.03 **Paradoxical insomnia**
AHA: Q4 2017

F51.04 **Psychophysiologic insomnia**
AHA: Q4 2017

F51.05 **Insomnia due to other mental disorder**
AHA: Q4 2017
Code also associated mental disorder

F51.09 **Other insomnia not due to a substance or known physiological condition**
AHA: Q4 2017

F51.1 **Hypersomnia not due to a substance or known physiological condition**
EXCLUDES2 alcohol related hypersomnia (F10.182, F10.282, F10.982)
drug-related hypersomnia (F11.182, F11.282, F11.982, F13.182, F13.282, F13.982, F14.182, F14.282, F14.982, F15.182, F15.282, F15.982, F19.182, F19.282, F19.982)
hypersomnia NOS (G47.10)
hypersomnia due to known physiological condition (G47.10)
idiopathic hypersomnia (G47.11, G47.12)
narcolepsy (G47.4-)

F51.11 **Primary hypersomnia**
AHA: Q4 2017

F51.12 **Insufficient sleep syndrome**
AHA: Q4 2017
EXCLUDES1 sleep deprivation (Z72.820)

F51.13 **Hypersomnia due to other mental disorder**
AHA: Q4 2017
Code also associated mental disorder

F51.19 **Other hypersomnia not due to a substance or known physiological condition**
AHA: Q4 2017

F51.3 **Sleepwalking [somnambulism]**
AHA: Q4 2017
Non-rapid eye movement sleep arousal disorders, sleepwalking type

---

POA Unacceptable principal diagnosis symbol per Medicare code edits   POA Code exempt from diagnosis present on admission requirement
❓ Questionable admission   cc Complication or comorbidity   MCC Major complication or comorbidity   CC/MCC CC/MCC exclusion
HCC HCC diagnosis code   RxHCC RxHCC diagnosis code   MACRA code   **DEFINITION** Describes condition/terminology
TIP Coding guidance   👁 Official Guideline Reference   Z1 Z code as first-listed diagnosis

F51.4 Sleep terrors [night terrors]
AHA: Q4 2017
Non-rapid eye movement sleep arousal disorders, sleep terror type

F51.5 Nightmare disorder
AHA: Q4 2017
Dream anxiety disorder

F51.8 Other sleep disorders not due to a substance or known physiological condition
AHA: Q4 2017

F51.9 Sleep disorder not due to a substance or known physiological condition, unspecified
AHA: Q4 2017
Emotional sleep disorder NOS

4ᵗʰ F52 Sexual dysfunction not due to a substance or known physiological condition
EXCLUDES2 Dhat syndrome (F48.8)

F52.0 Hypoactive sexual desire disorder
AHA: Q4 2017
Lack or loss of sexual desire
Male hypoactive sexual desire disorder
Sexual anhedonia
EXCLUDES1 decreased libido (R68.82)

F52.1 Sexual aversion disorder
AHA: Q4 2017
Sexual aversion and lack of sexual enjoyment

5ᵗʰ F52.2 Sexual arousal disorders
Failure of genital response

F52.21 Male erectile disorder ♂
AHA: Q4 2017
Erectile disorder
Psychogenic impotence
EXCLUDES1 impotence of organic origin (N52.-)
impotence NOS (N52.-)

F52.22 Female sexual arousal disorder ♀
AHA: Q4 2017
Female sexual interest/arousal disorder

5ᵗʰ F52.3 Orgasmic disorder
Inhibited orgasm
Psychogenic anorgasmy

F52.31 Female orgasmic disorder ♀
AHA: Q4 2017

F52.32 Male orgasmic disorder ♂
AHA: Q4 2017
Delayed ejaculation

F52.4 Premature ejaculation ♂
AHA: Q4 2017

F52.5 Vaginismus not due to a substance or known physiological condition ♀
AHA: Q4 2017
Psychogenic vaginismus
EXCLUDES2 vaginismus (due to a known physiological condition) (N94.2)

F52.6 Dyspareunia not due to a substance or known physiological condition
AHA: Q4 2017
Genito-pelvic pain penetration disorder
Psychogenic dyspareunia
EXCLUDES2 dyspareunia (due to a known physiological condition) (N94.1-)

F52.8 Other sexual dysfunction not due to a substance or known physiological condition
AHA: Q4 2017
Excessive sexual drive
Nymphomania
Satyriasis

F52.9 Unspecified sexual dysfunction not due to a substance or known physiological condition
AHA: Q4 2017
Sexual dysfunction NOS

4ᵗʰ F53 Mental and behavioral disorders associated with the puerperium, not elsewhere classified
EXCLUDES1 mood disorders with psychotic features (F30.2, F31.2, F31.5, F31.64, F32.3, F33.3)
postpartum dysphoria (O90.6)
psychosis in schizophrenia, schizotypal, delusional, and other psychotic disorders (F20-F29)

F53.0 Postpartum depression M RxHCC ♀
AHA: Q4 2018
Postnatal depression, NOS
Postpartum depression, NOS

F53.1 Puerperal psychosis M HCC ♀
AHA: Q4 2018
Postpartum psychosis
Puerperal psychosis, NOS

F54 Psychological and behavioral factors associated with disorders or diseases classified elsewhere
AHA: Q4 2017
Psychological factors affecting physical conditions
☛ Code first the associated physical disorder, such as:
asthma (J45.-)
dermatitis (L23-L25)
gastric ulcer (K25.-)
mucous colitis (K58.-)
ulcerative colitis (K51.-)
urticaria (L50.-)
EXCLUDES2 tension-type headache (G44.2)

4ᵗʰ F55 Abuse of non-psychoactive substances
EXCLUDES2 abuse of psychoactive substances (F10-F19)

F55.0 Abuse of antacids
AHA: Q4 2017

F55.1 Abuse of herbal or folk remedies
AHA: Q4 2017

F55.2 Abuse of laxatives
AHA: Q4 2017

F55.3 Abuse of steroids or hormones
AHA: Q4 2017

F55.4 Abuse of vitamins
AHA: Q4 2017

F55.8 Abuse of other non-psychoactive substances
AHA: Q4 2017

F59 Unspecified behavioral syndromes associated with physiological disturbances and physical factors
AHA: Q4 2017
Psychogenic physiological dysfunction NOS

Disorders of adult personality and behavior (F60-F69)

4ᵗʰ F60 Specific personality disorders

F60.0 Paranoid personality disorder HCC
AHA: Q4 2017
Expansive paranoid personality (disorder)
Fanatic personality (disorder)
Querulant personality (disorder)
Paranoid personality (disorder)
Sensitive paranoid personality (disorder)
EXCLUDES2 paranoia (F22)
paranoia querulans (F22)
paranoid psychosis (F22)
paranoid schizophrenia (F20.0)
paranoid state (F22)

F60.1 Schizoid personality disorder HCC
AHA: Q4 2017
EXCLUDES2 Asperger's syndrome (F84.5)
delusional disorder (F22)
schizoid disorder of childhood (F84.5)
schizophrenia (F20.-)
schizotypal disorder (F21)

Unspecified Code   Other Specified Code   Manifestation Code   Ⓝ Newborn   Ⓟ Pediatric   Ⓜ Maternity   Ⓐ Adult   ♂ Male   ♀ Female
● New Code   ▲ Revised Code Title   ►◄ Revised Text   **NOTES**   *INCLUDES*   *EXCLUDES1* Not coded here   *EXCLUDES2* Not included here
4ᵗʰ 4ᵗʰ character required   5ᵗʰ 5ᵗʰ character required   6ᵗʰ 6ᵗʰ character required   7ᵗʰ 7ᵗʰ character required   Extension 'X' Alert
HAC Hospital-acquired condition (HAC) alert   AHA AHA Coding Clinic©   ☛ Code first alert

F60.2 **Antisocial personality disorder** [HCC]
AHA: Q4 2017
Amoral personality (disorder)
Asocial personality (disorder)
Dissocial personality disorder
Psychopathic personality (disorder)
Sociopathic personality (disorder)
[EXCLUDES1] *conduct disorders (F91.-)*
[EXCLUDES2] *borderline personality disorder (F60.3)*

F60.3 **Borderline personality disorder** [HCC] [RxHCC]
AHA: Q4 2017
Aggressive personality (disorder)
Emotionally unstable personality disorder
Explosive personality (disorder)
[EXCLUDES2] *antisocial personality disorder (F60.2)*

F60.4 **Histrionic personality disorder** [HCC]
AHA: Q4 2017
Hysterical personality (disorder)
Psychoinfantile personality (disorder)

F60.5 **Obsessive-compulsive personality disorder** [HCC] [RxHCC]
AHA: Q4 2017
Anankastic personality (disorder)
Compulsive personality (disorder)
Obsessional personality (disorder)
[EXCLUDES2] *obsessive-compulsive disorder (F42-)*

F60.6 **Avoidant personality disorder** [HCC]
AHA: Q4 2017
Anxious personality disorder

F60.7 **Dependent personality disorder** [HCC]
AHA: Q4 2017
Asthenic personality (disorder)
Inadequate personality (disorder)
Passive personality (disorder)

[5th] F60.8 **Other specific personality disorders**

F60.81 **Narcissistic personality disorder** [HCC]
AHA: Q4 2017

F60.89 **Other specific personality disorders** [HCC]
AHA: Q4 2017
Eccentric personality disorder
'Haltlose' type personality disorder
Immature personality disorder
Passive-aggressive personality disorder
Psychoneurotic personality disorder
Self-defeating personality disorder

F60.9 **Personality disorder, unspecified** [HCC]
AHA: Q4 2017
Character disorder NOS
Character neurosis NOS
Pathological personality NOS

[4th] F63 **Impulse disorders**
[EXCLUDES2] *habitual excessive use of alcohol or psychoactive substances (F10-F19)*
impulse disorders involving sexual behavior (F65.-)

F63.0 **Pathological gambling** [RxHCC]
AHA: Q4 2017
Compulsive gambling
Gambling disorder
[EXCLUDES1] *gambling and betting NOS (Z72.6)*
[EXCLUDES2] *excessive gambling by manic patients (F30, F31)*
gambling in antisocial personality disorder (F60.2)

F63.1 **Pyromania** [RxHCC]
AHA: Q4 2017
Pathological fire-setting
[EXCLUDES2] *fire-setting (by) (in):*
adult with antisocial personality disorder (F60.2)
alcohol or psychoactive substance intoxication (F10-F19)
conduct disorders (F91.-)
mental disorders due to known physiological condition (F01-F09)
schizophrenia (F20.-)

F63.2 **Kleptomania** [RxHCC]
AHA: Q4 2017
Pathological stealing
[EXCLUDES1] *shoplifting as the reason for observation for suspected mental disorder (Z03.8)*
[EXCLUDES2] *depressive disorder with stealing (F31-F33)*
stealing due to underlying mental condition-code to mental condition
stealing in mental disorders due to known physiological condition (F01-F09)

F63.3 **Trichotillomania** [RxHCC]
AHA: Q4 2017
Hair plucking
[EXCLUDES2] *other stereotyped movement disorder (F98.4)*

[5th] F63.8 **Other impulse disorders**

F63.81 **Intermittent explosive disorder** [RxHCC]
AHA: Q4 2017

F63.89 **Other impulse disorders** [CC] [RxHCC] [CC/MCC Exc]
AHA: Q4 2017

F63.9 **Impulse disorder, unspecified** [CC] [RxHCC] [CC/MCC Exc]
AHA: Q4 2017
Impulse control disorder NOS

[4th] F64 **Gender identity disorders**

F64.0 **Transsexualism**
AHA: Q4 2017, Q4 2016
Gender identity disorder in adolescence and adulthood
Gender dysphoria in adolescents and adults

F64.1 **Dual role transvestism**
AHA: Q4 2017, Q4 2016
Use additional code to identify sex reassignment status (Z87.890)
[EXCLUDES1] *gender identity disorder in childhood (F64.2)*
[EXCLUDES2] *fetishistic transvestism (F65.1)*

F64.2 **Gender identity disorder of childhood** [P]
AHA: Q4 2017
Gender dysphoria in children
[EXCLUDES1] *gender identity disorder in adolescence and adulthood (F64.0)*
[EXCLUDES2] *sexual maturation disorder (F66)*

F64.8 **Other gender identity disorders**
AHA: Q4 2017
Other specified gender dysphoria

F64.9 **Gender identity disorder, unspecified**
AHA: Q4 2017
Gender dysphoria, unspecified
Gender-role disorder NOS

[4th] F65 **Paraphilias**

F65.0 **Fetishism**
AHA: Q4 2017
Fetishistic disorder

F65.1 **Transvestic fetishism**
AHA: Q4 2017
Fetishistic transvestism
Transvestic disorder

F65.2 **Exhibitionism**
AHA: Q4 2017
Exhibitionistic disorder

F65.3 **Voyeurism**
AHA: Q4 2017
Voyeuristic disorder

F65.4 **Pedophilia**
AHA: Q4 2017
Pedophilic disorder

[5th] F65.5 **Sadomasochism**

F65.50 **Sadomasochism, unspecified**
AHA: Q4 2017

F65.51 **Sexual masochism**
AHA: Q4 2017
Sexual masochism disorder

[PDx] Unacceptable principal diagnosis symbol per Medicare code edits [POA] Code exempt from diagnosis present on admission requirement
[?] Questionable admission [CC] Complication or comorbidity [MCC] Major complication or comorbidity [CC/MCC Exc] CC/MCC exclusion
[HCC] HCC diagnosis code [RxHCC] RxHCC diagnosis code MACRA code **DEFINITION** Describes condition/terminology
TIP Coding guidance 👁 Official Guideline Reference [Z-1] Z code as first-listed diagnosis

When symbols appear on a code that requires a 7th character extension, refer to Appendix B to identify applicable 7th character codes.

F65.52 **Sexual sadism**
    AHA: Q4 2017
    Sexual sadism disorder

🔵 F65.8 **Other paraphilias**
    F65.81 **Frotteurism**
       AHA: Q4 2017
       Frotteuristic disorder
    F65.89 **Other paraphilias**
       AHA: Q4 2017
       Necrophilia
       Other specified paraphilic disorder

F65.9 **Paraphilia, unspecified**
    AHA: Q4 2017
    Paraphilic disorder, unspecified
    Sexual deviation NOS

F66 **Other sexual disorders**
    AHA: Q4 2017
    Sexual maturation disorder
    Sexual relationship disorder

🔵 F68 **Other disorders of adult personality and behavior**
  🔵 F68.1 Factitious disorder imposed on self
    👁 **See Official Guidelines** "Factitious Disorder" I.C.5.c
    Compensation neurosis
    Elaboration of physical symptoms for psychological reasons
    Hospital hopper syndrome
    Münchausen's syndrome
    Peregrinating patient
    EXCLUDES2 *factitial dermatitis (L98.1)*
       person feigning illness (with obvious motivation) (Z76.5)

    F68.10 **Factitious disorder** imposed on self, **unspecified**   CC RxHCC CC/MCC Exc
       AHA: Q4 2018, Q4 2017
    F68.11 **Factitious disorder imposed on self, with** predominantly psychological signs and symptoms   RxHCC
       AHA: Q4 2018, Q4 2017
    F68.12 **Factitious disorder imposed on self, with** predominantly physical signs and symptoms   CC RxHCC CC/MCC Exc
       AHA: Q4 2018, Q4 2017
    F68.13 **Factitious disorder imposed on self, with combined** psychological and physical signs and symptoms   RxHCC
       AHA: Q4 2018, Q4 2017

  F68.A **Factitious disorder** imposed on another   CC RxHCC CC/MCC Exc
    👁 **See Official Guidelines** "Factitious Disorder" I.C.5.c
    AHA: Q4 2018
    Factitious disorder by proxy
    Münchausen's by proxy

  F68.8 **Other specified disorders of adult personality and behavior**
    AHA: Q4 2017

F69 **Unspecified disorder of adult personality and behavior**   A
    AHA: Q4 2017

Intellectual Disabilities (F70-F79)

📖 **Code first** any associated physical or developmental disorders
    EXCLUDES1 *borderline intellectual functioning, IQ above 70 to 84 (R41.83)*

F70 Mild **intellectual disabilities**   RxHCC
    AHA: Q4 2017
    IQ level 50-55 to approximately 70
    Mild mental subnormality

F71 Moderate **intellectual disabilities**   RxHCC
    AHA: Q4 2017
    IQ level 35-40 to 50-55
    Moderate mental subnormality

F72 Severe **intellectual disabilities**   RxHCC
    AHA: Q4 2017
    IQ 20-25 to 35-40
    Severe mental subnormality

F73 Profound **intellectual disabilities**   RxHCC
    AHA: Q4 2017
    IQ level below 20-25
    Profound mental subnormality

F78 Other **intellectual disabilities**   RxHCC
    AHA: Q4 2017

F79 **Unspecified intellectual disabilities**   RxHCC
    AHA: Q4 2017
    Mental deficiency NOS
    Mental subnormality NOS

Pervasive and specific developmental disorders (F80-F89)

🔵 F80 **Specific developmental disorders of speech and language**
  F80.0 Phonological **disorder**
    AHA: Q4 2017
    Dyslalia
    Functional speech articulation disorder
    Lalling
    Lisping
    Phonological developmental disorder
    Speech articulation developmental disorder
    Speech-sound disorder
    EXCLUDES1 *speech articulation impairment due to aphasia NOS (R47.01)*
       speech articulation impairment due to apraxia (R48.2)
    EXCLUDES2 *speech articulation impairment due to hearing loss (F80.4)*
       speech articulation impairment due to intellectual disabilities (F70-F79)
       speech articulation impairment with expressive language developmental disorder (F80.1)
       speech articulation impairment with mixed receptive expressive language developmental disorder (F80.2)

  F80.1 Expressive language **disorder**
    AHA: Q4 2017
    Developmental dysphasia or aphasia, expressive type
    EXCLUDES1 *mixed receptive-expressive language disorder (F80.2)*
       dysphasia and aphasia NOS (R47.-)
    EXCLUDES2 *acquired aphasia with epilepsy [Landau-Kleffner] (G40.80-)*
       selective mutism (F94.0)
       intellectual disabilities (F70-F79)
       pervasive developmental disorders (F84.-)

  F80.2 Mixed receptive-expressive language **disorder**
    AHA: Q4 2017
    Developmental dysphasia or aphasia, receptive type
    Developmental Wernicke's aphasia
    EXCLUDES1 *central auditory processing disorder (H93.25)*
       dysphasia or aphasia NOS (R47.-)
       expressive language disorder (F80.1)
       expressive type dysphasia or aphasia (F80.1)
       word deafness (H93.25)
    EXCLUDES2 *acquired aphasia with epilepsy [Landau-Kleffner] (G40.80-)*
       pervasive developmental disorders (F84.-)
       selective mutism (F94.0)
       intellectual disabilities (F70-F79)

  F80.4 **Speech and language development delay** due to hearing loss
    AHA: Q4 2017
    Code also type of hearing loss (H90.-, H91.-)

Unspecified Code   Other Specified Code   Manifestation Code   N Newborn   P Pediatric   M Maternity   A Adult   ♂ Male   ♀ Female
● New Code   ▲ Revised Code Title   ►◄ Revised Text   **NOTES**   *INCLUDES*   *EXCLUDES1* Not coded here   *EXCLUDES2* Not included here
4th character required   5th character required   6th character required   7th character required   Extension 'X' Alert
HAC Hospital-acquired condition (HAC) alert   AHA AHA Coding Clinic©   📖 Code first alert

2020 ICD-10-CM   When symbols appear on a code that requires a 7th character extension, refer to Appendix B to identify applicable 7th character codes.   **567**

F80.8 Other developmental disorders of speech and language

F80.81 Childhood onset fluency disorder
AHA: Q4 2017
Cluttering NOS
Stuttering NOS
EXCLUDES1 adult onset fluency disorder (F98.5)
fluency disorder in conditions classified elsewhere (R47.82)
fluency disorder (stuttering) following cerebrovascular disease (I69. with final characters -23)

F80.82 Social pragmatic communication disorder
AHA: Q4 2017, Q4 2016
EXCLUDES1 Asperger's syndrome (F84.5)
autistic disorder (F84.0)

F80.89 Other developmental disorders of speech and language
AHA: Q1 2017, Q4 2017

F80.9 Developmental disorder of speech and language, unspecified
AHA: Q4 2017
Communication disorder NOS
Language disorder NOS

F81 Specific developmental disorders of scholastic skills

F81.0 Specific reading disorder
AHA: Q4 2017
'Backward reading'
Developmental dyslexia
Specific learning disorder, with impairment in reading
Specific reading retardation
EXCLUDES1 alexia NOS (R48.0)
dyslexia NOS (R48.0)

F81.2 Mathematics disorder
AHA: Q4 2017
Developmental acalculia
Developmental arithmetical disorder
Developmental Gerstmann's syndrome
Specific learning disorder, with impairment in mathematics
EXCLUDES1 acalculia NOS (R48.8)
EXCLUDES2 arithmetical difficulties associated with a reading disorder (F81.0)
arithmetical difficulties associated with a spelling disorder (F81.81)
arithmetical difficulties due to inadequate teaching (Z55.8)

F81.8 Other developmental disorders of scholastic skills

F81.81 Disorder of written expression
AHA: Q4 2017
Specific learning disorder, with impairment in written expression
Specific spelling disorder

F81.89 Other developmental disorders of scholastic skills
AHA: Q4 2017

F81.9 Developmental disorder of scholastic skills, unspecified
AHA: Q4 2017
Knowledge acquisition disability NOS
Learning disability NOS
Learning disorder NOS

F82 Specific developmental disorder of motor function
AHA: Q4 2017
Clumsy child syndrome
Developmental coordination disorder
Developmental dyspraxia
EXCLUDES1 abnormalities of gait and mobility (R26.-)
lack of coordination (R27.-)
EXCLUDES2 lack of coordination secondary to intellectual disabilities (F70-F79)

F84 Pervasive developmental disorders
Use additional code to identify any associated medical condition and intellectual disabilities.

F84.0 Autistic disorder
AHA: Q1 2017, Q4 2017
Autism spectrum disorder
Infantile autism
Infantile psychosis
Kanner's syndrome
EXCLUDES1 Asperger's syndrome (F84.5)

F84.2 Rett's syndrome
AHA: Q4 2017
EXCLUDES1 Asperger's syndrome (F84.5)
Autistic disorder (F84.0)
Other childhood disintegrative disorder (F84.3)

F84.3 Other childhood disintegrative disorder
AHA: Q4 2017
Dementia infantilis
Disintegrative psychosis
Heller's syndrome
Symbiotic psychosis
Use additional code to identify any associated neurological condition.
EXCLUDES1 Asperger's syndrome (F84.5)
Autistic disorder (F84.0)
Rett's syndrome (F84.2)

F84.5 Asperger's syndrome
AHA: Q4 2017
Asperger's disorder
Autistic psychopathy
Schizoid disorder of childhood

F84.8 Other pervasive developmental disorders
AHA: Q4 2017
Overactive disorder associated with intellectual disabilities and stereotyped movements

F84.9 Pervasive developmental disorder, unspecified
AHA: Q4 2017
Atypical autism

F88 Other disorders of psychological development
AHA: Q4 2017
Developmental agnosia
Global developmental delay
Other specified neurodevelopmental disorder

F89 Unspecified disorder of psychological development
AHA: Q4 2017
Developmental disorder NOS
Neurodevelopmental disorder NOS

Behavioral and emotional disorders with onset usually occurring in childhood and adolescence (F90-F98)

NOTES Codes within categories F90-F98 may be used regardless of the age of a patient. These disorders generally have onset within the childhood or adolescent years, but may continue throughout life or not be diagnosed until adulthood

F90 Attention-deficit hyperactivity disorders
INCLUDES attention deficit disorder with hyperactivity
attention deficit syndrome with hyperactivity
EXCLUDES2 anxiety disorders (F40.-, F41.-)
mood [affective] disorders (F30-F39)
pervasive developmental disorders (F84.-)
schizophrenia (F20.-)

F90.0 Attention-deficit hyperactivity disorder, predominantly inattentive type
AHA: Q4 2017
Attention-deficit/hyperactivity disorder, predominantly inattentive presentation

---

PDxn Unacceptable principal diagnosis symbol per Medicare code edits   PoN Code exempt from diagnosis present on admission requirement
? Questionable admission   CC Complication or comorbidity   MCC Major complication or comorbidity   CC/MCC Exc CC/MCC exclusion
HCC HCC diagnosis code   RxHCC RxHCC diagnosis code   MACRA code   **DEFINITION** Describes condition/terminology
TIP Coding guidance   👁 Official Guideline Reference   Z1 Z code as first-listed diagnosis

When symbols appear on a code that requires a 7th character extension, refer to Appendix B to identify applicable 7th character codes.   **2020 ICD-10-CM**

F90.1 **Attention-deficit hyperactivity disorder,** predominantly hyperactive type `RxHCC`
  AHA: Q4 2017
  Attention-deficit/hyperactivity disorder, predominantly hyperactive impulsive presentation

F90.2 **Attention-deficit hyperactivity disorder,** combined type `RxHCC`
  AHA: Q4 2017
  Attention-deficit/hyperactivity disorder, combined presentation

F90.8 **Attention-deficit hyperactivity disorder, other type** `RxHCC`
  AHA: Q4 2017

F90.9 **Attention-deficit hyperactivity disorder, unspecified type** `RxHCC`
  AHA: Q4 2017
  Attention-deficit hyperactivity disorder of childhood or adolescence NOS
  Attention-deficit hyperactivity disorder NOS

④ᵗʰ **F91 Conduct disorders**
  EXCLUDES1 antisocial behavior (Z72.81-)
      antisocial personality disorder (F60.2)
  EXCLUDES2 conduct problems associated with attention-deficit hyperactivity disorder (F90.-)
      mood [affective] disorders (F30-F39)
      pervasive developmental disorders (F84.-)
      schizophrenia (F20.-)

  F91.0 **Conduct disorder** confined to family context `RxHCC`
    AHA: Q4 2017

  F91.1 **Conduct disorder,** childhood-onset type `RxHCC`
    AHA: Q4 2017
    Unsocialized conduct disorder
    Conduct disorder, solitary aggressive type
    Unsocialized aggressive disorder

  F91.2 **Conduct disorder,** adolescent-onset type `RxHCC`
    AHA: Q4 2017
    Socialized conduct disorder
    Conduct disorder, group type

  F91.3 Oppositional defiant **disorder** `RxHCC`
    AHA: Q4 2017

  F91.8 **Other conduct disorders** `RxHCC`
    AHA: Q4 2017
    Other specified conduct disorder
    Other specified disruptive disorder

  F91.9 **Conduct disorder, unspecified** `RxHCC`
    AHA: Q4 2017
    Behavioral disorder NOS
    Conduct disorder NOS
    Disruptive behavior disorder NOS
    Disruptive disorder NOS

④ᵗʰ **F93 Emotional disorders with onset specific to childhood**
  F93.0 **Separation anxiety disorder of childhood**
    AHA: Q4 2017
    EXCLUDES2 mood [affective] disorders (F30-F39)
        nonpsychotic mental disorders (F40-F48)
        phobic anxiety disorder of childhood (F40.8)
        social phobia (F40.1)

  F93.8 **Other childhood emotional disorders**
    AHA: Q4 2017
    Identity disorder
    EXCLUDES2 gender identity disorder of childhood (F64.2)

  F93.9 **Childhood emotional disorder, unspecified**
    AHA: Q4 2017

④ᵗʰ **F94 Disorders of social functioning with onset specific to childhood and adolescence**
  F94.0 Selective **mutism**
    AHA: Q4 2017
    Elective mutism
    EXCLUDES2 pervasive developmental disorders (F84.-)
        schizophrenia (F20.-)
        specific developmental disorders of speech and language (F80.-)
        transient mutism as part of separation anxiety in young children (F93.0)

F94.1 Reactive **attachment disorder of childhood**
  AHA: Q4 2017
  Use additional code to identify any associated failure to thrive or growth retardation
  EXCLUDES1 disinhibited attachment disorder of childhood (F94.2)
      normal variation in pattern of selective attachment
  EXCLUDES2 Asperger's syndrome (F84.5)
      maltreatment syndromes (T74.-)
      sexual or physical abuse in childhood, resulting in psychosocial problems (Z62.81-)

F94.2 Disinhibited **attachment disorder of childhood**
  AHA: Q4 2017
  Affectionless psychopathy
  Institutional syndrome
  EXCLUDES1 reactive attachment disorder of childhood (F94.1)
  EXCLUDES2 Asperger's syndrome (F84.5)
      attention-deficit hyperactivity disorders (F90.-)
      hospitalism in children (F43.2-)

F94.8 **Other childhood disorders of social functioning**
  AHA: Q4 2017

F94.9 **Childhood disorder of social functioning, unspecified**
  AHA: Q4 2017

④ᵗʰ **F95 Tic disorder**
  F95.0 Transient **tic disorder**
    AHA: Q4 2017
    Provisional tic disorder

  F95.1 Chronic motor **or** vocal **tic disorder**
    AHA: Q4 2017

  F95.2 Tourette's **disorder** `RxHCC`
    AHA: Q4 2017
    Combined vocal and multiple motor tic disorder [de la Tourette]
    Tourette's syndrome

  F95.8 **Other tic disorders**
    AHA: Q4 2017

  F95.9 **Tic disorder, unspecified**
    AHA: Q4 2017
    Tic NOS

④ᵗʰ **F98 Other behavioral and emotional disorders with onset usually occurring in childhood and adolescence**
  EXCLUDES2 breath-holding spells (R06.89)
      gender identity disorder of childhood (F64.2)
      Kleine-Levin syndrome (G47.13)
      obsessive-compulsive disorder (F42-)
      sleep disorders not due to a substance or known physiological condition (F51.-)

  F98.0 Enuresis **not due to a substance or known physiological condition**
    AHA: Q4 2017
    Enuresis (primary) (secondary) of nonorganic origin
    Functional enuresis
    Psychogenic enuresis
    Urinary incontinence of nonorganic origin
    EXCLUDES1 enuresis NOS (R32)

  F98.1 Encopresis **not due to a substance or known physiological condition**
    AHA: Q4 2017
    Functional encopresis
    Incontinence of feces of nonorganic origin
    Psychogenic encopresis
    Use additional code to identify the cause of any coexisting constipation.
    EXCLUDES1 encopresis NOS (R15.-)

⑤ᵗʰ F98.2 **Other feeding disorders of infancy and childhood**
    EXCLUDES1 feeding difficulties (R63.3)
    EXCLUDES2 anorexia nervosa and other eating disorders (F50.-)
        feeding problems of newborn (P92.-)
        pica of infancy or childhood (F98.3)

Unspecified Code   Other Specified Code   Manifestation Code   Ⓝ Newborn   Ⓟ Pediatric   Ⓜ Maternity   Ⓐ Adult   ♂ Male   ♀ Female
● New Code   ▲ Revised Code Title   ▶◀ Revised Text   **NOTES**   *INCLUDES*   *EXCLUDES1* Not coded here   *EXCLUDES2* Not included here
④ᵗʰ 4ᵗʰ character required   ⑤ᵗʰ 5ᵗʰ character required   ⑥ᵗʰ 6ᵗʰ character required   ⑦ᵗʰ 7ᵗʰ character required   ⑦ Extension 'X' Alert
HAC Hospital-acquired condition (HAC) alert   **AHA** AHA Coding Clinic©   📷 Code first alert

F98.21 **Rumination disorder of infancy**
AHA: Q4 2017

F98.29 **Other feeding disorders of infancy and early childhood**
AHA: Q4 2017

F98.3 **Pica of infancy and childhood**
AHA: Q4 2017

F98.4 **Stereotyped movement disorders** [RxHCC]
AHA: Q4 2017
Stereotype/habit disorder
EXCLUDES1 abnormal involuntary movements (R25.-)
EXCLUDES2 compulsions in obsessive-compulsive disorder (F42-)
hair plucking (F63.3)
movement disorders of organic origin (G20-G25)
nail-biting (F98.8)
nose-picking (F98.8)
stereotypies that are part of a broader psychiatric condition (F01-F95)
thumb-sucking (F98.8)
tic disorders (F95.-)
trichotillomania (F63.3)

F98.5 **Adult onset fluency disorder**
AHA: Q4 2017
EXCLUDES1 childhood onset fluency disorder (F80.81)
dysphasia (R47.02)
fluency disorder in conditions classified elsewhere (R47.82)
fluency disorder (stuttering) following cerebrovascular disease (I69. with final characters -23)
tic disorders (F95.-)

F98.8 **Other specified behavioral and emotional disorders with onset usually occurring in childhood and adolescence**
AHA: Q4 2017
Excessive masturbation
Nail-biting
Nose-picking
Thumb-sucking

F98.9 **Unspecified behavioral and emotional disorders with onset usually occurring in childhood and adolescence**
AHA: Q4 2017

Unspecified mental disorder (F99)

F99 **Mental disorder, not otherwise specified**
AHA: Q4 2017, Q4 2016
Mental illness NOS
EXCLUDES1 unspecified mental disorder due to known physiological condition (F09)

PDx Unacceptable principal diagnosis symbol per Medicare code edits   Code exempt from diagnosis present on admission requirement
❓ Questionable admission   cc Complication or comorbidity   MCC Major complication or comorbidity   cc/mcc ex CC/MCC exclusion
HCC HCC diagnosis code   RxHCC RxHCC diagnosis code   MACRA code   **DEFINITION** Describes condition/terminology
TIP Coding guidance   👁 Official Guideline Reference   Z Z code as first-listed diagnosis

570

When symbols appear on a code that requires a 7th character extension, refer to Appendix B to identify applicable 7th character codes.

2020 ICD-10-CM

Chapter 6: Diseases of the Nervous System (G00-G99)

Anatomy of the Nervous System

Introduction

The nervous system (Figure 6.a) constitutes the body's control center and the communication network and directs the functions of multiple body organs and systems. It helps the individual to interpret external environmental events and respond to various environmental stimuli. The nervous system includes the following types and components:

1. The Central Nervous System (CNS)

The central nervous system is regarded as the control center of the entire nervous system. It is composed of the brain and the spinal cord. The CNS receives the body's sensations and information about the external environmental changes via receptors and sense organs, and directs the body to act accordingly in response to these external environmental stimuli.

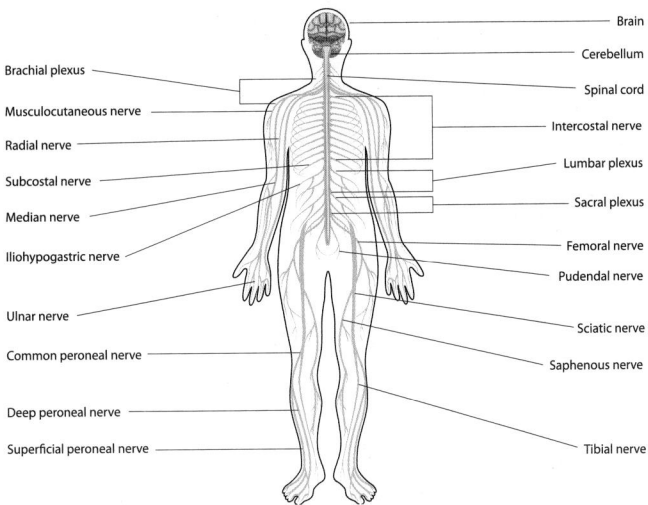

Figure 6.a Human Nervous System

2. The Peripheral Nervous System (PNS)

The peripheral nervous system is composed of the nerves that connect the brain and spinal cord with the glands, muscles and sensory receptors. The PNS can be further divided into the following subcategories:

a) The Afferent Peripheral System

The afferent peripheral system is composed of sensory (or afferent) neurons that transfer information to the brain and spinal cord via peripheral receptors.

b) The Efferent Peripheral System

The efferent peripheral system consists of the motor (or efferent) neurons that form a communication channel (for information transfer) between the brain, spinal cord, muscles and glands. This system of neurons is further divided into the following subcategories:

i) Somatic Nervous System

The somatic nervous system helps the individual to respond to the changes in the external environment by conducting the impulses from the brain and spinal cord to the skeletal muscle.

ii) Autonomic Nervous System

The autonomic nervous system (ANS) is an involuntary system of nerves that conduct impulses from the brain and spinal cord to the smooth muscles of the intestine, the cardiac muscles of the heart, and the endocrine glands. The organs of this particular system receive nerve fibers from the following divisions of the ANS:

(a) Sympathetic Division

The sympathetic division acts to mobilize the body's resources and induce the fight-or-flight response. This system uses norepinephrine as a neurotransmitter to speed up its activity through energy expenditure.

(b) Parasympathetic Division

The parasympathetic division facilitates the vegetative activities of human body (like digestion, urination and defecation).

3. The Spinal Cord (or Medulla Spinalis)

The spinal cord initiates as a continuation of the medulla oblongata of the brainstem. Its length varies between 16 to 18 inches and is made up of a series of 31 segments, each of which gives rise to a pair of spinal nerves. The human spinal cord is further protected by a series of connective tissue membranes that are known as the spinal meninges.

4. The Brain or Encephalon

The brain (Figure 6.b) is regarded as one of the largest organs of the body and weighs about 3 pounds in an average adult. The major parts of the human brain are described as follows:

a) The Brainstem

The brainstem is regarded as the posterior portion of the brain, which is structurally continuous with the spinal cord. It is composed of the medulla oblongata, the pons Varolii, and the midbrain.

b) The Diencephalon

The diencephalon is located between the two cerebral hemispheres, and superiorly to the midbrain. It surrounds the third ventricle of the brain and consists of the thalamus and hypothalamus regions.

c) The Cerebrum (or Telencephalon)

The cerebrum constitutes the bulk of the brain and is composed of the gray matter (or cerebral cortex), longitudinal fissure, and the right and left cerebral hemispheres. It is further subdivided into the frontal, parietal, occipital and temporal lobes.

d) The Cerebellum

The cerebellum is regarded as the second largest portion of the brain. It is located under the occipital lobes of the cerebrum, and behind the pons and medulla oblongata of brainstem. The two partially separated hemispheres of the cerebellum are connected together by a centrally constricted structure, which is known as the vermis. The cerebellum is constituted primarily by the white matter and a thin layer of gray matter on its surface, which is known as the cerebellar cortex. The cerebrospinal fluid (CSF) is a colorless fluid that fills up the subarachnoid space (or interval between the arachnoid membrane and pia mater) and the ventricular system inside and around the spinal cord and brain.

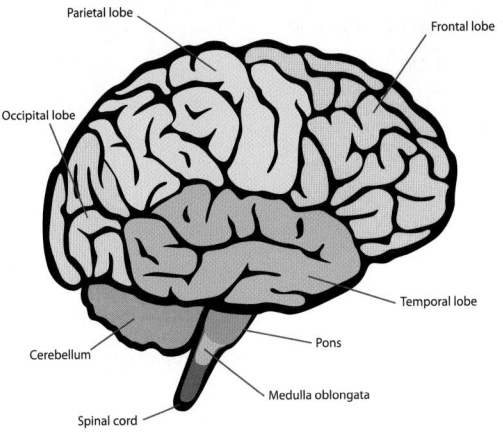

Figure 6.b Anatomy of the Brain

5. The Cranial Nerves

The cranial nerves (Figure 6.c, on the next page) are based on 12 pairs that remain attached to the brain and leave the skull through various foramina in the cranial base. The names of the various cranial nerves are listed below:

a) Olfactory (1st cranial nerve)

b) Optic (2nd cranial nerve)

c) Oculomotor (3rd cranial nerve)

d) Trochlear (4th cranial nerve)

e) Trigeminal (5th cranial nerve)

f) Abducens (6th cranial nerve)

g) The Facial (7th cranial nerve)

h) Acoustic (8th cranial nerve)

i) Glossopharyngeal (9th cranial nerve)

j) Vagus/Pneumogastric (10th cranial nerve)

k) Accessory (11th cranial nerve)

l) Hypoglossal (12th cranial nerve)

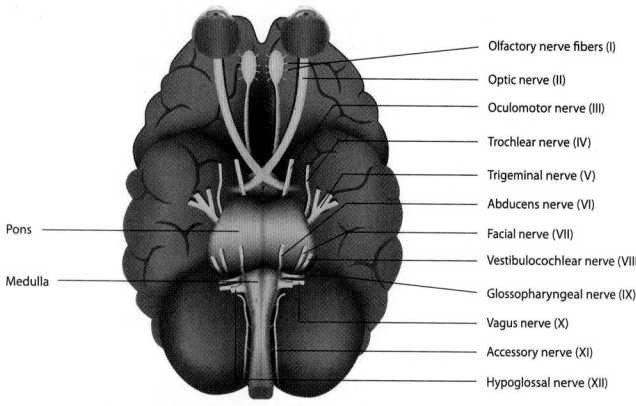

Figure 6.c The Cranial Nerves

6. **The Spinal Nerves**
   The 31 pairs of spinal nerves originate from the integration of the dorsal and ventral roots of the spinal nerves. These nerves carry the motor, sensory and the autonomic signals between the spinal cord and the body. They are also called mixed nerves as they consist of both motor and sensory fibers. The spinal nerves exit the vertebral column between the adjacent vertebrae. The naming convention of the spinal nerves is based on the region and level of the spinal cord from which these nerves arise. The division of the spinal nerves is documented below:

   a) 8 pairs of cervical nerves (C1-C8)

   b) 12 pairs of thoracic nerves (T1-T12)

   c) 5 pairs of lumbar nerves (L1-L5)

   d) 5 pairs of sacral nerves (S1-S5)

   e) 1 pair of coccygeal nerves (Cx)

7. **The Sympathetic Nerves**
   The sympathetic nerves are a part of the sympathetic nervous system, which innervates the striated muscles of the heart, the smooth muscles, and multiple glands of the body. The sympathetic nervous system is that division of the autonomic nervous system which prepares the body for stressful conditions requiring energy expenditure. The nerve fibers of this system originate from the thoracic and lumbar regions of the spinal cord. The axons of these nerves leave the spinal cord via the anterior root. They further pass near the spinal ganglion and integrate with the anterior rami of the spinal nerves.

Common Pathologies

Muscular Dystrophy (MD) (Figure 6.d)

A genetic disorder characterized by progressive muscle weakness, abnormal muscle protein, and death of muscle tissues and cells. MD is classified as both a myogenic and a nervous system disorder.

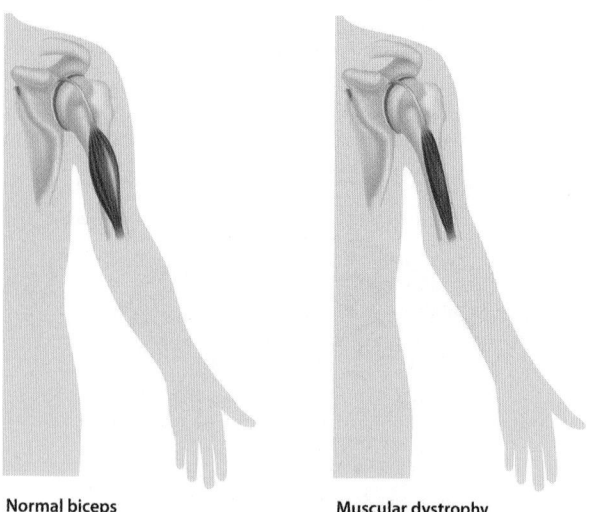

Figure 6.d Muscular Dystrophy (MD)

Spina Bifida
This is a type of birth defect of the brain, spine, or spinal cord, also known as the neural tube defect. It happens if the spinal column of the fetus doesn't close completely during the first month of pregnancy.

Parkinson's Disease (PD)
This is a progressive disorder of the nervous system that affects the movement and is known as a movement disorder.

Alzheimer's Disease (AD)
This is a brain disorder that seriously affects a person's ability to carry out daily activities. Alzheimer's disease is the most common form of dementia.

Strokes
This is a condition in which, due to lack of oxygen, the sudden death of brain cells occurs and can be caused by an obstruction in the blood flow to the brain. The more common kind, called ischemic stroke, is caused by a blood clot that blocks or plugs a blood vessel in the brain. The other kind, called hemorrhagic stroke (Figure 6.e), is caused by a blood vessel that breaks and bleeds into the brain. "Mini-strokes" or transient ischemic attacks (TIAs), occur when the blood supply to the brain is briefly interrupted.

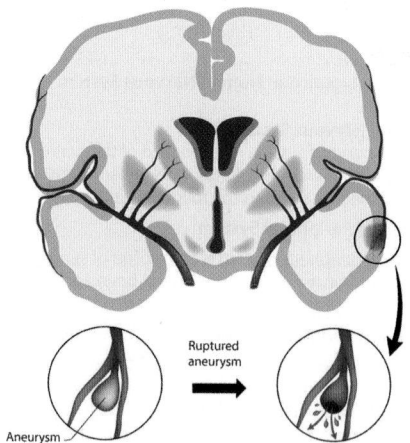

Figure 6.e Hemorrhagic Stroke

Malignant Brain Tumor
Cancer of the brain is usually called a malignant brain tumor.

Meningitis
The inflammation of the thin tissue that surrounds the brain and spinal cord, called the meninges, is known as Meningitis.

Epilepsy
This is a neurological condition that affects the nervous system. Epilepsy is also known as a seizure disorder that causes people to have recurring seizures.

Bell's Palsy
This condition occurs due to compression of a facial nerve.

Diseases of the nervous system (G00-G99)

> *EXCLUDES2* *certain conditions originating in the perinatal period (P04-P96)*
>
> *certain infectious and parasitic diseases (A00-B99)*
>
> *complications of pregnancy, childbirth and the puerperium (O00-O9A)*
>
> *congenital malformations, deformations, and chromosomal abnormalities (Q00-Q99)*
>
> *endocrine, nutritional and metabolic diseases (E00-E88)*
>
> *injury, poisoning and certain other consequences of external causes (S00-T88)*
>
> *neoplasms (C00-D49)*
>
> *symptoms, signs and abnormal clinical and laboratory findings, not elsewhere classified (R00-R94)*

This chapter contains the following blocks:

G00-G09 Inflammatory diseases of the central nervous system
G10-G14 Systemic atrophies primarily affecting the central nervous system
G20-G26 Extrapyramidal and movement disorders
G30-G32 Other degenerative diseases of the nervous system
G35-G37 Demyelinating diseases of the central nervous system
G40-G47 Episodic and paroxysmal disorders
G50-G59 Nerve, nerve root and plexus disorders
G60-G65 Polyneuropathies and other disorders of the peripheral nervous system
G70-G73 Diseases of myoneural junction and muscle
G80-G83 Cerebral palsy and other paralytic syndromes
G89-G99 Other disorders of the nervous system

Inflammatory diseases of the central nervous system (G00-G09)

G00 Bacterial meningitis, not elsewhere classified (Figure 6.1)

> *INCLUDES* *bacterial arachnoiditis*
> *bacterial leptomeningitis*
> *bacterial meningitis*
> *bacterial pachymeningitis*
>
> *EXCLUDES1* *bacterial meningoencephalitis (G04.2)*
> *bacterial meningomyelitis (G04.2)*

G00.0 Hemophilus meningitis
Meningitis due to Hemophilus influenzae

G00.1 Pneumococcal meningitis
Meningitis due to Streptococcal pneumoniae

G00.2 Streptococcal meningitis
Use additional code to further identify organism (B95.0-B95.5)

G00.3 Staphylococcal meningitis
Use additional code to further identify organism (B95.61-B95.8)

G00.8 Other bacterial meningitis
Meningitis due to Escherichia coli
Meningitis due to Friedländer's bacillus
Meningitis due to Klebsiella
Use additional code to further identify organism (B96.-)

G00.9 Bacterial meningitis, unspecified
Meningitis due to gram-negative bacteria, unspecified
Purulent meningitis NOS
Pyogenic meningitis NOS
Suppurative meningitis NOS

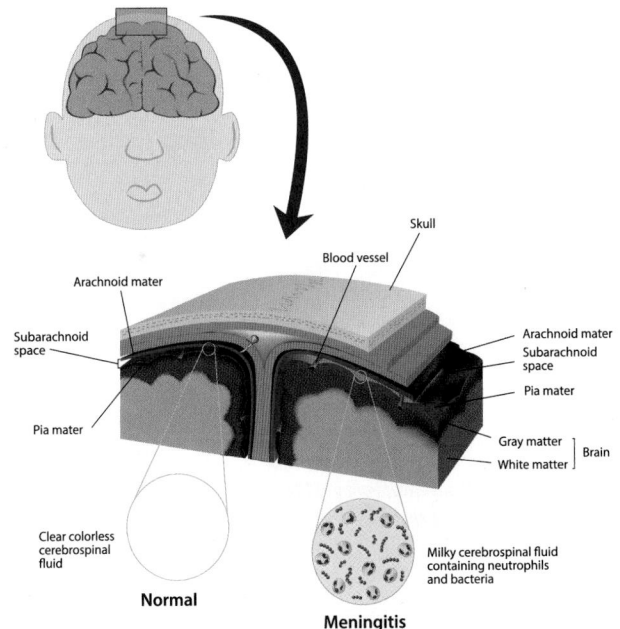

Figure 6.1 Meningitis

G01 Meningitis in bacterial diseases classified elsewhere

> ☞ Code first underlying disease
>
> *EXCLUDES1* *meningitis (in):*
> *gonococcal (A54.81)*
> *leptospirosis (A27.81)*
> *listeriosis (A32.11)*
> *Lyme disease (A69.21)*
> *meningococcal (A39.0)*
> *neurosyphilis (A52.13)*
> *tuberculosis (A17.0)*
> *meningoencephalitis and meningomyelitis in bacterial diseases classified elsewhere (G05)*

G02 Meningitis in other infectious and parasitic diseases classified elsewhere

> ☞ Code first underlying disease, such as:
> African trypanosomiasis (B56.-)
> poliovirus infection (A80.-)
>
> *EXCLUDES1* *candidal meningitis (B37.5)*
> *coccidioidomycosis meningitis (B38.4)*
> *cryptococcal meningitis (B45.1)*
> *herpesviral [herpes simplex] meningitis (B00.3)*
> *infectious mononucleosis complicated by meningitis (B27.- with fourth character 2)*
> *measles complicated by meningitis (B05.1)*
> *meningoencephalitis and meningomyelitis in other infectious and parasitic diseases classified elsewhere (G05)*
> *mumps meningitis (B26.1)*
> *rubella meningitis (B06.02)*
> *varicella [chickenpox] meningitis (B01.0)*
> *zoster meningitis (B02.1)*

G03 Meningitis due to other and unspecified causes

> *INCLUDES* *arachnoiditis NOS*
> *leptomeningitis NOS*
> *meningitis NOS*
> *pachymeningitis NOS*
>
> *EXCLUDES1* *meningoencephalitis (G04.-)*
> *meningomyelitis (G04.-)*

Unspecified Code   Other Specified Code   Manifestation Code   N Newborn   P Pediatric   M Maternity   A Adult   ♂ Male   ♀ Female
● New Code   ▲ Revised Code Title   ►◄ Revised Text   **NOTES**   *INCLUDES*   *EXCLUDES1* Not coded here   *EXCLUDES2* Not included here
4ᵗʰ character required   5ᵗʰ character required   6ᵗʰ character required   7ᵗʰ character required   Extension 'X' Alert
HAC Hospital-acquired condition (HAC) alert   **AHA** AHA Coding Clinic©   ☞ Code first alert

G03.0 Nonpyogenic meningitis   MCC CC/MCC Exc
     Aseptic meningitis
     Nonbacterial meningitis

G03.1 Chronic meningitis   CC CC/MCC Exc

G03.2 Benign recurrent meningitis [Mollaret]   CC CC/MCC Exc

G03.8 Meningitis due to other specified causes   MCC CC/MCC Exc

G03.9 Meningitis, unspecified   MCC CC/MCC Exc
     Arachnoiditis (spinal) NOS

G04 Encephalitis, myelitis and encephalomyelitis

   INCLUDES   acute ascending myelitis
           meningoencephalitis
           meningomyelitis

   EXCLUDES1 encephalopathy NOS (G93.40)

   EXCLUDES2 acute transverse myelitis (G37.3-)
            alcoholic encephalopathy (G31.2)
            benign myalgic encephalomyelitis (G93.3)
            multiple sclerosis (G35)
            subacute necrotizing myelitis (G37.4)
            toxic encephalitis (G92)
            toxic encephalopathy (G92)

   G04.0 Acute disseminated encephalitis and encephalomyelitis (ADEM)

     EXCLUDES1 acute necrotizing hemorrhagic encephalopathy (G04.3-)
             other noninfectious acute disseminated encephalomyelitis (noninfectious ADEM) (G04.81)

     G04.00 Acute disseminated encephalitis and encephalomyelitis, unspecified   MCC CC/MCC Exc

     G04.01 Postinfectious acute disseminated encephalitis and encephalomyelitis (postinfectious ADEM)   MCC CC/MCC Exc
         EXCLUDES1 post chickenpox encephalitis (B01.1)
               post measles encephalitis (B05.0)
               post measles myelitis (B05.1)

     G04.02 Postimmunization acute disseminated encephalitis, myelitis and encephalomyelitis   MCC
         Encephalitis, post immunization
         Encephalomyelitis, post immunization
         Use additional code to identify the vaccine (T50.A-, T50.B-, T50.Z-)

   G04.1 Tropical spastic paraplegia   CC HCC RxHCC CC/MCC Exc

   G04.2 Bacterial meningoencephalitis and meningomyelitis, not elsewhere classified   MCC CC/MCC Exc

   G04.3 Acute necrotizing hemorrhagic encephalopathy
     EXCLUDES1 acute disseminated encephalitis and encephalomyelitis (G04.0-)

     G04.30 Acute necrotizing hemorrhagic encephalopathy, unspecified   MCC

     G04.31 Postinfectious acute necrotizing hemorrhagic encephalopathy   MCC CC/MCC Exc

     G04.32 Postimmunization acute necrotizing hemorrhagic encephalopathy   MCC
         Use additional code to identify the vaccine (T50.A-, T50.B-, T50.Z-)

     G04.39 Other acute necrotizing hemorrhagic encephalopathy   MCC
         Code also underlying etiology, if applicable

   G04.8 Other encephalitis, myelitis and encephalomyelitis
     Code also any associated seizure (G40.-, R56.9)

     G04.81 Other encephalitis and encephalomyelitis   MCC CC/MCC Exc
         Noninfectious acute disseminated encephalomyelitis (noninfectious ADEM)

     G04.89 Other myelitis   HCC MCC RxHCC CC/MCC Exc

   G04.9 Encephalitis, myelitis and encephalomyelitis, unspecified

     G04.90 Encephalitis and encephalomyelitis, unspecified   MCC CC/MCC Exc
         Ventriculitis (cerebral) NOS

     G04.91 Myelitis, unspecified   HCC MCC RxHCC CC/MCC Exc

G05 Encephalitis, myelitis and encephalomyelitis in diseases classified elsewhere

   ☞ Code first underlying disease, such as:
     human immunodeficiency virus [HIV] disease (B20)
     poliovirus (A80.-)
     suppurative otitis media (H66.01-H66.4)
     trichinellosis (B75)

   EXCLUDES1 adenoviral encephalitis, myelitis and encephalomyelitis (A85.1)
            congenital toxoplasmosis encephalitis, myelitis and encephalomyelitis (P37.1)
            cytomegaloviral encephalitis, myelitis and encephalomyelitis (B25.8)
            encephalitis, myelitis and encephalomyelitis (in) measles (B05.0)
            encephalitis, myelitis and encephalomyelitis (in) systemic lupus erythematosus (M32.19)
            enteroviral encephalitis, myelitis and encephalomyelitis (A85.0)
            eosinophilic meningoencephalitis (B83.2)
            herpesviral [herpes simplex] encephalitis, myelitis and encephalomyelitis (B00.4)
            listerial encephalitis, myelitis and encephalomyelitis (A32.12)
            meningococcal encephalitis, myelitis and encephalomyelitis (A39.81)
            mumps encephalitis, myelitis and encephalomyelitis (B26.2)
            postchickenpox encephalitis, myelitis and encephalomyelitis (B01.1-)
            rubella encephalitis, myelitis and encephalomyelitis (B06.01)
            toxoplasmosis encephalitis, myelitis and encephalomyelitis (B58.2)
            zoster encephalitis, myelitis and encephalomyelitis (B02.0)

   G05.3 Encephalitis and encephalomyelitis in diseases classified elsewhere   MCC CC/MCC Exc
     Meningoencephalitis in diseases classified elsewhere

   G05.4 Myelitis in diseases classified elsewhere   HCC MCC RxHCC CC/MCC Exc
     Meningomyelitis in diseases classified elsewhere

G06 Intracranial and intraspinal abscess and granuloma
   Use additional code (B95-B97) to identify infectious agent.

   G06.0 Intracranial abscess and granuloma   MCC CC/MCC Exc
     Brain [any part] abscess (embolic)
     Cerebellar abscess (embolic)
     Cerebral abscess (embolic)
     Intracranial epidural abscess or granuloma
     Intracranial extradural abscess or granuloma
     Intracranial subdural abscess or granuloma
     Otogenic abscess (embolic)
     EXCLUDES1 tuberculous intracranial abscess and granuloma (A17.81)

   G06.1 Intraspinal abscess and granuloma   MCC CC/MCC Exc
     Abscess (embolic) of spinal cord [any part]
     Intraspinal epidural abscess or granuloma
     Intraspinal extradural abscess or granuloma
     Intraspinal subdural abscess or granuloma
     EXCLUDES1 tuberculous intraspinal abscess and granuloma (A17.81)

   G06.2 Extradural and subdural abscess, unspecified   MCC CC/MCC Exc

G07 Intracranial and intraspinal abscess and granuloma in diseases classified elsewhere   MCC CC/MCC Exc

   ☞ Code first underlying disease, such as:
     schistosomiasis granuloma of brain (B65.-)

   EXCLUDES1 abscess of brain:
         amebic (A06.6)
         chromomycotic (B43.1)
         gonococcal (A54.82)
         tuberculous (A17.81)
         tuberculoma of meninges (A17.1)

When symbols appear on a code that requires a 7th character extension, refer to Appendix B to identify applicable 7th character codes.   **2020 ICD-10-CM**

G08 **Intracranial and intraspinal phlebitis and thrombophlebitis** MCC CC/MCC Excl
Septic embolism of intracranial or intraspinal venous sinuses and veins
Septic endophlebitis of intracranial or intraspinal venous sinuses and veins
Septic phlebitis of intracranial or intraspinal venous sinuses and veins
Septic thrombophlebitis of intracranial or intraspinal venous sinuses and veins
Septic thrombosis of intracranial or intraspinal venous sinuses and veins
EXCLUDES1 intracranial phlebitis and thrombophlebitis complicating:
abortion, ectopic or molar pregnancy (O00-O07, O08.7)
pregnancy, childbirth and the puerperium (O22.5, O87.3)
nonpyogenic intracranial phlebitis and thrombophlebitis (I67.6)
EXCLUDES2 intracranial phlebitis and thrombophlebitis complicating nonpyogenic intraspinal phlebitis and thrombophlebitis (G95.1)

G09 **Sequelae of inflammatory diseases of central nervous system**
NOTES Category G09 is to be used to indicate conditions whose primary classification is to G00-G08 as the cause of sequelae, themselves classifiable elsewhere. The 'sequelae' include conditions specified as residuals.
☞ **Code first** condition resulting from (sequela) of inflammatory diseases of central nervous system

Systemic atrophies primarily affecting the central nervous system (G10-G14)

G10 **Huntington's disease** HCC RxHCC
Huntington's chorea
Huntington's dementia
Code also dementia in other diseases classified elsewhere without behavioral disturbance (F02.80)

4ᵗʰ G11 **Hereditary** ataxia
DEFINITION: Ataxia is lack of muscle coordination when attempting voluntary movement.
EXCLUDES2 cerebral palsy (G80.-)
hereditary and idiopathic neuropathy (G60.-)
metabolic disorders (E70-E88)
G11.0 Congenital nonprogressive **ataxia** HCC
G11.1 Early-onset cerebellar **ataxia** HCC
Early-onset cerebellar ataxia with essential tremor
Early-onset cerebellar ataxia with myoclonus [Hunt's ataxia]
Early-onset cerebellar ataxia with retained tendon reflexes
Friedreich's ataxia (autosomal recessive)
X-linked recessive spinocerebellar ataxia
G11.2 Late-onset cerebellar **ataxia** A HCC
G11.3 Cerebellar **ataxia** with defective DNA repair HCC
Ataxia telangiectasia [Louis-Bar]
EXCLUDES2 Cockayne's syndrome ▶(Q87.19)◀
other disorders of purine and pyrimidine metabolism (E79.-)
xeroderma pigmentosum (Q82.1)
G11.4 Hereditary spastic paraplegia HCC
G11.8 Other hereditary **ataxias** HCC
G11.9 **Hereditary ataxia, unspecified** HCC
Hereditary cerebellar ataxia NOS
Hereditary cerebellar degeneration
Hereditary cerebellar disease
Hereditary cerebellar syndrome

4ᵗʰ G12 **Spinal muscular atrophy and related syndromes**
G12.0 Infantile **spinal** muscular atrophy, type I [Werdnig-Hoffman] HCC RxHCC
G12.1 Other inherited **spinal** muscular atrophy HCC RxHCC
Adult form spinal muscular atrophy
Childhood form, type II spinal muscular atrophy
Distal spinal muscular atrophy
Juvenile form, type III spinal muscular atrophy [Kugelberg-Welander]
Progressive bulbar palsy of childhood [Fazio-Londe]
Scapuloperoneal form spinal muscular atrophy

5ᵗʰ G12.2 Motor neuron disease
G12.20 **Motor neuron disease, unspecified** HCC RxHCC
G12.21 Amyotrophic lateral sclerosis A HCC RxHCC
G12.22 Progressive bulbar palsy HCC RxHCC
G12.23 Primary **lateral** sclerosis CC HCC RxHCC CC/MCC Excl
G12.24 Familial **motor** neuron disease CC HCC RxHCC CC/MCC Excl
G12.25 Progressive **spinal** muscle atrophy CC HCC RxHCC CC/MCC Excl
G12.29 Other **motor** neuron disease HCC RxHCC
G12.8 **Other spinal muscular atrophies and related syndromes** HCC RxHCC
G12.9 **Spinal muscular atrophy, unspecified** HCC RxHCC

4ᵗʰ G13 **Systemic atrophies primarily affecting central nervous system in diseases classified elsewhere**
G13.0 **Paraneoplastic neuromyopathy and neuropathy** HCC RxHCC
Carcinomatous neuromyopathy
Sensorial paraneoplastic neuropathy [Denny Brown]
☞ **Code first** underlying neoplasm (C00-D49)
G13.1 **Other systemic atrophy primarily affecting central nervous system in neoplastic disease** HCC RxHCC
Paraneoplastic limbic encephalopathy
☞ **Code first** underlying neoplasm (C00-D49)
G13.2 **Systemic atrophy primarily affecting the central nervous system in myxedema** HCC RxHCC
☞ **Code first** underlying disease, such as:
hypothyroidism (E03.-)
myxedematous congenital iodine deficiency (E00.1)
G13.8 **Systemic atrophy primarily affecting central nervous system in other diseases classified elsewhere** HCC RxHCC
☞ **Code first** underlying disease

G14 **Postpolio syndrome**
INCLUDES postpolio myelitic syndrome
EXCLUDES1 sequelae of poliomyelitis (B91)

Extrapyramidal and movement disorders (G20-G26)

G20 **Parkinson's disease** HCC RxHCC
👁 **See Official Guidelines** "Etiology/manifestation convention" I.A.13
AHA: Q2 2017, Q2 2016
Hemiparkinsonism
Idiopathic Parkinsonism or Parkinson's disease
Paralysis agitans
Parkinsonism or Parkinson's disease NOS
Primary Parkinsonism or Parkinson's disease
EXCLUDES1 dementia with Parkinsonism (G31.83)

4ᵗʰ G21 **Secondary parkinsonism**
EXCLUDES1 dementia with Parkinsonism (G31.83)
Huntington's disease (G10)
Shy-Drager syndrome (G90.3)
syphilitic Parkinsonism (A52.19)
G21.0 Malignant neuroleptic **syndrome** MCC CC/MCC Excl
Use additional code for adverse effect, if applicable, to identify drug (T43.3X5, T43.4X5, T43.505, T43.595)
EXCLUDES1 neuroleptic induced parkinsonism (G21.11)
5ᵗʰ G21.1 Other drug-induced **secondary parkinsonism**
G21.11 Neuroleptic induced **parkinsonism** CC HCC RxHCC CC/MCC Excl
Use additional code for adverse effect, if applicable, to identify drug (T43.3X5, T43.4X5, T43.505, T43.595)
EXCLUDES1 malignant neuroleptic syndrome (G21.0)
G21.19 **Other drug induced secondary parkinsonism** CC HCC RxHCC CC/MCC Excl
Other medication-induced parkinsonism
Use additional code for adverse effect, if applicable, to identify drug (T36-T50 with fifth or sixth character 5)
G21.2 **Secondary parkinsonism due to other external agents** CC HCC RxHCC CC/MCC Excl
☞ **Code first** (T51-T65) to identify external agent
G21.3 Postencephalitic **parkinsonism** CC HCC RxHCC CC/MCC Excl
G21.4 Vascular **parkinsonism** HCC RxHCC
G21.8 Other secondary parkinsonism CC HCC RxHCC CC/MCC Excl
G21.9 **Secondary parkinsonism, unspecified** CC HCC RxHCC CC/MCC Excl

Unspecified Code   Other Specified Code   Manifestation Code   ℕ Newborn   ℙ Pediatric   𝕄 Maternity   𝔸 Adult   ♂ Male   ♀ Female
● New Code   ▲ Revised Code Title   ▶◀ Revised Text   **NOTES** *INCLUDES* *EXCLUDES1* Not coded here   *EXCLUDES2* Not included here
4ᵗʰ 4ᵗʰ character required   5ᵗʰ 5ᵗʰ character required   6ᵗʰ 6ᵗʰ character required   7ᵗʰ 7ᵗʰ character required   Extension 'X' Alert
HAC Hospital-acquired condition (HAC) alert   **AHA** AHA Coding Clinic©   ☞ Code first alert

4ᵗʰ G23 Other degenerative diseases of basal ganglia

EXCLUDES2 *multi-system degeneration of the autonomic nervous system (G90.3)*

G23.0 Hallervorden-Spatz disease cc🔒 HCC CC/MCC Exc
Pigmentary pallidal degeneration

G23.1 Progressive supranuclear ophthalmoplegia [Steele-Richardson-Olszewski] HCC
Progressive supranuclear palsy

G23.2 Striatonigral degeneration HCC

G23.8 Other specified degenerative diseases of basal ganglia cc🔒 HCC CC/MCC Exc
Calcification of basal ganglia

G23.9 Degenerative disease of basal ganglia, unspecified cc🔒 HCC CC/MCC Exc

4ᵗʰ G24 Dystonia

DEFINITION: Dystonia is a movement disorder that causes involuntary, often repetitive, movements and postures.

INCLUDES dyskinesia

EXCLUDES2 *athetoid cerebral palsy (G80.3)*

5ᵗʰ G24.0 Drug induced dystonia
Use additional code for adverse effect, if applicable, to identify drug (T36-T50 with fifth or sixth character 5)

G24.01 Drug induced subacute dyskinesia cc🔒 CC/MCC Exc
Drug induced blepharospasm
Drug induced orofacial dyskinesia
Neuroleptic induced tardive dyskinesia
Tardive dyskinesia

G24.02 Drug induced acute dystonia cc🔒 CC/MCC Exc
Acute dystonic reaction to drugs
Neuroleptic induced acute dystonia

G24.09 Other drug induced dystonia cc🔒 CC/MCC Exc

G24.1 Genetic torsion dystonia
Dystonia deformans progressiva
Dystonia musculorum deformans
Familial torsion dystonia
Idiopathic familial dystonia
Idiopathic (torsion) dystonia NOS
(Schwalbe-) Ziehen-Oppenheim disease

G24.2 Idiopathic nonfamilial dystonia cc🔒 CC/MCC Exc

G24.3 Spasmodic torticollis
EXCLUDES1 *congenital torticollis (Q68.0)*
hysterical torticollis (F44.4)
ocular torticollis (R29.891)
psychogenic torticollis (F45.8)
torticollis NOS (M43.6)
traumatic recurrent torticollis (S13.4)

G24.4 Idiopathic orofacial dystonia
Orofacial dyskinesia
EXCLUDES1 *drug induced orofacial dyskinesia (G24.01)*

G24.5 Blepharospasm
EXCLUDES1 *drug induced blepharospasm (G24.01)*

G24.8 Other dystonia
Acquired torsion dystonia NOS

G24.9 Dystonia, unspecified
Dyskinesia NOS

4ᵗʰ G25 Other extrapyramidal and movement disorders
EXCLUDES2 *sleep related movement disorders (G47.6-)*

G25.0 Essential tremor
Familial tremor
EXCLUDES1 *tremor NOS (R25.1)*

G25.1 Drug-induced tremor
Use additional code for adverse effect, if applicable, to identify drug (T36-T50 with fifth or sixth character 5)

G25.2 Other specified forms of tremor
Intention tremor

G25.3 Myoclonus
Drug-induced myoclonus
Palatal myoclonus
Use additional code for adverse effect, if applicable, to identify drug (T36-T50 with fifth or sixth character 5)

EXCLUDES1 *facial myokymia (G51.4)*
myoclonic epilepsy (G40.-)

G25.4 Drug-induced chorea
Use additional code for adverse effect, if applicable, to identify drug (T36-T50 with fifth or sixth character 5)

G25.5 Other chorea
Chorea NOS
EXCLUDES1 *chorea NOS with heart involvement (I02.0)*
Huntington's chorea (G10)
rheumatic chorea (I02.-)
Sydenham's chorea (I02.-)

5ᵗʰ G25.6 Drug induced tics and other tics of organic origin
G25.61 Drug induced tics
Use additional code for adverse effect, if applicable, to identify drug (T36-T50 with fifth or sixth character 5)
G25.69 Other tics of organic origin
EXCLUDES1 *habit spasm (F95.9)*
tic NOS (F95.9)
Tourette's syndrome (F95.2)

5ᵗʰ G25.7 Other and unspecified drug induced movement disorders
Use additional code for adverse effect, if applicable, to identify drug (T36-T50 with fifth or sixth character 5)
G25.70 Drug induced movement disorder, unspecified
G25.71 Drug induced akathisia
Drug induced acathisia
Neuroleptic induced acute akathisia
Tardive akathisia
G25.79 Other drug induced movement disorders

5ᵗʰ G25.8 Other specified extrapyramidal and movement disorders
G25.81 Restless legs syndrome
G25.82 Stiff-man syndrome cc🔒 CC/MCC Exc
G25.83 Benign shuddering attacks
G25.89 Other specified extrapyramidal and movement disorders

G25.9 Extrapyramidal and movement disorder, unspecified cc🔒 CC/MCC Exc

G26 Extrapyramidal and movement disorders in diseases classified elsewhere
📑 Code first underlying disease

Other degenerative diseases of the nervous system (G30-G32)

4ᵗʰ G30 Alzheimer's disease
INCLUDES *Alzheimer's dementia senile and presenile forms*
Use additional code to identify:
delirium, if applicable (F05)
dementia with behavioral disturbance (F02.81)
dementia without behavioral disturbance (F02.80)
EXCLUDES1 *senile degeneration of brain NEC (G31.1)*
senile dementia NOS (F03)
senility NOS (R41.81)

G30.0 Alzheimer's disease with early onset HCC RxHCC
G30.1 Alzheimer's disease with late onset A HCC RxHCC
G30.8 Other Alzheimer's disease HCC RxHCC
G30.9 Alzheimer's disease, unspecified HCC RxHCC
AHA: Q1 2017, Q2 2016

4ᵗʰ G31 Other degenerative diseases of nervous system, not elsewhere classified
Use additional ▶For codes G31.0-G31.83, G31.85-G31.9, use additional◀ code to identify:
dementia with behavioral disturbance (F02.81)
dementia without behavioral disturbance (F02.80)
EXCLUDES2 *Reye's syndrome (G93.7)*

5ᵗʰ G31.0 Frontotemporal dementia
G31.01 Pick's disease HCC RxHCC
Primary progressive aphasia
Progressive isolated aphasia
G31.09 Other frontotemporal dementia HCC RxHCC
Frontal dementia

POA🔒 Unacceptable principal diagnosis symbol per Medicare code edits POA🔒 Code exempt from diagnosis present on admission requirement
❓ Questionable admission cc🔒 Complication or comorbidity MCC Major complication or comorbidity CC/MCC Exc CC/MCC exclusion
HCC HCC diagnosis code RxHCC RxHCC diagnosis code MACRA MACRA code **DEFINITION** Describes condition/terminology
TIP Coding guidance 👁 Official Guideline Reference Z1 Z code as first-listed diagnosis

G31.1 **Senile degeneration of brain, not elsewhere classified** `HCC` `RxHCC`
  EXCLUDES1 *Alzheimer's disease (G30.-)*
    senility NOS (R41.81)

G31.2 **Degeneration of nervous system due to alcohol** `cc` `HCC` `RxHCC` `CC/MCC Exc`
  Alcoholic cerebellar ataxia
  Alcoholic cerebellar degeneration
  Alcoholic cerebral degeneration
  Alcoholic encephalopathy
  Dysfunction of the autonomic nervous system due to alcohol
  Code also associated alcoholism (F10.-)

5️⃣ G31.8 **Other specified degenerative diseases of nervous system**
  G31.81 **Alpers disease** `cc` `HCC` `RxHCC` `CC/MCC Exc`
    AHA: Q2 2017
    Grey-matter degeneration
  G31.82 **Leigh's disease** `cc` `HCC` `RxHCC` `CC/MCC Exc`
    Subacute necrotizing encephalopathy
  G31.83 **Dementia with Lewy bodies** `HCC` `RxHCC`
    AHA: Q2 2017, Q4 2016
    Dementia with Parkinsonism
    Lewy body dementia
    Lewy body disease
  G31.84 **Mild cognitive impairment, so stated**
    Mild neurocognitive disorder
    EXCLUDES1 *age related cognitive decline (R41.81)*
      altered mental status (R41.82)
      cerebral degeneration (G31.9)
      change in mental status (R41.82)
      cognitive deficits following (sequelae of) cerebral hemorrhage or infarction (I69.01-, I69.11-, I69.21-, I69.31-, I69.81-, I69.91-)
      cognitive impairment due to intracranial or head injury (S06.-)
      dementia (F01.-, F02.-, F03)
      mild memory disturbance (F06.8)
      neurologic neglect syndrome (R41.4)
      personality change, nonpsychotic (F68.8)
  G31.85 **Corticobasal degeneration** `HCC` `RxHCC`
  G31.89 **Other specified degenerative diseases of nervous system** `HCC` `RxHCC`
G31.9 **Degenerative disease of nervous system, unspecified** `HCC` `RxHCC`

4️⃣ G32 **Other degenerative disorders of nervous system in diseases classified elsewhere**
  G32.0 **Subacute combined degeneration of spinal cord in diseases classified elsewhere** `cc` `HCC` `RxHCC` `CC/MCC Exc`
    Dana-Putnam syndrome
    Sclerosis of spinal cord (combined) (dorsolateral) (posterolateral)
    ☞ **Code first** underlying disease, such as:
      anemia (D51.9)
      dietary (D51.3)
      pernicious (D51.0)
      vitamin B12 deficiency (E53.8)
    EXCLUDES1 *syphilitic combined degeneration of spinal cord (A52.11)*
  5️⃣ G32.8 **Other specified degenerative disorders of nervous system in diseases classified elsewhere**
    ☞ **Code first** underlying disease, such as:
      amyloidosis cerebral degeneration (E85.-)
      cerebral degeneration (due to) hypothyroidism (E00.0-E03.9)
      cerebral degeneration (due to) neoplasm (C00-D49)
      cerebral degeneration (due to) vitamin B deficiency, except thiamine (E52-E53.-)
    EXCLUDES1 *superior hemorrhagic polioencephalitis [Wernicke's encephalopathy] (E51.2)*
    G32.81 **Cerebellar ataxia in diseases classified elsewhere** `cc` `HCC` `CC/MCC Exc`
      ☞ **Code first** underlying disease, such as:
        celiac disease (with gluten ataxia) (K90.0)
        cerebellar ataxia (in) neoplastic disease (paraneoplastic cerebellar degeneration) (C00-D49)
        non-celiac gluten ataxia (M35.9)

    EXCLUDES1 *systemic atrophy primarily affecting the central nervous system in alcoholic cerebellar ataxia (G31.2)*
      systemic atrophy primarily affecting the central nervous system in myxedema (G13.2)
    G32.89 **Other specified degenerative disorders of nervous system in diseases classified elsewhere**
      Degenerative encephalopathy in diseases classified elsewhere

Demyelinating diseases of the central nervous system (G35-G37)

G35 **Multiple sclerosis** `HCC` `RxHCC`
  Disseminated multiple sclerosis
  Generalized multiple sclerosis
  Multiple sclerosis NOS
  Multiple sclerosis of brain stem
  Multiple sclerosis of cord

4️⃣ G36 **Other acute disseminated demyelination**
  EXCLUDES1 *postinfectious encephalitis and encephalomyelitis NOS (G04.01)*
  G36.0 **Neuromyelitis optica [Devic]** `cc` `HCC` `RxHCC` `CC/MCC Exc`
    Demyelination in optic neuritis
    EXCLUDES1 *optic neuritis NOS (H46)*
  G36.1 **Acute and subacute hemorrhagic leukoencephalitis [Hurst]** `cc` `HCC` `CC/MCC Exc`
  G36.8 **Other specified acute disseminated demyelination** `cc` `HCC` `CC/MCC Exc`
  G36.9 **Acute disseminated demyelination, unspecified** `cc` `HCC` `CC/MCC Exc`

4️⃣ G37 **Other demyelinating diseases of central nervous system**
  G37.0 **Diffuse sclerosis of central nervous system** `cc` `HCC` `RxHCC` `CC/MCC Exc`
    Periaxial encephalitis
    Schilder's disease
    EXCLUDES1 *X linked adrenoleukodystrophy (E71.52-)*
  G37.1 **Central demyelination of corpus callosum** `cc` `HCC` `CC/MCC Exc`
  G37.2 **Central pontine myelinolysis** `cc` `HCC` `CC/MCC Exc`
  G37.3 **Acute transverse myelitis in demyelinating disease of central nervous system** `cc` `HCC` `RxHCC` `CC/MCC Exc`
    Acute transverse myelitis NOS
    Acute transverse myelopathy
    EXCLUDES1 *multiple sclerosis (G35)*
      neuromyelitis optica [Devic] (G36.0)
  G37.4 **Subacute necrotizing myelitis of central nervous system** `HCC` `MCC` `RxHCC` `CC/MCC Exc`
  G37.5 **Concentric sclerosis [Balo] of central nervous system** `cc` `HCC` `RxHCC` `CC/MCC Exc`
  G37.8 **Other specified demyelinating diseases of central nervous system** `cc` `HCC` `CC/MCC Exc`
  G37.9 **Demyelinating disease of central nervous system, unspecified** `cc` `HCC` `CC/MCC Exc`

Episodic and paroxysmal disorders (G40-G47)

4️⃣ G40 **Epilepsy and recurrent seizures**
  NOTES The following terms are to be considered equivalent to intractable: pharmacoresistant (pharmacologically resistant), treatment resistant, refractory (medically) and poorly controlled
  EXCLUDES1 *conversion disorder with seizures (F44.5)*
    convulsions NOS (R56.9)
    post traumatic seizures (R56.1)
    seizure (convulsive) NOS (R56.9)
    seizure of newborn (P90)
  EXCLUDES2 *hippocampal sclerosis (G93.81)*
    mesial temporal sclerosis (G93.81)
    temporal sclerosis (G93.81)
    Todd's paralysis (G83.84)

Unspecified Code   Other Specified Code   Manifestation Code   🅽 Newborn   🅿 Pediatric   🅼 Maternity   🅐 Adult   ♂ Male   ♀ Female
● New Code   ▲ Revised Code Title   ►◄ Revised Text   **NOTES**   *INCLUDES*   *EXCLUDES1* Not coded here   *EXCLUDES2* Not included here
4️⃣ 4th character required   5️⃣ 5th character required   6️⃣ 6th character required   7️⃣ 7th character required   7️⃣ₓ Extension 'X' Alert
HAC Hospital-acquired condition (HAC) alert   **AHA** AHA Coding Clinic©   ☞ **Code first** alert

2020 ICD-10-CM   When symbols appear on a code that requires a 7th character extension, refer to Appendix B to identify applicable 7th character codes.   **577**

CHAPTER 6: DISEASES OF THE NERVOUS SYSTEM (G00-G99)

5ᵗʰ **G40.0 Localization-related (focal) (partial) idiopathic epilepsy and epileptic syndromes** with seizures of localized onset
Benign childhood epilepsy with centrotemporal EEG spikes
Childhood epilepsy with occipital EEG paroxysms
EXCLUDES1 adult onset localization-related epilepsy (G40.1-, G40.2-)

6ᵗʰ **G40.00 Localization-related (focal) (partial) idiopathic epilepsy and epileptic syndromes with seizures of localized onset,** not intractable
Localization-related (focal) (partial) idiopathic epilepsy and epileptic syndromes with seizures of localized onset without intractability
G40.001 Localization-related (focal) (partial) idiopathic epilepsy and epileptic syndromes with seizures of localized onset, not intractable, with status epilepticus cc🔒 HCC RxHCC CC/MCC Exc🔒

G40.009 Localization-related (focal) (partial) idiopathic epilepsy and epileptic syndromes with seizures of localized onset, not intractable, without status epilepticus cc🔒 HCC RxHCC CC/MCC Exc🔒
Localization-related (focal) (partial) idiopathic epilepsy and epileptic syndromes with seizures of localized onset NOS

6ᵗʰ **G40.01 Localization-related (focal) (partial) idiopathic epilepsy and epileptic syndromes with seizures of localized onset,** intractable
G40.011 Localization-related (focal) (partial) idiopathic epilepsy and epileptic syndromes with seizures of localized onset, intractable, with status epilepticus cc🔒 HCC RxHCC CC/MCC Exc🔒

G40.019 Localization-related (focal) (partial) idiopathic epilepsy and epileptic syndromes with seizures of localized onset, intractable, without status epilepticus cc🔒 HCC RxHCC CC/MCC Exc🔒

5ᵗʰ **G40.1 Localization-related (focal) (partial) symptomatic epilepsy and epileptic syndromes** with simple partial seizures
Attacks without alteration of consciousness
Epilepsia partialis continua [Kozhevnikof]
Simple partial seizures developing into secondarily generalized seizures

6ᵗʰ **G40.10 Localization-related (focal) (partial) symptomatic epilepsy and epileptic syndromes with simple partial seizures,** not intractable
Localization-related (focal) (partial) symptomatic epilepsy and epileptic syndromes with simple partial seizures without intractability
G40.101 Localization-related (focal) (partial) symptomatic epilepsy and epileptic syndromes with simple partial seizures, not intractable, with status epilepticus cc🔒 HCC RxHCC CC/MCC Exc🔒

G40.109 Localization-related (focal) (partial) symptomatic epilepsy and epileptic syndromes with simple partial seizures, not intractable, without status epilepticus cc🔒 HCC RxHCC CC/MCC Exc🔒
Localization-related (focal) (partial) symptomatic epilepsy and epileptic syndromes with simple partial seizures NOS

6ᵗʰ **G40.11 Localization-related (focal) (partial) symptomatic epilepsy and epileptic syndromes with simple partial seizures,** intractable
G40.111 Localization-related (focal) (partial) symptomatic epilepsy and epileptic syndromes with simple partial seizures, intractable, with status epilepticus cc🔒 HCC RxHCC CC/MCC Exc🔒

G40.119 Localization-related (focal) (partial) symptomatic epilepsy and epileptic syndromes with simple partial seizures, intractable, without status epilepticus cc🔒 HCC RxHCC CC/MCC Exc🔒

5ᵗʰ **G40.2 Localization-related (focal) (partial) symptomatic epilepsy and epileptic syndromes** with complex partial seizures
Attacks with alteration of consciousness, often with automatisms
Complex partial seizures developing into secondarily generalized seizures

6ᵗʰ **G40.20 Localization-related (focal) (partial) symptomatic epilepsy and epileptic syndromes with complex partial seizures,** not intractable
Localization-related (focal) (partial) symptomatic epilepsy and epileptic syndromes with complex partial seizures without intractability
G40.201 Localization-related (focal) (partial) symptomatic epilepsy and epileptic syndromes with complex partial seizures, not intractable, with status epilepticus cc🔒 HCC RxHCC CC/MCC Exc🔒

G40.209 Localization-related (focal) (partial) symptomatic epilepsy and epileptic syndromes with complex partial seizures, not intractable, without status epilepticus cc🔒 HCC RxHCC CC/MCC Exc🔒
Localization-related (focal) (partial) symptomatic epilepsy and epileptic syndromes with complex partial seizures NOS

6ᵗʰ **G40.21 Localization-related (focal) (partial) symptomatic epilepsy and epileptic syndromes with complex partial seizures,** intractable
G40.211 Localization-related (focal) (partial) symptomatic epilepsy and epileptic syndromes with complex partial seizures, intractable, with status epilepticus cc🔒 HCC RxHCC CC/MCC Exc🔒

G40.219 Localization-related (focal) (partial) symptomatic epilepsy and epileptic syndromes with complex partial seizures, intractable, without status epilepticus cc🔒 HCC RxHCC CC/MCC Exc🔒

5ᵗʰ **G40.3 Generalized idiopathic epilepsy and epileptic syndromes**
Code also MERRF syndrome, if applicable (E88.42)

6ᵗʰ **G40.30 Generalized idiopathic epilepsy and epileptic syndromes,** not intractable
Generalized idiopathic epilepsy and epileptic syndromes without intractability
G40.301 Generalized idiopathic epilepsy and epileptic syndromes, not intractable, with status epilepticus HCC MCC🔒 RxHCC CC/MCC Exc🔒

G40.309 Generalized idiopathic epilepsy and epileptic syndromes, not intractable, without status epilepticus HCC RxHCC
Generalized idiopathic epilepsy and epileptic syndromes NOS

6ᵗʰ **G40.31 Generalized idiopathic epilepsy and epileptic syndromes,** intractable
G40.311 Generalized idiopathic epilepsy and epileptic syndromes, intractable, with status epilepticus HCC MCC🔒 RxHCC CC/MCC Exc🔒

G40.319 Generalized idiopathic epilepsy and epileptic syndromes, intractable, without status epilepticus HCC MCC🔒 RxHCC CC/MCC Exc🔒

5ᵗʰ **G40.A Absence epileptic syndrome**
Childhood absence epilepsy [pyknolepsy]
Juvenile absence epilepsy
Absence epileptic syndrome, NOS

6ᵗʰ **G40.A0 Absence epileptic syndrome,** not intractable
G40.A01 Absence epileptic syndrome, not intractable, with status epilepticus HCC RxHCC

578

When symbols appear on a code that requires a 7th character extension, refer to Appendix B to identify applicable 7th character codes.

2020 ICD-10-CM

G40.A09 Absence epileptic syndrome, not intractable, without status epilepticus [HCC] [RxHCC]

[6th] G40.A1 Absence epileptic syndrome, intractable

G40.A11 Absence epileptic syndrome, intractable, with status epilepticus [CC] [HCC] [RxHCC] [CC/MCC Exc]

G40.A19 Absence epileptic syndrome, intractable, without status epilepticus [CC] [HCC] [RxHCC] [CC/MCC Exc]

[5th] G40.B Juvenile myoclonic epilepsy [impulsive petit mal]

[6th] G40.B0 Juvenile myoclonic epilepsy, not intractable

G40.B01 Juvenile myoclonic epilepsy, not intractable, with status epilepticus [CC] [HCC] [RxHCC] [CC/MCC Exc]

G40.B09 Juvenile myoclonic epilepsy, not intractable, without status epilepticus [CC] [HCC] [RxHCC] [CC/MCC Exc]

[6th] G40.B1 Juvenile myoclonic epilepsy, intractable

G40.B11 Juvenile myoclonic epilepsy, intractable, with status epilepticus [CC] [HCC] [RxHCC] [CC/MCC Exc]

G40.B19 Juvenile myoclonic epilepsy, intractable, without status epilepticus [CC] [HCC] [RxHCC] [CC/MCC Exc]

[5th] G40.4 Other generalized epilepsy and epileptic syndromes

Epilepsy with grand mal seizures on awakening
Epilepsy with myoclonic absences
Epilepsy with myoclonic-astatic seizures
Grand mal seizure NOS
Nonspecific atonic epileptic seizures
Nonspecific clonic epileptic seizures
Nonspecific myoclonic epileptic seizures
Nonspecific tonic epileptic seizures
Nonspecific tonic-clonic epileptic seizures
Symptomatic early myoclonic encephalopathy

[6th] G40.40 Other generalized epilepsy and epileptic syndromes, not intractable

Other generalized epilepsy and epileptic syndromes without intractability
Other generalized epilepsy and epileptic syndromes NOS

G40.401 Other generalized epilepsy and epileptic syndromes, not intractable, with status epilepticus [HCC] [RxHCC]

G40.409 Other generalized epilepsy and epileptic syndromes, not intractable, without status epilepticus [HCC] [RxHCC]

[6th] G40.41 Other generalized epilepsy and epileptic syndromes, intractable

G40.411 Other generalized epilepsy and epileptic syndromes, intractable, with status epilepticus [CC] [HCC] [RxHCC] [CC/MCC Exc]

G40.419 Other generalized epilepsy and epileptic syndromes, intractable, without status epilepticus [CC] [HCC] [RxHCC] [CC/MCC Exc]

[5th] G40.5 Epileptic seizures related to external causes

Epileptic seizures related to alcohol
Epileptic seizures related to drugs
Epileptic seizures related to hormonal changes
Epileptic seizures related to sleep deprivation
Epileptic seizures related to stress

Code also, if applicable, associated epilepsy and recurrent seizures (G40.-)

Use additional code for adverse effect, if applicable, to identify drug (T36-T50 with fifth or sixth character 5)

[6th] G40.50 Epileptic seizures related to external causes, not intractable

G40.501 Epileptic seizures related to external causes, not intractable, with status epilepticus [CC] [HCC] [RxHCC] [CC/MCC Exc]

G40.509 Epileptic seizures related to external causes, not intractable, without status epilepticus [CC] [HCC] [RxHCC] [CC/MCC Exc]

Epileptic seizures related to external causes, NOS

[5th] G40.8 Other epilepsy and recurrent seizures

Epilepsies and epileptic syndromes undetermined as to whether they are focal or generalized
Landau-Kleffner syndrome

[6th] G40.80 Other epilepsy

G40.801 Other epilepsy, not intractable, with status epilepticus [CC] [HCC] [RxHCC] [CC/MCC Exc]

Other epilepsy without intractability with status epilepticus

G40.802 Other epilepsy, not intractable, without status epilepticus [CC] [HCC] [RxHCC] [CC/MCC Exc]

Other epilepsy NOS
Other epilepsy without intractability without status epilepticus

G40.803 Other epilepsy, intractable, with status epilepticus [CC] [HCC] [RxHCC] [CC/MCC Exc]

G40.804 Other epilepsy, intractable, without status epilepticus [CC] [HCC] [RxHCC] [CC/MCC Exc]

[6th] G40.81 Lennox-Gastaut syndrome

G40.811 Lennox-Gastaut syndrome, not intractable, with status epilepticus [CC] [HCC] [RxHCC] [CC/MCC Exc]

G40.812 Lennox-Gastaut syndrome, not intractable, without status epilepticus [CC] [HCC] [RxHCC] [CC/MCC Exc]

G40.813 Lennox-Gastaut syndrome, intractable, with status epilepticus [CC] [HCC] [RxHCC] [CC/MCC Exc]

G40.814 Lennox-Gastaut syndrome, intractable, without status epilepticus [CC] [HCC] [RxHCC] [CC/MCC Exc]

[6th] G40.82 Epileptic spasms

Infantile spasms
Salaam attacks
West's syndrome

G40.821 Epileptic spasms, not intractable, with status epilepticus [CC] [HCC] [RxHCC] [CC/MCC Exc]

G40.822 Epileptic spasms, not intractable, without status epilepticus [CC] [HCC] [RxHCC] [CC/MCC Exc]

G40.823 Epileptic spasms, intractable, with status epilepticus [CC] [HCC] [RxHCC] [CC/MCC Exc]

G40.824 Epileptic spasms, intractable, without status epilepticus [CC] [HCC] [RxHCC] [CC/MCC Exc]

G40.89 Other seizures [CC] [HCC] [RxHCC] [CC/MCC Exc]

[EXCLUDES1] *post traumatic seizures (R56.1)*
recurrent seizures NOS (G40.909)
seizure NOS (R56.9)

[5th] G40.9 Epilepsy, unspecified

[6th] G40.90 Epilepsy, unspecified, not intractable

Epilepsy, unspecified, without intractability

G40.901 Epilepsy, unspecified, not intractable, with status epilepticus [HCC] [RxHCC]

G40.909 Epilepsy, unspecified, not intractable, without status epilepticus [HCC] [RxHCC]

Epilepsy NOS
Epileptic convulsions NOS
Epileptic fits NOS
Epileptic seizures NOS
Recurrent seizures NOS
Seizure disorder NOS

[6th] G40.91 Epilepsy, unspecified, intractable

Intractable seizure disorder NOS

G40.911 Epilepsy, unspecified, intractable, with status epilepticus [CC] [HCC] [RxHCC] [CC/MCC Exc]

G40.919 Epilepsy, unspecified, intractable, without status epilepticus [CC] [HCC] [RxHCC] [CC/MCC Exc]

G43 Migraine

NOTES The following terms are to be considered equivalent to intractable: pharmacoresistant (pharmacologically resistant), treatment resistant, refractory (medically) and poorly controlled

Use additional code for adverse effect, if applicable, to identify drug (T36-T50 with fifth or sixth character 5)

EXCLUDES1 headache NOS (R51)
     lower half migraine (G44.00)

EXCLUDES2 headache syndromes (G44.-)

G43.0 Migraine without aura
 Common migraine
 EXCLUDES1 chronic migraine without aura (G43.7-)

 G43.00 Migraine without aura, not intractable
  Migraine without aura without mention of refractory migraine

  G43.001 Migraine without aura, not intractable, with status migrainosus RxHCC

  G43.009 Migraine without aura, not intractable, without status migrainosus RxHCC
   Migraine without aura NOS

 G43.01 Migraine without aura, intractable
  Migraine without aura with refractory migraine

  G43.011 Migraine without aura, intractable, with status migrainosus RxHCC

  G43.019 Migraine without aura, intractable, without status migrainosus RxHCC

G43.1 Migraine with aura
 Basilar migraine
 Classical migraine
 Migraine equivalents
 Migraine preceded or accompanied by transient focal neurological phenomena
 Migraine triggered seizures
 Migraine with acute-onset aura
 Migraine with aura without headache (migraine equivalents)
 Migraine with prolonged aura
 Migraine with typical aura
 Retinal migraine
 Code also any associated seizure (G40.-, R56.9)
 EXCLUDES1 persistent migraine aura (G43.5-, G43.6-)

 G43.10 Migraine with aura, not intractable
  Migraine with aura without mention of refractory migraine

  G43.101 Migraine with aura, not intractable, with status migrainosus RxHCC

  G43.109 Migraine with aura, not intractable, without status migrainosus RxHCC
   Migraine with aura NOS

 G43.11 Migraine with aura, intractable
  Migraine with aura with refractory migraine

  G43.111 Migraine with aura, intractable, with status migrainosus RxHCC

  G43.119 Migraine with aura, intractable, without status migrainosus RxHCC

G43.4 Hemiplegic migraine
 Familial migraine
 Sporadic migraine

 G43.40 Hemiplegic migraine, not intractable
  Hemiplegic migraine without refractory migraine

  G43.401 Hemiplegic migraine, not intractable, with status migrainosus RxHCC

  G43.409 Hemiplegic migraine, not intractable, without status migrainosus RxHCC
   Hemiplegic migraine NOS

 G43.41 Hemiplegic migraine, intractable
  Hemiplegic migraine with refractory migraine

  G43.411 Hemiplegic migraine, intractable, with status migrainosus RxHCC

  G43.419 Hemiplegic migraine, intractable, without status migrainosus RxHCC

G43.5 Persistent migraine aura without cerebral infarction

 G43.50 Persistent migraine aura without cerebral infarction, not intractable
  Persistent migraine aura without cerebral infarction, without refractory migraine

  G43.501 Persistent migraine aura without cerebral infarction, not intractable, with status migrainosus RxHCC

  G43.509 Persistent migraine aura without cerebral infarction, not intractable, without status migrainosus RxHCC
   Persistent migraine aura NOS

 G43.51 Persistent migraine aura without cerebral infarction, intractable
  Persistent migraine aura without cerebral infarction, with refractory migraine

  G43.511 Persistent migraine aura without cerebral infarction, intractable, with status migrainosus RxHCC

  G43.519 Persistent migraine aura without cerebral infarction, intractable, without status migrainosus RxHCC

G43.6 Persistent migraine aura with cerebral infarction
 Code also the type of cerebral infarction (I63.-)

 G43.60 Persistent migraine aura with cerebral infarction, not intractable
  Persistent migraine aura with cerebral infarction, without refractory migraine

  G43.601 Persistent migraine aura with cerebral infarction, not intractable, with status migrainosus CC RxHCC CC/MCC Exc

  G43.609 Persistent migraine aura with cerebral infarction, not intractable, without status migrainosus CC RxHCC CC/MCC Exc

 G43.61 Persistent migraine aura with cerebral infarction, intractable
  Persistent migraine aura with cerebral infarction, with refractory migraine

  G43.611 Persistent migraine aura with cerebral infarction, intractable, with status migrainosus CC RxHCC CC/MCC Exc

  G43.619 Persistent migraine aura with cerebral infarction, intractable, without status migrainosus CC RxHCC CC/MCC Exc

G43.7 Chronic migraine without aura
 Transformed migraine
 EXCLUDES1 migraine without aura (G43.0-)

 G43.70 Chronic migraine without aura, not intractable
  Chronic migraine without aura, without refractory migraine

  G43.701 Chronic migraine without aura, not intractable, with status migrainosus RxHCC

  G43.709 Chronic migraine without aura, not intractable, without status migrainosus RxHCC
   Chronic migraine without aura NOS

 G43.71 Chronic migraine without aura, intractable
  Chronic migraine without aura, with refractory migraine

  G43.711 Chronic migraine without aura, intractable, with status migrainosus RxHCC

  G43.719 Chronic migraine without aura, intractable, without status migrainosus RxHCC

G43.A Cyclical vomiting
 EXCLUDES1 cyclical vomiting syndrome unrelated to migraine (R11.15)

 ▲ **G43.A0 Cyclical vomiting, ▶in migraine,◀** not intractable RxHCC
  Cyclical vomiting, without refractory migraine

 ▲ **G43.A1 Cyclical vomiting, ▶in migraine,◀** intractable RxHCC
  Cyclical vomiting, with refractory migraine

PDx Unacceptable principal diagnosis symbol per Medicare code edits   POA Code exempt from diagnosis present on admission requirement
? Questionable admission   CC Complication or comorbidity   MCC Major complication or comorbidity   CC/MCC Exc CC/MCC exclusion
HCC HCC diagnosis code   RxHCC RxHCC diagnosis code   MACRA MACRA code   **DEFINITION** Describes condition/terminology
TIP Coding guidance   👁 Official Guideline Reference   Z1 Z code as first-listed diagnosis

G43.B **Ophthalmoplegic migraine** ⑤ᵗʰ

  G43.B0 **Ophthalmoplegic migraine,** not intractable   RxHCC
    Ophthalmoplegic migraine, without refractory migraine

  G43.B1 **Ophthalmoplegic migraine,** intractable   RxHCC
    Ophthalmoplegic migraine, with refractory migraine

G43.C **Periodic headache syndromes in child or adult** ⑤ᵗʰ

  G43.C0 **Periodic headache syndromes in child or adult,** not intractable   RxHCC
    Periodic headache syndromes in child or adult, without refractory migraine

  G43.C1 **Periodic headache syndromes in child or adult,** intractable   RxHCC
    Periodic headache syndromes in child or adult, with refractory migraine

G43.D **Abdominal migraine** ⑤ᵗʰ

  G43.D0 **Abdominal migraine,** not intractable   RxHCC
    Abdominal migraine, without refractory migraine

  G43.D1 **Abdominal migraine,** intractable   RxHCC
    Abdominal migraine, with refractory migraine

G43.8 **Other migraine** ⑤ᵗʰ

  ⑥ᵗʰ G43.80 **Other migraine,** not intractable
    Other migraine, without refractory migraine

    G43.801 **Other migraine, not intractable, with status migrainosus**   RxHCC

    G43.809 **Other migraine, not intractable, without status migrainosus**   RxHCC

  ⑥ᵗʰ G43.81 **Other migraine,** intractable
    Other migraine, with refractory migraine

    G43.811 **Other migraine, intractable, with status migrainosus**   RxHCC

    G43.819 **Other migraine, intractable, without status migrainosus**   RxHCC

  ⑥ᵗʰ G43.82 **Menstrual migraine,** not intractable
    Menstrual headache, not intractable
    Menstrual migraine, without refractory migraine
    Menstrually related migraine, not intractable
    Pre-menstrual headache, not intractable
    Pre-menstrual migraine, not intractable
    Pure menstrual migraine, not intractable
    Code also associated premenstrual tension syndrome (N94.3)

    G43.821 **Menstrual migraine, not intractable, with status migrainosus**   RxHCC ♀

    G43.829 **Menstrual migraine, not intractable, without status migrainosus**   RxHCC ♀
      Menstrual migraine NOS

  ⑥ᵗʰ G43.83 **Menstrual migraine,** intractable
    Menstrual headache, intractable
    Menstrual migraine, with refractory migraine
    Menstrually related migraine, intractable
    Pre-menstrual headache, intractable
    Pre-menstrual migraine, intractable
    Pure menstrual migraine, intractable
    Code also associated premenstrual tension syndrome (N94.3)

    G43.831 **Menstrual migraine, intractable, with status migrainosus**   RxHCC ♀

    G43.839 **Menstrual migraine, intractable, without status migrainosus**   RxHCC ♀

G43.9 **Migraine,** unspecified ⑤ᵗʰ

  ⑥ᵗʰ G43.90 **Migraine, unspecified,** not intractable
    Migraine, unspecified, without refractory migraine

    G43.901 **Migraine, unspecified, not intractable, with status migrainosus**   RxHCC
      Status migrainosus NOS

    G43.909 **Migraine, unspecified, not intractable, without status migrainosus**   RxHCC
      Migraine NOS

  ⑥ᵗʰ G43.91 **Migraine, unspecified,** intractable
    Migraine, unspecified, with refractory migraine

    G43.911 **Migraine, unspecified, intractable, with status migrainosus**   RxHCC

    G43.919 **Migraine, unspecified, intractable, without status migrainosus**   RxHCC

④ᵗʰ G44 **Other headache syndromes**

  EXCLUDES1 headache NOS (R51)

  EXCLUDES2 atypical facial pain (G50.1)
    headache due to lumbar puncture (G97.1)
    migraines (G43.-)
    trigeminal neuralgia (G50.0)

  ⑤ᵗʰ G44.0 **Cluster headaches and other trigeminal autonomic cephalgias (TAC)**

    ⑥ᵗʰ G44.00 **Cluster headache syndrome,** unspecified
      Ciliary neuralgia
      Cluster headache NOS
      Histamine cephalgia
      Lower half migraine
      Migrainous neuralgia

      G44.001 **Cluster headache syndrome, unspecified, intractable**

      G44.009 **Cluster headache syndrome, unspecified,** not intractable
        Cluster headache syndrome NOS

    ⑥ᵗʰ G44.01 **Episodic cluster headache**

      G44.011 **Episodic cluster headache,** intractable

      G44.019 **Episodic cluster headache,** not intractable
        Episodic cluster headache NOS

    ⑥ᵗʰ G44.02 **Chronic cluster headache**

      G44.021 **Chronic cluster headache,** intractable

      G44.029 **Chronic cluster headache,** not intractable
        Chronic cluster headache NOS

    ⑥ᵗʰ G44.03 **Episodic paroxysmal hemicrania**
      Paroxysmal hemicrania NOS

      G44.031 **Episodic paroxysmal hemicrania,** intractable

      G44.039 **Episodic paroxysmal hemicrania,** not intractable
        Episodic paroxysmal hemicrania NOS

    ⑥ᵗʰ G44.04 **Chronic paroxysmal hemicrania**

      G44.041 **Chronic paroxysmal hemicrania,** intractable

      G44.049 **Chronic paroxysmal hemicrania,** not intractable
        Chronic paroxysmal hemicrania NOS

    ⑥ᵗʰ G44.05 **Short lasting unilateral neuralgiform headache** with conjunctival injection and tearing (SUNCT)

      G44.051 **Short lasting unilateral neuralgiform headache with conjunctival injection and tearing (SUNCT),** intractable

      G44.059 **Short lasting unilateral neuralgiform headache with conjunctival injection and tearing (SUNCT),** not intractable
        Short lasting unilateral neuralgiform headache with conjunctival injection and tearing (SUNCT) NOS

    ⑥ᵗʰ G44.09 **Other** trigeminal autonomic cephalgias (TAC)

      G44.091 **Other trigeminal autonomic cephalgias (TAC),** intractable

      G44.099 **Other trigeminal autonomic cephalgias (TAC),** not intractable

  G44.1 **Vascular headache, not elsewhere classified**

    EXCLUDES2 cluster headache (G44.0)
      complicated headache syndromes (G44.5-)
      drug-induced headache (G44.4-)
      migraine (G43.-)
      other specified headache syndromes (G44.8-)
      post-traumatic headache (G44.3-)
      tension-type headache (G44.2-)

  ⑤ᵗʰ G44.2 **Tension-type headache**

    ⑥ᵗʰ G44.20 **Tension-type headache,** unspecified

      G44.201 **Tension-type headache, unspecified,** intractable

Unspecified Code	Other Specified Code	Manifestation Code N Newborn P Pediatric M Maternity A Adult ♂ Male ♀ Female

● New Code   ▲ Revised Code Title   ▶◀ Revised Text   **NOTES**   *INCLUDES*   *EXCLUDES1* Not coded here   *EXCLUDES2* Not included here
④ᵗʰ 4ᵗʰ character required   ⑤ᵗʰ 5ᵗʰ character required   ⑥ᵗʰ 6ᵗʰ character required   ⑦ᵗʰ 7ᵗʰ character required   ⑦ᵡ Extension 'X' Alert
HAC Hospital-acquired condition (HAC) alert   **AHA** AHA Coding Clinic©   ☛ Code first alert

G44.209 **Tension-type headache, unspecified,** not intractable
Tension headache NOS

5ᵗʰ G44.21 Episodic tension-type headache
G44.211 **Episodic tension-type headache, intractable**
G44.219 **Episodic tension-type headache,** not intractable
Episodic tension-type headache NOS

5ᵗʰ G44.22 Chronic tension-type headache
G44.221 **Chronic tension-type headache, intractable**
G44.229 **Chronic tension-type headache,** not intractable
Chronic tension-type headache NOS

5ᵗʰ G44.3 Post-traumatic headache
5ᵗʰ G44.30 Post-traumatic headache, unspecified
G44.301 **Post-traumatic headache, unspecified, intractable**
G44.309 **Post-traumatic headache, unspecified,** not intractable
Post-traumatic headache NOS

6ᵗʰ G44.31 Acute post-traumatic headache
G44.311 **Acute post-traumatic headache, intractable**
G44.319 **Acute post-traumatic headache,** not intractable
Acute post-traumatic headache NOS

6ᵗʰ G44.32 Chronic post-traumatic headache
G44.321 **Chronic post-traumatic headache, intractable**
G44.329 **Chronic post-traumatic headache,** not intractable
Chronic post-traumatic headache NOS

5ᵗʰ G44.4 Drug-induced **headache,** not elsewhere classified
Medication overuse headache
Use additional code for adverse effect, if applicable, to identify drug (T36-T50 with fifth or sixth character 5)
G44.40 **Drug-induced headache, not elsewhere classified,** not intractable
G44.41 **Drug-induced headache, not elsewhere classified, intractable**

5ᵗʰ G44.5 Complicated **headache syndromes**
G44.51 Hemicrania continua
G44.52 New daily persistent **headache (NDPH)**
G44.53 Primary thunderclap **headache**
G44.59 Other complicated **headache syndrome**

5ᵗʰ G44.8 Other specified **headache syndromes**
G44.81 **Hypnic headache**
G44.82 **Headache associated** with sexual activity
Orgasmic headache
Preorgasmic headache
G44.83 Primary cough **headache**
G44.84 Primary exertional **headache**
G44.85 Primary stabbing **headache**
G44.89 Other **headache syndrome**

4ᵗʰ G45 Transient cerebral ischemic attacks and related syndromes
EXCLUDES1 neonatal cerebral ischemia (P91.0)
transient retinal artery occlusion (H34.0-)
G45.0 Vertebro-basilar artery **syndrome** RxHCC
G45.1 Carotid artery **syndrome (hemispheric)** RxHCC
G45.2 Multiple and bilateral precerebral artery **syndromes** RxHCC
G45.3 Amaurosis fugax
G45.4 Transient global amnesia
EXCLUDES1 amnesia NOS (R41.3)
G45.8 Other transient cerebral ischemic attacks and related syndromes cc RxHCC CC/MCC Exc
G45.9 **Transient cerebral ischemic attack, unspecified** cc RxHCC CC/MCC Exc
Spasm of cerebral artery
TIA
Transient cerebral ischemia NOS

4ᵗʰ G46 Vascular syndromes of brain **in cerebrovascular diseases**
☞ Code first underlying cerebrovascular disease (I60-I69)
G46.0 Middle **cerebral artery syndrome** cc RxHCC CC/MCC Exc
G46.1 Anterior **cerebral artery syndrome** cc RxHCC CC/MCC Exc
G46.2 Posterior **cerebral artery syndrome** cc RxHCC CC/MCC Exc
G46.3 Brain stem stroke **syndrome** RxHCC
Benedikt syndrome
Claude syndrome
Foville syndrome
Millard-Gubler syndrome
Wallenberg syndrome
Weber syndrome
G46.4 Cerebellar stroke **syndrome** RxHCC
G46.5 Pure motor lacunar **syndrome** RxHCC
AHA: Q4 2018
G46.6 Pure sensory lacunar **syndrome** RxHCC
AHA: Q4 2018
G46.7 Other **lacunar syndromes** RxHCC
AHA: Q4 2018
G46.8 **Other vascular syndromes of brain in cerebrovascular diseases** RxHCC

4ᵗʰ G47 Sleep disorders
EXCLUDES2 nightmares (F51.5)
nonorganic sleep disorders (F51.-)
sleep terrors (F51.4)
sleepwalking (F51.3)

5ᵗʰ G47.0 Insomnia
EXCLUDES2 alcohol related insomnia (F10.182, F10.282, F10.982)
drug-related insomnia (F11.182, F11.282, F11.982, F13.182, F13.282, F13.982, F14.182, F14.282, F14.982, F15.182, F15.282, F15.982, F19.182, F19.282, F19.982)
idiopathic insomnia (F51.01)
insomnia due to a mental disorder (F51.05)
insomnia not due to a substance or known physiological condition (F51.0-)
nonorganic insomnia (F51.0-)
primary insomnia (F51.01)
sleep apnea (G47.3-)
G47.00 **Insomnia, unspecified**
Insomnia NOS
G47.01 **Insomnia due to medical condition**
Code also associated medical condition
G47.09 **Other insomnia**

5ᵗʰ G47.1 Hypersomnia
EXCLUDES2 alcohol-related hypersomnia (F10.182, F10.282, F10.982)
drug-related hypersomnia (F11.182, F11.282, F11.982, F13.182, F13.282, F13.982, F14.182, F14.282, F14.982, F15.182, F15.282, F15.982, F19.182, F19.282, F19.982)
hypersomnia due to a mental disorder (F51.13)
hypersomnia not due to a substance or known physiological condition (F51.1-)
primary hypersomnia (F51.11)
sleep apnea (G47.3-)
G47.10 **Hypersomnia, unspecified**
Hypersomnia NOS
G47.11 **Idiopathic hypersomnia** with long sleep time
Idiopathic hypersomnia NOS
G47.12 **Idiopathic hypersomnia** without long sleep time
G47.13 **Recurrent hypersomnia**
Kleine-Levin syndrome
Menstrual related hypersomnia
G47.14 **Hypersomnia** due to medical condition
Code also associated medical condition
G47.19 **Other hypersomnia**

PDᵈˣ Unacceptable principal diagnosis symbol per Medicare code edits POA Code exempt from diagnosis present on admission requirement
❓ Questionable admission cc Complication or comorbidity MCC Major complication or comorbidity cc/MCC Exc CC/MCC exclusion
HCC HCC diagnosis code RxHCC RxHCC diagnosis code MACRA code **DEFINITION** Describes condition/terminology
TIP Coding guidance 👁 Official Guideline Reference Z1 Z code as first-listed diagnosis

582 When symbols appear on a code that requires a 7th character extension, refer to Appendix B to identify applicable 7th character codes. **2020 ICD-10-CM**

5ᵗʰ **G47.2 Circadian rhythm sleep disorders**
Disorders of the sleep wake schedule
Inversion of nyctohemeral rhythm
Inversion of sleep rhythm
    G47.20 Circadian rhythm sleep disorder, unspecified type
Sleep wake schedule disorder NOS
    G47.21 Circadian rhythm sleep disorder, delayed sleep phase type
Delayed sleep phase syndrome
    G47.22 Circadian rhythm sleep disorder, advanced sleep phase type
    G47.23 Circadian rhythm sleep disorder, irregular sleep wake type
Irregular sleep-wake pattern
    G47.24 Circadian rhythm sleep disorder, free running type
Circadian rhythm sleep disorder, non-24-hour sleep-wake type
    G47.25 Circadian rhythm sleep disorder, jet lag type
    G47.26 Circadian rhythm sleep disorder, shift work type
    G47.27 Circadian rhythm sleep disorder in conditions classified elsewhere
      ☛ **Code first** underlying condition
    G47.29 Other **circadian rhythm sleep disorder**

5ᵗʰ **G47.3 Sleep apnea**
Code also any associated underlying condition
EXCLUDES1 apnea NOS (R06.81)
      Cheyne-Stokes breathing (R06.3)
      pickwickian syndrome (E66.2)
      sleep apnea of newborn (P28.3)
    G47.30 Sleep apnea, unspecified
Sleep apnea NOS
    G47.31 Primary central **sleep apnea**
Idiopathic central sleep apnea
    G47.32 High altitude periodic breathing
    G47.33 Obstructive **sleep apnea (adult) (pediatric)**
Obstructive sleep apnea hypopnea
EXCLUDES1 obstructive sleep apnea of newborn (P28.3)
    G47.34 Idiopathic sleep related nonobstructive alveolar hypoventilation
Sleep related hypoxia
    G47.35 Congenital central alveolar hypoventilation syndrome
    G47.36 Sleep related hypoventilation **in conditions classified elsewhere**
Sleep related hypoxemia in conditions classified elsewhere
      ☛ **Code first** underlying condition
    G47.37 Central sleep apnea **in conditions classified elsewhere**
      ☛ **Code first** underlying condition
    G47.39 Other **sleep apnea**

5ᵗʰ **G47.4 Narcolepsy and cataplexy**
6ᵗʰ   **G47.41 Narcolepsy**
      G47.411 Narcolepsy with cataplexy   RxHCC
      G47.419 Narcolepsy without cataplexy   RxHCC
      Narcolepsy NOS
6ᵗʰ   **G47.42 Narcolepsy in conditions classified elsewhere**
      ☛ **Code first** underlying condition
      G47.421 Narcolepsy in conditions classified elsewhere with cataplexy   RxHCC
      G47.429 Narcolepsy in conditions classified elsewhere without cataplexy   RxHCC

5ᵗʰ **G47.5 Parasomnia**
EXCLUDES1 alcohol induced parasomnia (F10.182, F10.282, F10.982)
      drug induced parasomnia (F11.182, F11.282, F11.982, F13.182, F13.282, F13.982, F14.182, F14.282, F14.982, F15.182, F15.282, F15.982, F19.182, F19.282, F19.982)
      parasomnia not due to a substance or known physiological condition (F51.8)

    G47.50 Parasomnia, unspecified
Parasomnia NOS
    G47.51 Confusional arousals
    G47.52 REM sleep behavior **disorder**
    G47.53 Recurrent isolated **sleep paralysis**
    G47.54 Parasomnia in conditions classified elsewhere
      ☛ **Code first** underlying condition
    G47.59 Other **parasomnia**

5ᵗʰ **G47.6 Sleep related movement disorders**
EXCLUDES2 restless legs syndrome (G25.81)
    G47.61 Periodic limb movement disorder
    G47.62 Sleep related leg cramps
    G47.63 Sleep related bruxism
      👁 **See Official Guidelines** "Excludes Notes" I.A.12.a
      AHA: Q4 2016
      EXCLUDES1 psychogenic bruxism (F45.8)
    G47.69 Other **sleep related movement disorders**
  G47.8 Other **sleep disorders**
Other specified sleep-wake disorder
  G47.9 Sleep disorder, unspecified
Sleep disorder NOS
Unspecified sleep-wake disorder

Nerve, nerve root and plexus disorders (G50-G59)

EXCLUDES1 current traumatic nerve, nerve root and plexus disorders - see Injury, nerve by body region
    neuralgia NOS (M79.2)
    neuritis NOS (M79.2)
    peripheral neuritis in pregnancy (O26.82-)
    radiculitis NOS (M54.1-)

4ᵗʰ **G50 Disorders of** trigeminal nerve
INCLUDES disorders of 5th cranial nerve
  G50.0 Trigeminal neuralgia   RxHCC
Syndrome of paroxysmal facial pain
Tic douloureux
  G50.1 Atypical facial pain   RxHCC
  G50.8 Other disorders **of trigeminal nerve**   RxHCC
  G50.9 Disorder of trigeminal nerve, unspecified   RxHCC

4ᵗʰ **G51** Facial nerve **disorders**
INCLUDES disorders of 7th cranial nerve
  G51.0 Bell's palsy
Facial palsy
  G51.1 Geniculate ganglionitis
EXCLUDES1 postherpetic geniculate ganglionitis (B02.21)
  G51.2 Melkersson's **syndrome**
Melkersson-Rosenthal syndrome
5ᵗʰ   **G51.3** Clonic hemifacial spasm
    G51.31 Clonic hemifacial spasm, right
      AHA: Q4 2018
    G51.32 Clonic hemifacial spasm, left
      AHA: Q4 2018
    G51.33 Clonic hemifacial spasm, bilateral
      AHA: Q4 2018
    G51.39 Clonic hemifacial spasm, unspecified
      AHA: Q4 2018
  G51.4 Facial myokymia
  G51.8 Other disorders of facial nerve
  G51.9 Disorder of facial nerve, unspecified

4ᵗʰ **G52 Disorders of** other cranial nerves **(Figure 6.2)**
EXCLUDES2 disorders of acoustic [8th] nerve (H93.3)
    disorders of optic [2nd] nerve (H46, H47.0)
    paralytic strabismus due to nerve palsy (H49.0-H49.2)
  G52.0 Disorders of olfactory **nerve**
Disorders of 1st cranial nerve
  G52.1 Disorders of glossopharyngeal **nerve**
Disorder of 9th cranial nerve
Glossopharyngeal neuralgia

Unspecified Code   Other Specified Code   Manifestation Code Ⓝ Newborn Ⓟ Pediatric Ⓜ Maternity Ⓐ Adult ♂ Male ♀ Female
● New Code ▲ Revised Code Title ►◄ Revised Text **NOTES** *INCLUDES* EXCLUDES1 Not coded here EXCLUDES2 Not included here
4ᵗʰ 4ᵗʰ character required 5ᵗʰ 5ᵗʰ character required 6ᵗʰ 6ᵗʰ character required 7ᵗʰ 7ᵗʰ character required Extension 'X' Alert
HAC Hospital-acquired condition (HAC) alert **AHA** AHA Coding Clinic© ☛ **Code first** alert

2020 ICD-10-CM   When symbols appear on a code that requires a 7th character extension, refer to Appendix B to identify applicable 7th character codes.   **583**

G52.2 Disorders of vagus nerve
Disorders of pneumogastric [10th] nerve
G52.3 Disorders of hypoglossal nerve
Disorders of 12th cranial nerve
G52.7 Disorders of multiple cranial nerves
Polyneuritis cranialis
G52.8 Disorders of other specified cranial nerves
G52.9 Cranial nerve disorder, unspecified

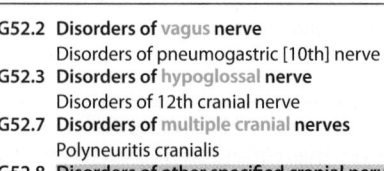

Olfactory bulb
Optic nerve
Oculomotor nerve
Trochlear nerve
Trigeminal nerve
Abducens nerve
Facial nerve
Vestibulocochlear nerve
Glossopharyngeal nerve
Hypoglossal nerve

Figure 6.2 The Cranial Nerves

G53 Cranial nerve disorders in diseases classified elsewhere
☞ **Code first** underlying disease, such as:
neoplasm (C00-D49)
EXCLUDES1 multiple cranial nerve palsy in sarcoidosis (D86.82)
multiple cranial nerve palsy in syphilis (A52.15)
postherpetic geniculate ganglionitis (B02.21)
postherpetic trigeminal neuralgia (B02.22)

G54 Nerve root and plexus disorders
EXCLUDES1 current traumatic nerve root and plexus disorders - see nerve injury by body region
intervertebral disc disorders (M50-M51)
neuralgia or neuritis NOS (M79.2)
neuritis or radiculitis brachial NOS (M54.13)
neuritis or radiculitis lumbar NOS (M54.16)
neuritis or radiculitis lumbosacral NOS (M54.17)
neuritis or radiculitis thoracic NOS (M54.14)
radiculitis NOS (M54.10)
radiculopathy NOS (M54.10)
spondylosis (M47.-)
G54.0 Brachial plexus disorders
Thoracic outlet syndrome
G54.1 Lumbosacral plexus disorders (Figure 6.3)
G54.2 Cervical root disorders, not elsewhere classified
G54.3 Thoracic root disorders, not elsewhere classified PDxIn
G54.4 Lumbosacral root disorders, not elsewhere classified
G54.5 Neuralgic amyotrophy
Parsonage-Aldren-Turner syndrome
Shoulder-girdle neuritis
EXCLUDES1 neuralgic amyotrophy in diabetes mellitus (E08-E13 with .44)
G54.6 Phantom limb syndrome with pain HCC
G54.7 Phantom limb syndrome without pain HCC
Phantom limb syndrome NOS
G54.8 Other nerve root and plexus disorders
G54.9 Nerve root and plexus disorder, unspecified

Anterior divisions
Posterior divisions

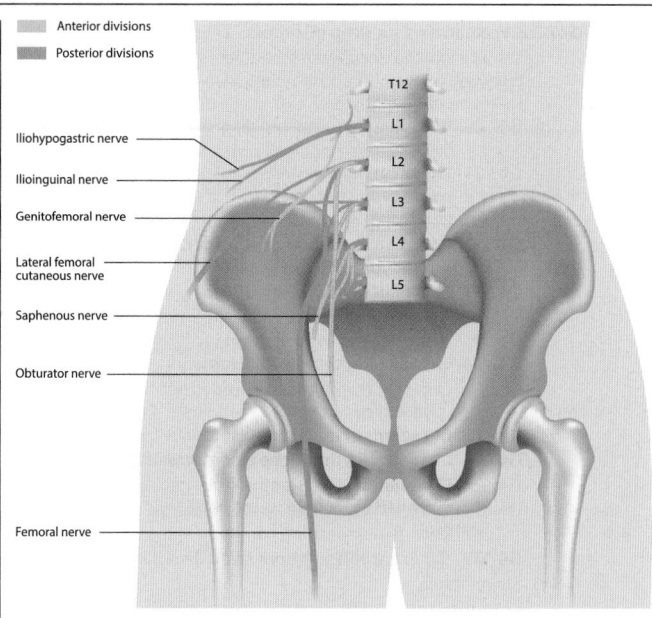

T12
L1
L2
L3
L4
L5

Iliohypogastric nerve
Ilioinguinal nerve
Genitofemoral nerve
Lateral femoral cutaneous nerve
Saphenous nerve
Obturator nerve
Femoral nerve

Figure 6.3 The Lumbar Plexus

G55 Nerve root and plexus compressions in diseases classified elsewhere
☞ **Code first** underlying disease, such as:
neoplasm (C00-D49)
EXCLUDES1 nerve root compression (due to) (in) ankylosing spondylitis (M45.-)
nerve root compression (due to) (in) dorsopathies (M53.-, M54.-)
nerve root compression (due to) (in) intervertebral disc disorders (M50.1.-, M51.1.-)
nerve root compression (due to) (in) spondylopathies (M46.-, M48.-)
nerve root compression (due to) (in) spondylosis (M47.0-M47.2.-)

G56 Mononeuropathies of upper limb
EXCLUDES1 current traumatic nerve disorder - see nerve injury by body region
G56.0 Carpal tunnel syndrome
G56.00 Carpal tunnel syndrome, unspecified upper limb
G56.01 Carpal tunnel syndrome, right upper limb
G56.02 Carpal tunnel syndrome, left upper limb
G56.03 Carpal tunnel syndrome, bilateral upper limbs
AHA: Q4 2016
G56.1 Other lesions of median nerve
G56.10 Other lesions of median nerve, unspecified upper limb
G56.11 Other lesions of median nerve, right upper limb
G56.12 Other lesions of median nerve, left upper limb
G56.13 Other lesions of median nerve, bilateral upper limbs
AHA: Q4 2016
G56.2 Lesion of ulnar nerve
Tardy ulnar nerve palsy
G56.20 Lesion of ulnar nerve, unspecified upper limb
G56.21 Lesion of ulnar nerve, right upper limb
G56.22 Lesion of ulnar nerve, left upper limb
G56.23 Lesion of ulnar nerve, bilateral upper limbs
AHA: Q4 2016
G56.3 Lesion of radial nerve
G56.30 Lesion of radial nerve, unspecified upper limb
G56.31 Lesion of radial nerve, right upper limb
G56.32 Lesion of radial nerve, left upper limb
G56.33 Lesion of radial nerve, bilateral upper limbs
AHA: Q4 2016

PDxIn Unacceptable principal diagnosis symbol per Medicare code edits   POA Code exempt from diagnosis present on admission requirement
? Questionable admission   ☾ Complication or comorbidity   MCC Major complication or comorbidity   CC/MCC Excl CC/MCC exclusion
HCC HCC diagnosis code   RxHCC RxHCC diagnosis code   MACRA MACRA code   **DEFINITION** Describes condition/terminology
TIP Coding guidance   ☜ Official Guideline Reference   Z1 Z code as first-listed diagnosis

584   When symbols appear on a code that requires a 7th character extension, refer to Appendix B to identify applicable 7th character codes.   **2020 ICD-10-CM**

[5th] **G56.4 Causalgia of upper limb**
Complex regional pain syndrome II of upper limb
[EXCLUDES1] *complex regional pain syndrome I of lower limb (G90.52-)*
complex regional pain syndrome I of upper limb (G90.51-)
complex regional pain syndrome II of lower limb (G57.7-)
reflex sympathetic dystrophy of lower limb (G90.52-)
reflex sympathetic dystrophy of upper limb (G90.51-)
G56.40 Causalgia of unspecified upper limb
G56.41 Causalgia of right upper limb
G56.42 Causalgia of left upper limb
G56.43 Causalgia of bilateral upper limbs
AHA: Q4 2016

[5th] **G56.8 Other specified mononeuropathies of upper limb**
Interdigital neuroma of upper limb
G56.80 Other specified mononeuropathies of unspecified upper limb
G56.81 Other specified mononeuropathies of right upper limb
G56.82 Other specified mononeuropathies of left upper limb
G56.83 Other specified mononeuropathies of bilateral upper limbs
AHA: Q4 2016

[5th] **G56.9 Unspecified mononeuropathy of upper limb**
G56.90 Unspecified mononeuropathy of unspecified upper limb
G56.91 Unspecified mononeuropathy of right upper limb
G56.92 Unspecified mononeuropathy of left upper limb
G56.93 Unspecified mononeuropathy of bilateral upper limbs
AHA: Q4 2016

[4th] **G57 Mononeuropathies of lower limb**
[EXCLUDES1] *current traumatic nerve disorder - see nerve injury by body region*

[5th] **G57.0 Lesion of sciatic nerve**
[EXCLUDES1] *sciatica NOS (M54.3-)*
[EXCLUDES2] *sciatica attributed to intervertebral disc disorder (M51.1.-)*
G57.00 Lesion of sciatic nerve, unspecified lower limb
G57.01 Lesion of sciatic nerve, right lower limb
G57.02 Lesion of sciatic nerve, left lower limb
G57.03 Lesion of sciatic nerve, bilateral lower limbs
AHA: Q4 2016

[5th] **G57.1 Meralgia paresthetica**
Lateral cutaneous nerve of thigh syndrome
G57.10 Meralgia paresthetica, unspecified lower limb
G57.11 Meralgia paresthetica, right lower limb
G57.12 Meralgia paresthetica, left lower limb
G57.13 Meralgia paresthetica, bilateral lower limbs
AHA: Q4 2016

[5th] **G57.2 Lesion of femoral nerve**
G57.20 Lesion of femoral nerve, unspecified lower limb
G57.21 Lesion of femoral nerve, right lower limb
G57.22 Lesion of femoral nerve, left lower limb
G57.23 Lesion of femoral nerve, bilateral lower limbs
AHA: Q4 2016

[5th] **G57.3 Lesion of lateral popliteal nerve**
Peroneal nerve palsy
G57.30 Lesion of lateral popliteal nerve, unspecified lower limb
G57.31 Lesion of lateral popliteal nerve, right lower limb
G57.32 Lesion of lateral popliteal nerve, left lower limb
G57.33 Lesion of lateral popliteal nerve, bilateral lower limbs
AHA: Q4 2016

[5th] **G57.4 Lesion of medial popliteal nerve**
G57.40 Lesion of medial popliteal nerve, unspecified lower limb
G57.41 Lesion of medial popliteal nerve, right lower limb
G57.42 Lesion of medial popliteal nerve, left lower limb
G57.43 Lesion of medial popliteal nerve, bilateral lower limbs
AHA: Q4 2016

[5th] **G57.5 Tarsal tunnel syndrome**
G57.50 Tarsal tunnel syndrome, unspecified lower limb
G57.51 Tarsal tunnel syndrome, right lower limb
G57.52 Tarsal tunnel syndrome, left lower limb
G57.53 Tarsal tunnel syndrome, bilateral lower limbs
AHA: Q4 2016

[5th] **G57.6 Lesion of plantar nerve**
Morton's metatarsalgia
G57.60 Lesion of plantar nerve, unspecified lower limb
G57.61 Lesion of plantar nerve, right lower limb
G57.62 Lesion of plantar nerve, left lower limb
G57.63 Lesion of plantar nerve, bilateral lower limbs
AHA: Q4 2016

[5th] **G57.7 Causalgia of lower limb**
Complex regional pain syndrome II of lower limb
[EXCLUDES1] *complex regional pain syndrome I of lower limb (G90.52-)*
complex regional pain syndrome I of upper limb (G90.51-)
complex regional pain syndrome II of upper limb (G56.4-)
reflex sympathetic dystrophy of lower limb (G90.52-)
reflex sympathetic dystrophy of upper limb (G90.51-)
G57.70 Causalgia of unspecified lower limb
G57.71 Causalgia of right lower limb
G57.72 Causalgia of left lower limb
G57.73 Causalgia of bilateral lower limbs
AHA: Q4 2016

[5th] **G57.8 Other specified mononeuropathies of lower limb**
Interdigital neuroma of lower limb
G57.80 Other specified mononeuropathies of unspecified lower limb
G57.81 Other specified mononeuropathies of right lower limb
G57.82 Other specified mononeuropathies of left lower limb
G57.83 Other specified mononeuropathies of bilateral lower limbs
AHA: Q4 2016

[5th] **G57.9 Unspecified mononeuropathy of lower limb**
G57.90 Unspecified mononeuropathy of unspecified lower limb
G57.91 Unspecified mononeuropathy of right lower limb
G57.92 Unspecified mononeuropathy of left lower limb
G57.93 Unspecified mononeuropathy of bilateral lower limbs
AHA: Q4 2016

[4th] **G58 Other mononeuropathies**
G58.0 Intercostal neuropathy
G58.7 Mononeuritis multiplex
G58.8 Other specified mononeuropathies
G58.9 Mononeuropathy, unspecified

G59 Mononeuropathy in diseases classified elsewhere
☞ Code first underlying disease
[EXCLUDES1] *diabetic mononeuropathy (E08-E13 with .41)*
syphilitic nerve paralysis (A52.19)
syphilitic neuritis (A52.15)
tuberculous mononeuropathy (A17.83)

Polyneuropathies and other disorders of the peripheral nervous system (G60-G65)

EXCLUDES1 *neuralgia NOS (M79.2)*
neuritis NOS (M79.2)
peripheral neuritis in pregnancy (O26.82-)
radiculitis NOS (M54.10)

G60　Hereditary and idiopathic neuropathy

G60.0 Hereditary motor and sensory **neuropathy**
Charcot-Marie-Tooth disease
Déjérine-Sottas disease
Hereditary motor and sensory neuropathy, types I-IV
Hypertrophic neuropathy of infancy
Peroneal muscular atrophy (axonal type) (hypertrophic type)
Roussy-Levy syndrome

G60.1　Refsum's disease　　　　　　　　CC CC/MCC Exc
Infantile Refsum disease

G60.2　Neuropathy in association with hereditary ataxia

G60.3 Idiopathic progressive **neuropathy**

G60.8 Other **hereditary and idiopathic neuropathies**
Dominantly inherited sensory neuropathy
Morvan's disease
Nelaton's syndrome
Recessively inherited sensory neuropathy

G60.9　Hereditary and idiopathic neuropathy, unspecified

G61 Inflammatory **polyneuropathy**

G61.0 Guillain-Barre **syndrome**　　　CC HCC RxHCC CC/MCC Exc
Acute (post-)infective polyneuritis
Miller Fisher Syndrome

G61.1 Serum **neuropathy**　　　　　　　　HCC RxHCC
Use additional code for adverse effect, if applicable, to identify serum (T50.-)

G61.8　Other inflammatory polyneuropathies

G61.81 Chronic inflammatory demyelinating **polyneuritis**　　CC HCC RxHCC CC/MCC Exc

G61.82 Multifocal motor neuropathy　　HCC RxHCC
AHA: Q4 2016
MMN

G61.89 Other **inflammatory polyneuropathies**　HCC RxHCC

G61.9　Inflammatory polyneuropathy, unspecified　HCC RxHCC

G62 Other and unspecified **polyneuropathies**

G62.0 Drug-induced **polyneuropathy**　　HCC RxHCC
Use additional code for adverse effect, if applicable, to identify drug (T36-T50 with fifth or sixth character 5)

G62.1 Alcoholic **polyneuropathy**　　　　HCC RxHCC

G62.2 Polyneuropathy due to other toxic agents　HCC RxHCC
☞ **Code first** (T51-T65) to identify toxic agent

G62.8 Other specified **polyneuropathies**

G62.81 Critical illness **polyneuropathy**　CC HCC RxHCC CC/MCC Exc
Acute motor neuropathy

G62.82 Radiation-induced **polyneuropathy**　HCC RxHCC
Use additional external cause code (W88-W90, X39.0-) to identify cause

G62.89 Other specified polyneuropathies
AHA: Q2 2016

G62.9　Polyneuropathy, unspecified
Neuropathy NOS

G63 Polyneuropathy in diseases classified elsewhere　HCC RxHCC
AHA: Q4 2012
☞ **Code first** underlying disease, such as:
amyloidosis (E85.-)
endocrine disease, except diabetes (E00-E07, E15-E16, E20-E34)
metabolic diseases (E70-E88)
neoplasm (C00-D49)
nutritional deficiency (E40-E64)
EXCLUDES1 *polyneuropathy (in):*
diabetes mellitus (E08-E13 with .42)
diphtheria (A36.83)
infectious mononucleosis (B27.0-B27.9 with 1)
Lyme disease (A69.22)

mumps (B26.84)
postherpetic (B02.23)
rheumatoid arthritis ▶(M05.5-)◀
scleroderma (M34.83)
systemic lupus erythematosus (M32.19)

G64　Other disorders of peripheral nervous system
Disorder of peripheral nervous system NOS

G65　Sequelae of inflammatory and toxic polyneuropathies
☞ **Code first** condition resulting from (sequela) of inflammatory and toxic polyneuropathies

G65.0　Sequelae of Guillain-Barré syndrome　HCC RxHCC

G65.1　Sequelae of other inflammatory **polyneuropathy**　HCC RxHCC

G65.2　Sequelae of toxic **polyneuropathy**　HCC RxHCC

Diseases of myoneural junction and muscle (G70-G73)

G70　Myasthenia gravis and other myoneural disorders
EXCLUDES1 *botulism (A05.1, A48.51-A48.52)*
transient neonatal myasthenia gravis (P94.0)

G70.0　Myasthenia gravis

G70.00　Myasthenia gravis without (acute) exacerbation　HCC RxHCC
Myasthenia gravis NOS

G70.01　Myasthenia gravis with (acute) exacerbation　HCC MCC RxHCC CC/MCC Exc
Myasthenia gravis in crisis

G70.1　Toxic myoneural disorders　　　HCC RxHCC
☞ **Code first** (T51-T65) to identify toxic agent

G70.2　Congenital and developmental myasthenia　HCC RxHCC

G70.8 Other specified **myoneural disorders**

G70.80　Lambert-Eaton syndrome, unspecified　CC HCC RxHCC CC/MCC Exc
Lambert-Eaton syndrome NOS

G70.81　Lambert-Eaton syndrome in disease classified elsewhere　CC HCC RxHCC CC/MCC Exc
☞ **Code first** underlying disease
EXCLUDES1 *Lambert-Eaton syndrome in neoplastic disease (G73.1)*

G70.89　Other specified myoneural disorders　HCC RxHCC

G70.9　Myoneural disorder, unspecified　HCC RxHCC

G71　Primary disorders of muscles
EXCLUDES2 *arthrogryposis multiplex congenita (Q74.3)*
metabolic disorders (E70-E88)
myositis (M60.-)

G71.0　Muscular dystrophy

G71.00　Muscular dystrophy, unspecified　HCC
AHA: Q4 2018

G71.01 Duchenne or Becker **muscular dystrophy**　HCC
AHA: Q4 2018
Autosomal recessive, childhood type, muscular dystrophy resembling Duchenne or Becker muscular dystrophy
Benign [Becker] muscular dystrophy
Severe [Duchenne] muscular dystrophy

G71.02 Facioscapulohumeral **muscular dystrophy**　HCC
AHA: Q4 2018
Scapulohumeral muscular dystrophy

G71.09 Other specified **muscular dystrophies**　HCC
AHA: Q4 2018
Benign scapuloperoneal muscular dystrophy with early contractures [Emery-Dreifuss]
Congenital muscular dystrophy NOS
Congenital muscular dystrophy with specific morphological abnormalities of the muscle fiber
Distal muscular dystrophy
Limb-girdle muscular dystrophy
Ocular muscular dystrophy
Oculopharyngeal muscular dystrophy
Scapuloperoneal muscular dystrophy

PDxN Unacceptable principal diagnosis symbol per Medicare code edits　　POA Code exempt from diagnosis present on admission requirement
❓ Questionable admission　CC Complication or comorbidity　MCC Major complication or comorbidity　CC/MCC Exc CC/MCC exclusion
HCC HCC diagnosis code　RxHCC RxHCC diagnosis code　MACRA code　**DEFINITION** Describes condition/terminology
TIP Coding guidance　👁 Official Guideline Reference　Z1 Z code as first-listed diagnosis

🔟 **G71.1** Myotonic **disorders**

    G71.11 **Myotonic muscular dystrophy**   HCC

        Dystrophia myotonica [Steinert]

        Myotonia atrophica

        Myotonic dystrophy

        Proximal myotonic myopathy (PROMM)

        Steinert disease

    G71.12 **Myotonia** congenita

        Acetazolamide responsive myotonia congenita

        Dominant myotonia congenita [Thomsen disease]

        Myotonia levior

        Recessive myotonia congenita [Becker disease]

    G71.13 **Myotonic** chondrodystrophy

        Chondrodystrophic myotonia

        Congenital myotonic chondrodystrophy

        Schwartz-Jampel disease

    G71.14 Drug induced **myotonia**

        Use additional code for adverse effect, if applicable, to identify drug (T36-T50 with fifth or sixth character 5)

    G71.19 Other specified myotonic disorders

        Myotonia fluctuans

        Myotonia permanens

        Neuromyotonia [Isaacs]

        Paramyotonia congenita (of von Eulenburg)

        Pseudomyotonia

        Symptomatic myotonia

G71.2 Congenital myopathies   cc HCC CC/MCC Exc

    Central core disease

    Fiber-type disproportion

    Minicore disease

    Multicore disease

    Myotubular (centronuclear) myopathy

    Nemaline myopathy

    EXCLUDES1 *arthrogryposis multiplex congenita (Q74.3)*

G71.3 Mitochondrial **myopathy, not elsewhere classified**

    EXCLUDES1 *Kearns-Sayre syndrome (H49.81)*

        Leber's disease (H47.21)

        Leigh's encephalopathy (G31.82)

        mitochondrial metabolism disorders (E88.4.-)

        Reye's syndrome (G93.7)

G71.8 Other primary **disorders of muscles**

G71.9 **Primary disorder of muscle, unspecified**

    Hereditary myopathy NOS

4️⃣ **G72** Other and unspecified **myopathies**

    EXCLUDES1 *arthrogryposis multiplex congenita (Q74.3)*

        dermatopolymyositis (M33.-)

        ischemic infarction of muscle (M62.2-)

        myositis (M60.-)

        polymyositis (M33.2.-)

G72.0 Drug-induced **myopathy**   cc CC/MCC Exc

    Use additional code for adverse effect, if applicable, to identify drug (T36-T50 with fifth or sixth character 5)

G72.1 Alcoholic **myopathy**   cc CC/MCC Exc

    Use additional code to identify alcoholism (F10.-)

G72.2 **Myopathy** due to other toxic agents   cc CC/MCC Exc

    📌 **Code first** (T51-T65) to identify toxic agent

G72.3 Periodic paralysis

    Familial periodic paralysis

    Hyperkalemic periodic paralysis (familial)

    Hypokalemic periodic paralysis (familial)

    Myotonic periodic paralysis (familial)

    Normokalemic paralysis (familial)

    Potassium sensitive periodic paralysis

    EXCLUDES1 *paramyotonia congenita (of von Eulenburg) (G71.19)*

🔟 **G72.4** Inflammatory and immune **myopathies, not elsewhere classified**

    G72.41 Inclusion body myositis [IBM]

    G72.49 Other **inflammatory and immune myopathies, not elsewhere classified**

        Inflammatory myopathy NOS

🔟 **G72.8** Other specified **myopathies**

    G72.81 Critical illness **myopathy**   cc CC/MCC Exc

        Acute necrotizing myopathy

        Acute quadriplegic myopathy

        Intensive care (ICU) myopathy

        Myopathy of critical illness

    G72.89 Other specified myopathies

G72.9 **Myopathy, unspecified**

4️⃣ **G73** **Disorders of myoneural junction and muscle in diseases classified elsewhere**

    G73.1 **Lambert-Eaton syndrome in neoplastic disease**   cc HCC RxHCC PDxIn CC/MCC Exc

        📌 **Code first** underlying neoplasm (C00-D49)

        EXCLUDES1 *Lambert-Eaton syndrome not associated with neoplasm (G70.80-G70.81)*

    G73.3 **Myasthenic syndromes in other diseases classified elsewhere**   cc HCC RxHCC CC/MCC Exc

        📌 **Code first** underlying disease, such as:

            neoplasm (C00-D49)

            thyrotoxicosis (E05.-)

    G73.7 **Myopathy in diseases classified elsewhere**

        📌 **Code first** underlying disease, such as:

            hyperparathyroidism (E21.0, E21.3)

            hypoparathyroidism (E20.-)

            glycogen storage disease (E74.0)

            lipid storage disorders (E75.-)

        EXCLUDES1 *myopathy in:*

            rheumatoid arthritis (M05.32)

            sarcoidosis (D86.87)

            scleroderma (M34.82)

            sicca syndrome [Sjögren] (M35.03)

            systemic lupus erythematosus (M32.19)

Cerebral palsy and other paralytic syndromes (G80-G83)

4️⃣ **G80** **Cerebral palsy**

    EXCLUDES1 *hereditary spastic paraplegia (G11.4)*

    G80.0 Spastic quadriplegic **cerebral palsy**   cc HCC CC/MCC Exc

        Congenital spastic paralysis (cerebral)

    G80.1 Spastic diplegic **cerebral palsy**   HCC

        Spastic cerebral palsy NOS

    G80.2 Spastic hemiplegic **cerebral palsy**   HCC

    G80.3 Athetoid **cerebral palsy**   HCC

        Double athetosis (syndrome)

        Dyskinetic cerebral palsy

        Dystonic cerebral palsy

        Vogt disease

    G80.4 Ataxic **cerebral palsy**   HCC

    G80.8 Other **cerebral palsy**   HCC

        Mixed cerebral palsy syndromes

    G80.9 **Cerebral palsy, unspecified**   HCC

        Cerebral palsy NOS

4️⃣ **G81** **Hemiplegia and hemiparesis**

    👁 **See Official Guidelines** "Dominant/nondominant side" I.C.6.a

    NOTES This category is to be used only when hemiplegia (complete)(incomplete) is reported without further specification, or is stated to be old or longstanding but of unspecified cause. The category is also for use in multiple coding to identify these types of hemiplegia resulting from any cause.

    EXCLUDES1 *congenital cerebral palsy (G80.-)*

        hemiplegia and hemiparesis due to sequela of cerebrovascular disease (I69.05-, I69.15-, I69.25-, I69.85-, I69.95-)

    🔟 **G81.0** Flaccid **hemiplegia**

        G81.00 **Flaccid hemiplegia affecting unspecified side**   cc HCC CC/MCC Exc

        G81.01 **Flaccid hemiplegia affecting** right **dominant side**   cc HCC CC/MCC Exc

---

G81.02 Flaccid hemiplegia affecting left dominant side ᴄᴄ⊘ ᴴᴄᴄ ᴄᴄ/ᴍᴄᴄ ᴇˣᴄ

G81.03 Flaccid hemiplegia affecting right nondominant side ᴄᴄ⊘ ᴴᴄᴄ ᴄᴄ/ᴍᴄᴄ ᴇˣᴄ

G81.04 Flaccid hemiplegia affecting left nondominant side ᴄᴄ⊘ ᴴᴄᴄ ᴄᴄ/ᴍᴄᴄ ᴇˣᴄ

G81.1 Spastic hemiplegia

G81.10 Spastic hemiplegia affecting unspecified side ᴄᴄ⊘ ᴴᴄᴄ ᴿˣᴴᴄᴄ ᴄᴄ/ᴍᴄᴄ ᴇˣᴄ

G81.11 Spastic hemiplegia affecting right dominant side ᴄᴄ⊘ ᴴᴄᴄ ᴿˣᴴᴄᴄ ᴄᴄ/ᴍᴄᴄ ᴇˣᴄ

G81.12 Spastic hemiplegia affecting left dominant side ᴄᴄ⊘ ᴴᴄᴄ ᴿˣᴴᴄᴄ ᴄᴄ/ᴍᴄᴄ ᴇˣᴄ

G81.13 Spastic hemiplegia affecting right nondominant side ᴄᴄ⊘ ᴴᴄᴄ ᴿˣᴴᴄᴄ ᴄᴄ/ᴍᴄᴄ ᴇˣᴄ

G81.14 Spastic hemiplegia affecting left nondominant side ᴄᴄ⊘ ᴴᴄᴄ ᴿˣᴴᴄᴄ ᴄᴄ/ᴍᴄᴄ ᴇˣᴄ

G81.9 Hemiplegia, unspecified

G81.90 Hemiplegia, unspecified affecting unspecified side ᴄᴄ⊘ ᴴᴄᴄ ᴄᴄ/ᴍᴄᴄ ᴇˣᴄ

G81.91 Hemiplegia, unspecified affecting right dominant side ᴄᴄ⊘ ᴴᴄᴄ ᴄᴄ/ᴍᴄᴄ ᴇˣᴄ

G81.92 Hemiplegia, unspecified affecting left dominant side ᴄᴄ⊘ ᴴᴄᴄ ᴄᴄ/ᴍᴄᴄ ᴇˣᴄ

G81.93 Hemiplegia, unspecified affecting right nondominant side ᴄᴄ⊘ ᴴᴄᴄ ᴄᴄ/ᴍᴄᴄ ᴇˣᴄ

G81.94 Hemiplegia, unspecified affecting left nondominant side ᴄᴄ⊘ ᴴᴄᴄ ᴄᴄ/ᴍᴄᴄ ᴇˣᴄ

AHA: Q1 2015

G82 Paraplegia (paraparesis) and quadriplegia (quadriparesis)

NOTES This category is to be used only when the listed conditions are reported without further specification, or are stated to be old or longstanding but of unspecified cause. The category is also for use in multiple coding to identify these conditions resulting from any cause

EXCLUDES1 congenital cerebral palsy (G80.-)

functional quadriplegia (R53.2)

hysterical paralysis (F44.4)

G82.2 Paraplegia

Paralysis of both lower limbs NOS
Paraparesis (lower) NOS
Paraplegia (lower) NOS

G82.20 Paraplegia, unspecified ᴄᴄ⊘ ᴴᴄᴄ ᴄᴄ/ᴍᴄᴄ ᴇˣᴄ

AHA: Q3 2017

G82.21 Paraplegia, complete ᴄᴄ⊘ ᴴᴄᴄ ᴄᴄ/ᴍᴄᴄ ᴇˣᴄ

G82.22 Paraplegia, incomplete ᴄᴄ⊘ ᴴᴄᴄ ᴄᴄ/ᴍᴄᴄ ᴇˣᴄ

G82.5 Quadriplegia

G82.50 Quadriplegia, unspecified ᴴᴄᴄ ᴍᴄᴄ⊘ ᴄᴄ/ᴍᴄᴄ ᴇˣᴄ

G82.51 Quadriplegia, C1-C4 complete ᴴᴄᴄ ᴍᴄᴄ⊘ ᴄᴄ/ᴍᴄᴄ ᴇˣᴄ

G82.52 Quadriplegia, C1-C4 incomplete ᴴᴄᴄ ᴍᴄᴄ⊘ ᴄᴄ/ᴍᴄᴄ ᴇˣᴄ

G82.53 Quadriplegia, C5-C7 complete ᴴᴄᴄ ᴍᴄᴄ⊘ ᴄᴄ/ᴍᴄᴄ ᴇˣᴄ

G82.54 Quadriplegia, C5-C7 incomplete ᴴᴄᴄ ᴍᴄᴄ⊘ ᴄᴄ/ᴍᴄᴄ ᴇˣᴄ

G83 Other paralytic syndromes

NOTES This category is to be used only when the listed conditions are reported without further specification, or are stated to be old or longstanding but of unspecified cause. The category is also for use in multiple coding to identify these conditions resulting from any cause.

INCLUDES paralysis (complete) (incomplete), except as in G80-G82

G83.0 Diplegia of upper limbs ᴄᴄ⊘ ᴴᴄᴄ ᴄᴄ/ᴍᴄᴄ ᴇˣᴄ

Diplegia (upper)
Paralysis of both upper limbs

G83.1 Monoplegia of lower limb

See Official Guidelines "Dominant/nondominant side" I.C.6.a

Paralysis of lower limb

EXCLUDES1 monoplegia of lower limbs due to sequela of cerebrovascular disease (I69.04-, I69.14-, I69.24-, I69.34-, I69.84-, I69.94-)

G83.10 Monoplegia of lower limb affecting unspecified side ᴴᴄᴄ

G83.11 Monoplegia of lower limb affecting right dominant side ᴴᴄᴄ

G83.12 Monoplegia of lower limb affecting left dominant side ᴴᴄᴄ

G83.13 Monoplegia of lower limb affecting right nondominant side ᴴᴄᴄ

G83.14 Monoplegia of lower limb affecting left nondominant side ᴴᴄᴄ

G83.2 Monoplegia of upper limb

See Official Guidelines "Dominant/nondominant side" I.C.6.a

Paralysis of upper limb

EXCLUDES1 monoplegia of upper limbs due to sequela of cerebrovascular disease (I69.03-, I69.13-, I69.23-, I69.33-, I69.83-, I69.93-)

G83.20 Monoplegia of upper limb affecting unspecified side ᴴᴄᴄ

G83.21 Monoplegia of upper limb affecting right dominant side ᴴᴄᴄ

G83.22 Monoplegia of upper limb affecting left dominant side ᴴᴄᴄ

G83.23 Monoplegia of upper limb affecting right nondominant side ᴴᴄᴄ

G83.24 Monoplegia of upper limb affecting left nondominant side ᴴᴄᴄ

G83.3 Monoplegia, unspecified

See Official Guidelines "Dominant/nondominant side" I.C.6.a

G83.30 Monoplegia, unspecified affecting unspecified side ᴴᴄᴄ

G83.31 Monoplegia, unspecified affecting right dominant side ᴴᴄᴄ

G83.32 Monoplegia, unspecified affecting left dominant side ᴴᴄᴄ

G83.33 Monoplegia, unspecified affecting right nondominant side ᴴᴄᴄ

G83.34 Monoplegia, unspecified affecting left nondominant side ᴴᴄᴄ

G83.4 Cauda equina syndrome ᴄᴄ⊘ ᴴᴄᴄ ᴿˣᴴᴄᴄ ᴄᴄ/ᴍᴄᴄ ᴇˣᴄ

Neurogenic bladder due to cauda equina syndrome

EXCLUDES1 cord bladder NOS (G95.89)

neurogenic bladder NOS (N31.9)

G83.5 Locked-in state ᴴᴄᴄ ᴍᴄᴄ⊘ ᴄᴄ/ᴍᴄᴄ ᴇˣᴄ

G83.8 Other specified paralytic syndromes

EXCLUDES1 paralytic syndromes due to current spinal cord injury-code to spinal cord injury (S14, S24, S34)

G83.81 Brown-Séquard syndrome ᴴᴄᴄ

G83.82 Anterior cord syndrome ᴴᴄᴄ

G83.83 Posterior cord syndrome ᴴᴄᴄ

G83.84 Todd's paralysis (postepileptic) ᴴᴄᴄ

G83.89 Other specified paralytic syndromes ᴴᴄᴄ

G83.9 Paralytic syndrome, unspecified ᴴᴄᴄ

Other disorders of the nervous system (G89-G99)

G89 Pain, not elsewhere classified

See Official Guidelines "Pain disorders related to psychological factors" I.C.5.a, "Pain - Category G89" I.C.6.b

TIP: Code first when the patient presents for pain control or pain management as the primary reason for visit.

Code also related psychological factors associated with pain (F45.42)

EXCLUDES1 generalized pain NOS (R52)

pain disorders exclusively related to psychological factors (F45.41)

pain NOS (R52)

EXCLUDES2 atypical face pain (G50.1)

headache syndromes (G44.-)

localized pain, unspecified type - code to pain by site, such as:

abdomen pain (R10.-)

ⁿᴾᴰ Unacceptable principal diagnosis symbol per Medicare code edits   ⁿᴾᴰ Code exempt from diagnosis present on admission requirement
❓ Questionable admission   ᴄᴄ⊘ Complication or comorbidity   ᴍᴄᴄ⊘ Major complication or comorbidity   ᴄᴄ/ᴍᴄᴄ⊘ CC/MCC exclusion
ᴴᴄᴄ HCC diagnosis code   ᴿˣᴴᴄᴄ RxHCC diagnosis code   MACRA code   **DEFINITION** Describes condition/terminology
TIP Coding guidance   ◉ Official Guideline Reference   ℤ¹ Z code as first-listed diagnosis

588   When symbols appear on a code that requires a 7th character extension, refer to Appendix B to identify applicable 7th character codes.   **2020 ICD-10-CM**

back pain (M54.9)

breast pain (N64.4)

chest pain (R07.1-R07.9)

ear pain (H92.0-)

eye pain (H57.1)

headache (R51)

joint pain (M25.5-)

limb pain (M79.6-)

lumbar region pain (M54.5)

painful urination (R30.9)

pelvic and perineal pain (R10.2)

shoulder pain (M25.51-)

spine pain (M54.-)

throat pain (R07.0)

tongue pain (K14.6)

tooth pain (K08.8)

renal colic (N23)

migraines (G43.-)

myalgia (M79.1-)

pain from prosthetic devices, implants, and grafts (T82.84, T83.84, T84.84, T85.84-)

phantom limb syndrome with pain (G54.6)

vulvar vestibulitis (N94.810)

vulvodynia (N94.81-)

G89.0 Central pain **syndrome**
  👁 **See Official Guidelines** "Chronic Pain Syndrome" I.C.6.b.6
  Déjérine-Roussy syndrome
  Myelopathic pain syndrome
  Thalamic pain syndrome (hyperesthetic)

5ᵗʰ G89.1 Acute pain, **not elsewhere classified**
  G89.11 Acute pain due to trauma
    👁 **See Official Guidelines** "Sequencing of Category G89 Codes with Site-specific Pain Codes" I.C.b.1.b.ii
  G89.12 Acute post-thoracotomy **pain**
    Post-thoracotomy pain NOS
  G89.18 Other **acute postprocedural pain**
    👁 **See Official Guidelines** "Pain due to medical devices" I.C.19.g.2, "Postoperative pain associated with specific postoperative complication" I.C.6.b.3.b
    Postoperative pain NOS
    Postprocedural pain NOS

5ᵗʰ G89.2 Chronic pain, **not elsewhere classified**
  👁 **See Official Guidelines** "Chronic pain" I.C.6.b.4
  TIP: There is no time frame defining when pain becomes chronic.
  EXCLUDES1 *causalgia, lower limb (G57.7-)*
    causalgia, upper limb (G56.4-)
    central pain syndrome (G89.0)
    chronic pain syndrome (G89.4)
    complex regional pain syndrome II, lower limb (G57.7-)
    complex regional pain syndrome II, upper limb (G56.4-)
    neoplasm related chronic pain (G89.3)
    reflex sympathetic dystrophy (G90.5-)
  G89.21 Chronic pain due to trauma
  G89.22 Chronic post-thoracotomy **pain**
  G89.28 Other **chronic postprocedural pain**
    👁 **See Official Guidelines** "Pain due to medical devices" I.C.19.g.2, "Postoperative pain associated with specific postoperative complication" I.C.6.b.3.b
    Other chronic postoperative pain
  G89.29 Other **chronic pain**
G89.3 Neoplasm related **pain (acute) (chronic)**
  Cancer associated pain
  Pain due to malignancy (primary) (secondary)
  Tumor associated pain
G89.4 Chronic **pain syndrome**
  Chronic pain associated with significant psychosocial dysfunction

4ᵗʰ G90 Disorders of autonomic **nervous system**
  EXCLUDES1 *dysfunction of the autonomic nervous system due to alcohol (G31.2)*
  5ᵗʰ G90.0 Idiopathic peripheral autonomic neuropathy
    G90.01 Carotid sinus syncope
      Carotid sinus syndrome
    G90.09 Other idiopathic **peripheral autonomic neuropathy**
      Idiopathic peripheral autonomic neuropathy NOS
  G90.1 Familial dysautonomia **[Riley-Day]** ⚕ HCC R:HCC CC/MCC Exc
  G90.2 Horner's **syndrome**
    Bernard(-Horner) syndrome
    Cervical sympathetic dystrophy or paralysis
  G90.3 Multi-system degeneration **of the autonomic nervous system** ⚕ HCC CC/MCC Exc
    Neurogenic orthostatic hypotension [Shy-Drager]
    EXCLUDES1 *orthostatic hypotension NOS (I95.1)*
  G90.4 Autonomic dysreflexia
    Use additional code to identify the cause, such as:
      fecal impaction (K56.41)
      pressure ulcer (pressure area) (L89.-)
      urinary tract infection (N39.0)
  5ᵗʰ G90.5 Complex regional pain syndrome I (CRPS I)
    Reflex sympathetic dystrophy
    EXCLUDES1 *causalgia of lower limb (G57.7-)*
      causalgia of upper limb (G56.4-)
      complex regional pain syndrome II of lower limb (G57.7-)
      complex regional pain syndrome II of upper limb (G56.4-)
    G90.50 Complex regional pain syndrome I, unspecified ⚕ CC/MCC Exc
    6ᵗʰ G90.51 Complex regional pain syndrome I of upper limb
      G90.511 Complex regional pain syndrome I of right upper limb ⚕ CC/MCC Exc
      G90.512 Complex regional pain syndrome I of left upper limb ⚕ CC/MCC Exc
      G90.513 Complex regional pain syndrome I of upper limb, bilateral ⚕ CC/MCC Exc
      G90.519 Complex regional pain syndrome I of unspecified upper limb ⚕ CC/MCC Exc
    6ᵗʰ G90.52 Complex regional pain syndrome I of lower limb
      G90.521 Complex regional pain syndrome I of right lower limb ⚕ CC/MCC Exc
      G90.522 Complex regional pain syndrome I of left lower limb ⚕ CC/MCC Exc
      G90.523 Complex regional pain syndrome I of lower limb, bilateral ⚕ CC/MCC Exc
      G90.529 Complex regional pain syndrome I of unspecified lower limb ⚕ CC/MCC Exc
    G90.59 Complex regional pain syndrome I of other specified site ⚕ CC/MCC Exc
  G90.8 Other disorders of autonomic nervous system
  G90.9 Disorder of the autonomic nervous system, unspecified
4ᵗʰ G91 Hydrocephalus
  INCLUDES *acquired hydrocephalus*
  EXCLUDES1 *Arnold-Chiari syndrome with hydrocephalus (Q07.-)*
    congenital hydrocephalus (Q03.-)
    spina bifida with hydrocephalus (Q05.-)
  G91.0 Communicating **hydrocephalus** ⚕ HCC CC/MCC Exc
    Secondary normal pressure hydrocephalus
  G91.1 Obstructive **hydrocephalus** ⚕ HCC CC/MCC Exc
  G91.2 (Idiopathic) normal pressure **hydrocephalus** ⚕ HCC CC/MCC Exc
    Normal pressure hydrocephalus NOS
  G91.3 Post-traumatic **hydrocephalus, unspecified** ⚕ HCC CC/MCC Exc
  G91.4 **Hydrocephalus in diseases classified elsewhere** HCC
    👈 **Code first** underlying condition, such as:
      congenital syphilis (A50.4-)
      neoplasm (C00-D49)
      plasminogen deficiency (E88.02)
    EXCLUDES1 *hydrocephalus due to congenital toxoplasmosis (P37.1)*

● Unspecified Code ■ Other Specified Code Manifestation Code N Newborn P Pediatric M Maternity A Adult ♂ Male ♀ Female

● New Code ▲ Revised Code Title ▶◀ Revised Text **NOTES** *INCLUDES* *EXCLUDES1* Not coded here *EXCLUDES2* Not included here
  4ᵗʰ 4ᵗʰ character required 5ᵗʰ 5ᵗʰ character required 6ᵗʰ 6ᵗʰ character required 7ᵗʰ 7ᵗʰ character required 7ˣ Extension 'X' Alert
  HAC Hospital-acquired condition (HAC) alert AHA AHA Coding Clinic© 👈 Code first alert

2020 ICD-10-CM When symbols appear on a code that requires a 7th character extension, refer to Appendix B to identify applicable 7th character codes. **589**

G91.8   Other hydrocephalus   CC° HCC CC/MCC Exc
G91.9   Hydrocephalus, unspecified   CC° HCC CC/MCC Exc
G92   Toxic encephalopathy   MCC° CC/MCC Exc
     AHA: Q1 2017
     Toxic encephalitis
     Toxic metabolic encephalopathy
     ☞ **Code first,** if applicable, drug induced (T36-T50)
        (T51-T65) to identify toxic agent
G93   Other disorders of brain
     G93.0   Cerebral cysts
            Arachnoid cyst
            Porencephalic cyst, acquired
            EXCLUDES1 acquired periventricular cysts of newborn (P91.1)
                        congenital cerebral cysts (Q04.6)
     G93.1   Anoxic brain damage, **not elsewhere classified**   CC° HCC CC/MCC Exc
            EXCLUDES1 cerebral anoxia due to anesthesia during labor and
                        delivery (O74.3)
                        cerebral anoxia due to anesthesia during the
                        puerperium (O89.2)
                        neonatal anoxia (P84)
     G93.2   Benign intracranial hypertension
            EXCLUDES1 hypertensive encephalopathy (I67.4)
     G93.3   Postviral fatigue syndrome
            Benign myalgic encephalomyelitis
            EXCLUDES1 chronic fatigue syndrome NOS (R53.82)
     G93.4   Other and unspecified encephalopathy
            EXCLUDES1 alcoholic encephalopathy (G31.2)
                        encephalopathy in diseases classified elsewhere
                        (G94)
                        hypertensive encephalopathy (I67.4)
                        toxic (metabolic) encephalopathy (G92)
            G93.40   Encephalopathy, unspecified   CC° CC/MCC Exc
                     AHA: Q2 2018, Q2 2017
            G93.41   Metabolic encephalopathy   MCC° CC/MCC Exc
                     AHA: Q2 2017, Q3 2016, Q3 2015
                     Septic encephalopathy
            G93.49   Other encephalopathy   CC° CC/MCC Exc
                     AHA: Q2 2018, Q4 2018, Q2 2017
                     Encephalopathy NEC
     G93.5   Compression of brain   CC° HCC CC/MCC Exc
            Arnold-Chiari type 1 compression of brain
            Compression of brain (stem)
            Herniation of brain (stem)
            EXCLUDES1 diffuse traumatic compression of brain (S06.2-)
                        focal traumatic compression of brain (S06.3-)
     G93.6   Cerebral edema   HCC MCC° CC/MCC Exc
            EXCLUDES1 cerebral edema due to birth injury (P11.0)
                        traumatic cerebral edema (S06.1-)
     G93.7   Reye's syndrome   P HCC MCC° RxHCC CC/MCC Exc
            ☞ **Code first** poisoning due to salicylates, if applicable (T39.0-,
               with sixth character 1-4)
            Use additional code for adverse effect due to salicylates, if
               applicable (T39.0-, with sixth character 5)
     G93.8   Other specified disorders of brain
            G93.81   Temporal sclerosis
                     Hippocampal sclerosis
                     Mesial temporal sclerosis
            G93.82   Brain death   CC° CC/MCC Exc
            G93.89   Other specified disorders of brain
                     AHA: Q4 2016
                     Postradiation encephalopathy
     G93.9   Disorder of brain, unspecified
G94   Other disorders of brain in diseases classified elsewhere
     AHA: Q2 2018, Q2 2017
     ☞ **Code first** underlying disease
     EXCLUDES1 encephalopathy in congenital syphilis (A50.49)
                 encephalopathy in influenza (J09.X9, J10.81, J11.81)
                 encephalopathy in syphilis (A52.19)
                 hydrocephalus in diseases classified elsewhere (G91.4)

G95   Other and unspecified diseases of spinal cord
     EXCLUDES2 myelitis (G04.-)
     G95.0   Syringomyelia and syringobulbia   CC° HCC RxHCC CC/MCC Exc
     G95.1   Vascular myelopathies
            EXCLUDES2 intraspinal phlebitis and thrombophlebitis, except
                        non-pyogenic (G08)
            G95.11   Acute infarction of spinal cord (embolic)   HCC MCC° RxHCC CC/MCC Exc
                     (nonembolic)
                     Anoxia of spinal cord
                     Arterial thrombosis of spinal cord
            G95.19   Other vascular myelopathies   CC° HCC RxHCC CC/MCC Exc
                     Edema of spinal cord
                     Hematomyelia
                     Nonpyogenic intraspinal phlebitis and
                        thrombophlebitis
                     Subacute necrotic myelopathy
     G95.2   Other and unspecified cord compression
            G95.20   Unspecified cord compression   CC° HCC RxHCC CC/MCC Exc
            G95.29   Other cord compression   CC° HCC RxHCC CC/MCC Exc
     G95.8   Other specified diseases of spinal cord
            EXCLUDES1 neurogenic bladder NOS (N31.9)
                        neurogenic bladder due to cauda equina syndrome
                        (G83.4)
                        neuromuscular dysfunction of bladder without
                        spinal cord lesion (N31.-)
            G95.81   Conus medullaris syndrome   CC° HCC RxHCC CC/MCC Exc
            G95.89   Other specified diseases of
                     spinal cord   CC° HCC RxHCC CC/MCC Exc
                     Cord bladder NOS
                     Drug-induced myelopathy
                     Radiation-induced myelopathy
                     EXCLUDES1 myelopathy NOS (G95.9)
     G95.9   Disease of spinal cord, unspecified   CC° HCC RxHCC CC/MCC Exc
            Myelopathy NOS
G96   Other disorders of central nervous system
     G96.0   Cerebrospinal fluid leak   CC° CC/MCC Exc
            AHA: Q2 2018
            EXCLUDES1 cerebrospinal fluid leak from spinal puncture (G97.0)
     G96.1   Disorders of meninges, not elsewhere classified
            G96.11   Dural tear   CC° CC/MCC Exc
                     EXCLUDES1 accidental puncture or laceration of dura
                                 during a procedure (G97.41)
            G96.12   Meningeal adhesions (cerebral) (spinal)
            G96.19   Other disorders of meninges, not elsewhere
                     classified
     G96.8   Other specified disorders of central nervous system
     G96.9   Disorder of central nervous system, unspecified
G97   Intraoperative and postprocedural complications and disorders of
     nervous system, not elsewhere classified
     EXCLUDES2 intraoperative and postprocedural cerebrovascular
                 infarction (I97.81-, I97.82-)
     G97.0   Cerebrospinal fluid leak from spinal puncture   CC° CC/MCC Exc
     G97.1   Other reaction to spinal and lumbar puncture
            Headache due to lumbar puncture
     G97.2   Intracranial hypotension following
            ventricular shunting   CC° CC/MCC Exc
     G97.3   Intraoperative hemorrhage and hematoma of a nervous
            system organ or structure complicating a procedure
            EXCLUDES1 intraoperative hemorrhage and hematoma of
                        a nervous system organ or structure due to
                        accidental puncture and laceration during a
                        procedure (G97.4-)
            G97.31   Intraoperative hemorrhage and hematoma of a
                     nervous system organ or structure complicating a
                     nervous system procedure   CC° CC/MCC Exc
            G97.32   Intraoperative hemorrhage and hematoma of a
                     nervous system organ or structure complicating
                     other procedure   CC° CC/MCC Exc
     G97.4   Accidental puncture and laceration of a nervous system
            organ or structure during a procedure

When symbols appear on a code that requires a 7th character extension, refer to Appendix B to identify applicable 7th character codes.
2020 ICD-10-CM

G97.41 **Accidental puncture or laceration of dura** during a procedure CC CC/MCC Exc
Incidental (inadvertent) durotomy

G97.48 **Accidental puncture and laceration of other nervous system organ or structure** during a nervous system procedure CC CC/MCC Exc

G97.49 **Accidental puncture and laceration of other nervous system organ or structure** during other procedure CC CC/MCC Exc

5ᵗʰ G97.5 Postprocedural hemorrhage **of a nervous system organ or structure following a procedure**

G97.51 **Postprocedural hemorrhage of a** nervous system **organ or structure following a** nervous system **procedure** CC CC/MCC Exc

G97.52 **Postprocedural hemorrhage of a nervous system organ or structure following** other **procedure** CC CC/MCC Exc

5ᵗʰ G97.6 Postprocedural hematoma and seroma **of a nervous system organ or structure following a procedure**

G97.61 **Postprocedural** hematoma **of a** nervous system **organ or structure following a** nervous system **procedure** CC CC/MCC Exc

G97.62 **Postprocedural hematoma of a nervous system organ or structure following** other **procedure** CC CC/MCC Exc

G97.63 **Postprocedural** seroma **of a** nervous system **organ or structure following a** nervous system **procedure** CC CC/MCC Exc

G97.64 **Postprocedural seroma of a nervous system organ or structure following** other **procedure** CC CC/MCC Exc

5ᵗʰ G97.8 Other intraoperative and postprocedural complications **and disorders of nervous system**
Use additional code to further specify disorder

G97.81 Other intraoperative **complications of nervous system** CC CC/MCC Exc

G97.82 Other postprocedural **complications and disorders of nervous system** CC CC/MCC Exc

4ᵗʰ **G98 Other disorders of nervous system not elsewhere classified**
INCLUDES   nervous system disorder NOS

G98.0 Neurogenic arthritis, **not elsewhere classified**
Nonsyphilitic neurogenic arthropathy NEC
Nonsyphilitic neurogenic spondylopathy NEC
EXCLUDES1 spondylopathy (in):
syringomyelia and syringobulbia (G95.0)
tabes dorsalis (A52.11)

G98.8 Other **disorders of nervous system**
Nervous system disorder NOS

4ᵗʰ **G99 Other disorders of nervous system in diseases classified elsewhere**

G99.0 Autonomic neuropathy **in diseases classified elsewhere** CC CC/MCC Exc
☞ **Code first** underlying disease, such as:
amyloidosis (E85.-)
gout (M1A.-, M10.-)
hyperthyroidism (E05.-)
EXCLUDES1 diabetic autonomic neuropathy (E08-E13 with .43)

G99.2 Myelopathy **in diseases classified elsewhere** CC HCC RHCC CC/MCC Exc
AHA: Q3 2018
☞ **Code first** underlying disease, such as:
neoplasm (C00-D49)
EXCLUDES1 myelopathy in:
intervertebral disease (M50.0-, M51.0-)
spondylosis (M47.0-, M47.1-)

G99.8 Other specified **disorders of nervous system in diseases classified elsewhere**
☞ **Code first** underlying disorder, such as:
amyloidosis (E85.-)
avitaminosis (E56.9)
EXCLUDES1 nervous system involvement in:
cysticercosis (B69.0)
rubella (B06.0-)
syphilis (A52.1-)

● Unspecified Code   Other Specified Code   Manifestation Code   ℕ Newborn   ℙ Pediatric   Ⅿ Maternity   🅐 Adult   ♂ Male   ♀ Female
● New Code   ▲ Revised Code Title   ▶◀ Revised Text   NOTES   INCLUDES   EXCLUDES1 Not coded here   EXCLUDES2 Not included here
4ᵗʰ 4ᵗʰ character required   5ᵗʰ 5ᵗʰ character required   6ᵗʰ 6ᵗʰ character required   7ᵗʰ 7ᵗʰ character required   ✗ Extension 'X' Alert
HAC Hospital-acquired condition (HAC) alert   AHA AHA Coding Clinic©   ☞ Code first alert

NOTES

Chapter 7: Diseases of the Eye and Adnexa (H00-H59)

Anatomy of the Eye

Introduction

Eyes (Figure 7.a) are regarded as the organs of sight. They are located in the orbits of the skull. The eyelids and eyelashes serve to protect the eyes from foreign objects. Blinking of the eyelids lubricates the surface of the eye by spreading tears that are produced by the lacrimal gland.

1. **The Organ of Sight**
   A typical human eye is in the form of a sphere and filled with the following two fluids:

   a) **Aqueous Humor:** The frontal portion of the lens of the eye is known as the anterior compartment that remains filled with fluid, which is called the aqueous humor.

   b) **Vitreous Humor:** The portion behind the lens of the eye is known as the posterior compartment that is filled with a fluid called the vitreous humor.

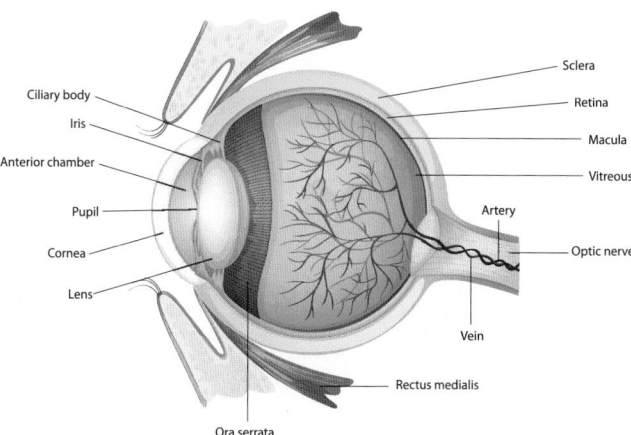

Figure 7.a Anatomy of the Eye

2. **The Other Parts of the Eye**
   a) **Ciliary Body and Muscle:** This is a ring of striated smooth muscle in the middle layer eye (vascular layer). It is triangular in the horizontal section and is coated by a double layer, the ciliary epithelium. The inner layer is transparent and covers the vitreous body and is a continuation of neural tissue of the retina. The outer layer is continuous with the retinal pigment epithelium and constitutes the cells of the dilator muscle.

   b) **Suspensory Ligament:** A series of fibers that connect the ciliary body of the eye with the lens, holding it in place. Suspensory ligaments are thin fibers that connect the ciliary body of the lens with the receptors. It is a thickening of Tenon's capsule, the dense connective tissue capsule surrounding the globe and separating it from orbital fat. Suspensory ligaments in the eye lens allow easy focusing.

   c) **Iris:** A thin, circular structure in the eye which covers the sclera. It is responsible for controlling the diameter and size of the pupils and thus the amount of light reaching the retina. In response to the amount of light entering the eye, muscles attached to the iris expand or contract the aperture at the center of the iris, known as the pupil.

   d) **Pupil:** The dark center opening in the middle of the iris is called the pupil. The pupil is a hole located in the center of the iris of the eye that allows light to enter the retina. The pupil changes size to adjust for the amount of light available.

   e) **Cornea:** The cornea is transparent and comprises the front part of the eye that covers the iris, pupil and anterior chamber. Together with the lens, the cornea refracts light accounting for approximately two-thirds of the eye's total optical power.

   f) **Lens:** The crystalline lens is a biconvex structure and is suspended behind the colored iris. The lens is behind the covering known as the cornea. The lens is more flat on its anterior side than on its posterior side.

   g) **Retina:** The vertebrate retina is 0.5 mm thick and lines the back of the eye. It is a light-sensitive layer of tissue, lining the inner surface of the eye. The optic nerve contains the ganglion cell axons running to the brain.

   h) **Retinal Arteries and Veins:** The retinal arteries and veins emerge from the nasal side of the optic disc. Vessels directed temporally have an arching course; those directed nasally have a radial course. Arteries are brighter red and narrower than veins.

   i) **Fovea Centralis:** The fovea is the depression in the inner retinal surface, about 1.5 mm wide and is specialized for maximum visual acuity. This is the thickest part of the retina. This part has the highest density of cones in the eye.

   j) **Optic Nerve:** The optic nerve is the second of twelve paired cranial nerves, but is considered to be part of the central nervous system as it is derived from an out-pouching of the diencephalon during embryonic development. It consists mainly of fibers derived from the ganglionic cells of the retina. Its fibers are covered with myelin produced by oligodendrocytes rather than Schwann cells.

   k) **Choroid Coat:** The choroid, also known as the choroidea or choroid coat, is the vascular layer of the eye containing connective tissue and lies between the retina and the sclera. It contains the retinal pigmented epithelial cells and provides oxygen and nourishment to the retina.

   l) **Sclera:** The posterior five-sixths of the connective tissue coat of the ocular globe is formed by sclera. It maintains the shape of the globe and provides an attachment for the extraocular muscle insertions. The sclera is perforated by many nerves and vessels passing through the posterior scleral foramen, the hole that is formed by the optic nerve. The inner layer of the sclera (lamina fusca) blends with the suprachoroidal and supraciliary lamellae of the uveal tract.

   m) **Blind Spot:** This is a small portion of the visual field of each eye where the optic nerve and blood vessels pass through to connect to the back of the eye and is also called an optic disk. There are no photoreceptors in the optic disk, therefore there is no image detection in this area. The blind spot of the right eye is located to the right of the center of vision and vice versa in the left eye.

   n) **Hyaloid Canal (or Cloquet's/Stilling's Canal):** This is a small transparent canal running through the vitreous body from the optical nerve disc to the lens. It is formed by pouch of the hyaloid membrane, which encloses the vitreous body. It is filled with lymph.

Common Pathologies

Cataract

Cataracts (Figure 7.b) are an eye disorder in which clouding of the lens occurs, which leads to blurry vision. It is an aging disorder. This disorder leads to dimness in eye vision, and if not treated can lead to blindness.

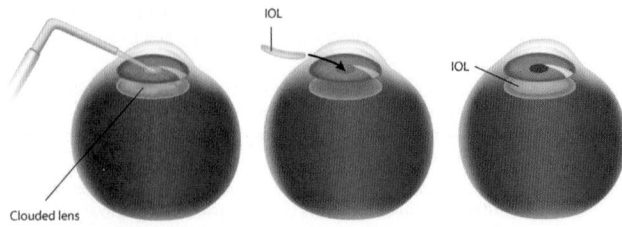

Clouded lens removed   **Intraocular lens (IOL implanted in place)**

Figure 7.b Cataract and Surgery to Remove the Cataract

Glaucoma (Figure 7.c)

In this disease, damage occurs to optic nerves due to increased intraocular pressure and leads to blindness.

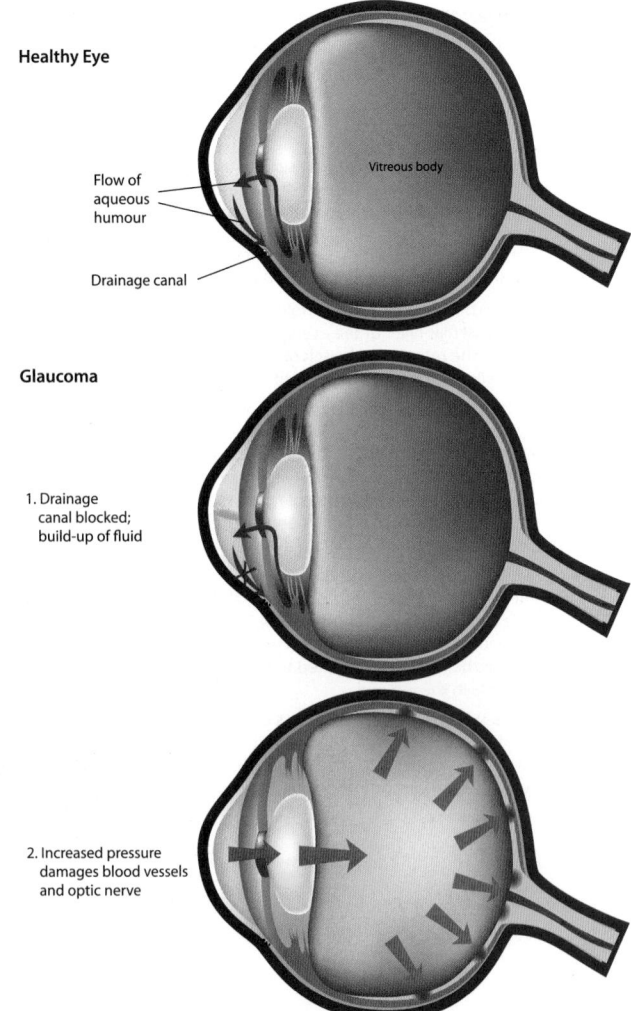

Figure 7.c Healthy Eye vs. Eye with Glaucoma

Strabismus (Figure 7.d)

A condition of the eye in which there is nonalignment between both eyes. This condition is commonly called squint.

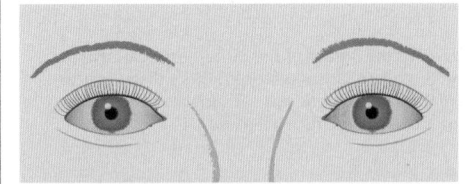

Normal

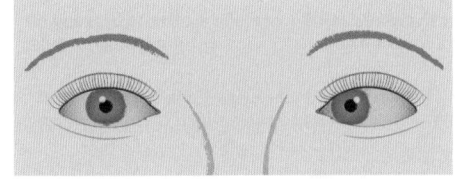

Esotropia - eye turns inward

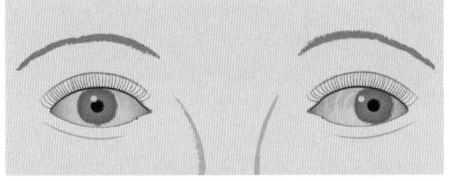

Exotropia - eye turns outward

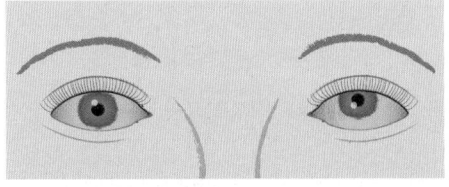

Hypertropia - eye turns upward

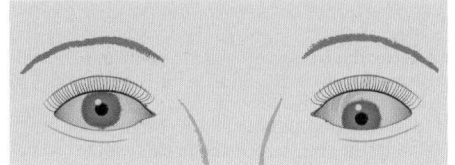

Hypotropia - eye turns downward

Figure 7.d Types of Strabismus

Macular Degeneration

This condition occurs because of degeneration in the macula of the eye due to aging and leads to blurry vision. It is a disease that destroys sharp, central vision. Central vision is required to see objects clearly and to do tasks such as reading and driving.

Conjunctivitis

An infection in the eye. The conjunctiva in the eye gets exposed to bacteria and other allergic irritants, which can lead to inflammation and infection. It is also known as pinkeye.

Optic Neuritis

This disorder occurs due to inflammation of the optic nerve. Pain and temporary vision loss are common.

Diseases of the eye and adnexa (H00-H59)

[NOTES] Use an external cause code following the code for the eye condition, if applicable, to identify the cause of the eye condition

[EXCLUDES2] *certain conditions originating in the perinatal period (P04-P96)*
certain infectious and parasitic diseases (A00-B99)
complications of pregnancy, childbirth and the puerperium (O00-O9A)
congenital malformations, deformations, and chromosomal abnormalities (Q00-Q99)
diabetes mellitus related eye conditions (E09.3-, E10.3-, E11.3-, E13.3-)
endocrine, nutritional and metabolic diseases (E00-E88)
injury (trauma) of eye and orbit (S05.-)
injury, poisoning and certain other consequences of external causes (S00-T88)
neoplasms (C00-D49)
symptoms, signs and abnormal clinical and laboratory findings, not elsewhere classified (R00-R94)
syphilis related eye disorders (A50.01, A50.3-, A51.43, A52.71)

This chapter contains the following blocks:

H00-H05	Disorders of eyelid, lacrimal system and orbit
H10-H11	Disorders of conjunctiva
H15-H22	Disorders of sclera, cornea, iris and ciliary body
H25-H28	Disorders of lens
H30-H36	Disorders of choroid and retina
H40-H42	Glaucoma
H43-H44	Disorders of vitreous body and globe
H46-H47	Disorders of optic nerve and visual pathways
H49-H52	Disorders of ocular muscles, binocular movement, accommodation and refraction
H53-H54	Visual disturbances and blindness
H55-H57	Other disorders of eye and adnexa
H59	Intraoperative and postprocedural complications and disorders of eye and adnexa, not elsewhere classified

Disorders of eyelid, lacrimal system and orbit (H00-H05)

[EXCLUDES2] *open wound of eyelid (S01.1-)*
superficial injury of eyelid (S00.1-, S00.2-)

④ **H00 Hordeolum and chalazion**
⑤ **H00.0 Hordeolum (externum) (internum) of eyelid**
⑥ **H00.01 Hordeolum externum**
Hordeolum NOS
Stye
H00.011 Hordeolum externum right upper eyelid
H00.012 Hordeolum externum right lower eyelid
H00.013 Hordeolum externum right eye, unspecified eyelid
H00.014 Hordeolum externum left upper eyelid
H00.015 Hordeolum externum left lower eyelid
H00.016 Hordeolum externum left eye, unspecified eyelid
H00.019 Hordeolum externum unspecified eye, unspecified eyelid
⑥ **H00.02 Hordeolum internum**
Infection of meibomian gland
H00.021 Hordeolum internum right upper eyelid
H00.022 Hordeolum internum right lower eyelid
H00.023 Hordeolum internum right eye, unspecified eyelid
H00.024 Hordeolum internum left upper eyelid
H00.025 Hordeolum internum left lower eyelid
H00.026 Hordeolum internum left eye, unspecified eyelid
H00.029 Hordeolum internum unspecified eye, unspecified eyelid
⑥ **H00.03 Abscess of eyelid**
Furuncle of eyelid
H00.031 Abscess of right upper eyelid
H00.032 Abscess of right lower eyelid
H00.033 Abscess of eyelid right eye, unspecified eyelid
H00.034 Abscess of left upper eyelid
H00.035 Abscess of left lower eyelid
H00.036 Abscess of eyelid left eye, unspecified eyelid
H00.039 Abscess of eyelid unspecified eye, unspecified eyelid
⑤ **H00.1 Chalazion**
Meibomian (gland) cyst
[EXCLUDES2] *infected meibomian gland (H00.02-)*
H00.11 Chalazion right upper eyelid
H00.12 Chalazion right lower eyelid
H00.13 Chalazion right eye, unspecified eyelid
H00.14 Chalazion left upper eyelid
H00.15 Chalazion left lower eyelid
H00.16 Chalazion left eye, unspecified eyelid
H00.19 Chalazion unspecified eye, unspecified eyelid
④ **H01 Other inflammation of eyelid**
⑤ **H01.0 Blepharitis (Figure 7.1)**
[EXCLUDES1] *blepharoconjunctivitis (H10.5-)*
⑥ **H01.00 Unspecified blepharitis**
H01.001 Unspecified blepharitis right upper eyelid
H01.002 Unspecified blepharitis right lower eyelid
H01.003 Unspecified blepharitis right eye, unspecified eyelid
H01.004 Unspecified blepharitis left upper eyelid
H01.005 Unspecified blepharitis left lower eyelid
H01.006 Unspecified blepharitis left eye, unspecified eyelid
H01.009 Unspecified blepharitis unspecified eye, unspecified eyelid
H01.00A Unspecified blepharitis right eye, upper and lower eyelids
H01.00B Unspecified blepharitis left eye, upper and lower eyelids

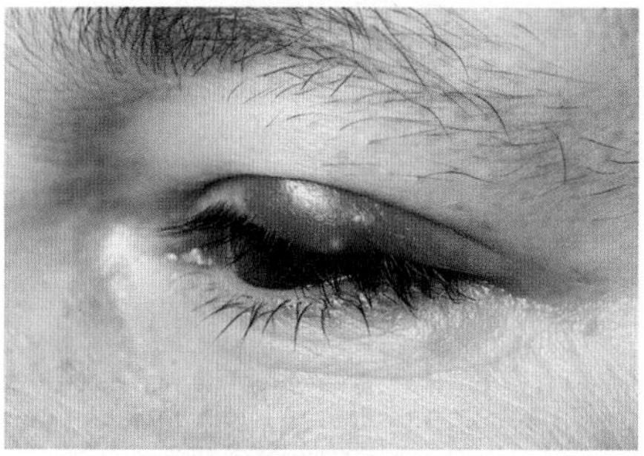

Figure 7.1 Blepharitis

⑥ **H01.01 Ulcerative blepharitis**
H01.011 Ulcerative blepharitis right upper eyelid
H01.012 Ulcerative blepharitis right lower eyelid
H01.013 Ulcerative blepharitis right eye, unspecified eyelid
H01.014 Ulcerative blepharitis left upper eyelid
H01.015 Ulcerative blepharitis left lower eyelid
H01.016 Ulcerative blepharitis left eye, unspecified eyelid
H01.019 Ulcerative blepharitis unspecified eye, unspecified eyelid
H01.01A Ulcerative blepharitis right eye, upper and lower eyelids

Unspecified Code | Other Specified Code | Manifestation Code | [N] Newborn | [P] Pediatric | [M] Maternity | [A] Adult | ♂ Male | ♀ Female
● New Code ▲ Revised Code Title ►◄ Revised Text [NOTES] [INCLUDES] [EXCLUDES1] Not coded here [EXCLUDES2] Not included here
④ 4th character required ⑤ 5th character required ⑥ 6th character required ⑦ 7th character required ⑦ Extension 'X' Alert
[HAC] Hospital-acquired condition (HAC) alert AHA AHA Coding Clinic© ☞ Code first alert

When symbols appear on a code that requires a 7th character extension, refer to Appendix B to identify applicable 7th character codes.

H01.01B Ulcerative blepharitis left eye, upper and lower eyelids

[6th] H01.02 Squamous blepharitis

H01.021 Squamous blepharitis right upper eyelid
H01.022 Squamous blepharitis right lower eyelid
H01.023 Squamous blepharitis right eye, unspecified eyelid
H01.024 Squamous blepharitis left upper eyelid
H01.025 Squamous blepharitis left lower eyelid
H01.026 Squamous blepharitis left eye, unspecified eyelid
H01.029 Squamous blepharitis unspecified eye, unspecified eyelid
H01.02A Squamous blepharitis right eye, upper and lower eyelids
H01.02B Squamous blepharitis left eye, upper and lower eyelids

[5th] H01.1 Noninfectious dermatoses of eyelid

[6th] H01.11 Allergic dermatitis of eyelid

Contact dermatitis of eyelid

H01.111 Allergic dermatitis of right upper eyelid
H01.112 Allergic dermatitis of right lower eyelid
H01.113 Allergic dermatitis of right eye, unspecified eyelid
H01.114 Allergic dermatitis of left upper eyelid
H01.115 Allergic dermatitis of left lower eyelid
H01.116 Allergic dermatitis of left eye, unspecified eyelid
H01.119 Allergic dermatitis of unspecified eye, unspecified eyelid

[6th] H01.12 Discoid lupus erythematosus of eyelid

H01.121 Discoid lupus erythematosus of right upper eyelid
H01.122 Discoid lupus erythematosus of right lower eyelid
H01.123 Discoid lupus erythematosus of right eye, unspecified eyelid
H01.124 Discoid lupus erythematosus of left upper eyelid
H01.125 Discoid lupus erythematosus of left lower eyelid
H01.126 Discoid lupus erythematosus of left eye, unspecified eyelid
H01.129 Discoid lupus erythematosus of unspecified eye, unspecified eyelid

[6th] H01.13 Eczematous dermatitis of eyelid

H01.131 Eczematous dermatitis of right upper eyelid
H01.132 Eczematous dermatitis of right lower eyelid
H01.133 Eczematous dermatitis of right eye, unspecified eyelid
H01.134 Eczematous dermatitis of left upper eyelid
H01.135 Eczematous dermatitis of left lower eyelid
H01.136 Eczematous dermatitis of left eye, unspecified eyelid
H01.139 Eczematous dermatitis of unspecified eye, unspecified eyelid

[6th] H01.14 Xeroderma of eyelid

H01.141 Xeroderma of right upper eyelid
H01.142 Xeroderma of right lower eyelid
H01.143 Xeroderma of right eye, unspecified eyelid
H01.144 Xeroderma of left upper eyelid
H01.145 Xeroderma of left lower eyelid
H01.146 Xeroderma of left eye, unspecified eyelid
H01.149 Xeroderma of unspecified eye, unspecified eyelid

H01.8 Other specified inflammations of eyelid

H01.9 Unspecified inflammation of eyelid

Inflammation of eyelid NOS

[4th] H02 Other disorders of eyelid

EXCLUDES1 *congenital malformations of eyelid (Q10.0-Q10.3)*

[5th] H02.0 Entropion and trichiasis of eyelid

[6th] H02.00 Unspecified entropion of eyelid

H02.001 Unspecified entropion of right upper eyelid
H02.002 Unspecified entropion of right lower eyelid
H02.003 Unspecified entropion of right eye, unspecified eyelid
H02.004 Unspecified entropion of left upper eyelid
H02.005 Unspecified entropion of left lower eyelid
H02.006 Unspecified entropion of left eye, unspecified eyelid
H02.009 Unspecified entropion of unspecified eye, unspecified eyelid

[6th] H02.01 Cicatricial entropion of eyelid

H02.011 Cicatricial entropion of right upper eyelid
H02.012 Cicatricial entropion of right lower eyelid
H02.013 Cicatricial entropion of right eye, unspecified eyelid
H02.014 Cicatricial entropion of left upper eyelid
H02.015 Cicatricial entropion of left lower eyelid
H02.016 Cicatricial entropion of left eye, unspecified eyelid
H02.019 Cicatricial entropion of unspecified eye, unspecified eyelid

[6th] H02.02 Mechanical entropion of eyelid

H02.021 Mechanical entropion of right upper eyelid
H02.022 Mechanical entropion of right lower eyelid
H02.023 Mechanical entropion of right eye, unspecified eyelid
H02.024 Mechanical entropion of left upper eyelid
H02.025 Mechanical entropion of left lower eyelid
H02.026 Mechanical entropion of left eye, unspecified eyelid
H02.029 Mechanical entropion of unspecified eye, unspecified eyelid

[6th] H02.03 Senile entropion of eyelid

H02.031 Senile entropion of right upper eyelid [A]
H02.032 Senile entropion of right lower eyelid [A]
H02.033 Senile entropion of right eye, unspecified eyelid [A]
H02.034 Senile entropion of left upper eyelid [A]
H02.035 Senile entropion of left lower eyelid [A]
H02.036 Senile entropion of left eye, unspecified eyelid [A]
H02.039 Senile entropion of unspecified eye, unspecified eyelid [A]

[6th] H02.04 Spastic entropion of eyelid

H02.041 Spastic entropion of right upper eyelid
H02.042 Spastic entropion of right lower eyelid
H02.043 Spastic entropion of right eye, unspecified eyelid
H02.044 Spastic entropion of left upper eyelid
H02.045 Spastic entropion of left lower eyelid
H02.046 Spastic entropion of left eye, unspecified eyelid
H02.049 Spastic entropion of unspecified eye, unspecified eyelid

[6th] H02.05 Trichiasis without entropion

DEFINITION: Trichiasis is the ingrowth of the eyelashes.

H02.051 Trichiasis without entropion right upper eyelid
H02.052 Trichiasis without entropion right lower eyelid
H02.053 Trichiasis without entropion right eye, unspecified eyelid

[PDx] Unacceptable principal diagnosis symbol per Medicare code edits [POA] Code exempt from diagnosis present on admission requirement
[?] Questionable admission [CC] Complication or comorbidity [MCC] Major complication or comorbidity [CC/MCC Exc] CC/MCC exclusion
[HCC] HCC diagnosis code [RxHCC] RxHCC diagnosis code MACRA code **DEFINITION** Describes condition/terminology
TIP Coding guidance 👁 Official Guideline Reference [Z1] Z code as first-listed diagnosis

H02.054 Trichiasis without entropion left upper eyelid

H02.055 Trichiasis without entropion left lower eyelid

H02.056 Trichiasis without entropion left eye, unspecified eyelid

H02.059 Trichiasis without entropion unspecified eye, unspecified eyelid

5ᵗʰ H02.1 Ectropion of eyelid

6ᵗʰ H02.10 Unspecified ectropion of eyelid

H02.101 Unspecified ectropion of right upper eyelid

H02.102 Unspecified ectropion of right lower eyelid

H02.103 Unspecified ectropion of right eye, unspecified eyelid

H02.104 Unspecified ectropion of left upper eyelid

H02.105 Unspecified ectropion of left lower eyelid

H02.106 Unspecified ectropion of left eye, unspecified eyelid

H02.109 Unspecified ectropion of unspecified eye, unspecified eyelid

6ᵗʰ H02.11 Cicatricial ectropion of eyelid

H02.111 Cicatricial ectropion of right upper eyelid

H02.112 Cicatricial ectropion of right lower eyelid

H02.113 Cicatricial ectropion of right eye, unspecified eyelid

H02.114 Cicatricial ectropion of left upper eyelid

H02.115 Cicatricial ectropion of left lower eyelid

H02.116 Cicatricial ectropion of left eye, unspecified eyelid

H02.119 Cicatricial ectropion of unspecified eye, unspecified eyelid

6ᵗʰ H02.12 Mechanical ectropion of eyelid

H02.121 Mechanical ectropion of right upper eyelid

H02.122 Mechanical ectropion of right lower eyelid

H02.123 Mechanical ectropion of right eye, unspecified eyelid

H02.124 Mechanical ectropion of left upper eyelid

H02.125 Mechanical ectropion of left lower eyelid

H02.126 Mechanical ectropion of left eye, unspecified eyelid

H02.129 Mechanical ectropion of unspecified eye, unspecified eyelid

6ᵗʰ H02.13 Senile ectropion of eyelid

H02.131 Senile ectropion of right upper eyelid ▲

H02.132 Senile ectropion of right lower eyelid ▲

H02.133 Senile ectropion of right eye, unspecified eyelid ▲

H02.134 Senile ectropion of left upper eyelid ▲

H02.135 Senile ectropion of left lower eyelid ▲

H02.136 Senile ectropion of left eye, unspecified eyelid ▲

H02.139 Senile ectropion of unspecified eye, unspecified eyelid ▲

6ᵗʰ H02.14 Spastic ectropion of eyelid

H02.141 Spastic ectropion of right upper eyelid

H02.142 Spastic ectropion of right lower eyelid

H02.143 Spastic ectropion of right eye, unspecified eyelid

H02.144 Spastic ectropion of left upper eyelid

H02.145 Spastic ectropion of left lower eyelid

H02.146 Spastic ectropion of left eye, unspecified eyelid

H02.149 Spastic ectropion of unspecified eye, unspecified eyelid

6ᵗʰ H02.15 Paralytic ectropion of eyelid

H02.151 Paralytic ectropion of right upper eyelid
AHA: Q4 2018

H02.152 Paralytic ectropion of right lower eyelid
AHA: Q4 2018

H02.153 Paralytic ectropion of right eye, unspecified eyelid
AHA: Q4 2018

H02.154 Paralytic ectropion of left upper eyelid
AHA: Q4 2018

H02.155 Paralytic ectropion of left lower eyelid
AHA: Q4 2018

H02.156 Paralytic ectropion of left eye, unspecified eyelid
AHA: Q4 2018

H02.159 Paralytic ectropion of unspecified eye, unspecified eyelid
AHA: Q4 2018

5ᵗʰ H02.2 Lagophthalmos

6ᵗʰ H02.20 Unspecified lagophthalmos

H02.201 Unspecified lagophthalmos right upper eyelid

H02.202 Unspecified lagophthalmos right lower eyelid

H02.203 Unspecified lagophthalmos right eye, unspecified eyelid

H02.204 Unspecified lagophthalmos left upper eyelid

H02.205 Unspecified lagophthalmos left lower eyelid

H02.206 Unspecified lagophthalmos left eye, unspecified eyelid

H02.209 Unspecified lagophthalmos unspecified eye, unspecified eyelid

H02.20A Unspecified lagophthalmos right eye, upper and lower eyelids
AHA: Q4 2018

H02.20B Unspecified lagophthalmos left eye, upper and lower eyelids
AHA: Q4 2018

H02.20C Unspecified lagophthalmos, bilateral, upper and lower eyelids
AHA: Q4 2018

6ᵗʰ H02.21 Cicatricial lagophthalmos

H02.211 Cicatricial lagophthalmos right upper eyelid

H02.212 Cicatricial lagophthalmos right lower eyelid

H02.213 Cicatricial lagophthalmos right eye, unspecified eyelid

H02.214 Cicatricial lagophthalmos left upper eyelid

H02.215 Cicatricial lagophthalmos left lower eyelid

H02.216 Cicatricial lagophthalmos left eye, unspecified eyelid

H02.219 Cicatricial lagophthalmos unspecified eye, unspecified eyelid

H02.21A Cicatricial lagophthalmos right eye, upper and lower eyelids
AHA: Q4 2018

H02.21B Cicatricial lagophthalmos left eye, upper and lower eyelids
AHA: Q4 2018

H02.21C Cicatricial lagophthalmos, bilateral, upper and lower eyelids
AHA: Q4 2018

6ᵗʰ H02.22 Mechanical lagophthalmos

H02.221 Mechanical lagophthalmos right upper eyelid

H02.222 Mechanical lagophthalmos right lower eyelid

H02.223 Mechanical lagophthalmos right eye, unspecified eyelid

H02.224 Mechanical lagophthalmos left upper eyelid

H02.225 Mechanical lagophthalmos left lower eyelid

Unspecified Code   Other Specified Code   Manifestation Code   ℕ Newborn   ℙ Pediatric   𝕄 Maternity   𝔸 Adult   ♂ Male   ♀ Female
● New Code   ▲ Revised Code Title   ▶◀ Revised Text   **NOTES**   *INCLUDES*   *EXCLUDES1* Not coded here   *EXCLUDES2* Not included here
4ᵗʰ character required   5ᵗʰ character required   6ᵗʰ character required   7ᵗʰ character required   Extension 'X' Alert
HAC Hospital-acquired condition (HAC) alert   **AHA** AHA Coding Clinic©   Code first alert

H02.226 **Mechanical lagophthalmos** left eye, unspecified eyelid

H02.229 **Mechanical lagophthalmos unspecified eye, unspecified eyelid**

H02.22A **Mechanical lagophthalmos** right eye, upper and lower **eyelids**
AHA: Q4 2018

H02.22B **Mechanical lagophthalmos** left eye, upper and lower **eyelids**
AHA: Q4 2018

H02.22C **Mechanical lagophthalmos,** bilateral, upper and lower **eyelids**
AHA: Q4 2018

H02.23 Paralytic **lagophthalmos**

H02.231 **Paralytic lagophthalmos** right upper eyelid

H02.232 **Paralytic lagophthalmos** right lower **eyelid**

H02.233 **Paralytic lagophthalmos** right eye, unspecified eyelid

H02.234 **Paralytic lagophthalmos** left upper **eyelid**

H02.235 **Paralytic lagophthalmos** left lower **eyelid**

H02.236 **Paralytic lagophthalmos** left eye, unspecified eyelid

H02.239 **Paralytic lagophthalmos unspecified eye, unspecified eyelid**

H02.23A **Paralytic lagophthalmos** right eye, upper and lower **eyelids**
AHA: Q4 2018

H02.23B **Paralytic lagophthalmos** left eye, upper and lower **eyelids**
AHA: Q4 2018

H02.23C **Paralytic lagophthalmos,** bilateral, upper and lower **eyelids**
AHA: Q4 2018

H02.3 Blepharochalasis
Pseudoptosis

H02.30 **Blepharochalasis unspecified eye, unspecified eyelid**

H02.31 **Blepharochalasis** right upper **eyelid**

H02.32 **Blepharochalasis** right lower **eyelid**

H02.33 **Blepharochalasis** right eye, unspecified eyelid

H02.34 **Blepharochalasis** left upper **eyelid**

H02.35 **Blepharochalasis** left lower **eyelid**

H02.36 **Blepharochalasis** left eye, unspecified eyelid

H02.4 Ptosis of eyelid

H02.40 Unspecified ptosis of eyelid

H02.401 **Unspecified ptosis of** right **eyelid**

H02.402 **Unspecified ptosis of** left **eyelid**

H02.403 **Unspecified ptosis of** bilateral **eyelids**

H02.409 **Unspecified ptosis of unspecified eyelid**

H02.41 Mechanical ptosis of eyelid

H02.411 **Mechanical ptosis of** right **eyelid**

H02.412 **Mechanical ptosis of** left **eyelid**

H02.413 **Mechanical ptosis of** bilateral **eyelids**

H02.419 **Mechanical ptosis of unspecified eyelid**

H02.42 Myogenic ptosis of eyelid

H02.421 **Myogenic ptosis of** right **eyelid**

H02.422 **Myogenic ptosis of** left **eyelid**

H02.423 **Myogenic ptosis of** bilateral **eyelids**

H02.429 **Myogenic ptosis of unspecified eyelid**

H02.43 Paralytic ptosis of eyelid
Neurogenic ptosis of eyelid

H02.431 **Paralytic ptosis of** right **eyelid**

H02.432 **Paralytic ptosis of** left **eyelid**

H02.433 **Paralytic ptosis of** bilateral **eyelids**

H02.439 **Paralytic ptosis unspecified eyelid**

H02.5 Other disorders affecting eyelid function
EXCLUDES2 blepharospasm (G24.5)
organic tic (G25.69)
psychogenic tic (F95.-)

H02.51 **Abnormal innervation syndrome**

H02.511 **Abnormal innervation syndrome** right upper **eyelid**

H02.512 **Abnormal innervation syndrome** right lower **eyelid**

H02.513 **Abnormal innervation syndrome** right eye, unspecified eyelid

H02.514 **Abnormal innervation syndrome** left upper **eyelid**

H02.515 **Abnormal innervation syndrome** left lower **eyelid**

H02.516 **Abnormal innervation syndrome** left eye, unspecified eyelid

H02.519 **Abnormal innervation syndrome unspecified eye, unspecified eyelid**

H02.52 Blepharophimosis
Ankyloblepharon

H02.521 **Blepharophimosis** right upper eyelid

H02.522 **Blepharophimosis** right lower eyelid

H02.523 **Blepharophimosis** right eye, unspecified eyelid

H02.524 **Blepharophimosis** left upper eyelid

H02.525 **Blepharophimosis** left lower eyelid

H02.526 **Blepharophimosis** left eye, unspecified eyelid

H02.529 **Blepharophimosis unspecified eye, unspecified lid**

H02.53 Eyelid retraction
Eyelid lag

H02.531 **Eyelid retraction** right upper eyelid

H02.532 **Eyelid retraction** right lower eyelid

H02.533 **Eyelid retraction** right eye, unspecified eyelid

H02.534 **Eyelid retraction** left upper eyelid

H02.535 **Eyelid retraction** left lower eyelid

H02.536 **Eyelid retraction** left eye, unspecified eyelid

H02.539 **Eyelid retraction unspecified eye, unspecified lid**

H02.59 Other disorders affecting eyelid function
Deficient blink reflex
Sensory disorders

H02.6 Xanthelasma of eyelid

H02.60 **Xanthelasma of unspecified eye, unspecified eyelid**

H02.61 **Xanthelasma of** right upper **eyelid**

H02.62 **Xanthelasma of** right lower **eyelid**

H02.63 **Xanthelasma of** right eye, unspecified eyelid

H02.64 **Xanthelasma of** left upper **eyelid**

H02.65 **Xanthelasma of** left lower **eyelid**

H02.66 **Xanthelasma of** left eye, unspecified eyelid

H02.7 Other and unspecified degenerative disorders of eyelid and periocular area

H02.70 **Unspecified degenerative disorders of eyelid and periocular area**

H02.71 Chloasma of eyelid and periocular area
Dyspigmentation of eyelid
Hyperpigmentation of eyelid

H02.711 **Chloasma of** right upper **eyelid and periocular area**

H02.712 **Chloasma of** right lower **eyelid and periocular area**

H02.713 **Chloasma of** right eye, unspecified eyelid and periocular area

H02.714 **Chloasma of** left upper **eyelid and periocular area**

H02.715 **Chloasma of** left lower **eyelid and periocular area**

H02.716 **Chloasma of** left eye, unspecified eyelid and periocular area

H02.719 **Chloasma of unspecified eye, unspecified eyelid and periocular area**

Unacceptable principal diagnosis symbol per Medicare code edits   Code exempt from diagnosis present on admission requirement
? Questionable admission   Complication or comorbidity   Major complication or comorbidity   CC/MCC exclusion
HCC HCC diagnosis code   RxHCC RxHCC diagnosis code   MACRA code   **DEFINITION** Describes condition/terminology
TIP Coding guidance   Official Guideline Reference   Z1 Z code as first-listed diagnosis

598   When symbols appear on a code that requires a 7th character extension, refer to Appendix B to identify applicable 7th character codes.   **2020 ICD-10-CM**

[6th] H02.72 Madarosis of eyelid and periocular area
Hypotrichosis of eyelid
H02.721 Madarosis of right upper eyelid and periocular area
H02.722 Madarosis of right lower eyelid and periocular area
H02.723 Madarosis of right eye, unspecified eyelid and periocular area
H02.724 Madarosis of left upper eyelid and periocular area
H02.725 Madarosis of left lower eyelid and periocular area
H02.726 Madarosis of left eye, unspecified eyelid and periocular area
H02.729 Madarosis of unspecified eye, unspecified eyelid and periocular area

[6th] H02.73 Vitiligo of eyelid and periocular area
Hypopigmentation of eyelid
H02.731 Vitiligo of right upper eyelid and periocular area
H02.732 Vitiligo of right lower eyelid and periocular area
H02.733 Vitiligo of right eye, unspecified eyelid and periocular area
H02.734 Vitiligo of left upper eyelid and periocular area
H02.735 Vitiligo of left lower eyelid and periocular area
H02.736 Vitiligo of left eye, unspecified eyelid and periocular area
H02.739 Vitiligo of unspecified eye, unspecified eyelid and periocular area

H02.79 Other degenerative disorders of eyelid and periocular area

[5th] H02.8 Other specified disorders of eyelid

[6th] H02.81 Retained foreign body in eyelid
Use additional code to identify the type of retained foreign body (Z18.-)
[EXCLUDES1] *laceration of eyelid with foreign body (S01.12-)*
retained intraocular foreign body (H44.6-, H44.7-)
superficial foreign body of eyelid and periocular area (S00.25-)
H02.811 Retained foreign body in right upper eyelid
H02.812 Retained foreign body in right lower eyelid
H02.813 Retained foreign body in right eye, unspecified eyelid
H02.814 Retained foreign body in left upper eyelid
H02.815 Retained foreign body in left lower eyelid
H02.816 Retained foreign body in left eye, unspecified eyelid
H02.819 Retained foreign body in unspecified eye, unspecified eyelid

[6th] H02.82 Cysts of eyelid
Sebaceous cyst of eyelid
H02.821 Cysts of right upper eyelid
H02.822 Cysts of right lower eyelid
H02.823 Cysts of right eye, unspecified eyelid
H02.824 Cysts of left upper eyelid
H02.825 Cysts of left lower eyelid
H02.826 Cysts of left eye, unspecified eyelid
H02.829 Cysts of unspecified eye, unspecified eyelid

[6th] H02.83 Dermatochalasis of eyelid
H02.831 Dermatochalasis of right upper eyelid
H02.832 Dermatochalasis of right lower eyelid
H02.833 Dermatochalasis of right eye, unspecified eyelid
H02.834 Dermatochalasis of left upper eyelid
H02.835 Dermatochalasis of left lower eyelid
H02.836 Dermatochalasis of left eye, unspecified eyelid
H02.839 Dermatochalasis of unspecified eye, unspecified eyelid

[6th] H02.84 Edema of eyelid
Hyperemia of eyelid
H02.841 Edema of right upper eyelid
H02.842 Edema of right lower eyelid
H02.843 Edema of right eye, unspecified eyelid
H02.844 Edema of left upper eyelid
H02.845 Edema of left lower eyelid
H02.846 Edema of left eye, unspecified eyelid
H02.849 Edema of unspecified eye, unspecified eyelid

[6th] H02.85 Elephantiasis of eyelid
H02.851 Elephantiasis of right upper eyelid
H02.852 Elephantiasis of right lower eyelid
H02.853 Elephantiasis of right eye, unspecified eyelid
H02.854 Elephantiasis of left upper eyelid
H02.855 Elephantiasis of left lower eyelid
H02.856 Elephantiasis of left eye, unspecified eyelid
H02.859 Elephantiasis of unspecified eye, unspecified eyelid

[6th] H02.86 Hypertrichosis of eyelid
H02.861 Hypertrichosis of right upper eyelid
H02.862 Hypertrichosis of right lower eyelid
H02.863 Hypertrichosis of right eye, unspecified eyelid
H02.864 Hypertrichosis of left upper eyelid
H02.865 Hypertrichosis of left lower eyelid
H02.866 Hypertrichosis of left eye, unspecified eyelid
H02.869 Hypertrichosis of unspecified eye, unspecified eyelid

[6th] H02.87 Vascular anomalies of eyelid
H02.871 Vascular anomalies of right upper eyelid
H02.872 Vascular anomalies of right lower eyelid
H02.873 Vascular anomalies of right eye, unspecified eyelid
H02.874 Vascular anomalies of left upper eyelid
H02.875 Vascular anomalies of left lower eyelid
H02.876 Vascular anomalies of left eye, unspecified eyelid
H02.879 Vascular anomalies of unspecified eye, unspecified eyelid

[6th] H02.88 Meibomian gland dysfunction of eyelid
H02.881 Meibomian gland dysfunction right upper eyelid
AHA: Q4 2018
H02.882 Meibomian gland dysfunction right lower eyelid
AHA: Q4 2018
H02.883 Meibomian gland dysfunction of right eye, unspecified eyelid
AHA: Q4 2018
H02.884 Meibomian gland dysfunction left upper eyelid
AHA: Q4 2018
H02.885 Meibomian gland dysfunction left lower eyelid
AHA: Q4 2018
H02.886 Meibomian gland dysfunction of left eye, unspecified eyelid
AHA: Q4 2018
H02.889 Meibomian gland dysfunction of unspecified eye, unspecified eyelid
AHA: Q4 2018

H02.88A Meibomian gland dysfunction right eye, upper and lower eyelids
AHA: Q4 2018

H02.88B Meibomian gland dysfunction left eye, upper and lower eyelids
AHA: Q4 2018

H02.89 Other specified disorders of eyelid
Hemorrhage of eyelid

H02.9 Unspecified disorder of eyelid
Disorder of eyelid NOS

H04 Disorders of lacrimal system (Figure 7.2)
EXCLUDES1 congenital malformations of lacrimal system (Q10.4-Q10.6)

H04.0 Dacryoadenitis
H04.00 Unspecified dacryoadenitis
H04.001 Unspecified dacryoadenitis, right lacrimal gland
H04.002 Unspecified dacryoadenitis, left lacrimal gland
H04.003 Unspecified dacryoadenitis, bilateral lacrimal glands
H04.009 Unspecified dacryoadenitis, unspecified lacrimal gland

H04.01 Acute dacryoadenitis
H04.011 Acute dacryoadenitis, right lacrimal gland
H04.012 Acute dacryoadenitis, left lacrimal gland
H04.013 Acute dacryoadenitis, bilateral lacrimal glands
H04.019 Acute dacryoadenitis, unspecified lacrimal gland

H04.02 Chronic dacryoadenitis
H04.021 Chronic dacryoadenitis, right lacrimal gland
H04.022 Chronic dacryoadenitis, left lacrimal gland
H04.023 Chronic dacryoadenitis, bilateral lacrimal gland
H04.029 Chronic dacryoadenitis, unspecified lacrimal gland

H04.03 Chronic enlargement of lacrimal gland
H04.031 Chronic enlargement of right lacrimal gland
H04.032 Chronic enlargement of left lacrimal gland
H04.033 Chronic enlargement of bilateral lacrimal glands
H04.039 Chronic enlargement of unspecified lacrimal gland

H04.1 Other disorders of lacrimal gland
H04.11 Dacryops
H04.111 Dacryops of right lacrimal gland
H04.112 Dacryops of left lacrimal gland
H04.113 Dacryops of bilateral lacrimal glands
H04.119 Dacryops of unspecified lacrimal gland

H04.12 Dry eye syndrome
Tear film insufficiency, NOS
H04.121 Dry eye syndrome of right lacrimal gland
H04.122 Dry eye syndrome of left lacrimal gland
H04.123 Dry eye syndrome of bilateral lacrimal glands
H04.129 Dry eye syndrome of unspecified lacrimal gland

H04.13 Lacrimal cyst
Lacrimal cystic degeneration
H04.131 Lacrimal cyst, right lacrimal gland
H04.132 Lacrimal cyst, left lacrimal gland
H04.133 Lacrimal cyst, bilateral lacrimal glands
H04.139 Lacrimal cyst, unspecified lacrimal gland

H04.14 Primary lacrimal gland atrophy
H04.141 Primary lacrimal gland atrophy, right lacrimal gland
H04.142 Primary lacrimal gland atrophy, left lacrimal gland

H04.143 Primary lacrimal gland atrophy, bilateral lacrimal glands
H04.149 Primary lacrimal gland atrophy, unspecified lacrimal gland

H04.15 Secondary lacrimal gland atrophy
H04.151 Secondary lacrimal gland atrophy, right lacrimal gland
H04.152 Secondary lacrimal gland atrophy, left lacrimal gland
H04.153 Secondary lacrimal gland atrophy, bilateral lacrimal glands
H04.159 Secondary lacrimal gland atrophy, unspecified lacrimal gland

H04.16 Lacrimal gland dislocation
H04.161 Lacrimal gland dislocation, right lacrimal gland
H04.162 Lacrimal gland dislocation, left lacrimal gland
H04.163 Lacrimal gland dislocation, bilateral lacrimal glands
H04.169 Lacrimal gland dislocation, unspecified lacrimal gland

H04.19 Other specified disorders of lacrimal gland

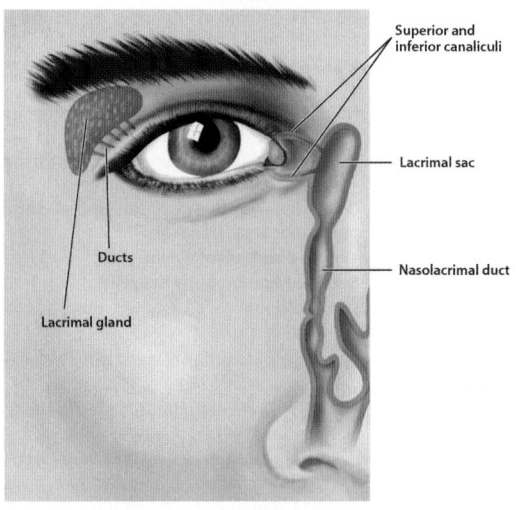

Figure 7.2 Lacrimal System

H04.2 Epiphora
H04.20 Unspecified epiphora
H04.201 Unspecified epiphora, right side
H04.202 Unspecified epiphora, left side
H04.203 Unspecified epiphora, bilateral
H04.209 Unspecified epiphora, unspecified side

H04.21 Epiphora due to excess lacrimation
H04.211 Epiphora due to excess lacrimation, right lacrimal gland
H04.212 Epiphora due to excess lacrimation, left lacrimal gland
H04.213 Epiphora due to excess lacrimation, bilateral lacrimal glands
H04.219 Epiphora due to excess lacrimation, unspecified lacrimal gland

H04.22 Epiphora due to insufficient drainage
H04.221 Epiphora due to insufficient drainage, right side
H04.222 Epiphora due to insufficient drainage, left side
H04.223 Epiphora due to insufficient drainage, bilateral
H04.229 Epiphora due to insufficient drainage, unspecified side

Unacceptable principal diagnosis symbol per Medicare code edits   Code exempt from diagnosis present on admission requirement
? Questionable admission   CC Complication or comorbidity   MCC Major complication or comorbidity   cc/mcc exc CC/MCC exclusion
HCC HCC diagnosis code   RxHCC RxHCC diagnosis code   MACRA MACRA code   DEFINITION Describes condition/terminology
TIP Coding guidance   Official Guideline Reference   Z1 Z code as first-listed diagnosis

600   When symbols appear on a code that requires a 7th character extension, refer to Appendix B to identify applicable 7th character codes.   2020 ICD-10-CM

[5th] H04.3 Acute and unspecified inflammation of lacrimal passages
[EXCLUDES1] *neonatal dacryocystitis (P39.1)*
[6th] H04.30 Unspecified dacryocystitis
H04.301 Unspecified dacryocystitis of right lacrimal passage
H04.302 Unspecified dacryocystitis of left lacrimal passage
H04.303 Unspecified dacryocystitis of bilateral lacrimal passages
H04.309 Unspecified dacryocystitis of unspecified lacrimal passage
[6th] H04.31 Phlegmonous dacryocystitis
H04.311 Phlegmonous dacryocystitis of right lacrimal passage
H04.312 Phlegmonous dacryocystitis of left lacrimal passage
H04.313 Phlegmonous dacryocystitis of bilateral lacrimal passages
H04.319 Phlegmonous dacryocystitis of unspecified lacrimal passage
[6th] H04.32 Acute dacryocystitis
Acute dacryopericystitis
H04.321 Acute dacryocystitis of right lacrimal passage
H04.322 Acute dacryocystitis of left lacrimal passage
H04.323 Acute dacryocystitis of bilateral lacrimal passages
H04.329 Acute dacryocystitis of unspecified lacrimal passage
[6th] H04.33 Acute lacrimal canaliculitis
H04.331 Acute lacrimal canaliculitis of right lacrimal passage
H04.332 Acute lacrimal canaliculitis of left lacrimal passage
H04.333 Acute lacrimal canaliculitis of bilateral lacrimal passages
H04.339 Acute lacrimal canaliculitis of unspecified lacrimal passage
[5th] H04.4 Chronic inflammation of lacrimal passages
[6th] H04.41 Chronic dacryocystitis
H04.411 Chronic dacryocystitis of right lacrimal passage
H04.412 Chronic dacryocystitis of left lacrimal passage
H04.413 Chronic dacryocystitis of bilateral lacrimal passages
H04.419 Chronic dacryocystitis of unspecified lacrimal passage
[6th] H04.42 Chronic lacrimal canaliculitis
H04.421 Chronic lacrimal canaliculitis of right lacrimal passage
H04.422 Chronic lacrimal canaliculitis of left lacrimal passage
H04.423 Chronic lacrimal canaliculitis of bilateral lacrimal passages
H04.429 Chronic lacrimal canaliculitis of unspecified lacrimal passage
[6th] H04.43 Chronic lacrimal mucocele
H04.431 Chronic lacrimal mucocele of right lacrimal passage
H04.432 Chronic lacrimal mucocele of left lacrimal passage
H04.433 Chronic lacrimal mucocele of bilateral lacrimal passages
H04.439 Chronic lacrimal mucocele of unspecified lacrimal passage
[5th] H04.5 Stenosis and insufficiency of lacrimal passages
[6th] H04.51 Dacryolith
H04.511 Dacryolith of right lacrimal passage
H04.512 Dacryolith of left lacrimal passage
H04.513 Dacryolith of bilateral lacrimal passages
H04.519 Dacryolith of unspecified lacrimal passage
[6th] H04.52 Eversion of lacrimal punctum
H04.521 Eversion of right lacrimal punctum
H04.522 Eversion of left lacrimal punctum
H04.523 Eversion of bilateral lacrimal punctum
H04.529 Eversion of unspecified lacrimal punctum
[6th] H04.53 Neonatal obstruction of nasolacrimal duct
[EXCLUDES1] *congenital stenosis and stricture of lacrimal duct (Q10.5)*
H04.531 Neonatal obstruction of right nasolacrimal duct [N]
H04.532 Neonatal obstruction of left nasolacrimal duct [N]
H04.533 Neonatal obstruction of bilateral nasolacrimal duct [N]
H04.539 Neonatal obstruction of unspecified nasolacrimal duct [N]
[6th] H04.54 Stenosis of lacrimal canaliculi
H04.541 Stenosis of right lacrimal canaliculi
H04.542 Stenosis of left lacrimal canaliculi
H04.543 Stenosis of bilateral lacrimal canaliculi
H04.549 Stenosis of unspecified lacrimal canaliculi
[6th] H04.55 Acquired stenosis of nasolacrimal duct
H04.551 Acquired stenosis of right nasolacrimal duct
H04.552 Acquired stenosis of left nasolacrimal duct
H04.553 Acquired stenosis of bilateral nasolacrimal duct
H04.559 Acquired stenosis of unspecified nasolacrimal duct
[6th] H04.56 Stenosis of lacrimal punctum
H04.561 Stenosis of right lacrimal punctum
H04.562 Stenosis of left lacrimal punctum
H04.563 Stenosis of bilateral lacrimal punctum
H04.569 Stenosis of unspecified lacrimal punctum
[6th] H04.57 Stenosis of lacrimal sac
H04.571 Stenosis of right lacrimal sac
H04.572 Stenosis of left lacrimal sac
H04.573 Stenosis of bilateral lacrimal sac
H04.579 Stenosis of unspecified lacrimal sac
[5th] H04.6 Other changes of lacrimal passages
[6th] H04.61 Lacrimal fistula
H04.611 Lacrimal fistula right lacrimal passage
H04.612 Lacrimal fistula left lacrimal passage
H04.613 Lacrimal fistula bilateral lacrimal passages
H04.619 Lacrimal fistula unspecified lacrimal passage
H04.69 Other changes of lacrimal passages
[5th] H04.8 Other disorders of lacrimal system
[6th] H04.81 Granuloma of lacrimal passages
H04.811 Granuloma of right lacrimal passage
H04.812 Granuloma of left lacrimal passage
H04.813 Granuloma of bilateral lacrimal passages
H04.819 Granuloma of unspecified lacrimal passage
H04.89 Other disorders of lacrimal system
H04.9 Disorder of lacrimal system, unspecified
[4th] H05 Disorders of orbit
[EXCLUDES1] *congenital malformation of orbit (Q10.7)*
[5th] H05.0 Acute inflammation of orbit
H05.00 Unspecified acute inflammation of orbit
[6th] H05.01 Cellulitis of orbit
Abscess of orbit
H05.011 Cellulitis of right orbit [CC] [CC/MCC Exc]
H05.012 Cellulitis of left orbit [CC] [CC/MCC Exc]
H05.013 Cellulitis of bilateral orbits [CC] [CC/MCC Exc]
H05.019 Cellulitis of unspecified orbit [CC] [CC/MCC Exc]
[6th] H05.02 Osteomyelitis of orbit

Unspecified Code Other Specified Code Manifestation Code [N] Newborn [P] Pediatric [M] Maternity [A] Adult ♂ Male ♀ Female
● New Code ▲ Revised Code Title ►◄ Revised Text [NOTES] [INCLUDES] [EXCLUDES1] Not coded here [EXCLUDES2] Not included here
[4th] 4th character required [5th] 5th character required [6th] 6th character required [7th] 7th character required [X] Extension 'X' Alert
[HAC] Hospital-acquired condition (HAC) alert AHA AHA Coding Clinic® ☞ Code first alert

H05.021 Osteomyelitis of right orbit [CC] [CC/MCC Exc]
H05.022 Osteomyelitis of left orbit [CC] [CC/MCC Exc]
H05.023 Osteomyelitis of bilateral orbits [CC] [CC/MCC Exc]
H05.029 Osteomyelitis of unspecified orbit [CC] [CC/MCC Exc]

(6) **H05.03 Periostitis of orbit**
H05.031 Periostitis of right orbit [CC] [CC/MCC Exc]
H05.032 Periostitis of left orbit [CC] [CC/MCC Exc]
H05.033 Periostitis of bilateral orbits [CC] [CC/MCC Exc]
H05.039 Periostitis of unspecified orbit [CC] [CC/MCC Exc]

(6) **H05.04 Tenonitis of orbit**
H05.041 Tenonitis of right orbit
H05.042 Tenonitis of left orbit
H05.043 Tenonitis of bilateral orbits
H05.049 Tenonitis of unspecified orbit

(5) **H05.1 Chronic inflammatory disorders of orbit**
H05.10 Unspecified chronic inflammatory disorders of orbit

(6) **H05.11 Granuloma of orbit**
Pseudotumor (inflammatory) of orbit
H05.111 Granuloma of right orbit
H05.112 Granuloma of left orbit
H05.113 Granuloma of bilateral orbits
H05.119 Granuloma of unspecified orbit

(6) **H05.12 Orbital myositis**
H05.121 Orbital myositis, right orbit
H05.122 Orbital myositis, left orbit
H05.123 Orbital myositis, bilateral
H05.129 Orbital myositis, unspecified orbit

(5) **H05.2 Exophthalmic conditions**
H05.20 Unspecified exophthalmos

(6) **H05.21 Displacement (lateral) of globe**
H05.211 Displacement (lateral) of globe, right eye
H05.212 Displacement (lateral) of globe, left eye
H05.213 Displacement (lateral) of globe, bilateral
H05.219 Displacement (lateral) of globe, unspecified eye

(6) **H05.22 Edema of orbit**
Orbital congestion
H05.221 Edema of right orbit
H05.222 Edema of left orbit
H05.223 Edema of bilateral orbit
H05.229 Edema of unspecified orbit

(6) **H05.23 Hemorrhage of orbit**
H05.231 Hemorrhage of right orbit
H05.232 Hemorrhage of left orbit
H05.233 Hemorrhage of bilateral orbit
H05.239 Hemorrhage of unspecified orbit

(6) **H05.24 Constant exophthalmos**
H05.241 Constant exophthalmos, right eye
H05.242 Constant exophthalmos, left eye
H05.243 Constant exophthalmos, bilateral
H05.249 Constant exophthalmos, unspecified eye

(6) **H05.25 Intermittent exophthalmos**
H05.251 Intermittent exophthalmos, right eye
H05.252 Intermittent exophthalmos, left eye
H05.253 Intermittent exophthalmos, bilateral
H05.259 Intermittent exophthalmos, unspecified eye

(6) **H05.26 Pulsating exophthalmos**
H05.261 Pulsating exophthalmos, right eye
H05.262 Pulsating exophthalmos, left eye
H05.263 Pulsating exophthalmos, bilateral
H05.269 Pulsating exophthalmos, unspecified eye

(5) **H05.3 Deformity of orbit**
EXCLUDES1 congenital deformity of orbit (Q10.7)
                    hypertelorism (Q75.2)
H05.30 Unspecified deformity of orbit

(6) **H05.31 Atrophy of orbit**
H05.311 Atrophy of right orbit
H05.312 Atrophy of left orbit

H05.313 Atrophy of bilateral orbit
H05.319 Atrophy of unspecified orbit

(6) **H05.32 Deformity of orbit due to bone disease**
Code also associated bone disease
H05.321 Deformity of right orbit due to bone disease
H05.322 Deformity of left orbit due to bone disease
H05.323 Deformity of bilateral orbits due to bone disease
H05.329 Deformity of unspecified orbit due to bone disease

(6) **H05.33 Deformity of orbit due to trauma or surgery**
H05.331 Deformity of right orbit due to trauma or surgery
H05.332 Deformity of left orbit due to trauma or surgery
H05.333 Deformity of bilateral orbits due to trauma or surgery
H05.339 Deformity of unspecified orbit due to trauma or surgery

(6) **H05.34 Enlargement of orbit**
H05.341 Enlargement of right orbit
H05.342 Enlargement of left orbit
H05.343 Enlargement of bilateral orbits
H05.349 Enlargement of unspecified orbit

(6) **H05.35 Exostosis of orbit**
H05.351 Exostosis of right orbit
H05.352 Exostosis of left orbit
H05.353 Exostosis of bilateral orbits
H05.359 Exostosis of unspecified orbit

(5) **H05.4 Enophthalmos**
(6) **H05.40 Unspecified enophthalmos**
H05.401 Unspecified enophthalmos, right eye
H05.402 Unspecified enophthalmos, left eye
H05.403 Unspecified enophthalmos, bilateral
H05.409 Unspecified enophthalmos, unspecified eye

(6) **H05.41 Enophthalmos due to atrophy of orbital tissue**
H05.411 Enophthalmos due to atrophy of orbital tissue, right eye
H05.412 Enophthalmos due to atrophy of orbital tissue, left eye
H05.413 Enophthalmos due to atrophy of orbital tissue, bilateral
H05.419 Enophthalmos due to atrophy of orbital tissue, unspecified eye

(6) **H05.42 Enophthalmos due to trauma or surgery**
H05.421 Enophthalmos due to trauma or surgery, right eye
H05.422 Enophthalmos due to trauma or surgery, left eye
H05.423 Enophthalmos due to trauma or surgery, bilateral
H05.429 Enophthalmos due to trauma or surgery, unspecified eye

(5) **H05.5 Retained (old) foreign body following penetrating wound of orbit**
Retrobulbar foreign body
Use additional code to identify the type of retained foreign body (Z18.-)
EXCLUDES1 current penetrating wound of orbit (S05.4-)
EXCLUDES2 retained foreign body of eyelid (H02.81-)
                    retained intraocular foreign body (H44.6-, H44.7-)
H05.50 Retained (old) foreign body following penetrating wound of unspecified orbit
H05.51 Retained (old) foreign body following penetrating wound of right orbit
H05.52 Retained (old) foreign body following penetrating wound of left orbit

---

[PDx] Unacceptable principal diagnosis symbol per Medicare code edits   [POA] Code exempt from diagnosis present on admission requirement
[?] Questionable admission   [CC] Complication or comorbidity   [MCC] Major complication or comorbidity   [CC/MCC Exc] CC/MCC exclusion
[HCC] HCC diagnosis code   [RxHCC] RxHCC diagnosis code   MACRA code   **DEFINITION** Describes condition/terminology
TIP Coding guidance   👁 Official Guideline Reference   [Z1] Z code as first-listed diagnosis

602   When symbols appear on a code that requires a 7th character extension, refer to Appendix B to identify applicable 7th character codes.   **2020 ICD-10-CM**

H05.53 Retained (old) foreign body following penetrating wound of bilateral orbits

🔵⁵ᵗʰ **H05.8** Other disorders of orbit

   🔵⁶ᵗʰ **H05.81** Cyst of orbit

     Encephalocele of orbit

     H05.811 Cyst of right orbit

     H05.812 Cyst of left orbit

     H05.813 Cyst of bilateral orbits

     H05.819 Cyst of unspecified orbit

   🔵⁶ᵗʰ **H05.82** Myopathy of extraocular muscles

     H05.821 Myopathy of extraocular muscles, right orbit

     H05.822 Myopathy of extraocular muscles, left orbit

     H05.823 Myopathy of extraocular muscles, bilateral

     H05.829 Myopathy of extraocular muscles, unspecified orbit

   H05.89 Other disorders of orbit

H05.9 Unspecified disorder of orbit

Disorders of conjunctiva (H10-H11)

🔵⁴ᵗʰ **H10** Conjunctivitis

   EXCLUDES1 keratoconjunctivitis (H16.2-)

🔵⁵ᵗʰ **H10.0** Mucopurulent conjunctivitis

   🔵⁶ᵗʰ **H10.01** Acute follicular conjunctivitis

     H10.011 Acute follicular conjunctivitis, right eye

     H10.012 Acute follicular conjunctivitis, left eye

     H10.013 Acute follicular conjunctivitis, bilateral

     H10.019 Acute follicular conjunctivitis, unspecified eye

   🔵⁶ᵗʰ **H10.02** Other mucopurulent conjunctivitis

     H10.021 Other mucopurulent conjunctivitis, right eye

     H10.022 Other mucopurulent conjunctivitis, left eye

     H10.023 Other mucopurulent conjunctivitis, bilateral

     H10.029 Other mucopurulent conjunctivitis, unspecified eye

🔵⁵ᵗʰ **H10.1** Acute atopic conjunctivitis

   Acute papillary conjunctivitis

   H10.10 Acute atopic conjunctivitis, unspecified eye

   H10.11 Acute atopic conjunctivitis, right eye

   H10.12 Acute atopic conjunctivitis, left eye

   H10.13 Acute atopic conjunctivitis, bilateral

🔵⁵ᵗʰ **H10.2** Other acute conjunctivitis

   🔵⁶ᵗʰ **H10.21** Acute toxic conjunctivitis

     Acute chemical conjunctivitis

     📌 Code first (T51-T65) to identify chemical and intent

     EXCLUDES1 burn and corrosion of eye and adnexa (T26.-)

     H10.211 Acute toxic conjunctivitis, right eye

     H10.212 Acute toxic conjunctivitis, left eye

     H10.213 Acute toxic conjunctivitis, bilateral

     H10.219 Acute toxic conjunctivitis, unspecified eye

   🔵⁶ᵗʰ **H10.22** Pseudomembranous conjunctivitis

     H10.221 Pseudomembranous conjunctivitis, right eye

     H10.222 Pseudomembranous conjunctivitis, left eye

     H10.223 Pseudomembranous conjunctivitis, bilateral

     H10.229 Pseudomembranous conjunctivitis, unspecified eye

   🔵⁶ᵗʰ **H10.23** Serous conjunctivitis, except viral

     EXCLUDES1 viral conjunctivitis (B30.-)

     H10.231 Serous conjunctivitis, except viral, right eye

     H10.232 Serous conjunctivitis, except viral, left eye

     H10.233 Serous conjunctivitis, except viral, bilateral

     H10.239 Serous conjunctivitis, except viral, unspecified eye

🔵⁵ᵗʰ **H10.3** Unspecified acute conjunctivitis

   EXCLUDES1 ophthalmia neonatorum NOS (P39.1)

   H10.30 Unspecified acute conjunctivitis, unspecified eye

   H10.31 Unspecified acute conjunctivitis, right eye

   H10.32 Unspecified acute conjunctivitis, left eye

   H10.33 Unspecified acute conjunctivitis, bilateral

🔵⁵ᵗʰ **H10.4** Chronic conjunctivitis

   🔵⁶ᵗʰ **H10.40** Unspecified chronic conjunctivitis

     H10.401 Unspecified chronic conjunctivitis, right eye

     H10.402 Unspecified chronic conjunctivitis, left eye

     H10.403 Unspecified chronic conjunctivitis, bilateral

     H10.409 Unspecified chronic conjunctivitis, unspecified eye

   🔵⁶ᵗʰ **H10.41** Chronic giant papillary conjunctivitis

     H10.411 Chronic giant papillary conjunctivitis, right eye

     H10.412 Chronic giant papillary conjunctivitis, left eye

     H10.413 Chronic giant papillary conjunctivitis, bilateral

     H10.419 Chronic giant papillary conjunctivitis, unspecified eye

   🔵⁶ᵗʰ **H10.42** Simple chronic conjunctivitis

     H10.421 Simple chronic conjunctivitis, right eye

     H10.422 Simple chronic conjunctivitis, left eye

     H10.423 Simple chronic conjunctivitis, bilateral

     H10.429 Simple chronic conjunctivitis, unspecified eye

   🔵⁶ᵗʰ **H10.43** Chronic follicular conjunctivitis

     H10.431 Chronic follicular conjunctivitis, right eye

     H10.432 Chronic follicular conjunctivitis, left eye

     H10.433 Chronic follicular conjunctivitis, bilateral

     H10.439 Chronic follicular conjunctivitis, unspecified eye

   H10.44 Vernal conjunctivitis

     EXCLUDES1 vernal keratoconjunctivitis with limbar and corneal involvement (H16.26-)

   H10.45 Other chronic allergic conjunctivitis

🔵⁵ᵗʰ **H10.5** Blepharoconjunctivitis

   🔵⁶ᵗʰ **H10.50** Unspecified blepharoconjunctivitis

     H10.501 Unspecified blepharoconjunctivitis, right eye

     H10.502 Unspecified blepharoconjunctivitis, left eye

     H10.503 Unspecified blepharoconjunctivitis, bilateral

     H10.509 Unspecified blepharoconjunctivitis, unspecified eye

   🔵⁶ᵗʰ **H10.51** Ligneous conjunctivitis

     Code also underlying condition if known, such as: plasminogen deficiency (E88.02)

     H10.511 Ligneous conjunctivitis, right eye

     H10.512 Ligneous conjunctivitis, left eye

     H10.513 Ligneous conjunctivitis, bilateral

     H10.519 Ligneous conjunctivitis, unspecified eye

   🔵⁶ᵗʰ **H10.52** Angular blepharoconjunctivitis

     H10.521 Angular blepharoconjunctivitis, right eye

     H10.522 Angular blepharoconjunctivitis, left eye

     H10.523 Angular blepharoconjunctivitis, bilateral

     H10.529 Angular blepharoconjunctivitis, unspecified eye

   🔵⁶ᵗʰ **H10.53** Contact blepharoconjunctivitis

     H10.531 Contact blepharoconjunctivitis, right eye

     H10.532 Contact blepharoconjunctivitis, left eye

H10.533 Contact blepharoconjunctivitis, bilateral
H10.539 Contact blepharoconjunctivitis, unspecified eye
- 5ᵗʰ H10.8 Other conjunctivitis
  - 6ᵗʰ H10.81 Pingueculitis
    - EXCLUDES1 pinguecula (H11.15-)
    H10.811 Pingueculitis, right eye
    H10.812 Pingueculitis, left eye
    H10.813 Pingueculitis, bilateral
    H10.819 Pingueculitis, unspecified eye
  - 6ᵗʰ H10.82 Rosacea conjunctivitis
    - ☞ Code first underlying rosacea dermatitis (L71.-)
    H10.821 Rosacea conjunctivitis, right eye
    AHA: Q4 2018
    H10.822 Rosacea conjunctivitis, left eye
    AHA: Q4 2018
    H10.823 Rosacea conjunctivitis, bilateral
    AHA: Q4 2018
    H10.829 Rosacea conjunctivitis, unspecified eye
    AHA: Q4 2018
  H10.89 Other conjunctivitis
  H10.9 Unspecified conjunctivitis
- 4ᵗʰ H11 Other disorders of conjunctiva
  - EXCLUDES1 keratoconjunctivitis (H16.2-)
  - 5ᵗʰ H11.0 Pterygium of eye (Figure 7.3)
    - DEFINITION: The conjunctival growths Pterygia are also sometimes called "Surfer's Eye."
    - EXCLUDES1 pseudopterygium (H11.81-)
    - 6ᵗʰ H11.00 Unspecified pterygium of eye
      H11.001 Unspecified pterygium of right eye
      H11.002 Unspecified pterygium of left eye
      H11.003 Unspecified pterygium of eye, bilateral
      H11.009 Unspecified pterygium of unspecified eye
    - 6ᵗʰ H11.01 Amyloid pterygium
      H11.011 Amyloid pterygium of right eye
      H11.012 Amyloid pterygium of left eye
      H11.013 Amyloid pterygium of eye, bilateral
      H11.019 Amyloid pterygium of unspecified eye
    - 6ᵗʰ H11.02 Central pterygium of eye
      H11.021 Central pterygium of right eye
      H11.022 Central pterygium of left eye
      H11.023 Central pterygium of eye, bilateral
      H11.029 Central pterygium of unspecified eye
    - 6ᵗʰ H11.03 Double pterygium of eye
      H11.031 Double pterygium of right eye
      H11.032 Double pterygium of left eye
      H11.033 Double pterygium of eye, bilateral
      H11.039 Double pterygium of unspecified eye
    - 6ᵗʰ H11.04 Peripheral pterygium of eye, stationary
      H11.041 Peripheral pterygium, stationary, right eye
      H11.042 Peripheral pterygium, stationary, left eye
      H11.043 Peripheral pterygium, stationary, bilateral
      H11.049 Peripheral pterygium, stationary, unspecified eye
    - 6ᵗʰ H11.05 Peripheral pterygium of eye, progressive
      H11.051 Peripheral pterygium, progressive, right eye
      H11.052 Peripheral pterygium, progressive, left eye
      H11.053 Peripheral pterygium, progressive, bilateral
      H11.059 Peripheral pterygium, progressive, unspecified eye
    - 6ᵗʰ H11.06 Recurrent pterygium of eye
      H11.061 Recurrent pterygium of right eye
      H11.062 Recurrent pterygium of left eye
      H11.063 Recurrent pterygium of eye, bilateral
      H11.069 Recurrent pterygium of unspecified eye

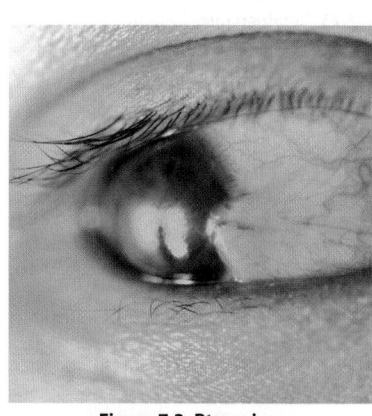

Figure 7.3 Pterygium

- 5ᵗʰ H11.1 Conjunctival degenerations and deposits
  - EXCLUDES2 pseudopterygium (H11.81)
  H11.10 Unspecified conjunctival degenerations
  - 6ᵗʰ H11.11 Conjunctival deposits
    H11.111 Conjunctival deposits, right eye
    H11.112 Conjunctival deposits, left eye
    H11.113 Conjunctival deposits, bilateral
    H11.119 Conjunctival deposits, unspecified eye
  - 6ᵗʰ H11.12 Conjunctival concretions
    H11.121 Conjunctival concretions, right eye
    H11.122 Conjunctival concretions, left eye
    H11.123 Conjunctival concretions, bilateral
    H11.129 Conjunctival concretions, unspecified eye
  - 6ᵗʰ H11.13 Conjunctival pigmentations
    Conjunctival argyrosis [argyria]
    H11.131 Conjunctival pigmentations, right eye
    H11.132 Conjunctival pigmentations, left eye
    H11.133 Conjunctival pigmentations, bilateral
    H11.139 Conjunctival pigmentations, unspecified eye
  - 6ᵗʰ H11.14 Conjunctival xerosis, unspecified
    - EXCLUDES1 xerosis of conjunctiva due to vitamin A deficiency (E50.0, E50.1)
    H11.141 Conjunctival xerosis, unspecified, right eye
    H11.142 Conjunctival xerosis, unspecified, left eye
    H11.143 Conjunctival xerosis, unspecified, bilateral
    H11.149 Conjunctival xerosis, unspecified, unspecified eye
  - 6ᵗʰ H11.15 Pinguecula
    - DEFINITION: Sun-caused non-cancerous bumps on the conjunctiva.
    - EXCLUDES1 pingueculitis (H10.81-)
    H11.151 Pinguecula, right eye
    H11.152 Pinguecula, left eye
    H11.153 Pinguecula, bilateral
    H11.159 Pinguecula, unspecified eye
- 5ᵗʰ H11.2 Conjunctival scars
  - 6ᵗʰ H11.21 Conjunctival adhesions and strands (localized)
    H11.211 Conjunctival adhesions and strands (localized), right eye
    H11.212 Conjunctival adhesions and strands (localized), left eye
    H11.213 Conjunctival adhesions and strands (localized), bilateral
    H11.219 Conjunctival adhesions and strands (localized), unspecified eye
  - 6ᵗʰ H11.22 Conjunctival granuloma
    H11.221 Conjunctival granuloma, right eye
    H11.222 Conjunctival granuloma, left eye
    H11.223 Conjunctival granuloma, bilateral
    H11.229 Conjunctival granuloma, unspecified

POA🚫 Unacceptable principal diagnosis symbol per Medicare code edits   POA Code exempt from diagnosis present on admission requirement
❓ Questionable admission   CC Complication or comorbidity   MCC Major complication or comorbidity   CC/MCC⊘ CC/MCC exclusion
HCC HCC diagnosis code   RxHCC RxHCC diagnosis code   MACRA code   **DEFINITION** Describes condition/terminology
TIP Coding guidance   👁 Official Guideline Reference   Z1 Z code as first-listed diagnosis

H11.23 Symblepharon
    H11.231 Symblepharon, right eye
    H11.232 Symblepharon, left eye
    H11.233 Symblepharon, bilateral
    H11.239 Symblepharon, unspecified eye
H11.24 Scarring of conjunctiva
    H11.241 Scarring of conjunctiva, right eye
    H11.242 Scarring of conjunctiva, left eye
    H11.243 Scarring of conjunctiva, bilateral
    H11.249 Scarring of conjunctiva, unspecified eye
H11.3 Conjunctival hemorrhage
Subconjunctival hemorrhage
    H11.30 Conjunctival hemorrhage, unspecified eye
    H11.31 Conjunctival hemorrhage, right eye
    H11.32 Conjunctival hemorrhage, left eye
    H11.33 Conjunctival hemorrhage, bilateral
H11.4 Other conjunctival vascular disorders and cysts
    H11.41 Vascular abnormalities of conjunctiva
    Conjunctival aneurysm
        H11.411 Vascular abnormalities of conjunctiva, right eye
        H11.412 Vascular abnormalities of conjunctiva, left eye
        H11.413 Vascular abnormalities of conjunctiva, bilateral
        H11.419 Vascular abnormalities of conjunctiva, unspecified eye
    H11.42 Conjunctival edema
        H11.421 Conjunctival edema, right eye
        H11.422 Conjunctival edema, left eye
        H11.423 Conjunctival edema, bilateral
        H11.429 Conjunctival edema, unspecified eye
    H11.43 Conjunctival hyperemia
        H11.431 Conjunctival hyperemia, right eye
        H11.432 Conjunctival hyperemia, left eye
        H11.433 Conjunctival hyperemia, bilateral
        H11.439 Conjunctival hyperemia, unspecified eye
    H11.44 Conjunctival cysts
        H11.441 Conjunctival cysts, right eye
        H11.442 Conjunctival cysts, left eye
        H11.443 Conjunctival cysts, bilateral
        H11.449 Conjunctival cysts, unspecified eye
H11.8 Other specified disorders of conjunctiva
    H11.81 Pseudopterygium of conjunctiva
        H11.811 Pseudopterygium of conjunctiva, right eye
        H11.812 Pseudopterygium of conjunctiva, left eye
        H11.813 Pseudopterygium of conjunctiva, bilateral
        H11.819 Pseudopterygium of conjunctiva, unspecified eye
    H11.82 Conjunctivochalasis
        H11.821 Conjunctivochalasis, right eye
        H11.822 Conjunctivochalasis, left eye
        H11.823 Conjunctivochalasis, bilateral
        H11.829 Conjunctivochalasis, unspecified eye
    H11.89 Other specified disorders of conjunctiva
H11.9 Unspecified disorder of conjunctiva

Disorders of sclera, cornea, iris and ciliary body (H15-H22)

H15 Disorders of sclera
    H15.0 Scleritis
        H15.00 Unspecified scleritis
            H15.001 Unspecified scleritis, right eye
            H15.002 Unspecified scleritis, left eye
            H15.003 Unspecified scleritis, bilateral
            H15.009 Unspecified scleritis, unspecified eye
        H15.01 Anterior scleritis
            H15.011 Anterior scleritis, right eye

H15.012 Anterior scleritis, left eye
H15.013 Anterior scleritis, bilateral
H15.019 Anterior scleritis, unspecified eye
H15.02 Brawny scleritis
    H15.021 Brawny scleritis, right eye
    H15.022 Brawny scleritis, left eye
    H15.023 Brawny scleritis, bilateral
    H15.029 Brawny scleritis, unspecified eye
H15.03 Posterior scleritis
Sclerotenonitis
    H15.031 Posterior scleritis, right eye
    H15.032 Posterior scleritis, left eye
    H15.033 Posterior scleritis, bilateral
    H15.039 Posterior scleritis, unspecified eye
H15.04 Scleritis with corneal involvement
    H15.041 Scleritis with corneal involvement, right eye
    H15.042 Scleritis with corneal involvement, left eye
    H15.043 Scleritis with corneal involvement, bilateral
    H15.049 Scleritis with corneal involvement, unspecified eye
H15.05 Scleromalacia perforans
    H15.051 Scleromalacia perforans, right eye
    H15.052 Scleromalacia perforans, left eye
    H15.053 Scleromalacia perforans, bilateral
    H15.059 Scleromalacia perforans, unspecified eye
H15.09 Other scleritis
Scleral abscess
    H15.091 Other scleritis, right eye
    H15.092 Other scleritis, left eye
    H15.093 Other scleritis, bilateral
    H15.099 Other scleritis, unspecified eye
H15.1 Episcleritis
    H15.10 Unspecified episcleritis
        H15.101 Unspecified episcleritis, right eye
        H15.102 Unspecified episcleritis, left eye
        H15.103 Unspecified episcleritis, bilateral
        H15.109 Unspecified episcleritis, unspecified eye
    H15.11 Episcleritis periodica fugax
        H15.111 Episcleritis periodica fugax, right eye
        H15.112 Episcleritis periodica fugax, left eye
        H15.113 Episcleritis periodica fugax, bilateral
        H15.119 Episcleritis periodica fugax, unspecified eye
    H15.12 Nodular episcleritis
        H15.121 Nodular episcleritis, right eye
        H15.122 Nodular episcleritis, left eye
        H15.123 Nodular episcleritis, bilateral
        H15.129 Nodular episcleritis, unspecified eye
H15.8 Other disorders of sclera
    EXCLUDES2 blue sclera (Q13.5)
                degenerative myopia (H44.2-)
    H15.81 Equatorial staphyloma
        H15.811 Equatorial staphyloma, right eye
        H15.812 Equatorial staphyloma, left eye
        H15.813 Equatorial staphyloma, bilateral
        H15.819 Equatorial staphyloma, unspecified eye
    H15.82 Localized anterior staphyloma
        H15.821 Localized anterior staphyloma, right eye
        H15.822 Localized anterior staphyloma, left eye
        H15.823 Localized anterior staphyloma, bilateral
        H15.829 Localized anterior staphyloma, unspecified eye
    H15.83 Staphyloma posticum
        H15.831 Staphyloma posticum, right eye
        H15.832 Staphyloma posticum, left eye
        H15.833 Staphyloma posticum, bilateral
        H15.839 Staphyloma posticum, unspecified eye

[6th] H15.84 Scleral ectasia
H15.841 Scleral ectasia, right eye
H15.842 Scleral ectasia, left eye
H15.843 Scleral ectasia, bilateral
H15.849 Scleral ectasia, unspecified eye
[6th] H15.85 Ring staphyloma
H15.851 Ring staphyloma, right eye
H15.852 Ring staphyloma, left eye
H15.853 Ring staphyloma, bilateral
H15.859 Ring staphyloma, unspecified eye
H15.89 Other disorders of sclera
H15.9 Unspecified disorder of sclera

[4th] H16 Keratitis
[5th] H16.0 Corneal ulcer
[6th] H16.00 Unspecified corneal ulcer
H16.001 Unspecified corneal ulcer, right eye
H16.002 Unspecified corneal ulcer, left eye
H16.003 Unspecified corneal ulcer, bilateral
H16.009 Unspecified corneal ulcer, unspecified eye
[6th] H16.01 Central corneal ulcer
H16.011 Central corneal ulcer, right eye
H16.012 Central corneal ulcer, left eye
H16.013 Central corneal ulcer, bilateral
H16.019 Central corneal ulcer, unspecified eye
[6th] H16.02 Ring corneal ulcer
H16.021 Ring corneal ulcer, right eye
H16.022 Ring corneal ulcer, left eye
H16.023 Ring corneal ulcer, bilateral
H16.029 Ring corneal ulcer, unspecified eye
[6th] H16.03 Corneal ulcer with hypopyon
H16.031 Corneal ulcer with hypopyon, right eye
H16.032 Corneal ulcer with hypopyon, left eye
H16.033 Corneal ulcer with hypopyon, bilateral
H16.039 Corneal ulcer with hypopyon, unspecified eye
[6th] H16.04 Marginal corneal ulcer
H16.041 Marginal corneal ulcer, right eye
H16.042 Marginal corneal ulcer, left eye
H16.043 Marginal corneal ulcer, bilateral
H16.049 Marginal corneal ulcer, unspecified eye
[6th] H16.05 Mooren's corneal ulcer
H16.051 Mooren's corneal ulcer, right eye
H16.052 Mooren's corneal ulcer, left eye
H16.053 Mooren's corneal ulcer, bilateral
H16.059 Mooren's corneal ulcer, unspecified eye
[6th] H16.06 Mycotic corneal ulcer
H16.061 Mycotic corneal ulcer, right eye
H16.062 Mycotic corneal ulcer, left eye
H16.063 Mycotic corneal ulcer, bilateral
H16.069 Mycotic corneal ulcer, unspecified eye
[6th] H16.07 Perforated corneal ulcer
H16.071 Perforated corneal ulcer, right eye
H16.072 Perforated corneal ulcer, left eye
H16.073 Perforated corneal ulcer, bilateral
H16.079 Perforated corneal ulcer, unspecified eye
[5th] H16.1 Other and unspecified superficial keratitis without conjunctivitis
[6th] H16.10 Unspecified superficial keratitis
H16.101 Unspecified superficial keratitis, right eye
H16.102 Unspecified superficial keratitis, left eye
H16.103 Unspecified superficial keratitis, bilateral
H16.109 Unspecified superficial keratitis, unspecified eye
[6th] H16.11 Macular keratitis
Areolar keratitis
Nummular keratitis
Stellate keratitis
Striate keratitis
H16.111 Macular keratitis, right eye
H16.112 Macular keratitis, left eye
H16.113 Macular keratitis, bilateral
H16.119 Macular keratitis, unspecified eye
[6th] H16.12 Filamentary keratitis
H16.121 Filamentary keratitis, right eye
H16.122 Filamentary keratitis, left eye
H16.123 Filamentary keratitis, bilateral
H16.129 Filamentary keratitis, unspecified eye
[6th] H16.13 Photokeratitis
Snow blindness
Welders keratitis
H16.131 Photokeratitis, right eye
H16.132 Photokeratitis, left eye
H16.133 Photokeratitis, bilateral
H16.139 Photokeratitis, unspecified eye
[6th] H16.14 Punctate keratitis
H16.141 Punctate keratitis, right eye
H16.142 Punctate keratitis, left eye
H16.143 Punctate keratitis, bilateral
H16.149 Punctate keratitis, unspecified eye
[5th] H16.2 Keratoconjunctivitis
[6th] H16.20 Unspecified keratoconjunctivitis
Superficial keratitis with conjunctivitis NOS
H16.201 Unspecified keratoconjunctivitis, right eye
H16.202 Unspecified keratoconjunctivitis, left eye
H16.203 Unspecified keratoconjunctivitis, bilateral
H16.209 Unspecified keratoconjunctivitis, unspecified eye
[6th] H16.21 Exposure keratoconjunctivitis
H16.211 Exposure keratoconjunctivitis, right eye
H16.212 Exposure keratoconjunctivitis, left eye
H16.213 Exposure keratoconjunctivitis, bilateral
H16.219 Exposure keratoconjunctivitis, unspecified eye
[6th] H16.22 Keratoconjunctivitis sicca, not specified as Sjögren's
EXCLUDES1 *Sjögren's syndrome (M35.01)*
H16.221 Keratoconjunctivitis sicca, not specified as Sjögren's, right eye
H16.222 Keratoconjunctivitis sicca, not specified as Sjögren's, left eye
H16.223 Keratoconjunctivitis sicca, not specified as Sjögren's, bilateral
H16.229 Keratoconjunctivitis sicca, not specified as Sjögren's, unspecified eye
[6th] H16.23 Neurotrophic keratoconjunctivitis
H16.231 Neurotrophic keratoconjunctivitis, right eye
H16.232 Neurotrophic keratoconjunctivitis, left eye
H16.233 Neurotrophic keratoconjunctivitis, bilateral
H16.239 Neurotrophic keratoconjunctivitis, unspecified eye
[6th] H16.24 Ophthalmia nodosa
H16.241 Ophthalmia nodosa, right eye
H16.242 Ophthalmia nodosa, left eye
H16.243 Ophthalmia nodosa, bilateral
H16.249 Ophthalmia nodosa, unspecified eye
[6th] H16.25 Phlyctenular keratoconjunctivitis
H16.251 Phlyctenular keratoconjunctivitis, right eye
H16.252 Phlyctenular keratoconjunctivitis, left eye
H16.253 Phlyctenular keratoconjunctivitis, bilateral
H16.259 Phlyctenular keratoconjunctivitis, unspecified eye
[6th] H16.26 Vernal keratoconjunctivitis, with limbar and corneal involvement
EXCLUDES1 *vernal conjunctivitis without limbar and corneal involvement (H10.44)*
H16.261 Vernal keratoconjunctivitis, with limbar and corneal involvement, right eye

PDx Unacceptable principal diagnosis symbol per Medicare code edits POA Code exempt from diagnosis present on admission requirement
[?] Questionable admission CC Complication or comorbidity MCC Major complication or comorbidity CC/MCC Excl CC/MCC exclusion
[HCC] HCC diagnosis code [RxHCC] RxHCC diagnosis code MACRA code DEFINITION Describes condition/terminology
TIP Coding guidance 👁 Official Guideline Reference [Z1] Z code as first-listed diagnosis

H16.262 Vernal keratoconjunctivitis, with limbar and corneal involvement, **left** eye

H16.263 Vernal keratoconjunctivitis, with limbar and corneal involvement, **bilateral**

H16.269 Vernal keratoconjunctivitis, with limbar and corneal involvement, unspecified eye

H16.29 Other keratoconjunctivitis

H16.291 Other keratoconjunctivitis, **right** eye

H16.292 Other keratoconjunctivitis, **left** eye

H16.293 Other keratoconjunctivitis, **bilateral**

H16.299 Other keratoconjunctivitis, **unspecified eye**

H16.3 Interstitial and deep keratitis

H16.30 Unspecified interstitial keratitis

H16.301 Unspecified interstitial keratitis, **right** eye

H16.302 Unspecified interstitial keratitis, **left** eye

H16.303 Unspecified interstitial keratitis, **bilateral**

H16.309 Unspecified interstitial keratitis, **unspecified eye**

H16.31 Corneal abscess

H16.311 Corneal abscess, **right** eye

H16.312 Corneal abscess, **left** eye

H16.313 Corneal abscess, **bilateral**

H16.319 Corneal abscess, **unspecified eye**

H16.32 Diffuse interstitial keratitis

Cogan's syndrome

H16.321 Diffuse interstitial keratitis, **right** eye

H16.322 Diffuse interstitial keratitis, **left** eye

H16.323 Diffuse interstitial keratitis, **bilateral**

H16.329 Diffuse interstitial keratitis, **unspecified eye**

H16.33 Sclerosing keratitis

H16.331 Sclerosing keratitis, **right** eye

H16.332 Sclerosing keratitis, **left** eye

H16.333 Sclerosing keratitis, **bilateral**

H16.339 Sclerosing keratitis, **unspecified eye**

H16.39 Other interstitial and deep keratitis

H16.391 Other interstitial and deep keratitis, **right eye**

H16.392 Other interstitial and deep keratitis, **left eye**

H16.393 Other interstitial and deep keratitis, **bilateral**

H16.399 Other interstitial and deep keratitis, **unspecified eye**

H16.4 Corneal neovascularization

H16.40 Unspecified corneal neovascularization

H16.401 Unspecified corneal neovascularization, **right eye**

H16.402 Unspecified corneal neovascularization, **left eye**

H16.403 Unspecified corneal neovascularization, **bilateral**

H16.409 Unspecified corneal neovascularization, **unspecified eye**

H16.41 Ghost vessels (corneal)

H16.411 Ghost vessels (corneal), **right** eye

H16.412 Ghost vessels (corneal), **left** eye

H16.413 Ghost vessels (corneal), **bilateral**

H16.419 Ghost vessels (corneal), **unspecified eye**

H16.42 Pannus (corneal)

H16.421 Pannus (corneal), **right** eye

H16.422 Pannus (corneal), **left** eye

H16.423 Pannus (corneal), **bilateral**

H16.429 Pannus (corneal), **unspecified eye**

H16.43 Localized vascularization of cornea

H16.431 Localized vascularization of cornea, **right eye**

H16.432 Localized vascularization of cornea, **left eye**

H16.433 Localized vascularization of cornea, **bilateral**

H16.439 Localized vascularization of cornea, **unspecified eye**

H16.44 Deep vascularization of cornea

H16.441 Deep vascularization of cornea, **right** eye

H16.442 Deep vascularization of cornea, **left** eye

H16.443 Deep vascularization of cornea, **bilateral**

H16.449 Deep vascularization of cornea, **unspecified eye**

H16.8 Other keratitis   PDxIn

H16.9 Unspecified keratitis

H17 Corneal scars and opacities

H17.0 Adherent leukoma

H17.00 Adherent leukoma, **unspecified eye**

H17.01 Adherent leukoma, **right** eye

H17.02 Adherent leukoma, **left** eye

H17.03 Adherent leukoma, **bilateral**

H17.1 Central corneal opacity

H17.10 Central corneal opacity, **unspecified eye**

H17.11 Central corneal opacity, **right** eye

H17.12 Central corneal opacity, **left** eye

H17.13 Central corneal opacity, **bilateral**

H17.8 Other corneal scars and opacities

H17.81 Minor opacity of cornea

Corneal nebula

H17.811 Minor opacity of cornea, **right** eye

H17.812 Minor opacity of cornea, **left** eye

H17.813 Minor opacity of cornea, **bilateral**

H17.819 Minor opacity of cornea, **unspecified eye**

H17.82 Peripheral opacity of cornea

H17.821 Peripheral opacity of cornea, **right** eye

H17.822 Peripheral opacity of cornea, **left** eye

H17.823 Peripheral opacity of cornea, **bilateral**

H17.829 Peripheral opacity of cornea, **unspecified eye**

H17.89 Other corneal scars and opacities

H17.9 Unspecified corneal scar and opacity

H18 Other disorders of cornea

H18.0 Corneal pigmentations and deposits

H18.00 Unspecified corneal deposit

H18.001 Unspecified corneal deposit, **right eye**

H18.002 Unspecified corneal deposit, **left eye**

H18.003 Unspecified corneal deposit, **bilateral**

H18.009 Unspecified corneal deposit, **unspecified eye**

H18.01 Anterior corneal pigmentations

Staehli's line

H18.011 Anterior corneal pigmentations, **right** eye

H18.012 Anterior corneal pigmentations, **left** eye

H18.013 Anterior corneal pigmentations, **bilateral**

H18.019 Anterior corneal pigmentations, **unspecified eye**

H18.02 Argentous corneal deposits

H18.021 Argentous corneal deposits, **right** eye

H18.022 Argentous corneal deposits, **left** eye

H18.023 Argentous corneal deposits, **bilateral**

H18.029 Argentous corneal deposits, **unspecified eye**

H18.03 Corneal deposits in metabolic disorders

Code also associated metabolic disorder

H18.031 Corneal deposits in metabolic disorders, **right eye**

H18.032 Corneal deposits in metabolic disorders, **left eye**

H18.033 Corneal deposits in metabolic disorders, **bilateral**

H18.039 Corneal deposits in metabolic disorders, **unspecified eye**

6️⃣ **H18.04** Kayser-Fleischer ring
Code also associated Wilson's disease (E83.01)
H18.041 Kayser-Fleischer ring, right eye
H18.042 Kayser-Fleischer ring, left eye
H18.043 Kayser-Fleischer ring, bilateral
H18.049 Kayser-Fleischer ring, unspecified eye

6️⃣ **H18.05** Posterior corneal pigmentations
Krukenberg's spindle
H18.051 Posterior corneal pigmentations, right eye
H18.052 Posterior corneal pigmentations, left eye
H18.053 Posterior corneal pigmentations, bilateral
H18.059 Posterior corneal pigmentations, unspecified eye

6️⃣ **H18.06** Stromal corneal pigmentations
Hematocornea
H18.061 Stromal corneal pigmentations, right eye
H18.062 Stromal corneal pigmentations, left eye
H18.063 Stromal corneal pigmentations, bilateral
H18.069 Stromal corneal pigmentations, unspecified eye

5️⃣ **H18.1** Bullous keratopathy
H18.10 Bullous keratopathy, unspecified eye
H18.11 Bullous keratopathy, right eye
H18.12 Bullous keratopathy, left eye
H18.13 Bullous keratopathy, bilateral

5️⃣ **H18.2** Other and unspecified corneal edema
H18.20 Unspecified corneal edema
6️⃣ **H18.21** Corneal edema secondary to contact lens
EXCLUDES2 other corneal disorders due to contact lens (H18.82-)
H18.211 Corneal edema secondary to contact lens, right eye
H18.212 Corneal edema secondary to contact lens, left eye
H18.213 Corneal edema secondary to contact lens, bilateral
H18.219 Corneal edema secondary to contact lens, unspecified eye

6️⃣ **H18.22** Idiopathic corneal edema
H18.221 Idiopathic corneal edema, right eye
H18.222 Idiopathic corneal edema, left eye
H18.223 Idiopathic corneal edema, bilateral
H18.229 Idiopathic corneal edema, unspecified eye

6️⃣ **H18.23** Secondary corneal edema
H18.231 Secondary corneal edema, right eye
H18.232 Secondary corneal edema, left eye
H18.233 Secondary corneal edema, bilateral
H18.239 Secondary corneal edema, unspecified eye

5️⃣ **H18.3** Changes of corneal membranes
H18.30 Unspecified corneal membrane change
6️⃣ **H18.31** Folds and rupture in Bowman's membrane
H18.311 Folds and rupture in Bowman's membrane, right eye
H18.312 Folds and rupture in Bowman's membrane, left eye
H18.313 Folds and rupture in Bowman's membrane, bilateral
H18.319 Folds and rupture in Bowman's membrane, unspecified eye

6️⃣ **H18.32** Folds in Descemet's membrane
H18.321 Folds in Descemet's membrane, right eye
H18.322 Folds in Descemet's membrane, left eye
H18.323 Folds in Descemet's membrane, bilateral
H18.329 Folds in Descemet's membrane, unspecified eye

6️⃣ **H18.33** Rupture in Descemet's membrane
H18.331 Rupture in Descemet's membrane, right eye
H18.332 Rupture in Descemet's membrane, left eye

H18.333 Rupture in Descemet's membrane, bilateral
H18.339 Rupture in Descemet's membrane, unspecified eye

5️⃣ **H18.4** Corneal degeneration
EXCLUDES1 Mooren's ulcer (H16.0-)
recurrent erosion of cornea (H18.83-)
H18.40 Unspecified corneal degeneration
6️⃣ **H18.41** Arcus senilis
Senile corneal changes
H18.411 Arcus senilis, right eye
H18.412 Arcus senilis, left eye
H18.413 Arcus senilis, bilateral
H18.419 Arcus senilis, unspecified eye

6️⃣ **H18.42** Band keratopathy
H18.421 Band keratopathy, right eye
H18.422 Band keratopathy, left eye
H18.423 Band keratopathy, bilateral
H18.429 Band keratopathy, unspecified eye
H18.43 Other calcerous corneal degeneration

6️⃣ **H18.44** Keratomalacia
EXCLUDES1 keratomalacia due to vitamin A deficiency (E50.4)
H18.441 Keratomalacia, right eye
H18.442 Keratomalacia, left eye
H18.443 Keratomalacia, bilateral
H18.449 Keratomalacia, unspecified eye

6️⃣ **H18.45** Nodular corneal degeneration
H18.451 Nodular corneal degeneration, right eye
H18.452 Nodular corneal degeneration, left eye
H18.453 Nodular corneal degeneration, bilateral
H18.459 Nodular corneal degeneration, unspecified eye

6️⃣ **H18.46** Peripheral corneal degeneration
H18.461 Peripheral corneal degeneration, right eye
H18.462 Peripheral corneal degeneration, left eye
H18.463 Peripheral corneal degeneration, bilateral
H18.469 Peripheral corneal degeneration, unspecified eye
H18.49 Other corneal degeneration

5️⃣ **H18.5** Hereditary corneal dystrophies
H18.50 Unspecified hereditary corneal dystrophies
H18.51 Endothelial corneal dystrophy
Fuchs' dystrophy
H18.52 Epithelial (juvenile) corneal dystrophy
H18.53 Granular corneal dystrophy
H18.54 Lattice corneal dystrophy
H18.55 Macular corneal dystrophy
H18.59 Other hereditary corneal dystrophies

5️⃣ **H18.6** Keratoconus
6️⃣ **H18.60** Keratoconus, unspecified
H18.601 Keratoconus, unspecified, right eye
H18.602 Keratoconus, unspecified, left eye
H18.603 Keratoconus, unspecified, bilateral
H18.609 Keratoconus, unspecified, unspecified eye

6️⃣ **H18.61** Keratoconus, stable
H18.611 Keratoconus, stable, right eye
H18.612 Keratoconus, stable, left eye
H18.613 Keratoconus, stable, bilateral
H18.619 Keratoconus, stable, unspecified eye

6️⃣ **H18.62** Keratoconus, unstable
Acute hydrops
H18.621 Keratoconus, unstable, right eye
H18.622 Keratoconus, unstable, left eye
H18.623 Keratoconus, unstable, bilateral
H18.629 Keratoconus, unstable, unspecified eye

5️⃣ **H18.7** Other and unspecified corneal deformities
EXCLUDES1 congenital malformations of cornea (Q13.3-Q13.4)
H18.70 Unspecified corneal deformity

PDXⁿ Unacceptable principal diagnosis symbol per Medicare code edits   PDX Code exempt from diagnosis present on admission requirement
❓ Questionable admission   CC Complication or comorbidity   MCC Major complication or comorbidity   CC/MCC Exc CC/MCC exclusion
HCC HCC diagnosis code   RxHCC RxHCC diagnosis code   MACRA code   **DEFINITION** Describes condition/terminology
TIP Coding guidance   👁 Official Guideline Reference   Z1 Z code as first-listed diagnosis

608   When symbols appear on a code that requires a 7th character extension, refer to Appendix B to identify applicable 7th character codes.   **2020 ICD-10-CM**

[6th] H18.71 Corneal ectasia
H18.711 Corneal ectasia, right eye
H18.712 Corneal ectasia, left eye
H18.713 Corneal ectasia, bilateral
H18.719 Corneal ectasia, unspecified eye
[6th] H18.72 Corneal staphyloma
H18.721 Corneal staphyloma, right eye
H18.722 Corneal staphyloma, left eye
H18.723 Corneal staphyloma, bilateral
H18.729 Corneal staphyloma, unspecified eye
[6th] H18.73 Descemetocele
H18.731 Descemetocele, right eye
H18.732 Descemetocele, left eye
H18.733 Descemetocele, bilateral
H18.739 Descemetocele, unspecified eye
[6th] H18.79 Other corneal deformities
H18.791 Other corneal deformities, right eye
H18.792 Other corneal deformities, left eye
H18.793 Other corneal deformities, bilateral
H18.799 Other corneal deformities, unspecified eye
[5th] H18.8 Other specified disorders of cornea
[6th] H18.81 Anesthesia and hypoesthesia of cornea
H18.811 Anesthesia and hypoesthesia of cornea, right eye
H18.812 Anesthesia and hypoesthesia of cornea, left eye
H18.813 Anesthesia and hypoesthesia of cornea, bilateral
H18.819 Anesthesia and hypoesthesia of cornea, unspecified eye
[6th] H18.82 Corneal disorder due to contact lens
[EXCLUDES2] *corneal edema due to contact lens (H18.21-)*
H18.821 Corneal disorder due to contact lens, right eye
H18.822 Corneal disorder due to contact lens, left eye
H18.823 Corneal disorder due to contact lens, bilateral
H18.829 Corneal disorder due to contact lens, unspecified eye
[6th] H18.83 Recurrent erosion of cornea
H18.831 Recurrent erosion of cornea, right eye
H18.832 Recurrent erosion of cornea, left eye
H18.833 Recurrent erosion of cornea, bilateral
H18.839 Recurrent erosion of cornea, unspecified eye
[6th] H18.89 Other specified disorders of cornea
H18.891 Other specified disorders of cornea, right eye
H18.892 Other specified disorders of cornea, left eye
H18.893 Other specified disorders of cornea, bilateral
H18.899 Other specified disorders of cornea, unspecified eye
H18.9 Unspecified disorder of cornea
[4th] H20 Iridocyclitis
[5th] H20.0 Acute and subacute iridocyclitis
Acute anterior uveitis
Acute cyclitis
Acute iritis
Subacute anterior uveitis
Subacute cyclitis
Subacute iritis
[EXCLUDES1] *iridocyclitis, iritis, uveitis (due to) (in) diabetes mellitus (E08-E13 with .39)*
iridocyclitis, iritis, uveitis (due to) (in) diphtheria (A36.89)
iridocyclitis, iritis, uveitis (due to) (in) gonococcal (A54.32)
iridocyclitis, iritis, uveitis (due to) (in) herpes (simplex) (B00.51)
iridocyclitis, iritis, uveitis (due to) (in) herpes zoster (B02.32)
iridocyclitis, iritis, uveitis (due to) (in) late congenital syphilis (A50.39)
iridocyclitis, iritis, uveitis (due to) (in) late syphilis (A52.71)
iridocyclitis, iritis, uveitis (due to) (in) sarcoidosis (D86.83)
iridocyclitis, iritis, uveitis (due to) (in) syphilis (A51.43)
iridocyclitis, iritis, uveitis (due to) (in) toxoplasmosis (B58.09)
iridocyclitis, iritis, uveitis (due to) (in) tuberculosis (A18.54)
H20.00 Unspecified acute and subacute iridocyclitis CC CC/MCC Exc
[6th] H20.01 Primary iridocyclitis
H20.011 Primary iridocyclitis, right eye CC CC/MCC Exc
H20.012 Primary iridocyclitis, left eye CC CC/MCC Exc
H20.013 Primary iridocyclitis, bilateral CC CC/MCC Exc
H20.019 Primary iridocyclitis, unspecified eye CC CC/MCC Exc
[6th] H20.02 Recurrent acute iridocyclitis
H20.021 Recurrent acute iridocyclitis, right eye CC CC/MCC Exc
H20.022 Recurrent acute iridocyclitis, left eye CC CC/MCC Exc
H20.023 Recurrent acute iridocyclitis, bilateral CC CC/MCC Exc
H20.029 Recurrent acute iridocyclitis, unspecified eye CC CC/MCC Exc
[6th] H20.03 Secondary infectious iridocyclitis
H20.031 Secondary infectious iridocyclitis, right eye CC CC/MCC Exc
H20.032 Secondary infectious iridocyclitis, left eye CC CC/MCC Exc
H20.033 Secondary infectious iridocyclitis, bilateral CC CC/MCC Exc
H20.039 Secondary infectious iridocyclitis, unspecified eye CC CC/MCC Exc
[6th] H20.04 Secondary noninfectious iridocyclitis
H20.041 Secondary noninfectious iridocyclitis, right eye
H20.042 Secondary noninfectious iridocyclitis, left eye
H20.043 Secondary noninfectious iridocyclitis, bilateral
H20.049 Secondary noninfectious iridocyclitis, unspecified eye
[6th] H20.05 Hypopyon
H20.051 Hypopyon, right eye
H20.052 Hypopyon, left eye
H20.053 Hypopyon, bilateral
H20.059 Hypopyon, unspecified eye
[5th] H20.1 Chronic iridocyclitis
Use additional code for any associated cataract (H26.21-)
[EXCLUDES2] *posterior cyclitis (H30.2-)*
H20.10 Chronic iridocyclitis, unspecified eye
H20.11 Chronic iridocyclitis, right eye
H20.12 Chronic iridocyclitis, left eye
H20.13 Chronic iridocyclitis, bilateral
[5th] H20.2 Lens-induced iridocyclitis
H20.20 Lens-induced iridocyclitis, unspecified eye
H20.21 Lens-induced iridocyclitis, right eye
H20.22 Lens-induced iridocyclitis, left eye
H20.23 Lens-induced iridocyclitis, bilateral

[5th] **H20.8 Other iridocyclitis**
[EXCLUDES2] *glaucomatocyclitis crises (H40.4-)*
posterior cyclitis (H30.2-)
sympathetic uveitis (H44.13-)
[6th] **H20.81 Fuchs' heterochromic cyclitis**
H20.811 **Fuchs' heterochromic cyclitis, right eye**
H20.812 **Fuchs' heterochromic cyclitis, left eye**
H20.813 **Fuchs' heterochromic cyclitis, bilateral**
H20.819 **Fuchs' heterochromic cyclitis, unspecified eye**
[6th] **H20.82 Vogt-Koyanagi syndrome**
H20.821 **Vogt-Koyanagi syndrome, right eye**
H20.822 **Vogt-Koyanagi syndrome, left eye**
H20.823 **Vogt-Koyanagi syndrome, bilateral**
H20.829 **Vogt-Koyanagi syndrome, unspecified eye**
H20.9 **Unspecified iridocyclitis** [CC] [CC/MCC Exc]
Uveitis NOS
[4th] **H21 Other disorders of iris and ciliary body**
[EXCLUDES2] *sympathetic uveitis (H44.1-)*
[5th] **H21.0 Hyphema**
[EXCLUDES1] *traumatic hyphema (S05.1-)*
H21.00 **Hyphema, unspecified eye**
H21.01 **Hyphema, right eye**
H21.02 **Hyphema, left eye**
H21.03 **Hyphema, bilateral**
[5th] **H21.1 Other vascular disorders of iris and ciliary body**
Neovascularization of iris or ciliary body
Rubeosis iridis
Rubeosis of iris
[6th] **H21.1X Other vascular disorders of iris and ciliary body**
H21.1X1 **Other vascular disorders of iris and ciliary body, right eye**
H21.1X2 **Other vascular disorders of iris and ciliary body, left eye**
H21.1X3 **Other vascular disorders of iris and ciliary body, bilateral**
H21.1X9 **Other vascular disorders of iris and ciliary body, unspecified eye**
[5th] **H21.2 Degeneration of iris and ciliary body**
[6th] **H21.21 Degeneration of chamber angle**
H21.211 **Degeneration of chamber angle, right eye**
H21.212 **Degeneration of chamber angle, left eye**
H21.213 **Degeneration of chamber angle, bilateral**
H21.219 **Degeneration of chamber angle, unspecified eye**
[6th] **H21.22 Degeneration of ciliary body**
H21.221 **Degeneration of ciliary body, right eye**
H21.222 **Degeneration of ciliary body, left eye**
H21.223 **Degeneration of ciliary body, bilateral**
H21.229 **Degeneration of ciliary body, unspecified eye**
[6th] **H21.23 Degeneration of iris (pigmentary)**
Translucency of iris
H21.231 **Degeneration of iris (pigmentary), right eye**
H21.232 **Degeneration of iris (pigmentary), left eye**
H21.233 **Degeneration of iris (pigmentary), bilateral**
H21.239 **Degeneration of iris (pigmentary), unspecified eye**
[6th] **H21.24 Degeneration of pupillary margin**
H21.241 **Degeneration of pupillary margin, right eye**
H21.242 **Degeneration of pupillary margin, left eye**
H21.243 **Degeneration of pupillary margin, bilateral**
H21.249 **Degeneration of pupillary margin, unspecified eye**
[6th] **H21.25 Iridoschisis**
H21.251 **Iridoschisis, right eye**
H21.252 **Iridoschisis, left eye**
H21.253 **Iridoschisis, bilateral**
H21.259 **Iridoschisis, unspecified eye**
[6th] **H21.26 Iris atrophy (essential) (progressive)**
H21.261 **Iris atrophy (essential) (progressive), right eye**
H21.262 **Iris atrophy (essential) (progressive), left eye**
H21.263 **Iris atrophy (essential) (progressive), bilateral**
H21.269 **Iris atrophy (essential) (progressive), unspecified eye**
[6th] **H21.27 Miotic pupillary cyst**
H21.271 **Miotic pupillary cyst, right eye**
H21.272 **Miotic pupillary cyst, left eye**
H21.273 **Miotic pupillary cyst, bilateral**
H21.279 **Miotic pupillary cyst, unspecified eye**
H21.29 **Other iris atrophy**
[5th] **H21.3 Cyst of iris, ciliary body and anterior chamber**
[EXCLUDES2] *miotic pupillary cyst (H21.27-)*
[6th] **H21.30 Idiopathic cysts of iris, ciliary body or anterior chamber**
Cyst of iris, ciliary body or anterior chamber NOS
H21.301 **Idiopathic cysts of iris, ciliary body or anterior chamber, right eye**
H21.302 **Idiopathic cysts of iris, ciliary body or anterior chamber, left eye**
H21.303 **Idiopathic cysts of iris, ciliary body or anterior chamber, bilateral**
H21.309 **Idiopathic cysts of iris, ciliary body or anterior chamber, unspecified eye**
[6th] **H21.31 Exudative cysts of iris or anterior chamber**
H21.311 **Exudative cysts of iris or anterior chamber, right eye**
H21.312 **Exudative cysts of iris or anterior chamber, left eye**
H21.313 **Exudative cysts of iris or anterior chamber, bilateral**
H21.319 **Exudative cysts of iris or anterior chamber, unspecified eye**
[6th] **H21.32 Implantation cysts of iris, ciliary body or anterior chamber**
H21.321 **Implantation cysts of iris, ciliary body or anterior chamber, right eye**
H21.322 **Implantation cysts of iris, ciliary body or anterior chamber, left eye**
H21.323 **Implantation cysts of iris, ciliary body or anterior chamber, bilateral**
H21.329 **Implantation cysts of iris, ciliary body or anterior chamber, unspecified eye**
[6th] **H21.33 Parasitic cyst of iris, ciliary body or anterior chamber**
H21.331 **Parasitic cyst of iris, ciliary body or anterior chamber, right eye** [CC] [CC/MCC Exc]
H21.332 **Parasitic cyst of iris, ciliary body or anterior chamber, left eye** [CC] [CC/MCC Exc]
H21.333 **Parasitic cyst of iris, ciliary body or anterior chamber, bilateral** [CC] [CC/MCC Exc]
H21.339 **Parasitic cyst of iris, ciliary body or anterior chamber, unspecified eye** [CC] [CC/MCC Exc]
[6th] **H21.34 Primary cyst of pars plana**
H21.341 **Primary cyst of pars plana, right eye**
H21.342 **Primary cyst of pars plana, left eye**
H21.343 **Primary cyst of pars plana, bilateral**
H21.349 **Primary cyst of pars plana, unspecified eye**
[6th] **H21.35 Exudative cyst of pars plana**
H21.351 **Exudative cyst of pars plana, right eye**
H21.352 **Exudative cyst of pars plana, left eye**
H21.353 **Exudative cyst of pars plana, bilateral**
H21.359 **Exudative cyst of pars plana, unspecified eye**

[PDx] Unacceptable principal diagnosis symbol per Medicare code edits [POA] Code exempt from diagnosis present on admission requirement
[?] Questionable admission [CC] Complication or comorbidity [MCC] Major complication or comorbidity [CC/MCC Exc] CC/MCC exclusion
[HCC] HCC diagnosis code [RxHCC] RxHCC diagnosis code MACRA code **DEFINITION** Describes condition/terminology
TIP Coding guidance 👁 Official Guideline Reference [Z1] Z code as first-listed diagnosis

[5th] H21.4 **Pupillary membranes**
Iris bombé
Pupillary occlusion
Pupillary seclusion
EXCLUDES1 *congenital pupillary membranes (Q13.8)*
H21.40 **Pupillary membranes, unspecified eye**
H21.41 **Pupillary membranes, right eye**
H21.42 **Pupillary membranes, left eye**
H21.43 **Pupillary membranes, bilateral**

[5th] H21.5 **Other and unspecified adhesions and disruptions of iris and ciliary body**
EXCLUDES1 *corectopia (Q13.2)*

[6th] H21.50 **Unspecified adhesions of iris**
Synechia (iris) NOS
H21.501 **Unspecified adhesions of iris, right eye**
H21.502 **Unspecified adhesions of iris, left eye**
H21.503 **Unspecified adhesions of iris, bilateral**
H21.509 **Unspecified adhesions of iris and ciliary body, unspecified eye**

[6th] H21.51 **Anterior synechiae (iris)**
H21.511 **Anterior synechiae (iris), right eye**
H21.512 **Anterior synechiae (iris), left eye**
H21.513 **Anterior synechiae (iris), bilateral**
H21.519 **Anterior synechiae (iris), unspecified eye**

[6th] H21.52 **Goniosynechiae**
H21.521 **Goniosynechiae, right eye**
H21.522 **Goniosynechiae, left eye**
H21.523 **Goniosynechiae, bilateral**
H21.529 **Goniosynechiae, unspecified eye**

[6th] H21.53 **Iridodialysis**
H21.531 **Iridodialysis, right eye**
H21.532 **Iridodialysis, left eye**
H21.533 **Iridodialysis, bilateral**
H21.539 **Iridodialysis, unspecified eye**

[6th] H21.54 **Posterior synechiae (iris)**
H21.541 **Posterior synechiae (iris), right eye**
H21.542 **Posterior synechiae (iris), left eye**
H21.543 **Posterior synechiae (iris), bilateral**
H21.549 **Posterior synechiae (iris), unspecified eye**

[6th] H21.55 **Recession of chamber angle**
H21.551 **Recession of chamber angle, right eye**
H21.552 **Recession of chamber angle, left eye**
H21.553 **Recession of chamber angle, bilateral**
H21.559 **Recession of chamber angle, unspecified eye**

[6th] H21.56 **Pupillary abnormalities**
Deformed pupil
Ectopic pupil
Rupture of sphincter, pupil
EXCLUDES1 *congenital deformity of pupil (Q13.2-)*
H21.561 **Pupillary abnormality, right eye**
H21.562 **Pupillary abnormality, left eye**
H21.563 **Pupillary abnormality, bilateral**
H21.569 **Pupillary abnormality, unspecified eye**

[5th] H21.8 **Other specified disorders of iris and ciliary body**
H21.81 **Floppy iris syndrome**
Intraoperative floppy iris syndrome (IFIS)
Use additional code for adverse effect, if applicable, to identify drug (T36-T50 with fifth or sixth character 5)
H21.82 **Plateau iris syndrome (post-iridectomy) (postprocedural)**
H21.89 **Other specified disorders of iris and ciliary body**

H21.9 **Unspecified disorder of iris and ciliary body**

H22 **Disorders of iris and ciliary body in diseases classified elsewhere**
☞ **Code first** underlying disease, such as:
gout (M1A.-, M10.-)
leprosy (A30.-)
parasitic disease (B89)

Disorders of lens (H25-H28)

[4th] H25 **Age-related cataract**
DEFINITION: A cataract is a clouding of the clear lens of the eye.
Senile cataract
EXCLUDES2 *capsular glaucoma with pseudoexfoliation of lens (H40.1-)*

[5th] H25.0 **Age-related incipient cataract**

[6th] H25.01 **Cortical age-related cataract**
H25.011 **Cortical age-related cataract, right eye** [A]
H25.012 **Cortical age-related cataract, left eye** [A]
H25.013 **Cortical age-related cataract, bilateral** [A]
H25.019 **Cortical age-related cataract, unspecified eye** [A]

[6th] H25.03 **Anterior subcapsular polar age-related cataract**
H25.031 **Anterior subcapsular polar age-related cataract, right eye** [A]
H25.032 **Anterior subcapsular polar age-related cataract, left eye** [A]
H25.033 **Anterior subcapsular polar age-related cataract, bilateral** [A]
H25.039 **Anterior subcapsular polar age-related cataract, unspecified eye** [A]

[6th] H25.04 **Posterior subcapsular polar age-related cataract**
H25.041 **Posterior subcapsular polar age-related cataract, right eye** [A]
H25.042 **Posterior subcapsular polar age-related cataract, left eye** [A]
H25.043 **Posterior subcapsular polar age-related cataract, bilateral** [A]
H25.049 **Posterior subcapsular polar age-related cataract, unspecified eye** [A]

[6th] H25.09 **Other age-related incipient cataract**
Coronary age-related cataract
Punctate age-related cataract
Water clefts
H25.091 **Other age-related incipient cataract, right eye** [A]
H25.092 **Other age-related incipient cataract, left eye** [A]
H25.093 **Other age-related incipient cataract, bilateral** [A]
H25.099 **Other age-related incipient cataract, unspecified eye** [A]

[5th] H25.1 **Age-related nuclear cataract**
Cataracta brunescens
Nuclear sclerosis cataract
H25.10 **Age-related nuclear cataract, unspecified eye** [A]
H25.11 **Age-related nuclear cataract, right eye** [A]
AHA: Q2 2019
H25.12 **Age-related nuclear cataract, left eye** [A]
AHA: Q1 2016
H25.13 **Age-related nuclear cataract, bilateral** [A]
AHA: Q1 2016

[5th] H25.2 **Age-related cataract, morgagnian type**
Age-related hypermature cataract
H25.20 **Age-related cataract, morgagnian type, unspecified eye** [A]
H25.21 **Age-related cataract, morgagnian type, right eye** [A]
H25.22 **Age-related cataract, morgagnian type, left eye** [A]
H25.23 **Age-related cataract, morgagnian type, bilateral** [A]

[5th] H25.8 **Other age-related cataract**

[6th] H25.81 **Combined forms of age-related cataract**
H25.811 **Combined forms of age-related cataract, right eye** [A]
H25.812 **Combined forms of age-related cataract, left eye** [A]
H25.813 **Combined forms of age-related cataract, bilateral** [A]
AHA: Q2 2019
H25.819 **Combined forms of age-related cataract, unspecified eye** [A]

H25.89 **Other age-related cataract** [A]

Unspecified Code | Other Specified Code | Manifestation Code | [N] Newborn | [P] Pediatric | [M] Maternity | [A] Adult | ♂ Male | ♀ Female
● New Code | ▲ Revised Code Title | ►◄ Revised Text | NOTES | INCLUDES | EXCLUDES1 Not coded here | EXCLUDES2 Not included here
[4th] 4th character required | [5th] 5th character required | [6th] 6th character required | [7th] 7th character required | [X] Extension 'X' Alert
[HAC] Hospital-acquired condition (HAC) alert | AHA AHA Coding Clinic© | ☞ Code first alert

When symbols appear on a code that requires a 7th character extension, refer to Appendix B to identify applicable 7th character codes.

H25.9 **Unspecified age-related cataract** 🄰

🔴 H26 Other **cataract**

　　EXCLUDES1 congenital cataract (Q12.0)

🔵 **H26.0** Infantile and juvenile **cataract**

　　🔵 **H26.00** Unspecified infantile and juvenile cataract

　　　　H26.001 **Unspecified infantile and juvenile cataract, right eye** 🄿

　　　　H26.002 **Unspecified infantile and juvenile cataract, left eye** 🄿

　　　　H26.003 **Unspecified infantile and juvenile cataract, bilateral** 🄿

　　　　H26.009 **Unspecified infantile and juvenile cataract, unspecified eye** 🄿

　　🔵 **H26.01** Infantile and juvenile cortical, lamellar, or zonular cataract

　　　　H26.011 **Infantile and juvenile cortical, lamellar, or zonular cataract, right eye** 🄿

　　　　H26.012 **Infantile and juvenile cortical, lamellar, or zonular cataract, left eye** 🄿

　　　　H26.013 **Infantile and juvenile cortical, lamellar, or zonular cataract, bilateral** 🄿

　　　　H26.019 **Infantile and juvenile cortical, lamellar, or zonular cataract, unspecified eye** 🄿

　　🔵 **H26.03** Infantile and juvenile nuclear **cataract**

　　　　H26.031 **Infantile and juvenile nuclear cataract, right eye** 🄿

　　　　H26.032 **Infantile and juvenile nuclear cataract, left eye** 🄿

　　　　H26.033 **Infantile and juvenile nuclear cataract, bilateral** 🄿

　　　　H26.039 **Infantile and juvenile nuclear cataract, unspecified eye** 🄿

　　🔵 **H26.04** Anterior subcapsular polar infantile and juvenile **cataract**

　　　　H26.041 **Anterior subcapsular polar infantile and juvenile cataract, right eye** 🄿

　　　　H26.042 **Anterior subcapsular polar infantile and juvenile cataract, left eye** 🄿

　　　　H26.043 **Anterior subcapsular polar infantile and juvenile cataract, bilateral** 🄿

　　　　H26.049 **Anterior subcapsular polar infantile and juvenile cataract, unspecified eye** 🄿

　　🔵 **H26.05** Posterior subcapsular polar infantile and juvenile **cataract**

　　　　H26.051 **Posterior subcapsular polar infantile and juvenile cataract, right eye** 🄿

　　　　H26.052 **Posterior subcapsular polar infantile and juvenile cataract, left eye** 🄿

　　　　H26.053 **Posterior subcapsular polar infantile and juvenile cataract, bilateral** 🄿

　　　　H26.059 **Posterior subcapsular polar infantile and juvenile cataract, unspecified eye** 🄿

　　🔵 **H26.06** Combined forms of infantile and juvenile cataract

　　　　H26.061 **Combined forms of infantile and juvenile cataract, right eye** 🄿

　　　　H26.062 **Combined forms of infantile and juvenile cataract, left eye** 🄿

　　　　H26.063 **Combined forms of infantile and juvenile cataract, bilateral** 🄿

　　　　H26.069 **Combined forms of infantile and juvenile cataract, unspecified eye** 🄿

　　　　H26.09 Other infantile and juvenile cataract 🄿

🔵 **H26.1** Traumatic **cataract**

　　Use **additional** code (Chapter 20) to identify external cause

　　🔵 **H26.10** Unspecified **traumatic cataract**

　　　　H26.101 **Unspecified traumatic cataract, right eye**

　　　　H26.102 **Unspecified traumatic cataract, left eye**

　　　　H26.103 **Unspecified traumatic cataract, bilateral**

　　　　H26.109 **Unspecified traumatic cataract, unspecified eye**

　　🔵 **H26.11** Localized **traumatic opacities**

　　　　H26.111 **Localized traumatic opacities, right eye**

　　　　H26.112 **Localized traumatic opacities, left eye**

　　　　H26.113 **Localized traumatic opacities, bilateral**

　　　　H26.119 **Localized traumatic opacities, unspecified eye**

　　🔵 **H26.12** Partially resolved **traumatic cataract**

　　　　H26.121 **Partially resolved traumatic cataract, right eye**

　　　　H26.122 **Partially resolved traumatic cataract, left eye**

　　　　H26.123 **Partially resolved traumatic cataract, bilateral**

　　　　H26.129 **Partially resolved traumatic cataract, unspecified eye**

　　🔵 **H26.13** Total **traumatic cataract**

　　　　H26.131 **Total traumatic cataract, right eye**

　　　　H26.132 **Total traumatic cataract, left eye**

　　　　H26.133 **Total traumatic cataract, bilateral**

　　　　H26.139 **Total traumatic cataract, unspecified eye**

🔵 **H26.2** Complicated **cataract**

　　H26.20 **Unspecified complicated cataract**

　　　　Cataracta complicata NOS

　　🔵 **H26.21** Cataract with neovascularization

　　　　Code also associated condition, such as:

　　　　　chronic iridocyclitis (H20.1-)

　　　　H26.211 **Cataract with neovascularization, right eye**

　　　　H26.212 **Cataract with neovascularization, left eye**

　　　　H26.213 **Cataract with neovascularization, bilateral**

　　　　H26.219 **Cataract with neovascularization, unspecified eye**

　　🔵 **H26.22** Cataract secondary to ocular disorders (degenerative) (inflammatory)

　　　　Code also associated ocular disorder

　　　　H26.221 **Cataract secondary to ocular disorders (degenerative) (inflammatory), right eye**

　　　　H26.222 **Cataract secondary to ocular disorders (degenerative) (inflammatory), left eye**

　　　　H26.223 **Cataract secondary to ocular disorders (degenerative) (inflammatory), bilateral**

　　　　H26.229 **Cataract secondary to ocular disorders (degenerative) (inflammatory), unspecified eye**

　　🔵 **H26.23** Glaucomatous flecks (subcapsular)

　　　　☞ **Code first** underlying glaucoma (H40-H42)

　　　　H26.231 **Glaucomatous flecks (subcapsular), right eye**

　　　　H26.232 **Glaucomatous flecks (subcapsular), left eye**

　　　　H26.233 **Glaucomatous flecks (subcapsular), bilateral**

　　　　H26.239 **Glaucomatous flecks (subcapsular), unspecified eye**

🔵 **H26.3** Drug-induced **cataract**

　　Toxic cataract

　　Use **additional** code for adverse effect, if applicable, to identify drug (T36-T50 with fifth or sixth character 5)

　　H26.30 **Drug-induced cataract, unspecified eye**

　　H26.31 **Drug-induced cataract, right eye**

　　H26.32 **Drug-induced cataract, left eye**

　　H26.33 **Drug-induced cataract, bilateral**

🔵 **H26.4** Secondary **cataract**

　　H26.40 **Unspecified secondary cataract**

　　🔵 **H26.41** Soemmering's **ring**

　　　　H26.411 **Soemmering's ring, right eye**

　　　　H26.412 **Soemmering's ring, left eye**

　　　　H26.413 **Soemmering's ring, bilateral**

　　　　H26.419 **Soemmering's ring, unspecified eye**

　　🔵 **H26.49** Other secondary **cataract**

　　　　H26.491 **Other secondary cataract, right eye**

🄿🔒 Unacceptable principal diagnosis symbol per Medicare code edits　　🔒 Code exempt from diagnosis present on admission requirement

❓ Questionable admission　　🔵 Complication or comorbidity　　ᴹᶜᶜ Major complication or comorbidity　　ᶜᶜ/ᴹᶜᶜᴱˣᶜ CC/MCC exclusion

🅷🅲🅲 HCC diagnosis code　　🆁🅷🅲🅲 RxHCC diagnosis code　　MACRA code　　**DEFINITION** Describes condition/terminology

TIP Coding guidance　　👁 Official Guideline Reference　　🆉🆁 Z code as first-listed diagnosis

H26.492 Other secondary cataract, left eye
AHA: Q2 2018
H26.493 Other secondary cataract, bilateral
H26.499 Other secondary cataract, unspecified eye
H26.8 Other specified cataract
H26.9 Unspecified cataract
4ᵗʰ H27 Other disorders of lens
EXCLUDES1 congenital lens malformations (Q12.-)
mechanical complications of intraocular lens implant (T85.2)
pseudophakia (Z96.1)
5ᵗʰ H27.0 Aphakia
Acquired absence of lens
Acquired aphakia
Aphakia due to trauma
EXCLUDES1 cataract extraction status (Z98.4-)
congenital absence of lens (Q12.3)
congenital aphakia (Q12.3)
H27.00 Aphakia, unspecified eye
H27.01 Aphakia, right eye
H27.02 Aphakia, left eye
H27.03 Aphakia, bilateral
5ᵗʰ H27.1 Dislocation of lens
H27.10 Unspecified dislocation of lens
6ᵗʰ H27.11 Subluxation of lens
H27.111 Subluxation of lens, right eye
H27.112 Subluxation of lens, left eye
H27.113 Subluxation of lens, bilateral
H27.119 Subluxation of lens, unspecified eye
6ᵗʰ H27.12 Anterior dislocation of lens
H27.121 Anterior dislocation of lens, right eye
H27.122 Anterior dislocation of lens, left eye
H27.123 Anterior dislocation of lens, bilateral
H27.129 Anterior dislocation of lens, unspecified eye
6ᵗʰ H27.13 Posterior dislocation of lens
H27.131 Posterior dislocation of lens, right eye
H27.132 Posterior dislocation of lens, left eye
H27.133 Posterior dislocation of lens, bilateral
H27.139 Posterior dislocation of lens, unspecified eye
H27.8 Other specified disorders of lens
H27.9 Unspecified disorder of lens
H28 Cataract in diseases classified elsewhere
☞ Code first underlying disease, such as:
hypoparathyroidism (E20.-)
myotonia (G71.1-)
myxedema (E03.-)
protein-calorie malnutrition (E40-E46)
EXCLUDES1 cataract in diabetes mellitus (E08.36, E09.36, E10.36, E11.36, E13.36)

Disorders of choroid and retina (H30-H36)

4ᵗʰ H30 Chorioretinal inflammation
5ᵗʰ H30.0 Focal chorioretinal inflammation
Focal chorioretinitis
Focal choroiditis
Focal retinitis
Focal retinochoroiditis
6ᵗʰ H30.00 Unspecified focal chorioretinal inflammation
Focal chorioretinitis NOS
Focal choroiditis NOS
Focal retinitis NOS
Focal retinochoroiditis NOS
H30.001 Unspecified focal chorioretinal inflammation, right eye
H30.002 Unspecified focal chorioretinal inflammation, left eye
H30.003 Unspecified focal chorioretinal inflammation, bilateral

H30.009 Unspecified focal chorioretinal inflammation, unspecified eye
6ᵗʰ H30.01 Focal chorioretinal inflammation, juxtapapillary
H30.011 Focal chorioretinal inflammation, juxtapapillary, right eye
H30.012 Focal chorioretinal inflammation, juxtapapillary, left eye
H30.013 Focal chorioretinal inflammation, juxtapapillary, bilateral
H30.019 Focal chorioretinal inflammation, juxtapapillary, unspecified eye
6ᵗʰ H30.02 Focal chorioretinal inflammation of posterior pole
H30.021 Focal chorioretinal inflammation of posterior pole, right eye
H30.022 Focal chorioretinal inflammation of posterior pole, left eye
H30.023 Focal chorioretinal inflammation of posterior pole, bilateral
H30.029 Focal chorioretinal inflammation of posterior pole, unspecified eye
6ᵗʰ H30.03 Focal chorioretinal inflammation, peripheral
H30.031 Focal chorioretinal inflammation, peripheral, right eye
H30.032 Focal chorioretinal inflammation, peripheral, left eye
H30.033 Focal chorioretinal inflammation, peripheral, bilateral
H30.039 Focal chorioretinal inflammation, peripheral, unspecified eye
6ᵗʰ H30.04 Focal chorioretinal inflammation, macular or paramacular
H30.041 Focal chorioretinal inflammation, macular or paramacular, right eye
H30.042 Focal chorioretinal inflammation, macular or paramacular, left eye
H30.043 Focal chorioretinal inflammation, macular or paramacular, bilateral
H30.049 Focal chorioretinal inflammation, macular or paramacular, unspecified eye
5ᵗʰ H30.1 Disseminated chorioretinal inflammation
Disseminated chorioretinitis
Disseminated choroiditis
Disseminated retinitis
Disseminated retinochoroiditis
EXCLUDES2 exudative retinopathy (H35.02-)
6ᵗʰ H30.10 Unspecified disseminated chorioretinal inflammation
Disseminated chorioretinitis NOS
Disseminated choroiditis NOS
Disseminated retinitis NOS
Disseminated retinochoroiditis NOS
H30.101 Unspecified disseminated chorioretinal inflammation, right eye CC CC/MCC Exc
H30.102 Unspecified disseminated chorioretinal inflammation, left eye CC CC/MCC Exc
H30.103 Unspecified disseminated chorioretinal inflammation, bilateral CC CC/MCC Exc
H30.109 Unspecified disseminated chorioretinal inflammation, unspecified eye CC CC/MCC Exc
6ᵗʰ H30.11 Disseminated chorioretinal inflammation of posterior pole
H30.111 Disseminated chorioretinal inflammation of posterior pole, right eye CC CC/MCC Exc
H30.112 Disseminated chorioretinal inflammation of posterior pole, left eye CC CC/MCC Exc
H30.113 Disseminated chorioretinal inflammation of posterior pole, bilateral CC CC/MCC Exc
H30.119 Disseminated chorioretinal inflammation of posterior pole, unspecified eye CC CC/MCC Exc
6ᵗʰ H30.12 Disseminated chorioretinal inflammation, peripheral

---

Unspecified Code   Other Specified Code   Manifestation Code   N Newborn   P Pediatric   M Maternity   A Adult   ♂ Male   ♀ Female
● New Code   ▲ Revised Code Title   ►◄ Revised Text   NOTES   INCLUDES   EXCLUDES1 Not coded here   EXCLUDES2 Not included here
4ᵗʰ 4ᵗʰ character required   5ᵗʰ 5ᵗʰ character required   6ᵗʰ 6ᵗʰ character required   7ᵗʰ 7ᵗʰ character required   Extension 'X' Alert
HAC Hospital-acquired condition (HAC) alert   AHA AHA Coding Clinic©   ☞ Code first alert

H30.121 Disseminated chorioretinal inflammation, peripheral **right** eye cc⊘ cc/mcc exc⊘

H30.122 Disseminated chorioretinal inflammation, peripheral, **left** eye cc⊘ cc/mcc exc⊘

H30.123 Disseminated chorioretinal inflammation, peripheral, **bilateral** cc⊘ cc/mcc exc⊘

H30.129 Disseminated chorioretinal inflammation, peripheral, **unspecified eye** cc⊘ cc/mcc exc⊘

6ᵗʰ H30.13 Disseminated chorioretinal inflammation, generalized

H30.131 Disseminated chorioretinal inflammation, generalized, **right** eye cc⊘ cc/mcc exc⊘

H30.132 Disseminated chorioretinal inflammation, generalized, **left** eye cc⊘ cc/mcc exc⊘

H30.133 Disseminated chorioretinal inflammation, generalized, **bilateral** cc⊘ cc/mcc exc⊘

H30.139 Disseminated chorioretinal inflammation, generalized, **unspecified eye** cc⊘ cc/mcc exc⊘

6ᵗʰ H30.14 Acute posterior multifocal placoid pigment epitheliopathy

H30.141 Acute posterior multifocal placoid pigment epitheliopathy, **right** eye cc⊘ cc/mcc exc⊘

H30.142 Acute posterior multifocal placoid pigment epitheliopathy, **left** eye cc⊘ cc/mcc exc⊘

H30.143 Acute posterior multifocal placoid pigment epitheliopathy, **bilateral** cc⊘ cc/mcc exc⊘

H30.149 Acute posterior multifocal placoid pigment epitheliopathy, unspecified eye cc⊘ cc/mcc exc⊘

5ᵗʰ H30.2 Posterior cyclitis
Pars planitis

H30.20 Posterior cyclitis, unspecified eye

H30.21 Posterior cyclitis, **right** eye

H30.22 Posterior cyclitis, **left** eye

H30.23 Posterior cyclitis, **bilateral**

5ᵗʰ H30.8 Other chorioretinal inflammations

6ᵗʰ H30.81 Harada's disease

H30.811 Harada's disease, **right** eye

H30.812 Harada's disease, **left** eye

H30.813 Harada's disease, **bilateral**

H30.819 Harada's disease, **unspecified eye**

6ᵗʰ H30.89 Other chorioretinal inflammations

H30.891 Other chorioretinal inflammations, **right** eye cc⊘ cc/mcc exc⊘

H30.892 Other chorioretinal inflammations, **left** eye cc⊘ cc/mcc exc⊘

H30.893 Other chorioretinal inflammations, **bilateral** cc⊘ cc/mcc exc⊘

H30.899 Other chorioretinal inflammations, **unspecified eye** cc⊘ cc/mcc exc⊘

5ᵗʰ H30.9 Unspecified chorioretinal inflammation
Chorioretinitis NOS
Choroiditis NOS
Neuroretinitis NOS
Retinitis NOS
Retinochoroiditis NOS

H30.90 Unspecified chorioretinal inflammation, unspecified eye cc⊘ cc/mcc exc⊘

H30.91 Unspecified chorioretinal inflammation, **right eye** cc⊘ cc/mcc exc⊘

H30.92 Unspecified chorioretinal inflammation, **left** eye cc⊘ cc/mcc exc⊘

H30.93 Unspecified chorioretinal inflammation, **bilateral** cc⊘ cc/mcc exc⊘

4ᵗʰ H31 Other disorders of choroid

5ᵗʰ H31.0 Chorioretinal scars

EXCLUDES2 postsurgical chorioretinal scars (H59.81-)

6ᵗʰ H31.00 Unspecified chorioretinal scars

H31.001 Unspecified chorioretinal scars, **right** eye

H31.002 Unspecified chorioretinal scars, **left** eye

H31.003 Unspecified chorioretinal scars, **bilateral**

H31.009 Unspecified chorioretinal scars, unspecified eye

6ᵗʰ H31.01 Macula scars of posterior pole (postinflammatory) (post-traumatic)

EXCLUDES1 postprocedural chorioretinal scar (H59.81-)

H31.011 Macula scars of posterior pole (postinflammatory) (post-traumatic), **right** eye

H31.012 Macula scars of posterior pole (postinflammatory) (post-traumatic), **left** eye

H31.013 Macula scars of posterior pole (postinflammatory) (post-traumatic), **bilateral**

H31.019 Macula scars of posterior pole (postinflammatory) (post-traumatic), **unspecified eye**

6ᵗʰ H31.02 Solar retinopathy

H31.021 Solar retinopathy, **right** eye

H31.022 Solar retinopathy, **left** eye

H31.023 Solar retinopathy, **bilateral**

H31.029 Solar retinopathy, **unspecified eye**

6ᵗʰ H31.09 Other chorioretinal scars

H31.091 Other chorioretinal scars, **right** eye

H31.092 Other chorioretinal scars, **left** eye

H31.093 Other chorioretinal scars, **bilateral**

H31.099 Other chorioretinal scars, unspecified eye

5ᵗʰ H31.1 Choroidal degeneration

EXCLUDES2 angioid streaks of macula (H35.33)

6ᵗʰ H31.10 Unspecified choroidal degeneration
Choroidal sclerosis NOS

H31.101 Choroidal degeneration, unspecified, **right** eye

H31.102 Choroidal degeneration, unspecified, **left** eye

H31.103 Choroidal degeneration, unspecified, **bilateral**

H31.109 Choroidal degeneration, unspecified, **unspecified eye**

6ᵗʰ H31.11 Age-related choroidal atrophy

H31.111 Age-related choroidal atrophy, **right** eye Ⓐ

H31.112 Age-related choroidal atrophy, **left** eye Ⓐ

H31.113 Age-related choroidal atrophy, **bilateral** Ⓐ

H31.119 Age-related choroidal atrophy, **unspecified eye** Ⓐ

6ᵗʰ H31.12 Diffuse secondary atrophy of choroid

H31.121 Diffuse secondary atrophy of choroid, **right** eye

H31.122 Diffuse secondary atrophy of choroid, **left** eye

H31.123 Diffuse secondary atrophy of choroid, **bilateral**

H31.129 Diffuse secondary atrophy of choroid, **unspecified eye**

5ᵗʰ H31.2 Hereditary choroidal dystrophy

EXCLUDES2 hyperornithinemia (E72.4)
ornithinemia (E72.4)

H31.20 Hereditary choroidal dystrophy, unspecified

H31.21 Choroideremia

H31.22 Choroidal dystrophy (central areolar) (generalized) (peripapillary)

H31.23 Gyrate atrophy, choroid

H31.29 Other hereditary choroidal dystrophy

5ᵗʰ H31.3 Choroidal hemorrhage and rupture

6ᵗʰ H31.30 Unspecified choroidal hemorrhage

H31.301 Unspecified choroidal hemorrhage, **right** eye

H31.302 Unspecified choroidal hemorrhage, **left** eye

H31.303 Unspecified choroidal hemorrhage, bilateral

H31.309 Unspecified choroidal hemorrhage, unspecified eye

6ᵗʰ H31.31 Expulsive choroidal hemorrhage

H31.311 Expulsive choroidal hemorrhage, right eye

H31.312 Expulsive choroidal hemorrhage, left eye

H31.313 Expulsive choroidal hemorrhage, bilateral

H31.319 Expulsive choroidal hemorrhage, unspecified eye

6ᵗʰ H31.32 Choroidal rupture

H31.321 Choroidal rupture, right eye CC⊘ CC/MCC Exc⊘

H31.322 Choroidal rupture, left eye CC⊘ CC/MCC Exc⊘

H31.323 Choroidal rupture, bilateral CC⊘ CC/MCC Exc⊘

H31.329 Choroidal rupture, unspecified eye CC⊘ CC/MCC Exc⊘

5ᵗʰ H31.4 Choroidal detachment

6ᵗʰ H31.40 Unspecified choroidal detachment

H31.401 Unspecified choroidal detachment, right eye CC⊘ CC/MCC Exc⊘

H31.402 Unspecified choroidal detachment, left eye CC⊘ CC/MCC Exc⊘

H31.403 Unspecified choroidal detachment, bilateral CC⊘ CC/MCC Exc⊘

H31.409 Unspecified choroidal detachment, unspecified eye CC⊘ CC/MCC Exc⊘

6ᵗʰ H31.41 Hemorrhagic choroidal detachment

H31.411 Hemorrhagic choroidal detachment, right eye CC⊘ CC/MCC Exc⊘

H31.412 Hemorrhagic choroidal detachment, left eye CC⊘ CC/MCC Exc⊘

H31.413 Hemorrhagic choroidal detachment, bilateral CC⊘ CC/MCC Exc⊘

H31.419 Hemorrhagic choroidal detachment, unspecified eye CC⊘ CC/MCC Exc⊘

6ᵗʰ H31.42 Serous choroidal detachment

H31.421 Serous choroidal detachment, right eye CC⊘ CC/MCC Exc⊘

H31.422 Serous choroidal detachment, left eye CC⊘ CC/MCC Exc⊘

H31.423 Serous choroidal detachment, bilateral CC⊘ CC/MCC Exc⊘

H31.429 Serous choroidal detachment, unspecified eye CC⊘ CC/MCC Exc⊘

H31.8 Other specified disorders of choroid

H31.9 Unspecified disorder of choroid

H32 Chorioretinal disorders in diseases classified elsewhere

☞ Code first underlying disease, such as:
congenital toxoplasmosis (P37.1)
histoplasmosis (B39.-)
leprosy (A30.-)
EXCLUDES1 chorioretinitis (in):
toxoplasmosis (acquired) (B58.01)
tuberculosis (A18.53)

4ᵗʰ H33 Retinal detachments and breaks
EXCLUDES1 detachment of retinal pigment epithelium (H35.72-, H35.73-)

5ᵗʰ H33.0 Retinal detachment with retinal break
Rhegmatogenous retinal detachment
EXCLUDES1 serous retinal detachment (without retinal break) (H33.2-)

6ᵗʰ H33.00 Unspecified retinal detachment with retinal break

H33.001 Unspecified retinal detachment with retinal break, right eye

H33.002 Unspecified retinal detachment with retinal break, left eye

H33.003 Unspecified retinal detachment with retinal break, bilateral

H33.009 Unspecified retinal detachment with retinal break, unspecified eye

6ᵗʰ H33.01 Retinal detachment with single break

H33.011 Retinal detachment with single break, right eye

H33.012 Retinal detachment with single break, left eye

H33.013 Retinal detachment with single break, bilateral

H33.019 Retinal detachment with single break, unspecified eye

6ᵗʰ H33.02 Retinal detachment with multiple breaks

H33.021 Retinal detachment with multiple breaks, right eye

H33.022 Retinal detachment with multiple breaks, left eye

H33.023 Retinal detachment with multiple breaks, bilateral

H33.029 Retinal detachment with multiple breaks, unspecified eye

6ᵗʰ H33.03 Retinal detachment with giant retinal tear

H33.031 Retinal detachment with giant retinal tear, right eye

H33.032 Retinal detachment with giant retinal tear, left eye

H33.033 Retinal detachment with giant retinal tear, bilateral

H33.039 Retinal detachment with giant retinal tear, unspecified eye

6ᵗʰ H33.04 Retinal detachment with retinal dialysis

H33.041 Retinal detachment with retinal dialysis, right eye

H33.042 Retinal detachment with retinal dialysis, left eye

H33.043 Retinal detachment with retinal dialysis, bilateral

H33.049 Retinal detachment with retinal dialysis, unspecified eye

6ᵗʰ H33.05 Total retinal detachment

H33.051 Total retinal detachment, right eye

H33.052 Total retinal detachment, left eye

H33.053 Total retinal detachment, bilateral

H33.059 Total retinal detachment, unspecified eye

5ᵗʰ H33.1 Retinoschisis and retinal cysts
EXCLUDES1 congenital retinoschisis (Q14.1)
microcystoid degeneration of retina (H35.42-)

6ᵗʰ H33.10 Unspecified retinoschisis

H33.101 Unspecified retinoschisis, right eye

H33.102 Unspecified retinoschisis, left eye

H33.103 Unspecified retinoschisis, bilateral

H33.109 Unspecified retinoschisis, unspecified eye

6ᵗʰ H33.11 Cyst of ora serrata

H33.111 Cyst of ora serrata, right eye

H33.112 Cyst of ora serrata, left eye

H33.113 Cyst of ora serrata, bilateral

H33.119 Cyst of ora serrata, unspecified eye

6ᵗʰ H33.12 Parasitic cyst of retina

H33.121 Parasitic cyst of retina, right eye CC⊘ CC/MCC Exc⊘

H33.122 Parasitic cyst of retina, left eye CC⊘ CC/MCC Exc⊘

H33.123 Parasitic cyst of retina, bilateral CC⊘ CC/MCC Exc⊘

H33.129 Parasitic cyst of retina, unspecified eye CC⊘ CC/MCC Exc⊘

6ᵗʰ H33.19 Other retinoschisis and retinal cysts
Pseudocyst of retina

H33.191 Other retinoschisis and retinal cysts, right eye

H33.192 Other retinoschisis and retinal cysts, left eye

H33.193 Other retinoschisis and retinal cysts, bilateral

H33.199 Other retinoschisis and retinal cysts, unspecified eye

H33.2 Serous **retinal detachment**
Retinal detachment NOS
Retinal detachment without retinal break
EXCLUDES1 central serous chorioretinopathy (H35.71-)
H33.20 Serous retinal detachment, unspecified eye cc⊘ CC/MCC Exc⊘
H33.21 Serous retinal detachment, right eye cc⊘ CC/MCC Exc⊘
H33.22 Serous retinal detachment, left eye cc⊘ CC/MCC Exc⊘
H33.23 Serous retinal detachment, bilateral cc⊘ CC/MCC Exc⊘

H33.3 Retinal breaks without detachment
EXCLUDES1 chorioretinal scars after surgery for detachment
(H59.81-)
peripheral retinal degeneration without break
(H35.4-)
H33.30 Unspecified **retinal break**
H33.301 Unspecified retinal break, right eye
H33.302 Unspecified retinal break, left eye
H33.303 Unspecified retinal break, bilateral
H33.309 Unspecified retinal break, unspecified eye
H33.31 Horseshoe tear **of retina without detachment**
Operculum of retina without detachment
H33.311 Horseshoe tear of retina without detachment, right eye
H33.312 Horseshoe tear of retina without detachment, left eye
H33.313 Horseshoe tear of retina without detachment, bilateral
H33.319 Horseshoe tear of retina without detachment, unspecified eye
H33.32 Round hole **of retina without detachment**
H33.321 Round hole, right eye
H33.322 Round hole, left eye
H33.323 Round hole, bilateral
H33.329 Round hole, unspecified eye
H33.33 Multiple defects **of retina without detachment**
H33.331 Multiple defects of retina without detachment, right eye
H33.332 Multiple defects of retina without detachment, left eye
H33.333 Multiple defects of retina without detachment, bilateral
H33.339 Multiple defects of retina without detachment, unspecified eye

H33.4 Traction **detachment of retina**
Proliferative vitreo-retinopathy with retinal detachment
H33.40 Traction detachment of retina, unspecified eye cc⊘ CC/MCC Exc⊘
H33.41 Traction detachment of retina, right eye cc⊘ CC/MCC Exc⊘
H33.42 Traction detachment of retina, left eye cc⊘ CC/MCC Exc⊘
H33.43 Traction detachment of retina, bilateral cc⊘ CC/MCC Exc⊘
H33.8 Other retinal detachments

H34 Retinal vascular occlusions
EXCLUDES1 amaurosis fugax (G45.3)
H34.0 Transient **retinal artery occlusion**
H34.00 Transient retinal artery occlusion, unspecified eye cc⊘ CC/MCC Exc⊘
H34.01 Transient retinal artery occlusion, right eye cc⊘ CC/MCC Exc⊘
H34.02 Transient retinal artery occlusion, left eye cc⊘ CC/MCC Exc⊘
H34.03 Transient retinal artery occlusion, bilateral cc⊘ CC/MCC Exc⊘
H34.1 Central **retinal artery occlusion**
H34.10 Central retinal artery occlusion, unspecified eye cc⊘ CC/MCC Exc⊘
H34.11 Central retinal artery occlusion, right eye cc⊘ CC/MCC Exc⊘
H34.12 Central retinal artery occlusion, left eye cc⊘ CC/MCC Exc⊘
H34.13 Central retinal artery occlusion, bilateral cc⊘ CC/MCC Exc⊘
H34.2 Other **retinal artery occlusions**
H34.21 Partial **retinal artery occlusion**
Hollenhorst's plaque
Retinal microembolism
H34.211 Partial retinal artery occlusion, right eye

H34.212 Partial retinal artery occlusion, left eye cc⊘ CC/MCC Exc⊘
H34.213 Partial retinal artery occlusion, bilateral cc⊘ CC/MCC Exc⊘
H34.219 Partial retinal artery occlusion, unspecified eye cc⊘ CC/MCC Exc⊘
H34.23 Retinal artery branch occlusion
H34.231 Retinal artery branch occlusion, right eye cc⊘ CC/MCC Exc⊘
H34.232 Retinal artery branch occlusion, left eye cc⊘ CC/MCC Exc⊘
H34.233 Retinal artery branch occlusion, bilateral cc⊘ CC/MCC Exc⊘
H34.239 Retinal artery branch occlusion, unspecified eye cc⊘ CC/MCC Exc⊘
H34.8 Other **retinal vascular occlusions**
H34.81 Central **retinal vein occlusion**
One of the following 7th characters is to be assigned to codes in subcategory H34.81 to designate the severity of the occlusion:
0 = with macular edema
1 = with retinal neovascularization
2 = stable
Old central retinal vein occlusion
H34.811 Central retinal vein occlusion, right eye cc⊘ CC/MCC Exc⊘
H34.812 Central retinal vein occlusion, left eye cc⊘ CC/MCC Exc⊘
H34.813 Central retinal vein occlusion, bilateral cc⊘ CC/MCC Exc⊘
H34.819 Central retinal vein occlusion, unspecified eye cc⊘ CC/MCC Exc⊘
H34.82 Venous engorgement
Incipient retinal vein occlusion
Partial retinal vein occlusion
H34.821 Venous engorgement, right eye
H34.822 Venous engorgement, left eye
H34.823 Venous engorgement, bilateral
H34.829 Venous engorgement, unspecified eye
H34.83 Tributary (branch) **retinal vein occlusion**
One of the following 7th characters is to be assigned to codes in subcategory H34.83 to designate the severity of the occlusion:
0 = with macular edema
1 = with retinal neovascularization
2 = stable
Old tributary (branch) retinal vein occlusion
H34.831 Tributary (branch) retinal vein occlusion, right eye
H34.832 Tributary (branch) retinal vein occlusion, left eye
H34.833 Tributary (branch) retinal vein occlusion, bilateral
H34.839 Tributary (branch) retinal vein occlusion, unspecified eye
H34.9 Unspecified retinal vascular occlusion

H35 Other retinal disorders
EXCLUDES2 diabetic retinal disorders (E08.311-E08.359, E09.311-E09.359, E10.311-E10.359, E11.311-E11.359, E13.311-E13.359)
H35.0 Background retinopathy **and retinal vascular changes**
👁 See Official Guidelines "Hypertensive Retinopathy" I.C.9.a.5
Code also any associated hypertension (I10.-)
H35.00 Unspecified background retinopathy
H35.01 Changes in retinal vascular appearance
Retinal vascular sheathing
H35.011 Changes in retinal vascular appearance, right eye
H35.012 Changes in retinal vascular appearance, left eye
H35.013 Changes in retinal vascular appearance, bilateral

PDxⓆ Unacceptable principal diagnosis symbol per Medicare code edits   PⓍ Code exempt from diagnosis present on admission requirement
❓ Questionable admission   cc⊘ Complication or comorbidity   MCC⊘ Major complication or comorbidity   CC/MCC Exc⊘ CC/MCC exclusion
HCC HCC diagnosis code   RxHCC RxHCC diagnosis code   MACRA MACRA code   **DEFINITION** Describes condition/terminology
TIP Coding guidance   👁 Official Guideline Reference   Z1 Z code as first-listed diagnosis

616   When symbols appear on a code that requires a 7th character extension, refer to Appendix B to identify applicable 7th character codes.   **2020 ICD-10-CM**

H35.019 Changes in retinal vascular appearance, unspecified eye

6️⃣ H35.02 Exudative retinopathy
Coats retinopathy
H35.021 Exudative retinopathy, right eye
H35.022 Exudative retinopathy, left eye
H35.023 Exudative retinopathy, bilateral
H35.029 Exudative retinopathy, unspecified eye

6️⃣ H35.03 Hypertensive retinopathy
H35.031 Hypertensive retinopathy, right eye
H35.032 Hypertensive retinopathy, left eye
H35.033 Hypertensive retinopathy, bilateral
H35.039 Hypertensive retinopathy, unspecified eye

6️⃣ H35.04 Retinal micro-aneurysms, unspecified
H35.041 Retinal micro-aneurysms, unspecified, right eye
H35.042 Retinal micro-aneurysms, unspecified, left eye
H35.043 Retinal micro-aneurysms, unspecified, bilateral
H35.049 Retinal micro-aneurysms, unspecified, unspecified eye

6️⃣ H35.05 Retinal neovascularization, unspecified
H35.051 Retinal neovascularization, unspecified, right eye
H35.052 Retinal neovascularization, unspecified, left eye
H35.053 Retinal neovascularization, unspecified, bilateral
H35.059 Retinal neovascularization, unspecified, unspecified eye

6️⃣ H35.06 Retinal vasculitis
Eales disease
Retinal perivasculitis
H35.061 Retinal vasculitis, right eye
H35.062 Retinal vasculitis, left eye
H35.063 Retinal vasculitis, bilateral
H35.069 Retinal vasculitis, unspecified eye

6️⃣ H35.07 Retinal telangiectasis
H35.071 Retinal telangiectasis, right eye
H35.072 Retinal telangiectasis, left eye
H35.073 Retinal telangiectasis, bilateral
H35.079 Retinal telangiectasis, unspecified eye

H35.09 Other intraretinal microvascular abnormalities
Retinal varices

5️⃣ H35.1 Retinopathy of prematurity
6️⃣ H35.10 Retinopathy of prematurity, unspecified
Retinopathy of prematurity NOS
H35.101 Retinopathy of prematurity, unspecified, right eye
H35.102 Retinopathy of prematurity, unspecified, left eye
H35.103 Retinopathy of prematurity, unspecified, bilateral
H35.109 Retinopathy of prematurity, unspecified, unspecified eye

6️⃣ H35.11 Retinopathy of prematurity, stage 0
H35.111 Retinopathy of prematurity, stage 0, right eye
H35.112 Retinopathy of prematurity, stage 0, left eye
H35.113 Retinopathy of prematurity, stage 0, bilateral
H35.119 Retinopathy of prematurity, stage 0, unspecified eye

6️⃣ H35.12 Retinopathy of prematurity, stage 1
H35.121 Retinopathy of prematurity, stage 1, right eye
H35.122 Retinopathy of prematurity, stage 1, left eye
H35.123 Retinopathy of prematurity, stage 1, bilateral

H35.129 Retinopathy of prematurity, stage 1, unspecified eye

6️⃣ H35.13 Retinopathy of prematurity, stage 2
H35.131 Retinopathy of prematurity, stage 2, right eye
H35.132 Retinopathy of prematurity, stage 2, left eye
H35.133 Retinopathy of prematurity, stage 2, bilateral
H35.139 Retinopathy of prematurity, stage 2, unspecified eye

6️⃣ H35.14 Retinopathy of prematurity, stage 3
H35.141 Retinopathy of prematurity, stage 3, right eye
H35.142 Retinopathy of prematurity, stage 3, left eye
H35.143 Retinopathy of prematurity, stage 3, bilateral
H35.149 Retinopathy of prematurity, stage 3, unspecified eye

6️⃣ H35.15 Retinopathy of prematurity, stage 4
H35.151 Retinopathy of prematurity, stage 4, right eye
H35.152 Retinopathy of prematurity, stage 4, left eye
H35.153 Retinopathy of prematurity, stage 4, bilateral
H35.159 Retinopathy of prematurity, stage 4, unspecified eye

6️⃣ H35.16 Retinopathy of prematurity, stage 5
H35.161 Retinopathy of prematurity, stage 5, right eye
H35.162 Retinopathy of prematurity, stage 5, left eye
H35.163 Retinopathy of prematurity, stage 5, bilateral
H35.169 Retinopathy of prematurity, stage 5, unspecified eye

6️⃣ H35.17 Retrolental fibroplasia
H35.171 Retrolental fibroplasia, right eye
H35.172 Retrolental fibroplasia, left eye
H35.173 Retrolental fibroplasia, bilateral
H35.179 Retrolental fibroplasia, unspecified eye

5️⃣ H35.2 Other non-diabetic proliferative retinopathy
Proliferative vitreo-retinopathy
EXCLUDES1 proliferative vitreo-retinopathy with retinal detachment (H33.4-)
H35.20 Other non-diabetic proliferative retinopathy, unspecified eye
H35.21 Other non-diabetic proliferative retinopathy, right eye
H35.22 Other non-diabetic proliferative retinopathy, left eye
H35.23 Other non-diabetic proliferative retinopathy, bilateral

5️⃣ H35.3 Degeneration of macula and posterior pole
H35.30 Unspecified macular degeneration 🅰
Age-related macular degeneration
6️⃣ H35.31 Nonexudative age-related macular degeneration
Atrophic age-related macular degeneration
Dry age-related macular degeneration
One of the following 7th characters is to be assigned to codes in subcategory H35.31 to designate the stage of the disease:
0 = stage unspecified
1 = early dry stage
2 = intermediate dry stage
3 = advanced atrophic without subfoveal involvement
advanced dry stage
4 = advanced atrophic with subfoveal involvement

Unspecified Code   Other Specified Code   Manifestation Code   Ⓝ Newborn   Ⓟ Pediatric   Ⓜ Maternity   🅰 Adult   ♂ Male   ♀ Female
● New Code   ▲ Revised Code Title   ▶◀ Revised Text   **NOTES**   *INCLUDES*   *EXCLUDES1* Not coded here   *EXCLUDES2* Not included here
4️⃣ 4th character required   5️⃣ 5th character required   6️⃣ 6th character required   7️⃣ 7th character required   ✖ Extension 'X' Alert
🅷🅰🅲 Hospital-acquired condition (HAC) alert   **AHA** AHA Coding Clinic©   📪 Code first alert

2020 ICD-10-CM   When symbols appear on a code that requires a 7th character extension, refer to Appendix B to identify applicable 7th character codes.   **617**

7️⃣ H35.311 **Nonexudative age-related macular degeneration,** right eye   A
     AHA: Q4 2016

7️⃣ H35.312 **Nonexudative age-related macular degeneration,** left eye   A
     AHA: Q4 2016

7️⃣ H35.313 **Nonexudative age-related macular degeneration,** bilateral   A
     AHA: Q4 2016

7️⃣ H35.319 **Nonexudative age-related macular degeneration, unspecified** eye   A
     AHA: Q4 2016

6️⃣ **H35.32** Exudative age-related **macular degeneration**
Wet age-related macular degeneration
One of the following 7th characters is to be assigned to codes in subcategory H35.32 to designate the stage of the disease:
     0 = stage unspecified
     1 = with active choroidal neovascularization
     2 = with inactive choroidal neovascularization with involuted or regressed neovascularization
     3 = with inactive scar

7️⃣ H35.321 **Exudative age-related macular degeneration,** right eye   A HCC
     AHA: Q4 2016

7️⃣ H35.322 **Exudative age-related macular degeneration,** left eye   A HCC
     AHA: Q4 2016

7️⃣ H35.323 **Exudative age-related macular degeneration,** bilateral   A HCC
     AHA: Q4 2016

7️⃣ H35.329 **Exudative age-related macular degeneration, unspecified** eye   A HCC
     AHA: Q4 2016

H35.33 Angioid streaks **of macula**

6️⃣ **H35.34** Macular cyst, **hole, or pseudohole**
   H35.341 **Macular cyst, hole, or pseudohole,** right eye
   H35.342 **Macular cyst, hole, or pseudohole,** left eye
   H35.343 **Macular cyst, hole, or pseudohole,** bilateral
   H35.349 **Macular cyst, hole, or pseudohole, unspecified eye**

6️⃣ **H35.35** Cystoid **macular degeneration**
   EXCLUDES1 cystoid macular edema following cataract surgery (H59.03-)
   H35.351 **Cystoid macular degeneration,** right eye
   H35.352 **Cystoid macular degeneration,** left eye
   H35.353 **Cystoid macular degeneration,** bilateral
   H35.359 **Cystoid macular degeneration, unspecified eye**

6️⃣ **H35.36** Drusen (degenerative) **of macula**
   H35.361 **Drusen (degenerative) of macula,** right eye
     AHA: Q4 2016
   H35.362 **Drusen (degenerative) of macula,** left eye
     AHA: Q4 2016
   H35.363 **Drusen (degenerative) of macula,** bilateral
     AHA: Q1 2017
   H35.369 **Drusen (degenerative) of macula, unspecified eye**

6️⃣ **H35.37** Puckering **of macula**
   H35.371 **Puckering of macula,** right eye
   H35.372 **Puckering of macula,** left eye
   H35.373 **Puckering of macula,** bilateral
   H35.379 **Puckering of macula, unspecified eye**

6️⃣ **H35.38** Toxic **maculopathy**
   ☞ **Code first** poisoning due to drug or toxin, if applicable (T36-T65 with fifth or sixth character 1-4 or 6)
   Use additional code for adverse effect, if applicable, to identify drug (T36-T50 with fifth or sixth character 5)

   H35.381 **Toxic maculopathy,** right eye
   H35.382 **Toxic maculopathy,** left eye
   H35.383 **Toxic maculopathy,** bilateral
   H35.389 **Toxic maculopathy, unspecified eye**

5️⃣ **H35.4** Peripheral **retinal degeneration**
   EXCLUDES1 hereditary retinal degeneration (dystrophy) (H35.5-)
          peripheral retinal degeneration with retinal break (H33.3-)

   H35.40 **Unspecified peripheral retinal degeneration**

6️⃣ **H35.41** Lattice **degeneration of retina**
   Palisade degeneration of retina
   H35.411 **Lattice degeneration of retina,** right eye
   H35.412 **Lattice degeneration of retina,** left eye
   H35.413 **Lattice degeneration of retina,** bilateral
   H35.419 **Lattice degeneration of retina, unspecified eye**

6️⃣ **H35.42** Microcystoid **degeneration of retina**
   H35.421 **Microcystoid degeneration of retina,** right eye
   H35.422 **Microcystoid degeneration of retina,** left eye
   H35.423 **Microcystoid degeneration of retina,** bilateral
   H35.429 **Microcystoid degeneration of retina, unspecified eye**

6️⃣ **H35.43** Paving stone **degeneration of retina**
   H35.431 **Paving stone degeneration of retina,** right eye
   H35.432 **Paving stone degeneration of retina,** left eye
   H35.433 **Paving stone degeneration of retina,** bilateral
   H35.439 **Paving stone degeneration of retina, unspecified eye**

6️⃣ **H35.44** Age-related reticular **degeneration of retina**
   H35.441 **Age-related reticular degeneration of retina,** left eye   A
   H35.442 **Age-related reticular degeneration of retina,** left eye   A
   H35.443 **Age-related reticular degeneration of retina,** bilateral   A
   H35.449 **Age-related reticular degeneration of retina, unspecified eye**   A

6️⃣ **H35.45** Secondary pigmentary **degeneration**
   H35.451 **Secondary pigmentary degeneration,** right eye
   H35.452 **Secondary pigmentary degeneration,** left eye
   H35.453 **Secondary pigmentary degeneration,** bilateral
   H35.459 **Secondary pigmentary degeneration, unspecified eye**

6️⃣ **H35.46** Secondary vitreoretinal **degeneration**
   H35.461 **Secondary vitreoretinal degeneration,** right eye
   H35.462 **Secondary vitreoretinal degeneration,** left eye
   H35.463 **Secondary vitreoretinal degeneration,** bilateral
   H35.469 **Secondary vitreoretinal degeneration, unspecified eye**

5️⃣ **H35.5** Hereditary **retinal dystrophy**
   EXCLUDES1 dystrophies primarily involving Bruch's membrane (H31.1-)

   H35.50 **Unspecified hereditary retinal dystrophy**
   H35.51 Vitreoretinal **dystrophy**
   H35.52 Pigmentary **retinal dystrophy**
     Albipunctate retinal dystrophy
     Retinitis pigmentosa
     Tapetoretinal dystrophy

Pᴅₓ Unacceptable principal diagnosis symbol per Medicare code edits   Pᴏᴀ Code exempt from diagnosis present on admission requirement
❓ Questionable admission   ᴄᴄ Complication or comorbidity   ᴍᴄᴄ Major complication or comorbidity   ᴄᴄ/ᴍᴄᴄ ᴇxᴄ CC/MCC exclusion
HCC HCC diagnosis code   RxHCC RxHCC diagnosis code   MACRA code   **DEFINITION** Describes condition/terminology
TIP Coding guidance   👁 Official Guideline Reference   Z Z code as first-listed diagnosis

618   When symbols appear on a code that requires a 7th character extension, refer to Appendix B to identify applicable 7th character codes.   **2020 ICD-10-CM**

H35.53 Other dystrophies primarily involving the sensory retina
Stargardt's disease

H35.54 Dystrophies primarily involving the retinal pigment epithelium
Vitelliform retinal dystrophy

5ᵗʰ H35.6 Retinal hemorrhage

H35.60 Retinal hemorrhage, unspecified eye

H35.61 Retinal hemorrhage, right eye

H35.62 Retinal hemorrhage, left eye

H35.63 Retinal hemorrhage, bilateral

5ᵗʰ H35.7 Separation of retinal layers
EXCLUDES1 retinal detachment (serous) (H33.2-)
rhegmatogenous retinal detachment (H33.0-)

H35.70 Unspecified separation of retinal layers CC CC/MCC Exc

6ᵗʰ H35.71 Central serous chorioretinopathy

H35.711 Central serous chorioretinopathy, right eye

H35.712 Central serous chorioretinopathy, left eye

H35.713 Central serous chorioretinopathy, bilateral

H35.719 Central serous chorioretinopathy, unspecified eye

6ᵗʰ H35.72 Serous detachment of retinal pigment epithelium

H35.721 Serous detachment of retinal pigment epithelium, right eye CC CC/MCC Exc

H35.722 Serous detachment of retinal pigment epithelium, left eye CC CC/MCC Exc

H35.723 Serous detachment of retinal pigment epithelium, bilateral CC CC/MCC Exc

H35.729 Serous detachment of retinal pigment epithelium, unspecified eye CC CC/MCC Exc

6ᵗʰ H35.73 Hemorrhagic detachment of retinal pigment epithelium

H35.731 Hemorrhagic detachment of retinal pigment epithelium, right eye CC CC/MCC Exc

H35.732 Hemorrhagic detachment of retinal pigment epithelium, left eye CC CC/MCC Exc

H35.733 Hemorrhagic detachment of retinal pigment epithelium, bilateral CC CC/MCC Exc

H35.739 Hemorrhagic detachment of retinal pigment epithelium, unspecified eye CC CC/MCC Exc

5ᵗʰ H35.8 Other specified retinal disorders
EXCLUDES2 retinal hemorrhage (H35.6-)

H35.81 Retinal edema
Retinal cotton wool spots

H35.82 Retinal ischemia CC CC/MCC Exc

H35.89 Other specified retinal disorders

H35.9 Unspecified retinal disorder

H36 Retinal disorders in diseases classified elsewhere
☞ Code first underlying disease, such as:
lipid storage disorders (E75.-)
sickle-cell disorders (D57.-)
EXCLUDES1 arteriosclerotic retinopathy (H35.0-)
diabetic retinopathy (E08.3-, E09.3-, E10.3-, E11.3-, E13.3-)

Glaucoma (H40-H42) (Figure 7.4)

4ᵗʰ H40 Glaucoma
👁 See Official Guidelines "Assigning Glaucoma Codes" I.C.7.a.1
EXCLUDES1 absolute glaucoma (H44.51-)
congenital glaucoma (Q15.0)
traumatic glaucoma due to birth injury (P15.3)

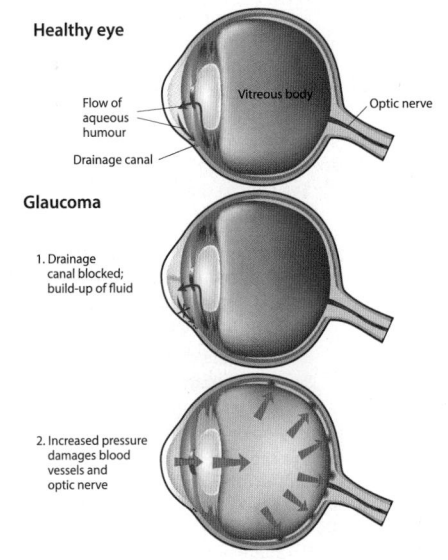

Figure 7.4 Glaucoma

5ᵗʰ H40.0 Glaucoma suspect

6ᵗʰ H40.00 Preglaucoma, unspecified

H40.001 Preglaucoma, unspecified, right eye

H40.002 Preglaucoma, unspecified, left eye

H40.003 Preglaucoma, unspecified, bilateral

H40.009 Preglaucoma, unspecified, unspecified eye

6ᵗʰ H40.01 Open angle with borderline findings, low risk
Open angle, low risk

H40.011 Open angle with borderline findings, low risk, right eye

H40.012 Open angle with borderline findings, low risk, left eye

H40.013 Open angle with borderline findings, low risk, bilateral

H40.019 Open angle with borderline findings, low risk, unspecified eye

6ᵗʰ H40.02 Open angle with borderline findings, high risk
Open angle, high risk

H40.021 Open angle with borderline findings, high risk, right eye

H40.022 Open angle with borderline findings, high risk, left eye

H40.023 Open angle with borderline findings, high risk, bilateral

H40.029 Open angle with borderline findings, high risk, unspecified eye

6ᵗʰ H40.03 Anatomical narrow angle
Primary angle closure suspect

H40.031 Anatomical narrow angle, right eye

H40.032 Anatomical narrow angle, left eye

H40.033 Anatomical narrow angle, bilateral

H40.039 Anatomical narrow angle, unspecified eye

6ᵗʰ H40.04 Steroid responder

H40.041 Steroid responder, right eye

H40.042 Steroid responder, left eye

H40.043 Steroid responder, bilateral

H40.049 Steroid responder, unspecified eye

6ᵗʰ H40.05 Ocular hypertension

H40.051 Ocular hypertension, right eye
H40.052 Ocular hypertension, left eye
H40.053 Ocular hypertension, bilateral
H40.059 Ocular hypertension, unspecified eye

6ᵗʰ H40.06 Primary angle closure without glaucoma damage

H40.061 Primary angle closure without glaucoma damage, right eye
H40.062 Primary angle closure without glaucoma damage, left eye
H40.063 Primary angle closure without glaucoma damage, bilateral
H40.069 Primary angle closure without glaucoma damage, unspecified eye

5ᵗʰ H40.1 Open-angle glaucoma

7ᵗʰ H40.10 Unspecified open-angle glaucoma   RxHCC

👁 See Official Guidelines "Bilateral glaucoma with same type and stage" I.C.7.a.2
AHA: Q4 2018
One of the following 7th characters is to be assigned to code H40.10 to designate the stage of glaucoma
0 = stage unspecified
1 = mild stage
2 = moderate stage
3 = severe stage
4 = indeterminate stage

6ᵗʰ H40.11 Primary open-angle glaucoma
Chronic simple glaucoma
One of the following 7th characters is to be assigned to each code in subcategory H40.11 to designate the stage of glaucoma
0 = stage unspecified
1 = mild stage
2 = moderate stage
3 = severe stage
4 = indeterminate stage

7ᵗʰ H40.111 Primary open-angle glaucoma, right eye   RxHCC
AHA: Q2 2019, Q4 2016
7ᵗʰ H40.112 Primary open-angle glaucoma, left eye   RxHCC
AHA: Q4 2016
7ᵗʰ H40.113 Primary open-angle glaucoma, bilateral   RxHCC
AHA: Q4 2016
7ᵗʰ H40.119 Primary open-angle glaucoma, unspecified eye   RxHCC
AHA: Q4 2016

6ᵗʰ H40.12 Low-tension glaucoma
One of the following 7th characters is to be assigned to each code in subcategory H40.12 to designate the stage of glaucoma
0 = stage unspecified
1 = mild stage
2 = moderate stage
3 = severe stage
4 = indeterminate stage

7ᵗʰ H40.121 Low-tension glaucoma, right eye   RxHCC PDxⁿ
7ᵗʰ H40.122 Low-tension glaucoma, left eye   RxHCC PDxⁿ
7ᵗʰ H40.123 Low-tension glaucoma, bilateral   RxHCC PDxⁿ
7ᵗʰ H40.129 Low-tension glaucoma, unspecified eye   RxHCC PDxⁿ

6ᵗʰ H40.13 Pigmentary glaucoma
One of the following 7th characters is to be assigned to each code in subcategory H40.13 to designate the stage of glaucoma
0 = stage unspecified
1 = mild stage
2 = moderate stage
3 = severe stage
4 = indeterminate stage

7ᵗʰ H40.131 Pigmentary glaucoma, right eye   RxHCC PDxⁿ
7ᵗʰ H40.132 Pigmentary glaucoma, left eye   RxHCC PDxⁿ

7ᵗʰ H40.133 Pigmentary glaucoma, bilateral   RxHCC PDxⁿ
7ᵗʰ H40.139 Pigmentary glaucoma, unspecified eye   RxHCC PDxⁿ

6ᵗʰ H40.14 Capsular glaucoma with pseudoexfoliation of lens
One of the following 7th characters is to be assigned to each code in subcategory H40.14 to designate the stage of glaucoma
0 = stage unspecified
1 = mild stage
2 = moderate stage
3 = severe stage
4 = indeterminate stage

7ᵗʰ H40.141 Capsular glaucoma with pseudoexfoliation of lens, right eye
7ᵗʰ H40.142 Capsular glaucoma with pseudoexfoliation of lens, left eye
7ᵗʰ H40.143 Capsular glaucoma with pseudoexfoliation of lens, bilateral
7ᵗʰ H40.149 Capsular glaucoma with pseudoexfoliation of lens, unspecified eye

6ᵗʰ H40.15 Residual stage of open-angle glaucoma
H40.151 Residual stage of open-angle glaucoma, right eye   RxHCC PDxⁿ
H40.152 Residual stage of open-angle glaucoma, left eye   RxHCC PDxⁿ
H40.153 Residual stage of open-angle glaucoma, bilateral   RxHCC PDxⁿ
H40.159 Residual stage of open-angle glaucoma, unspecified eye   RxHCC PDxⁿ

5ᵗʰ H40.2 Primary angle-closure glaucoma
EXCLUDES1 aqueous misdirection (H40.83-)
malignant glaucoma (H40.83-)

7ᵗʰ H40.20 Unspecified primary angle-closure glaucoma
👁 See Official Guidelines "Bilateral glaucoma with same type and stage" I.C.7.a.2
AHA: Q4 2018
One of the following 7th characters is to be assigned to code H40.20 to designate the stage of glaucoma
0 = stage unspecified
1 = mild stage
2 = moderate stage
3 = severe stage
4 = indeterminate stage

6ᵗʰ H40.21 Acute angle-closure glaucoma
Acute angle-closure glaucoma attack
Acute angle-closure glaucoma crisis
H40.211 Acute angle-closure glaucoma, right eye   cc CC/MCC Exc
H40.212 Acute angle-closure glaucoma, left eye   cc CC/MCC Exc
H40.213 Acute angle-closure glaucoma, bilateral   cc CC/MCC Exc
H40.219 Acute angle-closure glaucoma, unspecified eye   cc CC/MCC Exc

6ᵗʰ H40.22 Chronic angle-closure glaucoma
Chronic primary angle closure glaucoma
One of the following 7th characters is to be assigned to each code in subcategory H40.22 to designate the stage of glaucoma
0 = stage unspecified
1 = mild stage
2 = moderate stage
3 = severe stage
4 = indeterminate stage

7ᵗʰ H40.221 Chronic angle-closure glaucoma, right eye
7ᵗʰ H40.222 Chronic angle-closure glaucoma, left eye
7ᵗʰ H40.223 Chronic angle-closure glaucoma, bilateral
7ᵗʰ H40.229 Chronic angle-closure glaucoma, unspecified eye

6ᵗʰ H40.23 Intermittent angle-closure glaucoma

PDxⁿ Unacceptable principal diagnosis symbol per Medicare code edits   PDx Code exempt from diagnosis present on admission requirement
❓ Questionable admission   cc Complication or comorbidity   MCC Major complication or comorbidity   CC/MCC Exc CC/MCC exclusion
HCC HCC diagnosis code   RxHCC RxHCC diagnosis code   MACRA MACRA code   **DEFINITION** Describes condition/terminology
TIP Coding guidance   👁 Official Guideline Reference   Z1 Z code as first-listed diagnosis

H40.231 Intermittent angle-closure glaucoma, right eye

H40.232 Intermittent angle-closure glaucoma, left eye

H40.233 Intermittent angle-closure glaucoma, bilateral

H40.239 Intermittent angle-closure glaucoma, unspecified eye

6ᵗʰ H40.24 Residual stage of angle-closure glaucoma

H40.241 Residual stage of angle-closure glaucoma, right eye

H40.242 Residual stage of angle-closure glaucoma, left eye

H40.243 Residual stage of angle-closure glaucoma, bilateral

H40.249 Residual stage of angle-closure glaucoma, unspecified eye

5ᵗʰ H40.3 Glaucoma secondary to eye trauma

Code also underlying condition

One of the following 7th characters is to be assigned to each code in subcategory H40.3 to designate the stage of glaucoma

0 = stage unspecified
1 = mild stage
2 = moderate stage
3 = severe stage
4 = indeterminate stage

7ᵖ H40.30 Glaucoma secondary to eye trauma, unspecified eye

7ᵖ H40.31 Glaucoma secondary to eye trauma, right eye

7ᵖ H40.32 Glaucoma secondary to eye trauma, left eye

7ᵖ H40.33 Glaucoma secondary to eye trauma, bilateral

5ᵗʰ H40.4 Glaucoma secondary to eye inflammation

Code also underlying condition

One of the following 7th characters is to be assigned to each code in subcategory H40.4 to designate the stage of glaucoma

0 = stage unspecified
1 = mild stage
2 = moderate stage
3 = severe stage
4 = indeterminate stage

7ᵖ H40.40 Glaucoma secondary to eye inflammation, unspecified eye

7ᵖ H40.41 Glaucoma secondary to eye inflammation, right eye

7ᵖ H40.42 Glaucoma secondary to eye inflammation, left eye

7ᵖ H40.43 Glaucoma secondary to eye inflammation, bilateral

5ᵗʰ H40.5 Glaucoma secondary to other eye disorders

Code also underlying eye disorder

One of the following 7th characters is to be assigned to each code in subcategory H40.5 to designate the stage of glaucoma

0 = stage unspecified
1 = mild stage
2 = moderate stage
3 = severe stage
4 = indeterminate stage

7ᵖ H40.50 Glaucoma secondary to other eye disorders, unspecified eye

7ᵖ H40.51 Glaucoma secondary to other eye disorders, right eye

7ᵖ H40.52 Glaucoma secondary to other eye disorders, left eye

7ᵖ H40.53 Glaucoma secondary to other eye disorders, bilateral

5ᵗʰ H40.6 Glaucoma secondary to drugs

Use additional code for adverse effect, if applicable, to identify drug (T36-T50 with fifth or sixth character 5)

One of the following 7th characters is to be assigned to each code in subcategory H40.6 to designate the stage of glaucoma

0 = stage unspecified
1 = mild stage

2 = moderate stage
3 = severe stage
4 = indeterminate stage

7ᵖ H40.60 Glaucoma secondary to drugs, unspecified eye

7ᵖ H40.61 Glaucoma secondary to drugs, right eye

7ᵖ H40.62 Glaucoma secondary to drugs, left eye

7ᵖ H40.63 Glaucoma secondary to drugs, bilateral

5ᵗʰ H40.8 Other glaucoma

6ᵗʰ H40.81 Glaucoma with increased episcleral venous pressure

H40.811 Glaucoma with increased episcleral venous pressure, right eye

H40.812 Glaucoma with increased episcleral venous pressure, left eye

H40.813 Glaucoma with increased episcleral venous pressure, bilateral

H40.819 Glaucoma with increased episcleral venous pressure, unspecified eye

6ᵗʰ H40.82 Hypersecretion glaucoma

H40.821 Hypersecretion glaucoma, right eye

H40.822 Hypersecretion glaucoma, left eye

H40.823 Hypersecretion glaucoma, bilateral

H40.829 Hypersecretion glaucoma, unspecified eye

6ᵗʰ H40.83 Aqueous misdirection

Malignant glaucoma

H40.831 Aqueous misdirection, right eye

H40.832 Aqueous misdirection, left eye

H40.833 Aqueous misdirection, bilateral

H40.839 Aqueous misdirection, unspecified eye

H40.89 Other specified glaucoma

H40.9 Unspecified glaucoma

H42 Glaucoma in diseases classified elsewhere

☞ Code first underlying condition, such as:
amyloidosis (E85.-)
aniridia (Q13.1)
glaucoma (in) diabetes mellitus (E08.39, E09.39, E10.39, E11.39, E13.39)
Lowe's syndrome (E72.03)
Reiger's anomaly (Q13.81)
specified metabolic disorder (E70-E88)

EXCLUDES1 glaucoma (in) onchocerciasis (B73.02)
glaucoma (in) syphilis (A52.71)
glaucoma (in) tuberculous (A18.59)

Disorders of vitreous body and globe (H43-H44)

4ᵗʰ H43 Disorders of vitreous body

5ᵗʰ H43.0 Vitreous prolapse

EXCLUDES1 vitreous syndrome following cataract surgery (H59.0-)
traumatic vitreous prolapse (S05.2-)

H43.00 Vitreous prolapse, unspecified eye

H43.01 Vitreous prolapse, right eye

H43.02 Vitreous prolapse, left eye

H43.03 Vitreous prolapse, bilateral

5ᵗʰ H43.1 Vitreous hemorrhage

H43.10 Vitreous hemorrhage, unspecified eye HCC

H43.11 Vitreous hemorrhage, right eye HCC

H43.12 Vitreous hemorrhage, left eye HCC

H43.13 Vitreous hemorrhage, bilateral HCC

5ᵗʰ H43.2 Crystalline deposits in vitreous body

H43.20 Crystalline deposits in vitreous body, unspecified eye

H43.21 Crystalline deposits in vitreous body, right eye

H43.22 Crystalline deposits in vitreous body, left eye

H43.23 Crystalline deposits in vitreous body, bilateral

5ᵗʰ H43.3 Other vitreous opacities

6ᵗʰ H43.31 Vitreous membranes and strands

H43.311 Vitreous membranes and strands, right eye

Unspecified Code Other Specified Code Manifestation Code Ⓝ Newborn Ⓟ Pediatric Ⓜ Maternity Ⓐ Adult ♂ Male ♀ Female
● New Code ▲ Revised Code Title ▶◀ Revised Text **NOTES** *INCLUDES* *EXCLUDES1* Not coded here *EXCLUDES2* Not included here
4ᵗʰ 4ᵗʰ character required 5ᵗʰ 5ᵗʰ character required 6ᵗʰ 6ᵗʰ character required 7ᵖ 7ᵗʰ character required 7ᵖ Extension 'X' Alert
HAC Hospital-acquired condition (HAC) alert **AHA** AHA Coding Clinic© ☞ Code first alert

H43.312 Vitreous membranes and strands, left eye
H43.313 Vitreous membranes and strands, bilateral
H43.319 Vitreous membranes and strands, unspecified eye

6ᵗʰ **H43.39** Other vitreous opacities
Vitreous floaters
H43.391 Other vitreous opacities, right eye
H43.392 Other vitreous opacities, left eye
H43.393 Other vitreous opacities, bilateral
H43.399 Other vitreous opacities, unspecified eye

5ᵗʰ **H43.8** Other disorders of vitreous body
EXCLUDES1 proliferative vitreo-retinopathy with retinal detachment (H33.4-)
EXCLUDES2 vitreous abscess (H44.02-)

6ᵗʰ **H43.81** Vitreous degeneration
Vitreous detachment
H43.811 Vitreous degeneration, right eye
H43.812 Vitreous degeneration, left eye
H43.813 Vitreous degeneration, bilateral
H43.819 Vitreous degeneration, unspecified eye

6ᵗʰ **H43.82** Vitreomacular adhesion
Vitreomacular traction
H43.821 Vitreomacular adhesion, right eye **A**
H43.822 Vitreomacular adhesion, left eye **A**
H43.823 Vitreomacular adhesion, bilateral **A**
H43.829 Vitreomacular adhesion, unspecified eye **A**

H43.89 Other disorders of vitreous body
H43.9 Unspecified disorder of vitreous body

4ᵗʰ **H44** Disorders of globe
INCLUDES disorders affecting multiple structures of eye

5ᵗʰ **H44.0** Purulent endophthalmitis
Use additional code to identify organism
EXCLUDES1 bleb associated endophthalmitis (H59.4-)

6ᵗʰ **H44.00** Unspecified purulent endophthalmitis
H44.001 Unspecified purulent endophthalmitis, right eye CC CC/MCC Exc
H44.002 Unspecified purulent endophthalmitis, left eye CC CC/MCC Exc
H44.003 Unspecified purulent endophthalmitis, bilateral CC CC/MCC Exc
H44.009 Unspecified purulent endophthalmitis, unspecified eye CC CC/MCC Exc

6ᵗʰ **H44.01** Panophthalmitis (acute)
H44.011 Panophthalmitis (acute), right eye CC CC/MCC Exc
H44.012 Panophthalmitis (acute), left eye CC CC/MCC Exc
H44.013 Panophthalmitis (acute), bilateral CC CC/MCC Exc
H44.019 Panophthalmitis (acute), unspecified eye CC CC/MCC Exc

6ᵗʰ **H44.02** Vitreous abscess (chronic)
H44.021 Vitreous abscess (chronic), right eye CC CC/MCC Exc
H44.022 Vitreous abscess (chronic), left eye CC CC/MCC Exc
H44.023 Vitreous abscess (chronic), bilateral CC CC/MCC Exc
H44.029 Vitreous abscess (chronic), unspecified eye CC CC/MCC Exc

5ᵗʰ **H44.1** Other endophthalmitis
EXCLUDES1 bleb associated endophthalmitis (H59.4-)
EXCLUDES2 ophthalmia nodosa (H16.2-)

6ᵗʰ **H44.11** Panuveitis
H44.111 Panuveitis, right eye CC CC/MCC Exc
H44.112 Panuveitis, left eye CC CC/MCC Exc
H44.113 Panuveitis, bilateral CC CC/MCC Exc
H44.119 Panuveitis, unspecified eye CC CC/MCC Exc

6ᵗʰ **H44.12** Parasitic endophthalmitis, unspecified
H44.121 Parasitic endophthalmitis, unspecified, right eye CC CC/MCC Exc

H44.122 Parasitic endophthalmitis, unspecified, left eye CC CC/MCC Exc
H44.123 Parasitic endophthalmitis, unspecified, bilateral CC CC/MCC Exc
H44.129 Parasitic endophthalmitis, unspecified, unspecified eye CC CC/MCC Exc

6ᵗʰ **H44.13** Sympathetic uveitis
H44.131 Sympathetic uveitis, right eye CC CC/MCC Exc
H44.132 Sympathetic uveitis, left eye CC CC/MCC Exc
H44.133 Sympathetic uveitis, bilateral CC CC/MCC Exc
H44.139 Sympathetic uveitis, unspecified eye CC CC/MCC Exc

H44.19 Other endophthalmitis CC CC/MCC Exc

5ᵗʰ **H44.2** Degenerative myopia
Malignant myopia
H44.20 Degenerative myopia, unspecified eye
H44.21 Degenerative myopia, right eye
H44.22 Degenerative myopia, left eye
H44.23 Degenerative myopia, bilateral

6ᵗʰ **H44.2A** Degenerative myopia with choroidal neovascularization
Use additional code for any associated choroid disorders (H31.-)
H44.2A1 Degenerative myopia with choroidal neovascularization, right eye
H44.2A2 Degenerative myopia with choroidal neovascularization, left eye
H44.2A3 Degenerative myopia with choroidal neovascularization, bilateral eye
H44.2A9 Degenerative myopia with choroidal neovascularization, unspecified eye

6ᵗʰ **H44.2B** Degenerative myopia with macular hole
H44.2B1 Degenerative myopia with macular hole, right eye
H44.2B2 Degenerative myopia with macular hole, left eye
H44.2B3 Degenerative myopia with macular hole, bilateral eye
H44.2B9 Degenerative myopia with macular hole, unspecified eye

6ᵗʰ **H44.2C** Degenerative myopia with retinal detachment
Use additional code to identify the retinal detachment (H33.-)
H44.2C1 Degenerative myopia with retinal detachment, right eye
H44.2C2 Degenerative myopia with retinal detachment, left eye
H44.2C3 Degenerative myopia with retinal detachment, bilateral eye
H44.2C9 Degenerative myopia with retinal detachment, unspecified eye

6ᵗʰ **H44.2D** Degenerative myopia with foveoschisis
H44.2D1 Degenerative myopia with foveoschisis, right eye
H44.2D2 Degenerative myopia with foveoschisis, left eye
H44.2D3 Degenerative myopia with foveoschisis, bilateral eye
H44.2D9 Degenerative myopia with foveoschisis, unspecified eye

6ᵗʰ **H44.2E** Degenerative myopia with other maculopathy
H44.2E1 Degenerative myopia with other maculopathy, right eye
H44.2E2 Degenerative myopia with other maculopathy, left eye
H44.2E3 Degenerative myopia with other maculopathy, bilateral eye
H44.2E9 Degenerative myopia with other maculopathy, unspecified eye

5ᵗʰ **H44.3** Other and unspecified degenerative disorders of globe
H44.30 Unspecified degenerative disorder of globe

PDxⁿ Unacceptable principal diagnosis symbol per Medicare code edits   PDx Code exempt from diagnosis present on admission requirement
? Questionable admission   CC Complication or comorbidity   MCC Major complication or comorbidity   CC/MCC Exc CC/MCC exclusion
HCC HCC diagnosis code   RxHCC RxHCC diagnosis code   MACRA MACRA code   **DEFINITION** Describes condition/terminology
TIP Coding guidance   ⊙ Official Guideline Reference   Z1 Z code as first-listed diagnosis

622   When symbols appear on a code that requires a 7th character extension, refer to Appendix B to identify applicable 7th character codes.   **2020 ICD-10-CM**

H44.31 Chalcosis
- H44.311 Chalcosis, right eye
- H44.312 Chalcosis, left eye
- H44.313 Chalcosis, bilateral
- H44.319 Chalcosis, unspecified eye

H44.32 Siderosis of eye
- H44.321 Siderosis of eye, right eye
- H44.322 Siderosis of eye, left eye
- H44.323 Siderosis of eye, bilateral
- H44.329 Siderosis of eye, unspecified eye

H44.39 Other degenerative disorders of globe
- H44.391 Other degenerative disorders of globe, right eye
- H44.392 Other degenerative disorders of globe, left eye
- H44.393 Other degenerative disorders of globe, bilateral
- H44.399 Other degenerative disorders of globe, unspecified eye

H44.4 Hypotony of eye
- **H44.40** Unspecified hypotony of eye
- **H44.41** Flat anterior chamber hypotony of eye
  - H44.411 Flat anterior chamber hypotony of right eye
  - H44.412 Flat anterior chamber hypotony of left eye
  - H44.413 Flat anterior chamber hypotony of eye, bilateral
  - H44.419 Flat anterior chamber hypotony of unspecified eye
- **H44.42** Hypotony of eye due to ocular fistula
  - H44.421 Hypotony of right eye due to ocular fistula
  - H44.422 Hypotony of left eye due to ocular fistula
  - H44.423 Hypotony of eye due to ocular fistula, bilateral
  - H44.429 Hypotony of unspecified eye due to ocular fistula
- **H44.43** Hypotony of eye due to other ocular disorders
  - H44.431 Hypotony of eye due to other ocular disorders, right eye
  - H44.432 Hypotony of eye due to other ocular disorders, left eye
  - H44.433 Hypotony of eye due to other ocular disorders, bilateral
  - H44.439 Hypotony of eye due to other ocular disorders, unspecified eye
- **H44.44** Primary hypotony of eye
  - H44.441 Primary hypotony of right eye
  - H44.442 Primary hypotony of left eye
  - H44.443 Primary hypotony of eye, bilateral
  - H44.449 Primary hypotony of unspecified eye

H44.5 Degenerated conditions of globe
- **H44.50** Unspecified degenerated conditions of globe
- **H44.51** Absolute glaucoma
  - H44.511 Absolute glaucoma, right eye
  - H44.512 Absolute glaucoma, left eye
  - H44.513 Absolute glaucoma, bilateral
  - H44.519 Absolute glaucoma, unspecified eye
- **H44.52** Atrophy of globe
  - Phthisis bulbi
  - H44.521 Atrophy of globe, right eye
  - H44.522 Atrophy of globe, left eye
  - H44.523 Atrophy of globe, bilateral
  - H44.529 Atrophy of globe, unspecified eye
- **H44.53** Leucocoria
  - H44.531 Leucocoria, right eye
  - H44.532 Leucocoria, left eye
  - H44.533 Leucocoria, bilateral
  - H44.539 Leucocoria, unspecified eye

H44.6 Retained (old) intraocular foreign body, magnetic
Use additional code to identify magnetic foreign body (Z18.11)
EXCLUDES1 current intraocular foreign body (S05.-)
EXCLUDES2 retained foreign body in eyelid (H02.81-)
retained (old) foreign body following penetrating wound of orbit (H05.5-)
retained (old) intraocular foreign body, nonmagnetic (H44.7-)

H44.60 Unspecified retained (old) intraocular foreign body, magnetic
- H44.601 Unspecified retained (old) intraocular foreign body, magnetic, right eye
- H44.602 Unspecified retained (old) intraocular foreign body, magnetic, left eye
- H44.603 Unspecified retained (old) intraocular foreign body, magnetic, bilateral
- H44.609 Unspecified retained (old) intraocular foreign body, magnetic, unspecified eye

H44.61 Retained (old) magnetic foreign body in anterior chamber
- H44.611 Retained (old) magnetic foreign body in anterior chamber, right eye
- H44.612 Retained (old) magnetic foreign body in anterior chamber, left eye
- H44.613 Retained (old) magnetic foreign body in anterior chamber, bilateral
- H44.619 Retained (old) magnetic foreign body in anterior chamber, unspecified eye

H44.62 Retained (old) magnetic foreign body in iris or ciliary body
- H44.621 Retained (old) magnetic foreign body in iris or ciliary body, right eye
- H44.622 Retained (old) magnetic foreign body in iris or ciliary body, left eye
- H44.623 Retained (old) magnetic foreign body in iris or ciliary body, bilateral
- H44.629 Retained (old) magnetic foreign body in iris or ciliary body, unspecified eye

H44.63 Retained (old) magnetic foreign body in lens
- H44.631 Retained (old) magnetic foreign body in lens, right eye
- H44.632 Retained (old) magnetic foreign body in lens, left eye
- H44.633 Retained (old) magnetic foreign body in lens, bilateral
- H44.639 Retained (old) magnetic foreign body in lens, unspecified eye

H44.64 Retained (old) magnetic foreign body in posterior wall of globe
- H44.641 Retained (old) magnetic foreign body in posterior wall of globe, right eye
- H44.642 Retained (old) magnetic foreign body in posterior wall of globe, left eye
- H44.643 Retained (old) magnetic foreign body in posterior wall of globe, bilateral
- H44.649 Retained (old) magnetic foreign body in posterior wall of globe, unspecified eye

H44.65 Retained (old) magnetic foreign body in vitreous body
- H44.651 Retained (old) magnetic foreign body in vitreous body, right eye
- H44.652 Retained (old) magnetic foreign body in vitreous body, left eye
- H44.653 Retained (old) magnetic foreign body in vitreous body, bilateral
- H44.659 Retained (old) magnetic foreign body in vitreous body, unspecified eye

H44.69 Retained (old) intraocular foreign body, magnetic, in other or multiple sites

---

H44.691 Retained (old) intraocular foreign body, magnetic, in other or multiple sites, right eye
H44.692 Retained (old) intraocular foreign body, magnetic, in other or multiple sites, left eye
H44.693 Retained (old) intraocular foreign body, magnetic, in other or multiple sites, bilateral
H44.699 **Retained (old) intraocular foreign body, magnetic, in other or multiple sites, unspecified eye**

[5th] H44.7 Retained (old) intraocular foreign body, nonmagnetic
Use additional code to identify nonmagnetic foreign body (Z18.01-Z18.10, Z18.12, Z18.2-Z18.9)
[EXCLUDES1] *current intraocular foreign body (S05.-)*
[EXCLUDES2] *retained foreign body in eyelid (H02.81-)*
retained (old) foreign body following penetrating wound of orbit (H05.5-)
retained (old) intraocular foreign body, magnetic (H44.6-)

[6th] H44.70 Unspecified retained (old) intraocular foreign body, nonmagnetic
H44.701 Unspecified retained (old) intraocular foreign body, nonmagnetic, right eye
H44.702 Unspecified retained (old) intraocular foreign body, nonmagnetic, left eye
H44.703 Unspecified retained (old) intraocular foreign body, nonmagnetic, bilateral
H44.709 **Unspecified retained (old) intraocular foreign body, nonmagnetic, unspecified eye**
Retained (old) intraocular foreign body NOS

[6th] H44.71 Retained (nonmagnetic) (old) foreign body in anterior chamber
H44.711 Retained (nonmagnetic) (old) foreign body in anterior chamber, right eye
H44.712 Retained (nonmagnetic) (old) foreign body in anterior chamber, left eye
H44.713 Retained (nonmagnetic) (old) foreign body in anterior chamber, bilateral
H44.719 **Retained (nonmagnetic) (old) foreign body in anterior chamber, unspecified eye**

[6th] H44.72 Retained (nonmagnetic) (old) foreign body in iris or ciliary body
H44.721 Retained (nonmagnetic) (old) foreign body in iris or ciliary body, right eye
H44.722 Retained (nonmagnetic) (old) foreign body in iris or ciliary body, left eye
H44.723 Retained (nonmagnetic) (old) foreign body in iris or ciliary body, bilateral
H44.729 **Retained (nonmagnetic) (old) foreign body in iris or ciliary body, unspecified eye**

[6th] H44.73 Retained (nonmagnetic) (old) foreign body in lens
H44.731 Retained (nonmagnetic) (old) foreign body in lens, right eye
H44.732 Retained (nonmagnetic) (old) foreign body in lens, left eye
H44.733 Retained (nonmagnetic) (old) foreign body in lens, bilateral
H44.739 **Retained (nonmagnetic) (old) foreign body in lens, unspecified eye**

[6th] H44.74 Retained (nonmagnetic) (old) foreign body in posterior wall of globe
H44.741 Retained (nonmagnetic) (old) foreign body in posterior wall of globe, right eye
H44.742 Retained (nonmagnetic) (old) foreign body in posterior wall of globe, left eye
H44.743 Retained (nonmagnetic) (old) foreign body in posterior wall of globe, bilateral
H44.749 **Retained (nonmagnetic) (old) foreign body in posterior wall of globe, unspecified eye**

[6th] H44.75 Retained (nonmagnetic) (old) foreign body in vitreous body
H44.751 Retained (nonmagnetic) (old) foreign body in vitreous body, right eye
H44.752 Retained (nonmagnetic) (old) foreign body in vitreous body, left eye
H44.753 Retained (nonmagnetic) (old) foreign body in vitreous body, bilateral
H44.759 **Retained (nonmagnetic) (old) foreign body in vitreous body, unspecified eye**

[6th] H44.79 Retained (old) intraocular foreign body, nonmagnetic, in other or multiple sites
H44.791 Retained (old) intraocular foreign body, nonmagnetic, in other or multiple sites, right eye
H44.792 Retained (old) intraocular foreign body, nonmagnetic, in other or multiple sites, left eye
H44.793 Retained (old) intraocular foreign body, nonmagnetic, in other or multiple sites, bilateral
H44.799 **Retained (old) intraocular foreign body, nonmagnetic, in other or multiple sites, unspecified eye**

[5th] H44.8 Other disorders of globe
[6th] H44.81 Hemophthalmos
H44.811 Hemophthalmos, right eye
H44.812 Hemophthalmos, left eye
H44.813 Hemophthalmos, bilateral
H44.819 **Hemophthalmos, unspecified eye**
[6th] H44.82 Luxation of globe
H44.821 Luxation of globe, right eye
H44.822 Luxation of globe, left eye
H44.823 Luxation of globe, bilateral
H44.829 **Luxation of globe, unspecified eye**
H44.89 Other disorders of globe
H44.9 **Unspecified disorder of globe**

Disorders of optic nerve and visual pathways (H46-H47)

[4th] H46 Optic neuritis
[EXCLUDES2] *ischemic optic neuropathy (H47.01-)*
neuromyelitis optica [Devic] (G36.0)

[5th] H46.0 Optic papillitis
DEFINITION: Papillitis (optic neuritis) is inflammation and deterioration of the optic disk, a portion of the optic nerve.
H46.00 **Optic papillitis, unspecified eye** [CC] [CC/MCC Exc]
H46.01 Optic papillitis, right eye [CC] [CC/MCC Exc]
H46.02 Optic papillitis, left eye [CC] [CC/MCC Exc]
H46.03 Optic papillitis, bilateral [CC] [CC/MCC Exc]

[5th] H46.1 Retrobulbar neuritis
Retrobulbar neuritis NOS
[EXCLUDES1] *syphilitic retrobulbar neuritis (A52.15)*
H46.10 **Retrobulbar neuritis, unspecified eye** [CC] [CC/MCC Exc]
H46.11 Retrobulbar neuritis, right eye [CC] [CC/MCC Exc]
H46.12 Retrobulbar neuritis, left eye [CC] [CC/MCC Exc]
H46.13 Retrobulbar neuritis, bilateral [CC] [CC/MCC Exc]
H46.2 Nutritional optic neuropathy
H46.3 Toxic optic neuropathy
☞ Code first (T51-T65) to identify cause
H46.8 Other optic neuritis [CC] [CC/MCC Exc]
H46.9 **Unspecified optic neuritis** [CC] [CC/MCC Exc]

[4th] H47 Other disorders of optic [2nd] nerve and visual pathways
[5th] H47.0 Disorders of optic nerve, not elsewhere classified
[6th] H47.01 Ischemic optic neuropathy
H47.011 Ischemic optic neuropathy, right eye

[PDx] Unacceptable principal diagnosis symbol per Medicare code edits [POA] Code exempt from diagnosis present on admission requirement
[?] Questionable admission [CC] Complication or comorbidity [MCC] Major complication or comorbidity [CC/MCC Exc] CC/MCC exclusion
[HCC] HCC diagnosis code [RxHCC] RxHCC diagnosis code MACRA code **DEFINITION** Describes condition/terminology
TIP Coding guidance 👁 Official Guideline Reference [Z1] Z code as first-listed diagnosis

H47.012 Ischemic optic neuropathy, left eye
H47.013 Ischemic optic neuropathy, bilateral
H47.019 Ischemic optic neuropathy, unspecified eye

6th H47.02 Hemorrhage in optic nerve sheath
H47.021 Hemorrhage in optic nerve sheath, right eye
H47.022 Hemorrhage in optic nerve sheath, left eye
H47.023 Hemorrhage in optic nerve sheath, bilateral
H47.029 Hemorrhage in optic nerve sheath, unspecified eye

6th H47.03 Optic nerve hypoplasia
H47.031 Optic nerve hypoplasia, right eye
H47.032 Optic nerve hypoplasia, left eye
H47.033 Optic nerve hypoplasia, bilateral
H47.039 Optic nerve hypoplasia, unspecified eye

6th H47.09 Other disorders of optic nerve, not elsewhere classified
Compression of optic nerve
H47.091 Other disorders of optic nerve, not elsewhere classified, right eye
H47.092 Other disorders of optic nerve, not elsewhere classified, left eye
H47.093 Other disorders of optic nerve, not elsewhere classified, bilateral
H47.099 Other disorders of optic nerve, not elsewhere classified, unspecified eye

5th H47.1 Papilledema
H47.10 Unspecified papilledema   CC CC/MCC Exc
H47.11 Papilledema associated with increased intracranial pressure   CC CC/MCC Exc
H47.12 Papilledema associated with decreased ocular pressure
H47.13 Papilledema associated with retinal disorder

6th H47.14 Foster-Kennedy syndrome
H47.141 Foster-Kennedy syndrome, right eye
H47.142 Foster-Kennedy syndrome, left eye
H47.143 Foster-Kennedy syndrome, bilateral
H47.149 Foster-Kennedy syndrome, unspecified eye

5th H47.2 Optic atrophy
H47.20 Unspecified optic atrophy
6th H47.21 Primary optic atrophy
H47.211 Primary optic atrophy, right eye
H47.212 Primary optic atrophy, left eye
H47.213 Primary optic atrophy, bilateral
H47.219 Primary optic atrophy, unspecified eye
H47.22 Hereditary optic atrophy
Leber's optic atrophy
6th H47.23 Glaucomatous optic atrophy
H47.231 Glaucomatous optic atrophy, right eye
H47.232 Glaucomatous optic atrophy, left eye
H47.233 Glaucomatous optic atrophy, bilateral
H47.239 Glaucomatous optic atrophy, unspecified eye
6th H47.29 Other optic atrophy
Temporal pallor of optic disc
H47.291 Other optic atrophy, right eye
H47.292 Other optic atrophy, left eye
H47.293 Other optic atrophy, bilateral
H47.299 Other optic atrophy, unspecified eye

5th H47.3 Other disorders of optic disc
6th H47.31 Coloboma of optic disc
H47.311 Coloboma of optic disc, right eye
H47.312 Coloboma of optic disc, left eye
H47.313 Coloboma of optic disc, bilateral
H47.319 Coloboma of optic disc, unspecified eye
5th H47.32 Drusen of optic disc

H47.321 Drusen of optic disc, right eye
H47.322 Drusen of optic disc, left eye
H47.323 Drusen of optic disc, bilateral
H47.329 Drusen of optic disc, unspecified eye

6th H47.33 Pseudopapilledema of optic disc
H47.331 Pseudopapilledema of optic disc, right eye
H47.332 Pseudopapilledema of optic disc, left eye
H47.333 Pseudopapilledema of optic disc, bilateral
H47.339 Pseudopapilledema of optic disc, unspecified eye

6th H47.39 Other disorders of optic disc
H47.391 Other disorders of optic disc, right eye
H47.392 Other disorders of optic disc, left eye
H47.393 Other disorders of optic disc, bilateral
H47.399 Other disorders of optic disc, unspecified eye

5th H47.4 Disorders of optic chiasm
Code also underlying condition
H47.41 Disorders of optic chiasm in (due to) inflammatory disorders   CC CC/MCC Exc
H47.42 Disorders of optic chiasm in (due to) neoplasm   CC CC/MCC Exc
H47.43 Disorders of optic chiasm in (due to) vascular disorders   CC CC/MCC Exc
H47.49 Disorders of optic chiasm in (due to) other disorders   CC CC/MCC Exc

5th H47.5 Disorders of other visual pathways
Disorders of optic tracts, geniculate nuclei and optic radiations
Code also underlying condition
6th H47.51 Disorders of visual pathways in (due to) inflammatory disorders
H47.511 Disorders of visual pathways in (due to) inflammatory disorders, right side   CC CC/MCC Exc
H47.512 Disorders of visual pathways in (due to) inflammatory disorders, left side   CC CC/MCC Exc
H47.519 Disorders of visual pathways in (due to) inflammatory disorders, unspecified side   CC CC/MCC Exc
6th H47.52 Disorders of visual pathways in (due to) neoplasm
H47.521 Disorders of visual pathways in (due to) neoplasm, right side   CC CC/MCC Exc
H47.522 Disorders of visual pathways in (due to) neoplasm, left side   CC CC/MCC Exc
H47.529 Disorders of visual pathways in (due to) neoplasm, unspecified side   CC CC/MCC Exc
6th H47.53 Disorders of visual pathways in (due to) vascular disorders
H47.531 Disorders of visual pathways in (due to) vascular disorders, right side   CC CC/MCC Exc
H47.532 Disorders of visual pathways in (due to) vascular disorders, left side   CC CC/MCC Exc
H47.539 Disorders of visual pathways in (due to) vascular disorders, unspecified side   CC CC/MCC Exc

5th H47.6 Disorders of visual cortex
Code also underlying condition
EXCLUDES1 injury to visual cortex ►◄ S04.04-◄
6th H47.61 Cortical blindness
H47.611 Cortical blindness, right side of brain
H47.612 Cortical blindness, left side of brain
H47.619 Cortical blindness, unspecified side of brain
6th H47.62 Disorders of visual cortex in (due to) inflammatory disorders
H47.621 Disorders of visual cortex in (due to) inflammatory disorders, right side of brain   CC CC/MCC Exc
H47.622 Disorders of visual cortex in (due to) inflammatory disorders, left side of brain   CC CC/MCC Exc

---

Unspecified Code   Other Specified Code   Manifestation Code   N Newborn   P Pediatric   M Maternity   A Adult   ♂ Male   ♀ Female
● New Code   ▲ Revised Code Title   ►◄ Revised Text   NOTES   INCLUDES   EXCLUDES1   Not coded here   EXCLUDES2   Not included here
4th 4th character required   5th 5th character required   6th 6th character required   7th 7th character required   Extension 'X' Alert
HAC Hospital-acquired condition (HAC) alert   AHA AHA Coding Clinic©   ☞ Code first alert

H47.629 **Disorders of visual cortex in (due to) inflammatory disorders, unspecified side of brain** cc CC/MCC Exc

6th H47.63 **Disorders of visual cortex in (due to)** neoplasm

H47.631 **Disorders of visual cortex in (due to) neoplasm, right side of brain** cc CC/MCC Exc

H47.632 **Disorders of visual cortex in (due to) neoplasm, left side of brain** cc CC/MCC Exc

H47.639 **Disorders of visual cortex in (due to) neoplasm, unspecified side of brain** cc CC/MCC Exc

6th H47.64 **Disorders of visual cortex in (due to)** vascular disorders

H47.641 **Disorders of visual cortex in (due to) vascular disorders, right side of brain** cc CC/MCC Exc

H47.642 **Disorders of visual cortex in (due to) vascular disorders, left side of brain** cc CC/MCC Exc

H47.649 **Disorders of visual cortex in (due to) vascular disorders, unspecified side of brain** cc CC/MCC Exc

H47.9 **Unspecified disorder of visual pathways**

Disorders of ocular muscles, binocular movement, accommodation and refraction (H49-H52) (Figure 7.5)

EXCLUDES2 *nystagmus and other irregular eye movements (H55)*

4th H49 **Paralytic strabismus**

EXCLUDES2 *internal ophthalmoplegia (H52.51-)*

internuclear ophthalmoplegia (H51.2-)

progressive supranuclear ophthalmoplegia (G23.1)

5th H49.0 Third [oculomotor] nerve palsy

H49.00 **Third [oculomotor] nerve palsy, unspecified eye**

H49.01 **Third [oculomotor] nerve palsy, right eye**

H49.02 **Third [oculomotor] nerve palsy, left eye**

H49.03 **Third [oculomotor] nerve palsy, bilateral**

5th H49.1 Fourth [trochlear] nerve palsy

H49.10 **Fourth [trochlear] nerve palsy, unspecified eye**

H49.11 **Fourth [trochlear] nerve palsy, right eye**

H49.12 **Fourth [trochlear] nerve palsy, left eye**

H49.13 **Fourth [trochlear] nerve palsy, bilateral**

5th H49.2 Sixth [abducent] nerve palsy

H49.20 **Sixth [abducent] nerve palsy, unspecified eye**

H49.21 **Sixth [abducent] nerve palsy, right eye**

H49.22 **Sixth [abducent] nerve palsy, left eye**

H49.23 **Sixth [abducent] nerve palsy, bilateral**

5th H49.3 Total (external) ophthalmoplegia

H49.30 **Total (external) ophthalmoplegia, unspecified eye**

H49.31 **Total (external) ophthalmoplegia, right eye**

H49.32 **Total (external) ophthalmoplegia, left eye**

H49.33 **Total (external) ophthalmoplegia, bilateral**

5th H49.4 Progressive external ophthalmoplegia

EXCLUDES1 *Kearns-Sayre syndrome (H49.81-)*

H49.40 **Progressive external ophthalmoplegia, unspecified eye**

H49.41 **Progressive external ophthalmoplegia, right eye**

H49.42 **Progressive external ophthalmoplegia, left eye**

H49.43 **Progressive external ophthalmoplegia, bilateral**

5th H49.8 Other paralytic strabismus

6th H49.81 Kearns-Sayre syndrome

Progressive external ophthalmoplegia with pigmentary retinopathy

Use additional code for other manifestation, such as:

heart block (I45.9)

H49.811 **Kearns-Sayre syndrome, right eye** cc HCC RxHCC CC/MCC Exc

H49.812 **Kearns-Sayre syndrome, left eye** cc HCC RxHCC CC/MCC Exc

H49.813 **Kearns-Sayre syndrome, bilateral** cc HCC RxHCC CC/MCC Exc

H49.819 **Kearns-Sayre syndrome, unspecified eye** cc HCC RxHCC CC/MCC Exc

6th H49.88 Other paralytic strabismus

External ophthalmoplegia NOS

H49.881 **Other paralytic strabismus, right eye**

H49.882 **Other paralytic strabismus, left eye**

H49.883 **Other paralytic strabismus, bilateral**

H49.889 **Other paralytic strabismus, unspecified eye**

H49.9 **Unspecified paralytic strabismus**

4th H50 Other strabismus

5th H50.0 Esotropia

Convergent concomitant strabismus

EXCLUDES1 *intermittent esotropia (H50.31-, H50.32)*

H50.00 **Unspecified esotropia**

6th H50.01 Monocular esotropia

H50.011 **Monocular esotropia, right eye**

H50.012 **Monocular esotropia, left eye**

6th H50.02 Monocular esotropia with A pattern

H50.021 **Monocular esotropia with A pattern, right eye**

H50.022 **Monocular esotropia with A pattern, left eye**

6th H50.03 Monocular esotropia with V pattern

H50.031 **Monocular esotropia with V pattern, right eye**

H50.032 **Monocular esotropia with V pattern, left eye**

6th H50.04 Monocular esotropia with other noncomitancies

H50.041 **Monocular esotropia with other noncomitancies, right eye**

H50.042 **Monocular esotropia with other noncomitancies, left eye**

H50.05 Alternating esotropia

H50.06 Alternating esotropia with A pattern

H50.07 Alternating esotropia with V pattern

H50.08 Alternating esotropia with other noncomitancies

5th H50.1 Exotropia

Divergent concomitant strabismus

EXCLUDES1 *intermittent exotropia (H50.33-, H50.34)*

H50.10 **Unspecified exotropia**

6th H50.11 Monocular exotropia

H50.111 **Monocular exotropia, right eye**

H50.112 **Monocular exotropia, left eye**

6th H50.12 Monocular exotropia with A pattern

H50.121 **Monocular exotropia with A pattern, right eye**

H50.122 **Monocular exotropia with A pattern, left eye**

6th H50.13 Monocular exotropia with V pattern

H50.131 **Monocular exotropia with V pattern, right eye**

H50.132 **Monocular exotropia with V pattern, left eye**

6th H50.14 Monocular exotropia with other noncomitancies

H50.141 **Monocular exotropia with other noncomitancies, right eye**

H50.142 **Monocular exotropia with other noncomitancies, left eye**

H50.15 Alternating exotropia

H50.16 Alternating exotropia with A pattern

H50.17 Alternating exotropia with V pattern

H50.18 Alternating exotropia with other noncomitancies

5th H50.2 Vertical strabismus

Hypertropia

H50.21 **Vertical strabismus, right eye**

H50.22 **Vertical strabismus, left eye**

5th H50.3 Intermittent heterotropia

H50.30 **Unspecified intermittent heterotropia**

6th H50.31 Intermittent monocular esotropia

H50.311 Intermittent monocular esotropia, right eye
H50.312 Intermittent monocular esotropia, left eye
H50.32 Intermittent alternating esotropia
6th H50.33 Intermittent monocular exotropia
H50.331 Intermittent monocular exotropia, right eye
H50.332 Intermittent monocular exotropia, left eye
H50.34 Intermittent alternating exotropia
5th H50.4 Other and unspecified heterotropia
H50.40 Unspecified heterotropia
6th H50.41 Cyclotropia
H50.411 Cyclotropia, right eye
H50.412 Cyclotropia, left eye
H50.42 Monofixation syndrome
H50.43 Accommodative component in esotropia
5th H50.5 Heterophoria
H50.50 Unspecified heterophoria
H50.51 Esophoria
H50.52 Exophoria
H50.53 Vertical heterophoria
H50.54 Cyclophoria
H50.55 Alternating heterophoria
5th H50.6 Mechanical strabismus
H50.60 Mechanical strabismus, unspecified
6th H50.61 Brown's sheath syndrome
H50.611 Brown's sheath syndrome, right eye
H50.612 Brown's sheath syndrome, left eye
H50.69 Other mechanical strabismus
Strabismus due to adhesions
Traumatic limitation of duction of eye muscle
5th H50.8 Other specified strabismus
6th H50.81 Duane's syndrome
H50.811 Duane's syndrome, right eye
H50.812 Duane's syndrome, left eye
H50.89 Other specified strabismus
H50.9 Unspecified strabismus

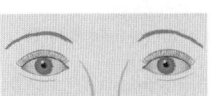
Normal

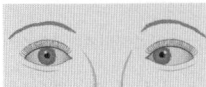
Esotropia - eye turns inward

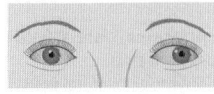
Exotropia - eye turns outward

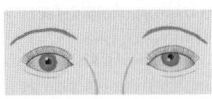
Hypertropia - eye turns upward

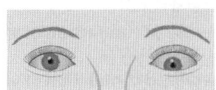
Hypotropia - eye turns downward

Figure 7.5 Types of Strabismus

4th H51 Other disorders of binocular movement
H51.0 Palsy (spasm) of conjugate gaze
5th H51.1 Convergence insufficiency and excess
H51.11 Convergence insufficiency
H51.12 Convergence excess
5th H51.2 Internuclear ophthalmoplegia
H51.20 Internuclear ophthalmoplegia, unspecified eye
H51.21 Internuclear ophthalmoplegia, right eye
H51.22 Internuclear ophthalmoplegia, left eye
H51.23 Internuclear ophthalmoplegia, bilateral

H51.8 Other specified disorders of binocular movement
H51.9 Unspecified disorder of binocular movement
4th H52 Disorders of refraction and accommodation
5th H52.0 Hypermetropia
H52.00 Hypermetropia, unspecified eye
H52.01 Hypermetropia, right eye
H52.02 Hypermetropia, left eye
H52.03 Hypermetropia, bilateral
5th H52.1 Myopia
EXCLUDES1 degenerative myopia (H44.2-)
H52.10 Myopia, unspecified eye
H52.11 Myopia, right eye
H52.12 Myopia, left eye
H52.13 Myopia, bilateral
5th H52.2 Astigmatism
6th H52.20 Unspecified astigmatism
H52.201 Unspecified astigmatism, right eye
H52.202 Unspecified astigmatism, left eye
H52.203 Unspecified astigmatism, bilateral
H52.209 Unspecified astigmatism, unspecified eye
6th H52.21 Irregular astigmatism
H52.211 Irregular astigmatism, right eye
H52.212 Irregular astigmatism, left eye
H52.213 Irregular astigmatism, bilateral
H52.219 Irregular astigmatism, unspecified eye
6th H52.22 Regular astigmatism
H52.221 Regular astigmatism, right eye
H52.222 Regular astigmatism, left eye
H52.223 Regular astigmatism, bilateral
H52.229 Regular astigmatism, unspecified eye
5th H52.3 Anisometropia and aniseikonia
H52.31 Anisometropia
H52.32 Aniseikonia
H52.4 Presbyopia
5th H52.5 Disorders of accommodation
6th H52.51 Internal ophthalmoplegia (complete) (total)
H52.511 Internal ophthalmoplegia (complete) (total), right eye
H52.512 Internal ophthalmoplegia (complete) (total), left eye
H52.513 Internal ophthalmoplegia (complete) (total), bilateral
H52.519 Internal ophthalmoplegia (complete) (total), unspecified eye
6th H52.52 Paresis of accommodation
H52.521 Paresis of accommodation, right eye
H52.522 Paresis of accommodation, left eye
H52.523 Paresis of accommodation, bilateral
H52.529 Paresis of accommodation, unspecified eye
6th H52.53 Spasm of accommodation
H52.531 Spasm of accommodation, right eye
H52.532 Spasm of accommodation, left eye
H52.533 Spasm of accommodation, bilateral
H52.539 Spasm of accommodation, unspecified eye
H52.6 Other disorders of refraction
H52.7 Unspecified disorder of refraction

Visual disturbances and blindness (H53-H54)

4th H53 Visual disturbances
5th H53.0 Amblyopia ex anopsia
DEFINITION: Amblyopia (lazy eye) is a sight disorder caused by the eye and brain not working together, resulting in decreased vision in an eye that otherwise appears normal.
EXCLUDES1 amblyopia due to vitamin A deficiency (E50.5)

Unspecified Code   Other Specified Code   Manifestation Code   N Newborn   P Pediatric   M Maternity   A Adult   ♂ Male   ♀ Female
● New Code   ▲ Revised Code Title   ▶◀ Revised Text   NOTES   INCLUDES   EXCLUDES1 Not coded here   EXCLUDES2 Not included here
4th 4th character required   5th 5th character required   6th 6th character required   7th 7th character required   Extension 'X' Alert
HAC Hospital-acquired condition (HAC) alert   AHA AHA Coding Clinic©   ☛ Code first alert

6ᵗʰ **H53.00** Unspecified amblyopia
    H53.001 **Unspecified amblyopia,** right **eye**
    H53.002 **Unspecified amblyopia,** left **eye**
    H53.003 **Unspecified amblyopia, bilateral**
    H53.009 **Unspecified amblyopia, unspecified eye**

6ᵗʰ **H53.01** Deprivation amblyopia
    H53.011 **Deprivation amblyopia,** right **eye**
    H53.012 **Deprivation amblyopia,** left **eye**
    H53.013 **Deprivation amblyopia, bilateral**
    H53.019 **Deprivation amblyopia, unspecified eye**

6ᵗʰ **H53.02** Refractive amblyopia
    H53.021 **Refractive amblyopia,** right **eye**
    H53.022 **Refractive amblyopia,** left **eye**
    H53.023 **Refractive amblyopia, bilateral**
    H53.029 **Refractive amblyopia, unspecified eye**

6ᵗʰ **H53.03** Strabismic amblyopia
    EXCLUDES1 strabismus (H50.-)
    H53.031 **Strabismic amblyopia,** right **eye**
    H53.032 **Strabismic amblyopia,** left **eye**
    H53.033 **Strabismic amblyopia, bilateral**
    H53.039 **Strabismic amblyopia, unspecified eye**

6ᵗʰ **H53.04** Amblyopia suspect
    H53.041 **Amblyopia suspect,** right **eye**
        AHA: Q4 2016
    H53.042 **Amblyopia suspect,** left **eye**
        AHA: Q4 2016
    H53.043 **Amblyopia suspect,** bilateral
        AHA: Q4 2016
    H53.049 **Amblyopia suspect, unspecified eye**
        AHA: Q4 2016

5ᵗʰ **H53.1** Subjective visual disturbances
    EXCLUDES1 subjective visual disturbances due to vitamin A deficiency (E50.5)
          visual hallucinations (R44.1)
    H53.10 **Unspecified subjective visual disturbances**
    H53.11 Day blindness
        Hemeralopia

6ᵗʰ **H53.12** Transient visual loss
    Scintillating scotoma
    EXCLUDES1 amaurosis fugax (G45.3-)
          transient retinal artery occlusion (H34.0-)
    H53.121 **Transient visual loss,** right **eye** cc cc/mcc exc
    H53.122 **Transient visual loss,** left **eye** cc cc/mcc exc
    H53.123 **Transient visual loss,** bilateral cc cc/mcc exc
    H53.129 **Transient visual loss, unspecified eye** cc cc/mcc exc

6ᵗʰ **H53.13** Sudden visual loss
    H53.131 **Sudden visual loss,** right **eye** cc cc/mcc exc
    H53.132 **Sudden visual loss,** left **eye** cc cc/mcc exc
    H53.133 **Sudden visual loss,** bilateral cc cc/mcc exc
    H53.139 **Sudden visual loss, unspecified eye** cc cc/mcc exc

6ᵗʰ **H53.14** Visual discomfort
    Asthenopia
    Photophobia
    H53.141 **Visual discomfort,** right **eye**
    H53.142 **Visual discomfort,** left **eye**
    H53.143 **Visual discomfort,** bilateral
    H53.149 **Visual discomfort, unspecified**
    H53.15 **Visual** distortions **of shape and size**
        Metamorphopsia
    H53.16 Psychophysical **visual disturbances**
    H53.19 **Other subjective visual disturbances**
        Visual halos

H53.2 **Diplopia**
    Double vision

5ᵗʰ **H53.3** Other and unspecified disorders of binocular vision
    H53.30 **Unspecified disorder of binocular vision**
    H53.31 **Abnormal retinal correspondence**
    H53.32 **Fusion with defective stereopsis**
    H53.33 **Simultaneous visual perception without fusion**
    H53.34 **Suppression of binocular vision**

5ᵗʰ **H53.4** Visual field defects
    H53.40 **Unspecified visual field defects**
    6ᵗʰ **H53.41** Scotoma involving central area
        Central scotoma
        H53.411 **Scotoma involving central area,** right **eye**
        H53.412 **Scotoma involving central area,** left **eye**
        H53.413 **Scotoma involving central area,** bilateral
        H53.419 **Scotoma involving central area, unspecified eye**
    6ᵗʰ **H53.42** Scotoma of blind spot area
        Enlarged blind spot
        H53.421 **Scotoma of blind spot area,** right **eye**
        H53.422 **Scotoma of blind spot area,** left **eye**
        H53.423 **Scotoma of blind spot area,** bilateral
        H53.429 **Scotoma of blind spot area, unspecified eye**
    6ᵗʰ **H53.43** Sector or arcuate defects
        Arcuate scotoma
        Bjerrum scotoma
        H53.431 **Sector or arcuate defects,** right **eye**
        H53.432 **Sector or arcuate defects,** left **eye**
        H53.433 **Sector or arcuate defects,** bilateral
        H53.439 **Sector or arcuate defects, unspecified eye**
    6ᵗʰ **H53.45** Other localized visual field defect
        Peripheral visual field defect
        Ring scotoma NOS
        Scotoma NOS
        H53.451 **Other localized visual field defect,** right **eye**
        H53.452 **Other localized visual field defect,** left **eye**
        H53.453 **Other localized visual field defect,** bilateral
        H53.459 **Other localized visual field defect, unspecified eye**
    6ᵗʰ **H53.46** Homonymous bilateral field defects
        Homonymous hemianopia
        Homonymous hemianopsia
        Quadrant anopia
        Quadrant anopsia
        H53.461 **Homonymous bilateral field defects,** right **side**
        H53.462 **Homonymous bilateral field defects,** left **side**
        H53.469 **Homonymous bilateral field defects, unspecified side**
            Homonymous bilateral field defects NOS
    H53.47 Heteronymous bilateral field defects
        Heteronymous hemianop(s)ia
    6ᵗʰ **H53.48** Generalized contraction of visual field
        H53.481 **Generalized contraction of visual field,** right **eye**
        H53.482 **Generalized contraction of visual field,** left **eye**
        H53.483 **Generalized contraction of visual field,** bilateral
        H53.489 **Generalized contraction of visual field, unspecified eye**

5ᵗʰ **H53.5** Color vision deficiencies
    Color blindness
    EXCLUDES2 day blindness (H53.11)
    H53.50 **Unspecified color vision deficiencies**
        Color blindness NOS
    H53.51 **Achromatopsia**
    H53.52 **Acquired color vision deficiency**
    H53.53 **Deuteranomaly**
        Deuteranopia

H53.54 **Protanomaly**
Protanopia
H53.55 **Tritanomaly**
Tritanopia
H53.59 Other color vision deficiencies
5ᵗʰ H53.6 **Night blindness**
EXCLUDES1 night blindness due to vitamin A deficiency (E50.5)
H53.60 **Unspecified night blindness**
H53.61 Abnormal dark adaptation curve
H53.62 Acquired night blindness
H53.63 Congenital night blindness
H53.69 **Other night blindness**
5ᵗʰ H53.7 **Vision** sensitivity deficiencies
H53.71 Glare sensitivity
H53.72 Impaired contrast sensitivity
H53.8 Other visual disturbances
H53.9 **Unspecified visual disturbance**
4ᵗʰ H54 Blindness and low vision
NOTES For definition of visual impairment categories *see* table below
☞ Code first any associated underlying cause of the blindness
EXCLUDES1 amaurosis fugax (G45.3)
5ᵗʰ H54.0 **Blindness,** both eyes
Visual impairment categories 3, 4, 5 in both eyes.
The appropriate 7th character is to be added to each code from subcategory H54.0*:
3 – blindness, left eye, category 3
4 – blindness, left eye, category 4
5 – blindness, left eye, category 5
6ᵗʰ H54.0X **Blindness,** both eyes, different category levels
7ᵗʰ H54.0X3 **Blindness** right eye, category 3
7ᵗʰ H54.0X4 **Blindness** right eye, category 4
7ᵗʰ H54.0X5 **Blindness** right eye, category 5
5ᵗʰ H54.1 **Blindness,** one eye, low vision other eye
Visual impairment categories 3, 4, 5 in one eye, with categories 1 or 2 in the other eye.
The appropriate 7th character is to be added to each code from subcategory H54.1*:
1 – low vision, left eye, category 1
2 – low vision, left eye, category 2
3 – blindness, left eye, category 3
4 – blindness, left eye, category 4
5 – blindness, left eye, category 5
H54.10 **Blindness, one eye, low vision other eye, unspecified eyes**
6ᵗʰ H54.11 **Blindness,** right eye, low vision left eye
7ᵗʰ H54.113 **Blindness** right eye category 3, low vision left eye
7ᵗʰ H54.114 **Blindness** right eye category 4, low vision left eye
7ᵗʰ H54.115 **Blindness** right eye category 5, low vision left eye
6ᵗʰ H54.12 **Blindness,** left eye, low vision right eye
7ᵗʰ H54.121 **Low vision** right eye category 1, blindness left eye
7ᵗʰ H54.122 **Low vision** right eye category 2, blindness left eye
5ᵗʰ H54.2 **Low vision,** both eyes
Visual impairment categories 1 or 2 in both eyes.
The appropriate 7th character is to be added to each code from subcategory H54.2*:
1 – low vision, left eye, category 1
2 – low vision, left eye, category 2
6ᵗʰ H54.2X **Low vision,** both eyes, different category levels
7ᵗʰ H54.2X1 **Low vision,** right eye, category 1
7ᵗʰ H54.2X2 **Low vision,** right eye, category 2
H54.3 Unqualified visual loss, both eyes
👁 **See Official Guidelines** "Blindness" I.C.7.b
AHA: Q4 2017
Visual impairment category 9 in both eyes.

5ᵗʰ H54.4 Blindness, one eye
Visual impairment categories 3, 4, 5 in one eye [normal vision in other eye]
The appropriate 7th character is to be added to each code from subcategory H54.4*:
A – normal vision, left eye
3 – category 3, normal vision right eye
4 – category 4, normal vision right eye
5 – category 5, normal vision right eye
H54.40 **Blindness, one eye, unspecified eye**
6ᵗʰ H54.41 **Blindness,** right eye, normal vision left eye
7ᵗʰ H54.413 **Blindness,** right eye, category 3
7ᵗʰ H54.414 **Blindness,** right eye, category 4
7ᵗʰ H54.415 **Blindness,** right eye, category 5
6ᵗʰ H54.42 **Blindness,** left eye, normal vision right eye
7ᵗʰ H54.42A **Blindness,** left eye, category 3-5
5ᵗʰ H54.5 Low vision, one eye
Visual impairment categories 1 or 2 in one eye [normal vision in other eye].
H54.50 **Low vision, one eye, unspecified eye**
6ᵗʰ H54.51 **Low vision,** right eye, normal vision left eye
7ᵗʰ H54.511 **Low vision,** right eye, category 1-2
The appropriate 7th character is to be added to each code from subcategory H54.511*:
A –category 1, normal vision, left eye
7ᵗʰ H54.512 **Low vision,** right eye, category 2
The appropriate 7th character is to be added to each code from subcategory H54.512*:
A – normal vision, left eye
6ᵗʰ H54.52 **Low vision,** left eye, normal vision right eye
The appropriate 7th character is to be added to each code from subcategory H54.52*:
1 – category 1, normal vision, right eye
2 – category 2, normal vision, right eye
7ᵗʰ H54.52A **Low vision,** left eye, category 1-2
5ᵗʰ H54.6 Unqualified visual loss, one eye
👁 **See Official Guidelines** "Blindness" I.C.7.b
Visual impairment category 9 in one eye [normal vision in other eye].
H54.60 **Unqualified visual loss, one eye, unspecified**
H54.61 **Unqualified visual loss,** right eye, normal vision left eye
H54.62 **Unqualified visual loss,** left eye, normal vision right eye
H54.7 **Unspecified visual loss**   PDxⓧ
👁 **See Official Guidelines** "Blindness" I.C.7.b
AHA: Q4 2017
Visual impairment category 9 NOS
H54.8 Legal blindness, as defined in USA
Blindness NOS according to USA definition
EXCLUDES1 legal blindness with specification of impairment level (H54.0-H54.7)
NOTES The table on the next page gives a classification of severity of visual impairment recommended by a WHO Study Group on the Prevention of Blindness, Geneva, 6-10 November 1972.
The term 'low vision' in category H54 comprises categories 1 and 2 of the table, the term 'blindness' categories 3, 4 and 5, and the term 'unqualified visual loss' category 9.
If the extent of the visual field is taken into account, patients with a field no greater than 10 but greater than 5 around central fixation should be placed in category 3 and patients with a field no greater than 5 around central fixation should be placed in category 4, even if the central acuity is not impaired.

Unspecified Code   Other Specified Code   Manifestation Code   **Ⓝ** Newborn   **Ⓟ** Pediatric   **Ⓜ** Maternity   **Ⓐ** Adult   ♂ Male   ♀ Female
● New Code   ▲ Revised Code Title   ►◄ Revised Text   **NOTES**   *INCLUDES*   *EXCLUDES1* Not coded here   *EXCLUDES2* Not included here
4ᵗʰ 4ᵗʰ character required   **5ᵗʰ** 5ᵗʰ character required   **6ᵗʰ** 6ᵗʰ character required   **7ᵗʰ** 7ᵗʰ character required   👁 Extension 'X' Alert
HAC Hospital-acquired condition (HAC) alert   **AHA** AHA Coding Clinic®   ☞ Code first alert

*CMS does not include 7ᵗʰ character options for several codes under category H54 and code H54.512 is missing as a 6-character code. The publisher added the 7ᵗʰ character options and code H54.512.
At press time, CMS did not issue an errata to correct these errors.

(Document 508 compliance requires all cells in the following table to be filled.)

Category of visual impairment	Visual acuity with best possible correction	
	Maximum less than:	Minimum equal to or better than:
	6/18	6/60
1	3/10 (0.3)	1/10 (0.1)
	20/70	20/200
	6/60	3/60
2	1/10 (0.1)	1/20 (0.5)
	20/200	20/400
	3/60	1/60 (finger counting at one meter)
3	1/20 (0.05)	1/50 (0.02)
	20/400	5/300 (20/1200)
	1/60 (finger counting at one meter)	Light perception
4	1/50 (0.02)	
	5/300	
5	No light perception	
9	Undetermined or unspecified	

Other disorders of eye and adnexa (H55-H57)

[4th] **H55 Nystagmus and other irregular eye movements**

[5th] **H55.0 Nystagmus**

- **H55.00 Unspecified nystagmus**
- **H55.01 Congenital nystagmus**
- **H55.02 Latent nystagmus**
- **H55.03 Visual deprivation nystagmus**
- **H55.04 Dissociated nystagmus**
- **H55.09 Other forms of nystagmus**

[5th] **H55.8 Other irregular eye movements**

- **H55.81 Saccadic eye movements**
- **H55.89 Other irregular eye movements**

[4th] **H57 Other disorders of eye and adnexa**

[5th] **H57.0 Anomalies of pupillary function**

- **H57.00 Unspecified anomaly of pupillary function**
- **H57.01 Argyll Robertson pupil, atypical**
  [EXCLUDES1] *syphilitic Argyll Robertson pupil (A52.19)*
- **H57.02 Anisocoria**
- **H57.03 Miosis**
- **H57.04 Mydriasis**

[6th] **H57.05 Tonic pupil**

- **H57.051 Tonic pupil, right eye**
- **H57.052 Tonic pupil, left eye**
- **H57.053 Tonic pupil, bilateral**
- **H57.059 Tonic pupil, unspecified eye**

- **H57.09 Other anomalies of pupillary function**

[5th] **H57.1 Ocular pain**

- **H57.10 Ocular pain, unspecified eye**
- **H57.11 Ocular pain, right eye**
- **H57.12 Ocular pain, left eye**
- **H57.13 Ocular pain, bilateral**

[5th] **H57.8 Other specified disorders of eye and adnexa**

[6th] **H57.81 Brow ptosis**

- **H57.811 Brow ptosis, right**
  AHA: Q4 2018
- **H57.812 Brow ptosis, left**
  AHA: Q4 2018
- **H57.813 Brow ptosis, bilateral**
  AHA: Q4 2018
- **H57.819 Brow ptosis, unspecified**
  AHA: Q4 2018

- **H57.89 Other specified disorders of eye and adnexa**

H57.9 Unspecified disorder of eye and adnexa [PDx]

Intraoperative and postprocedural complications and disorders of eye and adnexa, not elsewhere classified (H59)

[4th] **H59 Intraoperative and postprocedural complications and disorders of eye and adnexa, not elsewhere classified**

[EXCLUDES1] *mechanical complication of intraocular lens (T85.2)*
mechanical complication of other ocular prosthetic devices, implants and grafts (T85.3)
pseudophakia (Z96.1)
secondary cataracts (H26.4-)

[5th] **H59.0 Disorders of the eye following cataract surgery**

[6th] **H59.01 Keratopathy (bullous aphakic) following cataract surgery**

Vitreal corneal syndrome
Vitreous (touch) syndrome

- **H59.011 Keratopathy (bullous aphakic) following cataract surgery, right eye** [CC] [CC/MCC Exc]
- **H59.012 Keratopathy (bullous aphakic) following cataract surgery, left eye** [CC] [CC/MCC Exc]
- **H59.013 Keratopathy (bullous aphakic) following cataract surgery, bilateral** [CC] [CC/MCC Exc]
- **H59.019 Keratopathy (bullous aphakic) following cataract surgery, unspecified eye** [CC] [CC/MCC Exc]

[6th] **H59.02 Cataract (lens) fragments in eye following cataract surgery**

- **H59.021 Cataract (lens) fragments in eye following cataract surgery, right eye**
- **H59.022 Cataract (lens) fragments in eye following cataract surgery, left eye**
- **H59.023 Cataract (lens) fragments in eye following cataract surgery, bilateral**
- **H59.029 Cataract (lens) fragments in eye following cataract surgery, unspecified eye**

[6th] **H59.03 Cystoid macular edema following cataract surgery**

- **H59.031 Cystoid macular edema following cataract surgery, right eye** [CC] [CC/MCC Exc]
- **H59.032 Cystoid macular edema following cataract surgery, left eye** [CC] [CC/MCC Exc]
- **H59.033 Cystoid macular edema following cataract surgery, bilateral** [CC] [CC/MCC Exc]
- **H59.039 Cystoid macular edema following cataract surgery, unspecified eye** [CC] [CC/MCC Exc]

[6th] **H59.09 Other disorders of the eye following cataract surgery**

- **H59.091 Other disorders of the right eye following cataract surgery** [CC] [CC/MCC Exc]
- **H59.092 Other disorders of the left eye following cataract surgery** [CC] [CC/MCC Exc]
- **H59.093 Other disorders of the eye following cataract surgery, bilateral** [CC] [CC/MCC Exc]
- **H59.099 Other disorders of unspecified eye following cataract surgery** [CC] [CC/MCC Exc]

[5th] **H59.1 Intraoperative hemorrhage and hematoma of eye and adnexa complicating a procedure**

[EXCLUDES1] *intraoperative hemorrhage and hematoma of eye and adnexa due to accidental puncture or laceration during a procedure (H59.2-)*

[6th] **H59.11 Intraoperative hemorrhage and hematoma of eye and adnexa complicating an ophthalmic procedure**

- **H59.111 Intraoperative hemorrhage and hematoma of right eye and adnexa complicating an ophthalmic procedure** [CC] [CC/MCC Exc]

[PDx] Unacceptable principal diagnosis symbol per Medicare code edits [POA] Code exempt from diagnosis present on admission requirement
[?] Questionable admission [CC] Complication or comorbidity [MCC] Major complication or comorbidity [CC/MCC Exc] CC/MCC exclusion
[HCC] HCC diagnosis code [RxHCC] RxHCC diagnosis code MACRA code **DEFINITION** Describes condition/terminology
TIP Coding guidance 👁 Official Guideline Reference [Z1] Z code as first-listed diagnosis

H59.112 Intraoperative hemorrhage and hematoma of left eye and adnexa complicating an ophthalmic procedure CC CC/MCC Exc

H59.113 Intraoperative hemorrhage and hematoma of eye and adnexa complicating an ophthalmic procedure, bilateral CC CC/MCC Exc

H59.119 Intraoperative hemorrhage and hematoma of unspecified eye and adnexa complicating an ophthalmic procedure CC CC/MCC Exc

6ᵗʰ H59.12 Intraoperative hemorrhage and hematoma of eye and adnexa complicating other procedure

H59.121 Intraoperative hemorrhage and hematoma of right eye and adnexa complicating other procedure CC CC/MCC Exc

H59.122 Intraoperative hemorrhage and hematoma of left eye and adnexa complicating other procedure CC CC/MCC Exc

H59.123 Intraoperative hemorrhage and hematoma of eye and adnexa complicating other procedure, bilateral CC CC/MCC Exc

H59.129 Intraoperative hemorrhage and hematoma of unspecified eye and adnexa complicating other procedure CC CC/MCC Exc

5ᵗʰ H59.2 Accidental puncture and laceration of eye and adnexa during a procedure

6ᵗʰ H59.21 Accidental puncture and laceration of eye and adnexa during an ophthalmic procedure

H59.211 Accidental puncture and laceration of right eye and adnexa during an ophthalmic procedure CC CC/MCC Exc

H59.212 Accidental puncture and laceration of left eye and adnexa during an ophthalmic procedure CC CC/MCC Exc

H59.213 Accidental puncture and laceration of eye and adnexa during an ophthalmic procedure, bilateral CC CC/MCC Exc

H59.219 Accidental puncture and laceration of unspecified eye and adnexa during an ophthalmic procedure CC CC/MCC Exc

6ᵗʰ H59.22 Accidental puncture and laceration of eye and adnexa during other procedure

H59.221 Accidental puncture and laceration of right eye and adnexa during other procedure CC CC/MCC Exc

H59.222 Accidental puncture and laceration of left eye and adnexa during other procedure CC CC/MCC Exc

H59.223 Accidental puncture and laceration of eye and adnexa during other procedure, bilateral CC CC/MCC Exc

H59.229 Accidental puncture and laceration of unspecified eye and adnexa during other procedure CC CC/MCC Exc

5ᵗʰ H59.3 Postprocedural hemorrhage, hematoma, and seroma of eye and adnexa following a procedure

6ᵗʰ H59.31 Postprocedural hemorrhage of eye and adnexa following an ophthalmic procedure

H59.311 Postprocedural hemorrhage of right eye and adnexa following an ophthalmic procedure CC CC/MCC Exc

H59.312 Postprocedural hemorrhage of left eye and adnexa following an ophthalmic procedure CC CC/MCC Exc

H59.313 Postprocedural hemorrhage of eye and adnexa following an ophthalmic procedure, bilateral CC CC/MCC Exc

H59.319 Postprocedural hemorrhage of unspecified eye and adnexa following an ophthalmic procedure CC CC/MCC Exc

6ᵗʰ H59.32 Postprocedural hemorrhage of eye and adnexa following other procedure

H59.321 Postprocedural hemorrhage of right eye and adnexa following other procedure CC CC/MCC Exc

H59.322 Postprocedural hemorrhage of left eye and adnexa following other procedure CC CC/MCC Exc

H59.323 Postprocedural hemorrhage of eye and adnexa following other procedure, bilateral CC CC/MCC Exc

H59.329 Postprocedural hemorrhage of unspecified eye and adnexa following other procedure CC CC/MCC Exc

6ᵗʰ H59.33 Postprocedural hematoma of eye and adnexa following an ophthalmic procedure

H59.331 Postprocedural hematoma of right eye and adnexa following an ophthalmic procedure CC CC/MCC Exc

H59.332 Postprocedural hematoma of left eye and adnexa following an ophthalmic procedure CC CC/MCC Exc

H59.333 Postprocedural hematoma of eye and adnexa following an ophthalmic procedure, bilateral CC CC/MCC Exc

H59.339 Postprocedural hematoma of unspecified eye and adnexa following an ophthalmic procedure CC CC/MCC Exc

6ᵗʰ H59.34 Postprocedural hematoma of eye and adnexa following other procedure

H59.341 Postprocedural hematoma of right eye and adnexa following other procedure CC CC/MCC Exc

H59.342 Postprocedural hematoma of left eye and adnexa following other procedure CC CC/MCC Exc

H59.343 Postprocedural hematoma of eye and adnexa following other procedure, bilateral CC CC/MCC Exc

H59.349 Postprocedural hematoma of unspecified eye and adnexa following other procedure CC CC/MCC Exc

6ᵗʰ H59.35 Postprocedural seroma of eye and adnexa following an ophthalmic procedure

H59.351 Postprocedural seroma of right eye and adnexa following an ophthalmic procedure CC CC/MCC Exc

H59.352 Postprocedural seroma of left eye and adnexa following an ophthalmic procedure CC CC/MCC Exc

H59.353 Postprocedural seroma of eye and adnexa following an ophthalmic procedure, bilateral CC CC/MCC Exc

H59.359 Postprocedural seroma of unspecified eye and adnexa following an ophthalmic procedure CC CC/MCC Exc

6ᵗʰ H59.36 Postprocedural seroma of eye and adnexa following other procedure

H59.361 Postprocedural seroma of right eye and adnexa following other procedure CC CC/MCC Exc

H59.362 Postprocedural seroma of left eye and adnexa following other procedure CC CC/MCC Exc

H59.363 Postprocedural seroma of eye and adnexa following other procedure, bilateral CC CC/MCC Exc

H59.369 Postprocedural seroma of unspecified eye and adnexa following other procedure CC CC/MCC Exc

---

Unspecified Code   Other Specified Code   Manifestation Code   N Newborn   P Pediatric   M Maternity   A Adult   ♂ Male   ♀ Female
● New Code   ▲ Revised Code Title   ▶◀ Revised Text   NOTES   INCLUDES   EXCLUDES1 Not coded here   EXCLUDES2 Not included here
4ᵗʰ 4ᵗʰ character required   5ᵗʰ 5ᵗʰ character required   6ᵗʰ 6ᵗʰ character required   7ᵗʰ 7ᵗʰ character required   Extension 'X' Alert
HAC Hospital-acquired condition (HAC) alert   AHA AHA Coding Clinic©   ☛ Code first alert

⑤ⁿ **H59.4** Inflammation (infection) of postprocedural bleb

Postprocedural blebitis

EXCLUDES1 filtering (vitreous) bleb after glaucoma surgery status (Z98.83)

    H59.40 Inflammation (infection) of postprocedural bleb, unspecified

    H59.41 Inflammation (infection) of postprocedural bleb, stage 1

    H59.42 Inflammation (infection) of postprocedural bleb, stage 2

    H59.43 Inflammation (infection) of postprocedural bleb, stage 3

       Bleb endophthalmitis

⑤ⁿ **H59.8** Other intraoperative and postprocedural complications and disorders of eye and adnexa, not elsewhere classified

    ⑥ⁿ **H59.81** Chorioretinal scars after surgery for detachment

        H59.811 Chorioretinal scars after surgery for detachment, right eye   CC° CC/MCC Exc°

        H59.812 Chorioretinal scars after surgery for detachment, left eye   CC° CC/MCC Exc°

        H59.813 Chorioretinal scars after surgery for detachment, bilateral   CC° CC/MCC Exc°

        H59.819 Chorioretinal scars after surgery for detachment, unspecified eye   CC° CC/MCC Exc°

    H59.88 Other intraoperative complications of eye and adnexa, not elsewhere classified   CC° CC/MCC Exc°

    H59.89 Other postprocedural complications and disorders of eye and adnexa, not elsewhere classified   CC° CC/MCC Exc°

PDx° Unacceptable principal diagnosis symbol per Medicare code edits   POA° Code exempt from diagnosis present on admission requirement

❓ Questionable admission   CC° Complication or comorbidity   MCC° Major complication or comorbidity   CC/MCC Exc° CC/MCC exclusion

HCC HCC diagnosis code   RxHCC RxHCC diagnosis code   MACRA code   **DEFINITION** Describes condition/terminology

TIP Coding guidance   👁 Official Guideline Reference   Z1 Z code as first-listed diagnosis

When symbols appear on a code that requires a 7th character extension, refer to Appendix B to identify applicable 7th character codes.   **2020 ICD-10-CM**

Chapter 8: Diseases of the Ear and Mastoid Process (H60-H95)

Anatomy of the Ear

Introduction

The external, inner and middle ear (Figure 8.a) contain the organs of hearing and balance. The external ear extends from outside of the head to the eardrum. The middle ear is the air-filled chamber and located medially to the eardrum. It contains the auditory ossicles (the malleus, incus, and stapes). The external and middle ears are primarily involved in the process of hearing. The inner ear comprises of fluid-filled chambers, which serve to maintain balance (or equilibrium) and hearing. The various organs of a typical human ear are listed below:

1. **The External Ear**
   a) Auricle (or Pinna)
   b) External Auditory (or Auricular) Canal (or Ear Canal/External Auditory Meatus/External Acoustic Meatus)
   c) Surface of Eardrum

2. **The Middle Ear**
   a) Malleus
   b) Incus
   c) Stapes
   d) Tympanic Membrane (or Eardrum)
   e) Auditory/Eustachian Tube (or Pharyngotympanic Tube)

3. **The Inner Ear**
   a) Cochlea
   b) Vestibule
   c) Semicircular Canals

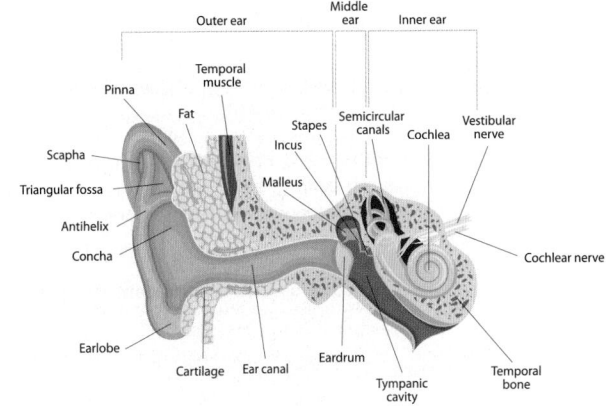

Figure 8.a Anatomy of the Ear

Common Pathologies

Swimmer's Ear
Swimmer's ear is an inflammation, irritation, or infection of the outer ear and ear canal. The medical term for swimmer's ear is otitis externa. Acute external otitis is commonly a bacterial infection caused by streptococcus, staphylococcus, or pseudomonas types of bacteria.

Otitis Media
Otitis media (Figure 8.b) is the medical term for middle ear infection. One symptom of acute otitis media is ear pain; other possible symptoms include fever and irritability (in infants) often with drainage of purulent material. After an acute infection, fluid (an effusion) may remain behind the ear drum (tympanic membrane) leading to otitis media with effusion chronic suppurative otitis media.

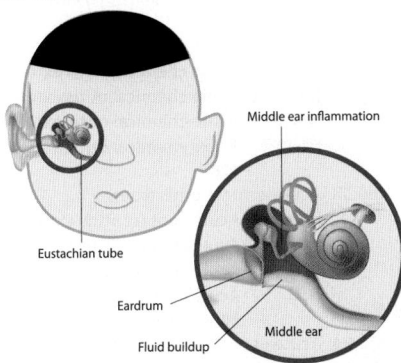

Figure 8.b Otitis Media

Ménière's Disease
Ménière's disease is a disorder of the inner ear that can affect hearing. It causes severe dizziness and a feeling of ear pressure or pain. It is characterized by episodes of vertigo, low-pitched tinnitus, and hearing loss. It usually affects just one ear. It may occur when the pressure of the fluid in part of the inner ear gets too high. The inner ear contains fluid-filled tubes called semicircular canals. These canals help to maintain position and balance.

Vestibular Neuritis
Vestibular neuritis is a disorder resulting from an acute infection of the nerves in the inner ear. This disrupts transmission of sensory information. Its main symptom is vertigo, which appears suddenly, often with nausea and vomiting.

This can be made worse by head movement. Vertigo usually lasts for several days or weeks. In rare cases it can take months to go away entirely. Vestibular neuritis does not lead to loss of hearing.

Cholesteatoma
Cholesteatoma can be congenital, but it more commonly occurs as a complication of chronic ear infection. An abnormal skin growth in the middle ear behind the eardrum is called cholesteatoma. Poor function in the eustachian tube leads to negative pressure in the middle ear. Over time, the cholesteatoma can increase in size and destroy the surrounding delicate bones of the middle ear leading to hearing loss.

Otosclerosis
Otosclerosis is an abnormal bone growth in the middle ear that causes hearing loss. This bone prevents structures within the ear from working properly and causes hearing loss. It is a condition that mainly affects the stapes, one of the tiny bony ossicles in the middle ear. It significantly involves the bone that surrounds the inner ear, called the otic capsule, and a sensory-type hearing loss occurs.

Acoustic Neuroma
An acoustic neuroma (Figure 8.c) is a benign tumor of the nerve that connects the ear to the brain. This nerve is called the vestibular cochlear nerve. It is also called vestibular schwannoma. The cause is generally unknown. If an acoustic tumor becomes large it will push on the surface of the brainstem but not really grow into brain tissue. Symptoms of acoustic neuroma are loss of hearing on one side, ringing in ears, dizziness and balance problems.

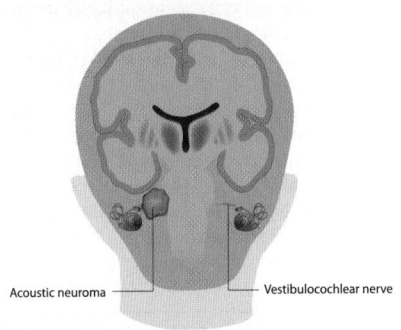

Figure 8.c Acoustic Neuroma

Diseases of the ear and mastoid process (H60-H95)

NOTES Use an external cause code following the code for the ear condition, if applicable, to identify the cause of the ear condition

EXCLUDES2 *certain conditions originating in the perinatal period (P04-P96)*
certain infectious and parasitic diseases (A00-B99)
complications of pregnancy, childbirth and the puerperium (O00-O9A)
congenital malformations, deformations and chromosomal abnormalities (Q00-Q99)
endocrine, nutritional and metabolic diseases (E00-E88)
injury, poisoning and certain other consequences of external causes (S00-T88)
neoplasms (C00-D49)
symptoms, signs and abnormal clinical and laboratory findings, not elsewhere classified (R00-R94)

This chapter contains the following blocks:

H60-H62	Diseases of external ear
H65-H75	Diseases of middle ear and mastoid
H80-H83	Diseases of inner ear
H90-H94	Other disorders of ear
H95	Intraoperative and postprocedural complications and disorders of ear and mastoid process, not elsewhere classified

Diseases of external ear (H60-H62) (Figure 8.1)

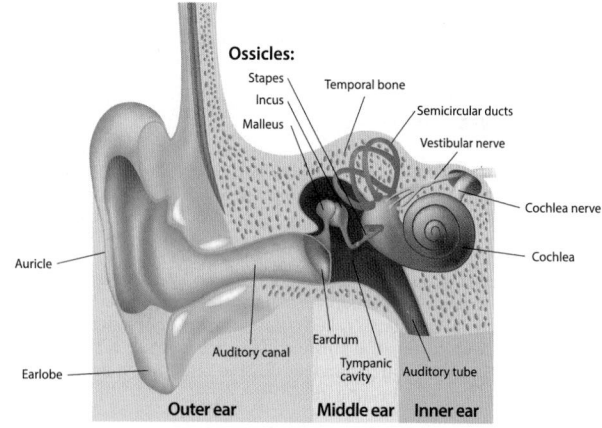

Ossicles:
Stapes
Incus
Malleus
Temporal bone
Semicircular ducts
Vestibular nerve
Cochlea nerve
Cochlea
Auricle
Auditory canal
Eardrum
Tympanic cavity
Auditory tube
Earlobe
Outer ear   Middle ear   Inner ear

Figure 8.1 Anatomy of the Ear

● H60 **Otitis externa**
   ● H60.0 Abscess **of external ear**
      Boil of external ear
      Carbuncle of auricle or external auditory canal
      Furuncle of external ear
      H60.00 **Abscess of external ear, unspecified ear**
      H60.01 **Abscess of** right **external ear**
      H60.02 **Abscess of** left **external ear**
      H60.03 **Abscess of external ear, bilateral**
   ● H60.1 Cellulitis **of external ear**
      Cellulitis of auricle
      Cellulitis of external auditory canal
      H60.10 **Cellulitis of external ear, unspecified ear**
      H60.11 **Cellulitis of** right **external ear**
      H60.12 **Cellulitis of** left **external ear**
      H60.13 **Cellulitis of external ear, bilateral**
   ● H60.2 Malignant otitis externa
      H60.20 **Malignant otitis externa, unspecified ear**   CC CC/MCC Exc
      H60.21 **Malignant otitis externa,** right **ear**   CC CC/MCC Exc
      H60.22 **Malignant otitis externa,** left **ear**   CC CC/MCC Exc
      H60.23 **Malignant otitis externa, bilateral**   CC CC/MCC Exc
   ● H60.3 Other infective **otitis externa**
      ● H60.31 Diffuse **otitis externa**

H60.311 **Diffuse otitis externa,** right **ear**
H60.312 **Diffuse otitis externa,** left **ear**
H60.313 **Diffuse otitis externa, bilateral**
H60.319 **Diffuse otitis externa, unspecified ear**
● H60.32 Hemorrhagic **otitis externa**
   H60.321 **Hemorrhagic otitis externa,** right **ear**
   H60.322 **Hemorrhagic otitis externa,** left **ear**
   H60.323 **Hemorrhagic otitis externa, bilateral**
   H60.329 **Hemorrhagic otitis externa, unspecified ear**
● H60.33 Swimmer's **ear**
   H60.331 **Swimmer's ear,** right **ear**
   H60.332 **Swimmer's ear,** left **ear**
   H60.333 **Swimmer's ear, bilateral**
   H60.339 **Swimmer's ear, unspecified ear**
● H60.39 Other infective otitis externa
   H60.391 **Other infective otitis externa,** right **ear**
   H60.392 **Other infective otitis externa,** left **ear**
   H60.393 **Other infective otitis externa, bilateral**
   H60.399 **Other infective otitis externa, unspecified ear**
● H60.4 **Cholesteatoma of external ear**
   Keratosis obturans of external ear (canal)
   EXCLUDES2 *cholesteatoma of middle ear (H71.-)*
      recurrent cholesteatoma of postmastoidectomy cavity (H95.0-)
   H60.40 **Cholesteatoma of external ear, unspecified ear**
   H60.41 **Cholesteatoma of** right **external ear**
   H60.42 **Cholesteatoma of** left **external ear**
   H60.43 **Cholesteatoma of external ear, bilateral**
● H60.5 Acute noninfective **otitis externa**
   ● H60.50 **Unspecified acute noninfective otitis externa**
      Acute otitis externa NOS
      H60.501 **Unspecified acute noninfective otitis externa,** right **ear**
      H60.502 **Unspecified acute noninfective otitis externa,** left **ear**
      H60.503 **Unspecified acute noninfective otitis externa, bilateral**
      H60.509 **Unspecified acute noninfective otitis externa, unspecified ear**
   ● H60.51 **Acute** actinic **otitis externa**
      H60.511 **Acute actinic otitis externa,** right **ear**
      H60.512 **Acute actinic otitis externa,** left **ear**
      H60.513 **Acute actinic otitis externa, bilateral**
      H60.519 **Acute actinic otitis externa, unspecified ear**
   ● H60.52 **Acute** chemical **otitis externa**
      H60.521 **Acute chemical otitis externa,** right **ear**
      H60.522 **Acute chemical otitis externa,** left **ear**
      H60.523 **Acute chemical otitis externa, bilateral**
      H60.529 **Acute chemical otitis externa, unspecified ear**
   ● H60.53 **Acute** contact **otitis externa**
      H60.531 **Acute contact otitis externa,** right **ear**
      H60.532 **Acute contact otitis externa,** left **ear**
      H60.533 **Acute contact otitis externa, bilateral**
      H60.539 **Acute contact otitis externa, unspecified ear**
   ● H60.54 **Acute** eczematoid **otitis externa**
      H60.541 **Acute eczematoid otitis externa,** right **ear**
      H60.542 **Acute eczematoid otitis externa,** left **ear**
      H60.543 **Acute eczematoid otitis externa, bilateral**
      H60.549 **Acute eczematoid otitis externa, unspecified ear**
   ● H60.55 **Acute** reactive **otitis externa**
      H60.551 **Acute reactive otitis externa,** right **ear**
      H60.552 **Acute reactive otitis externa,** left **ear**
      H60.553 **Acute reactive otitis externa, bilateral**
      H60.559 **Acute reactive otitis externa, unspecified ear**

PDx Unacceptable principal diagnosis symbol per Medicare code edits   POA Code exempt from diagnosis present on admission requirement
? Questionable admission   CC Complication or comorbidity   MCC Major complication or comorbidity   CC/MCC Exc CC/MCC exclusion
HCC HCC diagnosis code   RHCC RxHCC diagnosis code   MACRA code   **DEFINITION** Describes condition/terminology
TIP Coding guidance   ◉ Official Guideline Reference   Z1 Z code as first-listed diagnosis

⑥ H60.59 Other noninfective acute otitis externa
   H60.591 Other noninfective acute otitis externa, right ear
   H60.592 Other noninfective acute otitis externa, left ear
   H60.593 Other noninfective acute otitis externa, bilateral
   H60.599 Other noninfective acute otitis externa, unspecified ear
⑤ H60.6 Unspecified chronic otitis externa
  H60.60 Unspecified chronic otitis externa, unspecified ear
  H60.61 Unspecified chronic otitis externa, right ear
  H60.62 Unspecified chronic otitis externa, left ear
  H60.63 Unspecified chronic otitis externa, bilateral
⑤ H60.8 Other otitis externa
  ⑥ H60.8X Other otitis externa
   H60.8X1 Other otitis externa, right ear
   H60.8X2 Other otitis externa, left ear
   H60.8X3 Other otitis externa, bilateral
   H60.8X9 Other otitis externa, unspecified ear
⑤ H60.9 Unspecified otitis externa
  H60.90 Unspecified otitis externa, unspecified ear
  H60.91 Unspecified otitis externa, right ear
  H60.92 Unspecified otitis externa, left ear
  H60.93 Unspecified otitis externa, bilateral
④ H61 Other disorders of external ear
 ⑤ H61.0 Chondritis and perichondritis of external ear
  Chondrodermatitis nodularis chronica helicis
  Perichondritis of auricle
  Perichondritis of pinna
  ⑥ H61.00 Unspecified perichondritis of external ear
   H61.001 Unspecified perichondritis of right external ear
   H61.002 Unspecified perichondritis of left external ear
   H61.003 Unspecified perichondritis of external ear, bilateral
   H61.009 Unspecified perichondritis of external ear, unspecified ear
  ⑥ H61.01 Acute perichondritis of external ear
   H61.011 Acute perichondritis of right external ear
   H61.012 Acute perichondritis of left external ear
   H61.013 Acute perichondritis of external ear, bilateral
   H61.019 Acute perichondritis of external ear, unspecified ear
  ⑥ H61.02 Chronic perichondritis of external ear
   H61.021 Chronic perichondritis of right external ear
   H61.022 Chronic perichondritis of left external ear
   H61.023 Chronic perichondritis of external ear, bilateral
   H61.029 Chronic perichondritis of external ear, unspecified ear
  ⑥ H61.03 Chondritis of external ear
  Chondritis of auricle
  Chondritis of pinna
   H61.031 Chondritis of right external ear
   H61.032 Chondritis of left external ear
    AHA: Q1 2015
   H61.033 Chondritis of external ear, bilateral
   H61.039 Chondritis of external ear, unspecified ear
 ⑤ H61.1 Noninfective disorders of pinna
  EXCLUDES2 cauliflower ear (M95.1-)
   gouty tophi of ear (M1A.-)
  ⑥ H61.10 Unspecified noninfective disorders of pinna
  Disorder of pinna NOS
   H61.101 Unspecified noninfective disorders of pinna, right ear
   H61.102 Unspecified noninfective disorders of pinna, left ear

   H61.103 Unspecified noninfective disorders of pinna, bilateral
   H61.109 Unspecified noninfective disorders of pinna, unspecified ear
  ⑥ H61.11 Acquired deformity of pinna
  Acquired deformity of auricle
  EXCLUDES2 cauliflower ear (M95.1-)
   H61.111 Acquired deformity of pinna, right ear
   H61.112 Acquired deformity of pinna, left ear
   H61.113 Acquired deformity of pinna, bilateral
   H61.119 Acquired deformity of pinna, unspecified ear
  ⑥ H61.12 Hematoma of pinna
  Hematoma of auricle
   H61.121 Hematoma of pinna, right ear
   H61.122 Hematoma of pinna, left ear
   H61.123 Hematoma of pinna, bilateral
   H61.129 Hematoma of pinna, unspecified ear
  ⑥ H61.19 Other noninfective disorders of pinna
   H61.191 Noninfective disorders of pinna, right ear
   H61.192 Noninfective disorders of pinna, left ear
   H61.193 Noninfective disorders of pinna, bilateral
   H61.199 Noninfective disorders of pinna, unspecified ear
 ⑤ H61.2 Impacted cerumen
  Wax in ear
  H61.20 Impacted cerumen, unspecified ear ❓
  H61.21 Impacted cerumen, right ear ❓
  H61.22 Impacted cerumen, left ear ❓
  H61.23 Impacted cerumen, bilateral ❓
 ⑤ H61.3 Acquired stenosis of external ear canal
  Collapse of external ear canal
  EXCLUDES1 postprocedural stenosis of external ear canal (H95.81-)
  ⑥ H61.30 Acquired stenosis of external ear canal, unspecified
   H61.301 Acquired stenosis of right external ear canal, unspecified
   H61.302 Acquired stenosis of left external ear canal, unspecified
   H61.303 Acquired stenosis of external ear canal, unspecified, bilateral
   H61.309 Acquired stenosis of external ear canal, unspecified, unspecified ear
  ⑥ H61.31 Acquired stenosis of external ear canal secondary to trauma
   H61.311 Acquired stenosis of right external ear canal secondary to trauma
   H61.312 Acquired stenosis of left external ear canal secondary to trauma
   H61.313 Acquired stenosis of external ear canal secondary to trauma, bilateral
   H61.319 Acquired stenosis of external ear canal secondary to trauma, unspecified ear
  ⑥ H61.32 Acquired stenosis of external ear canal secondary to inflammation and infection
   H61.321 Acquired stenosis of right external ear canal secondary to inflammation and infection
   H61.322 Acquired stenosis of left external ear canal secondary to inflammation and infection
   H61.323 Acquired stenosis of external ear canal secondary to inflammation and infection, bilateral
   H61.329 Acquired stenosis of external ear canal secondary to inflammation and infection, unspecified ear
  ⑥ H61.39 Other acquired stenosis of external ear canal
   H61.391 Other acquired stenosis of right external ear canal
   H61.392 Other acquired stenosis of left external ear canal

H61.393   Other acquired stenosis of external ear canal, bilateral

H61.399   Other acquired stenosis of external ear canal, unspecified ear

H61.8 Other specified disorders of external ear

  H61.81 Exostosis of external canal

    H61.811   Exostosis of right external canal

    H61.812   Exostosis of left external canal

    H61.813   Exostosis of external canal, bilateral

    H61.819   Exostosis of external canal, unspecified ear

  H61.89 Other specified disorders of external ear

    H61.891   Other specified disorders of right external ear

    H61.892   Other specified disorders of left external ear

    H61.893   Other specified disorders of external ear, bilateral

    H61.899   Other specified disorders of external ear, unspecified ear

H61.9 Disorder of external ear, unspecified

  H61.90 Disorder of external ear, unspecified, unspecified ear

  H61.91 Disorder of right external ear, unspecified

  H61.92 Disorder of left external ear, unspecified

  H61.93 Disorder of external ear, unspecified, bilateral

H62 Disorders of external ear in diseases classified elsewhere

  H62.4 Otitis externa in other diseases classified elsewhere

    ☛ **Code first** underlying disease, such as:

      erysipelas (A46)

      impetigo (L01.0)

    EXCLUDES1 otitis externa (in):

        candidiasis (B37.84)

        herpes viral [herpes simplex] (B00.1)

        herpes zoster (B02.8)

    H62.40 **Otitis externa in other diseases classified elsewhere, unspecified ear**

    H62.41 **Otitis externa in other diseases classified elsewhere, right ear**

    H62.42 **Otitis externa in other diseases classified elsewhere, left ear**

    H62.43 **Otitis externa in other diseases classified elsewhere, bilateral**

  H62.8 Other disorders of external ear in diseases classified elsewhere

    ☛ **Code first** underlying disease, such as:

      gout (M1A.-, M10.-)

    H62.8X Other disorders of external ear in diseases classified elsewhere

      H62.8X1 **Other disorders of right external ear in diseases classified elsewhere**

      H62.8X2 **Other disorders of left external ear in diseases classified elsewhere**

      H62.8X3 **Other disorders of external ear in diseases classified elsewhere, bilateral**

      H62.8X9 **Other disorders of external ear in diseases classified elsewhere, unspecified ear**

Diseases of middle ear and mastoid (H65-H75)

H65 Nonsuppurative otitis media

  INCLUDES nonsuppurative otitis media with myringitis

  Use additional code for any associated perforated tympanic membrane (H72.-)

  Use additional code, ▶if applicable,◀ to identify:

    exposure to environmental tobacco smoke (Z77.22)

    exposure to tobacco smoke in the perinatal period (P96.81)

    history of tobacco dependence (Z87.891)

    infectious agent (B95-B97)

    occupational exposure to environmental tobacco smoke (Z57.31)

    tobacco dependence (F17.-)

    tobacco use (Z72.0)

H65.0 Acute serous otitis media

  Acute and subacute secretory otitis

  H65.00 **Acute serous otitis media, unspecified ear**

  H65.01 **Acute serous otitis media, right ear**

  H65.02 **Acute serous otitis media, left ear**

  H65.03 **Acute serous otitis media, bilateral**

  H65.04 **Acute serous otitis media, recurrent, right ear**

  H65.05 **Acute serous otitis media, recurrent, left ear**

  H65.06 **Acute serous otitis media, recurrent, bilateral**

  H65.07 **Acute serous otitis media, recurrent, unspecified ear**

H65.1 Other acute nonsuppurative otitis media

  EXCLUDES1 otitic barotrauma (T70.0)

        otitis media (acute) NOS (H66.9)

  H65.11 Acute and subacute allergic otitis media (mucoid) (sanguinous) (serous)

    H65.111 **Acute and subacute allergic otitis media (mucoid) (sanguinous) (serous), right ear**

    H65.112 **Acute and subacute allergic otitis media (mucoid) (sanguinous) (serous), left ear**

    H65.113 **Acute and subacute allergic otitis media (mucoid) (sanguinous) (serous), bilateral**

    H65.114 **Acute and subacute allergic otitis media (mucoid) (sanguinous) (serous), recurrent, right ear**

    H65.115 **Acute and subacute allergic otitis media (mucoid) (sanguinous) (serous), recurrent, left ear**

    H65.116 **Acute and subacute allergic otitis media (mucoid) (sanguinous) (serous), recurrent, bilateral**

    H65.117 **Acute and subacute allergic otitis media (mucoid) (sanguinous) (serous), recurrent, unspecified ear**

    H65.119 **Acute and subacute allergic otitis media (mucoid) (sanguinous) (serous), unspecified ear**

  H65.19 Other acute nonsuppurative otitis media

    Acute and subacute mucoid otitis media

    Acute and subacute nonsuppurative otitis media NOS

    Acute and subacute sanguinous otitis media

    Acute and subacute seromucinous otitis media

    H65.191 **Other acute nonsuppurative otitis media, right ear**

    H65.192 **Other acute nonsuppurative otitis media, left ear**

    H65.193 **Other acute nonsuppurative otitis media, bilateral**

    H65.194 **Other acute nonsuppurative otitis media, recurrent, right ear**

    H65.195 **Other acute nonsuppurative otitis media, recurrent, left ear**

    H65.196 **Other acute nonsuppurative otitis media, recurrent, bilateral**

    H65.197 **Other acute nonsuppurative otitis media recurrent, unspecified ear**

    H65.199 **Other acute nonsuppurative otitis media, unspecified ear**

H65.2 Chronic serous otitis media

  Chronic tubotympanal catarrh

  H65.20 **Chronic serous otitis media, unspecified ear**

  H65.21 **Chronic serous otitis media, right ear**

  H65.22 **Chronic serous otitis media, left ear**

  H65.23 **Chronic serous otitis media, bilateral**

H65.3 Chronic mucoid otitis media

  Chronic mucinous otitis media

  Chronic secretory otitis media

  Chronic transudative otitis media

  Glue ear

  EXCLUDES1 adhesive middle ear disease (H74.1)

  H65.30 **Chronic mucoid otitis media, unspecified ear**

  H65.31 **Chronic mucoid otitis media, right ear**

PDx Unacceptable principal diagnosis symbol per Medicare code edits   PDx Code exempt from diagnosis present on admission requirement

❓ Questionable admission   cc Complication or comorbidity   MCC Major complication or comorbidity   cc/MCC Exc CC/MCC exclusion

HCC HCC diagnosis code   RxHCC RxHCC diagnosis code   MACRA code   **DEFINITION** Describes condition/terminology

TIP Coding guidance   👁 Official Guideline Reference   Z1 Z code as first-listed diagnosis

636   When symbols appear on a code that requires a 7th character extension, refer to Appendix B to identify applicable 7th character codes.   **2020 ICD-10-CM**

TER 8: DISEA

H65.32 Chronic mucoid otitis media, left ear
H65.33 Chronic mucoid otitis media, bilateral

[5th] H65.4 Other chronic nonsuppurative otitis media

[6th] H65.41 Chronic allergic otitis media
H65.411 Chronic allergic otitis media, right ear
H65.412 Chronic allergic otitis media, left ear
H65.413 Chronic allergic otitis media, bilateral
H65.419 Chronic allergic otitis media, unspecified ear

[6th] H65.49 Other chronic nonsuppurative otitis media
Chronic exudative otitis media
Chronic nonsuppurative otitis media NOS
Chronic otitis media with effusion (nonpurulent)
Chronic seromucinous otitis media
H65.491 Other chronic nonsuppurative otitis media, right ear
H65.492 Other chronic nonsuppurative otitis media, left ear
H65.493 Other chronic nonsuppurative otitis media, bilateral
H65.499 Other chronic nonsuppurative otitis media, unspecified ear

[5th] H65.9 Unspecified nonsuppurative otitis media
Allergic otitis media NOS
Catarrhal otitis media NOS
Exudative otitis media NOS
Mucoid otitis media NOS
Otitis media with effusion (nonpurulent) NOS
Secretory otitis media NOS
Seromucinous otitis media NOS
Serous otitis media NOS
Transudative otitis media NOS
H65.90 Unspecified nonsuppurative otitis media, unspecified ear
H65.91 Unspecified nonsuppurative otitis media, right ear
H65.92 Unspecified nonsuppurative otitis media, left ear
H65.93 Unspecified nonsuppurative otitis media, bilateral

[4th] H66 Suppurative and unspecified otitis media
INCLUDES *suppurative and unspecified otitis media with myringitis*
Use additional code to identify:
exposure to environmental tobacco smoke (Z77.22)
exposure to tobacco smoke in the perinatal period (P96.81)
history of tobacco dependence (Z87.891)
occupational exposure to environmental tobacco smoke (Z57.31)
tobacco dependence (F17.-)
tobacco use (Z72.0)

[5th] H66.0 Acute suppurative otitis media

[6th] H66.00 Acute suppurative otitis media without spontaneous rupture of ear drum
H66.001 Acute suppurative otitis media without spontaneous rupture of ear drum, right ear
AHA: Q1 2016
H66.002 Acute suppurative otitis media without spontaneous rupture of ear drum, left ear
H66.003 Acute suppurative otitis media without spontaneous rupture of ear drum, bilateral
H66.004 Acute suppurative otitis media without spontaneous rupture of ear drum, recurrent, right ear
H66.005 Acute suppurative otitis media without spontaneous rupture of ear drum, recurrent, left ear
H66.006 Acute suppurative otitis media without spontaneous rupture of ear drum, recurrent, bilateral
H66.007 Acute suppurative otitis media without spontaneous rupture of ear drum, recurrent, unspecified ear
H66.009 Acute suppurative otitis media without spontaneous rupture of ear drum, unspecified ear

[6th] H66.01 Acute suppurative otitis media with spontaneous rupture of ear drum
H66.011 Acute suppurative otitis media with spontaneous rupture of ear drum, right ear
H66.012 Acute suppurative otitis media with spontaneous rupture of ear drum, left ear
H66.013 Acute suppurative otitis media with spontaneous rupture of ear drum, bilateral
H66.014 Acute suppurative otitis media with spontaneous rupture of ear drum, recurrent, right ear
H66.015 Acute suppurative otitis media with spontaneous rupture of ear drum, recurrent, left ear
H66.016 Acute suppurative otitis media with spontaneous rupture of ear drum, recurrent, bilateral
H66.017 Acute suppurative otitis media with spontaneous rupture of ear drum, recurrent, unspecified ear
H66.019 Acute suppurative otitis media with spontaneous rupture of ear drum, unspecified ear

[5th] H66.1 Chronic tubotympanic suppurative otitis media
Benign chronic suppurative otitis media
Chronic tubotympanic disease
Use additional code for any associated perforated tympanic membrane (H72.-)
H66.10 Chronic tubotympanic suppurative otitis media, unspecified
H66.11 Chronic tubotympanic suppurative otitis media, right ear
H66.12 Chronic tubotympanic suppurative otitis media, left ear
H66.13 Chronic tubotympanic suppurative otitis media, bilateral

[5th] H66.2 Chronic atticoantral suppurative otitis media
Chronic atticoantral disease
Use additional code for any associated perforated tympanic membrane (H72.-)
H66.20 Chronic atticoantral suppurative otitis media, unspecified ear
H66.21 Chronic atticoantral suppurative otitis media, right ear
H66.22 Chronic atticoantral suppurative otitis media, left ear
H66.23 Chronic atticoantral suppurative otitis media, bilateral

[5th] H66.3 Other chronic suppurative otitis media
Chronic suppurative otitis media NOS
Use additional code for any associated perforated tympanic membrane (H72.-)
EXCLUDES1 *tuberculous otitis media (A18.6)*

[6th] H66.3X Other chronic suppurative otitis media
H66.3X1 Other chronic suppurative otitis media, right ear
H66.3X2 Other chronic suppurative otitis media, left ear
H66.3X3 Other chronic suppurative otitis media, bilateral
H66.3X9 Other chronic suppurative otitis media, unspecified ear

[5th] H66.4 Suppurative otitis media, unspecified
Purulent otitis media NOS
Use additional code for any associated perforated tympanic membrane (H72.-)
H66.40 Suppurative otitis media, unspecified, unspecified ear
H66.41 Suppurative otitis media, unspecified, right ear
H66.42 Suppurative otitis media, unspecified, left ear
H66.43 Suppurative otitis media, unspecified, bilateral

Unspecified Code | Other Specified Code | Manifestation Code | [N] Newborn | [P] Pediatric | [M] Maternity | [A] Adult | ♂ Male | ♀ Female
● New Code | ▲ Revised Code Title | ▶◀ Revised Text | NOTES | INCLUDES | EXCLUDES1 Not coded here | EXCLUDES2 Not included here
[4th] 4th character required | [5th] 5th character required | [6th] 6th character required | [7th] 7th character required | [X] Extension 'X' Alert
[HAC] Hospital-acquired condition (HAC) alert | AHA AHA Coding Clinic© | ☛ Code first alert

5ᵗʰ H66.9 **Otitis media, unspecified**
　Otitis media NOS
　Acute otitis media NOS
　Chronic otitis media NOS
　Use additional code for any associated perforated tympanic
　　membrane (H72.-)
　H66.90 **Otitis media, unspecified, unspecified ear**
　H66.91 **Otitis media, unspecified,** right ear
　H66.92 **Otitis media, unspecified,** left ear
　H66.93 **Otitis media, unspecified,** bilateral

4ᵗʰ H67 **Otitis media in diseases classified elsewhere**
　☞ **Code first** underlying disease, such as:
　　plasminogen deficiency (E88.02)
　　viral disease NEC (B00-B34)
　Use additional code for any associated perforated tympanic
　　membrane (H72.-)
　　EXCLUDES1 otitis media in:
　　　influenza (J09.X9, J10.83, J11.83)
　　　measles (B05.3)
　　　scarlet fever (A38.0)
　　　tuberculosis (A18.6)
　H67.1 **Otitis media in diseases classified elsewhere,** right ear
　H67.2 **Otitis media in diseases classified elsewhere,** left ear
　H67.3 **Otitis media in diseases classified elsewhere,** bilateral
　H67.9 **Otitis media in diseases classified elsewhere, unspecified ear**

4ᵗʰ H68 **Eustachian salpingitis and obstruction**
　5ᵗʰ H68.0 **Eustachian** salpingitis
　　6ᵗʰ H68.00 **Unspecified Eustachian salpingitis**
　　　H68.001 **Unspecified Eustachian salpingitis,** right ear
　　　H68.002 **Unspecified Eustachian salpingitis,** left ear
　　　H68.003 **Unspecified Eustachian salpingitis,** bilateral
　　　H68.009 **Unspecified Eustachian salpingitis, unspecified ear**
　　6ᵗʰ H68.01 Acute **Eustachian salpingitis**
　　　H68.011 **Acute Eustachian salpingitis,** right ear
　　　H68.012 **Acute Eustachian salpingitis,** left ear
　　　H68.013 **Acute Eustachian salpingitis,** bilateral
　　　H68.019 **Acute Eustachian salpingitis, unspecified ear**
　　6ᵗʰ H68.02 Chronic **Eustachian salpingitis**
　　　H68.021 **Chronic Eustachian salpingitis,** right ear
　　　H68.022 **Chronic Eustachian salpingitis,** left ear
　　　H68.023 **Chronic Eustachian salpingitis,** bilateral
　　　H68.029 **Chronic Eustachian salpingitis, unspecified ear**
　5ᵗʰ H68.1 Obstruction **of Eustachian tube**
　　Stenosis of Eustachian tube
　　Stricture of Eustachian tube
　　6ᵗʰ H68.10 **Unspecified obstruction of Eustachian tube**
　　　H68.101 **Unspecified obstruction of Eustachian tube,** right ear
　　　H68.102 **Unspecified obstruction of Eustachian tube,** left ear
　　　H68.103 **Unspecified obstruction of Eustachian tube,** bilateral
　　　H68.109 **Unspecified obstruction of Eustachian tube, unspecified ear**
　　6ᵗʰ H68.11 Osseous **obstruction of Eustachian tube**
　　　H68.111 **Osseous obstruction of Eustachian tube,** right ear
　　　H68.112 **Osseous obstruction of Eustachian tube,** left ear
　　　H68.113 **Osseous obstruction of Eustachian tube,** bilateral
　　　H68.119 **Osseous obstruction of Eustachian tube, unspecified ear**
　　6ᵗʰ H68.12 Intrinsic cartilagenous **obstruction of Eustachian tube**

　　　H68.121 **Intrinsic cartilagenous obstruction of Eustachian tube,** right ear
　　　H68.122 **Intrinsic cartilagenous obstruction of Eustachian tube,** left ear
　　　H68.123 **Intrinsic cartilagenous obstruction of Eustachian tube,** bilateral
　　　H68.129 **Intrinsic cartilagenous obstruction of Eustachian tube, unspecified ear**
　　6ᵗʰ H68.13 Extrinsic cartilagenous **obstruction of Eustachian tube**
　　　Compression of Eustachian tube
　　　H68.131 **Extrinsic cartilagenous obstruction of Eustachian tube,** right ear
　　　H68.132 **Extrinsic cartilagenous obstruction of Eustachian tube,** left ear
　　　H68.133 **Extrinsic cartilagenous obstruction of Eustachian tube,** bilateral
　　　H68.139 **Extrinsic cartilagenous obstruction of Eustachian tube, unspecified ear**

4ᵗʰ H69 **Other and unspecified disorders of Eustachian tube**
　5ᵗʰ H69.0 Patulous **Eustachian tube**
　　H69.00 **Patulous Eustachian tube, unspecified ear**
　　H69.01 **Patulous Eustachian tube,** right ear
　　H69.02 **Patulous Eustachian tube,** left ear
　　H69.03 **Patulous Eustachian tube,** bilateral
　5ᵗʰ H69.8 **Other specified disorders of Eustachian tube**
　　H69.80 **Other specified disorders of Eustachian tube, unspecified ear**
　　H69.81 **Other specified disorders of Eustachian tube,** right ear
　　H69.82 **Other specified disorders of Eustachian tube,** left ear
　　H69.83 **Other specified disorders of Eustachian tube,** bilateral
　5ᵗʰ H69.9 **Unspecified Eustachian tube disorder**
　　H69.90 **Unspecified Eustachian tube disorder, unspecified ear**
　　H69.91 **Unspecified Eustachian tube disorder,** right ear
　　H69.92 **Unspecified Eustachian tube disorder,** left ear
　　H69.93 **Unspecified Eustachian tube disorder,** bilateral

4ᵗʰ H70 **Mastoiditis and related conditions**
　DEFINITION: Mastoiditis is a bacterial infection of the mastoid air cells
　　in the inner and middle ear, usually caused by untreated
　　acute otitis media (middle ear infection).
　5ᵗʰ H70.0 Acute **mastoiditis**
　　Abscess of mastoid
　　Empyema of mastoid
　　6ᵗʰ H70.00 **Acute mastoiditis** without complications
　　　H70.001 **Acute mastoiditis without complications,** right ear　🅒🅒 CC/MCC Exc
　　　H70.002 **Acute mastoiditis without complications,** left ear　🅒🅒 CC/MCC Exc
　　　H70.003 **Acute mastoiditis without complications,** bilateral　🅒🅒 CC/MCC Exc
　　　H70.009 **Acute mastoiditis without complications, unspecified ear**　🅒🅒 CC/MCC Exc
　　6ᵗʰ H70.01 Subperiosteal abscess **of mastoid**
　　　H70.011 **Subperiosteal abscess of mastoid,** right ear　🅒🅒 CC/MCC Exc
　　　H70.012 **Subperiosteal abscess of mastoid,** left ear　🅒🅒 CC/MCC Exc
　　　H70.013 **Subperiosteal abscess of mastoid,** bilateral　🅒🅒 CC/MCC Exc
　　　H70.019 **Subperiosteal abscess of mastoid, unspecified ear**　🅒🅒 CC/MCC Exc
　　6ᵗʰ H70.09 Acute mastoiditis with other complications
　　　H70.091 **Acute mastoiditis with other complications,** right ear　🅒🅒 CC/MCC Exc
　　　H70.092 **Acute mastoiditis with other complications,** left ear　🅒🅒 CC/MCC Exc
　　　H70.093 **Acute mastoiditis with other complications,** bilateral　🅒🅒 CC/MCC Exc

PDXⁿ Unacceptable principal diagnosis symbol per Medicare code edits　POA Code exempt from diagnosis present on admission requirement
❓ Questionable admission　🅒 Complication or comorbidity　MCC Major complication or comorbidity　CC/MCC Exc CC/MCC exclusion
HCC HCC diagnosis code　RxHCC RxHCC diagnosis code　MACRA MACRA code　**DEFINITION** Describes condition/terminology
TIP Coding guidance　👁 Official Guideline Reference　Z1 Z code as first-listed diagnosis

638　When symbols appear on a code that requires a 7th character extension, refer to Appendix B to identify applicable 7th character codes.　**2020 ICD-10-CM**

H70.099 Acute mastoiditis with other complications, unspecified ear ⟨CC⟩ ⟨CC/MCC Exc⟩

🔵5ᵗʰ H70.1 Chronic **mastoiditis**
Caries of mastoid
Fistula of mastoid
EXCLUDES1 *tuberculous mastoiditis (A18.03)*
H70.10 **Chronic mastoiditis, unspecified ear**
H70.11 **Chronic mastoiditis,** right **ear**
H70.12 **Chronic mastoiditis,** left **ear**
H70.13 **Chronic mastoiditis,** bilateral

🔵5ᵗʰ H70.2 Petrositis
Inflammation of petrous bone
🔵6ᵗʰ H70.20 **Unspecified petrositis**
H70.201 **Unspecified petrositis,** right **ear**
H70.202 **Unspecified petrositis,** left **ear**
H70.203 **Unspecified petrositis,** bilateral
H70.209 **Unspecified petrositis, unspecified ear**
🔵6ᵗʰ H70.21 Acute **petrositis**
H70.211 **Acute petrositis,** right **ear**
H70.212 **Acute petrositis,** left **ear**
H70.213 **Acute petrositis,** bilateral
H70.219 **Acute petrositis, unspecified ear**
🔵6ᵗʰ H70.22 Chronic petrositis
H70.221 **Chronic petrositis,** right **ear**
H70.222 **Chronic petrositis,** left **ear**
H70.223 **Chronic petrositis,** bilateral
H70.229 **Chronic petrositis, unspecified ear**

🔵5ᵗʰ H70.8 Other **mastoiditis and related conditions**
EXCLUDES1 *preauricular sinus and cyst (Q18.1)*
sinus, fistula, and cyst of branchial cleft (Q18.0)
🔵6ᵗʰ H70.81 Postauricular fistula
H70.811 **Postauricular fistula,** right **ear**
H70.812 **Postauricular fistula,** left **ear**
H70.813 **Postauricular fistula,** bilateral
H70.819 **Postauricular fistula, unspecified ear**
🔵6ᵗʰ H70.89 Other mastoiditis and related conditions
H70.891 **Other mastoiditis and related conditions,** right **ear**
H70.892 **Other mastoiditis and related conditions,** left **ear**
H70.893 **Other mastoiditis and related conditions,** bilateral
H70.899 **Other mastoiditis and related conditions, unspecified ear**

🔵5ᵗʰ H70.9 Unspecified **mastoiditis**
H70.90 **Unspecified mastoiditis, unspecified ear**
H70.91 **Unspecified mastoiditis,** right **ear**
H70.92 **Unspecified mastoiditis,** left **ear**
H70.93 **Unspecified mastoiditis,** bilateral

🔵4ᵗʰ H71 Cholesteatoma of middle ear
EXCLUDES2 *cholesteatoma of external ear (H60.4-)*
recurrent cholesteatoma of postmastoidectomy cavity (H95.0-)
🔵5ᵗʰ H71.0 Cholesteatoma of attic
H71.00 **Cholesteatoma of attic, unspecified ear**
H71.01 **Cholesteatoma of attic,** right **ear**
H71.02 **Cholesteatoma of attic,** left **ear**
H71.03 **Cholesteatoma of attic,** bilateral
🔵5ᵗʰ H71.1 Cholesteatoma of tympanum
H71.10 **Cholesteatoma of tympanum, unspecified ear**
H71.11 **Cholesteatoma of tympanum,** right **ear**
H71.12 **Cholesteatoma of tympanum,** left **ear**
H71.13 **Cholesteatoma of tympanum,** bilateral
🔵5ᵗʰ H71.2 Cholesteatoma of mastoid
H71.20 **Cholesteatoma of mastoid, unspecified ear**
H71.21 **Cholesteatoma of mastoid,** right **ear**
H71.22 **Cholesteatoma of mastoid,** left **ear**
H71.23 **Cholesteatoma of mastoid,** bilateral
🔵5ᵗʰ H71.3 Diffuse **cholesteatosis**

H71.30 **Diffuse cholesteatosis, unspecified ear**
H71.31 **Diffuse cholesteatosis,** right **ear**
H71.32 **Diffuse cholesteatosis,** left **ear**
H71.33 **Diffuse cholesteatosis,** bilateral
🔵5ᵗʰ H71.9 Unspecified cholesteatoma
H71.90 **Unspecified cholesteatoma, unspecified ear**
H71.91 **Unspecified cholesteatoma,** right **ear**
H71.92 **Unspecified cholesteatoma,** left **ear**
H71.93 **Unspecified cholesteatoma,** bilateral

🔵4ᵗʰ H72 Perforation **of tympanic membrane**
INCLUDES *persistent post-traumatic perforation of ear drum*
postinflammatory perforation of ear drum
📧 Code first any associated otitis media (H65.-, H66.1-, H66.2-, H66.3-, H66.4-, H66.9-, H67.-)
EXCLUDES1 *acute suppurative otitis media with rupture of the tympanic membrane (H66.01-)*
traumatic rupture of ear drum (S09.2-)
🔵5ᵗʰ H72.0 Central **perforation of tympanic membrane**
H72.00 **Central perforation of tympanic membrane, unspecified ear**
H72.01 **Central perforation of tympanic membrane,** right **ear**
H72.02 **Central perforation of tympanic membrane,** left **ear**
H72.03 **Central perforation of tympanic membrane,** bilateral
🔵5ᵗʰ H72.1 Attic **perforation of tympanic membrane**
Perforation of pars flaccida
H72.10 **Attic perforation of tympanic membrane, unspecified ear**
H72.11 **Attic perforation of tympanic membrane,** right **ear**
H72.12 **Attic perforation of tympanic membrane,** left **ear**
H72.13 **Attic perforation of tympanic membrane,** bilateral
🔵5ᵗʰ H72.2 Other marginal **perforations of tympanic membrane**
🔵6ᵗʰ H72.2X **Other marginal perforations of tympanic membrane**
H72.2X1 **Other marginal perforations of tympanic membrane,** right **ear**
H72.2X2 **Other marginal perforations of tympanic membrane,** left **ear**
H72.2X3 **Other marginal perforations of tympanic membrane,** bilateral
H72.2X9 **Other marginal perforations of tympanic membrane, unspecified ear**
🔵5ᵗʰ H72.8 Other perforations of tympanic membrane
🔵6ᵗʰ H72.81 Multiple **perforations of tympanic membrane**
H72.811 **Multiple perforations of tympanic membrane,** right **ear**
H72.812 **Multiple perforations of tympanic membrane,** left **ear**
H72.813 **Multiple perforations of tympanic membrane,** bilateral
H72.819 **Multiple perforations of tympanic membrane, unspecified ear**
🔵6ᵗʰ H72.82 Total **perforations of tympanic membrane**
H72.821 **Total perforations of tympanic membrane,** right **ear**
H72.822 **Total perforations of tympanic membrane,** left **ear**
H72.823 **Total perforations of tympanic membrane,** bilateral
H72.829 **Total perforations of tympanic membrane, unspecified ear**
🔵5ᵗʰ H72.9 Unspecified perforation of tympanic membrane
H72.90 **Unspecified perforation of tympanic membrane, unspecified ear**
H72.91 **Unspecified perforation of tympanic membrane,** right **ear**
H72.92 **Unspecified perforation of tympanic membrane,** left **ear**
H72.93 **Unspecified perforation of tympanic membrane,** bilateral

---

Unspecified Code   Other Specified Code   Manifestation Code   Ⓝ Newborn   Ⓟ Pediatric   Ⓜ Maternity   Ⓐ Adult   ♂ Male   ♀ Female
● New Code   ▲ Revised Code Title   ▶◀ Revised Text   NOTES   *INCLUDES*   *EXCLUDES1* Not coded here   *EXCLUDES2* Not included here
🔵4ᵗʰ 4ᵗʰ character required   🔵5ᵗʰ 5ᵗʰ character required   🔵6ᵗʰ 6ᵗʰ character required   🔵7ᵗʰ 7ᵗʰ character required   🔵 Extension 'X' Alert
HAC Hospital-acquired condition (HAC) alert   AHA AHA Coding Clinic©   📧 Code first alert

H73 - H75.0

CHAPTER 8: DISEASES OF THE EAR AND MASTOID PROCESS (H60-H95)

H73 Other disorders of tympanic membrane
- **H73.0 Acute myringitis**
  - EXCLUDES1 acute myringitis with otitis media (H65, H66)
  - **H73.00 Unspecified acute myringitis**
    - Acute tympanitis NOS
    - H73.001 Acute myringitis, right ear
    - H73.002 Acute myringitis, left ear
    - H73.003 Acute myringitis, bilateral
    - H73.009 Acute myringitis, unspecified ear
  - **H73.01 Bullous myringitis**
    - H73.011 Bullous myringitis, right ear
    - H73.012 Bullous myringitis, left ear
    - H73.013 Bullous myringitis, bilateral
    - H73.019 Bullous myringitis, unspecified ear
  - **H73.09 Other acute myringitis**
    - H73.091 Other acute myringitis, right ear
    - H73.092 Other acute myringitis, left ear
    - H73.093 Other acute myringitis, bilateral
    - H73.099 Other acute myringitis, unspecified ear
- **H73.1 Chronic myringitis**
  - Chronic tympanitis
  - EXCLUDES1 chronic myringitis with otitis media (H65, H66)
  - H73.10 Chronic myringitis, unspecified ear
  - H73.11 Chronic myringitis, right ear
  - H73.12 Chronic myringitis, left ear
  - H73.13 Chronic myringitis, bilateral
- **H73.2 Unspecified myringitis**
  - H73.20 Unspecified myringitis, unspecified ear
  - H73.21 Unspecified myringitis, right ear
  - H73.22 Unspecified myringitis, left ear
  - H73.23 Unspecified myringitis, bilateral
- **H73.8 Other specified disorders of tympanic membrane**
  - **H73.81 Atrophic flaccid tympanic membrane**
    - H73.811 Atrophic flaccid tympanic membrane, right ear
    - H73.812 Atrophic flaccid tympanic membrane, left ear
    - H73.813 Atrophic flaccid tympanic membrane, bilateral
    - H73.819 Atrophic flaccid tympanic membrane, unspecified ear
  - **H73.82 Atrophic nonflaccid tympanic membrane**
    - H73.821 Atrophic nonflaccid tympanic membrane, right ear
    - H73.822 Atrophic nonflaccid tympanic membrane, left ear
    - H73.823 Atrophic nonflaccid tympanic membrane, bilateral
    - H73.829 Atrophic nonflaccid tympanic membrane, unspecified ear
  - **H73.89 Other specified disorders of tympanic membrane**
    - H73.891 Other specified disorders of tympanic membrane, right ear
    - H73.892 Other specified disorders of tympanic membrane, left ear
    - H73.893 Other specified disorders of tympanic membrane, bilateral
    - H73.899 Other specified disorders of tympanic membrane, unspecified ear
- **H73.9 Unspecified disorder of tympanic membrane**
  - H73.90 Unspecified disorder of tympanic membrane, unspecified ear
  - H73.91 Unspecified disorder of tympanic membrane, right ear
  - H73.92 Unspecified disorder of tympanic membrane, left ear
  - H73.93 Unspecified disorder of tympanic membrane, bilateral

H74 Other disorders of middle ear mastoid
- EXCLUDES2 mastoiditis (H70.-)
- **H74.0 Tympanosclerosis**
  - H74.01 Tympanosclerosis, right ear
  - H74.02 Tympanosclerosis, left ear
  - H74.03 Tympanosclerosis, bilateral
  - H74.09 Tympanosclerosis, unspecified ear
- **H74.1 Adhesive middle ear disease**
  - Adhesive otitis
  - EXCLUDES1 glue ear (H65.3-)
  - H74.11 Adhesive right middle ear disease
  - H74.12 Adhesive left middle ear disease
  - H74.13 Adhesive middle ear disease, bilateral
  - H74.19 Adhesive middle ear disease, unspecified ear
- **H74.2 Discontinuity and dislocation of ear ossicles**
  - H74.20 Discontinuity and dislocation of ear ossicles, unspecified ear
  - H74.21 Discontinuity and dislocation of right ear ossicles
  - H74.22 Discontinuity and dislocation of left ear ossicles
  - H74.23 Discontinuity and dislocation of ear ossicles, bilateral
- **H74.3 Other acquired abnormalities of ear ossicles**
  - **H74.31 Ankylosis of ear ossicles**
    - H74.311 Ankylosis of ear ossicles, right ear
    - H74.312 Ankylosis of ear ossicles, left ear
    - H74.313 Ankylosis of ear ossicles, bilateral
    - H74.319 Ankylosis of ear ossicles, unspecified ear
  - **H74.32 Partial loss of ear ossicles**
    - H74.321 Partial loss of ear ossicles, right ear
    - H74.322 Partial loss of ear ossicles, left ear
    - H74.323 Partial loss of ear ossicles, bilateral
    - H74.329 Partial loss of ear ossicles, unspecified ear
  - **H74.39 Other acquired abnormalities of ear ossicles**
    - H74.391 Other acquired abnormalities of right ear ossicles
    - H74.392 Other acquired abnormalities of left ear ossicles
    - H74.393 Other acquired abnormalities of ear ossicles, bilateral
    - H74.399 Other acquired abnormalities of ear ossicles, unspecified ear
- **H74.4 Polyp of middle ear**
  - H74.40 Polyp of middle ear, unspecified ear
  - H74.41 Polyp of right middle ear
  - H74.42 Polyp of left middle ear
  - H74.43 Polyp of middle ear, bilateral
- **H74.8 Other specified disorders of middle ear and mastoid**
  - **H74.8X Other specified disorders of middle ear and mastoid**
    - H74.8X1 Other specified disorders of right middle ear and mastoid
    - H74.8X2 Other specified disorders of left middle ear and mastoid
    - H74.8X3 Other specified disorders of middle ear and mastoid, bilateral
    - H74.8X9 Other specified disorders of middle ear and mastoid, unspecified ear
- **H74.9 Unspecified disorder of middle ear and mastoid**
  - H74.90 Unspecified disorder of middle ear and mastoid, unspecified ear
  - H74.91 Unspecified disorder of right middle ear and mastoid
  - H74.92 Unspecified disorder of left middle ear and mastoid
  - H74.93 Unspecified disorder of middle ear and mastoid, bilateral

H75 Other disorders of middle ear and mastoid in diseases classified elsewhere
- Code first underlying disease
- **H75.0 Mastoiditis in infectious and parasitic diseases classified elsewhere**
  - EXCLUDES1 mastoiditis (in):
    - syphilis (A52.77)
    - tuberculosis (A18.03)

POAℹ Unacceptable principal diagnosis symbol per Medicare code edits   POA Code exempt from diagnosis present on admission requirement
❓ Questionable admission   ℭℭ Complication or comorbidity   MCC Major complication or comorbidity   CC/MCC CC/MCC exclusion
HCC HCC diagnosis code   RxHCC RxHCC diagnosis code   MACRA MACRA code   **DEFINITION** Describes condition/terminology
TIP Coding guidance   👁 Official Guideline Reference   Z1 Z code as first-listed diagnosis

H75.00 Mastoiditis in infectious and parasitic diseases classified elsewhere, unspecified ear
H75.01 Mastoiditis in infectious and parasitic diseases classified elsewhere, right ear
H75.02 Mastoiditis in infectious and parasitic diseases classified elsewhere, left ear
H75.03 Mastoiditis in infectious and parasitic diseases classified elsewhere, bilateral
H75.8 Other specified disorders of middle ear and mastoid in diseases classified elsewhere
H75.80 Other specified disorders of middle ear and mastoid in diseases classified elsewhere, unspecified ear
H75.81 Other specified disorders of right middle ear and mastoid in diseases classified elsewhere
H75.82 Other specified disorders of left middle ear and mastoid in diseases classified elsewhere
H75.83 Other specified disorders of middle ear and mastoid in diseases classified elsewhere, bilateral

Diseases of inner ear (H80-H83)

H80 Otosclerosis
DEFINITION: Otosclerosis is abnormal bone growth around the ossicles (bones) of the inner ear, which disrupts hearing.
INCLUDES Otospongiosis
H80.0 Otosclerosis involving oval window, nonobliterative
H80.00 Otosclerosis involving oval window, nonobliterative, unspecified ear
H80.01 Otosclerosis involving oval window, nonobliterative, right ear
H80.02 Otosclerosis involving oval window, nonobliterative, left ear
H80.03 Otosclerosis involving oval window, nonobliterative, bilateral
H80.1 Otosclerosis involving oval window, obliterative
H80.10 Otosclerosis involving oval window, obliterative, unspecified ear
H80.11 Otosclerosis involving oval window, obliterative, right ear
H80.12 Otosclerosis involving oval window, obliterative, left ear
H80.13 Otosclerosis involving oval window, obliterative, bilateral
H80.2 Cochlear otosclerosis
Otosclerosis involving otic capsule
Otosclerosis involving round window
H80.20 Cochlear otosclerosis, unspecified ear
H80.21 Cochlear otosclerosis, right ear
H80.22 Cochlear otosclerosis, left ear
H80.23 Cochlear otosclerosis, bilateral
H80.8 Other otosclerosis
H80.80 Other otosclerosis, unspecified ear
H80.81 Other otosclerosis, right ear
H80.82 Other otosclerosis, left ear
H80.83 Other otosclerosis, bilateral
H80.9 Unspecified otosclerosis
H80.90 Unspecified otosclerosis, unspecified ear
H80.91 Unspecified otosclerosis, right ear
H80.92 Unspecified otosclerosis, left ear
H80.93 Unspecified otosclerosis, bilateral
H81 Disorders of vestibular function
EXCLUDES1 epidemic vertigo (A88.1)
vertigo NOS (R42)
H81.0 Ménière's disease
Labyrinthine hydrops
Ménière's syndrome or vertigo
H81.01 Ménière's disease, right ear
H81.02 Ménière's disease, left ear
H81.03 Ménière's disease, bilateral
H81.09 Ménière's disease, unspecified ear

H81.1 Benign paroxysmal vertigo
H81.10 Benign paroxysmal vertigo, unspecified ear
H81.11 Benign paroxysmal vertigo, right ear
H81.12 Benign paroxysmal vertigo, left ear
H81.13 Benign paroxysmal vertigo, bilateral
H81.2 Vestibular neuronitis
H81.20 Vestibular neuronitis, unspecified ear
H81.21 Vestibular neuronitis, right ear
H81.22 Vestibular neuronitis, left ear
H81.23 Vestibular neuronitis, bilateral
H81.3 Other peripheral vertigo
H81.31 Aural vertigo
H81.311 Aural vertigo, right ear
H81.312 Aural vertigo, left ear
H81.313 Aural vertigo, bilateral
H81.319 Aural vertigo, unspecified ear
H81.39 Other peripheral vertigo
Lermoyez' syndrome
Otogenic vertigo
Peripheral vertigo NOS
H81.391 Other peripheral vertigo, right ear
H81.392 Other peripheral vertigo, left ear
H81.393 Other peripheral vertigo, bilateral
H81.399 Other peripheral vertigo, unspecified ear
H81.4 Vertigo of central origin
Central positional nystagmus
H81.8 Other disorders of vestibular function
H81.8X Other disorders of vestibular function
H81.8X1 Other disorders of vestibular function, right ear
H81.8X2 Other disorders of vestibular function, left ear
H81.8X3 Other disorders of vestibular function, bilateral
H81.8X9 Other disorders of vestibular function, unspecified ear
H81.9 Unspecified disorder of vestibular function
Vertiginous syndrome NOS
H81.90 Unspecified disorder of vestibular function, unspecified ear
H81.91 Unspecified disorder of vestibular function, right ear
H81.92 Unspecified disorder of vestibular function, left ear
H81.93 Unspecified disorder of vestibular function, bilateral
H82 Vertiginous syndromes in diseases classified elsewhere
Code first underlying disease
EXCLUDES1 epidemic vertigo (A88.1)
H82.1 Vertiginous syndromes in diseases classified elsewhere, right ear
H82.2 Vertiginous syndromes in diseases classified elsewhere, left ear
H82.3 Vertiginous syndromes in diseases classified elsewhere, bilateral
H82.9 Vertiginous syndromes in diseases classified elsewhere, unspecified ear
H83 Other diseases of inner ear
H83.0 Labyrinthitis
H83.01 Labyrinthitis, right ear
H83.02 Labyrinthitis, left ear
H83.03 Labyrinthitis, bilateral
H83.09 Labyrinthitis, unspecified ear
H83.1 Labyrinthine fistula
H83.11 Labyrinthine fistula, right ear
H83.12 Labyrinthine fistula, left ear
H83.13 Labyrinthine fistula, bilateral
H83.19 Labyrinthine fistula, unspecified ear
H83.2 Labyrinthine dysfunction
Labyrinthine hypersensitivity
Labyrinthine hypofunction
Labyrinthine loss of function

Unspecified Code Other Specified Code Manifestation Code N Newborn P Pediatric M Maternity A Adult ♂ Male ♀ Female
● New Code ▲ Revised Code Title ▶◀ Revised Text NOTES INCLUDES EXCLUDES1 Not coded here EXCLUDES2 Not included here
4th character required 5th character required 6th character required 7th character required Extension 'X' Alert
HAC Hospital-acquired condition (HAC) alert AHA AHA Coding Clinic© Code first alert

[6th] H83.2X Labyrinthine dysfunction
H83.2X1 Labyrinthine dysfunction, right ear
H83.2X2 Labyrinthine dysfunction, left ear
H83.2X3 Labyrinthine dysfunction, bilateral
H83.2X9 Labyrinthine dysfunction, unspecified ear

[5th] H83.3 Noise effects on inner ear
Acoustic trauma of inner ear
Noise-induced hearing loss of inner ear
[6th] H83.3X Noise effects on inner ear
H83.3X1 Noise effects on right inner ear
H83.3X2 Noise effects on left inner ear
H83.3X3 Noise effects on inner ear, bilateral
H83.3X9 Noise effects on inner ear, unspecified ear

[5th] H83.8 Other specified diseases of inner ear
[6th] H83.8X Other specified diseases of inner ear
H83.8X1 Other specified diseases of right inner ear
H83.8X2 Other specified diseases of left inner ear
H83.8X3 Other specified diseases of inner ear, bilateral
H83.8X9 Other specified diseases of inner ear, unspecified ear

[5th] H83.9 Unspecified disease of inner ear
H83.90 Unspecified disease of inner ear, unspecified ear
H83.91 Unspecified disease of right inner ear
H83.92 Unspecified disease of left inner ear
H83.93 Unspecified disease of inner ear, bilateral

Other disorders of ear (H90-H94)

[4th] H90 Conductive and sensorineural hearing loss
EXCLUDES1 *deaf nonspeaking NEC (H91.3)*
deafness NOS (H91.9-)
hearing loss NOS (H91.9-)
noise-induced hearing loss (H83.3-)
ototoxic hearing loss (H91.0-)
sudden (idiopathic) hearing loss (H91.2-)

H90.0 Conductive hearing loss, bilateral

[5th] H90.1 Conductive hearing loss, unilateral with unrestricted hearing on the contralateral side
H90.11 Conductive hearing loss, unilateral, right ear, with unrestricted hearing on the contralateral side
H90.12 Conductive hearing loss, unilateral, left ear, with unrestricted hearing on the contralateral side

H90.2 Conductive hearing loss, unspecified
Conductive deafness NOS

H90.3 Sensorineural hearing loss, bilateral

[5th] H90.4 Sensorineural hearing loss, unilateral with unrestricted hearing on the contralateral side
H90.41 Sensorineural hearing loss, unilateral, right ear, with unrestricted hearing on the contralateral side
H90.42 Sensorineural hearing loss, unilateral, left ear, with unrestricted hearing on the contralateral side

H90.5 Unspecified sensorineural hearing loss
Central hearing loss NOS
Congenital deafness NOS
Neural hearing loss NOS
Perceptive hearing loss NOS
Sensorineural deafness NOS
Sensory hearing loss NOS
EXCLUDES1 *abnormal auditory perception (H93.2-)*
psychogenic deafness (F44.6)

H90.6 Mixed conductive and sensorineural hearing loss, bilateral
AHA: Q2 2015

[5th] H90.7 Mixed conductive and sensorineural hearing loss, unilateral with unrestricted hearing on the contralateral side
H90.71 Mixed conductive and sensorineural hearing loss, unilateral, right ear, with unrestricted hearing on the contralateral side
H90.72 Mixed conductive and sensorineural hearing loss, unilateral, left ear, with unrestricted hearing on the contralateral side

H90.8 Mixed conductive and sensorineural hearing loss, unspecified

[5th] H90.A Conductive and sensorineural hearing loss with restricted hearing on the contralateral side
[6th] H90.A1 Conductive hearing loss, unilateral, with restricted hearing on the contralateral side
H90.A11 Conductive hearing loss, unilateral, right ear with restricted hearing on the contralateral side
AHA: Q4 2016
H90.A12 Conductive hearing loss, unilateral, left ear with restricted hearing on the contralateral side
AHA: Q4 2016
[6th] H90.A2 Sensorineural hearing loss, unilateral, with restricted hearing on the contralateral side
H90.A21 Sensorineural hearing loss, unilateral, right ear, with restricted hearing on the contralateral side
AHA: Q4 2016
H90.A22 Sensorineural hearing loss, unilateral, left ear, with restricted hearing on the contralateral side
AHA: Q4 2016
[6th] H90.A3 Mixed conductive and sensorineural hearing loss, unilateral with restricted hearing on the contralateral side
H90.A31 Mixed conductive and sensorineural hearing loss, unilateral, right ear with restricted hearing on the contralateral side
AHA: Q4 2016
H90.A32 Mixed conductive and sensorineural hearing loss, unilateral, left ear with restricted hearing on the contralateral side
AHA: Q4 2016

[4th] H91 Other and unspecified hearing loss
EXCLUDES1 *abnormal auditory perception (H93.2-)*
hearing loss as classified in H90.-
impacted cerumen (H61.2-)
noise-induced hearing loss (H83.3-)
psychogenic deafness (F44.6)
transient ischemic deafness (H93.01-)

[5th] H91.0 Ototoxic hearing loss
☞ **Code first** poisoning due to drug or toxin, if applicable (T36-T65 with fifth or sixth character 1-4 or 6)
Use additional code for adverse effect, if applicable, to identify drug (T36-T50 with fifth or sixth character 5)
H91.01 Ototoxic hearing loss, right ear
H91.02 Ototoxic hearing loss, left ear
H91.03 Ototoxic hearing loss, bilateral
H91.09 Ototoxic hearing loss, unspecified ear

[5th] H91.1 Presbycusis
Presbyacusia
H91.10 Presbycusis, unspecified ear
H91.11 Presbycusis, right ear
H91.12 Presbycusis, left ear
H91.13 Presbycusis, bilateral

[5th] H91.2 Sudden idiopathic hearing loss
Sudden hearing loss NOS
H91.20 Sudden idiopathic hearing loss, unspecified ear
H91.21 Sudden idiopathic hearing loss, right ear
H91.22 Sudden idiopathic hearing loss, left ear
H91.23 Sudden idiopathic hearing loss, bilateral

H91.3 Deaf nonspeaking, not elsewhere classified

[5th] H91.8 Other specified hearing loss
[6th] H91.8X Other specified hearing loss
H91.8X1 Other specified hearing loss, right ear
H91.8X2 Other specified hearing loss, left ear

[PDx] Unacceptable principal diagnosis symbol per Medicare code edits [POA] Code exempt from diagnosis present on admission requirement
[?] Questionable admission [CC] Complication or comorbidity [MCC] Major complication or comorbidity [CC/MCC Exc] CC/MCC exclusion
[HCC] HCC diagnosis code [RxHCC] RxHCC diagnosis code MACRA code **DEFINITION** Describes condition/terminology
TIP Coding guidance 👁 Official Guideline Reference [Z1] Z code as first-listed diagnosis

When symbols appear on a code that requires a 7th character extension, refer to Appendix B to identify applicable 7th character codes.

H83.2X - H91.8X2
CHAPTER 8: DISEASES OF THE EAR AND MASTOID PROCESS (H60-H95)

H91.8X3 **Other specified hearing loss, bilateral**

H91.8X9 **Other specified hearing loss, unspecified ear**

5ᵗʰ H91.9 Unspecified hearing loss

Deafness NOS

High frequency deafness

Low frequency deafness

H91.90 Unspecified hearing loss, unspecified ear

H91.91 Unspecified hearing loss, right ear

H91.92 Unspecified hearing loss, left ear

H91.93 Unspecified hearing loss, bilateral

4ᵗʰ H92 Otalgia and effusion of ear

5ᵗʰ H92.0 Otalgia

H92.01 Otalgia, right ear

H92.02 Otalgia, left ear

H92.03 Otalgia, bilateral

H92.09 Otalgia, unspecified ear

5ᵗʰ H92.1 Otorrhea

EXCLUDES1 *leakage of cerebrospinal fluid through ear (G96.0)*

H92.10 Otorrhea, unspecified ear

H92.11 Otorrhea, right ear

H92.12 Otorrhea, left ear

H92.13 Otorrhea, bilateral

5ᵗʰ H92.2 Otorrhagia

EXCLUDES1 *traumatic otorrhagia - code to injury*

H92.20 Otorrhagia, unspecified ear

H92.21 Otorrhagia, right ear

H92.22 Otorrhagia, left ear

H92.23 Otorrhagia, bilateral

4ᵗʰ H93 Other disorders of ear, not elsewhere classified

5ᵗʰ H93.0 Degenerative and vascular disorders of ear

EXCLUDES1 *presbycusis (H91.1)*

6ᵗʰ H93.01 Transient ischemic deafness

H93.011 Transient ischemic deafness, right ear

H93.012 Transient ischemic deafness, left ear

H93.013 Transient ischemic deafness, bilateral

H93.019 Transient ischemic deafness, unspecified ear

6ᵗʰ H93.09 Unspecified degenerative and vascular disorders of ear

H93.091 Unspecified degenerative and vascular disorders of right ear

H93.092 Unspecified degenerative and vascular disorders of left ear

H93.093 Unspecified degenerative and vascular disorders of ear, bilateral

H93.099 Unspecified degenerative and vascular disorders of unspecified ear

5ᵗʰ H93.1 Tinnitus

H93.11 Tinnitus, right ear

H93.12 Tinnitus, left ear

H93.13 Tinnitus, bilateral

H93.19 Tinnitus, unspecified ear

5ᵗʰ H93.A Pulsatile tinnitus

H93.A1 Pulsatile tinnitus, right ear

AHA: Q4 2016

H93.A2 Pulsatile tinnitus, left ear

AHA: Q4 2016

H93.A3 Pulsatile tinnitus, bilateral

AHA: Q4 2016

H93.A9 Pulsatile tinnitus, unspecified ear

AHA: Q4 2016

5ᵗʰ H93.2 Other abnormal auditory perceptions

EXCLUDES2 *auditory hallucinations (R44.0)*

6ᵗʰ H93.21 Auditory recruitment

H93.211 Auditory recruitment, right ear

H93.212 Auditory recruitment, left ear

H93.213 Auditory recruitment, bilateral

H93.219 Auditory recruitment, unspecified ear

6ᵗʰ H93.22 Diplacusis

H93.221 Diplacusis, right ear

H93.222 Diplacusis, left ear

H93.223 Diplacusis, bilateral

H93.229 Diplacusis, unspecified ear

6ᵗʰ H93.23 Hyperacusis

H93.231 Hyperacusis, right ear

H93.232 Hyperacusis, left ear

H93.233 Hyperacusis, bilateral

H93.239 Hyperacusis, unspecified ear

6ᵗʰ H93.24 Temporary auditory threshold shift

H93.241 Temporary auditory threshold shift, right ear

H93.242 Temporary auditory threshold shift, left ear

H93.243 Temporary auditory threshold shift, bilateral

H93.249 Temporary auditory threshold shift, unspecified ear

H93.25 Central auditory processing disorder

Congenital auditory imperception

Word deafness

EXCLUDES1 *mixed receptive-expressive language disorder (F80.2)*

6ᵗʰ H93.29 Other abnormal auditory perceptions

H93.291 Other abnormal auditory perceptions, right ear

H93.292 Other abnormal auditory perceptions, left ear

H93.293 Other abnormal auditory perceptions, bilateral

H93.299 Other abnormal auditory perceptions, unspecified ear

5ᵗʰ H93.3 Disorders of acoustic nerve

Disorder of 8th cranial nerve

EXCLUDES1 *acoustic neuroma (D33.3)*

syphilitic acoustic neuritis (A52.15)

6ᵗʰ H93.3X Disorders of acoustic nerve

H93.3X1 Disorders of right acoustic nerve

H93.3X2 Disorders of left acoustic nerve

H93.3X3 Disorders of bilateral acoustic nerves

H93.3X9 Disorders of unspecified acoustic nerve

5ᵗʰ H93.8 Other specified disorders of ear

6ᵗʰ H93.8X Other specified disorders of ear

H93.8X1 **Other specified disorders of right ear**

H93.8X2 **Other specified disorders of left ear**

H93.8X3 **Other specified disorders of ear, bilateral**

H93.8X9 **Other specified disorders of ear, unspecified ear**

5ᵗʰ H93.9 Unspecified disorder of ear

H93.90 Unspecified disorder of ear, unspecified ear   PDx In

H93.91 Unspecified disorder of right ear   PDx In

H93.92 Unspecified disorder of left ear   PDx In

H93.93 Unspecified disorder of ear, bilateral   PDx In

4ᵗʰ H94 Other disorders of ear in diseases classified elsewhere

5ᵗʰ H94.0 Acoustic neuritis in infectious and parasitic diseases classified elsewhere

☞ Code first underlying disease, such as:

parasitic disease (B65-B89)

EXCLUDES1 *acoustic neuritis (in):*

herpes zoster (B02.29)

syphilis (A52.15)

H94.00 **Acoustic neuritis in infectious and parasitic diseases classified elsewhere, unspecified ear**

H94.01 **Acoustic neuritis in infectious and parasitic diseases classified elsewhere, right ear**

H94.02 **Acoustic neuritis in infectious and parasitic diseases classified elsewhere, left ear**

H94.03 **Acoustic neuritis in infectious and parasitic diseases classified elsewhere, bilateral**

| Unspecified Code | Other Specified Code | Manifestation Code | N Newborn | P Pediatric | M Maternity | A Adult | ♂ Male | ♀ Female |

● New Code   ▲ Revised Code Title   ►◄ Revised Text   **NOTES** INCLUDES EXCLUDES1 Not coded here   EXCLUDES2 Not included here

4ᵗʰ 4ᵗʰ character required   5ᵗʰ 5ᵗʰ character required   6ᵗʰ 6ᵗʰ character required   7ᵗʰ 7ᵗʰ character required   7ᵗʰ Extension 'X' Alert

HAC Hospital-acquired condition (HAC) alert   AHA AHA Coding Clinic®   ☞ Code first alert

[5th] H94.8 Other specified disorders of ear in diseases classified elsewhere

☛ Code first underlying disease, such as:
congenital syphilis (A50.0)

[EXCLUDES1] *aural myiasis (B87.4)*
syphilitic labyrinthitis (A52.79)

H94.80 Other specified disorders of ear in diseases classified elsewhere, unspecified ear

H94.81 Other specified disorders of right ear in diseases classified elsewhere

H94.82 Other specified disorders of left ear in diseases classified elsewhere

H94.83 Other specified disorders of ear in diseases classified elsewhere, bilateral

Intraoperative and postprocedural complications and disorders of ear and mastoid process, not elsewhere classified (H95)

[4th] H95 Intraoperative and postprocedural complications and disorders of ear and mastoid process, not elsewhere classified

[5th] H95.0 Recurrent cholesteatoma of postmastoidectomy cavity

H95.00 Recurrent cholesteatoma of postmastoidectomy cavity, unspecified ear

H95.01 Recurrent cholesteatoma of postmastoidectomy cavity, right ear

H95.02 Recurrent cholesteatoma of postmastoidectomy cavity, left ear

H95.03 Recurrent cholesteatoma of postmastoidectomy cavity, bilateral ears

[5th] H95.1 Other disorders of ear and mastoid process following mastoidectomy

[6th] H95.11 Chronic inflammation of postmastoidectomy cavity

H95.111 Chronic inflammation of postmastoidectomy cavity, right ear

H95.112 Chronic inflammation of postmastoidectomy cavity, left ear

H95.113 Chronic inflammation of postmastoidectomy cavity, bilateral ears

H95.119 Chronic inflammation of postmastoidectomy cavity, unspecified ear

[6th] H95.12 Granulation of postmastoidectomy cavity

H95.121 Granulation of postmastoidectomy cavity, right ear

H95.122 Granulation of postmastoidectomy cavity, left ear

H95.123 Granulation of postmastoidectomy cavity, bilateral ears

H95.129 Granulation of postmastoidectomy cavity, unspecified ear

[6th] H95.13 Mucosal cyst of postmastoidectomy cavity

H95.131 Mucosal cyst of postmastoidectomy cavity, right ear

H95.132 Mucosal cyst of postmastoidectomy cavity, left ear

H95.133 Mucosal cyst of postmastoidectomy cavity, bilateral ears

H95.139 Mucosal cyst of postmastoidectomy cavity, unspecified ear

[6th] H95.19 Other disorders following mastoidectomy

H95.191 Other disorders following mastoidectomy, right ear

H95.192 Other disorders following mastoidectomy, left ear

H95.193 Other disorders following mastoidectomy, bilateral ears

H95.199 Other disorders following mastoidectomy, unspecified ear

[5th] H95.2 Intraoperative hemorrhage and hematoma of ear and mastoid process complicating a procedure

[EXCLUDES1] *intraoperative hemorrhage and hematoma of ear and mastoid process due to accidental puncture or laceration during a procedure (H95.3-)*

H95.21 Intraoperative hemorrhage and hematoma of ear and mastoid process complicating a procedure on the ear and mastoid process [CC] [CC/MCC Exc]

H95.22 Intraoperative hemorrhage and hematoma of ear and mastoid process complicating other procedure [CC] [CC/MCC Exc]

[5th] H95.3 Accidental puncture and laceration of ear and mastoid process during a procedure

H95.31 Accidental puncture and laceration of the ear and mastoid process during a procedure on the ear and mastoid process [CC] [CC/MCC Exc]

H95.32 Accidental puncture and laceration of the ear and mastoid process during other procedure [CC] [CC/MCC Exc]

[5th] H95.4 Postprocedural hemorrhage of ear and mastoid process following a procedure

H95.41 Postprocedural hemorrhage of ear and mastoid process following a procedure on the ear and mastoid process [CC] [CC/MCC Exc]

H95.42 Postprocedural hemorrhage of ear and mastoid process following other procedure [CC] [CC/MCC Exc]

[5th] H95.5 Postprocedural hematoma and seroma of ear and mastoid process following a procedure

H95.51 Postprocedural hematoma of ear and mastoid process following a procedure on the ear and mastoid process [CC] [CC/MCC Exc]

H95.52 Postprocedural hematoma of ear and mastoid process following other procedure [CC] [CC/MCC Exc]

H95.53 Postprocedural seroma of ear and mastoid process following a procedure on the ear and mastoid process [CC] [CC/MCC Exc]

H95.54 Postprocedural seroma of ear and mastoid process following other procedure [CC] [CC/MCC Exc]

[5th] H95.8 Other intraoperative and postprocedural complications and disorders of the ear and mastoid process, not elsewhere classified

[EXCLUDES2] *postprocedural complications and disorders following mastoidectomy (H95.0-, H95.1-)*

[6th] H95.81 Postprocedural stenosis of external ear canal

H95.811 Postprocedural stenosis of right external ear canal [CC] [CC/MCC Exc]

H95.812 Postprocedural stenosis of left external ear canal [CC] [CC/MCC Exc]

H95.813 Postprocedural stenosis of external ear canal, bilateral [CC] [CC/MCC Exc]

H95.819 Postprocedural stenosis of unspecified external ear canal [CC] [CC/MCC Exc]

H95.88 Other intraoperative complications and disorders of the ear and mastoid process, not elsewhere classified [CC] [CC/MCC Exc]

Use additional code, if applicable, to further specify disorder

H95.89 Other postprocedural complications and disorders of the ear and mastoid process, not elsewhere classified [CC] [CC/MCC Exc]

Use additional code, if applicable, to further specify disorder

Anatomy of the Cardiovascular System

Introduction

The human vascular system comprises a series of tubes (which are known as vessels) that travel in almost all parts of the human body. It is categorized into the blood vascular system and the lymphatic vascular system.

1. **Blood Vascular System**
   The blood vascular system (Figure 9.a) includes the heart and blood vessels required to facilitate the circulation of the colored fluid (blood) inside the body.

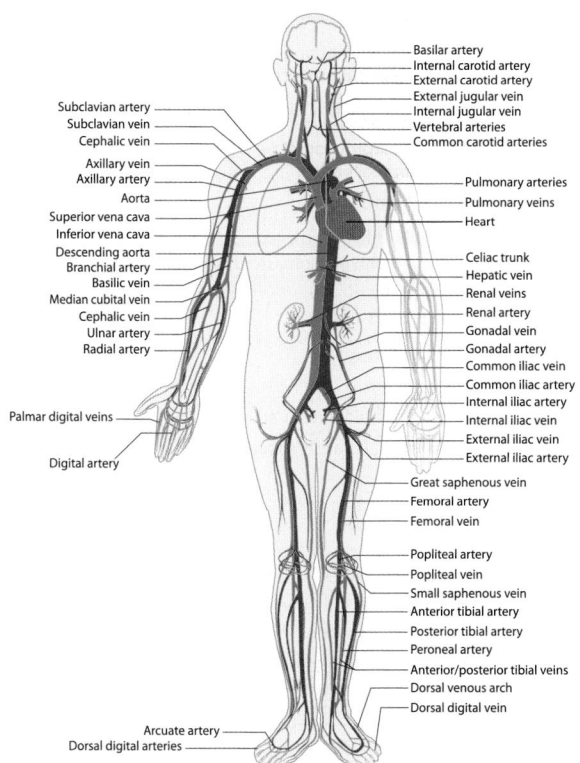

Figure 9.a Blood Vascular System - Arteries and Veins

a) **The Structure of Arteries**

   The arteries possess stronger and thicker walls than the corresponding veins and are based on the following components:

   i)   Tunica Intima

   ii) Tunica Media

   iii) Tunica Externa

b) **The Structure of Veins**

   The veins have a similar structure as that of the arteries. The components of a typical vein are described below:

   i)   Tunica Intima

   ii) Tunica Media

   iii) Tunica Externa

c) **The Blood**

   The blood is considered a uniquely specialized connective tissue that is composed of the formed elements (or the blood cells) and the fluid portion (or plasma). The formed elements of blood are based on the red blood cells (RBCs or erythrocytes), the white blood cells (WBCs or leukocytes) and the platelets (or thrombocytes). The blood contributes to about 8% of total body weight. The quantity of blood in an average human varies between 5 to 6 liters. The elements of blood are categorized below:

d) **Erythrocytes or Red Blood Cells**

   The red blood cells are the most common type of blood cells that contribute to about 95% of the blood cell volume.

e) **Leukocytes or White Blood Cells**

   The white blood cells can be divided into the following subcategories:

f) **Granular Leukocytes:**

   The granular leukocytes contain granules in their cytoplasm and can be further classified into the following three types:

   i)   neutrophils constitute about 60% to 70% of the white blood cells.

   ii) eosinophils constitute about 2% to 4% of the white blood cells.

   iii) basophils constitute about 0.5% to 1% of the white blood cells.

g) **Agranular Leukocytes**

   The agranular leukocytes do not contain granules in their cytoplasm and can be further classified into the following two types:

   i)   monocytes constitute about 3% to 8% of the white blood cells.

   ii) lymphocytes constitute about 20% to 25% of the white blood cells.

h) **Thrombocytes or Platelets**

   The platelets are small cell fragments that do not contain nucleus in their cytoplasm.

i) **Blood Plasma**

   The plasma is the fluid component of blood in which the blood cells usually remain suspended. The blood plasma is composed of 91% water, 7% proteins, and 2% solutes.

2. **Lymph Vascular System**
   The lymph vascular system includes the lymph glands and lymphatic vessels for circulating the colorless fluid (lymph) throughout the human body. Both of the blood vascular and the lymph vascular systems work in close association with each other for sustaining the human life cycle.

3. **The Thoracic Cavity**
   The thoracic cavity is enclosed by the thoracic wall and primarily contains the structures of the cardiovascular and respiratory systems.

   a) **The Pericardium**

      The heart and the roots of the great vessels are contained within the conical and fibro-serous sac, which is known as the pericardium. It is composed of two closely connected sacs, which are known as the fibrous pericardium (or the outer sac) and the serous pericardium (the inner sac).

   b) **The Heart**

      The heart is a hollow muscular organ that remains enclosed in the fibro-serous sac (or the pericardium) and is regarded as the central organ of the cardiovascular system. It lies between the lungs in the middle mediastinum and receives blood from the veins.

4. **The Chambers of the Heart**
   The human heart is based on the following four chambers (Figure 9.b):

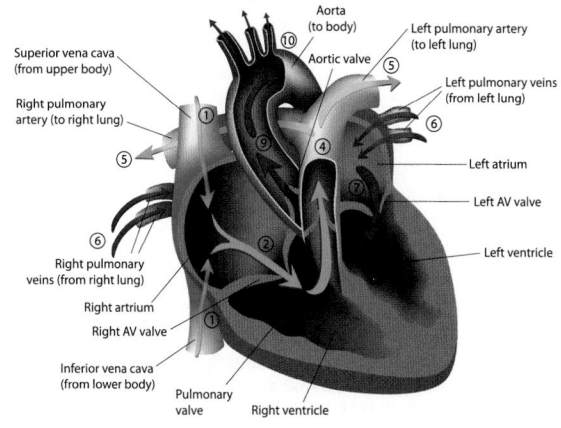

Figure 9.b Chambers of the Heart

a) **The Right Atrium:** The right border of the human heart is formed by the right atrium. The superior vena cava, inferior vena cava and coronary sinus provide venous blood supply to the right atrium of the heart.

The right atrium contains the following elements inside it:

i) Sinus Venarum
ii) Pectinate Muscles
iii) Opening of Superior Vena Cava
iv) Opening of Inferior Vena Cava
v) Opening of Coronary Sinus
vi) The Right Atrioventricular Orifice
vii) Interatrial Septum

b) **The Right Ventricle:** The inferior border of the human heart is constituted by the right ventricle.

c) **The Left Atrium:** The left atrium chiefly constitutes the base of the heart and utilizes the mitral valve to pump the oxygenated blood received from the pulmonary veins into the left ventricle of the heart. The interior of the left atrium is based on the following components:

i) Two superior and two inferior pulmonary veins that enter the posterior wall of the left atrium.
ii) A posteriorly directed interatrial septum that separates the right atrium from the left atrium of the heart.
iii) A smooth walled portion and a muscular auricle containing pectinate muscles.
iv) A comparatively thicker wall than the corresponding right atrium.
v) A left atrioventricular orifice that facilitates the discharge of oxygenated blood into the left ventricle.

d) **The Left Ventricle:** The left ventricle pumps the oxygenated blood (through the aortic valve) to the whole body through the aorta. The interior of the left ventricle is based on the following elements:

i) a double-leaflet/dual-flap mitral (bicuspid or left atrioventricular) valve, which is located between the left atrium and ventricle for guarding the left atrioventricular orifice.
ii) walls of the left ventricle, which are comparatively thicker than the corresponding right ventricle.
iii) conical cavity of the left ventricle that is comparatively longer than the corresponding right ventricle.
iv) anterior and posterior left ventricular papillary muscles that get attached to the cusps of the mitral valve through the tendinous cords (or the chordae tendineae).
v) aortic vestibule, which is a smooth-walled, nonmuscular, superoanterior outflow portion of the left ventricle that lies inferior to the aortic orifice and possesses fibrous walls.
vi) aortic orifice (or opening) is an opening of the left ventricle into the aorta. This valve is usually tricuspid (with three leaflets) and located posterior to the left side of the sternum at the level of the third intercostal space.
vii) inner surface of the left ventricle gives rise to the irregular, rounded and thick muscular ridges that are termed as the trabeculae carneae.

5. **The Cardiac Cycle**
The cardiac cycle is based on the synchronous pumping of the right and left chambers of the heart.

a) **The Arterial Supply of the Heart:** The heart is supplied by the following arteries:

i) right coronary artery (RCA)
ii) sino-atrial nodal artery
iii) right marginal artery
iv) posterior interventricular artery
v) atrioventricular nodal artery
vi) left coronary artery
vii) anterior interventricular artery (or Left Anterior Descending Artery)
viii) circumflex artery
ix) left marginal artery
x) posterior interventricular artery

b) **The Arteries:** The major types of arteries are described below:

i) pulmonary arteries- pulmonary arteries carry the oxygen deficient blood from the heart to the lungs for attaining oxygen.
ii) systemic arteries- systemic arteries transport the oxygenated blood to the rest of the body.

c) **The Aorta:** The aorta is divided into the following components:

i) ascending aorta
ii) arch of aorta
iii) descending aorta

d) **The Thoracic Aorta**

i) aortic intercostal arteries (nine pairs)
ii) left bronchial arteries (two in number)
iii) posterior mediastinal arteries
iv) pericardial arteries
v) superior phrenic arteries

e) **The Abdominal Aorta**

6. **The Arteries of the Head and Neck**
The major arteries that supply blood to the head and neck regions are the two common carotid arteries. These arteries travel through the neck and each one of them gets divided into the following branches:

a) **External Carotid Arteries**

b) **Ascending Pharyngeal Artery**

c) **Occipital Artery**

i) muscular branches
ii) sternocleidomastoid branch/sternocleidomastoid artery
iii) auricular branch
iv) meningeal or dural branch
v) descending branch

d) **Posterior Auricular Artery**

i) stylomastoid branch/stylomastoid artery
ii) auricular branch
iii) occipital branch

e) **Superior Thyroid Artery**

i) hyoid branch
ii) sternocleidomastoid branch/sternocleidomastoid artery
iii) superior laryngeal branch/superior laryngeal artery
iv) cricothyroid branch

f) **Lingual Artery**

i) hyoid branch
ii) dorsal lingual branches
iii) sublingual branch/sublingual artery
iv) deep lingual branch/deep lingual artery

g) **Facial (or External Maxillary) Artery**

Cervical Branches		Facial Branches	
i)	ascending palatine artery	i)	inferior labial artery
ii)	tonsillar branch	ii)	superior labial artery
iii)	glandular branches	iii)	lateral nasal branch
iv)	submental artery	iv)	angular artery
v)	muscular branches	v)	muscular branches

7. **The Internal Carotid Arteries**
The internal carotid arteries are the direct continuation of the common carotid arteries. However, the other portions of these arteries extend into the following arterial branches:

a) **The petrous portion of the internal carotid arteries gives rise to the following branches:**

i) caroticotympanic artery
ii) artery of the pterygoid canal (or vidian artery)

b) **The cavernous portion of the internal carotid arteries gives rise to the following branches:**

i) cavernous artery
ii) hypophyseal artery
iii) semilunar arterial branches
iv) anterior meningeal artery
v) ophthalmic artery

c) **Anterior Cerebral Artery**

i) anteromedial ganglionic branches
ii) inferior branches
iii) anterior branches
iv) middle branches
v) posterior branches

d) **The Middle Cerebral Artery**

   i) anterolateral ganglionic branches

   ii) inferior lateral frontal branch

   iii) ascending frontal branch

   iv) ascending parietal branch

   v) parietotemporal branch

   vi) temporal branches

e) **Posterior Communicating Artery**

f) **Anterior Choroidal Artery (or Choroid Artery)**

8. **The Arteries of the Upper Extremity**

   The Subclavian Artery divides into the following branches:

   a) **Vertebral Artery**

   The vertebral artery is divided into the following branches:

Cervical Branches	Cranial Branches
i) spinal branches	i) posterior meningeal branch
ii) muscular branches	ii) posterior/dorsal spinal artery
	iii) anterior/ventral spinal artery
	iv) posterior inferior cerebellar artery
	v) medullary arteries

   b) **Internal Thoracic (or Internal Mammary) Artery**

   i) pericardiacophrenic artery

   ii) anterior mediastinal arteries

   iii) pericardial branches

   iv) sternal branches

   v) anterior intercostal arteries

   vi) perforating branches

   vii) musculophrenic artery

   viii) superior epigastric artery

   c) **Thyrocervical Trunk (or Thyroid Axis)**

   i) inferior thyroid artery

   ii) inferior laryngeal artery

   iii) esophageal branches

   iv) tracheal artery

   v) ascending cervical artery

   vi) muscular branches

   d) **Suprascapular (or Transverse Scapular) Artery**

   i) suprasternal branch

   ii) acromial branch

   e) **Transverse Cervical Artery (or Transverse Artery of Neck)**

   i) ascending branch

   ii) descending branch

   f) **The costocervical trunk is the highest intercostal artery (superior intercostal), and it includes:**

   i) first posterior intercostal artery

   ii) second posterior intercostal artery

   iii) deep cervical artery

   iv) third arterial part

   g) **Axillary Artery**

   i) first part

   ii) second part

   iii) third part

   h) **Brachial Artery**

   i) muscular branches

   ii) human nutrient artery

   iii) profunda brachii artery (deep artery of the arm/superior profunda artery)

   iv) superior ulnar collateral artery (or inferior profunda artery)

   v) inferior ulnar collateral artery (or anastomotica magna artery)

i) **Radial Artery**

Branches of the Radial Artery in Forearm	Branches of the Radial Artery in Wrist	Branches of the Radial Artery in Hand
The Radial Recurrent Artery	The Posterior Radial Carpal Artery (The Dorsal Carpal Branch)	The Princeps Pollicis Artery
The Muscular (Arterial) Branches	The First Dorsal Metacarpal Artery	The Radialis Indicis Artery
The Anterior Radial Carpal Artery (The Volar Carpal Branch)		The Deep Palmar/Volar Arch
The Superficial Volar Artery (The Superficial Palmar Branch of Radial Artery)		The Palmar Interosseous (or Volar Metacarpal) Arteries
		The Perforating (Arterial) Branches
		The Recurrent (Arterial) Branches

j) **Ulnar Artery**

   The ulnar artery originates from the brachial artery and runs along the medial aspect (or ulnar side) of the forearm. A tabular representation of the arterial branches of ulnar artery is provided below:

Branches of the Ulnar Artery in Forearm	Branches of the Ulnar Artery in Wrist	Branches of the Ulnar Artery in Hand
The Anterior Ulnar Recurrent Artery	The Volar Carpal Branch (or Anterior Ulnar Carpal Artery)	The Deep Volar Branch (or Profunda Branch)
The Posterior Ulnar Recurrent Artery	The Dorsal Carpal Branch (or Posterior Ulnar Carpal Artery)	The Superficial Volar Arch (or Superficial Palmar Arch)
The Common Interosseous Artery (divides into the following two branches) i) The Volar Interosseous Artery (or Anterior Interosseous Artery) ii) The Dorsal Interosseous Artery (or Posterior Interosseous Artery)		
The Muscular (Arterial) Branches		

9. **Arteries of the Trunk**

   Arteries of the trunk are based on the following arteries:

   a) **The Descending Aorta**

   i) thoracic aorta

   ii) abdominal aorta

   b) **The Common Iliac Arteries**

   c) **Internal Iliac (or Hypogastric) Artery**

The Anterior Trunk	The Posterior Trunk
The Superior Vesical Artery	The Iliolumbar Artery-with the following branches:
The Middle Vesical Artery	
The Inferior Vesical Artery	i) The Lumbar (Arterial) Branch ii) The Iliac (Arterial) Branch
The Middle Hemorrhoidal Artery	The Superior and Inferior Lateral Sacral Arteries
The Uterine Artery (In Female)	
The Vaginal Artery (In Female)	The Superior Gluteal Artery (or Gluteal Artery)-with the following branches:
The Obturator Artery	
	i) The Superficial (Arterial) Branch ii) The Deep (Arterial) Branch

The Anterior Trunk	The Posterior Trunk
The Internal Pudendal Artery (Internal Pubic Artery)-with the following branches:	
The Muscular (Arterial) Branches	
The Inferior Hemorrhoidal Artery	
The Perineal (or Superficial Perineal) Artery	
The Artery of the Urethral Bulb	
The Urethral Artery	
The Deep Artery of the Penis (or Artery to the Corpus Cavernosum)	
The Dorsal Artery of the Penis	
The Inferior Gluteal Artery (Sciatic Artery)-with the following branches:	
The Muscular (Arterial) Branches	
The Coccygeal (Arterial) Branches	
The Arteria Comitans Nervi Ischiadici	
The Anastomotic (Arterial) Branch	
The Articular (Arterial) Branch	
The Cutaneous (Arterial) Branches	

d) **The External Iliac Artery divides into the inferior epigastric artery, which includes:**

   i)   muscular branches

   ii)   cutaneous branches

   iii) external spermatic branch (in males) and artery of round ligament of uterus (in females)

   iv) pubic branch

e) **Deep Iliac Circumflex Artery**

   i)   muscular branch

   ii)   cutaneous branch

10. The Arteries of the Lower Extremity

  a) **Femoral Artery**

The branches of the femoral artery are presented below in a tabular format:

The Branches of the Femoral Artery		
The Superficial Epigastric Artery		
The Superficial Iliac Circumflex Artery		
The Superficial External Pudendal Artery (or Superficial External Pubic Artery)		
The Deep External Pudendal Artery (or Deep External Pubic Artery)		
The Muscular (Arterial) Branches		
The Profunda Femoris Artery (or Deep Femoral Artery)		
Branches and Subordinate Branches of the Profunda Femoris Artery	The Lateral Femoral Circumflex Artery	
	Sub-Branches	The Ascending (Arterial) Branch
		The Descending (Arterial) Branch
		The Transverse (Arterial) Branch
	The Medial Femoral Circumflex Artery (or Internal Circumflex Artery)	
	Sub-Branches	The Superficial (Arterial) Branch
		The Deep (Arterial) Branch
		The Acetabular (Arterial) Branch
	The Perforating Arteries	
	Sub-Branches	The First Perforating Artery
		The Second Perforating Artery
		The Third Perforating Artery
	The Muscular (Arterial) Branches	
The Highest Genicular Artery (or Anastomotica Magna Artery)		

The Branches of the Femoral Artery	
Branches of the Highest Genicular Artery	The Saphenous (Arterial) Branch
	The Musculoarticular (Arterial) Branch

b) **Popliteal Artery**

A tabular presentation of the branches of the popliteal artery is given below:

Branches of the Popliteal Artery	
The Superior Muscular Branches	
The Sural Arteries (or Inferior Muscular Arteries)	
The Cutaneous Branches	
The Superior Genicular Arteries (or Superior Articular Arteries)	
Branches of the Superior Genicular Arteries	The Medial Superior Genicular Artery
	The Lateral Superior Genicular Artery
The Middle Genicular Artery (or Azygos Articular Artery)	
The Inferior Genicular Arteries (or Inferior Articular Arteries)	
Branches of the Inferior Genicular Arteries	The Medial Inferior Genicular Artery
	The Lateral Inferior Genicular Artery

c) **Anterior Tibial Artery**

   i)   Posterior Tibial Recurrent Artery

   ii)   Fibular Artery

   iii) Anterior Tibial Recurrent Artery

   iv) Muscular (Arterial) Branches

   v)   Anterior Medial Malleolar Artery (or Internal Malleolar Artery)

   vi) Anterior Lateral Malleolar Artery (or External Malleolar Artery)

d) **Dorsalis Pedis Artery (or Dorsal Artery of Foot)**

A tabular presentation of the branches of the dorsalis pedis artery is given below:

Branches of the Dorsalis Pedis Artery	
The lateral Tarsal Artery (or Tarsal Artery)	
The Medial Tarsal Arteries	
The Arcuate Artery (or Metatarsal Artery)	
Branches of Arcuate Artery	The Second Dorsal Metatarsal Artery
	The Third Dorsal Metatarsal Artery
	The Fourth Dorsal Metatarsal Artery
The First Dorsal Metatarsal Artery	
The Deep Plantar Artery (or Communicating Artery)	

e) **Posterior Tibial Artery**

The branching tree of the posterior tibial artery is presented below:

Branches of the Posterior Tibial Artery	
The Peroneal Artery	
Branches of Peroneal Artery	The Muscular (Arterial) Branches
	The Nutrient Artery of Fibula
	The Perforating Branch (or Anterior Peroneal Artery)
	The Communicating Branch of Peroneal Artery
	The Lateral Calcaneal Arteries (or External Calcaneal Arteries)
The Nutrient Artery of Tibia	
The Muscular Branches of the Posterior Tibial Artery	
The Posterior Medial Malleolar Artery (or Internal Malleolar Artery)	
The Communicating Branch of Posterior Tibial Artery	
The Medial Calcaneal Arteries (or Internal Calcaneal Arteries)	
The Medial Plantar Artery (or Internal Plantar Artery)	
The Lateral Plantar Artery (or External Plantar Artery)	

11. The Veins

The veins are the blood vessels that carry deoxygenated blood (Figure 9.c) from the body tissues towards the heart via capillaries. The veins can be categorized into the following classes:

a) **Pulmonary Veins**

The pulmonary veins carry oxygenated blood from the lungs to the left atrium of the heart. The pulmonary veins are of the following types:

  i)   right inferior pulmonary vein
  ii) right superior pulmonary vein
  iii) left inferior pulmonary vein
  iv) left superior pulmonary vein

b) **Systemic Veins**

The systemic veins deliver deoxygenated blood from the body tissues to the right atrium of the human heart.

c) **Superficial (or Cutaneous) Veins**

The superficial veins are found immediately beneath the skin between the layers of the superficial fascia.

d) **Deep Veins**

The deep veins are located under the deep fascia with their corresponding arteries.

e) **Systemic Veins**

The systemic veins are divided into the following groups:

  i)   veins of the heart
  ii) veins of the head and neck
  iii) veins of the upper extremity and thorax
  iv) veins of the lower extremity, abdomen, and pelvis

f) **Veins of the Heart**

  i)   great cardiac vein
  ii) small cardiac vein
  iii) middle cardiac vein
  iv) posterior vein of the left ventricle
  v)   oblique vein of the left atrium

g) **Veins of the Head and Neck**

  i)   frontal vein (or supratrochlear vein)
  ii)   supraorbital vein
  iii) angular vein
  iv)   anterior facial vein (or facial vein)
  v)   superficial temporal vein
  vi)   parotid veins
  vii) articular veins (from temporomandibular joint)
  viii) anterior auricular veins
  ix)   transverse facial veins
  x)   internal maxillary vein
  xi)   posterior facial vein (or temporomaxillary vein)
  xii) posterior auricular vein
  xiii) occipital vein

h) **Veins of the Neck**

  i)   external jugular vein
  ii) posterior external jugular vein
  iii) anterior jugular vein
  iv) internal jugular vein
  v)   vertebral vein
  vi) diploic veins
      (a) frontal diploic vein
      (b) anterior temporal diploic vein
      (c) posterior temporal diploic vein
      (d) occipital diploic vein

12. Veins of the Brain

a) **External Cerebral Veins**

  i)   superior cerebral veins
  ii) middle cerebral vein (or superficial sylvian vein)
  iii) inferior cerebral veins

b) **Internal Cerebral Veins (or Deep Cerebral Veins)**

c) **Terminal Vein**

d) **Great Cerebral Veins (or Great Vein of Galen)**

e) **Cerebellar Veins**

  i) superior cerebellar veins
  ii) inferior cerebellar veins

f) **Ophthalmic and Emissary Veins**

  i)   Ophthalmic veins are the veins that serve to perform the venous drainage of the orbit and pass through the superior orbital fissure to enter into the cavernous sinus.
  ii) superior ophthalmic veins
  iii) inferior ophthalmic veins
  iv) Emissary veins are those valveless veins that connect the dural venous sinuses with veins outside the cranium.

g) **Sinuses of the Dura Mater**

  i)   posterosuperior sinuses
  ii) superior sagittal sinus (or superior longitudinal sinus)
  iii) inferior sagittal sinus (or inferior sagittal sinus)
  iv) straight sinus (or tentorial sinus)
  v)   transverse sinuses (or lateral sinuses)

h) **Occipital Sinuses**

  i)   anteroinferior sinuses
  ii) cavernous sinuses
  iii) intercavernous sinuses
  iv) superior petrosal sinuses
  v)   inferior petrosal sinuses
  vi) basilar plexus (or transverse/basilar sinus)

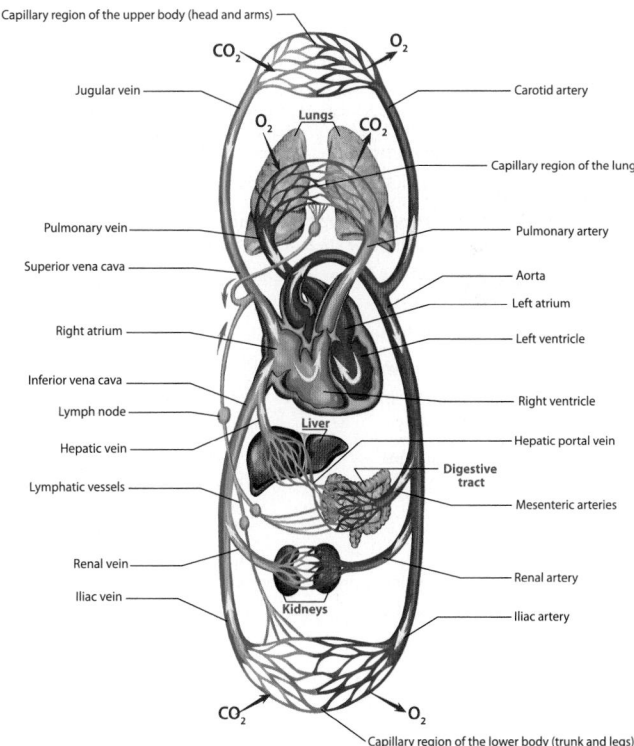

Figure 9.c Path of Oxygenated and De-oxygenated Blood Throughout the Circulatory System

13. Veins of the Upper Extremity, Thorax and Vertebral Column

The veins of the upper extremity are divided into the superficial and the deep veins.

a) **Superficial Veins of the Upper Extremity**

  i)   cephalic vein (or antecubital vein)
  ii) accessory cephalic vein
  iii) median cubital vein (or median basilic vein/antecubital vein)

    iv)   basilic vein

    v)   median antebrachial vein

    vi)   dorsal venous network of the hand

    vii) intercapitular veins

    viii) dorsal metacarpal veins

    ix)   dorsal digital veins

b) Deep Veins of the Upper Extremity

    i)   radial veins

    ii)   ulnar veins

    iii) brachial veins

    iv) axillary veins

    v)   subclavian veins

    vi) deep palmar venous arch

c) Veins of the Thorax

    i)   innominate veins (or brachiocephalic veins)

    ii)   internal mammary veins (or internal thoracic veins)

    iii) inferior thyroid veins

    iv) highest intercostal vein (or superior intercostal vein)

    v)   right superior intercostal vein

    vi) left superior intercostal vein

    vii) superior vena cava

    viii) azygos vein

    ix)   hemiazygos vein

    x)   accessory hemiazygos vein (or vena azygos minor superior)

    xi)   bronchial veins

d) Veins of the Vertebral Column

    i)   external vertebral venous plexuses (or extraspinal veins)

    ii)   anterior external vertebral plexuses

    iii) posterior external vertebral plexuses

    iv) internal vertebral venous plexus (or intraspinal veins)

    v)   basivertebral veins

    vi) intervertebral veins

    vii) veins of the medulla spinalis (or veins of spinal cord)

14. Veins of the Lower Extremity, Abdomen, and Pelvis

The veins of the lower extremity are arranged into the following groups:

a) Superficial Veins of the Lower Extremity

    i)   great saphenous vein

    ii)   small saphenous vein (or lesser saphenous vein)

b) Deep Veins of the Lower Extremity

    i)   posterior tibial veins

    ii)   peroneal veins

    iii) tibioperoneal trunk

    iv) anterior tibial veins

    v)   popliteal vein

    vi) femoral vein

    vii) deep femoral vein (or profunda femoris vein)

    viii) common femoral vein

    ix)   external iliac vein

c) Major Veins of Abdomen and Pelvis

    i)   ascending lumbar vein

    ii)   left gastric vein

    iii) right gastric vein

    iv) left gastro-omental vein

    v)   right gastro-omental vein

    vi) left hepatic vein

    vii) middle hepatic vein

    viii) right hepatic vein

    ix)   superior mesenteric vein

    x)   inferior phrenic veins

    xi)   inferior vena cava

    xii) left renal vein

    xiii) right renal vein

    xiv) splenic vein

    xv) suprarenal veins

    xvi) deep dorsal vein of clitoris

    xvii) deep dorsal vein of penis

    xviii) external pudendal veins

    xix) internal pudendal vein

    xx) ovarian vein

    xxi) pampiniform venous plexus

    xxii) prostatic venous plexus

    xxiii) rectal venous plexus

    xxiv) uterine venous plexus

    xxv) vaginal venous plexus

    xxvi) common iliac veins

    xxvii) middle sacral veins

    xxviii) vesical venous plexus

15. The Portal System of Veins

The hepatic portal system of the veins is responsible for the portal circulation, which denotes the passage of blood from the gastrointestinal tract and spleen through the portal vein to the liver.

The tributaries and sub-tributaries of the portal vein are presented below:

The Tributaries and Subtributaries of the Portal Vein		
The Lienal Vein		
The Tributaries of Lienal Vein	The Short Gastric Veins	
	The Left Gastroepiploic Vein	
	The Pancreatic Veins	
	The Inferior Mesenteric Vein	
	The Tributaries of Inferior Mesenteric Vein	The Sigmoid Veins
		The Left Colic Vein
The Superior Mesenteric Vein		
The Tributaries of Superior Mesenteric Vein	The Right Gastroepiploic Vein	
	The Pancreaticoduodenal Veins	
The Coronary Vein		
The Pyloric Vein		
The Cystic Vein		
The Paraumbilical Veins		

Common Pathologies

Angina pectoris

Commonly known as angina, angina pectoris chest pain is due to ischemia of the heart muscle, generally due to obstruction or spasm of the coronary arteries. The main cause of angina pectoris is coronary artery disease, due to atherosclerosis of the arteries feeding the heart.

Cardiomyopathy

Cardiomyopathy is a chronic disease of the heart muscle, in which the muscle is abnormally enlarged, thickened, and/or stiffened. The weakened heart muscle loses the ability to pump blood effectively, resulting in irregular heartbeats (arrhythmias) and possibly even heart failure.

Rheumatic Heart Disease

Rheumatic heart disease is a condition in which permanent damage to heart valves is caused by rheumatic fever. The heart valve is damaged by a disease process that generally begins with a strep throat caused by bacteria called Streptococcus, and may eventually cause rheumatic fever.

Arrhythmia

An arrhythmia is an abnormal rate or rhythm of the heartbeat. It can beat too fast, too slow, or with an irregular rhythm. If the heartbeat is fast it is called tachycardia and if is too slow, it is referred to as bradycardia.

Congenital Heart Defects

Congenital heart defects are abnormalities in the morphological or physiological functioning of the heart that are present at the time of birth. The primary cause is the incomplete or abnormal development of the fetal heart during the early weeks of pregnancy.

Hypertension

Hypertension or high blood pressure is a condition that exists when the force of blood pressing against the blood vessel walls is too high. Over time, hypertension can cause a myriad of complications within the body (Figure 9.d).

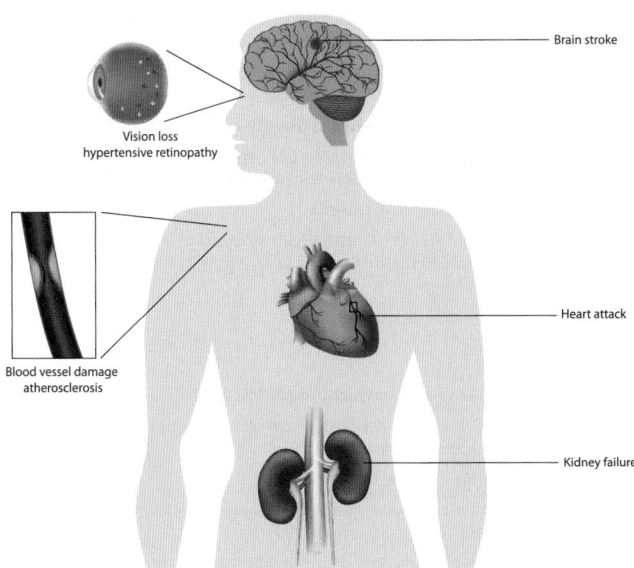

Figure 9.d Main Complications of Hypertension

Aortic Aneurysm

An aneurysm is an abnormal bulging or swelling of a portion of a blood vessel. The aorta, which can develop these abnormal bulges, is the large blood vessel that carries oxygen-rich blood away from the heart to the rest of the body.

Atherosclerosis

Atherosclerosis (Figure 9.e) is a disease of the arterial blood vessels (arteries), in which the walls of the blood vessels become thickened and hardened by "plaques." The plaques are composed of cholesterol and other lipids, inflammatory cells, and calcium deposits.

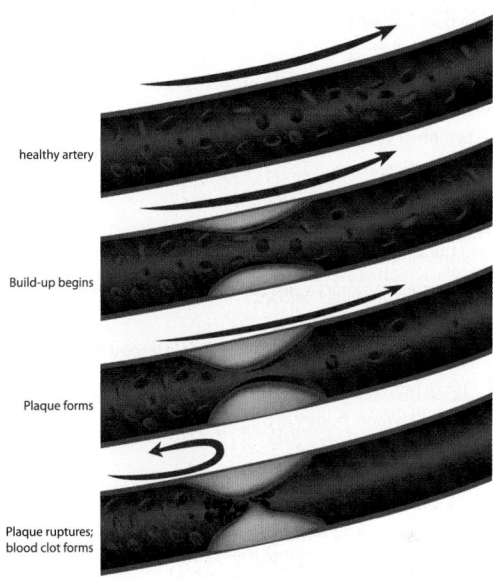

Figure 9.e Healthy Artery and Artery with Atherosclerosis

Deep Vein Thrombosis

Deep vein thrombosis (DVT) is a blood clot in a major vein that usually develops in the legs and/or pelvis.

Coronary Artery Disease

Coronary artery disease (CAD) is one of the common vascular diseases marked by accumulation of atherosclerotic plaque in the coronary blood vessels. As the plaque thickens, secondary changes may take place like enlargement of size and calcification that may lead to complete occlusion of the lumen of the coronary artery, resulting in inadequate supply of oxygen to the heart muscle.

Peripheral Vascular Disease

Peripheral vascular disease is a narrowing of blood vessels that restricts blood flow. It mostly occurs in the legs, but is sometimes seen in the arms.

Hypercholesterolemia

Hypercholesterolemia is the presence of high levels of cholesterol in the blood. It is a form of "hyperlipidemia" (elevated levels of lipids in the blood) and "hyperlipoproteinemia" (elevated levels of lipoproteins in the blood).

Lymphedema

A condition in which excess fluid collects in tissue and causes swelling. Lymphedema may occur in the arm or leg after lymph vessels or lymph nodes in the underarm or groin are removed.

Hodgkin's Lymphoma

This is a type of cancer of the lymphatic system. It can start almost anywhere in the body. It's believed to be caused by HIV, Epstein-Barr Syndrome, age, and family history.

Non-Hodgkin's Lymphoma

Non-Hodgkin's lymphoma is a cancer of the lymphoid system. It is divided into three types: high-grade, intermediate-grade and low-grade.

Lymphangitis

Lymphangitis is an inflammation of the lymphatics (lymph channels) due to an infection by a microbe or some chemical irritant. It occurs when an infection or inflammation occurs somewhere else and the microbe or the irritant is transported along with lymph fluid through the lymphatics.

Splenomegaly

Splenomegaly is a condition in which the spleen becomes enlarged, tender and painful. It can occur due to a number of reasons, ranging from certain infections to cancers.

Anatomy of the Lymphatic System

Introduction

The human lymphatic system (Figure 9.f) is closely linked with the blood and the vascular system. Both of these systems work in an intimate association with each other and transport vital fluids throughout the body via a system of vessels. The lymph capillaries and lymphatics are the special vessels that serve to transport a fluid (called lymph).

1. **The Lymphatic System**
   The human lymphatic system consists of the below mentioned components:
   a) The Lymph
   b) The Lymph Vessels
   c) The Lymph Nodes

   The lymph nodes (or lymph glands) are oval structures that are found along the length of lymphatics at various intervals. The lymph trunk is a specific lymph vessel containing lymph. The various types of lymph trunks are documented below:
   i) jugular lymph trunk
   ii) subclavian lymph trunk
   iii) bronchomediastinal lymph trunk
   iv) lumbar lymph trunk
   v) intestinal lymph trunk

   d) The Tonsils, Spleen, Thymus Gland and Peyer's Patches

   The most important function of the lymphatic system is to drain the protein containing fluid from the tissue spaces. The entire lymphatics of the body converge into one of the following major channels:
   i) thoracic duct (or the main collecting channel)
   ii) right lymphatic duct

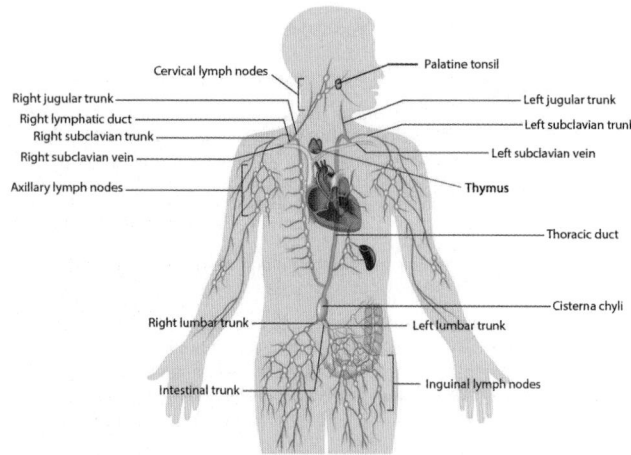

Right jugular trunk
Right lymphatic duct
Right subclavian trunk
Right subclavian vein
Axillary lymph nodes
Cervical lymph nodes
Palatine tonsil
Left jugular trunk
Left subclavian trunk
Left subclavian vein
Thymus
Thoracic duct
Cisterna chyli
Right lumbar trunk
Left lumbar trunk
Intestinal trunk
Inguinal lymph nodes

Figure 9.f Lymphatic System Anatomy

2. **Thoracic Duct**
   The thoracic duct is the largest lymphatic vessel in the body and constitutes an essential part of the lymphatic system. It is also called the alimentary duct, chyliferous duct, left lymphatic duct or Van Hoorne's canal.

3. **Lymphatics of the Head, Face and Neck**
   The entire lymph glands of the head are mostly extra-cranial, and arranged in the following groups:
   a) **Occipital Lymph Glands**

      The occipital lymph glands are two or three in number and located on the back of the head.
   b) **Posterior Auricular Lymph Glands (or Mastoid Glands)**

      The posterior auricular lymph glands are two in number and exist on the upper part of the sternomastoid muscle and mastoid portion of the temporal bone.
   c) **Anterior Auricular Lymph Glands (or Superficial Parotid/ Preauricular Glands)**

      The superficial parotid glands are present on the lateral surface of the parotid gland.

   d) **Parotid Lymph Glands (or Deep Parotid Glands)**

      The parotid lymph glands remain embedded in the deeper portions of the parotid gland.
   e) **Superficial Facial Lymph Glands**

      The superficial facial lymph glands are based on several lymph glands in the region of face. However, the major ones are described below:
      i) Infraorbital Lymph Glands (or Maxillary Glands): The infraorbital lymph glands remain scattered along the angle between the nose and cheek, and below the margin of the orbit.
      ii) Buccinator Lymph Glands: The buccinator lymph glands are found on the superficial surface of the anterior part of buccinator muscle, opposite to the angle of the mouth.
      iii) Supramandibular Lymph Glands: The supramandibular lymph glands lie on the outer surface of the mandible at the anterior border of the masseter muscle, between the external maxillary artery and the anterior facial vein.
   f) **The Deep Facial Lymph Glands (or Internal Maxillary Glands)**

      The deep facial lymph glands are found in association with the internal maxillary artery, on the outer surface of the external pterygoid muscle.
   g) **The Lingual Lymph Glands**

      The lingual lymph glands are based on two or three small nodules that exist on the lateral surfaces of the hypoglossal and genioglossus muscles.
   h) **The Retropharyngeal Glands**

      The retropharyngeal glands are located in the buccopharyngeal fascia behind the upper part of the pharynx.

4. **The Lymph Glands of the Neck**
   The lymph glands of the neck are divided into the following major groups:
   a) **The Submaxillary Glands**

      The submaxillary glands are a pair of salivary glands located on each side under the body of the mandible.
   b) **The Submental (or Suprahyoid Glands)**

      The submental glands are located beneath the chin, and between the anterior bellies of the two digastric muscles.
   c) **The Superficial Cervical Glands**

      The superficial cervical glands remain embedded in the deep fascia along the course of the external jugular vein, and superficial to the sternomastoid muscle.

5. **The Anterior Cervical Glands**
   The lymph glands of the anterior neck region are divisible into the following two groups:
   a) **Superficial Anterior Cervical Lymph Glands**

      The superficial anterior cervical lymph glands exist in association with the anterior jugular veins.
   b) **Deep Anterior Cervical Lymph Glands**

      The deep anterior cervical lymph glands are divisible into the following groups/types:
      i) infrahyoid glands obtain lymph fluid from the region of epiglottis and transport it to the deep cervical glands.
      ii) prelaryngeal gland obtains lymph from the anterior portion of the larynx, the isthmus, and the portions of the right and left lobes of the thyroid gland.
      iii) pretracheal lymph glands are the numerous small nodules that follow the course of the inferior thyroid veins.
      iv) paratracheal lymph glands lie in association with the branches of the superior and inferior thyroid arteries and the recurrent nerves.
   c) **Deep Cervical Glands**

      The deep cervical glands are the intercommunicating lymph vessels that remain positioned in the anterior and posterior triangles of the neck, and under the cover of the sternomastoid muscle. These glands are divisible into the following groups:
      i) superior deep cervical glands are located under the cover of the sternomastoid muscle, and lie in close association with the accessory nerve and internal jugular vein.
      ii) inferior deep cervical glands are located below the level of the omohyoid muscle.

d) **Lymphatic vessels of the scalp are distributed in the soft tissue envelope of the frontal, temporoparietal and the occipital regions of the cranium.**

e) **Lymphatic Vessels of the Ear divide into upper and lateral portions of the auricle and terminate into the anterior auricular glands.**

f) **Lymphatic vessels of the face are more widely distributed than the scalp vessels.**

6. **Lymphatic Vessels of the Eyelids and Conjunctiva**
The lymphatic vessels of the eyelids and conjunctiva form the following two groups:

a) **Medial Lymph Vessels**

The medial lymph vessels travel from the medial portions of the superior and inferior eyelids, and terminate to the submaxillary lymph glands.

b) **Lateral Lymph Vessels**

The lateral lymph vessels arise from the lateral parts of the eyelids, and terminate into the anterior auricular and the parotid lymph glands.

c) **Lymphatic Vessels of the Cheeks**

The superficial and deep lymphatic vessels of the cheeks usually communicate with the submaxillary glands.

d) **Lymphatic Vessels of the Lips**

The lymphatic vessels of the lips drain lymph fluid to the submental and submaxillary glands.

e) **Lymphatic Vessels of the Nose**

The lymphatic vessels from the external part of the nose drain lymph fluid to the anterior auricular and submaxillary glands.

f) **Lymphatic Vessels of the Nasal Cavities**

The lymphatic vessels from the anterior and posterior portions of the nasal cavities drain lymph fluid to the submaxillary, the retropharyngeal, and the superior deep cervical glands.

g) **Lymphatic Vessels of the Mouth**

The lymphatic vessels of the mouth can be divided into the following groups:

h) **Lymphatic Vessels of the Palatine Tonsil**

The lymphatic vessels of the palatine tonsil arise from the buccopharyngeal fascia and constrictor pharyngis superior and meet with the superior deep cervical glands.

i) **Lymphatic Vessels of the Tongue**

The lymphatic vessels of the tongue are divided into the following three groups:

i) anterior lymph vessels of the tongue drain lymph fluid from the tip and lower surface of the tongue to the submental glands.

ii) middle lymph vessels of the tongue drain lymph fluid from the anterior two third portion of the tongue to the submaxillary and medial superior deep cervical glands.

iii) posterior lymph vessels of the tongue drain lymph fluid from the portion of the tongue, which lies in the anterior wall of pharynx.

j) **Lymphatic Vessels of the Gums**

The lymph vessels of the anterior portion of mandibular gum drain lymph fluid to the submandibular gland. The lymph vessels from the inner portion of the mandibular gum also drain lymph fluid to the submaxillary glands.

k) **Lymphatic Vessels of the Teeth**

The lymph vessels of the teeth and mandible transport lymph fluid to the sub maxillary or the superior deep cervical glands.

7. **The Lymphatics of the Upper Extremity**
The lymph glands of the upper extremity are divisible into the following two groups:

a) **The Superficial Lymph Gland**

The superficial lymph glands of the upper extremity are of the following types:

i) supratrochlear lymph glands are situated above the medial epicondyle of humerus, and drain lymph fluid from the middle, ring and little fingers, and the portions of the hand and forearm.

ii) deltoideopectoral lymph glands are located in the groove between the pectoralis major and deltoid muscles.

b) **The Deep Lymph Glands**

The deep lymph glands are chiefly found in the axillary region, where they constitute several constant as well as variable groups.

i) lateral group of axillary lymph glands lies along the line of the great axillary vessels. These glands drain lymph fluid from the greater part of the upper extremity to the central and inferior deep cervical glands.

ii) anterior group of axillary lymph glands travels from third to sixth intercostal space, along the line of the lateral thoracic artery.

iii) posterior group of axillary lymph glands lies along the posterior wall of axilla, and follow the course of the subscapular vessels.

iv) central group of axillary lymph glands are located in the central part of the axilla, and along the line of the intercostobrachial nerve.

v) infra-clavicular group of axillary lymph glands is found between the upper border of the pectoralis minor muscle and the clavicle, along the medial side of the axillary artery.

c) **The Lymphatic Vessels of the Upper Extremity**

The lymphatic vessels of the upper extremity are divisible into the following two groups:

i) superficial lymph vessels of the upper extremity are located in the skin and subcutaneous tissues, and commence in the cutaneous plexuses on the volar aspects of the fingers and hand.

ii) deep lymph vessels of the upper extremity follow the course of the deeper blood vessels in the regions of the forearm and hand.

8. **Lymphatics of the Lower Extremity:**
The lymph glands of the lower extremity are divisible into the following groups:

a) **The Superficial Lymph Glands**

superficial lymph glands are found in the superficial fascia in subinguinal and inguinal regions. These glands are separable into the following groups:

i) inguinal lymph glands are located above the level of the inguinal ligament.

ii) superficial sublingual lymph glands are divisible into the proximal and distal groups.

b) **Deep Lymph Glands**

The deep lymph glands of the inferior extremity are divided into the following two groups:

i) popliteal lymph glands are located in the popliteal fossa.

ii) deep sublingual lymph glands are located in the femoral trigone.

c) **Lymphatic Vessels of the Lower Extremity**

The lymphatic vessels of the lower extremity are based on the following two groups:

i) superficial lymphatic vessels are located in the superficial fascia and divided into vessels of the medial group arises on the tibial side and dorsum of the foot, and terminates in the distal group of superficial subinguinal glands and vessels of the lateral group commences from the fibular side of the foot.

ii) deep lymphatic vessels of the lower extremity follow the course of the deep blood vessels, and terminate into the deep subinguinal and hypogastric glands.

9. **The Lymphatics of the Abdomen and Pelvis**
The lymph glands of the abdomen and pelvis are divisible into parietal lymph glands and visceral lymph glands.

a) **External Iliac Glands**

The external iliac group of glands pertains to the pelvic region, located along the course of the external iliac vessels, and constitutes the lateral, intermediate and medial chains.

b) **Common Iliac Glands:**

The common iliac glands of the pelvis are located on the sides of the common iliac artery and below the bifurcation of aorta.

c) **Epigastric Glands**

The epigastric glands of the anterior abdominal wall are divisible into the following types:

i) superior epigastric gland is located in the superficial fascia of the median part of the epigastric region.

ii) inferior epigastric glands are located along the course of the inferior epigastric artery.

d) **Circumflex Iliac Glands**

The circumflex iliac glands of the anterior abdominal wall follow the course of the deep circumflex iliac artery in the lateral aspect of groin.

e) **Hypogastric Glands**

The hypogastric glands of the pelvis are located along the course of the hypogastric vessels.

   i)   gluteal lymph glands

   ii) pubo-gluteal lymph glands

   iii) middle hemorrhoidal gland

   iv) inter-iliac glands

   v)   obturator gland

f) **Sacral Glands**

The sacral lymph glands of the pelvis are located along the anterior aspect of sacrum, between the anterior sacral foramina.

g) **Lumbar Glands**

The lumbar lymph glands are located behind the peritoneum of the posterior wall of the abdomen. The lumbar lymph glands are further separable into the following groups:

   i)   right lateral aortic glands

   ii) left lateral aortic glands

   iii) preaortic glands

   iv) retroaortic glands

h) **Superior Gastric Glands**

The superior gastric glands exist in association with the left gastric artery and constitute the following subdivisions:

   i)   anterior left gastric glands (or lower coronary glands)

   ii)   right paracardial glands

   iii) left paracardial glands

   iv)   posterior paracardial glands

   v)   posterior left gastric glands (or upper coronary glands)

   vi)   right gastric gland (or pyloric gland)

   vii) left suprapancreatic glands

   viii) right suprapancreatic glands

   ix)   subpyloric glands

   x)   biliary lymph glands

i) **Inferior Gastric Glands (or Right Gastroepiploic Glands)**

The inferior gastric glands are associated with the greater curvature of the stomach and follow the course of the right gastroepiploic artery.

j) **Hepatic Glands**

The hepatic lymph glands exist in the region of porta hepatis (or transverse fissure of the liver), between the layers of the lesser omentum.

k) **Pancreaticolienal Glands (or Splenic Glands)**

The pancreaticolienal glands are positioned in relation to the posterior surface and upper border of pancreas, and follow the course of the lienal (or splenic) artery.

l) **Mesenteric Glands**

The mesenteric lymph glands are located between the layers of the mesentery.

m) **Ileocolic glands**

The ileocolic glands are located around the ileocolic artery and form the following major groups:

   i)   ileal glands

   ii) anterior ileocolic glands

   iii) posterior ileocolic glands

   iv) right colic glands

n) **Mesocolic Glands**

The mesocolic glands exist in close association with the transverse colon.

o) **Inferior Mesenteric Glands**

The inferior mesenteric glands are located on the branches of the left colic and sigmoid arteries, the superior hemorrhoidal artery, and the muscular coat of the rectum.

10. **The Lymphatic Vessels of the Abdominal Viscera and the Superior and Posterior Walls of the Abdomen**

   a) Lymphatic Vessels of the Abdominal Part of the Alimentary Canal

   b) Lymphatic Vessels of the Stomach

   c) Lymphatic Vessels of the Duodenum

   d) Lymphatic Vessels of the Jejunum and Ileum (or the Lacteals)

   e) Lymphatic Vessels of the Cecum, Vermiform Process, and the Ascending Colon

   f) Lymphatic Vessels of the Right Colic Flexure and the Transverse Colon

   g) Lymphatic Vessels of the Left Colic Flexure, Descending Colon, Iliac Colon, and Pelvic Colon

   h) Lymphatic Vessels of the Liver

   i) Lymphatic Vessels of the Gall Bladder

   j) Lymphatic Vessels of the Pancreas

   k) Lymphatic Vessels of the Spleen

   l) Lymphatic Vessels of the Kidneys

   m) Lymphatic Vessels of the Ureters

   n) Lymphatic Vessels of the Suprarenal Glands

   o) Lymphatic Vessels of the Diaphragm

11. **The Lymphatic Vessels of the Pelvic Viscera**

   a) lymphatic Vessels of the Male Urethra

   b) Lymphatic Vessels of the Prostate

   c) Lymphatic Vessels of the Female Urethra

   d) Lymphatic Vessels of the Seminal Vesicle

   e) Lymphatic Vessels of the Ductus Deferens

   f) Lymphatic Vessels of the Urinary Bladder

   g) Lymphatic Vessels of the Ureter

   h) Lymphatic Vessels of the Vagina

   i) Lymphatic Vessels of the Uterus

   j) Lymphatic Vessels of the Uterine Tube

   k) Lymphatic Vessels of the Ovaries

   l) Lymphatic Vessels of the Testis and Epididymis

   m) Lymphatic Vessels of the Anus, Anal Canal and Rectum

12. **The Lymphatics of the Thorax**

The Lymph Glands of the thorax are separable into the following groups:

   a) **Sternal Lymph Glands**

   The sternal lymph glands are located at the margins of the sternum along the side of the internal mammary artery.

   b) **Intercostal Lymph Glands**

   The intercostal lymph glands are situated in the posterior portions of the intercostal spaces (in relation to the intercostal vessels), and in front of the heads of the ribs.

   c) **Anterior Mediastinal Lymph Glands**

   The anterior mediastinal lymph glands are located in the lower portion of the anterior mediastinum, and the anterior part of the superior mediastinal cavity.

   d) **Posterior Mediastinal Lymph Glands**

   The posterior mediastinal lymph glands exist along the thoracic part of the esophagus and the descending thoracic aorta.

   e) **Bronchial Lymph Glands**

   The bronchial lymph glands lie along the walls of the intrathoracic of the trachea, the bronchi and their intrapulmonary branches. These glands are further categorized into the following groups:

      i)   tracheobronchial lymph glands

      ii) lymph glands of the bifurcation (or intertracheobronchial lymph glands)

      iii) bronchopulmonary lymph glands

      iv) pulmonary lymph glands

13. **The Lymphatic Vessels of the Thorax**

These vessels are divisible into the following groups:

   a) **Intercostal Lymph Vessels**

   b) **Lymph Vessels of the Diaphragm**

   c) **Lymphatic Vessels of the Contents of the Thorax**

   The lymphatic vessels of the contents of the thorax are divisible into the following groups:

      i)   lymph vessels of the heart

      ii) lymph vessels of the pericardium

      iii) lymph vessels of the thymus

      iv) lymph vessels of the thoracic part of esophagus

      v)   lymph vessels of the pleura

      vi) lymph vessels of the lungs

Diseases of the circulatory system (I00-I99)

[EXCLUDES2] *certain conditions originating in the perinatal period (P04-P96)*
certain infectious and parasitic diseases (A00-B99)
complications of pregnancy, childbirth and the puerperium (O00-O9A)
congenital malformations, deformations, and chromosomal abnormalities (Q00-Q99)
endocrine, nutritional and metabolic diseases (E00-E88)
injury, poisoning and certain other consequences of external causes (S00-T88)
neoplasms (C00-D49)
symptoms, signs and abnormal clinical and laboratory findings, not elsewhere classified (R00-R94)
systemic connective tissue disorders (M30-M36)
transient cerebral ischemic attacks and related syndromes (G45.-)

This chapter contains the following blocks:

I00-I02	Acute rheumatic fever
I05-I09	Chronic rheumatic heart diseases
I10-I16	Hypertensive diseases
I20-I25	Ischemic heart diseases
I26-I28	Pulmonary heart disease and diseases of pulmonary circulation
I30-I52	Other forms of heart disease
I60-I69	Cerebrovascular diseases
I70-I79	Diseases of arteries, arterioles and capillaries
I80-I89	Diseases of veins, lymphatic vessels and lymph nodes, not elsewhere classified
I95-I99	Other and unspecified disorders of the circulatory system

Acute rheumatic fever (I00-I02)

I00 Rheumatic fever without heart involvement
AHA: Q4 2016
[INCLUDES] *arthritis, rheumatic, acute or subacute*
[EXCLUDES1] *rheumatic fever with heart involvement (I01.0 -I01.9)*

[4th] **I01 Rheumatic fever** with heart involvement
[EXCLUDES1] *chronic diseases of rheumatic origin (I05-I09) unless rheumatic fever is also present or there is evidence of reactivation or activity of the rheumatic process.*

I01.0 Acute rheumatic pericarditis [CC] [CC/MCC Exc]
Any condition in I00 with pericarditis
Rheumatic pericarditis (acute)
[EXCLUDES1] *acute pericarditis not specified as rheumatic (I30.-)*

I01.1 Acute rheumatic endocarditis [CC] [CC/MCC Exc]
Any condition in I00 with endocarditis or valvulitis
Acute rheumatic valvulitis

I01.2 Acute rheumatic myocarditis [CC] [CC/MCC Exc]
Any condition in I00 with myocarditis

I01.8 Other acute rheumatic heart disease [CC] [CC/MCC Exc]
Any condition in I00 with other or multiple types of heart involvement
Acute rheumatic pancarditis

I01.9 Acute rheumatic heart disease, unspecified [CC] [CC/MCC Exc]
Any condition in I00 with unspecified type of heart involvement
Rheumatic carditis, acute
Rheumatic heart disease, active or acute

[4th] **I02 Rheumatic** chorea
DEFINITION: Chorea is an abnormal involuntary movement resembling fidgeting or dancing.
[INCLUDES] *Sydenham's chorea*
[EXCLUDES1] *chorea NOS (G25.5)*
Huntington's chorea (G10)

I02.0 Rheumatic chorea with heart involvement [CC] [CC/MCC Exc]
Chorea NOS with heart involvement
Rheumatic chorea with heart involvement of any type classifiable under I01.-

I02.9 Rheumatic chorea without heart involvement [CC] [CC/MCC Exc]
Rheumatic chorea NOS

Chronic rheumatic heart diseases (I05-I09)

[4th] **I05 Rheumatic** mitral valve **diseases**
[INCLUDES] *conditions classifiable to both I05.0 and I05.2-I05.9, whether specified as rheumatic or not*
[EXCLUDES1] *mitral valve disease specified as nonrheumatic (I34.-)*
mitral valve disease with aortic and/or tricuspid valve involvement (I08.-)

I05.0 Rheumatic mitral stenosis
Mitral (valve) obstruction (rheumatic)

I05.1 Rheumatic mitral insufficiency
Rheumatic mitral incompetence
Rheumatic mitral regurgitation
[EXCLUDES1] *mitral insufficiency not specified as rheumatic (I34.0)*

I05.2 Rheumatic mitral stenosis with insufficiency
Rheumatic mitral stenosis with incompetence or regurgitation

I05.8 Other rheumatic mitral valve diseases
Rheumatic mitral (valve) failure

I05.9 Rheumatic mitral valve disease, unspecified
Rheumatic mitral (valve) disorder (chronic) NOS

[4th] **I06 Rheumatic** aortic valve **diseases**
[EXCLUDES1] *aortic valve disease not specified as rheumatic (I35.-)*
aortic valve disease with mitral and/or tricuspid valve involvement (I08.-)

I06.0 Rheumatic aortic stenosis
Rheumatic aortic (valve) obstruction

I06.1 Rheumatic aortic insufficiency
Rheumatic aortic incompetence
Rheumatic aortic regurgitation

I06.2 Rheumatic aortic stenosis with insufficiency
Rheumatic aortic stenosis with incompetence or regurgitation

I06.8 Other rheumatic aortic valve diseases

I06.9 Rheumatic aortic valve disease, unspecified
Rheumatic aortic (valve) disease NOS

[4th] **I07 Rheumatic** tricuspid valve **diseases**
[INCLUDES] *rheumatic tricuspid valve diseases specified as rheumatic or unspecified*
[EXCLUDES1] *tricuspid valve disease specified as nonrheumatic (I36.-)*
tricuspid valve disease with aortic and/or mitral valve involvement (I08.-)

I07.0 Rheumatic tricuspid stenosis
Tricuspid (valve) stenosis (rheumatic)

I07.1 Rheumatic tricuspid insufficiency
Tricuspid (valve) insufficiency (rheumatic)

I07.2 Rheumatic tricuspid stenosis and insufficiency

I07.8 Other rheumatic tricuspid valve diseases

I07.9 Rheumatic tricuspid valve disease, unspecified
Rheumatic tricuspid valve disorder NOS

[4th] **I08** Multiple valve **diseases**
[INCLUDES] *multiple valve diseases specified as rheumatic or unspecified*
[EXCLUDES1] *endocarditis, valve unspecified (I38)*
multiple valve disease specified a nonrheumatic (I34.-, I35.-, I36.-, I37.-, I38.-, Q22.-, Q23.-, Q24.8-)
rheumatic valve disease NOS (I09.1)

I08.0 Rheumatic disorders of both mitral **and** aortic **valves**
AHA: Q2 2019
Involvement of both mitral and aortic valves specified as rheumatic or unspecified

I08.1 Rheumatic disorders of both mitral **and** tricuspid **valves**

I08.2 Rheumatic disorders of both aortic **and** tricuspid **valves**

I08.3 Combined rheumatic disorders of mitral, aortic **and** tricuspid **valves**

I08.8 Other rheumatic multiple valve diseases

I08.9 Rheumatic multiple valve disease, unspecified

[4th] **I09 Other rheumatic heart diseases**

I09.0 Rheumatic myocarditis [CC] [CC/MCC Exc]
[EXCLUDES1] *myocarditis not specified as rheumatic (I51.4)*

I09.1 Rheumatic diseases of endocardium, valve unspecified
Rheumatic endocarditis (chronic)
Rheumatic valvulitis (chronic)
[EXCLUDES1] *endocarditis, valve unspecified (I38)*

Unspecified Code | Other Specified Code | Manifestation Code | [N] Newborn | [P] Pediatric | [M] Maternity | [A] Adult | ♂ Male | ♀ Female
● New Code | ▲ Revised Code Title | ►◄ Revised Text | [NOTES] | [INCLUDES] | [EXCLUDES1] Not coded here | [EXCLUDES2] Not included here
[4th] 4th character required | [5th] 5th character required | [6th] 6th character required | [7th] 7th character required | [X] Extension 'X' Alert
[HAC] Hospital-acquired condition (HAC) alert | AHA AHA Coding Clinic© | Code first alert

When symbols appear on a code that requires a 7th character extension, refer to Appendix B to identify applicable 7th character codes.

I09.2   Chronic **rheumatic** pericarditis   cc CC/MCC Exc
     Adherent pericardium, rheumatic
     Chronic rheumatic mediastinopericarditis
     Chronic rheumatic myopericarditis
     EXCLUDES1   chronic pericarditis not specified as rheumatic (I31.-)

I09.8   **Other specified rheumatic heart diseases**
     I09.81   **Rheumatic heart failure**   cc HCC RxHCC CC/MCC Exc
         Use additional code to identify type of heart failure (I50.-)
     I09.89   **Other specified rheumatic heart diseases**
         Rheumatic disease of pulmonary valve

I09.9   **Rheumatic heart disease, unspecified**
     Rheumatic carditis
     EXCLUDES1   rheumatoid carditis (M05.31)

Hypertensive diseases (I10-I16)

Use additional code to identify:
exposure to environmental tobacco smoke (Z77.22)
history of tobacco dependence (Z87.891)
occupational exposure to environmental tobacco smoke (Z57.31)
tobacco dependence (F17.-)
tobacco use (Z72.0)
EXCLUDES1   neonatal hypertension (P29.2)
         primary pulmonary hypertension (I27.0)
EXCLUDES2   hypertensive disease complicating pregnancy, childbirth and the
         puerperium (O10-O11, O13-O16)

I10   Essential **(primary) hypertension**   ? RxHCC
     AHA: Q2 2018, Q4 2016
     INCLUDES   high blood pressure
         hypertension (arterial) (benign) (essential) (malignant)
         (primary) (systemic)
     EXCLUDES1   hypertensive disease complicating pregnancy, childbirth and
         the puerperium (O10-O11, O13-O16)
     EXCLUDES2   essential (primary) hypertension involving vessels of brain
         (I60-I69)
         essential (primary) hypertension involving vessels of eye (H35.0-)

I11   **Hypertensive** heart **disease (Figure 9.1)**
     INCLUDES   any condition in I50.-, I51.4-I51.9 due to hypertension
     I11.0   **Hypertensive heart disease** with heart failure   HCC RxHCC
         AHA: Q1 2017
         Hypertensive heart failure
         Use additional code to identify type of heart failure (I50.-)
     I11.9   **Hypertensive heart disease** without heart failure   RxHCC
         AHA: Q2 2018
         Hypertensive heart disease NOS

I12   **Hypertensive** chronic kidney **disease**
     See Official Guidelines "Hypertensive Chronic Kidney Disease"
     I.C.9.a.2, "Hypertensive Heart and Chronic Kidney Disease" I.C.9.a.3
     INCLUDES   any condition in N18 and N26 - due to hypertension
         arteriosclerosis of kidney
         arteriosclerotic nephritis (chronic) (interstitial)
         hypertensive nephropathy
         nephrosclerosis
     EXCLUDES1   hypertension due to kidney disease (I15.0, I15.1)
         renovascular hypertension (I15.0)
         secondary hypertension (I15.-)
     EXCLUDES2   acute kidney failure (N17.-)
     I12.0   **Hypertensive chronic kidney disease with** stage 5 **chronic
         kidney disease or** end stage renal disease   cc HCC RxHCC CC/MCC Exc
         AHA: Q3 2016
         Use additional code to identify the stage of chronic kidney
         disease (N18.5, N18.6)
     I12.9   **Hypertensive chronic kidney disease with** stage 1 through
         stage 4 **chronic kidney disease, or unspecified chronic
         kidney disease**   RxHCC
         AHA: Q4 2018
         Hypertensive chronic kidney disease NOS
         Hypertensive renal disease NOS
         Use additional code to identify the stage of chronic kidney
         disease (N18.1-N18.4, N18.9)

I13   **Hypertensive** heart **and** chronic kidney **disease**
     See Official Guidelines "Hypertensive Heart and Chronic Kidney
     Disease" I.C.9.a.3
     INCLUDES   any condition in I11.- with any condition in I12.-
         cardiorenal disease
         cardiovascular renal disease
     I13.0   **Hypertensive heart and chronic kidney disease with heart
         failure and** stage 1 through stage 4 **chronic kidney disease,
         or unspecified chronic kidney disease**   cc HCC RxHCC CC/MCC Exc
         Use additional code to identify type of heart failure (I50.-)
         Use additional code to identify stage of chronic kidney disease
         (N18.1-N18.4, N18.9)
     I13.1   **Hypertensive** heart **and** chronic kidney **disease without**
         heart **failure**
         I13.10   **Hypertensive heart and chronic kidney disease
             without heart failure, with** stage 1 through stage 4
             **chronic kidney disease, or unspecified chronic
             kidney disease**   RxHCC
             Hypertensive heart disease and hypertensive chronic
             kidney disease NOS
             Use additional code to identify the stage of chronic
             kidney disease (N18.1-N18.4, N18.9)
         I13.11   **Hypertensive heart and chronic kidney disease
             without heart failure, with** stage 5 **chronic kidney
             disease, or** end stage renal disease   cc HCC RxHCC CC/MCC Exc
             Use additional code to identify the stage of chronic
             kidney disease (N18.5, N18.6)
     I13.2   **Hypertensive heart and chronic kidney disease** with heart
         failure **and with** stage 5 **chronic kidney disease,
         or** end stage renal disease   cc HCC RxHCC CC/MCC Exc
         Use additional code to identify type of heart failure (I50.-)
         Use additional code to identify the stage of chronic kidney
         disease (N18.5, N18.6)

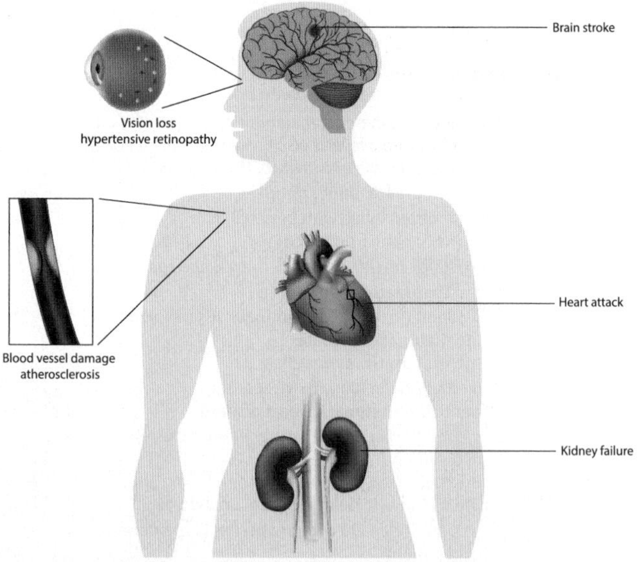

Figure 9.1 Complications of Hypertension

I15   Secondary **hypertension**
     Code also underlying condition
     EXCLUDES1   postprocedural hypertension (I97.3)
     EXCLUDES2   secondary hypertension involving vessels of brain (I60-I69)
         secondary hypertension involving vessels of eye (H35.0-)
     I15.0   Renovascular **hypertension**   RxHCC
     I15.1   **Hypertension secondary to other** renal disorders   RxHCC
         AHA: Q3 2016
     I15.2   **Hypertension secondary to** endocrine disorders   RxHCC
     I15.8   Other **secondary hypertension**   RxHCC
     I15.9   **Secondary hypertension, unspecified**   RxHCC

PDxⓈ Unacceptable principal diagnosis symbol per Medicare code edits   POA Code exempt from diagnosis present on admission requirement
? Questionable admission   cc Complication or comorbidity   MCC Major complication or comorbidity   CC/MCC Exc CC/MCC exclusion
HCC HCC diagnosis code   RxHCC RxHCC diagnosis code   MACRA code   **DEFINITION** Describes condition/terminology
TIP Coding guidance   Official Guideline Reference   Z1 Z code as first-listed diagnosis

I16 **Hypertensive** crisis

👁 **See Official Guidelines** "Hypertensive Crisis" I.C.9.a.10

Code also any identified hypertensive disease (I10-I15)

I16.0 **Hypertensive** urgency   RxHCC

     DEFINITION: A severe increase in blood pressure without corresponding organ damage.

     AHA: Q4 2016

I16.1 **Hypertensive** emergency   cc RxHCC

     DEFINITION: A severe increase in blood pressure with corresponding organ damage.

     AHA: Q4 2016

I16.9 **Hypertensive crisis, unspecified**   cc RxHCC

     AHA: Q4 2016

Ischemic heart diseases (I20-I25)

Use additional code to identify presence of hypertension (I10-I16)

I20 **Angina pectoris**

Use additional code to identify:

     exposure to environmental tobacco smoke (Z77.22)

     history of tobacco dependence (Z87.891)

     occupational exposure to environmental tobacco smoke (Z57.31)

     tobacco dependence (F17.-)

     tobacco use (Z72.0)

     EXCLUDES1 angina pectoris with atherosclerotic heart disease of native coronary arteries (I25.1-)

         atherosclerosis of coronary artery bypass graft(s) and coronary artery of transplanted heart with angina pectoris (I25.7-)

         postinfarction angina (I23.7)

I20.0 Unstable **angina**   cc HCC RxHCC CC/MCC Exc

     Accelerated angina

     Crescendo angina

     De novo effort angina

     Intermediate coronary syndrome

     Preinfarction syndrome

     Worsening effort angina

I20.1 **Angina pectoris** with documented spasm   cc HCC RxHCC CC/MCC Exc

     Angiospastic angina

     Prinzmetal angina

     Spasm-induced angina

     Variant angina

I20.8 Other forms **of angina pectoris**   HCC RxHCC

     Angina equivalent

     Angina of effort

     Coronary slow flow syndrome

     Stenocardia

     Stable angina

     Use additional code(s) for symptoms associated with angina equivalent

I20.9 **Angina pectoris, unspecified**   HCC RxHCC

     Angina NOS

     Anginal syndrome

     Cardiac angina

     Ischemic chest pain

I21 **Acute myocardial infarction**

👁 **See Official Guidelines** "Type 1 ST elevation myocardial infarction (STEMI) and non-ST elevation myocardial infarction (NSTEMI)" I.C.9.e.1, "Subsequent acute myocardial infarction" I.C.9.e.4

DEFINITION: (1) A Type 1 myocardial infarction is a spontaneous heart attack caused by plaque, erosion, fissure, rupture, or dissection. (2) A STEMI is an ST-elevation myocardial infarction with 100 percent blockage of a coronary artery. A STEMI is more severe than an NSTEMI.

INCLUDES   cardiac infarction

         coronary (artery) embolism

         coronary (artery) occlusion

         coronary (artery) rupture

         coronary (artery) thrombosis

         infarction of heart, myocardium, or ventricle

         myocardial infarction specified as acute or with a stated duration of 4 weeks (28 days) or less from onset

Use additional code, if applicable, to identify:

     exposure to environmental tobacco smoke (Z77.22)

     history of tobacco dependence (Z87.891)

     occupational exposure to environmental tobacco smoke (Z57.31)

     status post administration of tPA (rtPA) in a different facility within the last 24 hours prior to admission to current facility (Z92.82)

     tobacco dependence (F17.-)

     tobacco use (Z72.0)

     EXCLUDES2 old myocardial infarction (I25.2)

         postmyocardial infarction syndrome (I24.1)

         subsequent type 1 myocardial infarction (I22.-)

I21.0 ST elevation **(STEMI) myocardial infarction of** anterior wall

     Type 1 ST elevation myocardial infarction of anterior wall

I21.01 **ST elevation (STEMI) myocardial infarction involving** left main coronary artery   cc HCC RxHCC CC/MCC Exc

     AHA: Q4 2018, Q4 2017

I21.02 **ST elevation (STEMI) myocardial infarction involving** left anterior descending coronary artery   cc HCC RxHCC CC/MCC Exc

     AHA: Q4 2018, Q4 2017

     ST elevation (STEMI) myocardial infarction involving diagonal coronary artery

I21.09 **ST elevation (STEMI) myocardial infarction involving** other coronary artery **of anterior wall**   cc HCC RxHCC CC/MCC Exc

     AHA: Q4 2018, Q4 2017

     Acute transmural myocardial infarction of anterior wall

     Anteroapical transmural (Q wave) infarction (acute)

     Anterolateral transmural (Q wave) infarction (acute)

     Anteroseptal transmural (Q wave) infarction (acute)

     Transmural (Q wave) infarction (acute) (of) anterior (wall) NOS

I21.1 ST elevation **(STEMI) myocardial infarction of** inferior wall

     Type 1 ST elevation myocardial infarction of inferior wall

     👁 **See Official Guidelines** "Other Types of Myocardial Infarctions" I.C.9.e.5

I21.11 **ST elevation (STEMI) myocardial infarction involving** right coronary artery   cc HCC RxHCC CC/MCC Exc

     AHA: Q4 2018, Q4 2017

     Inferoposterior transmural (Q wave) infarction (acute)

I21.19 **ST elevation (STEMI) myocardial infarction involving** other coronary artery **of inferior wall**   cc HCC RxHCC CC/MCC Exc

     AHA: Q4 2018, Q4 2017

     Acute transmural myocardial infarction of inferior wall

     Inferolateral transmural (Q wave) infarction (acute)

     Transmural (Q wave) infarction (acute) (of) diaphragmatic wall

     Transmural (Q wave) infarction (acute) (of) inferior (wall) NOS

     EXCLUDES2 ST elevation (STEMI) myocardial infarction involving left circumflex coronary artery (I21.21)

I21.2 ST elevation **(STEMI) myocardial infarction of** other sites

     Type 1 ST elevation myocardial infarction of other sites

     👁 **See Official Guidelines** "Other Types of Myocardial Infarctions" I.C.9.e.5

I21.21 **ST elevation (STEMI) myocardial infarction involving** left circumflex coronary artery   cc HCC RxHCC CC/MCC Exc

     AHA: Q4 2018, Q4 2017

     ST elevation (STEMI) myocardial infarction involving oblique marginal coronary artery

I21.29 **ST elevation (STEMI) myocardial infarction involving** other sites   cc HCC RxHCC CC/MCC Exc

     AHA: Q4 2018, Q4 2017

     Acute transmural myocardial infarction of other sites

     Apical-lateral transmural (Q wave) infarction (acute)

     Basal-lateral transmural (Q wave) infarction (acute)

     High lateral transmural (Q wave) infarction (acute)

     Lateral (wall) NOS transmural (Q wave) infarction (acute)

     Posterior (true) transmural (Q wave) infarction (acute)

     Posterobasal transmural (Q wave) infarction (acute)

     Posterolateral transmural (Q wave) infarction (acute)

     Posteroseptal transmural (Q wave) infarction (acute)

     Septal transmural (Q wave) infarction (acute) NOS

Unspecified Code   Other Specified Code   Manifestation Code   N Newborn   P Pediatric   M Maternity   A Adult   ♂ Male   ♀ Female

● New Code   ▲ Revised Code Title   ▶◀ Revised Text   NOTES   INCLUDES   EXCLUDES1 Not coded here   EXCLUDES2 Not included here

4ᵗʰ character required   5ᵗʰ character required   6ᵗʰ character required   7ᵗʰ character required   Extension 'X' Alert

HAC Hospital-acquired condition (HAC) alert   AHA AHA Coding Clinic©   📣 Code first alert

2020 ICD-10-CM   When symbols appear on a code that requires a 7th character extension, refer to Appendix B to identify applicable 7th character codes.   **657**

I21.3 ST elevation **(STEMI) myocardial infarction of unspecified** site   cc◎ HCC RxHCC CC/MCC Exc

    👁 **See Official Guidelines** "Other Types of Myocardial Infarctions" I.C.9.e.5

    AHA: Q4 2017

    Acute transmural myocardial infarction of unspecified site

    Transmural (Q wave) myocardial infarction NOS

    Type 1 ST elevation myocardial infarction of unspecified site

I21.4 Non-ST elevation **(NSTEMI) myocardial infarction**   HCC MCC◎ RxHCC CC/MCC Exc

    👁 **See Official Guidelines** "Other Types of Myocardial Infarctions" I.C.9.e.5

    DEFINITION: An NSTEMI is a non-ST-elevation myocardial infarction caused by a severe narrowing of a coronary artery. The artery is not 100 percent blocked.

    AHA: Q4 2018, Q1 2017, Q4 2017, Q2 2015

    Acute subendocardial myocardial infarction

    Non-Q wave myocardial infarction NOS

    Nontransmural myocardial infarction NOS

    Type 1 non-ST elevation myocardial infarction

I21.9 Acute **myocardial infarction, unspecified**   HCC MCC◎ RxHCC CC/MCC Exc

    👁 **See Official Guidelines** "Acute myocardial infarction, unspecified" I.C.9.e.2, "Other Types of Myocardial Infarctions" I.C.9.e.5

    AHA: Q4 2018, Q4 2017

    Myocardial infarction (acute) NOS

🔟 **I21.A** Other **type of myocardial infarction**

    I21.A1 **Myocardial infarction** type 2   HCC MCC◎ RxHCC CC/MCC Exc

       👁 **See Official Guidelines** "Subsequent acute myocardial infarction" I.C.9.e.4, "Other Types of Myocardial Infarctions" I.C.9.e.5

       DEFINITION: A Type 2 myocardial infarction is a heart attack secondary to ischemia.

       AHA: Q4 2018, Q4 2017

       Myocardial infarction due to demand ischemia

       Myocardial infarction secondary to ischemic imbalance

       👉 **Code first** the underlying cause, such as:

          anemia (D50.0-D64.9)

          chronic obstructive pulmonary disease (J44.-)

          paroxysmal tachycardia (I47.0-I47.9)

          shock (R57.0-R57.9)

    I21.A9 Other **myocardial infarction type**   HCC MCC◎ RxHCC CC/MCC Exc

       👁 **See Official Guidelines** "Subsequent acute myocardial infarction" I.C.9.e.4

       DEFINITION: (1) A Type 3 myocardial infarction is sudden cardiac death. (2) A Type 4a-4c myocardial infarction is one related to percutaneous coronary intervention (PCI). (3) A Type 5 myocardial infarction is related to coronary artery bypass grafting (CABG).

       AHA: Q2 2019, Q4 2018, Q4 2017

       Myocardial infarction associated with revascularization procedure

       Myocardial infarction type 3

       Myocardial infarction type 4a

       Myocardial infarction type 4b

       Myocardial infarction type 4c

       Myocardial infarction type 5

       👉 **Code first,** if applicable, postprocedural myocardial infarction following cardiac surgery (I97.190), or postprocedural myocardial infarction during cardiac surgery (I97.790)

       Code also complication, if known and applicable, such as:

          (acute) stent occlusion (T82.897-)

          (acute) stent stenosis ▶(T82.855-)◀

          (acute) stent thrombosis (T82.867-)

          cardiac arrest due to underlying cardiac condition (I46.2)

          complication of percutaneous coronary intervention (PCI) (I97.89)

          occlusion of coronary artery bypass graft (T82.218-)

4ᵗʰ **I22** Subsequent **ST elevation (STEMI) and non-ST elevation (NSTEMI) myocardial infarction**

    👁 **See Official Guidelines** "Subsequent acute myocardial infarction" I.C.9.e.4

    DEFINITION: A STEMI is an ST-elevation myocardial infarction with 100 percent blockage of a coronary artery. A STEMI is more severe than an NSTEMI.

    TIP: Use a code from this category when a patient who has suffered a type 1 or unspecified acute myocardial infarction (AMI) has a new AMI within four weeks of the initial AMI.

    INCLUDES   acute myocardial infarction occurring within four weeks (28 days) of a previous acute myocardial infarction, regardless of site

          cardiac infarction

          coronary (artery) embolism

          coronary (artery) occlusion

          coronary (artery) rupture

          coronary (artery) thrombosis

          infarction of heart, myocardium, or ventricle

          recurrent myocardial infarction

          reinfarction of myocardium

          rupture of heart, myocardium, or ventricle

          subsequent type 1 myocardial infarction

Use additional code, if applicable, to identify:

    exposure to environmental tobacco smoke (Z77.22)

    history of tobacco dependence (Z87.891)

    occupational exposure to environmental tobacco smoke (Z57.31)

    status post administration of tPA (rtPA) in a different facility within the last 24 hours prior to admission to current facility (Z92.82)

    tobacco dependence (F17.-)

    tobacco use (Z72.0)

    EXCLUDES1   subsequent myocardial infarction, type 2 (I21.A1)

          subsequent myocardial infarction of other type (type 3) (type 4) (type 5) (I21.A9)

I22.0 **Subsequent** ST elevation **(STEMI) myocardial infarction of** anterior wall   cc◎ HCC RxHCC CC/MCC Exc

    Subsequent acute transmural myocardial infarction of anterior wall

    Subsequent transmural (Q wave) infarction (acute)(of) anterior (wall) NOS

    Subsequent anteroapical transmural (Q wave) infarction (acute)

    Subsequent anterolateral transmural (Q wave) infarction (acute)

    Subsequent anteroseptal transmural (Q wave) infarction (acute)

I22.1 **Subsequent** ST elevation **(STEMI) myocardial infarction of** inferior wall   cc◎ HCC RxHCC CC/MCC Exc

    AHA: Q4 2012

    Subsequent acute transmural myocardial infarction of inferior wall

    Subsequent transmural (Q wave) infarction (acute)(of) diaphragmatic wall

    Subsequent transmural (Q wave) infarction (acute)(of) inferior (wall) NOS

    Subsequent inferolateral transmural (Q wave) infarction (acute)

    Subsequent inferoposterior transmural (Q wave) infarction (acute)

I22.2 **Subsequent** non-ST elevation **(NSTEMI) myocardial infarction**   cc◎ HCC RxHCC CC/MCC Exc

    DEFINITION: An NSTEMI is a non-ST-elevation myocardial infarction caused by a severe narrowing of a coronary artery. The artery is not 100 percent blocked.

    Subsequent acute subendocardial myocardial infarction

    Subsequent non-Q wave myocardial infarction NOS

    Subsequent nontransmural myocardial infarction NOS

I22.8 **Subsequent** ST elevation **(STEMI) myocardial infarction of** other sites   cc◎ HCC RxHCC CC/MCC Exc

    Subsequent acute transmural myocardial infarction of other sites

    Subsequent apical-lateral transmural (Q wave) myocardial infarction (acute)

    Subsequent basal-lateral transmural (Q wave) myocardial infarction (acute)

    Subsequent high lateral transmural (Q wave) myocardial infarction (acute)

Subsequent transmural (Q wave) myocardial infarction (acute) (of) lateral (wall) NOS
Subsequent posterior (true) transmural (Q wave) myocardial infarction (acute)
Subsequent posterobasal transmural (Q wave) myocardial infarction (acute)
Subsequent posterolateral transmural (Q wave) myocardial infarction (acute)
Subsequent posteroseptal transmural (Q wave) myocardial infarction (acute)
Subsequent septal NOS transmural (Q wave) myocardial infarction (acute)

I22.9 **Subsequent ST elevation (STEMI) myocardial infarction of unspecified site** [CC] [HCC] [RxHCC] [CC/MCC Exc]
Subsequent acute myocardial infarction of unspecified site
Subsequent myocardial infarction (acute) NOS

[4th] I23 **Certain current complications following ST elevation (STEMI) and non-ST elevation (NSTEMI) myocardial infarction (within the 28 day period)**

I23.0 **Hemopericardium as current complication following acute myocardial infarction** [A] [CC] [HCC] [RxHCC]
[EXCLUDES1] *hemopericardium not specified as current complication following acute myocardial infarction (I31.2)*

I23.1 **Atrial septal defect as current complication following acute myocardial infarction** [A] [CC] [HCC] [RxHCC]
[EXCLUDES1] *acquired atrial septal defect not specified as current complication following acute myocardial infarction (I51.0)*

I23.2 **Ventricular septal defect as current complication following acute myocardial infarction** [A] [CC] [HCC] [RxHCC]
[EXCLUDES1] *acquired ventricular septal defect not specified as current complication following acute myocardial infarction (I51.0)*

I23.3 **Rupture of cardiac wall without hemopericardium as current complication following acute myocardial infarction** [A] [CC] [HCC] [RxHCC]
AHA: Q2 2017

I23.4 **Rupture of chordae tendineae as current complication following acute myocardial infarction** [HCC] [MCC] [RxHCC] [CC/MCC Exc]
[EXCLUDES1] *rupture of chordae tendineae not specified as current complication following acute myocardial infarction (I51.1)*

I23.5 **Rupture of papillary muscle as current complication following acute myocardial infarction** [HCC] [MCC] [RxHCC] [CC/MCC Exc]
[EXCLUDES1] *rupture of papillary muscle not specified as current complication following acute myocardial infarction (I51.2)*

I23.6 **Thrombosis of atrium, auricular appendage, and ventricle as current complications following acute myocardial infarction** [A] [CC] [HCC] [RxHCC]
[EXCLUDES1] *thrombosis of atrium, auricular appendage, and ventricle not specified as current complication following acute myocardial infarction (I51.3)*

I23.7 **Postinfarction angina** [A] [CC] [HCC] [RxHCC]
AHA: Q2 2015

I23.8 **Other current complications following acute myocardial infarction** [A] [CC] [HCC] [RxHCC]

[4th] I24 **Other acute ischemic heart diseases**
[EXCLUDES1] *angina pectoris (I20.-)*
transient myocardial ischemia in newborn (P29.4)

I24.0 **Acute coronary thrombosis not resulting in myocardial infarction** [CC] [HCC] [RxHCC] [CC/MCC Exc]
AHA: Q1 2013
Acute coronary (artery) (vein) embolism not resulting in myocardial infarction
Acute coronary (artery) (vein) occlusion not resulting in myocardial infarction
Acute coronary (artery) (vein) thromboembolism not resulting in myocardial infarction
[EXCLUDES1] *atherosclerotic heart disease (I25.1-)*

I24.1 **Dressler's syndrome** [CC] [HCC] [RxHCC] [CC/MCC Exc]
Postmyocardial infarction syndrome
[EXCLUDES1] *postinfarction angina (I23.7)*

I24.8 **Other forms of acute ischemic heart disease** [CC] [HCC] [RxHCC] [CC/MCC Exc]
👁 **See Official Guidelines** "Other Types of Myocardial Infarctions" I.C.9.e.5
AHA: Q4 2017
[EXCLUDES1] *myocardial infarction due to demand ischemia (I21.A1)*

I24.9 **Acute ischemic heart disease, unspecified** [CC] [HCC] [RxHCC] [CC/MCC Exc]
[EXCLUDES1] *ischemic heart disease (chronic) NOS (I25.9)*

[4th] I25 **Chronic ischemic heart disease**
Use additional code to identify:
chronic total occlusion of coronary artery (I25.82)
exposure to environmental tobacco smoke (Z77.22)
history of tobacco dependence (Z87.891)
occupational exposure to environmental tobacco smoke (Z57.31)
tobacco dependence (F17.-)
tobacco use (Z72.0)

[5th] I25.1 **Atherosclerotic heart disease of native coronary artery**
Atherosclerotic cardiovascular disease
Coronary (artery) atheroma
Coronary (artery) atherosclerosis
Coronary (artery) disease
Coronary (artery) sclerosis
Use additional code, if applicable, to identify:
coronary atherosclerosis due to calcified coronary lesion (I25.84)
coronary atherosclerosis due to lipid rich plaque (I25.83)
[EXCLUDES2] *atheroembolism (I75.-)*
atherosclerosis of coronary artery bypass graft(s) and transplanted heart (I25.7-)

I25.10 **Atherosclerotic heart disease of native coronary artery without angina pectoris** [A] [RxHCC]
AHA: Q2 2015
Atherosclerotic heart disease NOS

[6th] I25.11 **Atherosclerotic heart disease of native coronary artery with angina pectoris**
👁 **See Official Guidelines** "Atherosclerotic Coronary Artery Disease and Angina" I.C.9.b

I25.110 **Atherosclerotic heart disease of native coronary artery with unstable angina pectoris** [A] [CC] [HCC] [RxHCC] [CC/MCC Exc]
[EXCLUDES1] *unstable angina without atherosclerotic heart disease (I20.0)*

I25.111 **Atherosclerotic heart disease of native coronary artery with angina pectoris with documented spasm** [A] [HCC] [RxHCC]
[EXCLUDES1] *angina pectoris with documented spasm without atherosclerotic heart disease (I20.1)*

I25.118 **Atherosclerotic heart disease of native coronary artery with other forms of angina pectoris** [A] [HCC] [RxHCC]
AHA: Q2 2015
[EXCLUDES1] *other forms of angina pectoris without atherosclerotic heart disease (I20.8)*

I25.119 **Atherosclerotic heart disease of native coronary artery with unspecified angina pectoris** [A] [HCC] [RxHCC]
Atherosclerotic heart disease with angina NOS
Atherosclerotic heart disease with ischemic chest pain
[EXCLUDES1] *unspecified angina pectoris without atherosclerotic heart disease (I20.9)*

I25.2 **Old myocardial infarction** [POA] [RxHCC]
Healed myocardial infarction
Past myocardial infarction diagnosed by ECG or other investigation, but currently presenting no symptoms

I25.3 **Aneurysm of heart** [CC] [RxHCC] [CC/MCC Exc]
Mural aneurysm
Ventricular aneurysm

Unspecified Code Other Specified Code Manifestation Code [N] Newborn [P] Pediatric [M] Maternity [A] Adult ♂ Male ♀ Female
● New Code ▲ Revised Code Title ►◄ Revised Text [NOTES] [INCLUDES] [EXCLUDES1] Not coded here [EXCLUDES2] Not included here
[4th] 4th character required [5th] 5th character required [6th] 6th character required [7th] 7th character required [X] Extension 'X' Alert
[HAC] Hospital-acquired condition (HAC) alert AHA AHA Coding Clinic© Code first alert

I25.4 Coronary artery aneurysm **and dissection**
  I25.41 **Coronary artery** aneurysm `RxHCC`
    Coronary arteriovenous fistula, acquired
    EXCLUDES1 congenital coronary (artery) aneurysm (Q24.5)
  I25.42 **Coronary artery** dissection `MCC` `RxHCC` `CC/MCC Exc`
I25.5 **Ischemic** cardiomyopathy `RxHCC`
  EXCLUDES2 coronary atherosclerosis (I25.1-, I25.7-)
I25.6 Silent myocardial **ischemia** `RxHCC`
I25.7 **Atherosclerosis of** coronary artery bypass graft(s) **and coronary artery of** transplanted heart with angina pectoris
    👁 **See Official Guidelines** "Atherosclerotic Coronary Artery Disease and Angina" I.C.9.b
    Use additional code, if applicable, to identify:
    coronary atherosclerosis due to calcified coronary lesion (I25.84)
    coronary atherosclerosis due to lipid rich plaque (I25.83)
    EXCLUDES1 atherosclerosis of bypass graft(s) of transplanted heart without angina pectoris (I25.812)
    atherosclerosis of coronary artery bypass graft(s) without angina pectoris (I25.810)
    atherosclerosis of native coronary artery of transplanted heart without angina pectoris (I25.811)
  I25.70 **Atherosclerosis of coronary artery bypass graft(s),** unspecified, **with angina pectoris**
    I25.700 **Atherosclerosis of coronary artery bypass graft(s), unspecified, with** unstable angina **pectoris** `A` `cc` `HCC` `RxHCC` `CC/MCC Exc`
      EXCLUDES1 unstable angina pectoris without atherosclerosis of coronary artery bypass graft (I20.0)
    I25.701 **Atherosclerosis of coronary artery bypass graft(s), unspecified, with angina pectoris with** documented spasm `A` `HCC` `RxHCC`
      EXCLUDES1 angina pectoris with documented spasm without atherosclerosis of coronary artery bypass graft (I20.1)
    I25.708 **Atherosclerosis of coronary artery bypass graft(s), unspecified, with** other forms of angina **pectoris** `A` `HCC` `RxHCC`
      EXCLUDES1 other forms of angina pectoris without atherosclerosis of coronary artery bypass graft (I20.8)
    I25.709 **Atherosclerosis of coronary artery bypass graft(s), unspecified, with unspecified angina pectoris** `A` `HCC` `RxHCC`
      EXCLUDES1 unspecified angina pectoris without atherosclerosis of coronary artery bypass graft (I20.9)
  I25.71 **Atherosclerosis of** autologous vein **coronary artery bypass graft(s)** with angina pectoris
    I25.710 **Atherosclerosis of autologous vein coronary artery bypass graft(s) with** unstable angina **pectoris** `A` `cc` `HCC` `RxHCC` `CC/MCC Exc`
      EXCLUDES1 unstable angina without atherosclerosis of autologous vein coronary artery bypass graft(s) (I20.0)
      EXCLUDES2 embolism or thrombus of coronary artery bypass graft(s) (T82.8-)
    I25.711 **Atherosclerosis of autologous vein coronary artery bypass graft(s) with angina pectoris with** documented spasm `A` `cc` `HCC` `RxHCC` `CC/MCC Exc`
      EXCLUDES1 angina pectoris with documented spasm without atherosclerosis of autologous vein coronary artery bypass graft(s) (I20.1)

    I25.718 **Atherosclerosis of autologous vein coronary artery bypass graft(s) with** other forms of angina **pectoris** `A` `cc` `HCC` `RxHCC` `CC/MCC Exc`
      EXCLUDES1 other forms of angina pectoris without atherosclerosis of autologous vein coronary artery bypass graft(s) (I20.8)
    I25.719 **Atherosclerosis of autologous vein coronary artery bypass graft(s) with unspecified angina pectoris** `A` `cc` `HCC` `RxHCC` `CC/MCC Exc`
      EXCLUDES1 unspecified angina pectoris without atherosclerosis of autologous vein coronary artery bypass graft(s) (I20.9)
  I25.72 **Atherosclerosis of** autologous artery **coronary artery bypass graft(s) with angina pectoris**
    Atherosclerosis of internal mammary artery graft with angina pectoris
    I25.720 **Atherosclerosis of autologous artery coronary artery bypass graft(s) with** unstable angina **pectoris** `A` `cc` `HCC` `RxHCC` `CC/MCC Exc`
      EXCLUDES1 unstable angina without atherosclerosis of autologous artery coronary artery bypass graft(s) (I20.0)
    I25.721 **Atherosclerosis of autologous artery coronary artery bypass graft(s) with angina pectoris with** documented spasm `A` `cc` `HCC` `RxHCC` `CC/MCC Exc`
      EXCLUDES1 angina pectoris with documented spasm without atherosclerosis of autologous artery coronary artery bypass graft(s) (I20.1)
    I25.728 **Atherosclerosis of autologous artery coronary artery bypass graft(s) with** other forms of angina **pectoris** `A` `cc` `HCC` `RxHCC` `CC/MCC Exc`
      EXCLUDES1 other forms of angina pectoris without atherosclerosis of autologous artery coronary artery bypass graft(s) (I20.8)
    I25.729 **Atherosclerosis of autologous artery coronary artery bypass graft(s) with unspecified angina pectoris** `A` `cc` `HCC` `RxHCC` `CC/MCC Exc`
      EXCLUDES1 unspecified angina pectoris without atherosclerosis of autologous artery coronary artery bypass graft(s) (I20.9)
  I25.73 **Atherosclerosis of** nonautologous biological **coronary artery bypass graft(s)** with angina pectoris
    I25.730 **Atherosclerosis of nonautologous biological coronary artery bypass graft(s) with** unstable angina **pectoris** `A` `cc` `HCC` `RxHCC` `CC/MCC Exc`
      EXCLUDES1 unstable angina without atherosclerosis of nonautologous biological coronary artery bypass graft(s) (I20.0)
    I25.731 **Atherosclerosis of nonautologous biological coronary artery bypass graft(s) with angina pectoris with** documented spasm `A` `cc` `HCC` `RxHCC` `CC/MCC Exc`
      EXCLUDES1 angina pectoris with documented spasm without atherosclerosis of nonautologous biological coronary artery bypass graft(s) (I20.1)
    I25.738 **Atherosclerosis of nonautologous biological coronary artery bypass graft(s) with** other forms of angina **pectoris** `A` `cc` `HCC` `RxHCC` `CC/MCC Exc`

EXCLUDES1 *other forms of angina pectoris without atherosclerosis of nonautologous biological coronary artery bypass graft(s) (I20.8)*

I25.739 **Atherosclerosis of nonautologous biological coronary artery bypass graft(s) with unspecified angina pectoris** A cc HCC RxHCC CC/MCC Exc

EXCLUDES1 *unspecified angina pectoris without atherosclerosis of nonautologous biological coronary artery bypass graft(s) (I20.9)*

I25.75 **Atherosclerosis of** native coronary artery **of** transplanted heart with angina pectoris

EXCLUDES1 *atherosclerosis of native coronary artery of transplanted heart without angina pectoris (I25.811)*

I25.750 **Atherosclerosis of native coronary artery of transplanted heart with** unstable angina cc HCC RxHCC CC/MCC Exc

I25.751 **Atherosclerosis of native coronary artery of transplanted heart with angina pectoris with** documented spasm cc HCC RxHCC CC/MCC Exc

I25.758 **Atherosclerosis of native coronary artery of transplanted heart with** other forms of angina **pectoris** cc HCC RxHCC CC/MCC Exc

I25.759 **Atherosclerosis of native coronary artery of transplanted heart with unspecified angina pectoris** cc HCC RxHCC CC/MCC Exc

I25.76 **Atherosclerosis of** bypass graft **of coronary artery of** transplanted heart with angina pectoris

EXCLUDES1 *atherosclerosis of bypass graft of coronary artery of transplanted heart without angina pectoris (I25.812)*

I25.760 **Atherosclerosis of bypass graft of coronary artery of transplanted heart with** unstable angina A cc HCC RxHCC CC/MCC Exc

I25.761 **Atherosclerosis of bypass graft of coronary artery of transplanted heart with angina pectoris with** documented spasm A cc HCC RxHCC CC/MCC Exc

I25.768 **Atherosclerosis of bypass graft of coronary artery of transplanted heart with** other forms of angina **pectoris** A cc HCC RxHCC CC/MCC Exc

I25.769 **Atherosclerosis of bypass graft of coronary artery of transplanted heart with unspecified angina pectoris** A cc HCC RxHCC CC/MCC Exc

I25.79 **Atherosclerosis of** other coronary artery **bypass graft(s)** with angina pectoris

I25.790 **Atherosclerosis of other coronary artery bypass graft(s) with** unstable angina **pectoris** A cc HCC RxHCC CC/MCC Exc

EXCLUDES1 *unstable angina without atherosclerosis of other coronary artery bypass graft(s) (I20.0)*

I25.791 **Atherosclerosis of other coronary artery bypass graft(s) with angina pectoris with** documented spasm A cc HCC RxHCC

EXCLUDES1 *angina pectoris with documented spasm without atherosclerosis of other coronary artery bypass graft(s) (I20.1)*

I25.798 **Atherosclerosis of other coronary artery bypass graft(s) with** other forms of angina **pectoris** A cc HCC RxHCC

EXCLUDES1 *other forms of angina pectoris without atherosclerosis of other coronary artery bypass graft(s) (I20.8)*

I25.799 **Atherosclerosis of other coronary artery bypass graft(s) with unspecified angina pectoris** A cc HCC RxHCC

EXCLUDES1 *unspecified angina pectoris without atherosclerosis of other coronary artery bypass graft(s) (I20.9)*

I25.8 **Other forms** of chronic ischemic heart disease

I25.81 **Atherosclerosis of other coronary vessels** without angina pectoris

Use additional code, if applicable, to identify:
coronary atherosclerosis due to calcified coronary lesion (I25.84)
coronary atherosclerosis due to lipid rich plaque (I25.83)

EXCLUDES2 *atherosclerotic heart disease of native coronary artery without angina pectoris (I25.10)*

I25.810 **Atherosclerosis of** coronary artery bypass graft(s) **without angina pectoris** A cc RxHCC
AHA: Q4 2016
Atherosclerosis of coronary artery bypass graft NOS

EXCLUDES1 *atherosclerosis of coronary bypass graft(s) with angina pectoris (I25.70-I25.73-, I25.79-)*

I25.811 **Atherosclerosis of** native coronary artery of transplanted heart **without angina pectoris** cc RxHCC CC/MCC Exc
Atherosclerosis of native coronary artery of transplanted heart NOS

EXCLUDES1 *atherosclerosis of native coronary artery of transplanted heart with angina pectoris (I25.75-)*

I25.812 **Atherosclerosis of** bypass graft of coronary artery of transplanted heart **without angina pectoris** A cc RxHCC CC/MCC Exc
Atherosclerosis of bypass graft of transplanted heart NOS

EXCLUDES1 *atherosclerosis of bypass graft of transplanted heart with angina pectoris (I25.76)*

I25.82 **Chronic total occlusion** of coronary artery RxHCC PDxIn
AHA: Q3 2018
Complete occlusion of coronary artery
Total occlusion of coronary artery
☛ **Code first** coronary atherosclerosis (I25.1-, I25.7-, I25.81-)

EXCLUDES1 *acute coronary occlusion with myocardial infarction (I21.0-I21.9, I22.-)*
acute coronary occlusion without myocardial infarction (I24.0)

I25.83 **Coronary atherosclerosis** due to lipid rich plaque A RxHCC PDxIn
☛ **Code first** coronary atherosclerosis (I25.1-, I25.7-, I25.81-)

I25.84 **Coronary atherosclerosis** due to calcified coronary lesion RxHCC PDxIn
Coronary atherosclerosis due to severely calcified coronary lesion
☛ **Code first** coronary atherosclerosis (I25.1-, I25.7-, I25.81-)

I25.89 **Other forms of chronic ischemic heart disease** RxHCC

I25.9 **Chronic ischemic heart disease, unspecified** RxHCC
Ischemic heart disease (chronic) NOS

Unspecified Code   Other Specified Code   Manifestation Code   N Newborn   P Pediatric   M Maternity   A Adult   ♂ Male   ♀ Female
● New Code   ▲ Revised Code Title   ▶◀ Revised Text   NOTES   INCLUDES   EXCLUDES1 Not coded here   EXCLUDES2 Not included here
4th character required   5th character required   6th character required   7th character required   Extension 'X' Alert
HAC Hospital-acquired condition (HAC) alert   AHA AHA Coding Clinic©   ☛ Code first alert

2020 ICD-10-CM   When symbols appear on a code that requires a 7th character extension, refer to Appendix B to identify applicable 7th character codes.   **661**

Pulmonary heart disease and diseases of pulmonary circulation (I26-I28)

I26 Pulmonary embolism
- INCLUDES pulmonary (acute) (artery)(vein) infarction
  - pulmonary (acute) (artery)(vein) thromboembolism
  - pulmonary (acute) (artery)(vein) thrombosis
- EXCLUDES2 chronic pulmonary embolism (I27.82)
  - personal history of pulmonary embolism (Z86.711)
  - pulmonary embolism complicating abortion, ectopic or molar pregnancy (O00-O07, O08.2)
  - pulmonary embolism complicating pregnancy, childbirth and the puerperium (O88.-)
  - pulmonary embolism due to trauma (T79.0, T79.1)
  - pulmonary embolism due to complications of surgical and medical care (T80.0, T81.7-, T82.8-)
  - septic (non-pulmonary) arterial embolism (I76)

I26.0 Pulmonary embolism with acute cor pulmonale
- **I26.01 Septic pulmonary embolism with acute cor pulmonale** HCC MCC RxHCC PDxIn CC/MCC Exc
  - 🖝 Code first underlying infection
- **I26.02 Saddle embolus of pulmonary artery with acute cor pulmonale** HAC HCC MCC RxHCC CC/MCC Exc
- **I26.09 Other pulmonary embolism with acute cor pulmonale** HAC HCC MCC RxHCC CC/MCC Exc
  - Acute cor pulmonale NOS

I26.9 Pulmonary embolism without acute cor pulmonale
- **I26.90 Septic pulmonary embolism without acute cor pulmonale** HCC MCC RxHCC PDxIn CC/MCC Exc
  - 🖝 Code first underlying infection
- **I26.92 Saddle embolus of pulmonary artery without acute cor pulmonale** HAC HCC MCC RxHCC CC/MCC Exc
- **I26.93 Single subsegmental pulmonary embolism without acute cor pulmonale** MCC CC/MCC Exc
  - Subsegmental pulmonary embolism NOS
- **I26.94 Multiple subsegmental pulmonary emboli without acute cor pulmonale** MCC CC/MCC Exc
- **I26.99 Other pulmonary embolism without acute cor pulmonale** HAC HCC MCC RxHCC CC/MCC Exc
  - AHA: Q2 2019
  - Acute pulmonary embolism NOS
  - Pulmonary embolism NOS

I27 Other pulmonary heart diseases
- 👁 See Official Guidelines "Pulmonary Hypertension" I.C.9.a.11
- **I27.0 Primary pulmonary hypertension** CC HCC RxHCC CC/MCC Exc
  - DEFINITION: Pulmonary hypertension is a type of high blood pressure that affects the arteries of the lungs and the right side of the heart. The right ventricle must work harder to pump blood through the lungs.
  - TIP: Symptoms of pulmonary hypertension include shortness of breath, fatigue, fainting spells, chest pain or pressure, edema, cyanosis of the lips and/or skin, racing pulse, and palpitations.
  - Heritable pulmonary arterial hypertension
  - Idiopathic pulmonary arterial hypertension
  - Primary group 1 pulmonary hypertension
  - Primary pulmonary arterial hypertension
  - EXCLUDES1 persistent pulmonary hypertension of newborn (P29.30)
    - pulmonary hypertension NOS (I27.20)
    - secondary pulmonary arterial hypertension (I27.21)
    - secondary pulmonary hypertension (I27.29)
- **I27.1 Kyphoscoliotic heart disease** CC HCC RxHCC CC/MCC Exc
  - AHA: Q4 2018, Q4 2017
- **I27.2 Other secondary pulmonary hypertension**
  - Code also associated underlying condition
  - EXCLUDES1 Eisenmenger's syndrome (I27.83)
  - **I27.20 Pulmonary hypertension, unspecified** HCC RxHCC
    - Pulmonary hypertension NOS

I27.21 Secondary pulmonary arterial hypertension HCC RxHCC
- (Associated) (drug-induced) (toxin-induced) pulmonary arterial hypertension NOS
- (Associated) (drug-induced) (toxin-induced) (secondary) group 1 pulmonary hypertension
- Code also associated conditions if applicable, or adverse effects of drugs or toxins, such as:
  - adverse effect of appetite depressants (T50.5X5)
  - congenital heart disease (Q20-Q28)
  - human immunodeficiency virus [HIV] disease (B20)
  - polymyositis (M33.2-)
  - portal hypertension (K76.6)
  - rheumatoid arthritis (M05.-)
  - schistosomiasis (B65.-)
  - Sjögren syndrome (M35.0-)
  - systemic sclerosis (M34.-)

I27.22 Pulmonary hypertension due to left heart disease HCC RxHCC
- Group 2 pulmonary hypertension
- Code also associated left heart disease, if known, such as:
  - multiple valve disease (I08.-)
  - rheumatic mitral valve diseases (I05.-)
  - rheumatic aortic valve diseases (I06.-)

I27.23 Pulmonary hypertension due to lung diseases and hypoxia HCC RxHCC
- Group 3 pulmonary hypertension
- Code also associated lung disease, if known, such as:
  - bronchiectasis (J47.-)
  - cystic fibrosis with pulmonary manifestations (E84.0)
  - interstitial lung disease (J84.-)
  - pleural effusion (J90)
  - sleep apnea (G47.3-)

I27.24 Chronic thromboembolic pulmonary hypertension HCC RxHCC
- Group 4 pulmonary hypertension
- Code also associated pulmonary embolism, if applicable (I26.-, I27.82)

I27.29 Other secondary pulmonary hypertension HCC RxHCC
- Group 5 pulmonary hypertension
- Pulmonary hypertension with unclear multifactorial mechanisms
- Pulmonary hypertension due to hematologic disorders
- Pulmonary hypertension due to metabolic disorders
- Pulmonary hypertension due to other systemic disorders
- Code also other associated disorders, if known, such as:
  - chronic myeloid leukemia (C92.10- C92.22)
  - essential thrombocythemia (D47.3)
  - Gaucher disease (E75.22)
  - hypertensive chronic kidney disease with end stage renal disease (I12.0, I13.11, I13.2)
  - hyperthyroidism (E05.-)
  - hypothyroidism (E00-E03)
  - polycythemia vera (D45)
  - sarcoidosis (D86.-)

I27.8 Other specified pulmonary heart diseases
- **I27.81 Cor pulmonale (chronic)** CC HCC RxHCC CC/MCC Exc
  - Cor pulmonale NOS
  - EXCLUDES1 acute cor pulmonale (I26.0-)
- **I27.82 Chronic pulmonary embolism** CC HCC RxHCC CC/MCC Exc
  - Use additional code, if applicable, for associated long-term (current) use of anticoagulants (Z79.01)
  - EXCLUDES1 personal history of pulmonary embolism (Z86.711)
- **I27.83 Eisenmenger's syndrome** HCC RxHCC
  - Eisenmenger's complex
  - (Irreversible) Eisenmenger's disease

PDxIn Unacceptable principal diagnosis symbol per Medicare code edits   POA Code exempt from diagnosis present on admission requirement
❓ Questionable admission   CC Complication or comorbidity   MCC Major complication or comorbidity   CC/MCC CC/MCC exclusion
HCC HCC diagnosis code   RxHCC RxHCC diagnosis code   MACRA code   DEFINITION Describes condition/terminology
TIP Coding guidance   👁 Official Guideline Reference   Z1 Z code as first-listed diagnosis

662   When symbols appear on a code that requires a 7th character extension, refer to Appendix B to identify applicable 7th character codes.   2020 ICD-10-CM

Pulmonary hypertension with right to left shunt related to congenital heart disease

Code also underlying heart defect, if known, such as:
atrial septal defect (Q21.1)
Eisenmenger's defect (Q21.8)
patent ductus arteriosus (Q25.0)
ventricular septal defect (Q21.0)

I27.89 **Other specified pulmonary heart diseases** `HCC` `RxHCC`

I27.9 **Pulmonary heart disease, unspecified** `HCC` `RxHCC`
Chronic cardiopulmonary disease

4ᵗʰ **I28 Other diseases of pulmonary vessels**

I28.0 **Arteriovenous fistula of pulmonary vessels** `cc` `HCC` `RxHCC` `CC/MCC Exc`
EXCLUDES1 congenital arteriovenous fistula (Q25.72)

I28.1 **Aneurysm of pulmonary artery** `cc` `HCC` `RxHCC` `CC/MCC Exc`
EXCLUDES1 congenital aneurysm (Q25.79)
congenital arteriovenous aneurysm (Q25.72)

I28.8 **Other diseases of pulmonary vessels** `HCC` `RxHCC`
Pulmonary arteritis
Pulmonary endarteritis
Rupture of pulmonary vessels
Stenosis of pulmonary vessels
Stricture of pulmonary vessels

I28.9 **Disease of pulmonary vessels, unspecified** `HCC` `RxHCC`

Other forms of heart disease (I30-I52)

4ᵗʰ **I30 Acute pericarditis**
INCLUDES acute mediastinopericarditis
acute myopericarditis
acute pericardial effusion
acute pleuropericarditis
acute pneumopericarditis
EXCLUDES1 Dressler's syndrome (I24.1)
rheumatic pericarditis (acute) (I01.0)
viral pericarditis due to Coxsakie virus (B33.23)

I30.0 **Acute nonspecific idiopathic pericarditis** `cc` `CC/MCC Exc`

I30.1 **Infective pericarditis** `cc` `CC/MCC Exc`
Pneumococcal pericarditis
Pneumopyopericardium
Purulent pericarditis
Pyopericarditis
Pyopericardium
Pyopneumopericardium
Staphylococcal pericarditis
Streptococcal pericarditis
Suppurative pericarditis
Viral pericarditis
Use additional code (B95-B97) to identify infectious agent

I30.8 **Other forms of acute pericarditis** `cc` `CC/MCC Exc`

I30.9 **Acute pericarditis, unspecified** `cc` `CC/MCC Exc`

4ᵗʰ **I31 Other diseases of pericardium**
EXCLUDES1 diseases of pericardium specified as rheumatic (I09.2)
postcardiotomy syndrome (I97.0)
traumatic injury to pericardium (S26.-)

I31.0 **Chronic adhesive pericarditis** `cc` `CC/MCC Exc`
Accretio cordis
Adherent pericardium
Adhesive mediastinopericarditis

I31.1 **Chronic constrictive pericarditis** `cc` `CC/MCC Exc`
Concretio cordis
Pericardial calcification

I31.2 **Hemopericardium, not elsewhere classified** `cc` `CC/MCC Exc`
EXCLUDES1 hemopericardium as current complication following acute myocardial infarction (I23.0)

I31.3 **Pericardial effusion (noninflammatory)** `cc` `CC/MCC Exc`
AHA: Q1 2019
Chylopericardium
EXCLUDES1 acute pericardial effusion (I30.9)

I31.4 **Cardiac tamponade** `cc` `PDxIn` `CC/MCC Exc`
DEFINITION: Cardiac tamponade occurs with compression on the heart from an increase in pericardial fluid or blood. The increased pressure can lead to cardiac arrest if not treated.
☞ **Code first** underlying cause

I31.8 **Other specified diseases of pericardium** `cc` `CC/MCC Exc`
Epicardial plaques
Focal pericardial adhesions

I31.9 **Disease of pericardium, unspecified** `cc` `CC/MCC Exc`
Pericarditis (chronic) NOS

I32 Pericarditis in diseases classified elsewhere `cc` `CC/MCC Exc`
☞ **Code first** underlying disease
EXCLUDES1 pericarditis (in):
coxsackie (virus) (B33.23)
gonococcal (A54.83)
meningococcal (A39.53)
rheumatoid (arthritis) (M05.31)
syphilitic (A52.06)
systemic lupus erythematosus (M32.12)
tuberculosis (A18.84)

4ᵗʰ **I33 Acute and subacute endocarditis**
EXCLUDES1 acute rheumatic endocarditis (I01.1)
endocarditis NOS (I38)

I33.0 **Acute and subacute infective endocarditis** `MCC` `CC/MCC Exc`
Bacterial endocarditis (acute) (subacute)
Infective endocarditis (acute) (subacute) NOS
Endocarditis lenta (acute) (subacute)
Malignant endocarditis (acute) (subacute)
Purulent endocarditis (acute) (subacute)
Septic endocarditis (acute) (subacute)
Ulcerative endocarditis (acute) (subacute)
Vegetative endocarditis (acute) (subacute)
Use additional code (B95-B97) to identify infectious agent

I33.9 **Acute and subacute endocarditis, unspecified** `MCC` `CC/MCC Exc`
Acute endocarditis NOS
Acute myoendocarditis NOS
Acute periendocarditis NOS
Subacute endocarditis NOS
Subacute myoendocarditis NOS
Subacute periendocarditis NOS

4ᵗʰ **I34 Nonrheumatic mitral valve disorders**
EXCLUDES1 mitral valve disease (I05.9)
mitral valve failure (I05.8)
mitral valve stenosis (I05.0)
mitral valve disorder of unspecified cause with diseases of aortic and/or tricuspid valve(s) (I08.-)
mitral valve disorder of unspecified cause with mitral stenosis or obstruction (I05.0)
mitral valve disorder specified as congenital (Q23.2, Q23.9)
mitral valve disorder specified as rheumatic (I05.-)

I34.0 **Nonrheumatic mitral (valve) insufficiency**
Nonrheumatic mitral (valve) incompetence NOS
Nonrheumatic mitral (valve) regurgitation NOS

I34.1 **Nonrheumatic mitral (valve) prolapse**
Floppy nonrheumatic mitral valve syndrome
EXCLUDES1 Marfan's syndrome (Q87.4-)

I34.2 **Nonrheumatic mitral (valve) stenosis**

I34.8 **Other nonrheumatic mitral valve disorders**

I34.9 **Nonrheumatic mitral valve disorder, unspecified**

4ᵗʰ **I35 Nonrheumatic aortic valve disorders**
EXCLUDES1 aortic valve disorder of unspecified cause but with diseases of mitral and/or tricuspid valve(s) (I08.-)
aortic valve disorder specified as congenital (Q23.0, Q23.1)
aortic valve disorder specified as rheumatic (I06.-)
hypertrophic subaortic stenosis (I42.1)

I35.0 **Nonrheumatic aortic (valve) stenosis**

Unspecified Code Other Specified Code Manifestation Code Ⓝ Newborn Ⓟ Pediatric Ⓜ Maternity Ⓐ Adult ♂ Male ♀ Female
● New Code ▲ Revised Code Title ▶◀ Revised Text **NOTES** *INCLUDES* *EXCLUDES1* Not coded here *EXCLUDES2* Not included here
4ᵗʰ 4ᵗʰ character required 5ᵗʰ 5ᵗʰ character required 6ᵗʰ 6ᵗʰ character required 7ᵗʰ 7ᵗʰ character required Ⓧ Extension 'X' Alert
HAC Hospital-acquired condition (HAC) alert **AHA** AHA Coding Clinic© ☞ Code first alert

I35.1 **Nonrheumatic aortic (valve)** insufficiency
Nonrheumatic aortic (valve) incompetence NOS
Nonrheumatic aortic (valve) regurgitation NOS

I35.2 **Nonrheumatic aortic (valve)** stenosis with insufficiency

I35.8 **Other nonrheumatic aortic valve disorders**

I35.9 **Nonrheumatic aortic valve disorder, unspecified**

I36 **Nonrheumatic** tricuspid valve **disorders**

   EXCLUDES1 *tricuspid valve disorders of unspecified cause (I07.-)*

     tricuspid valve disorders specified as congenital (Q22.4, Q22.8, Q22.9)

     tricuspid valve disorders specified as rheumatic (I07.-)

     tricuspid valve disorders with aortic and/or mitral valve involvement (I08.-)

I36.0 **Nonrheumatic tricuspid (valve)** stenosis

I36.1 **Nonrheumatic tricuspid (valve)** insufficiency
Nonrheumatic tricuspid (valve) incompetence
Nonrheumatic tricuspid (valve) regurgitation

I36.2 **Nonrheumatic tricuspid (valve)** stenosis with insufficiency

I36.8 **Other nonrheumatic tricuspid valve disorders**

I36.9 **Nonrheumatic tricuspid valve disorder, unspecified**

I37 **Nonrheumatic** pulmonary valve **disorders**

   EXCLUDES1 *pulmonary valve disorder specified as congenital (Q22.1, Q22.2, Q22.3)*

     pulmonary valve disorder specified as rheumatic (I09.89)

I37.0 **Nonrheumatic pulmonary valve** stenosis

I37.1 **Nonrheumatic pulmonary valve** insufficiency
Nonrheumatic pulmonary valve incompetence
Nonrheumatic pulmonary valve regurgitation

I37.2 **Nonrheumatic pulmonary valve** stenosis with insufficiency

I37.8 **Other nonrheumatic pulmonary valve disorders**

I37.9 **Nonrheumatic pulmonary valve disorder, unspecified**

I38 **Endocarditis, valve unspecified**

   INCLUDES *endocarditis (chronic) NOS*
     valvular incompetence NOS
     valvular insufficiency NOS
     valvular regurgitation NOS
     valvular stenosis NOS
     valvulitis (chronic) NOS

   EXCLUDES1 *congenital insufficiency of cardiac valve NOS (Q24.8)*
     congenital stenosis of cardiac valve NOS (Q24.8)
     endocardial fibroelastosis (I42.4)
     endocarditis specified as rheumatic (I09.1)

I39 **Endocarditis and heart valve disorders in diseases classified elsewhere**

  ☞ **Code first** underlying disease, such as:
    Q fever (A78)

   EXCLUDES1 *endocardial involvement in:*
     candidiasis (B37.6)
     gonococcal infection (A54.83)
     Libman-Sacks disease (M32.11)
     listerosis (A32.82)
     meningococcal infection (A39.51)
     rheumatoid arthritis (M05.31)
     syphilis (A52.03)
     tuberculosis (A18.84)
     typhoid fever (A01.02)

I40 **Acute** myocarditis

   INCLUDES *subacute myocarditis*

   EXCLUDES1 *acute rheumatic myocarditis (I01.2)*

I40.0 **Infective myocarditis**
Septic myocarditis
Use additional code (B95-B97) to identify infectious agent

I40.1 **Isolated myocarditis**
Fiedler's myocarditis
Giant cell myocarditis
Idiopathic myocarditis

I40.8 **Other acute myocarditis**

I40.9 **Acute myocarditis, unspecified**

I41 **Myocarditis in diseases classified elsewhere**

  ☞ **Code first** underlying disease, such as:
    typhus (A75.0-A75.9)

   EXCLUDES1 *myocarditis (in):*
     Chagas' disease (chronic) (B57.2)
     acute (B57.0)
     coxsackie (virus) infection (B33.22)
     diphtheritic (A36.81)
     gonococcal (A54.83)
     influenzal (J09.X9, J10.82, J11.82)
     meningococcal (A39.52)
     mumps (B26.82)
     rheumatoid arthritis (M05.31)
     sarcoid (D86.85)
     syphilis (A52.06)
     toxoplasmosis (B58.81)
     tuberculous (A18.84)

I42 **Cardiomyopathy** (Figure 9.2)

   INCLUDES *myocardiopathy*

  ☞ **Code first** pre-existing cardiomyopathy complicating pregnancy and puerperium (O99.4)

   EXCLUDES2 *ischemic cardiomyopathy (I25.5)*
     peripartum cardiomyopathy (O90.3)
     ventricular hypertrophy (I51.7)

I42.0 **Dilated cardiomyopathy**
Congestive cardiomyopathy

I42.1 **Obstructive hypertrophic cardiomyopathy**
Hypertrophic subaortic stenosis (idiopathic)

I42.2 **Other hypertrophic cardiomyopathy**
Nonobstructive hypertrophic cardiomyopathy

I42.3 **Endomyocardial (eosinophilic) disease**
Endomyocardial (tropical) fibrosis
Löffler's endocarditis

I42.4 **Endocardial fibroelastosis**
Congenital cardiomyopathy
Elastomyofibrosis

I42.5 **Other restrictive cardiomyopathy**
Constrictive cardiomyopathy NOS

I42.6 **Alcoholic cardiomyopathy**
Code also presence of alcoholism (F10.-)

I42.7 **Cardiomyopathy** due to drug and external agent
  ☞ **Code first** poisoning due to drug or toxin, if applicable (T36-T65 with fifth or sixth character 1-4 or 6)
    Use additional code for adverse effect, if applicable, to identify drug (T36-T50 with fifth or sixth character 5)

I42.8 **Other cardiomyopathies**

I42.9 **Cardiomyopathy, unspecified**
Cardiomyopathy (primary) (secondary) NOS

I43 **Cardiomyopathy in diseases classified elsewhere**

  ☞ **Code first** underlying disease, such as:
    amyloidosis (E85.-)
    glycogen storage disease (E74.0)
    gout (M10.0-)
    thyrotoxicosis (E05.0-E05.9-)

   EXCLUDES1 *cardiomyopathy (in):*
     coxsackie (virus) (B33.24)
     diphtheria (A36.81)
     sarcoidosis (D86.85)
     tuberculosis (A18.84)

PDxⁿ Unacceptable principal diagnosis symbol per Medicare code edits   ₚₒₐ Code exempt from diagnosis present on admission requirement
❓ Questionable admission   ℭℭ Complication or comorbidity   MCC Major complication or comorbidity   CC/MCC Exc CC/MCC exclusion
HCC HCC diagnosis code   RxHCC RxHCC diagnosis code   MACRA code   **DEFINITION** Describes condition/terminology
TIP Coding guidance   👁 Official Guideline Reference   Z1 Z code as first-listed diagnosis

664   When symbols appear on a code that requires a 7th character extension, refer to Appendix B to identify applicable 7th character codes.   **2020 ICD-10-CM**

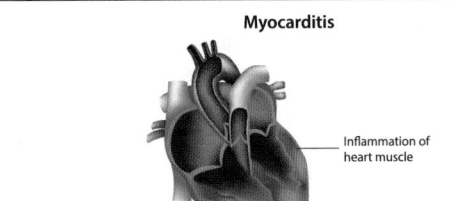

Myocarditis

Inflammation of heart muscle

Hypertrophic cardiomyopathy

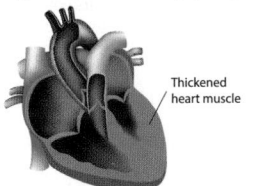

Thickened heart muscle

Dilated cardiomyopathy

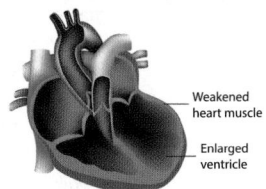

Weakened heart muscle

Enlarged ventricle

Figure 9.2 Myocarditis and Cardiomyopathy

I44 Atrioventricular **and** left bundle-branch block

I44.0 Atrioventricular block, first degree

I44.1 Atrioventricular block, second degree
Atrioventricular block, type I and II
Möbitz block, type I and II
Second degree block, type I and II
Wenckebach's block

I44.2 Atrioventricular block, complete
AHA: Q2 2019
Complete heart block NOS
Third degree block

I44.3 Other and unspecified atrioventricular block
Atrioventricular block NOS
I44.30 Unspecified atrioventricular block
I44.39 Other atrioventricular block

I44.4 Left anterior fascicular block

I44.5 Left posterior fascicular block

I44.6 Other and unspecified fascicular block
I44.60 Unspecified fascicular block
Left bundle-branch hemiblock NOS
I44.69 Other fascicular block

I44.7 Left bundle-branch block, unspecified

I45 Other conduction disorders

I45.0 Right fascicular block

I45.1 Other and unspecified right bundle-branch block
I45.10 Unspecified right bundle-branch block
Right bundle-branch block NOS
I45.19 Other right bundle-branch block

I45.2 Bifascicular block

I45.3 Trifascicular block

I45.4 Nonspecific intraventricular block
Bundle-branch block NOS

I45.5 Other specified heart block
Sinoatrial block
Sinoauricular block
EXCLUDES1 heart block NOS (I45.9)

I45.6 Pre-excitation syndrome
Accelerated atrioventricular conduction
Accessory atrioventricular conduction
Anomalous atrioventricular excitation
Lown-Ganong-Levine syndrome
Pre-excitation atrioventricular conduction
Wolff-Parkinson-White syndrome

I45.8 Other specified conduction disorders
I45.81 Long QT syndrome
I45.89 Other specified conduction disorders
Atrioventricular [AV] dissociation
Interference dissociation
Isorhythmic dissociation
Nonparoxysmal AV nodal tachycardia

I45.9 Conduction disorder, unspecified
Heart block NOS
Stokes-Adams syndrome

I46 Cardiac arrest
EXCLUDES1 cardiogenic shock (R57.0)

I46.2 Cardiac arrest due to underlying cardiac condition HCC
☞ Code first underlying cardiac condition

I46.8 Cardiac arrest due to other underlying condition
☞ Code first underlying condition

I46.9 Cardiac arrest, cause unspecified HCC

I47 Paroxysmal tachycardia
☞ Code first tachycardia complicating:
abortion or ectopic or molar pregnancy (O00-O07, O08.8)
obstetric surgery and procedures (O75.4)
EXCLUDES1 tachycardia NOS (R00.0)
sinoauricular tachycardia NOS (R00.0)
sinus [sinusal] tachycardia NOS (R00.0)

I47.0 Re-entry ventricular arrhythmia HCC

I47.1 Supraventricular tachycardia HCC RxHCC
Atrial (paroxysmal) tachycardia
Atrioventricular [AV] (paroxysmal) tachycardia
Atrioventricular re-entrant (nodal) tachycardia [AVNRT] [AVRT]
Junctional (paroxysmal) tachycardia
Nodal (paroxysmal) tachycardia

I47.2 Ventricular tachycardia HCC
AHA: Q3 2013

I47.9 Paroxysmal tachycardia, unspecified HCC RxHCC
Bouveret (-Hoffman) syndrome

I48 Atrial fibrillation and flutter

I48.0 Paroxysmal atrial fibrillation HCC RxHCC
AHA: Q3 2018

I48.1 Persistent atrial fibrillation
EXCLUDES1 Permanent atrial fibrillation (I48.21)

I48.11 Longstanding persistent atrial fibrillation
I48.19 Other persistent atrial fibrillation
Chronic persistent atrial fibrillation
Persistent atrial fibrillation, NOS

I48.2 Chronic atrial fibrillation
I48.20 Chronic atrial fibrillation, unspecified
EXCLUDES1 Chronic persistent atrial fibrillation (I48.19)
I48.21 Permanent atrial fibrillation

I48.3 Typical atrial flutter HCC RxHCC
Type I atrial flutter

I48.4 Atypical atrial flutter HCC RxHCC
Type II atrial flutter

I48.9 Unspecified atrial fibrillation and atrial flutter
I48.91 Unspecified atrial fibrillation HCC RxHCC
I48.92 Unspecified atrial flutter HCC RxHCC

I49 Other cardiac arrhythmias
☞ Code first cardiac arrhythmia complicating:
abortion or ectopic or molar pregnancy (O00-O07, O08.8)
obstetric surgery and procedures (O75.4)
EXCLUDES1 neonatal dysrhythmia (P29.1-)
sinoatrial bradycardia (R00.1)
sinus bradycardia (R00.1)
vagal bradycardia (R00.1)
EXCLUDES2 bradycardia NOS (R00.1)

I49.0 Ventricular fibrillation and flutter
I49.01 Ventricular fibrillation HCC
I49.02 Ventricular flutter HCC

I49.1 Atrial premature depolarization
Atrial premature beats

I49.2 Junctional premature depolarization HCC RxHCC

I49.3 Ventricular premature depolarization

I49.4 Other and unspecified premature depolarization
I49.40 Unspecified premature depolarization
Premature beats NOS

I49.49   Other premature depolarization
Ectopic beats
Extrasystoles
Extrasystolic arrhythmias
Premature contractions

I49.5   Sick sinus syndrome   HCC
AHA: Q1 2019
Tachycardia-bradycardia syndrome

I49.8   Other specified cardiac arrhythmias
Brugada syndrome
Coronary sinus rhythm disorder
Ectopic rhythm disorder
Nodal rhythm disorder

I49.9   Cardiac arrhythmia, unspecified
Arrhythmia (cardiac) NOS

I50   Heart failure
☞ **Code first** heart failure complicating abortion or ectopic or molar
pregnancy (O00-O07, O08.8)
heart failure due to hypertension (I11.0)
heart failure due to hypertension with chronic kidney disease (I13.-)
heart failure following surgery (I97.13-)
obstetric surgery and procedures (O75.4)
rheumatic heart failure (I09.81)
EXCLUDES1 neonatal cardiac failure (P29.0)
EXCLUDES2 cardiac arrest (I46.-)

I50.1   Left ventricular failure, unspecified   cc HCC RxHCC CC/MCC Exc
Cardiac asthma
Edema of lung with heart disease NOS
Edema of lung with heart failure
Left heart failure
Pulmonary edema with heart disease NOS
Pulmonary edema with heart failure
EXCLUDES1 edema of lung without heart disease or heart failure
(J81.-)

pulmonary edema without heart disease or failure
(J81.-)

I50.2   Systolic (congestive) heart failure
Heart failure with reduced ejection fraction [HFrEF]
Systolic left ventricular heart failure
Code also end stage heart failure, if applicable (I50.84)
EXCLUDES1 combined systolic (congestive) and diastolic
(congestive) heart failure (I50.4-)

**I50.20   Unspecified systolic (congestive) heart
failure**   cc HCC RxHCC CC/MCC Exc
**I50.21   Acute systolic (congestive) heart
failure**   HCC MCC RxHCC CC/MCC Exc
I50.22   Chronic systolic (congestive) heart failure   HCC RxHCC
**I50.23   Acute on chronic systolic (congestive)
heart failure**   HCC MCC RxHCC CC/MCC Exc

I50.3   Diastolic (congestive) heart failure
Diastolic left ventricular heart failure
Heart failure with normal ejection fraction
Heart failure with preserved ejection fraction [HFpEF]
Code also end stage heart failure, if applicable (I50.84)
EXCLUDES1 combined systolic (congestive) and diastolic
(congestive) heart failure (I50.4-)

**I50.30   Unspecified diastolic (congestive) heart
failure**   cc HCC RxHCC CC/MCC Exc
**I50.31   Acute diastolic (congestive) heart
failure**   HCC MCC RxHCC CC/MCC Exc
AHA: Q1 2017
I50.32   Chronic diastolic (congestive) heart failure HCC RxHCC
**I50.33   Acute on chronic diastolic (congestive)
heart failure**   HCC MCC RxHCC CC/MCC Exc

I50.4   Combined systolic (congestive) and diastolic (congestive)
heart failure
Combined systolic and diastolic left ventricular heart failure
Heart failure with reduced ejection fraction and diastolic
dysfunction
Code also end stage heart failure, if applicable (I50.84)

**I50.40   Unspecified combined systolic (congestive) and
diastolic (congestive) heart failure**   cc HCC RxHCC CC/MCC Exc
**I50.41   Acute combined systolic (congestive) and diastolic
(congestive) heart failure**   HCC MCC RxHCC CC/MCC Exc

**I50.42   Chronic combined systolic (congestive) and diastolic
(congestive) heart failure**   HCC RxHCC
**I50.43   Acute on chronic combined systolic (congestive)
and diastolic (congestive) heart
failure**   HCC MCC RxHCC CC/MCC Exc

I50.8   Other heart failure
DEFINITION: A result of left heart failure marked by swelling in
ankles, legs, abdomen.

I50.81   Right heart failure
Right ventricular failure
I50.810   Right heart failure, unspecified   HCC RxHCC
Right heart failure without mention of left
heart failure
Right ventricular failure NOS
I50.811   Acute right heart failure   HCC RxHCC
Acute isolated right heart failure
Acute (isolated) right ventricular failure
I50.812   Chronic right heart failure   HCC RxHCC
Chronic isolated right heart failure
Chronic (isolated) right ventricular failure
I50.813   Acute on chronic right heart failure   HCC RxHCC
Acute on chronic isolated right heart failure
Acute on chronic (isolated) right ventricular
failure
Acute decompensation of chronic (isolated)
right ventricular failure
Acute exacerbation of chronic (isolated)
right ventricular failure
**I50.814   Right heart failure due to left heart
failure**   HCC RxHCC
Right ventricular failure secondary to left
ventricular failure
Code also the type of left ventricular failure,
if known (I50.2-I50.43)
EXCLUDES1 Right heart failure with but not
due to left heart failure (I50.82)
I50.82   Biventricular heart failure   HCC RxHCC
Code also the type of left ventricular failure as systolic,
diastolic, or combined, if known (I50.2-I50.43)
I50.83   High output heart failure   HCC RxHCC
I50.84   End stage heart failure   HCC RxHCC
Stage D heart failure
Code also the type of heart failure as systolic,
diastolic, or combined, if known (I50.2-I50.43)
I50.89   Other heart failure   HCC RxHCC

I50.9   Heart failure, unspecified   HCC RxHCC
AHA: Q1 2017, Q2 2015
Cardiac, heart or myocardial failure NOS
Congestive heart disease
Congestive heart failure NOS
EXCLUDES2 fluid overload ▶unrelated to congestive heart
failure◀ (E87.70)

I51   Complications and ill-defined descriptions of heart disease
EXCLUDES1 any condition in I51.4-I51.9 due to hypertension (I11.-)
any condition in I51.4-I51.9 due to hypertension and chronic
kidney disease (I13.-)
heart disease specified as rheumatic (I00-I09)

I51.0   Cardiac septal defect, acquired   A cc
Acquired septal atrial defect (old)
Acquired septal auricular defect (old)
Acquired septal ventricular defect (old)
EXCLUDES1 cardiac septal defect as current complication
following acute myocardial infarction (I23.1, I23.2)

**I51.1   Rupture of chordae tendineae, not elsewhere
classified**   cc HCC RxHCC CC/MCC Exc
EXCLUDES1 rupture of chordae tendineae as current
complication following acute myocardial
infarction (I23.4)

**I51.2   Rupture of papillary muscle, not elsewhere
classified**   cc HCC RxHCC CC/MCC Exc
EXCLUDES1 rupture of papillary muscle as current complication
following acute myocardial infarction (I23.5)

PDX Unacceptable principal diagnosis symbol per Medicare code edits   POA Code exempt from diagnosis present on admission requirement
? Questionable admission   cc Complication or comorbidity   MCC Major complication or comorbidity   CC/MCC Exc CC/MCC exclusion
HCC HCC diagnosis code   RxHCC RxHCC diagnosis code   MACRA code   **DEFINITION** Describes condition/terminology
TIP Coding guidance   👁 Official Guideline Reference   Z1 Z code as first-listed diagnosis

666   When symbols appear on a code that requires a 7th character extension, refer to Appendix B to identify applicable 7th character codes.   **2020 ICD-10-CM**

I51.3 **Intracardiac thrombosis, not elsewhere classified** cc̄ CC/MCC Exc
AHA: Q1 2013
Apical thrombosis (old)
Atrial thrombosis (old)
Auricular thrombosis (old)
Mural thrombosis (old)
Ventricular thrombosis (old)
EXCLUDES1 intracardiac thrombosis as current complication
following acute myocardial infarction (I23.6)

I51.4 **Myocarditis, unspecified** HCC RxHCC
👁 See Official Guidelines "Hypertension with Heart Disease"
I.C.9.a.1
AHA: Q2 2018, Q4 2018, Q4 2017, Q4 2016
Chronic (interstitial) myocarditis
Myocardial fibrosis
Myocarditis NOS
EXCLUDES1 acute or subacute myocarditis (I40.-)

I51.5 **Myocardial degeneration** HCC RxHCC
👁 See Official Guidelines "Hypertension with Heart Disease"
I.C.9.a.1
AHA: Q2 2018, Q4 2018, Q4 2017, Q4 2016
Fatty degeneration of heart or myocardium
Myocardial disease
Senile degeneration of heart or myocardium

I51.7 **Cardiomegaly**
👁 See Official Guidelines "Hypertension with Heart Disease"
I.C.9.a.1
AHA: Q2 2018, Q4 2018, Q4 2017, Q4 2016
Cardiac dilatation
Cardiac hypertrophy
Ventricular dilatation

5ᵗʰ **I51.8** **Other ill-defined heart diseases**
I51.81 **Takotsubo syndrome** cc̄ CC/MCC Exc
AHA: Q2 2018, Q4 2017, Q4 2016
Reversible left ventricular dysfunction following
sudden emotional stress
Stress induced cardiomyopathy
Takotsubo cardiomyopathy
Transient left ventricular apical ballooning syndrome
I51.89 **Other ill-defined heart diseases**
👁 See Official Guidelines "Hypertension with Heart
Disease" I.C.9.a.1
AHA: Q2 2019, Q2 2018, Q4 2018, Q4 2017, Q4 2016
Carditis (acute)(chronic)
Pancarditis (acute)(chronic)

I51.9 **Heart disease, unspecified**
👁 See Official Guidelines "Hypertension with Heart Disease"
I.C.9.a.1
AHA: Q2 2018, Q4 2018, Q4 2017, Q4 2016

I52 **Other heart disorders in diseases classified elsewhere**
☞ Code first underlying disease, such as:
congenital syphilis (A50.5)
mucopolysaccharidosis (E76.3)
schistosomiasis (B65.0-B65.9)
EXCLUDES1 heart disease (in):
gonococcal infection (A54.83)
meningococcal infection (A39.50)
rheumatoid arthritis (M05.31)
syphilis (A52.06)

Cerebrovascular diseases (I60-I69)

Use additional code to identify presence of:
alcohol abuse and dependence (F10.-)
exposure to environmental tobacco smoke (Z77.22)
history of tobacco dependence (Z87.891)
hypertension (I10-I16)
occupational exposure to environmental tobacco smoke (Z57.31)
tobacco dependence (F17.-)
tobacco use (Z72.0)
EXCLUDES1 traumatic intracranial hemorrhage (S06.-)

4ᵗʰ **I60** **Nontraumatic subarachnoid hemorrhage (Figure 9.3)**
EXCLUDES1 syphilitic ruptured cerebral aneurysm (A52.05)
EXCLUDES2 sequelae of subarachnoid hemorrhage (I69.0-)

5ᵗʰ **I60.0** **Nontraumatic subarachnoid hemorrhage from** carotid
siphon and bifurcation
I60.00 **Nontraumatic subarachnoid hemorrhage from**
unspecified carotid siphon and
bifurcation HCC MCC CC/MCC Exc
I60.01 **Nontraumatic subarachnoid hemorrhage from** right
carotid siphon and bifurcation HCC MCC CC/MCC Exc
I60.02 **Nontraumatic subarachnoid hemorrhage from** left
carotid siphon and bifurcation HCC MCC CC/MCC Exc
5ᵗʰ **I60.1** **Nontraumatic subarachnoid hemorrhage from** middle
cerebral artery
I60.10 **Nontraumatic subarachnoid hemorrhage from**
unspecified middle cerebral artery HCC MCC CC/MCC Exc
I60.11 **Nontraumatic subarachnoid hemorrhage from** right
middle cerebral artery HCC MCC CC/MCC Exc
I60.12 **Nontraumatic subarachnoid hemorrhage from** left
middle cerebral artery HCC MCC CC/MCC Exc
I60.2 **Nontraumatic subarachnoid hemorrhage** from anterior
communicating artery HCC MCC CC/MCC Exc
5ᵗʰ **I60.3** **Nontraumatic subarachnoid hemorrhage from** posterior
communicating artery
I60.30 **Nontraumatic subarachnoid hemorrhage**
from unspecified posterior communicating
artery HCC MCC CC/MCC Exc
I60.31 **Nontraumatic subarachnoid hemorrhage from** right
posterior communicating artery HCC MCC CC/MCC Exc
I60.32 **Nontraumatic subarachnoid hemorrhage from** left
posterior communicating artery HCC MCC CC/MCC Exc
I60.4 **Nontraumatic subarachnoid hemorrhage from**
basilar artery HCC MCC CC/MCC Exc
5ᵗʰ **I60.5** **Nontraumatic subarachnoid hemorrhage from** vertebral artery
I60.50 **Nontraumatic subarachnoid hemorrhage from**
unspecified vertebral artery HCC MCC CC/MCC Exc
I60.51 **Nontraumatic subarachnoid hemorrhage from** right
vertebral artery HCC MCC CC/MCC Exc
I60.52 **Nontraumatic subarachnoid hemorrhage from** left
vertebral artery HCC MCC CC/MCC Exc
I60.6 **Nontraumatic subarachnoid hemorrhage from** other
intracranial arteries HCC MCC CC/MCC Exc
I60.7 **Nontraumatic subarachnoid hemorrhage from unspecified**
intracranial artery HCC MCC CC/MCC Exc
Ruptured (congenital) berry aneurysm
Ruptured (congenital) cerebral aneurysm
Subarachnoid hemorrhage (nontraumatic) from cerebral artery
NOS
Subarachnoid hemorrhage (nontraumatic) from
communicating artery NOS
EXCLUDES1 berry aneurysm, nonruptured (I67.1)
I60.8 **Other nontraumatic subarachnoid hemorrhage** HCC MCC CC/MCC Exc
Meningeal hemorrhage
Rupture of cerebral arteriovenous malformation
I60.9 **Nontraumatic subarachnoid hemorrhage,**
unspecified HCC MCC CC/MCC Exc
4ᵗʰ **I61** **Nontraumatic** intracerebral **hemorrhage**
EXCLUDES2 sequelae of intracerebral hemorrhage (I69.1-)
I61.0 **Nontraumatic intracerebral hemorrhage** in hemisphere,
subcortical HCC MCC CC/MCC Exc
AHA: Q4 2016
Deep intracerebral hemorrhage (nontraumatic)
I61.1 **Nontraumatic intracerebral hemorrhage** in hemisphere,
cortical HCC MCC CC/MCC Exc
Cerebral lobe hemorrhage (nontraumatic)
Superficial intracerebral hemorrhage (nontraumatic)
I61.2 **Nontraumatic intracerebral hemorrhage** in hemisphere,
unspecified HCC MCC CC/MCC Exc
I61.3 **Nontraumatic intracerebral hemorrhage** in
brain stem HCC MCC CC/MCC Exc
I61.4 **Nontraumatic intracerebral hemorrhage** in
cerebellum HCC MCC CC/MCC Exc
I61.5 **Nontraumatic intracerebral hemorrhage,**
intraventricular HCC MCC CC/MCC Exc
I61.6 **Nontraumatic intracerebral hemorrhage,**
multiple localized HCC MCC CC/MCC Exc

Unspecified Code   Other Specified Code   Manifestation Code   Ⓝ Newborn   Ⓟ Pediatric   Ⓜ Maternity   Ⓐ Adult   ♂ Male   ♀ Female
● New Code   ▲ Revised Code Title   ►◄ Revised Text   NOTES   INCLUDES   EXCLUDES1 Not coded here   EXCLUDES2 Not included here
4ᵗʰ 4ᵗʰ character required   **5ᵗʰ** 5ᵗʰ character required   **6ᵗʰ** 6ᵗʰ character required   **7ᵗʰ** 7ᵗʰ character required   👁 Extension 'X' Alert
HAC Hospital-acquired condition (HAC) alert   AHA AHA Coding Clinic©   ☞ Code first alert

I61.8   Other nontraumatic intracerebral hemorrhage   HCC MCC CC/MCC Exc

I61.9   Nontraumatic intracerebral hemorrhage, unspecified   HCC MCC CC/MCC Exc

I62   **Other and unspecified nontraumatic intracranial hemorrhage**

    EXCLUDES2   sequelae of intracranial hemorrhage (I69.2)

   I62.0   **Nontraumatic** subdural **hemorrhage**

     I62.00   **Nontraumatic subdural hemorrhage, unspecified**   HCC MCC CC/MCC Exc

     I62.01   **Nontraumatic** acute **subdural hemorrhage**   HCC MCC CC/MCC Exc

     I62.02   **Nontraumatic** subacute **subdural hemorrhage**   HCC MCC CC/MCC Exc

     I62.03   **Nontraumatic** chronic **subdural hemorrhage**   cc HCC CC/MCC Exc

   I62.1   **Nontraumatic** extradural **hemorrhage**   HCC MCC CC/MCC Exc

     Nontraumatic epidural hemorrhage

   I62.9   **Nontraumatic** intracranial **hemorrhage, unspecified**   cc HCC CC/MCC Exc

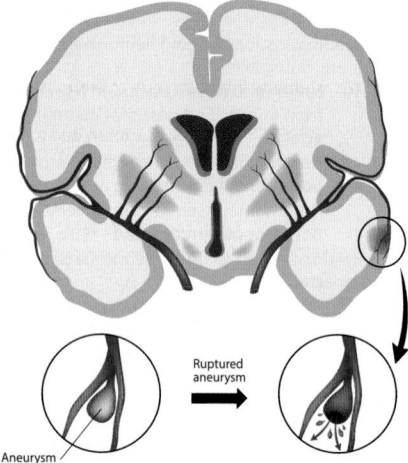

Figure 9.3 Nontraumatic Subarachnoid Hemorrhage

I63   Cerebral infarction (Figure 9.4)

    INCLUDES   occlusion and stenosis of cerebral and precerebral arteries, resulting in cerebral infarction

    Use additional code, if applicable, to identify status post administration of tPA (rtPA) in a different facility within the last 24 hours prior to admission to current facility (Z92.82)

    Use additional code, if known, to indicate National Institutes of Health Stroke Scale (NIHSS) score (R29.7-)

    EXCLUDES2   sequelae of cerebral infarction (I69.3-)

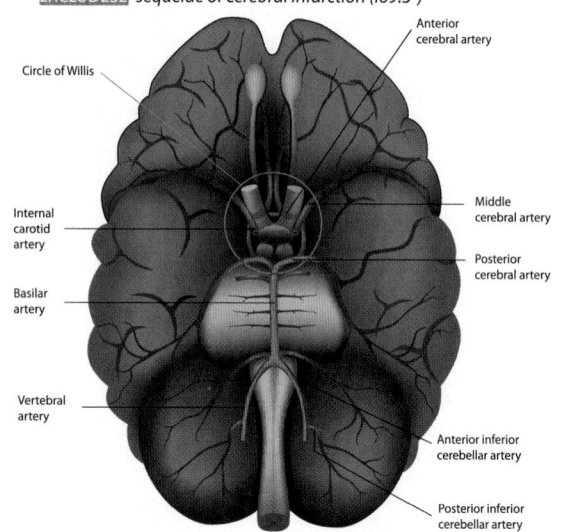

Figure 9.4 Blood Supply of the Brain

I63.0   **Cerebral infarction due to** thrombosis of precerebral arteries

   I63.00   **Cerebral infarction due to thrombosis of unspecified precerebral artery**   HCC MCC RxHCC CC/MCC Exc

   I63.01   **Cerebral infarction due to thrombosis of** vertebral artery

     I63.011   **Cerebral infarction due to thrombosis of** right **vertebral artery**   HCC MCC RxHCC CC/MCC Exc

     I63.012   **Cerebral infarction due to thrombosis of** left **vertebral artery**   HCC MCC RxHCC CC/MCC Exc

     I63.013   **Cerebral infarction due to thrombosis of bilateral vertebral arteries**   HCC MCC RxHCC CC/MCC Exc

     I63.019   **Cerebral infarction due to thrombosis of unspecified vertebral artery**   HCC MCC RxHCC CC/MCC Exc

   I63.02   **Cerebral infarction due to thrombosis of** basilar artery   HCC MCC RxHCC CC/MCC Exc

   I63.03   **Cerebral infarction due to thrombosis of** carotid artery

     I63.031   **Cerebral infarction due to thrombosis of** right **carotid artery**   HCC MCC RxHCC CC/MCC Exc

     I63.032   **Cerebral infarction due to thrombosis of** left **carotid artery**   HCC MCC RxHCC CC/MCC Exc

     I63.033   **Cerebral infarction due to thrombosis of** bilateral **carotid arteries**   HCC MCC RxHCC CC/MCC Exc

     I63.039   **Cerebral infarction due to thrombosis of unspecified carotid artery**   HCC MCC RxHCC CC/MCC Exc

   I63.09   **Cerebral infarction due to thrombosis of other precerebral artery**   HCC MCC RxHCC CC/MCC Exc

I63.1   **Cerebral infarction due to** embolism of precerebral arteries

   I63.10   **Cerebral infarction due to embolism of unspecified precerebral artery**   HCC MCC CC/MCC Exc

   I63.11   **Cerebral infarction due to embolism of** vertebral artery

     I63.111   **Cerebral infarction due to embolism of** right **vertebral artery**   HCC MCC RxHCC CC/MCC Exc

     I63.112   **Cerebral infarction due to embolism of** left **vertebral artery**   HCC MCC RxHCC CC/MCC Exc

     I63.113   **Cerebral infarction due to embolism of** bilateral **vertebral arteries**   HCC MCC RxHCC CC/MCC Exc

     I63.119   **Cerebral infarction due to embolism of unspecified vertebral artery**   HCC MCC RxHCC CC/MCC Exc

   I63.12   **Cerebral infarction due to embolism of basilar artery**   HCC MCC RxHCC CC/MCC Exc

   I63.13   **Cerebral infarction due to embolism of** carotid artery

     I63.131   **Cerebral infarction due to embolism of** right **carotid artery**   HCC MCC RxHCC CC/MCC Exc

     I63.132   **Cerebral infarction due to embolism of** left **carotid artery**   HCC MCC RxHCC CC/MCC Exc

     I63.133   **Cerebral infarction due to embolism of** bilateral **carotid arteries**   HCC MCC RxHCC CC/MCC Exc

     I63.139   **Cerebral infarction due to embolism of unspecified carotid artery**   HCC MCC RxHCC CC/MCC Exc

   I63.19   **Cerebral infarction due to embolism of other precerebral artery**   HCC MCC RxHCC CC/MCC Exc

I63.2   **Cerebral infarction due to** unspecified occlusion or stenosis of precerebral arteries

   I63.20   **Cerebral infarction due to unspecified occlusion or stenosis of unspecified precerebral arteries**   HCC MCC RxHCC CC/MCC Exc

   I63.21   **Cerebral infarction due to unspecified occlusion or stenosis of** vertebral arteries

     I63.211   **Cerebral infarction due to unspecified occlusion or stenosis of** right **vertebral artery**   HCC MCC RxHCC CC/MCC Exc

     I63.212   **Cerebral infarction due to unspecified occlusion or stenosis of** left **vertebral artery**   HCC MCC RxHCC CC/MCC Exc

     I63.213   **Cerebral infarction due to unspecified occlusion or stenosis of** bilateral **vertebral arteries**   HCC MCC RxHCC CC/MCC Exc

PDx Unacceptable principal diagnosis symbol per Medicare code edits   PDx Code exempt from diagnosis present on admission requirement

? Questionable admission   cc Complication or comorbidity   MCC Major complication or comorbidity   CC/MCC CC/MCC exclusion

HCC HCC diagnosis code   RxHCC RxHCC diagnosis code   MACRA code   **DEFINITION** Describes condition/terminology

TIP Coding guidance   👁 Official Guideline Reference   Z1 Z code as first-listed diagnosis

668

When symbols appear on a code that requires a 7th character extension, refer to Appendix B to identify applicable 7th character codes.

2020 ICD-10-CM

I63.219 Cerebral infarction due to unspecified occlusion or stenosis of unspecified vertebral artery HCC MCC RxHCC CC/MCC Exc

I63.22 Cerebral infarction due to unspecified occlusion or stenosis of basilar artery HCC MCC RxHCC CC/MCC Exc

I63.23 Cerebral infarction due to unspecified occlusion or stenosis of carotid arteries

I63.231 Cerebral infarction due to unspecified occlusion or stenosis of right carotid arteries HCC MCC RxHCC CC/MCC Exc

I63.232 Cerebral infarction due to unspecified occlusion or stenosis of left carotid arteries HCC MCC RxHCC CC/MCC Exc

I63.233 Cerebral infarction due to unspecified occlusion or stenosis of bilateral carotid arteries HCC MCC RxHCC CC/MCC Exc

I63.239 Cerebral infarction due to unspecified occlusion or stenosis of unspecified carotid artery HCC MCC RxHCC CC/MCC Exc

I63.29 Cerebral infarction due to unspecified occlusion or stenosis of other precerebral arteries HCC MCC RxHCC CC/MCC Exc

I63.3 Cerebral infarction due to thrombosis of cerebral arteries

I63.30 Cerebral infarction due to thrombosis of unspecified cerebral artery HCC MCC RxHCC CC/MCC Exc

I63.31 Cerebral infarction due to thrombosis of middle cerebral artery

I63.311 Cerebral infarction due to thrombosis of right middle cerebral artery HCC MCC RxHCC CC/MCC Exc

I63.312 Cerebral infarction due to thrombosis of left middle cerebral artery HCC MCC RxHCC CC/MCC Exc

I63.313 Cerebral infarction due to thrombosis of bilateral middle cerebral arteries HCC MCC RxHCC CC/MCC Exc

I63.319 Cerebral infarction due to thrombosis of unspecified middle cerebral artery HCC MCC RxHCC CC/MCC Exc

I63.32 Cerebral infarction due to thrombosis of anterior cerebral artery

I63.321 Cerebral infarction due to thrombosis of right anterior cerebral artery HCC MCC RxHCC CC/MCC Exc

I63.322 Cerebral infarction due to thrombosis of left anterior cerebral artery HCC MCC RxHCC CC/MCC Exc

I63.323 Cerebral infarction due to thrombosis of bilateral anterior cerebral arteries HCC MCC RxHCC CC/MCC Exc

I63.329 Cerebral infarction due to thrombosis of unspecified anterior cerebral artery HCC MCC RxHCC CC/MCC Exc

I63.33 Cerebral infarction due to thrombosis of posterior cerebral artery

I63.331 Cerebral infarction due to thrombosis of right posterior cerebral artery HCC MCC RxHCC CC/MCC Exc

I63.332 Cerebral infarction due to thrombosis of left posterior cerebral artery HCC MCC RxHCC CC/MCC Exc

I63.333 Cerebral infarction due to thrombosis of bilateral posterior cerebral arteries HCC MCC RxHCC CC/MCC Exc

I63.339 Cerebral infarction due to thrombosis of unspecified posterior cerebral artery HCC MCC RxHCC CC/MCC Exc

I63.34 Cerebral infarction due to thrombosis of cerebellar artery

I63.341 Cerebral infarction due to thrombosis of right cerebellar artery HCC MCC RxHCC CC/MCC Exc

I63.342 Cerebral infarction due to thrombosis of left cerebellar artery HCC MCC RxHCC CC/MCC Exc

I63.343 Cerebral infarction due to thrombosis of bilateral cerebellar arteries HCC MCC RxHCC CC/MCC Exc

I63.349 Cerebral infarction due to thrombosis of unspecified cerebellar artery HCC MCC RxHCC CC/MCC Exc

I63.39 Cerebral infarction due to thrombosis of other cerebral artery HCC MCC RxHCC CC/MCC Exc

I63.4 Cerebral infarction due to embolism of cerebral arteries

I63.40 Cerebral infarction due to embolism of unspecified cerebral artery HCC MCC RxHCC CC/MCC Exc

I63.41 Cerebral infarction due to embolism of middle cerebral artery

I63.411 Cerebral infarction due to embolism of right middle cerebral artery HCC MCC RxHCC CC/MCC Exc

I63.412 Cerebral infarction due to embolism of left middle cerebral artery HCC MCC RxHCC CC/MCC Exc

I63.413 Cerebral infarction due to embolism of bilateral middle cerebral arteries HCC MCC RxHCC CC/MCC Exc

I63.419 Cerebral infarction due to embolism of unspecified middle cerebral artery HCC MCC RxHCC CC/MCC Exc

I63.42 Cerebral infarction due to embolism of anterior cerebral artery

I63.421 Cerebral infarction due to embolism of right anterior cerebral artery HCC MCC RxHCC CC/MCC Exc

I63.422 Cerebral infarction due to embolism of left anterior cerebral artery HCC MCC RxHCC CC/MCC Exc

I63.423 Cerebral infarction due to embolism of bilateral anterior cerebral arteries HCC MCC RxHCC CC/MCC Exc

I63.429 Cerebral infarction due to embolism of unspecified anterior cerebral artery HCC MCC RxHCC CC/MCC Exc

I63.43 Cerebral infarction due to embolism of posterior cerebral artery

I63.431 Cerebral infarction due to embolism of right posterior cerebral artery HCC MCC RxHCC CC/MCC Exc

I63.432 Cerebral infarction due to embolism of left posterior cerebral artery HCC MCC RxHCC CC/MCC Exc

I63.433 Cerebral infarction due to embolism of bilateral posterior cerebral arteries HCC MCC RxHCC CC/MCC Exc

I63.439 Cerebral infarction due to embolism of unspecified posterior cerebral artery HCC MCC RxHCC CC/MCC Exc

I63.44 Cerebral infarction due to embolism of cerebellar artery

I63.441 Cerebral infarction due to embolism of right cerebellar artery HCC MCC RxHCC CC/MCC Exc

I63.442 Cerebral infarction due to embolism of left cerebellar artery HCC MCC RxHCC CC/MCC Exc

I63.443 Cerebral infarction due to embolism of bilateral cerebellar arteries HCC MCC RxHCC CC/MCC Exc

I63.449 Cerebral infarction due to embolism of unspecified cerebellar artery HCC MCC RxHCC CC/MCC Exc

I63.49 Cerebral infarction due to embolism of other cerebral artery HCC MCC RxHCC CC/MCC Exc

I63.5 Cerebral infarction due to unspecified occlusion or stenosis of cerebral arteries

I63.50 Cerebral infarction due to unspecified occlusion or stenosis of unspecified cerebral artery HCC MCC RxHCC CC/MCC Exc

I63.51 Cerebral infarction due to unspecified occlusion or stenosis of middle cerebral artery

I63.511 Cerebral infarction due to unspecified occlusion or stenosis of right middle cerebral artery HCC MCC RxHCC CC/MCC Exc

I63.512 Cerebral infarction due to unspecified occlusion or stenosis of left middle cerebral artery HCC MCC RxHCC CC/MCC Exc

---

Unspecified Code   Other Specified Code   Manifestation Code   N Newborn   P Pediatric   M Maternity   A Adult   ♂ Male   ♀ Female
● New Code   ▲ Revised Code Title   ►◄ Revised Text   NOTES   INCLUDES   EXCLUDES1 Not coded here   EXCLUDES2 Not included here
4th character required   5th character required   6th character required   7th character required   Extension 'X' Alert
HAC Hospital-acquired condition (HAC) alert   AHA AHA Coding Clinic©   ☛ Code first alert

I63.513   Cerebral infarction due to unspecified occlusion or stenosis of bilateral middle cerebral arteries   HCC MCC RxHCC CC/MCC Exc

I63.519   Cerebral infarction due to unspecified occlusion or stenosis of unspecified middle cerebral artery   HCC MCC RxHCC CC/MCC Exc

I63.52   Cerebral infarction due to unspecified occlusion or stenosis of anterior cerebral artery

   I63.521   Cerebral infarction due to unspecified occlusion or stenosis of right anterior cerebral artery   HCC MCC RxHCC CC/MCC Exc

   I63.522   Cerebral infarction due to unspecified occlusion or stenosis of left anterior cerebral artery   HCC MCC RxHCC CC/MCC Exc

   I63.523   Cerebral infarction due to unspecified occlusion or stenosis of bilateral anterior cerebral arteries   HCC MCC RxHCC CC/MCC Exc

   I63.529   Cerebral infarction due to unspecified occlusion or stenosis of unspecified anterior cerebral artery   HCC MCC RxHCC CC/MCC Exc

I63.53   Cerebral infarction due to unspecified occlusion or stenosis of posterior cerebral artery

   I63.531   Cerebral infarction due to unspecified occlusion or stenosis of right posterior cerebral artery   HCC MCC RxHCC CC/MCC Exc

   I63.532   Cerebral infarction due to unspecified occlusion or stenosis of left posterior cerebral artery   HCC MCC RxHCC CC/MCC Exc
     AHA: Q2 2017

   I63.533   Cerebral infarction due to unspecified occlusion or stenosis of bilateral posterior cerebral arteries   HCC MCC RxHCC CC/MCC Exc

   I63.539   Cerebral infarction due to unspecified occlusion or stenosis of unspecified posterior cerebral artery   HCC MCC RxHCC CC/MCC Exc

I63.54   Cerebral infarction due to unspecified occlusion or stenosis of cerebellar artery

   I63.541   Cerebral infarction due to unspecified occlusion or stenosis of right cerebellar artery   HCC MCC RxHCC CC/MCC Exc

   I63.542   Cerebral infarction due to unspecified occlusion or stenosis of left cerebellar artery   HCC MCC RxHCC CC/MCC Exc

   I63.543   Cerebral infarction due to unspecified occlusion or stenosis of bilateral cerebellar arteries   HCC MCC RxHCC CC/MCC Exc

   I63.549   Cerebral infarction due to unspecified occlusion or stenosis of unspecified cerebellar artery   HCC MCC RxHCC CC/MCC Exc

I63.59   Cerebral infarction due to unspecified occlusion or stenosis of other cerebral artery   HCC MCC RxHCC CC/MCC Exc

I63.6   Cerebral infarction due to cerebral venous thrombosis, nonpyogenic   HCC MCC RxHCC CC/MCC Exc

I63.8   Other cerebral infarction

   I63.81   Other cerebral infarction due to occlusion or stenosis of small artery   HCC MCC RxHCC CC/MCC Exc
     AHA: Q4 2018
     Lacunar infarction

   I63.89   Other cerebral infarction   HCC MCC RxHCC CC/MCC Exc
     AHA: Q4 2018

I63.9   Cerebral infarction, unspecified   HCC MCC RxHCC CC/MCC Exc
   AHA: Q4 2016, Q1 2015
   Stroke NOS
   EXCLUDES2   transient cerebral ischemic attacks and related syndromes (G45.-)

I65   **Occlusion and stenosis of precerebral arteries, not resulting in cerebral infarction**

   INCLUDES   embolism of precerebral artery
     narrowing of precerebral artery
     obstruction (complete) (partial) of precerebral artery
     thrombosis of precerebral artery

   EXCLUDES1   insufficiency, NOS, of precerebral artery (G45.-)
     insufficiency of precerebral arteries causing cerebral infarction (I63.0-I63.2)

I65.0   Occlusion and stenosis of vertebral artery

   I65.01   Occlusion and stenosis of right vertebral artery   RxHCC

   I65.02   Occlusion and stenosis of left vertebral artery   RxHCC

   I65.03   Occlusion and stenosis of bilateral vertebral arteries   CC RxHCC CC/MCC Exc

   I65.09   Occlusion and stenosis of unspecified vertebral artery   RxHCC

I65.1   Occlusion and stenosis of basilar artery   RxHCC

I65.2   Occlusion and stenosis of carotid artery

   I65.21   Occlusion and stenosis of right carotid artery   RxHCC

   I65.22   Occlusion and stenosis of left carotid artery   RxHCC

   I65.23   Occlusion and stenosis of bilateral carotid arteries   RxHCC
     AHA: Q2 2018

   I65.29   Occlusion and stenosis of unspecified carotid artery   RxHCC

I65.8   Occlusion and stenosis of other precerebral arteries   RxHCC

I65.9   Occlusion and stenosis of unspecified precerebral artery   RxHCC
   Occlusion and stenosis of precerebral artery NOS

I66   **Occlusion and stenosis of cerebral arteries, not resulting in cerebral infarction**

   INCLUDES   embolism of cerebral artery
     narrowing of cerebral artery
     obstruction (complete) (partial) of cerebral artery
     thrombosis of cerebral artery

   EXCLUDES1   Occlusion and stenosis of cerebral artery causing cerebral infarction (I63.3-I63.5)

I66.0   Occlusion and stenosis of middle cerebral artery

   I66.01   Occlusion and stenosis of right middle cerebral artery   RxHCC

   I66.02   Occlusion and stenosis of left middle cerebral artery   RxHCC

   I66.03   Occlusion and stenosis of bilateral middle cerebral arteries   RxHCC

   I66.09   Occlusion and stenosis of unspecified middle cerebral artery   RxHCC

I66.1   Occlusion and stenosis of anterior cerebral artery

   I66.11   Occlusion and stenosis of right anterior cerebral artery   RxHCC

   I66.12   Occlusion and stenosis of left anterior cerebral artery   RxHCC

   I66.13   Occlusion and stenosis of bilateral anterior cerebral arteries   RxHCC

   I66.19   Occlusion and stenosis of unspecified anterior cerebral artery   RxHCC

I66.2   Occlusion and stenosis of posterior cerebral artery

   I66.21   Occlusion and stenosis of right posterior cerebral artery   RxHCC

   I66.22   Occlusion and stenosis of left posterior cerebral artery   RxHCC

   I66.23   Occlusion and stenosis of bilateral posterior cerebral arteries   RxHCC

   I66.29   Occlusion and stenosis of unspecified posterior cerebral artery   RxHCC

I66.3   Occlusion and stenosis of cerebellar arteries   RxHCC

I66.8   Occlusion and stenosis of other cerebral arteries   RxHCC
   Occlusion and stenosis of perforating arteries

I66.9   Occlusion and stenosis of unspecified cerebral artery   RxHCC

I67   **Other cerebrovascular diseases**

   EXCLUDES2   sequelae of the listed conditions (I69.8)

I67.0   Dissection of cerebral arteries, nonruptured   HCC MCC CC/MCC Exc
   EXCLUDES1   ruptured cerebral arteries (I60.7)

I67.1   Cerebral aneurysm, nonruptured
   Cerebral aneurysm NOS
   Cerebral arteriovenous fistula, acquired
   Internal carotid artery aneurysm, intracranial portion
   Internal carotid artery aneurysm, NOS
   EXCLUDES1   congenital cerebral aneurysm, nonruptured (Q28.-)
     ruptured cerebral aneurysm (I60.7)

PDDx   Unacceptable principal diagnosis symbol per Medicare code edits   POA   Code exempt from diagnosis present on admission requirement
   ❓ Questionable admission   CC Complication or comorbidity   MCC Major complication or comorbidity   CC/MCC Exc CC/MCC exclusion
   HCC HCC diagnosis code   RxHCC RxHCC diagnosis code   MACRA code   **DEFINITION** Describes condition/terminology
   TIP Coding guidance   👁 Official Guideline Reference   Z Z code as first-listed diagnosis

I67.2 **Cerebral atherosclerosis** `A` `RxHCC`
Atheroma of cerebral and precerebral arteries

I67.3 **Progressive vascular leukoencephalopathy** `CC` `HCC` `RxHCC` `CC/MCC Exc`
Binswanger's disease

I67.4 **Hypertensive encephalopathy** `CC` `RxHCC` `CC/MCC Exc`
EXCLUDES2 insufficiency, NOS, of precerebral arteries (G45.2)

I67.5 **Moyamoya disease** `CC` `RxHCC` `CC/MCC Exc`

I67.6 **Nonpyogenic thrombosis of intracranial venous system** `CC` `RxHCC` `CC/MCC Exc`
Nonpyogenic thrombosis of cerebral vein
Nonpyogenic thrombosis of intracranial venous sinus
EXCLUDES1 nonpyogenic thrombosis of intracranial venous system causing infarction (I63.6)

I67.7 **Cerebral arteritis, not elsewhere classified** `CC` `RxHCC` `CC/MCC Exc`
Granulomatous angiitis of the nervous system
EXCLUDES1 allergic granulomatous angiitis (M30.1)

5th I67.8 **Other specified cerebrovascular diseases**

I67.81 **Acute cerebrovascular insufficiency** `CC` `RxHCC` `CC/MCC Exc`
Acute cerebrovascular insufficiency unspecified as to location or reversibility

I67.82 **Cerebral ischemia** `CC` `RxHCC` `CC/MCC Exc`
Chronic cerebral ischemia

I67.83 **Posterior reversible encephalopathy syndrome** `MCC` `CC/MCC Exc`
PRES

6th I67.84 **Cerebral vasospasm and vasoconstriction**

I67.841 **Reversible cerebrovascular vasoconstriction syndrome** `CC` `RxHCC` `CC/MCC Exc`
Call-Fleming syndrome
☛ **Code first** underlying condition, if applicable, such as eclampsia (O15.00-O15.9)

I67.848 **Other cerebrovascular vasospasm and vasoconstriction** `CC` `RxHCC` `CC/MCC Exc`

6th I67.85 **Hereditary cerebrovascular diseases**

I67.850 **Cerebral autosomal dominant arteriopathy with subcortical infarcts and leukoencephalopathy** `CC` `RxHCC` `CC/MCC Exc`
AHA: Q4 2018
CADASIL
Code also any associated diagnoses, such as:
epilepsy (G40.-)
stroke (I63.-)
vascular dementia (F01.-)

I67.858 **Other hereditary cerebrovascular disease** `CC` `RxHCC` `CC/MCC Exc`
AHA: Q4 2018

I67.89 **Other cerebrovascular disease** `RxHCC`

I67.9 **Cerebrovascular disease, unspecified** `RxHCC`

4th I68 **Cerebrovascular disorders in diseases classified elsewhere**

I68.0 **Cerebral amyloid angiopathy** `RxHCC`
☛ **Code first** underlying amyloidosis (E85.-)

I68.2 **Cerebral arteritis in other diseases classified elsewhere** `CC` `RxHCC` `CC/MCC Exc`
☛ **Code first** underlying disease
EXCLUDES1 cerebral arteritis (in):
listerosis (A32.89)
systemic lupus erythematosus (M32.19)
syphilis (A52.04)
tuberculosis (A18.89)

I68.8 **Other cerebrovascular disorders in diseases classified elsewhere** `RxHCC`
☛ **Code first** underlying disease
EXCLUDES1 syphilitic cerebral aneurysm (A52.05)

4th I69 **Sequelae of cerebrovascular disease**
👁 **See Official Guidelines** " Sequelae of Cerebrovascular disease" I.C.9.d.1-3
NOTES Category I69 is to be used to indicate conditions in I60-I67 as the cause of sequelae. The 'sequelae' include conditions specified as such or as residuals which may occur at any time after the onset of the causal condition.

EXCLUDES1 personal history of cerebral infarction without residual deficit (Z86.73)
personal history of prolonged reversible ischemic neurologic deficit (PRIND) (Z86.73)
personal history of reversible ischemic neurological deficit (RIND) (Z86.73)
sequelae of traumatic intracranial injury (S06.-)

5th I69.0 **Sequelae of nontraumatic subarachnoid hemorrhage**

I69.00 **Unspecified sequelae of nontraumatic subarachnoid hemorrhage** `POA`

6th I69.01 **Cognitive deficits following nontraumatic subarachnoid hemorrhage**

I69.010 **Attention and concentration deficit following nontraumatic subarachnoid hemorrhage** `POA`

I69.011 **Memory deficit following nontraumatic subarachnoid hemorrhage** `POA`

I69.012 **Visuospatial deficit and spatial neglect following nontraumatic subarachnoid hemorrhage** `POA`

I69.013 **Psychomotor deficit following nontraumatic subarachnoid hemorrhage** `POA`

I69.014 **Frontal lobe and executive function deficit following nontraumatic subarachnoid hemorrhage** `POA`

I69.015 **Cognitive social or emotional deficit following nontraumatic subarachnoid hemorrhage** `POA`

I69.018 **Other symptoms and signs involving cognitive functions following nontraumatic subarachnoid hemorrhage** `POA`

I69.019 **Unspecified symptoms and signs involving cognitive functions following nontraumatic subarachnoid hemorrhage** `POA`

6th I69.02 **Speech and language deficits following nontraumatic subarachnoid hemorrhage**

I69.020 **Aphasia following nontraumatic subarachnoid hemorrhage** `POA`

I69.021 **Dysphasia following nontraumatic subarachnoid hemorrhage** `POA`

I69.022 **Dysarthria following nontraumatic subarachnoid hemorrhage** `POA`

I69.023 **Fluency disorder following nontraumatic subarachnoid hemorrhage** `POA`
Stuttering following nontraumatic subarachnoid hemorrhage

I69.028 **Other speech and language deficits following nontraumatic subarachnoid hemorrhage** `POA`

6th I69.03 **Monoplegia of upper limb following nontraumatic subarachnoid hemorrhage**

I69.031 **Monoplegia of upper limb following nontraumatic subarachnoid hemorrhage affecting right dominant side** `POA` `HCC`

I69.032 **Monoplegia of upper limb following nontraumatic subarachnoid hemorrhage affecting left dominant side** `POA` `HCC`

I69.033 **Monoplegia of upper limb following nontraumatic subarachnoid hemorrhage affecting right non-dominant side** `POA` `HCC`

I69.034 **Monoplegia of upper limb following nontraumatic subarachnoid hemorrhage affecting left non-dominant side** `POA` `HCC`

I69.039 **Monoplegia of upper limb following nontraumatic subarachnoid hemorrhage affecting unspecified side** `POA` `HCC`

6th I69.04 **Monoplegia of lower limb following nontraumatic subarachnoid hemorrhage**

Unspecified Code Other Specified Code Manifestation Code N Newborn P Pediatric M Maternity A Adult ♂ Male ♀ Female
● New Code ▲ Revised Code Title ►◄ Revised Text NOTES INCLUDES EXCLUDES1 Not coded here EXCLUDES2 Not included here
4th 4th character required 5th 5th character required 6th 6th character required 7th 7th character required Extension 'X' Alert
HAC Hospital-acquired condition (HAC) alert AHA AHA Coding Clinic© ☛ Code first alert

I69.041 Monoplegia of lower limb following nontraumatic subarachnoid hemorrhage affecting right dominant side POA HCC

I69.042 Monoplegia of lower limb following nontraumatic subarachnoid hemorrhage affecting left dominant side POA HCC

I69.043 Monoplegia of lower limb following nontraumatic subarachnoid hemorrhage affecting right non-dominant side POA HCC

I69.044 Monoplegia of lower limb following nontraumatic subarachnoid hemorrhage affecting left non-dominant side POA HCC

I69.049 Monoplegia of lower limb following nontraumatic subarachnoid hemorrhage affecting unspecified side POA HCC

I69.05 Hemiplegia and hemiparesis following nontraumatic subarachnoid hemorrhage

I69.051 Hemiplegia and hemiparesis following nontraumatic subarachnoid hemorrhage affecting right dominant side CC POA HCC CC/MCC Exc

I69.052 Hemiplegia and hemiparesis following nontraumatic subarachnoid hemorrhage affecting left dominant side CC POA HCC CC/MCC Exc

I69.053 Hemiplegia and hemiparesis following nontraumatic subarachnoid hemorrhage affecting right non-dominant side CC POA HCC CC/MCC Exc

I69.054 Hemiplegia and hemiparesis following nontraumatic subarachnoid hemorrhage affecting left non-dominant side CC POA HCC CC/MCC Exc

I69.059 Hemiplegia and hemiparesis following nontraumatic subarachnoid hemorrhage affecting unspecified side CC POA HCC CC/MCC Exc

I69.06 Other paralytic syndrome following nontraumatic subarachnoid hemorrhage

Use additional code to identify type of paralytic syndrome, such as:
locked-in state (G83.5)
quadriplegia (G82.5-)

EXCLUDES1 hemiplegia/hemiparesis following nontraumatic subarachnoid hemorrhage (I69.05-)

monoplegia of lower limb following nontraumatic subarachnoid hemorrhage (I69.04-)

monoplegia of upper limb following nontraumatic subarachnoid hemorrhage (I69.03-)

I69.061 Other paralytic syndrome following nontraumatic subarachnoid hemorrhage affecting right dominant side POA HCC

I69.062 Other paralytic syndrome following nontraumatic subarachnoid hemorrhage affecting left dominant side POA HCC

I69.063 Other paralytic syndrome following nontraumatic subarachnoid hemorrhage affecting right non-dominant side POA HCC

I69.064 Other paralytic syndrome following nontraumatic subarachnoid hemorrhage affecting left non-dominant side POA HCC

I69.065 Other paralytic syndrome following nontraumatic subarachnoid hemorrhage, bilateral POA HCC

I69.069 Other paralytic syndrome following nontraumatic subarachnoid hemorrhage affecting unspecified side POA HCC

I69.09 Other sequelae of nontraumatic subarachnoid hemorrhage

I69.090 Apraxia following nontraumatic subarachnoid hemorrhage POA

I69.091 Dysphagia following nontraumatic subarachnoid hemorrhage POA

Use additional code to identify the type of dysphagia, if known (R13.1-)

I69.092 Facial weakness following nontraumatic subarachnoid hemorrhage POA

Facial droop following nontraumatic subarachnoid hemorrhage

I69.093 Ataxia following nontraumatic subarachnoid hemorrhage POA

I69.098 Other sequelae following nontraumatic subarachnoid hemorrhage POA

Alterations of sensation following nontraumatic subarachnoid hemorrhage

Disturbance of vision following nontraumatic subarachnoid hemorrhage

Use additional code to identify the sequelae

I69.1 Sequelae of nontraumatic intracerebral hemorrhage

I69.10 Unspecified sequelae of nontraumatic intracerebral hemorrhage POA

I69.11 Cognitive deficits following nontraumatic intracerebral hemorrhage

I69.110 Attention and concentration deficit following nontraumatic intracerebral hemorrhage POA

I69.111 Memory deficit following nontraumatic intracerebral hemorrhage POA

I69.112 Visuospatial deficit and spatial neglect following nontraumatic intracerebral hemorrhage POA

I69.113 Psychomotor deficit following nontraumatic intracerebral hemorrhage POA

I69.114 Frontal lobe and executive function deficit following nontraumatic intracerebral hemorrhage POA

I69.115 Cognitive social or emotional deficit following nontraumatic intracerebral hemorrhage POA

I69.118 Other symptoms and signs involving cognitive functions following nontraumatic intracerebral hemorrhage POA

I69.119 Unspecified symptoms and signs involving cognitive functions following nontraumatic intracerebral hemorrhage POA

I69.12 Speech and language deficits following nontraumatic intracerebral hemorrhage

I69.120 Aphasia following nontraumatic intracerebral hemorrhage POA

I69.121 Dysphasia following nontraumatic intracerebral hemorrhage POA

I69.122 Dysarthria following nontraumatic intracerebral hemorrhage POA

I69.123 Fluency disorder following nontraumatic intracerebral hemorrhage POA

Stuttering following nontraumatic intracerebral hemorrhage

I69.128 Other speech and language deficits following nontraumatic intracerebral hemorrhage POA

I69.13 Monoplegia of upper limb following nontraumatic intracerebral hemorrhage

I69.131 Monoplegia of upper limb following nontraumatic intracerebral hemorrhage affecting right dominant side POA HCC

I69.132 Monoplegia of upper limb following nontraumatic intracerebral hemorrhage affecting left dominant side POA HCC

I69.133 Monoplegia of upper limb following nontraumatic intracerebral hemorrhage affecting right non-dominant side POA HCC

POA=DX Unacceptable principal diagnosis symbol per Medicare code edits POA Code exempt from diagnosis present on admission requirement ？ Questionable admission CC Complication or comorbidity MCC Major complication or comorbidity CC/MCC Exc CC/MCC exclusion HCC HCC diagnosis code RxHCC RxHCC diagnosis code MACRA MACRA code DEFINITION Describes condition/terminology TIP Coding guidance 👁 Official Guideline Reference Z1 Z code as first-listed diagnosis

I69.134 Monoplegia of upper limb following nontraumatic intracerebral hemorrhage affecting left non-dominant side POA HCC

I69.139 Monoplegia of upper limb following nontraumatic intracerebral hemorrhage affecting unspecified side POA HCC

6ᵗʰ I69.14 Monoplegia of lower limb following nontraumatic intracerebral hemorrhage

I69.141 Monoplegia of lower limb following nontraumatic intracerebral hemorrhage affecting right dominant side POA HCC

I69.142 Monoplegia of lower limb following nontraumatic intracerebral hemorrhage affecting left dominant side POA HCC

I69.143 Monoplegia of lower limb following nontraumatic intracerebral hemorrhage affecting right non-dominant side POA HCC

I69.144 Monoplegia of lower limb following nontraumatic intracerebral hemorrhage affecting left non-dominant side POA HCC

I69.149 Monoplegia of lower limb following nontraumatic intracerebral hemorrhage affecting unspecified side POA HCC

6ᵗʰ I69.15 Hemiplegia and hemiparesis following nontraumatic intracerebral hemorrhage

I69.151 Hemiplegia and hemiparesis following nontraumatic intracerebral hemorrhage affecting right dominant side CC POA HCC CC/MCC Exc

I69.152 Hemiplegia and hemiparesis following nontraumatic intracerebral hemorrhage affecting left dominant side CC POA HCC CC/MCC Exc

I69.153 Hemiplegia and hemiparesis following nontraumatic intracerebral hemorrhage affecting right non-dominant side CC POA HCC CC/MCC Exc

I69.154 Hemiplegia and hemiparesis following nontraumatic intracerebral hemorrhage affecting left non-dominant side CC POA HCC CC/MCC Exc

I69.159 Hemiplegia and hemiparesis following nontraumatic intracerebral hemorrhage affecting unspecified side CC POA HCC CC/MCC Exc

6ᵗʰ I69.16 Other paralytic syndrome following nontraumatic intracerebral hemorrhage

Use additional code to identify type of paralytic syndrome, such as:
locked-in state (G83.5)
quadriplegia (G82.5-)

EXCLUDES1 hemiplegia/hemiparesis following nontraumatic intracerebral hemorrhage (I69.15-)
monoplegia of lower limb following nontraumatic intracerebral hemorrhage (I69.14-)
monoplegia of upper limb following nontraumatic intracerebral hemorrhage (I69.13-)

I69.161 Other paralytic syndrome following nontraumatic intracerebral hemorrhage affecting right dominant side POA HCC

I69.162 Other paralytic syndrome following nontraumatic intracerebral hemorrhage affecting left dominant side POA HCC

I69.163 Other paralytic syndrome following nontraumatic intracerebral hemorrhage affecting right non-dominant side POA HCC

I69.164 Other paralytic syndrome following nontraumatic intracerebral hemorrhage affecting left non-dominant side POA HCC

I69.165 Other paralytic syndrome following nontraumatic intracerebral hemorrhage, bilateral POA HCC

I69.169 Other paralytic syndrome following nontraumatic intracerebral hemorrhage affecting unspecified side POA HCC

6ᵗʰ I69.19 Other sequelae of nontraumatic intracerebral hemorrhage

I69.190 Apraxia following nontraumatic intracerebral hemorrhage POA

I69.191 Dysphagia following nontraumatic intracerebral hemorrhage POA

Use additional code to identify the type of dysphagia, if known (R13.1-)

I69.192 Facial weakness following nontraumatic intracerebral hemorrhage POA

Facial droop following nontraumatic intracerebral hemorrhage

I69.193 Ataxia following nontraumatic intracerebral hemorrhage POA

I69.198 Other sequelae of nontraumatic intracerebral hemorrhage POA

Alteration of sensations following nontraumatic intracerebral hemorrhage
Disturbance of vision following nontraumatic intracerebral hemorrhage
Use additional code to identify the sequelae

5ᵗʰ I69.2 Sequelae of other nontraumatic intracranial hemorrhage

I69.20 Unspecified sequelae of other nontraumatic intracranial hemorrhage POA

6ᵗʰ I69.21 Cognitive deficits following other nontraumatic intracranial hemorrhage

I69.210 Attention and concentration deficit following other nontraumatic intracranial hemorrhage POA

I69.211 Memory deficit following other nontraumatic intracranial hemorrhage POA

I69.212 Visuospatial deficit and spatial neglect following other nontraumatic intracranial hemorrhage POA

I69.213 Psychomotor deficit following other nontraumatic intracranial hemorrhage POA

I69.214 Frontal lobe and executive function deficit following other nontraumatic intracranial hemorrhage POA

I69.215 Cognitive social or emotional deficit following other nontraumatic intracranial hemorrhage POA

I69.218 Other symptoms and signs involving cognitive functions following other nontraumatic intracranial hemorrhage POA

I69.219 Unspecified symptoms and signs involving cognitive functions following other nontraumatic intracranial hemorrhage POA

6ᵗʰ I69.22 Speech and language deficits following other nontraumatic intracranial hemorrhage

I69.220 Aphasia following other nontraumatic intracranial hemorrhage POA

I69.221 Dysphasia following other nontraumatic intracranial hemorrhage POA

I69.222 Dysarthria following other nontraumatic intracranial hemorrhage POA

I69.223 Fluency disorder following other nontraumatic intracranial hemorrhage POA

Stuttering following other nontraumatic intracranial hemorrhage

I69.228 Other speech and language deficits following other nontraumatic intracranial hemorrhage POA

6ᵗʰ I69.23 Monoplegia of upper limb following other nontraumatic intracranial hemorrhage

I69.231 Monoplegia of upper limb following other nontraumatic intracranial hemorrhage affecting right dominant side POA HCC

I69.232 Monoplegia of upper limb following other nontraumatic intracranial hemorrhage affecting left dominant side ᴾᴼᴬ HCC

I69.233 Monoplegia of upper limb following other nontraumatic intracranial hemorrhage affecting right non-dominant side ᴾᴼᴬ HCC

I69.234 Monoplegia of upper limb following other nontraumatic intracranial hemorrhage affecting left non-dominant side ᴾᴼᴬ HCC

I69.239 Monoplegia of upper limb following other nontraumatic intracranial hemorrhage affecting unspecified side ᴾᴼᴬ HCC

6ᵗʰ I69.24 Monoplegia of lower limb following other nontraumatic intracranial hemorrhage

I69.241 Monoplegia of lower limb following other nontraumatic intracranial hemorrhage affecting right dominant side ᴾᴼᴬ HCC

I69.242 Monoplegia of lower limb following other nontraumatic intracranial hemorrhage affecting left dominant side ᴾᴼᴬ HCC

I69.243 Monoplegia of lower limb following other nontraumatic intracranial hemorrhage affecting right non-dominant side ᴾᴼᴬ HCC

I69.244 Monoplegia of lower limb following other nontraumatic intracranial hemorrhage affecting left non-dominant side ᴾᴼᴬ HCC

I69.249 Monoplegia of lower limb following other nontraumatic intracranial hemorrhage affecting unspecified side ᴾᴼᴬ HCC

6ᵗʰ I69.25 Hemiplegia and hemiparesis following other nontraumatic intracranial hemorrhage

I69.251 Hemiplegia and hemiparesis following other nontraumatic intracranial hemorrhage affecting right dominant side ᶜᶜ ᴾᴼᴬ HCC CC/MCC Exc

I69.252 Hemiplegia and hemiparesis following other nontraumatic intracranial hemorrhage affecting left dominant side ᶜᶜ ᴾᴼᴬ HCC CC/MCC Exc

I69.253 Hemiplegia and hemiparesis following other nontraumatic intracranial hemorrhage affecting right non-dominant side ᶜᶜ ᴾᴼᴬ HCC CC/MCC Exc

I69.254 Hemiplegia and hemiparesis following other nontraumatic intracranial hemorrhage affecting left non-dominant side ᶜᶜ ᴾᴼᴬ HCC CC/MCC Exc

I69.259 Hemiplegia and hemiparesis following other nontraumatic intracranial hemorrhage affecting unspecified side ᶜᶜ ᴾᴼᴬ HCC CC/MCC Exc

6ᵗʰ I69.26 Other paralytic syndrome following other nontraumatic intracranial hemorrhage
Use additional code to identify type of paralytic syndrome, such as:
locked-in state (G83.5)
quadriplegia (G82.5-)

EXCLUDES1 hemiplegia/hemiparesis following other nontraumatic intracranial hemorrhage (I69.25-)

monoplegia of lower limb following other nontraumatic intracranial hemorrhage (I69.24-)

monoplegia of upper limb following other nontraumatic intracranial hemorrhage (I69.23-)

I69.261 Other paralytic syndrome following other nontraumatic intracranial hemorrhage affecting right dominant side ᴾᴼᴬ HCC

I69.262 Other paralytic syndrome following other nontraumatic intracranial hemorrhage affecting left dominant side ᴾᴼᴬ HCC

I69.263 Other paralytic syndrome following other nontraumatic intracranial hemorrhage affecting right non-dominant side ᴾᴼᴬ HCC

I69.264 Other paralytic syndrome following other nontraumatic intracranial hemorrhage affecting left non-dominant side ᴾᴼᴬ HCC

I69.265 Other paralytic syndrome following other nontraumatic intracranial hemorrhage, bilateral ᴾᴼᴬ HCC

I69.269 Other paralytic syndrome following other nontraumatic intracranial hemorrhage affecting unspecified side ᴾᴼᴬ HCC

6ᵗʰ I69.29 Other sequelae of other nontraumatic intracranial hemorrhage

I69.290 Apraxia following other nontraumatic intracranial hemorrhage ᴾᴼᴬ

I69.291 Dysphagia following other nontraumatic intracranial hemorrhage ᴾᴼᴬ
Use additional code to identify the type of dysphagia, if known (R13.1-)

I69.292 Facial weakness following other nontraumatic intracranial hemorrhage ᴾᴼᴬ
Facial droop following other nontraumatic intracranial hemorrhage

I69.293 Ataxia following other nontraumatic intracranial hemorrhage ᴾᴼᴬ

I69.298 Other sequelae of other nontraumatic intracranial hemorrhage ᴾᴼᴬ
Alteration of sensation following other nontraumatic intracranial hemorrhage
Disturbance of vision following other nontraumatic intracranial hemorrhage
Use additional code to identify the sequelae

5ᵗʰ I69.3 Sequelae of cerebral infarction
Sequelae of stroke NOS

I69.30 Unspecified sequelae of cerebral infarction ᴾᴼᴬ

6ᵗʰ I69.31 Cognitive deficits following cerebral infarction

I69.310 Attention and concentration deficit following cerebral infarction ᴾᴼᴬ

I69.311 Memory deficit following cerebral infarction ᴾᴼᴬ

I69.312 Visuospatial deficit and spatial neglect following cerebral infarction ᴾᴼᴬ

I69.313 Psychomotor deficit following cerebral infarction ᴾᴼᴬ

I69.314 Frontal lobe and executive function deficit following cerebral infarction ᴾᴼᴬ

I69.315 Cognitive social or emotional deficit following cerebral infarction ᴾᴼᴬ

I69.318 Other symptoms and signs involving cognitive functions following cerebral infarction ᴾᴼᴬ

I69.319 Unspecified symptoms and signs involving cognitive functions following cerebral infarction ᴾᴼᴬ

6ᵗʰ I69.32 Speech and language deficits following cerebral infarction

I69.320 Aphasia following cerebral infarction ᴾᴼᴬ
AHA: Q4 2013

I69.321 Dysphasia following cerebral infarction ᴾᴼᴬ

I69.322 Dysarthria following cerebral infarction ᴾᴼᴬ
EXCLUDES2 transient ischemic attack (TIA) (G45.9)

I69.323 Fluency disorder following cerebral infarction ᴾᴼᴬ
Stuttering following cerebral infarction

I69.328 Other speech and language deficits following cerebral infarction ᴾᴼᴬ

6ᵗʰ I69.33 Monoplegia of upper limb following cerebral infarction

I69.331 Monoplegia of upper limb following cerebral infarction affecting right dominant side ᴾᴼᴬ HCC

I69.332 Monoplegia of upper limb following cerebral infarction affecting left dominant side ᴾᴼᴬ HCC

ᴾᴰˣ Unacceptable principal diagnosis symbol per Medicare code edits   ᴾᴼᴬ Code exempt from diagnosis present on admission requirement
❓ Questionable admission   ᶜᶜ Complication or comorbidity   ᴹᶜᶜ Major complication or comorbidity   ᶜᶜ/ᴹᶜᶜ Exc CC/MCC exclusion
HCC HCC diagnosis code   RxHCC RxHCC diagnosis code   MACRA code   **DEFINITION** Describes condition/terminology
TIP Coding guidance   👁 Official Guideline Reference   Ⓩ Z code as first-listed diagnosis

674   When symbols appear on a code that requires a 7th character extension, refer to Appendix B to identify applicable 7th character codes.   **2020 ICD-10-CM**

I69.333 **Monoplegia of upper limb following cerebral infarction affecting** right non-dominant side POA HCC

I69.334 **Monoplegia of upper limb following cerebral infarction affecting** left non-dominant side POA HCC

I69.339 **Monoplegia of upper limb following cerebral infarction affecting unspecified side** POA HCC

6th I69.34 **Monoplegia of lower limb following cerebral infarction**

I69.341 **Monoplegia of lower limb following cerebral infarction affecting** right dominant side POA HCC

I69.342 **Monoplegia of lower limb following cerebral infarction affecting** left dominant side POA HCC

I69.343 **Monoplegia of lower limb following cerebral infarction affecting** right non-dominant side POA HCC

I69.344 **Monoplegia of lower limb following cerebral infarction affecting** left non-dominant side POA HCC

I69.349 **Monoplegia of lower limb following cerebral infarction affecting unspecified side** POA HCC

6th I69.35 **Hemiplegia and hemiparesis following cerebral infarction**

I69.351 **Hemiplegia and hemiparesis following cerebral infarction affecting** right dominant side CC POA HCC CC/MCC Exc

AHA: Q1 2015

EXCLUDES2 transient ischemic attack (TIA) (G45.9)

I69.352 **Hemiplegia and hemiparesis following cerebral infarction affecting** left dominant side CC POA HCC CC/MCC Exc

I69.353 **Hemiplegia and hemiparesis following cerebral infarction affecting** right non-dominant side CC POA HCC CC/MCC Exc

I69.354 **Hemiplegia and hemiparesis following cerebral infarction affecting** left non-dominant side CC POA HCC CC/MCC Exc

I69.359 **Hemiplegia and hemiparesis following cerebral infarction affecting unspecified side** CC POA HCC CC/MCC Exc

6th I69.36 **Other paralytic syndrome following cerebral infarction**

Use additional code to identify type of paralytic syndrome, such as:
locked-in state (G83.5)
quadriplegia (G82.5-)

EXCLUDES1 hemiplegia/hemiparesis following cerebral infarction (I69.35-)

monoplegia of lower limb following cerebral infarction (I69.34-)

monoplegia of upper limb following cerebral infarction (I69.33-)

I69.361 **Other paralytic syndrome following cerebral infarction affecting** right dominant side POA HCC

I69.362 **Other paralytic syndrome following cerebral infarction affecting** left dominant side POA HCC

I69.363 **Other paralytic syndrome following cerebral infarction affecting** right non-dominant side POA HCC

I69.364 **Other paralytic syndrome following cerebral infarction affecting** left non-dominant side POA HCC

I69.365 **Other paralytic syndrome following cerebral infarction,** bilateral POA HCC

I69.369 **Other paralytic syndrome following cerebral infarction affecting unspecified side** POA HCC

6th I69.39 **Other sequelae** of cerebral infarction

I69.390 **Apraxia** following cerebral infarction POA

I69.391 **Dysphagia** following cerebral infarction POA

Use additional code to identify the type of dysphagia, if known (R13.1-)

I69.392 **Facial weakness** following cerebral infarction POA

Facial droop following cerebral infarction

I69.393 **Ataxia** following cerebral infarction POA

I69.398 **Other sequelae of cerebral infarction**

Alteration of sensation following cerebral infarction

Disturbance of vision following cerebral infarction

Use additional code to identify the sequelae

5th I69.8 **Sequelae of** other cerebrovascular diseases

EXCLUDES1 sequelae of traumatic intracranial injury (S06.-)

I69.80 **Unspecified sequelae of other cerebrovascular disease** POA

6th I69.81 **Cognitive deficits following other cerebrovascular disease**

I69.810 **Attention and concentration deficit following other cerebrovascular disease** POA

I69.811 **Memory deficit following other cerebrovascular disease** POA

I69.812 **Visuospatial deficit and spatial neglect following other cerebrovascular disease** POA

I69.813 **Psychomotor deficit following other cerebrovascular disease** POA

I69.814 **Frontal lobe and executive function deficit following other cerebrovascular disease** POA

I69.815 **Cognitive social or emotional deficit following other cerebrovascular disease** POA

I69.818 **Other symptoms and signs involving cognitive functions following other cerebrovascular disease** POA

I69.819 **Unspecified symptoms and signs involving cognitive functions following other cerebrovascular disease** POA

6th I69.82 **Speech and language deficits following other cerebrovascular disease**

I69.820 **Aphasia following other cerebrovascular disease** POA

I69.821 **Dysphasia following other cerebrovascular disease** POA

I69.822 **Dysarthria following other cerebrovascular disease** POA

I69.823 **Fluency disorder following other cerebrovascular disease** POA

Stuttering following other cerebrovascular disease

I69.828 **Other speech and language deficits following other cerebrovascular disease** POA

6th I69.83 **Monoplegia of upper limb following other cerebrovascular disease**

I69.831 **Monoplegia of upper limb following other cerebrovascular disease affecting** right dominant side POA HCC

I69.832 **Monoplegia of upper limb following other cerebrovascular disease affecting** left dominant side POA HCC

I69.833 **Monoplegia of upper limb following other cerebrovascular disease affecting** right non-dominant side POA HCC

I69.834 **Monoplegia of upper limb following other cerebrovascular disease affecting** left non-dominant side POA HCC

Unspecified Code   Other Specified Code   Manifestation Code   N Newborn   P Pediatric   M Maternity   A Adult   ♂ Male   ♀ Female
● New Code   ▲ Revised Code Title   ►◄ Revised Text   **NOTES** *INCLUDES* *EXCLUDES1* Not coded here   *EXCLUDES2* Not included here
4th 4th character required   5th 5th character required   6th 6th character required   7th 7th character required   Extension 'X' Alert
HAC Hospital-acquired condition (HAC) alert   **AHA** AHA Coding Clinic©   Code first alert

I69.839　Monoplegia of upper limb following other cerebrovascular disease affecting unspecified side ⓟₒₐ HCC

Ⓖ I69.84　Monoplegia of lower limb following other cerebrovascular disease

I69.841　Monoplegia of lower limb following other cerebrovascular disease affecting right dominant side ⓟₒₐ HCC

I69.842　Monoplegia of lower limb following other cerebrovascular disease affecting left dominant side ⓟₒₐ HCC

I69.843　Monoplegia of lower limb following other cerebrovascular disease affecting right non-dominant side ⓟₒₐ HCC

I69.844　Monoplegia of lower limb following other cerebrovascular disease affecting left non-dominant side ⓟₒₐ HCC

I69.849　Monoplegia of lower limb following other cerebrovascular disease affecting unspecified side ⓟₒₐ HCC

Ⓖ I69.85　Hemiplegia and hemiparesis following other cerebrovascular disease

I69.851　Hemiplegia and hemiparesis following other cerebrovascular disease affecting right dominant side cc ⓟₒₐ HCC CC/MCC Exc

I69.852　Hemiplegia and hemiparesis following other cerebrovascular disease affecting left dominant side cc ⓟₒₐ HCC CC/MCC Exc

I69.853　Hemiplegia and hemiparesis following other cerebrovascular disease affecting right non-dominant side cc ⓟₒₐ HCC CC/MCC Exc

I69.854　Hemiplegia and hemiparesis following other cerebrovascular disease affecting left non-dominant side cc ⓟₒₐ HCC CC/MCC Exc

I69.859　Hemiplegia and hemiparesis following other cerebrovascular disease affecting unspecified side cc ⓟₒₐ HCC CC/MCC Exc

Ⓖ I69.86　Other paralytic syndrome following other cerebrovascular disease

Use additional code to identify type of paralytic syndrome, such as:

locked-in state (G83.5)

quadriplegia (G82.5-)

EXCLUDES1　hemiplegia/hemiparesis following other cerebrovascular disease (I69.85-)

monoplegia of lower limb following other cerebrovascular disease (I69.84-)

monoplegia of upper limb following other cerebrovascular disease (I69.83-)

I69.861　Other paralytic syndrome following other cerebrovascular disease affecting right dominant side ⓟₒₐ HCC

I69.862　Other paralytic syndrome following other cerebrovascular disease affecting left dominant side ⓟₒₐ HCC

I69.863　Other paralytic syndrome following other cerebrovascular disease affecting right non-dominant side ⓟₒₐ HCC

I69.864　Other paralytic syndrome following other cerebrovascular disease affecting left non-dominant side ⓟₒₐ HCC

I69.865　Other paralytic syndrome following other cerebrovascular disease, bilateral ⓟₒₐ HCC

I69.869　Other paralytic syndrome following other cerebrovascular disease affecting unspecified side ⓟₒₐ HCC

Ⓖ I69.89　Other sequelae of other cerebrovascular disease

I69.890　Apraxia following other cerebrovascular disease ⓟₒₐ

I69.891　Dysphagia following other cerebrovascular disease ⓟₒₐ

Use additional code to identify the type of dysphagia, if known (R13.1-)

I69.892　Facial weakness following other cerebrovascular disease ⓟₒₐ

Facial droop following other cerebrovascular disease

I69.893　Ataxia following other cerebrovascular disease ⓟₒₐ

I69.898　Other sequelae of other cerebrovascular disease ⓟₒₐ

Alteration of sensation following other cerebrovascular disease

Disturbance of vision following other cerebrovascular disease

Use additional code to identify the sequelae

Ⓖ I69.9　Sequelae of unspecified cerebrovascular diseases

EXCLUDES1　sequelae of stroke (I69.3)

sequelae of traumatic intracranial injury (S06.-)

I69.90　Unspecified sequelae of unspecified cerebrovascular disease ⓟₒₐ

Ⓖ I69.91　Cognitive deficits following unspecified cerebrovascular disease

I69.910　Attention and concentration deficit following unspecified cerebrovascular disease

I69.911　Memory deficit following unspecified cerebrovascular disease

I69.912　Visuospatial deficit and spatial neglect following unspecified cerebrovascular disease

I69.913　Psychomotor deficit following unspecified cerebrovascular disease

I69.914　Frontal lobe and executive function deficit following unspecified cerebrovascular disease

I69.915　Cognitive social or emotional deficit following unspecified cerebrovascular disease

I69.918　Other symptoms and signs involving cognitive functions following unspecified cerebrovascular disease

I69.919　Unspecified symptoms and signs involving cognitive functions following unspecified cerebrovascular disease

Ⓖ I69.92　Speech and language deficits following unspecified cerebrovascular disease

I69.920　Aphasia following unspecified cerebrovascular disease ⓟₒₐ

I69.921　Dysphasia following unspecified cerebrovascular disease ⓟₒₐ

I69.922　Dysarthria following unspecified cerebrovascular disease ⓟₒₐ

I69.923　Fluency disorder following unspecified cerebrovascular disease ⓟₒₐ

Stuttering following unspecified cerebrovascular disease

I69.928　Other speech and language deficits following unspecified cerebrovascular disease ⓟₒₐ

Ⓖ I69.93　Monoplegia of upper limb following unspecified cerebrovascular disease

I69.931　Monoplegia of upper limb following unspecified cerebrovascular disease affecting right dominant side ⓟₒₐ HCC

I69.932　Monoplegia of upper limb following unspecified cerebrovascular disease affecting left dominant side ⓟₒₐ HCC

I69.933　Monoplegia of upper limb following unspecified cerebrovascular disease affecting right non-dominant side ⓟₒₐ HCC

I69.934　Monoplegia of upper limb following unspecified cerebrovascular disease affecting left non-dominant side ⓟₒₐ HCC

ⓟᴰⁿ Unacceptable principal diagnosis symbol per Medicare code edits　ⓟₒₐ Code exempt from diagnosis present on admission requirement
❓ Questionable admission　cc Complication or comorbidity　MCC Major complication or comorbidity　CC/MCC Exc CC/MCC exclusion
HCC HCC diagnosis code　RxHCC RxHCC diagnosis code　MACRA MACRA code　DEFINITION Describes condition/terminology
TIP Coding guidance　👁 Official Guideline Reference　Z1 Z code as first-listed diagnosis

I69.939 **Monoplegia of upper limb following unspecified cerebrovascular disease affecting unspecified side** POA HCC

6ᵗʰ I69.94 Monoplegia of lower limb following unspecified cerebrovascular disease

I69.941 **Monoplegia of lower limb following unspecified cerebrovascular disease affecting** right dominant side POA HCC

I69.942 **Monoplegia of lower limb following unspecified cerebrovascular disease affecting** left dominant side POA HCC

I69.943 **Monoplegia of lower limb following unspecified cerebrovascular disease affecting** right non-dominant side POA HCC

I69.944 **Monoplegia of lower limb following unspecified cerebrovascular disease affecting** left non-dominant side POA HCC

I69.949 **Monoplegia of lower limb following unspecified cerebrovascular disease affecting** unspecified side POA HCC

6ᵗʰ I69.95 Hemiplegia and hemiparesis following unspecified cerebrovascular disease

I69.951 **Hemiplegia and hemiparesis following unspecified cerebrovascular disease affecting** right dominant side CC POA HCC CC/MCC Exc

I69.952 **Hemiplegia and hemiparesis following unspecified cerebrovascular disease affecting** left dominant side CC POA HCC CC/MCC Exc

I69.953 **Hemiplegia and hemiparesis following unspecified cerebrovascular disease affecting** right non-dominant side CC POA HCC CC/MCC Exc

I69.954 **Hemiplegia and hemiparesis following unspecified cerebrovascular disease affecting** left non-dominant side CC POA HCC CC/MCC Exc

I69.959 **Hemiplegia and hemiparesis following unspecified cerebrovascular disease affecting** unspecified side CC POA HCC CC/MCC Exc

6ᵗʰ I69.96 Other paralytic syndrome following unspecified cerebrovascular disease

Use additional code to identify type of paralytic syndrome, such as:
locked-in state (G83.5)
quadriplegia (G82.5-)

EXCLUDES1 hemiplegia/hemiparesis following unspecified cerebrovascular disease (I69.95-)

monoplegia of lower limb following unspecified cerebrovascular disease (I69.94-)

monoplegia of upper limb following unspecified cerebrovascular disease (I69.93-)

I69.961 **Other paralytic syndrome following unspecified cerebrovascular disease affecting** right dominant side POA HCC

I69.962 **Other paralytic syndrome following unspecified cerebrovascular disease affecting** left dominant side POA HCC

I69.963 **Other paralytic syndrome following unspecified cerebrovascular disease affecting** right non-dominant side POA HCC

I69.964 **Other paralytic syndrome following unspecified cerebrovascular disease affecting** left non-dominant side POA HCC

I69.965 **Other paralytic syndrome following unspecified cerebrovascular disease,** bilateral POA HCC

I69.969 **Other paralytic syndrome following unspecified cerebrovascular disease affecting** unspecified side POA HCC

6ᵗʰ I69.99 Other sequelae of unspecified cerebrovascular disease

I69.990 Apraxia following unspecified cerebrovascular disease POA

I69.991 Dysphagia following unspecified cerebrovascular disease POA

Use additional code to identify the type of dysphagia, if known (R13.1-)

I69.992 **Facial weakness following unspecified cerebrovascular disease** POA

Facial droop following unspecified cerebrovascular disease

I69.993 Ataxia following unspecified cerebrovascular disease POA

I69.998 Other sequelae following unspecified cerebrovascular disease POA

Alteration in sensation following unspecified cerebrovascular disease
Disturbance of vision following unspecified cerebrovascular disease

Use additional code to identify the sequelae

Diseases of arteries, arterioles and capillaries (I70-I79)

4ᵗʰ **I70 Atherosclerosis (Figure 9.5)**

INCLUDES arteriolosclerosis
arterial degeneration
arteriosclerosis
arteriosclerotic vascular disease
arteriovascular degeneration
atheroma
endarteritis deformans or obliterans
senile arteritis
senile endarteritis
vascular degeneration

Use additional code to identify:
exposure to environmental tobacco smoke (Z77.22)
history of tobacco dependence (Z87.891)
occupational exposure to environmental tobacco smoke (Z57.31)
tobacco dependence (F17.-)
tobacco use (Z72.0)

EXCLUDES2 arteriosclerotic cardiovascular disease (I25.1-)
arteriosclerotic heart disease (I25.1-)
atheroembolism (I75.-)
cerebral atherosclerosis (I67.2)
coronary atherosclerosis (I25.1-)
mesenteric atherosclerosis (K55.1)
precerebral atherosclerosis (I67.2)
primary pulmonary atherosclerosis (I27.0)

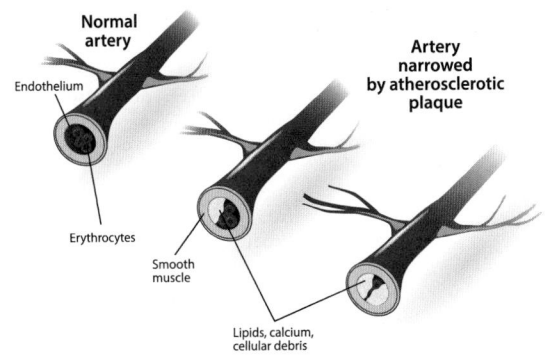

Figure 9.5 Atherosclerosis

Unspecified Code   Other Specified Code   Manifestation Code   Ⓝ Newborn   Ⓟ Pediatric   Ⓜ Maternity   Ⓐ Adult   ♂ Male   ♀ Female
● New Code   ▲ Revised Code Title   ►◄ Revised Text   NOTES   INCLUDES   EXCLUDES1 Not coded here   EXCLUDES2 Not included here
4ᵗʰ 4ᵗʰ character required   5ᵗʰ 5ᵗʰ character required   6ᵗʰ 6ᵗʰ character required   7ᵗʰ 7ᵗʰ character required   Extension 'X' Alert
HAC Hospital-acquired condition (HAC) alert   AHA AHA Coding Clinic©   ☞ Code first alert

2020 ICD-10-CM   When symbols appear on a code that requires a 7th character extension, refer to Appendix B to identify applicable 7th character codes.   **677**

I69.939 - I70

CHAPTER 9: DISEASES OF THE CIRCULATORY SYSTEM (I00-I99)

I70.0 Atherosclerosis of aorta 🅰 HCC RxHCC
I70.1 Atherosclerosis of renal artery 🅰 HCC RxHCC
Goldblatt's kidney
EXCLUDES2 atherosclerosis of renal arterioles (I12.-)
5ᵗʰ **I70.2** Atherosclerosis of native arteries of the extremities
Mönckeberg's (medial) sclerosis
Use additional code, if applicable, to identify chronic total occlusion of artery of extremity (I70.92)
EXCLUDES2 atherosclerosis of bypass graft of extremities (I70.30-I70.79)

6ᵗʰ **I70.20** Unspecified atherosclerosis of native arteries of extremities
I70.201 Unspecified atherosclerosis of native arteries of extremities, right leg 🅰 HCC RxHCC
I70.202 Unspecified atherosclerosis of native arteries of extremities, left leg 🅰 HCC RxHCC
I70.203 Unspecified atherosclerosis of native arteries of extremities, bilateral legs 🅰 HCC RxHCC
I70.208 Unspecified atherosclerosis of native arteries of extremities, other extremity 🅰 HCC RxHCC
I70.209 Unspecified atherosclerosis of native arteries of extremities, unspecified extremity 🅰 HCC RxHCC

6ᵗʰ **I70.21** Atherosclerosis of native arteries of extremities with intermittent claudication
I70.211 Atherosclerosis of native arteries of extremities with intermittent claudication, right leg 🅰 HCC RxHCC
I70.212 Atherosclerosis of native arteries of extremities with intermittent claudication, left leg 🅰 HCC RxHCC
I70.213 Atherosclerosis of native arteries of extremities with intermittent claudication, bilateral legs 🅰 HCC RxHCC
I70.218 Atherosclerosis of native arteries of extremities with intermittent claudication, other extremity 🅰 HCC RxHCC
I70.219 Atherosclerosis of native arteries of extremities with intermittent claudication, unspecified extremity 🅰 HCC RxHCC

6ᵗʰ **I70.22** Atherosclerosis of native arteries of extremities with rest pain
INCLUDES any condition classifiable to I70.21-
I70.221 Atherosclerosis of native arteries of extremities with rest pain, right leg 🅰 HCC RxHCC
I70.222 Atherosclerosis of native arteries of extremities with rest pain, left leg 🅰 HCC RxHCC
I70.223 Atherosclerosis of native arteries of extremities with rest pain, bilateral legs 🅰 HCC RxHCC
I70.228 Atherosclerosis of native arteries of extremities with rest pain, other extremity 🅰 HCC RxHCC
I70.229 Atherosclerosis of native arteries of extremities with rest pain, unspecified extremity 🅰 HCC RxHCC

6ᵗʰ **I70.23** Atherosclerosis of native arteries of right leg with ulceration
INCLUDES any condition classifiable to I70.211 and I70.221
Use additional code to identify severity of ulcer (L97.-)
I70.231 Atherosclerosis of native arteries of right leg with ulceration of thigh 🅰 HCC RxHCC
I70.232 Atherosclerosis of native arteries of right leg with ulceration of calf 🅰 HCC RxHCC
I70.233 Atherosclerosis of native arteries of right leg with ulceration of ankle 🅰 HCC RxHCC

I70.234 Atherosclerosis of native arteries of right leg with ulceration of heel and midfoot 🅰 HCC RxHCC
Atherosclerosis of native arteries of right leg with ulceration of plantar surface of midfoot
I70.235 Atherosclerosis of native arteries of right leg with ulceration of other part of foot 🅰 HCC RxHCC
Atherosclerosis of native arteries of right leg extremities with ulceration of toe
▲ **I70.238** Atherosclerosis of native arteries of right leg with ulceration of other part of lower leg 🅰 HCC RxHCC
I70.239 Atherosclerosis of native arteries of right leg with ulceration of unspecified site 🅰 HCC RxHCC

6ᵗʰ **I70.24** Atherosclerosis of native arteries of left leg with ulceration
INCLUDES any condition classifiable to I70.212 and I70.222
Use additional code to identify severity of ulcer (L97.-)
I70.241 Atherosclerosis of native arteries of left leg with ulceration of thigh 🅰 HCC RxHCC
I70.242 Atherosclerosis of native arteries of left leg with ulceration of calf 🅰 HCC RxHCC
I70.243 Atherosclerosis of native arteries of left leg with ulceration of ankle 🅰 HCC RxHCC
I70.244 Atherosclerosis of native arteries of left leg with ulceration of heel and midfoot 🅰 HCC RxHCC
Atherosclerosis of native arteries of left leg with ulceration of plantar surface of midfoot
I70.245 Atherosclerosis of native arteries of left leg with ulceration of other part of foot 🅰 HCC RxHCC
Atherosclerosis of native arteries of left leg extremities with ulceration of toe
▲ **I70.248** Atherosclerosis of native arteries of left leg with ulceration of other part of lower leg 🅰 HCC RxHCC
I70.249 Atherosclerosis of native arteries of left leg with ulceration of unspecified site 🅰 HCC RxHCC

I70.25 Atherosclerosis of native arteries of other extremities with ulceration 🅰 HCC RxHCC
INCLUDES any condition classifiable to I70.218 and I70.228
Use additional code to identify the severity of the ulcer (L98.49-)

6ᵗʰ **I70.26** Atherosclerosis of native arteries of extremities with gangrene
INCLUDES any condition classifiable to I70.21-, I70.22-, I70.23-, I70.24-, and I70.25-
Use additional code to identify the severity of any ulcer (L97.-, L98.49-), if applicable
I70.261 Atherosclerosis of native arteries of extremities with gangrene, right leg 🅰 cc HCC cc/mcc exc
I70.262 Atherosclerosis of native arteries of extremities with gangrene, left leg 🅰 cc HCC cc/mcc exc
I70.263 Atherosclerosis of native arteries of extremities with gangrene, bilateral legs 🅰 cc HCC cc/mcc exc
I70.268 Atherosclerosis of native arteries of extremities with gangrene, other extremity 🅰 cc HCC cc/mcc exc
I70.269 Atherosclerosis of native arteries of extremities with gangrene, unspecified extremity 🅰 cc HCC cc/mcc exc

---

PDxⁿ Unacceptable principal diagnosis symbol per Medicare code edits   PDx Code exempt from diagnosis present on admission requirement
❓ Questionable admission   cc Complication or comorbidity   MCC Major complication or comorbidity   cc/mcc exc CC/MCC exclusion
HCC HCC diagnosis code   RxHCC RxHCC diagnosis code   MACRA MACRA code   **DEFINITION** Describes condition/terminology
TIP Coding guidance   👁 Official Guideline Reference   Z1 Z code as first-listed diagnosis

When symbols appear on a code that requires a 7th character extension, refer to Appendix B to identify applicable 7th character codes.
2020 ICD-10-CM

⑥ I70.29 Other atherosclerosis of native arteries of extremities

    I70.291 **Other atherosclerosis of native arteries of extremities, right leg** 🅰 HCC RxHCC

    I70.292 **Other atherosclerosis of native arteries of extremities, left leg** 🅰 HCC RxHCC

    I70.293 **Other atherosclerosis of native arteries of extremities, bilateral legs** 🅰 HCC RxHCC

    I70.298 **Other atherosclerosis of native arteries of extremities, other extremity** 🅰 HCC RxHCC

    I70.299 **Other atherosclerosis of native arteries of extremities, unspecified extremity** 🅰 HCC RxHCC

⑤ I70.3 Atherosclerosis of unspecified type of bypass graft(s) of the extremities

    Use additional code, if applicable, to identify chronic total occlusion of artery of extremity (I70.92)

    EXCLUDES1 embolism or thrombus of bypass graft(s) of extremities (T82.8-)

    ⑥ I70.30 Unspecified atherosclerosis of unspecified type of bypass graft(s) of the extremities

        I70.301 **Unspecified atherosclerosis of unspecified type of bypass graft(s) of the extremities, right leg** 🅰 HCC RxHCC

        I70.302 **Unspecified atherosclerosis of unspecified type of bypass graft(s) of the extremities, left leg** 🅰 HCC RxHCC

        I70.303 **Unspecified atherosclerosis of unspecified type of bypass graft(s) of the extremities, bilateral legs** 🅰 HCC RxHCC

        I70.308 **Unspecified atherosclerosis of unspecified type of bypass graft(s) of the extremities, other extremity** 🅰 HCC RxHCC

        I70.309 **Unspecified atherosclerosis of unspecified type of bypass graft(s) of the extremities, unspecified extremity** 🅰 HCC RxHCC

    ⑥ I70.31 Atherosclerosis of unspecified type of bypass graft(s) of the extremities with intermittent claudication

        I70.311 **Atherosclerosis of unspecified type of bypass graft(s) of the extremities with intermittent claudication, right leg** 🅰 HCC RxHCC

        I70.312 **Atherosclerosis of unspecified type of bypass graft(s) of the extremities with intermittent claudication, left leg** 🅰 HCC RxHCC

        I70.313 **Atherosclerosis of unspecified type of bypass graft(s) of the extremities with intermittent claudication, bilateral legs** 🅰 HCC RxHCC

        I70.318 **Atherosclerosis of unspecified type of bypass graft(s) of the extremities with intermittent claudication, other extremity** 🅰 HCC RxHCC

        I70.319 **Atherosclerosis of unspecified type of bypass graft(s) of the extremities with intermittent claudication, unspecified extremity** 🅰 HCC RxHCC

    ⑥ I70.32 Atherosclerosis of unspecified type of bypass graft(s) of the extremities with rest pain

        INCLUDES any condition classifiable to I70.31-

        I70.321 **Atherosclerosis of unspecified type of bypass graft(s) of the extremities with rest pain, right leg** 🅰 HCC RxHCC

        I70.322 **Atherosclerosis of unspecified type of bypass graft(s) of the extremities with rest pain, left leg** 🅰 HCC RxHCC

        I70.323 **Atherosclerosis of unspecified type of bypass graft(s) of the extremities with rest pain, bilateral legs** 🅰 HCC RxHCC

        I70.328 **Atherosclerosis of unspecified type of bypass graft(s) of the extremities with rest pain, other extremity** 🅰 HCC RxHCC

    I70.329 **Atherosclerosis of unspecified type of bypass graft(s) of the extremities with rest pain, unspecified extremity** 🅰 HCC RxHCC

⑥ I70.33 Atherosclerosis of unspecified type of bypass graft(s) of the right leg with ulceration

    INCLUDES any condition classifiable to I70.311 and I70.321

    Use additional code to identify severity of ulcer (L97.-)

    I70.331 **Atherosclerosis of unspecified type of bypass graft(s) of the right leg with ulceration of thigh** 🅰 CC HCC RxHCC CC/MCC Exc

    I70.332 **Atherosclerosis of unspecified type of bypass graft(s) of the right leg with ulceration of calf** 🅰 CC HCC RxHCC CC/MCC Exc

    I70.333 **Atherosclerosis of unspecified type of bypass graft(s) of the right leg with ulceration of ankle** 🅰 CC HCC RxHCC CC/MCC Exc

    I70.334 **Atherosclerosis of unspecified type of bypass graft(s) of the right leg with ulceration of heel and midfoot** 🅰 CC HCC RxHCC CC/MCC Exc

        Atherosclerosis of unspecified type of bypass graft(s) of right leg with ulceration of plantar surface of midfoot

    I70.335 **Atherosclerosis of unspecified type of bypass graft(s) of the right leg with ulceration of other part of foot** 🅰 HCC RxHCC

        Atherosclerosis of unspecified type of bypass graft(s) of the right leg with ulceration of toe

    I70.338 **Atherosclerosis of unspecified type of bypass graft(s) of the right leg with ulceration of other part of lower leg** 🅰 CC HCC RxHCC CC/MCC Exc

    I70.339 **Atherosclerosis of unspecified type of bypass graft(s) of the right leg with ulceration of unspecified site** 🅰 CC HCC RxHCC CC/MCC Exc

⑥ I70.34 Atherosclerosis of unspecified type of bypass graft(s) of the left leg with ulceration

    INCLUDES any condition classifiable to I70.312 and I70.322

    Use additional code to identify severity of ulcer (L97.-)

    I70.341 **Atherosclerosis of unspecified type of bypass graft(s) of the left leg with ulceration of thigh** 🅰 CC HCC RxHCC CC/MCC Exc

    I70.342 **Atherosclerosis of unspecified type of bypass graft(s) of the left leg with ulceration of calf** 🅰 CC HCC RxHCC CC/MCC Exc

    I70.343 **Atherosclerosis of unspecified type of bypass graft(s) of the left leg with ulceration of ankle** 🅰 CC HCC RxHCC CC/MCC Exc

    I70.344 **Atherosclerosis of unspecified type of bypass graft(s) of the left leg with ulceration of heel and midfoot** 🅰 CC HCC RxHCC CC/MCC Exc

        Atherosclerosis of unspecified type of bypass graft(s) of left leg with ulceration of plantar surface of midfoot

    I70.345 **Atherosclerosis of unspecified type of bypass graft(s) of the left leg with ulceration of other part of foot** 🅰 HCC RxHCC

        Atherosclerosis of unspecified type of bypass graft(s) of the left leg with ulceration of toe

    I70.348 **Atherosclerosis of unspecified type of bypass graft(s) of the left leg with ulceration of other part of lower leg** 🅰 CC HCC RxHCC CC/MCC Exc

    I70.349 **Atherosclerosis of unspecified type of bypass graft(s) of the left leg with ulceration of unspecified site** 🅰 CC HCC RxHCC CC/MCC Exc

---

Unspecified Code Other Specified Code Manifestation Code Ⓝ Newborn Ⓟ Pediatric Ⓜ Maternity 🅰 Adult ♂ Male ♀ Female
● New Code ▲ Revised Code Title ▶◀ Revised Text **NOTES** *INCLUDES* *EXCLUDES1* Not coded here *EXCLUDES2* Not included here
④ 4th character required ⑤ 5th character required ⑥ 6th character required ⑦ 7th character required Extension 'X' Alert
HAC Hospital-acquired condition (HAC) alert **AHA** AHA Coding Clinic® 📧 Code first alert

I70.35 **Atherosclerosis of unspecified type of bypass graft(s) of other extremity with ulceration** A HCC RxHCC
INCLUDES   any condition classifiable to I70.318 and I70.328
Use additional code to identify severity of ulcer (L98.49-)

6ᵗʰ I70.36 **Atherosclerosis of unspecified type of bypass graft(s) of the extremities** with gangrene
INCLUDES   any condition classifiable to I70.31-, I70.32-, I70.33-, I70.34-, I70.35
Use additional code to identify the severity of any ulcer (L97.-, L98.49-), if applicable

I70.361 **Atherosclerosis of unspecified type of bypass graft(s) of the extremities with gangrene,** right leg A cc HCC CC/MCC Exc

I70.362 **Atherosclerosis of unspecified type of bypass graft(s) of the extremities with gangrene,** left leg A cc HCC CC/MCC Exc

I70.363 **Atherosclerosis of unspecified type of bypass graft(s) of the extremities with gangrene,** bilateral legs A cc HCC CC/MCC Exc

I70.368 **Atherosclerosis of unspecified type of bypass graft(s) of the extremities with gangrene,** other extremity A cc HCC CC/MCC Exc

I70.369 **Atherosclerosis of unspecified type of bypass graft(s) of the extremities with gangrene, unspecified extremity** A cc HCC CC/MCC Exc

6ᵗʰ I70.39 Other **atherosclerosis of unspecified type of bypass graft(s) of the extremities**

I70.391 **Other atherosclerosis of unspecified type of bypass graft(s) of the extremities,** right leg A HCC RxHCC

I70.392 **Other atherosclerosis of unspecified type of bypass graft(s) of the extremities,** left leg A HCC RxHCC

I70.393 **Other atherosclerosis of unspecified type of bypass graft(s) of the extremities,** bilateral legs A HCC RxHCC

I70.398 **Other atherosclerosis of unspecified type of bypass graft(s) of the extremities,** other extremity A HCC RxHCC

I70.399 **Other atherosclerosis of unspecified type of bypass graft(s) of the extremities, unspecified extremity** A HCC RxHCC

5ᵗʰ I70.4 **Atherosclerosis of** autologous vein bypass graft(s) of the extremities
Use additional code, if applicable, to identify chronic total occlusion of artery of extremity (I70.92)

6ᵗʰ I70.40 Unspecified **atherosclerosis of autologous vein bypass graft(s) of the extremities**

I70.401 **Unspecified atherosclerosis of autologous vein bypass graft(s) of the extremities,** right leg A HCC RxHCC

I70.402 **Unspecified atherosclerosis of autologous vein bypass graft(s) of the extremities,** left leg A HCC RxHCC

I70.403 **Unspecified atherosclerosis of autologous vein bypass graft(s) of the extremities,** bilateral legs A HCC RxHCC

I70.408 **Unspecified atherosclerosis of autologous vein bypass graft(s) of the extremities,** other extremity A HCC RxHCC

I70.409 **Unspecified atherosclerosis of autologous vein bypass graft(s) of the extremities, unspecified extremity** A HCC RxHCC

5ᵗʰ I70.41 **Atherosclerosis of autologous vein bypass graft(s) of the extremities** with intermittent claudication

I70.411 **Atherosclerosis of autologous vein bypass graft(s) of the extremities with intermittent claudication,** right leg A HCC RxHCC

I70.412 **Atherosclerosis of autologous vein bypass graft(s) of the extremities with intermittent claudication,** left leg A HCC RxHCC

I70.413 **Atherosclerosis of autologous vein bypass graft(s) of the extremities with intermittent claudication,** bilateral legs A HCC RxHCC

I70.418 **Atherosclerosis of autologous vein bypass graft(s) of the extremities with intermittent claudication, other extremity** A HCC RxHCC

I70.419 **Atherosclerosis of autologous vein bypass graft(s) of the extremities with intermittent claudication, unspecified extremity** A HCC RxHCC

6ᵗʰ I70.42 **Atherosclerosis of autologous vein bypass graft(s) of the extremities** with rest pain
INCLUDES   any condition classifiable to I70.41-

I70.421 **Atherosclerosis of autologous vein bypass graft(s) of the extremities with rest pain,** right leg A HCC RxHCC

I70.422 **Atherosclerosis of autologous vein bypass graft(s) of the extremities with rest pain,** left leg A HCC RxHCC

I70.423 **Atherosclerosis of autologous vein bypass graft(s) of the extremities with rest pain,** bilateral legs A HCC RxHCC

I70.428 **Atherosclerosis of autologous vein bypass graft(s) of the extremities with rest pain,** other extremity A HCC RxHCC

I70.429 **Atherosclerosis of autologous vein bypass graft(s) of the extremities with rest pain, unspecified extremity** A HCC RxHCC

6ᵗʰ I70.43 **Atherosclerosis of autologous vein bypass graft(s) of the** right leg with ulceration
INCLUDES   any condition classifiable to I70.411 and I70.421
Use additional code to identify severity of ulcer (L97.-)

I70.431 **Atherosclerosis of autologous vein bypass graft(s) of the** right leg **with ulceration of** thigh A cc HCC RxHCC CC/MCC Exc

I70.432 **Atherosclerosis of autologous vein bypass graft(s) of the** right leg **with ulceration of** calf A cc HCC RxHCC CC/MCC Exc

I70.433 **Atherosclerosis of autologous vein bypass graft(s) of the** right leg **with ulceration of** ankle A cc HCC RxHCC CC/MCC Exc

I70.434 **Atherosclerosis of autologous vein bypass graft(s) of the** right leg **with ulceration of** heel and midfoot A cc HCC RxHCC CC/MCC Exc
Atherosclerosis of autologous vein bypass graft(s) of right leg with ulceration of plantar surface of midfoot

I70.435 **Atherosclerosis of autologous vein bypass graft(s) of the** right leg **with ulceration of** other part of foot A HCC RxHCC
Atherosclerosis of autologous vein bypass graft(s) of right leg with ulceration of toe

I70.438 **Atherosclerosis of autologous vein bypass graft(s) of the** right leg **with ulceration of** other part of lower leg A cc HCC RxHCC CC/MCC Exc

I70.439 **Atherosclerosis of autologous vein bypass graft(s) of the** right leg **with ulceration of** unspecified site A cc HCC RxHCC CC/MCC Exc

6ᵗʰ I70.44 **Atherosclerosis of autologous vein bypass graft(s) of the** left leg with ulceration
INCLUDES   any condition classifiable to I70.412 and I70.422
Use additional code to identify severity of ulcer (L97.-)

I70.441 **Atherosclerosis of autologous vein bypass graft(s) of the** left leg **with ulceration of** thigh A cc HCC RxHCC CC/MCC Exc

PDxR Unacceptable principal diagnosis symbol per Medicare code edits   ⚑ Code exempt from diagnosis present on admission requirement
❓ Questionable admission   cc Complication or comorbidity   MCC Major complication or comorbidity   CC/MCC Exc CC/MCC exclusion
HCC HCC diagnosis code   RxHCC RxHCC diagnosis code   MACRA code   **DEFINITION** Describes condition/terminology
TIP Coding guidance   👁 Official Guideline Reference   Z1 Z code as first-listed diagnosis

680   When symbols appear on a code that requires a 7th character extension, refer to Appendix B to identify applicable 7th character codes.   **2020 ICD-10-CM**

I70.442   Atherosclerosis of autologous vein bypass graft(s) of the left leg with ulceration of calf   **A** cc⊘ HCC RxHCC CC/MCC Exc

I70.443   Atherosclerosis of autologous vein bypass graft(s) of the left leg with ulceration of ankle   **A** cc⊘ HCC RxHCC CC/MCC Exc

I70.444   Atherosclerosis of autologous vein bypass graft(s) of the left leg with ulceration of heel and midfoot   **A** cc⊘ HCC RxHCC CC/MCC Exc

Atherosclerosis of autologous vein bypass graft(s) of left leg with ulceration of plantar surface of midfoot

I70.445   Atherosclerosis of autologous vein bypass graft(s) of the left leg with ulceration of other part of foot   **A** HCC RxHCC

Atherosclerosis of autologous vein bypass graft(s) of left leg with ulceration of toe

I70.448   Atherosclerosis of autologous vein bypass graft(s) of the left leg with ulceration of other part of lower leg   **A** cc⊘ HCC RxHCC CC/MCC Exc

I70.449   Atherosclerosis of autologous vein bypass graft(s) of the left leg with ulceration of unspecified site   **A** cc⊘ HCC RxHCC CC/MCC Exc

I70.45   Atherosclerosis of autologous vein bypass graft(s) of other extremity with ulceration   **A** HCC RxHCC

    INCLUDES   any condition classifiable to I70.418, I70.428, and I70.438

    Use additional code to identify severity of ulcer (L98.49)

6th I70.46   Atherosclerosis of autologous vein bypass graft(s) of the extremities with gangrene

    INCLUDES   any condition classifiable to I70.41-, I70.42-, and I70.43-, I70.44-, I70.45

    Use additional code to identify the severity of any ulcer (L97.-, L98.49-), if applicable

I70.461   Atherosclerosis of autologous vein bypass graft(s) of the extremities with gangrene, right leg   **A** cc⊘ HCC CC/MCC Exc

I70.462   Atherosclerosis of autologous vein bypass graft(s) of the extremities with gangrene, left leg   **A** cc⊘ HCC CC/MCC Exc

I70.463   Atherosclerosis of autologous vein bypass graft(s) of the extremities with gangrene, bilateral legs   **A** cc⊘ HCC CC/MCC Exc

I70.468   Atherosclerosis of autologous vein bypass graft(s) of the extremities with gangrene, other extremity   **A** cc⊘ HCC CC/MCC Exc

I70.469   Atherosclerosis of autologous vein bypass graft(s) of the extremities with gangrene, unspecified extremity   **A** cc⊘ HCC CC/MCC Exc

6th I70.49   Other atherosclerosis of autologous vein bypass graft(s) of the extremities

I70.491   Other atherosclerosis of autologous vein bypass graft(s) of the extremities, right leg   **A** HCC RxHCC

I70.492   Other atherosclerosis of autologous vein bypass graft(s) of the extremities, left leg   **A** HCC RxHCC

I70.493   Other atherosclerosis of autologous vein bypass graft(s) of the extremities, bilateral legs   **A** HCC RxHCC

I70.498   Other atherosclerosis of autologous vein bypass graft(s) of the extremities, other extremity   **A** HCC RxHCC

I70.499   Other atherosclerosis of autologous vein bypass graft(s) of the extremities, unspecified extremity   **A** HCC RxHCC

5th I70.5   Atherosclerosis of nonautologous biological bypass graft(s) of the extremities

    Use additional code, if applicable, to identify chronic total occlusion of artery of extremity (I70.92)

6th I70.50   Unspecified atherosclerosis of nonautologous biological bypass graft(s) of the extremities

I70.501   Unspecified atherosclerosis of nonautologous biological bypass graft(s) of the extremities, right leg   **A** HCC RxHCC

I70.502   Unspecified atherosclerosis of nonautologous biological bypass graft(s) of the extremities, left leg   **A** HCC RxHCC

I70.503   Unspecified atherosclerosis of nonautologous biological bypass graft(s) of the extremities, bilateral legs   **A** HCC RxHCC

I70.508   Unspecified atherosclerosis of nonautologous biological bypass graft(s) of the extremities, other extremity   **A** HCC RxHCC

I70.509   Unspecified atherosclerosis of nonautologous biological bypass graft(s) of the extremities, unspecified extremity   **A** HCC RxHCC

6th I70.51   Atherosclerosis of nonautologous biological bypass graft(s) of the extremities intermittent claudication

I70.511   Atherosclerosis of nonautologous biological bypass graft(s) of the extremities with intermittent claudication, right leg   **A** HCC RxHCC

I70.512   Atherosclerosis of nonautologous biological bypass graft(s) of the extremities with intermittent claudication, left leg   **A** HCC RxHCC

I70.513   Atherosclerosis of nonautologous biological bypass graft(s) of the extremities with intermittent claudication, bilateral legs   **A** HCC RxHCC

I70.518   Atherosclerosis of nonautologous biological bypass graft(s) of the extremities with intermittent claudication, other extremity   **A** HCC RxHCC

I70.519   Atherosclerosis of nonautologous biological bypass graft(s) of the extremities with intermittent claudication, unspecified extremity   **A** HCC RxHCC

6th I70.52   Atherosclerosis of nonautologous biological bypass graft(s) of the extremities with rest pain

    INCLUDES   any condition classifiable to I70.51-

I70.521   Atherosclerosis of nonautologous biological bypass graft(s) of the extremities with rest pain, right leg   **A** HCC RxHCC

I70.522   Atherosclerosis of nonautologous biological bypass graft(s) of the extremities with rest pain, left leg   **A** HCC RxHCC

I70.523   Atherosclerosis of nonautologous biological bypass graft(s) of the extremities with rest pain, bilateral legs   **A** HCC RxHCC

I70.528   Atherosclerosis of nonautologous biological bypass graft(s) of the extremities with rest pain, other extremity   **A** HCC RxHCC

I70.529   Atherosclerosis of nonautologous biological bypass graft(s) of the extremities with rest pain, unspecified extremity   **A** HCC RxHCC

6th I70.53   Atherosclerosis of nonautologous biological bypass graft(s) of the right leg with ulceration

    INCLUDES   any condition classifiable to I70.511 and I70.521

    Use additional code to identify severity of ulcer (L97.-)

I70.531   Atherosclerosis of nonautologous biological bypass graft(s) of the right leg with ulceration of thigh   **A** cc⊘ HCC RxHCC CC/MCC Exc

I70.532   Atherosclerosis of nonautologous biological bypass graft(s) of the right leg with ulceration of calf   **A** cc⊘ HCC RxHCC CC/MCC Exc

---

Unspecified Code   Other Specified Code   Manifestation Code   **N** Newborn   **P** Pediatric   **M** Maternity   **A** Adult   ♂ Male   ♀ Female
● New Code   ▲ Revised Code Title   ►◄ Revised Text   **NOTES**   *INCLUDES*   *EXCLUDES1* Not coded here   *EXCLUDES2* Not included here
   4th 4th character required   5th 5th character required   6th 6th character required   7th 7th character required   ⊘ Extension 'X' Alert
   HAC Hospital-acquired condition (HAC) alert   **AHA** AHA Coding Clinic©   ☛ Code first alert

I70.533   **Atherosclerosis of nonautologous biological bypass graft(s) of the** right leg **with ulceration of** ankle   A cc HCC RxHCC CC/MCC Exc

I70.534   **Atherosclerosis of nonautologous biological bypass graft(s) of the** right leg **with ulceration of** heel and midfoot   A cc HCC RxHCC CC/MCC Exc

Atherosclerosis of nonautologous biological bypass graft(s) of right leg with ulceration of plantar surface of midfoot

I70.535   **Atherosclerosis of nonautologous biological bypass graft(s) of the** right leg **with ulceration of** other part of foot   A HCC RxHCC

Atherosclerosis of nonautologous biological bypass graft(s) of the right leg with ulceration of toe

I70.538   **Atherosclerosis of nonautologous biological bypass graft(s) of the** right leg **with ulceration of other part of lower leg**   A cc HCC RxHCC CC/MCC Exc

I70.539   **Atherosclerosis of nonautologous biological bypass graft(s) of the** right leg **with ulceration of unspecified site**   A cc HCC RxHCC CC/MCC Exc

5ᵗʰ **I70.54**   **Atherosclerosis of nonautologous biological bypass graft(s) of the** left leg with ulceration

INCLUDES   any condition classifiable to I70.512 and I70.522

Use additional code to identify severity of ulcer (L97.-)

I70.541   **Atherosclerosis of nonautologous biological bypass graft(s) of the** left leg **with ulceration of** thigh   A cc HCC RxHCC CC/MCC Exc

I70.542   **Atherosclerosis of nonautologous biological bypass graft(s) of the** left leg **with ulceration of** calf   A cc HCC RxHCC CC/MCC Exc

I70.543   **Atherosclerosis of nonautologous biological bypass graft(s) of the** left leg **with ulceration of** ankle   A cc HCC RxHCC CC/MCC Exc

I70.544   **Atherosclerosis of nonautologous biological bypass graft(s) of the** left leg **with ulceration of** heel and midfoot   A cc HCC RxHCC CC/MCC Exc

Atherosclerosis of nonautologous biological bypass graft(s) of left leg with ulceration of plantar surface of midfoot

I70.545   **Atherosclerosis of nonautologous biological bypass graft(s) of the** left leg **with ulceration of** other part of foot   A HCC RxHCC

Atherosclerosis of nonautologous biological bypass graft(s) of the left leg with ulceration of toe

I70.548   **Atherosclerosis of nonautologous biological bypass graft(s) of the** left leg **with ulceration of other part of lower leg**   A cc HCC RxHCC CC/MCC Exc

I70.549   **Atherosclerosis of nonautologous biological bypass graft(s) of the** left leg **with ulceration of unspecified site**   A cc HCC RxHCC CC/MCC Exc

I70.55   **Atherosclerosis of nonautologous biological bypass graft(s) of other extremity with ulceration**   A HCC RxHCC

INCLUDES   any condition classifiable to I70.518, I70.528, and I70.538

Use additional code to identify severity of ulcer (L98.49)

6ᵗʰ **I70.56**   **Atherosclerosis of nonautologous biological bypass graft(s) of the extremities** with gangrene

INCLUDES   any condition classifiable to I70.51-, I70.52-, and I70.53-, I70.54-, I70.55

Use additional code to identify the severity of any ulcer (L97.-, L98.49-), if applicable

I70.561   **Atherosclerosis of nonautologous biological bypass graft(s) of the extremities with gangrene,** right leg   A cc HCC CC/MCC Exc

I70.562   **Atherosclerosis of nonautologous biological bypass graft(s) of the extremities with gangrene,** left leg   A cc HCC CC/MCC Exc

I70.563   **Atherosclerosis of nonautologous biological bypass graft(s) of the extremities with gangrene,** bilateral legs   A cc HCC CC/MCC Exc

I70.568   **Atherosclerosis of nonautologous biological bypass graft(s) of the extremities with gangrene,** other extremity   A cc HCC CC/MCC Exc

I70.569   **Atherosclerosis of nonautologous biological bypass graft(s) of the extremities with gangrene, unspecified extremity**   A cc HCC CC/MCC Exc

6ᵗʰ **I70.59**   Other **atherosclerosis of nonautologous biological bypass graft(s) of the extremities**

I70.591   **Other atherosclerosis of nonautologous biological bypass graft(s) of the extremities,** right leg   A HCC RxHCC

I70.592   **Other atherosclerosis of nonautologous biological bypass graft(s) of the extremities,** left leg   A HCC RxHCC

I70.593   **Other atherosclerosis of nonautologous biological bypass graft(s) of the extremities,** bilateral legs   A HCC RxHCC

I70.598   **Other atherosclerosis of nonautologous biological bypass graft(s) of the extremities,** other extremity   A HCC RxHCC

I70.599   **Other atherosclerosis of nonautologous biological bypass graft(s) of the extremities, unspecified extremity**   A HCC RxHCC

5ᵗʰ **I70.6**   **Atherosclerosis of** nonbiological bypass graft(s) of the extremities

Use additional code, if applicable, to identify chronic total occlusion of artery of extremity (I70.92)

6ᵗʰ **I70.60**   Unspecified **atherosclerosis of nonbiological bypass graft(s) of the extremities**

I70.601   **Unspecified atherosclerosis of nonbiological bypass graft(s) of the extremities,** right leg   A HCC RxHCC

I70.602   **Unspecified atherosclerosis of nonbiological bypass graft(s) of the extremities,** left leg   A HCC RxHCC

I70.603   **Unspecified atherosclerosis of nonbiological bypass graft(s) of the extremities,** bilateral legs   A HCC RxHCC

I70.608   **Unspecified atherosclerosis of nonbiological bypass graft(s) of the extremities,** other extremity   A HCC RxHCC

I70.609   **Unspecified atherosclerosis of nonbiological bypass graft(s) of the extremities, unspecified extremity**   A HCC RxHCC

6ᵗʰ **I70.61**   **Atherosclerosis of nonbiological bypass graft(s) of the extremities** with intermittent claudication

I70.611   **Atherosclerosis of nonbiological bypass graft(s) of the extremities with intermittent claudication,** right leg   A HCC RxHCC

I70.612   **Atherosclerosis of nonbiological bypass graft(s) of the extremities with intermittent claudication,** left leg   A HCC RxHCC

I70.613   **Atherosclerosis of nonbiological bypass graft(s) of the extremities with intermittent claudication,** bilateral legs   A HCC RxHCC

I70.618   **Atherosclerosis of nonbiological bypass graft(s) of the extremities with intermittent claudication, other extremity**   A HCC RxHCC

PDx Unacceptable principal diagnosis symbol per Medicare code edits   PDx Code exempt from diagnosis present on admission requirement   ? Questionable admission   cc Complication or comorbidity   MCC Major complication or comorbidity   CC/MCC Exc CC/MCC exclusion   HCC HCC diagnosis code   RxHCC RxHCC diagnosis code   MACRA code   **DEFINITION** Describes condition/terminology   **TIP** Coding guidance   👁 Official Guideline Reference   Z1 Z code as first-listed diagnosis

682

When symbols appear on a code that requires a 7th character extension, refer to Appendix B to identify applicable 7th character codes.

2020 ICD-10-CM

I70.619   Atherosclerosis of nonbiological bypass graft(s) of the extremities with intermittent claudication, unspecified extremity   🄰 HCC RxHCC

⑥ᵗʰ I70.62   Atherosclerosis of nonbiological bypass graft(s) of the extremities with rest pain

     INCLUDES   any condition classifiable to I70.61-

I70.621   Atherosclerosis of nonbiological bypass graft(s) of the extremities with rest pain, right leg   🄰 HCC RxHCC

I70.622   Atherosclerosis of nonbiological bypass graft(s) of the extremities with rest pain, left leg   🄰 HCC RxHCC

I70.623   Atherosclerosis of nonbiological bypass graft(s) of the extremities with rest pain, bilateral legs   🄰 HCC RxHCC

I70.628   Atherosclerosis of nonbiological bypass graft(s) of the extremities with rest pain, other extremity   🄰 HCC RxHCC

I70.629   Atherosclerosis of nonbiological bypass graft(s) of the extremities with rest pain, unspecified extremity   🄰 HCC RxHCC

⑥ᵗʰ I70.63   Atherosclerosis of nonbiological bypass graft(s) of the right leg with ulceration

     INCLUDES   any condition classifiable to I70.611 and I70.621

     Use additional code to identify severity of ulcer (L97.-)

I70.631   Atherosclerosis of nonbiological bypass graft(s) of the right leg with ulceration of thigh   🄰 cᵒ HCC RxHCC CC/MCC Exc

I70.632   Atherosclerosis of nonbiological bypass graft(s) of the right leg with ulceration of calf   🄰 cᵒ HCC RxHCC CC/MCC Exc

I70.633   Atherosclerosis of nonbiological bypass graft(s) of the right leg with ulceration of ankle   🄰 cᵒ HCC RxHCC CC/MCC Exc

I70.634   Atherosclerosis of nonbiological bypass graft(s) of the right leg with ulceration of heel and midfoot   🄰 cᵒ HCC RxHCC CC/MCC Exc

Atherosclerosis of nonbiological bypass graft(s) of right leg with ulceration of plantar surface of midfoot

I70.635   Atherosclerosis of nonbiological bypass graft(s) of the right leg with ulceration of other part of foot   🄰 HCC RxHCC

Atherosclerosis of nonbiological bypass graft(s) of the right leg with ulceration of toe

I70.638   Atherosclerosis of nonbiological bypass graft(s) of the right leg with ulceration of other part of lower leg   🄰 cᵒ HCC RxHCC CC/MCC Exc

I70.639   Atherosclerosis of nonbiological bypass graft(s) of the right leg with ulceration of unspecified site   🄰 cᵒ HCC RxHCC CC/MCC Exc

⑥ᵗʰ I70.64   Atherosclerosis of nonbiological bypass graft(s) of the left leg with ulceration

     INCLUDES   any condition classifiable to I70.612 and I70.622

     Use additional code to identify severity of ulcer (L97.-)

I70.641   Atherosclerosis of nonbiological bypass graft(s) of the left leg with ulceration of thigh   🄰 cᵒ HCC RxHCC CC/MCC Exc

I70.642   Atherosclerosis of nonbiological bypass graft(s) of the left leg with ulceration of calf   🄰 cᵒ HCC RxHCC CC/MCC Exc

I70.643   Atherosclerosis of nonbiological bypass graft(s) of the left leg with ulceration of ankle   🄰 cᵒ HCC RxHCC CC/MCC Exc

I70.644   Atherosclerosis of nonbiological bypass graft(s) of the left leg with ulceration of heel and midfoot   🄰 cᵒ HCC RxHCC CC/MCC Exc

Atherosclerosis of nonbiological bypass graft(s) of left leg with ulceration of plantar surface of midfoot

I70.645   Atherosclerosis of nonbiological bypass graft(s) of the left leg with ulceration of other part of foot   🄰 HCC RxHCC

Atherosclerosis of nonbiological bypass graft(s) of the left leg with ulceration of toe

I70.648   Atherosclerosis of nonbiological bypass graft(s) of the left leg with ulceration of other part of lower leg   🄰 cᵒ HCC RxHCC CC/MCC Exc

I70.649   Atherosclerosis of nonbiological bypass graft(s) of the left leg with ulceration of unspecified site   🄰 cᵒ HCC RxHCC CC/MCC Exc

I70.65   Atherosclerosis of nonbiological bypass graft(s) of other extremity with ulceration   🄰 HCC RxHCC

     INCLUDES   any condition classifiable to I70.618 and I70.628

     Use additional code to identify severity of ulcer (L98.49)

⑥ᵗʰ I70.66   Atherosclerosis of nonbiological bypass graft(s) of the extremities with gangrene

     INCLUDES   any condition classifiable to I70.61-, I70.62-, I70.63-, I70.64-, I70.65

     Use additional code to identify the severity of any ulcer (L97.-, L98.49-), if applicable

I70.661   Atherosclerosis of nonbiological bypass graft(s) of the extremities with gangrene, right leg   🄰 cᵒ HCC CC/MCC Exc

I70.662   Atherosclerosis of nonbiological bypass graft(s) of the extremities with gangrene, left leg   🄰 cᵒ HCC CC/MCC Exc

I70.663   Atherosclerosis of nonbiological bypass graft(s) of the extremities with gangrene, bilateral legs   🄰 cᵒ HCC CC/MCC Exc

I70.668   Atherosclerosis of nonbiological bypass graft(s) of the extremities with gangrene, other extremity   🄰 cᵒ HCC CC/MCC Exc

I70.669   Atherosclerosis of nonbiological bypass graft(s) of the extremities with gangrene, unspecified extremity   🄰 cᵒ HCC CC/MCC Exc

⑥ᵗʰ I70.69   Other atherosclerosis of nonbiological bypass graft(s) of the extremities

I70.691   Other atherosclerosis of nonbiological bypass graft(s) of the extremities, right leg   🄰 HCC RxHCC

I70.692   Other atherosclerosis of nonbiological bypass graft(s) of the extremities, left leg   🄰 HCC RxHCC

I70.693   Other atherosclerosis of nonbiological bypass graft(s) of the extremities, bilateral legs   🄰 HCC RxHCC

I70.698   Other atherosclerosis of nonbiological bypass graft(s) of the extremities, other extremity   🄰 HCC RxHCC

I70.699   Other atherosclerosis of nonbiological bypass graft(s) of the extremities, unspecified extremity   🄰 HCC RxHCC

⑤ᵗʰ I70.7   Atherosclerosis of other type of bypass graft(s) of the extremities

     Use additional code, if applicable, to identify chronic total occlusion of artery of extremity (I70.92)

⑥ᵗʰ I70.70   Unspecified atherosclerosis of other type of bypass graft(s) of the extremities

I70.701   Unspecified atherosclerosis of other type of bypass graft(s) of the extremities, right leg   🄰 HCC RxHCC

I70.702   Unspecified atherosclerosis of other type of bypass graft(s) of the extremities, left leg   🄰 HCC RxHCC

I70.703   Unspecified atherosclerosis of other type of bypass graft(s) of the extremities, bilateral legs   🄰 HCC RxHCC

I70.708 Unspecified atherosclerosis of other type of bypass graft(s) of the extremities, other extremity 🅰 HCC RxHCC

I70.709 Unspecified atherosclerosis of other type of bypass graft(s) of the extremities, unspecified extremity 🅰 HCC RxHCC

6ᵗʰ I70.71 Atherosclerosis of other type of bypass graft(s) of the extremities with intermittent claudication

I70.711 Atherosclerosis of other type of bypass graft(s) of the extremities with intermittent claudication, right leg 🅰 HCC RxHCC

I70.712 Atherosclerosis of other type of bypass graft(s) of the extremities with intermittent claudication, left leg 🅰 HCC RxHCC

I70.713 Atherosclerosis of other type of bypass graft(s) of the extremities with intermittent claudication, bilateral legs 🅰 HCC RxHCC

I70.718 Atherosclerosis of other type of bypass graft(s) of the extremities with intermittent claudication, other extremity 🅰 HCC RxHCC

I70.719 Atherosclerosis of other type of bypass graft(s) of the extremities with intermittent claudication, unspecified extremity 🅰 HCC RxHCC

6ᵗʰ I70.72 Atherosclerosis of other type of bypass graft(s) of the extremities with rest pain

INCLUDES _any condition classifiable to I70.71-_

I70.721 Atherosclerosis of other type of bypass graft(s) of the extremities with rest pain, right leg 🅰 HCC RxHCC

I70.722 Atherosclerosis of other type of bypass graft(s) of the extremities with rest pain, left leg 🅰 HCC RxHCC

I70.723 Atherosclerosis of other type of bypass graft(s) of the extremities with rest pain, bilateral legs 🅰 HCC RxHCC

I70.728 Atherosclerosis of other type of bypass graft(s) of the extremities with rest pain, other extremity 🅰 HCC RxHCC

I70.729 Atherosclerosis of other type of bypass graft(s) of the extremities with rest pain, unspecified extremity 🅰 HCC RxHCC

6ᵗʰ I70.73 Atherosclerosis of other type of bypass graft(s) of the right leg with ulceration

INCLUDES _any condition classifiable to I70.711 and I70.721_

Use additional code to identify severity of ulcer (L97.-)

I70.731 Atherosclerosis of other type of bypass graft(s) of the right leg with ulceration of thigh 🅰 cc HCC RxHCC CC/MCC Exc

I70.732 Atherosclerosis of other type of bypass graft(s) of the right leg with ulceration of calf 🅰 cc HCC RxHCC CC/MCC Exc

I70.733 Atherosclerosis of other type of bypass graft(s) of the right leg with ulceration of ankle 🅰 cc HCC RxHCC CC/MCC Exc

I70.734 Atherosclerosis of other type of bypass graft(s) of the right leg with ulceration of heel and midfoot 🅰 cc HCC RxHCC CC/MCC Exc

Atherosclerosis of other type of bypass graft(s) of right leg with ulceration of plantar surface of midfoot

I70.735 Atherosclerosis of other type of bypass graft(s) of the right leg with ulceration of other part of foot 🅰 HCC RxHCC

Atherosclerosis of other type of bypass graft(s) of right leg with ulceration of toe

I70.738 Atherosclerosis of other type of bypass graft(s) of the right leg with ulceration of other part of lower leg 🅰 cc HCC RxHCC CC/MCC Exc

I70.739 Atherosclerosis of other type of bypass graft(s) of the right leg with ulceration of unspecified site 🅰 cc HCC RxHCC CC/MCC Exc

6ᵗʰ I70.74 Atherosclerosis of other type of bypass graft(s) of the left leg with ulceration

INCLUDES _any condition classifiable to I70.712 and I70.722_

Use additional code to identify severity of ulcer (L97.-)

I70.741 Atherosclerosis of other type of bypass graft(s) of the left leg with ulceration of thigh 🅰 cc HCC RxHCC CC/MCC Exc

I70.742 Atherosclerosis of other type of bypass graft(s) of the left leg with ulceration of calf 🅰 cc HCC RxHCC CC/MCC Exc

I70.743 Atherosclerosis of other type of bypass graft(s) of the left leg with ulceration of ankle 🅰 cc HCC RxHCC CC/MCC Exc

I70.744 Atherosclerosis of other type of bypass graft(s) of the left leg with ulceration of heel and midfoot 🅰 cc HCC RxHCC CC/MCC Exc

Atherosclerosis of other type of bypass graft(s) of left leg with ulceration of plantar surface of midfoot

I70.745 Atherosclerosis of other type of bypass graft(s) of the left leg with ulceration of other part of foot 🅰 HCC RxHCC

Atherosclerosis of other type of bypass graft(s) of left leg with ulceration of toe

I70.748 Atherosclerosis of other type of bypass graft(s) of the left leg with ulceration of other part of lower leg 🅰 cc HCC RxHCC CC/MCC Exc

I70.749 Atherosclerosis of other type of bypass graft(s) of the left leg with ulceration of unspecified site 🅰 cc HCC RxHCC CC/MCC Exc

I70.75 Atherosclerosis of other type of bypass graft(s) of other extremity with ulceration 🅰 HCC RxHCC

INCLUDES _any condition classifiable to I70.718 and I70.728_

Use additional code to identify severity of ulcer (L98.49)

6ᵗʰ I70.76 Atherosclerosis of other type of bypass graft(s) of the extremities with gangrene

INCLUDES _any condition classifiable to I70.71-, I70.72-, I70.73-, I70.74-, I70.75_

Use additional code to identify the severity of any ulcer (L97.-, L98.49-), if applicable

I70.761 Atherosclerosis of other type of bypass graft(s) of the extremities with gangrene, right leg 🅰 cc HCC CC/MCC Exc

I70.762 Atherosclerosis of other type of bypass graft(s) of the extremities with gangrene, left leg 🅰 cc HCC CC/MCC Exc

I70.763 Atherosclerosis of other type of bypass graft(s) of the extremities with gangrene, bilateral legs 🅰 cc HCC CC/MCC Exc

I70.768 Atherosclerosis of other type of bypass graft(s) of the extremities with gangrene, other extremity 🅰 cc HCC CC/MCC Exc

I70.769 Atherosclerosis of other type of bypass graft(s) of the extremities with gangrene, unspecified extremity 🅰 cc HCC CC/MCC Exc

6ᵗʰ I70.79 Other atherosclerosis of other type of bypass graft(s) of the extremities

I70.791 Other atherosclerosis of other type of bypass graft(s) of the extremities, right leg 🅰 HCC RxHCC

I70.792 Other atherosclerosis of other type of bypass graft(s) of the extremities, left leg 🅰 HCC RxHCC

I70.793 Other atherosclerosis of other type of bypass graft(s) of the extremities, bilateral legs 🅰 HCC RxHCC

PDx Unacceptable principal diagnosis symbol per Medicare code edits   PDx Code exempt from diagnosis present on admission requirement
❓ Questionable admission   cc Complication or comorbidity   MCC Major complication or comorbidity   CC/MCC Exc CC/MCC exclusion
HCC HCC diagnosis code   RxHCC RxHCC diagnosis code   MACRA code   **DEFINITION** Describes condition/terminology
TIP Coding guidance   👁 Official Guideline Reference   Z1 Z code as first-listed diagnosis

I70.798 **Other atherosclerosis of other type of bypass graft(s) of the extremities,** other extremity **A HCC RxHCC**

I70.799 Other atherosclerosis of other type of bypass graft(s) of the extremities, unspecified extremity **A HCC RxHCC**

I70.8 **Atherosclerosis of other arteries** **A**

⑤ I70.9 **Other and unspecified atherosclerosis**

I70.90 **Unspecified atherosclerosis** **A**

I70.91 Generalized **atherosclerosis** **A**

I70.92 **Chronic total occlusion of artery of the extremities** **A CC HCC RxHCC PDxIn CC/MCC Exc**

Complete occlusion of artery of the extremities

Total occlusion of artery of the extremities

☛ Code first atherosclerosis of arteries of the extremities (I70.2-, I70.3-, I70.4-, I70.5-, I70.6-, I70.7-)

④ **I71 Aortic aneurysm and dissection**

EXCLUDES1 aortic ectasia (I77.81-)

syphilitic aortic aneurysm (A52.01)

traumatic aortic aneurysm (S25.09, S35.09)

⑤ I71.0 **Dissection of aorta**

I71.00 **Dissection of unspecified site of aorta** **CC HCC CC/MCC Exc**

I71.01 **Dissection of thoracic aorta** **HCC MCC CC/MCC Exc**

I71.02 **Dissection of abdominal aorta** **HCC MCC CC/MCC Exc**

I71.03 **Dissection of thoracoabdominal aorta** **HCC MCC CC/MCC Exc**

I71.1 Thoracic **aortic aneurysm, ruptured** **HCC MCC CC/MCC Exc**

I71.2 Thoracic aortic aneurysm, without rupture **HCC**

I71.3 Abdominal **aortic aneurysm, ruptured (Figure 9.6)** **HCC MCC CC/MCC Exc**

I71.4 Abdominal aortic aneurysm, without rupture **HCC**

I71.5 Thoracoabdominal **aortic aneurysm, ruptured** **HCC MCC CC/MCC Exc**

I71.6 Thoracoabdominal **aortic aneurysm, without rupture** **HCC**

I71.8 **Aortic aneurysm of unspecified site, ruptured** **HCC MCC CC/MCC Exc**

Rupture of aorta NOS

I71.9 **Aortic aneurysm of unspecified site, without rupture** **HCC**

Aneurysm of aorta

Dilatation of aorta

Hyaline necrosis of aorta

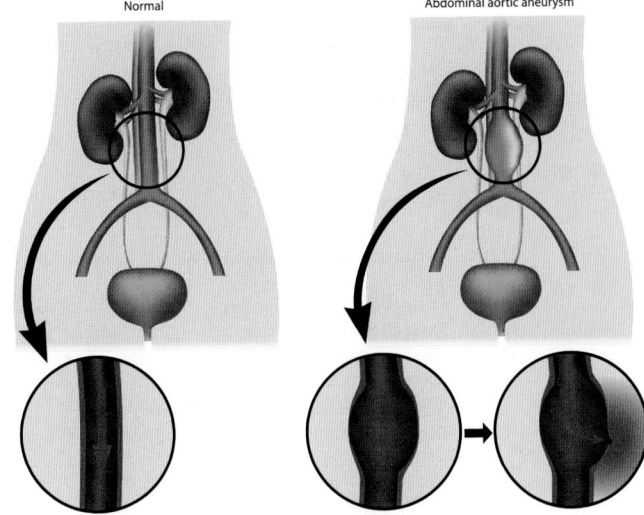

Normal   Abdominal aortic aneurysm

Figure 9.6 Ruptured Abdominal Aortic Aneurysm

④ **I72 Other aneurysm**

INCLUDES aneurysm (cirsoid) (false) (ruptured)

EXCLUDES2 acquired aneurysm (I77.0)

aneurysm (of) aorta (I71.-)

aneurysm (of) arteriovenous NOS (Q27.3-)

carotid artery dissection (I77.71)

cerebral (nonruptured) aneurysm (I67.1)

coronary aneurysm (I25.4)

coronary artery dissection (I25.42)

dissection of artery NEC (I77.79)

dissection of precerebral artery, congenital (nonruptured) (Q28.1)

heart aneurysm (I25.3)

iliac artery dissection (I77.72)

precerebral artery, congenital (nonruptured) (Q28.1)

pulmonary artery aneurysm (I28.1)

renal artery dissection (I77.73)

retinal aneurysm (H35.0)

ruptured cerebral aneurysm (I60.7)

varicose aneurysm (I77.0)

vertebral artery dissection (I77.74)

I72.0 **Aneurysm of carotid artery** **HCC**

Aneurysm of common carotid artery

Aneurysm of external carotid artery

Aneurysm of internal carotid artery, extracranial portion

EXCLUDES1 aneurysm of internal carotid artery, intracranial portion (I67.1)

aneurysm of internal carotid artery NOS (I67.1)

I72.1 **Aneurysm of artery of upper extremity** **HCC**

I72.2 **Aneurysm of renal artery** **HCC**

I72.3 **Aneurysm of iliac artery** **HCC**

I72.4 **Aneurysm of artery of lower extremity** **HCC**

AHA: Q2 2019

I72.5 **Aneurysm of other precerebral arteries** **HCC**

AHA: Q4 2016

Aneurysm of basilar artery (trunk)

EXCLUDES2 aneurysm of carotid artery (I72.0)

aneurysm of vertebral artery (I72.6)

dissection of carotid artery (I77.71)

dissection of other precerebral arteries (I77.75)

dissection of vertebral artery (I77.74)

I72.6 **Aneurysm of vertebral artery** **HCC**

AHA: Q4 2016

EXCLUDES2 dissection of vertebral artery (I77.74)

I72.8 **Aneurysm of other specified arteries** **HCC**

I72.9 **Aneurysm of unspecified site** **HCC**

④ **I73 Other peripheral vascular diseases**

EXCLUDES2 chilblains (T69.1)

frostbite (T33-T34)

immersion hand or foot (T69.0-)

spasm of cerebral artery (G45.9)

⑤ I73.0 Raynaud's syndrome

Raynaud's disease

Raynaud's phenomenon (secondary)

I73.00 **Raynaud's syndrome without gangrene**

I73.01 **Raynaud's syndrome with gangrene** **CC HCC CC/MCC Exc**

I73.1 **Thromboangiitis obliterans [Buerger's disease]** **HCC RxHCC**

⑤ I73.8 **Other specified peripheral vascular diseases**

EXCLUDES1 diabetic (peripheral) angiopathy (E08-E13 with .51-.52)

I73.81 **Erythromelalgia** **HCC RxHCC**

I73.89 **Other specified peripheral vascular diseases** **HCC RxHCC**

Acrocyanosis

Erythrocyanosis

Simple acroparesthesia [Schultze's type]

Vasomotor acroparesthesia [Nothnagel's type]

I73.9 **Peripheral vascular disease, unspecified** **HCC RxHCC**

AHA: Q4 2018

Intermittent claudication

Peripheral angiopathy NOS

Spasm of artery

EXCLUDES1 atherosclerosis of the extremities (I70.2--I70.7-)

④ **I74 Arterial embolism and thrombosis**

INCLUDES embolic infarction

embolic occlusion

thrombotic infarction

thrombotic occlusion

Unspecified Code   Other Specified Code   Manifestation Code   **N** Newborn   **P** Pediatric   **M** Maternity   **A** Adult   ♂ Male   ♀ Female

● New Code   ▲ Revised Code Title   ▶◀ Revised Text   **NOTES**   *INCLUDES*   *EXCLUDES1* Not coded here   *EXCLUDES2* Not included here

④ 4th character required   ⑤ 5th character required   ⑥ 6th character required   ⑦ 7th character required   ⑦ Extension 'X' Alert

HAC Hospital-acquired condition (HAC) alert   **AHA** AHA Coding Clinic©   ☛ Code first alert

☞ **Code first** embolism and thrombosis complicating abortion or ectopic or molar pregnancy (O00-O07, O08.2)

embolism and thrombosis complicating pregnancy, childbirth and the puerperium (O88.-)

EXCLUDES2 atheroembolism (I75.-)

basilar embolism and thrombosis (I63.0-I63.2, I65.1)

carotid embolism and thrombosis (I63.0-I63.2, I65.2)

cerebral embolism and thrombosis (I63.3-I63.5, I66.-)

coronary embolism and thrombosis (I21-I25)

mesenteric embolism and thrombosis (K55.0-)

ophthalmic embolism and thrombosis (H34.-)

precerebral embolism and thrombosis NOS (I63.0-I63.2, I65.9)

pulmonary embolism and thrombosis (I26.-)

renal embolism and thrombosis (N28.0)

retinal embolism and thrombosis (H34.-)

septic embolism and thrombosis (I76)

vertebral embolism and thrombosis (I63.0-I63.2, I65.0)

I74.0 Embolism and thrombosis of abdominal aorta

I74.01 Saddle embolus of abdominal aorta HCC MCC CC/MCC Exc

I74.09 Other arterial embolism and thrombosis of abdominal aorta cc HCC CC/MCC Exc

Aortic bifurcation syndrome

Aortoiliac obstruction

Leriche's syndrome

I74.1 Embolism and thrombosis of other and unspecified parts of aorta

I74.10 Embolism and thrombosis of unspecified parts of aorta cc HCC CC/MCC Exc

I74.11 Embolism and thrombosis of thoracic aorta cc HCC CC/MCC Exc

I74.19 Embolism and thrombosis of other parts of aorta cc HCC CC/MCC Exc

I74.2 Embolism and thrombosis of arteries of the upper extremities cc HCC CC/MCC Exc

I74.3 Embolism and thrombosis of arteries of the lower extremities cc HCC CC/MCC Exc

I74.4 Embolism and thrombosis of arteries of extremities, unspecified cc HCC CC/MCC Exc

Peripheral arterial embolism NOS

I74.5 Embolism and thrombosis of iliac artery cc HCC CC/MCC Exc

I74.8 Embolism and thrombosis of other arteries cc HCC CC/MCC Exc

I74.9 Embolism and thrombosis of unspecified artery cc HCC CC/MCC Exc

I75 Atheroembolism

INCLUDES atherothrombotic microembolism

cholesterol embolism

I75.0 Atheroembolism of extremities

I75.01 Atheroembolism of upper extremity

I75.011 Atheroembolism of right upper extremity cc HCC CC/MCC Exc

I75.012 Atheroembolism of left upper extremity cc HCC CC/MCC Exc

I75.013 Atheroembolism of bilateral upper extremities cc HCC CC/MCC Exc

I75.019 Atheroembolism of unspecified upper extremity cc HCC CC/MCC Exc

I75.02 Atheroembolism of lower extremity

I75.021 Atheroembolism of right lower extremity cc HCC CC/MCC Exc

I75.022 Atheroembolism of left lower extremity cc HCC CC/MCC Exc

I75.023 Atheroembolism of bilateral lower extremities cc HCC CC/MCC Exc

I75.029 Atheroembolism of unspecified lower extremity cc HCC CC/MCC Exc

I75.8 Atheroembolism of other sites

I75.81 Atheroembolism of kidney cc HCC CC/MCC Exc

Use additional code for any associated acute kidney failure and chronic kidney disease (N17.-, N18.-)

I75.89 Atheroembolism of other site cc HCC CC/MCC Exc

I76 Septic arterial embolism cc HCC PDxln CC/MCC Exc

☞ **Code first** underlying infection, such as:

infective endocarditis (I33.0)

lung abscess (J85.-)

Use additional code to identify the site of the embolism (I74.-)

EXCLUDES2 septic pulmonary embolism (I26.01, I26.90)

I77 Other disorders of arteries and arterioles

EXCLUDES2 collagen (vascular) diseases (M30-M36)

hypersensitivity angiitis (M31.0)

pulmonary artery (I28.-)

I77.0 Arteriovenous fistula, acquired HCC

Aneurysmal varix

Arteriovenous aneurysm, acquired

EXCLUDES1 arteriovenous aneurysm NOS (Q27.3-)

presence of arteriovenous shunt (fistula) for dialysis (Z99.2)

traumatic - see injury of blood vessel by body region

EXCLUDES2 cerebral (I67.1)

coronary (I25.4)

I77.1 Stricture of artery HCC

Narrowing of artery

I77.2 Rupture of artery cc HCC CC/MCC Exc

Erosion of artery

Fistula of artery

Ulcer of artery

EXCLUDES1 traumatic rupture of artery - see injury of blood vessel by body region

I77.3 Arterial fibromuscular dysplasia HCC

Fibromuscular hyperplasia (of) carotid artery

Fibromuscular hyperplasia (of) renal artery

I77.4 Celiac artery compression syndrome cc HCC CC/MCC Exc

I77.5 Necrosis of artery cc HCC CC/MCC Exc

I77.6 Arteritis, unspecified HCC

Aortitis NOS

Endarteritis NOS

EXCLUDES1 arteritis or endarteritis:

aortic arch (M31.4)

cerebral NEC (I67.7)

coronary (I25.89)

deformans (I70.-)

giant cell (M31.5, M31.6)

obliterans (I70.-)

senile (I70.-)

I77.7 Other arterial dissection

EXCLUDES2 dissection of aorta (I71.0-)

dissection of coronary artery (I25.42)

I77.70 Dissection of unspecified artery HCC MCC CC/MCC Exc

AHA: Q4 2016

I77.71 Dissection of carotid artery HCC MCC CC/MCC Exc

I77.72 Dissection of iliac artery HCC MCC CC/MCC Exc

I77.73 Dissection of renal artery HCC MCC CC/MCC Exc

I77.74 Dissection of vertebral artery HCC MCC CC/MCC Exc

EXCLUDES2 aneurysm of vertebral artery (I72.6)

I77.75 Dissection of other precerebral arteries HCC MCC CC/MCC Exc

AHA: Q4 2016

Dissection of basilar artery (trunk)

EXCLUDES2 aneurysm of carotid artery (I72.0)

aneurysm of other precerebral arteries (I72.5)

aneurysm of vertebral artery (I72.6)

dissection of carotid artery (I77.71)

dissection of vertebral artery (I77.74)

I77.76 Dissection of artery of upper extremity HCC MCC CC/MCC Exc

AHA: Q4 2016

I77.77 Dissection of artery of lower extremity HCC MCC CC/MCC Exc

AHA: Q4 2016

I77.79 Dissection of other specified artery HCC MCC CC/MCC Exc

AHA: Q4 2016

PDxln Unacceptable principal diagnosis symbol per Medicare code edits   POA Code exempt from diagnosis present on admission requirement
? Questionable admission   cc Complication or comorbidity   MCC Major complication or comorbidity   CC/MCC Exc CC/MCC exclusion
HCC HCC diagnosis code   RxHCC RxHCC diagnosis code   MACRA code MACRA code   **DEFINITION** Describes condition/terminology
TIP Coding guidance   👁 Official Guideline Reference   Z1 Z code as first-listed diagnosis

686

When symbols appear on a code that requires a 7th character extension, refer to Appendix B to identify applicable 7th character codes.

2020 ICD-10-CM

[5th] I77.8 Other specified disorders of arteries and arterioles
[6th] I77.81 Aortic ectasia
Ectasis aorta
EXCLUDES1 *aortic aneurysm and dissection (I71.0-)*
I77.810 Thoracic aortic ectasia [HCC]
I77.811 Abdominal aortic ectasia [HCC]
I77.812 Thoracoabdominal aortic ectasia [HCC]
I77.819 Aortic ectasia, unspecified site [HCC]
I77.89 Other specified disorders of arteries and arterioles [HCC]
I77.9 Disorder of arteries and arterioles, unspecified [HCC]
[4th] I78 Diseases of capillaries
I78.0 Hereditary hemorrhagic telangiectasia [HCC]
Rendu-Osler-Weber disease
I78.1 Nevus, non-neoplastic
AHA: Q1 2019
Araneus nevus
Senile nevus
Spider nevus
Stellar nevus
EXCLUDES1 *nevus NOS (D22.-)*
vascular NOS (Q82.5)
EXCLUDES2 *blue nevus (D22.-)*
flammeus nevus (Q82.5)
hairy nevus (D22.-)
melanocytic nevus (D22.-)
pigmented nevus (D22.-)
portwine nevus (Q82.5)
sanguineous nevus (Q82.5)
strawberry nevus (Q82.5)
verrucous nevus (Q82.5)
I78.8 Other diseases of capillaries
I78.9 Disease of capillaries, unspecified
[4th] I79 Disorders of arteries, arterioles and capillaries in diseases classified elsewhere
I79.0 Aneurysm of aorta in diseases classified elsewhere [HCC]
Code first underlying disease
EXCLUDES1 *syphilitic aneurysm (A52.01)*
I79.1 Aortitis in diseases classified elsewhere [HCC] [RxHCC]
Code first underlying disease
EXCLUDES1 *syphilitic aortitis (A52.02)*
I79.8 Other disorders of arteries, arterioles and capillaries in diseases classified elsewhere [HCC] [RxHCC]
Code first underlying disease, such as:
amyloidosis (E85.-)
EXCLUDES1 *diabetic (peripheral) angiopathy (E08-E13 with .51-.52)*
syphilitic endarteritis (A52.09)
tuberculous endarteritis (A18.89)

Diseases of veins, lymphatic vessels and lymph nodes, not elsewhere classified (I80-I89)

[4th] I80 Phlebitis and thrombophlebitis
INCLUDES *endophlebitis*
inflammation, vein
periphlebitis
suppurative phlebitis
Code first phlebitis and thrombophlebitis complicating abortion, ectopic or molar pregnancy (O00-O07, O08.7)
phlebitis and thrombophlebitis complicating pregnancy, childbirth and the puerperium (O22.-, O87.-)
EXCLUDES1 *venous embolism and thrombosis of lower extremities (I82.4-, I82.5-, I82.81-)*
[5th] I80.0 Phlebitis and thrombophlebitis of superficial vessels of lower extremities
Phlebitis and thrombophlebitis of femoropopliteal vein
I80.00 Phlebitis and thrombophlebitis of superficial vessels of unspecified lower extremity
I80.01 Phlebitis and thrombophlebitis of superficial vessels of right lower extremity
I80.02 Phlebitis and thrombophlebitis of superficial vessels of left lower extremity
I80.03 Phlebitis and thrombophlebitis of superficial vessels of lower extremities, bilateral
[5th] I80.1 Phlebitis and thrombophlebitis of femoral vein
Phlebitis and thrombophlebitis of common femoral vein
Phlebitis and thrombophlebitis of deep femoral vein
I80.10 Phlebitis and thrombophlebitis of unspecified femoral vein [CC] [HCC] [RxHCC] [CC/MCC Exc]
I80.11 Phlebitis and thrombophlebitis of right femoral vein [CC] [HCC] [RxHCC] [CC/MCC Exc]
I80.12 Phlebitis and thrombophlebitis of left femoral vein [CC] [HCC] [RxHCC] [CC/MCC Exc]
I80.13 Phlebitis and thrombophlebitis of femoral vein, bilateral [CC] [HCC] [RxHCC] [CC/MCC Exc]
[5th] I80.2 Phlebitis and thrombophlebitis of other and unspecified deep vessels of lower extremities
[6th] I80.20 Phlebitis and thrombophlebitis of unspecified deep vessels of lower extremities
I80.201 Phlebitis and thrombophlebitis of unspecified deep vessels of right lower extremity [CC] [HCC] [RxHCC] [CC/MCC Exc]
I80.202 Phlebitis and thrombophlebitis of unspecified deep vessels of left lower extremity [CC] [HCC] [RxHCC] [CC/MCC Exc]
I80.203 Phlebitis and thrombophlebitis of unspecified deep vessels of lower extremities, bilateral [CC] [HCC] [RxHCC] [CC/MCC Exc]
I80.209 Phlebitis and thrombophlebitis of unspecified deep vessels of unspecified lower extremity [CC] [HCC] [RxHCC] [CC/MCC Exc]
[6th] I80.21 Phlebitis and thrombophlebitis of iliac vein
Phlebitis and thrombophlebitis of common iliac vein
Phlebitis and thrombophlebitis of external iliac vein
Phlebitis and thrombophlebitis of internal iliac vein
I80.211 Phlebitis and thrombophlebitis of right iliac vein [CC] [HCC] [RxHCC] [CC/MCC Exc]
I80.212 Phlebitis and thrombophlebitis of left iliac vein [CC] [HCC] [RxHCC] [CC/MCC Exc]
I80.213 Phlebitis and thrombophlebitis of iliac vein, bilateral [CC] [HCC] [RxHCC] [CC/MCC Exc]
I80.219 Phlebitis and thrombophlebitis of unspecified iliac vein [CC] [HCC] [RxHCC] [CC/MCC Exc]
[6th] I80.22 Phlebitis and thrombophlebitis of popliteal vein
I80.221 Phlebitis and thrombophlebitis of right popliteal vein [CC] [HCC] [RxHCC] [CC/MCC Exc]
I80.222 Phlebitis and thrombophlebitis of left popliteal vein [CC] [HCC] [RxHCC] [CC/MCC Exc]
I80.223 Phlebitis and thrombophlebitis of popliteal vein, bilateral [CC] [HCC] [RxHCC] [CC/MCC Exc]
I80.229 Phlebitis and thrombophlebitis of unspecified popliteal vein [CC] [HCC] [RxHCC] [CC/MCC Exc]
[6th] I80.23 Phlebitis and thrombophlebitis of tibial vein
Phlebitis and thrombophlebitis of anterior tibial vein
Phlebitis and thrombophlebitis of posterior tibial vein
I80.231 Phlebitis and thrombophlebitis of right tibial vein [CC] [HCC] [RxHCC] [CC/MCC Exc]
I80.232 Phlebitis and thrombophlebitis of left tibial vein [CC] [HCC] [RxHCC] [CC/MCC Exc]
I80.233 Phlebitis and thrombophlebitis of tibial vein, bilateral [CC] [HCC] [RxHCC] [CC/MCC Exc]
I80.239 Phlebitis and thrombophlebitis of unspecified tibial vein [CC] [HCC] [RxHCC] [CC/MCC Exc]
● [6th] I80.24 Phlebitis and thrombophlebitis of peroneal vein
● I80.241 Phlebitis and thrombophlebitis of right peroneal vein [CC] [CC/MCC Exc]
● I80.242 Phlebitis and thrombophlebitis of left peroneal vein [CC] [CC/MCC Exc]

Unspecified Code | Other Specified Code | Manifestation Code | [N] Newborn | [P] Pediatric | [M] Maternity | [A] Adult | ♂ Male | ♀ Female
● New Code | ▲ Revised Code Title | ►◄ Revised Text | NOTES | INCLUDES | EXCLUDES1 Not coded here | EXCLUDES2 Not included here
[4th] 4th character required | [5th] 5th character required | [6th] 6th character required | [7th] 7th character required | [x7th] Extension 'X' Alert
[HAC] Hospital-acquired condition (HAC) alert | AHA AHA Coding Clinic® | Code first alert

● I80.243 **Phlebitis and thrombophlebitis of peroneal vein,** bilateral CC/MCC Exc

● I80.249 **Phlebitis and thrombophlebitis of unspecified peroneal vein** CC/MCC Exc

● 6ᵗʰ I80.25 **Phlebitis and thrombophlebitis of calf** muscular vein
Phlebitis and thrombophlebitis of calf muscular vein, NOS
Phlebitis and thrombophlebitis of gastrocnemial vein
Phlebitis and thrombophlebitis of soleal vein

● I80.251 **Phlebitis and thrombophlebitis of** right **calf muscular vein**

● I80.252 **Phlebitis and thrombophlebitis of** left **calf muscular vein**

● I80.253 **Phlebitis and thrombophlebitis of calf muscular vein,** bilateral

● I80.259 **Phlebitis and thrombophlebitis of unspecified calf muscular vein**

6ᵗʰ I80.29 **Phlebitis and thrombophlebitis of** other deep vessels of lower extremities

I80.291 **Phlebitis and thrombophlebitis of other deep vessels of** right **lower extremity** HCC RxHCC CC/MCC Exc

I80.292 **Phlebitis and thrombophlebitis of other deep vessels of** left **lower extremity** HCC RxHCC CC/MCC Exc

I80.293 **Phlebitis and thrombophlebitis of other deep vessels of lower extremity,** bilateral HCC RxHCC CC/MCC Exc

I80.299 **Phlebitis and thrombophlebitis of other deep vessels of unspecified lower extremity** HCC RxHCC CC/MCC Exc

I80.3 **Phlebitis and thrombophlebitis of lower extremities, unspecified**

I80.8 **Phlebitis and thrombophlebitis of other sites**

I80.9 **Phlebitis and thrombophlebitis of unspecified site**

I81 **Portal vein thrombosis** MCC CC/MCC Exc
Portal (vein) obstruction
EXCLUDES2 *hepatic vein thrombosis (I82.0)*
phlebitis of portal vein (K75.1)

4ᵗʰ I82 **Other** venous embolism **and** thrombosis
☞ **Code first** venous embolism and thrombosis complicating:
abortion, ectopic or molar pregnancy (O00-O07, O08.7)
pregnancy, childbirth and the puerperium (O22.-, O87.-)
EXCLUDES2 *venous embolism and thrombosis (of):*
cerebral (I63.6, I67.6)
coronary (I21-I25)
intracranial and intraspinal, septic or NOS (G08)
intracranial, nonpyogenic (I67.6)
intraspinal, nonpyogenic (G95.1)
mesenteric (K55.0-)
portal (I81)
pulmonary (I26.-)

I82.0 **Budd-Chiari syndrome** HCC MCC RxHCC CC/MCC Exc
Hepatic vein thrombosis

I82.1 **Thrombophlebitis migrans** CC/MCC Exc

5ᵗʰ I82.2 **Embolism and thrombosis of** vena cava and other thoracic veins

6ᵗʰ I82.21 **Embolism and thrombosis of** superior vena cava

I82.210 **Acute** embolism and thrombosis of superior **vena cava** HCC RxHCC CC/MCC Exc
Embolism and thrombosis of superior vena cava NOS

I82.211 **Chronic** embolism and thrombosis of superior **vena cava** HCC RxHCC CC/MCC Exc

6ᵗʰ I82.22 **Embolism and thrombosis of inferior vena cava**

I82.220 **Acute** embolism and thrombosis of inferior **vena cava** HCC MCC RxHCC CC/MCC Exc
Embolism and thrombosis of inferior vena cava NOS

I82.221 **Chronic** embolism and thrombosis of inferior **vena cava** HCC MCC RxHCC CC/MCC Exc

6ᵗʰ I82.29 **Embolism and thrombosis of** other thoracic veins
Embolism and thrombosis of brachiocephalic (innominate) vein

I82.290 **Acute** embolism and thrombosis of other **thoracic veins** HCC RxHCC CC/MCC Exc

I82.291 **Chronic** embolism and thrombosis of other thoracic veins HCC RxHCC CC/MCC Exc

I82.3 **Embolism and thrombosis of renal vein** HCC RxHCC CC/MCC Exc

5ᵗʰ I82.4 **Acute** embolism and thrombosis of deep veins of lower extremity

6ᵗʰ I82.40 **Acute embolism and thrombosis of** unspecified **deep veins of lower extremity**
Deep vein thrombosis NOS
DVT NOS
EXCLUDES1 *acute embolism and thrombosis of unspecified deep veins of distal lower extremity (I82.4Z-)*
acute embolism and thrombosis of unspecified deep veins of proximal lower extremity (I82.4Y-)

I82.401 **Acute embolism and thrombosis of unspecified deep veins of** right **lower extremity** HAC HCC RxHCC CC/MCC Exc

I82.402 **Acute embolism and thrombosis of unspecified deep veins of** left **lower extremity** HAC HCC RxHCC CC/MCC Exc

I82.403 **Acute embolism and thrombosis of unspecified deep veins of lower extremity,** bilateral HAC HCC RxHCC CC/MCC Exc

I82.409 **Acute embolism and thrombosis of unspecified deep veins of unspecified lower extremity** HAC HCC RxHCC CC/MCC Exc

6ᵗʰ I82.41 **Acute embolism and thrombosis of** femoral vein
Acute embolism and thrombosis of common femoral vein
Acute embolism and thrombosis of deep femoral vein

I82.411 **Acute embolism and thrombosis of** right **femoral vein** HAC HCC RxHCC CC/MCC Exc

I82.412 **Acute embolism and thrombosis of** left **femoral vein** HAC HCC RxHCC CC/MCC Exc

I82.413 **Acute embolism and thrombosis of femoral vein,** bilateral HAC HCC RxHCC CC/MCC Exc

I82.419 **Acute embolism and thrombosis of unspecified femoral vein** HAC HCC RxHCC CC/MCC Exc

6ᵗʰ I82.42 **Acute embolism and thrombosis of** iliac vein
Acute embolism and thrombosis of common iliac vein
Acute embolism and thrombosis of external iliac vein
Acute embolism and thrombosis of internal iliac vein

I82.421 **Acute embolism and thrombosis of** right **iliac vein** HAC HCC RxHCC CC/MCC Exc

I82.422 **Acute embolism and thrombosis of** left **iliac vein** HAC HCC RxHCC CC/MCC Exc

I82.423 **Acute embolism and thrombosis of iliac vein,** bilateral HAC HCC RxHCC CC/MCC Exc

I82.429 **Acute embolism and thrombosis of unspecified iliac vein** HAC HCC RxHCC CC/MCC Exc

6ᵗʰ I82.43 **Acute embolism and thrombosis of** popliteal vein

I82.431 **Acute embolism and thrombosis of** right **popliteal vein** HAC HCC RxHCC CC/MCC Exc

I82.432 **Acute embolism and thrombosis of** left **popliteal vein** HAC HCC RxHCC CC/MCC Exc

I82.433 **Acute embolism and thrombosis of popliteal vein,** bilateral HAC HCC RxHCC CC/MCC Exc

I82.439 **Acute embolism and thrombosis of unspecified popliteal vein** HAC HCC RxHCC CC/MCC Exc

6ᵗʰ I82.44 **Acute embolism and thrombosis of** tibial vein
Acute embolism and thrombosis of anterior tibial vein
Acute embolism and thrombosis of posterior tibial vein

PDx Unacceptable principal diagnosis symbol per Medicare code edits   PDx Code exempt from diagnosis present on admission requirement
? Questionable admission   CC Complication or comorbidity   MCC Major complication or comorbidity   CC/MCC Exc CC/MCC exclusion
HCC HCC diagnosis code   RxHCC RxHCC diagnosis code   MACRA code   **DEFINITION** Describes condition/terminology
TIP Coding guidance   👁 Official Guideline Reference   Z1 Z code as first-listed diagnosis

688   When symbols appear on a code that requires a 7th character extension, refer to Appendix B to identify applicable 7th character codes.   **2020 ICD-10-CM**

I82.441	Acute embolism and thrombosis of right tibial vein	cc⊘ HAC HCC RxHCC CC/MCC Exc
I82.442	Acute embolism and thrombosis of left tibial vein	cc⊘ HAC HCC RxHCC CC/MCC Exc
I82.443	Acute embolism and thrombosis of tibial vein, bilateral	cc⊘ HAC HCC RxHCC CC/MCC Exc
I82.449	Acute embolism and thrombosis of unspecified tibial vein	cc⊘ HAC HCC RxHCC CC/MCC Exc

● 6th **I82.45 Acute embolism and thrombosis of peroneal vein**

● I82.451	Acute embolism and thrombosis of right peroneal vein	cc⊘ CC/MCC Exc
● I82.452	Acute embolism and thrombosis of left peroneal vein	cc⊘ CC/MCC Exc
● I82.453	Acute embolism and thrombosis of peroneal vein, bilateral	cc⊘ CC/MCC Exc
● I82.459	Acute embolism and thrombosis of unspecified peroneal vein	cc⊘ CC/MCC Exc

● 6th **I82.46 Acute embolism and thrombosis of calf muscular vein**

Acute embolism and thrombosis of calf muscular vein, NOS

Acute embolism and thrombosis of gastrocnemial vein

Acute embolism and thrombosis of soleal vein

● I82.461	Acute embolism and thrombosis of right calf muscular vein	
● I82.462	Acute embolism and thrombosis of left calf muscular vein	
● I82.463	Acute embolism and thrombosis of calf muscular vein, bilateral	
● I82.469	Acute embolism and thrombosis of unspecified calf muscular vein	

6th **I82.49 Acute embolism and thrombosis of other specified deep vein of lower extremity**

I82.491	Acute embolism and thrombosis of other specified deep vein of right lower extremity	cc⊘ HAC HCC RxHCC CC/MCC Exc
I82.492	Acute embolism and thrombosis of other specified deep vein of left lower extremity	cc⊘ HAC HCC RxHCC CC/MCC Exc
I82.493	Acute embolism and thrombosis of other specified deep vein of lower extremity, bilateral	cc⊘ HAC HCC RxHCC CC/MCC Exc
I82.499	Acute embolism and thrombosis of other specified deep vein of unspecified lower extremity	cc⊘ HAC HCC RxHCC CC/MCC Exc

6th **I82.4Y Acute embolism and thrombosis of unspecified deep veins of proximal lower extremity**

Acute embolism and thrombosis of deep vein of thigh NOS

Acute embolism and thrombosis of deep vein of upper leg NOS

I82.4Y1	Acute embolism and thrombosis of unspecified deep veins of right proximal lower extremity	cc⊘ HAC HCC RxHCC CC/MCC Exc
I82.4Y2	Acute embolism and thrombosis of unspecified deep veins of left proximal lower extremity	cc⊘ HAC HCC RxHCC CC/MCC Exc
I82.4Y3	Acute embolism and thrombosis of unspecified deep veins of proximal lower extremity, bilateral	cc⊘ HAC HCC RxHCC CC/MCC Exc
I82.4Y9	Acute embolism and thrombosis of unspecified deep veins of unspecified proximal lower extremity	cc⊘ HAC HCC RxHCC CC/MCC Exc

6th **I82.4Z Acute embolism and thrombosis of unspecified deep veins of distal lower extremity**

Acute embolism and thrombosis of deep vein of calf NOS

Acute embolism and thrombosis of deep vein of lower leg NOS

I82.4Z1	Acute embolism and thrombosis of unspecified deep veins of right distal lower extremity	cc⊘ HAC HCC RxHCC CC/MCC Exc
I82.4Z2	Acute embolism and thrombosis of unspecified deep veins of left distal lower extremity	cc⊘ HAC HCC RxHCC CC/MCC Exc
I82.4Z3	Acute embolism and thrombosis of unspecified deep veins of distal lower extremity, bilateral	cc⊘ HAC HCC RxHCC CC/MCC Exc
I82.4Z9	Acute embolism and thrombosis of unspecified deep veins of unspecified distal lower extremity	cc⊘ HAC HCC RxHCC CC/MCC Exc

5th **I82.5 Chronic embolism and thrombosis of deep veins of lower extremity**

Use additional code, if applicable, for associated long-term (current) use of anticoagulants (Z79.01)

EXCLUDES1 *personal history of venous embolism and thrombosis (Z86.718)*

6th **I82.50 Chronic embolism and thrombosis of unspecified deep veins of lower extremity**

EXCLUDES1 *chronic embolism and thrombosis of unspecified deep veins of distal lower extremity (I82.5Z-)*

chronic embolism and thrombosis of unspecified deep veins of proximal lower extremity (I82.5Y-)

I82.501	Chronic embolism and thrombosis of unspecified deep veins of right lower extremity	cc⊘ HCC RxHCC CC/MCC Exc
I82.502	Chronic embolism and thrombosis of unspecified deep veins of left lower extremity	cc⊘ HCC RxHCC CC/MCC Exc
I82.503	Chronic embolism and thrombosis of unspecified deep veins of lower extremity, bilateral	cc⊘ HCC RxHCC CC/MCC Exc
I82.509	Chronic embolism and thrombosis of unspecified deep veins of unspecified lower extremity	cc⊘ HCC RxHCC CC/MCC Exc

6th **I82.51 Chronic embolism and thrombosis of femoral vein**

Chronic embolism and thrombosis of common femoral vein

Chronic embolism and thrombosis of deep femoral vein

I82.511	Chronic embolism and thrombosis of right femoral vein	cc⊘ HCC RxHCC CC/MCC Exc
I82.512	Chronic embolism and thrombosis of left femoral vein	cc⊘ HCC RxHCC CC/MCC Exc
I82.513	Chronic embolism and thrombosis of femoral vein, bilateral	cc⊘ HCC RxHCC CC/MCC Exc
I82.519	Chronic embolism and thrombosis of unspecified femoral vein	cc⊘ HCC RxHCC CC/MCC Exc

6th **I82.52 Chronic embolism and thrombosis of iliac vein**

Chronic embolism and thrombosis of common iliac vein

Chronic embolism and thrombosis of external iliac vein

Chronic embolism and thrombosis of internal iliac vein

I82.521	Chronic embolism and thrombosis of right iliac vein	cc⊘ HCC RxHCC CC/MCC Exc
I82.522	Chronic embolism and thrombosis of left iliac vein	cc⊘ HCC RxHCC CC/MCC Exc
I82.523	Chronic embolism and thrombosis of iliac vein, bilateral	cc⊘ HCC RxHCC CC/MCC Exc
I82.529	Chronic embolism and thrombosis of unspecified iliac vein	cc⊘ HCC RxHCC CC/MCC Exc

6th **I82.53 Chronic embolism and thrombosis of popliteal vein**

I82.531	Chronic embolism and thrombosis of right popliteal vein	cc⊘ HCC RxHCC CC/MCC Exc
I82.532	Chronic embolism and thrombosis of left popliteal vein	cc⊘ HCC RxHCC CC/MCC Exc
I82.533	Chronic embolism and thrombosis of popliteal vein, bilateral	cc⊘ HCC RxHCC CC/MCC Exc
I82.539	Chronic embolism and thrombosis of unspecified popliteal vein	cc⊘ HCC RxHCC CC/MCC Exc

I82.54 Chronic embolism and thrombosis of tibial vein
Chronic embolism and thrombosis of anterior tibial vein
Chronic embolism and thrombosis of posterior tibial vein

I82.541 Chronic embolism and thrombosis of right tibial vein ᶜᶜ HCC RxHCC CC/MCC Exc

I82.542 Chronic embolism and thrombosis of left tibial vein ᶜᶜ HCC RxHCC CC/MCC Exc

I82.543 Chronic embolism and thrombosis of tibial vein, bilateral ᶜᶜ HCC RxHCC CC/MCC Exc

I82.549 Chronic embolism and thrombosis of unspecified tibial vein ᶜᶜ HCC RxHCC CC/MCC Exc

I82.55 Chronic embolism and thrombosis of peroneal vein

I82.551 Chronic embolism and thrombosis of right peroneal vein ᶜᶜ CC/MCC Exc

I82.552 Chronic embolism and thrombosis of left peroneal vein ᶜᶜ CC/MCC Exc

I82.553 Chronic embolism and thrombosis of peroneal vein, bilateral ᶜᶜ CC/MCC Exc

I82.559 Chronic embolism and thrombosis of unspecified peroneal vein ᶜᶜ CC/MCC Exc

I82.56 Chronic embolism and thrombosis of calf muscular vein
Chronic embolism and thrombosis of calf muscular vein NOS
Chronic embolism and thrombosis of gastrocnemial vein
Chronic embolism and thrombosis of soleal vein

I82.561 Chronic embolism and thrombosis of right calf muscular vein

I82.562 Chronic embolism and thrombosis of left calf muscular vein

I82.563 Chronic embolism and thrombosis of calf muscular vein, bilateral

I82.569 Chronic embolism and thrombosis of unspecified calf muscular vein

I82.59 Chronic embolism and thrombosis of other specified deep vein of lower extremity

I82.591 Chronic embolism and thrombosis of other specified deep vein of right lower extremity ᶜᶜ HCC RxHCC CC/MCC Exc

I82.592 Chronic embolism and thrombosis of other specified deep vein of left lower extremity ᶜᶜ HCC RxHCC CC/MCC Exc

I82.593 Chronic embolism and thrombosis of other specified deep vein of lower extremity, bilateral ᶜᶜ HCC RxHCC CC/MCC Exc

I82.599 Chronic embolism and thrombosis of other specified deep vein of unspecified lower extremity ᶜᶜ HCC RxHCC CC/MCC Exc

I82.5Y Chronic embolism and thrombosis of unspecified deep veins of proximal lower extremity
Chronic embolism and thrombosis of deep veins of thigh NOS
Chronic embolism and thrombosis of deep veins of upper leg NOS

I82.5Y1 Chronic embolism and thrombosis of unspecified deep veins of right proximal lower extremity ᶜᶜ HCC RxHCC CC/MCC Exc

I82.5Y2 Chronic embolism and thrombosis of unspecified deep veins of left proximal lower extremity ᶜᶜ HCC RxHCC CC/MCC Exc

I82.5Y3 Chronic embolism and thrombosis of unspecified deep veins of proximal lower extremity, bilateral ᶜᶜ HCC RxHCC CC/MCC Exc

I82.5Y9 Chronic embolism and thrombosis of unspecified deep veins of unspecified proximal lower extremity ᶜᶜ HCC RxHCC CC/MCC Exc

I82.5Z Chronic embolism and thrombosis of unspecified deep veins of distal lower extremity
Chronic embolism and thrombosis of deep veins of calf NOS
Chronic embolism and thrombosis of deep veins of lower leg NOS

I82.5Z1 Chronic embolism and thrombosis of unspecified deep veins of right distal lower extremity ᶜᶜ HCC RxHCC CC/MCC Exc

I82.5Z2 Chronic embolism and thrombosis of unspecified deep veins of left distal lower extremity ᶜᶜ HCC RxHCC CC/MCC Exc

I82.5Z3 Chronic embolism and thrombosis of unspecified deep veins of distal lower extremity, bilateral ᶜᶜ HCC RxHCC CC/MCC Exc

I82.5Z9 Chronic embolism and thrombosis of unspecified deep veins of unspecified distal lower extremity ᶜᶜ HCC RxHCC CC/MCC Exc

I82.6 Acute embolism and thrombosis of veins of upper extremity

I82.60 Acute embolism and thrombosis of unspecified veins of upper extremity

I82.601 Acute embolism and thrombosis of unspecified veins of right upper extremity ᶜᶜ CC/MCC Exc

I82.602 Acute embolism and thrombosis of unspecified veins of left upper extremity ᶜᶜ CC/MCC Exc

I82.603 Acute embolism and thrombosis of unspecified veins of upper extremity, bilateral ᶜᶜ CC/MCC Exc

I82.609 Acute embolism and thrombosis of unspecified veins of unspecified upper extremity ᶜᶜ CC/MCC Exc

I82.61 Acute embolism and thrombosis of superficial veins of upper extremity
Acute embolism and thrombosis of antecubital vein
Acute embolism and thrombosis of basilic vein
Acute embolism and thrombosis of cephalic vein

I82.611 Acute embolism and thrombosis of superficial veins of right upper extremity ᶜᶜ CC/MCC Exc

I82.612 Acute embolism and thrombosis of superficial veins of left upper extremity ᶜᶜ CC/MCC Exc

I82.613 Acute embolism and thrombosis of superficial veins of upper extremity, bilateral ᶜᶜ CC/MCC Exc

I82.619 Acute embolism and thrombosis of superficial veins of unspecified upper extremity ᶜᶜ CC/MCC Exc

I82.62 Acute embolism and thrombosis of deep veins of upper extremity
Acute embolism and thrombosis of brachial vein
Acute embolism and thrombosis of radial vein
Acute embolism and thrombosis of ulnar vein

I82.621 Acute embolism and thrombosis of deep veins of right upper extremity ᶜᶜ HCC RxHCC CC/MCC Exc

I82.622 Acute embolism and thrombosis of deep veins of left upper extremity ᶜᶜ HCC RxHCC CC/MCC Exc

I82.623 Acute embolism and thrombosis of deep veins of upper extremity, bilateral ᶜᶜ HCC RxHCC CC/MCC Exc

I82.629 Acute embolism and thrombosis of deep veins of unspecified upper extremity ᶜᶜ HCC RxHCC CC/MCC Exc

I82.7 Chronic embolism and thrombosis of veins of upper extremity
Use additional code, if applicable, for associated long-term (current) use of anticoagulants (Z79.01)
EXCLUDES1 personal history of venous embolism and thrombosis (Z86.718)

I82.70 Chronic embolism and thrombosis of unspecified veins of upper extremity

I82.701 Chronic embolism and thrombosis of unspecified veins of right upper extremity ᶜᶜ CC/MCC Exc

---

ᴾᴰˣ Unacceptable principal diagnosis symbol per Medicare code edits   ᴾᴼˣ Code exempt from diagnosis present on admission requirement

❓ Questionable admission   ᶜᶜ Complication or comorbidity   ᴹᶜᶜ Major complication or comorbidity   ᶜᶜ/ᴹᶜᶜ CC/MCC exclusion

HCC HCC diagnosis code   RxHCC RxHCC diagnosis code   MACRA code   **DEFINITION** Describes condition/terminology

TIP Coding guidance   👁 Official Guideline Reference   Ⓩ Z code as first-listed diagnosis

690   When symbols appear on a code that requires a 7th character extension, refer to Appendix B to identify applicable 7th character codes.   **2020 ICD-10-CM**

I82.702 Chronic embolism and thrombosis of unspecified veins of left upper extremity cc⊘ CC/MCC Exc

I82.703 Chronic embolism and thrombosis of unspecified veins of upper extremity, bilateral cc⊘ CC/MCC Exc

I82.709 Chronic embolism and thrombosis of unspecified veins of unspecified upper extremity cc⊘ CC/MCC Exc

6ᵗʰ I82.71 Chronic embolism and thrombosis of superficial veins of upper extremity
Chronic embolism and thrombosis of antecubital vein
Chronic embolism and thrombosis of basilic vein
Chronic embolism and thrombosis of cephalic vein

I82.711 Chronic embolism and thrombosis of superficial veins of right upper extremity cc⊘ CC/MCC Exc

I82.712 Chronic embolism and thrombosis of superficial veins of left upper extremity cc⊘ CC/MCC Exc

I82.713 Chronic embolism and thrombosis of superficial veins of upper extremity, bilateral cc⊘ CC/MCC Exc

I82.719 Chronic embolism and thrombosis of superficial veins of unspecified upper extremity cc⊘ CC/MCC Exc

6ᵗʰ I82.72 Chronic embolism and thrombosis of deep veins of upper extremity
Chronic embolism and thrombosis of brachial vein
Chronic embolism and thrombosis of radial vein
Chronic embolism and thrombosis of ulnar vein

I82.721 Chronic embolism and thrombosis of deep veins of right upper extremity cc⊘ HCC RxHCC CC/MCC Exc

I82.722 Chronic embolism and thrombosis of deep veins of left upper extremity cc⊘ HCC RxHCC CC/MCC Exc

I82.723 Chronic embolism and thrombosis of deep veins of upper extremity, bilateral cc⊘ HCC RxHCC CC/MCC Exc

I82.729 Chronic embolism and thrombosis of deep veins of unspecified upper extremity cc⊘ HCC RxHCC CC/MCC Exc

5ᵗʰ I82.A Embolism and thrombosis of axillary vein

6ᵗʰ I82.A1 Acute embolism and thrombosis of axillary vein

I82.A11 Acute embolism and thrombosis of right axillary vein cc⊘ HCC RxHCC CC/MCC Exc

I82.A12 Acute embolism and thrombosis of left axillary vein cc⊘ HCC RxHCC CC/MCC Exc

I82.A13 Acute embolism and thrombosis of axillary vein, bilateral cc⊘ HCC RxHCC CC/MCC Exc

I82.A19 Acute embolism and thrombosis of unspecified axillary vein cc⊘ HCC RxHCC CC/MCC Exc

6ᵗʰ I82.A2 Chronic embolism and thrombosis of axillary vein

I82.A21 Chronic embolism and thrombosis of right axillary vein cc⊘ HCC RxHCC CC/MCC Exc

I82.A22 Chronic embolism and thrombosis of left axillary vein cc⊘ HCC RxHCC CC/MCC Exc

I82.A23 Chronic embolism and thrombosis of axillary vein, bilateral cc⊘ HCC RxHCC CC/MCC Exc

I82.A29 Chronic embolism and thrombosis of unspecified axillary vein cc⊘ HCC RxHCC CC/MCC Exc

5ᵗʰ I82.B Embolism and thrombosis of subclavian vein

6ᵗʰ I82.B1 Acute embolism and thrombosis of subclavian vein

I82.B11 Acute embolism and thrombosis of right subclavian vein cc⊘ HCC RxHCC CC/MCC Exc

I82.B12 Acute embolism and thrombosis of left subclavian vein cc⊘ HCC RxHCC CC/MCC Exc

I82.B13 Acute embolism and thrombosis of subclavian vein, bilateral cc⊘ HCC RxHCC CC/MCC Exc

I82.B19 Acute embolism and thrombosis of unspecified subclavian vein cc⊘ HCC RxHCC CC/MCC Exc

6ᵗʰ I82.B2 Chronic embolism and thrombosis of subclavian vein

I82.B21 Chronic embolism and thrombosis of right subclavian vein cc⊘ HCC RxHCC CC/MCC Exc

I82.B22 Chronic embolism and thrombosis of left subclavian vein cc⊘ HCC RxHCC CC/MCC Exc

I82.B23 Chronic embolism and thrombosis of subclavian vein, bilateral cc⊘ HCC RxHCC CC/MCC Exc

I82.B29 Chronic embolism and thrombosis of unspecified subclavian vein cc⊘ HCC RxHCC CC/MCC Exc

5ᵗʰ I82.C Embolism and thrombosis of internal jugular vein

6ᵗʰ I82.C1 Acute embolism and thrombosis of internal jugular vein

I82.C11 Acute embolism and thrombosis of right internal jugular vein cc⊘ HCC RxHCC CC/MCC Exc

I82.C12 Acute embolism and thrombosis of left internal jugular vein cc⊘ HCC RxHCC CC/MCC Exc

I82.C13 Acute embolism and thrombosis of internal jugular vein, bilateral cc⊘ HCC RxHCC CC/MCC Exc

I82.C19 Acute embolism and thrombosis of unspecified internal jugular vein cc⊘ HCC RxHCC CC/MCC Exc

6ᵗʰ I82.C2 Chronic embolism and thrombosis of internal jugular vein

I82.C21 Chronic embolism and thrombosis of right internal jugular vein cc⊘ HCC RxHCC CC/MCC Exc

I82.C22 Chronic embolism and thrombosis of left internal jugular vein cc⊘ HCC RxHCC CC/MCC Exc

I82.C23 Chronic embolism and thrombosis of internal jugular vein, bilateral cc⊘ HCC RxHCC CC/MCC Exc

I82.C29 Chronic embolism and thrombosis of unspecified internal jugular vein cc⊘ HCC RxHCC CC/MCC Exc

5ᵗʰ I82.8 Embolism and thrombosis of other specified veins
Use additional code, if applicable, for associated long-term (current) use of anticoagulants (Z79.01)

6ᵗʰ I82.81 Embolism and thrombosis of superficial veins of lower extremities
Embolism and thrombosis of saphenous vein (greater) (lesser)

I82.811 Embolism and thrombosis of superficial veins of right lower extremity cc⊘ CC/MCC Exc

I82.812 Embolism and thrombosis of superficial veins of left lower extremity cc⊘ CC/MCC Exc

I82.813 Embolism and thrombosis of superficial veins of lower extremities, bilateral cc⊘ CC/MCC Exc

I82.819 Embolism and thrombosis of superficial veins of unspecified lower extremity cc⊘ CC/MCC Exc

6ᵗʰ I82.89 Embolism and thrombosis of other specified veins

I82.890 Acute embolism and thrombosis of other specified veins cc⊘ CC/MCC Exc

I82.891 Chronic embolism and thrombosis of other specified veins cc⊘ CC/MCC Exc

5ᵗʰ I82.9 Embolism and thrombosis of unspecified vein

I82.90 Acute embolism and thrombosis of unspecified vein cc⊘ CC/MCC Exc
Embolism of vein NOS
Thrombosis (vein) NOS

I82.91 Chronic embolism and thrombosis of unspecified vein cc⊘ CC/MCC Exc

4ᵗʰ I83 Varicose veins of lower extremities (Figure 9.7)
EXCLUDES1 varicose veins complicating pregnancy (O22.0-)
varicose veins complicating the puerperium (O87.4)

Unspecified Code   Other Specified Code   Manifestation Code   ℕ Newborn   ℙ Pediatric   𝕄 Maternity   𝔸 Adult   ♂ Male   ♀ Female
● New Code   ▲ Revised Code Title   ▶◀ Revised Text   NOTES   INCLUDES   EXCLUDES1 Not coded here   EXCLUDES2 Not included here
4ᵗʰ 4ᵗʰ character required   5ᵗʰ 5ᵗʰ character required   6ᵗʰ 6ᵗʰ character required   7ᵗʰ 7ᵗʰ character required   7ᴮ Extension 'X' Alert
HAC Hospital-acquired condition (HAC) alert   AHA AHA Coding Clinic©   ☛ Code first alert

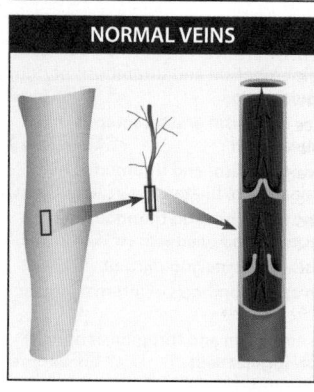
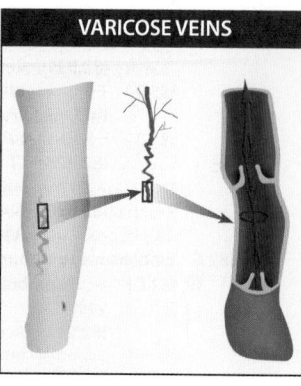

NORMAL VEINS

VARICOSE VEINS

Figure 9.7 Varicose Veins of Lower Extremities

5ᵗʰ **I83.0 Varicose veins of lower extremities** with ulcer
Use additional code to identify severity of ulcer (L97.-)

6ᵗʰ **I83.00 Varicose veins of** unspecified lower **extremity with ulcer**

I83.001 **Varicose veins of unspecified lower extremity with ulcer of** thigh A HCC

I83.002 **Varicose veins of unspecified lower extremity with ulcer of** calf A HCC

I83.003 **Varicose veins of unspecified lower extremity with ulcer of** ankle A HCC

I83.004 **Varicose veins of unspecified lower extremity with ulcer of** heel and midfoot A HCC
Varicose veins of unspecified lower extremity with ulcer of plantar surface of midfoot

I83.005 **Varicose veins of unspecified lower extremity with ulcer** other part of foot A HCC
Varicose veins of unspecified lower extremity with ulcer of toe

I83.008 **Varicose veins of unspecified lower extremity with ulcer** other part of lower leg A HCC

I83.009 **Varicose veins of unspecified lower extremity with ulcer of unspecified site** A HCC

5ᵗʰ **I83.01 Varicose veins of** right lower **extremity with ulcer**

I83.011 **Varicose veins of right lower extremity with ulcer of** thigh A HCC

I83.012 **Varicose veins of right lower extremity with ulcer of** calf A HCC

I83.013 **Varicose veins of right lower extremity with ulcer of** ankle A HCC

I83.014 **Varicose veins of right lower extremity with ulcer of** heel and midfoot A HCC
Varicose veins of right lower extremity with ulcer of plantar surface of midfoot

I83.015 **Varicose veins of right lower extremity with ulcer** other part of foot A HCC
Varicose veins of right lower extremity with ulcer of toe

I83.018 **Varicose veins of right lower extremity with** ulcer other part of lower leg A HCC

I83.019 **Varicose veins of right lower extremity with ulcer of unspecified site** A HCC

6ᵗʰ **I83.02 Varicose veins of** left lower **extremity with ulcer**

I83.021 **Varicose veins of left lower extremity with ulcer of** thigh A HCC

I83.022 **Varicose veins of left lower extremity with ulcer of** calf A HCC

I83.023 **Varicose veins of left lower extremity with ulcer of** ankle A HCC

I83.024 **Varicose veins of left lower extremity with ulcer of** heel and midfoot A HCC
Varicose veins of left lower extremity with ulcer of plantar surface of midfoot

I83.025 **Varicose veins of left lower extremity with ulcer** other part of foot A HCC
Varicose veins of left lower extremity with ulcer of toe

I83.028 **Varicose veins of left lower extremity with ulcer other part of lower leg** A HCC

I83.029 **Varicose veins of left lower extremity with ulcer of unspecified site** A HCC

5ᵗʰ **I83.1 Varicose veins of lower extremities** with inflammation

I83.10 **Varicose veins of unspecified** lower **extremity with inflammation** A

I83.11 **Varicose veins of** right lower **extremity with inflammation** A

I83.12 **Varicose veins of** left lower **extremity with inflammation** A

5ᵗʰ **I83.2 Varicose veins of lower extremities** with both ulcer and inflammation
Use additional code to identify severity of ulcer (L97.-)

6ᵗʰ **I83.20 Varicose veins of** unspecified lower **extremity with both ulcer and inflammation**

I83.201 **Varicose veins of unspecified lower extremity with both ulcer of** thigh **and inflammation** A CC HCC CC/MCC Exc

I83.202 **Varicose veins of unspecified lower extremity with both ulcer of** calf **and inflammation** A CC HCC CC/MCC Exc

I83.203 **Varicose veins of unspecified lower extremity with both ulcer of** ankle **and inflammation** A CC HCC CC/MCC Exc

I83.204 **Varicose veins of unspecified lower extremity with both ulcer of** heel and midfoot **and inflammation** A CC HCC CC/MCC Exc
Varicose veins of unspecified lower extremity with both ulcer of plantar surface of midfoot and inflammation

I83.205 **Varicose veins of unspecified lower extremity with both ulcer** other part of foot **and inflammation** A CC HCC CC/MCC Exc
Varicose veins of unspecified lower extremity with both ulcer of toe and inflammation

I83.208 **Varicose veins of unspecified lower extremity with both ulcer of other part of lower extremity and inflammation** A CC HCC CC/MCC Exc

I83.209 **Varicose veins of unspecified lower extremity with both ulcer of unspecified site and inflammation** A CC HCC CC/MCC Exc

6ᵗʰ **I83.21 Varicose veins of** right lower **extremity with both** ulcer and inflammation

I83.211 **Varicose veins of right lower extremity with both ulcer of** thigh **and inflammation** A CC HCC CC/MCC Exc

I83.212 **Varicose veins of right lower extremity with both ulcer of** calf **and inflammation** A CC HCC CC/MCC Exc

I83.213 **Varicose veins of right lower extremity with both ulcer of** ankle **and inflammation** A CC HCC CC/MCC Exc

I83.214 **Varicose veins of right lower extremity with both ulcer of** heel and midfoot **and inflammation** A CC HCC CC/MCC Exc
Varicose veins of right lower extremity with both ulcer of plantar surface of midfoot and inflammation

I83.215 **Varicose veins of right lower extremity with both ulcer** other part of foot **and inflammation** A CC HCC CC/MCC Exc
Varicose veins of right lower extremity with both ulcer of toe and inflammation

---

PDxⁿ Unacceptable principal diagnosis symbol per Medicare code edits   POA Code exempt from diagnosis present on admission requirement
? Questionable admission   CC Complication or comorbidity   MCC Major complication or comorbidity   CC/MCC Exc CC/MCC exclusion
HCC HCC diagnosis code   RxHCC RxHCC diagnosis code   MACRA code   **DEFINITION** Describes condition/terminology
TIP Coding guidance   👁 Official Guideline Reference   Z1 Z code as first-listed diagnosis

I83.218 **Varicose veins of right lower extremity with both ulcer of other part of lower extremity and inflammation** A cc⊘ HCC CC/MCC Exc⊘

I83.219 **Varicose veins of right lower extremity with both ulcer of unspecified site and inflammation** A cc⊘ HCC CC/MCC Exc⊘

6ᵗʰ I83.22 **Varicose veins of** left lower **extremity** with both ulcer and inflammation

I83.221 **Varicose veins of left lower extremity with both ulcer of** thigh **and inflammation** A cc⊘ HCC CC/MCC Exc⊘

I83.222 **Varicose veins of left lower extremity with both ulcer of** calf **and inflammation** A cc⊘ HCC CC/MCC Exc⊘

I83.223 **Varicose veins of left lower extremity with both ulcer of** ankle **and inflammation** A cc⊘ HCC CC/MCC Exc⊘

I83.224 **Varicose veins of left lower extremity with both ulcer of** heel and midfoot **and inflammation** A cc⊘ HCC CC/MCC Exc⊘
Varicose veins of left lower extremity with both ulcer of plantar surface of midfoot and inflammation

I83.225 **Varicose veins of left lower extremity with both ulcer** other part of foot **and inflammation** A cc⊘ HCC CC/MCC Exc⊘
Varicose veins of left lower extremity with both ulcer of toe and inflammation

I83.228 **Varicose veins of left lower extremity with both ulcer of other part of lower extremity and inflammation** A cc⊘ HCC CC/MCC Exc⊘

I83.229 **Varicose veins of left lower extremity with both ulcer of unspecified site and inflammation** A cc⊘ HCC CC/MCC Exc⊘

5ᵗʰ I83.8 **Varicose veins of lower extremities** with other complications

6ᵗʰ I83.81 **Varicose veins of lower extremities** with pain

I83.811 **Varicose veins of** right lower **extremity with pain** A

I83.812 **Varicose veins of** left lower **extremity with pain** A

I83.813 **Varicose veins of** bilateral lower **extremities with pain** A

I83.819 **Varicose veins of unspecified** lower **extremity with pain** A

6ᵗʰ I83.89 **Varicose veins of lower extremities** with other complications
Varicose veins of lower extremities with edema
Varicose veins of lower extremities with swelling

I83.891 **Varicose veins of** right lower **extremity with other complications** A

I83.892 **Varicose veins of** left lower **extremity with other complications** A

I83.893 **Varicose veins of** bilateral lower **extremities with other complications** A

I83.899 **Varicose veins of unspecified** lower **extremity with other complications** A

5ᵗʰ I83.9 Asymptomatic **varicose veins of** lower extremities
Phlebectasia of lower extremities
Varicose veins of lower extremities
Varix of lower extremities

I83.90 **Asymptomatic varicose veins of unspecified lower extremity** A
Varicose veins NOS

I83.91 **Asymptomatic varicose veins of** right lower **extremity** A

I83.92 **Asymptomatic varicose veins of** left lower **extremity** A

I83.93 **Asymptomatic varicose veins of** bilateral lower **extremities** A

4ᵗʰ I85 Esophageal varices
Use additional code to identify:
alcohol abuse and dependence (F10.-)

5ᵗʰ I85.0 Esophageal **varices**
Idiopathic esophageal varices
Primary esophageal varices

I85.00 **Esophageal varices** without bleeding cc⊘ HCC CC/MCC Exc⊘
Esophageal varices NOS

I85.01 **Esophageal varices** with bleeding HCC MCC⊘ CC/MCC Exc⊘

5ᵗʰ I85.1 Secondary esophageal **varices**
Esophageal varices secondary to alcoholic liver disease
Esophageal varices secondary to cirrhosis of liver
Esophageal varices secondary to schistosomiasis
Esophageal varices secondary to toxic liver disease
☛ **Code first** underlying disease

I85.10 **Secondary esophageal varices** without bleeding cc⊘ HCC CC/MCC Exc⊘

I85.11 **Secondary esophageal varices** with bleeding HCC MCC⊘ CC/MCC Exc⊘

4ᵗʰ I86 Varicose veins of other sites
EXCLUDES1 varicose veins of unspecified site (I83.9-)
EXCLUDES2 retinal varices (H35.0-)

I86.0 Sublingual **varices**

I86.1 Scrotal **varices** ♂
Varicocele

I86.2 Pelvic **varices**

I86.3 Vulval **varices** ♀
EXCLUDES1 vulval varices complicating childbirth and the puerperium (O87.8)
vulval varices complicating pregnancy (O22.1-)

I86.4 Gastric **varices**

I86.8 Varicose veins of other specified sites A
Varicose ulcer of nasal septum

4ᵗʰ I87 Other **disorders of veins**

5ᵗʰ I87.0 Postthrombotic syndrome
Chronic venous hypertension due to deep vein thrombosis
Postphlebitic syndrome
EXCLUDES1 chronic venous hypertension without deep vein thrombosis (I87.3-)

6ᵗʰ I87.00 **Postthrombotic syndrome** without complications
Asymptomatic Postthrombotic syndrome

I87.001 **Postthrombotic syndrome without complications of** right lower **extremity**

I87.002 **Postthrombotic syndrome without complications of** left lower **extremity**

I87.003 **Postthrombotic syndrome without complications of** bilateral lower **extremity**

I87.009 **Postthrombotic syndrome without complications of unspecified extremity**
Postthrombotic syndrome NOS

6ᵗʰ I87.01 **Postthrombotic syndrome** with ulcer
Use additional code to specify site and severity of ulcer (L97.-)

I87.011 **Postthrombotic syndrome with ulcer of** right lower **extremity** cc⊘ HCC CC/MCC Exc⊘

I87.012 **Postthrombotic syndrome with ulcer of** left lower **extremity** cc⊘ HCC CC/MCC Exc⊘

I87.013 **Postthrombotic syndrome with ulcer of** bilateral lower **extremity** cc⊘ HCC CC/MCC Exc⊘

I87.019 **Postthrombotic syndrome with ulcer of unspecified lower extremity** cc⊘ HCC CC/MCC Exc⊘

6ᵗʰ I87.02 **Postthrombotic syndrome** with inflammation

I87.021 **Postthrombotic syndrome with inflammation of** right lower **extremity**

I87.022 **Postthrombotic syndrome with inflammation of** left lower **extremity**

I87.023 **Postthrombotic syndrome with inflammation of** bilateral lower **extremity**

I87.029 **Postthrombotic syndrome with inflammation of unspecified lower extremity**

6ᵗʰ I87.03 **Postthrombotic syndrome** with ulcer and inflammation
Use additional code to specify site and severity of ulcer (L97.-)

● Unspecified Code		Other Specified Code		Manifestation Code		N Newborn	P Pediatric	M Maternity	A Adult	♂ Male	♀ Female

● New Code   ▲ Revised Code Title   ►◄ Revised Text   **NOTES**   *INCLUDES*   *EXCLUDES1* Not coded here   *EXCLUDES2* Not included here
4ᵗʰ 4ᵗʰ character required   5ᵗʰ 5ᵗʰ character required   6ᵗʰ 6ᵗʰ character required   7ᵗʰ 7ᵗʰ character required   7x Extension 'X' Alert
HAC Hospital-acquired condition (HAC) alert   **AHA** AHA Coding Clinic©   ☛ Code first alert

2020 ICD-10-CM   When symbols appear on a code that requires a 7th character extension, refer to Appendix B to identify applicable 7th character codes.   **693**

I83.218 - I87.03

CHAPTER 9: DISEASES OF THE CIRCULATORY SYSTEM (I00-I99)

I87.031 **Postthrombotic syndrome with ulcer and inflammation of right lower extremity** [CC] [HCC] [CC/MCC Exc]

I87.032 **Postthrombotic syndrome with ulcer and inflammation of left lower extremity** [CC] [HCC] [CC/MCC Exc]

I87.033 **Postthrombotic syndrome with ulcer and inflammation of bilateral lower extremity** [CC] [HCC] [CC/MCC Exc]

I87.039 **Postthrombotic syndrome with ulcer and inflammation of unspecified lower extremity** [CC] [HCC] [CC/MCC Exc]

[6th] I87.09 **Postthrombotic syndrome with other complications**

I87.091 **Postthrombotic syndrome with other complications of right lower extremity**

I87.092 **Postthrombotic syndrome with other complications of left lower extremity**

I87.093 **Postthrombotic syndrome with other complications of bilateral lower extremity**

I87.099 **Postthrombotic syndrome with other complications of unspecified lower extremity**

I87.1 **Compression of vein** [CC] [CC/MCC Exc]

Stricture of vein
Vena cava syndrome (inferior) (superior)

[EXCLUDES2] *compression of pulmonary vein (I28.8)*

I87.2 **Venous insufficiency (chronic) (peripheral)**

Stasis dermatitis

[EXCLUDES1] *stasis dermatitis with varicose veins of lower extremities (I83.1-, I83.2-)*

[5th] I87.3 **Chronic venous hypertension (idiopathic)**

Stasis edema

[EXCLUDES1] *chronic venous hypertension due to deep vein thrombosis (I87.0-)*
varicose veins of lower extremities (I83.-)

[6th] I87.30 **Chronic venous hypertension (idiopathic) without complications**

Asymptomatic chronic venous hypertension (idiopathic)

I87.301 **Chronic venous hypertension (idiopathic) without complications of right lower extremity**

I87.302 **Chronic venous hypertension (idiopathic) without complications of left lower extremity**

I87.303 **Chronic venous hypertension (idiopathic) without complications of bilateral lower extremity**

I87.309 **Chronic venous hypertension (idiopathic) without complications of unspecified lower extremity**

Chronic venous hypertension NOS

[6th] I87.31 **Chronic venous hypertension (idiopathic) with ulcer**

Use additional code to specify site and severity of ulcer (L97.-)

I87.311 **Chronic venous hypertension (idiopathic) with ulcer of right lower extremity** [CC] [HCC] [CC/MCC Exc]

I87.312 **Chronic venous hypertension (idiopathic) with ulcer of left lower extremity** [CC] [HCC] [CC/MCC Exc]

I87.313 **Chronic venous hypertension (idiopathic) with ulcer of bilateral lower extremity** [CC] [HCC] [CC/MCC Exc]

I87.319 **Chronic venous hypertension (idiopathic) with ulcer of unspecified lower extremity** [CC] [HCC] [CC/MCC Exc]

[6th] I87.32 **Chronic venous hypertension (idiopathic) with inflammation**

I87.321 **Chronic venous hypertension (idiopathic) with inflammation of right lower extremity**

I87.322 **Chronic venous hypertension (idiopathic) with inflammation of left lower extremity**

I87.323 **Chronic venous hypertension (idiopathic) with inflammation of bilateral lower extremity**

I87.329 **Chronic venous hypertension (idiopathic) with inflammation of unspecified lower extremity**

[6th] I87.33 **Chronic venous hypertension (idiopathic) with ulcer and inflammation**

Use additional code to specify site and severity of ulcer (L97.-)

I87.331 **Chronic venous hypertension (idiopathic) with ulcer and inflammation of right lower extremity** [CC] [HCC] [CC/MCC Exc]

I87.332 **Chronic venous hypertension (idiopathic) with ulcer and inflammation of left lower extremity** [CC] [HCC] [CC/MCC Exc]

I87.333 **Chronic venous hypertension (idiopathic) with ulcer and inflammation of bilateral lower extremity** [CC] [HCC] [CC/MCC Exc]

I87.339 **Chronic venous hypertension (idiopathic) with ulcer and inflammation of unspecified lower extremity** [CC] [HCC] [CC/MCC Exc]

[6th] I87.39 **Chronic venous hypertension (idiopathic) with other complications**

I87.391 **Chronic venous hypertension (idiopathic) with other complications of right lower extremity**

I87.392 **Chronic venous hypertension (idiopathic) with other complications of left lower extremity**

I87.393 **Chronic venous hypertension (idiopathic) with other complications of bilateral lower extremity**

I87.399 **Chronic venous hypertension (idiopathic) with other complications of unspecified lower extremity**

I87.8 **Other specified disorders of veins**

Phlebosclerosis
Venofibrosis

I87.9 **Disorder of vein, unspecified**

[4th] I88 **Nonspecific lymphadenitis**

[EXCLUDES1] *acute lymphadenitis, except mesenteric (L04.-)*
enlarged lymph nodes NOS (R59.-)
human immunodeficiency virus [HIV] disease resulting in generalized lymphadenopathy (B20)

I88.0 **Nonspecific mesenteric lymphadenitis**

Mesenteric lymphadenitis (acute)(chronic)

I88.1 **Chronic lymphadenitis, except mesenteric**

Adenitis
Lymphadenitis

I88.8 **Other nonspecific lymphadenitis**

I88.9 **Nonspecific lymphadenitis, unspecified**

Lymphadenitis NOS

[4th] I89 **Other noninfective disorders of lymphatic vessels and lymph nodes**

[EXCLUDES1] *chylocele, tunica vaginalis (nonfilarial) NOS (N50.89)*
enlarged lymph nodes NOS (R59.-)
filarial chylocele (B74.-)
hereditary lymphedema (Q82.0)

I89.0 **Lymphedema, not elsewhere classified**

Elephantiasis (nonfilarial) NOS
Lymphangiectasis
Obliteration, lymphatic vessel
Praecox lymphedema
Secondary lymphedema

[EXCLUDES1] *postmastectomy lymphedema (I97.2)*

I89.1 **Lymphangitis**

Chronic lymphangitis
Lymphangitis NOS
Subacute lymphangitis

[EXCLUDES1] *acute lymphangitis (L03.-)*

[PDx] Unacceptable principal diagnosis symbol per Medicare code edits [POA] Code exempt from diagnosis present on admission requirement
[?] Questionable admission [CC] Complication or comorbidity [MCC] Major complication or comorbidity [CC/MCC Exc] CC/MCC exclusion
[HCC] HCC diagnosis code [RxHCC] RxHCC diagnosis code MACRA code **DEFINITION** Describes condition/terminology
TIP Coding guidance 👁 Official Guideline Reference [Z1] Z code as first-listed diagnosis

When symbols appear on a code that requires a 7th character extension, refer to Appendix B to identify applicable 7th character codes.

I89.8 **Other specified noninfective disorders of lymphatic vessels and lymph nodes**
Chylocele (nonfilarial)
Chylous ascites
Chylous cyst
Lipomelanotic reticulosis
Lymph node or vessel fistula
Lymph node or vessel infarction
Lymph node or vessel rupture

I89.9 **Noninfective disorder of lymphatic vessels and lymph nodes, unspecified**
Disease of lymphatic vessels NOS

Other and unspecified disorders of the circulatory system (I95-I99)

4ᵗʰ I95 Hypotension
EXCLUDES1 cardiovascular collapse (R57.9)
maternal hypotension syndrome (O26.5-)
nonspecific low blood pressure reading NOS (R03.1)

I95.0 Idiopathic hypotension

I95.1 Orthostatic hypotension
Hypotension, postural
EXCLUDES1 neurogenic orthostatic hypotension [Shy-Drager] (G90.3)
orthostatic hypotension due to drugs (I95.2)

I95.2 **Hypotension** due to drugs
Orthostatic hypotension due to drugs
Use additional code for adverse effect, if applicable, to identify drug (T36-T50 with fifth or sixth character 5)

I95.3 **Hypotension of** hemodialysis
Intra-dialytic hypotension

5ᵗʰ I95.8 **Other hypotension**
I95.81 Postprocedural hypotension
I95.89 **Other hypotension**
Chronic hypotension

I95.9 **Hypotension, unspecified**

I96 Gangrene, not elsewhere classified   CC🔵 HCC CC/MCC Exc🔵
AHA: Q3 2018, Q4 2018
Gangrenous cellulitis
EXCLUDES1 gangrene in atherosclerosis of native arteries of the extremities (I70.26)
gangrene in hernia (K40.1, K40.4, K41.1, K41.4, K42.1, K43.1-, K44.1, K45.1, K46.1)
gangrene in other peripheral vascular diseases (I73.-)
gangrene of certain specified sites - see Alphabetical Index
gas gangrene (A48.0)
pyoderma gangrenosum (L88)
EXCLUDES2 gangrene in diabetes mellitus (E08-E13 with .52)

4ᵗʰ I97 Intraoperative and postprocedural complications and disorders of circulatory system, **not elsewhere classified**
EXCLUDES2 postprocedural shock (T81.1-)

I97.0 **Postcardiotomy syndrome**

5ᵗʰ I97.1 Other postprocedural cardiac functional disturbances
EXCLUDES2 acute pulmonary insufficiency following thoracic surgery (J95.1)
intraoperative cardiac functional disturbances (I97.7-)

6ᵗʰ I97.11 **Postprocedural cardiac** insufficiency
I97.110 **Postprocedural cardiac insufficiency following** cardiac surgery   CC🔵 CC/MCC Exc🔵
I97.111 **Postprocedural cardiac insufficiency following** other surgery   CC🔵 CC/MCC Exc🔵

6ᵗʰ I97.12 **Postprocedural cardiac** arrest
I97.120 **Postprocedural cardiac arrest following** cardiac surgery   CC🔵 CC/MCC Exc🔵
I97.121 **Postprocedural cardiac arrest following** other surgery   CC🔵 CC/MCC Exc🔵

6ᵗʰ I97.13 **Postprocedural heart** failure
Use additional code to identify the heart failure (I50.-)

I97.130 **Postprocedural heart failure following** cardiac surgery   CC🔵 CC/MCC Exc🔵
I97.131 **Postprocedural heart failure following** other surgery   CC🔵 CC/MCC Exc🔵

6ᵗʰ I97.19 Other postprocedural cardiac functional disturbances
Use additional code, if applicable, to further specify disorder

I97.190 **Other postprocedural cardiac functional disturbances following** cardiac surgery   CC🔵 CC/MCC Exc🔵
AHA: Q2 2019
Use additional code, if applicable, for type 4 or type 5 myocardial infarction, to further specify disorder

I97.191 **Other postprocedural cardiac functional disturbances following** other surgery   CC🔵 CC/MCC Exc🔵

I97.2 **Postmastectomy lymphedema syndrome**   🅰
Elephantiasis due to mastectomy
Obliteration of lymphatic vessels

I97.3 **Postprocedural hypertension**

5ᵗʰ I97.4 Intraoperative hemorrhage and hematoma of a circulatory system organ or structure complicating a procedure
EXCLUDES1 intraoperative hemorrhage and hematoma of a circulatory system organ or structure due to accidental puncture and laceration during a procedure (I97.5-)
EXCLUDES2 intraoperative cerebrovascular hemorrhage complicating a procedure (G97.3-)

6ᵗʰ I97.41 **Intraoperative hemorrhage and hematoma of a circulatory system organ or structure complicating a** circulatory system procedure
I97.410 **Intraoperative hemorrhage and hematoma of a circulatory system organ or structure complicating a** cardiac catheterization   CC🔵 CC/MCC Exc🔵
I97.411 **Intraoperative hemorrhage and hematoma of a circulatory system organ or structure complicating a** cardiac bypass   CC🔵 CC/MCC Exc🔵
I97.418 **Intraoperative hemorrhage and hematoma of a circulatory system organ or structure complicating** other circulatory system procedure   CC🔵 CC/MCC Exc🔵

I97.42 **Intraoperative hemorrhage and hematoma of a circulatory system organ or structure complicating** other procedure   CC🔵 CC/MCC Exc🔵
AHA: Q4 2016

5ᵗʰ I97.5 Accidental puncture and laceration of a circulatory system organ or structure during a procedure
EXCLUDES2 accidental puncture and laceration of brain during a procedure (G97.4-)

I97.51 **Accidental puncture and laceration of a circulatory system organ or structure during a** circulatory system procedure   CC🔵 CC/MCC Exc🔵
AHA: Q2 2019
I97.52 **Accidental puncture and laceration of a circulatory system organ or structure during** other procedure   CC🔵 CC/MCC Exc🔵

5ᵗʰ I97.6 Postprocedural hemorrhage, hematoma and seroma of a circulatory system organ or structure following a procedure
EXCLUDES2 postprocedural cerebrovascular hemorrhage complicating a procedure (G97.5-)

6ᵗʰ I97.61 **Postprocedural** hemorrhage **of a circulatory system organ or structure following a** circulatory system procedure
I97.610 **Postprocedural hemorrhage of a circulatory system organ or structure following a** cardiac catheterization   CC🔵 CC/MCC Exc🔵

Unspecified Code   Other Specified Code   Manifestation Code   ℕ Newborn   ℙ Pediatric   𝕄 Maternity   🅰 Adult   ♂ Male   ♀ Female
● New Code   ▲ Revised Code Title   ▶◀ Revised Text   **NOTES**   *INCLUDES*   *EXCLUDES1* Not coded here   *EXCLUDES2* Not included here
4ᵗʰ 4ᵗʰ character required   5ᵗʰ 5ᵗʰ character required   6ᵗʰ 6ᵗʰ character required   7ᵗʰ 7ᵗʰ character required   7ᵗʰ Extension 'X' Alert
HAC Hospital-acquired condition (HAC) alert   **AHA** AHA Coding Clinic©   📣 Code first alert

2020 ICD-10-CM   When symbols appear on a code that requires a 7th character extension, refer to Appendix B to identify applicable 7th character codes.   **695**

CHAPTER 9: DISEASES OF THE CIRCULATORY SYSTEM (I00-I99)

I89.8 - I97.610

I97.611   Postprocedural hemorrhage of a circulatory system organ or structure following cardiac bypass   cc RxHCC CC/MCC Exc

I97.618   Postprocedural hemorrhage of a circulatory system organ or structure following other circulatory system procedure   cc CC/MCC Exc

6ᵗʰ I97.62   Postprocedural hemorrhage, hematoma and seroma of a circulatory system organ or structure following other procedure

I97.620   Postprocedural hemorrhage of a circulatory system organ or structure following other procedure   cc CC/MCC Exc

I97.621   Postprocedural hematoma of a circulatory system organ or structure following other procedure   cc CC/MCC Exc

I97.622   Postprocedural seroma of a circulatory system organ or structure following other procedure   cc CC/MCC Exc

6ᵗʰ I97.63   Postprocedural hematoma of a circulatory system organ or structure following a circulatory system procedure

I97.630   Postprocedural hematoma of a circulatory system organ or structure following a cardiac catheterization   cc CC/MCC Exc

I97.631   Postprocedural hematoma of a circulatory system organ or structure following cardiac bypass   cc CC/MCC Exc

I97.638   Postprocedural hematoma of a circulatory system organ or structure following other circulatory system procedure   cc CC/MCC Exc

6ᵗʰ I97.64   Postprocedural seroma of a circulatory system organ or structure following a circulatory system procedure

I97.640   Postprocedural seroma of a circulatory system organ or structure following a cardiac catheterization   cc CC/MCC Exc

I97.641   Postprocedural seroma of a circulatory system organ or structure following cardiac bypass   cc CC/MCC Exc

I97.648   Postprocedural seroma of a circulatory system organ or structure following other circulatory system procedure   cc CC/MCC Exc

5ᵗʰ I97.7   Intraoperative cardiac functional disturbances

   EXCLUDES2   *acute pulmonary insufficiency following thoracic surgery (J95.1)*

     postprocedural cardiac functional disturbances (I97.1-)

6ᵗʰ I97.71   Intraoperative cardiac arrest

I97.710   Intraoperative cardiac arrest during cardiac surgery   cc CC/MCC Exc

I97.711   Intraoperative cardiac arrest during other surgery   cc CC/MCC Exc

6ᵗʰ I97.79   Other intraoperative cardiac functional disturbances

   Use additional code, if applicable, to further specify disorder

I97.790   Other intraoperative cardiac functional disturbances during cardiac surgery   cc CC/MCC Exc

I97.791   Other intraoperative cardiac functional disturbances during other surgery   cc CC/MCC Exc

5ᵗʰ I97.8   Other intraoperative and postprocedural complications and disorders of the circulatory system, not elsewhere classified

   Use additional code, if applicable, to further specify disorder

6ᵗʰ I97.81   Intraoperative cerebrovascular infarction

I97.810   Intraoperative cerebrovascular infarction during cardiac surgery   cc HCC RxHCC CC/MCC Exc

I97.811   Intraoperative cerebrovascular infarction during other surgery   cc HCC RxHCC CC/MCC Exc

6ᵗʰ I97.82   Postprocedural cerebrovascular infarction

I97.820   Postprocedural cerebrovascular infarction following cardiac surgery   cc HCC RxHCC CC/MCC Exc

I97.821   Postprocedural cerebrovascular infarction following other surgery   cc HCC RxHCC CC/MCC Exc

I97.88   Other intraoperative complications of the circulatory system, not elsewhere classified   cc CC/MCC Exc

I97.89   Other postprocedural complications and disorders of the circulatory system, not elsewhere classified   cc CC/MCC Exc

   AHA: Q2 2019

4ᵗʰ I99   Other and unspecified disorders of circulatory system

I99.8   Other disorder of circulatory system

I99.9   Unspecified disorder of circulatory system

PDxₘ Unacceptable principal diagnosis symbol per Medicare code edits   PDₓ Code exempt from diagnosis present on admission requirement

❓ Questionable admission   cc Complication or comorbidity   MCC Major complication or comorbidity   CC/MCC Exc CC/MCC exclusion

HCC HCC diagnosis code   RxHCC RxHCC diagnosis code   MACRA code   **DEFINITION** Describes condition/terminology

TIP Coding guidance   👁 Official Guideline Reference   Z1 Z code as first-listed diagnosis

Chapter 10: Diseases of the Respiratory System (J00-J99)

Anatomy of the Respiratory System

Introduction

The respiratory system, or respiratory tract, is responsible for the exchange of oxygen and carbon dioxide between the air we breathe and blood. It can be divided into the upper respiratory tract and the lower respiratory tract. The upper respiratory tract consists of the nose, nasal cavity, sinuses, larynx, and trachea, and the lower respiratory tract consisting of the bronchi and the lungs.

1. **An Outline of the Respiratory System**
   a) The human respiratory system (Figure 10.a) is based on the following organs:
      i) nose
      ii) pharynx
      iii) larynx
      iv) trachea
      v) bronchi
      vi) lungs
   b) The process of respiration involves the exchange of oxygen and carbon dioxide between the atmosphere, blood and cells.

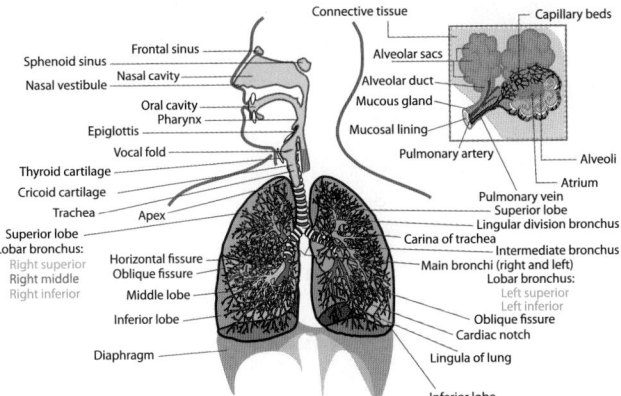

Figure 10.a Respiratory System Anatomy

2. **The Anatomy of the Nose**
   a) The nostrils or external nares are openings into the external nose.
   b) The internal nares serve to connect the internal nose with the throat or pharynx.
   c) The nasal septum divides the nose into the right and left nasal cavities.
   d) The internal nose contains three turbinate bones (superior, middle and inferior meatus).
   e) The olfactory receptors are located in the superior meatus.

3. **The Anatomy of the Pharynx**
   a) The pharynx is a resonating chamber for speech sounds and also provides a passage to both air and food.
   b) The nasopharynx, oropharynx and laryngopharynx are the parts of the pharynx.
   c) The nasopharynx surrounds the pharyngeal tonsils. It contains two internal nares and the openings of the eustachian tubes.
   d) The oropharynx surrounds the palatine and lingual tonsils and its opening (or fauces) provides connection to the mouth.
   e) The laryngopharynx gets connected with the larynx on anterior aspect and the esophagus posteriorly.

4. **The Anatomy of the Larynx**
   a) The larynx is also known as the voice box.
   b) The skeleton of the larynx is made up of nine cartilages. Three of them are single (thyroid, cricoid, and epiglottis) and the remaining three (arytenoid, corniculate, and cuneiform) are paired cartilages.
   c) The thyroid cartilage is also known as the Adam's apple. It is the largest single cartilage of the laryngeal skeleton.
   d) The cricoid cartilage connects with the first tracheal ring and is made up of a single ring of cartilage.

e) The epiglottis is a large and single leaf-shaped flap of elastic cartilage. It is lined with the mucous membrane and remains attached to the entrance of larynx. It pulls down over the glottis during the process of swallowing to obstruct the entrance of the fluids and food in the trachea.
   f) The arytenoid cartilages are formed by a pair of three ladle-shaped pyramids that remain attached to the laryngeal muscles and the vocal cords.
   g) The corniculate cartilages are based on two cone-shaped nodules of yellow elastic cartilage.
   h) The cuneiform cartilages are also known as the cartilages of Wrisberg. They are based on two rod-shaped pieces of yellow elastic cartilage.
   i) The mucous membrane of the larynx is divided into two pairs of folds. The vestibular folds (or false vocal cords) constitute the upper pair, while the vocal folds (or true vocal cords) form the lower pair of fold.
   j) The opening over the true vocal cords is known as the glottis.

5. **The Anatomy of the Trachea**
   a) The trachea is also known as the windpipe and located anteriorly to the esophagus.
   b) It begins at the larynx and gets divided into primary bronchi at the level of T4/T5 vertebrae.
   c) The trachea is lined by the respiratory epithelium and consists of a series of incomplete C-shaped cartilaginous rings.

6. **The Anatomy of the Bronchial Tree**
   a) The bronchial tree is based on right and left primary bronchi, secondary and tertiary bronchi, and the bronchioles.
   b) The right and left primary bronchi emanate from the trachea and merge with the right and left lungs.
   c) The primary bronchi further get branched into the secondary (or lobar) bronchi that penetrate into the lobes of the lungs.
   d) The secondary bronchi further get divided into the tertiary or segmental bronchi that penetrate into the segments of the lobes of the lungs.
   e) The bronchioles are the branches that emanate from the tertiary bronchi.

7. **The Anatomy of the Lungs**
   a) The lungs are the human organs of respiration.
   b) The right and left lungs are based on multiple lobes. The right lung contains three lobes, while the left lung is based on two lobes.
   c) The lungs are protected by the pleural membrane. The pleural membrane is further made up of two layers of serous membranes. The outer layer is known as the parietal pleura, while the inner layer is termed as the visceral pleura.
   d) The bronchopulmonary segment is a segment of lung tissue that is supplied by each of the tertiary bronchi. It is divided into multiple lobules that remain covered with the elastic connective tissue.
   e) A terminal bronchiole exists at the end of the conducting zone of the respiratory system.
   f) The microscopic respiratory bronchioles are the subdivisions of the terminal bronchioles. The atria or the alveolar ducts emanate from these respiratory bronchioles.
   g) The alveoli and alveolar sacs lie around the circumference of the alveolar ducts.
   h) The alveolar sac is made up of two or more alveoli with a common opening.
   i) The respiratory (or the alveolar capillary) membrane is a membrane that provides a medium for the movement of respiratory gases.

8. **The Process of Respiration**
   a) The respiration in humans is based on the following stages:
      i) Ventilation is also known as the breathing, which involves the movement of the ambient air into the alveoli of the lungs.
      ii) The process of pulmonary gas exchange is based on the exchange of respiratory gases between the alveoli and the pulmonary capillaries.
      iii) The gas process involves the transport of respiratory gases from the pulmonary capillaries to the peripheral capillaries in the organs via circulation.
      iv) Peripheral gas exchange is the process of exchange of respiratory gases between the tissue capillaries and the cells and mitochondria.
   b) Nasal breathing is the process of respiration that involves the inhalation and exhalation of the respiratory gases through the nose.

Common Pathologies

Sinusitis (Figure 10.b)

Inflammation of mucous membrane lining that lines the paranasal sinuses. This inflammation dries out the sinuses and can also cause dizziness and difficulty breathing. Using a humidifier can alleviate symptoms

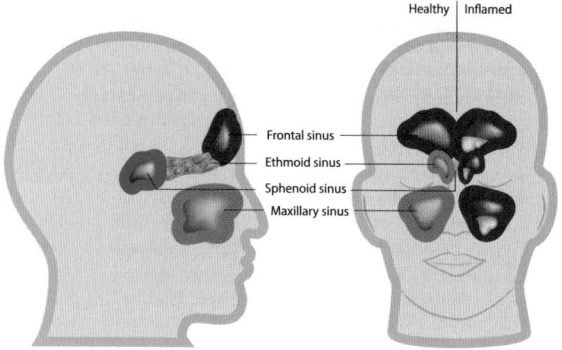

Figure 10.b Sinusitis

Epiglottitis

Inflammation of the epiglottis caused by H. Influenzae type B; characterized by fever and a severe sore throat and difficulty in swallowing.

Laryngitis

Inflammation of the larynx and vocal cords resulting in hoarseness of the voice (Dysphonia), and difficulty in swallowing (Dysphagia).

Pharyngitis

Inflammation of the pharynx, usually causing a sore throat. Acute Pharyngitis is a sudden, severe inflammation of the pharynx. Chronic Pharyngitis is a persistent throat inflammation that may be associated with the lymphoid granules in the pharyngeal mucosa.

Acute Bronchitis

Inflammation of the mucous membrane lining the bronchus, involves the trachea resulting in tracheobronchitis, chest tightness, fever, and a cough that progresses from nonproductive to productive.

Chronic Bronchitis

Inflammation of the bronchial mucous membrane characterized by cough, hyper-secretion of mucus, and expectoration of sputum over a long period of time and associated with increased vulnerability to bronchial infection.

Influenza

Influenza is a highly infectious respiratory disease. The disease is caused by certain strains of the influenza virus.

Pneumonia (Figure 10.c)

Pneumonia is an infection of the lung that can be caused by nearly any class of organism known to cause human infections. These include bacteria, amoebae, viruses, fungi, and parasites.

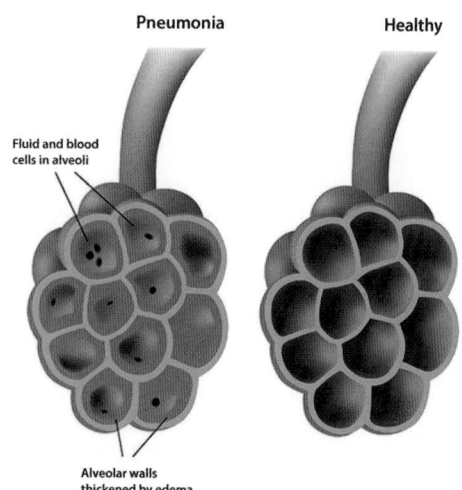

Figure 10.c Healthy Lung Alveoli and Alveoli with Pneumonia

Pulmonary Abscess

Lung abscess that is a collection of infectious material contained within a capsule in the lung, which results in coughing of bloody or foul-smelling sputum (breath foul-smelling). The most important preventative measure to avoid pulmonary abscess is to prevent aspiration.

Pulmonary Tuberculosis (TB)

Pulmonary tuberculosis is an infection (inflammation) caused by mycobacterium tuberculosis. Pathologic changes depend on the type of infection or "exposure" given below: Primary pulmonary TB (Primary Exposure), Secondary pulmonary TB (Reactivation) and Progressive pulmonary TB. The progression of tuberculosis is shown in Figure 10.d.

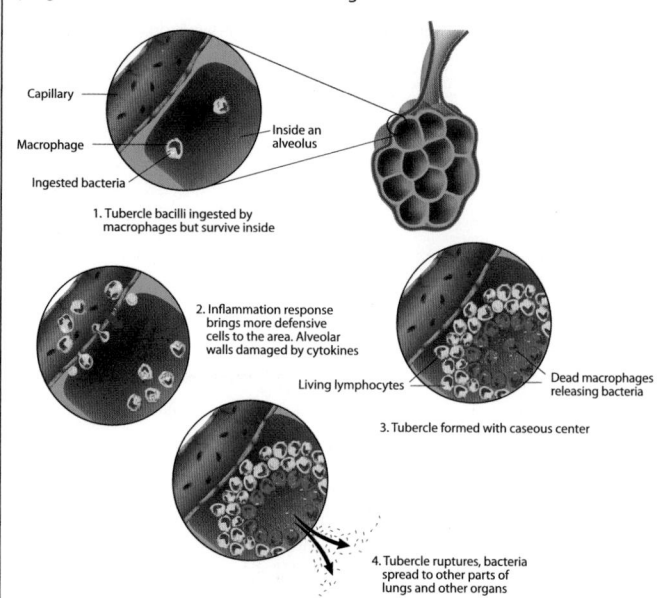

Figure 10.d Progression of Tuberculosis

Asthma

Asthma (Figure 10.e) is a common chronic inflammatory disease of the airways characterized by variable and recurring symptoms, reversible airflow obstruction, and bronchospasm. Common symptoms include wheezing, coughing, chest tightness, and shortness of breath.

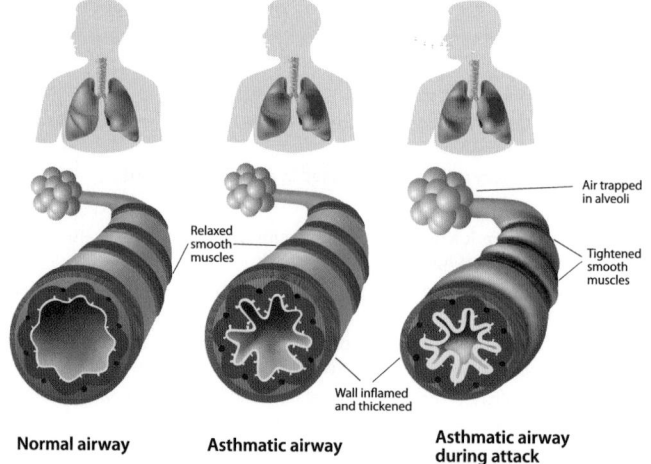

Figure 10.e Normal Airway and Asthmatic Airway

Cystic Fibrosis

Cystic Fibrosis (Figure 10.f) is an autosomal recessive genetic disorder that affects most critically the lungs, and also the pancreas, liver, and intestine. It is characterized by abnormal transport of chloride and sodium across an epithelium, leading to thick, viscous secretions.

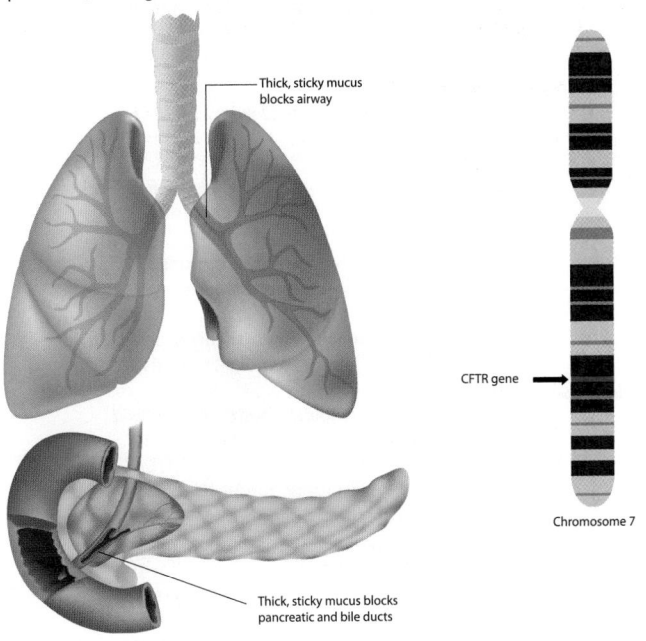

Figure 10.f Cystic Fibrosis

Chronic Obstructive Pulmonary Disease (COPD)

Chronic obstructive pulmonary disease (COPD) is a lung disease characterized by chronic obstruction of lung airflow that interferes with normal breathing and is not fully reversible. The more familiar terms 'chronic bronchitis' and 'emphysema' are no longer used, but are now included within the COPD diagnosis.

Emphysema

Emphysema is a chronic lung disease caused by damage to the alveoli, the tiny air sacs in the lung where exchange of oxygen and carbon dioxide takes place. With emphysema, damage to the alveoli results in air becoming trapped, causing them to expand and rupture.

Bronchiectasis

Bronchiectasis is a disease state defined by localized, irreversible dilation of part of the bronchial tree caused by destruction of the muscle and elastic tissue. It is classified as an obstructive lung disease, along with emphysema, bronchitis, asthma, and cystic fibrosis.

Diseases of the respiratory system (J00-J99)

NOTES When a respiratory condition is described as occurring in more than one site and is not specifically indexed, it should be classified to the lower anatomic site (e.g. tracheobronchitis to bronchitis in J40).

Use additional code, where applicable, to identify:

exposure to environmental tobacco smoke (Z77.22)

exposure to tobacco smoke in the perinatal period (P96.81)

history of tobacco dependence (Z87.891)

occupational exposure to environmental tobacco smoke (Z57.31)

tobacco dependence (F17.-)

tobacco use (Z72.0)

EXCLUDES2 *certain conditions originating in the perinatal period (P04-P96)*

certain infectious and parasitic diseases (A00-B99)

complications of pregnancy, childbirth and the puerperium (O00-O9A)

congenital malformations, deformations and chromosomal abnormalities (Q00-Q99)

endocrine, nutritional and metabolic diseases (E00-E88)

injury, poisoning and certain other consequences of external causes (S00-T88)

neoplasms (C00-D49)

smoke inhalation (T59.81-)

symptoms, signs and abnormal clinical and laboratory findings, not elsewhere classified (R00-R94)

This chapter contains the following blocks:

J00-J06	Acute upper respiratory infections
J09-J18	Influenza and pneumonia
J20-J22	Other acute lower respiratory infections
J30-J39	Other diseases of upper respiratory tract
J40-J47	Chronic lower respiratory diseases
J60-J70	Lung diseases due to external agents
J80-J84	Other respiratory diseases principally affecting the interstitium
J85-J86	Suppurative and necrotic conditions of the lower respiratory tract
J90-J94	Other diseases of the pleura
J95	Intraoperative and postprocedural complications and disorders of respiratory system, not elsewhere classified
J96-J99	Other diseases of the respiratory system

Acute upper respiratory infections (J00-J06)

EXCLUDES1 *chronic obstructive pulmonary disease with acute lower respiratory infection (J44.0)*

influenza virus with other respiratory manifestations (J09.X2, J10.1, J11.1)

J00 Acute nasopharyngitis [common cold]

Acute rhinitis

Coryza (acute)

Infective nasopharyngitis NOS

Infective rhinitis

Nasal catarrh, acute

Nasopharyngitis NOS

EXCLUDES1 *acute pharyngitis (J02.-)*

acute sore throat NOS (J02.9)

pharyngitis NOS (J02.9)

rhinitis NOS (J31.0)

sore throat NOS (J02.9)

EXCLUDES2 *allergic rhinitis (J30.1-J30.9)*

chronic pharyngitis (J31.2)

chronic rhinitis (J31.0)

chronic sore throat (J31.2)

nasopharyngitis, chronic (J31.1)

vasomotor rhinitis (J30.0)

J01 Acute sinusitis

INCLUDES *acute abscess of sinus*

acute empyema of sinus

acute infection of sinus

acute inflammation of sinus

acute suppuration of sinus

Use additional code (B95-B97) to identify infectious agent.

EXCLUDES1 *sinusitis NOS (J32.9)*

EXCLUDES2 *chronic sinusitis (J32.0-J32.8)*

J01.0 Acute maxillary sinusitis

Acute antritis

J01.00 **Acute maxillary sinusitis, unspecified**

J01.01 **Acute recurrent maxillary sinusitis**

J01.1 Acute frontal sinusitis

J01.10 **Acute frontal sinusitis, unspecified**

J01.11 **Acute recurrent frontal sinusitis**

J01.2 Acute ethmoidal sinusitis

J01.20 **Acute ethmoidal sinusitis, unspecified**

J01.21 **Acute recurrent ethmoidal sinusitis**

J01.3 Acute sphenoidal sinusitis

J01.30 **Acute sphenoidal sinusitis, unspecified**

J01.31 **Acute recurrent sphenoidal sinusitis**

J01.4 Acute pansinusitis

J01.40 **Acute pansinusitis, unspecified**

J01.41 **Acute recurrent pansinusitis**

J01.8 Other acute sinusitis

J01.80 **Other acute sinusitis**

Acute sinusitis involving more than one sinus but not pansinusitis

J01.81 **Other acute recurrent sinusitis**

Acute recurrent sinusitis involving more than one sinus but not pansinusitis

J01.9 Acute sinusitis, unspecified

J01.90 **Acute sinusitis, unspecified**

J01.91 **Acute recurrent sinusitis, unspecified**

J02 Acute pharyngitis

INCLUDES *acute sore throat*

EXCLUDES1 *acute laryngopharyngitis (J06.0)*

peritonsillar abscess (J36)

pharyngeal abscess (J39.1)

retropharyngeal abscess (J39.0)

EXCLUDES2 *chronic pharyngitis (J31.2)*

J02.0 Streptococcal pharyngitis

Septic pharyngitis

Streptococcal sore throat

EXCLUDES2 *scarlet fever (A38.-)*

J02.8 Acute pharyngitis due to other specified organisms

Use additional code (B95-B97) to identify infectious agent.

EXCLUDES1 *acute pharyngitis due to coxsackie virus (B08.5)*

acute pharyngitis due to gonococcus (A54.5)

acute pharyngitis due to herpes [simplex] virus (B00.2)

acute pharyngitis due to infectious mononucleosis (B27.-)

enteroviral vesicular pharyngitis (B08.5)

J02.9 Acute pharyngitis, unspecified

Gangrenous pharyngitis (acute)

Infective pharyngitis (acute) NOS

Pharyngitis (acute) NOS

Sore throat (acute) NOS

Suppurative pharyngitis (acute)

Ulcerative pharyngitis (acute)

J03 Acute tonsillitis

EXCLUDES1 *acute sore throat (J02.-)*

hypertrophy of tonsils (J35.1)

peritonsillar abscess (J36)

sore throat NOS (J02.9)

streptococcal sore throat (J02.0)

EXCLUDES2 *chronic tonsillitis (J35.0)*

When symbols appear on a code that requires a 7th character extension, refer to Appendix B to identify applicable 7th character codes.   **2020 ICD-10-CM**

5ᵗʰ **J03.0** Streptococcal **tonsillitis**

J03.00 Acute streptococcal tonsillitis, unspecified

J03.01 Acute recurrent streptococcal tonsillitis

5ᵗʰ **J03.8 Acute tonsillitis** due to other specified organisms

Use additional code (B95-B97) to identify infectious agent.

EXCLUDES1 *diphtheritic tonsillitis (A36.0)*

herpesviral pharyngotonsillitis (B00.2)

streptococcal tonsillitis (J03.0)

tuberculous tonsillitis (A15.8)

Vincent's tonsillitis (A69.1)

J03.80 Acute tonsillitis due to other specified organisms

J03.81 Acute recurrent tonsillitis due to other specified organisms

5ᵗʰ **J03.9 Acute tonsillitis, unspecified**

Follicular tonsillitis (acute)

Gangrenous tonsillitis (acute)

Infective tonsillitis (acute)

Tonsillitis (acute) NOS

Ulcerative tonsillitis (acute)

J03.90 Acute tonsillitis, unspecified

J03.91 Acute recurrent tonsillitis, unspecified

4ᵗʰ **J04 Acute laryngitis and tracheitis**

Use additional code (B95-B97) to identify infectious agent.

EXCLUDES1 *acute obstructive laryngitis [croup] and epiglottitis (J05.-)*

EXCLUDES2 *laryngismus (stridulus) (J38.5)*

J04.0 Acute laryngitis

Edematous laryngitis (acute)

Laryngitis (acute) NOS

Subglottic laryngitis (acute)

Suppurative laryngitis (acute)

Ulcerative laryngitis (acute)

EXCLUDES1 *acute obstructive laryngitis (J05.0)*

EXCLUDES2 *chronic laryngitis (J37.0)*

5ᵗʰ **J04.1 Acute** tracheitis

Acute viral tracheitis

Catarrhal tracheitis (acute)

Tracheitis (acute) NOS

EXCLUDES2 *chronic tracheitis (J42)*

J04.10 Acute tracheitis without obstruction

J04.11 Acute tracheitis with obstruction MCC⁰ CC/MCC Exc

J04.2 Acute laryngotracheitis

Laryngotracheitis NOS

Tracheitis (acute) with laryngitis (acute)

EXCLUDES1 *acute obstructive laryngotracheitis (J05.0)*

EXCLUDES2 *chronic laryngotracheitis (J37.1)*

5ᵗʰ **J04.3** Supraglottitis, **unspecified**

J04.30 Supraglottitis, unspecified, without obstruction

J04.31 Supraglottitis, unspecified, with obstruction MCC⁰ CC/MCC Exc

4ᵗʰ **J05 Acute obstructive laryngitis [croup] and epiglottitis**

Use additional code (B95-B97) to identify infectious agent.

J05.0 Acute obstructive laryngitis [croup]

Obstructive laryngitis (acute) NOS

Obstructive laryngotracheitis NOS

5ᵗʰ **J05.1 Acute** epiglottitis

EXCLUDES2 *epiglottitis, chronic (J37.0)*

J05.10 Acute epiglottitis without obstruction CC⁰ CC/MCC Exc

Epiglottitis NOS

J05.11 Acute epiglottitis with obstruction MCC⁰ CC/MCC Exc

4ᵗʰ **J06 Acute upper respiratory** infections of multiple and unspecified sites

EXCLUDES1 *acute respiratory infection NOS (J22)*

streptococcal pharyngitis (J02.0)

J06.0 Acute laryngopharyngitis

J06.9 Acute upper respiratory infection, unspecified

Upper respiratory disease, acute

Upper respiratory infection NOS

Use additional code (B95-B97) to identify infectious agent, if known, such as:

respiratory syncytial virus (RSV) (B97.4)

Influenza and pneumonia (J09-J18)

EXCLUDES2 *allergic or eosinophilic pneumonia (J82)*

aspiration pneumonia NOS (J69.0)

meconium pneumonia (P24.01)

neonatal aspiration pneumonia (P24.-)

pneumonia due to solids and liquids (J69.-)

congenital pneumonia (P23.9)

lipid pneumonia (J69.1)

rheumatic pneumonia (I00)

ventilator associated pneumonia (J95.851)

4ᵗʰ **J09 Influenza due to certain identified** influenza viruses

👁 **See Official Guidelines** "Influenza due to certain identified influenza viruses" I.C.10.c

EXCLUDES1 *influenza A/H1N1 (J10.-)*

influenza due to other identified influenza virus (J10.-)

influenza due to unidentified influenza virus (J11.-)

seasonal influenza due to other identified influenza virus (J10.-)

seasonal influenza due to unidentified influenza virus (J11.-)

5ᵗʰ **J09.X Influenza due to identified** novel influenza A virus

Avian influenza

Bird influenza

Influenza A/H5N1

Influenza of other animal origin, not bird or swine

Swine influenza virus (viruses that normally cause infections in pigs)

J09.X1 Influenza due to identified novel influenza A virus with pneumonia MCC⁰ CC/MCC Exc

Code also, if applicable, associated:

lung abscess (J85.1)

other specified type of pneumonia

J09.X2 Influenza due to identified novel influenza A virus with other respiratory manifestations

Influenza due to identified novel influenza A virus NOS

Influenza due to identified novel influenza A virus with laryngitis

Influenza due to identified novel influenza A virus with pharyngitis

Influenza due to identified novel influenza A virus with upper respiratory symptoms

Use additional code, if applicable, for associated:

pleural effusion (J91.8)

sinusitis (J01.-)

J09.X3 Influenza due to identified novel influenza A virus with gastrointestinal manifestations

Influenza due to identified novel influenza A virus gastroenteritis

EXCLUDES1 *'intestinal flu' [viral gastroenteritis] (A08.-)*

J09.X9 Influenza due to identified novel influenza A virus with other manifestations

Influenza due to identified novel influenza A virus with encephalopathy

Influenza due to identified novel influenza A virus with myocarditis

Influenza due to identified novel influenza A virus with otitis media

Use additional code to identify manifestation

4ᵗʰ **J10 Influenza due to** other identified influenza virus

👁 **See Official Guidelines** "Influenza due to certain identified influenza viruses" I.C.10.c

EXCLUDES1 *influenza due to avian influenza virus (J09.X-)*

influenza due to swine flu (J09.X-)

influenza due to unidentified influenza virus (J11.-)

5ᵗʰ **J10.0 Influenza due to other identified influenza virus** with pneumonia

Code also associated lung abscess, if applicable (J85.1)

J10.00 Influenza due to other identified influenza virus with unspecified type of pneumonia MCC⁰ CC/MCC Exc

J10.01 Influenza due to other identified influenza virus with the same other identified influenza virus pneumonia MCC⁰ CC/MCC Exc

---

Unspecified Code   Other Specified Code   Manifestation Code   N Newborn   P Pediatric   M Maternity   A Adult   ♂ Male   ♀ Female

● New Code   ▲ Revised Code Title   ▶◀ Revised Text   NOTES   INCLUDES   EXCLUDES1 Not coded here   EXCLUDES2 Not included here

4ᵗʰ 4ᵗʰ character required   5ᵗʰ 5ᵗʰ character required   6ᵗʰ 6ᵗʰ character required   7ᵗʰ 7ᵗʰ character required   Extension 'X' Alert

HAC Hospital-acquired condition (HAC) alert   AHA AHA Coding Clinic©   ☛ Code first alert

J10.08 **Influenza due to other identified influenza virus with other specified pneumonia** [MCC] [CC/MCC Exc]
Code also other specified type of pneumonia

J10.1 **Influenza due to other identified influenza virus** with other respiratory manifestations [CC] [CC/MCC Exc]
AHA: Q3 2016
Influenza due to other identified influenza virus NOS
Influenza due to other identified influenza virus with laryngitis
Influenza due to other identified influenza virus with pharyngitis
Influenza due to other identified influenza virus with upper respiratory symptoms
Use additional code for associated pleural effusion, if applicable (J91.8)
Use additional code for associated sinusitis, if applicable (J01.-)

J10.2 **Influenza due to other identified influenza virus** with gastrointestinal manifestations
Influenza due to other identified influenza virus gastroenteritis
[EXCLUDES1] *'intestinal flu' [viral gastroenteritis] (A08.-)*

[5th] J10.8 **Influenza due to other identified influenza virus** with other manifestations

J10.81 **Influenza due to other identified influenza virus** with encephalopathy

J10.82 **Influenza due to other identified influenza virus** with myocarditis

J10.83 **Influenza due to other identified influenza virus** with otitis media
Use additional code for any associated perforated tympanic membrane (H72.-)

J10.89 **Influenza due to other identified influenza virus** with other manifestations
Use additional codes to identify the manifestations

[4th] J11 **Influenza due to** unidentified influenza virus
👁 **See Official Guidelines** "Influenza due to certain identified influenza viruses" I.C.10.c

[5th] J11.0 **Influenza due to unidentified influenza virus** with pneumonia
Code also associated lung abscess, if applicable (J85.1)

J11.00 **Influenza due to unidentified influenza virus** with unspecified type of pneumonia [MCC] [CC/MCC Exc]
AHA: Q3 2016
Influenza with pneumonia NOS

J11.08 **Influenza due to unidentified influenza virus** with specified pneumonia [MCC] [CC/MCC Exc]
Code also other specified type of pneumonia

J11.1 **Influenza due to unidentified influenza virus** with other respiratory manifestations
Influenza NOS
Influenzal laryngitis NOS
Influenzal pharyngitis NOS
Influenza with upper respiratory symptoms NOS
Use additional code for associated pleural effusion, if applicable (J91.8)
Use additional code for associated sinusitis, if applicable (J01.-)

J11.2 **Influenza due to unidentified influenza virus** with gastrointestinal manifestations
Influenza gastroenteritis NOS
[EXCLUDES1] *'intestinal flu' [viral gastroenteritis] (A08.-)*

[5th] J11.8 **Influenza due to unidentified influenza virus** with other manifestations

J11.81 **Influenza due to unidentified influenza virus** with encephalopathy
Influenzal encephalopathy NOS

J11.82 **Influenza due to unidentified influenza virus** with myocarditis
Influenzal myocarditis NOS

J11.83 **Influenza due to unidentified influenza virus** with otitis media
Influenzal otitis media NOS
Use additional code for any associated perforated tympanic membrane (H72.-)

J11.89 **Influenza due to unidentified influenza virus** with other manifestations
Use additional codes to identify the manifestations

[4th] J12 Viral pneumonia, **not elsewhere classified**
[INCLUDES] *bronchopneumonia due to viruses other than influenza viruses*
☞ **Code first** associated influenza, if applicable (J09.X1, J10.0-, J11.0-)
Code also associated abscess, if applicable (J85.1)
[EXCLUDES1] *aspiration pneumonia due to anesthesia during labor and delivery (O74.0)*
aspiration pneumonia due to anesthesia during pregnancy (O29)
aspiration pneumonia due to anesthesia during puerperium (O89.0)
aspiration pneumonia due to solids and liquids (J69.-)
aspiration pneumonia NOS (J69.0)
congenital pneumonia (P23.0)
congenital rubella pneumonitis (P35.0)
interstitial pneumonia NOS (J84.9)
lipid pneumonia (J69.1)
neonatal aspiration pneumonia (P24.-)

J12.0 Adenoviral **pneumonia** [MCC] [CC/MCC Exc]

J12.1 Respiratory syncytial virus **pneumonia** [MCC] [CC/MCC Exc]
RSV pneumonia

J12.2 Parainfluenza virus **pneumonia** [MCC] [CC/MCC Exc]

J12.3 Human metapneumovirus **pneumonia** [MCC] [CC/MCC Exc]

[5th] J12.8 Other **viral pneumonia**

J12.81 **Pneumonia** due to SARS-associated coronavirus [MCC] [CC/MCC Exc]
Severe acute respiratory syndrome NOS

J12.89 Other **viral pneumonia** [MCC] [CC/MCC Exc]

J12.9 **Viral pneumonia, unspecified** [MCC] [CC/MCC Exc]

J13 **Pneumonia due to** Streptococcus pneumoniae [HCC] [MCC] [CC/MCC Exc]
👁 **See Official Guidelines** "Ventilator associated Pneumonia Develops after Admission" I.C.10.d.2
AHA: Q3 2018
Bronchopneumonia due to S. pneumoniae
☞ **Code first** associated influenza, if applicable (J09.X1, J10.0-, J11.0-)
Code also associated abscess, if applicable (J85.1)
[EXCLUDES1] *congenital pneumonia due to S. pneumoniae (P23.6)*
lobar pneumonia, unspecified organism (J18.1)
pneumonia due to other streptococci (J15.3-J15.4)

J14 **Pneumonia due to** Hemophilus influenzae [HCC] [MCC] [CC/MCC Exc]
Bronchopneumonia due to H. influenzae
☞ **Code first** associated influenza, if applicable (J09.X1, J10.0-, J11.0-)
Code also associated abscess, if applicable (J85.1)
[EXCLUDES1] *congenital pneumonia due to H. influenzae (P23.6)*

[4th] J15 Bacterial **pneumonia, not elsewhere classified**
[INCLUDES] *bronchopneumonia due to bacteria other than S. pneumoniae and H. influenzae*
☞ **Code first** associated influenza, if applicable (J09.X1, J10.0-, J11.0-)
Code also associated abscess, if applicable (J85.1)
[EXCLUDES1] *chlamydial pneumonia (J16.0)*
congenital pneumonia (P23.-)
Legionnaires' disease (A48.1)
spirochetal pneumonia (A69.8)

J15.0 **Pneumonia due to** Klebsiella pneumoniae [HCC] [MCC] [CC/MCC Exc]

J15.1 **Pneumonia due to** Pseudomonas [HCC] [MCC] [CC/MCC Exc]

[5th] J15.2 **Pneumonia due to** staphylococcus

J15.20 **Pneumonia due to staphylococcus, unspecified** [HCC] [MCC] [CC/MCC Exc]

[6th] J15.21 **Pneumonia due to** staphylococcus aureus

J15.211 **Pneumonia due to** Methicillin susceptible Staphylococcus aureus [HCC] [MCC] [CC/MCC Exc]
MSSA pneumonia
Pneumonia due to Staphylococcus aureus NOS

J15.212 **Pneumonia due to** Methicillin resistant Staphylococcus aureus [HCC] [MCC] [CC/MCC Exc]
👁 **See Official Guidelines** "Combination codes for MRSA infection" I.C.1.e.1.a

J15.29 **Pneumonia due to other** staphylococcus [HCC] [MCC] [CC/MCC Exc]

[PDx] Unacceptable principal diagnosis symbol per Medicare code edits [POA] Code exempt from diagnosis present on admission requirement
[?] Questionable admission [CC] Complication or comorbidity [MCC] Major complication or comorbidity [CC/MCC Exc] CC/MCC exclusion
[HCC] HCC diagnosis code [RxHCC] RxHCC diagnosis code MACRA code **DEFINITION** Describes condition/terminology
TIP Coding guidance 👁 Official Guideline Reference [Z1] Z code as first-listed diagnosis

J15.3 **Pneumonia due to** streptococcus, group B   HCC MCC CC/MCC Exc

J15.4 **Pneumonia due to** other streptococci   HCC MCC CC/MCC Exc

     EXCLUDES1 *pneumonia due to streptococcus, group B (J15.3)*

         pneumonia due to Streptococcus pneumoniae (J13)

J15.5 **Pneumonia due to** Escherichia coli   HCC MCC CC/MCC Exc

J15.6 **Pneumonia due to** other Gram-negative bacteria   HCC MCC CC/MCC Exc

     Pneumonia due to other aerobic Gram-negative bacteria

     Pneumonia due to Serratia marcescens

J15.7 **Pneumonia due to** Mycoplasma pneumoniae   MCC CC/MCC Exc

J15.8 **Pneumonia due to other specified** bacteria   HCC MCC CC/MCC Exc

J15.9 **Unspecified bacterial pneumonia**   MCC CC/MCC Exc

     AHA: Q4 2017

     Pneumonia due to gram-positive bacteria

J16 **Pneumonia due to** other infectious organisms, **not elsewhere classified**

     ☞ **Code first** associated influenza, if applicable (J09.X1, J10.0-, J11.0-)

     Code also associated abscess, if applicable (J85.1)

     EXCLUDES1 *congenital pneumonia (P23.-)*

         ornithosis (A70)

         pneumocystosis (B59)

         pneumonia NOS (J18.9)

J16.0 Chlamydial **pneumonia**   MCC CC/MCC Exc

J16.8 **Pneumonia due to other specified infectious organisms**   MCC CC/MCC Exc

J17 **Pneumonia in diseases classified elsewhere**   MCC CC/MCC Exc

     ☞ **Code first** underlying disease, such as:

     Q fever (A78)

     rheumatic fever (I00)

     schistosomiasis (B65.0-B65.9)

     EXCLUDES1 *candidial pneumonia (B37.1)*

         chlamydial pneumonia (J16.0)

         gonorrheal pneumonia (A54.84)

         histoplasmosis pneumonia (B39.0-B39.2)

         measles pneumonia (B05.2)

         nocardiosis pneumonia (A43.0)

         pneumocystosis (B59)

         pneumonia due to Pneumocystis carinii (B59)

         pneumonia due to Pneumocystis jiroveci (B59)

         pneumonia in actinomycosis (A42.0)

         pneumonia in anthrax (A22.1)

         pneumonia in ascariasis (B77.81)

         pneumonia in aspergillosis (B44.0-B44.1)

         pneumonia in coccidioidomycosis (B38.0-B38.2)

         pneumonia in cytomegalovirus disease (B25.0)

         pneumonia in toxoplasmosis (B58.3)

         rubella pneumonia (B06.81)

         salmonella pneumonia (A02.22)

         spirochetal infection NEC with pneumonia (A69.8)

         tularemia pneumonia (A21.2)

         typhoid fever with pneumonia (A01.03)

         varicella pneumonia (B01.2)

         whooping cough with pneumonia (A37 with fifth-character 1)

J18 **Pneumonia,** unspecified organism

     ☞ **Code first** associated influenza, if applicable (J09.X1, J10.0-, J11.0-)

     EXCLUDES1 *abscess of lung with pneumonia (J85.1)*

         aspiration pneumonia due to anesthesia during labor and delivery (O74.0)

         aspiration pneumonia due to anesthesia during pregnancy (O29)

         aspiration pneumonia due to anesthesia during puerperium (O89.0)

         aspiration pneumonia due to solids and liquids (J69.-)

         aspiration pneumonia NOS (J69.0)

         congenital pneumonia (P23.0)

         drug-induced interstitial lung disorder (J70.2-J70.4)

         interstitial pneumonia NOS (J84.9)

         lipid pneumonia (J69.1)

         neonatal aspiration pneumonia (P24.-)

         pneumonitis due to external agents (J67-J70)

         pneumonitis due to fumes and vapors (J68.0)

         usual interstitial pneumonia (J84.17)

J18.0 Bronchopneumonia, **unspecified organism**   MCC CC/MCC Exc

     EXCLUDES1 *hypostatic bronchopneumonia (J18.2)*

         lipid pneumonia (J69.1)

     EXCLUDES2 *acute bronchiolitis (J21.-)*

         chronic bronchiolitis (J44.9)

J18.1 Lobar pneumonia, **unspecified organism**   HCC MCC CC/MCC Exc

     AHA: Q3 2018, Q3 2016

J18.2 Hypostatic pneumonia, **unspecified organism**   CC/MCC Exc

     Hypostatic bronchopneumonia

     Passive pneumonia

J18.8 Other pneumonia, **unspecified organism**   MCC CC/MCC Exc

J18.9 **Pneumonia, unspecified organism**   MCC CC/MCC Exc

     AHA: Q1 2019, Q2 2019, Q3 2016

Other acute lower respiratory infections (J20-J22)

EXCLUDES2 *chronic obstructive pulmonary disease with acute lower respiratory infection (J44.0)*

J20 **Acute** bronchitis

     INCLUDES *acute and subacute bronchitis (with) bronchospasm*

         acute and subacute bronchitis (with) tracheitis

         acute and subacute bronchitis (with) tracheobronchitis, acute

         acute and subacute fibrinous bronchitis

         acute and subacute membranous bronchitis

         acute and subacute purulent bronchitis

         acute and subacute septic bronchitis

     EXCLUDES1 *bronchitis NOS (J40)*

         tracheobronchitis NOS (J40)

     EXCLUDES2 *acute bronchitis with bronchiectasis (J47.0)*

         acute bronchitis with chronic obstructive asthma (J44.0)

         acute bronchitis with chronic obstructive pulmonary disease (J44.0)

         allergic bronchitis NOS (J45.909-)

         bronchitis due to chemicals, fumes and vapors (J68.0)

         chronic bronchitis NOS (J42)

         chronic mucopurulent bronchitis (J41.1)

         chronic obstructive bronchitis (J44.-)

         chronic obstructive tracheobronchitis (J44.-)

         chronic simple bronchitis (J41.0)

         chronic tracheobronchitis (J42)

J20.0 **Acute bronchitis due to** Mycoplasma pneumoniae

J20.1 **Acute bronchitis due to** Hemophilus influenzae

J20.2 **Acute bronchitis due to** streptococcus

J20.3 **Acute bronchitis due to** coxsackievirus

J20.4 **Acute bronchitis due to** parainfluenza virus

J20.5 **Acute bronchitis due to** respiratory syncytial virus

     Acute bronchitis due to RSV

J20.6 **Acute bronchitis due to** rhinovirus

     AHA: Q3 2016

J20.7 **Acute bronchitis due to** echovirus

J20.8 **Acute bronchitis due to other specified** organisms

     AHA: Q3 2016

J20.9 **Acute bronchitis, unspecified**

     AHA: Q3 2016

J21 **Acute** bronchiolitis

     INCLUDES *acute bronchiolitis with bronchospasm*

     EXCLUDES2 *respiratory bronchiolitis interstitial lung disease (J84.115)*

J21.0 **Acute bronchiolitis due to** respiratory syncytial virus   CC/MCC Exc

     Acute bronchiolitis due to RSV

J21.1 **Acute bronchiolitis due to** human metapneumovirus   CC/MCC Exc

---

Unspecified Code   Other Specified Code   Manifestation Code   N Newborn   P Pediatric   M Maternity   A Adult   ♂ Male   ♀ Female

● New Code   ▲ Revised Code Title   ▶◀ Revised Text   NOTES   INCLUDES   EXCLUDES1 Not coded here   EXCLUDES2 Not included here

4th character required   5th character required   6th character required   7th character required   Extension 'X' Alert

HAC Hospital-acquired condition (HAC) alert   AHA AHA Coding Clinic©   ☞ Code first alert

J21.8 Acute bronchiolitis due to other specified organisms ᶜᶜ CC/MCC Exc

J21.9 Acute bronchiolitis, unspecified ᶜᶜ CC/MCC Exc
Bronchiolitis (acute)
EXCLUDES1 chronic bronchiolitis (J44.-)

J22 Unspecified acute lower respiratory infection
Acute (lower) respiratory (tract) infection NOS
EXCLUDES1 upper respiratory infection (acute) (J06.9)

Other diseases of upper respiratory tract (J30-J39)

J30 Vasomotor and allergic rhinitis
INCLUDES spasmodic rhinorrhea
EXCLUDES1 allergic rhinitis with asthma (bronchial) (J45.909)
rhinitis NOS (J31.0)

J30.0 Vasomotor rhinitis

J30.1 Allergic rhinitis due to pollen
Allergy NOS due to pollen
Hay fever
Pollinosis

J30.2 Other seasonal allergic rhinitis

J30.5 Allergic rhinitis due to food

J30.8 Other allergic rhinitis
J30.81 Allergic rhinitis due to animal (cat) (dog) hair and dander
J30.89 Other allergic rhinitis
Perennial allergic rhinitis

J30.9 Allergic rhinitis, unspecified

J31 Chronic rhinitis, nasopharyngitis and pharyngitis
Use additional code to identify:
exposure to environmental tobacco smoke (Z77.22)
exposure to tobacco smoke in the perinatal period (P96.81)
history of tobacco dependence (Z87.891)
occupational exposure to environmental tobacco smoke (Z57.31)
tobacco dependence (F17.-)
tobacco use (Z72.0)

J31.0 Chronic rhinitis
Atrophic rhinitis (chronic)
Granulomatous rhinitis (chronic)
Hypertrophic rhinitis (chronic)
Obstructive rhinitis (chronic)
Ozena
Purulent rhinitis (chronic)
Rhinitis (chronic) NOS
Ulcerative rhinitis (chronic)
EXCLUDES1 allergic rhinitis (J30.1-J30.9)
vasomotor rhinitis (J30.0)

J31.1 Chronic nasopharyngitis
EXCLUDES2 acute nasopharyngitis (J00)

J31.2 Chronic pharyngitis
Chronic sore throat
Atrophic pharyngitis (chronic)
Granular pharyngitis (chronic)
Hypertrophic pharyngitis (chronic)
EXCLUDES2 acute pharyngitis (J02.9)

J32 Chronic sinusitis (Figure 10.1)
INCLUDES sinus abscess
sinus empyema
sinus infection
sinus suppuration
Use additional code to identify:
exposure to environmental tobacco smoke (Z77.22)
exposure to tobacco smoke in the perinatal period (P96.81)
history of tobacco dependence (Z87.891)
infectious agent (B95-B97)
occupational exposure to environmental tobacco smoke (Z57.31)
tobacco dependence (F17.-)
tobacco use (Z72.0)
EXCLUDES2 acute sinusitis (J01.-)

J32.0 Chronic maxillary sinusitis
Antritis (chronic)
Maxillary sinusitis NOS

J32.1 Chronic frontal sinusitis
Frontal sinusitis NOS

J32.2 Chronic ethmoidal sinusitis
Ethmoidal sinusitis NOS
EXCLUDES1 Woakes' ethmoiditis (J33.1)

J32.3 Chronic sphenoidal sinusitis
Sphenoidal sinusitis NOS

J32.4 Chronic pansinusitis
Pansinusitis NOS

J32.8 Other chronic sinusitis
Sinusitis (chronic) involving more than one sinus but not pansinusitis

J32.9 Chronic sinusitis, unspecified
Sinusitis (chronic) NOS

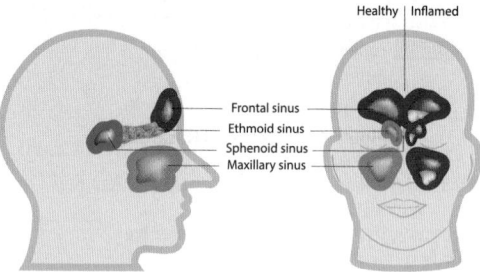

Healthy | Inflamed

Frontal sinus
Ethmoid sinus
Sphenoid sinus
Maxillary sinus

Figure 10.1 Chronic Sinusitis

J33 Nasal polyp
Use additional code to identify:
exposure to environmental tobacco smoke (Z77.22)
exposure to tobacco smoke in the perinatal period (P96.81)
history of tobacco dependence (Z87.891)
occupational exposure to environmental tobacco smoke (Z57.31)
tobacco dependence (F17.-)
tobacco use (Z72.0)
EXCLUDES1 adenomatous polyps (D14.0)

J33.0 Polyp of nasal cavity
Choanal polyp
Nasopharyngeal polyp

J33.1 Polypoid sinus degeneration
Woakes' syndrome or ethmoiditis

J33.8 Other polyp of sinus
Accessory polyp of sinus
Ethmoidal polyp of sinus
Maxillary polyp of sinus
Sphenoidal polyp of sinus

J33.9 Nasal polyp, unspecified

J34 Other and unspecified disorders of nose and nasal sinuses
EXCLUDES2 varicose ulcer of nasal septum (I86.8)

J34.0 Abscess, furuncle and carbuncle of nose
Cellulitis of nose
Necrosis of nose
Ulceration of nose

J34.1 Cyst and mucocele of nose and nasal sinus

J34.2 Deviated nasal septum (Figure 10.2)
Deflection or deviation of septum (nasal) (acquired)
EXCLUDES1 congenital deviated nasal septum (Q67.4)

J34.3 Hypertrophy of nasal turbinates

PDㅈ Unacceptable principal diagnosis symbol per Medicare code edits   PDㅈ Code exempt from diagnosis present on admission requirement
❓ Questionable admission   ᶜᶜ Complication or comorbidity   MCC Major complication or comorbidity   CC/MCC Exc CC/MCC exclusion
HCC HCC diagnosis code   RxHCC RxHCC diagnosis code   MACRA code   **DEFINITION** Describes condition/terminology
TIP Coding guidance   👁 Official Guideline Reference   Z Z code as first-listed diagnosis

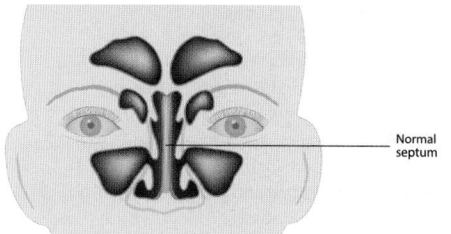

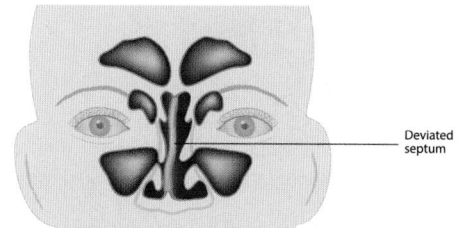

Figure 10.2 Deviated Nasal Septum

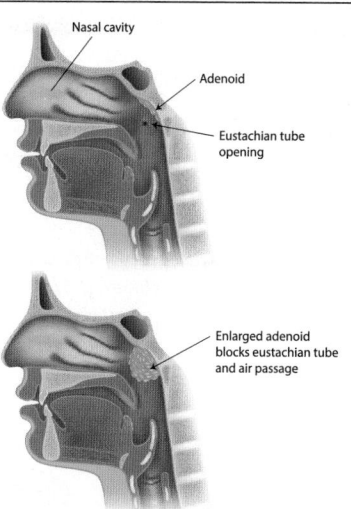

Figure 10.3 Adenoid Hypertrophy

5ᵗʰ **J34.8   Other specified disorders of nose and nasal sinuses**

J34.81   Nasal mucositis (ulcerative)

Code also type of associated therapy, such as:

antineoplastic and immunosuppressive drugs (T45.1X-)

radiological procedure and radiotherapy (Y84.2)

EXCLUDES2 *gastrointestinal mucositis (ulcerative) (K92.81)*

mucositis (ulcerative) of vagina and vulva (N76.81)

oral mucositis (ulcerative) (K12.3-)

J34.89   Other specified disorders of nose and nasal sinuses

Perforation of nasal septum NOS

Rhinolith

J34.9   Unspecified disorder of nose and nasal sinuses

4ᵗʰ **J35   Chronic diseases of** tonsils and adenoids

Use additional code to identify:

exposure to environmental tobacco smoke (Z77.22)

exposure to tobacco smoke in the perinatal period (P96.81)

history of tobacco dependence (Z87.891)

occupational exposure to environmental tobacco smoke (Z57.31)

tobacco dependence (F17.-)

tobacco use (Z72.0)

5ᵗʰ **J35.0   Chronic** tonsillitis and adenoiditis

EXCLUDES2 *acute tonsillitis (J03.-)*

J35.01   Chronic tonsillitis

J35.02   Chronic adenoiditis

J35.03   Chronic tonsillitis and adenoiditis

J35.1   Hypertrophy of tonsils

Enlargement of tonsils

EXCLUDES1 *hypertrophy of tonsils with tonsillitis (J35.0-)*

J35.2   Hypertrophy of adenoids **(Figure 10.3)**

Enlargement of adenoids

EXCLUDES1 *hypertrophy of adenoids with adenoiditis (J35.0-)*

J35.3   Hypertrophy of tonsils **with hypertrophy of** adenoids

EXCLUDES1 *hypertrophy of tonsils and adenoids with tonsillitis and adenoiditis (J35.03)*

J35.8   Other **chronic diseases of tonsils and adenoids**

Adenoid vegetations

Amygdalolith

Calculus, tonsil

Cicatrix of tonsil (and adenoid)

Tonsillar tag

Ulcer of tonsil

J35.9   Chronic disease of tonsils and adenoids, unspecified

Disease (chronic) of tonsils and adenoids NOS

J36   Peritonsillar abscess   CC CC/MCC Exc

INCLUDES   abscess of tonsil

peritonsillar cellulitis

quinsy

Use additional code (B95-B97) to identify infectious agent.

EXCLUDES1   *acute tonsillitis (J03.-)*

chronic tonsillitis (J35.0)

retropharyngeal abscess (J39.0)

tonsillitis NOS (J03.9-)

4ᵗʰ **J37   Chronic laryngitis and laryngotracheitis**

Use additional code to identify:

exposure to environmental tobacco smoke (Z77.22)

exposure to tobacco smoke in the perinatal period (P96.81)

history of tobacco dependence (Z87.891)

infectious agent (B95-B97)

occupational exposure to environmental tobacco smoke (Z57.31)

tobacco dependence (F17.-)

tobacco use (Z72.0)

J37.0   Chronic laryngitis

Catarrhal laryngitis

Hypertrophic laryngitis

Sicca laryngitis

EXCLUDES2   *acute laryngitis (J04.0)*

obstructive (acute) laryngitis (J05.0)

J37.1   Chronic laryngotracheitis

Laryngitis, chronic, with tracheitis (chronic)

Tracheitis, chronic, with laryngitis

EXCLUDES1   *chronic tracheitis (J42)*

EXCLUDES2   *acute laryngotracheitis (J04.2)*

acute tracheitis (J04.1)

2020 ICD-10-CM   When symbols appear on a code that requires a 7th character extension, refer to Appendix B to identify applicable 7th character codes.   **705**

CHAPTER 10: DISEASES OF THE RESPIRATORY SYSTEM (J00-J99)

🔵 J38 **Diseases of vocal cords and larynx, not elsewhere classified** (Figure 10.4)
Use additional code to identify:
exposure to environmental tobacco smoke (Z77.22)
exposure to tobacco smoke in the perinatal period (P96.81)
history of tobacco dependence (Z87.891)
occupational exposure to environmental tobacco smoke (Z57.31)
tobacco dependence (F17.-)
tobacco use (Z72.0)

EXCLUDES1 *congenital laryngeal stridor (P28.89)*
obstructive laryngitis (acute) (J05.0)
postprocedural subglottic stenosis (J95.5)
stridor (R06.1)
ulcerative laryngitis (J04.0)

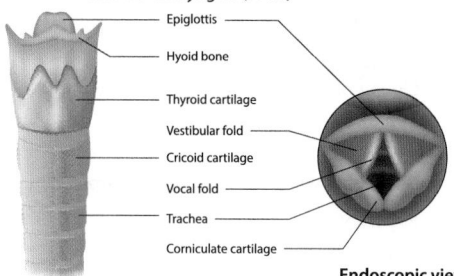

Anterior view   Endoscopic view

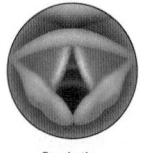   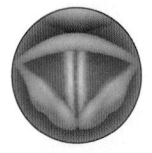

Respiration   Phonation

Figure 10.4 Larynx and Vocal Cords

🔵 J38.0 Paralysis of vocal cords and larynx
Laryngoplegia
Paralysis of glottis
J38.00 **Paralysis of vocal cords and larynx, unspecified**
J38.01 **Paralysis of vocal cords and larynx,** unilateral
J38.02 **Paralysis of vocal cords and larynx,** bilateral
J38.1 Polyp of vocal cord and larynx
EXCLUDES1 *adenomatous polyps (D14.1)*
J38.2 Nodules of vocal cords
Chorditis (fibrinous)(nodosa)(tuberosa)
Singer's nodes
Teacher's nodes
J38.3 Other diseases of vocal cords
Abscess of vocal cords
Cellulitis of vocal cords
Granuloma of vocal cords
Leukokeratosis of vocal cords
Leukoplakia of vocal cords
J38.4 Edema of larynx
Edema (of) glottis
Subglottic edema
Supraglottic edema
EXCLUDES1 *acute obstructive laryngitis [croup] (J05.0)*
edematous laryngitis (J04.0)
J38.5 **Laryngeal** spasm
Laryngismus (stridulus)
J38.6 Stenosis **of larynx**
J38.7 Other diseases **of larynx**
Abscess of larynx
Cellulitis of larynx
Disease of larynx NOS
Necrosis of larynx
Pachyderma of larynx

Perichondritis of larynx
Ulcer of larynx

🔵 J39 **Other diseases of** upper respiratory tract
EXCLUDES1 *acute respiratory infection NOS (J22)*
acute upper respiratory infection (J06.9)
upper respiratory inflammation due to chemicals, gases, fumes or vapors (J68.2)
J39.0 **Retropharyngeal and parapharyngeal** abscess cc° cc/mcc Exc
Peripharyngeal abscess
EXCLUDES1 *peritonsillar abscess (J36)*
J39.1 **Other** abscess **of pharynx** cc° cc/mcc Exc
Cellulitis of pharynx
Nasopharyngeal abscess
J39.2 **Other** diseases **of pharynx**
Cyst of pharynx
Edema of pharynx
EXCLUDES2 *chronic pharyngitis (J31.2)*
ulcerative pharyngitis (J02.9)
J39.3 **Upper respiratory tract hypersensitivity reaction, site unspecified**
EXCLUDES1 *hypersensitivity reaction of upper respiratory tract, such as:*
extrinsic allergic alveolitis (J67.9)
pneumoconiosis (J60-J67.9)
J39.8 **Other specified diseases of upper respiratory tract**
J39.9 **Disease of upper respiratory tract, unspecified**

Chronic lower respiratory diseases (J40-J47)

EXCLUDES1 *bronchitis due to chemicals, gases, fumes and vapors (J68.0)*
EXCLUDES2 *cystic fibrosis (E84.-)*
J40 Bronchitis, **not specified as acute or chronic**
Bronchitis NOS
Bronchitis with tracheitis NOS
Catarrhal bronchitis
Tracheobronchitis NOS
Use additional code to identify:
exposure to environmental tobacco smoke (Z77.22)
exposure to tobacco smoke in the perinatal period (P96.81)
history of tobacco dependence (Z87.891)
occupational exposure to environmental tobacco smoke (Z57.31)
tobacco dependence (F17.-)
tobacco use (Z72.0)
EXCLUDES1 *acute bronchitis (J20.-)*
allergic bronchitis NOS (J45.909-)
asthmatic bronchitis NOS (J45.9-)
bronchitis due to chemicals, gases, fumes and vapors (J68.0)
🔵 J41 **Simple and mucopurulent** chronic bronchitis
Use additional code to identify:
exposure to environmental tobacco smoke (Z77.22)
exposure to tobacco smoke in the perinatal period (P96.81)
history of tobacco dependence (Z87.891)
occupational exposure to environmental tobacco smoke (Z57.31)
tobacco dependence (F17.-)
tobacco use (Z72.0)
EXCLUDES1 *chronic bronchitis NOS (J42)*
chronic obstructive bronchitis (J44.-)
J41.0 Simple **chronic bronchitis** HCC RxHCC
J41.1 Mucopurulent **chronic bronchitis** HCC RxHCC
J41.8 Mixed simple and mucopurulent **chronic bronchitis** HCC RxHCC
J42 **Unspecified chronic bronchitis** HCC RxHCC
Chronic bronchitis NOS
Chronic tracheitis
Chronic tracheobronchitis
Use additional code to identify:
exposure to environmental tobacco smoke (Z77.22)
exposure to tobacco smoke in the perinatal period (P96.81)
history of tobacco dependence (Z87.891)

PDₓₓ Unacceptable principal diagnosis symbol per Medicare code edits   POA Code exempt from diagnosis present on admission requirement
❓ Questionable admission   CC° Complication or comorbidity   MCC° Major complication or comorbidity   CC/MCC Exc CC/MCC exclusion
HCC HCC diagnosis code   RxHCC RxHCC diagnosis code   MACRA MACRA code   **DEFINITION** Describes condition/terminology
TIP Coding guidance   👁 Official Guideline Reference   Zₓ Z code as first-listed diagnosis

706   When symbols appear on a code that requires a 7th character extension, refer to Appendix B to identify applicable 7th character codes.   **2020 ICD-10-CM**

occupational exposure to environmental tobacco smoke (Z57.31)
tobacco dependence (F17.-)
tobacco use (Z72.0)

EXCLUDES1 *chronic asthmatic bronchitis (J44.-)*
chronic bronchitis with airways obstruction (J44.-)
chronic emphysematous bronchitis (J44.-)
chronic obstructive pulmonary disease NOS (J44.9)
simple and mucopurulent chronic bronchitis (J41.-)

4ᵗʰ **J43** **Emphysema (Figure 10.5)**

Use additional code to identify:
exposure to environmental tobacco smoke (Z77.22)
history of tobacco dependence (Z87.891)
occupational exposure to environmental tobacco smoke (Z57.31)
tobacco dependence (F17.-)
tobacco use (Z72.0)

EXCLUDES1 *compensatory emphysema (J98.3)*
emphysema due to inhalation of chemicals, gases, fumes or vapors (J68.4)
emphysema with chronic (obstructive) bronchitis (J44.-)
emphysematous (obstructive) bronchitis (J44.-)
interstitial emphysema (J98.2)
mediastinal emphysema (J98.2)
neonatal interstitial emphysema (P25.0)
surgical (subcutaneous) emphysema (T81.82)
traumatic subcutaneous emphysema (T79.7)

J43.0 **Unilateral pulmonary emphysema [MacLeod's syndrome]** `HCC` `RxHCC`
Swyer-James syndrome
Unilateral emphysema
Unilateral hyperlucent lung
Unilateral pulmonary artery functional hypoplasia
Unilateral transparency of lung

J43.1 **Panlobular emphysema** `HCC` `RxHCC`
Panacinar emphysema

J43.2 **Centrilobular emphysema** `HCC` `RxHCC`

J43.8 **Other emphysema** `HCC` `RxHCC`

J43.9 **Emphysema, unspecified** `HCC` `RxHCC`
AHA: Q1 2019, Q4 2017
Bullous emphysema (lung)(pulmonary)
Emphysema (lung)(pulmonary) NOS
Emphysematous bleb
Vesicular emphysema (lung)(pulmonary)

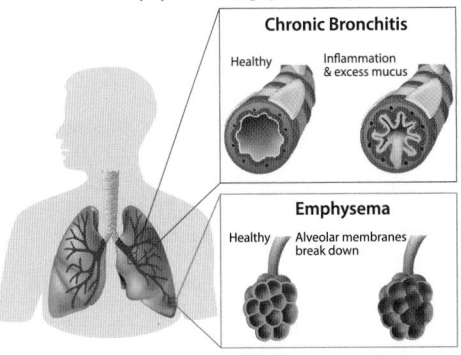

Figure 10.5 Chronic Bronchitis and Emphysema

4ᵗʰ **J44** **Other chronic obstructive pulmonary disease**

👁 **See Official Guidelines** "Acute exacerbation of chronic obstructive bronchitis and asthma" I.C.10.a.1

INCLUDES *asthma with chronic obstructive pulmonary disease*
chronic asthmatic (obstructive) bronchitis
chronic bronchitis with airways obstruction
chronic bronchitis with emphysema
chronic emphysematous bronchitis
chronic obstructive asthma
chronic obstructive bronchitis
chronic obstructive tracheobronchitis

Code also type of asthma, if applicable (J45.-)
Use additional code to identify:
exposure to environmental tobacco smoke (Z77.22)
history of tobacco dependence (Z87.891)
occupational exposure to environmental tobacco smoke (Z57.31)
tobacco dependence (F17.-)
tobacco use (Z72.0)

EXCLUDES1 *bronchiectasis (J47.-)*
chronic bronchitis NOS (J42)
chronic simple and mucopurulent bronchitis (J41.-)
chronic tracheitis (J42)
chronic tracheobronchitis (J42)
emphysema without chronic bronchitis (J43.-)

▲ **J44.0** **Chronic obstructive pulmonary disease with ▶(acute)◀ lower respiratory infection** `CC` `HCC` `RxHCC` `CC/MCC Exc`
AHA: Q1 2019, Q1 2017, Q2 2017, Q4 2017, Q3 2016
Code also to identify the infection

J44.1 **Chronic obstructive pulmonary disease with (acute) exacerbation** `CC` `HCC` `RxHCC` `CC/MCC Exc`
AHA: Q1 2019, Q1 2017, Q4 2017, Q3 2016
Decompensated COPD
Decompensated COPD with (acute) exacerbation
EXCLUDES2 *chronic obstructive pulmonary disease [COPD] with acute bronchitis (J44.0)*
lung diseases due to external agents (J60-J70)

J44.9 **Chronic obstructive pulmonary disease, unspecified** `HCC` `RxHCC`
AHA: Q1 2019, Q1 2017, Q4 2017, Q1 2016
Chronic obstructive airway disease NOS
Chronic obstructive lung disease NOS
EXCLUDES2 *lung diseases due to external agents (J60-J70)*

4ᵗʰ **J45** **Asthma**

👁 **See Official Guidelines** "Acute exacerbation of chronic obstructive bronchitis and asthma" I.C.10.a.1

INCLUDES *allergic (predominantly) asthma*
allergic bronchitis NOS
allergic rhinitis with asthma
atopic asthma
extrinsic allergic asthma
hay fever with asthma
idiosyncratic asthma
intrinsic nonallergic asthma
nonallergic asthma

Use additional code to identify:
exposure to environmental tobacco smoke (Z77.22)
exposure to tobacco smoke in the perinatal period (P96.81)
history of tobacco dependence (Z87.891)
occupational exposure to environmental tobacco smoke (Z57.31)
tobacco dependence (F17.-)
tobacco use (Z72.0)

EXCLUDES1 *detergent asthma (J69.8)*
eosinophilic asthma (J82)
miner's asthma (J60)
wheezing NOS (R06.2)
wood asthma (J67.8)

EXCLUDES2 *asthma with chronic obstructive pulmonary disease (J44.9)*
chronic asthmatic (obstructive) bronchitis (J44.9)
chronic obstructive asthma (J44.9)

5ᵗʰ **J45.2** **Mild intermittent asthma**

J45.20 **Mild intermittent asthma, uncomplicated** `RxHCC`
Mild intermittent asthma NOS

J45.21 **Mild intermittent asthma with (acute) exacerbation** `CC` `RxHCC` `CC/MCC Exc`

J45.22 **Mild intermittent asthma with status asthmaticus** `CC` `RxHCC` `CC/MCC Exc`

5ᵗʰ **J45.3** **Mild persistent asthma**

J45.30 **Mild persistent asthma, uncomplicated** `RxHCC`
Mild persistent asthma NOS

Unspecified Code Other Specified Code Manifestation Code N Newborn P Pediatric M Maternity A Adult ♂ Male ♀ Female
● New Code ▲ Revised Code Title ▶◀ Revised Text NOTES INCLUDES EXCLUDES1 Not coded here EXCLUDES2 Not included here
4ᵗʰ 4ᵗʰ character required 5ᵗʰ 5ᵗʰ character required 6ᵗʰ 6ᵗʰ character required 7ᵗʰ 7ᵗʰ character required Extension 'X' Alert
HAC Hospital-acquired condition (HAC) alert AHA AHA Coding Clinic© 📌 Code first alert

J45.31 Mild persistent asthma with (acute) exacerbation `cc` `RxHCC` `CC/MCC Exc`

J45.32 Mild persistent asthma with status asthmaticus `cc` `RxHCC` `CC/MCC Exc`

5ᵗʰ J45.4 Moderate persistent asthma

J45.40 Moderate persistent asthma, uncomplicated `RxHCC`
Moderate persistent asthma NOS

J45.41 Moderate persistent asthma with (acute) exacerbation `cc` `RxHCC` `CC/MCC Exc`
AHA: Q1 2017

J45.42 Moderate persistent asthma with status asthmaticus `cc` `RxHCC` `CC/MCC Exc`

5ᵗʰ J45.5 Severe persistent asthma

J45.50 Severe persistent asthma, uncomplicated `RxHCC`
Severe persistent asthma NOS

J45.51 Severe persistent asthma with (acute) exacerbation `MCC` `RxHCC` `CC/MCC Exc`

J45.52 Severe persistent asthma with status asthmaticus `cc` `RxHCC` `CC/MCC Exc`

5ᵗʰ J45.9 Other and unspecified asthma

6ᵗʰ J45.90 Unspecified asthma
Asthmatic bronchitis NOS
Childhood asthma NOS
Late onset asthma

J45.901 Unspecified asthma with (acute) exacerbation `cc` `RxHCC` `CC/MCC Exc`
AHA: Q4 2017

J45.902 Unspecified asthma with status asthmaticus `cc` `RxHCC` `CC/MCC Exc`

J45.909 Unspecified asthma, uncomplicated `RxHCC`
AHA: Q1 2017, Q4 2017
Asthma NOS
EXCLUDES2 *lung diseases due to external agents (J60-J70)*

6ᵗʰ J45.99 Other asthma
J45.990 Exercise induced bronchospasm `RxHCC`
J45.991 Cough variant asthma `RxHCC`
J45.998 Other asthma `RxHCC`

4ᵗʰ J47 Bronchiectasis
INCLUDES *bronchiolectasis*
Use additional code to identify:
exposure to environmental tobacco smoke (Z77.22)
exposure to tobacco smoke in the perinatal period (P96.81)
history of tobacco dependence (Z87.891)
occupational exposure to environmental tobacco smoke (Z57.31)
tobacco dependence (F17.-)
tobacco use (Z72.0)
EXCLUDES1 *congenital bronchiectasis (Q33.4)*
tuberculous bronchiectasis (current disease) (A15.0)

J47.0 Bronchiectasis with acute lower respiratory infection `cc` `HCC` `RxHCC` `CC/MCC Exc`
Bronchiectasis with acute bronchitis
Use additional code to identify the infection

J47.1 Bronchiectasis with (acute) exacerbation `cc` `HCC` `RxHCC` `CC/MCC Exc`

J47.9 Bronchiectasis, uncomplicated `HCC` `RxHCC`
Bronchiectasis NOS

Lung diseases due to external agents (J60-J70)

EXCLUDES2 *asthma (J45.-)*
malignant neoplasm of bronchus and lung (C34.-)

J60 Coalworker's pneumoconiosis `A` `HCC`
Anthracosilicosis
Anthracosis
Black lung disease
Coalworker's lung
EXCLUDES1 *coalworker pneumoconiosis with tuberculosis, any type in A15 (J65)*

J61 Pneumoconiosis due to asbestos and other mineral fibers `A` `HCC`
Asbestosis
EXCLUDES1 *pleural plaque with asbestosis (J92.0)*
pneumoconiosis with tuberculosis, any type in A15 (J65)

4ᵗʰ J62 Pneumoconiosis due to dust containing silica
INCLUDES *silicotic fibrosis (massive) of lung*
EXCLUDES1 *pneumoconiosis with tuberculosis, any type in A15 (J65)*

J62.0 Pneumoconiosis due to talc dust `HCC`

J62.8 Pneumoconiosis due to other dust containing silica `HCC`
Silicosis NOS

4ᵗʰ J63 Pneumoconiosis due to other inorganic dusts
EXCLUDES1 *pneumoconiosis with tuberculosis, any type in A15 (J65)*

J63.0 Aluminosis (of lung) `HCC`
J63.1 Bauxite fibrosis (of lung) `HCC`
J63.2 Berylliosis `HCC`
J63.3 Graphite fibrosis (of lung) `HCC`
J63.4 Siderosis `HCC`
J63.5 Stannosis `HCC`
J63.6 Pneumoconiosis due to other specified inorganic dusts `HCC`

J64 Unspecified pneumoconiosis `HCC`
EXCLUDES1 *pneumonoconiosis with tuberculosis, any type in A15 (J65)*

J65 Pneumoconiosis associated with tuberculosis `HCC`
Any condition in J60-J64 with tuberculosis, any type in A15
Silicotuberculosis

4ᵗʰ J66 Airway disease due to specific organic dust
EXCLUDES2 *allergic alveolitis (J67.-)*
asbestosis (J61)
bagassosis (J67.1)
farmer's lung (J67.0)
hypersensitivity pneumonitis due to organic dust (J67.-)
reactive airways dysfunction syndrome (J68.3)

J66.0 Byssinosis `HCC`
Airway disease due to cotton dust
J66.1 Flax-dressers' disease `HCC`
J66.2 Cannabinosis `HCC`
J66.8 Airway disease due to other specific organic dusts `HCC`

4ᵗʰ J67 Hypersensitivity pneumonitis due to organic dust
INCLUDES *allergic alveolitis and pneumonitis due to inhaled organic dust and particles of fungal, actinomycetic or other origin*
EXCLUDES1 *pneumonitis due to inhalation of chemicals, gases, fumes or vapors (J68.0)*

J67.0 Farmer's lung `HCC`
Harvester's lung
Haymaker's lung
Moldy hay disease

J67.1 Bagassosis `HCC`
Bagasse disease
Bagasse pneumonitis

J67.2 Bird fancier's lung `HCC`
Budgerigar fancier's disease or lung
Pigeon fancier's disease or lung

J67.3 Suberosis `HCC`
Corkhandler's disease or lung
Corkworker's disease or lung

J67.4 Maltworker's lung `HCC`
Alveolitis due to Aspergillus clavatus

J67.5 Mushroom-worker's lung `HCC`

J67.6 Maple-bark-stripper's lung `HCC`
Alveolitis due to Cryptostroma corticale
Cryptostromosis

J67.7 Air conditioner and humidifier lung `cc` `HCC` `CC/MCC Exc`
Allergic alveolitis due to fungal, thermophilic actinomycetes and other organisms growing in ventilation [air conditioning] systems

---

PDﬆ Unacceptable principal diagnosis symbol per Medicare code edits   ᴘᴏᴀ Code exempt from diagnosis present on admission requirement
❓ Questionable admission   `cc` Complication or comorbidity   `MCC` Major complication or comorbidity   `CC/MCC Exc` CC/MCC exclusion
`HCC` HCC diagnosis code   `RxHCC` RxHCC diagnosis code   MACRA code   **DEFINITION** Describes condition/terminology
TIP Coding guidance   👁 Official Guideline Reference   `Z1` Z code as first-listed diagnosis

When symbols appear on a code that requires a 7th character extension, refer to Appendix B to identify applicable 7th character codes.   **2020 ICD-10-CM**

J67.8 **Hypersensitivity pneumonitis due to** other
organic dusts   cc⃝ HCC CC/MCC Exc⃝
Cheese-washer's lung
Coffee-worker's lung
Fish-meal worker's lung
Furrier's lung
Sequoiosis

J67.9 **Hypersensitivity pneumonitis due to unspecified**
organic dust   cc⃝ HCC CC/MCC Exc⃝
Allergic alveolitis (extrinsic) NOS
Hypersensitivity pneumonitis NOS

④ᵗʰ **J68** Respiratory conditions **due to inhalation of chemicals, gases, fumes**
and vapors
☞ **Code first** (T51-T65) to identify cause
Use additional code to identify associated respiratory conditions,
such as:
acute respiratory failure (J96.0-)

J68.0 Bronchitis and pneumonitis **due to chemicals, gases, fumes**
and vapors   cc⃝ HCC CC/MCC Exc⃝
AHA: Q2 2019
Chemical bronchitis (acute)

J68.1 Pulmonary edema **due to chemicals, gases, fumes and**
vapors   HCC MCC⃝ CC/MCC Exc⃝
Chemical pulmonary edema (acute) (chronic)
EXCLUDES1 pulmonary edema (acute) (chronic) NOS (J81.-)

J68.2 Upper respiratory inflammation **due to chemicals, gases,**
fumes and vapors, not elsewhere classified   HCC

J68.3 Other acute and subacute respiratory conditions **due to**
chemicals, gases, fumes and vapors   HCC
Reactive airways dysfunction syndrome

J68.4 Chronic respiratory conditions **due to chemicals, gases,**
fumes and vapors   HCC
Emphysema (diffuse) (chronic) due to inhalation of chemicals,
gases, fumes and vapors
Obliterative bronchiolitis (chronic) (subacute) due to inhalation
of chemicals, gases, fumes and vapors
Pulmonary fibrosis (chronic) due to inhalation of chemicals,
gases, fumes and vapors
EXCLUDES1 chronic pulmonary edema due to chemicals, gases,
fumes and vapors (J68.1)

J68.8 Other respiratory conditions **due to chemicals, gases, fumes**
and vapors   HCC

J68.9 **Unspecified respiratory condition due to chemicals, gases,**
fumes and vapors   HCC

④ᵗʰ **J69** Pneumonitis **due to solids and liquids**
EXCLUDES1 neonatal aspiration syndromes (P24.-)
postprocedural pneumonitis (J95.4)

J69.0 **Pneumonitis due to inhalation of** food
and vomit   HCC MCC⃝ CC/MCC Exc⃝
AHA: Q2 2019, Q1 2017
Aspiration pneumonia NOS
Aspiration pneumonia (due to) food (regurgitated)
Aspiration pneumonia (due to) gastric secretions
Aspiration pneumonia (due to) milk
Aspiration pneumonia (due to) vomit
Code also any associated foreign body in respiratory tract
(T17.-)
EXCLUDES1 chemical pneumonitis due to anesthesia (J95.4)
obstetric aspiration pneumonitis (O74.0)

J69.1 **Pneumonitis due to inhalation of** oils
and essences   HCC MCC⃝ CC/MCC Exc⃝
Exogenous lipoid pneumonia
Lipid pneumonia NOS
☞ **Code first** (T51-T65) to identify substance
EXCLUDES1 endogenous lipoid pneumonia (J84.89)

J69.8 **Pneumonitis due to inhalation of** other solids
and liquids   HCC MCC⃝ CC/MCC Exc⃝
Pneumonitis due to aspiration of blood
Pneumonitis due to aspiration of detergent
☞ **Code first** (T51-T65) to identify substance

④ᵗʰ J70 Respiratory conditions **due to** other external agents
J70.0 Acute pulmonary manifestations due to
radiation   cc⃝ HCC RxHCC CC/MCC Exc⃝
Radiation pneumonitis
Use additional code (W88-W90, X39.0-) to identify the external
cause

J70.1 Chronic **and other pulmonary manifestations**
due to radiation   cc⃝ HCC RxHCC CC/MCC Exc⃝
Fibrosis of lung following radiation
Use additional code (W88-W90, X39.0-) to identify the external
cause

J70.2 Acute drug-induced **interstitial lung disorders**   HCC RxHCC
AHA: Q2 2019
Use additional code for adverse effect, if applicable, to identify
drug (T36-T50 with fifth or sixth character 5)
EXCLUDES1 interstitial pneumonia NOS (J84.9)
lymphoid interstitial pneumonia (J84.2)

J70.3 Chronic drug-induced **interstitial lung disorders**   HCC RxHCC
Use additional code for adverse effect, if applicable, to identify
drug (T36-T50 with fifth or sixth character 5)
EXCLUDES1 interstitial pneumonia NOS (J84.9)
lymphoid interstitial pneumonia (J84.2)

J70.4 Drug-induced **interstitial lung disorders, unspecified**   HCC RxHCC
AHA: Q2 2019
Use additional code for adverse effect, if applicable, to identify
drug (T36-T50 with fifth or sixth character 5)
EXCLUDES1 interstitial pneumonia NOS (J84.9)
lymphoid interstitial pneumonia (J84.2)

J70.5 **Respiratory conditions due to** smoke inhalation   HCC RxHCC
Smoke inhalation NOS
AHA: Q4 2013
EXCLUDES1 smoke inhalation due to chemicals, gases, fumes and
vapors (J68.9)

J70.8 **Respiratory conditions due to other specified**
external agents   HCC RxHCC
☞ **Code first** (T51-T65) to identify the external agent

J70.9 **Respiratory conditions due to unspecified**
external agent   HCC RxHCC
☞ **Code first** (T51-T65) to identify the external agent

Other respiratory diseases principally affecting the interstitium (J80-J84)

J80 **Acute respiratory distress syndrome**   HCC MCC⃝ CC/MCC Exc⃝
AHA: Q1 2017
Acute respiratory distress syndrome in adult or child
Adult hyaline membrane disease
EXCLUDES1 respiratory distress syndrome in newborn (perinatal) (P22.0)

④ᵗʰ J81 Pulmonary edema **(Figure 10.6)**
DEFINITION: Pulmonary edema occurs is abnormal buildup of fluid in
the alveolar sacs in the lungs.
Use additional code to identify:
exposure to environmental tobacco smoke (Z77.22)
history of tobacco dependence (Z87.891)
occupational exposure to environmental tobacco smoke (Z57.31)
tobacco dependence (F17.-)
tobacco use (Z72.0)
EXCLUDES1 chemical (acute) pulmonary edema (J68.1)
hypostatic pneumonia (J18.2)
passive pneumonia (J18.2)
pulmonary edema due to external agents (J60-J70)
pulmonary edema with heart disease NOS (I50.1)
pulmonary edema with heart failure (I50.1)

J81.0 Acute **pulmonary edema**   HCC MCC⃝ CC/MCC Exc⃝
Acute edema of lung

J81.1 Chronic **pulmonary edema**   cc⃝ CC/MCC Exc⃝
Pulmonary congestion (chronic) (passive)
Pulmonary edema NOS

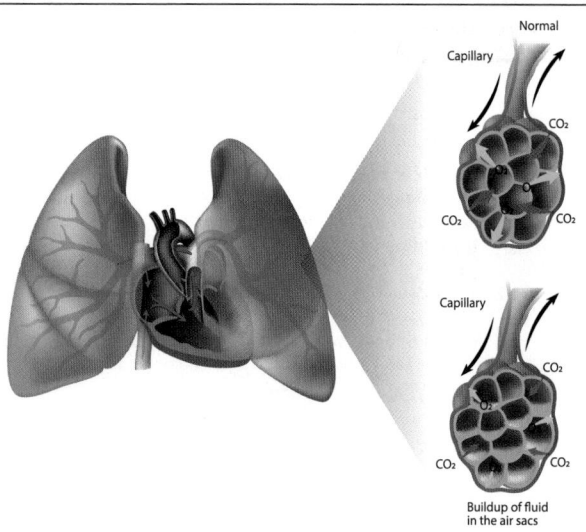

Normal

Capillary

CO_2

CO_2 / CO_2

Capillary

CO_2

O_2

CO_2 / CO_2

Buildup of fluid
in the air sacs

Figure 10.6 Pulmonary Edema

J82 Pulmonary eosinophilia, not elsewhere classified cc HCC CC/MCC Exc
Allergic pneumonia
Eosinophilic asthma
Eosinophilic pneumonia
Löffler's pneumonia
Tropical (pulmonary) eosinophilia NOS
EXCLUDES1 *pulmonary eosinophilia due to aspergillosis (B44.-)*
pulmonary eosinophilia due to drugs (J70.2-J70.4)
pulmonary eosinophilia due to specified parasitic infection (B50-B83)
pulmonary eosinophilia due to systemic connective tissue disorders (M30-M36)
pulmonary infiltrate NOS (R91.8)

J84 Other interstitial pulmonary diseases
EXCLUDES1 *drug-induced interstitial lung disorders (J70.2-J70.4)*
interstitial emphysema (J98.2)
EXCLUDES2 *lung diseases due to external agents (J60-J70)*

J84.0 Alveolar and parieto-alveolar conditions
J84.01 Alveolar proteinosis cc HCC RxHCC CC/MCC Exc
J84.02 Pulmonary alveolar microlithiasis cc HCC RxHCC CC/MCC Exc
J84.03 Idiopathic pulmonary hemosiderosis cc HCC RxHCC CC/MCC Exc
Essential brown induration of lung
☞ **Code first** underlying disease, such as:
disorders of iron metabolism (E83.1-)
EXCLUDES1 *acute idiopathic pulmonary hemorrhage in infants [AIPHI] (R04.81)*
J84.09 Other alveolar and parieto-alveolar conditions cc HCC RxHCC CC/MCC Exc

J84.1 Other interstitial pulmonary diseases with fibrosis
EXCLUDES1 *pulmonary fibrosis (chronic) due to inhalation of chemicals, gases, fumes or vapors (J68.4)*
pulmonary fibrosis (chronic) following radiation (J70.1)
J84.10 Pulmonary fibrosis, unspecified HCC RxHCC
Capillary fibrosis of lung
Cirrhosis of lung (chronic) NOS
Fibrosis of lung (atrophic) (chronic) (confluent) (massive) (perialveolar) (peribronchial) NOS
Induration of lung (chronic) NOS
Postinflammatory pulmonary fibrosis
J84.11 Idiopathic interstitial pneumonia
EXCLUDES1 *lymphoid interstitial pneumonia (J84.2)*
pneumocystis pneumonia (B59)
J84.111 Idiopathic interstitial pneumonia, not otherwise specified HCC RxHCC

J84.112 Idiopathic pulmonary fibrosis HCC RxHCC
Cryptogenic fibrosing alveolitis
Idiopathic fibrosing alveolitis
J84.113 Idiopathic non-specific interstitial pneumonitis HCC RxHCC
EXCLUDES1 *non-specific interstitial pneumonia NOS, or due to known underlying cause (J84.89)*
J84.114 Acute interstitial pneumonitis cc HCC RxHCC CC/MCC Exc
Hamman-Rich syndrome
EXCLUDES1 *pneumocystis pneumonia (B59)*
J84.115 Respiratory bronchiolitis interstitial lung disease HCC RxHCC
J84.116 Cryptogenic organizing pneumonia cc HCC RxHCC CC/MCC Exc
EXCLUDES1 *organizing pneumonia NOS, or due to known underlying cause (J84.89)*
J84.117 Desquamative interstitial pneumonia cc HCC RxHCC CC/MCC Exc

J84.17 Other interstitial pulmonary diseases with fibrosis in diseases classified elsewhere HCC RxHCC
Interstitial pneumonia (nonspecific) (usual) due to collagen vascular disease
Interstitial pneumonia (nonspecific) (usual) in diseases classified elsewhere
Organizing pneumonia due to collagen vascular disease
Organizing pneumonia in diseases classified elsewhere
☞ **Code first** underlying disease, such as:
progressive systemic sclerosis (M34.0)
rheumatoid arthritis (M05.00-M06.9)
systemic lupus erythematosis (M32.0-M32.9)

J84.2 Lymphoid interstitial pneumonia cc HCC RxHCC CC/MCC Exc
Lymphoid interstitial pneumonitis

J84.8 Other specified interstitial pulmonary diseases
EXCLUDES1 *exogenous lipoid pneumonia (J69.1)*
unspecified lipoid pneumonia (J69.1)
J84.81 Lymphangioleiomyomatosis HCC MCC RxHCC CC/MCC Exc
Lymphangiomyomatosis
J84.82 Adult pulmonary Langerhans cell histiocytosis A cc HCC RxHCC CC/MCC Exc
Adult PLCH
J84.83 Surfactant mutations of the lung HCC MCC RxHCC CC/MCC Exc
J84.84 Other interstitial lung diseases of childhood
J84.841 Neuroendocrine cell hyperplasia of infancy HCC MCC RxHCC CC/MCC Exc
J84.842 Pulmonary interstitial glycogenosis HCC MCC RxHCC CC/MCC Exc
J84.843 Alveolar capillary dysplasia with vein misalignment HCC MCC RxHCC CC/MCC Exc
J84.848 Other interstitial lung diseases of childhood HCC MCC RxHCC CC/MCC Exc

J84.89 Other specified interstitial pulmonary diseases HCC RxHCC
AHA: Q2 2019
Endogenous lipoid pneumonia
Interstitial pneumonitis
Non-specific interstitial pneumonitis NOS
Organizing pneumonia NOS
☞ **Code first,** if applicable:
poisoning due to drug or toxin (T51-T65 with fifth or sixth character to indicate intent), for toxic pneumonopathy
underlying cause of pneumonopathy, if known
Use additional code, for adverse effect, to identify drug (T36-T50 with fifth or sixth character 5), if drug-induced

PDxⁿ Unacceptable principal diagnosis symbol per Medicare code edits PDx Code exempt from diagnosis present on admission requirement
? Questionable admission cc Complication or comorbidity MCC Major complication or comorbidity cc/MCC Exc CC/MCC exclusion
HCC HCC diagnosis code RxHCC RxHCC diagnosis code MACRA code **DEFINITION** Describes condition/terminology
TIP Coding guidance 👁 Official Guideline Reference Z1 Z code as first-listed diagnosis

710 When symbols appear on a code that requires a 7th character extension, refer to Appendix B to identify applicable 7th character codes. **2020 ICD-10-CM**

[EXCLUDES1] *cryptogenic organizing pneumonia (J84.116)*
idiopathic non-specific interstitial pneumonitis (J84.113)
lipoid pneumonia, exogenous or unspecified (J69.1)
lymphoid interstitial pneumonia (J84.2)

J84.9 Interstitial pulmonary disease, unspecified [HCC] [RxHCC]
Interstitial pneumonia NOS

Suppurative and necrotic conditions of the lower respiratory tract (J85-J86)

[4th] **J85 Abscess of lung and mediastinum**
Use additional code (B95-B97) to identify infectious agent.
J85.0 Gangrene and necrosis of lung [HCC] [MCC] [CC/MCC Exc]
J85.1 Abscess of lung with pneumonia [HCC] [MCC] [CC/MCC Exc]
Code also the type of pneumonia
J85.2 Abscess of lung without pneumonia [HCC] [MCC] [CC/MCC Exc]
Abscess of lung NOS
J85.3 Abscess of mediastinum [HCC] [MCC] [CC/MCC Exc]

[4th] **J86 Pyothorax**
Use additional code (B95-B97) to identify infectious agent.
[EXCLUDES1] *abscess of lung (J85.-)*
pyothorax due to tuberculosis (A15.6)
J86.0 Pyothorax with fistula [HCC] [MCC] [CC/MCC Exc]
Bronchocutaneous fistula
Bronchopleural fistula
Hepatopleural fistula
Mediastinal fistula
Pleural fistula
Thoracic fistula
Any condition classifiable to J86.9 with fistula
J86.9 Pyothorax without fistula [HCC] [MCC] [CC/MCC Exc]
Abscess of pleura
Abscess of thorax
Empyema (chest) (lung) (pleura)
Fibrinopurulent pleurisy
Purulent pleurisy
Pyopneumothorax
Septic pleurisy
Seropurulent pleurisy
Suppurative pleurisy

Other diseases of the pleura (J90-J94)

J90 Pleural effusion, not elsewhere classified [CC] [CC/MCC Exc]
Encysted pleurisy
Pleural effusion NOS
Pleurisy with effusion (exudative) (serous)
[EXCLUDES1] *chylous (pleural) effusion (J94.0)*
malignant pleural effusion (J91.0))
pleurisy NOS (R09.1)
tuberculous pleural effusion (A15.6)

[4th] **J91 Pleural effusion in conditions classified elsewhere**
[EXCLUDES2] *pleural effusion in heart failure (I50.-)*
pleural effusion in systemic lupus erythematosus (M32.13)
J91.0 Malignant pleural effusion [CC] [CC/MCC Exc]
☞ **Code first** underlying neoplasm
J91.8 Pleural effusion in other conditions classified elsewhere [CC] [CC/MCC Exc]
AHA: Q2 2015
☞ **Code first** underlying disease, such as:
filariasis (B74.0-B74.9)
influenza (J09.X2, J10.1, J11.1)

[4th] **J92 Pleural plaque**
[INCLUDES] *pleural thickening*
J92.0 Pleural plaque with presence of asbestos
J92.9 Pleural plaque without asbestos
Pleural plaque NOS

[4th] **J93 Pneumothorax and air leak**
[EXCLUDES1] *congenital or perinatal pneumothorax (P25.1)*
postprocedural air leak (J95.812)
postprocedural pneumothorax (J95.811)
traumatic pneumothorax (S27.0)
tuberculous (current disease) pneumothorax (A15.-)
pyopneumothorax (J86.-)
J93.0 Spontaneous tension pneumothorax [MCC] [CC/MCC Exc]
[5th] **J93.1 Other spontaneous pneumothorax**
J93.11 Primary spontaneous pneumothorax [CC] [CC/MCC Exc]
J93.12 Secondary spontaneous pneumothorax [CC] [PDx] [CC/MCC Exc]
☞ **Code first** underlying condition, such as:
catamenial pneumothorax due to endometriosis (N80.8)
cystic fibrosis (E84.-)
eosinophilic pneumonia (J82)
lymphangioleiomyomatosis (J84.81)
malignant neoplasm of bronchus and lung (C34.-)
Marfan's syndrome (Q87.4)
pneumonia due to Pneumocystis carinii (B59)
secondary malignant neoplasm of lung (C78.0-)
spontaneous rupture of the esophagus (K22.3)
[5th] **J93.8 Other pneumothorax and air leak**
J93.81 Chronic pneumothorax [CC] [CC/MCC Exc]
J93.82 Other air leak [CC] [CC/MCC Exc]
Persistent air leak
J93.83 Other pneumothorax [CC] [CC/MCC Exc]
Acute pneumothorax
Spontaneous pneumothorax NOS
J93.9 Pneumothorax, unspecified [CC] [CC/MCC Exc]
Pneumothorax NOS

[4th] **J94 Other pleural conditions**
[EXCLUDES1] *pleurisy NOS (R09.1)*
traumatic hemopneumothorax (S27.2)
traumatic hemothorax (S27.1)
tuberculous pleural conditions (current disease) (A15.-)
J94.0 Chylous effusion [CC] [CC/MCC Exc]
Chyliform effusion
J94.1 Fibrothorax
J94.2 Hemothorax [CC] [CC/MCC Exc]
Hemopneumothorax
J94.8 Other specified pleural conditions [CC]
Hydropneumothorax
Hydrothorax
J94.9 Pleural condition, unspecified

Intraoperative and postprocedural complications and disorders of respiratory system, not elsewhere classified (J95)

[4th] **J95 Intraoperative and postprocedural complications and disorders of respiratory system, not elsewhere classified**
[EXCLUDES2] *aspiration pneumonia (J69.-)*
emphysema (subcutaneous) resulting from a procedure (T81.82)
hypostatic pneumonia (J18.2)
pulmonary manifestations due to radiation (J70.0-J70.1)
[5th] **J95.0 Tracheostomy complications**
J95.00 Unspecified tracheostomy complication [CC] [HCC] [CC/MCC Exc]
J95.01 Hemorrhage from tracheostomy stoma [CC] [HCC] [CC/MCC Exc]
J95.02 Infection of tracheostomy stoma [CC] [HCC] [CC/MCC Exc]
Use additional code to identify type of infection, such as:
cellulitis of neck (L03.221)
sepsis (A40, A41.-)
J95.03 Malfunction of tracheostomy stoma [CC] [HCC] [CC/MCC Exc]
Mechanical complication of tracheostomy stoma
Obstruction of tracheostomy airway
Tracheal stenosis due to tracheostomy

Unspecified Code | Other Specified Code | Manifestation Code | [N] Newborn | [P] Pediatric | [M] Maternity | [A] Adult | ♂ Male | ♀ Female
● New Code ▲ Revised Code Title ►◄ Revised Text [NOTES] [INCLUDES] [EXCLUDES1] Not coded here [EXCLUDES2] Not included here
[4th] 4th character required [5th] 5th character required [6th] 6th character required [7th] 7th character required [X] Extension 'X' Alert
[HAC] Hospital-acquired condition (HAC) alert **AHA** AHA Coding Clinic© ☞ **Code first** alert

J95.04 Tracheo-esophageal fistula **following tracheostomy** [CC] [HCC] [CC/MCC Exc]

J95.09 Other **tracheostomy complication** [CC] [HCC] [CC/MCC Exc]

J95.1 **Acute pulmonary insufficiency following** thoracic surgery [CC] [HCC] [CC/MCC Exc]
[EXCLUDES2] *Functional disturbances following cardiac surgery (I97.0, I97.1-)*

J95.2 **Acute pulmonary insufficiency following** nonthoracic surgery [HCC] [MCC] [CC/MCC Exc]
[EXCLUDES2] *Functional disturbances following cardiac surgery (I97.0, I97.1-)*

J95.3 Chronic pulmonary insufficiency **following surgery** [HCC] [MCC] [CC/MCC Exc]
[EXCLUDES2] *Functional disturbances following cardiac surgery (I97.0, I97.1-)*

J95.4 Chemical pneumonitis **due to anesthesia** [CC] [CC/MCC Exc]
Mendelson's syndrome
Postprocedural aspiration pneumonia
Use additional code for adverse effect, if applicable, to identify drug (T41.- with fifth or sixth character 5)
[EXCLUDES1] *aspiration pneumonitis due to anesthesia complicating labor and delivery (O74.0)*
aspiration pneumonitis due to anesthesia complicating pregnancy (O29)
aspiration pneumonitis due to anesthesia complicating the puerperium (O89.01)

J95.5 **Postprocedural** subglottic stenosis [CC] [CC/MCC Exc]

[5th] J95.6 **Intraoperative hemorrhage and hematoma of a respiratory system organ or structure** complicating a procedure
[EXCLUDES1] *intraoperative hemorrhage and hematoma of a respiratory system organ or structure due to accidental puncture and laceration during procedure (J95.7-)*

J95.61 **Intraoperative hemorrhage and hematoma of a respiratory system organ or structure complicating a** respiratory system procedure [CC] [CC/MCC Exc]

J95.62 **Intraoperative hemorrhage and hematoma of a respiratory system organ or structure** complicating other procedure [CC] [CC/MCC Exc]

[5th] J95.7 **Accidental puncture and laceration of a respiratory system organ or structure** during a procedure
[EXCLUDES2] *postprocedural pneumothorax (J95.811)*

J95.71 **Accidental puncture and laceration of a respiratory system organ or structure** during a respiratory system procedure [CC] [CC/MCC Exc]

J95.72 **Accidental puncture and laceration of a respiratory system organ or structure** during other procedure [CC] [CC/MCC Exc]

[5th] J95.8 Other **intraoperative and postprocedural complications and disorders of respiratory system, not elsewhere classified**

[6th] J95.81 Postprocedural **pneumothorax and air leak**

J95.811 **Postprocedural** pneumothorax [CC] [HAC] [CC/MCC Exc]

J95.812 **Postprocedural** air leak [CC] [CC/MCC Exc]

[6th] J95.82 **Postprocedural** respiratory failure
[EXCLUDES1] *Respiratory failure in other conditions (J96.-)*

J95.821 Acute **postprocedural respiratory failure** [CC] [HCC] [CC/MCC Exc]
Postprocedural respiratory failure NOS

J95.822 Acute and chronic **postprocedural respiratory failure** [HCC] [MCC] [CC/MCC Exc]

[6th] J95.83 **Postprocedural** hemorrhage **of a respiratory system organ or structure** following a procedure

J95.830 **Postprocedural hemorrhage of a respiratory system organ or structure** following a respiratory system procedure [CC] [CC/MCC Exc]

J95.831 **Postprocedural hemorrhage of a respiratory system organ or structure** following other procedure [CC] [CC/MCC Exc]

J95.84 Transfusion-related acute lung injury (TRALI) [CC] [CC/MCC Exc]

[6th] J95.85 **Complication of** respirator [ventilator]

J95.850 Mechanical complication **of respirator** [CC] [HCC] [CC/MCC Exc]
[EXCLUDES1] *encounter for respirator [ventilator] dependence during power failure (Z99.12)*

J95.851 Ventilator associated pneumonia [CC] [HCC] [CC/MCC Exc]
👁 **See Official Guidelines** "Documentation of Ventilator associated Pneumonia" I.C.10.d.1
AHA: Q1 2017
Ventilator associated pneumonitis
Use additional code to identify the organism, if known (B95.-, B96.-, B97.-)
[EXCLUDES1] *ventilator lung in newborn (P27.8)*

J95.859 Other complication **of respirator [ventilator]** [CC] [HCC] [CC/MCC Exc]

[6th] J95.86 **Postprocedural** hematoma and seroma **of a respiratory system organ or structure following a procedure**

J95.860 **Postprocedural** hematoma **of a** respiratory system **organ or structure following a** respiratory system **procedure** [CC] [CC/MCC Exc]

J95.861 **Postprocedural** hematoma **of a respiratory system organ or structure following** other **procedure** [CC] [CC/MCC Exc]

J95.862 **Postprocedural** seroma **of a** respiratory system **organ or structure following a** respiratory system **procedure** [CC] [CC/MCC Exc]

J95.863 **Postprocedural** seroma **of a respiratory system organ or structure following** other **procedure** [CC] [CC/MCC Exc]

J95.88 Other intraoperative complications **of respiratory system, not elsewhere classified** [CC] [CC/MCC Exc]

J95.89 Other postprocedural complications **and disorders of respiratory system, not elsewhere classified** [CC] [CC/MCC Exc]
Use additional code to identify disorder, such as:
aspiration pneumonia (J69.-)
bacterial or viral pneumonia (J12-J18)
[EXCLUDES2] *acute pulmonary insufficiency following thoracic surgery (J95.1)*
postprocedural subglottic stenosis (J95.5)

Other diseases of the respiratory system (J96-J99)

[4th] J96 **Respiratory failure, not elsewhere classified**
👁 **See Official Guidelines** "Acute respiratory failure as principal diagnosis" I.C.10.b.1
[EXCLUDES1] *acute respiratory distress syndrome (J80)*
cardiorespiratory failure (R09.2)
newborn respiratory distress syndrome (P22.0)
postprocedural respiratory failure (J95.82-)
respiratory arrest (R09.2)
respiratory arrest of newborn (P28.81)
respiratory failure of newborn (P28.5)

[5th] J96.0 Acute **respiratory failure**

J96.00 **Acute respiratory failure, unspecified whether with hypoxia or hypercapnia** [HCC] [MCC] [CC/MCC Exc]
AHA: Q3 2016

J96.01 **Acute respiratory failure** with hypoxia [HCC] [MCC] [CC/MCC Exc]

J96.02 **Acute respiratory failure** with hypercapnia [HCC] [MCC] [CC/MCC Exc]

[PDx] Unacceptable principal diagnosis symbol per Medicare code edits [POA] Code exempt from diagnosis present on admission requirement
[?] Questionable admission [CC] Complication or comorbidity [MCC] Major complication or comorbidity [CC/MCC Exc] CC/MCC exclusion
[HCC] HCC diagnosis code [RxHCC] RxHCC diagnosis code MACRA code **DEFINITION** Describes condition/terminology
TIP Coding guidance 👁 Official Guideline Reference [Z-1] Z code as first-listed diagnosis

J96.1   Chronic respiratory failure
   👁 See Official Guidelines "Status" I.C.21.c.3
   J96.10   **Chronic respiratory failure, unspecified whether with hypoxia or hypercapnia**   cͨ HCC CC/MCC Exc
     AHA: Q1 2016, Q1 2015
   J96.11   **Chronic respiratory failure with hypoxia**   cͨ HCC CC/MCC Exc
     AHA: Q4 2013
   J96.12   **Chronic respiratory failure with hypercapnia**   cͨ HCC CC/MCC Exc

J96.2   Acute and chronic respiratory failure
   👁 See Official Guidelines "Acute respiratory failure as principal diagnosis" I.C.10.b.1
   Acute on chronic respiratory failure
   J96.20   **Acute and chronic respiratory failure, unspecified whether with hypoxia or hypercapnia**   HCC MCCᶜ CC/MCC Exc
   J96.21   **Acute and chronic respiratory failure with hypoxia**   HCC MCCᶜ CC/MCC Exc
   J96.22   **Acute and chronic respiratory failure with hypercapnia**   HCC MCCᶜ CC/MCC Exc

J96.9   Respiratory failure, unspecified
   J96.90   **Respiratory failure, unspecified, unspecified whether with hypoxia or hypercapnia**   HCC MCCᶜ CC/MCC Exc
   J96.91   **Respiratory failure, unspecified with hypoxia**   HCC MCCᶜ CC/MCC Exc
   J96.92   **Respiratory failure, unspecified with hypercapnia**   HCC MCCᶜ CC/MCC Exc

J98   Other respiratory disorders
   Use additional code to identify:
   exposure to environmental tobacco smoke (Z77.22)
   exposure to tobacco smoke in the perinatal period (P96.81)
   history of tobacco dependence (Z87.891)
   occupational exposure to environmental tobacco smoke (Z57.31)
   tobacco dependence (F17.-)
   tobacco use (Z72.0)
   EXCLUDES1   newborn apnea (P28.4)
      newborn sleep apnea (P28.3)
   EXCLUDES2   apnea NOS (R06.81)
      sleep apnea (G47.3-)

   J98.0   Diseases of bronchus, not elsewhere classified
     J98.01   Acute bronchospasm   cͨ CC/MCC Exc
       EXCLUDES1   acute bronchiolitis with bronchospasm (J21.-)
         acute bronchitis with bronchospasm (J20.-)
         asthma (J45.-)
         exercise induced bronchospasm (J45.990)
     J98.09   Other diseases of bronchus, not elsewhere classified
       Broncholithiasis
       Calcification of bronchus
       Stenosis of bronchus
       Tracheobronchial collapse
       Tracheobronchial dyskinesia
       Ulcer of bronchus

   J98.1   Pulmonary collapse
     EXCLUDES1   therapeutic collapse of lung status (Z98.3)
     J98.11   Atelectasis   cͨ CC/MCC Exc
       EXCLUDES1   newborn atelectasis
         tuberculous atelectasis (current disease) (A15)
     J98.19   Other pulmonary collapse   cͨ CC/MCC Exc

   J98.2   Interstitial emphysema   HCC RxHCC
     Mediastinal emphysema
     EXCLUDES1   emphysema NOS (J43.9)
       emphysema in newborn (P25.0)
       surgical emphysema (subcutaneous) (T81.82)
       traumatic subcutaneous emphysema (T79.7)
   J98.3   Compensatory emphysema   HCC RxHCC

J98.4   Other disorders of lung
   AHA: Q4 2017
   Calcification of lung
   Cystic lung disease (acquired)
   Lung disease NOS
   Pulmolithiasis
   EXCLUDES1   acute interstitial pneumonitis (J84.114)
      pulmonary insufficiency following surgery (J95.1-J95.2)

J98.5   Diseases of mediastinum, not elsewhere classified
   EXCLUDES2   abscess of mediastinum (J85.3)
   J98.51   Mediastinitis   HAC MCCᶜ
     AHA: Q4 2016
     ☞ Code first underlying condition, if applicable, such as postoperative mediastinitis (T81.-)
   J98.59   Other diseases of mediastinum, not elsewhere classified   HAC MCCᶜ
     AHA: Q4 2016
     Fibrosis of mediastinum
     Hernia of mediastinum
     Retraction of mediastinum

J98.6   Disorders of diaphragm
   Diaphragmatitis
   Paralysis of diaphragm
   Relaxation of diaphragm
   EXCLUDES1   congenital malformation of diaphragm NEC (Q79.1)
      congenital diaphragmatic hernia (Q79.0)
   EXCLUDES2   diaphragmatic hernia (K44.-)

J98.8   Other specified respiratory disorders
J98.9   Respiratory disorder, unspecified
   Respiratory disease (chronic) NOS

J99   Respiratory disorders in diseases classified elsewhere   HCC RxHCC
  ☞ Code first underlying disease, such as:
   amyloidosis (E85.-)
   ankylosing spondylitis (M45)
   congenital syphilis (A50.5)
   cryoglobulinemia (D89.1)
   early congenital syphilis (A50.0)
   plasminogen deficiency (E88.02)
   schistosomiasis (B65.0-B65.9)
   EXCLUDES1   respiratory disorders in:
     amebiasis (A06.5)
     blastomycosis (B40.0-B40.2)
     candidiasis (B37.1)
     coccidioidomycosis (B38.0-B38.2)
     cystic fibrosis with pulmonary manifestations (E84.0)
     dermatomyositis (M33.01, M33.11)
     histoplasmosis (B39.0-B39.2)
     late syphilis (A52.72, A52.73)
     polymyositis (M33.21)
     sicca syndrome (M35.02)
     systemic lupus erythematosus (M32.13)
     systemic sclerosis (M34.81)
     Wegener's granulomatosis (M31.30-M31.31)

Unspecified Code   Other Specified Code   Manifestation Code   N Newborn   P Pediatric   M Maternity   A Adult   ♂ Male   ♀ Female
● New Code   ▲ Revised Code Title   ►◄ Revised Text   **NOTES**   *INCLUDES*   *EXCLUDES1* Not coded here   *EXCLUDES2* Not included here
4ᵗʰ character required   5ᵗʰ character required   6ᵗʰ character required   7ᵗʰ character required   Extension 'X' Alert
HAC Hospital-acquired condition (HAC) alert   AHA AHA Coding Clinic©   ☞ Code first alert

NOTES

Anatomy of the Digestive System

Introduction

The digestive system, or digestive tract, is responsible for breaking down food into nutrients that can be readily absorbed into the bloodstream. The digestive tract begins at the mouth and ends at the anus. Many accessory glands support the digestive tract and secrete enzymes for digestion.

1. **An Overview of the Digestive System**
    a) The process of digestion involves the breaking down of food into the simpler substances that can be utilized by multiple cells of the body for producing high energy (or ATP) molecules.
    b) The digestive system is based on the processes of ingestion, peristalsis, digestion, absorption and defecation.
    c) The mouth, pharynx, esophagus, stomach, small and large intestines, and anus are regarded as the organs of the digestive tract.
    d) The teeth, tongue, salivary glands, liver, gall bladder and pancreas are known as the accessory or subordinate organs of the digestive tract.
    e) The mucosa, submucosa, muscularis and adventitia (or serosa) are the coats (or tunics) of the digestive tract.

2. **The Anatomy of the Oral Cavity**
    a) The oral cavity is also known as the mouth (Figure 11.a) and is the first portion of the alimentary canal that receives food and saliva.
    b) The functions of the oral cavity are listed below:
        i) taste (through the taste buds on tongue).
        ii) mechanical breakdown of the food by the teeth.
        iii) chemical digestion of carbohydrates by the salivary enzyme amylase.
    c) The oral cavity is composed of the following components:
        i) mucus membrane that lines the oral cavity.
        ii) tongue that forms the floor of the oral cavity.
        iii) hard and soft palate that forms the roof of the oral cavity.
        iv) cheeks that form the sides of the oral cavity.

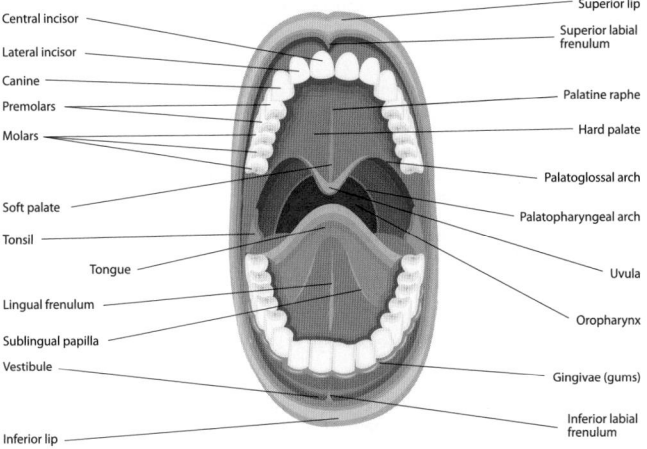

Figure 11.a Human Mouth

Central incisor, Lateral incisor, Canine, Premolars, Molars, Soft palate, Tonsil, Tongue, Lingual frenulum, Sublingual papilla, Vestibule, Inferior lip, Superior lip, Superior labial frenulum, Palatine raphe, Hard palate, Palatoglossal arch, Palatopharyngeal arch, Uvula, Oropharynx, Gingivae (gums), Inferior labial frenulum

    d) The salivary glands (Figure 11.b) are the exocrine glands that produce saliva. The parotid, submandibular (or submaxillary) and the sublingual glands are the three pairs of salivary glands.
    e) A typical human tooth is made up of dentin and consists of the following components:
        i) crown, which remains covered with enamel.
        ii) neck (or cervix).
        iii) root.
        iv) periodontal ligament, which fixates the tooth into its alveolar socket.

3. **The Anatomy of the Pharynx**
    a) The pharynx is the part of the throat that remains situated behind the nasal cavity and mouth and is a common passageway for food and air.

    b) The nasopharynx, oropharynx and laryngopharynx are the three parts of the pharynx.
    c) The pharynx is a part of both the digestive and respiratory systems and facilitates the process of speech production and swallowing (or deglutition).

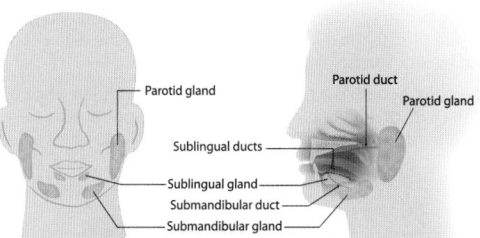

Parotid gland, Parotid duct, Parotid gland, Sublingual ducts, Sublingual gland, Submandibular duct, Submandibular gland

Figure 11.b The Salivary Glands

4. **The Anatomy of the Esophagus**
    a) The esophagus is a muscular tube for transporting the food from the pharynx to the stomach through the esophageal hiatus (or opening in the diaphragm).
    b) The food is propelled into the stomach via the lower esophageal sphincter. The movement of food is caused by the peristalsis (or symmetrical contraction and relaxation) of the smooth muscles.

5. **The Anatomy of the Stomach**
    a) The stomach is a muscular and hollow organ of the digestive tract and facilitates the second phase of digestion. It is positioned between the esophagus and the small intestine.
    b) The stomach aids in the digestion of food by performing the chemical breakdown of proteins through the protein-digesting enzyme pepsin.
    c) The stomach is based on the following four parts:
        i) cardia
        ii) fundus
        iii) body
        iv) pylorus
    d) The partially digested food (or chyme) is transported to the small intestine from the stomach.
    e) There are three kind of secretory cells in the gastric glands of the stomach mucosa.
        i) zymogenic cells, which secrete pepsinogen.
        ii) parietal cells, which secrete hydrochloric acid.
        iii) mucous cells, which secrete mucus.
    f) The stomach contains the below mentioned two sphincters (to retain the food contents inside it):
        i) esophageal sphincter, which is located in the cardiac region of the stomach.
        ii) pyloric sphincter, which demarcates the stomach from the small intestine.

6. **The Anatomy of the Pancreas**
    a) The pancreas (Figure 11.c, on the next page) is a glandular organ of both the digestive and endocrine systems.
    b) The pancreas is an endocrine as well as exocrine gland, and secretes hormones (like insulin, glucagon, and somatostatin) and the pancreatic juice (which contains several digestive enzymes). The digestive enzymes of the pancreatic juice facilitate the breakdown of the carbohydrates, proteins, and lipids in the chyme (or the partially digested food).
    c) The pancreas contains two types of the parenchymal tissues:
        i) pancreatic acini, which produce the digestive enzymes into the duodenum of the small intestine.
        ii) pancreatic islets of Langerhans, which secrete insulin and glucagon hormones into the blood for maintaining blood sugar levels.

7. **The Anatomy of the Liver**
    a) The liver (Figure 11.c, on the next page) is the largest glandular organ of the human body. It weighs about 1500g and is divided into the right and left lobes.

b) The lobules are the functional units of the liver.

c) The primary function of the liver is the storage of glycogen and secretion of bile. It also produces heparin, prothrombin, and thrombin.

d) The Kupffer cells (or stellate macrophages) of the liver perform phagocytosis of the bacteria and the worn out blood cells.

e) The liver stores various elements like copper, iron, and vitamins A, D, E, and K. It also helps to detoxify the poisonous substances in the human body, and produces bile salts for the emulsification (or break down) of the body fats.

f) The liver lobules facilitate the production of bile, which is then stored and concentrated in gall bladder.

g) The common bile duct carries the bile from the liver and gallbladder (Figure 11.c) to the duodenum. It is formed by the union of the cystic and hepatic ducts.

h) The porta hepatis is a transverse fissure in the middle visceral surface of the liver that gives passage to the hepatic portal vein, hepatic artery, hepatic nerve plexus, hepatic ducts, and the lymphatic vessels.

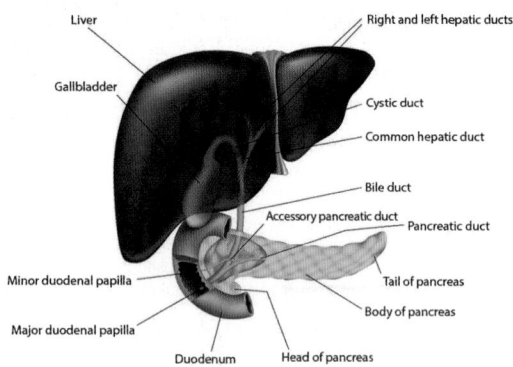

Figure 11.c Liver, Gallbladder, and Pancreas

8. The Anatomy of the Small Intestine

a) The small intestine extends from the pylorus of the stomach to the ileocecal junction. It is divided into the duodenum, jejunum and ileum.

b) The ileocecal valve serves to connect the small intestine with the large intestine.

c) The small intestine is involved in the completion of absorption of the digested food through the intestinal digestive enzymes, which are secreted by the intestinal glands (or the crypts of Lieberkuhn).

d) The Brunner's glands (or pancreal glands/duodenal glands) are the compound tubular submucosal glands of the duodenum that secrete alkaline mucus.

9. The Anatomy of the Large Intestine

a) The large intestine performs the following functions:

   i) reabsorption of water.

   ii) absorption and manufacture of vitamins.

   iii) formation and expulsion of feces.

b) The large intestine is based on cecum, colon, rectum, and anus.

c) The colon is divided into the following parts:

   i) ascending colon

   ii) right colic (or hepatic) flexure

   iii) transverse colon

   iv) left colic (or splenic) flexure

   v) descending colon

   vi) sigmoid colon

d) The rectum terminates at the anus. The dilated portion of the rectum where feces are stored (before their elimination through the anal canal) is termed as the rectal ampulla.

Common Pathologies

Appendicitis (Figure 11.d)
Inflammation of the appendix, which is usually acute and caused by the blocking of the appendix.

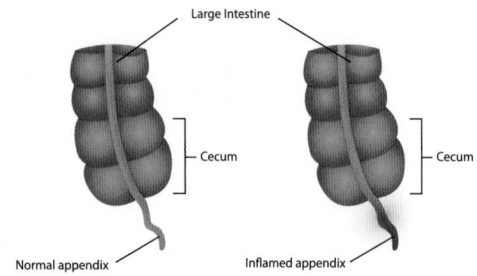

Figure 11.d Appendicitis

Ascites
Condition of abnormal accumulation of serous fluid in the peritoneal cavity.

Cirrhosis of Liver (Figure 11.e)
This is a chronic liver disease, which is characterized by destruction of liver cells that ultimately leads to ineffective liver function and jaundice.

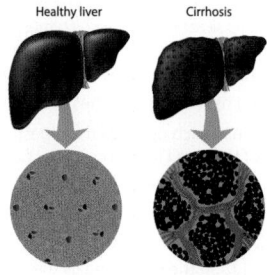

Figure 11.e Cirrhosis of the Liver

Diverticular Disease
This is a condition in which bulging pouches (known as diverticula) in the gastrointestinal (GI) tract push the mucosal lining through the surrounding muscle.

Dysentery
This is a condition that leads to inflammation of the intestine, especially of the colon, which may be caused by chemical irritants, bacteria, protozoa, or parasites.

Fistula
This is a condition in which there is an abnormal passage from one organ to another, or from a hollow organ to the surface.

Gastroesophageal Reflux Disease (GERD)
This is a condition that causes backflow (reflux) of gastric contents into the esophagus due to malfunction of the lower esophageal sphincter (LES).

Hematochezia
This is a condition marked by the passage of stools containing bright red blood.

Hemorrhoid (Figure 11.f)
This is a condition that causes a mass of enlarged, twisted varicose veins in the mucous membrane inside (internal) or just outside (external) the rectum; also known as piles.

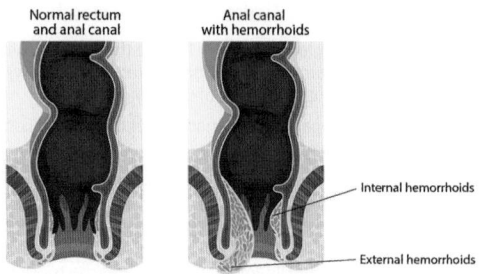

Figure 11.f Hemorrhoids

Hernia

This is a condition caused by the protrusion or projection of an organ or a part of an organ through the wall of the cavity that normally contains it. If a hernia protrudes through the diaphragm it is called a Hiatal hernia (Figure 11.g).

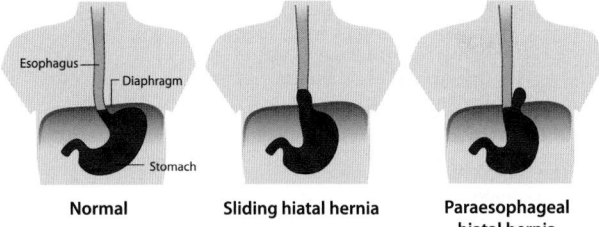

Normal   Sliding hiatal hernia   Paraesophageal hiatal hernia

Figure 11.g Hiatal Hernia

Inflammatory Bowel Disease (IBD) (Figure 11.h)

This is a condition in which ulceration of the colon mucosa occurs. Ulcerative colitis and Crohn's disease are forms of IBD.

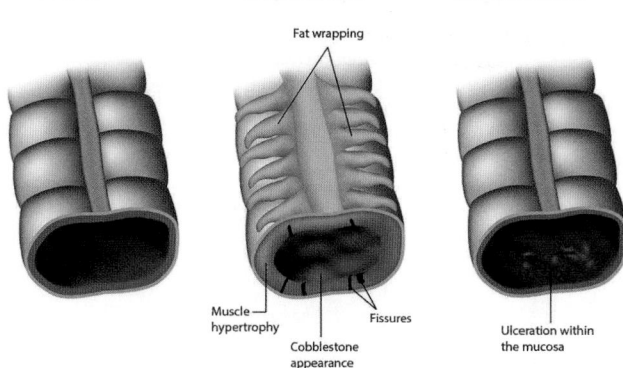

Figure 11.h Inflammatory Bowel Disease

Crohn's Disease

This is the condition of chronic IBD that usually affects the ileum but may affect any portion of the intestinal tract.

Ulcerative Colitis

This is the condition of chronic IBD of the colon characterized by episodes of diarrhea, rectal bleeding, and pain.

Irritable Bowel Syndrome (IBS)

This is the condition characterized by gastrointestinal signs and symptoms, including constipation, diarrhea, gas, and bloating, all in the absence of organic pathology; also called spastic colon.

Jaundice

This is the condition in which yellow discoloration of the skin, mucous membranes, and sclerae of the eyes is caused by excessive levels of bilirubin in the blood (hyperbilirubinemia).

Obesity

This is the condition in which a person accumulates an amount of fat that exceeds the body's skeletal and physical standards, usually an increase of 20 percent or more above ideal body weight.

Morbid Obesity

Condition of more severe obesity in which a person has a body mass index (BMI) of 40 or greater, which is generally 100 or more pounds over ideal body weight.

Polyp

A polyp is a small tumorlike, benign growth that projects from a mucous membrane surface.

Polyposis

This is a condition in which polyps develop in the intestinal tract.

Peptic Ulcer (Figure 11.i)

This condition is also known as peptic ulcer disease; these are the painful ulcers that usually arise in duodenum.

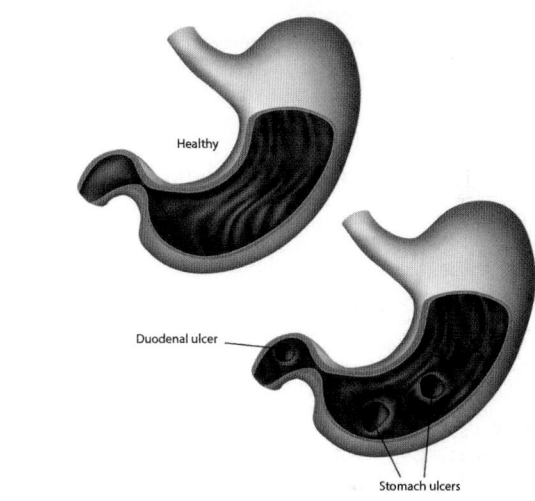

Figure 11.i Peptic Ulcer

Volvulus

This is a condition in which the bowel twists on itself, causing obstruction.

Diseases of the digestive system (K00-K95)

EXCLUDES2 *certain conditions originating in the perinatal period (P04-P96)*

certain infectious and parasitic diseases (A00-B99)

complications of pregnancy, childbirth and the puerperium (O00-O9A)

congenital malformations, deformations and chromosomal abnormalities (Q00-Q99)

endocrine, nutritional and metabolic diseases (E00-E88)

injury, poisoning and certain other consequences of external causes (S00-T88)

neoplasms (C00-D49)

symptoms, signs and abnormal clinical and laboratory findings, not elsewhere classified (R00-R94)

This chapter contains the following blocks:

K00-K14 Diseases of oral cavity and salivary glands
K20-K31 Diseases of esophagus, stomach and duodenum
K35-K38 Diseases of appendix
K40-K46 Hernia
K50-K52 Noninfective enteritis and colitis
K55-K64 Other diseases of intestines
K65-K68 Diseases of peritoneum and retroperitoneum
K70-K77 Diseases of liver
K80-K87 Disorders of gallbladder, biliary tract and pancreas
K90-K95 Other diseases of the digestive system

Diseases of oral cavity and salivary glands (K00-K14)

🔼 **K00 Disorders of tooth development and eruption (Figure 11.1)**

EXCLUDES2 *embedded and impacted teeth (K01.-)*

K00.0 Anodontia
Hypodontia
Oligodontia
EXCLUDES1 *acquired absence of teeth (K08.1-)*

K00.1 Supernumerary teeth
Distomolar
Fourth molar
Mesiodens
Paramolar
Supplementary teeth
EXCLUDES2 *supernumerary roots (K00.2)*

K00.2 Abnormalities of size and form of teeth
Concrescence of teeth
Fusion of teeth
Gemination of teeth
Dens evaginatus
Dens in dente
Dens invaginatus
Enamel pearls
Macrodontia
Microdontia
Peg-shaped [conical] teeth
Supernumerary roots
Taurodontism
Tuberculum paramolare
EXCLUDES1 *abnormalities of teeth due to congenital syphilis (A50.5)*

tuberculum Carabelli, which is regarded as a normal variation and should not be coded

K00.3 Mottled teeth
Dental fluorosis
Mottling of enamel
Nonfluoride enamel opacities
EXCLUDES2 *deposits [accretions] on teeth (K03.6)*

K00.4 Disturbances in tooth formation
Aplasia and hypoplasia of cementum
Dilaceration of tooth
Enamel hypoplasia (neonatal) (postnatal) (prenatal)
Regional odontodysplasia
Turner's tooth

EXCLUDES1 *Hutchinson's teeth and mulberry molars in congenital syphilis (A50.5)*

EXCLUDES2 *mottled teeth (K00.3)*

K00.5 Hereditary disturbances in tooth structure, not elsewhere classified
Amelogenesis imperfecta
Dentinogenesis imperfecta
Odontogenesis imperfecta
Dentinal dysplasia
Shell teeth

K00.6 Disturbances in tooth eruption
Dentia praecox
Natal tooth
Neonatal tooth
Premature eruption of tooth
Premature shedding of primary [deciduous] tooth
Prenatal teeth
Retained [persistent] primary tooth
EXCLUDES2 *embedded and impacted teeth (K01.-)*

K00.7 Teething syndrome

K00.8 Other disorders of tooth development
Color changes during tooth formation
Intrinsic staining of teeth NOS
EXCLUDES2 *posteruptive color changes (K03.7)*

K00.9 Disorder of tooth development, unspecified
Disorder of odontogenesis NOS

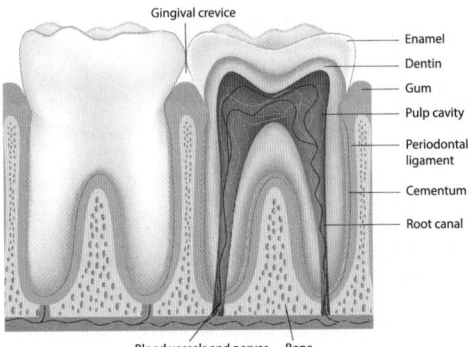

Figure 11.1 Tooth Anatomy

🔼 **K01 Embedded and impacted teeth**
EXCLUDES1 *abnormal position of fully erupted teeth (M26.3-)*
K01.0 Embedded teeth
K01.1 Impacted teeth

🔼 **K02 Dental caries**

DEFINITION: Dental caries means tooth decay or cavities.

INCLUDES *caries of dentine*

dental cavities

early childhood caries

pre-eruptive caries

recurrent caries (dentino enamel junction) (enamel) (to the pulp)

tooth decay

K02.3 Arrested dental caries
Arrested coronal and root caries

🔽 **K02.5 Dental caries on pit and fissure surface**
Dental caries on chewing surface of tooth

K02.51 Dental caries on pit and fissure surface limited to enamel
White spot lesions [initial caries] on pit and fissure surface of tooth

K02.52 Dental caries on pit and fissure surface penetrating into dentin
Primary dental caries, cervical origin

K02.53 Dental caries on pit and fissure surface penetrating into pulp

---

PDfin🅍 Unacceptable principal diagnosis symbol per Medicare code edits   POA🅝 Code exempt from diagnosis present on admission requirement
❓ Questionable admission   cᶜ Complication or comorbidity   MCC🅜 Major complication or comorbidity   cc/mcc excl CC/MCC exclusion
HCC HCC diagnosis code   RxHCC RxHCC diagnosis code   MACRA code   DEFINITION Describes condition/terminology
TIP Coding guidance   👁 Official Guideline Reference   Z1 Z code as first-listed diagnosis

When symbols appear on a code that requires a 7th character extension, refer to Appendix B to identify applicable 7th character codes.
2020 ICD-10-CM

(5ᵗʰ) **K02.6 Dental caries on** smooth surface
    K02.61 Dental caries on smooth surface limited to enamel
      White spot lesions [initial caries] on smooth surface of tooth
    K02.62 Dental caries on smooth surface penetrating into dentin
    K02.63 Dental caries on smooth surface penetrating into pulp
K02.7 Dental root **caries**
K02.9 Dental caries, unspecified
(4ᵗʰ) **K03** Other **diseases of hard tissues of teeth**
    EXCLUDES2 *bruxism (F45.8)*
      dental caries (K02.-)
      teeth-grinding NOS (F45.8)
K03.0 Excessive attrition of teeth
  Approximal wear of teeth
  Occlusal wear of teeth
K03.1 Abrasion of teeth
  Dentifrice abrasion of teeth
  Habitual abrasion of teeth
  Occupational abrasion of teeth
  Ritual abrasion of teeth
  Traditional abrasion of teeth
  Wedge defect NOS
K03.2 Erosion of teeth
  Erosion of teeth due to diet
  Erosion of teeth due to drugs and medicaments
  Erosion of teeth due to persistent vomiting
  Erosion of teeth NOS
  Idiopathic erosion of teeth
  Occupational erosion of teeth
K03.3 Pathological resorption of teeth
  Internal granuloma of pulp
  Resorption of teeth (external)
K03.4 Hypercementosis
  Cementation hyperplasia
K03.5 Ankylosis of teeth
K03.6 Deposits [accretions] on teeth
  Betel deposits [accretions] on teeth
  Black deposits [accretions] on teeth
  Extrinsic staining of teeth NOS
  Green deposits [accretions] on teeth
  Materia alba deposits [accretions] on teeth
  Orange deposits [accretions] on teeth
  Staining of teeth NOS
  Subgingival dental calculus
  Supragingival dental calculus
  Tobacco deposits [accretions] on teeth
K03.7 Posteruptive color changes of dental hard tissues
  EXCLUDES2 *deposits [accretions] on teeth (K03.6)*
(5ᵗʰ) **K03.8** Other **specified diseases of hard tissues of teeth**
    K03.81 Cracked tooth
      EXCLUDES1 *asymptomatic craze lines in enamel - omit code*
        broken or fractured tooth due to trauma (S02.5)
    K03.89 Other specified diseases of hard tissues of teeth
K03.9 Disease of hard tissues of teeth, unspecified
(4ᵗʰ) **K04 Diseases of pulp and periapical tissues**
  (5ᵗʰ) **K04.0 Pulpitis**
    Acute pulpitis
    Chronic (hyperplastic) (ulcerative) pulpitis
    K04.01 Reversible pulpitis
    K04.02 Irreversible pulpitis   CC CC/MCC Exc.
  K04.1 Necrosis of pulp
    Pulpal gangrene
  K04.2 Pulp degeneration
    Denticles
    Pulpal calcifications
    Pulpal stones
  K04.3 Abnormal hard tissue formation in pulp
    Secondary or irregular dentine

K04.4 Acute apical periodontitis of pulpal origin
  Acute apical periodontitis NOS
  EXCLUDES1 *acute periodontitis (K05.2-)*
K04.5 Chronic apical periodontitis
  Apical or periapical granuloma
  Apical periodontitis NOS
  EXCLUDES1 *chronic periodontitis (K05.3-)*
K04.6 Periapical abscess with sinus
  Dental abscess with sinus
  Dentoalveolar abscess with sinus
K04.7 Periapical abscess without sinus
  Dental abscess without sinus
  Dentoalveolar abscess without sinus
K04.8 Radicular cyst
  Apical (periodontal) cyst
  Periapical cyst
  Residual radicular cyst
  EXCLUDES2 *lateral periodontal cyst (K09.0)*
(5ᵗʰ) **K04.9** Other **and unspecified diseases of pulp and periapical tissues**
    K04.90 Unspecified diseases of pulp and periapical tissues
    K04.99 Other **diseases of pulp and periapical tissues**
(4ᵗʰ) **K05** Gingivitis **and** periodontal diseases
  Use additional code to identify:
  alcohol abuse and dependence (F10.-)
  exposure to environmental tobacco smoke (Z77.22)
  exposure to tobacco smoke in the perinatal period (P96.81)
  history of tobacco dependence (Z87.891)
  occupational exposure to environmental tobacco smoke (Z57.31)
  tobacco dependence (F17.-)
  tobacco use (Z72.0)
  (5ᵗʰ) **K05.0 Acute gingivitis**
    EXCLUDES1 *acute necrotizing ulcerative gingivitis (A69.1)*
      herpesviral [herpes simplex] gingivostomatitis (B00.2)
    K05.00 Acute gingivitis, plaque induced
      Acute gingivitis NOS
      Plaque induced gingival disease
    K05.01 Acute gingivitis, non-plaque induced
  (5ᵗʰ) **K05.1** Chronic **gingivitis**
    Desquamative gingivitis (chronic)
    Gingivitis (chronic) NOS
    Hyperplastic gingivitis (chronic)
    Pregnancy associated gingivitis
    Simple marginal gingivitis (chronic)
    Ulcerative gingivitis (chronic)
    ☛ **Code first,** if applicable, diseases of the digestive system complicating pregnancy (O99.61-)
    K05.10 Chronic gingivitis, plaque induced
      Chronic gingivitis NOS
      Gingivitis NOS
    K05.11 Chronic gingivitis, non-plaque induced
  (5ᵗʰ) **K05.2** Aggressive **periodontitis**
    Acute pericoronitis
    EXCLUDES1 *acute apical periodontitis (K04.4)*
      periapical abscess (K04.7)
      periapical abscess with sinus (K04.6)
    K05.20 Aggressive periodontitis, unspecified
    (6ᵗʰ) **K05.21 Aggressive periodontitis,** localized
      Periodontal abscess
      K05.211 Aggressive periodontitis, localized, slight
      K05.212 Aggressive periodontitis, localized, moderate
      K05.213 Aggressive periodontitis, localized, severe
      K05.219 Aggressive periodontitis, localized, unspecified severity
    (6ᵗʰ) **K05.22 Aggressive periodontitis,** generalized
      K05.221 Aggressive periodontitis, generalized, slight

K05.222 **Aggressive periodontitis, generalized,** moderate
K05.223 **Aggressive periodontitis, generalized,** severe
K05.229 **Aggressive periodontitis, generalized, unspecified severity**

[5th] K05.3 Chronic **periodontitis**
Chronic pericoronitis
Complex periodontitis
Periodontitis NOS
Simplex periodontitis
[EXCLUDES1] *chronic apical periodontitis (K04.5)*
K05.30 **Chronic periodontitis, unspecified**
[6th] K05.31 **Chronic periodontitis**, localized
K05.311 **Chronic periodontitis, localized,** slight
K05.312 **Chronic periodontitis, localized,** moderate
K05.313 **Chronic periodontitis, localized,** severe
K05.319 **Chronic periodontitis, localized, unspecified severity**
[6th] K05.32 **Chronic periodontitis,** generalized
K05.321 **Chronic periodontitis, generalized,** slight
K05.322 **Chronic periodontitis, generalized,** moderate
K05.323 **Chronic periodontitis, generalized,** severe
K05.329 **Chronic periodontitis, generalized, unspecified severity**

K05.4 **Periodontosis**
Juvenile periodontosis

K05.5 **Other periodontal diseases**
Combined periodontic-endodontic lesion
Narrow gingival width (of periodontal soft tissue)
[EXCLUDES2] *leukoplakia of gingiva (K13.21)*

K05.6 **Periodontal disease, unspecified**

[4th] K06 **Other disorders of gingiva and edentulous alveolar ridge**
[EXCLUDES2] *acute gingivitis (K05.0)*
atrophy of edentulous alveolar ridge (K08.2)
chronic gingivitis (K05.1)
gingivitis NOS (K05.1)

[5th] K06.0 **Gingival** recession
Gingival recession (postinfective) (postprocedural)
[6th] K06.01 **Gingival recession,** localized
K06.010 **Localized gingival recession, unspecified**
Localized gingival recession, NOS
K06.011 **Localized gingival recession,** minimal
K06.012 **Localized gingival recession,** moderate
K06.013 **Localized gingival recession,** severe
[6th] K06.02 **Gingival recession,** generalized
K06.020 **Generalized gingival recession, unspecified**
Generalized gingival recession, NOS
K06.021 **Generalized gingival recession,** minimal
K06.022 **Generalized gingival recession,** moderate
K06.023 **Generalized gingival recession,** severe

K06.1 **Gingival** enlargement
Gingival fibromatosis

K06.2 **Gingival and edentulous alveolar ridge lesions associated with** trauma
Irritative hyperplasia of edentulous ridge [denture hyperplasia]
Use additional code (Chapter 20) to identify external cause or denture status (Z97.2)

K06.3 **Horizontal alveolar bone loss**

K06.8 **Other specified disorders of gingiva and edentulous alveolar ridge**
Fibrous epulis
Flabby alveolar ridge
Giant cell epulis
Peripheral giant cell granuloma of gingiva
Pyogenic granuloma of gingiva
Vertical ridge deficiency
[EXCLUDES2] *gingival cyst (K09.0)*

K06.9 **Disorder of gingiva and edentulous alveolar ridge, unspecified**

[4th] K08 **Other disorders of teeth and supporting structures**
[EXCLUDES2] *dentofacial anomalies [including malocclusion] (M26.-)*
disorders of jaw (M27.-)

K08.0 **Exfoliation of teeth due to systemic causes**
Code also underlying systemic condition

[5th] K08.1 **Complete loss of teeth**
Acquired loss of teeth, complete
[EXCLUDES1] *congenital absence of teeth (K00.0)*
exfoliation of teeth due to systemic causes (K08.0)
partial loss of teeth (K08.4-)
[6th] K08.10 **Complete loss of teeth,** unspecified cause
K08.101 **Complete loss of teeth, unspecified cause,** class I
K08.102 **Complete loss of teeth, unspecified cause,** class II
K08.103 **Complete loss of teeth, unspecified cause,** class III
K08.104 **Complete loss of teeth, unspecified cause,** class IV
K08.109 **Complete loss of teeth, unspecified cause, unspecified class**
Edentulism NOS
[6th] K08.11 **Complete loss of teeth** due to trauma
K08.111 **Complete loss of teeth due to trauma,** class I
K08.112 **Complete loss of teeth due to trauma,** class II
K08.113 **Complete loss of teeth due to trauma,** class III
K08.114 **Complete loss of teeth due to trauma,** class IV
K08.119 **Complete loss of teeth due to trauma, unspecified class**
[6th] K08.12 **Complete loss of teeth due to** periodontal diseases
K08.121 **Complete loss of teeth due to periodontal diseases,** class I
K08.122 **Complete loss of teeth due to periodontal diseases,** class II
K08.123 **Complete loss of teeth due to periodontal diseases,** class III
K08.124 **Complete loss of teeth due to periodontal diseases,** class IV
K08.129 **Complete loss of teeth due to periodontal diseases, unspecified class**
[6th] K08.13 **Complete loss of teeth due to** caries
K08.131 **Complete loss of teeth due to caries,** class I
K08.132 **Complete loss of teeth due to caries,** class II
K08.133 **Complete loss of teeth due to caries,** class III
K08.134 **Complete loss of teeth due to caries,** class IV
K08.139 **Complete loss of teeth due to caries, unspecified class**
[6th] K08.19 **Complete loss of teeth due to** other specified cause
K08.191 **Complete loss of teeth due to other specified cause,** class I
K08.192 **Complete loss of teeth due to other specified cause,** class II
K08.193 **Complete loss of teeth due to other specified cause,** class III
K08.194 **Complete loss of teeth due to other specified cause,** class IV
K08.199 **Complete loss of teeth due to other specified cause, unspecified class**

[5th] K08.2 **Atrophy of edentulous alveolar ridge**
K08.20 **Unspecified atrophy of edentulous alveolar ridge**
Atrophy of the mandible NOS
Atrophy of the maxilla NOS
K08.21 Minimal **atrophy of the** mandible
Minimal atrophy of the edentulous mandible

[PDx] Unacceptable principal diagnosis symbol per Medicare code edits [POA] Code exempt from diagnosis present on admission requirement
[?] Questionable admission [CC] Complication or comorbidity [MCC] Major complication or comorbidity [CC/MCC Excl] CC/MCC exclusion
[HCC] HCC diagnosis code [RxHCC] RxHCC diagnosis code MACRA code **DEFINITION** Describes condition/terminology
TIP Coding guidance 👁 Official Guideline Reference [Z1] Z code as first-listed diagnosis

K08.22 Moderate **atrophy of the** mandible
Moderate atrophy of the edentulous mandible
K08.23 Severe **atrophy of the** mandible
Severe atrophy of the edentulous mandible
K08.24 Minimal **atrophy of** maxilla
Minimal atrophy of the edentulous maxilla
K08.25 Moderate **atrophy of the** maxilla
Moderate atrophy of the edentulous maxilla
K08.26 Severe **atrophy of the** maxilla
Severe atrophy of the edentulous maxilla
K08.3 **Retained dental root**
⑤ K08.4 **Partial loss of teeth**
Acquired loss of teeth, partial
EXCLUDES1 *complete loss of teeth (K08.1-)*
congenital absence of teeth (K00.0)
EXCLUDES2 *exfoliation of teeth due to systemic causes (K08.0)*
⑥ K08.40 **Partial loss of teeth,** unspecified cause
K08.401 **Partial loss of teeth, unspecified cause,** class I
K08.402 **Partial loss of teeth, unspecified cause,** class II
K08.403 **Partial loss of teeth, unspecified cause,** class III
K08.404 **Partial loss of teeth, unspecified cause,** class IV
K08.409 **Partial loss of teeth, unspecified cause, unspecified class**
Tooth extraction status NOS
⑥ K08.41 **Partial loss of teeth due to** trauma
K08.411 **Partial loss of teeth due to trauma,** class I
K08.412 **Partial loss of teeth due to trauma,** class II
K08.413 **Partial loss of teeth due to trauma,** class III
K08.414 **Partial loss of teeth due to trauma,** class IV
K08.419 **Partial loss of teeth due to trauma, unspecified class**
⑥ K08.42 **Partial loss of teeth due to** periodontal diseases
K08.421 **Partial loss of teeth due to periodontal diseases,** class I
K08.422 **Partial loss of teeth due to periodontal diseases,** class II
K08.423 **Partial loss of teeth due to periodontal diseases,** class III
K08.424 **Partial loss of teeth due to periodontal diseases,** class IV
K08.429 **Partial loss of teeth due to periodontal diseases, unspecified class**
⑥ K08.43 **Partial loss of teeth due to** caries
K08.431 **Partial loss of teeth due to caries,** class I
K08.432 **Partial loss of teeth due to caries,** class II
K08.433 **Partial loss of teeth due to caries,** class III
K08.434 **Partial loss of teeth due to caries,** class IV
K08.439 **Partial loss of teeth due to caries, unspecified class**
⑥ K08.49 **Partial loss of teeth due to** other specified cause
K08.491 **Partial loss of teeth due to other specified cause,** class I
K08.492 **Partial loss of teeth due to other specified cause,** class II
K08.493 **Partial loss of teeth due to other specified cause,** class III
K08.494 **Partial loss of teeth due to other specified cause,** class IV
K08.499 **Partial loss of teeth due to other specified cause, unspecified class**
⑤ K08.5 **Unsatisfactory restoration of tooth**
Defective bridge, crown, filling
Defective dental restoration
EXCLUDES1 *dental restoration status (Z98.811)*
EXCLUDES2 *endosseous dental implant failure (M27.6-)*
unsatisfactory endodontic treatment (M27.5-)

K08.50 **Unsatisfactory restoration of tooth, unspecified**
Defective dental restoration NOS
K08.51 **Open restoration margins of tooth**
Dental restoration failure of marginal integrity
Open margin on tooth restoration
Poor gingival margin to tooth restoration
K08.52 **Unrepairable overhanging of dental restorative materials**
Overhanging of tooth restoration
⑥ K08.53 **Fractured dental restorative material**
EXCLUDES1 *cracked tooth (K03.81)*
traumatic fracture of tooth (S02.5)
K08.530 **Fractured dental restorative material** without loss of material
K08.531 **Fractured dental restorative material** with loss of material
K08.539 **Fractured dental restorative material, unspecified**
K08.54 **Contour of existing restoration of tooth biologically incompatible with oral health**
Dental restoration failure of periodontal anatomical integrity
Unacceptable contours of existing restoration of tooth
Unacceptable morphology of existing restoration of tooth
K08.55 **Allergy to existing dental restorative material**
Use **additional** code to identify the specific type of allergy
K08.56 **Poor aesthetic of existing restoration of tooth**
Dental restoration aesthetically inadequate or displeasing
K08.59 **Other unsatisfactory restoration of tooth**
Other defective dental restoration
⑤ K08.8 **Other specified disorders of teeth and supporting structures**
K08.81 Primary **occlusal trauma**
K08.82 Secondary **occlusal trauma**
K08.89 Other specified disorders of teeth and supporting structures
Enlargement of alveolar ridge NOS
Insufficient anatomic crown height
Insufficient clinical crown length
Irregular alveolar process
Toothache NOS
K08.9 **Disorder of teeth and supporting structures, unspecified**
④ K09 **Cysts of oral region, not elsewhere classified**
INCLUDES *lesions showing histological features both of aneurysmal cyst and of another fibro-osseous lesion*
EXCLUDES2 *cysts of jaw (M27.0-, M27.4-)*
radicular cyst (K04.8)
K09.0 Developmental odontogenic **cysts**
Dentigerous cyst
Eruption cyst
Follicular cyst
Gingival cyst
Lateral periodontal cyst
Primordial cyst
EXCLUDES2 *keratocysts (D16.4, D16.5)*
odontogenic keratocystic tumors (D16.4, D16.5)
K09.1 Developmental (nonodontogenic) **cysts of oral region**
Cyst (of) incisive canal
Cyst (of) palatine of papilla
Globulomaxillary cyst
Median palatal cyst
Nasoalveolar cyst
Nasolabial cyst
Nasopalatine duct cyst
K09.8 **Other cysts of oral region, not elsewhere classified**
Dermoid cyst
Epidermoid cyst
Lymphoepithelial cyst
Epstein's pearl
K09.9 **Cyst of oral region, unspecified**

● Unspecified Code   Other Specified Code   Manifestation Code   Ⓝ Newborn   Ⓟ Pediatric   Ⓜ Maternity   Ⓐ Adult   ♂ Male   ♀ Female
● New Code   ▲ Revised Code Title   ►◄ Revised Text   **NOTES**   *INCLUDES*   EXCLUDES1 Not coded here   EXCLUDES2 Not included here
④ 4th character required   ⑤ 5th character required   ⑥ 6th character required   ⑦ 7th character required   ⑦ Extension 'X' Alert
HAC Hospital-acquired condition (HAC) alert   **AHA** AHA Coding Clinic©   📢 Code first alert

2020 ICD-10-CM   When symbols appear on a code that requires a 7th character extension, refer to Appendix B to identify applicable 7th character codes.   721

K11 Diseases of salivary glands (Figure 11.2)
 Use additional code to identify:
  alcohol abuse and dependence (F10.-)
  exposure to environmental tobacco smoke (Z77.22)
  exposure to tobacco smoke in the perinatal period (P96.81)
  history of tobacco dependence (Z87.891)
  occupational exposure to environmental tobacco smoke (Z57.31)
  tobacco dependence (F17.-)
  tobacco use (Z72.0)

K11.0 Atrophy of salivary gland
K11.1 Hypertrophy of salivary gland
K11.2 Sialoadenitis
   Parotitis
   EXCLUDES1 *epidemic parotitis (B26.-)*
        mumps (B26.-)
        uveoparotid fever [Heerfordt] (D86.89)
  K11.20 Sialoadenitis, unspecified
  K11.21 Acute sialoadenitis
       EXCLUDES1 *acute recurrent sialoadenitis (K11.22)*
  K11.22 Acute recurrent sialoadenitis
  K11.23 Chronic sialoadenitis
K11.3 Abscess of salivary gland
K11.4 Fistula of salivary gland
   EXCLUDES1 *congenital fistula of salivary gland (Q38.4)*
K11.5 Sialolithiasis
   Calculus of salivary gland or duct
   Stone of salivary gland or duct
K11.6 Mucocele of salivary gland
   Mucous extravasation cyst of salivary gland
   Mucous retention cyst of salivary gland
   Ranula
K11.7 Disturbances of salivary secretion
   Hypoptyalism
   Ptyalism
   Xerostomia
   EXCLUDES2 *dry mouth NOS (R68.2)*
K11.8 Other diseases of salivary glands
   Benign lymphoepithelial lesion of salivary gland
   Mikulicz' disease
   Necrotizing sialometaplasia
   Sialectasia
   Stenosis of salivary duct
   Stricture of salivary duct
   EXCLUDES1 *sicca syndrome [Sjögren] (M35.0-)*
K11.9 Disease of salivary gland, unspecified
   Sialoadenopathy NOS

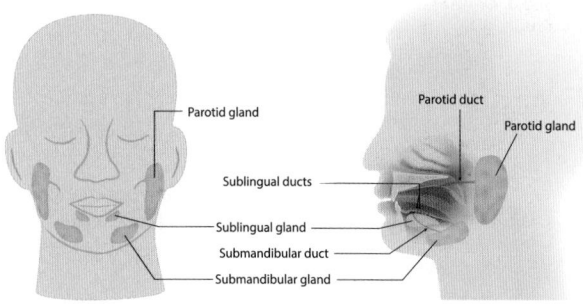

Figure 11.2 Salivary Glands

K12 Stomatitis and related lesions
 Use additional code to identify:
  alcohol abuse and dependence (F10.-)
  exposure to environmental tobacco smoke (Z77.22)
  exposure to tobacco smoke in the perinatal period (P96.81)
  history of tobacco dependence (Z87.891)

  occupational exposure to environmental tobacco smoke (Z57.31)
  tobacco dependence (F17.-)
  tobacco use (Z72.0)
 EXCLUDES1 *cancrum oris (A69.0)*
      cheilitis (K13.0)
      gangrenous stomatitis (A69.0)
      herpesviral [herpes simplex] gingivostomatitis (B00.2)
      noma (A69.0)

K12.0 Recurrent oral aphthae
   Aphthous stomatitis (major) (minor)
   Bednar's aphthae
   Periadenitis mucosa necrotica recurrens
   Recurrent aphthous ulcer
   Stomatitis herpetiformis
K12.1 Other forms of stomatitis
   Stomatitis NOS
   Denture stomatitis
   Ulcerative stomatitis
   Vesicular stomatitis
   EXCLUDES1 *acute necrotizing ulcerative stomatitis (A69.1)*
        Vincent's stomatitis (A69.1)
K12.2 Cellulitis and abscess of mouth   CC CC/MCC Exc
   Cellulitis of mouth (floor)
   Submandibular abscess
   EXCLUDES2 *abscess of salivary gland (K11.3)*
        abscess of tongue (K14.0)
        periapical abscess (K04.6-K04.7)
        periodontal abscess (K05.21)
        peritonsillar abscess (J36)
K12.3 Oral mucositis (ulcerative)
   Mucositis (oral) (oropharyngeal)
   EXCLUDES2 *gastrointestinal mucositis (ulcerative) (K92.81)*
        mucositis (ulcerative) of vagina and vulva (N76.81)
        nasal mucositis (ulcerative) (J34.81)
  K12.30 Oral mucositis (ulcerative), unspecified
  K12.31 Oral mucositis (ulcerative) due to antineoplastic therapy
       Use additional code for adverse effect, if applicable, to identify antineoplastic and immunosuppressive drugs (T45.1X5)
       Use additional code for other antineoplastic therapy, such as:
         radiological procedure and radiotherapy (Y84.2)
  K12.32 Oral mucositis (ulcerative) due to other drugs
       Use additional code for adverse effect, if applicable, to identify drug (T36-T50 with fifth or sixth character 5)
  K12.33 Oral mucositis (ulcerative) due to radiation
       Use additional external cause code (W88-W90, X39.0-) to identify cause
  K12.39 Other oral mucositis (ulcerative)
       Viral oral mucositis (ulcerative)
K13 Other diseases of lip and oral mucosa
 INCLUDES *epithelial disturbances of tongue*
 Use additional code to identify:
  alcohol abuse and dependence (F10.-)
  exposure to environmental tobacco smoke (Z77.22)
  exposure to tobacco smoke in the perinatal period (P96.81)
  history of tobacco dependence (Z87.891)
  occupational exposure to environmental tobacco smoke (Z57.31)
  tobacco dependence (F17.-)
  tobacco use (Z72.0)
 EXCLUDES2 *certain disorders of gingiva and edentulous alveolar ridge (K05-K06)*
      cysts of oral region (K09.-)
      diseases of tongue (K14.-)
      stomatitis and related lesions (K12.-)

K13.0 Diseases of lips
Abscess of lips
Angular cheilitis
Cellulitis of lips
Cheilitis NOS
Cheilodynia
Cheilosis
Exfoliative cheilitis
Fistula of lips
Glandular cheilitis
Hypertrophy of lips
Perlèche NEC
[EXCLUDES1] *ariboflavinosis (E53.0)*
cheilitis due to radiation-related disorders (L55-L59)
congenital fistula of lips (Q38.0)
congenital hypertrophy of lips (Q18.6)
Perlèche due to candidiasis (B37.83)
Perlèche due to riboflavin deficiency (E53.0)

K13.1 Cheek and lip biting

[5th] **K13.2 Leukoplakia and other disturbances of oral epithelium, including tongue**
[EXCLUDES1] *carcinoma in situ of oral epithelium (D00.0-)*
hairy leukoplakia (K13.3)

K13.21 Leukoplakia of oral mucosa, including tongue
Leukokeratosis of oral mucosa
Leukoplakia of gingiva, lips, tongue
[EXCLUDES1] *hairy leukoplakia (K13.3)*
leukokeratosis nicotina palati (K13.24)

K13.22 Minimal keratinized residual ridge mucosa
Minimal keratinization of alveolar ridge mucosa

K13.23 Excessive keratinized residual ridge mucosa
Excessive keratinization of alveolar ridge mucosa

K13.24 Leukokeratosis nicotina palati
Smoker's palate

K13.29 Other disturbances of oral epithelium, including tongue
Erythroplakia of mouth or tongue
Focal epithelial hyperplasia of mouth or tongue
Leukoedema of mouth or tongue
Other oral epithelium disturbances

K13.3 Hairy leukoplakia

K13.4 Granuloma and granuloma-like lesions of oral mucosa
Eosinophilic granuloma
Granuloma pyogenicum
Verrucous xanthoma

K13.5 Oral submucous fibrosis
Submucous fibrosis of tongue

K13.6 Irritative hyperplasia of oral mucosa
[EXCLUDES2] *irritative hyperplasia of edentulous ridge [denture hyperplasia] (K06.2)*

[5th] **K13.7 Other and unspecified lesions of oral mucosa**

K13.70 Unspecified lesions of oral mucosa

K13.79 Other lesions of oral mucosa
Focal oral mucinosis

[4th] **K14 Diseases of tongue (Figure 11.3)**
Use additional code to identify:
alcohol abuse and dependence (F10.-)
exposure to environmental tobacco smoke (Z77.22)
history of tobacco dependence (Z87.891)
occupational exposure to environmental tobacco smoke (Z57.31)
tobacco dependence (F17.-)
tobacco use (Z72.0)
[EXCLUDES2] *erythroplakia (K13.29)*
focal epithelial hyperplasia (K13.29)
leukedema of tongue (K13.29)
leukoplakia of tongue (K13.21)
hairy leukoplakia (K13.3)
macroglossia (congenital) (Q38.2)
submucous fibrosis of tongue (K13.5)

K14.0 Glossitis
Abscess of tongue
Ulceration (traumatic) of tongue
[EXCLUDES1] *atrophic glossitis (K14.4)*

K14.1 Geographic tongue
Benign migratory glossitis
Glossitis areata exfoliativa

K14.2 Median rhomboid glossitis

K14.3 Hypertrophy of tongue papillae
Black hairy tongue
Coated tongue
Hypertrophy of foliate papillae
Lingua villosa nigra

K14.4 Atrophy of tongue papillae
Atrophic glossitis

K14.5 Plicated tongue
Fissured tongue
Furrowed tongue
Scrotal tongue
[EXCLUDES1] *fissured tongue, congenital (Q38.3)*

K14.6 Glossodynia
Glossopyrosis
Painful tongue

K14.8 Other diseases of tongue
Atrophy of tongue
Crenated tongue
Enlargement of tongue
Glossocele
Glossoptosis
Hypertrophy of tongue

K14.9 Disease of tongue, unspecified
Glossopathy NOS

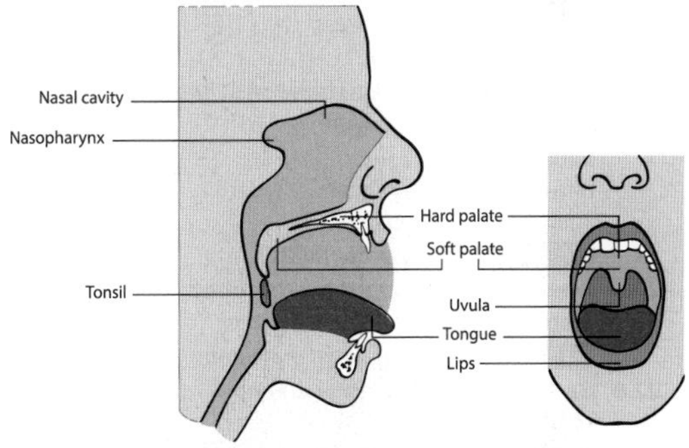

Figure 11.3 Mouth

Diseases of esophagus, stomach and duodenum (K20-K31)

[EXCLUDES2] *hiatus hernia (K44.-)*

[4th] **K20 Esophagitis**
Use additional code to identify:
alcohol abuse and dependence (F10.-)
[EXCLUDES1] *erosion of esophagus (K22.1-)*
esophagitis with gastro-esophageal reflux disease (K21.0)
reflux esophagitis (K21.0)
ulcerative esophagitis (K22.1-)
[EXCLUDES2] *eosinophilic gastritis or gastroenteritis (K52.81)*

K20.0 Eosinophilic esophagitis [RxHCC]

K20.8 Other esophagitis [RxHCC]
Abscess of esophagus

K20.9 Esophagitis, unspecified [RxHCC]
Esophagitis NOS

[4th] **K21 Gastro-esophageal reflux disease**
[EXCLUDES1] *newborn esophageal reflux (P78.83)*

K21.0 Gastro-esophageal reflux disease with esophagitis [RxHCC]
Reflux esophagitis

K21.9 Gastro-esophageal reflux disease without esophagitis [RxHCC]
AHA: Q1 2016
Esophageal reflux NOS

K22 Other diseases of esophagus
> *EXCLUDES2* esophageal varices (I85.-)

K22.0 Achalasia of cardia   RxHCC
> Achalasia NOS
> Cardiospasm
> *EXCLUDES1* congenital cardiospasm (Q39.5)

K22.1 Ulcer of esophagus
> Barrett's ulcer
> Erosion of esophagus
> Fungal ulcer of esophagus
> Peptic ulcer of esophagus
> Ulcer of esophagus due to ingestion of chemicals
> Ulcer of esophagus due to ingestion of drugs and medicaments
> Ulcerative esophagitis
> ☞ **Code first** poisoning due to drug or toxin, if applicable (T36-T65 with fifth or sixth character 1-4 or 6)
> **Use additional** code for adverse effect, if applicable, to identify drug (T36-T50 with fifth or sixth character 5)
> *EXCLUDES1* Barrett's esophagus (K22.7-)

   K22.10 Ulcer of esophagus without bleeding   CC CC/MCC Exc
> Ulcer of esophagus NOS

   K22.11 Ulcer of esophagus with bleeding   MCC CC/MCC Exc
> **AHA:** Q3 2018
> *EXCLUDES2* bleeding esophageal varices (I85.01, I85.11)

K22.2 Esophageal obstruction   RxHCC
> Compression of esophagus
> Constriction of esophagus
> Stenosis of esophagus
> Stricture of esophagus
> *EXCLUDES1* congenital stenosis or stricture of esophagus (Q39.3)

K22.3 Perforation of esophagus   MCC RxHCC CC/MCC Exc
> Rupture of esophagus
> *EXCLUDES1* traumatic perforation of (thoracic) esophagus (S27.8-)

K22.4 Dyskinesia of esophagus   RxHCC
> Corkscrew esophagus
> Diffuse esophageal spasm
> Spasm of esophagus
> *EXCLUDES1* cardiospasm (K22.0)

K22.5 Diverticulum of esophagus, acquired   RxHCC
> Esophageal pouch, acquired
> *EXCLUDES1* diverticulum of esophagus (congenital) (Q39.6)

K22.6 Gastro-esophageal laceration-hemorrhage syndrome   MCC CC/MCC Exc
> Mallory-Weiss syndrome

K22.7 Barrett's esophagus
> Barrett's disease
> Barrett's syndrome
> *EXCLUDES1* Barrett's ulcer (K22.1)
> > malignant neoplasm of esophagus (C15.-)

   K22.70 Barrett's esophagus without dysplasia   RxHCC
> Barrett's esophagus NOS

   K22.71 Barrett's esophagus with dysplasia

      K22.710 Barrett's esophagus with low grade dysplasia   RxHCC

      K22.711 Barrett's esophagus with high grade dysplasia   RxHCC

      K22.719 Barrett's esophagus with dysplasia, unspecified   RxHCC

K22.8 Other specified diseases of esophagus   RxHCC
> Hemorrhage of esophagus NOS
> *EXCLUDES2* esophageal varices (I85.-)
> > Paterson-Kelly syndrome (D50.1)

K22.9 Disease of esophagus, unspecified   RxHCC

K23 Disorders of esophagus in diseases classified elsewhere   RxHCC
> ☞ **Code first** underlying disease, such as:
> congenital syphilis (A50.5)
> *EXCLUDES1* late syphilis (A52.79)
> > megaesophagus due to Chagas' disease (B57.31)
> > tuberculosis (A18.83)

K25 Gastric ulcer
> *INCLUDES* erosion (acute) of stomach
> > pylorus ulcer (peptic)
> > stomach ulcer (peptic)
> **Use additional** code to identify:
> alcohol abuse and dependence (F10.-)
> *EXCLUDES1* acute gastritis (K29.0-)
> > peptic ulcer NOS (K27.-)

K25.0 Acute gastric ulcer with hemorrhage   MCC CC/MCC Exc

K25.1 Acute gastric ulcer with perforation   HCC MCC CC/MCC Exc

K25.2 Acute gastric ulcer with both hemorrhage and perforation   HCC MCC CC/MCC Exc

K25.3 Acute gastric ulcer without hemorrhage or perforation   CC CC/MCC Exc

K25.4 Chronic or unspecified gastric ulcer with hemorrhage   MCC CC/MCC Exc
> **AHA:** Q3 2017

K25.5 Chronic or unspecified gastric ulcer with perforation   HCC MCC CC/MCC Exc

K25.6 Chronic or unspecified gastric ulcer with both hemorrhage and perforation   HCC MCC CC/MCC Exc

K25.7 Chronic gastric ulcer without hemorrhage or perforation   CC CC/MCC Exc

K25.9 Gastric ulcer, unspecified as acute or chronic, without hemorrhage or perforation   CC CC/MCC Exc

K26 Duodenal ulcer
> *INCLUDES* erosion (acute) of duodenum
> > duodenum ulcer (peptic)
> > postpyloric ulcer (peptic)
> **Use additional** code to identify:
> alcohol abuse and dependence (F10.-)
> *EXCLUDES1* peptic ulcer NOS (K27.-)

K26.0 Acute duodenal ulcer with hemorrhage   MCC CC/MCC Exc

K26.1 Acute duodenal ulcer with perforation   HCC MCC CC/MCC Exc

K26.2 Acute duodenal ulcer with both hemorrhage and perforation   HCC MCC CC/MCC Exc

K26.3 Acute duodenal ulcer without hemorrhage or perforation   CC CC/MCC Exc

K26.4 Chronic or unspecified duodenal ulcer with hemorrhage   MCC CC/MCC Exc
> **AHA:** Q1 2016

K26.5 Chronic or unspecified duodenal ulcer with perforation   HCC MCC CC/MCC Exc

K26.6 Chronic or unspecified duodenal ulcer with both hemorrhage and perforation   HCC MCC CC/MCC Exc

K26.7 Chronic duodenal ulcer without hemorrhage or perforation

K26.9 Duodenal ulcer, unspecified as acute or chronic, without hemorrhage or perforation

K27 Peptic ulcer, site unspecified
> *INCLUDES* gastroduodenal ulcer NOS
> > peptic ulcer NOS
> **Use additional** code to identify:
> alcohol abuse and dependence (F10.-)
> *EXCLUDES1* peptic ulcer of newborn (P78.82)

K27.0 Acute peptic ulcer, site unspecified, with hemorrhage   MCC CC/MCC Exc

K27.1 Acute peptic ulcer, site unspecified, with perforation   HCC MCC CC/MCC Exc

K27.2 Acute peptic ulcer, site unspecified, with both hemorrhage and perforation   HCC MCC CC/MCC Exc

K27.3 Acute peptic ulcer, site unspecified, without hemorrhage or perforation   CC CC/MCC Exc

K27.4 Chronic or unspecified peptic ulcer, site unspecified, with hemorrhage   MCC CC/MCC Exc

K27.5 Chronic or unspecified peptic ulcer, site unspecified, with perforation   HCC MCC CC/MCC Exc

K27.6 Chronic or unspecified peptic ulcer, site unspecified, with both hemorrhage and perforation   HCC MCC CC/MCC Exc

---

Unacceptable principal diagnosis symbol per Medicare code edits   Code exempt from diagnosis present on admission requirement
   ❓ Questionable admission   CC Complication or comorbidity   MCC Major complication or comorbidity   CC/MCC Exc CC/MCC exclusion
HCC HCC diagnosis code   RxHCC RxHCC diagnosis code   MACRA code   **DEFINITION** Describes condition/terminology
TIP Coding guidance   👁 Official Guideline Reference   Z Z code as first-listed diagnosis

724   When symbols appear on a code that requires a 7th character extension, refer to Appendix B to identify applicable 7th character codes.   **2020 ICD-10-CM**

K27.7 Chronic **peptic ulcer, site unspecified,** without hemorrhage or perforation

K27.9 **Peptic ulcer, site unspecified, unspecified as acute or chronic,** without hemorrhage or perforation

🔟 **K28** Gastrojejunal **ulcer**

> *INCLUDES* anastomotic ulcer (peptic) or erosion
> gastrocolic ulcer (peptic) or erosion
> gastrointestinal ulcer (peptic) or erosion
> gastrojejunal ulcer (peptic) or erosion
> jejunal ulcer (peptic) or erosion
> marginal ulcer (peptic) or erosion
> stomal ulcer (peptic) or erosion

> Use additional code to identify:
> alcohol abuse and dependence (F10.-)

> *EXCLUDES1* primary ulcer of small intestine (K63.3)

K28.0 Acute **gastrojejunal ulcer** with hemorrhage

K28.1 Acute **gastrojejunal ulcer** with perforation

K28.2 Acute **gastrojejunal ulcer** with both hemorrhage and perforation

K28.3 Acute **gastrojejunal ulcer without hemorrhage or perforation**

K28.4 Chronic **or unspecified gastrojejunal ulcer** with hemorrhage

K28.5 Chronic **or unspecified gastrojejunal ulcer** with perforation

K28.6 Chronic **or unspecified gastrojejunal ulcer** with both hemorrhage and perforation

K28.7 Chronic **gastrojejunal ulcer** without hemorrhage or perforation

K28.9 **Gastrojejunal ulcer, unspecified as acute or chronic, without hemorrhage or perforation**

🔟 **K29** Gastritis and duodenitis

> *EXCLUDES1* eosinophilic gastritis or gastroenteritis (K52.81)
> Zollinger-Ellison syndrome (E16.4)

5️⃣ **K29.0** Acute **gastritis**

> Use additional code to identify:
> alcohol abuse and dependence (F10.-)

> *EXCLUDES1* erosion (acute) of stomach (K25.-)

K29.00 **Acute gastritis** without bleeding

K29.01 **Acute gastritis** with bleeding

5️⃣ **K29.2** Alcoholic **gastritis**

> Use additional code to identify:
> alcohol abuse and dependence (F10.-)

K29.20 **Alcoholic gastritis** without bleeding

K29.21 **Alcoholic gastritis** with bleeding

5️⃣ **K29.3** Chronic superficial **gastritis**

K29.30 **Chronic superficial gastritis** without bleeding

K29.31 **Chronic superficial gastritis** with bleeding

5️⃣ **K29.4** Chronic atrophic **gastritis**

> Gastric atrophy

K29.40 **Chronic atrophic gastritis** without bleeding

K29.41 **Chronic atrophic gastritis** with bleeding

5️⃣ **K29.5** Unspecified chronic **gastritis**

> Chronic antral gastritis
> Chronic fundal gastritis

K29.50 **Unspecified chronic gastritis** without bleeding

K29.51 **Unspecified chronic gastritis** with bleeding

5️⃣ **K29.6** Other **gastritis**

> Giant hypertrophic gastritis
> Granulomatous gastritis
> Ménétrier's disease

K29.60 **Other gastritis** without bleeding

K29.61 **Other gastritis** with bleeding

5️⃣ **K29.7** Gastritis, **unspecified**

K29.70 **Gastritis, unspecified,** without bleeding

K29.71 **Gastritis, unspecified,** with bleeding

5️⃣ **K29.8** Duodenitis

K29.80 **Duodenitis** without bleeding

K29.81 **Duodenitis** with bleeding

> **AHA:** Q3 2018

5️⃣ **K29.9** Gastroduodenitis, **unspecified**

K29.90 **Gastroduodenitis, unspecified,** without bleeding

K29.91 **Gastroduodenitis, unspecified,** with bleeding

K30 **Functional dyspepsia**

> Indigestion

> *EXCLUDES1* dyspepsia NOS (R10.13)
> heartburn (R12)
> nervous dyspepsia (F45.8)
> neurotic dyspepsia (F45.8)
> psychogenic dyspepsia (F45.8)

🔟 **K31** Other **diseases of stomach and duodenum**

> *INCLUDES* functional disorders of stomach

> *EXCLUDES2* diabetic gastroparesis (E08.43, E09.43, E10.43, E11.43, E13.43)
> diverticulum of duodenum (K57.00-K57.13)

K31.0 **Acute dilatation of stomach**

> Acute distention of stomach

K31.1 **Adult hypertrophic pyloric stenosis**

> Pyloric stenosis NOS

> *EXCLUDES1* congenital or infantile pyloric stenosis (Q40.0)

K31.2 **Hourglass stricture and stenosis of stomach**

> *EXCLUDES1* congenital hourglass stomach (Q40.2)
> hourglass contraction of stomach (K31.89)

K31.3 **Pylorospasm, not elsewhere classified**

> *EXCLUDES1* congenital or infantile pylorospasm (Q40.0)
> neurotic pylorospasm (F45.8)
> psychogenic pylorospasm (F45.8)

K31.4 **Gastric diverticulum**

> *EXCLUDES1* congenital diverticulum of stomach (Q40.2)

K31.5 **Obstruction of duodenum**

> Constriction of duodenum
> Duodenal ileus (chronic)
> Stenosis of duodenum
> Stricture of duodenum
> Volvulus of duodenum

> *EXCLUDES1* congenital stenosis of duodenum (Q41.0)

K31.6 **Fistula of stomach and duodenum**

> Gastrocolic fistula
> Gastrojejunocolic fistula

K31.7 **Polyp of stomach and duodenum**

> *EXCLUDES1* adenomatous polyp of stomach (D13.1)

5️⃣ **K31.8** Other **specified diseases of stomach and duodenum**

6️⃣ **K31.81** Angiodysplasia of stomach and duodenum

K31.811 **Angiodysplasia of stomach and duodenum with bleeding**

K31.819 **Angiodysplasia of stomach and duodenum without bleeding**

> Angiodysplasia of stomach and duodenum NOS

K31.82 **Dieulafoy lesion (hemorrhagic) of stomach and duodenum**

> *EXCLUDES2* Dieulafoy lesion of intestine (K63.81)

K31.83 **Achlorhydria**

K31.84 **Gastroparesis**

> **AHA:** Q4 2013
> Gastroparalysis

> ☞ **Code first** underlying disease, if known, such as:
> anorexia nervosa (F50.0-)
> diabetes mellitus (E08.43, E09.43, E10.43, E11.43, E13.43)
> scleroderma (M34.-)

K31.89 Other **diseases of stomach and duodenum**

> **AHA:** Q1 2017

K31.9 **Disease of stomach and duodenum, unspecified**

Diseases of appendix (K35-K38)

K35 Acute appendicitis (Figure 11.4)

  K35.2 **Acute appendicitis** with generalized peritonitis

    Appendicitis (acute) with generalized (diffuse) peritonitis following rupture or perforation of appendix

    K35.20 **Acute appendicitis with generalized peritonitis, without abscess**

      AHA: Q4 2018

      (Acute) appendicitis with generalized peritonitis NOS

    K35.21 **Acute appendicitis with generalized peritonitis, with abscess**

      AHA: Q4 2018

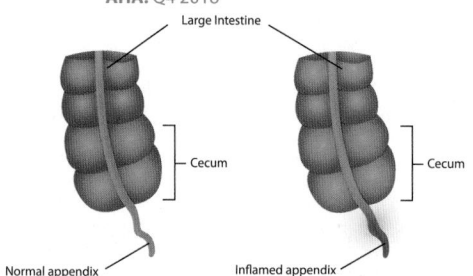

Large Intestine

Cecum — Cecum

Normal appendix — Inflamed appendix

Figure 11.4 Acute Appendicitis

  K35.3 **Acute appendicitis** with localized peritonitis

    K35.30 **Acute appendicitis with localized peritonitis, without perforation or gangrene**

      AHA: Q4 2018

      Acute appendicitis with localized peritonitis NOS

    K35.31 **Acute appendicitis with localized peritonitis and gangrene,** without perforation

      AHA: Q4 2018

    K35.32 **Acute appendicitis with perforation and localized peritonitis,** without abscess

      AHA: Q4 2018

      (Acute) appendicitis with perforation NOS

      Perforated appendix NOS

      Ruptured appendix (with localized peritonitis) NOS

    K35.33 **Acute appendicitis with perforation and localized peritonitis,** with abscess

      AHA: Q4 2018

      (Acute) appendicitis with (peritoneal) abscess NOS

      Ruptured appendix with localized peritonitis and abscess

  K35.8 Other and unspecified acute appendicitis

    K35.80 **Unspecified acute appendicitis**   CC⊘ CC/MCC Exc

      Acute appendicitis NOS

      Acute appendicitis without (localized) (generalized) peritonitis

    K35.89 Other acute appendicitis

      K35.890 **Other acute appendicitis** without perforation or gangrene   CC⊘ CC/MCC Exc

        AHA: Q4 2018

      K35.891 **Other acute appendicitis without perforation,** with gangrene   CC⊘ CC/MCC Exc

        AHA: Q4 2018

        (Acute) appendicitis with gangrene NOS

K36 **Other appendicitis**

  Chronic appendicitis

  Recurrent appendicitis

K37 **Unspecified appendicitis**

  EXCLUDES 1 -unspecified appendicitis with peritonitis (K35.2-, K35.3-)

K38 Other diseases of appendix

  K38.0 **Hyperplasia of appendix**

  K38.1 **Appendicular concretions**

    Fecalith of appendix

    Stercolith of appendix

  K38.2 **Diverticulum of appendix**

  K38.3 **Fistula of appendix**

  K38.8 **Other specified diseases of appendix**

    Intussusception of appendix

  K38.9 **Disease of appendix, unspecified**

Hernia (K40-K46)

  NOTES Hernia with both gangrene and obstruction is classified to hernia with gangrene.

  INCLUDES *acquired hernia*

    congenital [except diaphragmatic or hiatus] hernia

    recurrent hernia

K40 Inguinal **hernia**

  INCLUDES *bubonocele*

    direct inguinal hernia

    double inguinal hernia

    indirect inguinal hernia

    inguinal hernia NOS

    oblique inguinal hernia

    scrotal hernia

  K40.0 Bilateral **inguinal hernia,** with obstruction, without gangrene

    Inguinal hernia (bilateral) causing obstruction without gangrene

    Incarcerated inguinal hernia (bilateral) without gangrene

    Irreducible inguinal hernia (bilateral) without gangrene

    Strangulated inguinal hernia (bilateral) without gangrene

    K40.00 **Bilateral inguinal hernia, with obstruction, without gangrene,** not specified as recurrent   CC⊘ CC/MCC Exc

      Bilateral inguinal hernia, with obstruction, without gangrene NOS

    K40.01 **Bilateral inguinal hernia, with obstruction, without gangrene,** recurrent   CC⊘ CC/MCC Exc

  K40.1 Bilateral **inguinal hernia,** with gangrene

    K40.10 **Bilateral inguinal hernia, with gangrene,** not specified as recurrent   MCC⊘ CC/MCC Exc

      Bilateral inguinal hernia, with gangrene NOS

    K40.11 **Bilateral inguinal hernia, with gangrene,** recurrent   MCC⊘ CC/MCC Exc

  K40.2 Bilateral **inguinal hernia,** without obstruction or gangrene

    K40.20 **Bilateral inguinal hernia, without obstruction or gangrene,** not specified as recurrent

      Bilateral inguinal hernia NOS

    K40.21 **Bilateral inguinal hernia, without obstruction or gangrene,** recurrent

  K40.3 Unilateral **inguinal hernia,** with obstruction, without gangrene

    Inguinal hernia (unilateral) causing obstruction without gangrene

    Incarcerated inguinal hernia (unilateral) without gangrene

    Irreducible inguinal hernia (unilateral) without gangrene

    Strangulated inguinal hernia (unilateral) without gangrene

    K40.30 **Unilateral inguinal hernia, with obstruction, without gangrene,** not specified as recurrent   CC⊘ CC/MCC Exc

      Inguinal hernia, with obstruction NOS

      Unilateral inguinal hernia, with obstruction, without gangrene NOS

    K40.31 **Unilateral inguinal hernia, with obstruction, without gangrene,** recurrent   CC⊘ CC/MCC Exc

  K40.4 Unilateral **inguinal hernia,** with gangrene

    K40.40 **Unilateral inguinal hernia, with gangrene,** not specified as recurrent   MCC⊘ CC/MCC Exc

      Inguinal hernia with gangrene NOS

      Unilateral inguinal hernia with gangrene NOS

    K40.41 **Unilateral inguinal hernia, with gangrene,** recurrent   MCC⊘ CC/MCC Exc

  K40.9 Unilateral **inguinal hernia,** without obstruction or gangrene

    K40.90 **Unilateral inguinal hernia, without obstruction or gangrene,** not specified as recurrent

      Inguinal hernia NOS

      Unilateral inguinal hernia NOS

    K40.91 **Unilateral inguinal hernia, without obstruction or gangrene,** recurrent

K41 Femoral **hernia**

  K41.0 Bilateral **femoral hernia,** with obstruction, without gangrene

    Femoral hernia (bilateral) causing obstruction, without gangrene

    Incarcerated femoral hernia (bilateral), without gangrene

    Irreducible femoral hernia (bilateral), without gangrene

    Strangulated femoral hernia (bilateral), without gangrene

---

PDx Unacceptable principal diagnosis symbol per Medicare code edits   POA Code exempt from diagnosis present on admission requirement

  ❓ Questionable admission   CC Complication or comorbidity   MCC Major complication or comorbidity   CC/MCC Exc CC/MCC exclusion

  HCC HCC diagnosis code   RxHCC RxHCC diagnosis code   MACRA code   **DEFINITION** Describes condition/terminology

  TIP Coding guidance   👁 Official Guideline Reference   Z1 Z code as first-listed diagnosis

K41.00 Bilateral femoral hernia, with obstruction, without gangrene, not specified as recurrent cc⊘ CC/MCC Exc⊘
Bilateral femoral hernia, with obstruction, without gangrene NOS

K41.01 Bilateral femoral hernia, with obstruction, without gangrene, recurrent cc⊘ CC/MCC Exc⊘

🗣 **K41.1** Bilateral femoral hernia, with gangrene

K41.10 Bilateral femoral hernia, with gangrene, not specified as recurrent MCC⊘ CC/MCC Exc⊘
Bilateral femoral hernia, with gangrene NOS

K41.11 Bilateral femoral hernia, with gangrene, recurrent MCC⊘ CC/MCC Exc⊘

🗣 **K41.2** Bilateral femoral hernia, without obstruction or gangrene

K41.20 Bilateral femoral hernia, without obstruction or gangrene, not specified as recurrent
Bilateral femoral hernia NOS

K41.21 Bilateral femoral hernia, without obstruction or gangrene, recurrent

🗣 **K41.3** Unilateral femoral hernia, with obstruction, without gangrene
Femoral hernia (unilateral) causing obstruction, without gangrene
Incarcerated femoral hernia (unilateral), without gangrene
Irreducible femoral hernia (unilateral), without gangrene
Strangulated femoral hernia (unilateral), without gangrene

K41.30 Unilateral femoral hernia, with obstruction, without gangrene, not specified as recurrent cc⊘ CC/MCC Exc⊘
Femoral hernia, with obstruction NOS
Unilateral femoral hernia, with obstruction NOS

K41.31 Unilateral femoral hernia, with obstruction, without gangrene, recurrent cc⊘ CC/MCC Exc⊘

🗣 **K41.4** Unilateral femoral hernia, with gangrene

K41.40 Unilateral femoral hernia, with gangrene, not specified as recurrent MCC⊘ CC/MCC Exc⊘
Femoral hernia, with gangrene NOS
Unilateral femoral hernia, with gangrene NOS

K41.41 Unilateral femoral hernia, with gangrene, recurrent MCC⊘ CC/MCC Exc⊘

🗣 **K41.9** Unilateral femoral hernia, without obstruction or gangrene

K41.90 Unilateral femoral hernia, without obstruction or gangrene, not specified as recurrent
Femoral hernia NOS
Unilateral femoral hernia NOS

K41.91 Unilateral femoral hernia, without obstruction or gangrene, recurrent

④ᵗʰ **K42** Umbilical hernia

INCLUDES paraumbilical hernia

EXCLUDES1 omphalocele (Q79.2)

K42.0 Umbilical hernia with obstruction, without gangrene cc⊘ CC/MCC Exc⊘
Umbilical hernia causing obstruction, without gangrene
Incarcerated umbilical hernia, without gangrene
Irreducible umbilical hernia, without gangrene
Strangulated umbilical hernia, without gangrene

K42.1 Umbilical hernia with gangrene MCC⊘ CC/MCC Exc⊘
Gangrenous umbilical hernia

K42.9 Umbilical hernia without obstruction or gangrene
Umbilical hernia NOS

④ᵗʰ **K43** Ventral hernia

K43.0 Incisional hernia with obstruction, without gangrene cc⊘ CC/MCC Exc⊘
Incisional hernia causing obstruction, without gangrene
Incarcerated incisional hernia, without gangrene
Irreducible incisional hernia, without gangrene
Strangulated incisional hernia, without gangrene

K43.1 Incisional hernia with gangrene MCC⊘ CC/MCC Exc⊘
Gangrenous incisional hernia

K43.2 Incisional hernia without obstruction or gangrene
Incisional hernia NOS

K43.3 Parastomal hernia with obstruction, without gangrene cc⊘ CC/MCC Exc⊘
Incarcerated parastomal hernia, without gangrene
Irreducible parastomal hernia, without gangrene
Parastomal hernia causing obstruction, without gangrene
Strangulated parastomal hernia, without gangrene

K43.4 Parastomal hernia with gangrene MCC⊘ CC/MCC Exc⊘
Gangrenous parastomal hernia

K43.5 Parastomal hernia without obstruction or gangrene
Parastomal hernia NOS

K43.6 Other and unspecified ventral hernia with obstruction, without gangrene cc⊘ CC/MCC Exc⊘
Epigastric hernia causing obstruction, without gangrene
Hypogastric hernia causing obstruction, without gangrene
Incarcerated epigastric hernia without gangrene
Incarcerated hypogastric hernia without gangrene
Incarcerated midline hernia without gangrene
Incarcerated spigelian hernia without gangrene
Incarcerated subxiphoid hernia without gangrene
Irreducible epigastric hernia without gangrene
Irreducible hypogastric hernia without gangrene
Irreducible midline hernia without gangrene
Irreducible spigelian hernia without gangrene
Irreducible subxiphoid hernia without gangrene
Midline hernia causing obstruction, without gangrene
Spigelian hernia causing obstruction, without gangrene
Strangulated epigastric hernia without gangrene
Strangulated hypogastric hernia without gangrene
Strangulated midline hernia without gangrene
Strangulated spigelian hernia without gangrene
Strangulated subxiphoid hernia without gangrene
Subxiphoid hernia causing obstruction, without gangrene

K43.7 Other and unspecified ventral hernia with gangrene MCC⊘ CC/MCC Exc⊘
Any condition listed under K43.6 specified as gangrenous

K43.9 Ventral hernia without obstruction or gangrene
Epigastric hernia
Ventral hernia NOS

④ᵗʰ **K44** Diaphragmatic hernia

INCLUDES hiatus hernia (esophageal) (sliding)
paraesophageal hernia

EXCLUDES1 congenital diaphragmatic hernia (Q79.0)
congenital hiatus hernia (Q40.1)

K44.0 Diaphragmatic hernia with obstruction, without gangrene cc⊘ CC/MCC Exc⊘
Diaphragmatic hernia causing obstruction
Incarcerated diaphragmatic hernia
Irreducible diaphragmatic hernia
Strangulated diaphragmatic hernia

K44.1 Diaphragmatic hernia with gangrene MCC⊘ CC/MCC Exc⊘
Gangrenous diaphragmatic hernia

K44.9 Diaphragmatic hernia without obstruction or gangrene
Diaphragmatic hernia NOS

④ᵗʰ **K45** Other abdominal hernia

INCLUDES abdominal hernia, specified site NEC
lumbar hernia
obturator hernia
pudendal hernia
retroperitoneal hernia
sciatic hernia

K45.0 Other specified abdominal hernia with obstruction, without gangrene cc⊘ CC/MCC Exc⊘
Other specified abdominal hernia causing obstruction
Other specified incarcerated abdominal hernia
Other specified irreducible abdominal hernia
Other specified strangulated abdominal hernia

K45.1 Other specified abdominal hernia with gangrene MCC⊘ CC/MCC Exc⊘
Any condition listed under K45 specified as gangrenous

K45.8 Other specified abdominal hernia without obstruction or gangrene

④ᵗʰ **K46** Unspecified abdominal hernia

INCLUDES enterocele
epiplocele
hernia NOS
interstitial hernia
intestinal hernia
intra-abdominal hernia

EXCLUDES1 vaginal enterocele (N81.5)

Unspecified Code   Other Specified Code   Manifestation Code   Ⓝ Newborn   Ⓟ Pediatric   Ⓜ Maternity   Ⓐ Adult   ♂ Male   ♀ Female
● New Code   ▲ Revised Code Title   ▶◀ Revised Text   **NOTES**   *INCLUDES*   *EXCLUDES1* Not coded here   *EXCLUDES2* Not included here
④ᵗʰ 4ᵗʰ character required   🗣 5ᵗʰ character required   ⑥ᵗʰ 6ᵗʰ character required   ⑦ 7ᵗʰ character required   ⑦ Extension 'X' Alert
HAC Hospital-acquired condition (HAC) alert   **AHA** AHA Coding Clinic®   ☞ Code first alert

K46.0 **Unspecified abdominal hernia with obstruction, without gangrene** `CC` `CC/MCC Exc`
Unspecified abdominal hernia causing obstruction
Unspecified incarcerated abdominal hernia
Unspecified irreducible abdominal hernia
Unspecified strangulated abdominal hernia

K46.1 **Unspecified abdominal hernia with gangrene** `MCC` `CC/MCC Exc`
Any condition listed under K46 specified as gangrenous

K46.9 **Unspecified abdominal hernia without obstruction or gangrene**
Abdominal hernia NOS

Noninfective enteritis and colitis (K50-K52)(Figure 11.5)

INCLUDES   noninfective inflammatory bowel disease
EXCLUDES1 irritable bowel syndrome (K58.-)
           megacolon (K59.3-)

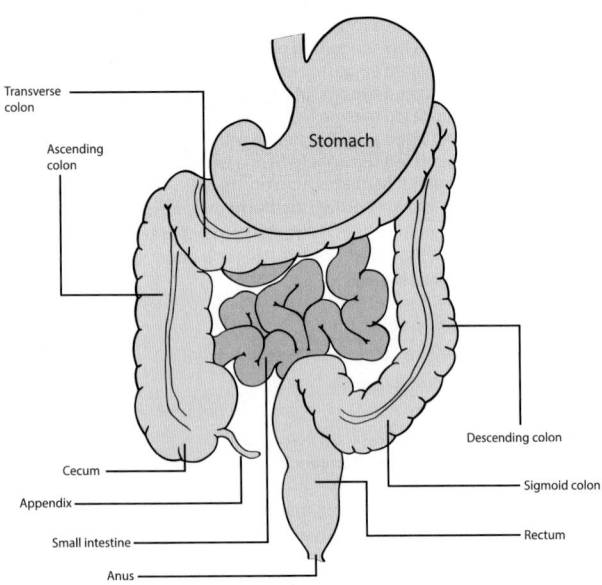

Transverse colon
Ascending colon
Stomach
Cecum
Appendix
Small intestine
Anus
Descending colon
Sigmoid colon
Rectum

Figure 11.5 Large and Small Intestine

4ᵗʰ **K50** Crohn's disease [regional enteritis]
INCLUDES   granulomatous enteritis
Use additional code to identify manifestations, such as:
pyoderma gangrenosum (L88)
EXCLUDES1 ulcerative colitis (K51.-)

5ᵗʰ **K50.0** Crohn's disease of small intestine
Crohn's disease [regional enteritis] of duodenum
Crohn's disease [regional enteritis] of ileum
Crohn's disease [regional enteritis] of jejunum
Regional ileitis
Terminal ileitis
EXCLUDES1 Crohn's disease of both small and large intestine (K50.8-)

K50.00 **Crohn's disease of small intestine** without complications `HCC` `RxHCC`

6ᵗʰ **K50.01** **Crohn's disease of small intestine** with complications
K50.011 **Crohn's disease of small intestine with** rectal bleeding `HCC` `RxHCC`
K50.012 **Crohn's disease of small intestine with** intestinal obstruction `HCC` `RxHCC`
K50.013 **Crohn's disease of small intestine with** fistula `HCC` `RxHCC`
K50.014 **Crohn's disease of small intestine with** abscess `HCC` `RxHCC`
AHA: Q4 2012
K50.018 **Crohn's disease of small intestine with other complication** `HCC` `RxHCC`
K50.019 **Crohn's disease of small intestine with unspecified complications** `HCC` `RxHCC`

5ᵗʰ **K50.1** Crohn's disease of large intestine
Crohn's disease [regional enteritis] of colon
Crohn's disease [regional enteritis] of large bowel
Crohn's disease [regional enteritis] of rectum
Granulomatous colitis
Regional colitis
EXCLUDES1 Crohn's disease of both small and large intestine (K50.8)

K50.10 **Crohn's disease of large intestine** without complications `HCC` `RxHCC`

6ᵗʰ **K50.11** **Crohn's disease of large intestine** with complications
K50.111 **Crohn's disease of large intestine with** rectal bleeding `HCC` `RxHCC`
K50.112 **Crohn's disease of large intestine with** intestinal obstruction `HCC` `RxHCC`
K50.113 **Crohn's disease of large intestine with** fistula `HCC` `RxHCC`
K50.114 **Crohn's disease of large intestine with** abscess `HCC` `RxHCC`
AHA: Q4 2012
K50.118 **Crohn's disease of large intestine with other complication** `HCC` `RxHCC`
K50.119 **Crohn's disease of large intestine with unspecified complications** `HCC` `RxHCC`

5ᵗʰ **K50.8** Crohn's disease of both small and large intestine
K50.80 **Crohn's disease of both small and large intestine** without complications `HCC` `RxHCC`

6ᵗʰ **K50.81** **Crohn's disease of both small and large intestine** with complications
K50.811 **Crohn's disease of both small and large intestine with** rectal bleeding `HCC` `RxHCC`
K50.812 **Crohn's disease of both small and large intestine with** intestinal obstruction `HCC` `RxHCC`
K50.813 **Crohn's disease of both small and large intestine with** fistula `HCC` `RxHCC`
K50.814 **Crohn's disease of both small and large intestine with** abscess `HCC` `RxHCC`
AHA: Q4 2012
K50.818 **Crohn's disease of both small and large intestine with other complication** `HCC` `RxHCC`
K50.819 **Crohn's disease of both small and large intestine with unspecified complications** `HCC` `RxHCC`

5ᵗʰ **K50.9** Crohn's disease, unspecified
K50.90 **Crohn's disease, unspecified,** without complications `HCC` `RxHCC`
Crohn's disease NOS
Regional enteritis NOS

6ᵗʰ **K50.91** **Crohn's disease, unspecified, with complications**
K50.911 **Crohn's disease, unspecified,** with rectal bleeding `HCC` `RxHCC`
K50.912 **Crohn's disease, unspecified,** with intestinal obstruction `HCC` `RxHCC`
K50.913 **Crohn's disease, unspecified,** with fistula `HCC` `RxHCC`
K50.914 **Crohn's disease, unspecified,** with abscess `HCC` `RxHCC`
AHA: Q4 2012
K50.918 **Crohn's disease, unspecified,** with other complication `HCC` `RxHCC`
K50.919 **Crohn's disease, unspecified,** with unspecified complications `HCC` `RxHCC`

4ᵗʰ **K51** Ulcerative colitis
Use additional code to identify manifestations, such as:
pyoderma gangrenosum (L88)
EXCLUDES1 Crohn's disease [regional enteritis] (K50.-)

5ᵗʰ **K51.0** Ulcerative (chronic) pancolitis
Backwash ileitis
K51.00 **Ulcerative (chronic) pancolitis without complications** `HCC` `RxHCC`
Ulcerative (chronic) pancolitis NOS

[6th] **K51.01 Ulcerative (chronic) pancolitis** with complications

- K51.011 **Ulcerative (chronic) pancolitis with** rectal bleeding [HCC] [RxHCC]
- K51.012 **Ulcerative (chronic) pancolitis with** intestinal obstruction [HCC] [RxHCC]
- K51.013 **Ulcerative (chronic) pancolitis with** fistula [HCC] [RxHCC]
- K51.014 **Ulcerative (chronic) pancolitis with** abscess [HCC] [RxHCC]
- K51.018 **Ulcerative (chronic) pancolitis with other complication** [HCC] [RxHCC]
- K51.019 **Ulcerative (chronic) pancolitis with unspecified complications** [HCC] [RxHCC]

[5th] **K51.2 Ulcerative (chronic)** proctitis

- K51.20 **Ulcerative (chronic) proctitis without complications** [HCC] [RxHCC]
  Ulcerative (chronic) proctitis NOS

[6th] **K51.21 Ulcerative (chronic) proctitis** with complications

- K51.211 **Ulcerative (chronic) proctitis with** rectal bleeding [HCC] [RxHCC]
- K51.212 **Ulcerative (chronic) proctitis with** intestinal obstruction [CC] [HCC] [RxHCC] [CC/MCC Exc]
- K51.213 **Ulcerative (chronic) proctitis with** fistula [HCC] [RxHCC]
- K51.214 **Ulcerative (chronic) proctitis with** abscess [HCC] [RxHCC]
- K51.218 **Ulcerative (chronic) proctitis with other complication** [HCC] [RxHCC]
- K51.219 **Ulcerative (chronic) proctitis with unspecified complications** [HCC] [RxHCC]

[5th] **K51.3 Ulcerative (chronic)** rectosigmoiditis

- K51.30 **Ulcerative (chronic) rectosigmoiditis** without complications [HCC] [RxHCC]
  Ulcerative (chronic) rectosigmoiditis NOS

[6th] **K51.31 Ulcerative (chronic) rectosigmoiditis** with complications

- K51.311 **Ulcerative (chronic) rectosigmoiditis with** rectal bleeding [HCC] [RxHCC]
- K51.312 **Ulcerative (chronic) rectosigmoiditis with** intestinal obstruction [HCC] [RxHCC]
- K51.313 **Ulcerative (chronic) rectosigmoiditis with** fistula [HCC] [RxHCC]
- K51.314 **Ulcerative (chronic) rectosigmoiditis with** abscess [HCC] [RxHCC]
- K51.318 **Ulcerative (chronic) rectosigmoiditis with** other complication [HCC] [RxHCC]
- K51.319 **Ulcerative (chronic) rectosigmoiditis with unspecified complications** [HCC] [RxHCC]

[5th] **K51.4** Inflammatory polyps **of colon**

[EXCLUDES1] *adenomatous polyp of colon (D12.6)*
polyposis of colon (D12.6)
polyps of colon NOS (K63.5)

- K51.40 **Inflammatory polyps of colon** without complications [HCC] [RxHCC]
  Inflammatory polyps of colon NOS

[6th] **K51.41 Inflammatory polyps of colon** with complications

- K51.411 **Inflammatory polyps of colon with** rectal bleeding [HCC] [RxHCC]
- K51.412 **Inflammatory polyps of colon with** intestinal obstruction [HCC] [RxHCC]
- K51.413 **Inflammatory polyps of colon with** fistula [CC] [HCC] [RxHCC] [CC/MCC Exc]
- K51.414 **Inflammatory polyps of colon with** abscess [HCC] [RxHCC]
- K51.418 **Inflammatory polyps of colon with other complication** [HCC] [RxHCC]
- K51.419 **Inflammatory polyps of colon with unspecified complications** [HCC] [RxHCC]

[5th] **K51.5** Left **sided colitis**

Left hemicolitis

- K51.50 **Left sided colitis** without complications [HCC] [RxHCC]
  Left sided colitis NOS

[6th] **K51.51 Left sided colitis** with complications

- K51.511 **Left sided colitis with** rectal bleeding [HCC] [RxHCC]
- K51.512 **Left sided colitis with** intestinal obstruction [HCC] [RxHCC]
- K51.513 **Left sided colitis with** fistula [HCC] [RxHCC]
- K51.514 **Left sided colitis with** abscess [HCC] [RxHCC]
- K51.518 **Left sided colitis with other complication** [HCC] [RxHCC]
- K51.519 **Left sided colitis with unspecified complications** [HCC] [RxHCC]

[5th] **K51.8** Other **ulcerative colitis**

- K51.80 **Other ulcerative colitis** without complications [HCC] [RxHCC]

[6th] **K51.81 Other ulcerative colitis** with complications

- K51.811 **Other ulcerative colitis with rectal** bleeding [CC] [HCC] [RxHCC] [CC/MCC Exc]
- K51.812 **Other ulcerative colitis with intestinal** obstruction [CC] [HCC] [RxHCC] [CC/MCC Exc]
- K51.813 **Other ulcerative colitis with** fistula [CC] [HCC] [RxHCC] [CC/MCC Exc]
- K51.814 **Other ulcerative colitis with** abscess [CC] [HCC] [RxHCC] [CC/MCC Exc]
- K51.818 **Other ulcerative colitis with other complication** [CC] [HCC] [RxHCC] [CC/MCC Exc]
- K51.819 **Other ulcerative colitis with unspecified complications** [CC] [HCC] [RxHCC] [CC/MCC Exc]

[5th] **K51.9 Ulcerative colitis, unspecified**

- K51.90 **Ulcerative colitis, unspecified, without complications** [HCC] [RxHCC]

[6th] **K51.91 Ulcerative colitis, unspecified,** with complications

- K51.911 **Ulcerative colitis, unspecified** with rectal bleeding [CC] [HCC] [RxHCC] [CC/MCC Exc]
- K51.912 **Ulcerative colitis, unspecified** with intestinal obstruction [CC] [HCC] [RxHCC] [CC/MCC Exc]
- K51.913 **Ulcerative colitis, unspecified** with fistula [CC] [HCC] [RxHCC] [CC/MCC Exc]
- K51.914 **Ulcerative colitis, unspecified** with abscess [CC] [HCC] [RxHCC] [CC/MCC Exc]
- K51.918 **Ulcerative colitis, unspecified with other complication** [CC] [HCC] [RxHCC] [CC/MCC Exc]
- K51.919 **Ulcerative colitis, unspecified with unspecified complications** [CC] [HCC] [RxHCC] [CC/MCC Exc]

[4th] **K52 Other and unspecified noninfective gastroenteritis and colitis**

- **K52.0 Gastroenteritis and colitis** due to radiation [CC] [CC/MCC Exc]
- **K52.1** Toxic **gastroenteritis and colitis** [CC] [CC/MCC Exc]
  AHA: Q1 2019
  Drug-induced gastroenteritis and colitis
  ☛ **Code first** (T51-T65) to identify toxic agent
  Use additional code for adverse effect, if applicable, to identify drug (T36-T50 with fifth or sixth character 5)

[5th] **K52.2** Allergic and dietetic **gastroenteritis and colitis**

Food hypersensitivity gastroenteritis or colitis
Use additional code to identify type of food allergy (Z91.01-, Z91.02-)

[EXCLUDES2] *allergic eosinophilic colitis (K52.82)*
allergic eosinophilic esophagitis (K20.0)
allergic eosinophilic gastritis (K52.81)
allergic eosinophilic gastroenteritis (K52.81)
food protein-induced proctocolitis (K52.82)

- K52.21 **Food protein-induced** enterocolitis syndrome
  AHA: Q4 2016
  FPIES
  Use additional code for hypovolemic shock, if present (R57.1)
- K52.22 **Food protein-induced** enteropathy
  AHA: Q4 2016
- K52.29 Other **allergic and dietetic gastroenteritis and colitis**
  AHA: Q4 2016
  Food hypersensitivity gastroenteritis or colitis
  Immediate gastrointestinal hypersensitivity

Unspecified Code | Other Specified Code | Manifestation Code | [N] Newborn | [P] Pediatric | [M] Maternity | [A] Adult | ♂ Male | ♀ Female
● New Code | ▲ Revised Code Title | ►◄ Revised Text | [NOTES] | [INCLUDES] | [EXCLUDES1] Not coded here | [EXCLUDES2] Not included here
[4th] 4th character required | [5th] 5th character required | [6th] 6th character required | [7th] 7th character required | [X] Extension 'X' Alert
[HAC] Hospital-acquired condition (HAC) alert | **AHA** AHA Coding Clinic© | ☛ **Code first alert**

K52.3 Indeterminate **colitis**
AHA: Q4 2016
Colonic inflammatory bowel disease unclassified (IBDU)
EXCLUDES1 unspecified colitis (K52.9)

K52.8 Other specified noninfective gastroenteritis and colitis
K52.81 Eosinophilic gastritis or gastroenteritis
Eosinophilic enteritis
EXCLUDES2 eosinophilic esophagitis (K20.0)
K52.82 Eosinophilic colitis
Allergic proctocolitis
Food-induced eosinophilic proctocolitis
Food protein-induced proctocolitis
Milk protein-induced proctocolitis
K52.83 Microscopic **colitis**
K52.831 Collagenous **colitis**
AHA: Q4 2016
K52.832 Lymphocytic **colitis**
AHA: Q4 2016
K52.838 Other **microscopic colitis**
AHA: Q4 2016
K52.839 **Microscopic colitis, unspecified**
AHA: Q4 2016
K52.89 Other specified noninfective gastroenteritis and colitis
AHA: Q1 2019
K52.9 Noninfective gastroenteritis and colitis, unspecified
Colitis NOS
Enteritis NOS
Gastroenteritis NOS
Ileitis NOS
Jejunitis NOS
Sigmoiditis NOS
EXCLUDES1 diarrhea NOS (R19.7)
functional diarrhea (K59.1)
infectious gastroenteritis and colitis NOS (A09)
neonatal diarrhea (noninfective) (P78.3)
psychogenic diarrhea (F45.8)

Other diseases of intestines (K55-K64)

K55 Vascular disorders of intestine
EXCLUDES1 necrotizing enterocolitis of newborn (P77.-)
K55.0 Acute vascular disorders of intestine
Infarction of appendices epiploicae
Mesenteric (artery) (vein) embolism
Mesenteric (artery) (vein) infarction
Mesenteric (artery) (vein) thrombosis
K55.01 Acute (reversible) ischemia of small **intestine**
K55.011 Focal (segmental) acute (reversible) ischemia of small intestine HCC MCC CC/MCC Exc
K55.012 Diffuse **acute (reversible) ischemia of small intestine** HCC MCC CC/MCC Exc
K55.019 **Acute (reversible) ischemia of small intestine,** extent **unspecified** HCC MCC CC/MCC Exc
K55.02 Acute infarction of small intestine
Gangrene of small intestine
Necrosis of small intestine
K55.021 Focal (segmental) acute infarction of small intestine HCC MCC CC/MCC Exc
K55.022 Diffuse **acute infarction of small intestine** HCC MCC CC/MCC Exc
K55.029 **Acute infarction of small intestine,** extent **unspecified** HCC MCC CC/MCC Exc
K55.03 Acute (reversible) ischemia of large **intestine**
Acute fulminant ischemic colitis
Subacute ischemic colitis
K55.031 Focal (segmental) acute (reversible) **ischemia of large intestine** HCC MCC CC/MCC Exc
K55.032 Diffuse **acute (reversible) ischemia of large intestine** HCC MCC CC/MCC Exc
K55.039 **Acute (reversible) ischemia of large intestine,** extent **unspecified** HCC MCC CC/MCC Exc
K55.04 Acute infarction of large intestine
Gangrene of large intestine
Necrosis of large intestine
K55.041 Focal (segmental) acute infarction of large intestine HCC MCC CC/MCC Exc

K55.042 Diffuse **acute infarction of large intestine** HCC MCC CC/MCC Exc
K55.049 **Acute infarction of large intestine,** extent **unspecified** HCC MCC CC/MCC Exc
K55.05 Acute (reversible) ischemia of intestine, part unspecified
K55.051 Focal (segmental) **acute (reversible) ischemia of intestine, part unspecified** HCC MCC CC/MCC Exc
K55.052 Diffuse **acute (reversible) ischemia of intestine, part unspecified** HCC MCC CC/MCC Exc
K55.059 **Acute (reversible) ischemia of intestine, part** and **extent unspecified** HCC MCC CC/MCC Exc
K55.06 Acute infarction of intestine, part unspecified
Acute intestinal infarction
Gangrene of intestine
Necrosis of intestine
K55.061 Focal (segmental) acute infarction of **intestine, part unspecified** HCC MCC CC/MCC Exc
K55.062 Diffuse **acute infarction of intestine, part unspecified** HCC MCC CC/MCC Exc
K55.069 **Acute infarction of intestine, part** and extent **unspecified** HCC MCC CC/MCC Exc
K55.1 Chronic **vascular disorders of intestine** HCC
Chronic ischemic colitis
Chronic ischemic enteritis
Chronic ischemic enterocolitis
Ischemic stricture of intestine
Mesenteric atherosclerosis
Mesenteric vascular insufficiency
K55.2 Angiodysplasia **of colon**
K55.20 Angiodysplasia **of colon** without hemorrhage
K55.21 Angiodysplasia **of colon** with hemorrhage MCC CC/MCC Exc
AHA: Q3 2018
K55.3 Necrotizing enterocolitis
EXCLUDES1 necrotizing enterocolitis of newborn (P77.-)
EXCLUDES2 necrotizing enterocolitis due to Clostridium difficile (A04.7-)
K55.30 **Necrotizing enterocolitis, unspecified** HCC MCC CC/MCC Exc
AHA: Q4 2016
Necrotizing enterocolitis, NOS
K55.31 Stage 1 **necrotizing enterocolitis** HCC MCC CC/MCC Exc
AHA: Q4 2016
Necrotizing enterocolitis without pneumatosis, without perforation
K55.32 Stage 2 **necrotizing enterocolitis** HCC MCC CC/MCC Exc
AHA: Q4 2016
Necrotizing enterocolitis with pneumatosis, without perforation
K55.33 Stage 3 **necrotizing enterocolitis** HCC MCC CC/MCC Exc
AHA: Q4 2016
Necrotizing enterocolitis with perforation
Necrotizing enterocolitis with pneumatosis and perforation
K55.8 Other vascular disorders of intestine HCC
K55.9 Vascular disorder of intestine, unspecified HCC
Ischemic colitis
Ischemic enteritis
Ischemic enterocolitis
K56 Paralytic ileus and intestinal obstruction without hernia
EXCLUDES1 congenital stricture or stenosis of intestine (Q41-Q42)
cystic fibrosis with meconium ileus (E84.11)
ischemic stricture of intestine (K55.1)
meconium ileus NOS (P76.0)
neonatal intestinal obstructions classifiable to P76.-
obstruction of duodenum (K31.5)
postprocedural intestinal obstruction (K91.3-)
stenosis of anus or rectum (K62.4)
K56.0 Paralytic ileus CC HCC CC/MCC Exc
Paralysis of bowel
Paralysis of colon
Paralysis of intestine

PDxₓ Unacceptable principal diagnosis symbol per Medicare code edits   POA Code exempt from diagnosis present on admission requirement
? Questionable admission   CC Complication or comorbidity   MCC Major complication or comorbidity   CC/MCC Exc CC/MCC exclusion
HCC HCC diagnosis code   RxHCC RxHCC diagnosis code   MACRA code   **DEFINITION** Describes condition/terminology
TIP Coding guidance   Official Guideline Reference   Z1 Z code as first-listed diagnosis

EXCLUDES1 *gallstone ileus (K56.3)*

ileus NOS (K56.7)

obstructive ileus NOS (K56.69-)

K56.1 **Intussusception** cc HCC CC/MCC Exc

Intussusception or invagination of bowel

Intussusception or invagination of colon

Intussusception or invagination of intestine

Intussusception or invagination of rectum

EXCLUDES2 *intussusception of appendix (K38.8)*

K56.2 **Volvulus** cc HCC CC/MCC Exc

Strangulation of colon or intestine

Torsion of colon or intestine

Twist of colon or intestine

EXCLUDES2 *volvulus of duodenum (K31.5)*

K56.3 **Gallstone ileus** cc HCC CC/MCC Exc

Obstruction of intestine by gallstone

5th **K56.4** **Other impaction of intestine**

K56.41 **Fecal impaction** cc HCC CC/MCC Exc

EXCLUDES1 *constipation (K59.0-)*

incomplete defecation (R15.0)

K56.49 **Other impaction of intestine** cc HCC CC/MCC Exc

5th **K56.5** **Intestinal adhesions [bands]** with obstruction **(postinfection)**

Abdominal hernia due to adhesions with obstruction

Peritoneal adhesions [bands] with intestinal obstruction
(postinfection)

K56.50 **Intestinal adhesions [bands], unspecified as to partial versus complete obstruction** cc HCC CC/MCC Exc

AHA: Q4 2017

Intestinal adhesions with obstruction NOS

K56.51 **Intestinal adhesions [bands], with** partial **obstruction** cc HCC CC/MCC Exc

AHA: Q4 2017

Intestinal adhesions with incomplete obstruction

K56.52 **Intestinal adhesions [bands] with** complete **obstruction** cc HCC CC/MCC Exc

AHA: Q4 2017

5th **K56.6** **Other and unspecified intestinal obstruction**

6th **K56.60** Unspecified **intestinal obstruction**

EXCLUDES1 *intestinal obstruction due to specified condition-code to condition*

K56.600 Partial **intestinal obstruction, unspecified as to cause** cc HCC CC/MCC Exc

AHA: Q4 2017

Incomplete intestinal obstruction, NOS

K56.601 Complete **intestinal obstruction, unspecified as to cause** cc HCC CC/MCC Exc

AHA: Q4 2017

K56.609 **Unspecified intestinal obstruction, unspecified as to partial versus complete obstruction** cc HCC CC/MCC Exc

AHA: Q4 2017

Intestinal obstruction NOS

6th **K56.69** **Other intestinal obstruction**

Enterostenosis NOS

Obstructive ileus NOS

Occlusion of colon or intestine NOS

Stenosis of colon or intestine NOS

Stricture of colon or intestine NOS

EXCLUDES1 *intestinal obstruction due to specified condition-code to condition*

K56.690 Other partial **intestinal obstruction** cc HCC CC/MCC Exc

AHA: Q4 2017

Other incomplete intestinal obstruction

K56.691 Other complete **intestinal obstruction** cc HCC CC/MCC Exc

AHA: Q4 2017

K56.699 **Other intestinal obstruction unspecified as to partial versus complete obstruction** cc HCC CC/MCC Exc

AHA: Q4 2017

Other intestinal obstruction, NEC

K56.7 **Ileus, unspecified** cc HCC CC/MCC Exc

AHA: Q1 2017

EXCLUDES1 *obstructive ileus (K56.69-)*

EXCLUDES2 *intestinal obstruction with hernia (K40-K46)*

4th **K57** **Diverticular disease of intestine (Figure 11.6)**

Code also if applicable peritonitis K65.-

EXCLUDES1 *congenital diverticulum of intestine (Q43.8)*

Meckel's diverticulum (Q43.0)

EXCLUDES2 *diverticulum of appendix (K38.2)*

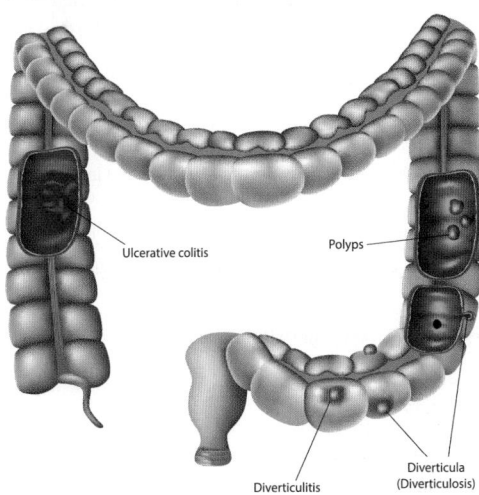

Ulcerative colitis

Polyps

Diverticulitis

Diverticula
(Diverticulosis)

Figure 11.6 Noncancerous Colon Disorders

5th **K57.0** **Diverticulitis of** small intestine with perforation and abscess

Diverticulitis of small intestine with peritonitis

EXCLUDES1 *diverticulitis of both small and large intestine with perforation and abscess (K57.4-)*

K57.00 **Diverticulitis of small intestine with perforation and abscess** without bleeding cc CC/MCC Exc

K57.01 **Diverticulitis of small intestine with perforation and abscess** with bleeding MCC CC/MCC Exc

5th **K57.1** **Diverticular disease of** small intestine without perforation or abscess

EXCLUDES1 *diverticular disease of both small and large intestine without perforation or abscess (K57.5-)*

K57.10 Diverticulosis **of small intestine without perforation or abscess** without bleeding

Diverticular disease of small intestine NOS

K57.11 Diverticulosis **of small intestine without perforation or abscess** with bleeding MCC CC/MCC Exc

K57.12 Diverticulitis **of small intestine without perforation or abscess** without bleeding

K57.13 Diverticulitis **of small intestine without perforation or abscess** with bleeding MCC CC/MCC Exc

5th **K57.2** **Diverticulitis of** large intestine with perforation and abscess

Diverticulitis of colon with peritonitis

EXCLUDES1 *diverticulitis of both small and large intestine with perforation and abscess (K57.4-)*

K57.20 **Diverticulitis of large intestine with perforation and abscess** without bleeding cc CC/MCC Exc

K57.21 **Diverticulitis of large intestine with perforation and abscess** with bleeding MCC CC/MCC Exc

5th **K57.3** **Diverticular disease of** large intestine without perforation or abscess

EXCLUDES1 *diverticular disease of both small and large intestine without perforation or abscess (K57.5-)*

K57.30 Diverticulosis **of large intestine without perforation or abscess** without bleeding

Diverticular disease of colon NOS

K57.31 Diverticulosis **of large intestine without perforation or abscess** with bleeding cc CC/MCC Exc

AHA: Q3 2018

K57.32 Diverticulitis of large intestine without perforation or abscess without bleeding cc cc/mcc Exc

K57.33 Diverticulitis of large intestine without perforation or abscess with bleeding cc cc/mcc Exc

5ᵗʰ **K57.4 Diverticulitis of both** small and large intestine with perforation and abscess

Diverticulitis of both small and large intestine with peritonitis

K57.40 **Diverticulitis of both small and large intestine with perforation and abscess** without bleeding cc cc/mcc Exc

K57.41 **Diverticulitis of both small and large intestine with perforation and abscess** with bleeding mcc cc/mcc Exc

5ᵗʰ **K57.5 Diverticular disease of** both small and large intestine without perforation or abscess

K57.50 **Diverticulosis of both small and large intestine without perforation or abscess** without bleeding

Diverticular disease of both small and large intestine NOS

K57.51 Diverticulosis **of both small and large intestine without perforation or abscess with bleeding** mcc cc/mcc Exc

K57.52 Diverticulitis **of both small and large intestine without perforation or abscess without bleeding** cc cc/mcc Exc

K57.53 Diverticulitis **of both small and large intestine without perforation or abscess with bleeding** mcc cc/mcc Exc

5ᵗʰ **K57.8 Diverticulitis of intestine, part unspecified, with perforation and abscess**

Diverticulitis of intestine NOS with peritonitis

K57.80 **Diverticulitis of intestine, part unspecified, with perforation and abscess** without bleeding cc cc/mcc Exc

K57.81 **Diverticulitis of intestine, part unspecified, with perforation and abscess** with bleeding mcc cc/mcc Exc

5ᵗʰ **K57.9 Diverticular disease of intestine, part unspecified, without perforation or abscess**

K57.90 **Diverticulosis of intestine, part unspecified, without perforation or abscess** without bleeding

Diverticular disease of intestine NOS

K57.91 **Diverticulosis of intestine, part unspecified, without perforation or abscess** with bleeding mcc cc/mcc Exc

K57.92 **Diverticulitis of intestine, part unspecified, without perforation or abscess** without bleeding cc cc/mcc Exc

K57.93 **Diverticulitis of intestine, part unspecified, without perforation or abscess** with bleeding mcc cc/mcc Exc

4ᵗʰ **K58 Irritable bowel syndrome**

INCLUDES irritable colon

spastic colon

K58.0 **Irritable bowel syndrome** with diarrhea

K58.1 **Irritable bowel syndrome** with constipation

AHA: Q4 2016

K58.2 Mixed **irritable bowel syndrome**

AHA: Q4 2016

K58.8 Other **irritable bowel syndrome**

AHA: Q4 2016

K58.9 **Irritable bowel syndrome** without diarrhea

Irritable bowel syndrome NOS

4ᵗʰ **K59 Other functional intestinal disorders**

EXCLUDES1 change in bowel habit NOS (R19.4)

intestinal malabsorption (K90.-)

psychogenic intestinal disorders (F45.8)

EXCLUDES2 functional disorders of stomach (K31.-)

5ᵗʰ **K59.0 Constipation**

EXCLUDES1 fecal impaction (K56.41)

incomplete defecation (R15.0)

K59.00 **Constipation, unspecified**

K59.01 Slow transit **constipation**

K59.02 Outlet dysfunction **constipation**

K59.03 Drug induced **constipation**

AHA: Q4 2016

Use additional code for adverse effect, if applicable, to identify drug (T36-T50) with fifth or sixth character 5

K59.04 Chronic idiopathic **constipation**

AHA: Q4 2016

Functional constipation

K59.09 Other **constipation**

Chronic constipation

K59.1 **Functional diarrhea**

EXCLUDES1 diarrhea NOS (R19.7)

irritable bowel syndrome with diarrhea (K58.0)

K59.2 **Neurogenic bowel, not elsewhere classified** cc cc/mcc Exc

5ᵗʰ **K59.3 Megacolon, not elsewhere classified**

Dilatation of colon

☞ **Code first,** if applicable (T51-T65) to identify toxic agent

EXCLUDES1 congenital megacolon (aganglionic) (Q43.1)

megacolon (due to) (in) Chagas' disease (B57.32)

megacolon (due to) (in) Clostridium difficile (A04.7-)

megacolon (due to) (in) Hirschsprung's disease (Q43.1)

K59.31 Toxic **megacolon** cc HCC cc/mcc Exc

AHA: Q4 2016

K59.39 Other **megacolon** cc cc/mcc Exc

AHA: Q4 2016

Megacolon NOS

K59.4 **Anal spasm**

Proctalgia fugax

K59.8 **Other specified functional intestinal disorders**

Atony of colon

Pseudo-obstruction (acute) (chronic) of intestine

K59.9 **Functional intestinal disorder, unspecified**

4ᵗʰ **K60 Fissure and fistula of anal and rectal regions (Figure 11.7)**

EXCLUDES1 fissure and fistula of anal and rectal regions with abscess or cellulitis (K61.-)

EXCLUDES2 anal sphincter tear (healed) (nontraumatic) (old) (K62.81)

K60.0 Acute **anal fissure**

K60.1 Chronic **anal fissure**

K60.2 **Anal fissure, unspecified**

K60.3 Anal **fistula**

K60.4 Rectal **fistula**

Fistula of rectum to skin

EXCLUDES1 rectovaginal fistula (N82.3)

vesicorectal fistula (N32.1)

K60.5 Anorectal **fistula**

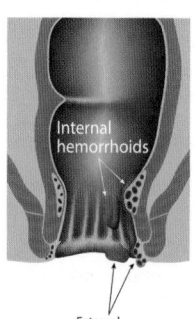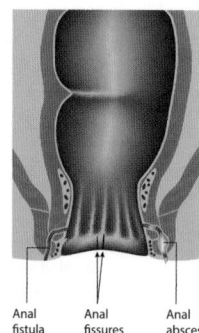

Internal hemorrhoids

External hemorrhoids

Anal fistula

Anal fissures

Anal abscess

Figure 11.7 Anal Disorders

4ᵗʰ **K61 Abscess of anal and rectal regions**

INCLUDES abscess of anal and rectal regions

cellulitis of anal and rectal regions

K61.0 Anal **abscess**

AHA: Q4 2018

Perianal abscess

EXCLUDES2 intrasphincteric abscess (K61.4)

K61.1 Rectal **abscess**

AHA: Q4 2012

Perirectal abscess

EXCLUDES1 ischiorectal abscess (K61.39)

K61.2 Anorectal **abscess**

5ᵗʰ K61.3 Ischiorectal **abscess**

    K61.31 Horseshoe **abscess**

        AHA: Q4 2018

    K61.39 Other ischiorectal **abscess**

        AHA: Q4 2018

        Abscess of ischiorectal fossa

        Ischiorectal abscess, NOS

K61.4 Intrasphincteric **abscess**

    AHA: Q4 2018

    Intersphincteric abscess

K61.5 Supralevator **abscess**

    AHA: Q4 2018

4ᵗʰ K62 Other diseases of anus and rectum

    INCLUDES anal canal

    EXCLUDES2 colostomy and enterostomy malfunction (K94.0-, K94.1-)

              fecal incontinence (R15.-)

              hemorrhoids (K64.-)

K62.0 **Anal polyp**

K62.1 **Rectal polyp**

    AHA: Q1 2018

    EXCLUDES1 adenomatous polyp (D12.8)

K62.2 **Anal prolapse**

    Prolapse of anal canal

K62.3 **Rectal prolapse**

    Prolapse of rectal mucosa

K62.4 **Stenosis of anus and rectum**

    AHA: Q2 2019

    Stricture of anus (sphincter)

K62.5 **Hemorrhage of anus and rectum**

    AHA: Q1 2019

    EXCLUDES1 gastrointestinal bleeding NOS (K92.2)

              melena (K92.1)

              neonatal rectal hemorrhage (P54.2)

K62.6 **Ulcer of anus and rectum**

    Solitary ulcer of anus and rectum

    Stercoral ulcer of anus and rectum

    EXCLUDES1 fissure and fistula of anus and rectum (K60.-)

              ulcerative colitis (K51.-)

K62.7 **Radiation proctitis**

    AHA: Q1 2019

    Use additional code to identify the type of radiation (W90.-)

5ᵗʰ K62.8 **Other specified diseases of anus and rectum**

    EXCLUDES2 ulcerative proctitis (K51.2)

    K62.81 **Anal sphincter tear (healed) (nontraumatic) (old)**

        Tear of anus, nontraumatic

        Use additional code for any associated fecal incontinence (R15.-)

        EXCLUDES2 anal fissure (K60.-)

              anal sphincter tear (healed) (old) complicating delivery (O34.7-)

              traumatic tear of anal sphincter (S31.831)

    K62.82 **Dysplasia of anus**

        Anal intraepithelial neoplasia I and II (AIN I and II) (histologically confirmed)

        Dysplasia of anus NOS

        Mild and moderate dysplasia of anus (histologically confirmed)

        EXCLUDES1 abnormal results from anal cytologic examination without histologic confirmation (R85.61-)

              anal intraepithelial neoplasia III (D01.3)

              carcinoma in situ of anus (D01.3)

              HGSIL of anus (R85.613)

              severe dysplasia of anus (D01.3)

    K62.89 **Other specified diseases of anus and rectum**

        Proctitis NOS

        Use additional code for any associated fecal incontinence (R15.-)

K62.9 **Disease of anus and rectum, unspecified**

4ᵗʰ K63 Other diseases of intestine

K63.0 Abscess **of intestine** CC✎ CC/MCC Exc

    EXCLUDES1 abscess of intestine with Crohn's disease (K50.014, K50.114, K50.814, K50.914,)

              abscess of intestine with diverticular disease (K57.0, K57.2, K57.4, K57.8)

              abscess of intestine with ulcerative colitis (K51.014, K51.214, K51.314, K51.414, K51.514, K51.814, K51.914)

    EXCLUDES2 abscess of anal and rectal regions (K61.-)

              abscess of appendix (K35.3-)

K63.1 Perforation **of intestine (nontraumatic)** CC✎ HCC CC/MCC Exc

    Perforation (nontraumatic) of rectum

    EXCLUDES1 perforation (nontraumatic) of duodenum (K26.-)

              perforation (nontraumatic) of intestine with diverticular disease (K57.0, K57.2, K57.4, K57.8)

    EXCLUDES2 perforation (nontraumatic) of appendix (K35.2-, K35.3-)

K63.2 Fistula **of intestine** CC✎ CC/MCC Exc

    AHA: Q3 2017

    EXCLUDES1 fistula of duodenum (K31.6)

              fistula of intestine with Crohn's disease (K50.013, K50.113, K50.813, K50.913,)

              fistula of intestine with ulcerative colitis (K51.013, K51.213, K51.313, K51.413, K51.513, K51.813, K51.913)

    EXCLUDES2 fistula of anal and rectal regions (K60.-)

              fistula of appendix (K38.3)

              intestinal-genital fistula, female (N82.2-N82.4)

              vesicointestinal fistula (N32.1)

K63.3 Ulcer **of intestine** CC✎ CC/MCC Exc

    Primary ulcer of small intestine

    EXCLUDES1 duodenal ulcer (K26.-)

              gastrointestinal ulcer (K28.-)

              gastrojejunal ulcer (K28.-)

              jejunal ulcer (K28.-)

              peptic ulcer, site unspecified (K27.-)

              ulcer of intestine with perforation (K63.1)

              ulcer of anus or rectum (K62.6)

              ulcerative colitis (K51.-)

K63.4 Enteroptosis

K63.5 Polyp **of colon**

    AHA: Q1 2019, Q1 2017, Q2 2015

    EXCLUDES1 adenomatous polyp of colon ▶(D12.-)◀

              inflammatory polyp of colon (K51.4-)

              polyposis of colon (D12.6)

5ᵗʰ K63.8 Other **specified diseases of intestine**

    K63.81 **Dieulafoy lesion of intestine** MCC✎ CC/MCC Exc

        EXCLUDES2 Dieulafoy lesion of stomach and duodenum (K31.82)

    K63.89 **Other specified diseases of intestine**

K63.9 **Disease of intestine, unspecified**

4ᵗʰ K64 Hemorrhoids and perianal venous thrombosis

    INCLUDES piles

    EXCLUDES1 hemorrhoids complicating childbirth and the puerperium (O87.2)

              hemorrhoids complicating pregnancy (O22.4)

K64.0 First degree **hemorrhoids**

    Grade/stage I hemorrhoids

    Hemorrhoids (bleeding) without prolapse outside of anal canal

K64.1 Second degree **hemorrhoids**

    Grade/stage II hemorrhoids

    Hemorrhoids (bleeding) that prolapse with straining, but retract spontaneously

K64.2 Third degree **hemorrhoids**

    Grade/stage III hemorrhoids

    Hemorrhoids (bleeding) that prolapse with straining and require manual replacement back inside anal canal

---

Unspecified Code Other Specified Code Manifestation Code **N** Newborn **P** Pediatric **M** Maternity **A** Adult ♂ Male ♀ Female

● New Code ▲ Revised Code Title ▶◀ Revised Text **NOTES** *INCLUDES* *EXCLUDES1* Not coded here *EXCLUDES2* Not included here

4ᵗʰ 4ᵗʰ character required **5ᵗʰ** 5ᵗʰ character required **6ᵗʰ** 6ᵗʰ character required **7ᵗʰ** 7ᵗʰ character required **7ᵗʰ** Extension 'X' Alert

HAC Hospital-acquired condition (HAC) alert **AHA** AHA Coding Clinic© ☛ Code first alert

K64.3 Fourth degree hemorrhoids
Grade/stage IV hemorrhoids
Hemorrhoids (bleeding) with prolapsed tissue that cannot be
  manually replaced

K64.4 Residual hemorrhoidal skin tags
External hemorrhoids, NOS
Skin tags of anus

K64.5 Perianal venous thrombosis
External hemorrhoids with thrombosis
Perianal hematoma
Thrombosed hemorrhoids NOS

K64.8 Other hemorrhoids
AHA: Q3 2018
Internal hemorrhoids, without mention of degree
Prolapsed hemorrhoids, degree not specified

K64.9 Unspecified hemorrhoids
Hemorrhoids (bleeding) NOS
Hemorrhoids (bleeding) without mention of degree

Diseases of peritoneum and retroperitoneum (K65-K68)

K65 Peritonitis
Use additional code (B95-B97), to identify infectious agent, if known
Code also if applicable diverticular disease of intestine (K57.-)
EXCLUDES1 *acute appendicitis with generalized peritonitis (K35.2-)*
  aseptic peritonitis (T81.6)
  benign paroxysmal peritonitis (E85.0)
  chemical peritonitis (T81.6)
  gonococcal peritonitis (A54.85)
  neonatal peritonitis (P78.0-P78.1)
  pelvic peritonitis, female (N73.3-N73.5)
  periodic familial peritonitis (E85.0)
  peritonitis due to talc or other foreign substance (T81.6)
  peritonitis in chlamydia (A74.81)
  peritonitis in diphtheria (A36.89)
  peritonitis in syphilis (late) (A52.74)
  peritonitis in tuberculosis (A18.31)
  peritonitis with or following abortion or ectopic or molar
    pregnancy (O00-O07, O08.0)
  peritonitis with or following appendicitis (K35.-)
  puerperal peritonitis (O85)
  retroperitoneal infections (K68.-)

K65.0 Generalized (acute) peritonitis
Pelvic peritonitis (acute), male
Subphrenic peritonitis (acute)
Suppurative peritonitis (acute)

K65.1 Peritoneal abscess
AHA: Q1 2019
Abdominopelvic abscess
Abscess (of) omentum
Abscess (of) peritoneum
Mesenteric abscess
Retrocecal abscess
Subdiaphragmatic abscess
Subhepatic abscess
Subphrenic abscess

K65.2 Spontaneous bacterial peritonitis
EXCLUDES1 *bacterial peritonitis NOS (K65.9)*

K65.3 Choleperitonitis
Peritonitis due to bile

K65.4 Sclerosing mesenteritis
Fat necrosis of peritoneum
(Idiopathic) sclerosing mesenteric fibrosis
Mesenteric lipodystrophy
Mesenteric panniculitis
Retractile mesenteritis

K65.8 Other peritonitis
Chronic proliferative peritonitis
Peritonitis due to urine

K65.9 Peritonitis, unspecified
Bacterial peritonitis NOS

K66 Other disorders of peritoneum
EXCLUDES2 *ascites (R18.-)*
  peritoneal effusion (chronic) (R18.8)

K66.0 Peritoneal adhesions (postprocedural) (postinfection)
Adhesions (of) abdominal (wall)
Adhesions (of) diaphragm
Adhesions (of) intestine
Adhesions (of) male pelvis
Adhesions (of) omentum
Adhesions (of) stomach
Adhesive bands
Mesenteric adhesions
EXCLUDES1 *female pelvic adhesions [bands] (N73.6)*
  peritoneal adhesions with intestinal obstruction
    (K56.5-)

K66.1 Hemoperitoneum
EXCLUDES1 *traumatic hemoperitoneum (S36.8-)*

K66.8 Other specified disorders of peritoneum

K66.9 Disorder of peritoneum, unspecified

K67 Disorders of peritoneum in infectious diseases classified elsewhere
Code first underlying disease, such as:
congenital syphilis (A50.0)
helminthiasis (B65.0 -B83.9)
EXCLUDES1 *peritonitis in chlamydia (A74.81)*
  peritonitis in diphtheria (A36.89)
  peritonitis in gonococcal (A54.85)
  peritonitis in syphilis (late) (A52.74)
  peritonitis in tuberculosis (A18.31)

K68 Disorders of retroperitoneum
K68.1 Retroperitoneal abscess
K68.11 Postprocedural retroperitoneal abscess
EXCLUDES2 *infection following procedure (T81.4-)*
K68.12 Psoas muscle abscess
K68.19 Other retroperitoneal abscess
AHA: Q1 2019
K68.9 Other disorders of retroperitoneum

Diseases of liver (K70-K77)

EXCLUDES1 *jaundice NOS (R17)*
EXCLUDES2 *hemochromatosis (E83.11-)*
  Reye's syndrome (G93.7)
  viral hepatitis (B15-B19)
  Wilson's disease (E83.0)

K70 Alcoholic liver disease
Use additional code to identify:
alcohol abuse and dependence (F10.-)
K70.0 Alcoholic fatty liver
K70.1 Alcoholic hepatitis
K70.10 Alcoholic hepatitis without ascites
K70.11 Alcoholic hepatitis with ascites
K70.2 Alcoholic fibrosis and sclerosis of liver
K70.3 Alcoholic cirrhosis of liver
Alcoholic cirrhosis NOS
K70.30 Alcoholic cirrhosis of liver without ascites
K70.31 Alcoholic cirrhosis of liver with ascites
AHA: Q1 2018
K70.4 Alcoholic hepatic failure
Acute alcoholic hepatic failure
Alcoholic hepatic failure NOS
Chronic alcoholic hepatic failure
Subacute alcoholic hepatic failure
K70.40 Alcoholic hepatic failure without coma
K70.41 Alcoholic hepatic failure with coma
K70.9 Alcoholic liver disease, unspecified

K71 Toxic liver disease
INCLUDES *drug-induced idiosyncratic (unpredictable) liver disease*
  drug-induced toxic (predictable) liver disease

PDIN Unacceptable principal diagnosis symbol per Medicare code edits   POA Code exempt from diagnosis present on admission requirement
? Questionable admission   CC Complication or comorbidity   MCC Major complication or comorbidity   CC/MCC Exc CC/MCC exclusion
HCC HCC diagnosis code   RxHCC RxHCC diagnosis code   MACRA code   **DEFINITION** Describes condition/terminology
TIP Coding guidance   👁 Official Guideline Reference   Z1 Z code as first-listed diagnosis

☞ **Code first** poisoning due to drug or toxin, if applicable (T36-T65 with fifth or sixth character 1-4 or 6)

Use additional code for adverse effect, if applicable, to identify drug (T36-T50 with fifth or sixth character 5)

EXCLUDES2 *alcoholic liver disease (K70.-)*

Budd-Chiari syndrome (I82.0)

K71.0 **Toxic liver disease with** cholestasis

Cholestasis with hepatocyte injury

'Pure' cholestasis

5ᵗʰ K71.1 **Toxic liver disease with** hepatic necrosis

Hepatic failure (acute) (chronic) due to drugs

    K71.10 **Toxic liver disease with hepatic necrosis,** without coma

    K71.11 **Toxic liver disease with hepatic necrosis, with coma** HCC MCC CC/MCC Exc

K71.2 **Toxic liver disease with** acute hepatitis

K71.3 **Toxic liver disease with** chronic persistent hepatitis

K71.4 **Toxic liver disease with** chronic lobular hepatitis

5ᵗʰ K71.5 **Toxic liver disease with** chronic active hepatitis

Toxic liver disease with lupoid hepatitis

    K71.50 **Toxic liver disease with chronic active hepatitis** without ascites

    K71.51 **Toxic liver disease with chronic active hepatitis** with ascites

      AHA: Q1 2018

K71.6 **Toxic liver disease with** hepatitis, not elsewhere classified

K71.7 **Toxic liver disease with** fibrosis and cirrhosis **of liver**

K71.8 **Toxic liver disease with other disorders of liver**

Toxic liver disease with focal nodular hyperplasia

Toxic liver disease with hepatic granulomas

Toxic liver disease with peliosis hepatis

Toxic liver disease with veno-occlusive disease of liver

K71.9 **Toxic liver disease, unspecified**

4ᵗʰ K72 **Hepatic failure, not elsewhere classified**

INCLUDES *fulminant hepatitis NEC, with hepatic failure*

hepatic encephalopathy NOS

liver (cell) necrosis with hepatic failure

malignant hepatitis NEC, with hepatic failure

yellow liver atrophy or dystrophy

EXCLUDES1 *alcoholic hepatic failure (K70.4)*

hepatic failure with toxic liver disease (K71.1-)

icterus of newborn (P55-P59)

postprocedural hepatic failure (K91.82)

EXCLUDES2 *hepatic failure complicating abortion or ectopic or molar pregnancy (O00-O07, O08.8)*

hepatic failure complicating pregnancy, childbirth and the puerperium (O26.6-)

viral hepatitis with hepatic coma (B15-B19)

5ᵗʰ K72.0 Acute and subacute **hepatic failure**

Acute non-viral hepatitis NOS

    K72.00 **Acute and subacute hepatic failure** without coma MCC CC/MCC Exc

      AHA: Q2 2015

    K72.01 **Acute and subacute hepatic failure** with coma HCC MCC CC/MCC Exc

5ᵗʰ K72.1 Chronic **hepatic failure**

    K72.10 **Chronic hepatic failure** without coma HCC

      AHA: Q1 2017

    K72.11 **Chronic hepatic failure** with coma HCC MCC CC/MCC Exc

5ᵗʰ K72.9 **Hepatic failure, unspecified**

    K72.90 **Hepatic failure, unspecified without coma** HCC

      AHA: Q4 2018, Q2 2016

    K72.91 **Hepatic failure, unspecified with coma** HCC MCC CC/MCC Exc

      Hepatic coma NOS

4ᵗʰ K73 **Chronic hepatitis, not elsewhere classified**

EXCLUDES1 *alcoholic hepatitis (chronic) (K70.1-)*

drug-induced hepatitis (chronic) (K71.-)

granulomatous hepatitis (chronic) NEC (K75.3)

reactive, nonspecific hepatitis (chronic) (K75.2)

viral hepatitis (chronic) (B15-B19)

K73.0 **Chronic** persistent **hepatitis, not elsewhere classified** HCC

K73.1 **Chronic** lobular **hepatitis, not elsewhere classified** HCC

K73.2 **Chronic** active **hepatitis, not elsewhere classified** HCC

K73.8 **Other chronic hepatitis, not elsewhere classified** HCC

K73.9 **Chronic hepatitis, unspecified** HCC

4ᵗʰ K74 **Fibrosis and cirrhosis of liver (Figure 11.8)**

Code also, if applicable, viral hepatitis (acute) (chronic) (B15-B19)

EXCLUDES1 *alcoholic cirrhosis (of liver) (K70.3)*

alcoholic fibrosis of liver (K70.2)

cardiac sclerosis of liver (K76.1)

cirrhosis (of liver) with toxic liver disease (K71.7)

congenital cirrhosis (of liver) (P78.81)

pigmentary cirrhosis (of liver) (E83.110)

K74.0 **Hepatic** fibrosis

K74.1 **Hepatic** sclerosis

K74.2 **Hepatic** fibrosis with hepatic sclerosis

K74.3 Primary **biliary cirrhosis** HCC

Chronic nonsuppurative destructive cholangitis

Primary biliary cholangitis

EXCLUDES2 *primary ▶sclerosing◀ cholangitis (K83.01)*

K74.4 Secondary **biliary cirrhosis** HCC

K74.5 **Biliary cirrhosis, unspecified** HCC

5ᵗʰ K74.6 **Other and unspecified cirrhosis of liver**

    K74.60 **Unspecified cirrhosis of liver** HCC

      AHA: Q1 2018

      Cirrhosis (of liver) NOS

    K74.69 **Other cirrhosis of liver** HCC

      Cryptogenic cirrhosis (of liver)

      Macronodular cirrhosis (of liver)

      Micronodular cirrhosis (of liver)

      Mixed type cirrhosis (of liver)

      Portal cirrhosis (of liver)

      Postnecrotic cirrhosis (of liver)

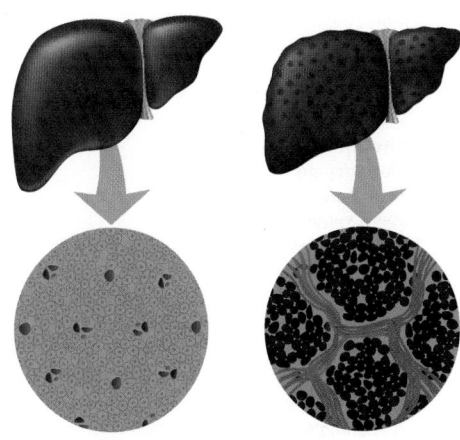

Healthy liver   Cirrhosis

Figure 11.8 Cirrhosis of the Liver

4ᵗʰ K75 **Other inflammatory liver diseases**

EXCLUDES2 *toxic liver disease (K71.-)*

K75.0 **Abscess of liver** MCC CC/MCC Exc

Cholangitic hepatic abscess

Hematogenic hepatic abscess

Hepatic abscess NOS

Lymphogenic hepatic abscess

Pylephlebitic hepatic abscess

EXCLUDES1 *amebic liver abscess (A06.4)*

cholangitis without liver abscess (K83.09)

pylephlebitis without liver abscess (K75.1)

EXCLUDES2 *acute or subacute hepatitis NOS (B17.9)*

acute or subacute non-viral hepatitis (K72.0)

chronic hepatitis NEC (K73.8)

K75.1 Phlebitis of portal vein ꜰᴄᴄ ᴄᴄ/ᴍᴄᴄ ᴇxᶜ
Pylephlebitis
EXCLUDES1 *pylephlebitic liver abscess (K75.0)*

K75.2 Nonspecific reactive hepatitis
EXCLUDES1 *acute or subacute hepatitis (K72.0-)*
chronic hepatitis NEC (K73.-)
viral hepatitis (B15-B19)

K75.3 Granulomatous hepatitis, not elsewhere classified
EXCLUDES1 *acute or subacute hepatitis (K72.0-)*
chronic hepatitis NEC (K73.-)
viral hepatitis (B15-B19)

K75.4 Autoimmune hepatitis ʜᴄᴄ
Lupoid hepatitis NEC

🆂⁵ᵗʰ **K75.8 Other specified inflammatory liver diseases**
K75.81 Nonalcoholic steatohepatitis (NASH)
K75.89 Other specified inflammatory liver diseases

K75.9 Inflammatory liver disease, unspecified
AHA: Q2 2015
Hepatitis NOS
EXCLUDES1 *acute or subacute hepatitis (K72.0-)*
chronic hepatitis NEC (K73.-)
viral hepatitis (B15-B19)

⁴ᵗʰ **K76 Other diseases of liver**
EXCLUDES2 *alcoholic liver disease (K70.-)*
amyloid degeneration of liver (E85.-)
cystic disease of liver (congenital) (Q44.6)
hepatic vein thrombosis (I82.0)
hepatomegaly NOS (R16.0)
pigmentary cirrhosis (of liver) (E83.110)
portal vein thrombosis (I81)
toxic liver disease (K71.-)

K76.0 Fatty (change of) liver, not elsewhere classified
Nonalcoholic fatty liver disease (NAFLD)
EXCLUDES1 *nonalcoholic steatohepatitis (NASH) (K75.81)*

K76.1 Chronic passive congestion of liver ᴄᴄ ᴄᴄ/ᴍᴄᴄ ᴇxᶜ
Cardiac cirrhosis
Cardiac sclerosis

K76.2 Central hemorrhagic necrosis of liver ᴍᴄᴄ ᴄᴄ/ᴍᴄᴄ ᴇxᶜ
EXCLUDES1 *liver necrosis with hepatic failure (K72.-)*

K76.3 Infarction of liver ᴍᴄᴄ ᴄᴄ/ᴍᴄᴄ ᴇxᶜ

K76.4 Peliosis hepatis
Hepatic angiomatosis

K76.5 Hepatic veno-occlusive disease
EXCLUDES1 *Budd-Chiari syndrome (I82.0)*

K76.6 Portal hypertension ᴄᴄ ʜᴄᴄ ᴄᴄ/ᴍᴄᴄ ᴇxᶜ
Use additional code for any associated complications, such as:
portal hypertensive gastropathy (K31.89)

K76.7 Hepatorenal syndrome ʜᴄᴄ ᴍᴄᴄ ᴄᴄ/ᴍᴄᴄ ᴇxᶜ
EXCLUDES1 *hepatorenal syndrome following labor and delivery (O90.4)*
postprocedural hepatorenal syndrome (K91.83)

🆂⁵ᵗʰ **K76.8 Other specified diseases of liver**
K76.81 Hepatopulmonary syndrome ʜᴄᴄ ᴘᴅxɴ
☞ **Code first** underlying liver disease, such as:
alcoholic cirrhosis of liver (K70.3-)
cirrhosis of liver without mention of alcohol (K74.6-)

K76.89 Other specified diseases of liver
Cyst (simple) of liver
Focal nodular hyperplasia of liver
Hepatoptosis

K76.9 Liver disease, unspecified

K77 Liver disorders in diseases classified elsewhere ᴄᴄ
☞ **Code first** underlying disease, such as:
amyloidosis (E85.-)
congenital syphilis (A50.0, A50.5)
congenital toxoplasmosis (P37.1)
schistosomiasis (B65.0-B65.9)

EXCLUDES1 *alcoholic hepatitis (K70.1-)*
alcoholic liver disease (K70.-)
cytomegaloviral hepatitis (B25.1)
herpesviral [herpes simplex] hepatitis (B00.81)
infectious mononucleosis with liver disease (B27.0-B27.9 with .9)
mumps hepatitis (B26.81)
sarcoidosis with liver disease (D86.89)
secondary syphilis with liver disease (A51.45)
syphilis (late) with liver disease (A52.74)
toxoplasmosis (acquired) hepatitis (B58.1)
tuberculosis with liver disease (A18.83)

Disorders of gallbladder, biliary tract and pancreas (K80-K87)

⁴ᵗʰ **K80 Cholelithiasis (Figure 11.9)**
DEFINITION: Cholelithiasis is the presence of gallstones, which are concretions that form in the biliary tract (usually, the gallbladder).
EXCLUDES1 *retained cholelithiasis following cholecystectomy (K91.86)*

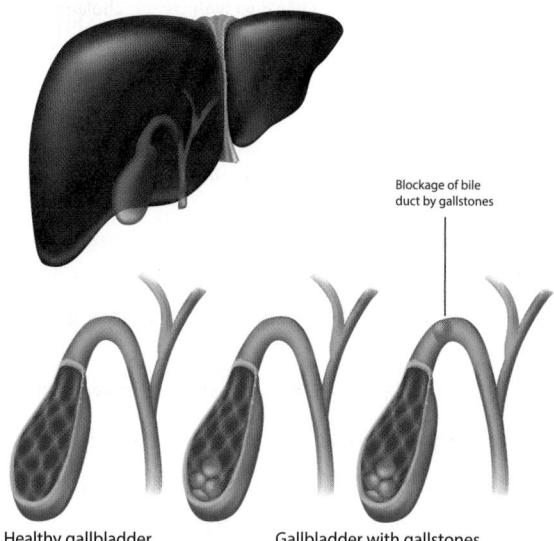

Blockage of bile duct by gallstones

Healthy gallbladder   Gallbladder with gallstones

Figure 11.9 Gallstones

🆂⁵ᵗʰ **K80.0 Calculus of gallbladder with acute cholecystitis**
Any condition listed in K80.2 with acute cholecystitis
Use additional code if applicable for associated gangrene of gallbladder (K82.A1), or perforation of gallbladder (K82.A2)
K80.00 Calculus of gallbladder with acute cholecystitis without obstruction
AHA: Q4 2018
K80.01 Calculus of gallbladder with acute cholecystitis with obstruction ᴄᴄ ᴄᴄ/ᴍᴄᴄ ᴇxᶜ

🆂⁵ᵗʰ **K80.1 Calculus of gallbladder with other cholecystitis**
Use additional code if applicable for associated gangrene of gallbladder (K82.A1), or perforation of gallbladder (K82.A2)
K80.10 Calculus of gallbladder with chronic cholecystitis without obstruction
Cholelithiasis with cholecystitis NOS
K80.11 Calculus of gallbladder with chronic cholecystitis with obstruction ᴄᴄ ᴄᴄ/ᴍᴄᴄ ᴇxᶜ
K80.12 Calculus of gallbladder with acute and chronic cholecystitis without obstruction
K80.13 Calculus of gallbladder with acute and chronic cholecystitis with obstruction ᴄᴄ ᴄᴄ/ᴍᴄᴄ ᴇxᶜ
K80.18 Calculus of gallbladder with other cholecystitis without obstruction
K80.19 Calculus of gallbladder with other cholecystitis with obstruction ᴄᴄ ᴄᴄ/ᴍᴄᴄ ᴇxᶜ

ᴘᴅxɴ Unacceptable principal diagnosis symbol per Medicare code edits   ᴘᴏᴀ Code exempt from diagnosis present on admission requirement
❓ Questionable admission   ᴄᴄ Complication or comorbidity   ᴍᴄᴄ Major complication or comorbidity   ᴄᴄ/ᴍᴄᴄ ᴇxᶜ CC/MCC exclusion
ʜᴄᴄ HCC diagnosis code   ʀxʜᴄᴄ RxHCC diagnosis code   MACRA code   **DEFINITION** Describes condition/terminology
TIP Coding guidance   👁 Official Guideline Reference   🆉 Z code as first-listed diagnosis

736   When symbols appear on a code that requires a 7th character extension, refer to Appendix B to identify applicable 7th character codes.   **2020 ICD-10-CM**

[5th] **K80.2 Calculus of gallbladder without cholecystitis**
Cholecystolithiasis without cholecystitis
Cholelithiasis (without cholecystitis)
Colic (recurrent) of gallbladder (without cholecystitis)
Gallstone (impacted) of cystic duct (without cholecystitis)
Gallstone (impacted) of gallbladder (without cholecystitis)
K80.20 Calculus of gallbladder without cholecystitis without obstruction
K80.21 Calculus of gallbladder without cholecystitis with obstruction [CC] [CC/MCC Exc]

[5th] **K80.3 Calculus of bile duct with cholangitis**
Any condition listed in K80.5 with cholangitis
K80.30 Calculus of bile duct with cholangitis, unspecified, without obstruction [CC] [CC/MCC Exc]
K80.31 Calculus of bile duct with cholangitis, unspecified, with obstruction [CC] [CC/MCC Exc]
K80.32 Calculus of bile duct with acute cholangitis without obstruction [CC] [CC/MCC Exc]
K80.33 Calculus of bile duct with acute cholangitis with obstruction [CC] [CC/MCC Exc]
K80.34 Calculus of bile duct with chronic cholangitis without obstruction [CC] [CC/MCC Exc]
K80.35 Calculus of bile duct with chronic cholangitis with obstruction [CC] [CC/MCC Exc]
K80.36 Calculus of bile duct with acute and chronic cholangitis without obstruction [CC] [CC/MCC Exc]
K80.37 Calculus of bile duct with acute and chronic cholangitis with obstruction [CC] [CC/MCC Exc]

[5th] **K80.4 Calculus of bile duct with cholecystitis**
Any condition listed in K80.5 with cholecystitis (with cholangitis)
Use additional code if applicable for associated gangrene of gallbladder (K82.A1), or perforation of gallbladder (K82.A2)
K80.40 Calculus of bile duct with cholecystitis, unspecified, without obstruction [CC] [CC/MCC Exc]
K80.41 Calculus of bile duct with cholecystitis, unspecified, with obstruction [CC] [CC/MCC Exc]
AHA: Q1 2019
K80.42 Calculus of bile duct with acute cholecystitis without obstruction [CC] [CC/MCC Exc]
K80.43 Calculus of bile duct with acute cholecystitis with obstruction [CC] [CC/MCC Exc]
K80.44 Calculus of bile duct with chronic cholecystitis without obstruction [CC] [CC/MCC Exc]
K80.45 Calculus of bile duct with chronic cholecystitis with obstruction [CC] [CC/MCC Exc]
K80.46 Calculus of bile duct with acute and chronic cholecystitis without obstruction [CC] [CC/MCC Exc]
K80.47 Calculus of bile duct with acute and chronic cholecystitis with obstruction [CC] [CC/MCC Exc]

[5th] **K80.5 Calculus of bile duct without cholangitis or cholecystitis**
Choledocholithiasis (without cholangitis or cholecystitis)
Gallstone (impacted) of bile duct NOS (without cholangitis or cholecystitis)
Gallstone (impacted) of common duct (without cholangitis or cholecystitis)
Gallstone (impacted) of hepatic duct (without cholangitis or cholecystitis)
Hepatic cholelithiasis (without cholangitis or cholecystitis)
Hepatic colic (recurrent) (without cholangitis or cholecystitis)
K80.50 Calculus of bile duct without cholangitis or cholecystitis without obstruction [CC] [CC/MCC Exc]
K80.51 Calculus of bile duct without cholangitis or cholecystitis with obstruction [CC] [CC/MCC Exc]

[5th] **K80.6 Calculus of gallbladder and bile duct with cholecystitis**
Use additional code if applicable for associated gangrene of gallbladder (K82.A1), or perforation of gallbladder (K82.A2)
K80.60 Calculus of gallbladder and bile duct with cholecystitis, unspecified, without obstruction [CC] [CC/MCC Exc]
K80.61 Calculus of gallbladder and bile duct with cholecystitis, unspecified, with obstruction [CC] [CC/MCC Exc]
K80.62 Calculus of gallbladder and bile duct with acute cholecystitis without obstruction [CC] [CC/MCC Exc]
K80.63 Calculus of gallbladder and bile duct with acute cholecystitis with obstruction [CC] [CC/MCC Exc]
K80.64 Calculus of gallbladder and bile duct with chronic cholecystitis without obstruction [CC] [CC/MCC Exc]
K80.65 Calculus of gallbladder and bile duct with chronic cholecystitis with obstruction [CC] [CC/MCC Exc]
K80.66 Calculus of gallbladder and bile duct with acute and chronic cholecystitis without obstruction [CC] [CC/MCC Exc]
K80.67 Calculus of gallbladder and bile duct with acute and chronic cholecystitis with obstruction [CC] [CC/MCC Exc]

[5th] **K80.7 Calculus of gallbladder and bile duct without cholecystitis**
K80.70 Calculus of gallbladder and bile duct without cholecystitis without obstruction [CC] [CC/MCC Exc]
K80.71 Calculus of gallbladder and bile duct without cholecystitis with obstruction [CC] [CC/MCC Exc]

[5th] **K80.8 Other cholelithiasis**
K80.80 Other cholelithiasis without obstruction
K80.81 Other cholelithiasis with obstruction [CC] [CC/MCC Exc]

[4th] **K81 Cholecystitis**
Use additional code if applicable for associated gangrene of gallbladder (K82.A1), or perforation of gallbladder (K82.A2)
[EXCLUDES1] *cholecystitis with cholelithiasis (K80.-)*
K81.0 Acute cholecystitis [CC] [CC/MCC Exc]
Abscess of gallbladder
Angiocholecystitis
Emphysematous (acute) cholecystitis
Empyema of gallbladder
Gangrene of gallbladder
Gangrenous cholecystitis
Suppurative cholecystitis
K81.1 Chronic cholecystitis
K81.2 Acute cholecystitis with chronic cholecystitis [CC] [CC/MCC Exc]
K81.9 Cholecystitis, unspecified

[4th] **K82 Other diseases of gallbladder**
[EXCLUDES1] *nonvisualization of gallbladder (R93.2)*
postcholecystectomy syndrome (K91.5)
K82.0 Obstruction of gallbladder [CC] [CC/MCC Exc]
Occlusion of cystic duct or gallbladder without cholelithiasis
Stenosis of cystic duct or gallbladder without cholelithiasis
Stricture of cystic duct or gallbladder without cholelithiasis
[EXCLUDES1] *obstruction of gallbladder with cholelithiasis (K80.-)*
K82.1 Hydrops of gallbladder
Mucocele of gallbladder
K82.2 Perforation of gallbladder [CC] [CC/MCC Exc]
Rupture of cystic duct or gallbladder
[EXCLUDES1] *Perforation of gallbladder in cholecystitis (K82.A2)*
K82.3 Fistula of gallbladder [CC] [CC/MCC Exc]
Cholecystocolic fistula
Cholecystoduodenal fistula
K82.4 Cholesterolosis of gallbladder
Strawberry gallbladder
[EXCLUDES1] *cholesterolosis of gallbladder with cholecystitis (K81.-)*
cholesterolosis of gallbladder with cholelithiasis (K80.-)
K82.8 Other specified diseases of gallbladder
Adhesions of cystic duct or gallbladder
Atrophy of cystic duct or gallbladder
Cyst of cystic duct or gallbladder
Dyskinesia of cystic duct or gallbladder
Hypertrophy of cystic duct or gallbladder
Nonfunctioning of cystic duct or gallbladder
Ulcer of cystic duct or gallbladder
K82.9 Disease of gallbladder, unspecified
[5th] **K82.A Disorders of gallbladder in diseases classified elsewhere**
☛ **Code first** the type of cholecystitis (K81.-), or cholelithiasis with cholecystitis (K80.00-K80.19, K80.40-K80.47, K80.60-K80.67)
K82.A1 Gangrene of gallbladder in cholecystitis
AHA: Q4 2018
K82.A2 Perforation of gallbladder in cholecystitis [CC] [CC/MCC Exc]
AHA: Q4 2018

Unspecified Code | Other Specified Code | Manifestation Code | [N] Newborn | [P] Pediatric | [M] Maternity | [A] Adult | ♂ Male | ♀ Female
● New Code | ▲ Revised Code Title | ►◄ Revised Text | [NOTES] | *INCLUDES* | [EXCLUDES1] Not coded here | [EXCLUDES2] Not included here
[4th] 4th character required | [5th] 5th character required | [6th] 6th character required | [7th] 7th character required | [x7th] Extension 'X' Alert
[HAC] Hospital-acquired condition (HAC) alert | **AHA** AHA Coding Clinic© | ☛ Code first alert

4ᵀʰ **K83** **Other diseases of biliary tract**
   EXCLUDES1 *postcholecystectomy syndrome (K91.5)*
   EXCLUDES2 *conditions involving the gallbladder (K81-K82)*
      conditions involving the cystic duct (K81-K82)

5ᵀʰ **K83.0** **Cholangitis**
   EXCLUDES1 *cholangitic liver abscess (K75.0)*
      cholangitis with choledocholithiasis (K80.3-, K80.4-)
   EXCLUDES2 *chronic nonsuppurative destructive cholangitis (K74.3)*
      primary biliary cholangitis (K74.3)
      primary biliary cirrhosis (K74.3)

   K83.01 **Primary sclerosing cholangitis**   CC CC/MCC Exc
      AHA: Q4 2018
   K83.09 **Other cholangitis**   CC CC/MCC Exc
      AHA: Q4 2018
      Ascending cholangitis
      Cholangitis NOS
      Primary cholangitis
      Recurrent cholangitis
      Sclerosing cholangitis
      Secondary cholangitis
      Stenosing cholangitis
      Suppurative cholangitis

K83.1 **Obstruction of bile duct**   MCC CC/MCC Exc
   AHA: Q1 2016
   Occlusion of bile duct without cholelithiasis
   Stenosis of bile duct without cholelithiasis
   Stricture of bile duct without cholelithiasis
   EXCLUDES1 *congenital obstruction of bile duct (Q44.3)*
      obstruction of bile duct with cholelithiasis (K80.-)

K83.2 **Perforation of bile duct**   MCC CC/MCC Exc
   Rupture of bile duct

K83.3 **Fistula of bile duct**   CC CC/MCC Exc
   AHA: Q1 2019
   Choledochoduodenal fistula

K83.4 **Spasm of sphincter of Oddi**

K83.5 **Biliary cyst**

K83.8 **Other specified diseases of biliary tract**
   Adhesions of biliary tract
   Atrophy of biliary tract
   Hypertrophy of biliary tract
   Ulcer of biliary tract

K83.9 **Disease of biliary tract, unspecified**

4ᵀʰ **K85** **Acute pancreatitis (Figure 11.10)**
   INCLUDES   *acute (recurrent) pancreatitis*
      subacute pancreatitis

5ᵀʰ **K85.0** **Idiopathic acute pancreatitis**
   K85.00 **Idiopathic acute pancreatitis** without necrosis or infection   MCC CC/MCC Exc
   K85.01 **Idiopathic acute pancreatitis** with uninfected necrosis   MCC CC/MCC Exc
   K85.02 **Idiopathic acute pancreatitis** with infected necrosis   MCC CC/MCC Exc

5ᵀʰ **K85.1** **Biliary acute pancreatitis**
   Gallstone pancreatitis
   K85.10 **Biliary acute pancreatitis** without necrosis or infection   MCC CC/MCC Exc
   K85.11 **Biliary acute pancreatitis** with uninfected necrosis   MCC CC/MCC Exc
   K85.12 **Biliary acute pancreatitis** with infected necrosis   MCC CC/MCC Exc

5ᵀʰ **K85.2** **Alcohol induced acute pancreatitis**
   EXCLUDES2 *alcohol induced chronic pancreatitis (K86.0)*
   K85.20 **Alcohol induced acute pancreatitis** without necrosis or infection   MCC CC/MCC Exc
   K85.21 **Alcohol induced acute pancreatitis** with uninfected necrosis   MCC CC/MCC Exc
   K85.22 **Alcohol induced acute pancreatitis** with infected necrosis   MCC CC/MCC Exc

5ᵀʰ **K85.3** **Drug induced acute pancreatitis**
   Use additional code for adverse effect, if applicable, to identify drug (T36-T50 with fifth or sixth character 5)
   Use additional code to identify drug abuse and dependence (F11.-F17.-)
   K85.30 **Drug induced acute pancreatitis** without necrosis or infection   MCC CC/MCC Exc
   K85.31 **Drug induced acute pancreatitis** with uninfected necrosis   MCC CC/MCC Exc
   K85.32 **Drug induced acute pancreatitis** with infected necrosis   MCC CC/MCC Exc

5ᵀʰ **K85.8** **Other acute pancreatitis**
   K85.80 **Other acute pancreatitis** without necrosis or infection   MCC CC/MCC Exc
   K85.81 **Other acute pancreatitis** with uninfected necrosis   MCC CC/MCC Exc
   K85.82 **Other acute pancreatitis** with infected necrosis   MCC CC/MCC Exc

5ᵀʰ **K85.9** **Acute pancreatitis, unspecified**
   Pancreatitis NOS

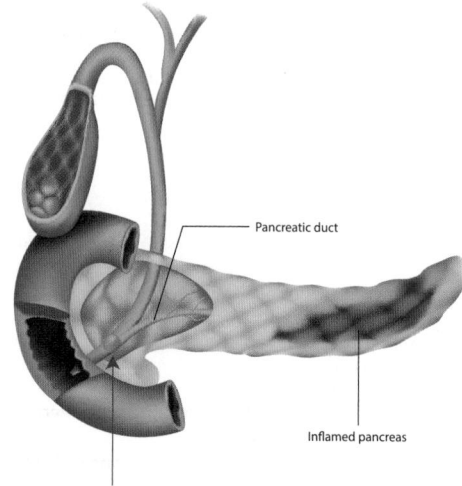

      Pancreatic duct
      Inflamed pancreas
Gallstone blocks pancreatic duct

Figure 11.10 Acute Pancreatitis

   K85.90 **Acute pancreatitis** without necrosis or infection, unspecified   MCC CC/MCC Exc
   K85.91 **Acute pancreatitis** with uninfected necrosis, unspecified   MCC CC/MCC Exc
   K85.92 **Acute pancreatitis** with infected necrosis, unspecified   MCC CC/MCC Exc

4ᵀʰ **K86** **Other diseases of pancreas**
   EXCLUDES2 *fibrocystic disease of pancreas (E84.-)*
      islet cell tumor (of pancreas) (D13.7)
      pancreatic steatorrhea (K90.3)

K86.0 **Alcohol-induced chronic pancreatitis**   HCC RxHCC
   Use additional code to identify:
      alcohol abuse and dependence (F10.-)
   Code also exocrine pancreatic insufficiency (K86.81)
   EXCLUDES2 *alcohol induced acute pancreatitis (K85.2-)*

K86.1 **Other chronic pancreatitis**   HCC RxHCC
   Chronic pancreatitis NOS
   Infectious chronic pancreatitis
   Recurrent chronic pancreatitis
   Relapsing chronic pancreatitis
   Code also exocrine pancreatic insufficiency (K86.81)

K86.2 **Cyst of pancreas**   RxHCC

K86.3 **Pseudocyst of pancreas**   RxHCC

5ᵀʰ **K86.8** **Other specified diseases of pancreas**
   K86.81 **Exocrine pancreatic insufficiency**   RxHCC
      AHA: Q4 2016

K86.89 **Other specified diseases of pancreas** `RxHCC`
    AHA: Q4 2016
    Aseptic pancreatic necrosis, unrelated to acute pancreatitis
    Atrophy of pancreas
    Calculus of pancreas
    Cirrhosis of pancreas
    Fibrosis of pancreas
    Pancreatic fat necrosis, unrelated to acute pancreatitis
    Pancreatic infantilism
    Pancreatic necrosis NOS, unrelated to acute pancreatitis

K86.9 **Disease of pancreas, unspecified** `RxHCC`

K87 **Disorders of gallbladder, biliary tract and pancreas in diseases classified elsewhere** `RxHCC`
  ☞ **Code first** underlying disease
    EXCLUDES1 *cytomegaloviral pancreatitis (B25.2)*
        mumps pancreatitis (B26.3)
        syphilitic gallbladder (A52.74)
        syphilitic pancreas (A52.74)
        tuberculosis of gallbladder (A18.83)
        tuberculosis of pancreas (A18.83)

Other diseases of the digestive system (K90-K95)

4ᵗʰ K90 **Intestinal malabsorption**
    EXCLUDES1 *intestinal malabsorption following gastrointestinal surgery (K91.2)*

K90.0 **Celiac disease** `RxHCC`
    Celiac disease with steatorrhea
    Celiac gluten-sensitive enteropathy
    Nontropical sprue
    Use additional code for associated disorders including:
      dermatitis herpetiformis (L13.0)
      gluten ataxia (G32.81)
    Code also exocrine pancreatic insufficiency (K86.81)

K90.1 **Tropical sprue** `RxHCC`
    Sprue NOS
    Tropical steatorrhea

K90.2 **Blind loop syndrome, not elsewhere classified** `RxHCC`
    Blind loop syndrome NOS
    EXCLUDES1 *congenital blind loop syndrome (Q43.8)*
         postsurgical blind loop syndrome (K91.2)

K90.3 **Pancreatic steatorrhea** `RxHCC`

5ᵗʰ K90.4 **Other malabsorption due to intolerance**
    EXCLUDES2 *celiac gluten-sensitive enteropathy (K90.0)*
         lactose intolerance (E73.-)

K90.41 **Non-celiac gluten sensitivity**
    AHA: Q4 2016
    Gluten sensitivity NOS
    Non-celiac gluten sensitive enteropathy

K90.49 **Malabsorption due to intolerance, not elsewhere classified** `RxHCC`
    AHA: Q4 2016
    Malabsorption due to intolerance to carbohydrate
    Malabsorption due to intolerance to fat
    Malabsorption due to intolerance to protein
    Malabsorption due to intolerance to starch

5ᵗʰ K90.8 **Other intestinal malabsorption**
  K90.81 **Whipple's disease** `RxHCC`
  K90.89 **Other intestinal malabsorption** `RxHCC`

K90.9 **Intestinal malabsorption, unspecified** `RxHCC`
    AHA: Q4 2017

4ᵗʰ K91 **Intraoperative and postprocedural complications and disorders of digestive system, not elsewhere classified**
    EXCLUDES2 *complications of artificial opening of digestive system (K94.-)*
         complications of bariatric procedures (K95.-)
         gastrojejunal ulcer (K28.-)
         postprocedural (radiation) retroperitoneal abscess (K68.11)
         radiation colitis (K52.0)
         radiation gastroenteritis (K52.0)
         radiation proctitis (K62.7)

K91.0 **Vomiting following gastrointestinal surgery**

K91.1 **Postgastric surgery syndromes**
    Dumping syndrome
    Postgastrectomy syndrome
    Postvagotomy syndrome

K91.2 **Postsurgical malabsorption, not elsewhere classified** `RxHCC`
    Postsurgical blind loop syndrome
    EXCLUDES1 *malabsorption osteomalacia in adults (M83.2)*
         malabsorption osteoporosis, postsurgical (M80.8-, M81.8)

5ᵗʰ K91.3 **Postprocedural intestinal obstruction**
  K91.30 **Postprocedural intestinal obstruction, unspecified as to partial versus complete** `CC` `CC/MCC Exc`
    AHA: Q4 2017
    Postprocedural intestinal obstruction NOS
  K91.31 **Postprocedural partial intestinal obstruction** `CC` `CC/MCC Exc`
    AHA: Q4 2017
    Postprocedural incomplete intestinal obstruction
  K91.32 **Postprocedural complete intestinal obstruction** `MCC` `CC/MCC Exc`
    AHA: Q4 2017

K91.5 **Postcholecystectomy syndrome**

5ᵗʰ K91.6 **Intraoperative hemorrhage and hematoma of a digestive system organ or structure complicating a procedure**
    EXCLUDES1 *intraoperative hemorrhage and hematoma of a digestive system organ or structure due to accidental puncture and laceration during a procedure (K91.7-)*
  K91.61 **Intraoperative hemorrhage and hematoma of a digestive system organ or structure complicating a digestive system procedure** `CC` `CC/MCC Exc`
  K91.62 **Intraoperative hemorrhage and hematoma of a digestive system organ or structure complicating other procedure** `CC` `CC/MCC Exc`

5ᵗʰ K91.7 **Accidental puncture and laceration of a digestive system organ or structure during a procedure**
  K91.71 **Accidental puncture and laceration of a digestive system organ or structure during a digestive system procedure** `CC` `CC/MCC Exc`
  K91.72 **Accidental puncture and laceration of a digestive system organ or structure during other procedure** `CC` `CC/MCC Exc`
    AHA: Q2 2019

5ᵗʰ K91.8 **Other intraoperative and postprocedural complications and disorders of digestive system**
  K91.81 **Other intraoperative complications of digestive system** `CC` `CC/MCC Exc`
  K91.82 **Postprocedural hepatic failure** `CC` `CC/MCC Exc`
  K91.83 **Postprocedural hepatorenal syndrome** `CC` `CC/MCC Exc`
  6ᵗʰ K91.84 **Postprocedural hemorrhage of a digestive system organ or structure following a procedure**
    K91.840 **Postprocedural hemorrhage of a digestive system organ or structure following a digestive system procedure** `CC` `CC/MCC Exc`
      AHA: Q1 2016
    K91.841 **Postprocedural hemorrhage of a digestive system organ or structure following other procedure** `CC` `CC/MCC Exc`
  6ᵗʰ K91.85 **Complications of intestinal pouch**
    K91.850 **Pouchitis** `CC` `HCC` `CC/MCC Exc`
      Inflammation of internal ileoanal pouch
    K91.858 **Other complications of intestinal pouch** `CC` `HCC` `CC/MCC Exc`
      AHA: Q2 2019
  K91.86 **Retained cholelithiasis following cholecystectomy** `CC` `CC/MCC Exc`
  6ᵗʰ K91.87 **Postprocedural hematoma and seroma of a digestive system organ or structure following a procedure**
    K91.870 **Postprocedural hematoma of a digestive system organ or structure following a digestive system procedure** `CC` `CC/MCC Exc`

Unspecified Code   Other Specified Code   Manifestation Code   N Newborn   P Pediatric   M Maternity   A Adult   ♂ Male   ♀ Female
● New Code   ▲ Revised Code Title   ►◄ Revised Text   NOTES   INCLUDES   EXCLUDES1 Not coded here   EXCLUDES2 Not included here
4ᵗʰ 4ᵗʰ character required   5ᵗʰ 5ᵗʰ character required   6ᵗʰ 6ᵗʰ character required   7ᵗʰ 7ᵗʰ character required   Extension 'X' Alert
HAC Hospital-acquired condition (HAC) alert   AHA AHA Coding Clinic©   ☞ Code first alert

K91.871 Postprocedural hematoma of a digestive system organ or structure following other procedure `cc` `CC/MCC Exc`

K91.872 Postprocedural seroma of a digestive system organ or structure following a digestive system procedure `cc` `CC/MCC Exc`

K91.873 Postprocedural seroma of a digestive system organ or structure following other procedure `cc` `CC/MCC Exc`

K91.89 Other postprocedural complications and disorders of digestive system `cc` `CC/MCC Exc`

AHA: Q1 2017

Use additional code, if applicable, to further specify disorder

EXCLUDES2 postprocedural retroperitoneal abscess (K68.11)

K92 Other diseases of digestive system

EXCLUDES1 neonatal gastrointestinal hemorrhage (P54.0-P54.3)

K92.0 Hematemesis

K92.1 Melena `cc` `CC/MCC Exc`

EXCLUDES1 occult blood in feces (R19.5)

K92.2 Gastrointestinal hemorrhage, unspecified `cc` `CC/MCC Exc`

Gastric hemorrhage NOS

Intestinal hemorrhage NOS

EXCLUDES1 acute hemorrhagic gastritis (K29.01)

hemorrhage of anus and rectum (K62.5)

angiodysplasia of stomach with hemorrhage (K31.811)

diverticular disease with hemorrhage (K57.-)

gastritis and duodenitis with hemorrhage (K29.-)

peptic ulcer with hemorrhage (K25-K28)

K92.8 Other specified diseases of the digestive system

K92.81 Gastrointestinal mucositis (ulcerative) `cc` `CC/MCC Exc`

Code also type of associated therapy, such as:

antineoplastic and immunosuppressive drugs (T45.1X-)

radiological procedure and radiotherapy (Y84.2)

EXCLUDES2 mucositis (ulcerative) of vagina and vulva (N76.81)

nasal mucositis (ulcerative) (J34.81)

oral mucositis (ulcerative) (K12.3-)

K92.89 Other specified diseases of the digestive system

K92.9 Disease of digestive system, unspecified

K94 Complications of artificial openings of the digestive system

K94.0 Colostomy complications

K94.00 Colostomy complication, unspecified `HCC`

K94.01 Colostomy hemorrhage `cc` `HCC` `CC/MCC Exc`

K94.02 Colostomy infection `cc` `HCC` `CC/MCC Exc`

Use additional code to specify type of infection, such as:

cellulitis of abdominal wall (L03.311)

sepsis (A40.-, A41.-)

K94.03 Colostomy malfunction `cc` `HCC` `CC/MCC Exc`

Mechanical complication of colostomy

K94.09 Other complications of colostomy `cc` `HCC` `CC/MCC Exc`

K94.1 Enterostomy complications

K94.10 Enterostomy complication, unspecified `HCC`

K94.11 Enterostomy hemorrhage `cc` `HCC` `CC/MCC Exc`

K94.12 Enterostomy infection `cc` `HCC` `CC/MCC Exc`

Use additional code to specify type of infection, such as:

cellulitis of abdominal wall (L03.311)

sepsis (A40.-, A41.-)

K94.13 Enterostomy malfunction `cc` `HCC` `CC/MCC Exc`

Mechanical complication of enterostomy

K94.19 Other complications of enterostomy `cc` `HCC` `CC/MCC Exc`

K94.2 Gastrostomy complications

K94.20 Gastrostomy complication, unspecified `HCC`

K94.21 Gastrostomy hemorrhage `HCC`

K94.22 Gastrostomy infection `cc` `HCC` `CC/MCC Exc`

Use additional code to specify type of infection, such as:

cellulitis of abdominal wall (L03.311)

sepsis (A40.-, A41.-)

K94.23 Gastrostomy malfunction `cc` `HCC` `CC/MCC Exc`

AHA: Q1 2019

Mechanical complication of gastrostomy

K94.29 Other complications of gastrostomy `HCC`

K94.3 Esophagostomy complications

K94.30 Esophagostomy complications, unspecified `cc` `HCC` `CC/MCC Exc`

K94.31 Esophagostomy hemorrhage `cc` `HCC` `CC/MCC Exc`

K94.32 Esophagostomy infection `cc` `HCC` `CC/MCC Exc`

Use additional code to identify the infection

K94.33 Esophagostomy malfunction `cc` `HCC` `CC/MCC Exc`

Mechanical complication of esophagostomy

K94.39 Other complications of esophagostomy `cc` `HCC` `CC/MCC Exc`

K95 Complications of bariatric procedures

K95.0 Complications of gastric band procedure

K95.01 Infection due to gastric band procedure `cc` `HAC` `CC/MCC Exc`

Use additional code to specify type of infection or organism, such as:

bacterial and viral infectious agents (B95.-, B96.-)

cellulitis of abdominal wall (L03.311)

sepsis (A40.-, A41.-)

K95.09 Other complications of gastric band procedure `cc` `CC/MCC Exc`

Use additional code, if applicable, to further specify complication

K95.8 Complications of other bariatric procedure

EXCLUDES1 complications of gastric band surgery (K95.0-)

K95.81 Infection due to other bariatric procedure `cc` `HAC` `CC/MCC Exc`

Use additional code to specify type of infection or organism, such as:

bacterial and viral infectious agents (B95.-, B96.-)

cellulitis of abdominal wall (L03.311)

sepsis (A40.-, A41.-)

K95.89 Other complications of other bariatric procedure `cc` `CC/MCC Exc`

Use additional code, if applicable, to further specify complication

---

`PDx` Unacceptable principal diagnosis symbol per Medicare code edits   `PDx` Code exempt from diagnosis present on admission requirement
? Questionable admission   `cc` Complication or comorbidity   `MCC` Major complication or comorbidity   `CC/MCC Exc` CC/MCC exclusion
`HCC` HCC diagnosis code   `RxHCC` RxHCC diagnosis code   MACRA code   **DEFINITION** Describes condition/terminology
TIP Coding guidance   👁 Official Guideline Reference   `Z1` Z code as first-listed diagnosis

Chapter 12: Diseases of the Skin and Subcutaneous Tissue (L00-L99)

Anatomy of the Integumentary System

Introduction

The integumentary system (Figure 12.a) is composed of the common integument (or skin) and its appendages. The skin covers the body and proves to be an effective barrier to most harmful chemicals that can cause damage to our internal body system. It contains the peripheral endings of various sensory nerves and plays an important role in the regulation of our body temperature. The various layers/components of the skin (from outside to inside) are listed below:

1. **The Epidermis**
   a) Stratum Corneum
   b) Stratum Lucidum
   c) Stratum Granulosum
   d) Stratum Spinosum
   e) Stratum Germinativum (or Basal Layer/Stratum Basale)

2. **The Dermis (or Corium)**
   a) Papillary Layer of Dermis
   b) Reticular Layer of Dermis

3. **The Subcutaneous Tissue/Superficial Fascia (or Hypodermis)**

4. **The Appendages of the Skin**
   a) Hair (for protection and sensation)
   b) Nails (for protection)
   c) Sebaceous Glands (or the glands that secrete sebum onto hair follicle)
   d) Sweat Glands (or the glands that secrete sweat) and ducts
      i) eccrine sweat glands (or the glands secreting sweat with faint odor)
      ii) apocrine sweat glands (or the glands secreting sweat with strong odor)
   e) Arrector Pili (or smooth muscles that pull hairs straight)

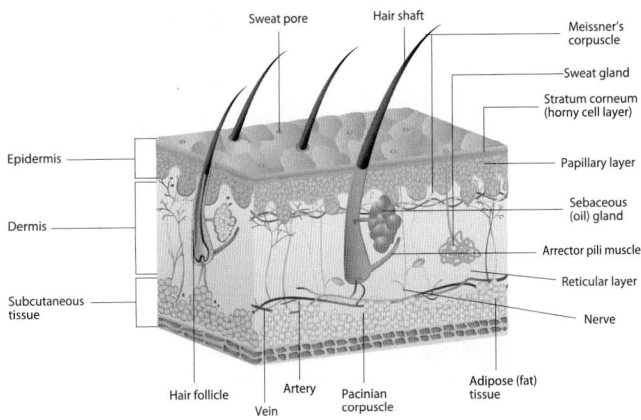

Figure 12.a Integumentary System Anatomy

Common Pathologies

Cellulitis
It is a noncontiguous inflammation of the skin and deeper tissues. It causes diffuse inflammation of connective tissue with severe inflammation of dermal and subcutaneous layers of the skin. Skin in the infected area will become red, hot, irritated and painful. Group A strep (streptococcal) bacteria are the most common cause of cellulitis.

Impetigo
Impetigo is a highly contagious skin infection which causes sores and blisters. This contagious superficial skin infection is generally caused by one of two bacteria: Staphylococcus aureus or Streptococcus pyogenes. Symptoms start with red or pimple-like sores surrounded by red skin.

Folliculitis
It is the infection and inflammation of one or more hair follicles. It usually is caused by bacteria. It can occur anywhere on the skin. Numerous smooth little red bumps form around hair follicles and are most commonly seen on the chest, back, buttocks and legs.

Acne
Acne vulgaris (Figure 12.b) is a common human skin disease. Human skin has pores which connect to oil glands located under the skin. A small hair grows through the follicle out of the skin. Pimples form when hair follicles under the skin clog up. Acne lesions heal slowly, and when one begins to resolve, others seem to crop up.

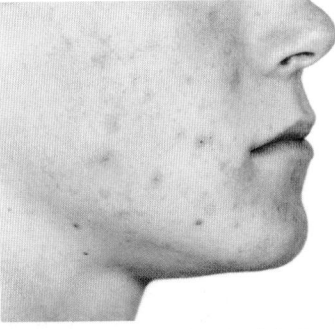

Figure 12.b Acne Vulgaris of the Face

Herpes Simplex (Figure 12.c)
Herpes is an infection that is caused by a herpes simplex virus (HSV). Oral herpes is the most common form of infection followed by genital herpes. Main symptoms of herpes are tingling, itching and burning.

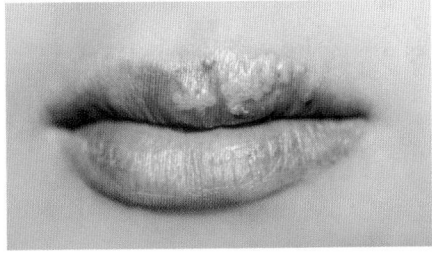

Figure 12.c Herpes Simplex of the Upper Lip

Verrucae
A verruca is a type of wart that is found on the soles of your feet, though they can also appear around the toes. Warts are rough lumps that often develop on the skin of the hands and feet. It is a small growth on the sole of the foot often with tiny black dots on the surface.

Scabies
Scabies is a contagious and itchy skin infection caused by the mite Sarcoptes scabiei. The mite is a tiny and usually not directly visible parasite which burrows under the patient's skin, causing intense allergic itching. Direct skin-to-skin contact is the mode of transmission. Scabies can also be spread by sharing towels, bed sheets, and other personal belongings. Scabies causes severe itching that is usually worse at night and a rash with tiny blisters. It spreads quickly in crowded conditions.

Ringworm
Ringworm is a type of fungal skin infection which is caused by fungi called tinea. It is a common highly contagious skin infection that causes a ring-like red rash on the skin. The rash can appear almost anywhere on the body, with the scalp, feet and groin being most common sites.

Chicken Pox (Figure 12.d)

Chicken pox is a viral infection in which extremely itchy blisters develop all over the body. It is a highly contagious disease caused by primary infection with varicella zoster virus. The classic symptoms of this disease are an uncomfortable itchy rash, fever, headache, tiredness and loss of appetite. The rash turns into fluid-filled blisters and eventually into scabs. It usually shows up on the face, chest, and back and then spreads to the rest of the body. If the virus becomes active again, it can cause a painful infection called shingles.

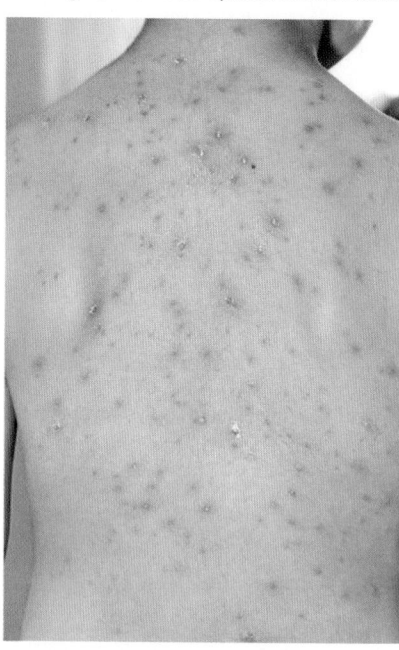

Figure 12.d Chicken Pox Shown on the Back

Psoriasis (Figure 12.e)

Psoriasis is a chronic skin problem that causes skin cells to grow too quickly, resulting in thick, white, silvery patches of skin. This occurs when the immune system mistakenly attacks and destroys healthy body tissue. Bacteria or viral infections, stress, dry air, injury to the skin and some medicines may trigger the condition. It is a noncontagious skin condition that produces red papules that merge together into plaques of thickened scaling skin. Psoriasis commonly affects the skin of the elbows, knees, and scalp. Psoriasis symptoms improve or can go into remission.

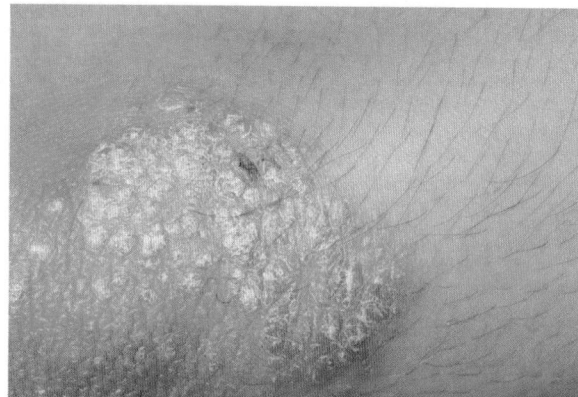

Figure 12.e Psoriasis Shown on the Elbow

Diseases of the skin and subcutaneous tissue (L00-L99)

| EXCLUDES2 | certain conditions originating in the perinatal period (P04-P96) |

certain conditions originating in the perinatal period (P04-P96)
certain infectious and parasitic diseases (A00-B99)
complications of pregnancy, childbirth and the puerperium (O00-O9A)
congenital malformations, deformations, and chromosomal abnormalities (Q00-Q99)
endocrine, nutritional and metabolic diseases (E00-E88)
lipomelanotic reticulosis (I89.8)
neoplasms (C00-D49)
symptoms, signs and abnormal clinical and laboratory findings, not elsewhere classified (R00-R94)
systemic connective tissue disorders (M30-M36)
viral warts (B07.-)

This chapter contains the following blocks:

L00-L08	Infections of the skin and subcutaneous tissue
L10-L14	Bullous disorders
L20-L30	Dermatitis and eczema
L40-L45	Papulosquamous disorders
L49-L54	Urticaria and erythema
L55-L59	Radiation-related disorders of the skin and subcutaneous tissue
L60-L75	Disorders of skin appendages
L76	Intraoperative and postprocedural complications of skin and subcutaneous tissue
L80-L99	Other disorders of the skin and subcutaneous tissue

Infections of the skin and subcutaneous tissue (L00-L08)

Use additional code (B95-B97) to identify infectious agent.

EXCLUDES2 hordeolum (H00.0)
infective dermatitis (L30.3)
local infections of skin classified in Chapter 1
lupus panniculitis (L93.2)
panniculitis NOS (M79.3)
panniculitis of neck and back (M54.0-)
Perlèche NOS (K13.0)
Perlèche due to candidiasis (B37.0)
Perlèche due to riboflavin deficiency (E53.0)
pyogenic granuloma (L98.0)
relapsing panniculitis [Weber-Christian] (M35.6)
viral warts (B07.-)
zoster (B02.-)

L00 Staphylococcal scalded skin syndrome
AHA: Q4 2016
Ritter's disease
Use additional code to identify percentage of skin exfoliation (L49.-)
EXCLUDES1 bullous impetigo (L01.03)
pemphigus neonatorum (L01.03)
toxic epidermal necrolysis [Lyell] (L51.2)

L01 Impetigo
DEFINITION: Impetigo is a common, contagious skin infection that mainly affects infants and children, and appears as red sores on the face, hands, and feet.
EXCLUDES1 impetigo herpetiformis (L40.1)
L01.0 Impetigo
Impetigo contagiosa
Impetigo vulgaris
L01.00 Impetigo, unspecified
Impetigo NOS
L01.01 Non-bullous impetigo
L01.02 Bockhart's impetigo
Impetigo follicularis
Perifolliculitis NOS
Superficial pustular perifolliculitis
L01.03 Bullous impetigo
Impetigo neonatorum
Pemphigus neonatorum

L01.09 Other impetigo
Ulcerative impetigo
L01.1 Impetiginization of other dermatoses
L02 Cutaneous abscess, furuncle and carbuncle
TIP: (1) A carbuncle is a severe abscess or boil in the skin, typically infected with staphylococcus bacteria. (2) A furuncle is a boil or a skin lesion caused by an infection around a hair follicle.
Use additional code to identify organism (B95-B96)
EXCLUDES2 abscess of anus and rectal regions (K61.-)
abscess of female genital organs (external) (N76.4)
abscess of male genital organs (external) (N48.2, N49.-)
L02.0 Cutaneous abscess, furuncle and carbuncle of face
EXCLUDES2 abscess of ear, external (H60.0)
abscess of eyelid (H00.0)
abscess of head [any part, except face] (L02.8)
abscess of lacrimal gland (H04.0)
abscess of lacrimal passages (H04.3)
abscess of mouth (K12.2)
abscess of nose (J34.0)
abscess of orbit (H05.0)
submandibular abscess (K12.2)
L02.01 Cutaneous abscess of face
L02.02 Furuncle of face
Boil of face
Folliculitis of face
L02.03 Carbuncle of face
L02.1 Cutaneous abscess, furuncle and carbuncle of neck
L02.11 Cutaneous abscess of neck
L02.12 Furuncle of neck
Boil of neck
Folliculitis of neck
L02.13 Carbuncle of neck
L02.2 Cutaneous abscess, furuncle and carbuncle of trunk
EXCLUDES1 non-newborn omphalitis (L08.82)
omphalitis of newborn (P38.-)
EXCLUDES2 abscess of breast (N61.1)
abscess of buttocks (L02.3)
abscess of female external genital organs (N76.4)
abscess of male external genital organs (N48.2, N49.-)
abscess of hip (L02.4)
L02.21 Cutaneous abscess of trunk
L02.211 Cutaneous abscess of abdominal wall
L02.212 Cutaneous abscess of back [any part, except buttock]
L02.213 Cutaneous abscess of chest wall
L02.214 Cutaneous abscess of groin
L02.215 Cutaneous abscess of perineum
L02.216 Cutaneous abscess of umbilicus
L02.219 Cutaneous abscess of trunk, unspecified
L02.22 Furuncle of trunk
Boil of trunk
Folliculitis of trunk
L02.221 Furuncle of abdominal wall
L02.222 Furuncle of back [any part, except buttock]
L02.223 Furuncle of chest wall
L02.224 Furuncle of groin
L02.225 Furuncle of perineum
L02.226 Furuncle of umbilicus
L02.229 Furuncle of trunk, unspecified
L02.23 Carbuncle of trunk
L02.231 Carbuncle of abdominal wall
L02.232 Carbuncle of back [any part, except buttock]
L02.233 Carbuncle of chest wall
L02.234 Carbuncle of groin
L02.235 Carbuncle of perineum

L02.236 **Carbuncle of** umbilicus
L02.239 **Carbuncle of trunk, unspecified**

5ᵗʰ L02.3 **Cutaneous abscess, furuncle and carbuncle of** buttock
EXCLUDES1 *pilonidal cyst with abscess (L05.01)*
L02.31 Cutaneous abscess **of buttock** cc cc/mcc exc
Cutaneous abscess of gluteal region
L02.32 **Furuncle of buttock**
Boil of buttock
Folliculitis of buttock
Furuncle of gluteal region
L02.33 **Carbuncle of buttock**
Carbuncle of gluteal region

5ᵗʰ L02.4 **Cutaneous abscess, furuncle and carbuncle of** limb
EXCLUDES2 *Cutaneous abscess, furuncle and carbuncle of groin (L02.214, L02.224, L02.234)*
Cutaneous abscess, furuncle and carbuncle of hand (L02.5-)
Cutaneous abscess, furuncle and carbuncle of foot (L02.6-)
6ᵗʰ L02.41 Cutaneous abscess **of limb**
L02.411 **Cutaneous abscess of** right **axilla** cc cc/mcc exc
L02.412 **Cutaneous abscess of** left **axilla** cc cc/mcc exc
L02.413 **Cutaneous abscess of** right **upper limb**
L02.414 **Cutaneous abscess of** left **upper limb**
L02.415 **Cutaneous abscess of** right **lower limb**
L02.416 **Cutaneous abscess of** left **lower limb**
L02.419 **Cutaneous abscess of limb, unspecified**
6ᵗʰ L02.42 Furuncle **of limb**
Boil of limb
Folliculitis of limb
L02.421 **Furuncle of** right **axilla**
L02.422 **Furuncle of** left **axilla**
L02.423 **Furuncle of** right **upper limb**
L02.424 **Furuncle of** left **upper limb**
L02.425 **Furuncle of** right **lower limb**
L02.426 **Furuncle of** left **lower limb**
L02.429 **Furuncle of limb, unspecified**
6ᵗʰ L02.43 Carbuncle **of limb**
L02.431 **Carbuncle of** right **axilla**
L02.432 **Carbuncle of** left **axilla**
L02.433 **Carbuncle of** right **upper limb**
L02.434 **Carbuncle of** left **upper limb**
L02.435 **Carbuncle of** right **lower limb**
L02.436 **Carbuncle of** left **lower limb**
L02.439 **Carbuncle of limb, unspecified**

5ᵗʰ L02.5 **Cutaneous abscess, furuncle and carbuncle of** hand
6ᵗʰ L02.51 Cutaneous abscess **of hand**
L02.511 **Cutaneous abscess of** right **hand**
L02.512 **Cutaneous abscess of** left **hand**
L02.519 **Cutaneous abscess of unspecified hand**
6ᵗʰ L02.52 Furuncle **hand**
Boil of hand
Folliculitis of hand
L02.521 **Furuncle** right **hand**
L02.522 **Furuncle** left **hand**
L02.529 **Furuncle unspecified hand**
6ᵗʰ L02.53 Carbuncle **of hand**
L02.531 **Carbuncle of** right **hand**
L02.532 **Carbuncle of** left **hand**
L02.539 **Carbuncle of unspecified hand**

5ᵗʰ L02.6 **Cutaneous abscess, furuncle and carbuncle of** foot
6ᵗʰ L02.61 Cutaneous abscess **of foot**
L02.611 **Cutaneous abscess of** right **foot** cc cc/mcc exc
L02.612 **Cutaneous abscess of** left **foot** cc cc/mcc exc
L02.619 **Cutaneous abscess of unspecified foot** cc cc/mcc exc
6ᵗʰ L02.62 Furuncle **of foot**
Boil of foot
Folliculitis of foot

L02.621 **Furuncle of** right **foot**
L02.622 **Furuncle of** left **foot**
L02.629 **Furuncle of unspecified foot**
6ᵗʰ L02.63 Carbuncle **of foot**
L02.631 **Carbuncle of** right **foot**
L02.632 **Carbuncle of** left **foot**
L02.639 **Carbuncle of unspecified foot**

5ᵗʰ L02.8 **Cutaneous abscess, furuncle and carbuncle of** other sites
6ᵗʰ L02.81 Cutaneous abscess **of other sites**
L02.811 **Cutaneous abscess of** head [any part, except face]
L02.818 **Cutaneous abscess of** other sites
6ᵗʰ L02.82 Furuncle **of other sites**
Boil of other sites
Folliculitis of other sites
L02.821 **Furuncle of** head [any part, except face]
L02.828 **Furuncle of** other sites
6ᵗʰ L02.83 Carbuncle **of other sites**
L02.831 **Carbuncle of** head [any part, except face]
L02.838 **Carbuncle of** other sites

5ᵗʰ L02.9 **Cutaneous abscess, furuncle and carbuncle,** unspecified
L02.91 Cutaneous abscess, **unspecified**
L02.92 Furuncle, **unspecified**
Boil NOS
Furunculosis NOS
L02.93 Carbuncle, **unspecified**

4ᵗʰ L03 **Cellulitis and acute lymphangitis**
EXCLUDES2 *cellulitis of anal and rectal region (K61.-)*
cellulitis of external auditory canal (H60.1)
cellulitis of eyelid (H00.0)
cellulitis of female external genital organs (N76.4)
cellulitis of lacrimal apparatus (H04.3)
cellulitis of male external genital organs (N48.2, N49.-)
cellulitis of mouth (K12.2)
cellulitis of nose (J34.0)
eosinophilic cellulitis [Wells] (L98.3)
febrile neutrophilic dermatosis [Sweet] (L98.2)
lymphangitis (chronic) (subacute) (I89.1)
5ᵗʰ L03.0 Cellulitis and acute lymphangitis **of finger and toe**
Infection of nail
Onychia
Paronychia
Perionychia
6ᵗʰ L03.01 Cellulitis of finger
Felon
Whitlow
EXCLUDES1 *herpetic whitlow (B00.89)*
L03.011 **Cellulitis of** right **finger**
L03.012 **Cellulitis of** left **finger**
L03.019 **Cellulitis of unspecified finger**
6ᵗʰ L03.02 **Acute lymphangitis of** finger
Hangnail with lymphangitis of finger
L03.021 **Acute lymphangitis of** right **finger**
L03.022 **Acute lymphangitis of** left **finger**
L03.029 **Acute lymphangitis of unspecified finger**
6ᵗʰ L03.03 **Cellulitis of** toe
L03.031 **Cellulitis of** right **toe**
L03.032 **Cellulitis of** left **toe**
L03.039 **Cellulitis of unspecified toe**
6ᵗʰ L03.04 **Acute lymphangitis of** toe
Hangnail with lymphangitis of toe
L03.041 **Acute lymphangitis of** right **toe**
L03.042 **Acute lymphangitis of** left **toe**
L03.049 **Acute lymphangitis of unspecified toe**
5ᵗʰ L03.1 **Cellulitis and acute lymphangitis of** other parts of limb
6ᵗʰ L03.11 Cellulitis **of other parts of limb**
EXCLUDES2 *cellulitis of fingers (L03.01-)*
cellulitis of toes (L03.03-)
groin (L03.314)

L03.111 **Cellulitis** of right **axilla** `cc` `CC/MCC Exc`
L03.112 **Cellulitis** of left **axilla** `cc` `CC/MCC Exc`
L03.113 **Cellulitis** of right **upper limb** `cc` `CC/MCC Exc`
L03.114 **Cellulitis** of left **upper limb** `cc` `CC/MCC Exc`
   AHA: Q1 2019
L03.115 **Cellulitis** of right **lower limb** `cc` `CC/MCC Exc`
L03.116 **Cellulitis** of left **lower limb** `cc` `CC/MCC Exc`
L03.119 **Cellulitis of unspecified part of limb** `cc` `CC/MCC Exc`

6th L03.12 Acute lymphangitis **of other parts of limb**
   EXCLUDES2 *acute lymphangitis of fingers (L03.2-)*
      acute lymphangitis of toes (L03.04-)
      acute lymphangitis of groin (L03.324)
L03.121 **Acute lymphangitis of** right **axilla** `cc` `CC/MCC Exc`
L03.122 **Acute lymphangitis of** left **axilla** `cc` `CC/MCC Exc`
L03.123 **Acute lymphangitis of** right **upper limb** `cc` `CC/MCC Exc`
L03.124 **Acute lymphangitis of** left **upper limb** `cc` `CC/MCC Exc`
L03.125 **Acute lymphangitis of** right **lower limb** `cc` `CC/MCC Exc`
L03.126 **Acute lymphangitis of** left **lower limb** `cc` `CC/MCC Exc`
L03.129 **Acute lymphangitis of unspecified part of limb** `cc` `CC/MCC Exc`

5th L03.2 **Cellulitis and acute lymphangitis of** face and neck
   6th L03.21 **Cellulitis and acute lymphangitis of face**
L03.211 Cellulitis **of face** `cc` `CC/MCC Exc`
   AHA: Q4 2013
   EXCLUDES2 *abscess of orbit (H05.01-)*
      cellulitis of ear (H60.1-)
      cellulitis of eyelid (H00.0-)
      cellulitis of head (L03.81)
      cellulitis of lacrimal apparatus (H04.3)
      cellulitis of lip (K13.0)
      cellulitis of mouth (K12.2)
      cellulitis of nose (internal) (J34.0)
      cellulitis of orbit (H05.01-)
      cellulitis of scalp (L03.81)
L03.212 Acute lymphangitis **of face** `cc`
L03.213 Periorbital **cellulitis** `cc` `CC/MCC Exc`
   AHA: Q4 2016
   Preseptal cellulitis
   6th L03.22 **Cellulitis and acute lymphangitis of neck**
L03.221 Cellulitis **of neck** `cc` `CC/MCC Exc`
L03.222 Acute lymphangitis **of neck** `cc` `CC/MCC Exc`

5th L03.3 **Cellulitis and acute lymphangitis of** trunk
   6th L03.31 Cellulitis **of trunk**
   EXCLUDES2 *cellulitis of anal and rectal regions (K61.-)*
      cellulitis of breast NOS (N61.0)
      cellulitis of female external genital organs (N76.4)
      cellulitis of male external genital organs (N48.2, N49.-)
      omphalitis of newborn (P38.-)
      puerperal cellulitis of breast (O91.2)
L03.311 **Cellulitis of** abdominal wall `cc` `CC/MCC Exc`
   EXCLUDES2 *cellulitis of umbilicus (L03.316)*
      cellulitis of groin (L03.314)
L03.312 **Cellulitis of** back [any part except buttock] `cc` `CC/MCC Exc`
L03.313 **Cellulitis of** chest wall `cc` `CC/MCC Exc`
L03.314 **Cellulitis of** groin `cc` `CC/MCC Exc`
L03.315 **Cellulitis of** perineum `cc` `CC/MCC Exc`
L03.316 **Cellulitis of** umbilicus `cc` `CC/MCC Exc`
L03.317 **Cellulitis of** buttock `cc` `CC/MCC Exc`
L03.319 **Cellulitis of trunk, unspecified** `cc` `CC/MCC Exc`

6th L03.32 Acute lymphangitis **of trunk**
L03.321 **Acute lymphangitis of** abdominal wall `cc` `CC/MCC Exc`
L03.322 **Acute lymphangitis of** back [any part except buttock] `cc` `CC/MCC Exc`
L03.323 **Acute lymphangitis of** chest wall `cc` `CC/MCC Exc`
L03.324 **Acute lymphangitis of** groin `cc` `CC/MCC Exc`
L03.325 **Acute lymphangitis of** perineum `cc` `CC/MCC Exc`
L03.326 **Acute lymphangitis of** umbilicus `cc` `CC/MCC Exc`
L03.327 **Acute lymphangitis of** buttock `cc` `CC/MCC Exc`
L03.329 **Acute lymphangitis of trunk, unspecified** `cc` `CC/MCC Exc`

5th L03.8 **Cellulitis and acute lymphangitis of** other sites
   6th L03.81 Cellulitis **of other sites**
L03.811 **Cellulitis of** head [any part, except face] `cc` `CC/MCC Exc`
   Cellulitis of scalp
   EXCLUDES2 *cellulitis of face (L03.211)*
L03.818 **Cellulitis of** other sites `cc` `CC/MCC Exc`
   6th L03.89 Acute lymphangitis **of other sites**
L03.891 **Acute lymphangitis of** head [any part, except face] `cc` `CC/MCC Exc`
L03.898 **Acute lymphangitis of** other sites `cc` `CC/MCC Exc`

5th L03.9 **Cellulitis and acute lymphangitis,** unspecified
L03.90 Cellulitis, **unspecified** `cc` `CC/MCC Exc`
L03.91 Acute lymphangitis, **unspecified** `cc` `CC/MCC Exc`
   EXCLUDES1 *lymphangitis NOS (I89.1)*

4th L04 **Acute lymphadenitis**
   INCLUDES *abscess (acute) of lymph nodes, except mesenteric*
      acute lymphadenitis, except mesenteric
   EXCLUDES1 *chronic or subacute lymphadenitis, except mesenteric (I88.1)*
      enlarged lymph nodes (R59.-)
      human immunodeficiency virus [HIV] disease resulting in generalized lymphadenopathy (B20)
      lymphadenitis NOS (I88.9)
      nonspecific mesenteric lymphadenitis (I88.0)
L04.0 **Acute lymphadenitis of** face, head and neck
L04.1 **Acute lymphadenitis of** trunk
L04.2 **Acute lymphadenitis of** upper limb
   Acute lymphadenitis of axilla
   Acute lymphadenitis of shoulder
L04.3 **Acute lymphadenitis of** lower limb
   Acute lymphadenitis of hip
   EXCLUDES2 *acute lymphadenitis of groin (L04.1)*
L04.8 **Acute lymphadenitis of** other sites
L04.9 **Acute lymphadenitis, unspecified**

4th L05 Pilonidal **cyst and sinus**
   5th L05.0 **Pilonidal cyst and sinus** with abscess
L05.01 **Pilonidal cyst with abscess** `cc` `CC/MCC Exc`
   Pilonidal abscess
   Pilonidal dimple with abscess
   Postanal dimple with abscess
   EXCLUDES2 *congenital sacral dimple (Q82.6)*
      parasacral dimple (Q82.6)
L05.02 **Pilonidal sinus with abscess** `cc` `CC/MCC Exc`
   Coccygeal fistula with abscess
   Coccygeal sinus with abscess
   Pilonidal fistula with abscess
   5th L05.9 **Pilonidal cyst and sinus** without abscess
L05.91 **Pilonidal cyst without abscess**
   Pilonidal dimple
   Postanal dimple
   Pilonidal cyst NOS
   EXCLUDES2 *congenital sacral dimple (Q82.6)*
      parasacral dimple (Q82.6)
L05.92 **Pilonidal sinus without abscess**
   Coccygeal fistula
   Coccygeal sinus without abscess
   Pilonidal fistula

Unspecified Code   Other Specified Code   Manifestation Code   N Newborn   P Pediatric   M Maternity   A Adult   ♂ Male   ♀ Female
● New Code   ▲ Revised Code Title   ►◄ Revised Text   NOTES   INCLUDES   EXCLUDES1 Not coded here   EXCLUDES2 Not included here
4th 4th character required   5th 5th character required   6th 6th character required   7th 7th character required   Extension 'X' Alert
HAC Hospital-acquired condition (HAC) alert   AHA AHA Coding Clinic©   📖 Code first alert

[4th] L08 Other local infections of skin and subcutaneous tissue
L08.0 Pyoderma
Dermatitis gangrenosa
Purulent dermatitis
Septic dermatitis
Suppurative dermatitis
[EXCLUDES1] *pyoderma gangrenosum (L88)*
pyoderma vegetans (L08.81)
L08.1 Erythrasma [CC] [CC/MCC Exc]
[5th] L08.8 Other specified local infections of the skin and subcutaneous tissue
L08.81 Pyoderma vegetans
[EXCLUDES1] *pyoderma gangrenosum (L88)*
pyoderma NOS (L08.0)
L08.82 Omphalitis not of newborn
[EXCLUDES1] *omphalitis of newborn (P38.-)*
L08.89 Other specified local infections of the skin and subcutaneous tissue
L08.9 Local infection of the skin and subcutaneous tissue, unspecified

Bullous disorders (L10-L14)

[EXCLUDES1] *benign familial pemphigus [Hailey-Hailey] (Q82.8)*
staphylococcal scalded skin syndrome (L00)
toxic epidermal necrolysis [Lyell] (L51.2)

[4th] L10 Pemphigus
DEFINITION: Pemphigus is a rare group of autoimmune diseases that cause blistering on the skin and mucous membranes.
[EXCLUDES1] *pemphigus neonatorum (L01.03)*
L10.0 Pemphigus vulgaris [CC] [RxHCC] [CC/MCC Exc]
L10.1 Pemphigus vegetans [CC] [RxHCC] [CC/MCC Exc]
L10.2 Pemphigus foliaceous [CC] [RxHCC] [CC/MCC Exc]
L10.3 Brazilian pemphigus [fogo selvagem] [CC] [RxHCC] [CC/MCC Exc]
L10.4 Pemphigus erythematosus [CC] [RxHCC] [CC/MCC Exc]
Senear-Usher syndrome
L10.5 Drug-induced pemphigus [CC] [RxHCC] [CC/MCC Exc]
Use additional code for adverse effect, if applicable, to identify drug (T36-T50 with fifth or sixth character 5)
[5th] L10.8 Other pemphigus
L10.81 Paraneoplastic pemphigus [CC] [RxHCC] [CC/MCC Exc]
L10.89 Other pemphigus [CC] [RxHCC] [CC/MCC Exc]
L10.9 Pemphigus, unspecified [CC] [RxHCC] [CC/MCC Exc]
[4th] L11 Other acantholytic disorders
L11.0 Acquired keratosis follicularis
[EXCLUDES1] *keratosis follicularis (congenital) [Darier-White] (Q82.8)*
L11.1 Transient acantholytic dermatosis [Grover]
L11.8 Other specified acantholytic disorders
L11.9 Acantholytic disorder, unspecified
[4th] L12 Pemphigoid
[EXCLUDES1] *herpes gestationis (O26.4-)*
impetigo herpetiformis (L40.1)
L12.0 Bullous pemphigoid [CC] [CC/MCC Exc]
L12.1 Cicatricial pemphigoid
Benign mucous membrane pemphigoid
L12.2 Chronic bullous disease of childhood [P]
Juvenile dermatitis herpetiformis
[5th] L12.3 Acquired epidermolysis bullosa
[EXCLUDES1] *epidermolysis bullosa (congenital) (Q81.-)*
L12.30 Acquired epidermolysis bullosa, unspecified [CC] [HCC] [CC/MCC Exc]
L12.31 Epidermolysis bullosa due to drug [CC] [HCC] [CC/MCC Exc]
Use additional code for adverse effect, if applicable, to identify drug (T36-T50 with fifth or sixth character 5)
L12.35 Other acquired epidermolysis bullosa [CC] [HCC] [CC/MCC Exc]
L12.8 Other pemphigoid [CC] [CC/MCC Exc]
L12.9 Pemphigoid, unspecified [CC] [CC/MCC Exc]

[4th] L13 Other bullous disorders
L13.0 Dermatitis herpetiformis
Duhring's disease
Hydroa herpetiformis
[EXCLUDES1] *juvenile dermatitis herpetiformis (L12.2)*
senile dermatitis herpetiformis (L12.0)
L13.1 Subcorneal pustular dermatitis
Sneddon-Wilkinson disease
L13.8 Other specified bullous disorders
L13.9 Bullous disorder, unspecified
L14 Bullous disorders in diseases classified elsewhere
☞ Code first underlying disease.

Dermatitis and eczema (L20-L30)

[NOTES] In this block the terms dermatitis and eczema are used synonymously and interchangeably.
[EXCLUDES2] *chronic (childhood) granulomatous disease (D71)*
dermatitis gangrenosa (L08.0)
dermatitis herpetiformis (L13.0)
dry skin dermatitis (L85.3)
factitial dermatitis (L98.1)
perioral dermatitis (L71.0)
radiation-related disorders of the skin and subcutaneous tissue (L55-L59)
stasis dermatitis (I87.2)

[4th] L20 Atopic dermatitis
L20.0 Besnier's prurigo
[5th] L20.8 Other atopic dermatitis
[EXCLUDES2] *circumscribed neurodermatitis (L28.0)*
L20.81 Atopic neurodermatitis
Diffuse neurodermatitis
L20.82 Flexural eczema
L20.83 Infantile (acute) (chronic) eczema [P]
L20.84 Intrinsic (allergic) eczema
L20.89 Other atopic dermatitis
L20.9 Atopic dermatitis, unspecified
[4th] L21 Seborrheic dermatitis
[EXCLUDES2] *infective dermatitis (L30.3)*
seborrheic keratosis (L82.-)
L21.0 Seborrhea capitis
AHA: Q1 2018
Cradle cap
L21.1 Seborrheic infantile dermatitis [P]
L21.8 Other seborrheic dermatitis
L21.9 Seborrheic dermatitis, unspecified
Seborrhea NOS
L22 Diaper dermatitis
Diaper erythema
Diaper rash
Psoriasiform diaper rash
[4th] L23 Allergic contact dermatitis
[EXCLUDES1] *allergy NOS (T78.40)*
contact dermatitis NOS (L25.9)
dermatitis NOS (L30.9)
[EXCLUDES2] *dermatitis due to substances taken internally (L27.-)*
dermatitis of eyelid (H01.1-)
diaper dermatitis (L22)
eczema of external ear (H60.5-)
irritant contact dermatitis (L24.-)
perioral dermatitis (L71.0)
radiation-related disorders of the skin and subcutaneous tissue (L55-L59)
L23.0 Allergic contact dermatitis due to metals
Allergic contact dermatitis due to chromium
Allergic contact dermatitis due to nickel
L23.1 Allergic contact dermatitis due to adhesives
L23.2 Allergic contact dermatitis due to cosmetics

[PDx] Unacceptable principal diagnosis symbol per Medicare code edits [POA] Code exempt from diagnosis present on admission requirement
[?] Questionable admission [CC] Complication or comorbidity [MCC] Major complication or comorbidity [CC/MCC Exc] CC/MCC exclusion
[HCC] HCC diagnosis code [RxHCC] RxHCC diagnosis code MACRA code DEFINITION Describes condition/terminology
TIP Coding guidance 👁 Official Guideline Reference [Z1] Z code as first-listed diagnosis

L23.3 **Allergic contact dermatitis** due to drugs in contact with skin
Use additional code for adverse effect, if applicable, to identify drug (T36-T50 with fifth or sixth character 5)
[EXCLUDES2] *dermatitis due to ingested drugs and medicaments (L27.0-L27.1)*

L23.4 **Allergic contact dermatitis** due to dyes

L23.5 **Allergic contact dermatitis** due to other chemical products
Allergic contact dermatitis due to cement
Allergic contact dermatitis due to insecticide
Allergic contact dermatitis due to plastic
Allergic contact dermatitis due to rubber

L23.6 **Allergic contact dermatitis** due to food in contact with the skin
[EXCLUDES2] *dermatitis due to ingested food (L27.2)*

L23.7 **Allergic contact dermatitis** due to plants, except food
[EXCLUDES2] *allergy NOS due to pollen (J30.1)*

[5th] L23.8 **Allergic contact dermatitis** due to other agents

L23.81 **Allergic contact dermatitis** due to animal (cat) (dog) dander
Allergic contact dermatitis due to animal (cat) (dog) hair

L23.89 **Allergic contact dermatitis** due to other agents

L23.9 **Allergic contact dermatitis, unspecified cause**
Allergic contact eczema NOS

[4th] L24 **Irritant contact dermatitis**
[EXCLUDES1] *allergy NOS (T78.40)*
contact dermatitis NOS (L25.9)
dermatitis NOS (L30.9)
[EXCLUDES2] *allergic contact dermatitis (L23.-)*
dermatitis due to substances taken internally (L27.-)
dermatitis of eyelid (H01.1-)
diaper dermatitis (L22)
eczema of external ear (H60.5-)
perioral dermatitis (L71.0)
radiation-related disorders of the skin and subcutaneous tissue (L55-L59)

L24.0 **Irritant contact dermatitis** due to detergents

L24.1 **Irritant contact dermatitis** due to oils and greases

L24.2 **Irritant contact dermatitis** due to solvents
Irritant contact dermatitis due to chlorocompound
Irritant contact dermatitis due to cyclohexane
Irritant contact dermatitis due to ester
Irritant contact dermatitis due to glycol
Irritant contact dermatitis due to hydrocarbon
Irritant contact dermatitis due to ketone

L24.3 **Irritant contact dermatitis** due to cosmetics

L24.4 **Irritant contact dermatitis** due to drugs in contact with skin
Use additional code for adverse effect, if applicable, to identify drug (T36-T50 with fifth or sixth character 5)

L24.5 **Irritant contact dermatitis** due to other chemical products
Irritant contact dermatitis due to cement
Irritant contact dermatitis due to insecticide
Irritant contact dermatitis due to plastic
Irritant contact dermatitis due to rubber

L24.6 **Irritant contact dermatitis** due to food in contact with skin
[EXCLUDES2] *dermatitis due to ingested food (L27.2)*

L24.7 **Irritant contact dermatitis** due to plants, except food
[EXCLUDES2] *allergy NOS to pollen (J30.1)*

[5th] L24.8 **Irritant contact dermatitis** due to other agents

L24.81 **Irritant contact dermatitis** due to metals
Irritant contact dermatitis due to chromium
Irritant contact dermatitis due to nickel

L24.89 **Irritant contact dermatitis** due to other agents
Irritant contact dermatitis due to dyes

L24.9 **Irritant contact dermatitis, unspecified cause**
Irritant contact eczema NOS

[4th] L25 **Unspecified contact dermatitis**
[EXCLUDES1] *allergic contact dermatitis (L23.-)*
allergy NOS (T78.40)
dermatitis NOS (L30.9)
irritant contact dermatitis (L24.-)
[EXCLUDES2] *dermatitis due to ingested substances (L27.-)*
dermatitis of eyelid (H01.1-)
eczema of external ear (H60.5-)
perioral dermatitis (L71.0)
radiation-related disorders of the skin and subcutaneous tissue (L55-L59)

L25.0 **Unspecified contact dermatitis** due to cosmetics

L25.1 **Unspecified contact dermatitis** due to drugs in contact with skin
Use additional code for adverse effect, if applicable, to identify drug (T36-T50 with fifth or sixth character 5)
[EXCLUDES2] *dermatitis due to ingested drugs and medicaments (L27.0-L27.1)*

L25.2 **Unspecified contact dermatitis** due to dyes

L25.3 **Unspecified contact dermatitis** due to other chemical products
Unspecified contact dermatitis due to cement
Unspecified contact dermatitis due to insecticide

L25.4 **Unspecified contact dermatitis** due to food in contact with skin
[EXCLUDES2] *dermatitis due to ingested food (L27.2)*

L25.5 **Unspecified contact dermatitis** due to plants, except food
[EXCLUDES1] *nettle rash (L50.9)*
[EXCLUDES2] *allergy NOS due to pollen (J30.1)*

L25.8 **Unspecified contact dermatitis** due to other agents

L25.9 **Unspecified contact dermatitis, unspecified cause**
Contact dermatitis (occupational) NOS
Contact eczema (occupational) NOS

L26 **Exfoliative dermatitis**
Hebra's pityriasis
[EXCLUDES1] *Ritter's disease (L00)*

[4th] L27 **Dermatitis** due to substances taken internally
[EXCLUDES1] *allergy NOS (T78.40)*
[EXCLUDES2] *adverse food reaction, except dermatitis (T78.0-T78.1)*
contact dermatitis (L23-L25)
drug photoallergic response (L56.1)
drug phototoxic response (L56.0)
urticaria (L50.-)

L27.0 Generalized **skin eruption** due to drugs and medicaments taken internally [CC] [CC/MCC Exc]
Use additional code for adverse effect, if applicable, to identify drug (T36-T50 with fifth or sixth character 5)

L27.1 Localized **skin eruption** due to drugs and medicaments taken internally [CC] [CC/MCC Exc]
Use additional code for adverse effect, if applicable, to identify drug (T36-T50 with fifth or sixth character 5)

L27.2 **Dermatitis** due to ingested food
[EXCLUDES2] *dermatitis due to food in contact with skin (L23.6, L24.6, L25.4)*

L27.8 **Dermatitis** due to other substances taken internally

L27.9 **Dermatitis due to unspecified substance taken internally**

[4th] L28 **Lichen simplex chronicus and prurigo**

L28.0 Lichen simplex chronicus
Circumscribed neurodermatitis
Lichen NOS

L28.1 Prurigo nodularis

L28.2 **Other prurigo**
Prurigo NOS
Prurigo Hebra
Prurigo mitis
Urticaria papulosa

[4th] L29 **Pruritus**
DEFINITION: Pruritus is itchy skin, which may be caused by dry skin, skin disease, and other conditions.
[EXCLUDES1] *neurotic excoriation (L98.1)*
psychogenic pruritus (F45.8)

L29.0 **Pruritus** ani

L29.1 **Pruritus** scroti ♂

L29.2 **Pruritus** vulvae ♀

L29.3 Anogenital **pruritus, unspecified**
L29.8 **Other pruritus**
L29.9 **Pruritus, unspecified**
Itch NOS

[4th] L30 Other and unspecified **dermatitis**
[EXCLUDES2] *contact dermatitis (L23-L25)*
dry skin dermatitis (L85.3)
small plaque parapsoriasis (L41.3)
stasis dermatitis (I87.2)
L30.0 Nummular **dermatitis**
L30.1 Dyshidrosis [pompholyx]
L30.2 Cutaneous autosensitization
Candidid [levurid]
Dermatophytid
Eczematid
L30.3 Infective **dermatitis**
Infectious eczematoid dermatitis
L30.4 Erythema intertrigo
L30.5 Pityriasis alba
AHA: Q1 2018
L30.8 **Other specified dermatitis**
L30.9 **Dermatitis, unspecified**
Eczema NOS

Papulosquamous disorders (L40-L45)

[4th] L40 Psoriasis
L40.0 **Psoriasis** vulgaris [RxHCC]
Nummular psoriasis
Plaque psoriasis
L40.1 Generalized pustular **psoriasis** [RxHCC]
Impetigo herpetiformis
Von Zumbusch's disease
L40.2 Acrodermatitis continua [RxHCC]
L40.3 Pustulosis palmaris et plantaris [RxHCC]
L40.4 Guttate **psoriasis** [RxHCC]
[5th] L40.5 Arthropathic **psoriasis**
L40.50 **Arthropathic psoriasis, unspecified** [HCC] [RxHCC]
L40.51 Distal interphalangeal **psoriatic arthropathy** [HCC] [RxHCC]
L40.52 **Psoriatic arthritis** mutilans [HCC] [RxHCC]
L40.53 **Psoriatic** spondylitis [HCC] [RxHCC]
L40.54 **Psoriatic** juvenile **arthropathy** [HCC] [RxHCC]
L40.59 **Other psoriatic arthropathy** [HCC] [RxHCC]
L40.8 **Other psoriasis** [RxHCC]
Flexural psoriasis
L40.9 **Psoriasis, unspecified** [RxHCC]

[4th] L41 Parapsoriasis
[EXCLUDES1] *poikiloderma vasculare atrophicans (L94.5)*
L41.0 Pityriasis lichenoides et varioliformis acuta [RxHCC]
Mucha-Habermann disease
L41.1 Pityriasis lichenoides chronica [RxHCC]
L41.3 Small plaque **parapsoriasis** [RxHCC]
L41.4 Large plaque **parapsoriasis** [RxHCC]
L41.5 Retiform **parapsoriasis** [RxHCC]
L41.8 **Other parapsoriasis** [RxHCC]
L41.9 **Parapsoriasis, unspecified** [RxHCC]

L42 Pityriasis rosea

[4th] L43 Lichen planus
[EXCLUDES1] *lichen planopilaris (L66.1)*
L43.0 Hypertrophic **lichen planus**
L43.1 Bullous **lichen planus**
L43.2 **Lichenoid** drug reaction
Use additional code for adverse effect, if applicable, to identify drug (T36-T50 with fifth or sixth character 5)
L43.3 Subacute (active) **lichen planus**
Lichen planus tropicus
L43.8 **Other lichen planus**
L43.9 **Lichen planus, unspecified**

[4th] L44 Other papulosquamous disorders
L44.0 Pityriasis rubra pilaris
L44.1 **Lichen** nitidus
L44.2 **Lichen** striatus
L44.3 **Lichen** ruber moniliformis
L44.4 Infantile papular acrodermatitis [Gianotti-Crosti] [P]
L44.8 **Other specified papulosquamous disorders**
L44.9 **Papulosquamous disorder, unspecified**

L45 **Papulosquamous disorders in diseases classified elsewhere**
☞ **Code first** underlying disease.

Urticaria and erythema (L49-L54)

[EXCLUDES1] *Lyme disease (A69.2-)*
rosacea (L71.-)

[4th] L49 **Exfoliation due to erythematous conditions according to** extent of body surface involved
☞ **Code first** erythematous condition causing exfoliation, such as:
Ritter's disease (L00)
(Staphylococcal) scalded skin ▶syndrome◀ (L00)
Stevens-Johnson syndrome (L51.1)
Stevens-Johnson syndrome-toxic epidermal necrolysis overlap syndrome (L51.3)
Toxic epidermal necrolysis (L51.2)
L49.0 **Exfoliation due to erythematous condition involving** less than 10 percent **of body surface** [PDx]
Exfoliation due to erythematous condition NOS
L49.1 **Exfoliation due to erythematous condition involving** 10-19 percent **of body surface** [PDx]
L49.2 **Exfoliation due to erythematous condition involving** 20-29 percent **of body surface** [PDx]
L49.3 **Exfoliation due to erythematous condition involving** 30-39 percent **of body surface** [CC] [PDx] [CC/MCC Exc]
L49.4 **Exfoliation due to erythematous condition involving** 40-49 percent **of body surface** [CC] [PDx] [CC/MCC Exc]
L49.5 **Exfoliation due to erythematous condition involving** 50-59 percent **of body surface** [CC] [PDx] [CC/MCC Exc]
L49.6 **Exfoliation due to erythematous condition involving** 60-69 percent **of body surface** [CC] [PDx] [CC/MCC Exc]
L49.7 **Exfoliation due to erythematous condition involving** 70-79 percent **of body surface** [CC] [PDx] [CC/MCC Exc]
L49.8 **Exfoliation due to erythematous condition involving** 80-89 percent **of body surface** [CC] [PDx] [CC/MCC Exc]
L49.9 **Exfoliation due to erythematous condition involving** 90 or more percent **of body surface** [CC] [PDx] [CC/MCC Exc]

[4th] L50 Urticaria (Figure 12.1)
[EXCLUDES1] *allergic contact dermatitis (L23.-)*
angioneurotic edema (T78.3)
giant urticaria (T78.3)
hereditary angio-edema (D84.1)
Quincke's edema (T78.3)
serum urticaria (T80.6-)
solar urticaria (L56.3)
urticaria neonatorum (P83.8)
urticaria papulosa (L28.2)
urticaria pigmentosa ▶(D47.01)◀
L50.0 Allergic **urticaria**
L50.1 Idiopathic **urticaria**
L50.2 **Urticaria** due to cold and heat
[EXCLUDES2] *familial cold urticaria (M04.2)*
L50.3 Dermatographic **urticaria**
L50.4 Vibratory **urticaria**
L50.5 Cholinergic **urticaria**
L50.6 Contact **urticaria**
L50.8 **Other urticaria**
Chronic urticaria
Recurrent periodic urticaria
L50.9 **Urticaria, unspecified**

[PDx] Unacceptable principal diagnosis symbol per Medicare code edits [POA] Code exempt from diagnosis present on admission requirement
[?] Questionable admission [CC] Complication or comorbidity [MCC] Major complication or comorbidity [CC/MCC Exc] CC/MCC exclusion
[HCC] HCC diagnosis code [RxHCC] RxHCC diagnosis code MACRA code **DEFINITION** Describes condition/terminology
TIP Coding guidance 👁 Official Guideline Reference [Z1] Z code as first-listed diagnosis

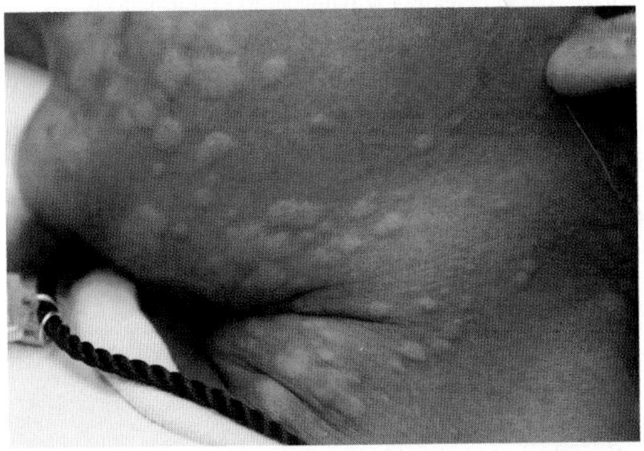

Figure 12.1 Urticaria

[4th] L51 Erythema multiforme
Use additional code for adverse effect, if applicable, to identify drug (T36-T50 with fifth or sixth character 5)
Use additional code to identify associated manifestations, such as:
arthropathy associated with dermatological disorders (M14.8-)
conjunctival edema (H11.42)
conjunctivitis (H10.22-)
corneal scars and opacities (H17.-)
corneal ulcer (H16.0-)
edema of eyelid (H02.84-)
inflammation of eyelid (H01.8)
keratoconjunctivitis sicca (H16.22-)
mechanical lagophthalmos (H02.22-)
stomatitis (K12.-)
symblepharon (H11.23-)
Use additional code to identify percentage of skin exfoliation (L49.-)
EXCLUDES1 *staphylococcal scalded skin syndrome (L00)*
Ritter's disease (L00)
L51.0 Nonbullous erythema multiforme
L51.1 Stevens-Johnson syndrome CC HCC CC/MCC Exc
L51.2 Toxic epidermal necrolysis [Lyell] CC HCC CC/MCC Exc
L51.3 Stevens-Johnson syndrome-toxic epidermal necrolysis overlap syndrome CC HCC CC/MCC Exc
SJS-TEN overlap syndrome
L51.8 Other erythema multiforme
L51.9 Erythema multiforme, unspecified
Erythema iris
Erythema multiforme major NOS
Erythema multiforme minor NOS
Herpes iris
L52 Erythema nodosum
EXCLUDES1 *tuberculous erythema nodosum (A18.4)*
[4th] L53 Other erythematous conditions
EXCLUDES1 *erythema ab igne (L59.0)*
erythema due to external agents in contact with skin (L23-L25)
erythema intertrigo (L30.4)
L53.0 Toxic erythema CC CC/MCC Exc
☞ Code first poisoning due to drug or toxin, if applicable (T36-T65 with fifth or sixth character 1-4 or 6)
Use additional code for adverse effect, if applicable, to identify drug (T36-T50 with fifth or sixth character 5)
EXCLUDES1 *neonatal erythema toxicum (P83.1)*
L53.1 Erythema annulare centrifugum CC CC/MCC Exc
L53.2 Erythema marginatum CC CC/MCC Exc
L53.3 Other chronic figurate erythema CC CC/MCC Exc
L53.8 Other specified erythematous conditions
L53.9 Erythematous condition, unspecified
Erythema NOS
Erythroderma NOS
L54 Erythema in diseases classified elsewhere
☞ Code first underlying disease.

Radiation-related disorders of the skin and subcutaneous tissue (L55-L59)

[4th] L55 Sunburn
L55.0 Sunburn of first degree
L55.1 Sunburn of second degree
L55.2 Sunburn of third degree
L55.9 Sunburn, unspecified
[4th] L56 Other acute skin changes due to ultraviolet radiation
Use additional code to identify the source of the ultraviolet radiation (W89, X32)
L56.0 Drug phototoxic response
Use additional code for adverse effect, if applicable, to identify drug (T36-T50 with fifth or sixth character 5)
L56.1 Drug photoallergic response
Use additional code for adverse effect, if applicable, to identify drug (T36-T50 with fifth or sixth character 5)
L56.2 Photocontact dermatitis [berloque dermatitis]
L56.3 Solar urticaria
L56.4 Polymorphous light eruption
L56.5 Disseminated superficial actinic porokeratosis (DSAP)
L56.8 Other specified acute skin changes due to ultraviolet radiation
L56.9 Acute skin change due to ultraviolet radiation, unspecified
[4th] L57 Skin changes due to chronic exposure to nonionizing radiation
Use additional code to identify the source of the ultraviolet radiation (W89)
L57.0 Actinic keratosis
Keratosis NOS
Senile keratosis
Solar keratosis
L57.1 Actinic reticuloid
L57.2 Cutis rhomboidalis nuchae
L57.3 Poikiloderma of Civatte
L57.4 Cutis laxa senilis
Elastosis senilis
L57.5 Actinic granuloma
L57.8 Other skin changes due to chronic exposure to nonionizing radiation
Farmer's skin
Sailor's skin
Solar dermatitis
L57.9 Skin changes due to chronic exposure to nonionizing radiation, unspecified
[4th] L58 Radiodermatitis
Use additional code to identify the source of the radiation (W88, W90)
L58.0 Acute radiodermatitis
L58.1 Chronic radiodermatitis
L58.9 Radiodermatitis, unspecified
[4th] L59 Other disorders of skin and subcutaneous tissue related to radiation
L59.0 Erythema ab igne [dermatitis ab igne]
L59.8 Other specified disorders of the skin and subcutaneous tissue related to radiation
AHA: Q1 2017
L59.9 Disorder of the skin and subcutaneous tissue related to radiation, unspecified

Disorders of skin appendages (L60-L75)

EXCLUDES1 *congenital malformations of integument (Q84.-)*
[4th] L60 Nail disorders
EXCLUDES2 *clubbing of nails (R68.3)*
onychia and paronychia (L03.0-)
L60.0 Ingrowing nail
L60.1 Onycholysis
L60.2 Onychogryphosis
L60.3 Nail dystrophy
L60.4 Beau's lines
L60.5 Yellow nail syndrome

Unspecified Code Other Specified Code Manifestation Code [N] Newborn [P] Pediatric [M] Maternity [A] Adult ♂ Male ♀ Female
● New Code ▲ Revised Code Title ►◄ Revised Text NOTES INCLUDES EXCLUDES1 Not coded here EXCLUDES2 Not included here
[4th] 4th character required [5th] 5th character required [6th] 6th character required [7th] 7th character required [x7th] Extension 'X' Alert
HAC Hospital-acquired condition (HAC) alert AHA AHA Coding Clinic© ☞ Code first alert

When symbols appear on a code that requires a 7th character extension, refer to Appendix B to identify applicable 7th character codes.

L60.8   Other nail disorders
L60.9   Nail disorder, unspecified
L62   Nail disorders in diseases classified elsewhere
☞ Code first underlying disease, such as:
pachydermoperiostosis (M89.4-)
L63   Alopecia areata (Figure 12.2)
DEFINITION: Alopecia areata is a form of hair loss caused by an autoimmune skin disease.
L63.0   Alopecia (capitis) totalis
L63.1   Alopecia universalis
L63.2   Ophiasis
L63.8   Other alopecia areata
L63.9   Alopecia areata, unspecified

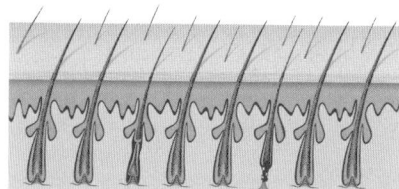
Healthy

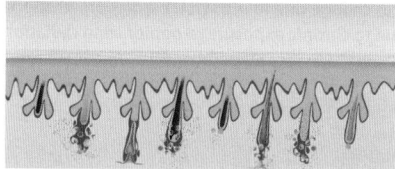
Alopecia areata

Figure 12.2 Alopecia Areata

L64   Androgenic alopecia
INCLUDES   male-pattern baldness
L64.0   Drug-induced androgenic alopecia
Use additional code for adverse effect, if applicable, to identify drug (T36-T50 with fifth or sixth character 5)
L64.8   Other androgenic alopecia
L64.9   Androgenic alopecia, unspecified
L65   Other nonscarring hair loss
Use additional code for adverse effect, if applicable, to identify drug (T36-T50 with fifth or sixth character 5)
EXCLUDES1   trichotillomania (F63.3)
L65.0   Telogen effluvium
L65.1   Anagen effluvium
L65.2   Alopecia mucinosa
L65.8   Other specified nonscarring hair loss
L65.9   Nonscarring hair loss, unspecified
Alopecia NOS
L66   Cicatricial alopecia [scarring hair loss]
L66.0   Pseudopelade
L66.1   Lichen planopilaris
Follicular lichen planus
L66.2   Folliculitis decalvans
L66.3   Perifolliculitis capitis abscedens
L66.4   Folliculitis ulerythematosa reticulata
L66.8   Other cicatricial alopecia
AHA: Q1 2015
L66.9   Cicatricial alopecia, unspecified
L67   Hair color and hair shaft abnormalities
EXCLUDES1   monilethrix (Q84.1)
pili annulati (Q84.1)
telogen effluvium (L65.0)
L67.0   Trichorrhexis nodosa
L67.1   Variations in hair color
Canities
Greyness, hair (premature)
Heterochromia of hair
Poliosis circumscripta, acquired
Poliosis NOS

L67.8   Other hair color and hair shaft abnormalities
Fragilitas crinium
L67.9   Hair color and hair shaft abnormality, unspecified
L68   Hypertrichosis
INCLUDES   excess hair
EXCLUDES1   congenital hypertrichosis (Q84.2)
persistent lanugo (Q84.2)
L68.0   Hirsutism
L68.1   Acquired hypertrichosis lanuginosa
L68.2   Localized hypertrichosis
L68.3   Polytrichia
L68.8   Other hypertrichosis
L68.9   Hypertrichosis, unspecified
L70   Acne
EXCLUDES2   acne keloid (L73.0)
L70.0   Acne vulgaris
L70.1   Acne conglobata
L70.2   Acne varioliformis
Acne necrotica miliaris
L70.3   Acne tropica
L70.4   Infantile acne   P
L70.5   Acné excoriée
Acné excoriée des jeunes filles
Picker's acne
L70.8   Other acne
L70.9   Acne, unspecified
L71   Rosacea
Use additional code for adverse effect, if applicable, to identify drug (T36-T50 with fifth or sixth character 5)
L71.0   Perioral dermatitis
L71.1   Rhinophyma
L71.8   Other rosacea
AHA: Q4 2018
L71.9   Rosacea, unspecified
L72   Follicular cysts of skin and subcutaneous tissue
L72.0   Epidermal cyst
L72.1   Pilar and trichodermal cyst
L72.11   Pilar cyst
L72.12   Trichodermal cyst
Trichilemmal (proliferating) cyst
L72.2   Steatocystoma multiplex
L72.3   Sebaceous cyst
EXCLUDES2   pilar cyst (L72.11)
trichilemmal (proliferating) cyst (L72.12)
L72.8   Other follicular cysts of the skin and subcutaneous tissue
L72.9   Follicular cyst of the skin and subcutaneous tissue, unspecified
L73   Other follicular disorders
L73.0   Acne keloid
L73.1   Pseudofolliculitis barbae
L73.2   Hidradenitis suppurativa
L73.8   Other specified follicular disorders
Sycosis barbae
L73.9   Follicular disorder, unspecified
L74   Eccrine sweat disorders
EXCLUDES2   generalized hyperhidrosis (R61)
L74.0   Miliaria rubra
L74.1   Miliaria crystallina
L74.2   Miliaria profunda
Miliaria tropicalis
L74.3   Miliaria, unspecified
L74.4   Anhidrosis
Hypohidrosis
L74.5   Focal hyperhidrosis
L74.51   Primary focal hyperhidrosis
L74.510   Primary focal hyperhidrosis, axilla
L74.511   Primary focal hyperhidrosis, face
L74.512   Primary focal hyperhidrosis, palms

PDx🔒 Unacceptable principal diagnosis symbol per Medicare code edits   PDx🔒 Code exempt from diagnosis present on admission requirement
❓ Questionable admission   CC Complication or comorbidity   MCC Major complication or comorbidity   CC/MCC Exc CC/MCC exclusion
HCC HCC diagnosis code   RxHCC RxHCC diagnosis code   MACRA code   DEFINITION Describes condition/terminology
TIP Coding guidance   👁 Official Guideline Reference   Z1 Z code as first-listed diagnosis

750   When symbols appear on a code that requires a 7th character extension, refer to Appendix B to identify applicable 7th character codes.   2020 ICD-10-CM

L74.513   Primary focal hyperhidrosis, soles
L74.519   Primary focal hyperhidrosis, unspecified
L74.52   Secondary focal hyperhidrosis
Frey's syndrome
L74.8   Other eccrine sweat disorders
L74.9   Eccrine sweat disorder, unspecified
Sweat gland disorder NOS

L75   Apocrine sweat disorders
EXCLUDES1   dyshidrosis (L30.1)
hidradenitis suppurativa (L73.2)
L75.0   Bromhidrosis
L75.1   Chromhidrosis
L75.2   Apocrine miliaria
Fox-Fordyce disease
L75.8   Other apocrine sweat disorders
L75.9   Apocrine sweat disorder, unspecified

Intraoperative and postprocedural complications of skin and subcutaneous tissue (L76)

L76   Intraoperative and postprocedural complications of skin and subcutaneous tissue
L76.0   Intraoperative hemorrhage and hematoma of skin and subcutaneous tissue complicating a procedure
EXCLUDES1   intraoperative hemorrhage and hematoma of skin and subcutaneous tissue due to accidental puncture and laceration during a procedure (L76.1-)
L76.01   Intraoperative hemorrhage and hematoma of skin and subcutaneous tissue complicating a dermatologic procedure
L76.02   Intraoperative hemorrhage and hematoma of skin and subcutaneous tissue complicating other procedure
L76.1   Accidental puncture and laceration of skin and subcutaneous tissue during a procedure
L76.11   Accidental puncture and laceration of skin and subcutaneous tissue during a dermatologic procedure
L76.12   Accidental puncture and laceration of skin and subcutaneous tissue during other procedure
L76.2   Postprocedural hemorrhage of skin and subcutaneous tissue following a procedure
L76.21   Postprocedural hemorrhage of skin and subcutaneous tissue following a dermatologic procedure
L76.22   Postprocedural hemorrhage of skin and subcutaneous tissue following other procedure
L76.3   Postprocedural hematoma and seroma of skin and subcutaneous tissue following a procedure
L76.31   Postprocedural hematoma of skin and subcutaneous tissue following a dermatologic procedure
L76.32   Postprocedural hematoma of skin and subcutaneous tissue following other procedure
L76.33   Postprocedural seroma of skin and subcutaneous tissue following a dermatologic procedure
L76.34   Postprocedural seroma of skin and subcutaneous tissue following other procedure
L76.8   Other intraoperative and postprocedural complications of skin and subcutaneous tissue
Use additional code, if applicable, to further specify disorder
L76.81   Other intraoperative complications of skin and subcutaneous tissue
L76.82   Other postprocedural complications of skin and subcutaneous tissue
AHA: Q3 2017

Other disorders of the skin and subcutaneous tissue (L80-L99)

L80   Vitiligo
EXCLUDES2   vitiligo of eyelids (H02.73-)
vitiligo of vulva (N90.89)
L81   Other disorders of pigmentation
EXCLUDES1   birthmark NOS (Q82.5)
Peutz-Jeghers syndrome (Q85.8)
EXCLUDES2   nevus - see Alphabetical Index
L81.0   Postinflammatory hyperpigmentation
L81.1   Chloasma
L81.2   Freckles
L81.3   Café au lait spots
L81.4   Other melanin hyperpigmentation
Lentigo
L81.5   Leukoderma, not elsewhere classified
L81.6   Other disorders of diminished melanin formation
L81.7   Pigmented purpuric dermatosis
Angioma serpiginosum
L81.8   Other specified disorders of pigmentation
Iron pigmentation
Tattoo pigmentation
L81.9   Disorder of pigmentation, unspecified
L82   Seborrheic keratosis
INCLUDES   basal cell papilloma
dermatosis papulosa nigra
Leser-Trélat disease
EXCLUDES2   seborrheic dermatitis (L21.-)
L82.0   Inflamed seborrheic keratosis
L82.1   Other seborrheic keratosis
Seborrheic keratosis NOS
L83   Acanthosis nigricans
Confluent and reticulated papillomatosis
L84   Corns and callosities
Callus
Clavus
L85   Other epidermal thickening
EXCLUDES2   hypertrophic disorders of the skin (L91.-)
L85.0   Acquired ichthyosis
EXCLUDES1   congenital ichthyosis (Q80.-)
L85.1   Acquired keratosis [keratoderma] palmaris et plantaris
EXCLUDES1   inherited keratosis palmaris et plantaris (Q82.8)
L85.2   Keratosis punctata (palmaris et plantaris)
L85.3   Xerosis cutis
Dry skin dermatitis
L85.8   Other specified epidermal thickening
Cutaneous horn
L85.9   Epidermal thickening, unspecified
L86   Keratoderma in diseases classified elsewhere
Code first underlying disease, such as:
Reiter's disease (M02.3-)
EXCLUDES1   gonococcal keratoderma (A54.89)
gonococcal keratosis (A54.89)
keratoderma due to vitamin A deficiency (E50.8)
keratosis due to vitamin A deficiency (E50.8)
xeroderma due to vitamin A deficiency (E50.8)
L87   Transepidermal elimination disorders
EXCLUDES1   granuloma annulare (perforating) (L92.0)
L87.0   Keratosis follicularis et parafollicularis in cutem penetrans
Kyrle disease
Hyperkeratosis follicularis penetrans
L87.1   Reactive perforating collagenosis
L87.2   Elastosis perforans serpiginosa
L87.8   Other transepidermal elimination disorders
L87.9   Transepidermal elimination disorder, unspecified
L88   Pyoderma gangrenosum
Phagedenic pyoderma
EXCLUDES1   dermatitis gangrenosa (L08.0)

L89 Pressure ulcer
- **See Official Guidelines** Pressure ulcer stages I.C.12.a.1, Unstageable pressure ulcers I.C.12.a.2
- INCLUDES
  - bed sore
  - decubitus ulcer
  - plaster ulcer
  - pressure area
  - pressure sore
- Code first any associated gangrene (I96)
- EXCLUDES2 decubitus (trophic) ulcer of cervix (uteri) (N86)
  - diabetic ulcers (E08.621, E08.622, E09.621, E09.622, E10.621, E10.622, E11.621, E11.622, E13.621, E13.622)
  - non-pressure chronic ulcer of skin (L97.-)
  - skin infections (L00-L08)
  - varicose ulcer (I83.0, I83.2)

L89.0 Pressure ulcer of elbow
- **L89.00 Pressure ulcer of unspecified elbow**
  - **L89.000 Pressure ulcer of unspecified elbow, unstageable**
  - **L89.001 Pressure ulcer of unspecified elbow, stage 1**
    - Healing pressure ulcer of unspecified elbow, stage 1
    - Pressure pre-ulcer skin changes limited to persistent focal edema, unspecified elbow
  - **L89.002 Pressure ulcer of unspecified elbow, stage 2**
    - Healing pressure ulcer of unspecified elbow, stage 2
    - Pressure ulcer with abrasion, blister, partial thickness skin loss involving epidermis and/or dermis, unspecified elbow
  - **L89.003 Pressure ulcer of unspecified elbow, stage 3**
    - Healing pressure ulcer of unspecified elbow, stage 3
    - Pressure ulcer with full thickness skin loss involving damage or necrosis of subcutaneous tissue, unspecified elbow
  - **L89.004 Pressure ulcer of unspecified elbow, stage 4**
    - Healing pressure ulcer of unspecified elbow, stage 4
    - Pressure ulcer with necrosis of soft tissues through to underlying muscle, tendon, or bone, unspecified elbow
  - **L89.006 Pressure-induced deep tissue damage of unspecified elbow**
  - **L89.009 Pressure ulcer of unspecified elbow, unspecified stage**
    - Healing pressure ulcer of elbow NOS
    - Healing pressure ulcer of unspecified elbow, unspecified stage
- **L89.01 Pressure ulcer of right elbow**
  - **L89.010 Pressure ulcer of right elbow, unstageable**
  - **L89.011 Pressure ulcer of right elbow, stage 1**
    - Healing pressure ulcer of right elbow, stage 1
    - Pressure pre-ulcer skin changes limited to persistent focal edema, right elbow
  - **L89.012 Pressure ulcer of right elbow, stage 2**
    - Healing pressure ulcer of right elbow, stage 2
    - Pressure ulcer with abrasion, blister, partial thickness skin loss involving epidermis and/or dermis, right elbow
  - **L89.013 Pressure ulcer of right elbow, stage 3**
    - Healing pressure ulcer of right elbow, stage 3
    - Pressure ulcer with full thickness skin loss involving damage or necrosis of subcutaneous tissue, right elbow

- **L89.014 Pressure ulcer of right elbow, stage 4**
  - Healing pressure ulcer of right elbow, stage 4
  - Pressure ulcer with necrosis of soft tissues through to underlying muscle, tendon, or bone, right elbow
- **L89.016 Pressure-induced deep tissue damage of right elbow**
- **L89.019 Pressure ulcer of right elbow, unspecified stage**
  - Healing pressure right of elbow NOS
  - Healing pressure ulcer of right elbow, unspecified stage

L89.02 Pressure ulcer of left elbow
- **L89.020 Pressure ulcer of left elbow, unstageable**
- **L89.021 Pressure ulcer of left elbow, stage 1**
  - Healing pressure ulcer of left elbow, stage 1
  - Pressure pre-ulcer skin changes limited to persistent focal edema, left elbow
- **L89.022 Pressure ulcer of left elbow, stage 2**
  - Healing pressure ulcer of left elbow, stage 2
  - Pressure ulcer with abrasion, blister, partial thickness skin loss involving epidermis and/or dermis, left elbow
- **L89.023 Pressure ulcer of left elbow, stage 3**
  - Healing pressure ulcer of left elbow, stage 3
  - Pressure ulcer with full thickness skin loss involving damage or necrosis of subcutaneous tissue, left elbow
- **L89.024 Pressure ulcer of left elbow, stage 4**
  - Healing pressure ulcer of left elbow, stage 4
  - Pressure ulcer with necrosis of soft tissues through to underlying muscle, tendon, or bone, left elbow
- **L89.026 Pressure-induced deep tissue damage of left elbow**
- **L89.029 Pressure ulcer of left elbow, unspecified stage**
  - Healing pressure ulcer of left of elbow NOS
  - Healing pressure ulcer of left elbow, unspecified stage

L89.1 Pressure ulcer of back
- **L89.10 Pressure ulcer of unspecified part of back**
  - **L89.100 Pressure ulcer of unspecified part of back, unstageable**
  - **L89.101 Pressure ulcer of unspecified part of back, stage 1**
    - Healing pressure ulcer of unspecified part of back, stage 1
    - Pressure pre-ulcer skin changes limited to persistent focal edema, unspecified part of back
  - **L89.102 Pressure ulcer of unspecified part of back, stage 2**
    - Healing pressure ulcer of unspecified part of back, stage 2
    - Pressure ulcer with abrasion, blister, partial thickness skin loss involving epidermis and/or dermis, unspecified part of back
  - **L89.103 Pressure ulcer of unspecified part of back, stage 3**
    - Healing pressure ulcer of unspecified part of back, stage 3
    - Pressure ulcer with full thickness skin loss involving damage or necrosis of subcutaneous tissue, unspecified part of back

L89.104 **Pressure ulcer of unspecified part of back, stage 4** CC HAC HCC CC/MCC Exc
Healing pressure ulcer of unspecified part of back, stage 4
Pressure ulcer with necrosis of soft tissues through to underlying muscle, tendon, or bone, unspecified part of back

● L89.106 **Pressure-induced deep tissue damage of unspecified part of back** CC CC/MCC Exc

L89.109 **Pressure ulcer of unspecified part of back, unspecified stage** CC CC/MCC Exc
Healing pressure ulcer of unspecified part of back NOS
Healing pressure ulcer of unspecified part of back, unspecified stage

[6th] L89.11 **Pressure ulcer of right upper back**
Pressure ulcer of right shoulder blade

L89.110 **Pressure ulcer of right upper back, unstageable** CC HCC CC/MCC Exc

L89.111 **Pressure ulcer of right upper back, stage 1** CC CC/MCC Exc
Healing pressure ulcer of right upper back, stage 1
Pressure pre-ulcer skin changes limited to persistent focal edema, right upper back

L89.112 **Pressure ulcer of right upper back, stage 2** CC HCC CC/MCC Exc
Healing pressure ulcer of right upper back, stage 2
Pressure ulcer with abrasion, blister, partial thickness skin loss involving epidermis and/or dermis, right upper back

L89.113 **Pressure ulcer of right upper back, stage 3** CC HAC HCC CC/MCC Exc
Healing pressure ulcer of right upper back, stage 3
Pressure ulcer with full thickness skin loss involving damage or necrosis of subcutaneous tissue, right upper back

L89.114 **Pressure ulcer of right upper back, stage 4** CC HAC HCC CC/MCC Exc
Healing pressure ulcer of right upper back, stage 4
Pressure ulcer with necrosis of soft tissues through to underlying muscle, tendon, or bone, right upper back

● L89.116 **Pressure-induced deep tissue damage of right upper back** CC CC/MCC Exc

L89.119 **Pressure ulcer of right upper back, unspecified stage** CC CC/MCC Exc
Healing pressure ulcer of right upper back NOS
Healing pressure ulcer of right upper back, unspecified stage

[6th] L89.12 **Pressure ulcer of left upper back**
Pressure ulcer of left shoulder blade

L89.120 **Pressure ulcer of left upper back, unstageable** CC HCC CC/MCC Exc

L89.121 **Pressure ulcer of left upper back, stage 1** CC CC/MCC Exc
Healing pressure ulcer of left upper back, stage 1
Pressure pre-ulcer skin changes limited to persistent focal edema, left upper back

L89.122 **Pressure ulcer of left upper back, stage 2** CC HCC CC/MCC Exc
Healing pressure ulcer of left upper back, stage 2
Pressure ulcer with abrasion, blister, partial thickness skin loss involving epidermis and/or dermis, left upper back

L89.123 **Pressure ulcer of left upper back, stage 3** CC HAC HCC CC/MCC Exc
Healing pressure ulcer of left upper back, stage 3
Pressure ulcer with full thickness skin loss involving damage or necrosis of subcutaneous tissue, left upper back

L89.124 **Pressure ulcer of left upper back, stage 4** CC HAC HCC CC/MCC Exc
Healing pressure ulcer of left upper back, stage 4
Pressure ulcer with necrosis of soft tissues through to underlying muscle, tendon, or bone, left upper back

● L89.126 **Pressure-induced deep tissue damage of left upper back** CC CC/MCC Exc

L89.129 **Pressure ulcer of left upper back, unspecified stage** CC CC/MCC Exc
Healing pressure ulcer of left upper back NOS
Healing pressure ulcer of left upper back, unspecified stage

[6th] L89.13 **Pressure ulcer of right lower back**

L89.130 **Pressure ulcer of right lower back, unstageable** CC HCC CC/MCC Exc

L89.131 **Pressure ulcer of right lower back, stage 1** CC CC/MCC Exc
Healing pressure ulcer of right lower back, stage 1
Pressure pre-ulcer skin changes limited to persistent focal edema, right lower back

L89.132 **Pressure ulcer of right lower back, stage 2** CC HCC CC/MCC Exc
Healing pressure ulcer of right lower back, stage 2
Pressure ulcer with abrasion, blister, partial thickness skin loss involving epidermis and/or dermis, right lower back

L89.133 **Pressure ulcer of right lower back, stage 3** CC HAC HCC CC/MCC Exc
Healing pressure ulcer of right lower back, stage 3
Pressure ulcer with full thickness skin loss involving damage or necrosis of subcutaneous tissue, right lower back

L89.134 **Pressure ulcer of right lower back, stage 4** CC HAC HCC CC/MCC Exc
Healing pressure ulcer of right lower back, stage 4
Pressure ulcer with necrosis of soft tissues through to underlying muscle, tendon, or bone, right lower back

● L89.136 **Pressure-induced deep tissue damage of right lower back** CC CC/MCC Exc

L89.139 **Pressure ulcer of right lower back, unspecified stage** CC CC/MCC Exc
Healing pressure ulcer of right lower back NOS
Healing pressure ulcer of right lower back, unspecified stage

[6th] L89.14 **Pressure ulcer of left lower back**

L89.140 **Pressure ulcer of left lower back, unstageable** CC HCC CC/MCC Exc

L89.141 **Pressure ulcer of left lower back, stage 1** CC CC/MCC Exc
Healing pressure ulcer of left lower back, stage 1
Pressure pre-ulcer skin changes limited to persistent focal edema, left lower back

Unspecified Code Other Specified Code Manifestation Code [N] Newborn [P] Pediatric [M] Maternity [A] Adult ♂ Male ♀ Female
● New Code ▲ Revised Code Title ►◄ Revised Text NOTES INCLUDES EXCLUDES1 Not coded here EXCLUDES2 Not included here
[4th] 4th character required [5th] 5th character required [6th] 6th character required [7th] 7th character required [x7] Extension 'X' Alert
HAC Hospital-acquired condition (HAC) alert AHA AHA Coding Clinic© Code first alert

L89.142 **Pressure ulcer of left lower back, stage 2** cc🔒 HCC CC/MCC Exc🔒

Healing pressure ulcer of left lower back, stage 2

Pressure ulcer with abrasion, blister, partial thickness skin loss involving epidermis and/or dermis, left lower back

L89.143 **Pressure ulcer of left lower back, stage 3** cc🔒 HAC HCC CC/MCC Exc🔒

Healing pressure ulcer of left lower back, stage 3

Pressure ulcer with full thickness skin loss involving damage or necrosis of subcutaneous tissue, left lower back

L89.144 **Pressure ulcer of left lower back, stage 4** cc🔒 HAC HCC CC/MCC Exc🔒

Healing pressure ulcer of left lower back, stage 4

Pressure ulcer with necrosis of soft tissues through to underlying muscle, tendon, or bone, left lower back

● **L89.146** **Pressure-induced** deep tissue damage **of left lower back** cc🔒 CC/MCC Exc🔒

L89.149 **Pressure ulcer of left lower back, unspecified stage** cc🔒 CC/MCC Exc🔒

Healing pressure ulcer of left lower back NOS

Healing pressure ulcer of left lower back, unspecified stage

6ᵗʰ **L89.15** **Pressure ulcer of** sacral region

Pressure ulcer of coccyx

Pressure ulcer of tailbone

L89.150 **Pressure ulcer of sacral region, unstageable** cc🔒 HCC CC/MCC Exc🔒

L89.151 **Pressure ulcer of sacral region, stage 1** cc🔒 CC/MCC Exc🔒

Healing pressure ulcer of sacral region, stage 1

Pressure pre-ulcer skin changes limited to persistent focal edema, sacral region

L89.152 **Pressure ulcer of sacral region, stage 2** cc🔒 HCC CC/MCC Exc🔒

Healing pressure ulcer of sacral region, stage 2

Pressure ulcer with abrasion, blister, partial thickness skin loss involving epidermis and/or dermis, sacral region

L89.153 **Pressure ulcer of sacral region, stage 3** cc🔒 HAC HCC CC/MCC Exc🔒

Healing pressure ulcer of sacral region, stage 3

Pressure ulcer with full thickness skin loss involving damage or necrosis of subcutaneous tissue, sacral region

L89.154 **Pressure ulcer of sacral region, stage 4** cc🔒 HAC HCC CC/MCC Exc🔒

Healing pressure ulcer of sacral region, stage 4

Pressure ulcer with necrosis of soft tissues through to underlying muscle, tendon, or bone, sacral region

● **L89.156** **Pressure-induced** deep tissue damage **of sacral region** cc🔒 CC/MCC Exc🔒

L89.159 **Pressure ulcer of sacral region, unspecified stage** cc🔒 CC/MCC Exc🔒

Healing pressure ulcer of sacral region NOS

Healing pressure ulcer of sacral region, unspecified stage

5ᵗʰ **L89.2** **Pressure ulcer of** hip

6ᵗʰ **L89.20** **Pressure ulcer of** unspecified **hip**

L89.200 **Pressure ulcer of unspecified hip, unstageable** cc🔒 HCC CC/MCC Exc🔒

L89.201 **Pressure ulcer of unspecified hip, stage 1** cc🔒 CC/MCC Exc🔒

Healing pressure ulcer of unspecified hip back, stage 1

Pressure pre-ulcer skin changes limited to persistent focal edema, unspecified hip

L89.202 **Pressure ulcer of unspecified hip, stage 2** cc🔒 HCC CC/MCC Exc🔒

Healing pressure ulcer of unspecified hip, stage 2

Pressure ulcer with abrasion, blister, partial thickness skin loss involving epidermis and/or dermis, unspecified hip

L89.203 **Pressure ulcer of unspecified hip, stage 3** cc🔒 HAC HCC CC/MCC Exc🔒

Healing pressure ulcer of unspecified hip, stage 3

Pressure ulcer with full thickness skin loss involving damage or necrosis of subcutaneous tissue, unspecified hip

L89.204 **Pressure ulcer of unspecified hip, stage 4** cc🔒 HAC HCC CC/MCC Exc🔒

Healing pressure ulcer of unspecified hip, stage 4

Pressure ulcer with necrosis of soft tissues through to underlying muscle, tendon, or bone, unspecified hip

● **L89.206** **Pressure-induced** deep tissue damage **of unspecified hip** cc🔒 CC/MCC Exc🔒

L89.209 **Pressure ulcer of unspecified hip, unspecified stage** cc🔒 CC/MCC Exc🔒

Healing pressure ulcer of unspecified hip NOS

Healing pressure ulcer of unspecified hip, unspecified stage

6ᵗʰ **L89.21** **Pressure ulcer of** right hip

L89.210 **Pressure ulcer of right hip, unstageable** cc🔒 HCC CC/MCC Exc🔒

L89.211 **Pressure ulcer of right hip, stage 1** cc🔒 CC/MCC Exc🔒

Healing pressure ulcer of right hip back, stage 1

Pressure pre-ulcer skin changes limited to persistent focal edema, right hip

L89.212 **Pressure ulcer of right hip, stage 2** cc🔒 HCC CC/MCC Exc🔒

Healing pressure ulcer of right hip, stage 2

Pressure ulcer with abrasion, blister, partial thickness skin loss involving epidermis and/or dermis, right hip

L89.213 **Pressure ulcer of right hip, stage 3** cc🔒 HAC HCC CC/MCC Exc🔒

Healing pressure ulcer of right hip, stage 3

Pressure ulcer with full thickness skin loss involving damage or necrosis of subcutaneous tissue, right hip

L89.214 **Pressure ulcer of right hip, stage 4** cc🔒 HAC HCC CC/MCC Exc🔒

Healing pressure ulcer of right hip, stage 4

Pressure ulcer with necrosis of soft tissues through to underlying muscle, tendon, or bone, right hip

● **L89.216** **Pressure-induced** deep tissue damage **of right hip** cc🔒 CC/MCC Exc🔒

L89.219 **Pressure ulcer of right hip, unspecified stage** cc🔒 CC/MCC Exc🔒

Healing pressure ulcer of right hip NOS

Healing pressure ulcer of right hip, unspecified stage

6ᵗʰ **L89.22** **Pressure ulcer of** left hip

L89.220 **Pressure ulcer of left hip, unstageable** cc🔒 HCC CC/MCC Exc🔒

L89.221 **Pressure ulcer of left hip, stage 1** cc🔒 CC/MCC Exc🔒

Healing pressure ulcer of left hip back, stage 1

Pressure pre-ulcer skin changes limited to persistent focal edema, left hip

---

PDXₙ Unacceptable principal diagnosis symbol per Medicare code edits   POX Code exempt from diagnosis present on admission requirement

❓ Questionable admission   cc🔒 Complication or comorbidity   MCC🔒 Major complication or comorbidity   CC/MCC🔒 CC/MCC exclusion

HCC HCC diagnosis code   RxHCC RxHCC diagnosis code   MACRA code   **DEFINITION** Describes condition/terminology

TIP Coding guidance   👁 Official Guideline Reference   Z1 Z code as first-listed diagnosis

L89.222 Pressure ulcer of left hip, stage 2 CC HCC CC/MCC Exc
Healing pressure ulcer of left hip, stage 2
Pressure ulcer with abrasion, blister, partial thickness skin loss involving epidermis and/or dermis, left hip

L89.223 Pressure ulcer of left hip, stage 3 CC HAC HCC CC/MCC Exc
Healing pressure ulcer of left hip, stage 3
Pressure ulcer with full thickness skin loss involving damage or necrosis of subcutaneous tissue, left hip

L89.224 Pressure ulcer of left hip, stage 4 CC HAC HCC CC/MCC Exc
Healing pressure ulcer of left hip, stage 4
Pressure ulcer with necrosis of soft tissues through to underlying muscle, tendon, or bone, left hip

● **L89.226 Pressure-induced deep tissue damage of left hip** CC CC/MCC Exc

L89.229 Pressure ulcer of left hip, unspecified stage CC CC/MCC Exc
Healing pressure ulcer of left hip NOS
Healing pressure ulcer of left hip, unspecified stage

5th **L89.3 Pressure ulcer of buttock**
6th **L89.30 Pressure ulcer of unspecified buttock**

L89.300 Pressure ulcer of unspecified buttock, unstageable CC HCC CC/MCC Exc

L89.301 Pressure ulcer of unspecified buttock, stage 1 CC CC/MCC Exc
Healing pressure ulcer of unspecified buttock, stage 1
Pressure pre-ulcer skin changes limited to persistent focal edema, unspecified buttock

L89.302 Pressure ulcer of unspecified buttock, stage 2 CC HCC CC/MCC Exc
Healing pressure ulcer of unspecified buttock, stage 2
Pressure ulcer with abrasion, blister, partial thickness skin loss involving epidermis and/or dermis, unspecified buttock

L89.303 Pressure ulcer of unspecified buttock, stage 3 CC HAC HCC CC/MCC Exc
Healing pressure ulcer of unspecified buttock, stage 3
Pressure ulcer with full thickness skin loss involving damage or necrosis of subcutaneous tissue, unspecified buttock

L89.304 Pressure ulcer of unspecified buttock, stage 4 CC HAC HCC CC/MCC Exc
Healing pressure ulcer of unspecified buttock, stage 4
Pressure ulcer with necrosis of soft tissues through to underlying muscle, tendon, or bone, unspecified buttock

● **L89.306 Pressure-induced deep tissue damage of unspecified buttock** CC CC/MCC Exc

L89.309 Pressure ulcer of unspecified buttock, unspecified stage CC CC/MCC Exc
Healing pressure ulcer of unspecified buttock NOS
Healing pressure ulcer of unspecified buttock, unspecified stage

6th **L89.31 Pressure ulcer of right buttock**

L89.310 Pressure ulcer of right buttock, unstageable CC HCC CC/MCC Exc

L89.311 Pressure ulcer of right buttock, stage 1 CC CC/MCC Exc
Healing pressure ulcer of right buttock, stage 1
Pressure pre-ulcer skin changes limited to persistent focal edema, right buttock

L89.312 Pressure ulcer of right buttock, stage 2 CC HCC CC/MCC Exc
Healing pressure ulcer of right buttock, stage 2
Pressure ulcer with abrasion, blister, partial thickness skin loss involving epidermis and/or dermis, right buttock

L89.313 Pressure ulcer of right buttock, stage 3 CC HAC HCC CC/MCC Exc
Healing pressure ulcer of right buttock, stage 3
Pressure ulcer with full thickness skin loss involving damage or necrosis of subcutaneous tissue, right buttock

L89.314 Pressure ulcer of right buttock, stage 4 CC HAC HCC CC/MCC Exc
Healing pressure ulcer of right buttock, stage 4
Pressure ulcer with necrosis of soft tissues through to underlying muscle, tendon, or bone, right buttock

● **L89.316 Pressure-induced deep tissue damage of right buttock** CC CC/MCC Exc

L89.319 Pressure ulcer of right buttock, unspecified stage CC CC/MCC Exc
Healing pressure ulcer of right buttock NOS
Healing pressure ulcer of right buttock, unspecified stage

6th **L89.32 Pressure ulcer of left buttock**

L89.320 Pressure ulcer of left buttock, unstageable CC HCC CC/MCC Exc

L89.321 Pressure ulcer of left buttock, stage 1 CC CC/MCC Exc
Healing pressure ulcer of left buttock, stage 1
Pressure pre-ulcer skin changes limited to persistent focal edema, left buttock

L89.322 Pressure ulcer of left buttock, stage 2 CC HCC CC/MCC Exc
Healing pressure ulcer of left buttock, stage 2
Pressure ulcer with abrasion, blister, partial thickness skin loss involving epidermis and/or dermis, left buttock

L89.323 Pressure ulcer of left buttock, stage 3 CC HAC HCC CC/MCC Exc
Healing pressure ulcer of left buttock, stage 3
Pressure ulcer with full thickness skin loss involving damage or necrosis of subcutaneous tissue, left buttock

L89.324 Pressure ulcer of left buttock, stage 4 CC HAC HCC CC/MCC Exc
Healing pressure ulcer of left buttock, stage 4
Pressure ulcer with necrosis of soft tissues through to underlying muscle, tendon, or bone, left buttock

● **L89.326 Pressure-induced deep tissue damage of left buttock** CC CC/MCC Exc

L89.329 Pressure ulcer of left buttock, unspecified stage CC CC/MCC Exc
Healing pressure ulcer of left buttock NOS
Healing pressure ulcer of left buttock, unspecified stage

5th **L89.4 Pressure ulcer of contiguous site of back, buttock and hip**

L89.40 Pressure ulcer of contiguous site of back, buttock and hip, unspecified stage CC CC/MCC Exc
Healing pressure ulcer of contiguous site of back, buttock and hip NOS
Healing pressure ulcer of contiguous site of back, buttock and hip, unspecified stage

L89.41 Pressure ulcer of contiguous site of back, buttock and hip, stage 1 CC CC/MCC Exc
Healing pressure ulcer of contiguous site of back, buttock and hip, stage 1
Pressure pre-ulcer skin changes limited to persistent focal edema, contiguous site of back, buttock and hip

Unspecified Code · Other Specified Code · Manifestation Code · N Newborn · P Pediatric · M Maternity · A Adult · ♂ Male · ♀ Female
● New Code ▲ Revised Code Title ►◄ Revised Text NOTES INCLUDES EXCLUDES1 Not coded here EXCLUDES2 Not included here
4th 4th character required 5th 5th character required 6th 6th character required 7th 7th character required Extension 'X' Alert
HAC Hospital-acquired condition (HAC) alert AHA AHA Coding Clinic© Code first alert

L89.42 **Pressure ulcer of contiguous site of back, buttock and hip,** stage 2   CC🄬 HCC CC/MCC Exc🄬

Healing pressure ulcer of contiguous site of back, buttock and hip, stage 2

Pressure ulcer with abrasion, blister, partial thickness skin loss involving epidermis and/or dermis, contiguous site of back, buttock and hip

L89.43 **Pressure ulcer of contiguous site of back, buttock and hip,** stage 3   CC🄬 HAC HCC CC/MCC Exc🄬

Healing pressure ulcer of contiguous site of back, buttock and hip, stage 3

Pressure ulcer with full thickness skin loss involving damage or necrosis of subcutaneous tissue, contiguous site of back, buttock and hip

L89.44 **Pressure ulcer of contiguous site of back, buttock and hip,** stage 4   CC🄬 HAC HCC CC/MCC Exc🄬

Healing pressure ulcer of contiguous site of back, buttock and hip, stage 4

Pressure ulcer with necrosis of soft tissues through to underlying muscle, tendon, or bone, contiguous site of back, buttock and hip

L89.45 **Pressure ulcer of contiguous site of back, buttock and hip,** unstageable   CC🄬 HCC CC/MCC Exc🄬

● L89.46 **Pressure-induced** deep tissue damage **of contiguous site of back, buttock and hip**   CC🄬 CC/MCC Exc🄬

5ᵗʰ L89.5 **Pressure ulcer of** ankle

6ᵗʰ L89.50 **Pressure ulcer of** unspecified **ankle**

L89.500 **Pressure ulcer of unspecified ankle,** unstageable   CC🄬 HCC CC/MCC Exc🄬

L89.501 **Pressure ulcer of unspecified ankle,** stage 1   CC🄬 CC/MCC Exc🄬

Healing pressure ulcer of unspecified ankle, stage 1

Pressure pre-ulcer skin changes limited to persistent focal edema, unspecified ankle

L89.502 **Pressure ulcer of unspecified ankle,** stage 2   CC🄬 HCC CC/MCC Exc🄬

Healing pressure ulcer of unspecified ankle, stage 2

Pressure ulcer with abrasion, blister, partial thickness skin loss involving epidermis and/or dermis, unspecified ankle

L89.503 **Pressure ulcer of unspecified ankle,** stage 3   CC🄬 HAC HCC CC/MCC Exc🄬

Healing pressure ulcer of unspecified ankle, stage 3

Pressure ulcer with full thickness skin loss involving damage or necrosis of subcutaneous tissue, unspecified ankle

L89.504 **Pressure ulcer of unspecified ankle,** stage 4   CC🄬 HAC HCC CC/MCC Exc🄬

Healing pressure ulcer of unspecified ankle, stage 4

Pressure ulcer with necrosis of soft tissues through to underlying muscle, tendon, or bone, unspecified ankle

● L89.506 **Pressure-induced** deep tissue damage **of unspecified ankle**   CC🄬 CC/MCC Exc🄬

L89.509 **Pressure ulcer of unspecified ankle, unspecified stage**   CC🄬 CC/MCC Exc🄬

Healing pressure ulcer of unspecified ankle NOS

Healing pressure ulcer of unspecified ankle, unspecified stage

6ᵗʰ L89.51 **Pressure ulcer of** right ankle

L89.510 **Pressure ulcer of right ankle,** unstageable   CC🄬 HCC CC/MCC Exc🄬

L89.511 **Pressure ulcer of right ankle,** stage 1   CC🄬 CC/MCC Exc🄬

Healing pressure ulcer of right ankle, stage 1

Pressure pre-ulcer skin changes limited to persistent focal edema, right ankle

L89.512 **Pressure ulcer of right ankle,** stage 2   CC🄬 HCC CC/MCC Exc🄬

Healing pressure ulcer of right ankle, stage 2

Pressure ulcer with abrasion, blister, partial thickness skin loss involving epidermis and/or dermis, right ankle

L89.513 **Pressure ulcer of right ankle,** stage 3   CC🄬 HAC HCC CC/MCC Exc🄬

Healing pressure ulcer of right ankle, stage 3

Pressure ulcer with full thickness skin loss involving damage or necrosis of subcutaneous tissue, right ankle

L89.514 **Pressure ulcer of right ankle,** stage 4   CC🄬 HAC HCC CC/MCC Exc🄬

Healing pressure ulcer of right ankle, stage 4

Pressure ulcer with necrosis of soft tissues through to underlying muscle, tendon, or bone, right ankle

● L89.516 **Pressure-induced** deep tissue damage **of right ankle**   CC🄬 CC/MCC Exc🄬

L89.519 **Pressure ulcer of right ankle, unspecified stage**   CC🄬 CC/MCC Exc🄬

Healing pressure ulcer of right ankle NOS

Healing pressure ulcer of right ankle, unspecified stage

6ᵗʰ L89.52 **Pressure ulcer of** left ankle

L89.520 **Pressure ulcer of left ankle,** unstageable   CC🄬 HCC CC/MCC Exc🄬

L89.521 **Pressure ulcer of left ankle,** stage 1   CC🄬 CC/MCC Exc🄬

Healing pressure ulcer of left ankle, stage 1

Pressure pre-ulcer skin changes limited to persistent focal edema, left ankle

L89.522 **Pressure ulcer of left ankle,** stage 2   CC🄬 HCC CC/MCC Exc🄬

Healing pressure ulcer of left ankle, stage 2

Pressure ulcer with abrasion, blister, partial thickness skin loss involving epidermis and/or dermis, left ankle

L89.523 **Pressure ulcer of left ankle,** stage 3   CC🄬 HAC HCC CC/MCC Exc🄬

Healing pressure ulcer of left ankle, stage 3

Pressure ulcer with full thickness skin loss involving damage or necrosis of subcutaneous tissue, left ankle

L89.524 **Pressure ulcer of left ankle,** stage 4   CC🄬 HAC HCC CC/MCC Exc🄬

Healing pressure ulcer of left ankle, stage 4

Pressure ulcer with necrosis of soft tissues through to underlying muscle, tendon, or bone, left ankle

● L89.526 **Pressure-induced** deep tissue damage **of left ankle**   CC🄬 CC/MCC Exc🄬

L89.529 **Pressure ulcer of left ankle, unspecified stage**   CC🄬 CC/MCC Exc🄬

Healing pressure ulcer of left ankle NOS

Healing pressure ulcer of left ankle, unspecified stage

5ᵗʰ L89.6 **Pressure ulcer of** heel

6ᵗʰ L89.60 **Pressure ulcer of** unspecified **heel**

L89.600 **Pressure ulcer of unspecified heel,** unstageable   CC🄬 HCC CC/MCC Exc🄬

L89.601 **Pressure ulcer of unspecified heel,** stage 1   CC🄬 CC/MCC Exc🄬

Healing pressure ulcer of unspecified heel, stage 1

Pressure pre-ulcer skin changes limited to persistent focal edema, unspecified heel

L89.602 **Pressure ulcer of unspecified heel,** stage 2   CC🄬 HCC CC/MCC Exc🄬

Healing pressure ulcer of unspecified heel, stage 2

Pressure ulcer with abrasion, blister, partial thickness skin loss involving epidermis and/or dermis, unspecified heel

---

PDₓ Unacceptable principal diagnosis symbol per Medicare code edits   POA Code exempt from diagnosis present on admission requirement
❓ Questionable admission   CC🄬 Complication or comorbidity   MCC🄬 Major complication or comorbidity   CC/MCC Exc CC/MCC exclusion
HCC HCC diagnosis code   RxHCC RxHCC diagnosis code   MACRA MACRA code   **DEFINITION** Describes condition/terminology
TIP Coding guidance   👁 Official Guideline Reference   Z1 Z code as first-listed diagnosis

L89.603 **Pressure ulcer of unspecified heel, stage 3** CC HAC HCC CC/MCC Exc
    Healing pressure ulcer of unspecified heel, stage 3
    Pressure ulcer with full thickness skin loss involving damage or necrosis of subcutaneous tissue, unspecified heel

L89.604 **Pressure ulcer of unspecified heel, stage 4** CC HAC HCC CC/MCC Exc
    Healing pressure ulcer of unspecified heel, stage 4
    Pressure ulcer with necrosis of soft tissues through to underlying muscle, tendon, or bone, unspecified heel

● **L89.606** **Pressure-induced deep tissue damage of unspecified heel** CC CC/MCC Exc

L89.609 **Pressure ulcer of unspecified heel, unspecified stage** CC CC/MCC Exc
    Healing pressure ulcer of unspecified heel NOS
    Healing pressure ulcer of unspecified heel, unspecified stage

6th **L89.61** **Pressure ulcer of right heel**

L89.610 **Pressure ulcer of right heel, unstageable** CC HCC CC/MCC Exc

L89.611 **Pressure ulcer of right heel, stage 1** CC CC/MCC Exc
    Healing pressure ulcer of right heel, stage 1
    Pressure pre-ulcer skin changes limited to persistent focal edema, right heel

L89.612 **Pressure ulcer of right heel, stage 2** CC HCC CC/MCC Exc
    Healing pressure ulcer of right heel, stage 2
    Pressure ulcer with abrasion, blister, partial thickness skin loss involving epidermis and/or dermis, right heel

L89.613 **Pressure ulcer of right heel, stage 3** CC HAC HCC CC/MCC Exc
    Healing pressure ulcer of right heel, stage 3
    Pressure ulcer with full thickness skin loss involving damage or necrosis of subcutaneous tissue, right heel

L89.614 **Pressure ulcer of right heel, stage 4** CC HAC HCC CC/MCC Exc
    Healing pressure ulcer of right heel, stage 4
    Pressure ulcer with necrosis of soft tissues through to underlying muscle, tendon, or bone, right heel

● **L89.616** **Pressure-induced deep tissue damage of right heel** CC CC/MCC Exc

L89.619 **Pressure ulcer of right heel, unspecified stage** CC CC/MCC Exc
    Healing pressure ulcer of right heel NOS
    Healing pressure ulcer of right heel, unspecified stage

6th **L89.62** **Pressure ulcer of left heel**

L89.620 **Pressure ulcer of left heel, unstageable** CC HCC CC/MCC Exc

L89.621 **Pressure ulcer of left heel, stage 1** CC CC/MCC Exc
    Healing pressure ulcer of left heel, stage 1
    Pressure pre-ulcer skin changes limited to persistent focal edema, left heel

L89.622 **Pressure ulcer of left heel, stage 2** CC HCC CC/MCC Exc
    AHA: Q4 2016
    Healing pressure ulcer of left heel, stage 2
    Pressure ulcer with abrasion, blister, partial thickness skin loss involving epidermis and/or dermis, left heel

L89.623 **Pressure ulcer of left heel, stage 3** CC HAC HCC CC/MCC Exc
    AHA: Q3 2018, Q4 2016
    Healing pressure ulcer of left heel, stage 3

    Pressure ulcer with full thickness skin loss involving damage or necrosis of subcutaneous tissue, left heel

L89.624 **Pressure ulcer of left heel, stage 4** CC HAC HCC CC/MCC Exc
    Healing pressure ulcer of left heel, stage 4
    Pressure ulcer with necrosis of soft tissues through to underlying muscle, tendon, or bone, left heel

● **L89.626** **Pressure-induced deep tissue damage of left heel** CC CC/MCC Exc

L89.629 **Pressure ulcer of left heel, unspecified stage** CC CC/MCC Exc
    Healing pressure ulcer of left heel NOS
    Healing pressure ulcer of left heel, unspecified stage

5th **L89.8** **Pressure ulcer of other site**

6th **L89.81** **Pressure ulcer of head**
    Pressure ulcer of face

L89.810 **Pressure ulcer of head, unstageable** CC HCC CC/MCC Exc

L89.811 **Pressure ulcer of head, stage 1** CC CC/MCC Exc
    Healing pressure ulcer of head, stage 1
    Pressure pre-ulcer skin changes limited to persistent focal edema, head

L89.812 **Pressure ulcer of head, stage 2** CC HCC CC/MCC Exc
    Healing pressure ulcer of head, stage 2
    Pressure ulcer with abrasion, blister, partial thickness skin loss involving epidermis and/or dermis, head

L89.813 **Pressure ulcer of head, stage 3** CC HAC HCC CC/MCC Exc
    Healing pressure ulcer of head, stage 3
    Pressure ulcer with full thickness skin loss involving damage or necrosis of subcutaneous tissue, head

L89.814 **Pressure ulcer of head, stage 4** CC HAC HCC CC/MCC Exc
    Healing pressure ulcer of head, stage 4
    Pressure ulcer with necrosis of soft tissues through to underlying muscle, tendon, or bone, head

● **L89.816** **Pressure-induced deep tissue damage of head** CC CC/MCC Exc

L89.819 **Pressure ulcer of head, unspecified stage** CC CC/MCC Exc
    Healing pressure ulcer of head NOS
    Healing pressure ulcer of head, unspecified stage

6th **L89.89** **Pressure ulcer of other site**

L89.890 **Pressure ulcer of other site, unstageable** CC HCC CC/MCC Exc

L89.891 **Pressure ulcer of other site, stage 1** CC CC/MCC Exc
    Healing pressure ulcer of other site, stage 1
    Pressure pre-ulcer skin changes limited to persistent focal edema, other site

L89.892 **Pressure ulcer of other site, stage 2** CC HCC CC/MCC Exc
    Healing pressure ulcer of other site, stage 2
    Pressure ulcer with abrasion, blister, partial thickness skin loss involving epidermis and/or dermis, other site

L89.893 **Pressure ulcer of other site, stage 3** CC HAC HCC CC/MCC Exc
    Healing pressure ulcer of other site, stage 3
    Pressure ulcer with full thickness skin loss involving damage or necrosis of subcutaneous tissue, other site

L89.894 **Pressure ulcer of other site, stage 4** CC HAC HCC CC/MCC Exc
    Healing pressure ulcer of other site, stage 4
    Pressure ulcer with necrosis of soft tissues through to underlying muscle, tendon, or bone, other site

---

Unspecified Code   Other Specified Code   Manifestation Code   N Newborn   P Pediatric   M Maternity   A Adult   ♂ Male   ♀ Female
● New Code   ▲ Revised Code Title   ►◄ Revised Text   **NOTES**   *INCLUDES*   *EXCLUDES1* Not coded here   *EXCLUDES2* Not included here
4th 4th character required   5th 5th character required   6th 6th character required   7th 7th character required   7th Extension 'X' Alert
HAC Hospital-acquired condition (HAC) alert   AHA AHA Coding Clinic®   ☛ Code first alert

● **L89.896** Pressure-induced deep tissue damage of other site CC CC/MCC Exc

L89.899 Pressure ulcer of other site, unspecified stage CC CC/MCC Exc

Healing pressure ulcer of other site NOS
Healing pressure ulcer of other site, unspecified stage

⑤ **L89.9** Pressure ulcer of unspecified site

L89.90 Pressure ulcer of unspecified site, unspecified stage CC CC/MCC Exc

Healing pressure ulcer of unspecified site NOS
Healing pressure ulcer of unspecified site, unspecified stage

L89.91 Pressure ulcer of unspecified site, stage 1 CC CC/MCC Exc

Healing pressure ulcer of unspecified site, stage 1
Pressure pre-ulcer skin changes limited to persistent focal edema, unspecified site

L89.92 Pressure ulcer of unspecified site, stage 2 CC HCC CC/MCC Exc

Healing pressure ulcer of unspecified site, stage 2
Pressure ulcer with abrasion, blister, partial thickness skin loss involving epidermis and/or dermis, unspecified site

L89.93 Pressure ulcer of unspecified site, stage 3 CC HAC HCC CC/MCC Exc

Healing pressure ulcer of unspecified site, stage 3
Pressure ulcer with full thickness skin loss involving damage or necrosis of subcutaneous tissue, unspecified site

L89.94 Pressure ulcer of unspecified site, stage 4 CC HAC HCC CC/MCC Exc

Healing pressure ulcer of unspecified site, stage 4
Pressure ulcer with necrosis of soft tissues through to underlying muscle, tendon, or bone, unspecified site

L89.95 Pressure ulcer of unspecified site, unstageable CC HCC CC/MCC Exc

● **L89.96** Pressure-induced deep tissue damage of unspecified site CC CC/MCC Exc

④ **L90** Atrophic disorders of skin

L90.0 Lichen sclerosus et atrophicus

EXCLUDES2 lichen sclerosus of external female genital organs (N90.4)

lichen sclerosus of external male genital organs (N48.0)

L90.1 Anetoderma of Schweninger-Buzzi

L90.2 Anetoderma of Jadassohn-Pellizzari

L90.3 Atrophoderma of Pasini and Pierini

L90.4 Acrodermatitis chronica atrophicans

L90.5 Scar conditions and fibrosis of skin

AHA: Q2 2016, Q1 2015
Adherent scar (skin)
Cicatrix
Disfigurement of skin due to scar
Fibrosis of skin NOS
Scar NOS

EXCLUDES2 hypertrophic scar (L91.0)

keloid scar (L91.0)

L90.6 Striae atrophicae

L90.8 Other atrophic disorders of skin

L90.9 Atrophic disorder of skin, unspecified

④ **L91** Hypertrophic disorders of skin

L91.0 Hypertrophic scar
Keloid
Keloid scar

EXCLUDES2 acne keloid (L73.0)

scar NOS (L90.5)

L91.8 Other hypertrophic disorders of the skin

L91.9 Hypertrophic disorder of the skin, unspecified

④ **L92** Granulomatous disorders of skin and subcutaneous tissue

EXCLUDES2 actinic granuloma (L57.5)

L92.0 Granuloma annulare
Perforating granuloma annulare

L92.1 Necrobiosis lipoidica, not elsewhere classified

EXCLUDES1 necrobiosis lipoidica associated with diabetes mellitus (E08-E13 with .620)

L92.2 Granuloma faciale [eosinophilic granuloma of skin]

L92.3 Foreign body granuloma of the skin and subcutaneous tissue

Use additional code to identify the type of retained foreign body (Z18.-)

L92.8 Other granulomatous disorders of the skin and subcutaneous tissue

L92.9 Granulomatous disorder of the skin and subcutaneous tissue, unspecified

EXCLUDES2 umbilical granuloma (P83.81)

④ **L93** Lupus erythematosus

Use additional code for adverse effect, if applicable, to identify drug (T36-T50 with fifth or sixth character 5)

EXCLUDES1 lupus exedens (A18.4)

lupus vulgaris (A18.4)

scleroderma (M34.-)

systemic lupus erythematosus (M32.-)

L93.0 Discoid lupus erythematosus
Lupus erythematosus NOS

L93.1 Subacute cutaneous lupus erythematosus

L93.2 Other local lupus erythematosus
Lupus erythematosus profundus
Lupus panniculitis

④ **L94** Other localized connective tissue disorders

EXCLUDES1 systemic connective tissue disorders (M30-M36)

L94.0 Localized scleroderma [morphea]
Circumscribed scleroderma

L94.1 Linear scleroderma
En coup de sabre lesion

L94.2 Calcinosis cutis

L94.3 Sclerodactyly

L94.4 Gottron's papules

L94.5 Poikiloderma vasculare atrophicans RxHCC

L94.6 Ainhum

L94.8 Other specified localized connective tissue disorders

L94.9 Localized connective tissue disorder, unspecified

④ **L95** Vasculitis limited to skin, not elsewhere classified

EXCLUDES1 angioma serpiginosum (L81.7)

Henoch(-Schönlein) purpura (D69.0)

hypersensitivity angiitis (M31.0)

lupus panniculitis (L93.2)

panniculitis NOS (M79.3)

panniculitis of neck and back (M54.0-)

polyarteritis nodosa (M30.0)

relapsing panniculitis (M35.6)

rheumatoid vasculitis (M05.2)

serum sickness (T80.6-)

urticaria (L50.-)

Wegener's granulomatosis (M31.3-)

L95.0 Livedoid vasculitis
Atrophie blanche (en plaque)

L95.1 Erythema elevatum diutinum

L95.8 Other vasculitis limited to the skin

L95.9 Vasculitis limited to the skin, unspecified

④ **L97** Non-pressure chronic ulcer of lower limb, not elsewhere classified

INCLUDES chronic ulcer of skin of lower limb NOS

non-healing ulcer of skin

non-infected sinus of skin

trophic ulcer NOS

tropical ulcer NOS

ulcer of skin of lower limb NOS

☞ **Code first** any associated underlying condition, such as:
any associated gangrene (I96)

PDx Unacceptable principal diagnosis symbol per Medicare code edits   POA Code exempt from diagnosis present on admission requirement
? Questionable admission   CC Complication or comorbidity   MCC Major complication or comorbidity   CC/MCC Exc CC/MCC exclusion
HCC HCC diagnosis code   RxHCC RxHCC diagnosis code   MACRA code   **DEFINITION** Describes condition/terminology
TIP Coding guidance   👁 Official Guideline Reference   Z1 Z code as first-listed diagnosis

When symbols appear on a code that requires a 7th character extension, refer to Appendix B to identify applicable 7th character codes.   **2020 ICD-10-CM**

atherosclerosis of the lower extremities (I70.23-, I70.24-, I70.33-, I70.34-, I70.43-, I70.44-, I70.53-, I70.54-, I70.63-, I70.64-, I70.73-, I70.74-)

chronic venous hypertension (I87.31-, I87.33-)

diabetic ulcers (E08.621, E08.622, E09.621, E09.622, E10.621, E10.622, E11.621, E11.622, E13.621, E13.622)

postphlebitic syndrome (I87.01-, I87.03-)

postthrombotic syndrome (I87.01-, I87.03-)

varicose ulcer (I83.0-, I83.2-)

EXCLUDES2 pressure ulcer (pressure area) (L89.-)

skin infections (L00-L08)

specific infections classified to A00-B99

5ᵗʰ **L97.1 Non-pressure chronic ulcer of** thigh

  6ᵗʰ **L97.10 Non-pressure chronic ulcer of** unspecified **thigh**

    L97.101 **Non-pressure chronic ulcer of unspecified thigh** limited to breakdown of skin   CC HCC RxHCC CC/MCC Exc

    L97.102 **Non-pressure chronic ulcer of unspecified thigh** with fat layer exposed   CC HCC RxHCC CC/MCC Exc

    L97.103 **Non-pressure chronic ulcer of unspecified thigh** with necrosis of muscle   CC HCC RxHCC CC/MCC Exc

    L97.104 **Non-pressure chronic ulcer of unspecified thigh** with necrosis of bone   CC HCC RxHCC CC/MCC Exc

    L97.105 **Non-pressure chronic ulcer of unspecified thigh** with muscle involvement without evidence of necrosis   CC HCC RxHCC CC/MCC Exc

    L97.106 **Non-pressure chronic ulcer of unspecified thigh** with bone involvement without evidence of necrosis   CC HCC RxHCC CC/MCC Exc

    L97.108 **Non-pressure chronic ulcer of unspecified thigh** with other specified severity   CC HCC RxHCC CC/MCC Exc

    L97.109 **Non-pressure chronic ulcer of unspecified thigh** with unspecified severity   CC HCC RxHCC CC/MCC Exc

  6ᵗʰ **L97.11 Non-pressure chronic ulcer of** right thigh

    L97.111 **Non-pressure chronic ulcer of right thigh** limited to breakdown of skin   CC HCC RxHCC CC/MCC Exc

    L97.112 **Non-pressure chronic ulcer of right thigh** with fat layer exposed   CC HCC RxHCC CC/MCC Exc

    L97.113 **Non-pressure chronic ulcer of right thigh** with necrosis of muscle   CC HCC RxHCC CC/MCC Exc

    L97.114 **Non-pressure chronic ulcer of right thigh** with necrosis of bone   CC HCC RxHCC CC/MCC Exc

    L97.115 **Non-pressure chronic ulcer of right thigh** with muscle involvement without evidence of necrosis   CC HCC RxHCC CC/MCC Exc

    L97.116 **Non-pressure chronic ulcer of right thigh** with bone involvement without evidence of necrosis   CC HCC RxHCC CC/MCC Exc

    L97.118 **Non-pressure chronic ulcer of right thigh** with other specified severity   CC HCC RxHCC CC/MCC Exc

    L97.119 **Non-pressure chronic ulcer of right thigh** with unspecified severity   CC HCC RxHCC CC/MCC Exc

  6ᵗʰ **L97.12 Non-pressure chronic ulcer of** left thigh

    L97.121 **Non-pressure chronic ulcer of left thigh** limited to breakdown of skin   CC HCC RxHCC CC/MCC Exc

    L97.122 **Non-pressure chronic ulcer of left thigh** with fat layer exposed   CC HCC RxHCC CC/MCC Exc

    L97.123 **Non-pressure chronic ulcer of left thigh** with necrosis of muscle   CC HCC RxHCC CC/MCC Exc

    L97.124 **Non-pressure chronic ulcer of left thigh** with necrosis of bone   CC HCC RxHCC CC/MCC Exc

    L97.125 **Non-pressure chronic ulcer of left thigh** with muscle involvement without evidence of necrosis   CC HCC RxHCC CC/MCC Exc

    L97.126 **Non-pressure chronic ulcer of left thigh** with bone involvement without evidence of necrosis   CC HCC RxHCC CC/MCC Exc

    L97.128 **Non-pressure chronic ulcer of left thigh with** other specified severity   CC HCC RxHCC CC/MCC Exc

    L97.129 **Non-pressure chronic ulcer of left thigh** with **unspecified** severity   CC HCC RxHCC CC/MCC Exc

5ᵗʰ **L97.2 Non-pressure chronic ulcer of** calf

  6ᵗʰ **L97.20 Non-pressure chronic ulcer of** unspecified **calf**

    L97.201 **Non-pressure chronic ulcer of unspecified calf** limited to breakdown of skin   CC HCC RxHCC CC/MCC Exc

    L97.202 **Non-pressure chronic ulcer of unspecified calf** with fat layer exposed   CC HCC RxHCC CC/MCC Exc

    L97.203 **Non-pressure chronic ulcer of unspecified calf** with necrosis of muscle   CC HCC RxHCC CC/MCC Exc

    L97.204 **Non-pressure chronic ulcer of unspecified calf** with necrosis of bone   CC HCC RxHCC CC/MCC Exc

    L97.205 **Non-pressure chronic ulcer of unspecified calf with** muscle involvement without evidence of necrosis   CC HCC RxHCC CC/MCC Exc

    L97.206 **Non-pressure chronic ulcer of unspecified calf** with bone involvement without evidence of necrosis   CC HCC RxHCC CC/MCC Exc

    L97.208 **Non-pressure chronic ulcer of unspecified calf with** other specified severity   CC HCC RxHCC CC/MCC Exc

    L97.209 **Non-pressure chronic ulcer of unspecified calf** with **unspecified** severity   CC HCC RxHCC CC/MCC Exc

  6ᵗʰ **L97.21 Non-pressure chronic ulcer of** right calf

    L97.211 **Non-pressure chronic ulcer of right calf** limited to breakdown of skin   CC HCC RxHCC CC/MCC Exc

    L97.212 **Non-pressure chronic ulcer of right calf** with fat layer exposed   CC HCC RxHCC CC/MCC Exc

    L97.213 **Non-pressure chronic ulcer of right calf** with necrosis of muscle   CC HCC RxHCC CC/MCC Exc

    L97.214 **Non-pressure chronic ulcer of right calf** with necrosis of bone   CC HCC RxHCC CC/MCC Exc

    L97.215 **Non-pressure chronic ulcer of right calf** with muscle involvement without evidence of necrosis   CC HCC RxHCC CC/MCC Exc

    L97.216 **Non-pressure chronic ulcer of right calf** with bone involvement without evidence of necrosis   CC HCC RxHCC CC/MCC Exc

    L97.218 **Non-pressure chronic ulcer of right calf with** other specified severity   CC HCC RxHCC CC/MCC Exc

    L97.219 **Non-pressure chronic ulcer of right calf** with **unspecified** severity   CC HCC RxHCC CC/MCC Exc

  6ᵗʰ **L97.22 Non-pressure chronic ulcer of** left calf

    L97.221 **Non-pressure chronic ulcer of left calf** limited to breakdown of skin   CC HCC RxHCC CC/MCC Exc

    L97.222 **Non-pressure chronic ulcer of left calf** with fat layer exposed   CC HCC RxHCC CC/MCC Exc

    L97.223 **Non-pressure chronic ulcer of left calf** with necrosis of muscle   CC HCC RxHCC CC/MCC Exc

    L97.224 **Non-pressure chronic ulcer of left calf** with necrosis of bone   CC HCC RxHCC CC/MCC Exc

    L97.225 **Non-pressure chronic ulcer of left calf** with muscle involvement without evidence of necrosis   CC HCC RxHCC CC/MCC Exc

    L97.226 **Non-pressure chronic ulcer of left calf** with bone involvement without evidence of necrosis   CC HCC RxHCC CC/MCC Exc

    L97.228 **Non-pressure chronic ulcer of left calf with** other specified severity   CC HCC RxHCC CC/MCC Exc

    L97.229 **Non-pressure chronic ulcer of left calf** with unspecified severity   CC HCC RxHCC CC/MCC Exc

---

Unspecified Code   Other Specified Code   Manifestation Code   N Newborn   P Pediatric   M Maternity   A Adult   ♂ Male   ♀ Female
● New Code   ▲ Revised Code Title   ▶◀ Revised Text   NOTES   INCLUDES   EXCLUDES1 Not coded here   EXCLUDES2 Not included here
4ᵗʰ 4ᵗʰ character required   5ᵗʰ 5ᵗʰ character required   6ᵗʰ 6ᵗʰ character required   7ᵗʰ 7ᵗʰ character required   7ˣ Extension 'X' Alert
HAC Hospital-acquired condition (HAC) alert   AHA AHA Coding Clinic©   ☛ Code first alert

L97.3 **Non-pressure chronic ulcer of** ankle

L97.30 **Non-pressure chronic ulcer of** unspecified **ankle**

L97.301 **Non-pressure chronic ulcer of unspecified ankle** limited to breakdown of skin `CC` `HCC` `RxHCC` `CC/MCC Exc`

L97.302 **Non-pressure chronic ulcer of unspecified ankle** with fat layer exposed `CC` `HCC` `RxHCC` `CC/MCC Exc`

L97.303 **Non-pressure chronic ulcer of unspecified ankle** with necrosis of muscle `CC` `HCC` `RxHCC` `CC/MCC Exc`

L97.304 **Non-pressure chronic ulcer of unspecified ankle** with necrosis of bone `CC` `HCC` `RxHCC` `CC/MCC Exc`

L97.305 **Non-pressure chronic ulcer of unspecified ankle** with muscle involvement without evidence of necrosis `CC` `HCC` `RxHCC` `CC/MCC Exc`

L97.306 **Non-pressure chronic ulcer of unspecified ankle** with bone involvement without evidence of necrosis `CC` `HCC` `RxHCC` `CC/MCC Exc`

L97.308 **Non-pressure chronic ulcer of unspecified ankle with other specified severity** `CC` `HCC` `RxHCC` `CC/MCC Exc`

L97.309 **Non-pressure chronic ulcer of unspecified ankle with unspecified severity** `CC` `HCC` `RxHCC` `CC/MCC Exc`

L97.31 **Non-pressure chronic ulcer of** right ankle

L97.311 **Non-pressure chronic ulcer of right ankle** limited to breakdown of skin `CC` `HCC` `RxHCC` `CC/MCC Exc`

L97.312 **Non-pressure chronic ulcer of right ankle** with fat layer exposed `CC` `HCC` `RxHCC` `CC/MCC Exc`

L97.313 **Non-pressure chronic ulcer of right ankle** with necrosis of muscle `CC` `HCC` `RxHCC` `CC/MCC Exc`

L97.314 **Non-pressure chronic ulcer of right ankle** with necrosis of bone `CC` `HCC` `RxHCC` `CC/MCC Exc`

L97.315 **Non-pressure chronic ulcer of right ankle** with muscle involvement without evidence of necrosis `CC` `HCC` `RxHCC` `CC/MCC Exc`

L97.316 **Non-pressure chronic ulcer of right ankle** with bone involvement without evidence of necrosis `CC` `HCC` `RxHCC` `CC/MCC Exc`

L97.318 **Non-pressure chronic ulcer of right ankle with other specified severity** `CC` `HCC` `RxHCC` `CC/MCC Exc`

L97.319 **Non-pressure chronic ulcer of right ankle** with unspecified severity `CC` `HCC` `RxHCC` `CC/MCC Exc`

L97.32 **Non-pressure chronic ulcer of** left ankle

L97.321 **Non-pressure chronic ulcer of left ankle** limited to breakdown of skin `CC` `HCC` `RxHCC` `CC/MCC Exc`

L97.322 **Non-pressure chronic ulcer of left ankle** with fat layer exposed `CC` `HCC` `RxHCC` `CC/MCC Exc`

L97.323 **Non-pressure chronic ulcer of left ankle** with necrosis of muscle `CC` `HCC` `RxHCC` `CC/MCC Exc`

L97.324 **Non-pressure chronic ulcer of left ankle** with necrosis of bone `CC` `HCC` `RxHCC` `CC/MCC Exc`

L97.325 **Non-pressure chronic ulcer of left ankle** with muscle involvement without evidence of necrosis `CC` `HCC` `RxHCC` `CC/MCC Exc`

L97.326 **Non-pressure chronic ulcer of left ankle** with bone involvement without evidence of necrosis `CC` `HCC` `RxHCC` `CC/MCC Exc`

L97.328 **Non-pressure chronic ulcer of left ankle with other specified severity** `CC` `HCC` `RxHCC` `CC/MCC Exc`

L97.329 **Non-pressure chronic ulcer of left ankle** with unspecified severity `CC` `HCC` `RxHCC` `CC/MCC Exc`

L97.4 **Non-pressure chronic ulcer of** heel and midfoot

Non-pressure chronic ulcer of plantar surface of midfoot

L97.40 **Non-pressure chronic ulcer of** unspecified **heel and midfoot**

L97.401 **Non-pressure chronic ulcer of unspecified heel and midfoot** limited to breakdown of skin `CC` `HCC` `RxHCC` `CC/MCC Exc`

L97.402 **Non-pressure chronic ulcer of unspecified heel and midfoot** with fat layer exposed `CC` `HCC` `RxHCC` `CC/MCC Exc`

L97.403 **Non-pressure chronic ulcer of unspecified heel and midfoot** with necrosis of muscle `CC` `HCC` `RxHCC` `CC/MCC Exc`

L97.404 **Non-pressure chronic ulcer of unspecified heel and midfoot** with necrosis of bone `CC` `HCC` `RxHCC` `CC/MCC Exc`

L97.405 **Non-pressure chronic ulcer of unspecified heel and midfoot** with muscle involvement without evidence of necrosis `CC` `HCC` `RxHCC` `CC/MCC Exc`

L97.406 **Non-pressure chronic ulcer of unspecified heel and midfoot** with bone involvement without evidence of necrosis `CC` `HCC` `RxHCC` `CC/MCC Exc`

L97.408 **Non-pressure chronic ulcer of unspecified heel and midfoot with other specified severity** `CC` `HCC` `RxHCC` `CC/MCC Exc`

L97.409 **Non-pressure chronic ulcer of unspecified heel and midfoot** with unspecified severity `CC` `HCC` `RxHCC` `CC/MCC Exc`

L97.41 **Non-pressure chronic ulcer of** right heel and midfoot

L97.411 **Non-pressure chronic ulcer of right heel and midfoot** limited to breakdown of skin `CC` `HCC` `RxHCC` `CC/MCC Exc`

L97.412 **Non-pressure chronic ulcer of right heel and midfoot** with fat layer exposed `CC` `HCC` `RxHCC` `CC/MCC Exc`

L97.413 **Non-pressure chronic ulcer of right heel and midfoot** with necrosis of muscle `CC` `HCC` `RxHCC` `CC/MCC Exc`

L97.414 **Non-pressure chronic ulcer of right heel and midfoot** with necrosis of bone `CC` `HCC` `RxHCC` `CC/MCC Exc`

L97.415 **Non-pressure chronic ulcer of right heel and midfoot** with muscle involvement without evidence of necrosis `CC` `HCC` `RxHCC` `CC/MCC Exc`

L97.416 **Non-pressure chronic ulcer of right heel and midfoot** with bone involvement without evidence of necrosis `CC` `HCC` `RxHCC` `CC/MCC Exc`

L97.418 **Non-pressure chronic ulcer of right heel and midfoot with other specified severity** `CC` `HCC` `RxHCC` `CC/MCC Exc`

L97.419 **Non-pressure chronic ulcer of right heel and midfoot** with unspecified severity `CC` `HCC` `RxHCC` `CC/MCC Exc`

L97.42 **Non-pressure chronic ulcer of** left heel and midfoot

L97.421 **Non-pressure chronic ulcer of left heel and midfoot limited to breakdown of skin** `CC` `HCC` `RxHCC` `CC/MCC Exc`

AHA: Q1 2016

L97.422 **Non-pressure chronic ulcer of left heel and midfoot** with fat layer exposed `CC` `HCC` `RxHCC` `CC/MCC Exc`

L97.423 **Non-pressure chronic ulcer of left heel and midfoot** with necrosis of muscle `CC` `HCC` `RxHCC` `CC/MCC Exc`

L97.424 **Non-pressure chronic ulcer of left heel and midfoot** with necrosis of bone `CC` `HCC` `RxHCC` `CC/MCC Exc`

L97.425 **Non-pressure chronic ulcer of left heel and midfoot** with muscle involvement without evidence of necrosis `CC` `HCC` `RxHCC` `CC/MCC Exc`

L97.426 **Non-pressure chronic ulcer of left heel and midfoot** with bone involvement without evidence of necrosis `CC` `HCC` `RxHCC` `CC/MCC Exc`

PDx **Unacceptable principal diagnosis symbol per Medicare code edits** POA **Code exempt from diagnosis present on admission requirement**
? Questionable admission CC Complication or comorbidity MCC Major complication or comorbidity CC/MCC Exc CC/MCC exclusion
HCC HCC diagnosis code RxHCC RxHCC diagnosis code MACRA MACRA code **DEFINITION** Describes condition/terminology
TIP Coding guidance 👁 Official Guideline Reference Z1 Z code as first-listed diagnosis

When symbols appear on a code that requires a 7th character extension, refer to Appendix B to identify applicable 7th character codes.

2020 ICD-10-CM

L97.428 **Non-pressure chronic ulcer of left heel and midfoot with other specified severity** CC HCC RxHCC CC/MCC Exc

L97.429 Non-pressure chronic ulcer of left heel and midfoot with **unspecified** severity CC HCC RxHCC CC/MCC Exc

5️⃣ **L97.5 Non-pressure chronic ulcer of** other part of foot
Non-pressure chronic ulcer of toe

6️⃣ **L97.50 Non-pressure chronic ulcer of other part of** unspecified foot

L97.501 **Non-pressure chronic ulcer of other part of unspecified foot** limited to breakdown of skin HCC RxHCC

L97.502 **Non-pressure chronic ulcer of other part of unspecified foot** with fat layer exposed HCC RxHCC

L97.503 **Non-pressure chronic ulcer of other part of unspecified foot** with necrosis of muscle HCC RxHCC

L97.504 **Non-pressure chronic ulcer of other part of unspecified foot** with necrosis of bone HCC RxHCC

L97.505 **Non-pressure chronic ulcer of other part of unspecified foot** with muscle involvement without evidence of necrosis CC HCC RxHCC CC/MCC Exc

L97.506 **Non-pressure chronic ulcer of other part of unspecified foot** with bone involvement without evidence of necrosis CC HCC RxHCC CC/MCC Exc

L97.508 **Non-pressure chronic ulcer of other part of unspecified foot with other specified severity** CC HCC RxHCC CC/MCC Exc

L97.509 **Non-pressure chronic ulcer of other part of unspecified foot** with **unspecified** severity HCC RxHCC

6️⃣ **L97.51 Non-pressure chronic ulcer of** other part of right foot

L97.511 **Non-pressure chronic ulcer of other part of right foot** limited to breakdown of skin HCC RxHCC

L97.512 **Non-pressure chronic ulcer of other part of right foot** with fat layer exposed HCC RxHCC

L97.513 **Non-pressure chronic ulcer of other part of right foot** with necrosis of muscle HCC RxHCC

L97.514 **Non-pressure chronic ulcer of other part of right foot** with necrosis of bone HCC RxHCC

L97.515 **Non-pressure chronic ulcer of other part of right foot with muscle involvement** without evidence of necrosis CC HCC RxHCC CC/MCC Exc

L97.516 **Non-pressure chronic ulcer of other part of right foot with bone involvement** without evidence of necrosis CC HCC RxHCC CC/MCC Exc

L97.518 **Non-pressure chronic ulcer of other part of right foot with other specified severity** CC HCC RxHCC CC/MCC Exc

L97.519 **Non-pressure chronic ulcer of other part of right foot** with **unspecified** severity HCC RxHCC

6️⃣ **L97.52 Non-pressure chronic ulcer of** other part of left foot

L97.521 **Non-pressure chronic ulcer of other part of left foot** limited to breakdown of skin HCC RxHCC

L97.522 **Non-pressure chronic ulcer of other part of left foot** with fat layer exposed HCC RxHCC

L97.523 **Non-pressure chronic ulcer of other part of left foot** with necrosis of muscle HCC RxHCC

L97.524 **Non-pressure chronic ulcer of other part of left foot** with necrosis of bone HCC RxHCC

L97.525 **Non-pressure chronic ulcer of other part of left foot** with muscle involvement without evidence of necrosis CC HCC RxHCC CC/MCC Exc

L97.526 **Non-pressure chronic ulcer of other part of left foot** with bone involvement without evidence of necrosis CC HCC RxHCC CC/MCC Exc

L97.528 **Non-pressure chronic ulcer of other part of left foot with other specified severity** CC HCC RxHCC CC/MCC Exc

L97.529 **Non-pressure chronic ulcer of other part of left foot** with **unspecified** severity HCC RxHCC

5️⃣ **L97.8 Non-pressure chronic ulcer of** other part of lower leg

5️⃣ **L97.80 Non-pressure chronic ulcer of other part of** unspecified **lower leg**

L97.801 **Non-pressure chronic ulcer of other part of unspecified lower leg** limited to breakdown of skin CC HCC RxHCC CC/MCC Exc

L97.802 **Non-pressure chronic ulcer of other part of unspecified lower leg** with fat layer exposed CC HCC RxHCC CC/MCC Exc

L97.803 **Non-pressure chronic ulcer of other part of unspecified lower leg** with necrosis of muscle CC HCC RxHCC CC/MCC Exc

L97.804 **Non-pressure chronic ulcer of other part of unspecified lower leg** with necrosis of bone CC HCC RxHCC CC/MCC Exc

L97.805 **Non-pressure chronic ulcer of other part of unspecified lower leg** with muscle involvement without evidence of necrosis CC HCC RxHCC CC/MCC Exc

L97.806 **Non-pressure chronic ulcer of other part of unspecified lower leg** with bone involvement without evidence of necrosis CC HCC RxHCC CC/MCC Exc

L97.808 **Non-pressure chronic ulcer of other part of unspecified lower leg with other specified severity** CC HCC RxHCC CC/MCC Exc

L97.809 **Non-pressure chronic ulcer of other part of unspecified lower leg** with **unspecified** severity CC HCC RxHCC CC/MCC Exc

6️⃣ **L97.81 Non-pressure chronic ulcer of** other part of right lower leg

L97.811 **Non-pressure chronic ulcer of other part of right lower leg** limited to breakdown of skin CC HCC RxHCC CC/MCC Exc

L97.812 **Non-pressure chronic ulcer of other part of right lower leg** with fat layer exposed CC HCC RxHCC CC/MCC Exc

L97.813 **Non-pressure chronic ulcer of other part of right lower leg** with necrosis of muscle CC HCC RxHCC CC/MCC Exc

L97.814 **Non-pressure chronic ulcer of other part of right lower leg** with necrosis of bone CC HCC RxHCC CC/MCC Exc

L97.815 **Non-pressure chronic ulcer of other part of right lower leg** with muscle involvement without evidence of necrosis CC HCC RxHCC CC/MCC Exc

L97.816 **Non-pressure chronic ulcer of other part of right lower leg** with bone involvement without evidence of necrosis CC HCC RxHCC CC/MCC Exc

L97.818 **Non-pressure chronic ulcer of other part of right lower leg with other specified severity** CC HCC RxHCC CC/MCC Exc

L97.819 **Non-pressure chronic ulcer of other part of right lower leg** with **unspecified** severity CC HCC RxHCC CC/MCC Exc

6️⃣ **L97.82 Non-pressure chronic ulcer of** other part of left lower leg

L97.821 **Non-pressure chronic ulcer of other part of left lower leg** limited to breakdown of skin CC HCC RxHCC CC/MCC Exc

L97.822 **Non-pressure chronic ulcer of other part of left lower leg** with fat layer exposed CC HCC RxHCC CC/MCC Exc

---

Unspecified Code   Other Specified Code   Manifestation Code   Ⓝ Newborn   Ⓟ Pediatric   Ⓜ Maternity   Ⓐ Adult   ♂ Male   ♀ Female
● New Code   ▲ Revised Code Title   ▶◀ Revised Text   **NOTES**   *INCLUDES*   *EXCLUDES1* Not coded here   *EXCLUDES2* Not included here
4️⃣ 4th character required   5️⃣ 5th character required   6️⃣ 6th character required   7️⃣ 7th character required   Extension 'X' Alert
HAC Hospital-acquired condition (HAC) alert   **AHA** AHA Coding Clinic©   ☛ Code first alert

L97.823 Non-pressure chronic ulcer of other part of left lower leg with necrosis of muscle ℗ HCC RxHCC CC/MCC Exc

L97.824 Non-pressure chronic ulcer of other part of left lower leg with necrosis of bone ℗ HCC RxHCC CC/MCC Exc

L97.825 Non-pressure chronic ulcer of other part of left lower leg with muscle involvement without evidence of necrosis ℗ HCC RxHCC CC/MCC Exc

L97.826 Non-pressure chronic ulcer of other part of left lower leg with bone involvement without evidence of necrosis ℗ HCC RxHCC CC/MCC Exc

L97.828 Non-pressure chronic ulcer of other part of left lower leg with other specified severity ℗ HCC RxHCC CC/MCC Exc

L97.829 Non-pressure chronic ulcer of other part of left lower leg with unspecified severity ℗ HCC RxHCC CC/MCC Exc

5th L97.9 Non-pressure chronic ulcer of unspecified part of lower leg

6th L97.90 Non-pressure chronic ulcer of unspecified part of unspecified lower leg

L97.901 Non-pressure chronic ulcer of unspecified part of unspecified lower leg limited to breakdown of skin ℗ HCC RxHCC CC/MCC Exc

L97.902 Non-pressure chronic ulcer of unspecified part of unspecified lower leg with fat layer exposed ℗ HCC RxHCC CC/MCC Exc

L97.903 Non-pressure chronic ulcer of unspecified part of unspecified lower leg with necrosis of muscle ℗ HCC RxHCC CC/MCC Exc

L97.904 Non-pressure chronic ulcer of unspecified part of unspecified lower leg with necrosis of bone ℗ HCC RxHCC CC/MCC Exc

L97.905 Non-pressure chronic ulcer of unspecified part of unspecified lower leg with muscle involvement without evidence of necrosis ℗ HCC RxHCC CC/MCC Exc

L97.906 Non-pressure chronic ulcer of unspecified part of unspecified lower leg with bone involvement without evidence of necrosis ℗ HCC RxHCC CC/MCC Exc

L97.908 Non-pressure chronic ulcer of unspecified part of unspecified lower leg with other specified severity ℗ HCC RxHCC CC/MCC Exc

L97.909 Non-pressure chronic ulcer of unspecified part of unspecified lower leg with unspecified severity ℗ HCC RxHCC CC/MCC Exc

6th L97.91 Non-pressure chronic ulcer of unspecified part of right lower leg

L97.911 Non-pressure chronic ulcer of unspecified part of right lower leg limited to breakdown of skin ℗ HCC RxHCC CC/MCC Exc

L97.912 Non-pressure chronic ulcer of unspecified part of right lower leg with fat layer exposed ℗ HCC RxHCC CC/MCC Exc

L97.913 Non-pressure chronic ulcer of unspecified part of right lower leg with necrosis of muscle ℗ HCC RxHCC CC/MCC Exc

L97.914 Non-pressure chronic ulcer of unspecified part of right lower leg with necrosis of bone ℗ HCC RxHCC CC/MCC Exc

L97.915 Non-pressure chronic ulcer of unspecified part of right lower leg with muscle involvement without evidence of necrosis ℗ HCC RxHCC CC/MCC Exc

L97.916 Non-pressure chronic ulcer of unspecified part of right lower leg with bone involvement without evidence of necrosis ℗ HCC RxHCC CC/MCC Exc

L97.918 Non-pressure chronic ulcer of unspecified part of right lower leg with other specified severity ℗ HCC RxHCC CC/MCC Exc

L97.919 Non-pressure chronic ulcer of unspecified part of right lower leg with unspecified severity ℗ HCC RxHCC CC/MCC Exc

6th L97.92 Non-pressure chronic ulcer of unspecified part of left lower leg

L97.921 Non-pressure chronic ulcer of unspecified part of left lower leg limited to breakdown of skin ℗ HCC RxHCC CC/MCC Exc

L97.922 Non-pressure chronic ulcer of unspecified part of left lower leg with fat layer exposed ℗ HCC RxHCC CC/MCC Exc

L97.923 Non-pressure chronic ulcer of unspecified part of left lower leg with necrosis of muscle ℗ HCC RxHCC CC/MCC Exc

L97.924 Non-pressure chronic ulcer of unspecified part of left lower leg with necrosis of bone ℗ HCC RxHCC CC/MCC Exc

L97.925 Non-pressure chronic ulcer of unspecified part of left lower leg with muscle involvement without evidence of necrosis ℗ HCC RxHCC CC/MCC Exc

L97.926 Non-pressure chronic ulcer of unspecified part of left lower leg with bone involvement without evidence of necrosis ℗ HCC RxHCC CC/MCC Exc

L97.928 Non-pressure chronic ulcer of unspecified part of left lower leg with other specified severity ℗ HCC RxHCC CC/MCC Exc

L97.929 Non-pressure chronic ulcer of unspecified part of left lower leg with unspecified severity ℗ HCC RxHCC CC/MCC Exc

4th L98 Other disorders of skin and subcutaneous tissue, not elsewhere classified

L98.0 Pyogenic granuloma

EXCLUDES2 pyogenic granuloma of gingiva (K06.8)

pyogenic granuloma of maxillary alveolar ridge (K04.5)

pyogenic granuloma of oral mucosa (K13.4)

L98.1 Factitial dermatitis

AHA: Q4 2016

Neurotic excoriation

EXCLUDES1 Excoriation (skin-picking) disorder (F42.4)

L98.2 Febrile neutrophilic dermatosis [Sweet]

L98.3 Eosinophilic cellulitis [Wells] ℗ CC/MCC Exc

5th L98.4 Non-pressure chronic ulcer of skin, not elsewhere classified

Chronic ulcer of skin NOS

Tropical ulcer NOS

Ulcer of skin NOS

EXCLUDES2 pressure ulcer (pressure area) (L89.-)

gangrene (I96)

skin infections (L00-L08)

specific infections classified to A00-B99

ulcer of lower limb NEC (L97.-)

varicose ulcer (I83.0-I82.2)

6th L98.41 Non-pressure chronic ulcer of buttock

L98.411 Non-pressure chronic ulcer of buttock limited to breakdown of skin HCC RxHCC

L98.412 Non-pressure chronic ulcer of buttock with fat layer exposed HCC RxHCC

L98.413 Non-pressure chronic ulcer of buttock with necrosis of muscle HCC RxHCC

L98.414 Non-pressure chronic ulcer of buttock with necrosis of bone HCC RxHCC

L98.415 Non-pressure chronic ulcer of buttock with muscle involvement without evidence of necrosis ℗ HCC RxHCC CC/MCC Exc

---

PDx Unacceptable principal diagnosis symbol per Medicare code edits POA Code exempt from diagnosis present on admission requirement
❓ Questionable admission ℗ Complication or comorbidity MCC Major complication or comorbidity CC/MCC Exc CC/MCC exclusion
HCC HCC diagnosis code RxHCC RxHCC diagnosis code MACRA code **DEFINITION** Describes condition/terminology
TIP Coding guidance 👁 Official Guideline Reference 1st Z code as first-listed diagnosis

L98.416   Non-pressure chronic ulcer of buttock with bone involvement without evidence of necrosis   cc⊘ HCC RxHCC CC/MCC Exc.

L98.418   Non-pressure chronic ulcer of buttock with other specified severity   cc⊘ HCC RxHCC CC/MCC Exc.

L98.419   Non-pressure chronic ulcer of buttock with unspecified severity   HCC RxHCC

6th   **L98.42**   Non-pressure chronic ulcer of back

L98.421   Non-pressure chronic ulcer of back limited to breakdown of skin   HCC RxHCC

L98.422   Non-pressure chronic ulcer of back with fat layer exposed   HCC RxHCC

L98.423   Non-pressure chronic ulcer of back with necrosis of muscle   HCC RxHCC

L98.424   Non-pressure chronic ulcer of back with necrosis of bone   HCC RxHCC

L98.425   Non-pressure chronic ulcer of back with muscle involvement without evidence of necrosis   cc⊘ HCC RxHCC CC/MCC Exc.

L98.426   Non-pressure chronic ulcer of back with bone involvement without evidence of necrosis   cc⊘ HCC RxHCC CC/MCC Exc.

L98.428   Non-pressure chronic ulcer of back with other specified severity   cc⊘ HCC RxHCC CC/MCC Exc.

L98.429   Non-pressure chronic ulcer of back with unspecified severity   HCC RxHCC

6th   **L98.49**   **Non-pressure chronic ulcer of skin of other sites**
Non-pressure chronic ulcer of skin NOS

L98.491   Non-pressure chronic ulcer of skin of other sites limited to breakdown of skin   HCC RxHCC

L98.492   Non-pressure chronic ulcer of skin of other sites with fat layer exposed   HCC RxHCC

L98.493   Non-pressure chronic ulcer of skin of other sites with necrosis of muscle   HCC RxHCC

L98.494   Non-pressure chronic ulcer of skin of other sites with necrosis of bone   HCC RxHCC

L98.495   Non-pressure chronic ulcer of skin of other sites with muscle involvement without evidence of necrosis   cc⊘ HCC RxHCC CC/MCC Exc.

L98.496   Non-pressure chronic ulcer of skin of other sites with bone involvement without evidence of necrosis   cc⊘ HCC RxHCC CC/MCC Exc.

L98.498   Non-pressure chronic ulcer of skin of other sites with other specified severity   cc⊘ HCC RxHCC CC/MCC Exc.

L98.499   Non-pressure chronic ulcer of skin of other sites with unspecified severity   HCC RxHCC

L98.5   **Mucinosis of the skin**
Focal mucinosis
Lichen myxedematosus
Reticular erythematous mucinosis
EXCLUDES1   focal oral mucinosis (K13.79)
         myxedema (E03.9)

L98.6   **Other infiltrative disorders of the skin and subcutaneous tissue**
EXCLUDES1   hyalinosis cutis et mucosae (E78.89)

L98.7   **Excessive and redundant skin and subcutaneous tissue**
AHA: Q4 2016
Loose or sagging skin following bariatric surgery weight loss
Loose or sagging skin following dietary weight loss
Loose or sagging skin, NOS
EXCLUDES2   acquired excess or redundant skin of eyelid (H02.3-)
         congenital excess or redundant skin of eyelid (Q10.3)
         skin changes due to chronic exposure to nonionizing radiation (L57.-)

L98.8   **Other specified disorders of the skin and subcutaneous tissue**

L98.9   **Disorder of the skin and subcutaneous tissue, unspecified**

L99   **Other disorders of skin and subcutaneous tissue in diseases classified elsewhere**
AHA: Q4 2016
☞ Code first underlying disease, such as:
     amyloidosis (E85.-)
EXCLUDES1   skin disorders in diabetes (E08-E13 with .62)
         skin disorders in gonorrhea (A54.89)
         skin disorders in syphilis (A51.31, A52.79)

Unspecified Code   Other Specified Code   Manifestation Code   N Newborn   P Pediatric   M Maternity   A Adult   ♂ Male   ♀ Female
● New Code   ▲ Revised Code Title   ►◄ Revised Text   NOTES   INCLUDES   EXCLUDES1 Not coded here   EXCLUDES2 Not included here
4th 4th character required   5th 5th character required   6th 6th character required   7th 7th character required   7x Extension 'X' Alert
HAC Hospital-acquired condition (HAC) alert   AHA AHA Coding Clinic®   ☞ Code first alert

NOTES

Chapter 13: Diseases of the Musculoskeletal System and Connective Tissue (M00-M99)

Anatomy of the Musculoskeletal System

Introduction

Osteology (Osteo: bone; logy: study) is the branch of anatomy that deals with the detailed analysis of structure, function and diseases of the skeletal elements. It constitutes the bony framework of the body. The human bony skeleton is composed of the below mentioned components (and is derived from the mesoderm, which is the primary germ cell layer).

Skeletal Region	Body Structure	Quantity of bones
Axial Skeleton (the trunk)	Skull	22
	Hyoid Bone	1
	Ribs & Sternum	25
	Vertebral Column	26
Appendicular Skeleton (the limbs)	Upper Extremities	64
	Lower Extremities	62
Auditory Ossicles		6

1. Structure of a Normal Human Bone

Bone is comprised of a rigid structure, which is based on dense connective tissue. A normal human bone is made up of the following essential macro and micro elements:

a) Periosteum
b) Medullary Membrane
c) Marrow
d) Blood Vessels and Nerves of Bone
e) Haversian Canals (Canals of Havers)
f) Lamellae
g) Lacunae
h) Canaliculi
i) Perichondrium
j) Osteoblasts
k) Osteoclasts
l) Medullary spaces
m) Epiphysis
n) Diaphysis
o) Metaphysis

2. The Vertebral Column

The vertebral column is composed of a continuous series of compact bones that articulate with each other via intervertebral discs, and are called vertebrae. The structure forms the dorsal aspect of the trunk. The vertebral column is also called spine. The spinal cord traverses through the spinal canal of the vertebral column. The individual vertebrae remain connected together by intervertebral discs. The cervical, thoracic, and lumbar vertebrae are termed true vertebrae. However, sacral and coccygeal ones are false vertebrae. The concept behind considering them as true or false is based on mobility of the individual vertebrae through intervertebral discs. Cervical, thoracic and lumbar vertebrae are moveable to some extent and therefore termed as true vertebral bodies. In contrast, the sacral-coccygeal section is rather fixed and thus not categorized as true vertebrae. Each vertebral segment is associated with a portion of spinal cord, which travels the entire vertebral column, and each spinal cord segment has specific physiology and functions. The vertebral bodies communicate with each other through the pads of elastic fibro-cartilage. These flexible pads constitute the intervertebral discs, which help in the movement of vertebral bodies and provide protection from trauma or shocks. However, the length of the adult vertebral column ranges from 60-70 cm. The entire vertebral column is based on a total of 33 vertebrae that are categorized in accordance with the occupied region.

a) **Cervical Vertebrae**

These are small and delicate bones, which are marked by the existence of a foramen in every transverse process. The cervical region is based on the seven cervical bones (C1-C7). However, the first cervical vertebra is known as Atlas and the second one is Axis.

b) **Thoracic Vertebrae**

Thoracic vertebrae are 12 in quantity (T1–T12), and communicate with the head (tubercles) of ribs in the thoracic region through articular facets of the transverse processes. Their body structure is similar to the shape of the heart, with nearly circular vertebral foramina.

c) **Lumbar Vertebrae**

These are five vertebrae (L1-L5), with kidney shaped bodies. Lumbar vertebrae are in fact the most toughest and robust in configuration. These are enlarged in size and marked by the absence of a transverse process foramen and vertebral facets. These are true vertebrae, thereby allowing flexion and extension movements via flexible intervertebral discs. Their broad lamellae, large bodies, long transverse processes, and strong pedicles make them suitable to support additional body weight as compared to other similar vertebrae.

d) **Sacral Vertebrae**

These are five vertebral bodies (S1-S5), which constitute a portion of the pelvic cavity. Sacral vertebral bodies consist of five separate segments that get fused together at maturity. As a matter of fact, these vertebrae lack intervertebral discs, which restrict their mobility and put them into the category of false vertebrae.

e) **Coccygeal Vertebrae**

The four coccygeal vertebrae constitute the human vestigial tail bone, in which vertebral bodies are fused together without the existence of any intervertebral disc. Movement of the individual vertebral bodies is restricted due to their interfusion. Hence, these are considered as false vertebrae. The number of bones in the coccygeal region may rarely vary between three to five vertebrae, in few individuals.

3. Thorax

The part of the trunk situated between the neck and abdomen constitutes the thorax. The thoracic cavity is bounded by ribs, sternum, costal cartilages, and the thoracic vertebrae. The thorax is also known as the chest region. The osseocartilaginous cage of the thorax covers and protects the prime organs of circulation and respiration. Furthermore, this osseocartilaginous cage is composed mainly of the ribcage, shoulder girdle, and spine.

The 12 thoracic vertebrae and certain component of the ribs constitute the posterior (back) wall of the thoracic cavity. However, the anterior (front) region is composed of sternum and the costal cartilages. The entire human chest (thorax) region contains multiple organs, muscles, bones, vasculature, internal and external structures. These contents include heart, lungs, thymus, pectoral muscles, scapula, sternum, ribs, aorta, trachea, diaphragm, and mammary glands etc.

4. Sternum (Chest or Breast Bone)

a) The sternum is a flat and long bone situated in the center of the thorax and forms the midline of the anterior thoracic cage. It articulates with both clavicles (collar bones) through its upper ends. It is composed of the following three (interfused) components:

i) manubrium
ii) body (gladiolus/corpus sterni)
iii) xiphoid process (processus xiphoideus/ensiform or xiphoid appendix) ribs.

b) Ribs are the elongated, flattened, lightweight, resilient, and twisted bones that are the essential constituent of the thoracic skeleton. The total number of ribs in the human body is 24 (12 on each side). The ribs can be classified as follows:

i) True ribs-These are also called vertebrosternal ribs. True ribs comprise the first seven ribs that communicate (to the dorsum) with the vertebral column as well as sternum (in front) via costal cartilages.

ii) False ribs-These are also called vertebrochondral ribs. False ribs comprise the eighth, ninth, and tenth ribs that are indirectly attached to the sternum through costal cartilages. The individual cartilages of each of these ribs are connected to the cartilage of the rib lying just above them.

iii) Floating ribs-These are also termed vertebral ribs. These ribs include the 11th and 12th ribs that are free at their anterior extremities (without any attachment with the sternum) and are connected to the vertebral bodies on their dorsal ends.

5. **The Skull**
The human skull is based on the skeleton of the head. Several bones of the skull integrate together to form the cranium (or the skull). The skull can be categorized as follows:

a) **The Brain Box or Brain Case (The Calvaria)**

The brain box constitutes the upper cranium and contains the brain.

b) **The Facial Skeleton**

The facial skeleton comprises the portion of skull (other than the brain box) and includes the mandible bone of the face.

The Composition of Human Skull

The Calvaria			
Paired Bones		**Unpaired Bones**	
i)	Parietal	i)	Frontal
ii)	Temporal	ii)	Occipital
		iii)	Sphenoid
		iv)	Ethmoid

The Facial Skeleton			
Paired Bones		**Unpaired Bones**	
i)	Maxilla	i)	Mandible
ii)	Zygomatic	ii)	Vomer
iii)	Nasal		
iv)	Lacrimal		
v)	Palatine		
vi)	Inferior Nasal Concha		

c) **The Facial Bones**

The facial skeleton comprises the lower and anterior portion of the human skull and includes the following bones:

i) nasal bones

ii) maxillae (upper jaw)

iii) lacrimal bone

iv) zygomatic bone

v) palatine bone

vi) inferior nasal concha

vii) vomer

viii) mandible (lower jaw)

ix) hyoid bone

6. **The Bones of the Upper Extremity**
a) **Clavicle**

The clavicle is also called the collar bone that forms the anterior portion of the shoulder girdle. The clavicles are two in number and called the right and left clavicles.

b) **Scapula**

The scapula is also called the shoulder blade and constitutes the back portion of the shoulder girdle. It is a flat bone that articulates with the clavicle and humerus. It also contains a triangular process that projects laterally and is called the acromion. Additionally, the upper part of the neck of the scapula contains a curved process, which is known as the coracoid process. The scapulae are two in number (right and left scapula).

c) **Humerus**

The humerus is the long bone of the arm that begins from the shoulder and ends up at the elbow. It is the largest bone of the upper extremity and consists of the following major components:

i) greater tubercle (greater tuberosity)

ii) lesser tubercle (lesser tuberosity)

iii) body or shaft (corpus humeri)

iv) anterior, lateral, and medial borders

v) medial and lateral epicondyles

vi) radial sulcus (musculospiral groove)

vii) lateral and medial supracondylar ridges

viii) deltoid tuberosity.

d) **Ulna**

The ulna is one of the two long and prismatic bones of the forearm that extends parallel with the radius. The ulna possesses a body and two extremities. The proximal or upper extremity contains olecranon and coronoid processes, and the semilunar and radial notches respectively. The body or shaft of the ulna is also known as the corpus ulnae. The lower or distal extremity is comprised of an articular eminence (the head of the ulna) and a nonarticular eminence (the styloid process).

e) **Radius**

The radius is one of the two long bones of the forearm that extends laterally with the ulna. Its lower end participates in the formation of the wrist joint and upper end helps to create the elbow joint. The upper or proximal extremity consists of a head, neck, and tuberosity. The body or shaft is also known as the corpus radii. The lateral surface of the lower extremity contains a conical projection, which is known as the styloid process.

f) **Carpus**

The carpus region of the hand contains the carpal bones, which consist of a total of eight bones positioned in proximal and distal rows to facilitate uninterrupted movement of the wrist joint. The carpal bones of the proximal row are: navicular, lunate, triangular, and pisiform. The bones of the distal row are: greater multangular, lesser multangular, capitate, and hamate.

g) **Metacarpus**

The metacarpus region of hand is based on cylindrical (metacarpal) bones that are five in number and constitute the intermediary portion of the bony skeleton of hand. The first through fifth metacarpal bones belong to the thumb, index, middle, ring and little fingers respectively.

h) **Phalanges of the Hand**

The phalanges (finger bones) of the hand constitute the fingers. These are 14 in number. Each finger consists of three phalanges. However, the thumb consists of only two phalanges. A single finger bone has a body, with two extremities. The finger bones serve to facilitate the basic functions of the hand, like-effective grasping of objects and writing, etc.

7. **The Bones of the Lower Extremity**
a) **Hip Bone**

The hip bone is also known as the coxal bone. It's based on three components: ilium, ischium, and pubis. The ilium holds the flank. It is the broad portion situated on top of the large cup-shaped articular cavity, the acetabulum. The ischium forms the lower back part of the hip bone that facilitates sitting. It's located downward from the acetabulum and is the strongest component of the hip bone, containing an enlarged opening, the obturator foramen. The pubis is the lower frontal portion of the hip bone, which is located medially below the acetabulum. It supports the internal organs of reproduction. The angle across the pubic symphysis is known as the pubic arch.

b) **Pelvis**

The pelvis consists of a bony ring that provides a connecting medium between the vertebral column and femurs. It is based on the following 4 bones:

i) The hip bones are two in number.

ii) The sacrum-The fused vertebrae that are five in number and connected to the hip bones.

iii) The coccyx-The fused vertebrae that are four in number and constitute the tailbone.

The space surrounded by the pelvic girdle is known as the pelvic cavity. The pelvic girdle bears the entire weight of the trunk and upper body while sitting and transfers this weight to the lower limbs during standing, walking, or running.

c) **Femur**

The femur is one of the two largest, longest, and strongest bones in the human skeleton that bears the load of the upper body via the pelvis in standing, walking, or running. It also participates in the formation of the hip and knee joints. The components of a normal femur bone are as follows:

The Upper (Proximal) Extremity consists of the following elements:

i) Head

ii) Neck

iii) Greater Trochanter

iv) Lesser Trochanter

The Body or Shaft-The body is cylindrical in shape, lies between the upper and lower extremities and is also known as corpus femoris.

The Lower (Distal) Extremity -The distal extremity is based on two projections (the lateral and medial condyles). These projections (condyles) are separated in front by an articular depression, known as the patellar surface. The same condyles are further interrupted from behind by a deep pit, which is termed as the intercondyloid fossa.

d) **Patella**

The knee cap (patella) is a flat, thick, circular-triangular, and dense cancellous articular bone that is situated on the frontal portion of the knee joint. The superior border is thick and forms the base of patella. The patella is further marked by medial and lateral borders. The apex of patella is a pointed region that provides attachment to the patellar ligament. The patella articulates with the femur through the patellofemoral joint.

e) **Tibia**

The tibia (shin bone) is located medially in the lower leg and is regarded as the largest and strongest bone of the skeleton after the femur. It also participates in the formation of the knee and ankle joints. The tibia is composed of the following elements:

i) upper (proximal) end – The proximal extremity is composed of the projections, which are known as the medial and lateral condyles. The condylar surfaces further merge to form an eminence on the frontal side, which is known as the tibial tuberosity.

ii) body or shaft of tibia – The shaft of the tibia is also known as corpus tibiae and contains the anterior crest (or border), the medial border, and the interosseous crest (or lateral border).

iii) lower (distal) end – The distal extremity contains the inferior articular surface, the anterior surface, the posterior surface, the lateral surface, and the medial surface. However, the medial surface extends medially to form a pyramidal process, which is termed as the medial malleolus.

f) **Fibula**

The fibula (calf bone) is located laterally in the lower leg and runs laterally with the adjacent shin bone (tibia). It's a thin and slender bone which is composed of a body with upper and lower extremities. The lower or distal extremity constitutes the lateral malleolus, which is also known as the external malleolus or malleolus lateralis.

g) **Tarsus**

The tarsus region of foot is based on the following seven tarsal bones:

i) calcaneus

ii) talus

iii) cuboid

iv) navicular

v) three cuneiforms

h) **Phalanges of the Foot**

The phalanges of the foot constitute the region of forefoot. These are also known as the toe bones. The great toe (hallux) contains two phalanges (proximal and distal). The proximal and distal phalangeal bones of the great toe articulate with each other to form the first interphalangeal joint. The proximal phalanges of the other toes articulate with their respective metatarsal heads to form the metatarsophalangeal joints.

8. **Syndesmology (The Articulations or Joints)**

Syndesmology is defined as the branch of anatomy that deals with the joints and their components (including ligaments). The junctions of bones, where multiple parts of the individual bones connect together, are called articulations or joints. These articulations are further supported by sheets of tough fibrous tissue that connect the joint bones together and are termed ligaments. Various components of the joints are listed below:

a) **Bones**

b) **Cartilages**

The cartilages are flexible nonvascular structures composed of connective tissue and found mainly in joints. A cartilage can be categorized into the following elements:

i) Hyaline cartilage

ii) White fibrocartilage

The white fibrocartilage can further be categorized into four subcategories:

a) interarticular fibrocartilage

b) connecting fibrocartilage

c) circumferential fibrocartilage

d) stratiform fibrocartilage

iii) Yellow or elastic fibrocartilage

c) **Articular Capsule**

The articular capsule is also known as the joint capsule that completely covers and protects the freely movable (synovial) joints.

d) **Mucous Sheaths**

The mucous sheaths cover a part of the fibroosseous canals and surface of the tendons that glide upon these canals to facilitate the movement of these tendons on their respective canals.

9. **Classification of Joints**

The joints can be classified into the following three classes:

a) Synarthroses (Immovable Joints)

b) Amphiarthroses (Slightly Movable Joints)

c) Diarthroses (Freely Movable Joints)

10. **Joints of the Trunk**

a) **Joints between Vertebral Bodies**

The articulations between the individual vertebral bodies are based on the amphiarthrodial (slightly movable) intervertebral joints that possess only a very slight degree of mobility.

b) **Joints between Vertebral Arches**

The articulations between the individual vertebral arches are carried out through the two pairs of articular processes. The articular processes of a typical vertebral arch connect together with the articular processes of the adjacent vertebral arch to form true diarthrosis of arthrodial variety.

c) **Joints of the Atlas with the Axis**

The atlas forms three diarthroses with the axis. Moreover, the articulations of the axis with the atlas are known as the Atlantoaxial articulations.

d) **Joints of the Vertebral Column with the Cranium**

The atlas forms two articulations (known as diarthrosis) with the occipital bone. The occipital condyles interact with the articular surfaces of the atlas to constitute diarthroses. The synovial stratum covers the articular capsules around the condyles of the occipital bone.

e) **Joints of the Mandible**

The temporomandibular articulation forms an arthrodial diarthrosis. The temporal mandibular fossa and mandibular condyle interact together to constitute the temporomandibular articulation.

f) **Joints of the Ribs with the Vertebrae**

The head and tubercle of a typical rib articulates with the vertebral column to form a costovertebral articulation.

g) **Joints of the Vertebral Column with the Pelvis**

The fifth lumbar vertebra connects with the sacrum to form the lumbosacral articulation. The inner lip of the iliac crest connects with the transverse processes of the fifth lumbar vertebra through iliolumbar ligament.

h) **Joints of the Pelvis**

The articulations of the pelvis are mainly based on the following types of joints:

i) symphysis pubis

The two pubic bones articulate with each other to constitute a joint, which is known as the symphysis pubis.

ii) sacroiliac articulation

The auricular surfaces of sacrum and ilium connect with each other to form an amphiarthrodial joint, which is termed as the sacroiliac articulation.

iii) sacrococcygeal symphysis

The apex of the sacrum and base of the coccyx articulate with each other to form an amphiarthrodial joint, which is known as the sacrococcygeal symphysis.

11. Joints of Upper Extremity

a) The Acromioclavicular Joint

The medial aspect of the acromion (of the scapula) connects with the acromial end of the clavicle to constitute the acromioclavicular articulation. However, this type of joint is categorized as an arthrodial diarthrosis.

b) The Shoulder Joint

The humeral articulation constitutes the shoulder joint, which is an enarthrodial (ball and socket) joint and considered as the largest joint of the upper limb. The shoulder joint offers an extended range of movement and is composed of the articular head of humerus and the shallow glenoid cavity of the scapula. The ligaments of the shoulder joint include the articular capsule (capsular ligament), glenoid labrum (glenoid ligament) as well as the glenohumeral, coracohumeral, and transverse humeral ligaments.

c) The Elbow Joint

The elbow articulation falls under the category of hinge joint (ginglymus diarthrosis). The elbow joint performs the flexion and extension movements around a transversely placed single axis. The elbow joint consists of the humerus, ulna, and radius bones. An elbow joint is formed when the trochlea of humerus connects with the semilunar notch of ulna and the capitulum of humerus interacts with the cup (shallow-depression or fovea) on the proximal aspect of the head of the radius. The articular surfaces of the elbow joint are enclosed by and interact with each other through a well-defined articular capsule.

d) The Radioulnar Joint

The radioulnar joint is based on two articulations positioned at the proximal and distal ends of the radius and ulna. These articulations facilitate the rotational movements of the radius around its longitudinal axis to constitute a uniaxial diarthrosis, which is known as lateral ginglymus.

e) The Radiocarpal Joint

The radiocarpal articulation is also known as the wrist joint, which is a type of condyloid articulation. The distal (lower) end of radius, discus articularis (the articular disc), and the proximal articular surfaces of navicular, lunate and triquetral bones (including their interosseous ligaments) together constitute the wrist articulation. Moreover, the wrist joint is completely encapsulated by the articular capsule.

f) The Intercarpal Joint

The carpal joints are based on the articulations between the carpal bones with limited range of movement. These joints consist of the arthrodial diarthroses and are therefore known as the gliding joints. The carpal bone articulations are characterized as follows:

i) Proximal Row (Carpal) Joint

ii) Distal Row (Carpal) Joint

iii) Transverse (Carpal) Joint

g) The Carpometacarpal joint

The Carpometacarpal (CMC) joints are based on the interaction between the carpal and metacarpal bones. However, the carpometacarpal articulation of the thumb region differs from the articulations of the other four metacarpal bones with the carpus. Therefore, the carpometacarpal articulations can be categorized as follows:

h) The Joints of the other Four Metacarpal Bones with the Carpus

These types of carpometacarpal articulations are formed by the connections between the bases of the second, third, fourth, and fifth medial metacarpal bones and the four bones of the distal carpal row.

i) The Intermetacarpal Joints

The four medial metacarpal bones articulate with each other to form the arthrodial diarthroses, which are known as the intermetacarpal joints.

j) The Metacarpophalangeal Joints

With the exception of the thumb, the spherical head of each metacarpal bone articulates with the shallow oval cavity on the base of the first phalanx to constitute the metacarpophalangeal joints. The metacarpophalangeal articulations facilitate flexion, extension, adduction, abduction, and circumduction type of joint movements.

k) The Joints of the Digits

The interphalangeal joints are categorized as hinge joints that are two in number for each finger and only one for the thumb. The interphalangeal joints can perform movements like flexion and extension.

12. Joints of the Lower Extremity

a) The Hip Joint

The coxal articulation constitutes the hip joint, which is a type of enarthrodial diarthrosis (ball and socket joint). The articular surfaces of the hip joint consists of the head of the femur and a cup shaped cavity (acetabulum) that connect together to constitute the coxal articulation. The hip joint can perform multi-axial movements like rotation, flexion, extension, abduction, and adduction. The hip joint cavity is completely encapsulated by an articular capsule or the capsular ligament. Other ligaments of the hip joint are described below:

i) iliofemoral ligament (ligamentum iliofemorale/Y-ligament/ligament of Bigelow)

ii) pubocapsular ligament (ligamentum pubocapsulare/pubofemoral ligament)

iii) ischiocapsular ligament (ligamentum ischiocapsulare/ischiocapsular band/ligament of Bertin)

iv) ligamentum teres femoris

v) glenoidal labrum (labrum glenoidale/cotyloid ligament)

vi) transverse acetabular ligament (ligamentum transversum acetabuli/transverse ligament)

b) The Knee Joint

The knee articulation/joint is considered as the largest articulation in the human body and related to the ginglymus (hinge) variety of diarthroses. However, its structure is more elaborate and complicated. The articular surfaces of the knee joint pertain to specific portions of the femur, tibia and patella bones. The ligaments associated with the knee joint are as follows:

i) articular capsule (capsula articularis/capsular ligament)

ii) ligamentum patellae (anterior ligament)

iii) oblique popliteal ligament (ligamentum popliteum obliquum/posterior ligament)

iv) tibial collateral ligament (ligamentum collaterale tibiale/internal lateral ligament)

v) fibular collateral ligament (ligamentum collaterale fibulare/external lateral or long external lateral ligament)

vi) anterior cruciate ligament (ligamentum cruciatum anterius/external crucial ligament)

vii) posterior cruciate ligament (ligamentum cruciatum posterius/internal crucial ligament)

viii) medial meniscus (meniscus medialis/internal semilunar fibrocartilage)

ix) lateral meniscus (meniscus lateralis/external semilunar fibrocartilage)

x) transverse ligament (ligamentum transversum genu)

xi) coronary ligaments

xii) synovial membrane encapsulates the upper border of the patella and the lower portion of the front of the femur. The movements associated with the knee joint are flexion, extension, internal, and external rotation.

c) The Joints between Tibia and Fibula

The articulations between the tibia and fibula constitute the tibiofibular joints. The fibula articulates with the tibia through its proximal and distal ends. The proximal tibiofibular joint is an arthrodial articulation between head of the fibula and lateral condyle of the tibia. The interosseous membrane acts as an accessory ligament to bind the shafts of tibia and fibula together. However, the tibiofibular syndesmosis constitutes the distal tibiofibular joint, which presents a series of ligaments that are accessory to the ankle joint.

d) The Talocrural Joint

The talocrural articulation constitutes the ankle joint, which is a ginglymus variety of diarthrosis. In other words, the ankle joint is a type of hinge joint. The ankle joint facilitates the movements like dorsiflexion and extension.

e) The Intertarsal Joints

The intertarsal articulations (joints) are diarthroses that facilitate the gliding movements of the foot. These joints can be categorized in the following manner:

i) talocalcaneal joint

ii) talocalcaneonavicular joint

iii) calcaneocuboid joint

iv)   cuneonavicular joint

v)   cuboideonavicular joint

vi)   intercuneiform and cuneocuboid joint

f)   **The Tarsometatarsal Joint**

The tarsometatarsal joints include the articular surfaces of the cuneiform, the cuboid, and the metatarsal bones. The articular facets of the three cuneiform and cuboid bones connect with the bases of the five metatarsal bones to constitute the tarsometatarsal articulations.

g)   **The Intermetatarsal Joint**

The articular facets on the bases of the four metatarsal bones connect with each other via dorsal, plantar, and interosseous ligaments to form the intermetatarsal joints. However, no ligament acts to connect the first metatarsal base with the second one.

h)   **The Metatarsophalangeal Joint**

The metatarsophalangeal joints are types of modified ball and socket articulations, wherein globular heads of metatarsal bones articulate with the shallow cups upon the bases of the first phalanges via plantar and collateral ligaments. These joints are encapsulated by an articular capsule.

i)   **The Joints of the Digits**

The articulations between the digits constitute the interphalangeal joints. The phalanges of the toes connect with each other to form the interphalangeal articulations. The great toe possesses only one interphalangeal joint. However, every other toe (except great toe) comprises of two interphalangeal joints.

13. The Muscular System

The muscle cells of the human body facilitate the movements of various body parts through their special function of contraction in response to a requisite external or internal stimulus. These muscle cells can be characterized under the below mentioned three different classes:

a)   **Striated Muscle Cells**

The striated muscle cells are those voluntary muscle cells that constitute the skeletal muscular system.

b)   **Non-Striated Muscle Cells**

The nonstriated muscle cells are those involuntary muscle cells that occur in the vessel walls and hollow viscera.

c)   **Cardiac Muscle Cells**

The cardiac muscle cells consist of those striated cells that constitute the substance of the heart. However, these muscle cells are involuntary in nature.

14. The Muscles of the Trunk

The muscles of the back are based on the following group of muscles:

a)   **Splenius**

The splenius muscles constitute the superficial layer of the intrinsic back muscles that occupy the back of neck and upper portion of the thoracic region. The splenius muscles overlap the vertical muscles like a bandage and have the following two types:

i)   splenius capitis

ii)   splenius cervicis

b)   **Sacrospinalis (Erector Spinae)**

The erector spinae muscles are positioned in a groove between the angle of the ribs and spinal processes on each side of the vertebral column. The erector spinae is divided into the following three muscle columns:

c)   **Iliocostalis**

The lateral column is further divided into the following muscle components:

i)   iliocostalis lumborum (iliocostalis/sacrolumbalis muscle)

ii)   iliocostalis dorsi (musculus accessorius)

iii)   iliocostalis cervicis (cervicalis ascendens)

d)   **Longissimus**

i)   longissimus dorsi

ii)   longissimus cervicis (transversalis cervicis)

iii)   longissimus capitis (trachelomastoid muscle)

e)   **Spinalis**

i)   spinalis dorsi

ii)   spinalis cervicis (spinalis coli)

iii)   spinalis capitis (biventer cervicis)

f)   **Semispinalis**

The semispinalis constitutes the deeper layer of intrinsic back muscles. These muscles originate from half of the vertebral column and are categorized into three distinct parts:

i)   semispinalis dorsi

ii)   semispinalis cervicis (semispinalis colli)

iii)   semispinalis capitis (complexus)

g)   **Multifidus (Multifidus Spinae)**

The multifidus consists of short triangular muscular bundles that remain apparent from sacrum to the axis.

h)   **Rotatores (Rotatores Spinae)**

It remains confined in the thoracic region.

i)   Interspinales and Intertransversarii (Intertransversales) are best developed and most distinct in the cervical region and considered as the smallest of the deep back muscles.

15. The Muscles of the Pelvis

The muscles of the pelvis include the following:

a)   Obturator Internus

b)   Piriformis

c)   Levator Ani (Pubococcygeus and Iliococcygeus)

d)   Coccygeus (Ischiococcygeus)

16. The Muscles of the Upper Extremity

a)   **The Muscles that Connect the Upper Extremity to the Vertebral Column are Defined Below:**

i)   trapezius

ii)   rhomboideus major

iii)   latissimus dorsi

iv)   rhomboideus minor

v)   levator scapulae

b)   **The Muscles Connecting the Upper Extremity to the Anterior and Lateral Thoracic Walls**

i)   pectoralis major

ii)   subclavius

iii)   pectoralis minor

iv)   serratus anterior

c)   **The Muscles of the Shoulder**

i)   Deltoid muscle originates from the lateral third portion of clavicle, the acromion, and the spine of scapula. However, it gets inserted into the deltoid tuberosity of humerus. This muscle facilitates the abduction and medial and lateral rotation of the arm.

ii)   Subscapularis muscle originates from the subscapular fossa that forms the ventral surface of scapula. However, it gets inserted into the lesser tubercle of humerus. The subscapularis helps to medially rotate and adduct the arm and fixes the humeral head in the glenoid cavity (of the scapula).

iii)   Supraspinatus muscle originates from the supraspinatus fossa of scapula and gets inserted into the superior facet of greater tubercle of humerus. This muscle assists the deltoid in the abduction of the arm.

iv)   Infraspinatus muscle arises from the infraspinatus fossa of scapula and gets inserted into the middle facet of the greater tubercle of humerus. This muscle helps in the lateral rotation of the arm and fixes the head of humerus into the glenoid cavity of scapula.

v)   Teres Minor muscle originates from the middle portion of lateral border of scapula and gets inserted into the inferior facet of greater tubercle of humerus. Like infraspinatus, teres minor muscle also helps in the lateral rotation of the arm and fixes the head of humerus into the glenoid cavity of scapula.

vi)   Teres Major muscle arises from the posterior surface of the inferior angle of scapula and gets inserted into the medial lip of the intertubercular groove of humerus. This muscle facilitates the adduction and medial rotation of the arm.

d)   **The Muscles of the Arm**

i)   coracobrachialis

ii)   biceps brachii

iii)   brachialis

iv)   triceps brachii

e) **The Muscles of the Anterior Compartment of the Forearm Superficial (First) Layer**

   i)   pronator teres

   ii)   flexor carpi radialis

   iii)   the palmaris longus

   iv)   flexor carpi ulnaris

f) **The Muscle of the Anterior Compartment of the Forearm Intermediate (Second) Layer**

   i)   flexor digitorum superficialis

g) **The Muscles of the Anterior Compartment of the Forearm Deep (Third) Layer**

   i)   flexor digitorum profundus

   ii)   flexor pollicis longus

   iii)   pronator quadrates

h) **The Muscles of the Posterior Compartment of Forearm of the Superficial Layer**

   i)   brachioradialis

   ii)   extensor carpi radialis longus

   iii)   extensor carpi radialis brevis

   iv)   extensor digitorum

   v)   extensor digiti minimi

   vi)   extensor carpi ulnaris

i) **The Muscles of the Posterior Compartment of the Forearm Deep Layer**

   i)   supinator

   ii)   abductor pollicis longus

   iii)   extensor pollicis longus

   iv)   extensor pollicis brevis

   v)   extensor indicis

j) **The Muscles of the Hand: Thenar Muscles**

   i)   opponens pollicis

   ii)   abductor pollicis brevis

   iii)   flexor pollicis brevis

   iv)   adductor pollicis

   Hypothenar Muscles

   i)   abductor digiti minimi

   ii)   flexor digiti minimi Brevis

   iii)   opponens digiti minimi

k) **The Short Muscles**

   i)   Lumbricals

   ii)   Dorsal Interossei

   iii)   Palmar Interossei

17. The Muscles of the Thigh

a) **Anterior Thigh Muscles**

The below mentioned anterior thigh muscles are based on the anterior compartment of thigh:

   i)   pectineus

   ii)   iliopsoas

   iii)   psoas major

   iv)   iliacus

   v)   femoris

   vi)   vastus lateralis

   vii)   vastus intermedius

   viii)   vastus medialis

b) **Medial Thigh Muscles**

   i)   adductor longus

   ii)   adductor brevis

   iii)   adductor magnus

   iv)   gracilis

   v)   obturator externus

c) **Gluteal Region Muscles**

   i)   gluteus maximus

   ii)   gluteus medius

   iii)   gluteus minimus

   iv)   tensor fasciae latae

   v)   piriformis

   vi)   obturator internus

   vii)   superior and inferior gemelli

   viii)   quadratus femoris

d) **Posterior Thigh Muscles**

   i)   semitendinosus

   ii)   semimembranosus

   iii)   biceps femoris (long head)

e) **The Muscles of the Anterior Compartment of the Leg**

   i)   tibialis anterior

   ii)   extensor hallucis longus

   iii)   extensor digitorum longus

   iv)   fibularis tertius

f) **The Muscles of the Lateral Compartment of the Leg**

   i)   fibularis longus

   ii)   fibularis brevis

g) **The Superficial Muscles of the Posterior Compartment of the Leg**

   i)   gastrocnemius

   ii)   soleus

   iii)   plantaris

h) **The Deep Muscles of the Leg**

   i)   Popliteus

   ii)   Flexor Hallucis Longus

   iii)   Flexor Digitorum Longus

   iv)   Tibialis Posterior

i) **First Layer Muscles of the Foot**

   i)   abductor hallucis

   ii)   flexor digitorum brevis

   iii)   abductor digiti minimi

j) **Second Layer Muscles of the Foot**

   i)   quadratus plantae

   ii)   lumbricals

k) **Third Layer Muscles of the Foot**

   i)   flexor hallucis brevis

   ii)   adductor hallucis

   iii)   flexor digiti minimi brevis

l) **Fourth Layer Muscles of the Foot**

   i)   plantar interossei (three muscles)

   ii)   dorsal interossei (four muscles)

m) **Muscles of the Dorsum of Foot**

   i)   extensor digitorum brevis

   ii)   extensor hallucis brevis

Common Pathologies

Rotator Cuff Tendinitis

Rotator cuff tendinitis, often with inflammation of the subacromial bursa overlying it, is the most common cause of shoulder pain other than trauma. In rotator cuff tendinitis, also known as impingement syndrome, the rotator cuff degenerates from rubbing against the acromion and/or the acromioclavicular joint. This results in irritation of the tendons and inflammation of the normally smooth bursa that line the tendons. Symptoms include pain, swelling, and tenderness at the front of the shoulder.

Frozen Shoulder

Frozen shoulder, also called adhesive capsulitis, causes pain and stiffness in the shoulder. It is characterized by progressive pain and global loss of motion in the shoulder. Movement of the shoulder is severely restricted. Pain is usually constant, worse at night. Inflammation of the capsule restricts movement of the bones in the shoulder joint. The pathophysiology of frozen shoulder is still unclear. As the condition progresses, the stiffness may continue to the point where range of motion can be severely limited.

De Quervain's Tenosynovitis

De Quervain's tenosynovitis is a painful condition affecting the tendons on the thumb side of wrist. Tendons include the extensor pollicis brevis and the abductor pollicis longus tendons. When the tendons swell, they rub against the walls of the narrow canal they pass through. Pain at the base of the thumb and in the lower arm results from the ongoing irritation. Pain is reproduced by stretching the tendons with the thumb inside a closed fist.

Carpal Tunnel Syndrome

Carpal tunnel syndrome is caused by compression of the median nerve at the wrist. Carpal tunnel is a narrow passageway of ligament and bones at the base of your hand. It contains nerve and tendons. Carpal tunnel syndrome results in a feeling of intermittent numbness of the thumb, index, and long fingers and the radial side of the ring finger. Symptoms are often worse at night or after use of vibrating tools or great force.

Dupuytren's Contracture

Dupuytren's contracture refers to a thickening of the underlying fibrous tissue beneath the skin of the palm of the hand and of the fingers. It involves the palmar fascia of the hand. The finger affected by contracture cannot be straightened completely, which can complicate everyday activities. The ring finger is affected most often.

Osteoarthrosis

Osteoarthrosis is a noninflammatory degenerative join disease. The cause of osteoarthritis (Figure 13.a) is unknown. Symptoms may include degeneration of the articular cartilage, hypertrophy of bone at the margins, changes in the synovial membrane, tenderness, stiffness, locking and sometimes an effusion. It can occur in multiple joints, but the symptoms will likely only be noticeable in just one or two joints. Primary symptoms of osteoarthritis include joint pain, stiffness upon arising, and locking of the joint with continued immobility.

Rheumatoid Arthritis

Rheumatoid arthritis (Figure 13.a) is a chronic autoimmune disease that progresses over time (Figure 13.b), resulting in disability. It is characterized by pain, swelling, and inflammation in the joints and surrounding tissues. It can also affect other organs in the body. The cause of rheumatoid arthritis is not known. It can affect any joint but is common in the wrist and fingers. It can be a disabling and painful condition, which can lead to substantial loss of functioning and mobility.

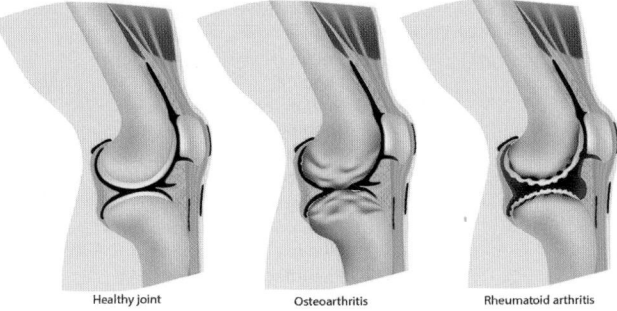

Figure 13.a   Common Types of Arthritis

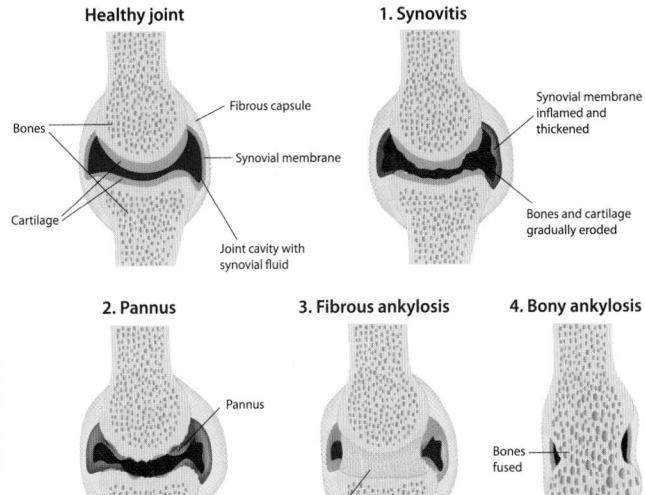

Figure 13.b   Stages of Rheumatoid Arthritis

Osteoporosis

Osteoporosis (Figure 13.c) is a systemic bone disease characterized as the diminishment of bone mass and damage of bone micro-structure. It is a silent disease. It causes bones to become weak and brittle. Its risk factors include aging, being female, low body weight, low sex hormones or menopause, smoking, and some medications. Hip, wrist, and spine fractures commonly result from osteoporosis.

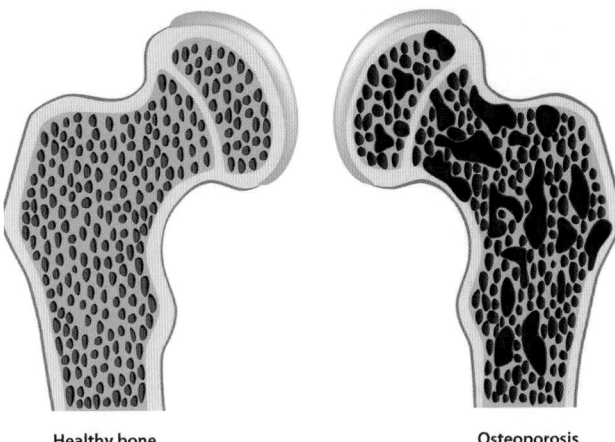

Figure 13.c   Osteoporosis

Septic Arthritis

Septic arthritis is the purulent invasion of a joint by an infectious agent which produces arthritis. Septic arthritis develops when bacteria or other tiny disease-causing microorganisms spread through the bloodstream to a joint. This inflammatory process, which is considered sterile because the skin remains unbroken, usually results from a bacterial infection in a location elsewhere in the body.

Meralgia Paresthetica

Meralgia paresthetica is a condition characterized by tingling, numbness and burning pain in the outer part of your thigh. Pain in the outer thigh is caused by injury to lateral cutaneous nerve of thigh. The nerve passes through the inguinal ligament, at its lateral end, at the level of the anterosuperior iliac spine, and becomes entrapped. It typically occurs in isolation

Diseases of the musculoskeletal system and connective tissue (M00-M99)

[NOTES] Use an external cause code following the code for the musculoskeletal condition, if applicable, to identify the cause of the musculoskeletal condition

[EXCLUDES2] *arthropathic psoriasis (L40.5-)*
certain conditions originating in the perinatal period (P04-P96)
certain infectious and parasitic diseases (A00-B99)
compartment syndrome (traumatic) (T79.A-)
complications of pregnancy, childbirth and the puerperium (O00-O9A)
congenital malformations, deformations, and chromosomal abnormalities (Q00-Q99)
endocrine, nutritional and metabolic diseases (E00-E88)
injury, poisoning and certain other consequences of external causes (S00-T88)
neoplasms (C00-D49)
symptoms, signs and abnormal clinical and laboratory findings, not elsewhere classified (R00-R94)

This chapter contains the following blocks:

M00-M02	Infectious arthropathies
M04	Autoinflammatory syndromes
M05-M14	Inflammatory polyarthropathies
M15-M19	Osteoarthritis
M20-M25	Other joint disorders
M26-M27	Dentofacial anomalies [including malocclusion] and other disorders of jaw
M30-M36	Systemic connective tissue disorders
M40-M43	Deforming dorsopathies
M45-M49	Spondylopathies
M50-M54	Other dorsopathies
M60-M63	Disorders of muscles
M65-M67	Disorders of synovium and tendon
M70-M79	Other soft tissue disorders
M80-M85	Disorders of bone density and structure
M86-M90	Other osteopathies
M91-M94	Chondropathies
M95	Other disorders of the musculoskeletal system and connective tissue
M96	Intraoperative and postprocedural complications and disorders of musculoskeletal system, not elsewhere classified
M97	Periprosthetic fracture around internal prosthetic joint
M99	Biomechanical lesions, not elsewhere classified

Arthropathies (M00-M25)

[INCLUDES] *Disorders affecting predominantly peripheral (limb) joints*

Infectious arthropathies (M00-M02)

[NOTES] This block comprises arthropathies due to microbiological agents. Distinction is made between the following types of etiological relationship:
a) direct infection of joint, where organisms invade synovial tissue and microbial antigen is present in the joint;
b) indirect infection, which may be of two types: a reactive arthropathy, where microbial infection of the body is established but neither organisms nor antigens can be identified in the joint, and a postinfective arthropathy, where microbial antigen is present but recovery of an organism is inconstant and evidence of local multiplication is lacking.

[4th] **M00 Pyogenic arthritis**
DEFINITION: Also known as infective arthritis occurring in a joint.

[5th] **M00.0 Staphylococcal arthritis and polyarthritis**
Use additional code (B95.61-B95.8) to identify bacterial agent
[EXCLUDES2] *infection and inflammatory reaction due to internal joint prosthesis (T84.5-)*

M00.00 Staphylococcal arthritis, unspecified joint [CC] [HCC] [CC/MCC Exc]

[6th] **M00.01 Staphylococcal arthritis, shoulder**
M00.011 Staphylococcal arthritis, right shoulder [CC] [HCC] [CC/MCC Exc]
M00.012 Staphylococcal arthritis, left shoulder [CC] [HCC] [CC/MCC Exc]
M00.019 Staphylococcal arthritis, unspecified shoulder [CC] [HCC] [CC/MCC Exc]

[6th] **M00.02 Staphylococcal arthritis, elbow**
M00.021 Staphylococcal arthritis, right elbow [CC] [HCC] [CC/MCC Exc]
M00.022 Staphylococcal arthritis, left elbow [CC] [HCC] [CC/MCC Exc]
M00.029 Staphylococcal arthritis, unspecified elbow [CC] [HCC] [CC/MCC Exc]

[6th] **M00.03 Staphylococcal arthritis, wrist**
Staphylococcal arthritis of carpal bones
M00.031 Staphylococcal arthritis, right wrist [CC] [HCC] [CC/MCC Exc]
M00.032 Staphylococcal arthritis, left wrist [CC] [HCC] [CC/MCC Exc]
M00.039 Staphylococcal arthritis, unspecified wrist [CC] [HCC] [CC/MCC Exc]

[6th] **M00.04 Staphylococcal arthritis, hand**
Staphylococcal arthritis of metacarpus and phalanges
M00.041 Staphylococcal arthritis, right hand [CC] [HCC] [CC/MCC Exc]
M00.042 Staphylococcal arthritis, left hand [CC] [HCC] [CC/MCC Exc]
M00.049 Staphylococcal arthritis, unspecified hand [CC] [HCC] [CC/MCC Exc]

[6th] **M00.05 Staphylococcal arthritis, hip**
M00.051 Staphylococcal arthritis, right hip [CC] [HCC] [CC/MCC Exc]
M00.052 Staphylococcal arthritis, left hip [CC] [HCC] [CC/MCC Exc]
M00.059 Staphylococcal arthritis, unspecified hip [CC] [HCC] [CC/MCC Exc]

[6th] **M00.06 Staphylococcal arthritis, knee**
M00.061 Staphylococcal arthritis, right knee [CC] [HCC] [CC/MCC Exc]
M00.062 Staphylococcal arthritis, left knee [CC] [HCC] [CC/MCC Exc]
M00.069 Staphylococcal arthritis, unspecified knee [CC] [HCC] [CC/MCC Exc]

[6th] **M00.07 Staphylococcal arthritis, ankle and foot**
Staphylococcal arthritis, tarsus, metatarsus and phalanges
M00.071 Staphylococcal arthritis, right ankle and foot [CC] [HCC] [CC/MCC Exc]
M00.072 Staphylococcal arthritis, left ankle and foot [CC] [HCC] [CC/MCC Exc]
M00.079 Staphylococcal arthritis, unspecified ankle and foot [CC] [HCC] [CC/MCC Exc]

M00.08 Staphylococcal arthritis, vertebrae [CC] [HCC] [CC/MCC Exc]
M00.09 Staphylococcal polyarthritis [CC] [HCC] [CC/MCC Exc]

[5th] **M00.1 Pneumococcal arthritis and polyarthritis**
M00.10 Pneumococcal arthritis, unspecified joint [CC] [HCC] [CC/MCC Exc]

[6th] **M00.11 Pneumococcal arthritis, shoulder**
M00.111 Pneumococcal arthritis, right shoulder [CC] [HCC] [CC/MCC Exc]
M00.112 Pneumococcal arthritis, left shoulder [CC] [HCC] [CC/MCC Exc]
M00.119 Pneumococcal arthritis, unspecified shoulder [CC] [HCC] [CC/MCC Exc]

[6th] **M00.12 Pneumococcal arthritis, elbow**
M00.121 Pneumococcal arthritis, right elbow [CC] [HCC] [CC/MCC Exc]
M00.122 Pneumococcal arthritis, left elbow [CC] [HCC] [CC/MCC Exc]
M00.129 Pneumococcal arthritis, unspecified elbow [CC] [HCC] [CC/MCC Exc]

[PDx] Unacceptable principal diagnosis symbol per Medicare code edits [POA] Code exempt from diagnosis present on admission requirement
[?] Questionable admission [CC] Complication or comorbidity [MCC] Major complication or comorbidity [CC/MCC Exc] CC/MCC exclusion
[HCC] HCC diagnosis code [RxHCC] RxHCC diagnosis code MACRA code **DEFINITION** Describes condition/terminology
TIP Coding guidance 👁 Official Guideline Reference [Z-1] Z code as first-listed diagnosis

6ᵗʰ **M00.13 Pneumococcal arthritis,** wrist
Pneumococcal arthritis of carpal bones
M00.131 **Pneumococcal arthritis,** right wrist cc HCC CC/MCC Exc
M00.132 **Pneumococcal arthritis,** left wrist cc HCC CC/MCC Exc
M00.139 **Pneumococcal arthritis, unspecified wrist** cc HCC CC/MCC Exc

6ᵗʰ **M00.14 Pneumococcal arthritis,** hand
Pneumococcal arthritis of metacarpus and phalanges
M00.141 **Pneumococcal arthritis,** right hand cc HCC CC/MCC Exc
M00.142 **Pneumococcal arthritis,** left hand cc HCC CC/MCC Exc
M00.149 **Pneumococcal arthritis, unspecified hand** cc HCC CC/MCC Exc

6ᵗʰ **M00.15 Pneumococcal arthritis,** hip
M00.151 **Pneumococcal arthritis,** right hip cc HCC CC/MCC Exc
M00.152 **Pneumococcal arthritis, left hip** cc HCC CC/MCC Exc
M00.159 **Pneumococcal arthritis, unspecified hip** cc HCC CC/MCC Exc

6ᵗʰ **M00.16 Pneumococcal arthritis,** knee
M00.161 **Pneumococcal arthritis,** right knee cc HCC CC/MCC Exc
M00.162 **Pneumococcal arthritis,** left knee cc HCC CC/MCC Exc
M00.169 **Pneumococcal arthritis, unspecified knee** cc HCC CC/MCC Exc

6ᵗʰ **M00.17 Pneumococcal arthritis,** ankle and foot
Pneumococcal arthritis, tarsus, metatarsus and phalanges
M00.171 **Pneumococcal arthritis,** right ankle and foot cc HCC CC/MCC Exc
M00.172 **Pneumococcal arthritis,** left ankle and foot cc HCC CC/MCC Exc
M00.179 **Pneumococcal arthritis, unspecified ankle and foot** cc HCC CC/MCC Exc

M00.18 **Pneumococcal arthritis,** vertebrae cc HCC CC/MCC Exc
M00.19 **Pneumococcal** polyarthritis cc HCC CC/MCC Exc

5ᵗʰ **M00.2** Other streptococcal **arthritis and polyarthritis**
Use additional code (B95.0-B95.2, B95.4-B95.5) to identify bacterial agent
M00.20 **Other streptococcal arthritis, unspecified joint** cc HCC CC/MCC Exc

6ᵗʰ **M00.21 Other streptococcal arthritis,** shoulder
M00.211 **Other streptococcal arthritis,** right shoulder cc HCC CC/MCC Exc
M00.212 **Other streptococcal arthritis,** left shoulder cc HCC CC/MCC Exc
M00.219 **Other streptococcal arthritis, unspecified shoulder** cc HCC CC/MCC Exc

6ᵗʰ **M00.22 Other streptococcal arthritis,** elbow
M00.221 **Other streptococcal arthritis,** right elbow cc HCC CC/MCC Exc
M00.222 **Other streptococcal arthritis,** left elbow cc HCC CC/MCC Exc
M00.229 **Other streptococcal arthritis, unspecified elbow** cc HCC CC/MCC Exc

6ᵗʰ **M00.23 Other streptococcal arthritis,** wrist
Other streptococcal arthritis of carpal bones
M00.231 **Other streptococcal arthritis,** right wrist cc HCC CC/MCC Exc
M00.232 **Other streptococcal arthritis,** left wrist cc HCC CC/MCC Exc
M00.239 **Other streptococcal arthritis, unspecified wrist** cc HCC CC/MCC Exc

6ᵗʰ **M00.24 Other streptococcal arthritis,** hand
Other streptococcal arthritis metacarpus and phalanges
M00.241 **Other streptococcal arthritis,** right hand cc HCC CC/MCC Exc

M00.242 **Other streptococcal arthritis,** left hand cc HCC CC/MCC Exc
M00.249 **Other streptococcal arthritis, unspecified hand** cc HCC CC/MCC Exc

6ᵗʰ **M00.25 Other streptococcal arthritis,** hip
M00.251 **Other streptococcal arthritis,** right hip cc HCC CC/MCC Exc
M00.252 **Other streptococcal arthritis,** left hip cc HCC CC/MCC Exc
M00.259 **Other streptococcal arthritis, unspecified hip** cc HCC CC/MCC Exc

6ᵗʰ **M00.26 Other streptococcal arthritis,** knee
M00.261 **Other streptococcal arthritis,** right knee cc HCC CC/MCC Exc
M00.262 **Other streptococcal arthritis,** left knee cc HCC CC/MCC Exc
M00.269 **Other streptococcal arthritis,** unspecified knee cc HCC CC/MCC Exc

6ᵗʰ **M00.27 Other streptococcal arthritis,** ankle and foot
Other streptococcal arthritis, tarsus, metatarsus and phalanges
M00.271 **Other streptococcal arthritis,** right ankle and foot cc HCC CC/MCC Exc
M00.272 **Other streptococcal arthritis,** left ankle and foot cc HCC CC/MCC Exc
M00.279 **Other streptococcal arthritis, unspecified ankle and foot** cc HCC CC/MCC Exc

M00.28 **Other streptococcal arthritis,** vertebrae cc HCC CC/MCC Exc
M00.29 **Other streptococcal** polyarthritis cc HCC CC/MCC Exc

5ᵗʰ **M00.8 Arthritis and polyarthritis** due to other bacteria
Use additional code (B96) to identify bacteria
M00.80 **Arthritis due to other bacteria, unspecified joint** cc HCC CC/MCC Exc

6ᵗʰ **M00.81 Arthritis due to other bacteria,** shoulder
M00.811 **Arthritis due to other bacteria,** right shoulder cc HCC CC/MCC Exc
M00.812 **Arthritis due to other bacteria,** left shoulder cc HCC CC/MCC Exc
M00.819 **Arthritis due to other bacteria, unspecified shoulder** cc HCC CC/MCC Exc

6ᵗʰ **M00.82 Arthritis due to other bacteria,** elbow
M00.821 **Arthritis due to other bacteria,** right elbow cc HCC CC/MCC Exc
M00.822 **Arthritis due to other bacteria,** left elbow cc HCC CC/MCC Exc
M00.829 **Arthritis due to other bacteria, unspecified elbow** cc HCC CC/MCC Exc

6ᵗʰ **M00.83 Arthritis due to other bacteria,** wrist
Arthritis due to other bacteria, carpal bones
M00.831 **Arthritis due to other bacteria,** right wrist cc HCC CC/MCC Exc
M00.832 **Arthritis due to other bacteria,** left wrist cc HCC CC/MCC Exc
M00.839 **Arthritis due to other bacteria, unspecified wrist** cc HCC CC/MCC Exc

6ᵗʰ **M00.84 Arthritis due to other bacteria,** hand
Arthritis due to other bacteria, metacarpus and phalanges
M00.841 **Arthritis due to other bacteria,** right hand cc HCC CC/MCC Exc
M00.842 **Arthritis due to other bacteria,** left hand cc HCC CC/MCC Exc
M00.849 **Arthritis due to other bacteria, unspecified hand** cc HCC CC/MCC Exc

6ᵗʰ **M00.85 Arthritis due to other bacteria,** hip
M00.851 **Arthritis due to other bacteria,** right hip cc HCC CC/MCC Exc
M00.852 **Arthritis due to other bacteria,** left hip cc HCC CC/MCC Exc
M00.859 **Arthritis due to other bacteria, unspecified hip** cc HCC CC/MCC Exc

---

Unspecified Code   Other Specified Code   Manifestation Code   Ⓝ Newborn   Ⓟ Pediatric   Ⓜ Maternity   Ⓐ Adult   ♂ Male   ♀ Female
● New Code   ▲ Revised Code Title   ►◄ Revised Text   **NOTES**   *INCLUDES*   *EXCLUDES1* Not coded here   *EXCLUDES2* Not included here
4ᵗʰ 4ᵗʰ character required   5ᵗʰ 5ᵗʰ character required   6ᵗʰ 6ᵗʰ character required   7ᵗʰ 7ᵗʰ character required   7ᵉˣ Extension 'X' Alert
HAC Hospital-acquired condition (HAC) alert   **AHA** AHA Coding Clinic©   📌 Code first alert

6ᵗʰ M00.86 **Arthritis due to other bacteria,** knee

M00.861 **Arthritis due to other bacteria,** right knee   cc HCC CC/MCC Exc

M00.862 **Arthritis due to other bacteria,** left knee   cc HCC CC/MCC Exc

M00.869 **Arthritis due to other bacteria, unspecified knee**   cc HCC CC/MCC Exc

6ᵗʰ M00.87 **Arthritis due to other bacteria,** ankle and foot

Arthritis due to other bacteria, tarsus, metatarsus, and phalanges

M00.871 **Arthritis due to other bacteria,** right ankle and foot   cc HCC CC/MCC Exc

M00.872 **Arthritis due to other bacteria,** left ankle and foot   cc HCC CC/MCC Exc

M00.879 **Arthritis due to other bacteria, unspecified ankle and foot**   cc HCC CC/MCC Exc

M00.88 **Arthritis due to other bacteria,** vertebrae   cc HCC CC/MCC Exc

M00.89 **Polyarthritis** due to other bacteria   cc HCC CC/MCC Exc

M00.9 **Pyogenic arthritis, unspecified**   cc HCC CC/MCC Exc

Infective arthritis NOS

4ᵗʰ M01 **Direct infections of joint in infectious and parasitic diseases classified elsewhere**

☞ **Code first** underlying disease, such as:

leprosy [Hansen's disease] (A30.-)

mycoses (B35-B49)

O'nyong-nyong fever (A92.1)

paratyphoid fever (A01.1-A01.4)

EXCLUDES1 *arthropathy in Lyme disease (A69.23)*

gonococcal arthritis (A54.42)

meningococcal arthritis (A39.83)

mumps arthritis (B26.85)

postinfective arthropathy (M02.-)

postmeningococcal arthritis (A39.84)

reactive arthritis (M02.3)

rubella arthritis (B06.82)

sarcoidosis arthritis (D86.86)

typhoid fever arthritis (A01.04)

tuberculosis arthritis (A18.01-A18.02)

5ᵗʰ M01.X **Direct infection of joint in infectious and parasitic diseases classified elsewhere**

M01.X0 **Direct infection of unspecified joint in infectious and parasitic diseases classified elsewhere**   cc HCC CC/MCC Exc

6ᵗʰ M01.X1 **Direct infection of** shoulder **joint in infectious and parasitic diseases classified elsewhere**

M01.X11 **Direct infection of** right **shoulder in infectious and parasitic diseases classified elsewhere**   cc HCC CC/MCC Exc

M01.X12 **Direct infection of** left **shoulder in infectious and parasitic diseases classified elsewhere**   cc HCC CC/MCC Exc

M01.X19 **Direct infection of unspecified shoulder in infectious and parasitic diseases classified elsewhere**   cc HCC CC/MCC Exc

6ᵗʰ M01.X2 **Direct infection of** elbow **in infectious and parasitic diseases classified elsewhere**

M01.X21 **Direct infection of** right **elbow in infectious and parasitic diseases classified elsewhere**   cc HCC CC/MCC Exc

M01.X22 **Direct infection of** left **elbow in infectious and parasitic diseases classified elsewhere**   cc HCC CC/MCC Exc

M01.X29 **Direct infection of unspecified elbow in infectious and parasitic diseases classified elsewhere**   cc HCC CC/MCC Exc

6ᵗʰ M01.X3 **Direct infection of** wrist **in infectious and parasitic diseases classified elsewhere**

Direct infection of carpal bones in infectious and parasitic diseases classified elsewhere

M01.X31 **Direct infection of** right **wrist in infectious and parasitic diseases classified elsewhere**   cc HCC CC/MCC Exc

M01.X32 **Direct infection of** left **wrist in infectious and parasitic diseases classified elsewhere**   cc HCC CC/MCC Exc

M01.X39 **Direct infection of unspecified wrist in infectious and parasitic diseases classified elsewhere**   cc HCC CC/MCC Exc

6ᵗʰ M01.X4 **Direct infection of** hand **in infectious and parasitic diseases classified elsewhere**

Direct infection of metacarpus and phalanges in infectious and parasitic diseases classified elsewhere

M01.X41 **Direct infection of** right **hand in infectious and parasitic diseases classified elsewhere**   cc HCC CC/MCC Exc

M01.X42 **Direct infection of** left **hand in infectious and parasitic diseases classified elsewhere**   cc HCC CC/MCC Exc

M01.X49 **Direct infection of unspecified hand in infectious and parasitic diseases classified elsewhere**   cc HCC CC/MCC Exc

6ᵗʰ M01.X5 **Direct infection of** hip **in infectious and parasitic diseases classified elsewhere**

M01.X51 **Direct infection of** right **hip in infectious and parasitic diseases classified elsewhere**   cc HCC CC/MCC Exc

M01.X52 **Direct infection of** left **hip in infectious and parasitic diseases classified elsewhere**   cc HCC CC/MCC Exc

M01.X59 **Direct infection of unspecified hip in infectious and parasitic diseases classified elsewhere**   cc HCC CC/MCC Exc

6ᵗʰ M01.X6 **Direct infection of** knee **in infectious and parasitic diseases classified elsewhere**

M01.X61 **Direct infection of** right **knee in infectious and parasitic diseases classified elsewhere**   cc HCC CC/MCC Exc

M01.X62 **Direct infection of** left **knee in infectious and parasitic diseases classified elsewhere**   cc HCC CC/MCC Exc

M01.X69 **Direct infection of unspecified knee in infectious and parasitic diseases classified elsewhere**   cc HCC CC/MCC Exc

6ᵗʰ M01.X7 **Direct infection of** ankle and foot **in infectious and parasitic diseases classified elsewhere**

Direct infection of tarsus, metatarsus and phalanges in infectious and parasitic diseases classified elsewhere

M01.X71 **Direct infection of** right **ankle and foot in infectious and parasitic diseases classified elsewhere**   cc HCC CC/MCC Exc

M01.X72 **Direct infection of** left **ankle and foot in infectious and parasitic diseases classified elsewhere**   cc HCC CC/MCC Exc

M01.X79 **Direct infection of unspecified ankle and foot in infectious and parasitic diseases classified elsewhere**   cc HCC CC/MCC Exc

M01.X8 **Direct infection of** vertebrae **in infectious and parasitic diseases classified elsewhere**   cc HCC CC/MCC Exc

M01.X9 **Direct infection of** multiple joints **in infectious and parasitic diseases classified elsewhere**   cc HCC CC/MCC Exc

4ᵗʰ M02 **Postinfective and reactive arthropathies**

☞ **Code first** underlying disease, such as:

congenital syphilis [Clutton's joints] (A50.5)

enteritis due to Yersinia enterocolitica (A04.6)

infective endocarditis (I33.0)

viral hepatitis (B15-B19)

EXCLUDES1 *Behçet's disease (M35.2)*

direct infections of joint in infectious and parasitic diseases classified elsewhere (M01.-)

postmeningococcal arthritis (A39.84)

mumps arthritis (B26.85)

rubella arthritis (B06.82)

syphilis arthritis (late) (A52.77)

rheumatic fever (I00)

tabetic arthropathy [Charcôt's] (A52.16)

774

When symbols appear on a code that requires a 7th character extension, refer to Appendix B to identify applicable 7th character codes.

2020 ICD-10-CM

5ᵗʰ **M02.0 Arthropathy** following intestinal bypass

M02.00 Arthropathy following intestinal bypass, unspecified site

6ᵗʰ **M02.01 Arthropathy following intestinal bypass,** shoulder

M02.011 Arthropathy following intestinal bypass, right shoulder

M02.012 Arthropathy following intestinal bypass, left shoulder

M02.019 Arthropathy following intestinal bypass, unspecified shoulder

6ᵗʰ **M02.02 Arthropathy following intestinal bypass,** elbow

M02.021 Arthropathy following intestinal bypass, right elbow

M02.022 Arthropathy following intestinal bypass, left elbow

M02.029 Arthropathy following intestinal bypass, unspecified elbow

6ᵗʰ **M02.03 Arthropathy following intestinal bypass,** wrist

Arthropathy following intestinal bypass, carpal bones

M02.031 Arthropathy following intestinal bypass, right wrist

M02.032 Arthropathy following intestinal bypass, left wrist

M02.039 Arthropathy following intestinal bypass, unspecified wrist

6ᵗʰ **M02.04 Arthropathy following intestinal bypass,** hand

Arthropathy following intestinal bypass, metacarpals and phalanges

M02.041 Arthropathy following intestinal bypass, right hand

M02.042 Arthropathy following intestinal bypass, left hand

M02.049 Arthropathy following intestinal bypass, unspecified hand

6ᵗʰ **M02.05 Arthropathy following intestinal bypass,** hip

M02.051 Arthropathy following intestinal bypass, right hip

M02.052 Arthropathy following intestinal bypass, left hip

M02.059 Arthropathy following intestinal bypass, unspecified hip

6ᵗʰ **M02.06 Arthropathy following intestinal bypass,** knee

M02.061 Arthropathy following intestinal bypass, right knee

M02.062 Arthropathy following intestinal bypass, left knee

M02.069 Arthropathy following intestinal bypass, unspecified knee

6ᵗʰ **M02.07 Arthropathy following intestinal bypass,** ankle and foot

Arthropathy following intestinal bypass, tarsus, metatarsus and phalanges

M02.071 Arthropathy following intestinal bypass, right ankle and foot

M02.072 Arthropathy following intestinal bypass, left ankle and foot

M02.079 Arthropathy following intestinal bypass, unspecified ankle and foot

M02.08 Arthropathy following intestinal bypass, vertebrae

M02.09 Arthropathy following intestinal bypass, multiple sites

5ᵗʰ **M02.1** Postdysenteric **arthropathy**

M02.10 Postdysenteric arthropathy, unspecified site HCC

6ᵗʰ **M02.11 Postdysenteric arthropathy,** shoulder

M02.111 Postdysenteric arthropathy, right shoulder HCC

M02.112 Postdysenteric arthropathy, left shoulder HCC

M02.119 Postdysenteric arthropathy, unspecified shoulder HCC

6ᵗʰ **M02.12 Postdysenteric arthropathy,** elbow

M02.121 Postdysenteric arthropathy, right elbow HCC

M02.122 Postdysenteric arthropathy, left elbow HCC

M02.129 Postdysenteric arthropathy, unspecified elbow HCC

6ᵗʰ **M02.13 Postdysenteric arthropathy,** wrist

Postdysenteric arthropathy, carpal bones

M02.131 Postdysenteric arthropathy, right wrist HCC

M02.132 Postdysenteric arthropathy, left wrist HCC

M02.139 Postdysenteric arthropathy, unspecified wrist HCC

6ᵗʰ **M02.14 Postdysenteric arthropathy,** hand

Postdysenteric arthropathy, metacarpus and phalanges

M02.141 Postdysenteric arthropathy, right hand HCC

M02.142 Postdysenteric arthropathy, left hand HCC

M02.149 Postdysenteric arthropathy, unspecified hand HCC

6ᵗʰ **M02.15 Postdysenteric arthropathy,** hip

M02.151 Postdysenteric arthropathy, right hip HCC

M02.152 Postdysenteric arthropathy, left hip HCC

M02.159 Postdysenteric arthropathy, unspecified hip HCC

6ᵗʰ **M02.16 Postdysenteric arthropathy,** knee

M02.161 Postdysenteric arthropathy, right knee HCC

M02.162 Postdysenteric arthropathy, left knee HCC

M02.169 Postdysenteric arthropathy, unspecified knee HCC

6ᵗʰ **M02.17 Postdysenteric arthropathy,** ankle and foot

Postdysenteric arthropathy, tarsus, metatarsus and phalanges

M02.171 Postdysenteric arthropathy, right ankle and foot HCC

M02.172 Postdysenteric arthropathy, left ankle and foot HCC

M02.179 Postdysenteric arthropathy, unspecified ankle and foot HCC

M02.18 Postdysenteric arthropathy, vertebrae HCC

M02.19 Postdysenteric arthropathy, multiple sites HCC

5ᵗʰ **M02.2** Postimmunization **arthropathy**

M02.20 Postimmunization arthropathy, unspecified site

6ᵗʰ **M02.21 Postimmunization arthropathy,** shoulder

M02.211 Postimmunization arthropathy, right shoulder

M02.212 Postimmunization arthropathy, left shoulder

M02.219 Postimmunization arthropathy, unspecified shoulder

6ᵗʰ **M02.22 Postimmunization arthropathy,** elbow

M02.221 Postimmunization arthropathy, right elbow

M02.222 Postimmunization arthropathy, left elbow

M02.229 Postimmunization arthropathy, unspecified elbow

6ᵗʰ **M02.23 Postimmunization arthropathy,** wrist

Postimmunization arthropathy, carpal bones

M02.231 Postimmunization arthropathy, right wrist

M02.232 Postimmunization arthropathy, left wrist

M02.239 Postimmunization arthropathy, unspecified wrist

6ᵗʰ **M02.24 Postimmunization arthropathy,** hand

Postimmunization arthropathy, metacarpus and phalanges

M02.241 Postimmunization arthropathy, right hand

M02.242 Postimmunization arthropathy, left hand

M02.249 Postimmunization arthropathy, unspecified hand

6ᵗʰ **M02.25 Postimmunization arthropathy,** hip

M02.251 Postimmunization arthropathy, right hip

M02.252 Postimmunization arthropathy, left hip

Unspecified Code　Other Specified Code　Manifestation Code　N Newborn　P Pediatric　M Maternity　A Adult　♂ Male　♀ Female
● New Code　▲ Revised Code Title　▶◀ Revised Text　**NOTES**　*INCLUDES*　*EXCLUDES1* Not coded here　*EXCLUDES2* Not included here
4ᵗʰ 4ᵗʰ character required　5ᵗʰ 5ᵗʰ character required　6ᵗʰ 6ᵗʰ character required　7ᵗʰ 7ᵗʰ character required　Ⓧ Extension 'X' Alert
HAC Hospital-acquired condition (HAC) alert　**AHA** AHA Coding Clinic©　☛ **Code first alert**

M02.259 Postimmunization arthropathy, unspecified hip

6ᵗʰ M02.26 Postimmunization arthropathy, knee

M02.261 Postimmunization arthropathy, right knee

M02.262 Postimmunization arthropathy, left knee

M02.269 Postimmunization arthropathy, unspecified knee

6ᵗʰ M02.27 Postimmunization arthropathy, ankle and foot

Postimmunization arthropathy, tarsus, metatarsus and phalanges

M02.271 Postimmunization arthropathy, right ankle and foot

M02.272 Postimmunization arthropathy, left ankle and foot

M02.279 Postimmunization arthropathy, unspecified ankle and foot

M02.28 Postimmunization arthropathy, vertebrae

M02.29 Postimmunization arthropathy, multiple sites

5ᵗʰ M02.3 Reiter's disease

Reactive arthritis

M02.30 Reiter's disease, unspecified site HCC RxHCC

6ᵗʰ M02.31 Reiter's disease, shoulder

M02.311 Reiter's disease, right shoulder HCC RxHCC

M02.312 Reiter's disease, left shoulder HCC RxHCC

M02.319 Reiter's disease, unspecified shoulder HCC RxHCC

6ᵗʰ M02.32 Reiter's disease, elbow

M02.321 Reiter's disease, right elbow HCC RxHCC

M02.322 Reiter's disease, left elbow HCC RxHCC

M02.329 Reiter's disease, unspecified elbow HCC RxHCC

6ᵗʰ M02.33 Reiter's disease, wrist

Reiter's disease, carpal bones

M02.331 Reiter's disease, right wrist HCC RxHCC

M02.332 Reiter's disease, left wrist HCC RxHCC

M02.339 Reiter's disease, unspecified wrist HCC RxHCC

6ᵗʰ M02.34 Reiter's disease, hand

Reiter's disease, metacarpus and phalanges

M02.341 Reiter's disease, right hand HCC RxHCC

M02.342 Reiter's disease, left hand HCC RxHCC

M02.349 Reiter's disease, unspecified hand HCC RxHCC

6ᵗʰ M02.35 Reiter's disease, hip

M02.351 Reiter's disease, right hip HCC RxHCC

M02.352 Reiter's disease, left hip HCC RxHCC

M02.359 Reiter's disease, unspecified hip HCC RxHCC

6ᵗʰ M02.36 Reiter's disease, knee

M02.361 Reiter's disease, right knee HCC RxHCC

M02.362 Reiter's disease, left knee HCC RxHCC

M02.369 Reiter's disease, unspecified knee HCC RxHCC

6ᵗʰ M02.37 Reiter's disease, ankle and foot

Reiter's disease, tarsus, metatarsus and phalanges

M02.371 Reiter's disease, right ankle and foot HCC RxHCC

M02.372 Reiter's disease, left ankle and foot HCC RxHCC

M02.379 Reiter's disease, unspecified ankle and foot HCC RxHCC

M02.38 Reiter's disease, vertebrae HCC RxHCC

M02.39 Reiter's disease, multiple sites HCC RxHCC

5ᵗʰ M02.8 Other reactive arthropathies

M02.80 Other reactive arthropathies, unspecified site HCC

6ᵗʰ M02.81 Other reactive arthropathies, shoulder

M02.811 Other reactive arthropathies, right shoulder HCC

M02.812 Other reactive arthropathies, left shoulder HCC

M02.819 Other reactive arthropathies, unspecified shoulder HCC

6ᵗʰ M02.82 Other reactive arthropathies, elbow

M02.821 Other reactive arthropathies, right elbow HCC

M02.822 Other reactive arthropathies, left elbow HCC

M02.829 Other reactive arthropathies, unspecified elbow HCC

6ᵗʰ M02.83 Other reactive arthropathies, wrist

Other reactive arthropathies, carpal bones

M02.831 Other reactive arthropathies, right wrist HCC

M02.832 Other reactive arthropathies, left wrist HCC

M02.839 Other reactive arthropathies, unspecified wrist HCC

6ᵗʰ M02.84 Other reactive arthropathies, hand

Other reactive arthropathies, metacarpus and phalanges

M02.841 Other reactive arthropathies, right hand HCC

M02.842 Other reactive arthropathies, left hand HCC

M02.849 Other reactive arthropathies, unspecified hand HCC

6ᵗʰ M02.85 Other reactive arthropathies, hip

M02.851 Other reactive arthropathies, right hip HCC

M02.852 Other reactive arthropathies, left hip HCC

M02.859 Other reactive arthropathies, unspecified hip HCC

6ᵗʰ M02.86 Other reactive arthropathies, knee

M02.861 Other reactive arthropathies, right knee HCC

M02.862 Other reactive arthropathies, left knee HCC

M02.869 Other reactive arthropathies, unspecified knee HCC

5ᵗʰ M02.87 Other reactive arthropathies, ankle and foot

Other reactive arthropathies, tarsus, metatarsus and phalanges

M02.871 Other reactive arthropathies, right ankle and foot HCC

M02.872 Other reactive arthropathies, left ankle and foot HCC

M02.879 Other reactive arthropathies, unspecified ankle and foot HCC

M02.88 Other reactive arthropathies, vertebrae HCC

M02.89 Other reactive arthropathies, multiple sites HCC

M02.9 Reactive arthropathy, unspecified HCC

Autoinflammatory syndromes (M04)

4ᵗʰ M04 Autoinflammatory syndromes

EXCLUDES2 Crohn's disease (K50.-)

M04.1 Periodic fever syndromes HCC RxHCC

AHA: Q4 2016

Familial Mediterranean fever

Hyperimmunoglobin D syndrome

Mevalonate kinase deficiency

Tumor necrosis factor receptor associated periodic syndrome [TRAPS]

M04.2 Cryopyrin-associated periodic syndromes HCC RxHCC

AHA: Q4 2016

Chronic infantile neurological, cutaneous and articular syndrome [CINCA]

Familial cold autoinflammatory syndrome

Familial cold urticaria

Muckle-Wells syndrome

Neonatal onset multisystemic inflammatory disorder [NOMID]

M04.8 Other autoinflammatory syndromes HCC RxHCC

AHA: Q4 2016

Blau syndrome

Deficiency of interleukin 1 receptor antagonist [DIRA]

Majeed syndrome

Periodic fever, aphthous stomatitis, pharyngitis, and adenopathy syndrome [PFAPA]

Pyogenic arthritis, pyoderma gangrenosum, and acne syndrome [PAPA]

M04.9 Autoinflammatory syndrome, unspecified HCC RxHCC

AHA: Q4 2016

PDxₓ Unacceptable principal diagnosis symbol per Medicare code edits   POA Code exempt from diagnosis present on admission requirement
❓ Questionable admission   CC Complication or comorbidity   MCC Major complication or comorbidity   CC/MCC Exc CC/MCC exclusion
HCC HCC diagnosis code   RxHCC RxHCC diagnosis code   MACRA code   **DEFINITION** Describes condition/terminology
TIP Coding guidance   👁 Official Guideline Reference   Z1 Z code as first-listed diagnosis

776   When symbols appear on a code that requires a 7th character extension, refer to Appendix B to identify applicable 7th character codes.   **2020 ICD-10-CM**

Inflammatory polyarthropathies (M05-M14)

🌀 **M05 Rheumatoid arthritis** with rheumatoid factor **(Figure 13.1)**

DEFINITION: Rheumatoid arthritis is an autoimmune condition that attacks the body's tissues.

EXCLUDES1 rheumatic fever (I00)

juvenile rheumatoid arthritis (M08.-)

rheumatoid arthritis of spine (M45.-)

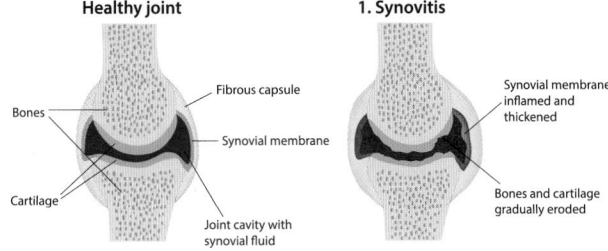

Healthy joint

Fibrous capsule
Bones
Synovial membrane
Cartilage
Joint cavity with synovial fluid

1. Synovitis

Synovial membrane inflamed and thickened

Bones and cartilage gradually eroded

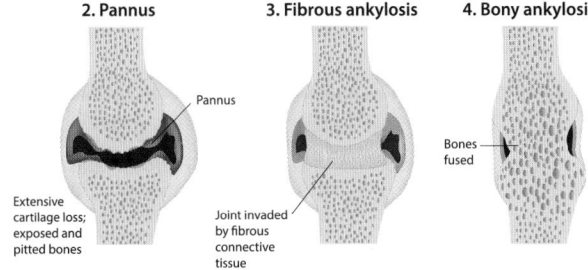

2. Pannus

Pannus

Extensive cartilage loss; exposed and pitted bones

3. Fibrous ankylosis

Joint invaded by fibrous connective tissue

4. Bony ankylosis

Bones fused

Figure 13.1 Stages of Rheumatoid Arthritis

🌀 **M05.0 Felty's syndrome**

DEFINITION: Felty's disease is an autoimmune disease that includes rheumatoid arthritis, splenomegaly, and neutropenia.

Rheumatoid arthritis with splenoadenomegaly and leukopenia

M05.00 Felty's syndrome, unspecified site HCC RxHCC

🌀 **M05.01 Felty's syndrome,** shoulder

M05.011 Felty's syndrome, right shoulder HCC RxHCC

M05.012 Felty's syndrome, left shoulder HCC RxHCC

M05.019 Felty's syndrome, unspecified shoulder HCC RxHCC

🌀 **M05.02 Felty's syndrome,** elbow

M05.021 Felty's syndrome, right elbow HCC RxHCC

M05.022 Felty's syndrome, left elbow HCC RxHCC

M05.029 Felty's syndrome, unspecified elbow HCC RxHCC

🌀 **M05.03 Felty's syndrome,** wrist

Felty's syndrome, carpal bones

M05.031 Felty's syndrome, right wrist HCC RxHCC

M05.032 Felty's syndrome, left wrist HCC RxHCC

M05.039 Felty's syndrome, unspecified wrist HCC RxHCC

🌀 **M05.04 Felty's syndrome,** hand

Felty's syndrome, metacarpus and phalanges

M05.041 Felty's syndrome, right hand HCC RxHCC

M05.042 Felty's syndrome, left hand HCC RxHCC

M05.049 Felty's syndrome, unspecified hand HCC RxHCC

🌀 **M05.05 Felty's syndrome,** hip

M05.051 Felty's syndrome, right hip HCC RxHCC

M05.052 Felty's syndrome, left hip HCC RxHCC

M05.059 Felty's syndrome, unspecified hip HCC RxHCC

🌀 **M05.06 Felty's syndrome,** knee

M05.061 Felty's syndrome, right knee HCC RxHCC

M05.062 Felty's syndrome, left knee HCC RxHCC

M05.069 Felty's syndrome, unspecified knee HCC RxHCC

🌀 **M05.07 Felty's syndrome,** ankle and foot

Felty's syndrome, tarsus, metatarsus and phalanges

M05.071 Felty's syndrome, right ankle and foot

M05.072 Felty's syndrome, left ankle and foot HCC RxHCC

M05.079 Felty's syndrome, unspecified ankle and foot HCC RxHCC

M05.09 Felty's syndrome, multiple sites HCC RxHCC

🌀 **M05.1 Rheumatoid** lung disease with rheumatoid arthritis

M05.10 Rheumatoid lung disease with rheumatoid arthritis of unspecified site HCC RxHCC

🌀 **M05.11 Rheumatoid lung disease with rheumatoid arthritis of** shoulder

M05.111 Rheumatoid lung disease with rheumatoid arthritis of right shoulder HCC RxHCC

M05.112 Rheumatoid lung disease with rheumatoid arthritis of left shoulder HCC RxHCC

M05.119 Rheumatoid lung disease with rheumatoid arthritis of unspecified shoulder HCC RxHCC

🌀 **M05.12 Rheumatoid lung disease with rheumatoid arthritis of** elbow

M05.121 Rheumatoid lung disease with rheumatoid arthritis of right elbow HCC RxHCC

M05.122 Rheumatoid lung disease with rheumatoid arthritis of left elbow HCC RxHCC

M05.129 Rheumatoid lung disease with rheumatoid arthritis of unspecified elbow HCC RxHCC

🌀 **M05.13 Rheumatoid lung disease with rheumatoid arthritis of** wrist

Rheumatoid lung disease with rheumatoid arthritis, carpal bones

M05.131 Rheumatoid lung disease with rheumatoid arthritis of right wrist HCC RxHCC

M05.132 Rheumatoid lung disease with rheumatoid arthritis of left wrist HCC RxHCC

M05.139 Rheumatoid lung disease with rheumatoid arthritis of unspecified wrist HCC RxHCC

🌀 **M05.14 Rheumatoid lung disease with rheumatoid arthritis of** hand

Rheumatoid lung disease with rheumatoid arthritis, metacarpus and phalanges

M05.141 Rheumatoid lung disease with rheumatoid arthritis of right hand HCC RxHCC

M05.142 Rheumatoid lung disease with rheumatoid arthritis of left hand HCC RxHCC

M05.149 Rheumatoid lung disease with rheumatoid arthritis of unspecified hand HCC RxHCC

🌀 **M05.15 Rheumatoid lung disease with rheumatoid arthritis of** hip

M05.151 Rheumatoid lung disease with rheumatoid arthritis of right hip HCC RxHCC

M05.152 Rheumatoid lung disease with rheumatoid arthritis of left hip HCC RxHCC

M05.159 Rheumatoid lung disease with rheumatoid arthritis of unspecified hip HCC RxHCC

🌀 **M05.16 Rheumatoid lung disease with rheumatoid arthritis of** knee

M05.161 Rheumatoid lung disease with rheumatoid arthritis of right knee HCC RxHCC

M05.162 Rheumatoid lung disease with rheumatoid arthritis of left knee HCC RxHCC

M05.169 Rheumatoid lung disease with rheumatoid arthritis of unspecified knee HCC RxHCC

🌀 **M05.17 Rheumatoid lung disease with rheumatoid arthritis of** ankle and foot

Rheumatoid lung disease with rheumatoid arthritis, tarsus, metatarsus and phalanges

M05.171 Rheumatoid lung disease with rheumatoid arthritis of right ankle and foot HCC RxHCC

M05.172 Rheumatoid lung disease with rheumatoid arthritis of left ankle and foot HCC RxHCC

M05.179 Rheumatoid lung disease with rheumatoid arthritis of unspecified ankle and foot HCC RxHCC

M05.19 Rheumatoid lung disease with rheumatoid arthritis of multiple sites HCC RxHCC

M05 - M05.19

CHAPTER 13: DISEASES OF THE MUSCULOSKELETAL SYSTEM AND CONNECTIVE TISSUE (M00-M99)

M05.2 Rheumatoid vasculitis with rheumatoid arthritis

    M05.20 **Rheumatoid vasculitis with rheumatoid arthritis of unspecified site** HCC RxHCC

    M05.21 **Rheumatoid vasculitis with rheumatoid arthritis of shoulder**

        M05.211 **Rheumatoid vasculitis with rheumatoid arthritis of right shoulder** HCC RxHCC

        M05.212 **Rheumatoid vasculitis with rheumatoid arthritis of left shoulder** HCC RxHCC

        M05.219 **Rheumatoid vasculitis with rheumatoid arthritis of unspecified shoulder** HCC RxHCC

    M05.22 **Rheumatoid vasculitis with rheumatoid arthritis of elbow**

        M05.221 **Rheumatoid vasculitis with rheumatoid arthritis of right elbow** HCC RxHCC

        M05.222 **Rheumatoid vasculitis with rheumatoid arthritis of left elbow** HCC RxHCC

        M05.229 **Rheumatoid vasculitis with rheumatoid arthritis of unspecified elbow** HCC RxHCC

    M05.23 **Rheumatoid vasculitis with rheumatoid arthritis of wrist**

        Rheumatoid vasculitis with rheumatoid arthritis, carpal bones

        M05.231 **Rheumatoid vasculitis with rheumatoid arthritis of right wrist** HCC RxHCC

        M05.232 **Rheumatoid vasculitis with rheumatoid arthritis of left wrist** HCC RxHCC

        M05.239 **Rheumatoid vasculitis with rheumatoid arthritis of unspecified wrist** HCC RxHCC

    M05.24 **Rheumatoid vasculitis with rheumatoid arthritis of hand**

        Rheumatoid vasculitis with rheumatoid arthritis, metacarpus and phalanges

        M05.241 **Rheumatoid vasculitis with rheumatoid arthritis of right hand** HCC RxHCC

        M05.242 **Rheumatoid vasculitis with rheumatoid arthritis of left hand** HCC RxHCC

        M05.249 **Rheumatoid vasculitis with rheumatoid arthritis of unspecified hand** HCC RxHCC

    M05.25 **Rheumatoid vasculitis with rheumatoid arthritis of hip**

        M05.251 **Rheumatoid vasculitis with rheumatoid arthritis of right hip** HCC RxHCC

        M05.252 **Rheumatoid vasculitis with rheumatoid arthritis of left hip** HCC RxHCC

        M05.259 **Rheumatoid vasculitis with rheumatoid arthritis of unspecified hip** HCC RxHCC

    M05.26 **Rheumatoid vasculitis with rheumatoid arthritis of knee**

        M05.261 **Rheumatoid vasculitis with rheumatoid arthritis of right knee** HCC RxHCC

        M05.262 **Rheumatoid vasculitis with rheumatoid arthritis of left knee** HCC RxHCC

        M05.269 **Rheumatoid vasculitis with rheumatoid arthritis of unspecified knee** HCC RxHCC

    M05.27 **Rheumatoid vasculitis with rheumatoid arthritis of ankle and foot**

        Rheumatoid vasculitis with rheumatoid arthritis, tarsus, metatarsus and phalanges

        M05.271 **Rheumatoid vasculitis with rheumatoid arthritis of right ankle and foot** HCC RxHCC

        M05.272 **Rheumatoid vasculitis with rheumatoid arthritis of left ankle and foot** HCC RxHCC

        M05.279 **Rheumatoid vasculitis with rheumatoid arthritis of unspecified ankle and foot** HCC RxHCC

    M05.29 **Rheumatoid vasculitis with rheumatoid arthritis of multiple sites** HCC RxHCC

M05.3 Rheumatoid heart disease with rheumatoid arthritis

    Rheumatoid carditis

    Rheumatoid endocarditis

    Rheumatoid myocarditis

    Rheumatoid pericarditis

    M05.30 **Rheumatoid heart disease with rheumatoid arthritis of unspecified site** HCC RxHCC

    M05.31 **Rheumatoid heart disease with rheumatoid arthritis of shoulder**

        M05.311 **Rheumatoid heart disease with rheumatoid arthritis of right shoulder** HCC RxHCC

        M05.312 **Rheumatoid heart disease with rheumatoid arthritis of left shoulder** HCC RxHCC

        M05.319 **Rheumatoid heart disease with rheumatoid arthritis of unspecified shoulder** HCC RxHCC

    M05.32 **Rheumatoid heart disease with rheumatoid arthritis of elbow**

        M05.321 **Rheumatoid heart disease with rheumatoid arthritis of right elbow** HCC RxHCC

        M05.322 **Rheumatoid heart disease with rheumatoid arthritis of left elbow** HCC RxHCC

        M05.329 **Rheumatoid heart disease with rheumatoid arthritis of unspecified elbow** HCC RxHCC

    M05.33 **Rheumatoid heart disease with rheumatoid arthritis of wrist**

        Rheumatoid heart disease with rheumatoid arthritis, carpal bones

        M05.331 **Rheumatoid heart disease with rheumatoid arthritis of right wrist** HCC RxHCC

        M05.332 **Rheumatoid heart disease with rheumatoid arthritis of left wrist** HCC RxHCC

        M05.339 **Rheumatoid heart disease with rheumatoid arthritis of unspecified wrist** HCC RxHCC

    M05.34 **Rheumatoid heart disease with rheumatoid arthritis of hand**

        Rheumatoid heart disease with rheumatoid arthritis, metacarpus and phalanges

        M05.341 **Rheumatoid heart disease with rheumatoid arthritis of right hand** HCC RxHCC

        M05.342 **Rheumatoid heart disease with rheumatoid arthritis of left hand** HCC RxHCC

        M05.349 **Rheumatoid heart disease with rheumatoid arthritis of unspecified hand** HCC RxHCC

    M05.35 **Rheumatoid heart disease with rheumatoid arthritis of hip**

        M05.351 **Rheumatoid heart disease with rheumatoid arthritis of right hip** HCC RxHCC

        M05.352 **Rheumatoid heart disease with rheumatoid arthritis of left hip** HCC RxHCC

        M05.359 **Rheumatoid heart disease with rheumatoid arthritis of unspecified hip** HCC RxHCC

    M05.36 **Rheumatoid heart disease with rheumatoid arthritis of knee**

        M05.361 **Rheumatoid heart disease with rheumatoid arthritis of right knee** HCC RxHCC

        M05.362 **Rheumatoid heart disease with rheumatoid arthritis of left knee** HCC RxHCC

        M05.369 **Rheumatoid heart disease with rheumatoid arthritis of unspecified knee** HCC RxHCC

    M05.37 **Rheumatoid heart disease with rheumatoid arthritis of ankle and foot**

        Rheumatoid heart disease with rheumatoid arthritis, tarsus, metatarsus and phalanges

        M05.371 **Rheumatoid heart disease with rheumatoid arthritis of right ankle and foot** HCC RxHCC

        M05.372 **Rheumatoid heart disease with rheumatoid arthritis of left ankle and foot** HCC RxHCC

        M05.379 **Rheumatoid heart disease with rheumatoid arthritis of unspecified ankle and foot** HCC RxHCC

PDx Unacceptable principal diagnosis symbol per Medicare code edits   POA Code exempt from diagnosis present on admission requirement   ❓ Questionable admission   CC Complication or comorbidity   MCC Major complication or comorbidity   CC/MCC CC/MCC exclusion   HCC HCC diagnosis code   RxHCC RxHCC diagnosis code   MACRA MACRA code   **DEFINITION** Describes condition/terminology   TIP Coding guidance   👁 Official Guideline Reference   Z1 Z code as first-listed diagnosis

778   When symbols appear on a code that requires a 7th character extension, refer to Appendix B to identify applicable 7th character codes.   **2020 ICD-10-CM**

M05.39 Rheumatoid heart disease with rheumatoid arthritis of multiple sites `HCC` `RxHCC`

5ᵗʰ **M05.4 Rheumatoid myopathy with rheumatoid arthritis**

M05.40 Rheumatoid myopathy with rheumatoid arthritis of unspecified site `HCC` `RxHCC`

6ᵗʰ M05.41 Rheumatoid myopathy with rheumatoid arthritis of shoulder

M05.411 Rheumatoid myopathy with rheumatoid arthritis of right shoulder `HCC` `RxHCC`

M05.412 Rheumatoid myopathy with rheumatoid arthritis of left shoulder `HCC` `RxHCC`

M05.419 Rheumatoid myopathy with rheumatoid arthritis of unspecified shoulder `HCC` `RxHCC`

6ᵗʰ M05.42 Rheumatoid myopathy with rheumatoid arthritis of elbow

M05.421 Rheumatoid myopathy with rheumatoid arthritis of right elbow `HCC` `RxHCC`

M05.422 Rheumatoid myopathy with rheumatoid arthritis of left elbow `HCC` `RxHCC`

M05.429 Rheumatoid myopathy with rheumatoid arthritis of unspecified elbow `HCC` `RxHCC`

6ᵗʰ M05.43 Rheumatoid myopathy with rheumatoid arthritis of wrist

Rheumatoid myopathy with rheumatoid arthritis, carpal bones

M05.431 Rheumatoid myopathy with rheumatoid arthritis of right wrist `HCC` `RxHCC`

M05.432 Rheumatoid myopathy with rheumatoid arthritis of left wrist `HCC` `RxHCC`

M05.439 Rheumatoid myopathy with rheumatoid arthritis of unspecified wrist `HCC` `RxHCC`

6ᵗʰ M05.44 Rheumatoid myopathy with rheumatoid arthritis of hand

Rheumatoid myopathy with rheumatoid arthritis, metacarpus and phalanges

M05.441 Rheumatoid myopathy with rheumatoid arthritis of right hand `HCC` `RxHCC`

M05.442 Rheumatoid myopathy with rheumatoid arthritis of left hand `HCC` `RxHCC`

M05.449 Rheumatoid myopathy with rheumatoid arthritis of unspecified hand `HCC` `RxHCC`

6ᵗʰ M05.45 Rheumatoid myopathy with rheumatoid arthritis of hip

M05.451 Rheumatoid myopathy with rheumatoid arthritis of right hip `HCC` `RxHCC`

M05.452 Rheumatoid myopathy with rheumatoid arthritis of left hip `HCC` `RxHCC`

M05.459 Rheumatoid myopathy with rheumatoid arthritis of unspecified hip `HCC` `RxHCC`

6ᵗʰ M05.46 Rheumatoid myopathy with rheumatoid arthritis of knee

M05.461 Rheumatoid myopathy with rheumatoid arthritis of right knee `HCC` `RxHCC`

M05.462 Rheumatoid myopathy with rheumatoid arthritis of left knee `HCC` `RxHCC`

M05.469 Rheumatoid myopathy with rheumatoid arthritis of unspecified knee `HCC` `RxHCC`

6ᵗʰ M05.47 Rheumatoid myopathy with rheumatoid arthritis of ankle and foot

Rheumatoid myopathy with rheumatoid arthritis, tarsus, metatarsus and phalanges

M05.471 Rheumatoid myopathy with rheumatoid arthritis of right ankle and foot `HCC` `RxHCC`

M05.472 Rheumatoid myopathy with rheumatoid arthritis of left ankle and foot `HCC` `RxHCC`

M05.479 Rheumatoid myopathy with rheumatoid arthritis of unspecified ankle and foot `HCC` `RxHCC`

M05.49 Rheumatoid myopathy with rheumatoid arthritis of multiple sites `HCC` `RxHCC`

5ᵗʰ **M05.5 Rheumatoid polyneuropathy with rheumatoid arthritis**

M05.50 Rheumatoid polyneuropathy with rheumatoid arthritis of unspecified site `HCC` `RxHCC`

6ᵗʰ M05.51 Rheumatoid polyneuropathy with rheumatoid arthritis of shoulder

M05.511 Rheumatoid polyneuropathy with rheumatoid arthritis of right shoulder `HCC` `RxHCC`

M05.512 Rheumatoid polyneuropathy with rheumatoid arthritis of left shoulder `HCC` `RxHCC`

M05.519 Rheumatoid polyneuropathy with rheumatoid arthritis of unspecified shoulder `HCC` `RxHCC`

6ᵗʰ M05.52 Rheumatoid polyneuropathy with rheumatoid arthritis of elbow

M05.521 Rheumatoid polyneuropathy with rheumatoid arthritis of right elbow `HCC` `RxHCC`

M05.522 Rheumatoid polyneuropathy with rheumatoid arthritis of left elbow `HCC` `RxHCC`

M05.529 Rheumatoid polyneuropathy with rheumatoid arthritis of unspecified elbow `HCC` `RxHCC`

6ᵗʰ M05.53 Rheumatoid polyneuropathy with rheumatoid arthritis of wrist

Rheumatoid polyneuropathy with rheumatoid arthritis, carpal bones

M05.531 Rheumatoid polyneuropathy with rheumatoid arthritis of right wrist `HCC` `RxHCC`

M05.532 Rheumatoid polyneuropathy with rheumatoid arthritis of left wrist `HCC` `RxHCC`

M05.539 Rheumatoid polyneuropathy with rheumatoid arthritis of unspecified wrist `HCC` `RxHCC`

6ᵗʰ M05.54 Rheumatoid polyneuropathy with rheumatoid arthritis of hand

Rheumatoid polyneuropathy with rheumatoid arthritis, metacarpus and phalanges

M05.541 Rheumatoid polyneuropathy with rheumatoid arthritis of right hand `HCC` `RxHCC`

M05.542 Rheumatoid polyneuropathy with rheumatoid arthritis of left hand `HCC` `RxHCC`

M05.549 Rheumatoid polyneuropathy with rheumatoid arthritis of unspecified hand `HCC` `RxHCC`

6ᵗʰ M05.55 Rheumatoid polyneuropathy with rheumatoid arthritis of hip

M05.551 Rheumatoid polyneuropathy with rheumatoid arthritis of right hip `HCC` `RxHCC`

M05.552 Rheumatoid polyneuropathy with rheumatoid arthritis of left hip `HCC` `RxHCC`

M05.559 Rheumatoid polyneuropathy with rheumatoid arthritis of unspecified hip `HCC` `RxHCC`

6ᵗʰ M05.56 Rheumatoid polyneuropathy with rheumatoid arthritis of knee

M05.561 Rheumatoid polyneuropathy with rheumatoid arthritis of right knee `HCC` `RxHCC`

M05.562 Rheumatoid polyneuropathy with rheumatoid arthritis of left knee `HCC` `RxHCC`

M05.569 Rheumatoid polyneuropathy with rheumatoid arthritis of unspecified knee `HCC` `RxHCC`

6ᵗʰ M05.57 Rheumatoid polyneuropathy with rheumatoid arthritis of ankle and foot

Rheumatoid polyneuropathy with rheumatoid arthritis, tarsus, metatarsus and phalanges

M05.571 Rheumatoid polyneuropathy with rheumatoid arthritis of right ankle and foot `HCC` `RxHCC`

M05.572 Rheumatoid polyneuropathy with rheumatoid arthritis of left ankle and foot `HCC` `RxHCC`

Unspecified Code Other Specified Code Manifestation Code Ⓝ Newborn Ⓟ Pediatric Ⓜ Maternity Ⓐ Adult ♂ Male ♀ Female
● New Code ▲ Revised Code Title ▶◀ Revised Text **NOTES** *INCLUDES* *EXCLUDES1* Not coded here *EXCLUDES2* Not included here
4ᵗʰ 4ᵗʰ character required 5ᵗʰ 5ᵗʰ character required 6ᵗʰ 6ᵗʰ character required 7ᵗʰ 7ᵗʰ character required 7ᵗʰ Extension 'X' Alert
HAC Hospital-acquired condition (HAC) alert **AHA** AHA Coding Clinic® ☞ Code first alert

M05.579 **Rheumatoid polyneuropathy with rheumatoid arthritis of unspecified ankle and foot** [HCC] [RxHCC]

M05.59 **Rheumatoid polyneuropathy with rheumatoid arthritis of multiple sites** [HCC] [RxHCC]

[5th] **M05.6 Rheumatoid arthritis with involvement of other organs and systems**

M05.60 **Rheumatoid arthritis of unspecified site with involvement of other organs and systems** [HCC] [RxHCC]

[6th] **M05.61 Rheumatoid arthritis of shoulder with involvement of other organs and systems**

M05.611 **Rheumatoid arthritis of right shoulder with involvement of other organs and systems** [HCC] [RxHCC]

M05.612 **Rheumatoid arthritis of left shoulder with involvement of other organs and systems** [HCC] [RxHCC]

M05.619 **Rheumatoid arthritis of unspecified shoulder with involvement of other organs and systems** [HCC] [RxHCC]

[6th] **M05.62 Rheumatoid arthritis of elbow with involvement of other organs and systems**

M05.621 **Rheumatoid arthritis of right elbow with involvement of other organs and systems** [HCC] [RxHCC]

M05.622 **Rheumatoid arthritis of left elbow with involvement of other organs and systems** [HCC] [RxHCC]

M05.629 **Rheumatoid arthritis of unspecified elbow with involvement of other organs and systems** [HCC] [RxHCC]

[6th] **M05.63 Rheumatoid arthritis of wrist with involvement of other organs and systems**

Rheumatoid arthritis of carpal bones with involvement of other organs and systems

M05.631 **Rheumatoid arthritis of right wrist with involvement of other organs and systems** [HCC] [RxHCC]

M05.632 **Rheumatoid arthritis of left wrist with involvement of other organs and systems** [HCC] [RxHCC]

M05.639 **Rheumatoid arthritis of unspecified wrist with involvement of other organs and systems** [HCC] [RxHCC]

[6th] **M05.64 Rheumatoid arthritis of hand with involvement of other organs and systems**

Rheumatoid arthritis of metacarpus and phalanges with involvement of other organs and systems

M05.641 **Rheumatoid arthritis of right hand with involvement of other organs and systems** [HCC] [RxHCC]

M05.642 **Rheumatoid arthritis of left hand with involvement of other organs and systems** [HCC] [RxHCC]

M05.649 **Rheumatoid arthritis of unspecified hand with involvement of other organs and systems** [HCC] [RxHCC]

[6th] **M05.65 Rheumatoid arthritis of hip with involvement of other organs and systems**

M05.651 **Rheumatoid arthritis of right hip with involvement of other organs and systems** [HCC] [RxHCC]

M05.652 **Rheumatoid arthritis of left hip with involvement of other organs and systems** [HCC] [RxHCC]

M05.659 **Rheumatoid arthritis of unspecified hip with involvement of other organs and systems** [HCC] [RxHCC]

[6th] **M05.66 Rheumatoid arthritis of knee with involvement of other organs and systems**

M05.661 **Rheumatoid arthritis of right knee with involvement of other organs and systems** [HCC] [RxHCC]

M05.662 **Rheumatoid arthritis of left knee with involvement of other organs and systems** [HCC] [RxHCC]

M05.669 **Rheumatoid arthritis of unspecified knee with involvement of other organs and systems** [HCC] [RxHCC]

[6th] **M05.67 Rheumatoid arthritis of ankle and foot with involvement of other organs and systems**

Rheumatoid arthritis of tarsus, metatarsus and phalanges with involvement of other organs and systems

M05.671 **Rheumatoid arthritis of right ankle and foot with involvement of other organs and systems** [HCC] [RxHCC]

M05.672 **Rheumatoid arthritis of left ankle and foot with involvement of other organs and systems** [HCC] [RxHCC]

M05.679 **Rheumatoid arthritis of unspecified ankle and foot with involvement of other organs and systems** [HCC] [RxHCC]

M05.69 **Rheumatoid arthritis of multiple sites with involvement of other organs and systems** [HCC] [RxHCC]

[5th] **M05.7 Rheumatoid arthritis with rheumatoid factor without organ or systems involvement**

M05.70 **Rheumatoid arthritis with rheumatoid factor of unspecified site without organ or systems involvement** [HCC] [RxHCC]

[6th] **M05.71 Rheumatoid arthritis with rheumatoid factor of shoulder without organ or systems involvement**

M05.711 **Rheumatoid arthritis with rheumatoid factor of right shoulder without organ or systems involvement** [HCC] [RxHCC]

M05.712 **Rheumatoid arthritis with rheumatoid factor of left shoulder without organ or systems involvement** [HCC] [RxHCC]

M05.719 **Rheumatoid arthritis with rheumatoid factor of unspecified shoulder without organ or systems involvement** [HCC] [RxHCC]

[6th] **M05.72 Rheumatoid arthritis with rheumatoid factor of elbow without organ or systems involvement**

M05.721 **Rheumatoid arthritis with rheumatoid factor of right elbow without organ or systems involvement** [HCC] [RxHCC]

M05.722 **Rheumatoid arthritis with rheumatoid factor of left elbow without organ or systems involvement** [HCC] [RxHCC]

M05.729 **Rheumatoid arthritis with rheumatoid factor of unspecified elbow without organ or systems involvement** [HCC] [RxHCC]

[6th] **M05.73 Rheumatoid arthritis with rheumatoid factor of wrist without organ or systems involvement**

M05.731 **Rheumatoid arthritis with rheumatoid factor of right wrist without organ or systems involvement** [HCC] [RxHCC]

M05.732 **Rheumatoid arthritis with rheumatoid factor of left wrist without organ or systems involvement** [HCC] [RxHCC]

M05.739 **Rheumatoid arthritis with rheumatoid factor of unspecified wrist without organ or systems involvement** [HCC] [RxHCC]

[6th] **M05.74 Rheumatoid arthritis with rheumatoid factor of hand without organ or systems involvement**

M05.741 **Rheumatoid arthritis with rheumatoid factor of right hand without organ or systems involvement** [HCC] [RxHCC]

M05.742 **Rheumatoid arthritis with rheumatoid factor of left hand without organ or systems involvement** [HCC] [RxHCC]

M05.749 **Rheumatoid arthritis with rheumatoid factor of unspecified hand without organ or systems involvement** [HCC] [RxHCC]

[PDx] Unacceptable principal diagnosis symbol per Medicare code edits [POA] Code exempt from diagnosis present on admission requirement
[?] Questionable admission [CC] Complication or comorbidity [MCC] Major complication or comorbidity [CC/MCC Exc] CC/MCC exclusion
[HCC] HCC diagnosis code [RxHCC] RxHCC diagnosis code MACRA code **DEFINITION** Describes condition/terminology
TIP Coding guidance 👁 Official Guideline Reference [Z-1] Z code as first-listed diagnosis

6th **M05.75 Rheumatoid arthritis with rheumatoid factor of** hip **without organ or systems involvement**

M05.751 Rheumatoid arthritis with rheumatoid factor of right hip without organ or systems involvement `HCC` `RxHCC`

M05.752 Rheumatoid arthritis with rheumatoid factor of left hip without organ or systems involvement `HCC` `RxHCC`

M05.759 Rheumatoid arthritis with rheumatoid factor of unspecified hip without organ or systems involvement `HCC` `RxHCC`

6th **M05.76 Rheumatoid arthritis with rheumatoid factor of** knee **without organ or systems involvement**

M05.761 Rheumatoid arthritis with rheumatoid factor of right knee without organ or systems involvement `HCC` `RxHCC`

M05.762 Rheumatoid arthritis with rheumatoid factor of left knee without organ or systems involvement `HCC` `RxHCC`

M05.769 Rheumatoid arthritis with rheumatoid factor of unspecified knee without organ or systems involvement `HCC` `RxHCC`

6th **M05.77 Rheumatoid arthritis with rheumatoid factor of** ankle and foot **without organ or systems involvement**

M05.771 Rheumatoid arthritis with rheumatoid factor of right ankle and foot without organ or systems involvement `HCC` `RxHCC`

M05.772 Rheumatoid arthritis with rheumatoid factor of left ankle and foot without organ or systems involvement `HCC` `RxHCC`

M05.779 Rheumatoid arthritis with rheumatoid factor of unspecified ankle and foot without organ or systems involvement `HCC` `RxHCC`

M05.79 Rheumatoid arthritis with rheumatoid factor of multiple sites **without organ or systems involvement** `HCC` `RxHCC`

5th **M05.8** Other **rheumatoid arthritis** with rheumatoid factor

M05.80 Other rheumatoid arthritis with rheumatoid factor of unspecified site `HCC` `RxHCC`

6th **M05.81 Other rheumatoid arthritis with rheumatoid factor of** shoulder

M05.811 Other rheumatoid arthritis with rheumatoid factor of right shoulder `HCC` `RxHCC`

M05.812 Other rheumatoid arthritis with rheumatoid factor of left shoulder `HCC` `RxHCC`

M05.819 Other rheumatoid arthritis with rheumatoid factor of unspecified shoulder `HCC` `RxHCC`

6th **M05.82 Other rheumatoid arthritis with rheumatoid factor of** elbow

M05.821 Other rheumatoid arthritis with rheumatoid factor of right elbow `HCC` `RxHCC`

M05.822 Other rheumatoid arthritis with rheumatoid factor of left elbow `HCC` `RxHCC`

M05.829 Other rheumatoid arthritis with rheumatoid factor of unspecified elbow `HCC` `RxHCC`

6th **M05.83 Other rheumatoid arthritis with rheumatoid factor of** wrist

M05.831 Other rheumatoid arthritis with rheumatoid factor of right wrist `HCC` `RxHCC`

M05.832 Other rheumatoid arthritis with rheumatoid factor of left wrist `HCC` `RxHCC`

M05.839 Other rheumatoid arthritis with rheumatoid factor of unspecified wrist `HCC` `RxHCC`

6th **M05.84 Other rheumatoid arthritis with rheumatoid factor of** hand

M05.841 Other rheumatoid arthritis with rheumatoid factor of right hand `HCC` `RxHCC`

M05.842 Other rheumatoid arthritis with rheumatoid factor of left hand `HCC` `RxHCC`

M05.849 Other rheumatoid arthritis with rheumatoid factor of unspecified hand `HCC` `RxHCC`

6th **M05.85 Other rheumatoid arthritis with rheumatoid factor of** hip

M05.851 Other rheumatoid arthritis with rheumatoid factor of right hip `HCC` `RxHCC`

M05.852 Other rheumatoid arthritis with rheumatoid factor of left hip `HCC` `RxHCC`

M05.859 Other rheumatoid arthritis with rheumatoid factor of unspecified hip `HCC` `RxHCC`

6th **M05.86 Other rheumatoid arthritis with rheumatoid factor of** knee

M05.861 Other rheumatoid arthritis with rheumatoid factor of right knee `HCC` `RxHCC`

M05.862 Other rheumatoid arthritis with rheumatoid factor of left knee `HCC` `RxHCC`

M05.869 Other rheumatoid arthritis with rheumatoid factor of unspecified knee `HCC` `RxHCC`

6th **M05.87 Other rheumatoid arthritis with rheumatoid factor of** ankle and foot

M05.871 Other rheumatoid arthritis with rheumatoid factor of right ankle and foot `HCC` `RxHCC`

M05.872 Other rheumatoid arthritis with rheumatoid factor of left ankle and foot `HCC` `RxHCC`

M05.879 Other rheumatoid arthritis with rheumatoid factor of unspecified ankle and foot `HCC` `RxHCC`

M05.89 Other rheumatoid arthritis with rheumatoid factor of multiple sites `HCC` `RxHCC`

M05.9 Rheumatoid arthritis with rheumatoid factor, unspecified `HCC` `RxHCC`

4th **M06 Other rheumatoid arthritis**

5th **M06.0 Rheumatoid arthritis** without rheumatoid factor

M06.00 Rheumatoid arthritis without rheumatoid factor, unspecified site `HCC` `RxHCC`

6th **M06.01 Rheumatoid arthritis without rheumatoid factor, shoulder**

M06.011 Rheumatoid arthritis without rheumatoid factor, right shoulder `HCC` `RxHCC`

M06.012 Rheumatoid arthritis without rheumatoid factor, left shoulder `HCC` `RxHCC`

M06.019 Rheumatoid arthritis without rheumatoid factor, unspecified shoulder `HCC` `RxHCC`

6th **M06.02 Rheumatoid arthritis without rheumatoid factor, elbow**

M06.021 Rheumatoid arthritis without rheumatoid factor, right elbow `HCC` `RxHCC`

M06.022 Rheumatoid arthritis without rheumatoid factor, left elbow `HCC` `RxHCC`

M06.029 Rheumatoid arthritis without rheumatoid factor, unspecified elbow `HCC` `RxHCC`

6th **M06.03 Rheumatoid arthritis without rheumatoid factor, wrist**

M06.031 Rheumatoid arthritis without rheumatoid factor, right wrist `HCC` `RxHCC`

M06.032 Rheumatoid arthritis without rheumatoid factor, left wrist `HCC` `RxHCC`

M06.039 Rheumatoid arthritis without rheumatoid factor, unspecified wrist `HCC` `RxHCC`

6th **M06.04 Rheumatoid arthritis without rheumatoid factor, hand**

M06.041 Rheumatoid arthritis without rheumatoid factor, right hand `HCC` `RxHCC`

M06.042 Rheumatoid arthritis without rheumatoid factor, left hand `HCC` `RxHCC`

Unspecified Code Other Specified Code Manifestation Code N Newborn P Pediatric M Maternity A Adult ♂ Male ♀ Female
● New Code ▲ Revised Code Title ►◄ Revised Text **NOTES** *INCLUDES* *EXCLUDES1* Not coded here *EXCLUDES2* Not included here
4th 4th character required 5th 5th character required 6th 6th character required 7th 7th character required Extension 'X' Alert
HAC Hospital-acquired condition (HAC) alert **AHA** AHA Coding Clinic© ☛ Code first alert

CHAPTER 13: DISEASES OF THE MUSCULOSKELETAL SYSTEM AND CONNECTIVE TISSUE (M00-M99)

M06.049 - M06.841

Chapter 13: Diseases of the Musculoskeletal System and Connective Tissue (M00-M99)

M06.049 - M06.841

Tabular List

M06.049 - M06.841

M06.049 Rheumatoid arthritis without rheumatoid factor, unspecified hand `HCC` `RxHCC`

6th M06.05 Rheumatoid arthritis without rheumatoid factor, hip

M06.051 Rheumatoid arthritis without rheumatoid factor, right hip `HCC` `RxHCC`

M06.052 Rheumatoid arthritis without rheumatoid factor, left hip `HCC` `RxHCC`

M06.059 Rheumatoid arthritis without rheumatoid factor, unspecified hip `HCC` `RxHCC`

6th M06.06 Rheumatoid arthritis without rheumatoid factor, knee

M06.061 Rheumatoid arthritis without rheumatoid factor, right knee `HCC` `RxHCC`

M06.062 Rheumatoid arthritis without rheumatoid factor, left knee `HCC` `RxHCC`

M06.069 Rheumatoid arthritis without rheumatoid factor, unspecified knee `HCC` `RxHCC`

6th M06.07 Rheumatoid arthritis without rheumatoid factor, ankle and foot

M06.071 Rheumatoid arthritis without rheumatoid factor, right ankle and foot `HCC` `RxHCC`

M06.072 Rheumatoid arthritis without rheumatoid factor, left ankle and foot `HCC` `RxHCC`

M06.079 Rheumatoid arthritis without rheumatoid factor, unspecified ankle and foot `HCC` `RxHCC`

M06.08 Rheumatoid arthritis without rheumatoid factor, vertebrae `HCC` `RxHCC`

M06.09 Rheumatoid arthritis without rheumatoid factor, multiple sites `HCC` `RxHCC`

M06.1 Adult-onset Still's disease `A` `HCC` `RxHCC`

EXCLUDES1 Still's disease NOS (M08.2-)

5th M06.2 Rheumatoid bursitis

M06.20 Rheumatoid bursitis, unspecified site `HCC` `RxHCC`

6th M06.21 Rheumatoid bursitis, shoulder

M06.211 Rheumatoid bursitis, right shoulder `HCC` `RxHCC`

M06.212 Rheumatoid bursitis, left shoulder `HCC` `RxHCC`

M06.219 Rheumatoid bursitis, unspecified shoulder `HCC` `RxHCC`

6th M06.22 Rheumatoid bursitis, elbow

M06.221 Rheumatoid bursitis, right elbow `HCC` `RxHCC`

M06.222 Rheumatoid bursitis, left elbow `HCC` `RxHCC`

M06.229 Rheumatoid bursitis, unspecified elbow `HCC` `RxHCC`

6th M06.23 Rheumatoid bursitis, wrist

M06.231 Rheumatoid bursitis, right wrist `HCC` `RxHCC`

M06.232 Rheumatoid bursitis, left wrist `HCC` `RxHCC`

M06.239 Rheumatoid bursitis, unspecified wrist `HCC` `RxHCC`

6th M06.24 Rheumatoid bursitis, hand

M06.241 Rheumatoid bursitis, right hand `HCC` `RxHCC`

M06.242 Rheumatoid bursitis, left hand `HCC` `RxHCC`

M06.249 Rheumatoid bursitis, unspecified hand `HCC` `RxHCC`

6th M06.25 Rheumatoid bursitis, hip

M06.251 Rheumatoid bursitis, right hip `HCC` `RxHCC`

M06.252 Rheumatoid bursitis, left hip `HCC` `RxHCC`

M06.259 Rheumatoid bursitis, unspecified hip `HCC` `RxHCC`

6th M06.26 Rheumatoid bursitis, knee

M06.261 Rheumatoid bursitis, right knee `HCC` `RxHCC`

M06.262 Rheumatoid bursitis, left knee `HCC` `RxHCC`

M06.269 Rheumatoid bursitis, unspecified knee `HCC` `RxHCC`

6th M06.27 Rheumatoid bursitis, ankle and foot

M06.271 Rheumatoid bursitis, right ankle and foot `HCC` `RxHCC`

M06.272 Rheumatoid bursitis, left ankle and foot `HCC` `RxHCC`

M06.279 Rheumatoid bursitis, unspecified ankle and foot `HCC` `RxHCC`

M06.28 Rheumatoid bursitis, vertebrae `HCC` `RxHCC`

M06.29 Rheumatoid bursitis, multiple sites `HCC` `RxHCC`

5th M06.3 Rheumatoid nodule

M06.30 Rheumatoid nodule, unspecified site `HCC` `RxHCC`

6th M06.31 Rheumatoid nodule, shoulder

M06.311 Rheumatoid nodule, right shoulder `HCC` `RxHCC`

M06.312 Rheumatoid nodule, left shoulder `HCC` `RxHCC`

M06.319 Rheumatoid nodule, unspecified shoulder `HCC` `RxHCC`

6th M06.32 Rheumatoid nodule, elbow

M06.321 Rheumatoid nodule, right elbow `HCC` `RxHCC`

M06.322 Rheumatoid nodule, left elbow `HCC` `RxHCC`

M06.329 Rheumatoid nodule, unspecified elbow `HCC` `RxHCC`

6th M06.33 Rheumatoid nodule, wrist

M06.331 Rheumatoid nodule, right wrist `HCC` `RxHCC`

M06.332 Rheumatoid nodule, left wrist `HCC` `RxHCC`

M06.339 Rheumatoid nodule, unspecified wrist `HCC` `RxHCC`

6th M06.34 Rheumatoid nodule, hand

M06.341 Rheumatoid nodule, right hand `HCC` `RxHCC`

M06.342 Rheumatoid nodule, left hand `HCC` `RxHCC`

M06.349 Rheumatoid nodule, unspecified hand `HCC` `RxHCC`

6th M06.35 Rheumatoid nodule, hip

M06.351 Rheumatoid nodule, right hip `HCC` `RxHCC`

M06.352 Rheumatoid nodule, left hip `HCC` `RxHCC`

M06.359 Rheumatoid nodule, unspecified hip `HCC` `RxHCC`

6th M06.36 Rheumatoid nodule, knee

M06.361 Rheumatoid nodule, right knee `HCC` `RxHCC`

M06.362 Rheumatoid nodule, left knee `HCC` `RxHCC`

M06.369 Rheumatoid nodule, unspecified knee `HCC` `RxHCC`

6th M06.37 Rheumatoid nodule, ankle and foot

M06.371 Rheumatoid nodule, right ankle and foot `HCC` `RxHCC`

M06.372 Rheumatoid nodule, left ankle and foot `HCC` `RxHCC`

M06.379 Rheumatoid nodule, unspecified ankle and foot `HCC` `RxHCC`

M06.38 Rheumatoid nodule, vertebrae `HCC` `RxHCC`

M06.39 Rheumatoid nodule, multiple sites `HCC` `RxHCC`

M06.4 Inflammatory polyarthropathy `HCC` `RxHCC`

EXCLUDES1 polyarthritis NOS (M13.0)

5th M06.8 Other specified rheumatoid arthritis

M06.80 Other specified rheumatoid arthritis, unspecified site `HCC` `RxHCC`

6th M06.81 Other specified rheumatoid arthritis, shoulder

M06.811 Other specified rheumatoid arthritis, right shoulder `HCC` `RxHCC`

M06.812 Other specified rheumatoid arthritis, left shoulder `HCC` `RxHCC`

M06.819 Other specified rheumatoid arthritis, unspecified shoulder `HCC` `RxHCC`

6th M06.82 Other specified rheumatoid arthritis, elbow

M06.821 Other specified rheumatoid arthritis, right elbow `HCC` `RxHCC`

M06.822 Other specified rheumatoid arthritis, left elbow `HCC` `RxHCC`

M06.829 Other specified rheumatoid arthritis, unspecified elbow `HCC` `RxHCC`

6th M06.83 Other specified rheumatoid arthritis, wrist

M06.831 Other specified rheumatoid arthritis, right wrist `HCC` `RxHCC`

M06.832 Other specified rheumatoid arthritis, left wrist `HCC` `RxHCC`

M06.839 Other specified rheumatoid arthritis, unspecified wrist `HCC` `RxHCC`

6th M06.84 Other specified rheumatoid arthritis, hand

M06.841 Other specified rheumatoid arthritis, right hand `HCC` `RxHCC`

PDx Unacceptable principal diagnosis symbol per Medicare code edits   POA Code exempt from diagnosis present on admission requirement
? Questionable admission   CC Complication or comorbidity   MCC Major complication or comorbidity   CC/MCC Excl CC/MCC exclusion
HCC HCC diagnosis code   RxHCC RxHCC diagnosis code   MACRA code   DEFINITION Describes condition/terminology
TIP Coding guidance   👁 Official Guideline Reference   Z1 Z code as first-listed diagnosis

782

When symbols appear on a code that requires a 7th character extension, refer to Appendix B to identify applicable 7th character codes.

2020 ICD-10-CM

M06.842 Other specified rheumatoid arthritis, left hand HCC RxHCC
M06.849 Other specified rheumatoid arthritis, unspecified hand HCC RxHCC
6ᵗʰ M06.85 Other specified rheumatoid arthritis, hip
M06.851 Other specified rheumatoid arthritis, right hip HCC RxHCC
M06.852 Other specified rheumatoid arthritis, left hip HCC RxHCC
M06.859 Other specified rheumatoid arthritis, unspecified hip HCC RxHCC
6ᵗʰ M06.86 Other specified rheumatoid arthritis, knee
M06.861 Other specified rheumatoid arthritis, right knee HCC RxHCC
M06.862 Other specified rheumatoid arthritis, left knee HCC RxHCC
M06.869 Other specified rheumatoid arthritis, unspecified knee HCC RxHCC
6ᵗʰ M06.87 Other specified rheumatoid arthritis, ankle and foot
M06.871 Other specified rheumatoid arthritis, right ankle and foot HCC RxHCC
M06.872 Other specified rheumatoid arthritis, left ankle and foot HCC RxHCC
M06.879 Other specified rheumatoid arthritis, unspecified ankle and foot HCC RxHCC
M06.88 Other specified rheumatoid arthritis, vertebrae HCC RxHCC
M06.89 Other specified rheumatoid arthritis, multiple sites HCC RxHCC
M06.9 Rheumatoid arthritis, unspecified HCC RxHCC
4ᵗʰ M07 Enteropathic arthropathies
DEFINITION: Enteropathic is a form of chronic inflammatory arthritis commonly associated with ulcerative colitis and Crohn's disease.
Code also associated enteropathy, such as:
regional enteritis [Crohn's disease] (K50.-)
ulcerative colitis (K51.-)
EXCLUDES1 psoriatic arthropathies (L40.5-)
5ᵗʰ M07.6 Enteropathic arthropathies
M07.60 Enteropathic arthropathies, unspecified site
6ᵗʰ M07.61 Enteropathic arthropathies, shoulder
M07.611 Enteropathic arthropathies, right shoulder
M07.612 Enteropathic arthropathies, left shoulder
M07.619 Enteropathic arthropathies, unspecified shoulder
6ᵗʰ M07.62 Enteropathic arthropathies, elbow
M07.621 Enteropathic arthropathies, right elbow
M07.622 Enteropathic arthropathies, left elbow
M07.629 Enteropathic arthropathies, unspecified elbow
6ᵗʰ M07.63 Enteropathic arthropathies, wrist
M07.631 Enteropathic arthropathies, right wrist
M07.632 Enteropathic arthropathies, left wrist
M07.639 Enteropathic arthropathies, unspecified wrist
6ᵗʰ M07.64 Enteropathic arthropathies, hand
M07.641 Enteropathic arthropathies, right hand
M07.642 Enteropathic arthropathies, left hand
M07.649 Enteropathic arthropathies, unspecified hand
6ᵗʰ M07.65 Enteropathic arthropathies, hip
M07.651 Enteropathic arthropathies, right hip
M07.652 Enteropathic arthropathies, left hip
M07.659 Enteropathic arthropathies, unspecified hip
6ᵗʰ M07.66 Enteropathic arthropathies, knee
M07.661 Enteropathic arthropathies, right knee
M07.662 Enteropathic arthropathies, left knee
M07.669 Enteropathic arthropathies, unspecified knee

6ᵗʰ M07.67 Enteropathic arthropathies, ankle and foot
M07.671 Enteropathic arthropathies, right ankle and foot
M07.672 Enteropathic arthropathies, left ankle and foot
M07.679 Enteropathic arthropathies, unspecified ankle and foot
M07.68 Enteropathic arthropathies, vertebrae
M07.69 Enteropathic arthropathies, multiple sites
4ᵗʰ M08 Juvenile arthritis
Code also any associated underlying condition, such as:
regional enteritis [Crohn's disease] (K50.-)
ulcerative colitis (K51.-)
EXCLUDES1 arthropathy in Whipple's disease (M14.8)
Felty's syndrome (M05.0)
juvenile dermatomyositis (M33.0-)
psoriatic juvenile arthropathy (L40.54)
5ᵗʰ M08.0 Unspecified juvenile rheumatoid arthritis
Juvenile rheumatoid arthritis with or without rheumatoid factor
M08.00 Unspecified juvenile rheumatoid arthritis of unspecified site HCC RxHCC
6ᵗʰ M08.01 Unspecified juvenile rheumatoid arthritis, shoulder
M08.011 Unspecified juvenile rheumatoid arthritis, right shoulder HCC RxHCC
M08.012 Unspecified juvenile rheumatoid arthritis, left shoulder HCC RxHCC
M08.019 Unspecified juvenile rheumatoid arthritis, unspecified shoulder HCC RxHCC
6ᵗʰ M08.02 Unspecified juvenile rheumatoid arthritis of elbow
M08.021 Unspecified juvenile rheumatoid arthritis, right elbow HCC RxHCC
M08.022 Unspecified juvenile rheumatoid arthritis, left elbow HCC RxHCC
M08.029 Unspecified juvenile rheumatoid arthritis, unspecified elbow HCC RxHCC
6ᵗʰ M08.03 Unspecified juvenile rheumatoid arthritis, wrist
M08.031 Unspecified juvenile rheumatoid arthritis, right wrist HCC RxHCC
M08.032 Unspecified juvenile rheumatoid arthritis, left wrist HCC RxHCC
M08.039 Unspecified juvenile rheumatoid arthritis, unspecified wrist HCC RxHCC
6ᵗʰ M08.04 Unspecified juvenile rheumatoid arthritis, hand
M08.041 Unspecified juvenile rheumatoid arthritis, right hand HCC RxHCC
M08.042 Unspecified juvenile rheumatoid arthritis, left hand HCC RxHCC
M08.049 Unspecified juvenile rheumatoid arthritis, unspecified hand HCC RxHCC
6ᵗʰ M08.05 Unspecified juvenile rheumatoid arthritis, hip
M08.051 Unspecified juvenile rheumatoid arthritis, right hip HCC RxHCC
M08.052 Unspecified juvenile rheumatoid arthritis, left hip HCC RxHCC
M08.059 Unspecified juvenile rheumatoid arthritis, unspecified hip HCC RxHCC
6ᵗʰ M08.06 Unspecified juvenile rheumatoid arthritis, knee
M08.061 Unspecified juvenile rheumatoid arthritis, right knee HCC RxHCC
M08.062 Unspecified juvenile rheumatoid arthritis, left knee HCC RxHCC
M08.069 Unspecified juvenile rheumatoid arthritis, unspecified knee HCC RxHCC
6ᵗʰ M08.07 Unspecified juvenile rheumatoid arthritis, ankle and foot
M08.071 Unspecified juvenile rheumatoid arthritis, right ankle and foot HCC RxHCC
M08.072 Unspecified juvenile rheumatoid arthritis, left ankle and foot HCC RxHCC

M08.079 **Unspecified juvenile rheumatoid arthritis, unspecified ankle and foot** HCC RxHCC

M08.08 **Unspecified juvenile rheumatoid arthritis,** vertebrae HCC RxHCC

M08.09 **Unspecified juvenile rheumatoid arthritis,** multiple sites HCC RxHCC

M08.1 **Juvenile** ankylosing spondylitis HCC RxHCC

     EXCLUDES1 ankylosing spondylitis in adults (M45.0-)

M08.2 **Juvenile rheumatoid arthritis** with systemic onset

     Still's disease NOS

     EXCLUDES1 adult-onset Still's disease (M06.1-)

M08.20 **Juvenile rheumatoid arthritis with systemic onset, unspecified site** HCC RxHCC

M08.21 **Juvenile rheumatoid arthritis with systemic onset,** shoulder

     M08.211 **Juvenile rheumatoid arthritis with systemic onset,** right **shoulder** HCC RxHCC

     M08.212 **Juvenile rheumatoid arthritis with systemic onset,** left **shoulder** HCC RxHCC

     M08.219 **Juvenile rheumatoid arthritis with systemic onset, unspecified shoulder** HCC RxHCC

M08.22 **Juvenile rheumatoid arthritis with systemic onset,** elbow

     M08.221 **Juvenile rheumatoid arthritis with systemic onset,** right **elbow** HCC RxHCC

     M08.222 **Juvenile rheumatoid arthritis with systemic onset,** left **elbow** HCC RxHCC

     M08.229 **Juvenile rheumatoid arthritis with systemic onset, unspecified elbow** HCC RxHCC

M08.23 **Juvenile rheumatoid arthritis with systemic onset,** wrist

     M08.231 **Juvenile rheumatoid arthritis with systemic onset,** right **wrist** HCC RxHCC

     M08.232 **Juvenile rheumatoid arthritis with systemic onset,** left **wrist** HCC RxHCC

     M08.239 **Juvenile rheumatoid arthritis with systemic onset, unspecified wrist** HCC RxHCC

M08.24 **Juvenile rheumatoid arthritis with systemic onset,** hand

     M08.241 **Juvenile rheumatoid arthritis with systemic onset,** right **hand** HCC RxHCC

     M08.242 **Juvenile rheumatoid arthritis with systemic onset,** left **hand** HCC RxHCC

     M08.249 **Juvenile rheumatoid arthritis with systemic onset, unspecified hand** HCC RxHCC

M08.25 **Juvenile rheumatoid arthritis with systemic onset,** hip

     M08.251 **Juvenile rheumatoid arthritis with systemic onset,** right **hip** HCC RxHCC

     M08.252 **Juvenile rheumatoid arthritis with systemic onset,** left **hip** HCC RxHCC

     M08.259 **Juvenile rheumatoid arthritis with systemic onset, unspecified hip** HCC RxHCC

M08.26 **Juvenile rheumatoid arthritis with systemic onset,** knee

     M08.261 **Juvenile rheumatoid arthritis with systemic onset,** right **knee** HCC RxHCC

     M08.262 **Juvenile rheumatoid arthritis with systemic onset,** left **knee** HCC RxHCC

     M08.269 **Juvenile rheumatoid arthritis with systemic onset, unspecified knee** HCC RxHCC

M08.27 **Juvenile rheumatoid arthritis with systemic onset,** ankle and foot

     M08.271 **Juvenile rheumatoid arthritis with systemic onset,** right **ankle and foot** HCC RxHCC

     M08.272 **Juvenile rheumatoid arthritis with systemic onset,** left **ankle and foot** HCC RxHCC

     M08.279 **Juvenile rheumatoid arthritis with systemic onset, unspecified ankle and foot** HCC RxHCC

M08.28 **Juvenile rheumatoid arthritis with systemic onset,** vertebrae HCC RxHCC

M08.29 **Juvenile rheumatoid arthritis with systemic onset,** multiple sites HCC RxHCC

M08.3 **Juvenile** rheumatoid polyarthritis (seronegative) HCC RxHCC

M08.4 **Pauciarticular** juvenile rheumatoid arthritis

M08.40 **Pauciarticular juvenile rheumatoid arthritis, unspecified site** HCC RxHCC

M08.41 **Pauciarticular juvenile rheumatoid arthritis,** shoulder

     M08.411 **Pauciarticular juvenile rheumatoid arthritis,** right **shoulder** HCC RxHCC

     M08.412 **Pauciarticular juvenile rheumatoid arthritis,** left **shoulder** HCC RxHCC

     M08.419 **Pauciarticular juvenile rheumatoid arthritis, unspecified shoulder** HCC RxHCC

M08.42 **Pauciarticular juvenile rheumatoid arthritis,** elbow

     M08.421 **Pauciarticular juvenile rheumatoid arthritis,** right **elbow** HCC RxHCC

     M08.422 **Pauciarticular juvenile rheumatoid arthritis,** left **elbow** HCC RxHCC

     M08.429 **Pauciarticular juvenile rheumatoid arthritis, unspecified elbow** HCC RxHCC

M08.43 **Pauciarticular juvenile rheumatoid arthritis,** wrist

     M08.431 **Pauciarticular juvenile rheumatoid arthritis,** right **wrist** HCC RxHCC

     M08.432 **Pauciarticular juvenile rheumatoid arthritis,** left **wrist** HCC RxHCC

     M08.439 **Pauciarticular juvenile rheumatoid arthritis, unspecified wrist** HCC RxHCC

M08.44 **Pauciarticular juvenile rheumatoid arthritis,** hand

     M08.441 **Pauciarticular juvenile rheumatoid arthritis,** right **hand** HCC RxHCC

     M08.442 **Pauciarticular juvenile rheumatoid arthritis,** left **hand** HCC RxHCC

     M08.449 **Pauciarticular juvenile rheumatoid arthritis, unspecified hand** HCC RxHCC

M08.45 **Pauciarticular juvenile rheumatoid arthritis,** hip

     M08.451 **Pauciarticular juvenile rheumatoid arthritis,** right **hip** HCC RxHCC

     M08.452 **Pauciarticular juvenile rheumatoid arthritis,** left **hip** HCC RxHCC

     M08.459 **Pauciarticular juvenile rheumatoid arthritis, unspecified hip** HCC RxHCC

M08.46 **Pauciarticular juvenile rheumatoid arthritis,** knee

     M08.461 **Pauciarticular juvenile rheumatoid arthritis,** right **knee** HCC RxHCC

     M08.462 **Pauciarticular juvenile rheumatoid arthritis,** left **knee** HCC RxHCC

     M08.469 **Pauciarticular juvenile rheumatoid arthritis, unspecified knee** HCC RxHCC

M08.47 **Pauciarticular juvenile rheumatoid arthritis,** ankle and foot

     M08.471 **Pauciarticular juvenile rheumatoid arthritis,** right **ankle and foot** HCC RxHCC

     M08.472 **Pauciarticular juvenile rheumatoid arthritis,** left **ankle and foot** HCC RxHCC

     M08.479 **Pauciarticular juvenile rheumatoid arthritis, unspecified ankle and foot** HCC RxHCC

M08.48 **Pauciarticular juvenile rheumatoid arthritis,** vertebrae HCC RxHCC

M08.8 **Other juvenile** arthritis

M08.80 **Other juvenile arthritis, unspecified site** HCC RxHCC

M08.81 **Other juvenile arthritis,** shoulder

     M08.811 **Other juvenile arthritis,** right **shoulder** HCC RxHCC

     M08.812 **Other juvenile arthritis,** left **shoulder** HCC RxHCC

     M08.819 **Other juvenile arthritis, unspecified shoulder** HCC RxHCC

M08.82 **Other juvenile arthritis,** elbow

     M08.821 **Other juvenile arthritis,** right **elbow** HCC RxHCC

PDx Unacceptable principal diagnosis symbol per Medicare code edits   Code exempt from diagnosis present on admission requirement

? Questionable admission   CC Complication or comorbidity   MCC Major complication or comorbidity   CC/MCC CC/MCC exclusion

HCC HCC diagnosis code   RxHCC RxHCC diagnosis code   MACRA code   **DEFINITION** Describes condition/terminology

TIP Coding guidance   Official Guideline Reference   Z1 Z code as first-listed diagnosis

M08.822 Other juvenile arthritis, left elbow [HCC] [RxHCC]
M08.829 Other juvenile arthritis, unspecified elbow [HCC] [RxHCC]

[6th] M08.83 Other juvenile arthritis, wrist
M08.831 Other juvenile arthritis, right wrist [HCC] [RxHCC]
M08.832 Other juvenile arthritis, left wrist [HCC] [RxHCC]
M08.839 Other juvenile arthritis, unspecified wrist [HCC] [RxHCC]

[6th] M08.84 Other juvenile arthritis, hand
M08.841 Other juvenile arthritis, right hand [HCC] [RxHCC]
M08.842 Other juvenile arthritis, left hand [HCC] [RxHCC]
M08.849 Other juvenile arthritis, unspecified hand [HCC] [RxHCC]

[6th] M08.85 Other juvenile arthritis, hip
M08.851 Other juvenile arthritis, right hip [HCC] [RxHCC]
M08.852 Other juvenile arthritis, left hip [HCC] [RxHCC]
M08.859 Other juvenile arthritis, unspecified hip [HCC] [RxHCC]

[6th] M08.86 Other juvenile arthritis, knee
M08.861 Other juvenile arthritis, right knee [HCC] [RxHCC]
M08.862 Other juvenile arthritis, left knee [HCC] [RxHCC]
M08.869 Other juvenile arthritis, unspecified knee [HCC] [RxHCC]

[6th] M08.87 Other juvenile arthritis, ankle and foot
M08.871 Other juvenile arthritis, right ankle and foot [HCC] [RxHCC]
M08.872 Other juvenile arthritis, left ankle and foot [HCC] [RxHCC]
M08.879 Other juvenile arthritis, unspecified ankle and foot [HCC] [RxHCC]

M08.88 Other juvenile arthritis, other specified site [HCC] [RxHCC]
Other juvenile arthritis, vertebrae

M08.89 Other juvenile arthritis, multiple sites [HCC] [RxHCC]

[5th] M08.9 Juvenile arthritis, unspecified
EXCLUDES1 *juvenile rheumatoid arthritis, unspecified (M08.0-)*

M08.90 Juvenile arthritis, unspecified, unspecified site [HCC] [RxHCC]

[6th] M08.91 Juvenile arthritis, unspecified, shoulder
M08.911 Juvenile arthritis, unspecified, right shoulder [HCC] [RxHCC]
M08.912 Juvenile arthritis, unspecified, left shoulder [HCC] [RxHCC]
M08.919 Juvenile arthritis, unspecified, unspecified shoulder [HCC] [RxHCC]

[6th] M08.92 Juvenile arthritis, unspecified, elbow
M08.921 Juvenile arthritis, unspecified, right elbow [HCC] [RxHCC]
M08.922 Juvenile arthritis, unspecified, left elbow [HCC] [RxHCC]
M08.929 Juvenile arthritis, unspecified, unspecified elbow [HCC] [RxHCC]

[6th] M08.93 Juvenile arthritis, unspecified, wrist
M08.931 Juvenile arthritis, unspecified, right wrist [HCC] [RxHCC]
M08.932 Juvenile arthritis, unspecified, left wrist [HCC] [RxHCC]
M08.939 Juvenile arthritis, unspecified, unspecified wrist [HCC] [RxHCC]

[6th] M08.94 Juvenile arthritis, unspecified, hand
M08.941 Juvenile arthritis, unspecified, right hand [HCC] [RxHCC]
M08.942 Juvenile arthritis, unspecified, left hand [HCC] [RxHCC]
M08.949 Juvenile arthritis, unspecified, unspecified hand [HCC] [RxHCC]

[6th] M08.95 Juvenile arthritis, unspecified, hip
M08.951 Juvenile arthritis, unspecified, right hip [HCC] [RxHCC]
M08.952 Juvenile arthritis, unspecified, left hip [HCC] [RxHCC]
M08.959 Juvenile arthritis, unspecified, unspecified hip [HCC] [RxHCC]

[6th] M08.96 Juvenile arthritis, unspecified, knee
M08.961 Juvenile arthritis, unspecified, right knee [HCC] [RxHCC]
M08.962 Juvenile arthritis, unspecified, left knee [HCC] [RxHCC]
M08.969 Juvenile arthritis, unspecified, unspecified knee [HCC] [RxHCC]

[6th] M08.97 Juvenile arthritis, unspecified, ankle and foot
M08.971 Juvenile arthritis, unspecified, right ankle and foot [HCC] [RxHCC]
M08.972 Juvenile arthritis, unspecified, left ankle and foot [HCC] [RxHCC]
M08.979 Juvenile arthritis, unspecified, unspecified ankle and foot [HCC] [RxHCC]

M08.98 Juvenile arthritis, unspecified, vertebrae [HCC] [RxHCC]
M08.99 Juvenile arthritis, unspecified, multiple sites [HCC] [RxHCC]

[4th] M1A Chronic gout
Use additional code to identify:
Autonomic neuropathy in diseases classified elsewhere (G99.0)
Calculus of urinary tract in diseases classified elsewhere (N22)
Cardiomyopathy in diseases classified elsewhere (I43)
Disorders of external ear in diseases classified elsewhere (H61.1-, H62.8-)
Disorders of iris and ciliary body in diseases classified elsewhere (H22)
Glomerular disorders in diseases classified elsewhere (N08)

EXCLUDES1 *gout NOS (M10.-)*
EXCLUDES2 *acute gout (M10.-)*

The appropriate 7th character is to be added to each code from category M1A
0 = without tophus (tophi)
1 = with tophus (tophi)

[5th] M1A.0 Idiopathic chronic gout
Chronic gouty bursitis
Primary chronic gout

[7th] M1A.00 Idiopathic chronic gout, unspecified site

[6th] M1A.01 Idiopathic chronic gout, shoulder
[7th] M1A.011 Idiopathic chronic gout, right shoulder
[7th] M1A.012 Idiopathic chronic gout, left shoulder
[7th] M1A.019 Idiopathic chronic gout, unspecified shoulder

[6th] M1A.02 Idiopathic chronic gout, elbow
[7th] M1A.021 Idiopathic chronic gout, right elbow
[7th] M1A.022 Idiopathic chronic gout, left elbow
[7th] M1A.029 Idiopathic chronic gout, unspecified elbow

[6th] M1A.03 Idiopathic chronic gout, wrist
[7th] M1A.031 Idiopathic chronic gout, right wrist
[7th] M1A.032 Idiopathic chronic gout, left wrist
[7th] M1A.039 Idiopathic chronic gout, unspecified wrist

[6th] M1A.04 Idiopathic chronic gout, hand
[7th] M1A.041 Idiopathic chronic gout, right hand
[7th] M1A.042 Idiopathic chronic gout, left hand
[7th] M1A.049 Idiopathic chronic gout, unspecified hand

[6th] M1A.05 Idiopathic chronic gout, hip
[7th] M1A.051 Idiopathic chronic gout, right hip
[7th] M1A.052 Idiopathic chronic gout, left hip
[7th] M1A.059 Idiopathic chronic gout, unspecified hip

[6th] M1A.06 Idiopathic chronic gout, knee
[7th] M1A.061 Idiopathic chronic gout, right knee
[7th] M1A.062 Idiopathic chronic gout, left knee
[7th] M1A.069 Idiopathic chronic gout, unspecified knee

[6th] M1A.07 Idiopathic chronic gout, ankle and foot
[7th] M1A.071 Idiopathic chronic gout, right ankle and foot
[7th] M1A.072 Idiopathic chronic gout, left ankle and foot
[7th] M1A.079 Idiopathic chronic gout, unspecified ankle and foot

- 🌀 **M1A.08 Idiopathic chronic gout,** vertebrae
- 🌀 **M1A.09 Idiopathic chronic gout,** multiple sites
- 5ᵗʰ **M1A.1 Lead-induced chronic gout**
  - ☛ Code first toxic effects of lead and its compounds (T56.0-)
  - 🌀 **M1A.10 Lead-induced chronic gout,** unspecified site
  - 6ᵗʰ **M1A.11 Lead-induced chronic gout,** shoulder
    - 7ᵗʰ **M1A.111 Lead-induced chronic gout,** right shoulder
    - 7ᵗʰ **M1A.112 Lead-induced chronic gout,** left shoulder
    - 7ᵗʰ **M1A.119 Lead-induced chronic gout,** unspecified shoulder
  - 6ᵗʰ **M1A.12 Lead-induced chronic gout,** elbow
    - 7ᵗʰ **M1A.121 Lead-induced chronic gout,** right elbow
    - 7ᵗʰ **M1A.122 Lead-induced chronic gout,** left elbow
    - 7ᵗʰ **M1A.129 Lead-induced chronic gout,** unspecified elbow
  - 6ᵗʰ **M1A.13 Lead-induced chronic gout,** wrist
    - 7ᵗʰ **M1A.131 Lead-induced chronic gout,** right wrist
    - 7ᵗʰ **M1A.132 Lead-induced chronic gout,** left wrist
    - 7ᵗʰ **M1A.139 Lead-induced chronic gout,** unspecified wrist
  - 6ᵗʰ **M1A.14 Lead-induced chronic gout,** hand
    - 7ᵗʰ **M1A.141 Lead-induced chronic gout,** right hand
    - 7ᵗʰ **M1A.142 Lead-induced chronic gout,** left hand
    - 7ᵗʰ **M1A.149 Lead-induced chronic gout,** unspecified hand
  - 6ᵗʰ **M1A.15 Lead-induced chronic gout,** hip
    - 7ᵗʰ **M1A.151 Lead-induced chronic gout,** right hip
    - 7ᵗʰ **M1A.152 Lead-induced chronic gout,** left hip
    - 7ᵗʰ **M1A.159 Lead-induced chronic gout,** unspecified hip
  - 6ᵗʰ **M1A.16 Lead-induced chronic gout,** knee
    - 7ᵗʰ **M1A.161 Lead-induced chronic gout,** right knee
    - 7ᵗʰ **M1A.162 Lead-induced chronic gout,** left knee
    - 7ᵗʰ **M1A.169 Lead-induced chronic gout,** unspecified knee
  - 6ᵗʰ **M1A.17 Lead-induced chronic gout,** ankle and foot
    - 7ᵗʰ **M1A.171 Lead-induced chronic gout,** right ankle and foot
    - 7ᵗʰ **M1A.172 Lead-induced chronic gout,** left ankle and foot
    - 7ᵗʰ **M1A.179 Lead-induced chronic gout,** unspecified ankle and foot
  - 🌀 **M1A.18 Lead-induced chronic gout,** vertebrae
  - 🌀 **M1A.19 Lead-induced chronic gout,** multiple sites
- 5ᵗʰ **M1A.2 Drug-induced chronic gout**
  - Use additional code for adverse effect, if applicable, to identify drug (T36-T50 with fifth or sixth character 5)
  - 🌀 **M1A.20 Drug-induced chronic gout,** unspecified site
  - 6ᵗʰ **M1A.21 Drug-induced chronic gout,** shoulder
    - 7ᵗʰ **M1A.211 Drug-induced chronic gout,** right shoulder
    - 7ᵗʰ **M1A.212 Drug-induced chronic gout,** left shoulder
    - 7ᵗʰ **M1A.219 Drug-induced chronic gout,** unspecified shoulder
  - 6ᵗʰ **M1A.22 Drug-induced chronic gout,** elbow
    - 7ᵗʰ **M1A.221 Drug-induced chronic gout,** right elbow
    - 7ᵗʰ **M1A.222 Drug-induced chronic gout,** left elbow
    - 7ᵗʰ **M1A.229 Drug-induced chronic gout,** unspecified elbow
  - 6ᵗʰ **M1A.23 Drug-induced chronic gout,** wrist
    - 7ᵗʰ **M1A.231 Drug-induced chronic gout,** right wrist
    - 7ᵗʰ **M1A.232 Drug-induced chronic gout,** left wrist
    - 7ᵗʰ **M1A.239 Drug-induced chronic gout,** unspecified wrist
  - 6ᵗʰ **M1A.24 Drug-induced chronic gout,** hand
    - 7ᵗʰ **M1A.241 Drug-induced chronic gout,** right hand
    - 7ᵗʰ **M1A.242 Drug-induced chronic gout,** left hand
    - 7ᵗʰ **M1A.249 Drug-induced chronic gout,** unspecified hand
  - 6ᵗʰ **M1A.25 Drug-induced chronic gout,** hip
    - 7ᵗʰ **M1A.251 Drug-induced chronic gout,** right hip
    - 7ᵗʰ **M1A.252 Drug-induced chronic gout,** left hip
    - 7ᵗʰ **M1A.259 Drug-induced chronic gout,** unspecified hip
  - 6ᵗʰ **M1A.26 Drug-induced chronic gout,** knee
    - 7ᵗʰ **M1A.261 Drug-induced chronic gout,** right knee
    - 7ᵗʰ **M1A.262 Drug-induced chronic gout,** left knee
    - 7ᵗʰ **M1A.269 Drug-induced chronic gout,** unspecified knee
  - 6ᵗʰ **M1A.27 Drug-induced chronic gout,** ankle and foot
    - 7ᵗʰ **M1A.271 Drug-induced chronic gout,** right ankle and foot
    - 7ᵗʰ **M1A.272 Drug-induced chronic gout,** left ankle and foot
    - 7ᵗʰ **M1A.279 Drug-induced chronic gout,** unspecified ankle and foot
  - 🌀 **M1A.28 Drug-induced chronic gout,** vertebrae
  - 🌀 **M1A.29 Drug-induced chronic gout,** multiple sites
- 5ᵗʰ **M1A.3 Chronic gout** due to renal impairment
  - ☛ Code first associated renal disease
  - 🌀 **M1A.30 Chronic gout due to renal impairment,** unspecified site
  - 6ᵗʰ **M1A.31 Chronic gout due to renal impairment,** shoulder
    - 7ᵗʰ **M1A.311 Chronic gout due to renal impairment,** right shoulder
    - 7ᵗʰ **M1A.312 Chronic gout due to renal impairment,** left shoulder
    - 7ᵗʰ **M1A.319 Chronic gout due to renal impairment,** unspecified shoulder
  - 6ᵗʰ **M1A.32 Chronic gout due to renal impairment,** elbow
    - 7ᵗʰ **M1A.321 Chronic gout due to renal impairment,** right elbow
    - 7ᵗʰ **M1A.322 Chronic gout due to renal impairment,** left elbow
    - 7ᵗʰ **M1A.329 Chronic gout due to renal impairment,** unspecified elbow
  - 6ᵗʰ **M1A.33 Chronic gout due to renal impairment,** wrist
    - 7ᵗʰ **M1A.331 Chronic gout due to renal impairment,** right wrist
    - 7ᵗʰ **M1A.332 Chronic gout due to renal impairment,** left wrist
    - 7ᵗʰ **M1A.339 Chronic gout due to renal impairment,** unspecified wrist
  - 6ᵗʰ **M1A.34 Chronic gout due to renal impairment,** hand
    - 7ᵗʰ **M1A.341 Chronic gout due to renal impairment,** right hand
    - 7ᵗʰ **M1A.342 Chronic gout due to renal impairment,** left hand
    - 7ᵗʰ **M1A.349 Chronic gout due to renal impairment,** unspecified hand
  - 6ᵗʰ **M1A.35 Chronic gout due to renal impairment,** hip
    - 7ᵗʰ **M1A.351 Chronic gout due to renal impairment,** right hip
    - 7ᵗʰ **M1A.352 Chronic gout due to renal impairment,** left hip
    - 7ᵗʰ **M1A.359 Chronic gout due to renal impairment,** unspecified hip
  - 6ᵗʰ **M1A.36 Chronic gout due to renal impairment,** knee
    - 7ᵗʰ **M1A.361 Chronic gout due to renal impairment,** right knee
    - 7ᵗʰ **M1A.362 Chronic gout due to renal impairment,** left knee
    - 7ᵗʰ **M1A.369 Chronic gout due to renal impairment,** unspecified knee
  - 6ᵗʰ **M1A.37 Chronic gout due to renal impairment,** ankle and foot
    - 7ᵗʰ **M1A.371 Chronic gout due to renal impairment,** right ankle and foot
    - 7ᵗʰ **M1A.372 Chronic gout due to renal impairment,** left ankle and foot
    - 7ᵗʰ **M1A.379 Chronic gout due to renal impairment,** unspecified ankle and foot

---

[7th] M1A.38 Chronic gout due to renal impairment, vertebrae
[7th] M1A.39 Chronic gout due to renal impairment, multiple sites
[5th] M1A.4 Other secondary chronic gout
☞ Code first associated condition
[7th] M1A.40 Other secondary chronic gout, unspecified site
[6th] M1A.41 Other secondary chronic gout, shoulder
[7th] M1A.411 Other secondary chronic gout, right shoulder
[7th] M1A.412 Other secondary chronic gout, left shoulder
[7th] M1A.419 Other secondary chronic gout, unspecified shoulder
[6th] M1A.42 Other secondary chronic gout, elbow
[7th] M1A.421 Other secondary chronic gout, right elbow
[7th] M1A.422 Other secondary chronic gout, left elbow
[7th] M1A.429 Other secondary chronic gout, unspecified elbow
[6th] M1A.43 Other secondary chronic gout, wrist
[7th] M1A.431 Other secondary chronic gout, right wrist
[7th] M1A.432 Other secondary chronic gout, left wrist
[7th] M1A.439 Other secondary chronic gout, unspecified wrist
[6th] M1A.44 Other secondary chronic gout, hand
[7th] M1A.441 Other secondary chronic gout, right hand
[7th] M1A.442 Other secondary chronic gout, left hand
[7th] M1A.449 Other secondary chronic gout, unspecified hand
[6th] M1A.45 Other secondary chronic gout, hip
[7th] M1A.451 Other secondary chronic gout, right hip
[7th] M1A.452 Other secondary chronic gout, left hip
[7th] M1A.459 Other secondary chronic gout, unspecified hip
[6th] M1A.46 Other secondary chronic gout, knee
[7th] M1A.461 Other secondary chronic gout, right knee
[7th] M1A.462 Other secondary chronic gout, left knee
[7th] M1A.469 Other secondary chronic gout, unspecified knee
[6th] M1A.47 Other secondary chronic gout, ankle and foot
[7th] M1A.471 Other secondary chronic gout, right ankle and foot
[7th] M1A.472 Other secondary chronic gout, left ankle and foot
[7th] M1A.479 Other secondary chronic gout, unspecified ankle and foot
[7th] M1A.48 Other secondary chronic gout, vertebrae
[7th] M1A.49 Other secondary chronic gout, multiple sites
[7th] M1A.9 Chronic gout, unspecified

[4th] M10 Gout
Acute gout
Gout attack
Gout flare
Podagra
Use additional code to identify:
Autonomic neuropathy in diseases classified elsewhere (G99.0)
Calculus of urinary tract in diseases classified elsewhere (N22)
Cardiomyopathy in diseases classified elsewhere (I43)
Disorders of external ear in diseases classified elsewhere (H61.1-, H62.8-)
Disorders of iris and ciliary body in diseases classified elsewhere (H22)
Glomerular disorders in diseases classified elsewhere (N08)
EXCLUDES2 *chronic gout (M1A.-)*
[5th] M10.0 Idiopathic gout
Gouty bursitis
Primary gout
M10.00 Idiopathic gout, unspecified site
[6th] M10.01 Idiopathic gout, shoulder
M10.011 Idiopathic gout, right shoulder
M10.012 Idiopathic gout, left shoulder
M10.019 Idiopathic gout, unspecified shoulder
[6th] M10.02 Idiopathic gout, elbow
M10.021 Idiopathic gout, right elbow
M10.022 Idiopathic gout, left elbow
M10.029 Idiopathic gout, unspecified elbow
[6th] M10.03 Idiopathic gout, wrist
M10.031 Idiopathic gout, right wrist
M10.032 Idiopathic gout, left wrist
M10.039 Idiopathic gout, unspecified wrist
[6th] M10.04 Idiopathic gout, hand
M10.041 Idiopathic gout, right hand
M10.042 Idiopathic gout, left hand
M10.049 Idiopathic gout, unspecified hand
[6th] M10.05 Idiopathic gout, hip
M10.051 Idiopathic gout, right hip
M10.052 Idiopathic gout, left hip
M10.059 Idiopathic gout, unspecified hip
[6th] M10.06 Idiopathic gout, knee
M10.061 Idiopathic gout, right knee
M10.062 Idiopathic gout, left knee
M10.069 Idiopathic gout, unspecified knee
[6th] M10.07 Idiopathic gout, ankle and foot
M10.071 Idiopathic gout, right ankle and foot
M10.072 Idiopathic gout, left ankle and foot
M10.079 Idiopathic gout, unspecified ankle and foot
M10.08 Idiopathic gout, vertebrae
M10.09 Idiopathic gout, multiple sites
[5th] M10.1 Lead-induced gout
☞ Code first toxic effects of lead and its compounds (T56.0-)
M10.10 Lead-induced gout, unspecified site
[6th] M10.11 Lead-induced gout, shoulder
M10.111 Lead-induced gout, right shoulder
M10.112 Lead-induced gout, left shoulder
M10.119 Lead-induced gout, unspecified shoulder
[6th] M10.12 Lead-induced gout, elbow
M10.121 Lead-induced gout, right elbow
M10.122 Lead-induced gout, left elbow
M10.129 Lead-induced gout, unspecified elbow
[6th] M10.13 Lead-induced gout, wrist
M10.131 Lead-induced gout, right wrist
M10.132 Lead-induced gout, left wrist
M10.139 Lead-induced gout, unspecified wrist
[6th] M10.14 Lead-induced gout, hand
M10.141 Lead-induced gout, right hand
M10.142 Lead-induced gout, left hand
M10.149 Lead-induced gout, unspecified hand
[6th] M10.15 Lead-induced gout, hip
M10.151 Lead-induced gout, right hip
M10.152 Lead-induced gout, left hip
M10.159 Lead-induced gout, unspecified hip
[6th] M10.16 Lead-induced gout, knee
M10.161 Lead-induced gout, right knee
M10.162 Lead-induced gout, left knee
M10.169 Lead-induced gout, unspecified knee
[6th] M10.17 Lead-induced gout, ankle and foot
M10.171 Lead-induced gout, right ankle and foot
M10.172 Lead-induced gout, left ankle and foot
M10.179 Lead-induced gout, unspecified ankle and foot
M10.18 Lead-induced gout, vertebrae
M10.19 Lead-induced gout, multiple sites
[5th] M10.2 Drug-induced gout
Use additional code for adverse effect, if applicable, to identify drug (T36-T50 with fifth or sixth character 5)
M10.20 Drug-induced gout, unspecified site
[6th] M10.21 Drug-induced gout, shoulder
M10.211 Drug-induced gout, right shoulder
M10.212 Drug-induced gout, left shoulder
M10.219 Drug-induced gout, unspecified shoulder

Unspecified Code Other Specified Code Manifestation Code [N] Newborn [P] Pediatric [M] Maternity [A] Adult ♂ Male ♀ Female
● New Code ▲ Revised Code Title ▶◀ Revised Text NOTES INCLUDES EXCLUDES1 Not coded here EXCLUDES2 Not included here
[4th] 4th character required [5th] 5th character required [6th] 6th character required [7th] 7th character required [7th] Extension 'X' Alert
[HAC] Hospital-acquired condition (HAC) alert AHA AHA Coding Clinic© ☞ Code first alert

🔵 M10.22 Drug-induced gout, elbow
    M10.221 Drug-induced gout, right elbow
    M10.222 Drug-induced gout, left elbow
    M10.229 Drug-induced gout, unspecified elbow
🔵 M10.23 Drug-induced gout, wrist
    M10.231 Drug-induced gout, right wrist
    M10.232 Drug-induced gout, left wrist
    M10.239 Drug-induced gout, unspecified wrist
🔵 M10.24 Drug-induced gout, hand
    M10.241 Drug-induced gout, right hand
    M10.242 Drug-induced gout, left hand
    M10.249 Drug-induced gout, unspecified hand
🔵 M10.25 Drug-induced gout, hip
    M10.251 Drug-induced gout, right hip
    M10.252 Drug-induced gout, left hip
    M10.259 Drug-induced gout, unspecified hip
🔵 M10.26 Drug-induced gout, knee
    M10.261 Drug-induced gout, right knee
    M10.262 Drug-induced gout, left knee
    M10.269 Drug-induced gout, unspecified knee
🔵 M10.27 Drug-induced gout, ankle and foot
    M10.271 Drug-induced gout, right ankle and foot
    M10.272 Drug-induced gout, left ankle and foot
    M10.279 Drug-induced gout, unspecified ankle and foot
M10.28 Drug-induced gout, vertebrae
M10.29 Drug-induced gout, multiple sites
🔵 M10.3 Gout due to renal impairment
    ☛ Code first associated renal disease
M10.30 Gout due to renal impairment, unspecified site
🔵 M10.31 Gout due to renal impairment, shoulder
    M10.311 Gout due to renal impairment, right shoulder
    M10.312 Gout due to renal impairment, left shoulder
    M10.319 Gout due to renal impairment, unspecified shoulder
🔵 M10.32 Gout due to renal impairment, elbow
    M10.321 Gout due to renal impairment, right elbow
    M10.322 Gout due to renal impairment, left elbow
    M10.329 Gout due to renal impairment, unspecified elbow
🔵 M10.33 Gout due to renal impairment, wrist
    M10.331 Gout due to renal impairment, right wrist
    M10.332 Gout due to renal impairment, left wrist
    M10.339 Gout due to renal impairment, unspecified wrist
🔵 M10.34 Gout due to renal impairment, hand
    M10.341 Gout due to renal impairment, right hand
    M10.342 Gout due to renal impairment, left hand
    M10.349 Gout due to renal impairment, unspecified hand
🔵 M10.35 Gout due to renal impairment, hip
    M10.351 Gout due to renal impairment, right hip
    M10.352 Gout due to renal impairment, left hip
    M10.359 Gout due to renal impairment, unspecified hip
🔵 M10.36 Gout due to renal impairment, knee
    M10.361 Gout due to renal impairment, right knee
    M10.362 Gout due to renal impairment, left knee
    M10.369 Gout due to renal impairment, unspecified knee
🔵 M10.37 Gout due to renal impairment, ankle and foot
    M10.371 Gout due to renal impairment, right ankle and foot
    M10.372 Gout due to renal impairment, left ankle and foot
    M10.379 Gout due to renal impairment, unspecified ankle and foot

M10.38 Gout due to renal impairment, vertebrae
M10.39 Gout due to renal impairment, multiple sites
🔵 M10.4 Other secondary gout
    ☛ Code first associated condition
M10.40 Other secondary gout, unspecified site
🔵 M10.41 Other secondary gout, shoulder
    M10.411 Other secondary gout, right shoulder
    M10.412 Other secondary gout, left shoulder
    M10.419 Other secondary gout, unspecified shoulder
🔵 M10.42 Other secondary gout, elbow
    M10.421 Other secondary gout, right elbow
    M10.422 Other secondary gout, left elbow
    M10.429 Other secondary gout, unspecified elbow
🔵 M10.43 Other secondary gout, wrist
    M10.431 Other secondary gout, right wrist
    M10.432 Other secondary gout, left wrist
    M10.439 Other secondary gout, unspecified wrist
🔵 M10.44 Other secondary gout, hand
    M10.441 Other secondary gout, right hand
    M10.442 Other secondary gout, left hand
    M10.449 Other secondary gout, unspecified hand
🔵 M10.45 Other secondary gout, hip
    M10.451 Other secondary gout, right hip
    M10.452 Other secondary gout, left hip
    M10.459 Other secondary gout, unspecified hip
🔵 M10.46 Other secondary gout, knee
    M10.461 Other secondary gout, right knee
    M10.462 Other secondary gout, left knee
    M10.469 Other secondary gout, unspecified knee
🔵 M10.47 Other secondary gout, ankle and foot
    M10.471 Other secondary gout, right ankle and foot
    M10.472 Other secondary gout, left ankle and foot
    M10.479 Other secondary gout, unspecified ankle and foot
M10.48 Other secondary gout, vertebrae
M10.49 Other secondary gout, multiple sites
M10.9 Gout, unspecified
    Gout NOS
🔵 M11 Other crystal arthropathies
🔵 M11.0 Hydroxyapatite deposition disease
M11.00 Hydroxyapatite deposition disease, unspecified site
🔵 M11.01 Hydroxyapatite deposition disease, shoulder
    M11.011 Hydroxyapatite deposition disease, right shoulder
    M11.012 Hydroxyapatite deposition disease, left shoulder
    M11.019 Hydroxyapatite deposition disease, unspecified shoulder
🔵 M11.02 Hydroxyapatite deposition disease, elbow
    M11.021 Hydroxyapatite deposition disease, right elbow
    M11.022 Hydroxyapatite deposition disease, left elbow
    M11.029 Hydroxyapatite deposition disease, unspecified elbow
🔵 M11.03 Hydroxyapatite deposition disease, wrist
    M11.031 Hydroxyapatite deposition disease, right wrist
    M11.032 Hydroxyapatite deposition disease, left wrist
    M11.039 Hydroxyapatite deposition disease, unspecified wrist
🔵 M11.04 Hydroxyapatite deposition disease, hand
    M11.041 Hydroxyapatite deposition disease, right hand
    M11.042 Hydroxyapatite deposition disease, left hand

When symbols appear on a code that requires a 7th character extension, refer to Appendix B to identify applicable 7th character codes.
2020 ICD-10-CM

M11.049 Hydroxyapatite deposition disease, unspecified hand

6th M11.05 Hydroxyapatite deposition disease, hip

M11.051 Hydroxyapatite deposition disease, right hip

M11.052 Hydroxyapatite deposition disease, left hip

M11.059 Hydroxyapatite deposition disease, unspecified hip

6th M11.06 Hydroxyapatite deposition disease, knee

M11.061 Hydroxyapatite deposition disease, right knee

M11.062 Hydroxyapatite deposition disease, left knee

M11.069 Hydroxyapatite deposition disease, unspecified knee

6th M11.07 Hydroxyapatite deposition disease, ankle and foot

M11.071 Hydroxyapatite deposition disease, right ankle and foot

M11.072 Hydroxyapatite deposition disease, left ankle and foot

M11.079 Hydroxyapatite deposition disease, unspecified ankle and foot

M11.08 Hydroxyapatite deposition disease, vertebrae

M11.09 Hydroxyapatite deposition disease, multiple sites

5th M11.1 Familial chondrocalcinosis

DEFINITION: Chondrocalcinosis is also known as pseudo gout.

M11.10 Familial chondrocalcinosis, unspecified site

6th M11.11 Familial chondrocalcinosis, shoulder

M11.111 Familial chondrocalcinosis, right shoulder

M11.112 Familial chondrocalcinosis, left shoulder

M11.119 Familial chondrocalcinosis, unspecified shoulder

6th M11.12 Familial chondrocalcinosis, elbow

M11.121 Familial chondrocalcinosis, right elbow

M11.122 Familial chondrocalcinosis, left elbow

M11.129 Familial chondrocalcinosis, unspecified elbow

6th M11.13 Familial chondrocalcinosis, wrist

M11.131 Familial chondrocalcinosis, right wrist

M11.132 Familial chondrocalcinosis, left wrist

M11.139 Familial chondrocalcinosis, unspecified wrist

6th M11.14 Familial chondrocalcinosis, hand

M11.141 Familial chondrocalcinosis, right hand

M11.142 Familial chondrocalcinosis, left hand

M11.149 Familial chondrocalcinosis, unspecified hand

6th M11.15 Familial chondrocalcinosis, hip

M11.151 Familial chondrocalcinosis, right hip

M11.152 Familial chondrocalcinosis, left hip

M11.159 Familial chondrocalcinosis, unspecified hip

6th M11.16 Familial chondrocalcinosis, knee

M11.161 Familial chondrocalcinosis, right knee

M11.162 Familial chondrocalcinosis, left knee

M11.169 Familial chondrocalcinosis, unspecified knee

6th M11.17 Familial chondrocalcinosis, ankle and foot

M11.171 Familial chondrocalcinosis, right ankle and foot

M11.172 Familial chondrocalcinosis, left ankle and foot

M11.179 Familial chondrocalcinosis, unspecified ankle and foot

M11.18 Familial chondrocalcinosis, vertebrae

M11.19 Familial chondrocalcinosis, multiple sites

5th M11.2 Other chondrocalcinosis

Chondrocalcinosis NOS

M11.20 Other chondrocalcinosis, unspecified site

6th M11.21 Other chondrocalcinosis, shoulder

M11.211 Other chondrocalcinosis, right shoulder

M11.212 Other chondrocalcinosis, left shoulder

M11.219 Other chondrocalcinosis, unspecified shoulder

6th M11.22 Other chondrocalcinosis, elbow

M11.221 Other chondrocalcinosis, right elbow

M11.222 Other chondrocalcinosis, left elbow

M11.229 Other chondrocalcinosis, unspecified elbow

6th M11.23 Other chondrocalcinosis, wrist

M11.231 Other chondrocalcinosis, right wrist

M11.232 Other chondrocalcinosis, left wrist

M11.239 Other chondrocalcinosis, unspecified wrist

6th M11.24 Other chondrocalcinosis, hand

M11.241 Other chondrocalcinosis, right hand

M11.242 Other chondrocalcinosis, left hand

M11.249 Other chondrocalcinosis, unspecified hand

6th M11.25 Other chondrocalcinosis, hip

M11.251 Other chondrocalcinosis, right hip

M11.252 Other chondrocalcinosis, left hip

M11.259 Other chondrocalcinosis, unspecified hip

6th M11.26 Other chondrocalcinosis, knee

M11.261 Other chondrocalcinosis, right knee

M11.262 Other chondrocalcinosis, left knee

AHA: Q3 2018

M11.269 Other chondrocalcinosis, unspecified knee

6th M11.27 Other chondrocalcinosis, ankle and foot

M11.271 Other chondrocalcinosis, right ankle and foot

M11.272 Other chondrocalcinosis, left ankle and foot

M11.279 Other chondrocalcinosis, unspecified ankle and foot

M11.28 Other chondrocalcinosis, vertebrae

M11.29 Other chondrocalcinosis, multiple sites

5th M11.8 Other specified crystal arthropathies

M11.80 Other specified crystal arthropathies, unspecified site

6th M11.81 Other specified crystal arthropathies, shoulder

M11.811 Other specified crystal arthropathies, right shoulder

M11.812 Other specified crystal arthropathies, left shoulder

M11.819 Other specified crystal arthropathies, unspecified shoulder

6th M11.82 Other specified crystal arthropathies, elbow

M11.821 Other specified crystal arthropathies, right elbow

M11.822 Other specified crystal arthropathies, left elbow

M11.829 Other specified crystal arthropathies, unspecified elbow

6th M11.83 Other specified crystal arthropathies, wrist

M11.831 Other specified crystal arthropathies, right wrist

M11.832 Other specified crystal arthropathies, left wrist

M11.839 Other specified crystal arthropathies, unspecified wrist

6th M11.84 Other specified crystal arthropathies, hand

M11.841 Other specified crystal arthropathies, right hand

M11.842 Other specified crystal arthropathies, left hand

M11.849 Other specified crystal arthropathies, unspecified hand

6th M11.85 Other specified crystal arthropathies, hip

M11.851 Other specified crystal arthropathies, right hip

Unspecified Code   Other Specified Code   Manifestation Code   N Newborn   P Pediatric   M Maternity   A Adult   ♂ Male   ♀ Female
● New Code   ▲ Revised Code Title   ►◄ Revised Text   **NOTES**   *INCLUDES*   *EXCLUDES1* Not coded here   *EXCLUDES2* Not included here
4th 4th character required   5th 5th character required   6th 6th character required   7th 7th character required   Extension 'X' Alert
HAC Hospital-acquired condition (HAC) alert   **AHA** AHA Coding Clinic©   ☛ Code first alert

M11.852 **Other specified crystal arthropathies, left hip**

M11.859 **Other specified crystal arthropathies, unspecified hip**

6ᵗʰ M11.86 Other specified crystal arthropathies, knee

M11.861 **Other specified crystal arthropathies, right knee**

M11.862 **Other specified crystal arthropathies, left knee**

M11.869 **Other specified crystal arthropathies, unspecified knee**

6ᵗʰ M11.87 Other specified crystal arthropathies, ankle and foot

M11.871 **Other specified crystal arthropathies, right ankle and foot**

M11.872 **Other specified crystal arthropathies, left ankle and foot**

M11.879 **Other specified crystal arthropathies, unspecified ankle and foot**

M11.88 **Other specified crystal arthropathies, vertebrae**

M11.89 **Other specified crystal arthropathies, multiple sites**

M11.9 **Crystal arthropathy, unspecified**

4ᵗʰ M12 Other and unspecified arthropathy

EXCLUDES1 arthrosis (M15-M19)

cricoarytenoid arthropathy (J38.7)

5ᵗʰ M12.0 Chronic postrheumatic arthropathy [Jaccoud]

M12.00 **Chronic postrheumatic arthropathy [Jaccoud], unspecified site** HCC RxHCC

5ᵗʰ M12.01 Chronic postrheumatic arthropathy [Jaccoud], shoulder

M12.011 **Chronic postrheumatic arthropathy [Jaccoud], right shoulder** HCC RxHCC

M12.012 **Chronic postrheumatic arthropathy [Jaccoud], left shoulder** HCC RxHCC

M12.019 **Chronic postrheumatic arthropathy [Jaccoud], unspecified shoulder** HCC RxHCC

5ᵗʰ M12.02 Chronic postrheumatic arthropathy [Jaccoud], elbow

M12.021 **Chronic postrheumatic arthropathy [Jaccoud], right elbow** HCC RxHCC

M12.022 **Chronic postrheumatic arthropathy [Jaccoud], left elbow** HCC RxHCC

M12.029 **Chronic postrheumatic arthropathy [Jaccoud], unspecified elbow** HCC RxHCC

6ᵗʰ M12.03 Chronic postrheumatic arthropathy [Jaccoud], wrist

M12.031 **Chronic postrheumatic arthropathy [Jaccoud], right wrist** HCC RxHCC

M12.032 **Chronic postrheumatic arthropathy [Jaccoud], left wrist** HCC RxHCC

M12.039 **Chronic postrheumatic arthropathy [Jaccoud], unspecified wrist** HCC RxHCC

6ᵗʰ M12.04 Chronic postrheumatic arthropathy [Jaccoud], hand

M12.041 **Chronic postrheumatic arthropathy [Jaccoud], right hand** HCC RxHCC

M12.042 **Chronic postrheumatic arthropathy [Jaccoud], left hand** HCC RxHCC

M12.049 **Chronic postrheumatic arthropathy [Jaccoud], unspecified hand** HCC RxHCC

6ᵗʰ M12.05 Chronic postrheumatic arthropathy [Jaccoud], hip

M12.051 **Chronic postrheumatic arthropathy [Jaccoud], right hip** HCC RxHCC

M12.052 **Chronic postrheumatic arthropathy [Jaccoud], left hip** HCC RxHCC

M12.059 **Chronic postrheumatic arthropathy [Jaccoud], unspecified hip** HCC RxHCC

6ᵗʰ M12.06 Chronic postrheumatic arthropathy [Jaccoud], knee

M12.061 **Chronic postrheumatic arthropathy [Jaccoud], right knee** HCC RxHCC

M12.062 **Chronic postrheumatic arthropathy [Jaccoud], left knee** HCC RxHCC

M12.069 **Chronic postrheumatic arthropathy [Jaccoud], unspecified knee** HCC RxHCC

6ᵗʰ M12.07 Chronic postrheumatic arthropathy [Jaccoud], ankle and foot

M12.071 **Chronic postrheumatic arthropathy [Jaccoud], right ankle and foot** HCC RxHCC

M12.072 **Chronic postrheumatic arthropathy [Jaccoud], left ankle and foot** HCC RxHCC

M12.079 **Chronic postrheumatic arthropathy [Jaccoud], unspecified ankle and foot** HCC RxHCC

M12.08 **Chronic postrheumatic arthropathy [Jaccoud], other specified site** HCC RxHCC

Chronic postrheumatic arthropathy [Jaccoud], vertebrae

M12.09 **Chronic postrheumatic arthropathy [Jaccoud], multiple sites** HCC RxHCC

5ᵗʰ M12.1 Kaschin-Beck disease

DEFINITION: Kaschin-Beck is a disorder of bones and joints of hands, fingers, elbows, knees and ankles of children and adolescents.

Osteochondroarthrosis deformans endemica

M12.10 **Kaschin-Beck disease, unspecified site**

6ᵗʰ M12.11 Kaschin-Beck disease, shoulder

M12.111 **Kaschin-Beck disease, right shoulder**

M12.112 **Kaschin-Beck disease, left shoulder**

M12.119 **Kaschin-Beck disease, unspecified shoulder**

6ᵗʰ M12.12 Kaschin-Beck disease, elbow

M12.121 **Kaschin-Beck disease, right elbow**

M12.122 **Kaschin-Beck disease, left elbow**

M12.129 **Kaschin-Beck disease, unspecified elbow**

6ᵗʰ M12.13 Kaschin-Beck disease, wrist

M12.131 **Kaschin-Beck disease, right wrist**

M12.132 **Kaschin-Beck disease, left wrist**

M12.139 **Kaschin-Beck disease, unspecified wrist**

6ᵗʰ M12.14 Kaschin-Beck disease, hand

M12.141 **Kaschin-Beck disease, right hand**

M12.142 **Kaschin-Beck disease, left hand**

M12.149 **Kaschin-Beck disease, unspecified hand**

6ᵗʰ M12.15 Kaschin-Beck disease, hip

M12.151 **Kaschin-Beck disease, right hip**

M12.152 **Kaschin-Beck disease, left hip**

M12.159 **Kaschin-Beck disease, unspecified hip**

6ᵗʰ M12.16 Kaschin-Beck disease, knee

M12.161 **Kaschin-Beck disease, right knee**

M12.162 **Kaschin-Beck disease, left knee**

M12.169 **Kaschin-Beck disease, unspecified knee**

6ᵗʰ M12.17 Kaschin-Beck disease, ankle and foot

M12.171 **Kaschin-Beck disease, right ankle and foot**

M12.172 **Kaschin-Beck disease, left ankle and foot**

M12.179 **Kaschin-Beck disease, unspecified ankle and foot**

M12.18 **Kaschin-Beck disease, vertebrae**

M12.19 **Kaschin-Beck disease, multiple sites**

5ᵗʰ M12.2 Villonodular synovitis (pigmented)

DEFINITION: Villonodular synovitis is a condition affecting the synovium (thin lining of a joint) causing it to thicken and overgrow.

M12.20 **Villonodular synovitis (pigmented), unspecified site**

6ᵗʰ M12.21 Villonodular synovitis (pigmented), shoulder

M12.211 **Villonodular synovitis (pigmented), right shoulder**

M12.212 **Villonodular synovitis (pigmented), left shoulder**

M12.219 **Villonodular synovitis (pigmented), unspecified shoulder**

6ᵗʰ M12.22 Villonodular synovitis (pigmented), elbow

M12.221 **Villonodular synovitis (pigmented), right elbow**

M12.222 **Villonodular synovitis (pigmented), left elbow**

PDx Unacceptable principal diagnosis symbol per Medicare code edits   POA Code exempt from diagnosis present on admission requirement
? Questionable admission   CC Complication or comorbidity   MCC Major complication or comorbidity   CC/MCC CC/MCC exclusion
HCC HCC diagnosis code   RxHCC RxHCC diagnosis code   MACRA code   **DEFINITION** Describes condition/terminology
TIP Coding guidance   👁 Official Guideline Reference   Z1 Z code as first-listed diagnosis

790   When symbols appear on a code that requires a 7th character extension, refer to Appendix B to identify applicable 7th character codes.   **2020 ICD-10-CM**

M12.229 Villonodular synovitis (pigmented), unspecified elbow

(6ᵗʰ) M12.23 Villonodular synovitis (pigmented), wrist

    M12.231 Villonodular synovitis (pigmented), right wrist

    M12.232 Villonodular synovitis (pigmented), left wrist

    M12.239 Villonodular synovitis (pigmented), unspecified wrist

(6ᵗʰ) M12.24 Villonodular synovitis (pigmented), hand

    M12.241 Villonodular synovitis (pigmented), right hand

    M12.242 Villonodular synovitis (pigmented), left hand

    M12.249 Villonodular synovitis (pigmented), unspecified hand

(6ᵗʰ) M12.25 Villonodular synovitis (pigmented), hip

    M12.251 Villonodular synovitis (pigmented), right hip

    M12.252 Villonodular synovitis (pigmented), left hip

    M12.259 Villonodular synovitis (pigmented), unspecified hip

(6ᵗʰ) M12.26 Villonodular synovitis (pigmented), knee

    M12.261 Villonodular synovitis (pigmented), right knee

    M12.262 Villonodular synovitis (pigmented), left knee

    M12.269 Villonodular synovitis (pigmented), unspecified knee

(6ᵗʰ) M12.27 Villonodular synovitis (pigmented), ankle and foot

    M12.271 Villonodular synovitis (pigmented), right ankle and foot

    M12.272 Villonodular synovitis (pigmented), left ankle and foot

    M12.279 Villonodular synovitis (pigmented), unspecified ankle and foot

M12.28 Villonodular synovitis (pigmented), other specified site

    Villonodular synovitis (pigmented), vertebrae

M12.29 Villonodular synovitis (pigmented), multiple sites

(5ᵗʰ) M12.3 Palindromic rheumatism

M12.30 Palindromic rheumatism, unspecified site

(6ᵗʰ) M12.31 Palindromic rheumatism, shoulder

    M12.311 Palindromic rheumatism, right shoulder

    M12.312 Palindromic rheumatism, left shoulder

    M12.319 Palindromic rheumatism, unspecified shoulder

(6ᵗʰ) M12.32 Palindromic rheumatism, elbow

    M12.321 Palindromic rheumatism, right elbow

    M12.322 Palindromic rheumatism, left elbow

    M12.329 Palindromic rheumatism, unspecified elbow

(6ᵗʰ) M12.33 Palindromic rheumatism, wrist

    M12.331 Palindromic rheumatism, right wrist

    M12.332 Palindromic rheumatism, left wrist

    M12.339 Palindromic rheumatism, unspecified wrist

(6ᵗʰ) M12.34 Palindromic rheumatism, hand

    M12.341 Palindromic rheumatism, right hand

    M12.342 Palindromic rheumatism, left hand

    M12.349 Palindromic rheumatism, unspecified hand

(6ᵗʰ) M12.35 Palindromic rheumatism, hip

    M12.351 Palindromic rheumatism, right hip

    M12.352 Palindromic rheumatism, left hip

    M12.359 Palindromic rheumatism, unspecified hip

(6ᵗʰ) M12.36 Palindromic rheumatism, knee

    M12.361 Palindromic rheumatism, right knee

    M12.362 Palindromic rheumatism, left knee

M12.369 Palindromic rheumatism, unspecified knee

(6ᵗʰ) M12.37 Palindromic rheumatism, ankle and foot

    M12.371 Palindromic rheumatism, right ankle and foot

    M12.372 Palindromic rheumatism, left ankle and foot

    M12.379 Palindromic rheumatism, unspecified ankle and foot

M12.38 Palindromic rheumatism, other specified site

    Palindromic rheumatism, vertebrae

M12.39 Palindromic rheumatism, multiple sites

(5ᵗʰ) M12.4 Intermittent hydrarthrosis

M12.40 Intermittent hydrarthrosis, unspecified site

(6ᵗʰ) M12.41 Intermittent hydrarthrosis, shoulder

    M12.411 Intermittent hydrarthrosis, right shoulder

    M12.412 Intermittent hydrarthrosis, left shoulder

    M12.419 Intermittent hydrarthrosis, unspecified shoulder

(6ᵗʰ) M12.42 Intermittent hydrarthrosis, elbow

    M12.421 Intermittent hydrarthrosis, right elbow

    M12.422 Intermittent hydrarthrosis, left elbow

    M12.429 Intermittent hydrarthrosis, unspecified elbow

(6ᵗʰ) M12.43 Intermittent hydrarthrosis, wrist

    M12.431 Intermittent hydrarthrosis, right wrist

    M12.432 Intermittent hydrarthrosis, left wrist

    M12.439 Intermittent hydrarthrosis, unspecified wrist

(6ᵗʰ) M12.44 Intermittent hydrarthrosis, hand

    M12.441 Intermittent hydrarthrosis, right hand

    M12.442 Intermittent hydrarthrosis, left hand

    M12.449 Intermittent hydrarthrosis, unspecified hand

(6ᵗʰ) M12.45 Intermittent hydrarthrosis, hip

    M12.451 Intermittent hydrarthrosis, right hip

    M12.452 Intermittent hydrarthrosis, left hip

    M12.459 Intermittent hydrarthrosis, unspecified hip

(6ᵗʰ) M12.46 Intermittent hydrarthrosis, knee

    M12.461 Intermittent hydrarthrosis, right knee

    M12.462 Intermittent hydrarthrosis, left knee

    M12.469 Intermittent hydrarthrosis, unspecified knee

(6ᵗʰ) M12.47 Intermittent hydrarthrosis, ankle and foot

    M12.471 Intermittent hydrarthrosis, right ankle and foot

    M12.472 Intermittent hydrarthrosis, left ankle and foot

    M12.479 Intermittent hydrarthrosis, unspecified ankle and foot

M12.48 Intermittent hydrarthrosis, other site

M12.49 Intermittent hydrarthrosis, multiple sites

(5ᵗʰ) M12.5 Traumatic arthropathy

    EXCLUDES1 current injury-see Alphabetic Index

        post-traumatic osteoarthritis of first carpometacarpal joint (M18.2-M18.3)

        post-traumatic osteoarthritis of hip (M16.4-M16.5)

        post-traumatic osteoarthritis of knee (M17.2-M17.3)

        post-traumatic osteoarthritis NOS (M19.1-)

        post-traumatic osteoarthritis of other single joints (M19.1-)

M12.50 Traumatic arthropathy, unspecified site

(6ᵗʰ) M12.51 Traumatic arthropathy, shoulder

    M12.511 Traumatic arthropathy, right shoulder

    M12.512 Traumatic arthropathy, left shoulder

    M12.519 Traumatic arthropathy, unspecified shoulder

(6ᵗʰ) M12.52 Traumatic arthropathy, elbow

    M12.521 Traumatic arthropathy, right elbow

M12.522 Traumatic arthropathy, left elbow
M12.529 Traumatic arthropathy, unspecified elbow
6ᵗʰ M12.53 Traumatic arthropathy, wrist
M12.531 Traumatic arthropathy, right wrist
M12.532 Traumatic arthropathy, left wrist
M12.539 Traumatic arthropathy, unspecified wrist
6ᵗʰ M12.54 Traumatic arthropathy, hand
M12.541 Traumatic arthropathy, right hand
M12.542 Traumatic arthropathy, left hand
M12.549 Traumatic arthropathy, unspecified hand
5ᵗʰ M12.55 Traumatic arthropathy, hip
M12.551 Traumatic arthropathy, right hip
M12.552 Traumatic arthropathy, left hip
AHA: Q1 2015
M12.559 Traumatic arthropathy, unspecified hip
6ᵗʰ M12.56 Traumatic arthropathy, knee
M12.561 Traumatic arthropathy, right knee
M12.562 Traumatic arthropathy, left knee
M12.569 Traumatic arthropathy, unspecified knee
5ᵗʰ M12.57 Traumatic arthropathy, ankle and foot
M12.571 Traumatic arthropathy, right ankle and foot
M12.572 Traumatic arthropathy, left ankle and foot
M12.579 Traumatic arthropathy, unspecified ankle and foot
M12.58 Traumatic arthropathy, other specified site
Traumatic arthropathy, vertebrae
M12.59 Traumatic arthropathy, multiple sites
5ᵗʰ M12.8 Other specific arthropathies, not elsewhere classified
Transient arthropathy
M12.80 Other specific arthropathies, not elsewhere classified, unspecified site
6ᵗʰ M12.81 Other specific arthropathies, not elsewhere classified, shoulder
M12.811 Other specific arthropathies, not elsewhere classified, right shoulder
M12.812 Other specific arthropathies, not elsewhere classified, left shoulder
M12.819 Other specific arthropathies, not elsewhere classified, unspecified shoulder
6ᵗʰ M12.82 Other specific arthropathies, not elsewhere classified, elbow
M12.821 Other specific arthropathies, not elsewhere classified, right elbow
M12.822 Other specific arthropathies, not elsewhere classified, left elbow
M12.829 Other specific arthropathies, not elsewhere classified, unspecified elbow
6ᵗʰ M12.83 Other specific arthropathies, not elsewhere classified, wrist
M12.831 Other specific arthropathies, not elsewhere classified, right wrist
M12.832 Other specific arthropathies, not elsewhere classified, left wrist
M12.839 Other specific arthropathies, not elsewhere classified, unspecified wrist
6ᵗʰ M12.84 Other specific arthropathies, not elsewhere classified, hand
M12.841 Other specific arthropathies, not elsewhere classified, right hand
M12.842 Other specific arthropathies, not elsewhere classified, left hand
M12.849 Other specific arthropathies, not elsewhere classified, unspecified hand
6ᵗʰ M12.85 Other specific arthropathies, not elsewhere classified, hip
M12.851 Other specific arthropathies, not elsewhere classified, right hip
M12.852 Other specific arthropathies, not elsewhere classified, left hip

M12.859 Other specific arthropathies, not elsewhere classified, unspecified hip
6ᵗʰ M12.86 Other specific arthropathies, not elsewhere classified, knee
M12.861 Other specific arthropathies, not elsewhere classified, right knee
M12.862 Other specific arthropathies, not elsewhere classified, left knee
M12.869 Other specific arthropathies, not elsewhere classified, unspecified knee
6ᵗʰ M12.87 Other specific arthropathies, not elsewhere classified, ankle and foot
M12.871 Other specific arthropathies, not elsewhere classified, right ankle and foot
M12.872 Other specific arthropathies, not elsewhere classified, left ankle and foot
M12.879 Other specific arthropathies, not elsewhere classified, unspecified ankle and foot
M12.88 Other specific arthropathies, not elsewhere classified, other specified site
Other specific arthropathies, not elsewhere classified, vertebrae
M12.89 Other specific arthropathies, not elsewhere classified, multiple sites
M12.9 Arthropathy, unspecified
4ᵗʰ M13 Other arthritis
EXCLUDES1 arthrosis (M15-M19)
osteoarthritis (M15-M19)
M13.0 Polyarthritis, unspecified
5ᵗʰ M13.1 Monoarthritis, not elsewhere classified
M13.10 Monoarthritis, not elsewhere classified, unspecified site
6ᵗʰ M13.11 Monoarthritis, not elsewhere classified, shoulder
M13.111 Monoarthritis, not elsewhere classified, right shoulder
M13.112 Monoarthritis, not elsewhere classified, left shoulder
M13.119 Monoarthritis, not elsewhere classified, unspecified shoulder
6ᵗʰ M13.12 Monoarthritis, not elsewhere classified, elbow
M13.121 Monoarthritis, not elsewhere classified, right elbow
M13.122 Monoarthritis, not elsewhere classified, left elbow
M13.129 Monoarthritis, not elsewhere classified, unspecified elbow
6ᵗʰ M13.13 Monoarthritis, not elsewhere classified, wrist
M13.131 Monoarthritis, not elsewhere classified, right wrist
M13.132 Monoarthritis, not elsewhere classified, left wrist
M13.139 Monoarthritis, not elsewhere classified, unspecified wrist
6ᵗʰ M13.14 Monoarthritis, not elsewhere classified, hand
M13.141 Monoarthritis, not elsewhere classified, right hand
M13.142 Monoarthritis, not elsewhere classified, left hand
M13.149 Monoarthritis, not elsewhere classified, unspecified hand
6ᵗʰ M13.15 Monoarthritis, not elsewhere classified, hip
M13.151 Monoarthritis, not elsewhere classified, right hip
M13.152 Monoarthritis, not elsewhere classified, left hip
M13.159 Monoarthritis, not elsewhere classified, unspecified hip
6ᵗʰ M13.16 Monoarthritis, not elsewhere classified, knee
M13.161 Monoarthritis, not elsewhere classified, right knee

PDx Unacceptable principal diagnosis symbol per Medicare code edits   PDx Code exempt from diagnosis present on admission requirement
❓ Questionable admission   ꞔᴄ Complication or comorbidity   ᴹᴄᴄ Major complication or comorbidity   ᴄᴄ/ᴍᴄᴄ ᴇˣᶜ CC/MCC exclusion
ᴴᶜᶜ HCC diagnosis code   ᴿˣᴴᶜᶜ RxHCC diagnosis code   MACRA code   **DEFINITION** Describes condition/terminology
TIP Coding guidance   👁 Official Guideline Reference   ᴢ¹ Z code as first-listed diagnosis

792   When symbols appear on a code that requires a 7th character extension, refer to Appendix B to identify applicable 7th character codes.   **2020 ICD-10-CM**

M13.162 Monoarthritis, not elsewhere classified, left knee

M13.169 Monoarthritis, not elsewhere classified, unspecified knee

🖐 M13.17 Monoarthritis, not elsewhere classified, ankle and foot

M13.171 Monoarthritis, not elsewhere classified, right ankle and foot

M13.172 Monoarthritis, not elsewhere classified, left ankle and foot

M13.179 Monoarthritis, not elsewhere classified, unspecified ankle and foot

🖐 M13.8 Other specified arthritis

Allergic arthritis

EXCLUDES1 osteoarthritis (M15-M19)

M13.80 Other specified arthritis, unspecified site

🖐 M13.81 Other specified arthritis, shoulder

M13.811 Other specified arthritis, right shoulder

M13.812 Other specified arthritis, left shoulder

M13.819 Other specified arthritis, unspecified shoulder

🖐 M13.82 Other specified arthritis, elbow

M13.821 Other specified arthritis, right elbow

M13.822 Other specified arthritis, left elbow

M13.829 Other specified arthritis, unspecified elbow

🖐 M13.83 Other specified arthritis, wrist

M13.831 Other specified arthritis, right wrist

M13.832 Other specified arthritis, left wrist

M13.839 Other specified arthritis, unspecified wrist

🖐 M13.84 Other specified arthritis, hand

M13.841 Other specified arthritis, right hand

M13.842 Other specified arthritis, left hand

M13.849 Other specified arthritis, unspecified hand

🖐 M13.85 Other specified arthritis, hip

M13.851 Other specified arthritis, right hip

M13.852 Other specified arthritis, left hip

M13.859 Other specified arthritis, unspecified hip

🖐 M13.86 Other specified arthritis, knee

M13.861 Other specified arthritis, right knee

M13.862 Other specified arthritis, left knee

M13.869 Other specified arthritis, unspecified knee

🖐 M13.87 Other specified arthritis, ankle and foot

M13.871 Other specified arthritis, right ankle and foot

M13.872 Other specified arthritis, left ankle and foot

M13.879 Other specified arthritis, unspecified ankle and foot

M13.88 Other specified arthritis, other site

M13.89 Other specified arthritis, multiple sites

🔵 M14 Arthropathies in other diseases classified elsewhere

EXCLUDES1 arthropathy in:

diabetes mellitus (E08-E13 with .61-)

hematological disorders (M36.2-M36.3)

hypersensitivity reactions (M36.4)

neoplastic disease (M36.1)

neurosyphilis (A52.16)

sarcoidosis (D86.86)

enteropathic arthropathies (M07.-)

juvenile psoriatic arthropathy (L40.54)

lipoid dermatoarthritis (E78.81)

🖐 M14.6 Charcôt's joint

Neuropathic arthropathy

EXCLUDES1 Charcôt's joint in diabetes mellitus (E08-E13 with .610)

Charcôt's joint in tabes dorsalis (A52.16)

M14.60 Charcôt's joint, unspecified site

🖐 M14.61 Charcôt's joint, shoulder

M14.611 Charcôt's joint, right shoulder

M14.612 Charcôt's joint, left shoulder

M14.619 Charcôt's joint, unspecified shoulder

🖐 M14.62 Charcôt's joint, elbow

M14.621 Charcôt's joint, right elbow

M14.622 Charcôt's joint, left elbow

M14.629 Charcôt's joint, unspecified elbow

🖐 M14.63 Charcôt's joint, wrist

M14.631 Charcôt's joint, right wrist

M14.632 Charcôt's joint, left wrist

M14.639 Charcôt's joint, unspecified wrist

🖐 M14.64 Charcôt's joint, hand

M14.641 Charcôt's joint, right hand

M14.642 Charcôt's joint, left hand

M14.649 Charcôt's joint, unspecified hand

🖐 M14.65 Charcôt's joint, hip

M14.651 Charcôt's joint, right hip

M14.652 Charcôt's joint, left hip

M14.659 Charcôt's joint, unspecified hip

🖐 M14.66 Charcôt's joint, knee

M14.661 Charcôt's joint, right knee

M14.662 Charcôt's joint, left knee

M14.669 Charcôt's joint, unspecified knee

🖐 M14.67 Charcôt's joint, ankle and foot

M14.671 Charcôt's joint, right ankle and foot

M14.672 Charcôt's joint, left ankle and foot

M14.679 Charcôt's joint, unspecified ankle and foot

M14.68 Charcôt's joint, vertebrae

M14.69 Charcôt's joint, multiple sites

🖐 M14.8 Arthropathies in other specified diseases classified elsewhere

☞ Code first underlying disease, such as:

amyloidosis (E85.-)

erythema multiforme (L51.-)

erythema nodosum (L52)

hemochromatosis (E83.11-)

hyperparathyroidism (E21.-)

hypothyroidism (E00-E03)

sickle-cell disorders (D57.-)

thyrotoxicosis [hyperthyroidism] (E05.-)

Whipple's disease (K90.81)

M14.80 Arthropathies in other specified diseases classified elsewhere, unspecified site

🖐 M14.81 Arthropathies in other specified diseases classified elsewhere, shoulder

M14.811 Arthropathies in other specified diseases classified elsewhere, right shoulder

M14.812 Arthropathies in other specified diseases classified elsewhere, left shoulder

M14.819 Arthropathies in other specified diseases classified elsewhere, unspecified shoulder

🖐 M14.82 Arthropathies in other specified diseases classified elsewhere, elbow

M14.821 Arthropathies in other specified diseases classified elsewhere, right elbow

M14.822 Arthropathies in other specified diseases classified elsewhere, left elbow

M14.829 Arthropathies in other specified diseases classified elsewhere, unspecified elbow

🖐 M14.83 Arthropathies in other specified diseases classified elsewhere, wrist

M14.831 Arthropathies in other specified diseases classified elsewhere, right wrist

M14.832 Arthropathies in other specified diseases classified elsewhere, left wrist

M14.839 Arthropathies in other specified diseases classified elsewhere, unspecified wrist

🖐 M14.84 Arthropathies in other specified diseases classified elsewhere, hand

M14.841 Arthropathies in other specified diseases classified elsewhere, right hand

M14.842 Arthropathies in other specified diseases classified elsewhere, left hand

M14.849 Arthropathies in other specified diseases classified elsewhere, unspecified hand

6ᵗʰ M14.85 Arthropathies in other specified diseases classified elsewhere, hip

M14.851 Arthropathies in other specified diseases classified elsewhere, right hip

M14.852 Arthropathies in other specified diseases classified elsewhere, left hip

M14.859 Arthropathies in other specified diseases classified elsewhere, unspecified hip

6ᵗʰ M14.86 Arthropathies in other specified diseases classified elsewhere, knee

M14.861 Arthropathies in other specified diseases classified elsewhere, right knee

M14.862 Arthropathies in other specified diseases classified elsewhere, left knee

M14.869 Arthropathies in other specified diseases classified elsewhere, unspecified knee

6ᵗʰ M14.87 Arthropathies in other specified diseases classified elsewhere, ankle and foot

M14.871 Arthropathies in other specified diseases classified elsewhere, right ankle and foot

M14.872 Arthropathies in other specified diseases classified elsewhere, left ankle and foot

M14.879 Arthropathies in other specified diseases classified elsewhere, unspecified ankle and foot

M14.88 Arthropathies in other specified diseases classified elsewhere, vertebrae

M14.89 Arthropathies in other specified diseases classified elsewhere, multiple sites

Osteoarthritis (M15-M19)

EXCLUDES2 osteoarthritis of spine (M47.-)

4ᵗʰ M15 Polyosteoarthritis

DEFINITION: Osteoarthritis is a common chronic, degenerative disorder caused by wear and tear on the joints.

INCLUDES arthritis of multiple sites

EXCLUDES1 bilateral involvement of single joint (M16-M19)

M15.0 Primary generalized (osteo)arthritis

M15.1 Heberden's nodes (with arthropathy)
Interphalangeal distal osteoarthritis

M15.2 Bouchard's nodes (with arthropathy)
Juxtaphalangeal distal osteoarthritis

M15.3 Secondary multiple arthritis
Post-traumatic polyosteoarthritis

M15.4 Erosive (osteo)arthritis

M15.8 Other polyosteoarthritis

M15.9 Polyosteoarthritis, unspecified
Generalized osteoarthritis NOS

4ᵗʰ M16 Osteoarthritis of hip

M16.0 Bilateral primary osteoarthritis of hip
AHA: Q2 2018, Q4 2016

5ᵗʰ M16.1 Unilateral primary osteoarthritis of hip
Primary osteoarthritis of hip NOS
M16.10 Unilateral primary osteoarthritis, unspecified hip
M16.11 Unilateral primary osteoarthritis, right hip
M16.12 Unilateral primary osteoarthritis, left hip

M16.2 Bilateral osteoarthritis resulting from hip dysplasia

5ᵗʰ M16.3 Unilateral osteoarthritis resulting from hip dysplasia
Dysplastic osteoarthritis of hip NOS
M16.30 Unilateral osteoarthritis resulting from hip dysplasia, unspecified hip
M16.31 Unilateral osteoarthritis resulting from hip dysplasia, right hip
M16.32 Unilateral osteoarthritis resulting from hip dysplasia, left hip

M16.4 Bilateral post-traumatic osteoarthritis of hip

5ᵗʰ M16.5 Unilateral post-traumatic osteoarthritis of hip
Post-traumatic osteoarthritis of hip NOS
M16.50 Unilateral post-traumatic osteoarthritis, unspecified hip
M16.51 Unilateral post-traumatic osteoarthritis, right hip
M16.52 Unilateral post-traumatic osteoarthritis, left hip

M16.6 Other bilateral secondary osteoarthritis of hip

M16.7 Other unilateral secondary osteoarthritis of hip
Secondary osteoarthritis of hip NOS

M16.9 Osteoarthritis of hip, unspecified

4ᵗʰ M17 Osteoarthritis of knee

M17.0 Bilateral primary osteoarthritis of knee

5ᵗʰ M17.1 Unilateral primary osteoarthritis of knee
Primary osteoarthritis of knee NOS
M17.10 Unilateral primary osteoarthritis, unspecified knee
AHA: Q4 2016
M17.11 Unilateral primary osteoarthritis, right knee
M17.12 Unilateral primary osteoarthritis, left knee
AHA: Q4 2016

M17.2 Bilateral post-traumatic osteoarthritis of knee

5ᵗʰ M17.3 Unilateral post-traumatic osteoarthritis of knee
Post-traumatic osteoarthritis of knee NOS
M17.30 Unilateral post-traumatic osteoarthritis, unspecified knee
M17.31 Unilateral post-traumatic osteoarthritis, right knee
M17.32 Unilateral post-traumatic osteoarthritis, left knee

M17.4 Other bilateral secondary osteoarthritis of knee

M17.5 Other unilateral secondary osteoarthritis of knee
Secondary osteoarthritis of knee NOS

M17.9 Osteoarthritis of knee, unspecified
AHA: Q4 2016

4ᵗʰ M18 Osteoarthritis of first carpometacarpal joint

M18.0 Bilateral primary osteoarthritis of first carpometacarpal joints

5ᵗʰ M18.1 Unilateral primary osteoarthritis of first carpometacarpal joint
Primary osteoarthritis of first carpometacarpal joint NOS
M18.10 Unilateral primary osteoarthritis of first carpometacarpal joint, unspecified hand
M18.11 Unilateral primary osteoarthritis of first carpometacarpal joint, right hand
M18.12 Unilateral primary osteoarthritis of first carpometacarpal joint, left hand

M18.2 Bilateral post-traumatic osteoarthritis of first carpometacarpal joints

5ᵗʰ M18.3 Unilateral post-traumatic osteoarthritis of first carpometacarpal joint
Post-traumatic osteoarthritis of first carpometacarpal joint NOS
M18.30 Unilateral post-traumatic osteoarthritis of first carpometacarpal joint, unspecified hand
M18.31 Unilateral post-traumatic osteoarthritis of first carpometacarpal joint, right hand
M18.32 Unilateral post-traumatic osteoarthritis of first carpometacarpal joint, left hand

M18.4 Other bilateral secondary osteoarthritis of first carpometacarpal joints

5ᵗʰ M18.5 Other unilateral secondary osteoarthritis of first carpometacarpal joint
Secondary osteoarthritis of first carpometacarpal joint NOS
M18.50 Other unilateral secondary osteoarthritis of first carpometacarpal joint, unspecified hand
M18.51 Other unilateral secondary osteoarthritis of first carpometacarpal joint, right hand
M18.52 Other unilateral secondary osteoarthritis of first carpometacarpal joint, left hand

M18.9 Osteoarthritis of first carpometacarpal joint, unspecified

4ᵗʰ M19 Other and unspecified osteoarthritis

EXCLUDES1 polyarthritis (M15.-)

EXCLUDES2 arthrosis of spine (M47.-)
hallux rigidus (M20.2)
osteoarthritis of spine (M47.-)

PDxⁿ Unacceptable principal diagnosis symbol per Medicare code edits   PDx Code exempt from diagnosis present on admission requirement

❓ Questionable admission   ꜀ᶜ Complication or comorbidity   ᴹᶜᶜ Major complication or comorbidity   ꜀ᶜ/ᴹᶜᶜ CC/MCC exclusion

HCC HCC diagnosis code   RxHCC RxHCC diagnosis code   MACRA code   **DEFINITION** Describes condition/terminology

TIP Coding guidance   👁 Official Guideline Reference   Z1 Z code as first-listed diagnosis

5ᵗʰ M19.0 Primary osteoarthritis of other joints
    6ᵗʰ M19.01 Primary osteoarthritis, shoulder
        M19.011 **Primary osteoarthritis, right shoulder**
            AHA: Q4 2016
        M19.012 **Primary osteoarthritis, left shoulder**
        M19.019 **Primary osteoarthritis, unspecified shoulder**
    6ᵗʰ M19.02 Primary osteoarthritis, elbow
        M19.021 **Primary osteoarthritis, right elbow**
        M19.022 **Primary osteoarthritis, left elbow**
        M19.029 **Primary osteoarthritis, unspecified elbow**
    6ᵗʰ M19.03 Primary osteoarthritis, wrist
        M19.031 **Primary osteoarthritis, right wrist**
        M19.032 **Primary osteoarthritis, left wrist**
        M19.039 **Primary osteoarthritis, unspecified wrist**
    6ᵗʰ M19.04 Primary osteoarthritis, hand
        EXCLUDES2 *primary osteoarthritis of first carpometacarpal joint (M18.0-, M18.1-)*
        M19.041 **Primary osteoarthritis, right hand**
        M19.042 **Primary osteoarthritis, left hand**
        M19.049 **Primary osteoarthritis, unspecified hand**
    6ᵗʰ M19.07 Primary osteoarthritis ankle and foot
        M19.071 **Primary osteoarthritis, right ankle and foot**
        M19.072 **Primary osteoarthritis, left ankle and foot**
        M19.079 **Primary osteoarthritis, unspecified ankle and foot**
5ᵗʰ M19.1 Post-traumatic osteoarthritis of other joints
    6ᵗʰ M19.11 Post-traumatic osteoarthritis, shoulder
        M19.111 **Post-traumatic osteoarthritis, right shoulder**
        M19.112 **Post-traumatic osteoarthritis, left shoulder**
        M19.119 **Post-traumatic osteoarthritis, unspecified shoulder**
    6ᵗʰ M19.12 Post-traumatic osteoarthritis, elbow
        M19.121 **Post-traumatic osteoarthritis, right elbow**
        M19.122 **Post-traumatic osteoarthritis, left elbow**
        M19.129 **Post-traumatic osteoarthritis, unspecified elbow**
    6ᵗʰ M19.13 Post-traumatic osteoarthritis, wrist
        M19.131 **Post-traumatic osteoarthritis, right wrist**
        M19.132 **Post-traumatic osteoarthritis, left wrist**
        M19.139 **Post-traumatic osteoarthritis, unspecified wrist**
    6ᵗʰ M19.14 Post-traumatic osteoarthritis, hand
        EXCLUDES2 *post-traumatic osteoarthritis of first carpometacarpal joint (M18.2-, M18.3-)*
        M19.141 **Post-traumatic osteoarthritis, right hand**
        M19.142 **Post-traumatic osteoarthritis, left hand**
        M19.149 **Post-traumatic osteoarthritis, unspecified hand**
    6ᵗʰ M19.17 Post-traumatic osteoarthritis, ankle and foot
        M19.171 **Post-traumatic osteoarthritis, right ankle and foot**
        M19.172 **Post-traumatic osteoarthritis, left ankle and foot**
        M19.179 **Post-traumatic osteoarthritis, unspecified ankle and foot**
5ᵗʰ M19.2 Secondary osteoarthritis of other joints
    6ᵗʰ M19.21 Secondary osteoarthritis, shoulder
        M19.211 **Secondary osteoarthritis, right shoulder**
        M19.212 **Secondary osteoarthritis, left shoulder**
        M19.219 **Secondary osteoarthritis, unspecified shoulder**
    6ᵗʰ M19.22 Secondary osteoarthritis, elbow
        M19.221 **Secondary osteoarthritis, right elbow**
        M19.222 **Secondary osteoarthritis, left elbow**
        M19.229 **Secondary osteoarthritis, unspecified elbow**

6ᵗʰ M19.23 Secondary osteoarthritis, wrist
    M19.231 **Secondary osteoarthritis, right wrist**
    M19.232 **Secondary osteoarthritis, left wrist**
    M19.239 **Secondary osteoarthritis, unspecified wrist**
6ᵗʰ M19.24 Secondary osteoarthritis, hand
    M19.241 **Secondary osteoarthritis, right hand**
    M19.242 **Secondary osteoarthritis, left hand**
    M19.249 **Secondary osteoarthritis, unspecified hand**
6ᵗʰ M19.27 Secondary osteoarthritis, ankle and foot
    M19.271 **Secondary osteoarthritis, right ankle and foot**
    M19.272 **Secondary osteoarthritis, left ankle and foot**
    M19.279 **Secondary osteoarthritis, unspecified ankle and foot**
5ᵗʰ M19.9 Osteoarthritis, unspecified site
    M19.90 **Unspecified osteoarthritis, unspecified site**
        AHA: Q4 2016
        Arthrosis NOS
        Arthritis NOS
        Osteoarthritis NOS
    M19.91 **Primary osteoarthritis, unspecified site**
        Primary osteoarthritis NOS
    M19.92 **Post-traumatic osteoarthritis, unspecified site**
        Post-traumatic osteoarthritis NOS
    M19.93 **Secondary osteoarthritis, unspecified site**
        Secondary osteoarthritis NOS

Other joint disorders (M20-M25)

EXCLUDES2 *joints of the spine (M40-M54)*
4ᵗʰ M20 Acquired deformities of fingers and toes
    EXCLUDES1 *acquired absence of fingers and toes (Z89.-)*
        congenital absence of fingers and toes (Q71.3-, Q72.3-)
        congenital deformities and malformations of fingers and toes (Q66.-, Q68-Q70, Q74.-)
    5ᵗʰ M20.0 Deformity of finger(s)
        EXCLUDES1 *clubbing of fingers (R68.3)*
            palmar fascial fibromatosis [Dupuytren] (M72.0)
            trigger finger (M65.3)
      6ᵗʰ M20.00 Unspecified deformity of finger(s)
        M20.001 **Unspecified deformity of right finger(s)**
        M20.002 **Unspecified deformity of left finger(s)**
        M20.009 **Unspecified deformity of unspecified finger(s)**
      6ᵗʰ M20.01 Mallet finger
        M20.011 **Mallet finger of right finger(s)**
        M20.012 **Mallet finger of left finger(s)**
        M20.019 **Mallet finger of unspecified finger(s)**
      6ᵗʰ M20.02 Boutonnière deformity
        M20.021 **Boutonnière deformity of right finger(s)**
        M20.022 **Boutonnière deformity of left finger(s)**
        M20.029 **Boutonnière deformity of unspecified finger(s)**
      6ᵗʰ M20.03 Swan-neck deformity
        M20.031 **Swan-neck deformity of right finger(s)**
        M20.032 **Swan-neck deformity of left finger(s)**
        M20.039 **Swan-neck deformity of unspecified finger(s)**
      6ᵗʰ M20.09 Other deformity of finger(s)
        M20.091 **Other deformity of right finger(s)**
        M20.092 **Other deformity of left finger(s)**
        M20.099 **Other deformity of finger(s), unspecified finger(s)**
    5ᵗʰ M20.1 Hallux valgus (acquired) (Figure 13.2)
        EXCLUDES2 *bunion (M21.6-)*
        M20.10 **Hallux valgus (acquired), unspecified foot**
        M20.11 **Hallux valgus (acquired), right foot**
        M20.12 **Hallux valgus (acquired), left foot**

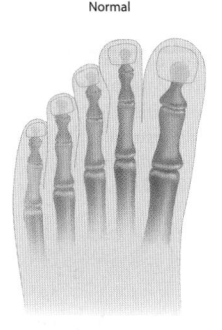 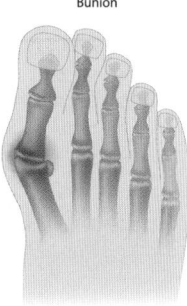

Normal   Bunion

Figure 13.2 Hallux Valgus (Bunion)

5ᵗʰ **M20.2** Hallux rigidus
   M20.20 Hallux rigidus, unspecified foot
   M20.21 Hallux rigidus, right **foot**
   M20.22 Hallux rigidus, left **foot**
5ᵗʰ **M20.3** Hallux varus (acquired)
   M20.30 Hallux varus (acquired), unspecified foot
   M20.31 Hallux varus (acquired), right **foot**
   M20.32 Hallux varus (acquired), left **foot**
5ᵗʰ **M20.4** Other hammer toe(s) (acquired)
   M20.40 Other hammer toe(s) (acquired), unspecified foot
   M20.41 Other hammer toe(s) (acquired), right **foot**
   M20.42 Other hammer toe(s) (acquired), left **foot**
5ᵗʰ **M20.5** Other deformities of toe(s) (acquired)
   6ᵗʰ **M20.5X** Other deformities of toe(s) (acquired)
      M20.5X1 Other deformities of toe(s) (acquired), right **foot**
      M20.5X2 Other deformities of toe(s) (acquired), left **foot**
      M20.5X9 Other deformities of toe(s) (acquired), unspecified foot
5ᵗʰ **M20.6** Acquired deformities of toe(s), unspecified
   M20.60 Acquired deformities of toe(s), unspecified, unspecified foot
   M20.61 Acquired deformities of toe(s), unspecified, right **foot**
   M20.62 Acquired deformities of toe(s), unspecified, left **foot**
4ᵗʰ **M21** Other acquired deformities of limbs
   EXCLUDES1 *acquired absence of limb (Z89.-)*
                  congenital absence of limbs (Q71-Q73)
                  congenital deformities and malformations of limbs (Q65-Q66, Q68-Q74)
   EXCLUDES2 *acquired deformities of fingers or toes (M20.-)*
                  coxa plana (M91.2)
5ᵗʰ **M21.0** Valgus deformity, not elsewhere classified
   EXCLUDES1 *metatarsus valgus (Q66.6)*
                  talipes calcaneovalgus ▶*(Q66.4-)*◀
   M21.00 Valgus deformity, not elsewhere classified, unspecified site
   6ᵗʰ **M21.02** Valgus deformity, not elsewhere classified, elbow
      Cubitus valgus
      M21.021 Valgus deformity, not elsewhere classified, right **elbow**
      M21.022 Valgus deformity, not elsewhere classified, left **elbow**
      M21.029 Valgus deformity, not elsewhere classified, unspecified elbow
   6ᵗʰ **M21.05** Valgus deformity, not elsewhere classified, hip
      M21.051 Valgus deformity, not elsewhere classified, right **hip**
      M21.052 Valgus deformity, not elsewhere classified, left **hip**
      M21.059 Valgus deformity, not elsewhere classified, unspecified hip

6ᵗʰ **M21.06** Valgus deformity, not elsewhere classified, knee
   Genu valgum
   Knock knee
   M21.061 Valgus deformity, not elsewhere classified, right **knee**
   M21.062 Valgus deformity, not elsewhere classified, left **knee**
   M21.069 Valgus deformity, not elsewhere classified, unspecified knee
6ᵗʰ **M21.07** Valgus deformity, not elsewhere classified, ankle
   M21.071 Valgus deformity, not elsewhere classified, right **ankle**
   M21.072 Valgus deformity, not elsewhere classified, left **ankle**
   M21.079 Valgus deformity, not elsewhere classified, unspecified ankle
5ᵗʰ **M21.1** Varus deformity, not elsewhere classified
   EXCLUDES1 *metatarsus varus* ▶*(Q66.22-)*◀
                  tibia vara (M92.5)
   M21.10 Varus deformity, not elsewhere classified, unspecified site
   6ᵗʰ **M21.12** Varus deformity, not elsewhere classified, elbow
      Cubitus varus, elbow
      M21.121 Varus deformity, not elsewhere classified, right **elbow**
      M21.122 Varus deformity, not elsewhere classified, left **elbow**
      M21.129 Varus deformity, not elsewhere classified, unspecified elbow
   6ᵗʰ **M21.15** Varus deformity, not elsewhere classified, hip
      M21.151 Varus deformity, not elsewhere classified, right **hip**
      M21.152 Varus deformity, not elsewhere classified, left **hip**
      M21.159 Varus deformity, not elsewhere classified, unspecified
   6ᵗʰ **M21.16** Varus deformity, not elsewhere classified, knee
      Bow leg
      Genu varum
      M21.161 Varus deformity, not elsewhere classified, right **knee**
      M21.162 Varus deformity, not elsewhere classified, left **knee**
      M21.169 Varus deformity, not elsewhere classified, unspecified knee
   6ᵗʰ **M21.17** Varus deformity, not elsewhere classified, ankle
      M21.171 Varus deformity, not elsewhere classified, right **ankle**
      M21.172 Varus deformity, not elsewhere classified, left **ankle**
      M21.179 Varus deformity, not elsewhere classified, unspecified ankle
5ᵗʰ **M21.2** Flexion deformity
   M21.20 Flexion deformity, unspecified site
   6ᵗʰ **M21.21** Flexion deformity, shoulder
      M21.211 Flexion deformity, right **shoulder**
      M21.212 Flexion deformity, left **shoulder**
      M21.219 Flexion deformity, unspecified shoulder
   6ᵗʰ **M21.22** Flexion deformity, elbow
      M21.221 Flexion deformity, right **elbow**
      M21.222 Flexion deformity, left **elbow**
      M21.229 Flexion deformity, unspecified elbow
   6ᵗʰ **M21.23** Flexion deformity, wrist
      M21.231 Flexion deformity, right **wrist**
      M21.232 Flexion deformity, left **wrist**
      M21.239 Flexion deformity, unspecified wrist
   6ᵗʰ **M21.24** Flexion deformity, finger joints
      M21.241 Flexion deformity, right **finger joints**
      M21.242 Flexion deformity, left **finger joints**
      M21.249 Flexion deformity, unspecified finger joints

PDN Unacceptable principal diagnosis symbol per Medicare code edits   POA Code exempt from diagnosis present on admission requirement
❓ Questionable admission   CC Complication or comorbidity   MCC Major complication or comorbidity   CC/MCC CC/MCC exclusion
HCC HCC diagnosis code   **RxHCC** RxHCC diagnosis code   MACRA MACRA code   **DEFINITION** Describes condition/terminology
TIP Coding guidance   👁 Official Guideline Reference   Z1 Z code as first-listed diagnosis

796   When symbols appear on a code that requires a 7th character extension, refer to Appendix B to identify applicable 7th character codes.   **2020 ICD-10-CM**

M21.25 Flexion deformity, hip
    M21.251 Flexion deformity, right hip
    M21.252 Flexion deformity, left hip
    M21.259 Flexion deformity, unspecified hip
M21.26 Flexion deformity, knee
    M21.261 Flexion deformity, right knee
    M21.262 Flexion deformity, left knee
    M21.269 Flexion deformity, unspecified knee
M21.27 Flexion deformity, ankle and toes
    M21.271 Flexion deformity, right ankle and toes
    M21.272 Flexion deformity, left ankle and toes
    M21.279 Flexion deformity, unspecified ankle and toes
M21.3 Wrist or foot drop (acquired)
  M21.33 Wrist drop (acquired)
    M21.331 Wrist drop, right wrist
    M21.332 Wrist drop, left wrist
    M21.339 Wrist drop, unspecified wrist
  M21.37 Foot drop (acquired)
    M21.371 Foot drop, right foot
    M21.372 Foot drop, left foot
    M21.379 Foot drop, unspecified foot
M21.4 Flat foot [pes planus] (acquired) (Figure 13.3)
    EXCLUDES1 congenital pes planus (Q66.5-)
  M21.40 Flat foot [pes planus] (acquired), unspecified foot
  M21.41 Flat foot [pes planus] (acquired), right foot
  M21.42 Flat foot [pes planus] (acquired), left foot

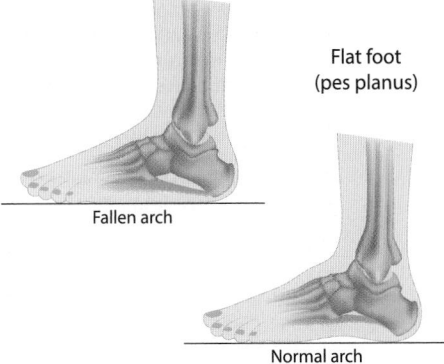

Flat foot
(pes planus)

Fallen arch

Normal arch

Figure 13.3 Normal Foot Arch and Fallen Foot Arch

M21.5 Acquired clawhand, clubhand, clawfoot and clubfoot
    EXCLUDES1 clubfoot, not specified as acquired (Q66.89)
  M21.51 Acquired clawhand
    M21.511 Acquired clawhand, right hand
    M21.512 Acquired clawhand, left hand
    M21.519 Acquired clawhand, unspecified hand
  M21.52 Acquired clubhand
    M21.521 Acquired clubhand, right hand
    M21.522 Acquired clubhand, left hand
    M21.529 Acquired clubhand, unspecified hand
  M21.53 Acquired clawfoot
    M21.531 Acquired clawfoot, right foot
    M21.532 Acquired clawfoot, left foot
    M21.539 Acquired clawfoot, unspecified foot
  M21.54 Acquired clubfoot
    M21.541 Acquired clubfoot, right foot
    M21.542 Acquired clubfoot, left foot
    M21.549 Acquired clubfoot, unspecified foot
M21.6 Other acquired deformities of foot
    EXCLUDES2 deformities of toe (acquired) (M20.1-M20.6-)
  M21.61 Bunion
    M21.611 Bunion of right foot
      AHA: Q4 2016

M21.612 Bunion of left foot
    AHA: Q4 2016
M21.619 Bunion of unspecified foot
    AHA: Q4 2016
M21.62 Bunionette
  M21.621 Bunionette of right foot
    AHA: Q4 2016
  M21.622 Bunionette of left foot
    AHA: Q4 2016
  M21.629 Bunionette of unspecified foot
    AHA: Q4 2016
M21.6X Other acquired deformities of foot
  M21.6X1 Other acquired deformities of right foot
  M21.6X2 Other acquired deformities of left foot
  M21.6X9 Other acquired deformities of unspecified foot
M21.7 Unequal limb length (acquired)
    NOTES The site used should correspond to the shorter limb
  M21.70 Unequal limb length (acquired), unspecified site
  M21.72 Unequal limb length (acquired), humerus
    M21.721 Unequal limb length (acquired), right humerus
    M21.722 Unequal limb length (acquired), left humerus
    M21.729 Unequal limb length (acquired), unspecified humerus
  M21.73 Unequal limb length (acquired), ulna and radius
    M21.731 Unequal limb length (acquired), right ulna
    M21.732 Unequal limb length (acquired), left ulna
    M21.733 Unequal limb length (acquired), right radius
    M21.734 Unequal limb length (acquired), left radius
    M21.739 Unequal limb length (acquired), unspecified ulna and radius
  M21.75 Unequal limb length (acquired), femur
    M21.751 Unequal limb length (acquired), right femur
    M21.752 Unequal limb length (acquired), left femur
    M21.759 Unequal limb length (acquired), unspecified femur
  M21.76 Unequal limb length (acquired), tibia and fibula
    M21.761 Unequal limb length (acquired), right tibia
    M21.762 Unequal limb length (acquired), left tibia
    M21.763 Unequal limb length (acquired), right fibula
    M21.764 Unequal limb length (acquired), left fibula
    M21.769 Unequal limb length (acquired), unspecified tibia and fibula
M21.8 Other specified acquired deformities of limbs
    EXCLUDES2 coxa plana (M91.2)
  M21.80 Other specified acquired deformities of unspecified limb
  M21.82 Other specified acquired deformities of upper arm
    M21.821 Other specified acquired deformities of right upper arm
    M21.822 Other specified acquired deformities of left upper arm
    M21.829 Other specified acquired deformities of unspecified upper arm
  M21.83 Other specified acquired deformities of forearm
    M21.831 Other specified acquired deformities of right forearm
    M21.832 Other specified acquired deformities of left forearm
    M21.839 Other specified acquired deformities of unspecified forearm
  M21.85 Other specified acquired deformities of thigh
    M21.851 Other specified acquired deformities of right thigh

---

Unspecified Code   Other Specified Code   Manifestation Code   **N** Newborn   **P** Pediatric   **M** Maternity   **A** Adult   ♂ Male   ♀ Female
● New Code   ▲ Revised Code Title   ►◄ Revised Text   **NOTES**   *INCLUDES*   *EXCLUDES1* Not coded here   *EXCLUDES2* Not included here
4th character required   5th character required   6th character required   7th character required   Extension 'X' Alert
HAC Hospital-acquired condition (HAC) alert   **AHA** AHA Coding Clinic©   Code first alert

M21.852 Other specified acquired deformities of left thigh
M21.859 Other specified acquired deformities of unspecified thigh
6ᵗʰ M21.86 Other specified acquired deformities of lower leg
M21.861 Other specified acquired deformities of right lower leg
M21.862 Other specified acquired deformities of left lower leg
M21.869 Other specified acquired deformities of unspecified lower leg
5ᵗʰ M21.9 Unspecified acquired deformity of limb and hand
M21.90 Unspecified acquired deformity of unspecified limb
6ᵗʰ M21.92 Unspecified acquired deformity of upper arm
M21.921 Unspecified acquired deformity of right upper arm
M21.922 Unspecified acquired deformity of left upper arm
M21.929 Unspecified acquired deformity of unspecified upper arm
6ᵗʰ M21.93 Unspecified acquired deformity of forearm
M21.931 Unspecified acquired deformity of right forearm
M21.932 Unspecified acquired deformity of left forearm
M21.939 Unspecified acquired deformity of unspecified forearm
6ᵗʰ M21.94 Unspecified acquired deformity of hand
M21.941 Unspecified acquired deformity of hand, right hand
M21.942 Unspecified acquired deformity of hand, left hand
M21.949 Unspecified acquired deformity of hand, unspecified hand
6ᵗʰ M21.95 Unspecified acquired deformity of thigh
M21.951 Unspecified acquired deformity of right thigh
M21.952 Unspecified acquired deformity of left thigh
M21.959 Unspecified acquired deformity of unspecified thigh
6ᵗʰ M21.96 Unspecified acquired deformity of lower leg
M21.961 Unspecified acquired deformity of right lower leg
M21.962 Unspecified acquired deformity of left lower leg
M21.969 Unspecified acquired deformity of unspecified lower leg
4ᵗʰ M22 Disorder of patella
EXCLUDES1 traumatic dislocation of patella (S83.0-)
5ᵗʰ M22.0 Recurrent dislocation of patella
M22.00 Recurrent dislocation of patella, unspecified knee
M22.01 Recurrent dislocation of patella, right knee
M22.02 Recurrent dislocation of patella, left knee
5ᵗʰ M22.1 Recurrent subluxation of patella
Incomplete dislocation of patella
M22.10 Recurrent subluxation of patella, unspecified knee
M22.11 Recurrent subluxation of patella, right knee
M22.12 Recurrent subluxation of patella, left knee
5ᵗʰ M22.2 Patellofemoral disorders
6ᵗʰ M22.2X Patellofemoral disorders
M22.2X1 Patellofemoral disorders, right knee
M22.2X2 Patellofemoral disorders, left knee
M22.2X9 Patellofemoral disorders, unspecified knee
5ᵗʰ M22.3 Other derangements of patella
6ᵗʰ M22.3X Other derangements of patella
M22.3X1 Other derangements of patella, right knee
M22.3X2 Other derangements of patella, left knee
M22.3X9 Other derangements of patella, unspecified knee

5ᵗʰ M22.4 Chondromalacia patellae
M22.40 Chondromalacia patellae, unspecified knee
M22.41 Chondromalacia patellae, right knee
M22.42 Chondromalacia patellae, left knee
5ᵗʰ M22.8 Other disorders of patella
6ᵗʰ M22.8X Other disorders of patella
M22.8X1 Other disorders of patella, right knee
M22.8X2 Other disorders of patella, left knee
M22.8X9 Other disorders of patella, unspecified knee
5ᵗʰ M22.9 Unspecified disorder of patella
M22.90 Unspecified disorder of patella, unspecified knee
M22.91 Unspecified disorder of patella, right knee
M22.92 Unspecified disorder of patella, left knee
4ᵗʰ M23 Internal derangement of knee
EXCLUDES1 ankylosis (M24.66)
current injury - see injury of knee and lower leg (S80-S89)
deformity of knee (M21.-)
osteochondritis dissecans (M93.2)
recurrent dislocation or subluxation of joints (M24.4)
recurrent dislocation or subluxation of patella (M22.0-M22.1)
5ᵗʰ M23.0 Cystic meniscus
6ᵗʰ M23.00 Cystic meniscus, unspecified meniscus
Cystic meniscus, unspecified lateral meniscus
Cystic meniscus, unspecified medial meniscus
M23.000 Cystic meniscus, unspecified lateral meniscus, right knee
M23.001 Cystic meniscus, unspecified lateral meniscus, left knee
M23.002 Cystic meniscus, unspecified lateral meniscus, unspecified knee
M23.003 Cystic meniscus, unspecified medial meniscus, right knee
M23.004 Cystic meniscus, unspecified medial meniscus, left knee
M23.005 Cystic meniscus, unspecified medial meniscus, unspecified knee
M23.006 Cystic meniscus, unspecified meniscus, right knee
M23.007 Cystic meniscus, unspecified meniscus, left knee
M23.009 Cystic meniscus, unspecified meniscus, unspecified knee
6ᵗʰ M23.01 Cystic meniscus, anterior horn of medial meniscus
M23.011 Cystic meniscus, anterior horn of medial meniscus, right knee
M23.012 Cystic meniscus, anterior horn of medial meniscus, left knee
M23.019 Cystic meniscus, anterior horn of medial meniscus, unspecified knee
6ᵗʰ M23.02 Cystic meniscus, posterior horn of medial meniscus
M23.021 Cystic meniscus, posterior horn of medial meniscus, right knee
M23.022 Cystic meniscus, posterior horn of medial meniscus, left knee
M23.029 Cystic meniscus, posterior horn of medial meniscus, unspecified knee
6ᵗʰ M23.03 Cystic meniscus, other medial meniscus
M23.031 Cystic meniscus, other medial meniscus, right knee
M23.032 Cystic meniscus, other medial meniscus, left knee
M23.039 Cystic meniscus, other medial meniscus, unspecified knee
6ᵗʰ M23.04 Cystic meniscus, anterior horn of lateral meniscus
M23.041 Cystic meniscus, anterior horn of lateral meniscus, right knee
M23.042 Cystic meniscus, anterior horn of lateral meniscus, left knee

---

M23.049 Cystic meniscus, anterior horn of lateral meniscus, unspecified knee

6ᵗʰ M23.05 Cystic meniscus, posterior horn of lateral meniscus

M23.051 Cystic meniscus, posterior horn of lateral meniscus, right knee

M23.052 Cystic meniscus, posterior horn of lateral meniscus, left knee

M23.059 Cystic meniscus, posterior horn of lateral meniscus, unspecified knee

6ᵗʰ M23.06 Cystic meniscus, other lateral meniscus

M23.061 Cystic meniscus, other lateral meniscus, right knee

M23.062 Cystic meniscus, other lateral meniscus, left knee

M23.069 Cystic meniscus, other lateral meniscus, unspecified knee

5ᵗʰ M23.2 Derangement of meniscus due to old tear or injury

Old bucket-handle tear

6ᵗʰ M23.20 Derangement of unspecified meniscus due to old tear or injury

Derangement of unspecified lateral meniscus due to old tear or injury

Derangement of unspecified medial meniscus due to old tear or injury

M23.200 Derangement of unspecified lateral meniscus due to old tear or injury, right knee

M23.201 Derangement of unspecified lateral meniscus due to old tear or injury, left knee

M23.202 Derangement of unspecified lateral meniscus due to old tear or injury, unspecified knee

M23.203 Derangement of unspecified medial meniscus due to old tear or injury, right knee

M23.204 Derangement of unspecified medial meniscus due to old tear or injury, left knee

M23.205 Derangement of unspecified medial meniscus due to old tear or injury, unspecified knee

M23.206 Derangement of unspecified meniscus due to old tear or injury, right knee

M23.207 Derangement of unspecified meniscus due to old tear or injury, left knee

M23.209 Derangement of unspecified meniscus due to old tear or injury, unspecified knee

6ᵗʰ M23.21 Derangement of anterior horn of medial meniscus due to old tear or injury

M23.211 Derangement of anterior horn of medial meniscus due to old tear or injury, right knee

M23.212 Derangement of anterior horn of medial meniscus due to old tear or injury, left knee

M23.219 Derangement of anterior horn of medial meniscus due to old tear or injury, unspecified knee

6ᵗʰ M23.22 Derangement of posterior horn of medial meniscus due to old tear or injury

M23.221 Derangement of posterior horn of medial meniscus due to old tear or injury, right knee

M23.222 Derangement of posterior horn of medial meniscus due to old tear or injury, left knee

M23.229 Derangement of posterior horn of medial meniscus due to old tear or injury, unspecified knee

6ᵗʰ M23.23 Derangement of other medial meniscus due to old tear or injury

M23.231 Derangement of other medial meniscus due to old tear or injury, right knee

M23.232 Derangement of other medial meniscus due to old tear or injury, left knee

M23.239 Derangement of other medial meniscus due to old tear or injury, unspecified knee

6ᵗʰ M23.24 Derangement of anterior horn of lateral meniscus due to old tear or injury

M23.241 Derangement of anterior horn of lateral meniscus due to old tear or injury, right knee

M23.242 Derangement of anterior horn of lateral meniscus due to old tear or injury, left knee

M23.249 Derangement of anterior horn of lateral meniscus due to old tear or injury, unspecified knee

6ᵗʰ M23.25 Derangement of posterior horn of lateral meniscus due to old tear or injury

M23.251 Derangement of posterior horn of lateral meniscus due to old tear or injury, right knee

M23.252 Derangement of posterior horn of lateral meniscus due to old tear or injury, left knee

M23.259 Derangement of posterior horn of lateral meniscus due to old tear or injury, unspecified knee

6ᵗʰ M23.26 Derangement of other lateral meniscus due to old tear or injury

M23.261 Derangement of other lateral meniscus due to old tear or injury, right knee

M23.262 Derangement of other lateral meniscus due to old tear or injury, left knee

M23.269 Derangement of other lateral meniscus due to old tear or injury, unspecified knee

5ᵗʰ M23.3 Other meniscus derangements

Degenerate meniscus

Detached meniscus

Retained meniscus

6ᵗʰ M23.30 Other meniscus derangements, unspecified meniscus

Other meniscus derangements, unspecified lateral meniscus

Other meniscus derangements, unspecified medial meniscus

M23.300 Other meniscus derangements, unspecified lateral meniscus, right knee

M23.301 Other meniscus derangements, unspecified lateral meniscus, left knee

M23.302 Other meniscus derangements, unspecified lateral meniscus, unspecified knee

M23.303 Other meniscus derangements, unspecified medial meniscus, right knee

M23.304 Other meniscus derangements, unspecified medial meniscus, left knee

M23.305 Other meniscus derangements, unspecified medial meniscus, unspecified knee

M23.306 Other meniscus derangements, unspecified meniscus, right knee

M23.307 Other meniscus derangements, unspecified meniscus, left knee

M23.309 Other meniscus derangements, unspecified meniscus, unspecified knee

6ᵗʰ M23.31 Other meniscus derangements, anterior horn of medial meniscus

M23.311 Other meniscus derangements, anterior horn of medial meniscus, right knee

M23.312 Other meniscus derangements, anterior horn of medial meniscus, left knee

---

Unspecified Code   Other Specified Code   Manifestation Code   N Newborn   P Pediatric   M Maternity   A Adult   ♂ Male   ♀ Female
● New Code   ▲ Revised Code Title   ▶◀ Revised Text   **NOTES**   *INCLUDES*   **EXCLUDES1** Not coded here   *EXCLUDES2* Not included here
4ᵗʰ 4ᵗʰ character required   5ᵗʰ 5ᵗʰ character required   6ᵗʰ 6ᵗʰ character required   7ᵗʰ 7ᵗʰ character required   Extension 'X' Alert
HAC Hospital-acquired condition (HAC) alert   **AHA** AHA Coding Clinic©   ☛ Code first alert

M23.319 Other meniscus derangements, anterior horn of medial meniscus, unspecified knee

6ᵗʰ M23.32 Other meniscus derangements, posterior horn of medial meniscus

M23.321 Other meniscus derangements, posterior horn of medial meniscus, right knee

M23.322 Other meniscus derangements, posterior horn of medial meniscus, left knee

M23.329 Other meniscus derangements, posterior horn of medial meniscus, unspecified knee

6ᵗʰ M23.33 Other meniscus derangements, other medial meniscus

M23.331 Other meniscus derangements, other medial meniscus, right knee

M23.332 Other meniscus derangements, other medial meniscus, left knee

M23.339 Other meniscus derangements, other medial meniscus, unspecified knee

6ᵗʰ M23.34 Other meniscus derangements, anterior horn of lateral meniscus

M23.341 Other meniscus derangements, anterior horn of lateral meniscus, right knee

M23.342 Other meniscus derangements, anterior horn of lateral meniscus, left knee

M23.349 Other meniscus derangements, anterior horn of lateral meniscus, unspecified knee

6ᵗʰ M23.35 Other meniscus derangements, posterior horn of lateral meniscus

M23.351 Other meniscus derangements, posterior horn of lateral meniscus, right knee

M23.352 Other meniscus derangements, posterior horn of lateral meniscus, left knee

M23.359 Other meniscus derangements, posterior horn of lateral meniscus, unspecified knee

6ᵗʰ M23.36 Other meniscus derangements, other lateral meniscus

M23.361 Other meniscus derangements, other lateral meniscus, right knee

M23.362 Other meniscus derangements, other lateral meniscus, left knee

M23.369 Other meniscus derangements, other lateral meniscus, unspecified knee

5ᵗʰ M23.4 Loose body in knee

M23.40 Loose body in knee, unspecified knee

M23.41 Loose body in knee, right knee

M23.42 Loose body in knee, left knee

5ᵗʰ M23.5 Chronic instability of knee

M23.50 Chronic instability of knee, unspecified knee

M23.51 Chronic instability of knee, right knee

M23.52 Chronic instability of knee, left knee

5ᵗʰ M23.6 Other spontaneous disruption of ligament(s) of knee

6ᵗʰ M23.60 Other spontaneous disruption of unspecified ligament of knee

M23.601 Other spontaneous disruption of unspecified ligament of right knee

M23.602 Other spontaneous disruption of unspecified ligament of left knee

M23.609 Other spontaneous disruption of unspecified ligament of unspecified knee

6ᵗʰ M23.61 Other spontaneous disruption of anterior cruciate ligament of knee

M23.611 Other spontaneous disruption of anterior cruciate ligament of right knee

M23.612 Other spontaneous disruption of anterior cruciate ligament of left knee

M23.619 Other spontaneous disruption of anterior cruciate ligament of unspecified knee

6ᵗʰ M23.62 Other spontaneous disruption of posterior cruciate ligament of knee

M23.621 Other spontaneous disruption of posterior cruciate ligament of right knee

M23.622 Other spontaneous disruption of posterior cruciate ligament of left knee

M23.629 Other spontaneous disruption of posterior cruciate ligament of unspecified knee

6ᵗʰ M23.63 Other spontaneous disruption of medial collateral ligament of knee

M23.631 Other spontaneous disruption of medial collateral ligament of right knee

M23.632 Other spontaneous disruption of medial collateral ligament of left knee

M23.639 Other spontaneous disruption of medial collateral ligament of unspecified knee

6ᵗʰ M23.64 Other spontaneous disruption of lateral collateral ligament of knee

M23.641 Other spontaneous disruption of lateral collateral ligament of right knee

M23.642 Other spontaneous disruption of lateral collateral ligament of left knee

M23.649 Other spontaneous disruption of lateral collateral ligament of unspecified knee

6ᵗʰ M23.67 Other spontaneous disruption of capsular ligament of knee

M23.671 Other spontaneous disruption of capsular ligament of right knee

M23.672 Other spontaneous disruption of capsular ligament of left knee

M23.679 Other spontaneous disruption of capsular ligament of unspecified knee

5ᵗʰ M23.8 Other internal derangements of knee

Laxity of ligament of knee
Snapping knee

6ᵗʰ M23.8X Other internal derangements of knee

M23.8X1 Other internal derangements of right knee

M23.8X2 Other internal derangements of left knee

M23.8X9 Other internal derangements of unspecified knee

5ᵗʰ M23.9 Unspecified internal derangement of knee

M23.90 Unspecified internal derangement of unspecified knee

M23.91 Unspecified internal derangement of right knee

M23.92 Unspecified internal derangement of left knee

4ᵗʰ M24 Other specific joint derangements

EXCLUDES1 current injury - see injury of joint by body region

EXCLUDES2 ganglion (M67.4)

snapping knee (M23.8-)

temporomandibular joint disorders (M26.6-)

5ᵗʰ M24.0 Loose body in joint

DEFINITION: A loose body in a joint consists of fragments of bone and/or cartilage that float in the joint. These can float freely, or cause the joint to lock or catch.

EXCLUDES2 loose body in knee (M23.4)

M24.00 Loose body in unspecified joint

6ᵗʰ M24.01 Loose body in shoulder

M24.011 Loose body in right shoulder

M24.012 Loose body in left shoulder

M24.019 Loose body in unspecified shoulder

6ᵗʰ M24.02 Loose body in elbow

M24.021 Loose body in right elbow

M24.022 Loose body in left elbow

M24.029 Loose body in unspecified elbow

6ᵗʰ M24.03 Loose body in wrist

M24.031 Loose body in right wrist

M24.032 Loose body in left wrist

M24.039 Loose body in unspecified wrist

6ᵗʰ M24.04 Loose body in finger joints

M24.041 Loose body in right finger joint(s)

M24.042 Loose body in left finger joint(s)

M24.049 Loose body in unspecified finger joint(s)

6ᵗʰ M24.05 Loose body in hip

M24.051 Loose body in right hip

M24.052 Loose body in left hip

M24.059 Loose body in unspecified hip

PDx🔒 Unacceptable principal diagnosis symbol per Medicare code edits   PDx🔒 Code exempt from diagnosis present on admission requirement

❓ Questionable admission   cᶜ Complication or comorbidity   MCC Major complication or comorbidity   cc/mcc exc CC/MCC exclusion

HCC HCC diagnosis code   RxHCC RxHCC diagnosis code   MACRA code   DEFINITION Describes condition/terminology

TIP Coding guidance   👁 Official Guideline Reference   Z1 Z code as first-listed diagnosis

800   When symbols appear on a code that requires a 7th character extension, refer to Appendix B to identify applicable 7th character codes.   2020 ICD-10-CM

[6th] M24.07 Loose body in ankle and toe joints
M24.071 Loose body in right ankle
M24.072 Loose body in left ankle
M24.073 Loose body in unspecified ankle
M24.074 Loose body in right toe joint(s)
M24.075 Loose body in left toe joint(s)
M24.076 Loose body in unspecified toe joints
M24.08 Loose body, other site

[5th] M24.1 Other articular cartilage disorders
EXCLUDES2 *chondrocalcinosis (M11.1, M11.2-)*
internal derangement of knee (M23.-)
metastatic calcification (E83.5)
ochronosis (E70.2)
M24.10 Other articular cartilage disorders, unspecified site
[6th] M24.11 Other articular cartilage disorders, shoulder
M24.111 Other articular cartilage disorders, right shoulder
M24.112 Other articular cartilage disorders, left shoulder
M24.119 Other articular cartilage disorders, unspecified shoulder
[6th] M24.12 Other articular cartilage disorders, elbow
M24.121 Other articular cartilage disorders, right elbow
M24.122 Other articular cartilage disorders, left elbow
M24.129 Other articular cartilage disorders, unspecified elbow
[6th] M24.13 Other articular cartilage disorders, wrist
M24.131 Other articular cartilage disorders, right wrist
M24.132 Other articular cartilage disorders, left wrist
M24.139 Other articular cartilage disorders, unspecified wrist
[6th] M24.14 Other articular cartilage disorders, hand
M24.141 Other articular cartilage disorders, right hand
M24.142 Other articular cartilage disorders, left hand
M24.149 Other articular cartilage disorders, unspecified hand
[6th] M24.15 Other articular cartilage disorders, hip
M24.151 Other articular cartilage disorders, right hip
M24.152 Other articular cartilage disorders, left hip
M24.159 Other articular cartilage disorders, unspecified hip
[6th] M24.17 Other articular cartilage disorders, ankle and foot
M24.171 Other articular cartilage disorders, right ankle
M24.172 Other articular cartilage disorders, left ankle
M24.173 Other articular cartilage disorders, unspecified ankle
M24.174 Other articular cartilage disorders, right foot
M24.175 Other articular cartilage disorders, left foot
M24.176 Other articular cartilage disorders, unspecified foot

[5th] M24.2 Disorder of ligament
Instability secondary to old ligament injury
Ligamentous laxity NOS
EXCLUDES1 *familial ligamentous laxity (M35.7)*
EXCLUDES2 *internal derangement of knee (M23.5-▶M23.8X9◀)*
M24.20 Disorder of ligament, unspecified site
[6th] M24.21 Disorder of ligament, shoulder
M24.211 Disorder of ligament, right shoulder
M24.212 Disorder of ligament, left shoulder
M24.219 Disorder of ligament, unspecified shoulder
[6th] M24.22 Disorder of ligament, elbow
M24.221 Disorder of ligament, right elbow
M24.222 Disorder of ligament, left elbow
M24.229 Disorder of ligament, unspecified elbow
[6th] M24.23 Disorder of ligament, wrist
M24.231 Disorder of ligament, right wrist
M24.232 Disorder of ligament, left wrist
M24.239 Disorder of ligament, unspecified wrist
[6th] M24.24 Disorder of ligament, hand
M24.241 Disorder of ligament, right hand
M24.242 Disorder of ligament, left hand
M24.249 Disorder of ligament, unspecified hand
[6th] M24.25 Disorder of ligament, hip
M24.251 Disorder of ligament, right hip
M24.252 Disorder of ligament, left hip
M24.259 Disorder of ligament, unspecified hip
[6th] M24.27 Disorder of ligament, ankle and foot
M24.271 Disorder of ligament, right ankle
M24.272 Disorder of ligament, left ankle
M24.273 Disorder of ligament, unspecified ankle
M24.274 Disorder of ligament, right foot
M24.275 Disorder of ligament, left foot
M24.276 Disorder of ligament, unspecified foot
M24.28 Disorder of ligament, vertebrae

[5th] M24.3 Pathological dislocation of joint, not elsewhere classified
EXCLUDES1 *congenital dislocation or displacement of joint- see congenital malformations and deformations of the musculoskeletal system (Q65-Q79)*
current injury - see injury of joints and ligaments by body region
recurrent dislocation of joint (M24.4-)
M24.30 Pathological dislocation of unspecified joint, not elsewhere classified
[6th] M24.31 Pathological dislocation of shoulder, not elsewhere classified
M24.311 Pathological dislocation of right shoulder, not elsewhere classified
M24.312 Pathological dislocation of left shoulder, not elsewhere classified
M24.319 Pathological dislocation of unspecified shoulder, not elsewhere classified
[6th] M24.32 Pathological dislocation of elbow, not elsewhere classified
M24.321 Pathological dislocation of right elbow, not elsewhere classified
M24.322 Pathological dislocation of left elbow, not elsewhere classified
M24.329 Pathological dislocation of unspecified elbow, not elsewhere classified
[6th] M24.33 Pathological dislocation of wrist, not elsewhere classified
M24.331 Pathological dislocation of right wrist, not elsewhere classified
M24.332 Pathological dislocation of left wrist, not elsewhere classified
M24.339 Pathological dislocation of unspecified wrist, not elsewhere classified
[6th] M24.34 Pathological dislocation of hand, not elsewhere classified
M24.341 Pathological dislocation of right hand, not elsewhere classified
M24.342 Pathological dislocation of left hand, not elsewhere classified
M24.349 Pathological dislocation of unspecified hand, not elsewhere classified
[6th] M24.35 Pathological dislocation of hip, not elsewhere classified
M24.351 Pathological dislocation of right hip, not elsewhere classified

Unspecified Code Other Specified Code Manifestation Code [N] Newborn [P] Pediatric [M] Maternity [A] Adult ♂ Male ♀ Female
● New Code ▲ Revised Code Title ▶◀ Revised Text NOTES INCLUDES EXCLUDES1 Not coded here EXCLUDES2 Not included here
[4th] 4th character required [5th] 5th character required [6th] 6th character required [7th] 7th character required [X] Extension 'X' Alert
[HAC] Hospital-acquired condition (HAC) alert AHA AHA Coding Clinic© ☞ Code first alert

M24.352 Pathological dislocation of left hip, not elsewhere classified

M24.359 Pathological dislocation of unspecified hip, not elsewhere classified

6ᵗʰ M24.36 Pathological dislocation of knee, not elsewhere classified

M24.361 Pathological dislocation of right knee, not elsewhere classified

M24.362 Pathological dislocation of left knee, not elsewhere classified

M24.369 Pathological dislocation of unspecified knee, not elsewhere classified

6ᵗʰ M24.37 Pathological dislocation of ankle and foot, not elsewhere classified

M24.371 Pathological dislocation of right ankle, not elsewhere classified

M24.372 Pathological dislocation of left ankle, not elsewhere classified

M24.373 Pathological dislocation of unspecified ankle, not elsewhere classified

M24.374 Pathological dislocation of right foot, not elsewhere classified

M24.375 Pathological dislocation of left foot, not elsewhere classified

M24.376 Pathological dislocation of unspecified foot, not elsewhere classified

5ᵗʰ M24.4 Recurrent dislocation of joint

Recurrent subluxation of joint

EXCLUDES2 recurrent dislocation of patella (M22.0-M22.1)

recurrent vertebral dislocation (M43.3-, M43.4, M43.5-)

M24.40 Recurrent dislocation, unspecified joint

6ᵗʰ M24.41 Recurrent dislocation, shoulder

M24.411 Recurrent dislocation, right shoulder

M24.412 Recurrent dislocation, left shoulder

M24.419 Recurrent dislocation, unspecified shoulder

6ᵗʰ M24.42 Recurrent dislocation, elbow

M24.421 Recurrent dislocation, right elbow

M24.422 Recurrent dislocation, left elbow

M24.429 Recurrent dislocation, unspecified elbow

6ᵗʰ M24.43 Recurrent dislocation, wrist

M24.431 Recurrent dislocation, right wrist

M24.432 Recurrent dislocation, left wrist

M24.439 Recurrent dislocation, unspecified wrist

6ᵗʰ M24.44 Recurrent dislocation, hand and finger(s)

M24.441 Recurrent dislocation, right hand

M24.442 Recurrent dislocation, left hand

M24.443 Recurrent dislocation, unspecified hand

M24.444 Recurrent dislocation, right finger

M24.445 Recurrent dislocation, left finger

M24.446 Recurrent dislocation, unspecified finger

6ᵗʰ M24.45 Recurrent dislocation, hip

M24.451 Recurrent dislocation, right hip

M24.452 Recurrent dislocation, left hip

M24.459 Recurrent dislocation, unspecified hip

6ᵗʰ M24.46 Recurrent dislocation, knee

M24.461 Recurrent dislocation, right knee

M24.462 Recurrent dislocation, left knee

M24.469 Recurrent dislocation, unspecified knee

6ᵗʰ M24.47 Recurrent dislocation, ankle, foot and toes

M24.471 Recurrent dislocation, right ankle

M24.472 Recurrent dislocation, left ankle

M24.473 Recurrent dislocation, unspecified ankle

M24.474 Recurrent dislocation, right foot

M24.475 Recurrent dislocation, left foot

M24.476 Recurrent dislocation, unspecified foot

M24.477 Recurrent dislocation, right toe(s)

M24.478 Recurrent dislocation, left toe(s)

M24.479 Recurrent dislocation, unspecified toe(s)

5ᵗʰ M24.5 Contracture of joint

DEFINITION: Joint contracture results from connective tissue (tendon, muscle, ligament) that becomes stiff or constricted.

EXCLUDES1 contracture of muscle without contracture of joint (M62.4-)

contracture of tendon (sheath) without contracture of joint (M62.4-)

Dupuytren's contracture (M72.0)

EXCLUDES2 acquired deformities of limbs (M20-M21)

M24.50 Contracture, unspecified joint

6ᵗʰ M24.51 Contracture, shoulder

M24.511 Contracture, right shoulder

M24.512 Contracture, left shoulder

M24.519 Contracture, unspecified shoulder

6ᵗʰ M24.52 Contracture, elbow

M24.521 Contracture, right elbow

M24.522 Contracture, left elbow

M24.529 Contracture, unspecified elbow

6ᵗʰ M24.53 Contracture, wrist

M24.531 Contracture, right wrist

M24.532 Contracture, left wrist

M24.539 Contracture, unspecified wrist

6ᵗʰ M24.54 Contracture, hand

M24.541 Contracture, right hand

M24.542 Contracture, left hand

M24.549 Contracture, unspecified hand

6ᵗʰ M24.55 Contracture, hip

M24.551 Contracture, right hip

AHA: Q2 2016

M24.552 Contracture, left hip

AHA: Q2 2016

M24.559 Contracture, unspecified hip

6ᵗʰ M24.56 Contracture, knee

M24.561 Contracture, right knee

AHA: Q2 2016

M24.562 Contracture, left knee

AHA: Q2 2016

M24.569 Contracture, unspecified knee

6ᵗʰ M24.57 Contracture, ankle and foot

M24.571 Contracture, right ankle

M24.572 Contracture, left ankle

M24.573 Contracture, unspecified ankle

M24.574 Contracture, right foot

M24.575 Contracture, left foot

M24.576 Contracture, unspecified foot

5ᵗʰ M24.6 Ankylosis of joint

EXCLUDES1 stiffness of joint without ankylosis (M25.6-)

EXCLUDES2 spine (M43.2-)

M24.60 Ankylosis, unspecified joint

6ᵗʰ M24.61 Ankylosis, shoulder

M24.611 Ankylosis, right shoulder

M24.612 Ankylosis, left shoulder

M24.619 Ankylosis, unspecified shoulder

6ᵗʰ M24.62 Ankylosis, elbow

M24.621 Ankylosis, right elbow

M24.622 Ankylosis, left elbow

M24.629 Ankylosis, unspecified elbow

6ᵗʰ M24.63 Ankylosis, wrist

M24.631 Ankylosis, right wrist

M24.632 Ankylosis, left wrist

M24.639 Ankylosis, unspecified wrist

6ᵗʰ M24.64 Ankylosis, hand

M24.641 Ankylosis, right hand

M24.642 Ankylosis, left hand

M24.649 Ankylosis, unspecified hand

PDXn Unacceptable principal diagnosis symbol per Medicare code edits PDX Code exempt from diagnosis present on admission requirement

? Questionable admission cc Complication or comorbidity MCC Major complication or comorbidity CC/MCC CC/MCC exclusion

HCC HCC diagnosis code RxHCC RxHCC diagnosis code MACRA MACRA code **DEFINITION** Describes condition/terminology

TIP Coding guidance 👁 Official Guideline Reference Z Z code as first-listed diagnosis

802

When symbols appear on a code that requires a 7th character extension, refer to Appendix B to identify applicable 7th character codes.

2020 ICD-10-CM

[6th] M24.65 Ankylosis, hip
M24.651 Ankylosis, right hip
M24.652 Ankylosis, left hip
M24.659 Ankylosis, unspecified hip
[6th] M24.66 Ankylosis, knee
M24.661 Ankylosis, right knee
M24.662 Ankylosis, left knee
M24.669 Ankylosis, unspecified knee
[6th] M24.67 Ankylosis, ankle and foot
M24.671 Ankylosis, right ankle
M24.672 Ankylosis, left ankle
M24.673 Ankylosis, unspecified ankle
M24.674 Ankylosis, right foot
M24.675 Ankylosis, left foot
M24.676 Ankylosis, unspecified foot
M24.7 Protrusio acetabuli
[5th] M24.8 Other specific joint derangements, not elsewhere classified
EXCLUDES2 *iliotibial band syndrome (M76.3)*
M24.80 Other specific joint derangements of unspecified joint, not elsewhere classified
[6th] M24.81 Other specific joint derangements of shoulder, not elsewhere classified
M24.811 Other specific joint derangements of right shoulder, not elsewhere classified
M24.812 Other specific joint derangements of left shoulder, not elsewhere classified
M24.819 Other specific joint derangements of unspecified shoulder, not elsewhere classified
[6th] M24.82 Other specific joint derangements of elbow, not elsewhere classified
M24.821 Other specific joint derangements of right elbow, not elsewhere classified
M24.822 Other specific joint derangements of left elbow, not elsewhere classified
M24.829 Other specific joint derangements of unspecified elbow, not elsewhere classified
[6th] M24.83 Other specific joint derangements of wrist, not elsewhere classified
M24.831 Other specific joint derangements of right wrist, not elsewhere classified
M24.832 Other specific joint derangements of left wrist, not elsewhere classified
M24.839 Other specific joint derangements of unspecified wrist, not elsewhere classified
[6th] M24.84 Other specific joint derangements of hand, not elsewhere classified
M24.841 Other specific joint derangements of right hand, not elsewhere classified
M24.842 Other specific joint derangements of left hand, not elsewhere classified
M24.849 Other specific joint derangements of unspecified hand, not elsewhere classified
[6th] M24.85 Other specific joint derangements of hip, not elsewhere classified
Irritable hip
M24.851 Other specific joint derangements of right hip, not elsewhere classified
M24.852 Other specific joint derangements of left hip, not elsewhere classified
M24.859 Other specific joint derangements of unspecified hip, not elsewhere classified
[6th] M24.87 Other specific joint derangements of ankle and foot, not elsewhere classified
M24.871 Other specific joint derangements of right ankle, not elsewhere classified
M24.872 Other specific joint derangements of left ankle, not elsewhere classified
M24.873 Other specific joint derangements of unspecified ankle, not elsewhere classified
M24.874 Other specific joint derangements of right foot, not elsewhere classified
M24.875 Other specific joint derangements left foot, not elsewhere classified
M24.876 Other specific joint derangements of unspecified foot, not elsewhere classified
M24.9 Joint derangement, unspecified
[4th] M25 Other joint disorder, not elsewhere classified
EXCLUDES2 *abnormality of gait and mobility (R26.-)*
acquired deformities of limb (M20-M21)
calcification of bursa (M71.4-)
calcification of shoulder (joint) (M75.3)
calcification of tendon (M65.2-)
difficulty in walking (R26.2)
temporomandibular joint disorder (M26.6-)
[5th] M25.0 Hemarthrosis
EXCLUDES1 *current injury - see injury of joint by body region*
hemophilic arthropathy (M36.2)
M25.00 Hemarthrosis, unspecified joint CC CC/MCC Exc
[6th] M25.01 Hemarthrosis, shoulder
M25.011 Hemarthrosis, right shoulder CC CC/MCC Exc
M25.012 Hemarthrosis, left shoulder CC CC/MCC Exc
M25.019 Hemarthrosis, unspecified shoulder CC CC/MCC Exc
[6th] M25.02 Hemarthrosis, elbow
M25.021 Hemarthrosis, right elbow CC CC/MCC Exc
M25.022 Hemarthrosis, left elbow CC CC/MCC Exc
M25.029 Hemarthrosis, unspecified elbow CC CC/MCC Exc
[6th] M25.03 Hemarthrosis, wrist
M25.031 Hemarthrosis, right wrist CC CC/MCC Exc
M25.032 Hemarthrosis, left wrist CC CC/MCC Exc
M25.039 Hemarthrosis, unspecified wrist CC CC/MCC Exc
[6th] M25.04 Hemarthrosis, hand
M25.041 Hemarthrosis, right hand CC CC/MCC Exc
M25.042 Hemarthrosis, left hand CC CC/MCC Exc
M25.049 Hemarthrosis, unspecified hand CC CC/MCC Exc
[6th] M25.05 Hemarthrosis, hip
M25.051 Hemarthrosis, right hip CC CC/MCC Exc
M25.052 Hemarthrosis, left hip CC CC/MCC Exc
M25.059 Hemarthrosis, unspecified hip CC CC/MCC Exc
[6th] M25.06 Hemarthrosis, knee
M25.061 Hemarthrosis, right knee CC CC/MCC Exc
M25.062 Hemarthrosis, left knee CC CC/MCC Exc
M25.069 Hemarthrosis, unspecified knee CC CC/MCC Exc
[6th] M25.07 Hemarthrosis, ankle and foot
M25.071 Hemarthrosis, right ankle CC CC/MCC Exc
M25.072 Hemarthrosis, left ankle CC CC/MCC Exc
M25.073 Hemarthrosis, unspecified ankle CC CC/MCC Exc
M25.074 Hemarthrosis, right foot CC CC/MCC Exc
M25.075 Hemarthrosis, left foot CC CC/MCC Exc
M25.076 Hemarthrosis, unspecified foot CC CC/MCC Exc
M25.08 Hemarthrosis, other specified site CC CC/MCC Exc
Hemarthrosis, vertebrae
[5th] M25.1 Fistula of joint
M25.10 Fistula, unspecified joint
[6th] M25.11 Fistula, shoulder
M25.111 Fistula, right shoulder
M25.112 Fistula, left shoulder
M25.119 Fistula, unspecified shoulder
[6th] M25.12 Fistula, elbow
M25.121 Fistula, right elbow
M25.122 Fistula, left elbow
M25.129 Fistula, unspecified elbow
[6th] M25.13 Fistula, wrist
M25.131 Fistula, right wrist
M25.132 Fistula, left wrist
M25.139 Fistula, unspecified wrist

Unspecified Code | Other Specified Code | Manifestation Code | [N] Newborn | [P] Pediatric | [M] Maternity | [A] Adult | ♂ Male | ♀ Female
● New Code ▲ Revised Code Title ►◄ Revised Text NOTES INCLUDES EXCLUDES1 Not coded here EXCLUDES2 Not included here
[4th] 4th character required [5th] 5th character required [6th] 6th character required [7th] 7th character required [7th] Extension 'X' Alert
[HAC] Hospital-acquired condition (HAC) alert AHA AHA Coding Clinic© ☞ Code first alert

[6th] **M25.14 Fistula, hand**
M25.141 Fistula, right hand
M25.142 Fistula, left hand
M25.149 Fistula, unspecified hand
[6th] **M25.15 Fistula, hip**
M25.151 Fistula, right hip
M25.152 Fistula, left hip
M25.159 Fistula, unspecified hip
[6th] **M25.16 Fistula, knee**
M25.161 Fistula, right knee
M25.162 Fistula, left knee
M25.169 Fistula, unspecified knee
[6th] **M25.17 Fistula, ankle and foot**
M25.171 Fistula, right ankle
M25.172 Fistula, left ankle
M25.173 Fistula, unspecified ankle
M25.174 Fistula, right foot
M25.175 Fistula, left foot
M25.176 Fistula, unspecified foot
M25.18 Fistula, other specified site
Fistula, vertebrae

[5th] **M25.2 Flail joint**
DEFINITION: A flail joint has lost stability and results in loss of function of the joint.
M25.20 Flail joint, unspecified joint
[6th] **M25.21 Flail joint, shoulder**
M25.211 Flail joint, right shoulder
M25.212 Flail joint, left shoulder
M25.219 Flail joint, unspecified shoulder
[6th] **M25.22 Flail joint, elbow**
M25.221 Flail joint, right elbow
M25.222 Flail joint, left elbow
M25.229 Flail joint, unspecified elbow
[6th] **M25.23 Flail joint, wrist**
M25.231 Flail joint, right wrist
M25.232 Flail joint, left wrist
M25.239 Flail joint, unspecified wrist
[6th] **M25.24 Flail joint, hand**
M25.241 Flail joint, right hand
M25.242 Flail joint, left hand
M25.249 Flail joint, unspecified hand
[6th] **M25.25 Flail joint, hip**
M25.251 Flail joint, right hip
M25.252 Flail joint, left hip
M25.259 Flail joint, unspecified hip
[6th] **M25.26 Flail joint, knee**
M25.261 Flail joint, right knee
M25.262 Flail joint, left knee
M25.269 Flail joint, unspecified knee
[6th] **M25.27 Flail joint, ankle and foot**
M25.271 Flail joint, right ankle and foot
M25.272 Flail joint, left ankle and foot
M25.279 Flail joint, unspecified ankle and foot
M25.28 Flail joint, other site

[5th] **M25.3 Other instability of joint**
EXCLUDES1 *instability of joint secondary to old ligament injury (M24.2-)*
instability of joint secondary to removal of joint prosthesis (M96.8-)
EXCLUDES2 *spinal instabilities (M53.2-)*
M25.30 Other instability, unspecified joint
[6th] **M25.31 Other instability, shoulder**
M25.311 Other instability, right shoulder
M25.312 Other instability, left shoulder
M25.319 Other instability, unspecified shoulder
[6th] **M25.32 Other instability, elbow**
M25.321 Other instability, right elbow
M25.322 Other instability, left elbow
M25.329 Other instability, unspecified elbow
[6th] **M25.33 Other instability, wrist**
M25.331 Other instability, right wrist
M25.332 Other instability, left wrist
M25.339 Other instability, unspecified wrist
[6th] **M25.34 Other instability, hand**
M25.341 Other instability, right hand
M25.342 Other instability, left hand
M25.349 Other instability, unspecified hand
[6th] **M25.35 Other instability, hip**
M25.351 Other instability, right hip
M25.352 Other instability, left hip
M25.359 Other instability, unspecified hip
[6th] **M25.36 Other instability, knee**
M25.361 Other instability, right knee
M25.362 Other instability, left knee
M25.369 Other instability, unspecified knee
[6th] **M25.37 Other instability, ankle and foot**
M25.371 Other instability, right ankle
M25.372 Other instability, left ankle
M25.373 Other instability, unspecified ankle
M25.374 Other instability, right foot
M25.375 Other instability, left foot
M25.376 Other instability, unspecified foot

[5th] **M25.4 Effusion of joint**
EXCLUDES1 *hydrarthrosis in yaws (A66.6)*
intermittent hydrarthrosis (M12.4-)
other infective (teno)synovitis (M65.1-)
M25.40 Effusion, unspecified joint
[6th] **M25.41 Effusion, shoulder**
M25.411 Effusion, right shoulder
M25.412 Effusion, left shoulder
M25.419 Effusion, unspecified shoulder
[6th] **M25.42 Effusion, elbow**
M25.421 Effusion, right elbow
M25.422 Effusion, left elbow
M25.429 Effusion, unspecified elbow
[6th] **M25.43 Effusion, wrist**
M25.431 Effusion, right wrist
M25.432 Effusion, left wrist
M25.439 Effusion, unspecified wrist
[6th] **M25.44 Effusion, hand**
M25.441 Effusion, right hand
M25.442 Effusion, left hand
M25.449 Effusion, unspecified hand
[6th] **M25.45 Effusion, hip**
M25.451 Effusion, right hip
M25.452 Effusion, left hip
M25.459 Effusion, unspecified hip
[6th] **M25.46 Effusion, knee**
M25.461 Effusion, right knee
M25.462 Effusion, left knee
M25.469 Effusion, unspecified knee
[6th] **M25.47 Effusion, ankle and foot**
M25.471 Effusion, right ankle
M25.472 Effusion, left ankle
M25.473 Effusion, unspecified ankle
M25.474 Effusion, right foot
M25.475 Effusion, left foot
M25.476 Effusion, unspecified foot
M25.48 Effusion, other site

[5th] **M25.5 Pain in joint**
EXCLUDES2 *pain in hand (M79.64-)*
pain in fingers (M79.64-)
pain in foot (M79.67-)
pain in limb (M79.6-)
pain in toes (M79.67-)
M25.50 Pain in unspecified joint

Unacceptable principal diagnosis symbol per Medicare code edits · Code exempt from diagnosis present on admission requirement
Questionable admission · Complication or comorbidity · Major complication or comorbidity · CC/MCC exclusion
HCC diagnosis code · RxHCC diagnosis code · MACRA code · DEFINITION Describes condition/terminology
TIP Coding guidance · Official Guideline Reference · Z code as first-listed diagnosis

M25.51 Pain in shoulder
    M25.511 Pain in right shoulder
    M25.512 Pain in left shoulder
    M25.519 Pain in unspecified shoulder
M25.52 Pain in elbow
    M25.521 Pain in right elbow
    M25.522 Pain in left elbow
    M25.529 Pain in unspecified elbow
M25.53 Pain in wrist
    M25.531 Pain in right wrist
    M25.532 Pain in left wrist
    M25.539 Pain in unspecified wrist
M25.54 Pain in joints of hand
    M25.541 Pain in joints of right hand
        AHA: Q4 2016
    M25.542 Pain in joints of left hand
        AHA: Q4 2016
    M25.549 Pain in joints of unspecified hand
        AHA: Q4 2016
        Pain in joints of hand NOS
M25.55 Pain in hip
    M25.551 Pain in right hip
    M25.552 Pain in left hip
    M25.559 Pain in unspecified hip
M25.56 Pain in knee
    M25.561 Pain in right knee
    M25.562 Pain in left knee
    M25.569 Pain in unspecified knee
M25.57 Pain in ankle and joints of foot
    M25.571 Pain in right ankle and joints of right foot
    M25.572 Pain in left ankle and joints of left foot
    M25.579 Pain in unspecified ankle and joints of unspecified foot
M25.6 Stiffness of joint, not elsewhere classified
    EXCLUDES1 ankylosis of joint (M24.6-)
              contracture of joint (M24.5-)
    M25.60 Stiffness of unspecified joint, not elsewhere classified
    M25.61 Stiffness of shoulder, not elsewhere classified
        M25.611 Stiffness of right shoulder, not elsewhere classified
        M25.612 Stiffness of left shoulder, not elsewhere classified
        M25.619 Stiffness of unspecified shoulder, not elsewhere classified
    M25.62 Stiffness of elbow, not elsewhere classified
        M25.621 Stiffness of right elbow, not elsewhere classified
        M25.622 Stiffness of left elbow, not elsewhere classified
        M25.629 Stiffness of unspecified elbow, not elsewhere classified
    M25.63 Stiffness of wrist, not elsewhere classified
        M25.631 Stiffness of right wrist, not elsewhere classified
        M25.632 Stiffness of left wrist, not elsewhere classified
        M25.639 Stiffness of unspecified wrist, not elsewhere classified
    M25.64 Stiffness of hand, not elsewhere classified
        M25.641 Stiffness of right hand, not elsewhere classified
        M25.642 Stiffness of left hand, not elsewhere classified
        M25.649 Stiffness of unspecified hand, not elsewhere classified
    M25.65 Stiffness of hip, not elsewhere classified
        M25.651 Stiffness of right hip, not elsewhere classified
        M25.652 Stiffness of left hip, not elsewhere classified

M25.659 Stiffness of unspecified hip, not elsewhere classified
M25.66 Stiffness of knee, not elsewhere classified
    M25.661 Stiffness of right knee, not elsewhere classified
    M25.662 Stiffness of left knee, not elsewhere classified
    M25.669 Stiffness of unspecified knee, not elsewhere classified
M25.67 Stiffness of ankle and foot, not elsewhere classified
    M25.671 Stiffness of right ankle, not elsewhere classified
    M25.672 Stiffness of left ankle, not elsewhere classified
    M25.673 Stiffness of unspecified ankle, not elsewhere classified
    M25.674 Stiffness of right foot, not elsewhere classified
    M25.675 Stiffness of left foot, not elsewhere classified
    M25.676 Stiffness of unspecified foot, not elsewhere classified
M25.7 Osteophyte
    DEFINITION: Osteophyte is a bony outgrowth along a joint margin - also called a bone spur.
    M25.70 Osteophyte, unspecified joint
    M25.71 Osteophyte, shoulder
        M25.711 Osteophyte, right shoulder
        M25.712 Osteophyte, left shoulder
        M25.719 Osteophyte, unspecified shoulder
    M25.72 Osteophyte, elbow
        M25.721 Osteophyte, right elbow
        M25.722 Osteophyte, left elbow
        M25.729 Osteophyte, unspecified elbow
    M25.73 Osteophyte, wrist
        M25.731 Osteophyte, right wrist
        M25.732 Osteophyte, left wrist
        M25.739 Osteophyte, unspecified wrist
    M25.74 Osteophyte, hand
        M25.741 Osteophyte, right hand
        M25.742 Osteophyte, left hand
        M25.749 Osteophyte, unspecified hand
    M25.75 Osteophyte, hip
        M25.751 Osteophyte, right hip
        M25.752 Osteophyte, left hip
        M25.759 Osteophyte, unspecified hip
    M25.76 Osteophyte, knee
        M25.761 Osteophyte, right knee
        M25.762 Osteophyte, left knee
        M25.769 Osteophyte, unspecified knee
    M25.77 Osteophyte, ankle and foot
        M25.771 Osteophyte, right ankle
        M25.772 Osteophyte, left ankle
        M25.773 Osteophyte, unspecified ankle
        M25.774 Osteophyte, right foot
        M25.775 Osteophyte, left foot
        M25.776 Osteophyte, unspecified foot
    M25.78 Osteophyte, vertebrae
M25.8 Other specified joint disorders
    M25.80 Other specified joint disorders, unspecified joint
    M25.81 Other specified joint disorders, shoulder
        M25.811 Other specified joint disorders, right shoulder
        M25.812 Other specified joint disorders, left shoulder
        M25.819 Other specified joint disorders, unspecified shoulder
    M25.82 Other specified joint disorders, elbow
        M25.821 Other specified joint disorders, right elbow
        M25.822 Other specified joint disorders, left elbow
        M25.829 Other specified joint disorders, unspecified elbow

Unspecified Code   Other Specified Code   Manifestation Code N Newborn P Pediatric M Maternity A Adult ♂ Male ♀ Female
● New Code ▲ Revised Code Title ►◄ Revised Text NOTES INCLUDES EXCLUDES1 Not coded here EXCLUDES2 Not included here
4th character required 5th character required 6th character required 7th character required Extension 'X' Alert
HAC Hospital-acquired condition (HAC) alert AHA AHA Coding Clinic© 📣 Code first alert

2020 ICD-10-CM   When symbols appear on a code that requires a 7th character extension, refer to Appendix B to identify applicable 7th character codes.   **805**

[6th] M25.83 Other specified joint disorders, wrist
- M25.831 Other specified joint disorders, right wrist
- M25.832 Other specified joint disorders, left wrist
- M25.839 Other specified joint disorders, unspecified wrist

[6th] M25.84 Other specified joint disorders, hand
- M25.841 Other specified joint disorders, right hand
- M25.842 Other specified joint disorders, left hand
- M25.849 Other specified joint disorders, unspecified hand

[6th] M25.85 Other specified joint disorders, hip
- M25.851 Other specified joint disorders, right hip
- M25.852 Other specified joint disorders, left hip
- M25.859 Other specified joint disorders, unspecified hip

[6th] M25.86 Other specified joint disorders, knee
- M25.861 Other specified joint disorders, right knee
- M25.862 Other specified joint disorders, left knee
- M25.869 Other specified joint disorders, unspecified knee

[6th] M25.87 Other specified joint disorders, ankle and foot
- M25.871 Other specified joint disorders, right ankle and foot
- M25.872 Other specified joint disorders, left ankle and foot
- M25.879 Other specified joint disorders, unspecified ankle and foot

M25.9 Joint disorder, unspecified

Dentofacial anomalies [including malocclusion] and other disorders of jaw (M26-M27)

[EXCLUDES1] *hemifacial atrophy or hypertrophy (Q67.4)*
unilateral condylar hyperplasia or hypoplasia (M27.8)

[4th] **M26 Dentofacial anomalies [including malocclusion]**

[5th] **M26.0 Major anomalies of jaw size**

[EXCLUDES1] *acromegaly (E22.0)*
Robin's syndrome (Q87.0)

- M26.00 Unspecified anomaly of jaw size
- M26.01 Maxillary hyperplasia
- M26.02 Maxillary hypoplasia
- M26.03 Mandibular hyperplasia
- M26.04 Mandibular hypoplasia
- M26.05 Macrogenia
- M26.06 Microgenia
- M26.07 Excessive tuberosity of jaw
  - Entire maxillary tuberosity
- M26.09 Other specified anomalies of jaw size

[5th] **M26.1 Anomalies of jaw-cranial base relationship**
- M26.10 Unspecified anomaly of jaw-cranial base relationship
- M26.11 Maxillary asymmetry
- M26.12 Other jaw asymmetry
- M26.19 Other specified anomalies of jaw-cranial base relationship

[5th] **M26.2 Anomalies of dental arch relationship**
- M26.20 Unspecified anomaly of dental arch relationship

[6th] M26.21 Malocclusion, Angle's class
- M26.211 Malocclusion, Angle's class I
  - Neutro-occlusion
- M26.212 Malocclusion, Angle's class II
  - Disto-occlusion Division I
  - Disto-occlusion Division II
- M26.213 Malocclusion, Angle's class III
  - Mesio-occlusion
- M26.219 Malocclusion, Angle's class, unspecified

[6th] M26.22 Open occlusal relationship
- M26.220 Open anterior occlusal relationship
  - Anterior open bite
- M26.221 Open posterior occlusal relationship
  - Posterior open bite

- M26.23 Excessive horizontal overlap
  - Excessive horizontal overjet
- M26.24 Reverse articulation
  - Crossbite (anterior) (posterior)
- M26.25 Anomalies of interarch distance
- M26.29 Other anomalies of dental arch relationship
  - Midline deviation of dental arch
  - Overbite (excessive) deep
  - Overbite (excessive) horizontal
  - Overbite (excessive) vertical
  - Posterior lingual occlusion of mandibular teeth

[5th] **M26.3 Anomalies of tooth position of fully erupted tooth or teeth**

[EXCLUDES2] *embedded and impacted teeth (K01.-)*

- M26.30 Unspecified anomaly of tooth position of fully erupted tooth or teeth
  - Abnormal spacing of fully erupted tooth or teeth NOS
  - Displacement of fully erupted tooth or teeth NOS
  - Transposition of fully erupted tooth or teeth NOS
- M26.31 Crowding of fully erupted teeth
- M26.32 Excessive spacing of fully erupted teeth
  - Diastema of fully erupted tooth or teeth NOS
- M26.33 Horizontal displacement of fully erupted tooth or teeth
  - Tipped tooth or teeth
  - Tipping of fully erupted tooth
- M26.34 Vertical displacement of fully erupted tooth or teeth
  - Extruded tooth
  - Infraeruption of tooth or teeth
  - Supraeruption of tooth or teeth
- M26.35 Rotation of fully erupted tooth or teeth
- M26.36 Insufficient interocclusal distance of fully erupted teeth (ridge)
  - Lack of adequate intermaxillary vertical dimension of fully erupted teeth
- M26.37 Excessive interocclusal distance of fully erupted teeth
  - Excessive intermaxillary vertical dimension of fully erupted teeth
  - Loss of occlusal vertical dimension of fully erupted teeth
- M26.39 Other anomalies of tooth position of fully erupted tooth or teeth

M26.4 Malocclusion, unspecified

[5th] **M26.5 Dentofacial functional abnormalities**

[EXCLUDES1] *bruxism (F45.8)*
teeth-grinding NOS (F45.8)

- M26.50 Dentofacial functional abnormalities, unspecified
- M26.51 Abnormal jaw closure
- M26.52 Limited mandibular range of motion
- M26.53 Deviation in opening and closing of the mandible
- M26.54 Insufficient anterior guidance
  - Insufficient anterior occlusal guidance
- M26.55 Centric occlusion maximum intercuspation discrepancy
  - [EXCLUDES1] *centric occlusion NOS (M26.59)*
- M26.56 Non-working side interference
  - Balancing side interference
- M26.57 Lack of posterior occlusal support
- M26.59 Other dentofacial functional abnormalities
  - Centric occlusion (of teeth) NOS
  - Malocclusion due to abnormal swallowing
  - Malocclusion due to mouth breathing
  - Malocclusion due to tongue, lip or finger habits

[5th] **M26.6 Temporomandibular joint disorders**

[EXCLUDES2] *current temporomandibular joint dislocation (S03.0)*
current temporomandibular joint sprain (S03.4)

[6th] M26.60 Temporomandibular joint disorder, unspecified
- M26.601 Right temporomandibular joint disorder, unspecified
- M26.602 Left temporomandibular joint disorder, unspecified

[PDx] Unacceptable principal diagnosis symbol per Medicare code edits [POA] Code exempt from diagnosis present on admission requirement
[?] Questionable admission [CC] Complication or comorbidity [MCC] Major complication or comorbidity [CC/MCC Exc] CC/MCC exclusion
[HCC] HCC diagnosis code [RxHCC] RxHCC diagnosis code MACRA code **DEFINITION** Describes condition/terminology
TIP Coding guidance 👁 Official Guideline Reference [Z1] Z code as first-listed diagnosis

When symbols appear on a code that requires a 7th character extension, refer to Appendix B to identify applicable 7th character codes.

M26.603 Bilateral temporomandibular joint disorder, unspecified

M26.609 Unspecified temporomandibular joint disorder, unspecified side

Temporomandibular joint disorder NOS

6ᵗʰ M26.61 Adhesions and ankylosis of temporomandibular joint

M26.611 Adhesions and ankylosis of right temporomandibular joint

M26.612 Adhesions and ankylosis of left temporomandibular joint

M26.613 Adhesions and ankylosis of bilateral temporomandibular joint

M26.619 Adhesions and ankylosis of temporomandibular joint, unspecified side

6ᵗʰ M26.62 Arthralgia of temporomandibular joint

M26.621 Arthralgia of right temporomandibular joint

M26.622 Arthralgia of left temporomandibular joint

M26.623 Arthralgia of bilateral temporomandibular joint

M26.629 Arthralgia of temporomandibular joint, unspecified side

6ᵗʰ M26.63 Articular disc disorder of temporomandibular joint

M26.631 Articular disc disorder of right temporomandibular joint

M26.632 Articular disc disorder of left temporomandibular joint

M26.633 Articular disc disorder of bilateral temporomandibular joint

M26.639 Articular disc disorder of temporomandibular joint, unspecified side

M26.69 Other specified disorders of temporomandibular joint

5ᵗʰ M26.7 Dental alveolar anomalies

M26.70 Unspecified alveolar anomaly

M26.71 Alveolar maxillary hyperplasia

M26.72 Alveolar mandibular hyperplasia

M26.73 Alveolar maxillary hypoplasia

M26.74 Alveolar mandibular hypoplasia

M26.79 Other specified alveolar anomalies

5ᵗʰ M26.8 Other dentofacial anomalies

M26.81 Anterior soft tissue impingement

Anterior soft tissue impingement on teeth

M26.82 Posterior soft tissue impingement

Posterior soft tissue impingement on teeth

M26.89 Other dentofacial anomalies

M26.9 Dentofacial anomaly, unspecified

4ᵗʰ M27 Other diseases of jaws

M27.0 Developmental disorders of jaws

Latent bone cyst of jaw
Stafne's cyst
Torus mandibularis
Torus palatinus

M27.1 Giant cell granuloma, central

Giant cell granuloma NOS

EXCLUDES1 peripheral giant cell granuloma (K06.8)

M27.2 Inflammatory conditions of jaws

Osteitis of jaw(s)
Osteomyelitis (neonatal) jaw(s)
Osteoradionecrosis jaw(s)
Periostitis jaw(s)
Sequestrum of jaw bone
Use additional code (W88-W90, X39.0) to identify radiation, if radiation-induced

EXCLUDES2 osteonecrosis of jaw due to drug (M87.180)

M27.3 Alveolitis of jaws

Alveolar osteitis
Dry socket

5ᵗʰ M27.4 Other and unspecified cysts of jaw

EXCLUDES1 cysts of oral region (K09.-)
latent bone cyst of jaw (M27.0)
Stafne's cyst (M27.0)

M27.40 Unspecified cyst of jaw

Cyst of jaw NOS

M27.49 Other cysts of jaw

Aneurysmal cyst of jaw
Hemorrhagic cyst of jaw
Traumatic cyst of jaw

5ᵗʰ M27.5 Periradicular pathology associated with previous endodontic treatment

M27.51 Perforation of root canal space due to endodontic treatment

M27.52 Endodontic overfill

M27.53 Endodontic underfill

M27.59 Other periradicular pathology associated with previous endodontic treatment

5ᵗʰ M27.6 Endosseous dental implant failure

M27.61 Osseointegration failure of dental implant

Hemorrhagic complications of dental implant placement
Iatrogenic osseointegration failure of dental implant
Osseointegration failure of dental implant due to complications of systemic disease
Osseointegration failure of dental implant due to poor bone quality
Pre-integration failure of dental implant NOS
Pre-osseointegration failure of dental implant

M27.62 Post-osseointegration biological failure of dental implant

Failure of dental implant due to lack of attached gingiva
Failure of dental implant due to occlusal trauma (caused by poor prosthetic design)
Failure of dental implant due to parafunctional habits
Failure of dental implant due to periodontal infection (peri-implantitis)
Failure of dental implant due to poor oral hygiene
Iatrogenic post-osseointegration failure of dental implant
Post-osseointegration failure of dental implant due to complications of systemic disease

M27.63 Post-osseointegration mechanical failure of dental implant

Failure of dental prosthesis causing loss of dental implant
Fracture of dental implant

EXCLUDES2 cracked tooth (K03.81)
fractured dental restorative material with loss of material (K08.531)
fractured dental restorative material without loss of material (K08.530)
fractured tooth (S02.5)

M27.69 Other endosseous dental implant failure

Dental implant failure NOS

M27.8 Other specified diseases of jaws

Cherubism
Exostosis
Fibrous dysplasia
Unilateral condylar hyperplasia
Unilateral condylar hypoplasia

EXCLUDES1 jaw pain (R68.84)

M27.9 Disease of jaws, unspecified

Unspecified Code   Other Specified Code   Manifestation Code   🅽 Newborn   🅿 Pediatric   🅼 Maternity   🅰 Adult   ♂ Male   ♀ Female
● New Code   ▲ Revised Code Title   ►◄ Revised Text   **NOTES**   *INCLUDES*   EXCLUDES1 Not coded here   EXCLUDES2 Not included here
4ᵗʰ 4ᵗʰ character required   5ᵗʰ 5ᵗʰ character required   6ᵗʰ 6ᵗʰ character required   7ᵗʰ 7ᵗʰ character required   7ˣ Extension 'X' Alert
HAC Hospital-acquired condition (HAC) alert   **AHA** AHA Coding Clinic®   📌 Code first alert

M26.603 - M27.9

CHAPTER 13: DISEASES OF THE MUSCULOSKELETAL SYSTEM AND CONNECTIVE TISSUE (M00-M99)

Systemic connective tissue disorders (M30-M36)

INCLUDES   autoimmune disease NOS
            collagen (vascular) disease NOS
            systemic autoimmune disease
            systemic collagen (vascular) disease

EXCLUDES1   autoimmune disease, single organ or single cell-type -code to
            relevant condition category

4ᵗʰ M30 **Polyarteritis nodosa and related conditions**

EXCLUDES1   microscopic polyarteritis (M31.7)

M30.0 **Polyarteritis nodosa**

M30.1 **Polyarteritis with lung involvement [Churg-Strauss]**

Allergic granulomatous angiitis

M30.2 **Juvenile polyarteritis**

M30.3 **Mucocutaneous lymph node syndrome [Kawasaki]**

M30.8 **Other conditions related to polyarteritis nodosa**

Polyangiitis overlap syndrome

4ᵗʰ M31 **Other necrotizing vasculopathies**

M31.0 **Hypersensitivity angiitis**

Goodpasture's syndrome

M31.1 **Thrombotic microangiopathy**

Thrombotic thrombocytopenic purpura

M31.2 **Lethal midline granuloma**

5ᵗʰ M31.3 **Wegener's granulomatosis**

Necrotizing respiratory granulomatosis

M31.30 **Wegener's granulomatosis** without renal involvement

Wegener's granulomatosis NOS

M31.31 **Wegener's granulomatosis** with renal involvement

M31.4 **Aortic arch syndrome [Takayasu]**

M31.5 **Giant cell arteritis with polymyalgia rheumatica**

M31.6 **Other giant cell arteritis**

M31.7 **Microscopic polyangiitis**

Microscopic polyarteritis

EXCLUDES1   polyarteritis nodosa (M30.0)

M31.8 **Other specified necrotizing vasculopathies**

Hypocomplementemic vasculitis
Septic vasculitis

M31.9 **Necrotizing vasculopathy, unspecified**

4ᵗʰ M32 **Systemic lupus erythematosus (SLE)**

EXCLUDES1   lupus erythematosus (discoid) (NOS) (L93.0)

M32.0 **Drug-induced systemic lupus erythematosus**

Use **additional** code for adverse effect, if applicable, to identify drug (T36-T50 with fifth or sixth character 5)

5ᵗʰ M32.1 Systemic **lupus erythematosus** with organ or system involvement

M32.10 **Systemic lupus erythematosus, organ or system involvement unspecified**

M32.11 Endocarditis **in systemic lupus erythematosus**

Libman-Sacks disease

M32.12 Pericarditis **in systemic lupus erythematosus**

Lupus pericarditis

M32.13 Lung involvement **in systemic lupus erythematosus**

Pleural effusion due to systemic lupus erythematosus

M32.14 Glomerular disease **in systemic lupus erythematosus**

AHA: Q4 2013

Lupus renal disease NOS

M32.15 Tubulo-interstitial nephropathy **in systemic lupus erythematosus**

M32.19 Other organ or system **involvement in systemic lupus erythematosus**

M32.8 Other forms **of systemic lupus erythematosus**

M32.9 **Systemic lupus erythematosus, unspecified**

AHA: Q3 2018

SLE NOS
Systemic lupus erythematosus NOS
Systemic lupus erythematosus without organ involvement

4ᵗʰ M33 **Dermatopolymyositis**

5ᵗʰ M33.0 Juvenile dermatomyositis

M33.00 **Juvenile dermatomyositis, organ involvement unspecified**

M33.01 **Juvenile dermatomyositis** with respiratory involvement

M33.02 **Juvenile dermatomyositis** with myopathy

M33.03 **Juvenile dermatomyositis** without myopathy

M33.09 **Juvenile dermatomyositis** with other organ involvement

5ᵗʰ M33.1 Other dermatomyositis

Adult dermatomyositis

M33.10 **Other dermatomyositis, organ involvement unspecified**

M33.11 **Other dermatomyositis** with respiratory involvement

M33.12 **Other dermatomyositis** with myopathy

M33.13 **Other dermatomyositis** without myopathy

Dermatomyositis NOS

M33.19 **Other dermatomyositis** with other organ involvement

5ᵗʰ M33.2 Polymyositis

M33.20 **Polymyositis, organ involvement unspecified**

M33.21 **Polymyositis** with respiratory involvement

M33.22 **Polymyositis** with myopathy

M33.29 **Polymyositis** with other organ involvement

5ᵗʰ M33.9 Dermatopolymyositis, unspecified

M33.90 **Dermatopolymyositis, unspecified, organ involvement unspecified**

M33.91 **Dermatopolymyositis, unspecified** with respiratory involvement

M33.92 **Dermatopolymyositis, unspecified** with myopathy

M33.93 **Dermatopolymyositis, unspecified** without myopathy

M33.99 **Dermatopolymyositis, unspecified** with other organ involvement

4ᵗʰ M34 **Systemic sclerosis [scleroderma]**

EXCLUDES1   circumscribed scleroderma (L94.0)
            neonatal scleroderma ▶(P83.88)◀

M34.0 Progressive **systemic sclerosis**

M34.1 CR(E)ST **syndrome**

Combination of calcinosis, Raynaud's phenomenon, esophageal dysfunction, sclerodactyly, telangiectasia

M34.2 **Systemic sclerosis** induced by drug and chemical

☛ **Code first** poisoning due to drug or toxin, if applicable (T36-T65 with fifth or sixth character 1-4 or 6)

Use **additional** code for adverse effect, if applicable, to identify drug (T36-T50 with fifth or sixth character 5)

5ᵗʰ M34.8 Other forms **of systemic sclerosis**

M34.81 **Systemic sclerosis** with lung involvement

M34.82 **Systemic sclerosis** with myopathy

M34.83 **Systemic sclerosis** with polyneuropathy

M34.89 Other **systemic sclerosis**

M34.9 **Systemic sclerosis, unspecified**

4ᵗʰ M35 **Other systemic involvement of connective tissue**

EXCLUDES1   reactive perforating collagenosis (L87.1)

Unacceptable principal diagnosis symbol per Medicare code edits   Code exempt from diagnosis present on admission requirement   ❓ Questionable admission   ℅ Complication or comorbidity   MCC Major complication or comorbidity   CC/MCC Exc CC/MCC exclusion   HCC HCC diagnosis code   RxHCC RxHCC diagnosis code   MACRA code   **DEFINITION** Describes condition/terminology   **TIP** Coding guidance   👁 Official Guideline Reference   ▥ Z code as first-listed diagnosis

808   When symbols appear on a code that requires a 7th character extension, refer to Appendix B to identify applicable 7th character codes.   **2020 ICD-10-CM**

[5th] **M35.0 Sicca syndrome [Sjögren]**

DEFINITION: Sicca syndrome is an autoimmune disease affecting connective tissues, most commonly rheumatoid arthritis.

M35.00 Sicca syndrome, unspecified [HCC] [RxHCC]

M35.01 Sicca syndrome with keratoconjunctivitis [HCC] [RxHCC]

M35.02 Sicca syndrome with lung involvement [HCC] [RxHCC]

M35.03 Sicca syndrome with myopathy [CC] [HCC] [RxHCC] [CC/MCC Exc]

M35.04 Sicca syndrome with tubulo-interstitial nephropathy [HCC] [RxHCC]

Renal tubular acidosis in sicca syndrome

M35.09 Sicca syndrome with other organ involvement [HCC] [RxHCC]

M35.1 Other overlap syndromes [CC] [HCC] [RxHCC] [CC/MCC Exc]

Mixed connective tissue disease

[EXCLUDES1] *polyangiitis overlap syndrome (M30.8)*

M35.2 Behçet's disease [CC] [HCC] [RxHCC] [CC/MCC Exc]

M35.3 Polymyalgia rheumatica [HCC]

[EXCLUDES1] *polymyalgia rheumatica with giant cell arteritis (M31.5)*

M35.4 Diffuse (eosinophilic) fasciitis

M35.5 Multifocal fibrosclerosis [CC] [HCC] [RxHCC] [CC/MCC Exc]

M35.6 Relapsing panniculitis [Weber-Christian]

[EXCLUDES1] *lupus panniculitis (L93.2)*
panniculitis NOS (M79.3-)

M35.7 Hypermobility syndrome

Familial ligamentous laxity

[EXCLUDES1] *Ehlers-Danlos syndrome ▶(Q79.6-)◀*
ligamentous laxity, NOS (M24.2-)

M35.8 Other specified systemic involvement of connective tissue [CC] [HCC] [RxHCC] [CC/MCC Exc]

M35.9 Systemic involvement of connective tissue, unspecified [HCC] [RxHCC]

Autoimmune disease (systemic) NOS
Collagen (vascular) disease NOS

[4th] **M36 Systemic disorders of connective tissue in diseases classified elsewhere**

[EXCLUDES2] *arthropathies in diseases classified elsewhere (M14.-)*

M36.0 Dermato(poly)myositis in neoplastic disease [CC] [HCC] [RxHCC] [CC/MCC Exc]

☞ **Code first** underlying neoplasm (C00-D49)

M36.1 Arthropathy in neoplastic disease

☞ **Code first** underlying neoplasm, such as:
leukemia (C91-C95)
malignant histiocytosis (C96.A)
multiple myeloma (C90.0)

M36.2 Hemophilic arthropathy

Hemarthrosis in hemophilic arthropathy

☞ **Code first** underlying disease, such as:
factor VIII deficiency (D66)
with vascular defect (D68.0)
factor IX deficiency (D67)
hemophilia (classical) (D66)
hemophilia B (D67)
hemophilia C (D68.1)

M36.3 Arthropathy in other blood disorders

M36.4 Arthropathy in hypersensitivity reactions classified elsewhere

☞ **Code first** underlying disease, such as:
Henoch (-Schönlein) purpura (D69.0)
serum sickness (T80.6-)

M36.8 Systemic disorders of connective tissue in other diseases classified elsewhere [HCC] [RxHCC]

☞ **Code first** underlying disease, such as:
alkaptonuria (E70.2)
hypogammaglobulinemia (D80.-)
ochronosis (E70.2)

Dorsopathies (M40-M54)

Deforming dorsopathies (M40-M43)

[4th] **M40 Kyphosis and lordosis**

DEFINITION: (1) Kyphosis is an abnormal curvature of the spine that causes a bowing or rounding of the back. It creates a hunchback appearance in the patient. (2) Lordosis is an inward curvature of the lumbar region of the spine. It is also known as swayback.

[EXCLUDES1] *congenital kyphosis and lordosis (Q76.4)*
kyphoscoliosis (M41.-)
postprocedural kyphosis and lordosis (M96.-)

[5th] **M40.0 Postural kyphosis**

[EXCLUDES1] *osteochondrosis of spine (M42.-)*

M40.00 Postural kyphosis, site unspecified
M40.03 Postural kyphosis, cervicothoracic region
M40.04 Postural kyphosis, thoracic region
M40.05 Postural kyphosis, thoracolumbar region

[5th] **M40.1 Other secondary kyphosis**

M40.10 Other secondary kyphosis, site unspecified
M40.12 Other secondary kyphosis, cervical region
M40.13 Other secondary kyphosis, cervicothoracic region
M40.14 Other secondary kyphosis, thoracic region
M40.15 Other secondary kyphosis, thoracolumbar region

[5th] **M40.2 Other and unspecified kyphosis**

[6th] **M40.20 Unspecified kyphosis**

M40.202 Unspecified kyphosis, cervical region
M40.203 Unspecified kyphosis, cervicothoracic region
M40.204 Unspecified kyphosis, thoracic region
M40.205 Unspecified kyphosis, thoracolumbar region
M40.209 Unspecified kyphosis, site unspecified

[6th] **M40.29 Other kyphosis**

M40.292 Other kyphosis, cervical region
M40.293 Other kyphosis, cervicothoracic region
M40.294 Other kyphosis, thoracic region
M40.295 Other kyphosis, thoracolumbar region
M40.299 Other kyphosis, site unspecified

[5th] **M40.3 Flatback syndrome**

M40.30 Flatback syndrome, site unspecified
M40.35 Flatback syndrome, thoracolumbar region
M40.36 Flatback syndrome, lumbar region
M40.37 Flatback syndrome, lumbosacral region

[5th] **M40.4 Postural lordosis**

Acquired lordosis

M40.40 Postural lordosis, site unspecified
M40.45 Postural lordosis, thoracolumbar region
M40.46 Postural lordosis, lumbar region
M40.47 Postural lordosis, lumbosacral region

[5th] **M40.5 Lordosis, unspecified**

M40.50 Lordosis, unspecified, site unspecified
M40.55 Lordosis, unspecified, thoracolumbar region
M40.56 Lordosis, unspecified, lumbar region
M40.57 Lordosis, unspecified, lumbosacral region

[4th] **M41 Scoliosis**

DEFINITION: Scoliosis is a lateral curvature of the spinal column. It can be both primary and secondary meaning a single curve or a curve with a second, compensating curve further down the spinal column.

[INCLUDES] *kyphoscoliosis*

[EXCLUDES1] *congenital scoliosis NOS (Q67.5)*
congenital scoliosis due to bony malformation (Q76.3)
postural congenital scoliosis (Q67.5)
kyphoscoliotic heart disease (I27.1)
postprocedural scoliosis (M96.-)

Unspecified Code Other Specified Code Manifestation Code [N] Newborn [P] Pediatric [M] Maternity [A] Adult ♂ Male ♀ Female
● New Code ▲ Revised Code Title ▶◀ Revised Text [NOTES] [INCLUDES] [EXCLUDES1] Not coded here [EXCLUDES2] Not included here
[4th] 4th character required [5th] 5th character required [6th] 6th character required [7th] 7th character required [X] Extension 'X' Alert
[HAC] Hospital-acquired condition (HAC) alert AHA AHA Coding Clinic© ☞ Code first alert

⑤ **M41.0** Infantile idiopathic scoliosis
    M41.00 Infantile idiopathic scoliosis, site unspecified
    M41.02 Infantile idiopathic scoliosis, cervical region
    M41.03 Infantile idiopathic scoliosis, cervicothoracic region
    M41.04 Infantile idiopathic scoliosis, thoracic region
    M41.05 Infantile idiopathic scoliosis, thoracolumbar region
    M41.06 Infantile idiopathic scoliosis, lumbar region
    M41.07 Infantile idiopathic scoliosis, lumbosacral region
    M41.08 Infantile idiopathic scoliosis, sacral and sacrococcygeal region

⑤ **M41.1** Juvenile and adolescent idiopathic scoliosis
  ⑥ **M41.11** Juvenile idiopathic scoliosis
    M41.112 Juvenile idiopathic scoliosis, cervical region
    M41.113 Juvenile idiopathic scoliosis, cervicothoracic region
    M41.114 Juvenile idiopathic scoliosis, thoracic region
    M41.115 Juvenile idiopathic scoliosis, thoracolumbar region
    M41.116 Juvenile idiopathic scoliosis, lumbar region
    M41.117 Juvenile idiopathic scoliosis, lumbosacral region
    M41.119 Juvenile idiopathic scoliosis, site unspecified
  ⑥ **M41.12** Adolescent scoliosis
    M41.122 Adolescent idiopathic scoliosis, cervical region
    M41.123 Adolescent idiopathic scoliosis, cervicothoracic region
    M41.124 Adolescent idiopathic scoliosis, thoracic region
    M41.125 Adolescent idiopathic scoliosis, thoracolumbar region
    M41.126 Adolescent idiopathic scoliosis, lumbar region
    M41.127 Adolescent idiopathic scoliosis, lumbosacral region
    M41.129 Adolescent idiopathic scoliosis, site unspecified

⑤ **M41.2** Other idiopathic scoliosis
    M41.20 Other idiopathic scoliosis, site unspecified
    M41.22 Other idiopathic scoliosis, cervical region
    M41.23 Other idiopathic scoliosis, cervicothoracic region
    M41.24 Other idiopathic scoliosis, thoracic region
    M41.25 Other idiopathic scoliosis, thoracolumbar region
    M41.26 Other idiopathic scoliosis, lumbar region
    M41.27 Other idiopathic scoliosis, lumbosacral region

⑤ **M41.3** Thoracogenic scoliosis
    M41.30 Thoracogenic scoliosis, site unspecified
    M41.34 Thoracogenic scoliosis, thoracic region
    M41.35 Thoracogenic scoliosis, thoracolumbar region

⑤ **M41.4** Neuromuscular scoliosis
  Scoliosis secondary to cerebral palsy, Friedreich's ataxia, poliomyelitis and other neuromuscular disorders
  Code also underlying condition
    M41.40 Neuromuscular scoliosis, site unspecified
    M41.41 Neuromuscular scoliosis, occipito-atlanto-axial region
    M41.42 Neuromuscular scoliosis, cervical region
    M41.43 Neuromuscular scoliosis, cervicothoracic region
    M41.44 Neuromuscular scoliosis, thoracic region
    M41.45 Neuromuscular scoliosis, thoracolumbar region
    M41.46 Neuromuscular scoliosis, lumbar region
    M41.47 Neuromuscular scoliosis, lumbosacral region

⑤ **M41.5** Other secondary scoliosis
    M41.50 Other secondary scoliosis, site unspecified
    M41.52 Other secondary scoliosis, cervical region
    M41.53 Other secondary scoliosis, cervicothoracic region
    M41.54 Other secondary scoliosis, thoracic region

    M41.55 Other secondary scoliosis, thoracolumbar region
    M41.56 Other secondary scoliosis, lumbar region
    M41.57 Other secondary scoliosis, lumbosacral region

⑤ **M41.8** Other forms of scoliosis
    M41.80 Other forms of scoliosis, site unspecified
    M41.82 Other forms of scoliosis, cervical region
    M41.83 Other forms of scoliosis, cervicothoracic region
    M41.84 Other forms of scoliosis, thoracic region
    M41.85 Other forms of scoliosis, thoracolumbar region
    M41.86 Other forms of scoliosis, lumbar region
    M41.87 Other forms of scoliosis, lumbosacral region

  M41.9 Scoliosis, unspecified

④ **M42** Spinal osteochondrosis
  ⑤ **M42.0** Juvenile osteochondrosis of spine
    Calvé's disease
    Scheuermann's disease
    EXCLUDES1 postural kyphosis (M40.0)
    M42.00 Juvenile osteochondrosis of spine, site unspecified
    M42.01 Juvenile osteochondrosis of spine, occipito-atlanto-axial region
    M42.02 Juvenile osteochondrosis of spine, cervical region
    M42.03 Juvenile osteochondrosis of spine, cervicothoracic region
    M42.04 Juvenile osteochondrosis of spine, thoracic region
    M42.05 Juvenile osteochondrosis of spine, thoracolumbar region
    M42.06 Juvenile osteochondrosis of spine, lumbar region
    M42.07 Juvenile osteochondrosis of spine, lumbosacral region
    M42.08 Juvenile osteochondrosis of spine, sacral and sacrococcygeal region
    M42.09 Juvenile osteochondrosis of spine, multiple sites in spine

  ⑤ **M42.1** Adult osteochondrosis of spine
    M42.10 Adult osteochondrosis of spine, site unspecified Ⓐ
    M42.11 Adult osteochondrosis of spine, occipito-atlanto-axial region Ⓐ
    M42.12 Adult osteochondrosis of spine, cervical region Ⓐ
    M42.13 Adult osteochondrosis of spine, cervicothoracic region Ⓐ
    M42.14 Adult osteochondrosis of spine, thoracic region Ⓐ
    M42.15 Adult osteochondrosis of spine, thoracolumbar region Ⓐ
    M42.16 Adult osteochondrosis of spine, lumbar region Ⓐ
    M42.17 Adult osteochondrosis of spine, lumbosacral region Ⓐ
    M42.18 Adult osteochondrosis of spine, sacral and sacrococcygeal region Ⓐ
    M42.19 Adult osteochondrosis of spine, multiple sites in spine Ⓐ

  M42.9 Spinal osteochondrosis, unspecified

④ **M43** Other deforming dorsopathies
  EXCLUDES1 congenital spondylolysis and spondylolisthesis (Q76.2)
    hemivertebra (Q76.3-Q76.4)
    Klippel-Feil syndrome (Q76.1)
    lumbarization and sacralization (Q76.4)
    platyspondylisis (Q76.4)
    spina bifida occulta (Q76.0)
    spinal curvature in osteoporosis (M80.-)
    spinal curvature in Paget's disease of bone [osteitis deformans] (M88.-)
  ⑤ **M43.0** Spondylolysis
    TIP: Spondylosis and spondylolisthesis cause low back pain. Spondylosis is a stress fracture or crack in the vertebrae. When the bone is weakened from the crack or fracture and slips out of place the condition is called spondylolisthesis.
    EXCLUDES1 congenital spondylolysis (Q76.2)
      spondylolisthesis (M43.1)

ᴾᴰˣ Unacceptable principal diagnosis symbol per Medicare code edits   ᴾᴼᴬ Code exempt from diagnosis present on admission requirement
❓ Questionable admission   ᶜᶜ Complication or comorbidity   ᴹᶜᶜ Major complication or comorbidity   ᶜᶜ/ᴹᶜᶜ ᴱˣᶜ CC/MCC exclusion
ᴴᶜᶜ HCC diagnosis code   ᴿˣᴴᶜᶜ RxHCC diagnosis code   MACRA code   **DEFINITION** Describes condition/terminology
TIP Coding guidance   ◉ Official Guideline Reference   Ⓩ¹ Z code as first-listed diagnosis

810   When symbols appear on a code that requires a 7th character extension, refer to Appendix B to identify applicable 7th character codes.   **2020 ICD-10-CM**

M43.00 Spondylolysis, site unspecified
M43.01 Spondylolysis, occipito-atlanto-axial region
M43.02 Spondylolysis, cervical region
M43.03 Spondylolysis, cervicothoracic region
M43.04 Spondylolysis, thoracic region
M43.05 Spondylolysis, thoracolumbar region
M43.06 Spondylolysis, lumbar region
M43.07 Spondylolysis, lumbosacral region
M43.08 Spondylolysis, sacral and sacrococcygeal region
M43.09 Spondylolysis, multiple sites in spine

5ᵗʰ M43.1 Spondylolisthesis
EXCLUDES1 acute traumatic of lumbosacral region (S33.1)
acute traumatic of sites other than lumbosacral-code to Fracture, vertebra, by region
congenital spondylolisthesis (Q76.2)
M43.10 Spondylolisthesis, site unspecified
M43.11 Spondylolisthesis, occipito-atlanto-axial region
M43.12 Spondylolisthesis, cervical region
M43.13 Spondylolisthesis, cervicothoracic region
M43.14 Spondylolisthesis, thoracic region
M43.15 Spondylolisthesis, thoracolumbar region
M43.16 Spondylolisthesis, lumbar region
AHA: Q3 2018
M43.17 Spondylolisthesis, lumbosacral region
M43.18 Spondylolisthesis, sacral and sacrococcygeal region
M43.19 Spondylolisthesis, multiple sites in spine

5ᵗʰ M43.2 Fusion of spine
Ankylosis of spinal joint
EXCLUDES1 ankylosing spondylitis (M45.0-)
congenital fusion of spine (Q76.4)
EXCLUDES2 arthrodesis status (Z98.1)
pseudoarthrosis after fusion or arthrodesis (M96.0)
M43.20 Fusion of spine, site unspecified
M43.21 Fusion of spine, occipito-atlanto-axial region
M43.22 Fusion of spine, cervical region
M43.23 Fusion of spine, cervicothoracic region
M43.24 Fusion of spine, thoracic region
M43.25 Fusion of spine, thoracolumbar region
M43.26 Fusion of spine, lumbar region
M43.27 Fusion of spine, lumbosacral region
M43.28 Fusion of spine, sacral and sacrococcygeal region
M43.3 Recurrent atlantoaxial dislocation with myelopathy
M43.4 Other recurrent atlantoaxial dislocation

5ᵗʰ M43.5 Other recurrent vertebral dislocation
EXCLUDES1 biomechanical lesions NEC (M99.-)
6ᵗʰ M43.5X Other recurrent vertebral dislocation
M43.5X2 Other recurrent vertebral dislocation, cervical region
M43.5X3 Other recurrent vertebral dislocation, cervicothoracic region
M43.5X4 Other recurrent vertebral dislocation, thoracic region
M43.5X5 Other recurrent vertebral dislocation, thoracolumbar region
M43.5X6 Other recurrent vertebral dislocation, lumbar region
M43.5X7 Other recurrent vertebral dislocation, lumbosacral region
M43.5X8 Other recurrent vertebral dislocation, sacral and sacrococcygeal region
M43.5X9 Other recurrent vertebral dislocation, site unspecified

M43.6 Torticollis
DEFINITION: Torticollis is a twisting of the neck due to tight neck muscles.
EXCLUDES1 congenital (sternomastoid) torticollis (Q68.0)
current injury - see Injury, of spine, by body region
ocular torticollis (R29.891)
psychogenic torticollis (F45.8)
spasmodic torticollis (G24.3)
torticollis due to birth injury (P15.2)

5ᵗʰ M43.8 Other specified deforming dorsopathies
EXCLUDES2 kyphosis and lordosis (M40.-)
scoliosis (M41.-)
6ᵗʰ M43.8X Other specified deforming dorsopathies
M43.8X1 Other specified deforming dorsopathies, occipito-atlanto-axial region
M43.8X2 Other specified deforming dorsopathies, cervical region
M43.8X3 Other specified deforming dorsopathies, cervicothoracic region
M43.8X4 Other specified deforming dorsopathies, thoracic region
M43.8X5 Other specified deforming dorsopathies, thoracolumbar region
M43.8X6 Other specified deforming dorsopathies, lumbar region
M43.8X7 Other specified deforming dorsopathies, lumbosacral region
M43.8X8 Other specified deforming dorsopathies, sacral and sacrococcygeal region
M43.8X9 Other specified deforming dorsopathies, site unspecified
M43.9 Deforming dorsopathy, unspecified
Curvature of spine NOS

Spondylopathies (M45-M49)

4ᵗʰ M45 Ankylosing spondylitis (Figure 13.4)
Rheumatoid arthritis of spine
EXCLUDES1 arthropathy in Reiter's disease (M02.3-)
juvenile (ankylosing) spondylitis (M08.1)
EXCLUDES2 Behçet's disease (M35.2)
M45.0 Ankylosing spondylitis of multiple sites in spine   HCC RxHCC
M45.1 Ankylosing spondylitis of occipito-atlanto-axial region   HCC RxHCC
M45.2 Ankylosing spondylitis of cervical region   HCC RxHCC
M45.3 Ankylosing spondylitis of cervicothoracic region   HCC RxHCC
M45.4 Ankylosing spondylitis of thoracic region   HCC RxHCC
M45.5 Ankylosing spondylitis of thoracolumbar region   HCC RxHCC
M45.6 Ankylosing spondylitis lumbar region   HCC RxHCC
M45.7 Ankylosing spondylitis of lumbosacral region   HCC RxHCC
M45.8 Ankylosing spondylitis sacral and sacrococcygeal region   HCC RxHCC
M45.9 Ankylosing spondylitis of unspecified sites in spine   HCC RxHCC

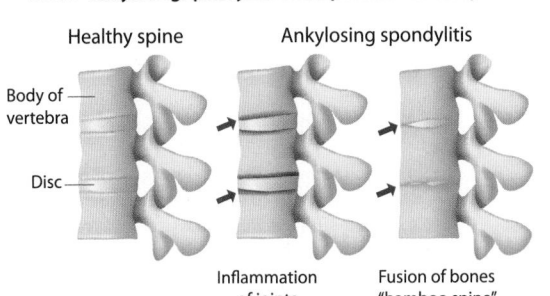

Figure 13.4 Healthy Spine Compared to Ankylosing Spondylitis

Unspecified Code   Other Specified Code   Manifestation Code   N Newborn   P Pediatric   M Maternity   A Adult   ♂ Male   ♀ Female
● New Code   ▲ Revised Code Title   ▶◀ Revised Text   NOTES   INCLUDES   EXCLUDES1 Not coded here   EXCLUDES2 Not included here
4ᵗʰ 4th character required   5ᵗʰ 5th character required   6ᵗʰ 6th character required   7ᵗʰ 7th character required   Extension 'X' Alert
HAC Hospital-acquired condition (HAC) alert   AHA AHA Coding Clinic©   ☛ Code first alert

M46 Other inflammatory spondylopathies
- **M46.0 Spinal enthesopathy**
  Disorder of ligamentous or muscular attachments of spine
  - M46.00 Spinal enthesopathy, site unspecified `HCC` `RxHCC`
  - M46.01 Spinal enthesopathy, occipito-atlanto-axial region `HCC` `RxHCC`
  - M46.02 Spinal enthesopathy, cervical region `HCC` `RxHCC`
  - M46.03 Spinal enthesopathy, cervicothoracic region `HCC` `RxHCC`
  - M46.04 Spinal enthesopathy, thoracic region `HCC` `RxHCC`
  - M46.05 Spinal enthesopathy, thoracolumbar region `HCC` `RxHCC`
  - M46.06 Spinal enthesopathy, lumbar region `HCC` `RxHCC`
  - M46.07 Spinal enthesopathy, lumbosacral region `HCC` `RxHCC`
  - M46.08 Spinal enthesopathy, sacral and sacrococcygeal region `HCC` `RxHCC`
  - M46.09 Spinal enthesopathy, multiple sites in spine `HCC` `RxHCC`
- **M46.1 Sacroiliitis, not elsewhere classified** `HCC` `RxHCC`
- **M46.2 Osteomyelitis of vertebra**
  - M46.20 Osteomyelitis of vertebra, site unspecified `cc` `HCC` `CC/MCC Exc`
  - M46.21 Osteomyelitis of vertebra, occipito-atlanto-axial region `cc` `HCC` `CC/MCC Exc`
  - M46.22 Osteomyelitis of vertebra, cervical region `cc` `HCC` `CC/MCC Exc`
  - M46.23 Osteomyelitis of vertebra, cervicothoracic region `cc` `HCC` `CC/MCC Exc`
  - M46.24 Osteomyelitis of vertebra, thoracic region `cc` `HCC` `CC/MCC Exc`
  - M46.25 Osteomyelitis of vertebra, thoracolumbar region `cc` `HCC` `CC/MCC Exc`
  - M46.26 Osteomyelitis of vertebra, lumbar region `cc` `HCC` `CC/MCC Exc`
  - M46.27 Osteomyelitis of vertebra, lumbosacral region `cc` `HCC` `CC/MCC Exc`
  - M46.28 Osteomyelitis of vertebra, sacral and sacrococcygeal region `cc` `HCC` `CC/MCC Exc`
- **M46.3 Infection of intervertebral disc (pyogenic)**
  Use additional code (B95-B97) to identify infectious agent.
  - M46.30 Infection of intervertebral disc (pyogenic), site unspecified `cc` `HCC` `CC/MCC Exc`
  - M46.31 Infection of intervertebral disc (pyogenic), occipito-atlanto-axial region `cc` `HCC` `CC/MCC Exc`
  - M46.32 Infection of intervertebral disc (pyogenic), cervical region `cc` `HCC` `CC/MCC Exc`
  - M46.33 Infection of intervertebral disc (pyogenic), cervicothoracic region `cc` `HCC` `CC/MCC Exc`
  - M46.34 Infection of intervertebral disc (pyogenic), thoracic region `cc` `HCC` `CC/MCC Exc`
  - M46.35 Infection of intervertebral disc (pyogenic), thoracolumbar region `cc` `HCC` `CC/MCC Exc`
  - M46.36 Infection of intervertebral disc (pyogenic), lumbar region `cc` `HCC` `CC/MCC Exc`
  - M46.37 Infection of intervertebral disc (pyogenic), lumbosacral region `cc` `HCC` `CC/MCC Exc`
  - M46.38 Infection of intervertebral disc (pyogenic), sacral and sacrococcygeal region `cc` `HCC` `CC/MCC Exc`
  - M46.39 Infection of intervertebral disc (pyogenic), multiple sites in spine `cc` `HCC` `CC/MCC Exc`
- **M46.4 Discitis, unspecified**
  - M46.40 Discitis, unspecified, site unspecified
  - M46.41 Discitis, unspecified, occipito-atlanto-axial region
  - M46.42 Discitis, unspecified, cervical region
  - M46.43 Discitis, unspecified, cervicothoracic region
  - M46.44 Discitis, unspecified, thoracic region
  - M46.45 Discitis, unspecified, thoracolumbar region
  - M46.46 Discitis, unspecified, lumbar region
  - M46.47 Discitis, unspecified, lumbosacral region
  - M46.48 Discitis, unspecified, sacral and sacrococcygeal region
  - M46.49 Discitis, unspecified, multiple sites in spine

- **M46.5 Other infective spondylopathies**
  - M46.50 Other infective spondylopathies, site unspecified `HCC` `RxHCC`
  - M46.51 Other infective spondylopathies, occipito-atlanto-axial region `HCC` `RxHCC`
  - M46.52 Other infective spondylopathies, cervical region `HCC` `RxHCC`
  - M46.53 Other infective spondylopathies, cervicothoracic region `HCC` `RxHCC`
  - M46.54 Other infective spondylopathies, thoracic region `HCC` `RxHCC`
  - M46.55 Other infective spondylopathies, thoracolumbar region `HCC` `RxHCC`
  - M46.56 Other infective spondylopathies, lumbar region `HCC` `RxHCC`
  - M46.57 Other infective spondylopathies, lumbosacral region `HCC` `RxHCC`
  - M46.58 Other infective spondylopathies, sacral and sacrococcygeal region `HCC` `RxHCC`
  - M46.59 Other infective spondylopathies, multiple sites in spine `HCC` `RxHCC`
- **M46.8 Other specified inflammatory spondylopathies**
  - M46.80 Other specified inflammatory spondylopathies, site unspecified `HCC` `RxHCC`
  - M46.81 Other specified inflammatory spondylopathies, occipito-atlanto-axial region `HCC` `RxHCC`
  - M46.82 Other specified inflammatory spondylopathies, cervical region `HCC` `RxHCC`
  - M46.83 Other specified inflammatory spondylopathies, cervicothoracic region `HCC` `RxHCC`
  - M46.84 Other specified inflammatory spondylopathies, thoracic region `HCC` `RxHCC`
  - M46.85 Other specified inflammatory spondylopathies, thoracolumbar region `HCC` `RxHCC`
  - M46.86 Other specified inflammatory spondylopathies, lumbar region `HCC` `RxHCC`
  - M46.87 Other specified inflammatory spondylopathies, lumbosacral region `HCC` `RxHCC`
  - M46.88 Other specified inflammatory spondylopathies, sacral and sacrococcygeal region `HCC` `RxHCC`
  - M46.89 Other specified inflammatory spondylopathies, multiple sites in spine `HCC` `RxHCC`
- **M46.9 Unspecified inflammatory spondylopathy**
  - M46.90 Unspecified inflammatory spondylopathy, site unspecified `HCC` `RxHCC`
  - M46.91 Unspecified inflammatory spondylopathy, occipito-atlanto-axial region `HCC` `RxHCC`
  - M46.92 Unspecified inflammatory spondylopathy, cervical region `HCC` `RxHCC`
  - M46.93 Unspecified inflammatory spondylopathy, cervicothoracic region `HCC` `RxHCC`
  - M46.94 Unspecified inflammatory spondylopathy, thoracic region `HCC` `RxHCC`
  - M46.95 Unspecified inflammatory spondylopathy, thoracolumbar region `HCC` `RxHCC`
  - M46.96 Unspecified inflammatory spondylopathy, lumbar region `HCC` `RxHCC`
  - M46.97 Unspecified inflammatory spondylopathy, lumbosacral region `HCC` `RxHCC`
  - M46.98 Unspecified inflammatory spondylopathy, sacral and sacrococcygeal region `HCC` `RxHCC`
  - M46.99 Unspecified inflammatory spondylopathy, multiple sites in spine `HCC` `RxHCC`

M47 Spondylosis (Figure 13.5)
- INCLUDES   arthrosis or osteoarthritis of spine
            degeneration of facet joints

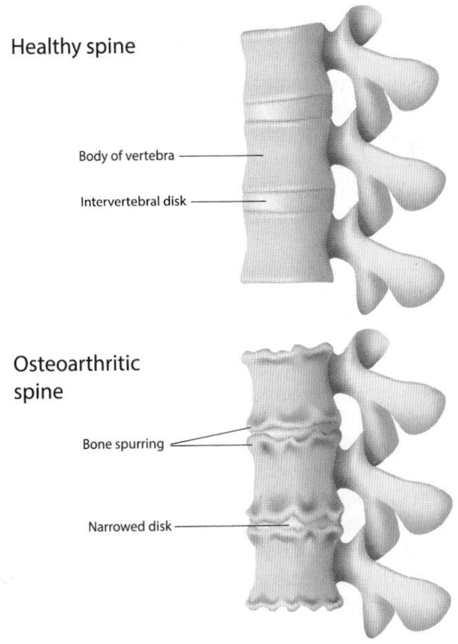
Healthy spine
Body of vertebra
Intervertebral disk
Osteoarthritic spine
Bone spurring
Narrowed disk

Figure 13.5 Osteoarthritic Spine

[5th] **M47.0 Anterior spinal and vertebral artery compression syndromes**
- [6th] **M47.01 Anterior spinal artery compression syndromes**
  - **M47.011 Anterior spinal artery compression syndromes, occipito-atlanto-axial region** [CC] [CC/MCC Exc]
  - **M47.012 Anterior spinal artery compression syndromes, cervical region** [CC] [CC/MCC Exc]
  - **M47.013 Anterior spinal artery compression syndromes, cervicothoracic region** [CC] [CC/MCC Exc]
  - **M47.014 Anterior spinal artery compression syndromes, thoracic region** [CC] [CC/MCC Exc]
  - **M47.015 Anterior spinal artery compression syndromes, thoracolumbar region** [CC] [CC/MCC Exc]
  - **M47.016 Anterior spinal artery compression syndromes, lumbar region** [CC] [CC/MCC Exc]
  - **M47.019 Anterior spinal artery compression syndromes, site unspecified** [CC] [CC/MCC Exc]
- [6th] **M47.02 Vertebral artery compression syndromes**
  - **M47.021 Vertebral artery compression syndromes, occipito-atlanto-axial region** [CC] [CC/MCC Exc]
  - **M47.022 Vertebral artery compression syndromes, cervical region** [CC] [CC/MCC Exc]
  - **M47.029 Vertebral artery compression syndromes, site unspecified** [CC] [CC/MCC Exc]

[5th] **M47.1 Other spondylosis with myelopathy**
Spondylogenic compression of spinal cord
[EXCLUDES1] *vertebral subluxation (M43.3-▶M43.5X9◀)*
- **M47.10 Other spondylosis with myelopathy, site unspecified** [CC] [CC/MCC Exc]
- **M47.11 Other spondylosis with myelopathy, occipito-atlanto-axial region** [CC] [CC/MCC Exc]
- **M47.12 Other spondylosis with myelopathy, cervical region** [CC] [CC/MCC Exc]
- **M47.13 Other spondylosis with myelopathy, cervicothoracic region** [CC] [CC/MCC Exc]
- **M47.14 Other spondylosis with myelopathy, thoracic region** [CC] [CC/MCC Exc]
- **M47.15 Other spondylosis with myelopathy, thoracolumbar region** [CC] [CC/MCC Exc]
- **M47.16 Other spondylosis with myelopathy, lumbar region** [CC] [CC/MCC Exc]

[5th] **M47.2 Other spondylosis with radiculopathy**
- **M47.20 Other spondylosis with radiculopathy, site unspecified**
- **M47.21 Other spondylosis with radiculopathy, occipito-atlanto-axial region**
- **M47.22 Other spondylosis with radiculopathy, cervical region**
- **M47.23 Other spondylosis with radiculopathy, cervicothoracic region**
- **M47.24 Other spondylosis with radiculopathy, thoracic region**
- **M47.25 Other spondylosis with radiculopathy, thoracolumbar region**
- **M47.26 Other spondylosis with radiculopathy, lumbar region**
- **M47.27 Other spondylosis with radiculopathy, lumbosacral region**
- **M47.28 Other spondylosis with radiculopathy, sacral and sacrococcygeal region**

[5th] **M47.8 Other spondylosis**
- [6th] **M47.81 Spondylosis without myelopathy or radiculopathy**
  - **M47.811 Spondylosis without myelopathy or radiculopathy, occipito-atlanto-axial region**
  - **M47.812 Spondylosis without myelopathy or radiculopathy, cervical region**
    AHA: Q2 2018
  - **M47.813 Spondylosis without myelopathy or radiculopathy, cervicothoracic region**
  - **M47.814 Spondylosis without myelopathy or radiculopathy, thoracic region**
  - **M47.815 Spondylosis without myelopathy or radiculopathy, thoracolumbar region**
  - **M47.816 Spondylosis without myelopathy or radiculopathy, lumbar region**
  - **M47.817 Spondylosis without myelopathy or radiculopathy, lumbosacral region**
  - **M47.818 Spondylosis without myelopathy or radiculopathy, sacral and sacrococcygeal region**
  - **M47.819 Spondylosis without myelopathy or radiculopathy, site unspecified**
- [6th] **M47.89 Other spondylosis**
  - **M47.891 Other spondylosis, occipito-atlanto-axial region**
  - **M47.892 Other spondylosis, cervical region**
  - **M47.893 Other spondylosis, cervicothoracic region**
  - **M47.894 Other spondylosis, thoracic region**
  - **M47.895 Other spondylosis, thoracolumbar region**
  - **M47.896 Other spondylosis, lumbar region**
  - **M47.897 Other spondylosis, lumbosacral region**
  - **M47.898 Other spondylosis, sacral and sacrococcygeal region**
  - **M47.899 Other spondylosis, site unspecified**

M47.9 Spondylosis, unspecified

[4th] **M48 Other spondylopathies**

[5th] **M48.0 Spinal stenosis**
Caudal stenosis
- **M48.00 Spinal stenosis, site unspecified**
- **M48.01 Spinal stenosis, occipito-atlanto-axial region**
- **M48.02 Spinal stenosis, cervical region**
  AHA: Q3 2018
- **M48.03 Spinal stenosis, cervicothoracic region**
- **M48.04 Spinal stenosis, thoracic region**
- **M48.05 Spinal stenosis, thoracolumbar region**
- [6th] **M48.06 Spinal stenosis, lumbar region**
  - **M48.061 Spinal stenosis, lumbar region without neurogenic claudication**
    AHA: Q3 2018
    Spinal stenosis, lumbar region NOS
  - **M48.062 Spinal stenosis, lumbar region with neurogenic claudication**
- **M48.07 Spinal stenosis, lumbosacral region**
  AHA: Q3 2018
- **M48.08 Spinal stenosis, sacral and sacrococcygeal region**

Unspecified Code | Other Specified Code | Manifestation Code | [N] Newborn | [P] Pediatric | [M] Maternity | [A] Adult | ♂ Male | ♀ Female
● New Code | ▲ Revised Code Title | ▶◀ Revised Text | [NOTES] | [INCLUDES] | [EXCLUDES1] Not coded here | [EXCLUDES2] Not included here
[4th] 4th character required | [5th] 5th character required | [6th] 6th character required | [7th] 7th character required | [X] Extension 'X' Alert
[HAC] Hospital-acquired condition (HAC) alert | AHA AHA Coding Clinic© | Code first alert

[5th] **M48.1** Ankylosing hyperostosis [Forestier]
Diffuse idiopathic skeletal hyperostosis [DISH]
M48.10 Ankylosing hyperostosis [Forestier], site unspecified
M48.11 Ankylosing hyperostosis [Forestier], occipito-atlanto-axial **region**
M48.12 Ankylosing hyperostosis [Forestier], cervical **region**
M48.13 Ankylosing hyperostosis [Forestier], cervicothoracic **region**
M48.14 Ankylosing hyperostosis [Forestier], thoracic **region**
M48.15 Ankylosing hyperostosis [Forestier], thoracolumbar **region**
M48.16 Ankylosing hyperostosis [Forestier], lumbar **region**
M48.17 Ankylosing hyperostosis [Forestier], lumbosacral **region**
M48.18 Ankylosing hyperostosis [Forestier], sacral and sacrococcygeal **region**
M48.19 Ankylosing hyperostosis [Forestier], multiple sites **in spine**

[5th] **M48.2** Kissing spine
M48.20 Kissing spine, site unspecified
M48.21 Kissing spine, occipito-atlanto-axial **region**
M48.22 Kissing spine, cervical **region**
M48.23 Kissing spine, cervicothoracic **region**
M48.24 Kissing spine, thoracic **region**
M48.25 Kissing spine, thoracolumbar **region**
M48.26 Kissing spine, lumbar **region**
M48.27 Kissing spine, lumbosacral **region**

[5th] **M48.3** Traumatic spondylopathy
M48.30 Traumatic spondylopathy, site unspecified [CC] [CC/MCC Exc]
M48.31 Traumatic spondylopathy, occipito-atlanto-axial **region** [CC] [CC/MCC Exc]
M48.32 Traumatic spondylopathy, cervical **region** [CC] [CC/MCC Exc]
M48.33 Traumatic spondylopathy, cervicothoracic **region** [CC] [CC/MCC Exc]
M48.34 Traumatic spondylopathy, thoracic **region** [CC] [CC/MCC Exc]
M48.35 Traumatic spondylopathy, thoracolumbar **region** [CC] [CC/MCC Exc]
M48.36 Traumatic spondylopathy, lumbar **region** [CC] [CC/MCC Exc]
M48.37 Traumatic spondylopathy, lumbosacral **region** [CC] [CC/MCC Exc]
M48.38 Traumatic spondylopathy, sacral and sacrococcygeal **region** [CC] [CC/MCC Exc]

[5th] **M48.4** Fatigue fracture **of vertebra**
Stress fracture of vertebra
[EXCLUDES1] *pathological fracture NOS (M84.4-)*
pathological fracture of vertebra due to neoplasm (M84.58)
pathological fracture of vertebra due to other diagnosis (M84.68)
pathological fracture of vertebra due to osteoporosis (M80.-)
traumatic fracture of vertebrae (S12.0-S12.3-, S22.0-, S32.0-)

The appropriate 7th character is to be added to each code from subcategory M48.4:
A = initial encounter for fracture
D = subsequent encounter for fracture with routine healing
G = subsequent encounter for fracture with delayed healing
S = sequela of fracture

[7th] **M48.40 Fatigue fracture of vertebra, site unspecified**
[7th] **M48.41 Fatigue fracture of vertebra,** occipito-atlanto-axial **region**
[7th] **M48.42 Fatigue fracture of vertebra,** cervical **region**
[7th] **M48.43 Fatigue fracture of vertebra,** cervicothoracic **region**
[7th] **M48.44 Fatigue fracture of vertebra,** thoracic **region**
[7th] **M48.45 Fatigue fracture of vertebra,** thoracolumbar **region**
[7th] **M48.46 Fatigue fracture of vertebra,** lumbar **region**
[7th] **M48.47 Fatigue fracture of vertebra,** lumbosacral **region**
[7th] **M48.48 Fatigue fracture of vertebra,** sacral and sacrococcygeal **region**

[5th] **M48.5** Collapsed vertebra, **not elsewhere classified**
Collapsed vertebra NOS
Compression fracture of vertebra NOS
Wedging of vertebra NOS
[EXCLUDES1] *current injury - see Injury of spine, by body region*
fatigue fracture of vertebra (M48.4)
pathological fracture of vertebra due to neoplasm (M84.58)
pathological fracture of vertebra due to other diagnosis (M84.68)
pathological fracture of vertebra due to osteoporosis (M80.-)
pathological fracture NOS (M84.4-)
stress fracture of vertebra (M48.4-)
traumatic fracture of vertebra (S12.-, S22.-, S32.-)

The appropriate 7th character is to be added to each code from subcategory M48.5:
A = initial encounter for fracture
D = subsequent encounter for fracture with routine healing
G = subsequent encounter for fracture with delayed healing
S = sequela of fracture

[7th] **M48.50 Collapsed vertebra, not elsewhere classified, site unspecified** [CC] [HCC] [RxHCC] [CC/MCC Exc]
[7th] **M48.51 Collapsed vertebra, not elsewhere classified,** occipito-atlanto-axial **region** [CC] [HCC] [RxHCC] [CC/MCC Exc]
[7th] **M48.52 Collapsed vertebra, not elsewhere classified,** cervical **region** [CC] [HCC] [RxHCC] [CC/MCC Exc]
[7th] **M48.53 Collapsed vertebra, not elsewhere classified,** cervicothoracic **region** [CC] [HCC] [RxHCC] [CC/MCC Exc]
[7th] **M48.54 Collapsed vertebra, not elsewhere classified,** thoracic **region** [CC] [HCC] [RxHCC] [CC/MCC Exc]
[7th] **M48.55 Collapsed vertebra, not elsewhere classified,** thoracolumbar **region** [CC] [HCC] [RxHCC] [CC/MCC Exc]
[7th] **M48.56 Collapsed vertebra, not elsewhere classified,** lumbar **region** [CC] [HCC] [RxHCC] [CC/MCC Exc]
[7th] **M48.57 Collapsed vertebra, not elsewhere classified,** lumbosacral **region** [CC] [HCC] [RxHCC] [CC/MCC Exc]
[7th] **M48.58 Collapsed vertebra, not elsewhere classified,** sacral and sacrococcygeal **region** [CC] [HCC] [RxHCC] [CC/MCC Exc]

[5th] **M48.8** Other specified **spondylopathies**
Ossification of posterior longitudinal ligament
[6th] **M48.8X Other specified spondylopathies**
M48.8X1 Other specified spondylopathies, occipito-atlanto-axial **region** [HCC] [RxHCC]
M48.8X2 Other specified spondylopathies, cervical **region** [HCC] [RxHCC]
M48.8X3 Other specified spondylopathies, cervicothoracic **region** [HCC] [RxHCC]
M48.8X4 Other specified spondylopathies, thoracic **region** [HCC] [RxHCC]
M48.8X5 Other specified spondylopathies, thoracolumbar **region** [HCC] [RxHCC]
M48.8X6 Other specified spondylopathies, lumbar **region** [HCC] [RxHCC]
M48.8X7 Other specified spondylopathies, lumbosacral **region** [HCC] [RxHCC]
M48.8X8 Other specified spondylopathies, sacral and sacrococcygeal **region** [HCC] [RxHCC]
M48.8X9 Other specified spondylopathies, site unspecified [HCC] [RxHCC]

M48.9 Spondylopathy, unspecified

[4th] **M49 Spondylopathies in diseases classified elsewhere**
[INCLUDES] *curvature of spine in diseases classified elsewhere*
deformity of spine in diseases classified elsewhere
kyphosis in diseases classified elsewhere
scoliosis in diseases classified elsewhere
spondylopathy in diseases classified elsewhere

[PDx] Unacceptable principal diagnosis symbol per Medicare code edits [POA] Code exempt from diagnosis present on admission requirement
[?] Questionable admission [CC] Complication or comorbidity [MCC] Major complication or comorbidity [CC/MCC Exc] CC/MCC exclusion
[HCC] HCC diagnosis code [RxHCC] RxHCC diagnosis code MACRA code **DEFINITION** Describes condition/terminology
TIP Coding guidance 👁 Official Guideline Reference [Z1] Z code as first-listed diagnosis

When symbols appear on a code that requires a 7th character extension, refer to Appendix B to identify applicable 7th character codes.

☞ **Code first** underlying disease, such as:
brucellosis (A23.-)
Charcot-Marie-Tooth disease (G60.0)
enterobacterial infections (A01-A04)
osteitis fibrosa cystica (E21.0)
EXCLUDES1 *curvature of spine in tuberculosis [Pott's] (A18.01)*
enteropathic arthropathies (M07.-)
gonococcal spondylitis (A54.41)
neuropathic [tabes dorsalis] spondylitis (A52.11)
neuropathic spondylopathy in syringomyelia (G95.0)
neuropathic spondylopathy in tabes dorsalis (A52.11)
nonsyphilitic neuropathic spondylopathy NEC (G98.0)
spondylitis in syphilis (acquired) (A52.77)
tuberculous spondylitis (A18.01)
typhoid fever spondylitis (A01.05)

5ᵗʰ **M49.8** Spondylopathy in diseases classified elsewhere

M49.80 **Spondylopathy in diseases classified elsewhere, site unspecified** HCC RxHCC

M49.81 **Spondylopathy in diseases classified elsewhere, occipito-atlanto-axial region** HCC RxHCC

M49.82 **Spondylopathy in diseases classified elsewhere, cervical region** HCC RxHCC

M49.83 **Spondylopathy in diseases classified elsewhere, cervicothoracic region** HCC RxHCC

M49.84 **Spondylopathy in diseases classified elsewhere, thoracic region** HCC RxHCC

M49.85 **Spondylopathy in diseases classified elsewhere, thoracolumbar region** HCC RxHCC

M49.86 **Spondylopathy in diseases classified elsewhere, lumbar region** HCC RxHCC

M49.87 **Spondylopathy in diseases classified elsewhere, lumbosacral region** HCC RxHCC

M49.88 **Spondylopathy in diseases classified elsewhere, sacral and sacrococcygeal region** HCC RxHCC

M49.89 **Spondylopathy in diseases classified elsewhere, multiple sites in spine** HCC RxHCC

Other dorsopathies (M50-M54)

EXCLUDES1 *current injury - see injury of spine by body region*
discitis NOS (M46.4-)

4ᵗʰ **M50** Cervical disc disorders
NOTES Code to the most superior level of disorder
INCLUDES *cervicothoracic disc disorders with cervicalgia*
cervicothoracic disc disorders

5ᵗʰ **M50.0** Cervical disc disorder with myelopathy
M50.00 **Cervical disc disorder with myelopathy, unspecified cervical region** CC CC/MCC Exc
M50.01 **Cervical disc disorder with myelopathy, high cervical region** CC CC/MCC Exc
AHA: Q1 2016
C2-C3 disc disorder with myelopathy
C3-C4 disc disorder with myelopathy
6ᵗʰ **M50.02** Cervical disc disorder with myelopathy, mid-cervical region
M50.020 **Cervical disc disorder with myelopathy, mid-cervical region, unspecified level** CC CC/MCC Exc
AHA: Q4 2016
M50.021 **Cervical disc disorder** at C4-C5 level **with myelopathy** CC CC/MCC Exc
AHA: Q4 2016
C4-C5 disc disorder with myelopathy
M50.022 **Cervical disc disorder** at C5-C6 level **with myelopathy** CC CC/MCC Exc
AHA: Q3 2018, Q4 2016
C5-C6 disc disorder with myelopathy
M50.023 **Cervical disc disorder** at C6-C7 level **with myelopathy** CC CC/MCC Exc
AHA: Q4 2016
C6-C7 disc disorder with myelopathy

M50.03 **Cervical disc disorder with myelopathy, cervicothoracic region** CC CC/MCC Exc
C7-T1 disc disorder with myelopathy
5ᵗʰ **M50.1** Cervical disc disorder with radiculopathy
EXCLUDES2 *brachial radiculitis NOS (M54.13)*
M50.10 **Cervical disc disorder with radiculopathy, unspecified cervical region**
M50.11 **Cervical disc disorder with radiculopathy, high cervical region**
C2-C3 disc disorder with radiculopathy
C3 radiculopathy due to disc disorder
C3-C4 disc disorder with radiculopathy
C4 radiculopathy due to disc disorder
6ᵗʰ **M50.12** Cervical disc disorder with radiculopathy, mid-cervical region
▲ **M50.120** **Mid-cervical disc disorder, unspecified ►level◄**
AHA: Q4 2016
M50.121 **Cervical disc disorder** at C4-C5 level **with radiculopathy**
AHA: Q4 2016
C4-C5 disc disorder with radiculopathy
C5 radiculopathy due to disc disorder
M50.122 **Cervical disc disorder** at C5-C6 level **with radiculopathy**
AHA: Q3 2018, Q4 2016
C5-C6 disc disorder with radiculopathy
C6 radiculopathy due to disc disorder
M50.123 **Cervical disc disorder** at C6-C7 level **with radiculopathy**
AHA: Q4 2016
C6-C7 disc disorder with radiculopathy
C7 radiculopathy due to disc disorder
M50.13 **Cervical disc disorder with radiculopathy, cervicothoracic region**
C7-T1 disc disorder with radiculopathy
C8 radiculopathy due to disc disorder
5ᵗʰ **M50.2** Other cervical disc displacement
M50.20 **Other cervical disc displacement, unspecified cervical region**
M50.21 **Other cervical disc displacement,** high cervical region
Other C2-C3 cervical disc displacement
Other C3-C4 cervical disc displacement
6ᵗʰ **M50.22** Other cervical disc displacement, mid-cervical region
M50.220 **Other cervical disc displacement, mid-cervical region, unspecified level**
M50.221 **Other cervical disc displacement** at C4-C5 level
Other C4-C5 cervical disc displacement
M50.222 **Other cervical disc displacement** at C5-C6 level
Other C5-C6 cervical disc displacement
M50.223 **Other cervical disc displacement** at C6-C7 level
Other C6-C7 cervical disc displacement
M50.23 **Other cervical disc displacement,** cervicothoracic region
Other C7-T1 cervical disc displacement
5ᵗʰ **M50.3** Other cervical disc degeneration
M50.30 **Other cervical disc degeneration, unspecified cervical region**
M50.31 **Other cervical disc degeneration,** high cervical **region**
Other C2-C3 cervical disc degeneration
Other C3-C4 cervical disc degeneration
6ᵗʰ **M50.32** Other cervical disc degeneration, mid-cervical region
M50.320 **Other cervical disc degeneration, mid-cervical region, unspecified** level
M50.321 **Other cervical disc degeneration** at C4-C5 level
Other C4-C5 cervical disc degeneration

● Unspecified Code   Other Specified Code   Manifestation Code   ℕ Newborn   ℙ Pediatric   Ⓜ Maternity   🄰 Adult   ♂ Male   ♀ Female
● New Code   ▲ Revised Code Title   ►◄ Revised Text   **NOTES** **INCLUDES** *EXCLUDES1* Not coded here   *EXCLUDES2* Not included here
4ᵗʰ 4ᵗʰ character required   5ᵗʰ 5ᵗʰ character required   6ᵗʰ 6ᵗʰ character required   7ᵗʰ 7ᵗʰ character required   Extension 'X' Alert
HAC Hospital-acquired condition (HAC) alert   AHA AHA Coding Clinic©   ☞ Code first alert

2020 ICD-10-CM   When symbols appear on a code that requires a 7th character extension, refer to Appendix B to identify applicable 7th character codes.   **815**

M50.322 **Other cervical disc degeneration at C5-C6 level**
Other C5-C6 cervical disc degeneration
M50.323 **Other cervical disc degeneration at C6-C7 level**
Other C6-C7 cervical disc degeneration
M50.33 **Other cervical disc degeneration, cervicothoracic region**
Other C7-T1 cervical disc degeneration
[5th] M50.8 **Other cervical disc disorders**
M50.80 **Other cervical disc disorders, unspecified cervical region**
M50.81 **Other cervical disc disorders, high cervical region**
Other C2-C3 cervical disc disorders
Other C3-C4 cervical disc disorders
[6th] M50.82 **Other cervical disc disorders, mid-cervical region**
M50.820 **Other cervical disc disorders, mid-cervical region, unspecified level**
M50.821 **Other cervical disc disorders at C4-C5 level**
Other C4-C5 cervical disc disorders
M50.822 **Other cervical disc disorders at C5-C6 level**
Other C5-C6 cervical disc disorders
M50.823 **Other cervical disc disorders at C6-C7 level**
Other C6-C7 cervical disc disorders
M50.83 **Other cervical disc disorders, cervicothoracic region**
Other C7-T1 cervical disc disorders
[5th] M50.9 **Cervical disc disorder, unspecified**
M50.90 **Cervical disc disorder, unspecified, unspecified cervical region**
M50.91 **Cervical disc disorder, unspecified, high cervical region**
C2-C3 cervical disc disorder, unspecified
C3-C4 cervical disc disorder, unspecified
[6th] M50.92 **Cervical disc disorder, unspecified, mid-cervical region**
M50.920 **Unspecified cervical disc disorder, mid-cervical region, unspecified level**
M50.921 **Unspecified cervical disc disorder at C4-C5 level**
Unspecified C4-C5 cervical disc disorder
M50.922 **Unspecified cervical disc disorder at C5-C6 level**
Unspecified C5-C6 cervical disc disorder
M50.923 **Unspecified cervical disc disorder at C6-C7 level**
Unspecified C6-C7 cervical disc disorder
M50.93 **Cervical disc disorder, unspecified, cervicothoracic region**
C7-T1 cervical disc disorder, unspecified
[4th] M51 **Thoracic, thoracolumbar, and lumbosacral intervertebral disc disorders**
EXCLUDES2 *cervical and cervicothoracic disc disorders (M50.-)*
sacral and sacrococcygeal disorders (M53.3)
[5th] M51.0 **Thoracic, thoracolumbar and lumbosacral intervertebral disc disorders with myelopathy**
M51.04 **Intervertebral disc disorders with myelopathy, thoracic region** CC CC/MCC Exc
M51.05 **Intervertebral disc disorders with myelopathy, thoracolumbar region** CC CC/MCC Exc
M51.06 **Intervertebral disc disorders with myelopathy, lumbar region** CC CC/MCC Exc
[5th] M51.1 **Thoracic, thoracolumbar and lumbosacral intervertebral disc disorders with radiculopathy**
Sciatica due to intervertebral disc disorder
EXCLUDES1 *lumbar radiculitis NOS (M54.16)*
sciatica NOS (M54.3)
M51.14 **Intervertebral disc disorders with radiculopathy, thoracic region**
M51.15 **Intervertebral disc disorders with radiculopathy, thoracolumbar region**
M51.16 **Intervertebral disc disorders with radiculopathy, lumbar region**
AHA: Q3 2018
M51.17 **Intervertebral disc disorders with radiculopathy, lumbosacral region**
[5th] M51.2 **Other thoracic, thoracolumbar and lumbosacral intervertebral disc displacement**
Lumbago due to displacement of intervertebral disc
M51.24 **Other intervertebral disc displacement, thoracic region**
M51.25 **Other intervertebral disc displacement, thoracolumbar region**
M51.26 **Other intervertebral disc displacement, lumbar region**
M51.27 **Other intervertebral disc displacement, lumbosacral region**
[5th] M51.3 **Other thoracic, thoracolumbar and lumbosacral intervertebral disc degeneration**
M51.34 **Other intervertebral disc degeneration, thoracic region**
M51.35 **Other intervertebral disc degeneration, thoracolumbar region**
M51.36 **Other intervertebral disc degeneration, lumbar region**
AHA: Q2 2018
M51.37 **Other intervertebral disc degeneration, lumbosacral region**
[5th] M51.4 **Schmorl's nodes**
M51.44 **Schmorl's nodes, thoracic region**
M51.45 **Schmorl's nodes, thoracolumbar region**
M51.46 **Schmorl's nodes, lumbar region**
M51.47 **Schmorl's nodes, lumbosacral region**
[5th] M51.8 **Other thoracic, thoracolumbar and lumbosacral intervertebral disc disorders**
M51.84 **Other intervertebral disc disorders, thoracic region**
M51.85 **Other intervertebral disc disorders, thoracolumbar region**
M51.86 **Other intervertebral disc disorders, lumbar region**
M51.87 **Other intervertebral disc disorders, lumbosacral region**
M51.9 **Unspecified thoracic, thoracolumbar and lumbosacral intervertebral disc disorder**
[4th] M53 **Other and unspecified dorsopathies, not elsewhere classified**
M53.0 **Cervicocranial syndrome**
Posterior cervical sympathetic syndrome
M53.1 **Cervicobrachial syndrome**
EXCLUDES2 *cervical disc disorder (M50.-)*
thoracic outlet syndrome (G54.0)
[5th] M53.2 **Spinal instabilities**
[6th] M53.2X **Spinal instabilities**
M53.2X1 **Spinal instabilities, occipito-atlanto-axial region**
M53.2X2 **Spinal instabilities, cervical region**
M53.2X3 **Spinal instabilities, cervicothoracic region**
M53.2X4 **Spinal instabilities, thoracic region**
M53.2X5 **Spinal instabilities, thoracolumbar region**
M53.2X6 **Spinal instabilities, lumbar region**
M53.2X7 **Spinal instabilities, lumbosacral region**
M53.2X8 **Spinal instabilities, sacral and sacrococcygeal region**
M53.2X9 **Spinal instabilities, site unspecified**
M53.3 **Sacrococcygeal disorders, not elsewhere classified**
Coccygodynia
[5th] M53.8 **Other specified dorsopathies**
M53.80 **Other specified dorsopathies, site unspecified**
M53.81 **Other specified dorsopathies, occipito-atlanto-axial region**
M53.82 **Other specified dorsopathies, cervical region**
M53.83 **Other specified dorsopathies, cervicothoracic region**
M53.84 **Other specified dorsopathies, thoracic region**
M53.85 **Other specified dorsopathies, thoracolumbar region**
M53.86 **Other specified dorsopathies, lumbar region**
M53.87 **Other specified dorsopathies, lumbosacral region**

[PDx] Unacceptable principal diagnosis symbol per Medicare code edits [POA] Code exempt from diagnosis present on admission requirement
[?] Questionable admission [CC] Complication or comorbidity [MCC] Major complication or comorbidity [CC/MCC Exc] CC/MCC exclusion
[HCC] HCC diagnosis code [RxHCC] RxHCC diagnosis code MACRA code **DEFINITION** Describes condition/terminology
TIP Coding guidance [Eye] Official Guideline Reference [Z1] Z code as first-listed diagnosis

M53.88 Other specified dorsopathies, sacral and sacrococcygeal region

M53.9 Dorsopathy, unspecified

🔵 M54 Dorsalgia

    EXCLUDES1 psychogenic dorsalgia (F45.41)

    🔵 M54.0 Panniculitis affecting regions of neck and back

        EXCLUDES1 lupus panniculitis (L93.2)

                panniculitis NOS (M79.3)

                relapsing [Weber-Christian] panniculitis (M35.6)

        M54.00 Panniculitis affecting regions of neck and back, site unspecified

        M54.01 Panniculitis affecting regions of neck and back, occipito-atlanto-axial region

        M54.02 Panniculitis affecting regions of neck and back, cervical region

        M54.03 Panniculitis affecting regions of neck and back, cervicothoracic region

        M54.04 Panniculitis affecting regions of neck and back, thoracic region

        M54.05 Panniculitis affecting regions of neck and back, thoracolumbar region

        M54.06 Panniculitis affecting regions of neck and back, lumbar region

        M54.07 Panniculitis affecting regions of neck and back, lumbosacral region

        M54.08 Panniculitis affecting regions of neck and back, sacral and sacrococcygeal region

        M54.09 Panniculitis affecting regions, neck and back, multiple sites in spine

    🔵 M54.1 Radiculopathy

        Brachial neuritis or radiculitis NOS

        Lumbar neuritis or radiculitis NOS

        Lumbosacral neuritis or radiculitis NOS

        Thoracic neuritis or radiculitis NOS

        Radiculitis NOS

        EXCLUDES1 neuralgia and neuritis NOS (M79.2)

                radiculopathy with cervical disc disorder (M50.1)

                radiculopathy with lumbar and other intervertebral disc disorder (M51.1-)

                radiculopathy with spondylosis (M47.2-)

        M54.10 Radiculopathy, site unspecified

            DEFINITION: Radiculopathy is a pinched nerve in the spine causing pain, weakness, and/or numbness.

        M54.11 Radiculopathy, occipito-atlanto-axial region

        M54.12 Radiculopathy, cervical region

            AHA: Q3 2018

        M54.13 Radiculopathy, cervicothoracic region

        M54.14 Radiculopathy, thoracic region

        M54.15 Radiculopathy, thoracolumbar region

        M54.16 Radiculopathy, lumbar region

            AHA: Q3 2018

        M54.17 Radiculopathy, lumbosacral region

        M54.18 Radiculopathy, sacral and sacrococcygeal region

    M54.2 Cervicalgia

        👁 See Official Guidelines "Sequencing of Category G89 Codes with Site-specific Pain Codes" I.C.6.b.1.b.ii

        EXCLUDES1 cervicalgia due to intervertebral cervical disc disorder (M50.-)

    🔵 M54.3 Sciatica

        EXCLUDES1 lesion of sciatic nerve (G57.0)

                sciatica due to intervertebral disc disorder (M51.1-)

                sciatica with lumbago (M54.4-)

        M54.30 Sciatica, unspecified side

        M54.31 Sciatica, right side

        M54.32 Sciatica, left side

    🔵 M54.4 Lumbago with sciatica

        EXCLUDES1 lumbago with sciatica due to intervertebral disc disorder (M51.1-)

M54.40 Lumbago with sciatica, unspecified side

M54.41 Lumbago with sciatica, right side

M54.42 Lumbago with sciatica, left side

    AHA: Q2 2016

M54.5 Low back pain

    Loin pain

    Lumbago NOS

    EXCLUDES1 low back strain (S39.012)

        lumbago due to intervertebral disc displacement (M51.2-)

        lumbago with sciatica (M54.4-)

M54.6 Pain in thoracic spine

    EXCLUDES1 pain in thoracic spine due to intervertebral disc disorder (M51.-)

🔵 M54.8 Other dorsalgia

    EXCLUDES1 dorsalgia in thoracic region (M54.6)

        low back pain (M54.5)

    M54.81 Occipital neuralgia

    M54.89 Other dorsalgia

M54.9 Dorsalgia, unspecified

    Backache NOS

    Back pain NOS

Soft tissue disorders (M60-M79)

Disorders of muscles (M60-M63)

EXCLUDES1 dermatopolymyositis (M33.-)

    muscular dystrophies and myopathies (G71-G72)

    myopathy in amyloidosis (E85.-)

    myopathy in polyarteritis nodosa (M30.0)

    myopathy in rheumatoid arthritis (M05.32)

    myopathy in scleroderma (M34.-)

    myopathy in Sjögren's syndrome (M35.03)

    myopathy in systemic lupus erythematosus (M32.-)

🔵 M60 Myositis

    EXCLUDES2 inclusion body myositis [IBM] (G72.41)

    🔵 M60.0 Infective myositis

        Tropical pyomyositis

        Use additional code (B95-B97) to identify infectious agent

        🔵 M60.00 Infective myositis, unspecified site

            M60.000 Infective myositis, unspecified right arm   CC CC/MCC Exc

                Infective myositis, right upper limb NOS

            M60.001 Infective myositis, unspecified left arm   CC CC/MCC Exc

                Infective myositis, left upper limb NOS

            M60.002 Infective myositis, unspecified arm   CC CC/MCC Exc

                Infective myositis, upper limb NOS

            M60.003 Infective myositis, unspecified right leg   CC CC/MCC Exc

                Infective myositis, right lower limb NOS

            M60.004 Infective myositis, unspecified left leg   CC CC/MCC Exc

                Infective myositis, left lower limb NOS

            M60.005 Infective myositis, unspecified leg   CC CC/MCC Exc

                Infective myositis, lower limb NOS

            M60.009 Infective myositis, unspecified site   CC CC/MCC Exc

        🔵 M60.01 Infective myositis, shoulder

            M60.011 Infective myositis, right shoulder   CC CC/MCC Exc

            M60.012 Infective myositis, left shoulder   CC CC/MCC Exc

            M60.019 Infective myositis, unspecified shoulder   CC CC/MCC Exc

        🔵 M60.02 Infective myositis, upper arm

            M60.021 Infective myositis, right upper arm   CC CC/MCC Exc

            M60.022 Infective myositis, left upper arm   CC CC/MCC Exc

            M60.029 Infective myositis, unspecified upper arm   CC CC/MCC Exc

Unspecified Code   Other Specified Code   Manifestation Code   N Newborn   P Pediatric   M Maternity   A Adult   ♂ Male   ♀ Female

● New Code   ▲ Revised Code Title   ►◄ Revised Text   **NOTES**   *INCLUDES*   *EXCLUDES1* Not coded here   *EXCLUDES2* Not included here

🔵 4th character required   🔵 5th character required   🔵 6th character required   🔵 7th character required   🔵 Extension 'X' Alert

HAC Hospital-acquired condition (HAC) alert   **AHA** AHA Coding Clinic©   📣 Code first alert

2020 ICD-10-CM   When symbols appear on a code that requires a 7th character extension, refer to Appendix B to identify applicable 7th character codes.   **817**

(6th) **M60.03** Infective myositis, forearm
  M60.031 Infective myositis, right forearm ⚐ CC/MCC Exc
  M60.032 Infective myositis, left forearm ⚐ CC/MCC Exc
  M60.039 Infective myositis, unspecified forearm ⚐ CC/MCC Exc
(6th) **M60.04** Infective myositis, hand and fingers
  M60.041 Infective myositis, right hand ⚐ CC/MCC Exc
  M60.042 Infective myositis, left hand ⚐ CC/MCC Exc
  M60.043 Infective myositis, unspecified hand ⚐ CC/MCC Exc
  M60.044 Infective myositis, right finger(s) ⚐ CC/MCC Exc
  M60.045 Infective myositis, left finger(s) ⚐ CC/MCC Exc
  M60.046 Infective myositis, unspecified finger(s) ⚐ CC/MCC Exc
(6th) **M60.05** Infective myositis, thigh
  M60.051 Infective myositis, right thigh ⚐ CC/MCC Exc
  M60.052 Infective myositis, left thigh ⚐ CC/MCC Exc
  M60.059 Infective myositis, unspecified thigh ⚐ CC/MCC Exc
(6th) **M60.06** Infective myositis, lower leg
  M60.061 Infective myositis, right lower leg ⚐ CC/MCC Exc
  M60.062 Infective myositis, left lower leg ⚐ CC/MCC Exc
  M60.069 Infective myositis, unspecified lower leg ⚐ CC/MCC Exc
(6th) **M60.07** Infective myositis, ankle, foot and toes
  M60.070 Infective myositis, right ankle ⚐ CC/MCC Exc
  M60.071 Infective myositis, left ankle ⚐ CC/MCC Exc
  M60.072 Infective myositis, unspecified ankle ⚐ CC/MCC Exc
  M60.073 Infective myositis, right foot ⚐ CC/MCC Exc
  M60.074 Infective myositis, left foot ⚐ CC/MCC Exc
  M60.075 Infective myositis, unspecified foot ⚐ CC/MCC Exc
  M60.076 Infective myositis, right toe(s) ⚐ CC/MCC Exc
  M60.077 Infective myositis, left toe(s) ⚐ CC/MCC Exc
  M60.078 Infective myositis, unspecified toe(s) ⚐ CC/MCC Exc
M60.08 Infective myositis, other site ⚐ CC/MCC Exc
M60.09 Infective myositis, multiple sites ⚐ CC/MCC Exc
(5th) **M60.1** Interstitial myositis
M60.10 Interstitial myositis of unspecified site
(6th) **M60.11** Interstitial myositis, shoulder
  M60.111 Interstitial myositis, right shoulder
  M60.112 Interstitial myositis, left shoulder
  M60.119 Interstitial myositis, unspecified shoulder
(6th) **M60.12** Interstitial myositis, upper arm
  M60.121 Interstitial myositis, right upper arm
  M60.122 Interstitial myositis, left upper arm
  M60.129 Interstitial myositis, unspecified upper arm
(6th) **M60.13** Interstitial myositis, forearm
  M60.131 Interstitial myositis, right forearm
  M60.132 Interstitial myositis, left forearm
  M60.139 Interstitial myositis, unspecified forearm
(6th) **M60.14** Interstitial myositis, hand
  M60.141 Interstitial myositis, right hand
  M60.142 Interstitial myositis, left hand
  M60.149 Interstitial myositis, unspecified hand
(6th) **M60.15** Interstitial myositis, thigh
  M60.151 Interstitial myositis, right thigh
  M60.152 Interstitial myositis, left thigh
  M60.159 Interstitial myositis, unspecified thigh
(6th) **M60.16** Interstitial myositis, lower leg
  M60.161 Interstitial myositis, right lower leg
  M60.162 Interstitial myositis, left lower leg
  M60.169 Interstitial myositis, unspecified lower leg
(6th) **M60.17** Interstitial myositis, ankle and foot
  M60.171 Interstitial myositis, right ankle and foot
  M60.172 Interstitial myositis, left ankle and foot

  M60.179 Interstitial myositis, unspecified ankle and foot
M60.18 Interstitial myositis, other site
M60.19 Interstitial myositis, multiple sites
(5th) **M60.2** Foreign body granuloma of soft tissue, not elsewhere classified
  Use additional code to identify the type of retained foreign body (Z18.-)
  EXCLUDES1 foreign body granuloma of skin and subcutaneous tissue (L92.3)
  M60.20 Foreign body granuloma of soft tissue, not elsewhere classified, unspecified site
(6th) **M60.21** Foreign body granuloma of soft tissue, not elsewhere classified, shoulder
  M60.211 Foreign body granuloma of soft tissue, not elsewhere classified, right shoulder
  M60.212 Foreign body granuloma of soft tissue, not elsewhere classified, left shoulder
  M60.219 Foreign body granuloma of soft tissue, not elsewhere classified, unspecified shoulder
(6th) **M60.22** Foreign body granuloma of soft tissue, not elsewhere classified, upper arm
  M60.221 Foreign body granuloma of soft tissue, not elsewhere classified, right upper arm
  M60.222 Foreign body granuloma of soft tissue, not elsewhere classified, left upper arm
  M60.229 Foreign body granuloma of soft tissue, not elsewhere classified, unspecified upper arm
(6th) **M60.23** Foreign body granuloma of soft tissue, not elsewhere classified, forearm
  M60.231 Foreign body granuloma of soft tissue, not elsewhere classified, right forearm
  M60.232 Foreign body granuloma of soft tissue, not elsewhere classified, left forearm
  M60.239 Foreign body granuloma of soft tissue, not elsewhere classified, unspecified forearm
(6th) **M60.24** Foreign body granuloma of soft tissue, not elsewhere classified, hand
  M60.241 Foreign body granuloma of soft tissue, not elsewhere classified, right hand
  M60.242 Foreign body granuloma of soft tissue, not elsewhere classified, left hand
  M60.249 Foreign body granuloma of soft tissue, not elsewhere classified, unspecified hand
(6th) **M60.25** Foreign body granuloma of soft tissue, not elsewhere classified, thigh
  M60.251 Foreign body granuloma of soft tissue, not elsewhere classified, right thigh
  M60.252 Foreign body granuloma of soft tissue, not elsewhere classified, left thigh
  M60.259 Foreign body granuloma of soft tissue, not elsewhere classified, unspecified thigh
(6th) **M60.26** Foreign body granuloma of soft tissue, not elsewhere classified, lower leg
  M60.261 Foreign body granuloma of soft tissue, not elsewhere classified, right lower leg
  M60.262 Foreign body granuloma of soft tissue, not elsewhere classified, left lower leg
  M60.269 Foreign body granuloma of soft tissue, not elsewhere classified, unspecified lower leg
(6th) **M60.27** Foreign body granuloma of soft tissue, not elsewhere classified, ankle and foot
  M60.271 Foreign body granuloma of soft tissue, not elsewhere classified, right ankle and foot
  M60.272 Foreign body granuloma of soft tissue, not elsewhere classified, left ankle and foot
  M60.279 Foreign body granuloma of soft tissue, not elsewhere classified, unspecified ankle and foot
M60.28 Foreign body granuloma of soft tissue, not elsewhere classified, other site

---

POA Unacceptable principal diagnosis symbol per Medicare code edits   POA Code exempt from diagnosis present on admission requirement
? Questionable admission   ⚐ Complication or comorbidity   MCC Major complication or comorbidity   CC/MCC Exc CC/MCC exclusion
HCC HCC diagnosis code   RHCC RxHCC diagnosis code   MACRA code   **DEFINITION** Describes condition/terminology
TIP Coding guidance   👁 Official Guideline Reference   Z1 Z code as first-listed diagnosis

[5th] M60.8 Other myositis
M60.80 Other myositis, unspecified site
[6th] M60.81 Other myositis shoulder
M60.811 Other myositis, right shoulder
M60.812 Other myositis, left shoulder
M60.819 Other myositis, unspecified shoulder
[6th] M60.82 Other myositis, upper arm
M60.821 Other myositis, right upper arm
M60.822 Other myositis, left upper arm
M60.829 Other myositis, unspecified upper arm
[6th] M60.83 Other myositis, forearm
M60.831 Other myositis, right forearm
M60.832 Other myositis, left forearm
M60.839 Other myositis, unspecified forearm
[6th] M60.84 Other myositis, hand
M60.841 Other myositis, right hand
M60.842 Other myositis, left hand
M60.849 Other myositis, unspecified hand
[6th] M60.85 Other myositis, thigh
M60.851 Other myositis, right thigh
M60.852 Other myositis, left thigh
M60.859 Other myositis, unspecified thigh
[6th] M60.86 Other myositis, lower leg
M60.861 Other myositis, right lower leg
M60.862 Other myositis, left lower leg
M60.869 Other myositis, unspecified lower leg
[6th] M60.87 Other myositis, ankle and foot
M60.871 Other myositis, right ankle and foot
M60.872 Other myositis, left ankle and foot
M60.879 Other myositis, unspecified ankle and foot
M60.88 Other myositis, other site
M60.89 Other myositis, multiple sites
M60.9 Myositis, unspecified
[4th] M61 Calcification and ossification of muscle
[5th] M61.0 Myositis ossificans traumatica
M61.00 Myositis ossificans traumatica, unspecified site
[6th] M61.01 Myositis ossificans traumatica, shoulder
M61.011 Myositis ossificans traumatica, right shoulder
M61.012 Myositis ossificans traumatica, left shoulder
M61.019 Myositis ossificans traumatica, unspecified shoulder
[6th] M61.02 Myositis ossificans traumatica, upper arm
M61.021 Myositis ossificans traumatica, right upper arm
M61.022 Myositis ossificans traumatica, left upper arm
M61.029 Myositis ossificans traumatica, unspecified upper arm
[6th] M61.03 Myositis ossificans traumatica, forearm
M61.031 Myositis ossificans traumatica, right forearm
M61.032 Myositis ossificans traumatica, left forearm
M61.039 Myositis ossificans traumatica, unspecified forearm
[6th] M61.04 Myositis ossificans traumatica, hand
M61.041 Myositis ossificans traumatica, right hand
M61.042 Myositis ossificans traumatica, left hand
M61.049 Myositis ossificans traumatica, unspecified hand
[6th] M61.05 Myositis ossificans traumatica, thigh
M61.051 Myositis ossificans traumatica, right thigh
M61.052 Myositis ossificans traumatica, left thigh
M61.059 Myositis ossificans traumatica, unspecified thigh
[6th] M61.06 Myositis ossificans traumatica, lower leg
M61.061 Myositis ossificans traumatica, right lower leg
M61.062 Myositis ossificans traumatica, left lower leg
M61.069 Myositis ossificans traumatica, unspecified lower leg
[6th] M61.07 Myositis ossificans traumatica, ankle and foot
M61.071 Myositis ossificans traumatica, right ankle and foot
M61.072 Myositis ossificans traumatica, left ankle and foot
M61.079 Myositis ossificans traumatica, unspecified ankle and foot
M61.08 Myositis ossificans traumatica, other site
M61.09 Myositis ossificans traumatica, multiple sites
[5th] M61.1 Myositis ossificans progressiva
Fibrodysplasia ossificans progressiva
M61.10 Myositis ossificans progressiva, unspecified site
[6th] M61.11 Myositis ossificans progressiva, shoulder
M61.111 Myositis ossificans progressiva, right shoulder
M61.112 Myositis ossificans progressiva, left shoulder
M61.119 Myositis ossificans progressiva, unspecified shoulder
[6th] M61.12 Myositis ossificans progressiva, upper arm
M61.121 Myositis ossificans progressiva, right upper arm
M61.122 Myositis ossificans progressiva, left upper arm
M61.129 Myositis ossificans progressiva, unspecified arm
[6th] M61.13 Myositis ossificans progressiva, forearm
M61.131 Myositis ossificans progressiva, right forearm
M61.132 Myositis ossificans progressiva, left forearm
M61.139 Myositis ossificans progressiva, unspecified forearm
[6th] M61.14 Myositis ossificans progressiva, hand and finger(s)
M61.141 Myositis ossificans progressiva, right hand
M61.142 Myositis ossificans progressiva, left hand
M61.143 Myositis ossificans progressiva, unspecified hand
M61.144 Myositis ossificans progressiva, right finger(s)
M61.145 Myositis ossificans progressiva, left finger(s)
M61.146 Myositis ossificans progressiva, unspecified finger(s)
[6th] M61.15 Myositis ossificans progressiva, thigh
M61.151 Myositis ossificans progressiva, right thigh
M61.152 Myositis ossificans progressiva, left thigh
M61.159 Myositis ossificans progressiva, unspecified thigh
[6th] M61.16 Myositis ossificans progressiva, lower leg
M61.161 Myositis ossificans progressiva, right lower leg
M61.162 Myositis ossificans progressiva, left lower leg
M61.169 Myositis ossificans progressiva, unspecified lower leg
[6th] M61.17 Myositis ossificans progressiva, ankle, foot and toe(s)
M61.171 Myositis ossificans progressiva, right ankle
M61.172 Myositis ossificans progressiva, left ankle
M61.173 Myositis ossificans progressiva, unspecified ankle
M61.174 Myositis ossificans progressiva, right foot
M61.175 Myositis ossificans progressiva, left foot

Unspecified Code Other Specified Code Manifestation Code [N] Newborn [P] Pediatric [M] Maternity [A] Adult ♂ Male ♀ Female
● New Code ▲ Revised Code Title ▶◀ Revised Text NOTES INCLUDES EXCLUDES1 Not coded here EXCLUDES2 Not included here
[4th] 4th character required [5th] 5th character required [6th] 6th character required [7th] 7th character required [x] Extension 'X' Alert
[HAC] Hospital-acquired condition (HAC) alert AHA AHA Coding Clinic© Code first alert

M61.176 Myositis ossificans progressiva, unspecified foot

M61.177 Myositis ossificans progressiva, right toe(s)

M61.178 Myositis ossificans progressiva, left toe(s)

M61.179 Myositis ossificans progressiva, unspecified toe(s)

M61.18 Myositis ossificans progressiva, other site

M61.19 Myositis ossificans progressiva, multiple sites

M61.2 Paralytic calcification and ossification of muscle

Myositis ossificans associated with quadriplegia or paraplegia

M61.20 Paralytic calcification and ossification of muscle, unspecified site

M61.21 Paralytic calcification and ossification of muscle, shoulder

M61.211 Paralytic calcification and ossification of muscle, right shoulder

M61.212 Paralytic calcification and ossification of muscle, left shoulder

M61.219 Paralytic calcification and ossification of muscle, unspecified shoulder

M61.22 Paralytic calcification and ossification of muscle, upper arm

M61.221 Paralytic calcification and ossification of muscle, right upper arm

M61.222 Paralytic calcification and ossification of muscle, left upper arm

M61.229 Paralytic calcification and ossification of muscle, unspecified upper arm

M61.23 Paralytic calcification and ossification of muscle, forearm

M61.231 Paralytic calcification and ossification of muscle, right forearm

M61.232 Paralytic calcification and ossification of muscle, left forearm

M61.239 Paralytic calcification and ossification of muscle, unspecified forearm

M61.24 Paralytic calcification and ossification of muscle, hand

M61.241 Paralytic calcification and ossification of muscle, right hand

M61.242 Paralytic calcification and ossification of muscle, left hand

M61.249 Paralytic calcification and ossification of muscle, unspecified hand

M61.25 Paralytic calcification and ossification of muscle, thigh

M61.251 Paralytic calcification and ossification of muscle, right thigh

M61.252 Paralytic calcification and ossification of muscle, left thigh

M61.259 Paralytic calcification and ossification of muscle, unspecified thigh

M61.26 Paralytic calcification and ossification of muscle, lower leg

M61.261 Paralytic calcification and ossification of muscle, right lower leg

M61.262 Paralytic calcification and ossification of muscle, left lower leg

M61.269 Paralytic calcification and ossification of muscle, unspecified lower leg

M61.27 Paralytic calcification and ossification of muscle, ankle and foot

M61.271 Paralytic calcification and ossification of muscle, right ankle and foot

M61.272 Paralytic calcification and ossification of muscle, left ankle and foot

M61.279 Paralytic calcification and ossification of muscle, unspecified ankle and foot

M61.28 Paralytic calcification and ossification of muscle, other site

M61.29 Paralytic calcification and ossification of muscle, multiple sites

M61.3 Calcification and ossification of muscles associated with burns

Myositis ossificans associated with burns

M61.30 Calcification and ossification of muscles associated with burns, unspecified site

M61.31 Calcification and ossification of muscles associated with burns, shoulder

M61.311 Calcification and ossification of muscles associated with burns, right shoulder

M61.312 Calcification and ossification of muscles associated with burns, left shoulder

M61.319 Calcification and ossification of muscles associated with burns, unspecified shoulder

M61.32 Calcification and ossification of muscles associated with burns, upper arm

M61.321 Calcification and ossification of muscles associated with burns, right upper arm

M61.322 Calcification and ossification of muscles associated with burns, left upper arm

M61.329 Calcification and ossification of muscles associated with burns, unspecified upper arm

M61.33 Calcification and ossification of muscles associated with burns, forearm

M61.331 Calcification and ossification of muscles associated with burns, right forearm

M61.332 Calcification and ossification of muscles associated with burns, left forearm

M61.339 Calcification and ossification of muscles associated with burns, unspecified forearm

M61.34 Calcification and ossification of muscles associated with burns, hand

M61.341 Calcification and ossification of muscles associated with burns, right hand

M61.342 Calcification and ossification of muscles associated with burns, left hand

M61.349 Calcification and ossification of muscles associated with burns, unspecified hand

M61.35 Calcification and ossification of muscles associated with burns, thigh

M61.351 Calcification and ossification of muscles associated with burns, right thigh

M61.352 Calcification and ossification of muscles associated with burns, left thigh

M61.359 Calcification and ossification of muscles associated with burns, unspecified thigh

M61.36 Calcification and ossification of muscles associated with burns, lower leg

M61.361 Calcification and ossification of muscles associated with burns, right lower leg

M61.362 Calcification and ossification of muscles associated with burns, left lower leg

M61.369 Calcification and ossification of muscles associated with burns, unspecified lower leg

M61.37 Calcification and ossification of muscles associated with burns, ankle and foot

M61.371 Calcification and ossification of muscles associated with burns, right ankle and foot

M61.372 Calcification and ossification of muscles associated with burns, left ankle and foot

M61.379 Calcification and ossification of muscles associated with burns, unspecified ankle and foot

M61.38 Calcification and ossification of muscles associated with burns, other site

M61.39 Calcification and ossification of muscles associated with burns, multiple sites

PDx Unacceptable principal diagnosis symbol per Medicare code edits · PDx Code exempt from diagnosis present on admission requirement

? Questionable admission · CC Complication or comorbidity · MCC Major complication or comorbidity · CC-MCC-EXC CC/MCC exclusion

HCC HCC diagnosis code · RxHCC RxHCC diagnosis code · MACRA code · **DEFINITION** Describes condition/terminology

TIP Coding guidance · Official Guideline Reference · Z1 Z code as first-listed diagnosis

820

When symbols appear on a code that requires a 7th character extension, refer to Appendix B to identify applicable 7th character codes.

2020 ICD-10-CM

M61.4 Other calcification of muscle
> EXCLUDES1 calcific tendinitis NOS (M65.2-)
> calcific tendinitis of shoulder (M75.3)

M61.40 Other calcification of muscle, unspecified site

M61.41 Other calcification of muscle, shoulder
- M61.411 Other calcification of muscle, right shoulder
- M61.412 Other calcification of muscle, left shoulder
- M61.419 Other calcification of muscle, unspecified shoulder

M61.42 Other calcification of muscle, upper arm
- M61.421 Other calcification of muscle, right upper arm
- M61.422 Other calcification of muscle, left upper arm
- M61.429 Other calcification of muscle, unspecified upper arm

M61.43 Other calcification of muscle, forearm
- M61.431 Other calcification of muscle, right forearm
- M61.432 Other calcification of muscle, left forearm
- M61.439 Other calcification of muscle, unspecified forearm

M61.44 Other calcification of muscle, hand
- M61.441 Other calcification of muscle, right hand
- M61.442 Other calcification of muscle, left hand
- M61.449 Other calcification of muscle, unspecified hand

M61.45 Other calcification of muscle, thigh
- M61.451 Other calcification of muscle, right thigh
- M61.452 Other calcification of muscle, left thigh
- M61.459 Other calcification of muscle, unspecified thigh

M61.46 Other calcification of muscle, lower leg
- M61.461 Other calcification of muscle, right lower leg
- M61.462 Other calcification of muscle, left lower leg
- M61.469 Other calcification of muscle, unspecified lower leg

M61.47 Other calcification of muscle, ankle and foot
- M61.471 Other calcification of muscle, right ankle and foot
- M61.472 Other calcification of muscle, left ankle and foot
- M61.479 Other calcification of muscle, unspecified ankle and foot

M61.48 Other calcification of muscle, other site
M61.49 Other calcification of muscle, multiple sites

M61.5 Other ossification of muscle
M61.50 Other ossification of muscle, unspecified site

M61.51 Other ossification of muscle, shoulder
- M61.511 Other ossification of muscle, right shoulder
- M61.512 Other ossification of muscle, left shoulder
- M61.519 Other ossification of muscle, unspecified shoulder

M61.52 Other ossification of muscle, upper arm
- M61.521 Other ossification of muscle, right upper arm
- M61.522 Other ossification of muscle, left upper arm
- M61.529 Other ossification of muscle, unspecified upper arm

M61.53 Other ossification of muscle, forearm
- M61.531 Other ossification of muscle, right forearm
- M61.532 Other ossification of muscle, left forearm
- M61.539 Other ossification of muscle, unspecified forearm

M61.54 Other ossification of muscle, hand
- M61.541 Other ossification of muscle, right hand
- M61.542 Other ossification of muscle, left hand
- M61.549 Other ossification of muscle, unspecified hand

M61.55 Other ossification of muscle, thigh
- M61.551 Other ossification of muscle, right thigh
- M61.552 Other ossification of muscle, left thigh
- M61.559 Other ossification of muscle, unspecified thigh

M61.56 Other ossification of muscle, lower leg
- M61.561 Other ossification of muscle, right lower leg
- M61.562 Other ossification of muscle, left lower leg
- M61.569 Other ossification of muscle, unspecified lower leg

M61.57 Other ossification of muscle, ankle and foot
- M61.571 Other ossification of muscle, right ankle and foot
- M61.572 Other ossification of muscle, left ankle and foot
- M61.579 Other ossification of muscle, unspecified ankle and foot

M61.58 Other ossification of muscle, other site
M61.59 Other ossification of muscle, multiple sites
M61.9 Calcification and ossification of muscle, unspecified

M62 Other disorders of muscle
> EXCLUDES1 alcoholic myopathy (G72.1)
> cramp and spasm (R25.2)
> drug-induced myopathy (G72.0)
> myalgia (M79.1-)
> stiff-man syndrome (G25.82)
> EXCLUDES2 nontraumatic hematoma of muscle (M79.81)

M62.0 Separation of muscle (nontraumatic)
> Diastasis of muscle
> EXCLUDES1 diastasis recti complicating pregnancy, labor and delivery (O71.8)
> traumatic separation of muscle- see strain of muscle by body region

M62.00 Separation of muscle (nontraumatic), unspecified site

M62.01 Separation of muscle (nontraumatic), shoulder
- M62.011 Separation of muscle (nontraumatic), right shoulder
- M62.012 Separation of muscle (nontraumatic), left shoulder
- M62.019 Separation of muscle (nontraumatic), unspecified shoulder

M62.02 Separation of muscle (nontraumatic), upper arm
- M62.021 Separation of muscle (nontraumatic), right upper arm
- M62.022 Separation of muscle (nontraumatic), left upper arm
- M62.029 Separation of muscle (nontraumatic), unspecified upper arm

M62.03 Separation of muscle (nontraumatic), forearm
- M62.031 Separation of muscle (nontraumatic), right forearm
- M62.032 Separation of muscle (nontraumatic), left forearm
- M62.039 Separation of muscle (nontraumatic), unspecified forearm

M62.04 Separation of muscle (nontraumatic), hand
- M62.041 Separation of muscle (nontraumatic), right hand
- M62.042 Separation of muscle (nontraumatic), left hand
- M62.049 Separation of muscle (nontraumatic), unspecified hand

Unspecified Code   Other Specified Code   Manifestation Code   N Newborn   P Pediatric   M Maternity   A Adult   ♂ Male   ♀ Female
● New Code   ▲ Revised Code Title   ►◄ Revised Text   NOTES   INCLUDES   EXCLUDES1 Not coded here   EXCLUDES2 Not included here
4ᵗʰ character required   5ᵗʰ character required   6ᵗʰ character required   7ᵗʰ character required   Extension 'X' Alert
HAC Hospital-acquired condition (HAC) alert   AHA AHA Coding Clinic©   ☞ Code first alert

CHAPTER 13: DISEASES OF THE MUSCULOSKELETAL SYSTEM AND CONNECTIVE TISSUE (M00-M99)

M62.05 - M62.279

6ᵗʰ **M62.05** Separation of muscle (nontraumatic), thigh

    M62.051 Separation of muscle (nontraumatic), right thigh

    M62.052 Separation of muscle (nontraumatic), left thigh

    M62.059 Separation of muscle (nontraumatic), unspecified thigh

6ᵗʰ **M62.06** Separation of muscle (nontraumatic), lower leg

    M62.061 Separation of muscle (nontraumatic), right lower leg

    M62.062 Separation of muscle (nontraumatic), left lower leg

    M62.069 Separation of muscle (nontraumatic), unspecified lower leg

6ᵗʰ **M62.07** Separation of muscle (nontraumatic), ankle and foot

    M62.071 Separation of muscle (nontraumatic), right ankle and foot

    M62.072 Separation of muscle (nontraumatic), left ankle and foot

    M62.079 Separation of muscle (nontraumatic), unspecified ankle and foot

M62.08 Separation of muscle (nontraumatic), other site

5ᵗʰ **M62.1** Other rupture of muscle (nontraumatic)

    EXCLUDES1 traumatic rupture of muscle - see strain of muscle by body region

    EXCLUDES2 rupture of tendon (M66.-)

M62.10 Other rupture of muscle (nontraumatic), unspecified site

6ᵗʰ **M62.11** Other rupture of muscle (nontraumatic), shoulder

    M62.111 Other rupture of muscle (nontraumatic), right shoulder

    M62.112 Other rupture of muscle (nontraumatic), left shoulder

    M62.119 Other rupture of muscle (nontraumatic), unspecified shoulder

6ᵗʰ **M62.12** Other rupture of muscle (nontraumatic), upper arm

    M62.121 Other rupture of muscle (nontraumatic), right upper arm

    M62.122 Other rupture of muscle (nontraumatic), left upper arm

    M62.129 Other rupture of muscle (nontraumatic), unspecified upper arm

6ᵗʰ **M62.13** Other rupture of muscle (nontraumatic), forearm

    M62.131 Other rupture of muscle (nontraumatic), right forearm

    M62.132 Other rupture of muscle (nontraumatic), left forearm

    M62.139 Other rupture of muscle (nontraumatic), unspecified forearm

5ᵗʰ **M62.14** Other rupture of muscle (nontraumatic), hand

    M62.141 Other rupture of muscle (nontraumatic), right hand

    M62.142 Other rupture of muscle (nontraumatic), left hand

    M62.149 Other rupture of muscle (nontraumatic), unspecified hand

6ᵗʰ **M62.15** Other rupture of muscle (nontraumatic), thigh

    M62.151 Other rupture of muscle (nontraumatic), right thigh

    M62.152 Other rupture of muscle (nontraumatic), left thigh

    M62.159 Other rupture of muscle (nontraumatic), unspecified thigh

6ᵗʰ **M62.16** Other rupture of muscle (nontraumatic), lower leg

    M62.161 Other rupture of muscle (nontraumatic), right lower leg

    M62.162 Other rupture of muscle (nontraumatic), left lower leg

    M62.169 Other rupture of muscle (nontraumatic), unspecified lower leg

6ᵗʰ **M62.17** Other rupture of muscle (nontraumatic), ankle and foot

    M62.171 Other rupture of muscle (nontraumatic), right ankle and foot

    M62.172 Other rupture of muscle (nontraumatic), left ankle and foot

    M62.179 Other rupture of muscle (nontraumatic), unspecified ankle and foot

M62.18 Other rupture of muscle (nontraumatic), other site

5ᵗʰ **M62.2** Nontraumatic ischemic infarction of muscle

    EXCLUDES1 compartment syndrome (traumatic) (T79.A-)

        nontraumatic compartment syndrome (M79.A-)

        traumatic ischemia of muscle (T79.6)

        rhabdomyolysis (M62.82)

        Volkmann's ischemic contracture (T79.6)

M62.20 Nontraumatic ischemic infarction of muscle, unspecified site

6ᵗʰ **M62.21** Nontraumatic ischemic infarction of muscle, shoulder

    M62.211 Nontraumatic ischemic infarction of muscle, right shoulder

    M62.212 Nontraumatic ischemic infarction of muscle, left shoulder

    M62.219 Nontraumatic ischemic infarction of muscle, unspecified shoulder

6ᵗʰ **M62.22** Nontraumatic ischemic infarction of muscle, upper arm

    M62.221 Nontraumatic ischemic infarction of muscle, right upper arm

    M62.222 Nontraumatic ischemic infarction of muscle, left upper arm

    M62.229 Nontraumatic ischemic infarction of muscle, unspecified upper arm

6ᵗʰ **M62.23** Nontraumatic ischemic infarction of muscle, forearm

    M62.231 Nontraumatic ischemic infarction of muscle, right forearm

    M62.232 Nontraumatic ischemic infarction of muscle, left forearm

    M62.239 Nontraumatic ischemic infarction of muscle, unspecified forearm

6ᵗʰ **M62.24** Nontraumatic ischemic infarction of muscle, hand

    M62.241 Nontraumatic ischemic infarction of muscle, right hand

    M62.242 Nontraumatic ischemic infarction of muscle, left hand

    M62.249 Nontraumatic ischemic infarction of muscle, unspecified hand

6ᵗʰ **M62.25** Nontraumatic ischemic infarction of muscle, thigh

    M62.251 Nontraumatic ischemic infarction of muscle, right thigh

    M62.252 Nontraumatic ischemic infarction of muscle, left thigh

    M62.259 Nontraumatic ischemic infarction of muscle, unspecified thigh

6ᵗʰ **M62.26** Nontraumatic ischemic infarction of muscle, lower leg

    M62.261 Nontraumatic ischemic infarction of muscle, right lower leg

    M62.262 Nontraumatic ischemic infarction of muscle, left lower leg

    M62.269 Nontraumatic ischemic infarction of muscle, unspecified lower leg

6ᵗʰ **M62.27** Nontraumatic ischemic infarction of muscle, ankle and foot

    M62.271 Nontraumatic ischemic infarction of muscle, right ankle and foot

    M62.272 Nontraumatic ischemic infarction of muscle, left ankle and foot

    M62.279 Nontraumatic ischemic infarction of muscle, unspecified ankle and foot

---

PDₓ Unacceptable principal diagnosis symbol per Medicare code edits   POA Code exempt from diagnosis present on admission requirement

❓ Questionable admission   CC Complication or comorbidity   MCC Major complication or comorbidity   CC/MCC EXC CC/MCC exclusion

HCC HCC diagnosis code   RxHCC RxHCC diagnosis code   MACRA code   **DEFINITION** Describes condition/terminology

TIP Coding guidance   👁 Official Guideline Reference   Z1 Z code as first-listed diagnosis

M62.28 Nontraumatic ischemic infarction of muscle, other site

M62.3 Immobility syndrome (paraplegic) cc© CC/MCC Exc

5ᵗʰ M62.4 Contracture of muscle
Contracture of tendon (sheath)
EXCLUDES1 contracture of joint (M24.5-)
M62.40 Contracture of muscle, unspecified site

6ᵗʰ M62.41 Contracture of muscle, shoulder
M62.411 Contracture of muscle, right shoulder
M62.412 Contracture of muscle, left shoulder
M62.419 Contracture of muscle, unspecified shoulder

6ᵗʰ M62.42 Contracture of muscle, upper arm
M62.421 Contracture of muscle, right upper arm
M62.422 Contracture of muscle, left upper arm
M62.429 Contracture of muscle, unspecified upper arm

6ᵗʰ M62.43 Contracture of muscle, forearm
M62.431 Contracture of muscle, right forearm
M62.432 Contracture of muscle, left forearm
M62.439 Contracture of muscle, unspecified forearm

6ᵗʰ M62.44 Contracture of muscle, hand
M62.441 Contracture of muscle, right hand
M62.442 Contracture of muscle, left hand
M62.449 Contracture of muscle, unspecified hand

6ᵗʰ M62.45 Contracture of muscle, thigh
M62.451 Contracture of muscle, right thigh
M62.452 Contracture of muscle, left thigh
M62.459 Contracture of muscle, unspecified thigh

6ᵗʰ M62.46 Contracture of muscle, lower leg
M62.461 Contracture of muscle, right lower leg
M62.462 Contracture of muscle, left lower leg
M62.469 Contracture of muscle, unspecified lower leg

6ᵗʰ M62.47 Contracture of muscle, ankle and foot
M62.471 Contracture of muscle, right ankle and foot
M62.472 Contracture of muscle, left ankle and foot
M62.479 Contracture of muscle, unspecified ankle and foot

M62.48 Contracture of muscle, other site
M62.49 Contracture of muscle, multiple sites

5ᵗʰ M62.5 Muscle wasting and atrophy, not elsewhere classified
Disuse atrophy NEC
EXCLUDES1 neuralgic amyotrophy (G54.5)
progressive muscular atrophy (G12.21)
sarcopenia (M62.84)
EXCLUDES2 pelvic muscle wasting (N81.84)
M62.50 Muscle wasting and atrophy, not elsewhere classified, unspecified site

6ᵗʰ M62.51 Muscle wasting and atrophy, not elsewhere classified, shoulder
M62.511 Muscle wasting and atrophy, not elsewhere classified, right shoulder
M62.512 Muscle wasting and atrophy, not elsewhere classified, left shoulder
M62.519 Muscle wasting and atrophy, not elsewhere classified, unspecified shoulder

6ᵗʰ M62.52 Muscle wasting and atrophy, not elsewhere classified, upper arm
M62.521 Muscle wasting and atrophy, not elsewhere classified, right upper arm
M62.522 Muscle wasting and atrophy, not elsewhere classified, left upper arm
M62.529 Muscle wasting and atrophy, not elsewhere classified, unspecified upper arm

6ᵗʰ M62.53 Muscle wasting and atrophy, not elsewhere classified, forearm
M62.531 Muscle wasting and atrophy, not elsewhere classified, right forearm
M62.532 Muscle wasting and atrophy, not elsewhere classified, left forearm
M62.539 Muscle wasting and atrophy, not elsewhere classified, unspecified forearm

6ᵗʰ M62.54 Muscle wasting and atrophy, not elsewhere classified, hand
M62.541 Muscle wasting and atrophy, not elsewhere classified, right hand
M62.542 Muscle wasting and atrophy, not elsewhere classified, left hand
M62.549 Muscle wasting and atrophy, not elsewhere classified, unspecified hand

6ᵗʰ M62.55 Muscle wasting and atrophy, not elsewhere classified, thigh
M62.551 Muscle wasting and atrophy, not elsewhere classified, right thigh
M62.552 Muscle wasting and atrophy, not elsewhere classified, left thigh
M62.559 Muscle wasting and atrophy, not elsewhere classified, unspecified thigh

6ᵗʰ M62.56 Muscle wasting and atrophy, not elsewhere classified, lower leg
M62.561 Muscle wasting and atrophy, not elsewhere classified, right lower leg
M62.562 Muscle wasting and atrophy, not elsewhere classified, left lower leg
M62.569 Muscle wasting and atrophy, not elsewhere classified, unspecified lower leg

6ᵗʰ M62.57 Muscle wasting and atrophy, not elsewhere classified, ankle and foot
M62.571 Muscle wasting and atrophy, not elsewhere classified, right ankle and foot
M62.572 Muscle wasting and atrophy, not elsewhere classified, left ankle and foot
M62.579 Muscle wasting and atrophy, not elsewhere classified, unspecified ankle and foot

M62.58 Muscle wasting and atrophy, not elsewhere classified, other site
M62.59 Muscle wasting and atrophy, not elsewhere classified, multiple sites

5ᵗʰ M62.8 Other specified disorders of muscle
EXCLUDES2 nontraumatic hematoma of muscle (M79.81)
M62.81 Muscle weakness (generalized)
EXCLUDES1 muscle weakness in sarcopenia (M62.84)
M62.82 Rhabdomyolysis cc© CC/MCC Exc
AHA: Q2 2019
EXCLUDES1 traumatic rhabdomyolysis (T79.6)

6ᵗʰ M62.83 Muscle spasm
M62.830 Muscle spasm of back
M62.831 Muscle spasm of calf
Charley-horse
M62.838 Other muscle spasm

M62.84 Sarcopenia
Age-related sarcopenia
☞ Code first underlying disease, if applicable, such as:
disorders of myoneural junction and muscle disease in diseases classified elsewhere (G73.-)
other and unspecified myopathies (G72.-)
primary disorders of muscles (G71.-)

M62.89 Other specified disorders of muscle
Muscle (sheath) hernia
M62.9 Disorder of muscle, unspecified

Unspecified Code   Other Specified Code   Manifestation Code   🄽 Newborn   🄿 Pediatric   🄼 Maternity   🄰 Adult   ♂ Male   ♀ Female
● New Code   ▲ Revised Code Title   ►◄ Revised Text   **NOTES**   *INCLUDES*   *EXCLUDES1* Not coded here   *EXCLUDES2* Not included here
4ᵗʰ 4ᵗʰ character required   5ᵗʰ 5ᵗʰ character required   6ᵗʰ 6ᵗʰ character required   7ᵗʰ 7ᵗʰ character required   7ᵗʰ Extension 'X' Alert
HAC Hospital-acquired condition (HAC) alert   **AHA** AHA Coding Clinic©   ☞ Code first alert

M63 Disorders of muscle in diseases classified elsewhere

☞ **Code first** underlying disease, such as:

leprosy (A30.-)
neoplasm (C49.-, C79.89, D21.-, D48.1)
schistosomiasis (B65.-)
trichinellosis (B75)

EXCLUDES1 myopathy in cysticercosis (B69.81)
myopathy in endocrine diseases (G73.7)
myopathy in metabolic diseases (G73.7)
myopathy in sarcoidosis (D86.87)
myopathy in secondary syphilis (A51.49)
myopathy in syphilis (late) (A52.78)
myopathy in toxoplasmosis (B58.82)
myopathy in tuberculosis (A18.09)

M63.8 Disorders of muscle in diseases classified elsewhere

M63.80 Disorders of muscle in diseases classified elsewhere, unspecified site

M63.81 Disorders of muscle in diseases classified elsewhere, shoulder

M63.811 Disorders of muscle in diseases classified elsewhere, right shoulder

M63.812 Disorders of muscle in diseases classified elsewhere, left shoulder

M63.819 Disorders of muscle in diseases classified elsewhere, unspecified shoulder

M63.82 Disorders of muscle in diseases classified elsewhere, upper arm

M63.821 Disorders of muscle in diseases classified elsewhere, right upper arm

M63.822 Disorders of muscle in diseases classified elsewhere, left upper arm

M63.829 Disorders of muscle in diseases classified elsewhere, unspecified upper arm

M63.83 Disorders of muscle in diseases classified elsewhere, forearm

M63.831 Disorders of muscle in diseases classified elsewhere, right forearm

M63.832 Disorders of muscle in diseases classified elsewhere, left forearm

M63.839 Disorders of muscle in diseases classified elsewhere, unspecified forearm

M63.84 Disorders of muscle in diseases classified elsewhere, hand

M63.841 Disorders of muscle in diseases classified elsewhere, right hand

M63.842 Disorders of muscle in diseases classified elsewhere, left hand

M63.849 Disorders of muscle in diseases classified elsewhere, unspecified hand

M63.85 Disorders of muscle in diseases classified elsewhere, thigh

M63.851 Disorders of muscle in diseases classified elsewhere, right thigh

M63.852 Disorders of muscle in diseases classified elsewhere, left thigh

M63.859 Disorders of muscle in diseases classified elsewhere, unspecified thigh

M63.86 Disorders of muscle in diseases classified elsewhere, lower leg

M63.861 Disorders of muscle in diseases classified elsewhere, right lower leg

M63.862 Disorders of muscle in diseases classified elsewhere, left lower leg

M63.869 Disorders of muscle in diseases classified elsewhere, unspecified lower leg

M63.87 Disorders of muscle in diseases classified elsewhere, ankle and foot

M63.871 Disorders of muscle in diseases classified elsewhere, right ankle and foot

M63.872 Disorders of muscle in diseases classified elsewhere, left ankle and foot

M63.879 Disorders of muscle in diseases classified elsewhere, unspecified ankle and foot

M63.88 Disorders of muscle in diseases classified elsewhere, other site

M63.89 Disorders of muscle in diseases classified elsewhere, multiple sites

Disorders of synovium and tendon (M65-M67)

M65 Synovitis and tenosynovitis

EXCLUDES1 chronic crepitant synovitis of hand and wrist (M70.0-)
current injury - see injury of ligament or tendon by body region
soft tissue disorders related to use, overuse and pressure (M70.-)

M65.0 Abscess of tendon sheath

Use additional code (B95-B96) to identify bacterial agent.

M65.00 Abscess of tendon sheath, unspecified site

M65.01 Abscess of tendon sheath, shoulder

M65.011 Abscess of tendon sheath, right shoulder

M65.012 Abscess of tendon sheath, left shoulder

M65.019 Abscess of tendon sheath, unspecified shoulder

M65.02 Abscess of tendon sheath, upper arm

M65.021 Abscess of tendon sheath, right upper arm

M65.022 Abscess of tendon sheath, left upper arm

M65.029 Abscess of tendon sheath, unspecified upper arm

M65.03 Abscess of tendon sheath, forearm

M65.031 Abscess of tendon sheath, right forearm

M65.032 Abscess of tendon sheath, left forearm

M65.039 Abscess of tendon sheath, unspecified forearm

M65.04 Abscess of tendon sheath, hand

M65.041 Abscess of tendon sheath, right hand

M65.042 Abscess of tendon sheath, left hand

M65.049 Abscess of tendon sheath, unspecified hand

M65.05 Abscess of tendon sheath, thigh

M65.051 Abscess of tendon sheath, right thigh

M65.052 Abscess of tendon sheath, left thigh

M65.059 Abscess of tendon sheath, unspecified thigh

M65.06 Abscess of tendon sheath, lower leg

M65.061 Abscess of tendon sheath, right lower leg

M65.062 Abscess of tendon sheath, left lower leg

M65.069 Abscess of tendon sheath, unspecified lower leg

M65.07 Abscess of tendon sheath, ankle and foot

M65.071 Abscess of tendon sheath, right ankle and foot

M65.072 Abscess of tendon sheath, left ankle and foot

M65.079 Abscess of tendon sheath, unspecified ankle and foot

M65.08 Abscess of tendon sheath, other site

M65.1 Other infective (teno)synovitis

M65.10 Other infective (teno)synovitis, unspecified site

M65.11 Other infective (teno)synovitis, shoulder

M65.111 Other infective (teno)synovitis, right shoulder

M65.112 Other infective (teno)synovitis, left shoulder

M65.119 Other infective (teno)synovitis, unspecified shoulder

M65.12 Other infective (teno)synovitis, elbow

M65.121 Other infective (teno)synovitis, right elbow

824

When symbols appear on a code that requires a 7th character extension, refer to Appendix B to identify applicable 7th character codes.

2020 ICD-10-CM

PDX Unacceptable principal diagnosis symbol per Medicare code edits   POA Code exempt from diagnosis present on admission requirement

❓ Questionable admission   CC Complication or comorbidity   MCC Major complication or comorbidity   CC/MCC EXC CC/MCC exclusion

HCC HCC diagnosis code   RxHCC RxHCC diagnosis code   MACRA code   **DEFINITION** Describes condition/terminology

TIP Coding guidance   👁 Official Guideline Reference   Z Z code as first-listed diagnosis

M65.122 Other infective (teno)synovitis, left elbow
M65.129 Other infective (teno)synovitis, unspecified elbow
[6th] M65.13 Other infective (teno)synovitis, wrist
M65.131 Other infective (teno)synovitis, right wrist
M65.132 Other infective (teno)synovitis, left wrist
M65.139 Other infective (teno)synovitis, unspecified wrist
[6th] M65.14 Other infective (teno)synovitis, hand
M65.141 Other infective (teno)synovitis, right hand
M65.142 Other infective (teno)synovitis, left hand
M65.149 Other infective (teno)synovitis, unspecified hand
[6th] M65.15 Other infective (teno)synovitis, hip
M65.151 Other infective (teno)synovitis, right hip
M65.152 Other infective (teno)synovitis, left hip
M65.159 Other infective (teno)synovitis, unspecified hip
[6th] M65.16 Other infective (teno)synovitis, knee
M65.161 Other infective (teno)synovitis, right knee
M65.162 Other infective (teno)synovitis, left knee
M65.169 Other infective (teno)synovitis, unspecified knee
[6th] M65.17 Other infective (teno)synovitis, ankle and foot
M65.171 Other infective (teno)synovitis, right ankle and foot
M65.172 Other infective (teno)synovitis, left ankle and foot
M65.179 Other infective (teno)synovitis, unspecified ankle and foot
M65.18 Other infective (teno)synovitis, other site
M65.19 Other infective (teno)synovitis, multiple sites
[5th] M65.2 Calcific tendinitis
EXCLUDES1 *tendinitis as classified in M75-M77*
calcified tendinitis of shoulder (M75.3)
M65.20 Calcific tendinitis, unspecified site
[6th] M65.22 Calcific tendinitis, upper arm
M65.221 Calcific tendinitis, right upper arm
M65.222 Calcific tendinitis, left upper arm
M65.229 Calcific tendinitis, unspecified upper arm
[6th] M65.23 Calcific tendinitis, forearm
M65.231 Calcific tendinitis, right forearm
M65.232 Calcific tendinitis, left forearm
M65.239 Calcific tendinitis, unspecified forearm
[6th] M65.24 Calcific tendinitis, hand
M65.241 Calcific tendinitis, right hand
M65.242 Calcific tendinitis, left hand
M65.249 Calcific tendinitis, unspecified hand
[6th] M65.25 Calcific tendinitis, thigh
M65.251 Calcific tendinitis, right thigh
M65.252 Calcific tendinitis, left thigh
M65.259 Calcific tendinitis, unspecified thigh
[6th] M65.26 Calcific tendinitis, lower leg
M65.261 Calcific tendinitis, right lower leg
M65.262 Calcific tendinitis, left lower leg
M65.269 Calcific tendinitis, unspecified lower leg
[6th] M65.27 Calcific tendinitis, ankle and foot
M65.271 Calcific tendinitis, right ankle and foot
M65.272 Calcific tendinitis, left ankle and foot
M65.279 Calcific tendinitis, unspecified ankle and foot
M65.28 Calcific tendinitis, other site
M65.29 Calcific tendinitis, multiple sites
[5th] M65.3 Trigger finger
DEFINITION: Trigger finger occurs when the tendon sheath of the finger is inflammed and causes the finger to stick in a bent position.
Nodular tendinous disease
M65.30 Trigger finger, unspecified finger
[6th] M65.31 Trigger thumb
M65.311 Trigger thumb, right thumb
M65.312 Trigger thumb, left thumb
M65.319 Trigger thumb, unspecified thumb
[6th] M65.32 Trigger finger, index finger
M65.321 Trigger finger, right index finger
M65.322 Trigger finger, left index finger
M65.329 Trigger finger, unspecified index finger
[6th] M65.33 Trigger finger, middle finger
M65.331 Trigger finger, right middle finger
M65.332 Trigger finger, left middle finger
M65.339 Trigger finger, unspecified middle finger
[6th] M65.34 Trigger finger, ring finger
M65.341 Trigger finger, right ring finger
M65.342 Trigger finger, left ring finger
M65.349 Trigger finger, unspecified ring finger
[6th] M65.35 Trigger finger, little finger
M65.351 Trigger finger, right little finger
M65.352 Trigger finger, left little finger
M65.359 Trigger finger, unspecified little finger
M65.4 Radial styloid tenosynovitis [de Quervain]
[5th] M65.8 Other synovitis and tenosynovitis
M65.80 Other synovitis and tenosynovitis, unspecified site
[6th] M65.81 Other synovitis and tenosynovitis, shoulder
M65.811 Other synovitis and tenosynovitis, right shoulder
M65.812 Other synovitis and tenosynovitis, left shoulder
M65.819 Other synovitis and tenosynovitis, unspecified shoulder
[6th] M65.82 Other synovitis and tenosynovitis, upper arm
M65.821 Other synovitis and tenosynovitis, right upper arm
M65.822 Other synovitis and tenosynovitis, left upper arm
M65.829 Other synovitis and tenosynovitis, unspecified upper arm
[6th] M65.83 Other synovitis and tenosynovitis, forearm
M65.831 Other synovitis and tenosynovitis, right forearm
M65.832 Other synovitis and tenosynovitis, left forearm
M65.839 Other synovitis and tenosynovitis, unspecified forearm
[6th] M65.84 Other synovitis and tenosynovitis, hand
M65.841 Other synovitis and tenosynovitis, right hand
M65.842 Other synovitis and tenosynovitis, left hand
M65.849 Other synovitis and tenosynovitis, unspecified hand
[6th] M65.85 Other synovitis and tenosynovitis, thigh
M65.851 Other synovitis and tenosynovitis, right thigh
M65.852 Other synovitis and tenosynovitis, left thigh
M65.859 Other synovitis and tenosynovitis, unspecified thigh
[6th] M65.86 Other synovitis and tenosynovitis, lower leg
M65.861 Other synovitis and tenosynovitis, right lower leg
M65.862 Other synovitis and tenosynovitis, left lower leg
M65.869 Other synovitis and tenosynovitis, unspecified lower leg
[6th] M65.87 Other synovitis and tenosynovitis, ankle and foot
M65.871 Other synovitis and tenosynovitis, right ankle and foot
M65.872 Other synovitis and tenosynovitis, left ankle and foot

Unspecified Code Other Specified Code Manifestation Code [N] Newborn [P] Pediatric [M] Maternity [A] Adult ♂ Male ♀ Female
● New Code ▲ Revised Code Title ►◄ Revised Text NOTES INCLUDES EXCLUDES1 Not coded here EXCLUDES2 Not included here
[4th] 4th character required [5th] 5th character required [6th] 6th character required [7th] 7th character required [7th] Extension 'X' Alert
[HAC] Hospital-acquired condition (HAC) alert AHA AHA Coding Clinic© ☛ Code first alert

M65.879 Other synovitis and tenosynovitis, unspecified ankle and foot

M65.88 Other synovitis and tenosynovitis, other site

M65.89 Other synovitis and tenosynovitis, multiple sites

M65.9 Synovitis and tenosynovitis, unspecified

4ᵗʰ M66 Spontaneous rupture of synovium and tendon

INCLUDES   rupture that occurs when a normal force is applied to tissues that are inferred to have less than normal strength

EXCLUDES2   rotator cuff syndrome (M75.1-)

     rupture where an abnormal force is applied to normal tissue - see injury of tendon by body region

M66.0 Rupture of popliteal cyst

5ᵗʰ M66.1 Rupture of synovium

Rupture of synovial cyst

EXCLUDES2 rupture of popliteal cyst (M66.0)

M66.10 Rupture of synovium, unspecified joint

6ᵗʰ M66.11 Rupture of synovium, shoulder

     M66.111 Rupture of synovium, right shoulder

     M66.112 Rupture of synovium, left shoulder

     M66.119 Rupture of synovium, unspecified shoulder

6ᵗʰ M66.12 Rupture of synovium, elbow

     M66.121 Rupture of synovium, right elbow

     M66.122 Rupture of synovium, left elbow

     M66.129 Rupture of synovium, unspecified elbow

6ᵗʰ M66.13 Rupture of synovium, wrist

     M66.131 Rupture of synovium, right wrist

     M66.132 Rupture of synovium, left wrist

     M66.139 Rupture of synovium, unspecified wrist

6ᵗʰ M66.14 Rupture of synovium, hand and fingers

     M66.141 Rupture of synovium, right hand

     M66.142 Rupture of synovium, left hand

     M66.143 Rupture of synovium, unspecified hand

     M66.144 Rupture of synovium, right finger(s)

     M66.145 Rupture of synovium, left finger(s)

     M66.146 Rupture of synovium, unspecified finger(s)

6ᵗʰ M66.15 Rupture of synovium, hip

     M66.151 Rupture of synovium, right hip

     M66.152 Rupture of synovium, left hip

     M66.159 Rupture of synovium, unspecified hip

6ᵗʰ M66.17 Rupture of synovium, ankle, foot and toes

     M66.171 Rupture of synovium, right ankle

     M66.172 Rupture of synovium, left ankle

     M66.173 Rupture of synovium, unspecified ankle

     M66.174 Rupture of synovium, right foot

     M66.175 Rupture of synovium, left foot

     M66.176 Rupture of synovium, unspecified foot

     M66.177 Rupture of synovium, right toe(s)

     M66.178 Rupture of synovium, left toe(s)

     M66.179 Rupture of synovium, unspecified toe(s)

M66.18 Rupture of synovium, other site

5ᵗʰ M66.2 Spontaneous rupture of extensor tendons

M66.20 Spontaneous rupture of extensor tendons, unspecified site

6ᵗʰ M66.21 Spontaneous rupture of extensor tendons, shoulder

     M66.211 Spontaneous rupture of extensor tendons, right shoulder

     M66.212 Spontaneous rupture of extensor tendons, left shoulder

     M66.219 Spontaneous rupture of extensor tendons, unspecified shoulder

6ᵗʰ M66.22 Spontaneous rupture of extensor tendons, upper arm

     M66.221 Spontaneous rupture of extensor tendons, right upper arm

     M66.222 Spontaneous rupture of extensor tendons, left upper arm

     M66.229 Spontaneous rupture of extensor tendons, unspecified upper arm

6ᵗʰ M66.23 Spontaneous rupture of extensor tendons, forearm

     M66.231 Spontaneous rupture of extensor tendons, right forearm

     M66.232 Spontaneous rupture of extensor tendons, left forearm

     M66.239 Spontaneous rupture of extensor tendons, unspecified forearm

6ᵗʰ M66.24 Spontaneous rupture of extensor tendons, hand

     M66.241 Spontaneous rupture of extensor tendons, right hand

     M66.242 Spontaneous rupture of extensor tendons, left hand

     M66.249 Spontaneous rupture of extensor tendons, unspecified hand

6ᵗʰ M66.25 Spontaneous rupture of extensor tendons, thigh

     M66.251 Spontaneous rupture of extensor tendons, right thigh

     M66.252 Spontaneous rupture of extensor tendons, left thigh

     M66.259 Spontaneous rupture of extensor tendons, unspecified thigh

6ᵗʰ M66.26 Spontaneous rupture of extensor tendons, lower leg

     M66.261 Spontaneous rupture of extensor tendons, right lower leg

     M66.262 Spontaneous rupture of extensor tendons, left lower leg

     M66.269 Spontaneous rupture of extensor tendons, unspecified lower leg

6ᵗʰ M66.27 Spontaneous rupture of extensor tendons, ankle and foot

     M66.271 Spontaneous rupture of extensor tendons, right ankle and foot

     M66.272 Spontaneous rupture of extensor tendons, left ankle and foot

     M66.279 Spontaneous rupture of extensor tendons, unspecified ankle and foot

M66.28 Spontaneous rupture of extensor tendons, other site

M66.29 Spontaneous rupture of extensor tendons, multiple sites

5ᵗʰ M66.3 Spontaneous rupture of flexor tendons

M66.30 Spontaneous rupture of flexor tendons, unspecified site

6ᵗʰ M66.31 Spontaneous rupture of flexor tendons, shoulder

     M66.311 Spontaneous rupture of flexor tendons, right shoulder

     M66.312 Spontaneous rupture of flexor tendons, left shoulder

     M66.319 Spontaneous rupture of flexor tendons, unspecified shoulder

6ᵗʰ M66.32 Spontaneous rupture of flexor tendons, upper arm

     M66.321 Spontaneous rupture of flexor tendons, right upper arm

     M66.322 Spontaneous rupture of flexor tendons, left upper arm

     M66.329 Spontaneous rupture of flexor tendons, unspecified upper arm

6ᵗʰ M66.33 Spontaneous rupture of flexor tendons, forearm

     M66.331 Spontaneous rupture of flexor tendons, right forearm

     M66.332 Spontaneous rupture of flexor tendons, left forearm

     M66.339 Spontaneous rupture of flexor tendons, unspecified forearm

6ᵗʰ M66.34 Spontaneous rupture of flexor tendons, hand

     M66.341 Spontaneous rupture of flexor tendons, right hand

     M66.342 Spontaneous rupture of flexor tendons, left hand

     M66.349 Spontaneous rupture of flexor tendons, unspecified hand

PDx Unacceptable principal diagnosis symbol per Medicare code edits   Code exempt from diagnosis present on admission requirement

❓ Questionable admission   Complication or comorbidity   MCC Major complication or comorbidity   CC/MCC CC/MCC exclusion

HCC HCC diagnosis code   RxHCC RxHCC diagnosis code   MACRA code   **DEFINITION** Describes condition/terminology

TIP Coding guidance   Official Guideline Reference   Z1 Z code as first-listed diagnosis

826

When symbols appear on a code that requires a 7th character extension, refer to Appendix B to identify applicable 7th character codes.

2020 ICD-10-CM

[6th] M66.35 Spontaneous rupture of flexor tendons, thigh
M66.351 Spontaneous rupture of flexor tendons, right thigh
M66.352 Spontaneous rupture of flexor tendons, left thigh
M66.359 Spontaneous rupture of flexor tendons, unspecified thigh
[6th] M66.36 Spontaneous rupture of flexor tendons, lower leg
M66.361 Spontaneous rupture of flexor tendons, right lower leg
M66.362 Spontaneous rupture of flexor tendons, left lower leg
M66.369 Spontaneous rupture of flexor tendons, unspecified lower leg
[6th] M66.37 Spontaneous rupture of flexor tendons, ankle and foot
M66.371 Spontaneous rupture of flexor tendons, right ankle and foot
M66.372 Spontaneous rupture of flexor tendons, left ankle and foot
M66.379 Spontaneous rupture of flexor tendons, unspecified ankle and foot
M66.38 Spontaneous rupture of flexor tendons, other site
M66.39 Spontaneous rupture of flexor tendons, multiple sites
[5th] M66.8 Spontaneous rupture of other tendons
M66.80 Spontaneous rupture of other tendons, unspecified site
[6th] M66.81 Spontaneous rupture of other tendons, shoulder
M66.811 Spontaneous rupture of other tendons, right shoulder
M66.812 Spontaneous rupture of other tendons, left shoulder
M66.819 Spontaneous rupture of other tendons, unspecified shoulder
[6th] M66.82 Spontaneous rupture of other tendons, upper arm
M66.821 Spontaneous rupture of other tendons, right upper arm
M66.822 Spontaneous rupture of other tendons, left upper arm
M66.829 Spontaneous rupture of other tendons, unspecified upper arm
[6th] M66.83 Spontaneous rupture of other tendons, forearm
M66.831 Spontaneous rupture of other tendons, right forearm
M66.832 Spontaneous rupture of other tendons, left forearm
M66.839 Spontaneous rupture of other tendons, unspecified forearm
[6th] M66.84 Spontaneous rupture of other tendons, hand
M66.841 Spontaneous rupture of other tendons, right hand
M66.842 Spontaneous rupture of other tendons, left hand
M66.849 Spontaneous rupture of other tendons, unspecified hand
[6th] M66.85 Spontaneous rupture of other tendons, thigh
M66.851 Spontaneous rupture of other tendons, right thigh
M66.852 Spontaneous rupture of other tendons, left thigh
M66.859 Spontaneous rupture of other tendons, unspecified thigh
[6th] M66.86 Spontaneous rupture of other tendons, lower leg
M66.861 Spontaneous rupture of other tendons, right lower leg
M66.862 Spontaneous rupture of other tendons, left lower leg
M66.869 Spontaneous rupture of other tendons, unspecified lower leg
[6th] M66.87 Spontaneous rupture of other tendons, ankle and foot
M66.871 Spontaneous rupture of other tendons, right ankle and foot
M66.872 Spontaneous rupture of other tendons, left ankle and foot
M66.879 Spontaneous rupture of other tendons, unspecified ankle and foot
▲ M66.88 Spontaneous rupture of other tendons, other ▶sites◀
M66.89 Spontaneous rupture of other tendons, multiple sites
M66.9 Spontaneous rupture of unspecified tendon
Rupture at musculotendinous junction, nontraumatic
[4th] M67 Other disorders of synovium and tendon
[EXCLUDES1] *palmar fascial fibromatosis [Dupuytren] (M72.0)*
tendinitis NOS (M77.9-)
xanthomatosis localized to tendons (E78.2)
[5th] M67.0 Short Achilles tendon (acquired)
M67.00 Short Achilles tendon (acquired), unspecified ankle
M67.01 Short Achilles tendon (acquired), right ankle
M67.02 Short Achilles tendon (acquired), left ankle
[5th] M67.2 Synovial hypertrophy, not elsewhere classified
[EXCLUDES1] *villonodular synovitis (pigmented) (M12.2-)*
M67.20 Synovial hypertrophy, not elsewhere classified, unspecified site
[6th] M67.21 Synovial hypertrophy, not elsewhere classified, shoulder
M67.211 Synovial hypertrophy, not elsewhere classified, right shoulder
M67.212 Synovial hypertrophy, not elsewhere classified, left shoulder
M67.219 Synovial hypertrophy, not elsewhere classified, unspecified shoulder
[6th] M67.22 Synovial hypertrophy, not elsewhere classified, upper arm
M67.221 Synovial hypertrophy, not elsewhere classified, right upper arm
M67.222 Synovial hypertrophy, not elsewhere classified, left upper arm
M67.229 Synovial hypertrophy, not elsewhere classified, unspecified upper arm
[6th] M67.23 Synovial hypertrophy, not elsewhere classified, forearm
M67.231 Synovial hypertrophy, not elsewhere classified, right forearm
M67.232 Synovial hypertrophy, not elsewhere classified, left forearm
M67.239 Synovial hypertrophy, not elsewhere classified, unspecified forearm
[6th] M67.24 Synovial hypertrophy, not elsewhere classified, hand
M67.241 Synovial hypertrophy, not elsewhere classified, right hand
M67.242 Synovial hypertrophy, not elsewhere classified, left hand
M67.249 Synovial hypertrophy, not elsewhere classified, unspecified hand
[6th] M67.25 Synovial hypertrophy, not elsewhere classified, thigh
M67.251 Synovial hypertrophy, not elsewhere classified, right thigh
M67.252 Synovial hypertrophy, not elsewhere classified, left thigh
M67.259 Synovial hypertrophy, not elsewhere classified, unspecified thigh
[6th] M67.26 Synovial hypertrophy, not elsewhere classified, lower leg
M67.261 Synovial hypertrophy, not elsewhere classified, right lower leg

Unspecified Code Other Specified Code Manifestation Code [N] Newborn [P] Pediatric [M] Maternity [A] Adult ♂ Male ♀ Female
● New Code ▲ Revised Code Title ▶◀ Revised Text [NOTES] [INCLUDES] [EXCLUDES1] Not coded here [EXCLUDES2] Not included here
[4th] 4th character required [5th] 5th character required [6th] 6th character required [7th] 7th character required [x] Extension 'X' Alert
[HAC] Hospital-acquired condition (HAC) alert AHA AHA Coding Clinic© ☞ Code first alert

M67.262 Synovial hypertrophy, not elsewhere classified, left lower leg

M67.269 Synovial hypertrophy, not elsewhere classified, unspecified lower leg

6ᵗʰ M67.27 Synovial hypertrophy, not elsewhere classified, ankle and foot

M67.271 Synovial hypertrophy, not elsewhere classified, right ankle and foot

M67.272 Synovial hypertrophy, not elsewhere classified, left ankle and foot

M67.279 Synovial hypertrophy, not elsewhere classified, unspecified ankle and foot

M67.28 Synovial hypertrophy, not elsewhere classified, other site

M67.29 Synovial hypertrophy, not elsewhere classified, multiple sites

5ᵗʰ M67.3 Transient synovitis

Toxic synovitis

EXCLUDES1 palindromic rheumatism (M12.3-)

M67.30 Transient synovitis, unspecified site

6ᵗʰ M67.31 Transient synovitis, shoulder

M67.311 Transient synovitis, right shoulder

M67.312 Transient synovitis, left shoulder

M67.319 Transient synovitis, unspecified shoulder

6ᵗʰ M67.32 Transient synovitis, elbow

M67.321 Transient synovitis, right elbow

M67.322 Transient synovitis, left elbow

M67.329 Transient synovitis, unspecified elbow

6ᵗʰ M67.33 Transient synovitis, wrist

M67.331 Transient synovitis, right wrist

M67.332 Transient synovitis, left wrist

M67.339 Transient synovitis, unspecified wrist

6ᵗʰ M67.34 Transient synovitis, hand

M67.341 Transient synovitis, right hand

M67.342 Transient synovitis, left hand

M67.349 Transient synovitis, unspecified hand

6ᵗʰ M67.35 Transient synovitis, hip

M67.351 Transient synovitis, right hip

M67.352 Transient synovitis, left hip

M67.359 Transient synovitis, unspecified hip

6ᵗʰ M67.36 Transient synovitis, knee

M67.361 Transient synovitis, right knee

M67.362 Transient synovitis, left knee

M67.369 Transient synovitis, unspecified knee

6ᵗʰ M67.37 Transient synovitis, ankle and foot

M67.371 Transient synovitis, right ankle and foot

M67.372 Transient synovitis, left ankle and foot

M67.379 Transient synovitis, unspecified ankle and foot

M67.38 Transient synovitis, other site

M67.39 Transient synovitis, multiple sites

5ᵗʰ M67.4 Ganglion

Ganglion of joint or tendon (sheath)

EXCLUDES1 ganglion in yaws (A66.6)

EXCLUDES2 cyst of bursa (M71.2-M71.3)

cyst of synovium (M71.2-M71.3)

M67.40 Ganglion, unspecified site

6ᵗʰ M67.41 Ganglion, shoulder

M67.411 Ganglion, right shoulder

M67.412 Ganglion, left shoulder

M67.419 Ganglion, unspecified shoulder

6ᵗʰ M67.42 Ganglion, elbow

M67.421 Ganglion, right elbow

M67.422 Ganglion, left elbow

M67.429 Ganglion, unspecified elbow

6ᵗʰ M67.43 Ganglion, wrist

M67.431 Ganglion, right wrist

M67.432 Ganglion, left wrist

M67.439 Ganglion, unspecified wrist

6ᵗʰ M67.44 Ganglion, hand

M67.441 Ganglion, right hand

M67.442 Ganglion, left hand

M67.449 Ganglion, unspecified hand

6ᵗʰ M67.45 Ganglion, hip

M67.451 Ganglion, right hip

M67.452 Ganglion, left hip

M67.459 Ganglion, unspecified hip

6ᵗʰ M67.46 Ganglion, knee

M67.461 Ganglion, right knee

M67.462 Ganglion, left knee

M67.469 Ganglion, unspecified knee

6ᵗʰ M67.47 Ganglion, ankle and foot

M67.471 Ganglion, right ankle and foot

M67.472 Ganglion, left ankle and foot

M67.479 Ganglion, unspecified ankle and foot

M67.48 Ganglion, other site

M67.49 Ganglion, multiple sites

5ᵗʰ M67.5 Plica syndrome

DEFINITION: Plica syndrome is an irritation or inflammation of the extension of the synovium (plica).

Plica knee

M67.50 Plica syndrome, unspecified knee

M67.51 Plica syndrome, right knee

M67.52 Plica syndrome, left knee

5ᵗʰ M67.8 Other specified disorders of synovium and tendon

M67.80 Other specified disorders of synovium and tendon, unspecified site

6ᵗʰ M67.81 Other specified disorders of synovium and tendon, shoulder

M67.811 Other specified disorders of synovium, right shoulder

M67.812 Other specified disorders of synovium, left shoulder

M67.813 Other specified disorders of tendon, right shoulder

M67.814 Other specified disorders of tendon, left shoulder

M67.819 Other specified disorders of synovium and tendon, unspecified shoulder

6ᵗʰ M67.82 Other specified disorders of synovium and tendon, elbow

M67.821 Other specified disorders of synovium, right elbow

M67.822 Other specified disorders of synovium, left elbow

M67.823 Other specified disorders of tendon, right elbow

M67.824 Other specified disorders of tendon, left elbow

M67.829 Other specified disorders of synovium and tendon, unspecified elbow

6ᵗʰ M67.83 Other specified disorders of synovium and tendon, wrist

M67.831 Other specified disorders of synovium, right wrist

M67.832 Other specified disorders of synovium, left wrist

M67.833 Other specified disorders of tendon, right wrist

M67.834 Other specified disorders of tendon, left wrist

▲ M67.839 Other specified disorders of synovium and tendon, unspecified ▶wrist◀

6ᵗʰ M67.84 Other specified disorders of synovium and tendon, hand

M67.841 Other specified disorders of synovium, right hand

M67.842 Other specified disorders of synovium, left hand

PDx̲ Unacceptable principal diagnosis symbol per Medicare code edits POA Code exempt from diagnosis present on admission requirement
❓ Questionable admission cc Complication or comorbidity MCC Major complication or comorbidity CC/MCC EXCL CC/MCC exclusion
HCC HCC diagnosis code RxHCC RxHCC diagnosis code MACRA code MACRA code DEFINITION Describes condition/terminology
TIP Coding guidance 👁 Official Guideline Reference Z1 Z code as first-listed diagnosis

When symbols appear on a code that requires a 7th character extension, refer to Appendix B to identify applicable 7th character codes.

M67.843 Other specified disorders of tendon, right hand

M67.844 Other specified disorders of tendon, left hand

M67.849 Other specified disorders of synovium and tendon, unspecified hand

M67.85 Other specified disorders of synovium and tendon, hip

M67.851 Other specified disorders of synovium, right hip

M67.852 Other specified disorders of synovium, left hip

M67.853 Other specified disorders of tendon, right hip

M67.854 Other specified disorders of tendon, left hip

M67.859 Other specified disorders of synovium and tendon, unspecified hip

M67.86 Other specified disorders of synovium and tendon, knee

M67.861 Other specified disorders of synovium, right knee

M67.862 Other specified disorders of synovium, left knee

M67.863 Other specified disorders of tendon, right knee

M67.864 Other specified disorders of tendon, left knee

M67.869 Other specified disorders of synovium and tendon, unspecified knee

M67.87 Other specified disorders of synovium and tendon, ankle and foot

M67.871 Other specified disorders of synovium, right ankle and foot

M67.872 Other specified disorders of synovium, left ankle and foot

M67.873 Other specified disorders of tendon, right ankle and foot

M67.874 Other specified disorders of tendon, left ankle and foot

M67.879 Other specified disorders of synovium and tendon, unspecified ankle and foot

M67.88 Other specified disorders of synovium and tendon, other site

M67.89 Other specified disorders of synovium and tendon, multiple sites

M67.9 Unspecified disorder of synovium and tendon

M67.90 Unspecified disorder of synovium and tendon, unspecified site

M67.91 Unspecified disorder of synovium and tendon, shoulder

M67.911 Unspecified disorder of synovium and tendon, right shoulder

M67.912 Unspecified disorder of synovium and tendon, left shoulder

M67.919 Unspecified disorder of synovium and tendon, unspecified shoulder

M67.92 Unspecified disorder of synovium and tendon, upper arm

M67.921 Unspecified disorder of synovium and tendon, right upper arm

M67.922 Unspecified disorder of synovium and tendon, left upper arm

M67.929 Unspecified disorder of synovium and tendon, unspecified upper arm

M67.93 Unspecified disorder of synovium and tendon, forearm

M67.931 Unspecified disorder of synovium and tendon, right forearm

M67.932 Unspecified disorder of synovium and tendon, left forearm

M67.939 Unspecified disorder of synovium and tendon, unspecified forearm

M67.94 Unspecified disorder of synovium and tendon, hand

M67.941 Unspecified disorder of synovium and tendon, right hand

M67.942 Unspecified disorder of synovium and tendon, left hand

M67.949 Unspecified disorder of synovium and tendon, unspecified hand

M67.95 Unspecified disorder of synovium and tendon, thigh

M67.951 Unspecified disorder of synovium and tendon, right thigh

M67.952 Unspecified disorder of synovium and tendon, left thigh

M67.959 Unspecified disorder of synovium and tendon, unspecified thigh

M67.96 Unspecified disorder of synovium and tendon, lower leg

M67.961 Unspecified disorder of synovium and tendon, right lower leg

M67.962 Unspecified disorder of synovium and tendon, left lower leg

M67.969 Unspecified disorder of synovium and tendon, unspecified lower leg

M67.97 Unspecified disorder of synovium and tendon, ankle and foot

M67.971 Unspecified disorder of synovium and tendon, right ankle and foot

M67.972 Unspecified disorder of synovium and tendon, left ankle and foot

M67.979 Unspecified disorder of synovium and tendon, unspecified ankle and foot

M67.98 Unspecified disorder of synovium and tendon, other site

M67.99 Unspecified disorder of synovium and tendon, multiple sites

Other soft tissue disorders (M70-M79)

M70 Soft tissue disorders related to use, overuse and pressure

INCLUDES soft tissue disorders of occupational origin

Use additional external cause code to identify activity causing disorder (Y93.-)

EXCLUDES1 bursitis NOS (M71.9-)

EXCLUDES2 bursitis of shoulder (M75.5)

enthesopathies (M76-M77)

pressure ulcer (pressure area) (L89.-)

M70.0 Crepitant synovitis (acute) (chronic) of hand and wrist

M70.03 Crepitant synovitis (acute) (chronic), wrist

M70.031 Crepitant synovitis (acute) (chronic), right wrist

M70.032 Crepitant synovitis (acute) (chronic), left wrist

M70.039 Crepitant synovitis (acute) (chronic), unspecified wrist

M70.04 Crepitant synovitis (acute) (chronic), hand

M70.041 Crepitant synovitis (acute) (chronic), right hand

M70.042 Crepitant synovitis (acute) (chronic), left hand

M70.049 Crepitant synovitis (acute) (chronic), unspecified hand

M70.1 Bursitis of hand

M70.10 Bursitis, unspecified hand

M70.11 Bursitis, right hand

M70.12 Bursitis, left hand

M70.2 Olecranon bursitis

M70.20 Olecranon bursitis, unspecified elbow

M70.21 Olecranon bursitis, right elbow

M70.22 Olecranon bursitis, left elbow

5ᵗʰ **M70.3** Other bursitis of elbow

M70.30 Other bursitis of elbow, unspecified elbow

M70.31 Other bursitis of elbow, right elbow

M70.32 Other bursitis of elbow, left elbow

5ᵗʰ **M70.4** Prepatellar bursitis

M70.40 Prepatellar bursitis, unspecified knee

M70.41 Prepatellar bursitis, right knee

M70.42 Prepatellar bursitis, left knee

5ᵗʰ **M70.5** Other bursitis of knee

M70.50 Other bursitis of knee, unspecified knee

M70.51 Other bursitis of knee, right knee

M70.52 Other bursitis of knee, left knee

5ᵗʰ **M70.6** Trochanteric bursitis

Trochanteric tendinitis

M70.60 Trochanteric bursitis, unspecified hip

M70.61 Trochanteric bursitis, right hip

M70.62 Trochanteric bursitis, left hip

5ᵗʰ **M70.7** Other bursitis of hip

Ischial bursitis

M70.70 Other bursitis of hip, unspecified hip

M70.71 Other bursitis of hip, right hip

M70.72 Other bursitis of hip, left hip

5ᵗʰ **M70.8** Other soft tissue disorders related to use, overuse and pressure

M70.80 Other soft tissue disorders related to use, overuse and pressure of unspecified site

6ᵗʰ **M70.81** Other soft tissue disorders related to use, overuse and pressure of shoulder

M70.811 Other soft tissue disorders related to use, overuse and pressure, right shoulder

M70.812 Other soft tissue disorders related to use, overuse and pressure, left shoulder

M70.819 Other soft tissue disorders related to use, overuse and pressure, unspecified shoulder

6ᵗʰ **M70.82** Other soft tissue disorders related to use, overuse and pressure of upper arm

M70.821 Other soft tissue disorders related to use, overuse and pressure, right upper arm

M70.822 Other soft tissue disorders related to use, overuse and pressure, left upper arm

M70.829 Other soft tissue disorders related to use, overuse and pressure, unspecified upper arms

6ᵗʰ **M70.83** Other soft tissue disorders related to use, overuse and pressure of forearm

M70.831 Other soft tissue disorders related to use, overuse and pressure, right forearm

M70.832 Other soft tissue disorders related to use, overuse and pressure, left forearm

M70.839 Other soft tissue disorders related to use, overuse and pressure, unspecified forearm

6ᵗʰ **M70.84** Other soft tissue disorders related to use, overuse and pressure of hand

M70.841 Other soft tissue disorders related to use, overuse and pressure, right hand

M70.842 Other soft tissue disorders related to use, overuse and pressure, left hand

M70.849 Other soft tissue disorders related to use, overuse and pressure, unspecified hand

6ᵗʰ **M70.85** Other soft tissue disorders related to use, overuse and pressure of thigh

M70.851 Other soft tissue disorders related to use, overuse and pressure, right thigh

M70.852 Other soft tissue disorders related to use, overuse and pressure, left thigh

M70.859 Other soft tissue disorders related to use, overuse and pressure, unspecified thigh

6ᵗʰ **M70.86** Other soft tissue disorders related to use, overuse and pressure lower leg

M70.861 Other soft tissue disorders related to use, overuse and pressure, right lower leg

M70.862 Other soft tissue disorders related to use, overuse and pressure, left lower leg

M70.869 Other soft tissue disorders related to use, overuse and pressure, unspecified leg

6ᵗʰ **M70.87** Other soft tissue disorders related to use, overuse and pressure of ankle and foot

M70.871 Other soft tissue disorders related to use, overuse and pressure, right ankle and foot

M70.872 Other soft tissue disorders related to use, overuse and pressure, left ankle and foot

M70.879 Other soft tissue disorders related to use, overuse and pressure, unspecified ankle and foot

M70.88 Other soft tissue disorders related to use, overuse and pressure other site

M70.89 Other soft tissue disorders related to use, overuse and pressure multiple sites

5ᵗʰ **M70.9** Unspecified soft tissue disorder related to use, overuse and pressure

M70.90 Unspecified soft tissue disorder related to use, overuse and pressure of unspecified site

6ᵗʰ **M70.91** Unspecified soft tissue disorder related to use, overuse and pressure of shoulder

M70.911 Unspecified soft tissue disorder related to use, overuse and pressure, right shoulder

M70.912 Unspecified soft tissue disorder related to use, overuse and pressure, left shoulder

M70.919 Unspecified soft tissue disorder related to use, overuse and pressure, unspecified shoulder

6ᵗʰ **M70.92** Unspecified soft tissue disorder related to use, overuse and pressure of upper arm

M70.921 Unspecified soft tissue disorder related to use, overuse and pressure, right upper arm

M70.922 Unspecified soft tissue disorder related to use, overuse and pressure, left upper arm

M70.929 Unspecified soft tissue disorder related to use, overuse and pressure, unspecified upper arm

6ᵗʰ **M70.93** Unspecified soft tissue disorder related to use, overuse and pressure of forearm

M70.931 Unspecified soft tissue disorder related to use, overuse and pressure, right forearm

M70.932 Unspecified soft tissue disorder related to use, overuse and pressure, left forearm

M70.939 Unspecified soft tissue disorder related to use, overuse and pressure, unspecified forearm

6ᵗʰ **M70.94** Unspecified soft tissue disorder related to use, overuse and pressure of hand

M70.941 Unspecified soft tissue disorder related to use, overuse and pressure, right hand

M70.942 Unspecified soft tissue disorder related to use, overuse and pressure, left hand

M70.949 Unspecified soft tissue disorder related to use, overuse and pressure, unspecified hand

6ᵗʰ **M70.95** Unspecified soft tissue disorder related to use, overuse and pressure of thigh

M70.951 Unspecified soft tissue disorder related to use, overuse and pressure, right thigh

M70.952 Unspecified soft tissue disorder related to use, overuse and pressure, left thigh

M70.959 Unspecified soft tissue disorder related to use, overuse and pressure, unspecified thigh

6ᵗʰ **M70.96** Unspecified soft tissue disorder related to use, overuse and pressure lower leg

---

PDₓ Unacceptable principal diagnosis symbol per Medicare code edits　POA Code exempt from diagnosis present on admission requirement

? Questionable admission　cc Complication or comorbidity　MCC Major complication or comorbidity　cc/mcc exc CC/MCC exclusion

HCC HCC diagnosis code　RxHCC RxHCC diagnosis code　MACRA code　**DEFINITION** Describes condition/terminology

TIP Coding guidance　👁 Official Guideline Reference　Z⁵ᵗ Z code as first-listed diagnosis

M70.961 Unspecified soft tissue disorder related to use, overuse and pressure, right lower leg

M70.962 Unspecified soft tissue disorder related to use, overuse and pressure, left lower leg

M70.969 Unspecified soft tissue disorder related to use, overuse and pressure, unspecified lower leg

🔟 M70.97 Unspecified soft tissue disorder related to use, overuse and pressure of ankle and foot

M70.971 Unspecified soft tissue disorder related to use, overuse and pressure, right ankle and foot

M70.972 Unspecified soft tissue disorder related to use, overuse and pressure, left ankle and foot

M70.979 Unspecified soft tissue disorder related to use, overuse and pressure, unspecified ankle and foot

M70.98 Unspecified soft tissue disorder related to use, overuse and pressure other

M70.99 Unspecified soft tissue disorder related to use, overuse and pressure multiple sites

🔟 M71 Other bursopathies

EXCLUDES1 bunion (M20.1)

bursitis related to use, overuse or pressure (M70.-)

enthesopathies (M76-M77)

🔟 M71.0 Abscess of bursa

Use additional code (B95.-, B96.-) to identify causative organism

M71.00 Abscess of bursa, unspecified site

🔟 M71.01 Abscess of bursa, shoulder

M71.011 Abscess of bursa, right shoulder

M71.012 Abscess of bursa, left shoulder

M71.019 Abscess of bursa, unspecified shoulder

🔟 M71.02 Abscess of bursa, elbow

M71.021 Abscess of bursa, right elbow

M71.022 Abscess of bursa, left elbow

M71.029 Abscess of bursa, unspecified elbow

🔟 M71.03 Abscess of bursa, wrist

M71.031 Abscess of bursa, right wrist

M71.032 Abscess of bursa, left wrist

M71.039 Abscess of bursa, unspecified wrist

🔟 M71.04 Abscess of bursa, hand

M71.041 Abscess of bursa, right hand

M71.042 Abscess of bursa, left hand

M71.049 Abscess of bursa, unspecified hand

🔟 M71.05 Abscess of bursa, hip

M71.051 Abscess of bursa, right hip

M71.052 Abscess of bursa, left hip

M71.059 Abscess of bursa, unspecified hip

🔟 M71.06 Abscess of bursa, knee

M71.061 Abscess of bursa, right knee

M71.062 Abscess of bursa, left knee

M71.069 Abscess of bursa, unspecified knee

🔟 M71.07 Abscess of bursa, ankle and foot

M71.071 Abscess of bursa, right ankle and foot

M71.072 Abscess of bursa, left ankle and foot

M71.079 Abscess of bursa, unspecified ankle and foot

M71.08 Abscess of bursa, other site

M71.09 Abscess of bursa, multiple sites

🔟 M71.1 Other infective bursitis

Use additional code (B95.-, B96.-) to identify causative organism

M71.10 Other infective bursitis, unspecified site

🔟 M71.11 Other infective bursitis, shoulder

M71.111 Other infective bursitis, right shoulder

M71.112 Other infective bursitis, left shoulder

M71.119 Other infective bursitis, unspecified shoulder

🔟 M71.12 Other infective bursitis, elbow

M71.121 Other infective bursitis, right elbow

M71.122 Other infective bursitis, left elbow

M71.129 Other infective bursitis, unspecified elbow

🔟 M71.13 Other infective bursitis, wrist

M71.131 Other infective bursitis, right wrist

M71.132 Other infective bursitis, left wrist

M71.139 Other infective bursitis, unspecified wrist

🔟 M71.14 Other infective bursitis, hand

M71.141 Other infective bursitis, right hand

M71.142 Other infective bursitis, left hand

M71.149 Other infective bursitis, unspecified hand

🔟 M71.15 Other infective bursitis, hip

M71.151 Other infective bursitis, right hip

M71.152 Other infective bursitis, left hip

M71.159 Other infective bursitis, unspecified hip

🔟 M71.16 Other infective bursitis, knee

M71.161 Other infective bursitis, right knee

M71.162 Other infective bursitis, left knee

M71.169 Other infective bursitis, unspecified knee

🔟 M71.17 Other infective bursitis, ankle and foot

M71.171 Other infective bursitis, right ankle and foot

M71.172 Other infective bursitis, left ankle and foot

M71.179 Other infective bursitis, unspecified ankle and foot

M71.18 Other infective bursitis, other site

M71.19 Other infective bursitis, multiple sites

🔟 M71.2 Synovial cyst of popliteal space [Baker]

EXCLUDES1 synovial cyst of popliteal space with rupture (M66.0)

M71.20 Synovial cyst of popliteal space [Baker], unspecified knee

M71.21 Synovial cyst of popliteal space [Baker], right knee

M71.22 Synovial cyst of popliteal space [Baker], left knee

🔟 M71.3 Other bursal cyst

Synovial cyst NOS

EXCLUDES1 synovial cyst with rupture (M66.1-)

M71.30 Other bursal cyst, unspecified site

🔟 M71.31 Other bursal cyst, shoulder

M71.311 Other bursal cyst, right shoulder

M71.312 Other bursal cyst, left shoulder

M71.319 Other bursal cyst, unspecified shoulder

🔟 M71.32 Other bursal cyst, elbow

M71.321 Other bursal cyst, right elbow

M71.322 Other bursal cyst, left elbow

M71.329 Other bursal cyst, unspecified elbow

🔟 M71.33 Other bursal cyst, wrist

M71.331 Other bursal cyst, right wrist

M71.332 Other bursal cyst, left wrist

M71.339 Other bursal cyst, unspecified wrist

🔟 M71.34 Other bursal cyst, hand

M71.341 Other bursal cyst, right hand

M71.342 Other bursal cyst, left hand

M71.349 Other bursal cyst, unspecified hand

🔟 M71.35 Other bursal cyst, hip

M71.351 Other bursal cyst, right hip

M71.352 Other bursal cyst, left hip

M71.359 Other bursal cyst, unspecified hip

🔟 M71.37 Other bursal cyst, ankle and foot

M71.371 Other bursal cyst, right ankle and foot

M71.372 Other bursal cyst, left ankle and foot

M71.379 Other bursal cyst, unspecified ankle and foot

M71.38 Other bursal cyst, other site

M71.39 Other bursal cyst, multiple sites

🔟 M71.4 Calcium deposit in bursa

EXCLUDES2 calcium deposit in bursa of shoulder (M75.3)

M71.40 Calcium deposit in bursa, unspecified site

M71.42 Calcium deposit in bursa, elbow
    M71.421 Calcium deposit in bursa, right elbow
    M71.422 Calcium deposit in bursa, left elbow
    M71.429 Calcium deposit in bursa, unspecified elbow

M71.43 Calcium deposit in bursa, wrist
    M71.431 Calcium deposit in bursa, right wrist
    M71.432 Calcium deposit in bursa, left wrist
    M71.439 Calcium deposit in bursa, unspecified wrist

M71.44 Calcium deposit in bursa, hand
    M71.441 Calcium deposit in bursa, right hand
    M71.442 Calcium deposit in bursa, left hand
    M71.449 Calcium deposit in bursa, unspecified hand

M71.45 Calcium deposit in bursa, hip
    M71.451 Calcium deposit in bursa, right hip
    M71.452 Calcium deposit in bursa, left hip
    M71.459 Calcium deposit in bursa, unspecified hip

M71.46 Calcium deposit in bursa, knee
    M71.461 Calcium deposit in bursa, right knee
    M71.462 Calcium deposit in bursa, left knee
    M71.469 Calcium deposit in bursa, unspecified knee

M71.47 Calcium deposit in bursa, ankle and foot
    M71.471 Calcium deposit in bursa, right ankle and foot
    M71.472 Calcium deposit in bursa, left ankle and foot
    M71.479 Calcium deposit in bursa, unspecified ankle and foot

M71.48 Calcium deposit in bursa, other site
M71.49 Calcium deposit in bursa, multiple sites

M71.5 Other bursitis, not elsewhere classified
    EXCLUDES1 bursitis NOS (M71.9-)
    EXCLUDES2 bursitis of shoulder (M75.5)
            bursitis of tibial collateral [Pellegrini-Stieda] (M76.4-)

M71.50 Other bursitis, not elsewhere classified, unspecified site

M71.52 Other bursitis, not elsewhere classified, elbow
    M71.521 Other bursitis, not elsewhere classified, right elbow
    M71.522 Other bursitis, not elsewhere classified, left elbow
    M71.529 Other bursitis, not elsewhere classified, unspecified elbow

M71.53 Other bursitis, not elsewhere classified, wrist
    M71.531 Other bursitis, not elsewhere classified, right wrist
    M71.532 Other bursitis, not elsewhere classified, left wrist
    M71.539 Other bursitis, not elsewhere classified, unspecified wrist

M71.54 Other bursitis, not elsewhere classified, hand
    M71.541 Other bursitis, not elsewhere classified, right hand
    M71.542 Other bursitis, not elsewhere classified, left hand
    M71.549 Other bursitis, not elsewhere classified, unspecified hand

M71.55 Other bursitis, not elsewhere classified, hip
    M71.551 Other bursitis, not elsewhere classified, right hip
    M71.552 Other bursitis, not elsewhere classified, left hip
    M71.559 Other bursitis, not elsewhere classified, unspecified hip

M71.56 Other bursitis, not elsewhere classified, knee
    M71.561 Other bursitis, not elsewhere classified, right knee
    M71.562 Other bursitis, not elsewhere classified, left knee
    M71.569 Other bursitis, not elsewhere classified, unspecified knee

M71.57 Other bursitis, not elsewhere classified, ankle and foot
    M71.571 Other bursitis, not elsewhere classified, right ankle and foot
    M71.572 Other bursitis, not elsewhere classified, left ankle and foot
    M71.579 Other bursitis, not elsewhere classified, unspecified ankle and foot

M71.58 Other bursitis, not elsewhere classified, other site

M71.8 Other specified bursopathies
M71.80 Other specified bursopathies, unspecified site
M71.81 Other specified bursopathies, shoulder
    M71.811 Other specified bursopathies, right shoulder
    M71.812 Other specified bursopathies, left shoulder
    M71.819 Other specified bursopathies, unspecified shoulder

M71.82 Other specified bursopathies, elbow
    M71.821 Other specified bursopathies, right elbow
    M71.822 Other specified bursopathies, left elbow
    M71.829 Other specified bursopathies, unspecified elbow

M71.83 Other specified bursopathies, wrist
    M71.831 Other specified bursopathies, right wrist
    M71.832 Other specified bursopathies, left wrist
    M71.839 Other specified bursopathies, unspecified wrist

M71.84 Other specified bursopathies, hand
    M71.841 Other specified bursopathies, right hand
    M71.842 Other specified bursopathies, left hand
    M71.849 Other specified bursopathies, unspecified hand

M71.85 Other specified bursopathies, hip
    M71.851 Other specified bursopathies, right hip
    M71.852 Other specified bursopathies, left hip
    M71.859 Other specified bursopathies, unspecified hip

M71.86 Other specified bursopathies, knee
    M71.861 Other specified bursopathies, right knee
    M71.862 Other specified bursopathies, left knee
    M71.869 Other specified bursopathies, unspecified knee

M71.87 Other specified bursopathies, ankle and foot
    M71.871 Other specified bursopathies, right ankle and foot
    M71.872 Other specified bursopathies, left ankle and foot
    M71.879 Other specified bursopathies, unspecified ankle and foot

M71.88 Other specified bursopathies, other site
M71.89 Other specified bursopathies, multiple sites

M71.9 Bursopathy, unspecified
    Bursitis NOS

M72 Fibroblastic disorders
    EXCLUDES2 retroperitoneal fibromatosis (D48.3)

M72.0 Palmar fascial fibromatosis [Dupuytren] 🄰
M72.1 Knuckle pads
M72.2 Plantar fascial fibromatosis
    Plantar fasciitis
M72.4 Pseudosarcomatous fibromatosis
    Nodular fasciitis
M72.6 Necrotizing fasciitis   HCC MCC CC/MCC Exc
    Use additional code (B95.-, B96.-) to identify causative organism

PDx Unacceptable principal diagnosis symbol per Medicare code edits   POA Code exempt from diagnosis present on admission requirement
? Questionable admission   cc Complication or comorbidity   MCC Major complication or comorbidity   cc/mcc exc CC/MCC exclusion
HCC HCC diagnosis code   RxHCC RxHCC diagnosis code   MACRA code   **DEFINITION** Describes condition/terminology
TIP Coding guidance   👁 Official Guideline Reference   Z1 Z code as first-listed diagnosis

832   When symbols appear on a code that requires a 7th character extension, refer to Appendix B to identify applicable 7th character codes.   **2020 ICD-10-CM**

M72.8 Other fibroblastic disorders
Abscess of fascia
Fasciitis NEC
Other infective fasciitis
Use additional code to (B95.-, B96.-) identify causative organism
EXCLUDES1 diffuse (eosinophilic) fasciitis (M35.4)
necrotizing fasciitis (M72.6)
nodular fasciitis (M72.4)
perirenal fasciitis NOS (N13.5)
perirenal fasciitis with infection (N13.6)
plantar fasciitis (M72.2)

M72.9 Fibroblastic disorder, unspecified
Fasciitis NOS
Fibromatosis NOS

M75 Shoulder lesions
EXCLUDES2 shoulder-hand syndrome (M89.0-)

M75.0 Adhesive capsulitis of shoulder
TIP: Shoulder impingement (frozen shoulder) that persists and left untreated can become Adhesive capsulitis.
Frozen shoulder
Periarthritis of shoulder
M75.00 Adhesive capsulitis of unspecified shoulder
M75.01 Adhesive capsulitis of right shoulder
M75.02 Adhesive capsulitis of left shoulder
AHA: Q2 2015

M75.1 Rotator cuff tear or rupture, not specified as traumatic
Rotator cuff syndrome
Supraspinatus tear or rupture, not specified as traumatic
Supraspinatus syndrome
EXCLUDES1 tear of rotator cuff, traumatic (S46.01-)

M75.10 Unspecified rotator cuff tear or rupture, not specified as traumatic
M75.100 Unspecified rotator cuff tear or rupture of unspecified shoulder, not specified as traumatic
M75.101 Unspecified rotator cuff tear or rupture of right shoulder, not specified as traumatic
M75.102 Unspecified rotator cuff tear or rupture of left shoulder, not specified as traumatic

M75.11 Incomplete rotator cuff tear or rupture not specified as traumatic
M75.110 Incomplete rotator cuff tear or rupture of unspecified shoulder, not specified as traumatic
M75.111 Incomplete rotator cuff tear or rupture of right shoulder, not specified as traumatic
M75.112 Incomplete rotator cuff tear or rupture of left shoulder, not specified as traumatic

M75.12 Complete rotator cuff tear or rupture not specified as traumatic
M75.120 Complete rotator cuff tear or rupture of unspecified shoulder, not specified as traumatic
M75.121 Complete rotator cuff tear or rupture of right shoulder, not specified as traumatic CC CC/MCC Exc
M75.122 Complete rotator cuff tear or rupture of left shoulder, not specified as traumatic CC CC/MCC Exc

M75.2 Bicipital tendinitis
M75.20 Bicipital tendinitis, unspecified shoulder
M75.21 Bicipital tendinitis, right shoulder
M75.22 Bicipital tendinitis, left shoulder

M75.3 Calcific tendinitis of shoulder
Calcified bursa of shoulder
M75.30 Calcific tendinitis of unspecified shoulder
M75.31 Calcific tendinitis of right shoulder
M75.32 Calcific tendinitis of left shoulder

M75.4 Impingement syndrome of shoulder
M75.40 Impingement syndrome of unspecified shoulder
M75.41 Impingement syndrome of right shoulder
M75.42 Impingement syndrome of left shoulder

M75.5 Bursitis of shoulder
M75.50 Bursitis of unspecified shoulder
M75.51 Bursitis of right shoulder
M75.52 Bursitis of left shoulder

M75.8 Other shoulder lesions
M75.80 Other shoulder lesions, unspecified shoulder
M75.81 Other shoulder lesions, right shoulder
M75.82 Other shoulder lesions, left shoulder

M75.9 Shoulder lesion, unspecified
M75.90 Shoulder lesion, unspecified, unspecified shoulder
M75.91 Shoulder lesion, unspecified, right shoulder
M75.92 Shoulder lesion, unspecified, left shoulder

M76 Enthesopathies, lower limb, excluding foot
EXCLUDES2 bursitis due to use, overuse and pressure (M70.-)
enthesopathies of ankle and foot (M77.5-)

M76.0 Gluteal tendinitis
M76.00 Gluteal tendinitis, unspecified hip
M76.01 Gluteal tendinitis, right hip
M76.02 Gluteal tendinitis, left hip

M76.1 Psoas tendinitis
M76.10 Psoas tendinitis, unspecified hip
M76.11 Psoas tendinitis, right hip
M76.12 Psoas tendinitis, left hip

M76.2 Iliac crest spur
M76.20 Iliac crest spur, unspecified hip
M76.21 Iliac crest spur, right hip
M76.22 Iliac crest spur, left hip

M76.3 Iliotibial band syndrome
M76.30 Iliotibial band syndrome, unspecified leg
M76.31 Iliotibial band syndrome, right leg
M76.32 Iliotibial band syndrome, left leg

M76.4 Tibial collateral bursitis [Pellegrini-Stieda]
M76.40 Tibial collateral bursitis [Pellegrini-Stieda], unspecified leg
M76.41 Tibial collateral bursitis [Pellegrini-Stieda], right leg
M76.42 Tibial collateral bursitis [Pellegrini-Stieda], left leg

M76.5 Patellar tendinitis
M76.50 Patellar tendinitis, unspecified knee
M76.51 Patellar tendinitis, right knee
M76.52 Patellar tendinitis, left knee

M76.6 Achilles tendinitis (Figure 13.6)
Achilles bursitis
M76.60 Achilles tendinitis, unspecified leg
M76.61 Achilles tendinitis, right leg
M76.62 Achilles tendinitis, left leg

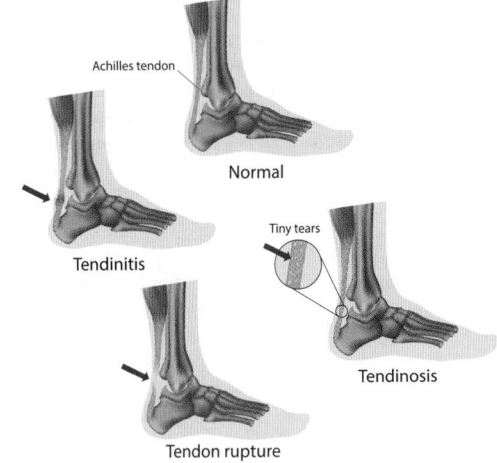

Achilles tendon

Normal

Tendinitis

Tiny tears

Tendinosis

Tendon rupture

Figure 13.6 Achilles Tendinitis

Unspecified Code   Other Specified Code   Manifestation Code   N Newborn   P Pediatric   M Maternity   A Adult   ♂ Male   ♀ Female
● New Code   ▲ Revised Code Title   ►◄ Revised Text   NOTES   INCLUDES   EXCLUDES1 Not coded here   EXCLUDES2 Not included here
4th character required   5th character required   6th character required   7th character required   7th Extension 'X' Alert
HAC Hospital-acquired condition (HAC) alert   AHA AHA Coding Clinic©   Code first alert

M76.7 Peroneal **tendinitis**
   M76.70 Peroneal tendinitis, unspecified leg
   M76.71 Peroneal tendinitis, right leg
   M76.72 Peroneal tendinitis, left leg
M76.8 Other specified enthesopathies **of lower limb, excluding foot**
   M76.81 Anterior tibial syndrome
      M76.811 Anterior tibial syndrome, right **leg**
      M76.812 Anterior tibial syndrome, left **leg**
      M76.819 Anterior tibial syndrome, unspecified **leg**
   M76.82 Posterior tibial tendinitis
      M76.821 Posterior tibial tendinitis, right **leg**
      M76.822 Posterior tibial tendinitis, left **leg**
      M76.829 Posterior tibial tendinitis, unspecified **leg**
   M76.89 Other specified enthesopathies of lower limb, excluding foot
      M76.891 Other specified enthesopathies of right lower limb, excluding foot
      M76.892 Other specified enthesopathies of left lower limb, excluding foot
      M76.899 Other specified enthesopathies of unspecified lower limb, excluding foot
M76.9 **Unspecified enthesopathy, lower limb, excluding foot**
M77 Other **enthesopathies**
   EXCLUDES1 bursitis NOS (M71.9-)
   EXCLUDES2 bursitis due to use, overuse and pressure (M70.-)
      osteophyte (M25.7)
      spinal enthesopathy (M46.0-)
M77.0 Medial **epicondylitis**
   M77.00 Medial epicondylitis, unspecified elbow
   M77.01 Medial epicondylitis, right **elbow**
   M77.02 Medial epicondylitis, left **elbow**
M77.1 Lateral **epicondylitis**
   Tennis elbow
   M77.10 Lateral epicondylitis, unspecified elbow
   M77.11 Lateral epicondylitis, right **elbow**
   M77.12 Lateral epicondylitis, left **elbow**
M77.2 Periarthritis **of wrist**
   M77.20 Periarthritis, unspecified wrist
   M77.21 Periarthritis, right **wrist**
   M77.22 Periarthritis, left **wrist**
M77.3 Calcaneal spur
   M77.30 Calcaneal spur, unspecified foot
   M77.31 Calcaneal spur, right **foot**
   M77.32 Calcaneal spur, left **foot**
M77.4 Metatarsalgia
   EXCLUDES1 Morton's metatarsalgia (G57.6)
   M77.40 Metatarsalgia, unspecified foot
   M77.41 Metatarsalgia, right **foot**
   M77.42 Metatarsalgia, left **foot**
▲ M77.5 Other enthesopathy of foot ▶and ankle◀
  ▲ M77.50 Other enthesopathy of unspecified foot ▶and ankle◀
  ▲ M77.51 Other enthesopathy of right foot ▶and ankle◀
  ▲ M77.52 Other enthesopathy of left foot ▶and ankle◀
M77.8 Other **enthesopathies, not elsewhere classified**
M77.9 **Enthesopathy, unspecified**
   Bone spur NOS
   Capsulitis NOS
   Periarthritis NOS
   Tendinitis NOS
M79 Other and unspecified soft tissue disorders, not elsewhere classified
   EXCLUDES1 psychogenic rheumatism (F45.8)
      soft tissue pain, psychogenic (F45.41)
M79.0 **Rheumatism, unspecified**
   EXCLUDES1 fibromyalgia (M79.7)
      palindromic rheumatism (M12.3-)
M79.1 Myalgia
   Myofascial pain syndrome
   EXCLUDES1 fibromyalgia (M79.7)
      myositis (M60.-)

M79.10 **Myalgia, unspecified site**
   AHA: Q4 2018
M79.11 **Myalgia of** mastication muscle
   AHA: Q4 2018
M79.12 **Myalgia of** auxiliary muscles, **head and neck**
   AHA: Q4 2018
M79.18 **Myalgia,** other site
   AHA: Q4 2018
M79.2 **Neuralgia and neuritis, unspecified**
   EXCLUDES1 brachial radiculitis NOS (M54.1)
      lumbosacral radiculitis NOS (M54.1)
      mononeuropathies (G56-G58)
      radiculitis NOS (M54.1)
      sciatica (M54.3-M54.4)
M79.3 **Panniculitis, unspecified**   CC CC/MCC Exc
   EXCLUDES1 lupus panniculitis (L93.2)
      neck and back panniculitis (M54.0-)
      relapsing [Weber-Christian] panniculitis (M35.6)
M79.4 **Hypertrophy of (infrapatellar) fat pad**
M79.5 **Residual foreign body in soft tissue**
   EXCLUDES1 foreign body granuloma of skin and subcutaneous tissue (L92.3)
      foreign body granuloma of soft tissue (M60.2-)
M79.6 Pain **in limb, hand, foot, fingers and toes**
   EXCLUDES2 pain in joint (M25.5-)
   M79.60 Pain in limb, unspecified
      M79.601 **Pain in** right arm
         Pain in right upper limb NOS
      M79.602 **Pain in** left arm
         Pain in left upper limb NOS
      M79.603 **Pain in arm, unspecified**
         Pain in upper limb NOS
      M79.604 **Pain in** right leg
         Pain in right lower limb NOS
      M79.605 **Pain in** left leg
         Pain in left lower limb NOS
      M79.606 **Pain in leg, unspecified**
         Pain in lower limb NOS
      M79.609 **Pain in unspecified limb**
         Pain in limb NOS
   M79.62 **Pain in** upper arm
      Pain in axillary region
      M79.621 **Pain in** right **upper arm**
      M79.622 **Pain in** left **upper arm**
      M79.629 **Pain in unspecified upper arm**
   M79.63 **Pain in** forearm
      M79.631 **Pain in** right **forearm**
      M79.632 **Pain in** left **forearm**
      M79.639 **Pain in unspecified forearm**
   M79.64 **Pain in** hand and fingers
      M79.641 **Pain in** right **hand**
      M79.642 **Pain in** left **hand**
      M79.643 **Pain in unspecified hand**
      M79.644 **Pain in** right **finger(s)**
      M79.645 **Pain in** left **finger(s)**
      M79.646 **Pain in unspecified finger(s)**
   M79.65 **Pain in** thigh
      M79.651 **Pain in** right **thigh**
      M79.652 **Pain in** left **thigh**
      M79.659 **Pain in unspecified thigh**
   M79.66 **Pain in** lower leg
      M79.661 **Pain in** right **lower leg**
      M79.662 **Pain in** left **lower leg**
      M79.669 **Pain in unspecified lower leg**
   M79.67 **Pain in** foot and toes
      M79.671 **Pain in** right **foot**
      M79.672 **Pain in** left **foot**
      M79.673 **Pain in unspecified foot**
      M79.674 **Pain in** right **toe(s)**

Unacceptable principal diagnosis symbol per Medicare code edits   Code exempt from diagnosis present on admission requirement
Questionable admission   Complication or comorbidity   Major complication or comorbidity   CC/MCC exclusion
HCC diagnosis code   RxHCC diagnosis code   MACRA code   **DEFINITION** Describes condition/terminology
TIP Coding guidance   Official Guideline Reference   Z code as first-listed diagnosis

834   When symbols appear on a code that requires a 7th character extension, refer to Appendix B to identify applicable 7th character codes.   **2020 ICD-10-CM**

M79.675 Pain in left toe(s)

M79.676 Pain in unspecified toe(s)

M79.7 Fibromyalgia
Fibromyositis
Fibrositis
Myofibrositis

5ᵗʰ M79.A Nontraumatic compartment syndrome

☞ Code first, if applicable, associated postprocedural complication

EXCLUDES1 compartment syndrome NOS (T79.A-)
fibromyalgia (M79.7)
nontraumatic ischemic infarction of muscle (M62.2-)
traumatic compartment syndrome (T79.A-)

6ᵗʰ M79.A1 Nontraumatic compartment syndrome of upper extremity
Nontraumatic compartment syndrome of shoulder, arm, forearm, wrist, hand, and fingers

M79.A11 Nontraumatic compartment syndrome of right upper extremity cc⊘ CC/MCC Exc

M79.A12 Nontraumatic compartment syndrome of left upper extremity cc⊘ CC/MCC Exc

M79.A19 Nontraumatic compartment syndrome of unspecified upper extremity cc⊘ CC/MCC Exc

6ᵗʰ M79.A2 Nontraumatic compartment syndrome of lower extremity
Nontraumatic compartment syndrome of hip, buttock, thigh, leg, foot, and toes

M79.A21 Nontraumatic compartment syndrome of right lower extremity cc⊘ CC/MCC Exc

M79.A22 Nontraumatic compartment syndrome of left lower extremity cc⊘ CC/MCC Exc

M79.A29 Nontraumatic compartment syndrome of unspecified lower extremity cc⊘ CC/MCC Exc

M79.A3 Nontraumatic compartment syndrome of abdomen cc⊘ CC/MCC Exc

M79.A9 Nontraumatic compartment syndrome of other sites cc⊘ CC/MCC Exc

5ᵗʰ M79.8 Other specified soft tissue disorders

M79.81 Nontraumatic hematoma of soft tissue
Nontraumatic hematoma of muscle
Nontraumatic seroma of muscle and soft tissue

M79.89 Other specified soft tissue disorders
Polyalgia

M79.9 Soft tissue disorder, unspecified

Osteopathies and chondropathies (M80-M94)

Disorders of bone density and structure (M80-M85) (Figure 13.7)

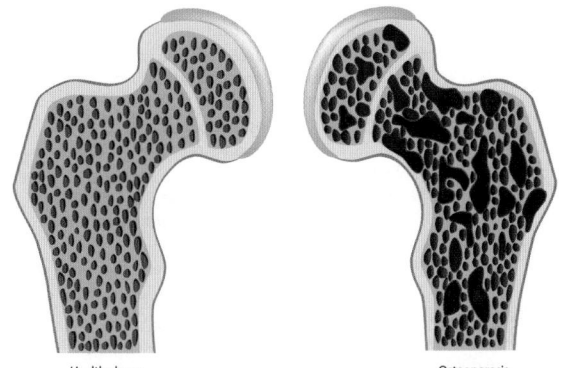

Healthy bone   Osteoporosis

Figure 13.7 Reduced Bone Matrix in Osteoporosis

4ᵗʰ M80 Osteoporosis with current pathological fracture

👁 See Official Guidelines "Osteoporosis with current pathological fracture" I.C.13.d.2, "Initial vs. Subsequent Encounter for Fractures" I.C.19.c.1

TIP: Osteoporosis occurs when the bone loses density and becomes thin or brittle. This can lead to fractures from falls or minor bumps and stresses.

INCLUDES osteoporosis with current fragility fracture

Use additional code to identify major osseous defect, if applicable (M89.7-)

EXCLUDES1 collapsed vertebra NOS (M48.5)
pathological fracture NOS (M84.4)
wedging of vertebra NOS (M48.5)

EXCLUDES2 personal history of (healed) osteoporosis fracture (Z87.310)

The appropriate 7th character is to be added to each code from category M80:

A = initial encounter for fracture
D = subsequent encounter for fracture with routine healing
G = subsequent encounter for fracture with delayed healing
K = subsequent encounter for fracture with nonunion
P = subsequent encounter for fracture with malunion
S = sequela

5ᵗʰ M80.0 Age-related osteoporosis with current pathological fracture
Involutional osteoporosis with current pathological fracture
Osteoporosis NOS with current pathological fracture
Postmenopausal osteoporosis with current pathological fracture
Senile osteoporosis with current pathological fracture

7ᵗʰ M80.00 Age-related osteoporosis with current pathological fracture, unspecified site A cc⊘ RxHCC CC/MCC Exc

6ᵗʰ M80.01 Age-related osteoporosis with current pathological fracture, shoulder

7ᵗʰ M80.011 Age-related osteoporosis with current pathological fracture, right shoulder A cc⊘ RxHCC CC/MCC Exc

7ᵗʰ M80.012 Age-related osteoporosis with current pathological fracture, left shoulder A cc⊘ RxHCC CC/MCC Exc

7ᵗʰ M80.019 Age-related osteoporosis with current pathological fracture, unspecified shoulder A cc⊘ RxHCC CC/MCC Exc

6ᵗʰ M80.02 Age-related osteoporosis with current pathological fracture, humerus

7ᵗʰ M80.021 Age-related osteoporosis with current pathological fracture, right humerus A cc⊘ RxHCC CC/MCC Exc

7ᵗʰ M80.022 Age-related osteoporosis with current pathological fracture, left humerus A cc⊘ RxHCC CC/MCC Exc

7ᵗʰ M80.029 Age-related osteoporosis with current pathological fracture, unspecified humerus A cc⊘ RxHCC CC/MCC Exc

6ᵗʰ M80.03 Age-related osteoporosis with current pathological fracture, forearm
Age-related osteoporosis with current pathological fracture of wrist

7ᵗʰ M80.031 Age-related osteoporosis with current pathological fracture, right forearm A cc⊘ RxHCC CC/MCC Exc

7ᵗʰ M80.032 Age-related osteoporosis with current pathological fracture, left forearm A cc⊘ RxHCC CC/MCC Exc

7ᵗʰ M80.039 Age-related osteoporosis with current pathological fracture, unspecified forearm A cc⊘ RxHCC CC/MCC Exc

6ᵗʰ M80.04 Age-related osteoporosis with current pathological fracture, hand

7ᵗʰ M80.041 Age-related osteoporosis with current pathological fracture, right hand A cc⊘ RxHCC CC/MCC Exc

---

Unspecified Code   Other Specified Code   Manifestation Code   N Newborn   P Pediatric   M Maternity   A Adult   ♂ Male   ♀ Female
● New Code   ▲ Revised Code Title   ▶◀ Revised Text   NOTES   INCLUDES   EXCLUDES1 Not coded here   EXCLUDES2 Not included here
4ᵗʰ 4ᵗʰ character required   5ᵗʰ 5ᵗʰ character required   6ᵗʰ 6ᵗʰ character required   7ᵗʰ 7ᵗʰ character required   ✗ Extension 'X' Alert
HAC Hospital-acquired condition (HAC) alert   AHA AHA Coding Clinic©   ☞ Code first alert

[7th] M80.042 **Age-related osteoporosis with current pathological fracture, left hand** [A] [CC] [RxHCC] [CC/MCC Exc]

[7th] M80.049 **Age-related osteoporosis with current pathological fracture, unspecified hand** [A] [CC] [RxHCC] [CC/MCC Exc]

[6th] **M80.05 Age-related osteoporosis with current pathological fracture, femur**

Age-related osteoporosis with current pathological fracture of hip

[7th] M80.051 **Age-related osteoporosis with current pathological fracture, right femur** [A] [CC] [HCC] [RxHCC] [CC/MCC Exc]

AHA: Q2 2018

[7th] M80.052 **Age-related osteoporosis with current pathological fracture, left femur** [A] [CC] [HCC] [RxHCC] [CC/MCC Exc]

[7th] M80.059 **Age-related osteoporosis with current pathological fracture, unspecified femur** [A] [CC] [HCC] [RxHCC] [CC/MCC Exc]

[6th] **M80.06 Age-related osteoporosis with current pathological fracture, lower leg**

[7th] M80.061 **Age-related osteoporosis with current pathological fracture, right lower leg** [A] [CC] [RxHCC] [CC/MCC Exc]

[7th] M80.062 **Age-related osteoporosis with current pathological fracture, left lower leg** [A] [CC] [RxHCC] [CC/MCC Exc]

[7th] M80.069 **Age-related osteoporosis with current pathological fracture, unspecified lower leg** [A] [CC] [RxHCC] [CC/MCC Exc]

[6th] **M80.07 Age-related osteoporosis with current pathological fracture, ankle and foot**

[7th] M80.071 **Age-related osteoporosis with current pathological fracture, right ankle and foot** [A] [CC] [RxHCC] [CC/MCC Exc]

[7th] M80.072 **Age-related osteoporosis with current pathological fracture, left ankle and foot** [A] [CC] [RxHCC] [CC/MCC Exc]

[7th] M80.079 **Age-related osteoporosis with current pathological fracture, unspecified ankle and foot** [A] [CC] [RxHCC] [CC/MCC Exc]

[7th] **M80.08 Age-related osteoporosis with current pathological fracture, vertebra(e)** [A] [CC] [HCC] [RxHCC] [CC/MCC Exc]

[5th] **M80.8 Other osteoporosis with current pathological fracture**

Drug-induced osteoporosis with current pathological fracture
Idiopathic osteoporosis with current pathological fracture
Osteoporosis of disuse with current pathological fracture
Postoophorectomy osteoporosis with current pathological fracture
Postsurgical malabsorption osteoporosis with current pathological fracture
Post-traumatic osteoporosis with current pathological fracture

Use additional code for adverse effect, if applicable, to identify drug (T36-T50 with fifth or sixth character 5)

[7th] **M80.80 Other osteoporosis with current pathological fracture, unspecified site** [CC] [RxHCC] [CC/MCC Exc]

[6th] **M80.81 Other osteoporosis with pathological fracture, shoulder**

[7th] M80.811 **Other osteoporosis with current pathological fracture, right shoulder** [CC] [RxHCC] [CC/MCC Exc]

[7th] M80.812 **Other osteoporosis with current pathological fracture, left shoulder** [CC] [RxHCC] [CC/MCC Exc]

[7th] M80.819 **Other osteoporosis with current pathological fracture, unspecified shoulder** [CC] [RxHCC] [CC/MCC Exc]

[6th] **M80.82 Other osteoporosis with current pathological fracture, humerus**

[7th] M80.821 **Other osteoporosis with current pathological fracture, right humerus** [CC] [RxHCC] [CC/MCC Exc]

[7th] M80.822 **Other osteoporosis with current pathological fracture, left humerus** [CC] [RxHCC] [CC/MCC Exc]

[7th] M80.829 **Other osteoporosis with current pathological fracture, unspecified humerus** [CC] [RxHCC] [CC/MCC Exc]

[6th] **M80.83 Other osteoporosis with current pathological fracture, forearm**

Other osteoporosis with current pathological fracture of wrist

[7th] M80.831 **Other osteoporosis with current pathological fracture, right forearm** [CC] [RxHCC] [CC/MCC Exc]

[7th] M80.832 **Other osteoporosis with current pathological fracture, left forearm** [CC] [RxHCC] [CC/MCC Exc]

[7th] M80.839 **Other osteoporosis with current pathological fracture, unspecified forearm** [CC] [RxHCC] [CC/MCC Exc]

[6th] **M80.84 Other osteoporosis with current pathological fracture, hand**

[7th] M80.841 **Other osteoporosis with current pathological fracture, right hand** [CC] [RxHCC] [CC/MCC Exc]

[7th] M80.842 **Other osteoporosis with current pathological fracture, left hand** [CC] [RxHCC] [CC/MCC Exc]

[7th] M80.849 **Other osteoporosis with current pathological fracture, unspecified hand** [CC] [RxHCC] [CC/MCC Exc]

[6th] **M80.85 Other osteoporosis with current pathological fracture, femur**

Other osteoporosis with current pathological fracture of hip

[7th] M80.851 **Other osteoporosis with current pathological fracture, right femur** [CC] [HCC] [RxHCC] [CC/MCC Exc]

[7th] M80.852 **Other osteoporosis with current pathological fracture, left femur** [CC] [HCC] [RxHCC] [CC/MCC Exc]

[7th] M80.859 **Other osteoporosis with current pathological fracture, unspecified femur** [CC] [HCC] [RxHCC] [CC/MCC Exc]

[6th] **M80.86 Other osteoporosis with current pathological fracture, lower leg**

[7th] M80.861 **Other osteoporosis with current pathological fracture, right lower leg** [CC] [RxHCC] [CC/MCC Exc]

[7th] M80.862 **Other osteoporosis with current pathological fracture, left lower leg** [CC] [RxHCC] [CC/MCC Exc]

[7th] M80.869 **Other osteoporosis with current pathological fracture, unspecified lower leg** [CC] [RxHCC] [CC/MCC Exc]

[6th] **M80.87 Other osteoporosis with current pathological fracture, ankle and foot**

[7th] M80.871 **Other osteoporosis with current pathological fracture, right ankle and foot** [CC] [RxHCC] [CC/MCC Exc]

[7th] M80.872 **Other osteoporosis with current pathological fracture, left ankle and foot** [CC] [RxHCC] [CC/MCC Exc]

[7th] M80.879 **Other osteoporosis with current pathological fracture, unspecified ankle and foot** [CC] [RxHCC] [CC/MCC Exc]

[7th] **M80.88 Other osteoporosis with current pathological fracture, vertebra(e)** [CC] [HCC] [RxHCC] [CC/MCC Exc]

[4th] **M81 Osteoporosis without current pathological fracture**

👁 **See Official Guidelines** "Osteoporosis" I.C.13.d, "Osteoporosis without current pathological fracture" I.C.13.d.1

Use additional code to identify:
major osseous defect, if applicable (M89.7-)
personal history of (healed) osteoporosis fracture, if applicable (Z87.310)

[PDx] Unacceptable principal diagnosis symbol per Medicare code edits [POA] Code exempt from diagnosis present on admission requirement
[?] Questionable admission [CC] Complication or comorbidity [MCC] Major complication or comorbidity [CC/MCC Exc] CC/MCC exclusion
[HCC] HCC diagnosis code [RxHCC] RxHCC diagnosis code MACRA code **DEFINITION** Describes condition/terminology
TIP Coding guidance 👁 Official Guideline Reference [Z1] Z code as first-listed diagnosis

[EXCLUDES1] *osteoporosis with current pathological fracture (M80.-)*
Sudeck's atrophy (M89.0)

M81.0 Age-related **osteoporosis without current pathological fracture** [A] [RxHCC]
Involutional osteoporosis without current pathological fracture
Osteoporosis NOS
Postmenopausal osteoporosis without current pathological fracture
Senile osteoporosis without current pathological fracture

M81.6 Localized **osteoporosis [Lequesne]** [RxHCC]
[EXCLUDES1] *Sudeck's atrophy (M89.0)*

M81.8 Other **osteoporosis without current pathological fracture** [RxHCC]
Drug-induced osteoporosis without current pathological fracture
Idiopathic osteoporosis without current pathological fracture
Osteoporosis of disuse without current pathological fracture
Postoophorectomy osteoporosis without current pathological fracture
Postsurgical malabsorption osteoporosis without current pathological fracture
Post-traumatic osteoporosis without current pathological fracture
Use additional code for adverse effect, if applicable, to identify drug (T36-T50 with fifth or sixth character 5)

[4th] **M83** Adult osteomalacia
[EXCLUDES1] *infantile and juvenile osteomalacia (E55.0)*
renal osteodystrophy (N25.0)
rickets (active) (E55.0)
rickets (active) sequelae (E64.3)
vitamin D-resistant osteomalacia (E83.3)
vitamin D-resistant rickets (active) (E83.3)

M83.0 Puerperal **osteomalacia** [M] [RxHCC] ♀
M83.1 Senile **osteomalacia** [A] [RxHCC]
M83.2 Adult **osteomalacia** due to malabsorption [A] [RxHCC]
Postsurgical malabsorption osteomalacia in adults
M83.3 Adult **osteomalacia** due to malnutrition [A] [RxHCC]
M83.4 Aluminum bone disease [RxHCC]
M83.5 **Other drug-induced osteomalacia in adults** [A] [RxHCC]
Use additional code for adverse effect, if applicable, to identify drug (T36-T50 with fifth or sixth character 5)
M83.8 Other **adult osteomalacia** [A] [RxHCC]
M83.9 **Adult osteomalacia, unspecified** [A] [RxHCC]

[4th] **M84** **Disorder of continuity of bone**
TIP: Pathologic fractures are the result of bone weakness or disease and not injury or trauma.
[EXCLUDES2] *traumatic fracture of bone-see fracture, by site*

[5th] **M84.3** Stress fracture
Fatigue fracture
March fracture
Stress fracture NOS
Stress reaction
Use additional external cause code(s) to identify the cause of the stress fracture
[EXCLUDES1] *pathological fracture NOS (M84.4.-)*
pathological fracture due to osteoporosis (M80.-)
traumatic fracture (S12.-, S22.-, S32.-, S42.-, S52.-, S62.-, S72.-, S82.-, S92.-)
[EXCLUDES2] *personal history of (healed) stress (fatigue) fracture (Z87.312)*
stress fracture of vertebra (M48.4-)

The appropriate 7th character is to be added to each code from subcategory M84.3:
A = initial encounter for fracture
D = subsequent encounter for fracture with routine healing
G = subsequent encounter for fracture with delayed healing
K = subsequent encounter for fracture with nonunion
P = subsequent encounter for fracture with malunion
S = sequela

[7th] **M84.30** **Stress fracture, unspecified site** CC CC/MCC Exc
[6th] **M84.31** **Stress fracture,** shoulder
[7th] **M84.311** **Stress fracture,** right **shoulder** CC CC/MCC Exc
[7th] **M84.312** **Stress fracture,** left **shoulder** CC CC/MCC Exc
[7th] **M84.319** **Stress fracture, unspecified shoulder** CC CC/MCC Exc
[6th] **M84.32** **Stress fracture,** humerus
[7th] **M84.321** **Stress fracture,** right **humerus** CC CC/MCC Exc
[7th] **M84.322** **Stress fracture,** left **humerus** CC CC/MCC Exc
[7th] **M84.329** **Stress fracture, unspecified humerus** CC CC/MCC Exc
[6th] **M84.33** **Stress fracture,** ulna and radius
[7th] **M84.331** **Stress fracture,** right ulna CC CC/MCC Exc
[7th] **M84.332** **Stress fracture,** left ulna CC CC/MCC Exc
[7th] **M84.333** **Stress fracture,** right radius CC CC/MCC Exc
[7th] **M84.334** **Stress fracture,** left radius CC CC/MCC Exc
[7th] **M84.339** **Stress fracture, unspecified ulna and radius** CC CC/MCC Exc
[6th] **M84.34** **Stress fracture,** hand and fingers
[7th] **M84.341** **Stress fracture,** right hand CC CC/MCC Exc
[7th] **M84.342** **Stress fracture,** left hand CC CC/MCC Exc
[7th] **M84.343** **Stress fracture, unspecified hand** CC CC/MCC Exc
[7th] **M84.344** **Stress fracture,** right finger(s) CC CC/MCC Exc
[7th] **M84.345** **Stress fracture,** left finger(s) CC CC/MCC Exc
[7th] **M84.346** **Stress fracture, unspecified finger(s)** CC CC/MCC Exc
[6th] **M84.35** **Stress fracture,** pelvis and femur
Stress fracture, hip
[7th] **M84.350** **Stress fracture, pelvis** CC CC/MCC Exc
[7th] **M84.351** **Stress fracture,** right femur CC CC/MCC Exc
[7th] **M84.352** **Stress fracture,** left femur CC CC/MCC Exc
[7th] **M84.353** **Stress fracture, unspecified femur** CC CC/MCC Exc
[7th] **M84.359** **Stress fracture, hip, unspecified** CC CC/MCC Exc
[6th] **M84.36** **Stress fracture,** tibia and fibula
[7th] **M84.361** **Stress fracture,** right tibia CC CC/MCC Exc
[7th] **M84.362** **Stress fracture,** left tibia CC CC/MCC Exc
[7th] **M84.363** **Stress fracture,** right fibula CC CC/MCC Exc
[7th] **M84.364** **Stress fracture,** left fibula CC CC/MCC Exc
[7th] **M84.369** **Stress fracture, unspecified tibia and fibula** CC CC/MCC Exc
[6th] **M84.37** **Stress fracture,** ankle, foot and toes
[7th] **M84.371** **Stress fracture,** right ankle CC CC/MCC Exc
[7th] **M84.372** **Stress fracture,** left ankle CC CC/MCC Exc
[7th] **M84.373** **Stress fracture, unspecified ankle** CC CC/MCC Exc
[7th] **M84.374** **Stress fracture,** right foot CC CC/MCC Exc
[7th] **M84.375** **Stress fracture,** left foot CC CC/MCC Exc
[7th] **M84.376** **Stress fracture, unspecified foot** CC CC/MCC Exc
[7th] **M84.377** **Stress fracture,** right toe(s) CC CC/MCC Exc
[7th] **M84.378** **Stress fracture,** left toe(s) CC CC/MCC Exc
[7th] **M84.379** **Stress fracture, unspecified toe(s)** CC CC/MCC Exc
[7th] **M84.38** **Stress fracture,** other site CC CC/MCC Exc
[EXCLUDES2] *stress fracture of vertebra (M48.4-)*

[5th] **M84.4** Pathological fracture, **not elsewhere classified**
Chronic fracture
Pathological fracture NOS
[EXCLUDES1] *collapsed vertebra NEC (M48.5)*
pathological fracture in neoplastic disease (M84.5-)
pathological fracture in osteoporosis (M80.-)
pathological fracture in other disease (M84.6-)
stress fracture (M84.3-)
traumatic fracture (S12.-, S22.-, S32.-, S42.-, S52.-, S62.-, S72.-, S82.-, S92.-)
[EXCLUDES2] *personal history of (healed) pathological fracture (Z87.311)*

Unspecified Code | Other Specified Code | Manifestation Code | [N] Newborn | [P] Pediatric | [M] Maternity | [A] Adult | ♂ Male | ♀ Female
● New Code | ▲ Revised Code Title | ►◄ Revised Text | [NOTES] | [INCLUDES] | [EXCLUDES1] Not coded here | [EXCLUDES2] Not included here
[4th] 4th character required | [5th] 5th character required | [6th] 6th character required | [7th] 7th character required | [X] Extension 'X' Alert
[HAC] Hospital-acquired condition (HAC) alert | AHA AHA Coding Clinic© | ☞ Code first alert

The appropriate 7th character is to be added to each code from subcategory M84.4:

A = initial encounter for fracture

D = subsequent encounter for fracture with routine healing

G = subsequent encounter for fracture with delayed healing

K = subsequent encounter for fracture with nonunion

P = subsequent encounter for fracture with malunion

S = sequela

🅦 M84.40 Pathological fracture, unspecified site cc RxHCC CC/MCC Exc

🅖 M84.41 Pathological fracture, shoulder

   🅦 M84.411 Pathological fracture, right shoulder cc RxHCC CC/MCC Exc

   🅦 M84.412 Pathological fracture, left shoulder cc RxHCC CC/MCC Exc

   🅦 M84.419 Pathological fracture, unspecified shoulder cc RxHCC CC/MCC Exc

🅖 M84.42 Pathological fracture, humerus

   🅦 M84.421 Pathological fracture, right humerus cc RxHCC CC/MCC Exc

   🅦 M84.422 Pathological fracture, left humerus cc RxHCC CC/MCC Exc

   🅦 M84.429 Pathological fracture, unspecified humerus cc RxHCC CC/MCC Exc

🅖 M84.43 Pathological fracture, ulna and radius

   🅦 M84.431 Pathological fracture, right ulna cc RxHCC CC/MCC Exc

   🅦 M84.432 Pathological fracture, left ulna cc RxHCC CC/MCC Exc

   🅦 M84.433 Pathological fracture, right radius cc RxHCC CC/MCC Exc

   🅦 M84.434 Pathological fracture, left radius cc RxHCC CC/MCC Exc

   🅦 M84.439 Pathological fracture, unspecified ulna and radius cc RxHCC CC/MCC Exc

🅖 M84.44 Pathological fracture, hand and fingers

   🅦 M84.441 Pathological fracture, right hand cc RxHCC CC/MCC Exc

   🅦 M84.442 Pathological fracture, left hand cc RxHCC CC/MCC Exc

   🅦 M84.443 Pathological fracture, unspecified hand cc RxHCC CC/MCC Exc

   🅦 M84.444 Pathological fracture, right finger(s) cc RxHCC CC/MCC Exc

   🅦 M84.445 Pathological fracture, left finger(s) cc RxHCC CC/MCC Exc

   🅦 M84.446 Pathological fracture, unspecified finger(s) cc RxHCC CC/MCC Exc

🅖 M84.45 Pathological fracture, femur and pelvis

   🅦 M84.451 Pathological fracture, right femur cc HCC CC/MCC Exc

   🅦 M84.452 Pathological fracture, left femur cc HCC RxHCC CC/MCC Exc

   🅦 M84.453 Pathological fracture, unspecified femur cc HCC RxHCC CC/MCC Exc

   🅦 M84.454 Pathological fracture, pelvis cc RxHCC CC/MCC Exc
       AHA: Q4 2016

   🅦 M84.459 Pathological fracture, hip, unspecified cc HCC RxHCC CC/MCC Exc

🅖 M84.46 Pathological fracture, tibia and fibula

   🅦 M84.461 Pathological fracture, right tibia cc RxHCC CC/MCC Exc

   🅦 M84.462 Pathological fracture, left tibia cc RxHCC CC/MCC Exc

   🅦 M84.463 Pathological fracture, right fibula cc RxHCC CC/MCC Exc

   🅦 M84.464 Pathological fracture, left fibula cc RxHCC CC/MCC Exc

   🅦 M84.469 Pathological fracture, unspecified tibia and fibula cc RxHCC CC/MCC Exc

🅖 M84.47 Pathological fracture, ankle, foot and toes

   🅦 M84.471 Pathological fracture, right ankle cc RxHCC CC/MCC Exc

   🅦 M84.472 Pathological fracture, left ankle cc RxHCC CC/MCC Exc

   🅦 M84.473 Pathological fracture, unspecified ankle cc RxHCC CC/MCC Exc

   🅦 M84.474 Pathological fracture, right foot cc RxHCC CC/MCC Exc

   🅦 M84.475 Pathological fracture, left foot cc RxHCC CC/MCC Exc

   🅦 M84.476 Pathological fracture, unspecified foot cc RxHCC CC/MCC Exc

   🅦 M84.477 Pathological fracture, right toe(s) cc RxHCC CC/MCC Exc

   🅦 M84.478 Pathological fracture, left toe(s) cc RxHCC CC/MCC Exc

   🅦 M84.479 Pathological fracture, unspecified toe(s) cc RxHCC CC/MCC Exc

🅦 M84.48 Pathological fracture, other site cc RxHCC CC/MCC Exc

🅕 M84.5 Pathological fracture in neoplastic disease

  👁 See Official Guidelines "Pathologic fracture due to a neoplasm" I.C.2.I.6

  Code also underlying neoplasm

The appropriate 7th character is to be added to each code from subcategory M84.5:

A = initial encounter for fracture

D = subsequent encounter for fracture with routine healing

G = subsequent encounter for fracture with delayed healing

K = subsequent encounter for fracture with nonunion

P = subsequent encounter for fracture with malunion

S = sequela

🅦 M84.50 Pathological fracture in neoplastic disease, unspecified site cc RxHCC CC/MCC Exc

🅖 M84.51 Pathological fracture in neoplastic disease, shoulder

   🅦 M84.511 Pathological fracture in neoplastic disease, right shoulder cc RxHCC CC/MCC Exc

   🅦 M84.512 Pathological fracture in neoplastic disease, left shoulder cc RxHCC CC/MCC Exc

   🅦 M84.519 Pathological fracture in neoplastic disease, unspecified shoulder cc RxHCC CC/MCC Exc

🅖 M84.52 Pathological fracture in neoplastic disease, humerus

   🅦 M84.521 Pathological fracture in neoplastic disease, right humerus cc RxHCC CC/MCC Exc

   🅦 M84.522 Pathological fracture in neoplastic disease, left humerus cc RxHCC CC/MCC Exc

   🅦 M84.529 Pathological fracture in neoplastic disease, unspecified humerus cc RxHCC CC/MCC Exc

🅖 M84.53 Pathological fracture in neoplastic disease, ulna and radius

   🅦 M84.531 Pathological fracture in neoplastic disease, right ulna cc RxHCC CC/MCC Exc

   🅦 M84.532 Pathological fracture in neoplastic disease, left ulna cc RxHCC CC/MCC Exc

   🅦 M84.533 Pathological fracture in neoplastic disease, right radius cc RxHCC CC/MCC Exc

   🅦 M84.534 Pathological fracture in neoplastic disease, left radius cc RxHCC CC/MCC Exc

   🅦 M84.539 Pathological fracture in neoplastic disease, unspecified ulna and radius cc RxHCC CC/MCC Exc

🅖 M84.54 Pathological fracture in neoplastic disease, hand

   🅦 M84.541 Pathological fracture in neoplastic disease, right hand cc RxHCC CC/MCC Exc

   🅦 M84.542 Pathological fracture in neoplastic disease, left hand cc RxHCC CC/MCC Exc

   🅦 M84.549 Pathological fracture in neoplastic disease, unspecified hand cc RxHCC CC/MCC Exc

🅖 M84.55 Pathological fracture in neoplastic disease, pelvis and femur

   🅦 M84.550 Pathological fracture in neoplastic disease, pelvis cc RxHCC CC/MCC Exc

   🅦 M84.551 Pathological fracture in neoplastic disease, right femur cc HCC RxHCC CC/MCC Exc

838

When symbols appear on a code that requires a 7th character extension, refer to Appendix B to identify applicable 7th character codes.

2020 ICD-10-CM

PDxR Unacceptable principal diagnosis symbol per Medicare code edits PDx Code exempt from diagnosis present on admission requirement ❓ Questionable admission cc Complication or comorbidity MCC Major complication or comorbidity CC/MCC Exc CC/MCC exclusion HCC HCC diagnosis code RxHCC RxHCC diagnosis code MACRA code **DEFINITION** Describes condition/terminology **TIP** Coding guidance 👁 Official Guideline Reference Z1 Z code as first-listed diagnosis

- [7th] M84.552 Pathological fracture in neoplastic disease, left femur [CC] [HCC] [RxHCC] [CC/MCC Exc]
- [7th] M84.553 Pathological fracture in neoplastic disease, unspecified femur [CC] [HCC] [RxHCC] [CC/MCC Exc]
- [7th] M84.559 Pathological fracture in neoplastic disease, hip, unspecified [CC] [HCC] [RxHCC] [CC/MCC Exc]
- [6th] M84.56 Pathological fracture in neoplastic disease, tibia and fibula
  - [7th] M84.561 Pathological fracture in neoplastic disease, right tibia [CC] [RxHCC] [CC/MCC Exc]
  - [7th] M84.562 Pathological fracture in neoplastic disease, left tibia [CC] [RxHCC] [CC/MCC Exc]
  - [7th] M84.563 Pathological fracture in neoplastic disease, right fibula [CC] [RxHCC] [CC/MCC Exc]
  - [7th] M84.564 Pathological fracture in neoplastic disease, left fibula [CC] [RxHCC] [CC/MCC Exc]
  - [7th] M84.569 Pathological fracture in neoplastic disease, unspecified tibia and fibula [CC] [RxHCC] [CC/MCC Exc]
- [6th] M84.57 Pathological fracture in neoplastic disease, ankle and foot
  - [7th] M84.571 Pathological fracture in neoplastic disease, right ankle [CC] [RxHCC] [CC/MCC Exc]
  - [7th] M84.572 Pathological fracture in neoplastic disease, left ankle [CC] [RxHCC] [CC/MCC Exc]
  - [7th] M84.573 Pathological fracture in neoplastic disease, unspecified ankle [CC] [RxHCC] [CC/MCC Exc]
  - [7th] M84.574 Pathological fracture in neoplastic disease, right foot [CC] [RxHCC] [CC/MCC Exc]
  - [7th] M84.575 Pathological fracture in neoplastic disease, left foot [CC] [RxHCC] [CC/MCC Exc]
  - [7th] M84.576 Pathological fracture in neoplastic disease, unspecified foot [CC] [RxHCC] [CC/MCC Exc]
- [7th] M84.58 Pathological fracture in neoplastic disease, other specified site [CC] [RxHCC] [CC/MCC Exc]
  - Pathological fracture in neoplastic disease, vertebrae

[5th] M84.6 Pathological fracture in other disease

Code also underlying condition

EXCLUDES1 *pathological fracture in osteoporosis (M80.-)*

The appropriate 7th character is to be added to each code from subcategory M84.6:

- A = initial encounter for fracture
- D = subsequent encounter for fracture with routine healing
- G = subsequent encounter for fracture with delayed healing
- K = subsequent encounter for fracture with nonunion
- P = subsequent encounter for fracture with malunion
- S = sequela

- [7th] M84.60 Pathological fracture in other disease, unspecified site [CC] [RxHCC] [CC/MCC Exc]
- [6th] M84.61 Pathological fracture in other disease, shoulder
  - [7th] M84.611 Pathological fracture in other disease, right shoulder [CC] [RxHCC] [CC/MCC Exc]
  - [7th] M84.612 Pathological fracture in other disease, left shoulder [CC] [RxHCC] [CC/MCC Exc]
  - [7th] M84.619 Pathological fracture in other disease, unspecified shoulder [CC] [RxHCC] [CC/MCC Exc]
- [6th] M84.62 Pathological fracture in other disease, humerus
  - [7th] M84.621 Pathological fracture in other disease, right humerus [CC] [RxHCC] [CC/MCC Exc]
  - [7th] M84.622 Pathological fracture in other disease, left humerus [CC] [RxHCC] [CC/MCC Exc]
  - [7th] M84.629 Pathological fracture in other disease, unspecified humerus [CC] [RxHCC] [CC/MCC Exc]
- [6th] M84.63 Pathological fracture in other disease, ulna and radius
  - [7th] M84.631 Pathological fracture in other disease, right ulna [CC] [RxHCC] [CC/MCC Exc]
  - [7th] M84.632 Pathological fracture in other disease, left ulna [CC] [RxHCC] [CC/MCC Exc]
  - [7th] M84.633 Pathological fracture in other disease, right radius [CC] [RxHCC] [CC/MCC Exc]
  - [7th] M84.634 Pathological fracture in other disease, left radius [CC] [RxHCC] [CC/MCC Exc]
  - [7th] M84.639 Pathological fracture in other disease, unspecified ulna and radius [CC] [RxHCC] [CC/MCC Exc]
- [6th] M84.64 Pathological fracture in other disease, hand
  - [7th] M84.641 Pathological fracture in other disease, right hand [CC] [RxHCC] [CC/MCC Exc]
  - [7th] M84.642 Pathological fracture in other disease, left hand [CC] [RxHCC] [CC/MCC Exc]
  - [7th] M84.649 Pathological fracture in other disease, unspecified hand [CC] [RxHCC] [CC/MCC Exc]
- [6th] M84.65 Pathological fracture in other disease, pelvis and femur
  - [7th] M84.650 Pathological fracture in other disease, pelvis [CC] [RxHCC] [CC/MCC Exc]
  - [7th] M84.651 Pathological fracture in other disease, right femur [CC] [HCC] [RxHCC] [CC/MCC Exc]
  - [7th] M84.652 Pathological fracture in other disease, left femur [CC] [HCC] [RxHCC] [CC/MCC Exc]
  - [7th] M84.653 Pathological fracture in other disease, unspecified femur [CC] [HCC] [RxHCC] [CC/MCC Exc]
  - [7th] M84.659 Pathological fracture in other disease, hip, unspecified [CC] [HCC] [RxHCC] [CC/MCC Exc]
- [6th] M84.66 Pathological fracture in other disease, tibia and fibula
  - [7th] M84.661 Pathological fracture in other disease, right tibia [CC] [RxHCC] [CC/MCC Exc]
  - [7th] M84.662 Pathological fracture in other disease, left tibia [CC] [RxHCC] [CC/MCC Exc]
  - [7th] M84.663 Pathological fracture in other disease, right fibula [CC] [RxHCC] [CC/MCC Exc]
  - [7th] M84.664 Pathological fracture in other disease, left fibula [CC] [RxHCC] [CC/MCC Exc]
  - [7th] M84.669 Pathological fracture in other disease, unspecified tibia and fibula [CC] [RxHCC] [CC/MCC Exc]
- [6th] M84.67 Pathological fracture in other disease, ankle and foot
  - [7th] M84.671 Pathological fracture in other disease, right ankle [CC] [RxHCC] [CC/MCC Exc]
  - [7th] M84.672 Pathological fracture in other disease, left ankle [CC] [RxHCC] [CC/MCC Exc]
  - [7th] M84.673 Pathological fracture in other disease, unspecified ankle [CC] [RxHCC] [CC/MCC Exc]
  - [7th] M84.674 Pathological fracture in other disease, right foot [CC] [RxHCC] [CC/MCC Exc]
  - [7th] M84.675 Pathological fracture in other disease, left foot [CC] [RxHCC] [CC/MCC Exc]
  - [7th] M84.676 Pathological fracture in other disease, unspecified foot [CC] [RxHCC] [CC/MCC Exc]
- [7th] M84.68 Pathological fracture in other disease, other site [CC] [RxHCC] [CC/MCC Exc]

[5th] M84.7 Nontraumatic fracture, not elsewhere classified

- [6th] M84.75 Atypical femoral fracture

  The appropriate 7th character is to be added to each code from M84.75:

  - A = initial encounter for fracture
  - D = subsequent encounter for fracture with routine healing
  - G = subsequent encounter for fracture with delayed healing
  - K = subsequent encounter for fracture with nonunion
  - P = subsequent encounter for fracture with malunion
  - S = sequela

  - [7th] M84.750 Atypical femoral fracture, unspecified [CC] [POA] [CC/MCC Exc]
  - [7th] M84.751 Incomplete atypical femoral fracture, right leg [CC] [POA] [CC/MCC Exc]

Unspecified Code | Other Specified Code | Manifestation Code | [N] Newborn | [P] Pediatric | [M] Maternity | [A] Adult | ♂ Male | ♀ Female
● New Code | ▲ Revised Code Title | ►◄ Revised Text | NOTES | INCLUDES | EXCLUDES1 Not coded here | EXCLUDES2 Not included here
[4th] 4th character required | [5th] 5th character required | [6th] 6th character required | [7th] 7th character required | [x] Extension 'X' Alert
[HAC] Hospital-acquired condition (HAC) alert | AHA AHA Coding Clinic© | Code first alert

When symbols appear on a code that requires a 7th character extension, refer to Appendix B to identify applicable 7th character codes.

[7th] M84.752 Incomplete atypical femoral fracture, left leg [CC] [POA] [CC/MCC Exc]

[7th] M84.753 Incomplete atypical femoral fracture, unspecified leg [CC] [POA] [CC/MCC Exc]

[7th] M84.754 Complete transverse atypical femoral fracture, right leg [CC] [POA] [HCC] [CC/MCC Exc]

[7th] M84.755 Complete transverse atypical femoral fracture, left leg [CC] [POA] [HCC] [CC/MCC Exc]

[7th] M84.756 Complete transverse atypical femoral fracture, unspecified leg [CC] [POA] [HCC] [CC/MCC Exc]

[7th] M84.757 Complete oblique atypical femoral fracture, right leg [CC] [POA] [HCC] [CC/MCC Exc]

[7th] M84.758 Complete oblique atypical femoral fracture, left leg [CC] [POA] [HCC] [CC/MCC Exc]

[7th] M84.759 Complete oblique atypical femoral fracture, unspecified leg [CC] [POA] [HCC] [CC/MCC Exc]

[5th] M84.8 Other disorders of continuity of bone

M84.80 Other disorders of continuity of bone, unspecified site

[6th] M84.81 Other disorders of continuity of bone, shoulder

M84.811 Other disorders of continuity of bone, right shoulder

M84.812 Other disorders of continuity of bone, left shoulder

M84.819 Other disorders of continuity of bone, unspecified shoulder

[6th] M84.82 Other disorders of continuity of bone, humerus

M84.821 Other disorders of continuity of bone, right humerus

M84.822 Other disorders of continuity of bone, left humerus

M84.829 Other disorders of continuity of bone, unspecified humerus

[6th] M84.83 Other disorders of continuity of bone, ulna and radius

M84.831 Other disorders of continuity of bone, right ulna

M84.832 Other disorders of continuity of bone, left ulna

M84.833 Other disorders of continuity of bone, right radius

M84.834 Other disorders of continuity of bone, left radius

M84.839 Other disorders of continuity of bone, unspecified ulna and radius

[6th] M84.84 Other disorders of continuity of bone, hand

M84.841 Other disorders of continuity of bone, right hand

M84.842 Other disorders of continuity of bone, left hand

M84.849 Other disorders of continuity of bone, unspecified hand

[6th] M84.85 Other disorders of continuity of bone, pelvic region and thigh

M84.851 Other disorders of continuity of bone, right pelvic region and thigh

M84.852 Other disorders of continuity of bone, left pelvic region and thigh

M84.859 Other disorders of continuity of bone, unspecified pelvic region and thigh

[6th] M84.86 Other disorders of continuity of bone, tibia and fibula

M84.861 Other disorders of continuity of bone, right tibia

M84.862 Other disorders of continuity of bone, left tibia

M84.863 Other disorders of continuity of bone, right fibula

M84.864 Other disorders of continuity of bone, left fibula

M84.869 Other disorders of continuity of bone, unspecified tibia and fibula

[6th] M84.87 Other disorders of continuity of bone, ankle and foot

M84.871 Other disorders of continuity of bone, right ankle and foot

M84.872 Other disorders of continuity of bone, left ankle and foot

M84.879 Other disorders of continuity of bone, unspecified ankle and foot

M84.88 Other disorders of continuity of bone, other site

M84.9 Disorder of continuity of bone, unspecified

[4th] M85 Other disorders of bone density and structure

[EXCLUDES1] *osteogenesis imperfecta (Q78.0)*
osteopetrosis (Q78.2)
osteopoikilosis (Q78.8)
polyostotic fibrous dysplasia (Q78.1)

[5th] M85.0 Fibrous dysplasia (monostotic)

[EXCLUDES2] *fibrous dysplasia of jaw (M27.8)*

M85.00 Fibrous dysplasia (monostotic), unspecified site

[6th] M85.01 Fibrous dysplasia (monostotic), shoulder

M85.011 Fibrous dysplasia (monostotic), right shoulder

M85.012 Fibrous dysplasia (monostotic), left shoulder

M85.019 Fibrous dysplasia (monostotic), unspecified shoulder

[6th] M85.02 Fibrous dysplasia (monostotic), upper arm

M85.021 Fibrous dysplasia (monostotic), right upper arm

M85.022 Fibrous dysplasia (monostotic), left upper arm

M85.029 Fibrous dysplasia (monostotic), unspecified upper arm

[6th] M85.03 Fibrous dysplasia (monostotic), forearm

M85.031 Fibrous dysplasia (monostotic), right forearm

M85.032 Fibrous dysplasia (monostotic), left forearm

M85.039 Fibrous dysplasia (monostotic), unspecified forearm

[6th] M85.04 Fibrous dysplasia (monostotic), hand

M85.041 Fibrous dysplasia (monostotic), right hand

M85.042 Fibrous dysplasia (monostotic), left hand

M85.049 Fibrous dysplasia (monostotic), unspecified hand

[6th] M85.05 Fibrous dysplasia (monostotic), thigh

M85.051 Fibrous dysplasia (monostotic), right thigh

M85.052 Fibrous dysplasia (monostotic), left thigh

M85.059 Fibrous dysplasia (monostotic), unspecified thigh

[6th] M85.06 Fibrous dysplasia (monostotic), lower leg

M85.061 Fibrous dysplasia (monostotic), right lower leg

M85.062 Fibrous dysplasia (monostotic), left lower leg

M85.069 Fibrous dysplasia (monostotic), unspecified lower leg

[6th] M85.07 Fibrous dysplasia (monostotic), ankle and foot

M85.071 Fibrous dysplasia (monostotic), right ankle and foot

M85.072 Fibrous dysplasia (monostotic), left ankle and foot

M85.079 Fibrous dysplasia (monostotic), unspecified ankle and foot

M85.08 Fibrous dysplasia (monostotic), other site

M85.09 Fibrous dysplasia (monostotic), multiple sites

[5th] M85.1 Skeletal fluorosis

M85.10 Skeletal fluorosis, unspecified site

[6th] M85.11 Skeletal fluorosis, shoulder

M85.111 Skeletal fluorosis, right shoulder

M85.112 Skeletal fluorosis, left shoulder

M85.119 Skeletal fluorosis, unspecified shoulder

[6th] M85.12 Skeletal fluorosis, upper arm
M85.121 Skeletal fluorosis, right upper arm
M85.122 Skeletal fluorosis, left upper arm
M85.129 Skeletal fluorosis, unspecified upper arm
[6th] M85.13 Skeletal fluorosis, forearm
M85.131 Skeletal fluorosis, right forearm
M85.132 Skeletal fluorosis, left forearm
M85.139 Skeletal fluorosis, unspecified forearm
[6th] M85.14 Skeletal fluorosis, hand
M85.141 Skeletal fluorosis, right hand
M85.142 Skeletal fluorosis, left hand
M85.149 Skeletal fluorosis, unspecified hand
[6th] M85.15 Skeletal fluorosis, thigh
M85.151 Skeletal fluorosis, right thigh
M85.152 Skeletal fluorosis, left thigh
M85.159 Skeletal fluorosis, unspecified thigh
[6th] M85.16 Skeletal fluorosis, lower leg
M85.161 Skeletal fluorosis, right lower leg
M85.162 Skeletal fluorosis, left lower leg
M85.169 Skeletal fluorosis, unspecified lower leg
[6th] M85.17 Skeletal fluorosis, ankle and foot
M85.171 Skeletal fluorosis, right ankle and foot
M85.172 Skeletal fluorosis, left ankle and foot
M85.179 Skeletal fluorosis, unspecified ankle and foot
M85.18 Skeletal fluorosis, other site
M85.19 Skeletal fluorosis, multiple sites
M85.2 Hyperostosis of skull
[5th] M85.3 Osteitis condensans
DEFINITION: Osteitis condensans is an increase in bone density and is typically an incidental finding on -ray.
M85.30 Osteitis condensans, unspecified site
[6th] M85.31 Osteitis condensans, shoulder
M85.311 Osteitis condensans, right shoulder
M85.312 Osteitis condensans, left shoulder
M85.319 Osteitis condensans, unspecified shoulder
[6th] M85.32 Osteitis condensans, upper arm
M85.321 Osteitis condensans, right upper arm
M85.322 Osteitis condensans, left upper arm
M85.329 Osteitis condensans, unspecified upper arm
[6th] M85.33 Osteitis condensans, forearm
M85.331 Osteitis condensans, right forearm
M85.332 Osteitis condensans, left forearm
M85.339 Osteitis condensans, unspecified forearm
[6th] M85.34 Osteitis condensans, hand
M85.341 Osteitis condensans, right hand
M85.342 Osteitis condensans, left hand
M85.349 Osteitis condensans, unspecified hand
[6th] M85.35 Osteitis condensans, thigh
M85.351 Osteitis condensans, right thigh
M85.352 Osteitis condensans, left thigh
M85.359 Osteitis condensans, unspecified thigh
[6th] M85.36 Osteitis condensans, lower leg
M85.361 Osteitis condensans, right lower leg
M85.362 Osteitis condensans, left lower leg
M85.369 Osteitis condensans, unspecified lower leg
[6th] M85.37 Osteitis condensans, ankle and foot
M85.371 Osteitis condensans, right ankle and foot
M85.372 Osteitis condensans, left ankle and foot
M85.379 Osteitis condensans, unspecified ankle and foot
M85.38 Osteitis condensans, other site
M85.39 Osteitis condensans, multiple sites
[5th] M85.4 Solitary bone cyst
EXCLUDES2 *solitary cyst of jaw (M27.4)*
M85.40 Solitary bone cyst, unspecified site
[6th] M85.41 Solitary bone cyst, shoulder
M85.411 Solitary bone cyst, right shoulder
M85.412 Solitary bone cyst, left shoulder
M85.419 Solitary bone cyst, unspecified shoulder
[6th] M85.42 Solitary bone cyst, humerus
M85.421 Solitary bone cyst, right humerus
M85.422 Solitary bone cyst, left humerus
M85.429 Solitary bone cyst, unspecified humerus
[6th] M85.43 Solitary bone cyst, ulna and radius
M85.431 Solitary bone cyst, right ulna and radius
M85.432 Solitary bone cyst, left ulna and radius
M85.439 Solitary bone cyst, unspecified ulna and radius
[6th] M85.44 Solitary bone cyst, hand
M85.441 Solitary bone cyst, right hand
M85.442 Solitary bone cyst, left hand
M85.449 Solitary bone cyst, unspecified hand
[6th] M85.45 Solitary bone cyst, pelvis
M85.451 Solitary bone cyst, right pelvis
M85.452 Solitary bone cyst, left pelvis
M85.459 Solitary bone cyst, unspecified pelvis
[6th] M85.46 Solitary bone cyst, tibia and fibula
M85.461 Solitary bone cyst, right tibia and fibula
M85.462 Solitary bone cyst, left tibia and fibula
M85.469 Solitary bone cyst, unspecified tibia and fibula
[6th] M85.47 Solitary bone cyst, ankle and foot
M85.471 Solitary bone cyst, right ankle and foot
M85.472 Solitary bone cyst, left ankle and foot
M85.479 Solitary bone cyst, unspecified ankle and foot
M85.48 Solitary bone cyst, other site
[5th] M85.5 Aneurysmal bone cyst
EXCLUDES2 *aneurysmal cyst of jaw (M27.4)*
M85.50 Aneurysmal bone cyst, unspecified site
[6th] M85.51 Aneurysmal bone cyst, shoulder
M85.511 Aneurysmal bone cyst, right shoulder
M85.512 Aneurysmal bone cyst, left shoulder
M85.519 Aneurysmal bone cyst, unspecified shoulder
[6th] M85.52 Aneurysmal bone cyst, upper arm
M85.521 Aneurysmal bone cyst, right upper arm
M85.522 Aneurysmal bone cyst, left upper arm
M85.529 Aneurysmal bone cyst, unspecified upper arm
[6th] M85.53 Aneurysmal bone cyst, forearm
M85.531 Aneurysmal bone cyst, right forearm
M85.532 Aneurysmal bone cyst, left forearm
M85.539 Aneurysmal bone cyst, unspecified forearm
[6th] M85.54 Aneurysmal bone cyst, hand
M85.541 Aneurysmal bone cyst, right hand
M85.542 Aneurysmal bone cyst, left hand
M85.549 Aneurysmal bone cyst, unspecified hand
[6th] M85.55 Aneurysmal bone cyst, thigh
M85.551 Aneurysmal bone cyst, right thigh
M85.552 Aneurysmal bone cyst, left thigh
M85.559 Aneurysmal bone cyst, unspecified thigh
[6th] M85.56 Aneurysmal bone cyst, lower leg
M85.561 Aneurysmal bone cyst, right lower leg
M85.562 Aneurysmal bone cyst, left lower leg
M85.569 Aneurysmal bone cyst, unspecified lower leg
[6th] M85.57 Aneurysmal bone cyst, ankle and foot
M85.571 Aneurysmal bone cyst, right ankle and foot
M85.572 Aneurysmal bone cyst, left ankle and foot
M85.579 Aneurysmal bone cyst, unspecified ankle and foot
M85.58 Aneurysmal bone cyst, other site

M85.59 Aneurysmal bone cyst, multiple sites

M85.6 Other cyst of bone

EXCLUDES1 cyst of jaw NEC (M27.4)

osteitis fibrosa cystica generalisata [von Recklinghausen's disease of bone] (E21.0)

M85.60 Other cyst of bone, unspecified site

M85.61 Other cyst of bone, shoulder
- M85.611 Other cyst of bone, right shoulder
- M85.612 Other cyst of bone, left shoulder
- M85.619 Other cyst of bone, unspecified shoulder

M85.62 Other cyst of bone, upper arm
- M85.621 Other cyst of bone, right upper arm
- M85.622 Other cyst of bone, left upper arm
- M85.629 Other cyst of bone, unspecified upper arm

M85.63 Other cyst of bone, forearm
- M85.631 Other cyst of bone, right forearm
- M85.632 Other cyst of bone, left forearm
- M85.639 Other cyst of bone, unspecified forearm

M85.64 Other cyst of bone, hand
- M85.641 Other cyst of bone, right hand
- M85.642 Other cyst of bone, left hand
- M85.649 Other cyst of bone, unspecified hand

M85.65 Other cyst of bone, thigh
- M85.651 Other cyst of bone, right thigh
- M85.652 Other cyst of bone, left thigh
- M85.659 Other cyst of bone, unspecified thigh

M85.66 Other cyst of bone, lower leg
- M85.661 Other cyst of bone, right lower leg
- M85.662 Other cyst of bone, left lower leg
- M85.669 Other cyst of bone, unspecified lower leg

M85.67 Other cyst of bone, ankle and foot
- M85.671 Other cyst of bone, right ankle and foot
- M85.672 Other cyst of bone, left ankle and foot
- M85.679 Other cyst of bone, unspecified ankle and foot

M85.68 Other cyst of bone, other site
M85.69 Other cyst of bone, multiple sites

M85.8 Other specified disorders of bone density and structure

DEFINITION: Hyperostosis is a hardening or calcification of bone.

Hyperostosis of bones, except skull
Osteosclerosis, acquired

EXCLUDES1 diffuse idiopathic skeletal hyperostosis [DISH] (M48.1)

osteosclerosis congenita (Q77.4)
osteosclerosis fragilitas (generalista) (Q78.2)
osteosclerosis myelofibrosis (D75.81)

M85.80 Other specified disorders of bone density and structure, unspecified site

M85.81 Other specified disorders of bone density and structure, shoulder
- M85.811 Other specified disorders of bone density and structure, right shoulder
- M85.812 Other specified disorders of bone density and structure, left shoulder
- M85.819 Other specified disorders of bone density and structure, unspecified shoulder

M85.82 Other specified disorders of bone density and structure, upper arm
- M85.821 Other specified disorders of bone density and structure, right upper arm
- M85.822 Other specified disorders of bone density and structure, left upper arm
- M85.829 Other specified disorders of bone density and structure, unspecified upper arm

M85.83 Other specified disorders of bone density and structure, forearm
- M85.831 Other specified disorders of bone density and structure, right forearm

M85.832 Other specified disorders of bone density and structure, left forearm
- M85.839 Other specified disorders of bone density and structure, unspecified forearm

M85.84 Other specified disorders of bone density and structure, hand
- M85.841 Other specified disorders of bone density and structure, right hand
- M85.842 Other specified disorders of bone density and structure, left hand
- M85.849 Other specified disorders of bone density and structure, unspecified hand

M85.85 Other specified disorders of bone density and structure, thigh
- M85.851 Other specified disorders of bone density and structure, right thigh
- M85.852 Other specified disorders of bone density and structure, left thigh
- M85.859 Other specified disorders of bone density and structure, unspecified thigh

M85.86 Other specified disorders of bone density and structure, lower leg
- M85.861 Other specified disorders of bone density and structure, right lower leg
- M85.862 Other specified disorders of bone density and structure, left lower leg
- M85.869 Other specified disorders of bone density and structure, unspecified lower leg

M85.87 Other specified disorders of bone density and structure, ankle and foot
- M85.871 Other specified disorders of bone density and structure, right ankle and foot
- M85.872 Other specified disorders of bone density and structure, left ankle and foot
- M85.879 Other specified disorders of bone density and structure, unspecified ankle and foot

M85.88 Other specified disorders of bone density and structure, other site
M85.89 Other specified disorders of bone density and structure, multiple sites

M85.9 Disorder of bone density and structure, unspecified

Other osteopathies (M86-M90)

EXCLUDES1 postprocedural osteopathies (M96.-)

M86 Osteomyelitis

Use additional code (B95-B97) to identify infectious agent
Use additional code to identify major osseous defect, if applicable (M89.7-)

EXCLUDES1 osteomyelitis due to:
echinococcus (B67.2)
gonococcus (A54.43)
salmonella (A02.24)

EXCLUDES2 ostemyelitis of:
orbit (H05.0-)
petrous bone (H70.2-)
vertebra (M46.2-)

M86.0 Acute hematogenous osteomyelitis
M86.00 Acute hematogenous osteomyelitis, unspecified site
M86.01 Acute hematogenous osteomyelitis, shoulder
- M86.011 Acute hematogenous osteomyelitis, right shoulder
- M86.012 Acute hematogenous osteomyelitis, left shoulder
- M86.019 Acute hematogenous osteomyelitis, unspecified shoulder
M86.02 Acute hematogenous osteomyelitis, humerus
- M86.021 Acute hematogenous osteomyelitis, right humerus

M86.022 Acute hematogenous osteomyelitis, left humerus CC [HCC] CC/MCC Exc

M86.029 Acute hematogenous osteomyelitis, unspecified humerus CC [HCC] CC/MCC Exc

[6th] M86.03 Acute hematogenous osteomyelitis, radius and ulna

M86.031 Acute hematogenous osteomyelitis, right radius and ulna CC [HCC] CC/MCC Exc

M86.032 Acute hematogenous osteomyelitis, left radius and ulna CC [HCC] CC/MCC Exc

M86.039 Acute hematogenous osteomyelitis, unspecified radius and ulna CC [HCC] CC/MCC Exc

[6th] M86.04 Acute hematogenous osteomyelitis, hand

M86.041 Acute hematogenous osteomyelitis, right hand CC [HCC] CC/MCC Exc

M86.042 Acute hematogenous osteomyelitis, left hand CC [HCC] CC/MCC Exc

M86.049 Acute hematogenous osteomyelitis, unspecified hand CC [HCC] CC/MCC Exc

[6th] M86.05 Acute hematogenous osteomyelitis, femur

M86.051 Acute hematogenous osteomyelitis, right femur CC [HCC] CC/MCC Exc

M86.052 Acute hematogenous osteomyelitis, left femur CC [HCC] CC/MCC Exc

M86.059 Acute hematogenous osteomyelitis, unspecified femur CC [HCC] CC/MCC Exc

[6th] M86.06 Acute hematogenous osteomyelitis, tibia and fibula

M86.061 Acute hematogenous osteomyelitis, right tibia and fibula CC [HCC] CC/MCC Exc

M86.062 Acute hematogenous osteomyelitis, left tibia and fibula CC [HCC] CC/MCC Exc

M86.069 Acute hematogenous osteomyelitis, unspecified tibia and fibula CC [HCC] CC/MCC Exc

[6th] M86.07 Acute hematogenous osteomyelitis, ankle and foot

M86.071 Acute hematogenous osteomyelitis, right ankle and foot CC [HCC] CC/MCC Exc

M86.072 Acute hematogenous osteomyelitis, left ankle and foot CC [HCC] CC/MCC Exc

M86.079 Acute hematogenous osteomyelitis, unspecified ankle and foot CC [HCC] CC/MCC Exc

M86.08 Acute hematogenous osteomyelitis, other sites CC [HCC] CC/MCC Exc

M86.09 Acute hematogenous osteomyelitis, multiple sites CC [HCC] CC/MCC Exc

[5th] M86.1 Other acute osteomyelitis

M86.10 Other acute osteomyelitis, unspecified site CC [HCC] CC/MCC Exc

[6th] M86.11 Other acute osteomyelitis, shoulder

M86.111 Other acute osteomyelitis, right shoulder CC [HCC] CC/MCC Exc

M86.112 Other acute osteomyelitis, left shoulder CC [HCC] CC/MCC Exc

M86.119 Other acute osteomyelitis, unspecified shoulder CC [HCC] CC/MCC Exc

[6th] M86.12 Other acute osteomyelitis, humerus

M86.121 Other acute osteomyelitis, right humerus CC [HCC] CC/MCC Exc

M86.122 Other acute osteomyelitis, left humerus CC [HCC] CC/MCC Exc

M86.129 Other acute osteomyelitis, unspecified humerus CC [HCC] CC/MCC Exc

[6th] M86.13 Other acute osteomyelitis, radius and ulna

M86.131 Other acute osteomyelitis, right radius and ulna CC [HCC] CC/MCC Exc

M86.132 Other acute osteomyelitis, left radius and ulna CC [HCC] CC/MCC Exc

M86.139 Other acute osteomyelitis, unspecified radius and ulna CC [HCC] CC/MCC Exc

[6th] M86.14 Other acute osteomyelitis, hand

M86.141 Other acute osteomyelitis, right hand CC [HCC] CC/MCC Exc

M86.142 Other acute osteomyelitis, left hand CC [HCC] CC/MCC Exc

M86.149 Other acute osteomyelitis, unspecified hand CC [HCC] CC/MCC Exc

[6th] M86.15 Other acute osteomyelitis, femur

M86.151 Other acute osteomyelitis, right femur CC [HCC] CC/MCC Exc

M86.152 Other acute osteomyelitis, left femur CC [HCC] CC/MCC Exc

M86.159 Other acute osteomyelitis, unspecified femur CC [HCC] CC/MCC Exc

[6th] M86.16 Other acute osteomyelitis, tibia and fibula

M86.161 Other acute osteomyelitis, right tibia and fibula CC [HCC] CC/MCC Exc

M86.162 Other acute osteomyelitis, left tibia and fibula CC [HCC] CC/MCC Exc

M86.169 Other acute osteomyelitis, unspecified tibia and fibula CC [HCC] CC/MCC Exc

[6th] M86.17 Other acute osteomyelitis, ankle and foot

M86.171 Other acute osteomyelitis, right ankle and foot CC [HCC] CC/MCC Exc

M86.172 Other acute osteomyelitis, left ankle and foot CC [HCC] CC/MCC Exc

M86.179 Other acute osteomyelitis, unspecified ankle and foot CC [HCC] CC/MCC Exc

M86.18 Other acute osteomyelitis, other site CC [HCC] CC/MCC Exc

M86.19 Other acute osteomyelitis, multiple sites CC [HCC] CC/MCC Exc

[5th] M86.2 Subacute osteomyelitis

M86.20 Subacute osteomyelitis, unspecified site CC [HCC] CC/MCC Exc

[6th] M86.21 Subacute osteomyelitis, shoulder

M86.211 Subacute osteomyelitis, right shoulder CC [HCC] CC/MCC Exc

M86.212 Subacute osteomyelitis, left shoulder CC [HCC] CC/MCC Exc

M86.219 Subacute osteomyelitis, unspecified shoulder CC [HCC] CC/MCC Exc

[6th] M86.22 Subacute osteomyelitis, humerus

M86.221 Subacute osteomyelitis, right humerus CC [HCC] CC/MCC Exc

M86.222 Subacute osteomyelitis, left humerus CC [HCC] CC/MCC Exc

M86.229 Subacute osteomyelitis, unspecified humerus CC [HCC] CC/MCC Exc

[6th] M86.23 Subacute osteomyelitis, radius and ulna

M86.231 Subacute osteomyelitis, right radius and ulna CC [HCC] CC/MCC Exc

M86.232 Subacute osteomyelitis, left radius and ulna CC [HCC] CC/MCC Exc

M86.239 Subacute osteomyelitis, unspecified radius and ulna CC [HCC] CC/MCC Exc

[6th] M86.24 Subacute osteomyelitis, hand

M86.241 Subacute osteomyelitis, right hand CC [HCC] CC/MCC Exc

M86.242 Subacute osteomyelitis, left hand CC [HCC] CC/MCC Exc

M86.249 Subacute osteomyelitis, unspecified hand CC [HCC] CC/MCC Exc

[6th] M86.25 Subacute osteomyelitis, femur

M86.251 Subacute osteomyelitis, right femur CC [HCC] CC/MCC Exc

M86.252 Subacute osteomyelitis, left femur CC [HCC] CC/MCC Exc

M86.259 Subacute osteomyelitis, unspecified femur CC [HCC] CC/MCC Exc

[6th] M86.26 Subacute osteomyelitis, tibia and fibula

M86.261 Subacute osteomyelitis, right tibia and fibula CC [HCC] CC/MCC Exc

M86.262 Subacute osteomyelitis, left tibia and fibula CC [HCC] CC/MCC Exc

M86.269 Subacute osteomyelitis, unspecified tibia and fibula CC [HCC] CC/MCC Exc

[6th] M86.27 Subacute osteomyelitis, ankle and foot

M86.271 Subacute osteomyelitis, right ankle and foot CC [HCC] CC/MCC Exc

Unspecified Code | Other Specified Code | Manifestation Code | [N] Newborn | [P] Pediatric | [M] Maternity | [A] Adult | ♂ Male | ♀ Female
● New Code | ▲ Revised Code Title | ►◄ Revised Text | [NOTES] | INCLUDES | [EXCLUDES1] Not coded here | [EXCLUDES2] Not included here
[4th] 4th character required | [5th] 5th character required | [6th] 6th character required | [7th] 7th character required | [7th] Extension 'X' Alert
[HAC] Hospital-acquired condition (HAC) alert | AHA AHA Coding Clinic© | Code first alert

M86.272 Subacute osteomyelitis, left ankle and foot ᴄᴄ HCC CC/MCC Exc

M86.279 Subacute osteomyelitis, unspecified ankle and foot ᴄᴄ HCC CC/MCC Exc

M86.28 Subacute osteomyelitis, other site ᴄᴄ HCC CC/MCC Exc

M86.29 Subacute osteomyelitis, multiple sites ᴄᴄ HCC CC/MCC Exc

M86.3 Chronic multifocal osteomyelitis

M86.30 Chronic multifocal osteomyelitis, unspecified site ᴄᴄ HCC CC/MCC Exc

M86.31 Chronic multifocal osteomyelitis, shoulder

M86.311 Chronic multifocal osteomyelitis, right shoulder ᴄᴄ HCC CC/MCC Exc

M86.312 Chronic multifocal osteomyelitis, left shoulder ᴄᴄ HCC CC/MCC Exc

M86.319 Chronic multifocal osteomyelitis, unspecified shoulder ᴄᴄ HCC CC/MCC Exc

M86.32 Chronic multifocal osteomyelitis, humerus

M86.321 Chronic multifocal osteomyelitis, right humerus ᴄᴄ HCC CC/MCC Exc

M86.322 Chronic multifocal osteomyelitis, left humerus ᴄᴄ HCC CC/MCC Exc

M86.329 Chronic multifocal osteomyelitis, unspecified humerus ᴄᴄ HCC CC/MCC Exc

M86.33 Chronic multifocal osteomyelitis, radius and ulna

M86.331 Chronic multifocal osteomyelitis, right radius and ulna ᴄᴄ HCC CC/MCC Exc

M86.332 Chronic multifocal osteomyelitis, left radius and ulna ᴄᴄ HCC CC/MCC Exc

M86.339 Chronic multifocal osteomyelitis, unspecified radius and ulna ᴄᴄ HCC CC/MCC Exc

M86.34 Chronic multifocal osteomyelitis, hand

M86.341 Chronic multifocal osteomyelitis, right hand ᴄᴄ HCC CC/MCC Exc

M86.342 Chronic multifocal osteomyelitis, left hand ᴄᴄ HCC CC/MCC Exc

M86.349 Chronic multifocal osteomyelitis, unspecified hand ᴄᴄ HCC CC/MCC Exc

M86.35 Chronic multifocal osteomyelitis, femur

M86.351 Chronic multifocal osteomyelitis, right femur ᴄᴄ HCC CC/MCC Exc

M86.352 Chronic multifocal osteomyelitis, left femur ᴄᴄ HCC CC/MCC Exc

M86.359 Chronic multifocal osteomyelitis, unspecified femur ᴄᴄ HCC CC/MCC Exc

M86.36 Chronic multifocal osteomyelitis, tibia and fibula

M86.361 Chronic multifocal osteomyelitis, right tibia and fibula ᴄᴄ HCC CC/MCC Exc

M86.362 Chronic multifocal osteomyelitis, left tibia and fibula ᴄᴄ HCC CC/MCC Exc

M86.369 Chronic multifocal osteomyelitis, unspecified tibia and fibula ᴄᴄ HCC CC/MCC Exc

M86.37 Chronic multifocal osteomyelitis, ankle and foot

M86.371 Chronic multifocal osteomyelitis, right ankle and foot ᴄᴄ HCC CC/MCC Exc

M86.372 Chronic multifocal osteomyelitis, left ankle and foot ᴄᴄ HCC CC/MCC Exc

M86.379 Chronic multifocal osteomyelitis, unspecified ankle and foot ᴄᴄ HCC CC/MCC Exc

M86.38 Chronic multifocal osteomyelitis, other site ᴄᴄ HCC CC/MCC Exc

M86.39 Chronic multifocal osteomyelitis, multiple sites ᴄᴄ HCC CC/MCC Exc

M86.4 Chronic osteomyelitis with draining sinus

M86.40 Chronic osteomyelitis with draining sinus, unspecified site ᴄᴄ HCC CC/MCC Exc

M86.41 Chronic osteomyelitis with draining sinus, shoulder

M86.411 Chronic osteomyelitis with draining sinus, right shoulder ᴄᴄ HCC CC/MCC Exc

M86.412 Chronic osteomyelitis with draining sinus, left shoulder ᴄᴄ HCC CC/MCC Exc

M86.419 Chronic osteomyelitis with draining sinus, unspecified shoulder ᴄᴄ HCC CC/MCC Exc

M86.42 Chronic osteomyelitis with draining sinus, humerus

M86.421 Chronic osteomyelitis with draining sinus, right humerus ᴄᴄ HCC CC/MCC Exc

M86.422 Chronic osteomyelitis with draining sinus, left humerus ᴄᴄ HCC CC/MCC Exc

M86.429 Chronic osteomyelitis with draining sinus, unspecified humerus ᴄᴄ HCC CC/MCC Exc

M86.43 Chronic osteomyelitis with draining sinus, radius and ulna

M86.431 Chronic osteomyelitis with draining sinus, right radius and ulna ᴄᴄ HCC CC/MCC Exc

M86.432 Chronic osteomyelitis with draining sinus, left radius and ulna ᴄᴄ HCC CC/MCC Exc

M86.439 Chronic osteomyelitis with draining sinus, unspecified radius and ulna ᴄᴄ HCC CC/MCC Exc

M86.44 Chronic osteomyelitis with draining sinus, hand

M86.441 Chronic osteomyelitis with draining sinus, right hand ᴄᴄ HCC CC/MCC Exc

M86.442 Chronic osteomyelitis with draining sinus, left hand ᴄᴄ HCC CC/MCC Exc

M86.449 Chronic osteomyelitis with draining sinus, unspecified hand ᴄᴄ HCC CC/MCC Exc

M86.45 Chronic osteomyelitis with draining sinus, femur

M86.451 Chronic osteomyelitis with draining sinus, right femur ᴄᴄ HCC CC/MCC Exc

M86.452 Chronic osteomyelitis with draining sinus, left femur ᴄᴄ HCC CC/MCC Exc

M86.459 Chronic osteomyelitis with draining sinus, unspecified femur ᴄᴄ HCC CC/MCC Exc

M86.46 Chronic osteomyelitis with draining sinus, tibia and fibula

M86.461 Chronic osteomyelitis with draining sinus, right tibia and fibula ᴄᴄ HCC CC/MCC Exc

M86.462 Chronic osteomyelitis with draining sinus, left tibia and fibula ᴄᴄ HCC CC/MCC Exc

M86.469 Chronic osteomyelitis with draining sinus, unspecified tibia and fibula ᴄᴄ HCC CC/MCC Exc

M86.47 Chronic osteomyelitis with draining sinus, ankle and foot

M86.471 Chronic osteomyelitis with draining sinus, right ankle and foot ᴄᴄ HCC CC/MCC Exc

M86.472 Chronic osteomyelitis with draining sinus, left ankle and foot ᴄᴄ HCC CC/MCC Exc

M86.479 Chronic osteomyelitis with draining sinus, unspecified ankle and foot ᴄᴄ HCC CC/MCC Exc

M86.48 Chronic osteomyelitis with draining sinus, other site ᴄᴄ HCC CC/MCC Exc

M86.49 Chronic osteomyelitis with draining sinus, multiple sites ᴄᴄ HCC CC/MCC Exc

M86.5 Other chronic hematogenous osteomyelitis

M86.50 Other chronic hematogenous osteomyelitis, unspecified site ᴄᴄ HCC CC/MCC Exc

M86.51 Other chronic hematogenous osteomyelitis, shoulder

M86.511 Other chronic hematogenous osteomyelitis, right shoulder ᴄᴄ HCC CC/MCC Exc

M86.512 Other chronic hematogenous osteomyelitis, left shoulder ᴄᴄ HCC CC/MCC Exc

M86.519 Other chronic hematogenous osteomyelitis, unspecified shoulder ᴄᴄ HCC CC/MCC Exc

M86.52 Other chronic hematogenous osteomyelitis, humerus

M86.521 Other chronic hematogenous osteomyelitis, right humerus ᴄᴄ HCC CC/MCC Exc

M86.522 Other chronic hematogenous osteomyelitis, left humerus ᴄᴄ HCC CC/MCC Exc

M86.529 Other chronic hematogenous osteomyelitis, unspecified humerus ᴄᴄ HCC CC/MCC Exc

---

PDncn Unacceptable principal diagnosis symbol per Medicare code edits   POA Code exempt from diagnosis present on admission requirement

❓ Questionable admission   ᴄᴄ Complication or comorbidity   MCC Major complication or comorbidity   CC/MCC Exc CC/MCC exclusion

HCC HCC diagnosis code   RxHCC RxHCC diagnosis code   MACRA MACRA code   **DEFINITION** Describes condition/terminology

TIP Coding guidance   👁 Official Guideline Reference   Z1 Z code as first-listed diagnosis

When symbols appear on a code that requires a 7th character extension, refer to Appendix B to identify applicable 7th character codes.   **2020 ICD-10-CM**

[6th] **M86.53 Other chronic hematogenous osteomyelitis,** radius and ulna
- **M86.531 Other chronic hematogenous osteomyelitis,** right **radius and ulna** [CC] [HCC] [CC/MCC Exc]
- **M86.532 Other chronic hematogenous osteomyelitis,** left **radius and ulna** [CC] [HCC] [CC/MCC Exc]
- **M86.539 Other chronic hematogenous osteomyelitis, unspecified radius and ulna** [CC] [HCC] [CC/MCC Exc]

[6th] **M86.54 Other chronic hematogenous osteomyelitis,** hand
- **M86.541 Other chronic hematogenous osteomyelitis,** right **hand** [CC] [HCC] [CC/MCC Exc]
- **M86.542 Other chronic hematogenous osteomyelitis,** left **hand** [CC] [HCC] [CC/MCC Exc]
- **M86.549 Other chronic hematogenous osteomyelitis, unspecified hand** [CC] [HCC] [CC/MCC Exc]

[6th] **M86.55 Other chronic hematogenous osteomyelitis,** femur
- **M86.551 Other chronic hematogenous osteomyelitis,** right **femur** [CC] [HCC] [CC/MCC Exc]
- **M86.552 Other chronic hematogenous osteomyelitis,** left **femur** [CC] [HCC] [CC/MCC Exc]
- **M86.559 Other chronic hematogenous osteomyelitis, unspecified femur** [CC] [HCC] [CC/MCC Exc]

[6th] **M86.56 Other chronic hematogenous osteomyelitis,** tibia and fibula
- **M86.561 Other chronic hematogenous osteomyelitis,** right **tibia and fibula** [CC] [HCC] [CC/MCC Exc]
- **M86.562 Other chronic hematogenous osteomyelitis,** left **tibia and fibula** [CC] [HCC] [CC/MCC Exc]
- **M86.569 Other chronic hematogenous osteomyelitis, unspecified tibia and fibula** [CC] [HCC] [CC/MCC Exc]

[6th] **M86.57 Other chronic hematogenous osteomyelitis,** ankle and foot
- **M86.571 Other chronic hematogenous osteomyelitis,** right **ankle and foot** [CC] [HCC] [CC/MCC Exc]
- **M86.572 Other chronic hematogenous osteomyelitis,** left **ankle and foot** [CC] [HCC] [CC/MCC Exc]
- **M86.579 Other chronic hematogenous osteomyelitis, unspecified ankle and foot** [CC] [HCC] [CC/MCC Exc]

M86.58 Other chronic hematogenous osteomyelitis, other site [CC] [HCC] [CC/MCC Exc]

M86.59 Other chronic hematogenous osteomyelitis, multiple sites [CC] [HCC] [CC/MCC Exc]

[5th] **M86.6** Other chronic **osteomyelitis**

M86.60 Other chronic osteomyelitis, unspecified site [CC] [HCC] [CC/MCC Exc]

[6th] **M86.61 Other chronic osteomyelitis,** shoulder
- **M86.611 Other chronic osteomyelitis,** right **shoulder** [CC] [HCC] [CC/MCC Exc]
- **M86.612 Other chronic osteomyelitis,** left **shoulder** [CC] [HCC] [CC/MCC Exc]
- **M86.619 Other chronic osteomyelitis, unspecified shoulder** [CC] [HCC] [CC/MCC Exc]

[6th] **M86.62** Other **chronic osteomyelitis,** humerus
- **M86.621 Other chronic osteomyelitis,** right humerus [CC] [HCC] [CC/MCC Exc]
- **M86.622 Other chronic osteomyelitis,** left humerus [CC] [HCC] [CC/MCC Exc]
- **M86.629 Other chronic osteomyelitis, unspecified humerus** [CC] [HCC] [CC/MCC Exc]

[6th] **M86.63 Other chronic osteomyelitis,** radius and ulna
- **M86.631 Other chronic osteomyelitis,** right **radius and ulna** [CC] [HCC] [CC/MCC Exc]
- **M86.632 Other chronic osteomyelitis,** left **radius and ulna** [CC] [HCC] [CC/MCC Exc]
- **M86.639 Other chronic osteomyelitis, unspecified radius and ulna** [CC] [HCC] [CC/MCC Exc]

[6th] **M86.64 Other chronic osteomyelitis,** hand
- **M86.641 Other chronic osteomyelitis,** right **hand** [CC] [HCC] [CC/MCC Exc]
- **M86.642 Other chronic osteomyelitis,** left **hand** [CC] [HCC] [CC/MCC Exc]
- **M86.649 Other chronic osteomyelitis, unspecified hand** [CC] [HCC] [CC/MCC Exc]

[6th] **M86.65 Other chronic osteomyelitis,** thigh
- **M86.651 Other chronic osteomyelitis,** right **thigh** [CC] [HCC] [CC/MCC Exc]
- **M86.652 Other chronic osteomyelitis,** left **thigh** [CC] [HCC] [CC/MCC Exc]
- **M86.659 Other chronic osteomyelitis, unspecified thigh** [CC] [HCC] [CC/MCC Exc]

[6th] **M86.66 Other chronic osteomyelitis,** tibia and fibula
- **M86.661 Other chronic osteomyelitis,** right **tibia and fibula** [CC] [HCC] [CC/MCC Exc]
- **M86.662 Other chronic osteomyelitis,** left **tibia and fibula** [CC] [HCC] [CC/MCC Exc]
- **M86.669 Other chronic osteomyelitis, unspecified tibia and fibula** [CC] [HCC] [CC/MCC Exc]

[6th] **M86.67 Other chronic osteomyelitis,** ankle and foot
- **M86.671 Other chronic osteomyelitis,** right **ankle and foot** [CC] [HCC] [CC/MCC Exc]
  AHA: Q1 2016
- **M86.672 Other chronic osteomyelitis,** left **ankle and foot** [CC] [HCC] [CC/MCC Exc]
- **M86.679 Other chronic osteomyelitis, unspecified ankle and foot** [CC] [HCC] [CC/MCC Exc]

M86.68 Other chronic osteomyelitis, other site [CC] [HCC] [CC/MCC Exc]

M86.69 Other chronic osteomyelitis, multiple sites [CC] [HCC] [CC/MCC Exc]

[5th] **M86.8** Other **osteomyelitis**

Brodie's abscess

[6th] **M86.8X Other osteomyelitis**
- **M86.8X0 Other osteomyelitis,** multiple sites [CC] [HCC] [CC/MCC Exc]
- **M86.8X1 Other osteomyelitis,** shoulder [CC] [HCC] [CC/MCC Exc]
- **M86.8X2 Other osteomyelitis,** upper arm [CC] [HCC] [CC/MCC Exc]
- **M86.8X3 Other osteomyelitis,** forearm [CC] [HCC] [CC/MCC Exc]
- **M86.8X4 Other osteomyelitis,** hand [CC] [HCC] [CC/MCC Exc]
- **M86.8X5 Other osteomyelitis,** thigh [CC] [HCC] [CC/MCC Exc]
- **M86.8X6 Other osteomyelitis,** lower leg [CC] [HCC] [CC/MCC Exc]
- **M86.8X7 Other osteomyelitis,** ankle and foot [CC] [HCC] [CC/MCC Exc]
- **M86.8X8 Other osteomyelitis,** other site [CC] [HCC] [CC/MCC Exc]
- **M86.8X9 Other osteomyelitis, unspecified sites** [CC] [HCC] [CC/MCC Exc]

M86.9 Osteomyelitis, unspecified [CC] [HCC] [CC/MCC Exc]

Infection of bone NOS

Periostitis without osteomyelitis

[4th] **M87 Osteonecrosis**

[INCLUDES] *avascular necrosis of bone*

Use additional code to identify major osseous defect, if applicable (M89.7-)

[EXCLUDES1] *juvenile osteonecrosis (M91-M92)*
osteochondropathies (M90-M93)

[5th] **M87.0** Idiopathic aseptic necrosis of bone

M87.00 Idiopathic aseptic necrosis of unspecified bone [CC] [HCC] [RxHCC] [CC/MCC Exc]

[6th] **M87.01 Idiopathic aseptic necrosis of** shoulder

Idiopathic aseptic necrosis of clavicle and scapula
- **M87.011 Idiopathic aseptic necrosis of** right **shoulder** [CC] [HCC] [RxHCC] [CC/MCC Exc]
- **M87.012 Idiopathic aseptic necrosis of** left **shoulder** [CC] [HCC] [RxHCC] [CC/MCC Exc]

Unspecified Code | Other Specified Code | Manifestation Code | [N] Newborn | [P] Pediatric | [M] Maternity | [A] Adult | ♂ Male | ♀ Female
● New Code ▲ Revised Code Title ►◄ Revised Text [NOTES] [INCLUDES] [EXCLUDES1] Not coded here [EXCLUDES2] Not included here
[4th] 4th character required [5th] 5th character required [6th] 6th character required [7th] 7th character required [X] Extension 'X' Alert
[HAC] Hospital-acquired condition (HAC) alert AHA AHA Coding Clinic© ☛ Code first alert

M87.019 Idiopathic aseptic necrosis of unspecified shoulder

6ᵗʰ M87.02 Idiopathic aseptic necrosis of humerus
M87.021 Idiopathic aseptic necrosis of right humerus
M87.022 Idiopathic aseptic necrosis of left humerus
M87.029 Idiopathic aseptic necrosis of unspecified humerus

6ᵗʰ M87.03 Idiopathic aseptic necrosis of radius, ulna and carpus
M87.031 Idiopathic aseptic necrosis of right radius
M87.032 Idiopathic aseptic necrosis of left radius
M87.033 Idiopathic aseptic necrosis of unspecified radius
M87.034 Idiopathic aseptic necrosis of right ulna
M87.035 Idiopathic aseptic necrosis of left ulna
M87.036 Idiopathic aseptic necrosis of unspecified ulna
M87.037 Idiopathic aseptic necrosis of right carpus
M87.038 Idiopathic aseptic necrosis of left carpus
M87.039 Idiopathic aseptic necrosis of unspecified carpus

6ᵗʰ M87.04 Idiopathic aseptic necrosis of hand and fingers
Idiopathic aseptic necrosis of metacarpals and phalanges of hands
M87.041 Idiopathic aseptic necrosis of right hand
M87.042 Idiopathic aseptic necrosis of left hand
M87.043 Idiopathic aseptic necrosis of unspecified hand
M87.044 Idiopathic aseptic necrosis of right finger(s)
M87.045 Idiopathic aseptic necrosis of left finger(s)
M87.046 Idiopathic aseptic necrosis of unspecified finger(s)

6ᵗʰ M87.05 Idiopathic aseptic necrosis of pelvis and femur
M87.050 Idiopathic aseptic necrosis of pelvis
M87.051 Idiopathic aseptic necrosis of right femur
M87.052 Idiopathic aseptic necrosis of left femur
M87.059 Idiopathic aseptic necrosis of unspecified femur
Idiopathic aseptic necrosis of hip NOS

6ᵗʰ M87.06 Idiopathic aseptic necrosis of tibia and fibula
M87.061 Idiopathic aseptic necrosis of right tibia
M87.062 Idiopathic aseptic necrosis of left tibia
M87.063 Idiopathic aseptic necrosis of unspecified tibia
M87.064 Idiopathic aseptic necrosis of right fibula
M87.065 Idiopathic aseptic necrosis of left fibula
M87.066 Idiopathic aseptic necrosis of unspecified fibula

6ᵗʰ M87.07 Idiopathic aseptic necrosis of ankle, foot and toes
Idiopathic aseptic necrosis of metatarsus, tarsus, and phalanges of toes
M87.071 Idiopathic aseptic necrosis of right ankle

M87.072 Idiopathic aseptic necrosis of left ankle
M87.073 Idiopathic aseptic necrosis of unspecified ankle
M87.074 Idiopathic aseptic necrosis of right foot
M87.075 Idiopathic aseptic necrosis of left foot
M87.076 Idiopathic aseptic necrosis of unspecified foot
M87.077 Idiopathic aseptic necrosis of right toe(s)
M87.078 Idiopathic aseptic necrosis of left toe(s)
M87.079 Idiopathic aseptic necrosis of unspecified toe(s)
M87.08 Idiopathic aseptic necrosis of bone, other site
M87.09 Idiopathic aseptic necrosis of bone, multiple sites

5ᵗʰ M87.1 Osteonecrosis due to drugs
Use additional code for adverse effect, if applicable, to identify drug (T36-T50 with fifth or sixth character 5)
M87.10 Osteonecrosis due to drugs, unspecified bone

6ᵗʰ M87.11 Osteonecrosis due to drugs, shoulder
M87.111 Osteonecrosis due to drugs, right shoulder
M87.112 Osteonecrosis due to drugs, left shoulder
M87.119 Osteonecrosis due to drugs, unspecified shoulder

6ᵗʰ M87.12 Osteonecrosis due to drugs, humerus
M87.121 Osteonecrosis due to drugs, right humerus
M87.122 Osteonecrosis due to drugs, left humerus
M87.129 Osteonecrosis due to drugs, unspecified humerus

6ᵗʰ M87.13 Osteonecrosis due to drugs of radius, ulna and carpus
M87.131 Osteonecrosis due to drugs of right radius
M87.132 Osteonecrosis due to drugs of left radius
M87.133 Osteonecrosis due to drugs of unspecified radius
M87.134 Osteonecrosis due to drugs of right ulna
M87.135 Osteonecrosis due to drugs of left ulna
M87.136 Osteonecrosis due to drugs of unspecified ulna
M87.137 Osteonecrosis due to drugs of right carpus
M87.138 Osteonecrosis due to drugs of left carpus
M87.139 Osteonecrosis due to drugs of unspecified carpus

6ᵗʰ M87.14 Osteonecrosis due to drugs, hand and fingers
M87.141 Osteonecrosis due to drugs, right hand
M87.142 Osteonecrosis due to drugs, left hand
M87.143 Osteonecrosis due to drugs, unspecified hand
M87.144 Osteonecrosis due to drugs, right finger(s)
M87.145 Osteonecrosis due to drugs, left finger(s)
M87.146 Osteonecrosis due to drugs, unspecified finger(s)

[6th] M87.15 Osteonecrosis due to drugs, pelvis and femur
- M87.150 Osteonecrosis due to drugs, pelvis [CC] [HCC] [RxHCC] [CC/MCC Exc]
- M87.151 Osteonecrosis due to drugs, right femur [CC] [HCC] [RxHCC] [CC/MCC Exc]
- M87.152 Osteonecrosis due to drugs, left femur [CC] [HCC] [RxHCC] [CC/MCC Exc]
- M87.159 Osteonecrosis due to drugs, unspecified femur [CC] [HCC] [RxHCC] [CC/MCC Exc]

[6th] M87.16 Osteonecrosis due to drugs, tibia and fibula
- M87.161 Osteonecrosis due to drugs, right tibia [CC] [HCC] [RxHCC] [CC/MCC Exc]
- M87.162 Osteonecrosis due to drugs, left tibia [CC] [HCC] [RxHCC] [CC/MCC Exc]
- M87.163 Osteonecrosis due to drugs, unspecified tibia [CC] [HCC] [RxHCC] [CC/MCC Exc]
- M87.164 Osteonecrosis due to drugs, right fibula [CC] [HCC] [RxHCC] [CC/MCC Exc]
- M87.165 Osteonecrosis due to drugs, left fibula [CC] [HCC] [RxHCC] [CC/MCC Exc]
- M87.166 Osteonecrosis due to drugs, unspecified fibula [CC] [HCC] [RxHCC] [CC/MCC Exc]

[6th] M87.17 Osteonecrosis due to drugs, ankle, foot and toes
- M87.171 Osteonecrosis due to drugs, right ankle [CC] [HCC] [RxHCC] [CC/MCC Exc]
- M87.172 Osteonecrosis due to drugs, left ankle [CC] [HCC] [RxHCC] [CC/MCC Exc]
- M87.173 Osteonecrosis due to drugs, unspecified ankle [CC] [HCC] [RxHCC] [CC/MCC Exc]
- M87.174 Osteonecrosis due to drugs, right foot [CC] [HCC] [RxHCC] [CC/MCC Exc]
- M87.175 Osteonecrosis due to drugs, left foot [CC] [HCC] [RxHCC] [CC/MCC Exc]
- M87.176 Osteonecrosis due to drugs, unspecified foot [CC] [HCC] [RxHCC] [CC/MCC Exc]
- M87.177 Osteonecrosis due to drugs, right toe(s) [CC] [HCC] [RxHCC] [CC/MCC Exc]
- M87.178 Osteonecrosis due to drugs, left toe(s) [CC] [HCC] [RxHCC] [CC/MCC Exc]
- M87.179 Osteonecrosis due to drugs, unspecified toe(s) [CC] [HCC] [RxHCC] [CC/MCC Exc]

[6th] M87.18 Osteonecrosis due to drugs, other site
- M87.180 Osteonecrosis due to drugs, jaw [CC] [HCC] [RxHCC] [CC/MCC Exc]
- M87.188 Osteonecrosis due to drugs, other site [CC] [HCC] [RxHCC] [CC/MCC Exc]

M87.19 Osteonecrosis due to drugs, multiple sites [CC] [HCC] [RxHCC] [CC/MCC Exc]

[5th] M87.2 Osteonecrosis due to previous trauma

M87.20 Osteonecrosis due to previous trauma, unspecified bone [CC] [HCC] [RxHCC] [CC/MCC Exc]

[6th] M87.21 Osteonecrosis due to previous trauma, shoulder
- M87.211 Osteonecrosis due to previous trauma, right shoulder [CC] [HCC] [RxHCC] [CC/MCC Exc]
- M87.212 Osteonecrosis due to previous trauma, left shoulder [CC] [HCC] [RxHCC] [CC/MCC Exc]
- M87.219 Osteonecrosis due to previous trauma, unspecified shoulder [CC] [HCC] [RxHCC] [CC/MCC Exc]

[6th] M87.22 Osteonecrosis due to previous trauma, humerus
- M87.221 Osteonecrosis due to previous trauma, right humerus [CC] [HCC] [RxHCC] [CC/MCC Exc]
- M87.222 Osteonecrosis due to previous trauma, left humerus [CC] [HCC] [RxHCC] [CC/MCC Exc]
- M87.229 Osteonecrosis due to previous trauma, unspecified humerus [CC] [HCC] [RxHCC] [CC/MCC Exc]

[6th] M87.23 Osteonecrosis due to previous trauma of radius, ulna and carpus
- M87.231 Osteonecrosis due to previous trauma of right radius [CC] [HCC] [RxHCC] [CC/MCC Exc]
- M87.232 Osteonecrosis due to previous trauma of left radius [CC] [HCC] [RxHCC] [CC/MCC Exc]
- M87.233 Osteonecrosis due to previous trauma of unspecified radius [CC] [HCC] [RxHCC] [CC/MCC Exc]
- M87.234 Osteonecrosis due to previous trauma of right ulna [CC] [HCC] [RxHCC] [CC/MCC Exc]
- M87.235 Osteonecrosis due to previous trauma of left ulna [CC] [HCC] [RxHCC] [CC/MCC Exc]
- M87.236 Osteonecrosis due to previous trauma of unspecified ulna [CC] [HCC] [RxHCC] [CC/MCC Exc]
- M87.237 Osteonecrosis due to previous trauma of right carpus [CC] [HCC] [RxHCC] [CC/MCC Exc]
- M87.238 Osteonecrosis due to previous trauma of left carpus [CC] [HCC] [RxHCC] [CC/MCC Exc]
- M87.239 Osteonecrosis due to previous trauma of unspecified carpus [CC] [HCC] [RxHCC] [CC/MCC Exc]

[6th] M87.24 Osteonecrosis due to previous trauma, hand and fingers
- M87.241 Osteonecrosis due to previous trauma, right hand [CC] [HCC] [RxHCC] [CC/MCC Exc]
- M87.242 Osteonecrosis due to previous trauma, left hand [CC] [HCC] [RxHCC] [CC/MCC Exc]
- M87.243 Osteonecrosis due to previous trauma, unspecified hand [CC] [HCC] [RxHCC] [CC/MCC Exc]
- M87.244 Osteonecrosis due to previous trauma, right finger(s) [CC] [HCC] [RxHCC] [CC/MCC Exc]
- M87.245 Osteonecrosis due to previous trauma, left finger(s) [CC] [HCC] [RxHCC] [CC/MCC Exc]
- M87.246 Osteonecrosis due to previous trauma, unspecified finger(s) [CC] [HCC] [RxHCC] [CC/MCC Exc]

[6th] M87.25 Osteonecrosis due to previous trauma, pelvis and femur
- M87.250 Osteonecrosis due to previous trauma, pelvis [CC] [HCC] [RxHCC] [CC/MCC Exc]
- M87.251 Osteonecrosis due to previous trauma, right femur [CC] [HCC] [RxHCC] [CC/MCC Exc]
- M87.252 Osteonecrosis due to previous trauma, left femur [CC] [HCC] [RxHCC] [CC/MCC Exc]
- M87.256 Osteonecrosis due to previous trauma, unspecified femur [CC] [HCC] [RxHCC] [CC/MCC Exc]

[6th] M87.26 Osteonecrosis due to previous trauma, tibia and fibula
- M87.261 Osteonecrosis due to previous trauma, right tibia [CC] [HCC] [RxHCC] [CC/MCC Exc]
- M87.262 Osteonecrosis due to previous trauma, left tibia [CC] [HCC] [RxHCC] [CC/MCC Exc]
- M87.263 Osteonecrosis due to previous trauma, unspecified tibia [CC] [HCC] [RxHCC] [CC/MCC Exc]
- M87.264 Osteonecrosis due to previous trauma, right fibula [CC] [HCC] [RxHCC] [CC/MCC Exc]
- M87.265 Osteonecrosis due to previous trauma, left fibula [CC] [HCC] [RxHCC] [CC/MCC Exc]
- M87.266 Osteonecrosis due to previous trauma, unspecified fibula [CC] [HCC] [RxHCC] [CC/MCC Exc]

[6th] M87.27 Osteonecrosis due to previous trauma, ankle, foot and toes
- M87.271 Osteonecrosis due to previous trauma, right ankle [CC] [HCC] [RxHCC] [CC/MCC Exc]
- M87.272 Osteonecrosis due to previous trauma, left ankle [CC] [HCC] [RxHCC] [CC/MCC Exc]
- M87.273 Osteonecrosis due to previous trauma, unspecified ankle [CC] [HCC] [RxHCC] [CC/MCC Exc]
- M87.274 Osteonecrosis due to previous trauma, right foot [CC] [HCC] [RxHCC] [CC/MCC Exc]
- M87.275 Osteonecrosis due to previous trauma, left foot [CC] [HCC] [RxHCC] [CC/MCC Exc]
- M87.276 Osteonecrosis due to previous trauma, unspecified foot [CC] [HCC] [RxHCC] [CC/MCC Exc]
- M87.277 Osteonecrosis due to previous trauma, right toe(s) [CC] [HCC] [RxHCC] [CC/MCC Exc]
- M87.278 Osteonecrosis due to previous trauma, left toe(s) [CC] [HCC] [RxHCC] [CC/MCC Exc]
- M87.279 Osteonecrosis due to previous trauma, unspecified toe(s) [CC] [HCC] [RxHCC] [CC/MCC Exc]

Unspecified Code Other Specified Code Manifestation Code [N] Newborn [P] Pediatric [M] Maternity [A] Adult ♂ Male ♀ Female
● New Code ▲ Revised Code Title ►◄ Revised Text [NOTES] *INCLUDES* [*EXCLUDES1*] Not coded here [*EXCLUDES2*] Not included here
[4th] 4th character required [5th] 5th character required [6th] 6th character required [7th] 7th character required [x] Extension 'X' Alert
[HAC] Hospital-acquired condition (HAC) alert AHA AHA Coding Clinic© ☛ Code first alert

M87.28 Osteonecrosis due to previous trauma, other site ◨ HCC RxHCC CC/MCC Exc

M87.29 Osteonecrosis due to previous trauma, multiple sites ◨ HCC RxHCC CC/MCC Exc

5ᵗʰ M87.3 Other secondary osteonecrosis

M87.30 Other secondary osteonecrosis, unspecified bone ◨ HCC RxHCC CC/MCC Exc

6ᵗʰ M87.31 Other secondary osteonecrosis, shoulder

M87.311 Other secondary osteonecrosis, right shoulder ◨ HCC RxHCC CC/MCC Exc

M87.312 Other secondary osteonecrosis, left shoulder ◨ HCC RxHCC CC/MCC Exc

M87.319 Other secondary osteonecrosis, unspecified shoulder ◨ HCC RxHCC CC/MCC Exc

6ᵗʰ M87.32 Other secondary osteonecrosis, humerus

M87.321 Other secondary osteonecrosis, right humerus ◨ HCC RxHCC CC/MCC Exc

M87.322 Other secondary osteonecrosis, left humerus ◨ HCC RxHCC CC/MCC Exc

M87.329 Other secondary osteonecrosis, unspecified humerus ◨ HCC RxHCC CC/MCC Exc

6ᵗʰ M87.33 Other secondary osteonecrosis of radius, ulna and carpus

M87.331 Other secondary osteonecrosis of right radius ◨ HCC RxHCC CC/MCC Exc

M87.332 Other secondary osteonecrosis of left radius ◨ HCC RxHCC CC/MCC Exc

M87.333 Other secondary osteonecrosis of unspecified radius ◨ HCC RxHCC CC/MCC Exc

M87.334 Other secondary osteonecrosis of right ulna ◨ HCC RxHCC CC/MCC Exc

M87.335 Other secondary osteonecrosis of left ulna ◨ HCC RxHCC CC/MCC Exc

M87.336 Other secondary osteonecrosis of unspecified ulna ◨ HCC RxHCC CC/MCC Exc

M87.337 Other secondary osteonecrosis of right carpus ◨ HCC RxHCC CC/MCC Exc

M87.338 Other secondary osteonecrosis of left carpus ◨ HCC RxHCC CC/MCC Exc

M87.339 Other secondary osteonecrosis of unspecified carpus ◨ HCC RxHCC CC/MCC Exc

6ᵗʰ M87.34 Other secondary osteonecrosis, hand and fingers

M87.341 Other secondary osteonecrosis, right hand ◨ HCC RxHCC CC/MCC Exc

M87.342 Other secondary osteonecrosis, left hand ◨ HCC RxHCC CC/MCC Exc

M87.343 Other secondary osteonecrosis, unspecified hand ◨ HCC RxHCC CC/MCC Exc

M87.344 Other secondary osteonecrosis, right finger(s) ◨ HCC RxHCC CC/MCC Exc

M87.345 Other secondary osteonecrosis, left finger(s) ◨ HCC RxHCC CC/MCC Exc

M87.346 Other secondary osteonecrosis, unspecified finger(s) ◨ HCC RxHCC CC/MCC Exc

6ᵗʰ M87.35 Other secondary osteonecrosis, pelvis and femur

M87.350 Other secondary osteonecrosis, pelvis ◨ HCC RxHCC CC/MCC Exc

M87.351 Other secondary osteonecrosis, right femur ◨ HCC RxHCC CC/MCC Exc

M87.352 Other secondary osteonecrosis, left femur ◨ HCC RxHCC CC/MCC Exc

M87.353 Other secondary osteonecrosis, unspecified femur ◨ HCC RxHCC CC/MCC Exc

6ᵗʰ M87.36 Other secondary osteonecrosis, tibia and fibula

M87.361 Other secondary osteonecrosis, right tibia ◨ HCC RxHCC CC/MCC Exc

M87.362 Other secondary osteonecrosis, left tibia ◨ HCC RxHCC CC/MCC Exc

M87.363 Other secondary osteonecrosis, unspecified tibia ◨ HCC RxHCC CC/MCC Exc

M87.364 Other secondary osteonecrosis, right fibula ◨ HCC RxHCC CC/MCC Exc

M87.365 Other secondary osteonecrosis, left fibula ◨ HCC RxHCC CC/MCC Exc

M87.366 Other secondary osteonecrosis, unspecified fibula ◨ HCC RxHCC CC/MCC Exc

6ᵗʰ M87.37 Other secondary osteonecrosis, ankle and foot

M87.371 Other secondary osteonecrosis, right ankle ◨ HCC RxHCC CC/MCC Exc

M87.372 Other secondary osteonecrosis, left ankle ◨ HCC RxHCC CC/MCC Exc

M87.373 Other secondary osteonecrosis, unspecified ankle ◨ HCC RxHCC CC/MCC Exc

M87.374 Other secondary osteonecrosis, right foot ◨ HCC RxHCC CC/MCC Exc

M87.375 Other secondary osteonecrosis, left foot ◨ HCC RxHCC CC/MCC Exc

M87.376 Other secondary osteonecrosis, unspecified foot ◨ HCC RxHCC CC/MCC Exc

M87.377 Other secondary osteonecrosis, right toe(s) ◨ HCC RxHCC CC/MCC Exc

M87.378 Other secondary osteonecrosis, left toe(s) ◨ HCC RxHCC CC/MCC Exc

M87.379 Other secondary osteonecrosis, unspecified toe(s) ◨ HCC RxHCC CC/MCC Exc

M87.38 Other secondary osteonecrosis, other site ◨ HCC RxHCC CC/MCC Exc

M87.39 Other secondary osteonecrosis, multiple sites ◨ HCC RxHCC CC/MCC Exc

5ᵗʰ M87.8 Other osteonecrosis

M87.80 Other osteonecrosis, unspecified bone ◨ HCC RxHCC CC/MCC Exc

5ᵗʰ M87.81 Other osteonecrosis, shoulder

M87.811 Other osteonecrosis, right shoulder ◨ HCC RxHCC CC/MCC Exc

M87.812 Other osteonecrosis, left shoulder ◨ HCC RxHCC CC/MCC Exc

M87.819 Other osteonecrosis, unspecified shoulder ◨ HCC RxHCC CC/MCC Exc

6ᵗʰ M87.82 Other osteonecrosis, humerus

M87.821 Other osteonecrosis, right humerus ◨ HCC RxHCC CC/MCC Exc

M87.822 Other osteonecrosis, left humerus ◨ HCC RxHCC CC/MCC Exc

M87.829 Other osteonecrosis, unspecified humerus ◨ HCC RxHCC CC/MCC Exc

6ᵗʰ M87.83 Other osteonecrosis of radius, ulna and carpus

M87.831 Other osteonecrosis of right radius ◨ HCC RxHCC CC/MCC Exc

M87.832 Other osteonecrosis of left radius ◨ HCC RxHCC CC/MCC Exc

M87.833 Other osteonecrosis of unspecified radius ◨ HCC RxHCC CC/MCC Exc

M87.834 Other osteonecrosis of right ulna ◨ HCC RxHCC CC/MCC Exc

M87.835 Other osteonecrosis of left ulna ◨ HCC RxHCC CC/MCC Exc

M87.836 Other osteonecrosis of unspecified ulna ◨ HCC RxHCC CC/MCC Exc

M87.837 Other osteonecrosis of right carpus ◨ HCC RxHCC CC/MCC Exc

M87.838 Other osteonecrosis of left carpus ◨ HCC RxHCC CC/MCC Exc

M87.839 Other osteonecrosis of unspecified carpus ◨ HCC RxHCC CC/MCC Exc

6ᵗʰ M87.84 Other osteonecrosis, hand and fingers

M87.841 Other osteonecrosis, right hand ◨ HCC RxHCC CC/MCC Exc

M87.842 Other osteonecrosis, left hand ◨ HCC RxHCC CC/MCC Exc

M87.843 Other osteonecrosis, unspecified hand ◨ HCC RxHCC CC/MCC Exc

M87.844 Other osteonecrosis, right finger(s) ◨ HCC RxHCC CC/MCC Exc

---

PDₓ Unacceptable principal diagnosis symbol per Medicare code edits   ◙ Code exempt from diagnosis present on admission requirement

☑ Questionable admission   ◨ Complication or comorbidity   MCC Major complication or comorbidity   CC/MCC Exc CC/MCC exclusion

HCC HCC diagnosis code   RxHCC RxHCC diagnosis code   MACRA code   **DEFINITION** Describes condition/terminology

TIP Coding guidance   👁 Official Guideline Reference   Zₓₛₜ Z code as first-listed diagnosis

M87.845 Other osteonecrosis, left finger(s) CC⁰ **HCC** **RxHCC** CC/MCC Exc⁰
M87.849 Other osteonecrosis, unspecified finger(s) CC⁰ **HCC** **RxHCC** CC/MCC Exc⁰
6ᵗʰ M87.85 Other osteonecrosis, pelvis and femur
M87.850 Other osteonecrosis, pelvis CC⁰ **HCC** **RxHCC** CC/MCC Exc⁰
M87.851 Other osteonecrosis, right femur CC⁰ **HCC** **RxHCC** CC/MCC Exc⁰
M87.852 Other osteonecrosis, left femur CC⁰ **HCC** **RxHCC** CC/MCC Exc⁰
M87.859 Other osteonecrosis, unspecified femur CC⁰ **HCC** **RxHCC** CC/MCC Exc⁰
6ᵗʰ M87.86 Other osteonecrosis, tibia and fibula
M87.861 Other osteonecrosis, right tibia CC⁰ **HCC** **RxHCC** CC/MCC Exc⁰
M87.862 Other osteonecrosis, left tibia CC⁰ **HCC** **RxHCC** CC/MCC Exc⁰
M87.863 Other osteonecrosis, unspecified tibia CC⁰ **HCC** **RxHCC** CC/MCC Exc⁰
M87.864 Other osteonecrosis, right fibula CC⁰ **HCC** **RxHCC** CC/MCC Exc⁰
M87.865 Other osteonecrosis, left fibula CC⁰ **HCC** **RxHCC** CC/MCC Exc⁰
M87.869 Other osteonecrosis, unspecified fibula CC⁰ **HCC** **RxHCC** CC/MCC Exc⁰
6ᵗʰ M87.87 Other osteonecrosis, ankle, foot and toes
M87.871 Other osteonecrosis, right ankle CC⁰ **HCC** **RxHCC** CC/MCC Exc⁰
M87.872 Other osteonecrosis, left ankle CC⁰ **HCC** **RxHCC** CC/MCC Exc⁰
M87.873 Other osteonecrosis, unspecified ankle CC⁰ **HCC** **RxHCC** CC/MCC Exc⁰
M87.874 Other osteonecrosis, right foot CC⁰ **HCC** **RxHCC** CC/MCC Exc⁰
M87.875 Other osteonecrosis, left foot CC⁰ **HCC** **RxHCC** CC/MCC Exc⁰
M87.876 Other osteonecrosis, unspecified foot CC⁰ **HCC** **RxHCC** CC/MCC Exc⁰
M87.877 Other osteonecrosis, right toe(s) CC⁰ **HCC** **RxHCC** CC/MCC Exc⁰
M87.878 Other osteonecrosis, left toe(s) CC⁰ **HCC** **RxHCC** CC/MCC Exc⁰
M87.879 Other osteonecrosis, unspecified toe(s) CC⁰ **HCC** **RxHCC** CC/MCC Exc⁰
M87.88 Other osteonecrosis, other site CC⁰ **HCC** **RxHCC** CC/MCC Exc⁰
M87.89 Other osteonecrosis, multiple sites CC⁰ **HCC** **RxHCC** CC/MCC Exc⁰
M87.9 Osteonecrosis, unspecified CC⁰ **HCC** **RxHCC** CC/MCC Exc⁰
Necrosis of bone NOS
4ᵗʰ M88 Osteitis deformans [Paget's disease of bone]
EXCLUDES1 osteitis deformans in neoplastic disease (M90.6)
M88.0 Osteitis deformans of skull
M88.1 Osteitis deformans of vertebrae
5ᵗʰ M88.8 Osteitis deformans of other bones
6ᵗʰ M88.81 Osteitis deformans of shoulder
M88.811 Osteitis deformans of right shoulder
M88.812 Osteitis deformans of left shoulder
M88.819 Osteitis deformans of unspecified shoulder
6ᵗʰ M88.82 Osteitis deformans of upper arm
M88.821 Osteitis deformans of right upper arm
M88.822 Osteitis deformans of left upper arm
M88.829 Osteitis deformans of unspecified upper arm
6ᵗʰ M88.83 Osteitis deformans of forearm
M88.831 Osteitis deformans of right forearm
M88.832 Osteitis deformans of left forearm
M88.839 Osteitis deformans of unspecified forearm
6ᵗʰ M88.84 Osteitis deformans of hand
M88.841 Osteitis deformans of right hand
M88.842 Osteitis deformans of left hand
M88.849 Osteitis deformans of unspecified hand

6ᵗʰ M88.85 Osteitis deformans of thigh
M88.851 Osteitis deformans of right thigh
M88.852 Osteitis deformans of left thigh
M88.859 Osteitis deformans of unspecified thigh
6ᵗʰ M88.86 Osteitis deformans of lower leg
M88.861 Osteitis deformans of right lower leg
M88.862 Osteitis deformans of left lower leg
M88.869 Osteitis deformans of unspecified lower leg
6ᵗʰ M88.87 Osteitis deformans of ankle and foot
M88.871 Osteitis deformans of right ankle and foot
M88.872 Osteitis deformans of left ankle and foot
M88.879 Osteitis deformans of unspecified ankle and foot
M88.88 Osteitis deformans of other bones
EXCLUDES2 osteitis deformans of skull (M88.0)
osteitis deformans of vertebrae (M88.1)
M88.89 Osteitis deformans of multiple sites
M88.9 Osteitis deformans of unspecified bone
4ᵗʰ M89 Other disorders of bone
5ᵗʰ M89.0 Algoneurodystrophy
DEFINITION: Algoneurodystrophy is a form of complex regional pain syndrome, also known as reflex sympathetic dystrophy.
Shoulder-hand syndrome
Sudeck's atrophy
EXCLUDES1 causalgia, lower limb (G57.7-)
causalgia, upper limb (G56.4-)
complex regional pain syndrome II, lower limb (G57.7-)
complex regional pain syndrome II, upper limb (G56.4-)
reflex sympathetic dystrophy (G90.5-)
M89.00 Algoneurodystrophy, unspecified site
6ᵗʰ M89.01 Algoneurodystrophy, shoulder
M89.011 Algoneurodystrophy, right shoulder
M89.012 Algoneurodystrophy, left shoulder
M89.019 Algoneurodystrophy, unspecified shoulder
6ᵗʰ M89.02 Algoneurodystrophy, upper arm
M89.021 Algoneurodystrophy, right upper arm
M89.022 Algoneurodystrophy, left upper arm
M89.029 Algoneurodystrophy, unspecified upper arm
6ᵗʰ M89.03 Algoneurodystrophy, forearm
M89.031 Algoneurodystrophy, right forearm
M89.032 Algoneurodystrophy, left forearm
M89.039 Algoneurodystrophy, unspecified forearm
6ᵗʰ M89.04 Algoneurodystrophy, hand
M89.041 Algoneurodystrophy, right hand
M89.042 Algoneurodystrophy, left hand
M89.049 Algoneurodystrophy, unspecified hand
6ᵗʰ M89.05 Algoneurodystrophy, thigh
M89.051 Algoneurodystrophy, right thigh
M89.052 Algoneurodystrophy, left thigh
M89.059 Algoneurodystrophy, unspecified thigh
6ᵗʰ M89.06 Algoneurodystrophy, lower leg
M89.061 Algoneurodystrophy, right lower leg
M89.062 Algoneurodystrophy, left lower leg
M89.069 Algoneurodystrophy, unspecified lower leg
6ᵗʰ M89.07 Algoneurodystrophy, ankle and foot
M89.071 Algoneurodystrophy, right ankle and foot
M89.072 Algoneurodystrophy, left ankle and foot
M89.079 Algoneurodystrophy, unspecified ankle and foot
M89.08 Algoneurodystrophy, other site
M89.09 Algoneurodystrophy, multiple sites

Unspecified Code | Other Specified Code | Manifestation Code | N Newborn | P Pediatric | M Maternity | A Adult | ♂ Male | ♀ Female
● New Code ▲ Revised Code Title ►◄ Revised Text **NOTES** *INCLUDES* *EXCLUDES1* Not coded here *EXCLUDES2* Not included here
4ᵗʰ 4ᵗʰ character required 5ᵗʰ 5ᵗʰ character required 6ᵗʰ 6ᵗʰ character required 7ᵗʰ 7ᵗʰ character required ⑦ Extension 'X' Alert
HAC Hospital-acquired condition (HAC) alert **AHA** AHA Coding Clinic© ☞ Code first alert

[5th] M89.1 Physeal arrest
Arrest of growth plate
Epiphyseal arrest
Growth plate arrest
[6th] M89.12 Physeal arrest, humerus
M89.121 Complete physeal arrest, right proximal humerus
M89.122 Complete physeal arrest, left proximal humerus
M89.123 Partial physeal arrest, right proximal humerus
M89.124 Partial physeal arrest, left proximal humerus
M89.125 Complete physeal arrest, right distal humerus
M89.126 Complete physeal arrest, left distal humerus
M89.127 Partial physeal arrest, right distal humerus
M89.128 Partial physeal arrest, left distal humerus
M89.129 Physeal arrest, humerus, unspecified
[6th] M89.13 Physeal arrest, forearm
M89.131 Complete physeal arrest, right distal radius
M89.132 Complete physeal arrest, left distal radius
M89.133 Partial physeal arrest, right distal radius
M89.134 Partial physeal arrest, left distal radius
M89.138 Other physeal arrest of forearm
M89.139 Physeal arrest, forearm, unspecified
[6th] M89.15 Physeal arrest, femur
M89.151 Complete physeal arrest, right proximal femur
M89.152 Complete physeal arrest, left proximal femur
M89.153 Partial physeal arrest, right proximal femur
M89.154 Partial physeal arrest, left proximal femur
M89.155 Complete physeal arrest, right distal femur
M89.156 Complete physeal arrest, left distal femur
M89.157 Partial physeal arrest, right distal femur
M89.158 Partial physeal arrest, left distal femur
M89.159 Physeal arrest, femur, unspecified
[6th] M89.16 Physeal arrest, lower leg
M89.160 Complete physeal arrest, right proximal tibia
M89.161 Complete physeal arrest, left proximal tibia
M89.162 Partial physeal arrest, right proximal tibia
M89.163 Partial physeal arrest, left proximal tibia
M89.164 Complete physeal arrest, right distal tibia
M89.165 Complete physeal arrest, left distal tibia
M89.166 Partial physeal arrest, right distal tibia
M89.167 Partial physeal arrest, left distal tibia
M89.168 Other physeal arrest of lower leg
M89.169 Physeal arrest, lower leg, unspecified
M89.18 Physeal arrest, other site
[5th] M89.2 Other disorders of bone development and growth
M89.20 Other disorders of bone development and growth, unspecified site
[6th] M89.21 Other disorders of bone development and growth, shoulder
M89.211 Other disorders of bone development and growth, right shoulder
M89.212 Other disorders of bone development and growth, left shoulder
M89.219 Other disorders of bone development and growth, unspecified shoulder
[6th] M89.22 Other disorders of bone development and growth, humerus
M89.221 Other disorders of bone development and growth, right humerus
M89.222 Other disorders of bone development and growth, left humerus
M89.229 Other disorders of bone development and growth, unspecified humerus
[6th] M89.23 Other disorders of bone development and growth, ulna and radius
M89.231 Other disorders of bone development and growth, right ulna
M89.232 Other disorders of bone development and growth, left ulna
M89.233 Other disorders of bone development and growth, right radius
M89.234 Other disorders of bone development and growth, left radius
M89.239 Other disorders of bone development and growth, unspecified ulna and radius
[6th] M89.24 Other disorders of bone development and growth, hand
M89.241 Other disorders of bone development and growth, right hand
M89.242 Other disorders of bone development and growth, left hand
M89.249 Other disorders of bone development and growth, unspecified hand
[6th] M89.25 Other disorders of bone development and growth, femur
M89.251 Other disorders of bone development and growth, right femur
M89.252 Other disorders of bone development and growth, left femur
M89.259 Other disorders of bone development and growth, unspecified femur
[6th] M89.26 Other disorders of bone development and growth, tibia and fibula
M89.261 Other disorders of bone development and growth, right tibia
M89.262 Other disorders of bone development and growth, left tibia
M89.263 Other disorders of bone development and growth, right fibula
M89.264 Other disorders of bone development and growth, left fibula
M89.269 Other disorders of bone development and growth, unspecified lower leg
[6th] M89.27 Other disorders of bone development and growth, ankle and foot
M89.271 Other disorders of bone development and growth, right ankle and foot
M89.272 Other disorders of bone development and growth, left ankle and foot
M89.279 Other disorders of bone development and growth, unspecified ankle and foot
M89.28 Other disorders of bone development and growth, other site
M89.29 Other disorders of bone development and growth, multiple sites
[5th] M89.3 Hypertrophy of bone
M89.30 Hypertrophy of bone, unspecified site
[6th] M89.31 Hypertrophy of bone, shoulder
M89.311 Hypertrophy of bone, right shoulder
M89.312 Hypertrophy of bone, left shoulder
M89.319 Hypertrophy of bone, unspecified shoulder
[6th] M89.32 Hypertrophy of bone, humerus
M89.321 Hypertrophy of bone, right humerus
M89.322 Hypertrophy of bone, left humerus
M89.329 Hypertrophy of bone, unspecified humerus
[6th] M89.33 Hypertrophy of bone, ulna and radius
M89.331 Hypertrophy of bone, right ulna
M89.332 Hypertrophy of bone, left ulna

M89.333 Hypertrophy of bone, right radius
M89.334 Hypertrophy of bone, left radius
M89.339 Hypertrophy of bone, unspecified ulna and radius
[6th] M89.34 Hypertrophy of bone, hand
M89.341 Hypertrophy of bone, right hand
M89.342 Hypertrophy of bone, left hand
M89.349 Hypertrophy of bone, unspecified hand
[6th] M89.35 Hypertrophy of bone, femur
M89.351 Hypertrophy of bone, right femur
M89.352 Hypertrophy of bone, left femur
M89.359 Hypertrophy of bone, unspecified femur
[6th] M89.36 Hypertrophy of bone, tibia and fibula
M89.361 Hypertrophy of bone, right tibia
M89.362 Hypertrophy of bone, left tibia
M89.363 Hypertrophy of bone, right fibula
M89.364 Hypertrophy of bone, left fibula
M89.369 Hypertrophy of bone, unspecified tibia and fibula
[6th] M89.37 Hypertrophy of bone, ankle and foot
M89.371 Hypertrophy of bone, right ankle and foot
M89.372 Hypertrophy of bone, left ankle and foot
M89.379 Hypertrophy of bone, unspecified ankle and foot
M89.38 Hypertrophy of bone, other site
M89.39 Hypertrophy of bone, multiple sites
[5th] M89.4 Other hypertrophic osteoarthropathy
Marie-Bamberger disease
Pachydermoperiostosis
M89.40 Other hypertrophic osteoarthropathy, unspecified site
[6th] M89.41 Other hypertrophic osteoarthropathy, shoulder
M89.411 Other hypertrophic osteoarthropathy, right shoulder
M89.412 Other hypertrophic osteoarthropathy, left shoulder
M89.419 Other hypertrophic osteoarthropathy, unspecified shoulder
[6th] M89.42 Other hypertrophic osteoarthropathy, upper arm
M89.421 Other hypertrophic osteoarthropathy, right upper arm
M89.422 Other hypertrophic osteoarthropathy, left upper arm
M89.429 Other hypertrophic osteoarthropathy, unspecified upper arm
[6th] M89.43 Other hypertrophic osteoarthropathy, forearm
M89.431 Other hypertrophic osteoarthropathy, right forearm
M89.432 Other hypertrophic osteoarthropathy, left forearm
M89.439 Other hypertrophic osteoarthropathy, unspecified forearm
[6th] M89.44 Other hypertrophic osteoarthropathy, hand
M89.441 Other hypertrophic osteoarthropathy, right hand
M89.442 Other hypertrophic osteoarthropathy, left hand
M89.449 Other hypertrophic osteoarthropathy, unspecified hand
[6th] M89.45 Other hypertrophic osteoarthropathy, thigh
M89.451 Other hypertrophic osteoarthropathy, right thigh
M89.452 Other hypertrophic osteoarthropathy, left thigh
M89.459 Other hypertrophic osteoarthropathy, unspecified thigh
[6th] M89.46 Other hypertrophic osteoarthropathy, lower leg
M89.461 Other hypertrophic osteoarthropathy, right lower leg
M89.462 Other hypertrophic osteoarthropathy, left lower leg
M89.469 Other hypertrophic osteoarthropathy, unspecified lower leg
[6th] M89.47 Other hypertrophic osteoarthropathy, ankle and foot
M89.471 Other hypertrophic osteoarthropathy, right ankle and foot
M89.472 Other hypertrophic osteoarthropathy, left ankle and foot
M89.479 Other hypertrophic osteoarthropathy, unspecified ankle and foot
M89.48 Other hypertrophic osteoarthropathy, other site
M89.49 Other hypertrophic osteoarthropathy, multiple sites
[5th] M89.5 Osteolysis
Use additional code to identify major osseous defect, if applicable (M89.7-)
[EXCLUDES2] *periprosthetic osteolysis of internal prosthetic joint (T84.05-)*
M89.50 Osteolysis, unspecified site
[6th] M89.51 Osteolysis, shoulder
M89.511 Osteolysis, right shoulder
M89.512 Osteolysis, left shoulder
M89.519 Osteolysis, unspecified shoulder
[6th] M89.52 Osteolysis, upper arm
M89.521 Osteolysis, right upper arm
M89.522 Osteolysis, left upper arm
M89.529 Osteolysis, unspecified upper arm
[6th] M89.53 Osteolysis, forearm
M89.531 Osteolysis, right forearm
M89.532 Osteolysis, left forearm
M89.539 Osteolysis, unspecified forearm
[6th] M89.54 Osteolysis, hand
M89.541 Osteolysis, right hand
M89.542 Osteolysis, left hand
M89.549 Osteolysis, unspecified hand
[6th] M89.55 Osteolysis, thigh
M89.551 Osteolysis, right thigh
M89.552 Osteolysis, left thigh
M89.559 Osteolysis, unspecified thigh
[6th] M89.56 Osteolysis, lower leg
M89.561 Osteolysis, right lower leg
M89.562 Osteolysis, left lower leg
M89.569 Osteolysis, unspecified lower leg
[6th] M89.57 Osteolysis, ankle and foot
M89.571 Osteolysis, right ankle and foot
M89.572 Osteolysis, left ankle and foot
M89.579 Osteolysis, unspecified ankle and foot
M89.58 Osteolysis, other site
M89.59 Osteolysis, multiple sites
[5th] M89.6 Osteopathy after poliomyelitis
Use additional code (B91) to identify previous poliomyelitis
[EXCLUDES1] *postpolio syndrome (G14)*
M89.60 Osteopathy after poliomyelitis, unspecified site [HCC]
[6th] M89.61 Osteopathy after poliomyelitis, shoulder
M89.611 Osteopathy after poliomyelitis, right shoulder [HCC]
M89.612 Osteopathy after poliomyelitis, left shoulder [HCC]
M89.619 Osteopathy after poliomyelitis, unspecified shoulder [HCC]
[6th] M89.62 Osteopathy after poliomyelitis, upper arm
M89.621 Osteopathy after poliomyelitis, right upper arm [HCC]
M89.622 Osteopathy after poliomyelitis, left upper arm [HCC]
M89.629 Osteopathy after poliomyelitis, unspecified upper arm [HCC]
[6th] M89.63 Osteopathy after poliomyelitis, forearm
M89.631 Osteopathy after poliomyelitis, right forearm [HCC]

Unspecified Code | Other Specified Code | Manifestation Code | [N] Newborn | [P] Pediatric | [M] Maternity | [A] Adult | ♂ Male | ♀ Female
● New Code | ▲ Revised Code Title | ►◄ Revised Text | [NOTES] | *INCLUDES* | [EXCLUDES1] Not coded here | [EXCLUDES2] Not included here
[4th] 4th character required | [5th] 5th character required | [6th] 6th character required | [7th] 7th character required | [X] Extension 'X' Alert
[HAC] Hospital-acquired condition (HAC) alert | AHA AHA Coding Clinic© | Code first alert

When symbols appear on a code that requires a 7th character extension, refer to Appendix B to identify applicable 7th character codes.

M89.632 Osteopathy after poliomyelitis, left forearm **HCC**

M89.639 Osteopathy after poliomyelitis, unspecified forearm **HCC**

M89.64 Osteopathy after poliomyelitis, hand

M89.641 Osteopathy after poliomyelitis, right hand **HCC**

M89.642 Osteopathy after poliomyelitis, left hand **HCC**

M89.649 Osteopathy after poliomyelitis, unspecified hand **HCC**

M89.65 Osteopathy after poliomyelitis, thigh

M89.651 Osteopathy after poliomyelitis, right thigh **HCC**

M89.652 Osteopathy after poliomyelitis, left thigh **HCC**

M89.659 Osteopathy after poliomyelitis, unspecified thigh **HCC**

M89.66 Osteopathy after poliomyelitis, lower leg

M89.661 Osteopathy after poliomyelitis, right lower leg **HCC**

M89.662 Osteopathy after poliomyelitis, left lower leg **HCC**

M89.669 Osteopathy after poliomyelitis, unspecified lower leg **HCC**

M89.67 Osteopathy after poliomyelitis, ankle and foot

M89.671 Osteopathy after poliomyelitis, right ankle and foot **HCC**

M89.672 Osteopathy after poliomyelitis, left ankle and foot **HCC**

M89.679 Osteopathy after poliomyelitis, unspecified ankle and foot **HCC**

M89.68 Osteopathy after poliomyelitis, other site **HCC**

M89.69 Osteopathy after poliomyelitis, multiple sites **HCC**

M89.7 Major osseous defect

TIP: List first the code that describes the cause of the defect.

☞ **Code first** underlying disease, if known, such as:
aseptic necrosis of bone (M87.-)
malignant neoplasm of bone (C40.-)
osteolysis (M89.5)
osteomyelitis (M86.-)
osteonecrosis (M87.-)
osteoporosis (M80.-, M81.-)
periprosthetic osteolysis (T84.05-)

M89.70 Major osseous defect, unspecified site

M89.71 Major osseous defect, shoulder region
Major osseous defect clavicle or scapula

M89.711 Major osseous defect, right shoulder region

M89.712 Major osseous defect, left shoulder region

M89.719 Major osseous defect, unspecified shoulder region

M89.72 Major osseous defect, humerus

M89.721 Major osseous defect, right humerus

M89.722 Major osseous defect, left humerus

M89.729 Major osseous defect, unspecified humerus

M89.73 Major osseous defect, forearm
Major osseous defect of radius and ulna

M89.731 Major osseous defect, right forearm

M89.732 Major osseous defect, left forearm

M89.739 Major osseous defect, unspecified forearm

M89.74 Major osseous defect, hand
Major osseous defect of carpus, fingers, metacarpus

M89.741 Major osseous defect, right hand

M89.742 Major osseous defect, left hand

M89.749 Major osseous defect, unspecified hand

M89.75 Major osseous defect, pelvic region and thigh
Major osseous defect of femur and pelvis

M89.751 Major osseous defect, right pelvic region and thigh

M89.752 Major osseous defect, left pelvic region and thigh

M89.759 Major osseous defect, unspecified pelvic region and thigh

M89.76 Major osseous defect, lower leg
Major osseous defect of fibula and tibia

M89.761 Major osseous defect, right lower leg

M89.762 Major osseous defect, left lower leg

M89.769 Major osseous defect, unspecified lower leg

M89.77 Major osseous defect, ankle and foot
Major osseous defect of metatarsus, tarsus, toes

M89.771 Major osseous defect, right ankle and foot

M89.772 Major osseous defect, left ankle and foot

M89.779 Major osseous defect, unspecified ankle and foot

M89.78 Major osseous defect, other site

M89.79 Major osseous defect, multiple sites

M89.8 Other specified disorders of bone
Infantile cortical hyperostoses
Post-traumatic subperiosteal ossification

M89.8X Other specified disorders of bone

M89.8X0 Other specified disorders of bone, multiple sites

M89.8X1 Other specified disorders of bone, shoulder

M89.8X2 Other specified disorders of bone, upper arm

M89.8X3 Other specified disorders of bone, forearm

M89.8X4 Other specified disorders of bone, hand

M89.8X5 Other specified disorders of bone, thigh

M89.8X6 Other specified disorders of bone, lower leg

M89.8X7 Other specified disorders of bone, ankle and foot

M89.8X8 Other specified disorders of bone, other site

M89.8X9 Other specified disorders of bone, unspecified site

M89.9 Disorder of bone, unspecified

M90 Osteopathies in diseases classified elsewhere

EXCLUDES1 osteochondritis, osteomyelitis, and osteopathy (in):
cryptococcosis (B45.3)
diabetes mellitus (E08-E13 with .69-)
gonococcal (A54.43)
neurogenic syphilis (A52.11)
renal osteodystrophy (N25.0)
salmonellosis (A02.24)
secondary syphilis (A51.46)
syphilis (late) (A52.77)

M90.5 Osteonecrosis in diseases classified elsewhere

☞ **Code first** underlying disease, such as:
caisson disease (T70.3)
hemoglobinopathy (D50-D64)

M90.50 Osteonecrosis in diseases classified elsewhere, unspecified site cc HCC RxHCC CC/MCC Exc

M90.51 Osteonecrosis in diseases classified elsewhere, shoulder

M90.511 Osteonecrosis in diseases classified elsewhere, right shoulder cc HCC RxHCC CC/MCC Exc

M90.512 Osteonecrosis in diseases classified elsewhere, left shoulder cc HCC RxHCC CC/MCC Exc

M90.519 Osteonecrosis in diseases classified elsewhere, unspecified shoulder cc HCC RxHCC CC/MCC Exc

M90.52 Osteonecrosis in diseases classified elsewhere, upper arm

M90.521 Osteonecrosis in diseases classified elsewhere, right upper arm cc HCC RxHCC CC/MCC Exc

PDx Unacceptable principal diagnosis symbol per Medicare code edits   PDx Code exempt from diagnosis present on admission requirement
❓ Questionable admission   cc Complication or comorbidity   MCC Major complication or comorbidity   CC/MCC CC/MCC exclusion
HCC HCC diagnosis code   RxHCC RxHCC diagnosis code   MACRA code   **DEFINITION** Describes condition/terminology
TIP Coding guidance   👁 Official Guideline Reference   Z Z code as first-listed diagnosis

852   When symbols appear on a code that requires a 7th character extension, refer to Appendix B to identify applicable 7th character codes.   **2020 ICD-10-CM**

M90.522 Osteonecrosis in diseases classified elsewhere, left upper arm [CC] [HCC] [RxHCC] [CC/MCC Exc]
M90.529 Osteonecrosis in diseases classified elsewhere, unspecified upper arm [CC] [HCC] [RxHCC] [CC/MCC Exc]

[6th] M90.53 Osteonecrosis in diseases classified elsewhere, forearm
M90.531 Osteonecrosis in diseases classified elsewhere, right forearm [CC] [HCC] [RxHCC] [CC/MCC Exc]
M90.532 Osteonecrosis in diseases classified elsewhere, left forearm [CC] [HCC] [RxHCC] [CC/MCC Exc]
M90.539 Osteonecrosis in diseases classified elsewhere, unspecified forearm [CC] [HCC] [RxHCC] [CC/MCC Exc]

[6th] M90.54 Osteonecrosis in diseases classified elsewhere, hand
M90.541 Osteonecrosis in diseases classified elsewhere, right hand [CC] [HCC] [RxHCC] [CC/MCC Exc]
M90.542 Osteonecrosis in diseases classified elsewhere, left hand [CC] [HCC] [RxHCC] [CC/MCC Exc]
M90.549 Osteonecrosis in diseases classified elsewhere, unspecified hand [CC] [HCC] [RxHCC] [CC/MCC Exc]

[6th] M90.55 Osteonecrosis in diseases classified elsewhere, thigh
M90.551 Osteonecrosis in diseases classified elsewhere, right thigh [CC] [HCC] [RxHCC] [CC/MCC Exc]
M90.552 Osteonecrosis in diseases classified elsewhere, left thigh [CC] [HCC] [RxHCC] [CC/MCC Exc]
M90.559 Osteonecrosis in diseases classified elsewhere, unspecified thigh [CC] [HCC] [RxHCC] [CC/MCC Exc]

[6th] M90.56 Osteonecrosis in diseases classified elsewhere, lower leg
M90.561 Osteonecrosis in diseases classified elsewhere, right lower leg [CC] [HCC] [RxHCC] [CC/MCC Exc]
M90.562 Osteonecrosis in diseases classified elsewhere, left lower leg [CC] [HCC] [RxHCC] [CC/MCC Exc]
M90.569 Osteonecrosis in diseases classified elsewhere, unspecified lower leg [CC] [HCC] [RxHCC] [CC/MCC Exc]

[6th] M90.57 Osteonecrosis in diseases classified elsewhere, ankle and foot
M90.571 Osteonecrosis in diseases classified elsewhere, right ankle and foot [CC] [HCC] [RxHCC] [CC/MCC Exc]
M90.572 Osteonecrosis in diseases classified elsewhere, left ankle and foot [CC] [HCC] [RxHCC] [CC/MCC Exc]
M90.579 Osteonecrosis in diseases classified elsewhere, unspecified ankle and foot [CC] [HCC] [RxHCC] [CC/MCC Exc]

M90.58 Osteonecrosis in diseases classified elsewhere, other site [CC] [HCC] [RxHCC] [CC/MCC Exc]
M90.59 Osteonecrosis in diseases classified elsewhere, multiple sites [CC] [HCC] [RxHCC] [CC/MCC Exc]

[5th] M90.6 Osteitis deformans in neoplastic diseases
Osteitis deformans in malignant neoplasm of bone
☞ **Code first** the neoplasm (C40.-, C41.-)
[EXCLUDES1] *osteitis deformans [Paget's disease of bone] (M88.-)*
M90.60 Osteitis deformans in neoplastic diseases, unspecified site

[6th] M90.61 Osteitis deformans in neoplastic diseases, shoulder
M90.611 Osteitis deformans in neoplastic diseases, right shoulder
M90.612 Osteitis deformans in neoplastic diseases, left shoulder
M90.619 Osteitis deformans in neoplastic diseases, unspecified shoulder

[6th] M90.62 Osteitis deformans in neoplastic diseases, upper arm
M90.621 Osteitis deformans in neoplastic diseases, right upper arm
M90.622 Osteitis deformans in neoplastic diseases, left upper arm
M90.629 Osteitis deformans in neoplastic diseases, unspecified upper arm

[6th] M90.63 Osteitis deformans in neoplastic diseases, forearm
M90.631 Osteitis deformans in neoplastic diseases, right forearm
M90.632 Osteitis deformans in neoplastic diseases, left forearm
M90.639 Osteitis deformans in neoplastic diseases, unspecified forearm

[6th] M90.64 Osteitis deformans in neoplastic diseases, hand
M90.641 Osteitis deformans in neoplastic diseases, right hand
M90.642 Osteitis deformans in neoplastic diseases, left hand
M90.649 Osteitis deformans in neoplastic diseases, unspecified hand

[6th] M90.65 Osteitis deformans in neoplastic diseases, thigh
M90.651 Osteitis deformans in neoplastic diseases, right thigh
M90.652 Osteitis deformans in neoplastic diseases, left thigh
M90.659 Osteitis deformans in neoplastic diseases, unspecified thigh

[6th] M90.66 Osteitis deformans in neoplastic diseases, lower leg
M90.661 Osteitis deformans in neoplastic diseases, right lower leg
M90.662 Osteitis deformans in neoplastic diseases, left lower leg
M90.669 Osteitis deformans in neoplastic diseases, unspecified lower leg

[6th] M90.67 Osteitis deformans in neoplastic diseases, ankle and foot
M90.671 Osteitis deformans in neoplastic diseases, right ankle and foot
M90.672 Osteitis deformans in neoplastic diseases, left ankle and foot
M90.679 Osteitis deformans in neoplastic diseases, unspecified ankle and foot

M90.68 Osteitis deformans in neoplastic diseases, other site
M90.69 Osteitis deformans in neoplastic diseases, multiple sites

[5th] M90.8 Osteopathy in diseases classified elsewhere
☞ **Code first** underlying disease, such as:
rickets (E55.0)
vitamin-D-resistant rickets (E83.3)
M90.80 Osteopathy in diseases classified elsewhere, unspecified site

[6th] M90.81 Osteopathy in diseases classified elsewhere, shoulder
M90.811 Osteopathy in diseases classified elsewhere, right shoulder
M90.812 Osteopathy in diseases classified elsewhere, left shoulder
M90.819 Osteopathy in diseases classified elsewhere, unspecified shoulder

[6th] M90.82 Osteopathy in diseases classified elsewhere, upper arm
M90.821 Osteopathy in diseases classified elsewhere, right upper arm
M90.822 Osteopathy in diseases classified elsewhere, left upper arm
M90.829 Osteopathy in diseases classified elsewhere, unspecified upper arm

[6th] M90.83 Osteopathy in diseases classified elsewhere, forearm
M90.831 Osteopathy in diseases classified elsewhere, right forearm
M90.832 Osteopathy in diseases classified elsewhere, left forearm

Unspecified Code   Other Specified Code   Manifestation Code   [N] Newborn   [P] Pediatric   [M] Maternity   [A] Adult   ♂ Male   ♀ Female
● New Code   ▲ Revised Code Title   ►◄ Revised Text   [NOTES]   *INCLUDES*   [EXCLUDES1] Not coded here   [EXCLUDES2] Not included here
[4th] 4th character required   [5th] 5th character required   [6th] 6th character required   [7th] 7th character required   [7th] Extension 'X' Alert
[HAC] Hospital-acquired condition (HAC) alert   **AHA** AHA Coding Clinic©   ☞ **Code first** alert

M90.839 Osteopathy in diseases classified elsewhere, unspecified forearm

🔟 M90.84 Osteopathy in diseases classified elsewhere, hand

    M90.841 Osteopathy in diseases classified elsewhere, right hand

    M90.842 Osteopathy in diseases classified elsewhere, left hand

    M90.849 Osteopathy in diseases classified elsewhere, unspecified hand

🔟 M90.85 Osteopathy in diseases classified elsewhere, thigh

    M90.851 Osteopathy in diseases classified elsewhere, right thigh

    M90.852 Osteopathy in diseases classified elsewhere, left thigh

    M90.859 Osteopathy in diseases classified elsewhere, unspecified thigh

🔟 M90.86 Osteopathy in diseases classified elsewhere, lower leg

    M90.861 Osteopathy in diseases classified elsewhere, right lower leg

    M90.862 Osteopathy in diseases classified elsewhere, left lower leg

    M90.869 Osteopathy in diseases classified elsewhere, unspecified lower leg

🔟 M90.87 Osteopathy in diseases classified elsewhere, ankle and foot

    M90.871 Osteopathy in diseases classified elsewhere, right ankle and foot

    M90.872 Osteopathy in diseases classified elsewhere, left ankle and foot

    M90.879 Osteopathy in diseases classified elsewhere, unspecified ankle and foot

M90.88 Osteopathy in diseases classified elsewhere, other site

M90.89 Osteopathy in diseases classified elsewhere, multiple sites

Chondropathies (M91-M94)

EXCLUDES1 postprocedural chondropathies (M96.-)

🔟 M91 Juvenile osteochondrosis of hip and pelvis

    EXCLUDES1 slipped upper femoral epiphysis (nontraumatic) (M93.0)

M91.0 Juvenile osteochondrosis of pelvis

Osteochondrosis (juvenile) of acetabulum

Osteochondrosis (juvenile) of iliac crest [Buchanan]

Osteochondrosis (juvenile) of ischiopubic synchondrosis [van Neck]

Osteochondrosis (juvenile) of symphysis pubis [Pierson]

🔟 M91.1 Juvenile osteochondrosis of head of femur [Legg-Calvé-Perthes]

    M91.10 Juvenile osteochondrosis of head of femur [Legg-Calvé-Perthes], unspecified leg

    M91.11 Juvenile osteochondrosis of head of femur [Legg-Calvé-Perthes], right leg

    M91.12 Juvenile osteochondrosis of head of femur [Legg-Calvé-Perthes], left leg

🔟 M91.2 Coxa plana

Hip deformity due to previous juvenile osteochondrosis

    M91.20 Coxa plana, unspecified hip

    M91.21 Coxa plana, right hip

    M91.22 Coxa plana, left hip

🔟 M91.3 Pseudocoxalgia

    M91.30 Pseudocoxalgia, unspecified hip

    M91.31 Pseudocoxalgia, right hip

    M91.32 Pseudocoxalgia, left hip

🔟 M91.4 Coxa magna

    M91.40 Coxa magna, unspecified hip

    M91.41 Coxa magna, right hip

    M91.42 Coxa magna, left hip

🔟 M91.8 Other juvenile osteochondrosis of hip and pelvis

Juvenile osteochondrosis after reduction of congenital dislocation of hip

    M91.80 Other juvenile osteochondrosis of hip and pelvis, unspecified leg

    M91.81 Other juvenile osteochondrosis of hip and pelvis, right leg

    M91.82 Other juvenile osteochondrosis of hip and pelvis, left leg

🔟 M91.9 Juvenile osteochondrosis of hip and pelvis, unspecified

    M91.90 Juvenile osteochondrosis of hip and pelvis, unspecified, unspecified leg

    M91.91 Juvenile osteochondrosis of hip and pelvis, unspecified, right leg

    M91.92 Juvenile osteochondrosis of hip and pelvis, unspecified, left leg

🔟 M92 Other juvenile osteochondrosis

🔟 M92.0 Juvenile osteochondrosis of humerus

Osteochondrosis (juvenile) of capitulum of humerus [Panner]

Osteochondrosis (juvenile) of head of humerus [Haas]

    M92.00 Juvenile osteochondrosis of humerus, unspecified arm

    M92.01 Juvenile osteochondrosis of humerus, right arm

    M92.02 Juvenile osteochondrosis of humerus, left arm

🔟 M92.1 Juvenile osteochondrosis of radius and ulna

Osteochondrosis (juvenile) of lower ulna [Burns]

Osteochondrosis (juvenile) of radial head [Brailsford]

    M92.10 Juvenile osteochondrosis of radius and ulna, unspecified arm

    M92.11 Juvenile osteochondrosis of radius and ulna, right arm

    M92.12 Juvenile osteochondrosis of radius and ulna, left arm

🔟 M92.2 Juvenile osteochondrosis, hand

🔟 M92.20 Unspecified juvenile osteochondrosis, hand

    M92.201 Unspecified juvenile osteochondrosis, right hand

    M92.202 Unspecified juvenile osteochondrosis, left hand

    M92.209 Unspecified juvenile osteochondrosis, unspecified hand

🔟 M92.21 Osteochondrosis (juvenile) of carpal lunate [Kienböck]

    M92.211 Osteochondrosis (juvenile) of carpal lunate [Kienböck], right hand

    M92.212 Osteochondrosis (juvenile) of carpal lunate [Kienböck], left hand

    M92.219 Osteochondrosis (juvenile) of carpal lunate [Kienböck], unspecified hand

🔟 M92.22 Osteochondrosis (juvenile) of metacarpal heads [Mauclaire]

    M92.221 Osteochondrosis (juvenile) of metacarpal heads [Mauclaire], right hand

    M92.222 Osteochondrosis (juvenile) of metacarpal heads [Mauclaire], left hand

    M92.229 Osteochondrosis (juvenile) of metacarpal heads [Mauclaire], unspecified hand

🔟 M92.29 Other juvenile osteochondrosis, hand

    M92.291 Other juvenile osteochondrosis, right hand

    M92.292 Other juvenile osteochondrosis, left hand

    M92.299 Other juvenile osteochondrosis, unspecified hand

🔟 M92.3 Other juvenile osteochondrosis, upper limb

    M92.30 Other juvenile osteochondrosis, unspecified upper limb

    M92.31 Other juvenile osteochondrosis, right upper limb

    M92.32 Other juvenile osteochondrosis, left upper limb

🔟 M92.4 Juvenile osteochondrosis of patella

Osteochondrosis (juvenile) of primary patellar center [Köhler]

Osteochondrosis (juvenile) of secondary patellar center [Sinding Larsen]

PDₓ Unacceptable principal diagnosis symbol per Medicare code edits   PDₓ Code exempt from diagnosis present on admission requirement

❓ Questionable admission   cc Complication or comorbidity   MCC Major complication or comorbidity   cc/MCC EXC CC/MCC exclusion

HCC HCC diagnosis code   RxHCC RxHCC diagnosis code   MACRA code MACRA code   **DEFINITION** Describes condition/terminology

TIP Coding guidance   👁 Official Guideline Reference   Z1 Z code as first-listed diagnosis

854   When symbols appear on a code that requires a 7th character extension, refer to Appendix B to identify applicable 7th character codes.   **2020 ICD-10-CM**

M92.40 **Juvenile osteochondrosis of patella, unspecified knee**
M92.41 **Juvenile osteochondrosis of patella, right knee**
M92.42 **Juvenile osteochondrosis of patella, left knee**

[5th] M92.5 **Juvenile osteochondrosis of tibia and fibula**
Osteochondrosis (juvenile) of proximal tibia [Blount]
Osteochondrosis (juvenile) of tibial tubercle [Osgood-Schlatter]
Tibia vara
M92.50 **Juvenile osteochondrosis of tibia and fibula, unspecified leg**
M92.51 **Juvenile osteochondrosis of tibia and fibula, right leg**
M92.52 **Juvenile osteochondrosis of tibia and fibula, left leg**

[5th] M92.6 **Juvenile osteochondrosis of tarsus**
Osteochondrosis (juvenile) of calcaneum [Sever]
Osteochondrosis (juvenile) of os tibiale externum [Haglund]
Osteochondrosis (juvenile) of talus [Diaz]
Osteochondrosis (juvenile) of tarsal navicular [Köhler]
M92.60 **Juvenile osteochondrosis of tarsus, unspecified ankle**
M92.61 **Juvenile osteochondrosis of tarsus, right ankle**
M92.62 **Juvenile osteochondrosis of tarsus, left ankle**

[5th] M92.7 **Juvenile osteochondrosis of metatarsus**
Osteochondrosis (juvenile) of fifth metatarsus [Iselin]
Osteochondrosis (juvenile) of second metatarsus [Freiberg]
M92.70 **Juvenile osteochondrosis of metatarsus, unspecified foot**
M92.71 **Juvenile osteochondrosis of metatarsus, right foot**
M92.72 **Juvenile osteochondrosis of metatarsus, left foot**

M92.8 **Other specified juvenile osteochondrosis**
Calcaneal apophysitis

M92.9 **Juvenile osteochondrosis, unspecified**
Juvenile apophysitis NOS
Juvenile epiphysitis NOS
Juvenile osteochondritis NOS
Juvenile osteochondrosis NOS

[4th] **M93 Other osteochondropathies**
[EXCLUDES2] *osteochondrosis of spine (M42.-)*

[5th] M93.0 **Slipped upper femoral epiphysis (nontraumatic)**
Use additional code for associated chondrolysis (M94.3)

[6th] M93.00 **Unspecified slipped upper femoral epiphysis (nontraumatic)**
M93.001 **Unspecified slipped upper femoral epiphysis (nontraumatic), right hip**
M93.002 **Unspecified slipped upper femoral epiphysis (nontraumatic), left hip**
M93.003 **Unspecified slipped upper femoral epiphysis (nontraumatic), unspecified hip**

[6th] M93.01 **Acute slipped upper femoral epiphysis (nontraumatic)**
M93.011 **Acute slipped upper femoral epiphysis (nontraumatic), right hip**
M93.012 **Acute slipped upper femoral epiphysis (nontraumatic), left hip**
M93.013 **Acute slipped upper femoral epiphysis (nontraumatic), unspecified hip**

[6th] M93.02 **Chronic slipped upper femoral epiphysis (nontraumatic)**
M93.021 **Chronic slipped upper femoral epiphysis (nontraumatic), right hip**
M93.022 **Chronic slipped upper femoral epiphysis (nontraumatic), left hip**
M93.023 **Chronic slipped upper femoral epiphysis (nontraumatic), unspecified hip**

[6th] M93.03 **Acute on chronic slipped upper femoral epiphysis (nontraumatic)**
M93.031 **Acute on chronic slipped upper femoral epiphysis (nontraumatic), right hip**
M93.032 **Acute on chronic slipped upper femoral epiphysis (nontraumatic), left hip**
M93.033 **Acute on chronic slipped upper femoral epiphysis (nontraumatic), unspecified hip**

M93.1 **Kienböck's disease of adults** [A]
Adult osteochondrosis of carpal lunates

[5th] M93.2 **Osteochondritis dissecans**
M93.20 **Osteochondritis dissecans of unspecified site**

[6th] M93.21 **Osteochondritis dissecans of shoulder**
M93.211 **Osteochondritis dissecans, right shoulder**
M93.212 **Osteochondritis dissecans, left shoulder**
M93.219 **Osteochondritis dissecans, unspecified shoulder**

[6th] M93.22 **Osteochondritis dissecans of elbow**
M93.221 **Osteochondritis dissecans, right elbow**
M93.222 **Osteochondritis dissecans, left elbow**
M93.229 **Osteochondritis dissecans, unspecified elbow**

[6th] M93.23 **Osteochondritis dissecans of wrist**
M93.231 **Osteochondritis dissecans, right wrist**
M93.232 **Osteochondritis dissecans, left wrist**
M93.239 **Osteochondritis dissecans, unspecified wrist**

[6th] M93.24 **Osteochondritis dissecans of joints of hand**
M93.241 **Osteochondritis dissecans, joints of right hand**
M93.242 **Osteochondritis dissecans, joints of left hand**
M93.249 **Osteochondritis dissecans, joints of unspecified hand**

[6th] M93.25 **Osteochondritis dissecans of hip**
M93.251 **Osteochondritis dissecans, right hip**
M93.252 **Osteochondritis dissecans, left hip**
M93.259 **Osteochondritis dissecans, unspecified hip**

[6th] M93.26 **Osteochondritis dissecans knee**
M93.261 **Osteochondritis dissecans, right knee**
M93.262 **Osteochondritis dissecans, left knee**
M93.269 **Osteochondritis dissecans, unspecified knee**

[6th] M93.27 **Osteochondritis dissecans of ankle and joints of foot**
M93.271 **Osteochondritis dissecans, right ankle and joints of right foot**
M93.272 **Osteochondritis dissecans, left ankle and joints of left foot**
M93.279 **Osteochondritis dissecans, unspecified ankle and joints of foot**

M93.28 **Osteochondritis dissecans other site**
M93.29 **Osteochondritis dissecans multiple sites**

[5th] M93.8 **Other specified osteochondropathies**
M93.80 **Other specified osteochondropathies of unspecified site**

[6th] M93.81 **Other specified osteochondropathies of shoulder**
M93.811 **Other specified osteochondropathies, right shoulder**
M93.812 **Other specified osteochondropathies, left shoulder**
M93.819 **Other specified osteochondropathies, unspecified shoulder**

[6th] M93.82 **Other specified osteochondropathies of upper arm**
M93.821 **Other specified osteochondropathies, right upper arm**
M93.822 **Other specified osteochondropathies, left upper arm**
M93.829 **Other specified osteochondropathies, unspecified upper arm**

[6th] M93.83 **Other specified osteochondropathies of forearm**
M93.831 **Other specified osteochondropathies, right forearm**
M93.832 **Other specified osteochondropathies, left forearm**
M93.839 **Other specified osteochondropathies, unspecified forearm**

Unspecified Code | Other Specified Code | Manifestation Code | [N] Newborn | [P] Pediatric | [M] Maternity | [A] Adult | ♂ Male | ♀ Female
● New Code | ▲ Revised Code Title | ►◄ Revised Text | [NOTES] | [INCLUDES] | [EXCLUDES1] Not coded here | [EXCLUDES2] Not included here
[4th] 4th character required | [5th] 5th character required | [6th] 6th character required | [7th] 7th character required | [X] Extension 'X' Alert
[HAC] Hospital-acquired condition (HAC) alert | AHA AHA Coding Clinic© | ☞ Code first alert

When symbols appear on a code that requires a 7th character extension, refer to Appendix B to identify applicable 7th character codes.

6️⃣ **M93.84** Other specified osteochondropathies of hand

    M93.841 **Other specified osteochondropathies, right hand**

    M93.842 **Other specified osteochondropathies, left hand**

    M93.849 **Other specified osteochondropathies, unspecified hand**

6️⃣ **M93.85** Other specified osteochondropathies of thigh

    M93.851 **Other specified osteochondropathies, right thigh**

    M93.852 **Other specified osteochondropathies, left thigh**

    M93.859 **Other specified osteochondropathies, unspecified thigh**

6️⃣ **M93.86** Other specified osteochondropathies lower leg

    M93.861 **Other specified osteochondropathies, right lower leg**

    M93.862 **Other specified osteochondropathies, left lower leg**

    M93.869 **Other specified osteochondropathies, unspecified lower leg**

6️⃣ **M93.87** Other specified osteochondropathies of ankle and foot

    M93.871 **Other specified osteochondropathies, right ankle and foot**

    M93.872 **Other specified osteochondropathies, left ankle and foot**

    M93.879 **Other specified osteochondropathies, unspecified ankle and foot**

    M93.88 **Other specified osteochondropathies other**

    M93.89 **Other specified osteochondropathies multiple sites**

5️⃣ **M93.9** Osteochondropathy, unspecified

    Apophysitis NOS
    Epiphysitis NOS
    Osteochondritis NOS
    Osteochondrosis NOS

    M93.90 **Osteochondropathy, unspecified of unspecified site**

6️⃣ **M93.91** Osteochondropathy, unspecified of shoulder

    M93.911 **Osteochondropathy, unspecified, right shoulder**

    M93.912 **Osteochondropathy, unspecified, left shoulder**

    M93.919 **Osteochondropathy, unspecified, unspecified shoulder**

6️⃣ **M93.92** Osteochondropathy, unspecified of upper arm

    M93.921 **Osteochondropathy, unspecified, right upper arm**

    M93.922 **Osteochondropathy, unspecified, left upper arm**

    M93.929 **Osteochondropathy, unspecified, unspecified upper arm**

6️⃣ **M93.93** Osteochondropathy, unspecified of forearm

    M93.931 **Osteochondropathy, unspecified, right forearm**

    M93.932 **Osteochondropathy, unspecified, left forearm**

    M93.939 **Osteochondropathy, unspecified, unspecified forearm**

6️⃣ **M93.94** Osteochondropathy, unspecified of hand

    M93.941 **Osteochondropathy, unspecified, right hand**

    M93.942 **Osteochondropathy, unspecified, left hand**

    M93.949 **Osteochondropathy, unspecified, unspecified hand**

6️⃣ **M93.95** Osteochondropathy, unspecified of thigh

    M93.951 **Osteochondropathy, unspecified, right thigh**

    M93.952 **Osteochondropathy, unspecified, left thigh**

    M93.959 **Osteochondropathy, unspecified, unspecified thigh**

6️⃣ **M93.96** Osteochondropathy, unspecified lower leg

    M93.961 **Osteochondropathy, unspecified, right lower leg**

    M93.962 **Osteochondropathy, unspecified, left lower leg**

    M93.969 **Osteochondropathy, unspecified, unspecified lower leg**

6️⃣ **M93.97** Osteochondropathy, unspecified of ankle and foot

    M93.971 **Osteochondropathy, unspecified, right ankle and foot**

    M93.972 **Osteochondropathy, unspecified, left ankle and foot**

    M93.979 **Osteochondropathy, unspecified, unspecified ankle and foot**

    M93.98 **Osteochondropathy, unspecified other**

    M93.99 **Osteochondropathy, unspecified multiple sites**

4️⃣ **M94** Other disorders of cartilage

    M94.0 **Chondrocostal junction syndrome [Tietze]**

    Costochondritis

    M94.1 **Relapsing polychondritis**

5️⃣ **M94.2** Chondromalacia

    EXCLUDES1 chondromalacia patellae (M22.4)

    M94.20 **Chondromalacia, unspecified site**

6️⃣ **M94.21** Chondromalacia, shoulder

    M94.211 **Chondromalacia, right shoulder**

    M94.212 **Chondromalacia, left shoulder**

    M94.219 **Chondromalacia, unspecified shoulder**

6️⃣ **M94.22** Chondromalacia, elbow

    M94.221 **Chondromalacia, right elbow**

    M94.222 **Chondromalacia, left elbow**

    M94.229 **Chondromalacia, unspecified elbow**

6️⃣ **M94.23** Chondromalacia, wrist

    M94.231 **Chondromalacia, right wrist**

    M94.232 **Chondromalacia, left wrist**

    M94.239 **Chondromalacia, unspecified wrist**

6️⃣ **M94.24** Chondromalacia, joints of hand

    M94.241 **Chondromalacia, joints of right hand**

    M94.242 **Chondromalacia, joints of left hand**

    M94.249 **Chondromalacia, joints of unspecified hand**

6️⃣ **M94.25** Chondromalacia, hip

    M94.251 **Chondromalacia, right hip**

    M94.252 **Chondromalacia, left hip**

    M94.259 **Chondromalacia, unspecified hip**

6️⃣ **M94.26** Chondromalacia, knee

    TIP: Commonly known as runner's knee.

    M94.261 **Chondromalacia, right knee**

    M94.262 **Chondromalacia, left knee**

    M94.269 **Chondromalacia, unspecified knee**

6️⃣ **M94.27** Chondromalacia, ankle and joints of foot

    M94.271 **Chondromalacia, right ankle and joints of right foot**

    M94.272 **Chondromalacia, left ankle and joints of left foot**

    M94.279 **Chondromalacia, unspecified ankle and joints of foot**

    M94.28 **Chondromalacia, other site**

    M94.29 **Chondromalacia, multiple sites**

5️⃣ **M94.3** Chondrolysis

    DEFINITION: Chondrolysis is an abrupt loss of cartilage in a joint due to a severe type of arthritis.

    ☞ Code first any associated slipped upper femoral epiphysis (nontraumatic) (M93.0-)

6️⃣ **M94.35** Chondrolysis, hip

    M94.351 **Chondrolysis, right hip**

    M94.352 **Chondrolysis, left hip**

    M94.359 **Chondrolysis, unspecified hip**

ᴾᴰˣ Unacceptable principal diagnosis symbol per Medicare code edits ᴾᴼᴬ Code exempt from diagnosis present on admission requirement
❓ Questionable admission © Complication or comorbidity ᴹᶜᶜ Major complication or comorbidity ᶜᶜ/ᴹᶜᶜ ᴱˣᶜ CC/MCC exclusion
ᴴᶜᶜ HCC diagnosis code ᴿˣᴴᶜᶜ RxHCC diagnosis code MACRA code **DEFINITION** Describes condition/terminology
TIP Coding guidance 👁 Official Guideline Reference ᶻ¹ Z code as first-listed diagnosis

856   When symbols appear on a code that requires a 7th character extension, refer to Appendix B to identify applicable 7th character codes.   **2020 ICD-10-CM**

M94.8 Other specified disorders of cartilage
    M94.8X Other specified disorders of cartilage
        M94.8X0 Other specified disorders of cartilage, multiple sites
        M94.8X1 Other specified disorders of cartilage, shoulder
        M94.8X2 Other specified disorders of cartilage, upper arm
        M94.8X3 Other specified disorders of cartilage, forearm
        M94.8X4 Other specified disorders of cartilage, hand
        M94.8X5 Other specified disorders of cartilage, thigh
        M94.8X6 Other specified disorders of cartilage, lower leg
        M94.8X7 Other specified disorders of cartilage, ankle and foot
        M94.8X8 Other specified disorders of cartilage, other site
        M94.8X9 Other specified disorders of cartilage, unspecified sites
M94.9 Disorder of cartilage, unspecified

Other disorders of the musculoskeletal system and connective tissue (M95)

M95 Other acquired deformities of musculoskeletal system and connective tissue
    EXCLUDES2 *acquired absence of limbs and organs (Z89-Z90)*
        acquired deformities of limbs (M20-M21)
        congenital malformations and deformations of the musculoskeletal system (Q65-Q79)
        deforming dorsopathies (M40-M43)
        dentofacial anomalies [including malocclusion] (M26.-)
        postprocedural musculoskeletal disorders (M96.-)
    M95.0 Acquired deformity of nose
        EXCLUDES2 *deviated nasal septum (J34.2)*
    M95.1 Cauliflower ear
        EXCLUDES2 *other acquired deformities of ear (H61.1)*
        M95.10 Cauliflower ear, unspecified ear
        M95.11 Cauliflower ear, right ear
        M95.12 Cauliflower ear, left ear
    M95.2 Other acquired deformity of head
    M95.3 Acquired deformity of neck
    M95.4 Acquired deformity of chest and rib
    M95.5 Acquired deformity of pelvis
        EXCLUDES1 *maternal care for known or suspected disproportion (O33.-)*
    M95.8 Other specified acquired deformities of musculoskeletal system
    M95.9 Acquired deformity of musculoskeletal system, unspecified

Intraoperative and postprocedural complications and disorders of musculoskeletal system, not elsewhere classified (M96)

M96 Intraoperative and postprocedural complications and disorders of musculoskeletal system, not elsewhere classified
    EXCLUDES2 *arthropathy following intestinal bypass (M02.0-)*
        complications of internal orthopedic prosthetic devices, implants and grafts (T84.-)
        disorders associated with osteoporosis (M80)
        periprosthetic fracture around internal prosthetic joint (M97.-)
        presence of functional implants and other devices (Z96-Z97)

M96.0 Pseudarthrosis after fusion or arthrodesis
M96.1 Postlaminectomy syndrome, not elsewhere classified
M96.2 Postradiation kyphosis
M96.3 Postlaminectomy kyphosis
M96.4 Postsurgical lordosis
M96.5 Postradiation scoliosis
M96.6 Fracture of bone following insertion of orthopedic implant, joint prosthesis, or bone plate
    TIP: This category of code is used when a fracture occurs at the time of surgery - not to be confused with Category T84 which is used for a mechanical complication of a prosthesis.
    Intraoperative fracture of bone during insertion of orthopedic implant, joint prosthesis, or bone plate
    EXCLUDES2 *complication of internal orthopedic devices, implants or grafts (T84.-)*
    M96.62 Fracture of humerus following insertion of orthopedic implant, joint prosthesis, or bone plate
        M96.621 Fracture of humerus following insertion of orthopedic implant, joint prosthesis, or bone plate, right arm
        M96.622 Fracture of humerus following insertion of orthopedic implant, joint prosthesis, or bone plate, left arm
        M96.629 Fracture of humerus following insertion of orthopedic implant, joint prosthesis, or bone plate, unspecified arm
    M96.63 Fracture of radius or ulna following insertion of orthopedic implant, joint prosthesis, or bone plate
        M96.631 Fracture of radius or ulna following insertion of orthopedic implant, joint prosthesis, or bone plate, right arm
        M96.632 Fracture of radius or ulna following insertion of orthopedic implant, joint prosthesis, or bone plate, left arm
        M96.639 Fracture of radius or ulna following insertion of orthopedic implant, joint prosthesis, or bone plate, unspecified arm
    M96.65 Fracture of pelvis following insertion of orthopedic implant, joint prosthesis, or bone plate
    M96.66 Fracture of femur following insertion of orthopedic implant, joint prosthesis, or bone plate
        M96.661 Fracture of femur following insertion of orthopedic implant, joint prosthesis, or bone plate, right leg
        M96.662 Fracture of femur following insertion of orthopedic implant, joint prosthesis, or bone plate, left leg
        M96.669 Fracture of femur following insertion of orthopedic implant, joint prosthesis, or bone plate, unspecified leg
    M96.67 Fracture of tibia or fibula following insertion of orthopedic implant, joint prosthesis, or bone plate
        M96.671 Fracture of tibia or fibula following insertion of orthopedic implant, joint prosthesis, or bone plate, right leg
        M96.672 Fracture of tibia or fibula following insertion of orthopedic implant, joint prosthesis, or bone plate, left leg
        M96.679 Fracture of tibia or fibula following insertion of orthopedic implant, joint prosthesis, or bone plate, unspecified leg
    M96.69 Fracture of other bone following insertion of orthopedic implant, joint prosthesis, or bone plate

---

5ᵗʰ **M96.8** Other intraoperative and postprocedural complications and disorders of musculoskeletal system, not elsewhere classified

  6ᵗʰ **M96.81** Intraoperative hemorrhage and hematoma of a musculoskeletal structure complicating a procedure

    EXCLUDES1 intraoperative hemorrhage and hematoma of a musculoskeletal structure due to accidental puncture and laceration during a procedure (M96.82-)

    M96.810 Intraoperative hemorrhage and hematoma of a musculoskeletal structure complicating a musculoskeletal system procedure `CC` `CC/MCC Exc`

    M96.811 Intraoperative hemorrhage and hematoma of a musculoskeletal structure complicating other procedure `CC` `CC/MCC Exc`

  6ᵗʰ **M96.82** Accidental puncture and laceration of a musculoskeletal structure during a procedure

    M96.820 Accidental puncture and laceration of a musculoskeletal structure during a musculoskeletal system procedure `CC` `CC/MCC Exc`

    M96.821 Accidental puncture and laceration of a musculoskeletal structure during other procedure `CC` `CC/MCC Exc`

  6ᵗʰ **M96.83** Postprocedural hemorrhage of a musculoskeletal structure following a procedure

    M96.830 Postprocedural hemorrhage of a musculoskeletal structure following a musculoskeletal system procedure `CC` `CC/MCC Exc`

    M96.831 Postprocedural hemorrhage of a musculoskeletal structure following other procedure `CC` `CC/MCC Exc`

  6ᵗʰ **M96.84** Postprocedural hematoma and seroma of a musculoskeletal structure following a procedure

    M96.840 Postprocedural hematoma of a musculoskeletal structure following a musculoskeletal system procedure `CC` `CC/MCC Exc`

    M96.841 Postprocedural hematoma of a musculoskeletal structure following other procedure `CC` `CC/MCC Exc`

    AHA: Q4 2016

    M96.842 Postprocedural seroma of a musculoskeletal structure following a musculoskeletal system procedure `CC` `CC/MCC Exc`

    M96.843 Postprocedural seroma of a musculoskeletal structure following other procedure `CC` `CC/MCC Exc`

    AHA: Q3 2018

  M96.89 Other intraoperative and postprocedural complications and disorders of the musculoskeletal system `CC` `CC/MCC Exc`

    Instability of joint secondary to removal of joint prosthesis

    Use additional code, if applicable, to further specify disorder

Periprosthetic fracture around internal prosthetic joint (M97)

4ᵗʰ **M97** Periprosthetic fracture around internal prosthetic joint

  EXCLUDES2 fracture of bone following insertion of orthopedic implant, joint prosthesis or bone plate (M96.6-)

    breakage (fracture) of prosthetic joint (T84.01-)

The appropriate 7th character is to be added to each code from category M97

  A = initial encounter

  D = subsequent encounter

  S = sequela

5ᵗʰ **M97.0** Periprosthetic fracture around internal prosthetic hip joint

  7ᵗʰ **M97.01** Periprosthetic fracture around internal prosthetic right hip joint `CC` `POA` `HCC` `CC/MCC Exc`

    AHA: Q4 2016

  7ᵗʰ **M97.02** Periprosthetic fracture around internal prosthetic left hip joint `CC` `POA` `HCC` `CC/MCC Exc`

5ᵗʰ **M97.1** Periprosthetic fracture around internal prosthetic knee joint

  7ᵗʰ **M97.11** Periprosthetic fracture around internal prosthetic right knee joint `CC` `POA` `CC/MCC Exc`

  7ᵗʰ **M97.12** Periprosthetic fracture around internal prosthetic left knee joint `CC` `POA` `CC/MCC Exc`

5ᵗʰ **M97.2** Periprosthetic fracture around internal prosthetic ankle joint

  7ᵗʰ **M97.21** Periprosthetic fracture around internal prosthetic right ankle joint `CC` `POA` `CC/MCC Exc`

  7ᵗʰ **M97.22** Periprosthetic fracture around internal prosthetic left ankle joint `CC` `POA` `CC/MCC Exc`

5ᵗʰ **M97.3** Periprosthetic fracture around internal prosthetic shoulder joint

  7ᵗʰ **M97.31** Periprosthetic fracture around internal prosthetic right shoulder joint `CC` `POA` `CC/MCC Exc`

  7ᵗʰ **M97.32** Periprosthetic fracture around internal prosthetic left shoulder joint `CC` `POA` `CC/MCC Exc`

5ᵗʰ **M97.4** Periprosthetic fracture around internal prosthetic elbow joint

  7ᵗʰ **M97.41** Periprosthetic fracture around internal prosthetic right elbow joint `CC` `POA` `CC/MCC Exc`

  7ᵗʰ **M97.42** Periprosthetic fracture around internal prosthetic left elbow joint `CC` `POA` `CC/MCC Exc`

7ᵗʰ **M97.8** Periprosthetic fracture around other internal prosthetic joint `CC` `POA` `CC/MCC Exc`

  AHA: Q4 2016

  Periprosthetic fracture around internal prosthetic finger joint

  Periprosthetic fracture around internal prosthetic spinal joint

  Periprosthetic fracture around internal prosthetic toe joint

  Periprosthetic fracture around internal prosthetic wrist joint

  Use additional code to identify the joint (Z96.6-)

7ᵗʰ **M97.9** Periprosthetic fracture around unspecified internal prosthetic joint `CC` `POA` `CC/MCC Exc`

Biomechanical lesions, not elsewhere classified (M99)

4ᵗʰ **M99** Biomechanical lesions, not elsewhere classified

  DEFINITION: Biomechanical lesion is a pathologic condition involving loss of tissue or lessor joint function.

  NOTES This category should not be used if the condition can be classified elsewhere.

5ᵗʰ **M99.0** Segmental and somatic dysfunction

  M99.00 Segmental and somatic dysfunction of head region

  M99.01 Segmental and somatic dysfunction of cervical region

  M99.02 Segmental and somatic dysfunction of thoracic region

  M99.03 Segmental and somatic dysfunction of lumbar region

  M99.04 Segmental and somatic dysfunction of sacral region

  M99.05 Segmental and somatic dysfunction of pelvic region

  M99.06 Segmental and somatic dysfunction of lower extremity

  M99.07 Segmental and somatic dysfunction of upper extremity

  M99.08 Segmental and somatic dysfunction of rib cage

  M99.09 Segmental and somatic dysfunction of abdomen and other regions

5ᵗʰ **M99.1** Subluxation complex (vertebral)

  M99.10 Subluxation complex (vertebral) of head region `CC` `HAC` `CC/MCC Exc`

  M99.11 Subluxation complex (vertebral) of cervical region `CC` `HAC` `CC/MCC Exc`

  M99.12 Subluxation complex (vertebral) of thoracic region

  M99.13 Subluxation complex (vertebral) of lumbar region

  M99.14 Subluxation complex (vertebral) of sacral region

  M99.15 Subluxation complex (vertebral) of pelvic region

`PDxN` Unacceptable principal diagnosis symbol per Medicare code edits   `POA` Code exempt from diagnosis present on admission requirement

`?` Questionable admission   `CC` Complication or comorbidity   `MCC` Major complication or comorbidity   `CC/MCC Exc` CC/MCC exclusion

`HCC` HCC diagnosis code   `RxHCC` RxHCC diagnosis code   MACRA code   **DEFINITION** Describes condition/terminology

TIP Coding guidance   👁 Official Guideline Reference   `Z1` Z code as first-listed diagnosis

858   When symbols appear on a code that requires a 7th character extension, refer to Appendix B to identify applicable 7th character codes.   **2020 ICD-10-CM**

M99.16 Subluxation complex (vertebral) of lower extremity
M99.17 Subluxation complex (vertebral) of upper extremity
M99.18 Subluxation complex (vertebral) of rib cage [CC] [HAC] CC/MCC Exc
M99.19 Subluxation complex (vertebral) of abdomen and other regions

[5th] M99.2 Subluxation stenosis of neural canal
M99.20 Subluxation stenosis of neural canal of head region
M99.21 Subluxation stenosis of neural canal of cervical region
M99.22 Subluxation stenosis of neural canal of thoracic region
M99.23 Subluxation stenosis of neural canal of lumbar region
M99.24 Subluxation stenosis of neural canal of sacral region
M99.25 Subluxation stenosis of neural canal of pelvic region
M99.26 Subluxation stenosis of neural canal of lower extremity
M99.27 Subluxation stenosis of neural canal of upper extremity
M99.28 Subluxation stenosis of neural canal of rib cage
M99.29 Subluxation stenosis of neural canal of abdomen and other regions

[5th] M99.3 Osseous stenosis of neural canal
M99.30 Osseous stenosis of neural canal of head region
M99.31 Osseous stenosis of neural canal of cervical region
M99.32 Osseous stenosis of neural canal of thoracic region
M99.33 Osseous stenosis of neural canal of lumbar region
M99.34 Osseous stenosis of neural canal of sacral region
M99.35 Osseous stenosis of neural canal of pelvic region
M99.36 Osseous stenosis of neural canal of lower extremity
M99.37 Osseous stenosis of neural canal of upper extremity
M99.38 Osseous stenosis of neural canal of rib cage
M99.39 Osseous stenosis of neural canal of abdomen and other regions

[5th] M99.4 Connective tissue stenosis of neural canal
M99.40 Connective tissue stenosis of neural canal of head region
M99.41 Connective tissue stenosis of neural canal of cervical region
M99.42 Connective tissue stenosis of neural canal of thoracic region
M99.43 Connective tissue stenosis of neural canal of lumbar region
M99.44 Connective tissue stenosis of neural canal of sacral region
M99.45 Connective tissue stenosis of neural canal of pelvic region
M99.46 Connective tissue stenosis of neural canal of lower extremity
M99.47 Connective tissue stenosis of neural canal of upper extremity
M99.48 Connective tissue stenosis of neural canal of rib cage
M99.49 Connective tissue stenosis of neural canal of abdomen and other regions

[5th] M99.5 Intervertebral disc stenosis of neural canal
M99.50 Intervertebral disc stenosis of neural canal of head region
M99.51 Intervertebral disc stenosis of neural canal of cervical region
M99.52 Intervertebral disc stenosis of neural canal of thoracic region
M99.53 Intervertebral disc stenosis of neural canal of lumbar region
M99.54 Intervertebral disc stenosis of neural canal of sacral region
M99.55 Intervertebral disc stenosis of neural canal of pelvic region
M99.56 Intervertebral disc stenosis of neural canal of lower extremity
M99.57 Intervertebral disc stenosis of neural canal of upper extremity
M99.58 Intervertebral disc stenosis of neural canal of rib cage
M99.59 Intervertebral disc stenosis of neural canal of abdomen and other regions

[5th] M99.6 Osseous and subluxation stenosis of intervertebral foramina
M99.60 Osseous and subluxation stenosis of intervertebral foramina of head region
M99.61 Osseous and subluxation stenosis of intervertebral foramina of cervical region
M99.62 Osseous and subluxation stenosis of intervertebral foramina of thoracic region
M99.63 Osseous and subluxation stenosis of intervertebral foramina of lumbar region
M99.64 Osseous and subluxation stenosis of intervertebral foramina of sacral region
M99.65 Osseous and subluxation stenosis of intervertebral foramina of pelvic region
M99.66 Osseous and subluxation stenosis of intervertebral foramina of lower extremity
M99.67 Osseous and subluxation stenosis of intervertebral foramina of upper extremity
M99.68 Osseous and subluxation stenosis of intervertebral foramina of rib cage
M99.69 Osseous and subluxation stenosis of intervertebral foramina of abdomen and other regions

[5th] M99.7 Connective tissue and disc stenosis of intervertebral foramina
M99.70 Connective tissue and disc stenosis of intervertebral foramina of head region
M99.71 Connective tissue and disc stenosis of intervertebral foramina of cervical region
M99.72 Connective tissue and disc stenosis of intervertebral foramina of thoracic region
M99.73 Connective tissue and disc stenosis of intervertebral foramina of lumbar region
M99.74 Connective tissue and disc stenosis of intervertebral foramina of sacral region
M99.75 Connective tissue and disc stenosis of intervertebral foramina of pelvic region
M99.76 Connective tissue and disc stenosis of intervertebral foramina of lower extremity
M99.77 Connective tissue and disc stenosis of intervertebral foramina of upper extremity
M99.78 Connective tissue and disc stenosis of intervertebral foramina of rib cage
M99.79 Connective tissue and disc stenosis of intervertebral foramina of abdomen and other regions

[5th] M99.8 Other biomechanical lesions
M99.80 Other biomechanical lesions of head region
M99.81 Other biomechanical lesions of cervical region
M99.82 Other biomechanical lesions of thoracic region
M99.83 Other biomechanical lesions of lumbar region
M99.84 Other biomechanical lesions of sacral region
M99.85 Other biomechanical lesions of pelvic region
M99.86 Other biomechanical lesions of lower extremity
M99.87 Other biomechanical lesions of upper extremity
M99.88 Other biomechanical lesions of rib cage
M99.89 Other biomechanical lesions of abdomen and other regions

M99.9 Biomechanical lesion, unspecified

NOTES

Anatomy of the Male Reproductive System

Introduction

The male reproductive system includes the external genitalia, and accessory ducts and glands, that function to procreate offspring.

1. **The male reproductive system (Figure 14.a) includes the following:**
    a) The primary sex organs (or the Testes/Male Gonads) that produce sperms and the male sex hormones.
    b) The accessory organs (or the scrotum and ducts) that support the testes and transport the sperm.
    c) The accessory glands that produce secretions for constituting the semen.
    d) The penis, which acts as a transporting and supporting structure of the male reproductive system

2. **The anatomy of structures/components of the male reproductive system is further described below:**
    a) **Scrotum**
        i)   It is an extension from the abdominal wall that supports the testes.
        ii) It is divided into two lateral pouches via a septum, and each pouch contains a single testis.
        iii) The scrotal sac serves to provide protection to the sperms from the changes in the external environment.
    b) **The Testes**
        i)   The testes are covered by a capsule of connective tissue, which is known as the tunica albuginea.
        ii) The tunica albuginea travels inwards to constitute a series of compartments, which are known as lobules.
        iii) A single lobule carries convoluted seminiferous tubules for spermatogenesis.
        iv) Male sex hormone (testosterone) is produced by the interstitial cells of Leydig that remain located in the individual lobules.
    c) **The Spermatozoa (or Mature Sperm Cell)**
        i)   A typical sperm cell is composed of a head, a middle piece, and a tail (or flagellum).
        ii) Spermatozoa can survive up to a period of 48 hours in the female reproductive tract. Approximately three hundred million spermatozoa are produced on a daily basis in a male.
    d) **The Ducts of the Male Reproductive System**
        i)   Convoluted seminiferous tubules of the testis contain the mature sperm cells.
        ii) A tightly coiled structure (or epididymis) is positioned on the posterior border of the testis.
        iii) The straightened epididymis is known as the ductus deferens (or vas deferens).
        iv) The spermatic cord is a sheath that contains the vas deferens and empties into the ejaculatory duct.
        v)   The urethra is regarded as the terminal duct of the male reproductive system. The ejaculatory duct ejects the spermatozoa

into the urethra. Moreover, the urethra provides a common passage for both sperm and urine.
        vi) The urethra traverses through the prostate gland, urogenital diaphragm, and penis.
    e) **The Accessory Glands**
        i)   Paired seminal vesicles generate the alkaline viscous part of the semen and transfer it to the ejaculatory duct.
        ii) The prostate gland produces the semen that provides a medium to the sperm cells for swimming.
        iii) Bulbourethral glands (or Cowper's glands) generate the viscous mucus that acts as a lubricant for sexual intercourse.
    f) **Semen**
        i)   Semen is a milky fluid, which is a mixture of the matured sperm cells and secretions of the accessory glands.
        ii) It provides a transport medium for the sperm.
    g) **The Penis**
        i)   It acts to transport the matured sperms to the female reproductive tract.
        ii) It is composed of a shaft, and the terminal point of the shaft is known as the glans penis (or head). The head of the penis is covered with loose skin, which is called the prepuce or foreskin.

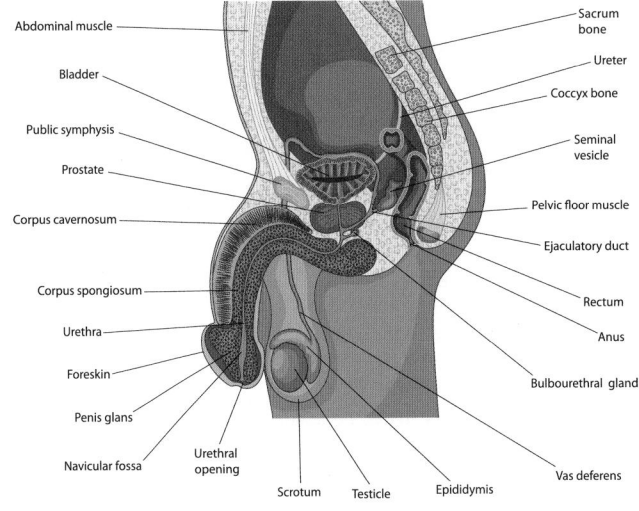

Figure 14.a Male Reproductive System Anatomy

Common Pathologies

Benign Prostate Hyperplasia
Benign prostate hyperplasia (BPH) (Figure 14.b) is a noncancerous enlargement of the prostate gland, typically in older males. It compresses the urethra and makes urination difficult. BPH symptoms are also known as lower urinary tract symptoms, or LUTS.

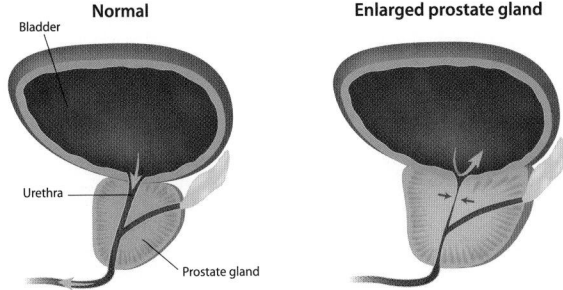

Figure 14.b Benign Prostatic Hyperplasia

Gynecomastia
Gynecomastia refers to enlargement of the male breast, common in adolescents and the elderly, which is due to an imbalance of sex hormones.

Hypospadias
Hypospadias is a medical condition present from birth in some males in which the opening of the urethra is on the underside of the penis instead of at its tip.

Orchitis
Orchitis, an inflammation of the testicles, results from infection with bacteria or the mumps virus. It can affect one or both testes.

Torsion of Testis
Testicular torsion is a painful condition in which the spermatic cord, which supplies blood to a testicle, twists and obstructs blood flow.

Hydrocele
Hydrocele refers to an abnormal accumulation of fluid in a sac-type structure, such as a testicle.

Phimosis
Phimosis is a painful condition in which the foreskin, or prepuce, cannot be retracted from the head, or glans, of the penis due to scarring or stricture.

Balanitis
Balanitis causes redness, swelling, and pain of the foreskin, or prepuce, due to inflammation or bacterial infection.

Anatomy of the Urinary System

Introduction

The urinary system, or urinary tract, is responsible for the regulation and elimination of water and solutes within the body.

1. **An Outline of the Urinary System (Figure 14.c)**
    a) Two Kidneys
    b) Two Ureters
    c) The Urinary Bladder
    d) The Urethra
    e) The urinary system maintains the state of homeostasis by regulating water and solutes in the human body.
    f) Kidneys produce the urine and function as the major filtering organs of the urinary system.
    g) Urine is composed of components like urea, water, ions, and toxic wastes that need to be regulated in the human body by the entire urinary system.

2. **The Functions of Kidneys**
    a) Excretion
    b) Maintenance of blood volume and concentration
    c) pH regulation
    d) Maintenance of blood pressure
    e) Maintenance of erythrocyte concentration
    f) The conversion of vitamin D to its active form (or calciferol).

3. **The Anatomy of Kidneys**
    a) Kidneys are situated between the parietal peritoneum and posterior wall of abdomen.
    b) There is a notch (known as hilum) located in the concave center of each kidney. The ureter exits the kidney, and blood vessels, lymph vessels and nerves enter and leave the kidney through the hilum.
    c) The kidney is surrounded by the following three layers:
        i) The innermost layer of the kidney is known as the renal capsule. It acts as a barrier against trauma and infection.
        ii) Adipose capsule is the middle layer of the kidney. It is made up of fatty tissue and protects the kidney from blows.
        iii) The renal fascia is the outermost layer of the kidney. It serves to attach the kidney to the abdominal wall.
    d) Cortex is the outer region of the kidney.
    e) Medulla is the inner area of the kidney.
    f) Renal pyramids are striated triangular structures that are found within the medulla. The bases of these pyramids face toward the cortex. However, their tips point to the center of the kidney and are known as the renal papillae.
    g) The renal columns constitute the cortical material that extends between the pyramids.
    h) The parenchyma of the kidney is formed by the cortex and renal pyramids.

i) The parenchyma is further composed of the microscopic units or nephrons, which are the structural and functional units of the kidneys.

j) The minor calyx is a funnel-shaped structure that surrounds the tip of each renal pyramid. The function of this minor calyx is to collect the urine from the ducts of the renal pyramids. The minor calyces integrate to constitute the major calyces.

k) The renal pelvis is the large collecting funnel that is formed by a bunch of major calyces. The renal pelvis is further narrowed and extended to constitute the ureter.

4. **The Ureter**
    a) It is the extension of the renal pelvis of the kidney and communicates with the urinary bladder.
    b) They are two in number and carry urine from the renal pelvis to the urinary bladder.
    c) Urine is expelled from the bladder by the act of micturition.

5. **The Urethra**
    a) It is a thin walled tube that connects the floor of the urinary bladder to the genitals for the expulsion of fluids (urine, semen, etc.) out of the body.
    b) It is located in the wall of the vagina and above the vaginal opening in females. The female urethral orifice is the opening of the urethra and situated between the vaginal opening and clitoris.
    c) It lies below the bladder in males and travels through the prostate gland and penis.
    d) The opening at the tip of the male penis is known as the male urethral orifice.
    e) The external urethral sphincter is a striated muscle and provides voluntary control of urination.

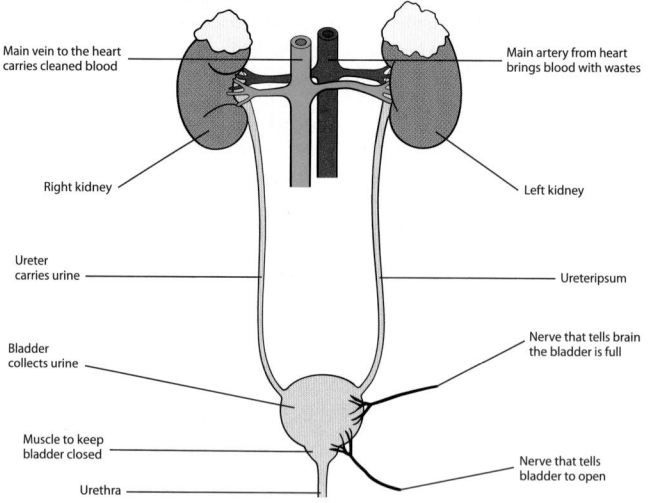

Figure 14.c Urinary System Anatomy

Common Pathologies

Glomerulonephritis

Glomerulonephritis, also known as nephritic syndrome, is a disease of the kidney, characterized by inflammation of the glomeruli, small structures through which the kidney filters urine. Inflammation of the glomeruli prevents the kidneys from being able to filter the urine. Fluid and toxins then build up in the body and can lead to chronic renal failure, also known as chronic kidney failure (CKD).

Acute Renal Failure

Acute renal failure refers to the inability of the kidneys to filter waste products, resulting in the buildup of toxic substances in the blood.

Chronic Kidney Disease

Chronic kidney disease, or CKD, is a condition of gradual loss of kidney function, described in five stages, with stage 1 being the least severe and stage 5 being end stage renal disease, requiring dialysis or kidney transplant for treatment.

Bladder Cancer

Bladder cancer (Figure 14.d) is an abnormal growth of cells in the bladder, typically beginning in the lining of the bladder and then spreading throughout the bladder and to adjacent organs.

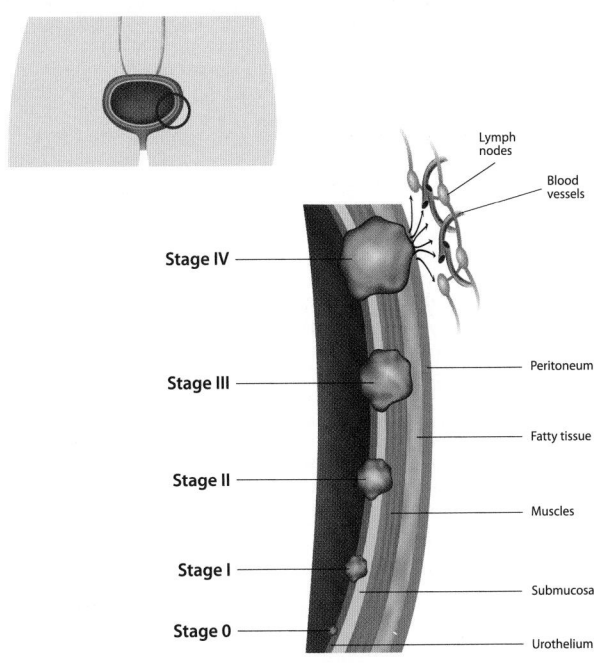

Figure 14.d Bladder Cancer

Interstitial Cystitis

Interstitial cystitis is an inflammatory condition of the bladder that results in ongoing pain and feeling the need to urinate urgently and frequently.

Cystocele

A cystocele (Figure 14.e) is a condition that occurs when the tough fibrous wall between a woman's bladder and her vagina weakens, allowing the bladder to droop into the vagina.

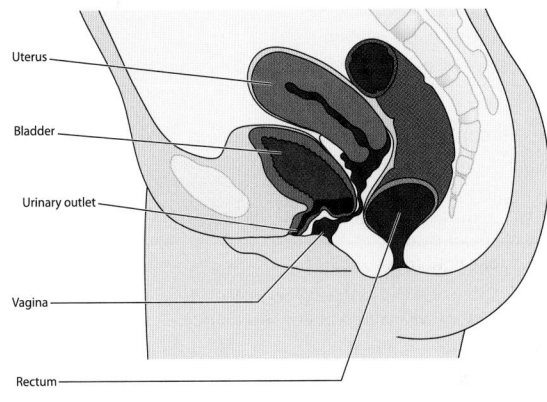

Figure 14.e Cystocele

UTI

A urinary tract infection, or UTI, is a bacterial infection of one or more structures in the urinary tract, typically involving the bladder or urethra.

Kidney Stones

A kidney stone, also known as a calculus, results from a buildup of mineral salts or other such material in the kidney. Kidney stones vary in size. Larger stones can block the flow of urine, resulting in severe pain and blood in the urine.

Diseases of the genitourinary system (N00-N99)

EXCLUDES2   certain conditions originating in the perinatal period (P04-P96)

certain infectious and parasitic diseases (A00-B99)

complications of pregnancy, childbirth and the puerperium (O00-O9A)

congenital malformations, deformations and chromosomal abnormalities (Q00-Q99)

endocrine, nutritional and metabolic diseases (E00-E88)

injury, poisoning and certain other consequences of external causes (S00-T88)

neoplasms (C00-D49)

symptoms, signs and abnormal clinical and laboratory findings, not elsewhere classified (R00-R94)

This chapter contains the following blocks:

N00-N08   Glomerular diseases
N10-N16   Renal tubulo-interstitial diseases
N17-N19   Acute kidney failure and chronic kidney disease
N20-N23   Urolithiasis
N25-N29   Other disorders of kidney and ureter
N30-N39   Other diseases of the urinary system
N40-N53   Diseases of male genital organs
N60-N65   Disorders of breast
N70-N77   Inflammatory diseases of female pelvic organs
N80-N98   Noninflammatory disorders of female genital tract
N99   Intraoperative and postprocedural complications and disorders of genitourinary system, not elsewhere classified

Glomerular diseases (N00-N08)

Code also any associated kidney failure (N17-N19).

EXCLUDES1   hypertensive chronic kidney disease (I12.-)

N00   Acute nephritic syndrome

INCLUDES   acute glomerular disease

acute glomerulonephritis

acute nephritis

EXCLUDES1   acute tubulo-interstitial nephritis (N10)

nephritic syndrome NOS (N05.-)

N00.0   **Acute nephritic syndrome** with minor glomerular abnormality   MCC CC/MCC Exc

Acute nephritic syndrome with minimal change lesion

N00.1   **Acute nephritic syndrome** with focal and segmental glomerular lesions   MCC CC/MCC Exc

Acute nephritic syndrome with focal and segmental hyalinosis
Acute nephritic syndrome with focal and segmental sclerosis
Acute nephritic syndrome with focal glomerulonephritis

N00.2   **Acute nephritic syndrome** with diffuse membranous glomerulonephritis   MCC CC/MCC Exc

N00.3   **Acute nephritic syndrome** with diffuse mesangial proliferative glomerulonephritis   MCC CC/MCC Exc

N00.4   **Acute nephritic syndrome** with diffuse endocapillary proliferative glomerulonephritis   MCC CC/MCC Exc

N00.5   **Acute nephritic syndrome** with diffuse mesangiocapillary glomerulonephritis   MCC CC/MCC Exc

Acute nephritic syndrome with membranoproliferative glomerulonephritis, types 1 and 3, or NOS

N00.6   **Acute nephritic syndrome** with dense deposit disease   MCC CC/MCC Exc

Acute nephritic syndrome with membranoproliferative glomerulonephritis, type 2

N00.7   **Acute nephritic syndrome** with diffuse crescentic glomerulonephritis   MCC CC/MCC Exc

Acute nephritic syndrome with extracapillary glomerulonephritis

N00.8   **Acute nephritic syndrome** with other morphologic changes   MCC CC/MCC Exc

Acute nephritic syndrome with proliferative glomerulonephritis NOS

N00.9   **Acute nephritic syndrome with unspecified morphologic changes**   MCC CC/MCC Exc

N01   Rapidly progressive nephritic syndrome

INCLUDES   rapidly progressive glomerular disease

rapidly progressive glomerulonephritis

rapidly progressive nephritis

EXCLUDES1   nephritic syndrome NOS (N05.-)

N01.0   **Rapidly progressive nephritic syndrome** with minor glomerular abnormality   MCC CC/MCC Exc

Rapidly progressive nephritic syndrome with minimal change lesion

N01.1   **Rapidly progressive nephritic syndrome** with focal and segmental glomerular lesions   MCC CC/MCC Exc

Rapidly progressive nephritic syndrome with focal and segmental hyalinosis
Rapidly progressive nephritic syndrome with focal and segmental sclerosis
Rapidly progressive nephritic syndrome with focal glomerulonephritis

N01.2   **Rapidly progressive nephritic syndrome** with diffuse membranous glomerulonephritis   MCC CC/MCC Exc

N01.3   **Rapidly progressive nephritic syndrome** with diffuse mesangial proliferative glomerulonephritis   MCC CC/MCC Exc

N01.4   **Rapidly progressive nephritic syndrome** with diffuse endocapillary proliferative glomerulonephritis   MCC CC/MCC Exc

N01.5   **Rapidly progressive nephritic syndrome** with diffuse mesangiocapillary glomerulonephritis   MCC CC/MCC Exc

Rapidly progressive nephritic syndrome with membranoproliferative glomerulonephritis, types 1 and 3, or NOS

N01.6   **Rapidly progressive nephritic syndrome** with dense deposit disease   MCC CC/MCC Exc

Rapidly progressive nephritic syndrome with membranoproliferative glomerulonephritis, type 2

N01.7   **Rapidly progressive nephritic syndrome** with diffuse crescentic glomerulonephritis   MCC CC/MCC Exc

Rapidly progressive nephritic syndrome with extracapillary glomerulonephritis

N01.8   **Rapidly progressive nephritic syndrome** with other morphologic changes   MCC CC/MCC Exc

Rapidly progressive nephritic syndrome with proliferative glomerulonephritis NOS

N01.9   **Rapidly progressive nephritic syndrome with unspecified morphologic changes**   MCC CC/MCC Exc

N02   Recurrent and persistent hematuria

EXCLUDES1   acute cystitis with hematuria (N30.01)

hematuria NOS (R31.9)

hematuria not associated with specified morphologic lesions (R31.-)

N02.0   **Recurrent and persistent hematuria** with minor glomerular abnormality   CC CC/MCC Exc

Recurrent and persistent hematuria with minimal change lesion

N02.1   **Recurrent and persistent hematuria** with focal and segmental glomerular lesions   CC CC/MCC Exc

Recurrent and persistent hematuria with focal and segmental hyalinosis
Recurrent and persistent hematuria with focal and segmental sclerosis
Recurrent and persistent hematuria with focal glomerulonephritis

N02.2   **Recurrent and persistent hematuria** with diffuse membranous glomerulonephritis   CC CC/MCC Exc

N02.3   **Recurrent and persistent hematuria** with diffuse mesangial proliferative glomerulonephritis   CC CC/MCC Exc

N02.4   **Recurrent and persistent hematuria** with diffuse endocapillary proliferative glomerulonephritis   CC CC/MCC Exc

N02.5   **Recurrent and persistent hematuria** with diffuse mesangiocapillary glomerulonephritis   CC CC/MCC Exc

Recurrent and persistent hematuria with membranoproliferative glomerulonephritis, types 1 and 3, or NOS

PDⁿ   Unacceptable principal diagnosis symbol per Medicare code edits   POA   Code exempt from diagnosis present on admission requirement
❓ Questionable admission   cc Complication or comorbidity   MCC Major complication or comorbidity   CC/MCC Exc CC/MCC exclusion
HCC HCC diagnosis code   RxHCC RxHCC diagnosis code   MACRA code   **DEFINITION** Describes condition/terminology
TIP Coding guidance   👁 Official Guideline Reference   Z Z code as first-listed diagnosis

N02.6 **Recurrent and persistent hematuria** with dense deposit disease `CC` `CC/MCC Exc`

Recurrent and persistent hematuria with membranoproliferative glomerulonephritis, type 2

N02.7 **Recurrent and persistent hematuria** with diffuse crescentic glomerulonephritis `CC` `CC/MCC Exc`

Recurrent and persistent hematuria with extracapillary glomerulonephritis

N02.8 **Recurrent and persistent hematuria** with other morphologic changes `CC` `CC/MCC Exc`

Recurrent and persistent hematuria with proliferative glomerulonephritis NOS

N02.9 **Recurrent and persistent hematuria with unspecified morphologic changes** `CC` `CC/MCC Exc`

AHA: Q2 2017

🔵 N03 Chronic **nephritic syndrome**

INCLUDES   chronic glomerular disease

chronic glomerulonephritis

chronic nephritis

EXCLUDES1   chronic tubulo-interstitial nephritis (N11.-)

diffuse sclerosing glomerulonephritis (N05.8-)

nephritic syndrome NOS (N05.-)

N03.0 **Chronic nephritic syndrome** with minor glomerular abnormality `CC` `CC/MCC Exc`

Chronic nephritic syndrome with minimal change lesion

N03.1 **Chronic nephritic syndrome** with focal and segmental glomerular lesions `CC` `CC/MCC Exc`

Chronic nephritic syndrome with focal and segmental hyalinosis

Chronic nephritic syndrome with focal and segmental sclerosis

Chronic nephritic syndrome with focal glomerulonephritis

N03.2 **Chronic nephritic syndrome** with diffuse membranous glomerulonephritis `CC` `CC/MCC Exc`

N03.3 **Chronic nephritic syndrome** with diffuse mesangial proliferative glomerulonephritis `CC` `CC/MCC Exc`

N03.4 **Chronic nephritic syndrome** with diffuse endocapillary proliferative glomerulonephritis `CC` `CC/MCC Exc`

N03.5 **Chronic nephritic syndrome** with diffuse mesangiocapillary glomerulonephritis `CC` `CC/MCC Exc`

Chronic nephritic syndrome with membranoproliferative glomerulonephritis, types 1 and 3, or NOS

N03.6 **Chronic nephritic syndrome** with dense deposit disease `CC` `CC/MCC Exc`

Chronic nephritic syndrome with membranoproliferative glomerulonephritis, type 2

N03.7 **Chronic nephritic syndrome** with diffuse crescentic glomerulonephritis `CC` `CC/MCC Exc`

Chronic nephritic syndrome with extracapillary glomerulonephritis

N03.8 **Chronic nephritic syndrome** with other morphologic changes `CC` `CC/MCC Exc`

Chronic nephritic syndrome with proliferative glomerulonephritis NOS

N03.9 **Chronic nephritic syndrome with unspecified morphologic changes** `CC` `CC/MCC Exc`

🔵 N04 Nephrotic **syndrome**

INCLUDES   congenital nephrotic syndrome

lipoid nephrosis

N04.0 **Nephrotic syndrome** with minor glomerular abnormality `CC` `CC/MCC Exc`

Nephrotic syndrome with minimal change lesion

N04.1 **Nephrotic syndrome** with focal and segmental glomerular lesions `CC` `CC/MCC Exc`

Nephrotic syndrome with focal and segmental hyalinosis

Nephrotic syndrome with focal and segmental sclerosis

Nephrotic syndrome with focal glomerulonephritis

N04.2 **Nephrotic syndrome** with diffuse membranous glomerulonephritis `CC` `CC/MCC Exc`

N04.3 **Nephrotic syndrome** with diffuse mesangial proliferative glomerulonephritis `CC` `CC/MCC Exc`

N04.4 **Nephrotic syndrome** with diffuse endocapillary proliferative glomerulonephritis

N04.5 **Nephrotic syndrome** with diffuse mesangiocapillary glomerulonephritis `CC` `CC/MCC Exc`

Nephrotic syndrome with membranoproliferative glomerulonephritis, types 1 and 3, or NOS

N04.6 **Nephrotic syndrome** with dense deposit disease `CC` `CC/MCC Exc`

Nephrotic syndrome with membranoproliferative glomerulonephritis, type 2

N04.7 **Nephrotic syndrome** with diffuse crescentic glomerulonephritis `CC` `CC/MCC Exc`

Nephrotic syndrome with extracapillary glomerulonephritis

N04.8 **Nephrotic syndrome with other morphologic changes** `CC` `CC/MCC Exc`

Nephrotic syndrome with proliferative glomerulonephritis NOS

N04.9 **Nephrotic syndrome with unspecified morphologic changes** `CC` `CC/MCC Exc`

🔵 N05 Unspecified nephritic syndrome

INCLUDES   glomerular disease NOS

glomerulonephritis NOS

nephritis NOS

nephropathy NOS and renal disease NOS with morphological lesion specified in .0-.8

EXCLUDES1   nephropathy NOS with no stated morphological lesion (N28.9)

renal disease NOS with no stated morphological lesion (N28.9)

tubulo-interstitial nephritis NOS (N12)

N05.0 **Unspecified nephritic syndrome** with minor glomerular abnormality

Unspecified nephritic syndrome with minimal change lesion

N05.1 **Unspecified nephritic syndrome** with focal and segmental glomerular lesions

Unspecified nephritic syndrome with focal and segmental hyalinosis

Unspecified nephritic syndrome with focal and segmental sclerosis

Unspecified nephritic syndrome with focal glomerulonephritis

N05.2 **Unspecified nephritic syndrome** with diffuse membranous glomerulonephritis `CC` `CC/MCC Exc`

N05.3 **Unspecified nephritic syndrome** with diffuse mesangial proliferative glomerulonephritis `CC` `CC/MCC Exc`

N05.4 **Unspecified nephritic syndrome** with diffuse endocapillary proliferative glomerulonephritis `CC` `CC/MCC Exc`

N05.5 **Unspecified nephritic syndrome** with diffuse mesangiocapillary glomerulonephritis `CC` `CC/MCC Exc`

Unspecified nephritic syndrome with membranoproliferative glomerulonephritis, types 1 and 3, or NOS

N05.6 **Unspecified nephritic syndrome** with dense deposit disease

Unspecified nephritic syndrome with membranoproliferative glomerulonephritis, type 2

N05.7 **Unspecified nephritic syndrome** with diffuse crescentic glomerulonephritis

Unspecified nephritic syndrome with extracapillary glomerulonephritis

N05.8 **Unspecified nephritic syndrome** with other morphologic changes

Unspecified nephritic syndrome with proliferative glomerulonephritis NOS

N05.9 **Unspecified nephritic syndrome** with unspecified morphologic changes

🔵 N06 Isolated proteinuria with specified morphological lesion

EXCLUDES1   Proteinuria not associated with specific morphologic lesions (R80.0)

N06.0 **Isolated proteinuria** with minor glomerular abnormality

Isolated proteinuria with minimal change lesion

N06.1 **Isolated proteinuria** with focal and segmental glomerular lesions

Isolated proteinuria with focal and segmental hyalinosis

Isolated proteinuria with focal and segmental sclerosis

Isolated proteinuria with focal glomerulonephritis

N06.2 **Isolated proteinuria** with diffuse membranous glomerulonephritis `CC` `CC/MCC Exc`

Unspecified Code   Other Specified Code   Manifestation Code   Ⓝ Newborn   Ⓟ Pediatric   Ⓜ Maternity   Ⓐ Adult   ♂ Male   ♀ Female

● New Code   ▲ Revised Code Title   ▶◀ Revised Text   **NOTES**   INCLUDES   EXCLUDES1 Not coded here   EXCLUDES2 Not included here

🔵 4th character required   🔵 5th character required   🔵 6th character required   🔵 7th character required   ⊗ Extension 'X' Alert

HAC Hospital-acquired condition (HAC) alert   **AHA** AHA Coding Clinic©   📧 Code first alert

2020 ICD-10-CM   When symbols appear on a code that requires a 7th character extension, refer to Appendix B to identify applicable 7th character codes.   **865**

N06.3 Isolated **proteinuria** with diffuse mesangial proliferative glomerulonephritis   CC CC/MCC Exc

N06.4 Isolated **proteinuria** with diffuse endocapillary proliferative glomerulonephritis   CC CC/MCC Exc

N06.5 Isolated **proteinuria** with diffuse mesangiocapillary glomerulonephritis   CC CC/MCC Exc

Isolated proteinuria with membranoproliferative glomerulonephritis, types 1 and 3, or NOS

N06.6 Isolated **proteinuria** with dense deposit disease

Isolated proteinuria with membranoproliferative glomerulonephritis, type 2

N06.7 Isolated **proteinuria** with diffuse crescentic glomerulonephritis

Isolated proteinuria with extracapillary glomerulonephritis

N06.8 Isolated **proteinuria** with other morphologic lesion

Isolated proteinuria with proliferative glomerulonephritis NOS

N06.9 Isolated **proteinuria with unspecified morphologic lesion**

4ᵗʰ **N07** **Hereditary nephropathy, not elsewhere classified**

EXCLUDES2 Alport's syndrome (Q87.81-)
hereditary amyloid nephropathy (E85.-)
nail patella syndrome (Q87.2)
non-neuropathic heredofamilial amyloidosis (E85.-)

N07.0 **Hereditary nephropathy, not elsewhere classified** with minor glomerular abnormality

Hereditary nephropathy, not elsewhere classified with minimal change lesion

N07.1 **Hereditary nephropathy, not elsewhere classified** with focal and segmental glomerular lesions

Hereditary nephropathy, not elsewhere classified with focal and segmental hyalinosis

Hereditary nephropathy, not elsewhere classified with focal and segmental sclerosis

Hereditary nephropathy, not elsewhere classified with focal glomerulonephritis

N07.2 **Hereditary nephropathy, not elsewhere classified** with diffuse membranous glomerulonephritis   CC CC/MCC Exc

N07.3 **Hereditary nephropathy, not elsewhere classified** with diffuse mesangial proliferative glomerulonephritis   CC CC/MCC Exc

N07.4 **Hereditary nephropathy, not elsewhere classified** with diffuse endocapillary proliferative glomerulonephritis   CC CC/MCC Exc

N07.5 **Hereditary nephropathy, not elsewhere classified** with diffuse mesangiocapillary glomerulonephritis   CC CC/MCC Exc

Hereditary nephropathy, not elsewhere classified with membranoproliferative glomerulonephritis, types 1 and 3, or NOS

N07.6 **Hereditary nephropathy, not elsewhere classified** with dense deposit disease

Hereditary nephropathy, not elsewhere classified with membranoproliferative glomerulonephritis, type 2

N07.7 **Hereditary nephropathy, not elsewhere classified** with diffuse crescentic glomerulonephritis

Hereditary nephropathy, not elsewhere classified with extracapillary glomerulonephritis

N07.8 **Hereditary nephropathy, not elsewhere classified** with other morphologic lesions

Hereditary nephropathy, not elsewhere classified with proliferative glomerulonephritis NOS

N07.9 **Hereditary nephropathy, not elsewhere classified with unspecified morphologic lesions**

N08 **Glomerular disorders in diseases classified elsewhere**

Glomerulonephritis
Nephritis
Nephropathy

☞ **Code first** underlying disease, such as:
amyloidosis (E85.-)
congenital syphilis (A50.5)
cryoglobulinemia (D89.1)
disseminated intravascular coagulation (D65)
gout (M1A.-, M10.-)
microscopic polyangiitis (M31.7)
multiple myeloma (C90.0-)

sepsis (A40.0-A41.9)
sickle-cell disease (D57.0-D57.8)

EXCLUDES1 glomerulonephritis, nephritis and nephropathy (in):
antiglomerular basement membrane disease (M31.0)
diabetes (E08-E13 with .21)
gonococcal (A54.21)
Goodpasture's syndrome (M31.0)
hemolytic-uremic syndrome (D59.3)
lupus (M32.14)
mumps (B26.83)
syphilis (A52.75)
systemic lupus erythematosus (M32.14)
Wegener's granulomatosis (M31.31)
pyelonephritis in diseases classified elsewhere (N16)
renal tubulo-interstitial disorders classified elsewhere (N16)

Renal tubulo-interstitial diseases (N10-N16)

INCLUDES pyelonephritis

EXCLUDES1 pyeloureteritis cystica (N28.85)

N10 Acute **pyelonephritis**   HAC

Acute infectious interstitial nephritis
Acute pyelitis
Acute tubulo-interstitial nephritis
Hemoglobin nephrosis
Myoglobin nephrosis

Use additional code (B95-B97), to identify infectious agent.

4ᵗʰ **N11** Chronic **tubulo-interstitial nephritis**

INCLUDES chronic infectious interstitial nephritis
chronic pyelitis
chronic pyelonephritis

Use additional code (B95-B97), to identify infectious agent.

N11.0 Nonobstructive **reflux-associated chronic pyelonephritis**

Pyelonephritis (chronic) associated with (vesicoureteral) reflux

EXCLUDES1 vesicoureteral reflux NOS (N13.70)

N11.1 Chronic obstructive **pyelonephritis**   CC CC/MCC Exc

Pyelonephritis (chronic) associated with anomaly of pelviureteric junction

Pyelonephritis (chronic) associated with anomaly of pyeloureteric junction

Pyelonephritis (chronic) associated with crossing of vessel

Pyelonephritis (chronic) associated with kinking of ureter

Pyelonephritis (chronic) associated with obstruction of ureter

Pyelonephritis (chronic) associated with stricture of pelviureteric junction

Pyelonephritis (chronic) associated with stricture of ureter

EXCLUDES1 calculous pyelonephritis (N20.9)
obstructive uropathy (N13.-)

N11.8 Other chronic **tubulo-interstitial nephritis**   CC CC/MCC Exc

Nonobstructive chronic pyelonephritis NOS

N11.9 Chronic **tubulo-interstitial nephritis, unspecified**   CC HAC CC/MCC Exc

Chronic interstitial nephritis NOS
Chronic pyelitis NOS
Chronic pyelonephritis NOS

N12 **Tubulo-interstitial nephritis, not specified as acute or chronic**   CC HAC CC/MCC Exc

Interstitial nephritis NOS
Pyelitis NOS
Pyelonephritis NOS

EXCLUDES1 calculous pyelonephritis (N20.9)

4ᵗʰ **N13** **Obstructive and reflux uropathy**

EXCLUDES2 calculus of kidney and ureter without hydronephrosis (N20.-)
congenital obstructive defects of renal pelvis and ureter (Q62.0-Q62.3)
hydronephrosis with ureteropelvic junction obstruction (Q62.11)
obstructive pyelonephritis (N11.1)

PDx Unacceptable principal diagnosis symbol per Medicare code edits   POA Code exempt from diagnosis present on admission requirement
❓ Questionable admission   CC Complication or comorbidity   MCC Major complication or comorbidity   CC/MCC Exc CC/MCC exclusion
HCC HCC diagnosis code   RxHCC RxHCC diagnosis code   MACRA code   **DEFINITION** Describes condition/terminology
TIP Coding guidance   👁 Official Guideline Reference   Z Z code as first-listed diagnosis

N13.0 Hydronephrosis with ureteropelvic junction obstruction CC CC/MCC Exc
  AHA: Q4 2016
  Hydronephrosis due to acquired occlusion of ureteropelvic junction
  EXCLUDES2 *Hydronephrosis with ureteropelvic junction obstruction due to calculus (N13.2)*

N13.1 Hydronephrosis with ureteral stricture, not elsewhere classified CC CC/MCC Exc
  EXCLUDES1 *Hydronephrosis with ureteral stricture with infection (N13.6)*

N13.2 Hydronephrosis with renal and ureteral calculous obstruction CC CC/MCC Exc
  EXCLUDES1 *Hydronephrosis with renal and ureteral calculous obstruction with infection (N13.6)*

5ᵗʰ N13.3 Other and unspecified hydronephrosis
  EXCLUDES1 *hydronephrosis with infection (N13.6)*
  N13.30 Unspecified hydronephrosis CC CC/MCC Exc
  N13.39 Other hydronephrosis CC CC/MCC Exc

N13.4 Hydroureter CC CC/MCC Exc
  EXCLUDES1 *congenital hydroureter (Q62.3-)*
    hydroureter with infection (N13.6)
    vesicoureteral-reflux with hydroureter (N13.73-)

N13.5 Crossing vessel and stricture of ureter without hydronephrosis
  AHA: Q4 2016
  Kinking and stricture of ureter without hydronephrosis
  EXCLUDES1 *Crossing vessel and stricture of ureter without hydronephrosis with infection (N13.6)*

N13.6 Pyonephrosis CC HAC CC/MCC Exc
  AHA: Q2 2018
  Conditions in N13.0-N13.5 with infection
  Obstructive uropathy with infection
  Use additional code (B95-B97), to identify infectious agent.

5ᵗʰ N13.7 Vesicoureteral-reflux
  EXCLUDES1 *reflux-associated pyelonephritis (N11.0)*
  N13.70 Vesicoureteral-reflux, unspecified
    Vesicoureteral-reflux NOS
  N13.71 Vesicoureteral-reflux without reflux nephropathy
  6ᵗʰ N13.72 Vesicoureteral-reflux with reflux nephropathy without hydroureter
    N13.721 Vesicoureteral-reflux with reflux nephropathy without hydroureter, unilateral
    N13.722 Vesicoureteral-reflux with reflux nephropathy without hydroureter, bilateral
    N13.729 Vesicoureteral-reflux with reflux nephropathy without hydroureter, unspecified
  6ᵗʰ N13.73 Vesicoureteral-reflux with reflux nephropathy with hydroureter
    N13.731 Vesicoureteral-reflux with reflux nephropathy with hydroureter, unilateral
    N13.732 Vesicoureteral-reflux with reflux nephropathy with hydroureter, bilateral
    N13.739 Vesicoureteral-reflux with reflux nephropathy with hydroureter, unspecified

N13.8 Other obstructive and reflux uropathy CC CC/MCC Exc
  Urinary tract obstruction due to specified cause
  ☞ **Code first,** if applicable, any causal condition, such as:
    enlarged prostate (N40.1)

N13.9 Obstructive and reflux uropathy, unspecified
  Urinary tract obstruction NOS

4ᵗʰ N14 Drug- and heavy-metal-induced tubulo-interstitial and tubular conditions
  ☞ **Code first** poisoning due to drug or toxin, if applicable (T36-T65 with fifth or sixth character 1-4 or 6)
  Use additional code for adverse effect, if applicable, to identify drug (T36-T50 with fifth or sixth character 5)

N14.0 Analgesic nephropathy
N14.1 Nephropathy induced by other drugs, medicaments and biological substances
N14.2 Nephropathy induced by unspecified drug, medicament or biological substance
N14.3 Nephropathy induced by heavy metals
N14.4 Toxic nephropathy, not elsewhere classified

4ᵗʰ N15 Other renal tubulo-interstitial diseases
  N15.0 Balkan nephropathy
    Balkan endemic nephropathy
  N15.1 Renal and perinephric abscess HAC MCC CC/MCC Exc
  N15.8 Other specified renal tubulo-interstitial diseases
  N15.9 Renal tubulo-interstitial disease, unspecified
    Infection of kidney NOS
    EXCLUDES1 *urinary tract infection NOS (N39.0)*

N16 Renal tubulo-interstitial disorders in diseases classified elsewhere
  Pyelonephritis
  Tubulo-interstitial nephritis
  ☞ **Code first** underlying disease, such as:
    brucellosis (A23.0-A23.9)
    cryoglobulinemia (D89.1)
    glycogen storage disease (E74.0)
    leukemia (C91-C95)
    lymphoma (C81.0-C85.9, C96.0-C96.9)
    multiple myeloma (C90.0-)
    sepsis (A40.0-A41.9)
    Wilson's disease (E83.0)
  EXCLUDES1 *diphtheritic pyelonephritis and tubulo-interstitial nephritis (A36.84)*
    pyelonephritis and tubulo-interstitial nephritis in candidiasis (B37.49)
    pyelonephritis and tubulo-interstitial nephritis in cystinosis (E72.04)
    pyelonephritis and tubulo-interstitial nephritis in salmonella infection (A02.25)
    pyelonephritis and tubulo-interstitial nephritis in sarcoidosis (D86.84)
    pyelonephritis and tubulo-interstitial nephritis in sicca syndrome [Sjogren's] (M35.04)
    pyelonephritis and tubulo-interstitial nephritis in systemic lupus erythematosus (M32.15)
    pyelonephritis and tubulo-interstitial nephritis in toxoplasmosis (B58.83)
    renal tubular degeneration in diabetes (E08-E13 with .29)
    syphilitic pyelonephritis and tubulo-interstitial nephritis (A52.75)

Acute kidney failure and chronic kidney disease (N17-N19)

EXCLUDES2 *congenital renal failure (P96.0)*
  drug- and heavy-metal-induced tubulo-interstitial and tubular conditions (N14.-)
  extrarenal uremia (R39.2)
  hemolytic-uremic syndrome (D59.3)
  hepatorenal syndrome (K76.7)
  postpartum hepatorenal syndrome (O90.4)
  posttraumatic renal failure (T79.5)
  prerenal uremia (R39.2)
  renal failure complicating abortion or ectopic or molar pregnancy (O00-O07, O08.4)
  renal failure following labor and delivery (O90.4)
  renal failure postprocedural (N99.0)

4ᵗʰ N17 Acute kidney failure
  Code also associated underlying condition
  EXCLUDES1 *posttraumatic renal failure (T79.5)*
  N17.0 Acute kidney failure with tubular necrosis HCC MCC CC/MCC Exc
    Acute tubular necrosis
    Renal tubular necrosis
    Tubular necrosis NOS

Unspecified Code   Other Specified Code   Manifestation Code   N Newborn   P Pediatric   M Maternity   A Adult   ♂ Male   ♀ Female
● New Code   ▲ Revised Code Title   ►◄ Revised Text   **NOTES**   *INCLUDES*   *EXCLUDES1* Not coded here   *EXCLUDES2* Not included here
4ᵗʰ 4ᵗʰ character required   5ᵗʰ 5ᵗʰ character required   6ᵗʰ 6ᵗʰ character required   7ᵗʰ 7ᵗʰ character required   ⊗ Extension 'X' Alert
HAC Hospital-acquired condition (HAC) alert   **AHA** AHA Coding Clinic©   ☞ **Code first** alert

N17.1 **Acute kidney failure** with acute cortical necrosis ⬛HCC ⬛MCC ⬛CC/MCC Exc
Acute cortical necrosis
Cortical necrosis NOS
Renal cortical necrosis

N17.2 **Acute kidney failure** with medullary necrosis ⬛HCC ⬛MCC ⬛CC/MCC Exc
Medullary [papillary] necrosis NOS
Acute medullary [papillary] necrosis
Renal medullary [papillary] necrosis

N17.8 **Other acute kidney failure** ⬛CC ⬛HCC ⬛CC/MCC Exc

N17.9 **Acute kidney failure, unspecified** ⬛CC ⬛HCC ⬛CC/MCC Exc
AHA: Q2 2019
Acute kidney injury (nontraumatic)
EXCLUDES2 traumatic kidney injury (S37.0-)

🔵 N18 Chronic **kidney disease (CKD)**
👁 **See Official Guidelines** "Hypertensive Chronic Kidney Disease" I.C.9.a.2, "Hypertensive Heart and Chronic Kidney Disease" I.C.9.a.3, "Stages of chronic kidney disease" I.C.14.a.1
☞ **Code first** any associated:
diabetic chronic kidney disease (E08.22, E09.22, E10.22, E11.22, E13.22)
hypertensive chronic kidney disease (I12.-, I13.-)
Use additional code to identify kidney transplant status, if applicable, (Z94.0)

N18.1 **Chronic kidney disease,** stage 1

N18.2 **Chronic kidney disease,** stage 2 (mild)

N18.3 **Chronic kidney disease,** stage 3 (moderate) ⬛HCC

N18.4 **Chronic kidney disease,** stage 4 (severe) ⬛HCC ⬛RxHCC
AHA: Q1 2013

N18.5 **Chronic kidney disease,** stage 5 ⬛HCC ⬛RxHCC
EXCLUDES1 chronic kidney disease, stage 5 requiring chronic dialysis (N18.6)

N18.6 End stage **renal disease** ⬛CC ⬛HCC ⬛RxHCC ⬛CC/MCC Exc
AHA: Q1 2016, Q3 2016
Chronic kidney disease requiring chronic dialysis
Use additional code to identify dialysis status (Z99.2)

N18.9 **Chronic kidney disease, unspecified**
AHA: Q4 2018
Chronic renal disease
Chronic renal failure NOS
Chronic renal insufficiency
Chronic uremia NOS
Diffuse sclerosing glomerulonephritis NOS

N19 **Unspecified kidney failure**
Uremia NOS
EXCLUDES1 acute kidney failure (N17.-)
chronic kidney disease (N18.-)
chronic uremia (N18.9)
extrarenal uremia (R39.2)
prerenal uremia (R39.2)
renal insufficiency (acute) (N28.9)
uremia of newborn (P96.0)

Urolithiasis (N20-N23)

🔵 N20 **Calculus of** kidney and ureter **(Figure 14.1)**
Calculous pyelonephritis
EXCLUDES1 nephrocalcinosis (E83.5)
that with hydronephrosis (N13.2)

N20.0 **Calculus of** kidney
Nephrolithiasis NOS
Renal calculus
Renal stone
Staghorn calculus
Stone in kidney

N20.1 **Calculus of** ureter ⬛CC ⬛CC/MCC Exc
AHA: Q3 2016
Ureteric stone

N20.2 **Calculus of** kidney with calculus of ureter ⬛CC ⬛CC/MCC Exc
AHA: Q2 2015

N20.9 **Urinary calculus, unspecified**

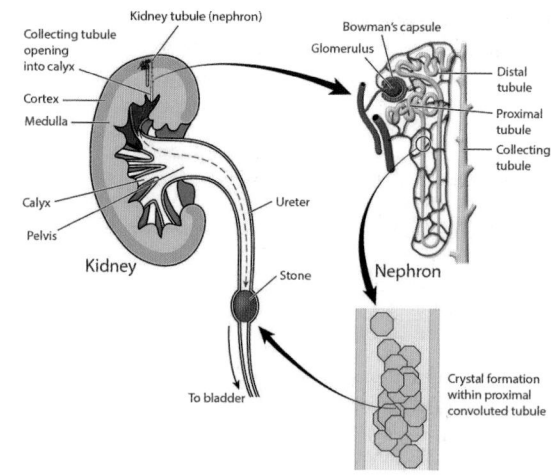

Figure 14.1 Renal Calculus Formation

🔵 N21 **Calculus of** lower urinary tract
INCLUDES calculus of lower urinary tract with cystitis and urethritis

N21.0 **Calculus in** bladder
AHA: Q2 2015
Calculus in diverticulum of bladder
Urinary bladder stone
EXCLUDES2 staghorn calculus (N20.0)

N21.1 **Calculus in** urethra
EXCLUDES2 calculus of prostate (N42.0)

N21.8 **Other** lower urinary tract calculus

N21.9 **Calculus of lower urinary tract, unspecified**
EXCLUDES1 calculus of urinary tract NOS (N20.9)

N22 **Calculus of urinary tract in diseases classified elsewhere**
☞ **Code first** underlying disease, such as:
gout (M1A.-, M10.-)
schistosomiasis (B65.0-B65.9)

N23 **Unspecified renal colic**

Other disorders of kidney and ureter (N25-N29)

EXCLUDES2 disorders of kidney and ureter with urolithiasis (N20-N23)

🔵 N25 **Disorders resulting from impaired renal tubular function**

N25.0 **Renal osteodystrophy** ⬛RxHCC
Azotemic osteodystrophy
Phosphate-losing tubular disorders
Renal rickets
Renal short stature
EXCLUDES2 metabolic disorders classifiable to E70-E88

N25.1 **Nephrogenic diabetes insipidus** ⬛CC ⬛HCC ⬛RxHCC ⬛CC/MCC Exc
EXCLUDES1 diabetes insipidus NOS (E23.2)

🔵 N25.8 **Other disorders resulting from impaired renal tubular function**

N25.81 **Secondary hyperparathyroidism of renal origin** ⬛CC ⬛HCC ⬛RxHCC ⬛CC/MCC Exc
EXCLUDES1 secondary hyperparathyroidism, non-renal (E21.1)
EXCLUDES2 metabolic disorders classifiable to E70-E88

N25.89 **Other disorders resulting from impaired renal tubular function**
Hypokalemic nephropathy
Lightwood-Albright syndrome
Renal tubular acidosis NOS

N25.9 **Disorder resulting from impaired renal tubular function, unspecified**

PDxⁿ Unacceptable principal diagnosis symbol per Medicare code edits   POA Code exempt from diagnosis present on admission requirement
❓ Questionable admission   ⬛CC Complication or comorbidity   ⬛MCC Major complication or comorbidity   ⬛CC/MCC Exc CC/MCC exclusion
⬛HCC HCC diagnosis code   ⬛RxHCC RxHCC diagnosis code   MACRA code   **DEFINITION** Describes condition/terminology
TIP Coding guidance   👁 Official Guideline Reference   Z Z code as first-listed diagnosis

4️⃣ **N26** **Unspecified contracted kidney**
    EXCLUDES1 contracted kidney due to hypertension (I12.-)
        diffuse sclerosing glomerulonephritis (N05.8.-)
        hypertensive nephrosclerosis (arteriolar) (arteriosclerotic) (I12.-)
        small kidney of unknown cause (N27.-)
    N26.1 **Atrophy of kidney (terminal)**
    N26.2 **Page kidney**   RxHCC
    N26.9 **Renal sclerosis, unspecified**

4️⃣ **N27** **Small kidney of unknown cause**
    INCLUDES oligonephronia
    N27.0 **Small kidney, unilateral**
    N27.1 **Small kidney, bilateral**
    N27.9 **Small kidney, unspecified**

4️⃣ **N28** **Other disorders of kidney and ureter, not elsewhere classified**
    N28.0 **Ischemia and infarction of kidney**   CC HCC CC/MCC Exc
        Renal artery embolism
        Renal artery obstruction
        Renal artery occlusion
        Renal artery thrombosis
        Renal infarct
        EXCLUDES1 atherosclerosis of renal artery (extrarenal part) (I70.1)
            congenital stenosis of renal artery (Q27.1)
            Goldblatt's kidney (I70.1)
    N28.1 **Cyst of kidney, acquired**
        Cyst (multiple) (solitary) of kidney (acquired)
        EXCLUDES1 cystic kidney disease (congenital) (Q61.-)
    5️⃣ **N28.8** **Other specified disorders of kidney and ureter**
        EXCLUDES1 hydroureter (N13.4)
            ureteric stricture with hydronephrosis (N13.1)
            ureteric stricture without hydronephrosis (N13.5)
        N28.81 **Hypertrophy of kidney**
        N28.82 **Megaloureter**
        N28.83 **Nephroptosis**
        N28.84 **Pyelitis cystica**   CC HAC CC/MCC Exc
        N28.85 **Pyeloureteritis cystica**   CC HAC CC/MCC Exc
        N28.86 **Ureteritis cystica**   CC HAC CC/MCC Exc
        N28.89 **Other specified disorders of kidney and ureter**
    N28.9 **Disorder of kidney and ureter, unspecified**
        AHA: Q1 2016
        Nephropathy NOS
        Renal disease (acute) NOS
        Renal insufficiency (acute)
        EXCLUDES1 chronic renal insufficiency (N18.9)
            unspecified nephritic syndrome (N05.-)

N29 **Other disorders of kidney and ureter in diseases classified elsewhere**
    ☛ Code first underlying disease, such as:
        amyloidosis (E85.-)
        nephrocalcinosis (E83.5)
        schistosomiasis (B65.0-B65.9)
    EXCLUDES1 disorders of kidney and ureter in:
        cystinosis (E72.0)
        gonorrhea (A54.21)
        syphilis (A52.75)
        tuberculosis (A18.11)

Other diseases of the urinary system (N30-N39)

    EXCLUDES1 urinary infection (complicating):
        abortion or ectopic or molar pregnancy (O00-O07, O08.8)
        pregnancy, childbirth and the puerperium (O23.-, O75.3, O86.2-)

4️⃣ **N30** **Cystitis**
    Use additional code to identify infectious agent (B95-B97)
    EXCLUDES1 prostatocystitis (N41.3)

5️⃣ **N30.0** **Acute cystitis**
    EXCLUDES1 irradiation cystitis (N30.4-)
        trigonitis (N30.3-)
    N30.00 **Acute cystitis** without hematuria   HAC
    N30.01 **Acute cystitis** with hematuria   HAC
5️⃣ **N30.1** Interstitial cystitis (chronic)
    N30.10 **Interstitial cystitis (chronic)** without hematuria
    N30.11 **Interstitial cystitis (chronic)** with hematuria
5️⃣ **N30.2** Other chronic cystitis
    N30.20 **Other chronic cystitis** without hematuria
    N30.21 **Other chronic cystitis** with hematuria
5️⃣ **N30.3** Trigonitis
    Urethrotrigonitis
    N30.30 **Trigonitis** without hematuria
    N30.31 **Trigonitis** with hematuria
5️⃣ **N30.4** Irradiation cystitis
    N30.40 **Irradiation cystitis** without hematuria   CC CC/MCC Exc
    N30.41 **Irradiation cystitis** with hematuria   CC CC/MCC Exc
5️⃣ **N30.8** Other cystitis
    Abscess of bladder
    N30.80 **Other cystitis** without hematuria
    N30.81 **Other cystitis** with hematuria
5️⃣ **N30.9** Cystitis, unspecified
    N30.90 **Cystitis, unspecified** without hematuria
    N30.91 **Cystitis, unspecified** with hematuria

4️⃣ **N31** **Neuromuscular dysfunction of bladder, not elsewhere classified**
    Use additional code to identify any associated urinary incontinence (N39.3-N39.4-)
    EXCLUDES1 cord bladder NOS (G95.89)
        neurogenic bladder due to cauda equina syndrome (G83.4)
        neuromuscular dysfunction due to spinal cord lesion (G95.89)
    N31.0 **Uninhibited neuropathic bladder, not elsewhere classified**
    N31.1 **Reflex neuropathic bladder, not elsewhere classified**
    N31.2 **Flaccid neuropathic bladder, not elsewhere classified**
        Atonic (motor) (sensory) neuropathic bladder
        Autonomous neuropathic bladder
        Nonreflex neuropathic bladder
    N31.8 **Other neuromuscular dysfunction of bladder**
    N31.9 **Neuromuscular dysfunction of bladder, unspecified**
        Neurogenic bladder dysfunction NOS

4️⃣ **N32** **Other disorders of bladder**
    EXCLUDES2 calculus of bladder (N21.0)
        cystocele (N81.1-)
        hernia or prolapse of bladder, female (N81.1-)
    N32.0 **Bladder-neck obstruction**
        Bladder-neck stenosis (acquired)
        EXCLUDES1 congenital bladder-neck obstruction (Q64.3-)
    N32.1 **Vesicointestinal fistula**   CC CC/MCC Exc
        Vesicorectal fistula
    N32.2 **Vesical fistula, not elsewhere classified**   CC CC/MCC Exc
        EXCLUDES1 fistula between bladder and female genital tract (N82.0-N82.1)
    N32.3 **Diverticulum of bladder**
        EXCLUDES1 congenital diverticulum of bladder (Q64.6)
            diverticulitis of bladder (N30.8-)
    5️⃣ **N32.8** **Other specified disorders of bladder**
        N32.81 **Overactive bladder**
            Detrusor muscle hyperactivity
            EXCLUDES1 frequent urination due to specified bladder condition- code to condition
        N32.89 **Other specified disorders of bladder**
            Bladder hemorrhage
            Bladder hypertrophy
            Calcified bladder
            Contracted bladder
    N32.9 **Bladder disorder, unspecified**

N33 **Bladder disorders in diseases classified elsewhere**
☞ **Code first** underlying disease, such as:
schistosomiasis (B65.0-B65.9)
EXCLUDES1 bladder disorder in syphilis (A52.76)
bladder disorder in tuberculosis (A18.12)
candidal cystitis (B37.41)
chlamydial cystitis (A56.01)
cystitis in gonorrhea (A54.01)
cystitis in neurogenic bladder (N31.-)
diphtheritic cystitis (A36.85)
syphilitic cystitis (A52.76)
trichomonal cystitis (A59.03)

4ᵗʰ **N34** **Urethritis and urethral syndrome**
Use additional code (B95-B97), to identify infectious agent.
EXCLUDES2 Reiter's disease (M02.3-)
urethritis in diseases with a predominantly sexual mode of transmission (A50-A64)
urethrotrigonitis (N30.3-)
N34.0 **Urethral abscess**   CC HAC CC/MCC Exc
Abscess (of) Cowper's gland
Abscess (of) Littré's gland
Abscess (of) urethral (gland)
Periurethral abscess
EXCLUDES1 urethral caruncle (N36.2)
N34.1 **Nonspecific urethritis**
Nongonococcal urethritis
Nonvenereal urethritis
N34.2 **Other urethritis**
Meatitis, urethral
Postmenopausal urethritis
Ulcer of urethra (meatus)
Urethritis NOS
N34.3 **Urethral syndrome, unspecified**

4ᵗʰ **N35** **Urethral stricture**
EXCLUDES1 congenital urethral stricture (Q64.3-)
postprocedural urethral stricture (N99.1-)
5ᵗʰ **N35.0** Post-traumatic **urethral stricture**
Urethral stricture due to injury
EXCLUDES1 postprocedural urethral stricture (N99.1-)
6ᵗʰ **N35.01** **Post-traumatic urethral stricture,** male
N35.010 **Post-traumatic urethral stricture, male, meatal** ♂
N35.011 **Post-traumatic** bulbous **urethral stricture** ♂
N35.012 **Post-traumatic** membranous **urethral stricture** ♂
N35.013 **Post-traumatic** anterior **urethral stricture** ♂
N35.014 **Post-traumatic urethral stricture, male, unspecified** ♂
N35.016 **Post-traumatic urethral stricture, male,** overlapping sites ♂
AHA: Q4 2018
6ᵗʰ **N35.02** **Post-traumatic urethral stricture,** female
N35.021 **Urethral stricture** due to childbirth ♀
N35.028 **Other post-traumatic urethral stricture, female** ♀
5ᵗʰ **N35.1** Postinfective **urethral stricture, not elsewhere classified**
EXCLUDES1 urethral stricture associated with schistosomiasis (B65.-, N29)
gonococcal urethral stricture (A54.01)
syphilitic urethral stricture (A52.76)
6ᵗʰ **N35.11** **Postinfective urethral stricture, not elsewhere classified,** male
N35.111 **Postinfective urethral stricture, not elsewhere classified, male,** meatal ♂
N35.112 **Postinfective** bulbous **urethral stricture, not elsewhere classified, male** ♂

N35.113 **Postinfective** membranous **urethral stricture, not elsewhere classified, male** ♂
N35.114 **Postinfective** anterior **urethral stricture, not elsewhere classified, male** ♂
N35.116 **Postinfective urethral stricture, not elsewhere classified, male,** overlapping sites ♂
AHA: Q4 2018
N35.119 **Postinfective urethral stricture, not elsewhere classified, male, unspecified** ♂
N35.12 **Postinfective urethral stricture, not elsewhere classified,** female ♀
5ᵗʰ **N35.8** **Other urethral stricture**
EXCLUDES1 postprocedural urethral stricture (N99.1-)
6ᵗʰ **N35.81** Other **urethral stricture,** male
N35.811 **Other urethral stricture, male,** meatal ♂
AHA: Q4 2018
N35.812 **Other urethral** bulbous **stricture, male** ♂
AHA: Q4 2018
N35.813 **Other** membranous **urethral stricture, male** ♂
AHA: Q4 2018
▲ **N35.814** **Other anterior urethral stricture, male** ♂
AHA: Q4 2018
N35.816 **Other urethral stricture, male,** overlapping sites ♂
AHA: Q4 2018
N35.819 **Other urethral stricture, male, unspecified site** ♂
AHA: Q4 2018
N35.82 Other **urethral stricture,** female ♀
AHA: Q4 2018
5ᵗʰ **N35.9** **Urethral stricture,** unspecified
6ᵗʰ **N35.91** **Urethral stricture,** unspecified, male
N35.911 **Unspecified urethral stricture, male,** meatal ♂
AHA: Q4 2018
N35.912 **Unspecified** bulbous **urethral stricture, male** ♂
AHA: Q4 2018
N35.913 **Unspecified** membranous **urethral stricture, male** ♂
AHA: Q4 2018
N35.914 **Unspecified** anterior **urethral stricture, male** ♂
AHA: Q4 2018
N35.916 **Unspecified urethral stricture, male,** overlapping sites ♂
AHA: Q4 2018
N35.919 **Unspecified urethral stricture, male, unspecified site** ♂
AHA: Q4 2018
Pinhole meatus NOS
Urethral stricture NOS
N35.92 **Unspecified urethral stricture,** female ♀
AHA: Q4 2018
4ᵗʰ **N36** **Other disorders of urethra**
N36.0 **Urethral** fistula   CC CC/MCC Exc
Urethroperineal fistula
Urethrorectal fistula
Urinary fistula NOS
EXCLUDES1 urethroscrotal fistula (N50.89)
urethrovaginal fistula (N82.1)
urethrovesicovaginal fistula (N82.1)
N36.1 **Urethral** diverticulum
N36.2 **Urethral** caruncle
5ᵗʰ **N36.4** **Urethral** functional and muscular disorders
Use additional code to identify associated urinary stress incontinence (N39.3)
N36.41 Hypermobility of urethra
N36.42 **Intrinsic sphincter deficiency (ISD)**

PDxᴹᴵᴿ Unacceptable principal diagnosis symbol per Medicare code edits   PDx Code exempt from diagnosis present on admission requirement
❓ Questionable admission   CC Complication or comorbidity   MCC Major complication or comorbidity   CC/MCC Exc CC/MCC exclusion
HCC HCC diagnosis code   RxHCC RxHCC diagnosis code   MACRA MACRA code   **DEFINITION** Describes condition/terminology
TIP Coding guidance   👁 Official Guideline Reference   Z1 Z code as first-listed diagnosis

N36.43 Combined hypermobility of urethra and intrinsic sphincter deficiency
N36.44 Muscular disorders of urethra
Bladder sphincter dyssynergy
N36.5 Urethral false passage
N36.8 Other specified disorders of urethra
EXCLUDES1 congenital urethrocele (Q64.7)
female urethrocele (N81.0)
N36.9 Urethral disorder, unspecified
N37 Urethral disorders in diseases classified elsewhere
☞ Code first underlying disease
EXCLUDES1 urethritis (in):
candidal infection (B37.41)
chlamydial (A56.01)
gonorrhea (A54.01)
syphilis (A52.76)
trichomonal infection (A59.03)
tuberculosis (A18.13)
N39 Other disorders of urinary system
EXCLUDES2 hematuria NOS (R31.-)
recurrent or persistent hematuria (N02.-)
recurrent or persistent hematuria with specified morphological lesion (N02.-)
proteinuria NOS (R80.-)
N39.0 Urinary tract infection, site not specified   CC HAC CC/MCC Exc
AHA: Q1 2018, Q2 2018
Use additional code (B95-B97), to identify infectious agent.
EXCLUDES1 candidiasis of urinary tract (B37.4-)
neonatal urinary tract infection (P39.3)
pyuria (R82.81)
urinary tract infection of specified site, such as:
cystitis (N30.-)
urethritis (N34.-)
N39.3 Stress incontinence (female) (male)
Code also any associated overactive bladder (N32.81)
EXCLUDES1 mixed incontinence (N39.46)
N39.4 Other specified urinary incontinence
Code also any associated overactive bladder (N32.81)
EXCLUDES1 enuresis NOS (R32)
functional urinary incontinence (R39.81)
urinary incontinence associated with cognitive impairment (R39.81)
urinary incontinence NOS (R32)
urinary incontinence of nonorganic origin (F98.0)
N39.41 Urge incontinence
EXCLUDES1 mixed incontinence (N39.46)
N39.42 Incontinence without sensory awareness
AHA: Q4 2016
Insensible (urinary) incontinence
N39.43 Post-void dribbling
N39.44 Nocturnal enuresis
N39.45 Continuous leakage
N39.46 Mixed incontinence
Urge and stress incontinence
N39.49 Other specified urinary incontinence
N39.490 Overflow incontinence
N39.491 Coital incontinence
AHA: Q4 2016
N39.492 Postural (urinary) incontinence
AHA: Q4 2016
N39.498 Other specified urinary incontinence
Reflex incontinence
Total incontinence
N39.8 Other specified disorders of urinary system
N39.9 Disorder of urinary system, unspecified

Diseases of male genital organs (N40-N53)

N40 Benign prostatic hyperplasia (Figure 14.2)
DEFINITION: (1) Prostatic hyperplasia is prostate enlargement caused by an overgrowth of prostatic cells or tissue that tends to cause urinary symptoms. (2) Prostatic hypertrophy is prostate enlargement caused by an enlargement of prostate cells without significant new prostate tissue.
INCLUDES adenofibromatous hypertrophy of prostate
benign hypertrophy of the prostate
benign prostatic hypertrophy
BPH
enlarged prostate
nodular prostate
polyp of prostate
EXCLUDES1 benign neoplasms of prostate (adenoma, benign) (fibroadenoma) (fibroma) (myoma) (D29.1)
EXCLUDES2 malignant neoplasm of prostate (C61)

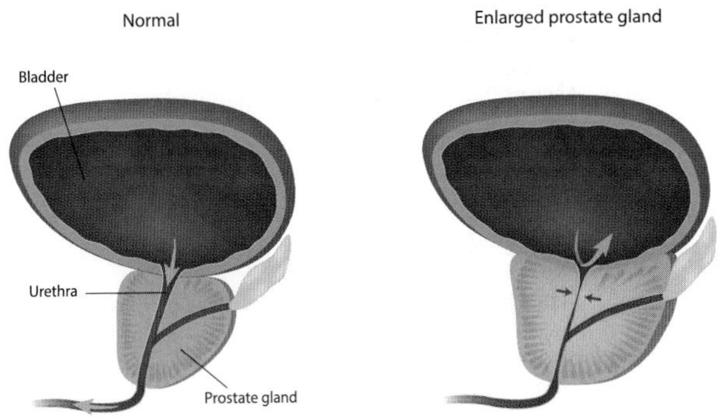

Figure 14.2 Benign Prostatic Hyperplasia

N40.0 Benign prostatic hyperplasia without lower urinary tract symptoms   A ♂
Enlarged prostate without LUTS
Enlarged prostate NOS
N40.1 Benign prostatic hyperplasia with lower urinary tract symptoms   A ♂
AHA: Q4 2018
Enlarged prostate with LUTS
Use additional code for associated symptoms, when specified:
incomplete bladder emptying (R39.14)
nocturia (R35.1)
straining on urination (R39.16)
urinary frequency (R35.0)
urinary hesitancy (R39.11)
urinary incontinence (N39.4-)
urinary obstruction (N13.8)
urinary retention (R33.8)
urinary urgency (R39.15)
weak urinary stream (R39.12)
N40.2 Nodular prostate without lower urinary tract symptoms   A ♂
Nodular prostate without LUTS
N40.3 Nodular prostate with lower urinary tract symptoms   A ♂
Use additional code for associated symptoms, when specified:
incomplete bladder emptying (R39.14)
nocturia (R35.1)
straining on urination (R39.16)
urinary frequency (R35.0)
urinary hesitancy (R39.11)
urinary incontinence (N39.4-)
urinary obstruction (N13.8)
urinary retention (R33.8)
urinary urgency (R39.15)
weak urinary stream (R39.12)

Unspecified Code   Other Specified Code   Manifestation Code   N Newborn   P Pediatric   M Maternity   A Adult   ♂ Male   ♀ Female
● New Code   ▲ Revised Code Title   ►◄ Revised Text   NOTES   INCLUDES   EXCLUDES1 Not coded here   EXCLUDES2 Not included here
④ 4th character required   ⑤ 5th character required   ⑥ 6th character required   ⑦ 7th character required   ⑦ˣ Extension 'X' Alert
HAC Hospital-acquired condition (HAC) alert   AHA AHA Coding Clinic®   ☞ Code first alert

N41 Inflammatory diseases of prostate
Use additional code (B95-B97), to identify infectious agent.
N41.0 Acute prostatitis   A ♂
N41.1 Chronic prostatitis   A ♂
N41.2 Abscess of prostate   A cc ♂ CC/MCC Exc
N41.3 Prostatocystitis   A ♂
N41.4 Granulomatous prostatitis   A ♂
N41.8 Other inflammatory diseases of prostate   A ♂
N41.9 Inflammatory disease of prostate, unspecified   A ♂
    Prostatitis NOS

N42 Other and unspecified disorders of prostate
N42.0 Calculus of prostate   A ♂
    Prostatic stone
N42.1 Congestion and hemorrhage of prostate   A ♂
    EXCLUDES1 enlarged prostate (N40.-)
           hematuria (R31.-)
           hyperplasia of prostate (N40.-)
           inflammatory diseases of prostate (N41.-)
N42.3 Dysplasia of prostate
   N42.30 Unspecified dysplasia of prostate   ♂
       AHA: Q4 2016
   N42.31 Prostatic intraepithelial neoplasia   ♂
       AHA: Q4 2016
       PIN
       Prostatic intraepithelial neoplasia I (PIN I)
       Prostatic intraepithelial neoplasia II (PIN II)
       EXCLUDES1 prostatic intraepithelial neoplasia III (PIN III)
              (D07.5)
   N42.32 Atypical small acinar proliferation of prostate   ♂
       AHA: Q4 2016
   N42.39 Other dysplasia of prostate   ♂
       AHA: Q4 2016
N42.8 Other specified disorders of prostate
   N42.81 Prostatodynia syndrome   A ♂
       Painful prostate syndrome
   N42.82 Prostatosis syndrome   A ♂
   N42.83 Cyst of prostate   A ♂
   N42.89 Other specified disorders of prostate   A ♂
N42.9 Disorder of prostate, unspecified   A ♂

N43 Hydrocele and spermatocele
INCLUDES hydrocele of spermatic cord, testis or tunica vaginalis
EXCLUDES1 congenital hydrocele (P83.5)
N43.0 Encysted hydrocele   ♂
N43.1 Infected hydrocele   cc ♂ CC/MCC Exc
    Use additional code (B95-B97), to identify infectious agent.
N43.2 Other hydrocele   ♂
N43.3 Hydrocele, unspecified   ♂
N43.4 Spermatocele of epididymis
    Spermatic cyst
   N43.40 Spermatocele of epididymis, unspecified   ♂
   N43.41 Spermatocele of epididymis, single   ♂
   N43.42 Spermatocele of epididymis, multiple   ♂

N44 Noninflammatory disorders of testis
N44.0 Torsion of testis
   N44.00 Torsion of testis, unspecified   cc ♂ CC/MCC Exc
   N44.01 Extravaginal torsion of spermatic cord   cc ♂ CC/MCC Exc
   N44.02 Intravaginal torsion of spermatic cord   cc ♂ CC/MCC Exc
       Torsion of spermatic cord NOS
   N44.03 Torsion of appendix testis   cc ♂ CC/MCC Exc
   N44.04 Torsion of appendix epididymis   cc ♂ CC/MCC Exc
N44.1 Cyst of tunica albuginea testis   ♂
N44.2 Benign cyst of testis   ♂
N44.8 Other noninflammatory disorders of the testis   ♂

N45 Orchitis and epididymitis
Use additional code (B95-B97), to identify infectious agent.
N45.1 Epididymitis   ♂
N45.2 Orchitis   ♂
N45.3 Epididymo-orchitis   ♂
N45.4 Abscess of epididymis or testis   cc ♂ CC/MCC Exc

N46 Male infertility
EXCLUDES1 vasectomy status (Z98.52)
N46.0 Azoospermia
    Absolute male infertility
    Male infertility due to germinal (cell) aplasia
    Male infertility due to spermatogenic arrest (complete)
   N46.01 Organic azoospermia   A ♂
       Azoospermia NOS
   N46.02 Azoospermia due to extratesticular causes
       Code also associated cause
     N46.021 Azoospermia due to drug therapy   A ♂
     N46.022 Azoospermia due to infection   A ♂
     N46.023 Azoospermia due to obstruction of efferent ducts   A ♂
     N46.024 Azoospermia due to radiation   A ♂
     N46.025 Azoospermia due to systemic disease   A ♂
     N46.029 Azoospermia due to other extratesticular causes   A ♂
N46.1 Oligospermia
    Male infertility due to germinal cell desquamation
    Male infertility due to hypospermatogenesis
    Male infertility due to incomplete spermatogenic arrest
   N46.11 Organic oligospermia   A ♂
       Oligospermia NOS
   N46.12 Oligospermia due to extratesticular causes
       Code also associated cause
     N46.121 Oligospermia due to drug therapy   A ♂
     N46.122 Oligospermia due to infection   A ♂
     N46.123 Oligospermia due to obstruction of efferent ducts   A ♂
     N46.124 Oligospermia due to radiation   A ♂
     N46.125 Oligospermia due to systemic disease   A ♂
     N46.129 Oligospermia due to other extratesticular causes   A ♂
N46.8 Other male infertility   A ♂
N46.9 Male infertility, unspecified   A ♂

N47 Disorders of prepuce
N47.0 Adherent prepuce, newborn   N ♂
N47.1 Phimosis   ♂
N47.2 Paraphimosis   ♂
N47.3 Deficient foreskin   ♂
N47.4 Benign cyst of prepuce   ♂
N47.5 Adhesions of prepuce and glans penis   ♂
N47.6 Balanoposthitis   ♂
    Use additional code (B95-B97), to identify infectious agent.
    EXCLUDES1 balanitis (N48.1)
N47.7 Other inflammatory diseases of prepuce   ♂
    Use additional code (B95-B97), to identify infectious agent.
N47.8 Other disorders of prepuce   ♂

N48 Other disorders of penis
N48.0 Leukoplakia of penis   ♂
    Balanitis xerotica obliterans
    Kraurosis of penis
    Lichen sclerosus of external male genital organs
    EXCLUDES1 carcinoma in situ of penis (D07.4)
N48.1 Balanitis   ♂
    Use additional code (B95-B97), to identify infectious agent.
    EXCLUDES1 amebic balanitis (A06.8)
           balanitis xerotica obliterans (N48.0)
           candidal balanitis (B37.42)
           gonococcal balanitis (A54.23)
           herpesviral [herpes simplex] balanitis (A60.01)
N48.2 Other inflammatory disorders of penis
    Use additional code (B95-B97), to identify infectious agent.
    EXCLUDES1 balanitis (N48.1)
           balanitis xerotica obliterans (N48.0)
           balanoposthitis (N47.6)
   N48.21 Abscess of corpus cavernosum and penis   ♂

PDxlₐ Unacceptable principal diagnosis symbol per Medicare code edits   PDx Code exempt from diagnosis present on admission requirement
❓ Questionable admission   cc Complication or comorbidity   MCC Major complication or comorbidity   CC/MCC Exc CC/MCC exclusion
HCC HCC diagnosis code   RxHCC RxHCC diagnosis code   MACRA code   **DEFINITION** Describes condition/terminology
TIP Coding guidance   👁 Official Guideline Reference   Z1 Z code as first-listed diagnosis

N48.22 Cellulitis of corpus cavernosum and penis ♂
N48.29 Other inflammatory disorders of penis ♂
🄓 N48.3 Priapism
Painful erection
☞ Code first underlying cause
N48.30 Priapism, unspecified CC ♂ CC/MCC Exc
N48.31 Priapism due to trauma CC ♂ CC/MCC Exc
N48.32 Priapism due to disease classified
elsewhere CC ♂ CC/MCC Exc
N48.33 Priapism, drug-induced CC ♂ CC/MCC Exc
N48.39 Other priapism CC ♂ CC/MCC Exc
N48.5 Ulcer of penis ♂
N48.6 Induration penis plastica
Peyronie's disease
Plastic induration of penis
🄓 N48.8 Other specified disorders of penis
N48.81 Thrombosis of superficial vein of penis ♂
N48.82 Acquired torsion of penis ♂
Acquired torsion of penis NOS
EXCLUDES1 congenital torsion of penis (Q55.63)
N48.83 Acquired buried penis ♂
EXCLUDES1 congenital hidden penis (Q55.64)
N48.89 Other specified disorders of penis ♂
N48.9 Disorder of penis, unspecified ♂
🄭 N49 Inflammatory disorders of male genital organs, not elsewhere
classified
Use additional code (B95-B97), to identify infectious agent.
EXCLUDES1 inflammation of penis (N48.1, N48.2-)
orchitis and epididymitis (N45.-)
N49.0 Inflammatory disorders of seminal vesicle ♂
Vesiculitis NOS
N49.1 Inflammatory disorders of spermatic cord, tunica
vaginalis and vas deferens ♂
Vasitis
N49.2 Inflammatory disorders of scrotum ♂
N49.3 Fournier gangrene ♂
N49.8 Inflammatory disorders of other specified male genital
organs ♂
Inflammation of multiple sites in male genital organs
N49.9 Inflammatory disorder of unspecified male genital organ ♂
Abscess of unspecified male genital organ
Boil of unspecified male genital organ
Carbuncle of unspecified male genital organ
Cellulitis of unspecified male genital organ
🄭 N50 Other and unspecified disorders of male genital organs
EXCLUDES2 torsion of testis (N44.0-)
N50.0 Atrophy of testis ♂
N50.1 Vascular disorders of male genital organs ♂
Hematocele, NOS, of male genital organs
Hemorrhage of male genital organs
Thrombosis of male genital organs
N50.3 Cyst of epididymis ♂
🄓 N50.8 Other specified disorders of male genital organs
🄮 N50.81 Testicular pain
N50.811 Right testicular pain ♂
AHA: Q4 2016
N50.812 Left testicular pain ♂
AHA: Q4 2016
N50.819 Testicular pain, unspecified ♂
AHA: Q4 2016
N50.82 Scrotal pain ♂
AHA: Q4 2016
N50.89 Other specified disorders of the male
genital organs ♂
AHA: Q4 2016
Atrophy of scrotum, seminal vesicle, spermatic cord,
tunica vaginalis and vas deferens
Chylocele, tunica vaginalis (nonfilarial) NOS
Edema of scrotum, seminal vesicle, spermatic cord,
tunica vaginalis and vas deferens

Hypertrophy of scrotum, seminal vesicle, spermatic
cord, tunica vaginalis and vas deferens
Stricture of spermatic cord, tunica vaginalis, and vas
deferens
Ulcer of scrotum, seminal vesicle, spermatic cord,
testis, tunica vaginalis and vas deferens
Urethroscrotal fistula
N50.9 Disorder of male genital organs, unspecified ♂
N51 Disorders of male genital organs in diseases classified elsewhere ♂
☞ Code first underlying disease, such as:
filariasis (B74.0-B74.9)
EXCLUDES1 amebic balanitis (A06.8)
candidal balanitis (B37.42)
gonococcal balanitis (A54.23)
gonococcal prostatitis (A54.22)
herpesviral [herpes simplex] balanitis (A60.01)
trichomonal prostatitis (A59.02)
tuberculous prostatitis (A18.14)
🄭 N52 Male erectile dysfunction
EXCLUDES1 psychogenic impotence (F52.21)
🄓 N52.0 Vasculogenic erectile dysfunction
N52.01 Erectile dysfunction due to arterial
insufficiency A ♂
N52.02 Corporo-venous occlusive erectile dysfunction A ♂
N52.03 Combined arterial insufficiency and corporo-venous
occlusive erectile dysfunction A ♂
N52.1 Erectile dysfunction due to diseases classified
elsewhere A ♂
☞ Code first underlying disease
N52.2 Drug-induced erectile dysfunction A ♂
🄓 N52.3 Postprocedural erectile dysfunction
N52.31 Erectile dysfunction following radical
prostatectomy A ♂
N52.32 Erectile dysfunction following radical
cystectomy A ♂
N52.33 Erectile dysfunction following urethral surgery A ♂
N52.34 Erectile dysfunction following simple
prostatectomy A ♂
N52.35 Erectile dysfunction following radiation
therapy A ♂
AHA: Q4 2016
N52.36 Erectile dysfunction following interstitial seed
therapy A ♂
AHA: Q4 2016
N52.37 Erectile dysfunction following prostate ablative
therapy A ♂
AHA: Q4 2016
Erectile dysfunction following cryotherapy
Erectile dysfunction following other prostate ablative
therapies
Erectile dysfunction following ultrasound ablative
therapies
N52.39 Other and unspecified postprocedural erectile
dysfunction A ♂
N52.8 Other male erectile dysfunction A ♂
N52.9 Male erectile dysfunction, unspecified A ♂
Impotence NOS
🄭 N53 Other male sexual dysfunction
EXCLUDES1 psychogenic sexual dysfunction (F52.-)
🄓 N53.1 Ejaculatory dysfunction
EXCLUDES1 premature ejaculation (F52.4)
N53.11 Retarded ejaculation ♂
N53.12 Painful ejaculation ♂
N53.13 Anejaculatory orgasm ♂
N53.14 Retrograde ejaculation ♂
N53.19 Other ejaculatory dysfunction ♂
Ejaculatory dysfunction NOS
N53.8 Other male sexual dysfunction ♂
N53.9 Unspecified male sexual dysfunction ♂

Disorders of breast (N60-N65)

EXCLUDES1 *disorders of breast associated with childbirth (O91-O92)*

4ᵗʰ **N60** **Benign mammary dysplasia**

INCLUDES *fibrocystic mastopathy*

5ᵗʰ **N60.0** **Solitary cyst of breast**

Cyst of breast

N60.01 **Solitary cyst of** right **breast**

N60.02 **Solitary cyst of** left **breast**

N60.09 **Solitary cyst of unspecified breast**

5ᵗʰ **N60.1** **Diffuse cystic mastopathy**

Cystic breast

Fibrocystic disease of breast

EXCLUDES1 *diffuse cystic mastopathy with epithelial proliferation (N60.3-)*

N60.11 **Diffuse cystic mastopathy of** right **breast** 🅰

N60.12 **Diffuse cystic mastopathy of** left **breast** 🅰

N60.19 **Diffuse cystic mastopathy of unspecified breast** 🅰

5ᵗʰ **N60.2** **Fibroadenosis of breast**

Adenofibrosis of breast

EXCLUDES2 *fibroadenoma of breast (D24.-)*

N60.21 **Fibroadenosis of** right **breast**

N60.22 **Fibroadenosis of** left **breast**

N60.29 **Fibroadenosis of unspecified breast**

5ᵗʰ **N60.3** **Fibrosclerosis of breast**

Cystic mastopathy with epithelial proliferation

N60.31 **Fibrosclerosis of** right **breast**

N60.32 **Fibrosclerosis of** left **breast**

N60.39 **Fibrosclerosis of unspecified breast**

5ᵗʰ **N60.4** **Mammary duct ectasia**

N60.41 **Mammary duct ectasia of** right **breast**

N60.42 **Mammary duct ectasia of** left **breast**

N60.49 **Mammary duct ectasia of unspecified breast**

5ᵗʰ **N60.8** **Other benign mammary dysplasias**

N60.81 **Other benign mammary dysplasias of** right **breast**

N60.82 **Other benign mammary dysplasias of** left **breast**

N60.89 **Other benign mammary dysplasias of unspecified breast**

5ᵗʰ **N60.9** **Unspecified benign mammary dysplasia**

N60.91 **Unspecified benign mammary dysplasia of** right **breast**

N60.92 **Unspecified benign mammary dysplasia of** left **breast**

N60.99 **Unspecified benign mammary dysplasia of unspecified breast**

4ᵗʰ **N61** **Inflammatory disorders of breast**

EXCLUDES1 *inflammatory carcinoma of breast (C50.9)*

inflammatory disorder of breast associated with childbirth (O91.-)

neonatal infective mastitis (P39.0)

thrombophlebitis of breast [Mondor's disease] (I80.8)

N61.0 **Mastitis without abscess**

Infective mastitis (acute) (nonpuerperal) (subacute)

Mastitis (acute) (nonpuerperal) (subacute) NOS

Cellulitis (acute) (nonpuerperal) (subacute) of breast NOS

Cellulitis (acute) (nonpuerperal) (subacute) of nipple NOS

N61.1 **Abscess of the breast and nipple**

Abscess (acute) (chronic) (nonpuerperal) of areola

Abscess (acute) (chronic) (nonpuerperal) of breast

Carbuncle of breast

Mastitis with abscess

N62 **Hypertrophy of breast**

Gynecomastia

Hypertrophy of breast NOS

Massive pubertal hypertrophy of breast

EXCLUDES1 *breast engorgement of newborn (P83.4)*

disproportion of reconstructed breast (N65.1)

4ᵗʰ **N63** **Unspecified lump in breast**

Nodule(s) NOS in breast

N63.0 **Unspecified lump in unspecified breast**

5ᵗʰ **N63.1** **Unspecified lump in the** right **breast**

N63.10 **Unspecified lump in the right breast, unspecified quadrant**

N63.11 **Unspecified lump in the right breast, upper outer quadrant**

N63.12 **Unspecified lump in the right breast, upper inner quadrant**

N63.13 **Unspecified lump in the right breast, lower outer quadrant**

N63.14 **Unspecified lump in the right breast, lower inner quadrant**

● N63.15 **Unspecified lump in the right breast, overlapping quadrants**

5ᵗʰ **N63.2** **Unspecified lump in the** left **breast**

N63.20 **Unspecified lump in the left breast, unspecified quadrant**

N63.21 **Unspecified lump in the left breast, upper outer quadrant**

N63.22 **Unspecified lump in the left breast, upper inner quadrant**

N63.23 **Unspecified lump in the left breast, lower outer quadrant**

N63.24 **Unspecified lump in the left breast, lower inner quadrant**

● N63.25 **Unspecified lump in the left breast, overlapping quadrants**

5ᵗʰ **N63.3** **Unspecified lump in axillary tail**

N63.31 **Unspecified lump in axillary tail of the** right **breast**

N63.32 **Unspecified lump in axillary tail of the** left **breast**

5ᵗʰ **N63.4** **Unspecified lump in breast, subareolar**

N63.41 **Unspecified lump in** right **breast, subareolar**

N63.42 **Unspecified lump in** left **breast, subareolar**

4ᵗʰ **N64** **Other disorders of breast**

EXCLUDES2 *mechanical complication of breast prosthesis and implant (T85.4-)*

N64.0 **Fissure and fistula of nipple**

N64.1 **Fat necrosis of breast** PDxↃ

Fat necrosis (segmental) of breast

☞ **Code first** breast necrosis due to breast graft (T85.898)

N64.2 **Atrophy of breast**

N64.3 **Galactorrhea not associated with childbirth**

N64.4 **Mastodynia**

5ᵗʰ **N64.5** **Other signs and symptoms in breast**

EXCLUDES2 *abnormal findings on diagnostic imaging of breast (R92.-)*

N64.51 **Induration of breast**

N64.52 **Nipple discharge**

EXCLUDES1 *abnormal findings in nipple discharge (R89.-)*

N64.53 **Retraction of nipple**

N64.59 **Other signs and symptoms in breast**

5ᵗʰ **N64.8** **Other specified disorders of breast**

N64.81 **Ptosis of breast** 🅰

EXCLUDES1 *ptosis of native breast in relation to reconstructed breast (N65.1)*

N64.82 **Hypoplasia of breast** 🅰

Micromastia

EXCLUDES1 *congenital absence of breast (Q83.0)*

hypoplasia of native breast in relation to reconstructed breast (N65.1)

N64.89 **Other specified disorders of breast**

AHA: Q1 2019, Q1 2018

Galactocele

Subinvolution of breast (postlactational)

N64.9 **Disorder of breast, unspecified**

AHA: Q1 2018

4ᵗʰ **N65** **Deformity and disproportion of reconstructed breast**

N65.0 **Deformity of reconstructed breast** 🅰

Contour irregularity in reconstructed breast

Excess tissue in reconstructed breast

Misshapen reconstructed breast

PDxↃ Unacceptable principal diagnosis symbol per Medicare code edits Ↄ Code exempt from diagnosis present on admission requirement

❓ Questionable admission ℂℂ Complication or comorbidity ℳℂℂ Major complication or comorbidity ℂℂ/ℳℂℂ CC/MCC exclusion

ℍℂℂ HCC diagnosis code Rxℍℂℂ RxHCC diagnosis code MACRA code **DEFINITION** Describes condition/terminology

TIP Coding guidance 👁 Official Guideline Reference ℤ1 Z code as first-listed diagnosis

N65.1 Disproportion of reconstructed breast   🅰
Breast asymmetry between native breast and reconstructed breast
Disproportion between native breast and reconstructed breast

Inflammatory diseases of female pelvic organs (N70-N77)

EXCLUDES1   *inflammatory diseases of female pelvic organs complicating:*
abortion or ectopic or molar pregnancy (O00-O07, O08.0)
pregnancy, childbirth and the puerperium (O23.-, O75.3, O85, O86.-)

🔵 **N70 Salpingitis and oophoritis**
INCLUDES   *abscess (of) fallopian tube*
abscess (of) ovary
pyosalpinx
salpingo-oophoritis
tubo-ovarian abscess
tubo-ovarian inflammatory disease
Use additional code (B95-B97), to identify infectious agent.
EXCLUDES1   *gonococcal infection (A54.24)*
tuberculous infection (A18.17)

🔵 **N70.0 Acute salpingitis and oophoritis**
     N70.01 Acute salpingitis   CC ♀ CC/MCC Exc
     N70.02 Acute oophoritis   CC ♀ CC/MCC Exc
     N70.03 Acute salpingitis and oophoritis   CC ♀ CC/MCC Exc
🔵 **N70.1 Chronic salpingitis and oophoritis**
     Hydrosalpinx
     N70.11 Chronic salpingitis   ♀
     N70.12 Chronic oophoritis   ♀
     N70.13 Chronic salpingitis and oophoritis   ♀
🔵 **N70.9 Salpingitis and oophoritis, unspecified**
     N70.91 Salpingitis, unspecified   ♀
     N70.92 Oophoritis, unspecified   ♀
     N70.93 Salpingitis and oophoritis, unspecified   ♀

🔵 **N71 Inflammatory disease of uterus, except cervix**
INCLUDES   *endo (myo) metritis*
metritis
myometritis
pyometra
uterine abscess
Use additional code (B95-B97), to identify infectious agent.
EXCLUDES1   *hyperplastic endometritis (N85.0-)*
infection of uterus following delivery (O85, O86.-)
    N71.0 Acute inflammatory disease of uterus   CC ♀ CC/MCC Exc
    N71.1 Chronic inflammatory disease of uterus   ♀
    N71.9 Inflammatory disease of uterus, unspecified   ♀

    N72 Inflammatory disease of cervix uteri
INCLUDES   *cervicitis (with or without erosion or ectropion)*
endocervicitis (with or without erosion or ectropion)
exocervicitis (with or without erosion or ectropion)
Use additional code (B95-B97), to identify infectious agent.
EXCLUDES1   *erosion and ectropion of cervix without cervicitis (N86)*

🔵 **N73 Other female pelvic inflammatory diseases**
Use additional code (B95-B97), to identify infectious agent.
    N73.0 Acute parametritis and pelvic cellulitis   CC ♀ CC/MCC Exc
     Abscess of broad ligament
     Abscess of parametrium
     Pelvic cellulitis, female
    N73.1 Chronic parametritis and pelvic cellulitis   ♀
     Any condition in N73.0 specified as chronic
     EXCLUDES1   *tuberculous parametritis and pelvic cellulitis (A18.17)*
    N73.2 Unspecified parametritis and pelvic cellulitis   ♀
     Any condition in N73.0 unspecified whether acute or chronic
    N73.3 Female acute pelvic peritonitis   MCC ♀ CC/MCC Exc
    N73.4 Female chronic pelvic peritonitis   CC ♀ CC/MCC Exc
     EXCLUDES1   *tuberculous pelvic (female) peritonitis (A18.17)*
    N73.5 Female pelvic peritonitis, unspecified   ♀

    N73.6 Female pelvic peritoneal adhesions (postinfective)   ♀
     EXCLUDES2   *postprocedural pelvic peritoneal adhesions (N99.4)*
    N73.8 Other specified female pelvic inflammatory diseases   ♀
    N73.9 Female pelvic inflammatory disease, unspecified   ♀
     Female pelvic infection or inflammation NOS

    N74 Female pelvic inflammatory disorders in diseases classified elsewhere   ♀
☞ **Code first** underlying disease
EXCLUDES1   *chlamydial cervicitis (A56.02)*
chlamydial pelvic inflammatory disease (A56.11)
gonococcal cervicitis (A54.03)
gonococcal pelvic inflammatory disease (A54.24)
herpesviral [herpes simplex] cervicitis (A60.03)
herpesviral [herpes simplex] pelvic inflammatory disease (A60.09)
syphilitic cervicitis (A52.76)
syphilitic pelvic inflammatory disease (A52.76)
trichomonal cervicitis (A59.09)
tuberculous cervicitis (A18.16)
tuberculous pelvic inflammatory disease (A18.17)

🔵 **N75 Diseases of Bartholin's gland**
    N75.0 Cyst of Bartholin's gland   ♀
    N75.1 Abscess of Bartholin's gland   CC ♀ CC/MCC Exc
    N75.8 Other diseases of Bartholin's gland   ♀
     Bartholinitis
    N75.9 Disease of Bartholin's gland, unspecified   ♀

🔵 **N76 Other inflammation of vagina and vulva**
Use additional code (B95-B97), to identify infectious agent.
EXCLUDES2   *senile (atrophic) vaginitis (N95.2)*
vulvar vestibulitis (N94.810)
    N76.0 Acute vaginitis   ♀
     Acute vulvovaginitis
     Vaginitis NOS
     Vulvovaginitis NOS
    N76.1 Subacute and chronic vaginitis   ♀
     Chronic vulvovaginitis
     Subacute vulvovaginitis
    N76.2 Acute vulvitis   ♀
     Vulvitis NOS
    N76.3 Subacute and chronic vulvitis   ♀
    N76.4 Abscess of vulva   ♀
     Furuncle of vulva
    N76.5 Ulceration of vagina   ♀
    N76.6 Ulceration of vulva   ♀
🔵 **N76.8 Other specified inflammation of vagina and vulva**
     N76.81 Mucositis (ulcerative) of vagina and vulva   CC ♀ CC/MCC Exc
      Code also type of associated therapy, such as:
       antineoplastic and immunosuppressive drugs (T45.1X-)
       radiological procedure and radiotherapy (Y84.2)
      EXCLUDES2   *gastrointestinal mucositis (ulcerative) (K92.81)*
nasal mucositis (ulcerative) (J34.81)
oral mucositis (ulcerative) (K12.3-)
     N76.89 Other specified inflammation of vagina and vulva   ♀

🔵 **N77 Vulvovaginal ulceration and inflammation in diseases classified elsewhere**
    N77.0 Ulceration of vulva in diseases classified elsewhere   ♀
☞ **Code first** underlying disease, such as:
     Behçet's disease (M35.2)
     EXCLUDES1   *ulceration of vulva in gonococcal infection (A54.02)*
ulceration of vulva in herpesviral [herpes simplex] infection (A60.04)
ulceration of vulva in syphilis (A51.0)
ulceration of vulva in tuberculosis (A18.18)
    N77.1 Vaginitis, vulvitis and vulvovaginitis in diseases classified elsewhere   ♀
☞ **Code first** underlying disease, such as:
     pinworm (B80)

Unspecified Code   Other Specified Code   Manifestation Code   Ⓝ Newborn   Ⓟ Pediatric   Ⓜ Maternity   🅰 Adult   ♂ Male   ♀ Female
● New Code   ▲ Revised Code Title   ▶◀ Revised Text   NOTES   INCLUDES   EXCLUDES1 Not coded here   EXCLUDES2 Not included here
🔵 4th character required   🔵 5th character required   🔵 6th character required   🔵 7th character required   🔵 Extension 'X' Alert
HAC Hospital-acquired condition (HAC) alert   AHA AHA Coding Clinic©   ☞ Code first alert

EXCLUDES1 *candidal vulvovaginitis (B37.3)*
chlamydial vulvovaginitis (A56.02)
gonococcal vulvovaginitis (A54.02)
herpesviral [herpes simplex] vulvovaginitis (A60.04)
trichomonal vulvovaginitis (A59.01)
tuberculous vulvovaginitis (A18.18)
vulvovaginitis in early syphilis (A51.0)
vulvovaginitis in late syphilis (A52.76)

Noninflammatory disorders of female genital tract (N80-N98)

N80 Endometriosis
  N80.0 **Endometriosis of** uterus ♀
      Adenomyosis
      EXCLUDES1 *stromal endometriosis (D39.0)*
  N80.1 **Endometriosis of** ovary ♀
  N80.2 **Endometriosis of** fallopian tube ♀
  N80.3 **Endometriosis of** pelvic peritoneum ♀
  N80.4 **Endometriosis of** rectovaginal septum and vagina ♀
  N80.5 **Endometriosis of** intestine ♀
  N80.6 **Endometriosis in** cutaneous scar ♀
  N80.8 **Other endometriosis**
      Endometriosis of thorax
  N80.9 **Endometriosis, unspecified** ♀
N81 Female genital prolapse
  EXCLUDES1 *genital prolapse complicating pregnancy, labor or delivery (O34.5-)*
      prolapse and hernia of ovary and fallopian tube (N83.4-)
      prolapse of vaginal vault after hysterectomy (N99.3)
  N81.0 **Urethrocele** ♀
      EXCLUDES1 *urethrocele with cystocele (N81.1-)*
          urethrocele with prolapse of uterus (N81.2-N81.4)
  N81.1 **Cystocele**
      Cystocele with urethrocele
      Cystourethrocele
      EXCLUDES1 *cystocele with prolapse of uterus (N81.2-N81.4)*
      N81.10 **Cystocele, unspecified** ♀
          Prolapse of (anterior) vaginal wall NOS
      N81.11 **Cystocele,** midline ♀
      N81.12 **Cystocele,** lateral ♀
          Paravaginal cystocele
  N81.2 Incomplete **uterovaginal prolapse** ♀
      First degree uterine prolapse
      Prolapse of cervix NOS
      Second degree uterine prolapse
      EXCLUDES1 *cervical stump prolapse (N81.85)*
  N81.3 Complete **uterovaginal prolapse** ♀
      Procidentia (uteri) NOS
      Third degree uterine prolapse
  N81.4 **Uterovaginal prolapse, unspecified** ♀
      Prolapse of uterus NOS
  N81.5 **Vaginal** enterocele ♀
      EXCLUDES1 *enterocele with prolapse of uterus (N81.2-N81.4)*
  N81.6 **Rectocele** ♀
      Prolapse of posterior vaginal wall
      Use additional code for any associated fecal incontinence, if applicable (R15.-)
      EXCLUDES2 *perineocele (N81.81)*
          rectal prolapse (K62.3)
          rectocele with prolapse of uterus (N81.2-N81.4)
  N81.8 Other **female genital prolapse**
      N81.81 **Perineocele** ♀
      N81.82 **Incompetence or weakening of** pubocervical **tissue** ♀
      N81.83 **Incompetence or weakening of** rectovaginal **tissue** ♀
      N81.84 **Pelvic muscle wasting** ♀
          Disuse atrophy of pelvic muscles and anal sphincter

      N81.85 **Cervical stump prolapse** ♀
      N81.89 **Other female genital prolapse** ♀
          Deficient perineum
          Old laceration of muscles of pelvic floor
  N81.9 **Female genital prolapse, unspecified** ♀
N82 Fistulae involving female genital tract
  EXCLUDES1 *vesicointestinal fistulae (N32.1)*
  N82.0 Vesicovaginal **fistula** cc♀ CC/MCC Exc
  N82.1 **Other female urinary-genital tract fistulae** cc♀ CC/MCC Exc
      AHA: Q3 2017
      Cervicovesical fistula
      Ureterovaginal fistula
      Urethrovaginal fistula
      Uteroureteric fistula
      Uterovesical fistula
  N82.2 **Fistula of vagina to** small intestine cc♀ CC/MCC Exc
  N82.3 **Fistula of vagina to** large intestine cc♀ CC/MCC Exc
      Rectovaginal fistula
  N82.4 **Other female intestinal-genital tract fistulae** cc♀ CC/MCC Exc
      Intestinouterine fistula
  N82.5 **Female** genital tract-skin **fistulae** cc♀ CC/MCC Exc
      Uterus to abdominal wall fistula
      Vaginoperineal fistula
  N82.8 **Other female genital tract fistulae** cc♀ CC/MCC Exc
  N82.9 **Female genital tract fistula, unspecified** cc♀ CC/MCC Exc
N83 Noninflammatory disorders of ovary, fallopian tube and broad ligament
  EXCLUDES2 *hydrosalpinx (N70.1-)*
  N83.0 **Follicular cyst of ovary**
      Cyst of graafian follicle
      Hemorrhagic follicular cyst (of ovary)
      N83.00 **Follicular cyst of ovary, unspecified side** ♀
      N83.01 **Follicular cyst of** right **ovary** ♀
      N83.02 **Follicular cyst of** left **ovary** ♀
  N83.1 **Corpus luteum cyst**
      Hemorrhagic corpus luteum cyst
      N83.10 **Corpus luteum cyst of ovary, unspecified side** ♀
      N83.11 **Corpus luteum cyst of** right **ovary** ♀
      N83.12 **Corpus luteum cyst of** left **ovary** ♀
  N83.2 Other and unspecified **ovarian cysts**
      EXCLUDES1 *developmental ovarian cyst (Q50.1)*
          neoplastic ovarian cyst (D27.-)
          polycystic ovarian syndrome (E28.2)
          Stein-Leventhal syndrome (E28.2)
      N83.20 **Unspecified ovarian cysts**
          N83.201 **Unspecified ovarian cyst,** right **side** ♀
          N83.202 **Unspecified ovarian cyst,** left **side** ♀
          N83.209 **Unspecified ovarian cyst, unspecified side** ♀
              Ovarian cyst, NOS
      N83.29 **Other ovarian cysts**
          Retention cyst of ovary
          Simple cyst of ovary
          N83.291 **Other ovarian cyst,** right **side** ♀
          N83.292 **Other ovarian cyst,** left **side** ♀
          N83.299 **Other ovarian cyst, unspecified side** ♀
  N83.3 Acquired atrophy **of ovary and fallopian tube**
      N83.31 **Acquired atrophy of** ovary
          N83.311 **Acquired atrophy of** right **ovary** ♀
          N83.312 **Acquired atrophy of** left **ovary** ♀
          N83.319 **Acquired atrophy of ovary, unspecified side** ♀
              Acquired atrophy of ovary, NOS
      N83.32 **Acquired atrophy of** fallopian tube
          N83.321 **Acquired atrophy of** right **fallopian tube** ♀
          N83.322 **Acquired atrophy of** left **fallopian tube** ♀
          N83.329 **Acquired atrophy of fallopian tube, unspecified side** ♀
              Acquired atrophy of fallopian tube, NOS

PDx Unacceptable principal diagnosis symbol per Medicare code edits   POA Code exempt from diagnosis present on admission requirement
? Questionable admission   cc Complication or comorbidity   MCC Major complication or comorbidity   CC/MCC Exc CC/MCC exclusion
HCC HCC diagnosis code   RxHCC RxHCC diagnosis code   MACRA code   **DEFINITION** Describes condition/terminology
TIP Coding guidance   👁 Official Guideline Reference   Z1 Z code as first-listed diagnosis

6th N83.33 Acquired atrophy of ovary and fallopian tube

N83.331 Acquired atrophy of right ovary and fallopian tube ♀

N83.332 Acquired atrophy of left ovary and fallopian tube ♀

N83.339 Acquired atrophy of ovary and fallopian tube, unspecified side ♀

Acquired atrophy of ovary and fallopian tube, NOS

5th N83.4 Prolapse and hernia of ovary and fallopian tube

N83.40 Prolapse and hernia of ovary and fallopian tube, unspecified side ♀

Prolapse and hernia of ovary and fallopian tube, NOS

N83.41 Prolapse and hernia of right ovary and fallopian tube ♀

N83.42 Prolapse and hernia of left ovary and fallopian tube ♀

5th N83.5 Torsion of ovary, ovarian pedicle and fallopian tube

Torsion of accessory tube

6th N83.51 Torsion of ovary and ovarian pedicle

N83.511 Torsion of right ovary and ovarian pedicle CC ♀ CC/MCC Exc

N83.512 Torsion of left ovary and ovarian pedicle CC ♀ CC/MCC Exc

N83.519 Torsion of ovary and ovarian pedicle, unspecified side CC ♀ CC/MCC Exc

Torsion of ovary and ovarian pedicle, NOS

6th N83.52 Torsion of fallopian tube

Torsion of hydatid of Morgagni

N83.521 Torsion of right fallopian tube CC ♀ CC/MCC Exc

N83.522 Torsion of left fallopian tube CC ♀ CC/MCC Exc

N83.529 Torsion of fallopian tube, unspecified side CC ♀ CC/MCC Exc

Torsion of fallopian tube, NOS

N83.53 Torsion of ovary, ovarian pedicle and fallopian tube CC ♀ CC/MCC Exc

N83.6 Hematosalpinx ♀

EXCLUDES1 hematosalpinx (with) (in):
hematocolpos (N89.7)
hematometra (N85.7)
tubal pregnancy (O00.1-)

N83.7 Hematoma of broad ligament ♀

N83.8 Other noninflammatory disorders of ovary, fallopian tube and broad ligament ♀

Broad ligament laceration syndrome [Allen-Masters]

N83.9 Noninflammatory disorder of ovary, fallopian tube and broad ligament, unspecified ♀

4th N84 Polyp of female genital tract

EXCLUDES1 adenomatous polyp (D28.-)
placental polyp (O90.89)

N84.0 Polyp of corpus uteri ♀

Polyp of endometrium
Polyp of uterus NOS
EXCLUDES1 polypoid endometrial hyperplasia (N85.0-)

N84.1 Polyp of cervix uteri ♀

Mucous polyp of cervix

N84.2 Polyp of vagina ♀

N84.3 Polyp of vulva ♀

Polyp of labia

N84.8 Polyp of other parts of female genital tract ♀

N84.9 Polyp of female genital tract, unspecified ♀

4th N85 Other noninflammatory disorders of uterus, except cervix

EXCLUDES1 endometriosis (N80.-)
inflammatory diseases of uterus (N71.-)
noninflammatory disorders of cervix, except malposition (N86-N88)
polyp of corpus uteri (N84.0)
uterine prolapse (N81.-)

5th N85.0 Endometrial hyperplasia

N85.00 Endometrial hyperplasia, unspecified ♀

Hyperplasia (adenomatous) (cystic) (glandular) of endometrium
Hyperplastic endometritis

N85.01 Benign endometrial hyperplasia ♀

Endometrial hyperplasia (complex) (simple) without atypia

N85.02 Endometrial intraepithelial neoplasia [EIN] ♀

Endometrial hyperplasia with atypia
EXCLUDES1 malignant neoplasm of endometrium (with endometrial intraepithelial neoplasia [EIN]) (C54.1)

N85.2 Hypertrophy of uterus ♀

Bulky or enlarged uterus
EXCLUDES1 puerperal hypertrophy of uterus (O90.89)

N85.3 Subinvolution of uterus ♀

EXCLUDES1 puerperal subinvolution of uterus (O90.89)

N85.4 Malposition of uterus ♀

Anteversion of uterus
Retroflexion of uterus
Retroversion of uterus
EXCLUDES1 malposition of uterus complicating pregnancy, labor or delivery (O34.5-, O65.5)

N85.5 Inversion of uterus ♀

EXCLUDES1 current obstetric trauma (O71.2)
postpartum inversion of uterus (O71.2)

N85.6 Intrauterine synechiae ♀

N85.7 Hematometra ♀

Hematosalpinx with hematometra
EXCLUDES1 hematometra with hematocolpos (N89.7)

N85.8 Other specified noninflammatory disorders of uterus ♀

Atrophy of uterus, acquired
Fibrosis of uterus NOS

N85.9 Noninflammatory disorder of uterus, unspecified ♀

Disorder of uterus NOS

N86 Erosion and ectropion of cervix uteri ♀

Decubitus (trophic) ulcer of cervix
Eversion of cervix
EXCLUDES1 erosion and ectropion of cervix with cervicitis (N72)

4th N87 Dysplasia of cervix uteri

DEFINITION: Precancerous condition of abnormal cells on the cervix or within the endocervical canal.

EXCLUDES1 abnormal results from cervical cytologic examination without histologic confirmation (R87.61-)
carcinoma in situ of cervix uteri (D06.-)
cervical intraepithelial neoplasia III [CIN III] (D06.-)
HGSIL of cervix (R87.613)
severe dysplasia of cervix uteri (D06.-)

N87.0 Mild cervical dysplasia ♀

Cervical intraepithelial neoplasia I [CIN I]

N87.1 Moderate cervical dysplasia ♀

Cervical intraepithelial neoplasia II [CIN II]

N87.9 Dysplasia of cervix uteri, unspecified ♀

Anaplasia of cervix
Cervical atypism
Cervical dysplasia NOS

4th N88 Other noninflammatory disorders of cervix uteri

EXCLUDES2 inflammatory disease of cervix (N72)
polyp of cervix (N84.1)

N88.0 Leukoplakia of cervix uteri ♀

N88.1 Old laceration of cervix uteri ♀

Adhesions of cervix
EXCLUDES1 current obstetric trauma (O71.3)

N88.2 Stricture and stenosis of cervix uteri ♀

EXCLUDES1 stricture and stenosis of cervix uteri complicating labor (O65.5)

N88.3 **Incompetence** of cervix uteri ♀
Investigation and management of (suspected) cervical
incompetence in a nonpregnant woman
EXCLUDES1 *cervical incompetence complicating pregnancy
(O34.3-)*

N88.4 **Hypertrophic elongation of cervix uteri** ♀

N88.8 **Other specified noninflammatory disorders of cervix uteri** ♀
EXCLUDES1 *current obstetric trauma (O71.3)*

N88.9 **Noninflammatory disorder of cervix uteri, unspecified** ♀

4ᵗʰ N89 Other **noninflammatory disorders of vagina**
EXCLUDES1 *abnormal results from vaginal cytologic examination
without histologic confirmation (R87.62-)*
carcinoma in situ of vagina (D07.2)
HGSIL of vagina (R87.623)
inflammation of vagina (N76.-)
senile (atrophic) vaginitis (N95.2)
severe dysplasia of vagina (D07.2)
trichomonal leukorrhea (A59.00)
vaginal intraepithelial neoplasia [VAIN], grade III (D07.2)

N89.0 **Mild vaginal dysplasia** ♀
Vaginal intraepithelial neoplasia [VAIN], grade I

N89.1 **Moderate vaginal dysplasia** ♀
Vaginal intraepithelial neoplasia [VAIN], grade II

N89.3 **Dysplasia of vagina, unspecified** ♀

N89.4 **Leukoplakia of vagina** ♀

N89.5 **Stricture and atresia of vagina** ♀
Vaginal adhesions
Vaginal stenosis
EXCLUDES1 *congenital atresia or stricture (Q52.4)*
postprocedural adhesions of vagina (N99.2)

N89.6 **Tight hymenal ring** ♀
Rigid hymen
Tight introitus
EXCLUDES1 *imperforate hymen (Q52.3)*

N89.7 **Hematocolpos** ♀
AHA: Q4 2016
Hematocolpos with hematometra or hematosalpinx

N89.8 **Other specified noninflammatory disorders of vagina** ♀
Leukorrhea NOS
Old vaginal laceration
Pessary ulcer of vagina
EXCLUDES1 *current obstetric trauma (O70.-, O71.4, O71.7-O71.8)*
*old laceration involving muscles of pelvic floor
(N81.8)*

N89.9 **Noninflammatory disorder of vagina, unspecified** ♀

4ᵗʰ N90 Other **noninflammatory disorders of vulva and perineum**
EXCLUDES1 *anogenital (venereal) warts (A63.0)*
carcinoma in situ of vulva (D07.1)
condyloma acuminatum (A63.0)
current obstetric trauma (O70.-, O71.7-O71.8)
inflammation of vulva (N76.-)
severe dysplasia of vulva (D07.1)
vulvar intraepithelial neoplasm III [VIN III] (D07.1)

N90.0 **Mild vulvar dysplasia** ♀
Vulvar intraepithelial neoplasia [VIN], grade I

N90.1 **Moderate vulvar dysplasia** ♀
Vulvar intraepithelial neoplasia [VIN], grade II

N90.3 **Dysplasia of vulva, unspecified** ♀

N90.4 **Leukoplakia of vulva** ♀
Dystrophy of vulva
Kraurosis of vulva
Lichen sclerosus of external female genital organs

N90.5 **Atrophy of vulva** ♀
Stenosis of vulva

5ᵗʰ N90.6 **Hypertrophy of vulva**
N90.60 **Unspecified hypertrophy of vulva** ♀
AHA: Q4 2016
Unspecified hypertrophy of labia

N90.61 **Childhood asymmetric labium majus enlargement** ♀
AHA: Q4 2016
CALME

N90.69 **Other specified hypertrophy of vulva** ♀
AHA: Q4 2016
Other specified hypertrophy of labia

N90.7 **Vulvar cyst** ♀

5ᵗʰ N90.8 Other specified **noninflammatory disorders of vulva and perineum**

6ᵗʰ N90.81 **Female genital mutilation status**
Female genital cutting status

N90.810 **Female genital mutilation status, unspecified** ♀
Female genital cutting status, unspecified
Female genital mutilation status NOS

N90.811 **Female genital mutilation Type I status** ♀
Clitorectomy status
Female genital cutting Type I status

N90.812 **Female genital mutilation Type II status** ♀
Clitorectomy with excision of labia minora status
Female genital cutting Type II status

N90.813 **Female genital mutilation Type III status** ♀
Female genital cutting Type III status
Infibulation status

N90.818 **Other female genital mutilation status** ♀
Female genital cutting Type IV status
Female genital mutilation Type IV status
Other female genital cutting status

N90.89 **Other specified noninflammatory disorders of vulva and perineum** ♀
Adhesions of vulva
Hypertrophy of clitoris

N90.9 **Noninflammatory disorder of vulva and perineum, unspecified** ♀

4ᵗʰ N91 **Absent, scanty and rare menstruation**
EXCLUDES1 *ovarian dysfunction (E28.-)*

N91.0 **Primary amenorrhea** ♀
N91.1 **Secondary amenorrhea** ♀
N91.2 **Amenorrhea, unspecified** ♀
N91.3 **Primary oligomenorrhea** ♀
N91.4 **Secondary oligomenorrhea** ♀
N91.5 **Oligomenorrhea, unspecified** ♀
Hypomenorrhea NOS

4ᵗʰ N92 **Excessive, frequent and irregular menstruation**
EXCLUDES1 *postmenopausal bleeding (N95.0)*
precocious puberty (menstruation) (E30.1)

N92.0 **Excessive and frequent menstruation with regular cycle** ♀
Heavy periods NOS
Menorrhagia NOS
Polymenorrhea

N92.1 **Excessive and frequent menstruation with irregular cycle** ♀
Irregular intermenstrual bleeding
Irregular, shortened intervals between menstrual bleeding
Menometrorrhagia
Metrorrhagia

N92.2 **Excessive menstruation at puberty** P ♀
Excessive bleeding associated with onset of menstrual periods
Pubertal menorrhagia
Puberty bleeding

N92.3 **Ovulation bleeding** ♀
Regular intermenstrual bleeding

N92.4 **Excessive bleeding in the premenopausal period** ♀
Climacteric menorrhagia or metrorrhagia
Menopausal menorrhagia or metrorrhagia
Perimenopausal bleeding
Perimenopausal menorrhagia or metrorrhagia
Preclimacteric menorrhagia or metrorrhagia
Premenopausal menorrhagia or metrorrhagia

N92.5 **Other specified irregular menstruation** ♀

N92.6 Irregular menstruation, unspecified ♀
Irregular bleeding NOS
Irregular periods NOS
EXCLUDES1 irregular menstruation with:
lengthened intervals or scanty bleeding
(N91.3-N91.5)
shortened intervals or excessive bleeding (N92.1)

4ᵗʰ **N93 Other abnormal uterine and vaginal bleeding**
EXCLUDES1 neonatal vaginal hemorrhage (P54.6)
precocious puberty (menstruation) (E30.1)
pseudomenses (P54.6)
N93.0 Postcoital and contact bleeding ♀
N93.1 Pre-pubertal vaginal bleeding ♀
AHA: Q4 2016
N93.8 Other specified abnormal uterine and vaginal bleeding
Dysfunctional or functional uterine or vaginal bleeding NOS
N93.9 Abnormal uterine and vaginal bleeding, unspecified ♀

4ᵗʰ **N94 Pain and other conditions associated with female genital organs and menstrual cycle**
N94.0 Mittelschmerz ♀
5ᵗʰ **N94.1 Dyspareunia**
EXCLUDES1 psychogenic dyspareunia (F52.6)
N94.10 Unspecified dyspareunia ♀
AHA: Q4 2016
N94.11 Superficial (introital) dyspareunia ♀
AHA: Q4 2016
N94.12 Deep dyspareunia ♀
AHA: Q4 2016
N94.19 Other specified dyspareunia ♀
AHA: Q4 2016
N94.2 Vaginismus ♀
EXCLUDES1 psychogenic vaginismus (F52.5)
N94.3 Premenstrual tension syndrome ♀
AHA: Q4 2016
Code also associated menstrual migraine (G43.82-, G43.83-)
EXCLUDES1 Premenstrual dysphoric disorder (F32.81)
N94.4 Primary dysmenorrhea ♀
N94.5 Secondary dysmenorrhea ♀
N94.6 Dysmenorrhea, unspecified ♀
EXCLUDES1 psychogenic dysmenorrhea (F45.8)
5ᵗʰ **N94.8 Other specified conditions associated with female genital organs and menstrual cycle**
6ᵗʰ **N94.81 Vulvodynia**
N94.810 Vulvar vestibulitis ♀
N94.818 Other vulvodynia ♀
N94.819 Vulvodynia, unspecified ♀
Vulvodynia NOS
N94.89 Other specified conditions associated with female genital organs and menstrual cycle ♀
N94.9 Unspecified condition associated with female genital organs and menstrual cycle ♀

4ᵗʰ **N95 Menopausal and other perimenopausal disorders**
Menopausal and other perimenopausal disorders due to naturally occurring (age-related) menopause and perimenopause
EXCLUDES1 excessive bleeding in the premenopausal period (N92.4)
menopausal and perimenopausal disorders due to artificial or premature menopause (E89.4-, E28.31-)
premature menopause (E28.31-)
EXCLUDES2 postmenopausal osteoporosis (M81.0-)
postmenopausal osteoporosis with current pathological fracture (M80.0-)
postmenopausal urethritis (N34.2)
N95.0 Postmenopausal bleeding ♀
N95.1 Menopausal and female climacteric states ♀
Symptoms such as flushing, sleeplessness, headache, lack of concentration, associated with natural (age-related) menopause
Use additional code for associated symptoms

EXCLUDES1 asymptomatic menopausal state (Z78.0)
symptoms associated with artificial menopause (E89.41)
symptoms associated with premature menopause (E28.310)
N95.2 Postmenopausal atrophic vaginitis ♀
Senile (atrophic) vaginitis
N95.8 Other specified menopausal and perimenopausal disorders ♀
N95.9 Unspecified menopausal and perimenopausal disorder ♀

N96 Recurrent pregnancy loss
Investigation or care in a nonpregnant woman with history of recurrent pregnancy loss
EXCLUDES1 recurrent pregnancy loss with current pregnancy (O26.2-)

4ᵗʰ **N97 Female infertility**
INCLUDES inability to achieve a pregnancy
sterility, female NOS
EXCLUDES1 female infertility associated with:
hypopituitarism (E23.0)
Stein-Leventhal syndrome (E28.2)
EXCLUDES2 incompetence of cervix uteri (N88.3)
N97.0 Female infertility associated with anovulation ♀
N97.1 Female infertility of tubal origin ♀
Female infertility associated with congenital anomaly of tube
Female infertility due to tubal block
Female infertility due to tubal occlusion
Female infertility due to tubal stenosis
N97.2 Female infertility of uterine origin ♀
Female infertility associated with congenital anomaly of uterus
Female infertility due to nonimplantation of ovum
N97.8 Female infertility of other origin ♀
N97.9 Female infertility, unspecified ♀

4ᵗʰ **N98 Complications associated with artificial fertilization**
N98.0 Infection associated with artificial insemination cc ♀ CC/MCC Exc
N98.1 Hyperstimulation of ovaries cc ♀ CC/MCC Exc
Hyperstimulation of ovaries NOS
Hyperstimulation of ovaries associated with induced ovulation
N98.2 Complications of attempted introduction of fertilized ovum following in vitro fertilization cc ♀ CC/MCC Exc
N98.3 Complications of attempted introduction of embryo in embryo transfer cc ♀ CC/MCC Exc
N98.8 Other complications associated with artificial fertilization cc ♀ CC/MCC Exc
N98.9 Complication associated with artificial fertilization, unspecified cc ♀ CC/MCC Exc

Intraoperative and postprocedural complications and disorders of genitourinary system, not elsewhere classified (N99)

4ᵗʰ **N99 Intraoperative and postprocedural complications and disorders of genitourinary system, not elsewhere classified**
EXCLUDES2 irradiation cystitis (N30.4-)
postoophorectomy osteoporosis with current pathological fracture (M80.8-)
postoophorectomy osteoporosis without current pathological fracture (M81.8)
N99.0 Postprocedural (acute) (chronic) kidney failure
Use additional code to type of kidney disease
5ᵗʰ **N99.1 Postprocedural urethral stricture**
Postcatheterization urethral stricture
6ᵗʰ **N99.11 Postprocedural urethral stricture, male**
N99.110 Postprocedural urethral stricture, male, meatal ♂
N99.111 Postprocedural bulbous urethral stricture, male ♂
N99.112 Postprocedural membranous urethral stricture, male ♂

Unspecified Code   Other Specified Code   Manifestation Code   N Newborn   P Pediatric   M Maternity   A Adult   ♂ Male   ♀ Female
● New Code   ▲ Revised Code Title   ►◄ Revised Text   **NOTES**   *INCLUDES*   *EXCLUDES1* Not coded here   *EXCLUDES2* Not included here
4ᵗʰ 4ᵗʰ character required   5ᵗʰ 5ᵗʰ character required   6ᵗʰ 6ᵗʰ character required   7ᵗʰ 7ᵗʰ character required   Extension 'X' Alert
HAC Hospital-acquired condition (HAC) alert   **AHA** AHA Coding Clinic©   ☛ Code first alert

N99.113 **Postprocedural** anterior bulbous **urethral stricture, male** ♂

AHA: Q4 2016

N99.114 **Postprocedural urethral stricture, male, unspecified** ♂

N99.115 **Postprocedural** fossa navicularis **urethral stricture** ♂

AHA: Q4 2016

N99.116 **Postprocedural urethral stricture, male, overlapping sites** ♂

AHA: Q4 2018

N99.12 **Postprocedural urethral stricture,** female ♀

N99.2 **Postprocedural** adhesions of vagina ♀

N99.3 Prolapse of vaginal vault **after hysterectomy** ♀

N99.4 **Postprocedural** pelvic peritoneal adhesions

EXCLUDES2 pelvic peritoneal adhesions NOS (N73.6)

postinfective pelvic peritoneal adhesions (N73.6)

5ᵗʰ N99.5 **Complications of stoma of urinary tract**

EXCLUDES2 mechanical complication of urinary catheter (T83.0-)

6ᵗʰ N99.51 **Complication of** cystostomy

N99.510 **Cystostomy** hemorrhage cᶜ HCC CC/MCC Exc

N99.511 **Cystostomy** infection cᶜ HCC CC/MCC Exc

N99.512 **Cystostomy** malfunction cᶜ HCC CC/MCC Exc

N99.518 **Other cystostomy complication** cᶜ HCC CC/MCC Exc

6ᵗʰ N99.52 **Complication of** incontinent external stoma **of urinary tract**

N99.520 Hemorrhage **of incontinent external stoma of urinary tract** HCC

N99.521 Infection **of incontinent external stoma of urinary tract** HCC

AHA: Q4 2016

N99.522 Malfunction **of incontinent external stoma of urinary tract** HCC

N99.523 Herniation **of incontinent stoma of urinary tract** HCC

AHA: Q4 2016

N99.524 Stenosis **of incontinent stoma of urinary tract** HCC

AHA: Q4 2016

N99.528 Other complication **of incontinent external stoma of urinary tract** HCC

6ᵗʰ N99.53 **Complication of** continent stoma **of urinary tract**

N99.530 Hemorrhage **of continent stoma of urinary tract** HCC

N99.531 Infection **of continent stoma of urinary tract** HCC

N99.532 Malfunction **of continent stoma of urinary tract** HCC

N99.533 Herniation **of continent stoma of urinary tract** HCC

AHA: Q4 2016

N99.534 Stenosis **of continent stoma of urinary tract** HCC

AHA: Q4 2016

N99.538 Other complication **of continent stoma of urinary tract** HCC

5ᵗʰ N99.6 Intraoperative hemorrhage and hematoma **of a genitourinary system organ or structure complicating a procedure**

EXCLUDES1 intraoperative hemorrhage and hematoma of a genitourinary system organ or structure due to accidental puncture or laceration during a procedure (N99.7-)

N99.61 **Intraoperative hemorrhage and hematoma of a genitourinary system organ or structure complicating a** genitourinary system procedure cᶜ CC/MCC Exc

N99.62 **Intraoperative hemorrhage and hematoma of a genitourinary system organ or structure complicating** other procedure cᶜ CC/MCC Exc

5ᵗʰ N99.7 Accidental puncture and laceration **of a genitourinary system organ or structure during a procedure**

N99.71 **Accidental puncture and laceration of a genitourinary system organ or structure during a** genitourinary system procedure cᶜ CC/MCC Exc

N99.72 **Accidental puncture and laceration of a genitourinary system organ or structure during** other procedure cᶜ CC/MCC Exc

5ᵗʰ N99.8 Other **intraoperative and postprocedural complications and disorders of genitourinary system**

N99.81 **Other** intraoperative complications **of genitourinary system**

6ᵗʰ N99.82 Postprocedural hemorrhage **of a genitourinary system organ or structure following a procedure**

N99.820 **Postprocedural hemorrhage of a genitourinary system organ or structure following a** genitourinary system procedure cᶜ CC/MCC Exc

N99.821 **Postprocedural hemorrhage of a genitourinary system organ or structure following** other procedure cᶜ CC/MCC Exc

N99.83 Residual ovary syndrome ♀

6ᵗʰ N99.84 Postprocedural hematoma and seroma **of a genitourinary system organ or structure following a procedure**

N99.840 **Postprocedural** hematoma **of a genitourinary system organ or structure following a** genitourinary system procedure cᶜ CC/MCC Exc

N99.841 **Postprocedural** hematoma **of a genitourinary system organ or structure following** other procedure cᶜ CC/MCC Exc

N99.842 **Postprocedural** seroma **of a genitourinary system organ or structure following a** genitourinary system procedure cᶜ CC/MCC Exc

N99.843 **Postprocedural** seroma **of a genitourinary system organ or structure following** other procedure cᶜ CC/MCC Exc

N99.85 **Post endometrial** ablation syndrome ♀

N99.89 **Other postprocedural** complications and disorders **of genitourinary system**

PDxㅤ Unacceptable principal diagnosis symbol per Medicare code edits ㅤPDx Code exempt from diagnosis present on admission requirement

❓ Questionable admission cᶜ Complication or comorbidity ᴹᶜᶜ Major complication or comorbidity CC/MCC Exc CC/MCC exclusion

HCC HCC diagnosis code RxHCC RxHCC diagnosis code MACRA code **DEFINITION** Describes condition/terminology

TIP Coding guidance 👁 Official Guideline Reference Z1 Z code as first-listed diagnosis

880

When symbols appear on a code that requires a 7th character extension, refer to Appendix B to identify applicable 7th character codes.

2020 ICD-10-CM

Anatomy of the Female Reproductive System

Introduction

The female reproductive system includes the external genitalia, and accessory ducts and glands, that function to procreate offspring.

1. **The female reproductive system includes the following:**
   a) The ovaries or female gonads are the primary sex organs of the female reproductive system.
   b) The uterine (or fallopian) tubes, uterus, vagina and external genitalia serve as the accessory organs of the female reproductive system.
   c) The accessory glands act to produce the mucus for providing lubrication during sexual intercourse.

2. **The anatomy of structures/components of the female reproductive system is further described below:**
   a) **The Ovaries**
      i) Ovaries are the paired glands in the upper pelvic cavity and remain located on each side of the uterus.
      ii) Capsule of the ovary is termed as the tunica albuginea. The outer region of the ovarian capsule is known as the cortex, which contains the ovarian follicles (or eggs).
      iii) Ovaries facilitate the discharge of eggs in ovulation and secrete the female sex hormones estrogen and progesterone.
   b) **The Uterine (or Fallopian) Tubes**
      i) Fallopian tubes are two in number and serve to transport the ova from the ovaries to the uterus.
      ii) The open end of the fallopian tube is of the shape of a funnel and is known as the infundibulum. The infundibulum is surrounded by the fimbriae, which form a fringe of fingerlike projections.
   c) **The Uterus**
      i) The uterus is known as the site of menstruation and fetal development.
      ii) The uterus is a pear-shaped organ. The dome shaped part of the uterus above the uterine tubes is known as the fundus. The major tapering portion of the uterus is called the body. However, the narrow inferior part of the uterus is known as the cervix (or cervix uteri/neck of uterus).
      iii) The uterine cavity forms the interior of the body of uterus. The interior portion of the cervix is known as the cervical canal.
      iv) The internal os is the opening between the uterine wall and the cervical canal. The external os is the opening between the cervical canal and the vagina.
      v) The endometrium is the innermost layer of the uterine wall and forms the site of implantation of the fertilized egg.
      vi) The myometrium is the middle layer of the wall of uterus and composed of the smooth muscle.
      vii) The perimetrium (or visceral peritoneum) is the outermost layer of the uterine wall.
   d) **The Vagina**
      i) It provides a passage for the menstrual flow. It is the lower part of the birth canal and serves as a receptacle for the penis during sexual intercourse.
      ii) Its attachment to the cervix is surrounded by a recess, which is known as the fornix.
   e) **The External Genitalia of the Female**
      i) The external genitalia of the female are known as the vulva (or pudendum).
      ii) The mons pubis (or veneris) is a rounded eminence of adipose or fatty tissue upon the pubic symphysis.
      iii) The outer fatty folds of the vulva that extend from the mons pubis are known as the labia majora.
      iv) Inner and highly vascular connective tissue folds of the vulva are known as the labia minora. These folds lack hairs and are also known as the nymphae.
      v) The small mass of erectile tissue at the anterior junction of labia minora is known as the clitoris. The clitoris remains covered with a skin layer, which is known as the prepuce. The glans is the exposed part of the clitoris.
      vi) The vestibule is an opening between the folds of the labia minora. This opening contains a thin fold of tissue (or the hymen) that gets ruptured at the time of the first sexual intercourse.
      vii) The vestibule is further linked to the vaginal and urethral orifices.
      viii) Lesser vestibular or Skene's glands secrete mucus, and the openings of their ducts lie on each side of the urethral orifice.
      ix) Bartholin's or greater vestibular glands generate mucus to facilitate the process of sexual intercourse. The openings of these glands lie on each side of the vaginal orifice.
   f) **The Perineum**
      i) The perineum is a region between the thighs and buttocks of both males and females. This area marks the boundary of the pelvic outlet and provides passage to the urogenital ducts and rectum.
      ii) The perineum is further divided into an anterior urogenital triangle containing the external genitalia, and a posterior anal triangle containing the anus.
   g) **The Menstrual Cycle**
      i) The menstrual cycle is also known by the names of menstruation or menses.
      ii) The menstrual cycle is divided into the menstrual, proliferative, and secretory phases.
      iii) The shedding of the endometrial lining of uterus, blood, and tissue fluid occurs during the menstrual phase of the menstrual cycle.
      iv) The proliferative phase of the menstrual cycle is also known as the follicular phase. The lining of the uterus grows and proliferates during this phase. The process of ovulation also starts in the follicular phase, wherein the egg ruptures from the Graafian follicle and the rising estrogen levels cause the endometrial lining of the uterus to thicken. The follicle eventually collapses and gets transformed to the corpus luteum.
      v) The estrogen and progesterone hormones are secreted during the secretory phase of the menstrual cycle. The fertilization and implantation process can occur in this stage after the hymen rupture during the first sexual intercourse. The corpus luteum degenerates and gets transformed to corpus albicans if the fertilization and implantation processes do not occur during this phase.
      vi) Following fertilization, the development of placenta is started. The placenta facilitates the secretion of estrogen and progesterone hormones to support the pregnancy and breast development for the production of milk inside the mammary glands.
   h) **The Mammary Glands**
      i) They serve to produce milk in females and are found in both males and females.
      ii) The mammary ducts expand into milk storage sinuses (or ampullae) near the nipple.
      iii) The areola is a circular pigmented area around the nipple.
      iv) They facilitate the process of lactation (which includes milk production and its ejection from the nipple).
   i) **Pregnancy and Embryonic Development**
      i) Pregnancy is initiated with the formation of a viable zygote (or fertilized egg) by the union of the male sperm and the female ovum (or fertilization).
      ii) Fertilization occurs in the outer third portion of the fallopian tube.
      iii) The zygote travels down the uterine tube and forms the blastocyst or blastula through mitotic division.
      iv) The zygote eventually gets transformed to the chorionic vesicle in the uterine cavity. This chorionic vesicle secretes the chorionic gonadotropin hormone that gets embedded in the endometrial lining and maintains it via hormones.
      v) The ectoderm forms the outer layer of the germ cells and develops into skin and nervous system.
      vi) The endoderm initially consists of the flattened cells that form the epithelial linings of the internal organs.

vii) The mesoderm induces the formation of coelom (or the fluid-filled cavity within the mesoderm) and gives rise to muscles, bones, cartilages, connective tissues, and other structures.

viii) The chorionic villi are the projections of the trophoblast (or the fluid-filled sphere of the blastocyst). These chorionic villi communicate with the uterine tissue to form the placenta.

ix) The amnion is the fluid filled sac that surrounds and protects the embryo as the placenta is formed.

x) The umbilical cord or birth cord is the stalk that connects the fetus (or embryo) to the placenta.

xi) The placenta serves to exchange oxygen, nutrients, and wastes between the embryo and the mother.

xii) With the ongoing pregnancy, the uterus expands in the abdominal cavity for accommodating the growing fetus.

xiii) Childbirth (or parturition) is induced by uterine contractions, and this process is termed as the labor.

xiv) The dilation stage involves the complete dilation of the cervix by the head of the fetus. The amniotic fluid (or bag of waters) is also released during the rupture of the amnion.

xv) The child moves out through the cervix and vagina during the expulsion stage.

xvi) The placental stage (or afterbirth) is marked by the detachment of the placenta from the uterus following the birth.

Common Pathologies

Dysfunctional Uterine Bleeding (DUB)
Dysfunctional uterine bleeding, or DUB, refers to bleeding originating from the uterus due to changes in hormone levels, common in adolescents and women nearing menopause.

Endometriosis
Endometriosis is a condition in which the tissue that lines the inside of the uterus, known as the endometrium, grows outside of the uterus, including on other organs in the pelvis.

Fibroids
Uterine Fibroids (Figure 15.a), also known as myomas or leiomyomas, are solid, benign tumors made of fibrous tissue that develop and grow in the muscular walls of the uterus. They tend to form during a woman's childbearing years and may grow fast or slow. Symptoms include heavy or prolonged menstrual bleeding, pelvic pain, and urinary symptoms due to pressure on the bladder. There are four types of fibroids: intramural, subserosal, submucosal, and cervical.

i) Intramural
These are located in the wall of the uterus. These are the most common types of fibroids.

ii) Subserosal
These are located outside the wall of the uterus. They may grow in the form stalks, called pedunculated fibroids. Subserosal fibroids can become quite large.

iii) Submucosal
These are located in the muscle beneath the lining of the uterus wall.

iv) Cervical
These are located in the neck of the womb (the cervix).

Gonorrhea
Gonorrhea is a sexually transmitted disease, or STD, that results from infection with the bacterium Neisseria gonorrhoeae. It damages the reproductive system and can be passed from mother to baby during delivery.

Urinary Incontinence
Urinary incontinence refers to the inability to hold urine. It is often caused by weakness of the external sphincter muscle of the urethra, the duct through which urine exits the body. It is more common in women.

Polycystic Ovarian Syndrome (PCOS)
Polycystic ovarian syndrome, or PCOS, is characterized by small cysts on the ovaries and is associated with a hormone imbalance that results in a variety of symptoms, which may include infertility. PCOS is also known as Stein-Leventhal syndrome.

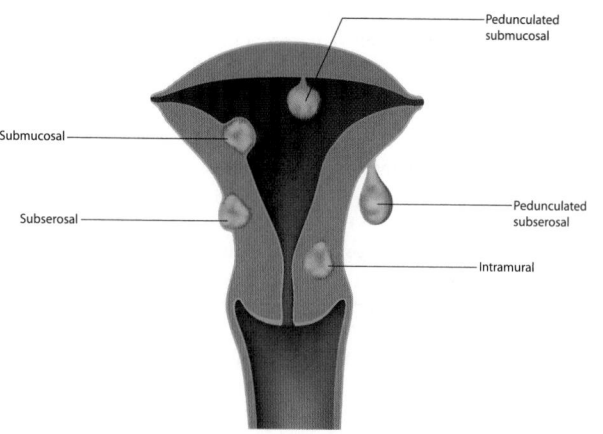

Figure 15.a   Uterine Fibroids

Pregnancy, childbirth and the puerperium (O00-O9A)

◉ See Official Guidelines "Codes from chapter 15 and sequencing priority" I.C.15.a.1

NOTES CODES FROM THIS CHAPTER ARE FOR USE ONLY ON MATERNAL RECORDS, NEVER ON NEWBORN RECORDS
Codes from this chapter are for use for conditions related to or aggravated by the pregnancy, childbirth, or by the puerperium (maternal causes or obstetric causes)
Trimesters are counted from the first day of the last menstrual period. They are defined as follows:
1st trimester- less than 14 weeks 0 days
2nd trimester- 14 weeks 0 days to less than 28 weeks 0 days
3rd trimester- 28 weeks 0 days until delivery

Use additional code from category Z3A, Weeks of gestation, to identify the specific week of the pregnancy, if known.

EXCLUDES1 supervision of normal pregnancy (Z34.-)

EXCLUDES2 mental and behavioral disorders associated with the puerperium (F53.-)
obstetrical tetanus (A34)
postpartum necrosis of pituitary gland (E23.0)
puerperal osteomalacia (M83.0)

This chapter contains the following blocks:

O00-O08 Pregnancy with abortive outcome
O09 Supervision of high risk pregnancy
O10-O16 Edema, proteinuria and hypertensive disorders in pregnancy, childbirth and the puerperium
O20-O29 Other maternal disorders predominantly related to pregnancy
O30-O48 Maternal care related to the fetus and amniotic cavity and possible delivery problems
O60-O77 Complications of labor and delivery
O80-O82 Encounter for delivery
O85-O92 Complications predominantly related to the puerperium
O94-O9A Other obstetric conditions, not elsewhere classified

Pregnancy with abortive outcome (O00-O08)

EXCLUDES1 continuing pregnancy in multiple gestation after abortion of one fetus or more (O31.1-, O31.3-)

④ **O00 Ectopic pregnancy**
DEFINITION: Pregnancy implanted outside of the uterus.
TIP: Code selection requires laterality.
INCLUDES ruptured ectopic pregnancy
Use additional code from category O08 to identify any associated complication

⑤ **O00.0 Abdominal pregnancy**
EXCLUDES1 maternal care for viable fetus in abdominal pregnancy (O36.7-)
O00.00 Abdominal pregnancy without intrauterine pregnancy Ⓜ ℃ ♀ CC/MCC Exc
AHA: Q4 2016
Abdominal pregnancy NOS
O00.01 Abdominal pregnancy with intrauterine pregnancy Ⓜ ℃ ♀ CC/MCC Exc
AHA: Q4 2016

⑤ **O00.1 Tubal pregnancy**
Fallopian pregnancy
Rupture of (fallopian) tube due to pregnancy
Tubal abortion
⑥ **O00.10 Tubal pregnancy** without intrauterine pregnancy
Tubal pregnancy NOS
O00.101 Right tubal pregnancy without intrauterine pregnancy Ⓜ ℃ ♀ CC/MCC Exc
O00.102 Left tubal pregnancy without intrauterine pregnancy Ⓜ ℃ ♀ CC/MCC Exc
O00.109 Unspecified tubal pregnancy without intrauterine pregnancy Ⓜ ℃ ♀ CC/MCC Exc
⑥ **O00.11 Tubal pregnancy** with intrauterine pregnancy
O00.111 Right tubal pregnancy with intrauterine pregnancy Ⓜ ℃ ♀ CC/MCC Exc
O00.112 Left tubal pregnancy with intrauterine pregnancy Ⓜ ℃ ♀ CC/MCC Exc

O00.119 Unspecified tubal pregnancy with intrauterine pregnancy Ⓜ ℃ ♀ CC/MCC Exc
⑤ **O00.2 Ovarian pregnancy**
⑥ **O00.20 Ovarian pregnancy** without intrauterine pregnancy
Ovarian pregnancy NOS
O00.201 Right ovarian pregnancy without intrauterine pregnancy Ⓜ ℃ ♀ CC/MCC Exc
O00.202 Left ovarian pregnancy without intrauterine pregnancy Ⓜ ℃ ♀ CC/MCC Exc
O00.209 Unspecified ovarian pregnancy without intrauterine pregnancy Ⓜ ℃ ♀ CC/MCC Exc
⑥ **O00.21 Ovarian pregnancy** with intrauterine pregnancy
O00.211 Right ovarian pregnancy with intrauterine pregnancy Ⓜ ℃ ♀ CC/MCC Exc
O00.212 Left ovarian pregnancy with intrauterine pregnancy Ⓜ ℃ ♀ CC/MCC Exc
O00.219 Unspecified ovarian pregnancy with intrauterine pregnancy Ⓜ ℃ ♀ CC/MCC Exc
⑤ **O00.8 Other ectopic pregnancy**
Cervical pregnancy
Cornual pregnancy
Intraligamentous pregnancy
Mural pregnancy
O00.80 Other ectopic pregnancy without intrauterine pregnancy Ⓜ ℃ ♀ CC/MCC Exc
AHA: Q4 2016
Other ectopic pregnancy NOS
O00.81 Other ectopic pregnancy with intrauterine pregnancy Ⓜ ℃ ♀ CC/MCC Exc
AHA: Q4 2016
⑤ **O00.9 Ectopic pregnancy, unspecified**
O00.90 Unspecified ectopic pregnancy without intrauterine pregnancy Ⓜ ℃ ♀ CC/MCC Exc
AHA: Q4 2016
Ectopic pregnancy NOS
O00.91 Unspecified ectopic pregnancy with intrauterine pregnancy Ⓜ ℃ ♀ CC/MCC Exc
AHA: Q4 2016

④ **O01 Hydatidiform mole**
DEFINITION: A clump or mass of tissue that does not develop into a fetus.
Use additional code from category O08 to identify any associated complication.
EXCLUDES1 chorioadenoma (destruens) (D39.2)
malignant hydatidiform mole (D39.2)
O01.0 Classical hydatidiform mole Ⓜ ♀
Complete hydatidiform mole
O01.1 Incomplete and partial hydatidiform mole Ⓜ ♀
O01.9 Hydatidiform mole, unspecified Ⓜ ♀
Trophoblastic disease NOS
Vesicular mole NOS

④ **O02 Other abnormal products of conception**
Use additional code from category O08 to identify any associated complication.
EXCLUDES1 papyraceous fetus (O31.0-)
O02.0 Blighted ovum and nonhydatidiform mole Ⓜ ♀
Carneous mole
Fleshy mole
Intrauterine mole NOS
Molar pregnancy NEC
Pathological ovum
O02.1 Missed abortion Ⓜ ♀
DEFINITION: Early fetal death, before completion of 20 weeks of gestation, with retention of dead fetus
EXCLUDES1 failed induced abortion (O07.-)
fetal death (intrauterine) (late) (O36.4)
missed abortion with blighted ovum (O02.0)
missed abortion with hydatidiform mole (O01.-)
missed abortion with nonhydatidiform (O02.0)
missed abortion with other abnormal products of conception (O02.8-)
missed delivery (O36.4)
stillbirth (P95)

Unspecified Code   Other Specified Code   Manifestation Code   Ⓝ Newborn   Ⓟ Pediatric   Ⓜ Maternity   Ⓐ Adult   ♂ Male   ♀ Female
● New Code   ▲ Revised Code Title   ►◄ Revised Text   **NOTES** INCLUDES EXCLUDES1 Not coded here   EXCLUDES2 Not included here
④ 4th character required   ⑤ 5th character required   ⑥ 6th character required   ⑦ 7th character required   ⑦ Extension 'X' Alert
HAC Hospital-acquired condition (HAC) alert   **AHA** AHA Coding Clinic©   ☛ Code first alert

O02.8 **Other specified abnormal products of conception**

EXCLUDES1 *abnormal products of conception with blighted ovum (O02.0)*

abnormal products of conception with hydatidiform mole (O01.-)

abnormal products of conception with nonhydatidiform mole (O02.0)

O02.81 **Inappropriate change in quantitative human chorionic gonadotropin (hCG) in early pregnancy** M ♀

Biochemical pregnancy

Chemical pregnancy

Inappropriate level of quantitative human chorionic gonadotropin (hCG) for gestational age in early pregnancy

O02.89 **Other abnormal products of conception** M ♀

O02.9 **Abnormal product of conception, unspecified** M ♀

O03 Spontaneous abortion

DEFINITION: Miscarriage, with symptoms of cramping, bleeding, expulsion of tissue.

NOTES Incomplete abortion includes retained products of conception following spontaneous abortion

INCLUDES *miscarriage*

O03.0 Genital tract and pelvic infection **following** incomplete **spontaneous abortion** M CC ♀ CC/MCC Exc

Endometritis following incomplete spontaneous abortion

Oophoritis following incomplete spontaneous abortion

Parametritis following incomplete spontaneous abortion

Pelvic peritonitis following incomplete spontaneous abortion

Salpingitis following incomplete spontaneous abortion

Salpingo-oophoritis following incomplete spontaneous abortion

EXCLUDES1 *sepsis following incomplete spontaneous abortion (O03.37)*

urinary tract infection following incomplete spontaneous abortion (O03.38)

O03.1 Delayed or excessive hemorrhage **following** incomplete **spontaneous abortion** M ♀

Afibrinogenemia following incomplete spontaneous abortion

Defibrination syndrome following incomplete spontaneous abortion

Hemolysis following incomplete spontaneous abortion

Intravascular coagulation following incomplete spontaneous abortion

O03.2 Embolism **following** incomplete **spontaneous abortion** M MCC ♀ CC/MCC Exc

Air embolism following incomplete spontaneous abortion

Amniotic fluid embolism following incomplete spontaneous abortion

Blood-clot embolism following incomplete spontaneous abortion

Embolism NOS following incomplete spontaneous abortion

Fat embolism following incomplete spontaneous abortion

Pulmonary embolism following incomplete spontaneous abortion

Pyemic embolism following incomplete spontaneous abortion

Septic or septicopyemic embolism following incomplete spontaneous abortion

Soap embolism following incomplete spontaneous abortion

O03.3 Other **and** unspecified complications **following** incomplete **spontaneous abortion**

O03.30 **Unspecified complication following incomplete spontaneous abortion** M CC ♀ CC/MCC Exc

O03.31 Shock **following incomplete spontaneous abortion** M MCC ♀ CC/MCC Exc

Circulatory collapse following incomplete spontaneous abortion

Shock (postprocedural) following incomplete spontaneous abortion

EXCLUDES1 *shock due to infection following incomplete spontaneous abortion (O03.37)*

O03.32 **Renal failure following incomplete spontaneous abortion** M MCC ♀ CC/MCC Exc

Kidney failure (acute) following incomplete spontaneous abortion

Oliguria following incomplete spontaneous abortion

Renal shutdown following incomplete spontaneous abortion

Renal tubular necrosis following incomplete spontaneous abortion

Uremia following incomplete spontaneous abortion

O03.33 Metabolic disorder **following incomplete spontaneous abortion** M CC ♀ CC/MCC Exc

O03.34 Damage to pelvic organs **following incomplete spontaneous abortion** M CC ♀ CC/MCC Exc

Laceration, perforation, tear or chemical damage of bladder following incomplete spontaneous abortion

Laceration, perforation, tear or chemical damage of bowel following incomplete spontaneous abortion

Laceration, perforation, tear or chemical damage of broad ligament following incomplete spontaneous abortion

Laceration, perforation, tear or chemical damage of cervix following incomplete spontaneous abortion

Laceration, perforation, tear or chemical damage of periurethral tissue following incomplete spontaneous abortion

Laceration, perforation, tear or chemical damage of uterus following incomplete spontaneous abortion

Laceration, perforation, tear or chemical damage of vagina following incomplete spontaneous abortion

O03.35 **Other** venous **complications following incomplete spontaneous abortion** M CC ♀ CC/MCC Exc

O03.36 Cardiac arrest **following incomplete spontaneous abortion** M CC ♀ CC/MCC Exc

O03.37 Sepsis **following incomplete spontaneous abortion** M CC ♀ CC/MCC Exc

Use additional code to identify infectious agent (B95-B97)

Use additional code to identify severe sepsis, if applicable (R65.2-)

EXCLUDES1 *septic or septicopyemic embolism following incomplete spontaneous abortion (O03.2)*

O03.38 Urinary tract infection **following incomplete spontaneous abortion** M CC ♀ CC/MCC Exc

Cystitis following incomplete spontaneous abortion

O03.39 **Incomplete spontaneous abortion with other** complications M CC ♀ CC/MCC Exc

O03.4 Incomplete spontaneous abortion without complication M ♀

See Official Guidelines "Retained Product of Conception following an abortion" I.C.15.q.2

AHA: Q4 2017

O03.5 **Genital tract and pelvic infection following complete or unspecified spontaneous abortion** M CC ♀ CC/MCC Exc

Endometritis following complete or unspecified spontaneous abortion

Oophoritis following complete or unspecified spontaneous abortion

Parametritis following complete or unspecified spontaneous abortion

Pelvic peritonitis following complete or unspecified spontaneous abortion

Salpingitis following complete or unspecified spontaneous abortion

Salpingo-oophoritis following complete or unspecified spontaneous abortion

EXCLUDES1 *sepsis following complete or unspecified spontaneous abortion (O03.87)*

urinary tract infection following complete or unspecified spontaneous abortion (O03.88)

O03.6 **Delayed or excessive hemorrhage following complete or unspecified spontaneous abortion** M ♀

Afibrinogenemia following complete or unspecified spontaneous abortion

---

1st 1st trimester 2nd 2nd trimester 3rd 3rd trimester PDx Unacceptable principal diagnosis symbol per Medicare code edits

POA Code exempt from diagnosis present on admission requirement ❓ Questionable admission CC Complication or comorbidity

MCC Major complication or comorbidity CC/MCC Exc CC/MCC exclusion HCC HCC diagnosis code RxHCC RxHCC diagnosis code MACRA code

DEFINITION Describes condition/terminology **TIP** Coding guidance 👁 Official Guideline Reference Z1 Z code as first-listed diagnosis

884

When symbols appear on a code that requires a 7th character extension, refer to Appendix B to identify applicable 7th character codes.

2020 ICD-10-CM

Defibrination syndrome following complete or unspecified spontaneous abortion

Hemolysis following complete or unspecified spontaneous abortion

Intravascular coagulation following complete or unspecified spontaneous abortion

O03.7 **Embolism following complete or unspecified spontaneous abortion** 🅼 cc♀ ♀ CC/MCC Exc

Air embolism following complete or unspecified spontaneous abortion

Amniotic fluid embolism following complete or unspecified spontaneous abortion

Blood-clot embolism following complete or unspecified spontaneous abortion

Embolism NOS following complete or unspecified spontaneous abortion

Fat embolism following complete or unspecified spontaneous abortion

Pulmonary embolism following complete or unspecified spontaneous abortion

Pyemic embolism following complete or unspecified spontaneous abortion

Septic or septicopyemic embolism following complete or unspecified spontaneous abortion

Soap embolism following complete or unspecified spontaneous abortion

🏵 **O03.8** Other and unspecified complications **following** complete or unspecified **spontaneous abortion**

O03.80 **Unspecified complication following complete or unspecified spontaneous abortion** 🅼 cc♀ ♀ CC/MCC Exc

O03.81 Shock **following complete or unspecified spontaneous abortion** 🅼 MCC♀ ♀ CC/MCC Exc

Circulatory collapse following complete or unspecified spontaneous abortion

Shock (postprocedural) following complete or unspecified spontaneous abortion

EXCLUDES1 *shock due to infection following complete or unspecified spontaneous abortion (O03.87)*

O03.82 Renal failure **following complete or unspecified spontaneous abortion** 🅼 MCC♀ ♀ CC/MCC Exc

Kidney failure (acute) following complete or unspecified spontaneous abortion

Oliguria following complete or unspecified spontaneous abortion

Renal shutdown following complete or unspecified spontaneous abortion

Renal tubular necrosis following complete or unspecified spontaneous abortion

Uremia following complete or unspecified spontaneous abortion

O03.83 Metabolic disorder **following complete or unspecified spontaneous abortion** 🅼 cc♀ ♀ CC/MCC Exc

O03.84 Damage to pelvic organs **following complete or unspecified spontaneous abortion** 🅼 cc♀ ♀ CC/MCC Exc

Laceration, perforation, tear or chemical damage of bladder following complete or unspecified spontaneous abortion

Laceration, perforation, tear or chemical damage of bowel following complete or unspecified spontaneous abortion

Laceration, perforation, tear or chemical damage of broad ligament following complete or unspecified spontaneous abortion

Laceration, perforation, tear or chemical damage of cervix following complete or unspecified spontaneous abortion

Laceration, perforation, tear or chemical damage of periurethral tissue following complete or unspecified spontaneous abortion

Laceration, perforation, tear or chemical damage of uterus following complete or unspecified spontaneous abortion

Laceration, perforation, tear or chemical damage of vagina following complete or unspecified spontaneous abortion

O03.85 **Other** venous **complications following complete or unspecified spontaneous abortion** 🅼 cc♀ ♀ CC/MCC Exc

O03.86 Cardiac arrest **following complete or unspecified spontaneous abortion** 🅼 cc♀ ♀ CC/MCC Exc

O03.87 Sepsis **following complete or unspecified spontaneous abortion** 🅼 cc♀ ♀ CC/MCC Exc

Use additional code to identify infectious agent (B95-B97)

Use additional code to identify severe sepsis, if applicable (R65.2-)

EXCLUDES1 *septic or septicopyemic embolism following complete or unspecified spontaneous abortion (O03.7)*

O03.88 Urinary tract infection **following complete or unspecified spontaneous abortion** 🅼 cc♀ ♀ CC/MCC Exc

Cystitis following complete or unspecified spontaneous abortion

O03.89 **Complete or unspecified spontaneous abortion** with other complications 🅼 cc♀ ♀ CC/MCC Exc

O03.9 **Complete or unspecified spontaneous abortion** without complication 🅼 ♀

Miscarriage NOS

Spontaneous abortion NOS

🅰 **O04** Complications **following (induced)** termination of pregnancy

👁 **See Official Guidelines** "Complications leading to abortion" I.C.15.q.3

INCLUDES *complications following (induced) termination of pregnancy*

EXCLUDES1 *encounter for elective termination of pregnancy, uncomplicated (Z33.2)*

failed attempted termination of pregnancy (O07.-)

O04.5 Genital tract and pelvic infection **following (induced) termination of pregnancy** 🅼 cc♀ ♀ CC/MCC Exc

Endometritis following (induced) termination of pregnancy

Oophoritis following (induced) termination of pregnancy

Parametritis following (induced) termination of pregnancy

Pelvic peritonitis following (induced) termination of pregnancy

Salpingitis following (induced) termination of pregnancy

Salpingo-oophoritis following (induced) termination of pregnancy

EXCLUDES1 *sepsis following (induced) termination of pregnancy (O04.87)*

urinary tract infection following (induced) termination of pregnancy (O04.88)

O04.6 Delayed or excessive hemorrhage **following (induced) termination of pregnancy** 🅼 ♀

Afibrinogenemia following (induced) termination of pregnancy

Defibrination syndrome following (induced) termination of pregnancy

Hemolysis following (induced) termination of pregnancy

Intravascular coagulation following (induced) termination of pregnancy

O04.7 Embolism **following (induced) termination of pregnancy** 🅼 MCC♀ ♀ CC/MCC Exc

Air embolism following (induced) termination of pregnancy

Amniotic fluid embolism following (induced) termination of pregnancy

Blood-clot embolism following (induced) termination of pregnancy

Embolism NOS following (induced) termination of pregnancy

Fat embolism following (induced) termination of pregnancy

Pulmonary embolism following (induced) termination of pregnancy

Pyemic embolism following (induced) termination of pregnancy

Septic or septicopyemic embolism following (induced) termination of pregnancy

Soap embolism following (induced) termination of pregnancy

🏵 **O04.8** **(Induced) termination of pregnancy** with other and unspecified complications

O04.80 **(Induced) termination of pregnancy with unspecified complications** 🅼 cc♀ ♀ CC/MCC Exc

Unspecified Code   Other Specified Code   Manifestation Code   🅽 Newborn   🅿 Pediatric   🅼 Maternity   🅰 Adult   ♂ Male   ♀ Female
● New Code   ▲ Revised Code Title   ►◄ Revised Text   **NOTES**   *INCLUDES*   *EXCLUDES1* Not coded here   *EXCLUDES2* Not included here
🅸 4th character required   🅕 5th character required   🅖 6th character required   🅗 7th character required   🅧 Extension 'X' Alert
HAC Hospital-acquired condition (HAC) alert   **AHA** AHA Coding Clinic®   📑 Code first alert

2020 ICD-10-CM   When symbols appear on a code that requires a 7th character extension, refer to Appendix B to identify applicable 7th character codes.   **885**

O04.81 Shock **following (induced) termination of pregnancy** Ⓜ MCC ♀ CC/MCC Exc

Circulatory collapse following (induced) termination of pregnancy

Shock (postprocedural) following (induced) termination of pregnancy

EXCLUDES1 *shock due to infection following (induced) termination of pregnancy (O04.87)*

O04.82 Renal failure **following (induced) termination of pregnancy** Ⓜ MCC ♀ CC/MCC Exc

Kidney failure (acute) following (induced) termination of pregnancy

Oliguria following (induced) termination of pregnancy

Renal shutdown following (induced) termination of pregnancy

Renal tubular necrosis following (induced) termination of pregnancy

Uremia following (induced) termination of pregnancy

O04.83 Metabolic disorder **following (induced) termination of pregnancy** Ⓜ CC ♀ CC/MCC Exc

O04.84 Damage to pelvic organs **following (induced) termination of pregnancy** Ⓜ CC ♀ CC/MCC Exc

Laceration, perforation, tear or chemical damage of bladder following (induced) termination of pregnancy

Laceration, perforation, tear or chemical damage of bowel following (induced) termination of pregnancy

Laceration, perforation, tear or chemical damage of broad ligament following (induced) termination of pregnancy

Laceration, perforation, tear or chemical damage of cervix following (induced) termination of pregnancy

Laceration, perforation, tear or chemical damage of periurethral tissue following (induced) termination of pregnancy

Laceration, perforation, tear or chemical damage of uterus following (induced) termination of pregnancy

Laceration, perforation, tear or chemical damage of vagina following (induced) termination of pregnancy

O04.85 Other venous **complications following (induced) termination of pregnancy** Ⓜ CC ♀ CC/MCC Exc

O04.86 Cardiac arrest **following (induced) termination of pregnancy** Ⓜ CC ♀ CC/MCC Exc

O04.87 Sepsis **following (induced) termination of pregnancy** Ⓜ CC ♀ CC/MCC Exc

Use additional code to identify infectious agent (B95-B97)

Use additional code to identify severe sepsis, if applicable (R65.2-)

EXCLUDES1 *septic or septicopyemic embolism following (induced) termination of pregnancy (O04.7)*

O04.88 Urinary tract infection **following (induced) termination of pregnancy** Ⓜ CC ♀ CC/MCC Exc

Cystitis following (induced) termination of pregnancy

O04.89 (Induced) termination of pregnancy with other **complications** Ⓜ CC ♀ CC/MCC Exc

🔵 **O07** Failed attempted termination **of pregnancy**

👁 **See Official Guidelines** "Complications leading to abortion" I.C.15.q.3

INCLUDES *failure of attempted induction of termination of pregnancy*

incomplete elective abortion

EXCLUDES1 *incomplete spontaneous abortion (O03.0-)*

O07.0 Genital tract and pelvic infection **following failed attempted termination of pregnancy** Ⓜ CC ♀ CC/MCC Exc

Endometritis following failed attempted termination of pregnancy

Oophoritis following failed attempted termination of pregnancy

Parametritis following failed attempted termination of pregnancy

Pelvic peritonitis following failed attempted termination of pregnancy

Salpingitis following failed attempted termination of pregnancy

Salpingo-oophoritis following failed attempted termination of pregnancy

EXCLUDES1 *sepsis following failed attempted termination of pregnancy (O07.37)*

urinary tract infection following failed attempted termination of pregnancy (O07.38)

O07.1 Delayed or excessive hemorrhage **following failed attempted termination of pregnancy** Ⓜ CC ♀ CC/MCC Exc

Afibrinogenemia following failed attempted termination of pregnancy

Defibrination syndrome following failed attempted termination of pregnancy

Hemolysis following failed attempted termination of pregnancy

Intravascular coagulation following failed attempted termination of pregnancy

O07.2 Embolism **following failed attempted termination of pregnancy** Ⓜ MCC ♀ CC/MCC Exc

Air embolism following failed attempted termination of pregnancy

Amniotic fluid embolism following failed attempted termination of pregnancy

Blood-clot embolism following failed attempted termination of pregnancy

Embolism NOS following failed attempted termination of pregnancy

Fat embolism following failed attempted termination of pregnancy

Pulmonary embolism following failed attempted termination of pregnancy

Pyemic embolism following failed attempted termination of pregnancy

Septic or septicopyemic embolism following failed attempted termination of pregnancy

Soap embolism following failed attempted termination of pregnancy

5ᵗʰ **O07.3** Failed attempted termination of pregnancy with other and unspecified complications

O07.30 Failed attempted termination of pregnancy with unspecified complications Ⓜ CC ♀ CC/MCC Exc

O07.31 Shock **following failed attempted termination of pregnancy** Ⓜ MCC ♀ CC/MCC Exc

Circulatory collapse following failed attempted termination of pregnancy

Shock (postprocedural) following failed attempted termination of pregnancy

EXCLUDES1 *shock due to infection following failed attempted termination of pregnancy (O07.37)*

O07.32 Renal failure **following failed attempted termination of pregnancy** Ⓜ MCC ♀ CC/MCC Exc

Kidney failure (acute) following failed attempted termination of pregnancy

Oliguria following failed attempted termination of pregnancy

Renal shutdown following failed attempted termination of pregnancy

Renal tubular necrosis following failed attempted termination of pregnancy

Uremia following failed attempted termination of pregnancy

O07.33 Metabolic disorder **following failed attempted termination of pregnancy** Ⓜ CC ♀ CC/MCC Exc

O07.34 Damage to pelvic organs **following failed attempted termination of pregnancy** Ⓜ CC ♀ CC/MCC Exc

Laceration, perforation, tear or chemical damage of bladder following failed attempted termination of pregnancy

Laceration, perforation, tear or chemical damage of bowel following failed attempted termination of pregnancy

886

When symbols appear on a code that requires a 7th character extension, refer to Appendix B to identify applicable 7th character codes.

2020 ICD-10-CM

1st 1st trimester   2nd 2nd trimester   3rd 3rd trimester   PDx Unacceptable principal diagnosis symbol per Medicare code edits

POA Code exempt from diagnosis present on admission requirement   ❓ Questionable admission   CC Complication or comorbidity

MCC Major complication or comorbidity   CC/MCC Exc CC/MCC exclusion   HCC HCC diagnosis code   RxHCC RxHCC diagnosis code   MACRA code

DEFINITION Describes condition/terminology   **TIP** Coding guidance   👁 Official Guideline Reference   Z1 Z code as first-listed diagnosis

Laceration, perforation, tear or chemical damage of broad ligament following failed attempted termination of pregnancy
Laceration, perforation, tear or chemical damage of cervix following failed attempted termination of pregnancy
Laceration, perforation, tear or chemical damage of periurethral tissue following failed attempted termination of pregnancy
Laceration, perforation, tear or chemical damage of uterus following failed attempted termination of pregnancy
Laceration, perforation, tear or chemical damage of vagina following failed attempted termination of pregnancy

O07.35 Other venous complications following failed attempted termination of pregnancy [M] [CC] ♀ [CC/MCC Exc]

O07.36 Cardiac arrest following failed attempted termination of pregnancy [M] [CC] ♀ [CC/MCC Exc]

O07.37 Sepsis following failed attempted termination of pregnancy [M] [CC] ♀ [CC/MCC Exc]
Use additional code (B95-B97), to identify infectious agent
Use additional code (R65.2-) to identify severe sepsis, if applicable
[EXCLUDES1] *septic or septicopyemic embolism following failed attempted termination of pregnancy (O07.2)*

O07.38 Urinary tract infection following failed attempted termination of pregnancy [M] [CC] ♀ [CC/MCC Exc]
Cystitis following failed attempted termination of pregnancy

O07.39 Failed attempted termination of pregnancy with other complications [M] [CC] ♀ [CC/MCC Exc]

O07.4 Failed attempted termination of pregnancy without complication [M] ♀
👁 **See Official Guidelines** "Retained Product of Conception following an abortion" I.C.15.q.2
AHA: Q4 2017

[4th] **O08 Complications following ectopic and molar pregnancy**
👁 **See Official Guidelines** "Complications leading to abortion" I.C.15.q.3
This category is for use with categories O00-O02 to identify any associated complications

O08.0 Genital tract and pelvic infection following ectopic and molar pregnancy [M] [CC] ♀ [CC/MCC Exc]
Endometritis following ectopic and molar pregnancy
Oophoritis following ectopic and molar pregnancy
Parametritis following ectopic and molar pregnancy
Pelvic peritonitis following ectopic and molar pregnancy
Salpingitis following ectopic and molar pregnancy
Salpingo-oophoritis following ectopic and molar pregnancy
[EXCLUDES1] *sepsis following ectopic and molar pregnancy (O08.82)*
urinary tract infection (O08.83)

O08.1 Delayed or excessive hemorrhage following ectopic and molar pregnancy [M] [CC] ♀ [CC/MCC Exc]
Afibrinogenemia following ectopic and molar pregnancy
Defibrination syndrome following ectopic and molar pregnancy
Hemolysis following ectopic and molar pregnancy
Intravascular coagulation following ectopic and molar pregnancy
[EXCLUDES1] *delayed or excessive hemorrhage due to incomplete abortion (O03.1)*

O08.2 Embolism following ectopic and molar pregnancy [M] [MCC] ♀ [CC/MCC Exc]
Air embolism following ectopic and molar pregnancy
Amniotic fluid embolism following ectopic and molar pregnancy
Blood-clot embolism following ectopic and molar pregnancy
Embolism NOS following ectopic and molar pregnancy
Fat embolism following ectopic and molar pregnancy
Pulmonary embolism following ectopic and molar pregnancy
Pyemic embolism following ectopic and molar pregnancy
Septic or septicopyemic embolism following ectopic and molar pregnancy
Soap embolism following ectopic and molar pregnancy

O08.3 Shock following ectopic and molar pregnancy [M] [MCC] ♀ [CC/MCC Exc]
Circulatory collapse following ectopic and molar pregnancy
Shock (postprocedural) following ectopic and molar pregnancy
[EXCLUDES1] *shock due to infection following ectopic and molar pregnancy (O08.82)*

O08.4 Renal failure following ectopic and molar pregnancy [M] [MCC] ♀ [CC/MCC Exc]
Kidney failure (acute) following ectopic and molar pregnancy
Oliguria following ectopic and molar pregnancy
Renal shutdown following ectopic and molar pregnancy
Renal tubular necrosis following ectopic and molar pregnancy
Uremia following ectopic and molar pregnancy

O08.5 Metabolic disorders following an ectopic and molar pregnancy [M] [CC] ♀ [CC/MCC Exc]

O08.6 Damage to pelvic organs and tissues following an ectopic and molar pregnancy [M] [CC] ♀ [CC/MCC Exc]
Laceration, perforation, tear or chemical damage of bladder following an ectopic and molar pregnancy
Laceration, perforation, tear or chemical damage of bowel following an ectopic and molar pregnancy
Laceration, perforation, tear or chemical damage of broad ligament following an ectopic and molar pregnancy
Laceration, perforation, tear or chemical damage of cervix following an ectopic and molar pregnancy
Laceration, perforation, tear or chemical damage of periurethral tissue following an ectopic and molar pregnancy
Laceration, perforation, tear or chemical damage of uterus following an ectopic and molar pregnancy
Laceration, perforation, tear or chemical damage of vagina following an ectopic and molar pregnancy

O08.7 Other venous complications following an ectopic and molar pregnancy [M] [CC] ♀ [CC/MCC Exc]

[5th] **O08.8 Other complications following an ectopic and molar pregnancy**

O08.81 Cardiac arrest following an ectopic and molar pregnancy [M] [CC] ♀ [CC/MCC Exc]

O08.82 Sepsis following ectopic and molar pregnancy [M] [CC] ♀ [CC/MCC Exc]
Use additional code (B95-B97), to identify infectious agent
Use additional code (R65.2-) to identify severe sepsis, if applicable
[EXCLUDES1] *septic or septicopyemic embolism following ectopic and molar pregnancy (O08.2)*

O08.83 Urinary tract infection following an ectopic and molar pregnancy [M] [CC] ♀ [CC/MCC Exc]
Cystitis following an ectopic and molar pregnancy

O08.89 Other complications following an ectopic and molar pregnancy [M] [CC] ♀ [CC/MCC Exc]

O08.9 Unspecified complication following an ectopic and molar pregnancy [M] [CC] ♀ [CC/MCC Exc]

Supervision of high risk pregnancy (O09)

[4th] **O09 Supervision of high risk pregnancy**
👁 **See Official Guidelines** "Supervision of High-Risk Pregnancy" I.C.15.b.2

[5th] **O09.0 Supervision of pregnancy with history of infertility**

O09.00 Supervision of pregnancy with history of infertility, unspecified trimester [M] [POA] ♀ [PDx]

O09.01 Supervision of pregnancy with history of infertility, first trimester [1st] [M] [POA] ♀ [PDx]

O09.02 Supervision of pregnancy with history of infertility, second trimester [2nd] [M] [POA] ♀ [PDx]

O09.03 Supervision of pregnancy with history of infertility, third trimester [3rd] [M] [POA] ♀ [PDx]

O09.1 Supervision of pregnancy with history of ectopic pregnancy

> **O09.10 Supervision of pregnancy with history of ectopic pregnancy, unspecified trimester** M PoA ♀ PDxIn
> AHA: Q4 2016

> **O09.11 Supervision of pregnancy with history of ectopic pregnancy, first trimester** 1st M PoA ♀ PDxIn
> AHA: Q4 2016

> **O09.12 Supervision of pregnancy with history of ectopic pregnancy, second trimester** 2nd M PoA ♀ PDxIn
> AHA: Q4 2016

> **O09.13 Supervision of pregnancy with history of ectopic pregnancy, third trimester** 3rd M PoA ♀ PDxIn
> AHA: Q4 2016

O09.A Supervision of pregnancy with history of molar pregnancy

> **O09.A0 Supervision of pregnancy with history of molar pregnancy, unspecified trimester** M PoA ♀ PDxIn
> AHA: Q4 2016

> **O09.A1 Supervision of pregnancy with history of molar pregnancy, first trimester** 1st M PoA ♀ PDxIn
> AHA: Q4 2016

> **O09.A2 Supervision of pregnancy with history of molar pregnancy, second trimester** 2nd M PoA ♀ PDxIn
> AHA: Q4 2016

> **O09.A3 Supervision of pregnancy with history of molar pregnancy, third trimester** 3rd M PoA ♀ PDxIn
> AHA: Q4 2016

O09.2 Supervision of pregnancy with other poor reproductive or obstetric history

> EXCLUDES2 *pregnancy care for patient with history of recurrent pregnancy loss (O26.2-)*

> **O09.21 Supervision of pregnancy** with history of pre-term labor

> > **O09.211 Supervision of pregnancy with history of pre-term labor, first trimester** 1st M PoA ♀ PDxIn

> > **O09.212 Supervision of pregnancy with history of pre-term labor, second trimester** 2nd M PoA ♀ PDxIn

> > **O09.213 Supervision of pregnancy with history of pre-term labor, third trimester** 3rd M PoA ♀ PDxIn

> > **O09.219 Supervision of pregnancy with history of pre-term labor, unspecified trimester** M PoA ♀ PDxIn

> **O09.29 Supervision of pregnancy with other poor reproductive or obstetric history**
> Supervision of pregnancy with history of neonatal death
> Supervision of pregnancy with history of stillbirth

> > **O09.291 Supervision of pregnancy with other poor reproductive or obstetric history, first trimester** 1st M PoA ♀ PDxIn

> > **O09.292 Supervision of pregnancy with other poor reproductive or obstetric history, second trimester** 2nd M PoA ♀ PDxIn

> > **O09.293 Supervision of pregnancy with other poor reproductive or obstetric history, third trimester** 3rd M PoA ♀ PDxIn

> > **O09.299 Supervision of pregnancy with other poor reproductive or obstetric history, unspecified trimester** M PoA ♀ PDxIn

O09.3 Supervision of pregnancy with insufficient antenatal care
Supervision of concealed pregnancy
Supervision of hidden pregnancy

> **O09.30 Supervision of pregnancy with insufficient antenatal care, unspecified trimester** M PoA ♀ PDxIn

> **O09.31 Supervision of pregnancy with insufficient antenatal care, first trimester** 1st M PoA ♀ PDxIn

> **O09.32 Supervision of pregnancy with insufficient antenatal care, second trimester** 2nd M PoA ♀ PDxIn

> **O09.33 Supervision of pregnancy with insufficient antenatal care, third trimester** 3rd M PoA ♀ PDxIn

O09.4 Supervision of pregnancy with grand multiparity

> **O09.40 Supervision of pregnancy with grand multiparity, unspecified trimester** M PoA ♀ PDxIn

> **O09.41 Supervision of pregnancy with grand multiparity, first trimester** 1st M PoA ♀ PDxIn

> **O09.42 Supervision of pregnancy with grand multiparity, second trimester** 2nd M PoA ♀ PDxIn

> **O09.43 Supervision of pregnancy with grand multiparity, third trimester** 3rd M PoA ♀ PDxIn

O09.5 Supervision of elderly primigravida and multigravida
Pregnancy for a female 35 years and older at expected date of delivery

> **O09.51 Supervision of** elderly primigravida

> > **O09.511 Supervision of elderly primigravida, first trimester** 1st M PoA ♀ PDxIn

> > **O09.512 Supervision of elderly primigravida, second trimester** 2nd M PoA ♀ PDxIn

> > **O09.513 Supervision of elderly primigravida, third trimester** 3rd M PoA ♀ PDxIn

> > **O09.519 Supervision of elderly primigravida, unspecified trimester** M PoA ♀ PDxIn

> **O09.52 Supervision of** elderly multigravida

> > **O09.521 Supervision of elderly multigravida, first trimester** 1st M PoA ♀ PDxIn

> > **O09.522 Supervision of elderly multigravida, second trimester** 2nd M PoA ♀ PDxIn

> > **O09.523 Supervision of elderly multigravida, third trimester** 3rd M PoA ♀ PDxIn
> > AHA: Q4 2016

> > **O09.529 Supervision of elderly multigravida, unspecified trimester** M PoA ♀ PDxIn

O09.6 Supervision of young primigravida and multigravida
Supervision of pregnancy for a female less than 16 years old at expected date of delivery

> **O09.61 Supervision of** young primigravida

> > **O09.611 Supervision of young primigravida, first trimester** 1st M PoA ♀ PDxIn

> > **O09.612 Supervision of young primigravida, second trimester** 2nd M PoA ♀ PDxIn

> > **O09.613 Supervision of young primigravida, third trimester** 3rd M PoA ♀ PDxIn

> > **O09.619 Supervision of young primigravida, unspecified trimester** M PoA ♀ PDxIn

> **O09.62 Supervision of** young multigravida

> > **O09.621 Supervision of young multigravida, first trimester** 1st M PoA ♀ PDxIn

> > **O09.622 Supervision of young multigravida, second trimester** 2nd M PoA ♀ PDxIn

> > **O09.623 Supervision of young multigravida, third trimester** 3rd M PoA ♀ PDxIn

> > **O09.629 Supervision of young multigravida, unspecified trimester** M PoA ♀ PDxIn

O09.7 Supervision of high risk pregnancy due to social problems

> **O09.70 Supervision of high risk pregnancy due to social problems, unspecified trimester** M PoA ♀ PDxIn

> **O09.71 Supervision of high risk pregnancy due to social problems, first trimester** 1st M PoA ♀ PDxIn

> **O09.72 Supervision of high risk pregnancy due to social problems, second trimester** 2nd M PoA ♀ PDxIn

> **O09.73 Supervision of high risk pregnancy due to social problems, third trimester** 3rd M PoA ♀ PDxIn

O09.8 Supervision of other high risk pregnancies

> **O09.81 Supervision of pregnancy** resulting from assisted reproductive technology
> Supervision of pregnancy resulting from in-vitro fertilization
> EXCLUDES2 *gestational carrier status (Z33.3)*

> > **O09.811 Supervision of pregnancy resulting from assisted reproductive technology, first trimester** 1st M PoA ♀ PDxIn

> > **O09.812 Supervision of pregnancy resulting from assisted reproductive technology, second trimester** 2nd M PoA ♀ PDxIn

---

1st 1st trimester 2nd 2nd trimester 3rd 3rd trimester PDxIn Unacceptable principal diagnosis symbol per Medicare code edits
PoA Code exempt from diagnosis present on admission requirement ❓ Questionable admission ⟲ Complication or comorbidity
MCC Major complication or comorbidity CC/MCC Ex CC/MCC exclusion HCC HCC diagnosis code RxHCC RxHCC diagnosis code MACRA code
DEFINITION Describes condition/terminology **TIP** Coding guidance ◉ Official Guideline Reference Z1 Z code as first-listed diagnosis

O09.813 Supervision of pregnancy resulting from assisted reproductive technology, third trimester 3rd M ♀ PDxIn

O09.819 Supervision of pregnancy resulting from assisted reproductive technology, unspecified trimester M ♀ PDxIn

6th **O09.82** Supervision of pregnancy with history of in utero procedure during previous pregnancy

O09.821 Supervision of pregnancy with history of in utero procedure during previous pregnancy, first trimester 1st M PoA ♀ PDxIn

O09.822 Supervision of pregnancy with history of in utero procedure during previous pregnancy, second trimester 2nd M PoA ♀ PDxIn

O09.823 Supervision of pregnancy with history of in utero procedure during previous pregnancy, third trimester 3rd M PoA ♀ PDxIn

O09.829 Supervision of pregnancy with history of in utero procedure during previous pregnancy, unspecified trimester M PoA ♀ PDxIn

EXCLUDES1 supervision of pregnancy affected by in utero procedure during current pregnancy (O35.7)

6th **O09.89** Supervision of other high risk pregnancies

O09.891 Supervision of other high risk pregnancies, first trimester 1st M PoA ♀ PDxIn

O09.892 Supervision of other high risk pregnancies, second trimester 2nd M PoA ♀ PDxIn

O09.893 Supervision of other high risk pregnancies, third trimester 3rd M PoA ♀ PDxIn

O09.899 Supervision of other high risk pregnancies, unspecified trimester M PoA ♀ PDxIn

5th **O09.9** Supervision of high risk pregnancy, unspecified

O09.90 Supervision of high risk pregnancy, unspecified, unspecified trimester M PoA ♀ PDxIn

O09.91 Supervision of high risk pregnancy, unspecified, first trimester 1st M PoA ♀ PDxIn

O09.92 Supervision of high risk pregnancy, unspecified, second trimester 2nd M PoA ♀ PDxIn

O09.93 Supervision of high risk pregnancy, unspecified, third trimester 3rd M PoA ♀ PDxIn

Edema, proteinuria and hypertensive disorders in pregnancy, childbirth and the puerperium (O10-O16)

4th **O10** Pre-existing hypertension complicating pregnancy, childbirth and the puerperium

👁 **See Official Guidelines** "Pre-existing hypertension in pregnancy" I.C.15.d

INCLUDES pre-existing hypertension with pre-existing proteinuria complicating pregnancy, childbirth and the puerperium

EXCLUDES2 pre-existing hypertension with superimposed pre-eclampsia complicating pregnancy, childbirth and the puerperium (O11.-)

5th **O10.0** Pre-existing essential hypertension complicating pregnancy, childbirth and the puerperium

Any condition in I10 specified as a reason for obstetric care during pregnancy, childbirth or the puerperium

6th **O10.01** Pre-existing essential hypertension complicating pregnancy

O10.011 Pre-existing essential hypertension complicating pregnancy, first trimester 1st M cc ♀ CC/MCC Exc

O10.012 Pre-existing essential hypertension complicating pregnancy, second trimester 2nd M cc ♀ CC/MCC Exc

O10.013 Pre-existing essential hypertension complicating pregnancy, third trimester 3rd M cc ♀ CC/MCC Exc

O10.019 Pre-existing essential hypertension complicating pregnancy, unspecified trimester M ♀

O10.02 Pre-existing essential hypertension complicating childbirth M cc ♀ CC/MCC Exc

O10.03 Pre-existing essential hypertension complicating the puerperium M ♀

5th **O10.1** Pre-existing hypertensive heart disease complicating pregnancy, childbirth and the puerperium

Any condition in I11 specified as a reason for obstetric care during pregnancy, childbirth or the puerperium

Use additional code from I11 to identify the type of hypertensive heart disease

6th **O10.11** Pre-existing hypertensive heart disease complicating pregnancy

O10.111 Pre-existing hypertensive heart disease complicating pregnancy, first trimester 1st M ♀

O10.112 Pre-existing hypertensive heart disease complicating pregnancy, second trimester 2nd M ♀

O10.113 Pre-existing hypertensive heart disease complicating pregnancy, third trimester 3rd M ♀

O10.119 Pre-existing hypertensive heart disease complicating pregnancy, unspecified trimester M ♀

O10.12 Pre-existing hypertensive heart disease complicating childbirth M ♀

O10.13 Pre-existing hypertensive heart disease complicating the puerperium M ♀

5th **O10.2** Pre-existing hypertensive chronic kidney disease complicating pregnancy, childbirth and the puerperium

Any condition in I12 specified as a reason for obstetric care during pregnancy, childbirth or the puerperium

Use additional code from I12 to identify the type of hypertensive chronic kidney disease

6th **O10.21** Pre-existing hypertensive chronic kidney disease complicating pregnancy

O10.211 Pre-existing hypertensive chronic kidney disease complicating pregnancy, first trimester 1st M ♀

O10.212 Pre-existing hypertensive chronic kidney disease complicating pregnancy, second trimester 2nd M ♀

O10.213 Pre-existing hypertensive chronic kidney disease complicating pregnancy, third trimester 3rd M ♀

O10.219 Pre-existing hypertensive chronic kidney disease complicating pregnancy, unspecified trimester M ♀

O10.22 Pre-existing hypertensive chronic kidney disease complicating childbirth M ♀

O10.23 Pre-existing hypertensive chronic kidney disease complicating the puerperium M ♀

5th **O10.3** Pre-existing hypertensive heart and chronic kidney disease complicating pregnancy, childbirth and the puerperium

Any condition in I13 specified as a reason for obstetric care during pregnancy, childbirth or the puerperium

Use additional code from I13 to identify the type of hypertensive heart and chronic kidney disease

6th **O10.31** Pre-existing hypertensive heart and chronic kidney disease complicating pregnancy

O10.311 Pre-existing hypertensive heart and chronic kidney disease complicating pregnancy, first trimester 1st M ♀

O10.312 Pre-existing hypertensive heart and chronic kidney disease complicating pregnancy, second trimester 2nd M ♀

Unspecified Code	Other Specified Code	Manifestation Code	N Newborn	P Pediatric	M Maternity	A Adult	♂ Male	♀ Female

● New Code ▲ Revised Code Title ▶◀ Revised Text NOTES INCLUDES EXCLUDES1 Not coded here EXCLUDES2 Not included here

4th 4th character required 5th 5th character required 6th 6th character required 7th 7th character required 7th Extension 'X' Alert

HAC Hospital-acquired condition (HAC) alert AHA AHA Coding Clinic© 📌 Code first alert

O10.313 Pre-existing hypertensive heart and chronic kidney disease complicating pregnancy, third trimester 3rd M ♀

O10.319 Pre-existing hypertensive heart and chronic kidney disease complicating pregnancy, unspecified trimester M ♀

O10.32 Pre-existing hypertensive heart and chronic kidney disease complicating childbirth M ♀

O10.33 Pre-existing hypertensive heart and chronic kidney disease complicating the puerperium M ♀

5th O10.4 Pre-existing secondary hypertension complicating pregnancy, childbirth and the puerperium

Any condition in I15 specified as a reason for obstetric care during pregnancy, childbirth or the puerperium

Use additional code from I15 to identify the type of secondary hypertension

6th O10.41 Pre-existing secondary hypertension complicating pregnancy

O10.411 Pre-existing secondary hypertension complicating pregnancy, first trimester 1st M cc ♀ CC/MCC Exc

O10.412 Pre-existing secondary hypertension complicating pregnancy, second trimester 2nd M cc ♀ CC/MCC Exc

O10.413 Pre-existing secondary hypertension complicating pregnancy, third trimester 3rd M cc ♀ CC/MCC Exc

O10.419 Pre-existing secondary hypertension complicating pregnancy, unspecified trimester M ♀

O10.42 Pre-existing secondary hypertension complicating childbirth M MCC ♀ CC/MCC Exc

O10.43 Pre-existing secondary hypertension complicating the puerperium M cc ♀ CC/MCC Exc

5th O10.9 Unspecified pre-existing hypertension complicating pregnancy, childbirth and the puerperium

6th O10.91 Unspecified pre-existing hypertension complicating pregnancy

O10.911 Unspecified pre-existing hypertension complicating pregnancy, first trimester 1st M cc ♀ CC/MCC Exc

O10.912 Unspecified pre-existing hypertension complicating pregnancy, second trimester 2nd M cc ♀ CC/MCC Exc

O10.913 Unspecified pre-existing hypertension complicating pregnancy, third trimester 3rd M cc ♀ CC/MCC Exc

O10.919 Unspecified pre-existing hypertension complicating pregnancy, unspecified trimester M ♀

O10.92 Unspecified pre-existing hypertension complicating childbirth M cc ♀ CC/MCC Exc

O10.93 Unspecified pre-existing hypertension complicating the puerperium M ♀

4th O11 Pre-existing hypertension with pre-eclampsia

INCLUDES conditions in O10 complicated by pre-eclampsia
pre-eclampsia superimposed pre-existing hypertension

Use additional code from O10 to identify the type of hypertension

O11.1 Pre-existing hypertension with pre-eclampsia, first trimester 1st M MCC ♀ CC/MCC Exc

O11.2 Pre-existing hypertension with pre-eclampsia, second trimester 2nd M MCC ♀ CC/MCC Exc

O11.3 Pre-existing hypertension with pre-eclampsia, third trimester 3rd M MCC ♀ CC/MCC Exc

O11.4 Pre-existing hypertension with pre-eclampsia, complicating childbirth M ♀

O11.5 Pre-existing hypertension with pre-eclampsia, complicating the puerperium M ♀

O11.9 Pre-existing hypertension with pre-eclampsia, unspecified trimester M ♀

4th O12 Gestational [pregnancy-induced] edema and proteinuria without hypertension

5th O12.0 Gestational edema

O12.00 Gestational edema, unspecified trimester M ♀

O12.01 Gestational edema, first trimester 1st M ♀

O12.02 Gestational edema, second trimester 2nd M ♀

O12.03 Gestational edema, third trimester 3rd M ♀

O12.04 Gestational edema, complicating childbirth M ♀

O12.05 Gestational edema, complicating the puerperium M ♀

5th O12.1 Gestational proteinuria

O12.10 Gestational proteinuria, unspecified trimester M ♀

O12.11 Gestational proteinuria, first trimester 1st M cc ♀ CC/MCC Exc

O12.12 Gestational proteinuria, second trimester 2nd M cc ♀ CC/MCC Exc

O12.13 Gestational proteinuria, third trimester 3rd M cc ♀ CC/MCC Exc

O12.14 Gestational proteinuria, complicating childbirth M ♀

O12.15 Gestational proteinuria, complicating the puerperium M ♀

5th O12.2 Gestational edema with proteinuria

O12.20 Gestational edema with proteinuria, unspecified trimester M ♀

O12.21 Gestational edema with proteinuria, first trimester 1st M cc ♀ CC/MCC Exc

O12.22 Gestational edema with proteinuria, second trimester 2nd M cc ♀ CC/MCC Exc

O12.23 Gestational edema with proteinuria, third trimester 3rd M cc ♀ CC/MCC Exc

O12.24 Gestational edema with proteinuria, complicating childbirth M ♀

O12.25 Gestational edema with proteinuria, complicating the puerperium M ♀

4th O13 Gestational [pregnancy-induced] hypertension without significant proteinuria

See Official Guidelines "Hypertension, Transient" I.C.9.a.7

INCLUDES gestational hypertension NOS
transient hypertension of pregnancy

O13.1 Gestational [pregnancy-induced] hypertension without significant proteinuria, first trimester 1st M ♀

O13.2 Gestational [pregnancy-induced] hypertension without significant proteinuria, second trimester 2nd M ♀

O13.3 Gestational [pregnancy-induced] hypertension without significant proteinuria, third trimester 3rd M ♀

O13.4 Gestational [pregnancy-induced] hypertension without significant proteinuria, complicating childbirth M ♀

O13.5 Gestational [pregnancy-induced] hypertension without significant proteinuria, complicating the puerperium M ♀

O13.9 Gestational [pregnancy-induced] hypertension without significant proteinuria, unspecified trimester M ♀

4th O14 Pre-eclampsia

See Official Guidelines "Hypertension, Transient" I.C.9.a.7

DEFINITION: Excessive weight gain, elevated BP, swelling of hands and feet, elevated albumin and creatinine in urine.

EXCLUDES1 pre-existing hypertension with pre-eclampsia (O11)

5th O14.0 Mild to moderate pre-eclampsia

O14.00 Mild to moderate pre-eclampsia, unspecified trimester M ♀

O14.02 Mild to moderate pre-eclampsia, second trimester 2nd M cc ♀ CC/MCC Exc

O14.03 Mild to moderate pre-eclampsia, third trimester 3rd M cc ♀ CC/MCC Exc

O14.04 Mild to moderate pre-eclampsia, complicating childbirth M ♀
AHA: Q2 2019

O14.05 Mild to moderate pre-eclampsia, complicating the puerperium M ♀

5th O14.1 Severe pre-eclampsia

EXCLUDES1 HELLP syndrome (O14.2-)

O14.10 Severe pre-eclampsia, unspecified trimester M ♀

1st 1st trimester 2nd 2nd trimester 3rd 3rd trimester PDx Unacceptable principal diagnosis symbol per Medicare code edits
PoA Code exempt from diagnosis present on admission requirement ? Questionable admission cc Complication or comorbidity
MCC Major complication or comorbidity CC/MCC Exc CC/MCC exclusion HCC HCC diagnosis code RxHCC RxHCC diagnosis code MACRA code
DEFINITION Describes condition/terminology TIP Coding guidance Official Guideline Reference Z1 Z code as first-listed diagnosis

890

When symbols appear on a code that requires a 7th character extension, refer to Appendix B to identify applicable 7th character codes.

2020 ICD-10-CM

O14.12 **Severe pre-eclampsia,** second trimester   2nd M MCC ♀ CC/MCC Exc

O14.13 **Severe pre-eclampsia,** third trimester   3rd M MCC ♀ CC/MCC Exc

O14.14 **Severe pre-eclampsia** complicating childbirth   M ♀

O14.15 **Severe pre-eclampsia, complicating the puerperium**   M ♀

5th O14.2 HELLP syndrome

Severe pre-eclampsia with hemolysis, elevated liver enzymes and low platelet count (HELLP)

O14.20 **HELLP syndrome (HELLP), unspecified trimester**   M ♀

O14.22 **HELLP syndrome (HELLP),** second trimester   2nd M MCC ♀ CC/MCC Exc

O14.23 **HELLP syndrome (HELLP),** third trimester   3rd M MCC ♀ CC/MCC Exc

O14.24 **HELLP syndrome,** complicating childbirth   M ♀

O14.25 **HELLP syndrome,** complicating the puerperium   M ♀

5th O14.9 Unspecified pre-eclampsia

O14.90 **Unspecified pre-eclampsia, unspecified trimester**   M ♀

O14.92 **Unspecified pre-eclampsia,** second trimester   2nd M CC ♀ CC/MCC Exc

O14.93 **Unspecified pre-eclampsia,** third trimester   3rd M CC ♀ CC/MCC Exc

O14.94 **Unspecified pre-eclampsia,** complicating childbirth   M ♀

O14.95 **Unspecified pre-eclampsia,** complicating the puerperium   M ♀

4th O15 Eclampsia

INCLUDES convulsions following conditions in O10-O14 and O16

5th O15.0 Eclampsia complicating pregnancy

O15.00 **Eclampsia complicating pregnancy, unspecified trimester**   M ♀

O15.02 **Eclampsia complicating pregnancy,** second trimester   2nd M MCC ♀ CC/MCC Exc

O15.03 **Eclampsia complicating pregnancy,** third trimester   3rd M MCC ♀ CC/MCC Exc

O15.1 **Eclampsia complicating** labor   M MCC ♀ CC/MCC Exc

O15.2 **Eclampsia complicating the** puerperium   M MCC ♀ CC/MCC Exc

O15.9 **Eclampsia, unspecified as to time period**   M ♀
Eclampsia NOS

4th O16 Unspecified maternal hypertension

O16.1 **Unspecified maternal hypertension,** first trimester   1st M CC ♀ CC/MCC Exc

O16.2 **Unspecified maternal hypertension,** second trimester   2nd M CC ♀ CC/MCC Exc

O16.3 **Unspecified maternal hypertension,** third trimester   3rd M CC ♀ CC/MCC Exc

O16.4 **Unspecified maternal hypertension,** complicating childbirth   M ♀

O16.5 **Unspecified maternal hypertension,** complicating the puerperium   M ♀

O16.9 **Unspecified maternal hypertension, unspecified trimester**   M ♀

Other maternal disorders predominantly related to pregnancy (O20-O29)

EXCLUDES2 maternal care related to the fetus and amniotic cavity and possible delivery problems (O30-O48)

maternal diseases classifiable elsewhere but complicating pregnancy, labor and delivery, and the puerperium (O98-O99)

4th O20 Hemorrhage in early pregnancy

INCLUDES hemorrhage before completion of 20 weeks gestation

EXCLUDES1 pregnancy with abortive outcome (O00-O08)

O20.0 **Threatened abortion**   M CC ♀ CC/MCC Exc
Hemorrhage specified as due to threatened abortion

O20.8 **Other hemorrhage in early pregnancy**   M ♀

O20.9 **Hemorrhage in early pregnancy, unspecified**   M CC ♀ CC/MCC Exc

4th O21 **Excessive vomiting in pregnancy**

O21.0 Mild **hyperemesis gravidarum**   M ♀
Hyperemesis gravidarum, mild or unspecified, starting before the end of the 20th week of gestation

O21.1 **Hyperemesis gravidarum** with metabolic disturbance   M ♀
Hyperemesis gravidarum, starting before the end of the 20th week of gestation, with metabolic disturbance such as carbohydrate depletion
Hyperemesis gravidarum, starting before the end of the 20th week of gestation, with metabolic disturbance such as dehydration
Hyperemesis gravidarum, starting before the end of the 20th week of gestation, with metabolic disturbance such as electrolyte imbalance

O21.2 Late **vomiting of pregnancy**   M ♀
Excessive vomiting starting after 20 completed weeks of gestation

O21.8 **Other vomiting complicating pregnancy**   M ♀
Vomiting due to diseases classified elsewhere, complicating pregnancy
Use additional code, to identify cause.

O21.9 **Vomiting of pregnancy, unspecified**   M ♀

4th O22 **Venous complications and hemorrhoids in pregnancy**

EXCLUDES1 venous complications of:
abortion NOS (O03.9)
ectopic or molar pregnancy (O08.7)
failed attempted abortion (O07.35)
induced abortion (O04.85)
spontaneous abortion (O03.89)

EXCLUDES2 obstetric pulmonary embolism (O88.-)
venous complications and hemorrhoids of childbirth and the puerperium (O87.-)

5th O22.0 Varicose veins of lower extremity **in pregnancy**
Varicose veins NOS in pregnancy

O22.00 **Varicose veins of lower extremity in pregnancy, unspecified trimester**   M ♀

O22.01 **Varicose veins of lower extremity in pregnancy,** first trimester   1st M ♀

O22.02 **Varicose veins of lower extremity in pregnancy,** second trimester   2nd M ♀

O22.03 **Varicose veins of lower extremity in pregnancy,** third trimester   3rd M ♀

5th O22.1 Genital varices **in pregnancy**
DEFINITION: Varices are enlarged veins.
Perineal varices in pregnancy
Vaginal varices in pregnancy
Vulval varices in pregnancy

O22.10 **Genital varices in pregnancy, unspecified trimester**   M ♀

O22.11 **Genital varices in pregnancy,** first trimester   1st M ♀

O22.12 **Genital varices in pregnancy,** second trimester   2nd M ♀

O22.13 **Genital varices in pregnancy,** third trimester   3rd M ♀

5th O22.2 Superficial thrombophlebitis **in pregnancy**
Phlebitis in pregnancy NOS
Thrombophlebitis of legs in pregnancy
Thrombosis in pregnancy NOS
Use additional code to identify the superficial thrombophlebitis (I80.0-)

O22.20 **Superficial thrombophlebitis in pregnancy, unspecified trimester**   M CC ♀ CC/MCC Exc

O22.21 **Superficial thrombophlebitis in pregnancy,** first trimester   1st M CC ♀ CC/MCC Exc

O22.22 **Superficial thrombophlebitis in pregnancy,** second trimester   2nd M CC ♀ CC/MCC Exc

O22.23 **Superficial thrombophlebitis in pregnancy,** third trimester   3rd M CC ♀ CC/MCC Exc

5th O22.3 Deep phlebothrombosis **in pregnancy**
Deep vein thrombosis, antepartum
Use additional code to identify the deep vein thrombosis (I82.4-, I82.5-, I82.62-, I82.72-)
Use additional code, if applicable, for associated long-term (current) use of anticoagulants (Z79.01)

CHAPTER 15: PREGNANCY, CHILDBIRTH AND THE PUERPERIUM (O00-O9A)

O22.30 Deep phlebothrombosis in pregnancy, unspecified trimester ☒ ⚲ CC/MCC Exc

O22.31 Deep phlebothrombosis in pregnancy, first trimester 1st ☒ MCC ⚲ CC/MCC Exc

O22.32 Deep phlebothrombosis in pregnancy, second trimester 2nd ☒ MCC ⚲ CC/MCC Exc

O22.33 Deep phlebothrombosis in pregnancy, third trimester 3rd ☒ MCC ⚲ CC/MCC Exc

5th **O22.4** Hemorrhoids in pregnancy

O22.40 Hemorrhoids in pregnancy, unspecified trimester ☒ cc ⚲ CC/MCC Exc

O22.41 Hemorrhoids in pregnancy, first trimester 1st ☒ cc ⚲ CC/MCC Exc

O22.42 Hemorrhoids in pregnancy, second trimester 2nd ☒ cc ⚲ CC/MCC Exc

O22.43 Hemorrhoids in pregnancy, third trimester 3rd ☒ cc ⚲ CC/MCC Exc

5th **O22.5** Cerebral venous thrombosis in pregnancy

Cerebrovenous sinus thrombosis in pregnancy

O22.50 Cerebral venous thrombosis in pregnancy, unspecified trimester ☒ cc ⚲ CC/MCC Exc

O22.51 Cerebral venous thrombosis in pregnancy, first trimester 1st ☒ cc ⚲ CC/MCC Exc

O22.52 Cerebral venous thrombosis in pregnancy, second trimester 2nd ☒ cc ⚲ CC/MCC Exc

O22.53 Cerebral venous thrombosis in pregnancy, third trimester 3rd ☒ cc ⚲ CC/MCC Exc

5th **O22.8** Other venous complications in pregnancy

6th **O22.8X** Other venous complications in pregnancy

O22.8X1 Other venous complications in pregnancy, first trimester 1st ☒ cc ⚲ CC/MCC Exc

O22.8X2 Other venous complications in pregnancy, second trimester 2nd ☒ cc ⚲ CC/MCC Exc

O22.8X3 Other venous complications in pregnancy, third trimester 3rd ☒ cc ⚲ CC/MCC Exc

O22.8X9 Other venous complications in pregnancy, unspecified trimester ☒ cc ⚲ CC/MCC Exc

5th **O22.9** Venous complication in pregnancy, unspecified

Gestational phlebitis NOS

Gestational phlebopathy NOS

Gestational thrombosis NOS

O22.90 Venous complication in pregnancy, unspecified, unspecified trimester ☒ cc ⚲ CC/MCC Exc

O22.91 Venous complication in pregnancy, unspecified, first trimester 1st ☒ ⚲

O22.92 Venous complication in pregnancy, unspecified, second trimester 2nd ☒ ⚲

O22.93 Venous complication in pregnancy, unspecified, third trimester 3rd ☒ ⚲

4th **O23** Infections of genitourinary tract in pregnancy

Use additional code to identify organism (B95.-, B96.-)

EXCLUDES2 gonococcal infections complicating pregnancy, childbirth and the puerperium (O98.2)

infections with a predominantly sexual mode of transmission NOS complicating pregnancy, childbirth and the puerperium (O98.3)

syphilis complicating pregnancy, childbirth and the puerperium (O98.1)

tuberculosis of genitourinary system complicating pregnancy, childbirth and the puerperium (O98.0)

venereal disease NOS complicating pregnancy, childbirth and the puerperium (O98.3)

5th **O23.0** Infections of kidney in pregnancy

Pyelonephritis in pregnancy

O23.00 Infections of kidney in pregnancy, unspecified trimester ☒ ⚲

O23.01 Infections of kidney in pregnancy, first trimester 1st ☒ cc ⚲ CC/MCC Exc

O23.02 Infections of kidney in pregnancy, second trimester 2nd ☒ cc ⚲ CC/MCC Exc

O23.03 Infections of kidney in pregnancy, third trimester 3rd ☒ cc ⚲ CC/MCC Exc

5th **O23.1** Infections of bladder in pregnancy

O23.10 Infections of bladder in pregnancy, unspecified trimester ☒ ⚲

O23.11 Infections of bladder in pregnancy, first trimester 1st ☒ cc ⚲ CC/MCC Exc

O23.12 Infections of bladder in pregnancy, second trimester 2nd ☒ cc ⚲ CC/MCC Exc

O23.13 Infections of bladder in pregnancy, third trimester 3rd ☒ cc ⚲ CC/MCC Exc

5th **O23.2** Infections of urethra in pregnancy

O23.20 Infections of urethra in pregnancy, unspecified trimester ☒ ⚲

O23.21 Infections of urethra in pregnancy, first trimester 1st ☒ cc ⚲ CC/MCC Exc

O23.22 Infections of urethra in pregnancy, second trimester 2nd ☒ cc ⚲ CC/MCC Exc

O23.23 Infections of urethra in pregnancy, third trimester 3rd ☒ cc ⚲ CC/MCC Exc

5th **O23.3** Infections of other parts of urinary tract in pregnancy

O23.30 Infections of other parts of urinary tract in pregnancy, unspecified trimester ☒ ⚲

O23.31 Infections of other parts of urinary tract in pregnancy, first trimester 1st ☒ cc ⚲ CC/MCC Exc

O23.32 Infections of other parts of urinary tract in pregnancy, second trimester 2nd ☒ cc ⚲ CC/MCC Exc

O23.33 Infections of other parts of urinary tract in pregnancy, third trimester 3rd ☒ cc ⚲ CC/MCC Exc

5th **O23.4** Unspecified infection of urinary tract in pregnancy

O23.40 Unspecified infection of urinary tract in pregnancy, unspecified trimester ☒ ⚲

O23.41 Unspecified infection of urinary tract in pregnancy, first trimester 1st ☒ cc ⚲ CC/MCC Exc

O23.42 Unspecified infection of urinary tract in pregnancy, second trimester 2nd ☒ cc ⚲ CC/MCC Exc

O23.43 Unspecified infection of urinary tract in pregnancy, third trimester 3rd ☒ cc ⚲ CC/MCC Exc

AHA: Q2 2018

5th **O23.5** Infections of the genital tract in pregnancy

6th **O23.51** Infection of cervix in pregnancy

O23.511 Infections of cervix in pregnancy, first trimester 1st cc ⚲ CC/MCC Exc

O23.512 Infections of cervix in pregnancy, second trimester 2nd cc ⚲ CC/MCC Exc

O23.513 Infections of cervix in pregnancy, third trimester 3rd ☒ cc ⚲ CC/MCC Exc

O23.519 Infections of cervix in pregnancy, unspecified trimester ☒ ⚲

6th **O23.52** Salpingo-oophoritis in pregnancy

Oophoritis in pregnancy

Salpingitis in pregnancy

O23.521 Salpingo-oophoritis in pregnancy, first trimester 1st ☒ cc ⚲ CC/MCC Exc

O23.522 Salpingo-oophoritis in pregnancy, second trimester 2nd ☒ cc ⚲ CC/MCC Exc

O23.523 Salpingo-oophoritis in pregnancy, third trimester 3rd ☒ cc ⚲ CC/MCC Exc

O23.529 Salpingo-oophoritis in pregnancy, unspecified trimester ☒ ⚲

6th **O23.59** Infection of other part of genital tract in pregnancy

O23.591 Infection of other part of genital tract in pregnancy, first trimester 1st cc ⚲ CC/MCC Exc

O23.592 Infection of other part of genital tract in pregnancy, second trimester 2nd ☒ cc ⚲ CC/MCC Exc

O23.593 Infection of other part of genital tract in pregnancy, third trimester 3rd ☒ cc ⚲ CC/MCC Exc

O23.599 Infection of other part of genital tract in pregnancy, unspecified trimester ☒ ⚲

1st 1st trimester 2nd 2nd trimester 3rd 3rd trimester PDx Unacceptable principal diagnosis symbol per Medicare code edits
PoA Code exempt from diagnosis present on admission requirement ❓ Questionable admission cc Complication or comorbidity
MCC Major complication or comorbidity CC/MCC Exc CC/MCC exclusion HCC HCC diagnosis code RxHCC RxHCC diagnosis code MACRA code
DEFINITION Describes condition/terminology **TIP** Coding guidance ◉ Official Guideline Reference Z Z code as first-listed diagnosis

When symbols appear on a code that requires a 7th character extension, refer to Appendix B to identify applicable 7th character codes.

2020 ICD-10-CM

[5th] **O23.9 Unspecified genitourinary tract infection in pregnancy**
Genitourinary tract infection in pregnancy NOS
O23.90 Unspecified genitourinary tract infection in pregnancy, unspecified trimester [M] ♀
O23.91 Unspecified genitourinary tract infection in pregnancy, first trimester [1st] [M] CC ♀ CC/MCC Exc
O23.92 Unspecified genitourinary tract infection in pregnancy, second trimester [2nd] [M] CC ♀ CC/MCC Exc
O23.93 Unspecified genitourinary tract infection in pregnancy, third trimester [3rd] [M] CC ♀ CC/MCC Exc

[4th] **O24 Diabetes mellitus in pregnancy, childbirth, and the puerperium**
👁 **See Official Guidelines** "Diabetes mellitus in pregnancy" I.C.15.g

[5th] **O24.0 Pre-existing type 1 diabetes mellitus, in pregnancy, childbirth and the puerperium**
Juvenile onset diabetes mellitus, in pregnancy, childbirth and the puerperium
Ketosis-prone diabetes mellitus in pregnancy, childbirth and the puerperium
Use additional code from category E10 to further identify any manifestations

[6th] **O24.01 Pre-existing type 1 diabetes mellitus, in pregnancy**
O24.011 Pre-existing type 1 diabetes mellitus, in pregnancy, first trimester [1st] [M] CC ♀ CC/MCC Exc
O24.012 Pre-existing type 1 diabetes mellitus, in pregnancy, second trimester [2nd] [M] CC ♀ CC/MCC Exc
O24.013 Pre-existing type 1 diabetes mellitus, in pregnancy, third trimester [3rd] [M] CC ♀ CC/MCC Exc
O24.019 Pre-existing type 1 diabetes mellitus, in pregnancy, unspecified trimester [M] CC ♀ CC/MCC Exc

O24.02 Pre-existing type 1 diabetes mellitus, in childbirth [M] CC ♀ CC/MCC Exc
O24.03 Pre-existing type 1 diabetes mellitus, in the puerperium [M] CC ♀ CC/MCC Exc

[5th] **O24.1 Pre-existing type 2 diabetes mellitus, in pregnancy, childbirth and the puerperium**
Insulin-resistant diabetes mellitus in pregnancy, childbirth and the puerperium
Use additional code (for):
from category E11 to further identify any manifestations
long-term (current) use of insulin (Z79.4)

[6th] **O24.11 Pre-existing type 2 diabetes mellitus, in pregnancy**
O24.111 Pre-existing type 2 diabetes mellitus, in pregnancy, first trimester [1st] [M] CC ♀ CC/MCC Exc
O24.112 Pre-existing type 2 diabetes mellitus, in pregnancy, second trimester [2nd] [M] CC ♀ CC/MCC Exc
O24.113 Pre-existing type 2 diabetes mellitus, in pregnancy, third trimester [3rd] [M] CC ♀ CC/MCC Exc
O24.119 Pre-existing type 2 diabetes mellitus, in pregnancy, unspecified trimester [M] CC ♀ CC/MCC Exc

O24.12 Pre-existing type 2 diabetes mellitus, in childbirth [M] CC ♀ CC/MCC Exc
O24.13 Pre-existing type 2 diabetes mellitus, in the puerperium [M] CC ♀ CC/MCC Exc

[5th] **O24.3 Unspecified pre-existing diabetes mellitus in pregnancy, childbirth and the puerperium**
Use additional code (for):
from category E11 to further identify any manifestation
long-term (current) use of insulin (Z79.4)

[6th] **O24.31 Unspecified pre-existing diabetes mellitus in pregnancy**
O24.311 Unspecified pre-existing diabetes mellitus in pregnancy, first trimester [1st] [M] CC ♀ CC/MCC Exc
O24.312 Unspecified pre-existing diabetes mellitus in pregnancy, second trimester [2nd] [M] CC ♀ CC/MCC Exc
O24.313 Unspecified pre-existing diabetes mellitus in pregnancy, third trimester [3rd] [M] CC ♀ CC/MCC Exc
O24.319 Unspecified pre-existing diabetes mellitus in pregnancy, unspecified trimester [M] CC ♀ CC/MCC Exc

O24.32 Unspecified pre-existing diabetes mellitus in childbirth [M] CC ♀ CC/MCC Exc
O24.33 Unspecified pre-existing diabetes mellitus in the puerperium [M] CC ♀ CC/MCC Exc

[5th] **O24.4 Gestational diabetes mellitus**
👁 **See Official Guidelines** "Gestational (pregnancy induced) diabetes" I.C.15.i
TIP: Do not report Z79.4 or Z79.84 with codes in this category.
Diabetes mellitus arising in pregnancy
Gestational diabetes mellitus NOS

[6th] **O24.41 Gestational diabetes mellitus in pregnancy**
O24.410 Gestational diabetes mellitus in pregnancy, diet controlled [M] ♀
O24.414 Gestational diabetes mellitus in pregnancy, insulin controlled [M] CC ♀ CC/MCC Exc
O24.415 Gestational diabetes mellitus in pregnancy, controlled by oral hypoglycemic drugs [M] CC ♀ CC/MCC Exc
AHA: Q4 2016
Gestational diabetes mellitus in pregnancy, controlled by oral antidiabetic drugs
O24.419 Gestational diabetes mellitus in pregnancy, unspecified control [M] ♀
AHA: Q4 2015

[6th] **O24.42 Gestational diabetes mellitus in childbirth**
O24.420 Gestational diabetes mellitus in childbirth, diet controlled [M] ♀
O24.424 Gestational diabetes mellitus in childbirth, insulin controlled [M] CC ♀ CC/MCC Exc
O24.425 Gestational diabetes mellitus in childbirth, controlled by oral hypoglycemic drugs [M] CC ♀ CC/MCC Exc
AHA: Q4 2016
Gestational diabetes mellitus in childbirth, controlled by oral antidiabetic drugs
O24.429 Gestational diabetes mellitus in childbirth, unspecified control [M] ♀

[6th] **O24.43 Gestational diabetes mellitus in the puerperium**
O24.430 Gestational diabetes mellitus in the puerperium, diet controlled [M] ♀
O24.434 Gestational diabetes mellitus in the puerperium, insulin controlled [M] CC ♀ CC/MCC Exc
O24.435 Gestational diabetes mellitus in puerperium, controlled by oral hypoglycemic drugs [M] CC ♀ CC/MCC Exc
AHA: Q4 2016
Gestational diabetes mellitus in puerperium, controlled by oral antidiabetic drugs
O24.439 Gestational diabetes mellitus in the puerperium, unspecified control [M] ♀

[5th] **O24.8 Other pre-existing diabetes mellitus in pregnancy, childbirth, and the puerperium**
Use additional code (for):
from categories E08, E09 and E13 to further identify any manifestation
long-term (current) use of insulin (Z79.4)

[6th] **O24.81 Other pre-existing diabetes mellitus in pregnancy**
O24.811 Other pre-existing diabetes mellitus in pregnancy, first trimester [1st] [M] CC ♀ CC/MCC Exc
O24.812 Other pre-existing diabetes mellitus in pregnancy, second trimester [2nd] [M] CC ♀ CC/MCC Exc
O24.813 Other pre-existing diabetes mellitus in pregnancy, third trimester [3rd] [M] CC ♀ CC/MCC Exc

Unspecified Code Other Specified Code Manifestation Code [N] Newborn [P] Pediatric [M] Maternity [A] Adult ♂ Male ♀ Female
● New Code ▲ Revised Code Title ▶◀ Revised Text NOTES INCLUDES EXCLUDES1 Not coded here EXCLUDES2 Not included here
[4th] 4th character required [5th] 5th character required [6th] 6th character required [7th] 7th character required [X] Extension 'X' Alert
[HAC] Hospital-acquired condition (HAC) alert AHA AHA Coding Clinic© ☛ Code first alert

When symbols appear on a code that requires a 7th character extension, refer to Appendix B to identify applicable 7th character codes.

O24.819 **Other pre-existing diabetes mellitus in pregnancy, unspecified trimester** M cc ♀ CC/MCC Exc

O24.82 **Other pre-existing diabetes mellitus in childbirth** M cc ♀ CC/MCC Exc

O24.83 **Other pre-existing diabetes mellitus in the puerperium** M cc ♀ CC/MCC Exc

O24.9 Unspecified **diabetes mellitus in pregnancy, childbirth and the puerperium**
Use additional code for long-term (current) use of insulin (Z79.4)

O24.91 **Unspecified diabetes mellitus in** pregnancy

O24.911 **Unspecified diabetes mellitus in pregnancy,** first trimester 1st M cc ♀ CC/MCC Exc

O24.912 **Unspecified diabetes mellitus in pregnancy,** second trimester 2nd M cc ♀ CC/MCC Exc

O24.913 **Unspecified diabetes mellitus in pregnancy,** third trimester 3rd M cc ♀ CC/MCC Exc

O24.919 **Unspecified diabetes mellitus in pregnancy, unspecified trimester** M cc ♀ CC/MCC Exc

O24.92 **Unspecified diabetes mellitus in childbirth** M cc ♀ CC/MCC Exc

O24.93 **Unspecified diabetes mellitus in the puerperium** M cc ♀ CC/MCC Exc

O25 Malnutrition **in pregnancy, childbirth and the puerperium**

O25.1 **Malnutrition in** pregnancy

O25.10 **Malnutrition in pregnancy, unspecified trimester** M ♀

O25.11 **Malnutrition in pregnancy,** first trimester 1st M ♀

O25.12 **Malnutrition in pregnancy,** second trimester 2nd M ♀

O25.13 **Malnutrition in pregnancy,** third trimester 3rd M ♀

O25.2 **Malnutrition in** childbirth M ♀

O25.3 **Malnutrition in the** puerperium M ♀

O26 Maternal care **for other conditions predominantly related to pregnancy**

O26.0 Excessive weight gain **in pregnancy**
EXCLUDES2 gestational edema (O12.0, O12.2)

O26.00 **Excessive weight gain in pregnancy, unspecified trimester** M ♀

O26.01 **Excessive weight gain in pregnancy,** first trimester 1st M ♀

O26.02 **Excessive weight gain in pregnancy,** second trimester 2nd M ♀

O26.03 **Excessive weight gain in pregnancy,** third trimester 3rd M ♀

O26.1 Low weight gain **in pregnancy**

O26.10 **Low weight gain in pregnancy, unspecified trimester** M ♀

O26.11 **Low weight gain in pregnancy,** first trimester 1st M ♀

O26.12 **Low weight gain in pregnancy,** second trimester 2nd M ♀

O26.13 **Low weight gain in pregnancy,** third trimester 3rd M ♀

O26.2 **Pregnancy care for patient with recurrent pregnancy loss**
DEFINITION: More than 3 pregnancy losses.

O26.20 **Pregnancy care for patient with recurrent pregnancy loss, unspecified trimester** M ♀

O26.21 **Pregnancy care for patient with recurrent pregnancy loss,** first trimester 1st M ♀

O26.22 **Pregnancy care for patient with recurrent pregnancy loss,** second trimester 2nd M ♀

O26.23 **Pregnancy care for patient with recurrent pregnancy loss,** third trimester 3rd M ♀

O26.3 Retained intrauterine contraceptive device **in pregnancy**

O26.30 **Retained intrauterine contraceptive device in pregnancy, unspecified trimester** M ♀

O26.31 **Retained intrauterine contraceptive device in pregnancy,** first trimester 1st M ♀

O26.32 **Retained intrauterine contraceptive device in pregnancy,** second trimester 2nd M ♀

O26.33 **Retained intrauterine contraceptive device in pregnancy,** third trimester 3rd M ♀

O26.4 **Herpes gestationis**

O26.40 **Herpes gestationis, unspecified trimester** M ♀

O26.41 **Herpes gestationis,** first trimester 1st M ♀

O26.42 **Herpes gestationis,** second trimester 2nd M ♀

O26.43 **Herpes gestationis,** third trimester 3rd M ♀

O26.5 **Maternal hypotension syndrome**
Supine hypotensive syndrome

O26.50 **Maternal hypotension syndrome, unspecified trimester** M ♀

O26.51 **Maternal hypotension syndrome,** first trimester 1st M ♀

O26.52 **Maternal hypotension syndrome,** second trimester 2nd M ♀

O26.53 **Maternal hypotension syndrome,** third trimester 3rd M ♀

O26.6 Liver and biliary tract disorders **in pregnancy, childbirth and the puerperium**
Use additional code to identify the specific disorder
EXCLUDES2 hepatorenal syndrome following labor and delivery (O90.4)

O26.61 **Liver and biliary tract disorders in** pregnancy

O26.611 **Liver and biliary tract disorders in pregnancy,** first trimester 1st M cc ♀ CC/MCC Exc

O26.612 **Liver and biliary tract disorders in pregnancy,** second trimester 2nd M cc ♀ CC/MCC Exc

O26.613 **Liver and biliary tract disorders in pregnancy,** third trimester 3rd M cc ♀ CC/MCC Exc

O26.619 **Liver and biliary tract disorders in pregnancy, unspecified trimester** M ♀

O26.62 **Liver and biliary tract disorders in childbirth** M cc ♀ CC/MCC Exc

O26.63 **Liver and biliary tract disorders in the puerperium** M ♀

O26.7 Subluxation of symphysis (pubis) **in pregnancy, childbirth and the puerperium**
EXCLUDES1 traumatic separation of symphysis (pubis) during childbirth (O71.6)

O26.71 **Subluxation of symphysis (pubis) in** pregnancy

O26.711 **Subluxation of symphysis (pubis) in pregnancy,** first trimester 1st M ♀

O26.712 **Subluxation of symphysis (pubis) in pregnancy,** second trimester 2nd M ♀

O26.713 **Subluxation of symphysis (pubis) in pregnancy,** third trimester 3rd M ♀

O26.719 **Subluxation of symphysis (pubis) in pregnancy, unspecified trimester** M ♀

O26.72 **Subluxation of symphysis (pubis) in** childbirth M ♀

O26.73 **Subluxation of symphysis (pubis) in the puerperium** M ♀

O26.8 Other specified **pregnancy related conditions**

O26.81 **Pregnancy related** exhaustion and fatigue

O26.811 **Pregnancy related exhaustion and fatigue,** first trimester 1st M ♀

O26.812 **Pregnancy related exhaustion and fatigue,** second trimester 2nd M ♀

O26.813 **Pregnancy related exhaustion and fatigue,** third trimester 3rd M ♀

O26.819 **Pregnancy related exhaustion and fatigue, unspecified trimester** M ♀

O26.82 **Pregnancy related** peripheral neuritis

O26.821 **Pregnancy related peripheral neuritis,** first trimester 1st M ♀

O26.822 **Pregnancy related peripheral neuritis,** second trimester 2nd M ♀

O26.823 **Pregnancy related peripheral neuritis,** third trimester 3rd M ♀

1st 1st trimester 2nd 2nd trimester 3rd 3rd trimester PDx Unacceptable principal diagnosis symbol per Medicare code edits POA Code exempt from diagnosis present on admission requirement ❓ Questionable admission cc Complication or comorbidity MCC Major complication or comorbidity CC/MCC Exc CC/MCC exclusion HCC HCC diagnosis code RxHCC RxHCC diagnosis code MACRA code DEFINITION Describes condition/terminology TIP Coding guidance Official Guideline Reference Z1 Z code as first-listed diagnosis

894

When symbols appear on a code that requires a 7th character extension, refer to Appendix B to identify applicable 7th character codes.

2020 ICD-10-CM

O26.829 **Pregnancy related peripheral neuritis, unspecified trimester** M ♀

🜄 O26.83 **Pregnancy related** renal disease
Use additional code to identify the specific disorder

O26.831 **Pregnancy related renal disease, first trimester** 1st M cc ♀ CC/MCC Excl

O26.832 **Pregnancy related renal disease, second trimester** 2nd M cc ♀ CC/MCC Excl

O26.833 **Pregnancy related renal disease, third trimester** 3rd M cc ♀ CC/MCC Excl

O26.839 **Pregnancy related renal disease, unspecified trimester** M ♀

🜄 O26.84 Uterine size-date discrepancy **complicating pregnancy**
EXCLUDES1 encounter for suspected problem with fetal growth ruled out (Z03.74)

O26.841 **Uterine size-date discrepancy, first trimester** 1st M ♀

O26.842 **Uterine size-date discrepancy, second trimester** 2nd M ♀

O26.843 **Uterine size-date discrepancy, third trimester** 3rd M ♀

O26.849 **Uterine size-date discrepancy, unspecified trimester** M ♀

🜄 O26.85 Spotting **complicating pregnancy**

O26.851 **Spotting complicating pregnancy, first trimester** 1st M ♀

O26.852 **Spotting complicating pregnancy, second trimester** 2nd M ♀

O26.853 **Spotting complicating pregnancy, third trimester** 3rd M ♀

O26.859 **Spotting complicating pregnancy, unspecified trimester** M ♀

O26.86 **Pruritic urticarial papules and plaques of pregnancy (PUPPP)** M ♀
Polymorphic eruption of pregnancy

🜄 O26.87 **Cervical shortening**
EXCLUDES1 encounter for suspected cervical shortening ruled out (Z03.75)

O26.872 **Cervical shortening, second trimester** 2nd M cc ♀ CC/MCC Excl

O26.873 **Cervical shortening, third trimester** 3rd M cc ♀ CC/MCC Excl

O26.879 **Cervical shortening, unspecified trimester** M cc ♀ CC/MCC Excl

🜄 O26.89 Other specified **pregnancy related conditions**

O26.891 **Other specified pregnancy related conditions, first trimester** 1st M ♀

O26.892 **Other specified pregnancy related conditions, second trimester** 2nd M ♀

O26.893 **Other specified pregnancy related conditions, third trimester** 3rd M ♀
AHA: Q3 2015

O26.899 **Other specified pregnancy related conditions, unspecified trimester** M ♀

🜅 O26.9 **Pregnancy related conditions,** unspecified

O26.90 **Pregnancy related conditions, unspecified, unspecified trimester** M ♀

O26.91 **Pregnancy related conditions, unspecified, first trimester** 1st M ♀

O26.92 **Pregnancy related conditions, unspecified, second trimester** 2nd M ♀

O26.93 **Pregnancy related conditions, unspecified, third trimester** 3rd M ♀

🜃 O28 **Abnormal findings on antenatal screening of mother**
EXCLUDES1 diagnostic findings classified elsewhere - see Alphabetical Index

O28.0 **Abnormal** hematological **finding on antenatal screening of mother** M ♀

O28.1 **Abnormal** biochemical **finding on antenatal screening of mother** M ♀

O28.2 **Abnormal** cytological **finding on antenatal screening of mother** M ♀

O28.3 **Abnormal** ultrasonic **finding on antenatal screening of mother** M ♀
AHA: Q4 2016

O28.4 **Abnormal** radiological **finding on antenatal screening of mother** M ♀

O28.5 **Abnormal** chromosomal and genetic **finding on antenatal screening of mother** M ♀

O28.8 Other abnormal findings **on antenatal screening of mother** M ♀

O28.9 **Unspecified abnormal findings on antenatal screening of mother** M ♀

🜃 O29 **Complications of anesthesia during pregnancy**
INCLUDES maternal complications arising from the administration of a general, regional or local anesthetic, analgesic or other sedation during pregnancy
Use additional code, if necessary, to identify the complication
EXCLUDES2 complications of anesthesia during labor and delivery (O74.-)
complications of anesthesia during the puerperium (O89.-)

🜅 O29.0 Pulmonary **complications of anesthesia during pregnancy**

🜄 O29.01 Aspiration pneumonitis **due to anesthesia during pregnancy**
Inhalation of stomach contents or secretions NOS due to anesthesia during pregnancy
Mendelson's syndrome due to anesthesia during pregnancy

O29.011 **Aspiration pneumonitis due to anesthesia during pregnancy,** first trimester 1st M ♀

O29.012 **Aspiration pneumonitis due to anesthesia during pregnancy,** second trimester 2nd M ♀

O29.013 **Aspiration pneumonitis due to anesthesia during pregnancy,** third trimester 3rd M ♀

O29.019 **Aspiration pneumonitis due to anesthesia during pregnancy, unspecified trimester** M ♀

🜄 O29.02 Pressure collapse of lung **due to anesthesia during pregnancy**

O29.021 **Pressure collapse of lung due to anesthesia during pregnancy,** first trimester 1st M ♀

O29.022 **Pressure collapse of lung due to anesthesia during pregnancy,** second trimester 2nd M ♀

O29.023 **Pressure collapse of lung due to anesthesia during pregnancy,** third trimester 3rd M ♀

O29.029 **Pressure collapse of lung due to anesthesia during pregnancy, unspecified trimester** M ♀

🜄 O29.09 Other pulmonary complications **of anesthesia during pregnancy**

O29.091 **Other pulmonary complications of anesthesia during pregnancy,** first trimester 1st M ♀

O29.092 **Other pulmonary complications of anesthesia during pregnancy,** second trimester 2nd M ♀

O29.093 **Other pulmonary complications of anesthesia during pregnancy,** third trimester 3rd M ♀

O29.099 **Other pulmonary complications of anesthesia during pregnancy, unspecified trimester** M ♀

🜅 O29.1 Cardiac complications of anesthesia **during pregnancy**

🜄 O29.11 Cardiac arrest **due to anesthesia during pregnancy**

O29.111 **Cardiac arrest due to anesthesia during pregnancy,** first trimester 1st M ♀

O29.112 **Cardiac arrest due to anesthesia during pregnancy,** second trimester 2nd M ♀

Unspecified Code   Other Specified Code   Manifestation Code   N Newborn   P Pediatric   M Maternity   A Adult   ♂ Male   ♀ Female
● New Code   ▲ Revised Code Title   ►◄ Revised Text   NOTES   INCLUDES   EXCLUDES1 Not coded here   EXCLUDES2 Not included here
🜃 4th character required   🜅 5th character required   🜄 6th character required   🝛 7th character required   🝙 Extension 'X' Alert
HAC Hospital-acquired condition (HAC) alert   AHA AHA Coding Clinic©   ☛ Code first alert

2020 ICD-10-CM   When symbols appear on a code that requires a 7th character extension, refer to Appendix B to identify applicable 7th character codes.   895

O29.113 **Cardiac arrest due to anesthesia during pregnancy, third trimester** 3rd M ♀

O29.119 **Cardiac arrest due to anesthesia during pregnancy, unspecified trimester** M ♀

6ᵗʰ O29.12 Cardiac failure due to anesthesia during pregnancy

O29.121 **Cardiac failure due to anesthesia during pregnancy, first trimester** 1st M ♀

O29.122 **Cardiac failure due to anesthesia during pregnancy, second trimester** 2nd M ♀

O29.123 **Cardiac failure due to anesthesia during pregnancy, third trimester** 3rd M ♀

O29.129 **Cardiac failure due to anesthesia during pregnancy, unspecified trimester** M ♀

6ᵗʰ O29.19 Other cardiac complications of anesthesia during pregnancy

O29.191 **Other cardiac complications of anesthesia during pregnancy, first trimester** 1st M ♀

O29.192 **Other cardiac complications of anesthesia during pregnancy, second trimester** 2nd M ♀

O29.193 **Other cardiac complications of anesthesia during pregnancy, third trimester** 3rd M ♀

O29.199 **Other cardiac complications of anesthesia during pregnancy, unspecified trimester** M ♀

5ᵗʰ O29.2 Central nervous system complications of anesthesia during pregnancy

6ᵗʰ O29.21 Cerebral anoxia due to anesthesia during pregnancy

O29.211 **Cerebral anoxia due to anesthesia during pregnancy, first trimester** 1st M ♀

O29.212 **Cerebral anoxia due to anesthesia during pregnancy, second trimester** 2nd M ♀

O29.213 **Cerebral anoxia due to anesthesia during pregnancy, third trimester** 3rd M ♀

O29.219 **Cerebral anoxia due to anesthesia during pregnancy, unspecified trimester** M ♀

6ᵗʰ O29.29 Other central nervous system complications of anesthesia during pregnancy

O29.291 **Other central nervous system complications of anesthesia during pregnancy, first trimester** 1st M ♀

O29.292 **Other central nervous system complications of anesthesia during pregnancy, second trimester** 2nd M ♀

O29.293 **Other central nervous system complications of anesthesia during pregnancy, third trimester** 3rd M ♀

O29.299 **Other central nervous system complications of anesthesia during pregnancy, unspecified trimester** M ♀

5ᵗʰ O29.3 Toxic reaction to local anesthesia during pregnancy

6ᵗʰ O29.3X Toxic reaction to local anesthesia during pregnancy

O29.3X1 **Toxic reaction to local anesthesia during pregnancy, first trimester** 1st M ♀

O29.3X2 **Toxic reaction to local anesthesia during pregnancy, second trimester** 2nd M ♀

O29.3X3 **Toxic reaction to local anesthesia during pregnancy, third trimester** 3rd M ♀

O29.3X9 **Toxic reaction to local anesthesia during pregnancy, unspecified trimester** M ♀

5ᵗʰ O29.4 Spinal and epidural anesthesia induced headache during pregnancy

O29.40 **Spinal and epidural anesthesia induced headache during pregnancy, unspecified trimester** M ♀

O29.41 **Spinal and epidural anesthesia induced headache during pregnancy, first trimester** 1st M ♀

O29.42 **Spinal and epidural anesthesia induced headache during pregnancy, second trimester** 2nd M ♀

O29.43 **Spinal and epidural anesthesia induced headache during pregnancy, third trimester** 3rd M ♀

5ᵗʰ O29.5 Other complications of spinal and epidural anesthesia during pregnancy

6ᵗʰ O29.5X Other complications of spinal and epidural anesthesia during pregnancy

O29.5X1 **Other complications of spinal and epidural anesthesia during pregnancy, first trimester** 1st M ♀

O29.5X2 **Other complications of spinal and epidural anesthesia during pregnancy, second trimester** 2nd M ♀

O29.5X3 **Other complications of spinal and epidural anesthesia during pregnancy, third trimester** 3rd M ♀

O29.5X9 **Other complications of spinal and epidural anesthesia during pregnancy, unspecified trimester** M ♀

5ᵗʰ O29.6 Failed or difficult intubation for anesthesia during pregnancy

O29.60 **Failed or difficult intubation for anesthesia during pregnancy, unspecified trimester** M ♀

O29.61 **Failed or difficult intubation for anesthesia during pregnancy, first trimester** 1st M ♀

O29.62 **Failed or difficult intubation for anesthesia during pregnancy, second trimester** 2nd M ♀

O29.63 **Failed or difficult intubation for anesthesia during pregnancy, third trimester** 3rd M ♀

5ᵗʰ O29.8 Other complications of anesthesia during pregnancy

6ᵗʰ O29.8X Other complications of anesthesia during pregnancy

O29.8X1 **Other complications of anesthesia during pregnancy, first trimester** 1st M ♀

O29.8X2 **Other complications of anesthesia during pregnancy, second trimester** 2nd M ♀

O29.8X3 **Other complications of anesthesia during pregnancy, third trimester** 3rd M ♀

O29.8X9 **Other complications of anesthesia during pregnancy, unspecified trimester** M ♀

5ᵗʰ O29.9 Unspecified complication of anesthesia during pregnancy

O29.90 **Unspecified complication of anesthesia during pregnancy, unspecified trimester** M ♀

O29.91 **Unspecified complication of anesthesia during pregnancy, first trimester** 1st M ♀

O29.92 **Unspecified complication of anesthesia during pregnancy, second trimester** 2nd M ♀

O29.93 **Unspecified complication of anesthesia during pregnancy, third trimester** 3rd M ♀

Maternal care related to the fetus and amniotic cavity and possible delivery problems (O30-O48)

4ᵗʰ O30 **Multiple gestation**

Code also any complications specific to multiple gestation

5ᵗʰ O30.0 Twin pregnancy

6ᵗʰ O30.00 **Twin pregnancy, unspecified number of placenta and unspecified number of amniotic sacs**

O30.001 **Twin pregnancy, unspecified number of placenta and unspecified number of amniotic sacs, first trimester** 1st M ♀

O30.002 **Twin pregnancy, unspecified number of placenta and unspecified number of amniotic sacs, second trimester** 2nd M ♀

O30.003 **Twin pregnancy, unspecified number of placenta and unspecified number of amniotic sacs, third trimester** 3rd M ♀

O30.009 **Twin pregnancy, unspecified number of placenta and unspecified number of amniotic sacs, unspecified trimester** M ♀

6ᵗʰ O30.01 **Twin pregnancy, monochorionic/monoamniotic**

Twin pregnancy, one placenta, one amniotic sac

EXCLUDES1 conjoined twins (O30.02-)

O30.011 **Twin pregnancy, monochorionic/monoamniotic, first trimester** 1st M ♀

O30.012 **Twin pregnancy, monochorionic/monoamniotic, second trimester** 2nd M ♀

1st 1st trimester   2nd 2nd trimester   3rd 3rd trimester   PDx Unacceptable principal diagnosis symbol per Medicare code edits
PDx Code exempt from diagnosis present on admission requirement   ❓ Questionable admission   cc Complication or comorbidity
MCC Major complication or comorbidity   CC/MCC CC/MCC exclusion   HCC HCC diagnosis code   RxHCC RxHCC diagnosis code   MACRA code
DEFINITION Describes condition/terminology   **TIP** Coding guidance   ◉ Official Guideline Reference   Z1 Z code as first-listed diagnosis

896   When symbols appear on a code that requires a 7th character extension, refer to Appendix B to identify applicable 7th character codes.   **2020 ICD-10-CM**

O30.013 Twin pregnancy, monochorionic/monoamniotic, third trimester `3rd` `M` ♀

O30.019 Twin pregnancy, monochorionic/monoamniotic, unspecified trimester `M` ♀

`6th` O30.02 Conjoined twin pregnancy

O30.021 Conjoined twin pregnancy, first trimester `1st` `M` ♀

O30.022 Conjoined twin pregnancy, second trimester `2nd` `M` ♀

O30.023 Conjoined twin pregnancy, third trimester `3rd` `M` `cc` ♀ `CC/MCC Exc`

O30.029 Conjoined twin pregnancy, unspecified trimester `M` ♀

`6th` O30.03 Twin pregnancy, monochorionic/diamniotic
Twin pregnancy, one placenta, two amniotic sacs

O30.031 Twin pregnancy, monochorionic/diamniotic, first trimester `1st` `M` ♀

O30.032 Twin pregnancy, monochorionic/diamniotic, second trimester `2nd` `M` ♀

O30.033 Twin pregnancy, monochorionic/diamniotic, third trimester `3rd` `M` ♀

O30.039 Twin pregnancy, monochorionic/diamniotic, unspecified trimester `M` ♀

`6th` O30.04 Twin pregnancy, dichorionic/diamniotic
Twin pregnancy, two placentae, two amniotic sacs

O30.041 Twin pregnancy, dichorionic/diamniotic, first trimester `1st` `M` ♀

O30.042 Twin pregnancy, dichorionic/diamniotic, second trimester `2nd` `M` ♀

O30.043 Twin pregnancy, dichorionic/diamniotic, third trimester `3rd` `M` ♀

O30.049 Twin pregnancy, dichorionic/diamniotic, unspecified trimester `M` ♀

`6th` O30.09 Twin pregnancy, unable to determine number of placenta and number of amniotic sacs

O30.091 Twin pregnancy, unable to determine number of placenta and number of amniotic sacs, first trimester `1st` `M` ♀

O30.092 Twin pregnancy, unable to determine number of placenta and number of amniotic sacs, second trimester `2nd` `M` ♀

O30.093 Twin pregnancy, unable to determine number of placenta and number of amniotic sacs, third trimester `3rd` `M` ♀

O30.099 Twin pregnancy, unable to determine number of placenta and number of amniotic sacs, unspecified trimester `M` ♀

`5th` O30.1 Triplet pregnancy

`6th` O30.10 Triplet pregnancy, unspecified number of placenta and unspecified number of amniotic sacs

O30.101 Triplet pregnancy, unspecified number of placenta and unspecified number of amniotic sacs, first trimester `1st` `M` `cc` ♀ `CC/MCC Exc`

O30.102 Triplet pregnancy, unspecified number of placenta and unspecified number of amniotic sacs, second trimester `2nd` `M` `cc` ♀ `CC/MCC Exc`

O30.103 Triplet pregnancy, unspecified number of placenta and unspecified number of amniotic sacs, third trimester `3rd` `M` `cc` ♀ `CC/MCC Exc`
AHA: Q2 2016

O30.109 Triplet pregnancy, unspecified number of placenta and unspecified number of amniotic sacs, unspecified trimester `M` ♀

`6th` O30.11 Triplet pregnancy with two or more monochorionic fetuses

O30.111 Triplet pregnancy with two or more monochorionic fetuses, first trimester `1st` `M` `cc` ♀ `CC/MCC Exc`

O30.112 Triplet pregnancy with two or more monochorionic fetuses, second trimester `2nd` `M` `cc` ♀ `CC/MCC Exc`

O30.113 Triplet pregnancy with two or more monochorionic fetuses, third trimester `3rd` `M` `cc` ♀ `CC/MCC Exc`

O30.119 Triplet pregnancy with two or more monochorionic fetuses, unspecified trimester `M` ♀

`6th` O30.12 Triplet pregnancy with two or more monoamniotic fetuses

O30.121 Triplet pregnancy with two or more monoamniotic fetuses, first trimester `1st` `M` `cc` ♀ `CC/MCC Exc`

O30.122 Triplet pregnancy with two or more monoamniotic fetuses, second trimester `2nd` `M` `cc` ♀ `CC/MCC Exc`

O30.123 Triplet pregnancy with two or more monoamniotic fetuses, third trimester `3rd` `M` `cc` ♀ `CC/MCC Exc`

O30.129 Triplet pregnancy with two or more monoamniotic fetuses, unspecified trimester `M` ♀

`6th` O30.13 Triplet pregnancy, trichorionic/triamniotic

O30.131 Triplet pregnancy, trichorionic/triamniotic, first trimester `1st` `M` `cc` ♀ `CC/MCC Exc`

O30.132 Triplet pregnancy, trichorionic/triamniotic, second trimester `2nd` `M` `cc` ♀ `CC/MCC Exc`

O30.133 Triplet pregnancy, trichorionic/triamniotic, third trimester `3rd` `M` `cc` ♀ `CC/MCC Exc`

O30.139 Triplet pregnancy, trichorionic/triamniotic, unspecified trimester `M` ♀

`6th` O30.19 Triplet pregnancy, unable to determine number of placenta and number of amniotic sacs

O30.191 Triplet pregnancy, unable to determine number of placenta and number of amniotic sacs, first trimester `1st` `M` `cc` ♀ `CC/MCC Exc`

O30.192 Triplet pregnancy, unable to determine number of placenta and number of amniotic sacs, second trimester `2nd` `M` `cc` ♀ `CC/MCC Exc`

O30.193 Triplet pregnancy, unable to determine number of placenta and number of amniotic sacs, third trimester `3rd` `M` `cc` ♀ `CC/MCC Exc`

O30.199 Triplet pregnancy, unable to determine number of placenta and number of amniotic sacs, unspecified trimester `M` ♀

`5th` O30.2 Quadruplet pregnancy

`6th` O30.20 Quadruplet pregnancy, unspecified number of placenta and unspecified number of amniotic sacs

O30.201 Quadruplet pregnancy, unspecified number of placenta and unspecified number of amniotic sacs, first trimester `1st` `M` `cc` ♀ `CC/MCC Exc`

O30.202 Quadruplet pregnancy, unspecified number of placenta and unspecified number of amniotic sacs, second trimester `2nd` `M` `cc` ♀ `CC/MCC Exc`

O30.203 Quadruplet pregnancy, unspecified number of placenta and unspecified number of amniotic sacs, third trimester `3rd` `M` `cc` ♀ `CC/MCC Exc`

O30.209 Quadruplet pregnancy, unspecified number of placenta and unspecified number of amniotic sacs, unspecified trimester `M` ♀

`6th` O30.21 Quadruplet pregnancy with two or more monochorionic fetuses

O30.211 Quadruplet pregnancy with two or more monochorionic fetuses, first trimester `1st` `M` `cc` ♀ `CC/MCC Exc`

Unspecified Code Other Specified Code Manifestation Code `N` Newborn `P` Pediatric `M` Maternity `A` Adult ♂ Male ♀ Female
● New Code ▲ Revised Code Title ►◄ Revised Text **NOTES** *INCLUDES* *EXCLUDES1* Not coded here *EXCLUDES2* Not included here
`4th` 4th character required `5th` 5th character required `6th` 6th character required `7th` 7th character required `7x` Extension 'X' Alert
`HAC` Hospital-acquired condition (HAC) alert **AHA** AHA Coding Clinic© `☞` Code first alert

O30.212 Quadruplet pregnancy with two or more monochorionic fetuses, second trimester **2nd** M cc Q CC/MCC Exc

O30.213 Quadruplet pregnancy with two or more monochorionic fetuses, third trimester **3rd** M cc Q CC/MCC Exc

O30.219 Quadruplet pregnancy with two or more monochorionic fetuses, unspecified trimester M Q

6th O30.22 Quadruplet pregnancy with two or more monoamniotic fetuses

O30.221 Quadruplet pregnancy with two or more monoamniotic fetuses, first trimester **1st** M cc Q CC/MCC Exc

O30.222 Quadruplet pregnancy with two or more monoamniotic fetuses, second trimester **2nd** M cc Q CC/MCC Exc

O30.223 Quadruplet pregnancy with two or more monoamniotic fetuses, third trimester **3rd** M cc Q CC/MCC Exc

O30.229 Quadruplet pregnancy with two or more monoamniotic fetuses, unspecified trimester M Q

6th O30.23 Quadruplet pregnancy, quadrachorionic/quadra-amniotic

O30.231 Quadruplet pregnancy, quadrachorionic/quadra-amniotic, first trimester **1st** M cc Q CC/MCC Exc

O30.232 Quadruplet pregnancy, quadrachorionic/quadra-amniotic, second trimester **2nd** M cc Q CC/MCC Exc

O30.233 Quadruplet pregnancy, quadrachorionic/quadra-amniotic, third trimester **3rd** M cc Q CC/MCC Exc

O30.239 Quadruplet pregnancy, quadrachorionic/quadra-amniotic, unspecified trimester M Q

6th O30.29 Quadruplet pregnancy, unable to determine number of placenta and number of amniotic sacs

O30.291 Quadruplet pregnancy, unable to determine number of placenta and number of amniotic sacs, first trimester **1st** M cc Q CC/MCC Exc

O30.292 Quadruplet pregnancy, unable to determine number of placenta and number of amniotic sacs, second trimester **2nd** M cc Q CC/MCC Exc

O30.293 Quadruplet pregnancy, unable to determine number of placenta and number of amniotic sacs, third trimester **3rd** M cc Q CC/MCC Exc

O30.299 Quadruplet pregnancy, unable to determine number of placenta and number of amniotic sacs, unspecified trimester M Q

5th O30.8 Other specified multiple gestation

Multiple gestation pregnancy greater then quadruplets

6th O30.80 Other specified multiple gestation, unspecified number of placenta and unspecified number of amniotic sacs

O30.801 Other specified multiple gestation, unspecified number of placenta and unspecified number of amniotic sacs, first trimester **1st** M cc Q CC/MCC Exc

O30.802 Other specified multiple gestation, unspecified number of placenta and unspecified number of amniotic sacs, second trimester **2nd** M cc Q CC/MCC Exc

O30.803 Other specified multiple gestation, unspecified number of placenta and unspecified number of amniotic sacs, third trimester **3rd** M cc Q CC/MCC Exc

O30.809 Other specified multiple gestation, unspecified number of placenta and

unspecified number of amniotic sacs, unspecified trimester M Q

6th O30.81 Other specified multiple gestation with two or more monochorionic fetuses

O30.811 Other specified multiple gestation with two or more monochorionic fetuses, first trimester **1st** M cc Q CC/MCC Exc

O30.812 Other specified multiple gestation with two or more monochorionic fetuses, second trimester **2nd** M cc Q CC/MCC Exc

O30.813 Other specified multiple gestation with two or more monochorionic fetuses, third trimester **3rd** M cc Q CC/MCC Exc

O30.819 Other specified multiple gestation with two or more monochorionic fetuses, unspecified trimester M Q

6th O30.82 Other specified multiple gestation with two or more monoamniotic fetuses

O30.821 Other specified multiple gestation with two or more monoamniotic fetuses, first trimester **1st** M cc Q CC/MCC Exc

O30.822 Other specified multiple gestation with two or more monoamniotic fetuses, second trimester **2nd** M cc Q CC/MCC Exc

O30.823 Other specified multiple gestation with two or more monoamniotic fetuses, third trimester **3rd** M cc Q CC/MCC Exc

O30.829 Other specified multiple gestation with two or more monoamniotic fetuses, unspecified trimester M Q

6th O30.83 Other specified multiple gestation, number of chorions and amnions are both equal to the number of fetuses

Pentachorionic, penta-amniotic pregnancy (quintuplets)
Hexachorionic, hexa-amniotic pregnancy (sextuplets)
Heptachorionic, hepta-amniotic pregnancy (septuplets)

O30.831 Other specified multiple gestation, number of chorions and amnions are both equal to the number of fetuses, first trimester **1st** M Q CC/MCC Exc

O30.832 Other specified multiple gestation, number of chorions and amnions are both equal to the number of fetuses, second trimester **2nd** M Q CC/MCC Exc

O30.833 Other specified multiple gestation, number of chorions and amnions are both equal to the number of fetuses, third trimester **3rd** M Q CC/MCC Exc

O30.839 Other specified multiple gestation, number of chorions and amnions are both equal to the number of fetuses, unspecified trimester M Q

6th O30.89 Other specified multiple gestation, unable to determine number of placenta and number of amniotic sacs

O30.891 Other specified multiple gestation, unable to determine number of placenta and number of amniotic sacs, first trimester **1st** M cc Q CC/MCC Exc

O30.892 Other specified multiple gestation, unable to determine number of placenta and number of amniotic sacs, second trimester **2nd** M cc Q CC/MCC Exc

O30.893 Other specified multiple gestation, unable to determine number of placenta and number of amniotic sacs, third trimester **3rd** M cc Q CC/MCC Exc

O30.899 Other specified multiple gestation, unable to determine number of placenta and number of amniotic sacs, unspecified trimester M Q

1st 1st trimester **2nd** 2nd trimester **3rd** 3rd trimester PDx Unacceptable principal diagnosis symbol per Medicare code edits
PDx Code exempt from diagnosis present on admission requirement ? Questionable admission cc Complication or comorbidity
MCC Major complication or comorbidity CC/MCC Exc CC/MCC exclusion HCC HCC diagnosis code RxHCC RxHCC diagnosis code MACRA code
DEFINITION Describes condition/terminology **TIP** Coding guidance 👁 Official Guideline Reference Z1 Z code as first-listed diagnosis

When symbols appear on a code that requires a 7th character extension, refer to Appendix B to identify applicable 7th character codes. **2020 ICD-10-CM**

O30.9 Multiple gestation, unspecified
Multiple pregnancy NOS
O30.90 Multiple gestation, unspecified, unspecified trimester M ♀
O30.91 Multiple gestation, unspecified, first trimester 1st M ♀
O30.92 Multiple gestation, unspecified, second trimester 2nd M ♀
O30.93 Multiple gestation, unspecified, third trimester 3rd M ♀

O31 Complications specific to multiple gestation
See Official Guidelines "7th character for Fetus Identification" I.C.15. a.6
EXCLUDES2 delayed delivery of second twin, triplet, etc. (O63.2)
malpresentation of one fetus or more (O32.9)
placental transfusion syndromes (O43.0-)
One of the following 7th characters is to be assigned to each code under category O31. 7th character 0 is for single gestations and multiple gestations where the fetus is unspecified. 7th characters 1 through 9 are for cases of multiple gestations to identify the fetus for which the code applies. The appropriate code from category O30, Multiple gestation, must also be assigned when assigning a code from category O31 that has a 7th character of 1 through 9.
0 = not applicable or unspecified
1 = fetus 1
2 = fetus 2
3 = fetus 3
4 = fetus 4
5 = fetus 5
9 = other fetus

O31.0 Papyraceous fetus
DEFINITION: Remains of expired fetus and is being compressed by the live twin.
Fetus compressus
O31.00 Papyraceous fetus, unspecified trimester M ♀
O31.01 Papyraceous fetus, first trimester 1st M ♀
O31.02 Papyraceous fetus, second trimester 2nd M ♀
O31.03 Papyraceous fetus, third trimester 3rd M ♀

O31.1 Continuing pregnancy after spontaneous abortion of one fetus or more
O31.10 Continuing pregnancy after spontaneous abortion of one fetus or more, unspecified trimester M ♀
O31.11 Continuing pregnancy after spontaneous abortion of one fetus or more, first trimester 1st M ♀
O31.12 Continuing pregnancy after spontaneous abortion of one fetus or more, second trimester 2nd M ♀
O31.13 Continuing pregnancy after spontaneous abortion of one fetus or more, third trimester 3rd M ♀

O31.2 Continuing pregnancy after intrauterine death of one fetus or more
O31.20 Continuing pregnancy after intrauterine death of one fetus or more, unspecified trimester M ♀
O31.21 Continuing pregnancy after intrauterine death of one fetus or more, first trimester 1st M ♀
O31.22 Continuing pregnancy after intrauterine death of one fetus or more, second trimester 2nd M ♀
O31.23 Continuing pregnancy after intrauterine death of one fetus or more, third trimester 3rd M ♀

O31.3 Continuing pregnancy after elective fetal reduction of one fetus or more
Continuing pregnancy after selective termination of one fetus or more
O31.30 Continuing pregnancy after elective fetal reduction of one fetus or more, unspecified trimester M ♀
O31.31 Continuing pregnancy after elective fetal reduction of one fetus or more, first trimester 1st M ♀
O31.32 Continuing pregnancy after elective fetal reduction of one fetus or more, second trimester 2nd M ♀
O31.33 Continuing pregnancy after elective fetal reduction of one fetus or more, third trimester 3rd M ♀

O31.8 Other complications specific to multiple gestation
O31.8X Other complications specific to multiple gestation
O31.8X1 Other complications specific to multiple gestation, first trimester 1st M cc ♀ CC/MCC Exc
O31.8X2 Other complications specific to multiple gestation, second trimester 2nd M cc ♀ CC/MCC Exc
O31.8X3 Other complications specific to multiple gestation, third trimester 3rd M cc ♀ CC/MCC Exc
O31.8X9 Other complications specific to multiple gestation, unspecified trimester M ♀

O32 Maternal care for malpresentation of fetus
See Official Guidelines "7th character for Fetus Identification" I.C.15. a.6
TIP: Normal fetal position for delivery is occiput anterior - head down, baby's body facing mother's back.
INCLUDES the listed conditions as a reason for observation, hospitalization or other obstetric care of the mother, or for cesarean delivery before onset of labor
EXCLUDES1 malpresentation of fetus with obstructed labor (O64.-)
One of the following 7th characters is to be assigned to each code under category O32. 7th character 0 is for single gestations and multiple gestations where the fetus is unspecified. 7th characters 1 through 9 are for cases of multiple gestations to identify the fetus for which the code applies. The appropriate code from category O30, Multiple gestation, must also be assigned when assigning a code from category O32 that has a 7th character of 1 through 9.
0 = not applicable or unspecified
1 = fetus 1
2 = fetus 2
3 = fetus 3
4 = fetus 4
5 = fetus 5
9 = other fetus

O32.0 Maternal care for unstable lie M ♀
O32.1 Maternal care for breech presentation M ♀
Maternal care for buttocks presentation
Maternal care for complete breech
Maternal care for frank breech
EXCLUDES1 footling presentation (O32.8)
incomplete breech (O32.8)
O32.2 Maternal care for transverse and oblique lie M ♀
Maternal care for oblique presentation
Maternal care for transverse presentation
O32.3 Maternal care for face, brow and chin presentation M ♀
O32.4 Maternal care for high head at term M ♀
Maternal care for failure of head to enter pelvic brim
O32.6 Maternal care for compound presentation M ♀
O32.8 Maternal care for other malpresentation of fetus M ♀
Maternal care for footling presentation
Maternal care for incomplete breech
O32.9 Maternal care for malpresentation of fetus, unspecified M ♀

O33 Maternal care for disproportion
See Official Guidelines "7th character for Fetus Identification" I.C.15. a.6
INCLUDES the listed conditions as a reason for observation, hospitalization or other obstetric care of the mother, or for cesarean delivery before onset of labor
EXCLUDES1 disproportion with obstructed labor (O65-O66)
O33.0 Maternal care for disproportion due to deformity of maternal pelvic bones M cc ♀ CC/MCC Exc
Maternal care for disproportion due to pelvic deformity causing disproportion NOS
O33.1 Maternal care for disproportion due to generally contracted pelvis M ♀
Maternal care for disproportion due to contracted pelvis NOS causing disproportion
O33.2 Maternal care for disproportion due to inlet contraction of pelvis M ♀
Maternal care for disproportion due to inlet contraction (pelvis) causing disproportion

O33.3 - O34.212

CHAPTER 15: PREGNANCY, CHILDBIRTH AND THE PUERPERIUM (O00-O9A)

O33.3 Maternal care for disproportion due to outlet contraction of pelvis M ♀

Maternal care for disproportion due to mid-cavity contraction (pelvis)

Maternal care for disproportion due to outlet contraction (pelvis)

One of the following 7th characters is to be assigned to code O33.3. 7th character 0 is for single gestations and multiple gestations where the fetus is unspecified. 7th characters 1 through 9 are for cases of multiple gestations to identify the fetus for which the code applies. The appropriate code from category O30, Multiple gestation, must also be assigned when assigning code O33.3 with a 7th character of 1 through 9.

0 = not applicable or unspecified
1 = fetus 1
2 = fetus 2
3 = fetus 3
4 = fetus 4
5 = fetus 5
9 = other fetus

O33.4 Maternal care for disproportion of mixed maternal and fetal origin M ♀

One of the following 7th characters is to be assigned to code O33.4. 7th character 0 is for single gestations and multiple gestations where the fetus is unspecified. 7th characters 1 through 9 are for cases of multiple gestations to identify the fetus for which the code applies. The appropriate code from category O30, Multiple gestation, must also be assigned when assigning code O33.4 with a 7th character of 1 through 9.

0 = not applicable or unspecified
1 = fetus 1
2 = fetus 2
3 = fetus 3
4 = fetus 4
5 = fetus 5
9 = other fetus

O33.5 Maternal care for disproportion due to unusually large fetus M ♀

Maternal care for disproportion due to disproportion of fetal origin with normally formed fetus

Maternal care for disproportion due to fetal disproportion NOS

One of the following 7th characters is to be assigned to code O33.5. 7th character 0 is for single gestations and multiple gestations where the fetus is unspecified. 7th characters 1 through 9 are for cases of multiple gestations to identify the fetus for which the code applies. The appropriate code from category O30, Multiple gestation, must also be assigned when assigning code O33.5 with a 7th character of 1 through 9.

0 = not applicable or unspecified
1 = fetus 1
2 = fetus 2
3 = fetus 3
4 = fetus 4
5 = fetus 5
9 = other fetus

O33.6 Maternal care for disproportion due to hydrocephalic fetus M ♀

One of the following 7th characters is to be assigned to code O33.6. 7th character 0 is for single gestations and multiple gestations where the fetus is unspecified. 7th characters 1 through 9 are for cases of multiple gestations to identify the fetus for which the code applies. The appropriate code from category O30, Multiple gestation, must also be assigned when assigning code O33.6 with a 7th character of 1 through 9.

0 = not applicable or unspecified
1 = fetus 1
2 = fetus 2
3 = fetus 3
4 = fetus 4

5 = fetus 5
9 = other fetus

O33.7 Maternal care for disproportion due to other fetal deformities M ♀

AHA: Q4 2016

Maternal care for disproportion due to fetal ascites

Maternal care for disproportion due to fetal hydrops

Maternal care for disproportion due to fetal meningomyelocele

Maternal care for disproportion due to fetal sacral teratoma

Maternal care for disproportion due to fetal tumor

One of the following 7th characters is to be assigned to code O33.7. 7th character 0 is for single gestations and multiple gestations where the fetus is unspecified. 7th characters 1 through 9 are for cases of multiple gestations to identify the fetus for which the code applies. The appropriate code from category O30, Multiple gestation, must also be assigned when assigning code O33.7 with a 7th character of 1 through 9.

0 = not applicable or unspecified
1 = fetus 1
2 = fetus 2
3 = fetus 3
4 = fetus 4
5 = fetus 5
9 = other fetus

EXCLUDES1 obstructed labor due to other fetal deformities (O66.3)

O33.8 **Maternal care for disproportion of other origin** M ♀

O33.9 **Maternal care for disproportion, unspecified** M ♀

Maternal care for disproportion due to cephalopelvic disproportion NOS

Maternal care for disproportion due to fetopelvic disproportion NOS

O34 Maternal care for abnormality of pelvic organs

INCLUDES the listed conditions as a reason for hospitalization or other obstetric care of the mother, or for cesarean delivery before onset of labor

☞ **Code first** any associated obstructed labor (O65.5)

Use additional code for specific condition

O34.0 Maternal care for congenital malformation of uterus

Maternal care for double uterus

Maternal care for uterus bicornis

O34.00 **Maternal care for unspecified congenital malformation of uterus, unspecified trimester** M ♀

O34.01 **Maternal care for unspecified congenital malformation of uterus,** first trimester 1st M ♀

O34.02 **Maternal care for unspecified congenital malformation of uterus,** second trimester 2nd M ♀

O34.03 **Maternal care for unspecified congenital malformation of uterus,** third trimester 3rd M ♀

O34.1 Maternal care for benign tumor of corpus uteri

EXCLUDES2 maternal care for benign tumor of cervix (O34.4-)

maternal care for malignant neoplasm of uterus (O9A.1-)

O34.10 **Maternal care for benign tumor of corpus uteri, unspecified trimester** M ♀

O34.11 **Maternal care for benign tumor of corpus uteri,** first trimester 1st M ♀

O34.12 **Maternal care for benign tumor of corpus uteri,** second trimester 2nd M ♀

O34.13 **Maternal care for benign tumor of corpus uteri,** third trimester 3rd M ♀

O34.2 Maternal care due to uterine scar from previous surgery

O34.21 **Maternal care for scar** from previous cesarean delivery

O34.211 **Maternal care for** low transverse **scar from previous cesarean delivery** M ♀

AHA: Q3 2018, Q4 2016

O34.212 **Maternal care for** vertical **scar from previous cesarean delivery** M ♀

AHA: Q4 2016

1st 1st trimester 2nd 2nd trimester 3rd 3rd trimester Unacceptable principal diagnosis symbol per Medicare code edits
Code exempt from diagnosis present on admission requirement ? Questionable admission Complication or comorbidity
MCC Major complication or comorbidity CC/MCC CC/MCC exclusion HCC HCC diagnosis code RxHCC RxHCC diagnosis code MACRA code
DEFINITION Describes condition/terminology TIP Coding guidance Official Guideline Reference Z code as first-listed diagnosis

900   When symbols appear on a code that requires a 7th character extension, refer to Appendix B to identify applicable 7th character codes.   2020 ICD-10-CM

Maternal care for classical scar from previous cesarean delivery
O34.219 Maternal care for unspecified type scar from previous cesarean delivery M ♀
AHA: Q3 2018, Q4 2016
O34.29 Maternal care due to uterine scar from other previous surgery M ♀
AHA: Q4 2016
Maternal care due to uterine scar from other transmural uterine incision

O34.3 Maternal care for cervical incompetence
Maternal care for cerclage with or without cervical incompetence
Maternal care for Shirodkar suture with or without cervical incompetence
O34.30 Maternal care for cervical incompetence, unspecified trimester M ♀
O34.31 Maternal care for cervical incompetence, first trimester 1st M MCC ♀ CC/MCC Exc
O34.32 Maternal care for cervical incompetence, second trimester 2nd M MCC ♀ CC/MCC Exc
O34.33 Maternal care for cervical incompetence, third trimester 3rd M MCC ♀ CC/MCC Exc

O34.4 Maternal care for other abnormalities of cervix
O34.40 Maternal care for other abnormalities of cervix, unspecified trimester M ♀
O34.41 Maternal care for other abnormalities of cervix, first trimester 1st M ♀
O34.42 Maternal care for other abnormalities of cervix, second trimester 2nd M ♀
O34.43 Maternal care for other abnormalities of cervix, third trimester 3rd M ♀

O34.5 Maternal care for other abnormalities of gravid uterus
O34.51 Maternal care for incarceration of gravid uterus
O34.511 Maternal care for incarceration of gravid uterus, first trimester 1st M ♀
O34.512 Maternal care for incarceration of gravid uterus, second trimester 2nd M ♀
O34.513 Maternal care for incarceration of gravid uterus, third trimester 3rd M ♀
O34.519 Maternal care for incarceration of gravid uterus, unspecified trimester M ♀
O34.52 Maternal care for prolapse of gravid uterus
O34.521 Maternal care for prolapse of gravid uterus, first trimester 1st M ♀
O34.522 Maternal care for prolapse of gravid uterus, second trimester 2nd M ♀
O34.523 Maternal care for prolapse of gravid uterus, third trimester 3rd M ♀
O34.529 Maternal care for prolapse of gravid uterus, unspecified trimester M ♀
O34.53 Maternal care for retroversion of gravid uterus
O34.531 Maternal care for retroversion of gravid uterus, first trimester 1st M ♀
O34.532 Maternal care for retroversion of gravid uterus, second trimester 2nd M ♀
O34.533 Maternal care for retroversion of gravid uterus, third trimester 3rd M ♀
O34.539 Maternal care for retroversion of gravid uterus, unspecified trimester M ♀
O34.59 Maternal care for other abnormalities of gravid uterus
O34.591 Maternal care for other abnormalities of gravid uterus, first trimester 1st M ♀
O34.592 Maternal care for other abnormalities of gravid uterus, second trimester 2nd M ♀
O34.593 Maternal care for other abnormalities of gravid uterus, third trimester 3rd M ♀
O34.599 Maternal care for other abnormalities of gravid uterus, unspecified trimester M ♀

O34.6 Maternal care for abnormality of vagina

EXCLUDES2 maternal care for vaginal varices in pregnancy (O22.1-)
O34.60 Maternal care for abnormality of vagina, unspecified trimester M ♀
O34.61 Maternal care for abnormality of vagina, first trimester 1st M ♀
O34.62 Maternal care for abnormality of vagina, second trimester 2nd M ♀
O34.63 Maternal care for abnormality of vagina, third trimester 3rd M ♀

O34.7 Maternal care for abnormality of vulva and perineum
EXCLUDES2 maternal care for perineal and vulval varices in pregnancy (O22.1-)
O34.70 Maternal care for abnormality of vulva and perineum, unspecified trimester M ♀
O34.71 Maternal care for abnormality of vulva and perineum, first trimester 1st M ♀
O34.72 Maternal care for abnormality of vulva and perineum, second trimester 2nd M ♀
O34.73 Maternal care for abnormality of vulva and perineum, third trimester 3rd M ♀

O34.8 Maternal care for other abnormalities of pelvic organs
O34.80 Maternal care for other abnormalities of pelvic organs, unspecified trimester M ♀
O34.81 Maternal care for other abnormalities of pelvic organs, first trimester 1st M ♀
O34.82 Maternal care for other abnormalities of pelvic organs, second trimester 2nd M ♀
O34.83 Maternal care for other abnormalities of pelvic organs, third trimester 3rd M ♀

O34.9 Maternal care for abnormality of pelvic organ, unspecified
O34.90 Maternal care for abnormality of pelvic organ, unspecified, unspecified trimester M ♀
O34.91 Maternal care for abnormality of pelvic organ, unspecified, first trimester 1st M ♀
O34.92 Maternal care for abnormality of pelvic organ, unspecified, second trimester 2nd M ♀
O34.93 Maternal care for abnormality of pelvic organ, unspecified, third trimester 3rd M ♀

O35 Maternal care for known or suspected fetal abnormality and damage
See Official Guidelines "7th character for Fetus Identification" I.C.15. a.6 "Codes from Categories O35 and O36" I.C.15.e.1
INCLUDES the listed conditions in the fetus as a reason for hospitalization or other obstetric care to the mother, or for termination of pregnancy
Code also any associated maternal condition
EXCLUDES1 encounter for suspected maternal and fetal conditions ruled out (Z03.7-)
One of the following 7th characters is to be assigned to each code under category O35. 7th character 0 is for single gestations and multiple gestations where the fetus is unspecified. 7th characters 1 through 9 are for cases of multiple gestations to identify the fetus for which the code applies. The appropriate code from category O30, Multiple gestation, must also be assigned when assigning a code from category O35 that has a 7th character of 1 through 9.
0 = not applicable or unspecified
1 = fetus 1
2 = fetus 2
3 = fetus 3
4 = fetus 4
5 = fetus 5
9 = other fetus

O35.0 Maternal care for (suspected) central nervous system malformation in fetus M ♀
Maternal care for fetal anencephaly
Maternal care for fetal hydrocephalus
Maternal care for fetal spina bifida
EXCLUDES2 chromosomal abnormality in fetus (O35.1)
O35.1 Maternal care for (suspected) chromosomal abnormality in fetus M ♀

O35.2 Maternal care for (suspected) hereditary disease in fetus M ♀
> *EXCLUDES2* chromosomal abnormality in fetus (O35.1)

O35.3 Maternal care for (suspected) damage to fetus from viral disease in mother M ♀
AHA: Q4 2016
Maternal care for damage to fetus from maternal cytomegalovirus infection
Maternal care for damage to fetus from maternal rubella

O35.4 Maternal care for (suspected) damage to fetus from alcohol M ♀

O35.5 Maternal care for (suspected) damage to fetus by drugs M ♀
Maternal care for damage to fetus from drug addiction

O35.6 Maternal care for (suspected) damage to fetus by radiation M ♀

O35.7 Maternal care for (suspected) damage to fetus by other medical procedures M ♀
Maternal care for damage to fetus by amniocentesis
Maternal care for damage to fetus by biopsy procedures
Maternal care for damage to fetus by hematological investigation
Maternal care for damage to fetus by intrauterine contraceptive device
Maternal care for damage to fetus by intrauterine surgery

O35.8 Maternal care for other (suspected) fetal abnormality and damage M ♀
Maternal care for damage to fetus from maternal listeriosis
Maternal care for damage to fetus from maternal toxoplasmosis

O35.9 Maternal care for (suspected) fetal abnormality and damage, unspecified M ♀

O36 Maternal care for other fetal problems
> See Official Guidelines "7th character for Fetus Identification" I.C.15. a.6 "Codes from Categories O35 and O36" I.C.15.e.1
> *INCLUDES* the listed conditions in the fetus as a reason for hospitalization or other obstetric care of the mother, or for termination of pregnancy
> *EXCLUDES1* encounter for suspected maternal and fetal conditions ruled out (Z03.7-)
> placental transfusion syndromes (O43.0-)
> *EXCLUDES2* labor and delivery complicated by fetal stress (O77.-)

One of the following 7th characters is to be assigned to each code under category O36. 7th character 0 is for single gestations and multiple gestations where the fetus is unspecified. 7th characters 1 through 9 are for cases of multiple gestations to identify the fetus for which the code applies. The appropriate code from category O30, Multiple gestation, must also be assigned when assigning a code from category O36 that has a 7th character of 1 through 9.

> 0 = not applicable or unspecified
> 1 = fetus 1
> 2 = fetus 2
> 3 = fetus 3
> 4 = fetus 4
> 5 = fetus 5
> 9 = other fetus

O36.0 Maternal care for rhesus isoimmunization
Maternal care for Rh incompatibility (with hydrops fetalis)

O36.01 Maternal care for anti-D [Rh] antibodies

O36.011 Maternal care for anti-D [Rh] antibodies, first trimester 1st M cc ♀ CC/MCC Exc

O36.012 Maternal care for anti-D [Rh] antibodies, second trimester 2nd M cc ♀ CC/MCC Exc

O36.013 Maternal care for anti-D [Rh] antibodies, third trimester 3rd M cc ♀ CC/MCC Exc

O36.019 Maternal care for anti-D [Rh] antibodies, unspecified trimester M ♀

O36.09 Maternal care for other rhesus isoimmunization

O36.091 Maternal care for other rhesus isoimmunization, first trimester 1st M cc ♀ CC/MCC Exc

O36.092 Maternal care for other rhesus isoimmunization, second trimester 2nd M cc ♀ CC/MCC Exc

O36.093 Maternal care for other rhesus isoimmunization, third trimester 3rd M cc ♀ CC/MCC Exc

O36.099 Maternal care for other rhesus isoimmunization, unspecified trimester M ♀

O36.1 Maternal care for other isoimmunization
Maternal care for ABO isoimmunization

O36.11 Maternal care for Anti-A sensitization
Maternal care for isoimmunization NOS (with hydrops fetalis)

O36.111 Maternal care for Anti-A sensitization, first trimester 1st M ♀

O36.112 Maternal care for Anti-A sensitization, second trimester 2nd M ♀

O36.113 Maternal care for Anti-A sensitization, third trimester 3rd M ♀

O36.119 Maternal care for Anti-A sensitization, unspecified trimester M ♀

O36.19 Maternal care for other isoimmunization
Maternal care for Anti-B sensitization

O36.191 Maternal care for other isoimmunization, first trimester 1st M cc ♀ CC/MCC Exc

O36.192 Maternal care for other isoimmunization, second trimester 2nd M ♀

O36.193 Maternal care for other isoimmunization, third trimester 3rd M ♀

O36.199 Maternal care for other isoimmunization, unspecified trimester M ♀

O36.2 Maternal care for hydrops fetalis
Maternal care for hydrops fetalis NOS
Maternal care for hydrops fetalis not associated with isoimmunization
> *EXCLUDES1* hydrops fetalis associated with ABO isoimmunization (O36.1-)
> hydrops fetalis associated with rhesus isoimmunization (O36.0-)

O36.20 Maternal care for hydrops fetalis, unspecified trimester M ♀

O36.21 Maternal care for hydrops fetalis, first trimester 1st M ♀

O36.22 Maternal care for hydrops fetalis, second trimester 2nd M ♀

O36.23 Maternal care for hydrops fetalis, third trimester 3rd M ♀

O36.4 Maternal care for intrauterine death M cc ♀ CC/MCC Exc
DEFINITION: Loss of pregnancy, greater than 20 weeks.
Maternal care for intrauterine fetal death NOS
Maternal care for intrauterine fetal death after completion of 20 weeks of gestation
Maternal care for late fetal death
Maternal care for missed delivery
> *EXCLUDES1* missed abortion (O02.1)
> stillbirth (P95)

O36.5 Maternal care for known or suspected poor fetal growth

O36.51 Maternal care for known or suspected placental insufficiency

O36.511 Maternal care for known or suspected placental insufficiency, first trimester 1st M ♀

O36.512 Maternal care for known or suspected placental insufficiency, second trimester 2nd M ♀

O36.513 Maternal care for known or suspected placental insufficiency, third trimester 3rd M ♀

O36.519 Maternal care for known or suspected placental insufficiency, unspecified trimester M ♀

1st 1st trimester 2nd 2nd trimester 3rd 3rd trimester PDx Unacceptable principal diagnosis symbol per Medicare code edits
POA Code exempt from diagnosis present on admission requirement ❓ Questionable admission cc Complication or comorbidity
MCC Major complication or comorbidity CC/MCC CC/MCC exclusion HCC HCC diagnosis code RxHCC RxHCC diagnosis code MACRA code
DEFINITION Describes condition/terminology **TIP** Coding guidance Official Guideline Reference Z1 Z code as first-listed diagnosis

902   When symbols appear on a code that requires a 7th character extension, refer to Appendix B to identify applicable 7th character codes.   2020 ICD-10-CM

O36.59 **Maternal care for other known or suspected poor fetal growth**
Maternal care for known or suspected light-for-dates NOS
Maternal care for known or suspected small-for-dates NOS

O36.591 **Maternal care for other known or suspected poor fetal growth, first trimester** 1st M ♀

O36.592 **Maternal care for other known or suspected poor fetal growth, second trimester** 2nd M ♀

O36.593 **Maternal care for other known or suspected poor fetal growth, third trimester** 3rd M ♀

O36.599 **Maternal care for other known or suspected poor fetal growth, unspecified trimester** M ♀

O36.6 **Maternal care for excessive fetal growth**
Maternal care for known or suspected large-for-dates

O36.60 **Maternal care for excessive fetal growth, unspecified trimester** M ♀

O36.61 **Maternal care for excessive fetal growth, first trimester** 1st M ♀

O36.62 **Maternal care for excessive fetal growth, second trimester** 2nd M ♀

O36.63 **Maternal care for excessive fetal growth, third trimester** 3rd M ♀

O36.7 **Maternal care for viable fetus in abdominal pregnancy**

O36.70 **Maternal care for viable fetus in abdominal pregnancy, unspecified trimester** M ♀

O36.71 **Maternal care for viable fetus in abdominal pregnancy, first trimester** 1st M ♀

O36.72 **Maternal care for viable fetus in abdominal pregnancy, second trimester** 2nd M ♀

O36.73 **Maternal care for viable fetus in abdominal pregnancy, third trimester** 3rd M ♀

O36.8 **Maternal care for other specified fetal problems**

O36.80 **Pregnancy with inconclusive fetal viability** M ♀ PDxIn
AHA: Q2 2019
Encounter to determine fetal viability of pregnancy

O36.81 **Decreased fetal movements**

O36.812 **Decreased fetal movements, second trimester** 2nd M ♀

O36.813 **Decreased fetal movements, third trimester** 3rd M ♀

O36.819 **Decreased fetal movements, unspecified trimester** M ♀

O36.82 **Fetal anemia and thrombocytopenia**

O36.821 **Fetal anemia and thrombocytopenia, first trimester** 1st M ♀

O36.822 **Fetal anemia and thrombocytopenia, second trimester** 2nd M ♀

O36.823 **Fetal anemia and thrombocytopenia, third trimester** 3rd M ♀

O36.829 **Fetal anemia and thrombocytopenia, unspecified trimester** M ♀

O36.83 **Maternal care for abnormalities of the fetal heart rate or rhythm**
Maternal care for depressed fetal heart rate tones
Maternal care for fetal bradycardia
Maternal care for fetal heart rate abnormal variability
Maternal care for fetal heart rate decelerations
Maternal care for fetal heart rate irregularity
Maternal care for fetal tachycardia
Maternal care for non-reassuring fetal heart rate or rhythm

O36.831 **Maternal care for abnormalities of the fetal heart rate or rhythm, first trimester** 1st M ♀

O36.832 **Maternal care for abnormalities of the fetal heart rate or rhythm, second trimester** 2nd M ♀

O36.833 **Maternal care for abnormalities of the fetal heart rate or rhythm, third trimester** 3rd M ♀

O36.839 **Maternal care for abnormalities of the fetal heart rate or rhythm, unspecified trimester** M ♀

O36.89 **Maternal care for other specified fetal problems**

O36.891 **Maternal care for other specified fetal problems, first trimester** 1st M ♀

O36.892 **Maternal care for other specified fetal problems, second trimester** 2nd M ♀

O36.893 **Maternal care for other specified fetal problems, third trimester** 3rd M ♀

O36.899 **Maternal care for other specified fetal problems, unspecified trimester** M ♀

O36.9 **Maternal care for fetal problem, unspecified**

O36.90 **Maternal care for fetal problem, unspecified, unspecified trimester** M ♀

O36.91 **Maternal care for fetal problem, unspecified, first trimester** 1st M ♀

O36.92 **Maternal care for fetal problem, unspecified, second trimester** 2nd M ♀

O36.93 **Maternal care for fetal problem, unspecified, third trimester** 3rd M ♀

O40 **Polyhydramnios**
See Official Guidelines "7th character for Fetus Identification" I.C.15. a.6
DEFINITION: Excessive amniotic fluid.
INCLUDES hydramnios
EXCLUDES1 encounter for suspected maternal and fetal conditions ruled out (Z03.7-)
One of the following 7th characters is to be assigned to each code under category O40. 7th character 0 is for single gestations and multiple gestations where the fetus is unspecified. 7th characters 1 through 9 are for cases of multiple gestations to identify the fetus for which the code applies. The appropriate code from category O30, Multiple gestation, must also be assigned when assigning a code from category O40 that has a 7th character of 1 through 9.
0 = not applicable or unspecified
1 = fetus 1
2 = fetus 2
3 = fetus 3
4 = fetus 4
5 = fetus 5
9 = other fetus

O40.1 **Polyhydramnios,** first trimester 1st M ♀
O40.2 **Polyhydramnios,** second trimester 2nd M ♀
O40.3 **Polyhydramnios,** third trimester 3rd M ♀
O40.9 **Polyhydramnios,** unspecified trimester M ♀

O41 **Other disorders of amniotic fluid and membranes**
See Official Guidelines "7th character for Fetus Identification" I.C.15. a.6
EXCLUDES1 encounter for suspected maternal and fetal conditions ruled out (Z03.7-)
One of the following 7th characters is to be assigned to each code under category O41. 7th character 0 is for single gestations and multiple gestations where the fetus is unspecified. 7th characters 1 through 9 are for cases of multiple gestations to identify the fetus for which the code applies. The appropriate code from category O30, Multiple gestation, must also be assigned when assigning a code from category O41 that has a 7th character of 1 through 9.
0 = not applicable or unspecified
1 = fetus 1
2 = fetus 2
3 = fetus 3
4 = fetus 4
5 = fetus 5
9 = other fetus

O41.0 **Oligohydramnios**
DEFINITION: Decreased amniotic fluid.
Oligohydramnios without rupture of membranes

Unspecified Code Other Specified Code Manifestation Code N Newborn P Pediatric M Maternity A Adult ♂ Male ♀ Female
● New Code ▲ Revised Code Title ►◄ Revised Text NOTES INCLUDES EXCLUDES1 Not coded here EXCLUDES2 Not included here
4th character required 5th character required 6th character required 7th character required Extension 'X' Alert
HAC Hospital-acquired condition (HAC) alert AHA AHA Coding Clinic© Code first alert

2020 ICD-10-CM   When symbols appear on a code that requires a 7th character extension, refer to Appendix B to identify applicable 7th character codes.   903

O41.00 – O43 (left margin)

CHAPTER 15: PREGNANCY, CHILDBIRTH AND THE PUERPERIUM (O00-O9A) (left margin)

7th **O41.00** Oligohydramnios, unspecified trimester M ♀

7th **O41.01** Oligohydramnios, first trimester 1st M cc ♀ CC/MCC Exc

7th **O41.02** Oligohydramnios, second trimester 2nd M cc ♀ CC/MCC Exc

7th **O41.03** Oligohydramnios, third trimester 3rd M cc ♀ CC/MCC Exc

5th **O41.1** Infection of amniotic sac and membranes

6th **O41.10** Infection of amniotic sac and membranes, unspecified

7th **O41.101** Infection of amniotic sac and membranes, unspecified, first trimester 1st MCC ♀ CC/MCC Exc

7th **O41.102** Infection of amniotic sac and membranes, unspecified, second trimester 2nd M MCC ♀ CC/MCC Exc

7th **O41.103** Infection of amniotic sac and membranes, unspecified, third trimester 3rd M MCC ♀ CC/MCC Exc

7th **O41.109** Infection of amniotic sac and membranes, unspecified, unspecified trimester M ♀

6th **O41.12** Chorioamnionitis

7th **O41.121** Chorioamnionitis, first trimester 1st M MCC ♀ CC/MCC Exc

7th **O41.122** Chorioamnionitis, second trimester 2nd M MCC ♀ CC/MCC Exc

7th **O41.123** Chorioamnionitis, third trimester 3rd M MCC ♀ CC/MCC Exc

7th **O41.129** Chorioamnionitis, unspecified trimester M ♀

6th **O41.14** Placentitis

7th **O41.141** Placentitis, first trimester 1st M MCC ♀ CC/MCC Exc

7th **O41.142** Placentitis, second trimester 2nd M MCC ♀ CC/MCC Exc

7th **O41.143** Placentitis, third trimester 3rd M MCC ♀ CC/MCC Exc

7th **O41.149** Placentitis, unspecified trimester M ♀

5th **O41.8** Other specified disorders of amniotic fluid and membranes

6th **O41.8X** Other specified disorders of amniotic fluid and membranes

7th **O41.8X1** Other specified disorders of amniotic fluid and membranes, first trimester 1st ♀

7th **O41.8X2** Other specified disorders of amniotic fluid and membranes, second trimester 2nd M ♀

7th **O41.8X3** Other specified disorders of amniotic fluid and membranes, third trimester 3rd M ♀

7th **O41.8X9** Other specified disorders of amniotic fluid and membranes, unspecified trimester M ♀

5th **O41.9** Disorder of amniotic fluid and membranes, unspecified

7th **O41.90** Disorder of amniotic fluid and membranes, unspecified, unspecified trimester M ♀

7th **O41.91** Disorder of amniotic fluid and membranes, unspecified, first trimester 1st M ♀

7th **O41.92** Disorder of amniotic fluid and membranes, unspecified, second trimester 2nd M ♀

7th **O41.93** Disorder of amniotic fluid and membranes, unspecified, third trimester 3rd M ♀

4th **O42** Premature rupture of membranes

5th **O42.0** Premature rupture of membranes, onset of labor within 24 hours of rupture

O42.00 Premature rupture of membranes, onset of labor within 24 hours of rupture, unspecified weeks of gestation M ♀

6th **O42.01** Preterm premature rupture of membranes, onset of labor within 24 hours of rupture

Premature rupture of membranes before 37 completed weeks of gestation

O42.011 Preterm premature rupture of membranes, onset of labor within 24 hours of rupture, first trimester 1st M ♀

O42.012 Preterm premature rupture of membranes, onset of labor within 24 hours of rupture, second trimester 2nd M ♀

O42.013 Preterm premature rupture of membranes, onset of labor within 24 hours of rupture, third trimester 3rd M ♀

O42.019 Preterm premature rupture of membranes, onset of labor within 24 hours of rupture, unspecified trimester M ♀

O42.02 Full-term premature rupture of membranes, onset of labor within 24 hours of rupture M ♀

Premature rupture of membranes at or after 37 completed weeks of gestation, onset of labor within 24 hours of rupture

5th **O42.1** Premature rupture of membranes, onset of labor more than 24 hours following rupture

O42.10 Premature rupture of membranes, onset of labor more than 24 hours following rupture, unspecified weeks of gestation M ♀

6th **O42.11** Preterm premature rupture of membranes, onset of labor more than 24 hours following rupture

Premature rupture of membranes before 37 completed weeks of gestation

O42.111 Preterm premature rupture of membranes, onset of labor more than 24 hours following rupture, first trimester 1st M ♀

O42.112 Preterm premature rupture of membranes, onset of labor more than 24 hours following rupture, second trimester 2nd M ♀

O42.113 Preterm premature rupture of membranes, onset of labor more than 24 hours following rupture, third trimester 3rd M ♀

O42.119 Preterm premature rupture of membranes, onset of labor more than 24 hours following rupture, unspecified trimester M ♀

O42.12 Full-term premature rupture of membranes, onset of labor more than 24 hours following rupture M ♀

Premature rupture of membranes at or after 37 completed weeks of gestation, onset of labor more than 24 hours following rupture

5th **O42.9** Premature rupture of membranes, unspecified as to length of time between rupture and onset of labor

O42.90 Premature rupture of membranes, unspecified as to length of time between rupture and onset of labor, unspecified weeks of gestation M ♀

6th **O42.91** Preterm premature rupture of membranes, unspecified as to length of time between rupture and onset of labor

Premature rupture of membranes before 37 completed weeks of gestation

O42.911 Preterm premature rupture of membranes, unspecified as to length of time between rupture and onset of labor, first trimester 1st M ♀

O42.912 Preterm premature rupture of membranes, unspecified as to length of time between rupture and onset of labor, second trimester 2nd M ♀

O42.913 Preterm premature rupture of membranes, unspecified as to length of time between rupture and onset of labor, third trimester 3rd M ♀

O42.919 Preterm premature rupture of membranes, unspecified as to length of time between rupture and onset of labor, unspecified trimester M ♀

O42.92 Full-term premature rupture of membranes, unspecified as to length of time between rupture and onset of labor M ♀

Premature rupture of membranes at or after 37 completed weeks of gestation, unspecified as to length of time between rupture and onset of labor

4th **O43** Placental disorders

EXCLUDES2 maternal care for poor fetal growth due to placental insufficiency (O36.5-)

placenta previa (O44.-)

placental polyp (O90.89)

placentitis (O41.14-)

premature separation of placenta [abruptio placentae] (O45.-)

1st 1st trimester 2nd 2nd trimester 3rd 3rd trimester PDx Unacceptable principal diagnosis symbol per Medicare code edits
POA Code exempt from diagnosis present on admission requirement ? Questionable admission cc Complication or comorbidity
MCC Major complication or comorbidity CC/MCC Exc CC/MCC exclusion HCC HCC diagnosis code RxHCC RxHCC diagnosis code MACRA code
DEFINITION Describes condition/terminology **TIP** Coding guidance ◉ Official Guideline Reference Z1 Z code as first-listed diagnosis

When symbols appear on a code that requires a 7th character extension, refer to Appendix B to identify applicable 7th character codes.
2020 ICD-10-CM

5ᵗʰ O43.0 Placental transfusion syndromes

6ᵗʰ O43.01 Fetomaternal placental transfusion syndrome
Maternofetal placental transfusion syndrome

    O43.011 Fetomaternal placental transfusion syndrome, first trimester 1st Ⓜ ♀

    O43.012 Fetomaternal placental transfusion syndrome, second trimester 2nd Ⓜ ♀

    O43.013 Fetomaternal placental transfusion syndrome, third trimester 3rd Ⓜ ♀

    O43.019 Fetomaternal placental transfusion syndrome, unspecified trimester Ⓜ ♀

6ᵗʰ O43.02 Fetus-to-fetus placental transfusion syndrome

    O43.021 Fetus-to-fetus placental transfusion syndrome, first trimester 1st Ⓜ ♀

    O43.022 Fetus-to-fetus placental transfusion syndrome, second trimester 2nd Ⓜ ♀

    O43.023 Fetus-to-fetus placental transfusion syndrome, third trimester 3rd Ⓜ ♀

    O43.029 Fetus-to-fetus placental transfusion syndrome, unspecified trimester Ⓜ ♀

5ᵗʰ O43.1 Malformation of placenta

6ᵗʰ O43.10 Malformation of placenta, unspecified
Abnormal placenta NOS

    O43.101 Malformation of placenta, unspecified, first trimester 1st Ⓜ ♀

    O43.102 Malformation of placenta, unspecified, second trimester 2nd Ⓜ ♀

    O43.103 Malformation of placenta, unspecified, third trimester 3rd Ⓜ ♀

    O43.109 Malformation of placenta, unspecified, unspecified trimester Ⓜ ♀

6ᵗʰ O43.11 Circumvallate placenta

    O43.111 Circumvallate placenta, first trimester 1st Ⓜ ♀

    O43.112 Circumvallate placenta, second trimester 2nd Ⓜ ♀

    O43.113 Circumvallate placenta, third trimester 3rd Ⓜ ♀

    O43.119 Circumvallate placenta, unspecified trimester Ⓜ ♀

6ᵗʰ O43.12 Velamentous insertion of umbilical cord

    O43.121 Velamentous insertion of umbilical cord, first trimester 1st Ⓜ ♀

    O43.122 Velamentous insertion of umbilical cord, second trimester 2nd Ⓜ ♀

    O43.123 Velamentous insertion of umbilical cord, third trimester 3rd Ⓜ ♀

    O43.129 Velamentous insertion of umbilical cord, unspecified trimester Ⓜ ♀

6ᵗʰ O43.19 Other malformation of placenta

    O43.191 Other malformation of placenta, first trimester 1st Ⓜ ♀

    O43.192 Other malformation of placenta, second trimester 2nd Ⓜ ♀

    O43.193 Other malformation of placenta, third trimester 3rd Ⓜ ♀

    O43.199 Other malformation of placenta, unspecified trimester Ⓜ ♀

5ᵗʰ O43.2 Morbidly adherent placenta
Code also associated third stage postpartum hemorrhage, if applicable (O72.0)
EXCLUDES1 retained placenta (O73.-)

6ᵗʰ O43.21 Placenta accreta

    O43.211 Placenta accreta, first trimester 1st Ⓜ ♀

    O43.212 Placenta accreta, second trimester 2nd Ⓜ ♀

    O43.213 Placenta accreta, third trimester 3rd Ⓜ ♀

    O43.219 Placenta accreta, unspecified trimester Ⓜ ♀

6ᵗʰ O43.22 Placenta increta

    O43.221 Placenta increta, first trimester 1st Ⓜ ♀

    O43.222 Placenta increta, second trimester 2nd Ⓜ ♀

    O43.223 Placenta increta, third trimester 3rd Ⓜ ♀

    O43.229 Placenta increta, unspecified trimester Ⓜ ♀

6ᵗʰ O43.23 Placenta percreta

    O43.231 Placenta percreta, first trimester 1st Ⓜ ♀

    O43.232 Placenta percreta, second trimester 2nd Ⓜ ♀

    O43.233 Placenta percreta, third trimester 3rd Ⓜ ♀

    O43.239 Placenta percreta, unspecified trimester Ⓜ ♀

5ᵗʰ O43.8 Other placental disorders

6ᵗʰ O43.81 Placental infarction

    O43.811 Placental infarction, first trimester 1st Ⓜ ♀

    O43.812 Placental infarction, second trimester 2nd Ⓜ ♀

    O43.813 Placental infarction, third trimester 3rd Ⓜ ♀

    O43.819 Placental infarction, unspecified trimester Ⓜ ♀

6ᵗʰ O43.89 Other placental disorders
Placental dysfunction

    O43.891 Other placental disorders, first trimester 1st Ⓜ ♀

    O43.892 Other placental disorders, second trimester 2nd Ⓜ ♀

    O43.893 Other placental disorders, third trimester 3rd Ⓜ ♀

    O43.899 Other placental disorders, unspecified trimester Ⓜ ♀

5ᵗʰ O43.9 Unspecified placental disorder

    O43.90 Unspecified placental disorder, unspecified trimester Ⓜ ♀

    O43.91 Unspecified placental disorder, first trimester 1st Ⓜ ♀

    O43.92 Unspecified placental disorder, second trimester 2nd Ⓜ ♀

    O43.93 Unspecified placental disorder, third trimester 3rd Ⓜ ♀

4ᵗʰ O44 Placenta previa

5ᵗʰ O44.0 Complete placenta previa NOS or without hemorrhage
Placenta previa NOS

    O44.00 Complete placenta previa NOS or without hemorrhage, unspecified trimester Ⓜ ♀

    O44.01 Complete placenta previa NOS or without hemorrhage, first trimester 1st Ⓜ c✎ ♀ CC/MCC Exc.

    O44.02 Complete placenta previa NOS or without hemorrhage, second trimester 2nd Ⓜ c✎ ♀ CC/MCC Exc.

    O44.03 Complete placenta previa NOS or without hemorrhage, third trimester 3rd Ⓜ c✎ ♀ CC/MCC Exc.

5ᵗʰ O44.1 Complete placenta previa with hemorrhage
EXCLUDES1 labor and delivery complicated by hemorrhage from vasa previa (O69.4)

    O44.10 Complete placenta previa with hemorrhage, unspecified trimester Ⓜ ♀

    O44.11 Complete placenta previa with hemorrhage, first trimester 1st Ⓜ MCC✎ ♀ CC/MCC Exc.

    O44.12 Complete placenta previa with hemorrhage, second trimester 2nd Ⓜ MCC✎ ♀ CC/MCC Exc.

    O44.13 Complete placenta previa with hemorrhage, third trimester 3rd Ⓜ MCC✎ ♀ CC/MCC Exc.

5ᵗʰ O44.2 Partial placenta previa without hemorrhage
Marginal placenta previa, NOS or without hemorrhage

    O44.20 Partial placenta previa NOS or without hemorrhage, unspecified trimester Ⓜ ♀

    O44.21 Partial placenta previa NOS or without hemorrhage, first trimester 1st Ⓜ c✎ ♀ CC/MCC Exc.

    O44.22 Partial placenta previa NOS or without hemorrhage, second trimester 2nd Ⓜ c✎ ♀ CC/MCC Exc.

    O44.23 Partial placenta previa NOS or without hemorrhage, third trimester 3rd Ⓜ c✎ ♀ CC/MCC Exc.

5ᵗʰ O44.3 Partial placenta previa with hemorrhage
Marginal placenta previa with hemorrhage

Unspecified Code   Other Specified Code   Manifestation Code   Ⓝ Newborn   Ⓟ Pediatric   Ⓜ Maternity   Ⓐ Adult   ♂ Male   ♀ Female
● New Code   ▲ Revised Code Title   ►◄ Revised Text   **NOTES**   *INCLUDES*   *EXCLUDES1* Not coded here   *EXCLUDES2* Not included here
4ᵗʰ 4ᵗʰ character required   5ᵗʰ 5ᵗʰ character required   6ᵗʰ 6ᵗʰ character required   7ᵗʰ 7ᵗʰ character required   Extension 'X' Alert
HAC Hospital-acquired condition (HAC) alert   **AHA** AHA Coding Clinic©   🖝 Code first alert

O44.30 **Partial placenta previa with hemorrhage, unspecified trimester** M ♀

O44.31 **Partial placenta previa with hemorrhage,** first trimester 1st M ♀ CC/MCC Exc

O44.32 **Partial placenta previa with hemorrhage,** second trimester 2nd MCC ♀ CC/MCC Exc

O44.33 **Partial placenta previa with hemorrhage,** third trimester 3rd MCC ♀ CC/MCC Exc

5th O44.4 **Low lying placenta** NOS or without hemorrhage
Low implantation of placenta NOS or without hemorrhage

O44.40 **Low lying placenta NOS or without hemorrhage, unspecified trimester** M ♀

O44.41 **Low lying placenta NOS or without hemorrhage,** first trimester 1st M CC ♀ CC/MCC Exc

O44.42 **Low lying placenta NOS or without hemorrhage,** second trimester 2nd M CC ♀ CC/MCC Exc

O44.43 **Low lying placenta NOS or without hemorrhage,** third trimester 3rd M CC ♀ CC/MCC Exc

5th O44.5 **Low lying placenta** with hemorrhage
Low implantation of placenta with hemorrhage

O44.50 **Low lying placenta with hemorrhage, unspecified trimester** M ♀

O44.51 **Low lying placenta with hemorrhage,** first trimester 1st M ♀ CC/MCC Exc

O44.52 **Low lying placenta with hemorrhage,** second trimester 2nd MCC ♀ CC/MCC Exc

O44.53 **Low lying placenta with hemorrhage,** third trimester 3rd M MCC ♀ CC/MCC Exc

4th O45 **Premature separation of placenta [abruptio placentae]**

5th O45.0 **Premature separation of placenta** with coagulation defect

6th O45.00 **Premature separation of placenta with coagulation defect, unspecified**

O45.001 **Premature separation of placenta with coagulation defect, unspecified,** first trimester 1st MCC ♀ CC/MCC Exc

O45.002 **Premature separation of placenta with coagulation defect, unspecified,** second trimester 2nd M MCC ♀ CC/MCC Exc

O45.003 **Premature separation of placenta with coagulation defect, unspecified,** third trimester 3rd MCC ♀ CC/MCC Exc

O45.009 **Premature separation of placenta with coagulation defect, unspecified trimester** M ♀

6th O45.01 **Premature separation of placenta** with afibrinogenemia
Premature separation of placenta with hypofibrinogenemia

O45.011 **Premature separation of placenta with afibrinogenemia,** first trimester 1st M MCC ♀ CC/MCC Exc

O45.012 **Premature separation of placenta with afibrinogenemia,** second trimester 2nd MCC ♀ CC/MCC Exc

O45.013 **Premature separation of placenta with afibrinogenemia,** third trimester 3rd M MCC ♀ CC/MCC Exc

O45.019 **Premature separation of placenta with afibrinogenemia, unspecified trimester** M ♀

6th O45.02 **Premature separation of placenta** with disseminated intravascular coagulation

O45.021 **Premature separation of placenta with disseminated intravascular coagulation,** first trimester 1st M MCC ♀ CC/MCC Exc

O45.022 **Premature separation of placenta with disseminated intravascular coagulation,** second trimester 2nd M MCC ♀ CC/MCC Exc

O45.023 **Premature separation of placenta with disseminated intravascular coagulation,** third trimester 3rd M MCC ♀ CC/MCC Exc

O45.029 **Premature separation of placenta with disseminated intravascular coagulation, unspecified trimester** M ♀

6th O45.09 **Premature separation of placenta** with other coagulation defect

O45.091 **Premature separation of placenta with other coagulation defect,** first trimester 1st MCC ♀ CC/MCC Exc

O45.092 **Premature separation of placenta with other coagulation defect,** second trimester 2nd M MCC ♀ CC/MCC Exc

O45.093 **Premature separation of placenta with other coagulation defect,** third trimester 3rd MCC ♀ CC/MCC Exc

O45.099 **Premature separation of placenta with other coagulation defect, unspecified trimester** M ♀

5th O45.8 **Other premature separation** of placenta

6th O45.8X **Other premature separation of placenta**

O45.8X1 **Other premature separation of placenta,** first trimester 1st M MCC ♀ CC/MCC Exc

O45.8X2 **Other premature separation of placenta,** second trimester 2nd M MCC ♀ CC/MCC Exc

O45.8X3 **Other premature separation of placenta,** third trimester 3rd M MCC ♀ CC/MCC Exc

O45.8X9 **Other premature separation of placenta, unspecified trimester** M ♀

5th O45.9 **Premature separation of placenta,** unspecified
Abruptio placentae NOS

O45.90 **Premature separation of placenta, unspecified, unspecified trimester** M ♀

O45.91 **Premature separation of placenta, unspecified,** first trimester 1st M MCC ♀ CC/MCC Exc

O45.92 **Premature separation of placenta, unspecified,** second trimester 2nd M MCC ♀ CC/MCC Exc

O45.93 **Premature separation of placenta, unspecified,** third trimester 3rd M MCC ♀ CC/MCC Exc

4th O46 **Antepartum hemorrhage, not elsewhere classified**
EXCLUDES1 hemorrhage in early pregnancy (O20.-)
intrapartum hemorrhage NEC (O67.-)
placenta previa (O44.-)
premature separation of placenta [abruptio placentae] (O45.-)

5th O46.0 **Antepartum hemorrhage** with coagulation defect

6th O46.00 **Antepartum hemorrhage with coagulation defect, unspecified**

O46.001 **Antepartum hemorrhage with coagulation defect, unspecified,** first trimester 1st M MCC ♀ CC/MCC Exc

O46.002 **Antepartum hemorrhage with coagulation defect, unspecified,** second trimester 2nd M MCC ♀ CC/MCC Exc

O46.003 **Antepartum hemorrhage with coagulation defect, unspecified, third trimester** 3rd M MCC ♀ CC/MCC Exc

O46.009 **Antepartum hemorrhage with coagulation defect, unspecified trimester** M ♀

6th O46.01 **Antepartum hemorrhage** with afibrinogenemia
Antepartum hemorrhage with hypofibrinogenemia

O46.011 **Antepartum hemorrhage with afibrinogenemia,** first trimester 1st M MCC ♀ CC/MCC Exc

O46.012 **Antepartum hemorrhage with afibrinogenemia,** second trimester 2nd M MCC ♀ CC/MCC Exc

O46.013 **Antepartum hemorrhage with afibrinogenemia,** third trimester 3rd M MCC ♀ CC/MCC Exc

O46.019 **Antepartum hemorrhage with afibrinogenemia, unspecified trimester** M ♀

1st 1st trimester 2nd 2nd trimester 3rd 3rd trimester PDx Unacceptable principal diagnosis symbol per Medicare code edits
POA Code exempt from diagnosis present on admission requirement ? Questionable admission CC Complication or comorbidity
MCC Major complication or comorbidity CC/MCC Exc CC/MCC exclusion HCC HCC diagnosis code RxHCC RxHCC diagnosis code MACRA code
DEFINITION Describes condition/terminology **TIP** Coding guidance ◉ Official Guideline Reference Z1 Z code as first-listed diagnosis

6ᵗʰ O46.02 **Antepartum hemorrhage** with disseminated intravascular coagulation

　O46.021 **Antepartum hemorrhage with disseminated intravascular coagulation, first trimester** 1st M MCC♀ ♀ CC/MCC Exc

　O46.022 **Antepartum hemorrhage with disseminated intravascular coagulation, second trimester** 2nd M MCC♀ ♀ CC/MCC Exc

　O46.023 **Antepartum hemorrhage with disseminated intravascular coagulation, third trimester** 3rd M MCC♀ ♀ CC/MCC Exc

　O46.029 **Antepartum hemorrhage with disseminated intravascular coagulation, unspecified trimester** M ♀

6ᵗʰ O46.09 **Antepartum hemorrhage with other coagulation defect**

　O46.091 **Antepartum hemorrhage with other coagulation defect, first trimester** 1st M MCC♀ ♀ CC/MCC Exc

　O46.092 **Antepartum hemorrhage with other coagulation defect, second trimester** 2nd M MCC♀ ♀ CC/MCC Exc

　O46.093 **Antepartum hemorrhage with other coagulation defect, third trimester** 3rd M MCC♀ ♀ CC/MCC Exc

　O46.099 **Antepartum hemorrhage with other coagulation defect, unspecified trimester** M ♀

5ᵗʰ O46.8 **Other** antepartum hemorrhage

　6ᵗʰ O46.8X **Other** antepartum hemorrhage

　　O46.8X1 **Other antepartum hemorrhage, first trimester** 1st M ♀

　　O46.8X2 **Other antepartum hemorrhage, second trimester** 2nd M ♀

　　O46.8X3 **Other antepartum hemorrhage, third trimester** 3rd M ♀

　　O46.8X9 **Other antepartum hemorrhage, unspecified trimester** M ♀

5ᵗʰ O46.9 **Antepartum hemorrhage,** unspecified

　O46.90 **Antepartum hemorrhage, unspecified, unspecified trimester** M ♀

　O46.91 **Antepartum hemorrhage, unspecified, first trimester** 1st M ♀

　O46.92 **Antepartum hemorrhage, unspecified, second trimester** 2nd M ♀

　O46.93 **Antepartum hemorrhage, unspecified, third trimester** 3rd M ♀

4ᵗʰ O47 **False labor**

　INCLUDES *Braxton Hicks contractions*

　　　　　 threatened labor

　EXCLUDES1 *preterm labor (O60.-)*

　5ᵗʰ O47.0 **False labor** before 37 completed weeks of gestation

　　O47.00 **False labor before 37 completed weeks of gestation, unspecified trimester** M ♀

　　O47.02 **False labor before 37 completed weeks of gestation, second trimester** 2nd M CC♀ ♀ CC/MCC Exc

　　O47.03 **False labor before 37 completed weeks of gestation, third trimester** 3rd M CC♀ ♀ CC/MCC Exc

　O47.1 **False labor** at or after 37 completed weeks of gestation 3rd M CC♀ ♀ CC/MCC Exc

　O47.9 **False labor, unspecified** M ♀

4ᵗʰ O48 **Late pregnancy**

　O48.0 **Post-term** pregnancy M ♀

　　Pregnancy over 40 completed weeks to 42 completed weeks gestation

　O48.1 **Prolonged** pregnancy M ♀

　　Pregnancy which has advanced beyond 42 completed weeks gestation

Complications of labor and delivery (O60-O77)

4ᵗʰ O60 **Preterm labor**

　INCLUDES *onset (spontaneous) of labor before 37 completed weeks of gestation*

　EXCLUDES1 *false labor (O47.0-)*

　　　　　 threatened labor NOS (O47.0-)

　5ᵗʰ O60.0 **Preterm labor** without delivery

　　O60.00 **Preterm labor without delivery, unspecified trimester** M ♀

　　O60.02 **Preterm labor without delivery, second trimester** 2nd M MCC♀ ♀ CC/MCC Exc

　　O60.03 **Preterm labor without delivery, third trimester** 3rd M MCC♀ ♀ CC/MCC Exc

　5ᵗʰ O60.1 **Preterm labor** with preterm delivery

　　　👁 **See Official Guidelines** "7th character for Fetus Identification" I.C.15. a.6

　　One of the following 7th characters is to be assigned to each code under subcategory O60.1. 7th character 0 is for single gestations and multiple gestations where the fetus is unspecified. 7th characters 1 through 9 are for cases of multiple gestations to identify the fetus for which the code applies. The appropriate code from category O30, Multiple gestation, must also be assigned when assigning a code from subcategory O60.1 that has a 7th character of 1 through 9.

　　　0 = not applicable or unspecified
　　　1 = fetus 1
　　　2 = fetus 2
　　　3 = fetus 3
　　　4 = fetus 4
　　　5 = fetus 5
　　　9 = other fetus

　　7ᵗʰ O60.10 **Preterm labor with preterm delivery, unspecified trimester** M CC♀ ♀ CC/MCC Exc
　　　Preterm labor with delivery NOS

　　7ᵗʰ O60.12 **Preterm labor** second trimester **with preterm delivery** second trimester 2nd M MCC♀ ♀ CC/MCC Exc

　　7ᵗʰ O60.13 **Preterm labor** second trimester **with preterm delivery** third trimester 2nd 3rd M MCC♀ ♀ CC/MCC Exc

　　7ᵗʰ O60.14 **Preterm labor** third trimester **with preterm delivery** third trimester 3rd M MCC♀ ♀ CC/MCC Exc
　　　AHA: Q2 2016

　5ᵗʰ O60.2 **Term delivery** with preterm labor

　　　👁 **See Official Guidelines** "7th character for Fetus Identification" I.C.15. a.6

　　One of the following 7th characters is to be assigned to each code under subcategory O60.2. 7th character 0 is for single gestations and multiple gestations where the fetus is unspecified. 7th characters 1 through 9 are for cases of multiple gestations to identify the fetus for which the code applies. The appropriate code from category O30, Multiple gestation, must also be assigned when assigning a code from subcategory O60.2 that has a 7th character of 1 through 9.

　　　0 = not applicable or unspecified
　　　1 = fetus 1
　　　2 = fetus 2
　　　3 = fetus 3
　　　4 = fetus 4
　　　5 = fetus 5
　　　9 = other fetus

　　7ᵗʰ O60.20 **Term delivery with preterm labor, unspecified trimester** M CC♀ ♀ CC/MCC Exc

　　7ᵗʰ O60.22 **Term delivery with preterm labor, second trimester** 2nd M MCC♀ ♀ CC/MCC Exc

　　7ᵗʰ O60.23 **Term delivery with preterm labor, third trimester** 3rd M MCC♀ ♀ CC/MCC Exc

4ᵗʰ O61 **Failed induction of labor**

　O61.0 **Failed** medical **induction of labor** M ♀
　　Failed induction (of labor) by oxytocin
　　Failed induction (of labor) by prostaglandins

　O61.1 **Failed** instrumental **induction of labor** M ♀
　　Failed mechanical induction (of labor)
　　Failed surgical induction (of labor)

　Unspecified Code　Other Specified Code　Manifestation Code　N Newborn　P Pediatric　M Maternity　A Adult　♂ Male　♀ Female
　● New Code　▲ Revised Code Title　►◄ Revised Text　NOTES　INCLUDES　EXCLUDES1 Not coded here　EXCLUDES2 Not included here
　　4ᵗʰ 4ᵗʰ character required　5ᵗʰ 5ᵗʰ character required　6ᵗʰ 6ᵗʰ character required　7ᵗʰ 7ᵗʰ character required　👁 Extension 'X' Alert
　　HAC Hospital-acquired condition (HAC) alert　AHA AHA Coding Clinic©　☛ Code first alert

2020 ICD-10-CM　　When symbols appear on a code that requires a 7th character extension, refer to Appendix B to identify applicable 7th character codes.　　**907**

O61.8 Other failed induction of labor [M] ♀
O61.9 Failed induction of labor, unspecified [M] ♀

[4th] **O62 Abnormalities of forces of labor**

O62.0 **Primary inadequate contractions** [M] ♀
- Failure of cervical dilatation
- Primary hypotonic uterine dysfunction
- Uterine inertia during latent phase of labor

O62.1 **Secondary uterine inertia** [M] ♀
- Arrested active phase of labor
- Secondary hypotonic uterine dysfunction

O62.2 **Other uterine inertia** [M] ♀
- Atony of uterus without hemorrhage
- Atony of uterus NOS
- Desultory labor
- Hypotonic uterine dysfunction NOS
- Irregular labor
- Poor contractions
- Slow slope active phase of labor
- Uterine inertia NOS

EXCLUDES1 *atony of uterus with hemorrhage (postpartum) (O72.1)*
postpartum atony of uterus without hemorrhage (O75.89)

O62.3 **Precipitate labor** [M] ♀

O62.4 **Hypertonic, incoordinate, and prolonged uterine contractions** [M] ♀
- Cervical spasm
- Contraction ring dystocia
- Dyscoordinate labor
- Hour-glass contraction of uterus
- Hypertonic uterine dysfunction
- Incoordinate uterine action
- Tetanic contractions
- Uterine dystocia NOS
- Uterine spasm

EXCLUDES1 *dystocia (fetal) (maternal) NOS (O66.9)*

O62.8 **Other abnormalities of forces of labor** [M] ♀
O62.9 **Abnormality of forces of labor, unspecified** [M] ♀

[4th] **O63 Long labor**

O63.0 Prolonged first stage **(of labor)** [M] ♀
O63.1 Prolonged second stage **(of labor)** [M] ♀
O63.2 Delayed delivery **of second twin, triplet, etc.** [M] ♀
O63.9 **Long labor, unspecified** [M] [CC] ♀ [CC/MCC Exc]
- Prolonged labor NOS

[4th] **O64 Obstructed labor due to malposition and malpresentation of fetus**

👁 **See Official Guidelines** "7th character for Fetus Identification" I.C.15. a.6

One of the following 7th characters is to be assigned to each code under category O64. 7th character 0 is for single gestations and multiple gestations where the fetus is unspecified. 7th characters 1 through 9 are for cases of multiple gestations to identify the fetus for which the code applies. The appropriate code from category O30, Multiple gestation, must also be assigned when assigning a code from category O64 that has a 7th character of 1 through 9.

- **0 = not applicable or unspecified**
- **1 = fetus 1**
- **2 = fetus 2**
- **3 = fetus 3**
- **4 = fetus 4**
- **5 = fetus 5**
- **9 = other fetus**

[7th] O64.0 **Obstructed labor due to** incomplete rotation of fetal head [M] ♀
- Deep transverse arrest
- Obstructed labor due to persistent occipitoiliac (position)
- Obstructed labor due to persistent occipitoposterior (position)
- Obstructed labor due to persistent occipitosacral (position)
- Obstructed labor due to persistent occipitotransverse (position)

[7th] O64.1 **Obstructed labor due to** breech presentation [M] ♀
- Obstructed labor due to buttocks presentation
- Obstructed labor due to complete breech presentation
- Obstructed labor due to frank breech presentation

[7th] O64.2 **Obstructed labor due to** face presentation [M] ♀
- Obstructed labor due to chin presentation

[7th] O64.3 **Obstructed labor due to** brow presentation [M] ♀

[7th] O64.4 **Obstructed labor due to** shoulder presentation [M] ♀
- Prolapsed arm

EXCLUDES1 *impacted shoulders (O66.0)*
shoulder dystocia (O66.0)

[7th] O64.5 **Obstructed labor due to** compound presentation [M] ♀

[7th] O64.8 **Obstructed labor due to** other malposition and malpresentation [M] ♀
- Obstructed labor due to footling presentation
- Obstructed labor due to incomplete breech presentation

[7th] O64.9 **Obstructed labor due to malposition and malpresentation, unspecified** [M] ♀

[4th] **O65 Obstructed labor due to maternal pelvic abnormality**

O65.0 **Obstructed labor due to** deformed pelvis [M] ♀
O65.1 **Obstructed labor due to** generally contracted pelvis [M] ♀
O65.2 **Obstructed labor due to** pelvic inlet contraction [M] ♀
O65.3 **Obstructed labor due to** pelvic outlet and mid-cavity contraction [M] ♀
O65.4 **Obstructed labor due to** fetopelvic disproportion, **unspecified** [M] ♀

EXCLUDES1 *dystocia due to abnormality of fetus (O66.2-O66.3)*

O65.5 **Obstructed labor due to** abnormality of maternal pelvic organs [M] ♀
- Obstructed labor due to conditions listed in O34.-

Use additional code to identify abnormality of pelvic organs O34.-

O65.8 **Obstructed labor due to** other maternal pelvic abnormalities [M] ♀
O65.9 **Obstructed labor due to maternal pelvic abnormality, unspecified** [M] ♀

[4th] **O66 Other obstructed labor**

O66.0 **Obstructed labor due to** shoulder dystocia [M] ♀
- Impacted shoulders

O66.1 **Obstructed labor due to** locked twins [M] ♀
O66.2 **Obstructed labor due to** unusually large fetus [M] ♀
O66.3 **Obstructed labor due to other** abnormalities of fetus [M] ♀
- Dystocia due to fetal ascites
- Dystocia due to fetal hydrops
- Dystocia due to fetal meningomyelocele
- Dystocia due to fetal sacral teratoma
- Dystocia due to fetal tumor
- Dystocia due to hydrocephalic fetus

Use additional code to identify cause of obstruction

[5th] O66.4 **Failed trial of labor**

O66.40 **Failed trial of labor, unspecified** [M] ♀
O66.41 **Failed** attempted vaginal birth after previous cesarean delivery [M] ♀

☞ **Code first** rupture of uterus, if applicable (O71.0-, O71.1)

O66.5 **Attempted application of** vacuum extractor and forceps [M] [POA] ♀
- Attempted application of vacuum or forceps, with subsequent delivery by forceps or cesarean delivery

O66.6 **Obstructed labor due to** other multiple fetuses [M] ♀
O66.8 **Other specified obstructed labor** [M] ♀

Use additional code to identify cause of obstruction

O66.9 **Obstructed labor, unspecified** [M] ♀
- Dystocia NOS
- Fetal dystocia NOS
- Maternal dystocia NOS

[4th] **O67 Labor and delivery** complicated by intrapartum hemorrhage, **not elsewhere classified**

EXCLUDES1 *antepartum hemorrhage NEC (O46.-)*
placenta previa (O44.-)
premature separation of placenta [abruptio placentae] (O45.-)

EXCLUDES2 *postpartum hemorrhage (O72.-)*

[1st] 1st trimester [2nd] 2nd trimester [3rd] 3rd trimester [PDx] Unacceptable principal diagnosis symbol per Medicare code edits
[POA] Code exempt from diagnosis present on admission requirement [?] Questionable admission [CC] Complication or comorbidity
[MCC] Major complication or comorbidity [CC/MCC Exc] CC/MCC exclusion [HCC] HCC diagnosis code [RxHCC] RxHCC diagnosis code MACRA code
DEFINITION Describes condition/terminology **TIP** Coding guidance 👁 Official Guideline Reference [Z1] Z code as first-listed diagnosis

O67.0 **Intrapartum hemorrhage** with coagulation defect   M MCC ♀ CC/MCC Exc

    Intrapartum hemorrhage (excessive) associated with afibrinogenemia

    Intrapartum hemorrhage (excessive) associated with disseminated intravascular coagulation

    Intrapartum hemorrhage (excessive) associated with hyperfibrinolysis

    Intrapartum hemorrhage (excessive) associated with hypofibrinogenemia

O67.8 Other **intrapartum hemorrhage**   M ♀

    Excessive intrapartum hemorrhage

O67.9 **Intrapartum hemorrhage, unspecified**   M ♀

O68 **Labor and delivery complicated by** abnormality of fetal acid-base balance   M CC ♀ CC/MCC Exc

    Fetal acidemia complicating labor and delivery

    Fetal acidosis complicating labor and delivery

    Fetal alkalosis complicating labor and delivery

    Fetal metabolic acidemia complicating labor and delivery

    EXCLUDES1   *fetal stress NOS (O77.9)*

        labor and delivery complicated by electrocardiographic evidence of fetal stress (O77.8)

        labor and delivery complicated by ultrasonic evidence of fetal stress (O77.8)

    EXCLUDES2   *abnormality in fetal heart rate or rhythm (O76)*

        labor and delivery complicated by meconium in amniotic fluid (O77.0)

O69 **Labor and delivery complicated by** umbilical cord complications

    👁 See Official Guidelines "7th character for Fetus Identification" I.C.15. a.6

    One of the following 7th characters is to be assigned to each code under category O69. 7th character 0 is for single gestations and multiple gestations where the fetus is unspecified. 7th characters 1 through 9 are for cases of multiple gestations to identify the fetus for which the code applies. The appropriate code from category O30, Multiple gestation, must also be assigned when assigning a code from category O69 that has a 7th character of 1 through 9.

        0 = not applicable or unspecified

        1 = fetus 1

        2 = fetus 2

        3 = fetus 3

        4 = fetus 4

        5 = fetus 5

        9 = other fetus

  7ᵗʰ O69.0 **Labor and delivery complicated by** prolapse of cord   M ♀

  7ᵗʰ O69.1 **Labor and delivery complicated by** cord around neck, with compression   M ♀

    EXCLUDES1   *labor and delivery complicated by cord around neck, without compression (O69.81)*

  7ᵗʰ O69.2 **Labor and delivery complicated by** other cord entanglement, with compression   M ♀

    Labor and delivery complicated by compression of cord NOS

    Labor and delivery complicated by entanglement of cords of twins in monoamniotic sac

    Labor and delivery complicated by knot in cord

    EXCLUDES1   *labor and delivery complicated by other cord entanglement, without compression (O69.82)*

  7ᵗʰ O69.3 **Labor and delivery complicated by** short cord   M ♀

  7ᵗʰ O69.4 **Labor and delivery complicated by** vasa previa   M ♀

    Labor and delivery complicated by hemorrhage from vasa previa

  7ᵗʰ O69.5 **Labor and delivery complicated by** vascular lesion of cord   M ♀

    Labor and delivery complicated by cord bruising

    Labor and delivery complicated by cord hematoma

    Labor and delivery complicated by thrombosis of umbilical vessels

  5ᵗʰ O69.8 **Labor and delivery complicated by** other cord complications

    7ᵗʰ O69.81 **Labor and delivery complicated by** cord around neck, without compression   M ♀

    7ᵗʰ O69.82 **Labor and delivery complicated by** other cord entanglement, without compression   M ♀

    7ᵗʰ O69.89 **Labor and delivery complicated by** other cord complications   M ♀

  7ᵗʰ O69.9 **Labor and delivery complicated by** cord complication, unspecified   M ♀

O70 **Perineal laceration during delivery**

    INCLUDES   *episiotomy extended by laceration*

    EXCLUDES1   *obstetric high vaginal laceration alone (O71.4)*

  O70.0 **First degree** perineal laceration during delivery   M ♀

    Perineal laceration, rupture or tear involving fourchette during delivery

    Perineal laceration, rupture or tear involving labia during delivery

    Perineal laceration, rupture or tear involving skin during delivery

    Perineal laceration, rupture or tear involving vagina during delivery

    Perineal laceration, rupture or tear involving vulva during delivery

    Slight perineal laceration, rupture or tear during delivery

  O70.1 **Second degree** perineal laceration during delivery   M ♀

    AHA: Q2 2016

    Perineal laceration, rupture or tear during delivery as in O70.0, also involving pelvic floor

    Perineal laceration, rupture or tear during delivery as in O70.0, also involving perineal muscles

    Perineal laceration, rupture or tear during delivery as in O70.0, also involving vaginal muscles

    EXCLUDES1   *perineal laceration involving anal sphincter (O70.2)*

  5ᵗʰ O70.2 **Third degree** perineal laceration during delivery

    Perineal laceration, rupture or tear during delivery as in O70.1, also involving anal sphincter

    Perineal laceration, rupture or tear during delivery as in O70.1, also involving rectovaginal septum

    Perineal laceration, rupture or tear during delivery as in O70.1, also involving sphincter NOS

    EXCLUDES1   *anal sphincter tear during delivery without third degree perineal laceration (O70.4)*

        perineal laceration involving anal or rectal mucosa (O70.3)

    O70.20 **Third degree perineal laceration during delivery, unspecified**   M CC ♀ CC/MCC Exc

        AHA: Q4 2016

    O70.21 **Third degree perineal laceration during delivery, IIIa**   M CC ♀ CC/MCC Exc

        AHA: Q4 2016

        Third degree perineal laceration during delivery with less than 50% of external anal sphincter (EAS) thickness torn

    O70.22 **Third degree perineal laceration during delivery, IIIb**   M CC ♀ CC/MCC Exc

        AHA: Q4 2016

        Third degree perineal laceration during delivery with more than 50% external anal sphincter (EAS) thickness torn

    O70.23 **Third degree perineal laceration during delivery, IIIc**   M CC ♀ CC/MCC Exc

        AHA: Q4 2016

        Third degree perineal laceration during delivery with both external anal sphincter (EAS) and internal anal sphincter (IAS) torn

  O70.3 **Fourth degree** perineal laceration during delivery   M CC ♀ CC/MCC Exc

    Perineal laceration, rupture or tear during delivery as in O70.2, also involving anal mucosa

    Perineal laceration, rupture or tear during delivery as in O70.2, also involving rectal mucosa

  O70.4 **Anal sphincter tear** complicating delivery, not associated with third degree laceration   M CC ♀ CC/MCC Exc

    EXCLUDES1   *anal sphincter tear with third degree perineal laceration (O70.2)*

  O70.9 **Perineal laceration during delivery, unspecified**   M ♀

O71 **Other obstetric trauma**

    INCLUDES   *obstetric damage from instruments*

Unspecified Code   Other Specified Code   Manifestation Code   N Newborn   P Pediatric   M Maternity   A Adult   ♂ Male   ♀ Female

● New Code   ▲ Revised Code Title   ►◄ Revised Text   **NOTES**   *INCLUDES*   *EXCLUDES1* Not coded here   *EXCLUDES2* Not included here

4ᵗʰ character required   5ᵗʰ character required   6ᵗʰ character required   7ᵗʰ character required   Extension 'X' Alert

HAC Hospital-acquired condition (HAC) alert   **AHA** AHA Coding Clinic©   📌 Code first alert

2020 ICD-10-CM   When symbols appear on a code that requires a 7th character extension, refer to Appendix B to identify applicable 7th character codes.   **909**

O71.0 Rupture of uterus (spontaneous) before onset of labor
  EXCLUDES1 disruption of (current) cesarean delivery wound (O90.0)
  laceration of uterus, NEC (O71.81)

  O71.00 Rupture of uterus before onset of labor, unspecified trimester M ♀

  O71.02 Rupture of uterus before onset of labor, second trimester   2nd M MCC ♀ CC/MCC Exc

  O71.03 Rupture of uterus before onset of labor, third trimester   3rd MCC ♀ CC/MCC Exc

O71.1 Rupture of uterus during labor   M MCC ♀ CC/MCC Exc
  Rupture of uterus not stated as occurring before onset of labor
  EXCLUDES1 disruption of cesarean delivery wound (O90.0)
  laceration of uterus, NEC (O71.81)

O71.2 Postpartum inversion of uterus   M CC ♀ CC/MCC Exc

O71.3 Obstetric laceration of cervix   M CC ♀ CC/MCC Exc
  Annular detachment of cervix

O71.4 Obstetric high vaginal laceration **alone**   M CC ♀ CC/MCC Exc
  Laceration of vaginal wall without perineal laceration
  EXCLUDES1 obstetric high vaginal laceration with perineal laceration (O70.-)

O71.5 Other obstetric injury to pelvic organs   M CC ♀ CC/MCC Exc
  Obstetric injury to bladder
  Obstetric injury to urethra
  EXCLUDES2 obstetric periurethral trauma (O71.82)

O71.6 Obstetric damage to pelvic joints and ligaments   M CC ♀ CC/MCC Exc
  Obstetric avulsion of inner symphyseal cartilage
  Obstetric damage to coccyx
  Obstetric traumatic separation of symphysis (pubis)

O71.7 Obstetric hematoma of pelvis   M CC ♀ CC/MCC Exc
  Obstetric hematoma of perineum
  Obstetric hematoma of vagina
  Obstetric hematoma of vulva

O71.8 Other specified obstetric trauma

  O71.81 Laceration of uterus, not elsewhere classified M ♀

  O71.82 Other specified trauma to perineum and vulva M ♀
  Obstetric periurethral trauma

  O71.89 Other specified obstetric trauma M ♀

O71.9 Obstetric trauma, unspecified M ♀

O72 Postpartum hemorrhage
  INCLUDES hemorrhage after delivery of fetus or infant

  O72.0 Third-stage hemorrhage   M CC ♀ CC/MCC Exc
  Hemorrhage associated with retained, trapped or adherent placenta
  Retained placenta NOS
  Code also type of adherent placenta (O43.2-)

  O72.1 Other immediate postpartum hemorrhage   M CC ♀ CC/MCC Exc
  Hemorrhage following delivery of placenta
  Postpartum hemorrhage (atonic) NOS
  Uterine atony with hemorrhage
  EXCLUDES1 uterine atony NOS (O62.2)
  uterine atony without hemorrhage (O62.2)
  postpartum atony of uterus without hemorrhage (O75.89)

  O72.2 Delayed and secondary postpartum hemorrhage   M CC ♀ CC/MCC Exc
  Hemorrhage associated with retained portions of placenta or membranes after the first 24 hours following delivery of placenta
  Retained products of conception NOS, following delivery

  O72.3 Postpartum coagulation defects   M ♀
  Postpartum afibrinogenemia
  Postpartum fibrinolysis

O73 Retained placenta and membranes, without hemorrhage
  EXCLUDES1 placenta accreta (O43.21-)
  placenta increta (O43.22-)
  placenta percreta (O43.23-)

  O73.0 Retained placenta **without hemorrhage**   M ♀
  Adherent placenta, without hemorrhage
  Trapped placenta without hemorrhage

  O73.1 Retained portions of placenta and membranes, **without hemorrhage**   M ♀
  Retained products of conception following delivery, without hemorrhage

O74 Complications of anesthesia during labor and delivery
  INCLUDES maternal complications arising from the administration of a general, regional or local anesthetic, analgesic or other sedation during labor and delivery
  Use additional code, if applicable, to identify specific complication

  O74.0 Aspiration pneumonitis due to anesthesia during labor and delivery   M ♀
  Inhalation of stomach contents or secretions NOS due to anesthesia during labor and delivery
  Mendelson's syndrome due to anesthesia during labor and delivery

  O74.1 Other pulmonary complications of anesthesia during labor and delivery   M ♀

  O74.2 Cardiac complications of anesthesia during labor and delivery   M ♀

  O74.3 Central nervous system complications of anesthesia during labor and delivery   M ♀

  O74.4 Toxic reaction to local anesthesia during labor and delivery   M ♀

  O74.5 Spinal and epidural anesthesia-induced headache during labor and delivery   M ♀

  O74.6 Other complications of spinal and epidural anesthesia during labor and delivery   M ♀

  O74.7 Failed or difficult intubation for anesthesia during labor and delivery   M ♀

  O74.8 Other complications of anesthesia during labor and delivery   M ♀

  O74.9 Complication of anesthesia during labor and delivery, unspecified   M ♀

O75 Other complications of labor and delivery, not elsewhere classified
  EXCLUDES2 puerperal (postpartum) infection (O86.-)
  puerperal (postpartum) sepsis (O85)

  O75.0 Maternal distress during labor and delivery   M ♀

  O75.1 Shock during or following labor and delivery   M MCC ♀ CC/MCC Exc
  Obstetric shock following labor and delivery

  O75.2 Pyrexia during labor, not elsewhere classified   M CC ♀ CC/MCC Exc

  O75.3 Other infection during labor   M MCC ♀ CC/MCC Exc
  Sepsis during labor
  Use additional code (B95-B97), to identify infectious agent

  O75.4 Other complications of obstetric surgery and procedures   M ♀
  Cardiac arrest following obstetric surgery or procedures
  Cardiac failure following obstetric surgery or procedures
  Cerebral anoxia following obstetric surgery or procedures
  Pulmonary edema following obstetric surgery or procedures
  Use additional code to identify specific complication
  EXCLUDES2 complications of anesthesia during labor and delivery (O74.-)
  disruption of obstetrical (surgical) wound (O90.0-O90.1)
  hematoma of obstetrical (surgical) wound (O90.2)
  infection of obstetrical (surgical) wound (O86.0-)

  O75.5 Delayed delivery after artificial rupture of membranes   M ♀

  O75.8 Other specified complications of labor and delivery

  O75.81 Maternal exhaustion complicating labor and delivery   M ♀

  O75.82 Onset (spontaneous) of labor after 37 completed weeks of gestation but before 39 completed weeks gestation, with delivery by (planned) cesarean section   3rd M ♀
  Delivery by (planned) cesarean section occurring after 37 completed weeks of gestation but before 39 completed weeks gestation due to (spontaneous) onset of labor
  ☞ **Code first** to specify reason for planned cesarean section such as:
  cephalopelvic disproportion (normally formed fetus) (O33.9)
  previous cesarean delivery (O34.21)

1st 1st trimester   2nd 2nd trimester   3rd 3rd trimester   PDx Unacceptable principal diagnosis symbol per Medicare code edits
PoA Code exempt from diagnosis present on admission requirement   ❓ Questionable admission   CC Complication or comorbidity
MCC Major complication or comorbidity   CC/MCC Exc CC/MCC exclusion   HCC HCC diagnosis code   RxHCC RxHCC diagnosis code   MACRA code
DEFINITION Describes condition/terminology   **TIP** Coding guidance   ◈ Official Guideline Reference   Z1 Z code as first-listed diagnosis

910   When symbols appear on a code that requires a 7th character extension, refer to Appendix B to identify applicable 7th character codes.   **2020 ICD-10-CM**

O75.89 Other specified complications of labor and delivery M ♀

O75.9 Complication of labor and delivery, unspecified M ♀

O76 Abnormality in fetal heart rate and rhythm complicating labor and delivery M CC ♀ CC/MCC Exc

AHA: Q4 2013

Depressed fetal heart rate tones complicating labor and delivery
Fetal bradycardia complicating labor and delivery
Fetal heart rate decelerations complicating labor and delivery
Fetal heart rate irregularity complicating labor and delivery
Fetal heart rate abnormal variability complicating labor and delivery
Fetal tachycardia complicating labor and delivery
Non-reassuring fetal heart rate or rhythm complicating labor and delivery

EXCLUDES1 *fetal stress NOS (O77.9)*
labor and delivery complicated by electrocardiographic evidence of fetal stress (O77.8)
labor and delivery complicated by ultrasonic evidence of fetal stress (O77.8)

EXCLUDES2 *fetal metabolic acidemia (O68)*
other fetal stress (O77.0-O77.1)

4th O77 Other fetal stress complicating labor and delivery

O77.0 Labor and delivery complicated by meconium in amniotic fluid M ♀
AHA: Q4 2013

O77.1 Fetal stress in labor or delivery due to drug administration M ♀

O77.8 Labor and delivery complicated by other evidence of fetal stress M ♀
Labor and delivery complicated by electrocardiographic evidence of fetal stress
Labor and delivery complicated by ultrasonic evidence of fetal stress
EXCLUDES1 *abnormality of fetal acid-base balance (O68)*
abnormality in fetal heart rate or rhythm (O76)
fetal metabolic acidemia (O68)

O77.9 Labor and delivery complicated by fetal stress, unspecified M ♀
EXCLUDES1 *abnormality of fetal acid-base balance (O68)*
abnormality in fetal heart rate or rhythm (O76)
fetal metabolic acidemia (O68)

Encounter for delivery (O80-O82)

O80 Encounter for full-term uncomplicated delivery M POA ♀

See Official Guidelines "Normal Delivery, Code O80" I.C.15.n

DEFINITION: Full term is greater than 37 weeks.

AHA: Q4 2016

Delivery requiring minimal or no assistance, with or without episiotomy, without fetal manipulation [e.g., rotation version] or instrumentation [forceps] of a spontaneous, cephalic, vaginal, full-term, single, live-born infant. This code is for use as a single diagnosis code and is not to be used with any other code from chapter 15.

Use additional code to indicate outcome of delivery (Z37.0)

O82 Encounter for cesarean delivery without indication M ♀

TIP: Used when documentation does not support medical necessity for cesarean (patient convenience).

Use additional code to indicate outcome of delivery (Z37.0)

Complications predominantly related to the puerperium (O85-O92)

EXCLUDES2 *mental and behavioral disorders associated with the puerperium (F53.-)*
obstetrical tetanus (A34)
puerperal osteomalacia (M83.0)

O85 Puerperal sepsis M MCC ♀ CC/MCC Exc

See Official Guidelines "Puerperal sepsis" I.C.15.k

AHA: Q4 2018

Postpartum sepsis
Puerperal peritonitis
Puerperal pyemia
Use additional code (B95-B97), to identify infectious agent
Use additional code (R65.2-) to identify severe sepsis, if applicable

EXCLUDES1 *fever of unknown origin following delivery (O86.4)*
genital tract infection following delivery (O86.1-)
obstetric pyemic and septic embolism (O88.3-)
puerperal septic thrombophlebitis (O86.81)
urinary tract infection following delivery (O86.2-)

EXCLUDES2 *sepsis during labor (O75.3)*

4th O86 Other puerperal infections

Use additional code (B95-B97), to identify infectious agent

EXCLUDES2 *infection during labor (O75.3)*
obstetrical tetanus (A34)

5th O86.0 Infection of obstetric surgical wound
Infected cesarean delivery wound following delivery
Infected perineal repair following delivery
EXCLUDES1 *complications of procedures, not elsewhere classified (T81.4-)*
postprocedural fever NOS (R50.82)
postprocedural retroperitoneal abscess (K68.11)

O86.00 Infection of obstetric surgical wound, unspecified M ♀
See Official Guidelines "Sepsis due to a postprocedural infection" I.C.1.d.5.b
AHA: Q2 2019, Q4 2018

O86.01 Infection of obstetric surgical wound, superficial incisional site M ♀
See Official Guidelines "Sepsis due to a postprocedural infection" I.C.1.d.5.b
AHA: Q4 2018
Subcutaneous abscess following an obstetrical procedure
Stitch abscess following an obstetrical procedure

O86.02 Infection of obstetric surgical wound, deep incisional site M ♀
See Official Guidelines "Sepsis due to a postprocedural infection" I.C.1.d.5.b
AHA: Q4 2018
Intramuscular abscess following an obstetrical procedure
Sub-fascial abscess following ▶an obstetrical◀ procedure

O86.03 Infection of obstetric surgical wound, organ and space site M ♀
See Official Guidelines "Sepsis due to a postprocedural infection" I.C.1.d.5.b
AHA: Q2 2019, Q4 2018
Intraabdominal abscess following an obstetrical procedure
Subphrenic abscess following an obstetrical procedure

O86.04 Sepsis following an obstetrical procedure M MCC ♀ CC/MCC Exc
See Official Guidelines "Sepsis due to a postprocedural infection" I.C.1.d.5.b
AHA: Q2 2019, Q4 2018
Use additional code to identify the sepsis

O86.09 Infection of obstetric surgical wound, other surgical site M ♀
AHA: Q4 2018

5th O86.1 Other infection of genital tract following delivery

O86.11 Cervicitis following delivery M CC ♀ CC/MCC Exc

O86.12 Endometritis following delivery M CC ♀ CC/MCC Exc

O86.13 Vaginitis following delivery M CC ♀ CC/MCC Exc

O86.19 Other infection of genital tract following delivery M CC ♀ CC/MCC Exc

5th O86.2 Urinary tract infection following delivery

O86.20 Urinary tract infection following delivery, unspecified M CC ♀ CC/MCC Exc
Puerperal urinary tract infection NOS

O86.21 Infection of kidney following delivery M CC ♀ CC/MCC Exc

O86.22 Infection of bladder following delivery M CC ♀ CC/MCC Exc
Infection of urethra following delivery

O86.29 Other urinary tract infection following delivery M CC ♀ CC/MCC Exc

Unspecified Code | Other Specified Code | Manifestation Code | N Newborn | P Pediatric | M Maternity | A Adult | ♂ Male | ♀ Female
● New Code | ▲ Revised Code Title | ▶◀ Revised Text | NOTES | INCLUDES | EXCLUDES1 Not coded here | EXCLUDES2 Not included here
4th character required | 5th character required | 6th character required | 7th character required | Extension 'X' Alert
HAC Hospital-acquired condition (HAC) alert | AHA AHA Coding Clinic© | Code first alert

O86.4 Pyrexia of unknown origin following delivery M cc♀ cc/mcc exc
Puerperal infection NOS following delivery
Puerperal pyrexia NOS following delivery
EXCLUDES2 pyrexia during labor (O75.2)

O86.8 Other specified puerperal infections
O86.81 Puerperal septic thrombophlebitis M mcc♀ cc/mcc exc
O86.89 Other specified puerperal infections M mcc♀ cc/mcc exc

O87 Venous complications and hemorrhoids in the puerperium
INCLUDES venous complications in labor, delivery and the puerperium
EXCLUDES2 obstetric embolism (O88.-)
puerperal septic thrombophlebitis (O86.81)
venous complications in pregnancy (O22.-)

O87.0 Superficial thrombophlebitis in the puerperium M cc♀ cc/mcc exc
Puerperal phlebitis NOS
Puerperal thrombosis NOS
O87.1 Deep phlebothrombosis in the puerperium M mcc♀ cc/mcc exc
Deep vein thrombosis, postpartum
Pelvic thrombophlebitis, postpartum
Use additional code to identify the deep vein thrombosis
(I82.4-, I82.5-, I82.62-. I82.72-)
Use additional code, if applicable, for associated long-term
(current) use of anticoagulants (Z79.01)
O87.2 Hemorrhoids in the puerperium M cc♀ cc/mcc exc
O87.3 Cerebral venous thrombosis in the puerperium M cc♀ cc/mcc exc
Cerebrovenous sinus thrombosis in the puerperium
O87.4 Varicose veins of lower extremity in the puerperium M ♀
O87.8 Other venous complications in the puerperium M cc♀ cc/mcc exc
Genital varices in the puerperium
O87.9 Venous complication in the puerperium, unspecified M ♀
Puerperal phlebopathy NOS

O88 Obstetric embolism
EXCLUDES1 embolism complicating abortion NOS (O03.2)
embolism complicating ectopic or molar pregnancy (O08.2)
embolism complicating failed attempted abortion (O07.2)
embolism complicating induced abortion (O04.7)
embolism complicating spontaneous abortion (O03.2, O03.7)

O88.0 Obstetric air embolism
O88.01 Obstetric air embolism in pregnancy
O88.011 Air embolism in pregnancy, first trimester 1st M mcc♀ cc/mcc exc
O88.012 Air embolism in pregnancy, second trimester 2nd M mcc♀ cc/mcc exc
O88.013 Air embolism in pregnancy, third trimester 3rd M mcc♀ cc/mcc exc
O88.019 Air embolism in pregnancy, unspecified trimester M ♀
O88.02 Air embolism in childbirth M mcc♀ cc/mcc exc
O88.03 Air embolism in the puerperium M mcc♀ cc/mcc exc
O88.1 Amniotic fluid embolism
Anaphylactoid syndrome in pregnancy
O88.11 Amniotic fluid embolism in pregnancy
O88.111 Amniotic fluid embolism in pregnancy, first trimester 1st M mcc♀ cc/mcc exc
O88.112 Amniotic fluid embolism in pregnancy, second trimester 2nd M mcc♀ cc/mcc exc
O88.113 Amniotic fluid embolism in pregnancy, third trimester 3rd M mcc♀ cc/mcc exc
O88.119 Amniotic fluid embolism in pregnancy, unspecified trimester M ♀
O88.12 Amniotic fluid embolism in childbirth M mcc♀ cc/mcc exc
O88.13 Amniotic fluid embolism in the puerperium M mcc♀ cc/mcc exc
O88.2 Obstetric thromboembolism
O88.21 Thromboembolism in pregnancy
Obstetric (pulmonary) embolism NOS
O88.211 Thromboembolism in pregnancy, first trimester 1st M mcc♀ cc/mcc exc
O88.212 Thromboembolism in pregnancy, second trimester 2nd M mcc♀ cc/mcc exc

O88.213 Thromboembolism in pregnancy, third trimester 3rd M mcc♀ cc/mcc exc
O88.219 Thromboembolism in pregnancy, unspecified trimester M ♀
O88.22 Thromboembolism in childbirth M mcc♀ cc/mcc exc
O88.23 Thromboembolism in the puerperium M mcc♀ cc/mcc exc
Puerperal (pulmonary) embolism NOS
O88.3 Obstetric pyemic and septic embolism
O88.31 Pyemic and septic embolism in pregnancy
O88.311 Pyemic and septic embolism in pregnancy, first trimester 1st M mcc♀ cc/mcc exc
O88.312 Pyemic and septic embolism in pregnancy, second trimester 2nd M mcc♀ cc/mcc exc
O88.313 Pyemic and septic embolism in pregnancy, third trimester 3rd M cc♀ cc/mcc exc
O88.319 Pyemic and septic embolism in pregnancy, unspecified trimester M cc♀ cc/mcc exc
O88.32 Pyemic and septic embolism in childbirth M mcc♀ cc/mcc exc
O88.33 Pyemic and septic embolism in the puerperium M mcc♀ cc/mcc exc
O88.8 Other obstetric embolism
Obstetric fat embolism
O88.81 Other embolism in pregnancy
O88.811 Other embolism in pregnancy, first trimester 1st M mcc♀ cc/mcc exc
O88.812 Other embolism in pregnancy, second trimester 2nd M mcc♀ cc/mcc exc
O88.813 Other embolism in pregnancy, third trimester 3rd M mcc♀ cc/mcc exc
O88.819 Other embolism in pregnancy, unspecified trimester M ♀
O88.82 Other embolism in childbirth M mcc♀ cc/mcc exc
O88.83 Other embolism in the puerperium M mcc♀ cc/mcc exc

O89 Complications of anesthesia during the puerperium
INCLUDES maternal complications arising from the administration of a general, regional or local anesthetic, analgesic or other sedation during the puerperium
Use additional code, if applicable, to identify specific complication
O89.0 Pulmonary complications of anesthesia during the puerperium
O89.01 Aspiration pneumonitis due to anesthesia during the puerperium M ♀
Inhalation of stomach contents or secretions NOS due to anesthesia during the puerperium
Mendelson's syndrome due to anesthesia during the puerperium
O89.09 Other pulmonary complications of anesthesia during the puerperium M ♀
O89.1 Cardiac complications of anesthesia during the puerperium M ♀
O89.2 Central nervous system complications of anesthesia during the puerperium M ♀
O89.3 Toxic reaction to local anesthesia during the puerperium M ♀
O89.4 Spinal and epidural anesthesia-induced headache during the puerperium M ♀
O89.5 Other complications of spinal and epidural anesthesia during the puerperium M ♀
O89.6 Failed or difficult intubation for anesthesia during the puerperium M ♀
O89.8 Other complications of anesthesia during the puerperium M ♀
O89.9 Complication of anesthesia during the puerperium, unspecified M ♀
O90 Complications of the puerperium, not elsewhere classified
O90.0 Disruption of cesarean delivery wound M ♀
Dehiscence of cesarean delivery wound
EXCLUDES1 rupture of uterus (spontaneous) before onset of labor (O71.0-)
rupture of uterus during labor (O71.1)

1st 1st trimester 2nd 2nd trimester 3rd 3rd trimester PDx Unacceptable principal diagnosis symbol per Medicare code edits
POA Code exempt from diagnosis present on admission requirement [?] Questionable admission cc Complication or comorbidity
mcc Major complication or comorbidity cc/mcc exc CC/MCC exclusion HCC HCC diagnosis code RxHCC RxHCC diagnosis code MACRA code
DEFINITION Describes condition/terminology **TIP** Coding guidance ◉ Official Guideline Reference Z1 Z code as first-listed diagnosis

When symbols appear on a code that requires a 7th character extension, refer to Appendix B to identify applicable 7th character codes. **2020 ICD-10-CM**

O90.1 **Disruption of** perineal obstetric wound   Ⓜ ♀
Disruption of wound of episiotomy
Disruption of wound of perineal laceration
Secondary perineal tear

O90.2 Hematoma **of obstetric wound**   Ⓜ ♀

O90.3 **Peripartum** cardiomyopathy   Ⓜ MCC⊘ ♀ CC/MCC Exc
👁 **See Official Guidelines** "Pregnancy associated cardiomyopathy" I.C.15.0.5
Conditions in I42.- arising during pregnancy and the puerperium
EXCLUDES1 *pre-existing heart disease complicating pregnancy and the puerperium (O99.4-)*

O90.4 **Postpartum** acute kidney failure   Ⓜ MCC⊘ ♀ CC/MCC Exc
Hepatorenal syndrome following labor and delivery

O90.5 **Postpartum** thyroiditis   Ⓜ ♀

O90.6 **Postpartum** mood disturbance   Ⓜ ♀
Postpartum blues
Postpartum dysphoria
Postpartum sadness
EXCLUDES1 *postpartum depression (F53.0)*
puerperal psychosis (F53.1)

5ᵗʰ O90.8 **Other complications of the puerperium, not elsewhere classified**
O90.81 **Anemia of the puerperium**   Ⓜ ♀
Postpartum anemia NOS
EXCLUDES1 *pre-existing anemia complicating the puerperium (O99.03)*
O90.89 **Other complications of the puerperium, not elsewhere classified**   Ⓜ ♀
Placental polyp

O90.9 **Complication of the puerperium, unspecified**   Ⓜ ♀

4ᵗʰ O91 Infections of breast **associated with pregnancy, the puerperium and lactation**
Use additional **code to identify infection**

5ᵗʰ O91.0 **Infection of nipple associated with pregnancy, the puerperium and lactation**
6ᵗʰ O91.01 **Infection of nipple associated with** pregnancy
Gestational abscess of nipple
O91.011 **Infection of nipple associated with pregnancy,** first trimester   1st Ⓜ ♀
O91.012 **Infection of nipple associated with pregnancy,** second trimester   2nd Ⓜ ♀
O91.013 **Infection of nipple associated with pregnancy,** third trimester   3rd Ⓜ ♀
O91.019 **Infection of nipple associated with pregnancy, unspecified trimester**   Ⓜ ♀
O91.02 **Infection of nipple associated with the puerperium**   Ⓜ ♀
Puerperal abscess of nipple
O91.03 **Infection of nipple associated with** lactation   Ⓜ ♀
Abscess of nipple associated with lactation

5ᵗʰ O91.1 Abscess of breast **associated with pregnancy, the puerperium and lactation**
6ᵗʰ O91.11 **Abscess of breast associated** with pregnancy
Gestational mammary abscess
Gestational purulent mastitis
Gestational subareolar abscess
O91.111 **Abscess of breast associated with pregnancy,** first trimester   1st Ⓜ ♀
O91.112 **Abscess of breast associated with pregnancy,** second trimester   2nd Ⓜ ♀
O91.113 **Abscess of breast associated with pregnancy,** third trimester   3rd Ⓜ ♀
O91.119 **Abscess of breast associated with pregnancy, unspecified trimester**   Ⓜ ♀
O91.12 **Abscess of breast associated** with the puerperium   Ⓜ ♀
Puerperal mammary abscess
Puerperal purulent mastitis
Puerperal subareolar abscess

O91.13 **Abscess of breast associated** with lactation   Ⓜ ♀
Mammary abscess associated with lactation
Purulent mastitis associated with lactation
Subareolar abscess associated with lactation

5ᵗʰ O91.2 Nonpurulent mastitis **associated with pregnancy, the puerperium and lactation**
6ᵗʰ O91.21 **Nonpurulent mastitis associated** with pregnancy
Gestational interstitial mastitis
Gestational lymphangitis of breast
Gestational mastitis NOS
Gestational parenchymatous mastitis
O91.211 **Nonpurulent mastitis associated with pregnancy,** first trimester   1st Ⓜ ♀
O91.212 **Nonpurulent mastitis associated with pregnancy,** second trimester   2nd Ⓜ ♀
O91.213 **Nonpurulent mastitis associated with pregnancy,** third trimester   3rd Ⓜ ♀
O91.219 **Nonpurulent mastitis associated with pregnancy, unspecified trimester**   Ⓜ ♀
O91.22 **Nonpurulent mastitis associated** with the puerperium   Ⓜ ♀
Puerperal interstitial mastitis
Puerperal lymphangitis of breast
Puerperal mastitis NOS
Puerperal parenchymatous mastitis
O91.23 **Nonpurulent mastitis associated** with lactation   Ⓜ ♀
Interstitial mastitis associated with lactation
Lymphangitis of breast associated with lactation
Mastitis NOS associated with lactation
Parenchymatous mastitis associated with lactation

4ᵗʰ O92 Other disorders of breast **and disorders of lactation associated with pregnancy and the puerperium**
5ᵗʰ O92.0 Retracted nipple **associated with pregnancy, the puerperium, and lactation**
6ᵗʰ O92.01 **Retracted nipple associated** with pregnancy
O92.011 **Retracted nipple associated with pregnancy,** first trimester   1st Ⓜ ♀
O92.012 **Retracted nipple associated with pregnancy,** second trimester   2nd Ⓜ ♀
O92.013 **Retracted nipple associated with pregnancy,** third trimester   3rd Ⓜ ♀
O92.019 **Retracted nipple associated with pregnancy, unspecified trimester**   Ⓜ ♀
O92.02 **Retracted nipple associated** with the puerperium   Ⓜ ♀
O92.03 **Retracted nipple associated** with lactation   Ⓜ ♀

5ᵗʰ O92.1 Cracked nipple **associated with pregnancy, the puerperium, and lactation**
Fissure of nipple, gestational or puerperal
6ᵗʰ O92.11 **Cracked nipple associated** with pregnancy
O92.111 **Cracked nipple associated with pregnancy,** first trimester   1st Ⓜ ♀
O92.112 **Cracked nipple associated with pregnancy,** second trimester   2nd Ⓜ ♀
O92.113 **Cracked nipple associated with pregnancy,** third trimester   3rd Ⓜ ♀
O92.119 **Cracked nipple associated with pregnancy, unspecified trimester**   Ⓜ ♀
O92.12 **Cracked nipple associated** with the puerperium   Ⓜ ♀
O92.13 **Cracked nipple associated** with lactation   Ⓜ ♀

5ᵗʰ O92.2 Other and unspecified disorders of breast **associated with pregnancy and the puerperium**
O92.20 **Unspecified disorder of breast associated with pregnancy and the puerperium**   Ⓜ ♀
O92.29 Other **disorders of breast associated with pregnancy and the puerperium**   Ⓜ ♀

O92.3 **Agalactia**   Ⓜ ♀
DEFINITION: Failure of secretion of milk.
Primary agalactia
EXCLUDES1 *Elective agalactia (O92.5)*
Secondary agalactia (O92.5)
Therapeutic agalactia (O92.5)

O92.4 **Hypogalactia** M ♀

O92.5 **Suppressed lactation** M ♀
Elective agalactia
Secondary agalactia
Therapeutic agalactia
EXCLUDES1 *primary agalactia (O92.3)*

O92.6 **Galactorrhea** M ♀

O92.7 **Other and unspecified disorders of** lactation
   O92.70 **Unspecified disorders of lactation** M ♀
   O92.79 **Other disorders of** lactation M ♀
      Puerperal galactocele

Other obstetric conditions, not elsewhere classified (O94-O9A)

O94 **Sequelae of complication of pregnancy, childbirth, and the puerperium** M POA ♀ PDxIn
   👁 **See Official Guidelines** "Code O94" I.C.15.p.1
   NOTES   This category is to be used to indicate conditions in O00-O77.-, O85-O94 and O98-O9A.- as the cause of late effects. The sequelae include conditions specified as such, or as late effects, which may occur at any time after the puerperium
   👉 **Code first** condition resulting from (sequela) of complication of pregnancy, childbirth, and the puerperium

O98 **Maternal infectious and parasitic diseases classifiable elsewhere but complicating pregnancy, childbirth and the puerperium**
   INCLUDES   *the listed conditions when complicating the pregnant state, when aggravated by the pregnancy, or as a reason for obstetric care*
   Use additional code (Chapter 1), to identify specific infectious or parasitic disease
   EXCLUDES2 *herpes gestationis (O26.4-)*
      infectious carrier state (O99.82-, O99.83-)
      obstetrical tetanus (A34)
      puerperal infection (O86.-)
      puerperal sepsis (O85)
      when the reason for maternal care is that the disease is known or suspected to have affected the fetus (O35-O36)

O98.0 **Tuberculosis complicating pregnancy, childbirth and the puerperium**
Conditions in A15-A19
   O98.01 **Tuberculosis complicating** pregnancy
      O98.011 **Tuberculosis complicating pregnancy, first trimester** 1st M cc ♀ CC/MCC Exc
      O98.012 **Tuberculosis complicating pregnancy, second trimester** 2nd M cc ♀ CC/MCC Exc
      O98.013 **Tuberculosis complicating pregnancy, third trimester** 3rd M cc ♀ CC/MCC Exc
      O98.019 **Tuberculosis complicating pregnancy, unspecified trimester** M ♀
   O98.02 **Tuberculosis complicating** childbirth M cc ♀ CC/MCC Exc
   O98.03 **Tuberculosis complicating the puerperium** M cc ♀ CC/MCC Exc

O98.1 **Syphilis complicating pregnancy, childbirth and the puerperium**
Conditions in A50-A53
   O98.11 **Syphilis complicating** pregnancy
      O98.111 **Syphilis complicating pregnancy, first trimester** 1st M cc ♀ CC/MCC Exc
      O98.112 **Syphilis complicating pregnancy, second trimester** 2nd M cc ♀ CC/MCC Exc
      O98.113 **Syphilis complicating pregnancy, third trimester** 3rd M cc ♀ CC/MCC Exc
      O98.119 **Syphilis complicating pregnancy, unspecified trimester** M ♀
   O98.12 **Syphilis complicating** childbirth M cc ♀ CC/MCC Exc
   O98.13 **Syphilis complicating the** puerperium M cc ♀ CC/MCC Exc

O98.2 **Gonorrhea complicating pregnancy, childbirth and the puerperium**
Conditions in A54.-
   O98.21 **Gonorrhea complicating** pregnancy

      O98.211 **Gonorrhea complicating pregnancy, first trimester** 1st M cc ♀ CC/MCC Exc
      O98.212 **Gonorrhea complicating pregnancy, second trimester** 2nd M cc ♀ CC/MCC Exc
      O98.213 **Gonorrhea complicating pregnancy, third trimester** 3rd M cc ♀ CC/MCC Exc
      O98.219 **Gonorrhea complicating pregnancy, unspecified trimester** M ♀
   O98.22 **Gonorrhea complicating** childbirth M cc ♀ CC/MCC Exc
   O98.23 **Gonorrhea complicating the puerperium** M cc ♀ CC/MCC Exc

O98.3 **Other infections with a predominantly sexual mode of transmission complicating pregnancy, childbirth and the puerperium**
Conditions in A55-A64
   O98.31 **Other infections with a predominantly sexual mode of transmission complicating** pregnancy
      O98.311 **Other infections with a predominantly sexual mode of transmission complicating pregnancy, first trimester** 1st M ♀
      O98.312 **Other infections with a predominantly sexual mode of transmission complicating pregnancy, second trimester** 2nd M ♀
      O98.313 **Other infections with a predominantly sexual mode of transmission complicating pregnancy, third trimester** 3rd M ♀
      O98.319 **Other infections with a predominantly sexual mode of transmission complicating pregnancy, unspecified trimester** M ♀
   O98.32 **Other infections with a predominantly sexual mode of transmission complicating** childbirth M ♀
   O98.33 **Other infections with a predominantly sexual mode of transmission complicating the** puerperium M ♀

O98.4 **Viral hepatitis complicating pregnancy, childbirth and the puerperium**
Conditions in B15-B19
   O98.41 **Viral hepatitis complicating** pregnancy
      O98.411 **Viral hepatitis complicating pregnancy, first trimester** 1st M cc ♀ CC/MCC Exc
      O98.412 **Viral hepatitis complicating pregnancy, second trimester** 2nd M cc ♀ CC/MCC Exc
      O98.413 **Viral hepatitis complicating pregnancy, third trimester** 3rd M cc ♀ CC/MCC Exc
      O98.419 **Viral hepatitis complicating pregnancy, unspecified trimester** M ♀
   O98.42 **Viral hepatitis complicating** childbirth M cc ♀ CC/MCC Exc
   O98.43 **Viral hepatitis complicating the puerperium** M cc ♀ CC/MCC Exc

O98.5 **Other viral diseases complicating pregnancy, childbirth and the puerperium**
Conditions in A80-B09, B25-B34, R87.81-, R87.82-
   EXCLUDES1 *human immunodeficiency virus [HIV] disease complicating pregnancy, childbirth and the puerperium (O98.7-)*
   O98.51 **Other viral diseases complicating** pregnancy
      O98.511 **Other viral diseases complicating pregnancy, first trimester** 1st M cc ♀ CC/MCC Exc
      O98.512 **Other viral diseases complicating pregnancy, second trimester** 2nd M cc ♀ CC/MCC Exc
         AHA: Q4 2016
      O98.513 **Other viral diseases complicating pregnancy, third trimester** 3rd M cc ♀ CC/MCC Exc
         AHA: Q4 2016
      O98.519 **Other viral diseases complicating pregnancy, unspecified trimester** M ♀
   O98.52 **Other viral diseases complicating** childbirth M ♀
   O98.53 **Other viral diseases complicating the** puerperium M cc ♀ CC/MCC Exc

O98.6 **Protozoal diseases complicating pregnancy, childbirth and the puerperium**
Conditions in B50-B64

1st 1st trimester   2nd 2nd trimester   3rd 3rd trimester   PDxIn Unacceptable principal diagnosis symbol per Medicare code edits
POA Code exempt from diagnosis present on admission requirement   ❓ Questionable admission   cc Complication or comorbidity
MCC Major complication or comorbidity   CC/MCC Exc CC/MCC exclusion   HCC HCC diagnosis code   RxHCC RxHCC diagnosis code   MACRA code
DEFINITION Describes condition/terminology   **TIP** Coding guidance   👁 Official Guideline Reference   Z Z code as first-listed diagnosis

914   When symbols appear on a code that requires a 7th character extension, refer to Appendix B to identify applicable 7th character codes.   **2020 ICD-10-CM**

[6th] **O98.61 Protozoal diseases complicating pregnancy**

O98.611 Protozoal diseases complicating pregnancy, first trimester [1st] [M] [CC] ♀ [CC/MCC Exc]

O98.612 Protozoal diseases complicating pregnancy, second trimester [2nd] [M] [CC] ♀ [CC/MCC Exc]

O98.613 Protozoal diseases complicating pregnancy, third trimester [3rd] [M] [CC] ♀ [CC/MCC Exc]

O98.619 Protozoal diseases complicating pregnancy, unspecified trimester [M] ♀

O98.62 Protozoal diseases complicating childbirth [M] [CC] ♀ [CC/MCC Exc]

O98.63 Protozoal diseases complicating the puerperium [M] [CC] ♀ [CC/MCC Exc]

[5th] **O98.7** Human immunodeficiency virus [HIV] disease **complicating pregnancy, childbirth and the puerperium**

See Official Guidelines "HIV Infection in Pregnancy, Childbirth and the Puerperium" I.C.1.a.2.g

Use additional code to identify the type of HIV disease:
- Acquired immune deficiency syndrome (AIDS) (B20)
- Asymptomatic HIV status (Z21)
- HIV positive NOS (Z21)
- Symptomatic HIV disease (B20)

[6th] **O98.71 Human immunodeficiency virus [HIV] disease complicating** pregnancy

O98.711 Human immunodeficiency virus [HIV] disease complicating pregnancy, first trimester [1st] [M] [CC] ♀ [CC/MCC Exc]

O98.712 Human immunodeficiency virus [HIV] disease complicating pregnancy, second trimester [2nd] [M] [CC] ♀ [CC/MCC Exc]

O98.713 Human immunodeficiency virus [HIV] disease complicating pregnancy, third trimester [3rd] [M] [CC] ♀ [CC/MCC Exc]

O98.719 Human immunodeficiency virus [HIV] disease complicating pregnancy, unspecified trimester [M] ♀

O98.72 Human immunodeficiency virus [HIV] disease complicating childbirth [M] [CC] ♀ [CC/MCC Exc]

O98.73 Human immunodeficiency virus [HIV] disease complicating the puerperium [M] [CC] ♀ [CC/MCC Exc]

[5th] **O98.8** Other maternal infectious and parasitic diseases **complicating pregnancy, childbirth and the puerperium**

[6th] **O98.81 Other maternal infectious and parasitic diseases complicating** pregnancy

O98.811 Other maternal infectious and parasitic diseases complicating pregnancy, first trimester [1st] [M] [CC] ♀ [CC/MCC Exc]

O98.812 Other maternal infectious and parasitic diseases complicating pregnancy, second trimester [2nd] [M] [CC] ♀ [CC/MCC Exc]

O98.813 Other maternal infectious and parasitic diseases complicating pregnancy, third trimester [3rd] [M] [CC] ♀ [CC/MCC Exc]

O98.819 Other maternal infectious and parasitic diseases complicating pregnancy, unspecified trimester [M] ♀

O98.82 Other maternal infectious and parasitic diseases complicating childbirth [M] [CC] ♀ [CC/MCC Exc]

O98.83 Other maternal infectious and parasitic diseases complicating the puerperium [M] [CC] ♀ [CC/MCC Exc]

[5th] **O98.9** Unspecified maternal infectious and parasitic disease **complicating pregnancy, childbirth and the puerperium**

[6th] **O98.91 Unspecified maternal infectious and parasitic disease complicating** pregnancy

O98.911 Unspecified maternal infectious and parasitic disease complicating pregnancy, first trimester [1st] [M] [CC] ♀ [CC/MCC Exc]

O98.912 Unspecified maternal infectious and parasitic disease complicating pregnancy, second trimester [2nd] [M] [CC] ♀ [CC/MCC Exc]

O98.913 Unspecified maternal infectious and parasitic disease complicating pregnancy, third trimester [3rd] [M] [CC] ♀ [CC/MCC Exc]

O98.919 Unspecified maternal infectious and parasitic disease complicating pregnancy, unspecified trimester [M] ♀

O98.92 Unspecified maternal infectious and parasitic disease complicating childbirth [M] [CC] ♀ [CC/MCC Exc]

O98.93 Unspecified maternal infectious and parasitic disease complicating the puerperium [M] [CC] ♀ [CC/MCC Exc]

[4th] **O99** Other maternal diseases classifiable elsewhere **but complicating pregnancy, childbirth and the puerperium**

[INCLUDES] *conditions which complicate the pregnant state, are aggravated by the pregnancy or are a main reason for obstetric care*

Use additional code to identify specific condition

[EXCLUDES2] *when the reason for maternal care is that the condition is known or suspected to have affected the fetus (O35-O36)*

[5th] **O99.0** Anemia **complicating pregnancy, childbirth and the puerperium**

Conditions in D50-D64

[EXCLUDES1] *anemia arising in the puerperium (O90.81)*
postpartum anemia NOS (O90.81)

[6th] **O99.01 Anemia complicating** pregnancy

O99.011 Anemia complicating pregnancy, first trimester [1st] [M] ♀

O99.012 Anemia complicating pregnancy, second trimester [2nd] [M] ♀

O99.013 Anemia complicating pregnancy, third trimester [3rd] [M] ♀

O99.019 Anemia complicating pregnancy, unspecified trimester [M] ♀

O99.02 Anemia complicating childbirth [M] ♀

O99.03 Anemia complicating the puerperium [M] ♀

[EXCLUDES1] *postpartum anemia not pre-existing prior to delivery (O90.81)*

[5th] **O99.1** Other diseases of the blood and blood-forming organs **and certain disorders** involving the immune mechanism **complicating pregnancy, childbirth and the puerperium**

Conditions in D65-D89

[EXCLUDES1] *hemorrhage with coagulation defects (O45.-, O46.0-, O67.0, O72.3)*

[6th] **O99.11 Other diseases of the blood and blood-forming organs and certain disorders involving the immune mechanism complicating** pregnancy

O99.111 Other diseases of the blood and blood-forming organs and certain disorders involving the immune mechanism complicating pregnancy, first trimester [1st] [M] [CC] ♀ [CC/MCC Exc]

O99.112 Other diseases of the blood and blood-forming organs and certain disorders involving the immune mechanism complicating pregnancy, second trimester [2nd] [M] [CC] ♀ [CC/MCC Exc]

O99.113 Other diseases of the blood and blood-forming organs and certain disorders involving the immune mechanism complicating pregnancy, third trimester [3rd] [M] [CC] ♀ [CC/MCC Exc]

O99.119 Other diseases of the blood and blood-forming organs and certain disorders involving the immune mechanism complicating pregnancy, unspecified trimester [M] [CC] ♀ [CC/MCC Exc]

O99.12 Other diseases of the blood and blood-forming organs and certain disorders involving the immune mechanism complicating childbirth [M] [CC] ♀ [CC/MCC Exc]

O99.13 Other diseases of the blood and blood-forming organs and certain disorders involving the immune mechanism complicating the puerperium [M] [CC] ♀ [CC/MCC Exc]

Unspecified Code | Other Specified Code | Manifestation Code | [N] Newborn | [P] Pediatric | [M] Maternity | [A] Adult | ♂ Male | ♀ Female
● New Code | ▲ Revised Code Title | ►◄ Revised Text | [NOTES] | [INCLUDES] | [EXCLUDES1] Not coded here | [EXCLUDES2] Not included here
[4th] 4th character required | [5th] 5th character required | [6th] 6th character required | [7th] 7th character required | [X] Extension 'X' Alert
[HAC] Hospital-acquired condition (HAC) alert | AHA AHA Coding Clinic© | Code first alert

5ᵗʰ O99.2 Endocrine, nutritional and metabolic diseases complicating pregnancy, childbirth and the puerperium
Conditions in E00-E88
EXCLUDES2 diabetes mellitus (O24.-)
malnutrition (O25.-)
postpartum thyroiditis (O90.5)

6ᵗʰ O99.21 Obesity complicating pregnancy, childbirth, and the puerperium
Use additional code to identify the type of obesity (E66.-)

O99.210 **Obesity complicating pregnancy, unspecified trimester** M ♀

O99.211 **Obesity complicating pregnancy, first trimester** 1st M ♀

O99.212 **Obesity complicating pregnancy, second trimester** 2nd M ♀

O99.213 **Obesity complicating pregnancy, third trimester** 3rd M ♀

O99.214 **Obesity complicating childbirth** M ♀
AHA: Q4 2018

O99.215 **Obesity complicating the puerperium** M ♀

6ᵗʰ O99.28 Other endocrine, nutritional and metabolic diseases complicating pregnancy, childbirth and the puerperium

O99.280 **Endocrine, nutritional and metabolic diseases complicating pregnancy, unspecified trimester** M ♀

O99.281 **Endocrine, nutritional and metabolic diseases complicating pregnancy, first trimester** 1st M ♀

O99.282 **Endocrine, nutritional and metabolic diseases complicating pregnancy, second trimester** 2nd M ♀

O99.283 **Endocrine, nutritional and metabolic diseases complicating pregnancy, third trimester** 3rd M ♀

O99.284 **Endocrine, nutritional and metabolic diseases complicating childbirth** M ♀

O99.285 **Endocrine, nutritional and metabolic diseases complicating the puerperium** M ♀

5ᵗʰ O99.3 Mental disorders and diseases of the nervous system complicating pregnancy, childbirth and the puerperium

6ᵗʰ O99.31 Alcohol use complicating pregnancy, childbirth, and the puerperium
👁 See Official Guidelines "Alcohol use during pregnancy, childbirth and the puerperium" I.C.15.l.1
Use additional code(s) from F10 to identify manifestations of the alcohol use

O99.310 **Alcohol use complicating pregnancy, unspecified trimester** M ♀

O99.311 **Alcohol use complicating pregnancy, first trimester** 1st M ♀

O99.312 **Alcohol use complicating pregnancy, second trimester** 2nd M ♀

O99.313 **Alcohol use complicating pregnancy, third trimester** 3rd M ♀

O99.314 **Alcohol use complicating childbirth** M ♀

O99.315 **Alcohol use complicating the puerperium** M ♀

6ᵗʰ O99.32 Drug use complicating pregnancy, childbirth, and the puerperium
Use additional code(s) from F11-F16 and F18-F19 to identify manifestations of the drug use

O99.320 **Drug use complicating pregnancy, unspecified trimester** M ♀
AHA: Q2 2018

O99.321 **Drug use complicating pregnancy, first trimester** 1st M cc ♀ CC/MCC Exc
AHA: Q2 2018

O99.322 **Drug use complicating pregnancy, second trimester** 2nd M cc ♀ CC/MCC Exc
AHA: Q2 2018

O99.323 **Drug use complicating pregnancy, third trimester** 3rd M cc ♀ CC/MCC Exc
AHA: Q2 2018

O99.324 **Drug use complicating childbirth** M cc ♀ CC/MCC Exc
AHA: Q2 2018

O99.325 **Drug use complicating the puerperium** M cc ♀ CC/MCC Exc
AHA: Q2 2018

6ᵗʰ O99.33 Tobacco use disorder complicating pregnancy, childbirth, and the puerperium
👁 See Official Guidelines "Tobacco use during pregnancy, childbirth and the puerperium" I.C.15.l.2
Smoking complicating pregnancy, childbirth, and the puerperium
Use additional code from category F17 to identify type of tobacco nicotine dependence

O99.330 **Smoking (tobacco) complicating pregnancy, unspecified trimester** M ♀

O99.331 **Smoking (tobacco) complicating pregnancy, first trimester** 1st M ♀

O99.332 **Smoking (tobacco) complicating pregnancy, second trimester** 2nd M ♀

O99.333 **Smoking (tobacco) complicating pregnancy, third trimester** 3rd M ♀

O99.334 **Smoking (tobacco) complicating childbirth** M ♀

O99.335 **Smoking (tobacco) complicating the puerperium** M ♀

6ᵗʰ O99.34 Other mental disorders complicating pregnancy, childbirth, and the puerperium
Conditions in F01-F09, ▶F20-F99 and F54-F99◀
EXCLUDES2 postpartum mood disturbance (O90.6)
postnatal psychosis (F53.1)
puerperal psychosis (F53.1)

O99.340 **Other mental disorders complicating pregnancy, unspecified trimester** M ♀

O99.341 **Other mental disorders complicating pregnancy, first trimester** 1st M ♀

O99.342 **Other mental disorders complicating pregnancy, second trimester** 2nd M ♀

O99.343 **Other mental disorders complicating pregnancy, third trimester** 3rd M ♀

O99.344 **Other mental disorders complicating childbirth** M ♀

O99.345 **Other mental disorders complicating the puerperium** M ♀
AHA: Q4 2018

6ᵗʰ O99.35 Diseases of the nervous system complicating pregnancy, childbirth, and the puerperium
Conditions in G00-G99
EXCLUDES2 pregnancy related peripheral neuritis (O26.8-)

O99.350 **Diseases of the nervous system complicating pregnancy, unspecified trimester** M ♀

O99.351 **Diseases of the nervous system complicating pregnancy, first trimester** 1st M ♀

O99.352 **Diseases of the nervous system complicating pregnancy, second trimester** 2nd M ♀

O99.353 **Diseases of the nervous system complicating pregnancy, third trimester** 3rd M ♀

O99.354 **Diseases of the nervous system complicating childbirth** M cc ♀ CC/MCC Exc

O99.355 **Diseases of the nervous system complicating the puerperium** M cc ♀ CC/MCC Exc

---

1st 1st trimester   2nd 2nd trimester   3rd 3rd trimester   PDx Unacceptable principal diagnosis symbol per Medicare code edits
PoA Code exempt from diagnosis present on admission requirement   ❓ Questionable admission   cc Complication or comorbidity
mcc Major complication or comorbidity   CC/MCC Exc CC/MCC exclusion   HCC HCC diagnosis code   RxHCC RxHCC diagnosis code   MACRA code
DEFINITION Describes condition/terminology   TIP Coding guidance   👁 Official Guideline Reference   Z1 Z code as first-listed diagnosis

5ᵗʰ O99.4 Diseases of the circulatory system complicating pregnancy, childbirth and the puerperium
Conditions in I00-I99
EXCLUDES1 peripartum cardiomyopathy (O90.3)
EXCLUDES2 hypertensive disorders (O10-O16)
obstetric embolism (O88.-)
venous complications and cerebrovenous sinus thrombosis in labor, childbirth and the puerperium (O87.-)
venous complications and cerebrovenous sinus thrombosis in pregnancy (O22.-)

6ᵗʰ O99.41 Diseases of the circulatory system complicating pregnancy
O99.411 Diseases of the circulatory system complicating pregnancy, first trimester 1st M cc Q CC/MCC Exc
O99.412 Diseases of the circulatory system complicating pregnancy, second trimester 2nd M cc Q CC/MCC Exc
O99.413 Diseases of the circulatory system complicating pregnancy, third trimester 3rd M cc Q CC/MCC Exc
O99.419 Diseases of the circulatory system complicating pregnancy, unspecified trimester M Q

O99.42 Diseases of the circulatory system complicating childbirth M MCC Q CC/MCC Exc
O99.43 Diseases of the circulatory system complicating the puerperium M cc Q CC/MCC Exc

5ᵗʰ O99.5 Diseases of the respiratory system complicating pregnancy, childbirth and the puerperium
Conditions in J00-J99

6ᵗʰ O99.51 Diseases of the respiratory system complicating pregnancy
O99.511 Diseases of the respiratory system complicating pregnancy, first trimester 1st M Q
O99.512 Diseases of the respiratory system complicating pregnancy, second trimester 2nd M Q
O99.513 Diseases of the respiratory system complicating pregnancy, third trimester 3rd M Q
O99.519 Diseases of the respiratory system complicating pregnancy, unspecified trimester M Q

O99.52 Diseases of the respiratory system complicating childbirth M Q
O99.53 Diseases of the respiratory system complicating the puerperium M Q

5ᵗʰ O99.6 Diseases of the digestive system complicating pregnancy, childbirth and the puerperium
Conditions in K00-K93
EXCLUDES2 hemorrhoids in pregnancy (O22.4-)
liver and biliary tract disorders in pregnancy, childbirth and the puerperium (O26.6-)

6ᵗʰ O99.61 Diseases of the digestive system complicating pregnancy
O99.611 Diseases of the digestive system complicating pregnancy, first trimester 1st M Q
O99.612 Diseases of the digestive system complicating pregnancy, second trimester 2nd M Q
O99.613 Diseases of the digestive system complicating pregnancy, third trimester 3rd M Q
O99.619 Diseases of the digestive system complicating pregnancy, unspecified trimester M Q

O99.62 Diseases of the digestive system complicating childbirth M Q

O99.63 Diseases of the digestive system complicating the puerperium M Q

5ᵗʰ O99.7 Diseases of the skin and subcutaneous tissue complicating pregnancy, childbirth and the puerperium
Conditions in L00-L99
EXCLUDES2 herpes gestationis (O26.4)
pruritic urticarial papules and plaques of pregnancy (PUPPP) (O26.86)

6ᵗʰ O99.71 Diseases of the skin and subcutaneous tissue complicating pregnancy
O99.711 Diseases of the skin and subcutaneous tissue complicating pregnancy, first trimester 1st M Q
O99.712 Diseases of the skin and subcutaneous tissue complicating pregnancy, second trimester 2nd M Q
O99.713 Diseases of the skin and subcutaneous tissue complicating pregnancy, third trimester 3rd M Q
O99.719 Diseases of the skin and subcutaneous tissue complicating pregnancy, unspecified trimester M Q

O99.72 Diseases of the skin and subcutaneous tissue complicating childbirth M Q
O99.73 Diseases of the skin and subcutaneous tissue complicating the puerperium M Q

5ᵗʰ O99.8 Other specified diseases and conditions complicating pregnancy, childbirth and the puerperium
Conditions in D00-D48, H00-H95, M00-N99, and Q00-Q99
Use additional code to identify condition
EXCLUDES2 genitourinary infections in pregnancy (O23.-)
infection of genitourinary tract following delivery (O86.1-►O86.4◄)
malignant neoplasm complicating pregnancy, childbirth and the puerperium (O9A.1-)
maternal care for known or suspected abnormality of maternal pelvic organs (O34.-)
postpartum acute kidney failure (O90.4)
traumatic injuries in pregnancy (O9A.2-)

6ᵗʰ O99.81 Abnormal glucose complicating pregnancy, childbirth and the puerperium
See Official Guidelines "Gestational (pregnancy induced) diabetes" I.C.15.i
EXCLUDES1 gestational diabetes (O24.4-)
O99.810 Abnormal glucose complicating pregnancy M Q
O99.814 Abnormal glucose complicating childbirth M Q
O99.815 Abnormal glucose complicating the puerperium M Q

6ᵗʰ O99.82 Streptococcus B carrier state complicating pregnancy, childbirth and the puerperium
EXCLUDES1 Carrier of streptococcus group B (GBS) in a nonpregnant woman (Z22.330)
O99.820 Streptococcus B carrier state complicating pregnancy M Q PDxIn
O99.824 Streptococcus B carrier state complicating childbirth M Q
AHA: Q2 2019
O99.825 Streptococcus B carrier state complicating the puerperium M Q PDxIn

6ᵗʰ O99.83 Other infection carrier state complicating pregnancy, childbirth and the puerperium
Use additional code to identify the carrier state (Z22.-)
O99.830 Other infection carrier state complicating pregnancy M cc Q CC/MCC Exc
O99.834 Other infection carrier state complicating childbirth M cc Q CC/MCC Exc
O99.835 Other infection carrier state complicating the puerperium M cc Q CC/MCC Exc

---

Unspecified Code   Other Specified Code   Manifestation Code   N Newborn   P Pediatric   M Maternity   A Adult   ♂ Male   ♀ Female
● New Code   ▲ Revised Code Title   ►◄ Revised Text   NOTES   INCLUDES   EXCLUDES1 Not coded here   EXCLUDES2 Not included here
4ᵗʰ 4ᵗʰ character required   5ᵗʰ 5ᵗʰ character required   6ᵗʰ 6ᵗʰ character required   7ᵗʰ 7ᵗʰ character required   Extension 'X' Alert
HAC Hospital-acquired condition (HAC) alert   AHA AHA Coding Clinic©   Code first alert

🔟 **O99.84** Bariatric surgery status complicating pregnancy, childbirth and the puerperium
Gastric banding status complicating pregnancy, childbirth and the puerperium
Gastric bypass status for obesity complicating pregnancy, childbirth and the puerperium
Obesity surgery status complicating pregnancy, childbirth and the puerperium

O99.840 Bariatric surgery status complicating pregnancy, unspecified trimester M ♀

O99.841 Bariatric surgery status complicating pregnancy, first trimester 1st M ♀

O99.842 Bariatric surgery status complicating pregnancy, second trimester 2nd M ♀

O99.843 Bariatric surgery status complicating pregnancy, third trimester 3rd M ♀

O99.844 Bariatric surgery status complicating childbirth M ♀

O99.845 Bariatric surgery status complicating the puerperium M ♀

O99.89 Other specified diseases and conditions complicating pregnancy, childbirth and the puerperium M ♀

🔟 **O9A** Maternal malignant neoplasms, traumatic injuries and abuse classifiable elsewhere but complicating pregnancy, childbirth and the puerperium

🔟 **O9A.1** Malignant neoplasm complicating pregnancy, childbirth and the puerperium
👁 **See Official Guidelines** "Malignant neoplasm in a pregnant patient" I.C.2.l.3
Conditions in C00-C96
Use additional code to identify neoplasm
EXCLUDES2 maternal care for benign tumor of corpus uteri (O34.1-)
maternal care for benign tumor of cervix (O34.4-)

🔟 **O9A.11** Malignant neoplasm complicating pregnancy

O9A.111 Malignant neoplasm complicating pregnancy, first trimester 1st M ♀

O9A.112 Malignant neoplasm complicating pregnancy, second trimester 2nd M ♀

O9A.113 Malignant neoplasm complicating pregnancy, third trimester 3rd M ♀

O9A.119 Malignant neoplasm complicating pregnancy, unspecified trimester M ♀

O9A.12 Malignant neoplasm complicating childbirth M ♀

O9A.13 Malignant neoplasm complicating the puerperium M ♀
AHA: Q3 2015

🔟 **O9A.2** Injury, poisoning and certain other consequences of external causes complicating pregnancy, childbirth and the puerperium
👁 **See Official Guidelines** "Poisoning, toxic effects, adverse effects and underdosing in a pregnant patient" I.C.15.m
Conditions in S00-T88, except T74 and T76
Use additional code(s) to identify the injury or poisoning
EXCLUDES2 physical, sexual and psychological abuse complicating pregnancy, childbirth and the puerperium (O9A.3-, O9A.4-, O9A.5-)

🔟 **O9A.21** Injury, poisoning and certain other consequences of external causes complicating pregnancy

O9A.211 Injury, poisoning and certain other consequences of external causes complicating pregnancy, first trimester 1st M ♀

O9A.212 Injury, poisoning and certain other consequences of external causes complicating pregnancy, second trimester 2nd M ♀

O9A.213 Injury, poisoning and certain other consequences of external causes complicating pregnancy, third trimester 3rd M ♀

O9A.219 Injury, poisoning and certain other consequences of external causes complicating pregnancy, unspecified trimester M ♀

O9A.22 Injury, poisoning and certain other consequences of external causes complicating childbirth M ♀

O9A.23 Injury, poisoning and certain other consequences of external causes complicating the puerperium M ♀

🔟 **O9A.3** Physical abuse complicating pregnancy, childbirth and the puerperium
👁 **See Official Guidelines** "Abuse in a pregnant patient" I.C.15.r
Conditions in T74.11 or T76.11
Use additional code (if applicable):
to identify any associated current injury due to physical abuse
to identify the perpetrator of abuse (Y07.-)
EXCLUDES2 sexual abuse complicating pregnancy, childbirth and the puerperium (O9A.4)

🔟 **O9A.31** Physical abuse complicating pregnancy

O9A.311 Physical abuse complicating pregnancy, first trimester 1st M ♀

O9A.312 Physical abuse complicating pregnancy, second trimester 2nd M ♀

O9A.313 Physical abuse complicating pregnancy, third trimester 3rd M ♀

O9A.319 Physical abuse complicating pregnancy, unspecified trimester M ♀

O9A.32 Physical abuse complicating childbirth M ♀

O9A.33 Physical abuse complicating the puerperium M ♀

🔟 **O9A.4** Sexual abuse complicating pregnancy, childbirth and the puerperium
👁 **See Official Guidelines** "Abuse in a pregnant patient" I.C.15.r
Conditions in T74.21 or T76.21
Use additional code (if applicable):
to identify any associated current injury due to sexual abuse
to identify the perpetrator of abuse (Y07.-)

🔟 **O9A.41** Sexual abuse complicating pregnancy

O9A.411 Sexual abuse complicating pregnancy, first trimester 1st M ♀

O9A.412 Sexual abuse complicating pregnancy, second trimester 2nd M ♀

O9A.413 Sexual abuse complicating pregnancy, third trimester 3rd M ♀

O9A.419 Sexual abuse complicating pregnancy, unspecified trimester M ♀

O9A.42 Sexual abuse complicating childbirth M ♀

O9A.43 Sexual abuse complicating the puerperium M ♀

🔟 **O9A.5** Psychological abuse complicating pregnancy, childbirth and the puerperium
👁 **See Official Guidelines** "Abuse in a pregnant patient" I.C.15.r
Conditions in T74.31 or T76.31
Use additional code to identify the perpetrator of abuse (Y07.-)

🔟 **O9A.51** Psychological abuse complicating pregnancy

O9A.511 Psychological abuse complicating pregnancy, first trimester 1st M ♀

O9A.512 Psychological abuse complicating pregnancy, second trimester 2nd M ♀

O9A.513 Psychological abuse complicating pregnancy, third trimester 3rd M ♀

O9A.519 Psychological abuse complicating pregnancy, unspecified trimester M ♀

O9A.52 Psychological abuse complicating childbirth M ♀

O9A.53 Psychological abuse complicating the puerperium M ♀

1st 1st trimester 2nd 2nd trimester 3rd 3rd trimester PDx Unacceptable principal diagnosis symbol per Medicare code edits
POA Code exempt from diagnosis present on admission requirement ❓ Questionable admission ℗ Complication or comorbidity
MCC Major complication or comorbidity CC/MCC Exc CC/MCC exclusion HCC HCC diagnosis code RxHCC RxHCC diagnosis code MACRA code
DEFINITION Describes condition/terminology **TIP** Coding guidance 👁 Official Guideline Reference Z1 Z code as first-listed diagnosis

When symbols appear on a code that requires a 7th character extension, refer to Appendix B to identify applicable 7th character codes.

2020 ICD-10-CM

Chapter 16: Certain Conditions Originating in the Perinatal Period (P00-P96)

Certain conditions originating in the perinatal period (P00-P96)

[NOTES] Codes from this chapter are for use on newborn records only, never on maternal records

[INCLUDES] *conditions that have their origin in the fetal or perinatal period (before birth through the first 28 days after birth) even if morbidity occurs later*

[EXCLUDES2] *congenital malformations, deformations and chromosomal abnormalities (Q00-Q99)*

endocrine, nutritional and metabolic diseases (E00-E88)

injury, poisoning and certain other consequences of external causes (S00-T88)

neoplasms (C00-D49)

tetanus neonatorum (A33)

This chapter contains the following blocks:

P00-P04 Newborn affected by maternal factors and by complications of pregnancy, labor, and delivery
P05-P08 Disorders of newborn related to length of gestation and fetal growth
P09 Abnormal findings on neonatal screening
P10-P15 Birth trauma
P19-P29 Respiratory and cardiovascular disorders specific to the perinatal period
P35-P39 Infections specific to the perinatal period
P50-P61 Hemorrhagic and hematological disorders of newborn
P70-P74 Transitory endocrine and metabolic disorders specific to newborn
P76-P78 Digestive system disorders of newborn
P80-P83 Conditions involving the integument and temperature regulation of newborn
P84 Other problems with newborn
P90-P96 Other disorders originating in the perinatal period

Newborn affected by maternal factors and by complications of pregnancy, labor, and delivery (P00-P04)

[NOTES] These codes are for use when the listed maternal conditions are specified as the cause of confirmed morbidity or potential morbidity which have their origin in the perinatal period (before birth through the first 28 days after birth).

[4] **P00 Newborn affected by maternal conditions that may be unrelated to present pregnancy**

☛ **Code first** any current condition in newborn

[EXCLUDES2] *encounter for observation of newborn for suspected diseases and conditions ruled out (Z05.-)*

newborn affected by maternal complications of pregnancy (P01.-)

newborn affected by maternal endocrine and metabolic disorders (P70-P74)

newborn affected by noxious substances transmitted via placenta or breast milk (P04.-)

P00.0 Newborn affected by maternal hypertensive disorders [POA]
AHA: Q4 2017
Newborn affected by maternal conditions classifiable to O10-O11, O13-O16

P00.1 Newborn affected by maternal renal and urinary tract diseases [POA]
AHA: Q4 2017
Newborn affected by maternal conditions classifiable to N00-N39

P00.2 Newborn affected by maternal infectious and parasitic diseases [POA]
AHA: Q2 2019, Q4 2017, Q3 2015
Newborn affected by maternal infectious disease classifiable to A00-B99, J09 and J10

[EXCLUDES1] *maternal genital tract or other localized infections (P00.8)*

[EXCLUDES2] *infections specific to the perinatal period (P35-P39)*

P00.3 Newborn affected by other maternal circulatory and respiratory diseases [POA]
AHA: Q4 2017
Newborn affected by maternal conditions classifiable to I00-I99, J00-J99, Q20-Q34 and not included in P00.0, P00.2

P00.4 Newborn affected by maternal nutritional disorders [POA]
AHA: Q4 2017
Newborn affected by maternal disorders classifiable to E40-E64
Maternal malnutrition NOS

P00.5 Newborn affected by maternal injury [POA]
AHA: Q4 2017
Newborn affected by maternal conditions classifiable to O9A.2-

P00.6 Newborn affected by surgical procedure on mother [POA]
AHA: Q4 2017
Newborn affected by amniocentesis

[EXCLUDES1] *Cesarean delivery for present delivery (P03.4)*

damage to placenta from amniocentesis, Cesarean delivery or surgical induction (P02.1)

previous surgery to uterus or pelvic organs (P03.89)

[EXCLUDES2] *newborn affected by complication of (fetal) intrauterine procedure (P96.5)*

P00.7 Newborn affected by other medical procedures on mother, not elsewhere classified [POA]
AHA: Q4 2017
Newborn affected by radiation to mother

[EXCLUDES1] *damage to placenta from amniocentesis, cesarean delivery or surgical induction (P02.1)*

newborn affected by other complications of labor and delivery (P03.-)

[5] **P00.8 Newborn affected by other maternal conditions**

P00.81 Newborn affected by periodontal disease in mother [POA]
AHA: Q4 2017

P00.89 Newborn affected by other maternal conditions [POA]
AHA: Q2 2019, Q4 2017
Newborn affected by conditions classifiable to T80-T88
Newborn affected by maternal genital tract or other localized infections
Newborn affected by maternal systemic lupus erythematosus

P00.9 Newborn affected by unspecified maternal condition [POA]
AHA: Q4 2017

[4] **P01 Newborn affected by maternal complications of pregnancy (Figure 16.1)**

☛ **Code first** any current condition in newborn

[EXCLUDES2] *encounter for observation of newborn for suspected diseases and conditions ruled out (Z05.-)*

P01.0 Newborn affected by incompetent cervix
AHA: Q4 2017

P01.1 Newborn affected by premature rupture of membranes
AHA: Q4 2017

P01.2 Newborn affected by oligohydramnios
AHA: Q4 2017

[EXCLUDES1] *oligohydramnios due to premature rupture of membranes (P01.1)*

P01.3 Newborn affected by polyhydramnios
AHA: Q4 2017
Newborn affected by hydramnios

P01.4 Newborn affected by ectopic pregnancy
AHA: Q4 2017
Newborn affected by abdominal pregnancy

P01.5 Newborn affected by multiple pregnancy
AHA: Q4 2017
Newborn affected by triplet (pregnancy)
Newborn affected by twin (pregnancy)

Unspecified Code | Other Specified Code | Manifestation Code | [N] Newborn | [P] Pediatric | [M] Maternity | [A] Adult | ♂ Male | ♀ Female
● New Code | ▲ Revised Code Title | ▶◀ Revised Text | [NOTES] | [INCLUDES] | [EXCLUDES1] Not coded here | [EXCLUDES2] Not included here
[4] 4th character required | [5] 5th character required | [6] 6th character required | [7] 7th character required | [7] Extension 'X' Alert
[HAC] Hospital-acquired condition (HAC) alert | AHA AHA Coding Clinic© | ☛ Code first alert

P01.6 **Newborn affected by maternal death**
AHA: Q4 2017

P01.7 **Newborn affected by malpresentation before labor**
AHA: Q4 2017
Newborn affected by breech presentation before labor
Newborn affected by external version before labor
Newborn affected by face presentation before labor
Newborn affected by transverse lie before labor
Newborn affected by unstable lie before labor

P01.8 **Newborn affected by other maternal complications of pregnancy**
AHA: Q4 2017

P01.9 **Newborn affected by maternal complication of pregnancy, unspecified**
AHA: Q4 2017

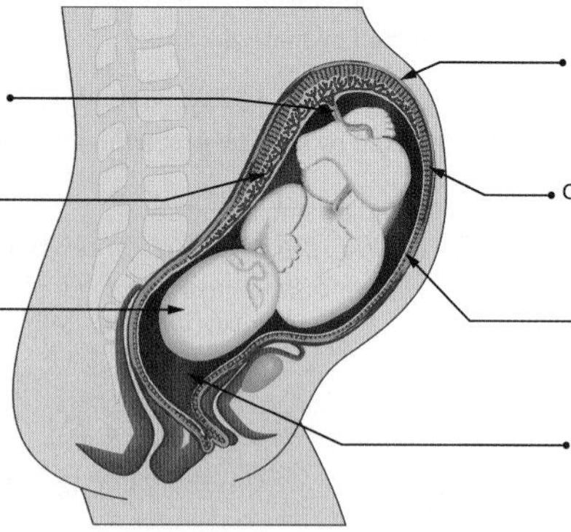
Wall of the uterus
Umbilical cord
Placenta
Chorion
Fetus
Amnion
Amniotic cavity

Figure 16.1 Anatomy of Uterine Cavity

4th P02 **Newborn affected by complications of placenta, cord and membranes**
Code first any current condition in newborn
EXCLUDES2 encounter for observation of newborn for suspected diseases and conditions ruled out (Z05.-)

P02.0 **Newborn affected by placenta previa**
AHA: Q4 2017

P02.1 **Newborn affected by other forms of placental separation and hemorrhage**
AHA: Q4 2017
Newborn affected by abruptio placenta
Newborn affected by accidental hemorrhage
Newborn affected by antepartum hemorrhage
Newborn affected by damage to placenta from amniocentesis, cesarean delivery or surgical induction
Newborn affected by maternal blood loss
Newborn affected by premature separation of placenta

5th P02.2 **Newborn affected by other and unspecified morphological and functional abnormalities of placenta**

P02.20 **Newborn affected by unspecified morphological and functional abnormalities of placenta**
AHA: Q4 2017

P02.29 **Newborn affected by other morphological and functional abnormalities of placenta**
AHA: Q4 2017
Newborn affected by placental dysfunction
Newborn affected by placental infarction
Newborn affected by placental insufficiency

P02.3 **Newborn affected by placental transfusion syndromes**
AHA: Q4 2017
Newborn affected by placental and cord abnormalities resulting in twin-to-twin or other transplacental transfusion

P02.4 **Newborn affected by prolapsed cord**
AHA: Q4 2017

P02.5 **Newborn affected by other compression of umbilical cord**
AHA: Q4 2017
Newborn affected by umbilical cord (tightly) around neck
Newborn affected by entanglement of umbilical cord
Newborn affected by knot in umbilical cord

5th P02.6 **Newborn affected by other and unspecified conditions of umbilical cord**

P02.60 **Newborn affected by unspecified conditions of umbilical cord**
AHA: Q4 2017

P02.69 **Newborn affected by other conditions of umbilical cord**
AHA: Q4 2017
Newborn affected by short umbilical cord
Newborn affected by vasa previa
EXCLUDES1 newborn affected by single umbilical artery (Q27.0)

5th P02.7 **Newborn affected by chorioamnionitis**

P02.70 **Newborn affected by fetal inflammatory response syndrome** HCC
AHA: Q4 2018
Newborn affected by FIRS

P02.78 **Newborn affected by other conditions from chorioamnionitis**
AHA: Q4 2018
Newborn affected by amnionitis
Newborn affected by membranitis
Newborn affected by placentitis

P02.8 **Newborn affected by other abnormalities of membranes**
AHA: Q4 2017

P02.9 **Newborn affected by abnormality of membranes, unspecified**
AHA: Q4 2017

4th P03 **Newborn affected by other complications of labor and delivery**
Code first any current condition in newborn
EXCLUDES2 encounter for observation of newborn for suspected diseases and conditions ruled out (Z05.-)

P03.0 **Newborn affected by breech delivery and extraction**
AHA: Q4 2017

P03.1 **Newborn affected by other malpresentation, malposition and disproportion during labor and delivery**
AHA: Q4 2017
Newborn affected by contracted pelvis
Newborn affected by conditions classifiable to O64-O66
Newborn affected by persistent occipitoposterior
Newborn affected by transverse lie

P03.2 **Newborn affected by forceps delivery**
AHA: Q4 2017

P03.3 **Newborn affected by delivery by vacuum extractor [ventouse]**
AHA: Q4 2017

P03.4 **Newborn affected by Cesarean delivery**
AHA: Q4 2017

P03.5 **Newborn affected by precipitate delivery**
AHA: Q4 2017
Newborn affected by rapid second stage

P03.6 **Newborn affected by abnormal uterine contractions**
AHA: Q4 2017
Newborn affected by conditions classifiable to O62.-, except O62.3
Newborn affected by hypertonic labor
Newborn affected by uterine inertia

5th P03.8 **Newborn affected by other specified complications of labor and delivery**

6th P03.81 **Newborn affected by abnormality in fetal (intrauterine) heart rate or rhythm**
EXCLUDES1 neonatal cardiac dysrhythmia (P29.1-)

P03.810 **Newborn affected by abnormality in fetal (intrauterine) heart rate or rhythm before the onset of labor**
AHA: Q4 2017

P03.811 **Newborn affected by abnormality in fetal (intrauterine) heart rate or rhythm during labor**
AHA: Q4 2017

P03.819 **Newborn affected by abnormality in fetal (intrauterine) heart rate or rhythm, unspecified as to time of onset**
AHA: Q4 2017

PDx Unacceptable principal diagnosis symbol per Medicare code edits POA Code exempt from diagnosis present on admission requirement
? Questionable admission CC Complication or comorbidity MCC Major complication or comorbidity CC/MCC Exc CC/MCC exclusion
HCC HCC diagnosis code RxHCC RxHCC diagnosis code MACRA code **DEFINITION** Describes condition/terminology
TIP Coding guidance Official Guideline Reference Z1 Z code as first-listed diagnosis

P03.82 Meconium passage during delivery
AHA: Q4 2017
EXCLUDES1 meconium aspiration (P24.00, P24.01)
meconium staining (P96.83)

P03.89 Newborn affected by other specified complications of labor and delivery
AHA: Q4 2017
Newborn affected by abnormality of maternal soft tissues
Newborn affected by conditions classifiable to O60-O75 and by procedures used in labor and delivery not included in P02.- and P03.0-P03.6
Newborn affected by induction of labor

P03.9 Newborn affected by complication of labor and delivery, unspecified
AHA: Q4 2017

⁴ᵗʰ P04 Newborn affected by noxious substances transmitted via placenta or breast milk
INCLUDES nonteratogenic effects of substances transmitted via placenta
EXCLUDES2 congenital malformations (Q00-Q99)
encounter for observation of newborn for suspected diseases and conditions ruled out (Z05.-)
neonatal jaundice from excessive hemolysis due to drugs or toxins transmitted from mother (P58.4)
newborn in contact with and (suspected) exposures hazardous to health not transmitted via placenta or breast milk (Z77.-)

P04.0 Newborn affected by maternal anesthesia and analgesia in pregnancy, labor and delivery
AHA: Q4 2018, Q4 2017
Newborn affected by reactions and intoxications from maternal opiates and tranquilizers administered for procedures during pregnancy or labor and delivery
EXCLUDES2 newborn affected by other maternal medication (P04.1-)

⁵ᵗʰ P04.1 Newborn affected by other maternal medication
☞ Code first withdrawal symptoms from maternal use of drugs of addiction, if applicable (P96.1)
EXCLUDES1 dysmorphism due to warfarin (Q86.2)
fetal hydantoin syndrome (Q86.1)
EXCLUDES2 maternal anesthesia and analgesia in pregnancy, labor and delivery (P04.0)
maternal use of drugs of addiction (P04.4-)

P04.11 Newborn affected by maternal antineoplastic chemotherapy
AHA: Q4 2018

P04.12 Newborn affected by maternal cytotoxic drugs
AHA: Q4 2018

P04.13 Newborn affected by maternal use of anticonvulsants
AHA: Q4 2018

P04.14 Newborn affected by maternal use of opiates
AHA: Q4 2018

P04.15 Newborn affected by maternal use of antidepressants
AHA: Q4 2018

P04.16 Newborn affected by maternal use of amphetamines
AHA: Q4 2018

P04.17 Newborn affected by maternal use of sedative-hypnotics
AHA: Q4 2018

P04.1A Newborn affected by maternal use of anxiolytics
AHA: Q4 2018

P04.18 Newborn affected by other maternal medication
AHA: Q4 2018

P04.19 Newborn affected by maternal use of unspecified medication
AHA: Q4 2018

P04.2 Newborn affected by maternal use of tobacco
AHA: Q4 2017
Newborn affected by exposure in utero to tobacco smoke
EXCLUDES2 newborn exposure to environmental tobacco smoke (P96.81)

P04.3 Newborn affected by maternal use of alcohol
AHA: Q4 2017
EXCLUDES1 fetal alcohol syndrome (Q86.0)

⁵ᵗʰ P04.4 Newborn affected by maternal use of drugs of addiction
P04.40 Newborn affected by maternal use of unspecified drugs of addiction
AHA: Q4 2018

P04.41 Newborn affected by maternal use of cocaine
AHA: Q4 2017

P04.42 Newborn affected by maternal use of hallucinogens
AHA: Q4 2018
EXCLUDES2 newborn affected by other maternal medication (P04.1-)

P04.49 Newborn affected by maternal use of other drugs of addiction
AHA: Q4 2017
EXCLUDES2 newborn affected by maternal anesthesia and analgesia (P04.0)
withdrawal symptoms from maternal use of drugs of addiction (P96.1)

P04.5 Newborn affected by maternal use of nutritional chemical substances
AHA: Q4 2017

P04.6 Newborn affected by maternal exposure to environmental chemical substances
AHA: Q4 2017

⁵ᵗʰ P04.8 Newborn affected by other maternal noxious substances
P04.81 Newborn affected by maternal use of cannabis
AHA: Q4 2018

P04.89 Newborn affected by other maternal noxious substances
AHA: Q4 2018

P04.9 Newborn affected by maternal noxious substance, unspecified
AHA: Q4 2017

Disorders of newborn related to length of gestation and fetal growth (P05-P08)

⁴ᵗʰ P05 Disorders of newborn related to slow fetal growth and fetal malnutrition

⁵ᵗʰ P05.0 Newborn light for gestational age
Newborn light-for-dates
Weight below but length above 10th percentile for gestational age

P05.00 Newborn light for gestational age, unspecified weight

P05.01 Newborn light for gestational age, less than 500 grams

P05.02 Newborn light for gestational age, 500-749 grams

P05.03 Newborn light for gestational age, 750-999 grams

P05.04 Newborn light for gestational age, 1000-1249 grams

P05.05 Newborn light for gestational age, 1250-1499 grams

P05.06 Newborn light for gestational age, 1500-1749 grams

P05.07 Newborn light for gestational age, 1750-1999 grams

P05.08 Newborn light for gestational age, 2000-2499 grams

P05.09 Newborn light for gestational age, 2500 grams and over
AHA: Q4 2016
Newborn light for gestational age, other

⁵ᵗʰ P05.1 Newborn small for gestational age
Newborn small-and-light-for-dates
Newborn small-for-dates
Weight and length below 10th percentile for gestational age

P05.10 Newborn small for gestational age, unspecified weight

Unspecified Code   Other Specified Code   Manifestation Code   Ⓝ Newborn   Ⓟ Pediatric   Ⓜ Maternity   Ⓐ Adult   ♂ Male   ♀ Female
● New Code   ▲ Revised Code Title   ▶◀ Revised Text   **NOTES**   INCLUDES   EXCLUDES1 Not coded here   EXCLUDES2 Not included here
④ 4ᵗʰ character required   ⑤ 5ᵗʰ character required   ⑥ 6ᵗʰ character required   ⑦ 7ᵗʰ character required   ⑦ Extension 'X' Alert
HAC Hospital-acquired condition (HAC) alert   AHA AHA Coding Clinic©   ☞ Code first alert

P05.11 **Newborn small for gestational age,** less than 500 grams

P05.12 **Newborn small for gestational age,** 500-749 grams

P05.13 **Newborn small for gestational age,** 750-999 grams

P05.14 **Newborn small for gestational age,** 1000-1249 grams

P05.15 **Newborn small for gestational age,** 1250-1499 grams

P05.16 **Newborn small for gestational age,** 1500-1749 grams

P05.17 **Newborn small for gestational age,** 1750-1999 grams

P05.18 **Newborn small for gestational age,** 2000-2499 grams

P05.19 **Newborn small for gestational age, other**
AHA: Q4 2016
Newborn small for gestational age, 2500 grams and over

P05.2 **Newborn affected by** fetal (intrauterine) malnutrition **not light or small for gestational age**
Infant, not light or small for gestational age, showing signs of fetal malnutrition, such as dry, peeling skin and loss of subcutaneous tissue
EXCLUDES1 *newborn affected by fetal malnutrition with light for gestational age (P05.0-)*
newborn affected by fetal malnutrition with small for gestational age (P05.1-)

P05.9 **Newborn affected by slow intrauterine growth, unspecified**
Newborn affected by fetal growth retardation NOS

P07 **Disorders of newborn related to short gestation and low birth weight, not elsewhere classified**
👁 See Official Guidelines "Low birth weight and immaturity status" I.C.16.e
NOTES When both birth weight and gestational age of the newborn are available, both should be coded with birth weight sequenced before gestational age
INCLUDES *the listed conditions, without further specification, as the cause of morbidity or additional care, in newborn*

P07.0 Extremely low **birth weight newborn**
Newborn birth weight 999 g. or less
EXCLUDES1 *low birth weight due to slow fetal growth and fetal malnutrition (P05.-)*

P07.00 **Extremely low birth weight newborn, unspecified weight**

P07.01 **Extremely low birth weight newborn,** less than 500 grams

P07.02 **Extremely low birth weight newborn,** 500-749 grams

P07.03 **Extremely low birth weight newborn,** 750-999 grams

P07.1 Other low **birth weight newborn**
Newborn birth weight 1000-2499 g.
EXCLUDES1 *low birth weight due to slow fetal growth and fetal malnutrition (P05.-)*

P07.10 **Other low birth weight newborn, unspecified weight**

P07.14 **Other low birth weight newborn,** 1000-1249 grams

P07.15 **Other low birth weight newborn,** 1250-1499 grams

P07.16 **Other low birth weight newborn,** 1500-1749 grams

P07.17 **Other low birth weight newborn,** 1750-1999 grams

P07.18 **Other low birth weight newborn,** 2000-2499 grams

P07.2 Extreme immaturity **of newborn**
Less than 28 completed weeks (less than 196 completed days) of gestation.

P07.20 **Extreme immaturity of newborn, unspecified weeks of gestation**
Gestational age less than 28 completed weeks NOS

P07.21 **Extreme immaturity of newborn, gestational age** less than 23 completed weeks
Extreme immaturity of newborn, gestational age less than 23 weeks, 0 days

P07.22 **Extreme immaturity of newborn, gestational age** 23 completed weeks
Extreme immaturity of newborn, gestational age 23 weeks, 0 days through 23 weeks, 6 days

P07.23 **Extreme immaturity of newborn, gestational age** 24 completed weeks
Extreme immaturity of newborn, gestational age 24 weeks, 0 days through 24 weeks, 6 days

P07.24 **Extreme immaturity of newborn, gestational age** 25 completed weeks
Extreme immaturity of newborn, gestational age 25 weeks, 0 days through 25 weeks, 6 days

P07.25 **Extreme immaturity of newborn, gestational age** 26 completed weeks
Extreme immaturity of newborn, gestational age 26 weeks, 0 days through 26 weeks, 6 days

P07.26 **Extreme immaturity of newborn, gestational age** 27 completed weeks
Extreme immaturity of newborn, gestational age 27 weeks, 0 days through 27 weeks, 6 days

P07.3 Preterm [premature] newborn [other]
28 completed weeks or more but less than 37 completed weeks (196 completed days but less than 259 completed days) of gestation.
Prematurity NOS

P07.30 **Preterm newborn, unspecified weeks of gestation**

P07.31 **Preterm newborn, gestational age** 28 completed weeks
Preterm newborn, gestational age 28 weeks, 0 days through 28 weeks, 6 days

P07.32 **Preterm newborn, gestational age** 29 completed weeks
Preterm newborn, gestational age 29 weeks, 0 days through 29 weeks, 6 days

P07.33 **Preterm newborn, gestational age** 30 completed weeks
Preterm newborn, gestational age 30 weeks, 0 days through 30 weeks, 6 days

P07.34 **Preterm newborn, gestational age** 31 completed weeks
Preterm newborn, gestational age 31 weeks, 0 days through 31 weeks, 6 days

P07.35 **Preterm newborn, gestational age** 32 completed weeks
Preterm newborn, gestational age 32 weeks, 0 days through 32 weeks, 6 days

P07.36 **Preterm newborn, gestational age** 33 completed weeks
Preterm newborn, gestational age 33 weeks, 0 days through 33 weeks, 6 days

P07.37 **Preterm newborn, gestational age** 34 completed weeks
AHA: Q2 2017
Preterm newborn, gestational age 34 weeks, 0 days through 34 weeks, 6 days

P07.38 **Preterm newborn, gestational age** 35 completed weeks
Preterm newborn, gestational age 35 weeks, 0 days through 35 weeks, 6 days

P07.39 **Preterm newborn, gestational age** 36 completed weeks
AHA: Q3 2017
Preterm newborn, gestational age 36 weeks, 0 days through 36 weeks, 6 days

P08 **Disorders of newborn related to long gestation and high birth weight**
NOTES When both birth weight and gestational age of the newborn are available, priority of assignment should be given to birth weight
INCLUDES *the listed conditions, without further specification, as causes of morbidity or additional care, in newborn*

PDxⁿ Unacceptable principal diagnosis symbol per Medicare code edits   PDx Code exempt from diagnosis present on admission requirement
❓ Questionable admission   CC Complication or comorbidity   MCC Major complication or comorbidity   CC/MCC Excl CC/MCC exclusion
HCC HCC diagnosis code   RHCC RxHCC diagnosis code   MACRA code   **DEFINITION** Describes condition/terminology
TIP Coding guidance   👁 Official Guideline Reference   Z1 Z code as first-listed diagnosis

P08.0 Exceptionally large newborn baby
Usually implies a birth weight of 4500 g. or more
EXCLUDES1 syndrome of infant of diabetic mother (P70.1)
syndrome of infant of mother with gestational diabetes (P70.0)

P08.1 Other heavy for gestational age newborn
Other newborn heavy- or large-for-dates regardless of period of gestation
Usually implies a birth weight of 4000 g. to 4499 g.
EXCLUDES1 newborn with a birth weight of 4500 or more (P08.0)
syndrome of infant of diabetic mother (P70.1)
syndrome of infant of mother with gestational diabetes (P70.0).

🔵 **P08.2** Late newborn, not heavy for gestational age
P08.21 Post-term newborn
Newborn with gestation period over 40 completed weeks to 42 completed weeks
P08.22 Prolonged gestation of newborn
Newborn with gestation period over 42 completed weeks (294 days or more), not heavy- or large-for-dates.
Postmaturity NOS

Abnormal findings on neonatal screening (P09)

P09 Abnormal findings on neonatal screening
Use additional code to identify signs, symptoms and conditions associated with the screening
EXCLUDES2 nonspecific serologic evidence of human immunodeficiency virus [HIV] (R75)

Birth trauma (P10-P15)

🔵 **P10** Intracranial laceration and hemorrhage **due to birth injury**
EXCLUDES1 intracranial hemorrhage of newborn NOS (P52.9)
intracranial hemorrhage of newborn due to anoxia or hypoxia (P52.-)
nontraumatic intracranial hemorrhage of newborn (P52.-)

P10.0 Subdural hemorrhage **due to birth injury**   MCC CC/MCC Exc
Subdural hematoma (localized) due to birth injury
EXCLUDES1 subdural hemorrhage accompanying tentorial tear (P10.4)

P10.1 Cerebral hemorrhage **due to birth injury**   MCC CC/MCC Exc
P10.2 Intraventricular hemorrhage **due to birth injury**   CC CC/MCC Exc
P10.3 Subarachnoid hemorrhage **due to birth injury**   MCC CC/MCC Exc
P10.4 Tentorial tear **due to birth injury**   MCC CC/MCC Exc
P10.8 Other intracranial lacerations and hemorrhages due to birth injury   MCC CC/MCC Exc
P10.9 Unspecified intracranial laceration and hemorrhage due to birth injury   MCC CC/MCC Exc

🔵 **P11** Other birth injuries to central nervous system
P11.0 Cerebral edema **due to birth injury**   MCC CC/MCC Exc
P11.1 Other specified brain damage due to birth injury
P11.2 Unspecified brain damage due to birth injury   MCC CC/MCC Exc
P11.3 Birth injury to facial nerve
Facial palsy due to birth injury
P11.4 Birth injury to other cranial nerves
P11.5 Birth injury to spine and spinal cord
Fracture of spine due to birth injury
P11.9 Birth injury to central nervous system, unspecified   MCC CC/MCC Exc

🔵 **P12** Birth injury to scalp
P12.0 Cephalhematoma **due to birth injury**
P12.1 Chignon (from vacuum extraction) **due to birth injury**
P12.2 Epicranial subaponeurotic hemorrhage **due to birth injury**   CC CC/MCC Exc
Subgaleal hemorrhage
P12.3 Bruising of scalp **due to birth injury**
P12.4 Injury of scalp of newborn due to monitoring equipment
Sampling incision of scalp of newborn
Scalp clip (electrode) injury of newborn

🔵 **P12.8** Other **birth injuries to scalp**
P12.81 Caput succedaneum
P12.89 Other birth injuries to scalp
P12.9 Birth injury to scalp, unspecified

🔵 **P13** Birth injury to skeleton
EXCLUDES2 birth injury to spine (P11.5)
P13.0 Fracture of skull **due to birth injury**
P13.1 Other birth injuries to skull
EXCLUDES1 cephalhematoma (P12.0)
P13.2 Birth injury to femur
P13.3 Birth injury to other long bones
P13.4 Fracture of clavicle **due to birth injury**
P13.8 Birth injuries to other parts of skeleton
P13.9 Birth injury to skeleton, unspecified

🔵 **P14** Birth injury to peripheral nervous system
P14.0 Erb's paralysis **due to birth injury**
P14.1 Klumpke's paralysis **due to birth injury**
P14.2 Phrenic nerve paralysis **due to birth injury**
P14.3 Other brachial plexus **birth injuries**
P14.8 Birth injuries to other parts of peripheral nervous system
P14.9 Birth injury to peripheral nervous system, unspecified

🔵 **P15** Other birth injuries
P15.0 Birth injury to liver
Rupture of liver due to birth injury
P15.1 Birth injury to spleen
Rupture of spleen due to birth injury
P15.2 Sternomastoid **injury due to birth injury**
P15.3 Birth injury to eye
Subconjunctival hemorrhage due to birth injury
Traumatic glaucoma due to birth injury
P15.4 Birth injury to face
Facial congestion due to birth injury
P15.5 Birth injury to external genitalia
P15.6 Subcutaneous fat necrosis **due to birth injury**
P15.8 Other specified birth injuries
P15.9 Birth injury, unspecified

Respiratory and cardiovascular disorders specific to the perinatal period (P19-P29)

🔵 **P19** Metabolic acidemia in newborn
INCLUDES metabolic acidemia in newborn
P19.0 Metabolic acidemia in newborn first noted before onset of labor
P19.1 Metabolic acidemia in newborn first noted during labor
P19.2 Metabolic acidemia noted at birth
P19.9 Metabolic acidemia, unspecified

🔵 **P22** Respiratory distress of newborn
P22.0 Respiratory distress syndrome of newborn   MCC CC/MCC Exc
AHA: Q2 2019
Cardiorespiratory distress syndrome of newborn
Hyaline membrane disease
Idiopathic respiratory distress syndrome [IRDS or RDS] of newborn
Pulmonary hypoperfusion syndrome
Respiratory distress syndrome, type I
EXCLUDES2 respiratory arrest of newborn (P28.81)
respiratory failure of newborn NOS (P28.5)

P22.1 Transient tachypnea of newborn
Idiopathic tachypnea of newborn
Respiratory distress syndrome, type II
Wet lung syndrome
P22.8 Other respiratory distress of newborn
EXCLUDES1 respiratory arrest of newborn (P28.81)
respiratory failure of newborn NOS (P28.5)
P22.9 Respiratory distress of newborn, unspecified
EXCLUDES1 respiratory arrest of newborn (P28.81)
respiratory failure of newborn NOS (P28.5)

Unspecified Code   Other Specified Code   Manifestation Code   N Newborn   P Pediatric   M Maternity   A Adult   ♂ Male   ♀ Female
● New Code   ▲ Revised Code Title   ►◄ Revised Text   **NOTES**   *INCLUDES*   *EXCLUDES1* Not coded here   *EXCLUDES2* Not included here
🔵 4th character required   🔵 5th character required   🔵 6th character required   🔵 7th character required   🔵 Extension 'X' Alert
HAC Hospital-acquired condition (HAC) alert   **AHA** AHA Coding Clinic©   📣 Code first alert

P23 Congenital pneumonia

INCLUDES infective pneumonia acquired in utero or during birth
EXCLUDES1 neonatal pneumonia resulting from aspiration (P24.-)

P23.0 Congenital pneumonia due to viral agent MCC CC/MCC Exc
Use additional code (B97) to identify organism
EXCLUDES1 congenital rubella pneumonitis (P35.0)

P23.1 Congenital pneumonia due to Chlamydia MCC CC/MCC Exc

P23.2 Congenital pneumonia due to staphylococcus MCC CC/MCC Exc

P23.3 Congenital pneumonia due to streptococcus, group B MCC CC/MCC Exc

P23.4 Congenital pneumonia due to Escherichia coli MCC CC/MCC Exc

P23.5 Congenital pneumonia due to Pseudomonas MCC CC/MCC Exc

P23.6 Congenital pneumonia due to other bacterial agents MCC CC/MCC Exc
Congenital pneumonia due to Hemophilus influenzae
Congenital pneumonia due to Klebsiella pneumoniae
Congenital pneumonia due to Mycoplasma
Congenital pneumonia due to Streptococcus, except group B
Use additional code (B95-B96) to identify organism

P23.8 Congenital pneumonia due to other organisms MCC CC/MCC Exc

P23.9 Congenital pneumonia, unspecified MCC CC/MCC Exc

P24 Neonatal aspiration

INCLUDES aspiration in utero and during delivery

P24.0 Meconium aspiration
EXCLUDES1 meconium passage (without aspiration) during delivery (P03.82)
meconium staining (P96.83)

P24.00 Meconium aspiration without respiratory symptoms
Meconium aspiration NOS

P24.01 Meconium aspiration with respiratory symptoms MCC CC/MCC Exc
Meconium aspiration pneumonia
Meconium aspiration pneumonitis
Meconium aspiration syndrome NOS
Use additional code to identify any secondary pulmonary hypertension, if applicable (I27.2-)

P24.1 Neonatal aspiration of (clear) amniotic fluid and mucus
Neonatal aspiration of liquor (amnii)

P24.10 Neonatal aspiration of (clear) amniotic fluid and mucus without respiratory symptoms
Neonatal aspiration of amniotic fluid and mucus NOS

P24.11 Neonatal aspiration of (clear) amniotic fluid and mucus with respiratory symptoms MCC CC/MCC Exc
Neonatal aspiration of amniotic fluid and mucus with pneumonia
Neonatal aspiration of amniotic fluid and mucus with pneumonitis
Use additional code to identify any secondary pulmonary hypertension, if applicable (I27.2-)

P24.2 Neonatal aspiration of blood

P24.20 Neonatal aspiration of blood without respiratory symptoms
Neonatal aspiration of blood NOS

P24.21 Neonatal aspiration of blood with respiratory symptoms MCC CC/MCC Exc
Neonatal aspiration of blood with pneumonia
Neonatal aspiration of blood with pneumonitis
Use additional code to identify any secondary pulmonary hypertension, if applicable (I27.2-)

P24.3 Neonatal aspiration of milk and regurgitated food
Neonatal aspiration of stomach contents

P24.30 Neonatal aspiration of milk and regurgitated food without respiratory symptoms
Neonatal aspiration of milk and regurgitated food NOS

P24.31 Neonatal aspiration of milk and regurgitated food with respiratory symptoms MCC CC/MCC Exc
Neonatal aspiration of milk and regurgitated food with pneumonia
Neonatal aspiration of milk and regurgitated food with pneumonitis
Use additional code to identify any secondary pulmonary hypertension, if applicable (I27.2-)

P24.8 Other neonatal aspiration

P24.80 Other neonatal aspiration without respiratory symptoms
Neonatal aspiration NEC

P24.81 Other neonatal aspiration with respiratory symptoms MCC CC/MCC Exc
Neonatal aspiration pneumonia NEC
Neonatal aspiration with pneumonitis NEC
Neonatal aspiration with pneumonia NOS
Neonatal aspiration with pneumonitis NOS
Use additional code to identify any secondary pulmonary hypertension, if applicable (I27.2-)

P24.9 Neonatal aspiration, unspecified

P25 Interstitial emphysema and related conditions originating in the perinatal period

P25.0 Interstitial emphysema originating in the perinatal period MCC CC/MCC Exc

P25.1 Pneumothorax originating in the perinatal period MCC CC/MCC Exc

P25.2 Pneumomediastinum originating in the perinatal period MCC CC/MCC Exc

P25.3 Pneumopericardium originating in the perinatal period MCC CC/MCC Exc

P25.8 Other conditions related to interstitial emphysema originating in the perinatal period MCC CC/MCC Exc

P26 Pulmonary hemorrhage originating in the perinatal period

EXCLUDES1 acute idiopathic hemorrhage in infants over 28 days old (R04.81)

P26.0 Tracheobronchial hemorrhage originating in the perinatal period MCC CC/MCC Exc

P26.1 Massive pulmonary hemorrhage originating in the perinatal period MCC CC/MCC Exc

P26.8 Other pulmonary hemorrhages originating in the perinatal period MCC CC/MCC Exc

P26.9 Unspecified pulmonary hemorrhage originating in the perinatal period MCC CC/MCC Exc

P27 Chronic respiratory disease originating in the perinatal period

EXCLUDES2 respiratory distress of newborn (P22.0-P22.9)

P27.0 Wilson-Mikity syndrome MCC CC/MCC Exc
Pulmonary dysmaturity

P27.1 Bronchopulmonary dysplasia originating in the perinatal period MCC CC/MCC Exc

P27.8 Other chronic respiratory diseases originating in the perinatal period MCC CC/MCC Exc
Congenital pulmonary fibrosis
Ventilator lung in newborn

P27.9 Unspecified chronic respiratory disease originating in the perinatal period MCC CC/MCC Exc

P28 Other respiratory conditions originating in the perinatal period

EXCLUDES1 congenital malformations of the respiratory system (Q30-Q34)

P28.0 Primary atelectasis of newborn CC CC/MCC Exc
Primary failure to expand terminal respiratory units
Pulmonary hypoplasia associated with short gestation
Pulmonary immaturity NOS

P28.1 Other and unspecified atelectasis of newborn

P28.10 Unspecified atelectasis of newborn CC CC/MCC Exc
Atelectasis of newborn NOS

P28.11 Resorption atelectasis without respiratory distress syndrome CC CC/MCC Exc
EXCLUDES1 resorption atelectasis with respiratory distress syndrome (P22.0)

P28.19 Other atelectasis of newborn CC CC/MCC Exc
Partial atelectasis of newborn
Secondary atelectasis of newborn

P28.2 Cyanotic attacks of newborn CC CC/MCC Exc
EXCLUDES1 apnea of newborn (P28.3-P28.4)

P28.3 Primary sleep apnea of newborn CC CC/MCC Exc
Central sleep apnea of newborn
Obstructive sleep apnea of newborn
Sleep apnea of newborn NOS

---

924   When symbols appear on a code that requires a 7th character extension, refer to Appendix B to identify applicable 7th character codes.   **2020 ICD-10-CM**

CHAPTER 16: CERTAIN CONDITIONS ORIGINATING IN THE PERINATAL PERIOD (P00-P96)

P23 - P28.3

P28.4 Other apnea of newborn ⓒⓒ CC/MCC Exc
Apnea of prematurity
Obstructive apnea of newborn
EXCLUDES1 obstructive sleep apnea of newborn (P28.3)

P28.5 Respiratory failure of newborn MCC CC/MCC Exc
AHA: Q2 2019
EXCLUDES1 respiratory arrest of newborn (P28.81)
respiratory distress of newborn (P22.0-)

5ᵗʰ **P28.8 Other specified respiratory conditions of newborn**
P28.81 Respiratory arrest of newborn MCC CC/MCC Exc
AHA: Q2 2017
P28.89 Other specified respiratory conditions of newborn
Congenital laryngeal stridor
Sniffles in newborn
Snuffles in newborn
EXCLUDES1 early congenital syphilitic rhinitis (A50.05)

P28.9 Respiratory condition of newborn, unspecified
Respiratory depression in newborn

4ᵗʰ **P29 Cardiovascular disorders originating in the perinatal period**
EXCLUDES1 congenital malformations of the circulatory system (Q20-Q28)
P29.0 Neonatal cardiac failure
5ᵗʰ **P29.1 Neonatal cardiac dysrhythmia**
P29.11 Neonatal tachycardia
P29.12 Neonatal bradycardia
P29.2 Neonatal hypertension
5ᵗʰ **P29.3 Persistent fetal circulation**
P29.30 Pulmonary hypertension of newborn POA MCC CC/MCC Exc
Persistent pulmonary hypertension of newborn
P29.38 Other persistent fetal circulation POA MCC CC/MCC Exc
Delayed closure of ductus arteriosus
P29.4 Transient myocardial ischemia in newborn
5ᵗʰ **P29.8 Other cardiovascular disorders originating in the perinatal period**
P29.81 Cardiac arrest of newborn MCC CC/MCC Exc
P29.89 Other cardiovascular disorders originating in the perinatal period
P29.9 Cardiovascular disorder originating in the perinatal period, unspecified

Infections specific to the perinatal period (P35-P39)

Infections acquired in utero, during birth via the umbilicus, or during the first 28 days after birth
EXCLUDES2 asymptomatic human immunodeficiency virus [HIV] infection status (Z21)
congenital gonococcal infection (A54.-)
congenital pneumonia (P23.-)
congenital syphilis (A50.-)
human immunodeficiency virus [HIV] disease (B20)
infant botulism (A48.51)
infectious diseases not specific to the perinatal period (A00-B99, J09, J10.-)
intestinal infectious disease (A00-A09)
laboratory evidence of human immunodeficiency virus [HIV] (R75)
tetanus neonatorum (A33)

4ᵗʰ **P35 Congenital viral diseases**
INCLUDES infections acquired in utero or during birth
P35.0 Congenital rubella syndrome ⓒⓒ CC/MCC Exc
Congenital rubella pneumonitis
P35.1 Congenital cytomegalovirus **infection** MCC CC/MCC Exc
P35.2 Congenital herpesviral [herpes simplex] **infection** MCC CC/MCC Exc
P35.3 Congenital viral hepatitis MCC CC/MCC Exc
P35.4 Congenital Zika virus **disease** MCC CC/MCC Exc
AHA: Q4 2018
Use additional code to identify manifestations of congenital Zika virus disease
P35.8 Other congenital viral diseases MCC CC/MCC Exc
AHA: Q4 2016
Congenital varicella [chickenpox]
P35.9 Congenital viral disease, unspecified MCC CC/MCC Exc

4ᵗʰ **P36 Bacterial sepsis of newborn**
👁 See Official Guidelines "Bacterial Sepsis of Newborn" I.C.16.f
INCLUDES congenital sepsis
Use additional code(s), if applicable, to identify severe sepsis (R65.2-) and associated acute organ dysfunction(s)
P36.0 Sepsis of newborn due to streptococcus, group B HCC MCC CC/MCC Exc
5ᵗʰ **P36.1 Sepsis of newborn due to other and unspecified** streptococci
P36.10 Sepsis of newborn due to unspecified streptococci HCC MCC CC/MCC Exc
P36.19 Sepsis of newborn due to other streptococci HCC MCC CC/MCC Exc
P36.2 Sepsis of newborn due to Staphylococcus aureus HCC MCC CC/MCC Exc
5ᵗʰ **P36.3 Sepsis of newborn due to other and unspecified** staphylococci
P36.30 Sepsis of newborn due to unspecified staphylococci HCC MCC CC/MCC Exc
P36.39 Sepsis of newborn due to other staphylococci HCC MCC CC/MCC Exc
P36.4 Sepsis of newborn due to Escherichia coli HCC MCC CC/MCC Exc
P36.5 Sepsis of newborn due to anaerobes HCC MCC CC/MCC Exc
P36.8 Other bacterial sepsis of newborn HCC MCC CC/MCC Exc
Use additional code from category B96 to identify organism
P36.9 Bacterial sepsis of newborn, unspecified HCC MCC CC/MCC Exc

4ᵗʰ **P37 Other congenital infectious and parasitic diseases**
EXCLUDES2 congenital syphilis (A50.-)
infectious neonatal diarrhea (A00-A09)
necrotizing enterocolitis in newborn (P77.-)
noninfectious neonatal diarrhea (P78.3)
ophthalmia neonatorum due to gonococcus (A54.31)
tetanus neonatorum (A33)
P37.0 Congenital tuberculosis MCC CC/MCC Exc
P37.1 Congenital toxoplasmosis MCC CC/MCC Exc
Hydrocephalus due to congenital toxoplasmosis
P37.2 Neonatal (disseminated) listeriosis MCC CC/MCC Exc
P37.3 Congenital falciparum malaria MCC CC/MCC Exc
P37.4 Other congenital malaria MCC CC/MCC Exc
P37.5 Neonatal candidiasis
P37.8 Other specified congenital infectious and parasitic diseases MCC CC/MCC Exc
P37.9 Congenital infectious or parasitic disease, unspecified MCC CC/MCC Exc

4ᵗʰ **P38 Omphalitis of newborn**
DEFINITION: Omphalitis is inflammation of the umbilical cord stump in the neonatal newborn period, most commonly caused by bacterial infection.
EXCLUDES1 omphalitis not of newborn (L08.82)
tetanus omphalitis (A33)
umbilical hemorrhage of newborn (P51.-)
P38.1 Omphalitis with mild hemorrhage ⓒⓒ CC/MCC Exc
P38.9 Omphalitis without hemorrhage ⓒⓒ CC/MCC Exc
Omphalitis of newborn NOS

4ᵗʰ **P39 Other infections specific to the perinatal period**
Use additional code to identify organism or specific infection
P39.0 Neonatal infective mastitis ⓒⓒ CC/MCC Exc
EXCLUDES1 breast engorgement of newborn (P83.4)
noninfective mastitis of newborn (P83.4)
P39.1 Neonatal conjunctivitis and dacryocystitis
Neonatal chlamydial conjunctivitis
Ophthalmia neonatorum NOS
EXCLUDES1 gonococcal conjunctivitis (A54.31)
P39.2 Intra-amniotic infection affecting newborn, not elsewhere classified ⓒⓒ CC/MCC Exc
P39.3 Neonatal urinary tract infection ⓒⓒ CC/MCC Exc
P39.4 Neonatal skin infection ⓒⓒ CC/MCC Exc
Neonatal pyoderma
EXCLUDES1 pemphigus neonatorum (L00)
staphylococcal scalded skin syndrome (L00)

Unspecified Code Other Specified Code Manifestation Code Ⓝ Newborn Ⓟ Pediatric Ⓜ Maternity Ⓐ Adult ♂ Male ♀ Female
● New Code ▲ Revised Code Title ▶◀ Revised Text **NOTES** *INCLUDES* *EXCLUDES1* Not coded here *EXCLUDES2* Not included here
4ᵗʰ 4ᵗʰ character required 5ᵗʰ 5ᵗʰ character required 6ᵗʰ 6ᵗʰ character required 7ᵗʰ 7ᵗʰ character required 7ˣ Extension 'X' Alert
HAC Hospital-acquired condition (HAC) alert **AHA** AHA Coding Clinic© 📕 Code first alert

P39.8 **Other specified infections specific to the perinatal period** CC CC/MCC Exc

P39.9 **Infection specific to the perinatal period, unspecified** CC CC/MCC Exc

Hemorrhagic and hematological disorders of newborn (P50-P61)

EXCLUDES1 *congenital stenosis and stricture of bile ducts (Q44.3)*
Crigler-Najjar syndrome (E80.5)
Dubin-Johnson syndrome (E80.6)
Gilbert syndrome (E80.4)
hereditary hemolytic anemias (D55-D58)

P50 **Newborn affected by intrauterine (fetal)** blood loss
EXCLUDES1 *congenital anemia from intrauterine (fetal) blood loss (P61.3)*

P50.0 **Newborn affected by intrauterine (fetal) blood loss from** vasa previa

P50.1 **Newborn affected by intrauterine (fetal) blood loss from** ruptured cord

P50.2 **Newborn affected by intrauterine (fetal) blood loss from** placenta

P50.3 **Newborn affected by hemorrhage into** co-twin

P50.4 **Newborn affected by hemorrhage into** maternal circulation

P50.5 **Newborn affected by intrauterine (fetal) blood loss from** cut end of co-twin's cord

P50.8 **Newborn affected by other intrauterine (fetal) blood loss**

P50.9 **Newborn affected by intrauterine (fetal) blood loss, unspecified**
Newborn affected by fetal hemorrhage NOS

P51 **Umbilical hemorrhage of newborn**
EXCLUDES1 *omphalitis with mild hemorrhage (P38.1)*
umbilical hemorrhage from cut end of co-twins cord (P50.5)

P51.0 **Massive umbilical hemorrhage of newborn**

P51.8 **Other umbilical hemorrhages of newborn**
Slipped umbilical ligature NOS

P51.9 **Umbilical hemorrhage of newborn, unspecified**

P52 **Intracranial nontraumatic hemorrhage of newborn**
INCLUDES *intracranial hemorrhage due to anoxia or hypoxia*
EXCLUDES1 *intracranial hemorrhage due to birth injury (P10.-)*
intracranial hemorrhage due to other injury (S06.-)

P52.0 **Intraventricular (nontraumatic) hemorrhage, grade 1, of newborn** CC CC/MCC Exc
Subependymal hemorrhage (without intraventricular extension)
Bleeding into germinal matrix

P52.1 **Intraventricular (nontraumatic) hemorrhage, grade 2, of newborn** CC CC/MCC Exc
Subependymal hemorrhage with intraventricular extension
Bleeding into ventricle

P52.2 **Intraventricular (nontraumatic) hemorrhage, grade 3 and grade 4, of newborn**

P52.21 **Intraventricular (nontraumatic) hemorrhage, grade 3, of newborn** MCC CC/MCC Exc
Subependymal hemorrhage with intraventricular extension with enlargement of ventricle

P52.22 **Intraventricular (nontraumatic) hemorrhage, grade 4, of newborn** MCC CC/MCC Exc
Bleeding into cerebral cortex
Subependymal hemorrhage with intracerebral extension

P52.3 **Unspecified intraventricular (nontraumatic) hemorrhage of newborn** CC CC/MCC Exc

P52.4 **Intracerebral (nontraumatic) hemorrhage of newborn** MCC CC/MCC Exc

P52.5 **Subarachnoid (nontraumatic) hemorrhage of newborn** MCC CC/MCC Exc

P52.6 **Cerebellar (nontraumatic) and posterior fossa hemorrhage of newborn** MCC CC/MCC Exc

P52.8 **Other intracranial (nontraumatic) hemorrhages of newborn** MCC CC/MCC Exc

P52.9 **Intracranial (nontraumatic) hemorrhage of newborn, unspecified** CC CC/MCC Exc

P53 **Hemorrhagic disease of newborn**
AHA: Q4 2004
Vitamin K deficiency of newborn

P54 **Other neonatal hemorrhages**
EXCLUDES1 *newborn affected by (intrauterine) blood loss (P50.-)*
pulmonary hemorrhage originating in the perinatal period (P26.-)

P54.0 **Neonatal hematemesis**
EXCLUDES1 *neonatal hematemesis due to swallowed maternal blood (P78.2)*

P54.1 **Neonatal melena** MCC CC/MCC Exc
EXCLUDES1 *neonatal melena due to swallowed maternal blood (P78.2)*

P54.2 **Neonatal rectal hemorrhage** MCC CC/MCC Exc

P54.3 **Other neonatal gastrointestinal hemorrhage** MCC CC/MCC Exc

P54.4 **Neonatal adrenal hemorrhage** CC CC/MCC Exc

P54.5 **Neonatal cutaneous hemorrhage**
Neonatal bruising
Neonatal ecchymoses
Neonatal petechiae
Neonatal superficial hematomata
EXCLUDES2 *bruising of scalp due to birth injury (P12.3)*
cephalhematoma due to birth injury (P12.0)

P54.6 **Neonatal vaginal hemorrhage** ♀
Neonatal pseudomenses

P54.8 **Other specified neonatal hemorrhages**

P54.9 **Neonatal hemorrhage, unspecified**

P55 **Hemolytic disease of newborn**

P55.0 **Rh isoimmunization of newborn**

P55.1 **ABO isoimmunization of newborn**
AHA: Q3 2015

P55.8 **Other hemolytic diseases of newborn**
AHA: Q3 2018

P55.9 **Hemolytic disease of newborn, unspecified**

P56 **Hydrops fetalis due to hemolytic disease**
EXCLUDES1 *hydrops fetalis NOS (P83.2)*

P56.0 **Hydrops fetalis due to isoimmunization** MCC CC/MCC Exc

P56.9 **Hydrops fetalis due to other and unspecified hemolytic disease**

P56.90 **Hydrops fetalis due to unspecified hemolytic disease** MCC CC/MCC Exc

P56.99 **Hydrops fetalis due to other hemolytic disease** MCC CC/MCC Exc

P57 **Kernicterus**
DEFINITION: Kernicterus is a rare, preventable brain damage in newborns with jaundice (excessive bilirubin in the blood).

P57.0 **Kernicterus due to isoimmunization** MCC CC/MCC Exc

P57.8 **Other specified kernicterus** MCC CC/MCC Exc
EXCLUDES1 *Crigler-Najjar syndrome (E80.5)*

P57.9 **Kernicterus, unspecified** MCC CC/MCC Exc

P58 **Neonatal jaundice due to other excessive hemolysis**
EXCLUDES1 *jaundice due to isoimmunization (P55-P57)*

P58.0 **Neonatal jaundice due to bruising**

P58.1 **Neonatal jaundice due to bleeding**

P58.2 **Neonatal jaundice due to infection**

P58.3 **Neonatal jaundice due to polycythemia**

P58.4 **Neonatal jaundice due to drugs or toxins transmitted from mother or given to newborn**
☛ Code first poisoning due to drug or toxin, if applicable (T36-T65 with fifth or sixth character 1-4 or 6)
Use additional code for adverse effect, if applicable, to identify drug (T36-T50 with fifth or sixth character 5)

P58.41 **Neonatal jaundice due to drugs or toxins transmitted from mother**

P58.42 **Neonatal jaundice due to drugs or toxins given to newborn**

PDx Unacceptable principal diagnosis symbol per Medicare code edits   POA Code exempt from diagnosis present on admission requirement
? Questionable admission   CC Complication or comorbidity   MCC Major complication or comorbidity   CC/MCC Exc CC/MCC exclusion
HCC HCC diagnosis code   RxHCC RxHCC diagnosis code   MACRA MACRA code   DEFINITION Describes condition/terminology
TIP Coding guidance   👁 Official Guideline Reference   Z1 Z code as first-listed diagnosis

926   When symbols appear on a code that requires a 7th character extension, refer to Appendix B to identify applicable 7th character codes.   **2020 ICD-10-CM**

P58.5 Neonatal jaundice due to swallowed maternal blood

P58.8 Neonatal jaundice due to other specified excessive hemolysis

P58.9 Neonatal jaundice due to excessive hemolysis, unspecified

P59 Neonatal jaundice from other and unspecified causes
EXCLUDES1 jaundice due to inborn errors of metabolism (E70-E88)
kernicterus (P57.-)

P59.0 Neonatal jaundice associated with preterm delivery
Hyperbilirubinemia of prematurity
Jaundice due to delayed conjugation associated with preterm delivery

P59.1 Inspissated bile syndrome   MCC CC/MCC Exc

P59.2 Neonatal jaundice from other and unspecified hepatocellular damage
EXCLUDES1 congenital viral hepatitis (P35.3)

P59.20 Neonatal jaundice from unspecified hepatocellular damage   MCC CC/MCC Exc

P59.29 Neonatal jaundice from other hepatocellular damage
Neonatal giant cell hepatitis
Neonatal (idiopathic) hepatitis

P59.3 Neonatal jaundice from breast milk inhibitor

P59.8 Neonatal jaundice from other specified causes

P59.9 Neonatal jaundice, unspecified
AHA: Q3 2015
Neonatal physiological jaundice (intense)(prolonged) NOS

P60 Disseminated intravascular coagulation of newborn   MCC CC/MCC Exc
Defibrination syndrome of newborn

P61 Other perinatal hematological disorders
EXCLUDES1 transient hypogammaglobulinemia of infancy (D80.7)

P61.0 Transient neonatal thrombocytopenia   MCC CC/MCC Exc
Neonatal thrombocytopenia due to exchange transfusion
Neonatal thrombocytopenia due to idiopathic maternal thrombocytopenia
Neonatal thrombocytopenia due to isoimmunization

P61.1 Polycythemia neonatorum

P61.2 Anemia of prematurity   CC CC/MCC Exc

P61.3 Congenital anemia from fetal blood loss   CC CC/MCC Exc

P61.4 Other congenital anemias, not elsewhere classified   CC CC/MCC Exc
Congenital anemia NOS

P61.5 Transient neonatal neutropenia   MCC CC/MCC Exc
EXCLUDES1 congenital neutropenia (nontransient) (D70.0)

P61.6 Other transient neonatal disorders of coagulation

P61.8 Other specified perinatal hematological disorders

P61.9 Perinatal hematological disorder, unspecified

Transitory endocrine and metabolic disorders specific to newborn (P70-P74)

INCLUDES transitory endocrine and metabolic disturbances caused by the infant's response to maternal endocrine and metabolic factors, or its adjustment to extrauterine environment

P70 Transitory disorders of carbohydrate metabolism specific to newborn

P70.0 Syndrome of infant of mother with gestational diabetes
Newborn (with hypoglycemia) affected by maternal gestational diabetes
EXCLUDES1 newborn (with hypoglycemia) affected by maternal (pre-existing) diabetes mellitus (P70.1)
syndrome of infant of a diabetic mother (P70.1)

P70.1 Syndrome of infant of a diabetic mother
Newborn (with hypoglycemia) affected by maternal (pre-existing) diabetes mellitus
EXCLUDES1 newborn (with hypoglycemia) affected by maternal gestational diabetes (P70.0)
syndrome of infant of mother with gestational diabetes (P70.0)

P70.2 Neonatal diabetes mellitus   CC CC/MCC Exc

P70.3 Iatrogenic neonatal hypoglycemia

P70.4 Other neonatal hypoglycemia
Transitory neonatal hypoglycemia

P70.8 Other transitory disorders of carbohydrate metabolism of newborn   CC CC/MCC Exc

P70.9 Transitory disorder of carbohydrate metabolism of newborn, unspecified

P71 Transitory neonatal disorders of calcium and magnesium metabolism

P71.0 Cow's milk hypocalcemia in newborn   CC CC/MCC Exc

P71.1 Other neonatal hypocalcemia   CC CC/MCC Exc
EXCLUDES1 neonatal hypoparathyroidism (P71.4)

P71.2 Neonatal hypomagnesemia   CC CC/MCC Exc

P71.3 Neonatal tetany without calcium or magnesium deficiency   CC CC/MCC Exc
Neonatal tetany NOS

P71.4 Transitory neonatal hypoparathyroidism   CC CC/MCC Exc

P71.8 Other transitory neonatal disorders of calcium and magnesium metabolism   CC CC/MCC Exc
AHA: Q4 2016

P71.9 Transitory neonatal disorder of calcium and magnesium metabolism, unspecified   CC CC/MCC Exc

P72 Other transitory neonatal endocrine disorders
EXCLUDES1 congenital hypothyroidism with or without goiter (E03.0-E03.1)
dyshormonogenetic goiter (E07.1)
Pendred's syndrome (E07.1)

P72.0 Neonatal goiter, not elsewhere classified   CC CC/MCC Exc
Transitory congenital goiter with normal functioning

P72.1 Transitory neonatal hyperthyroidism   CC CC/MCC Exc
Neonatal thyrotoxicosis

P72.2 Other transitory neonatal disorders of thyroid function, not elsewhere classified   CC CC/MCC Exc
Transitory neonatal hypothyroidism

P72.8 Other specified transitory neonatal endocrine disorders   CC CC/MCC Exc

P72.9 Transitory neonatal endocrine disorder, unspecified

P74 Other transitory neonatal electrolyte and metabolic disturbances

P74.0 Late metabolic acidosis of newborn   MCC CC/MCC Exc
EXCLUDES1 (fetal) metabolic acidosis of newborn (P19)

P74.1 Dehydration of newborn

P74.2 Disturbances of sodium balance of newborn
P74.21 Hypernatremia of newborn
AHA: Q4 2018
P74.22 Hyponatremia of newborn
AHA: Q4 2018

P74.3 Disturbances of potassium balance of newborn
P74.31 Hyperkalemia of newborn
AHA: Q4 2018
P74.32 Hypokalemia of newborn
AHA: Q4 2018

P74.4 Other transitory electrolyte disturbances of newborn
P74.41 Alkalosis of newborn   CC CC/MCC Exc
AHA: Q4 2018
Hyperbicarbonatemia

P74.42 Disturbances of chlorine balance of newborn
P74.421 Hyperchloremia of newborn
AHA: Q4 2018
Hyperchloremic metabolic acidosis
EXCLUDES2 late metabolic acidosis of the newborn ▶(P74.0)◀
P74.422 Hypochloremia of newborn
AHA: Q4 2018

P74.49 Other transitory electrolyte disturbance of newborn
AHA: Q4 2018

P74.5 Transitory tyrosinemia of newborn   CC CC/MCC Exc

P74.6 Transitory hyperammonemia of newborn   CC CC/MCC Exc

P74.8 Other transitory metabolic disturbances of newborn   CC CC/MCC Exc
Amino-acid metabolic disorders described as transitory

P74.9 Transitory metabolic disturbance of newborn, unspecified

Digestive system disorders of newborn (P76-P78)

P76 Other intestinal obstruction of newborn

P76.0 Meconium plug syndrome
Meconium ileus NOS
EXCLUDES1 meconium ileus in cystic fibrosis (E84.11)

P76.1 Transitory ileus of newborn CC CC/MCC Exc
EXCLUDES1 Hirschsprung's disease (Q43.1)

P76.2 Intestinal obstruction due to inspissated milk

P76.8 Other specified intestinal obstruction of newborn
EXCLUDES1 intestinal obstruction classifiable to K56.-

P76.9 Intestinal obstruction of newborn, unspecified

P77 Necrotizing enterocolitis of newborn

P77.1 Stage 1 necrotizing enterocolitis in newborn MCC CC/MCC Exc
Necrotizing enterocolitis without pneumatosis, without perforation

P77.2 Stage 2 necrotizing enterocolitis in newborn MCC CC/MCC Exc
Necrotizing enterocolitis with pneumatosis, without perforation

P77.3 Stage 3 necrotizing enterocolitis in newborn MCC CC/MCC Exc
Necrotizing enterocolitis with perforation
Necrotizing enterocolitis with pneumatosis and perforation

P77.9 Necrotizing enterocolitis in newborn, unspecified MCC CC/MCC Exc
Necrotizing enterocolitis in newborn, NOS

P78 Other perinatal digestive system disorders
EXCLUDES1 cystic fibrosis (E84.0-E84.9)
neonatal gastrointestinal hemorrhages (P54.0-P54.3)

P78.0 Perinatal intestinal perforation MCC CC/MCC Exc
Meconium peritonitis

P78.1 Other neonatal peritonitis
Neonatal peritonitis NOS

P78.2 Neonatal hematemesis and melena due to swallowed maternal blood

P78.3 Noninfective neonatal diarrhea
Neonatal diarrhea NOS

P78.8 Other specified perinatal digestive system disorders

P78.81 Congenital cirrhosis (of liver)

P78.82 Peptic ulcer of newborn

P78.83 Newborn esophageal reflux
Neonatal esophageal reflux

P78.84 Gestational alloimmune liver disease POA
GALD
Neonatal hemochromatosis
EXCLUDES1 hemochromatosis (E83.11-)

P78.89 Other specified perinatal digestive system disorders

P78.9 Perinatal digestive system disorder, unspecified

Conditions involving the integument and temperature regulation of newborn (P80-P83)

P80 Hypothermia of newborn

P80.0 Cold injury syndrome
Severe and usually chronic hypothermia associated with a pink flushed appearance, edema and neurological and biochemical abnormalities.
EXCLUDES1 mild hypothermia of newborn (P80.8)

P80.8 Other hypothermia of newborn
Mild hypothermia of newborn

P80.9 Hypothermia of newborn, unspecified

P81 Other disturbances of temperature regulation of newborn

P81.0 Environmental hyperthermia of newborn

P81.8 Other specified disturbances of temperature regulation of newborn

P81.9 Disturbance of temperature regulation of newborn, unspecified
Fever of newborn NOS

P83 Other conditions of integument specific to newborn
EXCLUDES1 congenital malformations of skin and integument (Q80-Q84)
hydrops fetalis due to hemolytic disease (P56.-)
neonatal skin infection (P39.4)
staphylococcal scalded skin syndrome (L00)
EXCLUDES2 cradle cap (L21.0)
diaper [napkin] dermatitis (L22)

P83.0 Sclerema neonatorum CC CC/MCC Exc

P83.1 Neonatal erythema toxicum

P83.2 Hydrops fetalis not due to hemolytic disease MCC CC/MCC Exc
Hydrops fetalis NOS

P83.3 Other and unspecified edema specific to newborn

P83.30 Unspecified edema specific to newborn CC CC/MCC Exc

P83.39 Other edema specific to newborn CC CC/MCC Exc

P83.4 Breast engorgement of newborn
Noninfective mastitis of newborn

P83.5 Congenital hydrocele ♂

P83.6 Umbilical polyp of newborn

P83.8 Other specified conditions of integument specific to newborn

P83.81 Umbilical granuloma POA
EXCLUDES2 Granulomatous disorder of the skin and subcutaneous tissue, unspecified (L92.9)

P83.88 Other specified conditions of integument specific to newborn POA
Bronze baby syndrome
Neonatal scleroderma
Urticaria neonatorum

P83.9 Condition of the integument specific to newborn, unspecified

Other problems with newborn (P84)

P84 Other problems with newborn
Acidemia of newborn
Acidosis of newborn
Anoxia of newborn NOS
Asphyxia of newborn NOS
Hypercapnia of newborn
Hypoxemia of newborn
Hypoxia of newborn NOS
Mixed metabolic and respiratory acidosis of newborn
EXCLUDES1 intracranial hemorrhage due to anoxia or hypoxia (P52.-)
hypoxic ischemic encephalopathy [HIE] (P91.6-)
late metabolic acidosis of newborn (P74.0)

Other disorders originating in the perinatal period (P90-P96)

P90 Convulsions of newborn MCC CC/MCC Exc
AHA: Q2 2018
EXCLUDES1 benign myoclonic epilepsy in infancy (G40.3-)
benign neonatal convulsions (familial) (G40.3-)

P91 Other disturbances of cerebral status of newborn

P91.0 Neonatal cerebral ischemia MCC CC/MCC Exc

P91.1 Acquired periventricular cysts of newborn MCC CC/MCC Exc

P91.2 Neonatal cerebral leukomalacia MCC CC/MCC Exc
Periventricular leukomalacia

P91.3 Neonatal cerebral irritability MCC CC/MCC Exc

P91.4 Neonatal cerebral depression MCC CC/MCC Exc

P91.5 Neonatal coma MCC CC/MCC Exc

P91.6 Hypoxic ischemic encephalopathy [HIE]
EXCLUDES1 Neonatal cerebral depression (P91.4)
Neonatal cerebral irritability (P91.3)
Neonatal coma (P91.5)

P91.60 Hypoxic ischemic encephalopathy [HIE], unspecified CC CC/MCC Exc

P91.61 Mild hypoxic ischemic encephalopathy [HIE] CC CC/MCC Exc

---

POA Unacceptable principal diagnosis symbol per Medicare code edits   POA Code exempt from diagnosis present on admission requirement
❓ Questionable admission   CC Complication or comorbidity   MCC Major complication or comorbidity   CC/MCC Exc CC/MCC exclusion
HCC HCC diagnosis code   RxHCC RxHCC diagnosis code   MACRA code   **DEFINITION** Describes condition/terminology
TIP Coding guidance   👁 Official Guideline Reference   Z1 Z code as first-listed diagnosis

P91.62 Moderate hypoxic ischemic encephalopathy
[HIE] CC CC/MCC Exc

P91.63 Severe hypoxic ischemic encephalopathy
[HIE] MCC CC/MCC Exc

5th **P91.8** **Other specified disturbances of cerebral status of newborn**

6th **P91.81** **Neonatal encephalopathy**

P91.811 **Neonatal encephalopathy in diseases classified elsewhere** POA

☞ **Code first** underlying condition, if known, such as:
congenital cirrhosis (of liver) (P78.81)
intracranial nontraumatic hemorrhage of newborn (P52.-)
kernicterus (P57.-)

P91.819 **Neonatal encephalopathy, unspecified** POA

P91.88 **Other specified disturbances of cerebral status of newborn** POA

P91.9 **Disturbance of cerebral status of newborn, unspecified**

4th **P92** **Feeding problems of newborn**

EXCLUDES1 eating disorders (F50.-)
feeding problems in child over 28 days old (R63.3)

5th **P92.0** **Vomiting of newborn**

EXCLUDES1 vomiting of child over 28 days old (R11.-)

P92.01 Bilious **vomiting of newborn** MCC CC/MCC Exc

EXCLUDES1 bilious vomiting in child over 28 days old (R11.14)

P92.09 **Other vomiting of newborn**

EXCLUDES1 regurgitation of food in newborn (P92.1)

P92.1 Regurgitation and rumination **of newborn**

P92.2 Slow feeding **of newborn**

P92.3 Underfeeding **of newborn**

P92.4 Overfeeding **of newborn**

P92.5 Neonatal difficulty in feeding at breast
AHA: Q1 2017, Q3 2016

P92.6 Failure to thrive **in newborn**

EXCLUDES1 failure to thrive in child over 28 days old (R62.51)

P92.8 **Other feeding problems of newborn**

P92.9 **Feeding problem of newborn, unspecified**

4th **P93** **Reactions and intoxications due to drugs administered to newborn**

INCLUDES reactions and intoxications due to drugs administered to fetus affecting newborn

EXCLUDES1 jaundice due to drugs or toxins transmitted from mother or given to newborn (P58.4-)
reactions and intoxications from maternal opiates, tranquilizers and other medication (P04.0-P04.1, P04.4-)
withdrawal symptoms from maternal use of drugs of addiction (P96.1)
withdrawal symptoms from therapeutic use of drugs in newborn (P96.2)

P93.0 **Grey baby syndrome** CC CC/MCC Exc
Grey syndrome from chloramphenicol administration in newborn

P93.8 **Other reactions and intoxications due to drugs administered to newborn** CC CC/MCC Exc
Use additional code for adverse effect, if applicable, to identify drug (T36-T50 with fifth or sixth character 5)

4th **P94** **Disorders of muscle tone of newborn**

P94.0 Transient neonatal myasthenia gravis CC CC/MCC Exc

EXCLUDES1 myasthenia gravis (G70.0)

P94.1 **Congenital** hypertonia

P94.2 **Congenital** hypotonia
Floppy baby syndrome, unspecified

P94.8 **Other disorders of muscle tone of newborn**

P94.9 **Disorder of muscle tone of newborn, unspecified**

P95 **Stillbirth**

👁 **See Official Guidelines** "Stillbirth" I.C.16.g
Deadborn fetus NOS
Fetal death of unspecified cause
Stillbirth NOS

EXCLUDES1 maternal care for intrauterine death (O36.4)
missed abortion (O02.1)
outcome of delivery, stillbirth (Z37.1, Z37.3, Z37.4, Z37.7)

4th **P96** **Other conditions originating in the perinatal period**

P96.0 **Congenital renal failure**
Uremia of newborn

P96.1 **Neonatal withdrawal symptoms from maternal use of drugs of addiction** CC CC/MCC Exc
AHA: Q4 2018
Drug withdrawal syndrome in infant of dependent mother
Neonatal abstinence syndrome

EXCLUDES1 reactions and intoxications from maternal opiates and tranquilizers administered during labor and delivery (P04.0)

P96.2 **Withdrawal symptoms from therapeutic use of drugs in newborn** CC CC/MCC Exc

P96.3 **Wide cranial sutures of newborn**
Neonatal craniotabes

P96.5 **Complication to newborn due to (fetal) intrauterine procedure**

EXCLUDES2 newborn affected by amniocentesis (P00.6)

5th **P96.8** **Other specified conditions originating in the perinatal period**

P96.81 **Exposure to (parental) (environmental) tobacco smoke in the perinatal period**

EXCLUDES2 newborn affected by in utero exposure to tobacco (P04.2)
exposure to environmental tobacco smoke after the perinatal period (Z77.22)

P96.82 **Delayed separation of umbilical cord**

P96.83 **Meconium staining**

EXCLUDES1 meconium aspiration (P24.00, P24.01)
meconium passage during delivery (P03.82)

P96.89 **Other specified conditions originating in the perinatal period**
Use additional code to specify condition

P96.9 **Condition originating in the perinatal period, unspecified**
Congenital debility NOS

NOTES

Chapter 17: Congenital Malformations, Deformations, and Chromosomal Abnormalities (Q00-Q99)

Congenital malformations, deformations, and chromosomal abnormalities (Q00-Q99)

👁 **See Official Guidelines** "Chapter 17: Congenital malformations, deformation, and chromosomal abnormalities (Q00-Q99)" I.C.17

NOTES Codes from this chapter are not for use on maternal records

EXCLUDES2 inborn errors of metabolism (E70-E88)

This chapter contains the following blocks:

Q00-Q07 Congenital malformations of the nervous system
Q10-Q18 Congenital malformations of eye, ear, face and neck
Q20-Q28 Congenital malformations of the circulatory system
Q30-Q34 Congenital malformations of the respiratory system
Q35-Q37 Cleft lip and cleft palate
Q38-Q45 Other congenital malformations of the digestive system
Q50-Q56 Congenital malformations of genital organs
Q60-Q64 Congenital malformations of the urinary system
Q65-Q79 Congenital malformations and deformations of the musculoskeletal system
Q80-Q89 Other congenital malformations
Q90-Q99 Chromosomal abnormalities, not elsewhere classified

Congenital malformations of the nervous system (Q00-Q07)

Q00 Anencephaly and similar malformations
    Q00.0 Anencephaly
      Acephaly
      Acrania
      Amyelencephaly
      Hemianencephaly
      Hemicephaly
    Q00.1 Craniorachischisis
    Q00.2 Iniencephaly

Q01 Encephalocele
    INCLUDES Arnold-Chiari syndrome, type III
           encephalocystocele
           encephalomyelocele
           hydroencephalocele
           hydromeningocele, cranial
           meningocele, cerebral
           meningoencephalocele
    EXCLUDES1 Meckel-Gruber syndrome (Q61.9)
    Q01.0 Frontal encephalocele
    Q01.1 Nasofrontal encephalocele
    Q01.2 Occipital encephalocele
    Q01.8 Encephalocele of other sites
    Q01.9 Encephalocele, unspecified

Q02 Microcephaly
    AHA: Q4 2018, Q4 2016
    INCLUDES hydromicrocephaly
           micrencephalon
    ☛ **Code first**, if applicable, congenital Zika virus disease
    EXCLUDES1 Meckel-Gruber syndrome (Q61.9)

Q03 Congenital hydrocephalus
    INCLUDES hydrocephalus in newborn
    EXCLUDES1 Arnold-Chiari syndrome, type II (Q07.0-)
           acquired hydrocephalus (G91.-)
           hydrocephalus due to congenital toxoplasmosis (P37.1)
           hydrocephalus with spina bifida (Q05.0-Q05.4)
    Q03.0 Malformations of aqueduct of Sylvius
      Anomaly of aqueduct of Sylvius
      Obstruction of aqueduct of Sylvius, congenital
      Stenosis of aqueduct of Sylvius

    Q03.1 Atresia of foramina of Magendie and Luschka
      Dandy-Walker syndrome
    Q03.8 Other congenital hydrocephalus
    Q03.9 Congenital hydrocephalus, unspecified

Q04 Other congenital malformations of brain
    EXCLUDES1 cyclopia (Q87.0)
           macrocephaly (Q75.3)
    Q04.0 Congenital malformations of corpus callosum
      Agenesis of corpus callosum
    Q04.1 Arhinencephaly
    Q04.2 Holoprosencephaly
    Q04.3 Other reduction deformities of brain
      Absence of part of brain
      Agenesis of part of brain
      Agyria
      Aplasia of part of brain
      Hydranencephaly
      Hypoplasia of part of brain
      Lissencephaly
      Microgyria
      Pachygyria
      EXCLUDES1 congenital malformations of corpus callosum (Q04.0)
    Q04.4 Septo-optic dysplasia of brain
    Q04.5 Megalencephaly
    Q04.6 Congenital cerebral cysts
      Porencephaly
      Schizencephaly
      EXCLUDES1 acquired porencephalic cyst (G93.0)
    Q04.8 Other specified congenital malformations of brain
      Arnold-Chiari syndrome, type IV
      Macrogyria
    Q04.9 Congenital malformation of brain, unspecified
      Congenital anomaly NOS of brain
      Congenital deformity NOS of brain
      Congenital disease or lesion NOS of brain
      Multiple anomalies NOS of brain, congenital

Q05 Spina bifida
    INCLUDES hydromeningocele (spinal)
           meningocele (spinal)
           meningomyelocele
           myelocele
           myelomeningocele
           rachischisis
           spina bifida (aperta)(cystica)
           syringomyelocele
    Use additional code for any associated paraplegia (paraparesis) (G82.2-)
    EXCLUDES1 Arnold-Chiari syndrome, type II (Q07.0-)
           spina bifida occulta (Q76.0)
    Q05.0 Cervical spina bifida with hydrocephalus
    Q05.1 Thoracic spina bifida with hydrocephalus
      Dorsal spina bifida with hydrocephalus
      Thoracolumbar spina bifida with hydrocephalus
    Q05.2 Lumbar spina bifida with hydrocephalus
      Lumbosacral spina bifida with hydrocephalus
    Q05.3 Sacral spina bifida with hydrocephalus
    Q05.4 Unspecified spina bifida with hydrocephalus
    Q05.5 Cervical spina bifida without hydrocephalus
    Q05.6 Thoracic spina bifida without hydrocephalus
      Dorsal spina bifida NOS
      Thoracolumbar spina bifida NOS

Unspecified Code   Other Specified Code   Manifestation Code   **N** Newborn   **P** Pediatric   **M** Maternity   **A** Adult   ♂ Male   ♀ Female
● New Code   ▲ Revised Code Title   ▶◀ Revised Text   **NOTES**   *INCLUDES*   *EXCLUDES1* Not coded here   *EXCLUDES2* Not included here
4ᵗʰ 4ᵗʰ character required   **5ᵗʰ** 5ᵗʰ character required   **6ᵗʰ** 6ᵗʰ character required   **7ᵗʰ** 7ᵗʰ character required   **X7** Extension 'X' Alert
HAC Hospital-acquired condition (HAC) alert   **AHA** AHA Coding Clinic©   ☛ Code first alert

Q05.7   Lumbar **spina bifida** without hydrocephalus   POA HCC RxHCC
     Lumbosacral spina bifida NOS

Q05.8   Sacral **spina bifida** without hydrocephalus   POA HCC RxHCC

Q05.9   **Spina bifida, unspecified**   POA HCC RxHCC

4ᵗʰ Q06   Other **congenital malformations of** spinal cord

Q06.0   **Amyelia**   POA HCC RxHCC

Q06.1   **Hypoplasia and dysplasia of spinal cord**   POA HCC RxHCC
     Atelomyelia
     Myelatelia
     Myelodysplasia of spinal cord

Q06.2   **Diastematomyelia**   POA HCC RxHCC

Q06.3   **Other congenital cauda equina malformations**   POA HCC RxHCC

Q06.4   **Hydromyelia**   POA HCC RxHCC
     Hydrorachis

Q06.8   **Other specified congenital malformations of spinal cord**   POA HCC RxHCC

Q06.9   **Congenital malformation of spinal cord, unspecified**   POA HCC RxHCC
     Congenital anomaly NOS of spinal cord
     Congenital deformity NOS of spinal cord
     Congenital disease or lesion NOS of spinal cord

4ᵗʰ Q07   Other **congenital malformations of** nervous system

    EXCLUDES2   congenital central alveolar hypoventilation syndrome (G47.35)
          familial dysautonomia [Riley-Day] (G90.1)
          neurofibromatosis (nonmalignant) (Q85.0-)

5ᵗʰ Q07.0   **Arnold-Chiari syndrome**
     Arnold-Chiari syndrome, type II

     EXCLUDES1   Arnold-Chiari syndrome, type III (Q01.-)
              Arnold-Chiari syndrome, type IV (Q04.8)

    Q07.00   **Arnold-Chiari syndrome** without spina bifida or hydrocephalus   POA HCC RxHCC

    Q07.01   **Arnold-Chiari syndrome** with spina bifida   POA HCC RxHCC

    Q07.02   **Arnold-Chiari syndrome** with hydrocephalus   CC POA HCC RxHCC

    Q07.03   **Arnold-Chiari syndrome** with spina bifida and hydrocephalus   CC POA HCC RxHCC

Q07.8   **Other specified congenital malformations of nervous system**   POA HCC RxHCC
     Agenesis of nerve
     Displacement of brachial plexus
     Jaw-winking syndrome
     Marcus Gunn's syndrome

Q07.9   **Congenital malformation of nervous system, unspecified**   POA HCC RxHCC
     Congenital anomaly NOS of nervous system
     Congenital deformity NOS of nervous system
     Congenital disease or lesion NOS of nervous system

Congenital malformations of eye, ear, face and neck (Q10-Q18)

    EXCLUDES2   cleft lip and cleft palate (Q35-Q37)
          congenital malformation of cervical spine (Q05.0, Q05.5, Q67.5, Q76.0-Q76.4)
          congenital malformation of larynx (Q31.-)
          congenital malformation of lip NEC (Q38.0)
          congenital malformation of nose (Q30.-)
          congenital malformation of parathyroid gland (Q89.2)
          congenital malformation of thyroid gland (Q89.2)

4ᵗʰ Q10   **Congenital malformations of** eyelid, lacrimal apparatus and orbit

    EXCLUDES1   cryptophthalmos NOS (Q11.2)
             cryptophthalmos syndrome (Q87.0)

Q10.0   **Congenital** ptosis   POA

Q10.1   **Congenital** ectropion   POA

Q10.2   **Congenital** entropion   POA

Q10.3   Other **congenital malformations of eyelid**   POA
     Ablepharon
     Blepharophimosis, congenital
     Coloboma of eyelid

     Congenital absence or agenesis of cilia
     Congenital absence or agenesis of eyelid
     Congenital accessory eyelid
     Congenital accessory eye muscle
     Congenital malformation of eyelid NOS

Q10.4   Absence and agenesis of lacrimal apparatus   POA
     Congenital absence of punctum lacrimale

Q10.5   **Congenital** stenosis and stricture of lacrimal duct   POA

Q10.6   Other **congenital malformations of lacrimal apparatus**   POA
     Congenital malformation of lacrimal apparatus NOS

Q10.7   **Congenital malformation of** orbit   POA

4ᵗʰ Q11   **Anophthalmos, microphthalmos and macrophthalmos**

Q11.0   **Cystic eyeball**   POA

     DEFINITION: Congenital cystic eye (CCE or cystic eyeball) is a rare ocular malformation in which the eye does not develop in utero, and is replaced by fluid-filled tissue.

Q11.1   **Other anophthalmos**   POA
     Anophthalmos NOS
     Agenesis of eye
     Aplasia of eye

Q11.2   **Microphthalmos**   POA
     Cryptophthalmos NOS
     Dysplasia of eye
     Hypoplasia of eye
     Rudimentary eye

     EXCLUDES1   cryptophthalmos syndrome (Q87.0)

Q11.3   **Macrophthalmos**   POA

     EXCLUDES1   macrophthalmos in congenital glaucoma (Q15.0)

4ᵗʰ Q12   **Congenital** lens malformations

Q12.0   **Congenital** cataract   POA

Q12.1   **Congenital** displaced lens   POA

Q12.2   **Coloboma of lens**   POA

Q12.3   **Congenital** aphakia   POA

Q12.4   **Spherophakia**   POA

Q12.8   Other **congenital lens malformations**   POA
     Microphakia

Q12.9   **Congenital lens malformation, unspecified**   POA

4ᵗʰ Q13   **Congenital malformations of** anterior segment of eye

Q13.0   **Coloboma** of iris   POA
     Coloboma NOS

Q13.1   Absence of iris   POA
     Aniridia
     Use additional code for associated glaucoma (H42)

Q13.2   Other **congenital malformations of iris**   POA
     Anisocoria, congenital
     Atresia of pupil
     Congenital malformation of iris NOS
     Corectopia

Q13.3   **Congenital** corneal opacity   POA

Q13.4   Other **congenital corneal malformations**   POA
     Congenital malformation of cornea NOS
     Microcornea
     Peter's anomaly

Q13.5   Blue sclera   POA

5ᵗʰ Q13.8   Other **congenital malformations of anterior segment of eye**

    Q13.81   **Rieger's anomaly**   POA
        Use additional code for associated glaucoma (H42)

    Q13.89   **Other congenital malformations of anterior segment of eye**   POA

Q13.9   **Congenital malformation of anterior segment of eye, unspecified**   POA

4ᵗʰ Q14   **Congenital malformations of** posterior segment of eye

    EXCLUDES2   optic nerve hypoplasia (H47.03-)

Q14.0   **Congenital malformation of** vitreous humor   POA
     Congenital vitreous opacity

Q14.1   **Congenital malformation of** retina   POA
     Congenital retinal aneurysm

Q14.2   **Congenital malformation of** optic disc   POA
     Coloboma of optic disc

Q14.3   **Congenital malformation of** choroid   POA

POA   Unacceptable principal diagnosis symbol per Medicare code edits   POA   Code exempt from diagnosis present on admission requirement
❓   Questionable admission   CC   Complication or comorbidity   MCC   Major complication or comorbidity   CC/MCC EXC   CC/MCC exclusion
HCC   HCC diagnosis code   RxHCC   RxHCC diagnosis code   MACRA code   **DEFINITION**   Describes condition/terminology
TIP   Coding guidance   👁   Official Guideline Reference   Z   Z code as first-listed diagnosis

When symbols appear on a code that requires a 7th character extension, refer to Appendix B to identify applicable 7th character codes.

2020 ICD-10-CM

Q14.8 **Other** congenital malformations of posterior segment of eye POA
Coloboma of the fundus
Q14.9 **Congenital malformation of posterior segment of eye, unspecified** POA
Q15 **Other** congenital malformations of **eye**
EXCLUDES1 congenital nystagmus (H55.01)
ocular albinism (E70.31-)
optic nerve hypoplasia (H47.03-)
retinitis pigmentosa (H35.52)
Q15.0 **Congenital** glaucoma POA
Axenfeld's anomaly
Buphthalmos
Glaucoma of childhood
Glaucoma of newborn
Hydrophthalmos
Keratoglobus, congenital, with glaucoma
Macrocornea with glaucoma
Macrophthalmos in congenital glaucoma
Megalocornea with glaucoma
Q15.8 **Other specified congenital malformations of eye** POA
Q15.9 **Congenital malformation of eye, unspecified** POA
Congenital anomaly of eye
Congenital deformity of eye
Q16 **Congenital malformations of** ear causing impairment of hearing
EXCLUDES1 congenital deafness (H90.-)
Q16.0 **Congenital** absence of (ear) auricle POA
Q16.1 **Congenital** absence, atresia and stricture of auditory canal (external) POA
Congenital atresia or stricture of osseous meatus
Q16.2 **Absence of eustachian tube** POA
Q16.3 **Congenital malformation of** ear ossicles POA
Congenital fusion of ear ossicles
Q16.4 **Other congenital malformations of middle ear** POA
Congenital malformation of middle ear NOS
Q16.5 **Congenital malformation of** inner ear POA
Congenital anomaly of membranous labyrinth
Congenital anomaly of organ of Corti
Q16.9 **Congenital malformation of ear causing impairment of hearing, unspecified** POA
Congenital absence of ear NOS
Q17 **Other** congenital malformations of **ear**
EXCLUDES1 congenital malformations of ear with impairment of hearing (Q16.0-Q16.9)
preauricular sinus (Q18.1)
Q17.0 **Accessory auricle** POA
Accessory tragus
Polyotia
Preauricular appendage or tag
Supernumerary ear
Supernumerary lobule
Q17.1 **Macrotia** POA
Q17.2 **Microtia** POA
Q17.3 **Other misshapen ear** POA
Pointed ear
Q17.4 **Misplaced ear** POA
Low-set ears
EXCLUDES1 cervical auricle (Q18.2)
Q17.5 **Prominent ear** POA
Bat ear
Q17.8 **Other specified congenital malformations of ear** POA
Congenital absence of lobe of ear
Q17.9 **Congenital malformation of ear, unspecified** POA
Congenital anomaly of ear NOS
Q18 **Other** congenital malformations of **face and neck**
EXCLUDES1 cleft lip and cleft palate (Q35-Q37)
conditions classified to Q67.0-Q67.4
congenital malformations of skull and face bones (Q75.-)
cyclopia (Q87.0)
dentofacial anomalies [including malocclusion] (M26.-)

malformation syndromes affecting facial appearance (Q87.0)
persistent thyroglossal duct (Q89.2)
Q18.0 **Sinus, fistula and cyst of branchial** cleft POA
Branchial vestige
Q18.1 **Preauricular sinus and cyst** POA
Fistula of auricle, congenital
Cervicoaural fistula
Q18.2 **Other branchial** cleft **malformations** POA
Branchial cleft malformation NOS
Cervical auricle
Otocephaly
Q18.3 **Webbing of neck** POA
Pterygium colli
Q18.4 **Macrostomia** POA
Q18.5 **Microstomia** POA
Q18.6 **Macrocheilia** POA
Hypertrophy of lip, congenital
Q18.7 **Microcheilia** POA
Q18.8 **Other specified congenital malformations of face and neck** POA
Medial cyst of face and neck
Medial fistula of face and neck
Medial sinus of face and neck
Q18.9 **Congenital malformation of face and neck, unspecified** POA
Congenital anomaly NOS of face and neck

Congenital malformations of the circulatory system (Q20-Q28)

Q20 **Congenital malformations of** cardiac chambers and connections
EXCLUDES1 dextrocardia with situs inversus (Q89.3)
mirror-image atrial arrangement with situs inversus (Q89.3)
Q20.0 **Common arterial trunk** POA MCC
Persistent truncus arteriosus
EXCLUDES1 aortic septal defect (Q21.4)
Q20.1 **Double** outlet right **ventricle** POA MCC
Taussig-Bing syndrome
Q20.2 **Double** outlet left **ventricle** POA MCC
Q20.3 **Discordant** ventriculoarterial connection POA MCC
Dextrotransposition of aorta
Transposition of great vessels (complete)
Q20.4 **Double** inlet **ventricle** POA MCC
Common ventricle
Cor triloculare biatriatum
Single ventricle
Q20.5 **Discordant** atrioventricular connection CC POA
Corrected transposition
Levotransposition
Ventricular inversion
Q20.6 **Isomerism of atrial appendages** POA
Isomerism of atrial appendages with asplenia or polysplenia
Q20.8 **Other congenital malformations of cardiac chambers and connections** POA
Cor binoculare
Q20.9 **Congenital malformation of cardiac chambers and connections, unspecified** POA
Q21 **Congenital malformations of** cardiac septa
EXCLUDES1 acquired cardiac septal defect (I51.0)
Q21.0 Ventricular **septal defect** POA
Roger's disease
Q21.1 Atrial **septal defect** POA
Coronary sinus defect
Patent or persistent foramen ovale
Patent or persistent ostium secundum defect (type II)
Patent or persistent sinus venosus defect
Q21.2 Atrioventricular **septal defect** POA
Common atrioventricular canal
Endocardial cushion defect
Ostium primum atrial septal defect (type I)
Q21.3 Tetralogy of Fallot POA MCC
Ventricular septal defect with pulmonary stenosis or atresia, dextroposition of aorta and hypertrophy of right ventricle.

Unspecified Code Other Specified Code Manifestation Code N Newborn P Pediatric M Maternity A Adult ♂ Male ♀ Female
● New Code ▲ Revised Code Title ►◄ Revised Text NOTES INCLUDES EXCLUDES1 Not coded here EXCLUDES2 Not included here
4ᵗʰ 4th character required 5ᵗʰ 5th character required 6ᵗʰ 6th character required 7ᵗʰ 7th character required Extension 'X' Alert
HAC Hospital-acquired condition (HAC) alert AHA AHA Coding Clinic© Code first alert

Q21.4 **Aortopulmonary** septal defect
Aortic septal defect
Aortopulmonary window

Q21.8 **Other congenital malformations of cardiac septa**
Eisenmenger's defect
Pentalogy of Fallot
Code also if applicable:
Eisenmenger's complex (I27.83)
Eisenmenger's syndrome (I27.83)

Q21.9 **Congenital malformation of cardiac septum, unspecified**
Septal (heart) defect NOS

Q22 Congenital malformations of pulmonary and tricuspid valves

Q22.0 **Pulmonary** valve atresia

Q22.1 **Congenital pulmonary valve** stenosis

Q22.2 **Congenital pulmonary valve** insufficiency
Congenital pulmonary valve regurgitation

Q22.3 **Other congenital malformations of pulmonary valve**
Congenital malformation of pulmonary valve NOS
Supernumerary cusps of pulmonary valve

Q22.4 **Congenital** tricuspid stenosis
Congenital tricuspid atresia

Q22.5 Ebstein's anomaly

Q22.6 **Hypoplastic** right heart syndrome

Q22.8 **Other congenital malformations of tricuspid valve**

Q22.9 **Congenital malformation of tricuspid valve, unspecified**

Q23 Congenital malformations of aortic and mitral valves

Q23.0 **Congenital** stenosis of aortic valve
Congenital aortic atresia
Congenital aortic stenosis NOS
EXCLUDES1 congenital stenosis of aortic valve in hypoplastic left heart syndrome (Q23.4)
congenital subaortic stenosis (Q24.4)
supravalvular aortic stenosis (congenital) (Q25.3)

Q23.1 **Congenital** insufficiency of aortic valve
Bicuspid aortic valve
Congenital aortic insufficiency

Q23.2 **Congenital** mitral stenosis
Congenital mitral atresia

Q23.3 **Congenital** mitral insufficiency

Q23.4 Hypoplastic left heart syndrome

Q23.8 **Other congenital malformations of aortic and mitral valves**

Q23.9 **Congenital malformation of aortic and mitral valves, unspecified**

Q24 Other congenital malformations of heart
EXCLUDES1 endocardial fibroelastosis (I42.4)

Q24.0 **Dextrocardia**
EXCLUDES1 dextrocardia with situs inversus (Q89.3)
isomerism of atrial appendages (with asplenia or polysplenia) (Q20.6)
mirror-image atrial arrangement with situs inversus (Q89.3)

Q24.1 **Levocardia**

Q24.2 **Cor triatriatum**

Q24.3 Pulmonary infundibular stenosis
Subvalvular pulmonic stenosis

Q24.4 Congenital subaortic stenosis

Q24.5 **Malformation of coronary vessels**
Congenital coronary (artery) aneurysm

Q24.6 **Congenital heart block**

Q24.8 **Other specified congenital malformations of heart**
Congenital diverticulum of left ventricle
Congenital malformation of myocardium
Congenital malformation of pericardium
Malposition of heart
Uhl's disease

Q24.9 **Congenital malformation of heart, unspecified**
Congenital anomaly of heart
Congenital disease of heart

Q25 Congenital malformations of great arteries

Q25.0 Patent ductus arteriosus
Patent ductus Botallo
Persistent ductus arteriosus

Q25.1 Coarctation of aorta
AHA: Q4 2016
Coarctation of aorta (preductal) (postductal)
Stenosis of aorta

Q25.2 Atresia of aorta

Q25.21 **Interruption of aortic** arch
AHA: Q4 2016
Atresia of aortic arch

Q25.29 Other atresia of aorta
AHA: Q4 2016
Atresia of aorta

Q25.3 Supravalvular aortic stenosis
EXCLUDES1 congenital aortic stenosis NOS (Q23.0)
congenital stenosis of aortic valve (Q23.0)

Q25.4 **Other congenital malformations of aorta**
EXCLUDES1 hypoplasia of aorta in hypoplastic left heart syndrome (Q23.4)

Q25.40 **Congenital malformation of aorta unspecified**
AHA: Q4 2016

Q25.41 Absence and aplasia of aorta
AHA: Q4 2016

Q25.42 Hypoplasia of aorta
AHA: Q4 2016

Q25.43 Congenital aneurysm of aorta
AHA: Q4 2016
Congenital aneurysm of aortic root
Congenital aneurysm of aortic sinus

Q25.44 Congenital dilation of aorta
AHA: Q4 2016

Q25.45 Double aortic arch
AHA: Q4 2016
Vascular ring of aorta

Q25.46 Tortuous aortic arch
AHA: Q4 2016
Persistent convolutions of aortic arch

Q25.47 Right aortic arch
AHA: Q4 2016
Persistent right aortic arch

Q25.48 Anomalous origin of subclavian artery
AHA: Q4 2016

Q25.49 Other congenital malformations of aorta
AHA: Q4 2016
Aortic arch
Bovine arch

Q25.5 Atresia of pulmonary artery

Q25.6 Stenosis of pulmonary artery
Supravalvular pulmonary stenosis

Q25.7 **Other congenital malformations of** pulmonary artery

Q25.71 Coarctation of pulmonary artery

Q25.72 **Congenital pulmonary** arteriovenous malformation
Congenital pulmonary arteriovenous aneurysm

Q25.79 **Other congenital malformations of pulmonary artery**
Aberrant pulmonary artery
Agenesis of pulmonary artery
Congenital aneurysm of pulmonary artery
Congenital anomaly of pulmonary artery
Hypoplasia of pulmonary artery

Q25.8 **Other congenital malformations of other great arteries**

Q25.9 **Congenital malformation of great arteries, unspecified**

Q26 Congenital malformations of great veins

Q26.0 **Congenital** stenosis of vena cava
Congenital stenosis of vena cava (inferior)(superior)

Q26.1 Persistent left superior vena cava

When symbols appear on a code that requires a 7th character extension, refer to Appendix B to identify applicable 7th character codes.

Q26.2 Total anomalous **pulmonary venous connection** cc POA CC/MCC Exc
Total anomalous pulmonary venous return [TAPVR], subdiaphragmatic
Total anomalous pulmonary venous return [TAPVR], supradiaphragmatic

Q26.3 Partial anomalous **pulmonary venous connection** cc POA CC/MCC Exc
Partial anomalous pulmonary venous return

Q26.4 **Anomalous pulmonary venous connection, unspecified** cc POA CC/MCC Exc

Q26.5 Anomalous portal **venous connection** POA

Q26.6 Portal vein-hepatic artery fistula POA

Q26.8 **Other congenital malformations of great veins** cc POA CC/MCC Exc
Absence of vena cava (inferior) (superior)
Azygos continuation of inferior vena cava
Persistent left posterior cardinal vein
Scimitar syndrome

Q26.9 **Congenital malformation of great vein, unspecified** cc POA CC/MCC Exc
Congenital anomaly of vena cava (inferior) (superior) NOS

Q27 Other congenital malformations of peripheral vascular system
EXCLUDES2 anomalies of cerebral and precerebral vessels (Q28.0-Q28.3)
anomalies of coronary vessels (Q24.5)
anomalies of pulmonary artery (Q25.5-Q25.7)
congenital retinal aneurysm (Q14.1)
hemangioma and lymphangioma (D18.-)

Q27.0 **Congenital** absence and hypoplasia of umbilical artery POA
Single umbilical artery

Q27.1 **Congenital** renal artery stenosis POA

Q27.2 **Other congenital malformations of** renal artery POA
Congenital malformation of renal artery NOS
Multiple renal arteries

Q27.3 **Arteriovenous malformation (peripheral)**
Arteriovenous aneurysm
EXCLUDES1 acquired arteriovenous aneurysm (I77.0)
EXCLUDES2 arteriovenous malformation of cerebral vessels (Q28.2)
arteriovenous malformation of precerebral vessels (Q28.0)

Q27.30 **Arteriovenous malformation, site unspecified** cc POA CC/MCC Exc

Q27.31 **Arteriovenous malformation of** vessel of upper limb POA

Q27.32 **Arteriovenous malformation of** vessel of lower limb POA

Q27.33 **Arteriovenous malformation of** digestive system vessel POA
AHA: Q3 2018

Q27.34 **Arteriovenous malformation of** renal vessel POA

Q27.39 **Arteriovenous malformation,** other site POA

Q27.4 **Congenital** phlebectasia cc POA CC/MCC Exc

Q27.8 **Other specified congenital malformations of peripheral vascular system** POA
Absence of peripheral vascular system
Atresia of peripheral vascular system
Congenital aneurysm (peripheral)
Congenital stricture, artery
Congenital varix
EXCLUDES1 arteriovenous malformation (Q27.3-)

Q27.9 **Congenital malformation of peripheral vascular system, unspecified** POA
Anomaly of artery or vein NOS

Q28 Other **congenital malformations of** circulatory system
EXCLUDES1 congenital aneurysm NOS (Q27.8)
congenital coronary aneurysm (Q24.5)
ruptured cerebral arteriovenous malformation (I60.8)
ruptured malformation of precerebral vessels (I72.0)
EXCLUDES2 congenital peripheral aneurysm (Q27.8)
congenital pulmonary aneurysm (Q25.79)
congenital retinal aneurysm (Q14.1)

Q28.0 Arteriovenous **malformation of** precerebral vessels cc POA CC/MCC Exc
Congenital arteriovenous precerebral aneurysm (nonruptured)

Q28.1 Other **malformations of** precerebral vessels cc POA CC/MCC Exc
Congenital malformation of precerebral vessels NOS
Congenital precerebral aneurysm (nonruptured)

Q28.2 Arteriovenous **malformation of** cerebral vessels POA MCC CC/MCC Exc
Arteriovenous malformation of brain NOS
Congenital arteriovenous cerebral aneurysm (nonruptured)

Q28.3 Other **malformations of** cerebral vessels POA MCC CC/MCC Exc
Congenital cerebral aneurysm (nonruptured)
Congenital malformation of cerebral vessels NOS
Developmental venous anomaly

Q28.8 **Other specified congenital malformations of circulatory system** cc POA CC/MCC Exc
Congenital aneurysm, specified site NEC
Spinal vessel anomaly

Q28.9 **Congenital malformation of circulatory system, unspecified** cc POA CC/MCC Exc

Congenital malformations of the respiratory system (Q30-Q34)

Q30 **Congenital malformations of** nose
EXCLUDES1 congenital deviation of nasal septum (Q67.4)

Q30.0 **Choanal atresia** POA
Atresia of nares (anterior) (posterior)
Congenital stenosis of nares (anterior) (posterior)

Q30.1 Agenesis and underdevelopment **of nose** POA
Congenital absent of nose

Q30.2 Fissured, notched and cleft **nose** POA

Q30.3 Congenital perforated **nasal septum** POA

Q30.8 **Other congenital malformations of nose** POA
Accessory nose
Congenital anomaly of nasal sinus wall

Q30.9 **Congenital malformation of nose, unspecified** POA

Q31 Congenital malformations of larynx
EXCLUDES1 congenital laryngeal stridor NOS (P28.89)

Q31.0 Web **of larynx** POA
Glottic web of larynx
Subglottic web of larynx
Web of larynx NOS

Q31.1 Congenital subglottic stenosis cc POA CC/MCC Exc

Q31.2 **Laryngeal** hypoplasia cc POA CC/MCC Exc

Q31.3 Laryngocele cc POA CC/MCC Exc

Q31.5 Congenital laryngomalacia cc POA CC/MCC Exc

Q31.8 **Other congenital malformations of larynx** cc POA CC/MCC Exc
Absence of larynx
Agenesis of larynx
Atresia of larynx
Congenital cleft thyroid cartilage
Congenital fissure of epiglottis
Congenital stenosis of larynx NEC
Posterior cleft of cricoid cartilage

Q31.9 **Congenital malformation of larynx, unspecified** cc POA CC/MCC Exc

Q32 Congenital malformations of trachea and bronchus
EXCLUDES1 congenital bronchiectasis (Q33.4)

Q32.0 **Congenital** tracheomalacia cc POA CC/MCC Exc

Q32.1 **Other congenital malformations of** trachea cc POA CC/MCC Exc
Atresia of trachea
Congenital anomaly of tracheal cartilage
Congenital dilatation of trachea
Congenital malformation of trachea
Congenital stenosis of trachea
Congenital tracheocele

Q32.2 **Congenital** bronchomalacia cc POA CC/MCC Exc

Q32.3 **Congenital** stenosis of bronchus cc POA CC/MCC Exc

Q32.4 **Other congenital malformations of** bronchus cc POA CC/MCC Exc
Absence of bronchus
Agenesis of bronchus
Atresia of bronchus
Congenital diverticulum of bronchus
Congenital malformation of bronchus NOS

Q33 **Congenital malformations of** lung

Q33.0 **Congenital** cystic **lung** CC POA CC/MCC Exc
Congenital cystic lung disease
Congenital honeycomb lung
Congenital polycystic lung disease
EXCLUDES1 cystic fibrosis (E84.0)
cystic lung disease, acquired or unspecified (J98.4)

Q33.1 Accessory **lobe of lung** POA
Azygos lobe (fissured), lung

Q33.2 Sequestration **of lung** POA MCC CC/MCC Exc

Q33.3 Agenesis **of lung** POA MCC CC/MCC Exc
Congenital absence of lung (lobe)

Q33.4 **Congenital** bronchiectasis CC POA CC/MCC Exc

Q33.5 Ectopic tissue **in lung**

Q33.6 **Congenital** hypoplasia and dysplasia **of lung** POA MCC CC/MCC Exc
EXCLUDES1 pulmonary hypoplasia associated with short gestation (P28.0)

Q33.8 **Other congenital malformations of lung** POA

Q33.9 **Congenital malformation of lung, unspecified** POA

Q34 Other **congenital malformations of** respiratory system
EXCLUDES2 congenital central alveolar hypoventilation syndrome (G47.35)

Q34.0 **Anomaly of** pleura POA

Q34.1 **Congenital cyst of** mediastinum POA

Q34.8 **Other specified congenital malformations of respiratory system** POA
Atresia of nasopharynx

Q34.9 **Congenital malformation of respiratory system, unspecified** POA
Congenital absence of respiratory system
Congenital anomaly of respiratory system NOS

Cleft lip and cleft palate (Q35-Q37)

Use additional code to identify associated malformation of the nose (Q30.2)
EXCLUDES1 Robin's syndrome (Q87.0)

Q35 **Cleft** palate
INCLUDES fissure of palate
palatoschisis
EXCLUDES1 cleft palate with cleft lip (Q37.-)

Q35.1 Cleft hard **palate** POA

Q35.3 Cleft soft **palate** POA

Q35.5 Cleft hard **palate** with cleft soft **palate** POA

Q35.7 Cleft uvula POA

Q35.9 **Cleft palate, unspecified** POA
Cleft palate NOS

Q36 **Cleft** lip
INCLUDES cheiloschisis
congenital fissure of lip
harelip
labium leporinum
EXCLUDES1 cleft lip with cleft palate (Q37.-)

Q36.0 **Cleft lip,** bilateral POA

Q36.1 **Cleft lip,** median POA

Q36.9 **Cleft lip,** unilateral POA
Cleft lip NOS

Q37 **Cleft palate** with cleft lip
INCLUDES cheilopalatoschisis

Q37.0 **Cleft** hard **palate with** bilateral **cleft lip** POA

Q37.1 **Cleft** hard **palate with** unilateral **cleft lip** POA
Cleft hard palate with cleft lip NOS

Q37.2 **Cleft** soft **palate with** bilateral **cleft lip** POA

Q37.3 **Cleft** soft **palate with** unilateral **cleft lip** POA
Cleft soft palate with cleft lip NOS

Q37.4 **Cleft** hard and soft **palate with** bilateral **cleft lip** POA

Q37.5 **Cleft** hard and soft **palate with** unilateral **cleft lip** POA
Cleft hard and soft palate with cleft lip NOS

Q37.8 **Unspecified** cleft **palate with** bilateral **cleft lip** POA

Q37.9 **Unspecified** cleft **palate with** unilateral **cleft lip** POA
Cleft palate with cleft lip NOS

Other congenital malformations of the digestive system (Q38-Q45)

Q38 Other **congenital malformations of** tongue, mouth and pharynx
EXCLUDES1 dentofacial anomalies (M26.-)
macrostomia (Q18.4)
microstomia (Q18.5)

Q38.0 **Congenital malformations of** lips, **not elsewhere classified** POA
Congenital fistula of lip
Congenital malformation of lip NOS
Van der Woude's syndrome
EXCLUDES1 cleft lip (Q36.-)
cleft lip with cleft palate (Q37.-)
macrocheilia (Q18.6)
microcheilia (Q18.7)

Q38.1 Ankyloglossia POA
Tongue tie

Q38.2 Macroglossia POA
Congenital hypertrophy of tongue

Q38.3 **Other congenital malformations of** tongue POA
Aglossia
Bifid tongue
Congenital adhesion of tongue
Congenital fissure of tongue
Congenital malformation of tongue NOS
Double tongue
Hypoglossia
Hypoplasia of tongue
Microglossia

Q38.4 **Congenital malformations of** salivary glands and ducts POA
Atresia of salivary glands and ducts
Congenital absence of salivary glands and ducts
Congenital accessory salivary glands and ducts
Congenital fistula of salivary gland

Q38.5 **Congenital malformations of** palate, **not elsewhere classified** POA
Congenital absence of uvula
Congenital malformation of palate NOS
Congenital high arched palate
EXCLUDES1 cleft palate (Q35.-)
cleft palate with cleft lip (Q37.-)

Q38.6 Other **congenital malformations of** mouth POA
Congenital malformation of mouth NOS

Q38.7 **Congenital** pharyngeal pouch POA
Congenital diverticulum of pharynx
EXCLUDES1 pharyngeal pouch syndrome (D82.1)

Q38.8 **Other congenital malformations of** pharynx POA
Congenital malformation of pharynx NOS
Imperforate pharynx

Q39 **Congenital malformations of** esophagus

Q39.0 Atresia **of esophagus** without fistula POA MCC CC/MCC Exc
Atresia of esophagus NOS

Q39.1 Atresia **of esophagus** with tracheo-esophageal fistula POA MCC CC/MCC Exc
Atresia of esophagus with broncho-esophageal fistula

Q39.2 **Congenital** tracheo-esophageal fistula without atresia POA MCC CC/MCC Exc
Congenital tracheo-esophageal fistula NOS

Q39.3 **Congenital** stenosis and stricture **of esophagus** POA MCC CC/MCC Exc

Q39.4 **Esophageal** web CC POA CC/MCC Exc

Q39.5 **Congenital** dilatation **of esophagus** CC POA CC/MCC Exc
Congenital cardiospasm

Q39.6 **Congenital** diverticulum **of esophagus** CC POA CC/MCC Exc
Congenital esophageal pouch

Q39.8 **Other congenital** malformations **of esophagus** CC POA CC/MCC Exc
Congenital absence of esophagus
Congenital displacement of esophagus
Congenital duplication of esophagus

Q39.9 **Congenital malformation of esophagus, unspecified** CC POA CC/MCC Exc

---

PDx Unacceptable principal diagnosis symbol per Medicare code edits POA Code exempt from diagnosis present on admission requirement
? Questionable admission CC Complication or comorbidity MCC Major complication or comorbidity CC/MCC Exc CC/MCC exclusion
HCC HCC diagnosis code RxHCC RxHCC diagnosis code MACRA code **DEFINITION** Describes condition/terminology
TIP Coding guidance 👁 Official Guideline Reference Z1 Z code as first-listed diagnosis

4ᵗʰ Q40 Other congenital malformations of upper alimentary tract

Q40.0 **Congenital hypertrophic pyloric stenosis** POA
    Congenital or infantile constriction
    Congenital or infantile hypertrophy
    Congenital or infantile spasm
    Congenital or infantile stenosis
    Congenital or infantile stricture

Q40.1 **Congenital hiatus hernia** POA
    Congenital displacement of cardia through esophageal hiatus
    EXCLUDES1 congenital diaphragmatic hernia (Q79.0)

Q40.2 **Other specified congenital malformations of stomach** POA
    Congenital displacement of stomach
    Congenital diverticulum of stomach
    Congenital hourglass stomach
    Congenital duplication of stomach
    Megalogastria
    Microgastria

Q40.3 **Congenital malformation of stomach, unspecified** POA

Q40.8 **Other specified congenital malformations of upper alimentary tract** POA

Q40.9 **Congenital malformation of upper alimentary tract, unspecified** POA
    Congenital anomaly of upper alimentary tract
    Congenital deformity of upper alimentary tract

4ᵗʰ Q41 Congenital absence, atresia and stenosis of small intestine

INCLUDES congenital obstruction, occlusion or stricture of small intestine or intestine NOS

EXCLUDES1 cystic fibrosis with intestinal manifestation (E84.11)
      meconium ileus NOS (without cystic fibrosis) (P76.0)

Q41.0 **Congenital absence, atresia and stenosis of duodenum** CC POA CC/MCC Exc

Q41.1 **Congenital absence, atresia and stenosis of jejunum** CC POA CC/MCC Exc
    Apple peel syndrome
    Imperforate jejunum

Q41.2 **Congenital absence, atresia and stenosis of ileum** CC POA CC/MCC Exc

Q41.8 **Congenital absence, atresia and stenosis of other specified parts of small intestine** CC POA CC/MCC Exc

Q41.9 **Congenital absence, atresia and stenosis of small intestine, part unspecified** CC POA CC/MCC Exc
    Congenital absence, atresia and stenosis of intestine NOS

4ᵗʰ Q42 Congenital absence, atresia and stenosis of large intestine

INCLUDES congenital obstruction, occlusion and stricture of large intestine

Q42.0 **Congenital absence, atresia and stenosis of rectum with fistula** CC POA CC/MCC Exc

Q42.1 **Congenital absence, atresia and stenosis of rectum without fistula** CC POA CC/MCC Exc
    Imperforate rectum

Q42.2 **Congenital absence, atresia and stenosis of anus with fistula** CC POA CC/MCC Exc

Q42.3 **Congenital absence, atresia and stenosis of anus without fistula** CC POA CC/MCC Exc
    Imperforate anus

Q42.8 **Congenital absence, atresia and stenosis of other parts of large intestine** CC POA CC/MCC Exc

Q42.9 **Congenital absence, atresia and stenosis of large intestine, part unspecified** CC POA CC/MCC Exc

4ᵗʰ Q43 Other congenital malformations of intestine

Q43.0 **Meckel's diverticulum (displaced) (hypertrophic)** POA
    Persistent omphalomesenteric duct
    Persistent vitelline duct

Q43.1 **Hirschsprung's disease** CC POA CC/MCC Exc
    Aganglionosis
    Congenital (aganglionic) megacolon

Q43.2 **Other congenital functional disorders of colon** CC POA CC/MCC Exc
    Congenital dilatation of colon

Q43.3 **Congenital malformations of intestinal fixation** CC POA CC/MCC Exc
    Congenital omental, anomalous adhesions [bands]
    Congenital peritoneal adhesions [bands]
    Incomplete rotation of cecum and colon
    Insufficient rotation of cecum and colon

    Jackson's membrane
    Malrotation of colon
    Rotation failure of cecum and colon
    Universal mesentery

Q43.4 **Duplication of intestine** CC POA CC/MCC Exc

Q43.5 **Ectopic anus** CC POA CC/MCC Exc

Q43.6 **Congenital fistula of rectum and anus** CC POA CC/MCC Exc
    EXCLUDES1 congenital fistula of anus with absence, atresia and stenosis (Q42.2)
      congenital fistula of rectum with absence, atresia and stenosis (Q42.0)
      congenital rectovaginal fistula (Q52.2)
      congenital urethrorectal fistula (Q64.73)
      pilonidal fistula or sinus (L05.-)

Q43.7 **Persistent cloaca** CC POA CC/MCC Exc
    Cloaca NOS

Q43.8 **Other specified congenital malformations of intestine** CC POA CC/MCC Exc
    Congenital blind loop syndrome
    Congenital diverticulitis, colon
    Congenital diverticulum, intestine
    Dolichocolon
    Megaloappendix
    Megaloduodenum
    Microcolon
    Transposition of appendix
    Transposition of colon
    Transposition of intestine

Q43.9 **Congenital malformation of intestine, unspecified** CC POA CC/MCC Exc

4ᵗʰ Q44 Congenital malformations of gallbladder, bile ducts and liver

Q44.0 **Agenesis, aplasia and hypoplasia of gallbladder** CC POA CC/MCC Exc
    Congenital absence of gallbladder

Q44.1 **Other congenital malformations of gallbladder** CC POA CC/MCC Exc
    Congenital malformation of gallbladder NOS
    Intrahepatic gallbladder

Q44.2 **Atresia of bile ducts** POA MCC CC/MCC Exc

Q44.3 **Congenital stenosis and stricture of bile ducts** POA MCC CC/MCC Exc

Q44.4 **Choledochal cyst** CC POA CC/MCC Exc

Q44.5 **Other congenital malformations of bile ducts** CC POA CC/MCC Exc
    Accessory hepatic duct
    Biliary duct duplication
    Congenital malformation of bile duct NOS
    Cystic duct duplication

Q44.6 **Cystic disease of liver** CC POA CC/MCC Exc
    Fibrocystic disease of liver

Q44.7 **Other congenital malformations of liver** CC POA CC/MCC Exc
    Accessory liver
    Alagille's syndrome
    Congenital absence of liver
    Congenital hepatomegaly
    Congenital malformation of liver NOS

4ᵗʰ Q45 Other congenital malformations of digestive system

EXCLUDES2 congenital diaphragmatic hernia (Q79.0)
      congenital hiatus hernia (Q40.1)

Q45.0 **Agenesis, aplasia and hypoplasia of pancreas** CC POA CC/MCC Exc
    Congenital absence of pancreas

Q45.1 **Annular pancreas** CC POA CC/MCC Exc

Q45.2 **Congenital pancreatic cyst** CC POA CC/MCC Exc

Q45.3 **Other congenital malformations of pancreas and pancreatic duct** CC POA CC/MCC Exc
    Accessory pancreas
    Congenital malformation of pancreas or pancreatic duct NOS
    EXCLUDES1 congenital diabetes mellitus (E10.-)
      cystic fibrosis (E84.0-E84.9)
      fibrocystic disease of pancreas (E84.-)
      neonatal diabetes mellitus (P70.2)

Q45.8 **Other specified congenital malformations of digestive system** POA
    Absence (complete) (partial) of alimentary tract NOS
    Duplication of digestive system
    Malposition, congenital of digestive system

Unspecified Code   Other Specified Code   Manifestation Code   Ⓝ Newborn   Ⓟ Pediatric   Ⓜ Maternity   Ⓐ Adult   ♂ Male   ♀ Female
● New Code   ▲ Revised Code Title   ▶◀ Revised Text   **NOTES**   *INCLUDES*   *EXCLUDES1* Not coded here   *EXCLUDES2* Not included here
4ᵗʰ 4ᵗʰ character required   5ᵗʰ 5ᵗʰ character required   6ᵗʰ 6ᵗʰ character required   7ᵗʰ 7ᵗʰ character required   7ᵗʰ Extension 'X' Alert
HAC Hospital-acquired condition (HAC) alert   **AHA** AHA Coding Clinic©   📖 Code first alert

Q45.9 **Congenital malformation of digestive system, unspecified** POA⊘
Congenital anomaly of digestive system
Congenital deformity of digestive system

Congenital malformations of genital organs (Q50-Q56)

EXCLUDES1 androgen insensitivity syndrome (E34.5-)

syndromes associated with anomalies in the number and form of chromosomes (Q90-Q99)

4ᵗʰ **Q50 Congenital malformations of** ovaries, fallopian tubes and broad ligaments

5ᵗʰ Q50.0 **Congenital absence of** ovary

EXCLUDES1 Turner's syndrome (Q96.-)

Q50.01 **Congenital absence of ovary,** unilateral POA⊘ ♀
Q50.02 **Congenital absence of ovary,** bilateral POA⊘ ♀
Q50.1 **Developmental ovarian** cyst POA⊘ ♀
Q50.2 **Congenital** torsion **of ovary** POA⊘ ♀

5ᵗʰ Q50.3 **Other congenital malformations of** ovary
Q50.31 Accessory **ovary** POA⊘ ♀
Q50.32 **Ovarian** streak POA⊘ ♀
46, XX with streak gonads
Q50.39 **Other congenital malformation of ovary** POA⊘ ♀
Congenital malformation of ovary NOS
Q50.4 **Embryonic cyst of** fallopian tube POA⊘ ♀
Fimbrial cyst
Q50.5 **Embryonic cyst of** broad ligament POA⊘ ♀
Epoophoron cyst
Parovarian cyst
Q50.6 **Other congenital malformations of fallopian tube and broad ligament** POA⊘ ♀
Absence of fallopian tube and broad ligament
Accessory fallopian tube and broad ligament
Atresia of fallopian tube and broad ligament
Congenital malformation of fallopian tube or broad ligament NOS

4ᵗʰ **Q51 Congenital malformations of** uterus and cervix
Q51.0 Agenesis and aplasia **of** uterus POA⊘ ♀
Congenital absence of uterus

5ᵗʰ Q51.1 Doubling **of** uterus **with doubling of cervix and vagina**
Q51.10 **Doubling of uterus with doubling of cervix and vagina** without obstruction POA⊘ ♀
Doubling of uterus with doubling of cervix and vagina NOS
Q51.11 **Doubling of uterus with doubling of cervix and vagina** with obstruction POA⊘ ♀

5ᵗʰ Q51.2 Other doubling **of uterus**
Doubling of uterus NOS
Septate uterus
Q51.20 **Other doubling of uterus, unspecified** POA⊘ ♀
AHA: Q4 2018
Septate uterus, unspecified
Q51.21 **Other** complete **doubling of uterus** POA⊘ ♀
AHA: Q4 2018
Complete septate uterus
Q51.22 **Other** partial **doubling of uterus** POA⊘ ♀
AHA: Q4 2018
Partial septate uterus
Q51.28 Other doubling of uterus, other specified POA⊘ ♀
AHA: Q4 2018
Septate uterus, other specified
Q51.3 Bicornate **uterus** POA⊘ ♀
Bicornate uterus, complete or partial
Q51.4 Unicornate **uterus** POA⊘ ♀
Unicornate uterus with or without a separate uterine horn
Uterus with only one functioning horn
Q51.5 Agenesis and aplasia of cervix POA⊘ ♀
Congenital absence of cervix
Q51.6 Embryonic cyst **of cervix** POA⊘ ♀
Q51.7 **Congenital** fistulae **between** uterus and digestive and urinary tracts POA⊘ ♀

5ᵗʰ Q51.8 Other **congenital malformations of uterus and cervix**
6ᵗʰ Q51.81 **Other congenital malformations of uterus**
Q51.810 Arcuate **uterus** POA⊘ ♀
Arcuatus uterus
Q51.811 Hypoplasia **of uterus** POA⊘ ♀
Q51.818 **Other congenital malformations of uterus** POA⊘ ♀
Müllerian anomaly of uterus NEC
6ᵗʰ Q51.82 **Other congenital malformations of** cervix
Q51.820 **Cervical** duplication POA⊘ ♀
Q51.821 Hypoplasia **of cervix** POA⊘ ♀
Q51.828 **Other congenital malformations of cervix** POA⊘ ♀
Q51.9 **Congenital malformation of uterus and cervix, unspecified** POA⊘ ♀

4ᵗʰ **Q52 Other congenital malformations of** female genitalia
Q52.0 **Congenital** absence of vagina POA⊘ ♀
Vaginal agenesis, total or partial

5ᵗʰ Q52.1 Doubling of vagina
EXCLUDES1 doubling of vagina with doubling of uterus and cervix (Q51.1-)
Q52.10 **Doubling of vagina, unspecified** POA⊘ ♀
Septate vagina NOS
Q52.11 Transverse **vaginal septum** POA⊘ ♀
6ᵗʰ Q52.12 Longitudinal **vaginal septum**
Q52.120 **Longitudinal vaginal septum,** nonobstructing POA⊘ ♀
AHA: Q4 2016
Q52.121 **Longitudinal vaginal septum,** obstructing, right side POA⊘ ♀
AHA: Q4 2016
Q52.122 **Longitudinal vaginal septum,** obstructing, left side POA⊘ ♀
AHA: Q4 2016
Q52.123 **Longitudinal vaginal septum,** microperforate, right side POA⊘ ♀
AHA: Q4 2016
Q52.124 **Longitudinal vaginal septum,** microperforate, left side POA⊘ ♀
AHA: Q4 2016
Q52.129 Other and **unspecified longitudinal vaginal septum** POA⊘ ♀
AHA: Q4 2016
Q52.2 **Congenital** rectovaginal fistula POA⊘ ♀
EXCLUDES1 cloaca (Q43.7)
Q52.3 Imperforate hymen POA⊘ ♀
Q52.4 **Other congenital malformations of vagina** POA⊘ ♀
Canal of Nuck cyst, congenital
Congenital malformation of vagina NOS
Embryonic vaginal cyst
Gartner's duct cyst
Q52.5 Fusion of labia POA⊘ ♀
Q52.6 **Congenital malformation of** clitoris POA⊘ ♀
5ᵗʰ Q52.7 Other and unspecified **congenital malformations of** vulva
Q52.70 **Unspecified congenital malformations of vulva** POA⊘ ♀
Congenital malformation of vulva NOS
Q52.71 **Congenital** absence **of vulva** POA⊘ ♀
Q52.79 **Other congenital malformations of vulva** POA⊘ ♀
Congenital cyst of vulva
Q52.8 **Other specified congenital malformations of female genitalia** POA⊘ ♀
Q52.9 **Congenital malformation of female genitalia, unspecified** POA⊘ ♀

4ᵗʰ **Q53 Undescended and ectopic** testicle
5ᵗʰ Q53.0 Ectopic testis
Q53.00 **Ectopic testis, unspecified** POA⊘ ♂
Q53.01 **Ectopic testis,** unilateral POA⊘ ♂
Q53.02 **Ectopic testes,** bilateral POA⊘ ♂
5ᵗʰ Q53.1 Undescended **testicle,** unilateral
Q53.10 **Unspecified undescended testicle, unilateral** POA⊘ ♂

POA⊘ Unacceptable principal diagnosis symbol per Medicare code edits   POA⊘ Code exempt from diagnosis present on admission requirement
❓ Questionable admission   ℅ Complication or comorbidity   MCC Major complication or comorbidity   CC/MCC EXC CC/MCC exclusion
HCC HCC diagnosis code   RxHCC RxHCC diagnosis code   MACRA code   **DEFINITION** Describes condition/terminology
TIP Coding guidance   👁 Official Guideline Reference   Z1 Z code as first-listed diagnosis

[6th] **Q53.11** Abdominal **testis, unilateral**
- **Q53.111** Unilateral **intraabdominal testis** POA ♂
- **Q53.112** Unilateral **inguinal testis** POA ♂

Q53.12 Ectopic perineal **testis, unilateral** POA ♂
Q53.13 Unilateral **high scrotal testis** POA ♂

[5th] **Q53.2** Undescended **testicle,** bilateral
Q53.20 Undescended testicle, unspecified, bilateral POA ♂
[6th] **Q53.21** Abdominal **testis,** bilateral
- **Q53.211** Bilateral **intraabdominal testes** POA ♂
- **Q53.212** Bilateral **inguinal testes** POA ♂

Q53.22 Ectopic perineal **testis,** bilateral POA ♂
Q53.23 Bilateral **high scrotal testes** POA ♂

Q53.9 Undescended testicle, unspecified POA ♂
Cryptorchism NOS

[4th] **Q54 Hypospadias**
[EXCLUDES1] *epispadias (Q64.0)*

Q54.0 Hypospadias, balanic POA ♂
Hypospadias, coronal
Hypospadias, glandular
Q54.1 Hypospadias, penile POA ♂
Q54.2 Hypospadias, penoscrotal POA ♂
Q54.3 Hypospadias, perineal POA ♂
Q54.4 Congenital chordee POA ♂
Chordee without hypospadias
Q54.8 Other **hypospadias** POA ♂
Hypospadias with intersex state
Q54.9 Hypospadias, unspecified POA ♂

[4th] **Q55 Other congenital malformations of** male genital organs
[EXCLUDES1] *congenital hydrocele (P83.5)*
hypospadias (Q54.-)

Q55.0 Absence and aplasia of testis POA ♂
Monorchism
Q55.1 Hypoplasia of testis and scrotum POA ♂
Fusion of testes

[5th] **Q55.2 Other and unspecified congenital malformations of** testis and scrotum
Q55.20 Unspecified congenital malformations of testis and scrotum POA ♂
Congenital malformation of testis or scrotum NOS
Q55.21 Polyorchism POA ♂
Q55.22 Retractile **testis** POA ♂
Q55.23 Scrotal transposition POA ♂
Q55.29 Other congenital malformations of testis and scrotum POA ♂

Q55.3 Atresia of vas deferens POA ♂
☛ **Code first** any associated cystic fibrosis (E84.-)
Q55.4 Other congenital malformations of vas deferens, epididymis, seminal vesicles and prostate POA ♂
Absence or aplasia of prostate
Absence or aplasia of spermatic cord
Congenital malformation of vas deferens, epididymis, seminal vesicles or prostate NOS
Q55.5 Congenital absence and aplasia of penis POA ♂

[5th] **Q55.6** Other **congenital malformations of** penis
Q55.61 Curvature **of penis (lateral)** POA ♂
Q55.62 Hypoplasia **of penis** POA ♂
Micropenis
Q55.63 Congenital torsion **of penis** POA ♂
[EXCLUDES1] *acquired torsion of penis (N48.82)*
Q55.64 Hidden **penis** POA ♂
Buried penis
Concealed penis
[EXCLUDES1] *acquired buried penis (N48.83)*
Q55.69 Other congenital malformation of penis POA ♂
Congenital malformation of penis NOS

Q55.7 Congenital vasocutaneous fistula POA ♂
Q55.8 Other specified congenital malformations of male genital organs POA ♂
Q55.9 Congenital malformation of male genital organ, unspecified POA ♂
Congenital anomaly of male genital organ
Congenital deformity of male genital organ

[4th] **Q56 Indeterminate sex and pseudohermaphroditism**
[EXCLUDES1] *46,XX true hermaphrodite (Q99.1)*
androgen insensitivity syndrome (E34.5-)
chimera 46,XX/46,XY true hermaphrodite (Q99.0)
female pseudohermaphroditism with adrenocortical disorder (E25.-)
pseudohermaphroditism with specified chromosomal anomaly (Q96-Q99)
pure gonadal dysgenesis (Q99.1)

Q56.0 Hermaphroditism, **not elsewhere classified** POA
Ovotestis
Q56.1 Male pseudohermaphroditism, **not elsewhere classified** POA ♂
46, XY with streak gonads
Male pseudohermaphroditism NOS
Q56.2 Female pseudohermaphroditism, **not elsewhere classified** POA ♀
Female pseudohermaphroditism NOS
Q56.3 Pseudohermaphroditism, unspecified POA
Q56.4 Indeterminate sex, unspecified POA
Ambiguous genitalia

Congenital malformations of the urinary system (Q60-Q64)

[4th] **Q60 Renal agenesis and other** reduction defects of kidney
[INCLUDES] *congenital absence of kidney*
congenital atrophy of kidney
infantile atrophy of kidney

Q60.0 Renal agenesis, unilateral POA
Q60.1 Renal agenesis, bilateral POA
Q60.2 Renal agenesis, unspecified POA
Q60.3 Renal hypoplasia, unilateral POA
Q60.4 Renal hypoplasia, bilateral POA
Q60.5 Renal hypoplasia, unspecified POA
Q60.6 Potter's syndrome POA

[4th] **Q61** Cystic kidney **disease**
[EXCLUDES1] *acquired cyst of kidney (N28.1)*
Potter's syndrome (Q60.6)

[5th] **Q61.0 Congenital renal** cyst
Q61.00 Congenital renal cyst, unspecified POA
Cyst of kidney NOS (congenital)
Q61.01 Congenital single **renal cyst** POA
Q61.02 Congenital multiple **renal cysts** POA

[5th] **Q61.1** Polycystic **kidney,** infantile type
Polycystic kidney, autosomal recessive
Q61.11 Cystic dilatation of collecting ducts POA
Q61.19 Other polycystic kidney, infantile type POA

Q61.2 Polycystic **kidney,** adult type POA
Polycystic kidney, autosomal dominant
Q61.3 Polycystic kidney, unspecified POA
AHA: Q3 2016
Q61.4 Renal dysplasia POA
Multicystic dysplastic kidney
Multicystic kidney (development)
Multicystic kidney disease
Multicystic renal dysplasia
[EXCLUDES1] *polycystic kidney disease (Q61.11-Q61.3)*
Q61.5 Medullary cystic **kidney** POA
Nephronopthisis
Sponge kidney NOS
Q61.8 Other cystic kidney diseases CC POA CC/MCC Exc
Fibrocystic kidney
Fibrocystic renal degeneration or disease
Q61.9 Cystic kidney disease, unspecified CC POA CC/MCC Exc
Meckel-Gruber syndrome

Unspecified Code | Other Specified Code | Manifestation Code | [N] Newborn | [P] Pediatric | [M] Maternity | [A] Adult | ♂ Male | ♀ Female
● New Code | ▲ Revised Code Title | ►◄ Revised Text | [NOTES] | [INCLUDES] | [EXCLUDES1] Not coded here | [EXCLUDES2] Not included here
[4th] 4th character required | [5th] 5th character required | [6th] 6th character required | [7th] 7th character required | [x] Extension 'X' Alert
[HAC] Hospital-acquired condition (HAC) alert | AHA AHA Coding Clinic© | ☛ Code first alert

Q62 **Congenital obstructive defects of** renal pelvis **and congenital malformations of** ureter

Q62.0 **Congenital** hydronephrosis

Q62.1 **Congenital** occlusion of ureter
Atresia and stenosis of ureter

Q62.10 **Congenital occlusion of ureter, unspecified**

Q62.11 **Congenital occlusion of** ureteropelvic junction

Q62.12 **Congenital occlusion of** ureterovesical orifice

Q62.2 **Congenital** megaureter
Congenital dilatation of ureter

Q62.3 Other **obstructive defects of** renal pelvis and ureter

Q62.31 **Congenital** ureterocele, orthotopic

Q62.32 Cecoureterocele
Ectopic ureterocele

Q62.39 **Other obstructive defects of renal pelvis and ureter**
Ureteropelvic junction obstruction NOS

Q62.4 Agenesis of ureter
Congenital absence ureter

Q62.5 Duplication of ureter
Accessory ureter
Double ureter

Q62.6 Malposition of ureter

Q62.60 **Malposition of ureter, unspecified**

Q62.61 **Deviation of ureter**

Q62.62 **Displacement of ureter**

Q62.63 **Anomalous implantation of ureter**
Ectopia of ureter
Ectopic ureter

Q62.69 **Other malposition of ureter**

Q62.7 **Congenital** vesico-uretero-renal reflux

Q62.8 **Other congenital malformations of ureter**
Anomaly of ureter NOS

Q63 Other **congenital malformations of** kidney

EXCLUDES1 congenital nephrotic syndrome (N04.-)

Q63.0 Accessory kidney

Q63.1 Lobulated, fused and horseshoe kidney

Q63.2 Ectopic kidney
Congenital displaced kidney
Malrotation of kidney

Q63.3 Hyperplastic and giant kidney
Compensatory hypertrophy of kidney

Q63.8 **Other specified congenital malformations of kidney**
Congenital renal calculi

Q63.9 **Congenital malformation of kidney, unspecified**

Q64 Other **congenital malformations of** urinary system

Q64.0 Epispadias

EXCLUDES1 hypospadias (Q54.-)

Q64.1 Exstrophy of urinary bladder

Q64.10 Exstrophy of urinary bladder, unspecified
Ectopia vesicae

Q64.11 Supravesical fissure of urinary bladder

Q64.12 Cloacal exstrophy of urinary bladder

Q64.19 **Other exstrophy of urinary bladder**
Extroversion of bladder

Q64.2 **Congenital** posterior urethral valves

Q64.3 Other **atresia and stenosis of** urethra and bladder neck

Q64.31 **Congenital** bladder neck obstruction
Congenital obstruction of vesicourethral orifice

Q64.32 **Congenital** stricture of urethra

Q64.33 **Congenital** stricture of urinary meatus

Q64.39 **Other atresia and stenosis of urethra and bladder neck**
Atresia and stenosis of urethra and bladder neck NOS

Q64.4 Malformation of urachus
Cyst of urachus
Patent urachus
Prolapse of urachus

Q64.5 **Congenital** absence of bladder and urethra

Q64.6 **Congenital** diverticulum of bladder

Q64.7 Other and unspecified **congenital malformations of** bladder and urethra

EXCLUDES1 congenital prolapse of bladder (mucosa) (Q79.4)

Q64.70 **Unspecified congenital malformation of bladder and urethra**
Malformation of bladder or urethra NOS

Q64.71 **Congenital** prolapse of urethra

Q64.72 **Congenital** prolapse of urinary meatus

Q64.73 **Congenital** urethrorectal fistula

Q64.74 Double **urethra**

Q64.75 Double urinary meatus

Q64.79 **Other congenital malformations of bladder and urethra**

Q64.8 **Other specified congenital malformations of urinary system**

Q64.9 **Congenital malformation of urinary system, unspecified**
Congenital anomaly NOS of urinary system
Congenital deformity NOS of urinary system

Congenital malformations and deformations of the musculoskeletal system (Q65-Q79)

Q65 **Congenital deformities of** hip

EXCLUDES1 clicking hip (R29.4)

Q65.0 **Congenital** dislocation of hip, unilateral

Q65.00 **Congenital dislocation of unspecified hip, unilateral**

Q65.01 **Congenital dislocation of** right hip, unilateral

Q65.02 **Congenital dislocation of** left hip, unilateral

Q65.1 **Congenital dislocation of hip,** bilateral

Q65.2 **Congenital dislocation of hip,** unspecified

Q65.3 **Congenital** partial dislocation of hip, unilateral

Q65.30 **Congenital partial dislocation of unspecified hip, unilateral**

Q65.31 **Congenital partial dislocation of** right hip, unilateral

Q65.32 **Congenital partial dislocation of** left hip, unilateral

Q65.4 **Congenital partial dislocation of hip,** bilateral

Q65.5 **Congenital partial dislocation of hip,** unspecified

Q65.6 **Congenital** unstable hip
Congenital dislocatable hip

Q65.8 Other **congenital deformities of** hip

Q65.81 **Congenital** coxa valga

Q65.82 **Congenital** coxa vara

Q65.89 **Other specified congenital deformities of hip**
Anteversion of femoral neck
Congenital acetabular dysplasia

Q65.9 **Congenital deformity of hip, unspecified**

Q66 **Congenital deformities of** feet

EXCLUDES1 reduction defects of feet (Q72.-)
valgus deformities (acquired) (M21.0-)
varus deformities (acquired) (M21.1-)

Q66.0 **Congenital** talipes equinovarus

Q66.00 **Congenital talipes equinovarus, unspecified foot**

Q66.01 **Congenital talipes equinovarus,** right foot

Q66.02 **Congenital talipes equinovarus,** left foot

Q66.1 **Congenital** talipes calcaneovarus

Q66.10 **Congenital talipes calcaneovarus, unspecified foot**

Q66.11 **Congenital talipes calcaneovarus,** right **foot**

Q66.12 **Congenital talipes calcaneovarus,** left **foot**

Q66.2 **Congenital** metatarsus (primus) varus

Q66.21 **Congenital metatarsus** primus varus

Q66.211 **Congenital metatarsus primus varus,** right foot

Q66.212 **Congenital metatarsus primus varus,** left **foot**

- Q66.219 **Congenital metatarsus primus varus, unspecified foot** POA
- 6th Q66.22 **Congenital metatarsus** adductus
    Congenital metatarsus varus
- Q66.221 **Congenital metatarsus adductus, right foot** POA
- Q66.222 **Congenital metatarsus adductus, left foot** POA
- Q66.229 **Congenital metatarsus adductus, unspecified foot** POA
- 5th Q66.3 **Other congenital varus deformities of feet**
    Hallux varus, congenital
- Q66.30 **Other congenital varus deformities of feet, unspecified foot** POA
- Q66.31 **Other congenital varus deformities of feet, right foot** POA
- Q66.32 **Other congenital varus deformities of feet, left foot** POA
- 5th Q66.4 **Congenital** talipes calcaneovalgus
- Q66.40 **Congenital talipes calcaneovalgus, unspecified foot** POA
- Q66.41 **Congenital talipes calcaneovalgus,** right **foot** POA
- Q66.42 **Congenital talipes calcaneovalgus,** left **foot** POA
- 5th Q66.5 **Congenital** pes planus
    Congenital flat foot
    Congenital rigid flat foot
    Congenital spastic (everted) flat foot
    EXCLUDES1 *pes planus, acquired (M21.4)*
    Q66.50 **Congenital pes planus, unspecified foot** POA
    Q66.51 **Congenital pes planus,** right **foot** POA
    Q66.52 **Congenital pes planus,** left **foot** POA
- Q66.6 **Other congenital valgus deformities of** feet POA
    Congenital metatarsus valgus
- 5th Q66.7 **Congenital** pes cavus
- Q66.70 **Congenital pes cavus, unspecified foot** POA
- Q66.71 **Congenital pes cavus,** right **foot** POA
- Q66.72 **Congenital pes cavus,** left **foot** POA
- 5th Q66.8 Other **congenital deformities of** feet
    Q66.80 **Congenital vertical talus deformity, unspecified foot** POA
    Q66.81 **Congenital vertical talus deformity,** right **foot** POA
    Q66.82 **Congenital vertical talus deformity,** left **foot** POA
    Q66.89 Other specified congenital deformities of feet POA
        Congenital asymmetric talipes
        Congenital clubfoot NOS
        Congenital talipes NOS
        Congenital tarsal coalition
        Hammer toe, congenital
- 5th Q66.9 **Congenital deformity of feet, unspecified**
- Q66.90 **Congenital deformity of feet, unspecified, unspecified foot** POA
- Q66.91 **Congenital deformity of feet, unspecified, right foot** POA
- Q66.92 **Congenital deformity of feet, unspecified, left foot** POA
- 4th Q67 **Congenital musculoskeletal deformities of** head, face, spine and chest
    EXCLUDES1 *congenital malformation syndromes classified to Q87.-*
        Potter's syndrome (Q60.6)
    Q67.0 **Congenital** facial asymmetry POA
    Q67.1 **Congenital** compression facies POA
    Q67.2 Dolichocephaly POA
    Q67.3 Plagiocephaly POA
    Q67.4 **Other congenital deformities of** skull, face and jaw POA
        Congenital depressions in skull
        Congenital hemifacial atrophy or hypertrophy
        Deviation of nasal septum, congenital
        Squashed or bent nose, congenital
        EXCLUDES1 *dentofacial anomalies [including malocclusion] (M26.-)*
            syphilitic saddle nose (A50.5)

Q67.5 **Congenital deformity of** spine   CC POA CC/MCC Exc
    Congenital postural scoliosis
    Congenital scoliosis NOS
    EXCLUDES1 *infantile idiopathic scoliosis (M41.0)*
        scoliosis due to congenital bony malformation (Q76.3)
Q67.6 Pectus excavatum POA
    Congenital funnel chest
Q67.7 Pectus carinatum POA
    Congenital pigeon chest
Q67.8 **Other congenital deformities of** chest   CC POA CC/MCC Exc
    Congenital deformity of chest wall NOS
- 4th Q68 Other **congenital** musculoskeletal **deformities**
    EXCLUDES1 *reduction defects of limb(s) (Q71-Q73)*
    EXCLUDES2 *congenital myotonic chondrodystrophy (G71.13)*
    Q68.0 **Congenital deformity of** sternocleidomastoid muscle POA
        Congenital contracture of sternocleidomastoid (muscle)
        Congenital (sternomastoid) torticollis
        Sternomastoid tumor (congenital)
    Q68.1 **Congenital deformity of** finger(s) and hand   CC POA CC/MCC Exc
        Congenital clubfinger
        Spade-like hand (congenital)
    Q68.2 **Congenital deformity of** knee POA
        Congenital dislocation of knee
        Congenital genu recurvatum
    Q68.3 **Congenital bowing of** femur POA
        EXCLUDES1 *anteversion of femur (neck) (Q65.89)*
    Q68.4 **Congenital bowing of** tibia and fibula POA
    Q68.5 **Congenital bowing of long bones of leg, unspecified** POA
    Q68.6 Discoid meniscus POA
    Q68.8 **Other specified congenital musculoskeletal deformities** POA
        Congenital deformity of clavicle
        Congenital deformity of elbow
        Congenital deformity of forearm
        Congenital deformity of scapula
        Congenital deformity of wrist
        Congenital dislocation of elbow
        Congenital dislocation of shoulder
        Congenital dislocation of wrist
- 4th Q69 Polydactyly
    Q69.0 **Accessory** finger(s) POA
    Q69.1 **Accessory** thumb(s) POA
    Q69.2 **Accessory** toe(s) POA
        Accessory hallux
    Q69.9 **Polydactyly, unspecified** POA
        Supernumerary digit(s) NOS
- 4th Q70 Syndactyly
    - 5th Q70.0 Fused fingers
        Complex syndactyly of fingers with synostosis
        Q70.00 **Fused fingers, unspecified hand** POA
        Q70.01 **Fused fingers,** right **hand** POA
        Q70.02 **Fused fingers,** left **hand** POA
        Q70.03 **Fused fingers,** bilateral POA
    - 5th Q70.1 Webbed fingers
        Simple syndactyly of fingers without synostosis
        Q70.10 **Webbed fingers, unspecified hand** POA
        Q70.11 **Webbed fingers,** right **hand** POA
        Q70.12 **Webbed fingers,** left **hand** POA
        Q70.13 **Webbed fingers,** bilateral POA
    - 5th Q70.2 Fused toes
        Complex syndactyly of toes with synostosis
        Q70.20 **Fused toes, unspecified foot** POA
        Q70.21 **Fused toes,** right **foot** POA
        Q70.22 **Fused toes,** left **foot** POA
        Q70.23 **Fused toes,** bilateral POA
    - 5th Q70.3 Webbed toes
        Simple syndactyly of toes without synostosis
        Q70.30 **Webbed toes, unspecified foot** POA
        Q70.31 **Webbed toes,** right **foot** POA
        Q70.32 **Webbed toes,** left **foot** POA
        Q70.33 **Webbed toes,** bilateral POA

Unspecified Code	Other Specified Code	Manifestation Code	N Newborn	P Pediatric	M Maternity	A Adult	♂ Male	♀ Female

● New Code   ▲ Revised Code Title   ►◄ Revised Text   **NOTES**   *INCLUDES*   EXCLUDES1 Not coded here   EXCLUDES2 Not included here
4th 4th character required   5th 5th character required   6th 6th character required   7th 7th character required   Extension 'X' Alert
HAC Hospital-acquired condition (HAC) alert   **AHA** AHA Coding Clinic©   📖 Code first alert

Q70.4 Polysyndactyly, unspecified
> EXCLUDES1 specified syndactyly of hand and feet - code to specified conditions (Q70.0- -Q70.3-)

Q70.9 Syndactyly, unspecified
Symphalangy NOS

4ᵗʰ **Q71 Reduction defects of upper limb**

5ᵗʰ **Q71.0 Congenital complete absence of upper limb**
Q71.00 Congenital complete absence of unspecified upper limb
Q71.01 Congenital complete absence of right upper limb
Q71.02 Congenital complete absence of left upper limb
Q71.03 Congenital complete absence of upper limb, bilateral

5ᵗʰ **Q71.1 Congenital absence of upper arm and forearm with hand present**
Q71.10 Congenital absence of unspecified upper arm and forearm with hand present
Q71.11 Congenital absence of right upper arm and forearm with hand present
Q71.12 Congenital absence of left upper arm and forearm with hand present
Q71.13 Congenital absence of upper arm and forearm with hand present, bilateral

5ᵗʰ **Q71.2 Congenital absence of both forearm and hand**
Q71.20 Congenital absence of both forearm and hand, unspecified upper limb
Q71.21 Congenital absence of both forearm and hand, right upper limb
Q71.22 Congenital absence of both forearm and hand, left upper limb
Q71.23 Congenital absence of both forearm and hand, bilateral

5ᵗʰ **Q71.3 Congenital absence of hand and finger**
Q71.30 Congenital absence of unspecified hand and finger
Q71.31 Congenital absence of right hand and finger
Q71.32 Congenital absence of left hand and finger
Q71.33 Congenital absence of hand and finger, bilateral

5ᵗʰ **Q71.4 Longitudinal reduction defect of radius**
Clubhand (congenital)
Radial clubhand
Q71.40 Longitudinal reduction defect of unspecified radius
Q71.41 Longitudinal reduction defect of right radius
Q71.42 Longitudinal reduction defect of left radius
Q71.43 Longitudinal reduction defect of radius, bilateral

5ᵗʰ **Q71.5 Longitudinal reduction defect of ulna**
Q71.50 Longitudinal reduction defect of unspecified ulna
Q71.51 Longitudinal reduction defect of right ulna
Q71.52 Longitudinal reduction defect of left ulna
Q71.53 Longitudinal reduction defect of ulna, bilateral

5ᵗʰ **Q71.6 Lobster-claw hand**
Q71.60 Lobster-claw hand, unspecified hand
Q71.61 Lobster-claw right hand
Q71.62 Lobster-claw left hand
Q71.63 Lobster-claw hand, bilateral

5ᵗʰ **Q71.8 Other reduction defects of upper limb**
6ᵗʰ **Q71.81 Congenital shortening of upper limb**
Q71.811 Congenital shortening of right upper limb
Q71.812 Congenital shortening of left upper limb
Q71.813 Congenital shortening of upper limb, bilateral
Q71.819 Congenital shortening of unspecified upper limb
6ᵗʰ **Q71.89 Other reduction defects of upper limb**
Q71.891 Other reduction defects of right upper limb
Q71.892 Other reduction defects of left upper limb

Q71.893 Other reduction defects of upper limb, bilateral
Q71.899 Other reduction defects of unspecified upper limb

5ᵗʰ **Q71.9 Unspecified reduction defect of upper limb**
Q71.90 Unspecified reduction defect of unspecified upper limb
Q71.91 Unspecified reduction defect of right upper limb
Q71.92 Unspecified reduction defect of left upper limb
Q71.93 Unspecified reduction defect of upper limb, bilateral

4ᵗʰ **Q72 Reduction defects of lower limb**

5ᵗʰ **Q72.0 Congenital complete absence of lower limb**
Q72.00 Congenital complete absence of unspecified lower limb
Q72.01 Congenital complete absence of right lower limb
Q72.02 Congenital complete absence of left lower limb
Q72.03 Congenital complete absence of lower limb, bilateral

5ᵗʰ **Q72.1 Congenital absence of thigh and lower leg with foot present**
Q72.10 Congenital absence of unspecified thigh and lower leg with foot present
Q72.11 Congenital absence of right thigh and lower leg with foot present
Q72.12 Congenital absence of left thigh and lower leg with foot present
Q72.13 Congenital absence of thigh and lower leg with foot present, bilateral

5ᵗʰ **Q72.2 Congenital absence of both lower leg and foot**
Q72.20 Congenital absence of both lower leg and foot, unspecified lower limb
Q72.21 Congenital absence of both lower leg and foot, right lower limb
Q72.22 Congenital absence of both lower leg and foot, left lower limb
Q72.23 Congenital absence of both lower leg and foot, bilateral

5ᵗʰ **Q72.3 Congenital absence of foot and toe(s)**
Q72.30 Congenital absence of unspecified foot and toe(s)
Q72.31 Congenital absence of right foot and toe(s)
Q72.32 Congenital absence of left foot and toe(s)
Q72.33 Congenital absence of foot and toe(s), bilateral

5ᵗʰ **Q72.4 Longitudinal reduction defect of femur**
Proximal femoral focal deficiency
Q72.40 Longitudinal reduction defect of unspecified femur
Q72.41 Longitudinal reduction defect of right femur
Q72.42 Longitudinal reduction defect of left femur
Q72.43 Longitudinal reduction defect of femur, bilateral

5ᵗʰ **Q72.5 Longitudinal reduction defect of tibia**
Q72.50 Longitudinal reduction defect of unspecified tibia
Q72.51 Longitudinal reduction defect of right tibia
Q72.52 Longitudinal reduction defect of left tibia
Q72.53 Longitudinal reduction defect of tibia, bilateral

5ᵗʰ **Q72.6 Longitudinal reduction defect of fibula**
Q72.60 Longitudinal reduction defect of unspecified fibula
Q72.61 Longitudinal reduction defect of right fibula
Q72.62 Longitudinal reduction defect of left fibula
Q72.63 Longitudinal reduction defect of fibula, bilateral

5ᵗʰ **Q72.7 Split foot**
Q72.70 Split foot, unspecified lower limb
Q72.71 Split foot, right lower limb
Q72.72 Split foot, left lower limb
Q72.73 Split foot, bilateral

5ᵗʰ **Q72.8 Other reduction defects of lower limb**
6ᵗʰ **Q72.81 Congenital shortening of lower limb**
Q72.811 Congenital shortening of right lower limb
Q72.812 Congenital shortening of left lower limb

POA̲ Unacceptable principal diagnosis symbol per Medicare code edits   POA̲ Code exempt from diagnosis present on admission requirement
❓ Questionable admission   CC Complication or comorbidity   MCC Major complication or comorbidity   CC/MCC EXC CC/MCC exclusion
HCC HCC diagnosis code   RxHCC RxHCC diagnosis code   MACRA code   **DEFINITION** Describes condition/terminology
TIP Coding guidance   👁 Official Guideline Reference   Z1 Z code as first-listed diagnosis

942   When symbols appear on a code that requires a 7th character extension, refer to Appendix B to identify applicable 7th character codes.   **2020 ICD-10-CM**

Q72.813 **Congenital shortening of lower limb,** bilateral POA

Q72.819 **Congenital shortening of unspecified** lower limb POA

🔯 Q72.89 Other **reduction defects of** lower limb

Q72.891 **Other reduction defects of** right **lower** limb POA

Q72.892 **Other reduction defects of** left **lower** limb POA

Q72.893 **Other reduction defects of lower limb,** bilateral POA

Q72.899 **Other reduction defects of unspecified** lower limb POA

🔯 Q72.9 **Unspecified reduction defect of** lower limb

Q72.90 **Unspecified reduction defect of unspecified** lower limb POA

Q72.91 **Unspecified reduction defect of** right **lower limb** POA

Q72.92 **Unspecified reduction defect of** left **lower limb** POA

Q72.93 **Unspecified reduction defect of lower limb,** bilateral POA

🔯 Q73 **Reduction defects of** unspecified limb

Q73.0 **Congenital absence of unspecified limb(s)** POA
Amelia NOS

Q73.1 Phocomelia, **unspecified limb(s)** POA
Phocomelia NOS

Q73.8 Other reduction defects **of unspecified limb(s)** POA
Longitudinal reduction deformity of unspecified limb(s)
Ectromelia of limb NOS
Hemimelia of limb NOS
Reduction defect of limb NOS

🔯 Q74 Other **congenital malformations of** limb(s)

EXCLUDES1 polydactyly (Q69.-)
reduction defect of limb (Q71-Q73)
syndactyly (Q70.-)

Q74.0 **Other congenital malformations of** upper limb(s), including shoulder girdle POA
Accessory carpal bones
Cleidocranial dysostosis
Congenital pseudarthrosis of clavicle
Macrodactylia (fingers)
Madelung's deformity
Radioulnar synostosis
Sprengel's deformity
Triphalangeal thumb

Q74.1 **Congenital malformation of** knee POA
Congenital absence of patella
Congenital dislocation of patella
Congenital genu valgum
Congenital genu varum
Rudimentary patella
EXCLUDES1 congenital dislocation of knee (Q68.2)
congenital genu recurvatum (Q68.2)
nail patella syndrome (Q87.2)

Q74.2 **Other congenital malformations of** lower limb(s), including pelvic girdle POA
Congenital fusion of sacroiliac joint
Congenital malformation of ankle joint
Congenital malformation of sacroiliac joint
EXCLUDES1 anteversion of femur (neck) (Q65.89)

Q74.3 Arthrogryposis multiplex **congenita** CC POA CC/MCC Exc

Q74.8 **Other specified congenital malformations of limb(s)** POA

Q74.9 **Unspecified congenital malformation of limb(s)** POA
Congenital anomaly of limb(s) NOS

🔯 Q75 Other **congenital malformations of** skull and face bones
EXCLUDES1 congenital malformation of face NOS (Q18.-)
congenital malformation syndromes classified to Q87.-
dentofacial anomalies [including malocclusion] (M26.-)

musculoskeletal deformities of head and face (Q67.0-Q67.4)
skull defects associated with congenital anomalies of brain such as:
anencephaly (Q00.0)
encephalocele (Q01.-)
hydrocephalus (Q03.-)
microcephaly (Q02)

Q75.0 **Craniosynostosis** POA
Acrocephaly
Imperfect fusion of skull
Oxycephaly
Trigonocephaly

Q75.1 **Craniofacial dysostosis** POA
Crouzon's disease

Q75.2 **Hypertelorism** POA

Q75.3 **Macrocephaly** POA

Q75.4 **Mandibulofacial dysostosis** POA
Franceschetti syndrome
Treacher Collins syndrome

Q75.5 **Oculomandibular dysostosis** POA

Q75.8 **Other specified congenital malformations of skull and face bones** POA
Absence of skull bone, congenital
Congenital deformity of forehead
Platybasia

Q75.9 **Congenital malformation of skull and face bones, unspecified** POA
Congenital anomaly of face bones NOS
Congenital anomaly of skull NOS

🔯 Q76 **Congenital malformations of** spine and bony thorax
EXCLUDES1 congenital musculoskeletal deformities of spine and chest (Q67.5-Q67.8)

Q76.0 **Spina bifida occulta** POA
EXCLUDES1 meningocele (spinal) (Q05.-)
spina bifida (aperta) (cystica) (Q05.-)

Q76.1 **Klippel-Feil syndrome** POA
Cervical fusion syndrome

Q76.2 **Congenital spondylolisthesis** POA
Congenital spondylolysis
EXCLUDES1 spondylolisthesis (acquired) (M43.1-)
spondylolysis (acquired) (M43.0-)

Q76.3 **Congenital scoliosis due to congenital bony malformation** CC POA CC/MCC Exc
Hemivertebra fusion or failure of segmentation with scoliosis

🔯 Q76.4 Other **congenital malformations of** spine, not associated with scoliosis

🔯 Q76.41 **Congenital** kyphosis

Q76.411 **Congenital kyphosis,** occipito-atlanto-axial **region** POA

Q76.412 **Congenital kyphosis,** cervical **region** POA

Q76.413 **Congenital kyphosis,** cervicothoracic **region** POA

Q76.414 **Congenital kyphosis,** thoracic **region** POA

Q76.415 **Congenital kyphosis,** thoracolumbar **region** POA

Q76.419 **Congenital kyphosis, unspecified region** POA

🔯 Q76.42 **Congenital** lordosis

Q76.425 **Congenital lordosis,** thoracolumbar **region** CC POA CC/MCC Exc

Q76.426 **Congenital lordosis,** lumbar **region** CC POA CC/MCC Exc

Q76.427 **Congenital lordosis,** lumbosacral **region** CC POA CC/MCC Exc

Q76.428 **Congenital lordosis,** sacral and sacrococcygeal **region** CC POA CC/MCC Exc

Q76.429 **Congenital lordosis, unspecified region** CC POA CC/MCC Exc

Unspecified Code   Other Specified Code   Manifestation Code   🅽 Newborn   🅿 Pediatric   🅼 Maternity   🅰 Adult   ♂ Male   ♀ Female
● New Code   ▲ Revised Code Title   ►◄ Revised Text   **NOTES**   INCLUDES   EXCLUDES1 Not coded here   EXCLUDES2 Not included here
🔯 4ᵗʰ character required   🔯 5ᵗʰ character required   🔯 6ᵗʰ character required   🔯 7ᵗʰ character required   🔯 Extension 'X' Alert
HAC Hospital-acquired condition (HAC) alert   **AHA** AHA Coding Clinic©   📣 Code first alert

2020 ICD-10-CM   When symbols appear on a code that requires a 7th character extension, refer to Appendix B to identify applicable 7th character codes.   **943**

Q76.49 **Other congenital malformations of spine, not associated with scoliosis** POA
  Congenital absence of vertebra NOS
  Congenital fusion of spine NOS
  Congenital malformation of lumbosacral (joint) (region) NOS
  Congenital malformation of spine NOS
  Hemivertebra NOS
  Malformation of spine NOS
  Platyspondylisis NOS
  Supernumerary vertebra NOS

Q76.5 Cervical rib POA
  Supernumerary rib in cervical region

Q76.6 **Other congenital malformations of** ribs CC POA CC/MCC Exc
  Accessory rib
  Congenital absence of rib
  Congenital fusion of ribs
  Congenital malformation of ribs NOS
  EXCLUDES1 short rib syndrome (Q77.2)

Q76.7 **Congenital malformation of** sternum CC POA CC/MCC Exc
  Congenital absence of sternum
  Sternum bifidum

Q76.8 **Other congenital malformations of** bony thorax CC POA CC/MCC Exc

Q76.9 **Congenital malformation of bony thorax, unspecified** CC POA CC/MCC Exc

Q77 **Osteochondrodysplasia with defects of growth of tubular bones and spine**
  EXCLUDES1 mucopolysaccharidosis (E76.0-E76.3)
  EXCLUDES2 congenital myotonic chondrodystrophy (G71.13)

Q77.0 **Achondrogenesis** POA
  Hypochondrogenesis

Q77.1 **Thanatophoric short stature** POA

Q77.2 **Short rib syndrome** CC POA CC/MCC Exc
  Asphyxiating thoracic dysplasia [Jeune]

Q77.3 **Chondrodysplasia punctata** POA
  EXCLUDES1 Rhizomelic chondrodysplasia punctata (E71.43)

Q77.4 **Achondroplasia** POA
  Hypochondroplasia
  Osteosclerosis congenita

Q77.5 **Diastrophic dysplasia** POA

Q77.6 **Chondroectodermal dysplasia** POA
  Ellis-van Creveld syndrome

Q77.7 **Spondyloepiphyseal dysplasia** POA

Q77.8 **Other osteochondrodysplasia with defects of growth of tubular bones and spine** POA

Q77.9 **Osteochondrodysplasia with defects of growth of tubular bones and spine, unspecified** POA

Q78 Other **osteochondrodysplasias**
  EXCLUDES2 congenital myotonic chondrodystrophy (G71.13)

Q78.0 **Osteogenesis imperfecta** CC POA CC/MCC Exc
  Fragilitas ossium
  Osteopsathyrosis

Q78.1 **Polyostotic fibrous dysplasia** POA
  Albright(-McCune)(-Sternberg) syndrome

Q78.2 **Osteopetrosis** CC POA CC/MCC Exc
  Albers-Schönberg syndrome
  Osteosclerosis NOS

Q78.3 **Progressive diaphyseal dysplasia** POA
  Camurati-Engelmann syndrome

Q78.4 **Enchondromatosis** POA
  Maffucci's syndrome
  Ollier's disease

Q78.5 **Metaphyseal dysplasia** POA
  Pyle's syndrome

Q78.6 **Multiple congenital exostoses** POA
  Diaphyseal aclasis

Q78.8 Other specified **osteochondrodysplasias** POA
  Osteopoikilosis

Q78.9 **Osteochondrodysplasia, unspecified** POA
  Chondrodystrophy NOS
  Osteodystrophy NOS

Q79 **Congenital malformations of musculoskeletal system, not elsewhere classified**
  EXCLUDES2 congenital (sternomastoid) torticollis (Q68.0)

Q79.0 **Congenital diaphragmatic hernia** POA MCC CC/MCC Exc
  EXCLUDES1 congenital hiatus hernia (Q40.1)

Q79.1 **Other congenital malformations of diaphragm** POA MCC CC/MCC Exc
  Absence of diaphragm
  Congenital malformation of diaphragm NOS
  Eventration of diaphragm

Q79.2 **Exomphalos** POA MCC CC/MCC Exc
  Omphalocele
  EXCLUDES1 umbilical hernia (K42.-)

Q79.3 **Gastroschisis** POA MCC CC/MCC Exc

Q79.4 **Prune belly syndrome** CC POA CC/MCC Exc
  Congenital prolapse of bladder mucosa
  Eagle-Barrett syndrome

Q79.5 Other **congenital malformations of** abdominal wall
  EXCLUDES1 umbilical hernia (K42.-)

  Q79.51 **Congenital hernia of bladder** CC POA CC/MCC Exc

  Q79.59 **Other congenital malformations of abdominal wall** CC POA CC/MCC Exc

▲ Q79.6 Ehlers-Danlos ▶syndromes◀

  ● Q79.60 **Ehlers-Danlos syndrome, unspecified** POA

  ● Q79.61 Classical **Ehlers-Danlos syndrome** POA
    Classical EDS (cEDS)

  ● Q79.62 Hypermobile **Ehlers-Danlos syndrome** POA
    Hypermobile EDS (hEDS)

  ● Q79.63 Vascular **Ehlers-Danlos syndrome** POA
    Vascular EDS (vEDS)

  ● Q79.69 Other **Ehlers-Danlos syndromes** POA

Q79.8 **Other congenital malformations of musculoskeletal system** POA
  Absence of muscle
  Absence of tendon
  Accessory muscle
  Amyotrophia congenita
  Congenital constricting bands
  Congenital shortening of tendon
  Poland syndrome

Q79.9 **Congenital malformation of musculoskeletal system, unspecified** POA
  Congenital anomaly of musculoskeletal system NOS
  Congenital deformity of musculoskeletal system NOS

Other congenital malformations (Q80-Q89)

Q80 **Congenital ichthyosis**
  EXCLUDES1 Refsum's disease (G60.1)

Q80.0 **Ichthyosis** vulgaris POA

Q80.1 X-linked **ichthyosis** POA

Q80.2 Lamellar **ichthyosis** POA
  Collodion baby

Q80.3 **Congenital** bullous **ichthyosiform erythroderma** POA

Q80.4 **Harlequin fetus** POA

Q80.8 **Other congenital ichthyosis** POA

Q80.9 **Congenital ichthyosis, unspecified** POA

Q81 **Epidermolysis bullosa**

Q81.0 **Epidermolysis bullosa** simplex POA
  EXCLUDES1 Cockayne's syndrome ▶(Q87.19)◀

Q81.1 **Epidermolysis bullosa** letalis POA
  Herlitz' syndrome

Q81.2 **Epidermolysis bullosa** dystrophica POA

Q81.8 **Other epidermolysis bullosa** POA

Q81.9 **Epidermolysis bullosa, unspecified** POA

Q82 Other **congenital malformations of** skin
  EXCLUDES1 acrodermatitis enteropathica (E83.2)
    congenital erythropoietic porphyria (E80.0)
    pilonidal cyst or sinus (L05.-)
    Sturge-Weber (-Dimitri) syndrome (Q85.8)

Q82.0 **Hereditary lymphedema** POA

POA Unacceptable principal diagnosis symbol per Medicare code edits POA Code exempt from diagnosis present on admission requirement
❓ Questionable admission CC Complication or comorbidity MCC Major complication or comorbidity CC/MCC Exc CC/MCC exclusion
HCC HCC diagnosis code RxHCC RxHCC diagnosis code MACRA MACRA code **DEFINITION** Describes condition/terminology
TIP Coding guidance 👁 Official Guideline Reference Z1 Z code as first-listed diagnosis

944 When symbols appear on a code that requires a 7th character extension, refer to Appendix B to identify applicable 7th character codes. **2020 ICD-10-CM**

Q82.1 **Xeroderma pigmentosum** [POA]
Q82.2 **Congenital cutaneous mastocytosis** [POA]
AHA: Q4 2017
Congenital diffuse cutaneous mastocytosis
Congenital maculopapular cutaneous mastocytosis
Congenital urticaria pigmentosa
[EXCLUDES1] *cutaneous mastocytosis NOS (D47.01)*
diffuse cutaneous mastocytosis (with onset after newborn period) (D47.01)
malignant mastocytosis (C96.2-)
systemic mastocytosis (D47.02)
urticaria pigmentosa (non-congenital) (with onset after newborn period) (D47.01)
Q82.3 **Incontinentia pigmenti** [POA]
Q82.4 **Ectodermal dysplasia (anhidrotic)** [POA]
[EXCLUDES1] *Ellis-van Creveld syndrome (Q77.6)*
Q82.5 **Congenital non-neoplastic nevus** [POA]
Birthmark NOS
Flammeus Nevus
Portwine Nevus
Sanguineous Nevus
Strawberry Nevus
Vascular Nevus NOS
Verrucous Nevus
[EXCLUDES2] *Café au lait spots (L81.3)*
lentigo (L81.4)
nevus NOS (D22.-)
araneus nevus (I78.1)
melanocytic nevus (D22.-)
pigmented nevus (D22.-)
spider nevus (I78.1)
stellar nevus (I78.1)
Q82.6 **Congenital sacral dimple** [POA]
AHA: Q4 2016
Parasacral dimple
[EXCLUDES2] *pilonidal cyst with abscess (L05.01)*
pilonidal cyst without abscess (L05.91)
Q82.8 **Other specified congenital malformations of skin** [POA]
AHA: Q1 2016
Abnormal palmar creases
Accessory skin tags
Benign familial pemphigus [Hailey-Hailey]
Congenital poikiloderma
Cutis laxa (hyperelastica)
Dermatoglyphic anomalies
Inherited keratosis palmaris et plantaris
Keratosis follicularis [Darier-White]
[EXCLUDES1] *Ehlers-Danlos syndrome ▶(Q79.6-)◀*
Q82.9 **Congenital malformation of skin, unspecified** [POA]

[4th] Q83 **Congenital malformations of breast**
[EXCLUDES2] *absence of pectoral muscle (Q79.8)*
hypoplasia of breast (N64.82)
micromastia (N64.82)
Q83.0 **Congenital absence of breast with absent nipple** [POA]
Q83.1 **Accessory breast** [POA]
Supernumerary breast
Q83.2 **Absent nipple** [POA]
Q83.3 **Accessory nipple** [POA]
Supernumerary nipple
Q83.8 **Other congenital malformations of breast** [POA]
Q83.9 **Congenital malformation of breast, unspecified** [POA]

[4th] Q84 **Other congenital malformations of integument**
Q84.0 **Congenital alopecia** [POA]
Congenital atrichosis
Q84.1 **Congenital morphological disturbances of hair, not elsewhere classified** [POA]
Beaded hair
Monilethrix
Pili annulati
[EXCLUDES1] *Menkes' kinky hair syndrome (E83.0)*
Q84.2 **Other congenital malformations of hair** [POA]
Congenital hypertrichosis
Congenital malformation of hair NOS
Persistent lanugo
Q84.3 **Anonychia** [POA]
[EXCLUDES1] *nail patella syndrome (Q87.2)*
Q84.4 **Congenital leukonychia** [POA]
Q84.5 **Enlarged and hypertrophic nails** [POA]
Congenital onychauxis
Pachyonychia
Q84.6 **Other congenital malformations of nails** [POA]
Congenital clubnail
Congenital koilonychia
Congenital malformation of nail NOS
Q84.8 **Other specified congenital malformations of integument** [POA]
Aplasia cutis congenita
Q84.9 **Congenital malformation of integument, unspecified** [POA]
Congenital anomaly of integument NOS
Congenital deformity of integument NOS

[4th] Q85 **Phakomatoses, not elsewhere classified**
[EXCLUDES1] *ataxia telangiectasia [Louis-Bar] (G11.3)*
familial dysautonomia [Riley-Day] (G90.1)
[5th] Q85.0 **Neurofibromatosis (nonmalignant)**
Q85.00 **Neurofibromatosis, unspecified** [POA] [HCC]
Q85.01 **Neurofibromatosis, type 1** [POA] [HCC]
Von Recklinghausen disease
Q85.02 **Neurofibromatosis, type 2** [POA] [HCC]
Acoustic neurofibromatosis
Q85.03 **Schwannomatosis** [POA] [HCC]
Q85.09 **Other neurofibromatosis** [POA] [HCC]
Q85.1 **Tuberous sclerosis** [CC] [POA] [HCC] [RxHCC] [CC/MCC Exc]
Bourneville's disease
Epiloia
Q85.8 **Other phakomatoses, not elsewhere classified** [CC] [POA] [HCC] [RxHCC] [CC/MCC Exc]
Peutz-Jeghers Syndrome
Sturge-Weber(-Dimitri) syndrome
von Hippel-Lindau syndrome
[EXCLUDES1] *Meckel-Gruber syndrome (Q61.9)*
Q85.9 **Phakomatosis, unspecified** [CC] [POA] [HCC] [RxHCC] [CC/MCC Exc]
Hamartosis NOS

[4th] Q86 **Congenital malformation syndromes due to known exogenous causes, not elsewhere classified**
[EXCLUDES2] *iodine-deficiency-related hypothyroidism (E00-E02)*
nonteratogenic effects of substances transmitted via placenta or breast milk (P04.-)
Q86.0 **Fetal alcohol syndrome (dysmorphic)** [POA]
Q86.1 **Fetal hydantoin syndrome** [POA]
Meadow's syndrome
Q86.2 **Dysmorphism due to warfarin** [POA]
Q86.8 **Other congenital malformation syndromes due to known exogenous causes** [POA]

[4th] Q87 **Other specified congenital malformation syndromes affecting multiple systems**
Use additional code(s) to identify all associated manifestations
Q87.0 **Congenital malformation syndromes predominantly affecting facial appearance** [POA]
Acrocephalopolysyndactyly
Acrocephalosyndactyly [Apert]
Cryptophthalmos syndrome
Cyclopia
Goldenhar syndrome
Moebius syndrome
Oro-facial-digital syndrome
Robin syndrome
Whistling face
[5th] Q87.1 **Congenital malformation syndromes predominantly associated with short stature**
[EXCLUDES1] *Ellis-van Creveld syndrome (Q77.6)*
Smith-Lemli-Opitz syndrome (E78.72)
● Q87.11 **Prader-Willi syndrome** [POA]

Unspecified Code Other Specified Code Manifestation Code [N] Newborn [P] Pediatric [M] Maternity [A] Adult ♂ Male ♀ Female
● New Code ▲ Revised Code Title ▶◀ Revised Text [NOTES] [INCLUDES] [EXCLUDES1] Not coded here [EXCLUDES2] Not included here
[4th] 4th character required [5th] 5th character required [6th] 6th character required [7th] 7th character required [7th] Extension 'X' Alert
[HAC] Hospital-acquired condition (HAC) alert AHA AHA Coding Clinic© Code first alert

● **Q87.19 Other congenital** malformation **syndromes predominantly associated with short stature** POA
Aarskog syndrome
Cockayne syndrome
De Lange syndrome
Dubowitz syndrome
Noonan syndrome
Robinow-Silverman-Smith syndrome
Russell-Silver syndrome
Seckel syndrome

Q87.2 Congenital malformation syndromes predominantly involving limbs POA
Holt-Oram syndrome
Klippel-Trenaunay-Weber syndrome
Nail patella syndrome
Rubinstein-Taybi syndrome
Sirenomelia syndrome
Thrombocytopenia with absent radius [TAR] syndrome
VATER syndrome

Q87.3 Congenital malformation syndromes involving early overgrowth POA
Beckwith-Wiedemann syndrome
Sotos syndrome
Weaver syndrome

5ᵗʰ **Q87.4 Marfan's syndrome**
Q87.40 Marfan's syndrome, unspecified CC POA RxHCC
6ᵗʰ **Q87.41 Marfan's syndrome with** cardiovascular manifestations
Q87.410 Marfan's syndrome with aortic dilation CC POA RxHCC
Q87.418 Marfan's syndrome with other cardiovascular manifestations CC POA RxHCC
Q87.42 Marfan's syndrome with ocular manifestations CC POA RxHCC
Q87.43 Marfan's syndrome with skeletal manifestation CC POA RxHCC

Q87.5 Other congenital malformation syndromes with other skeletal changes CC POA

5ᵗʰ **Q87.8 Other specified congenital malformation syndromes, not elsewhere classified**
EXCLUDES1 Zellweger syndrome (E71.510)
Q87.81 Alport syndrome POA
Use additional code to identify stage of chronic kidney disease (N18.1-N18.6)
Q87.82 Arterial tortuosity syndrome POA RxHCC
AHA: Q4 2016
Q87.89 Other specified congenital malformation syndromes, not elsewhere classified POA
Laurence-Moon (-Bardet)-Biedl syndrome

4ᵗʰ **Q89 Other** congenital malformations, not elsewhere classified
5ᵗʰ **Q89.0 Congenital absence and malformations of** spleen
EXCLUDES1 isomerism of atrial appendages (with asplenia or polysplenia) (Q20.6)
Q89.01 Asplenia (congenital) POA
Q89.09 Congenital malformations of spleen POA
Congenital splenomegaly
Q89.1 Congenital malformations of adrenal gland POA
EXCLUDES1 adrenogenital disorders (E25.-)
congenital adrenal hyperplasia (E25.0)
Q89.2 Congenital malformations of other endocrine glands POA
Congenital malformation of parathyroid or thyroid gland
Persistent thyroglossal duct
Thyroglossal cyst
EXCLUDES1 congenital goiter (E03.0)
congenital hypothyroidism (E03.1)
Q89.3 Situs inversus POA
Dextrocardia with situs inversus
Mirror-image atrial arrangement with situs inversus
Situs inversus or transversus abdominalis
Situs inversus or transversus thoracis
Transposition of abdominal viscera
Transposition of thoracic viscera

EXCLUDES1 dextrocardia NOS (Q24.0)
Q89.4 Conjoined twins POA MCC CC/MCC Exc
Craniopagus
Dicephaly
Pygopagus
Thoracopagus
Q89.7 Multiple congenital malformations, not elsewhere classified POA
Multiple congenital anomalies NOS
Multiple congenital deformities NOS
EXCLUDES1 congenital malformation syndromes affecting multiple systems (Q87.-)
Q89.8 Other specified congenital malformations POA
Use additional code(s) to identify all associated manifestations
Q89.9 Congenital malformation, unspecified POA
Congenital anomaly NOS
Congenital deformity NOS

Chromosomal abnormalities, not elsewhere classified (Q90-Q99)

EXCLUDES2 mitochondrial metabolic disorders (E88.4-)
4ᵗʰ **Q90 Down syndrome**
Use additional code(s) to identify any associated physical conditions and degree of intellectual disabilities (F70-F79)
Q90.0 Trisomy 21, nonmosaicism **(meiotic nondisjunction)** POA
Q90.1 Trisomy 21, mosaicism **(mitotic nondisjunction)** POA
Q90.2 Trisomy 21, translocation POA
Q90.9 Down syndrome, unspecified POA
Trisomy 21 NOS
4ᵗʰ **Q91 Trisomy 18 and Trisomy 13**
Q91.0 Trisomy 18, nonmosaicism **(meiotic nondisjunction)** POA RxHCC
Q91.1 Trisomy 18, mosaicism **(mitotic nondisjunction)** POA RxHCC
Q91.2 Trisomy 18, translocation POA RxHCC
Q91.3 Trisomy 18, unspecified POA RxHCC
Q91.4 Trisomy 13, nonmosaicism **(meiotic nondisjunction)** POA RxHCC
Q91.5 Trisomy 13, mosaicism **(mitotic nondisjunction)** POA RxHCC
Q91.6 Trisomy 13, translocation POA RxHCC
Q91.7 Trisomy 13, unspecified POA RxHCC
4ᵗʰ **Q92 Other** trisomies and partial trisomies of the autosomes, not elsewhere classified
INCLUDES unbalanced translocations and insertions
EXCLUDES1 trisomies of chromosomes 13, 18, 21 (Q90-Q91)
Q92.0 Whole chromosome trisomy, nonmosaicism **(meiotic nondisjunction)** POA RxHCC
Q92.1 Whole chromosome trisomy, mosaicism **(mitotic nondisjunction)** POA RxHCC
Q92.2 Partial trisomy POA RxHCC
Less than whole arm duplicated
Whole arm or more duplicated
EXCLUDES1 partial trisomy due to unbalanced translocation (Q92.5)
Q92.5 Duplications with other complex rearrangements POA RxHCC
Partial trisomy due to unbalanced translocations
Code also any associated deletions due to unbalanced translocations, inversions and insertions (Q93.7)
5ᵗʰ **Q92.6 Marker chromosomes**
Trisomies due to dicentrics
Trisomies due to extra rings
Trisomies due to isochromosomes
Individual with marker heterochromatin
Q92.61 Marker chromosomes in normal **individual** POA RxHCC
Q92.62 Marker chromosomes in abnormal **individual** POA RxHCC
Q92.7 Triploidy and polyploidy POA RxHCC
Q92.8 Other specified trisomies and partial trisomies of autosomes POA RxHCC
Duplications identified by fluorescence in situ hybridization (FISH)
Duplications identified by in situ hybridization (ISH)
Duplications seen only at prometaphase
Q92.9 Trisomy and partial trisomy of autosomes, unspecified POA RxHCC

POA Unacceptable principal diagnosis symbol per Medicare code edits   POA Code exempt from diagnosis present on admission requirement
❓ Questionable admission   CC Complication or comorbidity   MCC Major complication or comorbidity   CC/MCC Exc CC/MCC exclusion
HCC HCC diagnosis code   RxHCC RxHCC diagnosis code   MACRA code   **DEFINITION** Describes condition/terminology
TIP Coding guidance   👁 Official Guideline Reference   Z1 Z code as first-listed diagnosis

4ᵗʰ **Q93 Monosomies and deletions from the autosomes, not elsewhere classified**

Q93.0 Whole **chromosome monosomy,** nonmosaicism **(meiotic nondisjunction)** `POA` `RxHCC`

Q93.1 Whole **chromosome monosomy,** mosaicism **(mitotic nondisjunction)** `POA` `RxHCC`

Q93.2 Chromosome replaced with ring, **dicentric or isochromosome** `POA` `RxHCC`

Q93.3 Deletion of short arm of chromosome 4 `POA` `RxHCC`
Wolff-Hirschorn syndrome

Q93.4 Deletion of short arm of chromosome 5
Cri-du-chat syndrome

5ᵗʰ **Q93.5 Other deletions of** part of a chromosome

Q93.51 Angelman **syndrome** `CC` `POA` `RxHCC` `CC/MCC Exc`
AHA: Q4 2018

Q93.59 Other deletions of part of a chromosome `CC` `POA` `RxHCC` `CC/MCC Exc`
AHA: Q4 2018

Q93.7 Deletions with other complex rearrangements `POA` `RxHCC`
Deletions due to unbalanced translocations, inversions and insertions
Code also any associated duplications due to unbalanced translocations, inversions and insertions (Q92.5)

5ᵗʰ **Q93.8 Other deletions from the autosomes**

Q93.81 Velo-cardio-facial syndrome `CC` `POA` `RxHCC` `CC/MCC Exc`
Deletion 22q11.2

Q93.82 Williams **syndrome** `CC` `POA` `RxHCC` `CC/MCC Exc`
AHA: Q4 2018

Q93.88 Other microdeletions `CC` `POA` `RxHCC` `CC/MCC Exc`
Miller-Dieker syndrome
Smith-Magenis syndrome

Q93.89 Other deletions from the autosomes `CC` `POA` `RxHCC` `CC/MCC Exc`
Deletions identified by fluorescence in situ hybridization (FISH)
Deletions identified by in situ hybridization (ISH)
Deletions seen only at prometaphase

Q93.9 Deletion from autosomes, unspecified `CC` `POA` `RxHCC` `CC/MCC Exc`

4ᵗʰ **Q95 Balanced rearrangements and structural markers, not elsewhere classified**

INCLUDES Robertsonian and balanced reciprocal translocations and insertions

Q95.0 Balanced translocation and insertion in normal **individual** `POA`

Q95.1 Chromosome inversion in normal **individual** `POA`

Q95.2 Balanced autosomal rearrangement in abnormal **individual** `POA` `RxHCC`

Q95.3 Balanced sex/autosomal rearrangement in abnormal **individual** `POA` `RxHCC`

Q95.5 Individual with autosomal fragile site `POA`

Q95.8 Other balanced rearrangements and structural markers `POA`

Q95.9 Balanced rearrangement and structural marker, unspecified `POA`

4ᵗʰ **Q96 Turner's syndrome**

EXCLUDES1 Noonan syndrome ▶(Q87.19)◀

Q96.0 Karyotype 45, X `POA` ♀

Q96.1 Karyotype 46, X iso (Xq) `POA` ♀
Karyotype 46, isochromosome Xq

Q96.2 Karyotype 46, X with abnormal sex chromosome, except iso (Xq) `POA` ♀
Karyotype 46, X with abnormal sex chromosome, except isochromosome Xq

Q96.3 Mosaicism, 45, X/46, XX or XY `POA` ♀

Q96.4 Mosaicism, 45, X/other cell line(s) with abnormal sex chromosome `POA` ♀

Q96.8 Other variants of Turner's syndrome `POA` ♀

Q96.9 Turner's syndrome, unspecified `POA` ♀

4ᵗʰ **Q97 Other sex chromosome abnormalities,** female phenotype, **not elsewhere classified**

EXCLUDES1 Turner's syndrome (Q96.-)

Q97.0 Karyotype 47, XXX `POA` ♀

Q97.1 Female with more than three X chromosomes `POA` ♀

Q97.2 Mosaicism, lines with various numbers of X chromosomes `POA` ♀

Q97.3 Female with 46, XY karyotype `POA` ♀

Q97.8 Other specified sex chromosome abnormalities, female phenotype `POA` ♀

Q97.9 Sex chromosome abnormality, female phenotype, unspecified `POA` ♀

4ᵗʰ **Q98 Other sex chromosome abnormalities,** male phenotype, **not elsewhere classified**

Q98.0 Klinefelter syndrome karyotype 47, XXY `POA` ♂

Q98.1 Klinefelter syndrome, male with more than two X chromosomes `POA` ♂

Q98.3 Other male with 46, XX karyotype `POA` ♂

Q98.4 Klinefelter syndrome, unspecified `POA` ♂

Q98.5 Karyotype 47, XYY `POA`

Q98.6 Male with structurally abnormal sex chromosome `POA` ♂

Q98.7 Male with sex chromosome mosaicism `POA` ♂

Q98.8 Other specified sex chromosome abnormalities, male phenotype `POA` ♂

Q98.9 Sex chromosome abnormality, male phenotype, unspecified `POA` ♂

4ᵗʰ **Q99 Other** chromosome abnormalities, not elsewhere classified

Q99.0 Chimera 46, XX/46, XY `POA`
Chimera 46, XX/46, XY true hermaphrodite

Q99.1 46, XX true hermaphrodite `POA`
46, XX with streak gonads
46, XY with streak gonads
Pure gonadal dysgenesis

Q99.2 Fragile X chromosome `POA` `RxHCC`
Fragile X syndrome

Q99.8 Other specified chromosome abnormalities `POA`

Q99.9 Chromosomal abnormality, unspecified `POA`

Unspecified Code   Other Specified Code   Manifestation Code   Ⓝ Newborn   Ⓟ Pediatric   Ⓜ Maternity   Ⓐ Adult   ♂ Male   ♀ Female
● **New Code** ▲ Revised Code Title ▶◀ Revised Text **NOTES** *INCLUDES* *EXCLUDES1* Not coded here *EXCLUDES2* Not included here
4ᵗʰ 4ᵗʰ character required   5ᵗʰ 5ᵗʰ character required   6ᵗʰ 6ᵗʰ character required   7ᵗʰ 7ᵗʰ character required   7ᵗʰ Extension 'X' Alert
`HAC` Hospital-acquired condition (HAC) alert   **AHA** AHA Coding Clinic©   ☛ Code first alert

2020 ICD-10-CM   When symbols appear on a code that requires a 7th character extension, refer to Appendix B to identify applicable 7th character codes.   **947**

Q93 - Q99.9   CHAPTER 17: CONGENITAL MALFORMATIONS, DEFORMATIONS, AND CHROMOSOMAL ABNORMALITIES (Q00-Q99)

NOTES

Chapter 18: Symptoms, Signs, and Abnormal Clinical and Laboratory Findings, Not Elsewhere Classified (R00-R99)

Symptoms, signs, and abnormal clinical and laboratory findings, not elsewhere classified (R00-R99)

[NOTES] This chapter includes symptoms, signs, abnormal results of clinical or other investigative procedures, and ill-defined conditions regarding which no diagnosis classifiable elsewhere is recorded.

Signs and symptoms that point rather definitely to a given diagnosis have been assigned to a category in other chapters of the classification. In general, categories in this chapter include the less well-defined conditions and symptoms that, without the necessary study of the case to establish a final diagnosis, point perhaps equally to two or more diseases or to two or more systems of the body. Practically all categories in the chapter could be designated 'not otherwise specified', 'unknown etiology' or 'transient'. The Alphabetical Index should be consulted to determine which symptoms and signs are to be allocated here and which to other chapters. The residual subcategories, numbered .8, are generally provided for other relevant symptoms that cannot be allocated elsewhere in the classification.

The conditions and signs or symptoms included in categories R00-R94 consist of:

(a) cases for which no more specific diagnosis can be made even after all the facts bearing on the case have been investigated;

(b) signs or symptoms existing at the time of initial encounter that proved to be transient and whose causes could not be determined;

(c) provisional diagnosis in a patient who failed to return for further investigation or care;

(d) cases referred elsewhere for investigation or treatment before the diagnosis was made;

(e) cases in which a more precise diagnosis was not available for any other reason;

(f) certain symptoms, for which supplementary information is provided, that represent important problems in medical care in their own right.

[EXCLUDES2] *abnormal findings on antenatal screening of mother (O28.-)*
certain conditions originating in the perinatal period (P04-P96)
signs and symptoms classified in the body system chapters
signs and symptoms of breast (N63, N64.5)

This chapter contains the following blocks:

R00-R09	Symptoms and signs involving the circulatory and respiratory systems
R10-R19	Symptoms and signs involving the digestive system and abdomen
R20-R23	Symptoms and signs involving the skin and subcutaneous tissue
R25-R29	Symptoms and signs involving the nervous and musculoskeletal systems
R30-R39	Symptoms and signs involving the genitourinary system
R40-R46	Symptoms and signs involving cognition, perception, emotional state and behavior
R47-R49	Symptoms and signs involving speech and voice
R50-R69	General symptoms and signs
R70-R79	Abnormal findings on examination of blood, without diagnosis
R80-R82	Abnormal findings on examination of urine, without diagnosis
R83-R89	Abnormal findings on examination of other body fluids, substances and tissues, without diagnosis
R90-R94	Abnormal findings on diagnostic imaging and in function studies, without diagnosis
R97	Abnormal tumor markers
R99	Ill-defined and unknown cause of mortality

Symptoms and signs involving the circulatory and respiratory systems (R00-R09)

See Official Guidelines "Signs and symptoms" I.B.4

R00 Abnormalities of heart beat [4th]
[EXCLUDES1] *abnormalities originating in the perinatal period (P29.1-)*
[EXCLUDES2] *specified arrhythmias (I47-I49)*

R00.0 Tachycardia, unspecified
Rapid heart beat
Sinoauricular tachycardia NOS
Sinus [sinusal] tachycardia NOS
[EXCLUDES1] *neonatal tachycardia (P29.11)*
paroxysmal tachycardia (I47.-)

R00.1 Bradycardia, unspecified
Sinoatrial bradycardia
Sinus bradycardia
Slow heart beat
Vagal bradycardia
Use additional code for adverse effect, if applicable, to identify drug (T36-T50 with fifth or sixth character 5)
[EXCLUDES1] *neonatal bradycardia (P29.12)*

R00.2 Palpitations
Awareness of heart beat

R00.8 Other abnormalities of heart beat

R00.9 Unspecified abnormalities of heart beat

R01 Cardiac murmurs and other cardiac sounds [4th]
[EXCLUDES1] *cardiac murmurs and sounds originating in the perinatal period (P29.8)*

R01.0 Benign and innocent cardiac murmurs
Functional cardiac murmur

R01.1 Cardiac murmur, unspecified
Cardiac bruit NOS
Heart murmur NOS
Systolic murmur NOS

R01.2 Other cardiac sounds
Cardiac dullness, increased or decreased
Precordial friction

R03 Abnormal blood-pressure reading, without diagnosis [4th]

R03.0 Elevated blood-pressure **reading, without diagnosis of hypertension** [?]
See Official Guidelines "Hypertension, Transient" I.C.9.a.7
[NOTES] This category is to be used to record an episode of elevated blood pressure in a patient in whom no formal diagnosis of hypertension has been made, or as an isolated incidental finding.

R03.1 Nonspecific low blood-pressure **reading**
[EXCLUDES1] *hypotension (I95.-)*
maternal hypotension syndrome (O26.5-)
neurogenic orthostatic hypotension (G90.3)

R04 Hemorrhage from respiratory passages [4th]

R04.0 Epistaxis [CC] [CC/MCC Exc]
AHA: Q4 2018
Hemorrhage from nose
Nosebleed

R04.1 Hemorrhage from throat [CC] [CC/MCC Exc]
[EXCLUDES2] *hemoptysis (R04.2)*

R04.2 Hemoptysis [CC] [CC/MCC Exc]
AHA: Q4 2013
Blood-stained sputum
Cough with hemorrhage

R04.8 Hemorrhage from other sites in respiratory passages [5th]

R04.81 Acute idiopathic pulmonary hemorrhage in infants [P] [CC] [CC/MCC Exc]
AIPHI
Acute idiopathic hemorrhage in infants over 28 days old
[EXCLUDES1] *perinatal pulmonary hemorrhage (P26.-)*
von Willebrand's disease (D68.0)

Unspecified Code | Other Specified Code | Manifestation Code | [N] Newborn | [P] Pediatric | [M] Maternity | [A] Adult | ♂ Male | ♀ Female
● New Code | ▲ Revised Code Title | ►◄ Revised Text | [NOTES] | INCLUDES | [EXCLUDES1] Not coded here | [EXCLUDES2] Not included here
[4th] 4th character required | [5th] 5th character required | [6th] 6th character required | [7th] 7th character required | [x] Extension 'X' Alert
[HAC] Hospital-acquired condition (HAC) alert | **AHA** AHA Coding Clinic© | ☞ Code first alert

When symbols appear on a code that requires a 7th character extension, refer to Appendix B to identify applicable 7th character codes.

R04.89   Hemorrhage from other sites in respiratory passages CC CC/MCC Exc

Pulmonary hemorrhage NOS

R04.9   **Hemorrhage from respiratory passages, unspecified** CC CC/MCC Exc

R05   **Cough**

AHA: Q2 2016

EXCLUDES1 cough with hemorrhage (R04.2)

smoker's cough (J41.0)

R06   **Abnormalities of breathing**

EXCLUDES1 acute respiratory distress syndrome (J80)

respiratory arrest (R09.2)

respiratory arrest of newborn (P28.81)

respiratory distress syndrome of newborn (P22.-)

respiratory failure (J96.-)

respiratory failure of newborn (P28.5)

R06.0   **Dyspnea**

EXCLUDES1 tachypnea NOS (R06.82)

transient tachypnea of newborn (P22.1)

R06.00   **Dyspnea, unspecified**

AHA: Q1 2017

R06.01   **Orthopnea**

R06.02   **Shortness of breath**

R06.03   **Acute respiratory distress**

R06.09   **Other forms of dyspnea**

R06.1   **Stridor**

EXCLUDES1 congenital laryngeal stridor (P28.89)

laryngismus (stridulus) (J38.5)

R06.2   **Wheezing**

AHA: Q2 2016

EXCLUDES1 Asthma (J45.-)

R06.3   **Periodic breathing**   CC CC/MCC Exc

Cheyne-Stokes breathing

R06.4   **Hyperventilation**

EXCLUDES1 psychogenic hyperventilation (F45.8)

R06.5   **Mouth breathing**

EXCLUDES2 dry mouth NOS (R68.2)

R06.6   **Hiccough**

EXCLUDES1 psychogenic hiccough (F45.8)

R06.7   **Sneezing**

R06.8   **Other abnormalities of breathing**

R06.81   **Apnea, not elsewhere classified**

Apnea NOS

EXCLUDES1 apnea (of) newborn (P28.4)

sleep apnea (G47.3-)

sleep apnea of newborn (primary) (P28.3)

R06.82   **Tachypnea, not elsewhere classified**

Tachypnea NOS

EXCLUDES1 transitory tachypnea of newborn (P22.1)

R06.83   **Snoring**

R06.89   **Other abnormalities of breathing**

Breath-holding (spells)

Sighing

R06.9   **Unspecified abnormalities of breathing**

R07   **Pain in throat and chest**

EXCLUDES1 epidemic myalgia (B33.0)

EXCLUDES2 jaw pain R68.84

pain in breast (N64.4)

R07.0   **Pain in throat**

EXCLUDES1 chronic sore throat (J31.2)

sore throat (acute) NOS (J02.9)

EXCLUDES2 dysphagia (R13.1-)

pain in neck (M54.2)

R07.1   **Chest pain on breathing**

Painful respiration

R07.2   **Precordial pain**

R07.8   **Other chest pain**

R07.81   **Pleurodynia**

Pleurodynia NOS

EXCLUDES1 epidemic pleurodynia (B33.0)

R07.82   **Intercostal pain**

R07.89   **Other chest pain**

Anterior chest-wall pain NOS

R07.9   **Chest pain, unspecified**

R09   **Other symptoms and signs involving the circulatory and respiratory system**

EXCLUDES1 acute respiratory distress syndrome (J80)

respiratory arrest of newborn (P28.81)

respiratory distress syndrome of newborn (P22.0)

respiratory failure (J96.-)

respiratory failure of newborn (P28.5)

R09.0   **Asphyxia and hypoxemia**

EXCLUDES1 asphyxia due to carbon monoxide (T58.-)

asphyxia due to foreign body in respiratory tract (T17.-)

birth (intrauterine) asphyxia (P84)

hyperventilation (R06.4)

traumatic asphyxia (T71.-)

EXCLUDES2 hypercapnia (R06.89)

R09.01   **Asphyxia**   CC CC/MCC Exc

R09.02   **Hypoxemia**

R09.1   **Pleurisy**

EXCLUDES1 pleurisy with effusion (J90)

R09.2   **Respiratory arrest**   HCC MCC CC/MCC Exc

Cardiorespiratory failure

EXCLUDES1 cardiac arrest (I46.-)

respiratory arrest of newborn (P28.81)

respiratory distress of newborn (P22.0)

respiratory failure (J96.-)

respiratory failure of newborn (P28.5)

respiratory insufficiency (R06.89)

respiratory insufficiency of newborn (P28.5)

R09.3   **Abnormal sputum**

Abnormal amount of sputum

Abnormal color of sputum

Abnormal odor of sputum

Excessive sputum

EXCLUDES1 blood-stained sputum (R04.2)

R09.8   **Other specified symptoms and signs involving the circulatory and respiratory systems**

R09.81   **Nasal congestion**

R09.82   **Postnasal drip**

R09.89   **Other specified symptoms and signs involving the circulatory and respiratory systems**

Bruit (arterial)

Abnormal chest percussion

Feeling of foreign body in throat

Friction sounds in chest

Chest tympany

Choking sensation

Rales

Weak pulse

EXCLUDES2 foreign body in throat (T17.2-)

wheezing (R06.2)

Symptoms and signs involving the digestive system and abdomen (R10-R19)

EXCLUDES2 congenital or infantile pylorospasm (Q40.0)

gastrointestinal hemorrhage (K92.0-K92.2)

intestinal obstruction (K56.-)

newborn gastrointestinal hemorrhage (P54.0-P54.3)

newborn intestinal obstruction (P76.-)

pylorospasm (K31.3)

signs and symptoms involving the urinary system (R30-R39)

symptoms referable to female genital organs (N94.-)

symptoms referable to male genital organs (N48-N50)

R10   **Abdominal and pelvic pain**

EXCLUDES1 renal colic (N23)

EXCLUDES2 dorsalgia (M54.-)

flatulence and related conditions (R14.-)

PDx Unacceptable principal diagnosis symbol per Medicare code edits   PDx Code exempt from diagnosis present on admission requirement

? Questionable admission   CC Complication or comorbidity   MCC Major complication or comorbidity   CC/MCC CC/MCC exclusion

HCC HCC diagnosis code   RxHCC RxHCC diagnosis code   MACRA MACRA code   **DEFINITION** Describes condition/terminology

TIP Coding guidance   👁 Official Guideline Reference   Z1 Z code as first-listed diagnosis

R10.0 **Acute** abdomen
Severe abdominal pain (generalized) (with abdominal rigidity)
EXCLUDES1 *abdominal rigidity NOS (R19.3)*
generalized abdominal pain NOS (R10.84)
localized abdominal pain (R10.1-R10.3-)

R10.1 **Pain** localized **to** upper abdomen
R10.10 **Upper abdominal pain, unspecified**
R10.11 **Right** upper quadrant pain
R10.12 **Left** upper quadrant pain
R10.13 **Epigastric pain**
Dyspepsia
EXCLUDES1 *functional dyspepsia (K30)*

R10.2 **Pelvic and** perineal **pain**
EXCLUDES1 *vulvodynia (N94.81)*

R10.3 **Pain** localized **to other parts of** lower abdomen
R10.30 **Lower abdominal pain, unspecified**
R10.31 **Right lower quadrant pain**
R10.32 **Left lower quadrant pain**
R10.33 Periumbilical **pain**

R10.8 Other abdominal **pain**
R10.81 **Abdominal** tenderness
Abdominal tenderness NOS
R10.811 **Right upper** quadrant abdominal tenderness
R10.812 **Left upper** quadrant abdominal tenderness
R10.813 **Right lower** quadrant abdominal tenderness
R10.814 **Left lower** quadrant abdominal tenderness
R10.815 Periumbilic **abdominal tenderness**
R10.816 **Epigastric abdominal tenderness**
R10.817 Generalized **abdominal tenderness**
R10.819 **Abdominal tenderness, unspecified site**
R10.82 Rebound **abdominal tenderness**
R10.821 **Right upper** quadrant rebound abdominal tenderness
R10.822 **Left upper** quadrant rebound abdominal tenderness
R10.823 **Right lower** quadrant rebound abdominal tenderness
R10.824 **Left lower** quadrant rebound abdominal tenderness
R10.825 Periumbilic **rebound abdominal tenderness**
R10.826 **Epigastric** rebound abdominal tenderness
R10.827 Generalized **rebound abdominal tenderness**
R10.829 **Rebound abdominal tenderness, unspecified site**
R10.83 Colic **P**
Colic NOS
Infantile colic
EXCLUDES1 *colic in adult and child over 12 months old (R10.84)*
R10.84 Generalized **abdominal pain**
EXCLUDES1 *generalized abdominal pain associated with acute abdomen (R10.0)*

R10.9 **Unspecified abdominal pain**

R11 **Nausea and vomiting**
EXCLUDES1 *cyclical vomiting associated with migraine (G43.A-)*
excessive vomiting in pregnancy (O21.-)
hematemesis (K92.0)
neonatal hematemesis (P54.0)
newborn vomiting (P92.0-)
psychogenic vomiting (F50.89)
vomiting associated with bulimia nervosa (F50.2)
vomiting following gastrointestinal surgery (K91.0)

R11.0 **Nausea**
Nausea NOS
Nausea without vomiting
R11.1 **Vomiting**
R11.10 **Vomiting, unspecified**
Vomiting NOS
R11.11 **Vomiting** without nausea
R11.12 Projectile **vomiting**
R11.13 **Vomiting of** fecal matter
R11.14 Bilious **vomiting**
Bilious emesis
R11.15 Cyclical **vomiting syndrome** unrelated to migraine
Cyclic vomiting syndrome NOS
Persistent vomiting
EXCLUDES1 *cyclical vomiting in migraine (G43.A-)*
EXCLUDES2 *bulimia nervosa (F50.2)*
diabetes mellitus due to underlying condition (E08.-)
R11.2 **Nausea with vomiting, unspecified**
Persistent nausea with vomiting NOS

R12 **Heartburn**
EXCLUDES1 *dyspepsia NOS (R10.13)*
functional dyspepsia (K30)

R13 **Aphagia and dysphagia**
R13.0 **Aphagia** CC CC/MCC Exc
Inability to swallow
EXCLUDES1 *psychogenic aphagia (F50.9)*
R13.1 **Dysphagia**
☞ **Code first,** if applicable, dysphagia following cerebrovascular disease (I69. with final characters -91)
EXCLUDES1 *psychogenic dysphagia (F45.8)*
R13.10 **Dysphagia, unspecified**
Difficulty in swallowing NOS
R13.11 **Dysphagia,** oral phase
R13.12 **Dysphagia,** oropharyngeal phase
R13.13 **Dysphagia,** pharyngeal phase
R13.14 **Dysphagia,** pharyngoesophageal phase
R13.19 Other **dysphagia**
Cervical dysphagia
Neurogenic dysphagia

R14 **Flatulence and related conditions**
EXCLUDES1 *psychogenic aerophagy (F45.8)*
R14.0 **Abdominal distension (gaseous)**
Bloating
Tympanites (abdominal) (intestinal)
R14.1 **Gas pain**
R14.2 **Eructation**
R14.3 **Flatulence**

R15 **Fecal incontinence**
INCLUDES encopresis NOS
EXCLUDES1 *fecal incontinence of nonorganic origin (F98.1)*
R15.0 **Incomplete defecation**
EXCLUDES1 *constipation (K59.0-)*
fecal impaction (K56.41)
R15.1 **Fecal smearing**
Fecal soiling
R15.2 **Fecal urgency**
R15.9 **Full incontinence of feces**
Fecal incontinence NOS

R16 **Hepatomegaly and splenomegaly, not elsewhere classified**
R16.0 Hepatomegaly, **not elsewhere classified**
Hepatomegaly NOS
R16.1 Splenomegaly, **not elsewhere classified**
Splenomegaly NOS
R16.2 Hepatomegaly with splenomegaly, **not elsewhere classified**
Hepatosplenomegaly NOS

R17 **Unspecified jaundice** CC CC/MCC Exc
EXCLUDES1 *neonatal jaundice (P55, P57-P59)*

R18 **Ascites**

    INCLUDES   fluid in peritoneal cavity

    EXCLUDES1 ascites in alcoholic cirrhosis (K70.31)

        ascites in alcoholic hepatitis (K70.11)

        ascites in toxic liver disease with chronic active hepatitis (K71.51)

    R18.0 **Malignant** ascites   CC PDxIn CC/MCC Exc

      ☞ **Code first** malignancy, such as:

        malignant neoplasm of ovary (C56.-)

        secondary malignant neoplasm of retroperitoneum and peritoneum (C78.6)

    R18.8 **Other** ascites   CC CC/MCC Exc

      AHA: Q1 2018

      Ascites NOS

      Peritoneal effusion (chronic)

R19 **Other symptoms and signs involving the digestive system and abdomen**

    EXCLUDES1 acute abdomen (R10.0)

    R19.0 **Intra-abdominal and pelvic swelling, mass and lump**

        EXCLUDES1 abdominal distension (gaseous) (R14.-)

            ascites (R18.-)

      R19.00 **Intra-abdominal and pelvic swelling, mass and lump, unspecified site**

      R19.01 **Right upper quadrant** abdominal swelling, mass and lump

      R19.02 **Left upper quadrant** abdominal swelling, mass and lump

      R19.03 **Right lower quadrant** abdominal swelling, mass and lump

      R19.04 **Left lower quadrant** abdominal swelling, mass and lump

      R19.05 **Periumbilic** swelling, mass or lump

        Diffuse or generalized umbilical swelling or mass

      R19.06 **Epigastric** swelling, mass or lump

      R19.07 **Generalized** intra-abdominal and pelvic swelling, mass and lump

        Diffuse or generalized intra-abdominal swelling or mass NOS

        Diffuse or generalized pelvic swelling or mass NOS

      R19.09 **Other** intra-abdominal and pelvic swelling, mass and lump

    R19.1 **Abnormal bowel sounds**

      R19.11 **Absent** bowel sounds

      R19.12 **Hyperactive** bowel sounds

      R19.15 **Other** abnormal bowel sounds

        Abnormal bowel sounds NOS

    R19.2 **Visible peristalsis**

      Hyperperistalsis

    R19.3 **Abdominal rigidity**

      EXCLUDES1 abdominal rigidity with severe abdominal pain (R10.0)

      R19.30 **Abdominal rigidity, unspecified site**

      R19.31 **Right upper quadrant** abdominal rigidity

      R19.32 **Left upper quadrant** abdominal rigidity

      R19.33 **Right lower quadrant** abdominal rigidity

      R19.34 **Left lower quadrant** abdominal rigidity

      R19.35 **Periumbilic** abdominal rigidity

      R19.36 **Epigastric** abdominal rigidity

      R19.37 **Generalized** abdominal rigidity

    R19.4 **Change in bowel habit**

      EXCLUDES1 constipation (K59.0-)

            functional diarrhea (K59.1)

    R19.5 **Other fecal abnormalities**

      AHA: Q1 2019

      Abnormal stool color

      Bulky stools

      Mucus in stools

      Occult blood in feces

      Occult blood in stools

      EXCLUDES1 melena (K92.1)

            neonatal melena (P54.1)

R19.6 **Halitosis**

R19.7 **Diarrhea, unspecified**

    Diarrhea NOS

    EXCLUDES1 functional diarrhea (K59.1)

        neonatal diarrhea (P78.3)

        psychogenic diarrhea (F45.8)

R19.8 **Other specified symptoms and signs involving the digestive system and abdomen**

Symptoms and signs involving the skin and subcutaneous tissue (R20-R23)

    EXCLUDES2 symptoms relating to breast (N64.4-N64.5)

R20 **Disturbances of skin sensation**

    EXCLUDES1 dissociative anesthesia and sensory loss (F44.6)

        psychogenic disturbances (F45.8)

    R20.0 **Anesthesia** of skin

    R20.1 **Hypoesthesia** of skin

    R20.2 **Paresthesia** of skin

      Formication

      Pins and needles

      Tingling skin

      EXCLUDES1 acroparesthesia (I73.8)

    R20.3 **Hyperesthesia**

    R20.8 **Other** disturbances of skin sensation

    R20.9 **Unspecified disturbances of skin sensation**

R21 **Rash and other nonspecific skin eruption**

    INCLUDES   rash NOS

    EXCLUDES1 specified type of rash- code to condition

        vesicular eruption (R23.8)

R22 **Localized swelling, mass and lump of skin and subcutaneous tissue**

    INCLUDES   subcutaneous nodules (localized)(superficial)

    EXCLUDES1 abnormal findings on diagnostic imaging (R90-R93)

        edema (R60.-)

        enlarged lymph nodes (R59.-)

        localized adiposity (E65)

        swelling of joint (M25.4-)

    R22.0 **Localized swelling, mass and lump, head**

    R22.1 **Localized swelling, mass and lump, neck**

    R22.2 **Localized swelling, mass and lump, trunk**

      EXCLUDES1 intra-abdominal or pelvic mass and lump (R19.0-)

        intra-abdominal or pelvic swelling (R19.0-)

      EXCLUDES2 breast mass and lump (N63)

    R22.3 **Localized swelling, mass and lump, upper limb**

      R22.30 **Localized swelling, mass and lump, unspecified upper limb**

      R22.31 **Localized swelling, mass and lump, right upper limb**

      R22.32 **Localized swelling, mass and lump, left upper limb**

      R22.33 **Localized swelling, mass and lump, upper limb, bilateral**

    R22.4 **Localized swelling, mass and lump, lower limb**

      R22.40 **Localized swelling, mass and lump, unspecified lower limb**

      R22.41 **Localized swelling, mass and lump, right lower limb**

      R22.42 **Localized swelling, mass and lump, left lower limb**

      R22.43 **Localized swelling, mass and lump, lower limb, bilateral**

    R22.9 **Localized swelling, mass and lump, unspecified**

R23 **Other skin changes**

    R23.0 **Cyanosis**

      EXCLUDES1 acrocyanosis (I73.8)

        cyanotic attacks of newborn (P28.2)

    R23.1 **Pallor**

      Clammy skin

    R23.2 **Flushing**

      Excessive blushing

      ☞ **Code first,** if applicable, menopausal and female climacteric states (N95.1)

PDxIn Unacceptable principal diagnosis symbol per Medicare code edits   POX Code exempt from diagnosis present on admission requirement

? Questionable admission   CC Complication or comorbidity   MCC Major complication or comorbidity   CC/MCC Exc CC/MCC exclusion

HCC HCC diagnosis code   RxHCC RxHCC diagnosis code   MACRA code   **DEFINITION** Describes condition/terminology

TIP Coding guidance   👁 Official Guideline Reference   Z Z code as first-listed diagnosis

When symbols appear on a code that requires a 7th character extension, refer to Appendix B to identify applicable 7th character codes.

2020 ICD-10-CM

R23.3 **Spontaneous ecchymoses**
Petechiae
EXCLUDES1 *ecchymoses of newborn (P54.5)*
purpura (D69.-)
R23.4 **Changes in skin texture**
Desquamation of skin
Induration of skin
Scaling of skin
EXCLUDES1 *epidermal thickening NOS (L85.9)*
R23.8 Other **skin changes**
R23.9 **Unspecified skin changes**

Symptoms and signs involving the nervous and musculoskeletal systems (R25-R29)

R25 **Abnormal involuntary movements**
EXCLUDES1 *specific movement disorders (G20-G26)*
stereotyped movement disorders (F98.4)
tic disorders (F95.-)
R25.0 **Abnormal head movements**
R25.1 **Tremor, unspecified**
EXCLUDES1 *chorea NOS (G25.5)*
essential tremor (G25.0)
hysterical tremor (F44.4)
intention tremor (G25.2)
R25.2 **Cramp and spasm**
EXCLUDES2 *carpopedal spasm (R29.0)*
charley-horse (M62.831)
infantile spasms (G40.4-)
muscle spasm of back (M62.830)
muscle spasm of calf (M62.831)
R25.3 **Fasciculation**
Twitching NOS
R25.8 Other **abnormal involuntary movements**
R25.9 **Unspecified abnormal involuntary movements**
R26 **Abnormalities of gait and mobility**
EXCLUDES1 *ataxia NOS (R27.0)*
hereditary ataxia (G11.-)
locomotor (syphilitic) ataxia (A52.11)
immobility syndrome (paraplegic) (M62.3)
R26.0 Ataxic **gait**
Staggering gait
R26.1 Paralytic **gait**
Spastic gait
R26.2 Difficulty **in walking, not elsewhere classified**
AHA: Q2 2016
EXCLUDES1 *falling (R29.6)*
unsteadiness on feet (R26.81)
R26.8 Other **abnormalities of gait and mobility**
R26.81 **Unsteadiness on feet**
R26.89 **Other abnormalities of gait and mobility**
R26.9 **Unspecified abnormalities of gait and mobility**
R27 **Other lack of coordination**
EXCLUDES1 *ataxic gait (R26.0)*
hereditary ataxia (G11.-)
vertigo NOS (R42)
R27.0 **Ataxia, unspecified**
EXCLUDES1 *ataxia following cerebrovascular disease (I69. with final characters -93)*
R27.8 Other **lack of coordination**
R27.9 **Unspecified lack of coordination**
R29 **Other symptoms and signs involving the nervous and musculoskeletal systems**
R29.0 **Tetany** CC CC/MCC Exc
Carpopedal spasm
EXCLUDES1 *hysterical tetany (F44.5)*
neonatal tetany (P71.3)
parathyroid tetany (E20.9)
post-thyroidectomy tetany (E89.2)

R29.1 **Meningismus** CC CC/MCC Exc
R29.2 **Abnormal reflex**
EXCLUDES2 *abnormal pupillary reflex (H57.0)*
hyperactive gag reflex (J39.2)
vasovagal reaction or syncope (R55)
R29.3 **Abnormal posture**
R29.4 **Clicking hip**
EXCLUDES1 *congenital deformities of hip (Q65.-)*
R29.5 **Transient paralysis** CC CC/MCC Exc
Code first any associated spinal cord injury (S14.0, S14.1-, S24.0, S24.1-, S34.0-, S34.1-)
EXCLUDES1 *transient ischemic attack (G45.9)*
R29.6 **Repeated falls**
See Official Guidelines "Repeated falls" I.C.18.d
AHA: Q2 2016
Falling
Tendency to fall
EXCLUDES2 *at risk for falling (Z91.81)*
history of falling (Z91.81)
R29.7 National Institutes of Health Stroke Scale (NIHSS) score
See Official Guidelines "NIHSS Stroke Scale: I.C.18.i
Code first the type of cerebral infarction (I63-)
R29.70 **NIHSS score** 0-9
R29.700 **NIHSS score** 0 PDxIn
R29.701 **NIHSS score** 1 PDxIn
R29.702 **NIHSS score** 2 PDxIn
R29.703 **NIHSS score** 3 PDxIn
R29.704 **NIHSS score** 4 PDxIn
R29.705 **NIHSS score** 5 PDxIn
R29.706 **NIHSS score** 6 PDxIn
R29.707 **NIHSS score** 7 PDxIn
R29.708 **NIHSS score** 8 PDxIn
R29.709 **NIHSS score** 9 PDxIn
R29.71 **NIHSS score** 10-19
R29.710 **NIHSS score** 10 PDxIn
R29.711 **NIHSS score** 11 PDxIn
R29.712 **NIHSS score** 12 PDxIn
R29.713 **NIHSS score** 13 PDxIn
R29.714 **NIHSS score** 14 PDxIn
R29.715 **NIHSS score** 15 PDxIn
R29.716 **NIHSS score** 16 PDxIn
R29.717 **NIHSS score** 17 PDxIn
R29.718 **NIHSS score** 18 PDxIn
R29.719 **NIHSS score** 19 PDxIn
R29.72 **NIHSS score** 20-29
R29.720 **NIHSS score** 20 PDxIn
R29.721 **NIHSS score** 21 PDxIn
R29.722 **NIHSS score** 22 PDxIn
R29.723 **NIHSS score** 23 PDxIn
R29.724 **NIHSS score** 24 PDxIn
R29.725 **NIHSS score** 25 PDxIn
R29.726 **NIHSS score** 26 PDxIn
R29.727 **NIHSS score** 27 PDxIn
R29.728 **NIHSS score** 28 PDxIn
R29.729 **NIHSS score** 29 PDxIn
R29.73 **NIHSS score** 30-39
R29.730 **NIHSS score** 30 PDxIn
AHA: Q4 2016
R29.731 **NIHSS score** 31 PDxIn
R29.732 **NIHSS score** 32 PDxIn
R29.733 **NIHSS score** 33 PDxIn
R29.734 **NIHSS score** 34 PDxIn
R29.735 **NIHSS score** 35 PDxIn
R29.736 **NIHSS score** 36 PDxIn
R29.737 **NIHSS score** 37 PDxIn
R29.738 **NIHSS score** 38 PDxIn
R29.739 **NIHSS score** 39 PDxIn

Unspecified Code   Other Specified Code   Manifestation Code   N Newborn   P Pediatric   M Maternity   A Adult   ♂ Male   ♀ Female
● New Code   ▲ Revised Code Title   ►◄ Revised Text   NOTES   INCLUDES   EXCLUDES1 Not coded here   EXCLUDES2 Not included here
4th character required   5th character required   6th character required   7th character required   Extension 'X' Alert
HAC Hospital-acquired condition (HAC) alert   AHA AHA Coding Clinic©   Code first alert

[6th] **R29.74 NIHSS score 40-42**
- **R29.740 NIHSS score 40** PDx
- **R29.741 NIHSS score 41** PDx
- **R29.742 NIHSS score 42** PDx

[5th] **R29.8 Other symptoms and signs involving the nervous and musculoskeletal systems**

[6th] **R29.81 Other symptoms and signs involving the nervous system**
- **R29.810 Facial weakness**
  Facial droop
  EXCLUDES1 *Bell's palsy (G51.0)*
  facial weakness following cerebrovascular disease (I69. with final characters -92)
- **R29.818 Other symptoms and signs involving the nervous system**

[6th] **R29.89 Other symptoms and signs involving the musculoskeletal system**
EXCLUDES2 *pain in limb (M79.6-)*
- **R29.890 Loss of height**
  EXCLUDES1 *osteoporosis (M80-M81)*
- **R29.891 Ocular torticollis**
  EXCLUDES1 *congenital (sternomastoid) torticollis Q68.0*
  psychogenic torticollis (F45.8)
  spasmodic torticollis (G24.3)
  torticollis due to birth injury (P15.8)
  torticollis NOS M43.6
- **R29.898 Other symptoms and signs involving the musculoskeletal system**

[5th] **R29.9 Unspecified symptoms and signs involving the nervous and musculoskeletal systems**
- **R29.90 Unspecified symptoms and signs involving the nervous system**
- **R29.91 Unspecified symptoms and signs involving the musculoskeletal system**

Symptoms and signs involving the genitourinary system (R30-R39)

[4th] **R30 Pain associated with micturition**
EXCLUDES1 *psychogenic pain associated with micturition (F45.8)*
- **R30.0 Dysuria**
  Strangury
- **R30.1 Vesical tenesmus**
- **R30.9 Painful micturition, unspecified**
  Painful urination NOS

[4th] **R31 Hematuria**
EXCLUDES1 *hematuria included with underlying conditions, such as:*
acute cystitis with hematuria (N30.01)
recurrent and persistent hematuria in glomerular diseases (N02.-)
- **R31.0 Gross hematuria**
  AHA: Q1 2017
- **R31.1 Benign essential microscopic hematuria**

[5th] **R31.2 Other microscopic hematuria**
- **R31.21 Asymptomatic microscopic hematuria**
  AHA: Q4 2016
  AMH
- **R31.29 Other microscopic hematuria**
  AHA: Q4 2016
- **R31.9 Hematuria, unspecified**

R32 Unspecified urinary incontinence
Enuresis NOS
EXCLUDES1 *functional urinary incontinence (R39.81)*
nonorganic enuresis (F98.0)
stress incontinence and other specified urinary incontinence (N39.3-N39.4-)
urinary incontinence associated with cognitive impairment (R39.81)

[4th] **R33 Retention of urine**
EXCLUDES1 *psychogenic retention of urine (F45.8)*
- **R33.0 Drug induced retention of urine**
  Use additional code for adverse effect, if applicable, to identify drug (T36-T50 with fifth or sixth character 5)
- **R33.8 Other retention of urine**
  AHA: Q4 2018
  ☞ **Code first,** if applicable, any causal condition, such as:
  enlarged prostate (N40.1)
- **R33.9 Retention of urine, unspecified**

R34 Anuria and oliguria
EXCLUDES1 *anuria and oliguria complicating abortion or ectopic or molar pregnancy (O00-O07, O08.4)*
anuria and oliguria complicating pregnancy (O26.83-)
anuria and oliguria complicating the puerperium (O90.4)

[4th] **R35 Polyuria**
☞ **Code first,** if applicable, any causal condition, such as:
enlarged prostate (N40.1)
EXCLUDES1 *psychogenic polyuria (F45.8)*
- **R35.0 Frequency of micturition**
- **R35.1 Nocturia**
- **R35.8 Other polyuria**
  Polyuria NOS

[4th] **R36 Urethral discharge**
- **R36.0 Urethral discharge without blood**
- **R36.1 Hematospermia** ♂
- **R36.9 Urethral discharge, unspecified**
  Penile discharge NOS
  Urethrorrhea

R37 Sexual dysfunction, unspecified

[4th] **R39 Other and unspecified symptoms and signs involving the genitourinary system**
- **R39.0 Extravasation of urine** CC CC/MCC Exc

[5th] **R39.1 Other difficulties with micturition**
☞ **Code first,** if applicable, any causal condition, such as:
enlarged prostate (N40.1)
- **R39.11 Hesitancy of micturition**
- **R39.12 Poor urinary stream**
  Weak urinary steam
- **R39.13 Splitting of urinary stream**
- **R39.14 Feeling of incomplete bladder emptying**
- **R39.15 Urgency of urination**
  EXCLUDES1 *urge incontinence (N39.41, N39.46)*
- **R39.16 Straining to void**

[6th] **R39.19 Other difficulties with micturition**
- **R39.191 Need to immediately re-void**
  AHA: Q4 2016
- **R39.192 Position dependent micturition**
  AHA: Q4 2016
- **R39.198 Other difficulties with micturition**
  AHA: Q4 2016

- **R39.2 Extrarenal uremia**
  Prerenal uremia
  EXCLUDES1 *uremia NOS (N19)*

[5th] **R39.8 Other symptoms and signs involving the genitourinary system**
- **R39.81 Functional urinary incontinence**
  Urinary incontinence due to cognitive impairment, or severe physical disability or immobility
  EXCLUDES1 *stress incontinence and other specified urinary incontinence (N39.3-N39.4-)*
  urinary incontinence NOS (R32)
- **R39.82 Chronic bladder pain**
  AHA: Q4 2016
- **R39.83 Unilateral non-palpable testicle** ♂
- **R39.84 Bilateral non-palpable testicles** ♂
- **R39.89 Other symptoms and signs involving the genitourinary system**
  AHA: Q4 2016
- **R39.9 Unspecified symptoms and signs involving the genitourinary system**

PDx Unacceptable principal diagnosis symbol per Medicare code edits POA Code exempt from diagnosis present on admission requirement
[?] Questionable admission CC Complication or comorbidity MCC Major complication or comorbidity CC/MCC Exc CC/MCC exclusion
[HCC] HCC diagnosis code [RxHCC] RxHCC diagnosis code MACRA code **DEFINITION** Describes condition/terminology
TIP Coding guidance 👁 Official Guideline Reference [Z-1] Z code as first-listed diagnosis

Symptoms and signs involving cognition, perception, emotional state and behavior (R40-R46)

EXCLUDES2 symptoms and signs constituting part of a pattern of mental disorder (F01-F99)

4ᵗʰ R40 Somnolence, stupor and coma

EXCLUDES1 neonatal coma (P91.5)
somnolence, stupor and coma in diabetes (E08-E13)
somnolence, stupor and coma in hepatic failure (K72.-)
somnolence, stupor and coma in hypoglycemia (nondiabetic) (E15)

R40.0 Somnolence
Drowsiness
EXCLUDES1 coma (R40.2-)

R40.1 Stupor
Catatonic stupor
Semicoma
EXCLUDES1 catatonic schizophrenia (F20.2)
coma (R40.2-)
depressive stupor (F31-F33)
dissociative stupor (F44.2)
manic stupor (F30.2)

5ᵗʰ R40.2 Coma
👁 See Official Guidelines "Coma scale" I.C.18.e
☞ Code first any associated:
fracture of skull (S02.-)
intracranial injury (S06.-)
NOTES One code from each subcategory, R40.21-R40.23, is required to complete the coma scale.

R40.20 Unspecified coma HCC MCC° CC/MCC Exc
Coma NOS
Unconsciousness NOS

6ᵗʰ R40.21 Coma scale, eyes open
The following appropriate 7th character is to be added to subcategory R40.21-:
0 = unspecified time
1 = in the field [EMT or ambulance]
2 = at arrival to emergency department
3 = at hospital admission
4 = 24 hours or more after hospital admission

7ᵗʰ R40.211 Coma scale, eyes open, never HCC MCC° PDxIn CC/MCC Exc
AHA: Q4 2017
Coma scale eye opening score of 1

7ᵗʰ R40.212 Coma scale, eyes open, to pain HCC MCC° PDxIn CC/MCC Exc
AHA: Q4 2017
Coma scale eye opening score of 2

7ᵗʰ R40.213 Coma scale, eyes open, to sound PDxIn
AHA: Q4 2017
Coma scale eye opening score of 3

7ᵗʰ R40.214 Coma scale, eyes open, spontaneous PDxIn
AHA: Q4 2017
Coma scale eye opening score of 4

6ᵗʰ R40.22 Coma scale, best verbal response
The following appropriate 7th character is to be added to subcategory R40.22-:
0 = unspecified time
1 = in the field [EMT or ambulance]
2 = at arrival to emergency department
3 = at hospital admission
4 = 24 hours or more after hospital admission

7ᵗʰ R40.221 Coma scale, best verbal response, none HCC MCC° PDxIn CC/MCC Exc
AHA: Q4 2017
Coma scale verbal score of 1

7ᵗʰ R40.222 Coma scale, best verbal response, incomprehensible words HCC MCC° PDxIn CC/MCC Exc
AHA: Q4 2017
Coma scale verbal score of 2
Incomprehensible sounds (2-5 years of age)
Moans/grunts to pain; restless (<2 years old)

7ᵗʰ R40.223 Coma scale, best verbal response, inappropriate words PDxIn
AHA: Q4 2017
Coma scale verbal score of 3
Inappropriate crying or screaming (< 2 years of age)
Screaming (2-5 years of age)

7ᵗʰ R40.224 Coma scale, best verbal response, confused conversation PDxIn
AHA: Q4 2017
Coma scale verbal score of 4
Inappropriate words (2-5 years of age)
Irritable cries (< 2 years of age)

7ᵗʰ R40.225 Coma scale, best verbal response, oriented PDxIn
AHA: Q4 2017
Coma scale verbal score of 5
Cooing or babbling or crying appropriately (< 2 years of age)
Uses appropriate words (2- 5 years of age)

6ᵗʰ R40.23 Coma scale, best motor response
The following appropriate 7th character is to be added to subcategory R40.23-:
0 = unspecified time
1 = in the field [EMT or ambulance]
2 = at arrival to emergency department
3 = at hospital admission
4 = 24 hours or more after hospital admission

7ᵗʰ R40.231 Coma scale, best motor response, none HCC MCC° PDxIn CC/MCC Exc
AHA: Q4 2017
Coma scale motor score of 1

7ᵗʰ R40.232 Coma scale, best motor response, extension HCC MCC° PDxIn CC/MCC Exc
AHA: Q4 2017
Abnormal extensor posturing to pain or noxious stimuli (< 2 years of age)
Coma scale motor score of 2
Extensor posturing to pain or noxious stimuli (2-5 years of age)

7ᵗʰ R40.233 Coma scale, best motor response, abnormal flexion PDxIn
AHA: Q4 2017
Abnormal flexure posturing to pain or noxious stimuli (2-5 years of age)
Coma scale motor score of 3
Flexion/decorticate posturing (< 2 years of age)

7ᵗʰ R40.234 Coma scale, best motor response, flexion withdrawal HCC MCC° PDxIn CC/MCC Exc
AHA: Q4 2017
Coma scale motor score of 4
Withdraws from pain or noxious stimuli (2-5 years of age)

7ᵗʰ R40.235 Coma scale, best motor response, localizes pain PDxIn
AHA: Q4 2017
Coma scale motor score of 5
Localizes pain (2-5 years of age)
Withdraws to touch (< 2 years of age)

7ᵗʰ R40.236 Coma scale, best motor response, obeys commands PDxIn
AHA: Q4 2017
Coma scale motor score of 6
Normal or spontaneous movement (< 2 years of age)
Obeys commands (2-5 years of age)

6ᵗʰ R40.24 Glasgow coma scale, total score
👁 See Official Guidelines "Coma scale" I.C.18.e
NOTES Assign a code from subcategory R40.24, when only the total coma score is documented.

Unspecified Code   Other Specified Code   Manifestation Code   N Newborn   P Pediatric   M Maternity   A Adult   ♂ Male   ♀ Female
● New Code   ▲ Revised Code Title   ►◄ Revised Text   NOTES   INCLUDES   EXCLUDES1 Not coded here   EXCLUDES2 Not included here
4ᵗʰ 4ᵗʰ character required   5ᵗʰ 5ᵗʰ character required   6ᵗʰ 6ᵗʰ character required   7ᵗʰ 7ᵗʰ character required   👁 Extension 'X' Alert
HAC Hospital-acquired condition (HAC) alert   AHA AHA Coding Clinic©   ☞ Code first alert

The following appropriate 7th character is to be added to subcategory R40.24-:
- 0 = unspecified time
- 1 = in the field [EMT or ambulance]
- 2 = at arrival to emergency department
- 3 = at hospital admission
- 4 = 24 hours or more after hospital admission

7ᵗʰ **R40.241 Glasgow coma scale** score 13-15   PDxIn

7ᵗʰ **R40.242 Glasgow coma scale** score 9-12   PDxIn

7ᵗʰ **R40.243 Glasgow coma scale** score 3-8   HCC PDxIn

7ᵗʰ **R40.244 Other coma,** without documented Glasgow coma scale score, or with partial score reported   HCC PDxIn

R40.3 Persistent vegetative state   cc HCC CC/MCC Exc

R40.4 Transient alteration of awareness

4ᵗʰ **R41 Other symptoms and signs involving cognitive functions and awareness**

EXCLUDES1 dissociative [conversion] disorders (F44.-)

mild cognitive impairment, so stated (G31.84)

R41.0 Disorientation, unspecified

AHA: Q2 2019, Q4 2016

Confusion NOS

Delirium NOS

R41.1 Anterograde amnesia

R41.2 Retrograde amnesia

R41.3 Other amnesia

Amnesia NOS

Memory loss NOS

EXCLUDES1 amnestic disorder due to known physiologic condition (F04)

amnestic syndrome due to psychoactive substance use (F10-F19 with 5th character .6)

mild memory disturbance due to known physiological condition (F06.8)

transient global amnesia (G45.4)

R41.4 Neurologic neglect syndrome   cc CC/MCC Exc

Asomatognosia

Hemi-akinesia

Hemi-inattention

Hemispatial neglect

Left-sided neglect

Sensory neglect

Visuospatial neglect

EXCLUDES1 visuospatial deficit (R41.842)

5ᵗʰ **R41.8 Other symptoms and signs involving cognitive functions and awareness**

R41.81 Age-related cognitive decline   A

Senility NOS

R41.82 Altered mental status, unspecified

Change in mental status NOS

EXCLUDES1 altered level of consciousness (R40.-)

altered mental status due to known condition - code to condition

delirium NOS (R41.0)

R41.83 Borderline intellectual functioning   PDxIn

IQ level 71 to 84

EXCLUDES1 intellectual disabilities (F70-F79)

5ᵗʰ **R41.84 Other specified cognitive deficit**

EXCLUDES1 cognitive deficits as sequelae of cerebrovascular disease (I69.01-, I69.11-, I69.21-, I69.31-, I69.81-, I69.91-)

R41.840 Attention and concentration deficit

EXCLUDES1 attention-deficit hyperactivity disorders (F90.-)

R41.841 Cognitive communication deficit

R41.842 Visuospatial deficit

R41.843 Psychomotor deficit

R41.844 Frontal lobe and executive function deficit

R41.89 Other symptoms and signs involving cognitive functions and awareness

Anosognosia

R41.9 Unspecified symptoms and signs involving cognitive functions and awareness

Unspecified neurocognitive disorder

R42 Dizziness and giddiness

AHA: Q4 2015

Light-headedness

Vertigo NOS

EXCLUDES1 vertiginous syndromes (H81.-)

vertigo from infrasound (T75.23)

4ᵗʰ **R43 Disturbances of smell and taste**

R43.0 Anosmia

R43.1 Parosmia

R43.2 Parageusia

R43.8 Other disturbances of smell and taste

Mixed disturbance of smell and taste

R43.9 Unspecified disturbances of smell and taste

4ᵗʰ **R44 Other symptoms and signs involving general sensations and perceptions**

EXCLUDES1 alcoholic hallucinations (F1.5)

hallucinations in drug psychosis (F11-F19 with .5)

hallucinations in mood disorders with psychotic symptoms (F30.2, F31.5, F32.3, F33.3)

hallucinations in schizophrenia, schizotypal and delusional disorders (F20-F29)

EXCLUDES2 disturbances of skin sensation (R20.-)

R44.0 Auditory hallucinations   cc CC/MCC Exc

R44.1 Visual hallucinations

R44.2 Other hallucinations   cc CC/MCC Exc

R44.3 Hallucinations, unspecified   cc CC/MCC Exc

R44.8 Other symptoms and signs involving general sensations and perceptions

R44.9 Unspecified symptoms and signs involving general sensations and perceptions

4ᵗʰ **R45 Symptoms and signs involving emotional state**

R45.0 Nervousness

Nervous tension

R45.1 Restlessness and agitation

R45.2 Unhappiness

R45.3 Demoralization and apathy

EXCLUDES1 anhedonia (R45.84)

R45.4 Irritability and anger

R45.5 Hostility

R45.6 Violent behavior

R45.7 State of emotional shock and stress, unspecified

5ᵗʰ **R45.8 Other symptoms and signs involving emotional state**

R45.81 Low self-esteem

R45.82 Worries

R45.83 Excessive crying of child, adolescent or adult

EXCLUDES1 excessive crying of infant (baby) R68.11

R45.84 Anhedonia

6ᵗʰ **R45.85 Homicidal and suicidal ideations**

EXCLUDES1 suicide attempt (T14.91)

R45.850 Homicidal ideations   PDxIn

R45.851 Suicidal ideations   cc CC/MCC Exc

R45.86 Emotional lability

R45.87 Impulsiveness

R45.89 Other symptoms and signs involving emotional state

4ᵗʰ **R46 Symptoms and signs involving appearance and behavior**

EXCLUDES1 appearance and behavior in schizophrenia, schizotypal and delusional disorders (F20-F29)

mental and behavioral disorders (F01-F99)

R46.0 Very low level of personal hygiene

R46.1 Bizarre personal appearance

R46.2 Strange and inexplicable behavior

R46.3 Overactivity

R46.4 Slowness and poor responsiveness

EXCLUDES1 stupor (R40.1)

R46.5 Suspiciousness and marked evasiveness
R46.6 Undue concern and preoccupation with stressful events
R46.7 Verbosity and circumstantial detail obscuring reason for contact
[5th] R46.8 Other symptoms and signs involving appearance and behavior
R46.81 Obsessive-compulsive behavior PDx
[EXCLUDES1] *obsessive-compulsive disorder (F42-)*
R46.89 Other symptoms and signs involving appearance and behavior PDx

Symptoms and signs involving speech and voice (R47-R49)

[4th] R47 Speech disturbances, not elsewhere classified
[EXCLUDES1] *autism (F84.0)*
cluttering (F80.81)
specific developmental disorders of speech and language (F80.-)
stuttering (F80.81)
[5th] R47.0 Dysphasia and aphasia
R47.01 Aphasia CC CC/MCC Exc
[EXCLUDES1] *aphasia following cerebrovascular disease (I69. with final characters -20)*
progressive isolated aphasia (G31.01)
R47.02 Dysphasia
[EXCLUDES1] *dysphasia following cerebrovascular disease (I69. with final characters -21)*
R47.1 Dysarthria and anarthria
[EXCLUDES1] *dysarthria following cerebrovascular disease (I69. with final characters -22)*
[5th] R47.8 Other speech disturbances
[EXCLUDES1] *dysarthria following cerebrovascular disease (I69. with final characters -28)*
R47.81 Slurred speech
R47.82 Fluency disorder in conditions classified elsewhere
Stuttering in conditions classified elsewhere
☛ Code first underlying disease or condition, such as:
Parkinson's disease (G20)
[EXCLUDES1] *adult onset fluency disorder (F98.5)*
childhood onset fluency disorder (F80.81)
fluency disorder (stuttering) following cerebrovascular disease (I69. with final characters -23)
R47.89 Other speech disturbances
R47.9 Unspecified speech disturbances
[4th] R48 Dyslexia and other symbolic dysfunctions, not elsewhere classified
[EXCLUDES1] *specific developmental disorders of scholastic skills (F81.-)*
R48.0 Dyslexia and alexia
R48.1 Agnosia
Astereognosia (astereognosis)
Autotopagnosia
[EXCLUDES1] *visual object agnosia (R48.3)*
R48.2 Apraxia
[EXCLUDES1] *apraxia following cerebrovascular disease (I69. with final characters -90)*
R48.3 Visual agnosia
Prosopagnosia
Simultanagnosia (asimultagnosia)
R48.8 Other symbolic dysfunctions
AHA: Q1 2017
Acalculia
Agraphia
R48.9 Unspecified symbolic dysfunctions
[4th] R49 Voice and resonance disorders
[EXCLUDES1] *psychogenic voice and resonance disorders (F44.4)*
R49.0 Dysphonia
Hoarseness
R49.1 Aphonia
Loss of voice
[5th] R49.2 Hypernasality and hyponasality
R49.21 Hypernasality
R49.22 Hyponasality
R49.8 Other voice and resonance disorders
R49.9 Unspecified voice and resonance disorder
Change in voice NOS
Resonance disorder NOS

General symptoms and signs (R50-R69)

[4th] R50 Fever of other and unknown origin
[EXCLUDES1] *chills without fever (R68.83)*
febrile convulsions (R56.0-)
fever of unknown origin during labor (O75.2)
fever of unknown origin in newborn (P81.9)
hypothermia due to illness (R68.0)
malignant hyperthermia due to anesthesia (T88.3)
puerperal pyrexia NOS (O86.4)
R50.2 Drug induced fever CC CC/MCC Exc
Use additional code for adverse effect, if applicable, to identify drug (T36-T50 with fifth or sixth character 5)
[EXCLUDES1] *postvaccination (postimmunization) fever (R50.83)*
[5th] R50.8 Other specified fever
R50.81 Fever presenting with conditions classified elsewhere
AHA: Q2 2019
☛ Code first underlying condition when associated fever is present, such as with:
leukemia (C91-C95)
neutropenia (D70.-)
sickle-cell disease (D57.-)
R50.82 Postprocedural fever CC CC/MCC Exc
[EXCLUDES1] *postprocedural infection (T81.4-)*
posttransfusion fever (R50.84)
postvaccination (postimmunization) fever (R50.83)
R50.83 Postvaccination fever
Postimmunization fever
R50.84 Febrile nonhemolytic transfusion reaction
FNHTR
Posttransfusion fever
R50.9 Fever, unspecified
Fever NOS
Fever of unknown origin [FUO]
Fever with chills
Fever with rigors
Hyperpyrexia NOS
Persistent fever
Pyrexia NOS
R51 Headache
Facial pain NOS
[EXCLUDES1] *atypical face pain (G50.1)*
migraine and other headache syndromes (G43-G44)
trigeminal neuralgia (G50.0)
R52 Pain, unspecified
Acute pain NOS
Generalized pain NOS
Pain NOS
[EXCLUDES1] *acute and chronic pain, not elsewhere classified (G89.-)*
localized pain, unspecified type - code to pain by site, such as:
abdomen pain (R10.-)
back pain (M54.9)
breast pain (N64.4)
chest pain (R07.1-R07.9)
ear pain (H92.0-)
eye pain (H57.1)
headache (R51)

Unspecified Code | Other Specified Code | Manifestation Code | [N] Newborn | [P] Pediatric | [M] Maternity | [A] Adult | ♂ Male | ♀ Female
● New Code ▲ Revised Code Title ►◄ Revised Text [NOTES] INCLUDES [EXCLUDES1] Not coded here [EXCLUDES2] Not included here
[4th] 4th character required [5th] 5th character required [6th] 6th character required [7th] 7th character required [7th] Extension 'X' Alert
[HAC] Hospital-acquired condition (HAC) alert AHA AHA Coding Clinic© ☛ Code first alert

R53 - R58

CHAPTER 18: SYMPTOMS, SIGNS, AND ABNORMAL CLINICAL AND LABORATORY FINDINGS, NOT ELSEWHERE CLASSIFIED (R00-R99)

joint pain (M25.5-)

limb pain (M79.6-)

lumbar region pain (M54.5)

pelvic and perineal pain (R10.2)

shoulder pain (M25.51-)

spine pain (M54.-)

throat pain (R07.0)

tongue pain (K14.6)

tooth pain (K08.8)

renal colic (N23)

pain disorders exclusively related to psychological factors (F45.41)

R53 Malaise and fatigue

R53.0 Neoplastic (malignant) related fatigue

☞ **Code first** associated neoplasm

R53.1 Weakness

Asthenia NOS

EXCLUDES1 age-related weakness (R54)

muscle weakness (M62.8-)

sarcopenia (M62.84)

senile asthenia (R54)

R53.2 Functional quadriplegia HCC MCC CC/MCC Exc

AHA: Q2 2016

Complete immobility due to severe physical disability or frailty

EXCLUDES1 frailty NOS (R54)

hysterical paralysis (F44.4)

immobility syndrome (M62.3)

neurologic quadriplegia (G82.5-)

quadriplegia (G82.50)

R53.8 Other malaise and fatigue

EXCLUDES1 combat exhaustion and fatigue (F43.0)

congenital debility (P96.9)

exhaustion and fatigue due to excessive exertion (T73.3)

exhaustion and fatigue due to exposure (T73.2)

exhaustion and fatigue due to heat (T67.-)

exhaustion and fatigue due to pregnancy (O26.8-)

exhaustion and fatigue due to recurrent depressive episode (F33)

exhaustion and fatigue due to senile debility (R54)

R53.81 Other malaise

Chronic debility

Debility NOS

General physical deterioration

Malaise NOS

Nervous debility

EXCLUDES1 age-related physical debility (R54)

R53.82 Chronic fatigue, unspecified

Chronic fatigue syndrome NOS

EXCLUDES1 postviral fatigue syndrome (G93.3)

R53.83 Other fatigue

Fatigue NOS

Lack of energy

Lethargy

Tiredness

EXCLUDES2 exhaustion and fatigue due to depressive episode (F32.-)

R54 Age-related physical debility A

Frailty

Old age

Senescence

Senile asthenia

Senile debility

EXCLUDES1 age-related cognitive decline (R41.81)

sarcopenia (M62.84)

senile psychosis (F03)

senility NOS (R41.81)

R55 Syncope and collapse

Blackout

Fainting

Vasovagal attack

EXCLUDES1 cardiogenic shock (R57.0)

carotid sinus syncope (G90.01)

heat syncope (T67.1)

neurocirculatory asthenia (F45.8)

neurogenic orthostatic hypotension (G90.3)

orthostatic hypotension (I95.1)

postprocedural shock (T81.1-)

psychogenic syncope (F48.8)

shock NOS (R57.9)

shock complicating or following abortion or ectopic or molar pregnancy (O00-O07, O08.3)

shock complicating or following labor and delivery (O75.1)

Stokes-Adams attack (I45.9)

unconsciousness NOS (R40.2-)

R56 Convulsions, not elsewhere classified

EXCLUDES1 dissociative convulsions and seizures (F44.5)

epileptic convulsions and seizures (G40.-)

newborn convulsions and seizures (P90)

R56.0 Febrile convulsions

R56.00 Simple febrile convulsions CC HCC RxHCC CC/MCC Exc

Febrile convulsion NOS

Febrile seizure NOS

R56.01 Complex febrile convulsions CC HCC RxHCC CC/MCC Exc

Atypical febrile seizure

Complex febrile seizure

Complicated febrile seizure

EXCLUDES1 status epilepticus (G40.901)

R56.1 Post traumatic seizures CC HCC RxHCC CC/MCC Exc

EXCLUDES1 post traumatic epilepsy (G40.-)

R56.9 Unspecified convulsions HCC RxHCC

Convulsion disorder

Fit NOS

Recurrent convulsions

Seizure(s) (convulsive) NOS

R57 Shock, not elsewhere classified

EXCLUDES1 anaphylactic shock NOS (T78.2)

anaphylactic reaction or shock due to adverse food reaction (T78.0-)

anaphylactic shock due to adverse effect of correct drug or medicament properly administered (T88.6)

anaphylactic shock due to serum (T80.5-)

anesthetic shock (T88.3)

electric shock (T75.4)

obstetric shock (O75.1)

postprocedural shock (T81.1-)

psychic shock (F43.0)

shock complicating or following ectopic or molar pregnancy (O00-O07, O08.3)

shock due to lightning (T75.01)

traumatic shock (T79.4)

toxic shock syndrome (A48.3)

R57.0 Cardiogenic shock HCC MCC CC/MCC Exc

EXCLUDES2 septic shock (R65.21)

R57.1 Hypovolemic shock HCC MCC CC/MCC Exc

AHA: Q2 2019

R57.8 Other shock HCC MCC CC/MCC Exc

R57.9 Shock, unspecified CC HCC CC/MCC Exc

Failure of peripheral circulation NOS

R58 Hemorrhage, not elsewhere classified CC CC/MCC Exc

Hemorrhage NOS

EXCLUDES1 hemorrhage included with underlying conditions, such as:

acute duodenal ulcer with hemorrhage (K26.0)

acute gastritis with bleeding (K29.01)

ulcerative enterocolitis with rectal bleeding (K51.01)

PDHx Unacceptable principal diagnosis symbol per Medicare code edits   PDHx Code exempt from diagnosis present on admission requirement
❓ Questionable admission   CC Complication or comorbidity   MCC Major complication or comorbidity   CC/MCC Exc CC/MCC exclusion
HCC HCC diagnosis code   RxHCC RxHCC diagnosis code   MACRA code   **DEFINITION** Describes condition/terminology
TIP Coding guidance   👁 Official Guideline Reference   Z1 Z code as first-listed diagnosis

R59 Enlarged lymph nodes
   INCLUDES swollen glands
   EXCLUDES1 lymphadenitis NOS (I88.9)
         acute lymphadenitis (L04.-)
         chronic lymphadenitis (I88.1)
         mesenteric (acute) (chronic) lymphadenitis (I88.0)

  R59.0 Localized **enlarged lymph nodes**

  R59.1 Generalized **enlarged lymph nodes**
     Lymphadenopathy NOS

  R59.9 Enlarged lymph nodes, unspecified

R60 Edema, not elsewhere classified
   EXCLUDES1 angioneurotic edema (T78.3)
         ascites (R18.-)
         cerebral edema (G93.6)
         cerebral edema due to birth injury (P11.0)
         edema of larynx (J38.4)
         edema of nasopharynx (J39.2)
         edema of pharynx (J39.2)
         gestational edema (O12.0-)
         hereditary edema (Q82.0)
         hydrops fetalis NOS (P83.2)
         hydrothorax (J94.8)
         hydrops fetalis NOS (P83.2)
         newborn edema (P83.3)
         pulmonary edema (J81.-)

  R60.0 Localized **edema**

  R60.1 Generalized **edema**   CC CC/MCC Exc
     EXCLUDES2 nutritional edema (E40-E46)

  R60.9 Edema, unspecified
     Fluid retention NOS

  R61 Generalized hyperhidrosis
     Excessive sweating
     Night sweats
     Secondary hyperhidrosis
   ☞ **Code first,** if applicable, menopausal and female climacteric states (N95.1)
     EXCLUDES1 focal (primary) (secondary) hyperhidrosis (L74.5-)
         Frey's syndrome (L74.52)
         localized (primary) (secondary) hyperhidrosis (L74.5-)

R62 Lack of expected normal physiological development in childhood and adults
   EXCLUDES1 delayed puberty (E30.0)
         gonadal dysgenesis (Q99.1)
         hypopituitarism (E23.0)

  R62.0 Delayed milestone **in childhood**   P
     Delayed attainment of expected physiological developmental stage
     Late talker
     Late walker

  R62.5 Other and unspecified lack of expected normal physiological development **in childhood**
     EXCLUDES1 HIV disease resulting in failure to thrive (B20)
         physical retardation due to malnutrition (E45)

    R62.50 Unspecified lack of expected normal physiological development in childhood
       Infantilism NOS

    R62.51 Failure to thrive (child)   P
       AHA: Q4 2018
       Failure to gain weight
       EXCLUDES1 failure to thrive in child under 28 days old (P92.6)

    R62.52 Short stature (child)
       Lack of growth
       Physical retardation
       Short stature NOS
       EXCLUDES1 short stature due to endocrine disorder (E34.3)

    R62.59 Other lack of expected normal physiological development in childhood

  R62.7 Adult failure to thrive   A CC CC/MCC Exc

R63 Symptoms and signs concerning food and fluid intake
   EXCLUDES1 bulimia NOS (F50.2)

  R63.0 Anorexia
     Loss of appetite
     EXCLUDES1 anorexia nervosa (F50.0-)
         loss of appetite of nonorganic origin (F50.89)

  R63.1 Polydipsia
     Excessive thirst

  R63.2 Polyphagia
     Excessive eating
     Hyperalimentation NOS

  R63.3 Feeding difficulties   CC CC/MCC Exc
     AHA: Q1 2017, Q3 2016
     Feeding problem (elderly) (infant) NOS
     Picky eater
     EXCLUDES1 eating disorders (F50.-)
         feeding problems of newborn (P92.-)
         infant feeding disorder of nonorganic origin (F98.2-)

  R63.4 Abnormal weight loss

  R63.5 Abnormal weight gain
     EXCLUDES1 excessive weight gain in pregnancy (O26.0-)
         obesity (E66.-)

  R63.6 Underweight
     Use additional code to identify body mass index (BMI), if known (Z68.-)
     EXCLUDES1 abnormal weight loss (R63.4)
         anorexia nervosa (F50.0-)
         malnutrition (E40-E46)

  R63.8 Other symptoms and signs concerning food and fluid intake

 R64 Cachexia   CC HCC CC/MCC Exc
     AHA: Q3 2017
     Wasting syndrome
   ☞ **Code first** underlying condition, if known
     EXCLUDES1 abnormal weight loss (R63.4)
         nutritional marasmus (E41)

R65 Symptoms and signs specifically associated with systemic inflammation and infection
   👁 **See Official Guidelines** "Sepsis and severe sepsis associated with a noninfectious process" I.C.1.d.6

  R65.1 Systemic inflammatory response syndrome (SIRS) of non-infectious origin
   ☞ **Code first** underlying condition, such as:
     heatstroke ►(T67.0-)◄
     injury and trauma (S00-T88)
     EXCLUDES1 sepsis- code to infection
         severe sepsis (R65.2)

    R65.10 Systemic inflammatory response syndrome (SIRS) of non-infectious origin without acute organ dysfunction   CC HCC PDxIn CC/MCC Exc
       👁 **See Official Guidelines** "SIRS due to Non-infectious Process" I.C.18.g
       AHA: Q2 2019
       Systemic inflammatory response syndrome (SIRS) NOS

    R65.11 Systemic inflammatory response syndrome (SIRS) of non-infectious origin with acute organ dysfunction   CC HCC PDxIn CC/MCC Exc
       👁 **See Official Guidelines** "SIRS due to Non-infectious Process" I.C.18.g
       Use additional code to identify specific acute organ dysfunction, such as:
       acute kidney failure (N17.-)
       acute respiratory failure (J96.0-)
       critical illness myopathy (G72.81)
       critical illness polyneuropathy (G62.81)
       disseminated intravascular coagulopathy [DIC] (D65)
       encephalopathy (metabolic) (septic) (G93.41)
       hepatic failure (K72.0-)

Unspecified Code   Other Specified Code   Manifestation Code   N Newborn   P Pediatric   M Maternity   A Adult   ♂ Male   ♀ Female
● New Code   ▲ Revised Code Title   ►◄ Revised Text   **NOTES**   *INCLUDES*   *EXCLUDES1* Not coded here   *EXCLUDES2* Not included here
④ 4th character required   ⑤ 5th character required   ⑥ 6th character required   ⑦ 7th character required   ⑦ Extension 'X' Alert
HAC Hospital-acquired condition (HAC) alert   **AHA** AHA Coding Clinic©   ☞ Code first alert

R65.2 Severe sepsis

    See Official Guidelines "Sepsis" I.C.1.d.1.a, "Sepsis" I.C.1.d.1.a.iv, "Severe sepsis" I.C.1.d.1.b, "Severe shock" I.C.1.d.2.a, "Sequencing of severe sepsis" I.C.1.d.3, "Sepsis and severe sepsis with a localized infection" I.C.1.d.4, "Sepsis due to a postprocedural infection" I.C.1.d.5.b, "Sepsis and septic shock complicating abortion, pregnancy, childbirth and the puerperium" I.C.15.j

    Infection with associated acute organ dysfunction

    Sepsis with acute organ dysfunction

    Sepsis with multiple organ dysfunction

    Systemic inflammatory response syndrome due to infectious process with acute organ dysfunction

    Code first underlying infection, such as:

        infection following a procedure (T81.4-)

        infections following infusion, transfusion and therapeutic injection (T80.2-)

        puerperal sepsis (O85)

        sepsis following complete or unspecified spontaneous abortion (O03.87)

        sepsis following ectopic and molar pregnancy (O08.82)

        sepsis following incomplete spontaneous abortion (O03.37)

        sepsis following (induced) termination of pregnancy (O04.87)

        sepsis NOS (A41.9)

    Use additional code to identify specific acute organ dysfunction, such as:

        acute kidney failure (N17.-)

        acute respiratory failure (J96.0-)

        critical illness myopathy (G72.81)

        critical illness polyneuropathy (G62.81)

        disseminated intravascular coagulopathy [DIC] (D65)

        encephalopathy (metabolic) (septic) (G93.41)

        hepatic failure (K72.0-)

    R65.20 Severe sepsis without septic shock `HCC` `MCC` `PDxin` `CC/MCC Exc`

        AHA: Q4 2018, Q3 2016

        Severe sepsis NOS

    R65.21 Severe sepsis with septic shock `HCC` `MCC` `PDxin` `CC/MCC Exc`

        See Official Guidelines "Postprocedural infection and postprocedural septic shock" I.C.1.d.5.c

        AHA: Q4 2018

R68 Other general symptoms and signs

    R68.0 Hypothermia, not associated with low environmental temperature

        EXCLUDES1 hypothermia NOS (accidental) (T68)

            hypothermia due to anesthesia (T88.51)

            hypothermia due to low environmental temperature (T68)

            newborn hypothermia (P80.-)

    R68.1 Nonspecific symptoms peculiar to infancy

        EXCLUDES1 colic, infantile (R10.83)

            neonatal cerebral irritability (P91.3)

            teething syndrome (K00.7)

    R68.11 Excessive crying of infant (baby) `P`

        EXCLUDES1 excessive crying of child, adolescent, or adult (R45.83)

    R68.12 Fussy infant (baby) `P`

        Irritable infant

    R68.13 Apparent life threatening event in infant (ALTE) `P`

        Apparent life threatening event in newborn

        Brief resolved unexplained event (BRUE)

        Code first confirmed diagnosis, if known

        Use additional code(s) for associated signs and symptoms if no confirmed diagnosis established, or if signs and symptoms are not associated routinely with confirmed diagnosis, or provide additional information for cause of ALTE

    R68.19 Other nonspecific symptoms peculiar to infancy `P`

    R68.2 Dry mouth, unspecified

        EXCLUDES1 dry mouth due to dehydration (E86.0)

            dry mouth due to sicca syndrome [Sjögren] (M35.0-)

            salivary gland hyposecretion (K11.7)

R68.3 Clubbing of fingers

    Clubbing of nails

    EXCLUDES1 congenital clubfinger (Q68.1)

R68.8 Other general symptoms and signs

    R68.81 Early satiety

    R68.82 Decreased libido `A`

        Decreased sexual desire

    R68.83 Chills (without fever)

        Chills NOS

        EXCLUDES1 chills with fever (R50.9)

    R68.84 Jaw pain

        Mandibular pain

        Maxilla pain

        EXCLUDES1 temporomandibular joint arthralgia (M26.62-)

    R68.89 Other general symptoms and signs

R69 Illness, unspecified

    Unknown and unspecified cases of morbidity

Abnormal findings on examination of blood, without diagnosis (R70-R79)

    EXCLUDES2 abnormal findings on antenatal screening of mother (O28.-)

        abnormalities of lipids (E78.-)

        abnormalities of platelets and thrombocytes (D69.-)

        abnormalities of white blood cells classified elsewhere (D70-D72)

        coagulation hemorrhagic disorders (D65-D68)

        diagnostic abnormal findings classified elsewhere - see Alphabetical Index

        hemorrhagic and hematological disorders of newborn (P50-P61)

R70 Elevated erythrocyte sedimentation rate and abnormality of plasma viscosity

    R70.0 Elevated erythrocyte sedimentation rate

    R70.1 Abnormal plasma viscosity

R71 Abnormality of red blood cells

    EXCLUDES1 anemias (D50-D64)

        anemia of premature infant (P61.2)

        benign (familial) polycythemia (D75.0)

        congenital anemias (P61.2-P61.4)

        newborn anemia due to isoimmunization (P55.-)

        polycythemia neonatorum (P61.1)

        polycythemia NOS (D75.1)

        polycythemia vera (D45)

        secondary polycythemia (D75.1)

    R71.0 Precipitous drop in hematocrit `CC` `CC/MCC Exc`

        Drop (precipitous) in hemoglobin

        Drop in hematocrit

    R71.8 Other abnormality of red blood cells

        Abnormal red-cell morphology NOS

        Abnormal red-cell volume NOS

        Anisocytosis

        Poikilocytosis

R73 Elevated blood glucose level

    EXCLUDES1 diabetes mellitus (E08-E13)

        diabetes mellitus in pregnancy, childbirth and the puerperium (O24.-)

        neonatal disorders (P70.0-P70.2)

        postsurgical hypoinsulinemia (E89.1)

    R73.0 Abnormal glucose

        EXCLUDES1 abnormal glucose in pregnancy (O99.81-)

            diabetes mellitus (E08-E13)

            dysmetabolic syndrome X (E88.81)

            gestational diabetes (O24.4-)

            glycosuria (R81)

            hypoglycemia (E16.2)

    R73.01 Impaired fasting glucose

        Elevated fasting glucose

`PDxin` Unacceptable principal diagnosis symbol per Medicare code edits   `POAex` Code exempt from diagnosis present on admission requirement
   `?` Questionable admission   `CC` Complication or comorbidity   `MCC` Major complication or comorbidity   `CC/MCC Exc` CC/MCC exclusion
   `HCC` HCC diagnosis code   `RxHCC` RxHCC diagnosis code   MACRA code   **DEFINITION** Describes condition/terminology
   TIP Coding guidance   Official Guideline Reference   `Z1` Z code as first-listed diagnosis

960   When symbols appear on a code that requires a 7th character extension, refer to Appendix B to identify applicable 7th character codes.   **2020 ICD-10-CM**

R73.02 **Impaired glucose tolerance (oral)**
Elevated glucose tolerance
R73.03 **Prediabetes**
AHA: Q4 2016
Latent diabetes
R73.09 **Other abnormal glucose**
AHA: Q4 2016
Abnormal glucose NOS
Abnormal non-fasting glucose tolerance
R73.9 **Hyperglycemia, unspecified**

[4th] R74 **Abnormal serum enzyme levels**
R74.0 **Nonspecific elevation of levels of transaminase and lactic acid dehydrogenase [LDH]**
R74.8 **Abnormal levels of other serum enzymes**
AHA: Q2 2019
Abnormal level of acid phosphatase
Abnormal level of alkaline phosphatase
Abnormal level of amylase
Abnormal level of lipase [triacylglycerol lipase]
R74.9 **Abnormal serum enzyme level, unspecified**

R75 **Inconclusive laboratory evidence of human immunodeficiency virus [HIV]**
See Official Guidelines "Patients with inconclusive HIV serology" I.C.1.a.2.e, "Previously diagnosed HIV-related illness" I.C.1.a.2.f
Nonconclusive HIV-test finding in infants
EXCLUDES1 *asymptomatic human immunodeficiency virus [HIV] infection status (Z21)*
human immunodeficiency virus [HIV] disease (B20)

[4th] R76 **Other abnormal immunological findings in serum**
R76.0 **Raised antibody titer**
EXCLUDES1 *isoimmunization in pregnancy (O36.0-O36.1)*
isoimmunization affecting newborn (P55.-)
[5th] R76.1 **Nonspecific reaction to test for tuberculosis**
R76.11 **Nonspecific reaction to tuberculin skin test without active tuberculosis**
Abnormal result of Mantoux test
PPD positive
Tuberculin (skin test) positive
Tuberculin (skin test) reactor
EXCLUDES1 *nonspecific reaction to cell mediated immunity measurement of gamma interferon antigen response without active tuberculosis (R76.12)*
R76.12 **Nonspecific reaction to cell mediated immunity measurement of gamma interferon antigen response without active tuberculosis**
Nonspecific reaction to QuantiFERON-TB test (QFT) without active tuberculosis
EXCLUDES1 *nonspecific reaction to tuberculin skin test without active tuberculosis (R76.11)*
positive tuberculin skin test (R76.11)
R76.8 **Other specified abnormal immunological findings in serum**
Raised level of immunoglobulins NOS
R76.9 **Abnormal immunological finding in serum, unspecified**

[4th] R77 **Other abnormalities of plasma proteins**
EXCLUDES1 *disorders of plasma-protein metabolism (E88.0-)*
R77.0 **Abnormality of albumin**
R77.1 **Abnormality of globulin**
Hyperglobulinemia NOS
R77.2 **Abnormality of alphafetoprotein**
R77.8 **Other specified abnormalities of plasma proteins**
AHA: Q2 2019
R77.9 **Abnormality of plasma protein, unspecified**
AHA: Q2 2019

[4th] R78 **Findings of drugs and other substances, not normally found in blood**
Use additional code to identify the any retained foreign body, if applicable (Z18.-)
EXCLUDES1 *mental or behavioral disorders due to psychoactive substance use (F10-F19)*
R78.0 **Finding of alcohol in blood**
Use additional external cause code (Y90.-), for detail regarding alcohol level.
R78.1 **Finding of opiate drug in blood**
R78.2 **Finding of cocaine in blood**
R78.3 **Finding of hallucinogen in blood**
R78.4 **Finding of other drugs of addictive potential in blood**
R78.5 **Finding of other psychotropic drug in blood**
R78.6 **Finding of steroid agent in blood**
[5th] R78.7 **Finding of abnormal level of heavy metals in blood**
R78.71 **Abnormal lead level in blood**
EXCLUDES1 *lead poisoning (T56.0-)*
R78.79 **Finding of abnormal level of heavy metals in blood**
[5th] R78.8 **Finding of other specified substances, not normally found in blood**
R78.81 **Bacteremia** MCC CC/MCC Exc
EXCLUDES1 *sepsis-code to specified infection*
R78.89 **Finding of other specified substances, not normally found in blood**
Finding of abnormal level of lithium in blood
R78.9 **Finding of unspecified substance, not normally found in blood**

[4th] R79 **Other abnormal findings of blood chemistry**
Use additional code to identify any retained foreign body, if applicable (Z18.-)
EXCLUDES1 *asymptomatic hyperuricemia (E79.0)*
hyperglycemia NOS (R73.9)
hypoglycemia NOS (E16.2)
neonatal hypoglycemia (P70.3-P70.4)
specific findings indicating disorder of amino-acid metabolism (E70-E72)
specific findings indicating disorder of carbohydrate metabolism (E73-E74)
specific findings indicating disorder of lipid metabolism (E75.-)
R79.0 **Abnormal level of blood mineral**
Abnormal blood level of cobalt
Abnormal blood level of copper
Abnormal blood level of iron
Abnormal blood level of magnesium
Abnormal blood level of mineral NEC
Abnormal blood level of zinc
EXCLUDES1 *abnormal level of lithium (R78.89)*
disorders of mineral metabolism (E83.-)
neonatal hypomagnesemia (P71.2)
nutritional mineral deficiency (E58-E61)
R79.1 **Abnormal coagulation profile**
Abnormal or prolonged bleeding time
Abnormal or prolonged coagulation time
Abnormal or prolonged partial thromboplastin time [PTT]
Abnormal or prolonged prothrombin time [PT]
EXCLUDES1 *coagulation defects (D68.-)*
EXCLUDES2 *abnormality of fluid, electrolyte or acid-base balance (E86-E87)*
[5th] R79.8 **Other specified abnormal findings of blood chemistry**
R79.81 **Abnormal blood-gas level**
R79.82 **Elevated C-reactive protein (CRP)**
R79.89 **Other specified abnormal findings of blood chemistry**
AHA: Q2 2019
R79.9 **Abnormal finding of blood chemistry, unspecified**

Abnormal findings on examination of urine, without diagnosis (R80-R82)

EXCLUDES1 *abnormal findings on antenatal screening of mother (O28.-)*
diagnostic abnormal findings classified elsewhere - see Alphabetical Index
specific findings indicating disorder of amino-acid metabolism (E70-E72)
specific findings indicating disorder of carbohydrate metabolism (E73-E74)

[4th] R80 Proteinuria
[EXCLUDES1] *gestational proteinuria (O12.1-)*
R80.0 Isolated **proteinuria**
Idiopathic proteinuria
[EXCLUDES1] *isolated proteinuria with specific morphological lesion (N06.-)*
R80.1 **Persistent proteinuria, unspecified**
R80.2 **Orthostatic proteinuria, unspecified**
Postural proteinuria
R80.3 Bence Jones **proteinuria**
R80.8 Other **proteinuria**
R80.9 **Proteinuria, unspecified**
Albuminuria NOS

R81 **Glycosuria**
[EXCLUDES1] *renal glycosuria (E74.8)*

[4th] R82 **Other and unspecified abnormal findings in urine**
[INCLUDES] *chromoabnormalities in urine*
Use additional code to identify any retained foreign body, if applicable (Z18.-)
[EXCLUDES2] *hematuria (R31.-)*
R82.0 **Chyluria** [CC]
[EXCLUDES1] *filarial chyluria (B74.-)*
R82.1 **Myoglobinuria** [CC]
R82.2 **Biliuria**
R82.3 **Hemoglobinuria**
[EXCLUDES1] *hemoglobinuria due to hemolysis from external causes NEC (D59.6)*
hemoglobinuria due to paroxysmal nocturnal [Marchiafava-Micheli] (D59.5)
R82.4 **Acetonuria**
Ketonuria
R82.5 **Elevated urine levels of drugs, medicaments and biological substances**
Elevated urine levels of catecholamines
Elevated urine levels of indoleacetic acid
Elevated urine levels of 17-ketosteroids
Elevated urine levels of steroids
R82.6 **Abnormal urine levels of substances chiefly nonmedicinal as to source**
Abnormal urine level of heavy metals
[5th] R82.7 **Abnormal findings on microbiological examination of urine**
[EXCLUDES1] *colonization status (Z22.-)*
R82.71 Bacteriuria
AHA: Q4 2016
R82.79 Other **abnormal findings on microbiological examination of urine**
AHA: Q4 2016
Positive culture findings of urine
[5th] R82.8 **Abnormal findings on cytological and histological examination of urine**
● R82.81 Pyuria
Sterile pyuria
● R82.89 Other **abnormal findings on cytological and histological examination of urine**
[5th] R82.9 **Other and unspecified abnormal findings in urine**
R82.90 **Unspecified abnormal findings in urine**
R82.91 **Other chromoabnormalities of urine**
Chromoconversion (dipstick)
Idiopathic dipstick converts positive for blood with no cellular forms in sediment
[EXCLUDES1] *hemoglobinuria (R82.3)*
myoglobinuria (R82.1)
[6th] R82.99 **Other abnormal findings in urine**
R82.991 Hypocitraturia
AHA: Q4 2018
R82.992 Hyperoxaluria
AHA: Q4 2018
[EXCLUDES1] *Primary hyperoxaluria (E72.53)*
▲ R82.993 ▶Hyperuricosuria◀
AHA: Q4 2018
R82.994 Hypercalciuria
AHA: Q4 2018
Idiopathic hypercalciuria
R82.998 **Other** abnormal **findings in** urine
AHA: Q4 2018
Cells and casts in urine
Crystalluria
Melanuria

Abnormal findings on examination of other body fluids, substances and tissues, without diagnosis (R83-R89)

[EXCLUDES1] *abnormal findings on antenatal screening of mother (O28.-)*
diagnostic abnormal findings classified elsewhere - see Alphabetical Index
[EXCLUDES2] *abnormal findings on examination of blood, without diagnosis (R70-R79)*
abnormal findings on examination of urine, without diagnosis (R80-R82)
abnormal tumor markers (R97.-)

[4th] R83 **Abnormal findings in** cerebrospinal fluid
R83.0 **Abnormal level of** enzymes **in cerebrospinal fluid**
R83.1 **Abnormal level of** hormones **in cerebrospinal fluid**
R83.2 **Abnormal level of** other drugs, medicaments and biological substances **in cerebrospinal fluid**
R83.3 **Abnormal level of** substances chiefly nonmedicinal **as to source in cerebrospinal fluid**
R83.4 **Abnormal** immunological **findings in cerebrospinal fluid**
R83.5 **Abnormal** microbiological **findings in cerebrospinal fluid**
Positive culture findings in cerebrospinal fluid
[EXCLUDES1] *colonization status (Z22.-)*
R83.6 **Abnormal** cytological **findings in cerebrospinal fluid**
R83.8 Other abnormal findings **in cerebrospinal fluid**
Abnormal chromosomal findings in cerebrospinal fluid
R83.9 **Unspecified abnormal finding in cerebrospinal fluid**

[4th] R84 **Abnormal findings in specimens from** respiratory organs and thorax
[INCLUDES] *abnormal findings in bronchial washings*
abnormal findings in nasal secretions
abnormal findings in pleural fluid
abnormal findings in sputum
abnormal findings in throat scrapings
[EXCLUDES1] *blood-stained sputum (R04.2)*
R84.0 **Abnormal level of** enzymes **in specimens from respiratory organs and thorax**
R84.1 **Abnormal level of** hormones **in specimens from respiratory organs and thorax**
R84.2 **Abnormal level of other** drugs, medicaments and biological substances **in specimens from respiratory organs and thorax**
R84.3 **Abnormal level of** substances chiefly nonmedicinal **as to source in specimens from respiratory organs and thorax**
R84.4 **Abnormal** immunological **findings in specimens from respiratory organs and thorax**
R84.5 **Abnormal** microbiological **findings in specimens from respiratory organs and thorax**
Positive culture findings in specimens from respiratory organs and thorax
[EXCLUDES1] *colonization status (Z22.-)*
R84.6 **Abnormal** cytological **findings in specimens from respiratory organs and thorax**
R84.7 **Abnormal** histological **findings in specimens from respiratory organs and thorax**
R84.8 Other abnormal findings **in specimens from respiratory organs and thorax**
Abnormal chromosomal findings in specimens from respiratory organs and thorax
R84.9 **Unspecified abnormal finding in specimens from respiratory organs and thorax**

[4th] R85 **Abnormal findings in** specimens **from** digestive organs and abdominal cavity
[INCLUDES] *abnormal findings in peritoneal fluid*
abnormal findings in saliva

[PDx] Unacceptable principal diagnosis symbol per Medicare code edits [POA] Code exempt from diagnosis present on admission requirement
[?] Questionable admission [CC] Complication or comorbidity [MCC] Major complication or comorbidity [CC/MCC Exc] CC/MCC exclusion
[HCC] HCC diagnosis code [RxHCC] RxHCC diagnosis code MACRA code **DEFINITION** Describes condition/terminology
TIP Coding guidance 👁 Official Guideline Reference [Z-1] Z code as first-listed diagnosis

EXCLUDES1 *cloudy peritoneal dialysis effluent (R88.0)*

fecal abnormalities (R19.5)

R85.0 **Abnormal level of** enzymes **in specimens from digestive organs and abdominal cavity**

R85.1 **Abnormal level of** hormones **in specimens from digestive organs and abdominal cavity**

R85.2 **Abnormal level of** other drugs, medicaments and biological substances **in specimens from digestive organs and abdominal cavity**

R85.3 **Abnormal level of** substances chiefly nonmedicinal **as to source in specimens from digestive organs and abdominal cavity**

R85.4 **Abnormal** immunological **findings in specimens from digestive organs and abdominal cavity**

R85.5 **Abnormal** microbiological **findings in specimens from digestive organs and abdominal cavity**

Positive culture findings in specimens from digestive organs and abdominal cavity

EXCLUDES1 *colonization status (Z22.-)*

5ᵗʰ R85.6 **Abnormal** cytological **findings in specimens from digestive organs and abdominal cavity**

6ᵗʰ R85.61 **Abnormal cytologic smear of** anus

EXCLUDES1 *abnormal cytological findings in specimens from other digestive organs and abdominal cavity (R85.69)*

carcinoma in situ of anus (histologically confirmed) (D01.3)

anal intraepithelial neoplasia I [AIN I] (K62.82)

anal intraepithelial neoplasia II [AIN II] (K62.82)

anal intraepithelial neoplasia III [AIN III] (D01.3)

dysplasia (mild) (moderate) of anus (histologically confirmed) (K62.82)

severe dysplasia of anus (histologically confirmed) (D01.3)

EXCLUDES2 *anal high risk human papillomavirus (HPV) DNA test positive (R85.81)*

anal low risk human papillomavirus (HPV) DNA test positive (R85.82)

R85.610 Atypical **squamous cells of** undetermined significance **on cytologic smear of anus** (ASC-US)

R85.611 Atypical **squamous cells cannot exclude** high grade **squamous intraepithelial lesion on cytologic smear of anus** (ASC-H)

R85.612 Low grade **squamous intraepithelial lesion on cytologic smear of anus** (LGSIL)

R85.613 High grade **squamous intraepithelial lesion on cytologic smear of anus** (HGSIL)

R85.614 **Cytologic evidence of** malignancy **on smear of anus**

R85.615 Unsatisfactory **cytologic smear of anus**

Inadequate sample of cytologic smear of anus

R85.616 Satisfactory **anal smear but** lacking transformation zone

R85.618 **Other abnormal cytological findings on specimens from anus**

R85.619 **Unspecified abnormal cytological findings in specimens from anus**

Abnormal anal cytology NOS

Atypical glandular cells of anus NOS

R85.69 **Abnormal cytological findings in specimens from other digestive organs and abdominal cavity**

R85.7 **Abnormal** histological **findings in specimens from digestive organs and abdominal cavity**

5ᵗʰ R85.8 Other **abnormal findings in specimens from digestive organs and abdominal cavity**

R85.81 **Anal** high risk human papillomavirus **(HPV) DNA test positive**

EXCLUDES1 *anogenital warts due to human papillomavirus (HPV) (A63.0)*

condyloma acuminatum (A63.0)

R85.82 **Anal** low risk human papillomavirus **(HPV) DNA test positive**

Use additional code for associated human papillomavirus (B97.7)

R85.89 Other abnormal findings **in specimens from digestive organs and abdominal cavity**

Abnormal chromosomal findings in specimens from digestive organs and abdominal cavity

R85.9 **Unspecified abnormal finding in specimens from digestive organs and abdominal cavity**

4ᵗʰ R86 **Abnormal findings in specimens from** male genital organs

INCLUDES *abnormal findings in prostatic secretions*

abnormal findings in semen, seminal fluid

abnormal spermatozoa

EXCLUDES1 *azoospermia (N46.0-)*

oligospermia (N46.1-)

R86.0 **Abnormal level of** enzymes **in specimens from male genital organs** ♂

R86.1 **Abnormal level of** hormones **in specimens from male genital organs** ♂

R86.2 **Abnormal level of** other drugs, medicaments and biological substances **in specimens from male genital organs** ♂

R86.3 **Abnormal level of** substances chiefly nonmedicinal **as to source in specimens from male genital organs** ♂

R86.4 **Abnormal** immunological **findings in specimens from male genital organs** ♂

R86.5 **Abnormal** microbiological **findings in specimens from male genital organs** ♂

Positive culture findings in specimens from male genital organs

EXCLUDES1 *colonization status (Z22.-)*

R86.6 **Abnormal** cytological **findings in specimens from male genital organs** ♂

R86.7 **Abnormal** histological **findings in specimens from male genital organs** ♂

R86.8 Other abnormal findings **in specimens from male genital organs** ♂

Abnormal chromosomal findings in specimens from male genital organs

R86.9 **Unspecified abnormal finding in specimens from male genital organs** ♂

4ᵗʰ R87 **Abnormal findings in specimens from** female genital organs

INCLUDES *abnormal findings in secretion and smears from cervix uteri*

abnormal findings in secretion and smears from vagina

abnormal findings in secretion and smears from vulva

R87.0 **Abnormal level of** enzymes **in specimens from female genital organs** ♀

R87.1 **Abnormal level of** hormones **in specimens from female genital organs** ♀

R87.2 **Abnormal level of** other drugs, medicaments and biological substances **in specimens from female genital organs** ♀

R87.3 **Abnormal level of** substances chiefly nonmedicinal **as to source in specimens from female genital organs** ♀

R87.4 **Abnormal** immunological **findings in specimens from female genital organs** ♀

R87.5 **Abnormal** microbiological **findings in specimens from female genital organs** ♀

Positive culture findings in specimens from female genital organs

EXCLUDES1 *colonization status (Z22.-)*

5ᵗʰ R87.6 **Abnormal** cytological **findings in specimens from female genital organs**

6ᵗʰ R87.61 **Abnormal cytological findings in specimens from** cervix uteri

---

Unspecified Code   Other Specified Code   Manifestation Code   Ⓝ Newborn   Ⓟ Pediatric   Ⓜ Maternity   Ⓐ Adult   ♂ Male   ♀ Female
● New Code   ▲ Revised Code Title   ▶◀ Revised Text   **NOTES**   *INCLUDES*   EXCLUDES1 Not coded here   EXCLUDES2 Not included here
4ᵗʰ 4ᵗʰ character required   5ᵗʰ 5ᵗʰ character required   6ᵗʰ 6ᵗʰ character required   7ᵗʰ 7ᵗʰ character required   7ᵗʰ Extension 'X' Alert
HAC Hospital-acquired condition (HAC) alert   **AHA** AHA Coding Clinic©   ☛ Code first alert

[EXCLUDES1] *abnormal cytological findings in specimens from other female genital organs (R87.69)*
abnormal cytological findings in specimens from vagina (R87.62-)
carcinoma in situ of cervix uteri (histologically confirmed) (D06.-)
cervical intraepithelial neoplasia I [CIN I] (N87.0)
cervical intraepithelial neoplasia II [CIN II] (N87.1)
cervical intraepithelial neoplasia III [CIN III] (D06.-)
dysplasia (mild) (moderate) of cervix uteri (histologically confirmed) (N87.-)
severe dysplasia of cervix uteri (histologically confirmed) (D06.-)

[EXCLUDES2] *cervical high risk human papillomavirus (HPV) DNA test positive (R87.810)*
cervical low risk human papillomavirus (HPV) DNA test positive (R87.820)

R87.610 Atypical **squamous cells of** undetermined significance **on cytologic smear of cervix** (ASC-US) ♀

R87.611 Atypical **squamous cells cannot exclude** high grade **squamous intraepithelial lesion on cytologic smear of cervix** (ASC-H) ♀

R87.612 Low grade **squamous intraepithelial lesion on cytologic smear of cervix (LGSIL)** ♀

R87.613 High grade **squamous intraepithelial lesion on cytologic smear of cervix** (HGSIL) ♀

R87.614 **Cytologic evidence of** malignancy **on smear of cervix** ♀

R87.615 Unsatisfactory **cytologic smear of cervix** ♀
Inadequate sample of cytologic smear of cervix

R87.616 Satisfactory **cervical smear but** lacking transformation zone ♀

R87.618 Other abnormal cytological findings **on specimens from cervix uteri** ♀

R87.619 **Unspecified abnormal cytological findings in specimens from cervix uteri** ♀
Abnormal cervical cytology NOS
Abnormal Papanicolaou smear of cervix NOS
Abnormal thin preparation smear of cervix NOS
Atypical endocervical cells of cervix NOS
Atypical endometrial cells of cervix NOS
Atypical glandular cells of cervix NOS

[6th] **R87.62** **Abnormal cytological findings in specimens from** vagina
Use additional code to identify acquired absence of uterus and cervix, if applicable (Z90.71-)

[EXCLUDES1] *abnormal cytological findings in specimens from cervix uteri (R87.61-)*
abnormal cytological findings in specimens from other female genital organs (R87.69)
carcinoma in situ of vagina (histologically confirmed) (D07.2)
vaginal intraepithelial neoplasia I [VAIN I] (N89.0)
vaginal intraepithelial neoplasia II [VAIN II] (N89.1)
vaginal intraepithelial neoplasia III [VAIN III] (D07.2)
dysplasia (mild) (moderate) of vagina (histologically confirmed) (N89.-)
severe dysplasia of vagina (histologically confirmed) (D07.2)

[EXCLUDES2] *vaginal high risk human papillomavirus (HPV) DNA test positive (R87.811)*
vaginal low risk human papillomavirus (HPV) DNA test positive (R87.821)

R87.620 Atypical **squamous cells of** undetermined significance **on cytologic smear of vagina** (ASC-US) ♀

R87.621 Atypical **squamous cells cannot exclude** high grade **squamous intraepithelial lesion on cytologic smear of vagina** (ASC-H) ♀

R87.622 Low grade **squamous intraepithelial lesion on cytologic smear of vagina (LGSIL)** ♀

R87.623 High grade **squamous intraepithelial lesion on cytologic smear of vagina** (HGSIL) ♀

R87.624 **Cytologic evidence of** malignancy **on smear of vagina** ♀

R87.625 Unsatisfactory **cytologic smear of vagina** ♀
Inadequate sample of cytologic smear of vagina

R87.628 Other abnormal cytological findings **on specimens from vagina** ♀

R87.629 **Unspecified abnormal cytological findings in specimens from vagina** ♀
Abnormal Papanicolaou smear of vagina NOS
Abnormal thin preparation smear of vagina NOS
Abnormal vaginal cytology NOS
Atypical endocervical cells of vagina NOS
Atypical endometrial cells of vagina NOS
Atypical glandular cells of vagina NOS

R87.69 **Abnormal cytological findings in specimens from other female genital organs** ♀
Abnormal cytological findings in specimens from female genital organs NOS

[EXCLUDES1] *dysplasia of vulva (histologically confirmed) (N90.0-N90.3)*

R87.7 **Abnormal histological findings in specimens from** female genital organs ♀

[EXCLUDES1] *carcinoma in situ (histologically confirmed) of female genital organs (D06-D07.3)*
cervical intraepithelial neoplasia I [CIN I] (N87.0)
cervical intraepithelial neoplasia II [CIN II] (N87.1)
cervical intraepithelial neoplasia III [CIN III] (D06.-)
dysplasia (mild) (moderate) of cervix uteri (histologically confirmed) (N87.-)
dysplasia (mild) (moderate) of vagina (histologically confirmed) (N89.-)
vaginal intraepithelial neoplasia I [VAIN I] (N89.0)
vaginal intraepithelial neoplasia II [VAIN II] (N89.1)
vaginal intraepithelial neoplasia III [VAIN III] (D07.2)
severe dysplasia of cervix uteri (histologically confirmed) (D06.-)
severe dysplasia of vagina (histologically confirmed) (D07.2)

[5th] **R87.8** Other **abnormal findings in specimens from female genital organs**

[6th] **R87.81** High risk human papillomavirus **(HPV) DNA test positive from female genital organs**

[EXCLUDES1] *anogenital warts due to human papillomavirus (HPV) (A63.0)*
condyloma acuminatum (A63.0)

R87.810 Cervical **high risk human papillomavirus (HPV) DNA test positive** ♀

R87.811 Vaginal **high risk human papillomavirus (HPV) DNA test positive** ♀

[6th] **R87.82** Low risk human papillomavirus **(HPV) DNA test positive from female genital organs**
Use additional code for associated human papillomavirus (B97.7)

Unacceptable principal diagnosis symbol per Medicare code edits; Code exempt from diagnosis present on admission requirement
[?] Questionable admission; [CC] Complication or comorbidity; [MCC] Major complication or comorbidity; [CC/MCC Exc] CC/MCC exclusion
[HCC] HCC diagnosis code; [RxHCC] RxHCC diagnosis code; MACRA code; **DEFINITION** Describes condition/terminology
TIP Coding guidance; Official Guideline Reference; [Z1] Z code as first-listed diagnosis

R87.820 Cervical low risk human papillomavirus (HPV) DNA test positive ♀
R87.821 Vaginal low risk human papillomavirus (HPV) DNA test positive ♀
R87.89 Other abnormal findings in specimens from female genital organs ♀
Abnormal chromosomal findings in specimens from female genital organs
R87.9 Unspecified abnormal finding in specimens from female genital organs ♀

[4th] R88 Abnormal findings in other body fluids and substances
R88.0 Cloudy (hemodialysis) (peritoneal) dialysis effluent
R88.8 Abnormal findings in other body fluids and substances

[4th] R89 Abnormal findings in specimens from other organs, systems and tissues
INCLUDES *abnormal findings in nipple discharge*
abnormal findings in synovial fluid
abnormal findings in wound secretions
R89.0 Abnormal level of enzymes in specimens from other organs, systems and tissues
R89.1 Abnormal level of hormones in specimens from other organs, systems and tissues
R89.2 Abnormal level of other drugs, medicaments and biological substances in specimens from other organs, systems and tissues
R89.3 Abnormal level of substances chiefly nonmedicinal as to source in specimens from other organs, systems and tissues
R89.4 Abnormal immunological findings in specimens from other organs, systems and tissues
R89.5 Abnormal microbiological findings in specimens from other organs, systems and tissues
Positive culture findings in specimens from other organs, systems and tissues
EXCLUDES1 *colonization status (Z22.-)*
R89.6 Abnormal cytological findings in specimens from other organs, systems and tissues
R89.7 Abnormal histological findings in specimens from other organs, systems and tissues
R89.8 Other abnormal findings in specimens from other organs, systems and tissues
Abnormal chromosomal findings in specimens from other organs, systems and tissues
R89.9 Unspecified abnormal finding in specimens from other organs, systems and tissues

Abnormal findings on diagnostic imaging and in function studies, without diagnosis (R90-R94)

INCLUDES *nonspecific abnormal findings on diagnostic imaging by computerized axial tomography [CAT scan]*
nonspecific abnormal findings on diagnostic imaging by magnetic resonance imaging [MRI][NMR]
nonspecific abnormal findings on diagnostic imaging by positron emission tomography [PET scan]
nonspecific abnormal findings on diagnostic imaging by thermography
nonspecific abnormal findings on diagnostic imaging by ultrasound [echogram]
nonspecific abnormal findings on diagnostic imaging by X-ray examination
EXCLUDES1 *abnormal findings on antenatal screening of mother (O28.-)*
diagnostic abnormal findings classified elsewhere - see Alphabetical Index

[4th] R90 Abnormal findings on diagnostic imaging of central nervous system
R90.0 Intracranial space-occupying lesion found on diagnostic imaging of central nervous system
[5th] R90.8 Other abnormal findings on diagnostic imaging of central nervous system
R90.81 Abnormal echoencephalogram
R90.82 White matter disease, unspecified
R90.89 Other abnormal findings on diagnostic imaging of central nervous system
Other cerebrovascular abnormality found on diagnostic imaging of central nervous system

[4th] R91 Abnormal findings on diagnostic imaging of lung
R91.1 Solitary pulmonary nodule
Coin lesion lung
Solitary pulmonary nodule, subsegmental branch of the bronchial tree
R91.8 Other nonspecific abnormal finding of lung field
Lung mass NOS found on diagnostic imaging of lung
Pulmonary infiltrate NOS
Shadow, lung

[4th] R92 Abnormal and inconclusive findings on diagnostic imaging of breast
R92.0 Mammographic microcalcification found on diagnostic imaging of breast
EXCLUDES2 *mammographic calcification (calculus) found on diagnostic imaging of breast (R92.1)*
R92.1 Mammographic calcification found on diagnostic imaging of breast
Mammographic calculus found on diagnostic imaging of breast
R92.2 Inconclusive mammogram
AHA: Q1 2015
Dense breasts NOS
Inconclusive mammogram NEC
Inconclusive mammography due to dense breasts
Inconclusive mammography NEC
R92.8 Other abnormal and inconclusive findings on diagnostic imaging of breast

[4th] R93 Abnormal findings on diagnostic imaging of other body structures
R93.0 Abnormal findings on diagnostic imaging of skull and head, not elsewhere classified
EXCLUDES1 *intracranial space-occupying lesion found on diagnostic imaging (R90.0)*
R93.1 Abnormal findings on diagnostic imaging of heart and coronary circulation
Abnormal echocardiogram NOS
Abnormal heart shadow
R93.2 Abnormal findings on diagnostic imaging of liver and biliary tract
Nonvisualization of gallbladder
R93.3 Abnormal findings on diagnostic imaging of other parts of digestive tract
[5th] R93.4 Abnormal findings on diagnostic imaging of urinary organs
EXCLUDES2 *hypertrophy of kidney (N28.81)*
R93.41 Abnormal radiologic findings on diagnostic imaging of renal pelvis, ureter, or bladder
AHA: Q4 2016
Filling defect of bladder found on diagnostic imaging
Filling defect of renal pelvis found on diagnostic imaging
Filling defect of ureter found on diagnostic imaging
[6th] R93.42 Abnormal radiologic findings on diagnostic imaging of kidney
R93.421 Abnormal radiologic findings on diagnostic imaging of right kidney
AHA: Q4 2016
R93.422 Abnormal radiologic findings on diagnostic imaging of left kidney
AHA: Q4 2016
R93.429 Abnormal radiologic findings on diagnostic imaging of unspecified kidney
AHA: Q4 2016
R93.49 Abnormal radiologic findings on diagnostic imaging of other urinary organs
AHA: Q4 2016
R93.5 Abnormal findings on diagnostic imaging of other abdominal regions, including retroperitoneum
R93.6 Abnormal findings on diagnostic imaging of limbs
EXCLUDES2 *abnormal finding in skin and subcutaneous tissue (R93.8-)*

Unspecified Code Other Specified Code Manifestation Code [N] Newborn [P] Pediatric [M] Maternity [A] Adult ♂ Male ♀ Female
● New Code ▲ Revised Code Title ►◄ Revised Text NOTES INCLUDES EXCLUDES1 Not coded here EXCLUDES2 Not included here
[4th] 4th character required [5th] 5th character required [6th] 6th character required [7th] 7th character required [7th] Extension 'X' Alert
[HAC] Hospital-acquired condition (HAC) alert AHA AHA Coding Clinic© ☛ Code first alert

R93.7 **Abnormal findings on diagnostic imaging of other parts of musculoskeletal system**
[EXCLUDES2] *abnormal findings on diagnostic imaging of skull (R93.0)*

[5th] R93.8 **Abnormal findings on diagnostic imaging of other specified body structures**

[6th] R93.81 **Abnormal radiologic findings on diagnostic imaging of testis**

R93.811 **Abnormal radiologic findings on diagnostic imaging of right testicle** ♂
AHA: Q4 2018

R93.812 **Abnormal radiologic findings on diagnostic imaging of left testicle** ♂
AHA: Q4 2018

R93.813 **Abnormal radiologic findings on diagnostic imaging of testicles, bilateral** ♂
AHA: Q4 2018

R93.819 **Abnormal radiologic findings on diagnostic imaging of unspecified testicle** ♂
AHA: Q4 2018

R93.89 **Abnormal findings on diagnostic imaging of other specified body structures**
AHA: Q4 2018
Abnormal finding by radioisotope localization of placenta
Abnormal radiological finding in skin and subcutaneous tissue
Mediastinal shift

R93.9 **Diagnostic imaging inconclusive due to excess body fat of patient**

[4th] R94 **Abnormal results of function studies**
[INCLUDES] *abnormal results of radionuclide [radioisotope] uptake studies*
abnormal results of scintigraphy

[5th] R94.0 **Abnormal results of function studies of central nervous system**

R94.01 **Abnormal electroencephalogram [EEG]**

R94.02 **Abnormal brain scan**

R94.09 **Abnormal results of other function studies of central nervous system**

[5th] R94.1 **Abnormal results of function studies of peripheral nervous system and special senses**

[6th] R94.11 **Abnormal results of function studies of eye**

R94.110 **Abnormal electro-oculogram [EOG]**

R94.111 **Abnormal electroretinogram [ERG]**
Abnormal retinal function study

R94.112 **Abnormal visually evoked potential [VEP]**

R94.113 **Abnormal oculomotor study**

R94.118 **Abnormal results of other function studies of eye**

[6th] R94.12 **Abnormal results of function studies of ear and other special senses**

R94.120 **Abnormal auditory function study**
AHA: Q3 2016

R94.121 **Abnormal vestibular function study**

R94.128 **Abnormal results of other function studies of ear and other special senses**

[6th] R94.13 **Abnormal results of function studies of peripheral nervous system**

R94.130 **Abnormal response to nerve stimulation, unspecified**

R94.131 **Abnormal electromyogram [EMG]**
[EXCLUDES1] *electromyogram of eye (R94.113)*

R94.138 **Abnormal results of other function studies of peripheral nervous system**

R94.2 **Abnormal results of pulmonary function studies**
Reduced ventilatory capacity
Reduced vital capacity

[5th] R94.3 **Abnormal results of cardiovascular function studies**

R94.30 **Abnormal result of cardiovascular function study, unspecified**

R94.31 **Abnormal electrocardiogram [ECG] [EKG]**
[EXCLUDES1] *long QT syndrome (I45.81)*

R94.39 **Abnormal result of other cardiovascular function study**
Abnormal electrophysiological intracardiac studies
Abnormal phonocardiogram
Abnormal vectorcardiogram

R94.4 **Abnormal results of kidney function studies**
Abnormal renal function test

R94.5 **Abnormal results of liver function studies**

R94.6 **Abnormal results of thyroid function studies**

R94.7 **Abnormal results of other endocrine function studies**
[EXCLUDES2] *abnormal glucose (R73.0-)*

R94.8 **Abnormal results of function studies of other organs and systems**
Abnormal basal metabolic rate [BMR]
Abnormal bladder function test
Abnormal splenic function test

Abnormal tumor markers (R97)

[4th] R97 **Abnormal tumor markers**
Elevated tumor associated antigens [TAA]
Elevated tumor specific antigens [TSA]

R97.0 **Elevated carcinoembryonic antigen [CEA]**

R97.1 **Elevated cancer antigen 125 [CA 125]**

[5th] R97.2 **Elevated prostate specific antigen [PSA]**

R97.20 **Elevated prostate specific antigen [PSA]** [A] [?] ♂
AHA: Q4 2016

R97.21 **Rising PSA following treatment for malignant neoplasm of prostate** [A] [?] ♂
AHA: Q4 2016

R97.8 **Other abnormal tumor markers**

Ill-defined and unknown cause of mortality (R99)

R99 **Ill-defined and unknown cause of mortality**
AHA: Q4 2016
Death (unexplained) NOS
Unspecified cause of mortality
👁 **See Official Guidelines** "Codes or codes from A00.0 through T88.9, Z00-Z99.8" I.B3

Chapter 19: Injury, Poisoning, and Certain Other Consequences of External Causes (S00-T88)

Injury, poisoning, and certain other consequences of external causes (S00-T88)

👁 **See Official Guidelines** "Pain due to medical devices" I.C.19.g.2

NOTES Use secondary code(s) from Chapter 20, External causes of morbidity, to indicate cause of injury. Codes within the T section that include the external cause do not require an additional external cause code.

Use additional code to identify any retained foreign body, if applicable (Z18.-)

EXCLUDES1 birth trauma (P10-P15)
obstetric trauma (O70-O71)

This chapter contains the following blocks:

S00-S09 Injuries to the head
S10-S19 Injuries to the neck
S20-S29 Injuries to the thorax
S30-S39 Injuries to the abdomen, lower back, lumbar spine, pelvis and external genitals
S40-S49 Injuries to the shoulder and upper arm
S50-S59 Injuries to the elbow and forearm
S60-S69 Injuries to the wrist, hand and fingers
S70-S79 Injuries to the hip and thigh
S80-S89 Injuries to the knee and lower leg
S90-S99 Injuries to the ankle and foot
T07 Injuries involving multiple body regions
T14 Injury of unspecified body region
T15-T19 Effects of foreign body entering through natural orifice
T20-T25 Burns and corrosions of external body surface, specified by site
T26-T28 Burns and corrosions confined to eye and internal organs
T30-T32 Burns and corrosions of multiple and unspecified body regions
T33-T34 Frostbite
T36-T50 Poisoning by, adverse effect of and underdosing of drugs, medicaments and biological substances
T51-T65 Toxic effects of substances chiefly nonmedicinal as to source
T66-T78 Other and unspecified effects of external causes
T79 Certain early complications of trauma
T80-T88 Complications of surgical and medical care, not elsewhere classified

NOTES The chapter uses the S-section for coding different types of injuries related to single body regions and the T-section to cover injuries to unspecified body regions as well as poisoning and certain other consequences of external causes.

Injuries to the head (S00-S09)

INCLUDES injuries of ear
injuries of eye
injuries of face [any part]
injuries of gum
injuries of jaw
injuries of oral cavity
injuries of palate
injuries of periocular area
injuries of scalp
injuries of temporomandibular joint area
injuries of tongue
injuries of tooth

Code also for any associated infection

EXCLUDES2 burns and corrosions (T20-T32)
effects of foreign body in ear (T16)
effects of foreign body in larynx (T17.3)
effects of foreign body in mouth NOS (T18.0)
effects of foreign body in nose (T17.0-T17.1)
effects of foreign body in pharynx (T17.2)
effects of foreign body on external eye (T15.-)
frostbite (T33-T34)
insect bite or sting, venomous (T63.4)

4️⃣ **S00** Superficial injury **of head**

EXCLUDES1 diffuse cerebral contusion (S06.2-)
focal cerebral contusion (S06.3-)
injury of eye and orbit (S05.-)
open wound of head (S01.-)

The appropriate 7th character is to be added to each code from category S00
A = initial encounter
D = subsequent encounter
S = sequela

5️⃣ **S00.0** Superficial injury **of scalp**
7️⃣ S00.00 **Unspecified superficial injury of scalp** POA
7️⃣ S00.01 Abrasion **of scalp** POA
7️⃣ S00.02 Blister **(nonthermal) of scalp** POA
7️⃣ S00.03 Contusion **of scalp** POA
Bruise of scalp
Hematoma of scalp
7️⃣ S00.04 External constriction of part **of scalp** POA
7️⃣ S00.05 **Superficial** foreign body **of scalp** POA
Splinter in the scalp
7️⃣ S00.06 Insect bite **(nonvenomous) of scalp** POA
7️⃣ S00.07 Other **superficial bite of scalp** POA
EXCLUDES1 open bite of scalp (S01.05)

5️⃣ **S00.1** Contusion **of eyelid and periocular area**
Black eye
EXCLUDES2 contusion of eyeball and orbital tissues (S05.1)
7️⃣ S00.10 **Contusion of unspecified eyelid and periocular area** POA
7️⃣ S00.11 **Contusion of** right **eyelid and periocular area** POA
7️⃣ S00.12 **Contusion of** left **eyelid and periocular area** POA

5️⃣ **S00.2** Other and unspecified superficial injuries of eyelid and periocular area
EXCLUDES2 superficial injury of conjunctiva and cornea (S05.0-)
6️⃣ S00.20 Unspecified **superficial injury of eyelid and periocular area**
7️⃣ S00.201 **Unspecified superficial injury of** right **eyelid and periocular area** POA
7️⃣ S00.202 **Unspecified superficial injury of** left **eyelid and periocular area** POA
7️⃣ S00.209 **Unspecified superficial injury of unspecified eyelid and periocular area** POA
6️⃣ S00.21 Abrasion **of eyelid and periocular area**
7️⃣ S00.211 **Abrasion of** right **eyelid and periocular area** POA
7️⃣ S00.212 **Abrasion of** left **eyelid and periocular area** POA
7️⃣ S00.219 **Abrasion of unspecified eyelid and periocular area** POA
6️⃣ S00.22 Blister **(nonthermal) of eyelid and periocular area**
7️⃣ S00.221 **Blister (nonthermal) of** right **eyelid and periocular area** POA
7️⃣ S00.222 **Blister (nonthermal) of** left **eyelid and periocular area** POA
7️⃣ S00.229 **Blister (nonthermal) of unspecified eyelid and periocular area** POA
6️⃣ S00.24 External constriction **of eyelid and periocular area**
7️⃣ S00.241 **External constriction of** right **eyelid and periocular area** POA

Unspecified Code Other Specified Code Manifestation Code N Newborn P Pediatric M Maternity A Adult ♂ Male ♀ Female
● New Code ▲ Revised Code Title ▶◀ Revised Text **NOTES** INCLUDES EXCLUDES1 Not coded here EXCLUDES2 Not included here
4️⃣ 4th character required 5️⃣ 5th character required 6️⃣ 6th character required 7️⃣ 7th character required Extension 'X' Alert
HAC Hospital-acquired condition (HAC) alert AHA AHA Coding Clinic© 📕 Code first alert

2020 ICD-10-CM When symbols appear on a code that requires a 7th character extension, refer to Appendix B to identify applicable 7th character codes. **967**

S00.242 **External constriction of** left **eyelid and periocular area**

S00.249 **External constriction of unspecified eyelid and periocular area**

S00.25 **Superficial** foreign body **of eyelid and periocular area**
Splinter of eyelid and periocular area
EXCLUDES2 *retained foreign body in eyelid (H02.81-)*

S00.251 **Superficial foreign body of** right **eyelid and periocular area**

S00.252 **Superficial foreign body of** left **eyelid and periocular area**

S00.259 **Superficial foreign body of unspecified eyelid and periocular area**

S00.26 Insect bite (nonvenomous) of eyelid and periocular area

S00.261 **Insect bite (nonvenomous) of** right **eyelid and periocular area**

S00.262 **Insect bite (nonvenomous) of** left **eyelid and periocular area**

S00.269 **Insect bite (nonvenomous) of unspecified eyelid and periocular area**

S00.27 Other **superficial bite of eyelid and periocular area**
EXCLUDES1 *open bite of eyelid and periocular area (S01.15)*

S00.271 **Other superficial bite of** right **eyelid and periocular area**

S00.272 **Other superficial bite of** left **eyelid and periocular area**

S00.279 **Other superficial bite of unspecified eyelid and periocular area**

S00.3 **Superficial injury of** nose

S00.30 **Unspecified superficial injury of nose**

S00.31 Abrasion **of nose**

S00.32 Blister (nonthermal) **of nose**

S00.33 Contusion **of nose**
Bruise of nose
Hematoma of nose

S00.34 External constriction **of nose**

S00.35 **Superficial** foreign body **of nose**
Splinter in the nose

S00.36 Insect bite (nonvenomous) **of nose**

S00.37 Other **superficial bite of nose**
EXCLUDES1 *open bite of nose (S01.25)*

S00.4 **Superficial injury of** ear

S00.40 Unspecified **superficial injury of** ear

S00.401 **Unspecified superficial injury of** right **ear**

S00.402 **Unspecified superficial injury of** left **ear**

S00.409 **Unspecified superficial injury of unspecified ear**

S00.41 Abrasion **of ear**

S00.411 **Abrasion of** right **ear**

S00.412 **Abrasion of** left **ear**

S00.419 **Abrasion of unspecified ear**

S00.42 Blister (nonthermal) **of ear**

S00.421 **Blister (nonthermal) of** right **ear**

S00.422 **Blister (nonthermal) of** left **ear**

S00.429 **Blister (nonthermal) of unspecified ear**

S00.43 Contusion **of ear**
Bruise of ear
Hematoma of ear

S00.431 **Contusion of** right **ear**

S00.432 **Contusion of** left **ear**

S00.439 **Contusion of unspecified ear**

S00.44 External constriction **of ear**

S00.441 **External constriction of** right **ear**

S00.442 **External constriction of** left **ear**

S00.449 **External constriction of unspecified ear**

S00.45 **Superficial** foreign body **of ear**
Splinter in the ear

S00.451 **Superficial foreign body of** right **ear**

S00.452 **Superficial foreign body of** left **ear**

S00.459 **Superficial foreign body of unspecified ear**

S00.46 Insect bite (nonvenomous) **of ear**

S00.461 **Insect bite (nonvenomous) of** right **ear**

S00.462 **Insect bite (nonvenomous) of** left **ear**

S00.469 **Insect bite (nonvenomous) of unspecified ear**

S00.47 Other **superficial bite of ear**
EXCLUDES1 *open bite of ear (S01.35)*

S00.471 **Other superficial bite of** right **ear**

S00.472 **Other superficial bite of** left **ear**

S00.479 **Other superficial bite of unspecified ear**

S00.5 **Superficial injury of** lip and oral cavity

S00.50 Unspecified **superficial injury of lip and oral cavity**

S00.501 **Unspecified superficial injury of lip**

S00.502 **Unspecified superficial injury of oral cavity**

S00.51 Abrasion **of lip and oral cavity**

S00.511 **Abrasion of** lip

S00.512 **Abrasion of** oral cavity

S00.52 Blister (nonthermal) **of lip and oral cavity**

S00.521 **Blister (nonthermal) of** lip

S00.522 **Blister (nonthermal) of** oral cavity

S00.53 Contusion **of lip and oral cavity**

S00.531 **Contusion of** lip
Bruise of lip
Hematoma of lip

S00.532 **Contusion of** oral cavity
Bruise of oral cavity
Hematoma of oral cavity

S00.54 External constriction **of lip and oral cavity**

S00.541 **External constriction of** lip

S00.542 **External constriction of** oral cavity

S00.55 **Superficial** foreign body **of lip and oral cavity**

S00.551 **Superficial foreign body of** lip
Splinter of lip and oral cavity

S00.552 **Superficial foreign body of** oral cavity
Splinter of lip and oral cavity

S00.56 Insect bite (nonvenomous) **of lip and oral cavity**

S00.561 **Insect bite (nonvenomous) of** lip

S00.562 **Insect bite (nonvenomous) of** oral cavity

S00.57 Other **superficial bite of lip and oral cavity**

S00.571 **Other superficial bite of** lip
EXCLUDES1 *open bite of lip (S01.551)*

S00.572 **Other superficial bite of** oral cavity
EXCLUDES1 *open bite of oral cavity (S01.552)*

S00.8 **Superficial injury of other parts of head**
Superficial injuries of face [any part]

S00.80 **Unspecified superficial injury of other part of head**

S00.81 Abrasion **of other part of head**

S00.82 Blister (nonthermal) **of other part of head**

S00.83 Contusion **of other part of head**
Bruise of other part of head
Hematoma of other part of head

S00.84 External constriction **of other part of head**

S00.85 Superficial foreign body **of other part of head**
Splinter in other part of head

S00.86 Insect bite (nonvenomous) **of other part of head**

S00.87 Other **superficial bite of other part of head**
EXCLUDES1 *open bite of other part of head (S01.85)*

S00.9 **Superficial injury of unspecified part of head**

S00.90 **Unspecified superficial injury of unspecified part of head**

PDA Unacceptable principal diagnosis symbol per Medicare code edits   POA Code exempt from diagnosis present on admission requirement
❓ Questionable admission   CC Complication or comorbidity   MCC Major complication or comorbidity   CC/MCC EXC CC/MCC exclusion
HCC HCC diagnosis code   RxHCC RxHCC diagnosis code   MACRA code   **DEFINITION** Describes condition/terminology
TIP Coding guidance   👁 Official Guideline Reference   Z1 Z code as first-listed diagnosis

968   When symbols appear on a code that requires a 7th character extension, refer to Appendix B to identify applicable 7th character codes.   **2020 ICD-10-CM**

7ᵗʰ S00.91 Abrasion of unspecified part of head · POA

7ᵗʰ S00.92 Blister (nonthermal) of unspecified part of head · POA

7ᵗʰ S00.93 Contusion of unspecified part of head · POA
Bruise of head
Hematoma of head

7ᵗʰ S00.94 External constriction of unspecified part of head · POA

7ᵗʰ S00.95 Superficial foreign body of unspecified part of head · POA
Splinter of head

7ᵗʰ S00.96 Insect bite (nonvenomous) of unspecified part of head · POA

7ᵗʰ S00.97 Other superficial bite of unspecified part of head · POA
EXCLUDES1 open bite of head (S01.95)

4ᵗʰ S01 Open wound of head
Code also any associated:
injury of cranial nerve (S04.-)
injury of muscle and tendon of head (S09.1-)
intracranial injury (S06.-)
wound infection
EXCLUDES1 open skull fracture (S02.- with 7th character B)
EXCLUDES2 injury of eye and orbit (S05.-)
traumatic amputation of part of head (S08.-)

The appropriate 7th character is to be added to each code from category S01
A = initial encounter
D = subsequent encounter
S = sequela

5ᵗʰ S01.0 Open wound of scalp
EXCLUDES1 avulsion of scalp (S08.0)

7ᵗʰ S01.00 Unspecified open wound of scalp · POA

7ᵗʰ S01.01 Laceration without foreign body of scalp · POA

7ᵗʰ S01.02 Laceration with foreign body of scalp · POA
AHA: Q1 2015

7ᵗʰ S01.03 Puncture wound without foreign body of scalp · POA

7ᵗʰ S01.04 Puncture wound with foreign body of scalp · POA

7ᵗʰ S01.05 Open bite of scalp · POA
Bite of scalp NOS
EXCLUDES1 superficial bite of scalp (S00.06, S00.07-)

5ᵗʰ S01.1 Open wound of eyelid and periocular area
Open wound of eyelid and periocular area with or without involvement of lacrimal passages

6ᵗʰ S01.10 Unspecified open wound of eyelid and periocular area

7ᵗʰ S01.101 Unspecified open wound of right eyelid and periocular area · CC POA CC/MCC Exc.

7ᵗʰ S01.102 Unspecified open wound of left eyelid and periocular area · CC POA CC/MCC Exc.

7ᵗʰ S01.109 Unspecified open wound of unspecified eyelid and periocular area · CC POA CC/MCC Exc.

6ᵗʰ S01.11 Laceration without foreign body of eyelid and periocular area

7ᵗʰ S01.111 Laceration without foreign body of right eyelid and periocular area

7ᵗʰ S01.112 Laceration without foreign body of left eyelid and periocular area

7ᵗʰ S01.119 Laceration without foreign body of unspecified eyelid and periocular area · POA

6ᵗʰ S01.12 Laceration with foreign body of eyelid and periocular area

7ᵗʰ S01.121 Laceration with foreign body of right eyelid and periocular area

7ᵗʰ S01.122 Laceration with foreign body of left eyelid and periocular area · POA

7ᵗʰ S01.129 Laceration with foreign body of unspecified eyelid and periocular area · POA

6ᵗʰ S01.13 Puncture wound without foreign body of eyelid and periocular area

7ᵗʰ S01.131 Puncture wound without foreign body of right eyelid and periocular area · POA

7ᵗʰ S01.132 Puncture wound without foreign body of left eyelid and periocular area · POA

7ᵗʰ S01.139 Puncture wound without foreign body of unspecified eyelid and periocular area · POA

6ᵗʰ S01.14 Puncture wound with foreign body of eyelid and periocular area

7ᵗʰ S01.141 Puncture wound with foreign body of right eyelid and periocular area · POA

7ᵗʰ S01.142 Puncture wound with foreign body of left eyelid and periocular area · POA

7ᵗʰ S01.149 Puncture wound with foreign body of unspecified eyelid and periocular area · POA

6ᵗʰ S01.15 Open bite of eyelid and periocular area
Bite of eyelid and periocular area NOS
EXCLUDES1 superficial bite of eyelid and periocular area (S00.26, S00.27)

7ᵗʰ S01.151 Open bite of right eyelid and periocular area · POA

7ᵗʰ S01.152 Open bite of left eyelid and periocular area · POA

7ᵗʰ S01.159 Open bite of unspecified eyelid and periocular area · POA

5ᵗʰ S01.2 Open wound of nose

7ᵗʰ S01.20 Unspecified open wound of nose · POA

7ᵗʰ S01.21 Laceration without foreign body of nose · POA
AHA: Q1 2015

7ᵗʰ S01.22 Laceration with foreign body of nose · POA

7ᵗʰ S01.23 Puncture wound without foreign body of nose · POA

7ᵗʰ S01.24 Puncture wound with foreign body of nose · POA

7ᵗʰ S01.25 Open bite of nose · POA
Bite of nose NOS
EXCLUDES1 superficial bite of nose (S00.36, S00.37)

5ᵗʰ S01.3 Open wound of ear

6ᵗʰ S01.30 Unspecified open wound of ear

7ᵗʰ S01.301 Unspecified open wound of right ear · POA

7ᵗʰ S01.302 Unspecified open wound of left ear · POA

7ᵗʰ S01.309 Unspecified open wound of unspecified ear · POA

6ᵗʰ S01.31 Laceration without foreign body of ear

7ᵗʰ S01.311 Laceration without foreign body of right ear · POA

7ᵗʰ S01.312 Laceration without foreign body of left ear · POA

7ᵗʰ S01.319 Laceration without foreign body of unspecified ear · POA

6ᵗʰ S01.32 Laceration with foreign body of ear

7ᵗʰ S01.321 Laceration with foreign body of right ear · POA

7ᵗʰ S01.322 Laceration with foreign body of left ear · POA

7ᵗʰ S01.329 Laceration with foreign body of unspecified ear · POA

6ᵗʰ S01.33 Puncture wound without foreign body of ear

7ᵗʰ S01.331 Puncture wound without foreign body of right ear · POA

7ᵗʰ S01.332 Puncture wound without foreign body of left ear · POA

7ᵗʰ S01.339 Puncture wound without foreign body of unspecified ear · POA

6ᵗʰ S01.34 Puncture wound with foreign body of ear

7ᵗʰ S01.341 Puncture wound with foreign body of right ear · POA

7ᵗʰ S01.342 Puncture wound with foreign body of left ear · POA

7ᵗʰ S01.349 Puncture wound with foreign body of unspecified ear · POA

6ᵗʰ S01.35 Open bite of ear
Bite of ear NOS
EXCLUDES1 superficial bite of ear (S00.46, S00.47)

7ᵗʰ S01.351 Open bite of right ear · POA

7ᵗʰ S01.352 Open bite of left ear · POA

7ᵗʰ S01.359 Open bite of unspecified ear · POA

Unspecified Code	Other Specified Code	Manifestation Code	N Newborn	P Pediatric	M Maternity	A Adult	♂ Male	♀ Female

● New Code ▲ Revised Code Title ►◄ Revised Text NOTES INCLUDES EXCLUDES1 Not coded here EXCLUDES2 Not included here
4ᵗʰ 4ᵗʰ character required 5ᵗʰ 5ᵗʰ character required 6ᵗʰ 6ᵗʰ character required 7ᵗʰ 7ᵗʰ character required ⊗ Extension 'X' Alert
HAC Hospital-acquired condition (HAC) alert AHA AHA Coding Clinic® ☞ Code first alert

S01.4 Open wound of cheek and temporomandibular area
  S01.40 Unspecified open wound of cheek and temporomandibular area
    S01.401 Unspecified open wound of right cheek and temporomandibular area POA
    S01.402 Unspecified open wound of left cheek and temporomandibular area POA
    S01.409 Unspecified open wound of unspecified cheek and temporomandibular area POA
  S01.41 Laceration without foreign body of cheek and temporomandibular area
    S01.411 Laceration without foreign body of right cheek and temporomandibular area POA
      AHA: Q1 2015
    S01.412 Laceration without foreign body of left cheek and temporomandibular area POA
    S01.419 Laceration without foreign body of unspecified cheek and temporomandibular area POA
  S01.42 Laceration with foreign body of cheek and temporomandibular area
    S01.421 Laceration with foreign body of right cheek and temporomandibular area POA
    S01.422 Laceration with foreign body of left cheek and temporomandibular area POA
    S01.429 Laceration with foreign body of unspecified cheek and temporomandibular area POA
  S01.43 Puncture wound without foreign body of cheek and temporomandibular area
    S01.431 Puncture wound without foreign body of right cheek and temporomandibular area POA
    S01.432 Puncture wound without foreign body of left cheek and temporomandibular area POA
    S01.439 Puncture wound without foreign body of unspecified cheek and temporomandibular area POA
  S01.44 Puncture wound with foreign body of cheek and temporomandibular area
    S01.441 Puncture wound with foreign body of right cheek and temporomandibular area POA
    S01.442 Puncture wound with foreign body of left cheek and temporomandibular area POA
    S01.449 Puncture wound with foreign body of unspecified cheek and temporomandibular area POA
  S01.45 Open bite of cheek and temporomandibular area
    Bite of cheek and temporomandibular area NOS
    EXCLUDES2 superficial bite of cheek and temporomandibular area (S00.86, S00.87)
    S01.451 Open bite of right cheek and temporomandibular area POA
    S01.452 Open bite of left cheek and temporomandibular area POA
    S01.459 Open bite of unspecified cheek and temporomandibular area POA
S01.5 Open wound of lip and oral cavity
  EXCLUDES2 tooth dislocation (S03.2)
           tooth fracture (S02.5)
  S01.50 Unspecified open wound of lip and oral cavity
    S01.501 Unspecified open wound of lip POA
    S01.502 Unspecified open wound of oral cavity POA
  S01.51 Laceration of lip and oral cavity without foreign body
    S01.511 Laceration without foreign body of lip POA
    S01.512 Laceration without foreign body of oral cavity POA
  S01.52 Laceration of lip and oral cavity with foreign body
    S01.521 Laceration with foreign body of lip POA

S01.522 Laceration with foreign body of oral cavity POA
S01.53 Puncture wound of lip and oral cavity without foreign body
  S01.531 Puncture wound without foreign body of lip POA
  S01.532 Puncture wound without foreign body of oral cavity POA
S01.54 Puncture wound of lip and oral cavity with foreign body
  S01.541 Puncture wound with foreign body of lip POA
  S01.542 Puncture wound with foreign body of oral cavity POA
S01.55 Open bite of lip and oral cavity
  S01.551 Open bite of lip POA
    Bite of lip NOS
    EXCLUDES1 superficial bite of lip (S00.571)
  S01.552 Open bite of oral cavity POA
    Bite of oral cavity NOS
    EXCLUDES1 superficial bite of oral cavity (S00.572)
S01.8 Open wound of other parts of head
  S01.80 Unspecified open wound of other part of head POA
  S01.81 Laceration without foreign body of other part of head POA
  S01.82 Laceration with foreign body of other part of head POA
  S01.83 Puncture wound without foreign body of other part of head POA
  S01.84 Puncture wound with foreign body of other part of head POA
  S01.85 Open bite of other part of head POA
    Bite of other part of head NOS
    EXCLUDES1 superficial bite of other part of head (S00.87)
S01.9 Open wound of unspecified part of head
  S01.90 Unspecified open wound of unspecified part of head POA
  S01.91 Laceration without foreign body of unspecified part of head POA
  S01.92 Laceration with foreign body of unspecified part of head POA
  S01.93 Puncture wound without foreign body of unspecified part of head POA
  S01.94 Puncture wound with foreign body of unspecified part of head POA
  S01.95 Open bite of unspecified part of head POA
    Bite of head NOS
    EXCLUDES1 superficial bite of head NOS (S00.97)
S02 Fracture of skull and facial bones
  See Official Guidelines "Coding of Traumatic Fractures" I.C.19.c
  NOTES A fracture not indicated as open or closed should be coded to closed.
  Code also any associated intracranial injury (S06.-)
  The appropriate 7th character is to be added to each code from category S02
    A = initial encounter for closed fracture
    B = initial encounter for open fracture
    D = subsequent encounter for fracture with routine healing
    G = subsequent encounter for fracture with delayed healing
    K = subsequent encounter for fracture with nonunion
    S = sequela
  S02.0 Fracture of vault of skull CC POA HAC HCC MCC CC/MCC Exc
    Fracture of frontal bone
    Fracture of parietal bone
  S02.1 Fracture of base of skull
    EXCLUDES2 lateral orbital wall (S02.84-)
             medial orbital wall (S02.83-)
             orbital floor (S02.3-)

[6th] S02.10 Unspecified fracture of base of skull
- [7th] S02.101 Fracture of base of skull, right side [CC] [POA] [HAC] [HCC] [MCC] [CC/MCC Exc]
- [7th] S02.102 Fracture of base of skull, left side [CC] [POA] [HAC] [HCC] [MCC] [CC/MCC Exc]
- [7th] S02.109 Fracture of base of skull, unspecified side [CC] [POA] [HAC] [HCC] [MCC] [CC/MCC Exc]

[6th] S02.11 Fracture of occiput
- [7th] S02.110 Type I occipital condyle fracture, unspecified side [CC] [POA] [HAC] [HCC] [MCC] [CC/MCC Exc]
- [7th] S02.111 Type II occipital condyle fracture, unspecified side [CC] [POA] [HAC] [HCC] [MCC] [CC/MCC Exc]
- [7th] S02.112 Type III occipital condyle fracture, unspecified side [CC] [POA] [HAC] [HCC] [MCC] [CC/MCC Exc]
- [7th] S02.113 Unspecified occipital condyle fracture [CC] [POA] [HAC] [HCC] [MCC] [CC/MCC Exc]
- [7th] S02.118 Other fracture of occiput, unspecified side [CC] [POA] [HAC] [HCC] [MCC] [CC/MCC Exc]
- [7th] S02.119 Unspecified fracture of occiput [CC] [POA] [HAC] [HCC] [MCC] [CC/MCC Exc]
- [7th] S02.11A Type I occipital condyle fracture, right side [CC] [POA] [HAC] [HCC] [MCC] [CC/MCC Exc]
- [7th] S02.11B Type I occipital condyle fracture, left side [CC] [POA] [HAC] [HCC] [MCC] [CC/MCC Exc]
- [7th] S02.11C Type II occipital condyle fracture, right side [CC] [POA] [HAC] [HCC] [MCC] [CC/MCC Exc]
- [7th] S02.11D Type II occipital condyle fracture, left side [CC] [POA] [HAC] [HCC] [MCC] [CC/MCC Exc]
- [7th] S02.11E Type III occipital condyle fracture, right side [CC] [POA] [HAC] [HCC] [MCC] [CC/MCC Exc]
- [7th] S02.11F Type III occipital condyle fracture, left side [CC] [POA] [HAC] [HCC] [MCC] [CC/MCC Exc]
- [7th] S02.11G Other fracture of occiput, right side [CC] [POA] [HAC] [HCC] [MCC] [CC/MCC Exc]
- [7th] S02.11H Other fracture of occiput, left side [CC] [POA] [HAC] [HCC] [MCC] [CC/MCC Exc]

● [6th] S02.12 Fracture of orbital roof
- ● [7th] S02.121 Fracture of orbital roof, right side [CC] [MCC] [CC/MCC Exc]
- ● [7th] S02.122 Fracture of orbital roof, left side [CC] [MCC] [CC/MCC Exc]
- ● [7th] S02.129 Fracture of orbital roof, unspecified side [CC] [MCC] [CC/MCC Exc]

[7th] S02.19 Other fracture of base of skull [CC] [POA] [HAC] [HCC] [MCC] [CC/MCC Exc]
Fracture of anterior fossa of base of skull
Fracture of ethmoid sinus
Fracture of frontal sinus
Fracture of middle fossa of base of skull
Fracture of posterior fossa of base of skull
Fracture of sphenoid
Fracture of temporal bone

[7th] S02.2 Fracture of nasal bones [CC] [POA] [HAC] [CC/MCC Exc]

[5th] S02.3 Fracture of orbital floor
Fracture of inferior orbital wall
[EXCLUDES1] *orbit NOS ►(S02.85)◄*
[EXCLUDES2] *lateral orbital wall (S02.84-)*
medial orbital wall (S02.83-)
orbital roof (S02.1-)
- [7th] S02.30 Fracture of orbital floor, unspecified side [CC] [POA] [HAC] [HCC] [CC/MCC Exc]
- [7th] S02.31 Fracture of orbital floor, right side [CC] [POA] [HAC] [HCC] [CC/MCC Exc]
- [7th] S02.32 Fracture of orbital floor, left side [CC] [POA] [HAC] [HCC] [CC/MCC Exc]

[5th] S02.4 Fracture of malar, maxillary and zygoma bones
Fracture of superior maxilla
Fracture of upper jaw (bone)
Fracture of zygomatic process of temporal bone

[6th] S02.40 Fracture of malar, maxillary and zygoma bones, unspecified
- [7th] S02.400 Malar fracture, unspecified side [CC] [POA] [HAC] [HCC] [CC/MCC Exc]
- [7th] S02.401 Maxillary fracture, unspecified side [CC] [POA] [HAC] [HCC] [CC/MCC Exc]
- [7th] S02.402 Zygomatic fracture, unspecified side [CC] [POA] [HAC] [HCC] [CC/MCC Exc]
- [7th] S02.40A Malar fracture, right side [CC] [POA] [HAC] [HCC] [CC/MCC Exc]
- [7th] S02.40B Malar fracture, left side [CC] [POA] [HAC] [HCC] [CC/MCC Exc]
- [7th] S02.40C Maxillary fracture, right side [CC] [POA] [HAC] [HCC] [CC/MCC Exc]
- [7th] S02.40D Maxillary fracture, left side [CC] [POA] [HAC] [HCC] [CC/MCC Exc]
- [7th] S02.40E Zygomatic fracture, right side [CC] [POA] [HAC] [HCC] [CC/MCC Exc]
- [7th] S02.40F Zygomatic fracture, left side [CC] [POA] [HAC] [HCC] [CC/MCC Exc]

[6th] S02.41 LeFort fracture
- [7th] S02.411 LeFort I fracture [CC] [POA] [HAC] [HCC] [CC/MCC Exc]
- [7th] S02.412 LeFort II fracture [CC] [POA] [HAC] [HCC] [CC/MCC Exc]
- [7th] S02.413 LeFort III fracture [CC] [POA] [HAC] [HCC] [CC/MCC Exc]

[7th] S02.42 Fracture of alveolus of maxilla [CC] [POA] [HAC] [HCC] [CC/MCC Exc]

[7th] S02.5 Fracture of tooth (traumatic) [CC] [POA] [CC/MCC Exc]
Broken tooth
[EXCLUDES1] *cracked tooth (nontraumatic) (K03.81)*

[5th] S02.6 Fracture of mandible
Fracture of lower jaw (bone)

[6th] S02.60 Fracture of mandible, unspecified
- [7th] S02.600 Fracture of unspecified part of body of mandible, unspecified side [CC] [POA] [HAC] [HCC] [CC/MCC Exc]
- [7th] S02.601 Fracture of unspecified part of body of right mandible [CC] [POA] [HAC] [HCC] [CC/MCC Exc]
- [7th] S02.602 Fracture of unspecified part of body of left mandible [CC] [POA] [HAC] [HCC] [CC/MCC Exc]
- [7th] S02.609 Fracture of mandible, unspecified [CC] [POA] [HAC] [HCC] [CC/MCC Exc]

[6th] S02.61 Fracture of condylar process of mandible
- [7th] S02.610 Fracture of condylar process of mandible, unspecified side [CC] [POA] [HAC] [HCC] [CC/MCC Exc]
- [7th] S02.611 Fracture of condylar process of right mandible [CC] [POA] [HAC] [HCC] [CC/MCC Exc]
- [7th] S02.612 Fracture of condylar process of left mandible [CC] [POA] [HAC] [HCC] [CC/MCC Exc]

[6th] S02.62 Fracture of subcondylar process of mandible
- [7th] S02.620 Fracture of subcondylar process of mandible, unspecified side [CC] [POA] [HAC] [HCC] [CC/MCC Exc]
- [7th] S02.621 Fracture of subcondylar process of right mandible [CC] [POA] [HAC] [HCC] [CC/MCC Exc]
- [7th] S02.622 Fracture of subcondylar process of left mandible [CC] [POA] [HAC] [HCC] [CC/MCC Exc]

[6th] S02.63 Fracture of coronoid process of mandible
- [7th] S02.630 Fracture of coronoid process of mandible, unspecified side [CC] [POA] [HAC] [HCC] [CC/MCC Exc]
- [7th] S02.631 Fracture of coronoid process of right mandible [CC] [POA] [HAC] [HCC] [CC/MCC Exc]
- [7th] S02.632 Fracture of coronoid process of left mandible [CC] [POA] [HAC] [HCC] [CC/MCC Exc]

[6th] S02.64 Fracture of ramus of mandible
- [7th] S02.640 Fracture of ramus of mandible, unspecified side [CC] [POA] [HAC] [HCC] [CC/MCC Exc]
- [7th] S02.641 Fracture of ramus of right mandible [CC] [POA] [HAC] [HCC] [CC/MCC Exc]
- [7th] S02.642 Fracture of ramus of left mandible [CC] [POA] [HAC] [HCC] [CC/MCC Exc]

[6th] S02.65 Fracture of angle of mandible
- [7th] S02.650 Fracture of angle of mandible, unspecified side [CC] [POA] [HAC] [HCC] [CC/MCC Exc]
- [7th] S02.651 Fracture of angle of right mandible [CC] [POA] [HAC] [HCC] [CC/MCC Exc]
- [7th] S02.652 Fracture of angle of left mandible [CC] [POA] [HAC] [HCC] [CC/MCC Exc]

[7th] S02.66 Fracture of symphysis of mandible [CC] [POA] [HAC] [HCC] [CC/MCC Exc]

Unspecified Code | Other Specified Code | Manifestation Code | [N] Newborn | [P] Pediatric | [M] Maternity | [A] Adult | ♂ Male | ♀ Female
● New Code | ▲ Revised Code Title | ►◄ Revised Text | [NOTES] | [INCLUDES] | [EXCLUDES1] Not coded here | [EXCLUDES2] Not included here
[4th] 4th character required | [5th] 5th character required | [6th] 6th character required | [7th] 7th character required | [7th] Extension 'X' Alert
[HAC] Hospital-acquired condition (HAC) alert | AHA AHA Coding Clinic© | Code first alert

6ᵗʰ S02.67 Fracture of alveolus of mandible

　　7ᵗʰ **S02.670 Fracture of alveolus of mandible, unspecified side** CC PQA HAC HCC CC/MCC Exc

　　7ᵗʰ **S02.671 Fracture of alveolus of** right **mandible** CC PQA HAC HCC CC/MCC Exc

　　7ᵗʰ **S02.672 Fracture of alveolus of** left **mandible** CC PQA HAC HCC CC/MCC Exc

　7ᵗʰ **S02.69 Fracture of mandible of other specified site** CC PQA HAC HCC CC/MCC Exc

5ᵗʰ **S02.8 Fractures of** other specified skull and facial bones

　　Fracture of palate

　　EXCLUDES2 fracture of orbital floor (S02.3-)

　　　　　　fracture of orbital roof (S02.12-)

　7ᵗʰ **S02.80 Fracture of other specified skull and facial bones, unspecified side** CC PQA HAC HCC CC/MCC Exc

　7ᵗʰ **S02.81 Fracture of other specified skull and facial bones, right side** CC PQA HAC HCC CC/MCC Exc

　7ᵗʰ **S02.82 Fracture of other specified skull and facial bones, left side** CC PQA HAC HCC CC/MCC Exc

● 6ᵗʰ **S02.83 Fracture of** medial orbital wall

　　EXCLUDES2 orbital floor (S02.3-)

　　　　　　orbital roof (S02.12-)

　● 7ᵗʰ **S02.831 Fracture of medial orbital wall, right side** CC CC/MCC Exc

　● 7ᵗʰ **S02.832 Fracture of medial orbital wall, left side** CC CC/MCC Exc

　● 7ᵗʰ **S02.839 Fracture of medial orbital wall, unspecified side** CC CC/MCC Exc

● 6ᵗʰ **S02.84 Fracture of** lateral orbital wall

　　EXCLUDES2 orbital floor (S02.3-)

　　　　　　orbital roof (S02.12-)

　● 7ᵗʰ **S02.841 Fracture of lateral orbital wall, right side** CC CC/MCC Exc

　● 7ᵗʰ **S02.842 Fracture of lateral orbital wall, left side** CC CC/MCC Exc

　● 7ᵗʰ **S02.849 Fracture of lateral orbital wall, unspecified side** CC CC/MCC Exc

● 7ᵗʰ **S02.85 Fracture of orbit, unspecified** CC CC/MCC Exc

　　Fracture of orbit NOS

　　Fracture of orbit wall NOS

　　EXCLUDES1 lateral orbital wall (S02.84-)

　　　　　　medial orbital wall (S02.83-)

　　　　　　orbital floor (S02.3-)

　　　　　　orbital roof (S02.12-)

5ᵗʰ **S02.9 Fracture of** unspecified skull and facial bones

　7ᵗʰ **S02.91 Unspecified fracture of** skull CC PQA HAC HCC MCC CC/MCC Exc

　7ᵗʰ **S02.92 Unspecified fracture of facial bones** CC PQA HAC HCC CC/MCC Exc

4ᵗʰ **S03 Dislocation and sprain of joints and ligaments of head**

　INCLUDES avulsion of joint (capsule) or ligament of head

　　　　　laceration of cartilage, joint (capsule) or ligament of head

　　　　　sprain of cartilage, joint (capsule) or ligament of head

　　　　　traumatic hemarthrosis of joint or ligament of head

　　　　　traumatic rupture of joint or ligament of head

　　　　　traumatic subluxation of joint or ligament of head

　　　　　traumatic tear of joint or ligament of head

　Code also any associated open wound

　EXCLUDES2 Strain of muscle or tendon of head (S09.1)

　The appropriate 7th character is to be added to each code from category S03

　　A = initial encounter

　　D = subsequent encounter

　　S = sequela

5ᵗʰ **S03.0 Dislocation of** jaw

　　Dislocation of jaw (cartilage) (meniscus)

　　Dislocation of mandible

　　Dislocation of temporomandibular (joint)

　7ᵗʰ **S03.00 Dislocation of jaw, unspecified side** PQA

7ᵗʰ **S03.01 Dislocation of jaw,** right side PQA

7ᵗʰ **S03.02 Dislocation of jaw,** left side PQA

7ᵗʰ **S03.03 Dislocation of jaw,** bilateral PQA

7ᵗʰ **S03.1 Dislocation of** septal cartilage of nose PQA

7ᵗʰ **S03.2 Dislocation of** tooth PQA

5ᵗʰ **S03.4 Sprain of** jaw

　　Sprain of temporomandibular (joint) (ligament)

　7ᵗʰ **S03.40 Sprain of jaw, unspecified side** PQA

　7ᵗʰ **S03.41 Sprain of jaw,** right side PQA

　7ᵗʰ **S03.42 Sprain of jaw,** left side PQA

　7ᵗʰ **S03.43 Sprain of jaw,** bilateral PQA

7ᵗʰ **S03.8 Sprain of joints and ligaments of** other **parts of** head PQA

7ᵗʰ **S03.9 Sprain of joints and ligaments of unspecified parts of head** PQA

4ᵗʰ **S04 Injury of** cranial nerve **(Figure 19.1)**

　The selection of side should be based on the side of the body being affected

　☞ **Code first** any associated intracranial injury (S06.-)

　Code also any associated:

　　open wound of head (S01.-)

　　skull fracture (S02.-)

　The appropriate 7th character is to be added to each code from category S04

　　A = initial encounter

　　D = subsequent encounter

　　S = sequela

5ᵗʰ **S04.0 Injury of** optic nerve **and** pathways

　　Use additional code to identify any visual field defect or blindness (H53.4-, H54.-)

　6ᵗʰ **S04.01 Injury of optic** nerve

　　Injury of 2nd cranial nerve

　　7ᵗʰ **S04.011 Injury of optic nerve,** right eye CC PQA CC/MCC Exc

　　7ᵗʰ **S04.012 Injury of optic nerve,** left eye CC PQA CC/MCC Exc

　　7ᵗʰ **S04.019 Injury of optic nerve, unspecified eye** CC PQA CC/MCC Exc

　　　Injury of optic nerve NOS

　7ᵗʰ **S04.02 Injury of optic** chiasm CC PQA CC/MCC Exc

　6ᵗʰ **S04.03 Injury of optic** tract **and** pathways

　　Injury of optic radiation

　　7ᵗʰ **S04.031 Injury of optic tract and pathways, right side** CC PQA CC/MCC Exc

　　7ᵗʰ **S04.032 Injury of optic tract and pathways, left side** CC PQA CC/MCC Exc

　　7ᵗʰ **S04.039 Injury of optic tract and pathways, unspecified side** CC PQA CC/MCC Exc

　　　Injury of optic tract and pathways NOS

　6ᵗʰ **S04.04 Injury of** visual cortex

　　7ᵗʰ **S04.041 Injury of visual cortex,** right side CC PQA CC/MCC Exc

　　7ᵗʰ **S04.042 Injury of visual cortex,** left side CC PQA CC/MCC Exc

　　7ᵗʰ **S04.049 Injury of visual cortex, unspecified side** CC PQA CC/MCC Exc

　　　Injury of visual cortex NOS

5ᵗʰ **S04.1 Injury of** oculomotor **nerve**

　　Injury of 3rd cranial nerve

　7ᵗʰ **S04.10 Injury of oculomotor nerve, unspecified side** CC PQA CC/MCC Exc

　7ᵗʰ **S04.11 Injury of oculomotor nerve,** right side CC PQA CC/MCC Exc

　7ᵗʰ **S04.12 Injury of oculomotor nerve,** left side CC PQA CC/MCC Exc

5ᵗʰ **S04.2 Injury of** trochlear **nerve**

　　Injury of 4th cranial nerve

　7ᵗʰ **S04.20 Injury of trochlear nerve, unspecified side** CC PQA CC/MCC Exc

　7ᵗʰ **S04.21 Injury of trochlear nerve,** right side CC PQA CC/MCC Exc

　7ᵗʰ **S04.22 Injury of trochlear nerve,** left side CC PQA CC/MCC Exc

5ᵗʰ **S04.3 Injury of** trigeminal **nerve**

　　Injury of 5th cranial nerve

　7ᵗʰ **S04.30 Injury of trigeminal nerve, unspecified side** CC PQA CC/MCC Exc

　7ᵗʰ **S04.31 Injury of trigeminal nerve,** right side CC PQA CC/MCC Exc

　7ᵗʰ **S04.32 Injury of trigeminal nerve,** left side CC PQA CC/MCC Exc

5ᵗʰ **S04.4 Injury of** abducent **nerve**

　　Injury of 6th cranial nerve

　7ᵗʰ **S04.40 Injury of abducent nerve, unspecified side** CC PQA CC/MCC Exc

PQA Unacceptable principal diagnosis symbol per Medicare code edits　PQ Code exempt from diagnosis present on admission requirement

? Questionable admission　CC Complication or comorbidity　MCC Major complication or comorbidity　CC/MCC Exc CC/MCC exclusion

HCC HCC diagnosis code　RxHCC RxHCC diagnosis code　MACRA code　**DEFINITION** Describes condition/terminology

TIP Coding guidance　👁 Official Guideline Reference　Z1 Z code as first-listed diagnosis

S04.41 Injury of abducent nerve, right side
S04.42 Injury of abducent nerve, left side
S04.5 Injury of facial nerve
Injury of 7th cranial nerve
S04.50 Injury of facial nerve, unspecified side
S04.51 Injury of facial nerve, right side
S04.52 Injury of facial nerve, left side
S04.6 Injury of acoustic nerve
Injury of auditory nerve
Injury of 8th cranial nerve
S04.60 Injury of acoustic nerve, unspecified side
S04.61 Injury of acoustic nerve, right side
S04.62 Injury of acoustic nerve, left side
S04.7 Injury of accessory nerve
Injury of 11th cranial nerve
S04.70 Injury of accessory nerve, unspecified side
S04.71 Injury of accessory nerve, right side
S04.72 Injury of accessory nerve, left side
S04.8 Injury of other cranial nerves
S04.81 Injury of olfactory [1st] nerve
S04.811 Injury of olfactory [1st] nerve, right side
S04.812 Injury of olfactory [1st] nerve, left side
S04.819 Injury of olfactory [1st] nerve, unspecified side
S04.89 Injury of other cranial nerves
Injury of vagus [10th] nerve
S04.891 Injury of other cranial nerves, right side
S04.892 Injury of other cranial nerves, left side
S04.899 Injury of other cranial nerves, unspecified side
S04.9 Injury of unspecified cranial nerve

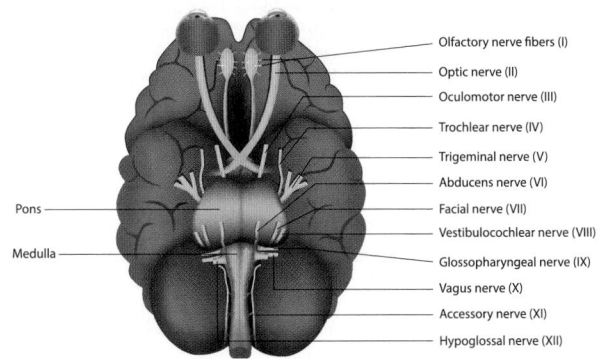

Olfactory nerve fibers (I)
Optic nerve (II)
Oculomotor nerve (III)
Trochlear nerve (IV)
Trigeminal nerve (V)
Abducens nerve (VI)
Pons
Facial nerve (VII)
Vestibulocochlear nerve (VIII)
Medulla
Glossopharyngeal nerve (IX)
Vagus nerve (X)
Accessory nerve (XI)
Hypoglossal nerve (XII)

Figure 19.1 Cranial Nerves

S05 Injury of eye and orbit
INCLUDES   open wound of eye and orbit
EXCLUDES2   2nd cranial [optic] nerve injury (S04.0-)
            3rd cranial [oculomotor] nerve injury (S04.1-)
            open wound of eyelid and periocular area (S01.1-)
            orbital bone fracture (S02.1-, S02.3-, S02.8-)
            superficial injury of eyelid (S00.1-S00.2)

The appropriate 7th character is to be added to each code from category S05
    A = initial encounter
    D = subsequent encounter
    S = sequela

S05.0 Injury of conjunctiva and corneal abrasion without foreign body
    EXCLUDES1 foreign body in conjunctival sac (T15.1)
              foreign body in cornea (T15.0)

S05.00 Injury of conjunctiva and corneal abrasion without foreign body, unspecified eye
S05.01 Injury of conjunctiva and corneal abrasion without foreign body, right eye
S05.02 Injury of conjunctiva and corneal abrasion without foreign body, left eye
S05.1 Contusion of eyeball and orbital tissues
Traumatic hyphema
    EXCLUDES2 black eye NOS (S00.1)
              contusion of eyelid and periocular area (S00.1)
S05.10 Contusion of eyeball and orbital tissues, unspecified eye
S05.11 Contusion of eyeball and orbital tissues, right eye
S05.12 Contusion of eyeball and orbital tissues, left eye
S05.2 Ocular laceration and rupture with prolapse or loss of intraocular tissue
S05.20 Ocular laceration and rupture with prolapse or loss of intraocular tissue, unspecified eye
S05.21 Ocular laceration and rupture with prolapse or loss of intraocular tissue, right eye
S05.22 Ocular laceration and rupture with prolapse or loss of intraocular tissue, left eye
S05.3 Ocular laceration without prolapse or loss of intraocular tissue
Laceration of eye NOS
S05.30 Ocular laceration without prolapse or loss of intraocular tissue, unspecified eye
S05.31 Ocular laceration without prolapse or loss of intraocular tissue, right eye
S05.32 Ocular laceration without prolapse or loss of intraocular tissue, left eye
S05.4 Penetrating wound of orbit with or without foreign body
    EXCLUDES2 retained (old) foreign body following penetrating wound in orbit (H05.5-)
S05.40 Penetrating wound of orbit with or without foreign body, unspecified eye
S05.41 Penetrating wound of orbit with or without foreign body, right eye
S05.42 Penetrating wound of orbit with or without foreign body, left eye
S05.5 Penetrating wound with foreign body of eyeball
    EXCLUDES2 retained (old) intraocular foreign body (H44.6-, H44.7)
S05.50 Penetrating wound with foreign body of unspecified eyeball
S05.51 Penetrating wound with foreign body of right eyeball
S05.52 Penetrating wound with foreign body of left eyeball
S05.6 Penetrating wound without foreign body of eyeball
Ocular penetration NOS
S05.60 Penetrating wound without foreign body of unspecified eyeball
S05.61 Penetrating wound without foreign body of right eyeball
S05.62 Penetrating wound without foreign body of left eyeball
S05.7 Avulsion of eye
Traumatic enucleation
S05.70 Avulsion of unspecified eye
S05.71 Avulsion of right eye
S05.72 Avulsion of left eye
S05.8 Other injuries of eye and orbit
Lacrimal duct injury
S05.8X Other injuries of eye and orbit
S05.8X1 Other injuries of right eye and orbit
S05.8X2 Other injuries of left eye and orbit
S05.8X9 Other injuries of unspecified eye and orbit

Unspecified Code   Other Specified Code   Manifestation Code   N Newborn   P Pediatric   M Maternity   A Adult   ♂ Male   ♀ Female
● New Code   ▲ Revised Code Title   ▶◀ Revised Text   NOTES   INCLUDES   EXCLUDES1 Not coded here   EXCLUDES2 Not included here
4th 4th character required   5th 5th character required   6th 6th character required   7th 7th character required   7x Extension 'X' Alert
HAC Hospital-acquired condition (HAC) alert   AHA AHA Coding Clinic©   ☛ Code first alert

[5th] **S05.9 Unspecified injury of eye and orbit**
Injury of eye NOS
[7th] **S05.90 Unspecified injury of unspecified eye and orbit** POA
[7th] **S05.91 Unspecified injury of right eye and orbit** CC POA CC/MCC Exc
[7th] **S05.92 Unspecified injury of left eye and orbit** CC POA CC/MCC Exc

[4th] **S06 Intracranial injury**
[INCLUDES] *traumatic brain injury*
Code also any associated:
open wound of head (S01.-)
skull fracture (S02.-)
[EXCLUDES1] *head injury NOS (S09.90)*
The appropriate 7th character is to be added to each code from category S06
A = initial encounter
D = subsequent encounter
S = sequela
[NOTES] 7th characters D and S do not apply to codes in category S06 with 6th character 7 - death due to brain injury prior to regaining consciousness, or 8 - death due to other cause prior to regaining consciousness.

[5th] **S06.0 Concussion**
Commotio cerebri
[EXCLUDES1] *concussion with other intracranial injuries classified in subcategories S06.1- to S06.6-, S06.81- and S06.82- code to specified intracranial injury*
[6th] **S06.0X Concussion**
[7th] **S06.0X0 Concussion without loss of consciousness** CC POA HCC CC/MCC Exc
[7th] **S06.0X1 Concussion with loss of consciousness of 30 minutes or less** CC POA HAC HCC CC/MCC Exc
[7th] **S06.0X9 Concussion with loss of consciousness of unspecified duration** CC POA HAC HCC CC/MCC Exc
AHA: Q4 2016
Concussion NOS

[5th] **S06.1 Traumatic cerebral edema**
Diffuse traumatic cerebral edema
Focal traumatic cerebral edema
[6th] **S06.1X Traumatic cerebral edema**
[7th] **S06.1X0 Traumatic cerebral edema without loss of consciousness** POA HCC MCC CC/MCC Exc
AHA: Q1 2015
[7th] **S06.1X1 Traumatic cerebral edema with loss of consciousness of 30 minutes or less** POA HAC HCC MCC CC/MCC Exc
[7th] **S06.1X2 Traumatic cerebral edema with loss of consciousness of 31 minutes to 59 minutes** POA HAC HCC MCC CC/MCC Exc
[7th] **S06.1X3 Traumatic cerebral edema with loss of consciousness of 1 hour to 5 hours 59 minutes** POA HAC HCC MCC CC/MCC Exc
[7th] **S06.1X4 Traumatic cerebral edema with loss of consciousness of 6 hours to 24 hours** POA HAC HCC MCC CC/MCC Exc
[7th] **S06.1X5 Traumatic cerebral edema with loss of consciousness greater than 24 hours with return to pre-existing conscious level** POA HAC HCC MCC CC/MCC Exc
[7th] **S06.1X6 Traumatic cerebral edema with loss of consciousness greater than 24 hours without return to pre-existing conscious level with patient surviving** POA HAC HCC MCC CC/MCC Exc
[7th] **S06.1X7 Traumatic cerebral edema with loss of consciousness of any duration with death due to brain injury prior to regaining consciousness** HAC MCC CC/MCC Exc
[7th] **S06.1X8 Traumatic cerebral edema with loss of consciousness of any duration with death due to other cause prior to regaining consciousness** HAC MCC CC/MCC Exc
[7th] **S06.1X9 Traumatic cerebral edema with loss of consciousness of unspecified duration** POA HAC HCC MCC CC/MCC Exc
Traumatic cerebral edema NOS

[5th] **S06.2 Diffuse traumatic brain injury**
Diffuse axonal brain injury
[EXCLUDES1] *traumatic diffuse cerebral edema (S06.1X-)*
[6th] **S06.2X Diffuse traumatic brain injury**
[7th] **S06.2X0 Diffuse traumatic brain injury without loss of consciousness** POA HCC
[7th] **S06.2X1 Diffuse traumatic brain injury with loss of consciousness of 30 minutes or less** CC POA HAC HCC CC/MCC Exc
[7th] **S06.2X2 Diffuse traumatic brain injury with loss of consciousness of 31 minutes to 59 minutes** CC POA HAC HCC CC/MCC Exc
[7th] **S06.2X3 Diffuse traumatic brain injury with loss of consciousness of 1 hour to 5 hours 59 minutes** CC POA HAC HCC CC/MCC Exc
[7th] **S06.2X4 Diffuse traumatic brain injury with loss of consciousness of 6 hours to 24 hours** CC POA HAC HCC CC/MCC Exc
[7th] **S06.2X5 Diffuse traumatic brain injury with loss of consciousness greater than 24 hours with return to pre-existing conscious levels** CC POA HAC HCC CC/MCC Exc
[7th] **S06.2X6 Diffuse traumatic brain injury with loss of consciousness greater than 24 hours without return to pre-existing conscious level with patient surviving** POA HAC HCC MCC CC/MCC Exc
[7th] **S06.2X7 Diffuse traumatic brain injury with loss of consciousness of any duration with death due to brain injury prior to regaining consciousness** HAC MCC CC/MCC Exc
[7th] **S06.2X8 Diffuse traumatic brain injury with loss of consciousness of any duration with death due to other cause prior to regaining consciousness** HAC MCC CC/MCC Exc
[7th] **S06.2X9 Diffuse traumatic brain injury with loss of consciousness of unspecified duration** CC POA HAC HCC CC/MCC Exc
Diffuse traumatic brain injury NOS

[5th] **S06.3 Focal traumatic brain injury**
[EXCLUDES1] *any condition classifiable to S06.4-S06.6*
focal cerebral edema (S06.1)
[6th] **S06.30 Unspecified focal traumatic brain injury**
[7th] **S06.300 Unspecified focal traumatic brain injury without loss of consciousness** POA HCC
[7th] **S06.301 Unspecified focal traumatic brain injury with loss of consciousness of 30 minutes or less** CC POA HAC HCC CC/MCC Exc
[7th] **S06.302 Unspecified focal traumatic brain injury with loss of consciousness of 31 minutes to 59 minutes** CC POA HAC HCC CC/MCC Exc
[7th] **S06.303 Unspecified focal traumatic brain injury with loss of consciousness of 1 hour to 5 hours 59 minutes** CC POA HAC HCC CC/MCC Exc
[7th] **S06.304 Unspecified focal traumatic brain injury with loss of consciousness of 6 hours to 24 hours** CC POA HAC HCC CC/MCC Exc
[7th] **S06.305 Unspecified focal traumatic brain injury with loss of consciousness greater than 24 hours with return to pre-existing conscious level** CC POA HAC HCC CC/MCC Exc
[7th] **S06.306 Unspecified focal traumatic brain injury with loss of consciousness greater than 24 hours without return to pre-existing conscious level with patient surviving** POA HAC HCC MCC CC/MCC Exc

PDx Unacceptable principal diagnosis symbol per Medicare code edits · POA Code exempt from diagnosis present on admission requirement
[?] Questionable admission · CC Complication or comorbidity · MCC Major complication or comorbidity · CC/MCC Exc CC/MCC exclusion
HCC HCC diagnosis code · RxHCC RxHCC diagnosis code · MACRA code · **DEFINITION** Describes condition/terminology
TIP Coding guidance · 👁 Official Guideline Reference · [Z-1] Z code as first-listed diagnosis

⑦ **S06.307** Unspecified focal traumatic brain injury **with loss of consciousness of** any duration with death due to brain injury prior to regaining consciousness HAC MCC CC/MCC Exc

⑦ **S06.308** Unspecified focal traumatic brain injury **with loss of consciousness of** any duration with death due to other cause prior to regaining consciousness HAC MCC CC/MCC Exc

⑦ **S06.309** Unspecified focal traumatic brain injury **with loss of consciousness of unspecified duration** CC POA HAC HCC CC/MCC Exc

Unspecified focal traumatic brain injury NOS

⑥ **S06.31** Contusion and laceration of right cerebrum

⑦ **S06.310** Contusion and laceration of **right cerebrum** without loss of consciousness POA HAC HCC MCC CC/MCC Exc

⑦ **S06.311** Contusion and laceration of right **cerebrum with loss of consciousness of** 30 minutes or less POA HAC HCC MCC CC/MCC Exc

⑦ **S06.312** Contusion and laceration of **right cerebrum with loss of consciousness of** 31 minutes to 59 minutes POA HAC HCC MCC CC/MCC Exc

⑦ **S06.313** Contusion and laceration of **right cerebrum with loss of consciousness of** 1 hour to 5 hours 59 minutes POA HAC HCC MCC CC/MCC Exc

⑦ **S06.314** Contusion and laceration of right **cerebrum with loss of consciousness of** 6 hours to 24 hours POA HAC HCC MCC CC/MCC Exc

⑦ **S06.315** Contusion and laceration of right **cerebrum with loss of consciousness** greater than 24 hours with return to pre-existing conscious level POA HAC HCC MCC CC/MCC Exc

⑦ **S06.316** Contusion and laceration of right **cerebrum with loss of consciousness** greater than 24 hours without return to pre-existing conscious level with patient surviving POA HAC HCC MCC CC/MCC Exc

⑦ **S06.317** Contusion and laceration of right **cerebrum with loss of consciousness of** any duration with death due to brain injury prior to regaining consciousness HAC MCC CC/MCC Exc

⑦ **S06.318** Contusion and laceration of right **cerebrum with loss of consciousness of** any duration with death due to other cause prior to regaining consciousness HAC MCC CC/MCC Exc

⑦ **S06.319** Contusion and laceration of right **cerebrum with loss of consciousness of unspecified duration** POA HAC HCC MCC CC/MCC Exc

Contusion and laceration of right cerebrum NOS

⑥ **S06.32** Contusion and laceration of left cerebrum

⑦ **S06.320** Contusion and laceration of **left cerebrum** without loss of consciousness POA HAC HCC MCC CC/MCC Exc

⑦ **S06.321** Contusion and laceration of left cerebrum **with loss of consciousness of** 30 minutes or less POA HAC HCC MCC CC/MCC Exc

⑦ **S06.322** Contusion and laceration of left cerebrum **with loss of consciousness of** 31 minutes to 59 minutes POA HAC HCC MCC CC/MCC Exc

⑦ **S06.323** Contusion and laceration of left cerebrum **with loss of consciousness of** 1 hour to 5 hours 59 minutes POA HAC HCC MCC CC/MCC Exc

⑦ **S06.324** Contusion and laceration of left cerebrum **with loss of consciousness of** 6 hours to 24 hours POA HAC HCC MCC CC/MCC Exc

⑦ **S06.325** Contusion and laceration of left cerebrum **with loss of consciousness** greater than 24 hours with return to pre-existing conscious level POA HAC HCC MCC CC/MCC Exc

⑦ **S06.326** Contusion and laceration of left cerebrum **with loss of consciousness** greater than 24 hours without return to pre-existing conscious level with patient surviving POA HAC HCC MCC CC/MCC Exc

⑦ **S06.327** Contusion and laceration of left cerebrum **with loss of consciousness of** any duration with death due to brain injury prior to regaining consciousness HAC MCC CC/MCC Exc

⑦ **S06.328** Contusion and laceration of left cerebrum **with loss of consciousness of** any duration with death due to other cause prior to regaining consciousness HAC MCC CC/MCC Exc

⑦ **S06.329** Contusion and laceration of left cerebrum **with loss of consciousness of unspecified duration** POA HAC HCC MCC CC/MCC Exc

Contusion and laceration of left cerebrum NOS

⑥ **S06.33** Contusion and laceration of cerebrum, unspecified

⑦ **S06.330** Contusion and laceration of **cerebrum, unspecified,** without loss of consciousness POA HAC HCC MCC CC/MCC Exc

⑦ **S06.331** Contusion and laceration of cerebrum, **unspecified, with loss of consciousness of** 30 minutes or less POA HAC HCC MCC CC/MCC Exc

⑦ **S06.332** Contusion and laceration of **cerebrum, unspecified, with loss of consciousness of 31 minutes to 59 minutes** POA HAC HCC MCC CC/MCC Exc

⑦ **S06.333** Contusion and laceration of **cerebrum, unspecified, with loss of consciousness of 1 hour to 5 hours 59 minutes** POA HAC HCC MCC CC/MCC Exc

⑦ **S06.334** Contusion and laceration of cerebrum, **unspecified, with loss of consciousness of 6 hours to 24 hours** POA HAC HCC MCC CC/MCC Exc

⑦ **S06.335** Contusion and laceration of cerebrum, **unspecified, with loss of consciousness** greater than 24 hours with return to pre-existing conscious level POA HAC HCC MCC CC/MCC Exc

⑦ **S06.336** Contusion and laceration of cerebrum, **unspecified, with loss of consciousness** greater than 24 hours without return to pre-existing conscious level with patient surviving POA HAC HCC MCC CC/MCC Exc

⑦ **S06.337** Contusion and laceration of cerebrum, **unspecified, with loss of consciousness of** any duration with death due to brain injury prior to regaining consciousness HAC MCC CC/MCC Exc

⑦ **S06.338** Contusion and laceration of cerebrum, **unspecified, with loss of consciousness** of any duration with death due to other cause prior to regaining consciousness HAC MCC CC/MCC Exc

⑦ **S06.339** Contusion and laceration of cerebrum, **unspecified, with loss of consciousness of unspecified duration** POA HAC HCC MCC CC/MCC Exc

Contusion and laceration of cerebrum NOS

⑥ **S06.34** Traumatic hemorrhage of right cerebrum

Traumatic intracerebral hemorrhage and hematoma of right cerebrum

⑦ **S06.340** Traumatic hemorrhage of **right cerebrum** without loss of consciousness POA HAC HCC MCC CC/MCC Exc

AHA: Q1 2015

⑦ **S06.341** Traumatic hemorrhage of right cerebrum **with loss of consciousness of** 30 minutes or less POA HAC HCC MCC CC/MCC Exc

---

Unspecified Code   Other Specified Code   Manifestation Code   Ⓝ Newborn   Ⓟ Pediatric   Ⓜ Maternity   Ⓐ Adult   ♂ Male   ♀ Female
● New Code   ▲ Revised Code Title   ▶◀ Revised Text   **NOTES** *INCLUDES* *EXCLUDES1* Not coded here *EXCLUDES2* Not included here
④ 4th character required   ⑤ 5th character required   ⑥ 6th character required   ⑦ 7th character required   ⑦ Extension 'X' Alert
HAC Hospital-acquired condition (HAC) alert   **AHA** AHA Coding Clinic©   ☛ **Code first alert**

7th S06.342 Traumatic hemorrhage of right cerebrum with loss of consciousness of 31 minutes to 59 minutes POA HAC HCC MCC CC/MCC Exc

7th S06.343 Traumatic hemorrhage of right cerebrum with loss of consciousness of 1 hours to 5 hours 59 minutes POA HAC HCC MCC CC/MCC Exc

7th S06.344 Traumatic hemorrhage of right cerebrum with loss of consciousness of 6 hours to 24 hours POA HAC HCC MCC CC/MCC Exc

7th S06.345 Traumatic hemorrhage of right cerebrum with loss of consciousness greater than 24 hours with return to pre-existing conscious level POA HAC HCC MCC CC/MCC Exc

7th S06.346 Traumatic hemorrhage of right cerebrum with loss of consciousness greater than 24 hours without return to pre-existing conscious level with patient surviving POA HAC HCC MCC CC/MCC Exc

7th S06.347 Traumatic hemorrhage of right cerebrum with loss of consciousness of any duration with death due to brain injury prior to regaining consciousness HAC MCC CC/MCC Exc

7th S06.348 Traumatic hemorrhage of right cerebrum with loss of consciousness of any duration with death due to other cause prior to regaining consciousness HAC MCC CC/MCC Exc

7th S06.349 Traumatic hemorrhage of right cerebrum with loss of consciousness of unspecified duration POA HAC HCC MCC CC/MCC Exc
Traumatic hemorrhage of right cerebrum NOS

6th S06.35 Traumatic hemorrhage of left cerebrum
Traumatic intracerebral hemorrhage and hematoma of left cerebrum

7th S06.350 Traumatic hemorrhage of left cerebrum without loss of consciousness POA HAC HCC MCC CC/MCC Exc

7th S06.351 Traumatic hemorrhage of left cerebrum with loss of consciousness of 30 minutes or less POA HAC HCC MCC CC/MCC Exc

7th S06.352 Traumatic hemorrhage of left cerebrum with loss of consciousness of 31 minutes to 59 minutes POA HAC HCC MCC CC/MCC Exc

7th S06.353 Traumatic hemorrhage of left cerebrum with loss of consciousness of 1 hours to 5 hours 59 minutes POA HAC HCC MCC CC/MCC Exc

7th S06.354 Traumatic hemorrhage of left cerebrum with loss of consciousness of 6 hours to 24 hours POA HAC HCC MCC CC/MCC Exc

7th S06.355 Traumatic hemorrhage of left cerebrum with loss of consciousness greater than 24 hours with return to pre-existing conscious level POA HAC HCC MCC CC/MCC Exc

7th S06.356 Traumatic hemorrhage of left cerebrum with loss of consciousness greater than 24 hours without return to pre-existing conscious level with patient surviving POA HAC HCC MCC CC/MCC Exc

7th S06.357 Traumatic hemorrhage of left cerebrum with loss of consciousness of any duration with death due to brain injury prior to regaining consciousness HAC MCC CC/MCC Exc

7th S06.358 Traumatic hemorrhage of left cerebrum with loss of consciousness of any duration with death due to other cause prior to regaining consciousness HAC MCC CC/MCC Exc

7th S06.359 Traumatic hemorrhage of left cerebrum with loss of consciousness of unspecified duration POA HAC HCC MCC CC/MCC Exc
Traumatic hemorrhage of left cerebrum NOS

6th S06.36 Traumatic hemorrhage of cerebrum, unspecified
Traumatic intracerebral hemorrhage and hematoma, unspecified

7th S06.360 Traumatic hemorrhage of cerebrum, unspecified, without loss of consciousness POA HAC HCC MCC CC/MCC Exc

7th S06.361 Traumatic hemorrhage of cerebrum, unspecified, with loss of consciousness of 30 minutes or less POA HAC HCC MCC CC/MCC Exc

7th S06.362 Traumatic hemorrhage of cerebrum, unspecified, with loss of consciousness of 31 minutes to 59 minutes POA HAC HCC MCC CC/MCC Exc

7th S06.363 Traumatic hemorrhage of cerebrum, unspecified, with loss of consciousness of 1 hours to 5 hours 59 minutes POA HAC HCC MCC CC/MCC Exc

7th S06.364 Traumatic hemorrhage of cerebrum, unspecified, with loss of consciousness of 6 hours to 24 hours POA HAC HCC MCC CC/MCC Exc

7th S06.365 Traumatic hemorrhage of cerebrum, unspecified, with loss of consciousness greater than 24 hours with return to pre-existing conscious level POA HAC HCC MCC CC/MCC Exc

7th S06.366 Traumatic hemorrhage of cerebrum, unspecified, with loss of consciousness greater than 24 hours without return to pre-existing conscious level with patient surviving POA HAC HCC MCC CC/MCC Exc

7th S06.367 Traumatic hemorrhage of cerebrum, unspecified, with loss of consciousness of any duration with death due to brain injury prior to regaining consciousness HAC MCC CC/MCC Exc

7th S06.368 Traumatic hemorrhage of cerebrum, unspecified, with loss of consciousness of any duration with death due to other cause prior to regaining consciousness HAC MCC CC/MCC Exc

7th S06.369 Traumatic hemorrhage of cerebrum, unspecified, with loss of consciousness of unspecified duration POA HAC HCC MCC CC/MCC Exc
Traumatic hemorrhage of cerebrum NOS

6th S06.37 Contusion, laceration, and hemorrhage of cerebellum

7th S06.370 Contusion, laceration, and hemorrhage of cerebellum without loss of consciousness POA HAC HCC MCC

7th S06.371 Contusion, laceration, and hemorrhage of cerebellum with loss of consciousness of 30 minutes or less CC POA HAC HCC CC/MCC Exc

7th S06.372 Contusion, laceration, and hemorrhage of cerebellum with loss of consciousness of 31 minutes to 59 minutes CC POA HAC HCC CC/MCC Exc

7th S06.373 Contusion, laceration, and hemorrhage of cerebellum with loss of consciousness of 1 hour to 5 hours 59 minutes CC POA HAC HCC CC/MCC Exc

7th S06.374 Contusion, laceration, and hemorrhage of cerebellum with loss of consciousness of 6 hours to 24 hours CC POA HAC HCC CC/MCC Exc

7th S06.375 Contusion, laceration, and hemorrhage of cerebellum with loss of consciousness greater than 24 hours with return to pre-existing conscious level CC POA HAC HCC CC/MCC Exc

7th S06.376 Contusion, laceration, and hemorrhage of cerebellum with loss of consciousness greater than 24 hours without return to pre-existing conscious level with patient surviving POA HAC HCC MCC CC/MCC Exc

7th S06.377 Contusion, laceration, and hemorrhage of cerebellum with loss of consciousness of any duration with death due to brain injury prior to regaining consciousness HAC MCC CC/MCC Exc

[7th] **S06.378** Contusion, laceration, and hemorrhage of cerebellum with loss of consciousness of any duration with death due to other cause prior to regaining consciousness [HAC] [MCC] [CC/MCC Exc]

[7th] **S06.379** Contusion, laceration, and hemorrhage of cerebellum with loss of consciousness of unspecified duration [CC] [POA] [HAC] [HCC] [CC/MCC Exc]
Contusion, laceration, and hemorrhage of cerebellum NOS

[6th] **S06.38** Contusion, laceration, and hemorrhage of brainstem

[7th] **S06.380** Contusion, laceration, and hemorrhage of brainstem without loss of consciousness [POA] [HAC] [HCC] [MCC]

[7th] **S06.381** Contusion, laceration, and hemorrhage of brainstem with loss of consciousness of 30 minutes or less [CC] [POA] [HAC] [HCC] [CC/MCC Exc]

[7th] **S06.382** Contusion, laceration, and hemorrhage of brainstem with loss of consciousness of 31 minutes to 59 minutes [CC] [POA] [HAC] [HCC] [CC/MCC Exc]

[7th] **S06.383** Contusion, laceration, and hemorrhage of brainstem with loss of consciousness of 1 hour to 5 hours 59 minutes [CC] [POA] [HAC] [HCC] [CC/MCC Exc]

[7th] **S06.384** Contusion, laceration, and hemorrhage of brainstem with loss of consciousness of 6 hours to 24 hours [CC] [POA] [HAC] [HCC] [CC/MCC Exc]

[7th] **S06.385** Contusion, laceration, and hemorrhage of brainstem with loss of consciousness greater than 24 hours with return to pre-existing conscious level [CC] [POA] [HAC] [HCC] [CC/MCC Exc]

[7th] **S06.386** Contusion, laceration, and hemorrhage of brainstem with loss of consciousness greater than 24 hours without return to pre-existing conscious level with patient surviving [POA] [HAC] [HCC] [MCC] [CC/MCC Exc]

[7th] **S06.387** Contusion, laceration, and hemorrhage of brainstem with loss of consciousness of any duration with death due to brain injury prior to regaining consciousness [HAC] [MCC] [CC/MCC Exc]

[7th] **S06.388** Contusion, laceration, and hemorrhage of brainstem with loss of consciousness of any duration with death due to other cause prior to regaining consciousness [HAC] [MCC] [CC/MCC Exc]

[7th] **S06.389** Contusion, laceration, and hemorrhage of brainstem with loss of consciousness of unspecified duration [CC] [POA] [HAC] [HCC] [CC/MCC Exc]
Contusion, laceration, and hemorrhage of brainstem NOS

[5th] **S06.4** Epidural hemorrhage
Extradural hemorrhage NOS
Extradural hemorrhage (traumatic)

[6th] **S06.4X** Epidural hemorrhage

[7th] **S06.4X0** Epidural hemorrhage without loss of consciousness [POA] [HAC] [HCC] [MCC] [CC/MCC Exc]

[7th] **S06.4X1** Epidural hemorrhage with loss of consciousness of 30 minutes or less [POA] [HAC] [HCC] [MCC] [CC/MCC Exc]

[7th] **S06.4X2** Epidural hemorrhage with loss of consciousness of 31 minutes to 59 minutes [POA] [HAC] [HCC] [MCC] [CC/MCC Exc]

[7th] **S06.4X3** Epidural hemorrhage with loss of consciousness of 1 hour to 5 hours 59 minutes [POA] [HAC] [HCC] [MCC] [CC/MCC Exc]

[7th] **S06.4X4** Epidural hemorrhage with loss of consciousness of 6 hours to 24 hours [POA] [HAC] [HCC] [MCC] [CC/MCC Exc]

[7th] **S06.4X5** Epidural hemorrhage with loss of consciousness greater than 24 hours with return to pre-existing conscious level [POA] [HAC] [HCC] [MCC] [CC/MCC Exc]

[7th] **S06.4X6** Epidural hemorrhage with loss of consciousness greater than 24 hours without return to pre-existing conscious level with patient surviving [POA] [HAC] [HCC] [MCC] [CC/MCC Exc]

[7th] **S06.4X7** Epidural hemorrhage with loss of consciousness of any duration with death due to brain injury prior to regaining consciousness [HAC] [MCC] [CC/MCC Exc]

[7th] **S06.4X8** Epidural hemorrhage with loss of consciousness of any duration with death due to other causes prior to regaining consciousness [HAC] [MCC] [CC/MCC Exc]

[7th] **S06.4X9** Epidural hemorrhage with loss of consciousness of unspecified duration [POA] [HAC] [HCC] [MCC] [CC/MCC Exc]
Epidural hemorrhage NOS

[5th] **S06.5** Traumatic subdural hemorrhage

[6th] **S06.5X** Traumatic subdural hemorrhage

[7th] **S06.5X0** Traumatic subdural hemorrhage without loss of consciousness [POA] [HAC] [HCC] [MCC] [CC/MCC Exc]
AHA: Q2 2018, Q3 2015

[7th] **S06.5X1** Traumatic subdural hemorrhage with loss of consciousness of 30 minutes or less [POA] [HAC] [HCC] [MCC] [CC/MCC Exc]

[7th] **S06.5X2** Traumatic subdural hemorrhage with loss of consciousness of 31 minutes to 59 minutes [POA] [HAC] [HCC] [MCC] [CC/MCC Exc]

[7th] **S06.5X3** Traumatic subdural hemorrhage with loss of consciousness of 1 hour to 5 hours 59 minutes [POA] [HAC] [HCC] [MCC] [CC/MCC Exc]

[7th] **S06.5X4** Traumatic subdural hemorrhage with loss of consciousness of 6 hours to 24 hours [POA] [HAC] [HCC] [MCC] [CC/MCC Exc]

[7th] **S06.5X5** Traumatic subdural hemorrhage with loss of consciousness greater than 24 hours with return to pre-existing conscious level [POA] [HAC] [HCC] [MCC] [CC/MCC Exc]

[7th] **S06.5X6** Traumatic subdural hemorrhage with loss of consciousness greater than 24 hours without return to pre-existing conscious level with patient surviving [POA] [HAC] [HCC] [MCC] [CC/MCC Exc]

[7th] **S06.5X7** Traumatic subdural hemorrhage with loss of consciousness of any duration with death due to brain injury before regaining consciousness [HAC] [MCC] [CC/MCC Exc]

[7th] **S06.5X8** Traumatic subdural hemorrhage with loss of consciousness of any duration with death due to other cause before regaining consciousness [HAC] [MCC] [CC/MCC Exc]

[7th] **S06.5X9** Traumatic subdural hemorrhage with loss of consciousness of unspecified duration [POA] [HAC] [HCC] [MCC] [CC/MCC Exc]
Traumatic subdural hemorrhage NOS

[5th] **S06.6** Traumatic subarachnoid hemorrhage

[6th] **S06.6X** Traumatic subarachnoid hemorrhage

[7th] **S06.6X0** Traumatic subarachnoid hemorrhage without loss of consciousness [POA] [HAC] [HCC] [MCC] [CC/MCC Exc]
AHA: Q3 2015

[7th] **S06.6X1** Traumatic subarachnoid hemorrhage with loss of consciousness of 30 minutes or less [POA] [HAC] [HCC] [MCC] [CC/MCC Exc]

[7th] **S06.6X2** Traumatic subarachnoid hemorrhage with loss of consciousness of 31 minutes to 59 minutes [POA] [HAC] [HCC] [MCC] [CC/MCC Exc]

[7th] **S06.6X3** Traumatic subarachnoid hemorrhage with loss of consciousness of 1 hour to 5 hours 59 minutes [POA] [HAC] [HCC] [MCC] [CC/MCC Exc]

[7th] **S06.6X4** Traumatic subarachnoid hemorrhage with loss of consciousness of 6 hours to 24 hours [POA] [HAC] [HCC] [MCC] [CC/MCC Exc]

CHAPTER 19: INJURY, POISONING, AND CERTAIN OTHER CONSEQUENCES OF EXTERNAL CAUSES (S00-T88)

S06.6X5 - S06.894

7ᵗʰ **S06.6X5** **Traumatic subarachnoid hemorrhage with loss of consciousness** greater than 24 hours with return to pre-existing conscious level POA꜒ HAC HCC MCC꜒ CC/MCC Exc

7ᵗʰ **S06.6X6** **Traumatic subarachnoid hemorrhage with loss of consciousness** greater than 24 hours without return to pre-existing conscious level with patient surviving POA꜒ HAC HCC MCC꜒ CC/MCC Exc

7ᵗʰ **S06.6X7** **Traumatic subarachnoid hemorrhage with loss of consciousness of** any duration with death due to brain injury prior to regaining consciousness HAC MCC꜒ CC/MCC Exc

7ᵗʰ **S06.6X8** **Traumatic subarachnoid hemorrhage with loss of consciousness of** any duration with death due to other cause prior to regaining consciousness HAC MCC꜒ CC/MCC Exc

7ᵗʰ **S06.6X9** **Traumatic subarachnoid hemorrhage with loss of consciousness of unspecified duration** POA꜒ HAC HCC MCC꜒ CC/MCC Exc
  Traumatic subarachnoid hemorrhage NOS

5ᵗʰ **S06.8** **Other specified intracranial injuries**
  6ᵗʰ **S06.81** **Injury of** right **internal carotid artery, intracranial portion, not elsewhere classified**
    7ᵗʰ **S06.810** **Injury of right internal carotid artery, intracranial portion, not elsewhere classified** without loss of consciousness POA꜒ HCC
    7ᵗʰ **S06.811** **Injury of right internal carotid artery, intracranial portion, not elsewhere classified** with **loss of consciousness of** 30 minutes or less CC꜒ POA꜒ HAC HCC CC/MCC Exc
    7ᵗʰ **S06.812** **Injury of right internal carotid artery, intracranial portion, not elsewhere classified with loss of consciousness of** 31 minutes to 59 minutes CC꜒ POA꜒ HAC HCC CC/MCC Exc
    7ᵗʰ **S06.813** **Injury of right internal carotid artery, intracranial portion, not elsewhere classified with loss of consciousness of** 1 hour to 5 hours 59 minutes CC꜒ POA꜒ HAC HCC CC/MCC Exc
    7ᵗʰ **S06.814** **Injury of right internal carotid artery, intracranial portion, not elsewhere classified with loss of consciousness of** 6 hours to 24 hours CC꜒ POA꜒ HAC HCC CC/MCC Exc
    7ᵗʰ **S06.815** **Injury of right internal carotid artery, intracranial portion, not elsewhere classified with loss of consciousness** greater than 24 hours with return to pre-existing conscious level CC꜒ POA꜒ HAC HCC CC/MCC Exc
    7ᵗʰ **S06.816** **Injury of right internal carotid artery, intracranial portion, not elsewhere classified with loss of consciousness** greater than 24 hours without return to pre-existing conscious level with patient surviving POA꜒ HAC HCC MCC꜒ CC/MCC Exc
    7ᵗʰ **S06.817** **Injury of right internal carotid artery, intracranial portion, not elsewhere classified with loss of consciousness of** any duration with death due to brain injury prior to regaining consciousness HAC MCC꜒ CC/MCC Exc
    7ᵗʰ **S06.818** **Injury of right internal carotid artery, intracranial portion, not elsewhere classified with loss of consciousness of** any duration with death due to other cause prior to regaining consciousness HAC MCC꜒ CC/MCC Exc
    7ᵗʰ **S06.819** **Injury of right internal carotid artery, intracranial portion, not elsewhere classified with loss of consciousness of unspecified duration** CC꜒ POA꜒ HAC HCC CC/MCC Exc

  Injury of right internal carotid artery, intracranial portion, not elsewhere classified NOS

  6ᵗʰ **S06.82** **Injury of** left **internal carotid artery, intracranial portion, not elsewhere classified**
    7ᵗʰ **S06.820** **Injury of left internal carotid artery, intracranial portion, not elsewhere classified** without loss of consciousness POA꜒ HCC
    7ᵗʰ **S06.821** **Injury of left internal carotid artery, intracranial portion, not elsewhere classified with loss of consciousness of** 30 minutes or less CC꜒ POA꜒ HAC HCC CC/MCC Exc
    7ᵗʰ **S06.822** **Injury of left internal carotid artery, intracranial portion, not elsewhere classified with loss of consciousness of** 31 minutes to 59 minutes CC꜒ POA꜒ HAC HCC CC/MCC Exc
    7ᵗʰ **S06.823** **Injury of left internal carotid artery, intracranial portion, not elsewhere classified with loss of consciousness of** 1 hour to 5 hours 59 minutes CC꜒ POA꜒ HAC HCC CC/MCC Exc
    7ᵗʰ **S06.824** **Injury of left internal carotid artery, intracranial portion, not elsewhere classified with loss of consciousness of** 6 hours to 24 hours CC꜒ POA꜒ HAC HCC CC/MCC Exc
    7ᵗʰ **S06.825** **Injury of left internal carotid artery, intracranial portion, not elsewhere classified with loss of consciousness** greater than 24 hours with return to pre-existing conscious level CC꜒ POA꜒ HAC HCC CC/MCC Exc
    7ᵗʰ **S06.826** **Injury of left internal carotid artery, intracranial portion, not elsewhere classified with loss of consciousness** greater than 24 hours without return to pre-existing conscious level with patient surviving POA꜒ HAC HCC MCC꜒ CC/MCC Exc
    7ᵗʰ **S06.827** **Injury of left internal carotid artery, intracranial portion, not elsewhere classified with loss of consciousness of** any duration with death due to brain injury prior to regaining consciousness HAC MCC꜒ CC/MCC Exc
    7ᵗʰ **S06.828** **Injury of left internal carotid artery, intracranial portion, not elsewhere classified with loss of consciousness of** any duration with death due to other cause prior to regaining consciousness HAC MCC꜒ CC/MCC Exc
    7ᵗʰ **S06.829** **Injury of left internal carotid artery, intracranial portion, not elsewhere classified with loss of consciousness of unspecified duration** CC꜒ POA꜒ HAC HCC CC/MCC Exc

    Injury of left internal carotid artery, intracranial portion, not elsewhere classified NOS

  6ᵗʰ **S06.89** **Other** specified intracranial injury
    EXCLUDES1 concussion (S06.0X-)
    7ᵗʰ **S06.890** **Other specified intracranial injury** without loss of consciousness POA꜒ HCC
    7ᵗʰ **S06.891** **Other specified intracranial injury with loss of consciousness of 30 minutes or less** CC꜒ POA꜒ HAC HCC CC/MCC Exc
    7ᵗʰ **S06.892** **Other specified intracranial injury with loss of consciousness of 31 minutes to 59 minutes** CC꜒ POA꜒ HAC HCC CC/MCC Exc
    7ᵗʰ **S06.893** **Other specified intracranial injury with loss of consciousness of 1 hour to 5 hours 59 minutes** CC꜒ POA꜒ HAC HCC CC/MCC Exc
    7ᵗʰ **S06.894** **Other specified intracranial injury with loss of consciousness of 6 hours to 24 hours** CC꜒ POA꜒ HAC HCC CC/MCC Exc

---

POADisch Unacceptable principal diagnosis symbol per Medicare code edits   POA꜒ Code exempt from diagnosis present on admission requirement
❓ Questionable admission   CC Complication or comorbidity   MCC Major complication or comorbidity   CC/MCC Exc CC/MCC exclusion
HCC HCC diagnosis code   RxHCC RxHCC diagnosis code   MACRA code   **DEFINITION** Describes condition/terminology
TIP Coding guidance   👁 Official Guideline Reference   Z1 Z code as first-listed diagnosis

[7th] S06.895 Other specified intracranial injury with loss of consciousness greater than 24 hours with return to pre-existing conscious level [CC] [POA] [HAC] [HCC] [CC/MCC Exc]

[7th] S06.896 Other specified intracranial injury with loss of consciousness greater than 24 hours without return to pre-existing conscious level with patient surviving [POA] [HAC] [HCC] [MCC] [CC/MCC Exc]

[7th] S06.897 Other specified intracranial injury with loss of consciousness of any duration with death due to brain injury prior to regaining consciousness [HAC] [MCC] [CC/MCC Exc]

[7th] S06.898 Other specified intracranial injury with loss of consciousness of any duration with death due to other cause prior to regaining consciousness [HAC] [MCC] [CC/MCC Exc]

[7th] S06.899 Other specified intracranial injury with loss of consciousness of unspecified duration [CC] [POA] [HAC] [HCC] [CC/MCC Exc]

[5th] S06.9 Unspecified intracranial injury

Brain injury NOS

Head injury NOS with loss of consciousness

Traumatic brain injury NOS

[EXCLUDES1] *conditions classifiable to S06.0- to S06.8-code to specified intracranial injury*

head injury NOS (S09.90)

[6th] S06.9X Unspecified intracranial injury

[7th] S06.9X0 Unspecified intracranial injury without loss of consciousness [POA] [HCC]

[7th] S06.9X1 Unspecified intracranial injury with loss of consciousness of 30 minutes or less [CC] [POA] [HAC] [HCC] [CC/MCC Exc]

[7th] S06.9X2 Unspecified intracranial injury with loss of consciousness of 31 minutes to 59 minutes [CC] [POA] [HAC] [HCC] [CC/MCC Exc]

[7th] S06.9X3 Unspecified intracranial injury with loss of consciousness of 1 hour to 5 hours 59 minutes [CC] [POA] [HAC] [HCC] [CC/MCC Exc]

[7th] S06.9X4 Unspecified intracranial injury with loss of consciousness of 6 hours to 24 hours [CC] [POA] [HAC] [HCC] [CC/MCC Exc]

[7th] S06.9X5 Unspecified intracranial injury with loss of consciousness greater than 24 hours with return to pre-existing conscious level [CC] [POA] [HAC] [HCC] [CC/MCC Exc]

[7th] S06.9X6 Unspecified intracranial injury with loss of consciousness greater than 24 hours without return to pre-existing conscious level with patient surviving [POA] [HAC] [HCC] [MCC] [CC/MCC Exc]

[7th] S06.9X7 Unspecified intracranial injury with loss of consciousness of any duration with death due to brain injury prior to regaining consciousness [HAC] [MCC] [CC/MCC Exc]

[7th] S06.9X8 Unspecified intracranial injury with loss of consciousness of any duration with death due to other cause prior to regaining consciousness [HAC] [MCC] [CC/MCC Exc]

[7th] S06.9X9 Unspecified intracranial injury with loss of consciousness of unspecified duration [CC] [POA] [HAC] [HCC] [CC/MCC Exc]

[4th] S07 Crushing injury of head

Use additional code for all associated injuries, such as:

intracranial injuries (S06.-)

skull fractures (S02.-)

The appropriate 7th character is to be added to each code from category S07

A = initial encounter

D = subsequent encounter

S = sequela

[7th] S07.0 Crushing injury of face [CC] [POA] [HAC] [CC/MCC Exc]

[7th] S07.1 Crushing injury of skull [CC] [POA] [HAC] [CC/MCC Exc]

[7th] S07.8 Crushing injury of other parts of head [CC] [POA] [HAC] [CC/MCC Exc]

[7th] S07.9 Crushing injury of head, part unspecified [CC] [POA] [HAC] [CC/MCC Exc]

[4th] S08 Avulsion and traumatic amputation of part of head

An amputation not identified as partial or complete should be coded to complete

The appropriate 7th character is to be added to each code from category S08

A = initial encounter

D = subsequent encounter

S = sequela

[7th] S08.0 Avulsion of scalp [POA]

[5th] S08.1 Traumatic amputation of ear

[6th] S08.11 Complete traumatic amputation of ear

[7th] S08.111 Complete traumatic amputation of right ear [POA]

[7th] S08.112 Complete traumatic amputation of left ear [POA]

[7th] S08.119 Complete traumatic amputation of unspecified ear [POA]

[6th] S08.12 Partial traumatic amputation of ear

[7th] S08.121 Partial traumatic amputation of right ear [POA]

[7th] S08.122 Partial traumatic amputation of left ear [POA]

[7th] S08.129 Partial traumatic amputation of unspecified ear [POA]

[5th] S08.8 Traumatic amputation of other parts of head

[6th] S08.81 Traumatic amputation of nose

[7th] S08.811 Complete traumatic amputation of nose [POA]

[7th] S08.812 Partial traumatic amputation of nose [POA]

[7th] S08.89 Traumatic amputation of other parts of head [POA]

[4th] S09 Other and unspecified injuries of head

The appropriate 7th character is to be added to each code from category S09

A = initial encounter

D = subsequent encounter

S = sequela

[7th] S09.0 Injury of blood vessels of head, not elsewhere classified [CC] [POA] [CC/MCC Exc]

[EXCLUDES1] *injury of cerebral blood vessels (S06.-)*

injury of precerebral blood vessels (S15.-)

[5th] S09.1 Injury of muscle and tendon of head

Code also any associated open wound (S01.-)

[EXCLUDES2] *sprain to joints and ligament of head (S03.9)*

[7th] S09.10 Unspecified injury of muscle and tendon of head [POA]

Injury of muscle and tendon of head NOS

[7th] S09.11 Strain of muscle and tendon of head [POA]

[7th] S09.12 Laceration of muscle and tendon of head [POA]

[7th] S09.19 Other specified injury of muscle and tendon of head [POA]

[5th] S09.2 Traumatic rupture of ear drum

[EXCLUDES1] *traumatic rupture of ear drum due to blast injury (S09.31-)*

[7th] S09.20 Traumatic rupture of unspecified ear drum [CC] [POA] [CC/MCC Exc]

[7th] S09.21 Traumatic rupture of right ear drum [CC] [POA] [CC/MCC Exc]

[7th] S09.22 Traumatic rupture of left ear drum [CC] [POA] [CC/MCC Exc]

[5th] S09.3 Other specified and unspecified injury of middle and inner ear

[EXCLUDES1] *injury to ear NOS (S09.91-)*

[EXCLUDES2] *injury to external ear (S00.4-, S01.3-, S08.1-)*

[6th] S09.30 Unspecified injury of middle and inner ear

[7th] S09.301 Unspecified injury of right middle and inner ear [CC] [POA] [CC/MCC Exc]

[7th] S09.302 Unspecified injury of left middle and inner ear [CC] [POA] [CC/MCC Exc]

[7th] S09.309 Unspecified injury of unspecified middle and inner ear [CC] [POA] [CC/MCC Exc]

Unspecified Code   Other Specified Code   Manifestation Code   [N] Newborn   [P] Pediatric   [M] Maternity   [A] Adult   ♂ Male   ♀ Female
● New Code   ▲ Revised Code Title   ►◄ Revised Text   [NOTES]   [INCLUDES]   [EXCLUDES1] Not coded here   [EXCLUDES2] Not included here
[4th] 4th character required   [5th] 5th character required   [6th] 6th character required   [7th] 7th character required   [7th] Extension 'X' Alert
[HAC] Hospital-acquired condition (HAC) alert   AHA AHA Coding Clinic©   ☞ Code first alert

 When symbols appear on a code that requires a 7th character extension, refer to Appendix B to identify applicable 7th character codes.

S09.31 **Primary blast** injury of ear
Blast injury of ear NOS
- S09.311 **Primary blast injury of right ear**
- S09.312 **Primary blast injury of left ear**
- S09.313 **Primary blast injury of ear, bilateral**
- S09.319 **Primary blast injury of unspecified ear**

S09.39 Other specified injury of middle and inner ear
Secondary blast injury to ear
- S09.391 **Other specified injury of right middle and inner ear**
- S09.392 **Other specified injury of left middle and inner ear**
- S09.399 **Other specified injury of unspecified middle and inner ear**

S09.8 **Other specified injuries of head**

S09.9 Unspecified injury of face and head
- S09.90 **Unspecified injury of head**
  Head injury NOS
  EXCLUDES1 brain injury NOS (S06.9-)
  head injury NOS with loss of consciousness (S06.9-)
  intracranial injury NOS (S06.9-)
- S09.91 **Unspecified injury of ear**
  Injury of ear NOS
- S09.92 **Unspecified injury of nose**
  Injury of nose NOS
- S09.93 **Unspecified injury of face**
  Injury of face NOS

Injuries to the neck (S10-S19)

INCLUDES injuries of nape
injuries of supraclavicular region
injuries of throat
EXCLUDES2 burns and corrosions (T20-T32)
effects of foreign body in esophagus (T18.1)
effects of foreign body in larynx (T17.3)
effects of foreign body in pharynx (T17.2)
effects of foreign body in trachea (T17.4)
frostbite (T33-T34)
insect bite or sting, venomous (T63.4)

S10 **Superficial injury of neck**
The appropriate 7th character is to be added to each code from category S10
A = initial encounter
D = subsequent encounter
S = sequela

S10.0 **Contusion of** throat
Contusion of cervical esophagus
Contusion of larynx
Contusion of pharynx
Contusion of trachea

S10.1 **Other and unspecified superficial injuries of throat**
- S10.10 **Unspecified superficial injuries of throat**
- S10.11 Abrasion of throat
- S10.12 Blister (nonthermal) of throat
- S10.14 External constriction of part of throat
- S10.15 Superficial foreign body of throat
  Splinter in the throat
- S10.16 Insect bite (nonvenomous) of throat
- S10.17 Other superficial bite of throat
  EXCLUDES1 open bite of throat (S11.85)

S10.8 **Superficial injury of other specified parts of neck**
- S10.80 Unspecified superficial injury of other specified part of neck
- S10.81 Abrasion of other specified part of neck
- S10.82 Blister (nonthermal) of other specified part of neck
- S10.83 Contusion of other specified part of neck
- S10.84 External constriction of other specified part of neck
- S10.85 Superficial foreign body of other specified part of neck
  Splinter in other specified part of neck
- S10.86 Insect bite of other specified part of neck
- S10.87 Other superficial bite of other specified part of neck
  EXCLUDES1 open bite of other specified parts of neck (S11.85)

S10.9 **Superficial injury of** unspecified part of neck
- S10.90 **Unspecified superficial injury of unspecified part of neck**
- S10.91 Abrasion of unspecified part of neck
- S10.92 Blister (nonthermal) of unspecified part of neck
- S10.93 Contusion of unspecified part of neck
- S10.94 External constriction of unspecified part of neck
- S10.95 Superficial foreign body of unspecified part of neck
- S10.96 Insect bite of unspecified part of neck
- S10.97 Other superficial bite of unspecified part of neck

S11 **Open wound of** neck
Code also any associated:
spinal cord injury (S14.0, S14.1-)
wound infection
EXCLUDES2 open fracture of vertebra (S12.- with 7th character B)
The appropriate 7th character is to be added to each code from category S11
A = initial encounter
D = subsequent encounter
S = sequela

S11.0 **Open wound of** larynx and trachea
- S11.01 **Open wound of larynx**
  EXCLUDES2 open wound of vocal cord (S11.03)
  - S11.011 Laceration without foreign body of larynx
  - S11.012 Laceration with foreign body of larynx
  - S11.013 Puncture wound without foreign body of larynx
  - S11.014 Puncture wound with foreign body of larynx
  - S11.015 Open bite of larynx
    Bite of larynx NOS
  - S11.019 Unspecified open wound of larynx
- S11.02 **Open wound of** trachea
  Open wound of cervical trachea
  Open wound of trachea NOS
  EXCLUDES2 open wound of thoracic trachea (S27.5-)
  - S11.021 Laceration without foreign body of trachea
  - S11.022 Laceration with foreign body of trachea
  - S11.023 Puncture wound without foreign body of trachea
  - S11.024 Puncture wound with foreign body of trachea
  - S11.025 Open bite of trachea
    Bite of trachea NOS
  - S11.029 Unspecified open wound of trachea
- S11.03 **Open wound of** vocal cord
  - S11.031 Laceration without foreign body of vocal cord
  - S11.032 Laceration with foreign body of vocal cord

Unacceptable principal diagnosis symbol per Medicare code edits · Code exempt from diagnosis present on admission requirement · Questionable admission · Complication or comorbidity · Major complication or comorbidity · CC/MCC exclusion · HCC diagnosis code · RxHCC diagnosis code · MACRA code · DEFINITION Describes condition/terminology · TIP Coding guidance · Official Guideline Reference · Z code as first-listed diagnosis

980   When symbols appear on a code that requires a 7th character extension, refer to Appendix B to identify applicable 7th character codes.   2020 ICD-10-CM

[7th] S11.033 Puncture wound without foreign body of vocal cord [POA] [MCC] [CC/MCC Exc]
[7th] S11.034 Puncture wound with foreign body of vocal cord [POA] [MCC] [CC/MCC Exc]
[7th] S11.035 Open bite of vocal cord [POA] [MCC] [CC/MCC Exc]
Bite of vocal cord NOS
[7th] S11.039 Unspecified open wound of vocal cord [POA] [MCC] [CC/MCC Exc]

[5th] S11.1 Open wound of thyroid gland
[7th] S11.10 Unspecified open wound of thyroid gland [CC] [POA] [CC/MCC Exc]
[7th] S11.11 Laceration without foreign body of thyroid gland [CC] [POA] [CC/MCC Exc]
[7th] S11.12 Laceration with foreign body of thyroid gland [CC] [POA] [CC/MCC Exc]
[7th] S11.13 Puncture wound without foreign body of thyroid gland [CC] [POA] [CC/MCC Exc]
[7th] S11.14 Puncture wound with foreign body of thyroid gland [CC] [POA] [CC/MCC Exc]
[7th] S11.15 Open bite of thyroid gland [CC] [POA] [CC/MCC Exc]
Bite of thyroid gland NOS

[5th] S11.2 Open wound of pharynx and cervical esophagus
[EXCLUDES1] *open wound of esophagus NOS (S27.8-)*
[7th] S11.20 Unspecified open wound of pharynx and cervical esophagus [CC] [POA] [CC/MCC Exc]
[7th] S11.21 Laceration without foreign body of pharynx and cervical esophagus [CC] [POA] [CC/MCC Exc]
[7th] S11.22 Laceration with foreign body of pharynx and cervical esophagus [CC] [POA] [CC/MCC Exc]
[7th] S11.23 Puncture wound without foreign body of pharynx and cervical esophagus [CC] [POA] [CC/MCC Exc]
[7th] S11.24 Puncture wound with foreign body of pharynx and cervical esophagus [CC] [POA] [CC/MCC Exc]
[7th] S11.25 Open bite of pharynx and cervical esophagus [CC] [POA] [CC/MCC Exc]
Bite of pharynx and cervical esophagus NOS

[5th] S11.8 Open wound of other specified parts of neck
[7th] S11.80 Unspecified open wound of other specified part of neck [POA]
[7th] S11.81 Laceration without foreign body of other specified part of neck [POA]
[7th] S11.82 Laceration with foreign body of other specified part of neck [POA]
[7th] S11.83 Puncture wound without foreign body of other specified part of neck [POA]
[7th] S11.84 Puncture wound with foreign body of other specified part of neck [POA]
[7th] S11.85 Open bite of other specified part of neck [POA]
Bite of other specified part of neck NOS
[EXCLUDES1] *superficial bite of other specified part of neck (S10.87)*
[7th] S11.89 Other open wound of other specified part of neck [POA]

[5th] S11.9 Open wound of unspecified part of neck
[7th] S11.90 Unspecified open wound of unspecified part of neck [POA]
[7th] S11.91 Laceration without foreign body of unspecified part of neck [POA]
[7th] S11.92 Laceration with foreign body of unspecified part of neck [POA]
[7th] S11.93 Puncture wound without foreign body of unspecified part of neck [POA]
[7th] S11.94 Puncture wound with foreign body of unspecified part of neck [POA]
[7th] S11.95 Open bite of unspecified part of neck [POA]
Bite of neck NOS
[EXCLUDES1] *superficial bite of neck (S10.97)*

[4th] S12 Fracture of cervical vertebra and other parts of neck
See Official Guidelines "Coding of Traumatic Fractures" I.C.19.c
[NOTES] A fracture not indicated as displaced or nondisplaced should be coded to displaced.
A fracture not indicated as open or closed should be coded to closed.
[INCLUDES] *fracture of cervical neural arch*
fracture of cervical spine
fracture of cervical spinous process
fracture of cervical transverse process
fracture of cervical vertebral arch
fracture of neck

☞ Code first any associated cervical spinal cord injury (S14.0, S14.1-)

The appropriate 7th character is to be added to all codes from subcategories S12.0-S12.6
A = initial encounter for closed fracture
B = initial encounter for open fracture
D = subsequent encounter for fracture with routine healing
G = subsequent encounter for fracture with delayed healing
K = subsequent encounter for fracture with nonunion
S = sequela

[5th] S12.0 Fracture of first cervical vertebra
Atlas
[6th] S12.00 Unspecified fracture of first cervical vertebra
[7th] S12.000 Unspecified displaced fracture of first cervical vertebra [CC] [POA] [HAC] [HCC] [MCC] [CC/MCC Exc]
[7th] S12.001 Unspecified nondisplaced fracture of first cervical vertebra [CC] [POA] [HAC] [HCC] [MCC] [CC/MCC Exc]
[7th] S12.01 Stable burst fracture of first cervical vertebra [CC] [POA] [HAC] [HCC] [MCC] [CC/MCC Exc]
[7th] S12.02 Unstable burst fracture of first cervical vertebra [CC] [POA] [HAC] [HCC] [MCC] [CC/MCC Exc]
[6th] S12.03 Posterior arch fracture of first cervical vertebra
[7th] S12.030 Displaced posterior arch fracture of first cervical vertebra [CC] [POA] [HAC] [HCC] [MCC] [CC/MCC Exc]
[7th] S12.031 Nondisplaced posterior arch fracture of first cervical vertebra [CC] [POA] [HAC] [HCC] [MCC] [CC/MCC Exc]
[6th] S12.04 Lateral mass fracture of first cervical vertebra
[7th] S12.040 Displaced lateral mass fracture of first cervical vertebra [CC] [POA] [HAC] [HCC] [MCC] [CC/MCC Exc]
[7th] S12.041 Nondisplaced lateral mass fracture of first cervical vertebra [CC] [POA] [HAC] [HCC] [MCC] [CC/MCC Exc]
[6th] S12.09 Other fracture of first cervical vertebra
[7th] S12.090 Other displaced fracture of first cervical vertebra [CC] [POA] [HAC] [HCC] [MCC] [CC/MCC Exc]
[7th] S12.091 Other nondisplaced fracture of first cervical vertebra [CC] [POA] [HAC] [HCC] [MCC] [CC/MCC Exc]

[5th] S12.1 Fracture of second cervical vertebra
Axis
[6th] S12.10 Unspecified fracture of second cervical vertebra
[7th] S12.100 Unspecified displaced fracture of second cervical vertebra [CC] [POA] [HAC] [HCC] [MCC] [CC/MCC Exc]
[7th] S12.101 Unspecified nondisplaced fracture of second cervical vertebra [CC] [POA] [HAC] [HCC] [MCC] [CC/MCC Exc]
[6th] S12.11 Type II dens fracture
[7th] S12.110 Anterior displaced Type II dens fracture [CC] [POA] [HAC] [HCC] [MCC] [CC/MCC Exc]
[7th] S12.111 Posterior displaced Type II dens fracture [CC] [POA] [HAC] [HCC] [MCC] [CC/MCC Exc]
[7th] S12.112 Nondisplaced Type II dens fracture [CC] [POA] [HAC] [HCC] [MCC] [CC/MCC Exc]
[6th] S12.12 Other dens fracture
[7th] S12.120 Other displaced dens fracture [CC] [POA] [HAC] [HCC] [MCC] [CC/MCC Exc]
[7th] S12.121 Other nondisplaced dens fracture [CC] [POA] [HAC] [HCC] [MCC] [CC/MCC Exc]
[6th] S12.13 Unspecified traumatic spondylolisthesis of second cervical vertebra
[7th] S12.130 Unspecified traumatic displaced spondylolisthesis of second cervical vertebra [CC] [POA] [HAC] [HCC] [MCC] [CC/MCC Exc]
[7th] S12.131 Unspecified traumatic nondisplaced spondylolisthesis of second cervical vertebra [CC] [POA] [HAC] [HCC] [MCC] [CC/MCC Exc]
[7th] S12.14 Type III traumatic spondylolisthesis of second cervical vertebra [CC] [POA] [HAC] [HCC] [MCC] [CC/MCC Exc]

Unspecified Code | Other Specified Code | Manifestation Code | [N] Newborn | [P] Pediatric | [M] Maternity | [A] Adult | ♂ Male | ♀ Female
● New Code ▲ Revised Code Title ►◄ Revised Text [NOTES] [INCLUDES] [EXCLUDES1] Not coded here [EXCLUDES2] Not included here
[4th] 4th character required [5th] 5th character required [6th] 6th character required [7th] 7th character required [x] Extension 'X' Alert
[HAC] Hospital-acquired condition (HAC) alert AHA AHA Coding Clinic© ☞ Code first alert

6ᵗʰ **S12.15** Other traumatic spondylolisthesis of second cervical vertebra
- 7ᵗʰ **S12.150** **Other traumatic** displaced **spondylolisthesis of second cervical vertebra**
- 7ᵗʰ **S12.151** **Other traumatic** nondisplaced **spondylolisthesis of second cervical vertebra** cc poa HAC HCC MCC CC/MCC Exc

6ᵗʰ **S12.19** Other fracture of second cervical vertebra
- 7ᵗʰ **S12.190** **Other** displaced **fracture of second cervical vertebra** cc poa HAC HCC MCC CC/MCC Exc
- 7ᵗʰ **S12.191** **Other** nondisplaced **fracture of second cervical vertebra** cc poa HAC HCC MCC CC/MCC Exc

5ᵗʰ **S12.2** Fracture of third cervical vertebra
- 6ᵗʰ **S12.20** Unspecified fracture of third cervical vertebra
  - 7ᵗʰ **S12.200** **Unspecified** displaced **fracture of third cervical vertebra** cc poa HAC HCC MCC CC/MCC Exc
  - 7ᵗʰ **S12.201** **Unspecified** nondisplaced **fracture of third cervical vertebra** cc poa HAC HCC MCC CC/MCC Exc
- 6ᵗʰ **S12.23** Unspecified traumatic spondylolisthesis of third cervical vertebra
  - 7ᵗʰ **S12.230** **Unspecified traumatic** displaced **spondylolisthesis of third cervical vertebra** cc poa HAC HCC MCC CC/MCC Exc
  - 7ᵗʰ **S12.231** **Unspecified traumatic** nondisplaced **spondylolisthesis of third cervical vertebra** cc poa HAC HCC MCC CC/MCC Exc
- 7ᵗʰ **S12.24** Type III traumatic spondylolisthesis of third cervical vertebra cc poa HAC HCC MCC CC/MCC Exc
- 6ᵗʰ **S12.25** Other traumatic spondylolisthesis of third cervical vertebra
  - 7ᵗʰ **S12.250** **Other traumatic** displaced **spondylolisthesis of third cervical vertebra** cc poa HAC HCC MCC CC/MCC Exc
  - 7ᵗʰ **S12.251** **Other traumatic** nondisplaced **spondylolisthesis of third cervical vertebra** cc poa HAC HCC MCC CC/MCC Exc
- 6ᵗʰ **S12.29** Other fracture of third cervical vertebra
  - 7ᵗʰ **S12.290** **Other** displaced **fracture of third cervical vertebra** cc poa HAC HCC MCC CC/MCC Exc
  - 7ᵗʰ **S12.291** **Other** nondisplaced **fracture of third cervical vertebra** cc poa HAC HCC MCC CC/MCC Exc

5ᵗʰ **S12.3** Fracture of fourth cervical vertebra
- 6ᵗʰ **S12.30** Unspecified fracture of fourth cervical vertebra
  - 7ᵗʰ **S12.300** **Unspecified** displaced **fracture of fourth cervical vertebra** cc poa HAC HCC MCC CC/MCC Exc
  - 7ᵗʰ **S12.301** **Unspecified** nondisplaced **fracture of fourth cervical vertebra** cc poa HAC HCC MCC CC/MCC Exc
- 6ᵗʰ **S12.33** Unspecified traumatic spondylolisthesis of fourth cervical vertebra
  - 7ᵗʰ **S12.330** **Unspecified traumatic** displaced **spondylolisthesis of fourth cervical vertebra** cc poa HAC HCC MCC CC/MCC Exc
  - 7ᵗʰ **S12.331** **Unspecified traumatic** nondisplaced **spondylolisthesis of fourth cervical vertebra** cc poa HAC HCC MCC CC/MCC Exc
- 7ᵗʰ **S12.34** Type III traumatic spondylolisthesis of fourth cervical vertebra cc poa HAC HCC MCC CC/MCC Exc
- 6ᵗʰ **S12.35** Other traumatic spondylolisthesis of fourth cervical vertebra
  - 7ᵗʰ **S12.350** **Other traumatic** displaced **spondylolisthesis of fourth cervical vertebra** cc poa HAC HCC MCC CC/MCC Exc
  - 7ᵗʰ **S12.351** **Other traumatic** nondisplaced **spondylolisthesis of fourth cervical vertebra** cc poa HAC HCC MCC CC/MCC Exc
- 6ᵗʰ **S12.39** Other fracture of fourth cervical vertebra
  - 7ᵗʰ **S12.390** **Other** displaced **fracture of fourth cervical vertebra** cc poa HAC HCC MCC CC/MCC Exc
  - 7ᵗʰ **S12.391** **Other** nondisplaced **fracture of fourth cervical vertebra** cc poa HAC HCC MCC CC/MCC Exc

5ᵗʰ **S12.4** Fracture of fifth cervical vertebra
- 6ᵗʰ **S12.40** Unspecified fracture of fifth cervical vertebra
  - 7ᵗʰ **S12.400** **Unspecified** displaced **fracture of fifth cervical vertebra** cc poa HAC HCC MCC CC/MCC Exc
  - 7ᵗʰ **S12.401** **Unspecified** nondisplaced **fracture of fifth cervical vertebra** cc poa HAC HCC MCC CC/MCC Exc
- 6ᵗʰ **S12.43** Unspecified traumatic spondylolisthesis of fifth cervical vertebra
  - 7ᵗʰ **S12.430** **Unspecified traumatic** displaced **spondylolisthesis of fifth cervical vertebra** cc poa HAC HCC MCC CC/MCC Exc
  - 7ᵗʰ **S12.431** **Unspecified traumatic** nondisplaced **spondylolisthesis of fifth cervical vertebra** cc poa HAC HCC MCC CC/MCC Exc
- 7ᵗʰ **S12.44** Type III traumatic spondylolisthesis of fifth cervical vertebra
- 6ᵗʰ **S12.45** Other traumatic spondylolisthesis of fifth cervical vertebra
  - 7ᵗʰ **S12.450** **Other traumatic** displaced **spondylolisthesis of fifth cervical vertebra** cc poa HAC HCC MCC CC/MCC Exc
  - 7ᵗʰ **S12.451** **Other traumatic** nondisplaced **spondylolisthesis of fifth cervical vertebra** cc poa HAC HCC MCC CC/MCC Exc
- 6ᵗʰ **S12.49** Other fracture of fifth cervical vertebra
  - 7ᵗʰ **S12.490** **Other** displaced **fracture of fifth cervical vertebra** cc poa HAC HCC MCC CC/MCC Exc
  - 7ᵗʰ **S12.491** **Other** nondisplaced **fracture of fifth cervical vertebra** cc poa HAC HCC MCC CC/MCC Exc

5ᵗʰ **S12.5** Fracture of sixth cervical vertebra
- 6ᵗʰ **S12.50** Unspecified fracture of sixth cervical vertebra
  - 7ᵗʰ **S12.500** **Unspecified** displaced **fracture of sixth cervical vertebra** cc poa HAC HCC MCC CC/MCC Exc
  - 7ᵗʰ **S12.501** **Unspecified** nondisplaced **fracture of sixth cervical vertebra** cc poa HAC HCC MCC CC/MCC Exc
- 6ᵗʰ **S12.53** Unspecified traumatic spondylolisthesis of sixth cervical vertebra
  - 7ᵗʰ **S12.530** **Unspecified traumatic** displaced **spondylolisthesis of sixth cervical vertebra** cc poa HAC HCC MCC CC/MCC Exc
  - 7ᵗʰ **S12.531** **Unspecified traumatic** nondisplaced **spondylolisthesis of sixth cervical vertebra** cc poa HAC HCC MCC CC/MCC Exc
- 7ᵗʰ **S12.54** Type III traumatic spondylolisthesis of sixth cervical vertebra cc poa HAC HCC MCC CC/MCC Exc
- 6ᵗʰ **S12.55** Other traumatic spondylolisthesis of sixth cervical vertebra
  - 7ᵗʰ **S12.550** **Other traumatic** displaced **spondylolisthesis of sixth cervical vertebra** cc poa HAC HCC MCC CC/MCC Exc
  - 7ᵗʰ **S12.551** **Other traumatic** nondisplaced **spondylolisthesis of sixth cervical vertebra** cc poa HAC HCC MCC CC/MCC Exc
- 6ᵗʰ **S12.59** Other fracture of sixth cervical vertebra
  - 7ᵗʰ **S12.590** **Other** displaced **fracture of sixth cervical vertebra** cc poa HAC HCC MCC CC/MCC Exc
  - 7ᵗʰ **S12.591** **Other** nondisplaced **fracture of sixth cervical vertebra** cc poa HAC HCC MCC CC/MCC Exc

5ᵗʰ **S12.6** Fracture of seventh cervical vertebra
- 6ᵗʰ **S12.60** Unspecified fracture of seventh cervical vertebra
  - 7ᵗʰ **S12.600** **Unspecified** displaced **fracture of seventh cervical vertebra** cc poa HAC HCC MCC CC/MCC Exc
  - 7ᵗʰ **S12.601** **Unspecified** nondisplaced **fracture of seventh cervical vertebra** cc poa HAC HCC MCC CC/MCC Exc
- 6ᵗʰ **S12.63** Unspecified traumatic spondylolisthesis of seventh cervical vertebra
  - 7ᵗʰ **S12.630** **Unspecified traumatic** displaced **spondylolisthesis of seventh cervical vertebra** cc poa HAC HCC MCC CC/MCC Exc

---

poa🚫 Unacceptable principal diagnosis symbol per Medicare code edits   poa Code exempt from diagnosis present on admission requirement
? Questionable admission   cc Complication or comorbidity   MCC Major complication or comorbidity   CC/MCC Exc CC/MCC exclusion
HCC HCC diagnosis code   RxHCC RxHCC diagnosis code   MACRA code   **DEFINITION** Describes condition/terminology
TIP Coding guidance   👁 Official Guideline Reference   Z1 Z code as first-listed diagnosis

[7th] S12.631 **Unspecified traumatic nondisplaced spondylolisthesis of seventh cervical vertebra** [CC] [POA] [HAC] [HCC] [MCC] [CC/MCC Exc]

[7th] S12.64 **Type III traumatic spondylolisthesis of seventh cervical vertebra** [CC] [POA] [HAC] [HCC] [MCC] [CC/MCC Exc]

[6th] S12.65 **Other traumatic spondylolisthesis of seventh cervical vertebra**

[7th] S12.650 **Other traumatic displaced spondylolisthesis of seventh cervical vertebra** [CC] [POA] [HAC] [HCC] [MCC] [CC/MCC Exc]

[7th] S12.651 **Other traumatic nondisplaced spondylolisthesis of seventh cervical vertebra** [CC] [POA] [HAC] [HCC] [MCC] [CC/MCC Exc]

[6th] S12.69 **Other fracture of seventh cervical vertebra**

[7th] S12.690 **Other displaced fracture of seventh cervical vertebra** [CC] [POA] [HAC] [HCC] [MCC] [CC/MCC Exc]

[7th] S12.691 **Other nondisplaced fracture of seventh cervical vertebra** [CC] [POA] [HAC] [HCC] [MCC] [CC/MCC Exc]

[7th] S12.8 **Fracture of other parts of neck** [POA] [HAC] [HCC] [MCC] [CC/MCC Exc]

Hyoid bone
Larynx
Thyroid cartilage
Trachea

The appropriate 7th character is to be added to code S12.8
- **A = initial encounter**
- **D = subsequent encounter**
- **S = sequela**

[7th] S12.9 **Fracture of neck, unspecified** [CC] [POA] [HAC] [HCC] [CC/MCC Exc]

Fracture of neck NOS
Fracture of cervical spine NOS
Fracture of cervical vertebra NOS

The appropriate 7th character is to be added to code S12.9
- **A = initial encounter**
- **D = subsequent encounter**
- **S = sequela**

[4th] S13 **Dislocation and sprain of joints and ligaments at neck level**

INCLUDES *avulsion of joint or ligament at neck level*
laceration of cartilage, joint or ligament at neck level
sprain of cartilage, joint or ligament at neck level
traumatic hemarthrosis of joint or ligament at neck level
traumatic rupture of joint or ligament at neck level
traumatic subluxation of joint or ligament at neck level
traumatic tear of joint or ligament at neck level

Code also any associated open wound

EXCLUDES2 *strain of muscle or tendon at neck level (S16.1)*

The appropriate 7th character is to be added to each code from category S13
- **A = initial encounter**
- **D = subsequent encounter**
- **S = sequela**

[7th] S13.0 **Traumatic rupture of cervical intervertebral disc** [CC] [POA] [HAC] [CC/MCC Exc]

EXCLUDES1 *rupture or displacement (nontraumatic) of cervical intervertebral disc NOS (M50.-)*

[5th] S13.1 **Subluxation and dislocation of cervical vertebrae**

Code also any associated:
open wound of neck (S11.-)
spinal cord injury (S14.1-)

EXCLUDES2 *fracture of cervical vertebrae (S12.0-S12.3-)*

[6th] S13.10 **Subluxation and dislocation of unspecified cervical vertebrae**

[7th] S13.100 **Subluxation of unspecified cervical vertebrae** [CC] [POA] [HAC] [CC/MCC Exc]

[7th] S13.101 **Dislocation of unspecified cervical vertebrae** [CC] [POA] [HAC] [CC/MCC Exc]

[6th] S13.11 **Subluxation and dislocation of C0/C1 cervical vertebrae**

Subluxation and dislocation of atlantooccipital joint
Subluxation and dislocation of atloidooccipital joint
Subluxation and dislocation of occipitoatloid joint

[7th] S13.110 **Subluxation of C0/C1 cervical vertebrae** [CC] [POA] [HAC] [CC/MCC Exc]

[7th] S13.111 **Dislocation of C0/C1 cervical vertebrae** [CC] [POA] [HAC] [CC/MCC Exc]

[6th] S13.12 **Subluxation and dislocation of C1/C2 cervical vertebrae**

Subluxation and dislocation of atlantoaxial joint

[7th] S13.120 **Subluxation of C1/C2 cervical vertebrae** [CC] [POA] [HAC] [CC/MCC Exc]

[7th] S13.121 **Dislocation of C1/C2 cervical vertebrae** [CC] [POA] [HAC] [CC/MCC Exc]

[6th] S13.13 **Subluxation and dislocation of C2/C3 cervical vertebrae**

[7th] S13.130 **Subluxation of C2/C3 cervical vertebrae** [CC] [POA] [HAC] [CC/MCC Exc]

[7th] S13.131 **Dislocation of C2/C3 cervical vertebrae** [CC] [POA] [HAC] [CC/MCC Exc]

[6th] S13.14 **Subluxation and dislocation of C3/C4 cervical vertebrae**

[7th] S13.140 **Subluxation of C3/C4 cervical vertebrae** [CC] [POA] [HAC] [CC/MCC Exc]

[7th] S13.141 **Dislocation of C3/C4 cervical vertebrae** [CC] [POA] [HAC] [CC/MCC Exc]

[6th] S13.15 **Subluxation and dislocation of C4/C5 cervical vertebrae**

[7th] S13.150 **Subluxation of C4/C5 cervical vertebrae** [CC] [POA] [HAC] [CC/MCC Exc]

[7th] S13.151 **Dislocation of C4/C5 cervical vertebrae** [CC] [POA] [HAC] [CC/MCC Exc]

[6th] S13.16 **Subluxation and dislocation of C5/C6 cervical vertebrae**

[7th] S13.160 **Subluxation of C5/C6 cervical vertebrae** [CC] [POA] [HAC] [CC/MCC Exc]

[7th] S13.161 **Dislocation of C5/C6 cervical vertebrae** [CC] [POA] [HAC] [CC/MCC Exc]

[6th] S13.17 **Subluxation and dislocation of C6/C7 cervical vertebrae**

[7th] S13.170 **Subluxation of C6/C7 cervical vertebrae** [CC] [POA] [HAC] [CC/MCC Exc]

[7th] S13.171 **Dislocation of C6/C7 cervical vertebrae** [CC] [POA] [HAC] [CC/MCC Exc]

[6th] S13.18 **Subluxation and dislocation of C7/T1 cervical vertebrae**

[7th] S13.180 **Subluxation of C7/T1 cervical vertebrae** [CC] [POA] [HAC] [CC/MCC Exc]

[7th] S13.181 **Dislocation of C7/T1 cervical vertebrae** [CC] [POA] [HAC] [CC/MCC Exc]

[5th] S13.2 **Dislocation of other and unspecified parts of neck**

[7th] S13.20 **Dislocation of unspecified parts of neck** [CC] [POA] [HAC] [CC/MCC Exc]

[7th] S13.29 **Dislocation of other parts of neck** [CC] [POA] [HAC] [CC/MCC Exc]

[7th] S13.4 **Sprain of ligaments of cervical spine** [POA]

Sprain of anterior longitudinal (ligament), cervical
Sprain of atlanto-axial (joints)
Sprain of atlanto-occipital (joints)
Whiplash injury of cervical spine

[7th] S13.5 **Sprain of thyroid region** [POA]

Sprain of cricoarytenoid (joint) (ligament)
Sprain of cricothyroid (joint) (ligament)
Sprain of thyroid cartilage

[7th] S13.8 **Sprain of joints and ligaments of other parts of neck** [POA]

[7th] S13.9 **Sprain of joints and ligaments of unspecified parts of neck** [POA]

[4th] S14 **Injury of nerves and spinal cord at neck level**

NOTES Code to highest level of cervical cord injury.

Code also any associated:
fracture of cervical vertebra (S12.0--S12.6.-)
open wound of neck (S11.-)
transient paralysis (R29.5)

The appropriate 7th character is to be added to each code from category S14
- **A = initial encounter**
- **D = subsequent encounter**
- **S = sequela**

Unspecified Code | Other Specified Code | Manifestation Code | [N] Newborn | [P] Pediatric | [M] Maternity | [A] Adult | ♂ Male | ♀ Female
● New Code ▲ Revised Code Title ►◄ Revised Text **NOTES** *INCLUDES* *EXCLUDES1* Not coded here *EXCLUDES2* Not included here
[4th] 4th character required [5th] 5th character required [6th] 6th character required [7th] 7th character required [7th] Extension 'X' Alert
[HAC] Hospital-acquired condition (HAC) alert **AHA** AHA Coding Clinic© ☞ **Code first alert**

CHAPTER 19: INJURY, POISONING, AND CERTAIN OTHER CONSEQUENCES OF EXTERNAL CAUSES (S00-T88)

S14.0 - S15.001

- S14.0 Concussion and edema of cervical spinal cord
- S14.1 Other and unspecified injuries of cervical spinal cord
  - S14.10 Unspecified injury of cervical spinal cord
    - S14.101 Unspecified injury at C1 level of cervical spinal cord
    - S14.102 Unspecified injury at C2 level of cervical spinal cord
    - S14.103 Unspecified injury at C3 level of cervical spinal cord
    - S14.104 Unspecified injury at C4 level of cervical spinal cord
    - S14.105 Unspecified injury at C5 level of cervical spinal cord
    - S14.106 Unspecified injury at C6 level of cervical spinal cord
    - S14.107 Unspecified injury at C7 level of cervical spinal cord
    - S14.108 Unspecified injury at C8 level of cervical spinal cord
    - S14.109 Unspecified injury at unspecified level of cervical spinal cord
      Injury of cervical spinal cord NOS
  - S14.11 Complete lesion of cervical spinal cord
    - S14.111 Complete lesion at C1 level of cervical spinal cord
    - S14.112 Complete lesion at C2 level of cervical spinal cord
    - S14.113 Complete lesion at C3 level of cervical spinal cord
    - S14.114 Complete lesion at C4 level of cervical spinal cord
    - S14.115 Complete lesion at C5 level of cervical spinal cord
    - S14.116 Complete lesion at C6 level of cervical spinal cord
    - S14.117 Complete lesion at C7 level of cervical spinal cord
    - S14.118 Complete lesion at C8 level of cervical spinal cord
    - S14.119 Complete lesion at unspecified level of cervical spinal cord
  - S14.12 Central cord syndrome of cervical spinal cord
    - S14.121 Central cord syndrome at C1 level of cervical spinal cord
    - S14.122 Central cord syndrome at C2 level of cervical spinal cord
    - S14.123 Central cord syndrome at C3 level of cervical spinal cord
    - S14.124 Central cord syndrome at C4 level of cervical spinal cord
    - S14.125 Central cord syndrome at C5 level of cervical spinal cord
    - S14.126 Central cord syndrome at C6 level of cervical spinal cord
    - S14.127 Central cord syndrome at C7 level of cervical spinal cord
    - S14.128 Central cord syndrome at C8 level of cervical spinal cord
    - S14.129 Central cord syndrome at unspecified level of cervical spinal cord
  - S14.13 Anterior cord syndrome of cervical spinal cord
    - S14.131 Anterior cord syndrome at C1 level of cervical spinal cord
    - S14.132 Anterior cord syndrome at C2 level of cervical spinal cord
    - S14.133 Anterior cord syndrome at C3 level of cervical spinal cord
    - S14.134 Anterior cord syndrome at C4 level of cervical spinal cord
    - S14.135 Anterior cord syndrome at C5 level of cervical spinal cord
    - S14.136 Anterior cord syndrome at C6 level of cervical spinal cord
    - S14.137 Anterior cord syndrome at C7 level of cervical spinal cord
    - S14.138 Anterior cord syndrome at C8 level of cervical spinal cord
    - S14.139 Anterior cord syndrome at unspecified level of cervical spinal cord
  - S14.14 Brown-Séquard syndrome of cervical spinal cord
    - S14.141 Brown-Séquard syndrome at C1 level of cervical spinal cord
    - S14.142 Brown-Séquard syndrome at C2 level of cervical spinal cord
    - S14.143 Brown-Séquard syndrome at C3 level of cervical spinal cord
    - S14.144 Brown-Séquard syndrome at C4 level of cervical spinal cord
    - S14.145 Brown-Séquard syndrome at C5 level of cervical spinal cord
    - S14.146 Brown-Séquard syndrome at C6 level of cervical spinal cord
    - S14.147 Brown-Séquard syndrome at C7 level of cervical spinal cord
    - S14.148 Brown-Séquard syndrome at C8 level of cervical spinal cord
    - S14.149 Brown-Séquard syndrome at unspecified level of cervical spinal cord
  - S14.15 Other incomplete lesions of cervical spinal cord
    Incomplete lesion of cervical spinal cord NOS
    Posterior cord syndrome of cervical spinal cord
    - S14.151 Other incomplete lesion at C1 level of cervical spinal cord
    - S14.152 Other incomplete lesion at C2 level of cervical spinal cord
    - S14.153 Other incomplete lesion at C3 level of cervical spinal cord
    - S14.154 Other incomplete lesion at C4 level of cervical spinal cord
    - S14.155 Other incomplete lesion at C5 level of cervical spinal cord
    - S14.156 Other incomplete lesion at C6 level of cervical spinal cord
    - S14.157 Other incomplete lesion at C7 level of cervical spinal cord
    - S14.158 Other incomplete lesion at C8 level of cervical spinal cord
    - S14.159 Other incomplete lesion at unspecified level of cervical spinal cord
- S14.2 Injury of nerve root of cervical spine
- S14.3 Injury of brachial plexus
- S14.4 Injury of peripheral nerves of neck
- S14.5 Injury of cervical sympathetic nerves
- S14.8 Injury of other specified nerves of neck
- S14.9 Injury of unspecified nerves of neck
- S15 Injury of blood vessels at neck level
  Code also any associated open wound (S11.-)
  The appropriate 7th character is to be added to each code from category S15
  A = initial encounter
  D = subsequent encounter
  S = sequela
  - S15.0 Injury of carotid artery of neck
    Injury of carotid artery (common) (external) (internal, extracranial portion)
    Injury of carotid artery NOS
    EXCLUDES1 injury of internal carotid artery, intracranial portion (S06.8)
    - S15.00 Unspecified injury of carotid artery
      - S15.001 Unspecified injury of right carotid artery

Unacceptable principal diagnosis symbol per Medicare code edits   Code exempt from diagnosis present on admission requirement
? Questionable admission   Complication or comorbidity   MCC Major complication or comorbidity   CC/MCC CC/MCC exclusion
HCC HCC diagnosis code   RxHCC RxHCC diagnosis code   MACRA code   DEFINITION Describes condition/terminology
TIP Coding guidance   Official Guideline Reference   Z1 Z code as first-listed diagnosis

984   When symbols appear on a code that requires a 7th character extension, refer to Appendix B to identify applicable 7th character codes.   **2020 ICD-10-CM**

7️⃣ S15.002 Unspecified injury of left carotid artery ⚕ POA CC/MCC Exc

7️⃣ S15.009 Unspecified injury of unspecified carotid artery ⚕ POA CC/MCC Exc

6️⃣ S15.01 Minor laceration of carotid artery
  Incomplete transection of carotid artery
  Laceration of carotid artery NOS
  Superficial laceration of carotid artery

7️⃣ S15.011 Minor laceration of right carotid artery ⚕ POA CC/MCC Exc

7️⃣ S15.012 Minor laceration of left carotid artery ⚕ POA CC/MCC Exc

7️⃣ S15.019 Minor laceration of unspecified carotid artery ⚕ POA CC/MCC Exc

6️⃣ S15.02 Major laceration of carotid artery
  Complete transection of carotid artery
  Traumatic rupture of carotid artery

7️⃣ S15.021 Major laceration of right carotid artery ⚕ POA CC/MCC Exc

7️⃣ S15.022 Major laceration of left carotid artery ⚕ POA CC/MCC Exc

7️⃣ S15.029 Major laceration of unspecified carotid artery ⚕ POA CC/MCC Exc

6️⃣ S15.09 Other specified injury of carotid artery

7️⃣ S15.091 Other specified injury of right carotid artery ⚕ POA CC/MCC Exc

7️⃣ S15.092 Other specified injury of left carotid artery ⚕ POA CC/MCC Exc

7️⃣ S15.099 Other specified injury of unspecified carotid artery ⚕ POA CC/MCC Exc

5️⃣ S15.1 Injury of vertebral artery

6️⃣ S15.10 Unspecified injury of vertebral artery

7️⃣ S15.101 Unspecified injury of right vertebral artery ⚕ POA CC/MCC Exc

7️⃣ S15.102 Unspecified injury of left vertebral artery ⚕ POA CC/MCC Exc

7️⃣ S15.109 Unspecified injury of unspecified vertebral artery ⚕ POA CC/MCC Exc

6️⃣ S15.11 Minor laceration of vertebral artery
  Incomplete transection of vertebral artery
  Laceration of vertebral artery NOS
  Superficial laceration of vertebral artery

7️⃣ S15.111 Minor laceration of right vertebral artery ⚕ POA CC/MCC Exc

7️⃣ S15.112 Minor laceration of left vertebral artery ⚕ POA CC/MCC Exc

7️⃣ S15.119 Minor laceration of unspecified vertebral artery ⚕ POA CC/MCC Exc

6️⃣ S15.12 Major laceration of vertebral artery
  Complete transection of vertebral artery
  Traumatic rupture of vertebral artery

7️⃣ S15.121 Major laceration of right vertebral artery ⚕ POA CC/MCC Exc

7️⃣ S15.122 Major laceration of left vertebral artery ⚕ POA CC/MCC Exc

7️⃣ S15.129 Major laceration of unspecified vertebral artery ⚕ POA CC/MCC Exc

6️⃣ S15.19 Other specified injury of vertebral artery

7️⃣ S15.191 Other specified injury of right vertebral artery ⚕ POA CC/MCC Exc

7️⃣ S15.192 Other specified injury of left vertebral artery ⚕ POA CC/MCC Exc

7️⃣ S15.199 Other specified injury of unspecified vertebral artery ⚕ POA CC/MCC Exc

5️⃣ S15.2 Injury of external jugular vein

6️⃣ S15.20 Unspecified injury of external jugular vein

7️⃣ S15.201 Unspecified injury of right external jugular vein ⚕ POA CC/MCC Exc

7️⃣ S15.202 Unspecified injury of left external jugular vein ⚕ POA CC/MCC Exc

7️⃣ S15.209 Unspecified injury of unspecified external jugular vein ⚕ POA CC/MCC Exc

6️⃣ S15.21 Minor laceration of external jugular vein
  Incomplete transection of external jugular vein
  Laceration of external jugular vein NOS
  Superficial laceration of external jugular vein

7️⃣ S15.211 Minor laceration of right external jugular vein ⚕ POA CC/MCC Exc

7️⃣ S15.212 Minor laceration of left external jugular vein ⚕ POA CC/MCC Exc

7️⃣ S15.219 Minor laceration of unspecified external jugular vein ⚕ POA CC/MCC Exc

6️⃣ S15.22 Major laceration of external jugular vein
  Complete transection of external jugular vein
  Traumatic rupture of external jugular vein

7️⃣ S15.221 Major laceration of right external jugular vein ⚕ POA CC/MCC Exc

7️⃣ S15.222 Major laceration of left external jugular vein ⚕ POA CC/MCC Exc

7️⃣ S15.229 Major laceration of unspecified external jugular vein ⚕ POA CC/MCC Exc

6️⃣ S15.29 Other specified injury of external jugular vein

7️⃣ S15.291 Other specified injury of right external jugular vein ⚕ POA CC/MCC Exc

7️⃣ S15.292 Other specified injury of left external jugular vein ⚕ POA CC/MCC Exc

7️⃣ S15.299 Other specified injury of unspecified external jugular vein ⚕ POA CC/MCC Exc

5️⃣ S15.3 Injury of internal jugular vein

6️⃣ S15.30 Unspecified injury of internal jugular vein

7️⃣ S15.301 Unspecified injury of right internal jugular vein ⚕ POA CC/MCC Exc

7️⃣ S15.302 Unspecified injury of left internal jugular vein ⚕ POA CC/MCC Exc

7️⃣ S15.309 Unspecified injury of unspecified internal jugular vein ⚕ POA CC/MCC Exc

6️⃣ S15.31 Minor laceration of internal jugular vein
  Incomplete transection of internal jugular vein
  Laceration of internal jugular vein NOS
  Superficial laceration of internal jugular vein

7️⃣ S15.311 Minor laceration of right internal jugular vein ⚕ POA CC/MCC Exc

7️⃣ S15.312 Minor laceration of left internal jugular vein ⚕ POA CC/MCC Exc

7️⃣ S15.319 Minor laceration of unspecified internal jugular vein ⚕ POA CC/MCC Exc

6️⃣ S15.32 Major laceration of internal jugular vein
  Complete transection of internal jugular vein
  Traumatic rupture of internal jugular vein

7️⃣ S15.321 Major laceration of right internal jugular vein ⚕ POA CC/MCC Exc

7️⃣ S15.322 Major laceration of left internal jugular vein ⚕ POA CC/MCC Exc

7️⃣ S15.329 Major laceration of unspecified internal jugular vein ⚕ POA CC/MCC Exc

6️⃣ S15.39 Other specified injury of internal jugular vein

7️⃣ S15.391 Other specified injury of right internal jugular vein ⚕ POA CC/MCC Exc

7️⃣ S15.392 Other specified injury of left internal jugular vein ⚕ POA CC/MCC Exc

7️⃣ S15.399 Other specified injury of unspecified internal jugular vein ⚕ POA CC/MCC Exc

7️⃣ S15.8 Injury of other specified blood vessels at neck level ⚕ POA CC/MCC Exc

7️⃣ S15.9 Injury of unspecified blood vessel at neck level ⚕ POA CC/MCC Exc

4️⃣ S16 Injury of muscle, fascia and tendon at neck level
  Code also any associated open wound (S11.-)
  EXCLUDES2 sprain of joint or ligament at neck level (S13.9)
  The appropriate 7th character is to be added to each code from category S16
    A = initial encounter
    D = subsequent encounter
    S = sequela

S16.1 Strain of muscle, fascia and tendon at neck level

S16.2 Laceration of muscle, fascia and tendon at neck level

S16.8 Other specified injury of muscle, fascia and tendon at neck level

S16.9 Unspecified injury of muscle, fascia and tendon at neck level

S17 Crushing injury of neck
Use additional code for all associated injuries, such as:
injury of blood vessels (S15.-)
open wound of neck (S11.-)
spinal cord injury (S14.0, S14.1-)
vertebral fracture (S12.0--S12.3-)

The appropriate 7th character is to be added to each code from category S17
A = initial encounter
D = subsequent encounter
S = sequela

S17.0 Crushing injury of larynx and trachea   CC POA HAC CC/MCC Exc

S17.8 Crushing injury of other specified parts of neck   CC POA HAC CC/MCC Exc

S17.9 Crushing injury of neck, part unspecified   CC POA HAC CC/MCC Exc

S19 Other specified and unspecified injuries of neck

The appropriate 7th character is to be added to each code from category S19
A = initial encounter
D = subsequent encounter
S = sequela

S19.8 Other specified injuries of neck

S19.80 Other specified injuries of unspecified part of neck   POA

S19.81 Other specified injuries of larynx   POA

S19.82 Other specified injuries of cervical trachea   POA
EXCLUDES2 other specified injury of thoracic trachea (S27.5-)

S19.83 Other specified injuries of vocal cord   POA

S19.84 Other specified injuries of thyroid gland   POA

S19.85 Other specified injuries of pharynx and cervical esophagus   POA

S19.89 Other specified injuries of other specified part of neck   POA

S19.9 Unspecified injury of neck   POA

Injuries to the thorax (S20-S29)

INCLUDES   injuries of breast
injuries of chest (wall)
injuries of interscapular area
EXCLUDES2 burns and corrosions (T20-T32)
effects of foreign body in bronchus (T17.5)
effects of foreign body in esophagus (T18.1)
effects of foreign body in lung (T17.8)
effects of foreign body in trachea (T17.4)
frostbite (T33-T34)
injuries of axilla
injuries of clavicle
injuries of scapular region
injuries of shoulder
insect bite or sting, venomous (T63.4)

S20 Superficial injury of thorax
The appropriate 7th character is to be added to each code from category S20
A = initial encounter
D = subsequent encounter
S = sequela

S20.0 Contusion of breast

S20.00 Contusion of breast, unspecified breast   POA

S20.01 Contusion of right breast   POA

S20.02 Contusion of left breast   POA

S20.1 Other and unspecified superficial injuries of breast

S20.10 Unspecified superficial injuries of breast

S20.101 Unspecified superficial injuries of breast, right breast   POA

S20.102 Unspecified superficial injuries of breast, left breast   POA

S20.109 Unspecified superficial injuries of breast, unspecified breast   POA

S20.11 Abrasion of breast

S20.111 Abrasion of breast, right breast   POA

S20.112 Abrasion of breast, left breast   POA

S20.119 Abrasion of breast, unspecified breast   POA

S20.12 Blister (nonthermal) of breast

S20.121 Blister (nonthermal) of breast, right breast   POA

S20.122 Blister (nonthermal) of breast, left breast   POA

S20.129 Blister (nonthermal) of breast, unspecified breast   POA

S20.14 External constriction of part of breast

S20.141 External constriction of part of breast, right breast   POA

S20.142 External constriction of part of breast, left breast   POA

S20.149 External constriction of part of breast, unspecified breast   POA

S20.15 Superficial foreign body of breast
Splinter in the breast

S20.151 Superficial foreign body of breast, right breast   POA

S20.152 Superficial foreign body of breast, left breast   POA

S20.159 Superficial foreign body of breast, unspecified breast   POA

S20.16 Insect bite (nonvenomous) of breast

S20.161 Insect bite (nonvenomous) of breast, right breast   POA

S20.162 Insect bite (nonvenomous) of breast, left breast   POA

S20.169 Insect bite (nonvenomous) of breast, unspecified breast   POA

S20.17 Other superficial bite of breast
EXCLUDES1 open bite of breast (S21.05-)

S20.171 Other superficial bite of breast, right breast   POA

S20.172 Other superficial bite of breast, left breast   POA

S20.179 Other superficial bite of breast, unspecified breast   POA

S20.2 Contusion of thorax

S20.20 Contusion of thorax, unspecified   POA

S20.21 Contusion of front wall of thorax

S20.211 Contusion of right front wall of thorax   POA

S20.212 Contusion of left front wall of thorax   POA

S20.219 Contusion of unspecified front wall of thorax   POA

S20.22 Contusion of back wall of thorax

S20.221 Contusion of right back wall of thorax   POA

S20.222 Contusion of left back wall of thorax   POA

S20.229 Contusion of unspecified back wall of thorax   POA

S20.3 Other and unspecified superficial injuries of front wall of thorax

S20.30 Unspecified superficial injuries of front wall of thorax

S20.301 Unspecified superficial injuries of right front wall of thorax   POA

S20.302 Unspecified superficial injuries of left front wall of thorax   POA

S20.309 Unspecified superficial injuries of unspecified front wall of thorax   POA

POA Unacceptable principal diagnosis symbol per Medicare code edits   POA Code exempt from diagnosis present on admission requirement
? Questionable admission   CC Complication or comorbidity   MCC Major complication or comorbidity   CC/MCC Exc CC/MCC exclusion
HCC HCC diagnosis code   RxHCC RxHCC diagnosis code   MACRA MACRA code   **DEFINITION** Describes condition/terminology
TIP Coding guidance   Official Guideline Reference   Z1 Z code as first-listed diagnosis

When symbols appear on a code that requires a 7th character extension, refer to Appendix B to identify applicable 7th character codes.   **2020 ICD-10-CM**

- [6th] **S20.31 Abrasion of front wall of thorax**
  - [7th] **S20.311 Abrasion of right front wall of thorax** POA
  - [7th] **S20.312 Abrasion of left front wall of thorax** POA
  - [7th] **S20.319 Abrasion of unspecified front wall of thorax** POA
- [6th] **S20.32 Blister (nonthermal) of front wall of thorax**
  - [7th] **S20.321 Blister (nonthermal) of right front wall of thorax** POA
  - [7th] **S20.322 Blister (nonthermal) of left front wall of thorax** POA
  - [7th] **S20.329 Blister (nonthermal) of unspecified front wall of thorax** POA
- [6th] **S20.34 External constriction of front wall of thorax**
  - [7th] **S20.341 External constriction of right front wall of thorax** POA
  - [7th] **S20.342 External constriction of left front wall of thorax** POA
  - [7th] **S20.349 External constriction of unspecified front wall of thorax** POA
- [6th] **S20.35 Superficial foreign body of front wall of thorax**
  Splinter in front wall of thorax
  - [7th] **S20.351 Superficial foreign body of right front wall of thorax** POA
  - [7th] **S20.352 Superficial foreign body of left front wall of thorax** POA
  - [7th] **S20.359 Superficial foreign body of unspecified front wall of thorax** POA
- [6th] **S20.36 Insect bite (nonvenomous) of front wall of thorax**
  - [7th] **S20.361 Insect bite (nonvenomous) of right front wall of thorax** POA
  - [7th] **S20.362 Insect bite (nonvenomous) of left front wall of thorax** POA
  - [7th] **S20.369 Insect bite (nonvenomous) of unspecified front wall of thorax** POA
- [6th] **S20.37 Other superficial bite of front wall of thorax**
  [EXCLUDES1] *open bite of front wall of thorax (S21.14)*
  - [7th] **S20.371 Other superficial bite of right front wall of thorax** POA
  - [7th] **S20.372 Other superficial bite of left front wall of thorax** POA
  - [7th] **S20.379 Other superficial bite of unspecified front wall of thorax** POA

[5th] **S20.4 Other and unspecified superficial injuries of back wall of thorax**

- [6th] **S20.40 Unspecified superficial injuries of back wall of thorax**
  - [7th] **S20.401 Unspecified superficial injuries of right back wall of thorax** POA
  - [7th] **S20.402 Unspecified superficial injuries of left back wall of thorax** POA
  - [7th] **S20.409 Unspecified superficial injuries of unspecified back wall of thorax** POA
- [6th] **S20.41 Abrasion of back wall of thorax**
  - [7th] **S20.411 Abrasion of right back wall of thorax** POA
  - [7th] **S20.412 Abrasion of left back wall of thorax** POA
  - [7th] **S20.419 Abrasion of unspecified back wall of thorax** POA
- [6th] **S20.42 Blister (nonthermal) of back wall of thorax**
  - [7th] **S20.421 Blister (nonthermal) of right back wall of thorax** POA
  - [7th] **S20.422 Blister (nonthermal) of left back wall of thorax** POA
  - [7th] **S20.429 Blister (nonthermal) of unspecified back wall of thorax** POA
- [6th] **S20.44 External constriction of back wall of thorax**
  - [7th] **S20.441 External constriction of right back wall of thorax** POA
  - [7th] **S20.442 External constriction of left back wall of thorax** POA
  - [7th] **S20.449 External constriction of unspecified back wall of thorax** POA
- [6th] **S20.45 Superficial foreign body of back wall of thorax**
  Splinter of back wall of thorax
  - [7th] **S20.451 Superficial foreign body of right back wall of thorax** POA
  - [7th] **S20.452 Superficial foreign body of left back wall of thorax** POA
  - [7th] **S20.459 Superficial foreign body of unspecified back wall of thorax** POA
- [6th] **S20.46 Insect bite (nonvenomous) of back wall of thorax**
  - [7th] **S20.461 Insect bite (nonvenomous) of right back wall of thorax** POA
  - [7th] **S20.462 Insect bite (nonvenomous) of left back wall of thorax** POA
  - [7th] **S20.469 Insect bite (nonvenomous) of unspecified back wall of thorax** POA
- [6th] **S20.47 Other superficial bite of back wall of thorax**
  [EXCLUDES1] *open bite of back wall of thorax (S21.24)*
  - [7th] **S20.471 Other superficial bite of right back wall of thorax** POA
  - [7th] **S20.472 Other superficial bite of left back wall of thorax** POA
  - [7th] **S20.479 Other superficial bite of unspecified back wall of thorax** POA

[5th] **S20.9 Superficial injury of unspecified parts of thorax**

[EXCLUDES1] *contusion of thorax NOS (S20.20)*

- [7th] **S20.90 Unspecified superficial injury of unspecified parts of thorax** POA
  Superficial injury of thoracic wall NOS
- [7th] **S20.91 Abrasion of unspecified parts of thorax** POA
- [7th] **S20.92 Blister (nonthermal) of unspecified parts of thorax** POA
- [7th] **S20.94 External constriction of unspecified parts of thorax** POA
- [7th] **S20.95 Superficial foreign body of unspecified parts of thorax** POA
  Splinter in thorax NOS
- [7th] **S20.96 Insect bite (nonvenomous) of unspecified parts of thorax** POA
- [7th] **S20.97 Other superficial bite of unspecified parts of thorax** POA
  [EXCLUDES1] *open bite of thorax NOS (S21.95)*

[4th] **S21 Open wound of thorax**

Code also any associated injury, such as:
- injury of heart (S26.-)
- injury of intrathoracic organs (S27.-)
- rib fracture (S22.3-, S22.4-)
- spinal cord injury (S24.0-, S24.1-)
- traumatic hemopneumothorax (S27.3)
- traumatic hemothorax (S27.1)
- traumatic pneumothorax (S27.0)
- wound infection

[EXCLUDES1] *traumatic amputation (partial) of thorax (S28.1)*

The appropriate 7th character is to be added to each code from category S21
- **A = initial encounter**
- **D = subsequent encounter**
- **S = sequela**

[5th] **S21.0 Open wound of breast**

- [6th] **S21.00 Unspecified open wound of breast**
  - [7th] **S21.001 Unspecified open wound of right breast** POA
  - [7th] **S21.002 Unspecified open wound of left breast** POA
  - [7th] **S21.009 Unspecified open wound of unspecified breast** POA
- [6th] **S21.01 Laceration without foreign body of breast**
  - [7th] **S21.011 Laceration without foreign body of right breast** POA
  - [7th] **S21.012 Laceration without foreign body of left breast** POA
  - [7th] **S21.019 Laceration without foreign body of unspecified breast** POA

⑥ S21.02 Laceration with foreign body of breast
    ⑦ S21.021 Laceration with foreign body of right breast   POA
    ⑦ S21.022 Laceration with foreign body of left breast   POA
    ⑦ S21.029 Laceration with foreign body of unspecified breast   POA

⑥ S21.03 Puncture wound without foreign body of breast
    ⑦ S21.031 Puncture wound without foreign body of right breast   POA
    ⑦ S21.032 Puncture wound without foreign body of left breast   POA
    ⑦ S21.039 Puncture wound without foreign body of unspecified breast   POA

⑤ S21.04 Puncture wound with foreign body of breast
    ⑦ S21.041 Puncture wound with foreign body of right breast   POA
    ⑦ S21.042 Puncture wound with foreign body of left breast   POA
    ⑦ S21.049 Puncture wound with foreign body of unspecified breast   POA

⑤ S21.05 Open bite of breast
    Bite of breast NOS
    EXCLUDES1 superficial bite of breast (S20.17)
    ⑦ S21.051 Open bite of right breast   POA
    ⑦ S21.052 Open bite of left breast   POA
    ⑦ S21.059 Open bite of unspecified breast   POA

⑤ S21.1 Open wound of front wall of thorax without penetration into thoracic cavity
    Open wound of chest without penetration into thoracic cavity

⑥ S21.10 Unspecified open wound of front wall of thorax without penetration into thoracic cavity
    ⑦ S21.101 Unspecified open wound of right front wall of thorax without penetration into thoracic cavity   CC POA CC/MCC Exc
    ⑦ S21.102 Unspecified open wound of left front wall of thorax without penetration into thoracic cavity   CC POA CC/MCC Exc
    ⑦ S21.109 Unspecified open wound of unspecified front wall of thorax without penetration into thoracic cavity   CC POA CC/MCC Exc

⑥ S21.11 Laceration without foreign body of front wall of thorax without penetration into thoracic cavity
    ⑦ S21.111 Laceration without foreign body of right front wall of thorax without penetration into thoracic cavity   CC POA CC/MCC Exc
    ⑦ S21.112 Laceration without foreign body of left front wall of thorax without penetration into thoracic cavity   CC POA CC/MCC Exc
    ⑦ S21.119 Laceration without foreign body of unspecified front wall of thorax without penetration into thoracic cavity   CC POA CC/MCC Exc

⑥ S21.12 Laceration with foreign body of front wall of thorax without penetration into thoracic cavity
    ⑦ S21.121 Laceration with foreign body of right front wall of thorax without penetration into thoracic cavity   CC POA CC/MCC Exc
    ⑦ S21.122 Laceration with foreign body of left front wall of thorax without penetration into thoracic cavity   CC POA CC/MCC Exc
    ⑦ S21.129 Laceration with foreign body of unspecified front wall of thorax without penetration into thoracic cavity   CC POA CC/MCC Exc

⑥ S21.13 Puncture wound without foreign body of front wall of thorax without penetration into thoracic cavity
    ⑦ S21.131 Puncture wound without foreign body of right front wall of thorax without penetration into thoracic cavity   CC POA CC/MCC Exc
    ⑦ S21.132 Puncture wound without foreign body of left front wall of thorax without penetration into thoracic cavity   CC POA CC/MCC Exc

⑦ S21.139 Puncture wound without foreign body of unspecified front wall of thorax without penetration into thoracic cavity   CC POA CC/MCC Exc

⑥ S21.14 Puncture wound with foreign body of front wall of thorax without penetration into thoracic cavity
    ⑦ S21.141 Puncture wound with foreign body of right front wall of thorax without penetration into thoracic cavity   CC POA CC/MCC Exc
    ⑦ S21.142 Puncture wound with foreign body of left front wall of thorax without penetration into thoracic cavity   CC POA CC/MCC Exc
    ⑦ S21.149 Puncture wound with foreign body of unspecified front wall of thorax without penetration into thoracic cavity   CC POA CC/MCC Exc

⑥ S21.15 Open bite of front wall of thorax without penetration into thoracic cavity
    Bite of front wall of thorax NOS
    EXCLUDES1 superficial bite of front wall of thorax (S20.37)
    ⑦ S21.151 Open bite of right front wall of thorax without penetration into thoracic cavity   CC POA CC/MCC Exc
    ⑦ S21.152 Open bite of left front wall of thorax without penetration into thoracic cavity   CC POA CC/MCC Exc
    ⑦ S21.159 Open bite of unspecified front wall of thorax without penetration into thoracic cavity   CC POA CC/MCC Exc

⑤ S21.2 Open wound of back wall of thorax without penetration into thoracic cavity
⑥ S21.20 Unspecified open wound of back wall of thorax without penetration into thoracic cavity
    ⑦ S21.201 Unspecified open wound of right back wall of thorax without penetration into thoracic cavity   POA
    ⑦ S21.202 Unspecified open wound of left back wall of thorax without penetration into thoracic cavity   POA
    ⑦ S21.209 Unspecified open wound of unspecified back wall of thorax without penetration into thoracic cavity   POA

⑥ S21.21 Laceration without foreign body of back wall of thorax without penetration into thoracic cavity
    ⑦ S21.211 Laceration without foreign body of right back wall of thorax without penetration into thoracic cavity   POA
    ⑦ S21.212 Laceration without foreign body of left back wall of thorax without penetration into thoracic cavity   POA
    ⑦ S21.219 Laceration without foreign body of unspecified back wall of thorax without penetration into thoracic cavity   POA

⑥ S21.22 Laceration with foreign body of back wall of thorax without penetration into thoracic cavity
    ⑦ S21.221 Laceration with foreign body of right back wall of thorax without penetration into thoracic cavity   POA
    ⑦ S21.222 Laceration with foreign body of left back wall of thorax without penetration into thoracic cavity   POA
    ⑦ S21.229 Laceration with foreign body of unspecified back wall of thorax without penetration into thoracic cavity   POA

⑥ S21.23 Puncture wound without foreign body of back wall of thorax without penetration into thoracic cavity
    ⑦ S21.231 Puncture wound without foreign body of right back wall of thorax without penetration into thoracic cavity   POA
    ⑦ S21.232 Puncture wound without foreign body of left back wall of thorax without penetration into thoracic cavity   POA

PDxⁿ Unacceptable principal diagnosis symbol per Medicare code edits   Ⓢ Code exempt from diagnosis present on admission requirement
   ❓ Questionable admission   CC Complication or comorbidity   MCC Major complication or comorbidity   CC/MCC Exc CC/MCC exclusion
   HCC HCC diagnosis code   RxHCC RxHCC diagnosis code   MACRA code   **DEFINITION** Describes condition/terminology
   TIP Coding guidance   👁 Official Guideline Reference   Z1 Z code as first-listed diagnosis

When symbols appear on a code that requires a 7th character extension, refer to Appendix B to identify applicable 7th character codes.
    2020 ICD-10-CM

[7th] S21.239 Puncture wound without foreign body of unspecified back wall of thorax without penetration into thoracic cavity [POA]

[6th] S21.24 Puncture wound with foreign body of back wall of thorax without penetration into thoracic cavity

[7th] S21.241 Puncture wound with foreign body of right back wall of thorax without penetration into thoracic cavity [POA]

[7th] S21.242 Puncture wound with foreign body of left back wall of thorax without penetration into thoracic cavity [POA]

[7th] S21.249 Puncture wound with foreign body of unspecified back wall of thorax without penetration into thoracic cavity [POA]

[6th] S21.25 Open bite of back wall of thorax without penetration into thoracic cavity

Bite of back wall of thorax NOS

[EXCLUDES1] *superficial bite of back wall of thorax (S20.47)*

[7th] S21.251 Open bite of right back wall of thorax without penetration into thoracic cavity [POA]

[7th] S21.252 Open bite of left back wall of thorax without penetration into thoracic cavity [POA]

[7th] S21.259 Open bite of unspecified back wall of thorax without penetration into thoracic cavity [POA]

[5th] S21.3 Open wound of front wall of thorax with penetration into thoracic cavity

Open wound of chest with penetration into thoracic cavity

[6th] S21.30 Unspecified open wound of front wall of thorax with penetration into thoracic cavity

[7th] S21.301 Unspecified open wound of right front wall of thorax with penetration into thoracic cavity [POA] [MCC] [CC/MCC Exc]

[7th] S21.302 Unspecified open wound of left front wall of thorax with penetration into thoracic cavity [POA] [MCC] [CC/MCC Exc]

[7th] S21.309 Unspecified open wound of unspecified front wall of thorax with penetration into thoracic cavity [POA] [MCC] [CC/MCC Exc]

[6th] S21.31 Laceration without foreign body of front wall of thorax with penetration into thoracic cavity

[7th] S21.311 Laceration without foreign body of right front wall of thorax with penetration into thoracic cavity [POA] [MCC] [CC/MCC Exc]

[7th] S21.312 Laceration without foreign body of left front wall of thorax with penetration into thoracic cavity [POA] [MCC] [CC/MCC Exc]

[7th] S21.319 Laceration without foreign body of unspecified front wall of thorax with penetration into thoracic cavity [POA] [MCC] [CC/MCC Exc]

[6th] S21.32 Laceration with foreign body of front wall of thorax with penetration into thoracic cavity

[7th] S21.321 Laceration with foreign body of right front wall of thorax with penetration into thoracic cavity [POA] [MCC] [CC/MCC Exc]

[7th] S21.322 Laceration with foreign body of left front wall of thorax with penetration into thoracic cavity [POA] [MCC] [CC/MCC Exc]

[7th] S21.329 Laceration with foreign body of unspecified front wall of thorax with penetration into thoracic cavity [POA] [MCC] [CC/MCC Exc]

[6th] S21.33 Puncture wound without foreign body of front wall of thorax with penetration into thoracic cavity

[7th] S21.331 Puncture wound without foreign body of right front wall of thorax with penetration into thoracic cavity [POA] [MCC] [CC/MCC Exc]

[7th] S21.332 Puncture wound without foreign body of left front wall of thorax with penetration into thoracic cavity [POA] [MCC] [CC/MCC Exc]

[7th] S21.339 Puncture wound without foreign body of unspecified front wall of thorax with penetration into thoracic cavity [POA] [MCC] [CC/MCC Exc]

[6th] S21.34 Puncture wound with foreign body of front wall of thorax with penetration into thoracic cavity

[7th] S21.341 Puncture wound with foreign body of right front wall of thorax with penetration into thoracic cavity [POA] [MCC] [CC/MCC Exc]

[7th] S21.342 Puncture wound with foreign body of left front wall of thorax with penetration into thoracic cavity [POA] [MCC] [CC/MCC Exc]

[7th] S21.349 Puncture wound with foreign body of unspecified front wall of thorax with penetration into thoracic cavity [POA] [MCC] [CC/MCC Exc]

[6th] S21.35 Open bite of front wall of thorax with penetration into thoracic cavity

[EXCLUDES1] *superficial bite of front wall of thorax (S20.37)*

[7th] S21.351 Open bite of right front wall of thorax with penetration into thoracic cavity [POA] [MCC] [CC/MCC Exc]

[7th] S21.352 Open bite of left front wall of thorax with penetration into thoracic cavity [POA] [MCC] [CC/MCC Exc]

[7th] S21.359 Open bite of unspecified front wall of thorax with penetration into thoracic cavity [POA] [MCC] [CC/MCC Exc]

[5th] S21.4 Open wound of back wall of thorax with penetration into thoracic cavity

[6th] S21.40 Unspecified open wound of back wall of thorax with penetration into thoracic cavity

[7th] S21.401 Unspecified open wound of right back wall of thorax with penetration into thoracic cavity [POA] [MCC] [CC/MCC Exc]

[7th] S21.402 Unspecified open wound of left back wall of thorax with penetration into thoracic cavity [POA] [MCC] [CC/MCC Exc]

[7th] S21.409 Unspecified open wound of unspecified back wall of thorax with penetration into thoracic cavity [POA] [MCC] [CC/MCC Exc]

[6th] S21.41 Laceration without foreign body of back wall of thorax with penetration into thoracic cavity

[7th] S21.411 Laceration without foreign body of right back wall of thorax with penetration into thoracic cavity [POA] [MCC] [CC/MCC Exc]

[7th] S21.412 Laceration without foreign body of left back wall of thorax with penetration into thoracic cavity [POA] [MCC] [CC/MCC Exc]

[7th] S21.419 Laceration without foreign body of unspecified back wall of thorax with penetration into thoracic cavity [POA] [MCC] [CC/MCC Exc]

[6th] S21.42 Laceration with foreign body of back wall of thorax with penetration into thoracic cavity

[7th] S21.421 Laceration with foreign body of right back wall of thorax with penetration into thoracic cavity [POA] [MCC] [CC/MCC Exc]

[7th] S21.422 Laceration with foreign body of left back wall of thorax with penetration into thoracic cavity [POA] [MCC] [CC/MCC Exc]

[7th] S21.429 Laceration with foreign body of unspecified back wall of thorax with penetration into thoracic cavity [POA] [MCC] [CC/MCC Exc]

[6th] S21.43 Puncture wound without foreign body of back wall of thorax with penetration into thoracic cavity

[7th] S21.431 Puncture wound without foreign body of right back wall of thorax with penetration into thoracic cavity [POA] [MCC] [CC/MCC Exc]

[7th] S21.432 Puncture wound without foreign body of left back wall of thorax with penetration into thoracic cavity [POA] [MCC] [CC/MCC Exc]

[7th] S21.439 Puncture wound without foreign body of unspecified back wall of thorax with penetration into thoracic cavity [POA] [MCC] [CC/MCC Exc]

[6th] S21.44 Puncture wound with foreign body of back wall of thorax with penetration into thoracic cavity

[7th] S21.441 Puncture wound with foreign body of right back wall of thorax with penetration into thoracic cavity [POA] [MCC] [CC/MCC Exc]

S21.442 Puncture wound with foreign body of left back wall of thorax with penetration into thoracic cavity POA MCC CC/MCC Exc

S21.449 Puncture wound with foreign body of unspecified back wall of thorax with penetration into thoracic cavity POA MCC CC/MCC Exc

S21.45 Open bite of back wall of thorax with penetration into thoracic cavity
Bite of back wall of thorax NOS
EXCLUDES1 superficial bite of back wall of thorax (S20.47)

S21.451 Open bite of right back wall of thorax with penetration into thoracic cavity POA MCC CC/MCC Exc

S21.452 Open bite of left back wall of thorax with penetration into thoracic cavity POA MCC CC/MCC Exc

S21.459 Open bite of unspecified back wall of thorax with penetration into thoracic cavity POA MCC CC/MCC Exc

S21.9 Open wound of unspecified part of thorax
Open wound of thoracic wall NOS

S21.90 Unspecified open wound of unspecified part of thorax CC POA CC/MCC Exc

S21.91 Laceration without foreign body of unspecified part of thorax CC POA CC/MCC Exc

S21.92 Laceration with foreign body of unspecified part of thorax CC POA CC/MCC Exc

S21.93 Puncture wound without foreign body of unspecified part of thorax CC POA CC/MCC Exc

S21.94 Puncture wound with foreign body of unspecified part of thorax CC POA CC/MCC Exc

S21.95 Open bite of unspecified part of thorax CC POA CC/MCC Exc
EXCLUDES1 superficial bite of thorax (S20.97)

S22 Fracture of rib(s), sternum and thoracic spine
See Official Guidelines "Coding of Traumatic Fractures" I.C.19.c
NOTES A fracture not indicated as displaced or nondisplaced should be coded to displaced.
A fracture not indicated as open or closed should be coded to closed.
INCLUDES fracture of thoracic neural arch
fracture of thoracic spinous process
fracture of thoracic transverse process
fracture of thoracic vertebra
fracture of thoracic vertebral arch

Code first any associated:
injury of intrathoracic organ (S27.-)
spinal cord injury (S24.0-, S24.1-)
EXCLUDES1 transection of thorax (S28.1)
EXCLUDES2 fracture of clavicle (S42.0-)
fracture of scapula (S42.1-)

The appropriate 7th character is to be added to each code from category S22
A = initial encounter for closed fracture
B = initial encounter for open fracture
D = subsequent encounter for fracture with routine healing
G = subsequent encounter for fracture with delayed healing
K = subsequent encounter for fracture with nonunion
S = sequela

S22.0 Fracture of thoracic vertebra

S22.00 Fracture of unspecified thoracic vertebra

S22.000 Wedge compression fracture of unspecified thoracic vertebra CC POA HAC HCC MCC CC/MCC Exc

S22.001 Stable burst fracture of unspecified thoracic vertebra CC POA HAC HCC MCC CC/MCC Exc

S22.002 Unstable burst fracture of unspecified thoracic vertebra CC POA HAC HCC MCC CC/MCC Exc

S22.008 Other fracture of unspecified thoracic vertebra CC POA HAC HCC MCC CC/MCC Exc

S22.009 Unspecified fracture of unspecified thoracic vertebra CC POA HAC HCC MCC CC/MCC Exc

S22.01 Fracture of first thoracic vertebra

S22.010 Wedge compression fracture of first thoracic vertebra CC POA HAC HCC MCC CC/MCC Exc

S22.011 Stable burst fracture of first thoracic vertebra CC POA HAC HCC MCC CC/MCC Exc

S22.012 Unstable burst fracture of first thoracic vertebra CC POA HAC HCC MCC CC/MCC Exc

S22.018 Other fracture of first thoracic vertebra CC POA HAC HCC MCC CC/MCC Exc

S22.019 Unspecified fracture of first thoracic vertebra CC POA HAC HCC MCC CC/MCC Exc

S22.02 Fracture of second thoracic vertebra

S22.020 Wedge compression fracture of second thoracic vertebra CC POA HAC HCC MCC CC/MCC Exc

S22.021 Stable burst fracture of second thoracic vertebra CC POA HAC HCC MCC CC/MCC Exc

S22.022 Unstable burst fracture of second thoracic vertebra CC POA HAC HCC MCC CC/MCC Exc

S22.028 Other fracture of second thoracic vertebra CC POA HAC HCC MCC CC/MCC Exc

S22.029 Unspecified fracture of second thoracic vertebra CC POA HAC HCC MCC CC/MCC Exc

S22.03 Fracture of third thoracic vertebra

S22.030 Wedge compression fracture of third thoracic vertebra CC POA HAC HCC MCC CC/MCC Exc

S22.031 Stable burst fracture of third thoracic vertebra CC POA HAC HCC MCC CC/MCC Exc

S22.032 Unstable burst fracture of third thoracic vertebra CC POA HAC HCC MCC CC/MCC Exc

S22.038 Other fracture of third thoracic vertebra CC POA HAC HCC MCC CC/MCC Exc

S22.039 Unspecified fracture of third thoracic vertebra CC POA HAC HCC MCC CC/MCC Exc

S22.04 Fracture of fourth thoracic vertebra

S22.040 Wedge compression fracture of fourth thoracic vertebra CC POA HAC HCC MCC CC/MCC Exc

S22.041 Stable burst fracture of fourth thoracic vertebra CC POA HAC HCC MCC CC/MCC Exc

S22.042 Unstable burst fracture of fourth thoracic vertebra CC POA HAC HCC MCC CC/MCC Exc

S22.048 Other fracture of fourth thoracic vertebra CC POA HAC HCC MCC CC/MCC Exc

S22.049 Unspecified fracture of fourth thoracic vertebra CC POA HAC HCC MCC CC/MCC Exc

S22.05 Fracture of T5-T6 vertebra

S22.050 Wedge compression fracture of T5-T6 vertebra CC POA HAC HCC MCC CC/MCC Exc

S22.051 Stable burst fracture of T5-T6 vertebra CC POA HAC HCC MCC CC/MCC Exc

S22.052 Unstable burst fracture of T5-T6 vertebra CC POA HAC HCC MCC CC/MCC Exc

S22.058 Other fracture of T5-T6 vertebra CC POA HAC HCC MCC CC/MCC Exc

S22.059 Unspecified fracture of T5-T6 vertebra CC POA HAC HCC MCC CC/MCC Exc

S22.06 Fracture of T7-T8 vertebra

S22.060 Wedge compression fracture of T7-T8 vertebra CC POA HAC HCC MCC CC/MCC Exc

S22.061 Stable burst fracture of T7-T8 vertebra CC POA HAC HCC MCC CC/MCC Exc

S22.062 Unstable burst fracture of T7-T8 vertebra CC POA HAC HCC MCC CC/MCC Exc

S22.068 Other fracture of T7-T8 thoracic vertebra CC POA HAC HCC MCC CC/MCC Exc

S22.069 Unspecified fracture of T7-T8 vertebra CC POA HAC HCC MCC CC/MCC Exc

S22.07 Fracture of T9-T10 vertebra

S22.070 Wedge compression fracture of T9-T10 vertebra CC POA HAC HCC MCC CC/MCC Exc

---

POA Unacceptable principal diagnosis symbol per Medicare code edits POA Code exempt from diagnosis present on admission requirement
? Questionable admission CC Complication or comorbidity MCC Major complication or comorbidity CC/MCC Exc CC/MCC exclusion
HCC HCC diagnosis code RxHCC RxHCC diagnosis code MACRA MACRA code DEFINITION Describes condition/terminology
TIP Coding guidance Official Guideline Reference Z1 Z code as first-listed diagnosis

990
When symbols appear on a code that requires a 7th character extension, refer to Appendix B to identify applicable 7th character codes.
2020 ICD-10-CM

S22.071 Stable burst fracture of T9-T10 vertebra   CC POA HAC HCC MCC CC/MCC

S22.072 Unstable burst fracture of T9-T10 vertebra   CC POA HAC HCC MCC CC/MCC Exc

S22.078 Other fracture of T9-T10 vertebra   CC POA HAC HCC MCC CC/MCC Exc

S22.079 Unspecified fracture of T9-T10 vertebra   CC POA HAC HCC MCC CC/MCC Exc

S22.08 Fracture of T11-T12 vertebra

    S22.080 Wedge compression fracture of T11-T12 vertebra   CC POA HAC HCC MCC CC/MCC Exc

    S22.081 Stable burst fracture of T11-T12 vertebra   CC POA HAC HCC MCC CC/MCC Exc

    S22.082 Unstable burst fracture of T11-T12 vertebra   CC POA HAC HCC MCC CC/MCC Exc

    S22.088 Other fracture of T11-T12 vertebra   CC POA HAC HCC MCC CC/MCC Exc

    S22.089 Unspecified fracture of T11-T12 vertebra   CC POA HAC HCC MCC CC/MCC Exc

S22.2 Fracture of sternum

    S22.20 Unspecified fracture of sternum   CC POA HAC CC/MCC Exc

    S22.21 Fracture of manubrium   CC POA HAC MCC CC/MCC Exc

    S22.22 Fracture of body of sternum   CC POA HAC MCC CC/MCC Exc

    S22.23 Sternal manubrial dissociation   CC POA HAC MCC CC/MCC Exc

    S22.24 Fracture of xiphoid process   CC POA HAC MCC CC/MCC Exc

S22.3 Fracture of one rib

    S22.31 Fracture of one rib, right side   CC POA HAC MCC CC/MCC Exc

    S22.32 Fracture of one rib, left side   CC POA HAC MCC CC/MCC Exc

    S22.39 Fracture of one rib, unspecified side   CC POA HAC MCC CC/MCC Exc

S22.4 Multiple fractures of ribs

Fractures of two or more ribs

    EXCLUDES1 flail chest (S22.5-)

    S22.41 Multiple fractures of ribs, right side   CC POA HAC MCC CC/MCC Exc

    S22.42 Multiple fractures of ribs, left side   CC POA HAC MCC CC/MCC Exc

    S22.43 Multiple fractures of ribs, bilateral   CC POA HAC MCC CC/MCC Exc

    S22.49 Multiple fractures of ribs, unspecified side   CC POA HAC MCC CC/MCC Exc

S22.5 Flail chest   CC POA HAC MCC CC/MCC Exc

S22.9 Fracture of bony thorax, part unspecified   CC POA HAC MCC CC/MCC Exc

S23 Dislocation and sprain of joints and ligaments of thorax

   INCLUDES   avulsion of joint or ligament of thorax

            laceration of cartilage, joint or ligament of thorax

            sprain of cartilage, joint or ligament of thorax

            traumatic hemarthrosis of joint or ligament of thorax

            traumatic rupture of joint or ligament of thorax

            traumatic subluxation of joint or ligament of thorax

            traumatic tear of joint or ligament of thorax

Code also any associated open wound

EXCLUDES2 dislocation, sprain of sternoclavicular joint (S43.2, S43.6)

          strain of muscle or tendon of thorax (S29.01-)

The appropriate 7th character is to be added to each code from category S23

    A = initial encounter

    D = subsequent encounter

    S = sequela

S23.0 Traumatic rupture of thoracic intervertebral disc   POA

    EXCLUDES1 rupture or displacement (nontraumatic) of thoracic intervertebral disc NOS (M51.- with fifth character 4)

S23.1 Subluxation and dislocation of thoracic vertebra

Code also any associated

    open wound of thorax (S21.-)

    spinal cord injury (S24.0-, S24.1-)

    EXCLUDES2 fracture of thoracic vertebrae (S22.0-)

    S23.10 Subluxation and dislocation of unspecified thoracic vertebra

       S23.100 Subluxation of unspecified thoracic vertebra   POA

       S23.101 Dislocation of unspecified thoracic vertebra   POA

    S23.11 Subluxation and dislocation of T1/T2 thoracic vertebra

       S23.110 Subluxation of T1/T2 thoracic vertebra   POA

       S23.111 Dislocation of T1/T2 thoracic vertebra   POA

    S23.12 Subluxation and dislocation of T2/T3-T3/T4 thoracic vertebra

       S23.120 Subluxation of T2/T3 thoracic vertebra   POA

       S23.121 Dislocation of T2/T3 thoracic vertebra   POA

       S23.122 Subluxation of T3/T4 thoracic vertebra   POA

       S23.123 Dislocation of T3/T4 thoracic vertebra   POA

    S23.13 Subluxation and dislocation of T4/T5-T5/T6 thoracic vertebra

       S23.130 Subluxation of T4/T5 thoracic vertebra   POA

       S23.131 Dislocation of T4/T5 thoracic vertebra   POA

       S23.132 Subluxation of T5/T6 thoracic vertebra   POA

       S23.133 Dislocation of T5/T6 thoracic vertebra   POA

    S23.14 Subluxation and dislocation of T6/T7-T7/T8 thoracic vertebra

       S23.140 Subluxation of T6/T7 thoracic vertebra   POA

       S23.141 Dislocation of T6/T7 thoracic vertebra   POA

       S23.142 Subluxation of T7/T8 thoracic vertebra   POA

       S23.143 Dislocation of T7/T8 thoracic vertebra   POA

    S23.15 Subluxation and dislocation of T8/T9-T9/T10 thoracic vertebra

       S23.150 Subluxation of T8/T9 thoracic vertebra   POA

       S23.151 Dislocation of T8/T9 thoracic vertebra   POA

       S23.152 Subluxation of T9/T10 thoracic vertebra   POA

       S23.153 Dislocation of T9/T10 thoracic vertebra   POA

    S23.16 Subluxation and dislocation of T10/T11-T11/T12 thoracic vertebra

       S23.160 Subluxation of T10/T11 thoracic vertebra

       S23.161 Dislocation of T10/T11 thoracic vertebra   POA

       S23.162 Subluxation of T11/T12 thoracic vertebra

       S23.163 Dislocation of T11/T12 thoracic vertebra   POA

    S23.17 Subluxation and dislocation of T12/L1 thoracic vertebra

       S23.170 Subluxation of T12/L1 thoracic vertebra

       S23.171 Dislocation of T12/L1 thoracic vertebra

S23.2 Dislocation of other and unspecified parts of thorax

    S23.20 Dislocation of unspecified part of thorax   POA

    S23.29 Dislocation of other parts of thorax   POA

S23.3 Sprain of ligaments of thoracic spine   POA

S23.4 Sprain of ribs and sternum

    S23.41 Sprain of ribs   POA

    S23.42 Sprain of sternum

       S23.420 Sprain of sternoclavicular (joint) (ligament)   POA

       S23.421 Sprain of chondrosternal joint   POA

       S23.428 Other sprain of sternum   POA

       S23.429 Unspecified sprain of sternum   POA

S23.8 Sprain of other specified parts of thorax   POA

S23.9 Sprain of unspecified parts of thorax   POA

S24 Injury of nerves and spinal cord at thorax level

   NOTES   Code to highest level of thoracic spinal cord injury

          Injuries to the spinal cord (S24.0 and S24.1) refer to the cord level and not bone level injury, and can affect nerve roots at and below the level given.

Code also any associated:

   fracture of thoracic vertebra (S22.0-)

   open wound of thorax (S21.-)

   transient paralysis (R29.5)

EXCLUDES2 injury of brachial plexus (S14.3)

The appropriate 7th character is to be added to each code from category S24

    A = initial encounter

    D = subsequent encounter

    S = sequela

Unspecified Code   Other Specified Code   Manifestation Code   N Newborn   P Pediatric   M Maternity   A Adult   ♂ Male   ♀ Female
● New Code   ▲ Revised Code Title   ►◄ Revised Text   NOTES   INCLUDES   EXCLUDES1 Not coded here   EXCLUDES2 Not included here
4th character required   5th character required   6th character required   7th character required   Extension 'X' Alert
HAC Hospital-acquired condition (HAC) alert   AHA AHA Coding Clinic©   🖙 Code first alert

S24.0 Concussion and edema of thoracic spinal cord `POA` `HCC` `CC/MCC Exc`

S24.1 Other and unspecified injuries of thoracic spinal cord

    S24.10 Unspecified injury of thoracic spinal cord

        S24.101 Unspecified injury at T1 level of thoracic spinal cord `POA` `HAC` `HCC` `MCC` `CC/MCC Exc`

        S24.102 Unspecified injury at T2-T6 level of thoracic spinal cord `POA` `HAC` `HCC` `MCC` `CC/MCC Exc`

        S24.103 Unspecified injury at T7-T10 level of thoracic spinal cord `POA` `HAC` `HCC` `MCC` `CC/MCC Exc`

        S24.104 Unspecified injury at T11-T12 level of thoracic spinal cord `POA` `HAC` `HCC` `MCC` `CC/MCC Exc`

        S24.109 Unspecified injury at unspecified level of thoracic spinal cord `POA` `HCC`

            Injury of thoracic spinal cord NOS

    S24.11 Complete lesion of thoracic spinal cord

        S24.111 Complete lesion at T1 level of thoracic spinal cord `POA` `HAC` `HCC` `MCC` `CC/MCC Exc`

        S24.112 Complete lesion at T2-T6 level of thoracic spinal cord `POA` `HAC` `HCC` `MCC` `CC/MCC Exc`

        S24.113 Complete lesion at T7-T10 level of thoracic spinal cord `POA` `HAC` `HCC` `MCC` `CC/MCC Exc`

        S24.114 Complete lesion at T11-T12 level of thoracic spinal cord `POA` `HAC` `HCC` `MCC` `CC/MCC Exc`

        S24.119 Complete lesion at unspecified level of thoracic spinal cord `POA` `HCC`

    S24.13 Anterior cord syndrome of thoracic spinal cord

        S24.131 Anterior cord syndrome at T1 level of thoracic spinal cord `POA` `HAC` `HCC` `MCC` `CC/MCC Exc`

        S24.132 Anterior cord syndrome at T2-T6 level of thoracic spinal cord `POA` `HAC` `HCC` `MCC` `CC/MCC Exc`

        S24.133 Anterior cord syndrome at T7-T10 level of thoracic spinal cord `POA` `HAC` `HCC` `MCC` `CC/MCC Exc`

        S24.134 Anterior cord syndrome at T11-T12 level of thoracic spinal cord `POA` `HAC` `HCC` `MCC` `CC/MCC Exc`

        S24.139 Anterior cord syndrome at unspecified level of thoracic spinal cord `POA` `HCC`

    S24.14 Brown-Séquard syndrome of thoracic spinal cord

        S24.141 Brown-Séquard syndrome at T1 level of thoracic spinal cord `POA` `HCC` `MCC` `CC/MCC Exc`

        S24.142 Brown-Séquard syndrome at T2-T6 level of thoracic spinal cord `POA` `HCC` `MCC` `CC/MCC Exc`

        S24.143 Brown-Séquard syndrome at T7-T10 level of thoracic spinal cord `POA` `HCC` `MCC` `CC/MCC Exc`

        S24.144 Brown-Séquard syndrome at T11-T12 level of thoracic spinal cord `POA` `HCC` `MCC` `CC/MCC Exc`

        S24.149 Brown-Séquard syndrome at unspecified level of thoracic spinal cord `POA` `HCC`

    S24.15 Other incomplete lesions of thoracic spinal cord

        Incomplete lesion of thoracic spinal cord NOS
        Posterior cord syndrome of thoracic spinal cord

        S24.151 Other incomplete lesion at T1 level of thoracic spinal cord `POA` `HAC` `HCC` `MCC` `CC/MCC Exc`

        S24.152 Other incomplete lesion at T2-T6 level of thoracic spinal cord `POA` `HAC` `HCC` `MCC` `CC/MCC Exc`

        S24.153 Other incomplete lesion at T7-T10 level of thoracic spinal cord `POA` `HAC` `HCC` `MCC` `CC/MCC Exc`

        S24.154 Other incomplete lesion at T11-T12 level of thoracic spinal cord `POA` `HAC` `HCC` `MCC` `CC/MCC Exc`

        S24.159 Other incomplete lesion at unspecified level of thoracic spinal cord `POA` `HCC`

S24.2 Injury of nerve root of thoracic spine `POA`

S24.3 Injury of peripheral nerves of thorax `POA`

S24.4 Injury of thoracic sympathetic nervous system `POA`

    Injury of cardiac plexus
    Injury of esophageal plexus
    Injury of pulmonary plexus
    Injury of stellate ganglion
    Injury of thoracic sympathetic ganglion

S24.8 Injury of other specified nerves of thorax `POA`

S24.9 Injury of unspecified nerve of thorax `POA`

S25 Injury of blood vessels of thorax

    Code also any associated open wound (S21.-)

    The appropriate 7th character is to be added to each code from category S25

        A = initial encounter
        D = subsequent encounter
        S = sequela

S25.0 Injury of thoracic aorta

    Injury of aorta NOS

    S25.00 Unspecified injury of thoracic aorta `POA` `MCC` `CC/MCC Exc`

    S25.01 Minor laceration of thoracic aorta `POA` `MCC` `CC/MCC Exc`

        Incomplete transection of thoracic aorta
        Laceration of thoracic aorta NOS
        Superficial laceration of thoracic aorta

    S25.02 Major laceration of thoracic aorta `POA` `MCC` `CC/MCC Exc`

        Complete transection of thoracic aorta
        Traumatic rupture of thoracic aorta

    S25.09 Other specified injury of thoracic aorta `POA` `MCC` `CC/MCC Exc`

S25.1 Injury of innominate or subclavian artery

    S25.10 Unspecified injury of innominate or subclavian artery

        S25.101 Unspecified injury of right innominate or subclavian artery `POA` `MCC` `CC/MCC Exc`

        S25.102 Unspecified injury of left innominate or subclavian artery `POA` `MCC` `CC/MCC Exc`

        S25.109 Unspecified injury of unspecified innominate or subclavian artery `POA` `MCC` `CC/MCC Exc`

    S25.11 Minor laceration of innominate or subclavian artery

        Incomplete transection of innominate or subclavian artery
        Laceration of innominate or subclavian artery NOS
        Superficial laceration of innominate or subclavian artery

        S25.111 Minor laceration of right innominate or subclavian artery `POA` `MCC` `CC/MCC Exc`

        S25.112 Minor laceration of left innominate or subclavian artery `POA` `MCC` `CC/MCC Exc`

        S25.119 Minor laceration of unspecified innominate or subclavian artery `POA` `MCC` `CC/MCC Exc`

    S25.12 Major laceration of innominate or subclavian artery

        Complete transection of innominate or subclavian artery
        Traumatic rupture of innominate or subclavian artery

        S25.121 Major laceration of right innominate or subclavian artery `POA` `MCC` `CC/MCC Exc`

        S25.122 Major laceration of left innominate or subclavian artery `POA` `MCC` `CC/MCC Exc`

        S25.129 Major laceration of unspecified innominate or subclavian artery `POA` `MCC` `CC/MCC Exc`

    S25.19 Other specified injury of innominate or subclavian artery

        S25.191 Other specified injury of right innominate or subclavian artery `POA` `MCC` `CC/MCC Exc`

        S25.192 Other specified injury of left innominate or subclavian artery `POA` `MCC` `CC/MCC Exc`

        S25.199 Other specified injury of unspecified innominate or subclavian artery `POA` `MCC` `CC/MCC Exc`

S25.2 Injury of superior vena cava

    Injury of vena cava NOS

    S25.20 Unspecified injury of superior vena cava `POA` `MCC` `CC/MCC Exc`

    S25.21 Minor laceration of superior vena cava `POA` `MCC` `CC/MCC Exc`

        Incomplete transection of superior vena cava
        Laceration of superior vena cava NOS
        Superficial laceration of superior vena cava

    S25.22 Major laceration of superior vena cava `POA` `MCC` `CC/MCC Exc`

        Complete transection of superior vena cava
        Traumatic rupture of superior vena cava

992

When symbols appear on a code that requires a 7th character extension, refer to Appendix B to identify applicable 7th character codes.

2020 ICD-10-CM

7ᵗʰ **S25.29 Other specified injury of superior vena cava** POA MCC CC/MCC Exc

5ᵗʰ **S25.3 Injury of** innominate or subclavian vein
  6ᵗʰ **S25.30 Unspecified injury of innominate or subclavian vein**
    7ᵗʰ **S25.301 Unspecified injury of right innominate or subclavian vein**
    7ᵗʰ **S25.302 Unspecified injury of left innominate or subclavian vein** POA MCC CC/MCC Exc
    7ᵗʰ **S25.309 Unspecified injury of unspecified innominate or subclavian vein** POA MCC CC/MCC Exc
  6ᵗʰ **S25.31 Minor laceration of innominate or subclavian vein**
    Incomplete transection of innominate or subclavian vein
    Laceration of innominate or subclavian vein NOS
    Superficial laceration of innominate or subclavian vein
    7ᵗʰ **S25.311 Minor laceration of right innominate or subclavian vein** POA MCC CC/MCC Exc
    7ᵗʰ **S25.312 Minor laceration of left innominate or subclavian vein** POA MCC CC/MCC Exc
    7ᵗʰ **S25.319 Minor laceration of unspecified innominate or subclavian vein** POA MCC CC/MCC Exc
  6ᵗʰ **S25.32 Major laceration of innominate or subclavian vein**
    Complete transection of innominate or subclavian vein
    Traumatic rupture of innominate or subclavian vein
    7ᵗʰ **S25.321 Major laceration of right innominate or subclavian vein** POA MCC CC/MCC Exc
    7ᵗʰ **S25.322 Major laceration of left innominate or subclavian vein** POA MCC CC/MCC Exc
    7ᵗʰ **S25.329 Major laceration of unspecified innominate or subclavian vein** POA MCC CC/MCC Exc
  6ᵗʰ **S25.39 Other specified injury of innominate or subclavian vein**
    7ᵗʰ **S25.391 Other specified injury of right innominate or subclavian vein** POA MCC CC/MCC Exc
    7ᵗʰ **S25.392 Other specified injury of left innominate or subclavian vein** POA MCC CC/MCC Exc
    7ᵗʰ **S25.399 Other specified injury of unspecified innominate or subclavian vein** POA MCC CC/MCC Exc

5ᵗʰ **S25.4 Injury of** pulmonary blood vessels
  6ᵗʰ **S25.40 Unspecified injury of pulmonary blood vessels**
    7ᵗʰ **S25.401 Unspecified injury of right pulmonary blood vessels** POA MCC CC/MCC Exc
    7ᵗʰ **S25.402 Unspecified injury of left pulmonary blood vessels** POA MCC CC/MCC Exc
    7ᵗʰ **S25.409 Unspecified injury of unspecified pulmonary blood vessels** POA MCC CC/MCC Exc
  6ᵗʰ **S25.41 Minor laceration of pulmonary blood vessels**
    Incomplete transection of pulmonary blood vessels
    Laceration of pulmonary blood vessels NOS
    Superficial laceration of pulmonary blood vessels
    7ᵗʰ **S25.411 Minor laceration of right pulmonary blood vessels** POA MCC CC/MCC Exc
    7ᵗʰ **S25.412 Minor laceration of left pulmonary blood vessels** POA MCC CC/MCC Exc
    7ᵗʰ **S25.419 Minor laceration of unspecified pulmonary blood vessels** POA MCC CC/MCC Exc
  6ᵗʰ **S25.42 Major laceration of pulmonary blood vessels**
    Complete transection of pulmonary blood vessels
    Traumatic rupture of pulmonary blood vessels
    7ᵗʰ **S25.421 Major laceration of right pulmonary blood vessels** POA MCC CC/MCC Exc
    7ᵗʰ **S25.422 Major laceration of left pulmonary blood vessels** POA MCC CC/MCC Exc
    7ᵗʰ **S25.429 Major laceration of unspecified pulmonary blood vessels** POA MCC CC/MCC Exc
  6ᵗʰ **S25.49 Other specified injury of pulmonary blood vessels**
    7ᵗʰ **S25.491 Other specified injury of right pulmonary blood vessels** POA MCC CC/MCC Exc
    7ᵗʰ **S25.492 Other specified injury of left pulmonary blood vessels** POA MCC CC/MCC Exc

7ᵗʰ **S25.499 Other specified injury of unspecified pulmonary blood vessels** POA MCC CC/MCC Exc

5ᵗʰ **S25.5 Injury of** intercostal blood vessels
  6ᵗʰ **S25.50 Unspecified injury of intercostal blood vessels**
    7ᵗʰ **S25.501 Unspecified injury of intercostal blood vessels, right side**
    7ᵗʰ **S25.502 Unspecified injury of intercostal blood vessels, left side** CC POA CC/MCC Exc
    7ᵗʰ **S25.509 Unspecified injury of intercostal blood vessels, unspecified side** CC POA CC/MCC Exc
  6ᵗʰ **S25.51 Laceration of intercostal blood vessels**
    7ᵗʰ **S25.511 Laceration of intercostal blood vessels, right side** CC POA CC/MCC Exc
    7ᵗʰ **S25.512 Laceration of intercostal blood vessels, left side** CC POA CC/MCC Exc
    7ᵗʰ **S25.519 Laceration of intercostal blood vessels, unspecified side** CC POA CC/MCC Exc
  6ᵗʰ **S25.59 Other specified injury of intercostal blood vessels**
    7ᵗʰ **S25.591 Other specified injury of intercostal blood vessels, right side** CC POA CC/MCC Exc
    7ᵗʰ **S25.592 Other specified injury of intercostal blood vessels, left side** CC POA CC/MCC Exc
    7ᵗʰ **S25.599 Other specified injury of intercostal blood vessels, unspecified side** CC POA CC/MCC Exc

5ᵗʰ **S25.8 Injury of** other blood vessels of thorax
    Injury of azygos vein
    Injury of mammary artery or vein
  6ᵗʰ **S25.80 Unspecified injury of other blood vessels of thorax**
    7ᵗʰ **S25.801 Unspecified injury of other blood vessels of thorax, right side** CC POA CC/MCC Exc
    7ᵗʰ **S25.802 Unspecified injury of other blood vessels of thorax, left side** CC POA CC/MCC Exc
    7ᵗʰ **S25.809 Unspecified injury of other blood vessels of thorax, unspecified side** CC POA CC/MCC Exc
  6ᵗʰ **S25.81 Laceration of other blood vessels of thorax**
    7ᵗʰ **S25.811 Laceration of other blood vessels of thorax, right side** CC POA CC/MCC Exc
    7ᵗʰ **S25.812 Laceration of other blood vessels of thorax, left side** CC POA CC/MCC Exc
    7ᵗʰ **S25.819 Laceration of other blood vessels of thorax, unspecified side** CC POA CC/MCC Exc
  6ᵗʰ **S25.89 Other specified injury of other blood vessels of thorax**
    7ᵗʰ **S25.891 Other specified injury of other blood vessels of thorax, right side** CC POA CC/MCC Exc
    7ᵗʰ **S25.892 Other specified injury of other blood vessels of thorax, left side** CC POA CC/MCC Exc
    7ᵗʰ **S25.899 Other specified injury of other blood vessels of thorax, unspecified side** CC POA CC/MCC Exc

5ᵗʰ **S25.9 Injury of** unspecified blood vessel of thorax
    7ᵗʰ **S25.90 Unspecified injury of unspecified blood vessel of thorax** CC POA CC/MCC Exc
    7ᵗʰ **S25.91 Laceration of unspecified blood vessel of thorax** CC POA CC/MCC Exc
    7ᵗʰ **S25.99 Other specified injury of unspecified blood vessel of thorax** CC POA CC/MCC Exc

4ᵗʰ **S26 Injury of heart**
    Code also any associated:
      open wound of thorax (S21.-)
      traumatic hemopneumothorax (S27.2)
      traumatic hemothorax (S27.1)
      traumatic pneumothorax (S27.0)
    The appropriate 7th character is to be added to each code from category S26
      A = initial encounter
      D = subsequent encounter
      S = sequela
  5ᵗʰ **S26.0 Injury of heart** with hemopericardium
    7ᵗʰ **S26.00 Unspecified injury of heart with hemopericardium** CC POA CC/MCC Exc

Unspecified Code   Other Specified Code   Manifestation Code   N Newborn   P Pediatric   M Maternity   A Adult   ♂ Male   ♀ Female
● New Code   ▲ Revised Code Title   ▶◀ Revised Text   NOTES   INCLUDES   EXCLUDES1 Not coded here   EXCLUDES2 Not included here
4ᵗʰ 4ᵗʰ character required   5ᵗʰ 5ᵗʰ character required   6ᵗʰ 6ᵗʰ character required   7ᵗʰ 7ᵗʰ character required   Extension 'X' Alert
HAC Hospital-acquired condition (HAC) alert   AHA AHA Coding Clinic©   📪 Code first alert

2020 ICD-10-CM   When symbols appear on a code that requires a 7th character extension, refer to Appendix B to identify applicable 7th character codes.   **993**

- S26.01 Contusion of heart with hemopericardium
- S26.02 Laceration of heart with hemopericardium
    - S26.020 Mild laceration of heart with hemopericardium
      Laceration of heart without penetration of heart chamber
    - S26.021 Moderate laceration of heart with hemopericardium
      Laceration of heart with penetration of heart chamber
    - S26.022 Major laceration of heart with hemopericardium
      Laceration of heart with penetration of multiple heart chambers
  - S26.09 Other injury of heart with hemopericardium
- S26.1 Injury of heart without hemopericardium
  - S26.10 Unspecified injury of heart without hemopericardium
  - S26.11 Contusion of heart without hemopericardium
  - S26.12 Laceration of heart without hemopericardium
  - S26.19 Other injury of heart without hemopericardium
- S26.9 Injury of heart, unspecified with or without hemopericardium
  - S26.90 Unspecified injury of heart, unspecified with or without hemopericardium
  - S26.91 Contusion of heart, unspecified with or without hemopericardium
  - S26.92 Laceration of heart, unspecified with or without hemopericardium
    Laceration of heart NOS
  - S26.99 Other injury of heart, unspecified with or without hemopericardium

- S27 Injury of other and unspecified intrathoracic organs
  Code also any associated open wound of thorax (S21.-)
  EXCLUDES2 injury of cervical esophagus (S10-S19)
  injury of trachea (cervical) (S10-S19)

  The appropriate 7th character is to be added to each code from category S27
  A = initial encounter
  D = subsequent encounter
  S = sequela

  - S27.0 Traumatic pneumothorax
    EXCLUDES1 spontaneous pneumothorax (J93.-)
  - S27.1 Traumatic hemothorax
  - S27.2 Traumatic hemopneumothorax
  - S27.3 Other and unspecified injuries of lung
    - S27.30 Unspecified injury of lung
      - S27.301 Unspecified injury of lung, unilateral
      - S27.302 Unspecified injury of lung, bilateral
      - S27.309 Unspecified injury of lung, unspecified
    - S27.31 Primary blast injury of lung
      Blast injury of lung NOS
      - S27.311 Primary blast injury of lung, unilateral
      - S27.312 Primary blast injury of lung, bilateral
      - S27.319 Primary blast injury of lung, unspecified
    - S27.32 Contusion of lung
      - S27.321 Contusion of lung, unilateral
      - S27.322 Contusion of lung, bilateral
      - S27.329 Contusion of lung, unspecified

- S27.33 Laceration of lung
  - S27.331 Laceration of lung, unilateral
  - S27.332 Laceration of lung, bilateral
  - S27.339 Laceration of lung, unspecified
- S27.39 Other injuries of lung
  Secondary blast injury of lung
  - S27.391 Other injuries of lung, unilateral
  - S27.392 Other injuries of lung, bilateral
  - S27.399 Other injuries of lung, unspecified
- S27.4 Injury of bronchus
  - S27.40 Unspecified injury of bronchus
    - S27.401 Unspecified injury of bronchus, unilateral
    - S27.402 Unspecified injury of bronchus, bilateral
    - S27.409 Unspecified injury of bronchus, unspecified
  - S27.41 Primary blast injury of bronchus
    Blast injury of bronchus NOS
    - S27.411 Primary blast injury of bronchus, unilateral
    - S27.412 Primary blast injury of bronchus, bilateral
    - S27.419 Primary blast injury of bronchus, unspecified
  - S27.42 Contusion of bronchus
    - S27.421 Contusion of bronchus, unilateral
    - S27.422 Contusion of bronchus, bilateral
    - S27.429 Contusion of bronchus, unspecified
  - S27.43 Laceration of bronchus
    - S27.431 Laceration of bronchus, unilateral
    - S27.432 Laceration of bronchus, bilateral
    - S27.439 Laceration of bronchus, unspecified
  - S27.49 Other injury of bronchus
    Secondary blast injury of bronchus
    - S27.491 Other injury of bronchus, unilateral
    - S27.492 Other injury of bronchus, bilateral
    - S27.499 Other injury of bronchus, unspecified
- S27.5 Injury of thoracic trachea
  - S27.50 Unspecified injury of thoracic trachea
  - S27.51 Primary blast injury of thoracic trachea
    Blast injury of thoracic trachea NOS
  - S27.52 Contusion of thoracic trachea
  - S27.53 Laceration of thoracic trachea
  - S27.59 Other injury of thoracic trachea
    Secondary blast injury of thoracic trachea
- S27.6 Injury of pleura
  - S27.60 Unspecified injury of pleura
  - S27.63 Laceration of pleura
  - S27.69 Other injury of pleura
- S27.8 Injury of other specified intrathoracic organs
  - S27.80 Injury of diaphragm
    - S27.802 Contusion of diaphragm
    - S27.803 Laceration of diaphragm
    - S27.808 Other injury of diaphragm
    - S27.809 Unspecified injury of diaphragm
  - S27.81 Injury of esophagus (thoracic part)
    - S27.812 Contusion of esophagus (thoracic part)

PDxⁿ Unacceptable principal diagnosis symbol per Medicare code edits   Code exempt from diagnosis present on admission requirement
? Questionable admission   Complication or comorbidity   MCC Major complication or comorbidity   CC/MCC exclusion
HCC HCC diagnosis code   RxHCC RxHCC diagnosis code   MACRA code   **DEFINITION** Describes condition/terminology
TIP Coding guidance   Official Guideline Reference   Z1 Z code as first-listed diagnosis

When symbols appear on a code that requires a 7th character extension, refer to Appendix B to identify applicable 7th character codes.
2020 ICD-10-CM

7️⃣ S27.813 Laceration of esophagus (thoracic part) POA MCC CC/MCC Exc

7️⃣ S27.818 Other injury of esophagus (thoracic part) POA MCC CC/MCC Exc

7️⃣ S27.819 Unspecified injury of esophagus (thoracic part) POA MCC CC/MCC Exc

6️⃣ S27.89 Injury of other specified intrathoracic organs
Injury of lymphatic thoracic duct
Injury of thymus gland

7️⃣ S27.892 Contusion of other specified intrathoracic organs CC POA CC/MCC Exc

7️⃣ S27.893 Laceration of other specified intrathoracic organs CC POA CC/MCC Exc

7️⃣ S27.898 Other injury of other specified intrathoracic organs CC POA CC/MCC Exc

7️⃣ S27.899 Unspecified injury of other specified intrathoracic organs CC POA CC/MCC Exc

7️⃣ S27.9 Injury of unspecified intrathoracic organ CC POA CC/MCC Exc

4️⃣ S28 Crushing injury of thorax, and traumatic amputation of part of thorax

The appropriate 7th character is to be added to each code from category S28
A = initial encounter
D = subsequent encounter
S = sequela

7️⃣ S28.0 Crushed chest POA
Use additional code for all associated injuries
EXCLUDES1 flail chest (S22.5)

7️⃣ S28.1 Traumatic amputation (partial) of part of thorax, except breast CC POA CC/MCC Exc

5️⃣ S28.2 Traumatic amputation of breast

6️⃣ S28.21 Complete traumatic amputation of breast
Traumatic amputation of breast NOS

7️⃣ S28.211 Complete traumatic amputation of right breast POA

7️⃣ S28.212 Complete traumatic amputation of left breast POA

7️⃣ S28.219 Complete traumatic amputation of unspecified breast POA

6️⃣ S28.22 Partial traumatic amputation of breast

7️⃣ S28.221 Partial traumatic amputation of right breast POA

7️⃣ S28.222 Partial traumatic amputation of left breast POA

7️⃣ S28.229 Partial traumatic amputation of unspecified breast POA

4️⃣ S29 Other and unspecified injuries of thorax
Code also any associated open wound (S21.-)

The appropriate 7th character is to be added to each code from category S29
A = initial encounter
D = subsequent encounter
S = sequela

5️⃣ S29.0 Injury of muscle and tendon at thorax level

6️⃣ S29.00 Unspecified injury of muscle and tendon of thorax

7️⃣ S29.001 Unspecified injury of muscle and tendon of front wall of thorax POA

7️⃣ S29.002 Unspecified injury of muscle and tendon of back wall of thorax POA

7️⃣ S29.009 Unspecified injury of muscle and tendon of unspecified wall of thorax POA

6️⃣ S29.01 Strain of muscle and tendon of thorax

7️⃣ S29.011 Strain of muscle and tendon of front wall of thorax POA

7️⃣ S29.012 Strain of muscle and tendon of back wall of thorax POA

7️⃣ S29.019 Strain of muscle and tendon of unspecified wall of thorax POA

6️⃣ S29.02 Laceration of muscle and tendon of thorax

7️⃣ S29.021 Laceration of muscle and tendon of front wall of thorax CC POA CC/MCC Exc

7️⃣ S29.022 Laceration of muscle and tendon of back wall of thorax POA

7️⃣ S29.029 Laceration of muscle and tendon of unspecified wall of thorax CC POA CC/MCC Exc

6️⃣ S29.09 Other injury of muscle and tendon of thorax

7️⃣ S29.091 Other injury of muscle and tendon of front wall of thorax POA

7️⃣ S29.092 Other injury of muscle and tendon of back wall of thorax POA

7️⃣ S29.099 Other injury of muscle and tendon of unspecified wall of thorax POA

7️⃣ S29.8 Other specified injuries of thorax POA

7️⃣ S29.9 Unspecified injury of thorax POA

Injuries to the abdomen, lower back, lumbar spine, pelvis and external genitals (S30-S39)

INCLUDES injuries to the abdominal wall
injuries to the anus
injuries to the buttock
injuries to the external genitalia
injuries to the flank
injuries to the groin

EXCLUDES2 burns and corrosions (T20-T32)
effects of foreign body in anus and rectum (T18.5)
effects of foreign body in genitourinary tract (T19.-)
effects of foreign body in stomach, small intestine and colon (T18.2-T18.4)
frostbite (T33-T34)
insect bite or sting, venomous (T63.4)

4️⃣ S30 Superficial injury of abdomen, lower back, pelvis and external genitals

EXCLUDES2 superficial injury of hip (S70.-)

The appropriate 7th character is to be added to each code from category S30
A = initial encounter
D = subsequent encounter
S = sequela

7️⃣ S30.0 Contusion of lower back and pelvis POA
Contusion of buttock

7️⃣ S30.1 Contusion of abdominal wall POA
Contusion of flank
Contusion of groin

5️⃣ S30.2 Contusion of external genital organs

6️⃣ S30.20 Contusion of unspecified external genital organ

7️⃣ S30.201 Contusion of unspecified external genital organ, male POA ♂

7️⃣ S30.202 Contusion of unspecified external genital organ, female POA ♀

6️⃣ S30.21 Contusion of penis POA ♂

6️⃣ S30.22 Contusion of scrotum and testes POA ♂

6️⃣ S30.23 Contusion of vagina and vulva POA ♀

7️⃣ S30.3 Contusion of anus POA

5️⃣ S30.8 Other superficial injuries of abdomen, lower back, pelvis and external genitals

6️⃣ S30.81 Abrasion of abdomen, lower back, pelvis and external genitals

7️⃣ S30.810 Abrasion of lower back and pelvis POA

7️⃣ S30.811 Abrasion of abdominal wall POA

7️⃣ S30.812 Abrasion of penis POA ♂

7️⃣ S30.813 Abrasion of scrotum and testes POA ♂

7️⃣ S30.814 Abrasion of vagina and vulva POA ♀

7️⃣ S30.815 Abrasion of unspecified external genital organs, male POA ♂

7️⃣ S30.816 Abrasion of unspecified external genital organs, female POA ♀

7️⃣ S30.817 Abrasion of anus POA

6ᵗʰ **S30.82** Blister (nonthermal) of abdomen, lower back, pelvis and external genitals
- 7ᵗʰ **S30.820** Blister (nonthermal) of lower back and pelvis POA
- 7ᵗʰ **S30.821** Blister (nonthermal) of abdominal wall POA
- 7ᵗʰ **S30.822** Blister (nonthermal) of penis POA ♂
- 7ᵗʰ **S30.823** Blister (nonthermal) of scrotum and testes POA ♂
- 7ᵗʰ **S30.824** Blister (nonthermal) of vagina and vulva POA ♀
- 7ᵗʰ **S30.825** Blister (nonthermal) of unspecified external genital organs, male POA ♂
- 7ᵗʰ **S30.826** Blister (nonthermal) of unspecified external genital organs, female POA ♀
- 7ᵗʰ **S30.827** Blister (nonthermal) of anus POA

6ᵗʰ **S30.84** External constriction of abdomen, lower back, pelvis and external genitals
- 7ᵗʰ **S30.840** External constriction of lower back and pelvis POA
- 7ᵗʰ **S30.841** External constriction of abdominal wall POA
- 7ᵗʰ **S30.842** External constriction of penis POA ♂
  Hair tourniquet syndrome of penis
  Use additional cause code to identify the constricting item (W49.0-)
- 7ᵗʰ **S30.843** External constriction of scrotum and testes POA ♂
- 7ᵗʰ **S30.844** External constriction of vagina and vulva POA ♀
- 7ᵗʰ **S30.845** External constriction of unspecified external genital organs, male POA ♂
- 7ᵗʰ **S30.846** External constriction of unspecified external genital organs, female POA ♀

6ᵗʰ **S30.85** Superficial foreign body of abdomen, lower back, pelvis and external genitals
  Splinter in the abdomen, lower back, pelvis and external genitals
- 7ᵗʰ **S30.850** Superficial foreign body of lower back and pelvis POA
- 7ᵗʰ **S30.851** Superficial foreign body of abdominal wall POA
- 7ᵗʰ **S30.852** Superficial foreign body of penis POA ♂
- 7ᵗʰ **S30.853** Superficial foreign body of scrotum and testes POA ♂
- 7ᵗʰ **S30.854** Superficial foreign body of vagina and vulva POA ♀
- 7ᵗʰ **S30.855** Superficial foreign body of unspecified external genital organs, male POA ♂
- 7ᵗʰ **S30.856** Superficial foreign body of unspecified external genital organs, female POA ♀
- 7ᵗʰ **S30.857** Superficial foreign body of anus POA

6ᵗʰ **S30.86** Insect bite (nonvenomous) of abdomen, lower back, pelvis and external genitals
- 7ᵗʰ **S30.860** Insect bite (nonvenomous) of lower back and pelvis POA
- 7ᵗʰ **S30.861** Insect bite (nonvenomous) of abdominal wall POA
- 7ᵗʰ **S30.862** Insect bite (nonvenomous) of penis POA ♂
- 7ᵗʰ **S30.863** Insect bite (nonvenomous) of scrotum and testes POA ♂
- 7ᵗʰ **S30.864** Insect bite (nonvenomous) of vagina and vulva POA ♀
- 7ᵗʰ **S30.865** Insect bite (nonvenomous) of unspecified external genital organs, male POA ♂
- 7ᵗʰ **S30.866** Insect bite (nonvenomous) of unspecified external genital organs, female POA ♀
- 7ᵗʰ **S30.867** Insect bite (nonvenomous) of anus POA

6ᵗʰ **S30.87** Other superficial bite of abdomen, lower back, pelvis and external genitals
  EXCLUDES1 open bite of abdomen, lower back, pelvis and external genitals (S31.05, S31.15, S31.25, S31.35, S31.45, S31.55)
- 7ᵗʰ **S30.870** Other superficial bite of lower back and pelvis POA
- 7ᵗʰ **S30.871** Other superficial bite of abdominal wall POA
- 7ᵗʰ **S30.872** Other superficial bite of penis POA ♂
- 7ᵗʰ **S30.873** Other superficial bite of scrotum and testes POA ♂
- 7ᵗʰ **S30.874** Other superficial bite of vagina and vulva POA ♀
- 7ᵗʰ **S30.875** Other superficial bite of unspecified external genital organs, male POA ♂
- 7ᵗʰ **S30.876** Other superficial bite of unspecified external genital organs, female POA ♀
- 7ᵗʰ **S30.877** Other superficial bite of anus POA

5ᵗʰ **S30.9** Unspecified superficial injury of abdomen, lower back, pelvis and external genitals
- 7ᵗʰ **S30.91** Unspecified superficial injury of lower back and pelvis POA
- 7ᵗʰ **S30.92** Unspecified superficial injury of abdominal wall POA
- 7ᵗʰ **S30.93** Unspecified superficial injury of penis POA ♂
- 7ᵗʰ **S30.94** Unspecified superficial injury of scrotum and testes POA ♂
- 7ᵗʰ **S30.95** Unspecified superficial injury of vagina and vulva POA ♀
- 7ᵗʰ **S30.96** Unspecified superficial injury of unspecified external genital organs, male POA ♂
- 7ᵗʰ **S30.97** Unspecified superficial injury of unspecified external genital organs, female POA ♀
- 7ᵗʰ **S30.98** Unspecified superficial injury of anus POA

4ᵗʰ **S31** Open wound of abdomen, lower back, pelvis and external genitals
  Code also any associated:
    spinal cord injury (S24.0, S24.1-, S34.0-, S34.1-)
    wound infection
  EXCLUDES1 traumatic amputation of part of abdomen, lower back and pelvis (S38.2-, S38.3)
  EXCLUDES2 open wound of hip (S71.00-S71.02)
    open fracture of pelvis (S32.1--S32.9 with 7th character B)
  The appropriate 7th character is to be added to each code from category S31
    A = initial encounter
    D = subsequent encounter
    S = sequela

5ᵗʰ **S31.0** Open wound of lower back and pelvis
- 6ᵗʰ **S31.00** Unspecified open wound of lower back and pelvis
  - 7ᵗʰ **S31.000** Unspecified open wound of lower back and pelvis without penetration into retroperitoneum POA
    Unspecified open wound of lower back and pelvis NOS
  - 7ᵗʰ **S31.001** Unspecified open wound of lower back and pelvis with penetration into retroperitoneum POA MCC CC/MCC Exc
- 6ᵗʰ **S31.01** Laceration without foreign body of lower back and pelvis
  - 7ᵗʰ **S31.010** Laceration without foreign body of lower back and pelvis without penetration into retroperitoneum POA
    Laceration without foreign body of lower back and pelvis NOS
  - 7ᵗʰ **S31.011** Laceration without foreign body of lower back and pelvis with penetration into retroperitoneum POA MCC CC/MCC Exc
- 6ᵗʰ **S31.02** Laceration with foreign body of lower back and pelvis
  - 7ᵗʰ **S31.020** Laceration with foreign body of lower back and pelvis without penetration into retroperitoneum POA
    Laceration with foreign body of lower back and pelvis NOS
  - 7ᵗʰ **S31.021** Laceration with foreign body of lower back and pelvis with penetration into retroperitoneum POA MCC CC/MCC Exc

---

POA Unacceptable principal diagnosis symbol per Medicare code edits POA Code exempt from diagnosis present on admission requirement
? Questionable admission CC Complication or comorbidity MCC Major complication or comorbidity CC/MCC Exc CC/MCC exclusion
HCC HCC diagnosis code RxHCC RxHCC diagnosis code MACRA code **DEFINITION** Describes condition/terminology
TIP Coding guidance 👁 Official Guideline Reference Z1 Z code as first-listed diagnosis

996

When symbols appear on a code that requires a 7th character extension, refer to Appendix B to identify applicable 7th character codes.

2020 ICD-10-CM

6ᵗʰ S31.03 Puncture wound without foreign body of lower back and pelvis

  7ᵗʰ S31.030 Puncture wound without foreign body of lower back and pelvis without penetration into retroperitoneum POA

    Puncture wound without foreign body of lower back and pelvis NOS

  7ᵗʰ S31.031 Puncture wound without foreign body of lower back and pelvis with penetration into retroperitoneum POA MCC CC/MCC Exc.

6ᵗʰ S31.04 Puncture wound with foreign body of lower back and pelvis

  7ᵗʰ S31.040 Puncture wound with foreign body of lower back and pelvis without penetration into retroperitoneum POA

    Puncture wound with foreign body of lower back and pelvis NOS

  7ᵗʰ S31.041 Puncture wound with foreign body of lower back and pelvis with penetration into retroperitoneum POA MCC CC/MCC Exc.

6ᵗʰ S31.05 Open bite of lower back and pelvis

    Bite of lower back and pelvis NOS

    EXCLUDES1 superficial bite of lower back and pelvis (S30.860, S30.870)

  7ᵗʰ S31.050 Open bite of lower back and pelvis without penetration into retroperitoneum POA

    Open bite of lower back and pelvis NOS

  7ᵗʰ S31.051 Open bite of lower back and pelvis with penetration into retroperitoneum POA MCC CC/MCC Exc.

5ᵗʰ S31.1 Open wound of abdominal wall without penetration into peritoneal cavity

    Open wound of abdominal wall NOS

    EXCLUDES2 open wound of abdominal wall with penetration into peritoneal cavity (S31.6-)

6ᵗʰ S31.10 Unspecified open wound of abdominal wall without penetration into peritoneal cavity

  7ᵗʰ S31.100 Unspecified open wound of abdominal wall, right upper quadrant without penetration into peritoneal cavity POA

  7ᵗʰ S31.101 Unspecified open wound of abdominal wall, left upper quadrant without penetration into peritoneal cavity POA

  7ᵗʰ S31.102 Unspecified open wound of abdominal wall, epigastric region without penetration into peritoneal cavity POA

  7ᵗʰ S31.103 Unspecified open wound of abdominal wall, right lower quadrant without penetration into peritoneal cavity POA

  7ᵗʰ S31.104 Unspecified open wound of abdominal wall, left lower quadrant without penetration into peritoneal cavity POA

  7ᵗʰ S31.105 Unspecified open wound of abdominal wall, periumbilic region without penetration into peritoneal cavity POA

  7ᵗʰ S31.109 Unspecified open wound of abdominal wall, unspecified quadrant without penetration into peritoneal cavity POA

    Unspecified open wound of abdominal wall NOS

6ᵗʰ S31.11 Laceration without foreign body of abdominal wall without penetration into peritoneal cavity

  7ᵗʰ S31.110 Laceration without foreign body of abdominal wall, right upper quadrant without penetration into peritoneal cavity POA

  7ᵗʰ S31.111 Laceration without foreign body of abdominal wall, left upper quadrant without penetration into peritoneal cavity POA

  7ᵗʰ S31.112 Laceration without foreign body of abdominal wall, epigastric region without penetration into peritoneal cavity POA

  7ᵗʰ S31.113 Laceration without foreign body of abdominal wall, right lower quadrant without penetration into peritoneal cavity POA

  7ᵗʰ S31.114 Laceration without foreign body of abdominal wall, left lower quadrant without penetration into peritoneal cavity POA

  7ᵗʰ S31.115 Laceration without foreign body of abdominal wall, periumbilic region without penetration into peritoneal cavity POA

  7ᵗʰ S31.119 Laceration without foreign body of abdominal wall, unspecified quadrant without penetration into peritoneal cavity POA

6ᵗʰ S31.12 Laceration with foreign body of abdominal wall without penetration into peritoneal cavity

  7ᵗʰ S31.120 Laceration of abdominal wall with foreign body, right upper quadrant without penetration into peritoneal cavity POA

  7ᵗʰ S31.121 Laceration of abdominal wall with foreign body, left upper quadrant without penetration into peritoneal cavity POA

  7ᵗʰ S31.122 Laceration of abdominal wall with foreign body, epigastric region without penetration into peritoneal cavity POA

  7ᵗʰ S31.123 Laceration of abdominal wall with foreign body, right lower quadrant without penetration into peritoneal cavity POA

  7ᵗʰ S31.124 Laceration of abdominal wall with foreign body, left lower quadrant without penetration into peritoneal cavity POA

  7ᵗʰ S31.125 Laceration of abdominal wall with foreign body, periumbilic region without penetration into peritoneal cavity POA

  7ᵗʰ S31.129 Laceration of abdominal wall with foreign body, unspecified quadrant without penetration into peritoneal cavity POA

6ᵗʰ S31.13 Puncture wound of abdominal wall without foreign body without penetration into peritoneal cavity

  7ᵗʰ S31.130 Puncture wound of abdominal wall without foreign body, right upper quadrant without penetration into peritoneal cavity POA

  7ᵗʰ S31.131 Puncture wound of abdominal wall without foreign body, left upper quadrant without penetration into peritoneal cavity POA

  7ᵗʰ S31.132 Puncture wound of abdominal wall without foreign body, epigastric region without penetration into peritoneal cavity POA

  7ᵗʰ S31.133 Puncture wound of abdominal wall without foreign body, right lower quadrant without penetration into peritoneal cavity POA

  7ᵗʰ S31.134 Puncture wound of abdominal wall without foreign body, left lower quadrant without penetration into peritoneal cavity POA

  7ᵗʰ S31.135 Puncture wound of abdominal wall without foreign body, periumbilic region without penetration into peritoneal cavity POA

  7ᵗʰ S31.139 Puncture wound of abdominal wall without foreign body, unspecified quadrant without penetration into peritoneal cavity POA

Unspecified Code Other Specified Code Manifestation Code Ⓝ Newborn Ⓟ Pediatric Ⓜ Maternity Ⓐ Adult ♂ Male ♀ Female

● New Code ▲ Revised Code Title ▶◀ Revised Text NOTES INCLUDES EXCLUDES1 Not coded here EXCLUDES2 Not included here

4ᵗʰ 4ᵗʰ character required 5ᵗʰ 5ᵗʰ character required 6ᵗʰ 6ᵗʰ character required 7ᵗʰ 7ᵗʰ character required Ⓧ Extension 'X' Alert

HAC Hospital-acquired condition (HAC) alert AHA AHA Coding Clinic© 📖 Code first alert

[6th] **S31.14 Puncture wound of abdominal wall with foreign body without penetration into peritoneal cavity**

- [7th] **S31.140 Puncture wound of abdominal wall with foreign body, right upper quadrant without penetration into peritoneal cavity** [POA]
- [7th] **S31.141 Puncture wound of abdominal wall with foreign body, left upper quadrant without penetration into peritoneal cavity** [POA]
- [7th] **S31.142 Puncture wound of abdominal wall with foreign body, epigastric region without penetration into peritoneal cavity** [POA]
- [7th] **S31.143 Puncture wound of abdominal wall with foreign body, right lower quadrant without penetration into peritoneal cavity** [POA]
- [7th] **S31.144 Puncture wound of abdominal wall with foreign body, left lower quadrant without penetration into peritoneal cavity** [POA]
- [7th] **S31.145 Puncture wound of abdominal wall with foreign body, periumbilic region without penetration into peritoneal cavity** [POA]
- [7th] **S31.149 Puncture wound of abdominal wall with foreign body, unspecified quadrant without penetration into peritoneal cavity** [POA]

[6th] **S31.15 Open bite of abdominal wall without penetration into peritoneal cavity**
Bite of abdominal wall NOS
[EXCLUDES1] *superficial bite of abdominal wall (S30.871)*

- [7th] **S31.150 Open bite of abdominal wall, right upper quadrant without penetration into peritoneal cavity** [POA]
- [7th] **S31.151 Open bite of abdominal wall, left upper quadrant without penetration into peritoneal cavity** [POA]
- [7th] **S31.152 Open bite of abdominal wall, epigastric region without penetration into peritoneal cavity** [POA]
- [7th] **S31.153 Open bite of abdominal wall, right lower quadrant without penetration into peritoneal cavity** [POA]
- [7th] **S31.154 Open bite of abdominal wall, left lower quadrant without penetration into peritoneal cavity** [POA]
- [7th] **S31.155 Open bite of abdominal wall, periumbilic region without penetration into peritoneal cavity** [POA]
- [7th] **S31.159 Open bite of abdominal wall, unspecified quadrant without penetration into peritoneal cavity** [POA]

[5th] **S31.2 Open wound of penis**

- [7th] **S31.20 Unspecified open wound of penis** [POA] ♂
- [7th] **S31.21 Laceration without foreign body of penis** [POA] ♂
- [7th] **S31.22 Laceration with foreign body of penis** [POA] ♂
- [7th] **S31.23 Puncture wound without foreign body of penis** [POA] ♂
- [7th] **S31.24 Puncture wound with foreign body of penis** [POA] ♂
- [7th] **S31.25 Open bite of penis** [POA] ♂
  Bite of penis NOS
  [EXCLUDES1] *superficial bite of penis (S30.862, S30.872)*

[5th] **S31.3 Open wound of scrotum and testes**

- [7th] **S31.30 Unspecified open wound of scrotum and testes** [POA] ♂
- [7th] **S31.31 Laceration without foreign body of scrotum and testes** [POA] ♂
- [7th] **S31.32 Laceration with foreign body of scrotum and testes** [POA] ♂
- [7th] **S31.33 Puncture wound without foreign body of scrotum and testes** [POA] ♂
- [7th] **S31.34 Puncture wound with foreign body of scrotum and testes** [POA] ♂
- [7th] **S31.35 Open bite of scrotum and testes** [POA] ♂
  Bite of scrotum and testes NOS
  [EXCLUDES1] *superficial bite of scrotum and testes (S30.863, S30.873)*

[5th] **S31.4 Open wound of vagina and vulva**
[EXCLUDES1] *injury to vagina and vulva during delivery (O70.-, O71.4)*

- [7th] **S31.40 Unspecified open wound of vagina and vulva** [POA] ♀
- [7th] **S31.41 Laceration without foreign body of vagina and vulva** [POA] ♀
- [7th] **S31.42 Laceration with foreign body of vagina and vulva** [POA] ♀
- [7th] **S31.43 Puncture wound without foreign body of vagina and vulva** [POA] ♀
- [7th] **S31.44 Puncture wound with foreign body of vagina and vulva** [POA] ♀
- [7th] **S31.45 Open bite of vagina and vulva** [POA] ♀
  Bite of vagina and vulva NOS
  [EXCLUDES1] *superficial bite of vagina and vulva (S30.864, S30.874)*

[5th] **S31.5 Open wound of unspecified external genital organs**
[EXCLUDES1] *traumatic amputation of external genital organs (S38.21, S38.22)*

[6th] **S31.50 Unspecified open wound of unspecified external genital organs**

- [7th] **S31.501 Unspecified open wound of unspecified external genital organs, male** [POA] ♂
- [7th] **S31.502 Unspecified open wound of unspecified external genital organs, female** [POA] ♀

[6th] **S31.51 Laceration without foreign body of unspecified external genital organs**

- [7th] **S31.511 Laceration without foreign body of unspecified external genital organs, male** [POA] ♂
- [7th] **S31.512 Laceration without foreign body of unspecified external genital organs, female** [POA] ♀

[6th] **S31.52 Laceration with foreign body of unspecified external genital organs**

- [7th] **S31.521 Laceration with foreign body of unspecified external genital organs, male** [POA] ♂
- [7th] **S31.522 Laceration with foreign body of unspecified external genital organs, female** [POA] ♀

[6th] **S31.53 Puncture wound without foreign body of unspecified external genital organs**

- [7th] **S31.531 Puncture wound without foreign body of unspecified external genital organs, male** [POA] ♂
- [7th] **S31.532 Puncture wound without foreign body of unspecified external genital organs, female** [POA] ♀

[6th] **S31.54 Puncture wound with foreign body of unspecified external genital organs**

- [7th] **S31.541 Puncture wound with foreign body of unspecified external genital organs, male** [POA] ♂
- [7th] **S31.542 Puncture wound with foreign body of unspecified external genital organs, female** [POA] ♀

[6th] **S31.55 Open bite of unspecified external genital organs**
Bite of unspecified external genital organs NOS
[EXCLUDES1] *superficial bite of unspecified external genital organs (S30.865, S30.866, S30.875, S30.876)*

- [7th] **S31.551 Open bite of unspecified external genital organs, male** [POA] ♂
- [7th] **S31.552 Open bite of unspecified external genital organs, female** [POA] ♀

[PDx] Unacceptable principal diagnosis symbol per Medicare code edits [POA] Code exempt from diagnosis present on admission requirement
[?] Questionable admission [CC] Complication or comorbidity [MCC] Major complication or comorbidity [CC/MCC Exc] CC/MCC exclusion
[HCC] HCC diagnosis code [RxHCC] RxHCC diagnosis code MACRA code **DEFINITION** Describes condition/terminology
TIP Coding guidance 👁 Official Guideline Reference [Z1] Z code as first-listed diagnosis

5ᵗʰ **S31.6 Open wound of** abdominal wall with penetration into peritoneal cavity

  6ᵗʰ **S31.60** Unspecified **open wound of abdominal wall with penetration into peritoneal cavity**

    7ᵗʰ **S31.600 Unspecified open wound of abdominal wall,** right upper quadrant **with penetration into peritoneal cavity** POA MCC CC/MCC Exc

    7ᵗʰ **S31.601 Unspecified open wound of abdominal wall,** left upper quadrant **with penetration into peritoneal cavity** POA MCC CC/MCC Exc

    7ᵗʰ **S31.602 Unspecified open wound of abdominal wall,** epigastric region **with penetration into peritoneal cavity** POA MCC CC/MCC Exc

    7ᵗʰ **S31.603 Unspecified open wound of abdominal wall,** right lower quadrant **with penetration into peritoneal cavity** POA MCC CC/MCC Exc

    7ᵗʰ **S31.604 Unspecified open wound of abdominal wall,** left lower quadrant **with penetration into peritoneal cavity** POA MCC CC/MCC Exc

    7ᵗʰ **S31.605 Unspecified open wound of abdominal wall,** periumbilic region **with penetration into peritoneal cavity** POA MCC CC/MCC Exc

    7ᵗʰ **S31.609 Unspecified open wound of abdominal wall, unspecified quadrant with penetration into peritoneal cavity** POA MCC CC/MCC Exc

  6ᵗʰ **S31.61** Laceration without foreign body **of abdominal wall with penetration into peritoneal cavity**

    7ᵗʰ **S31.610 Laceration without foreign body of abdominal wall,** right upper quadrant **with penetration into peritoneal cavity** POA MCC CC/MCC Exc

    7ᵗʰ **S31.611 Laceration without foreign body of abdominal wall,** left upper quadrant **with penetration into peritoneal cavity** POA MCC CC/MCC Exc

    7ᵗʰ **S31.612 Laceration without foreign body of abdominal wall,** epigastric region **with penetration into peritoneal cavity** POA MCC CC/MCC Exc

    7ᵗʰ **S31.613 Laceration without foreign body of abdominal wall,** right lower quadrant **with penetration into peritoneal cavity** POA MCC CC/MCC Exc

      AHA: Q4 2015

    7ᵗʰ **S31.614 Laceration without foreign body of abdominal wall,** left lower quadrant **with penetration into peritoneal cavity** POA MCC CC/MCC Exc

    7ᵗʰ **S31.615 Laceration without foreign body of abdominal wall,** periumbilic region **with penetration into peritoneal cavity** POA MCC CC/MCC Exc

    7ᵗʰ **S31.619 Laceration without foreign body of abdominal wall, unspecified quadrant with penetration into peritoneal cavity** POA MCC CC/MCC Exc

  6ᵗʰ **S31.62** Laceration with foreign body **of abdominal wall with penetration into peritoneal cavity**

    7ᵗʰ **S31.620 Laceration with foreign body of abdominal wall,** right upper quadrant **with penetration into peritoneal cavity** POA MCC CC/MCC Exc

    7ᵗʰ **S31.621 Laceration with foreign body of abdominal wall,** left upper quadrant **with penetration into peritoneal cavity** POA MCC CC/MCC Exc

    7ᵗʰ **S31.622 Laceration with foreign body of abdominal wall,** epigastric region **with penetration into peritoneal cavity** POA MCC CC/MCC Exc

    7ᵗʰ **S31.623 Laceration with foreign body of abdominal wall,** right lower quadrant **with penetration into peritoneal cavity** POA MCC CC/MCC Exc

    7ᵗʰ **S31.624 Laceration with foreign body of abdominal wall,** left lower quadrant **with penetration into peritoneal cavity** POA MCC CC/MCC Exc

    7ᵗʰ **S31.625 Laceration with foreign body of abdominal wall,** periumbilic region **with penetration into peritoneal cavity** POA MCC CC/MCC Exc

    7ᵗʰ **S31.629 Laceration with foreign body of abdominal wall, unspecified quadrant with penetration into peritoneal cavity** POA MCC CC/MCC Exc

  6ᵗʰ **S31.63** Puncture wound without foreign body **of abdominal wall with penetration into peritoneal cavity**

    7ᵗʰ **S31.630 Puncture wound without foreign body of abdominal wall,** right upper quadrant **with penetration into peritoneal cavity** POA MCC CC/MCC Exc

    7ᵗʰ **S31.631 Puncture wound without foreign body of abdominal wall,** left upper quadrant **with penetration into peritoneal cavity** POA MCC CC/MCC Exc

    7ᵗʰ **S31.632 Puncture wound without foreign body of abdominal wall,** epigastric region **with penetration into peritoneal cavity** POA MCC CC/MCC Exc

    7ᵗʰ **S31.633 Puncture wound without foreign body of abdominal wall,** right lower quadrant **with penetration into peritoneal cavity** POA MCC CC/MCC Exc

    7ᵗʰ **S31.634 Puncture wound without foreign body of abdominal wall,** left lower quadrant **with penetration into peritoneal cavity** POA MCC CC/MCC Exc

    7ᵗʰ **S31.635 Puncture wound without foreign body of abdominal wall,** periumbilic region **with penetration into peritoneal cavity** POA MCC CC/MCC Exc

    7ᵗʰ **S31.639 Puncture wound without foreign body of abdominal wall, unspecified quadrant with penetration into peritoneal cavity** POA MCC CC/MCC Exc

  6ᵗʰ **S31.64** Puncture wound with foreign body **of abdominal wall with penetration into peritoneal cavity**

    7ᵗʰ **S31.640 Puncture wound with foreign body of abdominal wall,** right upper quadrant **with penetration into peritoneal cavity** POA MCC CC/MCC Exc

    7ᵗʰ **S31.641 Puncture wound with foreign body of abdominal wall,** left upper quadrant **with penetration into peritoneal cavity** POA MCC CC/MCC Exc

    7ᵗʰ **S31.642 Puncture wound with foreign body of abdominal wall,** epigastric region **with penetration into peritoneal cavity** POA MCC CC/MCC Exc

    7ᵗʰ **S31.643 Puncture wound with foreign body of abdominal wall,** right lower quadrant **with penetration into peritoneal cavity** POA MCC CC/MCC Exc

    7ᵗʰ **S31.644 Puncture wound with foreign body of abdominal wall,** left lower quadrant **with penetration into peritoneal cavity** POA MCC CC/MCC Exc

    7ᵗʰ **S31.645 Puncture wound with foreign body of abdominal wall,** periumbilic region **with penetration into peritoneal cavity** POA MCC CC/MCC Exc

---

Unspecified Code   Other Specified Code   Manifestation Code   N Newborn   P Pediatric   M Maternity   A Adult   ♂ Male   ♀ Female
● New Code   ▲ Revised Code Title   ▶◀ Revised Text   **NOTES**   *INCLUDES*   *EXCLUDES1* Not coded here   *EXCLUDES2* Not included here
4ᵗʰ character required   5ᵗʰ character required   6ᵗʰ character required   7ᵗʰ character required   Extension 'X' Alert
HAC Hospital-acquired condition (HAC) alert   **AHA** AHA Coding Clinic®   📌 Code first alert

S31.649 **Puncture wound with foreign body of abdominal wall, unspecified quadrant with penetration into peritoneal cavity** POA MCC CC/MCC Exc

S31.65 Open bite of abdominal wall with penetration into peritoneal cavity

EXCLUDES1 *superficial bite of abdominal wall (S30.861, S30.871)*

S31.650 **Open bite of abdominal wall, right upper quadrant with penetration into peritoneal cavity** POA MCC CC/MCC Exc

S31.651 **Open bite of abdominal wall, left upper quadrant with penetration into peritoneal cavity** POA MCC CC/MCC Exc

S31.652 **Open bite of abdominal wall, epigastric region with penetration into peritoneal cavity** POA MCC CC/MCC Exc

S31.653 **Open bite of abdominal wall, right lower quadrant with penetration into peritoneal cavity** POA MCC CC/MCC Exc

S31.654 **Open bite of abdominal wall, left lower quadrant with penetration into peritoneal cavity** POA MCC CC/MCC Exc

S31.655 **Open bite of abdominal wall, periumbilic region with penetration into peritoneal cavity** POA MCC CC/MCC Exc

S31.659 **Open bite of abdominal wall, unspecified quadrant with penetration into peritoneal cavity** POA MCC CC/MCC Exc

S31.8 Open wound of other parts of abdomen, lower back and pelvis

S31.80 **Open wound of unspecified buttock**

S31.801 Laceration without foreign body of unspecified buttock POA

S31.802 Laceration with foreign body of unspecified buttock POA

S31.803 Puncture wound without foreign body of unspecified buttock POA

S31.804 Puncture wound with foreign body of unspecified buttock POA

S31.805 Open bite of unspecified buttock POA
Bite of buttock NOS
EXCLUDES1 *superficial bite of buttock (S30.870)*

S31.809 **Unspecified open wound of unspecified buttock** POA

S31.81 **Open wound of right buttock**

S31.811 Laceration without foreign body of right buttock POA

S31.812 Laceration with foreign body of right buttock POA

S31.813 Puncture wound without foreign body of right buttock POA

S31.814 Puncture wound with foreign body of right buttock POA

S31.815 Open bite of right buttock POA
Bite of right buttock NOS
EXCLUDES1 *superficial bite of buttock (S30.870)*

S31.819 **Unspecified open wound of right buttock** POA

S31.82 **Open wound of left buttock**

S31.821 Laceration without foreign body of left buttock POA

S31.822 Laceration with foreign body of left buttock POA

S31.823 Puncture wound without foreign body of left buttock POA

S31.824 Puncture wound with foreign body of left buttock POA

S31.825 Open bite of left buttock POA
Bite of left buttock NOS
EXCLUDES1 *superficial bite of buttock (S30.870)*

S31.829 **Unspecified open wound of left buttock** POA

S31.83 **Open wound of anus**

S31.831 Laceration without foreign body of anus POA

S31.832 Laceration with foreign body of anus POA

S31.833 Puncture wound without foreign body of anus POA

S31.834 Puncture wound with foreign body of anus POA

S31.835 Open bite of anus POA
Bite of anus NOS
EXCLUDES1 *superficial bite of anus (S30.877)*

S31.839 **Unspecified open wound of anus** POA

S32 Fracture of lumbar spine and pelvis

👁 **See Official Guidelines** "Coding of Traumatic Fractures" I.C.19.c

NOTES A fracture not indicated as displaced or nondisplaced should be coded to displaced.
A fracture not indicated as opened or closed should be coded to closed.

INCLUDES *fracture of lumbosacral neural arch*
fracture of lumbosacral spinous process
fracture of lumbosacral transverse process
fracture of lumbosacral vertebra
fracture of lumbosacral vertebral arch

👉 **Code first** any associated spinal cord and spinal nerve injury (S34.-)

EXCLUDES1 *transection of abdomen (S38.3)*
EXCLUDES2 *fracture of hip NOS (S72.0-)*

The appropriate 7th character is to be added to each code from category S32

A = initial encounter for closed fracture
B = initial encounter for open fracture
D = subsequent encounter for fracture with routine healing
G = subsequent encounter for fracture with delayed healing
K = subsequent encounter for fracture with nonunion
S = sequela

S32.0 **Fracture of lumbar vertebra**
Fracture of lumbar spine NOS

S32.00 **Fracture of unspecified lumbar vertebra**

S32.000 Wedge compression fracture of unspecified lumbar vertebra CC POA HAC HCC MCC CC/MCC Exc

S32.001 Stable burst fracture of unspecified lumbar vertebra CC POA HAC HCC MCC CC/MCC Exc

S32.002 Unstable burst fracture of unspecified lumbar vertebra CC POA HAC HCC MCC CC/MCC Exc

S32.008 **Other fracture of unspecified lumbar vertebra** CC POA HAC HCC MCC CC/MCC Exc

S32.009 **Unspecified fracture of unspecified lumbar vertebra** CC POA HAC HCC MCC CC/MCC Exc

S32.01 **Fracture of first lumbar vertebra**

S32.010 Wedge compression fracture of first lumbar vertebra CC POA HAC HCC MCC CC/MCC Exc

S32.011 Stable burst fracture of first lumbar vertebra CC POA HAC HCC MCC CC/MCC Exc

S32.012 Unstable burst fracture of first lumbar vertebra CC POA HAC HCC MCC CC/MCC Exc

S32.018 Other fracture of first lumbar vertebra CC POA HAC HCC MCC CC/MCC Exc

S32.019 Unspecified fracture of first lumbar vertebra CC POA HAC HCC MCC CC/MCC Exc

S32.02 **Fracture of second lumbar vertebra**

S32.020 Wedge compression fracture of second lumbar vertebra CC POA HAC HCC MCC CC/MCC Exc

S32.021 Stable burst fracture of second lumbar vertebra CC POA HAC HCC MCC CC/MCC Exc

S32.022 Unstable burst fracture of second lumbar vertebra CC POA HAC HCC MCC CC/MCC Exc

S32.028 Other fracture of second lumbar vertebra CC POA HAC HCC MCC CC/MCC Exc

S32.029 Unspecified fracture of second lumbar vertebra CC POA HAC HCC MCC CC/MCC Exc

POA Unacceptable principal diagnosis symbol per Medicare code edits   POA Code exempt from diagnosis present on admission requirement
❓ Questionable admission   CC Complication or comorbidity   MCC Major complication or comorbidity   CC/MCC Exc CC/MCC exclusion
HCC HCC diagnosis code   RxHCC RxHCC diagnosis code   MACRA MACRA code   **DEFINITION** Describes condition/terminology
TIP Coding guidance   👁 Official Guideline Reference   Z Z code as first-listed diagnosis

1000   When symbols appear on a code that requires a 7th character extension, refer to Appendix B to identify applicable 7th character codes.   **2020 ICD-10-CM**

6ᵗʰ **S32.03 Fracture of** third lumbar **vertebra**
- 7ᵗʰ S32.030 Wedge compression **fracture of third lumbar vertebra** CC♀ POA HAC HCC MCC♀ CC/MCC Exc
- 7ᵗʰ S32.031 Stable burst **fracture of third lumbar vertebra** CC♀ POA HAC HCC MCC♀ CC/MCC Exc
- 7ᵗʰ S32.032 Unstable burst **fracture of third lumbar vertebra** CC♀ POA HAC HCC MCC♀ CC/MCC Exc
- 7ᵗʰ S32.038 Other **fracture of third lumbar vertebra** CC♀ POA HAC HCC MCC♀ CC/MCC Exc
- 7ᵗʰ S32.039 Unspecified **fracture of third lumbar vertebra** CC♀ POA HAC HCC MCC♀ CC/MCC Exc

6ᵗʰ **S32.04 Fracture of** fourth lumbar **vertebra**
- 7ᵗʰ S32.040 Wedge compression **fracture of fourth lumbar vertebra** CC♀ POA HAC HCC MCC♀ CC/MCC Exc
- 7ᵗʰ S32.041 Stable burst **fracture of fourth lumbar vertebra** CC♀ POA HAC HCC MCC♀ CC/MCC Exc
- 7ᵗʰ S32.042 Unstable burst **fracture of fourth lumbar vertebra** CC♀ POA HAC HCC MCC♀ CC/MCC Exc
- 7ᵗʰ S32.048 Other **fracture of fourth lumbar vertebra** CC♀ POA HAC HCC MCC♀ CC/MCC Exc
- 7ᵗʰ S32.049 Unspecified **fracture of fourth lumbar vertebra** CC♀ POA HAC HCC MCC♀ CC/MCC Exc

6ᵗʰ **S32.05 Fracture of** fifth lumbar **vertebra**
- 7ᵗʰ S32.050 Wedge compression **fracture of fifth lumbar vertebra** CC♀ POA HAC HCC MCC♀ CC/MCC Exc
- 7ᵗʰ S32.051 Stable burst **fracture of fifth lumbar vertebra** CC♀ POA HAC HCC MCC♀ CC/MCC Exc
- 7ᵗʰ S32.052 Unstable burst **fracture of fifth lumbar vertebra** CC♀ POA HAC HCC MCC♀ CC/MCC Exc
- 7ᵗʰ S32.058 Other **fracture of fifth lumbar vertebra** CC♀ POA HAC HCC MCC♀ CC/MCC Exc
- 7ᵗʰ S32.059 Unspecified **fracture of fifth lumbar vertebra** CC♀ POA HAC HCC MCC♀ CC/MCC Exc

5ᵗʰ **S32.1 Fracture of** sacrum

For vertical fractures, code to most medial fracture extension

Use two codes if both a vertical and transverse fracture are present

Code also any associated fracture of pelvic ring (S32.8-)
- 7ᵗʰ **S32.10 Unspecified fracture of sacrum** CC♀ POA HAC HCC MCC♀ CC/MCC Exc
- 6ᵗʰ **S32.11 Zone I fracture of sacrum**
  Vertical sacral ala fracture of sacrum
  - 7ᵗʰ S32.110 Nondisplaced **Zone I fracture of sacrum** CC♀ POA HAC HCC MCC♀ CC/MCC Exc
  - 7ᵗʰ S32.111 Minimally displaced **Zone I fracture of sacrum** CC♀ POA HAC HCC MCC♀ CC/MCC Exc
  - 7ᵗʰ S32.112 Severely displaced **Zone I fracture of sacrum** CC♀ POA HAC HCC MCC♀ CC/MCC Exc
  - 7ᵗʰ S32.119 Unspecified **Zone I fracture of sacrum** CC♀ POA HAC HCC MCC♀ CC/MCC Exc
- 6ᵗʰ **S32.12 Zone II fracture of sacrum**
  Vertical foraminal region fracture of sacrum
  - 7ᵗʰ S32.120 Nondisplaced **Zone II fracture of sacrum** CC♀ POA HAC HCC MCC♀ CC/MCC Exc
  - 7ᵗʰ S32.121 Minimally displaced **Zone II fracture of sacrum** CC♀ POA HAC HCC MCC♀ CC/MCC Exc
  - 7ᵗʰ S32.122 Severely displaced **Zone II fracture of sacrum** CC♀ POA HAC HCC MCC♀ CC/MCC Exc
  - 7ᵗʰ S32.129 Unspecified **Zone II fracture of sacrum** CC♀ POA HAC HCC MCC♀ CC/MCC Exc
- 6ᵗʰ **S32.13 Zone III fracture of sacrum**
  Vertical fracture into spinal canal region of sacrum
  - 7ᵗʰ S32.130 Nondisplaced **Zone III fracture of sacrum** CC♀ POA HAC HCC MCC♀ CC/MCC Exc
  - 7ᵗʰ S32.131 Minimally displaced **Zone III fracture of sacrum** CC♀ POA HAC HCC MCC♀ CC/MCC Exc
  - 7ᵗʰ S32.132 Severely displaced **Zone III fracture of sacrum** CC♀ POA HAC HCC MCC♀ CC/MCC Exc
  - 7ᵗʰ S32.139 Unspecified **Zone III fracture of sacrum** CC♀ POA HAC HCC MCC♀ CC/MCC Exc
- 7ᵗʰ **S32.14 Type 1 fracture of sacrum** CC♀ POA HAC HCC MCC♀ CC/MCC Exc
  Transverse flexion fracture of sacrum without displacement

- 7ᵗʰ **S32.15 Type 2 fracture of sacrum** CC♀ POA HAC HCC MCC♀ CC/MCC Exc
  Transverse flexion fracture of sacrum with posterior displacement
- 7ᵗʰ **S32.16 Type 3 fracture of sacrum** CC♀ POA HAC HCC MCC♀ CC/MCC Exc
  Transverse extension fracture of sacrum with anterior displacement
- 7ᵗʰ **S32.17 Type 4 fracture of sacrum** CC♀ POA HAC HCC MCC♀ CC/MCC Exc
  Transverse segmental comminution of upper sacrum
- 7ᵗʰ **S32.19 Other fracture of sacrum** CC♀ POA HAC HCC MCC♀ CC/MCC Exc

7ᵗʰ **S32.2 Fracture of** coccyx CC♀ POA HAC HCC MCC♀ CC/MCC Exc

5ᵗʰ **S32.3 Fracture of** ilium

EXCLUDES1 fracture of ilium with associated disruption of pelvic ring (S32.8-)
- 6ᵗʰ **S32.30 Unspecified fracture of ilium**
  - 7ᵗʰ S32.301 **Unspecified fracture of** right **ilium** CC♀ POA HAC HCC MCC♀ CC/MCC Exc
  - 7ᵗʰ S32.302 **Unspecified fracture of** left **ilium** CC♀ POA HAC HCC MCC♀ CC/MCC Exc
  - 7ᵗʰ S32.309 **Unspecified fracture of** unspecified **ilium** CC♀ POA HAC HCC MCC♀ CC/MCC Exc
- 6ᵗʰ **S32.31 Avulsion fracture of ilium**
  - 7ᵗʰ S32.311 Displaced **avulsion fracture of** right **ilium** CC♀ POA HAC HCC MCC♀ CC/MCC Exc
  - 7ᵗʰ S32.312 Displaced **avulsion fracture of** left **ilium** CC♀ POA HAC HCC MCC♀ CC/MCC Exc
  - 7ᵗʰ S32.313 Displaced **avulsion fracture of** unspecified **ilium** CC♀ POA HAC HCC MCC♀ CC/MCC Exc
  - 7ᵗʰ S32.314 Nondisplaced **avulsion fracture of** right **ilium** CC♀ POA HAC HCC MCC♀ CC/MCC Exc
  - 7ᵗʰ S32.315 Nondisplaced **avulsion fracture of** left **ilium** CC♀ POA HAC HCC MCC♀ CC/MCC Exc
  - 7ᵗʰ S32.316 Nondisplaced **avulsion fracture of** unspecified **ilium** CC♀ POA HAC HCC MCC♀ CC/MCC Exc
- 6ᵗʰ **S32.39 Other fracture of ilium**
  - 7ᵗʰ S32.391 **Other fracture of** right **ilium** CC♀ POA HAC HCC MCC♀ CC/MCC Exc
  - 7ᵗʰ S32.392 **Other fracture of** left **ilium** CC♀ POA HAC HCC MCC♀ CC/MCC Exc
  - 7ᵗʰ S32.399 **Other fracture of** unspecified **ilium** CC♀ POA HAC HCC MCC♀ CC/MCC Exc

5ᵗʰ **S32.4 Fracture of** acetabulum

Code also any associated fracture of pelvic ring (S32.8-)
- 6ᵗʰ **S32.40 Unspecified fracture of acetabulum**
  - 7ᵗʰ S32.401 **Unspecified fracture of** right **acetabulum** CC♀ POA HAC HCC MCC♀ CC/MCC Exc
  - 7ᵗʰ S32.402 **Unspecified fracture of** left **acetabulum** CC♀ POA HAC HCC MCC♀ CC/MCC Exc
  - 7ᵗʰ S32.409 **Unspecified fracture of unspecified acetabulum** CC♀ POA HAC HCC MCC♀ CC/MCC Exc
- 6ᵗʰ **S32.41 Fracture of** anterior wall **of acetabulum**
  - 7ᵗʰ S32.411 Displaced **fracture of anterior wall of** right **acetabulum** CC♀ POA HAC HCC MCC♀ CC/MCC Exc
  - 7ᵗʰ S32.412 Displaced **fracture of anterior wall of** left **acetabulum** CC♀ POA HAC HCC MCC♀ CC/MCC Exc
  - 7ᵗʰ S32.413 Displaced **fracture of anterior wall of unspecified acetabulum** CC♀ POA HAC HCC MCC♀ CC/MCC Exc
  - 7ᵗʰ S32.414 Nondisplaced **fracture of anterior wall of** right **acetabulum** CC♀ POA HAC HCC MCC♀ CC/MCC Exc
  - 7ᵗʰ S32.415 Nondisplaced **fracture of anterior wall of** left **acetabulum** CC♀ POA HAC HCC MCC♀ CC/MCC Exc
  - 7ᵗʰ S32.416 Nondisplaced **fracture of anterior wall of unspecified acetabulum** CC♀ POA HAC HCC MCC♀ CC/MCC Exc
- 6ᵗʰ **S32.42 Fracture of** posterior wall **of acetabulum**
  - 7ᵗʰ S32.421 Displaced **fracture of posterior wall of** right **acetabulum** CC♀ POA HAC HCC MCC♀ CC/MCC Exc
  - 7ᵗʰ S32.422 Displaced **fracture of posterior wall of** left **acetabulum** CC♀ POA HAC HCC MCC♀ CC/MCC Exc

● Unspecified Code	Other Specified Code	Manifestation Code	N Newborn	P Pediatric	M Maternity	A Adult	♂ Male	♀ Female

● New Code   ▲ Revised Code Title   ►◄ Revised Text   **NOTES**   *INCLUDES*   *EXCLUDES1* Not coded here   *EXCLUDES2* Not included here

4ᵗʰ 4ᵗʰ character required   5ᵗʰ 5ᵗʰ character required   6ᵗʰ 6ᵗʰ character required   7ᵗʰ 7ᵗʰ character required   7ᵗʰ Extension 'X' Alert

HAC Hospital-acquired condition (HAC) alert   **AHA** AHA Coding Clinic®   📌 **Code first alert**

7ᵗʰ S32.423 Displaced fracture of posterior wall of unspecified acetabulum ᶜᶜ ᴾᴼᴬ HAC HCC MCC CC/MCC Exc

7ᵗʰ S32.424 Nondisplaced fracture of posterior wall of right acetabulum ᶜᶜ ᴾᴼᴬ HAC HCC MCC CC/MCC Exc

7ᵗʰ S32.425 Nondisplaced fracture of posterior wall of left acetabulum ᶜᶜ ᴾᴼᴬ HAC HCC MCC CC/MCC Exc

7ᵗʰ S32.426 Nondisplaced fracture of posterior wall of unspecified acetabulum ᶜᶜ ᴾᴼᴬ HAC HCC MCC CC/MCC Exc

6ᵗʰ S32.43 Fracture of anterior column [iliopubic] of acetabulum

7ᵗʰ S32.431 Displaced fracture of anterior column [iliopubic] of right acetabulum ᶜᶜ ᴾᴼᴬ HAC HCC MCC CC/MCC Exc

7ᵗʰ S32.432 Displaced fracture of anterior column [iliopubic] of left acetabulum ᶜᶜ ᴾᴼᴬ HAC HCC MCC CC/MCC Exc

7ᵗʰ S32.433 Displaced fracture of anterior column [iliopubic] of unspecified acetabulum ᶜᶜ ᴾᴼᴬ HAC HCC MCC CC/MCC Exc

7ᵗʰ S32.434 Nondisplaced fracture of anterior column [iliopubic] of right acetabulum ᶜᶜ ᴾᴼᴬ HAC HCC MCC CC/MCC Exc

7ᵗʰ S32.435 Nondisplaced fracture of anterior column [iliopubic] of left acetabulum ᶜᶜ ᴾᴼᴬ HAC HCC MCC CC/MCC Exc

7ᵗʰ S32.436 Nondisplaced fracture of anterior column [iliopubic] of unspecified acetabulum ᶜᶜ ᴾᴼᴬ HAC HCC MCC CC/MCC Exc

6ᵗʰ S32.44 Fracture of posterior column [ilioischial] of acetabulum

7ᵗʰ S32.441 Displaced fracture of posterior column [ilioischial] of right acetabulum ᶜᶜ ᴾᴼᴬ HAC HCC MCC CC/MCC Exc

7ᵗʰ S32.442 Displaced fracture of posterior column [ilioischial] of left acetabulum ᶜᶜ ᴾᴼᴬ HAC HCC MCC CC/MCC Exc

7ᵗʰ S32.443 Displaced fracture of posterior column [ilioischial] of unspecified acetabulum ᶜᶜ ᴾᴼᴬ HAC HCC MCC CC/MCC Exc

7ᵗʰ S32.444 Nondisplaced fracture of posterior column [ilioischial] of right acetabulum ᶜᶜ ᴾᴼᴬ HAC HCC MCC CC/MCC Exc

7ᵗʰ S32.445 Nondisplaced fracture of posterior column [ilioischial] of left acetabulum ᶜᶜ ᴾᴼᴬ HAC HCC MCC CC/MCC Exc

7ᵗʰ S32.446 Nondisplaced fracture of posterior column [ilioischial] of unspecified acetabulum ᶜᶜ ᴾᴼᴬ HAC HCC MCC CC/MCC Exc

6ᵗʰ S32.45 Transverse fracture of acetabulum

7ᵗʰ S32.451 Displaced transverse fracture of right acetabulum ᶜᶜ ᴾᴼᴬ HAC HCC MCC CC/MCC Exc

7ᵗʰ S32.452 Displaced transverse fracture of left acetabulum ᶜᶜ ᴾᴼᴬ HAC HCC MCC CC/MCC Exc

7ᵗʰ S32.453 Displaced transverse fracture of unspecified acetabulum ᶜᶜ ᴾᴼᴬ HAC HCC MCC CC/MCC Exc

7ᵗʰ S32.454 Nondisplaced transverse fracture of right acetabulum ᶜᶜ ᴾᴼᴬ HAC HCC MCC CC/MCC Exc

7ᵗʰ S32.455 Nondisplaced transverse fracture of left acetabulum ᶜᶜ ᴾᴼᴬ HAC HCC MCC CC/MCC Exc

7ᵗʰ S32.456 Nondisplaced transverse fracture of unspecified acetabulum ᶜᶜ ᴾᴼᴬ HAC HCC MCC CC/MCC Exc

6ᵗʰ S32.46 Associated transverse-posterior fracture of acetabulum

7ᵗʰ S32.461 Displaced associated transverse-posterior fracture of right acetabulum ᶜᶜ ᴾᴼᴬ HAC HCC MCC CC/MCC Exc

7ᵗʰ S32.462 Displaced associated transverse-posterior fracture of left acetabulum ᶜᶜ ᴾᴼᴬ HAC HCC MCC CC/MCC Exc

7ᵗʰ S32.463 Displaced associated transverse-posterior fracture of unspecified acetabulum ᶜᶜ ᴾᴼᴬ HAC HCC MCC CC/MCC Exc

7ᵗʰ S32.464 Nondisplaced associated transverse-posterior fracture of right acetabulum ᶜᶜ ᴾᴼᴬ HAC HCC MCC CC/MCC Exc

7ᵗʰ S32.465 Nondisplaced associated transverse-posterior fracture of left acetabulum ᶜᶜ ᴾᴼᴬ HAC HCC MCC CC/MCC Exc

7ᵗʰ S32.466 Nondisplaced associated transverse-posterior fracture of unspecified acetabulum ᶜᶜ ᴾᴼᴬ HAC HCC MCC CC/MCC Exc

6ᵗʰ S32.47 Fracture of medial wall of acetabulum

7ᵗʰ S32.471 Displaced fracture of medial wall of right acetabulum ᶜᶜ ᴾᴼᴬ HAC HCC MCC CC/MCC Exc

7ᵗʰ S32.472 Displaced fracture of medial wall of left acetabulum ᶜᶜ ᴾᴼᴬ HAC HCC MCC CC/MCC Exc

7ᵗʰ S32.473 Displaced fracture of medial wall of unspecified acetabulum ᶜᶜ ᴾᴼᴬ HAC HCC MCC CC/MCC Exc

7ᵗʰ S32.474 Nondisplaced fracture of medial wall of right acetabulum ᶜᶜ ᴾᴼᴬ HAC HCC MCC CC/MCC Exc

7ᵗʰ S32.475 Nondisplaced fracture of medial wall of left acetabulum ᶜᶜ ᴾᴼᴬ HAC HCC MCC CC/MCC Exc

7ᵗʰ S32.476 Nondisplaced fracture of medial wall of unspecified acetabulum ᶜᶜ ᴾᴼᴬ HAC HCC MCC CC/MCC Exc

6ᵗʰ S32.48 Dome fracture of acetabulum

7ᵗʰ S32.481 Displaced dome fracture of right acetabulum ᶜᶜ ᴾᴼᴬ HAC HCC MCC CC/MCC Exc

7ᵗʰ S32.482 Displaced dome fracture of left acetabulum ᶜᶜ ᴾᴼᴬ HAC HCC MCC CC/MCC Exc

7ᵗʰ S32.483 Displaced dome fracture of unspecified acetabulum ᶜᶜ ᴾᴼᴬ HAC HCC MCC CC/MCC Exc

7ᵗʰ S32.484 Nondisplaced dome fracture of right acetabulum ᶜᶜ ᴾᴼᴬ HAC HCC MCC CC/MCC Exc

7ᵗʰ S32.485 Nondisplaced dome fracture of left acetabulum ᶜᶜ ᴾᴼᴬ HAC HCC MCC CC/MCC Exc

7ᵗʰ S32.486 Nondisplaced dome fracture of unspecified acetabulum ᶜᶜ ᴾᴼᴬ HAC HCC MCC CC/MCC Exc

6ᵗʰ S32.49 Other specified fracture of acetabulum

7ᵗʰ S32.491 Other specified fracture of right acetabulum ᶜᶜ ᴾᴼᴬ HAC HCC MCC CC/MCC Exc

7ᵗʰ S32.492 Other specified fracture of left acetabulum ᶜᶜ ᴾᴼᴬ HAC HCC MCC CC/MCC Exc

7ᵗʰ S32.499 Other specified fracture of unspecified acetabulum ᶜᶜ ᴾᴼᴬ HAC HCC MCC CC/MCC Exc

5ᵗʰ S32.5 Fracture of pubis

EXCLUDES1 fracture of pubis with associated disruption of pelvic ring (S32.8-)

6ᵗʰ S32.50 Unspecified fracture of pubis

7ᵗʰ S32.501 Unspecified fracture of right pubis ᴾᴼᴬ HAC HCC MCC CC/MCC Exc

7ᵗʰ S32.502 Unspecified fracture of left pubis ᴾᴼᴬ HAC HCC MCC CC/MCC Exc

7ᵗʰ S32.509 Unspecified fracture of unspecified pubis ᴾᴼᴬ HAC HCC MCC CC/MCC Exc

6ᵗʰ S32.51 Fracture of superior rim of pubis

7ᵗʰ S32.511 Fracture of superior rim of right pubis ᴾᴼᴬ HAC HCC MCC CC/MCC Exc

7ᵗʰ S32.512 Fracture of superior rim of left pubis ᴾᴼᴬ HAC HCC MCC CC/MCC Exc

7ᵗʰ S32.519 Fracture of superior rim of unspecified pubis ᴾᴼᴬ HAC HCC MCC CC/MCC Exc

6ᵗʰ S32.59 Other specified fracture of pubis

7ᵗʰ S32.591 Other specified fracture of right pubis ᴾᴼᴬ HAC HCC MCC CC/MCC Exc

7ᵗʰ S32.592 Other specified fracture of left pubis ᴾᴼᴬ HAC HCC MCC CC/MCC Exc

7ᵗʰ S32.599 Other specified fracture of unspecified pubis ᴾᴼᴬ HAC HCC MCC CC/MCC Exc

---

ᴾᴰˣ Unacceptable principal diagnosis symbol per Medicare code edits ᴾᴼᴬ Code exempt from diagnosis present on admission requirement
❓ Questionable admission ᶜᶜ Complication or comorbidity ᴹᶜᶜ Major complication or comorbidity ᶜᶜ/ᴹᶜᶜ CC/MCC exclusion
HCC HCC diagnosis code RxHCC RxHCC diagnosis code MACRA MACRA code **DEFINITION** Describes condition/terminology
TIP Coding guidance 👁 Official Guideline Reference Z1 Z code as first-listed diagnosis

When symbols appear on a code that requires a 7th character extension, refer to Appendix B to identify applicable 7th character codes.

S32.6 Fracture of ischium
> EXCLUDES1 *fracture of ischium with associated disruption of pelvic ring (S32.8-)*

S32.60 Unspecified fracture of ischium
- S32.601 **Unspecified fracture of** right **ischium** cc POA HAC HCC MCC CC/MCC Exc
- S32.602 **Unspecified fracture of** left **ischium** cc POA HAC HCC MCC CC/MCC Exc
- S32.609 **Unspecified fracture of unspecified ischium**

S32.61 Avulsion fracture of ischium
- S32.611 Displaced **avulsion fracture of** right **ischium** cc POA HAC HCC MCC CC/MCC Exc
- S32.612 Displaced **avulsion fracture of** left **ischium** cc POA HAC HCC MCC CC/MCC Exc
- S32.613 Displaced **avulsion fracture of unspecified ischium**
- S32.614 Nondisplaced **avulsion fracture of** right **ischium** cc POA HAC HCC MCC CC/MCC Exc
- S32.615 Nondisplaced **avulsion fracture of** left **ischium** cc POA HAC HCC MCC CC/MCC Exc
- S32.616 Nondisplaced **avulsion fracture of unspecified ischium**

S32.69 Other specified fracture of ischium
- S32.691 **Other specified fracture of** right **ischium** cc POA HAC HCC MCC CC/MCC Exc
- S32.692 **Other specified fracture of** left **ischium** cc POA HAC HCC MCC CC/MCC Exc
- S32.699 **Other specified fracture of unspecified ischium** cc POA HAC HCC MCC CC/MCC Exc

S32.8 Fracture of other parts of pelvis
> Code also any associated:
> fracture of acetabulum (S32.4-)
> sacral fracture (S32.1-)

S32.81 Multiple fractures of pelvis with disruption of pelvic ring
> Multiple pelvic fractures with disruption of pelvic circle
- S32.810 **Multiple fractures of pelvis with** stable **disruption of pelvic ring** cc POA HAC HCC MCC CC/MCC Exc
- S32.811 **Multiple fractures of pelvis with** unstable **disruption of pelvic ring** cc POA HAC HCC MCC CC/MCC Exc

- S32.82 **Multiple fractures of pelvis** without disruption of pelvic ring cc POA HAC HCC MCC CC/MCC Exc
> Multiple pelvic fractures without disruption of pelvic circle

- S32.89 **Fracture of** other **parts of pelvis** cc POA HAC HCC MCC CC/MCC Exc

- S32.9 **Fracture of unspecified parts of lumbosacral spine and pelvis** cc POA HAC HCC MCC CC/MCC Exc
> Fracture of lumbosacral spine NOS
> Fracture of pelvis NOS

S33 Dislocation and sprain of joints and ligaments of lumbar spine and pelvis
> INCLUDES avulsion of joint or ligament of lumbar spine and pelvis
> laceration of cartilage, joint or ligament of lumbar spine and pelvis
> sprain of cartilage, joint or ligament of lumbar spine and pelvis
> traumatic hemarthrosis of joint or ligament of lumbar spine and pelvis
> traumatic rupture of joint or ligament of lumbar spine and pelvis
> traumatic subluxation of joint or ligament of lumbar spine and pelvis
> traumatic tear of joint or ligament of lumbar spine and pelvis
> Code also any associated open wound
> EXCLUDES1 *nontraumatic rupture or displacement of lumbar intervertebral disc NOS (M51.-)*
> *obstetric damage to pelvic joints and ligaments (O71.6)*

> EXCLUDES2 *dislocation and sprain of joints and ligaments of hip (S73.-)*
> *strain of muscle of lower back and pelvis (S39.01-)*

The appropriate 7th character is to be added to each code from category S33
> A = initial encounter
> D = subsequent encounter
> S = sequela

- S33.0 Traumatic rupture of lumbar intervertebral disc POA
> EXCLUDES1 *rupture or displacement (nontraumatic) of lumbar intervertebral disc NOS (M51.- with fifth character 6)*

- S33.1 Subluxation and dislocation of lumbar vertebra
> Code also any associated:
> open wound of abdomen, lower back and pelvis (S31)
> spinal cord injury (S24.0, S24.1-, S34.0-, S34.1-)
> EXCLUDES2 *fracture of lumbar vertebrae (S32.0-)*

S33.10 Subluxation and dislocation of unspecified **lumbar vertebra**
- S33.100 Subluxation of unspecified lumbar vertebra POA
- S33.101 Dislocation of unspecified lumbar vertebra POA

S33.11 Subluxation and dislocation of L1/L2 **lumbar vertebra**
- S33.110 Subluxation of L1/L2 lumbar vertebra POA
- S33.111 Dislocation of L1/L2 lumbar vertebra POA

S33.12 Subluxation and dislocation of L2/L3 **lumbar vertebra**
- S33.120 Subluxation of L2/L3 lumbar vertebra POA
- S33.121 Dislocation of L2/L3 lumbar vertebra POA

S33.13 Subluxation and dislocation of L3/L4 **lumbar vertebra**
- S33.130 Subluxation of L3/L4 lumbar vertebra POA
- S33.131 Dislocation of L3/L4 lumbar vertebra POA

S33.14 Subluxation and dislocation of L4/L5 **lumbar vertebra**
- S33.140 Subluxation of L4/L5 lumbar vertebra POA
- S33.141 Dislocation of L4/L5 lumbar vertebra POA

- S33.2 Dislocation of sacroiliac and sacrococcygeal joint POA
- S33.3 Dislocation of other and unspecified parts of lumbar spine and pelvis
  - S33.30 **Dislocation of unspecified parts of lumbar spine and pelvis** POA
  - S33.39 **Dislocation of other parts of lumbar spine and pelvis** POA
- S33.4 Traumatic rupture of symphysis pubis POA
- S33.5 **Sprain of** ligaments of lumbar spine POA
- S33.6 **Sprain of** sacroiliac joint POA
- S33.8 **Sprain of** other parts of lumbar spine and pelvis POA
- S33.9 **Sprain of unspecified parts of lumbar spine and pelvis** POA

S34 Injury of lumbar and sacral spinal cord and nerves at abdomen, lower back and pelvis level
> NOTES Code to highest level of lumbar cord injury
> Injuries to the spinal cord (S34.0 and S34.1) refer to the cord level and not bone level injury, and can affect nerve roots at and below the level given.
> Code also any associated:
> fracture of vertebra (S22.0-, S32.0-)
> open wound of abdomen, lower back and pelvis (S31.-)
> transient paralysis (R29.5)

The appropriate 7th character is to be added to each code from category S34
> A = initial encounter
> D = subsequent encounter
> S = sequela

S34.0 Concussion and edema of lumbar and sacral spinal cord
- S34.01 **Concussion and edema of** lumbar **spinal cord** POA HCC MCC CC/MCC Exc
- S34.02 **Concussion and edema of** sacral **spinal cord** POA HCC MCC CC/MCC Exc
> Concussion and edema of conus medullaris

Unspecified Code   Other Specified Code   Manifestation Code   N Newborn   P Pediatric   M Maternity   A Adult   ♂ Male   ♀ Female
● New Code   ▲ Revised Code Title   ►◄ Revised Text   NOTES   INCLUDES   EXCLUDES1 Not coded here   EXCLUDES2 Not included here
4th character required   5th character required   6th character required   7th character required   Extension 'X' Alert
HAC Hospital-acquired condition (HAC) alert   AHA AHA Coding Clinic©   ☛ Code first alert

5ᵈ S34.1 Other and unspecified injury of lumbar and sacral spinal cord
  6ᵈ S34.10 Unspecified injury to lumbar spinal cord
    7ᵈ S34.101 Unspecified injury to L1 level of lumbar spinal cord POA HAC HCC MCC CC/MCC Exc
      Unspecified injury to lumbar spinal cord level 1
    7ᵈ S34.102 Unspecified injury to L2 level of lumbar spinal cord POA HAC HCC MCC CC/MCC Exc
      Unspecified injury to lumbar spinal cord level 2
    7ᵈ S34.103 Unspecified injury to L3 level of lumbar spinal cord POA HAC HCC MCC CC/MCC Exc
      Unspecified injury to lumbar spinal cord level 3
    7ᵈ S34.104 Unspecified injury to L4 level of lumbar spinal cord POA HAC HCC MCC CC/MCC Exc
      Unspecified injury to lumbar spinal cord level 4
    7ᵈ S34.105 Unspecified injury to L5 level of lumbar spinal cord POA HAC HCC MCC CC/MCC Exc
      Unspecified injury to lumbar spinal cord level 5
    7ᵈ S34.109 Unspecified injury to unspecified level of lumbar spinal cord POA HAC HCC MCC CC/MCC Exc
  6ᵈ S34.11 Complete lesion of lumbar spinal cord
    7ᵈ S34.111 Complete lesion of L1 level of lumbar spinal cord POA HAC HCC MCC CC/MCC Exc
      Complete lesion of lumbar spinal cord level 1
    7ᵈ S34.112 Complete lesion of L2 level of lumbar spinal cord POA HAC HCC MCC CC/MCC Exc
      Complete lesion of lumbar spinal cord level 2
    7ᵈ S34.113 Complete lesion of L3 level of lumbar spinal cord POA HAC HCC MCC CC/MCC Exc
      Complete lesion of lumbar spinal cord level 3
    7ᵈ S34.114 Complete lesion of L4 level of lumbar spinal cord POA HAC HCC MCC CC/MCC Exc
      Complete lesion of lumbar spinal cord level 4
    7ᵈ S34.115 Complete lesion of L5 level of lumbar spinal cord POA HAC HCC MCC CC/MCC Exc
      Complete lesion of lumbar spinal cord level 5
    7ᵈ S34.119 Complete lesion of unspecified level of lumbar spinal cord POA HAC HCC MCC CC/MCC Exc
  6ᵈ S34.12 Incomplete lesion of lumbar spinal cord
    7ᵈ S34.121 Incomplete lesion of L1 level of lumbar spinal cord POA HAC HCC MCC CC/MCC Exc
      Incomplete lesion of lumbar spinal cord level 1
    7ᵈ S34.122 Incomplete lesion of L2 level of lumbar spinal cord POA HAC HCC MCC CC/MCC Exc
      Incomplete lesion of lumbar spinal cord level 2
    7ᵈ S34.123 Incomplete lesion of L3 level of lumbar spinal cord POA HAC HCC MCC CC/MCC Exc
      Incomplete lesion of lumbar spinal cord level 3
    7ᵈ S34.124 Incomplete lesion of L4 level of lumbar spinal cord POA HAC HCC MCC CC/MCC Exc
      Incomplete lesion of lumbar spinal cord level 4
    7ᵈ S34.125 Incomplete lesion of L5 level of lumbar spinal cord POA HAC HCC MCC CC/MCC Exc
      Incomplete lesion of lumbar spinal cord level 5
    7ᵈ S34.129 Incomplete lesion of unspecified level of lumbar spinal cord POA HAC HCC MCC CC/MCC Exc
  6ᵈ S34.13 Other and unspecified injury to sacral spinal cord
    Other injury to conus medullaris

    7ᵈ S34.131 Complete lesion of sacral spinal cord POA HAC HCC MCC CC/MCC Exc
      Complete lesion of conus medullaris
    7ᵈ S34.132 Incomplete lesion of sacral spinal cord POA HAC HCC MCC CC/MCC Exc
      Incomplete lesion of conus medullaris
    7ᵈ S34.139 Unspecified injury to sacral spinal cord POA HAC HCC MCC CC/MCC Exc
      Unspecified injury of conus medullaris
  5ᵈ S34.2 Injury of nerve root of lumbar and sacral spine
    7ᵈ S34.21 Injury of nerve root of lumbar spine POA
    7ᵈ S34.22 Injury of nerve root of sacral spine POA
  7ᵈ S34.3 Injury of cauda equina POA HAC HCC MCC CC/MCC Exc
  7ᵈ S34.4 Injury of lumbosacral plexus POA
  7ᵈ S34.5 Injury of lumbar, sacral and pelvic sympathetic nerves POA
    Injury of celiac ganglion or plexus
    Injury of hypogastric plexus
    Injury of mesenteric plexus (inferior) (superior)
    Injury of splanchnic nerve
  7ᵈ S34.6 Injury of peripheral nerve(s) at abdomen, lower back and pelvis level POA
  7ᵈ S34.8 Injury of other nerves at abdomen, lower back and pelvis level POA
  7ᵈ S34.9 Injury of unspecified nerves at abdomen, lower back and pelvis level POA

4ᵈ S35 Injury of blood vessels at abdomen, lower back and pelvis level
  Code also any associated open wound (S31.-)
  The appropriate 7th character is to be added to each code from category S35
  A = initial encounter
  D = subsequent encounter
  S = sequela
  5ᵈ S35.0 Injury of abdominal aorta
    EXCLUDES1 injury of aorta NOS (S25.0)
    7ᵈ S35.00 Unspecified injury of abdominal aorta POA MCC CC/MCC Exc
    7ᵈ S35.01 Minor laceration of abdominal aorta POA MCC CC/MCC Exc
      Incomplete transection of abdominal aorta
      Laceration of abdominal aorta NOS
      Superficial laceration of abdominal aorta
    7ᵈ S35.02 Major laceration of abdominal aorta POA MCC CC/MCC Exc
      Complete transection of abdominal aorta
      Traumatic rupture of abdominal aorta
    7ᵈ S35.09 Other injury of abdominal aorta POA MCC CC/MCC Exc
  5ᵈ S35.1 Injury of inferior vena cava
    Injury of hepatic vein
    EXCLUDES1 injury of vena cava NOS (S25.2)
    7ᵈ S35.10 Unspecified injury of inferior vena cava POA MCC CC/MCC Exc
    7ᵈ S35.11 Minor laceration of inferior vena cava POA MCC CC/MCC Exc
      Incomplete transection of inferior vena cava
      Laceration of inferior vena cava NOS
      Superficial laceration of inferior vena cava
    7ᵈ S35.12 Major laceration of inferior vena cava POA MCC CC/MCC Exc
      Complete transection of inferior vena cava
      Traumatic rupture of inferior vena cava
    7ᵈ S35.19 Other injury of inferior vena cava POA MCC CC/MCC Exc
  5ᵈ S35.2 Injury of celiac or mesenteric artery and branches
    6ᵈ S35.21 Injury of celiac artery
      7ᵈ S35.211 Minor laceration of celiac artery POA MCC CC/MCC Exc
        Incomplete transection of celiac artery
        Laceration of celiac artery NOS
        Superficial laceration of celiac artery
      7ᵈ S35.212 Major laceration of celiac artery POA MCC CC/MCC Exc
        Complete transection of celiac artery
        Traumatic rupture of celiac artery
      7ᵈ S35.218 Other injury of celiac artery POA MCC CC/MCC Exc
      7ᵈ S35.219 Unspecified injury of celiac artery POA MCC CC/MCC Exc

When symbols appear on a code that requires a 7th character extension, refer to Appendix B to identify applicable 7th character codes.

2020 ICD-10-CM

[6th] **S35.22 Injury of superior mesenteric artery**
- [7th] **S35.221 Minor laceration of superior mesenteric artery** [POA] [MCC] [CC/MCC Exc]
  - Incomplete transection of superior mesenteric artery
  - Laceration of superior mesenteric artery NOS
  - Superficial laceration of superior mesenteric artery
- [7th] **S35.222 Major laceration of superior mesenteric artery** [POA] [MCC] [CC/MCC Exc]
  - Complete transection of superior mesenteric artery
  - Traumatic rupture of superior mesenteric artery
- [7th] **S35.228 Other injury of superior mesenteric artery** [POA] [MCC] [CC/MCC Exc]
- [7th] **S35.229 Unspecified injury of superior mesenteric artery** [POA] [MCC] [CC/MCC Exc]

[6th] **S35.23 Injury of inferior mesenteric artery**
- [7th] **S35.231 Minor laceration of inferior mesenteric artery** [POA] [MCC] [CC/MCC Exc]
  - Incomplete transection of inferior mesenteric artery
  - Laceration of inferior mesenteric artery NOS
  - Superficial laceration of inferior mesenteric artery
- [7th] **S35.232 Major laceration of inferior mesenteric artery** [POA] [MCC] [CC/MCC Exc]
  - Complete transection of inferior mesenteric artery
  - Traumatic rupture of inferior mesenteric artery
- [7th] **S35.238 Other injury of inferior mesenteric artery** [POA] [MCC] [CC/MCC Exc]
- [7th] **S35.239 Unspecified injury of inferior mesenteric artery** [POA] [MCC] [CC/MCC Exc]

[6th] **S35.29 Injury of branches of celiac and mesenteric artery**
- Injury of gastric artery
- Injury of gastroduodenal artery
- Injury of hepatic artery
- Injury of splenic artery
- [7th] **S35.291 Minor laceration of branches of celiac and mesenteric artery** [POA] [MCC] [CC/MCC Exc]
  - Incomplete transection of branches of celiac and mesenteric artery
  - Laceration of branches of celiac and mesenteric artery NOS
  - Superficial laceration of branches of celiac and mesenteric artery
- [7th] **S35.292 Major laceration of branches of celiac and mesenteric artery** [POA] [MCC] [CC/MCC Exc]
  - Complete transection of branches of celiac and mesenteric artery
  - Traumatic rupture of branches of celiac and mesenteric artery
- [7th] **S35.298 Other injury of branches of celiac and mesenteric artery** [POA] [MCC] [CC/MCC Exc]
- [7th] **S35.299 Unspecified injury of branches of celiac and mesenteric artery** [POA] [MCC] [CC/MCC Exc]

[5th] **S35.3 Injury of portal or splenic vein and branches**

[6th] **S35.31 Injury of portal vein**
- [7th] **S35.311 Laceration of portal vein** [POA] [MCC] [CC/MCC Exc]
- [7th] **S35.318 Other specified injury of portal vein** [POA] [MCC] [CC/MCC Exc]
- [7th] **S35.319 Unspecified injury of portal vein** [POA] [MCC] [CC/MCC Exc]

[6th] **S35.32 Injury of splenic vein**
- [7th] **S35.321 Laceration of splenic vein** [POA] [MCC] [CC/MCC Exc]
- [7th] **S35.328 Other specified injury of splenic vein** [POA] [MCC] [CC/MCC Exc]
- [7th] **S35.329 Unspecified injury of splenic vein** [POA] [MCC] [CC/MCC Exc]

[6th] **S35.33 Injury of superior mesenteric vein**
- [7th] **S35.331 Laceration of superior mesenteric vein** [POA] [MCC] [CC/MCC Exc]
- [7th] **S35.338 Other specified injury of superior mesenteric vein** [POA] [MCC] [CC/MCC Exc]
- [7th] **S35.339 Unspecified injury of superior mesenteric vein** [POA] [MCC] [CC/MCC Exc]

[6th] **S35.34 Injury of inferior mesenteric vein**
- [7th] **S35.341 Laceration of inferior mesenteric vein** [POA] [MCC] [CC/MCC Exc]
- [7th] **S35.348 Other specified injury of inferior mesenteric vein** [POA] [MCC] [CC/MCC Exc]
- [7th] **S35.349 Unspecified injury of inferior mesenteric vein** [POA] [MCC] [CC/MCC Exc]

[5th] **S35.4 Injury of renal blood vessels**

[6th] **S35.40 Unspecified injury of renal blood vessel**
- [7th] **S35.401 Unspecified injury of right renal artery** [POA] [MCC] [CC/MCC Exc]
- [7th] **S35.402 Unspecified injury of left renal artery** [POA] [MCC] [CC/MCC Exc]
- [7th] **S35.403 Unspecified injury of unspecified renal artery** [POA] [MCC] [CC/MCC Exc]
- [7th] **S35.404 Unspecified injury of right renal vein** [POA] [MCC] [CC/MCC Exc]
- [7th] **S35.405 Unspecified injury of left renal vein** [POA] [MCC] [CC/MCC Exc]
- [7th] **S35.406 Unspecified injury of unspecified renal vein** [POA] [MCC] [CC/MCC Exc]

[6th] **S35.41 Laceration of renal blood vessel**
- [7th] **S35.411 Laceration of right renal artery** [POA] [MCC] [CC/MCC Exc]
- [7th] **S35.412 Laceration of left renal artery** [POA] [MCC] [CC/MCC Exc]
- [7th] **S35.413 Laceration of unspecified renal artery** [POA] [MCC] [CC/MCC Exc]
- [7th] **S35.414 Laceration of right renal vein** [POA] [MCC] [CC/MCC Exc]
- [7th] **S35.415 Laceration of left renal vein** [POA] [MCC] [CC/MCC Exc]
- [7th] **S35.416 Laceration of unspecified renal vein** [POA] [MCC] [CC/MCC Exc]

[6th] **S35.49 Other specified injury of renal blood vessel**
- [7th] **S35.491 Other specified injury of right renal artery** [POA] [MCC] [CC/MCC Exc]
- [7th] **S35.492 Other specified injury of left renal artery** [POA] [MCC] [CC/MCC Exc]
- [7th] **S35.493 Other specified injury of unspecified renal artery** [POA] [MCC] [CC/MCC Exc]
- [7th] **S35.494 Other specified injury of right renal vein** [POA] [MCC] [CC/MCC Exc]
- [7th] **S35.495 Other specified injury of left renal vein** [POA] [MCC] [CC/MCC Exc]
- [7th] **S35.496 Other specified injury of unspecified renal vein** [POA] [MCC] [CC/MCC Exc]

[5th] **S35.5 Injury of iliac blood vessels**

[7th] **S35.50 Injury of unspecified iliac blood vessel(s)** [POA] [MCC] [CC/MCC Exc]

[6th] **S35.51 Injury of iliac artery or vein**
- Injury of hypogastric artery or vein
- [7th] **S35.511 Injury of right iliac artery** [POA] [MCC] [CC/MCC Exc]
- [7th] **S35.512 Injury of left iliac artery** [POA] [MCC] [CC/MCC Exc]
- [7th] **S35.513 Injury of unspecified iliac artery** [POA] [MCC] [CC/MCC Exc]
- [7th] **S35.514 Injury of right iliac vein** [POA] [MCC] [CC/MCC Exc]
- [7th] **S35.515 Injury of left iliac vein** [POA] [MCC] [CC/MCC Exc]
- [7th] **S35.516 Injury of unspecified iliac vein** [POA] [MCC] [CC/MCC Exc]

[6th] **S35.53 Injury of uterine artery or vein**
- [7th] **S35.531 Injury of right uterine artery** [CC] [POA] ♀ [CC/MCC Exc]
- [7th] **S35.532 Injury of left uterine artery** [CC] [POA] ♀ [CC/MCC Exc]
- [7th] **S35.533 Injury of unspecified uterine artery** [CC] [POA] ♀ [CC/MCC Exc]
- [7th] **S35.534 Injury of right uterine vein** [CC] [POA] ♀ [CC/MCC Exc]
- [7th] **S35.535 Injury of left uterine vein** [CC] [POA] ♀ [CC/MCC Exc]
- [7th] **S35.536 Injury of unspecified uterine vein** [CC] [POA] ♀ [CC/MCC Exc]

[7th] **S35.59 Injury of other iliac blood vessels** [POA] [MCC] [CC/MCC Exc]

5ᵗʰ S35.8 Injury of other blood vessels at abdomen, lower back and pelvis level

Injury of ovarian artery or vein

6ᵗʰ S35.8X Injury of other blood vessels at abdomen, lower back and pelvis level

7ᵗʰ S35.8X1 Laceration of other blood vessels at abdomen, lower back and pelvis level CC POA CC/MCC Exc

7ᵗʰ S35.8X8 Other specified injury of other blood vessels at abdomen, lower back and pelvis level CC POA CC/MCC Exc

7ᵗʰ S35.8X9 Unspecified injury of other blood vessels at abdomen, lower back and pelvis level CC/MCC Exc

5ᵗʰ S35.9 Injury of unspecified blood vessel at abdomen, lower back and pelvis level

7ᵗʰ S35.90 Unspecified injury of unspecified blood vessel at abdomen, lower back and pelvis level CC POA CC/MCC Exc

7ᵗʰ S35.91 Laceration of unspecified blood vessel at abdomen, lower back and pelvis level CC POA CC/MCC Exc

7ᵗʰ S35.99 Other specified injury of unspecified blood vessel at abdomen, lower back and pelvis level CC POA CC/MCC Exc

4ᵗʰ S36 Injury of intra-abdominal organs

Code also any associated open wound (S31.-)

The appropriate 7th character is to be added to each code from category S36

A = initial encounter

D = subsequent encounter

S = sequela

5ᵗʰ S36.0 Injury of spleen

7ᵗʰ S36.00 Unspecified injury of spleen CC POA CC/MCC Exc

6ᵗʰ S36.02 Contusion of spleen

7ᵗʰ S36.020 Minor contusion of spleen CC POA CC/MCC Exc

Contusion of spleen less than 2 cm

7ᵗʰ S36.021 Major contusion of spleen CC POA CC/MCC Exc

Contusion of spleen greater than 2 cm

7ᵗʰ S36.029 Unspecified contusion of spleen CC POA CC/MCC Exc

AHA: Q1 2015

6ᵗʰ S36.03 Laceration of spleen

7ᵗʰ S36.030 Superficial (capsular) laceration of spleen CC POA CC/MCC Exc

Laceration of spleen less than 1 cm

Minor laceration of spleen

7ᵗʰ S36.031 Moderate laceration of spleen POA MCC CC/MCC Exc

AHA: Q1 2015, Q2 2015

Laceration of spleen 1 to 3 cm

7ᵗʰ S36.032 Major laceration of spleen POA MCC CC/MCC Exc

Avulsion of spleen

Laceration of spleen greater than 3 cm

Massive laceration of spleen

Multiple moderate lacerations of spleen

Stellate laceration of spleen

7ᵗʰ S36.039 Unspecified laceration of spleen CC POA CC/MCC Exc

7ᵗʰ S36.09 Other injury of spleen CC POA CC/MCC Exc

5ᵗʰ S36.1 Injury of liver and gallbladder and bile duct

6ᵗʰ S36.11 Injury of liver

7ᵗʰ S36.112 Contusion of liver CC POA CC/MCC Exc

7ᵗʰ S36.113 Laceration of liver, unspecified degree CC POA CC/MCC Exc

7ᵗʰ S36.114 Minor laceration of liver CC POA CC/MCC Exc

Laceration involving capsule only, or, without significant involvement of hepatic parenchyma [i.e., less than 1 cm deep]

7ᵗʰ S36.115 Moderate laceration of liver POA MCC CC/MCC Exc

Laceration involving parenchyma but without major disruption of parenchyma [i.e., less than 10 cm long and less than 3 cm deep]

7ᵗʰ S36.116 Major laceration of liver POA MCC CC/MCC Exc

Laceration with significant disruption of hepatic parenchyma [i.e., greater than 10 cm long and 3 cm deep]

Multiple moderate lacerations, with or without hematoma

Stellate laceration of liver

7ᵗʰ S36.118 Other injury of liver CC POA CC/MCC Exc

7ᵗʰ S36.119 Unspecified injury of liver CC POA CC/MCC Exc

AHA: Q2 2015

6ᵗʰ S36.12 Injury of gallbladder

7ᵗʰ S36.122 Contusion of gallbladder CC POA CC/MCC Exc

7ᵗʰ S36.123 Laceration of gallbladder CC POA CC/MCC Exc

7ᵗʰ S36.128 Other injury of gallbladder CC POA CC/MCC Exc

7ᵗʰ S36.129 Unspecified injury of gallbladder CC POA CC/MCC Exc

7ᵗʰ S36.13 Injury of bile duct CC POA CC/MCC Exc

5ᵗʰ S36.2 Injury of pancreas

6ᵗʰ S36.20 Unspecified injury of pancreas

7ᵗʰ S36.200 Unspecified injury of head of pancreas CC POA CC/MCC Exc

7ᵗʰ S36.201 Unspecified injury of body of pancreas CC POA CC/MCC Exc

7ᵗʰ S36.202 Unspecified injury of tail of pancreas CC POA CC/MCC Exc

7ᵗʰ S36.209 Unspecified injury of unspecified part of pancreas CC POA CC/MCC Exc

6ᵗʰ S36.22 Contusion of pancreas

7ᵗʰ S36.220 Contusion of head of pancreas CC POA CC/MCC Exc

7ᵗʰ S36.221 Contusion of body of pancreas CC POA CC/MCC Exc

7ᵗʰ S36.222 Contusion of tail of pancreas CC POA CC/MCC Exc

7ᵗʰ S36.229 Contusion of unspecified part of pancreas CC POA CC/MCC Exc

6ᵗʰ S36.23 Laceration of pancreas, unspecified degree

7ᵗʰ S36.230 Laceration of head of pancreas, unspecified degree CC POA CC/MCC Exc

7ᵗʰ S36.231 Laceration of body of pancreas, unspecified degree CC POA CC/MCC Exc

7ᵗʰ S36.232 Laceration of tail of pancreas, unspecified degree CC POA CC/MCC Exc

7ᵗʰ S36.239 Laceration of unspecified part of pancreas, unspecified degree CC POA CC/MCC Exc

6ᵗʰ S36.24 Minor laceration of pancreas

7ᵗʰ S36.240 Minor laceration of head of pancreas CC POA CC/MCC Exc

7ᵗʰ S36.241 Minor laceration of body of pancreas CC POA CC/MCC Exc

7ᵗʰ S36.242 Minor laceration of tail of pancreas CC POA CC/MCC Exc

7ᵗʰ S36.249 Minor laceration of unspecified part of pancreas CC POA CC/MCC Exc

6ᵗʰ S36.25 Moderate laceration of pancreas

7ᵗʰ S36.250 Moderate laceration of head of pancreas CC POA CC/MCC Exc

7ᵗʰ S36.251 Moderate laceration of body of pancreas CC POA CC/MCC Exc

7ᵗʰ S36.252 Moderate laceration of tail of pancreas CC POA CC/MCC Exc

7ᵗʰ S36.259 Moderate laceration of unspecified part of pancreas CC POA CC/MCC Exc

6ᵗʰ S36.26 Major laceration of pancreas

7ᵗʰ S36.260 Major laceration of head of pancreas CC POA CC/MCC Exc

7ᵗʰ S36.261 Major laceration of body of pancreas CC POA CC/MCC Exc

7ᵗʰ S36.262 Major laceration of tail of pancreas CC POA CC/MCC Exc

7ᵗʰ S36.269 Major laceration of unspecified part of pancreas CC POA CC/MCC Exc

---

PDx Unacceptable principal diagnosis symbol per Medicare code edits   Code exempt from diagnosis present on admission requirement

❓ Questionable admission   CC Complication or comorbidity   MCC Major complication or comorbidity   CC/MCC CC/MCC exclusion

HCC HCC diagnosis code   RxHCC RxHCC diagnosis code   MACRA MACRA code   **DEFINITION** Describes condition/terminology

TIP Coding guidance   👁 Official Guideline Reference   Z1 Z code as first-listed diagnosis

[6th] S36.29 Other injury of pancreas
[7th] S36.290 Other injury of head of pancreas [CC] [POA] [CC/MCC Exc]
[7th] S36.291 Other injury of body of pancreas [CC] [POA] [CC/MCC Exc]
[7th] S36.292 Other injury of tail of pancreas [CC] [POA] [CC/MCC Exc]
[7th] S36.299 Other injury of unspecified part of pancreas [CC] [POA] [CC/MCC Exc]

[5th] S36.3 Injury of stomach
[7th] S36.30 Unspecified injury of stomach [CC] [POA] [CC/MCC Exc]
[7th] S36.32 Contusion of stomach [CC] [POA] [CC/MCC Exc]
[7th] S36.33 Laceration of stomach [CC] [POA] [CC/MCC Exc]
[7th] S36.39 Other injury of stomach [CC] [POA] [CC/MCC Exc]

[5th] S36.4 Injury of small intestine
[6th] S36.40 Unspecified injury of small intestine
[7th] S36.400 Unspecified injury of duodenum [CC] [POA] [CC/MCC Exc]
[7th] S36.408 Unspecified injury of other part of small intestine [CC] [POA] [CC/MCC Exc]
[7th] S36.409 Unspecified injury of unspecified part of small intestine [CC] [POA] [CC/MCC Exc]
[6th] S36.41 Primary blast injury of small intestine
Blast injury of small intestine NOS
[7th] S36.410 Primary blast injury of duodenum [CC] [POA] [CC/MCC Exc]
[7th] S36.418 Primary blast injury of other part of small intestine [CC] [POA] [CC/MCC Exc]
[7th] S36.419 Primary blast injury of unspecified part of small intestine [CC] [POA] [CC/MCC Exc]
[6th] S36.42 Contusion of small intestine
[7th] S36.420 Contusion of duodenum [CC] [POA] [CC/MCC Exc]
[7th] S36.428 Contusion of other part of small intestine [CC] [POA] [CC/MCC Exc]
[7th] S36.429 Contusion of unspecified part of small intestine [CC] [POA] [CC/MCC Exc]
[6th] S36.43 Laceration of small intestine
[7th] S36.430 Laceration of duodenum [CC] [POA] [CC/MCC Exc]
[7th] S36.438 Laceration of other part of small intestine [CC] [POA] [CC/MCC Exc]
[7th] S36.439 Laceration of unspecified part of small intestine [CC] [POA] [CC/MCC Exc]
[6th] S36.49 Other injury of small intestine
[7th] S36.490 Other injury of duodenum [CC] [POA] [CC/MCC Exc]
[7th] S36.498 Other injury of other part of small intestine [CC] [POA] [CC/MCC Exc]
[7th] S36.499 Other injury of unspecified part of small intestine [CC] [POA] [CC/MCC Exc]

[5th] S36.5 Injury of colon
EXCLUDES2 *injury of rectum (S36.6-)*
[6th] S36.50 Unspecified injury of colon
[7th] S36.500 Unspecified injury of ascending [right] colon [CC] [POA] [CC/MCC Exc]
[7th] S36.501 Unspecified injury of transverse colon [CC] [POA] [CC/MCC Exc]
[7th] S36.502 Unspecified injury of descending [left] colon [CC] [POA] [CC/MCC Exc]
[7th] S36.503 Unspecified injury of sigmoid colon [CC] [POA] [CC/MCC Exc]
[7th] S36.508 Unspecified injury of other part of colon [CC] [POA] [CC/MCC Exc]
[7th] S36.509 Unspecified injury of unspecified part of colon [CC] [POA] [CC/MCC Exc]
[6th] S36.51 Primary blast injury of colon
Blast injury of colon NOS
[7th] S36.510 Primary blast injury of ascending [right] colon [CC] [POA] [CC/MCC Exc]
[7th] S36.511 Primary blast injury of transverse colon [CC] [POA] [CC/MCC Exc]
[7th] S36.512 Primary blast injury of descending [left] colon [CC] [POA] [CC/MCC Exc]
[7th] S36.513 Primary blast injury of sigmoid colon [CC] [POA] [CC/MCC Exc]
[7th] S36.518 Primary blast injury of other part of colon [CC] [POA] [CC/MCC Exc]
[7th] S36.519 Primary blast injury of unspecified part of colon [CC] [POA] [CC/MCC Exc]
[6th] S36.52 Contusion of colon
[7th] S36.520 Contusion of ascending [right] colon [CC] [POA] [CC/MCC Exc]
[7th] S36.521 Contusion of transverse colon [CC] [POA] [CC/MCC Exc]
[7th] S36.522 Contusion of descending [left] colon [CC] [POA] [CC/MCC Exc]
[7th] S36.523 Contusion of sigmoid colon [CC] [POA] [CC/MCC Exc]
[7th] S36.528 Contusion of other part of colon [CC] [POA] [CC/MCC Exc]
[7th] S36.529 Contusion of unspecified part of colon [CC] [POA] [CC/MCC Exc]
[6th] S36.53 Laceration of colon
[7th] S36.530 Laceration of ascending [right] colon [CC] [POA] [CC/MCC Exc]
[7th] S36.531 Laceration of transverse colon [CC] [POA] [CC/MCC Exc]
[7th] S36.532 Laceration of descending [left] colon [CC] [POA] [CC/MCC Exc]
[7th] S36.533 Laceration of sigmoid colon [CC] [POA] [CC/MCC Exc]
[7th] S36.538 Laceration of other part of colon [CC] [POA] [CC/MCC Exc]
[7th] S36.539 Laceration of unspecified part of colon [CC] [POA] [CC/MCC Exc]
[6th] S36.59 Other injury of colon
Secondary blast injury of colon
[7th] S36.590 Other injury of ascending [right] colon [CC] [POA] [CC/MCC Exc]
[7th] S36.591 Other injury of transverse colon [CC] [POA] [CC/MCC Exc]
[7th] S36.592 Other injury of descending [left] colon [CC] [POA] [CC/MCC Exc]
[7th] S36.593 Other injury of sigmoid colon [CC] [POA] [CC/MCC Exc]
[7th] S36.598 Other injury of other part of colon [CC] [POA] [CC/MCC Exc]
[7th] S36.599 Other injury of unspecified part of colon [CC] [POA] [CC/MCC Exc]

[5th] S36.6 Injury of rectum
[7th] S36.60 Unspecified injury of rectum [CC] [POA] [CC/MCC Exc]
[7th] S36.61 Primary blast injury of rectum [CC] [POA] [CC/MCC Exc]
Blast injury of rectum NOS
[7th] S36.62 Contusion of rectum [CC] [POA] [CC/MCC Exc]
[7th] S36.63 Laceration of rectum [CC] [POA] [CC/MCC Exc]
[7th] S36.69 Other injury of rectum [CC] [POA] [CC/MCC Exc]
Secondary blast injury of rectum

[5th] S36.8 Injury of other intra-abdominal organs
[7th] S36.81 Injury of peritoneum [CC] [POA] [CC/MCC Exc]
[6th] S36.89 Injury of other intra-abdominal organs
Injury of retroperitoneum
[7th] S36.892 Contusion of other intra-abdominal organs [CC] [POA] [CC/MCC Exc]
[7th] S36.893 Laceration of other intra-abdominal organs [CC] [POA] [CC/MCC Exc]
[7th] S36.898 Other injury of other intra-abdominal organs [CC] [POA] [CC/MCC Exc]
[7th] S36.899 Unspecified injury of other intra-abdominal organs [CC] [POA] [CC/MCC Exc]

[5th] S36.9 Injury of unspecified intra-abdominal organ
[7th] S36.90 Unspecified injury of unspecified intra-abdominal organ [CC] [POA] [CC/MCC Exc]
[7th] S36.92 Contusion of unspecified intra-abdominal organ [CC] [POA] [CC/MCC Exc]
[7th] S36.93 Laceration of unspecified intra-abdominal organ [CC] [POA] [CC/MCC Exc]
[7th] S36.99 Other injury of unspecified intra-abdominal organ [CC] [POA] [CC/MCC Exc]

Unspecified Code Other Specified Code Manifestation Code [N] Newborn [P] Pediatric [M] Maternity [A] Adult ♂ Male ♀ Female
● New Code ▲ Revised Code Title ►◄ Revised Text NOTES INCLUDES EXCLUDES1 Not coded here EXCLUDES2 Not included here
[4th] 4th character required [5th] 5th character required [6th] 6th character required [7th] 7th character required [7th] Extension 'X' Alert
[HAC] Hospital-acquired condition (HAC) alert AHA AHA Coding Clinic© ☞ Code first alert

S37 Injury of urinary and pelvic organs
Code also any associated open wound (S31.-)
EXCLUDES1 obstetric trauma to pelvic organs (O71.-)
EXCLUDES2 injury of peritoneum (S36.81)
injury of retroperitoneum (S36.89-)

The appropriate 7th character is to be added to each code from category S37
A = initial encounter
D = subsequent encounter
S = sequela

S37.0 Injury of kidney
EXCLUDES2 acute kidney injury (nontraumatic) (N17.9)

S37.00 Unspecified injury of kidney
- S37.001 Unspecified injury of right kidney
- S37.002 Unspecified injury of left kidney
- S37.009 Unspecified injury of unspecified kidney

S37.01 Minor contusion of kidney
Contusion of kidney less than 2 cm
Contusion of kidney NOS
- S37.011 Minor contusion of right kidney
- S37.012 Minor contusion of left kidney
- S37.019 Minor contusion of unspecified kidney

S37.02 Major contusion of kidney
Contusion of kidney greater than 2 cm
- S37.021 Major contusion of right kidney
- S37.022 Major contusion of left kidney
- S37.029 Major contusion of unspecified kidney

S37.03 Laceration of kidney, unspecified degree
- S37.031 Laceration of right kidney, unspecified degree
- S37.032 Laceration of left kidney, unspecified degree
- S37.039 Laceration of unspecified kidney, unspecified degree

S37.04 Minor laceration of kidney
Laceration of kidney less than 1 cm
- S37.041 Minor laceration of right kidney
- S37.042 Minor laceration of left kidney
- S37.049 Minor laceration of unspecified kidney

S37.05 Moderate laceration of kidney
Laceration of kidney 1 to 3 cm
- S37.051 Moderate laceration of right kidney
- S37.052 Moderate laceration of left kidney
- S37.059 Moderate laceration of unspecified kidney

S37.06 Major laceration of kidney
Avulsion of kidney
Laceration of kidney greater than 3 cm
Massive laceration of kidney
Multiple moderate lacerations of kidney
Stellate laceration of kidney
- S37.061 Major laceration of right kidney
- S37.062 Major laceration of left kidney
- S37.069 Major laceration of unspecified kidney

S37.09 Other injury of kidney
- S37.091 Other injury of right kidney
- S37.092 Other injury of left kidney
- S37.099 Other injury of unspecified kidney

S37.1 Injury of ureter
- S37.10 Unspecified injury of ureter
- S37.12 Contusion of ureter

- S37.13 Laceration of ureter
- S37.19 Other injury of ureter

S37.2 Injury of bladder
- S37.20 Unspecified injury of bladder
- S37.22 Contusion of bladder
- S37.23 Laceration of bladder
- S37.29 Other injury of bladder

S37.3 Injury of urethra
- S37.30 Unspecified injury of urethra
- S37.32 Contusion of urethra
- S37.33 Laceration of urethra
- S37.39 Other injury of urethra

S37.4 Injury of ovary
S37.40 Unspecified injury of ovary
- S37.401 Unspecified injury of ovary, unilateral
- S37.402 Unspecified injury of ovary, bilateral
- S37.409 Unspecified injury of ovary, unspecified

S37.42 Contusion of ovary
- S37.421 Contusion of ovary, unilateral
- S37.422 Contusion of ovary, bilateral
- S37.429 Contusion of ovary, unspecified

S37.43 Laceration of ovary
- S37.431 Laceration of ovary, unilateral
- S37.432 Laceration of ovary, bilateral
- S37.439 Laceration of ovary, unspecified

S37.49 Other injury of ovary
- S37.491 Other injury of ovary, unilateral
- S37.492 Other injury of ovary, bilateral
- S37.499 Other injury of ovary, unspecified

S37.5 Injury of fallopian tube
S37.50 Unspecified injury of fallopian tube
- S37.501 Unspecified injury of fallopian tube, unilateral
- S37.502 Unspecified injury of fallopian tube, bilateral
- S37.509 Unspecified injury of fallopian tube, unspecified

S37.51 Primary blast injury of fallopian tube
Blast injury of fallopian tube NOS
- S37.511 Primary blast injury of fallopian tube, unilateral
- S37.512 Primary blast injury of fallopian tube, bilateral
- S37.519 Primary blast injury of fallopian tube, unspecified

S37.52 Contusion of fallopian tube
- S37.521 Contusion of fallopian tube, unilateral
- S37.522 Contusion of fallopian tube, bilateral
- S37.529 Contusion of fallopian tube, unspecified

S37.53 Laceration of fallopian tube
- S37.531 Laceration of fallopian tube, unilateral
- S37.532 Laceration of fallopian tube, bilateral
- S37.539 Laceration of fallopian tube, unspecified

S37.59 Other injury of fallopian tube
Secondary blast injury of fallopian tube
- S37.591 Other injury of fallopian tube, unilateral
- S37.592 Other injury of fallopian tube, bilateral
- S37.599 Other injury of fallopian tube, unspecified

S37.6 Injury of uterus
EXCLUDES1 injury to gravid uterus (O9A.2-)
injury to uterus during delivery (O71.-)
- S37.60 Unspecified injury of uterus

Unacceptable principal diagnosis symbol per Medicare code edits   Code exempt from diagnosis present on admission requirement
❓ Questionable admission   Complication or comorbidity   MCC Major complication or comorbidity   CC/MCC Exc CC/MCC exclusion
HCC HCC diagnosis code   RxHCC RxHCC diagnosis code   MACRA code   **DEFINITION** Describes condition/terminology
TIP Coding guidance   ⊚ Official Guideline Reference   Z1 Z code as first-listed diagnosis

[7th] S37.62 Contusion of uterus CC POA ♀ CC/MCC Exc
[7th] S37.63 Laceration of uterus CC POA ♀ CC/MCC Exc
[7th] S37.69 Other injury of uterus CC POA ♀ CC/MCC Exc
[5th] S37.8 Injury of other urinary and pelvic organs
[6th] S37.81 Injury of adrenal gland
[7th] S37.812 Contusion of adrenal gland CC POA CC/MCC Exc
[7th] S37.813 Laceration of adrenal gland CC POA CC/MCC Exc
[7th] S37.818 Other injury of adrenal gland CC POA CC/MCC Exc
[7th] S37.819 Unspecified injury of adrenal gland CC POA CC/MCC Exc
[6th] S37.82 Injury of prostate
[7th] S37.822 Contusion of prostate POA ♂
[7th] S37.823 Laceration of prostate POA ♂
[7th] S37.828 Other injury of prostate POA ♂
[7th] S37.829 Unspecified injury of prostate POA ♂
[6th] S37.89 Injury of other urinary and pelvic organ
[7th] S37.892 Contusion of other urinary and pelvic organ CC POA CC/MCC Exc
[7th] S37.893 Laceration of other urinary and pelvic organ CC POA CC/MCC Exc
[7th] S37.898 Other injury of other urinary and pelvic organ CC POA CC/MCC Exc
[7th] S37.899 Unspecified injury of other urinary and pelvic organ CC POA CC/MCC Exc
[5th] S37.9 Injury of unspecified urinary and pelvic organ
[7th] S37.90 Unspecified injury of unspecified urinary and pelvic organ CC POA CC/MCC Exc
[7th] S37.92 Contusion of unspecified urinary and pelvic organ CC POA CC/MCC Exc
[7th] S37.93 Laceration of unspecified urinary and pelvic organ CC POA CC/MCC Exc
[7th] S37.99 Other injury of unspecified urinary and pelvic organ CC POA CC/MCC Exc

[4th] **S38 Crushing injury and traumatic amputation of abdomen, lower back, pelvis and external genitals**

An amputation not identified as partial or complete should be coded to complete

The appropriate 7th character is to be added to each code from category S38
- A = initial encounter
- D = subsequent encounter
- S = sequela

[5th] S38.0 Crushing injury of external genital organs
Use additional code for any associated injuries
[6th] S38.00 Crushing injury of unspecified external genital organs
[7th] S38.001 Crushing injury of unspecified external genital organs, male POA ♂
[7th] S38.002 Crushing injury of unspecified external genital organs, female POA ♀
[7th] S38.01 Crushing injury of penis POA ♂
[7th] S38.02 Crushing injury of scrotum and testis POA ♂
[7th] S38.03 Crushing injury of vulva POA ♀
[7th] S38.1 Crushing injury of abdomen, lower back, and pelvis POA
Use additional code for all associated injuries, such as:
- fracture of thoracic or lumbar spine and pelvis (S22.0-, S32.-)
- injury to intra-abdominal organs (S36.-)
- injury to urinary and pelvic organs (S37.-)
- open wound of abdominal wall (S31.-)
- spinal cord injury (S34.0, S34.1-)

[EXCLUDES2] *crushing injury of external genital organs (S38.0-)*

[5th] S38.2 Traumatic amputation of external genital organs
[6th] S38.21 Traumatic amputation of female external genital organs
Traumatic amputation of clitoris
Traumatic amputation of labium (majus) (minus)
Traumatic amputation of vulva
[7th] S38.211 Complete traumatic amputation of female external genital organs POA ♀
[7th] S38.212 Partial traumatic amputation of female external genital organs POA ♀
[6th] S38.22 Traumatic amputation of penis
[7th] S38.221 Complete traumatic amputation of penis POA ♂
[7th] S38.222 Partial traumatic amputation of penis POA ♂
[6th] S38.23 Traumatic amputation of scrotum and testis
[7th] S38.231 Complete traumatic amputation of scrotum and testis POA ♂
[7th] S38.232 Partial traumatic amputation of scrotum and testis POA ♂
[7th] S38.3 Transection (partial) of abdomen POA

[4th] **S39 Other and unspecified injuries of abdomen, lower back, pelvis and external genitals**

Code also any associated open wound (S31.-)

[EXCLUDES2] *sprain of joints and ligaments of lumbar spine and pelvis (S33.-)*

The appropriate 7th character is to be added to each code from category S39
- A = initial encounter
- D = subsequent encounter
- S = sequela

[5th] S39.0 Injury of muscle, fascia and tendon of abdomen, lower back and pelvis
[6th] S39.00 Unspecified injury of muscle, fascia and tendon of abdomen, lower back and pelvis
[7th] S39.001 Unspecified injury of muscle, fascia and tendon of abdomen POA
[7th] S39.002 Unspecified injury of muscle, fascia and tendon of lower back POA
[7th] S39.003 Unspecified injury of muscle, fascia and tendon of pelvis POA
[6th] S39.01 Strain of muscle, fascia and tendon of abdomen, lower back and pelvis
[7th] S39.011 Strain of muscle, fascia and tendon of abdomen POA
[7th] S39.012 Strain of muscle, fascia and tendon of lower back POA
AHA: Q4 2016
[7th] S39.013 Strain of muscle, fascia and tendon of pelvis POA
[6th] S39.02 Laceration of muscle, fascia and tendon of abdomen, lower back and pelvis
[7th] S39.021 Laceration of muscle, fascia and tendon of abdomen POA
[7th] S39.022 Laceration of muscle, fascia and tendon of lower back POA
[7th] S39.023 Laceration of muscle, fascia and tendon of pelvis POA
[6th] S39.09 Other injury of muscle, fascia and tendon of abdomen, lower back and pelvis
[7th] S39.091 Other injury of muscle, fascia and tendon of abdomen POA
[7th] S39.092 Other injury of muscle, fascia and tendon of lower back POA
[7th] S39.093 Other injury of muscle, fascia and tendon of pelvis POA
[5th] S39.8 Other specified injuries of abdomen, lower back, pelvis and external genitals
[7th] S39.81 Other specified injuries of abdomen POA
[7th] S39.82 Other specified injuries of lower back POA
[7th] S39.83 Other specified injuries of pelvis POA
[6th] S39.84 Other specified injuries of external genitals
[7th] S39.840 Fracture of corpus cavernosum penis POA ♂
[7th] S39.848 Other specified injuries of external genitals POA
[5th] S39.9 Unspecified injury of abdomen, lower back, pelvis and external genitals
[7th] S39.91 Unspecified injury of abdomen POA
[7th] S39.92 Unspecified injury of lower back POA
[7th] S39.93 Unspecified injury of pelvis POA
[7th] S39.94 Unspecified injury of external genitals POA

Unspecified Code | Other Specified Code | Manifestation Code | [N] Newborn | [P] Pediatric | [M] Maternity | [A] Adult | ♂ Male | ♀ Female
● New Code ▲ Revised Code Title ►◄ Revised Text [NOTES] *INCLUDES* [EXCLUDES1] Not coded here [EXCLUDES2] Not included here
[4th] 4th character required [5th] 5th character required [6th] 6th character required [7th] 7th character required [x] Extension 'X' Alert
[HAC] Hospital-acquired condition (HAC) alert AHA AHA Coding Clinic© Code first alert

Injuries to the shoulder and upper arm (S40-S49)

INCLUDES   injuries of axilla
              injuries of scapular region
EXCLUDES2   burns and corrosions (T20-T32)
              frostbite (T33-T34)
              injuries of elbow (S50-S59)
              insect bite or sting, venomous (T63.4)

4ᵗʰ **S40** Superficial injury of shoulder and upper arm
The appropriate 7th character is to be added to each code from category S40
A = initial encounter
D = subsequent encounter
S = sequela

5ᵗʰ **S40.0** Contusion of shoulder and upper arm
  6ᵗʰ **S40.01** Contusion of shoulder
    7ᵗʰ **S40.011** Contusion of right shoulder POA
    7ᵗʰ **S40.012** Contusion of left shoulder POA
    7ᵗʰ **S40.019** Contusion of unspecified shoulder POA
  6ᵗʰ **S40.02** Contusion of upper arm
    7ᵗʰ **S40.021** Contusion of right upper arm POA
    7ᵗʰ **S40.022** Contusion of left upper arm POA
    7ᵗʰ **S40.029** Contusion of unspecified upper arm POA

5ᵗʰ **S40.2** Other superficial injuries of shoulder
  6ᵗʰ **S40.21** Abrasion of shoulder
    7ᵗʰ **S40.211** Abrasion of right shoulder POA
    7ᵗʰ **S40.212** Abrasion of left shoulder POA
    7ᵗʰ **S40.219** Abrasion of unspecified shoulder POA
  6ᵗʰ **S40.22** Blister (nonthermal) of shoulder
    7ᵗʰ **S40.221** Blister (nonthermal) of right shoulder POA
    7ᵗʰ **S40.222** Blister (nonthermal) of left shoulder POA
    7ᵗʰ **S40.229** Blister (nonthermal) of unspecified shoulder POA
  6ᵗʰ **S40.24** External constriction of shoulder
    7ᵗʰ **S40.241** External constriction of right shoulder POA
    7ᵗʰ **S40.242** External constriction of left shoulder POA
    7ᵗʰ **S40.249** External constriction of unspecified shoulder POA
  6ᵗʰ **S40.25** Superficial foreign body of shoulder
    Splinter in the shoulder
    7ᵗʰ **S40.251** Superficial foreign body of right shoulder POA
    7ᵗʰ **S40.252** Superficial foreign body of left shoulder POA
    7ᵗʰ **S40.259** Superficial foreign body of unspecified shoulder POA
  6ᵗʰ **S40.26** Insect bite (nonvenomous) of shoulder
    7ᵗʰ **S40.261** Insect bite (nonvenomous) of right shoulder POA
    7ᵗʰ **S40.262** Insect bite (nonvenomous) of left shoulder POA
    7ᵗʰ **S40.269** Insect bite (nonvenomous) of unspecified shoulder POA
  6ᵗʰ **S40.27** Other superficial bite of shoulder
    EXCLUDES1 open bite of shoulder (S41.05)
    7ᵗʰ **S40.271** Other superficial bite of right shoulder POA
    7ᵗʰ **S40.272** Other superficial bite of left shoulder POA
    7ᵗʰ **S40.279** Other superficial bite of unspecified shoulder POA

5ᵗʰ **S40.8** Other superficial injuries of upper arm
  6ᵗʰ **S40.81** Abrasion of upper arm
    7ᵗʰ **S40.811** Abrasion of right upper arm POA
    7ᵗʰ **S40.812** Abrasion of left upper arm POA
    7ᵗʰ **S40.819** Abrasion of unspecified upper arm POA
  6ᵗʰ **S40.82** Blister (nonthermal) of upper arm
    7ᵗʰ **S40.821** Blister (nonthermal) of right upper arm POA
    7ᵗʰ **S40.822** Blister (nonthermal) of left upper arm POA
    7ᵗʰ **S40.829** Blister (nonthermal) of unspecified upper arm POA

  6ᵗʰ **S40.84** External constriction of upper arm
    7ᵗʰ **S40.841** External constriction of right upper arm POA
    7ᵗʰ **S40.842** External constriction of left upper arm POA
    7ᵗʰ **S40.849** External constriction of unspecified upper arm POA
  6ᵗʰ **S40.85** Superficial foreign body of upper arm
    Splinter in the upper arm
    7ᵗʰ **S40.851** Superficial foreign body of right upper arm POA
    7ᵗʰ **S40.852** Superficial foreign body of left upper arm POA
    7ᵗʰ **S40.859** Superficial foreign body of unspecified upper arm POA
  6ᵗʰ **S40.86** Insect bite (nonvenomous) of upper arm
    7ᵗʰ **S40.861** Insect bite (nonvenomous) of right upper arm POA
    7ᵗʰ **S40.862** Insect bite (nonvenomous) of left upper arm POA
    7ᵗʰ **S40.869** Insect bite (nonvenomous) of unspecified upper arm POA
  6ᵗʰ **S40.87** Other superficial bite of upper arm
    EXCLUDES1 open bite of upper arm (S41.14)
    EXCLUDES2 other superficial bite of shoulder (S40.27-)
    7ᵗʰ **S40.871** Other superficial bite of right upper arm POA
    7ᵗʰ **S40.872** Other superficial bite of left upper arm POA
    7ᵗʰ **S40.879** Other superficial bite of unspecified upper arm POA

5ᵗʰ **S40.9** Unspecified superficial injury of shoulder and upper arm
  6ᵗʰ **S40.91** Unspecified superficial injury of shoulder
    7ᵗʰ **S40.911** Unspecified superficial injury of right shoulder POA
    7ᵗʰ **S40.912** Unspecified superficial injury of left shoulder POA
    7ᵗʰ **S40.919** Unspecified superficial injury of unspecified shoulder POA
  6ᵗʰ **S40.92** Unspecified superficial injury of upper arm
    7ᵗʰ **S40.921** Unspecified superficial injury of right upper arm POA
    7ᵗʰ **S40.922** Unspecified superficial injury of left upper arm POA
    7ᵗʰ **S40.929** Unspecified superficial injury of unspecified upper arm POA

4ᵗʰ **S41** Open wound of shoulder and upper arm
Code also any associated wound infection
EXCLUDES1 traumatic amputation of shoulder and upper arm (S48.-)
EXCLUDES2 open fracture of shoulder and upper arm (S42.- with 7th character B or C)
The appropriate 7th character is to be added to each code from category S41
A = initial encounter
D = subsequent encounter
S = sequela

5ᵗʰ **S41.0** Open wound of shoulder
  6ᵗʰ **S41.00** Unspecified open wound of shoulder
    7ᵗʰ **S41.001** Unspecified open wound of right shoulder POA
    7ᵗʰ **S41.002** Unspecified open wound of left shoulder POA
    7ᵗʰ **S41.009** Unspecified open wound of unspecified shoulder POA
  6ᵗʰ **S41.01** Laceration without foreign body of shoulder
    7ᵗʰ **S41.011** Laceration without foreign body of right shoulder POA
    7ᵗʰ **S41.012** Laceration without foreign body of left shoulder POA
    7ᵗʰ **S41.019** Laceration without foreign body of unspecified shoulder POA
  6ᵗʰ **S41.02** Laceration with foreign body of shoulder
    7ᵗʰ **S41.021** Laceration with foreign body of right shoulder POA

[7th] S41.022 Laceration with foreign body of left shoulder POA
[7th] S41.029 Laceration with foreign body of unspecified shoulder POA
[6th] S41.03 Puncture wound without foreign body of shoulder
[7th] S41.031 Puncture wound without foreign body of right shoulder POA
[7th] S41.032 Puncture wound without foreign body of left shoulder POA
[7th] S41.039 Puncture wound without foreign body of unspecified shoulder POA
[6th] S41.04 Puncture wound with foreign body of shoulder
[7th] S41.041 Puncture wound with foreign body of right shoulder POA
[7th] S41.042 Puncture wound with foreign body of left shoulder POA
[7th] S41.049 Puncture wound with foreign body of unspecified shoulder POA
[6th] S41.05 Open bite of shoulder
Bite of shoulder NOS
[EXCLUDES1] *superficial bite of shoulder (S40.27)*
[7th] S41.051 Open bite of right shoulder POA
[7th] S41.052 Open bite of left shoulder POA
[7th] S41.059 Open bite of unspecified shoulder POA
[5th] S41.1 Open wound of upper arm
[6th] S41.10 Unspecified open wound of upper arm
[7th] S41.101 Unspecified open wound of right upper arm POA
[7th] S41.102 Unspecified open wound of left upper arm POA
[7th] S41.109 Unspecified open wound of unspecified upper arm POA
[6th] S41.11 Laceration without foreign body of upper arm
[7th] S41.111 Laceration without foreign body of right upper arm POA
[7th] S41.112 Laceration without foreign body of left upper arm POA
[7th] S41.119 Laceration without foreign body of unspecified upper arm POA
[6th] S41.12 Laceration with foreign body of upper arm
[7th] S41.121 Laceration with foreign body of right upper arm POA
[7th] S41.122 Laceration with foreign body of left upper arm POA
[7th] S41.129 Laceration with foreign body of unspecified upper arm POA
[6th] S41.13 Puncture wound without foreign body of upper arm
[7th] S41.131 Puncture wound without foreign body of right upper arm POA
[7th] S41.132 Puncture wound without foreign body of left upper arm POA
[7th] S41.139 Puncture wound without foreign body of unspecified upper arm POA
[6th] S41.14 Puncture wound with foreign body of upper arm
[7th] S41.141 Puncture wound with foreign body of right upper arm POA
[7th] S41.142 Puncture wound with foreign body of left upper arm POA
[7th] S41.149 Puncture wound with foreign body of unspecified upper arm POA
[6th] S41.15 Open bite of upper arm
Bite of upper arm NOS
[EXCLUDES1] *superficial bite of upper arm (S40.87)*
[7th] S41.151 Open bite of right upper arm POA
[7th] S41.152 Open bite of left upper arm POA
[7th] S41.159 Open bite of unspecified upper arm POA
[4th] S42 Fracture of shoulder and upper arm
👁 **See Official Guidelines** "Coding of Traumatic Fractures" I.C.19.c
[NOTES] A fracture not indicated as displaced or nondisplaced should be coded to displaced.
A fracture not indicated as open or closed should be coded to closed.
[EXCLUDES1] *traumatic amputation of shoulder and upper arm (S48.-)*

The appropriate 7th character is to be added to all codes from category S42
A = initial encounter for closed fracture
B = initial encounter for open fracture
D = subsequent encounter for fracture with routine healing
G = subsequent encounter for fracture with delayed healing
K = subsequent encounter for fracture with nonunion
P = subsequent encounter for fracture with malunion
S = sequela

[5th] S42.0 Fracture of clavicle
[6th] S42.00 Fracture of unspecified part of clavicle
[7th] S42.001 Fracture of unspecified part of right clavicle CC POA HAC CC/MCC Exc
[7th] S42.002 Fracture of unspecified part of left clavicle CC POA HAC CC/MCC Exc
[7th] S42.009 Fracture of unspecified part of unspecified clavicle CC POA HAC CC/MCC Exc
[6th] S42.01 Fracture of sternal end of clavicle
[7th] S42.011 Anterior displaced fracture of sternal end of right clavicle CC POA HAC CC/MCC Exc
[7th] S42.012 Anterior displaced fracture of sternal end of left clavicle CC POA HAC CC/MCC Exc
[7th] S42.013 Anterior displaced fracture of sternal end of unspecified clavicle CC POA HAC CC/MCC Exc
Displaced fracture of sternal end of clavicle NOS
[7th] S42.014 Posterior displaced fracture of sternal end of right clavicle CC POA HAC CC/MCC Exc
[7th] S42.015 Posterior displaced fracture of sternal end of left clavicle CC POA HAC CC/MCC Exc
[7th] S42.016 Posterior displaced fracture of sternal end of unspecified clavicle CC POA HAC CC/MCC Exc
[7th] S42.017 Nondisplaced fracture of sternal end of right clavicle CC POA HAC CC/MCC Exc
[7th] S42.018 Nondisplaced fracture of sternal end of left clavicle CC POA HAC CC/MCC Exc
[7th] S42.019 Nondisplaced fracture of sternal end of unspecified clavicle CC POA HAC CC/MCC Exc
[6th] S42.02 Fracture of shaft of clavicle
[7th] S42.021 Displaced fracture of shaft of right clavicle CC POA HAC CC/MCC Exc
[7th] S42.022 Displaced fracture of shaft of left clavicle CC POA HAC CC/MCC Exc
[7th] S42.023 Displaced fracture of shaft of unspecified clavicle CC POA HAC CC/MCC Exc
[7th] S42.024 Nondisplaced fracture of shaft of right clavicle CC POA HAC CC/MCC Exc
[7th] S42.025 Nondisplaced fracture of shaft of left clavicle CC POA HAC CC/MCC Exc
[7th] S42.026 Nondisplaced fracture of shaft of unspecified clavicle CC POA HAC CC/MCC Exc
[6th] S42.03 Fracture of lateral end of clavicle
Fracture of acromial end of clavicle
[7th] S42.031 Displaced fracture of lateral end of right clavicle CC POA HAC CC/MCC Exc
[7th] S42.032 Displaced fracture of lateral end of left clavicle CC POA HAC CC/MCC Exc
[7th] S42.033 Displaced fracture of lateral end of unspecified clavicle CC POA HAC CC/MCC Exc
[7th] S42.034 Nondisplaced fracture of lateral end of right clavicle CC POA HAC CC/MCC Exc
[7th] S42.035 Nondisplaced fracture of lateral end of left clavicle CC POA HAC CC/MCC Exc
[7th] S42.036 Nondisplaced fracture of lateral end of unspecified clavicle CC POA HAC CC/MCC Exc

Unspecified Code · Other Specified Code · Manifestation Code · [N] Newborn · [P] Pediatric · [M] Maternity · [A] Adult · ♂ Male · ♀ Female
● New Code · ▲ Revised Code Title · ►◄ Revised Text · [NOTES] · *INCLUDES* · [EXCLUDES1] Not coded here · [EXCLUDES2] Not included here
[4th] 4th character required · [5th] 5th character required · [6th] 6th character required · [7th] 7th character required · [7th] Extension 'X' Alert
[HAC] Hospital-acquired condition (HAC) alert · AHA AHA Coding Clinic© · ☞ Code first alert

5ᵗʰ **S42.1** Fracture of scapula
- 6ᵗʰ **S42.10** Fracture of unspecified part of scapula
  - 7ᵗʰ **S42.101** Fracture of unspecified part of scapula, right shoulder ᴄᴄ ᴘᴏᴀ ᴴᴬᶜ ᴄᴄ/ᴍᴄᴄ ᴇxᴄ
  - 7ᵗʰ **S42.102** Fracture of unspecified part of scapula, left shoulder ᴄᴄ ᴘᴏᴀ ᴴᴬᶜ ᴄᴄ/ᴍᴄᴄ ᴇxᴄ
  - 7ᵗʰ **S42.109** Fracture of unspecified part of scapula, unspecified shoulder ᴄᴄ ᴘᴏᴀ ᴴᴬᶜ ᴄᴄ/ᴍᴄᴄ ᴇxᴄ
- 6ᵗʰ **S42.11** Fracture of body of scapula
  - 7ᵗʰ **S42.111** Displaced fracture of body of scapula, right shoulder ᴄᴄ ᴘᴏᴀ ᴴᴬᶜ ᴄᴄ/ᴍᴄᴄ ᴇxᴄ
  - 7ᵗʰ **S42.112** Displaced fracture of body of scapula, left shoulder ᴄᴄ ᴘᴏᴀ ᴴᴬᶜ ᴄᴄ/ᴍᴄᴄ ᴇxᴄ
  - 7ᵗʰ **S42.113** Displaced fracture of body of scapula, unspecified shoulder ᴄᴄ ᴘᴏᴀ ᴴᴬᶜ ᴄᴄ/ᴍᴄᴄ ᴇxᴄ
  - 7ᵗʰ **S42.114** Nondisplaced fracture of body of scapula, right shoulder ᴄᴄ ᴘᴏᴀ ᴴᴬᶜ ᴄᴄ/ᴍᴄᴄ ᴇxᴄ
  - 7ᵗʰ **S42.115** Nondisplaced fracture of body of scapula, left shoulder ᴄᴄ ᴘᴏᴀ ᴴᴬᶜ ᴄᴄ/ᴍᴄᴄ ᴇxᴄ
  - 7ᵗʰ **S42.116** Nondisplaced fracture of body of scapula, unspecified shoulder ᴄᴄ ᴘᴏᴀ ᴴᴬᶜ ᴄᴄ/ᴍᴄᴄ ᴇxᴄ
- 6ᵗʰ **S42.12** Fracture of acromial process
  - 7ᵗʰ **S42.121** Displaced fracture of acromial process, right shoulder ᴄᴄ ᴘᴏᴀ ᴴᴬᶜ ᴄᴄ/ᴍᴄᴄ ᴇxᴄ
  - 7ᵗʰ **S42.122** Displaced fracture of acromial process, left shoulder ᴄᴄ ᴘᴏᴀ ᴴᴬᶜ ᴄᴄ/ᴍᴄᴄ ᴇxᴄ
  - 7ᵗʰ **S42.123** Displaced fracture of acromial process, unspecified shoulder ᴄᴄ ᴘᴏᴀ ᴴᴬᶜ ᴄᴄ/ᴍᴄᴄ ᴇxᴄ
  - 7ᵗʰ **S42.124** Nondisplaced fracture of acromial process, right shoulder ᴄᴄ ᴘᴏᴀ ᴴᴬᶜ ᴄᴄ/ᴍᴄᴄ ᴇxᴄ
  - 7ᵗʰ **S42.125** Nondisplaced fracture of acromial process, left shoulder ᴄᴄ ᴘᴏᴀ ᴴᴬᶜ ᴄᴄ/ᴍᴄᴄ ᴇxᴄ
  - 7ᵗʰ **S42.126** Nondisplaced fracture of acromial process, unspecified shoulder ᴄᴄ ᴘᴏᴀ ᴴᴬᶜ ᴄᴄ/ᴍᴄᴄ ᴇxᴄ
- 6ᵗʰ **S42.13** Fracture of coracoid process
  - 7ᵗʰ **S42.131** Displaced fracture of coracoid process, right shoulder ᴄᴄ ᴘᴏᴀ ᴴᴬᶜ ᴄᴄ/ᴍᴄᴄ ᴇxᴄ
  - 7ᵗʰ **S42.132** Displaced fracture of coracoid process, left shoulder ᴄᴄ ᴘᴏᴀ ᴴᴬᶜ ᴄᴄ/ᴍᴄᴄ ᴇxᴄ
  - 7ᵗʰ **S42.133** Displaced fracture of coracoid process, unspecified shoulder ᴄᴄ ᴘᴏᴀ ᴴᴬᶜ ᴄᴄ/ᴍᴄᴄ ᴇxᴄ
  - 7ᵗʰ **S42.134** Nondisplaced fracture of coracoid process, right shoulder ᴄᴄ ᴘᴏᴀ ᴴᴬᶜ ᴄᴄ/ᴍᴄᴄ ᴇxᴄ
  - 7ᵗʰ **S42.135** Nondisplaced fracture of coracoid process, left shoulder ᴄᴄ ᴘᴏᴀ ᴴᴬᶜ ᴄᴄ/ᴍᴄᴄ ᴇxᴄ
  - 7ᵗʰ **S42.136** Nondisplaced fracture of coracoid process, unspecified shoulder ᴄᴄ ᴘᴏᴀ ᴴᴬᶜ ᴄᴄ/ᴍᴄᴄ ᴇxᴄ
- 6ᵗʰ **S42.14** Fracture of glenoid cavity of scapula
  - 7ᵗʰ **S42.141** Displaced fracture of glenoid cavity of scapula, right shoulder ᴄᴄ ᴘᴏᴀ ᴴᴬᶜ ᴄᴄ/ᴍᴄᴄ ᴇxᴄ
  - 7ᵗʰ **S42.142** Displaced fracture of glenoid cavity of scapula, left shoulder ᴄᴄ ᴘᴏᴀ ᴴᴬᶜ ᴄᴄ/ᴍᴄᴄ ᴇxᴄ
  - 7ᵗʰ **S42.143** Displaced fracture of glenoid cavity of scapula, unspecified shoulder ᴄᴄ ᴘᴏᴀ ᴴᴬᶜ ᴄᴄ/ᴍᴄᴄ ᴇxᴄ
  - 7ᵗʰ **S42.144** Nondisplaced fracture of glenoid cavity of scapula, right shoulder ᴄᴄ ᴘᴏᴀ ᴴᴬᶜ ᴄᴄ/ᴍᴄᴄ ᴇxᴄ
  - 7ᵗʰ **S42.145** Nondisplaced fracture of glenoid cavity of scapula, left shoulder ᴄᴄ ᴘᴏᴀ ᴴᴬᶜ ᴄᴄ/ᴍᴄᴄ ᴇxᴄ
  - 7ᵗʰ **S42.146** Nondisplaced fracture of glenoid cavity of scapula, unspecified shoulder ᴄᴄ ᴘᴏᴀ ᴴᴬᶜ ᴄᴄ/ᴍᴄᴄ ᴇxᴄ
- 6ᵗʰ **S42.15** Fracture of neck of scapula
  - 7ᵗʰ **S42.151** Displaced fracture of neck of scapula, right shoulder ᴄᴄ ᴘᴏᴀ ᴴᴬᶜ ᴄᴄ/ᴍᴄᴄ ᴇxᴄ
  - 7ᵗʰ **S42.152** Displaced fracture of neck of scapula, left shoulder ᴄᴄ ᴘᴏᴀ ᴴᴬᶜ ᴄᴄ/ᴍᴄᴄ ᴇxᴄ
  - 7ᵗʰ **S42.153** Displaced fracture of neck of scapula, unspecified shoulder ᴄᴄ ᴘᴏᴀ ᴴᴬᶜ ᴄᴄ/ᴍᴄᴄ ᴇxᴄ
  - 7ᵗʰ **S42.154** Nondisplaced fracture of neck of scapula, right shoulder ᴄᴄ ᴘᴏᴀ ᴴᴬᶜ ᴄᴄ/ᴍᴄᴄ ᴇxᴄ
  - 7ᵗʰ **S42.155** Nondisplaced fracture of neck of scapula, left shoulder ᴄᴄ ᴘᴏᴀ ᴴᴬᶜ ᴄᴄ/ᴍᴄᴄ ᴇxᴄ
  - 7ᵗʰ **S42.156** Nondisplaced fracture of neck of scapula, unspecified shoulder ᴄᴄ ᴘᴏᴀ ᴴᴬᶜ ᴄᴄ/ᴍᴄᴄ ᴇxᴄ
- 6ᵗʰ **S42.19** Fracture of other part of scapula
  - 7ᵗʰ **S42.191** Fracture of other part of scapula, right shoulder ᴄᴄ ᴘᴏᴀ ᴴᴬᶜ ᴄᴄ/ᴍᴄᴄ ᴇxᴄ
  - 7ᵗʰ **S42.192** Fracture of other part of scapula, left shoulder ᴄᴄ ᴘᴏᴀ ᴴᴬᶜ ᴄᴄ/ᴍᴄᴄ ᴇxᴄ
  - 7ᵗʰ **S42.199** Fracture of other part of scapula, unspecified shoulder ᴄᴄ ᴘᴏᴀ ᴴᴬᶜ ᴄᴄ/ᴍᴄᴄ ᴇxᴄ

5ᵗʰ **S42.2** Fracture of upper end of humerus
Fracture of proximal end of humerus
> *EXCLUDES2* fracture of shaft of humerus (S42.3-)
> physeal fracture of upper end of humerus (S49.0-)
- 6ᵗʰ **S42.20** Unspecified fracture of upper end of humerus
  - 7ᵗʰ **S42.201** Unspecified fracture of upper end of right humerus ᴄᴄ ᴘᴏᴀ ᴴᴬᶜ ᴍᴄᴄ ᴄᴄ/ᴍᴄᴄ ᴇxᴄ
  - 7ᵗʰ **S42.202** Unspecified fracture of upper end of left humerus ᴄᴄ ᴘᴏᴀ ᴴᴬᶜ ᴍᴄᴄ ᴄᴄ/ᴍᴄᴄ ᴇxᴄ
  - 7ᵗʰ **S42.209** Unspecified fracture of upper end of unspecified humerus ᴄᴄ ᴘᴏᴀ ᴴᴬᶜ ᴍᴄᴄ ᴄᴄ/ᴍᴄᴄ ᴇxᴄ
- 6ᵗʰ **S42.21** Unspecified fracture of surgical neck of humerus
  Fracture of neck of humerus NOS
  - 7ᵗʰ **S42.211** Unspecified displaced fracture of surgical neck of right humerus ᴄᴄ ᴘᴏᴀ ᴴᴬᶜ ᴍᴄᴄ ᴄᴄ/ᴍᴄᴄ ᴇxᴄ
  - 7ᵗʰ **S42.212** Unspecified displaced fracture of surgical neck of left humerus ᴄᴄ ᴘᴏᴀ ᴴᴬᶜ ᴍᴄᴄ ᴄᴄ/ᴍᴄᴄ ᴇxᴄ
  - 7ᵗʰ **S42.213** Unspecified displaced fracture of surgical neck of unspecified humerus ᴄᴄ ᴘᴏᴀ ᴴᴬᶜ ᴍᴄᴄ ᴄᴄ/ᴍᴄᴄ ᴇxᴄ
  - 7ᵗʰ **S42.214** Unspecified nondisplaced fracture of surgical neck of right humerus ᴄᴄ ᴘᴏᴀ ᴴᴬᶜ ᴍᴄᴄ ᴄᴄ/ᴍᴄᴄ ᴇxᴄ
  - 7ᵗʰ **S42.215** Unspecified nondisplaced fracture of surgical neck of left humerus ᴄᴄ ᴘᴏᴀ ᴴᴬᶜ ᴍᴄᴄ ᴄᴄ/ᴍᴄᴄ ᴇxᴄ
  - 7ᵗʰ **S42.216** Unspecified nondisplaced fracture of surgical neck of unspecified humerus ᴄᴄ ᴘᴏᴀ ᴴᴬᶜ ᴍᴄᴄ ᴄᴄ/ᴍᴄᴄ ᴇxᴄ
- 6ᵗʰ **S42.22** 2-part fracture of surgical neck of humerus
  - 7ᵗʰ **S42.221** 2-part displaced fracture of surgical neck of right humerus ᴄᴄ ᴘᴏᴀ ᴴᴬᶜ ᴍᴄᴄ ᴄᴄ/ᴍᴄᴄ ᴇxᴄ
  - 7ᵗʰ **S42.222** 2-part displaced fracture of surgical neck of left humerus ᴄᴄ ᴘᴏᴀ ᴴᴬᶜ ᴍᴄᴄ ᴄᴄ/ᴍᴄᴄ ᴇxᴄ
  - 7ᵗʰ **S42.223** 2-part displaced fracture of surgical neck of unspecified humerus ᴄᴄ ᴘᴏᴀ ᴴᴬᶜ ᴍᴄᴄ ᴄᴄ/ᴍᴄᴄ ᴇxᴄ
  - 7ᵗʰ **S42.224** 2-part nondisplaced fracture of surgical neck of right humerus ᴄᴄ ᴘᴏᴀ ᴴᴬᶜ ᴍᴄᴄ ᴄᴄ/ᴍᴄᴄ ᴇxᴄ
  - 7ᵗʰ **S42.225** 2-part nondisplaced fracture of surgical neck of left humerus ᴄᴄ ᴘᴏᴀ ᴴᴬᶜ ᴍᴄᴄ ᴄᴄ/ᴍᴄᴄ ᴇxᴄ
  - 7ᵗʰ **S42.226** 2-part nondisplaced fracture of surgical neck of unspecified humerus ᴄᴄ ᴘᴏᴀ ᴴᴬᶜ ᴍᴄᴄ ᴄᴄ/ᴍᴄᴄ ᴇxᴄ
- 6ᵗʰ **S42.23** 3-part fracture of surgical neck of humerus
  - 7ᵗʰ **S42.231** 3-part fracture of surgical neck of right humerus ᴄᴄ ᴘᴏᴀ ᴴᴬᶜ ᴍᴄᴄ ᴄᴄ/ᴍᴄᴄ ᴇxᴄ
  - 7ᵗʰ **S42.232** 3-part fracture of surgical neck of left humerus ᴄᴄ ᴘᴏᴀ ᴴᴬᶜ ᴍᴄᴄ ᴄᴄ/ᴍᴄᴄ ᴇxᴄ
  - 7ᵗʰ **S42.239** 3-part fracture of surgical neck of unspecified humerus ᴄᴄ ᴘᴏᴀ ᴴᴬᶜ ᴍᴄᴄ ᴄᴄ/ᴍᴄᴄ ᴇxᴄ
- 6ᵗʰ **S42.24** 4-part fracture of surgical neck of humerus
  - 7ᵗʰ **S42.241** 4-part fracture of surgical neck of right humerus ᴄᴄ ᴘᴏᴀ ᴴᴬᶜ ᴍᴄᴄ ᴄᴄ/ᴍᴄᴄ ᴇxᴄ
  - 7ᵗʰ **S42.242** 4-part fracture of surgical neck of left humerus ᴄᴄ ᴘᴏᴀ ᴴᴬᶜ ᴍᴄᴄ ᴄᴄ/ᴍᴄᴄ ᴇxᴄ
  - 7ᵗʰ **S42.249** 4-part fracture of surgical neck of unspecified humerus ᴄᴄ ᴘᴏᴀ ᴴᴬᶜ ᴍᴄᴄ ᴄᴄ/ᴍᴄᴄ ᴇxᴄ
- 6ᵗʰ **S42.25** Fracture of greater tuberosity of humerus
  - 7ᵗʰ **S42.251** Displaced fracture of greater tuberosity of right humerus ᴄᴄ ᴘᴏᴀ ᴴᴬᶜ ᴍᴄᴄ ᴄᴄ/ᴍᴄᴄ ᴇxᴄ

ᴘᴅx Unacceptable principal diagnosis symbol per Medicare code edits   ᴏ Code exempt from diagnosis present on admission requirement
🅿 Questionable admission   ᴄᴄ Complication or comorbidity   ᴍᴄᴄ Major complication or comorbidity   ᴄᴄ/ᴍᴄᴄ ᴇxᴄ CC/MCC exclusion
ᴴᶜᶜ HCC diagnosis code   ᴿˣᴴᶜᶜ RxHCC diagnosis code   MACRA code   **DEFINITION** Describes condition/terminology
TIP Coding guidance   👁 Official Guideline Reference   🅩 Z code as first-listed diagnosis

7️⃣ S42.252 Displaced fracture of greater tuberosity of left humerus CC POA HAC MCC CC/MCC Exc

7️⃣ S42.253 Displaced fracture of greater tuberosity of unspecified humerus CC POA HAC MCC CC/MCC Exc

7️⃣ S42.254 Nondisplaced fracture of greater tuberosity of right humerus CC POA HAC MCC CC/MCC Exc

7️⃣ S42.255 Nondisplaced fracture of greater tuberosity of left humerus CC POA HAC MCC CC/MCC Exc

7️⃣ S42.256 Nondisplaced fracture of greater tuberosity of unspecified humerus CC POA HAC MCC CC/MCC Exc

6️⃣ S42.26 Fracture of lesser tuberosity of humerus

7️⃣ S42.261 Displaced fracture of lesser tuberosity of right humerus CC POA HAC MCC CC/MCC Exc

7️⃣ S42.262 Displaced fracture of lesser tuberosity of left humerus CC POA HAC MCC CC/MCC Exc

7️⃣ S42.263 Displaced fracture of lesser tuberosity of unspecified humerus CC POA HAC MCC CC/MCC Exc

7️⃣ S42.264 Nondisplaced fracture of lesser tuberosity of right humerus CC POA HAC MCC CC/MCC Exc

7️⃣ S42.265 Nondisplaced fracture of lesser tuberosity of left humerus CC POA HAC MCC CC/MCC Exc

7️⃣ S42.266 Nondisplaced fracture of lesser tuberosity of unspecified humerus CC POA HAC MCC CC/MCC Exc

6️⃣ S42.27 Torus fracture of upper end of humerus

The appropriate 7th character is to be added to all codes in subcategory S42.27
A = initial encounter for closed fracture
D = subsequent encounter for fracture with routine healing
G = subsequent encounter for fracture with delayed healing
K = subsequent encounter for fracture with nonunion
P = subsequent encounter for fracture with malunion
S = sequela

7️⃣ S42.271 Torus fracture of upper end of right humerus CC POA HAC CC/MCC Exc

7️⃣ S42.272 Torus fracture of upper end of left humerus CC POA HAC CC/MCC Exc

7️⃣ S42.279 Torus fracture of upper end of unspecified humerus CC POA HAC CC/MCC Exc

6️⃣ S42.29 Other fracture of upper end of humerus
Fracture of anatomical neck of humerus
Fracture of articular head of humerus

7️⃣ S42.291 Other displaced fracture of upper end of right humerus CC POA HAC MCC CC/MCC Exc

7️⃣ S42.292 Other displaced fracture of upper end of left humerus CC POA HAC MCC CC/MCC Exc

7️⃣ S42.293 Other displaced fracture of upper end of unspecified humerus CC POA HAC MCC CC/MCC Exc

7️⃣ S42.294 Other nondisplaced fracture of upper end of right humerus CC POA HAC MCC CC/MCC Exc

7️⃣ S42.295 Other nondisplaced fracture of upper end of left humerus CC POA HAC MCC CC/MCC Exc
AHA: Q1 2019

7️⃣ S42.296 Other nondisplaced fracture of upper end of unspecified humerus CC POA HAC MCC CC/MCC Exc

5️⃣ S42.3 Fracture of shaft of humerus
Fracture of humerus NOS
Fracture of upper arm NOS
EXCLUDES2 physeal fractures of upper end of humerus (S49.0-)
physeal fractures of lower end of humerus (S49.1-)

6️⃣ S42.30 Unspecified fracture of shaft of humerus

7️⃣ S42.301 Unspecified fracture of shaft of humerus, right arm CC POA HAC MCC CC/MCC Exc

7️⃣ S42.302 Unspecified fracture of shaft of humerus, left arm CC POA HAC MCC CC/MCC Exc

7️⃣ S42.309 Unspecified fracture of shaft of humerus, unspecified arm CC POA HAC MCC CC/MCC Exc

6️⃣ S42.31 Greenstick fracture of shaft of humerus

The appropriate 7th character is to be added to all codes in subcategory S42.31
A = initial encounter for closed fracture
D = subsequent encounter for fracture with routine healing
G = subsequent encounter for fracture with delayed healing
K = subsequent encounter for fracture with nonunion
P = subsequent encounter for fracture with malunion
S = sequela

7️⃣ S42.311 Greenstick fracture of shaft of humerus, right arm CC POA HAC CC/MCC Exc

7️⃣ S42.312 Greenstick fracture of shaft of humerus, left arm CC POA HAC CC/MCC Exc

7️⃣ S42.319 Greenstick fracture of shaft of humerus, unspecified arm CC POA HAC CC/MCC Exc

6️⃣ S42.32 Transverse fracture of shaft of humerus

7️⃣ S42.321 Displaced transverse fracture of shaft of humerus, right arm CC POA HAC MCC CC/MCC Exc

7️⃣ S42.322 Displaced transverse fracture of shaft of humerus, left arm CC POA HAC MCC CC/MCC Exc

7️⃣ S42.323 Displaced transverse fracture of shaft of humerus, unspecified arm CC POA HAC MCC CC/MCC Exc

7️⃣ S42.324 Nondisplaced transverse fracture of shaft of humerus, right arm CC POA HAC MCC CC/MCC Exc

7️⃣ S42.325 Nondisplaced transverse fracture of shaft of humerus, left arm CC POA HAC MCC CC/MCC Exc

7️⃣ S42.326 Nondisplaced transverse fracture of shaft of humerus, unspecified arm CC POA HAC MCC CC/MCC Exc

6️⃣ S42.33 Oblique fracture of shaft of humerus

7️⃣ S42.331 Displaced oblique fracture of shaft of humerus, right arm CC POA HAC MCC CC/MCC Exc

7️⃣ S42.332 Displaced oblique fracture of shaft of humerus, left arm CC POA HAC MCC CC/MCC Exc

7️⃣ S42.333 Displaced oblique fracture of shaft of humerus, unspecified arm CC POA HAC MCC CC/MCC Exc

7️⃣ S42.334 Nondisplaced oblique fracture of shaft of humerus, right arm CC POA HAC MCC CC/MCC Exc

7️⃣ S42.335 Nondisplaced oblique fracture of shaft of humerus, left arm CC POA HAC MCC CC/MCC Exc

7️⃣ S42.336 Nondisplaced oblique fracture of shaft of humerus, unspecified arm CC POA HAC MCC CC/MCC Exc

6️⃣ S42.34 Spiral fracture of shaft of humerus

7️⃣ S42.341 Displaced spiral fracture of shaft of humerus, right arm CC POA HAC MCC CC/MCC Exc

7️⃣ S42.342 Displaced spiral fracture of shaft of humerus, left arm CC POA HAC MCC CC/MCC Exc

7️⃣ S42.343 Displaced spiral fracture of shaft of humerus, unspecified arm CC POA HAC MCC CC/MCC Exc

7️⃣ S42.344 Nondisplaced spiral fracture of shaft of humerus, right arm CC POA HAC MCC CC/MCC Exc

7️⃣ S42.345 Nondisplaced spiral fracture of shaft of humerus, left arm CC POA HAC MCC CC/MCC Exc

7️⃣ S42.346 Nondisplaced spiral fracture of shaft of humerus, unspecified arm CC POA HAC MCC CC/MCC Exc

6️⃣ S42.35 Comminuted fracture of shaft of humerus

7️⃣ S42.351 Displaced comminuted fracture of shaft of humerus, right arm CC POA HAC MCC CC/MCC Exc

7️⃣ S42.352 Displaced comminuted fracture of shaft of humerus, left arm CC POA HAC MCC CC/MCC Exc

7️⃣ S42.353 Displaced comminuted fracture of shaft of humerus, unspecified arm CC POA HAC MCC CC/MCC Exc

---

Unspecified Code   Other Specified Code   Manifestation Code   Ⓝ Newborn   Ⓟ Pediatric   Ⓜ Maternity   Ⓐ Adult   ♂ Male   ♀ Female
● New Code   ▲ Revised Code Title   ▶◀ Revised Text   NOTES   INCLUDES   EXCLUDES1 Not coded here   EXCLUDES2 Not included here
4️⃣ 4th character required   5️⃣ 5th character required   6️⃣ 6th character required   7️⃣ 7th character required   Extension 'X' Alert
HAC Hospital-acquired condition (HAC) alert   AHA AHA Coding Clinic©   📌 Code first alert

- 7ᵗʰ S42.354 Nondisplaced comminuted fracture of shaft of humerus, right arm ⚕ ᴘᴏᴀ HAC CC/MCC CC/MCC Exc
- 7ᵗʰ S42.355 Nondisplaced comminuted fracture of shaft of humerus, left arm ⚕ ᴘᴏᴀ HAC MCC CC/MCC Exc
- 7ᵗʰ S42.356 Nondisplaced comminuted fracture of shaft of humerus, unspecified arm ⚕ ᴘᴏᴀ HAC MCC CC/MCC Exc
- 6ᵗʰ S42.36 Segmental fracture of shaft of humerus
  - 7ᵗʰ S42.361 Displaced segmental fracture of shaft of humerus, right arm ⚕ ᴘᴏᴀ HAC MCC CC/MCC Exc
  - 7ᵗʰ S42.362 Displaced segmental fracture of shaft of humerus, left arm ⚕ ᴘᴏᴀ HAC MCC CC/MCC Exc
  - 7ᵗʰ S42.363 Displaced segmental fracture of shaft of humerus, unspecified arm ⚕ ᴘᴏᴀ HAC MCC CC/MCC Exc
  - 7ᵗʰ S42.364 Nondisplaced segmental fracture of shaft of humerus, right arm ⚕ ᴘᴏᴀ HAC MCC CC/MCC Exc
  - 7ᵗʰ S42.365 Nondisplaced segmental fracture of shaft of humerus, left arm ⚕ ᴘᴏᴀ HAC MCC CC/MCC Exc
  - 7ᵗʰ S42.366 Nondisplaced segmental fracture of shaft of humerus, unspecified arm ⚕ ᴘᴏᴀ HAC MCC CC/MCC Exc
- 6ᵗʰ S42.39 Other fracture of shaft of humerus
  - 7ᵗʰ S42.391 Other fracture of shaft of right humerus ⚕ ᴘᴏᴀ HAC MCC CC/MCC Exc
  - 7ᵗʰ S42.392 Other fracture of shaft of left humerus ⚕ ᴘᴏᴀ HAC MCC CC/MCC Exc
  - 7ᵗʰ S42.399 Other fracture of shaft of unspecified humerus ⚕ ᴘᴏᴀ HAC MCC CC/MCC Exc
- 5ᵗʰ S42.4 Fracture of lower end of humerus
  Fracture of distal end of humerus
  EXCLUDES2 fracture of shaft of humerus (S42.3-)
  physeal fracture of lower end of humerus (S49.1-)
  - 5ᵗʰ S42.40 Unspecified fracture of lower end of humerus
    Fracture of elbow NOS
    - 7ᵗʰ S42.401 Unspecified fracture of lower end of right humerus ⚕ ᴘᴏᴀ HAC MCC CC/MCC Exc
    - 7ᵗʰ S42.402 Unspecified fracture of lower end of left humerus ⚕ ᴘᴏᴀ HAC MCC CC/MCC Exc
    - 7ᵗʰ S42.409 Unspecified fracture of lower end of unspecified humerus ⚕ ᴘᴏᴀ HAC MCC CC/MCC Exc
  - 6ᵗʰ S42.41 Simple supracondylar fracture without intercondylar fracture of humerus
    - 7ᵗʰ S42.411 Displaced simple supracondylar fracture without intercondylar fracture of right humerus ⚕ ᴘᴏᴀ HAC MCC CC/MCC Exc
    - 7ᵗʰ S42.412 Displaced simple supracondylar fracture without intercondylar fracture of left humerus ⚕ ᴘᴏᴀ HAC MCC CC/MCC Exc
    - 7ᵗʰ S42.413 Displaced simple supracondylar fracture without intercondylar fracture of unspecified humerus ⚕ ᴘᴏᴀ HAC MCC CC/MCC Exc
    - 7ᵗʰ S42.414 Nondisplaced simple supracondylar fracture without intercondylar fracture of right humerus ⚕ ᴘᴏᴀ HAC MCC CC/MCC Exc
    - 7ᵗʰ S42.415 Nondisplaced simple supracondylar fracture without intercondylar fracture of left humerus ⚕ ᴘᴏᴀ HAC MCC CC/MCC Exc
    - 7ᵗʰ S42.416 Nondisplaced simple supracondylar fracture without intercondylar fracture of unspecified humerus ⚕ ᴘᴏᴀ HAC MCC CC/MCC Exc
  - 6ᵗʰ S42.42 Comminuted supracondylar fracture without intercondylar fracture of humerus
    - 7ᵗʰ S42.421 Displaced comminuted supracondylar fracture without intercondylar fracture of right humerus ⚕ ᴘᴏᴀ HAC MCC CC/MCC Exc
    - 7ᵗʰ S42.422 Displaced comminuted supracondylar fracture without intercondylar fracture of left humerus ⚕ ᴘᴏᴀ HAC MCC CC/MCC Exc

- 7ᵗʰ S42.423 Displaced comminuted supracondylar fracture without intercondylar fracture of unspecified humerus ⚕ ᴘᴏᴀ HAC MCC CC/MCC Exc
- 7ᵗʰ S42.424 Nondisplaced comminuted supracondylar fracture without intercondylar fracture of right humerus ⚕ ᴘᴏᴀ HAC MCC CC/MCC Exc
- 7ᵗʰ S42.425 Nondisplaced comminuted supracondylar fracture without intercondylar fracture of left humerus ⚕ ᴘᴏᴀ HAC MCC CC/MCC Exc
- 7ᵗʰ S42.426 Nondisplaced comminuted supracondylar fracture without intercondylar fracture of unspecified humerus ⚕ ᴘᴏᴀ HAC MCC CC/MCC Exc
- 6ᵗʰ S42.43 Fracture (avulsion) of lateral epicondyle of humerus
  - 7ᵗʰ S42.431 Displaced fracture (avulsion) of lateral epicondyle of right humerus ⚕ ᴘᴏᴀ HAC MCC CC/MCC Exc
  - 7ᵗʰ S42.432 Displaced fracture (avulsion) of lateral epicondyle of left humerus ⚕ ᴘᴏᴀ HAC MCC CC/MCC Exc
  - 7ᵗʰ S42.433 Displaced fracture (avulsion) of lateral epicondyle of unspecified humerus ⚕ ᴘᴏᴀ HAC MCC CC/MCC Exc
  - 7ᵗʰ S42.434 Nondisplaced fracture (avulsion) of lateral epicondyle of right humerus ⚕ ᴘᴏᴀ HAC MCC CC/MCC Exc
  - 7ᵗʰ S42.435 Nondisplaced fracture (avulsion) of lateral epicondyle of left humerus ⚕ ᴘᴏᴀ HAC MCC CC/MCC Exc
  - 7ᵗʰ S42.436 Nondisplaced fracture (avulsion) of lateral epicondyle of unspecified humerus ⚕ ᴘᴏᴀ HAC MCC CC/MCC Exc
- 6ᵗʰ S42.44 Fracture (avulsion) of medial epicondyle of humerus
  - 7ᵗʰ S42.441 Displaced fracture (avulsion) of medial epicondyle of right humerus ⚕ ᴘᴏᴀ HAC MCC CC/MCC Exc
  - 7ᵗʰ S42.442 Displaced fracture (avulsion) of medial epicondyle of left humerus ⚕ ᴘᴏᴀ HAC MCC CC/MCC Exc
  - 7ᵗʰ S42.443 Displaced fracture (avulsion) of medial epicondyle of unspecified humerus ⚕ ᴘᴏᴀ HAC MCC CC/MCC Exc
  - 7ᵗʰ S42.444 Nondisplaced fracture (avulsion) of medial epicondyle of right humerus ⚕ ᴘᴏᴀ HAC MCC CC/MCC Exc
  - 7ᵗʰ S42.445 Nondisplaced fracture (avulsion) of medial epicondyle of left humerus ⚕ ᴘᴏᴀ HAC MCC CC/MCC Exc
  - 7ᵗʰ S42.446 Nondisplaced fracture (avulsion) of medial epicondyle of unspecified humerus ⚕ ᴘᴏᴀ HAC MCC CC/MCC Exc
  - 7ᵗʰ S42.447 Incarcerated fracture (avulsion) of medial epicondyle of right humerus ⚕ ᴘᴏᴀ HAC MCC CC/MCC Exc
  - 7ᵗʰ S42.448 Incarcerated fracture (avulsion) of medial epicondyle of left humerus ⚕ ᴘᴏᴀ HAC MCC CC/MCC Exc
  - 7ᵗʰ S42.449 Incarcerated fracture (avulsion) of medial epicondyle of unspecified humerus ⚕ ᴘᴏᴀ HAC MCC CC/MCC Exc
- 6ᵗʰ S42.45 Fracture of lateral condyle of humerus
  Fracture of capitellum of humerus
  - 7ᵗʰ S42.451 Displaced fracture of lateral condyle of right humerus ⚕ ᴘᴏᴀ HAC MCC CC/MCC Exc
  - 7ᵗʰ S42.452 Displaced fracture of lateral condyle of left humerus ⚕ ᴘᴏᴀ HAC MCC CC/MCC Exc
  - 7ᵗʰ S42.453 Displaced fracture of lateral condyle of unspecified humerus ⚕ ᴘᴏᴀ HAC MCC CC/MCC Exc
  - 7ᵗʰ S42.454 Nondisplaced fracture of lateral condyle of right humerus ⚕ ᴘᴏᴀ HAC MCC CC/MCC Exc
  - 7ᵗʰ S42.455 Nondisplaced fracture of lateral condyle of left humerus ⚕ ᴘᴏᴀ HAC MCC CC/MCC Exc
  - 7ᵗʰ S42.456 Nondisplaced fracture of lateral condyle of unspecified humerus ⚕ ᴘᴏᴀ HAC MCC CC/MCC Exc

---

6ᵗʰ **S42.46** Fracture of medial condyle of humerus
Trochlea fracture of humerus

7ᵗʰ S42.461 Displaced fracture of medial condyle of right humerus `cc` `poa` `HAC` `MCC` `cc/MCC Exc`

7ᵗʰ S42.462 Displaced fracture of medial condyle of left humerus `cc` `poa` `HAC` `MCC` `cc/MCC Exc`

7ᵗʰ S42.463 Displaced fracture of medial condyle of unspecified humerus `cc` `poa` `HAC` `MCC` `cc/MCC Exc`

7ᵗʰ S42.464 Nondisplaced fracture of medial condyle of right humerus `cc` `poa` `HAC` `MCC` `cc/MCC Exc`

7ᵗʰ S42.465 Nondisplaced fracture of medial condyle of left humerus `cc` `poa` `HAC` `MCC` `cc/MCC Exc`

7ᵗʰ S42.466 Nondisplaced fracture of medial condyle of unspecified humerus `cc` `poa` `HAC` `MCC` `cc/MCC Exc`

6ᵗʰ **S42.47** Transcondylar fracture of humerus

7ᵗʰ S42.471 Displaced transcondylar fracture of right humerus `cc` `poa` `HAC` `MCC` `cc/MCC Exc`

7ᵗʰ S42.472 Displaced transcondylar fracture of left humerus `cc` `poa` `HAC` `MCC` `cc/MCC Exc`

7ᵗʰ S42.473 Displaced transcondylar fracture of unspecified humerus `cc` `poa` `HAC` `MCC` `cc/MCC Exc`

7ᵗʰ S42.474 Nondisplaced transcondylar fracture of right humerus `cc` `poa` `HAC` `MCC` `cc/MCC Exc`

7ᵗʰ S42.475 Nondisplaced transcondylar fracture of left humerus `cc` `poa` `HAC` `MCC` `cc/MCC Exc`

7ᵗʰ S42.476 Nondisplaced transcondylar fracture of unspecified humerus `cc` `poa` `HAC` `MCC` `cc/MCC Exc`

6ᵗʰ **S42.48** Torus fracture of lower end of humerus

The appropriate 7th character is to be added to all codes in subcategory S42.48

A = initial encounter for closed fracture

D = subsequent encounter for fracture with routine healing

G = subsequent encounter for fracture with delayed healing

K = subsequent encounter for fracture with nonunion

P = subsequent encounter for fracture with malunion

S = sequela

7ᵗʰ S42.481 Torus fracture of lower end of right humerus `cc` `poa` `HAC` `cc/MCC Exc`

7ᵗʰ S42.482 Torus fracture of lower end of left humerus `cc` `poa` `HAC` `cc/MCC Exc`

7ᵗʰ S42.489 Torus fracture of lower end of unspecified humerus `cc` `poa` `HAC` `cc/MCC Exc`

6ᵗʰ **S42.49** Other fracture of lower end of humerus

7ᵗʰ S42.491 Other displaced fracture of lower end of right humerus `cc` `poa` `HAC` `MCC` `cc/MCC Exc`

7ᵗʰ S42.492 Other displaced fracture of lower end of left humerus `cc` `poa` `HAC` `MCC` `cc/MCC Exc`

7ᵗʰ S42.493 Other displaced fracture of lower end of unspecified humerus `cc` `poa` `HAC` `MCC` `cc/MCC Exc`

7ᵗʰ S42.494 Other nondisplaced fracture of lower end of right humerus `cc` `poa` `HAC` `MCC` `cc/MCC Exc`

7ᵗʰ S42.495 Other nondisplaced fracture of lower end of left humerus `cc` `poa` `HAC` `MCC` `cc/MCC Exc`

7ᵗʰ S42.496 Other nondisplaced fracture of lower end of unspecified humerus `cc` `poa` `HAC` `MCC` `cc/MCC Exc`

5ᵗʰ **S42.9** Fracture of shoulder girdle, part unspecified
Fracture of shoulder NOS

7ᵗʰ S42.90 Fracture of unspecified shoulder girdle, part unspecified `cc` `poa` `HAC` `MCC` `cc/MCC Exc`

7ᵗʰ S42.91 Fracture of right shoulder girdle, part unspecified `cc` `poa` `HAC` `MCC` `cc/MCC Exc`

7ᵗʰ S42.92 Fracture of left shoulder girdle, part unspecified `cc` `poa` `HAC` `MCC` `cc/MCC Exc`

4ᵗʰ **S43** Dislocation and sprain of joints and ligaments of shoulder girdle

INCLUDES avulsion of joint or ligament of shoulder girdle
laceration of cartilage, joint or ligament of shoulder girdle
sprain of cartilage, joint or ligament of shoulder girdle

traumatic hemarthrosis of joint or ligament of shoulder girdle
traumatic rupture of joint or ligament of shoulder girdle
traumatic subluxation of joint or ligament of shoulder girdle
traumatic tear of joint or ligament of shoulder girdle

Code also any associated open wound

EXCLUDES2 strain of muscle, fascia and tendon of shoulder and upper arm (S46.-)

The appropriate 7th character is to be added to each code from category S43

A = initial encounter

D = subsequent encounter

S = sequela

5ᵗʰ **S43.0** Subluxation and dislocation of shoulder joint
Dislocation of glenohumeral joint
Subluxation of glenohumeral joint

6ᵗʰ **S43.00** Unspecified subluxation and dislocation of shoulder joint
Dislocation of humerus NOS
Subluxation of humerus NOS

7ᵗʰ S43.001 Unspecified subluxation of right shoulder joint `poa`

7ᵗʰ S43.002 Unspecified subluxation of left shoulder joint `poa`

7ᵗʰ S43.003 Unspecified subluxation of unspecified shoulder joint `poa`

7ᵗʰ S43.004 Unspecified dislocation of right shoulder joint `poa`

7ᵗʰ S43.005 Unspecified dislocation of left shoulder joint `poa`

7ᵗʰ S43.006 Unspecified dislocation of unspecified shoulder joint `poa`

6ᵗʰ **S43.01** Anterior subluxation and dislocation of humerus

7ᵗʰ S43.011 Anterior subluxation of right humerus `poa`

7ᵗʰ S43.012 Anterior subluxation of left humerus `poa`

7ᵗʰ S43.013 Anterior subluxation of unspecified humerus `poa`

7ᵗʰ S43.014 Anterior dislocation of right humerus `poa`

7ᵗʰ S43.015 Anterior dislocation of left humerus `poa`

7ᵗʰ S43.016 Anterior dislocation of unspecified humerus `poa`

6ᵗʰ **S43.02** Posterior subluxation and dislocation of humerus

7ᵗʰ S43.021 Posterior subluxation of right humerus `poa`

7ᵗʰ S43.022 Posterior subluxation of left humerus `poa`

7ᵗʰ S43.023 Posterior subluxation of unspecified humerus `poa`

7ᵗʰ S43.024 Posterior dislocation of right humerus `poa`

7ᵗʰ S43.025 Posterior dislocation of left humerus `poa`

7ᵗʰ S43.026 Posterior dislocation of unspecified humerus `poa`

6ᵗʰ **S43.03** Inferior subluxation and dislocation of humerus

7ᵗʰ S43.031 Inferior subluxation of right humerus `poa`

7ᵗʰ S43.032 Inferior subluxation of left humerus `poa`

7ᵗʰ S43.033 Inferior subluxation of unspecified humerus `poa`

7ᵗʰ S43.034 Inferior dislocation of right humerus `poa`

7ᵗʰ S43.035 Inferior dislocation of left humerus `poa`

7ᵗʰ S43.036 Inferior dislocation of unspecified humerus `poa`

6ᵗʰ **S43.08** Other subluxation and dislocation of shoulder joint

7ᵗʰ S43.081 Other subluxation of right shoulder joint `poa`

7ᵗʰ S43.082 Other subluxation of left shoulder joint `poa`

7ᵗʰ S43.083 Other subluxation of unspecified shoulder joint `poa`

7ᵗʰ S43.084 Other dislocation of right shoulder joint `poa`

7ᵗʰ S43.085 Other dislocation of left shoulder joint `poa`

7ᵗʰ S43.086 Other dislocation of unspecified shoulder joint `poa`

Unspecified Code Other Specified Code Manifestation Code Ⓝ Newborn Ⓟ Pediatric Ⓜ Maternity Ⓐ Adult ♂ Male ♀ Female
● New Code ▲ Revised Code Title ▶◀ Revised Text **NOTES** *INCLUDES* *EXCLUDES1* Not coded here *EXCLUDES2* Not included here
4ᵗʰ 4ᵗʰ character required 5ᵗʰ 5ᵗʰ character required 6ᵗʰ 6ᵗʰ character required 7ᵗʰ 7ᵗʰ character required Ⓧ Extension 'X' Alert
HAC Hospital-acquired condition (HAC) alert **AHA** AHA Coding Clinic© 📣 Code first alert

5ᵗʰ S43.1 Subluxation and dislocation of acromioclavicular joint
  6ᵗʰ S43.10 Unspecified dislocation of acromioclavicular joint
    7ᵗʰ S43.101 Unspecified dislocation of right acromioclavicular joint POA
    7ᵗʰ S43.102 Unspecified dislocation of left acromioclavicular joint POA
    7ᵗʰ S43.109 Unspecified dislocation of unspecified acromioclavicular joint POA
  6ᵗʰ S43.11 Subluxation of acromioclavicular joint
    7ᵗʰ S43.111 Subluxation of right acromioclavicular joint POA
    7ᵗʰ S43.112 Subluxation of left acromioclavicular joint POA
    7ᵗʰ S43.119 Subluxation of unspecified acromioclavicular joint POA
  6ᵗʰ S43.12 Dislocation of acromioclavicular joint, 100%-200% displacement
    7ᵗʰ S43.121 Dislocation of right acromioclavicular joint, 100%-200% displacement POA
    7ᵗʰ S43.122 Dislocation of left acromioclavicular joint, 100%-200% displacement POA
    7ᵗʰ S43.129 Dislocation of unspecified acromioclavicular joint, 100%-200% displacement POA
  6ᵗʰ S43.13 Dislocation of acromioclavicular joint, greater than 200% displacement
    7ᵗʰ S43.131 Dislocation of right acromioclavicular joint, greater than 200% displacement POA
    7ᵗʰ S43.132 Dislocation of left acromioclavicular joint, greater than 200% displacement POA
    7ᵗʰ S43.139 Dislocation of unspecified acromioclavicular joint, greater than 200% displacement POA
  6ᵗʰ S43.14 Inferior dislocation of acromioclavicular joint
    7ᵗʰ S43.141 Inferior dislocation of right acromioclavicular joint POA
    7ᵗʰ S43.142 Inferior dislocation of left acromioclavicular joint POA
    7ᵗʰ S43.149 Inferior dislocation of unspecified acromioclavicular joint POA
  6ᵗʰ S43.15 Posterior dislocation of acromioclavicular joint
    7ᵗʰ S43.151 Posterior dislocation of right acromioclavicular joint POA
    7ᵗʰ S43.152 Posterior dislocation of left acromioclavicular joint POA
    7ᵗʰ S43.159 Posterior dislocation of unspecified acromioclavicular joint POA
5ᵗʰ S43.2 Subluxation and dislocation of sternoclavicular joint
  6ᵗʰ S43.20 Unspecified subluxation and dislocation of sternoclavicular joint
    7ᵗʰ S43.201 Unspecified subluxation of right sternoclavicular joint CC POA HAC CC/MCC Exc
    7ᵗʰ S43.202 Unspecified subluxation of left sternoclavicular joint CC POA HAC CC/MCC Exc
    7ᵗʰ S43.203 Unspecified subluxation of unspecified sternoclavicular joint CC POA HAC CC/MCC Exc
    7ᵗʰ S43.204 Unspecified dislocation of right sternoclavicular joint CC POA HAC CC/MCC Exc
    7ᵗʰ S43.205 Unspecified dislocation of left sternoclavicular joint CC POA HAC CC/MCC Exc
    7ᵗʰ S43.206 Unspecified dislocation of unspecified sternoclavicular joint CC POA HAC CC/MCC Exc
  6ᵗʰ S43.21 Anterior subluxation and dislocation of sternoclavicular joint
    7ᵗʰ S43.211 Anterior subluxation of right sternoclavicular joint CC POA HAC CC/MCC Exc
    7ᵗʰ S43.212 Anterior subluxation of left sternoclavicular joint CC POA HAC CC/MCC Exc
    7ᵗʰ S43.213 Anterior subluxation of unspecified sternoclavicular joint CC POA HAC CC/MCC Exc
    7ᵗʰ S43.214 Anterior dislocation of right sternoclavicular joint CC POA HAC CC/MCC Exc

    7ᵗʰ S43.215 Anterior dislocation of left sternoclavicular joint CC POA HAC CC/MCC Exc
    7ᵗʰ S43.216 Anterior dislocation of unspecified sternoclavicular joint CC POA HAC CC/MCC Exc
  6ᵗʰ S43.22 Posterior subluxation and dislocation of sternoclavicular joint
    7ᵗʰ S43.221 Posterior subluxation of right sternoclavicular joint CC POA HAC CC/MCC Exc
    7ᵗʰ S43.222 Posterior subluxation of left sternoclavicular joint CC POA HAC CC/MCC Exc
    7ᵗʰ S43.223 Posterior subluxation of unspecified sternoclavicular joint CC POA HAC CC/MCC Exc
    7ᵗʰ S43.224 Posterior dislocation of right sternoclavicular joint CC POA HAC CC/MCC Exc
    7ᵗʰ S43.225 Posterior dislocation of left sternoclavicular joint CC POA HAC CC/MCC Exc
    7ᵗʰ S43.226 Posterior dislocation of unspecified sternoclavicular joint CC POA HAC CC/MCC Exc
5ᵗʰ S43.3 Subluxation and dislocation of other and unspecified parts of shoulder girdle
  6ᵗʰ S43.30 Subluxation and dislocation of unspecified parts of shoulder girdle
      Dislocation of shoulder girdle NOS
      Subluxation of shoulder girdle NOS
    7ᵗʰ S43.301 Subluxation of unspecified parts of right shoulder girdle POA
    7ᵗʰ S43.302 Subluxation of unspecified parts of left shoulder girdle POA
    7ᵗʰ S43.303 Subluxation of unspecified parts of unspecified shoulder girdle POA
    7ᵗʰ S43.304 Dislocation of unspecified parts of right shoulder girdle POA
    7ᵗʰ S43.305 Dislocation of unspecified parts of left shoulder girdle POA
    7ᵗʰ S43.306 Dislocation of unspecified parts of unspecified shoulder girdle POA
  6ᵗʰ S43.31 Subluxation and dislocation of scapula
    7ᵗʰ S43.311 Subluxation of right scapula POA
    7ᵗʰ S43.312 Subluxation of left scapula POA
    7ᵗʰ S43.313 Subluxation of unspecified scapula POA
    7ᵗʰ S43.314 Dislocation of right scapula POA
    7ᵗʰ S43.315 Dislocation of left scapula POA
    7ᵗʰ S43.316 Dislocation of unspecified scapula POA
  6ᵗʰ S43.39 Subluxation and dislocation of other parts of shoulder girdle
    7ᵗʰ S43.391 Subluxation of other parts of right shoulder girdle POA
    7ᵗʰ S43.392 Subluxation of other parts of left shoulder girdle POA
    7ᵗʰ S43.393 Subluxation of other parts of unspecified shoulder girdle POA
    7ᵗʰ S43.394 Dislocation of other parts of right shoulder girdle POA
    7ᵗʰ S43.395 Dislocation of other parts of left shoulder girdle POA
    7ᵗʰ S43.396 Dislocation of other parts of unspecified shoulder girdle POA
5ᵗʰ S43.4 Sprain of shoulder joint
  6ᵗʰ S43.40 Unspecified sprain of shoulder joint
    7ᵗʰ S43.401 Unspecified sprain of right shoulder joint POA
    7ᵗʰ S43.402 Unspecified sprain of left shoulder joint POA
    7ᵗʰ S43.409 Unspecified sprain of unspecified shoulder joint POA
  6ᵗʰ S43.41 Sprain of coracohumeral (ligament)
    7ᵗʰ S43.411 Sprain of right coracohumeral (ligament) POA
    7ᵗʰ S43.412 Sprain of left coracohumeral (ligament) POA
    7ᵗʰ S43.419 Sprain of unspecified coracohumeral (ligament) POA

POA Unacceptable principal diagnosis symbol per Medicare code edits   Code exempt from diagnosis present on admission requirement
? Questionable admission   CC Complication or comorbidity   MCC Major complication or comorbidity   CC/MCC Exc CC/MCC exclusion
HCC HCC diagnosis code   RxHCC RxHCC diagnosis code   MACRA MACRA code   **DEFINITION** Describes condition/terminology
TIP Coding guidance   Official Guideline Reference   Z1 Z code as first-listed diagnosis

[6th] S43.42 Sprain of rotator cuff capsule
EXCLUDES1 rotator cuff syndrome (complete) (incomplete), not specified as traumatic (M75.1-)
EXCLUDES2 injury of tendon of rotator cuff (S46.0-)
[7th] S43.421 Sprain of right rotator cuff capsule POA
[7th] S43.422 Sprain of left rotator cuff capsule POA
[7th] S43.429 Sprain of unspecified rotator cuff capsule POA
[6th] S43.43 Superior glenoid labrum lesion
SLAP lesion
[7th] S43.431 Superior glenoid labrum lesion of right shoulder POA
[7th] S43.432 Superior glenoid labrum lesion of left shoulder POA
[7th] S43.439 Superior glenoid labrum lesion of unspecified shoulder POA
[6th] S43.49 Other sprain of shoulder joint
[7th] S43.491 Other sprain of right shoulder joint POA
[7th] S43.492 Other sprain of left shoulder joint POA
[7th] S43.499 Other sprain of unspecified shoulder joint POA
[5th] S43.5 Sprain of acromioclavicular joint
Sprain of acromioclavicular ligament
[7th] S43.50 Sprain of unspecified acromioclavicular joint POA
[7th] S43.51 Sprain of right acromioclavicular joint POA
[7th] S43.52 Sprain of left acromioclavicular joint POA
[5th] S43.6 Sprain of sternoclavicular joint
[7th] S43.60 Sprain of unspecified sternoclavicular joint POA
[7th] S43.61 Sprain of right sternoclavicular joint POA
[7th] S43.62 Sprain of left sternoclavicular joint POA
[5th] S43.8 Sprain of other specified parts of shoulder girdle
[7th] S43.80 Sprain of other specified parts of unspecified shoulder girdle POA
[7th] S43.81 Sprain of other specified parts of right shoulder girdle POA
[7th] S43.82 Sprain of other specified parts of left shoulder girdle POA
[5th] S43.9 Sprain of unspecified parts of shoulder girdle
[7th] S43.90 Sprain of unspecified parts of unspecified shoulder girdle POA
Sprain of shoulder girdle NOS
[7th] S43.91 Sprain of unspecified parts of right shoulder girdle POA
[7th] S43.92 Sprain of unspecified parts of left shoulder girdle POA

[4th] S44 Injury of nerves at shoulder and upper arm level
Code also any associated open wound (S41.-)
EXCLUDES2 injury of brachial plexus (S14.3-)
The appropriate 7th character is to be added to each code from category S44
A = initial encounter
D = subsequent encounter
S = sequela
[5th] S44.0 Injury of ulnar nerve at upper arm level
EXCLUDES1 ulnar nerve NOS (S54.0)
[7th] S44.00 Injury of ulnar nerve at upper arm level, unspecified arm POA
[7th] S44.01 Injury of ulnar nerve at upper arm level, right arm POA
[7th] S44.02 Injury of ulnar nerve at upper arm level, left arm POA
[5th] S44.1 Injury of median nerve at upper arm level
EXCLUDES1 median nerve NOS (S54.1)
[7th] S44.10 Injury of median nerve at upper arm level, unspecified arm POA
[7th] S44.11 Injury of median nerve at upper arm level, right arm POA
[7th] S44.12 Injury of median nerve at upper arm level, left arm POA
[5th] S44.2 Injury of radial nerve at upper arm level
EXCLUDES1 radial nerve NOS (S54.2)
[7th] S44.20 Injury of radial nerve at upper arm level, unspecified arm POA
[7th] S44.21 Injury of radial nerve at upper arm level, right arm POA
[7th] S44.22 Injury of radial nerve at upper arm level, left arm POA
[5th] S44.3 Injury of axillary nerve
[7th] S44.30 Injury of axillary nerve, unspecified arm POA
[7th] S44.31 Injury of axillary nerve, right arm POA
[7th] S44.32 Injury of axillary nerve, left arm POA
[5th] S44.4 Injury of musculocutaneous nerve
[7th] S44.40 Injury of musculocutaneous nerve, unspecified arm POA
[7th] S44.41 Injury of musculocutaneous nerve, right arm POA
[7th] S44.42 Injury of musculocutaneous nerve, left arm POA
[5th] S44.5 Injury of cutaneous sensory nerve at shoulder and upper arm level
[7th] S44.50 Injury of cutaneous sensory nerve at shoulder and upper arm level, unspecified arm POA
[7th] S44.51 Injury of cutaneous sensory nerve at shoulder and upper arm level, right arm POA
[7th] S44.52 Injury of cutaneous sensory nerve at shoulder and upper arm level, left arm POA
[5th] S44.8 Injury of other nerves at shoulder and upper arm level
[6th] S44.8X Injury of other nerves at shoulder and upper arm level
[7th] S44.8X1 Injury of other nerves at shoulder and upper arm level, right arm POA
[7th] S44.8X2 Injury of other nerves at shoulder and upper arm level, left arm POA
[7th] S44.8X9 Injury of other nerves at shoulder and upper arm level, unspecified arm POA
[5th] S44.9 Injury of unspecified nerve at shoulder and upper arm level
[7th] S44.90 Injury of unspecified nerve at shoulder and upper arm level, unspecified arm POA
[7th] S44.91 Injury of unspecified nerve at shoulder and upper arm level, right arm POA
[7th] S44.92 Injury of unspecified nerve at shoulder and upper arm level, left arm POA

[4th] S45 Injury of blood vessels at shoulder and upper arm level
Code also any associated open wound (S41.-)
EXCLUDES2 injury of subclavian artery (S25.1)
injury of subclavian vein (S25.3)
The appropriate 7th character is to be added to each code from category S45
A = initial encounter
D = subsequent encounter
S = sequela
[5th] S45.0 Injury of axillary artery
[6th] S45.00 Unspecified injury of axillary artery
[7th] S45.001 Unspecified injury of axillary artery, right side POA MCC CC/MCC Exc
[7th] S45.002 Unspecified injury of axillary artery, left side POA MCC CC/MCC Exc
[7th] S45.009 Unspecified injury of axillary artery, unspecified side POA MCC CC/MCC Exc
[6th] S45.01 Laceration of axillary artery
[7th] S45.011 Laceration of axillary artery, right side POA MCC CC/MCC Exc
[7th] S45.012 Laceration of axillary artery, left side POA MCC CC/MCC Exc
[7th] S45.019 Laceration of axillary artery, unspecified side POA MCC CC/MCC Exc
[6th] S45.09 Other specified injury of axillary artery
[7th] S45.091 Other specified injury of axillary artery, right side POA MCC CC/MCC Exc
[7th] S45.092 Other specified injury of axillary artery, left side POA MCC CC/MCC Exc
[7th] S45.099 Other specified injury of axillary artery, unspecified side POA MCC CC/MCC Exc
[5th] S45.1 Injury of brachial artery
[6th] S45.10 Unspecified injury of brachial artery
[7th] S45.101 Unspecified injury of brachial artery, right side CC POA CC/MCC Exc

Unspecified Code | Other Specified Code | Manifestation Code | [N] Newborn | [P] Pediatric | [M] Maternity | [A] Adult | ♂ Male | ♀ Female
● New Code | ▲ Revised Code Title | ►◄ Revised Text | NOTES | INCLUDES | EXCLUDES1 Not coded here | EXCLUDES2 Not included here
[4th] 4th character required | [5th] 5th character required | [6th] 6th character required | [7th] 7th character required | [X] Extension 'X' Alert
[HAC] Hospital-acquired condition (HAC) alert | AHA AHA Coding Clinic© | ☞ Code first alert

S45.102 Unspecified injury of brachial artery, left side CC POA CC/MCC Exc

S45.109 Unspecified injury of brachial artery, unspecified side CC POA CC/MCC Exc

S45.11 Laceration of brachial artery

S45.111 Laceration of brachial artery, right side CC POA CC/MCC Exc

S45.112 Laceration of brachial artery, left side CC POA CC/MCC Exc

S45.119 Laceration of brachial artery, unspecified side CC POA CC/MCC Exc

S45.19 Other specified injury of brachial artery

S45.191 Other specified injury of brachial artery, right side CC POA CC/MCC Exc

S45.192 Other specified injury of brachial artery, left side CC POA CC/MCC Exc

S45.199 Other specified injury of brachial artery, unspecified side CC POA CC/MCC Exc

S45.2 Injury of axillary or brachial vein

S45.20 Unspecified injury of axillary or brachial vein

S45.201 Unspecified injury of axillary or brachial vein, right side CC POA CC/MCC Exc

S45.202 Unspecified injury of axillary or brachial vein, left side CC POA CC/MCC Exc

S45.209 Unspecified injury of axillary or brachial vein, unspecified side CC POA CC/MCC Exc

S45.21 Laceration of axillary or brachial vein

S45.211 Laceration of axillary or brachial vein, right side CC POA CC/MCC Exc

S45.212 Laceration of axillary or brachial vein, left side CC POA CC/MCC Exc

S45.219 Laceration of axillary or brachial vein, unspecified side CC POA CC/MCC Exc

S45.29 Other specified injury of axillary or brachial vein

S45.291 Other specified injury of axillary or brachial vein, right side CC POA CC/MCC Exc

S45.292 Other specified injury of axillary or brachial vein, left side CC POA CC/MCC Exc

S45.299 Other specified injury of axillary or brachial vein, unspecified side CC POA CC/MCC Exc

S45.3 Injury of superficial vein at shoulder and upper arm level

S45.30 Unspecified injury of superficial vein at shoulder and upper arm level

S45.301 Unspecified injury of superficial vein at shoulder and upper arm level, right arm CC POA CC/MCC Exc

S45.302 Unspecified injury of superficial vein at shoulder and upper arm level, left arm CC POA CC/MCC Exc

S45.309 Unspecified injury of superficial vein at shoulder and upper arm level, unspecified arm CC POA CC/MCC Exc

S45.31 Laceration of superficial vein at shoulder and upper arm level

S45.311 Laceration of superficial vein at shoulder and upper arm level, right arm CC POA CC/MCC Exc

S45.312 Laceration of superficial vein at shoulder and upper arm level, left arm CC POA CC/MCC Exc

S45.319 Laceration of superficial vein at shoulder and upper arm level, unspecified arm CC POA CC/MCC Exc

S45.39 Other specified injury of superficial vein at shoulder and upper arm level

S45.391 Other specified injury of superficial vein at shoulder and upper arm level, right arm CC POA CC/MCC Exc

S45.392 Other specified injury of superficial vein at shoulder and upper arm level, left arm CC POA CC/MCC Exc

S45.399 Other specified injury of superficial vein at shoulder and upper arm level, unspecified arm CC POA CC/MCC Exc

S45.8 Injury of other specified blood vessels at shoulder and upper arm level

S45.80 Unspecified injury of other specified blood vessels at shoulder and upper arm level

S45.801 Unspecified injury of other specified blood vessels at shoulder and upper arm level, right arm CC POA CC/MCC Exc

S45.802 Unspecified injury of other specified blood vessels at shoulder and upper arm level, left arm CC POA CC/MCC Exc

S45.809 Unspecified injury of other specified blood vessels at shoulder and upper arm level, unspecified arm CC POA CC/MCC Exc

S45.81 Laceration of other specified blood vessels at shoulder and upper arm level

S45.811 Laceration of other specified blood vessels at shoulder and upper arm level, right arm CC POA CC/MCC Exc

S45.812 Laceration of other specified blood vessels at shoulder and upper arm level, left arm CC POA CC/MCC Exc

S45.819 Laceration of other specified blood vessels at shoulder and upper arm level, unspecified arm CC POA CC/MCC Exc

S45.89 Other specified injury of other specified blood vessels at shoulder and upper arm level

S45.891 Other specified injury of other specified blood vessels at shoulder and upper arm level, right arm CC POA CC/MCC Exc

S45.892 Other specified injury of other specified blood vessels at shoulder and upper arm level, left arm CC POA CC/MCC Exc

S45.899 Other specified injury of other specified blood vessels at shoulder and upper arm level, unspecified arm CC POA CC/MCC Exc

S45.9 Injury of unspecified blood vessel at shoulder and upper arm level

S45.90 Unspecified injury of unspecified blood vessel at shoulder and upper arm level

S45.901 Unspecified injury of unspecified blood vessel at shoulder and upper arm level, right arm CC POA CC/MCC Exc

S45.902 Unspecified injury of unspecified blood vessel at shoulder and upper arm level, left arm CC POA CC/MCC Exc

S45.909 Unspecified injury of unspecified blood vessel at shoulder and upper arm level, unspecified arm CC POA CC/MCC Exc

S45.91 Laceration of unspecified blood vessel at shoulder and upper arm level

S45.911 Laceration of unspecified blood vessel at shoulder and upper arm level, right arm POA CC/MCC Exc

S45.912 Laceration of unspecified blood vessel at shoulder and upper arm level, left arm POA CC/MCC Exc

S45.919 Laceration of unspecified blood vessel at shoulder and upper arm level, unspecified arm POA CC/MCC Exc

S45.99 Other specified injury of unspecified blood vessel at shoulder and upper arm level

S45.991 Other specified injury of unspecified blood vessel at shoulder and upper arm level, right arm CC POA CC/MCC Exc

S45.992 Other specified injury of unspecified blood vessel at shoulder and upper arm level, left arm CC POA CC/MCC Exc

S45.999 Other specified injury of unspecified blood vessel at shoulder and upper arm level, unspecified arm CC POA CC/MCC Exc

---

PDin Unacceptable principal diagnosis symbol per Medicare code edits   POA Code exempt from diagnosis present on admission requirement
? Questionable admission   CC Complication or comorbidity   MCC Major complication or comorbidity   CC/MCC Exc CC/MCC exclusion
HCC HCC diagnosis code   RxHCC RxHCC diagnosis code   MACRA MACRA code   **DEFINITION** Describes condition/terminology
TIP Coding guidance   👁 Official Guideline Reference   Z1 Z code as first-listed diagnosis

S46 **Injury of muscle, fascia and tendon at shoulder and upper arm level**
   Code also any associated open wound (S41.-)
   EXCLUDES2 *injury of muscle, fascia and tendon at elbow (S56.-)*
   sprain of joints and ligaments of shoulder girdle (S43.9)

   The appropriate 7th character is to be added to each code from category S46
   A = initial encounter
   D = subsequent encounter
   S = sequela

S46.0 **Injury of muscle(s) and tendon(s) of** the rotator cuff of shoulder
   S46.00 **Unspecified injury of muscle(s) and tendon(s) of the rotator cuff of shoulder**
      S46.001 **Unspecified injury of muscle(s) and tendon(s) of the rotator cuff of** right shoulder POA
      S46.002 **Unspecified injury of muscle(s) and tendon(s) of the rotator cuff of** left shoulder POA
      S46.009 **Unspecified injury of muscle(s) and tendon(s) of the rotator cuff of unspecified shoulder** POA
   S46.01 **Strain of muscle(s) and tendon(s) of the rotator cuff of shoulder**
      S46.011 **Strain of muscle(s) and tendon(s) of the rotator cuff of** right shoulder POA
      S46.012 **Strain of muscle(s) and tendon(s) of the rotator cuff of** left shoulder POA
      S46.019 **Strain of muscle(s) and tendon(s) of the rotator cuff of unspecified shoulder** POA
   S46.02 **Laceration of muscle(s) and tendon(s) of the rotator cuff of shoulder**
      S46.021 **Laceration of muscle(s) and tendon(s) of the rotator cuff of** right shoulder CC POA CC/MCC Exc
      S46.022 **Laceration of muscle(s) and tendon(s) of the rotator cuff of** left shoulder CC POA CC/MCC Exc
      S46.029 **Laceration of muscle(s) and tendon(s) of the rotator cuff of unspecified shoulder** CC POA CC/MCC Exc
   S46.09 **Other injury of muscle(s) and tendon(s) of the rotator cuff of shoulder**
      S46.091 **Other injury of muscle(s) and tendon(s) of the rotator cuff of** right shoulder POA
      S46.092 **Other injury of muscle(s) and tendon(s) of the rotator cuff of** left shoulder POA
      S46.099 **Other injury of muscle(s) and tendon(s) of the rotator cuff of unspecified shoulder** POA

S46.1 **Injury of muscle, fascia and tendon of** long head of biceps
   S46.10 **Unspecified injury of muscle, fascia and tendon of long head of biceps**
      S46.101 **Unspecified injury of muscle, fascia and tendon of long head of biceps,** right arm POA
      S46.102 **Unspecified injury of muscle, fascia and tendon of long head of biceps,** left arm POA
      S46.109 **Unspecified injury of muscle, fascia and tendon of long head of biceps, unspecified arm** POA
   S46.11 **Strain of muscle, fascia and tendon of long head of biceps**
      S46.111 **Strain of muscle, fascia and tendon of long head of biceps,** right arm POA
      S46.112 **Strain of muscle, fascia and tendon of long head of biceps,** left arm POA
      S46.119 **Strain of muscle, fascia and tendon of long head of biceps, unspecified arm** POA
   S46.12 **Laceration of muscle, fascia and tendon of long head of biceps**
      S46.121 **Laceration of muscle, fascia and tendon of long head of biceps,** right arm CC POA CC/MCC Exc
      S46.122 **Laceration of muscle, fascia and tendon of long head of biceps,** left arm

      S46.129 **Laceration of muscle, fascia and tendon of long head of biceps, unspecified arm** CC POA CC/MCC Exc
   S46.19 **Other injury of muscle, fascia and tendon of long head of biceps**
      S46.191 **Other injury of muscle, fascia and tendon of long head of biceps,** right arm POA
      S46.192 **Other injury of muscle, fascia and tendon of long head of biceps,** left arm POA
      S46.199 **Other injury of muscle, fascia and tendon of long head of biceps, unspecified arm** POA

S46.2 **Injury of muscle, fascia and tendon of** other parts of biceps
   S46.20 **Unspecified injury of muscle, fascia and tendon of other parts of biceps**
      S46.201 **Unspecified injury of muscle, fascia and tendon of other parts of biceps,** right arm POA
      S46.202 **Unspecified injury of muscle, fascia and tendon of other parts of biceps,** left arm POA
      S46.209 **Unspecified injury of muscle, fascia and tendon of other parts of biceps, unspecified arm** POA
   S46.21 **Strain of muscle, fascia and tendon of other parts of biceps**
      S46.211 **Strain of muscle, fascia and tendon of other parts of biceps,** right arm POA
      S46.212 **Strain of muscle, fascia and tendon of other parts of biceps,** left arm POA
      S46.219 **Strain of muscle, fascia and tendon of other parts of biceps, unspecified arm** POA
   S46.22 **Laceration of muscle, fascia and tendon of other parts of biceps**
      S46.221 **Laceration of muscle, fascia and tendon of other parts of biceps,** right arm CC POA CC/MCC Exc
      S46.222 **Laceration of muscle, fascia and tendon of other parts of biceps,** left arm CC POA CC/MCC Exc
      S46.229 **Laceration of muscle, fascia and tendon of other parts of biceps, unspecified arm** CC POA CC/MCC Exc
   S46.29 **Other injury of muscle, fascia and tendon of other parts of biceps**
      S46.291 **Other injury of muscle, fascia and tendon of other parts of biceps,** right arm POA
      S46.292 **Other injury of muscle, fascia and tendon of other parts of biceps,** left arm POA
      S46.299 **Other injury of muscle, fascia and tendon of other parts of biceps, unspecified arm** POA

S46.3 **Injury of muscle, fascia and tendon of** triceps
   S46.30 **Unspecified injury of muscle, fascia and tendon of triceps**
      S46.301 **Unspecified injury of muscle, fascia and tendon of triceps,** right arm POA
      S46.302 **Unspecified injury of muscle, fascia and tendon of triceps,** left arm POA
      S46.309 **Unspecified injury of muscle, fascia and tendon of triceps, unspecified arm** POA
   S46.31 **Strain of muscle, fascia and tendon of triceps**
      S46.311 **Strain of muscle, fascia and tendon of triceps,** right arm POA
      S46.312 **Strain of muscle, fascia and tendon of triceps,** left arm POA
      S46.319 **Strain of muscle, fascia and tendon of triceps, unspecified arm** POA
   S46.32 **Laceration of muscle, fascia and tendon of triceps**
      S46.321 **Laceration of muscle, fascia and tendon of triceps,** right arm CC POA CC/MCC Exc
      S46.322 **Laceration of muscle, fascia and tendon of triceps,** left arm CC POA CC/MCC Exc
      S46.329 **Laceration of muscle, fascia and tendon of triceps, unspecified arm** CC POA CC/MCC Exc

---

● Unspecified Code	Other Specified Code	Manifestation Code	Ⓝ Newborn	Ⓟ Pediatric	Ⓜ Maternity	Ⓐ Adult	♂ Male	♀ Female
● New Code	▲ Revised Code Title	►◄ Revised Text	**NOTES**	*INCLUDES*	*EXCLUDES1* Not coded here	*EXCLUDES2* Not included here

4th character required   5th character required   6th character required   7th character required   Extension 'X' Alert
HAC Hospital-acquired condition (HAC) alert   AHA AHA Coding Clinic©   ☛ Code first alert

6ᵗʰ S46.39 Other injury of muscle, fascia and tendon of triceps
- 7ᵗʰ S46.391 Other injury of muscle, fascia and tendon of triceps, right arm POA
- 7ᵗʰ S46.392 Other injury of muscle, fascia and tendon of triceps, left arm POA
- 7ᵗʰ S46.399 Other injury of muscle, fascia and tendon of triceps, unspecified arm POA

5ᵗʰ S46.8 Injury of other muscles, fascia and tendons at shoulder and upper arm level
- 6ᵗʰ S46.80 Unspecified injury of other muscles, fascia and tendons at shoulder and upper arm level
  - 7ᵗʰ S46.801 Unspecified injury of other muscles, fascia and tendons at shoulder and upper arm level, right arm POA
  - 7ᵗʰ S46.802 Unspecified injury of other muscles, fascia and tendons at shoulder and upper arm level, left arm POA
  - 7ᵗʰ S46.809 Unspecified injury of other muscles, fascia and tendons at shoulder and upper arm level, unspecified arm POA
- 6ᵗʰ S46.81 Strain of other muscles, fascia and tendons at shoulder and upper arm level
  - 7ᵗʰ S46.811 Strain of other muscles, fascia and tendons at shoulder and upper arm level, right arm POA
  - 7ᵗʰ S46.812 Strain of other muscles, fascia and tendons at shoulder and upper arm level, left arm POA
  - 7ᵗʰ S46.819 Strain of other muscles, fascia and tendons at shoulder and upper arm level, unspecified arm POA
- 6ᵗʰ S46.82 Laceration of other muscles, fascia and tendons at shoulder and upper arm level
  - 7ᵗʰ S46.821 Laceration of other muscles, fascia and tendons at shoulder and upper arm level, right arm CC POA CC/MCC Exc
  - 7ᵗʰ S46.822 Laceration of other muscles, fascia and tendons at shoulder and upper arm level, left arm CC POA CC/MCC Exc
  - 7ᵗʰ S46.829 Laceration of other muscles, fascia and tendons at shoulder and upper arm level, unspecified arm CC POA CC/MCC Exc
- 6ᵗʰ S46.89 Other injury of other muscles, fascia and tendons at shoulder and upper arm level
  - 7ᵗʰ S46.891 Other injury of other muscles, fascia and tendons at shoulder and upper arm level, right arm POA
  - 7ᵗʰ S46.892 Other injury of other muscles, fascia and tendons at shoulder and upper arm level, left arm POA
  - 7ᵗʰ S46.899 Other injury of other muscles, fascia and tendons at shoulder and upper arm level, unspecified arm POA

5ᵗʰ S46.9 Injury of unspecified muscle, fascia and tendon at shoulder and upper arm level
- 6ᵗʰ S46.90 Unspecified injury of unspecified muscle, fascia and tendon at shoulder and upper arm level
  - 7ᵗʰ S46.901 Unspecified injury of unspecified muscle, fascia and tendon at shoulder and upper arm level, right arm POA
  - 7ᵗʰ S46.902 Unspecified injury of unspecified muscle, fascia and tendon at shoulder and upper arm level, left arm POA
  - 7ᵗʰ S46.909 Unspecified injury of unspecified muscle, fascia and tendon at shoulder and upper arm level, unspecified arm POA
- 6ᵗʰ S46.91 Strain of unspecified muscle, fascia and tendon at shoulder and upper arm level
  - 7ᵗʰ S46.911 Strain of unspecified muscle, fascia and tendon at shoulder and upper arm level, right arm POA

- 7ᵗʰ S46.912 Strain of unspecified muscle, fascia and tendon at shoulder and upper arm level, left arm POA
- 7ᵗʰ S46.919 Strain of unspecified muscle, fascia and tendon at shoulder and upper arm level, unspecified arm POA

6ᵗʰ S46.92 Laceration of unspecified muscle, fascia and tendon at shoulder and upper arm level
- 7ᵗʰ S46.921 Laceration of unspecified muscle, fascia and tendon at shoulder and upper arm level, right arm CC POA CC/MCC Exc
- 7ᵗʰ S46.922 Laceration of unspecified muscle, fascia and tendon at shoulder and upper arm level, left arm CC POA CC/MCC Exc
- 7ᵗʰ S46.929 Laceration of unspecified muscle, fascia and tendon at shoulder and upper arm level, unspecified arm CC POA CC/MCC Exc

6ᵗʰ S46.99 Other injury of unspecified muscle, fascia and tendon at shoulder and upper arm level
- 7ᵗʰ S46.991 Other injury of unspecified muscle, fascia and tendon at shoulder and upper arm level, right arm POA
- 7ᵗʰ S46.992 Other injury of unspecified muscle, fascia and tendon at shoulder and upper arm level, left arm POA
- 7ᵗʰ S46.999 Other injury of unspecified muscle, fascia and tendon at shoulder and upper arm level, unspecified arm POA

4ᵗʰ S47 Crushing injury of shoulder and upper arm
Use additional code for all associated injuries
EXCLUDES2 crushing injury of elbow (S57.0-)
The appropriate 7th character is to be added to each code from category S47
  A = initial encounter
  D = subsequent encounter
  S = sequela
- 7ᵗʰ S47.1 Crushing injury of right shoulder and upper arm POA
- 7ᵗʰ S47.2 Crushing injury of left shoulder and upper arm POA
- 7ᵗʰ S47.9 Crushing injury of shoulder and upper arm, unspecified arm POA

4ᵗʰ S48 Traumatic amputation of shoulder and upper arm
An amputation not identified as partial or complete should be coded to complete
EXCLUDES1 traumatic amputation at elbow level (S58.0)
The appropriate 7th character is to be added to each code from category S48
  A = initial encounter
  D = subsequent encounter
  S = sequela
- 5ᵗʰ S48.0 Traumatic amputation at shoulder joint
  - 6ᵗʰ S48.01 Complete traumatic amputation at shoulder joint
    - 7ᵗʰ S48.011 Complete traumatic amputation at right shoulder joint CC POA HCC CC/MCC Exc
    - 7ᵗʰ S48.012 Complete traumatic amputation at left shoulder joint CC POA HCC CC/MCC Exc
    - 7ᵗʰ S48.019 Complete traumatic amputation at unspecified shoulder joint CC POA HCC CC/MCC Exc
  - 6ᵗʰ S48.02 Partial traumatic amputation at shoulder joint
    - 7ᵗʰ S48.021 Partial traumatic amputation at right shoulder joint CC POA HCC CC/MCC Exc
    - 7ᵗʰ S48.022 Partial traumatic amputation at left shoulder joint CC POA HCC CC/MCC Exc
    - 7ᵗʰ S48.029 Partial traumatic amputation at unspecified shoulder joint CC POA HCC CC/MCC Exc
- 5ᵗʰ S48.1 Traumatic amputation at level between shoulder and elbow
  - 6ᵗʰ S48.11 Complete traumatic amputation at level between shoulder and elbow
    - 7ᵗʰ S48.111 Complete traumatic amputation at level between right shoulder and elbow CC POA HCC CC/MCC Exc

POA Unacceptable principal diagnosis symbol per Medicare code edits   POA Code exempt from diagnosis present on admission requirement
? Questionable admission   CC Complication or comorbidity   MCC Major complication or comorbidity   CC/MCC Exc CC/MCC exclusion
HCC HCC diagnosis code   RxHCC RxHCC diagnosis code   MACRA code   DEFINITION Describes condition/terminology
TIP Coding guidance   👁 Official Guideline Reference   Z1 Z code as first-listed diagnosis

⑦ **S48.112** Complete traumatic amputation at level between left shoulder and elbow   CC° POA HCC CC/MCC Exc

⑦ **S48.119** Complete traumatic amputation at level between unspecified shoulder and elbow   CC° POA HCC CC/MCC Exc

⑥ **S48.12** Partial traumatic amputation at level between shoulder and elbow

⑦ **S48.121** Partial traumatic amputation at level between right shoulder and elbow   CC° POA HCC CC/MCC Exc

⑦ **S48.122** Partial traumatic amputation at level between left shoulder and elbow   CC° POA HCC CC/MCC Exc

⑦ **S48.129** Partial traumatic amputation at level between unspecified shoulder and elbow   CC° POA HCC CC/MCC Exc

⑤ **S48.9** Traumatic amputation of shoulder and upper arm, level unspecified

⑥ **S48.91** Complete traumatic amputation of shoulder and upper arm, level unspecified

⑦ **S48.911** Complete traumatic amputation of right shoulder and upper arm, level unspecified   CC° POA HCC CC/MCC Exc

⑦ **S48.912** Complete traumatic amputation of left shoulder and upper arm, level unspecified   CC° POA HCC CC/MCC Exc

⑦ **S48.919** Complete traumatic amputation of unspecified shoulder and upper arm, level unspecified   CC° POA HCC CC/MCC Exc

⑥ **S48.92** Partial traumatic amputation of shoulder and upper arm, level unspecified

⑦ **S48.921** Partial traumatic amputation of right shoulder and upper arm, level unspecified   CC° POA HCC CC/MCC Exc

⑦ **S48.922** Partial traumatic amputation of left shoulder and upper arm, level unspecified   CC° POA HCC CC/MCC Exc

⑦ **S48.929** Partial traumatic amputation of unspecified shoulder and upper arm, level unspecified   CC° POA HCC CC/MCC Exc

④ **S49** Other and unspecified injuries of shoulder and upper arm

👁 See Official Guidelines "Coding of Traumatic Fractures" I.C.19.c

The appropriate 7th character is to be added to each code from subcategories S49.0 and S49.1

A = initial encounter for closed fracture
D = subsequent encounter for fracture with routine healing
G = subsequent encounter for fracture with delayed healing
K = subsequent encounter for fracture with nonunion
P = subsequent encounter for fracture with malunion
S = sequela

⑤ **S49.0** Physeal fracture of upper end of humerus

⑥ **S49.00** Unspecified physeal fracture of upper end of humerus

⑦ **S49.001** Unspecified physeal fracture of upper end of humerus, right arm   CC° POA HAC CC/MCC Exc

⑦ **S49.002** Unspecified physeal fracture of upper end of humerus, left arm   CC° POA HAC CC/MCC Exc

⑦ **S49.009** Unspecified physeal fracture of upper end of humerus, unspecified arm   CC° POA HAC CC/MCC Exc

⑥ **S49.01** Salter-Harris Type I physeal fracture of upper end of humerus

⑦ **S49.011** Salter-Harris Type I physeal fracture of upper end of humerus, right arm   CC° POA HAC CC/MCC Exc

⑦ **S49.012** Salter-Harris Type I physeal fracture of upper end of humerus, left arm   CC° POA HAC CC/MCC Exc

⑦ **S49.019** Salter-Harris Type I physeal fracture of upper end of humerus, unspecified arm   CC° POA HAC CC/MCC Exc

⑥ **S49.02** Salter-Harris Type II physeal fracture of upper end of humerus

⑦ **S49.021** Salter-Harris Type II physeal fracture of upper end of humerus, right arm   CC° POA HAC CC/MCC Exc

⑦ **S49.022** Salter-Harris Type II physeal fracture of upper end of humerus, left arm   CC° POA HAC CC/MCC Exc

⑦ **S49.029** Salter-Harris Type II physeal fracture of upper end of humerus, unspecified arm   CC° POA HAC CC/MCC Exc

⑥ **S49.03** Salter-Harris Type III physeal fracture of upper end of humerus

⑦ **S49.031** Salter-Harris Type III physeal fracture of upper end of humerus, right arm   CC° POA HAC CC/MCC Exc

⑦ **S49.032** Salter-Harris Type III physeal fracture of upper end of humerus, left arm   CC° POA HAC CC/MCC Exc

⑦ **S49.039** Salter-Harris Type III physeal fracture of upper end of humerus, unspecified arm   CC° POA HAC CC/MCC Exc

⑥ **S49.04** Salter-Harris Type IV physeal fracture of upper end of humerus

⑦ **S49.041** Salter-Harris Type IV physeal fracture of upper end of humerus, right arm   CC° POA HAC CC/MCC Exc

⑦ **S49.042** Salter-Harris Type IV physeal fracture of upper end of humerus, left arm   CC° POA HAC CC/MCC Exc

⑦ **S49.049** Salter-Harris Type IV physeal fracture of upper end of humerus, unspecified arm   CC° POA HAC CC/MCC Exc

⑥ **S49.09** Other physeal fracture of upper end of humerus

⑦ **S49.091** Other physeal fracture of upper end of humerus, right arm   CC° POA HAC CC/MCC Exc

⑦ **S49.092** Other physeal fracture of upper end of humerus, left arm   CC° POA HAC CC/MCC Exc

⑦ **S49.099** Other physeal fracture of upper end of humerus, unspecified arm   CC° POA HAC CC/MCC Exc

⑤ **S49.1** Physeal fracture of lower end of humerus

⑥ **S49.10** Unspecified physeal fracture of lower end of humerus

⑦ **S49.101** Unspecified physeal fracture of lower end of humerus, right arm   CC° POA HAC CC/MCC Exc

⑦ **S49.102** Unspecified physeal fracture of lower end of humerus, left arm   CC° POA HAC CC/MCC Exc

⑦ **S49.109** Unspecified physeal fracture of lower end of humerus, unspecified arm   CC° POA HAC CC/MCC Exc

⑥ **S49.11** Salter-Harris Type I physeal fracture of lower end of humerus

⑦ **S49.111** Salter-Harris Type I physeal fracture of lower end of humerus, right arm   CC° POA HAC CC/MCC Exc

⑦ **S49.112** Salter-Harris Type I physeal fracture of lower end of humerus, left arm   CC° POA HAC CC/MCC Exc

⑦ **S49.119** Salter-Harris Type I physeal fracture of lower end of humerus, unspecified arm   CC° POA HAC CC/MCC Exc

⑥ **S49.12** Salter-Harris Type II physeal fracture of lower end of humerus

⑦ **S49.121** Salter-Harris Type II physeal fracture of lower end of humerus, right arm   CC° POA HAC CC/MCC Exc

⑦ **S49.122** Salter-Harris Type II physeal fracture of lower end of humerus, left arm   CC° POA HAC CC/MCC Exc

⑦ **S49.129** Salter-Harris Type II physeal fracture of lower end of humerus, unspecified arm   CC° POA HAC CC/MCC Exc

---

Unspecified Code   Other Specified Code   Manifestation Code   Ⓝ Newborn   Ⓟ Pediatric   Ⓜ Maternity   Ⓐ Adult   ♂ Male   ♀ Female
● New Code   ▲ Revised Code Title   ►◄ Revised Text   **NOTES**   *INCLUDES*   *EXCLUDES1* Not coded here   *EXCLUDES2* Not included here
④ 4th character required   ⑤ 5th character required   ⑥ 6th character required   ⑦ 7th character required   ⑩ Extension 'X' Alert
HAC Hospital-acquired condition (HAC) alert   **AHA** AHA Coding Clinic©   📯 Code first alert

6ᵗʰ **S49.13** Salter-Harris Type III physeal fracture of lower end of humerus
- 7ᵗʰ **S49.131** Salter-Harris Type III physeal fracture of lower end of humerus, right arm CC POA HAC CC/MCC Exc
- 7ᵗʰ **S49.132** Salter-Harris Type III physeal fracture of lower end of humerus, left arm CC POA HAC CC/MCC Exc
- 7ᵗʰ **S49.139** Salter-Harris Type III physeal fracture of lower end of humerus, unspecified arm CC POA HAC CC/MCC Exc

6ᵗʰ **S49.14** Salter-Harris Type IV physeal fracture of lower end of humerus
- 7ᵗʰ **S49.141** Salter-Harris Type IV physeal fracture of lower end of humerus, right arm CC POA HAC CC/MCC Exc
- 7ᵗʰ **S49.142** Salter-Harris Type IV physeal fracture of lower end of humerus, left arm CC POA HAC CC/MCC Exc
- 7ᵗʰ **S49.149** Salter-Harris Type IV physeal fracture of lower end of humerus, unspecified arm CC POA HAC CC/MCC Exc

6ᵗʰ **S49.19** Other physeal fracture of lower end of humerus
- 7ᵗʰ **S49.191** Other physeal fracture of lower end of humerus, right arm CC POA HAC CC/MCC Exc
- 7ᵗʰ **S49.192** Other physeal fracture of lower end of humerus, left arm CC POA HAC CC/MCC Exc
- 7ᵗʰ **S49.199** Other physeal fracture of lower end of humerus, unspecified arm CC POA HAC CC/MCC Exc

5ᵗʰ **S49.8** Other specified injuries of shoulder and upper arm
The appropriate 7th character is to be added to each code in subcategory S49.8
A = initial encounter
D = subsequent encounter
S = sequela
- 7ᵗʰ **S49.80** Other specified injuries of shoulder and upper arm, unspecified arm POA
- 7ᵗʰ **S49.81** Other specified injuries of right shoulder and upper arm POA
- 7ᵗʰ **S49.82** Other specified injuries of left shoulder and upper arm POA

5ᵗʰ **S49.9** Unspecified injury of shoulder and upper arm
The appropriate 7th character is to be added to each code in subcategory S49.9
A = initial encounter
D = subsequent encounter
S = sequela
- 7ᵗʰ **S49.90** Unspecified injury of shoulder and upper arm, unspecified arm POA
- 7ᵗʰ **S49.91** Unspecified injury of right shoulder and upper arm POA
- 7ᵗʰ **S49.92** Unspecified injury of left shoulder and upper arm POA

Injuries to the elbow and forearm (S50-S59)

EXCLUDES2 burns and corrosions (T20-T32)
frostbite (T33-T34)
injuries of wrist and hand (S60-S69)
insect bite or sting, venomous (T63.4)

4ᵗʰ **S50** Superficial injury of elbow and forearm
EXCLUDES2 superficial injury of wrist and hand (S60.-)
The appropriate 7th character is to be added to each code from category S50
A = initial encounter
D = subsequent encounter
S = sequela

5ᵗʰ **S50.0** Contusion of elbow
- 7ᵗʰ **S50.00** Contusion of unspecified elbow POA
- 7ᵗʰ **S50.01** Contusion of right elbow POA
- 7ᵗʰ **S50.02** Contusion of left elbow POA

5ᵗʰ **S50.1** Contusion of forearm
- 7ᵗʰ **S50.10** Contusion of unspecified forearm POA
- 7ᵗʰ **S50.11** Contusion of right forearm POA
- 7ᵗʰ **S50.12** Contusion of left forearm POA

5ᵗʰ **S50.3** Other superficial injuries of elbow
- 6ᵗʰ **S50.31** Abrasion of elbow
  - 7ᵗʰ **S50.311** Abrasion of right elbow POA
  - 7ᵗʰ **S50.312** Abrasion of left elbow POA
  - 7ᵗʰ **S50.319** Abrasion of unspecified elbow POA
- 6ᵗʰ **S50.32** Blister (nonthermal) of elbow
  - 7ᵗʰ **S50.321** Blister (nonthermal) of right elbow POA
  - 7ᵗʰ **S50.322** Blister (nonthermal) of left elbow POA
  - 7ᵗʰ **S50.329** Blister (nonthermal) of unspecified elbow POA
- 6ᵗʰ **S50.34** External constriction of elbow
  - 7ᵗʰ **S50.341** External constriction of right elbow POA
  - 7ᵗʰ **S50.342** External constriction of left elbow POA
  - 7ᵗʰ **S50.349** External constriction of unspecified elbow POA
- 6ᵗʰ **S50.35** Superficial foreign body of elbow
  Splinter in the elbow
  - 7ᵗʰ **S50.351** Superficial foreign body of right elbow POA
  - 7ᵗʰ **S50.352** Superficial foreign body of left elbow POA
  - 7ᵗʰ **S50.359** Superficial foreign body of unspecified elbow POA
- 6ᵗʰ **S50.36** Insect bite (nonvenomous) of elbow
  - 7ᵗʰ **S50.361** Insect bite (nonvenomous) of right elbow POA
  - 7ᵗʰ **S50.362** Insect bite (nonvenomous) of left elbow POA
  - 7ᵗʰ **S50.369** Insect bite (nonvenomous) of unspecified elbow POA
- 6ᵗʰ **S50.37** Other superficial bite of elbow
  EXCLUDES1 open bite of elbow (S51.04)
  - 7ᵗʰ **S50.371** Other superficial bite of right elbow POA
  - 7ᵗʰ **S50.372** Other superficial bite of left elbow POA
  - 7ᵗʰ **S50.379** Other superficial bite of unspecified elbow POA

5ᵗʰ **S50.8** Other superficial injuries of forearm
- 6ᵗʰ **S50.81** Abrasion of forearm
  - 7ᵗʰ **S50.811** Abrasion of right forearm POA
  - 7ᵗʰ **S50.812** Abrasion of left forearm POA
  - 7ᵗʰ **S50.819** Abrasion of unspecified forearm POA
- 6ᵗʰ **S50.82** Blister (nonthermal) of forearm
  - 7ᵗʰ **S50.821** Blister (nonthermal) of right forearm POA
  - 7ᵗʰ **S50.822** Blister (nonthermal) of left forearm POA
  - 7ᵗʰ **S50.829** Blister (nonthermal) of unspecified forearm POA
- 6ᵗʰ **S50.84** External constriction of forearm
  - 7ᵗʰ **S50.841** External constriction of right forearm POA
  - 7ᵗʰ **S50.842** External constriction of left forearm POA
  - 7ᵗʰ **S50.849** External constriction of unspecified forearm POA
- 6ᵗʰ **S50.85** Superficial foreign body of forearm
  Splinter in the forearm
  - 7ᵗʰ **S50.851** Superficial foreign body of right forearm POA
  - 7ᵗʰ **S50.852** Superficial foreign body of left forearm POA
  - 7ᵗʰ **S50.859** Superficial foreign body of unspecified forearm POA
- 6ᵗʰ **S50.86** Insect bite (nonvenomous) of forearm
  - 7ᵗʰ **S50.861** Insect bite (nonvenomous) of right forearm POA
  - 7ᵗʰ **S50.862** Insect bite (nonvenomous) of left forearm POA
  - 7ᵗʰ **S50.869** Insect bite (nonvenomous) of unspecified forearm POA
- 6ᵗʰ **S50.87** Other superficial bite of forearm
  EXCLUDES1 open bite of forearm (S51.84)
  - 7ᵗʰ **S50.871** Other superficial bite of right forearm POA
  - 7ᵗʰ **S50.872** Other superficial bite of left forearm POA

POA⃠ Unacceptable principal diagnosis symbol per Medicare code edits POA Code exempt from diagnosis present on admission requirement
 ❓ Questionable admission CC Complication or comorbidity MCC Major complication or comorbidity CC/MCC Exc CC/MCC exclusion
 HCC HCC diagnosis code RxHCC RxHCC diagnosis code MACRA MACRA code **DEFINITION** Describes condition/terminology
 TIP Coding guidance 👁 Official Guideline Reference Z1 Z code as first-listed diagnosis

S50.879 Other superficial bite of unspecified forearm POA

S50.9 Unspecified superficial injury of elbow and forearm
- **S50.90** Unspecified superficial injury of elbow
  - **S50.901** Unspecified superficial injury of right elbow POA
  - **S50.902** Unspecified superficial injury of left elbow POA
  - **S50.909** Unspecified superficial injury of unspecified elbow POA
- **S50.91** Unspecified superficial injury of forearm
  - **S50.911** Unspecified superficial injury of right forearm POA
  - **S50.912** Unspecified superficial injury of left forearm POA
  - **S50.919** Unspecified superficial injury of unspecified forearm POA

S51 Open wound of elbow and forearm
Code also any associated wound infection
EXCLUDES1 open fracture of elbow and forearm (S52.- with open fracture 7th character)
traumatic amputation of elbow and forearm (S58.-)
EXCLUDES2 open wound of wrist and hand (S61.-)
The appropriate 7th character is to be added to each code from category S51
A = initial encounter
D = subsequent encounter
S = sequela

S51.0 Open wound of elbow
- **S51.00** Unspecified open wound of elbow
  - **S51.001** Unspecified open wound of right elbow POA
    AHA: Q4 2012
  - **S51.002** Unspecified open wound of left elbow POA
  - **S51.009** Unspecified open wound of unspecified elbow POA
    Open wound of elbow NOS
- **S51.01** Laceration without foreign body of elbow
  - **S51.011** Laceration without foreign body of right elbow POA
  - **S51.012** Laceration without foreign body of left elbow POA
  - **S51.019** Laceration without foreign body of unspecified elbow POA
- **S51.02** Laceration with foreign body of elbow
  - **S51.021** Laceration with foreign body of right elbow POA
  - **S51.022** Laceration with foreign body of left elbow POA
  - **S51.029** Laceration with foreign body of unspecified elbow POA
- **S51.03** Puncture wound without foreign body of elbow
  - **S51.031** Puncture wound without foreign body of right elbow POA
  - **S51.032** Puncture wound without foreign body of left elbow POA
  - **S51.039** Puncture wound without foreign body of unspecified elbow POA
- **S51.04** Puncture wound with foreign body of elbow
  - **S51.041** Puncture wound with foreign body of right elbow POA
  - **S51.042** Puncture wound with foreign body of left elbow POA
  - **S51.049** Puncture wound with foreign body of unspecified elbow POA
- **S51.05** Open bite of elbow
  Bite of elbow NOS
  EXCLUDES1 superficial bite of elbow (S50.36, S50.37)
  - **S51.051** Open bite, right elbow POA
  - **S51.052** Open bite, left elbow POA
  - **S51.059** Open bite, unspecified elbow POA

S51.8 Open wound of forearm
EXCLUDES2 open wound of elbow (S51.0-)
- **S51.80** Unspecified open wound of forearm
  - **S51.801** Unspecified open wound of right forearm POA
  - **S51.802** Unspecified open wound of left forearm POA
  - **S51.809** Unspecified open wound of unspecified forearm POA
    Open wound of forearm NOS
- **S51.81** Laceration without foreign body of forearm
  - **S51.811** Laceration without foreign body of right forearm POA
  - **S51.812** Laceration without foreign body of left forearm POA
  - **S51.819** Laceration without foreign body of unspecified forearm POA
- **S51.82** Laceration with foreign body of forearm
  - **S51.821** Laceration with foreign body of right forearm POA
  - **S51.822** Laceration with foreign body of left forearm POA
  - **S51.829** Laceration with foreign body of unspecified forearm POA
- **S51.83** Puncture wound without foreign body of forearm
  - **S51.831** Puncture wound without foreign body of right forearm POA
  - **S51.832** Puncture wound without foreign body of left forearm POA
  - **S51.839** Puncture wound without foreign body of unspecified forearm POA
- **S51.84** Puncture wound with foreign body of forearm
  - **S51.841** Puncture wound with foreign body of right forearm POA
  - **S51.842** Puncture wound with foreign body of left forearm POA
  - **S51.849** Puncture wound with foreign body of unspecified forearm POA
- **S51.85** Open bite of forearm
  Bite of forearm NOS
  EXCLUDES1 superficial bite of forearm (S50.86, S50.87)
  - **S51.851** Open bite of right forearm POA
  - **S51.852** Open bite of left forearm POA
  - **S51.859** Open bite of unspecified forearm POA

S52 Fracture of forearm
See Official Guidelines "Coding of Traumatic Fractures" I.C.19.c
NOTES A fracture not indicated as displaced or nondisplaced should be coded to displaced
A fracture not indicated as open or closed should be coded to closed
The open fracture designations are based on the Gustilo open fracture classification
EXCLUDES1 traumatic amputation of forearm (S58.-)
EXCLUDES2 fracture at wrist and hand level (S62.-)
The appropriate 7th character is to be added to all codes from category S52
A = initial encounter for closed fracture
B = initial encounter for open fracture type I or II
    initial encounter for open fracture NOS
C = initial encounter for open fracture type IIIA, IIIB, or IIIC
D = subsequent encounter for closed fracture with routine healing
E = subsequent encounter for open fracture type I or II with routine healing
F = subsequent encounter for open fracture type IIIA, IIIB, or IIIC with routine healing
G = subsequent encounter for closed fracture with delayed healing
H = subsequent encounter for open fracture type I or II with delayed healing
J = subsequent encounter for open fracture type IIIA, IIIB, or IIIC with delayed healing

Unspecified Code — Other Specified Code — Manifestation Code — N Newborn — P Pediatric — M Maternity — A Adult — Male — Female — ● New Code — ▲ Revised Code Title — ►◄ Revised Text — NOTES — INCLUDES — EXCLUDES1 Not coded here — EXCLUDES2 Not included here — 4th character required — 5th character required — 6th character required — 7th character required — Extension 'X' Alert — HAC Hospital-acquired condition (HAC) alert — AHA AHA Coding Clinic© — Code first alert

2020 ICD-10-CM   When symbols appear on a code that requires a 7th character extension, refer to Appendix B to identify applicable 7th character codes.   1023

K = subsequent encounter for closed fracture with nonunion

M = subsequent encounter for open fracture type I or II with nonunion

N = subsequent encounter for open fracture type IIIA, IIIB, or IIIC with nonunion

P = subsequent encounter for closed fracture with malunion

Q = subsequent encounter for open fracture type I or II with malunion

R = subsequent encounter for open fracture type IIIA, IIIB, or IIIC with malunion

S = sequela

5ᵗʰ **S52.0 Fracture of** upper end of ulna

Fracture of proximal end of ulna

EXCLUDES2 fracture of elbow NOS (S42.40-)

fractures of shaft of ulna (S52.2-)

6ᵗʰ **S52.00** Unspecified **fracture of upper end of ulna**

7ᵗʰ **S52.001 Unspecified fracture of upper end of** right **ulna** cᶜ ᴘᴏᴀ HAC ᴍᴄᴄ ᴄᴄ/ᴍᴄᴄ ᴇxᶜ

7ᵗʰ **S52.002 Unspecified fracture of upper end of** left **ulna** cᶜ ᴘᴏᴀ HAC ᴍᴄᴄ ᴄᴄ/ᴍᴄᴄ ᴇxᶜ

7ᵗʰ **S52.009 Unspecified fracture of upper end of unspecified ulna** cᶜ ᴘᴏᴀ HAC ᴍᴄᴄ ᴄᴄ/ᴍᴄᴄ ᴇxᶜ

6ᵗʰ **S52.01** Torus **fracture of upper end of ulna**

The appropriate 7th character is to be added to all codes in subcategory S52.01

A = initial encounter for closed fracture

D = subsequent encounter for fracture with routine healing

G = subsequent encounter for fracture with delayed healing

K = subsequent encounter for fracture with nonunion

P = subsequent encounter for fracture with malunion

S = sequela

7ᵗʰ **S52.011 Torus fracture of upper end of** right **ulna** cᶜ ᴘᴏᴀ HAC ᴄᴄ/ᴍᴄᴄ ᴇxᶜ

7ᵗʰ **S52.012 Torus fracture of upper end of** left **ulna** cᶜ ᴘᴏᴀ HAC ᴄᴄ/ᴍᴄᴄ ᴇxᶜ

7ᵗʰ **S52.019 Torus fracture of upper end of unspecified ulna** cᶜ ᴘᴏᴀ HAC ᴄᴄ/ᴍᴄᴄ ᴇxᶜ

6ᵗʰ **S52.02 Fracture of** olecranon process without intraarticular extension **of ulna**

7ᵗʰ **S52.021** Displaced **fracture of olecranon process without intraarticular extension of** right **ulna** cᶜ ᴘᴏᴀ HAC ᴍᴄᴄ ᴄᴄ/ᴍᴄᴄ ᴇxᶜ

7ᵗʰ **S52.022** Displaced **fracture of olecranon process without intraarticular extension of** left **ulna** cᶜ ᴘᴏᴀ HAC ᴍᴄᴄ ᴄᴄ/ᴍᴄᴄ ᴇxᶜ

7ᵗʰ **S52.023** Displaced **fracture of olecranon process without intraarticular extension of unspecified ulna** cᶜ ᴘᴏᴀ HAC ᴍᴄᴄ ᴄᴄ/ᴍᴄᴄ ᴇxᶜ

7ᵗʰ **S52.024** Nondisplaced **fracture of olecranon process without intraarticular extension of** right **ulna** cᶜ ᴘᴏᴀ HAC ᴍᴄᴄ ᴄᴄ/ᴍᴄᴄ ᴇxᶜ

7ᵗʰ **S52.025** Nondisplaced **fracture of olecranon process without intraarticular extension of** left **ulna** cᶜ ᴘᴏᴀ HAC ᴍᴄᴄ ᴄᴄ/ᴍᴄᴄ ᴇxᶜ

7ᵗʰ **S52.026** Nondisplaced **fracture of olecranon process without intraarticular extension of unspecified ulna** cᶜ ᴘᴏᴀ HAC ᴍᴄᴄ ᴄᴄ/ᴍᴄᴄ ᴇxᶜ

6ᵗʰ **S52.03 Fracture of** olecranon process with intraarticular extension **of ulna**

7ᵗʰ **S52.031** Displaced **fracture of olecranon process with intraarticular extension of right ulna** cᶜ ᴘᴏᴀ HAC ᴍᴄᴄ ᴄᴄ/ᴍᴄᴄ ᴇxᶜ

7ᵗʰ **S52.032** Displaced **fracture of olecranon process with intraarticular extension of** left **ulna** cᶜ ᴘᴏᴀ HAC ᴍᴄᴄ ᴄᴄ/ᴍᴄᴄ ᴇxᶜ

7ᵗʰ **S52.033** Displaced **fracture of olecranon process with intraarticular extension of unspecified ulna** cᶜ ᴘᴏᴀ HAC ᴍᴄᴄ ᴄᴄ/ᴍᴄᴄ ᴇxᶜ

7ᵗʰ **S52.034** Nondisplaced **fracture of olecranon process with intraarticular extension of** right **ulna** cᶜ ᴘᴏᴀ HAC ᴍᴄᴄ ᴄᴄ/ᴍᴄᴄ ᴇxᶜ

7ᵗʰ **S52.035** Nondisplaced **fracture of olecranon process with intraarticular extension of** left **ulna** cᶜ ᴘᴏᴀ HAC ᴍᴄᴄ ᴄᴄ/ᴍᴄᴄ ᴇxᶜ

7ᵗʰ **S52.036** Nondisplaced **fracture of olecranon process with intraarticular extension of unspecified ulna** cᶜ ᴘᴏᴀ HAC ᴍᴄᴄ ᴄᴄ/ᴍᴄᴄ ᴇxᶜ

6ᵗʰ **S52.04 Fracture of** coronoid process **of ulna**

7ᵗʰ **S52.041** Displaced **fracture of coronoid process of** right **ulna** cᶜ ᴘᴏᴀ HAC ᴍᴄᴄ ᴄᴄ/ᴍᴄᴄ ᴇxᶜ

7ᵗʰ **S52.042** Displaced **fracture of coronoid process of** left **ulna** cᶜ ᴘᴏᴀ HAC ᴍᴄᴄ ᴄᴄ/ᴍᴄᴄ ᴇxᶜ

7ᵗʰ **S52.043** Displaced **fracture of coronoid process of unspecified ulna** cᶜ ᴘᴏᴀ HAC ᴍᴄᴄ ᴄᴄ/ᴍᴄᴄ ᴇxᶜ

7ᵗʰ **S52.044** Nondisplaced **fracture of coronoid process of** right **ulna** cᶜ ᴘᴏᴀ HAC ᴍᴄᴄ ᴄᴄ/ᴍᴄᴄ ᴇxᶜ

7ᵗʰ **S52.045** Nondisplaced **fracture of coronoid process of** left **ulna** cᶜ ᴘᴏᴀ HAC ᴍᴄᴄ ᴄᴄ/ᴍᴄᴄ ᴇxᶜ

7ᵗʰ **S52.046** Nondisplaced **fracture of coronoid process of unspecified ulna** cᶜ ᴘᴏᴀ HAC ᴍᴄᴄ ᴄᴄ/ᴍᴄᴄ ᴇxᶜ

6ᵗʰ **S52.09** Other **fracture of upper end of ulna**

7ᵗʰ **S52.091 Other fracture of upper end of** right **ulna** cᶜ ᴘᴏᴀ HAC ᴍᴄᴄ ᴄᴄ/ᴍᴄᴄ ᴇxᶜ

7ᵗʰ **S52.092 Other fracture of upper end of** left **ulna** cᶜ ᴘᴏᴀ HAC ᴍᴄᴄ ᴄᴄ/ᴍᴄᴄ ᴇxᶜ

7ᵗʰ **S52.099 Other fracture of upper end of unspecified ulna** cᶜ ᴘᴏᴀ HAC ᴍᴄᴄ ᴄᴄ/ᴍᴄᴄ ᴇxᶜ

5ᵗʰ **S52.1 Fracture of** upper end of radius

Fracture of proximal end of radius

EXCLUDES2 physeal fractures of upper end of radius (S59.2-)

fracture of shaft of radius (S52.3-)

6ᵗʰ **S52.10** Unspecified **fracture of upper end of radius**

7ᵗʰ **S52.101 Unspecified fracture of upper end of** right **radius** cᶜ ᴘᴏᴀ HAC ᴍᴄᴄ ᴄᴄ/ᴍᴄᴄ ᴇxᶜ

7ᵗʰ **S52.102 Unspecified fracture of upper end of** left **radius** cᶜ ᴘᴏᴀ HAC ᴍᴄᴄ ᴄᴄ/ᴍᴄᴄ ᴇxᶜ

7ᵗʰ **S52.109 Unspecified fracture of upper end of unspecified radius** cᶜ ᴘᴏᴀ HAC ᴍᴄᴄ ᴄᴄ/ᴍᴄᴄ ᴇxᶜ

6ᵗʰ **S52.11** Torus **fracture of upper end of radius**

The appropriate 7th character is to be added to all codes in subcategory S52.11

A = initial encounter for closed fracture

D = subsequent encounter for fracture with routine healing

G = subsequent encounter for fracture with delayed healing

K = subsequent encounter for fracture with nonunion

P = subsequent encounter for fracture with malunion

S = sequela

7ᵗʰ **S52.111 Torus fracture of upper end of** right **radius** cᶜ ᴘᴏᴀ HAC ᴄᴄ/ᴍᴄᴄ ᴇxᶜ

7ᵗʰ **S52.112 Torus fracture of upper end of** left **radius** cᶜ ᴘᴏᴀ HAC ᴄᴄ/ᴍᴄᴄ ᴇxᶜ

7ᵗʰ **S52.119 Torus fracture of upper end of unspecified radius** cᶜ ᴘᴏᴀ HAC ᴄᴄ/ᴍᴄᴄ ᴇxᶜ

6ᵗʰ **S52.12 Fracture of** head of radius

7ᵗʰ **S52.121** Displaced **fracture of head of right radius** cᶜ ᴘᴏᴀ HAC ᴍᴄᴄ ᴄᴄ/ᴍᴄᴄ ᴇxᶜ

7ᵗʰ **S52.122** Displaced **fracture of head of** left **radius** cᶜ ᴘᴏᴀ HAC ᴍᴄᴄ ᴄᴄ/ᴍᴄᴄ ᴇxᶜ

7ᵗʰ **S52.123** Displaced **fracture of head of unspecified radius** cᶜ ᴘᴏᴀ HAC ᴍᴄᴄ ᴄᴄ/ᴍᴄᴄ ᴇxᶜ

7ᵗʰ **S52.124** Nondisplaced **fracture of head of** right **radius** cᶜ ᴘᴏᴀ HAC ᴍᴄᴄ ᴄᴄ/ᴍᴄᴄ ᴇxᶜ

7ᵗʰ **S52.125** Nondisplaced **fracture of head of** left **radius** cᶜ ᴘᴏᴀ HAC ᴍᴄᴄ ᴄᴄ/ᴍᴄᴄ ᴇxᶜ

ᴘᴏᴀ Unacceptable principal diagnosis symbol per Medicare code edits   ᴘᴏᴀ Code exempt from diagnosis present on admission requirement

❓ Questionable admission   cᶜ Complication or comorbidity   ᴍᴄᴄ Major complication or comorbidity   ᴄᴄ/ᴍᴄᴄᴇxᶜ CC/MCC exclusion

HCC HCC diagnosis code   RxHCC RxHCC diagnosis code   MACRA MACRA code   **DEFINITION** Describes condition/terminology

TIP Coding guidance   👁 Official Guideline Reference   Z1 Z code as first-listed diagnosis

- [7th] S52.126 Nondisplaced fracture of head of unspecified radius CC POA HAC MCC CC/MCC Exc
- [6th] S52.13 Fracture of neck of radius
  - [7th] S52.131 Displaced fracture of neck of right radius CC POA HAC MCC CC/MCC Exc
  - [7th] S52.132 Displaced fracture of neck of left radius CC POA HAC MCC CC/MCC Exc
  - [7th] S52.133 Displaced fracture of neck of unspecified radius CC POA HAC MCC CC/MCC Exc
  - [7th] S52.134 Nondisplaced fracture of neck of right radius CC POA HAC MCC CC/MCC Exc
  - [7th] S52.135 Nondisplaced fracture of neck of left radius CC POA HAC MCC CC/MCC Exc
  - [7th] S52.136 Nondisplaced fracture of neck of unspecified radius CC POA HAC MCC CC/MCC Exc
- [6th] S52.18 Other fracture of upper end of radius
  - [7th] S52.181 Other fracture of upper end of right radius CC POA HAC MCC CC/MCC Exc
  - [7th] S52.182 Other fracture of upper end of left radius CC POA HAC MCC CC/MCC Exc
  - [7th] S52.189 Other fracture of upper end of unspecified radius CC POA HAC MCC CC/MCC Exc

[5th] S52.2 Fracture of shaft of ulna

- [6th] S52.20 Unspecified fracture of shaft of ulna
  - Fracture of ulna NOS
  - [7th] S52.201 Unspecified fracture of shaft of right ulna CC POA HAC MCC CC/MCC Exc
  - [7th] S52.202 Unspecified fracture of shaft of left ulna CC POA HAC MCC CC/MCC Exc
  - [7th] S52.209 Unspecified fracture of shaft of unspecified ulna CC POA HAC MCC CC/MCC Exc
- [6th] S52.21 Greenstick fracture of shaft of ulna
  - The appropriate 7th character is to be added to all codes in subcategory S52.21
    - A = initial encounter for closed fracture
    - D = subsequent encounter for fracture with routine healing
    - G = subsequent encounter for fracture with delayed healing
    - K = subsequent encounter for fracture with nonunion
    - P = subsequent encounter for fracture with malunion
    - S = sequela
  - [7th] S52.211 Greenstick fracture of shaft of right ulna CC POA HAC CC/MCC Exc
  - [7th] S52.212 Greenstick fracture of shaft of left ulna CC POA HAC CC/MCC Exc
  - [7th] S52.219 Greenstick fracture of shaft of unspecified ulna CC POA HAC CC/MCC Exc
- [6th] S52.22 Transverse fracture of shaft of ulna
  - [7th] S52.221 Displaced transverse fracture of shaft of right ulna CC POA HAC MCC CC/MCC Exc
  - [7th] S52.222 Displaced transverse fracture of shaft of left ulna CC POA HAC MCC CC/MCC Exc
  - [7th] S52.223 Displaced transverse fracture of shaft of unspecified ulna CC POA HAC MCC CC/MCC Exc
  - [7th] S52.224 Nondisplaced transverse fracture of shaft of right ulna CC POA HAC MCC CC/MCC Exc
  - [7th] S52.225 Nondisplaced transverse fracture of shaft of left ulna CC POA HAC MCC CC/MCC Exc
  - [7th] S52.226 Nondisplaced transverse fracture of shaft of unspecified ulna CC POA HAC MCC CC/MCC Exc
- [6th] S52.23 Oblique fracture of shaft of ulna
  - [7th] S52.231 Displaced oblique fracture of shaft of right ulna CC POA HAC MCC CC/MCC Exc
  - [7th] S52.232 Displaced oblique fracture of shaft of left ulna CC POA HAC MCC CC/MCC Exc
  - [7th] S52.233 Displaced oblique fracture of shaft of unspecified ulna CC POA HAC MCC CC/MCC Exc
  - [7th] S52.234 Nondisplaced oblique fracture of shaft of right ulna CC POA HAC MCC CC/MCC Exc
  - [7th] S52.235 Nondisplaced oblique fracture of shaft of left ulna CC POA HAC MCC CC/MCC Exc
  - [7th] S52.236 Nondisplaced oblique fracture of shaft of unspecified ulna CC POA HAC MCC CC/MCC Exc
- [6th] S52.24 Spiral fracture of shaft of ulna
  - [7th] S52.241 Displaced spiral fracture of shaft of ulna, right arm CC POA HAC MCC CC/MCC Exc
  - [7th] S52.242 Displaced spiral fracture of shaft of ulna, left arm CC POA HAC MCC CC/MCC Exc
  - [7th] S52.243 Displaced spiral fracture of shaft of ulna, unspecified arm CC POA HAC MCC CC/MCC Exc
  - [7th] S52.244 Nondisplaced spiral fracture of shaft of ulna, right arm CC POA HAC MCC CC/MCC Exc
  - [7th] S52.245 Nondisplaced spiral fracture of shaft of ulna, left arm CC POA HAC MCC CC/MCC Exc
  - [7th] S52.246 Nondisplaced spiral fracture of shaft of ulna, unspecified arm CC POA HAC MCC CC/MCC Exc
- [6th] S52.25 Comminuted fracture of shaft of ulna
  - [7th] S52.251 Displaced comminuted fracture of shaft of ulna, right arm CC POA HAC MCC CC/MCC Exc
  - [7th] S52.252 Displaced comminuted fracture of shaft of ulna, left arm CC POA HAC MCC CC/MCC Exc
  - [7th] S52.253 Displaced comminuted fracture of shaft of ulna, unspecified arm CC POA HAC MCC CC/MCC Exc
  - [7th] S52.254 Nondisplaced comminuted fracture of shaft of ulna, right arm CC POA HAC MCC CC/MCC Exc
  - [7th] S52.255 Nondisplaced comminuted fracture of shaft of ulna, left arm CC POA HAC MCC CC/MCC Exc
  - [7th] S52.256 Nondisplaced comminuted fracture of shaft of ulna, unspecified arm CC POA HAC MCC CC/MCC Exc
- [6th] S52.26 Segmental fracture of shaft of ulna
  - [7th] S52.261 Displaced segmental fracture of shaft of ulna, right arm CC POA HAC MCC CC/MCC Exc
  - [7th] S52.262 Displaced segmental fracture of shaft of ulna, left arm CC POA HAC MCC CC/MCC Exc
  - [7th] S52.263 Displaced segmental fracture of shaft of ulna, unspecified arm CC POA HAC MCC CC/MCC Exc
  - [7th] S52.264 Nondisplaced segmental fracture of shaft of ulna, right arm CC POA HAC MCC CC/MCC Exc
  - [7th] S52.265 Nondisplaced segmental fracture of shaft of ulna, left arm CC POA HAC MCC CC/MCC Exc
  - [7th] S52.266 Nondisplaced segmental fracture of shaft of ulna, unspecified arm CC POA HAC MCC CC/MCC Exc
- [6th] S52.27 Monteggia's fracture of ulna
  - Fracture of upper shaft of ulna with dislocation of radial head
  - [7th] S52.271 Monteggia's fracture of right ulna CC POA HAC MCC CC/MCC Exc
  - [7th] S52.272 Monteggia's fracture of left ulna CC POA HAC MCC CC/MCC Exc
  - [7th] S52.279 Monteggia's fracture of unspecified ulna CC POA HAC MCC CC/MCC Exc
- [6th] S52.28 Bent bone of ulna
  - [7th] S52.281 Bent bone of right ulna CC POA HAC MCC CC/MCC Exc
  - [7th] S52.282 Bent bone of left ulna CC POA HAC MCC CC/MCC Exc
  - [7th] S52.283 Bent bone of unspecified ulna CC POA HAC MCC CC/MCC Exc
- [6th] S52.29 Other fracture of shaft of ulna
  - [7th] S52.291 Other fracture of shaft of right ulna CC POA HAC MCC CC/MCC Exc
  - [7th] S52.292 Other fracture of shaft of left ulna CC POA HAC MCC CC/MCC Exc
  - [7th] S52.299 Other fracture of shaft of unspecified ulna CC POA HAC MCC CC/MCC Exc

[5th] S52.3 Fracture of shaft of radius

- [6th] S52.30 Unspecified fracture of shaft of radius
  - [7th] S52.301 Unspecified fracture of shaft of right radius CC POA HAC MCC CC/MCC Exc
  - [7th] S52.302 Unspecified fracture of shaft of left radius CC POA HAC MCC CC/MCC Exc
  - [7th] S52.309 Unspecified fracture of shaft of unspecified radius CC POA HAC MCC CC/MCC Exc

Unspecified Code | Other Specified Code | Manifestation Code | [N] Newborn | [P] Pediatric | [M] Maternity | [A] Adult | ♂ Male | ♀ Female
● New Code | ▲ Revised Code Title | ►◄ Revised Text | NOTES | INCLUDES | EXCLUDES1 Not coded here | EXCLUDES2 Not included here
[4th] 4th character required | [5th] 5th character required | [6th] 6th character required | [7th] 7th character required | [X] Extension 'X' Alert
HAC Hospital-acquired condition (HAC) alert | AHA AHA Coding Clinic© | ☞ Code first alert

When symbols appear on a code that requires a 7th character extension, refer to Appendix B to identify applicable 7th character codes.

S52.31 Greenstick fracture of shaft of radius

The appropriate 7th character is to be added to all codes in subcategory S52.31

A = initial encounter for closed fracture

D = subsequent encounter for fracture with routine healing

G = subsequent encounter for fracture with delayed healing

K = subsequent encounter for fracture with nonunion

P = subsequent encounter for fracture with malunion

S = sequela

S52.311 Greenstick fracture of shaft of radius, right arm `cc` `POA` `HAC` `MCC` `CC/MCC Exc`

S52.312 Greenstick fracture of shaft of radius, left arm `cc` `POA` `HAC` `MCC` `CC/MCC Exc`

S52.319 Greenstick fracture of shaft of radius, unspecified arm `cc` `POA` `HAC` `MCC` `CC/MCC Exc`

S52.32 Transverse fracture of shaft of radius

S52.321 Displaced transverse fracture of shaft of right radius `cc` `POA` `HAC` `MCC` `CC/MCC Exc`

S52.322 Displaced transverse fracture of shaft of left radius `cc` `POA` `HAC` `MCC` `CC/MCC Exc`

S52.323 Displaced transverse fracture of shaft of unspecified radius `cc` `POA` `HAC` `MCC` `CC/MCC Exc`

S52.324 Nondisplaced transverse fracture of shaft of right radius `cc` `POA` `HAC` `MCC` `CC/MCC Exc`

S52.325 Nondisplaced transverse fracture of shaft of left radius `cc` `POA` `HAC` `MCC` `CC/MCC Exc`

S52.326 Nondisplaced transverse fracture of shaft of unspecified radius `cc` `POA` `HAC` `MCC` `CC/MCC Exc`

S52.33 Oblique fracture of shaft of radius

S52.331 Displaced oblique fracture of shaft of right radius `cc` `POA` `HAC` `MCC` `CC/MCC Exc`

S52.332 Displaced oblique fracture of shaft of left radius `cc` `POA` `HAC` `MCC` `CC/MCC Exc`

S52.333 Displaced oblique fracture of shaft of unspecified radius `cc` `POA` `HAC` `MCC` `CC/MCC Exc`

S52.334 Nondisplaced oblique fracture of shaft of right radius `cc` `POA` `HAC` `MCC` `CC/MCC Exc`

S52.335 Nondisplaced oblique fracture of shaft of left radius `cc` `POA` `HAC` `MCC` `CC/MCC Exc`

S52.336 Nondisplaced oblique fracture of shaft of unspecified radius `cc` `POA` `HAC` `MCC` `CC/MCC Exc`

S52.34 Spiral fracture of shaft of radius

S52.341 Displaced spiral fracture of shaft of radius, right arm `cc` `POA` `HAC` `MCC` `CC/MCC Exc`

S52.342 Displaced spiral fracture of shaft of radius, left arm `cc` `POA` `HAC` `MCC` `CC/MCC Exc`

S52.343 Displaced spiral fracture of shaft of radius, unspecified arm `cc` `POA` `HAC` `MCC` `CC/MCC Exc`

S52.344 Nondisplaced spiral fracture of shaft of radius, right arm `cc` `POA` `HAC` `MCC` `CC/MCC Exc`

S52.345 Nondisplaced spiral fracture of shaft of radius, left arm `cc` `POA` `HAC` `MCC` `CC/MCC Exc`

S52.346 Nondisplaced spiral fracture of shaft of radius, unspecified arm `cc` `POA` `HAC` `MCC` `CC/MCC Exc`

S52.35 Comminuted fracture of shaft of radius

S52.351 Displaced comminuted fracture of shaft of radius, right arm `cc` `POA` `HAC` `MCC` `CC/MCC Exc`

S52.352 Displaced comminuted fracture of shaft of radius, left arm `cc` `POA` `HAC` `MCC` `CC/MCC Exc`

S52.353 Displaced comminuted fracture of shaft of radius, unspecified arm `cc` `POA` `HAC` `MCC` `CC/MCC Exc`

S52.354 Nondisplaced comminuted fracture of shaft of radius, right arm `cc` `POA` `HAC` `MCC` `CC/MCC Exc`

S52.355 Nondisplaced comminuted fracture of shaft of radius, left arm `cc` `POA` `HAC` `MCC` `CC/MCC Exc`

S52.356 Nondisplaced comminuted fracture of shaft of radius, unspecified arm `cc` `POA` `HAC` `MCC` `CC/MCC Exc`

S52.36 Segmental fracture of shaft of radius

S52.361 Displaced segmental fracture of shaft of radius, right arm `cc` `POA` `HAC` `MCC` `CC/MCC Exc`

S52.362 Displaced segmental fracture of shaft of radius, left arm `cc` `POA` `HAC` `MCC` `CC/MCC Exc`

S52.363 Displaced segmental fracture of shaft of radius, unspecified arm `cc` `POA` `HAC` `MCC` `CC/MCC Exc`

S52.364 Nondisplaced segmental fracture of shaft of radius, right arm `cc` `POA` `HAC` `MCC` `CC/MCC Exc`

S52.365 Nondisplaced segmental fracture of shaft of radius, left arm `cc` `POA` `HAC` `MCC` `CC/MCC Exc`

S52.366 Nondisplaced segmental fracture of shaft of radius, unspecified arm `cc` `POA` `HAC` `MCC` `CC/MCC Exc`

S52.37 Galeazzi's fracture

Fracture of lower shaft of radius with radioulnar joint dislocation

S52.371 Galeazzi's fracture of right radius `cc` `POA` `HAC` `MCC` `CC/MCC Exc`

S52.372 Galeazzi's fracture of left radius `cc` `POA` `HAC` `MCC` `CC/MCC Exc`

S52.379 Galeazzi's fracture of unspecified radius `cc` `POA` `HAC` `MCC` `CC/MCC Exc`

S52.38 Bent bone of radius

S52.381 Bent bone of right radius `cc` `POA` `HAC` `MCC` `CC/MCC Exc`

S52.382 Bent bone of left radius `cc` `POA` `HAC` `MCC` `CC/MCC Exc`

S52.389 Bent bone of unspecified radius `cc` `POA` `HAC` `MCC` `CC/MCC Exc`

S52.39 Other fracture of shaft of radius

S52.391 Other fracture of shaft of radius, right arm `cc` `POA` `HAC` `MCC` `CC/MCC Exc`

S52.392 Other fracture of shaft of radius, left arm `cc` `POA` `HAC` `MCC` `CC/MCC Exc`

S52.399 Other fracture of shaft of radius, unspecified arm `cc` `POA` `HAC` `MCC` `CC/MCC Exc`

S52.5 Fracture of lower end of radius

Fracture of distal end of radius

EXCLUDES2 physeal fractures of lower end of radius (S59.2-)

S52.50 Unspecified fracture of the lower end of radius

S52.501 Unspecified fracture of the lower end of right radius `cc` `POA` `HAC` `MCC` `CC/MCC Exc`

S52.502 Unspecified fracture of the lower end of left radius `cc` `POA` `HAC` `MCC` `CC/MCC Exc`

S52.509 Unspecified fracture of the lower end of unspecified radius `cc` `POA` `HAC` `MCC` `CC/MCC Exc`

S52.51 Fracture of radial styloid process

S52.511 Displaced fracture of right radial styloid process `cc` `POA` `HAC` `MCC` `CC/MCC Exc`

S52.512 Displaced fracture of left radial styloid process `cc` `POA` `HAC` `MCC` `CC/MCC Exc`

S52.513 Displaced fracture of unspecified radial styloid process `cc` `POA` `HAC` `MCC` `CC/MCC Exc`

S52.514 Nondisplaced fracture of right radial styloid process `cc` `POA` `HAC` `MCC` `CC/MCC Exc`

S52.515 Nondisplaced fracture of left radial styloid process `cc` `POA` `HAC` `MCC` `CC/MCC Exc`

S52.516 Nondisplaced fracture of unspecified radial styloid process `cc` `POA` `HAC` `MCC` `CC/MCC Exc`

S52.52 Torus fracture of lower end of radius

The appropriate 7th character is to be added to all codes in subcategory S52.52

A = initial encounter for closed fracture

D = subsequent encounter for fracture with routine healing

G = subsequent encounter for fracture with delayed healing

K = subsequent encounter for fracture with nonunion

P = subsequent encounter for fracture with malunion

S = sequela

`POA` Unacceptable principal diagnosis symbol per Medicare code edits `POA` Code exempt from diagnosis present on admission requirement

`?` Questionable admission `cc` Complication or comorbidity `MCC` Major complication or comorbidity `CC/MCC Exc` CC/MCC exclusion

`HCC` HCC diagnosis code `RxHCC` RxHCC diagnosis code `MACRA` MACRA code **DEFINITION** Describes condition/terminology

TIP Coding guidance `👁` Official Guideline Reference `Z1` Z code as first-listed diagnosis

1026 When symbols appear on a code that requires a 7th character extension, refer to Appendix B to identify applicable 7th character codes. **2020 ICD-10-CM**

⑦ᵗʰ S52.521   Torus fracture of lower end of right
              radius   CC꜀ POA HAC CC/MCC Exc
⑦ᵗʰ S52.522   Torus fracture of lower end of left
              radius   CC꜀ POA HAC CC/MCC Exc
⑦ᵗʰ S52.529   Torus fracture of lower end of unspecified
              radius   CC꜀ POA HAC CC/MCC Exc
⑥ᵗʰ S52.53   Colles' fracture
              DEFINITION: A fracture of the distal radius with
                          displacement of the distal bone.
⑦ᵗʰ S52.531   Colles' fracture of right
              radius   CC꜀ POA HAC MCC꜀ CC/MCC Exc
⑦ᵗʰ S52.532   Colles' fracture of left
              radius   CC꜀ POA HAC MCC꜀ CC/MCC Exc
              AHA: Q2 2016
⑦ᵗʰ S52.539   Colles' fracture of unspecified
              radius   CC꜀ POA HAC MCC꜀ CC/MCC Exc
⑥ᵗʰ S52.54   Smith's fracture
              DEFINITION: A fracture of the distal radius with
                          displacement of the bone fragment
                          toward the palmar aspect. This is a
                          reverse Colles' fracture.
⑦ᵗʰ S52.541   Smith's fracture of right
              radius   CC꜀ POA HAC MCC꜀ CC/MCC Exc
⑦ᵗʰ S52.542   Smith's fracture of left
              radius   CC꜀ POA HAC MCC꜀ CC/MCC Exc
⑦ᵗʰ S52.549   Smith's fracture of unspecified
              radius   CC꜀ POA HAC MCC꜀ CC/MCC Exc
⑥ᵗʰ S52.55   Other extraarticular fracture of lower end of radius
⑦ᵗʰ S52.551   Other extraarticular fracture of lower end
              of right radius   CC꜀ POA HAC MCC꜀ CC/MCC Exc
⑦ᵗʰ S52.552   Other extraarticular fracture of lower end
              of left radius   CC꜀ POA HAC MCC꜀ CC/MCC Exc
⑦ᵗʰ S52.559   Other extraarticular fracture of lower end
              of unspecified radius   CC꜀ POA HAC MCC꜀ CC/MCC Exc
⑥ᵗʰ S52.56   Barton's fracture
⑦ᵗʰ S52.561   Barton's fracture of right
              radius   CC꜀ POA HAC MCC꜀ CC/MCC Exc
⑦ᵗʰ S52.562   Barton's fracture of left
              radius   CC꜀ POA HAC MCC꜀ CC/MCC Exc
⑦ᵗʰ S52.569   Barton's fracture of unspecified
              radius   CC꜀ POA HAC MCC꜀ CC/MCC Exc
⑥ᵗʰ S52.57   Other intraarticular fracture of lower end of radius
⑦ᵗʰ S52.571   Other intraarticular fracture of lower end
              of right radius   CC꜀ POA HAC MCC꜀ CC/MCC Exc
⑦ᵗʰ S52.572   Other intraarticular fracture of lower end
              of left radius   CC꜀ POA HAC MCC꜀ CC/MCC Exc
⑦ᵗʰ S52.579   Other intraarticular fracture of lower end
              of unspecified radius   CC꜀ POA HAC MCC꜀ CC/MCC Exc
⑥ᵗʰ S52.59   Other fractures of lower end of radius
⑦ᵗʰ S52.591   Other fractures of lower end of right
              radius   CC꜀ POA HAC MCC꜀ CC/MCC Exc
⑦ᵗʰ S52.592   Other fractures of lower end of left
              radius   CC꜀ POA HAC MCC꜀ CC/MCC Exc
⑦ᵗʰ S52.599   Other fractures of lower end of
              unspecified radius   CC꜀ POA HAC MCC꜀ CC/MCC Exc
⑤ᵗʰ S52.6   Fracture of lower end of ulna
⑥ᵗʰ S52.60   Unspecified fracture of lower end of ulna
⑦ᵗʰ S52.601   Unspecified fracture of lower end of right
              ulna   CC꜀ POA HAC MCC꜀ CC/MCC Exc
⑦ᵗʰ S52.602   Unspecified fracture of lower end of left
              ulna   CC꜀ POA HAC MCC꜀ CC/MCC Exc
⑦ᵗʰ S52.609   Unspecified fracture of lower end of
              unspecified ulna   CC꜀ POA HAC MCC꜀ CC/MCC Exc
⑥ᵗʰ S52.61   Fracture of ulna styloid process
⑦ᵗʰ S52.611   Displaced fracture of right ulna styloid
              process   CC꜀ POA HAC MCC꜀ CC/MCC Exc
⑦ᵗʰ S52.612   Displaced fracture of left ulna styloid
              process   CC꜀ POA HAC MCC꜀ CC/MCC Exc
⑦ᵗʰ S52.613   Displaced fracture of unspecified ulna
              styloid process   CC꜀ POA HAC MCC꜀ CC/MCC Exc
⑦ᵗʰ S52.614   Nondisplaced fracture of right ulna styloid
              process   CC꜀ POA HAC MCC꜀ CC/MCC Exc

⑦ᵗʰ S52.615   Nondisplaced fracture of left ulna styloid
              process   CC꜀ POA HAC MCC꜀ CC/MCC Exc
⑦ᵗʰ S52.616   Nondisplaced fracture of unspecified ulna
              styloid process   CC꜀ POA HAC MCC꜀ CC/MCC Exc
⑥ᵗʰ S52.62   Torus fracture of lower end of ulna
              The appropriate 7th character is to be added to all
              codes in subcategory S52.62
                  A = initial encounter for closed fracture
                  D = subsequent encounter for fracture with
                      routine healing
                  G = subsequent encounter for fracture with
                      delayed healing
                  K = subsequent encounter for fracture with
                      nonunion
                  P = subsequent encounter for fracture with
                      malunion
                  S = sequela
⑦ᵗʰ S52.621   Torus fracture of lower end of right
              ulna   CC꜀ POA HAC CC/MCC Exc
⑦ᵗʰ S52.622   Torus fracture of lower end of left
              ulna   CC꜀ POA HAC CC/MCC Exc
⑦ᵗʰ S52.629   Torus fracture of lower end of unspecified
              ulna   CC꜀ POA HAC CC/MCC Exc
⑥ᵗʰ S52.69   Other fracture of lower end of ulna
⑦ᵗʰ S52.691   Other fracture of lower end of right
              ulna   CC꜀ POA HAC MCC꜀ CC/MCC Exc
⑦ᵗʰ S52.692   Other fracture of lower end of left
              ulna   CC꜀ POA HAC MCC꜀ CC/MCC Exc
⑦ᵗʰ S52.699   Other fracture of lower end of unspecified
              ulna   CC꜀ POA HAC MCC꜀ CC/MCC Exc
⑤ᵗʰ S52.9   Unspecified fracture of forearm
⑦ᵗʰ S52.90   Unspecified fracture of unspecified
              forearm   CC꜀ POA HAC MCC꜀ CC/MCC Exc
⑦ᵗʰ S52.91   Unspecified fracture of right
              forearm   CC꜀ POA HAC MCC꜀ CC/MCC Exc
⑦ᵗʰ S52.92   Unspecified fracture of left
              forearm   CC꜀ POA HAC MCC꜀ CC/MCC Exc
④ᵗʰ S53   Dislocation and sprain of joints and ligaments of elbow
       INCLUDES   avulsion of joint or ligament of elbow
                  laceration of cartilage, joint or ligament of elbow
                  sprain of cartilage, joint or ligament of elbow
                  traumatic hemarthrosis of joint or ligament of elbow
                  traumatic rupture of joint or ligament of elbow
                  traumatic subluxation of joint or ligament of elbow
                  traumatic tear of joint or ligament of elbow
       Code also any associated open wound
       EXCLUDES2 strain of muscle, fascia and tendon at forearm level (S56.-)
       The appropriate 7th character is to be added to each code from
       category S53
           A = initial encounter
           D = subsequent encounter
           S = sequela
⑤ᵗʰ S53.0   Subluxation and dislocation of radial head
              Dislocation of radiohumeral joint
              Subluxation of radiohumeral joint
              EXCLUDES1 Monteggia's fracture-dislocation (S52.27-)
⑥ᵗʰ S53.00   Unspecified subluxation and dislocation of radial
              head
⑦ᵗʰ S53.001   Unspecified subluxation of right radial
              head   POA
⑦ᵗʰ S53.002   Unspecified subluxation of left radial
              head   POA
⑦ᵗʰ S53.003   Unspecified subluxation of unspecified
              radial head   POA
⑦ᵗʰ S53.004   Unspecified dislocation of right radial
              head   POA
⑦ᵗʰ S53.005   Unspecified dislocation of left radial
              head   POA
⑦ᵗʰ S53.006   Unspecified dislocation of unspecified
              radial head   POA

Unspecified Code   Other Specified Code   Manifestation Code   Ⓝ Newborn   Ⓟ Pediatric   Ⓜ Maternity   Ⓐ Adult   ♂ Male   ♀ Female
● New Code   ▲ Revised Code Title   ►◄ Revised Text   NOTES   INCLUDES   EXCLUDES1 Not coded here   EXCLUDES2 Not included here
④ᵗʰ 4th character required   ⑤ᵗʰ 5th character required   ⑥ᵗʰ 6th character required   ⑦ᵗʰ 7th character required   ⑦ Extension 'X' Alert
HAC Hospital-acquired condition (HAC) alert   AHA AHA Coding Clinic®   ☞ Code first alert

6ᵗʰ **S53.01** Anterior **subluxation and dislocation of radial head**
Anteriomedial subluxation and dislocation of radial head
- 7ᵗʰ **S53.011** Anterior subluxation of right radial head PDxᴏ̸ᴀ
- 7ᵗʰ **S53.012** Anterior subluxation of left radial head PDxᴏ̸ᴀ
- 7ᵗʰ **S53.013** Anterior subluxation of unspecified radial head PDxᴏ̸ᴀ
- 7ᵗʰ **S53.014** Anterior dislocation of right radial head PDxᴏ̸ᴀ
- 7ᵗʰ **S53.015** Anterior dislocation of left radial head PDxᴏ̸ᴀ
- 7ᵗʰ **S53.016** Anterior dislocation of unspecified radial head PDxᴏ̸ᴀ

6ᵗʰ **S53.02** Posterior **subluxation and dislocation of radial head**
Posteriolateral subluxation and dislocation of radial head
- 7ᵗʰ **S53.021** Posterior subluxation of right radial head PDxᴏ̸ᴀ
- 7ᵗʰ **S53.022** Posterior subluxation of left radial head PDxᴏ̸ᴀ
- 7ᵗʰ **S53.023** Posterior subluxation of unspecified radial head PDxᴏ̸ᴀ
- 7ᵗʰ **S53.024** Posterior dislocation of right radial head PDxᴏ̸ᴀ
- 7ᵗʰ **S53.025** Posterior dislocation of left radial head PDxᴏ̸ᴀ
- 7ᵗʰ **S53.026** Posterior dislocation of unspecified radial head PDxᴏ̸ᴀ

6ᵗʰ **S53.03** Nursemaid's **elbow**
- 7ᵗʰ **S53.031** Nursemaid's elbow, right elbow PDxᴏ̸ᴀ
  AHA: Q1 2015
- 7ᵗʰ **S53.032** Nursemaid's elbow, left elbow PDxᴏ̸ᴀ
- 7ᵗʰ **S53.033** Nursemaid's elbow, unspecified elbow PDxᴏ̸ᴀ

6ᵗʰ **S53.09** Other **subluxation and dislocation of radial head**
- 7ᵗʰ **S53.091** Other subluxation of right radial head PDxᴏ̸ᴀ
- 7ᵗʰ **S53.092** Other subluxation of left radial head PDxᴏ̸ᴀ
- 7ᵗʰ **S53.093** Other subluxation of unspecified radial head PDxᴏ̸ᴀ
- 7ᵗʰ **S53.094** Other dislocation of right radial head PDxᴏ̸ᴀ
- 7ᵗʰ **S53.095** Other dislocation of left radial head PDxᴏ̸ᴀ
- 7ᵗʰ **S53.096** Other dislocation of unspecified radial head PDxᴏ̸ᴀ

5ᵗʰ **S53.1 Subluxation and dislocation of** ulnohumeral joint
Subluxation and dislocation of elbow NOS
EXCLUDES1 dislocation of radial head alone (S53.0-)

6ᵗʰ **S53.10** Unspecified **subluxation and dislocation of ulnohumeral joint**
- 7ᵗʰ **S53.101** Unspecified subluxation of right ulnohumeral joint ᴏ̸ᴀ
- 7ᵗʰ **S53.102** Unspecified subluxation of left ulnohumeral joint ᴏ̸ᴀ
- 7ᵗʰ **S53.103** Unspecified subluxation of unspecified ulnohumeral joint ᴏ̸ᴀ
- 7ᵗʰ **S53.104** Unspecified dislocation of right ulnohumeral joint ᴏ̸ᴀ
- 7ᵗʰ **S53.105** Unspecified dislocation of left ulnohumeral joint ᴏ̸ᴀ
- 7ᵗʰ **S53.106** Unspecified dislocation of unspecified ulnohumeral joint ᴏ̸ᴀ

6ᵗʰ **S53.11** Anterior **subluxation and dislocation of ulnohumeral joint**
- 7ᵗʰ **S53.111** Anterior subluxation of right ulnohumeral joint ᴏ̸ᴀ
- 7ᵗʰ **S53.112** Anterior subluxation of left ulnohumeral joint ᴏ̸ᴀ
- 7ᵗʰ **S53.113** Anterior subluxation of unspecified ulnohumeral joint ᴏ̸ᴀ
- 7ᵗʰ **S53.114** Anterior dislocation of right ulnohumeral joint ᴏ̸ᴀ
  AHA: Q4 2012
- 7ᵗʰ **S53.115** Anterior dislocation of left ulnohumeral joint ᴏ̸ᴀ
- 7ᵗʰ **S53.116** Anterior dislocation of unspecified ulnohumeral joint ᴏ̸ᴀ

6ᵗʰ **S53.12** Posterior **subluxation and dislocation of ulnohumeral joint**

- 7ᵗʰ **S53.121** Posterior subluxation of right ulnohumeral joint ᴏ̸ᴀ
- 7ᵗʰ **S53.122** Posterior subluxation of left ulnohumeral joint ᴏ̸ᴀ
- 7ᵗʰ **S53.123** Posterior subluxation of unspecified ulnohumeral joint ᴏ̸ᴀ
- 7ᵗʰ **S53.124** Posterior dislocation of right ulnohumeral joint ᴏ̸ᴀ
- 7ᵗʰ **S53.125** Posterior dislocation of left ulnohumeral joint ᴏ̸ᴀ
- 7ᵗʰ **S53.126** Posterior dislocation of unspecified ulnohumeral joint ᴏ̸ᴀ

6ᵗʰ **S53.13** Medial **subluxation and dislocation of ulnohumeral joint**
- 7ᵗʰ **S53.131** Medial subluxation of right ulnohumeral joint ᴏ̸ᴀ
- 7ᵗʰ **S53.132** Medial subluxation of left ulnohumeral joint ᴏ̸ᴀ
- 7ᵗʰ **S53.133** Medial subluxation of unspecified ulnohumeral joint ᴏ̸ᴀ
- 7ᵗʰ **S53.134** Medial dislocation of right ulnohumeral joint ᴏ̸ᴀ
- 7ᵗʰ **S53.135** Medial dislocation of left ulnohumeral joint ᴏ̸ᴀ
- 7ᵗʰ **S53.136** Medial dislocation of unspecified ulnohumeral joint ᴏ̸ᴀ

6ᵗʰ **S53.14** Lateral **subluxation and dislocation of ulnohumeral joint**
- 7ᵗʰ **S53.141** Lateral subluxation of right ulnohumeral joint ᴏ̸ᴀ
- 7ᵗʰ **S53.142** Lateral subluxation of left ulnohumeral joint ᴏ̸ᴀ
- 7ᵗʰ **S53.143** Lateral subluxation of unspecified ulnohumeral joint ᴏ̸ᴀ
- 7ᵗʰ **S53.144** Lateral dislocation of right ulnohumeral joint ᴏ̸ᴀ
- 7ᵗʰ **S53.145** Lateral dislocation of left ulnohumeral joint ᴏ̸ᴀ
- 7ᵗʰ **S53.146** Lateral dislocation of unspecified ulnohumeral joint ᴏ̸ᴀ

6ᵗʰ **S53.19** Other **subluxation and dislocation of ulnohumeral joint**
- 7ᵗʰ **S53.191** Other subluxation of right ulnohumeral joint ᴏ̸ᴀ
- 7ᵗʰ **S53.192** Other subluxation of left ulnohumeral joint ᴏ̸ᴀ
- 7ᵗʰ **S53.193** Other subluxation of unspecified ulnohumeral joint ᴏ̸ᴀ
- 7ᵗʰ **S53.194** Other dislocation of right ulnohumeral joint ᴏ̸ᴀ
- 7ᵗʰ **S53.195** Other dislocation of left ulnohumeral joint ᴏ̸ᴀ
- 7ᵗʰ **S53.196** Other dislocation of unspecified ulnohumeral joint ᴏ̸ᴀ

5ᵗʰ **S53.2 Traumatic rupture of** radial collateral ligament
EXCLUDES1 sprain of radial collateral ligament NOS (S53.43-)
- 7ᵗʰ **S53.20 Traumatic rupture of unspecified radial collateral ligament** ᴏ̸ᴀ
- 7ᵗʰ **S53.21 Traumatic rupture of** right **radial collateral ligament** ᴏ̸ᴀ
- 7ᵗʰ **S53.22 Traumatic rupture of** left **radial collateral ligament** ᴏ̸ᴀ

5ᵗʰ **S53.3 Traumatic rupture of** ulnar collateral ligament
EXCLUDES1 sprain of ulnar collateral ligament (S53.44-)
- 7ᵗʰ **S53.30 Traumatic rupture of unspecified ulnar collateral ligament** ᴏ̸ᴀ
- 7ᵗʰ **S53.31 Traumatic rupture of** right **ulnar collateral ligament** ᴏ̸ᴀ
- 7ᵗʰ **S53.32 Traumatic rupture of** left **ulnar collateral ligament** ᴏ̸ᴀ

5ᵗʰ **S53.4 Sprain of** elbow
EXCLUDES2 traumatic rupture of radial collateral ligament (S53.2-)
traumatic rupture of ulnar collateral ligament (S53.3-)

PDxᴏ̸ᴀ Unacceptable principal diagnosis symbol per Medicare code edits   ᴏ̸ᴀ Code exempt from diagnosis present on admission requirement
? Questionable admission   ᴄᴄ Complication or comorbidity   ᴍᴄᴄ Major complication or comorbidity   ᴄᴄ/ᴍᴄᴄ ᴇxᴄ CC/MCC exclusion
ᴴᴄᴄ HCC diagnosis code   ᴿxᴴᴄᴄ RxHCC diagnosis code   MACRA code   **DEFINITION** Describes condition/terminology
TIP Coding guidance   👁 Official Guideline Reference   Z1 Z code as first-listed diagnosis

6️⃣ **S53.40** Unspecified sprain of elbow
  7️⃣ **S53.401** Unspecified sprain of right elbow 🔲POA
  7️⃣ **S53.402** Unspecified sprain of left elbow 🔲POA
  7️⃣ **S53.409** Unspecified sprain of unspecified elbow 🔲POA
    Sprain of elbow NOS
6️⃣ **S53.41** Radiohumeral (joint) sprain
  7️⃣ **S53.411** Radiohumeral (joint) sprain of right elbow 🔲POA
  7️⃣ **S53.412** Radiohumeral (joint) sprain of left elbow 🔲POA
  7️⃣ **S53.419** Radiohumeral (joint) sprain of unspecified elbow 🔲POA
6️⃣ **S53.42** Ulnohumeral (joint) sprain
  7️⃣ **S53.421** Ulnohumeral (joint) sprain of right elbow 🔲POA
  7️⃣ **S53.422** Ulnohumeral (joint) sprain of left elbow 🔲POA
  7️⃣ **S53.429** Ulnohumeral (joint) sprain of unspecified elbow 🔲POA
6️⃣ **S53.43** Radial collateral ligament sprain
  7️⃣ **S53.431** Radial collateral ligament sprain of right elbow 🔲POA
  7️⃣ **S53.432** Radial collateral ligament sprain of left elbow 🔲POA
  7️⃣ **S53.439** Radial collateral ligament sprain of unspecified elbow 🔲POA
6️⃣ **S53.44** Ulnar collateral ligament sprain
  7️⃣ **S53.441** Ulnar collateral ligament sprain of right elbow 🔲POA
  7️⃣ **S53.442** Ulnar collateral ligament sprain of left elbow 🔲POA
  7️⃣ **S53.449** Ulnar collateral ligament sprain of unspecified elbow 🔲POA
6️⃣ **S53.49** Other sprain of elbow
  7️⃣ **S53.491** Other sprain of right elbow 🔲POA
  7️⃣ **S53.492** Other sprain of left elbow 🔲POA
  7️⃣ **S53.499** Other sprain of unspecified elbow 🔲POA

4️⃣ **S54** Injury of nerves at forearm level
  Code also any associated open wound (S51.-)
  EXCLUDES2 injury of nerves at wrist and hand level (S64.-)
  The appropriate 7th character is to be added to each code from category S54
    A = initial encounter
    D = subsequent encounter
    S = sequela
5️⃣ **S54.0** Injury of ulnar nerve at forearm level
    Injury of ulnar nerve NOS
  7️⃣ **S54.00** Injury of ulnar nerve at forearm level, unspecified arm 🔲POA
  7️⃣ **S54.01** Injury of ulnar nerve at forearm level, right arm 🔲POA
  7️⃣ **S54.02** Injury of ulnar nerve at forearm level, left arm 🔲POA
5️⃣ **S54.1** Injury of median nerve at forearm level
    Injury of median nerve NOS
  7️⃣ **S54.10** Injury of median nerve at forearm level, unspecified arm 🔲POA
  7️⃣ **S54.11** Injury of median nerve at forearm level, right arm 🔲POA
  7️⃣ **S54.12** Injury of median nerve at forearm level, left arm 🔲POA
5️⃣ **S54.2** Injury of radial nerve at forearm level
    Injury of radial nerve NOS
  7️⃣ **S54.20** Injury of radial nerve at forearm level, unspecified arm 🔲POA
  7️⃣ **S54.21** Injury of radial nerve at forearm level, right arm 🔲POA
  7️⃣ **S54.22** Injury of radial nerve at forearm level, left arm 🔲POA
5️⃣ **S54.3** Injury of cutaneous sensory nerve at forearm level
  7️⃣ **S54.30** Injury of cutaneous sensory nerve at forearm level, unspecified arm 🔲POA
  7️⃣ **S54.31** Injury of cutaneous sensory nerve at forearm level, right arm 🔲POA
  7️⃣ **S54.32** Injury of cutaneous sensory nerve at forearm level, left arm 🔲POA
5️⃣ **S54.8** Injury of other nerves at forearm level

6️⃣ **S54.8X** Injury of other nerves at forearm level
  7️⃣ **S54.8X1** Injury of other nerves at forearm level, right arm 🔲POA
  7️⃣ **S54.8X2** Injury of other nerves at forearm level, left arm 🔲POA
  7️⃣ **S54.8X9** Injury of other nerves at forearm level, unspecified arm 🔲POA
5️⃣ **S54.9** Injury of unspecified nerve at forearm level
  7️⃣ **S54.90** Injury of unspecified nerve at forearm level, unspecified arm 🔲POA
  7️⃣ **S54.91** Injury of unspecified nerve at forearm level, right arm 🔲POA
  7️⃣ **S54.92** Injury of unspecified nerve at forearm level, left arm 🔲POA

4️⃣ **S55** Injury of blood vessels at forearm level
  Code also any associated open wound (S51.-)
  EXCLUDES2 injury of blood vessels at wrist and hand level (S65.-)
    injury of brachial vessels (S45.1-S45.2)
  The appropriate 7th character is to be added to each code from category S55
    A = initial encounter
    D = subsequent encounter
    S = sequela
5️⃣ **S55.0** Injury of ulnar artery at forearm level
  6️⃣ **S55.00** Unspecified injury of ulnar artery at forearm level
    7️⃣ **S55.001** Unspecified injury of ulnar artery at forearm level, right arm ♂ 🔲POA CC/MCC Exc
    7️⃣ **S55.002** Unspecified injury of ulnar artery at forearm level, left arm ♂ 🔲POA CC/MCC Exc
    7️⃣ **S55.009** Unspecified injury of ulnar artery at forearm level, unspecified arm ♂ 🔲POA CC/MCC Exc
  6️⃣ **S55.01** Laceration of ulnar artery at forearm level
    7️⃣ **S55.011** Laceration of ulnar artery at forearm level, right arm ♂ 🔲POA CC/MCC Exc
    7️⃣ **S55.012** Laceration of ulnar artery at forearm level, left arm ♂ 🔲POA CC/MCC Exc
    7️⃣ **S55.019** Laceration of ulnar artery at forearm level, unspecified arm ♂ 🔲POA CC/MCC Exc
  6️⃣ **S55.09** Other specified injury of ulnar artery at forearm level
    7️⃣ **S55.091** Other specified injury of ulnar artery at forearm level, right arm ♂ 🔲POA CC/MCC Exc
    7️⃣ **S55.092** Other specified injury of ulnar artery at forearm level, left arm ♂ 🔲POA CC/MCC Exc
    7️⃣ **S55.099** Other specified injury of ulnar artery at forearm level, unspecified arm ♂ 🔲POA CC/MCC Exc
5️⃣ **S55.1** Injury of radial artery at forearm level
  6️⃣ **S55.10** Unspecified injury of radial artery at forearm level
    7️⃣ **S55.101** Unspecified injury of radial artery at forearm level, right arm ♂ 🔲POA CC/MCC Exc
    7️⃣ **S55.102** Unspecified injury of radial artery at forearm level, left arm ♂ 🔲POA CC/MCC Exc
    7️⃣ **S55.109** Unspecified injury of radial artery at forearm level, unspecified arm ♂ 🔲POA CC/MCC Exc
  6️⃣ **S55.11** Laceration of radial artery at forearm level
    7️⃣ **S55.111** Laceration of radial artery at forearm level, right arm ♂ 🔲POA CC/MCC Exc
    7️⃣ **S55.112** Laceration of radial artery at forearm level, left arm ♂ 🔲POA CC/MCC Exc
    7️⃣ **S55.119** Laceration of radial artery at forearm level, unspecified arm ♂ 🔲POA CC/MCC Exc
  6️⃣ **S55.19** Other specified injury of radial artery at forearm level
    7️⃣ **S55.191** Other specified injury of radial artery at forearm level, right arm ♂ 🔲POA CC/MCC Exc
    7️⃣ **S55.192** Other specified injury of radial artery at forearm level, left arm ♂ 🔲POA CC/MCC Exc
    7️⃣ **S55.199** Other specified injury of radial artery at forearm level, unspecified arm ♂ 🔲POA CC/MCC Exc
5️⃣ **S55.2** Injury of vein at forearm level
  6️⃣ **S55.20** Unspecified injury of vein at forearm level

| Unspecified Code | Other Specified Code | Manifestation Code | Ⓝ Newborn | Ⓟ Pediatric | Ⓜ Maternity | Ⓐ Adult | ♂ Male | ♀ Female |

● New Code　▲ Revised Code Title　▶◀ Revised Text　**NOTES**　*INCLUDES*　*EXCLUDES1* Not coded here　*EXCLUDES2* Not included here
4️⃣ 4th character required　5️⃣ 5th character required　6️⃣ 6th character required　7️⃣ 7th character required　⑦ Extension 'X' Alert
HAC Hospital-acquired condition (HAC) alert　**AHA** AHA Coding Clinic®　☛ Code first alert

[7th] S55.201 Unspecified injury of vein at forearm level, right arm CC POA CC/MCC Exc
[7th] S55.202 Unspecified injury of vein at forearm level, left arm CC POA CC/MCC Exc
[7th] S55.209 Unspecified injury of vein at forearm level, unspecified arm CC POA CC/MCC Exc

[6th] S55.21 Laceration of vein at forearm level
[7th] S55.211 Laceration of vein at forearm level, right arm CC POA CC/MCC Exc
[7th] S55.212 Laceration of vein at forearm level, left arm CC POA CC/MCC Exc
[7th] S55.219 Laceration of vein at forearm level, unspecified arm CC POA CC/MCC Exc

[6th] S55.29 Other specified injury of vein at forearm level
[7th] S55.291 Other specified injury of vein at forearm level, right arm CC POA CC/MCC Exc
[7th] S55.292 Other specified injury of vein at forearm level, left arm CC POA CC/MCC Exc
[7th] S55.299 Other specified injury of vein at forearm level, unspecified arm CC POA CC/MCC Exc

[5th] S55.8 Injury of other blood vessels at forearm level
[6th] S55.80 Unspecified injury of other blood vessels at forearm level
[7th] S55.801 Unspecified injury of other blood vessels at forearm level, right arm CC POA CC/MCC Exc
[7th] S55.802 Unspecified injury of other blood vessels at forearm level, left arm CC POA CC/MCC Exc
[7th] S55.809 Unspecified injury of other blood vessels at forearm level, unspecified arm CC POA CC/MCC Exc

[6th] S55.81 Laceration of other blood vessels at forearm level
[7th] S55.811 Laceration of other blood vessels at forearm level, right arm CC POA CC/MCC Exc
[7th] S55.812 Laceration of other blood vessels at forearm level, left arm CC POA CC/MCC Exc
[7th] S55.819 Laceration of other blood vessels at forearm level, unspecified arm CC POA CC/MCC Exc

[6th] S55.89 Other specified injury of other blood vessels at forearm level
[7th] S55.891 Other specified injury of other blood vessels at forearm level, right arm CC POA CC/MCC Exc
[7th] S55.892 Other specified injury of other blood vessels at forearm level, left arm CC POA CC/MCC Exc
[7th] S55.899 Other specified injury of other blood vessels at forearm level, unspecified arm CC POA CC/MCC Exc

[5th] S55.9 Injury of unspecified blood vessel at forearm level
[6th] S55.90 Unspecified injury of unspecified blood vessel at forearm level
[7th] S55.901 Unspecified injury of unspecified blood vessel at forearm level, right arm CC POA CC/MCC Exc
[7th] S55.902 Unspecified injury of unspecified blood vessel at forearm level, left arm CC POA CC/MCC Exc
[7th] S55.909 Unspecified injury of unspecified blood vessel at forearm level, unspecified arm CC POA CC/MCC Exc

[6th] S55.91 Laceration of unspecified blood vessel at forearm level
[7th] S55.911 Laceration of unspecified blood vessel at forearm level, right arm CC POA CC/MCC Exc
[7th] S55.912 Laceration of unspecified blood vessel at forearm level, left arm CC POA CC/MCC Exc
[7th] S55.919 Laceration of unspecified blood vessel at forearm level, unspecified arm CC POA CC/MCC Exc

[6th] S55.99 Other specified injury of unspecified blood vessel at forearm level
[7th] S55.991 Other specified injury of unspecified blood vessel at forearm level, right arm CC POA CC/MCC Exc
[7th] S55.992 Other specified injury of unspecified blood vessel at forearm level, left arm CC POA CC/MCC Exc
[7th] S55.999 Other specified injury of unspecified blood vessel at forearm level, unspecified arm CC POA CC/MCC Exc

[4th] S56 Injury of muscle, fascia and tendon at forearm level

Code also any associated open wound (S51.-)

[EXCLUDES2] *injury of muscle, fascia and tendon at or below wrist (S66.-)*
sprain of joints and ligaments of elbow (S53.4-)

The appropriate 7th character is to be added to each code from category S56
A = initial encounter
D = subsequent encounter
S = sequela

[5th] S56.0 Injury of flexor muscle, fascia and tendon of thumb at forearm level
[6th] S56.00 Unspecified injury of flexor muscle, fascia and tendon of thumb at forearm level
[7th] S56.001 Unspecified injury of flexor muscle, fascia and tendon of right thumb at forearm level POA
[7th] S56.002 Unspecified injury of flexor muscle, fascia and tendon of left thumb at forearm level POA
[7th] S56.009 Unspecified injury of flexor muscle, fascia and tendon of unspecified thumb at forearm level POA

[6th] S56.01 Strain of flexor muscle, fascia and tendon of thumb at forearm level
[7th] S56.011 Strain of flexor muscle, fascia and tendon of right thumb at forearm level POA
[7th] S56.012 Strain of flexor muscle, fascia and tendon of left thumb at forearm level POA
[7th] S56.019 Strain of flexor muscle, fascia and tendon of unspecified thumb at forearm level POA

[6th] S56.02 Laceration of flexor muscle, fascia and tendon of thumb at forearm level
[7th] S56.021 Laceration of flexor muscle, fascia and tendon of right thumb at forearm level CC POA CC/MCC Exc
[7th] S56.022 Laceration of flexor muscle, fascia and tendon of left thumb at forearm level CC POA CC/MCC Exc
[7th] S56.029 Laceration of flexor muscle, fascia and tendon of unspecified thumb at forearm level CC POA CC/MCC Exc

[6th] S56.09 Other injury of flexor muscle, fascia and tendon of thumb at forearm level
[7th] S56.091 Other injury of flexor muscle, fascia and tendon of right thumb at forearm level POA
[7th] S56.092 Other injury of flexor muscle, fascia and tendon of left thumb at forearm level POA
[7th] S56.099 Other injury of flexor muscle, fascia and tendon of unspecified thumb at forearm level POA

[5th] S56.1 Injury of flexor muscle, fascia and tendon of other and unspecified finger at forearm level
[6th] S56.10 Unspecified injury of flexor muscle, fascia and tendon of other and unspecified finger at forearm level
[7th] S56.101 Unspecified injury of flexor muscle, fascia and tendon of right index finger at forearm level POA
[7th] S56.102 Unspecified injury of flexor muscle, fascia and tendon of left index finger at forearm level POA
[7th] S56.103 Unspecified injury of flexor muscle, fascia and tendon of right middle finger at forearm level POA

PDx Unacceptable principal diagnosis symbol per Medicare code edits · POA Code exempt from diagnosis present on admission requirement
? Questionable admission · CC Complication or comorbidity · MCC Major complication or comorbidity · CC/MCC Exc CC/MCC exclusion
[HCC] HCC diagnosis code · [RxHCC] RxHCC diagnosis code · MACRA code · **DEFINITION** Describes condition/terminology
TIP Coding guidance · 👁 Official Guideline Reference · [Z1] Z code as first-listed diagnosis

[7th] S56.104 Unspecified injury of flexor muscle, fascia and tendon of left middle finger at forearm level POA
[7th] S56.105 Unspecified injury of flexor muscle, fascia and tendon of right ring finger at forearm level POA
[7th] S56.106 Unspecified injury of flexor muscle, fascia and tendon of left ring finger at forearm level POA
[7th] S56.107 Unspecified injury of flexor muscle, fascia and tendon of right little finger at forearm level POA
[7th] S56.108 Unspecified injury of flexor muscle, fascia and tendon of left little finger at forearm level POA
[7th] S56.109 Unspecified injury of flexor muscle, fascia and tendon of unspecified finger at forearm level POA

[6th] S56.11 Strain of flexor muscle, fascia and tendon of other and unspecified finger at forearm level
[7th] S56.111 Strain of flexor muscle, fascia and tendon of right index finger at forearm level POA
[7th] S56.112 Strain of flexor muscle, fascia and tendon of left index finger at forearm level POA
[7th] S56.113 Strain of flexor muscle, fascia and tendon of right middle finger at forearm level POA
[7th] S56.114 Strain of flexor muscle, fascia and tendon of left middle finger at forearm level POA
[7th] S56.115 Strain of flexor muscle, fascia and tendon of right ring finger at forearm level POA
[7th] S56.116 Strain of flexor muscle, fascia and tendon of left ring finger at forearm level POA
[7th] S56.117 Strain of flexor muscle, fascia and tendon of right little finger at forearm level POA
[7th] S56.118 Strain of flexor muscle, fascia and tendon of left little finger at forearm level POA
[7th] S56.119 Strain of flexor muscle, fascia and tendon of finger of unspecified finger at forearm level POA

[6th] S56.12 Laceration of flexor muscle, fascia and tendon of other and unspecified finger at forearm level
[7th] S56.121 Laceration of flexor muscle, fascia and tendon of right index finger at forearm level CC POA CC/MCC Exc
[7th] S56.122 Laceration of flexor muscle, fascia and tendon of left index finger at forearm level CC POA CC/MCC Exc
[7th] S56.123 Laceration of flexor muscle, fascia and tendon of right middle finger at forearm level CC POA CC/MCC Exc
[7th] S56.124 Laceration of flexor muscle, fascia and tendon of left middle finger at forearm level CC POA CC/MCC Exc
[7th] S56.125 Laceration of flexor muscle, fascia and tendon of right ring finger at forearm level CC POA CC/MCC Exc
[7th] S56.126 Laceration of flexor muscle, fascia and tendon of left ring finger at forearm level CC POA CC/MCC Exc
[7th] S56.127 Laceration of flexor muscle, fascia and tendon of right little finger at forearm level CC POA CC/MCC Exc
[7th] S56.128 Laceration of flexor muscle, fascia and tendon of left little finger at forearm level CC POA CC/MCC Exc
[7th] S56.129 Laceration of flexor muscle, fascia and tendon of unspecified finger at forearm level CC POA CC/MCC Exc

[6th] S56.19 Other injury of flexor muscle, fascia and tendon of other and unspecified finger at forearm level
[7th] S56.191 Other injury of flexor muscle, fascia and tendon of right index finger at forearm level POA
[7th] S56.192 Other injury of flexor muscle, fascia and tendon of left index finger at forearm level POA
[7th] S56.193 Other injury of flexor muscle, fascia and tendon of right middle finger at forearm level POA
[7th] S56.194 Other injury of flexor muscle, fascia and tendon of left middle finger at forearm level POA
[7th] S56.195 Other injury of flexor muscle, fascia and tendon of right ring finger at forearm level POA
[7th] S56.196 Other injury of flexor muscle, fascia and tendon of left ring finger at forearm level POA
[7th] S56.197 Other injury of flexor muscle, fascia and tendon of right little finger at forearm level POA
[7th] S56.198 Other injury of flexor muscle, fascia and tendon of left little finger at forearm level POA
[7th] S56.199 Other injury of flexor muscle, fascia and tendon of unspecified finger at forearm level POA

[5th] S56.2 Injury of other flexor muscle, fascia and tendon at forearm level
[6th] S56.20 Unspecified injury of other flexor muscle, fascia and tendon at forearm level
[7th] S56.201 Unspecified injury of other flexor muscle, fascia and tendon at forearm level, right arm POA
[7th] S56.202 Unspecified injury of other flexor muscle, fascia and tendon at forearm level, left arm POA
[7th] S56.209 Unspecified injury of other flexor muscle, fascia and tendon at forearm level, unspecified arm POA

[6th] S56.21 Strain of other flexor muscle, fascia and tendon at forearm level
[7th] S56.211 Strain of other flexor muscle, fascia and tendon at forearm level, right arm POA
[7th] S56.212 Strain of other flexor muscle, fascia and tendon at forearm level, left arm POA
[7th] S56.219 Strain of other flexor muscle, fascia and tendon at forearm level, unspecified arm POA

[6th] S56.22 Laceration of other flexor muscle, fascia and tendon at forearm level
[7th] S56.221 Laceration of other flexor muscle, fascia and tendon at forearm level, right arm CC POA CC/MCC Exc
[7th] S56.222 Laceration of other flexor muscle, fascia and tendon at forearm level, left arm CC POA CC/MCC Exc
[7th] S56.229 Laceration of other flexor muscle, fascia and tendon at forearm level, unspecified arm CC POA CC/MCC Exc

[6th] S56.29 Other injury of other flexor muscle, fascia and tendon at forearm level
[7th] S56.291 Other injury of other flexor muscle, fascia and tendon at forearm level, right arm POA
[7th] S56.292 Other injury of other flexor muscle, fascia and tendon at forearm level, left arm POA
[7th] S56.299 Other injury of other flexor muscle, fascia and tendon at forearm level, unspecified arm POA

[5th] S56.3 Injury of extensor or abductor muscles, fascia and tendons of thumb at forearm level
[6th] S56.30 Unspecified injury of extensor or abductor muscles, fascia and tendons of thumb at forearm level
[7th] S56.301 Unspecified injury of extensor or abductor muscles, fascia and tendons of right thumb at forearm level POA

Unspecified Code | Other Specified Code | Manifestation Code | [N] Newborn | [P] Pediatric | [M] Maternity | [A] Adult | ♂ Male | ♀ Female
● New Code | ▲ Revised Code Title | ►◄ Revised Text | NOTES | INCLUDES | EXCLUDES1 Not coded here | EXCLUDES2 Not included here
[4th] 4th character required | [5th] 5th character required | [6th] 6th character required | [7th] 7th character required | [X] Extension 'X' Alert
[HAC] Hospital-acquired condition (HAC) alert | AHA AHA Coding Clinic© | ☞ Code first alert

7th S56.302 Unspecified injury of extensor or abductor muscles, fascia and tendons of left thumb at forearm level POA

7th S56.309 Unspecified injury of extensor or abductor muscles, fascia and tendons of unspecified thumb at forearm level POA

6th S56.31 Strain of extensor or abductor muscles, fascia and tendons of thumb at forearm level

7th S56.311 Strain of extensor or abductor muscles, fascia and tendons of right thumb at forearm level POA

7th S56.312 Strain of extensor or abductor muscles, fascia and tendons of left thumb at forearm level POA

7th S56.319 Strain of extensor or abductor muscles, fascia and tendons of unspecified thumb at forearm level POA

6th S56.32 Laceration of extensor or abductor muscles, fascia and tendons of thumb at forearm level

7th S56.321 Laceration of extensor or abductor muscles, fascia and tendons of right thumb at forearm level CC POA CC/MCC Exc

7th S56.322 Laceration of extensor or abductor muscles, fascia and tendons of left thumb at forearm level CC POA CC/MCC Exc

7th S56.329 Laceration of extensor or abductor muscles, fascia and tendons of unspecified thumb at forearm level CC POA CC/MCC Exc

6th S56.39 Other injury of extensor or abductor muscles, fascia and tendons of thumb at forearm level

7th S56.391 Other injury of extensor or abductor muscles, fascia and tendons of right thumb at forearm level POA

7th S56.392 Other injury of extensor or abductor muscles, fascia and tendons of left thumb at forearm level POA

7th S56.399 Other injury of extensor or abductor muscles, fascia and tendons of unspecified thumb at forearm level POA

5th S56.4 Injury of extensor muscle, fascia and tendon of other and unspecified finger at forearm level

6th S56.40 Unspecified injury of extensor muscle, fascia and tendon of other and unspecified finger at forearm level

7th S56.401 Unspecified injury of extensor muscle, fascia and tendon of right index finger at forearm level POA

7th S56.402 Unspecified injury of extensor muscle, fascia and tendon of left index finger at forearm level POA

7th S56.403 Unspecified injury of extensor muscle, fascia and tendon of right middle finger at forearm level POA

7th S56.404 Unspecified injury of extensor muscle, fascia and tendon of left middle finger at forearm level POA

7th S56.405 Unspecified injury of extensor muscle, fascia and tendon of right ring finger at forearm level POA

7th S56.406 Unspecified injury of extensor muscle, fascia and tendon of left ring finger at forearm level POA

7th S56.407 Unspecified injury of extensor muscle, fascia and tendon of right little finger at forearm level POA

7th S56.408 Unspecified injury of extensor muscle, fascia and tendon of left little finger at forearm level POA

7th S56.409 Unspecified injury of extensor muscle, fascia and tendon of unspecified finger at forearm level POA

6th S56.41 Strain of extensor muscle, fascia and tendon of other and unspecified finger at forearm level

7th S56.411 Strain of extensor muscle, fascia and tendon of right index finger at forearm level POA

7th S56.412 Strain of extensor muscle, fascia and tendon of left index finger at forearm level POA

7th S56.413 Strain of extensor muscle, fascia and tendon of right middle finger at forearm level POA

7th S56.414 Strain of extensor muscle, fascia and tendon of left middle finger at forearm level POA

7th S56.415 Strain of extensor muscle, fascia and tendon of right ring finger at forearm level POA

7th S56.416 Strain of extensor muscle, fascia and tendon of left ring finger at forearm level POA

7th S56.417 Strain of extensor muscle, fascia and tendon of right little finger at forearm level POA

7th S56.418 Strain of extensor muscle, fascia and tendon of left little finger at forearm level POA

7th S56.419 Strain of extensor muscle, fascia and tendon of finger, unspecified finger at forearm level POA

6th S56.42 Laceration of extensor muscle, fascia and tendon of other and unspecified finger at forearm level

7th S56.421 Laceration of extensor muscle, fascia and tendon of right index finger at forearm level CC POA CC/MCC Exc

7th S56.422 Laceration of extensor muscle, fascia and tendon of left index finger at forearm level CC POA CC/MCC Exc

7th S56.423 Laceration of extensor muscle, fascia and tendon of right middle finger at forearm level CC POA CC/MCC Exc

7th S56.424 Laceration of extensor muscle, fascia and tendon of left middle finger at forearm level CC POA CC/MCC Exc

7th S56.425 Laceration of extensor muscle, fascia and tendon of right ring finger at forearm level CC POA CC/MCC Exc

7th S56.426 Laceration of extensor muscle, fascia and tendon of left ring finger at forearm level CC POA CC/MCC Exc

7th S56.427 Laceration of extensor muscle, fascia and tendon of right little finger at forearm level CC POA CC/MCC Exc

7th S56.428 Laceration of extensor muscle, fascia and tendon of left little finger at forearm level CC POA CC/MCC Exc

7th S56.429 Laceration of extensor muscle, fascia and tendon of unspecified finger at forearm level CC POA CC/MCC Exc

6th S56.49 Other injury of extensor muscle, fascia and tendon of other and unspecified finger at forearm level

7th S56.491 Other injury of extensor muscle, fascia and tendon of right index finger at forearm level POA

7th S56.492 Other injury of extensor muscle, fascia and tendon of left index finger at forearm level POA

7th S56.493 Other injury of extensor muscle, fascia and tendon of right middle finger at forearm level POA

7th S56.494 Other injury of extensor muscle, fascia and tendon of left middle finger at forearm level POA

7th S56.495 Other injury of extensor muscle, fascia and tendon of right ring finger at forearm level POA

PDx Unacceptable principal diagnosis symbol per Medicare code edits   Code exempt from diagnosis present on admission requirement

? Questionable admission   CC Complication or comorbidity   MCC Major complication or comorbidity   CC/MCC Exc CC/MCC exclusion

HCC HCC diagnosis code   RxHCC RxHCC diagnosis code   MACRA code   DEFINITION Describes condition/terminology

TIP Coding guidance   Official Guideline Reference   Z1 Z code as first-listed diagnosis

7️⃣ S56.496 Other injury of extensor muscle, fascia and tendon of left ring finger at forearm level POA

7️⃣ S56.497 Other injury of extensor muscle, fascia and tendon of right little finger at forearm level POA

7️⃣ S56.498 Other injury of extensor muscle, fascia and tendon of left little finger at forearm level POA

7️⃣ S56.499 Other injury of extensor muscle, fascia and tendon of unspecified finger at forearm level POA

5️⃣ S56.5 Injury of other extensor muscle, fascia and tendon at forearm level

6️⃣ S56.50 Unspecified injury of other extensor muscle, fascia and tendon at forearm level

7️⃣ S56.501 Unspecified injury of other extensor muscle, fascia and tendon at forearm level, right arm POA

7️⃣ S56.502 Unspecified injury of other extensor muscle, fascia and tendon at forearm level, left arm POA

7️⃣ S56.509 Unspecified injury of other extensor muscle, fascia and tendon at forearm level, unspecified arm POA

6️⃣ S56.51 Strain of other extensor muscle, fascia and tendon at forearm level

7️⃣ S56.511 Strain of other extensor muscle, fascia and tendon at forearm level, right arm POA

7️⃣ S56.512 Strain of other extensor muscle, fascia and tendon at forearm level, left arm POA

7️⃣ S56.519 Strain of other extensor muscle, fascia and tendon at forearm level, unspecified arm POA

6️⃣ S56.52 Laceration of other extensor muscle, fascia and tendon at forearm level

7️⃣ S56.521 Laceration of other extensor muscle, fascia and tendon at forearm level, right arm CC POA CC/MCC Exc

7️⃣ S56.522 Laceration of other extensor muscle, fascia and tendon at forearm level, left arm CC POA CC/MCC Exc

7️⃣ S56.529 Laceration of other extensor muscle, fascia and tendon at forearm level, unspecified arm CC POA CC/MCC Exc

6️⃣ S56.59 Other injury of other extensor muscle, fascia and tendon at forearm level

7️⃣ S56.591 Other injury of other extensor muscle, fascia and tendon at forearm level, right arm POA

7️⃣ S56.592 Other injury of other extensor muscle, fascia and tendon at forearm level, left arm POA

7️⃣ S56.599 Other injury of other extensor muscle, fascia and tendon at forearm level, unspecified arm POA

5️⃣ S56.8 Injury of other muscles, fascia and tendons at forearm level

6️⃣ S56.80 Unspecified injury of other muscles, fascia and tendons at forearm level

7️⃣ S56.801 Unspecified injury of other muscles, fascia and tendons at forearm level, right arm POA

7️⃣ S56.802 Unspecified injury of other muscles, fascia and tendons at forearm level, left arm POA

7️⃣ S56.809 Unspecified injury of other muscles, fascia and tendons at forearm level, unspecified arm POA

6️⃣ S56.81 Strain of other muscles, fascia and tendons at forearm level

7️⃣ S56.811 Strain of other muscles, fascia and tendons at forearm level, right arm POA

7️⃣ S56.812 Strain of other muscles, fascia and tendons at forearm level, left arm POA

7️⃣ S56.819 Strain of other muscles, fascia and tendons at forearm level, unspecified arm POA

6️⃣ S56.82 Laceration of other muscles, fascia and tendons at forearm level

7️⃣ S56.821 Laceration of other muscles, fascia and tendons at forearm level, right arm CC POA CC/MCC Exc

7️⃣ S56.822 Laceration of other muscles, fascia and tendons at forearm level, left arm CC POA CC/MCC Exc

7️⃣ S56.829 Laceration of other muscles, fascia and tendons at forearm level, unspecified arm CC POA CC/MCC Exc

6️⃣ S56.89 Other injury of other muscles, fascia and tendons at forearm level

7️⃣ S56.891 Other injury of other muscles, fascia and tendons at forearm level, right arm POA

7️⃣ S56.892 Other injury of other muscles, fascia and tendons at forearm level, left arm POA

7️⃣ S56.899 Other injury of other muscles, fascia and tendons at forearm level, unspecified arm POA

5️⃣ S56.9 Injury of unspecified muscles, fascia and tendons at forearm level

6️⃣ S56.90 Unspecified injury of unspecified muscles, fascia and tendons at forearm level

7️⃣ S56.901 Unspecified injury of unspecified muscles, fascia and tendons at forearm level, right arm POA

7️⃣ S56.902 Unspecified injury of unspecified muscles, fascia and tendons at forearm level, left arm POA

7️⃣ S56.909 Unspecified injury of unspecified muscles, fascia and tendons at forearm level, unspecified arm POA

6️⃣ S56.91 Strain of unspecified muscles, fascia and tendons at forearm level

7️⃣ S56.911 Strain of unspecified muscles, fascia and tendons at forearm level, right arm POA

7️⃣ S56.912 Strain of unspecified muscles, fascia and tendons at forearm level, left arm POA

7️⃣ S56.919 Strain of unspecified muscles, fascia and tendons at forearm level, unspecified arm POA

6️⃣ S56.92 Laceration of unspecified muscles, fascia and tendons at forearm level

7️⃣ S56.921 Laceration of unspecified muscles, fascia and tendons at forearm level, right arm CC POA CC/MCC Exc

7️⃣ S56.922 Laceration of unspecified muscles, fascia and tendons at forearm level, left arm CC POA CC/MCC Exc

7️⃣ S56.929 Laceration of unspecified muscles, fascia and tendons at forearm level, unspecified arm CC POA CC/MCC Exc

6️⃣ S56.99 Other injury of unspecified muscles, fascia and tendons at forearm level

7️⃣ S56.991 Other injury of unspecified muscles, fascia and tendons at forearm level, right arm POA

7️⃣ S56.992 Other injury of unspecified muscles, fascia and tendons at forearm level, left arm POA

7️⃣ S56.999 Other injury of unspecified muscles, fascia and tendons at forearm level, unspecified arm POA

4️⃣ **S57 Crushing injury of elbow and forearm**
Use additional code(s) for all associated injuries
EXCLUDES2 crushing injury of wrist and hand (S67.-)
The appropriate 7th character is to be added to each code from category S57
A = initial encounter
D = subsequent encounter
S = sequela

Unspecified Code | Other Specified Code | Manifestation Code | Ⓝ Newborn | Ⓟ Pediatric | Ⓜ Maternity | Ⓐ Adult | ♂ Male | ♀ Female
● New Code ▲ Revised Code Title ▶◀ Revised Text **NOTES** *INCLUDES* *EXCLUDES1* Not coded here *EXCLUDES2* Not included here
4️⃣ 4th character required 5️⃣ 5th character required 6️⃣ 6th character required 7️⃣ 7th character required Ⓧ Extension 'X' Alert
HAC Hospital-acquired condition (HAC) alert **AHA** AHA Coding Clinic© ☞ Code first alert

[5th] S57.0 Crushing injury of elbow
- [7th] S57.00 Crushing injury of unspecified elbow [POA]
- [7th] S57.01 Crushing injury of right elbow [POA]
- [7th] S57.02 Crushing injury of left elbow [POA]

[5th] S57.8 Crushing injury of forearm
- [7th] S57.80 Crushing injury of unspecified forearm [POA]
- [7th] S57.81 Crushing injury of right forearm [POA]
- [7th] S57.82 Crushing injury of left forearm [POA]

[4th] S58 Traumatic amputation of elbow and forearm

An amputation not identified as partial or complete should be coded to complete

[EXCLUDES1] *traumatic amputation of wrist and hand (S68.-)*

The appropriate 7th character is to be added to each code from category S58
- A = initial encounter
- D = subsequent encounter
- S = sequela

[5th] S58.0 Traumatic amputation at elbow level
- [6th] S58.01 Complete traumatic amputation at elbow level
  - [7th] S58.011 Complete traumatic amputation at elbow level, right arm [CC] [POA] [HCC] [CC/MCC Exc]
  - [7th] S58.012 Complete traumatic amputation at elbow level, left arm [CC] [POA] [HCC] [CC/MCC Exc]
  - [7th] S58.019 Complete traumatic amputation at elbow level, unspecified arm [CC] [POA] [HCC] [CC/MCC Exc]
- [6th] S58.02 Partial traumatic amputation at elbow level
  - [7th] S58.021 Partial traumatic amputation at elbow level, right arm [CC] [POA] [HCC] [CC/MCC Exc]
  - [7th] S58.022 Partial traumatic amputation at elbow level, left arm [CC] [POA] [HCC] [CC/MCC Exc]
  - [7th] S58.029 Partial traumatic amputation at elbow level, unspecified arm [CC] [POA] [HCC] [CC/MCC Exc]

[5th] S58.1 Traumatic amputation at level between elbow and wrist
- [6th] S58.11 Complete traumatic amputation at level between elbow and wrist
  - [7th] S58.111 Complete traumatic amputation at level between elbow and wrist, right arm [CC] [POA] [HCC] [CC/MCC Exc]
  - [7th] S58.112 Complete traumatic amputation at level between elbow and wrist, left arm [CC] [POA] [HCC] [CC/MCC Exc]
  - [7th] S58.119 Complete traumatic amputation at level between elbow and wrist, unspecified arm [CC] [POA] [HCC] [CC/MCC Exc]
- [6th] S58.12 Partial traumatic amputation at level between elbow and wrist
  - [7th] S58.121 Partial traumatic amputation at level between elbow and wrist, right arm [CC] [POA] [HCC] [CC/MCC Exc]
  - [7th] S58.122 Partial traumatic amputation at level between elbow and wrist, left arm [CC] [POA] [HCC] [CC/MCC Exc]
  - [7th] S58.129 Partial traumatic amputation at level between elbow and wrist, unspecified arm [CC] [POA] [HCC] [CC/MCC Exc]

[5th] S58.9 Traumatic amputation of forearm, level unspecified

[EXCLUDES1] *traumatic amputation of wrist (S68.-)*
- [6th] S58.91 Complete traumatic amputation of forearm, level unspecified
  - [7th] S58.911 Complete traumatic amputation of right forearm, level unspecified [CC] [POA] [HCC] [CC/MCC Exc]
  - [7th] S58.912 Complete traumatic amputation of left forearm, level unspecified [CC] [POA] [HCC] [CC/MCC Exc]
  - [7th] S58.919 Complete traumatic amputation of unspecified forearm, level unspecified [CC] [POA] [HCC] [CC/MCC Exc]
- [6th] S58.92 Partial traumatic amputation of forearm, level unspecified
  - [7th] S58.921 Partial traumatic amputation of right forearm, level unspecified [CC] [POA] [HCC] [CC/MCC Exc]
  - [7th] S58.922 Partial traumatic amputation of left forearm, level unspecified [CC] [POA] [HCC] [CC/MCC Exc]
  - [7th] S58.929 Partial traumatic amputation of unspecified forearm, level unspecified [CC] [POA] [HCC] [CC/MCC Exc]

[4th] S59 Other and unspecified injuries of elbow and forearm

👁 See Official Guidelines "Coding of Traumatic Fractures" I.C.19.c

[EXCLUDES2] *other and unspecified injuries of wrist and hand (S69.-)*

The appropriate 7th character is to be added to each code from subcategories S59.0, S59.1, and S59.2
- A = initial encounter for closed fracture
- D = subsequent encounter for fracture with routine healing
- G = subsequent encounter for fracture with delayed healing
- K = subsequent encounter for fracture with nonunion
- P = subsequent encounter for fracture with malunion
- S = sequela

[5th] S59.0 Physeal fracture of lower end of ulna
- [6th] S59.00 Unspecified physeal fracture of lower end of ulna
  - [7th] S59.001 Unspecified physeal fracture of lower end of ulna, right arm [CC] [POA] [HAC] [CC/MCC Exc]
  - [7th] S59.002 Unspecified physeal fracture of lower end of ulna, left arm [CC] [POA] [HAC] [CC/MCC Exc]
  - [7th] S59.009 Unspecified physeal fracture of lower end of ulna, unspecified arm [CC] [POA] [HAC] [CC/MCC Exc]
- [6th] S59.01 Salter-Harris Type I physeal fracture of lower end of ulna
  - [7th] S59.011 Salter-Harris Type I physeal fracture of lower end of ulna, right arm [CC] [POA] [HAC] [CC/MCC Exc]
  - [7th] S59.012 Salter-Harris Type I physeal fracture of lower end of ulna, left arm [CC] [POA] [HAC] [CC/MCC Exc]
  - [7th] S59.019 Salter-Harris Type I physeal fracture of lower end of ulna, unspecified arm [CC] [POA] [HAC] [CC/MCC Exc]
- [6th] S59.02 Salter-Harris Type II physeal fracture of lower end of ulna
  - [7th] S59.021 Salter-Harris Type II physeal fracture of lower end of ulna, right arm [CC] [POA] [HAC] [CC/MCC Exc]
  - [7th] S59.022 Salter-Harris Type II physeal fracture of lower end of ulna, left arm [CC] [POA] [HAC] [CC/MCC Exc]
  - [7th] S59.029 Salter-Harris Type II physeal fracture of lower end of ulna, unspecified arm [CC] [POA] [HAC] [CC/MCC Exc]
- [6th] S59.03 Salter-Harris Type III physeal fracture of lower end of ulna
  - [7th] S59.031 Salter-Harris Type III physeal fracture of lower end of ulna, right arm [CC] [POA] [HAC] [CC/MCC Exc]
  - [7th] S59.032 Salter-Harris Type III physeal fracture of lower end of ulna, left arm [CC] [POA] [HAC] [CC/MCC Exc]
  - [7th] S59.039 Salter-Harris Type III physeal fracture of lower end of ulna, unspecified arm [CC] [POA] [HAC] [CC/MCC Exc]
- [6th] S59.04 Salter-Harris Type IV physeal fracture of lower end of ulna
  - [7th] S59.041 Salter-Harris Type IV physeal fracture of lower end of ulna, right arm [CC] [POA] [HAC] [CC/MCC Exc]
  - [7th] S59.042 Salter-Harris Type IV physeal fracture of lower end of ulna, left arm [CC] [POA] [HAC] [CC/MCC Exc]
  - [7th] S59.049 Salter-Harris Type IV physeal fracture of lower end of ulna, unspecified arm [CC] [POA] [HAC] [CC/MCC Exc]
- [6th] S59.09 Other physeal fracture of lower end of ulna
  - [7th] S59.091 Other physeal fracture of lower end of ulna, right arm [CC] [POA] [HAC] [CC/MCC Exc]
  - [7th] S59.092 Other physeal fracture of lower end of ulna, left arm [CC] [POA] [HAC] [CC/MCC Exc]
  - [7th] S59.099 Other physeal fracture of lower end of ulna, unspecified arm [CC] [POA] [HAC] [CC/MCC Exc]

[5th] S59.1 Physeal fracture of upper end of radius
- [6th] S59.10 Unspecified physeal fracture of upper end of radius
  - [7th] S59.101 Unspecified physeal fracture of upper end of radius, right arm [CC] [POA] [CC/MCC Exc]

[PDx] Unacceptable principal diagnosis symbol per Medicare code edits [POA] Code exempt from diagnosis present on admission requirement
[?] Questionable admission [CC] Complication or comorbidity [MCC] Major complication or comorbidity [CC/MCC Exc] CC/MCC exclusion
[HCC] HCC diagnosis code [RxHCC] RxHCC diagnosis code MACRA code **DEFINITION** Describes condition/terminology
TIP Coding guidance 👁 Official Guideline Reference [Z1] Z code as first-listed diagnosis

- [7th] S59.102 Unspecified physeal fracture of upper end of radius, left arm [CC] [POA] [CC/MCC Exc]
- [7th] S59.109 Unspecified physeal fracture of upper end of radius, unspecified arm [CC] [POA] [CC/MCC Exc]

[6th] S59.11 Salter-Harris Type I physeal fracture of upper end of radius
- [7th] S59.111 Salter-Harris Type I physeal fracture of upper end of radius, right arm [CC] [POA] [CC/MCC Exc]
- [7th] S59.112 Salter-Harris Type I physeal fracture of upper end of radius, left arm [CC] [POA] [CC/MCC Exc]
- [7th] S59.119 Salter-Harris Type I physeal fracture of upper end of radius, unspecified arm [CC] [POA] [CC/MCC Exc]

[6th] S59.12 Salter-Harris Type II physeal fracture of upper end of radius
- [7th] S59.121 Salter-Harris Type II physeal fracture of upper end of radius, right arm [CC] [POA] [CC/MCC Exc]
- [7th] S59.122 Salter-Harris Type II physeal fracture of upper end of radius, left arm [CC] [POA] [CC/MCC Exc]
- [7th] S59.129 Salter-Harris Type II physeal fracture of upper end of radius, unspecified arm [CC] [POA] [CC/MCC Exc]

[6th] S59.13 Salter-Harris Type III physeal fracture of upper end of radius
- [7th] S59.131 Salter-Harris Type III physeal fracture of upper end of radius, right arm [CC] [POA] [CC/MCC Exc]
- [7th] S59.132 Salter-Harris Type III physeal fracture of upper end of radius, left arm [CC] [POA] [CC/MCC Exc]
- [7th] S59.139 Salter-Harris Type III physeal fracture of upper end of radius, unspecified arm [CC] [POA] [CC/MCC Exc]

[6th] S59.14 Salter-Harris Type IV physeal fracture of upper end of radius
- [7th] S59.141 Salter-Harris Type IV physeal fracture of upper end of radius, right arm [CC] [POA] [CC/MCC Exc]
- [7th] S59.142 Salter-Harris Type IV physeal fracture of upper end of radius, left arm [CC] [POA] [CC/MCC Exc]
- [7th] S59.149 Salter-Harris Type IV physeal fracture of upper end of radius, unspecified arm [CC] [POA] [CC/MCC Exc]

[6th] S59.19 Other physeal fracture of upper end of radius
- [7th] S59.191 Other physeal fracture of upper end of radius, right arm [CC] [POA] [CC/MCC Exc]
- [7th] S59.192 Other physeal fracture of upper end of radius, left arm [CC] [POA] [CC/MCC Exc]
- [7th] S59.199 Other physeal fracture of upper end of radius, unspecified arm [CC] [POA] [CC/MCC Exc]

[5th] S59.2 Physeal fracture of lower end of radius

[6th] S59.20 Unspecified physeal fracture of lower end of radius
- [7th] S59.201 Unspecified physeal fracture of lower end of radius, right arm [CC] [POA] [HAC] [CC/MCC Exc]
- [7th] S59.202 Unspecified physeal fracture of lower end of radius, left arm [CC] [POA] [HAC] [CC/MCC Exc]
- [7th] S59.209 Unspecified physeal fracture of lower end of radius, unspecified arm [CC] [POA] [HAC] [CC/MCC Exc]

[6th] S59.21 Salter-Harris Type I physeal fracture of lower end of radius
- [7th] S59.211 Salter-Harris Type I physeal fracture of lower end of radius, right arm [CC] [POA] [HAC] [CC/MCC Exc]
- [7th] S59.212 Salter-Harris Type I physeal fracture of lower end of radius, left arm [CC] [POA] [HAC] [CC/MCC Exc]
- [7th] S59.219 Salter-Harris Type I physeal fracture of lower end of radius, unspecified arm [CC] [POA] [HAC] [CC/MCC Exc]

[6th] S59.22 Salter-Harris Type II physeal fracture of lower end of radius
- [7th] S59.221 Salter-Harris Type II physeal fracture of lower end of radius, right arm [CC] [POA] [HAC] [CC/MCC Exc]
- [7th] S59.222 Salter-Harris Type II physeal fracture of lower end of radius, left arm [CC] [POA] [HAC] [CC/MCC Exc]
- [7th] S59.229 Salter-Harris Type II physeal fracture of lower end of radius, unspecified arm [CC] [POA] [HAC] [CC/MCC Exc]

[6th] S59.23 Salter-Harris Type III physeal fracture of lower end of radius
- [7th] S59.231 Salter-Harris Type III physeal fracture of lower end of radius, right arm [CC] [POA] [HAC] [CC/MCC Exc]
- [7th] S59.232 Salter-Harris Type III physeal fracture of lower end of radius, left arm [CC] [POA] [HAC] [CC/MCC Exc]
- [7th] S59.239 Salter-Harris Type III physeal fracture of lower end of radius, unspecified arm [CC] [POA] [HAC] [CC/MCC Exc]

[6th] S59.24 Salter-Harris Type IV physeal fracture of lower end of radius
- [7th] S59.241 Salter-Harris Type IV physeal fracture of lower end of radius, right arm [CC] [POA] [HAC] [CC/MCC Exc]
- [7th] S59.242 Salter-Harris Type IV physeal fracture of lower end of radius, left arm [CC] [POA] [HAC] [CC/MCC Exc]
- [7th] S59.249 Salter-Harris Type IV physeal fracture of lower end of radius, unspecified arm [CC] [POA] [HAC] [CC/MCC Exc]

[6th] S59.29 Other physeal fracture of lower end of radius
- [7th] S59.291 Other physeal fracture of lower end of radius, right arm [CC] [POA] [HAC] [CC/MCC Exc]
- [7th] S59.292 Other physeal fracture of lower end of radius, left arm [CC] [POA] [HAC] [CC/MCC Exc]
- [7th] S59.299 Other physeal fracture of lower end of radius, unspecified arm [CC] [POA] [HAC] [CC/MCC Exc]

[5th] S59.8 Other specified injuries of elbow and forearm

The appropriate 7th character is to be added to each code in subcategory S59.8
- A = initial encounter
- D = subsequent encounter
- S = sequela

[6th] S59.80 Other specified injuries of elbow
- [7th] S59.801 Other specified injuries of right elbow [POA]
- [7th] S59.802 Other specified injuries of left elbow [POA]
- [7th] S59.809 Other specified injuries of unspecified elbow [POA]

[6th] S59.81 Other specified injuries of forearm
- [7th] S59.811 Other specified injuries right forearm [POA]
- [7th] S59.812 Other specified injuries left forearm [POA]
- [7th] S59.819 Other specified injuries unspecified forearm [POA]

[5th] S59.9 Unspecified injury of elbow and forearm

The appropriate 7th character is to be added to each code in subcategory S59.9
- A = initial encounter
- D = subsequent encounter
- S = sequela

[6th] S59.90 Unspecified injury of elbow
- [7th] S59.901 Unspecified injury of right elbow [POA]
- [7th] S59.902 Unspecified injury of left elbow [POA]
- [7th] S59.909 Unspecified injury of unspecified elbow [POA]

[6th] S59.91 Unspecified injury of forearm
- [7th] S59.911 Unspecified injury of right forearm [POA]
- [7th] S59.912 Unspecified injury of left forearm [POA]
- [7th] S59.919 Unspecified injury of unspecified forearm [POA]

Unspecified Code | Other Specified Code | Manifestation Code | [N] Newborn | [P] Pediatric | [M] Maternity | [A] Adult | ♂ Male | ♀ Female
● New Code | ▲ Revised Code Title | ►◄ Revised Text | [NOTES] | *INCLUDES* | [EXCLUDES1] Not coded here | [EXCLUDES2] Not included here
[4th] 4th character required | [5th] 5th character required | [6th] 6th character required | [7th] 7th character required | [x7th] Extension 'X' Alert
[HAC] Hospital-acquired condition (HAC) alert | AHA AHA Coding Clinic© | ☞ Code first alert

Injuries to the wrist, hand and fingers (S60-S69)

EXCLUDES2 burns and corrosions (T20-T32)
frostbite (T33-T34)
insect bite or sting, venomous (T63.4)

S60 **Superficial injury of wrist, hand and fingers**
The appropriate 7th character is to be added to each code from category S60
A = initial encounter
D = subsequent encounter
S = sequela

S60.0 **Contusion of** finger without damage to nail
EXCLUDES1 contusion involving nail (matrix) (S60.1)

S60.00 **Contusion of unspecified finger without damage to nail** POA
Contusion of finger(s) NOS

S60.01 **Contusion of** thumb **without damage to nail**
S60.011 **Contusion of** right **thumb without damage to nail** POA
S60.012 **Contusion of** left **thumb without damage to nail** POA
S60.019 **Contusion of unspecified thumb without damage to nail** POA

S60.02 **Contusion of** index finger **without damage to nail**
S60.021 **Contusion of** right **index finger without damage to nail** POA
S60.022 **Contusion of** left **index finger without damage to nail** POA
S60.029 **Contusion of unspecified index finger without damage to nail** POA

S60.03 **Contusion of** middle finger **without damage to nail**
S60.031 **Contusion of** right **middle finger without damage to nail** POA
S60.032 **Contusion of** left **middle finger without damage to nail** POA
S60.039 **Contusion of unspecified middle finger without damage to nail** POA

S60.04 **Contusion of** ring finger **without damage to nail**
S60.041 **Contusion of** right **ring finger without damage to nail** POA
S60.042 **Contusion of** left **ring finger without damage to nail** POA
S60.049 **Contusion of unspecified ring finger without damage to nail** POA

S60.05 **Contusion of** little finger **without damage to nail**
S60.051 **Contusion of** right **little finger without damage to nail** POA
S60.052 **Contusion of** left **little finger without damage to nail** POA
S60.059 **Contusion of unspecified little finger without damage to nail** POA

S60.1 **Contusion of** finger with damage to nail
S60.10 **Contusion of unspecified finger with damage to nail** POA
S60.11 **Contusion of** thumb **with damage to nail**
S60.111 **Contusion of** right **thumb with damage to nail** POA
S60.112 **Contusion of** left **thumb with damage to nail** POA
S60.119 **Contusion of unspecified thumb with damage to nail** POA

S60.12 **Contusion of** index finger **with damage to nail**
S60.121 **Contusion of** right **index finger with damage to nail** POA
S60.122 **Contusion of** left **index finger with damage to nail** POA
S60.129 **Contusion of unspecified index finger with damage to nail** POA

S60.13 **Contusion of** middle finger **with damage to nail**
S60.131 **Contusion of** right **middle finger with damage to nail** POA

S60.132 **Contusion of** left **middle finger with damage to nail** POA
S60.139 **Contusion of unspecified middle finger with damage to nail** POA

S60.14 **Contusion of** ring finger **with damage to nail**
S60.141 **Contusion of** right **ring finger with damage to nail** POA
S60.142 **Contusion of** left **ring finger with damage to nail** POA
S60.149 **Contusion of unspecified ring finger with damage to nail** POA

S60.15 **Contusion of** little finger **with damage to nail**
S60.151 **Contusion of** right **little finger with damage to nail** POA
S60.152 **Contusion of** left **little finger with damage to nail** POA
S60.159 **Contusion of unspecified little finger with damage to nail** POA

S60.2 **Contusion of** wrist and hand
EXCLUDES2 contusion of fingers (S60.0-, S60.1-)
S60.21 **Contusion of** wrist
S60.211 **Contusion of** right **wrist** POA
S60.212 **Contusion of** left **wrist** POA
S60.219 **Contusion of unspecified wrist** POA

S60.22 **Contusion of** hand
S60.221 **Contusion of** right **hand** POA
S60.222 **Contusion of** left **hand** POA
S60.229 **Contusion of unspecified hand** POA

S60.3 Other **superficial injuries of thumb**
S60.31 Abrasion **of thumb**
S60.311 **Abrasion of** right **thumb** POA
S60.312 **Abrasion of** left **thumb** POA
S60.319 **Abrasion of unspecified thumb** POA

S60.32 Blister (nonthermal) **of thumb**
S60.321 **Blister (nonthermal) of** right **thumb** POA
S60.322 **Blister (nonthermal) of** left **thumb** POA
S60.329 **Blister (nonthermal) of unspecified thumb** POA

S60.34 External constriction **of thumb**
Hair tourniquet syndrome of thumb
Use additional cause code to identify the constricting item (W49.0-)
S60.341 **External constriction of** right **thumb** POA
S60.342 **External constriction of** left **thumb** POA
S60.349 **External constriction of unspecified thumb** POA

S60.35 Superficial foreign body **of thumb**
Splinter in the thumb
S60.351 **Superficial foreign body of** right **thumb** POA
S60.352 **Superficial foreign body of** left **thumb** POA
S60.359 **Superficial foreign body of unspecified thumb** POA

S60.36 Insect bite (nonvenomous) **of thumb**
S60.361 **Insect bite (nonvenomous) of** right **thumb** POA
S60.362 **Insect bite (nonvenomous) of** left **thumb** POA
S60.369 **Insect bite (nonvenomous) of unspecified thumb** POA

S60.37 Other superficial bite **of thumb**
EXCLUDES1 open bite of thumb (S61.05-, S61.15-)
S60.371 **Other superficial bite of** right **thumb** POA
S60.372 **Other superficial bite of** left **thumb** POA
S60.379 **Other superficial bite of unspecified thumb** POA

S60.39 Other superficial injuries **of thumb**
S60.391 **Other superficial injuries of** right **thumb** POA
S60.392 **Other superficial injuries of** left **thumb** POA
S60.399 **Other superficial injuries of unspecified thumb** POA

POA Unacceptable principal diagnosis symbol per Medicare code edits POA Code exempt from diagnosis present on admission requirement
? Questionable admission CC Complication or comorbidity MCC Major complication or comorbidity CC/MCC CC/MCC exclusion
HCC HCC diagnosis code RxHCC RxHCC diagnosis code MACRA MACRA code **DEFINITION** Describes condition/terminology
TIP Coding guidance Official Guideline Reference Z1 Z code as first-listed diagnosis

1036 When symbols appear on a code that requires a 7th character extension, refer to Appendix B to identify applicable 7th character codes. **2020 ICD-10-CM**

[5th] S60.4 Other superficial injuries of other fingers
[6th] S60.41 Abrasion of fingers
[7th] S60.410 Abrasion of right index finger [POA]
[7th] S60.411 Abrasion of left index finger [POA]
[7th] S60.412 Abrasion of right middle finger [POA]
[7th] S60.413 Abrasion of left middle finger [POA]
[7th] S60.414 Abrasion of right ring finger [POA]
[7th] S60.415 Abrasion of left ring finger [POA]
[7th] S60.416 Abrasion of right little finger [POA]
[7th] S60.417 Abrasion of left little finger [POA]
[7th] S60.418 Abrasion of other finger [POA]
Abrasion of specified finger with unspecified laterality
[7th] S60.419 Abrasion of unspecified finger [POA]
[6th] S60.42 Blister (nonthermal) of fingers
[7th] S60.420 Blister (nonthermal) of right index finger [POA]
[7th] S60.421 Blister (nonthermal) of left index finger [POA]
[7th] S60.422 Blister (nonthermal) of right middle finger [POA]
[7th] S60.423 Blister (nonthermal) of left middle finger [POA]
[7th] S60.424 Blister (nonthermal) of right ring finger [POA]
[7th] S60.425 Blister (nonthermal) of left ring finger [POA]
[7th] S60.426 Blister (nonthermal) of right little finger [POA]
[7th] S60.427 Blister (nonthermal) of left little finger [POA]
[7th] S60.428 Blister (nonthermal) of other finger [POA]
Blister (nonthermal) of specified finger with unspecified laterality
[7th] S60.429 Blister (nonthermal) of unspecified finger [POA]
[6th] S60.44 External constriction of fingers
Hair tourniquet syndrome of finger
Use additional cause code to identify the constricting item (W49.0-)
[7th] S60.440 External constriction of right index finger [POA]
[7th] S60.441 External constriction of left index finger [POA]
[7th] S60.442 External constriction of right middle finger [POA]
[7th] S60.443 External constriction of left middle finger [POA]
[7th] S60.444 External constriction of right ring finger [POA]
[7th] S60.445 External constriction of left ring finger [POA]
[7th] S60.446 External constriction of right little finger [POA]
[7th] S60.447 External constriction of left little finger [POA]
[7th] S60.448 External constriction of other finger [POA]
External constriction of specified finger with unspecified laterality
[7th] S60.449 External constriction of unspecified finger [POA]
[6th] S60.45 Superficial foreign body of fingers
Splinter in the finger(s)
[7th] S60.450 Superficial foreign body of right index finger [POA]
[7th] S60.451 Superficial foreign body of left index finger [POA]
[7th] S60.452 Superficial foreign body of right middle finger [POA]
[7th] S60.453 Superficial foreign body of left middle finger [POA]
[7th] S60.454 Superficial foreign body of right ring finger [POA]
[7th] S60.455 Superficial foreign body of left ring finger [POA]
[7th] S60.456 Superficial foreign body of right little finger [POA]
[7th] S60.457 Superficial foreign body of left little finger [POA]
[7th] S60.458 Superficial foreign body of other finger [POA]
Superficial foreign body of specified finger with unspecified laterality
[7th] S60.459 Superficial foreign body of unspecified finger [POA]
[6th] S60.46 Insect bite (nonvenomous) of fingers
[7th] S60.460 Insect bite (nonvenomous) of right index finger [POA]
[7th] S60.461 Insect bite (nonvenomous) of left index finger [POA]
[7th] S60.462 Insect bite (nonvenomous) of right middle finger [POA]
[7th] S60.463 Insect bite (nonvenomous) of left middle finger [POA]
[7th] S60.464 Insect bite (nonvenomous) of right ring finger [POA]
[7th] S60.465 Insect bite (nonvenomous) of left ring finger [POA]
[7th] S60.466 Insect bite (nonvenomous) of right little finger [POA]
[7th] S60.467 Insect bite (nonvenomous) of left little finger [POA]
[7th] S60.468 Insect bite (nonvenomous) of other finger [POA]
Insect bite (nonvenomous) of specified finger with unspecified laterality
[7th] S60.469 Insect bite (nonvenomous) of unspecified finger [POA]
[6th] S60.47 Other superficial bite of fingers
EXCLUDES1 *open bite of fingers (S61.25-, S61.35-)*
[7th] S60.470 Other superficial bite of right index finger [POA]
[7th] S60.471 Other superficial bite of left index finger [POA]
[7th] S60.472 Other superficial bite of right middle finger [POA]
[7th] S60.473 Other superficial bite of left middle finger [POA]
[7th] S60.474 Other superficial bite of right ring finger [POA]
[7th] S60.475 Other superficial bite of left ring finger [POA]
[7th] S60.476 Other superficial bite of right little finger [POA]
[7th] S60.477 Other superficial bite of left little finger [POA]
[7th] S60.478 Other superficial bite of other finger [POA]
Other superficial bite of specified finger with unspecified laterality
[7th] S60.479 Other superficial bite of unspecified finger [POA]
[5th] S60.5 Other superficial injuries of hand
EXCLUDES2 *superficial injuries of fingers (S60.3-, S60.4-)*
[6th] S60.51 Abrasion of hand
[7th] S60.511 Abrasion of right hand [POA]
[7th] S60.512 Abrasion of left hand [POA]
[7th] S60.519 Abrasion of unspecified hand [POA]
[6th] S60.52 Blister (nonthermal) of hand
[7th] S60.521 Blister (nonthermal) of right hand [POA]
[7th] S60.522 Blister (nonthermal) of left hand [POA]
[7th] S60.529 Blister (nonthermal) of unspecified hand [POA]
[6th] S60.54 External constriction of hand
[7th] S60.541 External constriction of right hand [POA]
[7th] S60.542 External constriction of left hand [POA]
[7th] S60.549 External constriction of unspecified hand [POA]
[6th] S60.55 Superficial foreign body of hand
Splinter in the hand
[7th] S60.551 Superficial foreign body of right hand [POA]
[7th] S60.552 Superficial foreign body of left hand [POA]
[7th] S60.559 Superficial foreign body of unspecified hand [POA]
[6th] S60.56 Insect bite (nonvenomous) of hand
[7th] S60.561 Insect bite (nonvenomous) of right hand [POA]
[7th] S60.562 Insect bite (nonvenomous) of left hand [POA]

Unspecified Code Other Specified Code Manifestation Code [N] Newborn [P] Pediatric [M] Maternity [A] Adult ♂ Male ♀ Female
● New Code ▲ Revised Code Title ►◄ Revised Text NOTES INCLUDES EXCLUDES1 Not coded here EXCLUDES2 Not included here
[4th] 4th character required [5th] 5th character required [6th] 6th character required [7th] 7th character required [X] Extension 'X' Alert
[HAC] Hospital-acquired condition (HAC) alert AHA AHA Coding Clinic© ☞ Code first alert

[7th] S60.569 Insect bite (nonvenomous) of unspecified hand POA
[6th] S60.57 Other superficial bite of hand
[EXCLUDES1] open bite of hand (S61.45-)
[7th] S60.571 Other superficial bite of hand of right hand POA
[7th] S60.572 Other superficial bite of hand of left hand POA
[7th] S60.579 Other superficial bite of hand of unspecified hand POA
[5th] S60.8 Other superficial injuries of wrist
[6th] S60.81 Abrasion of wrist
[7th] S60.811 Abrasion of right wrist POA
[7th] S60.812 Abrasion of left wrist POA
[7th] S60.819 Abrasion of unspecified wrist POA
[6th] S60.82 Blister (nonthermal) of wrist
[7th] S60.821 Blister (nonthermal) of right wrist POA
[7th] S60.822 Blister (nonthermal) of left wrist POA
[7th] S60.829 Blister (nonthermal) of unspecified wrist POA
[6th] S60.84 External constriction of wrist
[7th] S60.841 External constriction of right wrist POA
[7th] S60.842 External constriction of left wrist POA
[7th] S60.849 External constriction of unspecified wrist POA
[6th] S60.85 Superficial foreign body of wrist
Splinter in the wrist
[7th] S60.851 Superficial foreign body of right wrist POA
[7th] S60.852 Superficial foreign body of left wrist POA
[7th] S60.859 Superficial foreign body of unspecified wrist POA
[6th] S60.86 Insect bite (nonvenomous) of wrist
[7th] S60.861 Insect bite (nonvenomous) of right wrist POA
[7th] S60.862 Insect bite (nonvenomous) of left wrist POA
[7th] S60.869 Insect bite (nonvenomous) of unspecified wrist POA
[6th] S60.87 Other superficial bite of wrist
[EXCLUDES1] open bite of wrist (S61.55)
[7th] S60.871 Other superficial bite of right wrist POA
[7th] S60.872 Other superficial bite of left wrist POA
[7th] S60.879 Other superficial bite of unspecified wrist POA
[5th] S60.9 Unspecified superficial injury of wrist, hand and fingers
[6th] S60.91 Unspecified superficial injury of wrist
[7th] S60.911 Unspecified superficial injury of right wrist POA
[7th] S60.912 Unspecified superficial injury of left wrist POA
[7th] S60.919 Unspecified superficial injury of unspecified wrist POA
[6th] S60.92 Unspecified superficial injury of hand
[7th] S60.921 Unspecified superficial injury of right hand POA
[7th] S60.922 Unspecified superficial injury of left hand POA
[7th] S60.929 Unspecified superficial injury of unspecified hand POA
[6th] S60.93 Unspecified superficial injury of thumb
[7th] S60.931 Unspecified superficial injury of right thumb POA
[7th] S60.932 Unspecified superficial injury of left thumb POA
[7th] S60.939 Unspecified superficial injury of unspecified thumb POA
[6th] S60.94 Unspecified superficial injury of other fingers
[7th] S60.940 Unspecified superficial injury of right index finger POA
[7th] S60.941 Unspecified superficial injury of left index finger POA
[7th] S60.942 Unspecified superficial injury of right middle finger POA
[7th] S60.943 Unspecified superficial injury of left middle finger POA
[7th] S60.944 Unspecified superficial injury of right ring finger POA
[7th] S60.945 Unspecified superficial injury of left ring finger POA
[7th] S60.946 Unspecified superficial injury of right little finger POA
[7th] S60.947 Unspecified superficial injury of left little finger POA
[7th] S60.948 Unspecified superficial injury of other finger POA
Unspecified superficial injury of specified finger with unspecified laterality
[7th] S60.949 Unspecified superficial injury of unspecified finger POA

[4th] S61 Open wound of wrist, hand and fingers
Code also any associated wound infection
[EXCLUDES1] open fracture of wrist, hand and finger (S62.- with 7th character B)
traumatic amputation of wrist and hand (S68.-)
The appropriate 7th character is to be added to each code from category S61
A = initial encounter
D = subsequent encounter
S = sequela
[5th] S61.0 Open wound of thumb without damage to nail
[EXCLUDES1] open wound of thumb with damage to nail (S61.1-)
[6th] S61.00 Unspecified open wound of thumb without damage to nail
[7th] S61.001 Unspecified open wound of right thumb without damage to nail POA
[7th] S61.002 Unspecified open wound of left thumb without damage to nail POA
[7th] S61.009 Unspecified open wound of unspecified thumb without damage to nail POA
[6th] S61.01 Laceration without foreign body of thumb without damage to nail
[7th] S61.011 Laceration without foreign body of right thumb without damage to nail POA
[7th] S61.012 Laceration without foreign body of left thumb without damage to nail POA
[7th] S61.019 Laceration without foreign body of unspecified thumb without damage to nail POA
[6th] S61.02 Laceration with foreign body of thumb without damage to nail
[7th] S61.021 Laceration with foreign body of right thumb without damage to nail POA
[7th] S61.022 Laceration with foreign body of left thumb without damage to nail POA
[7th] S61.029 Laceration with foreign body of unspecified thumb without damage to nail POA
[6th] S61.03 Puncture wound without foreign body of thumb without damage to nail
[7th] S61.031 Puncture wound without foreign body of right thumb without damage to nail POA
[7th] S61.032 Puncture wound without foreign body of left thumb without damage to nail POA
[7th] S61.039 Puncture wound without foreign body of unspecified thumb without damage to nail POA
[6th] S61.04 Puncture wound with foreign body of thumb without damage to nail
[7th] S61.041 Puncture wound with foreign body of right thumb without damage to nail POA
[7th] S61.042 Puncture wound with foreign body of left thumb without damage to nail POA

PDx Unacceptable principal diagnosis symbol per Medicare code edits POA Code exempt from diagnosis present on admission requirement
[?] Questionable admission CC Complication or comorbidity MCC Major complication or comorbidity CC/MCC Excl CC/MCC exclusion
[HCC] HCC diagnosis code [RxHCC] RxHCC diagnosis code MACRA code **DEFINITION** Describes condition/terminology
TIP Coding guidance 👁 Official Guideline Reference [Z-1] Z code as first-listed diagnosis

⑦ᵗʰ S61.049 **Puncture wound with foreign body of unspecified thumb without damage to nail** POA

⑥ᵗʰ S61.05 Open bite of thumb without damage to nail
Bite of thumb NOS
EXCLUDES1 *superficial bite of thumb (S60.36-, S60.37-)*

⑦ᵗʰ S61.051 **Open bite of** right **thumb without damage to nail** POA

⑦ᵗʰ S61.052 **Open bite of** left **thumb without damage to nail** POA

⑦ᵗʰ S61.059 **Open bite of unspecified thumb without damage to nail** POA

⑤ᵗʰ S61.1 **Open wound of** thumb with damage to nail

⑥ᵗʰ S61.10 Unspecified **open wound of thumb with damage to nail**

⑦ᵗʰ S61.101 **Unspecified open wound of** right **thumb with damage to nail** POA

⑦ᵗʰ S61.102 **Unspecified open wound of** left **thumb with damage to nail** POA

⑦ᵗʰ S61.109 **Unspecified open wound of unspecified thumb with damage to nail** POA

⑥ᵗʰ S61.11 Laceration without foreign body **of thumb with damage to nail**

⑦ᵗʰ S61.111 **Laceration without foreign body of** right **thumb with damage to nail** POA

⑦ᵗʰ S61.112 **Laceration without foreign body of** left **thumb with damage to nail** POA

⑦ᵗʰ S61.119 **Laceration without foreign body of unspecified thumb with damage to nail** POA

⑥ᵗʰ S61.12 Laceration with foreign body **of thumb with damage to nail**

⑦ᵗʰ S61.121 **Laceration with foreign body of** right **thumb with damage to nail** POA

⑦ᵗʰ S61.122 **Laceration with foreign body of** left **thumb with damage to nail** POA

⑦ᵗʰ S61.129 **Laceration with foreign body of unspecified thumb with damage to nail** POA

⑥ᵗʰ S61.13 Puncture wound without foreign body **of thumb with damage to nail**

⑦ᵗʰ S61.131 **Puncture wound without foreign body of** right **thumb with damage to nail** POA

⑦ᵗʰ S61.132 **Puncture wound without foreign body of** left **thumb with damage to nail** POA

⑦ᵗʰ S61.139 **Puncture wound without foreign body of unspecified thumb with damage to nail** POA

⑥ᵗʰ S61.14 Puncture wound with foreign body **of thumb with damage to nail**

⑦ᵗʰ S61.141 **Puncture wound with foreign body of** right **thumb with damage to nail** POA

⑦ᵗʰ S61.142 **Puncture wound with foreign body of** left **thumb with damage to nail** POA

⑦ᵗʰ S61.149 **Puncture wound with foreign body of unspecified thumb with damage to nail** POA

⑥ᵗʰ S61.15 Open bite of thumb with damage to nail
Bite of thumb with damage to nail NOS
EXCLUDES1 *superficial bite of thumb (S60.36-, S60.37-)*

⑦ᵗʰ S61.151 **Open bite of** right **thumb with damage to nail** POA

⑦ᵗʰ S61.152 **Open bite of** left **thumb with damage to nail** POA

⑦ᵗʰ S61.159 **Open bite of unspecified thumb with damage to nail** POA

⑤ᵗʰ S61.2 **Open wound of** other finger without damage to nail
EXCLUDES1 *open wound of finger involving nail (matrix) (S61.3-)*
EXCLUDES2 *open wound of thumb without damage to nail (S61.0-)*

⑥ᵗʰ S61.20 Unspecified **open wound of other finger without damage to nail**

⑦ᵗʰ S61.200 **Unspecified open wound of** right index **finger without damage to nail** POA

⑦ᵗʰ S61.201 **Unspecified open wound of** left index **finger without damage to nail** POA

⑦ᵗʰ S61.202 **Unspecified open wound of** right middle **finger without damage to nail** POA

⑦ᵗʰ S61.203 **Unspecified open wound of** left middle **finger without damage to nail** POA

⑦ᵗʰ S61.204 **Unspecified open wound of** right ring **finger without damage to nail** POA

⑦ᵗʰ S61.205 **Unspecified open wound of** left ring **finger without damage to nail** POA

⑦ᵗʰ S61.206 **Unspecified open wound of** right little **finger without damage to nail** POA

⑦ᵗʰ S61.207 **Unspecified open wound of** left little **finger without damage to nail** POA

⑦ᵗʰ S61.208 **Unspecified open wound of** other **finger without damage to nail** POA
Unspecified open wound of specified finger with unspecified laterality without damage to nail

⑦ᵗʰ S61.209 **Unspecified open wound of unspecified finger without damage to nail** POA

⑥ᵗʰ S61.21 Laceration without foreign body **of finger without damage to nail**

⑦ᵗʰ S61.210 **Laceration without foreign body of** right index **finger without damage to nail** POA

⑦ᵗʰ S61.211 **Laceration without foreign body of** left index **finger without damage to nail** POA

⑦ᵗʰ S61.212 **Laceration without foreign body of** right middle **finger without damage to nail** POA

⑦ᵗʰ S61.213 **Laceration without foreign body of** left middle **finger without damage to nail** POA

⑦ᵗʰ S61.214 **Laceration without foreign body of** right ring **finger without damage to nail** POA

⑦ᵗʰ S61.215 **Laceration without foreign body of** left ring **finger without damage to nail** POA

⑦ᵗʰ S61.216 **Laceration without foreign body of** right little **finger without damage to nail** POA

⑦ᵗʰ S61.217 **Laceration without foreign body of** left little **finger without damage to nail** POA

⑦ᵗʰ S61.218 **Laceration without foreign body of** other **finger without damage to nail** POA
Laceration without foreign body of specified finger with unspecified laterality without damage to nail

⑦ᵗʰ S61.219 **Laceration without foreign body of unspecified finger without damage to nail** POA

⑥ᵗʰ S61.22 Laceration with foreign body **of finger without damage to nail**

⑦ᵗʰ S61.220 **Laceration with foreign body of** right index **finger without damage to nail** POA

⑦ᵗʰ S61.221 **Laceration with foreign body of** left index **finger without damage to nail** POA

⑦ᵗʰ S61.222 **Laceration with foreign body of** right middle **finger without damage to nail** POA

⑦ᵗʰ S61.223 **Laceration with foreign body of** left middle **finger without damage to nail** POA

⑦ᵗʰ S61.224 **Laceration with foreign body of** right ring **finger without damage to nail** POA

⑦ᵗʰ S61.225 **Laceration with foreign body of** left ring **finger without damage to nail** POA

⑦ᵗʰ S61.226 **Laceration with foreign body of** right little **finger without damage to nail** POA

⑦ᵗʰ S61.227 **Laceration with foreign body of** left little **finger without damage to nail** POA

⑦ᵗʰ S61.228 **Laceration with foreign body of** other **finger without damage to nail** POA
Laceration with foreign body of specified finger with unspecified laterality without damage to nail

⑦ᵗʰ S61.229 **Laceration with foreign body of unspecified finger without damage to nail** POA

Unspecified Code	Other Specified Code	Manifestation Code	Ⓝ Newborn	Ⓟ Pediatric	Ⓜ Maternity	Ⓐ Adult	♂ Male	♀ Female

● New Code   ▲ Revised Code Title   ▶◀ Revised Text   **NOTES**   *INCLUDES*   *EXCLUDES1* Not coded here   *EXCLUDES2* Not included here
④ᵗʰ 4ᵗʰ character required   ⑤ᵗʰ 5ᵗʰ character required   ⑥ᵗʰ 6ᵗʰ character required   ⑦ᵗʰ 7ᵗʰ character required   ⑦ Extension 'X' Alert
HAC Hospital-acquired condition (HAC) alert   **AHA** AHA Coding Clinic©   ☛ Code first alert

6ᵗʰ **S61.23** Puncture wound without foreign body of finger without damage to nail

  7ᵗʰ **S61.230** Puncture wound without foreign body of right index finger without damage to nail

  7ᵗʰ **S61.231** Puncture wound without foreign body of left index finger without damage to nail POA

  7ᵗʰ **S61.232** Puncture wound without foreign body of right middle finger without damage to nail

  7ᵗʰ **S61.233** Puncture wound without foreign body of left middle finger without damage to nail

  7ᵗʰ **S61.234** Puncture wound without foreign body of right ring finger without damage to nail POA

  7ᵗʰ **S61.235** Puncture wound without foreign body of left ring finger without damage to nail POA

  7ᵗʰ **S61.236** Puncture wound without foreign body of right little finger without damage to nail POA

  7ᵗʰ **S61.237** Puncture wound without foreign body of left little finger without damage to nail POA

  7ᵗʰ **S61.238** Puncture wound without foreign body of other finger without damage to nail POA

    Puncture wound without foreign body of specified finger with unspecified laterality without damage to nail

  7ᵗʰ **S61.239** Puncture wound without foreign body of unspecified finger without damage to nail POA

6ᵗʰ **S61.24** Puncture wound with foreign body of finger without damage to nail

  7ᵗʰ **S61.240** Puncture wound with foreign body of right index finger without damage to nail POA

  7ᵗʰ **S61.241** Puncture wound with foreign body of left index finger without damage to nail POA

  7ᵗʰ **S61.242** Puncture wound with foreign body of right middle finger without damage to nail POA

  7ᵗʰ **S61.243** Puncture wound with foreign body of left middle finger without damage to nail POA

  7ᵗʰ **S61.244** Puncture wound with foreign body of right ring finger without damage to nail POA

  7ᵗʰ **S61.245** Puncture wound with foreign body of left ring finger without damage to nail POA

  7ᵗʰ **S61.246** Puncture wound with foreign body of right little finger without damage to nail POA

  7ᵗʰ **S61.247** Puncture wound with foreign body of left little finger without damage to nail POA

  7ᵗʰ **S61.248** Puncture wound with foreign body of other finger without damage to nail POA

    Puncture wound with foreign body of specified finger with unspecified laterality without damage to nail

  7ᵗʰ **S61.249** Puncture wound with foreign body of unspecified finger without damage to nail POA

6ᵗʰ **S61.25** Open bite of finger without damage to nail

  Bite of finger without damage to nail NOS

  EXCLUDES1 superficial bite of finger (S60.46-, S60.47-)

  7ᵗʰ **S61.250** Open bite of right index finger without damage to nail POA

  7ᵗʰ **S61.251** Open bite of left index finger without damage to nail POA

  7ᵗʰ **S61.252** Open bite of right middle finger without damage to nail POA

  7ᵗʰ **S61.253** Open bite of left middle finger without damage to nail POA

  7ᵗʰ **S61.254** Open bite of right ring finger without damage to nail POA

  7ᵗʰ **S61.255** Open bite of left ring finger without damage to nail

  7ᵗʰ **S61.256** Open bite of right little finger without damage to nail POA

  7ᵗʰ **S61.257** Open bite of left little finger without damage to nail POA

  7ᵗʰ **S61.258** Open bite of other finger without damage to nail POA

    Open bite of specified finger with unspecified laterality without damage to nail

  7ᵗʰ **S61.259** Open bite of unspecified finger without damage to nail POA

5ᵗʰ **S61.3** Open wound of other finger with damage to nail

6ᵗʰ **S61.30** Unspecified open wound of finger with damage to nail

  7ᵗʰ **S61.300** Unspecified open wound of right index finger with damage to nail POA

  7ᵗʰ **S61.301** Unspecified open wound of left index finger with damage to nail POA

  7ᵗʰ **S61.302** Unspecified open wound of right middle finger with damage to nail POA

  7ᵗʰ **S61.303** Unspecified open wound of left middle finger with damage to nail POA

  7ᵗʰ **S61.304** Unspecified open wound of right ring finger with damage to nail POA

  7ᵗʰ **S61.305** Unspecified open wound of left ring finger with damage to nail POA

  7ᵗʰ **S61.306** Unspecified open wound of right little finger with damage to nail POA

  7ᵗʰ **S61.307** Unspecified open wound of left little finger with damage to nail POA

  7ᵗʰ **S61.308** Unspecified open wound of other finger with damage to nail POA

    Unspecified open wound of specified finger with unspecified laterality with damage to nail

  7ᵗʰ **S61.309** Unspecified open wound of unspecified finger with damage to nail POA

6ᵗʰ **S61.31** Laceration without foreign body of finger with damage to nail

  7ᵗʰ **S61.310** Laceration without foreign body of right index finger with damage to nail POA

  7ᵗʰ **S61.311** Laceration without foreign body of left index finger with damage to nail POA

  7ᵗʰ **S61.312** Laceration without foreign body of right middle finger with damage to nail POA

  7ᵗʰ **S61.313** Laceration without foreign body of left middle finger with damage to nail POA

  7ᵗʰ **S61.314** Laceration without foreign body of right ring finger with damage to nail POA

  7ᵗʰ **S61.315** Laceration without foreign body of left ring finger with damage to nail POA

  7ᵗʰ **S61.316** Laceration without foreign body of right little finger with damage to nail POA

  7ᵗʰ **S61.317** Laceration without foreign body of left little finger with damage to nail POA

  7ᵗʰ **S61.318** Laceration without foreign body of other finger with damage to nail POA

    Laceration without foreign body of specified finger with unspecified laterality with damage to nail

  7ᵗʰ **S61.319** Laceration without foreign body of unspecified finger with damage to nail POA

6ᵗʰ **S61.32** Laceration with foreign body of finger with damage to nail

  7ᵗʰ **S61.320** Laceration with foreign body of right index finger with damage to nail POA

  7ᵗʰ **S61.321** Laceration with foreign body of left index finger with damage to nail POA

  7ᵗʰ **S61.322** Laceration with foreign body of right middle finger with damage to nail POA

  7ᵗʰ **S61.323** Laceration with foreign body of left middle finger with damage to nail POA

7ᵀ **S61.324** Laceration with foreign body of right ring finger with damage to nail POA

7ᵀ **S61.325** Laceration with foreign body of left ring finger with damage to nail POA

7ᵀ **S61.326** Laceration with foreign body of right little finger with damage to nail POA

7ᵀ **S61.327** Laceration with foreign body of left little finger with damage to nail POA

7ᵀ **S61.328** Laceration with foreign body of other finger with damage to nail POA
Laceration with foreign body of specified finger with unspecified laterality with damage to nail

7ᵀ **S61.329** Laceration with foreign body of unspecified finger with damage to nail POA

6ᵀ **S61.33** Puncture wound without foreign body of finger with damage to nail

7ᵀ **S61.330** Puncture wound without foreign body of right index finger with damage to nail POA

7ᵀ **S61.331** Puncture wound without foreign body of left index finger with damage to nail POA

7ᵀ **S61.332** Puncture wound without foreign body of right middle finger with damage to nail POA

7ᵀ **S61.333** Puncture wound without foreign body of left middle finger with damage to nail POA

7ᵀ **S61.334** Puncture wound without foreign body of right ring finger with damage to nail POA

7ᵀ **S61.335** Puncture wound without foreign body of left ring finger with damage to nail POA

7ᵀ **S61.336** Puncture wound without foreign body of right little finger with damage to nail POA

7ᵀ **S61.337** Puncture wound without foreign body of left little finger with damage to nail POA

7ᵀ **S61.338** Puncture wound without foreign body of other finger with damage to nail POA
Puncture wound without foreign body of specified finger with unspecified laterality with damage to nail

7ᵀ **S61.339** Puncture wound without foreign body of unspecified finger with damage to nail POA

6ᵀ **S61.34** Puncture wound with foreign body of finger with damage to nail

7ᵀ **S61.340** Puncture wound with foreign body of right index finger with damage to nail POA

7ᵀ **S61.341** Puncture wound with foreign body of left index finger with damage to nail POA

7ᵀ **S61.342** Puncture wound with foreign body of right middle finger with damage to nail POA

7ᵀ **S61.343** Puncture wound with foreign body of left middle finger with damage to nail POA

7ᵀ **S61.344** Puncture wound with foreign body of right ring finger with damage to nail POA

7ᵀ **S61.345** Puncture wound with foreign body of left ring finger with damage to nail POA

7ᵀ **S61.346** Puncture wound with foreign body of right little finger with damage to nail POA

7ᵀ **S61.347** Puncture wound with foreign body of left little finger with damage to nail POA

7ᵀ **S61.348** Puncture wound with foreign body of other finger with damage to nail POA
Puncture wound with foreign body of specified finger with unspecified laterality with damage to nail

7ᵀ **S61.349** Puncture wound with foreign body of unspecified finger with damage to nail POA

6ᵀ **S61.35** Open bite of finger with damage to nail
Bite of finger with damage to nail NOS
EXCLUDES1 superficial bite of finger (S60.46-, S60.47-)

7ᵀ **S61.350** Open bite of right index finger with damage to nail POA

7ᵀ **S61.351** Open bite of left index finger with damage to nail POA

7ᵀ **S61.352** Open bite of right middle finger with damage to nail POA

7ᵀ **S61.353** Open bite of left middle finger with damage to nail POA

7ᵀ **S61.354** Open bite of right ring finger with damage to nail POA

7ᵀ **S61.355** Open bite of left ring finger with damage to nail POA

7ᵀ **S61.356** Open bite of right little finger with damage to nail POA

7ᵀ **S61.357** Open bite of left little finger with damage to nail POA

7ᵀ **S61.358** Open bite of other finger with damage to nail POA
Open bite of specified finger with unspecified laterality with damage to nail

7ᵀ **S61.359** Open bite of unspecified finger with damage to nail POA

5ᵀ **S61.4** Open wound of hand

6ᵀ **S61.40** Unspecified open wound of hand

7ᵀ **S61.401** Unspecified open wound of right hand POA

7ᵀ **S61.402** Unspecified open wound of left hand POA

7ᵀ **S61.409** Unspecified open wound of unspecified hand POA

6ᵀ **S61.41** Laceration without foreign body of hand

7ᵀ **S61.411** Laceration without foreign body of right hand POA

7ᵀ **S61.412** Laceration without foreign body of left hand POA

7ᵀ **S61.419** Laceration without foreign body of unspecified hand POA

6ᵀ **S61.42** Laceration with foreign body of hand

7ᵀ **S61.421** Laceration with foreign body of right hand POA

7ᵀ **S61.422** Laceration with foreign body of left hand POA

7ᵀ **S61.429** Laceration with foreign body of unspecified hand POA

6ᵀ **S61.43** Puncture wound without foreign body of hand

7ᵀ **S61.431** Puncture wound without foreign body of right hand POA

7ᵀ **S61.432** Puncture wound without foreign body of left hand POA

7ᵀ **S61.439** Puncture wound without foreign body of unspecified hand POA

6ᵀ **S61.44** Puncture wound with foreign body of hand

7ᵀ **S61.441** Puncture wound with foreign body of right hand POA

7ᵀ **S61.442** Puncture wound with foreign body of left hand POA

7ᵀ **S61.449** Puncture wound with foreign body of unspecified hand POA

6ᵀ **S61.45** Open bite of hand
Bite of hand NOS
EXCLUDES1 superficial bite of hand (S60.56-, S60.57-)

7ᵀ **S61.451** Open bite of right hand POA

7ᵀ **S61.452** Open bite of left hand POA

7ᵀ **S61.459** Open bite of unspecified hand POA

5ᵀ **S61.5** Open wound of wrist

6ᵀ **S61.50** Unspecified open wound of wrist

7ᵀ **S61.501** Unspecified open wound of right wrist POA

7ᵀ **S61.502** Unspecified open wound of left wrist POA

7ᵀ **S61.509** Unspecified open wound of unspecified wrist POA

6ᵀ **S61.51** Laceration without foreign body of wrist

7ᵀ **S61.511** Laceration without foreign body of right wrist POA

7ᵀ **S61.512** Laceration without foreign body of left wrist POA

7ᵀ **S61.519** Laceration without foreign body of unspecified wrist POA

[6th] S61.52 Laceration with foreign body of wrist
[7th] S61.521 Laceration with foreign body of right wrist [POA]
[7th] S61.522 Laceration with foreign body of left wrist [POA]
[7th] S61.529 Laceration with foreign body of unspecified wrist [POA]
[6th] S61.53 Puncture wound without foreign body of wrist
[7th] S61.531 Puncture wound without foreign body of right wrist [POA]
[7th] S61.532 Puncture wound without foreign body of left wrist [POA]
[7th] S61.539 Puncture wound without foreign body of unspecified wrist [POA]
[6th] S61.54 Puncture wound with foreign body of wrist
[7th] S61.541 Puncture wound with foreign body of right wrist [POA]
[7th] S61.542 Puncture wound with foreign body of left wrist [POA]
[7th] S61.549 Puncture wound with foreign body of unspecified wrist [POA]
[6th] S61.55 Open bite of wrist
Bite of wrist NOS
[EXCLUDES1] *superficial bite of wrist (S60.86-, S60.87-)*
[7th] S61.551 Open bite of right wrist [POA]
[7th] S61.552 Open bite of left wrist [POA]
[7th] S61.559 Open bite of unspecified wrist [POA]

[4th] S62 Fracture at wrist and hand level
👁 See Official Guidelines "Coding of Traumatic Fractures" I.C.19.c
[NOTES] A fracture not indicated as displaced or nondisplaced should be coded to displaced
A fracture not indicated as open or closed should be coded to closed
[EXCLUDES1] *traumatic amputation of wrist and hand (S68.-)*
[EXCLUDES2] *fracture of distal parts of ulna and radius (S52.-)*
The appropriate 7th character is to be added to each code from category S62
A = initial encounter for closed fracture
B = initial encounter for open fracture
D = subsequent encounter for fracture with routine healing
G = subsequent encounter for fracture with delayed healing
K = subsequent encounter for fracture with nonunion
P = subsequent encounter for fracture with malunion
S = sequela

[5th] S62.0 Fracture of navicular [scaphoid] bone of wrist
[6th] S62.00 Unspecified fracture of navicular [scaphoid] bone of wrist
[7th] S62.001 Unspecified fracture of navicular [scaphoid] bone of right wrist [CC] [POA] [HAC] [CC/MCC Exc]
[7th] S62.002 Unspecified fracture of navicular [scaphoid] bone of left wrist [CC] [POA] [HAC] [CC/MCC Exc]
AHA: Q4 2012
[7th] S62.009 Unspecified fracture of navicular [scaphoid] bone of unspecified wrist [CC] [POA] [HAC] [CC/MCC Exc]
[6th] S62.01 Fracture of distal pole of navicular [scaphoid] bone of wrist
Fracture of volar tuberosity of navicular [scaphoid] bone of wrist
[7th] S62.011 Displaced fracture of distal pole of navicular [scaphoid] bone of right wrist [CC] [POA] [HAC] [CC/MCC Exc]
[7th] S62.012 Displaced fracture of distal pole of navicular [scaphoid] bone of left wrist [CC] [POA] [HAC] [CC/MCC Exc]
[7th] S62.013 Displaced fracture of distal pole of navicular [scaphoid] bone of unspecified wrist [CC] [POA] [HAC] [CC/MCC Exc]
[7th] S62.014 Nondisplaced fracture of distal pole of navicular [scaphoid] bone of right wrist [CC] [POA] [HAC] [CC/MCC Exc]
[7th] S62.015 Nondisplaced fracture of distal pole of navicular [scaphoid] bone of left wrist [CC] [POA] [HAC] [CC/MCC Exc]
[7th] S62.016 Nondisplaced fracture of distal pole of navicular [scaphoid] bone of unspecified wrist [CC] [POA] [HAC] [CC/MCC Exc]
[6th] S62.02 Fracture of middle third of navicular [scaphoid] bone of wrist
[7th] S62.021 Displaced fracture of middle third of navicular [scaphoid] bone of right wrist [CC] [POA] [HAC] [CC/MCC Exc]
[7th] S62.022 Displaced fracture of middle third of navicular [scaphoid] bone of left wrist [CC] [POA] [HAC] [CC/MCC Exc]
[7th] S62.023 Displaced fracture of middle third of navicular [scaphoid] bone of unspecified wrist [CC] [POA] [HAC] [CC/MCC Exc]
[7th] S62.024 Nondisplaced fracture of middle third of navicular [scaphoid] bone of right wrist [CC] [POA] [HAC] [CC/MCC Exc]
[7th] S62.025 Nondisplaced fracture of middle third of navicular [scaphoid] bone of left wrist [CC] [POA] [HAC] [CC/MCC Exc]
[7th] S62.026 Nondisplaced fracture of middle third of navicular [scaphoid] bone of unspecified wrist [CC] [POA] [HAC] [CC/MCC Exc]
[6th] S62.03 Fracture of proximal third of navicular [scaphoid] bone of wrist
[7th] S62.031 Displaced fracture of proximal third of navicular [scaphoid] bone of right wrist [CC] [POA] [HAC] [CC/MCC Exc]
[7th] S62.032 Displaced fracture of proximal third of navicular [scaphoid] bone of left wrist [CC] [POA] [HAC] [CC/MCC Exc]
[7th] S62.033 Displaced fracture of proximal third of navicular [scaphoid] bone of unspecified wrist [CC] [POA] [HAC] [CC/MCC Exc]
[7th] S62.034 Nondisplaced fracture of proximal third of navicular [scaphoid] bone of right wrist [CC] [POA] [HAC] [CC/MCC Exc]
[7th] S62.035 Nondisplaced fracture of proximal third of navicular [scaphoid] bone of left wrist [CC] [POA] [HAC] [CC/MCC Exc]
[7th] S62.036 Nondisplaced fracture of proximal third of navicular [scaphoid] bone of unspecified wrist [CC] [POA] [HAC] [CC/MCC Exc]

[5th] S62.1 Fracture of other and unspecified carpal bone(s)
[EXCLUDES2] *fracture of scaphoid of wrist (S62.0-)*
[6th] S62.10 Fracture of unspecified carpal bone
Fracture of wrist NOS
[7th] S62.101 Fracture of unspecified carpal bone, right wrist [CC] [POA] [HAC] [CC/MCC Exc]
[7th] S62.102 Fracture of unspecified carpal bone, left wrist [CC] [POA] [HAC] [CC/MCC Exc]
AHA: Q4 2012
[7th] S62.109 Fracture of unspecified carpal bone, unspecified wrist [CC] [POA] [HAC] [CC/MCC Exc]
[6th] S62.11 Fracture of triquetrum [cuneiform] bone of wrist
[7th] S62.111 Displaced fracture of triquetrum [cuneiform] bone, right wrist [CC] [POA] [HAC] [CC/MCC Exc]
[7th] S62.112 Displaced fracture of triquetrum [cuneiform] bone, left wrist [CC] [POA] [HAC] [CC/MCC Exc]
[7th] S62.113 Displaced fracture of triquetrum [cuneiform] bone, unspecified wrist [CC] [POA] [HAC] [CC/MCC Exc]
[7th] S62.114 Nondisplaced fracture of triquetrum [cuneiform] bone, right wrist [CC] [POA] [HAC] [CC/MCC Exc]
[7th] S62.115 Nondisplaced fracture of triquetrum [cuneiform] bone, left wrist [CC] [POA] [HAC] [CC/MCC Exc]

[PDx] Unacceptable principal diagnosis symbol per Medicare code edits [POA] Code exempt from diagnosis present on admission requirement
[?] Questionable admission [CC] Complication or comorbidity [MCC] Major complication or comorbidity [CC/MCC Exc] CC/MCC exclusion
[HCC] HCC diagnosis code [RxHCC] RxHCC diagnosis code MACRA code **DEFINITION** Describes condition/terminology
TIP Coding guidance 👁 Official Guideline Reference [Z1] Z code as first-listed diagnosis

When symbols appear on a code that requires a 7th character extension, refer to Appendix B to identify applicable 7th character codes.

⑦ S62.116 Nondisplaced fracture of triquetrum [cuneiform] bone, unspecified wrist   CC POA HAC CC/MCC Exc

⑥ S62.12 Fracture of lunate [semilunar]

  ⑦ S62.121 Displaced fracture of lunate [semilunar], right wrist   CC POA HAC CC/MCC Exc

  ⑦ S62.122 Displaced fracture of lunate [semilunar], left wrist   CC POA HAC CC/MCC Exc

  ⑦ S62.123 Displaced fracture of lunate [semilunar], unspecified wrist   CC POA HAC CC/MCC Exc

  ⑦ S62.124 Nondisplaced fracture of lunate [semilunar], right wrist

  ⑦ S62.125 Nondisplaced fracture of lunate [semilunar], left wrist   CC POA HAC CC/MCC Exc

  ⑦ S62.126 Nondisplaced fracture of lunate [semilunar], unspecified wrist   CC POA HAC CC/MCC Exc

⑥ S62.13 Fracture of capitate [os magnum] bone

  ⑦ S62.131 Displaced fracture of capitate [os magnum] bone, right wrist   CC POA HAC CC/MCC Exc

  ⑦ S62.132 Displaced fracture of capitate [os magnum] bone, left wrist   CC POA HAC CC/MCC Exc

  ⑦ S62.133 Displaced fracture of capitate [os magnum] bone, unspecified wrist   CC POA HAC CC/MCC Exc

  ⑦ S62.134 Nondisplaced fracture of capitate [os magnum] bone, right wrist   CC POA HAC CC/MCC Exc

  ⑦ S62.135 Nondisplaced fracture of capitate [os magnum] bone, left wrist   CC POA HAC CC/MCC Exc

  ⑦ S62.136 Nondisplaced fracture of capitate [os magnum] bone, unspecified wrist   CC POA HAC CC/MCC Exc

⑥ S62.14 Fracture of body of hamate [unciform] bone

Fracture of hamate [unciform] bone NOS

  ⑦ S62.141 Displaced fracture of body of hamate [unciform] bone, right wrist   CC POA HAC CC/MCC Exc

  ⑦ S62.142 Displaced fracture of body of hamate [unciform] bone, left wrist   CC POA HAC CC/MCC Exc

  ⑦ S62.143 Displaced fracture of body of hamate [unciform] bone, unspecified wrist   CC POA HAC CC/MCC Exc

  ⑦ S62.144 Nondisplaced fracture of body of hamate [unciform] bone, right wrist   CC POA HAC CC/MCC Exc

  ⑦ S62.145 Nondisplaced fracture of body of hamate [unciform] bone, left wrist   CC POA HAC CC/MCC Exc

  ⑦ S62.146 Nondisplaced fracture of body of hamate [unciform] bone, unspecified wrist   CC POA HAC CC/MCC Exc

⑥ S62.15 Fracture of hook process of hamate [unciform] bone

Fracture of unciform process of hamate [unciform] bone

  ⑦ S62.151 Displaced fracture of hook process of hamate [unciform] bone, right wrist   CC POA HAC CC/MCC Exc

  ⑦ S62.152 Displaced fracture of hook process of hamate [unciform] bone, left wrist   CC POA HAC CC/MCC Exc

  ⑦ S62.153 Displaced fracture of hook process of hamate [unciform] bone, unspecified wrist   CC POA HAC CC/MCC Exc

  ⑦ S62.154 Nondisplaced fracture of hook process of hamate [unciform] bone, right wrist   CC POA HAC CC/MCC Exc

  ⑦ S62.155 Nondisplaced fracture of hook process of hamate [unciform] bone, left wrist   CC POA HAC CC/MCC Exc

  ⑦ S62.156 Nondisplaced fracture of hook process of hamate [unciform] bone, unspecified wrist   CC POA HAC CC/MCC Exc

⑥ S62.16 Fracture of pisiform

  ⑦ S62.161 Displaced fracture of pisiform, right wrist   CC POA HAC CC/MCC Exc

  ⑦ S62.162 Displaced fracture of pisiform, left wrist   CC POA HAC CC/MCC Exc

  ⑦ S62.163 Displaced fracture of pisiform, unspecified wrist   CC POA HAC CC/MCC Exc

  ⑦ S62.164 Nondisplaced fracture of pisiform, right wrist   CC POA HAC CC/MCC Exc

  ⑦ S62.165 Nondisplaced fracture of pisiform, left wrist   CC POA HAC CC/MCC Exc

  ⑦ S62.166 Nondisplaced fracture of pisiform, unspecified wrist   CC POA HAC CC/MCC Exc

⑥ S62.17 Fracture of trapezium [larger multangular]

  ⑦ S62.171 Displaced fracture of trapezium [larger multangular], right wrist   CC POA HAC CC/MCC Exc

  ⑦ S62.172 Displaced fracture of trapezium [larger multangular], left wrist   CC POA HAC CC/MCC Exc

  ⑦ S62.173 Displaced fracture of trapezium [larger multangular], unspecified wrist   CC POA HAC CC/MCC Exc

  ⑦ S62.174 Nondisplaced fracture of trapezium [larger multangular], right wrist   CC POA HAC CC/MCC Exc

  ⑦ S62.175 Nondisplaced fracture of trapezium [larger multangular], left wrist   CC POA HAC CC/MCC Exc

  ⑦ S62.176 Nondisplaced fracture of trapezium [larger multangular], unspecified wrist   CC POA HAC CC/MCC Exc

⑥ S62.18 Fracture of trapezoid [smaller multangular]

  ⑦ S62.181 Displaced fracture of trapezoid [smaller multangular], right wrist   CC POA HAC CC/MCC Exc

  ⑦ S62.182 Displaced fracture of trapezoid [smaller multangular], left wrist   CC POA HAC CC/MCC Exc

  ⑦ S62.183 Displaced fracture of trapezoid [smaller multangular], unspecified wrist   CC POA HAC CC/MCC Exc

  ⑦ S62.184 Nondisplaced fracture of trapezoid [smaller multangular], right wrist   CC POA HAC CC/MCC Exc

  ⑦ S62.185 Nondisplaced fracture of trapezoid [smaller multangular], left wrist   CC POA HAC CC/MCC Exc

  ⑦ S62.186 Nondisplaced fracture of trapezoid [smaller multangular], unspecified wrist   CC POA HAC CC/MCC Exc

⑤ S62.2 Fracture of first metacarpal bone

  ⑥ S62.20 Unspecified fracture of first metacarpal bone

    ⑦ S62.201 Unspecified fracture of first metacarpal bone, right hand   CC POA HAC CC/MCC Exc

    ⑦ S62.202 Unspecified fracture of first metacarpal bone, left hand   CC POA HAC CC/MCC Exc

    ⑦ S62.209 Unspecified fracture of first metacarpal bone, unspecified hand   CC POA HAC CC/MCC Exc

  ⑥ S62.21 Bennett's fracture

    ⑦ S62.211 Bennett's fracture, right hand   CC POA HAC CC/MCC Exc

    ⑦ S62.212 Bennett's fracture, left hand   CC POA HAC CC/MCC Exc

    ⑦ S62.213 Bennett's fracture, unspecified hand   CC POA HAC CC/MCC Exc

  ⑥ S62.22 Rolando's fracture

    ⑦ S62.221 Displaced Rolando's fracture, right hand   CC POA HAC CC/MCC Exc

    ⑦ S62.222 Displaced Rolando's fracture, left hand   CC POA HAC CC/MCC Exc

    ⑦ S62.223 Displaced Rolando's fracture, unspecified hand   CC POA HAC CC/MCC Exc

    ⑦ S62.224 Nondisplaced Rolando's fracture, right hand   CC POA HAC CC/MCC Exc

    ⑦ S62.225 Nondisplaced Rolando's fracture, left hand   CC POA HAC CC/MCC Exc

    ⑦ S62.226 Nondisplaced Rolando's fracture, unspecified hand   CC POA HAC CC/MCC Exc

  ⑥ S62.23 Other fracture of base of first metacarpal bone

    ⑦ S62.231 Other displaced fracture of base of first metacarpal bone, right hand   POA HAC CC/MCC Exc

---

Unspecified Code   Other Specified Code   Manifestation Code   N Newborn   P Pediatric   M Maternity   A Adult   ♂ Male   ♀ Female
● New Code   ▲ Revised Code Title   ▶◀ Revised Text   **NOTES**   *INCLUDES*   *EXCLUDES1* Not coded here   *EXCLUDES2* Not included here
⑦ 4th character required   ⑤ 5th character required   ⑥ 6th character required   ⑦ 7th character required   ⑦ Extension 'X' Alert
HAC Hospital-acquired condition (HAC) alert   AHA AHA Coding Clinic©   ☛ Code first alert

S62.232 and S62.331 (side tab)

CHAPTER 19: INJURY, POISONING, AND CERTAIN OTHER CONSEQUENCES OF EXTERNAL CAUSES (S00-T88) (side tab)

7ᵗʰ S62.232 Other displaced fracture of base of first metacarpal bone, left hand cc poa HAC cc/mcc exc

7ᵗʰ S62.233 Other displaced fracture of base of first metacarpal bone, unspecified hand cc poa HAC cc/mcc exc

7ᵗʰ S62.234 Other nondisplaced fracture of base of first metacarpal bone, right hand cc poa HAC cc/mcc exc

7ᵗʰ S62.235 Other nondisplaced fracture of base of first metacarpal bone, left hand cc poa HAC cc/mcc exc

7ᵗʰ S62.236 Other nondisplaced fracture of base of first metacarpal bone, unspecified hand cc poa HAC cc/mcc exc

6ᵗʰ S62.24 Fracture of shaft of first metacarpal bone

7ᵗʰ S62.241 Displaced fracture of shaft of first metacarpal bone, right hand cc poa HAC cc/mcc exc

7ᵗʰ S62.242 Displaced fracture of shaft of first metacarpal bone, left hand cc poa HAC cc/mcc exc

7ᵗʰ S62.243 Displaced fracture of shaft of first metacarpal bone, unspecified hand cc poa HAC cc/mcc exc

7ᵗʰ S62.244 Nondisplaced fracture of shaft of first metacarpal bone, right hand cc poa HAC cc/mcc exc

7ᵗʰ S62.245 Nondisplaced fracture of shaft of first metacarpal bone, left hand cc poa HAC cc/mcc exc

7ᵗʰ S62.246 Nondisplaced fracture of shaft of first metacarpal bone, unspecified hand cc poa HAC cc/mcc exc

6ᵗʰ S62.25 Fracture of neck of first metacarpal bone

7ᵗʰ S62.251 Displaced fracture of neck of first metacarpal bone, right hand cc poa HAC cc/mcc exc

7ᵗʰ S62.252 Displaced fracture of neck of first metacarpal bone, left hand cc poa HAC cc/mcc exc

7ᵗʰ S62.253 Displaced fracture of neck of first metacarpal bone, unspecified hand cc poa HAC cc/mcc exc

7ᵗʰ S62.254 Nondisplaced fracture of neck of first metacarpal bone, right hand cc poa HAC cc/mcc exc

7ᵗʰ S62.255 Nondisplaced fracture of neck of first metacarpal bone, left hand cc poa HAC cc/mcc exc

7ᵗʰ S62.256 Nondisplaced fracture of neck of first metacarpal bone, unspecified hand cc poa HAC cc/mcc exc

6ᵗʰ S62.29 Other fracture of first metacarpal bone

7ᵗʰ S62.291 Other fracture of first metacarpal bone, right hand cc poa HAC cc/mcc exc

7ᵗʰ S62.292 Other fracture of first metacarpal bone, left hand cc poa HAC cc/mcc exc

7ᵗʰ S62.299 Other fracture of first metacarpal bone, unspecified hand cc poa HAC cc/mcc exc

5ᵗʰ S62.3 Fracture of other and unspecified metacarpal bone

EXCLUDES2 fracture of first metacarpal bone (S62.2-)

6ᵗʰ S62.30 Unspecified fracture of other metacarpal bone

7ᵗʰ S62.300 Unspecified fracture of second metacarpal bone, right hand cc poa HAC cc/mcc exc

7ᵗʰ S62.301 Unspecified fracture of second metacarpal bone, left hand cc poa HAC cc/mcc exc

7ᵗʰ S62.302 Unspecified fracture of third metacarpal bone, right hand cc poa HAC cc/mcc exc

7ᵗʰ S62.303 Unspecified fracture of third metacarpal bone, left hand cc poa HAC cc/mcc exc

7ᵗʰ S62.304 Unspecified fracture of fourth metacarpal bone, right hand cc poa HAC cc/mcc exc

7ᵗʰ S62.305 Unspecified fracture of fourth metacarpal bone, left hand cc poa HAC cc/mcc exc

7ᵗʰ S62.306 Unspecified fracture of fifth metacarpal bone, right hand cc poa HAC cc/mcc exc

7ᵗʰ S62.307 Unspecified fracture of fifth metacarpal bone, left hand cc poa HAC cc/mcc exc

7ᵗʰ S62.308 Unspecified fracture of other metacarpal bone cc poa HAC cc/mcc exc

Unspecified fracture of specified metacarpal bone with unspecified laterality

7ᵗʰ S62.309 Unspecified fracture of unspecified metacarpal bone

6ᵗʰ S62.31 Displaced fracture of base of other metacarpal bone

7ᵗʰ S62.310 Displaced fracture of base of second metacarpal bone, right hand cc poa HAC cc/mcc exc

7ᵗʰ S62.311 Displaced fracture of base of second metacarpal bone, left hand cc poa HAC cc/mcc exc

7ᵗʰ S62.312 Displaced fracture of base of third metacarpal bone, right hand cc poa HAC cc/mcc exc

7ᵗʰ S62.313 Displaced fracture of base of third metacarpal bone, left hand cc poa HAC cc/mcc exc

7ᵗʰ S62.314 Displaced fracture of base of fourth metacarpal bone, right hand cc poa HAC cc/mcc exc

7ᵗʰ S62.315 Displaced fracture of base of fourth metacarpal bone, left hand cc poa HAC cc/mcc exc

7ᵗʰ S62.316 Displaced fracture of base of fifth metacarpal bone, right hand cc poa HAC cc/mcc exc

7ᵗʰ S62.317 Displaced fracture of base of fifth metacarpal bone, left hand cc poa HAC cc/mcc exc

7ᵗʰ S62.318 Displaced fracture of base of other metacarpal bone cc poa HAC cc/mcc exc

Displaced fracture of base of specified metacarpal bone with unspecified laterality

7ᵗʰ S62.319 Displaced fracture of base of unspecified metacarpal bone cc poa HAC cc/mcc exc

6ᵗʰ S62.32 Displaced fracture of shaft of other metacarpal bone

7ᵗʰ S62.320 Displaced fracture of shaft of second metacarpal bone, right hand cc poa HAC cc/mcc exc

7ᵗʰ S62.321 Displaced fracture of shaft of second metacarpal bone, left hand cc poa HAC cc/mcc exc

7ᵗʰ S62.322 Displaced fracture of shaft of third metacarpal bone, right hand cc poa HAC cc/mcc exc

7ᵗʰ S62.323 Displaced fracture of shaft of third metacarpal bone, left hand cc poa HAC cc/mcc exc

7ᵗʰ S62.324 Displaced fracture of shaft of fourth metacarpal bone, right hand cc poa HAC cc/mcc exc

7ᵗʰ S62.325 Displaced fracture of shaft of fourth metacarpal bone, left hand cc poa HAC cc/mcc exc

7ᵗʰ S62.326 Displaced fracture of shaft of fifth metacarpal bone, right hand cc poa HAC cc/mcc exc

7ᵗʰ S62.327 Displaced fracture of shaft of fifth metacarpal bone, left hand cc poa HAC cc/mcc exc

7ᵗʰ S62.328 Displaced fracture of shaft of other metacarpal bone cc poa HAC cc/mcc exc

Displaced fracture of shaft of specified metacarpal bone with unspecified laterality

7ᵗʰ S62.329 Displaced fracture of shaft of unspecified metacarpal bone cc poa HAC cc/mcc exc

6ᵗʰ S62.33 Displaced fracture of neck of other metacarpal bone

7ᵗʰ S62.330 Displaced fracture of neck of second metacarpal bone, right hand cc poa HAC cc/mcc exc

7ᵗʰ S62.331 Displaced fracture of neck of second metacarpal bone, left hand cc poa HAC cc/mcc exc

PDxᴵⁿ Unacceptable principal diagnosis symbol per Medicare code edits   poa Code exempt from diagnosis present on admission requirement
? Questionable admission   cc Complication or comorbidity   mcc Major complication or comorbidity   cc/mcc exc CC/MCC exclusion
HCC HCC diagnosis code   RxHCC RxHCC diagnosis code   MACRA code   DEFINITION Describes condition/terminology
TIP Coding guidance   👁 Official Guideline Reference   Z1 Z code as first-listed diagnosis

1044   When symbols appear on a code that requires a 7th character extension, refer to Appendix B to identify applicable 7th character codes.   2020 ICD-10-CM

7ᵗʰ S62.332 **Displaced fracture of neck of** third **metacarpal bone,** right **hand** cᶜ pᵒᴬ **HAC** cc/mcc Exc

7ᵗʰ S62.333 **Displaced fracture of neck of** third **metacarpal bone,** left **hand** cᶜ pᵒᴬ **HAC** cc/mcc Exc

7ᵗʰ S62.334 **Displaced fracture of neck of** fourth **metacarpal bone,** right **hand** cᶜ pᵒᴬ **HAC** cc/mcc Exc

7ᵗʰ S62.335 **Displaced fracture of neck of** fourth **metacarpal bone,** left **hand** cᶜ pᵒᴬ **HAC** cc/mcc Exc

7ᵗʰ S62.336 **Displaced fracture of neck of** fifth **metacarpal bone,** right **hand** cᶜ pᵒᴬ **HAC** cc/mcc Exc

7ᵗʰ S62.337 **Displaced fracture of neck of** fifth **metacarpal bone,** left **hand** cᶜ pᵒᴬ **HAC** cc/mcc Exc

7ᵗʰ S62.338 **Displaced fracture of neck of** other **metacarpal bone** cᶜ pᵒᴬ **HAC** cc/mcc Exc

Displaced fracture of neck of specified metacarpal bone with unspecified laterality

7ᵗʰ S62.339 **Displaced fracture of neck of unspecified metacarpal bone** cᶜ pᵒᴬ **HAC** cc/mcc Exc

6ᵗʰ S62.34 Nondisplaced fracture of base **of other metacarpal bone**

7ᵗʰ S62.340 **Nondisplaced fracture of base of** second **metacarpal bone,** right **hand** cᶜ pᵒᴬ **HAC** cc/mcc Exc

7ᵗʰ S62.341 **Nondisplaced fracture of base of** second **metacarpal bone,** left **hand** cᶜ pᵒᴬ **HAC** cc/mcc Exc

7ᵗʰ S62.342 **Nondisplaced fracture of base of** third **metacarpal bone,** right **hand** cᶜ pᵒᴬ **HAC** cc/mcc Exc

7ᵗʰ S62.343 **Nondisplaced fracture of base of** third **metacarpal bone,** left **hand** cᶜ pᵒᴬ **HAC** cc/mcc Exc

7ᵗʰ S62.344 **Nondisplaced fracture of base of** fourth **metacarpal bone,** right **hand** cᶜ pᵒᴬ **HAC** cc/mcc Exc

7ᵗʰ S62.345 **Nondisplaced fracture of base of** fourth **metacarpal bone,** left **hand** cᶜ pᵒᴬ **HAC** cc/mcc Exc

7ᵗʰ S62.346 **Nondisplaced fracture of base of** fifth **metacarpal bone,** right **hand** cᶜ pᵒᴬ **HAC** cc/mcc Exc

7ᵗʰ S62.347 **Nondisplaced fracture of base of** fifth **metacarpal bone,** left **hand** cᶜ pᵒᴬ **HAC** cc/mcc Exc

7ᵗʰ S62.348 **Nondisplaced fracture of base of** other **metacarpal bone** cᶜ pᵒᴬ **HAC** cc/mcc Exc

Nondisplaced fracture of base of specified metacarpal bone with unspecified laterality

7ᵗʰ S62.349 **Nondisplaced fracture of base of unspecified metacarpal bone** cᶜ pᵒᴬ **HAC** cc/mcc Exc

6ᵗʰ S62.35 Nondisplaced fracture of shaft **of other metacarpal bone**

7ᵗʰ S62.350 **Nondisplaced fracture of shaft of** second **metacarpal bone,** right **hand** pᵒᴬ **HAC** cc/mcc Exc

7ᵗʰ S62.351 **Nondisplaced fracture of shaft of** second **metacarpal bone,** left **hand** cᶜ pᵒᴬ **HAC** cc/mcc Exc

7ᵗʰ S62.352 **Nondisplaced fracture of shaft of** third **metacarpal bone,** right **hand** cᶜ pᵒᴬ **HAC** cc/mcc Exc

7ᵗʰ S62.353 **Nondisplaced fracture of shaft of** third **metacarpal bone,** left **hand** cᶜ pᵒᴬ **HAC** cc/mcc Exc

7ᵗʰ S62.354 **Nondisplaced fracture of shaft of** fourth **metacarpal bone,** right **hand** cᶜ pᵒᴬ **HAC** cc/mcc Exc

7ᵗʰ S62.355 **Nondisplaced fracture of shaft of** fourth **metacarpal bone,** left **hand** cᶜ pᵒᴬ **HAC** cc/mcc Exc

7ᵗʰ S62.356 **Nondisplaced fracture of shaft of** fifth **metacarpal bone,** right **hand** cᶜ pᵒᴬ **HAC** cc/mcc Exc

7ᵗʰ S62.357 **Nondisplaced fracture of shaft of** fifth **metacarpal bone,** left **hand** cᶜ pᵒᴬ **HAC** cc/mcc Exc

7ᵗʰ S62.358 **Nondisplaced fracture of shaft of** other **metacarpal bone** cᶜ pᵒᴬ **HAC** cc/mcc Exc

Nondisplaced fracture of shaft of specified metacarpal bone with unspecified laterality

7ᵗʰ S62.359 **Nondisplaced fracture of shaft of unspecified metacarpal bone** cᶜ pᵒᴬ **HAC** cc/mcc Exc

6ᵗʰ S62.36 Nondisplaced fracture of neck **of other metacarpal bone**

7ᵗʰ S62.360 **Nondisplaced fracture of neck of** second **metacarpal bone,** right **hand** cᶜ pᵒᴬ **HAC** cc/mcc Exc

7ᵗʰ S62.361 **Nondisplaced fracture of neck of** second **metacarpal bone,** left **hand** cᶜ pᵒᴬ **HAC** cc/mcc Exc

7ᵗʰ S62.362 **Nondisplaced fracture of neck of** third **metacarpal bone,** right **hand** cᶜ pᵒᴬ **HAC** cc/mcc Exc

7ᵗʰ S62.363 **Nondisplaced fracture of neck of** third **metacarpal bone,** left **hand** cᶜ pᵒᴬ **HAC** cc/mcc Exc

7ᵗʰ S62.364 **Nondisplaced fracture of neck of** fourth **metacarpal bone,** right **hand** cᶜ pᵒᴬ **HAC** cc/mcc Exc

7ᵗʰ S62.365 **Nondisplaced fracture of neck of** fourth **metacarpal bone,** left **hand** cᶜ pᵒᴬ **HAC** cc/mcc Exc

7ᵗʰ S62.366 **Nondisplaced fracture of neck of** fifth **metacarpal bone,** right **hand** cᶜ pᵒᴬ **HAC** cc/mcc Exc

7ᵗʰ S62.367 **Nondisplaced fracture of neck of** fifth **metacarpal bone,** left **hand** cᶜ pᵒᴬ **HAC** cc/mcc Exc

7ᵗʰ S62.368 **Nondisplaced fracture of neck of** other **metacarpal bone** cᶜ pᵒᴬ **HAC** cc/mcc Exc

Nondisplaced fracture of neck of specified metacarpal bone with unspecified laterality

7ᵗʰ S62.369 **Nondisplaced fracture of neck of unspecified metacarpal bone** cᶜ pᵒᴬ **HAC** cc/mcc Exc

6ᵗʰ S62.39 Other fracture of other metacarpal bone

7ᵗʰ S62.390 **Other fracture of** second **metacarpal bone,** right **hand** cᶜ pᵒᴬ **HAC** cc/mcc Exc

7ᵗʰ S62.391 **Other fracture of** second **metacarpal bone,** left **hand** cᶜ pᵒᴬ **HAC** cc/mcc Exc

7ᵗʰ S62.392 **Other fracture of** third **metacarpal bone,** right **hand** cᶜ pᵒᴬ **HAC** cc/mcc Exc

7ᵗʰ S62.393 **Other fracture of** third **metacarpal bone,** left **hand** cᶜ pᵒᴬ **HAC** cc/mcc Exc

7ᵗʰ S62.394 **Other fracture of** fourth **metacarpal bone,** right **hand** cᶜ pᵒᴬ **HAC** cc/mcc Exc

7ᵗʰ S62.395 **Other fracture of** fourth **metacarpal bone,** left **hand** cᶜ pᵒᴬ **HAC** cc/mcc Exc

7ᵗʰ S62.396 **Other fracture of** fifth **metacarpal bone,** right **hand** cᶜ pᵒᴬ **HAC** cc/mcc Exc

7ᵗʰ S62.397 **Other fracture of** fifth **metacarpal bone,** left **hand** cᶜ pᵒᴬ **HAC** cc/mcc Exc

7ᵗʰ S62.398 **Other fracture of** other **metacarpal bone** cᶜ pᵒᴬ **HAC** cc/mcc Exc

Other fracture of specified metacarpal bone with unspecified laterality

7ᵗʰ S62.399 **Other fracture of unspecified metacarpal bone** cᶜ pᵒᴬ **HAC** cc/mcc Exc

5ᵗʰ S62.5 Fracture of thumb

6ᵗʰ S62.50 Fracture of unspecified phalanx of thumb

7ᵗʰ S62.501 **Fracture of unspecified phalanx of** right **thumb** cᶜ pᵒᴬ **HAC** cc/mcc Exc

7ᵗʰ S62.502 **Fracture of unspecified phalanx of** left **thumb** cᶜ pᵒᴬ **HAC** cc/mcc Exc

7ᵗʰ S62.509 **Fracture of unspecified phalanx of unspecified thumb** cᶜ pᵒᴬ **HAC** cc/mcc Exc

CHAPTER 19: INJURY, POISONING, AND CERTAIN OTHER CONSEQUENCES OF EXTERNAL CAUSES (S00-T88)

S62.51 - S62.648

6ᵗʰ **S62.51** Fracture of proximal phalanx of thumb
- 7ᵗʰ **S62.511** Displaced fracture of proximal phalanx of right **thumb** cc⊘ poⓧ HAC cc/mcc exc⊘
- 7ᵗʰ **S62.512** Displaced fracture of proximal phalanx of left **thumb** cc⊘ poⓧ HAC cc/mcc exc⊘
- 7ᵗʰ **S62.513** Displaced fracture of proximal phalanx of unspecified **thumb** cc⊘ poⓧ HAC cc/mcc exc⊘
- 7ᵗʰ **S62.514** Nondisplaced fracture of proximal phalanx of right **thumb** cc⊘ poⓧ HAC cc/mcc exc⊘
- 7ᵗʰ **S62.515** Nondisplaced fracture of proximal phalanx of left **thumb** cc⊘ poⓧ HAC cc/mcc exc⊘
- 7ᵗʰ **S62.516** Nondisplaced fracture of proximal phalanx of unspecified **thumb** cc⊘ poⓧ HAC cc/mcc exc⊘

6ᵗʰ **S62.52** Fracture of distal phalanx of thumb
- 7ᵗʰ **S62.521** Displaced fracture of distal phalanx of right **thumb** cc⊘ poⓧ HAC cc/mcc exc⊘
- 7ᵗʰ **S62.522** Displaced fracture of distal phalanx of left **thumb** cc⊘ poⓧ HAC cc/mcc exc⊘
- 7ᵗʰ **S62.523** Displaced fracture of distal phalanx of unspecified **thumb** cc⊘ poⓧ HAC cc/mcc exc⊘
- 7ᵗʰ **S62.524** Nondisplaced fracture of distal phalanx of right **thumb** cc⊘ poⓧ HAC cc/mcc exc⊘
- 7ᵗʰ **S62.525** Nondisplaced fracture of distal phalanx of left **thumb** cc⊘ poⓧ HAC cc/mcc exc⊘
- 7ᵗʰ **S62.526** Nondisplaced fracture of distal phalanx of unspecified **thumb** cc⊘ poⓧ HAC cc/mcc exc⊘

5ᵗʰ **S62.6** Fracture of other and unspecified finger(s)

EXCLUDES2 *fracture of thumb (S62.5-)*

6ᵗʰ **S62.60** Fracture of unspecified phalanx of finger
- 7ᵗʰ **S62.600** Fracture of unspecified phalanx of right index **finger** cc⊘ poⓧ HAC cc/mcc exc⊘
- 7ᵗʰ **S62.601** Fracture of unspecified phalanx of left index **finger** cc⊘ poⓧ HAC cc/mcc exc⊘
- 7ᵗʰ **S62.602** Fracture of unspecified phalanx of right middle **finger** cc⊘ poⓧ HAC cc/mcc exc⊘
- 7ᵗʰ **S62.603** Fracture of unspecified phalanx of left middle **finger** cc⊘ poⓧ HAC cc/mcc exc⊘
- 7ᵗʰ **S62.604** Fracture of unspecified phalanx of right ring **finger** cc⊘ poⓧ HAC cc/mcc exc⊘
- 7ᵗʰ **S62.605** Fracture of unspecified phalanx of left ring **finger** cc⊘ poⓧ HAC cc/mcc exc⊘
- 7ᵗʰ **S62.606** Fracture of unspecified phalanx of right little **finger** cc⊘ poⓧ HAC cc/mcc exc⊘
- 7ᵗʰ **S62.607** Fracture of unspecified phalanx of left little **finger** cc⊘ poⓧ HAC cc/mcc exc⊘
- 7ᵗʰ **S62.608** Fracture of unspecified phalanx of other **finger** cc⊘ poⓧ HAC cc/mcc exc⊘

  Fracture of unspecified phalanx of specified finger with unspecified laterality
- 7ᵗʰ **S62.609** Fracture of unspecified phalanx of unspecified **finger** cc⊘ poⓧ HAC cc/mcc exc⊘

6ᵗʰ **S62.61** Displaced fracture of proximal phalanx of finger
- 7ᵗʰ **S62.610** Displaced fracture of proximal phalanx of right index **finger** cc⊘ poⓧ HAC cc/mcc exc⊘
- 7ᵗʰ **S62.611** Displaced fracture of proximal phalanx of left index **finger** cc⊘ poⓧ HAC cc/mcc exc⊘
- 7ᵗʰ **S62.612** Displaced fracture of proximal phalanx of right middle **finger** cc⊘ poⓧ HAC cc/mcc exc⊘
- 7ᵗʰ **S62.613** Displaced fracture of proximal phalanx of left middle **finger** cc⊘ poⓧ HAC cc/mcc exc⊘
- 7ᵗʰ **S62.614** Displaced fracture of proximal phalanx of right ring **finger** cc⊘ poⓧ HAC cc/mcc exc⊘
- 7ᵗʰ **S62.615** Displaced fracture of proximal phalanx of left ring **finger** cc⊘ poⓧ HAC cc/mcc exc⊘
- 7ᵗʰ **S62.616** Displaced fracture of proximal phalanx of right little **finger** cc⊘ poⓧ HAC cc/mcc exc⊘
- 7ᵗʰ **S62.617** Displaced fracture of proximal phalanx of left little **finger** cc⊘ poⓧ HAC cc/mcc exc⊘
- 7ᵗʰ **S62.618** Displaced fracture of proximal phalanx of other **finger** cc⊘ poⓧ HAC cc/mcc exc⊘

  Displaced fracture of proximal phalanx of specified finger with unspecified laterality
- 7ᵗʰ **S62.619** Displaced fracture of proximal phalanx of unspecified **finger** cc⊘ poⓧ HAC cc/mcc exc⊘

6ᵗʰ **S62.62** Displaced fracture of middle phalanx of finger
- 7ᵗʰ **S62.620** Displaced fracture of middle phalanx of right index **finger** cc⊘ poⓧ HAC cc/mcc exc⊘
- 7ᵗʰ **S62.621** Displaced fracture of middle phalanx of left index **finger** cc⊘ poⓧ HAC cc/mcc exc⊘
- 7ᵗʰ **S62.622** Displaced fracture of middle phalanx of right middle **finger** cc⊘ poⓧ HAC cc/mcc exc⊘
- 7ᵗʰ **S62.623** Displaced fracture of middle phalanx of left middle **finger** cc⊘ poⓧ HAC cc/mcc exc⊘
- 7ᵗʰ **S62.624** Displaced fracture of middle phalanx of right ring **finger** cc⊘ poⓧ HAC cc/mcc exc⊘
- 7ᵗʰ **S62.625** Displaced fracture of middle phalanx of left ring **finger** cc⊘ poⓧ HAC cc/mcc exc⊘
- 7ᵗʰ **S62.626** Displaced fracture of middle phalanx of right little **finger** cc⊘ poⓧ HAC cc/mcc exc⊘
- 7ᵗʰ **S62.627** Displaced fracture of middle phalanx of left little **finger** cc⊘ poⓧ HAC cc/mcc exc⊘
- 7ᵗʰ **S62.628** Displaced fracture of middle phalanx of other **finger** cc⊘ poⓧ HAC cc/mcc exc⊘

  Displaced fracture of middle phalanx of specified finger with unspecified laterality
- 7ᵗʰ **S62.629** Displaced fracture of middle phalanx of unspecified **finger** cc⊘ poⓧ HAC cc/mcc exc⊘

6ᵗʰ **S62.63** Displaced fracture of distal phalanx of finger
- 7ᵗʰ **S62.630** Displaced fracture of distal phalanx of right index **finger** cc⊘ poⓧ HAC cc/mcc exc⊘
- 7ᵗʰ **S62.631** Displaced fracture of distal phalanx of left index **finger** cc⊘ poⓧ HAC cc/mcc exc⊘
- 7ᵗʰ **S62.632** Displaced fracture of distal phalanx of right middle **finger** cc⊘ poⓧ HAC cc/mcc exc⊘
- 7ᵗʰ **S62.633** Displaced fracture of distal phalanx of left middle **finger** cc⊘ poⓧ HAC cc/mcc exc⊘
- 7ᵗʰ **S62.634** Displaced fracture of distal phalanx of right ring **finger** cc⊘ poⓧ HAC cc/mcc exc⊘
- 7ᵗʰ **S62.635** Displaced fracture of distal phalanx of left ring **finger** cc⊘ poⓧ HAC cc/mcc exc⊘
- 7ᵗʰ **S62.636** Displaced fracture of distal phalanx of right little **finger** cc⊘ poⓧ HAC cc/mcc exc⊘
- 7ᵗʰ **S62.637** Displaced fracture of distal phalanx of left little **finger** cc⊘ poⓧ HAC cc/mcc exc⊘
- 7ᵗʰ **S62.638** Displaced fracture of distal phalanx of other **finger** cc⊘ poⓧ HAC cc/mcc exc⊘

  Displaced fracture of distal phalanx of specified finger with unspecified laterality
- 7ᵗʰ **S62.639** Displaced fracture of distal phalanx of unspecified **finger** cc⊘ poⓧ HAC cc/mcc exc⊘

6ᵗʰ **S62.64** Nondisplaced fracture of proximal phalanx of finger
- 7ᵗʰ **S62.640** Nondisplaced fracture of proximal phalanx of right index **finger** cc⊘ poⓧ HAC cc/mcc exc⊘
- 7ᵗʰ **S62.641** Nondisplaced fracture of proximal phalanx of left index **finger** cc⊘ poⓧ HAC cc/mcc exc⊘
- 7ᵗʰ **S62.642** Nondisplaced fracture of proximal phalanx of right middle **finger** cc⊘ poⓧ HAC cc/mcc exc⊘
- 7ᵗʰ **S62.643** Nondisplaced fracture of proximal phalanx of left middle **finger** cc⊘ poⓧ HAC cc/mcc exc⊘
- 7ᵗʰ **S62.644** Nondisplaced fracture of proximal phalanx of right ring **finger** cc⊘ poⓧ HAC cc/mcc exc⊘
- 7ᵗʰ **S62.645** Nondisplaced fracture of proximal phalanx of left ring **finger** cc⊘ poⓧ HAC cc/mcc exc⊘
- 7ᵗʰ **S62.646** Nondisplaced fracture of proximal phalanx of right little **finger** cc⊘ poⓧ HAC cc/mcc exc⊘
- 7ᵗʰ **S62.647** Nondisplaced fracture of proximal phalanx of left little **finger** cc⊘ poⓧ HAC cc/mcc exc⊘
- 7ᵗʰ **S62.648** Nondisplaced fracture of proximal phalanx of other **finger** cc⊘ poⓧ HAC cc/mcc exc⊘

  Nondisplaced fracture of proximal phalanx of specified finger with unspecified laterality

---

poⓧ Unacceptable principal diagnosis symbol per Medicare code edits ⓧ Code exempt from diagnosis present on admission requirement
❓ Questionable admission cc⊘ Complication or comorbidity mcc⊘ Major complication or comorbidity cc/mcc exc⊘ CC/MCC exclusion
HCC HCC diagnosis code RxHCC RxHCC diagnosis code MACRA code **DEFINITION** Describes condition/terminology
TIP Coding guidance 👁 Official Guideline Reference Ⓩ Z code as first-listed diagnosis

[7th] S62.649 **Nondisplaced fracture of proximal phalanx of unspecified finger** [CC] [POA] [HAC] [CC/MCC Exc]

[6th] S62.65 **Nondisplaced fracture of middle phalanx of finger**

[7th] S62.650 **Nondisplaced fracture of middle phalanx of right index finger** [CC] [POA] [HAC] [CC/MCC Exc]

[7th] S62.651 **Nondisplaced fracture of middle phalanx of left index finger** [CC] [POA] [HAC] [CC/MCC Exc]

[7th] S62.652 **Nondisplaced fracture of middle phalanx of right middle finger** [CC] [POA] [HAC] [CC/MCC Exc]

[7th] S62.653 **Nondisplaced fracture of middle phalanx of left middle finger** [CC] [POA] [HAC] [CC/MCC Exc]

[7th] S62.654 **Nondisplaced fracture of middle phalanx of right ring finger** [CC] [POA] [HAC] [CC/MCC Exc]

[7th] S62.655 **Nondisplaced fracture of middle phalanx of left ring finger** [CC] [POA] [HAC] [CC/MCC Exc]

[7th] S62.656 **Nondisplaced fracture of middle phalanx of right little finger** [CC] [POA] [HAC] [CC/MCC Exc]

[7th] S62.657 **Nondisplaced fracture of middle phalanx of left little finger** [CC] [POA] [HAC] [CC/MCC Exc]

[7th] S62.658 **Nondisplaced fracture of middle phalanx of other finger** [CC] [POA] [HAC] [CC/MCC Exc]
Nondisplaced fracture of middle phalanx of specified finger with unspecified laterality

[7th] S62.659 **Nondisplaced fracture of middle phalanx of unspecified finger** [CC] [POA] [HAC] [CC/MCC Exc]

[6th] S62.66 **Nondisplaced fracture of distal phalanx of finger**

[7th] S62.660 **Nondisplaced fracture of distal phalanx of right index finger** [CC] [POA] [HAC] [CC/MCC Exc]

[7th] S62.661 **Nondisplaced fracture of distal phalanx of left index finger** [CC] [POA] [HAC] [CC/MCC Exc]

[7th] S62.662 **Nondisplaced fracture of distal phalanx of right middle finger** [CC] [POA] [HAC] [CC/MCC Exc]

[7th] S62.663 **Nondisplaced fracture of distal phalanx of left middle finger** [CC] [POA] [HAC] [CC/MCC Exc]

[7th] S62.664 **Nondisplaced fracture of distal phalanx of right ring finger** [CC] [POA] [HAC] [CC/MCC Exc]

[7th] S62.665 **Nondisplaced fracture of distal phalanx of left ring finger** [CC] [POA] [HAC] [CC/MCC Exc]

[7th] S62.666 **Nondisplaced fracture of distal phalanx of right little finger** [CC] [POA] [HAC] [CC/MCC Exc]

[7th] S62.667 **Nondisplaced fracture of distal phalanx of left little finger** [CC] [POA] [HAC] [CC/MCC Exc]

[7th] S62.668 **Nondisplaced fracture of distal phalanx of other finger** [CC] [POA] [HAC] [CC/MCC Exc]
Nondisplaced fracture of distal phalanx of specified finger with unspecified laterality

[7th] S62.669 **Nondisplaced fracture of distal phalanx of unspecified finger** [CC] [POA] [HAC] [CC/MCC Exc]

[5th] S62.9 **Unspecified fracture of wrist and hand**

[7th] S62.90 **Unspecified fracture of unspecified wrist and hand** [CC] [POA] [HAC] [CC/MCC Exc]

[7th] S62.91 **Unspecified fracture of right wrist and hand** [CC] [POA] [HAC] [CC/MCC Exc]

[7th] S62.92 **Unspecified fracture of left wrist and hand** [CC] [POA] [HAC] [CC/MCC Exc]

[4th] S63 **Dislocation and sprain of joints and ligaments at wrist and hand level**

INCLUDES *avulsion of joint or ligament at wrist and hand level*
laceration of cartilage, joint or ligament at wrist and hand level
sprain of cartilage, joint or ligament at wrist and hand level
traumatic hemarthrosis of joint or ligament at wrist and hand level
traumatic rupture of joint or ligament at wrist and hand level
traumatic subluxation of joint or ligament at wrist and hand level
traumatic tear of joint or ligament at wrist and hand level

Code also any associated open wound

EXCLUDES2 *strain of muscle, fascia and tendon of wrist and hand (S66.-)*

The appropriate 7th character is to be added to each code from category S63
A = initial encounter
D = subsequent encounter
S = sequela

[5th] S63.0 **Subluxation and dislocation of wrist and hand joints**

[6th] S63.00 **Unspecified subluxation and dislocation of wrist and hand**
Dislocation of carpal bone NOS
Dislocation of distal end of radius NOS
Subluxation of carpal bone NOS
Subluxation of distal end of radius NOS

[7th] S63.001 **Unspecified subluxation of right wrist and hand** [POA]

[7th] S63.002 **Unspecified subluxation of left wrist and hand** [POA]

[7th] S63.003 **Unspecified subluxation of unspecified wrist and hand** [POA]

[7th] S63.004 **Unspecified dislocation of right wrist and hand** [POA]

[7th] S63.005 **Unspecified dislocation of left wrist and hand** [POA]

[7th] S63.006 **Unspecified dislocation of unspecified wrist and hand** [POA]

[6th] S63.01 **Subluxation and dislocation of distal radioulnar joint**

[7th] S63.011 **Subluxation of distal radioulnar joint of right wrist** [POA]

[7th] S63.012 **Subluxation of distal radioulnar joint of left wrist** [POA]

[7th] S63.013 **Subluxation of distal radioulnar joint of unspecified wrist** [POA]

[7th] S63.014 **Dislocation of distal radioulnar joint of right wrist** [POA]

[7th] S63.015 **Dislocation of distal radioulnar joint of left wrist** [POA]

[7th] S63.016 **Dislocation of distal radioulnar joint of unspecified wrist** [POA]

[6th] S63.02 **Subluxation and dislocation of radiocarpal joint**

[7th] S63.021 **Subluxation of radiocarpal joint of right wrist** [POA]

[7th] S63.022 **Subluxation of radiocarpal joint of left wrist** [POA]

[7th] S63.023 **Subluxation of radiocarpal joint of unspecified wrist** [POA]

[7th] S63.024 **Dislocation of radiocarpal joint of right wrist** [POA]

[7th] S63.025 **Dislocation of radiocarpal joint of left wrist** [POA]

[7th] S63.026 **Dislocation of radiocarpal joint of unspecified wrist** [POA]

[6th] S63.03 **Subluxation and dislocation of midcarpal joint**

[7th] S63.031 **Subluxation of midcarpal joint of right wrist** [POA]

[7th] S63.032 **Subluxation of midcarpal joint of left wrist** [POA]

[7th] S63.033 **Subluxation of midcarpal joint of unspecified wrist** [POA]

[7th] S63.034 **Dislocation of midcarpal joint of right wrist** [POA]

[7th] S63.035 **Dislocation of midcarpal joint of left wrist** [POA]

[7th] S63.036 **Dislocation of midcarpal joint of unspecified wrist** [POA]

[6th] S63.04 **Subluxation and dislocation of carpometacarpal joint of thumb**
EXCLUDES2 *interphalangeal subluxation and dislocation of thumb (S63.1-)*

[7th] S63.041 **Subluxation of carpometacarpal joint of right thumb** [POA]

[7th] S63.042 **Subluxation of carpometacarpal joint of left thumb** [POA]

Unspecified Code | Other Specified Code | Manifestation Code | [N] Newborn | [P] Pediatric | [M] Maternity | [A] Adult | ♂ Male | ♀ Female
● New Code | ▲ Revised Code Title | ►◄ Revised Text | NOTES | INCLUDES | EXCLUDES1 Not coded here | EXCLUDES2 Not included here
[4th] 4th character required | [5th] 5th character required | [6th] 6th character required | [7th] 7th character required | [x7th] Extension 'X' Alert
[HAC] Hospital-acquired condition (HAC) alert | AHA AHA Coding Clinic© | ☞ Code first alert

7ᵗʰ S63.043 Subluxation of carpometacarpal joint of unspecified thumb ᴾᴼᴬ

7ᵗʰ S63.044 Dislocation of carpometacarpal joint of right thumb ᴾᴼᴬ

7ᵗʰ S63.045 Dislocation of carpometacarpal joint of left thumb ᴾᴼᴬ

7ᵗʰ S63.046 Dislocation of carpometacarpal joint of unspecified thumb ᴾᴼᴬ

6ᵗʰ S63.05 Subluxation and dislocation of other carpometacarpal joint

EXCLUDES2 subluxation and dislocation of carpometacarpal joint of thumb (S63.04-)

7ᵗʰ S63.051 Subluxation of other carpometacarpal joint of right hand ᴾᴼᴬ

7ᵗʰ S63.052 Subluxation of other carpometacarpal joint of left hand ᴾᴼᴬ

7ᵗʰ S63.053 Subluxation of other carpometacarpal joint of unspecified hand ᴾᴼᴬ

7ᵗʰ S63.054 Dislocation of other carpometacarpal joint of right hand ᴾᴼᴬ

7ᵗʰ S63.055 Dislocation of other carpometacarpal joint of left hand ᴾᴼᴬ

7ᵗʰ S63.056 Dislocation of other carpometacarpal joint of unspecified hand ᴾᴼᴬ

6ᵗʰ S63.06 Subluxation and dislocation of metacarpal (bone), proximal end

7ᵗʰ S63.061 Subluxation of metacarpal (bone), proximal end of right hand ᴾᴼᴬ

7ᵗʰ S63.062 Subluxation of metacarpal (bone), proximal end of left hand ᴾᴼᴬ

7ᵗʰ S63.063 Subluxation of metacarpal (bone), proximal end of unspecified hand ᴾᴼᴬ

7ᵗʰ S63.064 Dislocation of metacarpal (bone), proximal end of right hand ᴾᴼᴬ

7ᵗʰ S63.065 Dislocation of metacarpal (bone), proximal end of left hand ᴾᴼᴬ

7ᵗʰ S63.066 Dislocation of metacarpal (bone), proximal end of unspecified hand ᴾᴼᴬ

6ᵗʰ S63.07 Subluxation and dislocation of distal end of ulna

7ᵗʰ S63.071 Subluxation of distal end of right ulna ᴾᴼᴬ

7ᵗʰ S63.072 Subluxation of distal end of left ulna ᴾᴼᴬ

7ᵗʰ S63.073 Subluxation of distal end of unspecified ulna ᴾᴼᴬ

7ᵗʰ S63.074 Dislocation of distal end of right ulna ᴾᴼᴬ

7ᵗʰ S63.075 Dislocation of distal end of left ulna ᴾᴼᴬ

7ᵗʰ S63.076 Dislocation of distal end of unspecified ulna ᴾᴼᴬ

6ᵗʰ S63.09 Other subluxation and dislocation of wrist and hand

7ᵗʰ S63.091 Other subluxation of right wrist and hand ᴾᴼᴬ

7ᵗʰ S63.092 Other subluxation of left wrist and hand ᴾᴼᴬ

7ᵗʰ S63.093 Other subluxation of unspecified wrist and hand ᴾᴼᴬ

7ᵗʰ S63.094 Other dislocation of right wrist and hand ᴾᴼᴬ

7ᵗʰ S63.095 Other dislocation of left wrist and hand ᴾᴼᴬ

7ᵗʰ S63.096 Other dislocation of unspecified wrist and hand ᴾᴼᴬ

5ᵗʰ S63.1 Subluxation and dislocation of thumb

6ᵗʰ S63.10 Unspecified subluxation and dislocation of thumb

7ᵗʰ S63.101 Unspecified subluxation of right thumb ᴾᴼᴬ

7ᵗʰ S63.102 Unspecified subluxation of left thumb ᴾᴼᴬ

7ᵗʰ S63.103 Unspecified subluxation of unspecified thumb ᴾᴼᴬ

7ᵗʰ S63.104 Unspecified dislocation of right thumb ᴾᴼᴬ

7ᵗʰ S63.105 Unspecified dislocation of left thumb ᴾᴼᴬ

7ᵗʰ S63.106 Unspecified dislocation of unspecified thumb ᴾᴼᴬ

6ᵗʰ S63.11 Subluxation and dislocation of metacarpophalangeal joint of thumb

7ᵗʰ S63.111 Subluxation of metacarpophalangeal joint of right thumb ᴾᴼᴬ

7ᵗʰ S63.112 Subluxation of metacarpophalangeal joint of left thumb ᴾᴼᴬ

7ᵗʰ S63.113 Subluxation of metacarpophalangeal joint of unspecified thumb ᴾᴼᴬ

7ᵗʰ S63.114 Dislocation of metacarpophalangeal joint of right thumb ᴾᴼᴬ

7ᵗʰ S63.115 Dislocation of metacarpophalangeal joint of left thumb ᴾᴼᴬ

7ᵗʰ S63.116 Dislocation of metacarpophalangeal joint of unspecified thumb ᴾᴼᴬ

6ᵗʰ S63.12 Subluxation and dislocation of interphalangeal joint of thumb

7ᵗʰ S63.121 Subluxation of interphalangeal joint of right thumb ᴾᴼᴬ

7ᵗʰ S63.122 Subluxation of interphalangeal joint of left thumb ᴾᴼᴬ

7ᵗʰ S63.123 Subluxation of interphalangeal joint of unspecified thumb ᴾᴼᴬ

7ᵗʰ S63.124 Dislocation of interphalangeal joint of right thumb ᴾᴼᴬ

7ᵗʰ S63.125 Dislocation of interphalangeal joint of left thumb ᴾᴼᴬ

7ᵗʰ S63.126 Dislocation of interphalangeal joint of unspecified thumb ᴾᴼᴬ

5ᵗʰ S63.2 Subluxation and dislocation of other finger(s)

EXCLUDES2 subluxation and dislocation of thumb (S63.1-)

6ᵗʰ S63.20 Unspecified subluxation of other finger

7ᵗʰ S63.200 Unspecified subluxation of right index finger ᴾᴼᴬ

7ᵗʰ S63.201 Unspecified subluxation of left index finger ᴾᴼᴬ

7ᵗʰ S63.202 Unspecified subluxation of right middle finger ᴾᴼᴬ

7ᵗʰ S63.203 Unspecified subluxation of left middle finger ᴾᴼᴬ

7ᵗʰ S63.204 Unspecified subluxation of right ring finger ᴾᴼᴬ

7ᵗʰ S63.205 Unspecified subluxation of left ring finger ᴾᴼᴬ

7ᵗʰ S63.206 Unspecified subluxation of right little finger ᴾᴼᴬ

7ᵗʰ S63.207 Unspecified subluxation of left little finger ᴾᴼᴬ

7ᵗʰ S63.208 Unspecified subluxation of other finger ᴾᴼᴬ
Unspecified subluxation of specified finger with unspecified laterality

7ᵗʰ S63.209 Unspecified subluxation of unspecified finger ᴾᴼᴬ

6ᵗʰ S63.21 Subluxation of metacarpophalangeal joint of finger

7ᵗʰ S63.210 Subluxation of metacarpophalangeal joint of right index finger ᴾᴼᴬ

7ᵗʰ S63.211 Subluxation of metacarpophalangeal joint of left index finger ᴾᴼᴬ

7ᵗʰ S63.212 Subluxation of metacarpophalangeal joint of right middle finger ᴾᴼᴬ

7ᵗʰ S63.213 Subluxation of metacarpophalangeal joint of left middle finger ᴾᴼᴬ

7ᵗʰ S63.214 Subluxation of metacarpophalangeal joint of right ring finger ᴾᴼᴬ

7ᵗʰ S63.215 Subluxation of metacarpophalangeal joint of left ring finger ᴾᴼᴬ

7ᵗʰ S63.216 Subluxation of metacarpophalangeal joint of right little finger ᴾᴼᴬ

7ᵗʰ S63.217 Subluxation of metacarpophalangeal joint of left little finger ᴾᴼᴬ

7ᵗʰ S63.218 Subluxation of metacarpophalangeal joint of other finger ᴾᴼᴬ
Subluxation of metacarpophalangeal joint of specified finger with unspecified laterality

---

ᴾᴼᴬ Unacceptable principal diagnosis symbol per Medicare code edits   ᴾᴼᴬ Code exempt from diagnosis present on admission requirement
? Questionable admission   ᶜᶜ Complication or comorbidity   ᴹᶜᶜ Major complication or comorbidity   ᶜᶜ/ᴹᶜᶜ ᴱˣᶜ CC/MCC exclusion
HCC HCC diagnosis code   RxHCC RxHCC diagnosis code   MACRA MACRA code   **DEFINITION** Describes condition/terminology
TIP Coding guidance   👁 Official Guideline Reference   Z1 Z code as first-listed diagnosis

7ᵗʰ **S63.219** Subluxation of metacarpophalangeal joint of unspecified finger POA

6ᵗʰ **S63.22** Subluxation of unspecified interphalangeal joint of finger

7ᵗʰ **S63.220** Subluxation of unspecified interphalangeal joint of right index finger POA

7ᵗʰ **S63.221** Subluxation of unspecified interphalangeal joint of left index finger POA

7ᵗʰ **S63.222** Subluxation of unspecified interphalangeal joint of right middle finger POA

7ᵗʰ **S63.223** Subluxation of unspecified interphalangeal joint of left middle finger POA

7ᵗʰ **S63.224** Subluxation of unspecified interphalangeal joint of right ring finger POA

7ᵗʰ **S63.225** Subluxation of unspecified interphalangeal joint of left ring finger POA

7ᵗʰ **S63.226** Subluxation of unspecified interphalangeal joint of right little finger POA

7ᵗʰ **S63.227** Subluxation of unspecified interphalangeal joint of left little finger POA

7ᵗʰ **S63.228** Subluxation of unspecified interphalangeal joint of other finger POA
Subluxation of unspecified interphalangeal joint of specified finger with unspecified laterality

7ᵗʰ **S63.229** Subluxation of unspecified interphalangeal joint of unspecified finger POA

6ᵗʰ **S63.23** Subluxation of proximal interphalangeal joint of finger

7ᵗʰ **S63.230** Subluxation of proximal interphalangeal joint of right index finger POA

7ᵗʰ **S63.231** Subluxation of proximal interphalangeal joint of left index finger POA

7ᵗʰ **S63.232** Subluxation of proximal interphalangeal joint of right middle finger POA

7ᵗʰ **S63.233** Subluxation of proximal interphalangeal joint of left middle finger POA

7ᵗʰ **S63.234** Subluxation of proximal interphalangeal joint of right ring finger POA

7ᵗʰ **S63.235** Subluxation of proximal interphalangeal joint of left ring finger POA

7ᵗʰ **S63.236** Subluxation of proximal interphalangeal joint of right little finger POA

7ᵗʰ **S63.237** Subluxation of proximal interphalangeal joint of left little finger POA

7ᵗʰ **S63.238** Subluxation of proximal interphalangeal joint of other finger POA
Subluxation of proximal interphalangeal joint of specified finger with unspecified laterality

7ᵗʰ **S63.239** Subluxation of proximal interphalangeal joint of unspecified finger POA

6ᵗʰ **S63.24** Subluxation of distal interphalangeal joint of finger

7ᵗʰ **S63.240** Subluxation of distal interphalangeal joint of right index finger POA

7ᵗʰ **S63.241** Subluxation of distal interphalangeal joint of left index finger POA

7ᵗʰ **S63.242** Subluxation of distal interphalangeal joint of right middle finger POA

7ᵗʰ **S63.243** Subluxation of distal interphalangeal joint of left middle finger POA

7ᵗʰ **S63.244** Subluxation of distal interphalangeal joint of right ring finger POA

7ᵗʰ **S63.245** Subluxation of distal interphalangeal joint of left ring finger POA

7ᵗʰ **S63.246** Subluxation of distal interphalangeal joint of right little finger POA

7ᵗʰ **S63.247** Subluxation of distal interphalangeal joint of left little finger POA

7ᵗʰ **S63.248** Subluxation of distal interphalangeal joint of other finger POA
Subluxation of distal interphalangeal joint of specified finger with unspecified laterality

7ᵗʰ **S63.249** Subluxation of distal interphalangeal joint of unspecified finger POA

6ᵗʰ **S63.25** Unspecified dislocation of other finger

7ᵗʰ **S63.250** Unspecified dislocation of right index finger POA

7ᵗʰ **S63.251** Unspecified dislocation of left index finger POA

7ᵗʰ **S63.252** Unspecified dislocation of right middle finger POA

7ᵗʰ **S63.253** Unspecified dislocation of left middle finger POA

7ᵗʰ **S63.254** Unspecified dislocation of right ring finger POA

7ᵗʰ **S63.255** Unspecified dislocation of left ring finger POA

7ᵗʰ **S63.256** Unspecified dislocation of right little finger POA

7ᵗʰ **S63.257** Unspecified dislocation of left little finger POA

7ᵗʰ **S63.258** Unspecified dislocation of other finger POA
Unspecified dislocation of specified finger with unspecified laterality

7ᵗʰ **S63.259** Unspecified dislocation of unspecified finger POA
Unspecified dislocation of unspecified finger with unspecified laterality

6ᵗʰ **S63.26** Dislocation of metacarpophalangeal joint of finger

7ᵗʰ **S63.260** Dislocation of metacarpophalangeal joint of right index finger POA

7ᵗʰ **S63.261** Dislocation of metacarpophalangeal joint of left index finger POA

7ᵗʰ **S63.262** Dislocation of metacarpophalangeal joint of right middle finger POA

7ᵗʰ **S63.263** Dislocation of metacarpophalangeal joint of left middle finger POA

7ᵗʰ **S63.264** Dislocation of metacarpophalangeal joint of right ring finger POA

7ᵗʰ **S63.265** Dislocation of metacarpophalangeal joint of left ring finger POA

7ᵗʰ **S63.266** Dislocation of metacarpophalangeal joint of right little finger POA

7ᵗʰ **S63.267** Dislocation of metacarpophalangeal joint of left little finger POA

7ᵗʰ **S63.268** Dislocation of metacarpophalangeal joint of other finger POA
Dislocation of metacarpophalangeal joint of specified finger with unspecified laterality

7ᵗʰ **S63.269** Dislocation of metacarpophalangeal joint of unspecified finger POA

6ᵗʰ **S63.27** Dislocation of unspecified interphalangeal joint of finger

7ᵗʰ **S63.270** Dislocation of unspecified interphalangeal joint of right index finger POA

7ᵗʰ **S63.271** Dislocation of unspecified interphalangeal joint of left index finger POA

7ᵗʰ **S63.272** Dislocation of unspecified interphalangeal joint of right middle finger POA

7ᵗʰ **S63.273** Dislocation of unspecified interphalangeal joint of left middle finger POA

7ᵗʰ **S63.274** Dislocation of unspecified interphalangeal joint of right ring finger POA

7ᵗʰ **S63.275** Dislocation of unspecified interphalangeal joint of left ring finger POA

7ᵗʰ **S63.276** Dislocation of unspecified interphalangeal joint of right little finger POA

Unspecified Code   Other Specified Code   Manifestation Code   N Newborn   P Pediatric   M Maternity   A Adult   ♂ Male   ♀ Female
● New Code   ▲ Revised Code Title   ▶◀ Revised Text   **NOTES**   *INCLUDES*   *EXCLUDES1* Not coded here   *EXCLUDES2* Not included here
4ᵗʰ 4ᵗʰ character required   5ᵗʰ 5ᵗʰ character required   6ᵗʰ 6ᵗʰ character required   7ᵗʰ 7ᵗʰ character required   Extension 'X' Alert
HAC Hospital-acquired condition (HAC) alert   **AHA** AHA Coding Clinic®   ☞ Code first alert

S63.277 Dislocation of unspecified interphalangeal joint of left little finger

S63.278 Dislocation of unspecified interphalangeal joint of other finger

Dislocation of unspecified interphalangeal joint of specified finger with unspecified laterality

S63.279 Dislocation of unspecified interphalangeal joint of unspecified finger

Dislocation of unspecified interphalangeal joint of unspecified finger without specified laterality

S63.28 Dislocation of proximal interphalangeal joint of finger

S63.280 Dislocation of proximal interphalangeal joint of right index finger

S63.281 Dislocation of proximal interphalangeal joint of left index finger

S63.282 Dislocation of proximal interphalangeal joint of right middle finger

S63.283 Dislocation of proximal interphalangeal joint of left middle finger

S63.284 Dislocation of proximal interphalangeal joint of right ring finger

S63.285 Dislocation of proximal interphalangeal joint of left ring finger

S63.286 Dislocation of proximal interphalangeal joint of right little finger

S63.287 Dislocation of proximal interphalangeal joint of left little finger

S63.288 Dislocation of proximal interphalangeal joint of other finger

Dislocation of proximal interphalangeal joint of specified finger with unspecified laterality

S63.289 Dislocation of proximal interphalangeal joint of unspecified finger

S63.29 Dislocation of distal interphalangeal joint of finger

S63.290 Dislocation of distal interphalangeal joint of right index finger

S63.291 Dislocation of distal interphalangeal joint of left index finger

S63.292 Dislocation of distal interphalangeal joint of right middle finger

S63.293 Dislocation of distal interphalangeal joint of left middle finger

S63.294 Dislocation of distal interphalangeal joint of right ring finger

S63.295 Dislocation of distal interphalangeal joint of left ring finger

S63.296 Dislocation of distal interphalangeal joint of right little finger

S63.297 Dislocation of distal interphalangeal joint of left little finger

S63.298 Dislocation of distal interphalangeal joint of other finger

Dislocation of distal interphalangeal joint of specified finger with unspecified laterality

S63.299 Dislocation of distal interphalangeal joint of unspecified finger

S63.3 Traumatic rupture of ligament of wrist

S63.30 Traumatic rupture of unspecified ligament of wrist

S63.301 Traumatic rupture of unspecified ligament of right wrist

S63.302 Traumatic rupture of unspecified ligament of left wrist

S63.309 Traumatic rupture of unspecified ligament of unspecified wrist

S63.31 Traumatic rupture of collateral ligament of wrist

S63.311 Traumatic rupture of collateral ligament of right wrist

S63.312 Traumatic rupture of collateral ligament of left wrist

S63.319 Traumatic rupture of collateral ligament of unspecified wrist

S63.32 Traumatic rupture of radiocarpal ligament

S63.321 Traumatic rupture of right radiocarpal ligament

S63.322 Traumatic rupture of left radiocarpal ligament

S63.329 Traumatic rupture of unspecified radiocarpal ligament

S63.33 Traumatic rupture of ulnocarpal (palmar) ligament

S63.331 Traumatic rupture of right ulnocarpal (palmar) ligament

S63.332 Traumatic rupture of left ulnocarpal (palmar) ligament

S63.339 Traumatic rupture of unspecified ulnocarpal (palmar) ligament

S63.39 Traumatic rupture of other ligament of wrist

S63.391 Traumatic rupture of other ligament of right wrist

S63.392 Traumatic rupture of other ligament of left wrist

S63.399 Traumatic rupture of other ligament of unspecified wrist

S63.4 Traumatic rupture of ligament of finger at metacarpophalangeal and interphalangeal joint(s)

S63.40 Traumatic rupture of unspecified ligament of finger at metacarpophalangeal and interphalangeal joint

S63.400 Traumatic rupture of unspecified ligament of right index finger at metacarpophalangeal and interphalangeal joint

S63.401 Traumatic rupture of unspecified ligament of left index finger at metacarpophalangeal and interphalangeal joint

S63.402 Traumatic rupture of unspecified ligament of right middle finger at metacarpophalangeal and interphalangeal joint

S63.403 Traumatic rupture of unspecified ligament of left middle finger at metacarpophalangeal and interphalangeal joint

S63.404 Traumatic rupture of unspecified ligament of right ring finger at metacarpophalangeal and interphalangeal joint

S63.405 Traumatic rupture of unspecified ligament of left ring finger at metacarpophalangeal and interphalangeal joint

S63.406 Traumatic rupture of unspecified ligament of right little finger at metacarpophalangeal and interphalangeal joint

S63.407 Traumatic rupture of unspecified ligament of left little finger at metacarpophalangeal and interphalangeal joint

S63.408 Traumatic rupture of unspecified ligament of other finger at metacarpophalangeal and interphalangeal joint

Traumatic rupture of unspecified ligament of specified finger with unspecified laterality at metacarpophalangeal and interphalangeal joint

S63.409 Traumatic rupture of unspecified ligament of unspecified finger at metacarpophalangeal and interphalangeal joint

S63.41 Traumatic rupture of collateral ligament of finger at metacarpophalangeal and interphalangeal joint

PDxIR: Unacceptable principal diagnosis symbol per Medicare code edits   Code exempt from diagnosis present on admission requirement
? Questionable admission   Complication or comorbidity   MCC Major complication or comorbidity   CC/MCC Exc CC/MCC exclusion
HCC HCC diagnosis code   RxHCC RxHCC diagnosis code   MACRA code   **DEFINITION** Describes condition/terminology
TIP Coding guidance   Official Guideline Reference   Z1 Z code as first-listed diagnosis

1050   When symbols appear on a code that requires a 7th character extension, refer to Appendix B to identify applicable 7th character codes.   **2020 ICD-10-CM**

7️⃣ S63.410 Traumatic rupture of collateral ligament of right index finger at metacarpophalangeal and interphalangeal joint POA

7️⃣ S63.411 Traumatic rupture of collateral ligament of left index finger at metacarpophalangeal and interphalangeal joint POA

7️⃣ S63.412 Traumatic rupture of collateral ligament of right middle finger at metacarpophalangeal and interphalangeal joint POA

7️⃣ S63.413 Traumatic rupture of collateral ligament of left middle finger at metacarpophalangeal and interphalangeal joint POA

7️⃣ S63.414 Traumatic rupture of collateral ligament of right ring finger at metacarpophalangeal and interphalangeal joint POA

7️⃣ S63.415 Traumatic rupture of collateral ligament of left ring finger at metacarpophalangeal and interphalangeal joint POA

7️⃣ S63.416 Traumatic rupture of collateral ligament of right little finger at metacarpophalangeal and interphalangeal joint POA

7️⃣ S63.417 Traumatic rupture of collateral ligament of left little finger at metacarpophalangeal and interphalangeal joint POA

7️⃣ S63.418 Traumatic rupture of collateral ligament of other finger at metacarpophalangeal and interphalangeal joint POA

Traumatic rupture of collateral ligament of specified finger with unspecified laterality at metacarpophalangeal and interphalangeal joint

7️⃣ S63.419 Traumatic rupture of collateral ligament of unspecified finger at metacarpophalangeal and interphalangeal joint POA

6️⃣ S63.42 Traumatic rupture of palmar ligament of finger at metacarpophalangeal and interphalangeal joint

7️⃣ S63.420 Traumatic rupture of palmar ligament of right index finger at metacarpophalangeal and interphalangeal joint POA

7️⃣ S63.421 Traumatic rupture of palmar ligament of left index finger at metacarpophalangeal and interphalangeal joint POA

7️⃣ S63.422 Traumatic rupture of palmar ligament of right middle finger at metacarpophalangeal and interphalangeal joint POA

7️⃣ S63.423 Traumatic rupture of palmar ligament of left middle finger at metacarpophalangeal and interphalangeal joint POA

7️⃣ S63.424 Traumatic rupture of palmar ligament of right ring finger at metacarpophalangeal and interphalangeal joint POA

7️⃣ S63.425 Traumatic rupture of palmar ligament of left ring finger at metacarpophalangeal and interphalangeal joint POA

7️⃣ S63.426 Traumatic rupture of palmar ligament of right little finger at metacarpophalangeal and interphalangeal joint POA

7️⃣ S63.427 Traumatic rupture of palmar ligament of left little finger at metacarpophalangeal and interphalangeal joint POA

7️⃣ S63.428 Traumatic rupture of palmar ligament of other finger at metacarpophalangeal and interphalangeal joint POA

Traumatic rupture of palmar ligament of specified finger with unspecified laterality at metacarpophalangeal and interphalangeal joint

7️⃣ S63.429 Traumatic rupture of palmar ligament of unspecified finger at metacarpophalangeal and interphalangeal joint POA

6️⃣ S63.43 Traumatic rupture of volar plate of finger at metacarpophalangeal and interphalangeal joint

7️⃣ S63.430 Traumatic rupture of volar plate of right index finger at metacarpophalangeal and interphalangeal joint POA

7️⃣ S63.431 Traumatic rupture of volar plate of left index finger at metacarpophalangeal and interphalangeal joint POA

7️⃣ S63.432 Traumatic rupture of volar plate of right middle finger at metacarpophalangeal and interphalangeal joint POA

7️⃣ S63.433 Traumatic rupture of volar plate of left middle finger at metacarpophalangeal and interphalangeal joint POA

7️⃣ S63.434 Traumatic rupture of volar plate of right ring finger at metacarpophalangeal and interphalangeal joint POA

7️⃣ S63.435 Traumatic rupture of volar plate of left ring finger at metacarpophalangeal and interphalangeal joint POA

7️⃣ S63.436 Traumatic rupture of volar plate of right little finger at metacarpophalangeal and interphalangeal joint POA

7️⃣ S63.437 Traumatic rupture of volar plate of left little finger at metacarpophalangeal and interphalangeal joint POA

7️⃣ S63.438 Traumatic rupture of volar plate of other finger at metacarpophalangeal and interphalangeal joint POA

Traumatic rupture of volar plate of specified finger with unspecified laterality at metacarpophalangeal and interphalangeal joint

7️⃣ S63.439 Traumatic rupture of volar plate of unspecified finger at metacarpophalangeal and interphalangeal joint POA

6️⃣ S63.49 Traumatic rupture of other ligament of finger at metacarpophalangeal and interphalangeal joint

7️⃣ S63.490 Traumatic rupture of other ligament of right index finger at metacarpophalangeal and interphalangeal joint POA

7️⃣ S63.491 Traumatic rupture of other ligament of left index finger at metacarpophalangeal and interphalangeal joint POA

7️⃣ S63.492 Traumatic rupture of other ligament of right middle finger at metacarpophalangeal and interphalangeal joint POA

7️⃣ S63.493 Traumatic rupture of other ligament of left middle finger at metacarpophalangeal and interphalangeal joint POA

7️⃣ S63.494 Traumatic rupture of other ligament of right ring finger at metacarpophalangeal and interphalangeal joint POA

7️⃣ S63.495 Traumatic rupture of other ligament of left ring finger at metacarpophalangeal and interphalangeal joint POA

7️⃣ S63.496 Traumatic rupture of other ligament of right little finger at metacarpophalangeal and interphalangeal joint POA

7️⃣ S63.497 Traumatic rupture of other ligament of left little finger at metacarpophalangeal and interphalangeal joint POA

7️⃣ S63.498 Traumatic rupture of other ligament of other finger at metacarpophalangeal and interphalangeal joint POA

Traumatic rupture of ligament of specified finger with unspecified laterality at metacarpophalangeal and interphalangeal joint

---

	Unspecified Code	Other Specified Code	Manifestation Code	N Newborn	P Pediatric	M Maternity	A Adult	♂ Male	♀ Female

● New Code ▲ Revised Code Title ▶◀ Revised Text **NOTES** *INCLUDES* *EXCLUDES1* Not coded here *EXCLUDES2* Not included here

4️⃣ 4th character required 5️⃣ 5th character required 6️⃣ 6th character required 7️⃣ 7th character required ⊘ Extension 'X' Alert

HAC Hospital-acquired condition (HAC) alert **AHA** AHA Coding Clinic© ☛ Code first alert

S63.499 - S63.92 *(side margin)*

CHAPTER 19: INJURY, POISONING, AND CERTAIN OTHER CONSEQUENCES OF EXTERNAL CAUSES (S00-T88) *(side margin)*

7ᵗʰ S63.499 Traumatic rupture of other ligament of unspecified finger at metacarpophalangeal and interphalangeal joint POA

5ᵗʰ S63.5 Other and unspecified sprain of wrist
  6ᵗʰ S63.50 Unspecified sprain of wrist
    S63.501 Unspecified sprain of right wrist POA
    7ᵗʰ S63.502 Unspecified sprain of left wrist POA
    7ᵗʰ S63.509 Unspecified sprain of unspecified wrist POA
  6ᵗʰ S63.51 Sprain of carpal (joint)
    7ᵗʰ S63.511 Sprain of carpal joint of right wrist POA
    7ᵗʰ S63.512 Sprain of carpal joint of left wrist POA
    7ᵗʰ S63.519 Sprain of carpal joint of unspecified wrist POA
  6ᵗʰ S63.52 Sprain of radiocarpal joint
    EXCLUDES1 traumatic rupture of radiocarpal ligament (S63.32-)
    7ᵗʰ S63.521 Sprain of radiocarpal joint of right wrist POA
    7ᵗʰ S63.522 Sprain of radiocarpal joint of left wrist POA
    7ᵗʰ S63.529 Sprain of radiocarpal joint of unspecified wrist POA
  6ᵗʰ S63.59 Other specified sprain of wrist
    7ᵗʰ S63.591 Other specified sprain of right wrist POA
    7ᵗʰ S63.592 Other specified sprain of left wrist POA
    7ᵗʰ S63.599 Other specified sprain of unspecified wrist POA

5ᵗʰ S63.6 Other and unspecified sprain of finger(s)
  EXCLUDES1 traumatic rupture of ligament of finger at metacarpophalangeal and interphalangeal joint(s) (S63.4-)
  6ᵗʰ S63.60 Unspecified sprain of thumb
    7ᵗʰ S63.601 Unspecified sprain of right thumb POA
    7ᵗʰ S63.602 Unspecified sprain of left thumb POA
    7ᵗʰ S63.609 Unspecified sprain of unspecified thumb POA
  6ᵗʰ S63.61 Unspecified sprain of other and unspecified finger(s)
    7ᵗʰ S63.610 Unspecified sprain of right index finger POA
    7ᵗʰ S63.611 Unspecified sprain of left index finger POA
    7ᵗʰ S63.612 Unspecified sprain of right middle finger POA
    7ᵗʰ S63.613 Unspecified sprain of left middle finger POA
    7ᵗʰ S63.614 Unspecified sprain of right ring finger POA
    7ᵗʰ S63.615 Unspecified sprain of left ring finger POA
    7ᵗʰ S63.616 Unspecified sprain of right little finger POA
    7ᵗʰ S63.617 Unspecified sprain of left little finger POA
    7ᵗʰ S63.618 Unspecified sprain of other finger POA
      Unspecified sprain of specified finger with unspecified laterality
    7ᵗʰ S63.619 Unspecified sprain of unspecified finger POA
  6ᵗʰ S63.62 Sprain of interphalangeal joint of thumb
    7ᵗʰ S63.621 Sprain of interphalangeal joint of right thumb POA
    7ᵗʰ S63.622 Sprain of interphalangeal joint of left thumb POA
    7ᵗʰ S63.629 Sprain of interphalangeal joint of unspecified thumb POA
  6ᵗʰ S63.63 Sprain of interphalangeal joint of other and unspecified finger(s)
    7ᵗʰ S63.630 Sprain of interphalangeal joint of right index finger POA
    7ᵗʰ S63.631 Sprain of interphalangeal joint of left index finger POA
    7ᵗʰ S63.632 Sprain of interphalangeal joint of right middle finger POA
    7ᵗʰ S63.633 Sprain of interphalangeal joint of left middle finger POA
    7ᵗʰ S63.634 Sprain of interphalangeal joint of right ring finger POA
    7ᵗʰ S63.635 Sprain of interphalangeal joint of left ring finger POA

7ᵗʰ S63.636 Sprain of interphalangeal joint of right little finger POA
7ᵗʰ S63.637 Sprain of interphalangeal joint of left little finger POA
7ᵗʰ S63.638 Sprain of interphalangeal joint of other finger POA
7ᵗʰ S63.639 Sprain of interphalangeal joint of unspecified finger POA

6ᵗʰ S63.64 Sprain of metacarpophalangeal joint of thumb
  7ᵗʰ S63.641 Sprain of metacarpophalangeal joint of right thumb POA
  7ᵗʰ S63.642 Sprain of metacarpophalangeal joint of left thumb POA
  7ᵗʰ S63.649 Sprain of metacarpophalangeal joint of unspecified thumb POA
6ᵗʰ S63.65 Sprain of metacarpophalangeal joint of other and unspecified finger(s)
  7ᵗʰ S63.650 Sprain of metacarpophalangeal joint of right index finger POA
  7ᵗʰ S63.651 Sprain of metacarpophalangeal joint of left index finger POA
  7ᵗʰ S63.652 Sprain of metacarpophalangeal joint of right middle finger POA
  7ᵗʰ S63.653 Sprain of metacarpophalangeal joint of left middle finger POA
  7ᵗʰ S63.654 Sprain of metacarpophalangeal joint of right ring finger POA
  7ᵗʰ S63.655 Sprain of metacarpophalangeal joint of left ring finger POA
  7ᵗʰ S63.656 Sprain of metacarpophalangeal joint of right little finger POA
  7ᵗʰ S63.657 Sprain of metacarpophalangeal joint of left little finger POA
  7ᵗʰ S63.658 Sprain of metacarpophalangeal joint of other finger POA
    Sprain of metacarpophalangeal joint of specified finger with unspecified laterality
  7ᵗʰ S63.659 Sprain of metacarpophalangeal joint of unspecified finger POA
6ᵗʰ S63.68 Other sprain of thumb
  7ᵗʰ S63.681 Other sprain of right thumb POA
  7ᵗʰ S63.682 Other sprain of left thumb POA
  7ᵗʰ S63.689 Other sprain of unspecified thumb POA
6ᵗʰ S63.69 Other sprain of other and unspecified finger(s)
  7ᵗʰ S63.690 Other sprain of right index finger POA
  7ᵗʰ S63.691 Other sprain of left index finger POA
  7ᵗʰ S63.692 Other sprain of right middle finger POA
  7ᵗʰ S63.693 Other sprain of left middle finger POA
  7ᵗʰ S63.694 Other sprain of right ring finger POA
  7ᵗʰ S63.695 Other sprain of left ring finger POA
  7ᵗʰ S63.696 Other sprain of right little finger POA
  7ᵗʰ S63.697 Other sprain of left little finger POA
  7ᵗʰ S63.698 Other sprain of other finger POA
    Other sprain of specified finger with unspecified laterality
  7ᵗʰ S63.699 Other sprain of unspecified finger POA

5ᵗʰ S63.8 Sprain of other part of wrist and hand
  6ᵗʰ S63.8X Sprain of other part of wrist and hand
    7ᵗʰ S63.8X1 Sprain of other part of right wrist and hand POA
    7ᵗʰ S63.8X2 Sprain of other part of left wrist and hand POA
    7ᵗʰ S63.8X9 Sprain of other part of unspecified wrist and hand POA
5ᵗʰ S63.9 Sprain of unspecified part of wrist and hand
  7ᵗʰ S63.90 Sprain of unspecified part of unspecified wrist and hand POA
  7ᵗʰ S63.91 Sprain of unspecified part of right wrist and hand POA
  7ᵗʰ S63.92 Sprain of unspecified part of left wrist and hand POA

POA↯ Unacceptable principal diagnosis symbol per Medicare code edits POA Code exempt from diagnosis present on admission requirement
? Questionable admission CC Complication or comorbidity MCC Major complication or comorbidity CC/MCC Exc CC/MCC exclusion
HCC HCC diagnosis code RxHCC RxHCC diagnosis code MACRA code **DEFINITION** Describes condition/terminology
TIP Coding guidance Official Guideline Reference Z1 Z code as first-listed diagnosis

4ᵗʰ **S64** Injury of nerves at wrist and hand level
    Code also any associated open wound (S61.-)
    The appropriate 7th character is to be added to each code from category S64
        A = initial encounter
        D = subsequent encounter
        S = sequela

  5ᵗʰ **S64.0** Injury of ulnar nerve at wrist and hand level
    7ᵗʰ **S64.00** Injury of ulnar nerve at wrist and hand level of unspecified arm **POA**
    7ᵗʰ **S64.01** Injury of ulnar nerve at wrist and hand level of right arm **POA**
    7ᵗʰ **S64.02** Injury of ulnar nerve at wrist and hand level of left arm **POA**

  5ᵗʰ **S64.1** Injury of median nerve at wrist and hand level
    7ᵗʰ **S64.10** Injury of median nerve at wrist and hand level of unspecified arm **POA**
    7ᵗʰ **S64.11** Injury of median nerve at wrist and hand level of right arm **POA**
    7ᵗʰ **S64.12** Injury of median nerve at wrist and hand level of left arm **POA**

  5ᵗʰ **S64.2** Injury of radial nerve at wrist and hand level
    7ᵗʰ **S64.20** Injury of radial nerve at wrist and hand level of unspecified arm **POA**
    7ᵗʰ **S64.21** Injury of radial nerve at wrist and hand level of right arm **POA**
    7ᵗʰ **S64.22** Injury of radial nerve at wrist and hand level of left arm **POA**

  5ᵗʰ **S64.3** Injury of digital nerve of thumb
    7ᵗʰ **S64.30** Injury of digital nerve of unspecified thumb **POA**
    7ᵗʰ **S64.31** Injury of digital nerve of right thumb **POA**
    7ᵗʰ **S64.32** Injury of digital nerve of left thumb **POA**

  5ᵗʰ **S64.4** Injury of digital nerve of other and unspecified finger
    7ᵗʰ **S64.40** Injury of digital nerve of unspecified finger **POA**
    6ᵗʰ **S64.49** Injury of digital nerve of other finger
      7ᵗʰ **S64.490** Injury of digital nerve of right index finger **POA**
      7ᵗʰ **S64.491** Injury of digital nerve of left index finger **POA**
      7ᵗʰ **S64.492** Injury of digital nerve of right middle finger **POA**
      7ᵗʰ **S64.493** Injury of digital nerve of left middle finger **POA**
      7ᵗʰ **S64.494** Injury of digital nerve of right ring finger **POA**
      7ᵗʰ **S64.495** Injury of digital nerve of left ring finger **POA**
      7ᵗʰ **S64.496** Injury of digital nerve of right little finger **POA**
      7ᵗʰ **S64.497** Injury of digital nerve of left little finger **POA**
      7ᵗʰ **S64.498** Injury of digital nerve of other finger **POA**
          Injury of digital nerve of specified finger with unspecified laterality

  5ᵗʰ **S64.8** Injury of other nerves at wrist and hand level
    6ᵗʰ **S64.8X** Injury of other nerves at wrist and hand level
      7ᵗʰ **S64.8X1** Injury of other nerves at wrist and hand level of right arm **POA**
      7ᵗʰ **S64.8X2** Injury of other nerves at wrist and hand level of left arm **POA**
      7ᵗʰ **S64.8X9** Injury of other nerves at wrist and hand level of unspecified arm **POA**

  5ᵗʰ **S64.9** Injury of unspecified nerve at wrist and hand level
    7ᵗʰ **S64.90** Injury of unspecified nerve at wrist and hand level of unspecified arm **POA**
    7ᵗʰ **S64.91** Injury of unspecified nerve at wrist and hand level of right arm **POA**
    7ᵗʰ **S64.92** Injury of unspecified nerve at wrist and hand level of left arm **POA**

4ᵗʰ **S65** Injury of blood vessels at wrist and hand level
    Code also any associated open wound (S61.-)
    The appropriate 7th character is to be added to each code from category S65
        A = initial encounter
        D = subsequent encounter
        S = sequela

5ᵗʰ **S65.0** Injury of ulnar artery at wrist and hand level
  6ᵗʰ **S65.00** Unspecified injury of ulnar artery at wrist and hand level
    7ᵗʰ **S65.001** Unspecified injury of ulnar artery at wrist and hand level of right arm **CC POA CC/MCC Excl**
    7ᵗʰ **S65.002** Unspecified injury of ulnar artery at wrist and hand level of left arm **CC POA CC/MCC Excl**
    7ᵗʰ **S65.009** Unspecified injury of ulnar artery at wrist and hand level of unspecified arm **CC POA CC/MCC Excl**

  6ᵗʰ **S65.01** Laceration of ulnar artery at wrist and hand level
    7ᵗʰ **S65.011** Laceration of ulnar artery at wrist and hand level of right arm **CC POA CC/MCC Excl**
    7ᵗʰ **S65.012** Laceration of ulnar artery at wrist and hand level of left arm **CC POA CC/MCC Excl**
    7ᵗʰ **S65.019** Laceration of ulnar artery at wrist and hand level of unspecified arm **CC POA CC/MCC Excl**

  6ᵗʰ **S65.09** Other specified injury of ulnar artery at wrist and hand level
    7ᵗʰ **S65.091** Other specified injury of ulnar artery at wrist and hand level of right arm **CC POA CC/MCC Excl**
    7ᵗʰ **S65.092** Other specified injury of ulnar artery at wrist and hand level of left arm **CC POA CC/MCC Excl**
    7ᵗʰ **S65.099** Other specified injury of ulnar artery at wrist and hand level of unspecified arm **CC POA CC/MCC Excl**

5ᵗʰ **S65.1** Injury of radial artery at wrist and hand level
  6ᵗʰ **S65.10** Unspecified injury of radial artery at wrist and hand level
    7ᵗʰ **S65.101** Unspecified injury of radial artery at wrist and hand level of right arm **CC POA CC/MCC Excl**
    7ᵗʰ **S65.102** Unspecified injury of radial artery at wrist and hand level of left arm **CC POA CC/MCC Excl**
    7ᵗʰ **S65.109** Unspecified injury of radial artery at wrist and hand level of unspecified arm **CC POA CC/MCC Excl**

  6ᵗʰ **S65.11** Laceration of radial artery at wrist and hand level
    7ᵗʰ **S65.111** Laceration of radial artery at wrist and hand level of right arm **CC POA CC/MCC Excl**
    7ᵗʰ **S65.112** Laceration of radial artery at wrist and hand level of left arm **CC POA CC/MCC Excl**
    7ᵗʰ **S65.119** Laceration of radial artery at wrist and hand level of unspecified arm **CC POA CC/MCC Excl**

  6ᵗʰ **S65.19** Other specified injury of radial artery at wrist and hand level
    7ᵗʰ **S65.191** Other specified injury of radial artery at wrist and hand level of right arm **CC POA CC/MCC Excl**
    7ᵗʰ **S65.192** Other specified injury of radial artery at wrist and hand level of left arm **CC POA CC/MCC Excl**
    7ᵗʰ **S65.199** Other specified injury of radial artery at wrist and hand level of unspecified arm **CC POA CC/MCC Excl**

5ᵗʰ **S65.2** Injury of superficial palmar arch
  6ᵗʰ **S65.20** Unspecified injury of superficial palmar arch
    7ᵗʰ **S65.201** Unspecified injury of superficial palmar arch of right hand **CC POA CC/MCC Excl**
    7ᵗʰ **S65.202** Unspecified injury of superficial palmar arch of left hand **CC POA CC/MCC Excl**
    7ᵗʰ **S65.209** Unspecified injury of superficial palmar arch of unspecified hand **CC POA CC/MCC Excl**

  6ᵗʰ **S65.21** Laceration of superficial palmar arch
    7ᵗʰ **S65.211** Laceration of superficial palmar arch of right hand **CC POA CC/MCC Excl**
    7ᵗʰ **S65.212** Laceration of superficial palmar arch of left hand **CC POA CC/MCC Excl**
    7ᵗʰ **S65.219** Laceration of superficial palmar arch of unspecified hand **CC POA CC/MCC Excl**

Unspecified Code	Other Specified Code	Manifestation Code	N Newborn	P Pediatric	M Maternity	A Adult	♂ Male	♀ Female

● New Code   ▲ Revised Code Title   ▶◀ Revised Text   **NOTES**   *INCLUDES*   *EXCLUDES1* Not coded here   *EXCLUDES2* Not included here
4ᵗʰ 4ᵗʰ character required   5ᵗʰ 5ᵗʰ character required   6ᵗʰ 6ᵗʰ character required   7ᵗʰ 7ᵗʰ character required   Extension 'X' Alert
HAC Hospital-acquired condition (HAC) alert   **AHA** AHA Coding Clinic©   ☞ **Code first alert**

[6th] S65.29 Other specified injury of superficial palmar arch
- [7th] S65.291 Other specified injury of superficial palmar arch of right hand [CC] [POA] [CC/MCC Exc]
- [7th] S65.292 Other specified injury of superficial palmar arch of left hand [CC] [POA] [CC/MCC Exc]
- [7th] S65.299 Other specified injury of superficial palmar arch of unspecified hand [CC] [POA] [CC/MCC Exc]

[5th] S65.3 Injury of deep palmar arch

[6th] S65.30 Unspecified injury of deep palmar arch
- [7th] S65.301 Unspecified injury of deep palmar arch of right hand [CC] [POA] [CC/MCC Exc]
- [7th] S65.302 Unspecified injury of deep palmar arch of left hand [CC] [POA] [CC/MCC Exc]
- [7th] S65.309 Unspecified injury of deep palmar arch of unspecified hand [CC] [POA] [CC/MCC Exc]

[6th] S65.31 Laceration of deep palmar arch
- [7th] S65.311 Laceration of deep palmar arch of right hand [CC] [POA] [CC/MCC Exc]
- [7th] S65.312 Laceration of deep palmar arch of left hand [CC] [POA] [CC/MCC Exc]
- [7th] S65.319 Laceration of deep palmar arch of unspecified hand [CC] [POA] [CC/MCC Exc]

[6th] S65.39 Other specified injury of deep palmar arch
- [7th] S65.391 Other specified injury of deep palmar arch of right hand [CC] [POA] [CC/MCC Exc]
- [7th] S65.392 Other specified injury of deep palmar arch of left hand [CC] [POA] [CC/MCC Exc]
- [7th] S65.399 Other specified injury of deep palmar arch of unspecified hand [CC] [POA] [CC/MCC Exc]

[5th] S65.4 Injury of blood vessel of thumb

[6th] S65.40 Unspecified injury of blood vessel of thumb
- [7th] S65.401 Unspecified injury of blood vessel of right thumb [CC] [POA] [CC/MCC Exc]
- [7th] S65.402 Unspecified injury of blood vessel of left thumb [CC] [POA] [CC/MCC Exc]
- [7th] S65.409 Unspecified injury of blood vessel of unspecified thumb [CC] [POA] [CC/MCC Exc]

[6th] S65.41 Laceration of blood vessel of thumb
- [7th] S65.411 Laceration of blood vessel of right thumb [CC] [POA] [CC/MCC Exc]
- [7th] S65.412 Laceration of blood vessel of left thumb [CC] [POA] [CC/MCC Exc]
- [7th] S65.419 Laceration of blood vessel of unspecified thumb [CC] [POA] [CC/MCC Exc]

[6th] S65.49 Other specified injury of blood vessel of thumb
- [7th] S65.491 Other specified injury of blood vessel of right thumb [CC] [POA] [CC/MCC Exc]
- [7th] S65.492 Other specified injury of blood vessel of left thumb [CC] [POA] [CC/MCC Exc]
- [7th] S65.499 Other specified injury of blood vessel of unspecified thumb [CC] [POA] [CC/MCC Exc]

[5th] S65.5 Injury of blood vessel of other and unspecified finger

[6th] S65.50 Unspecified injury of blood vessel of other and unspecified finger
- [7th] S65.500 Unspecified injury of blood vessel of right index finger [CC] [POA] [CC/MCC Exc]
- [7th] S65.501 Unspecified injury of blood vessel of left index finger [CC] [POA] [CC/MCC Exc]
- [7th] S65.502 Unspecified injury of blood vessel of right middle finger [CC] [POA] [CC/MCC Exc]
- [7th] S65.503 Unspecified injury of blood vessel of left middle finger [CC] [POA] [CC/MCC Exc]
- [7th] S65.504 Unspecified injury of blood vessel of right ring finger [CC] [POA] [CC/MCC Exc]
- [7th] S65.505 Unspecified injury of blood vessel of left ring finger [CC] [POA] [CC/MCC Exc]
- [7th] S65.506 Unspecified injury of blood vessel of right little finger [CC] [POA] [CC/MCC Exc]
- [7th] S65.507 Unspecified injury of blood vessel of left little finger [CC] [POA] [CC/MCC Exc]
- [7th] S65.508 Unspecified injury of blood vessel of other finger [CC] [POA] [CC/MCC Exc]
  Unspecified injury of blood vessel of specified finger with unspecified laterality
- [7th] S65.509 Unspecified injury of blood vessel of unspecified finger [CC] [POA] [CC/MCC Exc]

[6th] S65.51 Laceration of blood vessel of other and unspecified finger
- [7th] S65.510 Laceration of blood vessel of right index finger [CC] [POA] [CC/MCC Exc]
- [7th] S65.511 Laceration of blood vessel of left index finger [CC] [POA] [CC/MCC Exc]
- [7th] S65.512 Laceration of blood vessel of right middle finger [CC] [POA] [CC/MCC Exc]
- [7th] S65.513 Laceration of blood vessel of left middle finger [CC] [POA] [CC/MCC Exc]
- [7th] S65.514 Laceration of blood vessel of right ring finger [CC] [POA] [CC/MCC Exc]
- [7th] S65.515 Laceration of blood vessel of left ring finger [CC] [POA] [CC/MCC Exc]
- [7th] S65.516 Laceration of blood vessel of right little finger [CC] [POA] [CC/MCC Exc]
- [7th] S65.517 Laceration of blood vessel of left little finger [CC] [POA] [CC/MCC Exc]
- [7th] S65.518 Laceration of blood vessel of other finger [CC] [POA] [CC/MCC Exc]
  Laceration of blood vessel of specified finger with unspecified laterality
- [7th] S65.519 Laceration of blood vessel of unspecified finger [CC] [POA] [CC/MCC Exc]

[6th] S65.59 Other specified injury of blood vessel of other and unspecified finger
- [7th] S65.590 Other specified injury of blood vessel of right index finger [CC] [POA] [CC/MCC Exc]
- [7th] S65.591 Other specified injury of blood vessel of left index finger [CC] [POA] [CC/MCC Exc]
- [7th] S65.592 Other specified injury of blood vessel of right middle finger [CC] [POA] [CC/MCC Exc]
- [7th] S65.593 Other specified injury of blood vessel of left middle finger [CC] [POA] [CC/MCC Exc]
- [7th] S65.594 Other specified injury of blood vessel of right ring finger [CC] [POA] [CC/MCC Exc]
- [7th] S65.595 Other specified injury of blood vessel of left ring finger [CC] [POA] [CC/MCC Exc]
- [7th] S65.596 Other specified injury of blood vessel of right little finger [CC] [POA] [CC/MCC Exc]
- [7th] S65.597 Other specified injury of blood vessel of left little finger [CC] [POA] [CC/MCC Exc]
- [7th] S65.598 Other specified injury of blood vessel of other finger [CC] [POA] [CC/MCC Exc]
  Other specified injury of blood vessel of specified finger with unspecified laterality
- [7th] S65.599 Other specified injury of blood vessel of unspecified finger [CC] [POA] [CC/MCC Exc]

[5th] S65.8 Injury of other blood vessels at wrist and hand level

[6th] S65.80 Unspecified injury of other blood vessels at wrist and hand level
- [7th] S65.801 Unspecified injury of other blood vessels at wrist and hand level of right arm [CC] [POA] [CC/MCC Exc]
- [7th] S65.802 Unspecified injury of other blood vessels at wrist and hand level of left arm [CC] [POA] [CC/MCC Exc]
- [7th] S65.809 Unspecified injury of other blood vessels at wrist and hand level of unspecified arm [CC] [POA] [CC/MCC Exc]

[6th] S65.81 Laceration of other blood vessels at wrist and hand level
- [7th] S65.811 Laceration of other blood vessels at wrist and hand level of right arm [CC] [POA] [CC/MCC Exc]
- [7th] S65.812 Laceration of other blood vessels at wrist and hand level of left arm [CC] [POA] [CC/MCC Exc]

[PDx] Unacceptable principal diagnosis symbol per Medicare code edits [POA] Code exempt from diagnosis present on admission requirement
[?] Questionable admission [CC] Complication or comorbidity [MCC] Major complication or comorbidity [CC/MCC Exc] CC/MCC exclusion
[HCC] HCC diagnosis code [RxHCC] RxHCC diagnosis code MACRA code **DEFINITION** Describes condition/terminology
TIP Coding guidance 👁 Official Guideline Reference [Z-1] Z code as first-listed diagnosis

[7th] S65.819 Laceration of other blood vessels at wrist and hand level of unspecified arm CC POA CC/MCC Exc

[6th] S65.89 Other specified injury of other blood vessels at wrist and hand level

[7th] S65.891 Other specified injury of other blood vessels at wrist and hand level of right arm CC POA CC/MCC Exc

[7th] S65.892 Other specified injury of other blood vessels at wrist and hand level of left arm CC POA CC/MCC Exc

[7th] S65.899 Other specified injury of other blood vessels at wrist and hand level of unspecified arm CC POA CC/MCC Exc

[5th] S65.9 Injury of unspecified blood vessel at wrist and hand level

[6th] S65.90 Unspecified injury of unspecified blood vessel at wrist and hand level

[7th] S65.901 Unspecified injury of unspecified blood vessel at wrist and hand level of right arm CC POA CC/MCC Exc

[7th] S65.902 Unspecified injury of unspecified blood vessel at wrist and hand level of left arm CC POA CC/MCC Exc

[7th] S65.909 Unspecified injury of unspecified blood vessel at wrist and hand level of unspecified arm CC POA CC/MCC Exc

[6th] S65.91 Laceration of unspecified blood vessel at wrist and hand level

[7th] S65.911 Laceration of unspecified blood vessel at wrist and hand level of right arm CC POA CC/MCC Exc

[7th] S65.912 Laceration of unspecified blood vessel at wrist and hand level of left arm CC POA CC/MCC Exc

[7th] S65.919 Laceration of unspecified blood vessel at wrist and hand level of unspecified arm CC POA CC/MCC Exc

[6th] S65.99 Other specified injury of unspecified blood vessel at wrist and hand level

[7th] S65.991 Other specified injury of unspecified blood vessel at wrist and hand of right arm CC POA CC/MCC Exc

[7th] S65.992 Other specified injury of unspecified blood vessel at wrist and hand of left arm CC POA CC/MCC Exc

[7th] S65.999 Other specified injury of unspecified blood vessel at wrist and hand of unspecified arm CC POA CC/MCC Exc

[4th] S66 Injury of muscle, fascia and tendon at wrist and hand level

Code also any associated open wound (S61.-)

EXCLUDES2 *sprain of joints and ligaments of wrist and hand (S63.-)*

The appropriate 7th character is to be added to each code from category S66

A = initial encounter
D = subsequent encounter
S = sequela

[5th] S66.0 Injury of long flexor muscle, fascia and tendon of thumb at wrist and hand level

[6th] S66.00 Unspecified injury of long flexor muscle, fascia and tendon of thumb at wrist and hand level

[7th] S66.001 Unspecified injury of long flexor muscle, fascia and tendon of right thumb at wrist and hand level POA

[7th] S66.002 Unspecified injury of long flexor muscle, fascia and tendon of left thumb at wrist and hand level POA

[7th] S66.009 Unspecified injury of long flexor muscle, fascia and tendon of unspecified thumb at wrist and hand level POA

[6th] S66.01 Strain of long flexor muscle, fascia and tendon of thumb at wrist and hand level

[7th] S66.011 Strain of long flexor muscle, fascia and tendon of right thumb at wrist and hand level POA

[7th] S66.012 Strain of long flexor muscle, fascia and tendon of left thumb at wrist and hand level POA

[7th] S66.019 Strain of long flexor muscle, fascia and tendon of unspecified thumb at wrist and hand level POA

[6th] S66.02 Laceration of long flexor muscle, fascia and tendon of thumb at wrist and hand level

[7th] S66.021 Laceration of long flexor muscle, fascia and tendon of right thumb at wrist and hand level CC POA CC/MCC Exc

[7th] S66.022 Laceration of long flexor muscle, fascia and tendon of left thumb at wrist and hand level CC POA CC/MCC Exc

[7th] S66.029 Laceration of long flexor muscle, fascia and tendon of unspecified thumb at wrist and hand level CC POA CC/MCC Exc

[6th] S66.09 Other specified injury of long flexor muscle, fascia and tendon of thumb at wrist and hand level

[7th] S66.091 Other specified injury of long flexor muscle, fascia and tendon of right thumb at wrist and hand level POA

[7th] S66.092 Other specified injury of long flexor muscle, fascia and tendon of left thumb at wrist and hand level POA

[7th] S66.099 Other specified injury of long flexor muscle, fascia and tendon of unspecified thumb at wrist and hand level POA

[5th] S66.1 Injury of flexor muscle, fascia and tendon of other and unspecified finger at wrist and hand level

EXCLUDES2 *Injury of long flexor muscle, fascia and tendon of thumb at wrist and hand level (S66.0-)*

[6th] S66.10 Unspecified injury of flexor muscle, fascia and tendon of other and unspecified finger at wrist and hand level

[7th] S66.100 Unspecified injury of flexor muscle, fascia and tendon of right index finger at wrist and hand level POA

[7th] S66.101 Unspecified injury of flexor muscle, fascia and tendon of left index finger at wrist and hand level POA

[7th] S66.102 Unspecified injury of flexor muscle, fascia and tendon of right middle finger at wrist and hand level POA

[7th] S66.103 Unspecified injury of flexor muscle, fascia and tendon of left middle finger at wrist and hand level POA

[7th] S66.104 Unspecified injury of flexor muscle, fascia and tendon of right ring finger at wrist and hand level POA

[7th] S66.105 Unspecified injury of flexor muscle, fascia and tendon of left ring finger at wrist and hand level POA

[7th] S66.106 Unspecified injury of flexor muscle, fascia and tendon of right little finger at wrist and hand level POA

[7th] S66.107 Unspecified injury of flexor muscle, fascia and tendon of left little finger at wrist and hand level POA

[7th] S66.108 Unspecified injury of flexor muscle, fascia and tendon of other finger at wrist and hand level POA

Unspecified injury of flexor muscle, fascia and tendon of specified finger with unspecified laterality at wrist and hand level

[7th] S66.109 Unspecified injury of flexor muscle, fascia and tendon of unspecified finger at wrist and hand level POA

6ᵗʰ **S66.11** Strain of flexor muscle, fascia and tendon of other and unspecified finger at wrist and hand level

　7ᵗʰ **S66.110** Strain of flexor muscle, fascia and tendon of right index finger at wrist and hand level POA

　7ᵗʰ **S66.111** Strain of flexor muscle, fascia and tendon of left index finger at wrist and hand level POA

　7ᵗʰ **S66.112** Strain of flexor muscle, fascia and tendon of right middle finger at wrist and hand level POA

　7ᵗʰ **S66.113** Strain of flexor muscle, fascia and tendon of left middle finger at wrist and hand level POA

　7ᵗʰ **S66.114** Strain of flexor muscle, fascia and tendon of right ring finger at wrist and hand level POA

　7ᵗʰ **S66.115** Strain of flexor muscle, fascia and tendon of left ring finger at wrist and hand level POA

　7ᵗʰ **S66.116** Strain of flexor muscle, fascia and tendon of right little finger at wrist and hand level POA

　7ᵗʰ **S66.117** Strain of flexor muscle, fascia and tendon of left little finger at wrist and hand level POA

　7ᵗʰ **S66.118** Strain of flexor muscle, fascia and tendon of other finger at wrist and hand level POA
　　　Strain of flexor muscle, fascia and tendon of specified finger with unspecified laterality at wrist and hand level

　7ᵗʰ **S66.119** Strain of flexor muscle, fascia and tendon of unspecified finger at wrist and hand level POA

6ᵗʰ **S66.12** Laceration of flexor muscle, fascia and tendon of other and unspecified finger at wrist and hand level

　7ᵗʰ **S66.120** Laceration of flexor muscle, fascia and tendon of right index finger at wrist and hand level CC POA CC/MCC Exc

　7ᵗʰ **S66.121** Laceration of flexor muscle, fascia and tendon of left index finger at wrist and hand level CC POA CC/MCC Exc

　7ᵗʰ **S66.122** Laceration of flexor muscle, fascia and tendon of right middle finger at wrist and hand level CC POA CC/MCC Exc

　7ᵗʰ **S66.123** Laceration of flexor muscle, fascia and tendon of left middle finger at wrist and hand level CC POA CC/MCC Exc

　7ᵗʰ **S66.124** Laceration of flexor muscle, fascia and tendon of right ring finger at wrist and hand level CC POA CC/MCC Exc

　7ᵗʰ **S66.125** Laceration of flexor muscle, fascia and tendon of left ring finger at wrist and hand level CC POA CC/MCC Exc

　7ᵗʰ **S66.126** Laceration of flexor muscle, fascia and tendon of right little finger at wrist and hand level CC POA CC/MCC Exc

　7ᵗʰ **S66.127** Laceration of flexor muscle, fascia and tendon of left little finger at wrist and hand level CC POA CC/MCC Exc

　7ᵗʰ **S66.128** Laceration of flexor muscle, fascia and tendon of other finger at wrist and hand level CC POA CC/MCC Exc
　　　Laceration of flexor muscle, fascia and tendon of specified finger with unspecified laterality at wrist and hand level

　7ᵗʰ **S66.129** Laceration of flexor muscle, fascia and tendon of unspecified finger at wrist and hand level CC POA CC/MCC Exc

6ᵗʰ **S66.19** Other injury of flexor muscle, fascia and tendon of other and unspecified finger at wrist and hand level

　7ᵗʰ **S66.190** Other injury of flexor muscle, fascia and tendon of right index finger at wrist and hand level POA

　7ᵗʰ **S66.191** Other injury of flexor muscle, fascia and tendon of left index finger at wrist and hand level POA

　7ᵗʰ **S66.192** Other injury of flexor muscle, fascia and tendon of right middle finger at wrist and hand level POA

　7ᵗʰ **S66.193** Other injury of flexor muscle, fascia and tendon of left middle finger at wrist and hand level POA

　7ᵗʰ **S66.194** Other injury of flexor muscle, fascia and tendon of right ring finger at wrist and hand level POA

　7ᵗʰ **S66.195** Other injury of flexor muscle, fascia and tendon of left ring finger at wrist and hand level POA

　7ᵗʰ **S66.196** Other injury of flexor muscle, fascia and tendon of right little finger at wrist and hand level POA

　7ᵗʰ **S66.197** Other injury of flexor muscle, fascia and tendon of left little finger at wrist and hand level POA

　7ᵗʰ **S66.198** Other injury of flexor muscle, fascia and tendon of other finger at wrist and hand level POA
　　　Other injury of flexor muscle, fascia and tendon of specified finger with unspecified laterality at wrist and hand level

　7ᵗʰ **S66.199** Other injury of flexor muscle, fascia and tendon of unspecified finger at wrist and hand level POA

5ᵗʰ **S66.2** Injury of extensor muscle, fascia and tendon of thumb at wrist and hand level

6ᵗʰ **S66.20** Unspecified injury of extensor muscle, fascia and tendon of thumb at wrist and hand level

　7ᵗʰ **S66.201** Unspecified injury of extensor muscle, fascia and tendon of right thumb at wrist and hand level POA

　7ᵗʰ **S66.202** Unspecified injury of extensor muscle, fascia and tendon of left thumb at wrist and hand level POA

　7ᵗʰ **S66.209** Unspecified injury of extensor muscle, fascia and tendon of unspecified thumb at wrist and hand level POA

6ᵗʰ **S66.21** Strain of extensor muscle, fascia and tendon of thumb at wrist and hand level

　7ᵗʰ **S66.211** Strain of extensor muscle, fascia and tendon of right thumb at wrist and hand level POA

　7ᵗʰ **S66.212** Strain of extensor muscle, fascia and tendon of left thumb at wrist and hand level POA

　7ᵗʰ **S66.219** Strain of extensor muscle, fascia and tendon of unspecified thumb at wrist and hand level POA

6ᵗʰ **S66.22** Laceration of extensor muscle, fascia and tendon of thumb at wrist and hand level

　7ᵗʰ **S66.221** Laceration of extensor muscle, fascia and tendon of right thumb at wrist and hand level CC POA CC/MCC Exc

　7ᵗʰ **S66.222** Laceration of extensor muscle, fascia and tendon of left thumb at wrist and hand level CC POA CC/MCC Exc

　7ᵗʰ **S66.229** Laceration of extensor muscle, fascia and tendon of unspecified thumb at wrist and hand level CC POA CC/MCC Exc

---

POA Unacceptable principal diagnosis symbol per Medicare code edits　　POA Code exempt from diagnosis present on admission requirement
　? Questionable admission　　CC Complication or comorbidity　　MCC Major complication or comorbidity　　CC/MCC Exc CC/MCC exclusion
　HCC HCC diagnosis code　　RHCC RxHCC diagnosis code　　MACRA code　　**DEFINITION** Describes condition/terminology
　　TIP Coding guidance　　◉ Official Guideline Reference　　Z1 Z code as first-listed diagnosis

When symbols appear on a code that requires a 7th character extension, refer to Appendix B to identify applicable 7th character codes.
2020 ICD-10-CM

6️⃣ S66.29 Other specified injury of extensor muscle, fascia and tendon of thumb at wrist and hand level

  7️⃣ S66.291 Other specified injury of extensor muscle, fascia and tendon of right thumb at wrist and hand level POA

  7️⃣ S66.292 Other specified injury of extensor muscle, fascia and tendon of left thumb at wrist and hand level POA

  7️⃣ S66.299 Other specified injury of extensor muscle, fascia and tendon of unspecified thumb at wrist and hand level POA

5️⃣ S66.3 Injury of extensor muscle, fascia and tendon of other and unspecified finger at wrist and hand level

  EXCLUDES2 Injury of extensor muscle, fascia and tendon of thumb at wrist and hand level (S66.2-)

6️⃣ S66.30 Unspecified injury of extensor muscle, fascia and tendon of other and unspecified finger at wrist and hand level

  7️⃣ S66.300 Unspecified injury of extensor muscle, fascia and tendon of right index finger at wrist and hand level POA

  7️⃣ S66.301 Unspecified injury of extensor muscle, fascia and tendon of left index finger at wrist and hand level POA

  7️⃣ S66.302 Unspecified injury of extensor muscle, fascia and tendon of right middle finger at wrist and hand level POA

  7️⃣ S66.303 Unspecified injury of extensor muscle, fascia and tendon of left middle finger at wrist and hand level POA

  7️⃣ S66.304 Unspecified injury of extensor muscle, fascia and tendon of right ring finger at wrist and hand level POA

  7️⃣ S66.305 Unspecified injury of extensor muscle, fascia and tendon of left ring finger at wrist and hand level POA

  7️⃣ S66.306 Unspecified injury of extensor muscle, fascia and tendon of right little finger at wrist and hand level POA

  7️⃣ S66.307 Unspecified injury of extensor muscle, fascia and tendon of left little finger at wrist and hand level POA

  7️⃣ S66.308 Unspecified injury of extensor muscle, fascia and tendon of other finger at wrist and hand level POA

    Unspecified injury of extensor muscle, fascia and tendon of specified finger with unspecified laterality at wrist and hand level

  7️⃣ S66.309 Unspecified injury of extensor muscle, fascia and tendon of unspecified finger at wrist and hand level POA

6️⃣ S66.31 Strain of extensor muscle, fascia and tendon of other and unspecified finger at wrist and hand level

  7️⃣ S66.310 Strain of extensor muscle, fascia and tendon of right index finger at wrist and hand level POA

  7️⃣ S66.311 Strain of extensor muscle, fascia and tendon of left index finger at wrist and hand level POA

  7️⃣ S66.312 Strain of extensor muscle, fascia and tendon of right middle finger at wrist and hand level POA

  7️⃣ S66.313 Strain of extensor muscle, fascia and tendon of left middle finger at wrist and hand level POA

  7️⃣ S66.314 Strain of extensor muscle, fascia and tendon of right ring finger at wrist and hand level POA

  7️⃣ S66.315 Strain of extensor muscle, fascia and tendon of left ring finger at wrist and hand level POA

7️⃣ S66.316 Strain of extensor muscle, fascia and tendon of right little finger at wrist and hand level POA

7️⃣ S66.317 Strain of extensor muscle, fascia and tendon of left little finger at wrist and hand level POA

7️⃣ S66.318 Strain of extensor muscle, fascia and tendon of other finger at wrist and hand level POA

  Strain of extensor muscle, fascia and tendon of specified finger with unspecified laterality at wrist and hand level

7️⃣ S66.319 Strain of extensor muscle, fascia and tendon of unspecified finger at wrist and hand level POA

6️⃣ S66.32 Laceration of extensor muscle, fascia and tendon of other and unspecified finger at wrist and hand level

  7️⃣ S66.320 Laceration of extensor muscle, fascia and tendon of right index finger at wrist and hand level CC POA CC/MCC Exc

  7️⃣ S66.321 Laceration of extensor muscle, fascia and tendon of left index finger at wrist and hand level CC POA CC/MCC Exc

  7️⃣ S66.322 Laceration of extensor muscle, fascia and tendon of right middle finger at wrist and hand level CC POA CC/MCC Exc

  7️⃣ S66.323 Laceration of extensor muscle, fascia and tendon of left middle finger at wrist and hand level CC POA CC/MCC Exc

  7️⃣ S66.324 Laceration of extensor muscle, fascia and tendon of right ring finger at wrist and hand level CC POA CC/MCC Exc

  7️⃣ S66.325 Laceration of extensor muscle, fascia and tendon of left ring finger at wrist and hand level CC POA CC/MCC Exc

  7️⃣ S66.326 Laceration of extensor muscle, fascia and tendon of right little finger at wrist and hand level CC POA CC/MCC Exc

  7️⃣ S66.327 Laceration of extensor muscle, fascia and tendon of left little finger at wrist and hand level CC POA CC/MCC Exc

  7️⃣ S66.328 Laceration of extensor muscle, fascia and tendon of other finger at wrist and hand level CC POA CC/MCC Exc

    Laceration of extensor muscle, fascia and tendon of specified finger with unspecified laterality at wrist and hand level

  7️⃣ S66.329 Laceration of extensor muscle, fascia and tendon of unspecified finger at wrist and hand level CC POA CC/MCC Exc

6️⃣ S66.39 Other injury of extensor muscle, fascia and tendon of other and unspecified finger at wrist and hand level

  7️⃣ S66.390 Other injury of extensor muscle, fascia and tendon of right index finger at wrist and hand level POA

  7️⃣ S66.391 Other injury of extensor muscle, fascia and tendon of left index finger at wrist and hand level POA

  7️⃣ S66.392 Other injury of extensor muscle, fascia and tendon of right middle finger at wrist and hand level POA

  7️⃣ S66.393 Other injury of extensor muscle, fascia and tendon of left middle finger at wrist and hand level POA

  7️⃣ S66.394 Other injury of extensor muscle, fascia and tendon of right ring finger at wrist and hand level POA

  7️⃣ S66.395 Other injury of extensor muscle, fascia and tendon of left ring finger at wrist and hand level POA

Unspecified Code Other Specified Code Manifestation Code N Newborn P Pediatric M Maternity A Adult ♂ Male ♀ Female
● New Code ▲ Revised Code Title ▶◀ Revised Text **NOTES** *INCLUDES* *EXCLUDES1* Not coded here *EXCLUDES2* Not included here
4️⃣ 4th character required 5️⃣ 5th character required 6️⃣ 6th character required 7️⃣ 7th character required ⓧ Extension 'X' Alert
HAC Hospital-acquired condition (HAC) alert **AHA** AHA Coding Clinic© 📌 Code first alert

S66.396 Other injury of extensor muscle, fascia and tendon of right little finger at wrist and hand level POA

S66.397 Other injury of extensor muscle, fascia and tendon of left little finger at wrist and hand level POA

S66.398 Other injury of extensor muscle, fascia and tendon of other finger at wrist and hand level
Other injury of extensor muscle, fascia and tendon of specified finger with unspecified laterality at wrist and hand level

S66.399 Other injury of extensor muscle, fascia and tendon of unspecified finger at wrist and hand level POA

S66.4 Injury of intrinsic muscle, fascia and tendon of thumb at wrist and hand level

S66.40 Unspecified injury of intrinsic muscle, fascia and tendon of thumb at wrist and hand level

S66.401 Unspecified injury of intrinsic muscle, fascia and tendon of right thumb at wrist and hand level POA

S66.402 Unspecified injury of intrinsic muscle, fascia and tendon of left thumb at wrist and hand level POA

S66.409 Unspecified injury of intrinsic muscle, fascia and tendon of unspecified thumb at wrist and hand level POA

S66.41 Strain of intrinsic muscle, fascia and tendon of thumb at wrist and hand level

S66.411 Strain of intrinsic muscle, fascia and tendon of right thumb at wrist and hand level POA

S66.412 Strain of intrinsic muscle, fascia and tendon of left thumb at wrist and hand level POA

S66.419 Strain of intrinsic muscle, fascia and tendon of unspecified thumb at wrist and hand level POA

S66.42 Laceration of intrinsic muscle, fascia and tendon of thumb at wrist and hand level

S66.421 Laceration of intrinsic muscle, fascia and tendon of right thumb at wrist and hand level CC POA CC/MCC Exc

S66.422 Laceration of intrinsic muscle, fascia and tendon of left thumb at wrist and hand level CC POA CC/MCC Exc

S66.429 Laceration of intrinsic muscle, fascia and tendon of unspecified thumb at wrist and hand level CC POA CC/MCC Exc

S66.49 Other specified injury of intrinsic muscle, fascia and tendon of thumb at wrist and hand level

S66.491 Other specified injury of intrinsic muscle, fascia and tendon of right thumb at wrist and hand level POA

S66.492 Other specified injury of intrinsic muscle, fascia and tendon of left thumb at wrist and hand level POA

S66.499 Other specified injury of intrinsic muscle, fascia and tendon of unspecified thumb at wrist and hand level POA

S66.5 Injury of intrinsic muscle, fascia and tendon of other and unspecified finger at wrist and hand level
EXCLUDES2 injury of intrinsic muscle, fascia and tendon of thumb at wrist and hand level (S66.4-)

S66.50 Unspecified injury of intrinsic muscle, fascia and tendon of other and unspecified finger at wrist and hand level

S66.500 Unspecified injury of intrinsic muscle, fascia and tendon of right index finger at wrist and hand level POA

S66.501 Unspecified injury of intrinsic muscle, fascia and tendon of left index finger at wrist and hand level POA

S66.502 Unspecified injury of intrinsic muscle, fascia and tendon of right middle finger at wrist and hand level POA

S66.503 Unspecified injury of intrinsic muscle, fascia and tendon of left middle finger at wrist and hand level POA

S66.504 Unspecified injury of intrinsic muscle, fascia and tendon of right ring finger at wrist and hand level POA

S66.505 Unspecified injury of intrinsic muscle, fascia and tendon of left ring finger at wrist and hand level POA

S66.506 Unspecified injury of intrinsic muscle, fascia and tendon of right little finger at wrist and hand level POA

S66.507 Unspecified injury of intrinsic muscle, fascia and tendon of left little finger at wrist and hand level POA

S66.508 Unspecified injury of intrinsic muscle, fascia and tendon of other finger at wrist and hand level
Unspecified injury of intrinsic muscle, fascia and tendon of specified finger with unspecified laterality at wrist and hand level

S66.509 Unspecified injury of intrinsic muscle, fascia and tendon of unspecified finger at wrist and hand level POA

S66.51 Strain of intrinsic muscle, fascia and tendon of other and unspecified finger at wrist and hand level

S66.510 Strain of intrinsic muscle, fascia and tendon of right index finger at wrist and hand level POA

S66.511 Strain of intrinsic muscle, fascia and tendon of left index finger at wrist and hand level POA

S66.512 Strain of intrinsic muscle, fascia and tendon of right middle finger at wrist and hand level POA

S66.513 Strain of intrinsic muscle, fascia and tendon of left middle finger at wrist and hand level POA

S66.514 Strain of intrinsic muscle, fascia and tendon of right ring finger at wrist and hand level POA

S66.515 Strain of intrinsic muscle, fascia and tendon of left ring finger at wrist and hand level POA

S66.516 Strain of intrinsic muscle, fascia and tendon of right little finger at wrist and hand level POA

S66.517 Strain of intrinsic muscle, fascia and tendon of left little finger at wrist and hand level POA

S66.518 Strain of intrinsic muscle, fascia and tendon of other finger at wrist and hand level POA
Strain of intrinsic muscle, fascia and tendon of specified finger with unspecified laterality at wrist and hand level

S66.519 Strain of intrinsic muscle, fascia and tendon of unspecified finger at wrist and hand level POA

S66.52 Laceration of intrinsic muscle, fascia and tendon of other and unspecified finger at wrist and hand level

S66.520 Laceration of intrinsic muscle, fascia and tendon of right index finger at wrist and hand level CC POA CC/MCC Exc

---

POA Unacceptable principal diagnosis symbol per Medicare code edits   POA Code exempt from diagnosis present on admission requirement
? Questionable admission   CC Complication or comorbidity   MCC Major complication or comorbidity   CC/MCC CC/MCC exclusion
HCC HCC diagnosis code   RxHCC RxHCC diagnosis code   MACRA code   **DEFINITION** Describes condition/terminology
TIP Coding guidance   Official Guideline Reference   Z1 Z code as first-listed diagnosis

7ᵈ **S66.521** Laceration of intrinsic muscle, fascia and tendon of left index finger at wrist and hand level CC⬚ POA CC/MCC Exc

7ᵈ **S66.522** Laceration of intrinsic muscle, fascia and tendon of right middle finger at wrist and hand level CC⬚ POA CC/MCC Exc

7ᵈ **S66.523** Laceration of intrinsic muscle, fascia and tendon of left middle finger at wrist and hand level CC⬚ POA CC/MCC Exc

7ᵈ **S66.524** Laceration of intrinsic muscle, fascia and tendon of right ring finger at wrist and hand level CC⬚ POA CC/MCC Exc

7ᵈ **S66.525** Laceration of intrinsic muscle, fascia and tendon of left ring finger at wrist and hand level CC⬚ POA CC/MCC Exc

7ᵈ **S66.526** Laceration of intrinsic muscle, fascia and tendon of right little finger at wrist and hand level CC⬚ POA CC/MCC Exc

7ᵈ **S66.527** Laceration of intrinsic muscle, fascia and tendon of left little finger at wrist and hand level CC⬚ POA CC/MCC Exc

7ᵈ **S66.528** Laceration of intrinsic muscle, fascia and tendon of other finger at wrist and hand level CC⬚ POA CC/MCC Exc

   Laceration of intrinsic muscle, fascia and tendon of specified finger with unspecified laterality at wrist and hand level

7ᵈ **S66.529** Laceration of intrinsic muscle, fascia and tendon of unspecified finger at wrist and hand level CC⬚ POA CC/MCC Exc

6ᵈ **S66.59** Other injury of intrinsic muscle, fascia and tendon of other and unspecified finger at wrist and hand level

7ᵈ **S66.590** Other injury of intrinsic muscle, fascia and tendon of right index finger at wrist and hand level POA

7ᵈ **S66.591** Other injury of intrinsic muscle, fascia and tendon of left index finger at wrist and hand level POA

7ᵈ **S66.592** Other injury of intrinsic muscle, fascia and tendon of right middle finger at wrist and hand level POA

7ᵈ **S66.593** Other injury of intrinsic muscle, fascia and tendon of left middle finger at wrist and hand level POA

7ᵈ **S66.594** Other injury of intrinsic muscle, fascia and tendon of right ring finger at wrist and hand level POA

7ᵈ **S66.595** Other injury of intrinsic muscle, fascia and tendon of left ring finger at wrist and hand level POA

7ᵈ **S66.596** Other injury of intrinsic muscle, fascia and tendon of right little finger at wrist and hand level POA

7ᵈ **S66.597** Other injury of intrinsic muscle, fascia and tendon of left little finger at wrist and hand level POA

7ᵈ **S66.598** Other injury of intrinsic muscle, fascia and tendon of other finger at wrist and hand level POA

   Other injury of intrinsic muscle, fascia and tendon of specified finger with unspecified laterality at wrist and hand level

7ᵈ **S66.599** Other injury of intrinsic muscle, fascia and tendon of unspecified finger at wrist and hand level POA

5ᵈ **S66.8** Injury of other specified muscles, fascia and tendons at wrist and hand level

6ᵈ **S66.80** Unspecified injury of other specified muscles, fascia and tendons at wrist and hand level

7ᵈ **S66.801** Unspecified injury of other specified muscles, fascia and tendons at wrist and hand level, right hand POA

7ᵈ **S66.802** Unspecified injury of other specified muscles, fascia and tendons at wrist and hand level, left hand POA

7ᵈ **S66.809** Unspecified injury of other specified muscles, fascia and tendons at wrist and hand level, unspecified hand POA

6ᵈ **S66.81** Strain of other specified muscles, fascia and tendons at wrist and hand level

7ᵈ **S66.811** Strain of other specified muscles, fascia and tendons at wrist and hand level, right hand POA

7ᵈ **S66.812** Strain of other specified muscles, fascia and tendons at wrist and hand level, left hand POA

7ᵈ **S66.819** Strain of other specified muscles, fascia and tendons at wrist and hand level, unspecified hand POA

6ᵈ **S66.82** Laceration of other specified muscles, fascia and tendons at wrist and hand level

7ᵈ **S66.821** Laceration of other specified muscles, fascia and tendons at wrist and hand level, right hand CC⬚ POA CC/MCC Exc

7ᵈ **S66.822** Laceration of other specified muscles, fascia and tendons at wrist and hand level, left hand CC⬚ POA CC/MCC Exc

7ᵈ **S66.829** Laceration of other specified muscles, fascia and tendons at wrist and hand level, unspecified hand CC⬚ POA CC/MCC Exc

6ᵈ **S66.89** Other injury of other specified muscles, fascia and tendons at wrist and hand level

7ᵈ **S66.891** Other injury of other specified muscles, fascia and tendons at wrist and hand level, right hand POA

7ᵈ **S66.892** Other injury of other specified muscles, fascia and tendons at wrist and hand level, left hand POA

7ᵈ **S66.899** Other injury of other specified muscles, fascia and tendons at wrist and hand level, unspecified hand POA

5ᵈ **S66.9** Injury of unspecified muscle, fascia and tendon at wrist and hand level

6ᵈ **S66.90** Unspecified injury of unspecified muscle, fascia and tendon at wrist and hand level

7ᵈ **S66.901** Unspecified injury of unspecified muscle, fascia and tendon at wrist and hand level, right hand POA

7ᵈ **S66.902** Unspecified injury of unspecified muscle, fascia and tendon at wrist and hand level, left hand POA

7ᵈ **S66.909** Unspecified injury of unspecified muscle, fascia and tendon at wrist and hand level, unspecified hand POA

6ᵈ **S66.91** Strain of unspecified muscle, fascia and tendon at wrist and hand level

7ᵈ **S66.911** Strain of unspecified muscle, fascia and tendon at wrist and hand level, right hand POA

7ᵈ **S66.912** Strain of unspecified muscle, fascia and tendon at wrist and hand level, left hand POA

7ᵈ **S66.919** Strain of unspecified muscle, fascia and tendon at wrist and hand level, unspecified hand POA

6ᵈ **S66.92** Laceration of unspecified muscle, fascia and tendon at wrist and hand level

7ᵈ **S66.921** Laceration of unspecified muscle, fascia and tendon at wrist and hand level, right hand CC⬚ POA CC/MCC Exc

7ᵈ **S66.922** Laceration of unspecified muscle, fascia and tendon at wrist and hand level, left hand CC⬚ POA CC/MCC Exc

---

Unspecified Code	Other Specified Code	Manifestation Code	Ⓝ Newborn Ⓟ Pediatric Ⓜ Maternity Ⓐ Adult ♂ Male ♀ Female

● New Code ▲ Revised Code Title ►◄ Revised Text **NOTES** *INCLUDES* *EXCLUDES1* Not coded here *EXCLUDES2* Not included here

4ᵈ 4ᵗʰ character required 5ᵈ 5ᵗʰ character required 6ᵈ 6ᵗʰ character required 7ᵈ 7ᵗʰ character required ⊗ Extension 'X' Alert

HAC Hospital-acquired condition (HAC) alert **AHA** AHA Coding Clinic© 📖 Code first alert

7️⃣ **S66.929** Laceration of unspecified muscle, fascia and tendon at wrist and hand level, unspecified hand CC POA CC/MCC Exc

6️⃣ **S66.99** Other injury of unspecified muscle, fascia and tendon at wrist and hand level

7️⃣ **S66.991** Other injury of unspecified muscle, fascia and tendon at wrist and hand level, right hand POA

7️⃣ **S66.992** Other injury of unspecified muscle, fascia and tendon at wrist and hand level, left hand POA

7️⃣ **S66.999** Other injury of unspecified muscle, fascia and tendon at wrist and hand level, unspecified hand POA

4️⃣ **S67** Crushing injury of wrist, hand and fingers

Use additional code for all associated injuries, such as:
fracture of wrist and hand (S62.-)
open wound of wrist and hand (S61.-)

The appropriate 7th character is to be added to each code from category S67
A = initial encounter
D = subsequent encounter
S = sequela

5️⃣ **S67.0** Crushing injury of thumb

7️⃣ **S67.00** Crushing injury of unspecified thumb POA
7️⃣ **S67.01** Crushing injury of right thumb POA
7️⃣ **S67.02** Crushing injury of left thumb POA

5️⃣ **S67.1** Crushing injury of other and unspecified finger(s)
EXCLUDES2 crushing injury of thumb (S67.0-)

7️⃣ **S67.10** Crushing injury of unspecified finger(s) POA

6️⃣ **S67.19** Crushing injury of other finger(s)
7️⃣ **S67.190** Crushing injury of right index finger POA
7️⃣ **S67.191** Crushing injury of left index finger POA
7️⃣ **S67.192** Crushing injury of right middle finger POA
7️⃣ **S67.193** Crushing injury of left middle finger POA
7️⃣ **S67.194** Crushing injury of right ring finger POA
7️⃣ **S67.195** Crushing injury of left ring finger POA
7️⃣ **S67.196** Crushing injury of right little finger POA
7️⃣ **S67.197** Crushing injury of left little finger POA
7️⃣ **S67.198** Crushing injury of other finger POA
Crushing injury of specified finger with unspecified laterality

5️⃣ **S67.2** Crushing injury of hand
EXCLUDES2 crushing injury of fingers (S67.1-)
crushing injury of thumb (S67.0-)

7️⃣ **S67.20** Crushing injury of unspecified hand POA
7️⃣ **S67.21** Crushing injury of right hand POA
7️⃣ **S67.22** Crushing injury of left hand POA

5️⃣ **S67.3** Crushing injury of wrist
7️⃣ **S67.30** Crushing injury of unspecified wrist POA
7️⃣ **S67.31** Crushing injury of right wrist POA
7️⃣ **S67.32** Crushing injury of left wrist POA

5️⃣ **S67.4** Crushing injury of wrist and hand
EXCLUDES1 crushing injury of hand alone (S67.2-)
crushing injury of wrist alone (S67.3-)
EXCLUDES2 crushing injury of fingers (S67.1-)
crushing injury of thumb (S67.0-)

7️⃣ **S67.40** Crushing injury of unspecified wrist and hand POA
7️⃣ **S67.41** Crushing injury of right wrist and hand POA
7️⃣ **S67.42** Crushing injury of left wrist and hand POA

5️⃣ **S67.9** Crushing injury of unspecified part(s) of wrist, hand and fingers

7️⃣ **S67.90** Crushing injury of unspecified part(s) of unspecified wrist, hand and fingers POA
7️⃣ **S67.91** Crushing injury of unspecified part(s) of right wrist, hand and fingers POA
7️⃣ **S67.92** Crushing injury of unspecified part(s) of left wrist, hand and fingers POA

4️⃣ **S68** Traumatic amputation of wrist, hand and fingers
An amputation not identified as partial or complete should be coded to complete

The appropriate 7th character is to be added to each code from category S68
A = initial encounter
D = subsequent encounter
S = sequela

5️⃣ **S68.0** Traumatic metacarpophalangeal amputation of thumb
Traumatic amputation of thumb NOS

6️⃣ **S68.01** Complete traumatic metacarpophalangeal amputation of thumb
7️⃣ **S68.011** Complete traumatic metacarpophalangeal amputation of right thumb POA HCC
7️⃣ **S68.012** Complete traumatic metacarpophalangeal amputation of left thumb POA HCC
7️⃣ **S68.019** Complete traumatic metacarpophalangeal amputation of unspecified thumb POA HCC

6️⃣ **S68.02** Partial traumatic metacarpophalangeal amputation of thumb
7️⃣ **S68.021** Partial traumatic metacarpophalangeal amputation of right thumb POA HCC
7️⃣ **S68.022** Partial traumatic metacarpophalangeal amputation of left thumb POA HCC
7️⃣ **S68.029** Partial traumatic metacarpophalangeal amputation of unspecified thumb POA HCC

5️⃣ **S68.1** Traumatic metacarpophalangeal amputation of other and unspecified finger
Traumatic amputation of finger NOS
EXCLUDES2 traumatic metacarpophalangeal amputation of thumb (S68.0-)

6️⃣ **S68.11** Complete traumatic metacarpophalangeal amputation of other and unspecified finger
7️⃣ **S68.110** Complete traumatic metacarpophalangeal amputation of right index finger POA HCC
7️⃣ **S68.111** Complete traumatic metacarpophalangeal amputation of left index finger POA HCC
7️⃣ **S68.112** Complete traumatic metacarpophalangeal amputation of right middle finger POA HCC
7️⃣ **S68.113** Complete traumatic metacarpophalangeal amputation of left middle finger POA HCC
7️⃣ **S68.114** Complete traumatic metacarpophalangeal amputation of right ring finger POA HCC
7️⃣ **S68.115** Complete traumatic metacarpophalangeal amputation of left ring finger POA HCC
7️⃣ **S68.116** Complete traumatic metacarpophalangeal amputation of right little finger POA HCC
7️⃣ **S68.117** Complete traumatic metacarpophalangeal amputation of left little finger POA HCC
7️⃣ **S68.118** Complete traumatic metacarpophalangeal amputation of other finger POA HCC
Complete traumatic metacarpophalangeal amputation of specified finger with unspecified laterality
7️⃣ **S68.119** Complete traumatic metacarpophalangeal amputation of unspecified finger POA HCC

6️⃣ **S68.12** Partial traumatic metacarpophalangeal amputation of other and unspecified finger
7️⃣ **S68.120** Partial traumatic metacarpophalangeal amputation of right index finger POA HCC
7️⃣ **S68.121** Partial traumatic metacarpophalangeal amputation of left index finger POA HCC
7️⃣ **S68.122** Partial traumatic metacarpophalangeal amputation of right middle finger POA HCC
7️⃣ **S68.123** Partial traumatic metacarpophalangeal amputation of left middle finger POA HCC
7️⃣ **S68.124** Partial traumatic metacarpophalangeal amputation of right ring finger POA HCC
7️⃣ **S68.125** Partial traumatic metacarpophalangeal amputation of left ring finger POA HCC
7️⃣ **S68.126** Partial traumatic metacarpophalangeal amputation of right little finger POA HCC

POA Unacceptable principal diagnosis symbol per Medicare code edits   POA Code exempt from diagnosis present on admission requirement
❓ Questionable admission   CC Complication or comorbidity   MCC Major complication or comorbidity   CC/MCC Exc CC/MCC exclusion
HCC HCC diagnosis code   RxHCC RxHCC diagnosis code   MACRA code   DEFINITION Describes condition/terminology
TIP Coding guidance   👁 Official Guideline Reference   Z1 Z code as first-listed diagnosis

[7th] S68.127 Partial traumatic metacarpophalangeal amputation of left little finger [POA] [HCC]

[7th] S68.128 Partial traumatic metacarpophalangeal amputation of other finger [POA] [HCC]
Partial traumatic metacarpophalangeal amputation of specified finger with unspecified laterality

[7th] S68.129 Partial traumatic metacarpophalangeal amputation of unspecified finger [POA] [HCC]

[5th] S68.4 Traumatic amputation of hand at wrist level
Traumatic amputation of hand NOS
Traumatic amputation of wrist

[6th] S68.41 Complete traumatic amputation of hand at wrist level

[7th] S68.411 Complete traumatic amputation of right hand at wrist level [CC] [POA] [HCC] [CC/MCC Exc]

[7th] S68.412 Complete traumatic amputation of left hand at wrist level [CC] [POA] [HCC] [CC/MCC Exc]

[7th] S68.419 Complete traumatic amputation of unspecified hand at wrist level [CC] [POA] [HCC] [CC/MCC Exc]

[6th] S68.42 Partial traumatic amputation of hand at wrist level

[7th] S68.421 Partial traumatic amputation of right hand at wrist level [CC] [POA] [HCC] [CC/MCC Exc]

[7th] S68.422 Partial traumatic amputation of left hand at wrist level [CC] [POA] [HCC] [CC/MCC Exc]

[7th] S68.429 Partial traumatic amputation of unspecified hand at wrist level [CC] [POA] [HCC] [CC/MCC Exc]

[5th] S68.5 Traumatic transphalangeal amputation of thumb
Traumatic interphalangeal joint amputation of thumb

[6th] S68.51 Complete traumatic transphalangeal amputation of thumb

[7th] S68.511 Complete traumatic transphalangeal amputation of right thumb [POA] [HCC]

[7th] S68.512 Complete traumatic transphalangeal amputation of left thumb [POA] [HCC]

[7th] S68.519 Complete traumatic transphalangeal amputation of unspecified thumb [POA] [HCC]

[6th] S68.52 Partial traumatic transphalangeal amputation of thumb

[7th] S68.521 Partial traumatic transphalangeal amputation of right thumb [POA] [HCC]

[7th] S68.522 Partial traumatic transphalangeal amputation of left thumb [POA] [HCC]

[7th] S68.529 Partial traumatic transphalangeal amputation of unspecified thumb [POA] [HCC]

[5th] S68.6 Traumatic transphalangeal amputation of other and unspecified finger

[6th] S68.61 Complete traumatic transphalangeal amputation of other and unspecified finger(s)

[7th] S68.610 Complete traumatic transphalangeal amputation of right index finger [POA] [HCC]

[7th] S68.611 Complete traumatic transphalangeal amputation of left index finger [POA] [HCC]

[7th] S68.612 Complete traumatic transphalangeal amputation of right middle finger [POA] [HCC]

[7th] S68.613 Complete traumatic transphalangeal amputation of left middle finger [POA] [HCC]

[7th] S68.614 Complete traumatic transphalangeal amputation of right ring finger [POA] [HCC]

[7th] S68.615 Complete traumatic transphalangeal amputation of left ring finger [POA] [HCC]

[7th] S68.616 Complete traumatic transphalangeal amputation of right little finger [POA] [HCC]

[7th] S68.617 Complete traumatic transphalangeal amputation of left little finger [POA] [HCC]

[7th] S68.618 Complete traumatic transphalangeal amputation of other finger [POA] [HCC]
Complete traumatic transphalangeal amputation of specified finger with unspecified laterality

[7th] S68.619 Complete traumatic transphalangeal amputation of unspecified finger [POA] [HCC]

[6th] S68.62 Partial traumatic transphalangeal amputation of other and unspecified finger

[7th] S68.620 Partial traumatic transphalangeal amputation of right index finger [POA] [HCC]

[7th] S68.621 Partial traumatic transphalangeal amputation of left index finger [POA] [HCC]

[7th] S68.622 Partial traumatic transphalangeal amputation of right middle finger [POA] [HCC]

[7th] S68.623 Partial traumatic transphalangeal amputation of left middle finger [POA] [HCC]

[7th] S68.624 Partial traumatic transphalangeal amputation of right ring finger [POA] [HCC]

[7th] S68.625 Partial traumatic transphalangeal amputation of left ring finger [POA] [HCC]

[7th] S68.626 Partial traumatic transphalangeal amputation of right little finger [POA] [HCC]

[7th] S68.627 Partial traumatic transphalangeal amputation of left little finger [POA] [HCC]

[7th] S68.628 Partial traumatic transphalangeal amputation of other finger [POA] [HCC]
Partial traumatic transphalangeal amputation of specified finger with unspecified laterality

[7th] S68.629 Partial traumatic transphalangeal amputation of unspecified finger [POA] [HCC]

[5th] S68.7 Traumatic transmetacarpal amputation of hand

[6th] S68.71 Complete traumatic transmetacarpal amputation of hand

[7th] S68.711 Complete traumatic transmetacarpal amputation of right hand [CC] [POA] [HCC] [CC/MCC Exc]

[7th] S68.712 Complete traumatic transmetacarpal amputation of left hand [CC] [POA] [HCC] [CC/MCC Exc]

[7th] S68.719 Complete traumatic transmetacarpal amputation of unspecified hand [CC] [POA] [HCC] [CC/MCC Exc]

[6th] S68.72 Partial traumatic transmetacarpal amputation of hand

[7th] S68.721 Partial traumatic transmetacarpal amputation of right hand [CC] [POA] [HCC] [CC/MCC Exc]

[7th] S68.722 Partial traumatic transmetacarpal amputation of left hand [CC] [POA] [HCC] [CC/MCC Exc]

[7th] S68.729 Partial traumatic transmetacarpal amputation of unspecified hand [CC] [POA] [HCC] [CC/MCC Exc]

[4th] S69 Other and unspecified injuries of wrist, hand and finger(s)
The appropriate 7th character is to be added to each code from category S69
A = initial encounter
D = subsequent encounter
S = sequela

[5th] S69.8 Other specified injuries of wrist, hand and finger(s)

[7th] S69.80 Other specified injuries of unspecified wrist, hand and finger(s) [POA]

[7th] S69.81 Other specified injuries of right wrist, hand and finger(s) [POA]

[7th] S69.82 Other specified injuries of left wrist, hand and finger(s) [POA]

[5th] S69.9 Unspecified injury of wrist, hand and finger(s)

[7th] S69.90 Unspecified injury of unspecified wrist, hand and finger(s) [POA]

[7th] S69.91 Unspecified injury of right wrist, hand and finger(s) [POA]

[7th] S69.92 Unspecified injury of left wrist, hand and finger(s) [POA]

Unspecified Code | Other Specified Code | Manifestation Code | [N] Newborn | [P] Pediatric | [M] Maternity | [A] Adult | ♂ Male | ♀ Female
● New Code | ▲ Revised Code Title | ►◄ Revised Text | NOTES | INCLUDES | EXCLUDES1 Not coded here | EXCLUDES2 Not included here
[4th] 4th character required | [5th] 5th character required | [6th] 6th character required | [7th] 7th character required | [X] Extension 'X' Alert
[HAC] Hospital-acquired condition (HAC) alert | AHA AHA Coding Clinic© | Code first alert

Injuries to the hip and thigh (S70-S79)

EXCLUDES2 burns and corrosions (T20-T32)

frostbite (T33-T34)

snake bite (T63.0-)

venomous insect bite or sting (T63.4-)

4ᵗʰ **S70** Superficial injury of hip and thigh

The appropriate 7th character is to be added to each code from category S70

A = initial encounter

D = subsequent encounter

S = sequela

5ᵗʰ **S70.0** Contusion of hip

- 7ᵗʰ **S70.00** Contusion of unspecified hip POA
- 7ᵗʰ **S70.01** Contusion of right hip POA
- 7ᵗʰ **S70.02** Contusion of left hip POA

5ᵗʰ **S70.1** Contusion of thigh

- 7ᵗʰ **S70.10** Contusion of unspecified thigh POA
- 7ᵗʰ **S70.11** Contusion of right thigh POA
- 7ᵗʰ **S70.12** Contusion of left thigh POA

5ᵗʰ **S70.2** Other superficial injuries of hip

- 6ᵗʰ **S70.21** Abrasion of hip
  - 7ᵗʰ **S70.211** Abrasion, right hip POA
  - 7ᵗʰ **S70.212** Abrasion, left hip POA
  - 7ᵗʰ **S70.219** Abrasion, unspecified hip POA
- 6ᵗʰ **S70.22** Blister (nonthermal) of hip
  - 7ᵗʰ **S70.221** Blister (nonthermal), right hip POA
  - 7ᵗʰ **S70.222** Blister (nonthermal), left hip POA
  - 7ᵗʰ **S70.229** Blister (nonthermal), unspecified hip POA
- 6ᵗʰ **S70.24** External constriction of hip
  - 7ᵗʰ **S70.241** External constriction, right hip POA
  - 7ᵗʰ **S70.242** External constriction, left hip POA
  - 7ᵗʰ **S70.249** External constriction, unspecified hip POA
- 6ᵗʰ **S70.25** Superficial foreign body of hip
  Splinter in the hip
  - 7ᵗʰ **S70.251** Superficial foreign body, right hip POA
  - 7ᵗʰ **S70.252** Superficial foreign body, left hip POA
  - 7ᵗʰ **S70.259** Superficial foreign body, unspecified hip POA
- 6ᵗʰ **S70.26** Insect bite (nonvenomous) of hip
  - 7ᵗʰ **S70.261** Insect bite (nonvenomous), right hip POA
  - 7ᵗʰ **S70.262** Insect bite (nonvenomous), left hip POA
  - 7ᵗʰ **S70.269** Insect bite (nonvenomous), unspecified hip POA
- 6ᵗʰ **S70.27** Other superficial bite of hip
  EXCLUDES1 open bite of hip (S71.05-)
  - 7ᵗʰ **S70.271** Other superficial bite of hip, right hip POA
  - 7ᵗʰ **S70.272** Other superficial bite of hip, left hip POA
  - 7ᵗʰ **S70.279** Other superficial bite of hip, unspecified hip POA

5ᵗʰ **S70.3** Other superficial injuries of thigh

- 6ᵗʰ **S70.31** Abrasion of thigh
  - 7ᵗʰ **S70.311** Abrasion, right thigh POA
  - 7ᵗʰ **S70.312** Abrasion, left thigh POA
  - 7ᵗʰ **S70.319** Abrasion, unspecified thigh POA
- 6ᵗʰ **S70.32** Blister (nonthermal) of thigh
  - 7ᵗʰ **S70.321** Blister (nonthermal), right thigh POA
  - 7ᵗʰ **S70.322** Blister (nonthermal), left thigh POA
  - 7ᵗʰ **S70.329** Blister (nonthermal), unspecified thigh POA
- 6ᵗʰ **S70.34** External constriction of thigh
  - 7ᵗʰ **S70.341** External constriction, right thigh POA
  - 7ᵗʰ **S70.342** External constriction, left thigh POA
  - 7ᵗʰ **S70.349** External constriction, unspecified thigh POA
- 6ᵗʰ **S70.35** Superficial foreign body of thigh
  Splinter in the thigh
  - 7ᵗʰ **S70.351** Superficial foreign body, right thigh POA
  - 7ᵗʰ **S70.352** Superficial foreign body, left thigh POA
  - 7ᵗʰ **S70.359** Superficial foreign body, unspecified thigh POA

6ᵗʰ **S70.36** Insect bite (nonvenomous) of thigh

- 7ᵗʰ **S70.361** Insect bite (nonvenomous), right thigh POA
- 7ᵗʰ **S70.362** Insect bite (nonvenomous), left thigh POA
- 7ᵗʰ **S70.369** Insect bite (nonvenomous), unspecified thigh POA

6ᵗʰ **S70.37** Other superficial bite of thigh

EXCLUDES1 open bite of thigh (S71.15)

- 7ᵗʰ **S70.371** Other superficial bite of right thigh POA
- 7ᵗʰ **S70.372** Other superficial bite of left thigh POA
- 7ᵗʰ **S70.379** Other superficial bite of unspecified thigh POA

5ᵗʰ **S70.9** Unspecified superficial injury of hip and thigh

- 6ᵗʰ **S70.91** Unspecified superficial injury of hip
  - 7ᵗʰ **S70.911** Unspecified superficial injury of right hip POA
  - 7ᵗʰ **S70.912** Unspecified superficial injury of left hip POA
  - 7ᵗʰ **S70.919** Unspecified superficial injury of unspecified hip POA
- 6ᵗʰ **S70.92** Unspecified superficial injury of thigh
  - 7ᵗʰ **S70.921** Unspecified superficial injury of right thigh POA
  - 7ᵗʰ **S70.922** Unspecified superficial injury of left thigh POA
  - 7ᵗʰ **S70.929** Unspecified superficial injury of unspecified thigh POA

4ᵗʰ **S71** Open wound of hip and thigh

Code also any associated wound infection

EXCLUDES1 open fracture of hip and thigh (S72.-)

traumatic amputation of hip and thigh (S78.-)

EXCLUDES2 bite of venomous animal (T63.-)

open wound of ankle, foot and toes (S91.-)

open wound of knee and lower leg (S81.-)

The appropriate 7th character is to be added to each code from category S71

A = initial encounter

D = subsequent encounter

S = sequela

5ᵗʰ **S71.0** Open wound of hip

- 6ᵗʰ **S71.00** Unspecified open wound of hip
  - 7ᵗʰ **S71.001** Unspecified open wound, right hip POA
  - 7ᵗʰ **S71.002** Unspecified open wound, left hip POA
  - 7ᵗʰ **S71.009** Unspecified open wound, unspecified hip POA
- 6ᵗʰ **S71.01** Laceration without foreign body of hip
  - 7ᵗʰ **S71.011** Laceration without foreign body, right hip POA
  - 7ᵗʰ **S71.012** Laceration without foreign body, left hip POA
  - 7ᵗʰ **S71.019** Laceration without foreign body, unspecified hip POA
- 6ᵗʰ **S71.02** Laceration with foreign body of hip
  - 7ᵗʰ **S71.021** Laceration with foreign body, right hip POA
  - 7ᵗʰ **S71.022** Laceration with foreign body, left hip POA
  - 7ᵗʰ **S71.029** Laceration with foreign body, unspecified hip POA
- 6ᵗʰ **S71.03** Puncture wound without foreign body of hip
  - 7ᵗʰ **S71.031** Puncture wound without foreign body, right hip POA
  - 7ᵗʰ **S71.032** Puncture wound without foreign body, left hip POA
  - 7ᵗʰ **S71.039** Puncture wound without foreign body, unspecified hip POA
- 6ᵗʰ **S71.04** Puncture wound with foreign body of hip
  - 7ᵗʰ **S71.041** Puncture wound with foreign body, right hip POA
  - 7ᵗʰ **S71.042** Puncture wound with foreign body, left hip POA
  - 7ᵗʰ **S71.049** Puncture wound with foreign body, unspecified hip POA

POA Unacceptable principal diagnosis symbol per Medicare code edits   POA Code exempt from diagnosis present on admission requirement
❓ Questionable admission   cᶜ Complication or comorbidity   ᴹᶜᶜ Major complication or comorbidity   ᶜᶜ/ᴹᶜᶜ CC/MCC exclusion
HCC HCC diagnosis code   RxHCC RxHCC diagnosis code   MACRA MACRA code   **DEFINITION** Describes condition/terminology
TIP Coding guidance   👁 Official Guideline Reference   Z1 Z code as first-listed diagnosis

S71.05 Open bite of hip
Bite of hip NOS
EXCLUDES1 superficial bite of hip (S70.26, S70.27)
S71.051 Open bite, right hip POA
S71.052 Open bite, left hip POA
S71.059 Open bite, unspecified hip POA

S71.1 Open wound of thigh
S71.10 Unspecified open wound of thigh
S71.101 Unspecified open wound, right thigh POA
S71.102 Unspecified open wound, left thigh POA
S71.109 Unspecified open wound, unspecified thigh POA

S71.11 Laceration without foreign body of thigh
S71.111 Laceration without foreign body, right thigh POA
S71.112 Laceration without foreign body, left thigh POA
S71.119 Laceration without foreign body, unspecified thigh POA

S71.12 Laceration with foreign body of thigh
S71.121 Laceration with foreign body, right thigh POA
S71.122 Laceration with foreign body, left thigh POA
S71.129 Laceration with foreign body, unspecified thigh POA

S71.13 Puncture wound without foreign body of thigh
S71.131 Puncture wound without foreign body, right thigh POA
S71.132 Puncture wound without foreign body, left thigh POA
S71.139 Puncture wound without foreign body, unspecified thigh POA

S71.14 Puncture wound with foreign body of thigh
S71.141 Puncture wound with foreign body, right thigh POA
S71.142 Puncture wound with foreign body, left thigh POA
S71.149 Puncture wound with foreign body, unspecified thigh POA

S71.15 Open bite of thigh
Bite of thigh NOS
EXCLUDES1 superficial bite of thigh (S70.37-)
S71.151 Open bite, right thigh POA
S71.152 Open bite, left thigh POA
S71.159 Open bite, unspecified thigh POA

S72 Fracture of femur (Figure 19.2)
See Official Guidelines "Coding of Traumatic Fractures" I.C.19.c
NOTES A fracture not indicated as displaced or nondisplaced should be coded to displaced
A fracture not indicated as open or closed should be coded to closed
The open fracture designations are based on the Gustilo open fracture classification
EXCLUDES1 traumatic amputation of hip and thigh (S78.-)
EXCLUDES2 fracture of lower leg and ankle (S82.-)
fracture of foot (S92.-)
periprosthetic fracture of prosthetic implant of hip (M97.0-)

The appropriate 7th character is to be added to all codes from category S72
A = initial encounter for closed fracture
B = initial encounter for open fracture type I or II
initial encounter for open fracture NOS
C = initial encounter for open fracture type IIIA, IIIB, or IIIC
D = subsequent encounter for closed fracture with routine healing
E = subsequent encounter for open fracture type I or II with routine healing
F = subsequent encounter for open fracture type IIIA, IIIB, or IIIC with routine healing
G = subsequent encounter for closed fracture with delayed healing
H = subsequent encounter for open fracture type I or II with delayed healing

J = subsequent encounter for open fracture type IIIA, IIIB, or IIIC with delayed healing
K = subsequent encounter for closed fracture with nonunion
M = subsequent encounter for open fracture type I or II with nonunion
N = subsequent encounter for open fracture type IIIA, IIIB, or IIIC with nonunion
P = subsequent encounter for closed fracture with malunion
Q = subsequent encounter for open fracture type I or II with malunion
R = subsequent encounter for open fracture type IIIA, IIIB, or IIIC with malunion
S = sequela

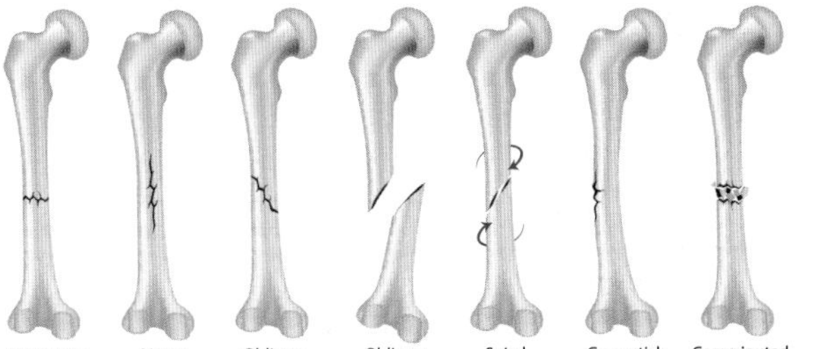

Figure 19.2 Types of Bone Fractures

Transverse, Linear, Oblique nondisplaced, Oblique displaced, Spiral, Greenstick, Comminuted

S72.0 Fracture of head and neck of femur
EXCLUDES2 physeal fracture of upper end of femur (S79.0-)
S72.00 Fracture of unspecified part of neck of femur
Fracture of hip NOS
Fracture of neck of femur NOS
S72.001 Fracture of unspecified part of neck of right femur
S72.002 Fracture of unspecified part of neck of left femur
AHA: Q1 2015, Q4 2015
S72.009 Fracture of unspecified part of neck of unspecified femur
S72.01 Unspecified intracapsular fracture of femur
Subcapital fracture of femur
S72.011 Unspecified intracapsular fracture of right femur
S72.012 Unspecified intracapsular fracture of left femur
S72.019 Unspecified intracapsular fracture of unspecified femur
S72.02 Fracture of epiphysis (separation) (upper) of femur
Transepiphyseal fracture of femur
EXCLUDES1 capital femoral epiphyseal fracture (pediatric) of femur (S79.01-)
Salter-Harris Type I physeal fracture of upper end of femur (S79.01-)
S72.021 Displaced fracture of epiphysis (separation) (upper) of right femur
S72.022 Displaced fracture of epiphysis (separation) (upper) of left femur
S72.023 Displaced fracture of epiphysis (separation) (upper) of unspecified femur
S72.024 Nondisplaced fracture of epiphysis (separation) (upper) of right femur
S72.025 Nondisplaced fracture of epiphysis (separation) (upper) of left femur
S72.026 Nondisplaced fracture of epiphysis (separation) (upper) of unspecified femur

S72.03 Midcervical fracture of femur
Transcervical fracture of femur NOS
- **S72.031** Displaced midcervical fracture of right femur `CC POA HAC HCC MCC CC/MCC Exc`
- **S72.032** Displaced midcervical fracture of left femur `CC POA HAC HCC MCC CC/MCC Exc`
- **S72.033** Displaced midcervical fracture of unspecified femur `CC POA HAC HCC MCC CC/MCC Exc`
- **S72.034** Nondisplaced midcervical fracture of right femur `CC POA HAC HCC MCC CC/MCC Exc`
- **S72.035** Nondisplaced midcervical fracture of left femur `CC POA HAC HCC MCC CC/MCC Exc`
- **S72.036** Nondisplaced midcervical fracture of unspecified femur `CC POA HAC HCC MCC CC/MCC Exc`

S72.04 Fracture of base of neck of femur
Cervicotrochanteric fracture of femur
- **S72.041** Displaced fracture of base of neck of right femur `CC POA HAC HCC MCC CC/MCC Exc`
- **S72.042** Displaced fracture of base of neck of left femur `CC POA HAC HCC MCC CC/MCC Exc`
- **S72.043** Displaced fracture of base of neck of unspecified femur `CC POA HAC HCC MCC CC/MCC Exc`
- **S72.044** Nondisplaced fracture of base of neck of right femur `CC POA HAC HCC MCC CC/MCC Exc`
- **S72.045** Nondisplaced fracture of base of neck of left femur `CC POA HAC HCC MCC CC/MCC Exc`
- **S72.046** Nondisplaced fracture of base of neck of unspecified femur `CC POA HAC HCC MCC CC/MCC Exc`

S72.05 Unspecified fracture of head of femur
Fracture of head of femur NOS
- **S72.051** Unspecified fracture of head of right femur `CC POA HAC HCC MCC CC/MCC Exc`
- **S72.052** Unspecified fracture of head of left femur `CC POA HAC HCC MCC CC/MCC Exc`
- **S72.059** Unspecified fracture of head of unspecified femur `CC POA HAC HCC MCC CC/MCC Exc`

S72.06 Articular fracture of head of femur
- **S72.061** Displaced articular fracture of head of right femur `CC POA HAC HCC MCC CC/MCC Exc`
- **S72.062** Displaced articular fracture of head of left femur `CC POA HAC HCC MCC CC/MCC Exc`
- **S72.063** Displaced articular fracture of head of unspecified femur `CC POA HAC HCC MCC CC/MCC Exc`
- **S72.064** Nondisplaced articular fracture of head of right femur `CC POA HAC HCC MCC CC/MCC Exc`
- **S72.065** Nondisplaced articular fracture of head of left femur `CC POA HAC HCC MCC CC/MCC Exc`
- **S72.066** Nondisplaced articular fracture of head of unspecified femur `CC POA HAC HCC MCC CC/MCC Exc`

S72.09 Other fracture of head and neck of femur
- **S72.091** Other fracture of head and neck of right femur `CC POA HAC HCC MCC CC/MCC Exc`
- **S72.092** Other fracture of head and neck of left femur `CC POA HAC HCC MCC CC/MCC Exc`
- **S72.099** Other fracture of head and neck of unspecified femur `CC POA HAC HCC MCC CC/MCC Exc`

S72.1 Pertrochanteric fracture
S72.10 Unspecified trochanteric fracture of femur
Fracture of trochanter NOS
- **S72.101** Unspecified trochanteric fracture of right femur `CC POA HAC HCC MCC CC/MCC Exc`
- **S72.102** Unspecified trochanteric fracture of left femur `CC POA HAC HCC MCC CC/MCC Exc`
- **S72.109** Unspecified trochanteric fracture of unspecified femur `CC POA HAC HCC MCC CC/MCC Exc`

S72.11 Fracture of greater trochanter of femur
- **S72.111** Displaced fracture of greater trochanter of right femur `CC POA HAC HCC MCC CC/MCC Exc`
- **S72.112** Displaced fracture of greater trochanter of left femur `CC POA HAC HCC MCC CC/MCC Exc`
- **S72.113** Displaced fracture of greater trochanter of unspecified femur `CC POA HAC HCC MCC CC/MCC Exc`

- **S72.114** Nondisplaced fracture of greater trochanter of right femur `CC POA HAC HCC MCC CC/MCC Exc`
- **S72.115** Nondisplaced fracture of greater trochanter of left femur `CC POA HAC HCC MCC CC/MCC Exc`
- **S72.116** Nondisplaced fracture of greater trochanter of unspecified femur `CC POA HAC HCC MCC CC/MCC Exc`

S72.12 Fracture of lesser trochanter of femur
- **S72.121** Displaced fracture of lesser trochanter of right femur `CC POA HAC HCC MCC CC/MCC Exc`
- **S72.122** Displaced fracture of lesser trochanter of left femur `CC POA HAC HCC MCC CC/MCC Exc`
- **S72.123** Displaced fracture of lesser trochanter of unspecified femur `CC POA HAC HCC MCC CC/MCC Exc`
- **S72.124** Nondisplaced fracture of lesser trochanter of right femur `CC POA HAC HCC MCC CC/MCC Exc`
- **S72.125** Nondisplaced fracture of lesser trochanter of left femur `CC POA HAC HCC MCC CC/MCC Exc`
- **S72.126** Nondisplaced fracture of lesser trochanter of unspecified femur `CC POA HAC HCC MCC CC/MCC Exc`

S72.13 Apophyseal fracture of femur
> **EXCLUDES1** chronic (nontraumatic) slipped upper femoral epiphysis (M93.0-)
- **S72.131** Displaced apophyseal fracture of right femur `CC POA HAC HCC MCC CC/MCC Exc`
- **S72.132** Displaced apophyseal fracture of left femur `CC POA HAC HCC MCC CC/MCC Exc`
- **S72.133** Displaced apophyseal fracture of unspecified femur `CC POA HAC HCC MCC CC/MCC Exc`
- **S72.134** Nondisplaced apophyseal fracture of right femur `CC POA HAC HCC MCC CC/MCC Exc`
- **S72.135** Nondisplaced apophyseal fracture of left femur `CC POA HAC HCC MCC CC/MCC Exc`
- **S72.136** Nondisplaced apophyseal fracture of unspecified femur `CC POA HAC HCC MCC CC/MCC Exc`

S72.14 Intertrochanteric fracture of femur
- **S72.141** Displaced intertrochanteric fracture of right femur `CC POA HAC HCC MCC CC/MCC Exc`
  - 👁 See Official Guidelines "Admissions/Encounters for Rehabilitation" II.K
  - **AHA:** Q4 2017, Q3 2016
- **S72.142** Displaced intertrochanteric fracture of left femur `CC POA HAC HCC MCC CC/MCC Exc`
- **S72.143** Displaced intertrochanteric fracture of unspecified femur `CC POA HAC HCC MCC CC/MCC Exc`
- **S72.144** Nondisplaced intertrochanteric fracture of right femur `CC POA HAC HCC MCC CC/MCC Exc`
- **S72.145** Nondisplaced intertrochanteric fracture of left femur `CC POA HAC HCC MCC CC/MCC Exc`
- **S72.146** Nondisplaced intertrochanteric fracture of unspecified femur `CC POA HAC HCC MCC CC/MCC Exc`

S72.2 Subtrochanteric fracture of femur
- **S72.21** Displaced subtrochanteric fracture of right femur `CC POA HAC HCC MCC CC/MCC Exc`
- **S72.22** Displaced subtrochanteric fracture of left femur `CC POA HAC HCC MCC CC/MCC Exc`
- **S72.23** Displaced subtrochanteric fracture of unspecified femur `CC POA HAC HCC MCC CC/MCC Exc`
- **S72.24** Nondisplaced subtrochanteric fracture of right femur `CC POA HAC HCC MCC CC/MCC Exc`
- **S72.25** Nondisplaced subtrochanteric fracture of left femur `CC POA HAC HCC MCC CC/MCC Exc`
- **S72.26** Nondisplaced subtrochanteric fracture of unspecified femur `CC POA HAC HCC MCC CC/MCC Exc`

S72.3 Fracture of shaft of femur
S72.30 Unspecified fracture of shaft of femur
- **S72.301** Unspecified fracture of shaft of right femur `CC POA HAC HCC MCC CC/MCC Exc`
- **S72.302** Unspecified fracture of shaft of left femur `CC POA HAC HCC MCC CC/MCC Exc`
- **S72.309** Unspecified fracture of shaft of unspecified femur `CC POA HAC HCC MCC CC/MCC Exc`

PDₓ Unacceptable principal diagnosis symbol per Medicare code edits   POA Code exempt from diagnosis present on admission requirement
? Questionable admission   CC Complication or comorbidity   MCC Major complication or comorbidity   CC/MCC Exc CC/MCC exclusion
HCC HCC diagnosis code   RxHCC RxHCC diagnosis code   MACRA code   **DEFINITION** Describes condition/terminology
TIP Coding guidance   👁 Official Guideline Reference   Z Z code as first-listed diagnosis

6ᵗʰ **S72.32** Transverse fracture of shaft of femur
  7ᵗʰ S72.321 Displaced **transverse fracture of shaft of** right **femur** cc POA HAC HCC MCC CC/MCC Exc
  7ᵗʰ S72.322 Displaced **transverse fracture of shaft of** left **femur** cc POA HAC HCC MCC CC/MCC Exc
  7ᵗʰ S72.323 Displaced **transverse fracture of shaft of unspecified femur** cc POA HAC HCC MCC CC/MCC Exc
  7ᵗʰ S72.324 Nondisplaced **transverse fracture of shaft of** right **femur** cc POA HAC HCC MCC CC/MCC Exc
  7ᵗʰ S72.325 Nondisplaced **transverse fracture of shaft of** left **femur** cc POA HAC HCC MCC CC/MCC Exc
  7ᵗʰ S72.326 Nondisplaced **transverse fracture of shaft of unspecified femur** cc POA HAC HCC MCC CC/MCC Exc

6ᵗʰ **S72.33** Oblique fracture of shaft of femur
  7ᵗʰ S72.331 Displaced **oblique fracture of shaft of** right **femur** cc POA HAC HCC MCC CC/MCC Exc
  7ᵗʰ S72.332 Displaced **oblique fracture of shaft of** left **femur** cc POA HAC HCC MCC CC/MCC Exc
  7ᵗʰ S72.333 Displaced **oblique fracture of shaft of unspecified femur** cc POA HAC HCC MCC CC/MCC Exc
  7ᵗʰ S72.334 Nondisplaced **oblique fracture of shaft of** right **femur** cc POA HAC HCC MCC CC/MCC Exc
  7ᵗʰ S72.335 Nondisplaced **oblique fracture of shaft of** left **femur** cc POA HAC HCC MCC CC/MCC Exc
  7ᵗʰ S72.336 Nondisplaced **oblique fracture of shaft of unspecified femur** cc POA HAC HCC MCC CC/MCC Exc

6ᵗʰ **S72.34** Spiral fracture of shaft of femur
  7ᵗʰ S72.341 Displaced **spiral fracture of shaft of** right **femur** cc POA HAC HCC MCC CC/MCC Exc
  7ᵗʰ S72.342 Displaced **spiral fracture of shaft of** left **femur** cc POA HAC HCC MCC CC/MCC Exc
  7ᵗʰ S72.343 Displaced **spiral fracture of shaft of unspecified femur** cc POA HAC HCC MCC CC/MCC Exc
  7ᵗʰ S72.344 Nondisplaced **spiral fracture of shaft of** right **femur** cc POA HAC HCC MCC CC/MCC Exc
  7ᵗʰ S72.345 Nondisplaced **spiral fracture of shaft of** left **femur** cc POA HAC HCC MCC CC/MCC Exc
  7ᵗʰ S72.346 Nondisplaced **spiral fracture of shaft of unspecified femur** cc POA HAC HCC MCC CC/MCC Exc

6ᵗʰ **S72.35** Comminuted fracture of shaft of femur
  7ᵗʰ S72.351 Displaced **comminuted fracture of shaft of** right **femur** cc POA HAC HCC MCC CC/MCC Exc
  7ᵗʰ S72.352 Displaced **comminuted fracture of shaft of** left **femur** cc POA HAC HCC MCC CC/MCC Exc
  7ᵗʰ S72.353 Displaced **comminuted fracture of shaft of unspecified femur** cc POA HAC HCC MCC CC/MCC Exc
  7ᵗʰ S72.354 Nondisplaced **comminuted fracture of shaft of** right **femur** cc POA HAC HCC MCC CC/MCC Exc
  7ᵗʰ S72.355 Nondisplaced **comminuted fracture of shaft of** left **femur** cc POA HAC HCC MCC CC/MCC Exc
  7ᵗʰ S72.356 Nondisplaced **comminuted fracture of shaft of unspecified femur** cc POA HAC HCC MCC CC/MCC Exc

6ᵗʰ **S72.36** Segmental fracture of shaft of femur
  7ᵗʰ S72.361 Displaced **segmental fracture of shaft of** right **femur** cc POA HAC HCC MCC CC/MCC Exc
  7ᵗʰ S72.362 Displaced **segmental fracture of shaft of** left **femur** cc POA HAC HCC MCC CC/MCC Exc
  7ᵗʰ S72.363 Displaced **segmental fracture of shaft of unspecified femur** cc POA HAC HCC MCC CC/MCC Exc
  7ᵗʰ S72.364 Nondisplaced **segmental fracture of shaft of** right **femur** cc POA HAC HCC MCC CC/MCC Exc
  7ᵗʰ S72.365 Nondisplaced **segmental fracture of shaft of** left **femur** cc POA HAC HCC MCC CC/MCC Exc
  7ᵗʰ S72.366 Nondisplaced **segmental fracture of shaft of unspecified femur** cc POA HAC HCC MCC CC/MCC Exc

6ᵗʰ **S72.39** Other fracture of shaft of femur
  7ᵗʰ S72.391 Other **fracture of shaft of** right **femur** cc POA HAC HCC MCC CC/MCC Exc
  7ᵗʰ S72.392 Other **fracture of shaft of** left **femur** cc POA HAC HCC MCC CC/MCC Exc
  7ᵗʰ S72.399 Other **fracture of shaft of unspecified femur** cc POA HAC HCC MCC CC/MCC Exc

5ᵗʰ **S72.4 Fracture of** lower end **of femur**
Fracture of distal end of femur
EXCLUDES2 *fracture of shaft of femur (S72.3-)*
physeal fracture of lower end of femur (S79.1-)

6ᵗʰ **S72.40** Unspecified fracture of lower end of femur
  7ᵗʰ S72.401 **Unspecified fracture of lower end of** right **femur** cc POA HAC HCC MCC CC/MCC Exc
    AHA: Q4 2016
  7ᵗʰ S72.402 **Unspecified fracture of lower end of** left **femur** cc POA HAC HCC MCC CC/MCC Exc
  7ᵗʰ S72.409 **Unspecified fracture of lower end of unspecified femur** cc POA HAC HCC MCC CC/MCC Exc

5ᵗʰ **S72.41** Unspecified condyle fracture of lower end of femur
Condyle fracture of femur NOS
  7ᵗʰ S72.411 Displaced **unspecified condyle fracture of lower end of** right **femur** cc POA HAC HCC MCC CC/MCC Exc
  7ᵗʰ S72.412 Displaced **unspecified condyle fracture of lower end of** left **femur** cc POA HAC HCC MCC CC/MCC Exc
  7ᵗʰ S72.413 Displaced **unspecified condyle fracture of lower end of unspecified femur** cc POA HAC HCC MCC CC/MCC Exc
  7ᵗʰ S72.414 Nondisplaced **unspecified condyle fracture of lower end of** right **femur** cc POA HAC HCC MCC CC/MCC Exc
  7ᵗʰ S72.415 Nondisplaced **unspecified condyle fracture of lower end of** left **femur** cc POA HAC HCC MCC CC/MCC Exc
  7ᵗʰ S72.416 Nondisplaced **unspecified condyle fracture of lower end of unspecified femur** cc POA HAC HCC MCC CC/MCC Exc

6ᵗʰ **S72.42 Fracture of** lateral condyle **of femur**
  7ᵗʰ S72.421 Displaced **fracture of lateral condyle of** right **femur** cc POA HAC HCC MCC CC/MCC Exc
  7ᵗʰ S72.422 Displaced **fracture of lateral condyle of** left **femur** cc POA HAC HCC MCC CC/MCC Exc
  7ᵗʰ S72.423 Displaced **fracture of lateral condyle of unspecified femur** cc POA HAC HCC MCC CC/MCC Exc
  7ᵗʰ S72.424 Nondisplaced **fracture of lateral condyle of** right **femur** cc POA HAC HCC MCC CC/MCC Exc
  7ᵗʰ S72.425 Nondisplaced **fracture of lateral condyle of** left **femur** cc POA HAC HCC MCC CC/MCC Exc
  7ᵗʰ S72.426 Nondisplaced **fracture of lateral condyle of unspecified femur** cc POA HAC HCC MCC CC/MCC Exc

6ᵗʰ **S72.43 Fracture of** medial condyle **of femur**
  7ᵗʰ S72.431 Displaced **fracture of medial condyle of** right **femur** cc POA HAC HCC MCC CC/MCC Exc
  7ᵗʰ S72.432 Displaced **fracture of medial condyle of** left **femur** cc POA HAC HCC MCC CC/MCC Exc
  7ᵗʰ S72.433 Displaced **fracture of medial condyle of unspecified femur** cc POA HAC HCC MCC CC/MCC Exc
  7ᵗʰ S72.434 Nondisplaced **fracture of medial condyle of** right **femur** cc POA HAC HCC MCC CC/MCC Exc
  7ᵗʰ S72.435 Nondisplaced **fracture of medial condyle of** left **femur** cc POA HAC HCC MCC CC/MCC Exc
  7ᵗʰ S72.436 Nondisplaced **fracture of medial condyle of unspecified femur** cc POA HAC HCC MCC CC/MCC Exc

6ᵗʰ **S72.44 Fracture of** lower epiphysis (separation) **of femur**
EXCLUDES1 *Salter-Harris Type I physeal fracture of lower end of femur (S79.11-)*
  7ᵗʰ S72.441 Displaced **fracture of lower epiphysis (separation) of** right **femur** cc POA HAC HCC MCC CC/MCC Exc
  7ᵗʰ S72.442 Displaced **fracture of lower epiphysis (separation) of** left **femur** cc POA HAC HCC MCC CC/MCC Exc
  7ᵗʰ S72.443 Displaced **fracture of lower epiphysis (separation) of unspecified femur** cc POA HAC HCC MCC CC/MCC Exc

---

Unspecified Code   Other Specified Code   Manifestation Code   Ⓝ Newborn   Ⓟ Pediatric   Ⓜ Maternity   Ⓐ Adult   ♂ Male   ♀ Female
● New Code   ▲ Revised Code Title   ►◄ Revised Text   **NOTES**   *INCLUDES*   *EXCLUDES1* Not coded here   *EXCLUDES2* Not included here
4ᵗʰ 4ᵗʰ character required   5ᵗʰ 5ᵗʰ character required   6ᵗʰ 6ᵗʰ character required   7ᵗʰ 7ᵗʰ character required   7ᵗʰ Extension 'X' Alert
HAC Hospital-acquired condition (HAC) alert   **AHA** AHA Coding Clinic©   📌 Code first alert

S72.444 axis Nondisplaced fracture of lower epiphysis (separation) of right femur ⚕ᴄᴄ ᴘᴏ̷ᴀ ᴴᴬᶜ ᴴᶜᶜ ᴹᶜᶜ ᴄᴄ/ᴍᴄᴄ ᴇxᴄ

S72.445 axis Nondisplaced fracture of lower epiphysis (separation) of left femur ⚕ᴄᴄ ᴘᴏ̷ᴀ ᴴᴬᶜ ᴴᶜᶜ ᴹᶜᶜ ᴄᴄ/ᴍᴄᴄ ᴇxᴄ

S72.446 axis Nondisplaced fracture of lower epiphysis (separation) of unspecified femur ⚕ᴄᴄ ᴘᴏ̷ᴀ ᴴᴬᶜ ᴴᶜᶜ ᴹᶜᶜ ᴄᴄ/ᴍᴄᴄ ᴇxᴄ

S72.45 Supracondylar fracture without intracondylar extension of lower end of femur
Supracondylar fracture of lower end of femur NOS
EXCLUDES1 *supracondylar fracture with intracondylar extension of lower end of femur (S72.46-)*

S72.451 axis Displaced supracondylar fracture without intracondylar extension of lower end of right femur ⚕ᴄᴄ ᴘᴏ̷ᴀ ᴴᴬᶜ ᴴᶜᶜ ᴹᶜᶜ ᴄᴄ/ᴍᴄᴄ ᴇxᴄ

S72.452 axis Displaced supracondylar fracture without intracondylar extension of lower end of left femur ⚕ᴄᴄ ᴘᴏ̷ᴀ ᴴᴬᶜ ᴴᶜᶜ ᴹᶜᶜ ᴄᴄ/ᴍᴄᴄ ᴇxᴄ

S72.453 axis Displaced supracondylar fracture without intracondylar extension of lower end of unspecified femur ⚕ᴄᴄ ᴘᴏ̷ᴀ ᴴᴬᶜ ᴴᶜᶜ ᴹᶜᶜ ᴄᴄ/ᴍᴄᴄ ᴇxᴄ

S72.454 axis Nondisplaced supracondylar fracture without intracondylar extension of lower end of right femur ⚕ᴄᴄ ᴘᴏ̷ᴀ ᴴᴬᶜ ᴴᶜᶜ ᴹᶜᶜ ᴄᴄ/ᴍᴄᴄ ᴇxᴄ

S72.455 axis Nondisplaced supracondylar fracture without intracondylar extension of lower end of left femur ⚕ᴄᴄ ᴘᴏ̷ᴀ ᴴᴬᶜ ᴴᶜᶜ ᴹᶜᶜ ᴄᴄ/ᴍᴄᴄ ᴇxᴄ

S72.456 axis Nondisplaced supracondylar fracture without intracondylar extension of lower end of unspecified femur ⚕ᴄᴄ ᴘᴏ̷ᴀ ᴴᴬᶜ ᴴᶜᶜ ᴹᶜᶜ ᴄᴄ/ᴍᴄᴄ ᴇxᴄ

S72.46 Supracondylar fracture with intracondylar extension of lower end of femur
EXCLUDES1 *supracondylar fracture without intracondylar extension of lower end of femur (S72.45-)*

S72.461 axis Displaced supracondylar fracture with intracondylar extension of lower end of right femur ⚕ᴄᴄ ᴘᴏ̷ᴀ ᴴᴬᶜ ᴴᶜᶜ ᴹᶜᶜ ᴄᴄ/ᴍᴄᴄ ᴇxᴄ

S72.462 axis Displaced supracondylar fracture with intracondylar extension of lower end of left femur ⚕ᴄᴄ ᴘᴏ̷ᴀ ᴴᴬᶜ ᴴᶜᶜ ᴹᶜᶜ ᴄᴄ/ᴍᴄᴄ ᴇxᴄ

S72.463 axis Displaced supracondylar fracture with intracondylar extension of lower end of unspecified femur ⚕ᴄᴄ ᴘᴏ̷ᴀ ᴴᴬᶜ ᴴᶜᶜ ᴹᶜᶜ ᴄᴄ/ᴍᴄᴄ ᴇxᴄ

S72.464 axis Nondisplaced supracondylar fracture with intracondylar extension of lower end of right femur ⚕ᴄᴄ ᴘᴏ̷ᴀ ᴴᴬᶜ ᴴᶜᶜ ᴹᶜᶜ ᴄᴄ/ᴍᴄᴄ ᴇxᴄ

S72.465 axis Nondisplaced supracondylar fracture with intracondylar extension of lower end of left femur ⚕ᴄᴄ ᴘᴏ̷ᴀ ᴴᴬᶜ ᴴᶜᶜ ᴹᶜᶜ ᴄᴄ/ᴍᴄᴄ ᴇxᴄ

S72.466 axis Nondisplaced supracondylar fracture with intracondylar extension of lower end of unspecified femur ⚕ᴄᴄ ᴘᴏ̷ᴀ ᴴᴬᶜ ᴴᶜᶜ ᴹᶜᶜ ᴄᴄ/ᴍᴄᴄ ᴇxᴄ

S72.47 Torus fracture of lower end of femur
The appropriate 7th character is to be added to all codes in subcategory S72.47
A = initial encounter for closed fracture
D = subsequent encounter for fracture with routine healing
G = subsequent encounter for fracture with delayed healing
K = subsequent encounter for fracture with nonunion
P = subsequent encounter for fracture with malunion
S = sequela

S72.471 axis Torus fracture of lower end of right femur ⚕ᴄᴄ ᴘᴏ̷ᴀ ᴴᴬᶜ ᴴᶜᶜ ᴄᴄ/ᴍᴄᴄ ᴇxᴄ

S72.472 axis Torus fracture of lower end of left femur ⚕ᴄᴄ ᴘᴏ̷ᴀ ᴴᴬᶜ ᴴᶜᶜ ᴄᴄ/ᴍᴄᴄ ᴇxᴄ

S72.479 axis **Torus fracture of lower end of unspecified femur** ⚕ᴄᴄ ᴘᴏ̷ᴀ ᴴᴬᶜ ᴴᶜᶜ ᴄᴄ/ᴍᴄᴄ ᴇxᴄ

S72.49 Other fracture of lower end of femur

S72.491 axis Other fracture of lower end of right femur ⚕ᴄᴄ ᴘᴏ̷ᴀ ᴴᴬᶜ ᴴᶜᶜ ᴹᶜᶜ ᴄᴄ/ᴍᴄᴄ ᴇxᴄ

S72.492 axis Other fracture of lower end of left femur ⚕ᴄᴄ ᴘᴏ̷ᴀ ᴴᴬᶜ ᴴᶜᶜ ᴹᶜᶜ ᴄᴄ/ᴍᴄᴄ ᴇxᴄ

S72.499 axis Other fracture of lower end of unspecified femur ⚕ᴄᴄ ᴘᴏ̷ᴀ ᴴᴬᶜ ᴴᶜᶜ ᴹᶜᶜ ᴄᴄ/ᴍᴄᴄ ᴇxᴄ

S72.8 Other fracture of femur

S72.8X Other fracture of femur

S72.8X1 axis Other fracture of right femur ⚕ᴄᴄ ᴘᴏ̷ᴀ ᴴᴬᶜ ᴴᶜᶜ ᴹᶜᶜ ᴄᴄ/ᴍᴄᴄ ᴇxᴄ

S72.8X2 axis Other fracture of left femur ⚕ᴄᴄ ᴘᴏ̷ᴀ ᴴᴬᶜ ᴴᶜᶜ ᴹᶜᶜ ᴄᴄ/ᴍᴄᴄ ᴇxᴄ

S72.8X9 axis Other fracture of unspecified femur ⚕ᴄᴄ ᴘᴏ̷ᴀ ᴴᴬᶜ ᴴᶜᶜ ᴹᶜᶜ ᴄᴄ/ᴍᴄᴄ ᴇxᴄ

S72.9 Unspecified fracture of femur
Fracture of thigh NOS
Fracture of upper leg NOS
EXCLUDES1 *fracture of hip NOS (S72.00-, S72.01-)*

S72.90 axis **Unspecified fracture of unspecified femur** ⚕ᴄᴄ ᴘᴏ̷ᴀ ᴴᴬᶜ ᴴᶜᶜ ᴹᶜᶜ ᴄᴄ/ᴍᴄᴄ ᴇxᴄ

S72.91 axis **Unspecified fracture of right femur** ⚕ᴄᴄ ᴘᴏ̷ᴀ ᴴᴬᶜ ᴴᶜᶜ ᴹᶜᶜ ᴄᴄ/ᴍᴄᴄ ᴇxᴄ

S72.92 axis **Unspecified fracture of left femur** ⚕ᴄᴄ ᴘᴏ̷ᴀ ᴴᴬᶜ ᴴᶜᶜ ᴹᶜᶜ ᴄᴄ/ᴍᴄᴄ ᴇxᴄ

S73 Dislocation and sprain of joint and ligaments of hip
INCLUDES   avulsion of joint or ligament of hip
             laceration of cartilage, joint or ligament of hip
             sprain of cartilage, joint or ligament of hip
             traumatic hemarthrosis of joint or ligament of hip
             traumatic rupture of joint or ligament of hip
             traumatic subluxation of joint or ligament of hip
             traumatic tear of joint or ligament of hip
Code also any associated open wound
EXCLUDES2 *strain of muscle, fascia and tendon of hip and thigh (S76.-)*
The appropriate 7th character is to be added to each code from category S73
A = initial encounter
D = subsequent encounter
S = sequela

S73.0 Subluxation and dislocation of hip
EXCLUDES2 *dislocation and subluxation of hip prosthesis (T84.020, T84.021)*

S73.00 Unspecified subluxation and dislocation of hip
Dislocation of hip NOS
Subluxation of hip NOS

S73.001 axis Unspecified subluxation of right hip ⚕ᴄᴄ ᴘᴏ̷ᴀ ᴴᴬᶜ ᴴᶜᶜ ᴄᴄ/ᴍᴄᴄ ᴇxᴄ

S73.002 axis Unspecified subluxation of left hip ⚕ᴄᴄ ᴘᴏ̷ᴀ ᴴᴬᶜ ᴴᶜᶜ ᴄᴄ/ᴍᴄᴄ ᴇxᴄ

S73.003 axis Unspecified subluxation of unspecified hip ⚕ᴄᴄ ᴘᴏ̷ᴀ ᴴᴬᶜ ᴴᶜᶜ ᴄᴄ/ᴍᴄᴄ ᴇxᴄ

S73.004 axis Unspecified dislocation of right hip ⚕ᴄᴄ ᴘᴏ̷ᴀ ᴴᴬᶜ ᴴᶜᶜ ᴄᴄ/ᴍᴄᴄ ᴇxᴄ

S73.005 axis Unspecified dislocation of left hip ⚕ᴄᴄ ᴘᴏ̷ᴀ ᴴᴬᶜ ᴴᶜᶜ ᴄᴄ/ᴍᴄᴄ ᴇxᴄ

S73.006 axis Unspecified dislocation of unspecified hip ⚕ᴄᴄ ᴘᴏ̷ᴀ ᴴᴬᶜ ᴴᶜᶜ ᴄᴄ/ᴍᴄᴄ ᴇxᴄ

S73.01 Posterior subluxation and dislocation of hip

S73.011 axis Posterior subluxation of right hip ⚕ᴄᴄ ᴘᴏ̷ᴀ ᴴᴬᶜ ᴴᶜᶜ ᴄᴄ/ᴍᴄᴄ ᴇxᴄ

S73.012 axis Posterior subluxation of left hip ⚕ᴄᴄ ᴘᴏ̷ᴀ ᴴᴬᶜ ᴴᶜᶜ ᴄᴄ/ᴍᴄᴄ ᴇxᴄ

S73.013 axis Posterior subluxation of unspecified hip ⚕ᴄᴄ ᴘᴏ̷ᴀ ᴴᴬᶜ ᴴᶜᶜ ᴄᴄ/ᴍᴄᴄ ᴇxᴄ

S73.014 axis Posterior dislocation of right hip ⚕ᴄᴄ ᴘᴏ̷ᴀ ᴴᴬᶜ ᴴᶜᶜ ᴄᴄ/ᴍᴄᴄ ᴇxᴄ

ᴘᴅx Unacceptable principal diagnosis symbol per Medicare code edits   ᴘᴏ̷ᴀ Code exempt from diagnosis present on admission requirement
? Questionable admission   ⚕ᴄᴄ Complication or comorbidity   ᴹᶜᶜ Major complication or comorbidity   ᴄᴄ/ᴍᴄᴄ Exᴄ CC/MCC exclusion
ᴴᶜᶜ HCC diagnosis code   ᴿxᴴᶜᶜ RxHCC diagnosis code   MACRA code   **DEFINITION** Describes condition/terminology
TIP Coding guidance   👁 Official Guideline Reference   🆉 Z code as first-listed diagnosis

1066   When symbols appear on a code that requires a 7th character extension, refer to Appendix B to identify applicable 7th character codes.   **2020 ICD-10-CM**

[7th] S73.015 Posterior dislocation of left hip [CC] [POA] [HAC] [HCC] [CC/MCC Exc]

[7th] S73.016 Posterior dislocation of unspecified hip [CC] [POA] [HAC] [HCC] [CC/MCC Exc]

[6th] S73.02 Obturator subluxation and dislocation of hip

[7th] S73.021 Obturator subluxation of right hip [CC] [POA] [HAC] [HCC] [CC/MCC Exc]

[7th] S73.022 Obturator subluxation of left hip [CC] [POA] [HAC] [HCC] [CC/MCC Exc]

[7th] S73.023 Obturator subluxation of unspecified hip [CC] [POA] [HAC] [HCC] [CC/MCC Exc]

[7th] S73.024 Obturator dislocation of right hip [CC] [POA] [HAC] [HCC] [CC/MCC Exc]

[7th] S73.025 Obturator dislocation of left hip [CC] [POA] [HAC] [HCC] [CC/MCC Exc]

[7th] S73.026 Obturator dislocation of unspecified hip [CC] [POA] [HAC] [HCC] [CC/MCC Exc]

[6th] S73.03 Other anterior subluxation and dislocation of hip

[7th] S73.031 Other anterior subluxation of right hip [CC] [POA] [HAC] [HCC] [CC/MCC Exc]

[7th] S73.032 Other anterior subluxation of left hip [CC] [POA] [HAC] [HCC] [CC/MCC Exc]

[7th] S73.033 Other anterior subluxation of unspecified hip [CC] [POA] [HAC] [HCC] [CC/MCC Exc]

[7th] S73.034 Other anterior dislocation of right hip [CC] [POA] [HAC] [HCC] [CC/MCC Exc]

[7th] S73.035 Other anterior dislocation of left hip [CC] [POA] [HAC] [HCC] [CC/MCC Exc]

[7th] S73.036 Other anterior dislocation of unspecified hip [CC] [POA] [HAC] [HCC] [CC/MCC Exc]

[6th] S73.04 Central subluxation and dislocation of hip

[7th] S73.041 Central subluxation of right hip [CC] [POA] [HAC] [HCC] [CC/MCC Exc]

[7th] S73.042 Central subluxation of left hip [CC] [POA] [HAC] [HCC] [CC/MCC Exc]

[7th] S73.043 Central subluxation of unspecified hip [CC] [POA] [HAC] [HCC] [CC/MCC Exc]

[7th] S73.044 Central dislocation of right hip [CC] [POA] [HAC] [HCC] [CC/MCC Exc]

[7th] S73.045 Central dislocation of left hip [CC] [POA] [HAC] [HCC] [CC/MCC Exc]

[7th] S73.046 Central dislocation of unspecified hip [CC] [POA] [HAC] [HCC] [CC/MCC Exc]

[5th] S73.1 Sprain of hip

[6th] S73.10 Unspecified sprain of hip

[7th] S73.101 Unspecified sprain of right hip [POA]

[7th] S73.102 Unspecified sprain of left hip [POA]

[7th] S73.109 Unspecified sprain of unspecified hip [POA]

[6th] S73.11 Iliofemoral ligament sprain of hip

[7th] S73.111 Iliofemoral ligament sprain of right hip [POA]

[7th] S73.112 Iliofemoral ligament sprain of left hip [POA]

[7th] S73.119 Iliofemoral ligament sprain of unspecified hip [POA]

[6th] S73.12 Ischiocapsular (ligament) sprain of hip

[7th] S73.121 Ischiocapsular ligament sprain of right hip [POA]

[7th] S73.122 Ischiocapsular ligament sprain of left hip [POA]

[7th] S73.129 Ischiocapsular ligament sprain of unspecified hip [POA]

[6th] S73.19 Other sprain of hip

[7th] S73.191 Other sprain of right hip [POA]

[7th] S73.192 Other sprain of left hip [POA]

[7th] S73.199 Other sprain of unspecified hip [POA]

[4th] S74 Injury of nerves at hip and thigh level

Code also any associated open wound (S71.-)

EXCLUDES2 *injury of nerves at ankle and foot level (S94.-)*
injury of nerves at lower leg level (S84.-)

The appropriate 7th character is to be added to each code from category S74

A = initial encounter
D = subsequent encounter
S = sequela

[5th] S74.0 Injury of sciatic nerve at hip and thigh level

[7th] S74.00 Injury of sciatic nerve at hip and thigh level, unspecified leg [POA]

[7th] S74.01 Injury of sciatic nerve at hip and thigh level, right leg [POA]

[7th] S74.02 Injury of sciatic nerve at hip and thigh level, left leg [POA]

[5th] S74.1 Injury of femoral nerve at hip and thigh level

[7th] S74.10 Injury of femoral nerve at hip and thigh level, unspecified leg [POA]

[7th] S74.11 Injury of femoral nerve at hip and thigh level, right leg [POA]

[7th] S74.12 Injury of femoral nerve at hip and thigh level, left leg [POA]

[5th] S74.2 Injury of cutaneous sensory nerve at hip and thigh level

[7th] S74.20 Injury of cutaneous sensory nerve at hip and thigh level, unspecified leg [POA]

[7th] S74.21 Injury of cutaneous sensory nerve at hip and high level, right leg [POA]

[7th] S74.22 Injury of cutaneous sensory nerve at hip and thigh level, left leg [POA]

[5th] S74.8 Injury of other nerves at hip and thigh level

[6th] S74.8X Injury of other nerves at hip and thigh level

[7th] S74.8X1 Injury of other nerves at hip and thigh level, right leg [POA]

[7th] S74.8X2 Injury of other nerves at hip and thigh level, left leg [POA]

[7th] S74.8X9 Injury of other nerves at hip and thigh level, unspecified leg [POA]

[5th] S74.9 Injury of unspecified nerve at hip and thigh level

[7th] S74.90 Injury of unspecified nerve at hip and thigh level, unspecified leg [POA]

[7th] S74.91 Injury of unspecified nerve at hip and thigh level, right leg [POA]

[7th] S74.92 Injury of unspecified nerve at hip and thigh level, left leg [POA]

[4th] S75 Injury of blood vessels at hip and thigh level

Code also any associated open wound (S71.-)

EXCLUDES2 *injury of blood vessels at lower leg level (S85.-)*
injury of popliteal artery (S85.0)

The appropriate 7th character is to be added to each code from category S75

A = initial encounter
D = subsequent encounter
S = sequela

[5th] S75.0 Injury of femoral artery

[6th] S75.00 Unspecified injury of femoral artery

[7th] S75.001 Unspecified injury of femoral artery, right leg [POA] [MCC] [CC/MCC Exc]

[7th] S75.002 Unspecified injury of femoral artery, left leg [POA] [MCC] [CC/MCC Exc]

[7th] S75.009 Unspecified injury of femoral artery, unspecified leg [POA] [MCC] [CC/MCC Exc]

[6th] S75.01 Minor laceration of femoral artery

Incomplete transection of femoral artery
Laceration of femoral artery NOS
Superficial laceration of femoral artery

[7th] S75.011 Minor laceration of femoral artery, right leg [POA] [MCC] [CC/MCC Exc]

Unspecified Code Other Specified Code Manifestation Code [N] Newborn [P] Pediatric [M] Maternity [A] Adult ♂ Male ♀ Female
● New Code ▲ Revised Code Title ►◄ Revised Text NOTES INCLUDES EXCLUDES1 Not coded here EXCLUDES2 Not included here
[4th] 4th character required [5th] 5th character required [6th] 6th character required [7th] 7th character required [X] Extension 'X' Alert
[HAC] Hospital-acquired condition (HAC) alert AHA AHA Coding Clinic© ☞ Code first alert

When symbols appear on a code that requires a 7th character extension, refer to Appendix B to identify applicable 7th character codes.

[7th] S75.012 Minor laceration of femoral artery, left leg POA MCC CC/MCC Exc
[7th] S75.019 Minor laceration of femoral artery, unspecified leg POA MCC CC/MCC Exc
[6th] S75.02 Major laceration of femoral artery
Complete transection of femoral artery
Traumatic rupture of femoral artery
[7th] S75.021 Major laceration of femoral artery, right leg POA MCC CC/MCC Exc
[7th] S75.022 Major laceration of femoral artery, left leg POA MCC CC/MCC Exc
[7th] S75.029 Major laceration of femoral artery, unspecified leg POA MCC CC/MCC Exc
[6th] S75.09 Other specified injury of femoral artery
[7th] S75.091 Other specified injury of femoral artery, right leg POA MCC CC/MCC Exc
[7th] S75.092 Other specified injury of femoral artery, left leg POA MCC CC/MCC Exc
[7th] S75.099 Other specified injury of femoral artery, unspecified leg POA MCC CC/MCC Exc
[5th] S75.1 Injury of femoral vein at hip and thigh level
[6th] S75.10 Unspecified injury of femoral vein at hip and thigh level
[7th] S75.101 Unspecified injury of femoral vein at hip and thigh level, right leg POA MCC CC/MCC Exc
[7th] S75.102 Unspecified injury of femoral vein at hip and thigh level, left leg POA MCC CC/MCC Exc
[7th] S75.109 Unspecified injury of femoral vein at hip and thigh level, unspecified leg POA MCC CC/MCC Exc
[6th] S75.11 Minor laceration of femoral vein at hip and thigh level
Incomplete transection of femoral vein at hip and thigh level
Laceration of femoral vein at hip and thigh level NOS
Superficial laceration of femoral vein at hip and thigh level
[7th] S75.111 Minor laceration of femoral vein at hip and thigh level, right leg POA MCC CC/MCC Exc
[7th] S75.112 Minor laceration of femoral vein at hip and thigh level, left leg POA MCC CC/MCC Exc
[7th] S75.119 Minor laceration of femoral vein at hip and thigh level, unspecified leg POA MCC CC/MCC Exc
[6th] S75.12 Major laceration of femoral vein at hip and thigh level
Complete transection of femoral vein at hip and thigh level
Traumatic rupture of femoral vein at hip and thigh level
[7th] S75.121 Major laceration of femoral vein at hip and thigh level, right leg POA MCC CC/MCC Exc
[7th] S75.122 Major laceration of femoral vein at hip and thigh level, left leg POA MCC CC/MCC Exc
[7th] S75.129 Major laceration of femoral vein at hip and thigh level, unspecified leg POA MCC CC/MCC Exc
[6th] S75.19 Other specified injury of femoral vein at hip and thigh level
[7th] S75.191 Other specified injury of femoral vein at hip and thigh level, right leg POA MCC CC/MCC Exc
[7th] S75.192 Other specified injury of femoral vein at hip and thigh level, left leg POA MCC CC/MCC Exc
[7th] S75.199 Other specified injury of femoral vein at hip and thigh level, unspecified leg POA MCC CC/MCC Exc
[5th] S75.2 Injury of greater saphenous vein at hip and thigh level
EXCLUDES1 *greater saphenous vein NOS (S85.3)*
[6th] S75.20 Unspecified injury of greater saphenous vein at hip and thigh level
[7th] S75.201 Unspecified injury of greater saphenous vein at hip and thigh level, right leg CC POA CC/MCC Exc
[7th] S75.202 Unspecified injury of greater saphenous vein at hip and thigh level, left leg CC POA CC/MCC Exc
[7th] S75.209 Unspecified injury of greater saphenous vein at hip and thigh level, unspecified leg CC POA CC/MCC Exc
[6th] S75.21 Minor laceration of greater saphenous vein at hip and thigh level
Incomplete transection of greater saphenous vein at hip and thigh level
Laceration of greater saphenous vein at hip and thigh level NOS
Superficial laceration of greater saphenous vein at hip and thigh level
[7th] S75.211 Minor laceration of greater saphenous vein at hip and thigh level, right leg CC POA CC/MCC Exc
[7th] S75.212 Minor laceration of greater saphenous vein at hip and thigh level, left leg CC POA CC/MCC Exc
[7th] S75.219 Minor laceration of greater saphenous vein at hip and thigh level, unspecified leg CC POA CC/MCC Exc
[6th] S75.22 Major laceration of greater saphenous vein at hip and thigh level
Complete transection of greater saphenous vein at hip and thigh level
Traumatic rupture of greater saphenous vein at hip and thigh level
[7th] S75.221 Major laceration of greater saphenous vein at hip and thigh level, right leg CC POA CC/MCC Exc
[7th] S75.222 Major laceration of greater saphenous vein at hip and thigh level, left leg CC POA CC/MCC Exc
[7th] S75.229 Major laceration of greater saphenous vein at hip and thigh level, unspecified leg CC POA CC/MCC Exc
[6th] S75.29 Other specified injury of greater saphenous vein at hip and thigh level
[7th] S75.291 Other specified injury of greater saphenous vein at hip and thigh level, right leg CC POA CC/MCC Exc
[7th] S75.292 Other specified injury of greater saphenous vein at hip and thigh level, left leg CC POA CC/MCC Exc
[7th] S75.299 Other specified injury of greater saphenous vein at hip and thigh level, unspecified leg CC POA CC/MCC Exc
[5th] S75.8 Injury of other blood vessels at hip and thigh level
[6th] S75.80 Unspecified injury of other blood vessels at hip and thigh level
[7th] S75.801 Unspecified injury of other blood vessels at hip and thigh level, right leg CC POA CC/MCC Exc
[7th] S75.802 Unspecified injury of other blood vessels at hip and thigh level, left leg CC POA CC/MCC Exc
[7th] S75.809 Unspecified injury of other blood vessels at hip and thigh level, unspecified leg CC POA CC/MCC Exc
[6th] S75.81 Laceration of other blood vessels at hip and thigh level
[7th] S75.811 Laceration of other blood vessels at hip and thigh level, right leg CC POA CC/MCC Exc
[7th] S75.812 Laceration of other blood vessels at hip and thigh level, left leg CC POA CC/MCC Exc
[7th] S75.819 Laceration of other blood vessels at hip and thigh level, unspecified leg CC POA CC/MCC Exc
[6th] S75.89 Other specified injury of other blood vessels at hip and thigh level
[7th] S75.891 Other specified injury of other blood vessels at hip and thigh level, right leg CC POA CC/MCC Exc

PDx Unacceptable principal diagnosis symbol per Medicare code edits POA Code exempt from diagnosis present on admission requirement
? Questionable admission CC Complication or comorbidity MCC Major complication or comorbidity CC/MCC Exc CC/MCC exclusion
HCC HCC diagnosis code RxHCC RxHCC diagnosis code MACRA code **DEFINITION** Describes condition/terminology
TIP Coding guidance 👁 Official Guideline Reference Z1 Z code as first-listed diagnosis

7️⃣ **S75.892** Other specified injury of other blood vessels at hip and thigh level, left leg CC⊘ POA CC/MCC Exc

7️⃣ **S75.899** Other specified injury of other blood vessels at hip and thigh level, unspecified leg CC⊘ POA CC/MCC Exc

5️⃣ **S75.9** Injury of unspecified blood vessel at hip and thigh level

6️⃣ **S75.90** Unspecified injury of unspecified blood vessel at hip and thigh level

7️⃣ **S75.901** Unspecified injury of unspecified blood vessel at hip and thigh level, right leg CC⊘ POA CC/MCC Exc

7️⃣ **S75.902** Unspecified injury of unspecified blood vessel at hip and thigh level, left leg CC⊘ POA CC/MCC Exc

7️⃣ **S75.909** Unspecified injury of unspecified blood vessel at hip and thigh level, unspecified leg CC⊘ POA CC/MCC Exc

6️⃣ **S75.91** Laceration of unspecified blood vessel at hip and thigh level

7️⃣ **S75.911** Laceration of unspecified blood vessel at hip and thigh level, right leg CC⊘ POA CC/MCC Exc

7️⃣ **S75.912** Laceration of unspecified blood vessel at hip and thigh level, left leg CC⊘ POA CC/MCC Exc

7️⃣ **S75.919** Laceration of unspecified blood vessel at hip and thigh level, unspecified leg CC⊘ POA CC/MCC Exc

6️⃣ **S75.99** Other specified injury of unspecified blood vessel at hip and thigh level

7️⃣ **S75.991** Other specified injury of unspecified blood vessel at hip and thigh level, right leg CC⊘ POA CC/MCC Exc

7️⃣ **S75.992** Other specified injury of unspecified blood vessel at hip and thigh level, left leg CC⊘ POA CC/MCC Exc

7️⃣ **S75.999** Other specified injury of unspecified blood vessel at hip and thigh level, unspecified leg CC⊘ POA CC/MCC Exc

4️⃣ **S76** Injury of muscle, fascia and tendon at hip and thigh level
Code also any associated open wound (S71.-)
EXCLUDES2 injury of muscle, fascia and tendon at lower leg level (S86)
sprain of joint and ligament of hip (S73.1)

The appropriate 7th character is to be added to each code from category S76
A = initial encounter
D = subsequent encounter
S = sequela

5️⃣ **S76.0** Injury of muscle, fascia and tendon of hip

6️⃣ **S76.00** Unspecified injury of muscle, fascia and tendon of hip

7️⃣ **S76.001** Unspecified injury of muscle, fascia and tendon of right hip POA

7️⃣ **S76.002** Unspecified injury of muscle, fascia and tendon of left hip POA

7️⃣ **S76.009** Unspecified injury of muscle, fascia and tendon of unspecified hip POA

6️⃣ **S76.01** Strain of muscle, fascia and tendon of hip

7️⃣ **S76.011** Strain of muscle, fascia and tendon of right hip POA

7️⃣ **S76.012** Strain of muscle, fascia and tendon of left hip POA

7️⃣ **S76.019** Strain of muscle, fascia and tendon of unspecified hip POA

6️⃣ **S76.02** Laceration of muscle, fascia and tendon of hip

7️⃣ **S76.021** Laceration of muscle, fascia and tendon of right hip CC⊘ POA CC/MCC Exc

7️⃣ **S76.022** Laceration of muscle, fascia and tendon of left hip CC⊘ POA CC/MCC Exc

7️⃣ **S76.029** Laceration of muscle, fascia and tendon of unspecified hip CC⊘ POA CC/MCC Exc

6️⃣ **S76.09** Other specified injury of muscle, fascia and tendon of hip

7️⃣ **S76.091** Other specified injury of muscle, fascia and tendon of right hip POA

7️⃣ **S76.092** Other specified injury of muscle, fascia and tendon of left hip POA

7️⃣ **S76.099** Other specified injury of muscle, fascia and tendon of unspecified hip POA

5️⃣ **S76.1** Injury of quadriceps muscle, fascia and tendon
Injury of patellar ligament (tendon)

6️⃣ **S76.10** Unspecified injury of quadriceps muscle, fascia and tendon

7️⃣ **S76.101** Unspecified injury of right quadriceps muscle, fascia and tendon POA

7️⃣ **S76.102** Unspecified injury of left quadriceps muscle, fascia and tendon POA

7️⃣ **S76.109** Unspecified injury of unspecified quadriceps muscle, fascia and tendon POA

6️⃣ **S76.11** Strain of quadriceps muscle, fascia and tendon

7️⃣ **S76.111** Strain of right quadriceps muscle, fascia and tendon POA

7️⃣ **S76.112** Strain of left quadriceps muscle, fascia and tendon POA

7️⃣ **S76.119** Strain of unspecified quadriceps muscle, fascia and tendon POA

6️⃣ **S76.12** Laceration of quadriceps muscle, fascia and tendon

7️⃣ **S76.121** Laceration of right quadriceps muscle, fascia and tendon CC⊘ POA CC/MCC Exc

7️⃣ **S76.122** Laceration of left quadriceps muscle, fascia and tendon CC⊘ POA CC/MCC Exc

7️⃣ **S76.129** Laceration of unspecified quadriceps muscle, fascia and tendon CC⊘ POA CC/MCC Exc

6️⃣ **S76.19** Other specified injury of quadriceps muscle, fascia and tendon

7️⃣ **S76.191** Other specified injury of right quadriceps muscle, fascia and tendon POA

7️⃣ **S76.192** Other specified injury of left quadriceps muscle, fascia and tendon POA

7️⃣ **S76.199** Other specified injury of unspecified quadriceps muscle, fascia and tendon POA

5️⃣ **S76.2** Injury of adductor muscle, fascia and tendon of thigh

6️⃣ **S76.20** Unspecified injury of adductor muscle, fascia and tendon of thigh

7️⃣ **S76.201** Unspecified injury of adductor muscle, fascia and tendon of right thigh POA

7️⃣ **S76.202** Unspecified injury of adductor muscle, fascia and tendon of left thigh POA

7️⃣ **S76.209** Unspecified injury of adductor muscle, fascia and tendon of unspecified thigh POA

6️⃣ **S76.21** Strain of adductor muscle, fascia and tendon of thigh

7️⃣ **S76.211** Strain of adductor muscle, fascia and tendon of right thigh POA

7️⃣ **S76.212** Strain of adductor muscle, fascia and tendon of left thigh POA

7️⃣ **S76.219** Strain of adductor muscle, fascia and tendon of unspecified thigh POA

6️⃣ **S76.22** Laceration of adductor muscle, fascia and tendon of thigh

7️⃣ **S76.221** Laceration of adductor muscle, fascia and tendon of right thigh CC⊘ POA CC/MCC Exc

7️⃣ **S76.222** Laceration of adductor muscle, fascia and tendon of left thigh CC⊘ POA CC/MCC Exc

7️⃣ **S76.229** Laceration of adductor muscle, fascia and tendon of unspecified thigh CC⊘ POA CC/MCC Exc

6️⃣ **S76.29** Other injury of adductor muscle, fascia and tendon of thigh

7️⃣ **S76.291** Other injury of adductor muscle, fascia and tendon of right thigh POA

7️⃣ **S76.292** Other injury of adductor muscle, fascia and tendon of left thigh POA

7️⃣ **S76.299** Other injury of adductor muscle, fascia and tendon of unspecified thigh POA

Unspecified Code   Other Specified Code   Manifestation Code   🆖 Newborn   🅿 Pediatric   🅼 Maternity   🅰 Adult   ♂ Male   ♀ Female
● New Code   ▲ Revised Code Title   ▶◀ Revised Text   **NOTES**   *INCLUDES*   *EXCLUDES1* Not coded here   *EXCLUDES2* Not included here
4️⃣ 4th character required   5️⃣ 5th character required   6️⃣ 6th character required   7️⃣ 7th character required   Ⓧ Extension 'X' Alert
HAC Hospital-acquired condition (HAC) alert   **AHA** AHA Coding Clinic©   📌 Code first alert

S76.3 Injury of muscle, fascia and tendon of the posterior muscle group at thigh level
- S76.30 Unspecified injury of muscle, fascia and tendon of the posterior muscle group at thigh level
  - S76.301 Unspecified injury of muscle, fascia and tendon of the posterior muscle group at thigh level, right thigh
  - S76.302 Unspecified injury of muscle, fascia and tendon of the posterior muscle group at thigh level, left thigh
  - S76.309 Unspecified injury of muscle, fascia and tendon of the posterior muscle group at thigh level, unspecified thigh
- S76.31 Strain of muscle, fascia and tendon of the posterior muscle group at thigh level
  - S76.311 Strain of muscle, fascia and tendon of the posterior muscle group at thigh level, right thigh
  - S76.312 Strain of muscle, fascia and tendon of the posterior muscle group at thigh level, left thigh
  - S76.319 Strain of muscle, fascia and tendon of the posterior muscle group at thigh level, unspecified thigh
- S76.32 Laceration of muscle, fascia and tendon of the posterior muscle group at thigh level
  - S76.321 Laceration of muscle, fascia and tendon of the posterior muscle group at thigh level, right thigh
  - S76.322 Laceration of muscle, fascia and tendon of the posterior muscle group at thigh level, left thigh
  - S76.329 Laceration of muscle, fascia and tendon of the posterior muscle group at thigh level, unspecified thigh
- S76.39 Other specified injury of muscle, fascia and tendon of the posterior muscle group at thigh level
  - S76.391 Other specified injury of muscle, fascia and tendon of the posterior muscle group at thigh level, right thigh
  - S76.392 Other specified injury of muscle, fascia and tendon of the posterior muscle group at thigh level, left thigh
  - S76.399 Other specified injury of muscle, fascia and tendon of the posterior muscle group at thigh level, unspecified thigh

S76.8 Injury of other specified muscles, fascia and tendons at thigh level
- S76.80 Unspecified injury of other specified muscles, fascia and tendons at thigh level
  - S76.801 Unspecified injury of other specified muscles, fascia and tendons at thigh level, right thigh
  - S76.802 Unspecified injury of other specified muscles, fascia and tendons at thigh level, left thigh
  - S76.809 Unspecified injury of other specified muscles, fascia and tendons at thigh level, unspecified thigh
- S76.81 Strain of other specified muscles, fascia and tendons at thigh level
  - S76.811 Strain of other specified muscles, fascia and tendons at thigh level, right thigh
  - S76.812 Strain of other specified muscles, fascia and tendons at thigh level, left thigh
  - S76.819 Strain of other specified muscles, fascia and tendons at thigh level, unspecified thigh
- S76.82 Laceration of other specified muscles, fascia and tendons at thigh level
  - S76.821 Laceration of other specified muscles, fascia and tendons at thigh level, right thigh

- S76.822 Laceration of other specified muscles, fascia and tendons at thigh level, left thigh
- S76.829 Laceration of other specified muscles, fascia and tendons at thigh level, unspecified thigh
- S76.89 Other injury of other specified muscles, fascia and tendons at thigh level
  - S76.891 Other injury of other specified muscles, fascia and tendons at thigh level, right thigh
  - S76.892 Other injury of other specified muscles, fascia and tendons at thigh level, left thigh
  - S76.899 Other injury of other specified muscles, fascia and tendons at thigh level, unspecified thigh

S76.9 Injury of unspecified muscles, fascia and tendons at thigh level
- S76.90 Unspecified injury of unspecified muscles, fascia and tendons at thigh level
  - S76.901 Unspecified injury of unspecified muscles, fascia and tendons at thigh level, right thigh
  - S76.902 Unspecified injury of unspecified muscles, fascia and tendons at thigh level, left thigh
  - S76.909 Unspecified injury of unspecified muscles, fascia and tendons at thigh level, unspecified thigh
- S76.91 Strain of unspecified muscles, fascia and tendons at thigh level
  - S76.911 Strain of unspecified muscles, fascia and tendons at thigh level, right thigh
  - S76.912 Strain of unspecified muscles, fascia and tendons at thigh level, left thigh
  - S76.919 Strain of unspecified muscles, fascia and tendons at thigh level, unspecified thigh
- S76.92 Laceration of unspecified muscles, fascia and tendons at thigh level
  - S76.921 Laceration of unspecified muscles, fascia and tendons at thigh level, right thigh
  - S76.922 Laceration of unspecified muscles, fascia and tendons at thigh level, left thigh
  - S76.929 Laceration of unspecified muscles, fascia and tendons at thigh level, unspecified thigh
- S76.99 Other specified injury of unspecified muscles, fascia and tendons at thigh level
  - S76.991 Other specified injury of unspecified muscles, fascia and tendons at thigh level, right thigh
  - S76.992 Other specified injury of unspecified muscles, fascia and tendons at thigh level, left thigh
  - S76.999 Other specified injury of unspecified muscles, fascia and tendons at thigh level, unspecified thigh

S77 Crushing injury of hip and thigh
Use additional code(s) for all associated injuries
EXCLUDES2 crushing injury of ankle and foot (S97.-)
crushing injury of lower leg (S87.-)
The appropriate 7th character is to be added to each code from category S77
A = initial encounter
D = subsequent encounter
S = sequela
- S77.0 Crushing injury of hip
  - S77.00 Crushing injury of unspecified hip

Unacceptable principal diagnosis symbol per Medicare code edits   Code exempt from diagnosis present on admission requirement

? Questionable admission   Complication or comorbidity   MCC Major complication or comorbidity   CC/MCC Exc CC/MCC exclusion

HCC HCC diagnosis code   RxHCC RxHCC diagnosis code   MACRA code   **DEFINITION** Describes condition/terminology

TIP Coding guidance   Official Guideline Reference   Z1 Z code as first-listed diagnosis

1070   When symbols appear on a code that requires a 7th character extension, refer to Appendix B to identify applicable 7th character codes.   **2020 ICD-10-CM**

[6th] S79.12 Salter-Harris Type II physeal fracture of lower end of femur
- [7th] S79.121 Salter-Harris Type II physeal fracture of lower end of right femur [CC] [POA] [HAC] [HCC] [CC/MCC Exc]
- [7th] S79.122 Salter-Harris Type II physeal fracture of lower end of left femur [CC] [POA] [HAC] [HCC] [CC/MCC Exc]
- [7th] S79.129 Salter-Harris Type II physeal fracture of lower end of unspecified femur [CC] [POA] [HAC] [HCC] [CC/MCC Exc]

[6th] S79.13 Salter-Harris Type III physeal fracture of lower end of femur
- [7th] S79.131 Salter-Harris Type III physeal fracture of lower end of right femur [CC] [POA] [HAC] [HCC] [CC/MCC Exc]
- [7th] S79.132 Salter-Harris Type III physeal fracture of lower end of left femur [CC] [POA] [HAC] [HCC] [CC/MCC Exc]
- [7th] S79.139 Salter-Harris Type III physeal fracture of lower end of unspecified femur [CC] [POA] [HAC] [HCC] [CC/MCC Exc]

[6th] S79.14 Salter-Harris Type IV physeal fracture of lower end of femur
- [7th] S79.141 Salter-Harris Type IV physeal fracture of lower end of right femur [CC] [POA] [HAC] [HCC] [CC/MCC Exc]
- [7th] S79.142 Salter-Harris Type IV physeal fracture of lower end of left femur [CC] [POA] [HAC] [HCC] [CC/MCC Exc]
- [7th] S79.149 Salter-Harris Type IV physeal fracture of lower end of unspecified femur [CC] [POA] [HAC] [HCC] [CC/MCC Exc]

[6th] S79.19 Other physeal fracture of lower end of femur
- [7th] S79.191 Other physeal fracture of lower end of right femur [CC] [POA] [HAC] [HCC] [CC/MCC Exc]
- [7th] S79.192 Other physeal fracture of lower end of left femur [CC] [POA] [HAC] [HCC] [CC/MCC Exc]
- [7th] S79.199 Other physeal fracture of lower end of unspecified femur [CC] [POA] [HAC] [HCC] [CC/MCC Exc]

[5th] S79.8 Other specified injuries of hip and thigh

The appropriate 7th character is to be added to each code in subcategory S79.8
A = initial encounter
D = subsequent encounter
S = sequela

[6th] S79.81 Other specified injuries of hip
- [7th] S79.811 Other specified injuries of right hip [POA]
- [7th] S79.812 Other specified injuries of left hip [POA]
- [7th] S79.819 Other specified injuries of unspecified hip [POA]

[6th] S79.82 Other specified injuries of thigh
- [7th] S79.821 Other specified injuries of right thigh [POA]
- [7th] S79.822 Other specified injuries of left thigh [POA]
- [7th] S79.829 Other specified injuries of unspecified thigh [POA]

[5th] S79.9 Unspecified injury of hip and thigh

The appropriate 7th character is to be added to each code in subcategory S79.9
A = initial encounter
D = subsequent encounter
S = sequela

[6th] S79.91 Unspecified injury of hip
- [7th] S79.911 Unspecified injury of right hip [POA]
- [7th] S79.912 Unspecified injury of left hip [POA]
- [7th] S79.919 Unspecified injury of unspecified hip [POA]

[6th] S79.92 Unspecified injury of thigh
- [7th] S79.921 Unspecified injury of right thigh [POA]
- [7th] S79.922 Unspecified injury of left thigh [POA]
- [7th] S79.929 Unspecified injury of unspecified thigh [POA]

Injuries to the knee and lower leg (S80-S89)

[EXCLUDES2] *burns and corrosions (T20-T32)*
frostbite (T33-T34)
injuries of ankle and foot, except fracture of ankle and malleolus (S90-S99)
insect bite or sting, venomous (T63.4)

[4th] S80 Superficial injury of knee and lower leg

[EXCLUDES2] *superficial injury of ankle and foot (S90.-)*

The appropriate 7th character is to be added to each code from category S80
A = initial encounter
D = subsequent encounter
S = sequela

[5th] S80.0 Contusion of knee
- [7th] S80.00 Contusion of unspecified knee [POA]
- [7th] S80.01 Contusion of right knee [POA]
- [7th] S80.02 Contusion of left knee [POA]

[5th] S80.1 Contusion of lower leg
- [7th] S80.10 Contusion of unspecified lower leg [POA]
- [7th] S80.11 Contusion of right lower leg [POA]
- [7th] S80.12 Contusion of left lower leg [POA]

[5th] S80.2 Other superficial injuries of knee

[6th] S80.21 Abrasion of knee
- [7th] S80.211 Abrasion, right knee [POA]
- [7th] S80.212 Abrasion, left knee [POA]
- [7th] S80.219 Abrasion, unspecified knee [POA]

[6th] S80.22 Blister (nonthermal) of knee
- [7th] S80.221 Blister (nonthermal), right knee [POA]
- [7th] S80.222 Blister (nonthermal), left knee [POA]
- [7th] S80.229 Blister (nonthermal), unspecified knee [POA]

[6th] S80.24 External constriction of knee
- [7th] S80.241 External constriction, right knee [POA]
- [7th] S80.242 External constriction, left knee [POA]
- [7th] S80.249 External constriction, unspecified knee [POA]

[6th] S80.25 Superficial foreign body of knee
Splinter in the knee
- [7th] S80.251 Superficial foreign body, right knee [POA]
- [7th] S80.252 Superficial foreign body, left knee [POA]
- [7th] S80.259 Superficial foreign body, unspecified knee [POA]

[6th] S80.26 Insect bite (nonvenomous) of knee
- [7th] S80.261 Insect bite (nonvenomous), right knee [POA]
- [7th] S80.262 Insect bite (nonvenomous), left knee [POA]
- [7th] S80.269 Insect bite (nonvenomous), unspecified knee [POA]

[6th] S80.27 Other superficial bite of knee

[EXCLUDES1] *open bite of knee (S81.05-)*
- [7th] S80.271 Other superficial bite of right knee [POA]
- [7th] S80.272 Other superficial bite of left knee [POA]
- [7th] S80.279 Other superficial bite of unspecified knee [POA]

[5th] S80.8 Other superficial injuries of lower leg

[6th] S80.81 Abrasion of lower leg
- [7th] S80.811 Abrasion, right lower leg [POA]
- [7th] S80.812 Abrasion, left lower leg [POA]
- [7th] S80.819 Abrasion, unspecified lower leg [POA]

[6th] S80.82 Blister (nonthermal) of lower leg
- [7th] S80.821 Blister (nonthermal), right lower leg [POA]
- [7th] S80.822 Blister (nonthermal), left lower leg [POA]
- [7th] S80.829 Blister (nonthermal), unspecified lower leg [POA]

[6th] S80.84 External constriction of lower leg
- [7th] S80.841 External constriction, right lower leg [POA]
- [7th] S80.842 External constriction, left lower leg [POA]
- [7th] S80.849 External constriction, unspecified lower leg [POA]

[PDx] Unacceptable principal diagnosis symbol per Medicare code edits [POA] Code exempt from diagnosis present on admission requirement
[?] Questionable admission [CC] Complication or comorbidity [MCC] Major complication or comorbidity [CC/MCC Exc] CC/MCC exclusion
[HCC] HCC diagnosis code [RxHCC] RxHCC diagnosis code MACRA code **DEFINITION** Describes condition/terminology
TIP Coding guidance 👁 Official Guideline Reference [Z1] Z code as first-listed diagnosis

CHAPTER 19: INJURY, POISONING, AND CERTAIN OTHER CONSEQUENCES OF EXTERNAL CAUSES (S00-T88)

S77.01 - S79.119

S77.01 Crushing injury of right hip
S77.02 Crushing injury of left hip

S77.1 Crushing injury of thigh
  S77.10 Crushing injury of unspecified thigh
  S77.11 Crushing injury of right thigh
  S77.12 Crushing injury of left thigh

S77.2 Crushing injury of hip with thigh
  S77.20 Crushing injury of unspecified hip with thigh
  S77.21 Crushing injury of right hip with thigh
  S77.22 Crushing injury of left hip with thigh

S78 Traumatic amputation of hip and thigh
An amputation not identified as partial or complete should be coded to complete
EXCLUDES1 traumatic amputation of knee (S88.0-)

The appropriate 7th character is to be added to each code from category S78
A = initial encounter
D = subsequent encounter
S = sequela

S78.0 Traumatic amputation at hip joint
  S78.01 Complete traumatic amputation at hip joint
    S78.011 Complete traumatic amputation at right hip joint
    S78.012 Complete traumatic amputation at left hip joint
    S78.019 Complete traumatic amputation at unspecified hip joint
  S78.02 Partial traumatic amputation at hip joint
    S78.021 Partial traumatic amputation at right hip joint
    S78.022 Partial traumatic amputation at left hip joint
    S78.029 Partial traumatic amputation at unspecified hip joint

S78.1 Traumatic amputation at level between hip and knee
EXCLUDES1 traumatic amputation of knee (S88.0-)
  S78.11 Complete traumatic amputation at level between hip and knee
    S78.111 Complete traumatic amputation at level between right hip and knee
    S78.112 Complete traumatic amputation at level between left hip and knee
    S78.119 Complete traumatic amputation at level between unspecified hip and knee
  S78.12 Partial traumatic amputation at level between hip and knee
    S78.121 Partial traumatic amputation at level between right hip and knee
    S78.122 Partial traumatic amputation at level between left hip and knee
    S78.129 Partial traumatic amputation at level between unspecified hip and knee

S78.9 Traumatic amputation of hip and thigh, level unspecified
  S78.91 Complete traumatic amputation of hip and thigh, level unspecified
    S78.911 Complete traumatic amputation of right hip and thigh, level unspecified
    S78.912 Complete traumatic amputation of left hip and thigh, level unspecified
    S78.919 Complete traumatic amputation of unspecified hip and thigh, level unspecified
  S78.92 Partial traumatic amputation of hip and thigh, level unspecified
    S78.921 Partial traumatic amputation of right hip and thigh, level unspecified
    S78.922 Partial traumatic amputation of left hip and thigh, level unspecified
    S78.929 Partial traumatic amputation of unspecified hip and thigh, level unspecified

S79 Other and unspecified injuries of hip and thigh
See Official Guidelines "Coding of Traumatic Fractures" I.C.19.c
NOTES A fracture not indicated as open or closed should be coded to closed

The appropriate 7th character is to be added to each code from subcategories S79.0 and S79.1
A = initial encounter for closed fracture
D = subsequent encounter for fracture with routine healing
G = subsequent encounter for fracture with delayed healing
K = subsequent encounter for fracture with nonunion
P = subsequent encounter for fracture with malunion
S = sequela

S79.0 Physeal fracture of upper end of femur
EXCLUDES1 apophyseal fracture of upper end of femur (S72.13-)
nontraumatic slipped upper femoral epiphysis (M93.0-)
  S79.00 Unspecified physeal fracture of upper end of femur
    S79.001 Unspecified physeal fracture of upper end of right femur
    S79.002 Unspecified physeal fracture of upper end of left femur
    S79.009 Unspecified physeal fracture of upper end of unspecified femur
  S79.01 Salter-Harris Type I physeal fracture of upper end of femur
      Acute on chronic slipped capital femoral epiphysis
      Acute slipped capital femoral epiphysis (traumatic)
    EXCLUDES1 Capital femoral epiphyseal fracture chronic slipped upper femoral epiphysis (nontraumatic) (M93.02-)
    S79.011 Salter-Harris Type I physeal fracture of upper end of right femur
    S79.012 Salter-Harris Type I physeal fracture of upper end of left femur
    S79.019 Salter-Harris Type I physeal fracture of upper end of unspecified femur
  S79.09 Other physeal fracture of upper end of femur
    S79.091 Other physeal fracture of upper end of right femur
    S79.092 Other physeal fracture of upper end of left femur
    S79.099 Other physeal fracture of upper end of unspecified femur

S79.1 Physeal fracture of lower end of femur
  S79.10 Unspecified physeal fracture of lower end of femur
    S79.101 Unspecified physeal fracture of lower end of right femur
    S79.102 Unspecified physeal fracture of lower end of left femur
    S79.109 Unspecified physeal fracture of lower end of unspecified femur
  S79.11 Salter-Harris Type I physeal fracture of lower end of femur
    S79.111 Salter-Harris Type I physeal fracture of lower end of right femur
    S79.112 Salter-Harris Type I physeal fracture of lower end of left femur
    S79.119 Salter-Harris Type I physeal fracture of lower end of unspecified femur

● New Code ▲ Revised Code Title ◄► Revised Text NOTES EXCLUDES1 Not coded here EXCLUDES2 Not included here
4th character required 5th character required 6th character required 7th character required Extension 'X' Alert Code first alert
Unspecified Code Other Specified Code Manifestation Code N Newborn P Pediatric M Maternity A Adult ♂ Male ♀ Female
HAC Hospital-acquired condition (HAC) alert AHA AHA Coding Clinic®

6ᵗʰ **S80.85** Superficial foreign body of lower leg
Splinter in the lower leg
7ᵗʰ **S80.851** Superficial foreign body, right lower leg Ⓟ POA
7ᵗʰ **S80.852** Superficial foreign body, left lower leg ⓅPOA
7ᵗʰ **S80.859** Superficial foreign body, unspecified lower leg ⓅPOA

6ᵗʰ **S80.86** Insect bite (nonvenomous) of lower leg
7ᵗʰ **S80.861** Insect bite (nonvenomous), right lower leg ⓅPOA
7ᵗʰ **S80.862** Insect bite (nonvenomous), left lower leg ⓅPOA
7ᵗʰ **S80.869** Insect bite (nonvenomous), unspecified lower leg ⓅPOA

6ᵗʰ **S80.87** Other superficial bite of lower leg
EXCLUDES1 open bite of lower leg (S81.85-)
7ᵗʰ **S80.871** Other superficial bite, right lower leg ⓅPOA
7ᵗʰ **S80.872** Other superficial bite, left lower leg ⓅPOA
7ᵗʰ **S80.879** Other superficial bite, unspecified lower leg ⓅPOA

5ᵗʰ **S80.9** Unspecified superficial injury of knee and lower leg
6ᵗʰ **S80.91** Unspecified superficial injury of knee
7ᵗʰ **S80.911** Unspecified superficial injury of right knee ⓅPOA
7ᵗʰ **S80.912** Unspecified superficial injury of left knee ⓅPOA
7ᵗʰ **S80.919** Unspecified superficial injury of unspecified knee ⓅPOA

6ᵗʰ **S80.92** Unspecified superficial injury of lower leg
7ᵗʰ **S80.921** Unspecified superficial injury of right lower leg ⓅPOA
7ᵗʰ **S80.922** Unspecified superficial injury of left lower leg ⓅPOA
7ᵗʰ **S80.929** Unspecified superficial injury of unspecified lower leg ⓅPOA

4ᵗʰ **S81** Open wound of knee and lower leg
Code also any associated wound infection
EXCLUDES1 open fracture of knee and lower leg (S82.-)
traumatic amputation of lower leg (S88.-)
EXCLUDES2 open wound of ankle and foot (S91.-)
The appropriate 7th character is to be added to each code from category S81
A = initial encounter
D = subsequent encounter
S = sequela

5ᵗʰ **S81.0** Open wound of knee
6ᵗʰ **S81.00** Unspecified open wound of knee
7ᵗʰ **S81.001** Unspecified open wound, right knee ⓅPOA
7ᵗʰ **S81.002** Unspecified open wound, left knee ⓅPOA
7ᵗʰ **S81.009** Unspecified open wound, unspecified knee ⓅPOA

6ᵗʰ **S81.01** Laceration without foreign body of knee
7ᵗʰ **S81.011** Laceration without foreign body, right knee ⓅPOA
7ᵗʰ **S81.012** Laceration without foreign body, left knee ⓅPOA
7ᵗʰ **S81.019** Laceration without foreign body, unspecified knee ⓅPOA

6ᵗʰ **S81.02** Laceration with foreign body of knee
7ᵗʰ **S81.021** Laceration with foreign body, right knee ⓅPOA
7ᵗʰ **S81.022** Laceration with foreign body, left knee ⓅPOA
7ᵗʰ **S81.029** Laceration with foreign body, unspecified knee ⓅPOA

6ᵗʰ **S81.03** Puncture wound without foreign body of knee
7ᵗʰ **S81.031** Puncture wound without foreign body, right knee ⓅPOA
7ᵗʰ **S81.032** Puncture wound without foreign body, left knee ⓅPOA

7ᵗʰ **S81.039** Puncture wound without foreign body, unspecified knee ⓅPOA

6ᵗʰ **S81.04** Puncture wound with foreign body of knee
7ᵗʰ **S81.041** Puncture wound with foreign body, right knee ⓅPOA
7ᵗʰ **S81.042** Puncture wound with foreign body, left knee ⓅPOA
7ᵗʰ **S81.049** Puncture wound with foreign body, unspecified knee ⓅPOA

6ᵗʰ **S81.05** Open bite of knee
Bite of knee NOS
EXCLUDES1 superficial bite of knee (S80.27-)
7ᵗʰ **S81.051** Open bite, right knee ⓅPOA
7ᵗʰ **S81.052** Open bite, left knee ⓅPOA
7ᵗʰ **S81.059** Open bite, unspecified knee ⓅPOA

5ᵗʰ **S81.8** Open wound of lower leg
6ᵗʰ **S81.80** Unspecified open wound of lower leg
7ᵗʰ **S81.801** Unspecified open wound, right lower leg ⓅPOA
7ᵗʰ **S81.802** Unspecified open wound, left lower leg ⓅPOA
7ᵗʰ **S81.809** Unspecified open wound, unspecified lower leg ⓅPOA

6ᵗʰ **S81.81** Laceration without foreign body of lower leg
7ᵗʰ **S81.811** Laceration without foreign body, right lower leg ⓅPOA
7ᵗʰ **S81.812** Laceration without foreign body, left lower leg ⓅPOA
7ᵗʰ **S81.819** Laceration without foreign body, unspecified lower leg ⓅPOA

6ᵗʰ **S81.82** Laceration with foreign body of lower leg
7ᵗʰ **S81.821** Laceration with foreign body, right lower leg ⓅPOA
7ᵗʰ **S81.822** Laceration with foreign body, left lower leg ⓅPOA
7ᵗʰ **S81.829** Laceration with foreign body, unspecified lower leg ⓅPOA

6ᵗʰ **S81.83** Puncture wound without foreign body of lower leg
7ᵗʰ **S81.831** Puncture wound without foreign body, right lower leg ⓅPOA
7ᵗʰ **S81.832** Puncture wound without foreign body, left lower leg ⓅPOA
7ᵗʰ **S81.839** Puncture wound without foreign body, unspecified lower leg ⓅPOA

6ᵗʰ **S81.84** Puncture wound with foreign body of lower leg
7ᵗʰ **S81.841** Puncture wound with foreign body, right lower leg ⓅPOA
AHA: Q3 2016
7ᵗʰ **S81.842** Puncture wound with foreign body, left lower leg ⓅPOA
7ᵗʰ **S81.849** Puncture wound with foreign body, unspecified lower leg ⓅPOA

6ᵗʰ **S81.85** Open bite of lower leg
Bite of lower leg NOS
EXCLUDES1 superficial bite of lower leg (S80.86-, S80.87-)
7ᵗʰ **S81.851** Open bite, right lower leg ⓅPOA
7ᵗʰ **S81.852** Open bite, left lower leg ⓅPOA
7ᵗʰ **S81.859** Open bite, unspecified lower leg ⓅPOA

4ᵗʰ **S82** Fracture of lower leg, including ankle
👁 **See Official Guidelines** "Coding of Traumatic Fractures" I.C.19.c
NOTES A fracture not indicated as displaced or nondisplaced should be coded to displaced
A fracture not indicated as open or closed should be coded to closed
The open fracture designations are based on the Gustilo open fracture classification
INCLUDES fracture of malleolus
EXCLUDES1 traumatic amputation of lower leg (S88.-)
EXCLUDES2 fracture of foot, except ankle (S92.-)
periprosthetic fracture of prosthetic implant of knee (M97.0-)

Unspecified Code   Other Specified Code   Manifestation Code   Ⓝ Newborn   Ⓟ Pediatric   Ⓜ Maternity   Ⓐ Adult   ♂ Male   ♀ Female
● New Code   ▲ Revised Code Title   ►◄ Revised Text   **NOTES**   *INCLUDES*   *EXCLUDES1* Not coded here   *EXCLUDES2* Not included here
4ᵗʰ 4ᵗʰ character required   5ᵗʰ 5ᵗʰ character required   6ᵗʰ 6ᵗʰ character required   7ᵗʰ 7ᵗʰ character required   Ⓧ Extension 'X' Alert
HAC Hospital-acquired condition (HAC) alert   **AHA** AHA Coding Clinic©   📧 Code first alert

The appropriate 7th character is to be added to all codes from category S82

A = initial encounter for closed fracture

B = initial encounter for open fracture type I or II
   initial encounter for open fracture NOS

C = initial encounter for open fracture type IIIA, IIIB, or IIIC

D = subsequent encounter for closed fracture with routine healing

E = subsequent encounter for open fracture type I or II with routine healing

F = subsequent encounter for open fracture type IIIA, IIIB, or IIIC with routine healing

G = subsequent encounter for closed fracture with delayed healing

H = subsequent encounter for open fracture type I or II with delayed healing

J = subsequent encounter for open fracture type IIIA, IIIB, or IIIC with delayed healing

K = subsequent encounter for closed fracture with nonunion

M = subsequent encounter for open fracture type I or II with nonunion

N = subsequent encounter for open fracture type IIIA, IIIB, or IIIC with nonunion

P = subsequent encounter for closed fracture with malunion

Q = subsequent encounter for open fracture type I or II with malunion

R = subsequent encounter for open fracture type IIIA, IIIB, or IIIC with malunion

S = sequela

S82.0 Fracture of patella
Knee cap

S82.00 Unspecified fracture of patella
- S82.001 Unspecified fracture of right patella
- S82.002 Unspecified fracture of left patella
- S82.009 Unspecified fracture of unspecified patella

S82.01 Osteochondral fracture of patella
- S82.011 Displaced osteochondral fracture of right patella
- S82.012 Displaced osteochondral fracture of left patella
- S82.013 Displaced osteochondral fracture of unspecified patella
- S82.014 Nondisplaced osteochondral fracture of right patella
- S82.015 Nondisplaced osteochondral fracture of left patella
- S82.016 Nondisplaced osteochondral fracture of unspecified patella

S82.02 Longitudinal fracture of patella
- S82.021 Displaced longitudinal fracture of right patella
- S82.022 Displaced longitudinal fracture of left patella
- S82.023 Displaced longitudinal fracture of unspecified patella
- S82.024 Nondisplaced longitudinal fracture of right patella
- S82.025 Nondisplaced longitudinal fracture of left patella
- S82.026 Nondisplaced longitudinal fracture of unspecified patella

S82.03 Transverse fracture of patella
- S82.031 Displaced transverse fracture of right patella
- S82.032 Displaced transverse fracture of left patella
- S82.033 Displaced transverse fracture of unspecified patella
- S82.034 Nondisplaced transverse fracture of right patella
- S82.035 Nondisplaced transverse fracture of left patella
- S82.036 Nondisplaced transverse fracture of unspecified patella

S82.04 Comminuted fracture of patella
- S82.041 Displaced comminuted fracture of right patella
- S82.042 Displaced comminuted fracture of left patella
- S82.043 Displaced comminuted fracture of unspecified patella
- S82.044 Nondisplaced comminuted fracture of right patella
- S82.045 Nondisplaced comminuted fracture of left patella
- S82.046 Nondisplaced comminuted fracture of unspecified patella

S82.09 Other fracture of patella
- S82.091 Other fracture of right patella
- S82.092 Other fracture of left patella
- S82.099 Other fracture of unspecified patella

S82.1 Fracture of upper end of tibia
Fracture of proximal end of tibia
EXCLUDES2 fracture of shaft of tibia (S82.2-)
   physeal fracture of upper end of tibia (S89.0-)

S82.10 Unspecified fracture of upper end of tibia
- S82.101 Unspecified fracture of upper end of right tibia
- S82.102 Unspecified fracture of upper end of left tibia
- S82.109 Unspecified fracture of upper end of unspecified tibia

S82.11 Fracture of tibial spine
- S82.111 Displaced fracture of right tibial spine
- S82.112 Displaced fracture of left tibial spine
- S82.113 Displaced fracture of unspecified tibial spine
- S82.114 Nondisplaced fracture of right tibial spine
- S82.115 Nondisplaced fracture of left tibial spine
- S82.116 Nondisplaced fracture of unspecified tibial spine

S82.12 Fracture of lateral condyle of tibia
- S82.121 Displaced fracture of lateral condyle of right tibia
- S82.122 Displaced fracture of lateral condyle of left tibia
- S82.123 Displaced fracture of lateral condyle of unspecified tibia
- S82.124 Nondisplaced fracture of lateral condyle of right tibia
- S82.125 Nondisplaced fracture of lateral condyle of left tibia
- S82.126 Nondisplaced fracture of lateral condyle of unspecified tibia

S82.13 Fracture of medial condyle of tibia
- S82.131 Displaced fracture of medial condyle of right tibia
- S82.132 Displaced fracture of medial condyle of left tibia

Legend: PDXᴺ Unacceptable principal diagnosis symbol per Medicare code edits · Code exempt from diagnosis present on admission requirement · Questionable admission · Complication or comorbidity · MCC Major complication or comorbidity · CC/MCC Exc CC/MCC exclusion · HCC HCC diagnosis code · RxHCC RxHCC diagnosis code · MACRA code · DEFINITION Describes condition/terminology · TIP Coding guidance · Official Guideline Reference · Z code as first-listed diagnosis

7ᵗʰ S82.133 Displaced fracture of medial condyle of unspecified tibia CC POA HAC MCC CC/MCC Exc

7ᵗʰ S82.134 Nondisplaced fracture of medial condyle of right tibia CC POA HAC MCC CC/MCC Exc

7ᵗʰ S82.135 Nondisplaced fracture of medial condyle of left tibia CC POA HAC MCC CC/MCC Exc

7ᵗʰ S82.136 Nondisplaced fracture of medial condyle of unspecified tibia CC POA HAC MCC CC/MCC Exc

6ᵗʰ S82.14 Bicondylar fracture of tibia
Fracture of tibial plateau NOS

7ᵗʰ S82.141 Displaced bicondylar fracture of right tibia CC POA HAC MCC CC/MCC Exc

7ᵗʰ S82.142 Displaced bicondylar fracture of left tibia CC POA HAC MCC CC/MCC Exc

7ᵗʰ S82.143 Displaced bicondylar fracture of unspecified tibia CC POA HAC MCC CC/MCC Exc

7ᵗʰ S82.144 Nondisplaced bicondylar fracture of right tibia CC POA HAC MCC CC/MCC Exc

7ᵗʰ S82.145 Nondisplaced bicondylar fracture of left tibia CC POA HAC MCC CC/MCC Exc

7ᵗʰ S82.146 Nondisplaced bicondylar fracture of unspecified tibia CC POA HAC MCC CC/MCC Exc

6ᵗʰ S82.15 Fracture of tibial tuberosity

7ᵗʰ S82.151 Displaced fracture of right tibial tuberosity CC POA HAC MCC CC/MCC Exc

7ᵗʰ S82.152 Displaced fracture of left tibial tuberosity CC POA HAC MCC CC/MCC Exc

7ᵗʰ S82.153 Displaced fracture of unspecified tibial tuberosity CC POA HAC MCC CC/MCC Exc

7ᵗʰ S82.154 Nondisplaced fracture of right tibial tuberosity CC POA HAC MCC CC/MCC Exc

7ᵗʰ S82.155 Nondisplaced fracture of left tibial tuberosity CC POA HAC MCC CC/MCC Exc

7ᵗʰ S82.156 Nondisplaced fracture of unspecified tibial tuberosity CC POA HAC MCC CC/MCC Exc

6ᵗʰ S82.16 Torus fracture of upper end of tibia
The appropriate 7th character is to be added to all codes in subcategory S82.16
A = initial encounter for closed fracture
D = subsequent encounter for fracture with routine healing
G = subsequent encounter for fracture with delayed healing
K = subsequent encounter for fracture with nonunion
P = subsequent encounter for fracture with malunion
S = sequela

7ᵗʰ S82.161 Torus fracture of upper end of right tibia CC POA HAC CC/MCC Exc

7ᵗʰ S82.162 Torus fracture of upper end of left tibia CC POA HAC CC/MCC Exc

7ᵗʰ S82.169 Torus fracture of upper end of unspecified tibia CC POA HAC CC/MCC Exc

6ᵗʰ S82.19 Other fracture of upper end of tibia

7ᵗʰ S82.191 Other fracture of upper end of right tibia CC POA HAC MCC CC/MCC Exc

7ᵗʰ S82.192 Other fracture of upper end of left tibia CC POA HAC MCC CC/MCC Exc

7ᵗʰ S82.199 Other fracture of upper end of unspecified tibia CC POA HAC MCC CC/MCC Exc

5ᵗʰ S82.2 Fracture of shaft of tibia

6ᵗʰ S82.20 Unspecified fracture of shaft of tibia
Fracture of tibia NOS

7ᵗʰ S82.201 Unspecified fracture of shaft of right tibia CC POA HAC MCC CC/MCC Exc

7ᵗʰ S82.202 Unspecified fracture of shaft of left tibia CC POA HAC MCC CC/MCC Exc

7ᵗʰ S82.209 Unspecified fracture of shaft of unspecified tibia CC POA HAC MCC CC/MCC Exc

6ᵗʰ S82.22 Transverse fracture of shaft of tibia

7ᵗʰ S82.221 Displaced transverse fracture of shaft of right tibia CC POA HAC MCC CC/MCC Exc

7ᵗʰ S82.222 Displaced transverse fracture of shaft of left tibia CC POA HAC MCC CC/MCC Exc

7ᵗʰ S82.223 Displaced transverse fracture of shaft of unspecified tibia CC POA HAC MCC CC/MCC Exc

7ᵗʰ S82.224 Nondisplaced transverse fracture of shaft of right tibia CC POA HAC MCC CC/MCC Exc

7ᵗʰ S82.225 Nondisplaced transverse fracture of shaft of left tibia CC POA HAC MCC CC/MCC Exc

7ᵗʰ S82.226 Nondisplaced transverse fracture of shaft of unspecified tibia CC POA HAC MCC CC/MCC Exc

6ᵗʰ S82.23 Oblique fracture of shaft of tibia

7ᵗʰ S82.231 Displaced oblique fracture of shaft of right tibia CC POA HAC MCC CC/MCC Exc

7ᵗʰ S82.232 Displaced oblique fracture of shaft of left tibia CC POA HAC MCC CC/MCC Exc

7ᵗʰ S82.233 Displaced oblique fracture of shaft of unspecified tibia CC POA HAC MCC CC/MCC Exc

7ᵗʰ S82.234 Nondisplaced oblique fracture of shaft of right tibia CC POA HAC MCC CC/MCC Exc
AHA: Q1 2015

7ᵗʰ S82.235 Nondisplaced oblique fracture of shaft of left tibia CC POA HAC MCC CC/MCC Exc

7ᵗʰ S82.236 Nondisplaced oblique fracture of shaft of unspecified tibia CC POA HAC MCC CC/MCC Exc

6ᵗʰ S82.24 Spiral fracture of shaft of tibia
Toddler fracture

7ᵗʰ S82.241 Displaced spiral fracture of shaft of right tibia CC POA HAC MCC CC/MCC Exc

7ᵗʰ S82.242 Displaced spiral fracture of shaft of left tibia CC POA HAC MCC CC/MCC Exc

7ᵗʰ S82.243 Displaced spiral fracture of shaft of unspecified tibia CC POA HAC MCC CC/MCC Exc

7ᵗʰ S82.244 Nondisplaced spiral fracture of shaft of right tibia CC POA HAC MCC CC/MCC Exc

7ᵗʰ S82.245 Nondisplaced spiral fracture of shaft of left tibia CC POA HAC MCC CC/MCC Exc

7ᵗʰ S82.246 Nondisplaced spiral fracture of shaft of unspecified tibia CC POA HAC MCC CC/MCC Exc

6ᵗʰ S82.25 Comminuted fracture of shaft of tibia

7ᵗʰ S82.251 Displaced comminuted fracture of shaft of right tibia CC POA HAC MCC CC/MCC Exc
AHA: Q2 2015

7ᵗʰ S82.252 Displaced comminuted fracture of shaft of left tibia CC POA HAC MCC CC/MCC Exc

7ᵗʰ S82.253 Displaced comminuted fracture of shaft of unspecified tibia CC POA HAC MCC CC/MCC Exc

7ᵗʰ S82.254 Nondisplaced comminuted fracture of shaft of right tibia CC POA HAC MCC CC/MCC Exc

7ᵗʰ S82.255 Nondisplaced comminuted fracture of shaft of left tibia CC POA HAC MCC CC/MCC Exc

7ᵗʰ S82.256 Nondisplaced comminuted fracture of shaft of unspecified tibia CC POA HAC MCC CC/MCC Exc

6ᵗʰ S82.26 Segmental fracture of shaft of tibia

7ᵗʰ S82.261 Displaced segmental fracture of shaft of right tibia CC POA HAC MCC CC/MCC Exc

7ᵗʰ S82.262 Displaced segmental fracture of shaft of left tibia CC POA HAC MCC CC/MCC Exc

7ᵗʰ S82.263 Displaced segmental fracture of shaft of unspecified tibia CC POA HAC MCC CC/MCC Exc

7ᵗʰ S82.264 Nondisplaced segmental fracture of shaft of right tibia CC POA HAC MCC CC/MCC Exc

7ᵗʰ S82.265 Nondisplaced segmental fracture of shaft of left tibia CC POA HAC MCC CC/MCC Exc

7ᵗʰ S82.266 Nondisplaced segmental fracture of shaft of unspecified tibia CC POA HAC MCC CC/MCC Exc

---

Unspecified Code Other Specified Code Manifestation Code N Newborn P Pediatric M Maternity A Adult ♂ Male ♀ Female
● New Code ▲ Revised Code Title ▶◀ Revised Text NOTES INCLUDES EXCLUDES1 Not coded here EXCLUDES2 Not included here
4ᵗʰ 4ᵗʰ character required 5ᵗʰ 5ᵗʰ character required 6ᵗʰ 6ᵗʰ character required 7ᵗʰ 7ᵗʰ character required Extension 'X' Alert
HAC Hospital-acquired condition (HAC) alert AHA AHA Coding Clinic© ☞ Code first alert

6ᵗʰ **S82.29** Other fracture of shaft of tibia

   7ᵗʰ S82.291 Other fracture of shaft of right tibia   CC POA HAC MCC CC/MCC Exc

   7ᵗʰ S82.292 Other fracture of shaft of left tibia   CC POA HAC MCC CC/MCC Exc

   7ᵗʰ S82.299 Other fracture of shaft of unspecified tibia   CC POA HAC MCC CC/MCC Exc

5ᵗʰ **S82.3** Fracture of lower end of tibia

   EXCLUDES1   bimalleolar fracture of lower leg (S82.84-)

        fracture of medial malleolus alone (S82.5-)

        Maisonneuve's fracture (S82.86-)

        pilon fracture of distal tibia (S82.87-)

        trimalleolar fractures of lower leg (S82.85-)

  6ᵗʰ **S82.30** Unspecified fracture of lower end of tibia

    7ᵗʰ S82.301 Unspecified fracture of lower end of right tibia   CC POA HAC CC/MCC Exc

    7ᵗʰ S82.302 Unspecified fracture of lower end of left tibia   CC POA HAC CC/MCC Exc

    7ᵗʰ S82.309 Unspecified fracture of lower end of unspecified tibia   CC POA HAC CC/MCC Exc

  6ᵗʰ **S82.31** Torus fracture of lower end of tibia

    The appropriate 7th character is to be added to all codes in subcategory S82.31

    A = initial encounter for closed fracture

    D = subsequent encounter for fracture with routine healing

    G = subsequent encounter for fracture with delayed healing

    K = subsequent encounter for fracture with nonunion

    P = subsequent encounter for fracture with malunion

    S = sequela

    7ᵗʰ S82.311 Torus fracture of lower end of right tibia   CC POA HAC CC/MCC Exc

    7ᵗʰ S82.312 Torus fracture of lower end of left tibia   CC POA HAC CC/MCC Exc

    7ᵗʰ S82.319 Torus fracture of lower end of unspecified tibia   CC POA HAC CC/MCC Exc

  6ᵗʰ **S82.39** Other fracture of lower end of tibia

    7ᵗʰ S82.391 Other fracture of lower end of right tibia   CC POA HAC CC/MCC Exc

    7ᵗʰ S82.392 Other fracture of lower end of left tibia   CC POA HAC CC/MCC Exc

    7ᵗʰ S82.399 Other fracture of lower end of unspecified tibia   CC POA HAC CC/MCC Exc

5ᵗʰ **S82.4** Fracture of shaft of fibula

   EXCLUDES2   fracture of lateral malleolus alone (S82.6-)

  6ᵗʰ **S82.40** Unspecified fracture of shaft of fibula

    7ᵗʰ S82.401 Unspecified fracture of shaft of right fibula   CC POA HAC MCC CC/MCC Exc

    7ᵗʰ S82.402 Unspecified fracture of shaft of left fibula   CC POA HAC MCC CC/MCC Exc

    7ᵗʰ S82.409 Unspecified fracture of shaft of unspecified fibula   CC POA HAC MCC CC/MCC Exc

  6ᵗʰ **S82.42** Transverse fracture of shaft of fibula

    7ᵗʰ S82.421 Displaced transverse fracture of shaft of right fibula   CC POA HAC MCC CC/MCC Exc

    7ᵗʰ S82.422 Displaced transverse fracture of shaft of left fibula   CC POA HAC MCC CC/MCC Exc

    7ᵗʰ S82.423 Displaced transverse fracture of shaft of unspecified fibula   CC POA HAC MCC CC/MCC Exc

    7ᵗʰ S82.424 Nondisplaced transverse fracture of shaft of right fibula   CC POA HAC MCC CC/MCC Exc

    7ᵗʰ S82.425 Nondisplaced transverse fracture of shaft of left fibula   CC POA HAC MCC CC/MCC Exc

    7ᵗʰ S82.426 Nondisplaced transverse fracture of shaft of unspecified fibula   CC POA HAC MCC CC/MCC Exc

6ᵗʰ **S82.43** Oblique fracture of shaft of fibula

   7ᵗʰ S82.431 Displaced oblique fracture of shaft of right fibula   CC POA HAC MCC CC/MCC Exc

   7ᵗʰ S82.432 Displaced oblique fracture of shaft of left fibula   CC POA HAC MCC CC/MCC Exc

   7ᵗʰ S82.433 Displaced oblique fracture of shaft of unspecified fibula   CC POA HAC MCC CC/MCC Exc

   7ᵗʰ S82.434 Nondisplaced oblique fracture of shaft of right fibula   CC POA HAC MCC CC/MCC Exc

   7ᵗʰ S82.435 Nondisplaced oblique fracture of shaft of left fibula   CC POA HAC MCC CC/MCC Exc

   7ᵗʰ S82.436 Nondisplaced oblique fracture of shaft of unspecified fibula   CC POA HAC MCC CC/MCC Exc

  6ᵗʰ **S82.44** Spiral fracture of shaft of fibula

    7ᵗʰ S82.441 Displaced spiral fracture of shaft of right fibula   CC POA HAC MCC CC/MCC Exc

    7ᵗʰ S82.442 Displaced spiral fracture of shaft of left fibula   CC POA HAC MCC CC/MCC Exc

    7ᵗʰ S82.443 Displaced spiral fracture of shaft of unspecified fibula   CC POA HAC MCC CC/MCC Exc

    7ᵗʰ S82.444 Nondisplaced spiral fracture of shaft of right fibula   CC POA HAC MCC CC/MCC Exc

    7ᵗʰ S82.445 Nondisplaced spiral fracture of shaft of left fibula   CC POA HAC MCC CC/MCC Exc

    7ᵗʰ S82.446 Nondisplaced spiral fracture of shaft of unspecified fibula   CC POA HAC MCC CC/MCC Exc

  6ᵗʰ **S82.45** Comminuted fracture of shaft of fibula

    7ᵗʰ S82.451 Displaced comminuted fracture of shaft of right fibula   CC POA HAC MCC CC/MCC Exc

    7ᵗʰ S82.452 Displaced comminuted fracture of shaft of left fibula   CC POA HAC MCC CC/MCC Exc

    7ᵗʰ S82.453 Displaced comminuted fracture of shaft of unspecified fibula   CC POA HAC MCC CC/MCC Exc

    7ᵗʰ S82.454 Nondisplaced comminuted fracture of shaft of right fibula   CC POA HAC MCC CC/MCC Exc

    7ᵗʰ S82.455 Nondisplaced comminuted fracture of shaft of left fibula   CC POA HAC MCC CC/MCC Exc

    7ᵗʰ S82.456 Nondisplaced comminuted fracture of shaft of unspecified fibula   CC POA HAC MCC CC/MCC Exc

  6ᵗʰ **S82.46** Segmental fracture of shaft of fibula

    7ᵗʰ S82.461 Displaced segmental fracture of shaft of right fibula   CC POA HAC MCC CC/MCC Exc

    7ᵗʰ S82.462 Displaced segmental fracture of shaft of left fibula   CC POA HAC MCC CC/MCC Exc

    7ᵗʰ S82.463 Displaced segmental fracture of shaft of unspecified fibula   CC POA HAC MCC CC/MCC Exc

    7ᵗʰ S82.464 Nondisplaced segmental fracture of shaft of right fibula   CC POA HAC MCC CC/MCC Exc

    7ᵗʰ S82.465 Nondisplaced segmental fracture of shaft of left fibula   CC POA HAC MCC CC/MCC Exc

    7ᵗʰ S82.466 Nondisplaced segmental fracture of shaft of unspecified fibula   CC POA HAC MCC CC/MCC Exc

  6ᵗʰ **S82.49** Other fracture of shaft of fibula

    7ᵗʰ S82.491 Other fracture of shaft of right fibula   CC POA HAC MCC CC/MCC Exc

    7ᵗʰ S82.492 Other fracture of shaft of left fibula   CC POA HAC MCC CC/MCC Exc

    7ᵗʰ S82.499 Other fracture of shaft of unspecified fibula   CC POA HAC MCC CC/MCC Exc

5ᵗʰ **S82.5** Fracture of medial malleolus

   EXCLUDES1   pilon fracture of distal tibia (S82.87-)

        Salter-Harris type III of lower end of tibia (S89.13-)

        Salter-Harris type IV of lower end of tibia (S89.14-)

  7ᵗʰ **S82.51** Displaced fracture of medial malleolus of right tibia   CC POA HAC CC/MCC Exc

  7ᵗʰ **S82.52** Displaced fracture of medial malleolus of left tibia   CC POA HAC CC/MCC Exc

---

POA꜀ Unacceptable principal diagnosis symbol per Medicare code edits   POA Code exempt from diagnosis present on admission requirement

❓ Questionable admission   CC Complication or comorbidity   MCC Major complication or comorbidity   CC/MCC CC/MCC exclusion

HCC HCC diagnosis code   RxHCC RxHCC diagnosis code   MACRA MACRA code   **DEFINITION** Describes condition/terminology

TIP Coding guidance   👁 Official Guideline Reference   Z1 Z code as first-listed diagnosis

[7th] S82.53 Displaced fracture of medial malleolus of unspecified tibia CC POA HAC CC/MCC Exc
[7th] S82.54 Nondisplaced fracture of medial malleolus of right tibia CC POA HAC CC/MCC Exc
[7th] S82.55 Nondisplaced fracture of medial malleolus of left tibia CC POA HAC CC/MCC Exc
[7th] S82.56 Nondisplaced fracture of medial malleolus of unspecified tibia CC POA HAC CC/MCC Exc

[5th] S82.6 Fracture of lateral malleolus

[EXCLUDES1] *pilon fracture of distal tibia (S82.87-)*

[7th] S82.61 Displaced fracture of lateral malleolus of right fibula CC POA HAC CC/MCC Exc
[7th] S82.62 Displaced fracture of lateral malleolus of left fibula CC POA HAC CC/MCC Exc
[7th] S82.63 Displaced fracture of lateral malleolus of unspecified fibula CC POA HAC CC/MCC Exc
[7th] S82.64 Nondisplaced fracture of lateral malleolus of right fibula CC POA HAC CC/MCC Exc
[7th] S82.65 Nondisplaced fracture of lateral malleolus of left fibula CC POA HAC CC/MCC Exc
[7th] S82.66 Nondisplaced fracture of lateral malleolus of unspecified fibula CC POA HAC CC/MCC Exc

[5th] S82.8 Other fractures of lower leg

[6th] S82.81 Torus fracture of upper end of fibula

The appropriate 7th character is to be added to all codes in subcategory S82.81

- A = initial encounter for closed fracture
- D = subsequent encounter for fracture with routine healing
- G = subsequent encounter for fracture with delayed healing
- K = subsequent encounter for fracture with nonunion
- P = subsequent encounter for fracture with malunion
- S = sequela

[7th] S82.811 Torus fracture of upper end of right fibula CC POA CC/MCC Exc
[7th] S82.812 Torus fracture of upper end of left fibula CC POA CC/MCC Exc
[7th] S82.819 Torus fracture of upper end of unspecified fibula CC POA CC/MCC Exc

[6th] S82.82 Torus fracture of lower end of fibula

The appropriate 7th character is to be added to all codes in subcategory S82.82

- A = initial encounter for closed fracture
- D = subsequent encounter for fracture with routine healing
- G = subsequent encounter for fracture with delayed healing
- K = subsequent encounter for fracture with nonunion
- P = subsequent encounter for fracture with malunion
- S = sequela

[7th] S82.821 Torus fracture of lower end of right fibula CC POA CC/MCC Exc
[7th] S82.822 Torus fracture of lower end of left fibula CC POA CC/MCC Exc
[7th] S82.829 Torus fracture of lower end of unspecified fibula CC POA CC/MCC Exc

[6th] S82.83 Other fracture of upper and lower end of fibula

[7th] S82.831 Other fracture of upper and lower end of right fibula CC POA HAC MCC CC/MCC Exc
[7th] S82.832 Other fracture of upper and lower end of left fibula CC POA HAC MCC CC/MCC Exc
[7th] S82.839 Other fracture of upper and lower end of unspecified fibula CC POA HAC MCC CC/MCC Exc

[6th] S82.84 Bimalleolar fracture of lower leg

[7th] S82.841 Displaced bimalleolar fracture of right lower leg CC POA HAC CC/MCC Exc
[7th] S82.842 Displaced bimalleolar fracture of left lower leg CC POA HAC CC/MCC Exc
[7th] S82.843 Displaced bimalleolar fracture of unspecified lower leg CC POA HAC CC/MCC Exc
[7th] S82.844 Nondisplaced bimalleolar fracture of right lower leg CC POA HAC CC/MCC Exc
[7th] S82.845 Nondisplaced bimalleolar fracture of left lower leg CC POA HAC CC/MCC Exc
[7th] S82.846 Nondisplaced bimalleolar fracture of unspecified lower leg CC POA HAC CC/MCC Exc

[6th] S82.85 Trimalleolar fracture of lower leg

[7th] S82.851 Displaced trimalleolar fracture of right lower leg CC POA HAC CC/MCC Exc
[7th] S82.852 Displaced trimalleolar fracture of left lower leg CC POA HAC CC/MCC Exc
[7th] S82.853 Displaced trimalleolar fracture of unspecified lower leg CC POA HAC CC/MCC Exc
[7th] S82.854 Nondisplaced trimalleolar fracture of right lower leg CC POA HAC CC/MCC Exc
[7th] S82.855 Nondisplaced trimalleolar fracture of left lower leg CC POA HAC CC/MCC Exc
[7th] S82.856 Nondisplaced trimalleolar fracture of unspecified lower leg CC POA HAC CC/MCC Exc

[6th] S82.86 Maisonneuve's fracture

[7th] S82.861 Displaced Maisonneuve's fracture of right leg CC POA HAC MCC CC/MCC Exc
[7th] S82.862 Displaced Maisonneuve's fracture of left leg CC POA HAC MCC CC/MCC Exc
[7th] S82.863 Displaced Maisonneuve's fracture of unspecified leg CC POA HAC MCC CC/MCC Exc
[7th] S82.864 Nondisplaced Maisonneuve's fracture of right leg CC POA HAC MCC CC/MCC Exc
[7th] S82.865 Nondisplaced Maisonneuve's fracture of left leg CC POA HAC MCC CC/MCC Exc
[7th] S82.866 Nondisplaced Maisonneuve's fracture of unspecified leg CC POA HAC MCC CC/MCC Exc

[6th] S82.87 Pilon fracture of tibia

[7th] S82.871 Displaced pilon fracture of right tibia CC POA HAC CC/MCC Exc
[7th] S82.872 Displaced pilon fracture of left tibia CC POA HAC CC/MCC Exc
[7th] S82.873 Displaced pilon fracture of unspecified tibia CC POA HAC CC/MCC Exc
[7th] S82.874 Nondisplaced pilon fracture of right tibia CC POA HAC CC/MCC Exc
[7th] S82.875 Nondisplaced pilon fracture of left tibia CC POA HAC CC/MCC Exc
[7th] S82.876 Nondisplaced pilon fracture of unspecified tibia CC POA HAC CC/MCC Exc

[6th] S82.89 Other fractures of lower leg

Fracture of ankle NOS

[7th] S82.891 Other fracture of right lower leg CC POA HAC CC/MCC Exc
[7th] S82.892 Other fracture of left lower leg CC POA HAC CC/MCC Exc
[7th] S82.899 Other fracture of unspecified lower leg CC POA HAC CC/MCC Exc

[5th] S82.9 Unspecified fracture of lower leg

[7th] S82.90 Unspecified fracture of unspecified lower leg CC POA HAC CC/MCC Exc
[7th] S82.91 Unspecified fracture of right lower leg CC POA HAC CC/MCC Exc
[7th] S82.92 Unspecified fracture of left lower leg CC POA HAC CC/MCC Exc

Unspecified Code Other Specified Code Manifestation Code [N] Newborn [P] Pediatric [M] Maternity [A] Adult ♂ Male ♀ Female
● New Code ▲ Revised Code Title ►◄ Revised Text [NOTES] *INCLUDES* [EXCLUDES1] Not coded here [EXCLUDES2] Not included here
[4th] 4th character required [5th] 5th character required [6th] 6th character required [7th] 7th character required [7th] Extension 'X' Alert
[HAC] Hospital-acquired condition (HAC) alert **AHA** AHA Coding Clinic© ☞ Code first alert

S83 Dislocation and sprain of joints and ligaments of knee

INCLUDES avulsion of joint or ligament of knee

laceration of cartilage, joint or ligament of knee

sprain of cartilage, joint or ligament of knee

traumatic hemarthrosis of joint or ligament of knee

traumatic rupture of joint or ligament of knee

traumatic subluxation of joint or ligament of knee

traumatic tear of joint or ligament of knee

Code also any associated open wound

EXCLUDES1 derangement of patella (M22.0-M22.3)

injury of patellar ligament (tendon) (S76.1-)

internal derangement of knee (M23.-)

old dislocation of knee (M24.36)

pathological dislocation of knee (M24.36)

recurrent dislocation of knee (M22.0)

EXCLUDES2 strain of muscle, fascia and tendon of lower leg (S86.-)

The appropriate 7th character is to be added to each code from category S83

A = initial encounter

D = subsequent encounter

S = sequela

S83.0 Subluxation and dislocation of patella

S83.00 Unspecified subluxation and dislocation of patella

S83.001 Unspecified subluxation of right patella POA

S83.002 Unspecified subluxation of left patella POA

S83.003 Unspecified subluxation of unspecified patella POA

S83.004 Unspecified dislocation of right patella POA

S83.005 Unspecified dislocation of left patella POA

S83.006 Unspecified dislocation of unspecified patella POA

S83.01 Lateral subluxation and dislocation of patella

S83.011 Lateral subluxation of right patella POA

S83.012 Lateral subluxation of left patella POA

S83.013 Lateral subluxation of unspecified patella POA

S83.014 Lateral dislocation of right patella POA

S83.015 Lateral dislocation of left patella POA

S83.016 Lateral dislocation of unspecified patella POA

S83.09 Other subluxation and dislocation of patella

S83.091 Other subluxation of right patella POA

S83.092 Other subluxation of left patella POA

S83.093 Other subluxation of unspecified patella POA

S83.094 Other dislocation of right patella POA

S83.095 Other dislocation of left patella POA

S83.096 Other dislocation of unspecified patella POA

S83.1 Subluxation and dislocation of knee

EXCLUDES2 instability of knee prosthesis (T84.022, T84.023)

S83.10 Unspecified subluxation and dislocation of knee

S83.101 Unspecified subluxation of right knee POA

S83.102 Unspecified subluxation of left knee POA

S83.103 Unspecified subluxation of unspecified knee POA

S83.104 Unspecified dislocation of right knee POA

S83.105 Unspecified dislocation of left knee POA

S83.106 Unspecified dislocation of unspecified knee POA

S83.11 Anterior subluxation and dislocation of proximal end of tibia

Posterior subluxation and dislocation of distal end of femur

S83.111 Anterior subluxation of proximal end of tibia, right knee POA

S83.112 Anterior subluxation of proximal end of tibia, left knee POA

S83.113 Anterior subluxation of proximal end of tibia, unspecified knee POA

S83.114 Anterior dislocation of proximal end of tibia, right knee POA

S83.115 Anterior dislocation of proximal end of tibia, left knee POA

S83.116 Anterior dislocation of proximal end of tibia, unspecified knee POA

S83.12 Posterior subluxation and dislocation of proximal end of tibia

Anterior dislocation of distal end of femur

S83.121 Posterior subluxation of proximal end of tibia, right knee POA

S83.122 Posterior subluxation of proximal end of tibia, left knee POA

S83.123 Posterior subluxation of proximal end of tibia, unspecified knee POA

S83.124 Posterior dislocation of proximal end of tibia, right knee POA

S83.125 Posterior dislocation of proximal end of tibia, left knee POA

S83.126 Posterior dislocation of proximal end of tibia, unspecified knee POA

S83.13 Medial subluxation and dislocation of proximal end of tibia

S83.131 Medial subluxation of proximal end of tibia, right knee POA

S83.132 Medial subluxation of proximal end of tibia, left knee POA

S83.133 Medial subluxation of proximal end of tibia, unspecified knee POA

S83.134 Medial dislocation of proximal end of tibia, right knee POA

S83.135 Medial dislocation of proximal end of tibia, left knee POA

S83.136 Medial dislocation of proximal end of tibia, unspecified knee POA

S83.14 Lateral subluxation and dislocation of proximal end of tibia

S83.141 Lateral subluxation of proximal end of tibia, right knee POA

S83.142 Lateral subluxation of proximal end of tibia, left knee POA

S83.143 Lateral subluxation of proximal end of tibia, unspecified knee POA

S83.144 Lateral dislocation of proximal end of tibia, right knee POA

S83.145 Lateral dislocation of proximal end of tibia, left knee POA

S83.146 Lateral dislocation of proximal end of tibia, unspecified knee POA

S83.19 Other subluxation and dislocation of knee

S83.191 Other subluxation of right knee POA

S83.192 Other subluxation of left knee POA

S83.193 Other subluxation of unspecified knee POA

S83.194 Other dislocation of right knee POA

S83.195 Other dislocation of left knee POA

S83.196 Other dislocation of unspecified knee POA

S83.2 Tear of meniscus, current injury

EXCLUDES1 old bucket-handle tear (M23.2)

S83.20 Tear of unspecified meniscus, current injury

Tear of meniscus of knee NOS

S83.200 Bucket-handle tear of unspecified meniscus, current injury, right knee POA

S83.201 Bucket-handle tear of unspecified meniscus, current injury, left knee POA

S83.202 Bucket-handle tear of unspecified meniscus, current injury, unspecified knee POA

S83.203 Other tear of unspecified meniscus, current injury, right knee POA

S83.204 Other tear of unspecified meniscus, current injury, left knee POA

PDxIR Unacceptable principal diagnosis symbol per Medicare code edits   POA Code exempt from diagnosis present on admission requirement
? Questionable admission   cc Complication or comorbidity   MCC Major complication or comorbidity   cc/MCC Excl CC/MCC exclusion
HCC HCC diagnosis code   RxHCC RxHCC diagnosis code   MACRA code   **DEFINITION** Describes condition/terminology
TIP Coding guidance   👁 Official Guideline Reference   Z51 Z code as first-listed diagnosis

1078   When symbols appear on a code that requires a 7th character extension, refer to Appendix B to identify applicable 7th character codes.   **2020 ICD-10-CM**

[7th] S83.205 Other tear of unspecified meniscus, current injury, unspecified knee POA
[7th] S83.206 Unspecified tear of unspecified meniscus, current injury, right knee POA
[7th] S83.207 Unspecified tear of unspecified meniscus, current injury, left knee POA
[7th] S83.209 Unspecified tear of unspecified meniscus, current injury, unspecified knee POA
[6th] S83.21 Bucket-handle tear of medial meniscus, current injury
[7th] S83.211 Bucket-handle tear of medial meniscus, current injury, right knee POA
[7th] S83.212 Bucket-handle tear of medial meniscus, current injury, left knee POA
[7th] S83.219 Bucket-handle tear of medial meniscus, current injury, unspecified knee POA
[6th] S83.22 Peripheral tear of medial meniscus, current injury
[7th] S83.221 Peripheral tear of medial meniscus, current injury, right knee POA
[7th] S83.222 Peripheral tear of medial meniscus, current injury, left knee POA
[7th] S83.229 Peripheral tear of medial meniscus, current injury, unspecified knee POA
[6th] S83.23 Complex tear of medial meniscus, current injury
[7th] S83.231 Complex tear of medial meniscus, current injury, right knee POA
[7th] S83.232 Complex tear of medial meniscus, current injury, left knee POA
AHA: Q2 2019
[7th] S83.239 Complex tear of medial meniscus, current injury, unspecified knee POA
[6th] S83.24 Other tear of medial meniscus, current injury
[7th] S83.241 Other tear of medial meniscus, current injury, right knee POA
[7th] S83.242 Other tear of medial meniscus, current injury, left knee POA
[7th] S83.249 Other tear of medial meniscus, current injury, unspecified knee POA
[6th] S83.25 Bucket-handle tear of lateral meniscus, current injury
[7th] S83.251 Bucket-handle tear of lateral meniscus, current injury, right knee POA
[7th] S83.252 Bucket-handle tear of lateral meniscus, current injury, left knee POA
[7th] S83.259 Bucket-handle tear of lateral meniscus, current injury, unspecified knee POA
[6th] S83.26 Peripheral tear of lateral meniscus, current injury
[7th] S83.261 Peripheral tear of lateral meniscus, current injury, right knee POA
[7th] S83.262 Peripheral tear of lateral meniscus, current injury, left knee POA
[7th] S83.269 Peripheral tear of lateral meniscus, current injury, unspecified knee POA
[6th] S83.27 Complex tear of lateral meniscus, current injury
[7th] S83.271 Complex tear of lateral meniscus, current injury, right knee POA
[7th] S83.272 Complex tear of lateral meniscus, current injury, left knee POA
[7th] S83.279 Complex tear of lateral meniscus, current injury, unspecified knee POA
[6th] S83.28 Other tear of lateral meniscus, current injury
[7th] S83.281 Other tear of lateral meniscus, current injury, right knee POA
[7th] S83.282 Other tear of lateral meniscus, current injury, left knee POA
[7th] S83.289 Other tear of lateral meniscus, current injury, unspecified knee POA
[5th] S83.3 Tear of articular cartilage of knee, current
[7th] S83.30 Tear of articular cartilage of unspecified knee, current POA
[7th] S83.31 Tear of articular cartilage of right knee, current POA
[7th] S83.32 Tear of articular cartilage of left knee, current POA
[5th] S83.4 Sprain of collateral ligament of knee
[6th] S83.40 Sprain of unspecified collateral ligament of knee
[7th] S83.401 Sprain of unspecified collateral ligament of right knee POA
[7th] S83.402 Sprain of unspecified collateral ligament of left knee POA
[7th] S83.409 Sprain of unspecified collateral ligament of unspecified knee POA
[6th] S83.41 Sprain of medial collateral ligament of knee
Sprain of tibial collateral ligament
[7th] S83.411 Sprain of medial collateral ligament of right knee POA
[7th] S83.412 Sprain of medial collateral ligament of left knee POA
[7th] S83.419 Sprain of medial collateral ligament of unspecified knee POA
[6th] S83.42 Sprain of lateral collateral ligament of knee
Sprain of fibular collateral ligament
[7th] S83.421 Sprain of lateral collateral ligament of right knee POA
[7th] S83.422 Sprain of lateral collateral ligament of left knee POA
[7th] S83.429 Sprain of lateral collateral ligament of unspecified knee POA
[5th] S83.5 Sprain of cruciate ligament of knee
[6th] S83.50 Sprain of unspecified cruciate ligament of knee
[7th] S83.501 Sprain of unspecified cruciate ligament of right knee POA
[7th] S83.502 Sprain of unspecified cruciate ligament of left knee POA
[7th] S83.509 Sprain of unspecified cruciate ligament of unspecified knee POA
[6th] S83.51 Sprain of anterior cruciate ligament of knee
[7th] S83.511 Sprain of anterior cruciate ligament of right knee POA
AHA: Q2 2016
[7th] S83.512 Sprain of anterior cruciate ligament of left knee POA
[7th] S83.519 Sprain of anterior cruciate ligament of unspecified knee POA
[6th] S83.52 Sprain of posterior cruciate ligament of knee
[7th] S83.521 Sprain of posterior cruciate ligament of right knee POA
[7th] S83.522 Sprain of posterior cruciate ligament of left knee POA
[7th] S83.529 Sprain of posterior cruciate ligament of unspecified knee POA
[5th] S83.6 Sprain of the superior tibiofibular joint and ligament
[7th] S83.60 Sprain of the superior tibiofibular joint and ligament, unspecified knee POA
[7th] S83.61 Sprain of the superior tibiofibular joint and ligament, right knee POA
[7th] S83.62 Sprain of the superior tibiofibular joint and ligament, left knee POA
[5th] S83.8 Sprain of other specified parts of knee
[6th] S83.8X Sprain of other specified parts of knee
[7th] S83.8X1 Sprain of other specified parts of right knee POA
[7th] S83.8X2 Sprain of other specified parts of left knee POA
[7th] S83.8X9 Sprain of other specified parts of unspecified knee POA
[5th] S83.9 Sprain of unspecified site of knee
[7th] S83.90 Sprain of unspecified site of unspecified knee POA
[7th] S83.91 Sprain of unspecified site of right knee POA
[7th] S83.92 Sprain of unspecified site of left knee POA
[4th] S84 Injury of nerves at lower leg level
Code also any associated open wound (S81.-)
EXCLUDES2 *injury of nerves at ankle and foot level (S94.-)*

Unspecified Code | Other Specified Code | Manifestation Code | [N] Newborn | [P] Pediatric | [M] Maternity | [A] Adult | ♂ Male | ♀ Female
● New Code ▲ Revised Code Title ►◄ Revised Text NOTES INCLUDES EXCLUDES1 Not coded here EXCLUDES2 Not included here
[4th] 4th character required [5th] 5th character required [6th] 6th character required [7th] 7th character required [7th] Extension 'X' Alert
[HAC] Hospital-acquired condition (HAC) alert AHA AHA Coding Clinic© ☞ Code first alert

The appropriate 7th character is to be added to each code from category S84
- A = initial encounter
- D = subsequent encounter
- S = sequela

5ᵗʰ **S84.0** Injury of tibial nerve at lower leg level
- 7ᵗʰ **S84.00** Injury of tibial nerve at lower leg level, unspecified leg — POA
- 7ᵗʰ **S84.01** Injury of tibial nerve at lower leg level, right leg — POA
- 7ᵗʰ **S84.02** Injury of tibial nerve at lower leg level, left leg — POA

5ᵗʰ **S84.1** Injury of peroneal nerve at lower leg level
- 7ᵗʰ **S84.10** Injury of peroneal nerve at lower leg level, unspecified leg — POA
- 7ᵗʰ **S84.11** Injury of peroneal nerve at lower leg level, right leg — POA
- 7ᵗʰ **S84.12** Injury of peroneal nerve at lower leg level, left leg — POA

5ᵗʰ **S84.2** Injury of cutaneous sensory nerve at lower leg level
- 7ᵗʰ **S84.20** Injury of cutaneous sensory nerve at lower leg level, unspecified leg — POA
- 7ᵗʰ **S84.21** Injury of cutaneous sensory nerve at lower leg level, right leg — POA
- 7ᵗʰ **S84.22** Injury of cutaneous sensory nerve at lower leg level, left leg — POA

5ᵗʰ **S84.8** Injury of other nerves at lower leg level
- 6ᵗʰ **S84.80** Injury of other nerves at lower leg level
  - 7ᵗʰ **S84.801** Injury of other nerves at lower leg level, right leg — POA
  - 7ᵗʰ **S84.802** Injury of other nerves at lower leg level, left leg — POA
  - 7ᵗʰ **S84.809** Injury of other nerves at lower leg level, unspecified leg — POA

5ᵗʰ **S84.9** Injury of unspecified nerve at lower leg level
- 7ᵗʰ **S84.90** Injury of unspecified nerve at lower leg level, unspecified leg — POA
- 7ᵗʰ **S84.91** Injury of unspecified nerve at lower leg level, right leg — POA
- 7ᵗʰ **S84.92** Injury of unspecified nerve at lower leg level, left leg — POA

4ᵗʰ **S85** Injury of blood vessels at lower leg level

Code also any associated open wound (S81.-)

EXCLUDES2 injury of blood vessels at ankle and foot level (S95.-)

The appropriate 7th character is to be added to each code from category S85
- A = initial encounter
- D = subsequent encounter
- S = sequela

5ᵗʰ **S85.0** Injury of popliteal artery
- 6ᵗʰ **S85.00** Unspecified injury of popliteal artery
  - 7ᵗʰ **S85.001** Unspecified injury of popliteal artery, right leg — POA MCC CC/MCC Exc
  - 7ᵗʰ **S85.002** Unspecified injury of popliteal artery, left leg — POA MCC CC/MCC Exc
  - 7ᵗʰ **S85.009** Unspecified injury of popliteal artery, unspecified leg — POA MCC CC/MCC Exc
- 6ᵗʰ **S85.01** Laceration of popliteal artery
  - 7ᵗʰ **S85.011** Laceration of popliteal artery, right leg — POA MCC CC/MCC Exc
  - 7ᵗʰ **S85.012** Laceration of popliteal artery, left leg — POA MCC CC/MCC Exc
  - 7ᵗʰ **S85.019** Laceration of popliteal artery, unspecified leg — POA MCC CC/MCC Exc
- 6ᵗʰ **S85.09** Other specified injury of popliteal artery
  - 7ᵗʰ **S85.091** Other specified injury of popliteal artery, right leg — POA MCC CC/MCC Exc
  - 7ᵗʰ **S85.092** Other specified injury of popliteal artery, left leg — POA MCC CC/MCC Exc
  - 7ᵗʰ **S85.099** Other specified injury of popliteal artery, unspecified leg — POA MCC CC/MCC Exc

5ᵗʰ **S85.1** Injury of tibial artery
- 6ᵗʰ **S85.10** Unspecified injury of unspecified tibial artery

Injury of tibial artery NOS

- 7ᵗʰ **S85.101** Unspecified injury of unspecified tibial artery, right leg — CC POA CC/MCC Exc
- 7ᵗʰ **S85.102** Unspecified injury of unspecified tibial artery, left leg — CC POA CC/MCC Exc
- 7ᵗʰ **S85.109** Unspecified injury of unspecified tibial artery, unspecified leg — CC POA CC/MCC Exc

- 6ᵗʰ **S85.11** Laceration of unspecified tibial artery
  - 7ᵗʰ **S85.111** Laceration of unspecified tibial artery, right leg — CC POA CC/MCC Exc
  - 7ᵗʰ **S85.112** Laceration of unspecified tibial artery, left leg — CC POA CC/MCC Exc
  - 7ᵗʰ **S85.119** Laceration of unspecified tibial artery, unspecified leg — CC POA CC/MCC Exc

- 6ᵗʰ **S85.12** Other specified injury of unspecified tibial artery
  - 7ᵗʰ **S85.121** Other specified injury of unspecified tibial artery, right leg — CC POA CC/MCC Exc
  - 7ᵗʰ **S85.122** Other specified injury of unspecified tibial artery, left leg — CC POA CC/MCC Exc
  - 7ᵗʰ **S85.129** Other specified injury of unspecified tibial artery, unspecified leg — CC POA CC/MCC Exc

- 6ᵗʰ **S85.13** Unspecified injury of anterior tibial artery
  - 7ᵗʰ **S85.131** Unspecified injury of anterior tibial artery, right leg — CC POA CC/MCC Exc
  - 7ᵗʰ **S85.132** Unspecified injury of anterior tibial artery, left leg — CC POA CC/MCC Exc
  - 7ᵗʰ **S85.139** Unspecified injury of anterior tibial artery, unspecified leg — CC POA CC/MCC Exc

- 6ᵗʰ **S85.14** Laceration of anterior tibial artery
  - 7ᵗʰ **S85.141** Laceration of anterior tibial artery, right leg — CC POA CC/MCC Exc
  - 7ᵗʰ **S85.142** Laceration of anterior tibial artery, left leg — CC POA CC/MCC Exc
  - 7ᵗʰ **S85.149** Laceration of anterior tibial artery, unspecified leg — CC POA CC/MCC Exc

- 6ᵗʰ **S85.15** Other specified injury of anterior tibial artery
  - 7ᵗʰ **S85.151** Other specified injury of anterior tibial artery, right leg — CC POA CC/MCC Exc
  - 7ᵗʰ **S85.152** Other specified injury of anterior tibial artery, left leg — CC POA CC/MCC Exc
  - 7ᵗʰ **S85.159** Other specified injury of anterior tibial artery, unspecified leg — CC POA CC/MCC Exc

- 6ᵗʰ **S85.16** Unspecified injury of posterior tibial artery
  - 7ᵗʰ **S85.161** Unspecified injury of posterior tibial artery, right leg — CC POA CC/MCC Exc
  - 7ᵗʰ **S85.162** Unspecified injury of posterior tibial artery, left leg — CC POA CC/MCC Exc
  - 7ᵗʰ **S85.169** Unspecified injury of posterior tibial artery, unspecified leg — CC POA CC/MCC Exc

- 6ᵗʰ **S85.17** Laceration of posterior tibial artery
  - 7ᵗʰ **S85.171** Laceration of posterior tibial artery, right leg — CC POA CC/MCC Exc
  - 7ᵗʰ **S85.172** Laceration of posterior tibial artery, left leg — CC POA CC/MCC Exc
  - 7ᵗʰ **S85.179** Laceration of posterior tibial artery, unspecified leg — CC POA CC/MCC Exc

- 6ᵗʰ **S85.18** Other specified injury of posterior tibial artery
  - 7ᵗʰ **S85.181** Other specified injury of posterior tibial artery, right leg — CC POA CC/MCC Exc
  - 7ᵗʰ **S85.182** Other specified injury of posterior tibial artery, left leg — CC POA CC/MCC Exc
  - 7ᵗʰ **S85.189** Other specified injury of posterior tibial artery, unspecified leg — CC POA CC/MCC Exc

5ᵗʰ **S85.2** Injury of peroneal artery
- 6ᵗʰ **S85.20** Unspecified injury of peroneal artery
  - 7ᵗʰ **S85.201** Unspecified injury of peroneal artery, right leg — CC POA CC/MCC Exc
  - 7ᵗʰ **S85.202** Unspecified injury of peroneal artery, left leg — CC POA CC/MCC Exc
  - 7ᵗʰ **S85.209** Unspecified injury of peroneal artery, unspecified leg — CC POA CC/MCC Exc

---

POA Unacceptable principal diagnosis symbol per Medicare code edits   Code exempt from diagnosis present on admission requirement
? Questionable admission   CC Complication or comorbidity   MCC Major complication or comorbidity   CC/MCC CC/MCC exclusion
HCC HCC diagnosis code   RxHCC RxHCC diagnosis code   MACRA MACRA code   **DEFINITION** Describes condition/terminology
TIP Coding guidance   Official Guideline Reference   Z1 Z code as first-listed diagnosis

6th S85.21 Laceration of peroneal artery
- 7th S85.211 Laceration of peroneal artery, right leg — CC POA CC/MCC Exc
- 7th S85.212 Laceration of peroneal artery, left leg — CC POA CC/MCC Exc
- 7th S85.219 Laceration of peroneal artery, unspecified leg — CC POA CC/MCC Exc

6th S85.29 Other specified injury of peroneal artery
- 7th S85.291 Other specified injury of peroneal artery, right leg — CC POA CC/MCC Exc
- 7th S85.292 Other specified injury of peroneal artery, left leg — CC POA CC/MCC Exc
- 7th S85.299 Other specified injury of peroneal artery, unspecified leg — CC POA CC/MCC Exc

5th S85.3 Injury of greater saphenous vein at lower leg level
Injury of greater saphenous vein NOS
Injury of saphenous vein NOS
- 6th S85.30 Unspecified injury of greater saphenous vein at lower leg level
  - 7th S85.301 Unspecified injury of greater saphenous vein at lower leg level, right leg — CC POA CC/MCC Exc
  - 7th S85.302 Unspecified injury of greater saphenous vein at lower leg level, left leg — CC POA CC/MCC Exc
  - 7th S85.309 Unspecified injury of greater saphenous vein at lower leg level, unspecified leg — CC POA CC/MCC Exc
- 6th S85.31 Laceration of greater saphenous vein at lower leg level
  - 7th S85.311 Laceration of greater saphenous vein at lower leg level, right leg — CC POA CC/MCC Exc
  - 7th S85.312 Laceration of greater saphenous vein at lower leg level, left leg — CC POA CC/MCC Exc
  - 7th S85.319 Laceration of greater saphenous vein at lower leg level, unspecified leg — CC POA CC/MCC Exc
- 6th S85.39 Other specified injury of greater saphenous vein at lower leg level
  - 7th S85.391 Other specified injury of greater saphenous vein at lower leg level, right leg — CC POA CC/MCC Exc
  - 7th S85.392 Other specified injury of greater saphenous vein at lower leg level, left leg — CC POA CC/MCC Exc
  - 7th S85.399 Other specified injury of greater saphenous vein at lower leg level, unspecified leg — CC POA CC/MCC Exc

5th S85.4 Injury of lesser saphenous vein at lower leg level
- 6th S85.40 Unspecified injury of lesser saphenous vein at lower leg level
  - 7th S85.401 Unspecified injury of lesser saphenous vein at lower leg level, right leg — CC POA CC/MCC Exc
  - 7th S85.402 Unspecified injury of lesser saphenous vein at lower leg level, left leg — CC POA CC/MCC Exc
  - 7th S85.409 Unspecified injury of lesser saphenous vein at lower leg level, unspecified leg — CC POA CC/MCC Exc
- 6th S85.41 Laceration of lesser saphenous vein at lower leg level
  - 7th S85.411 Laceration of lesser saphenous vein at lower leg level, right leg — CC POA CC/MCC Exc
  - 7th S85.412 Laceration of lesser saphenous vein at lower leg level, left leg — CC POA CC/MCC Exc
  - 7th S85.419 Laceration of lesser saphenous vein at lower leg level, unspecified leg — CC POA CC/MCC Exc
- 6th S85.49 Other specified injury of lesser saphenous vein at lower leg level
  - 7th S85.491 Other specified injury of lesser saphenous vein at lower leg level, right leg — CC POA CC/MCC Exc
  - 7th S85.492 Other specified injury of lesser saphenous vein at lower leg level, left leg — CC POA CC/MCC Exc
  - 7th S85.499 Other specified injury of lesser saphenous vein at lower leg level, unspecified leg — CC POA CC/MCC Exc

5th S85.5 Injury of popliteal vein
- 6th S85.50 Unspecified injury of popliteal vein
  - 7th S85.501 Unspecified injury of popliteal vein, right leg — POA MCC CC/MCC Exc
  - 7th S85.502 Unspecified injury of popliteal vein, left leg — POA MCC CC/MCC Exc
  - 7th S85.509 Unspecified injury of popliteal vein, unspecified leg — POA MCC CC/MCC Exc
- 6th S85.51 Laceration of popliteal vein
  - 7th S85.511 Laceration of popliteal vein, right leg — POA MCC CC/MCC Exc
  - 7th S85.512 Laceration of popliteal vein, left leg — POA MCC CC/MCC Exc
  - 7th S85.519 Laceration of popliteal vein, unspecified leg — POA MCC CC/MCC Exc
- 6th S85.59 Other specified injury of popliteal vein
  - 7th S85.591 Other specified injury of popliteal vein, right leg — POA MCC CC/MCC Exc
  - 7th S85.592 Other specified injury of popliteal vein, left leg — POA MCC CC/MCC Exc
  - 7th S85.599 Other specified injury of popliteal vein, unspecified leg — POA MCC CC/MCC Exc

5th S85.8 Injury of other blood vessels at lower leg level
- 6th S85.80 Unspecified injury of other blood vessels at lower leg level
  - 7th S85.801 Unspecified injury of other blood vessels at lower leg level, right leg — CC POA CC/MCC Exc
  - 7th S85.802 Unspecified injury of other blood vessels at lower leg level, left leg — CC POA CC/MCC Exc
  - 7th S85.809 Unspecified injury of other blood vessels at lower leg level, unspecified leg — CC POA CC/MCC Exc
- 6th S85.81 Laceration of other blood vessels at lower leg level
  - 7th S85.811 Laceration of other blood vessels at lower leg level, right leg — CC POA CC/MCC Exc
  - 7th S85.812 Laceration of other blood vessels at lower leg level, left leg — CC POA CC/MCC Exc
  - 7th S85.819 Laceration of other blood vessels at lower leg level, unspecified leg — CC POA CC/MCC Exc
- 6th S85.89 Other specified injury of other blood vessels at lower leg level
  - 7th S85.891 Other specified injury of other blood vessels at lower leg level, right leg — CC POA CC/MCC Exc
  - 7th S85.892 Other specified injury of other blood vessels at lower leg level, left leg — CC POA CC/MCC Exc
  - 7th S85.899 Other specified injury of other blood vessels at lower leg level, unspecified leg — CC POA CC/MCC Exc

5th S85.9 Injury of unspecified blood vessel at lower leg level
- 6th S85.90 Unspecified injury of unspecified blood vessel at lower leg level
  - 7th S85.901 Unspecified injury of unspecified blood vessel at lower leg level, right leg — CC POA CC/MCC Exc
  - 7th S85.902 Unspecified injury of unspecified blood vessel at lower leg level, left leg — CC POA CC/MCC Exc
  - 7th S85.909 Unspecified injury of unspecified blood vessel at lower leg level, unspecified leg — CC POA CC/MCC Exc
- 6th S85.91 Laceration of unspecified blood vessel at lower leg level
  - 7th S85.911 Laceration of unspecified blood vessel at lower leg level, right leg — CC POA CC/MCC Exc
  - 7th S85.912 Laceration of unspecified blood vessel at lower leg level, left leg — CC POA CC/MCC Exc
  - 7th S85.919 Laceration of unspecified blood vessel at lower leg level, unspecified leg — CC POA CC/MCC Exc
- 6th S85.99 Other specified injury of unspecified blood vessel at lower leg level
  - 7th S85.991 Other specified injury of unspecified blood vessel at lower leg level, right leg — CC POA CC/MCC Exc

---

Unspecified Code   Other Specified Code   Manifestation Code   N Newborn   P Pediatric   M Maternity   A Adult   ♂ Male   ♀ Female
● New Code   ▲ Revised Code Title   ▶◀ Revised Text   **NOTES**   *INCLUDES*   *EXCLUDES1* Not coded here   *EXCLUDES2* Not included here
4th 4th character required   5th 5th character required   6th 6th character required   7th 7th character required   Extension 'X' Alert
HAC Hospital-acquired condition (HAC) alert   AHA AHA Coding Clinic©   ☛ Code first alert

[7th] S85.992 Other specified injury of unspecified blood vessel at lower leg level, left leg CC POA CC/MCC Exc

[7th] S85.999 Other specified injury of unspecified blood vessel at lower leg level, unspecified leg CC POA CC/MCC Exc

[4th] **S86 Injury of muscle, fascia and tendon at lower leg level**

Code also any associated open wound (S81.-)

[EXCLUDES2] *injury of muscle, fascia and tendon at ankle (S96.-)*
injury of patellar ligament (tendon) (S76.1-)
sprain of joints and ligaments of knee (S83.-)

The appropriate 7th character is to be added to each code from category S86
- A = initial encounter
- D = subsequent encounter
- S = sequela

[5th] S86.0 Injury of Achilles tendon
- [6th] S86.00 Unspecified injury of Achilles tendon
  - [7th] S86.001 Unspecified injury of right Achilles tendon POA
  - [7th] S86.002 Unspecified injury of left Achilles tendon POA
  - [7th] S86.009 Unspecified injury of unspecified Achilles tendon POA
- [6th] S86.01 Strain of Achilles tendon
  - [7th] S86.011 Strain of right Achilles tendon POA
  - [7th] S86.012 Strain of left Achilles tendon POA
  - [7th] S86.019 Strain of unspecified Achilles tendon POA
- [6th] S86.02 Laceration of Achilles tendon
  - [7th] S86.021 Laceration of right Achilles tendon CC POA CC/MCC Exc
  - [7th] S86.022 Laceration of left Achilles tendon CC POA CC/MCC Exc
  - [7th] S86.029 Laceration of unspecified Achilles tendon CC POA CC/MCC Exc
- [6th] S86.09 Other specified injury of Achilles tendon
  - [7th] S86.091 Other specified injury of right Achilles tendon POA
  - [7th] S86.092 Other specified injury of left Achilles tendon POA
  - [7th] S86.099 Other specified injury of unspecified Achilles tendon POA

[5th] S86.1 Injury of other muscle(s) and tendon(s) of posterior muscle group at lower leg level
- [6th] S86.10 Unspecified injury of other muscle(s) and tendon(s) of posterior muscle group at lower leg level
  - [7th] S86.101 Unspecified injury of other muscle(s) and tendon(s) of posterior muscle group at lower leg level, right leg POA
  - [7th] S86.102 Unspecified injury of other muscle(s) and tendon(s) of posterior muscle group at lower leg level, left leg POA
  - [7th] S86.109 Unspecified injury of other muscle(s) and tendon(s) of posterior muscle group at lower leg level, unspecified leg POA
- [6th] S86.11 Strain of other muscle(s) and tendon(s) of posterior muscle group at lower leg level
  - [7th] S86.111 Strain of other muscle(s) and tendon(s) of posterior muscle group at lower leg level, right leg POA
  - [7th] S86.112 Strain of other muscle(s) and tendon(s) of posterior muscle group at lower leg level, left leg POA
  - [7th] S86.119 Strain of other muscle(s) and tendon(s) of posterior muscle group at lower leg level, unspecified leg POA
- [6th] S86.12 Laceration of other muscle(s) and tendon(s) of posterior muscle group at lower leg level
  - [7th] S86.121 Laceration of other muscle(s) and tendon(s) of posterior muscle group at lower leg level, right leg CC POA CC/MCC Exc
  - [7th] S86.122 Laceration of other muscle(s) and tendon(s) of posterior muscle group at lower leg level, left leg CC POA CC/MCC Exc
  - [7th] S86.129 Laceration of other muscle(s) and tendon(s) of posterior muscle group at lower leg level, unspecified leg CC POA CC/MCC Exc
- [6th] S86.19 Other injury of other muscle(s) and tendon(s) of posterior muscle group at lower leg level
  - [7th] S86.191 Other injury of other muscle(s) and tendon(s) of posterior muscle group at lower leg level, right leg POA
  - [7th] S86.192 Other injury of other muscle(s) and tendon(s) of posterior muscle group at lower leg level, left leg POA
  - [7th] S86.199 Other injury of other muscle(s) and tendon(s) of posterior muscle group at lower leg level, unspecified leg POA

[5th] S86.2 Injury of muscle(s) and tendon(s) of anterior muscle group at lower leg level
- [6th] S86.20 Unspecified injury of muscle(s) and tendon(s) of anterior muscle group at lower leg level
  - [7th] S86.201 Unspecified injury of muscle(s) and tendon(s) of anterior muscle group at lower leg level, right leg POA
  - [7th] S86.202 Unspecified injury of muscle(s) and tendon(s) of anterior muscle group at lower leg level, left leg POA
  - [7th] S86.209 Unspecified injury of muscle(s) and tendon(s) of anterior muscle group at lower leg level, unspecified leg POA
- [6th] S86.21 Strain of muscle(s) and tendon(s) of anterior muscle group at lower leg level
  - [7th] S86.211 Strain of muscle(s) and tendon(s) of anterior muscle group at lower leg level, right leg POA
  - [7th] S86.212 Strain of muscle(s) and tendon(s) of anterior muscle group at lower leg level, left leg POA
  - [7th] S86.219 Strain of muscle(s) and tendon(s) of anterior muscle group at lower leg level, unspecified leg POA
- [6th] S86.22 Laceration of muscle(s) and tendon(s) of anterior muscle group at lower leg level
  - [7th] S86.221 Laceration of muscle(s) and tendon(s) of anterior muscle group at lower leg level, right leg CC POA CC/MCC Exc
  - [7th] S86.222 Laceration of muscle(s) and tendon(s) of anterior muscle group at lower leg level, left leg CC POA CC/MCC Exc
  - [7th] S86.229 Laceration of muscle(s) and tendon(s) of anterior muscle group at lower leg level, unspecified leg CC POA CC/MCC Exc
- [6th] S86.29 Other injury of muscle(s) and tendon(s) of anterior muscle group at lower leg level
  - [7th] S86.291 Other injury of muscle(s) and tendon(s) of anterior muscle group at lower leg level, right leg POA
  - [7th] S86.292 Other injury of muscle(s) and tendon(s) of anterior muscle group at lower leg level, left leg POA
  - [7th] S86.299 Other injury of muscle(s) and tendon(s) of anterior muscle group at lower leg level, unspecified leg POA

[5th] S86.3 Injury of muscle(s) and tendon(s) of peroneal muscle group at lower leg level
- [6th] S86.30 Unspecified injury of muscle(s) and tendon(s) of peroneal muscle group at lower leg level
  - [7th] S86.301 Unspecified injury of muscle(s) and tendon(s) of peroneal muscle group at lower leg level, right leg POA
  - [7th] S86.302 Unspecified injury of muscle(s) and tendon(s) of peroneal muscle group at lower leg level, left leg POA

PDx Unacceptable principal diagnosis symbol per Medicare code edits; POA Code exempt from diagnosis present on admission requirement
[?] Questionable admission; CC Complication or comorbidity; MCC Major complication or comorbidity; CC/MCC Exc CC/MCC exclusion
[HCC] HCC diagnosis code; [RxHCC] RxHCC diagnosis code; MACRA code; **DEFINITION** Describes condition/terminology
TIP Coding guidance; Official Guideline Reference; [Z-1] Z code as first-listed diagnosis

[7th] S86.309 Unspecified injury of muscle(s) and tendon(s) of peroneal muscle group at lower leg level, unspecified leg POA

[6th] S86.31 Strain of muscle(s) and tendon(s) of peroneal muscle group at lower leg level

[7th] S86.311 Strain of muscle(s) and tendon(s) of peroneal muscle group at lower leg level, right leg POA

[7th] S86.312 Strain of muscle(s) and tendon(s) of peroneal muscle group at lower leg level, left leg POA

[7th] S86.319 Strain of muscle(s) and tendon(s) of peroneal muscle group at lower leg level, unspecified leg POA

[6th] S86.32 Laceration of muscle(s) and tendon(s) of peroneal muscle group at lower leg level

[7th] S86.321 Laceration of muscle(s) and tendon(s) of peroneal muscle group at lower leg level, right leg CC POA CC/MCC Exc

[7th] S86.322 Laceration of muscle(s) and tendon(s) of peroneal muscle group at lower leg level, left leg CC POA CC/MCC Exc

[7th] S86.329 Laceration of muscle(s) and tendon(s) of peroneal muscle group at lower leg level, unspecified leg CC POA CC/MCC Exc

[6th] S86.39 Other injury of muscle(s) and tendon(s) of peroneal muscle group at lower leg level

[7th] S86.391 Other injury of muscle(s) and tendon(s) of peroneal muscle group at lower leg level, right leg POA

[7th] S86.392 Other injury of muscle(s) and tendon(s) of peroneal muscle group at lower leg level, left leg POA

[7th] S86.399 Other injury of muscle(s) and tendon(s) of peroneal muscle group at lower leg level, unspecified leg POA

[5th] S86.8 Injury of other muscles and tendons at lower leg level

[6th] S86.80 Unspecified injury of other muscles and tendons at lower leg level

[7th] S86.801 Unspecified injury of other muscle(s) and tendon(s) at lower leg level, right leg POA

[7th] S86.802 Unspecified injury of other muscle(s) and tendon(s) at lower leg level, left leg POA

[7th] S86.809 Unspecified injury of other muscle(s) and tendon(s) at lower leg level, unspecified leg POA

[6th] S86.81 Strain of other muscles and tendons at lower leg level

[7th] S86.811 Strain of other muscle(s) and tendon(s) at lower leg level, right leg POA

[7th] S86.812 Strain of other muscle(s) and tendon(s) at lower leg level, left leg POA

[7th] S86.819 Strain of other muscle(s) and tendon(s) at lower leg level, unspecified leg POA

[6th] S86.82 Laceration of other muscles and tendons at lower leg level

[7th] S86.821 Laceration of other muscle(s) and tendon(s) at lower leg level, right leg CC POA CC/MCC Exc

[7th] S86.822 Laceration of other muscle(s) and tendon(s) at lower leg level, left leg CC POA CC/MCC Exc

[7th] S86.829 Laceration of other muscle(s) and tendon(s) at lower leg level, unspecified leg CC POA CC/MCC Exc

[6th] S86.89 Other injury of other muscles and tendons at lower leg level

[7th] S86.891 Other injury of other muscle(s) and tendon(s) at lower leg level, right leg POA

[7th] S86.892 Other injury of other muscle(s) and tendon(s) at lower leg level, left leg POA

[7th] S86.899 Other injury of other muscle(s) and tendon(s) at lower leg level, unspecified leg POA

[5th] S86.9 Injury of unspecified muscle and tendon at lower leg level

[6th] S86.90 Unspecified injury of unspecified muscle and tendon at lower leg level

[7th] S86.901 Unspecified injury of unspecified muscle(s) and tendon(s) at lower leg level, right leg POA

[7th] S86.902 Unspecified injury of unspecified muscle(s) and tendon(s) at lower leg level, left leg POA

[7th] S86.909 Unspecified injury of unspecified muscle(s) and tendon(s) at lower leg level, unspecified leg POA

[6th] S86.91 Strain of unspecified muscle and tendon at lower leg level

[7th] S86.911 Strain of unspecified muscle(s) and tendon(s) at lower leg level, right leg POA

[7th] S86.912 Strain of unspecified muscle(s) and tendon(s) at lower leg level, left leg POA

[7th] S86.919 Strain of unspecified muscle(s) and tendon(s) at lower leg level, unspecified leg POA

[6th] S86.92 Laceration of unspecified muscle and tendon at lower leg level

[7th] S86.921 Laceration of unspecified muscle(s) and tendon(s) at lower leg level, right leg CC POA CC/MCC Exc

[7th] S86.922 Laceration of unspecified muscle(s) and tendon(s) at lower leg level, left leg CC POA CC/MCC Exc

[7th] S86.929 Laceration of unspecified muscle(s) and tendon(s) at lower leg level, unspecified leg CC POA CC/MCC Exc

[6th] S86.99 Other injury of unspecified muscle and tendon at lower leg level

[7th] S86.991 Other injury of unspecified muscle(s) and tendon(s) at lower leg level, right leg POA

[7th] S86.992 Other injury of unspecified muscle(s) and tendon(s) at lower leg level, left leg POA

[7th] S86.999 Other injury of unspecified muscle(s) and tendon(s) at lower leg level, unspecified leg POA

[4th] S87 Crushing injury of lower leg

Use additional code(s) for all associated injuries

EXCLUDES2 *crushing injury of ankle and foot (S97.-)*

The appropriate 7th character is to be added to each code from category S87

A = initial encounter
D = subsequent encounter
S = sequela

[5th] S87.0 Crushing injury of knee

[7th] S87.00 Crushing injury of unspecified knee POA

[7th] S87.01 Crushing injury of right knee POA

[7th] S87.02 Crushing injury of left knee POA

[5th] S87.8 Crushing injury of lower leg

[7th] S87.80 Crushing injury of unspecified lower leg POA

[7th] S87.81 Crushing injury of right lower leg POA

[7th] S87.82 Crushing injury of left lower leg POA

[4th] S88 Traumatic amputation of lower leg

An amputation not identified as partial or complete should be coded to complete

EXCLUDES1 *traumatic amputation of ankle and foot (S98.-)*

The appropriate 7th character is to be added to each code from category S88

A = initial encounter
D = subsequent encounter
S = sequela

[5th] S88.0 Traumatic amputation at knee level

[6th] S88.01 Complete traumatic amputation at knee level

Unspecified Code Other Specified Code Manifestation Code [N] Newborn [P] Pediatric [M] Maternity [A] Adult ♂ Male ♀ Female
● New Code ▲ Revised Code Title ►◄ Revised Text NOTES INCLUDES EXCLUDES1 Not coded here EXCLUDES2 Not included here
[4th] 4th character required [5th] 5th character required [6th] 6th character required [7th] 7th character required [x7th] Extension 'X' Alert
[HAC] Hospital-acquired condition (HAC) alert AHA AHA Coding Clinic© ☛ Code first alert

7ᵗʰ S88.011 Complete traumatic amputation at knee level, **right** lower leg cᶜ Pᴏᴀ HCC CC/MCC Exc

7ᵗʰ S88.012 Complete traumatic amputation at knee level, **left** lower leg cᶜ Pᴏᴀ HCC CC/MCC Exc

7ᵗʰ S88.019 Complete traumatic amputation at knee level, **unspecified** lower leg cᶜ Pᴏᴀ HCC CC/MCC Exc

6ᵗʰ S88.02 **Partial** traumatic amputation at knee level

7ᵗʰ S88.021 Partial traumatic amputation at knee level, **right** lower leg cᶜ Pᴏᴀ HCC CC/MCC Exc

7ᵗʰ S88.022 Partial traumatic amputation at knee level, **left** lower leg cᶜ Pᴏᴀ HCC CC/MCC Exc

7ᵗʰ S88.029 Partial traumatic amputation at knee level, **unspecified** lower leg cᶜ Pᴏᴀ HCC CC/MCC Exc

5ᵗʰ S88.1 Traumatic amputation at level **between knee and ankle**

6ᵗʰ S88.11 **Complete** traumatic amputation at level between knee and ankle

7ᵗʰ S88.111 Complete traumatic amputation at level between knee and ankle, **right** lower leg cᶜ Pᴏᴀ HCC CC/MCC Exc

7ᵗʰ S88.112 Complete traumatic amputation at level between knee and ankle, **left** lower leg cᶜ Pᴏᴀ HCC CC/MCC Exc

7ᵗʰ S88.119 Complete traumatic amputation at level between knee and ankle, **unspecified** lower leg cᶜ Pᴏᴀ HCC CC/MCC Exc

6ᵗʰ S88.12 **Partial** traumatic amputation at level between knee and ankle

7ᵗʰ S88.121 Partial traumatic amputation at level between knee and ankle, **right** lower leg cᶜ Pᴏᴀ HCC CC/MCC Exc

7ᵗʰ S88.122 Partial traumatic amputation at level between knee and ankle, **left** lower leg cᶜ Pᴏᴀ HCC CC/MCC Exc

7ᵗʰ S88.129 Partial traumatic amputation at level between knee and ankle, **unspecified** lower leg cᶜ Pᴏᴀ HCC CC/MCC Exc

5ᵗʰ S88.9 Traumatic amputation of lower leg, **level unspecified**

6ᵗʰ S88.91 **Complete** traumatic amputation of lower leg, level unspecified

7ᵗʰ S88.911 Complete traumatic amputation of **right** lower leg, level unspecified cᶜ Pᴏᴀ HCC CC/MCC Exc

7ᵗʰ S88.912 Complete traumatic amputation of **left** lower leg, level unspecified cᶜ Pᴏᴀ HCC CC/MCC Exc

7ᵗʰ S88.919 Complete traumatic amputation of unspecified lower leg, level unspecified cᶜ Pᴏᴀ HCC CC/MCC Exc

6ᵗʰ S88.92 **Partial** traumatic amputation of lower leg, level unspecified

7ᵗʰ S88.921 Partial traumatic amputation of **right** lower leg, level unspecified cᶜ Pᴏᴀ HCC CC/MCC Exc

7ᵗʰ S88.922 Partial traumatic amputation of **left** lower leg, level unspecified cᶜ Pᴏᴀ HCC CC/MCC Exc

7ᵗʰ S88.929 Partial traumatic amputation of unspecified lower leg, level unspecified cᶜ Pᴏᴀ HCC CC/MCC Exc

4ᵗʰ S89 **Other** and **unspecified** injuries of lower leg

👁 See Official Guidelines "Coding of Traumatic Fractures" I.C.19.c

NOTES A fracture not indicated as open or closed should be coded to closed

EXCLUDES2 *other and unspecified injuries of ankle and foot (S99.-)*

The appropriate 7th character is to be added to each code from subcategories S89.0, S89.1, S89.2, and S89.3

A = initial encounter for closed fracture

D = subsequent encounter for fracture with routine healing

G = subsequent encounter for fracture with delayed healing

K = subsequent encounter for fracture with nonunion

P = subsequent encounter for fracture with malunion

S = sequela

5ᵗʰ S89.0 Physeal fracture of **upper end of tibia**

6ᵗʰ S89.00 **Unspecified** physeal fracture of upper end of tibia

7ᵗʰ S89.001 Unspecified physeal fracture of upper end of **right** tibia cᶜ Pᴏᴀ HAC CC/MCC Exc

7ᵗʰ S89.002 Unspecified physeal fracture of upper end of **left** tibia cᶜ Pᴏᴀ HAC CC/MCC Exc

7ᵗʰ S89.009 Unspecified physeal fracture of upper end of unspecified tibia cᶜ Pᴏᴀ HAC CC/MCC Exc

6ᵗʰ S89.01 **Salter-Harris Type I** physeal fracture of upper end of tibia

7ᵗʰ S89.011 Salter-Harris Type I physeal fracture of upper end of **right** tibia cᶜ Pᴏᴀ HAC CC/MCC Exc

7ᵗʰ S89.012 Salter-Harris Type I physeal fracture of upper end of **left** tibia cᶜ Pᴏᴀ HAC CC/MCC Exc

7ᵗʰ S89.019 Salter-Harris Type I physeal fracture of upper end of unspecified tibia cᶜ Pᴏᴀ HAC CC/MCC Exc

6ᵗʰ S89.02 **Salter-Harris Type II** physeal fracture of upper end of tibia

7ᵗʰ S89.021 Salter-Harris Type II physeal fracture of upper end of **right** tibia cᶜ Pᴏᴀ HAC CC/MCC Exc

7ᵗʰ S89.022 Salter-Harris Type II physeal fracture of upper end of **left** tibia cᶜ Pᴏᴀ HAC CC/MCC Exc

7ᵗʰ S89.029 Salter-Harris Type II physeal fracture of upper end of unspecified tibia cᶜ Pᴏᴀ HAC CC/MCC Exc

5ᵗʰ S89.03 **Salter-Harris Type III** physeal fracture of upper end of tibia

7ᵗʰ S89.031 Salter-Harris Type III physeal fracture of upper end of **right** tibia cᶜ Pᴏᴀ HAC CC/MCC Exc

7ᵗʰ S89.032 Salter-Harris Type III physeal fracture of upper end of **left** tibia cᶜ Pᴏᴀ HAC CC/MCC Exc

7ᵗʰ S89.039 Salter-Harris Type III physeal fracture of upper end of unspecified tibia cᶜ Pᴏᴀ HAC CC/MCC Exc

6ᵗʰ S89.04 **Salter-Harris Type IV** physeal fracture of upper end of tibia

7ᵗʰ S89.041 Salter-Harris Type IV physeal fracture of upper end of **right** tibia cᶜ Pᴏᴀ HAC CC/MCC Exc

7ᵗʰ S89.042 Salter-Harris Type IV physeal fracture of upper end of **left** tibia cᶜ Pᴏᴀ HAC CC/MCC Exc

7ᵗʰ S89.049 Salter-Harris Type IV physeal fracture of upper end of unspecified tibia cᶜ Pᴏᴀ HAC CC/MCC Exc

6ᵗʰ S89.09 **Other** physeal fracture of upper end of tibia

7ᵗʰ S89.091 Other physeal fracture of upper end of **right** tibia cᶜ Pᴏᴀ HAC CC/MCC Exc

7ᵗʰ S89.092 Other physeal fracture of upper end of **left** tibia cᶜ Pᴏᴀ HAC CC/MCC Exc

7ᵗʰ S89.099 Other physeal fracture of upper end of unspecified tibia cᶜ Pᴏᴀ HAC CC/MCC Exc

5ᵗʰ S89.1 Physeal fracture of **lower end of tibia**

6ᵗʰ S89.10 **Unspecified** physeal fracture of lower end of tibia

7ᵗʰ S89.101 Unspecified physeal fracture of lower end of **right** tibia cᶜ Pᴏᴀ CC/MCC Exc

7ᵗʰ S89.102 Unspecified physeal fracture of lower end of **left** tibia cᶜ Pᴏᴀ CC/MCC Exc

7ᵗʰ S89.109 Unspecified physeal fracture of lower end of unspecified tibia cᶜ Pᴏᴀ CC/MCC Exc

6ᵗʰ S89.11 **Salter-Harris Type I** physeal fracture of lower end of tibia

7ᵗʰ S89.111 Salter-Harris Type I physeal fracture of lower end of **right** tibia cᶜ Pᴏᴀ CC/MCC Exc

7ᵗʰ S89.112 Salter-Harris Type I physeal fracture of lower end of **left** tibia cᶜ Pᴏᴀ CC/MCC Exc

7ᵗʰ S89.119 Salter-Harris Type I physeal fracture of lower end of unspecified tibia cᶜ Pᴏᴀ CC/MCC Exc

6ᵗʰ S89.12 **Salter-Harris Type II** physeal fracture of lower end of tibia

7ᵗʰ S89.121 Salter-Harris Type II physeal fracture of lower end of **right** tibia cᶜ Pᴏᴀ CC/MCC Exc

7ᵗʰ S89.122 Salter-Harris Type II physeal fracture of lower end of **left** tibia cᶜ Pᴏᴀ CC/MCC Exc

7ᵗʰ S89.129 Salter-Harris Type II physeal fracture of lower end of unspecified tibia cᶜ Pᴏᴀ CC/MCC Exc

[6th] S89.13 Salter-Harris Type III physeal fracture of lower end of tibia
[EXCLUDES1] *fracture of medial malleolus (adult) (S82.5-)*
- [7th] S89.131 Salter-Harris Type III physeal fracture of lower end of right tibia CC POA CC/MCC Exc
- [7th] S89.132 Salter-Harris Type III physeal fracture of lower end of left tibia CC POA CC/MCC Exc
- [7th] S89.139 Salter-Harris Type III physeal fracture of lower end of unspecified tibia CC POA CC/MCC Exc

[6th] S89.14 Salter-Harris Type IV physeal fracture of lower end of tibia
[EXCLUDES1] *fracture of medial malleolus (adult) (S82.5-)*
- [7th] S89.141 Salter-Harris Type IV physeal fracture of lower end of right tibia CC POA CC/MCC Exc
- [7th] S89.142 Salter-Harris Type IV physeal fracture of lower end of left tibia CC POA CC/MCC Exc
- [7th] S89.149 Salter-Harris Type IV physeal fracture of lower end of unspecified tibia CC POA CC/MCC Exc

[6th] S89.19 Other physeal fracture of lower end of tibia
- [7th] S89.191 Other physeal fracture of lower end of right tibia CC POA CC/MCC Exc
- [7th] S89.192 Other physeal fracture of lower end of left tibia CC POA CC/MCC Exc
- [7th] S89.199 Other physeal fracture of lower end of unspecified tibia CC POA CC/MCC Exc

[5th] S89.2 Physeal fracture of upper end of fibula

[6th] S89.20 Unspecified physeal fracture of upper end of fibula
- [7th] S89.201 Unspecified physeal fracture of upper end of right fibula CC POA CC/MCC Exc
- [7th] S89.202 Unspecified physeal fracture of upper end of left fibula CC POA CC/MCC Exc
- [7th] S89.209 Unspecified physeal fracture of upper end of unspecified fibula CC POA CC/MCC Exc

[6th] S89.21 Salter-Harris Type I physeal fracture of upper end of fibula
- [7th] S89.211 Salter-Harris Type I physeal fracture of upper end of right fibula CC POA CC/MCC Exc
- [7th] S89.212 Salter-Harris Type I physeal fracture of upper end of left fibula CC POA CC/MCC Exc
- [7th] S89.219 Salter-Harris Type I physeal fracture of upper end of unspecified fibula CC POA CC/MCC Exc

[6th] S89.22 Salter-Harris Type II physeal fracture of upper end of fibula
- [7th] S89.221 Salter-Harris Type II physeal fracture of upper end of right fibula CC POA CC/MCC Exc
- [7th] S89.222 Salter-Harris Type II physeal fracture of upper end of left fibula CC POA CC/MCC Exc
- [7th] S89.229 Salter-Harris Type II physeal fracture of upper end of unspecified fibula CC POA CC/MCC Exc

[6th] S89.29 Other physeal fracture of upper end of fibula
- [7th] S89.291 Other physeal fracture of upper end of right fibula CC POA CC/MCC Exc
- [7th] S89.292 Other physeal fracture of upper end of left fibula CC POA CC/MCC Exc
- [7th] S89.299 Other physeal fracture of upper end of unspecified fibula CC POA CC/MCC Exc

[5th] S89.3 Physeal fracture of lower end of fibula

[6th] S89.30 Unspecified physeal fracture of lower end of fibula
- [7th] S89.301 Unspecified physeal fracture of lower end of right fibula CC POA CC/MCC Exc
- [7th] S89.302 Unspecified physeal fracture of lower end of left fibula CC POA CC/MCC Exc
- [7th] S89.309 Unspecified physeal fracture of lower end of unspecified fibula CC POA CC/MCC Exc

[6th] S89.31 Salter-Harris Type I physeal fracture of lower end of fibula
- [7th] S89.311 Salter-Harris Type I physeal fracture of lower end of right fibula CC POA CC/MCC Exc
- [7th] S89.312 Salter-Harris Type I physeal fracture of lower end of left fibula CC POA CC/MCC Exc
- [7th] S89.319 Salter-Harris Type I physeal fracture of lower end of unspecified fibula CC POA CC/MCC Exc

[6th] S89.32 Salter-Harris Type II physeal fracture of lower end of fibula
- [7th] S89.321 Salter-Harris Type II physeal fracture of lower end of right fibula CC POA CC/MCC Exc
- [7th] S89.322 Salter-Harris Type II physeal fracture of lower end of left fibula CC POA CC/MCC Exc
- [7th] S89.329 Salter-Harris Type II physeal fracture of lower end of unspecified fibula CC POA CC/MCC Exc

[6th] S89.39 Other physeal fracture of lower end of fibula
- [7th] S89.391 Other physeal fracture of lower end of right fibula CC POA CC/MCC Exc
- [7th] S89.392 Other physeal fracture of lower end of left fibula CC POA CC/MCC Exc
- [7th] S89.399 Other physeal fracture of lower end of unspecified fibula CC POA CC/MCC Exc

[5th] S89.8 Other specified injuries of lower leg
The appropriate 7th character is to be added to each code in subcategory S89.8
A = initial encounter
D = subsequent encounter
S = sequela
- [7th] S89.80 Other specified injuries of unspecified lower leg POA
- [7th] S89.81 Other specified injuries of right lower leg POA
- [7th] S89.82 Other specified injuries of left lower leg POA

[5th] S89.9 Unspecified injury of lower leg
The appropriate 7th character is to be added to each code in subcategory S89.9
A = initial encounter
D = subsequent encounter
S = sequela
- [7th] S89.90 Unspecified injury of unspecified lower leg POA
- [7th] S89.91 Unspecified injury of right lower leg POA
- [7th] S89.92 Unspecified injury of left lower leg POA

Injuries to the ankle and foot (S90-S99)

[EXCLUDES2] *burns and corrosions (T20-T32)*
fracture of ankle and malleolus (S82.-)
frostbite (T33-T34)
insect bite or sting, venomous (T63.4)

[4th] S90 Superficial injury of ankle, foot and toes
The appropriate 7th character is to be added to each code from category S90
A = initial encounter
D = subsequent encounter
S = sequela

[5th] S90.0 Contusion of ankle
- [7th] S90.00 Contusion of unspecified ankle POA
- [7th] S90.01 Contusion of right ankle POA
- [7th] S90.02 Contusion of left ankle POA

[5th] S90.1 Contusion of toe without damage to nail

[6th] S90.11 Contusion of great toe without damage to nail
- [7th] S90.111 Contusion of right great toe without damage to nail POA
- [7th] S90.112 Contusion of left great toe without damage to nail POA
- [7th] S90.119 Contusion of unspecified great toe without damage to nail POA

[6th] S90.12 Contusion of lesser toe without damage to nail
- [7th] S90.121 Contusion of right lesser toe(s) without damage to nail POA
- [7th] S90.122 Contusion of left lesser toe(s) without damage to nail POA
- [7th] S90.129 Contusion of unspecified lesser toe(s) without damage to nail POA
  Contusion of toe NOS

[5th] S90.2 Contusion of toe with damage to nail

[6th] S90.21 Contusion of great toe with damage to nail
- [7th] S90.211 Contusion of right great toe with damage to nail POA

Unspecified Code | Other Specified Code | Manifestation Code | [N] Newborn | [P] Pediatric | [M] Maternity | [A] Adult | ♂ Male | ♀ Female
● New Code | ▲ Revised Code Title | ►◄ Revised Text | NOTES | INCLUDES | EXCLUDES1 Not coded here | EXCLUDES2 Not included here
[4th] 4th character required | [5th] 5th character required | [6th] 6th character required | [7th] 7th character required | [7th] Extension 'X' Alert
[HAC] Hospital-acquired condition (HAC) alert | AHA AHA Coding Clinic© | ☞ Code first alert

S90.212 Contusion of left great toe with damage to nail

S90.219 Contusion of unspecified great toe with damage to nail

6ᵗʰ S90.22 Contusion of lesser toe with damage to nail

S90.221 Contusion of right lesser toe(s) with damage to nail

S90.222 Contusion of left lesser toe(s) with damage to nail

S90.229 Contusion of unspecified lesser toe(s) with damage to nail

5ᵗʰ S90.3 Contusion of foot

EXCLUDES2 contusion of toes (S90.1-, S90.2-)

S90.30 Contusion of unspecified foot
Contusion of foot NOS

S90.31 Contusion of right foot

S90.32 Contusion of left foot

5ᵗʰ S90.4 Other superficial injuries of toe

6ᵗʰ S90.41 Abrasion of toe

S90.411 Abrasion, right great toe

S90.412 Abrasion, left great toe

S90.413 Abrasion, unspecified great toe

S90.414 Abrasion, right lesser toe(s)

S90.415 Abrasion, left lesser toe(s)

S90.416 Abrasion, unspecified lesser toe(s)

6ᵗʰ S90.42 Blister (nonthermal) of toe

S90.421 Blister (nonthermal), right great toe

S90.422 Blister (nonthermal), left great toe

S90.423 Blister (nonthermal), unspecified great toe

S90.424 Blister (nonthermal), right lesser toe(s)

S90.425 Blister (nonthermal), left lesser toe(s)

S90.426 Blister (nonthermal), unspecified lesser toe(s)

6ᵗʰ S90.44 External constriction of toe
Hair tourniquet syndrome of toe

S90.441 External constriction, right great toe

S90.442 External constriction, left great toe

S90.443 External constriction, unspecified great toe

S90.444 External constriction, right lesser toe(s)

S90.445 External constriction, left lesser toe(s)

S90.446 External constriction, unspecified lesser toe(s)

6ᵗʰ S90.45 Superficial foreign body of toe
Splinter in the toe

S90.451 Superficial foreign body, right great toe

S90.452 Superficial foreign body, left great toe

S90.453 Superficial foreign body, unspecified great toe

S90.454 Superficial foreign body, right lesser toe(s)

S90.455 Superficial foreign body, left lesser toe(s)

S90.456 Superficial foreign body, unspecified lesser toe(s)

6ᵗʰ S90.46 Insect bite (nonvenomous) of toe

S90.461 Insect bite (nonvenomous), right great toe

S90.462 Insect bite (nonvenomous), left great toe

S90.463 Insect bite (nonvenomous), unspecified great toe

S90.464 Insect bite (nonvenomous), right lesser toe(s)

S90.465 Insect bite (nonvenomous), left lesser toe(s)

S90.466 Insect bite (nonvenomous), unspecified lesser toe(s)

6ᵗʰ S90.47 Other superficial bite of toe

EXCLUDES1 open bite of toe (S91.15-, S91.25-)

S90.471 Other superficial bite of right great toe

S90.472 Other superficial bite of left great toe

S90.473 Other superficial bite of unspecified great toe

S90.474 Other superficial bite of right lesser toe(s)

S90.475 Other superficial bite of left lesser toe(s)

S90.476 Other superficial bite of unspecified lesser toe(s)

5ᵗʰ S90.5 Other superficial injuries of ankle

6ᵗʰ S90.51 Abrasion of ankle

S90.511 Abrasion, right ankle

S90.512 Abrasion, left ankle

S90.519 Abrasion, unspecified ankle

6ᵗʰ S90.52 Blister (nonthermal) of ankle

S90.521 Blister (nonthermal), right ankle

S90.522 Blister (nonthermal), left ankle

S90.529 Blister (nonthermal), unspecified ankle

6ᵗʰ S90.54 External constriction of ankle

S90.541 External constriction, right ankle

S90.542 External constriction, left ankle

S90.549 External constriction, unspecified ankle

6ᵗʰ S90.55 Superficial foreign body of ankle
Splinter in the ankle

S90.551 Superficial foreign body, right ankle

S90.552 Superficial foreign body, left ankle

S90.559 Superficial foreign body, unspecified ankle

6ᵗʰ S90.56 Insect bite (nonvenomous) of ankle

S90.561 Insect bite (nonvenomous), right ankle

S90.562 Insect bite (nonvenomous), left ankle

S90.569 Insect bite (nonvenomous), unspecified ankle

6ᵗʰ S90.57 Other superficial bite of ankle

EXCLUDES1 open bite of ankle (S91.05-)

S90.571 Other superficial bite of ankle, right ankle

S90.572 Other superficial bite of ankle, left ankle

S90.579 Other superficial bite of ankle, unspecified ankle

5ᵗʰ S90.8 Other superficial injuries of foot

6ᵗʰ S90.81 Abrasion of foot

S90.811 Abrasion, right foot

S90.812 Abrasion, left foot

S90.819 Abrasion, unspecified foot

6ᵗʰ S90.82 Blister (nonthermal) of foot

S90.821 Blister (nonthermal), right foot

S90.822 Blister (nonthermal), left foot

S90.829 Blister (nonthermal), unspecified foot

6ᵗʰ S90.84 External constriction of foot

S90.841 External constriction, right foot

S90.842 External constriction, left foot

S90.849 External constriction, unspecified foot

6ᵗʰ S90.85 Superficial foreign body of foot
Splinter in the foot

S90.851 Superficial foreign body, right foot

S90.852 Superficial foreign body, left foot

S90.859 Superficial foreign body, unspecified foot

6ᵗʰ S90.86 Insect bite (nonvenomous) of foot

S90.861 Insect bite (nonvenomous), right foot

S90.862 Insect bite (nonvenomous), left foot

S90.869 Insect bite (nonvenomous), unspecified foot

6ᵗʰ S90.87 Other superficial bite of foot

EXCLUDES1 open bite of foot (S91.35-)

S90.871 Other superficial bite of right foot

S90.872 Other superficial bite of left foot

S90.879 Other superficial bite of unspecified foot

- [5th] S90.9 Unspecified superficial injury of ankle, foot and toe
  - [6th] S90.91 Unspecified superficial injury of ankle
    - [7th] S90.911 Unspecified superficial injury of right ankle [POA]
    - [7th] S90.912 Unspecified superficial injury of left ankle [POA]
    - [7th] S90.919 Unspecified superficial injury of unspecified ankle [POA]
  - [6th] S90.92 Unspecified superficial injury of foot
    - [7th] S90.921 Unspecified superficial injury of right foot [POA]
    - [7th] S90.922 Unspecified superficial injury of left foot [POA]
    - [7th] S90.929 Unspecified superficial injury of unspecified foot [POA]
  - [6th] S90.93 Unspecified superficial injury of toes
    - [7th] S90.931 Unspecified superficial injury of right great toe [POA]
    - [7th] S90.932 Unspecified superficial injury of left great toe [POA]
    - [7th] S90.933 Unspecified superficial injury of unspecified great toe [POA]
    - [7th] S90.934 Unspecified superficial injury of right lesser toe(s) [POA]
    - [7th] S90.935 Unspecified superficial injury of left lesser toe(s) [POA]
    - [7th] S90.936 Unspecified superficial injury of unspecified lesser toe(s) [POA]

[4th] **S91 Open wound of ankle, foot and toes**

Code also any associated wound infection

[EXCLUDES1] *open fracture of ankle, foot and toes (S92.-with 7th character B)*
traumatic amputation of ankle and foot (S98.-)

The appropriate 7th character is to be added to each code from category S91
- A = initial encounter
- D = subsequent encounter
- S = sequela

- [5th] S91.0 Open wound of ankle
  - [6th] S91.00 Unspecified open wound of ankle
    - [7th] S91.001 Unspecified open wound, right ankle [POA]
    - [7th] S91.002 Unspecified open wound, left ankle [POA]
    - [7th] S91.009 Unspecified open wound, unspecified ankle [POA]
  - [6th] S91.01 Laceration without foreign body of ankle
    - [7th] S91.011 Laceration without foreign body, right ankle [POA]
    - [7th] S91.012 Laceration without foreign body, left ankle [POA]
    - [7th] S91.019 Laceration without foreign body, unspecified ankle [POA]
  - [6th] S91.02 Laceration with foreign body of ankle
    - [7th] S91.021 Laceration with foreign body, right ankle [POA]
    - [7th] S91.022 Laceration with foreign body, left ankle [POA]
    - [7th] S91.029 Laceration with foreign body, unspecified ankle [POA]
  - [6th] S91.03 Puncture wound without foreign body of ankle
    - [7th] S91.031 Puncture wound without foreign body, right ankle [POA]
    - [7th] S91.032 Puncture wound without foreign body, left ankle [POA]
    - [7th] S91.039 Puncture wound without foreign body, unspecified ankle [POA]
  - [6th] S91.04 Puncture wound with foreign body of ankle
    - [7th] S91.041 Puncture wound with foreign body, right ankle [POA]
    - [7th] S91.042 Puncture wound with foreign body, left ankle [POA]
    - [7th] S91.049 Puncture wound with foreign body, unspecified ankle [POA]
  - [6th] S91.05 Open bite of ankle

    [EXCLUDES1] *superficial bite of ankle (S90.56-, S90.57-)*
    - [7th] S91.051 Open bite, right ankle [POA]
    - [7th] S91.052 Open bite, left ankle [POA]
    - [7th] S91.059 Open bite, unspecified ankle [POA]
- [5th] S91.1 Open wound of toe without damage to nail
  - [6th] S91.10 Unspecified open wound of toe without damage to nail
    - [7th] S91.101 Unspecified open wound of right great toe without damage to nail [POA]
    - [7th] S91.102 Unspecified open wound of left great toe without damage to nail [POA]
    - [7th] S91.103 Unspecified open wound of unspecified great toe without damage to nail [POA]
    - [7th] S91.104 Unspecified open wound of right lesser toe(s) without damage to nail [POA]
    - [7th] S91.105 Unspecified open wound of left lesser toe(s) without damage to nail [POA]
    - [7th] S91.106 Unspecified open wound of unspecified lesser toe(s) without damage to nail [POA]
    - [7th] S91.109 Unspecified open wound of unspecified toe(s) without damage to nail [POA]
  - [6th] S91.11 Laceration without foreign body of toe without damage to nail
    - [7th] S91.111 Laceration without foreign body of right great toe without damage to nail [POA]
    - [7th] S91.112 Laceration without foreign body of left great toe without damage to nail [POA]
    - [7th] S91.113 Laceration without foreign body of unspecified great toe without damage to nail [POA]
    - [7th] S91.114 Laceration without foreign body of right lesser toe(s) without damage to nail [POA]
    - [7th] S91.115 Laceration without foreign body of left lesser toe(s) without damage to nail [POA]
    - [7th] S91.116 Laceration without foreign body of unspecified lesser toe(s) without damage to nail [POA]
    - [7th] S91.119 Laceration without foreign body of unspecified toe without damage to nail [POA]
  - [6th] S91.12 Laceration with foreign body of toe without damage to nail
    - [7th] S91.121 Laceration with foreign body of right great toe without damage to nail [POA]
    - [7th] S91.122 Laceration with foreign body of left great toe without damage to nail [POA]
    - [7th] S91.123 Laceration with foreign body of unspecified great toe without damage to nail [POA]
    - [7th] S91.124 Laceration with foreign body of right lesser toe(s) without damage to nail [POA]
    - [7th] S91.125 Laceration with foreign body of left lesser toe(s) without damage to nail [POA]
    - [7th] S91.126 Laceration with foreign body of unspecified lesser toe(s) without damage to nail [POA]
    - [7th] S91.129 Laceration with foreign body of unspecified toe(s) without damage to nail [POA]
  - [6th] S91.13 Puncture wound without foreign body of toe without damage to nail
    - [7th] S91.131 Puncture wound without foreign body of right great toe without damage to nail [POA]
    - [7th] S91.132 Puncture wound without foreign body of left great toe without damage to nail [POA]
    - [7th] S91.133 Puncture wound without foreign body of unspecified great toe without damage to nail [POA]
    - [7th] S91.134 Puncture wound without foreign body of right lesser toe(s) without damage to nail [POA]
    - [7th] S91.135 Puncture wound without foreign body of left lesser toe(s) without damage to nail [POA]

Unspecified Code | Other Specified Code | Manifestation Code | [N] Newborn | [P] Pediatric | [M] Maternity | [A] Adult | ♂ Male | ♀ Female
● New Code | ▲ Revised Code Title | ►◄ Revised Text | [NOTES] | [INCLUDES] | [EXCLUDES1] Not coded here | [EXCLUDES2] Not included here
[4th] 4th character required | [5th] 5th character required | [6th] 6th character required | [7th] 7th character required | [X] Extension 'X' Alert
[HAC] Hospital-acquired condition (HAC) alert | AHA AHA Coding Clinic© | ☞ Code first alert

When symbols appear on a code that requires a 7th character extension, refer to Appendix B to identify applicable 7th character codes.

7️⃣ **S91.136** Puncture wound without foreign body of unspecified lesser toe(s) without damage to nail POA

7️⃣ **S91.139** Puncture wound without foreign body of unspecified toe(s) without damage to nail POA

6️⃣ **S91.14** Puncture wound with foreign body of toe without damage to nail

7️⃣ **S91.141** Puncture wound with foreign body of right great toe without damage to nail POA

7️⃣ **S91.142** Puncture wound with foreign body of left great toe without damage to nail POA

7️⃣ **S91.143** Puncture wound with foreign body of unspecified great toe without damage to nail POA

7️⃣ **S91.144** Puncture wound with foreign body of right lesser toe(s) without damage to nail POA

7️⃣ **S91.145** Puncture wound with foreign body of left lesser toe(s) without damage to nail POA

7️⃣ **S91.146** Puncture wound with foreign body of unspecified lesser toe(s) without damage to nail POA

7️⃣ **S91.149** Puncture wound with foreign body of unspecified toe(s) without damage to nail POA

6️⃣ **S91.15** Open bite of toe without damage to nail
Bite of toe NOS
EXCLUDES1 superficial bite of toe (S90.46-, S90.47-)

7️⃣ **S91.151** Open bite of right great toe without damage to nail POA

7️⃣ **S91.152** Open bite of left great toe without damage to nail POA

7️⃣ **S91.153** Open bite of unspecified great toe without damage to nail POA

7️⃣ **S91.154** Open bite of right lesser toe(s) without damage to nail POA

7️⃣ **S91.155** Open bite of left lesser toe(s) without damage to nail POA

7️⃣ **S91.156** Open bite of unspecified lesser toe(s) without damage to nail POA

7️⃣ **S91.159** Open bite of unspecified toe(s) without damage to nail POA

5️⃣ **S91.2** Open wound of toe with damage to nail

6️⃣ **S91.20** Unspecified open wound of toe with damage to nail

7️⃣ **S91.201** Unspecified open wound of right great toe with damage to nail POA

7️⃣ **S91.202** Unspecified open wound of left great toe with damage to nail POA

7️⃣ **S91.203** Unspecified open wound of unspecified great toe with damage to nail POA

7️⃣ **S91.204** Unspecified open wound of right lesser toe(s) with damage to nail POA

7️⃣ **S91.205** Unspecified open wound of left lesser toe(s) with damage to nail POA

7️⃣ **S91.206** Unspecified open wound of unspecified lesser toe(s) with damage to nail POA

7️⃣ **S91.209** Unspecified open wound of unspecified toe(s) with damage to nail POA

6️⃣ **S91.21** Laceration without foreign body of toe with damage to nail

7️⃣ **S91.211** Laceration without foreign body of right great toe with damage to nail POA

7️⃣ **S91.212** Laceration without foreign body of left great toe with damage to nail POA

7️⃣ **S91.213** Laceration without foreign body of unspecified great toe with damage to nail POA

7️⃣ **S91.214** Laceration without foreign body of right lesser toe(s) with damage to nail POA

7️⃣ **S91.215** Laceration without foreign body of left lesser toe(s) with damage to nail POA

7️⃣ **S91.216** Laceration without foreign body of unspecified lesser toe(s) with damage to nail POA

7️⃣ **S91.219** Laceration without foreign body of unspecified toe(s) with damage to nail POA

6️⃣ **S91.22** Laceration with foreign body of toe with damage to nail

7️⃣ **S91.221** Laceration with foreign body of right great toe with damage to nail POA

7️⃣ **S91.222** Laceration with foreign body of left great toe with damage to nail POA

7️⃣ **S91.223** Laceration with foreign body of unspecified great toe with damage to nail POA

7️⃣ **S91.224** Laceration with foreign body of right lesser toe(s) with damage to nail POA

7️⃣ **S91.225** Laceration with foreign body of left lesser toe(s) with damage to nail POA

7️⃣ **S91.226** Laceration with foreign body of unspecified lesser toe(s) with damage to nail POA

7️⃣ **S91.229** Laceration with foreign body of unspecified toe(s) with damage to nail POA

6️⃣ **S91.23** Puncture wound without foreign body of toe with damage to nail

7️⃣ **S91.231** Puncture wound without foreign body of right great toe with damage to nail POA

7️⃣ **S91.232** Puncture wound without foreign body of left great toe with damage to nail POA

7️⃣ **S91.233** Puncture wound without foreign body of unspecified great toe with damage to nail POA

7️⃣ **S91.234** Puncture wound without foreign body of right lesser toe(s) with damage to nail POA

7️⃣ **S91.235** Puncture wound without foreign body of left lesser toe(s) with damage to nail POA

7️⃣ **S91.236** Puncture wound without foreign body of unspecified lesser toe(s) with damage to nail POA

7️⃣ **S91.239** Puncture wound without foreign body of unspecified toe(s) with damage to nail POA

6️⃣ **S91.24** Puncture wound with foreign body of toe with damage to nail

7️⃣ **S91.241** Puncture wound with foreign body of right great toe with damage to nail POA

7️⃣ **S91.242** Puncture wound with foreign body of left great toe with damage to nail POA

7️⃣ **S91.243** Puncture wound with foreign body of unspecified great toe with damage to nail POA

7️⃣ **S91.244** Puncture wound with foreign body of right lesser toe(s) with damage to nail POA

7️⃣ **S91.245** Puncture wound with foreign body of left lesser toe(s) with damage to nail POA

7️⃣ **S91.246** Puncture wound with foreign body of unspecified lesser toe(s) with damage to nail POA

7️⃣ **S91.249** Puncture wound with foreign body of unspecified toe(s) with damage to nail POA

6️⃣ **S91.25** Open bite of toe with damage to nail
Bite of toe with damage to nail NOS
EXCLUDES1 superficial bite of toe (S90.46-, S90.47-)

7️⃣ **S91.251** Open bite of right great toe with damage to nail POA

7️⃣ **S91.252** Open bite of left great toe with damage to nail POA

7️⃣ **S91.253** Open bite of unspecified great toe with damage to nail POA

7️⃣ **S91.254** Open bite of right lesser toe(s) with damage to nail POA

7️⃣ **S91.255** Open bite of left lesser toe(s) with damage to nail POA

7️⃣ S91.256 **Open bite** of unspecified lesser toe(s) with **damage to nail** POA

7️⃣ S91.259 **Open bite** of unspecified toe(s) with **damage to nail** POA

5️⃣ S91.3 Open wound of foot

  6️⃣ S91.30 Unspecified open wound of foot

    7️⃣ S91.301 **Unspecified open wound**, right **foot** POA

    7️⃣ S91.302 **Unspecified open wound**, left **foot** POA

    7️⃣ S91.309 **Unspecified open wound, unspecified foot** POA

  6️⃣ S91.31 Laceration without foreign body of foot

    7️⃣ S91.311 **Laceration without foreign body,** right **foot** POA

    7️⃣ S91.312 **Laceration without foreign body,** left **foot** POA

    7️⃣ S91.319 **Laceration without foreign body, unspecified foot** POA

  6️⃣ S91.32 Laceration with foreign body of foot

    7️⃣ S91.321 **Laceration with foreign body,** right **foot** POA

    7️⃣ S91.322 **Laceration with foreign body,** left **foot** POA

    7️⃣ S91.329 **Laceration with foreign body, unspecified foot** POA

  6️⃣ S91.33 Puncture wound without foreign body of foot

    7️⃣ S91.331 **Puncture wound without foreign body,** right **foot** POA

    7️⃣ S91.332 **Puncture wound without foreign body,** left **foot** POA

    7️⃣ S91.339 **Puncture wound without foreign body, unspecified foot** POA

  6️⃣ S91.34 Puncture wound with foreign body of foot

    7️⃣ S91.341 **Puncture wound with foreign body,** right **foot** POA

    7️⃣ S91.342 **Puncture wound with foreign body,** left **foot** POA

    7️⃣ S91.349 **Puncture wound with foreign body, unspecified foot** POA

  6️⃣ S91.35 Open bite of foot

    EXCLUDES1 superficial bite of foot (S90.86-, S90.87-)

    7️⃣ S91.351 **Open bite,** right **foot** POA

    7️⃣ S91.352 **Open bite,** left **foot** POA

    7️⃣ S91.359 **Open bite, unspecified foot** POA

4️⃣ S92 Fracture of foot and toe, **except ankle**

  👁 See Official Guidelines "Coding of Traumatic Fractures" I.C.19.c

  NOTES A fracture not indicated as displaced or nondisplaced should be coded to displaced.

    A fracture not indicated as open or closed should be coded to closed.

  EXCLUDES1 traumatic amputation of ankle and foot (S98.-)

  EXCLUDES2 fracture of ankle (S82.-)

    fracture of malleolus (S82.-)

The appropriate 7th character is to be added to each code from category S92

  A = initial encounter for closed fracture

  B = initial encounter for open fracture

  D = subsequent encounter for fracture with routine healing

  G = subsequent encounter for fracture with delayed healing

  K = subsequent encounter for fracture with nonunion

  P = subsequent encounter for fracture with malunion

  S = sequela

5️⃣ S92.0 **Fracture of** calcaneus

  Heel bone

  Os calcis

  EXCLUDES2 Physeal fracture of calcaneus (S99.0-)

  6️⃣ S92.00 Unspecified fracture of calcaneus

    7️⃣ S92.001 **Unspecified fracture of** right **calcaneus** ✔ POA HAC CC/MCC Exc

    7️⃣ S92.002 **Unspecified fracture of** left **calcaneus** ✔ POA HAC CC/MCC Exc

    7️⃣ S92.009 **Unspecified fracture of unspecified calcaneus** ✔ POA HAC CC/MCC Exc

6️⃣ S92.01 **Fracture of** body of calcaneus

  7️⃣ S92.011 Displaced **fracture of body of** right **calcaneus** ✔ POA HAC CC/MCC Exc

  7️⃣ S92.012 Displaced **fracture of body of** left **calcaneus** ✔ POA HAC CC/MCC Exc

  7️⃣ S92.013 Displaced **fracture of body of unspecified calcaneus** ✔ POA HAC CC/MCC Exc

  7️⃣ S92.014 Nondisplaced **fracture of body of** right **calcaneus** ✔ POA HAC CC/MCC Exc

  7️⃣ S92.015 Nondisplaced **fracture of body of** left **calcaneus** ✔ POA HAC CC/MCC Exc

  7️⃣ S92.016 Nondisplaced **fracture of body of unspecified calcaneus** ✔ POA HAC CC/MCC Exc

6️⃣ S92.02 **Fracture of** anterior process of calcaneus

  7️⃣ S92.021 Displaced **fracture of anterior process of** right **calcaneus** ✔ POA HAC CC/MCC Exc

  7️⃣ S92.022 Displaced **fracture of anterior process of** left **calcaneus** ✔ POA HAC CC/MCC Exc

  7️⃣ S92.023 Displaced **fracture of anterior process of unspecified calcaneus** ✔ POA HAC CC/MCC Exc

  7️⃣ S92.024 Nondisplaced **fracture of anterior process of** right **calcaneus** ✔ POA HAC CC/MCC Exc

  7️⃣ S92.025 Nondisplaced **fracture of anterior process of** left **calcaneus** ✔ POA HAC CC/MCC Exc

  7️⃣ S92.026 Nondisplaced **fracture of anterior process of unspecified calcaneus** ✔ POA HAC CC/MCC Exc

6️⃣ S92.03 Avulsion **fracture of** tuberosity of calcaneus

  7️⃣ S92.031 Displaced **avulsion fracture of tuberosity of** right **calcaneus** ✔ POA HAC CC/MCC Exc

  7️⃣ S92.032 Displaced **avulsion fracture of tuberosity of** left **calcaneus** ✔ POA HAC CC/MCC Exc

  7️⃣ S92.033 Displaced **avulsion fracture of tuberosity of unspecified calcaneus** ✔ POA HAC CC/MCC Exc

  7️⃣ S92.034 Nondisplaced **avulsion fracture of tuberosity of** right **calcaneus** ✔ POA HAC CC/MCC Exc

  7️⃣ S92.035 Nondisplaced **avulsion fracture of tuberosity of** left **calcaneus** ✔ POA HAC CC/MCC Exc

  7️⃣ S92.036 Nondisplaced **avulsion fracture of tuberosity of unspecified calcaneus** ✔ POA HAC CC/MCC Exc

6️⃣ S92.04 Other **fracture of** tuberosity of calcaneus

  7️⃣ S92.041 Displaced **other fracture of tuberosity of** right **calcaneus** ✔ POA HAC CC/MCC Exc

  7️⃣ S92.042 Displaced **other fracture of tuberosity of** left **calcaneus** ✔ POA HAC CC/MCC Exc

  7️⃣ S92.043 Displaced **other fracture of tuberosity of unspecified calcaneus** ✔ POA HAC CC/MCC Exc

  7️⃣ S92.044 Nondisplaced **other fracture of tuberosity of** right **calcaneus** ✔ POA HAC CC/MCC Exc

  7️⃣ S92.045 Nondisplaced **other fracture of tuberosity of** left **calcaneus** ✔ POA HAC CC/MCC Exc

  7️⃣ S92.046 Nondisplaced **other fracture of tuberosity of unspecified calcaneus** ✔ POA HAC CC/MCC Exc

6️⃣ S92.05 Other extraarticular **fracture of** calcaneus

  7️⃣ S92.051 Displaced **other extraarticular fracture of** right **calcaneus** ✔ POA HAC CC/MCC Exc

  7️⃣ S92.052 Displaced **other extraarticular fracture of** left **calcaneus** ✔ POA HAC CC/MCC Exc

  7️⃣ S92.053 Displaced **other extraarticular fracture of unspecified calcaneus** ✔ POA HAC CC/MCC Exc

  7️⃣ S92.054 Nondisplaced **other extraarticular fracture of** right **calcaneus** ✔ POA HAC CC/MCC Exc

  7️⃣ S92.055 Nondisplaced **other extraarticular fracture of** left **calcaneus** ✔ POA HAC CC/MCC Exc

  7️⃣ S92.056 Nondisplaced **other extraarticular fracture of unspecified calcaneus** ✔ POA HAC CC/MCC Exc

6️⃣ S92.06 Intraarticular **fracture of** calcaneus

  7️⃣ S92.061 Displaced **intraarticular fracture of** right **calcaneus** ✔ POA HAC CC/MCC Exc

  7️⃣ S92.062 Displaced **intraarticular fracture of** left **calcaneus** ✔ POA HAC CC/MCC Exc

---

Unspecified Code   Other Specified Code   Manifestation Code   N Newborn   P Pediatric   M Maternity   A Adult   ♂ Male   ♀ Female

● New Code   ▲ Revised Code Title   ▶◀ Revised Text   **NOTES**   *INCLUDES*   *EXCLUDES1* Not coded here   *EXCLUDES2* Not included here

4️⃣ 4th character required   5️⃣ 5th character required   6️⃣ 6th character required   7️⃣ 7th character required   Extension 'X' Alert

HAC Hospital-acquired condition (HAC) alert   **AHA** AHA Coding Clinic®   📖 Code first alert

7ᵗʰ S92.063 Displaced **intraarticular fracture of unspecified calcaneus** cc᷉ poÅ HAC CC/MCC Exc

7ᵗʰ S92.064 Nondisplaced **intraarticular fracture of right calcaneus** cc᷉ poÅ HAC CC/MCC Exc

7ᵗʰ S92.065 Nondisplaced **intraarticular fracture of left calcaneus** cc᷉ poÅ HAC CC/MCC Exc

7ᵗʰ S92.066 Nondisplaced **intraarticular fracture of unspecified calcaneus** cc᷉ poÅ HAC CC/MCC Exc

5ᵗʰ S92.1 Fracture of talus
Astragalus

6ᵗʰ S92.10 Unspecified fracture of talus

7ᵗʰ S92.101 **Unspecified fracture of right talus** cc᷉ poÅ HAC CC/MCC Exc

7ᵗʰ S92.102 **Unspecified fracture of left talus** cc᷉ poÅ HAC CC/MCC Exc

7ᵗʰ S92.109 **Unspecified fracture of unspecified talus** cc᷉ poÅ HAC CC/MCC Exc

6ᵗʰ S92.11 Fracture of neck of talus

7ᵗʰ S92.111 Displaced **fracture of neck of right talus** cc᷉ poÅ HAC CC/MCC Exc

7ᵗʰ S92.112 Displaced **fracture of neck of left talus** cc᷉ poÅ HAC CC/MCC Exc

7ᵗʰ S92.113 Displaced **fracture of neck of unspecified talus** cc᷉ poÅ HAC CC/MCC Exc

7ᵗʰ S92.114 Nondisplaced **fracture of neck of right talus** cc᷉ poÅ HAC CC/MCC Exc

7ᵗʰ S92.115 Nondisplaced **fracture of neck of left talus** cc᷉ poÅ HAC CC/MCC Exc

7ᵗʰ S92.116 Nondisplaced **fracture of neck of unspecified talus** cc᷉ poÅ HAC CC/MCC Exc

6ᵗʰ S92.12 Fracture of body of talus

7ᵗʰ S92.121 Displaced **fracture of body of right talus** cc᷉ poÅ HAC CC/MCC Exc

7ᵗʰ S92.122 Displaced **fracture of body of left talus** cc᷉ poÅ HAC CC/MCC Exc

7ᵗʰ S92.123 Displaced **fracture of body of unspecified talus** cc᷉ poÅ HAC CC/MCC Exc

7ᵗʰ S92.124 Nondisplaced **fracture of body of right talus** cc᷉ poÅ HAC CC/MCC Exc

7ᵗʰ S92.125 Nondisplaced **fracture of body of left talus** cc᷉ poÅ HAC CC/MCC Exc

7ᵗʰ S92.126 Nondisplaced **fracture of body of unspecified talus** cc᷉ poÅ HAC CC/MCC Exc

6ᵗʰ S92.13 Fracture of posterior process of talus

7ᵗʰ S92.131 Displaced **fracture of posterior process of right talus** cc᷉ poÅ HAC CC/MCC Exc

7ᵗʰ S92.132 Displaced **fracture of posterior process of left talus** cc᷉ poÅ HAC CC/MCC Exc

7ᵗʰ S92.133 Displaced **fracture of posterior process of unspecified talus** cc᷉ poÅ HAC CC/MCC Exc

7ᵗʰ S92.134 Nondisplaced **fracture of posterior process of right talus** cc᷉ poÅ HAC CC/MCC Exc

7ᵗʰ S92.135 Nondisplaced **fracture of posterior process of left talus** cc᷉ poÅ HAC CC/MCC Exc

7ᵗʰ S92.136 Nondisplaced **fracture of posterior process of unspecified talus** cc᷉ poÅ HAC CC/MCC Exc

6ᵗʰ S92.14 Dome fracture of talus

EXCLUDES1 *osteochondritis dissecans (M93.2)*

7ᵗʰ S92.141 Displaced **dome fracture of right talus** cc᷉ poÅ HAC CC/MCC Exc

7ᵗʰ S92.142 Displaced **dome fracture of left talus** cc᷉ poÅ HAC CC/MCC Exc

7ᵗʰ S92.143 Displaced **dome fracture of unspecified talus** cc᷉ poÅ HAC CC/MCC Exc

7ᵗʰ S92.144 Nondisplaced **dome fracture of right talus** cc᷉ poÅ HAC CC/MCC Exc

7ᵗʰ S92.145 Nondisplaced **dome fracture of left talus** cc᷉ poÅ HAC CC/MCC Exc

7ᵗʰ S92.146 Nondisplaced **dome fracture of unspecified talus** cc᷉ poÅ HAC CC/MCC Exc

6ᵗʰ S92.15 Avulsion fracture (chip fracture) of talus

7ᵗʰ S92.151 Displaced **avulsion fracture (chip fracture) of right talus** cc᷉ poÅ HAC CC/MCC Exc

7ᵗʰ S92.152 Displaced **avulsion fracture (chip fracture) of left talus** cc᷉ poÅ HAC CC/MCC Exc

7ᵗʰ S92.153 Displaced **avulsion fracture (chip fracture) of unspecified talus** cc᷉ poÅ HAC CC/MCC Exc

7ᵗʰ S92.154 Nondisplaced **avulsion fracture (chip fracture) of right talus** cc᷉ poÅ HAC CC/MCC Exc

7ᵗʰ S92.155 Nondisplaced **avulsion fracture (chip fracture) of left talus** cc᷉ poÅ HAC CC/MCC Exc

7ᵗʰ S92.156 Nondisplaced **avulsion fracture (chip fracture) of unspecified talus** cc᷉ poÅ HAC CC/MCC Exc

6ᵗʰ S92.19 Other fracture of talus

7ᵗʰ S92.191 Other fracture of right talus cc᷉ poÅ HAC CC/MCC Exc

7ᵗʰ S92.192 Other fracture of left talus cc᷉ poÅ HAC CC/MCC Exc

7ᵗʰ S92.199 **Other fracture of unspecified talus** cc᷉ poÅ HAC CC/MCC Exc

5ᵗʰ S92.2 Fracture of other and unspecified tarsal bone(s)

6ᵗʰ S92.20 Fracture of unspecified tarsal bone(s)

7ᵗʰ S92.201 **Fracture of unspecified tarsal bone(s) of right foot** cc᷉ poÅ HAC CC/MCC Exc

7ᵗʰ S92.202 **Fracture of unspecified tarsal bone(s) of left foot** cc᷉ poÅ HAC CC/MCC Exc

7ᵗʰ S92.209 **Fracture of unspecified tarsal bone(s) of unspecified foot** cc᷉ poÅ HAC CC/MCC Exc

6ᵗʰ S92.21 Fracture of cuboid bone

7ᵗʰ S92.211 Displaced **fracture of cuboid bone of right foot** cc᷉ poÅ HAC CC/MCC Exc

7ᵗʰ S92.212 Displaced **fracture of cuboid bone of left foot** cc᷉ poÅ HAC CC/MCC Exc

7ᵗʰ S92.213 Displaced **fracture of cuboid bone of unspecified foot** cc᷉ poÅ HAC CC/MCC Exc

7ᵗʰ S92.214 Nondisplaced **fracture of cuboid bone of right foot** cc᷉ poÅ HAC CC/MCC Exc

7ᵗʰ S92.215 Nondisplaced **fracture of cuboid bone of left foot** cc᷉ poÅ HAC CC/MCC Exc

7ᵗʰ S92.216 Nondisplaced **fracture of cuboid bone of unspecified foot** cc᷉ poÅ HAC CC/MCC Exc

6ᵗʰ S92.22 Fracture of lateral cuneiform

7ᵗʰ S92.221 Displaced **fracture of lateral cuneiform of right foot** cc᷉ poÅ HAC CC/MCC Exc

7ᵗʰ S92.222 Displaced **fracture of lateral cuneiform of left foot** cc᷉ poÅ HAC CC/MCC Exc

7ᵗʰ S92.223 Displaced **fracture of lateral cuneiform of unspecified foot** cc᷉ poÅ HAC CC/MCC Exc

7ᵗʰ S92.224 Nondisplaced **fracture of lateral cuneiform of right foot** cc᷉ poÅ HAC CC/MCC Exc

7ᵗʰ S92.225 Nondisplaced **fracture of lateral cuneiform of left foot** cc᷉ poÅ HAC CC/MCC Exc

7ᵗʰ S92.226 Nondisplaced **fracture of lateral cuneiform of unspecified foot** cc᷉ poÅ HAC CC/MCC Exc

6ᵗʰ S92.23 Fracture of intermediate cuneiform

7ᵗʰ S92.231 Displaced **fracture of intermediate cuneiform of right foot** cc᷉ poÅ HAC CC/MCC Exc

7ᵗʰ S92.232 Displaced **fracture of intermediate cuneiform of left foot** cc᷉ poÅ HAC CC/MCC Exc

7ᵗʰ S92.233 Displaced **fracture of intermediate cuneiform of unspecified foot** cc᷉ poÅ HAC CC/MCC Exc

7ᵗʰ S92.234 Nondisplaced **fracture of intermediate cuneiform of right foot** cc᷉ poÅ HAC CC/MCC Exc

7ᵗʰ S92.235 Nondisplaced **fracture of intermediate cuneiform of left foot** cc᷉ poÅ HAC CC/MCC Exc

7ᵗʰ S92.236 Nondisplaced **fracture of intermediate cuneiform of unspecified foot** cc᷉ poÅ HAC CC/MCC Exc

6ᵗʰ S92.24 Fracture of medial cuneiform

7ᵗʰ S92.241 Displaced **fracture of medial cuneiform of right foot** cc᷉ poÅ HAC CC/MCC Exc

7ᵗʰ S92.242 Displaced **fracture of medial cuneiform of left foot** cc᷉ poÅ HAC CC/MCC Exc

---

poÅ-blk Unacceptable principal diagnosis symbol per Medicare code edits   poÅ Code exempt from diagnosis present on admission requirement
❓ Questionable admission   cc᷉ Complication or comorbidity   mcc Major complication or comorbidity   cc/mcc Exc CC/MCC exclusion
HCC HCC diagnosis code   RxHCC RxHCC diagnosis code   MACRA code   **DEFINITION** Describes condition/terminology
TIP Coding guidance   👁 Official Guideline Reference   Z1 Z code as first-listed diagnosis

1090   When symbols appear on a code that requires a 7th character extension, refer to Appendix B to identify applicable 7th character codes.   **2020 ICD-10-CM**

7️⃣ S92.243 Displaced **fracture of medial cuneiform of unspecified foot** CC POA HAC CC/MCC Exc

7️⃣ S92.244 Nondisplaced **fracture of medial cuneiform of** right **foot** CC POA HAC CC/MCC Exc

7️⃣ S92.245 Nondisplaced **fracture of medial cuneiform of** left **foot** CC POA HAC CC/MCC Exc

7️⃣ S92.246 Nondisplaced **fracture of medial cuneiform of unspecified foot** CC POA HAC CC/MCC Exc

6️⃣ S92.25 Fracture of navicular [scaphoid] of foot

7️⃣ S92.251 Displaced **fracture of navicular [scaphoid] of** right **foot** CC POA HAC CC/MCC Exc

7️⃣ S92.252 Displaced **fracture of navicular [scaphoid] of** left **foot** CC POA HAC CC/MCC Exc

7️⃣ S92.253 Displaced **fracture of navicular [scaphoid] of unspecified foot** CC POA HAC CC/MCC Exc

7️⃣ S92.254 Nondisplaced **fracture of navicular [scaphoid] of** right **foot** CC POA HAC CC/MCC Exc

7️⃣ S92.255 Nondisplaced **fracture of navicular [scaphoid] of** left **foot** CC POA HAC CC/MCC Exc

7️⃣ S92.256 Nondisplaced **fracture of navicular [scaphoid] of unspecified foot** CC POA HAC CC/MCC Exc

5️⃣ S92.3 Fracture of metatarsal bone(s)

EXCLUDES2 *Physeal fracture of metatarsal (S99.1-)*

6️⃣ S92.30 Fracture of unspecified metatarsal bone(s)

7️⃣ S92.301 **Fracture of unspecified metatarsal bone(s),** right **foot** CC POA HAC CC/MCC Exc

7️⃣ S92.302 **Fracture of unspecified metatarsal bone(s),** left **foot** CC POA HAC CC/MCC Exc

7️⃣ S92.309 **Fracture of unspecified metatarsal bone(s), unspecified foot** CC POA HAC CC/MCC Exc

6️⃣ S92.31 Fracture of first metatarsal bone

7️⃣ S92.311 Displaced **fracture of first metatarsal bone,** right **foot** CC POA HAC CC/MCC Exc

7️⃣ S92.312 Displaced **fracture of first metatarsal bone,** left **foot** CC POA HAC CC/MCC Exc

7️⃣ S92.313 Displaced **fracture of first metatarsal bone, unspecified foot** CC POA HAC CC/MCC Exc

7️⃣ S92.314 Nondisplaced **fracture of first metatarsal bone,** right **foot** CC POA HAC CC/MCC Exc

7️⃣ S92.315 Nondisplaced **fracture of first metatarsal bone,** left **foot** CC POA HAC CC/MCC Exc

7️⃣ S92.316 Nondisplaced **fracture of first metatarsal bone, unspecified foot** CC POA HAC CC/MCC Exc

6️⃣ S92.32 Fracture of second metatarsal bone

7️⃣ S92.321 Displaced **fracture of second metatarsal bone,** right **foot** CC POA HAC CC/MCC Exc

7️⃣ S92.322 Displaced **fracture of second metatarsal bone,** left **foot** CC POA HAC CC/MCC Exc

7️⃣ S92.323 Displaced **fracture of second metatarsal bone, unspecified foot** CC POA HAC CC/MCC Exc

7️⃣ S92.324 Nondisplaced **fracture of second metatarsal bone,** right **foot** CC POA HAC CC/MCC Exc

7️⃣ S92.325 Nondisplaced **fracture of second metatarsal bone,** left **foot** CC POA HAC CC/MCC Exc

7️⃣ S92.326 Nondisplaced **fracture of second metatarsal bone, unspecified foot** CC POA HAC CC/MCC Exc

6️⃣ S92.33 Fracture of third metatarsal bone

7️⃣ S92.331 Displaced **fracture of third metatarsal bone,** right **foot** CC POA HAC CC/MCC Exc

AHA: Q1 2018

7️⃣ S92.332 Displaced **fracture of third metatarsal bone,** left **foot** CC POA HAC CC/MCC Exc

AHA: Q1 2018

7️⃣ S92.333 Displaced **fracture of third metatarsal bone, unspecified foot** CC POA HAC CC/MCC Exc

AHA: Q1 2018

7️⃣ S92.334 Nondisplaced **fracture of third metatarsal bone,** right **foot** CC POA HAC CC/MCC Exc

AHA: Q1 2018

7️⃣ S92.335 Nondisplaced **fracture of third metatarsal bone,** left **foot** CC POA HAC CC/MCC Exc

AHA: Q1 2018

7️⃣ S92.336 Nondisplaced **fracture of third metatarsal bone, unspecified foot** CC POA HAC CC/MCC Exc

AHA: Q1 2018

6️⃣ S92.34 Fracture of fourth metatarsal bone

7️⃣ S92.341 Displaced **fracture of fourth metatarsal bone,** right **foot** CC POA HAC CC/MCC Exc

7️⃣ S92.342 Displaced **fracture of fourth metatarsal bone,** left **foot** CC POA HAC CC/MCC Exc

7️⃣ S92.343 Displaced **fracture of fourth metatarsal bone, unspecified foot** CC POA HAC CC/MCC Exc

7️⃣ S92.344 Nondisplaced **fracture of fourth metatarsal bone,** right **foot** CC POA HAC CC/MCC Exc

7️⃣ S92.345 Nondisplaced **fracture of fourth metatarsal bone,** left **foot** CC POA HAC CC/MCC Exc

7️⃣ S92.346 Nondisplaced **fracture of fourth metatarsal bone, unspecified foot** CC POA HAC CC/MCC Exc

6️⃣ S92.35 Fracture of fifth metatarsal bone

7️⃣ S92.351 Displaced **fracture of fifth metatarsal bone,** right **foot** CC POA HAC CC/MCC Exc

7️⃣ S92.352 Displaced **fracture of fifth metatarsal bone,** left **foot** CC POA HAC CC/MCC Exc

7️⃣ S92.353 Displaced **fracture of fifth metatarsal bone, unspecified foot** CC POA HAC CC/MCC Exc

7️⃣ S92.354 Nondisplaced **fracture of fifth metatarsal bone,** right **foot** CC POA HAC CC/MCC Exc

7️⃣ S92.355 Nondisplaced **fracture of fifth metatarsal bone,** left **foot** CC POA HAC CC/MCC Exc

7️⃣ S92.356 Nondisplaced **fracture of fifth metatarsal bone, unspecified foot** CC POA HAC CC/MCC Exc

5️⃣ S92.4 Fracture of great toe

EXCLUDES2 *Physeal fracture of phalanx of toe (S99.2-)*

6️⃣ S92.40 Unspecified **fracture of great toe**

7️⃣ S92.401 Displaced **unspecified fracture of** right **great toe** CC POA CC/MCC Exc

7️⃣ S92.402 Displaced **unspecified fracture of** left **great toe** CC POA CC/MCC Exc

7️⃣ S92.403 Displaced **unspecified fracture of unspecified great toe** CC POA CC/MCC Exc

7️⃣ S92.404 Nondisplaced **unspecified fracture of** right **great toe** CC POA CC/MCC Exc

7️⃣ S92.405 Nondisplaced **unspecified fracture of** left **great toe** CC POA CC/MCC Exc

7️⃣ S92.406 Nondisplaced **unspecified fracture of unspecified great toe** CC POA CC/MCC Exc

6️⃣ S92.41 Fracture of proximal phalanx of great toe

7️⃣ S92.411 Displaced **fracture of proximal phalanx of** right **great toe** CC POA CC/MCC Exc

7️⃣ S92.412 Displaced **fracture of proximal phalanx of** left **great toe** CC POA CC/MCC Exc

7️⃣ S92.413 Displaced **fracture of proximal phalanx of unspecified great toe** CC POA CC/MCC Exc

7️⃣ S92.414 Nondisplaced **fracture of proximal phalanx of** right **great toe** CC POA CC/MCC Exc

7️⃣ S92.415 Nondisplaced **fracture of proximal phalanx of** left **great toe** CC POA CC/MCC Exc

7️⃣ S92.416 Nondisplaced **fracture of proximal phalanx of unspecified great toe** CC POA CC/MCC Exc

6️⃣ S92.42 Fracture of distal phalanx of great toe

7️⃣ S92.421 Displaced **fracture of distal phalanx of** right **great toe** CC POA CC/MCC Exc

7️⃣ S92.422 Displaced **fracture of distal phalanx of** left **great toe** CC POA CC/MCC Exc

7️⃣ S92.423 Displaced **fracture of distal phalanx of unspecified great toe** CC POA CC/MCC Exc

7️⃣ S92.424 Nondisplaced **fracture of distal phalanx of** right **great toe** CC POA CC/MCC Exc

7️⃣ S92.425 Nondisplaced **fracture of distal phalanx of** left **great toe** CC POA CC/MCC Exc

7️⃣ S92.426 Nondisplaced **fracture of distal phalanx of unspecified great toe** CC POA CC/MCC Exc

---

Unspecified Code   Other Specified Code   Manifestation Code   🅽 Newborn   🅿 Pediatric   🅼 Maternity   🅰 Adult   ♂ Male   ♀ Female
● New Code   ▲ Revised Code Title   ▶◀ Revised Text   **NOTES**   *INCLUDES*   *EXCLUDES1* Not coded here   *EXCLUDES2* Not included here
4️⃣ 4th character required   5️⃣ 5th character required   6️⃣ 6th character required   7️⃣ 7th character required   Extension 'X' Alert
HAC Hospital-acquired condition (HAC) alert   **AHA** AHA Coding Clinic©   ☛ Code first alert

- 6ᵗʰ **S92.49** Other fracture of great toe
  - 7ᵗʰ **S92.491** Other fracture of right great toe CC POA CC/MCC Exc
  - 7ᵗʰ **S92.492** Other fracture of left great toe CC POA CC/MCC Exc
  - 7ᵗʰ **S92.499** Other fracture of unspecified great toe CC POA CC/MCC Exc
- 5ᵗʰ **S92.5** Fracture of lesser toe(s)
  - EXCLUDES2 *Physeal fracture of phalanx of toe (S99.2-)*
  - 6ᵗʰ **S92.50** Unspecified fracture of lesser toe(s)
    - 7ᵗʰ **S92.501** Displaced unspecified fracture of right lesser toe(s) CC POA CC/MCC Exc
    - 7ᵗʰ **S92.502** Displaced unspecified fracture of left lesser toe(s) CC POA CC/MCC Exc
    - 7ᵗʰ **S92.503** Displaced unspecified fracture of unspecified lesser toe(s) CC POA CC/MCC Exc
    - 7ᵗʰ **S92.504** Nondisplaced unspecified fracture of right lesser toe(s) CC POA CC/MCC Exc
    - 7ᵗʰ **S92.505** Nondisplaced unspecified fracture of left lesser toe(s) CC POA CC/MCC Exc
    - 7ᵗʰ **S92.506** Nondisplaced unspecified fracture of unspecified lesser toe(s) CC POA CC/MCC Exc
  - 6ᵗʰ **S92.51** Fracture of proximal phalanx of lesser toe(s)
    - 7ᵗʰ **S92.511** Displaced fracture of proximal phalanx of right lesser toe(s) CC POA CC/MCC Exc
    - 7ᵗʰ **S92.512** Displaced fracture of proximal phalanx of left lesser toe(s) CC POA CC/MCC Exc
    - 7ᵗʰ **S92.513** Displaced fracture of proximal phalanx of unspecified lesser toe(s) CC POA CC/MCC Exc
    - 7ᵗʰ **S92.514** Nondisplaced fracture of proximal phalanx of right lesser toe(s) CC POA CC/MCC Exc
    - 7ᵗʰ **S92.515** Nondisplaced fracture of proximal phalanx of left lesser toe(s) CC POA CC/MCC Exc
    - 7ᵗʰ **S92.516** Nondisplaced fracture of proximal phalanx of unspecified lesser toe(s) CC POA CC/MCC Exc
  - 6ᵗʰ **S92.52** Fracture of middle phalanx of lesser toe(s)
    - 7ᵗʰ **S92.521** Displaced fracture of middle phalanx of right lesser toe(s) CC POA CC/MCC Exc
    - 7ᵗʰ **S92.522** Displaced fracture of middle phalanx of left lesser toe(s) CC POA CC/MCC Exc
    - 7ᵗʰ **S92.523** Displaced fracture of middle phalanx of unspecified lesser toe(s) CC POA CC/MCC Exc
    - 7ᵗʰ **S92.524** Nondisplaced fracture of middle phalanx of right lesser toe(s) CC POA CC/MCC Exc
    - 7ᵗʰ **S92.525** Nondisplaced fracture of middle phalanx of left lesser toe(s) CC POA CC/MCC Exc
    - 7ᵗʰ **S92.526** Nondisplaced fracture of middle phalanx of unspecified lesser toe(s) CC POA CC/MCC Exc
  - 6ᵗʰ **S92.53** Fracture of distal phalanx of lesser toe(s)
    - 7ᵗʰ **S92.531** Displaced fracture of distal phalanx of right lesser toe(s) CC POA CC/MCC Exc
    - 7ᵗʰ **S92.532** Displaced fracture of distal phalanx of left lesser toe(s) CC POA CC/MCC Exc
    - 7ᵗʰ **S92.533** Displaced fracture of distal phalanx of unspecified lesser toe(s) CC POA CC/MCC Exc
    - 7ᵗʰ **S92.534** Nondisplaced fracture of distal phalanx of right lesser toe(s) CC POA CC/MCC Exc
    - 7ᵗʰ **S92.535** Nondisplaced fracture of distal phalanx of left lesser toe(s) CC POA CC/MCC Exc
    - 7ᵗʰ **S92.536** Nondisplaced fracture of distal phalanx of unspecified lesser toe(s) CC POA CC/MCC Exc
  - 6ᵗʰ **S92.59** Other fracture of lesser toe(s)
    - 7ᵗʰ **S92.591** Other fracture of right lesser toe(s) CC POA CC/MCC Exc
    - 7ᵗʰ **S92.592** Other fracture of left lesser toe(s) CC POA CC/MCC Exc
    - 7ᵗʰ **S92.599** Other fracture of unspecified lesser toe(s) CC POA CC/MCC Exc
- 5ᵗʰ **S92.8** Other fracture of foot, except ankle
  - 6ᵗʰ **S92.81** Other fracture of foot
    - Sesamoid fracture of foot
    - 7ᵗʰ **S92.811** Other fracture of right foot CC POA HAC CC/MCC Exc

- 7ᵗʰ **S92.812** Other fracture of left foot CC POA HAC CC/MCC Exc
- 7ᵗʰ **S92.819** Other fracture of unspecified foot CC POA HAC CC/MCC Exc
- 5ᵗʰ **S92.9** Unspecified fracture of foot and toe
  - 6ᵗʰ **S92.90** Unspecified fracture of foot
    - 7ᵗʰ **S92.901** Unspecified fracture of right foot CC POA HAC CC/MCC Exc
    - 7ᵗʰ **S92.902** Unspecified fracture of left foot CC POA HAC CC/MCC Exc
    - 7ᵗʰ **S92.909** Unspecified fracture of unspecified foot CC POA HAC CC/MCC Exc
  - 6ᵗʰ **S92.91** Unspecified fracture of toe
    - 7ᵗʰ **S92.911** Unspecified fracture of right toe(s) CC POA CC/MCC Exc
    - 7ᵗʰ **S92.912** Unspecified fracture of left toe(s) CC POA CC/MCC Exc
    - 7ᵗʰ **S92.919** Unspecified fracture of unspecified toe(s) CC POA CC/MCC Exc

- 4ᵗʰ **S93** Dislocation and sprain of joints and ligaments at ankle, foot and toe level
  - INCLUDES avulsion of joint or ligament of ankle, foot and toe
    - laceration of cartilage, joint or ligament of ankle, foot and toe
    - sprain of cartilage, joint or ligament of ankle, foot and toe
    - traumatic hemarthrosis of joint or ligament of ankle, foot and toe
    - traumatic rupture of joint or ligament of ankle, foot and toe
    - traumatic subluxation of joint or ligament of ankle, foot and toe
    - traumatic tear of joint or ligament of ankle, foot and toe
  - Code also any associated open wound
  - EXCLUDES2 *strain of muscle and tendon of ankle and foot (S96.-)*
  - **The appropriate 7th character is to be added to each code from category S93**
    - **A = initial encounter**
    - **D = subsequent encounter**
    - **S = sequela**
  - 5ᵗʰ **S93.0** Subluxation and dislocation of ankle joint
    - Subluxation and dislocation of astragalus
    - Subluxation and dislocation of fibula, lower end
    - Subluxation and dislocation of talus
    - Subluxation and dislocation of tibia, lower end
    - 7ᵗʰ **S93.01** Subluxation of right ankle joint POA
    - 7ᵗʰ **S93.02** Subluxation of left ankle joint POA
    - 7ᵗʰ **S93.03** Subluxation of unspecified ankle joint POA
    - 7ᵗʰ **S93.04** Dislocation of right ankle joint POA
    - 7ᵗʰ **S93.05** Dislocation of left ankle joint POA
    - 7ᵗʰ **S93.06** Dislocation of unspecified ankle joint POA
  - 5ᵗʰ **S93.1** Subluxation and dislocation of toe
    - 6ᵗʰ **S93.10** Unspecified subluxation and dislocation of toe
      - Dislocation of toe NOS
      - Subluxation of toe NOS
      - 7ᵗʰ **S93.101** Unspecified subluxation of right toe(s) POA
      - 7ᵗʰ **S93.102** Unspecified subluxation of left toe(s) POA
      - 7ᵗʰ **S93.103** Unspecified subluxation of unspecified toe(s) POA
      - 7ᵗʰ **S93.104** Unspecified dislocation of right toe(s) POA
      - 7ᵗʰ **S93.105** Unspecified dislocation of left toe(s) POA
      - 7ᵗʰ **S93.106** Unspecified dislocation of unspecified toe(s) POA
    - 6ᵗʰ **S93.11** Dislocation of interphalangeal joint
      - 7ᵗʰ **S93.111** Dislocation of interphalangeal joint of right great toe POA
      - 7ᵗʰ **S93.112** Dislocation of interphalangeal joint of left great toe POA
      - 7ᵗʰ **S93.113** Dislocation of interphalangeal joint of unspecified great toe POA
      - 7ᵗʰ **S93.114** Dislocation of interphalangeal joint of right lesser toe(s) POA

PDx Unacceptable principal diagnosis symbol per Medicare code edits   POA Code exempt from diagnosis present on admission requirement
? Questionable admission   CC Complication or comorbidity   MCC Major complication or comorbidity   CC/MCC Exc CC/MCC exclusion
HCC HCC diagnosis code   RxHCC RxHCC diagnosis code   MACRA code   **DEFINITION** Describes condition/terminology
TIP Coding guidance   👁 Official Guideline Reference   Z1 Z code as first-listed diagnosis

[7th] S93.115 Dislocation of interphalangeal joint of left lesser toe(s) POA
[7th] S93.116 Dislocation of interphalangeal joint of unspecified lesser toe(s) POA
[7th] S93.119 Dislocation of interphalangeal joint of unspecified toe(s) POA
[6th] S93.12 Dislocation of metatarsophalangeal joint
[7th] S93.121 Dislocation of metatarsophalangeal joint of right great toe POA
[7th] S93.122 Dislocation of metatarsophalangeal joint of left great toe POA
[7th] S93.123 Dislocation of metatarsophalangeal joint of unspecified great toe POA
[7th] S93.124 Dislocation of metatarsophalangeal joint of right lesser toe(s) POA
[7th] S93.125 Dislocation of metatarsophalangeal joint of left lesser toe(s) POA
[7th] S93.126 Dislocation of metatarsophalangeal joint of unspecified lesser toe(s) POA
[7th] S93.129 Dislocation of metatarsophalangeal joint of unspecified toe(s) POA
[6th] S93.13 Subluxation of interphalangeal joint
[7th] S93.131 Subluxation of interphalangeal joint of right great toe POA
[7th] S93.132 Subluxation of interphalangeal joint of left great toe POA
[7th] S93.133 Subluxation of interphalangeal joint of unspecified great toe POA
[7th] S93.134 Subluxation of interphalangeal joint of right lesser toe(s) POA
[7th] S93.135 Subluxation of interphalangeal joint of left lesser toe(s) POA
[7th] S93.136 Subluxation of interphalangeal joint of unspecified lesser toe(s) POA
[7th] S93.139 Subluxation of interphalangeal joint of unspecified toe(s) POA
[6th] S93.14 Subluxation of metatarsophalangeal joint
[7th] S93.141 Subluxation of metatarsophalangeal joint of right great toe POA
[7th] S93.142 Subluxation of metatarsophalangeal joint of left great toe POA
[7th] S93.143 Subluxation of metatarsophalangeal joint of unspecified great toe POA
[7th] S93.144 Subluxation of metatarsophalangeal joint of right lesser toe(s) POA
[7th] S93.145 Subluxation of metatarsophalangeal joint of left lesser toe(s) POA
[7th] S93.146 Subluxation of metatarsophalangeal joint of unspecified lesser toe(s) POA
[7th] S93.149 Subluxation of metatarsophalangeal joint of unspecified toe(s) POA
[5th] S93.3 Subluxation and dislocation of foot
EXCLUDES2 *dislocation of toe (S93.1-)*
[6th] S93.30 Unspecified subluxation and dislocation of foot
Dislocation of foot NOS
Subluxation of foot NOS
[7th] S93.301 Unspecified subluxation of right foot POA
[7th] S93.302 Unspecified subluxation of left foot POA
[7th] S93.303 Unspecified subluxation of unspecified foot POA
[7th] S93.304 Unspecified dislocation of right foot POA
[7th] S93.305 Unspecified dislocation of left foot POA
[7th] S93.306 Unspecified dislocation of unspecified foot POA
[6th] S93.31 Subluxation and dislocation of tarsal joint
[7th] S93.311 Subluxation of tarsal joint of right foot POA
[7th] S93.312 Subluxation of tarsal joint of left foot POA
[7th] S93.313 Subluxation of tarsal joint of unspecified foot POA
[7th] S93.314 Dislocation of tarsal joint of right foot POA
[7th] S93.315 Dislocation of tarsal joint of left foot POA
[7th] S93.316 Dislocation of tarsal joint of unspecified foot POA
[6th] S93.32 Subluxation and dislocation of tarsometatarsal joint
[7th] S93.321 Subluxation of tarsometatarsal joint of right foot POA
[7th] S93.322 Subluxation of tarsometatarsal joint of left foot POA
[7th] S93.323 Subluxation of tarsometatarsal joint of unspecified foot POA
[7th] S93.324 Dislocation of tarsometatarsal joint of right foot POA
[7th] S93.325 Dislocation of tarsometatarsal joint of left foot POA
[7th] S93.326 Dislocation of tarsometatarsal joint of unspecified foot POA
[6th] S93.33 Other subluxation and dislocation of foot
[7th] S93.331 Other subluxation of right foot POA
[7th] S93.332 Other subluxation of left foot POA
[7th] S93.333 Other subluxation of unspecified foot POA
[7th] S93.334 Other dislocation of right foot POA
[7th] S93.335 Other dislocation of left foot POA
[7th] S93.336 Other dislocation of unspecified foot POA
[5th] S93.4 Sprain of ankle
EXCLUDES2 *injury of Achilles tendon (S86.0-)*
[6th] S93.40 Sprain of unspecified ligament of ankle
Sprain of ankle NOS
Sprained ankle NOS
[7th] S93.401 Sprain of unspecified ligament of right ankle POA
[7th] S93.402 Sprain of unspecified ligament of left ankle POA
[7th] S93.409 Sprain of unspecified ligament of unspecified ankle POA
[6th] S93.41 Sprain of calcaneofibular ligament
[7th] S93.411 Sprain of calcaneofibular ligament of right ankle POA
[7th] S93.412 Sprain of calcaneofibular ligament of left ankle POA
[7th] S93.419 Sprain of calcaneofibular ligament of unspecified ankle POA
[6th] S93.42 Sprain of deltoid ligament
[7th] S93.421 Sprain of deltoid ligament of right ankle POA
[7th] S93.422 Sprain of deltoid ligament of left ankle POA
[7th] S93.429 Sprain of deltoid ligament of unspecified ankle POA
[6th] S93.43 Sprain of tibiofibular ligament
[7th] S93.431 Sprain of tibiofibular ligament of right ankle POA
[7th] S93.432 Sprain of tibiofibular ligament of left ankle POA
[7th] S93.439 Sprain of tibiofibular ligament of unspecified ankle POA
[6th] S93.49 Sprain of other ligament of ankle
Sprain of internal collateral ligament
Sprain of talofibular ligament
[7th] S93.491 Sprain of other ligament of right ankle POA
[7th] S93.492 Sprain of other ligament of left ankle POA
[7th] S93.499 Sprain of other ligament of unspecified ankle POA
[5th] S93.5 Sprain of toe
[6th] S93.50 Unspecified sprain of toe
[7th] S93.501 Unspecified sprain of right great toe POA
[7th] S93.502 Unspecified sprain of left great toe POA
[7th] S93.503 Unspecified sprain of unspecified great toe POA
[7th] S93.504 Unspecified sprain of right lesser toe(s) POA
[7th] S93.505 Unspecified sprain of left lesser toe(s) POA
[7th] S93.506 Unspecified sprain of unspecified lesser toe(s) POA
[7th] S93.509 Unspecified sprain of unspecified toe(s) POA

[6th] S93.51 Sprain of interphalangeal joint of toe
[7th] S93.511 Sprain of interphalangeal joint of right great toe [POA]
[7th] S93.512 Sprain of interphalangeal joint of left great toe [POA]
[7th] S93.513 Sprain of interphalangeal joint of unspecified great toe [POA]
[7th] S93.514 Sprain of interphalangeal joint of right lesser toe(s) [POA]
[7th] S93.515 Sprain of interphalangeal joint of left lesser toe(s) [POA]
[7th] S93.516 Sprain of interphalangeal joint of unspecified lesser toe(s) [POA]
[7th] S93.519 Sprain of interphalangeal joint of unspecified toe(s) [POA]
[6th] S93.52 Sprain of metatarsophalangeal joint of toe
[7th] S93.521 Sprain of metatarsophalangeal joint of right great toe [POA]
[7th] S93.522 Sprain of metatarsophalangeal joint of left great toe [POA]
[7th] S93.523 Sprain of metatarsophalangeal joint of unspecified great toe [POA]
[7th] S93.524 Sprain of metatarsophalangeal joint of right lesser toe(s) [POA]
[7th] S93.525 Sprain of metatarsophalangeal joint of left lesser toe(s) [POA]
[7th] S93.526 Sprain of metatarsophalangeal joint of unspecified lesser toe(s) [POA]
[7th] S93.529 Sprain of metatarsophalangeal joint of unspecified toe(s) [POA]
[5th] S93.6 Sprain of foot
EXCLUDES2 *sprain of metatarsophalangeal joint of toe (S93.52-)*
sprain of toe (S93.5-)
[6th] S93.60 Unspecified sprain of foot
[7th] S93.601 Unspecified sprain of right foot [POA]
[7th] S93.602 Unspecified sprain of left foot [POA]
[7th] S93.609 Unspecified sprain of unspecified foot [POA]
[6th] S93.61 Sprain of tarsal ligament of foot
[7th] S93.611 Sprain of tarsal ligament of right foot [POA]
[7th] S93.612 Sprain of tarsal ligament of left foot [POA]
[7th] S93.619 Sprain of tarsal ligament of unspecified foot [POA]
[6th] S93.62 Sprain of tarsometatarsal ligament of foot
[7th] S93.621 Sprain of tarsometatarsal ligament of right foot [POA]
[7th] S93.622 Sprain of tarsometatarsal ligament of left foot [POA]
[7th] S93.629 Sprain of tarsometatarsal ligament of unspecified foot [POA]
[6th] S93.69 Other sprain of foot
[7th] S93.691 Other sprain of right foot [POA]
[7th] S93.692 Other sprain of left foot [POA]
[7th] S93.699 Other sprain of unspecified foot [POA]
[4th] S94 Injury of nerves at ankle and foot level
Code also any associated open wound (S91.-)
The appropriate 7th character is to be added to each code from category S94
A = initial encounter
D = subsequent encounter
S = sequela
[5th] S94.0 Injury of lateral plantar nerve
[7th] S94.00 Injury of lateral plantar nerve, unspecified leg [POA]
[7th] S94.01 Injury of lateral plantar nerve, right leg [POA]
[7th] S94.02 Injury of lateral plantar nerve, left leg [POA]
[5th] S94.1 Injury of medial plantar nerve
[7th] S94.10 Injury of medial plantar nerve, unspecified leg [POA]
[7th] S94.11 Injury of medial plantar nerve, right leg [POA]
[7th] S94.12 Injury of medial plantar nerve, left leg [POA]
[5th] S94.2 Injury of deep peroneal nerve at ankle and foot level
Injury of terminal, lateral branch of deep peroneal nerve
[7th] S94.20 Injury of deep peroneal nerve at ankle and foot level, unspecified leg [POA]
[7th] S94.21 Injury of deep peroneal nerve at ankle and foot level, right leg [POA]
[7th] S94.22 Injury of deep peroneal nerve at ankle and foot level, left leg [POA]
[5th] S94.3 Injury of cutaneous sensory nerve at ankle and foot level
[7th] S94.30 Injury of cutaneous sensory nerve at ankle and foot level, unspecified leg [POA]
[7th] S94.31 Injury of cutaneous sensory nerve at ankle and foot level, right leg [POA]
[7th] S94.32 Injury of cutaneous sensory nerve at ankle and foot level, left leg [POA]
[5th] S94.8 Injury of other nerves at ankle and foot level
[6th] S94.8X Injury of other nerves at ankle and foot level
[7th] S94.8X1 Injury of other nerves at ankle and foot level, right leg [POA]
[7th] S94.8X2 Injury of other nerves at ankle and foot level, left leg [POA]
[7th] S94.8X9 Injury of other nerves at ankle and foot level, unspecified leg [POA]
[5th] S94.9 Injury of unspecified nerve at ankle and foot level
[7th] S94.90 Injury of unspecified nerve at ankle and foot level, unspecified leg [POA]
[7th] S94.91 Injury of unspecified nerve at ankle and foot level, right leg [POA]
[7th] S94.92 Injury of unspecified nerve at ankle and foot level, left leg [POA]
[4th] S95 Injury of blood vessels at ankle and foot level
Code also any associated open wound (S91.-)
EXCLUDES2 *injury of posterior tibial artery and vein (S85.1-, S85.8-)*
The appropriate 7th character is to be added to each code from category S95
A = initial encounter
D = subsequent encounter
S = sequela
[5th] S95.0 Injury of dorsal artery of foot
[6th] S95.00 Unspecified injury of dorsal artery of foot
[7th] S95.001 Unspecified injury of dorsal artery of right foot [CC] [POA] [CC/MCC Exc]
[7th] S95.002 Unspecified injury of dorsal artery of left foot [CC] [POA] [CC/MCC Exc]
[7th] S95.009 Unspecified injury of dorsal artery of unspecified foot [CC] [POA] [CC/MCC Exc]
[6th] S95.01 Laceration of dorsal artery of foot
[7th] S95.011 Laceration of dorsal artery of right foot [CC] [POA] [CC/MCC Exc]
[7th] S95.012 Laceration of dorsal artery of left foot [CC] [POA] [CC/MCC Exc]
[7th] S95.019 Laceration of dorsal artery of unspecified foot [CC] [POA] [CC/MCC Exc]
[6th] S95.09 Other specified injury of dorsal artery of foot
[7th] S95.091 Other specified injury of dorsal artery of right foot [CC] [POA] [CC/MCC Exc]
[7th] S95.092 Other specified injury of dorsal artery of left foot [CC] [POA] [CC/MCC Exc]
[7th] S95.099 Other specified injury of dorsal artery of unspecified foot [CC] [POA] [CC/MCC Exc]
[5th] S95.1 Injury of plantar artery of foot
[6th] S95.10 Unspecified injury of plantar artery of foot
[7th] S95.101 Unspecified injury of plantar artery of right foot [CC] [POA] [CC/MCC Exc]
[7th] S95.102 Unspecified injury of plantar artery of left foot [CC] [POA] [CC/MCC Exc]
[7th] S95.109 Unspecified injury of plantar artery of unspecified foot [CC] [POA] [CC/MCC Exc]
[6th] S95.11 Laceration of plantar artery of foot
[7th] S95.111 Laceration of plantar artery of right foot [CC] [POA] [CC/MCC Exc]
[7th] S95.112 Laceration of plantar artery of left foot [CC] [POA] [CC/MCC Exc]

[PDx] Unacceptable principal diagnosis symbol per Medicare code edits [POA] Code exempt from diagnosis present on admission requirement
[?] Questionable admission [CC] Complication or comorbidity [MCC] Major complication or comorbidity [CC/MCC Exc] CC/MCC exclusion
[HCC] HCC diagnosis code [RxHCC] RxHCC diagnosis code MACRA code **DEFINITION** Describes condition/terminology
TIP Coding guidance 👁 Official Guideline Reference [Z-1] Z code as first-listed diagnosis

7️⃣ S95.119 Laceration of plantar artery of unspecified foot cc POA CC/MCC Exc

6️⃣ S95.19 Other specified injury of plantar artery of foot

7️⃣ S95.191 Other specified injury of plantar artery of right foot cc POA CC/MCC Exc

7️⃣ S95.192 Other specified injury of plantar artery of left foot cc POA CC/MCC Exc

7️⃣ S95.199 Other specified injury of plantar artery of unspecified foot cc POA CC/MCC Exc

5️⃣ S95.2 Injury of dorsal vein of foot

6️⃣ S95.20 Unspecified injury of dorsal vein of foot

7️⃣ S95.201 Unspecified injury of dorsal vein of right foot cc POA CC/MCC Exc

7️⃣ S95.202 Unspecified injury of dorsal vein of left foot cc POA CC/MCC Exc

7️⃣ S95.209 Unspecified injury of dorsal vein of unspecified foot cc POA CC/MCC Exc

6️⃣ S95.21 Laceration of dorsal vein of foot

7️⃣ S95.211 Laceration of dorsal vein of right foot cc POA CC/MCC Exc

7️⃣ S95.212 Laceration of dorsal vein of left foot cc POA CC/MCC Exc

7️⃣ S95.219 Laceration of dorsal vein of unspecified foot cc POA CC/MCC Exc

6️⃣ S95.29 Other specified injury of dorsal vein of foot

7️⃣ S95.291 Other specified injury of dorsal vein of right foot cc POA CC/MCC Exc

7️⃣ S95.292 Other specified injury of dorsal vein of left foot cc POA CC/MCC Exc

7️⃣ S95.299 Other specified injury of dorsal vein of unspecified foot cc POA CC/MCC Exc

5️⃣ S95.8 Injury of other blood vessels at ankle and foot level

6️⃣ S95.80 Unspecified injury of other blood vessels at ankle and foot level

7️⃣ S95.801 Unspecified injury of other blood vessels at ankle and foot level, right leg cc POA CC/MCC Exc

7️⃣ S95.802 Unspecified injury of other blood vessels at ankle and foot level, left leg cc POA CC/MCC Exc

7️⃣ S95.809 Unspecified injury of other blood vessels at ankle and foot level, unspecified leg cc POA CC/MCC Exc

6️⃣ S95.81 Laceration of other blood vessels at ankle and foot level

7️⃣ S95.811 Laceration of other blood vessels at ankle and foot level, right leg cc POA CC/MCC Exc

7️⃣ S95.812 Laceration of other blood vessels at ankle and foot level, left leg cc POA CC/MCC Exc

7️⃣ S95.819 Laceration of other blood vessels at ankle and foot level, unspecified leg cc POA CC/MCC Exc

6️⃣ S95.89 Other specified injury of other blood vessels at ankle and foot level

7️⃣ S95.891 Other specified injury of other blood vessels at ankle and foot level, right leg cc POA CC/MCC Exc

7️⃣ S95.892 Other specified injury of other blood vessels at ankle and foot level, left leg cc POA CC/MCC Exc

7️⃣ S95.899 Other specified injury of other blood vessels at ankle and foot level, unspecified leg cc POA CC/MCC Exc

5️⃣ S95.9 Injury of unspecified blood vessel at ankle and foot level

6️⃣ S95.90 Unspecified injury of unspecified blood vessel at ankle and foot level

7️⃣ S95.901 Unspecified injury of unspecified blood vessel at ankle and foot level, right leg cc POA CC/MCC Exc

7️⃣ S95.902 Unspecified injury of unspecified blood vessel at ankle and foot level, left leg cc POA CC/MCC Exc

7️⃣ S95.909 Unspecified injury of unspecified blood vessel at ankle and foot level, unspecified leg cc POA CC/MCC Exc

6️⃣ S95.91 Laceration of unspecified blood vessel at ankle and foot level

7️⃣ S95.911 Laceration of unspecified blood vessel at ankle and foot level, right leg cc POA CC/MCC Exc

7️⃣ S95.912 Laceration of unspecified blood vessel at ankle and foot level, left leg cc POA CC/MCC Exc

7️⃣ S95.919 Laceration of unspecified blood vessel at ankle and foot level, unspecified leg cc POA CC/MCC Exc

6️⃣ S95.99 Other specified injury of unspecified blood vessel at ankle and foot level

7️⃣ S95.991 Other specified injury of unspecified blood vessel at ankle and foot level, right leg cc POA CC/MCC Exc

7️⃣ S95.992 Other specified injury of unspecified blood vessel at ankle and foot level, left leg cc POA CC/MCC Exc

7️⃣ S95.999 Other specified injury of unspecified blood vessel at ankle and foot level, unspecified leg cc POA CC/MCC Exc

4️⃣ S96 Injury of muscle and tendon at ankle and foot level

Code also any associated open wound (S91.-)

EXCLUDES2 injury of Achilles tendon (S86.0-)

sprain of joints and ligaments of ankle and foot (S93.-)

The appropriate 7th character is to be added to each code from category S96

A = initial encounter

D = subsequent encounter

S = sequela

5️⃣ S96.0 Injury of muscle and tendon of long flexor muscle of toe at ankle and foot level

6️⃣ S96.00 Unspecified injury of muscle and tendon of long flexor muscle of toe at ankle and foot level

7️⃣ S96.001 Unspecified injury of muscle and tendon of long flexor muscle of toe at ankle and foot level, right foot POA

7️⃣ S96.002 Unspecified injury of muscle and tendon of long flexor muscle of toe at ankle and foot level, left foot POA

7️⃣ S96.009 Unspecified injury of muscle and tendon of long flexor muscle of toe at ankle and foot level, unspecified foot POA

6️⃣ S96.01 Strain of muscle and tendon of long flexor muscle of toe at ankle and foot level

7️⃣ S96.011 Strain of muscle and tendon of long flexor muscle of toe at ankle and foot level, right foot POA

7️⃣ S96.012 Strain of muscle and tendon of long flexor muscle of toe at ankle and foot level, left foot POA

7️⃣ S96.019 Strain of muscle and tendon of long flexor muscle of toe at ankle and foot level, unspecified foot POA

6️⃣ S96.02 Laceration of muscle and tendon of long flexor muscle of toe at ankle and foot level

7️⃣ S96.021 Laceration of muscle and tendon of long flexor muscle of toe at ankle and foot level, right foot cc POA CC/MCC Exc

7️⃣ S96.022 Laceration of muscle and tendon of long flexor muscle of toe at ankle and foot level, left foot cc POA CC/MCC Exc

7️⃣ S96.029 Laceration of muscle and tendon of long flexor muscle of toe at ankle and foot level, unspecified foot cc POA CC/MCC Exc

6️⃣ S96.09 Other injury of muscle and tendon of long flexor muscle of toe at ankle and foot level

7️⃣ S96.091 Other injury of muscle and tendon of long flexor muscle of toe at ankle and foot level, right foot POA

7️⃣ S96.092 Other injury of muscle and tendon of long flexor muscle of toe at ankle and foot level, left foot POA

Unspecified Code Other Specified Code Manifestation Code N Newborn P Pediatric M Maternity A Adult ♂ Male ♀ Female
● New Code ▲ Revised Code Title ▶◀ Revised Text NOTES INCLUDES EXCLUDES1 Not coded here EXCLUDES2 Not included here
4️⃣ 4th character required 5️⃣ 5th character required 6️⃣ 6th character required 7️⃣ 7th character required Ⓧ Extension 'X' Alert
HAC Hospital-acquired condition (HAC) alert AHA AHA Coding Clinic© ☛ Code first alert

S96.099 Other injury of muscle and tendon of long flexor muscle of toe at ankle and foot level, unspecified foot POA

S96.1 Injury of muscle and tendon of long extensor muscle of toe at ankle and foot level

S96.10 Unspecified injury of muscle and tendon of long extensor muscle of toe at ankle and foot level

S96.101 Unspecified injury of muscle and tendon of long extensor muscle of toe at ankle and foot level, right foot POA

S96.102 Unspecified injury of muscle and tendon of long extensor muscle of toe at ankle and foot level, left foot POA

S96.109 Unspecified injury of muscle and tendon of long extensor muscle of toe at ankle and foot level, unspecified foot POA

S96.11 Strain of muscle and tendon of long extensor muscle of toe at ankle and foot level

S96.111 Strain of muscle and tendon of long extensor muscle of toe at ankle and foot level, right foot POA

S96.112 Strain of muscle and tendon of long extensor muscle of toe at ankle and foot level, left foot POA

S96.119 Strain of muscle and tendon of long extensor muscle of toe at ankle and foot level, unspecified foot POA

S96.12 Laceration of muscle and tendon of long extensor muscle of toe at ankle and foot level

S96.121 Laceration of muscle and tendon of long extensor muscle of toe at ankle and foot level, right foot CC POA CC/MCC Exc

S96.122 Laceration of muscle and tendon of long extensor muscle of toe at ankle and foot level, left foot CC POA CC/MCC Exc

S96.129 Laceration of muscle and tendon of long extensor muscle of toe at ankle and foot level, unspecified foot POA CC/MCC Exc

S96.19 Other specified injury of muscle and tendon of long extensor muscle of toe at ankle and foot level

S96.191 Other specified injury of muscle and tendon of long extensor muscle of toe at ankle and foot level, right foot POA

S96.192 Other specified injury of muscle and tendon of long extensor muscle of toe at ankle and foot level, left foot POA

S96.199 Other specified injury of muscle and tendon of long extensor muscle of toe at ankle and foot level, unspecified foot POA

S96.2 Injury of intrinsic muscle and tendon at ankle and foot level

S96.20 Unspecified injury of intrinsic muscle and tendon at ankle and foot level

S96.201 Unspecified injury of intrinsic muscle and tendon at ankle and foot level, right foot POA

S96.202 Unspecified injury of intrinsic muscle and tendon at ankle and foot level, left foot POA

S96.209 Unspecified injury of intrinsic muscle and tendon at ankle and foot level, unspecified foot POA

S96.21 Strain of intrinsic muscle and tendon at ankle and foot level

S96.211 Strain of intrinsic muscle and tendon at ankle and foot level, right foot POA

S96.212 Strain of intrinsic muscle and tendon at ankle and foot level, left foot POA

S96.219 Strain of intrinsic muscle and tendon at ankle and foot level, unspecified foot POA

S96.22 Laceration of intrinsic muscle and tendon at ankle and foot level

S96.221 Laceration of intrinsic muscle and tendon at ankle and foot level, right foot CC POA CC/MCC Exc

S96.222 Laceration of intrinsic muscle and tendon at ankle and foot level, left foot CC POA CC/MCC Exc

S96.229 Laceration of intrinsic muscle and tendon at ankle and foot level, unspecified foot POA CC/MCC Exc

S96.29 Other specified injury of intrinsic muscle and tendon at ankle and foot level

S96.291 Other specified injury of intrinsic muscle and tendon at ankle and foot level, right foot POA

S96.292 Other specified injury of intrinsic muscle and tendon at ankle and foot level, left foot POA

S96.299 Other specified injury of intrinsic muscle and tendon at ankle and foot level, unspecified foot POA

S96.8 Injury of other specified muscles and tendons at ankle and foot level

S96.80 Unspecified injury of other specified muscles and tendons at ankle and foot level

S96.801 Unspecified injury of other specified muscles and tendons at ankle and foot level, right foot POA

S96.802 Unspecified injury of other specified muscles and tendons at ankle and foot level, left foot POA

S96.809 Unspecified injury of other specified muscles and tendons at ankle and foot level, unspecified foot POA

S96.81 Strain of other specified muscles and tendons at ankle and foot level

S96.811 Strain of other specified muscles and tendons at ankle and foot level, right foot POA

S96.812 Strain of other specified muscles and tendons at ankle and foot level, left foot POA

S96.819 Strain of other specified muscles and tendons at ankle and foot level, unspecified foot POA

S96.82 Laceration of other specified muscles and tendons at ankle and foot level

S96.821 Laceration of other specified muscles and tendons at ankle and foot level, right foot CC POA CC/MCC Exc

S96.822 Laceration of other specified muscles and tendons at ankle and foot level, left foot CC POA CC/MCC Exc

S96.829 Laceration of other specified muscles and tendons at ankle and foot level, unspecified foot CC POA CC/MCC Exc

S96.89 Other specified injury of other specified muscles and tendons at ankle and foot level

S96.891 Other specified injury of other specified muscles and tendons at ankle and foot level, right foot POA

S96.892 Other specified injury of other specified muscles and tendons at ankle and foot level, left foot POA

S96.899 Other specified injury of other specified muscles and tendons at ankle and foot level, unspecified foot POA

S96.9 Injury of unspecified muscle and tendon at ankle and foot level

S96.90 Unspecified injury of unspecified muscle and tendon at ankle and foot level

S96.901 Unspecified injury of unspecified muscle and tendon at ankle and foot level, right foot POA

S96.902 Unspecified injury of unspecified muscle and tendon at ankle and foot level, left foot POA

Unacceptable principal diagnosis symbol per Medicare code edits Code exempt from diagnosis present on admission requirement ❓ Questionable admission Complication or comorbidity MCC Major complication or comorbidity CC/MCC CC/MCC exclusion HCC HCC diagnosis code RHCC RxHCC diagnosis code MACRA code **DEFINITION** Describes condition/terminology **TIP** Coding guidance Official Guideline Reference Z Z code as first-listed diagnosis

1096 When symbols appear on a code that requires a 7th character extension, refer to Appendix B to identify applicable 7th character codes. **2020 ICD-10-CM**

[7th] S96.909 Unspecified injury of unspecified muscle and tendon at ankle and foot level, unspecified foot POA

[6th] S96.91 Strain of unspecified muscle and tendon at ankle and foot level

[7th] S96.911 Strain of unspecified muscle and tendon at ankle and foot level, right foot POA

[7th] S96.912 Strain of unspecified muscle and tendon at ankle and foot level, left foot POA

[7th] S96.919 Strain of unspecified muscle and tendon at ankle and foot level, unspecified foot POA

[6th] S96.92 Laceration of unspecified muscle and tendon at ankle and foot level

[7th] S96.921 Laceration of unspecified muscle and tendon at ankle and foot level, right foot CC POA CC/MCC Exc

[7th] S96.922 Laceration of unspecified muscle and tendon at ankle and foot level, left foot CC POA CC/MCC Exc

[7th] S96.929 Laceration of unspecified muscle and tendon at ankle and foot level, unspecified foot CC POA CC/MCC Exc

[6th] S96.99 Other specified injury of unspecified muscle and tendon at ankle and foot level

[7th] S96.991 Other specified injury of unspecified muscle and tendon at ankle and foot level, right foot POA

[7th] S96.992 Other specified injury of unspecified muscle and tendon at ankle and foot level, left foot POA

[7th] S96.999 Other specified injury of unspecified muscle and tendon at ankle and foot level, unspecified foot POA

[4th] S97 Crushing injury of ankle and foot

Use additional code(s) for all associated injuries

The appropriate 7th character is to be added to each code from category S97

A = initial encounter
D = subsequent encounter
S = sequela

[5th] S97.0 Crushing injury of ankle

[7th] S97.00 Crushing injury of unspecified ankle POA

[7th] S97.01 Crushing injury of right ankle POA

[7th] S97.02 Crushing injury of left ankle POA

[5th] S97.1 Crushing injury of toe

[6th] S97.10 Crushing injury of unspecified toe(s)

[7th] S97.101 Crushing injury of unspecified right toe(s) POA

[7th] S97.102 Crushing injury of unspecified left toe(s) POA

[7th] S97.109 Crushing injury of unspecified toe(s) POA

Crushing injury of toe NOS

[6th] S97.11 Crushing injury of great toe

[7th] S97.111 Crushing injury of right great toe POA

[7th] S97.112 Crushing injury of left great toe POA

[7th] S97.119 Crushing injury of unspecified great toe POA

[6th] S97.12 Crushing injury of lesser toe(s)

[7th] S97.121 Crushing injury of right lesser toe(s) POA

[7th] S97.122 Crushing injury of left lesser toe(s) POA

[7th] S97.129 Crushing injury of unspecified lesser toe(s) POA

[5th] S97.8 Crushing injury of foot

[7th] S97.80 Crushing injury of unspecified foot POA

Crushing injury of foot NOS

[7th] S97.81 Crushing injury of right foot POA

[7th] S97.82 Crushing injury of left foot POA

[4th] S98 Traumatic amputation of ankle and foot

An amputation not identified as partial or complete should be coded to complete

The appropriate 7th character is to be added to each code from category S98

A = initial encounter
D = subsequent encounter
S = sequela

[5th] S98.0 Traumatic amputation of foot at ankle level

[6th] S98.01 Complete traumatic amputation of foot at ankle level

[7th] S98.011 Complete traumatic amputation of right foot at ankle level CC POA HCC CC/MCC Exc

[7th] S98.012 Complete traumatic amputation of left foot at ankle level CC POA HCC CC/MCC Exc

[7th] S98.019 Complete traumatic amputation of unspecified foot at ankle level CC POA HCC CC/MCC Exc

[6th] S98.02 Partial traumatic amputation of foot at ankle level

[7th] S98.021 Partial traumatic amputation of right foot at ankle level CC POA HCC CC/MCC Exc

[7th] S98.022 Partial traumatic amputation of left foot at ankle level CC POA HCC CC/MCC Exc

[7th] S98.029 Partial traumatic amputation of unspecified foot at ankle level CC POA HCC CC/MCC Exc

[5th] S98.1 Traumatic amputation of one toe

[6th] S98.11 Complete traumatic amputation of great toe

[7th] S98.111 Complete traumatic amputation of right great toe POA HCC

[7th] S98.112 Complete traumatic amputation of left great toe POA HCC

[7th] S98.119 Complete traumatic amputation of unspecified great toe POA HCC

[6th] S98.12 Partial traumatic amputation of great toe

[7th] S98.121 Partial traumatic amputation of right great toe POA HCC

[7th] S98.122 Partial traumatic amputation of left great toe POA HCC

[7th] S98.129 Partial traumatic amputation of unspecified great toe POA HCC

[6th] S98.13 Complete traumatic amputation of one lesser toe

Traumatic amputation of toe NOS

[7th] S98.131 Complete traumatic amputation of one right lesser toe POA HCC

[7th] S98.132 Complete traumatic amputation of one left lesser toe POA HCC

[7th] S98.139 Complete traumatic amputation of one unspecified lesser toe POA HCC

[6th] S98.14 Partial traumatic amputation of one lesser toe

[7th] S98.141 Partial traumatic amputation of one right lesser toe POA HCC

[7th] S98.142 Partial traumatic amputation of one left lesser toe POA HCC

[7th] S98.149 Partial traumatic amputation of one unspecified lesser toe POA HCC

[5th] S98.2 Traumatic amputation of two or more lesser toes

[6th] S98.21 Complete traumatic amputation of two or more lesser toes

[7th] S98.211 Complete traumatic amputation of two or more right lesser toes POA HCC

[7th] S98.212 Complete traumatic amputation of two or more left lesser toes POA HCC

[7th] S98.219 Complete traumatic amputation of two or more unspecified lesser toes POA HCC

[6th] S98.22 Partial traumatic amputation of two or more lesser toes

[7th] S98.221 Partial traumatic amputation of two or more right lesser toes POA HCC

[7th] S98.222 Partial traumatic amputation of two or more left lesser toes POA HCC

[7th] S98.229 Partial traumatic amputation of two or more unspecified lesser toes POA HCC

[5th] S98.3 Traumatic amputation of midfoot

[6th] S98.31 Complete traumatic amputation of midfoot

[7th] S98.311 Complete traumatic amputation of right midfoot CC POA HCC CC/MCC Exc

[7th] S98.312 Complete traumatic amputation of left midfoot CC POA HCC CC/MCC Exc

S98.319 **Complete** traumatic amputation of unspecified midfoot ᶜᶜ ᴘᴼᴬ ᴴᶜᶜ ᶜᶜ/ᴹᶜᶜ ᴱˣᶜ

S98.32 **Partial** traumatic amputation of midfoot

S98.321 **Partial** traumatic amputation of right midfoot ᶜᶜ ᴘᴼᴬ ᴴᶜᶜ ᶜᶜ/ᴹᶜᶜ ᴱˣᶜ

S98.322 **Partial** traumatic amputation of left midfoot ᶜᶜ ᴘᴼᴬ ᴴᶜᶜ ᶜᶜ/ᴹᶜᶜ ᴱˣᶜ

S98.329 **Partial** traumatic amputation of unspecified midfoot ᶜᶜ ᴘᴼᴬ ᴴᶜᶜ ᶜᶜ/ᴹᶜᶜ ᴱˣᶜ

S98.9 **Traumatic amputation of** foot, level unspecified

S98.91 **Complete** traumatic amputation of foot, level unspecified

S98.911 **Complete** traumatic amputation of right foot, level unspecified ᶜᶜ ᴘᴼᴬ ᴴᶜᶜ ᶜᶜ/ᴹᶜᶜ ᴱˣᶜ

S98.912 **Complete** traumatic amputation of left foot, level unspecified ᶜᶜ ᴘᴼᴬ ᴴᶜᶜ ᶜᶜ/ᴹᶜᶜ ᴱˣᶜ

S98.919 **Complete** traumatic amputation of unspecified foot, level unspecified ᶜᶜ ᴘᴼᴬ ᴴᶜᶜ ᶜᶜ/ᴹᶜᶜ ᴱˣᶜ

S98.92 **Partial** traumatic amputation of foot, level unspecified

S98.921 **Partial** traumatic amputation of right foot, level unspecified ᶜᶜ ᴘᴼᴬ ᴴᶜᶜ ᶜᶜ/ᴹᶜᶜ ᴱˣᶜ

S98.922 **Partial** traumatic amputation of left foot, level unspecified ᶜᶜ ᴘᴼᴬ ᴴᶜᶜ ᶜᶜ/ᴹᶜᶜ ᴱˣᶜ

S98.929 **Partial** traumatic amputation of unspecified foot, level unspecified ᶜᶜ ᴘᴼᴬ ᴴᶜᶜ ᶜᶜ/ᴹᶜᶜ ᴱˣᶜ

S99 **Other** and unspecified injuries of ankle and foot

S99.0 **Physeal fracture of** calcaneus

The appropriate 7th character is to be added to each code from subcategories S99.0

A = initial encounter for closed fracture

B = initial encounter for open fracture

D = subsequent encounter for fracture with routine healing

G = subsequent encounter for fracture with delayed healing

K = subsequent encounter for fracture with nonunion

P = subsequent encounter for fracture with malunion

S = sequela

S99.00 **Unspecified** physeal fracture of calcaneus

S99.001 Unspecified physeal fracture of right calcaneus ᴘᴼᴬ

S99.002 Unspecified physeal fracture of left calcaneus ᴘᴼᴬ

S99.009 Unspecified physeal fracture of unspecified calcaneus ᴘᴼᴬ

S99.01 **Salter-Harris Type I** physeal fracture of calcaneus

S99.011 Salter-Harris Type I physeal fracture of right calcaneus ᴘᴼᴬ

S99.012 Salter-Harris Type I physeal fracture of left calcaneus ᴘᴼᴬ

S99.019 Salter-Harris Type I physeal fracture of unspecified calcaneus ᴘᴼᴬ

S99.02 **Salter-Harris Type II** physeal fracture of calcaneus

S99.021 Salter-Harris Type II physeal fracture of right calcaneus ᴘᴼᴬ

S99.022 Salter-Harris Type II physeal fracture of left calcaneus ᴘᴼᴬ

S99.029 Salter-Harris Type II physeal fracture of unspecified calcaneus ᴘᴼᴬ

S99.03 **Salter-Harris Type III** physeal fracture of calcaneus

S99.031 Salter-Harris Type III physeal fracture of right calcaneus ᴘᴼᴬ

S99.032 Salter-Harris Type III physeal fracture of left calcaneus ᴘᴼᴬ

S99.039 Salter-Harris Type III physeal fracture of unspecified calcaneus ᴘᴼᴬ

S99.04 **Salter-Harris Type IV** physeal fracture of calcaneus

S99.041 Salter-Harris Type IV physeal fracture of right calcaneus ᴘᴼᴬ

S99.042 Salter-Harris Type IV physeal fracture of left calcaneus ᴘᴼᴬ

S99.049 Salter-Harris Type IV physeal fracture of unspecified calcaneus ᴘᴼᴬ

S99.09 **Other** physeal fracture of calcaneus

S99.091 Other physeal fracture of right calcaneus ᴘᴼᴬ

S99.092 Other physeal fracture of left calcaneus ᴘᴼᴬ

S99.099 Other physeal fracture of unspecified calcaneus ᴘᴼᴬ

S99.1 **Physeal fracture of** metatarsal

The appropriate 7th character is to be added to each code from subcategories S99.1

A = initial encounter for closed fracture

B = initial encounter for open fracture

D = subsequent encounter for fracture with routine healing

G = subsequent encounter for fracture with delayed healing

K = subsequent encounter for fracture with nonunion

P = subsequent encounter for fracture with malunion

S = sequela

S99.10 **Unspecified** physeal fracture of metatarsal

S99.101 Unspecified physeal fracture of right metatarsal ᴘᴼᴬ

S99.102 Unspecified physeal fracture of left metatarsal ᴘᴼᴬ

S99.109 Unspecified physeal fracture of unspecified metatarsal ᴘᴼᴬ

S99.11 **Salter-Harris Type I** physeal fracture of metatarsal

S99.111 Salter-Harris Type I physeal fracture of right metatarsal ᴘᴼᴬ

S99.112 Salter-Harris Type I physeal fracture of left metatarsal ᴘᴼᴬ

AHA: Q1 2018

S99.119 Salter-Harris Type I physeal fracture of unspecified metatarsal ᴘᴼᴬ

S99.12 **Salter-Harris Type II** physeal fracture of metatarsal

S99.121 Salter-Harris Type II physeal fracture of right metatarsal ᴘᴼᴬ

S99.122 Salter-Harris Type II physeal fracture of left metatarsal ᴘᴼᴬ

S99.129 Salter-Harris Type II physeal fracture of unspecified metatarsal ᴘᴼᴬ

S99.13 **Salter-Harris Type III** physeal fracture of metatarsal

S99.131 Salter-Harris Type III physeal fracture of right metatarsal ᴘᴼᴬ

S99.132 Salter-Harris Type III physeal fracture of left metatarsal ᴘᴼᴬ

S99.139 Salter-Harris Type III physeal fracture of unspecified metatarsal ᴘᴼᴬ

S99.14 **Salter-Harris Type IV** physeal fracture of metatarsal

S99.141 Salter-Harris Type IV physeal fracture of right metatarsal ᴘᴼᴬ

S99.142 Salter-Harris Type IV physeal fracture of left metatarsal ᴘᴼᴬ

S99.149 Salter-Harris Type IV physeal fracture of unspecified metatarsal ᴘᴼᴬ

S99.19 **Other** physeal fracture of metatarsal

S99.191 Other physeal fracture of right metatarsal ᴘᴼᴬ

S99.192 Other physeal fracture of left metatarsal ᴘᴼᴬ

S99.199 Other physeal fracture of unspecified metatarsal ᴘᴼᴬ

ᴘᴰˣ Unacceptable principal diagnosis symbol per Medicare code edits   ᴘᴼᴬ Code exempt from diagnosis present on admission requirement
? Questionable admission   ᶜᶜ Complication or comorbidity   ᴹᶜᶜ Major complication or comorbidity   ᶜᶜ/ᴹᶜᶜ ᴱˣᶜ CC/MCC exclusion
ᴴᶜᶜ HCC diagnosis code   ᴿˣᴴᶜᶜ RxHCC diagnosis code   MACRA code   **DEFINITION** Describes condition/terminology
TIP Coding guidance   👁 Official Guideline Reference   🆉 Z code as first-listed diagnosis

1098   When symbols appear on a code that requires a 7th character extension, refer to Appendix B to identify applicable 7th character codes.   **2020 ICD-10-CM**

[5th] S99.2 Physeal fracture of phalanx of toe
The appropriate 7th character is to be added to each code from subcategories S99.2
A = initial encounter for closed fracture
B = initial encounter for open fracture
D = subsequent encounter for fracture with routine healing
G = subsequent encounter for fracture with delayed healing
K = subsequent encounter for fracture with nonunion
P = subsequent encounter for fracture with malunion
S = sequela

[6th] S99.20 Unspecified physeal fracture of phalanx of toe
[7th] S99.201 Unspecified physeal fracture of phalanx of right toe [POA]
[7th] S99.202 Unspecified physeal fracture of phalanx of left toe [POA]
[7th] S99.209 Unspecified physeal fracture of phalanx of unspecified toe [POA]

[6th] S99.21 Salter-Harris Type I physeal fracture of phalanx of toe
[7th] S99.211 Salter-Harris Type I physeal fracture of phalanx of right toe [POA]
[7th] S99.212 Salter-Harris Type I physeal fracture of phalanx of left toe [POA]
[7th] S99.219 Salter-Harris Type I physeal fracture of phalanx of unspecified toe [POA]

[6th] S99.22 Salter-Harris Type II physeal fracture of phalanx of toe
[7th] S99.221 Salter-Harris Type II physeal fracture of phalanx of right toe [POA]
[7th] S99.222 Salter-Harris Type II physeal fracture of phalanx of left toe [POA]
[7th] S99.229 Salter-Harris Type II physeal fracture of phalanx of unspecified toe [POA]

[6th] S99.23 Salter-Harris Type III physeal fracture of phalanx of toe
[7th] S99.231 Salter-Harris Type III physeal fracture of phalanx of right toe [POA]
[7th] S99.232 Salter-Harris Type III physeal fracture of phalanx of left toe [POA]
[7th] S99.239 Salter-Harris Type III physeal fracture of phalanx of unspecified toe [POA]

[6th] S99.24 Salter-Harris Type IV physeal fracture of phalanx of toe
[7th] S99.241 Salter-Harris Type IV physeal fracture of phalanx of right toe [POA]
[7th] S99.242 Salter-Harris Type IV physeal fracture of phalanx of left toe [POA]
[7th] S99.249 Salter-Harris Type IV physeal fracture of phalanx of unspecified toe [POA]

[6th] S99.29 Other physeal fracture of phalanx of toe
[7th] S99.291 Other physeal fracture of phalanx of right toe [POA]
[7th] S99.292 Other physeal fracture of phalanx of left toe [POA]
[7th] S99.299 Other physeal fracture of phalanx of unspecified toe [POA]

[5th] S99.8 Other specified injuries of ankle and foot
The appropriate 7th character is to be added to each code from subcategory S99.8
A = initial encounter
D = subsequent encounter
S = sequela

[6th] S99.81 Other specified injuries of ankle
[7th] S99.811 Other specified injuries of right ankle [POA]
[7th] S99.812 Other specified injuries of left ankle [POA]
[7th] S99.819 Other specified injuries of unspecified ankle [POA]

[6th] S99.82 Other specified injuries of foot
[7th] S99.821 Other specified injuries of right foot [POA]
[7th] S99.822 Other specified injuries of left foot [POA]
[7th] S99.829 Other specified injuries of unspecified foot [POA]

[5th] S99.9 Unspecified injury of ankle and foot
The appropriate 7th character is to be added to each code from subcategory S99.9
A = initial encounter
D = subsequent encounter
S = sequela

[6th] S99.91 Unspecified injury of ankle
[7th] S99.911 Unspecified injury of right ankle [POA]
[7th] S99.912 Unspecified injury of left ankle [POA]
[7th] S99.919 Unspecified injury of unspecified ankle [POA]

[6th] S99.92 Unspecified injury of foot
[7th] S99.921 Unspecified injury of right foot [POA]
[7th] S99.922 Unspecified injury of left foot [POA]
[7th] S99.929 Unspecified injury of unspecified foot [POA]

Injury, poisoning and certain other consequences of external causes (T07-T88)

Injuries involving multiple body regions (T07)

[EXCLUDES1] *burns and corrosions (T20-T32)*
frostbite (T33-T34)
insect bite or sting, venomous (T63.4)
sunburn (L55.-)

[7th] T07 Unspecified multiple injuries [POA]
See Official Guidelines "Coding of Injuries" I.C.19.b
The appropriate 7th character is to be added to code T07
A = initial encounter
D = subsequent encounter
S = sequela
[EXCLUDES1] *injury NOS (T14.90)*

Injury of unspecified body region (T14)

[4th] T14 Injury of unspecified body region
The appropriate 7th character is to be added to each code from category T14
A = initial encounter
D = subsequent encounter
S = sequela
[EXCLUDES1] *multiple unspecified injuries (T07)*

[7th] T14.8 Other injury of unspecified body region [POA]
Abrasion NOS
Contusion NOS
Crush injury NOS
Fracture NOS
Skin injury NOS
Vascular injury NOS
Wound NOS

[5th] T14.9 Unspecified injury
[7th] T14.90 Injury, unspecified [POA]
Injury NOS
[7th] T14.91 Suicide attempt [POA] [HCC]
Attempted suicide NOS

Effects of foreign body entering through natural orifice (T15-T19)

[EXCLUDES2] *foreign body accidentally left in operation wound (T81.5-)*
foreign body in penetrating wound - See open wound by body region
residual foreign body in soft tissue (M79.5)
splinter, without open wound - See superficial injury by body region

Unspecified Code Other Specified Code Manifestation Code [N] Newborn [P] Pediatric [M] Maternity [A] Adult ♂ Male ♀ Female
● New Code ▲ Revised Code Title ►◄ Revised Text [NOTES] *INCLUDES* [EXCLUDES1] Not coded here [EXCLUDES2] Not included here
[4th] 4th character required [5th] 5th character required [6th] 6th character required [7th] 7th character required [X] Extension 'X' Alert
[HAC] Hospital-acquired condition (HAC) alert AHA AHA Coding Clinic© ☞ Code first alert

T15 Foreign body on external eye

> EXCLUDES2 foreign body in penetrating wound of orbit and eye ball (S05.4-, S05.5-)
>
> open wound of eyelid and periocular area (S01.1-)
>
> retained foreign body in eyelid (H02.8-)
>
> retained (old) foreign body in penetrating wound of orbit and eye ball (H05.5-, H44.6-, H44.7-)
>
> superficial foreign body of eyelid and periocular area (S00.25-)

The appropriate 7th character is to be added to each code from category T15
A = initial encounter
D = subsequent encounter
S = sequela

T15.0 Foreign body in cornea
- **T15.00** Foreign body in cornea, unspecified eye
- **T15.01** Foreign body in cornea, right eye
- **T15.02** Foreign body in cornea, left eye

T15.1 Foreign body in conjunctival sac
- **T15.10** Foreign body in conjunctival sac, unspecified eye
- **T15.11** Foreign body in conjunctival sac, right eye
- **T15.12** Foreign body in conjunctival sac, left eye

T15.8 Foreign body in other and multiple parts of external eye
> Foreign body in lacrimal punctum
- **T15.80** Foreign body in other and multiple parts of external eye, unspecified eye
- **T15.81** Foreign body in other and multiple parts of external eye, right eye
- **T15.82** Foreign body in other and multiple parts of external eye, left eye

T15.9 Foreign body on external eye, part unspecified
- **T15.90** Foreign body on external eye, part unspecified, unspecified eye
- **T15.91** Foreign body on external eye, part unspecified, right eye
- **T15.92** Foreign body on external eye, part unspecified, left eye

T16 Foreign body in ear

> INCLUDES foreign body in auditory canal

The appropriate 7th character is to be added to each code from category T16
A = initial encounter
D = subsequent encounter
S = sequela

- **T16.1** Foreign body in right ear
- **T16.2** Foreign body in left ear
- **T16.9** Foreign body in ear, unspecified ear

T17 Foreign body in respiratory tract

The appropriate 7th character is to be added to each code from category T17
A = initial encounter
D = subsequent encounter
S = sequela

- **T17.0** Foreign body in nasal sinus
- **T17.1** Foreign body in nostril
  > Foreign body in nose NOS
- **T17.2** Foreign body in pharynx
  > Foreign body in nasopharynx
  > Foreign body in throat NOS
  - **T17.20** Unspecified foreign body in pharynx
    - **T17.200** Unspecified foreign body in pharynx causing asphyxiation
    - **T17.208** Unspecified foreign body in pharynx causing other injury
  - **T17.21** Gastric contents in pharynx
    > Aspiration of gastric contents into pharynx
    > Vomitus in pharynx
    - **T17.210** Gastric contents in pharynx causing asphyxiation

- **T17.218** Gastric contents in pharynx causing other injury
  - **T17.22** Food in pharynx
    > Bones in pharynx
    > Seeds in pharynx
    - **T17.220** Food in pharynx causing asphyxiation
    - **T17.228** Food in pharynx causing other injury
  - **T17.29** Other foreign object in pharynx
    - **T17.290** Other foreign object in pharynx causing asphyxiation
    - **T17.298** Other foreign object in pharynx causing other injury

T17.3 Foreign body in larynx
  - **T17.30** Unspecified foreign body in larynx
    - **T17.300** Unspecified foreign body in larynx causing asphyxiation
    - **T17.308** Unspecified foreign body in larynx causing other injury
  - **T17.31** Gastric contents in larynx
    > Aspiration of gastric contents into larynx
    > Vomitus in larynx
    - **T17.310** Gastric contents in larynx causing asphyxiation
    - **T17.318** Gastric contents in larynx causing other injury
  - **T17.32** Food in larynx
    > Bones in larynx
    > Seeds in larynx
    - **T17.320** Food in larynx causing asphyxiation
    - **T17.328** Food in larynx causing other injury
  - **T17.39** Other foreign object in larynx
    - **T17.390** Other foreign object in larynx causing asphyxiation
    - **T17.398** Other foreign object in larynx causing other injury

T17.4 Foreign body in trachea
  - **T17.40** Unspecified foreign body in trachea
    - **T17.400** Unspecified foreign body in trachea causing asphyxiation
    - **T17.408** Unspecified foreign body in trachea causing other injury
  - **T17.41** Gastric contents in trachea
    > Aspiration of gastric contents into trachea
    > Vomitus in trachea
    - **T17.410** Gastric contents in trachea causing asphyxiation
    - **T17.418** Gastric contents in trachea causing other injury
  - **T17.42** Food in trachea
    > Bones in trachea
    > Seeds in trachea
    - **T17.420** Food in trachea causing asphyxiation
    - **T17.428** Food in trachea causing other injury
  - **T17.49** Other foreign object in trachea
    - **T17.490** Other foreign object in trachea causing asphyxiation
    - **T17.498** Other foreign object in trachea causing other injury

T17.5 Foreign body in bronchus
  - **T17.50** Unspecified foreign body in bronchus
    - **T17.500** Unspecified foreign body in bronchus causing asphyxiation
    - **T17.508** Unspecified foreign body in bronchus causing other injury
  - **T17.51** Gastric contents in bronchus
    > Aspiration of gastric contents into bronchus
    > Vomitus in bronchus
    - **T17.510** Gastric contents in bronchus causing asphyxiation

---

Unacceptable principal diagnosis symbol per Medicare code edits   Code exempt from diagnosis present on admission requirement
? Questionable admission   Complication or comorbidity   MCC Major complication or comorbidity   CC/MCC CC/MCC exclusion
HCC HCC diagnosis code   RxHCC RxHCC diagnosis code   MACRA code   **DEFINITION** Describes condition/terminology
TIP Coding guidance   Official Guideline Reference   Z1 Z code as first-listed diagnosis

1100   When symbols appear on a code that requires a 7th character extension, refer to Appendix B to identify applicable 7th character codes.   **2020 ICD-10-CM**

[7th] T17.518 **Gastric contents in bronchus** causing other injury CC POA CC/MCC Exc

[6th] T17.52 Food **in bronchus**
Bones in bronchus
Seeds in bronchus

[7th] T17.520 **Food in bronchus** causing asphyxiation CC POA CC/MCC Exc

[7th] T17.528 **Food in bronchus** causing other injury CC POA CC/MCC Exc

[6th] T17.59 Other **foreign object in bronchus**

[7th] T17.590 **Other foreign object in bronchus** causing asphyxiation CC POA CC/MCC Exc

[7th] T17.598 **Other foreign object in bronchus** causing other injury CC POA CC/MCC Exc

[5th] T17.8 **Foreign body in** other parts of respiratory tract
Foreign body in bronchioles
Foreign body in lung

[6th] T17.80 Unspecified **foreign body in other parts of respiratory tract**

[7th] T17.800 **Unspecified foreign body in other parts of respiratory tract** causing asphyxiation CC POA CC/MCC Exc

[7th] T17.808 **Unspecified foreign body in other parts of respiratory tract** causing other injury CC POA CC/MCC Exc

[6th] T17.81 Gastric contents **in other parts of respiratory tract**
Aspiration of gastric contents into other parts of respiratory tract
Vomitus in other parts of respiratory tract

[7th] T17.810 **Gastric contents in other parts of respiratory tract** causing asphyxiation CC POA CC/MCC Exc

[7th] T17.818 **Gastric contents in other parts of respiratory tract** causing other injury CC POA CC/MCC Exc

[6th] T17.82 Food **in other parts of respiratory tract**
Bones in other parts of respiratory tract
Seeds in other parts of respiratory tract

[7th] T17.820 **Food in other parts of respiratory tract** causing asphyxiation CC POA CC/MCC Exc

[7th] T17.828 **Food in other parts of respiratory tract** causing other injury CC POA CC/MCC Exc

[6th] T17.89 Other **foreign object in other parts of respiratory tract**

[7th] T17.890 **Other foreign object in other parts of respiratory tract** causing asphyxiation CC POA CC/MCC Exc

[7th] T17.898 **Other foreign object in other parts of respiratory tract causing other injury** CC POA CC/MCC Exc

[5th] T17.9 **Foreign body in respiratory tract,** part unspecified

[6th] T17.90 Unspecified **foreign body in respiratory tract, part unspecified**

[7th] T17.900 **Unspecified foreign body in respiratory tract, part unspecified** causing asphyxiation CC POA CC/MCC Exc

[7th] T17.908 **Unspecified foreign body in respiratory tract, part unspecified** causing other injury POA

[6th] T17.91 Gastric contents **in respiratory tract, part unspecified**
Aspiration of gastric contents into respiratory tract, part unspecified
Vomitus in trachea respiratory tract, part unspecified

[7th] T17.910 **Gastric contents in respiratory tract, part unspecified** causing asphyxiation CC POA CC/MCC Exc

[7th] T17.918 **Gastric contents in respiratory tract, part unspecified** causing other injury POA

[6th] T17.92 Food **in respiratory tract, part unspecified**
Bones in respiratory tract, part unspecified
Seeds in respiratory tract, part unspecified

[7th] T17.920 **Food in respiratory tract, part unspecified** causing asphyxiation CC POA CC/MCC Exc

[7th] T17.928 **Food in respiratory tract, part unspecified** causing other injury POA

[6th] T17.99 Other **foreign object in respiratory tract, part unspecified**

[7th] T17.990 **Other foreign object in respiratory tract, part unspecified in** causing asphyxiation CC POA CC/MCC Exc

[7th] T17.998 **Other foreign object in respiratory tract, part unspecified** causing other injury POA

[4th] T18 **Foreign body in** alimentary tract
EXCLUDES2 *foreign body in pharynx (T17.2-)*
The appropriate 7th character is to be added to each code from category T18
A = initial encounter
D = subsequent encounter
S = sequela

[7th] T18.0 **Foreign body in** mouth POA

[5th] T18.1 **Foreign body in** esophagus
EXCLUDES2 *foreign body in respiratory tract (T17.-)*

[6th] T18.10 Unspecified **foreign body in esophagus**

[7th] T18.100 **Unspecified foreign body in esophagus** causing compression of trachea POA
Unspecified foreign body in esophagus causing obstruction of respiration

[7th] T18.108 **Unspecified foreign body in esophagus** causing other injury POA

[6th] T18.11 Gastric contents **in esophagus**
Vomitus in esophagus

[7th] T18.110 **Gastric contents in esophagus** causing compression of trachea POA
Gastric contents in esophagus causing obstruction of respiration

[7th] T18.118 **Gastric contents in esophagus** causing other injury POA

[6th] T18.12 Food **in esophagus**
Bones in esophagus
Seeds in esophagus

[7th] T18.120 **Food in esophagus** causing compression of trachea POA
Food in esophagus causing obstruction of respiration

[7th] T18.128 **Food in esophagus** causing other injury POA

[6th] T18.19 Other **foreign object in esophagus**

[7th] T18.190 **Other foreign object in esophagus** causing compression of trachea CC POA CC/MCC Exc
Other foreign body in esophagus causing obstruction of respiration

[7th] T18.198 **Other foreign object in esophagus** causing other injury POA

[7th] T18.2 **Foreign body in** stomach CC POA CC/MCC Exc

[7th] T18.3 **Foreign body in** small intestine POA

[7th] T18.4 **Foreign body in** colon POA

[7th] T18.5 **Foreign body in** anus and rectum POA
Foreign body in rectosigmoid (junction)

[7th] T18.8 **Foreign body in** other **parts of alimentary tract** POA

[7th] T18.9 **Foreign body of** alimentary tract**, part unspecified** POA
Foreign body in digestive system NOS
Swallowed foreign body NOS

[4th] T19 **Foreign body in** genitourinary tract
EXCLUDES2 *complications due to implanted mesh (T83.7-)*
mechanical complications of contraceptive device (intrauterine) (vaginal) (T83.3-)
presence of contraceptive device (intrauterine) (vaginal) (Z97.5)
The appropriate 7th character is to be added to each code from category T19
A = initial encounter
D = subsequent encounter
S = sequela

Unspecified Code | Other Specified Code | Manifestation Code | [N] Newborn | [P] Pediatric | [M] Maternity | [A] Adult | ♂ Male | ♀ Female
● New Code | ▲ Revised Code Title | ►◄ Revised Text | NOTES | INCLUDES | EXCLUDES1 Not coded here | EXCLUDES2 Not included here
[4th] 4th character required | [5th] 5th character required | [6th] 6th character required | [7th] 7th character required | [x7th] Extension 'X' Alert
[HAC] Hospital-acquired condition (HAC) alert | AHA AHA Coding Clinic© | ☞ Code first alert

T19.0 - T20.37

CHAPTER 19: INJURY, POISONING, AND CERTAIN OTHER CONSEQUENCES OF EXTERNAL CAUSES (S00-T88)

T19.0 **Foreign body in** urethra
T19.1 **Foreign body in** bladder
T19.2 **Foreign body in** vulva and vagina ♀
T19.3 **Foreign body in** uterus ♀
T19.4 **Foreign body in** penis ♂
T19.8 **Foreign body in** other **parts of genitourinary tract**
T19.9 **Foreign body in** genitourinary tract, **part unspecified**

Burns and corrosions (T20-T32)

INCLUDES burns (thermal) from electrical heating appliances
burns (thermal) from electricity
burns (thermal) from flame
burns (thermal) from friction
burns (thermal) from hot air and hot gases
burns (thermal) from hot objects
burns (thermal) from lightning
burns (thermal) from radiation
chemical burn [corrosion] (external) (internal)
scalds

EXCLUDES2 erythema [dermatitis] ab igne (L59.0)
radiation-related disorders of the skin and subcutaneous tissue (L55-L59)
sunburn (L55.-)

Burns and corrosions of external body surface, specified by site (T20-T25)

👁 **See Official Guidelines** "Coding of Burns and Corrosions" I.C.19.d

INCLUDES burns and corrosions of first degree [erythema]
burns and corrosions of second degree [blisters][epidermal loss]
burns and corrosions of third degree [deep necrosis of underlying tissue] [full-thickness skin loss]

Use additional code from category T31 or T32 to identify extent of body surface involved

T20 Burn and corrosion **of head, face, and neck**

EXCLUDES2 burn and corrosion of ear drum (T28.41, T28.91)
burn and corrosion of eye and adnexa (T26.-)
burn and corrosion of mouth and pharynx (T28.0)

The appropriate 7th character is to be added to each code from category T20
A = initial encounter
D = subsequent encounter
S = sequela

T20.0 **Burn of** unspecified **degree of head, face, and neck**
Use additional external cause code to identify the source, place and intent of the burn (X00-X19, X75-X77, X96-X98, Y92)

T20.00 **Burn of unspecified degree of head, face, and neck, unspecified site**
T20.01 **Burn of unspecified degree of ear [any part,** except ear drum]
EXCLUDES2 burn of ear drum (T28.41-)
T20.011 **Burn of unspecified degree of** right **ear [any part, except ear drum]**
T20.012 **Burn of unspecified degree of** left **ear [any part, except ear drum]**
T20.019 **Burn of unspecified degree of unspecified ear [any part, except ear drum]**
T20.02 **Burn of unspecified degree of** lip(s)
T20.03 **Burn of unspecified degree of** chin
T20.04 **Burn of unspecified degree of** nose (septum)
T20.05 **Burn of unspecified degree of** scalp [any part]
T20.06 **Burn of unspecified degree of** forehead and cheek
T20.07 **Burn of unspecified degree of** neck
T20.09 **Burn of unspecified degree of** multiple sites **of head, face, and neck**

T20.1 **Burn of** first degree **of head, face, and neck**
Use additional external cause code to identify the source, place and intent of the burn (X00-X19, X75-X77, X96-X98, Y92)

T20.10 **Burn of first degree of head, face, and neck, unspecified site**
T20.11 **Burn of first degree of** ear [any part, except ear drum]
EXCLUDES2 burn of ear drum (T28.41-)
T20.111 **Burn of first degree of** right **ear [any part, except ear drum]**
T20.112 **Burn of first degree of** left **ear [any part, except ear drum]**
T20.119 **Burn of first degree of unspecified ear [any part, except ear drum]**
T20.12 **Burn of first degree of** lip(s)
T20.13 **Burn of first degree of** chin
T20.14 **Burn of first degree of** nose (septum)
T20.15 **Burn of first degree of** scalp [any part]
T20.16 **Burn of first degree of** forehead and cheek
T20.17 **Burn of first degree of** neck
T20.19 **Burn of first degree of** multiple sites **of head, face, and neck**

T20.2 **Burn of** second degree **of head, face, and neck**
Use additional external cause code to identify the source, place and intent of the burn (X00-X19, X75-X77, X96-X98, Y92)

T20.20 **Burn of second degree of head, face, and neck, unspecified site**
T20.21 **Burn of second degree of** ear [any part, except ear drum]
EXCLUDES2 burn of ear drum (T28.41-)
T20.211 **Burn of second degree of** right **ear [any part, except ear drum]**
T20.212 **Burn of second degree of** left **ear [any part, except ear drum]**
T20.219 **Burn of second degree of unspecified ear [any part, except ear drum]**
T20.22 **Burn of second degree of** lip(s)
T20.23 **Burn of second degree of** chin
T20.24 **Burn of second degree of** nose (septum)
T20.25 **Burn of second degree of** scalp [any part]
AHA: Q1 2015
T20.26 **Burn of second degree of** forehead and cheek
T20.27 **Burn of second degree of** neck
T20.29 **Burn of second degree of** multiple sites **of head, face, and neck**

T20.3 **Burn of** third degree **of head, face, and neck**
Use additional external cause code to identify the source, place and intent of the burn (X00-X19, X75-X77, X96-X98, Y92)

T20.30 **Burn of third degree of head, face, and neck, unspecified site**
T20.31 **Burn of third degree of** ear [any part, except ear drum]
EXCLUDES2 burn of ear drum (T28.41-)
T20.311 **Burn of third degree of** right **ear [any part, except ear drum]**
T20.312 **Burn of third degree of** left **ear [any part, except ear drum]**
AHA: Q1 2015
T20.319 **Burn of third degree of unspecified ear [any part, except ear drum]**
T20.32 **Burn of third degree of** lip(s)
T20.33 **Burn of third degree of** chin
T20.34 **Burn of third degree of** nose (septum)
T20.35 **Burn of third degree of** scalp [any part]
T20.36 **Burn of third degree of** forehead and cheek
T20.37 **Burn of third degree of** neck

PDₓ Unacceptable principal diagnosis symbol per Medicare code edits POA Code exempt from diagnosis present on admission requirement
❓ Questionable admission cc Complication or comorbidity MCC Major complication or comorbidity CC/MCC Exc CC/MCC exclusion
HCC HCC diagnosis code RxHCC RxHCC diagnosis code MACRA code **DEFINITION** Describes condition/terminology
TIP Coding guidance 👁 Official Guideline Reference Z1 Z code as first-listed diagnosis

T20.39 Burn of third degree of multiple sites of head, face, and neck   CC POA HAC CC/MCC Exc

T20.4 Corrosion of unspecified degree of head, face, and neck
  Code first (T51-T65) to identify chemical and intent
  Use additional external cause code to identify place (Y92)

T20.40 Corrosion of unspecified degree of head, face, and neck, unspecified site   POA

T20.41 Corrosion of unspecified degree of ear [any part, except ear drum]

  EXCLUDES2 corrosion of ear drum (T28.91-)

T20.411 Corrosion of unspecified degree of right ear [any part, except ear drum]   POA

T20.412 Corrosion of unspecified degree of left ear [any part, except ear drum]   POA

T20.419 Corrosion of unspecified degree of unspecified ear [any part, except ear drum]   POA

T20.42 Corrosion of unspecified degree of lip(s)   POA

T20.43 Corrosion of unspecified degree of chin   POA

T20.44 Corrosion of unspecified degree of nose (septum)   POA

T20.45 Corrosion of unspecified degree of scalp [any part]   POA

T20.46 Corrosion of unspecified degree of forehead and cheek   POA

T20.47 Corrosion of unspecified degree of neck   POA

T20.49 Corrosion of unspecified degree of multiple sites of head, face, and neck   POA

T20.5 Corrosion of first degree of head, face, and neck
  Code first (T51-T65) to identify chemical and intent
  Use additional external cause code to identify place (Y92)

T20.50 Corrosion of first degree of head, face, and neck, unspecified site   POA

T20.51 Corrosion of first degree of ear [any part, except ear drum]

  EXCLUDES2 corrosion of ear drum (T28.91-)

T20.511 Corrosion of first degree of right ear [any part, except ear drum]   POA

T20.512 Corrosion of first degree of left ear [any part, except ear drum]   POA

T20.519 Corrosion of first degree of unspecified ear [any part, except ear drum]   POA

T20.52 Corrosion of first degree of lip(s)   POA

T20.53 Corrosion of first degree of chin   POA

T20.54 Corrosion of first degree of nose (septum)   POA

T20.55 Corrosion of first degree of scalp [any part]   POA

T20.56 Corrosion of first degree of forehead and cheek   POA

T20.57 Corrosion of first degree of neck   POA

T20.59 Corrosion of first degree of multiple sites of head, face, and neck   POA

T20.6 Corrosion of second degree of head, face, and neck
  Code first (T51-T65) to identify chemical and intent
  Use additional external cause code to identify place (Y92)

T20.60 Corrosion of second degree of head, face, and neck, unspecified site   POA

T20.61 Corrosion of second degree of ear [any part, except ear drum]

  EXCLUDES2 corrosion of ear drum (T28.91-)

T20.611 Corrosion of second degree of right ear [any part, except ear drum]   POA

T20.612 Corrosion of second degree of left ear [any part, except ear drum]   POA

T20.619 Corrosion of second degree of unspecified ear [any part, except ear drum]   POA

T20.62 Corrosion of second degree of lip(s)   POA

T20.63 Corrosion of second degree of chin   POA

T20.64 Corrosion of second degree of nose (septum)   POA

T20.65 Corrosion of second degree of scalp [any part]   POA

T20.66 Corrosion of second degree of forehead and cheek   POA

T20.67 Corrosion of second degree of neck   POA

T20.69 Corrosion of second degree of multiple sites of head, face, and neck   POA

T20.7 Corrosion of third degree of head, face, and neck
  Code first (T51-T65) to identify chemical and intent
  Use additional external cause code to identify place (Y92)

T20.70 Corrosion of third degree of head, face, and neck, unspecified site   CC POA HAC CC/MCC Exc

T20.71 Corrosion of third degree of ear [any part, except ear drum]

  EXCLUDES2 corrosion of ear drum (T28.91-)

T20.711 Corrosion of third degree of right ear [any part, except ear drum]   CC POA HAC CC/MCC Exc

T20.712 Corrosion of third degree of left ear [any part, except ear drum]   CC POA HAC CC/MCC Exc

T20.719 Corrosion of third degree of unspecified ear [any part, except ear drum]   CC POA HAC CC/MCC Exc

T20.72 Corrosion of third degree of lip(s)   CC POA HAC CC/MCC Exc

T20.73 Corrosion of third degree of chin   CC POA HAC CC/MCC Exc

T20.74 Corrosion of third degree of nose (septum)   CC POA HAC CC/MCC Exc

T20.75 Corrosion of third degree of scalp [any part]   CC POA HAC CC/MCC Exc

T20.76 Corrosion of third degree of forehead and cheek   CC POA HAC CC/MCC Exc

T20.77 Corrosion of third degree of neck   CC POA HAC CC/MCC Exc

T20.79 Corrosion of third degree of multiple sites of head, face, and neck   CC POA HAC CC/MCC Exc

T21 Burn and corrosion of trunk

  INCLUDES burns and corrosion of hip region

  EXCLUDES2 burns and corrosion of axilla (T22.- with fifth character 4)

  burns and corrosion of scapular region (T22.- with fifth character 6)

  burns and corrosion of shoulder (T22.- with fifth character 5)

The appropriate 7th character is to be added to each code from category T21

  A = initial encounter

  D = subsequent encounter

  S = sequela

T21.0 Burn of unspecified degree of trunk
  Use additional external cause code to identify the source, place and intent of the burn (X00-X19, X75-X77, X96-X98, Y92)

T21.00 Burn of unspecified degree of trunk, unspecified site   POA

T21.01 Burn of unspecified degree of chest wall   POA
  Burn of unspecified degree of breast

T21.02 Burn of unspecified degree of abdominal wall   POA
  Burn of unspecified degree of flank
  Burn of unspecified degree of groin

T21.03 Burn of unspecified degree of upper back   POA
  Burn of unspecified degree of interscapular region

T21.04 Burn of unspecified degree of lower back   POA

T21.05 Burn of unspecified degree of buttock   POA
  Burn of unspecified degree of anus

T21.06 Burn of unspecified degree of male genital region   POA ♂
  Burn of unspecified degree of penis
  Burn of unspecified degree of scrotum
  Burn of unspecified degree of testis

T21.07 Burn of unspecified degree of female genital region   POA ♀
  Burn of unspecified degree of labium (majus) (minus)
  Burn of unspecified degree of perineum
  Burn of unspecified degree of vulva

  EXCLUDES2 burn of vagina (T28.3)

T21.09 Burn of unspecified degree of other site of trunk   POA

T21.1 Burn of first degree of trunk
  Use additional external cause code to identify the source, place and intent of the burn (X00-X19, X75-X77, X96-X98, Y92)

T21.10 Burn of first degree of trunk, unspecified site   POA

Unspecified Code	Other Specified Code	Manifestation Code	N Newborn P Pediatric M Maternity A Adult ♂ Male ♀ Female

● New Code   ▲ Revised Code Title   ►◄ Revised Text   NOTES   INCLUDES   EXCLUDES1 Not coded here   EXCLUDES2 Not included here

4ᵗʰ 4th character required   5ᵗʰ 5th character required   6ᵗʰ 6th character required   7ᵗʰ 7th character required   Extension 'X' Alert

HAC Hospital-acquired condition (HAC) alert   AHA AHA Coding Clinic©   Code first alert

T21.11 **Burn of first degree of** chest wall   POA
   Burn of first degree of breast

T21.12 **Burn of first degree of** abdominal wall   POA
   Burn of first degree of flank
   Burn of first degree of groin

T21.13 **Burn of first degree of** upper back   POA
   Burn of first degree of interscapular region

T21.14 **Burn of first degree of** lower back   POA

T21.15 **Burn of first degree of** buttock   POA

T21.16 **Burn of first degree of** male genital region   POA ♂
   Burn of first degree of penis
   Burn of first degree of scrotum
   Burn of first degree of testis

T21.17 **Burn of first degree of** female genital region   POA ♀
   Burn of first degree of labium (majus) (minus)
   Burn of first degree of perineum
   Burn of first degree of vulva
   EXCLUDES2 *burn of vagina (T28.3)*

T21.19 **Burn of first degree of** other site of trunk   POA

T21.2 **Burn of** second degree **of trunk**
   Use additional external cause code to identify the source, place and intent of the burn (X00-X19, X75-X77, X96-X98, Y92)

T21.20 **Burn of second degree of trunk, unspecified site**   POA

T21.21 **Burn of second degree of** chest wall   POA
   Burn of second degree of breast

T21.22 **Burn of second degree of** abdominal wall   POA
   Burn of second degree of flank
   Burn of second degree of groin

T21.23 **Burn of second degree of** upper back   POA
   Burn of second degree of interscapular region

T21.24 **Burn of second degree of** lower back   POA

T21.25 **Burn of second degree of** buttock   POA
   Burn of second degree of anus

T21.26 **Burn of second degree of** male genital region   POA ♂
   Burn of second degree of penis
   Burn of second degree of scrotum
   Burn of second degree of testis

T21.27 **Burn of second degree of** female genital region   POA ♀
   Burn of second degree of labium (majus) (minus)
   Burn of second degree of perineum
   Burn of second degree of vulva
   EXCLUDES2 *burn of vagina (T28.3)*

T21.29 **Burn of second degree of** other site of trunk   POA

T21.3 **Burn of** third degree **of trunk**
   Use additional external cause code to identify the source, place and intent of the burn (X00-X19, X75-X77, X96-X98, Y92)

T21.30 **Burn of third degree of trunk, unspecified site**   CC POA HAC CC/MCC Exc

T21.31 **Burn of third degree of** chest wall   CC POA HAC CC/MCC Exc
   AHA: Q2 2016
   Burn of third degree of breast

T21.32 **Burn of third degree of** abdominal wall   CC POA HAC CC/MCC Exc
   Burn of third degree of flank
   Burn of third degree of groin

T21.33 **Burn of third degree of** upper back   CC POA HAC CC/MCC Exc
   Burn of third degree of interscapular region

T21.34 **Burn of third degree of** lower back   CC POA HAC CC/MCC Exc

T21.35 **Burn of third degree of** buttock   CC POA HAC CC/MCC Exc
   Burn of third degree of anus

T21.36 **Burn of third degree of** male genital region   CC POA HAC ♂ CC/MCC Exc
   Burn of third degree of penis
   Burn of third degree of scrotum
   Burn of third degree of testis

T21.37 **Burn of third degree of** female genital region   CC POA HAC ♀ CC/MCC Exc
   Burn of third degree of labium (majus) (minus)
   Burn of third degree of perineum
   Burn of third degree of vulva
   EXCLUDES2 *burn of vagina (T28.3)*

T21.39 **Burn of third degree of** other site of trunk   CC POA HAC CC/MCC Exc

T21.4 **Corrosion of** unspecified degree **of trunk**
   ☞ Code first (T51-T65) to identify chemical and intent
   Use additional external cause code to identify place (Y92)

T21.40 **Corrosion of unspecified degree of trunk, unspecified site**   POA

T21.41 **Corrosion of unspecified degree of** chest wall   POA
   Corrosion of unspecified degree of breast

T21.42 **Corrosion of unspecified degree of** abdominal wall   POA
   Corrosion of unspecified degree of flank
   Corrosion of unspecified degree of groin

T21.43 **Corrosion of unspecified degree of** upper back   POA
   Corrosion of unspecified degree of interscapular region

T21.44 **Corrosion of unspecified degree of** lower back   POA

T21.45 **Corrosion of unspecified degree of** buttock   POA
   Corrosion of unspecified degree of anus

T21.46 **Corrosion of unspecified degree of** male genital region   POA ♂
   Corrosion of unspecified degree of penis
   Corrosion of unspecified degree of scrotum
   Corrosion of unspecified degree of testis

T21.47 **Corrosion of unspecified degree of** female genital region   POA ♀
   Corrosion of unspecified degree of labium (majus) (minus)
   Corrosion of unspecified degree of perineum
   Corrosion of unspecified degree of vulva
   EXCLUDES2 *corrosion of vagina (T28.8)*

T21.49 **Corrosion of unspecified degree of other site of trunk**   POA

T21.5 **Corrosion of** first degree **of trunk**
   ☞ Code first (T51-T65) to identify chemical and intent
   Use additional external cause code to identify place (Y92)

T21.50 **Corrosion of first degree of trunk, unspecified site**   POA

T21.51 **Corrosion of first degree of** chest wall   POA
   Corrosion of first degree of breast

T21.52 **Corrosion of first degree of** abdominal wall   POA
   Corrosion of first degree of flank
   Corrosion of first degree of groin

T21.53 **Corrosion of first degree of** upper back   POA
   Corrosion of first degree of interscapular region

T21.54 **Corrosion of first degree of** lower back   POA

T21.55 **Corrosion of first degree of** buttock   POA
   Corrosion of first degree of anus

T21.56 **Corrosion of first degree of** male genital region   POA ♂
   Corrosion of first degree of penis
   Corrosion of first degree of scrotum
   Corrosion of first degree of testis

T21.57 **Corrosion of first degree of** female genital region   POA ♀
   Corrosion of first degree of labium (majus) (minus)
   Corrosion of first degree of perineum
   Corrosion of first degree of vulva
   EXCLUDES2 *corrosion of vagina (T28.8)*

T21.59 **Corrosion of first degree of** other site of trunk   POA

T21.6 **Corrosion of** second degree **of trunk**
   ☞ Code first (T51-T65) to identify chemical and intent
   Use additional external cause code to identify place (Y92)

T21.60 **Corrosion of second degree of trunk, unspecified site**   POA

T21.61 **Corrosion of second degree of** chest wall   POA
   Corrosion of second degree of breast

T21.62 **Corrosion of second degree of** abdominal wall   POA
   Corrosion of second degree of flank
   Corrosion of second degree of groin

T21.63 **Corrosion of second degree of** upper back   POA
   Corrosion of second degree of interscapular region

T21.64 **Corrosion of second degree of** lower back   POA

T21.65 **Corrosion of second degree of** buttock   POA
   Corrosion of second degree of anus

POA Unacceptable principal diagnosis symbol per Medicare code edits   POA Code exempt from diagnosis present on admission requirement
? Questionable admission   CC Complication or comorbidity   MCC Major complication or comorbidity   CC/MCC Exc CC/MCC exclusion
HCC HCC diagnosis code   RxHCC RxHCC diagnosis code   MACRA MACRA code   **DEFINITION** Describes condition/terminology
TIP Coding guidance   ◉ Official Guideline Reference   Z1 Z code as first-listed diagnosis

⑦ T21.66 **Corrosion of second degree of** male genital
region POA ♂
Corrosion of second degree of penis
Corrosion of second degree of scrotum
Corrosion of second degree of testis

⑦ T21.67 **Corrosion of second degree of** female genital
region POA ♀
Corrosion of second degree of labium (majus) (minus)
Corrosion of second degree of perineum
Corrosion of second degree of vulva
EXCLUDES2 corrosion of vagina (T28.8)

⑦ T21.69 **Corrosion of second degree of** other site of trunk POA

⑤ T21.7 **Corrosion of** third degree **of trunk**
☞ **Code first** (T51-T65) to identify chemical and intent
Use additional external cause code to identify place (Y92)

⑦ T21.70 **Corrosion of third degree of trunk,**
unspecified site CC POA HAC CC/MCC Exc

⑦ T21.71 **Corrosion of third degree of**
chest wall CC POA HAC CC/MCC Exc
Corrosion of third degree of breast

⑦ T21.72 **Corrosion of third degree of**
abdominal wall CC POA HAC CC/MCC Exc
Corrosion of third degree of flank
Corrosion of third degree of groin

⑦ T21.73 **Corrosion of third degree of**
upper back CC POA HAC CC/MCC Exc
Corrosion of third degree of interscapular region

⑦ T21.74 **Corrosion of third degree of**
lower back CC POA HAC CC/MCC Exc

⑦ T21.75 **Corrosion of third degree of** buttock CC POA HAC CC/MCC Exc
Corrosion of third degree of anus

⑦ T21.76 **Corrosion of third degree of** male genital
region CC POA HAC ♂ CC/MCC Exc
Corrosion of third degree of penis
Corrosion of third degree of scrotum
Corrosion of third degree of testis

⑦ T21.77 **Corrosion of third degree of** female genital
region CC POA HAC ♀ CC/MCC Exc
Corrosion of third degree of labium (majus) (minus)
Corrosion of third degree of perineum
Corrosion of third degree of vulva
EXCLUDES2 corrosion of vagina (T28.8)

⑦ T21.79 **Corrosion of third degree of** other site
of trunk CC POA HAC CC/MCC Exc

④ T22 **Burn and corrosion of shoulder and upper limb, except wrist and**
hand
EXCLUDES2 burn and corrosion of interscapular region (T21.-)
burn and corrosion of wrist and hand (T23.-)

The appropriate 7th character is to be added to each code from
category T22
A = initial encounter
D = subsequent encounter
S = sequela

⑤ T22.0 **Burn of** unspecified degree **of shoulder and upper limb,**
except wrist and hand
Use additional external cause code to identify the source,
place and intent of the burn (X00-X19, X75-X77, X96-X98,
Y92)

⑦ T22.00 **Burn of unspecified degree of shoulder and upper**
limb, except wrist and hand, unspecified site POA

⑥ T22.01 **Burn of unspecified degree of** forearm
⑦ T22.011 **Burn of unspecified degree of** right
forearm POA
⑦ T22.012 **Burn of unspecified degree of** left
forearm POA
⑦ T22.019 **Burn of unspecified degree of unspecified**
forearm POA

⑥ T22.02 **Burn of unspecified degree of** elbow
⑦ T22.021 **Burn of unspecified degree of**
right elbow POA
⑦ T22.022 **Burn of unspecified degree of** left elbow POA

⑦ T22.029 **Burn of unspecified degree of**
unspecified elbow POA

⑥ T22.03 **Burn of unspecified degree of** upper arm
⑦ T22.031 **Burn of unspecified degree of** right
upper arm POA
⑦ T22.032 **Burn of unspecified degree of** left
upper arm POA
⑦ T22.039 **Burn of unspecified degree of unspecified**
upper arm POA

⑥ T22.04 **Burn of unspecified degree of** axilla
⑦ T22.041 **Burn of unspecified degree of** right
axilla POA
⑦ T22.042 **Burn of unspecified degree of** left axilla POA
⑦ T22.049 **Burn of unspecified degree of unspecified**
axilla POA

⑥ T22.05 **Burn of unspecified degree of** shoulder
⑦ T22.051 **Burn of unspecified degree of** right
shoulder POA
⑦ T22.052 **Burn of unspecified degree of** left
shoulder POA
⑦ T22.059 **Burn of unspecified degree of unspecified**
shoulder POA

⑥ T22.06 **Burn of unspecified degree of** scapular region
⑦ T22.061 **Burn of unspecified degree of** right
scapular region POA
⑦ T22.062 **Burn of unspecified degree of** left scapular
region POA
⑦ T22.069 **Burn of unspecified degree of unspecified**
scapular region POA

⑥ T22.09 **Burn of unspecified degree of** multiple sites of
shoulder and upper limb, except wrist and hand
⑦ T22.091 **Burn of unspecified degree of multiple**
sites of right shoulder and upper limb,
except wrist and hand POA
⑦ T22.092 **Burn of unspecified degree of multiple**
sites of left shoulder and upper limb,
except wrist and hand POA
⑦ T22.099 **Burn of unspecified degree of multiple**
sites of unspecified shoulder and upper
limb, except wrist and hand POA

⑤ T22.1 **Burn of** first degree **of shoulder and upper limb, except wrist**
and hand
Use additional external cause code to identify the source,
place and intent of the burn (X00-X19, X75-X77, X96-X98,
Y92)

⑦ T22.10 **Burn of first degree of shoulder and upper limb,**
except wrist and hand, unspecified site POA

⑥ T22.11 **Burn of first degree of** forearm
⑦ T22.111 **Burn of first degree of** right forearm POA
⑦ T22.112 **Burn of first degree of** left forearm POA
⑦ T22.119 **Burn of first degree of unspecified**
forearm POA

⑥ T22.12 **Burn of first degree of** elbow
⑦ T22.121 **Burn of first degree of** right elbow POA
⑦ T22.122 **Burn of first degree of** left elbow POA
⑦ T22.129 **Burn of first degree of unspecified elbow** POA

⑥ T22.13 **Burn of first degree of** upper arm
⑦ T22.131 **Burn of first degree of** right upper arm POA
⑦ T22.132 **Burn of first degree of** left upper arm POA
⑦ T22.139 **Burn of first degree of unspecified**
upper arm POA

⑥ T22.14 **Burn of first degree of** axilla
⑦ T22.141 **Burn of first degree of** right axilla POA
⑦ T22.142 **Burn of first degree of** left axilla POA
⑦ T22.149 **Burn of first degree of unspecified axilla** POA

⑥ T22.15 **Burn of first degree of** shoulder
⑦ T22.151 **Burn of first degree of** right shoulder POA
⑦ T22.152 **Burn of first degree of** left shoulder POA
⑦ T22.159 **Burn of first degree of unspecified**
shoulder POA

⑥ T22.16 **Burn of first degree of** scapular region

Unspecified Code   Other Specified Code   Manifestation Code   N Newborn   P Pediatric   M Maternity   A Adult   ♂ Male   ♀ Female
● New Code   ▲ Revised Code Title   ►◄ Revised Text   **NOTES**   *INCLUDES*   *EXCLUDES1* Not coded here   *EXCLUDES2* Not included here
④ 4ᵗʰ character required   ⑤ 5ᵗʰ character required   ⑥ 6ᵗʰ character required   ⑦ 7ᵗʰ character required   ⑦ Extension 'X' Alert
HAC Hospital-acquired condition (HAC) alert   **AHA** AHA Coding Clinic©   ☞ Code first alert

T22.161 Burn of first degree of right scapular region

T22.162 Burn of first degree of left scapular region

T22.169 Burn of first degree of unspecified scapular region

T22.19 Burn of first degree of multiple sites of shoulder and upper limb, except wrist and hand

T22.191 Burn of first degree of multiple sites of right shoulder and upper limb, except wrist and hand

T22.192 Burn of first degree of multiple sites of left shoulder and upper limb, except wrist and hand

T22.199 Burn of first degree of multiple sites of unspecified shoulder and upper limb, except wrist and hand

T22.2 Burn of second degree of shoulder and upper limb, except wrist and hand

Use additional external cause code to identify the source, place and intent of the burn (X00-X19, X75-X77, X96-X98, Y92)

T22.20 Burn of second degree of shoulder and upper limb, except wrist and hand, unspecified site

T22.21 Burn of second degree of forearm

T22.211 Burn of second degree of right forearm
T22.212 Burn of second degree of left forearm
T22.219 Burn of second degree of unspecified forearm

T22.22 Burn of second degree of elbow

T22.221 Burn of second degree of right elbow
T22.222 Burn of second degree of left elbow
T22.229 Burn of second degree of unspecified elbow

T22.23 Burn of second degree of upper arm

T22.231 Burn of second degree of right upper arm
T22.232 Burn of second degree of left upper arm
T22.239 Burn of second degree of unspecified upper arm

T22.24 Burn of second degree of axilla

T22.241 Burn of second degree of right axilla
T22.242 Burn of second degree of left axilla
T22.249 Burn of second degree of unspecified axilla

T22.25 Burn of second degree of shoulder

T22.251 Burn of second degree of right shoulder
T22.252 Burn of second degree of left shoulder
T22.259 Burn of second degree of unspecified shoulder

T22.26 Burn of second degree of scapular region

T22.261 Burn of second degree of right scapular region

T22.262 Burn of second degree of left scapular region

T22.269 Burn of second degree of unspecified scapular region

T22.29 Burn of second degree of multiple sites of shoulder and upper limb, except wrist and hand

T22.291 Burn of second degree of multiple sites of right shoulder and upper limb, except wrist and hand

T22.292 Burn of second degree of multiple sites of left shoulder and upper limb, except wrist and hand

T22.299 Burn of second degree of multiple sites of unspecified shoulder and upper limb, except wrist and hand

T22.3 Burn of third degree of shoulder and upper limb, except wrist and hand

Use additional external cause code to identify the source, place and intent of the burn (X00-X19, X75-X77, X96-X98, Y92)

T22.30 Burn of third degree of shoulder and upper limb, except wrist and hand, unspecified site

T22.31 Burn of third degree of forearm

T22.311 Burn of third degree of right forearm

T22.312 Burn of third degree of left forearm

T22.319 Burn of third degree of unspecified forearm

T22.32 Burn of third degree of elbow

T22.321 Burn of third degree of right elbow

T22.322 Burn of third degree of left elbow

T22.329 Burn of third degree of unspecified elbow

T22.33 Burn of third degree of upper arm

T22.331 Burn of third degree of right upper arm

T22.332 Burn of third degree of left upper arm

T22.339 Burn of third degree of unspecified upper arm

T22.34 Burn of third degree of axilla

T22.341 Burn of third degree of right axilla

T22.342 Burn of third degree of left axilla

T22.349 Burn of third degree of unspecified axilla

T22.35 Burn of third degree of shoulder

T22.351 Burn of third degree of right shoulder

T22.352 Burn of third degree of left shoulder

T22.359 Burn of third degree of unspecified shoulder

T22.36 Burn of third degree of scapular region

T22.361 Burn of third degree of right scapular region

T22.362 Burn of third degree of left scapular region

T22.369 Burn of third degree of unspecified scapular region

T22.39 Burn of third degree of multiple sites of shoulder and upper limb, except wrist and hand

T22.391 Burn of third degree of multiple sites of right shoulder and upper limb, except wrist and hand

T22.392 Burn of third degree of multiple sites of left shoulder and upper limb, except wrist and hand

T22.399 Burn of third degree of multiple sites of unspecified shoulder and upper limb, except wrist and hand

T22.4 Corrosion of unspecified degree of shoulder and upper limb, except wrist and hand

Code first (T51-T65) to identify chemical and intent

Use additional external cause code to identify place (Y92)

T22.40 Corrosion of unspecified degree of shoulder and upper limb, except wrist and hand, unspecified site

T22.41 Corrosion of unspecified degree of forearm

T22.411 Corrosion of unspecified degree of right forearm

T22.412 Corrosion of unspecified degree of left forearm

T22.419 Corrosion of unspecified degree of unspecified forearm

PDx Unacceptable principal diagnosis symbol per Medicare code edits   Code exempt from diagnosis present on admission requirement
? Questionable admission   CC Complication or comorbidity   MCC Major complication or comorbidity   CC/MCC Exc CC/MCC exclusion
HCC HCC diagnosis code   RxHCC RxHCC diagnosis code   MACRA code   DEFINITION Describes condition/terminology
TIP Coding guidance   Official Guideline Reference   Z1 Z code as first-listed diagnosis

1106   When symbols appear on a code that requires a 7th character extension, refer to Appendix B to identify applicable 7th character codes.   2020 ICD-10-CM

6ᵗʰ **T22.42** Corrosion of unspecified degree of elbow
   7ᵗʰ **T22.421** Corrosion of unspecified degree of right elbow POA
   7ᵗʰ **T22.422** Corrosion of unspecified degree of left elbow POA
   7ᵗʰ **T22.429** Corrosion of unspecified degree of unspecified elbow POA

6ᵗʰ **T22.43** Corrosion of unspecified degree of upper arm
   7ᵗʰ **T22.431** Corrosion of unspecified degree of right upper arm POA
   7ᵗʰ **T22.432** Corrosion of unspecified degree of left upper arm POA
   7ᵗʰ **T22.439** Corrosion of unspecified degree of unspecified upper arm POA

6ᵗʰ **T22.44** Corrosion of unspecified degree of axilla
   7ᵗʰ **T22.441** Corrosion of unspecified degree of right axilla POA
   7ᵗʰ **T22.442** Corrosion of unspecified degree of left axilla POA
   7ᵗʰ **T22.449** Corrosion of unspecified degree of unspecified axilla POA

6ᵗʰ **T22.45** Corrosion of unspecified degree of shoulder
   7ᵗʰ **T22.451** Corrosion of unspecified degree of right shoulder POA
   7ᵗʰ **T22.452** Corrosion of unspecified degree of left shoulder POA
   7ᵗʰ **T22.459** Corrosion of unspecified degree of unspecified shoulder POA

6ᵗʰ **T22.46** Corrosion of unspecified degree of scapular region
   7ᵗʰ **T22.461** Corrosion of unspecified degree of right scapular region POA
   7ᵗʰ **T22.462** Corrosion of unspecified degree of left scapular region POA
   7ᵗʰ **T22.469** Corrosion of unspecified degree of unspecified scapular region POA

5ᵗʰ **T22.49** Corrosion of unspecified degree of multiple sites of shoulder and upper limb, except wrist and hand
   7ᵗʰ **T22.491** Corrosion of unspecified degree of multiple sites of right shoulder and upper limb, except wrist and hand POA
   7ᵗʰ **T22.492** Corrosion of unspecified degree of multiple sites of left shoulder and upper limb, except wrist and hand POA
   7ᵗʰ **T22.499** Corrosion of unspecified degree of multiple sites of unspecified shoulder and upper limb, except wrist and hand POA

5ᵗʰ **T22.5** Corrosion of first degree of shoulder and upper limb, except wrist and hand
  ☞ **Code first** (T51-T65) to identify chemical and intent
    Use additional external cause code to identify place (Y92)
7ᵗʰ **T22.50** Corrosion of first degree of shoulder and upper limb, except wrist and hand unspecified site POA
6ᵗʰ **T22.51** Corrosion of first degree of forearm
   7ᵗʰ **T22.511** Corrosion of first degree of right forearm POA
   7ᵗʰ **T22.512** Corrosion of first degree of left forearm POA
   7ᵗʰ **T22.519** Corrosion of first degree of unspecified forearm POA

6ᵗʰ **T22.52** Corrosion of first degree of elbow
   7ᵗʰ **T22.521** Corrosion of first degree of right elbow POA
   7ᵗʰ **T22.522** Corrosion of first degree of left elbow POA
   7ᵗʰ **T22.529** Corrosion of first degree of unspecified elbow POA

6ᵗʰ **T22.53** Corrosion of first degree of upper arm
   7ᵗʰ **T22.531** Corrosion of first degree of right upper arm POA
   7ᵗʰ **T22.532** Corrosion of first degree of left upper arm POA
   7ᵗʰ **T22.539** Corrosion of first degree of unspecified upper arm POA

6ᵗʰ **T22.54** Corrosion of first degree of axilla
   7ᵗʰ **T22.541** Corrosion of first degree of right axilla POA

7ᵗʰ **T22.542** Corrosion of first degree of left axilla POA
   7ᵗʰ **T22.549** Corrosion of first degree of unspecified axilla POA

6ᵗʰ **T22.55** Corrosion of first degree of shoulder
   7ᵗʰ **T22.551** Corrosion of first degree of right shoulder POA
   7ᵗʰ **T22.552** Corrosion of first degree of left shoulder POA
   7ᵗʰ **T22.559** Corrosion of first degree of unspecified shoulder POA

6ᵗʰ **T22.56** Corrosion of first degree of scapular region
   7ᵗʰ **T22.561** Corrosion of first degree of right scapular region POA
   7ᵗʰ **T22.562** Corrosion of first degree of left scapular region POA
   7ᵗʰ **T22.569** Corrosion of first degree of unspecified scapular region POA

6ᵗʰ **T22.59** Corrosion of first degree of multiple sites of shoulder and upper limb, except wrist and hand
   7ᵗʰ **T22.591** Corrosion of first degree of multiple sites of right shoulder and upper limb, except wrist and hand POA
   7ᵗʰ **T22.592** Corrosion of first degree of multiple sites of left shoulder and upper limb, except wrist and hand POA
   7ᵗʰ **T22.599** Corrosion of first degree of multiple sites of unspecified shoulder and upper limb, except wrist and hand POA

5ᵗʰ **T22.6** Corrosion of second degree of shoulder and upper limb, except wrist and hand
  ☞ **Code first** (T51-T65) to identify chemical and intent
    Use additional external cause code to identify place (Y92)
7ᵗʰ **T22.60** Corrosion of second degree of shoulder and upper limb, except wrist and hand, unspecified site POA
6ᵗʰ **T22.61** Corrosion of second degree of forearm
   7ᵗʰ **T22.611** Corrosion of second degree of right forearm POA
   7ᵗʰ **T22.612** Corrosion of second degree of left forearm POA
   7ᵗʰ **T22.619** Corrosion of second degree of unspecified forearm POA

6ᵗʰ **T22.62** Corrosion of second degree of elbow
   7ᵗʰ **T22.621** Corrosion of second degree of right elbow POA
   7ᵗʰ **T22.622** Corrosion of second degree of left elbow POA
   7ᵗʰ **T22.629** Corrosion of second degree of unspecified elbow POA

6ᵗʰ **T22.63** Corrosion of second degree of upper arm
   7ᵗʰ **T22.631** Corrosion of second degree of right upper arm POA
   7ᵗʰ **T22.632** Corrosion of second degree of left upper arm POA
   7ᵗʰ **T22.639** Corrosion of second degree of unspecified upper arm POA

6ᵗʰ **T22.64** Corrosion of second degree of axilla
   7ᵗʰ **T22.641** Corrosion of second degree of right axilla POA
   7ᵗʰ **T22.642** Corrosion of second degree of left axilla POA
   7ᵗʰ **T22.649** Corrosion of second degree of unspecified axilla POA

6ᵗʰ **T22.65** Corrosion of second degree of shoulder
   7ᵗʰ **T22.651** Corrosion of second degree of right shoulder POA
   7ᵗʰ **T22.652** Corrosion of second degree of left shoulder POA
   7ᵗʰ **T22.659** Corrosion of second degree of unspecified shoulder POA

6ᵗʰ **T22.66** Corrosion of second degree of scapular region
   7ᵗʰ **T22.661** Corrosion of second degree of right scapular region POA
   7ᵗʰ **T22.662** Corrosion of second degree of left scapular region POA

Unspecified Code   Other Specified Code   Manifestation Code   N Newborn   P Pediatric   M Maternity   A Adult   ♂ Male   ♀ Female
● New Code   ▲ Revised Code Title   ▶◀ Revised Text   **NOTES**   *INCLUDES*   *EXCLUDES1* Not coded here   *EXCLUDES2* Not included here
4ᵗʰ 4ᵗʰ character required   5ᵗʰ 5ᵗʰ character required   6ᵗʰ 6ᵗʰ character required   7ᵗʰ 7ᵗʰ character required   ⊗ Extension 'X' Alert
HAC Hospital-acquired condition (HAC) alert   **AHA** AHA Coding Clinic©   ☞ Code first alert

T22.669 - T23.09

CHAPTER 19: INJURY, POISONING, AND CERTAIN OTHER CONSEQUENCES OF EXTERNAL CAUSES (S00-T88)

7th **T22.669** Corrosion of second degree of unspecified scapular region POA

5th **T22.69** Corrosion of second degree of multiple sites of shoulder and upper limb, except wrist and hand

7th **T22.691** Corrosion of second degree of multiple sites of right shoulder and upper limb, except wrist and hand POA

7th **T22.692** Corrosion of second degree of multiple sites of left shoulder and upper limb, except wrist and hand POA

7th **T22.699** Corrosion of second degree of multiple sites of unspecified shoulder and upper limb, except wrist and hand POA

5th **T22.7** Corrosion of third degree of shoulder and upper limb, except wrist and hand

☞ **Code first** (T51-T65) to identify chemical and intent
Use additional external cause code to identify place (Y92)

7th **T22.70** Corrosion of third degree of shoulder and upper limb, except wrist and hand, unspecified site CC POA HAC CC/MCC Exc

6th **T22.71** Corrosion of third degree of forearm

7th **T22.711** Corrosion of third degree of right forearm CC POA HAC CC/MCC Exc

7th **T22.712** Corrosion of third degree of left forearm CC POA HAC CC/MCC Exc

7th **T22.719** Corrosion of third degree of unspecified forearm CC POA HAC CC/MCC Exc

6th **T22.72** Corrosion of third degree of elbow

7th **T22.721** Corrosion of third degree of right elbow CC POA HAC CC/MCC Exc

7th **T22.722** Corrosion of third degree of left elbow CC POA HAC CC/MCC Exc

7th **T22.729** Corrosion of third degree of unspecified elbow CC POA HAC CC/MCC Exc

6th **T22.73** Corrosion of third degree of upper arm

7th **T22.731** Corrosion of third degree of right upper arm CC POA HAC CC/MCC Exc

7th **T22.732** Corrosion of third degree of left upper arm CC POA HAC CC/MCC Exc

7th **T22.739** Corrosion of third degree of unspecified upper arm CC POA HAC CC/MCC Exc

6th **T22.74** Corrosion of third degree of axilla

7th **T22.741** Corrosion of third degree of right axilla CC POA HAC CC/MCC Exc

7th **T22.742** Corrosion of third degree of left axilla CC POA HAC CC/MCC Exc

7th **T22.749** Corrosion of third degree of unspecified axilla CC POA HAC CC/MCC Exc

6th **T22.75** Corrosion of third degree of shoulder

7th **T22.751** Corrosion of third degree of right shoulder CC POA HAC CC/MCC Exc

7th **T22.752** Corrosion of third degree of left shoulder CC POA HAC CC/MCC Exc

7th **T22.759** Corrosion of third degree of unspecified shoulder CC POA HAC CC/MCC Exc

6th **T22.76** Corrosion of third degree of scapular region

7th **T22.761** Corrosion of third degree of right scapular region CC POA HAC CC/MCC Exc

7th **T22.762** Corrosion of third degree of left scapular region CC POA HAC CC/MCC Exc

7th **T22.769** Corrosion of third degree of unspecified scapular region CC POA HAC CC/MCC Exc

6th **T22.79** Corrosion of third degree of multiple sites of shoulder and upper limb, except wrist and hand

7th **T22.791** Corrosion of third degree of multiple sites of right shoulder and upper limb, except wrist and hand CC POA HAC CC/MCC Exc

7th **T22.792** Corrosion of third degree of multiple sites of left shoulder and upper limb, except wrist and hand CC POA HAC CC/MCC Exc

7th **T22.799** Corrosion of third degree of multiple sites of unspecified shoulder and upper limb, except wrist and hand CC POA HAC CC/MCC Exc

4th **T23** Burn and corrosion of wrist and hand

The appropriate 7th character is to be added to each code from category T23

A = initial encounter
D = subsequent encounter
S = sequela

5th **T23.0** Burn of unspecified degree of wrist and hand

Use additional external cause code to identify the source, place and intent of the burn (X00-X19, X75-X77, X96-X98, Y92)

6th **T23.00** Burn of unspecified degree of hand, unspecified site

7th **T23.001** Burn of unspecified degree of right hand, unspecified site POA

7th **T23.002** Burn of unspecified degree of left hand, unspecified site POA

7th **T23.009** Burn of unspecified degree of unspecified hand, unspecified site POA

6th **T23.01** Burn of unspecified degree of thumb (nail)

7th **T23.011** Burn of unspecified degree of right thumb (nail) POA

7th **T23.012** Burn of unspecified degree of left thumb (nail) POA

7th **T23.019** Burn of unspecified degree of unspecified thumb (nail) POA

6th **T23.02** Burn of unspecified degree of single finger (nail) except thumb

7th **T23.021** Burn of unspecified degree of single right finger (nail) except thumb POA

7th **T23.022** Burn of unspecified degree of single left finger (nail) except thumb POA

7th **T23.029** Burn of unspecified degree of unspecified single finger (nail) except thumb POA

6th **T23.03** Burn of unspecified degree of multiple fingers (nail), not including thumb

7th **T23.031** Burn of unspecified degree of multiple right fingers (nail), not including thumb POA

7th **T23.032** Burn of unspecified degree of multiple left fingers (nail), not including thumb POA

7th **T23.039** Burn of unspecified degree of unspecified multiple fingers (nail), not including thumb POA

6th **T23.04** Burn of unspecified degree of multiple fingers (nail), including thumb

7th **T23.041** Burn of unspecified degree of multiple right fingers (nail), including thumb POA

7th **T23.042** Burn of unspecified degree of multiple left fingers (nail), including thumb POA

7th **T23.049** Burn of unspecified degree of unspecified multiple fingers (nail), including thumb POA

6th **T23.05** Burn of unspecified degree of palm

7th **T23.051** Burn of unspecified degree of right palm POA

7th **T23.052** Burn of unspecified degree of left palm POA

7th **T23.059** Burn of unspecified degree of unspecified palm POA

6th **T23.06** Burn of unspecified degree of back of hand

7th **T23.061** Burn of unspecified degree of back of right hand POA

7th **T23.062** Burn of unspecified degree of back of left hand POA

7th **T23.069** Burn of unspecified degree of back of unspecified hand POA

6th **T23.07** Burn of unspecified degree of wrist

7th **T23.071** Burn of unspecified degree of right wrist POA

7th **T23.072** Burn of unspecified degree of left wrist POA

7th **T23.079** Burn of unspecified degree of unspecified wrist POA

6th **T23.09** Burn of unspecified degree of multiple sites of wrist and hand

---

POA Unacceptable principal diagnosis symbol per Medicare code edits   POA Code exempt from diagnosis present on admission requirement

❓ Questionable admission   CC Complication or comorbidity   MCC Major complication or comorbidity   CC/MCC Exc CC/MCC exclusion

HCC HCC diagnosis code   RxHCC RxHCC diagnosis code   MACRA MACRA code   **DEFINITION** Describes condition/terminology

TIP Coding guidance   👁 Official Guideline Reference   Z1 Z code as first-listed diagnosis

1108   When symbols appear on a code that requires a 7th character extension, refer to Appendix B to identify applicable 7th character codes.   **2020 ICD-10-CM**

- [7th] T23.091 Burn of unspecified degree of multiple sites of right wrist and hand [POA]
- [7th] T23.092 Burn of unspecified degree of multiple sites of left wrist and hand [POA]
- [7th] T23.099 Burn of unspecified degree of multiple sites of unspecified wrist and hand [POA]

[5th] T23.1 Burn of first degree of wrist and hand

Use additional external cause code to identify the source, place and intent of the burn (X00-X19, X75-X77, X96-X98, Y92)

- [6th] T23.10 Burn of first degree of hand, unspecified site
  - [7th] T23.101 Burn of first degree of right hand, unspecified site [POA]
  - [7th] T23.102 Burn of first degree of left hand, unspecified site [POA]
  - [7th] T23.109 Burn of first degree of unspecified hand, unspecified site [POA]
- [6th] T23.11 Burn of first degree of thumb (nail)
  - [7th] T23.111 Burn of first degree of right thumb (nail) [POA]
  - [7th] T23.112 Burn of first degree of left thumb (nail) [POA]
  - [7th] T23.119 Burn of first degree of unspecified thumb (nail) [POA]
- [6th] T23.12 Burn of first degree of single finger (nail) except thumb
  - [7th] T23.121 Burn of first degree of single right finger (nail) except thumb [POA]
  - [7th] T23.122 Burn of first degree of single left finger (nail) except thumb [POA]
  - [7th] T23.129 Burn of first degree of unspecified single finger (nail) except thumb [POA]
- [6th] T23.13 Burn of first degree of multiple fingers (nail), not including thumb
  - [7th] T23.131 Burn of first degree of multiple right fingers (nail), not including thumb [POA]
  - [7th] T23.132 Burn of first degree of multiple left fingers (nail), not including thumb [POA]
  - [7th] T23.139 Burn of first degree of unspecified multiple fingers (nail), not including thumb [POA]
- [6th] T23.14 Burn of first degree of multiple fingers (nail), including thumb
  - [7th] T23.141 Burn of first degree of multiple right fingers (nail), including thumb [POA]
  - [7th] T23.142 Burn of first degree of multiple left fingers (nail), including thumb [POA]
  - [7th] T23.149 Burn of first degree of unspecified multiple fingers (nail), including thumb [POA]
- [6th] T23.15 Burn of first degree of palm
  - [7th] T23.151 Burn of first degree of right palm [POA]
  - [7th] T23.152 Burn of first degree of left palm [POA]
  - [7th] T23.159 Burn of first degree of unspecified palm [POA]
- [6th] T23.16 Burn of first degree of back of hand
  - [7th] T23.161 Burn of first degree of back of right hand [POA]
  - [7th] T23.162 Burn of first degree of back of left hand [POA]
  - [7th] T23.169 Burn of first degree of back of unspecified hand [POA]
- [6th] T23.17 Burn of first degree of wrist
  - [7th] T23.171 Burn of first degree of right wrist [POA]
  - [7th] T23.172 Burn of first degree of left wrist [POA]
  - [7th] T23.179 Burn of first degree of unspecified wrist [POA]
- [6th] T23.19 Burn of first degree of multiple sites of wrist and hand
  - [7th] T23.191 Burn of first degree of multiple sites of right wrist and hand [POA]
  - [7th] T23.192 Burn of first degree of multiple sites of left wrist and hand [POA]
  - [7th] T23.199 Burn of first degree of multiple sites of unspecified wrist and hand [POA]

[5th] T23.2 Burn of second degree of wrist and hand

Use additional external cause code to identify the source, place and intent of the burn (X00-X19, X75-X77, X96-X98, Y92)

- [6th] T23.20 Burn of second degree of hand, unspecified site
  - [7th] T23.201 Burn of second degree of right hand, unspecified site [POA]
  - [7th] T23.202 Burn of second degree of left hand, unspecified site [POA]
  - [7th] T23.209 Burn of second degree of unspecified hand, unspecified site [POA]
- [6th] T23.21 Burn of second degree of thumb (nail)
  - [7th] T23.211 Burn of second degree of right thumb (nail) [POA]
  - [7th] T23.212 Burn of second degree of left thumb (nail) [POA]
  - [7th] T23.219 Burn of second degree of unspecified thumb (nail) [POA]
- [6th] T23.22 Burn of second degree of single finger (nail) except thumb
  - [7th] T23.221 Burn of second degree of single right finger (nail) except thumb [POA]
  - [7th] T23.222 Burn of second degree of single left finger (nail) except thumb [POA]
  - [7th] T23.229 Burn of second degree of unspecified single finger (nail) except thumb [POA]
- [6th] T23.23 Burn of second degree of multiple fingers (nail), not including thumb
  - [7th] T23.231 Burn of second degree of multiple right fingers (nail), not including thumb [POA]
  - [7th] T23.232 Burn of second degree of multiple left fingers (nail), not including thumb [POA]
  - [7th] T23.239 Burn of second degree of unspecified multiple fingers (nail), not including thumb [POA]
- [6th] T23.24 Burn of second degree of multiple fingers (nail), including thumb
  - [7th] T23.241 Burn of second degree of multiple right fingers (nail), including thumb [POA]
  - [7th] T23.242 Burn of second degree of multiple left fingers (nail), including thumb [POA]
  - [7th] T23.249 Burn of second degree of unspecified multiple fingers (nail), including thumb [POA]
- [6th] T23.25 Burn of second degree of palm
  - [7th] T23.251 Burn of second degree of right palm [POA]
  - [7th] T23.252 Burn of second degree of left palm [POA]
  - [7th] T23.259 Burn of second degree of unspecified palm [POA]
- [6th] T23.26 Burn of second degree of back of hand
  - [7th] T23.261 Burn of second degree of back of right hand [POA]
  - [7th] T23.262 Burn of second degree of back of left hand [POA]
  - [7th] T23.269 Burn of second degree of back of unspecified hand [POA]
- [6th] T23.27 Burn of second degree of wrist
  - [7th] T23.271 Burn of second degree of right wrist [POA]
  - [7th] T23.272 Burn of second degree of left wrist [POA]
  - [7th] T23.279 Burn of second degree of unspecified wrist [POA]
- [6th] T23.29 Burn of second degree of multiple sites of wrist and hand
  - [7th] T23.291 Burn of second degree of multiple sites of right wrist and hand [POA]
  - [7th] T23.292 Burn of second degree of multiple sites of left wrist and hand [POA]
  - [7th] T23.299 Burn of second degree of multiple sites of unspecified wrist and hand [POA]

[5th] T23.3 Burn of third degree of wrist and hand

Use additional external cause code to identify the source, place and intent of the burn (X00-X19, X75-X77, X96-X98, Y92)

- [6th] T23.30 Burn of third degree of hand, unspecified site
  - [7th] T23.301 Burn of third degree of right hand, unspecified site [CC] [POA] [HAC] [CC/MCC Exc]
    AHA: Q1 2015
  - [7th] T23.302 Burn of third degree of left hand, unspecified site [CC] [POA] [HAC] [CC/MCC Exc]
    AHA: Q2 2016

Unspecified Code | Other Specified Code | Manifestation Code | [N] Newborn | [P] Pediatric | [M] Maternity | [A] Adult | ♂ Male | ♀ Female
● New Code | ▲ Revised Code Title | ►◄ Revised Text | [NOTES] | [INCLUDES] | [EXCLUDES1] Not coded here | [EXCLUDES2] Not included here
[4th] 4th character required | [5th] 5th character required | [6th] 6th character required | [7th] 7th character required | [x] Extension 'X' Alert
[HAC] Hospital-acquired condition (HAC) alert | AHA AHA Coding Clinic© | ☞ Code first alert

7ᵗʰ **T23.309** Burn of third degree of unspecified hand, unspecified site cc⊘ ᴘᴏₐ̸ HAC ᴄᴄ/ᴍᴄᴄ ᴇₓᴄ⊘

5ᵗʰ **T23.31** Burn of third degree of thumb (nail)

7ᵗʰ **T23.311** Burn of third degree of right thumb (nail)

7ᵗʰ **T23.312** Burn of third degree of left thumb (nail) cc⊘ ᴘᴏₐ̸ HAC ᴄᴄ/ᴍᴄᴄ ᴇₓᴄ⊘

7ᵗʰ **T23.319** Burn of third degree of unspecified thumb (nail)

6ᵗʰ **T23.32** Burn of third degree of single finger (nail) except thumb

7ᵗʰ **T23.321** Burn of third degree of single right finger (nail) except thumb

7ᵗʰ **T23.322** Burn of third degree of single left finger (nail) except thumb

7ᵗʰ **T23.329** Burn of third degree of unspecified single finger (nail) except thumb cc⊘ ᴘᴏₐ̸ HAC ᴄᴄ/ᴍᴄᴄ ᴇₓᴄ⊘

6ᵗʰ **T23.33** Burn of third degree of multiple fingers (nail), not including thumb

7ᵗʰ **T23.331** Burn of third degree of multiple right fingers (nail), not including thumb cc⊘ ᴘᴏₐ̸ HAC ᴄᴄ/ᴍᴄᴄ ᴇₓᴄ⊘

7ᵗʰ **T23.332** Burn of third degree of multiple left fingers (nail), not including thumb

7ᵗʰ **T23.339** Burn of third degree of unspecified multiple fingers (nail), not including thumb cc⊘ ᴘᴏₐ̸ HAC ᴄᴄ/ᴍᴄᴄ ᴇₓᴄ⊘

6ᵗʰ **T23.34** Burn of third degree of multiple fingers (nail), including thumb

7ᵗʰ **T23.341** Burn of third degree of multiple right fingers (nail), including thumb cc⊘ ᴘᴏₐ̸ HAC ᴄᴄ/ᴍᴄᴄ ᴇₓᴄ⊘

7ᵗʰ **T23.342** Burn of third degree of multiple left fingers (nail), including thumb

7ᵗʰ **T23.349** Burn of third degree of unspecified multiple fingers (nail), including thumb cc⊘ ᴘᴏₐ̸ HAC ᴄᴄ/ᴍᴄᴄ ᴇₓᴄ⊘

6ᵗʰ **T23.35** Burn of third degree of palm

7ᵗʰ **T23.351** Burn of third degree of right palm cc⊘ ᴘᴏₐ̸ HAC ᴄᴄ/ᴍᴄᴄ ᴇₓᴄ⊘

7ᵗʰ **T23.352** Burn of third degree of left palm cc⊘ ᴘᴏₐ̸ HAC ᴄᴄ/ᴍᴄᴄ ᴇₓᴄ⊘

7ᵗʰ **T23.359** Burn of third degree of unspecified palm cc⊘ ᴘᴏₐ̸ HAC ᴄᴄ/ᴍᴄᴄ ᴇₓᴄ⊘

6ᵗʰ **T23.36** Burn of third degree of back of hand

7ᵗʰ **T23.361** Burn of third degree of back of right hand cc⊘ ᴘᴏₐ̸ HAC ᴄᴄ/ᴍᴄᴄ ᴇₓᴄ⊘

7ᵗʰ **T23.362** Burn of third degree of back of left hand cc⊘ ᴘᴏₐ̸ HAC ᴄᴄ/ᴍᴄᴄ ᴇₓᴄ⊘

7ᵗʰ **T23.369** Burn of third degree of back of unspecified hand cc⊘ ᴘᴏₐ̸ HAC ᴄᴄ/ᴍᴄᴄ ᴇₓᴄ⊘

6ᵗʰ **T23.37** Burn of third degree of wrist

7ᵗʰ **T23.371** Burn of third degree of right wrist cc⊘ ᴘᴏₐ̸ HAC ᴄᴄ/ᴍᴄᴄ ᴇₓᴄ⊘

7ᵗʰ **T23.372** Burn of third degree of left wrist cc⊘ ᴘᴏₐ̸ HAC ᴄᴄ/ᴍᴄᴄ ᴇₓᴄ⊘

7ᵗʰ **T23.379** Burn of third degree of unspecified wrist cc⊘ ᴘᴏₐ̸ HAC ᴄᴄ/ᴍᴄᴄ ᴇₓᴄ⊘

6ᵗʰ **T23.39** Burn of third degree of multiple sites of wrist and hand

7ᵗʰ **T23.391** Burn of third degree of multiple sites of right wrist and hand cc⊘ ᴘᴏₐ̸ HAC ᴄᴄ/ᴍᴄᴄ ᴇₓᴄ⊘

7ᵗʰ **T23.392** Burn of third degree of multiple sites of left wrist and hand cc⊘ ᴘᴏₐ̸ HAC ᴄᴄ/ᴍᴄᴄ ᴇₓᴄ⊘

7ᵗʰ **T23.399** Burn of third degree of multiple sites of unspecified wrist and hand cc⊘ ᴘᴏₐ̸ HAC ᴄᴄ/ᴍᴄᴄ ᴇₓᴄ⊘

5ᵗʰ **T23.4** Corrosion of unspecified degree of wrist and hand

☞ **Code first** (T51-T65) to identify chemical and intent

Use additional external cause code to identify place (Y92)

6ᵗʰ **T23.40** Corrosion of unspecified degree of hand, unspecified site

7ᵗʰ **T23.401** Corrosion of unspecified degree of right hand, unspecified site ᴘᴏₐ̸

7ᵗʰ **T23.402** Corrosion of unspecified degree of left hand, unspecified site ᴘᴏₐ̸

7ᵗʰ **T23.409** Corrosion of unspecified degree of unspecified hand, unspecified site ᴘᴏₐ̸

6ᵗʰ **T23.41** Corrosion of unspecified degree of thumb (nail)

7ᵗʰ **T23.411** Corrosion of unspecified degree of right thumb (nail) ᴘᴏₐ̸

7ᵗʰ **T23.412** Corrosion of unspecified degree of left thumb (nail) ᴘᴏₐ̸

7ᵗʰ **T23.419** Corrosion of unspecified degree of unspecified thumb (nail) ᴘᴏₐ̸

6ᵗʰ **T23.42** Corrosion of unspecified degree of single finger (nail) except thumb

7ᵗʰ **T23.421** Corrosion of unspecified degree of single right finger (nail) except thumb ᴘᴏₐ̸

7ᵗʰ **T23.422** Corrosion of unspecified degree of single left finger (nail) except thumb ᴘᴏₐ̸

7ᵗʰ **T23.429** Corrosion of unspecified degree of unspecified single finger (nail) except thumb ᴘᴏₐ̸

6ᵗʰ **T23.43** Corrosion of unspecified degree of multiple fingers (nail), not including thumb

7ᵗʰ **T23.431** Corrosion of unspecified degree of multiple right fingers (nail), not including thumb ᴘᴏₐ̸

7ᵗʰ **T23.432** Corrosion of unspecified degree of multiple left fingers (nail), not including thumb ᴘᴏₐ̸

7ᵗʰ **T23.439** Corrosion of unspecified degree of unspecified multiple fingers (nail), not including thumb ᴘᴏₐ̸

6ᵗʰ **T23.44** Corrosion of unspecified degree of multiple fingers (nail), including thumb

7ᵗʰ **T23.441** Corrosion of unspecified degree of multiple right fingers (nail), including thumb ᴘᴏₐ̸

7ᵗʰ **T23.442** Corrosion of unspecified degree of multiple left fingers (nail), including thumb ᴘᴏₐ̸

7ᵗʰ **T23.449** Corrosion of unspecified degree of unspecified multiple fingers (nail), including thumb ᴘᴏₐ̸

6ᵗʰ **T23.45** Corrosion of unspecified degree of palm

7ᵗʰ **T23.451** Corrosion of unspecified degree of right palm ᴘᴏₐ̸

7ᵗʰ **T23.452** Corrosion of unspecified degree of left palm ᴘᴏₐ̸

7ᵗʰ **T23.459** Corrosion of unspecified degree of unspecified palm ᴘᴏₐ̸

6ᵗʰ **T23.46** Corrosion of unspecified degree of back of hand

7ᵗʰ **T23.461** Corrosion of unspecified degree of back of right hand ᴘᴏₐ̸

7ᵗʰ **T23.462** Corrosion of unspecified degree of back of left hand ᴘᴏₐ̸

7ᵗʰ **T23.469** Corrosion of unspecified degree of back of unspecified hand ᴘᴏₐ̸

6ᵗʰ **T23.47** Corrosion of unspecified degree of wrist

7ᵗʰ **T23.471** Corrosion of unspecified degree of right wrist ᴘᴏₐ̸

7ᵗʰ **T23.472** Corrosion of unspecified degree of left wrist ᴘᴏₐ̸

7ᵗʰ **T23.479** Corrosion of unspecified degree of unspecified wrist ᴘᴏₐ̸

6ᵗʰ **T23.49** Corrosion of unspecified degree of multiple sites of wrist and hand

7ᵗʰ **T23.491** Corrosion of unspecified degree of multiple sites of right wrist and hand ᴘᴏₐ̸

ᴘᴏₓ̸ Unacceptable principal diagnosis symbol per Medicare code edits   ᴘᴏₐ̸ Code exempt from diagnosis present on admission requirement

❓ Questionable admission   cc⊘ Complication or comorbidity   ᴍᴄᴄ⊘ Major complication or comorbidity   ᴄᴄ/ᴍᴄᴄ ᴇₓᴄ⊘ CC/MCC exclusion

HCC HCC diagnosis code   ᴿᴴᶜᶜ RxHCC diagnosis code   MACRA code   **DEFINITION** Describes condition/terminology

TIP Coding guidance   👁 Official Guideline Reference   Z1 Z code as first-listed diagnosis

[7th] T23.492 Corrosion of unspecified degree of multiple sites of left wrist and hand POA
[7th] T23.499 Corrosion of unspecified degree of multiple sites of unspecified wrist and hand POA
[5th] T23.5 Corrosion of first degree of wrist and hand
☛ Code first (T51-T65) to identify chemical and intent
Use additional external cause code to identify place (Y92)
[6th] T23.50 Corrosion of first degree of hand, unspecified site
[7th] T23.501 Corrosion of first degree of right hand, unspecified site POA
[7th] T23.502 Corrosion of first degree of left hand, unspecified site POA
[7th] T23.509 Corrosion of first degree of unspecified hand, unspecified site POA
[6th] T23.51 Corrosion of first degree of thumb (nail)
[7th] T23.511 Corrosion of first degree of right thumb (nail) POA
[7th] T23.512 Corrosion of first degree of left thumb (nail) POA
[7th] T23.519 Corrosion of first degree of unspecified thumb (nail) POA
[6th] T23.52 Corrosion of first degree of single finger (nail) except thumb
[7th] T23.521 Corrosion of first degree of single right finger (nail) except thumb POA
[7th] T23.522 Corrosion of first degree of single left finger (nail) except thumb POA
[7th] T23.529 Corrosion of first degree of unspecified single finger (nail) except thumb POA
[6th] T23.53 Corrosion of first degree of multiple fingers (nail), not including thumb
[7th] T23.531 Corrosion of first degree of multiple right fingers (nail), not including thumb POA
[7th] T23.532 Corrosion of first degree of multiple left fingers (nail), not including thumb POA
[7th] T23.539 Corrosion of first degree of unspecified multiple fingers (nail), not including thumb POA
[6th] T23.54 Corrosion of first degree of multiple fingers (nail), including thumb
[7th] T23.541 Corrosion of first degree of multiple right fingers (nail), including thumb POA
[7th] T23.542 Corrosion of first degree of multiple left fingers (nail), including thumb POA
[7th] T23.549 Corrosion of first degree of unspecified multiple fingers (nail), including thumb POA
[6th] T23.55 Corrosion of first degree of palm
[7th] T23.551 Corrosion of first degree of right palm POA
[7th] T23.552 Corrosion of first degree of left palm POA
[7th] T23.559 Corrosion of first degree of unspecified palm POA
[6th] T23.56 Corrosion of first degree of back of hand
[7th] T23.561 Corrosion of first degree of back of right hand POA
[7th] T23.562 Corrosion of first degree of back of left hand POA
[7th] T23.569 Corrosion of first degree of back of unspecified hand POA
[6th] T23.57 Corrosion of first degree of wrist
[7th] T23.571 Corrosion of first degree of right wrist POA
[7th] T23.572 Corrosion of first degree of left wrist POA
[7th] T23.579 Corrosion of first degree of unspecified wrist POA
[6th] T23.59 Corrosion of first degree of multiple sites of wrist and hand
[7th] T23.591 Corrosion of first degree of multiple sites of right wrist and hand POA
[7th] T23.592 Corrosion of first degree of multiple sites of left wrist and hand POA
[7th] T23.599 Corrosion of first degree of multiple sites of unspecified wrist and hand POA
[5th] T23.6 Corrosion of second degree of wrist and hand
☛ Code first (T51-T65) to identify chemical and intent
Use additional external cause code to identify place (Y92)
[6th] T23.60 Corrosion of second degree of hand, unspecified site
[7th] T23.601 Corrosion of second degree of right hand, unspecified site POA
[7th] T23.602 Corrosion of second degree of left hand, unspecified site POA
[7th] T23.609 Corrosion of second degree of unspecified hand, unspecified site POA
[6th] T23.61 Corrosion of second degree of thumb (nail)
[7th] T23.611 Corrosion of second degree of right thumb (nail) POA
[7th] T23.612 Corrosion of second degree of left thumb (nail) POA
[7th] T23.619 Corrosion of second degree of unspecified thumb (nail) POA
[6th] T23.62 Corrosion of second degree of single finger (nail) except thumb
[7th] T23.621 Corrosion of second degree of single right finger (nail) except thumb POA
[7th] T23.622 Corrosion of second degree of single left finger (nail) except thumb POA
[7th] T23.629 Corrosion of second degree of unspecified single finger (nail) except thumb POA
[6th] T23.63 Corrosion of second degree of multiple fingers (nail), not including thumb
[7th] T23.631 Corrosion of second degree of multiple right fingers (nail), not including thumb POA
[7th] T23.632 Corrosion of second degree of multiple left fingers (nail), not including thumb POA
[7th] T23.639 Corrosion of second degree of unspecified multiple fingers (nail), not including thumb POA
[6th] T23.64 Corrosion of second degree of multiple fingers (nail), including thumb
[7th] T23.641 Corrosion of second degree of multiple right fingers (nail), including thumb POA
[7th] T23.642 Corrosion of second degree of multiple left fingers (nail), including thumb POA
[7th] T23.649 Corrosion of second degree of unspecified multiple fingers (nail), including thumb POA
[6th] T23.65 Corrosion of second degree of palm
[7th] T23.651 Corrosion of second degree of right palm POA
[7th] T23.652 Corrosion of second degree of left palm POA
[7th] T23.659 Corrosion of second degree of unspecified palm POA
[6th] T23.66 Corrosion of second degree of back of hand
[7th] T23.661 Corrosion of second degree back of right hand POA
[7th] T23.662 Corrosion of second degree back of left hand POA
[7th] T23.669 Corrosion of second degree back of unspecified hand POA
[6th] T23.67 Corrosion of second degree of wrist
[7th] T23.671 Corrosion of second degree of right wrist POA
[7th] T23.672 Corrosion of second degree of left wrist POA
[7th] T23.679 Corrosion of second degree of unspecified wrist POA
[6th] T23.69 Corrosion of second degree of multiple sites of wrist and hand
[7th] T23.691 Corrosion of second degree of multiple sites of right wrist and hand POA
[7th] T23.692 Corrosion of second degree of multiple sites of left wrist and hand POA

[7th] T23.699 Corrosion of second degree of multiple sites of unspecified wrist and hand POA

[5th] T23.7 Corrosion of third degree of wrist and hand

☞ Code first (T51-T65) to identify chemical and intent

Use additional external cause code to identify place (Y92)

[6th] T23.70 Corrosion of third degree of hand, unspecified site

[7th] T23.701 Corrosion of third degree of right hand, unspecified site CC POA [HAC] CC/MCC Exc

[7th] T23.702 Corrosion of third degree of left hand, unspecified site CC POA [HAC] CC/MCC Exc

[7th] T23.709 Corrosion of third degree of unspecified hand, unspecified site CC POA [HAC] CC/MCC Exc

[6th] T23.71 Corrosion of third degree of thumb (nail)

[7th] T23.711 Corrosion of third degree of right thumb (nail) CC POA [HAC] CC/MCC Exc

[7th] T23.712 Corrosion of third degree of left thumb (nail) CC POA [HAC] CC/MCC Exc

[7th] T23.719 Corrosion of third degree of unspecified thumb (nail) CC POA [HAC] CC/MCC Exc

[6th] T23.72 Corrosion of third degree of single finger (nail) except thumb

[7th] T23.721 Corrosion of third degree of single right finger (nail) except thumb CC POA [HAC] CC/MCC Exc

[7th] T23.722 Corrosion of third degree of single left finger (nail) except thumb CC POA [HAC] CC/MCC Exc

[7th] T23.729 Corrosion of third degree of unspecified single finger (nail) except thumb CC POA [HAC] CC/MCC Exc

[6th] T23.73 Corrosion of third degree of multiple fingers (nail), not including thumb

[7th] T23.731 Corrosion of third degree of multiple right fingers (nail), not including thumb CC POA [HAC] CC/MCC Exc

[7th] T23.732 Corrosion of third degree of multiple left fingers (nail), not including thumb CC POA [HAC] CC/MCC Exc

[7th] T23.739 Corrosion of third degree of unspecified multiple fingers (nail), not including thumb CC POA [HAC] CC/MCC Exc

[6th] T23.74 Corrosion of third degree of multiple fingers (nail), including thumb

[7th] T23.741 Corrosion of third degree of multiple right fingers (nail), including thumb CC POA [HAC] CC/MCC Exc

[7th] T23.742 Corrosion of third degree of multiple left fingers (nail), including thumb CC POA [HAC] CC/MCC Exc

[7th] T23.749 Corrosion of third degree of unspecified multiple fingers (nail), including thumb CC POA [HAC] CC/MCC Exc

[6th] T23.75 Corrosion of third degree of palm

[7th] T23.751 Corrosion of third degree of right palm CC POA [HAC] CC/MCC Exc

[7th] T23.752 Corrosion of third degree of left palm CC POA [HAC] CC/MCC Exc

[7th] T23.759 Corrosion of third degree of unspecified palm CC POA [HAC] CC/MCC Exc

[6th] T23.76 Corrosion of third degree of back of hand

[7th] T23.761 Corrosion of third degree of back of right hand CC POA [HAC] CC/MCC Exc

[7th] T23.762 Corrosion of third degree of back of left hand CC POA [HAC] CC/MCC Exc

[7th] T23.769 Corrosion of third degree back of unspecified hand CC POA [HAC] CC/MCC Exc

[6th] T23.77 Corrosion of third degree of wrist

[7th] T23.771 Corrosion of third degree of right wrist CC POA [HAC] CC/MCC Exc

[7th] T23.772 Corrosion of third degree of left wrist CC POA [HAC] CC/MCC Exc

[7th] T23.779 Corrosion of third degree of unspecified wrist CC POA [HAC] CC/MCC Exc

[6th] T23.79 Corrosion of third degree of multiple sites of wrist and hand

[7th] T23.791 Corrosion of third degree of multiple sites of right wrist and hand CC POA [HAC] CC/MCC Exc

[7th] T23.792 Corrosion of third degree of multiple sites of left wrist and hand CC POA [HAC] CC/MCC Exc

[7th] T23.799 Corrosion of third degree of multiple sites of unspecified wrist and hand CC POA [HAC] CC/MCC Exc

[4th] T24 Burn and corrosion of lower limb, except ankle and foot

[EXCLUDES2] *burn and corrosion of ankle and foot (T25.-)*

burn and corrosion of hip region (T21.-)

The appropriate 7th character is to be added to each code from category T24

A = initial encounter

D = subsequent encounter

S = sequela

[5th] T24.0 Burn of unspecified degree of lower limb, except ankle and foot

Use additional external cause code to identify the source, place and intent of the burn (X00-X19, X75-X77, X96-X98, Y92)

[6th] T24.00 Burn of unspecified degree of unspecified site of lower limb, except ankle and foot

[7th] T24.001 Burn of unspecified degree of unspecified site of right lower limb, except ankle and foot POA

[7th] T24.002 Burn of unspecified degree of unspecified site of left lower limb, except ankle and foot POA

[7th] T24.009 Burn of unspecified degree of unspecified site of unspecified lower limb, except ankle and foot POA

[6th] T24.01 Burn of unspecified degree of thigh

[7th] T24.011 Burn of unspecified degree of right thigh POA

[7th] T24.012 Burn of unspecified degree of left thigh POA

[7th] T24.019 Burn of unspecified degree of unspecified thigh POA

[6th] T24.02 Burn of unspecified degree of knee

[7th] T24.021 Burn of unspecified degree of right knee POA

[7th] T24.022 Burn of unspecified degree of left knee POA

[7th] T24.029 Burn of unspecified degree of unspecified knee POA

[6th] T24.03 Burn of unspecified degree of lower leg

[7th] T24.031 Burn of unspecified degree of right lower leg POA

[7th] T24.032 Burn of unspecified degree of left lower leg POA

[7th] T24.039 Burn of unspecified degree of unspecified lower leg POA

[6th] T24.09 Burn of unspecified degree of multiple sites of lower limb, except ankle and foot

[7th] T24.091 Burn of unspecified degree of multiple sites of right lower limb, except ankle and foot POA

[7th] T24.092 Burn of unspecified degree of multiple sites of left lower limb, except ankle and foot POA

[7th] T24.099 Burn of unspecified degree of multiple sites of unspecified lower limb, except ankle and foot POA

[5th] T24.1 Burn of first degree of lower limb, except ankle and foot

Use additional external cause code to identify the source, place and intent of the burn (X00-X19, X75-X77, X96-X98, Y92)

[6th] T24.10 Burn of first degree of unspecified site of lower limb, except ankle and foot

[7th] T24.101 Burn of first degree of unspecified site of right lower limb, except ankle and foot POA

PDx Unacceptable principal diagnosis symbol per Medicare code edits POA Code exempt from diagnosis present on admission requirement
[?] Questionable admission CC Complication or comorbidity MCC Major complication or comorbidity CC/MCC Exc CC/MCC exclusion
[HCC] HCC diagnosis code [RxHCC] RxHCC diagnosis code MACRA code **DEFINITION** Describes condition/terminology
TIP Coding guidance 👁 Official Guideline Reference [Z1] Z code as first-listed diagnosis

7ᵗʰ **T24.102** Burn of first degree of unspecified site of left lower limb, except ankle and foot POA

7ᵗʰ **T24.109** Burn of first degree of unspecified site of unspecified lower limb, except ankle and foot POA

6ᵗʰ **T24.11** Burn of first degree of thigh
  7ᵗʰ **T24.111** Burn of first degree of right thigh POA
  7ᵗʰ **T24.112** Burn of first degree of left thigh POA
  7ᵗʰ **T24.119** Burn of first degree of unspecified thigh POA

6ᵗʰ **T24.12** Burn of first degree of knee
  7ᵗʰ **T24.121** Burn of first degree of right knee POA
  7ᵗʰ **T24.122** Burn of first degree of left knee POA
  7ᵗʰ **T24.129** Burn of first degree of unspecified knee POA

6ᵗʰ **T24.13** Burn of first degree of lower leg
  7ᵗʰ **T24.131** Burn of first degree of right lower leg POA
  7ᵗʰ **T24.132** Burn of first degree of left lower leg POA
  7ᵗʰ **T24.139** Burn of first degree of unspecified lower leg POA

6ᵗʰ **T24.19** Burn of first degree of multiple sites of lower limb, except ankle and foot
  7ᵗʰ **T24.191** Burn of first degree of multiple sites of right lower limb, except ankle and foot POA
  7ᵗʰ **T24.192** Burn of first degree of multiple sites of left lower limb, except ankle and foot POA
  7ᵗʰ **T24.199** Burn of first degree of multiple sites of unspecified lower limb, except ankle and foot POA

5ᵗʰ **T24.2** Burn of second degree of lower limb, except ankle and foot
Use additional external cause code to identify the source, place and intent of the burn (X00-X19, X75-X77, X96-X98, Y92)
  6ᵗʰ **T24.20** Burn of second degree of unspecified site of lower limb, except ankle and foot
    7ᵗʰ **T24.201** Burn of second degree of unspecified site of right lower limb, except ankle and foot POA
    7ᵗʰ **T24.202** Burn of second degree of unspecified site of left lower limb, except ankle and foot POA
    7ᵗʰ **T24.209** Burn of second degree of unspecified site of unspecified lower limb, except ankle and foot POA
  6ᵗʰ **T24.21** Burn of second degree of thigh
    7ᵗʰ **T24.211** Burn of second degree of right thigh POA
    7ᵗʰ **T24.212** Burn of second degree of left thigh POA
    7ᵗʰ **T24.219** Burn of second degree of unspecified thigh POA
  6ᵗʰ **T24.22** Burn of second degree of knee
    7ᵗʰ **T24.221** Burn of second degree of right knee POA
    7ᵗʰ **T24.222** Burn of second degree of left knee POA
    7ᵗʰ **T24.229** Burn of second degree of unspecified knee POA
  6ᵗʰ **T24.23** Burn of second degree of lower leg
    7ᵗʰ **T24.231** Burn of second degree of right lower leg POA
    7ᵗʰ **T24.232** Burn of second degree of left lower leg POA
    7ᵗʰ **T24.239** Burn of second degree of unspecified lower leg POA
  6ᵗʰ **T24.29** Burn of second degree of multiple sites of lower limb, except ankle and foot
    7ᵗʰ **T24.291** Burn of second degree of multiple sites of right lower limb, except ankle and foot POA
    7ᵗʰ **T24.292** Burn of second degree of multiple sites of left lower limb, except ankle and foot POA
    7ᵗʰ **T24.299** Burn of second degree of multiple sites of unspecified lower limb, except ankle and foot POA

5ᵗʰ **T24.3** Burn of third degree of lower limb, except ankle and foot
Use additional external cause code to identify the source, place and intent of the burn (X00-X19, X75-X77, X96-X98, Y92)
  6ᵗʰ **T24.30** Burn of third degree of unspecified site of lower limb, except ankle and foot

7ᵗʰ **T24.301** Burn of third degree of unspecified site of right lower limb, except ankle and foot POA HAC CC/MCC Exc
7ᵗʰ **T24.302** Burn of third degree of unspecified site of left lower limb, except ankle and foot POA HAC CC/MCC Exc
7ᵗʰ **T24.309** Burn of third degree of unspecified site of unspecified lower limb, except ankle and foot POA HAC CC/MCC Exc

6ᵗʰ **T24.31** Burn of third degree of thigh
  7ᵗʰ **T24.311** Burn of third degree of right thigh POA HAC CC/MCC Exc
    AHA: Q4 2018
  7ᵗʰ **T24.312** Burn of third degree of left thigh POA HAC CC/MCC Exc
  7ᵗʰ **T24.319** Burn of third degree of unspecified thigh POA HAC CC/MCC Exc

6ᵗʰ **T24.32** Burn of third degree of knee
  7ᵗʰ **T24.321** Burn of third degree of right knee POA HAC CC/MCC Exc
  7ᵗʰ **T24.322** Burn of third degree of left knee POA HAC CC/MCC Exc
  7ᵗʰ **T24.329** Burn of third degree of unspecified knee POA HAC CC/MCC Exc

6ᵗʰ **T24.33** Burn of third degree of lower leg
  7ᵗʰ **T24.331** Burn of third degree of right lower leg POA HAC CC/MCC Exc
  7ᵗʰ **T24.332** Burn of third degree of left lower leg POA HAC CC/MCC Exc
  7ᵗʰ **T24.339** Burn of third degree of unspecified lower leg POA HAC CC/MCC Exc

6ᵗʰ **T24.39** Burn of third degree of multiple sites of lower limb, except ankle and foot
  7ᵗʰ **T24.391** Burn of third degree of multiple sites of right lower limb, except ankle and foot POA HAC CC/MCC Exc
    AHA: Q2 2016
  7ᵗʰ **T24.392** Burn of third degree of multiple sites of left lower limb, except ankle and foot POA HAC CC/MCC Exc
    AHA: Q2 2016
  7ᵗʰ **T24.399** Burn of third degree of multiple sites of unspecified lower limb, except ankle and foot POA HAC CC/MCC Exc

5ᵗʰ **T24.4** Corrosion of unspecified degree of lower limb, except ankle and foot
Code first (T51-T65) to identify chemical and intent
Use additional external cause code to identify place (Y92)
  6ᵗʰ **T24.40** Corrosion of unspecified degree of unspecified site of lower limb, except ankle and foot
    7ᵗʰ **T24.401** Corrosion of unspecified degree of unspecified site of right lower limb, except ankle and foot POA
    7ᵗʰ **T24.402** Corrosion of unspecified degree of unspecified site of left lower limb, except ankle and foot POA
    7ᵗʰ **T24.409** Corrosion of unspecified degree of unspecified site of unspecified lower limb, except ankle and foot POA
  6ᵗʰ **T24.41** Corrosion of unspecified degree of thigh
    7ᵗʰ **T24.411** Corrosion of unspecified degree of right thigh POA
    7ᵗʰ **T24.412** Corrosion of unspecified degree of left thigh POA
    7ᵗʰ **T24.419** Corrosion of unspecified degree of unspecified thigh POA
  6ᵗʰ **T24.42** Corrosion of unspecified degree of knee
    7ᵗʰ **T24.421** Corrosion of unspecified degree of right knee POA
    7ᵗʰ **T24.422** Corrosion of unspecified degree of left knee POA
    7ᵗʰ **T24.429** Corrosion of unspecified degree of unspecified knee POA
  6ᵗʰ **T24.43** Corrosion of unspecified degree of lower leg
    7ᵗʰ **T24.431** Corrosion of unspecified degree of right lower leg POA

Unspecified Code   Other Specified Code   Manifestation Code   N Newborn   P Pediatric   M Maternity   A Adult   ♂ Male   ♀ Female
● New Code   ▲ Revised Code Title   ►◄ Revised Text   NOTES   INCLUDES   EXCLUDES1 Not coded here   EXCLUDES2 Not included here
4ᵗʰ character required   5ᵗʰ character required   6ᵗʰ character required   7ᵗʰ character required   Extension 'X' Alert
HAC Hospital-acquired condition (HAC) alert   AHA AHA Coding Clinic®   Code first alert

2020 ICD-10-CM   When symbols appear on a code that requires a 7th character extension, refer to Appendix B to identify applicable 7th character codes.   **1113**

7ᵈ **T24.432** Corrosion of unspecified degree of left lower leg **POA**

7ᵈ **T24.439** Corrosion of unspecified degree of unspecified lower leg **POA**

6ᵈ **T24.49** Corrosion of unspecified degree of multiple sites of lower limb, except ankle and foot

    7ᵈ **T24.491** Corrosion of unspecified degree of multiple sites of right lower limb, except ankle and foot **POA**

    7ᵈ **T24.492** Corrosion of unspecified degree of multiple sites of left lower limb, except ankle and foot **POA**

    7ᵈ **T24.499** Corrosion of unspecified degree of multiple sites of unspecified lower limb, except ankle and foot **POA**

5ᵈ **T24.5** Corrosion of first degree of lower limb, except ankle and foot

    ☛ **Code first** (T51-T65) to identify chemical and intent
    Use additional external cause code to identify place (Y92)

6ᵈ **T24.50** Corrosion of first degree of unspecified site of lower limb, except ankle and foot

    7ᵈ **T24.501** Corrosion of first degree of unspecified site of right lower limb, except ankle and foot **POA**

    7ᵈ **T24.502** Corrosion of first degree of unspecified site of left lower limb, except ankle and foot **POA**

    7ᵈ **T24.509** Corrosion of first degree of unspecified site of unspecified lower limb, except ankle and foot **POA**

6ᵈ **T24.51** Corrosion of first degree of thigh

    7ᵈ **T24.511** Corrosion of first degree of right thigh **POA**
    7ᵈ **T24.512** Corrosion of first degree of left thigh **POA**
    7ᵈ **T24.519** Corrosion of first degree of unspecified thigh **POA**

6ᵈ **T24.52** Corrosion of first degree of knee

    7ᵈ **T24.521** Corrosion of first degree of right knee **POA**
    7ᵈ **T24.522** Corrosion of first degree of left knee **POA**
    7ᵈ **T24.529** Corrosion of first degree of unspecified knee **POA**

6ᵈ **T24.53** Corrosion of first degree of lower leg

    7ᵈ **T24.531** Corrosion of first degree of right lower leg **POA**
    7ᵈ **T24.532** Corrosion of first degree of left lower leg **POA**
    7ᵈ **T24.539** Corrosion of first degree of unspecified lower leg **POA**

6ᵈ **T24.59** Corrosion of first degree of multiple sites of lower limb, except ankle and foot

    7ᵈ **T24.591** Corrosion of first degree of multiple sites of right lower limb, except ankle and foot **POA**

    7ᵈ **T24.592** Corrosion of first degree of multiple sites of left lower limb, except ankle and foot **POA**

    7ᵈ **T24.599** Corrosion of first degree of multiple sites of unspecified lower limb, except ankle and foot **POA**

5ᵈ **T24.6** Corrosion of second degree of lower limb, except ankle and foot

    ☛ **Code first** (T51-T65) to identify chemical and intent
    Use additional external cause code to identify place (Y92)

6ᵈ **T24.60** Corrosion of second degree of unspecified site of lower limb, except ankle and foot

    7ᵈ **T24.601** Corrosion of second degree of unspecified site of right lower limb, except ankle and foot **POA**

    7ᵈ **T24.602** Corrosion of second degree of unspecified site of left lower limb, except ankle and foot **POA**

    7ᵈ **T24.609** Corrosion of second degree of unspecified site of unspecified lower limb, except ankle and foot **POA**

6ᵈ **T24.61** Corrosion of second degree of thigh

    7ᵈ **T24.611** Corrosion of second degree of right thigh

    7ᵈ **T24.612** Corrosion of second degree of left thigh **POA**
    7ᵈ **T24.619** Corrosion of second degree of unspecified thigh **POA**

6ᵈ **T24.62** Corrosion of second degree of knee

    7ᵈ **T24.621** Corrosion of second degree of right knee **POA**
    7ᵈ **T24.622** Corrosion of second degree of left knee **POA**
    7ᵈ **T24.629** Corrosion of second degree of unspecified knee **POA**

6ᵈ **T24.63** Corrosion of second degree of lower leg

    7ᵈ **T24.631** Corrosion of second degree of right lower leg **POA**
    7ᵈ **T24.632** Corrosion of second degree of left lower leg **POA**
    7ᵈ **T24.639** Corrosion of second degree of unspecified lower leg **POA**

6ᵈ **T24.69** Corrosion of second degree of multiple sites of lower limb, except ankle and foot

    7ᵈ **T24.691** Corrosion of second degree of multiple sites of right lower limb, except ankle and foot **POA**

    7ᵈ **T24.692** Corrosion of second degree of multiple sites of left lower limb, except ankle and foot **POA**

    7ᵈ **T24.699** Corrosion of second degree of multiple sites of unspecified lower limb, except ankle and foot **POA**

5ᵈ **T24.7** Corrosion of third degree of lower limb, except ankle and foot

    ☛ **Code first** (T51-T65) to identify chemical and intent
    Use additional external cause code to identify place (Y92)

6ᵈ **T24.70** Corrosion of third degree of unspecified site of lower limb, except ankle and foot

    7ᵈ **T24.701** Corrosion of third degree of unspecified site of right lower limb, except ankle and foot ᴄᶜ **POA** **HAC** ᴄᴄ/ᴍᴄᴄ ᴇˣᶜ

    7ᵈ **T24.702** Corrosion of third degree of unspecified site of left lower limb, except ankle and foot ᴄᶜ **POA** **HAC** ᴄᴄ/ᴍᴄᴄ ᴇˣᶜ

    7ᵈ **T24.709** Corrosion of third degree of unspecified site of unspecified lower limb, except ankle and foot **POA** **HAC** ᴄᴄ/ᴍᴄᴄ ᴇˣᶜ

6ᵈ **T24.71** Corrosion of third degree of thigh

    7ᵈ **T24.711** Corrosion of third degree of right thigh ᴄᶜ **POA** **HAC** ᴄᴄ/ᴍᴄᴄ ᴇˣᶜ

    7ᵈ **T24.712** Corrosion of third degree of left thigh ᴄᶜ **POA** **HAC** ᴄᴄ/ᴍᴄᴄ ᴇˣᶜ

    7ᵈ **T24.719** Corrosion of third degree of unspecified thigh ᴄᶜ **POA** **HAC** ᴄᴄ/ᴍᴄᴄ ᴇˣᶜ

6ᵈ **T24.72** Corrosion of third degree of knee

    7ᵈ **T24.721** Corrosion of third degree of right knee ᴄᶜ **POA** **HAC** ᴄᴄ/ᴍᴄᴄ ᴇˣᶜ

    7ᵈ **T24.722** Corrosion of third degree of left knee ᴄᶜ **POA** **HAC** ᴄᴄ/ᴍᴄᴄ ᴇˣᶜ

    7ᵈ **T24.729** Corrosion of third degree of unspecified knee ᴄᶜ **POA** **HAC** ᴄᴄ/ᴍᴄᴄ ᴇˣᶜ

6ᵈ **T24.73** Corrosion of third degree of lower leg

    7ᵈ **T24.731** Corrosion of third degree of right lower leg ᴄᶜ **POA** **HAC** ᴄᴄ/ᴍᴄᴄ ᴇˣᶜ

    7ᵈ **T24.732** Corrosion of third degree of left lower leg ᴄᶜ **POA** **HAC** ᴄᴄ/ᴍᴄᴄ ᴇˣᶜ

    7ᵈ **T24.739** Corrosion of third degree of unspecified lower leg ᴄᶜ **POA** **HAC** ᴄᴄ/ᴍᴄᴄ ᴇˣᶜ

6ᵈ **T24.79** Corrosion of third degree of multiple sites of lower limb, except ankle and foot

    7ᵈ **T24.791** Corrosion of third degree of multiple sites of right lower limb, except ankle and foot ᴄᶜ **POA** **HAC** ᴄᴄ/ᴍᴄᴄ ᴇˣᶜ

    7ᵈ **T24.792** Corrosion of third degree of multiple sites of left lower limb, except ankle and foot ᴄᶜ **POA** **HAC** ᴄᴄ/ᴍᴄᴄ ᴇˣᶜ

7th T24.799 Corrosion of third degree of multiple sites of unspecified lower limb, except ankle and foot CC⊘ POA HAC CC/MCC Exc

4th T25 Burn and corrosion of ankle and foot

The appropriate 7th character is to be added to each code from category T25
A = initial encounter
D = subsequent encounter
S = sequela

5th T25.0 Burn of unspecified degree of ankle and foot
Use additional external cause code to identify the source, place and intent of the burn (X00-X19, X75-X77, X96-X98, Y92)

6th T25.01 Burn of unspecified degree of ankle
7th T25.011 Burn of unspecified degree of right ankle POA
7th T25.012 Burn of unspecified degree of left ankle POA
7th T25.019 Burn of unspecified degree of unspecified ankle POA

6th T25.02 Burn of unspecified degree of foot
EXCLUDES2 burn of unspecified degree of toe(s) (nail) (T25.03-)
7th T25.021 Burn of unspecified degree of right foot POA
7th T25.022 Burn of unspecified degree of left foot POA
7th T25.029 Burn of unspecified degree of unspecified foot POA

6th T25.03 Burn of unspecified degree of toe(s) (nail)
7th T25.031 Burn of unspecified degree of right toe(s) (nail) POA
7th T25.032 Burn of unspecified degree of left toe(s) (nail) POA
7th T25.039 Burn of unspecified degree of unspecified toe(s) (nail) POA

6th T25.09 Burn of unspecified degree of multiple sites of ankle and foot
7th T25.091 Burn of unspecified degree of multiple sites of right ankle and foot POA
7th T25.092 Burn of unspecified degree of multiple sites of left ankle and foot POA
7th T25.099 Burn of unspecified degree of multiple sites of unspecified ankle and foot POA

5th T25.1 Burn of first degree of ankle and foot
Use additional external cause code to identify the source, place and intent of the burn (X00-X19, X75-X77, X96-X98, Y92)

6th T25.11 Burn of first degree of ankle
7th T25.111 Burn of first degree of right ankle POA
7th T25.112 Burn of first degree of left ankle POA
7th T25.119 Burn of first degree of unspecified ankle POA

6th T25.12 Burn of first degree of foot
EXCLUDES2 burn of first degree of toe(s) (nail) (T25.13-)
7th T25.121 Burn of first degree of right foot POA
7th T25.122 Burn of first degree of left foot POA
7th T25.129 Burn of first degree of unspecified foot POA

6th T25.13 Burn of first degree of toe(s) (nail)
7th T25.131 Burn of first degree of right toe(s) (nail) POA
7th T25.132 Burn of first degree of left toe(s) (nail) POA
7th T25.139 Burn of first degree of unspecified toe(s) (nail) POA

6th T25.19 Burn of first degree of multiple sites of ankle and foot
7th T25.191 Burn of first degree of multiple sites of right ankle and foot POA
7th T25.192 Burn of first degree of multiple sites of left ankle and foot POA
7th T25.199 Burn of first degree of multiple sites of unspecified ankle and foot POA

5th T25.2 Burn of second degree of ankle and foot
Use additional external cause code to identify the source, place and intent of the burn (X00-X19, X75-X77, X96-X98, Y92)

6th T25.21 Burn of second degree of ankle
7th T25.211 Burn of second degree of right ankle POA
7th T25.212 Burn of second degree of left ankle POA
7th T25.219 Burn of second degree of unspecified ankle POA

6th T25.22 Burn of second degree of foot
EXCLUDES2 burn of second degree of toe(s) (nail) (T25.23-)
7th T25.221 Burn of second degree of right foot POA
7th T25.222 Burn of second degree of left foot POA
7th T25.229 Burn of second degree of unspecified foot POA

6th T25.23 Burn of second degree of toe(s) (nail)
7th T25.231 Burn of second degree of right toe(s) (nail) POA
7th T25.232 Burn of second degree of left toe(s) (nail) POA
7th T25.239 Burn of second degree of unspecified toe(s) (nail) POA

6th T25.29 Burn of second degree of multiple sites of ankle and foot
7th T25.291 Burn of second degree of multiple sites of right ankle and foot POA
7th T25.292 Burn of second degree of multiple sites of left ankle and foot POA
7th T25.299 Burn of second degree of multiple sites of unspecified ankle and foot POA

5th T25.3 Burn of third degree of ankle and foot
Use additional external cause code to identify the source, place and intent of the burn (X00-X19, X75-X77, X96-X98, Y92)

6th T25.31 Burn of third degree of ankle
7th T25.311 Burn of third degree of right ankle CC⊘ POA HAC CC/MCC Exc
7th T25.312 Burn of third degree of left ankle CC⊘ POA HAC CC/MCC Exc
7th T25.319 Burn of third degree of unspecified ankle CC⊘ POA HAC CC/MCC Exc

6th T25.32 Burn of third degree of foot
EXCLUDES2 burn of third degree of toe(s) (nail) (T25.33-)
7th T25.321 Burn of third degree of right foot CC⊘ POA HAC CC/MCC Exc
7th T25.322 Burn of third degree of left foot CC⊘ POA HAC CC/MCC Exc
7th T25.329 Burn of third degree of unspecified foot CC⊘ POA HAC CC/MCC Exc

6th T25.33 Burn of third degree of toe(s) (nail)
7th T25.331 Burn of third degree of right toe(s) (nail) CC⊘ POA HAC CC/MCC Exc
7th T25.332 Burn of third degree of left toe(s) (nail) CC⊘ POA HAC CC/MCC Exc
7th T25.339 Burn of third degree of unspecified toe(s) (nail) CC⊘ POA HAC CC/MCC Exc

6th T25.39 Burn of third degree of multiple sites of ankle and foot
7th T25.391 Burn of third degree of multiple sites of right ankle and foot CC⊘ POA HAC CC/MCC Exc
7th T25.392 Burn of third degree of multiple sites of left ankle and foot CC⊘ POA HAC CC/MCC Exc
7th T25.399 Burn of third degree of multiple sites of unspecified ankle and foot CC⊘ POA HAC CC/MCC Exc

5th T25.4 Corrosion of unspecified degree of ankle and foot
☞ Code first (T51-T65) to identify chemical and intent
Use additional external cause code to identify place (Y92)

6th T25.41 Corrosion of unspecified degree of ankle
7th T25.411 Corrosion of unspecified degree of right ankle POA
7th T25.412 Corrosion of unspecified degree of left ankle POA
7th T25.419 Corrosion of unspecified degree of unspecified ankle POA

Unspecified Code   Other Specified Code   Manifestation Code   N Newborn   P Pediatric   M Maternity   A Adult   ♂ Male   ♀ Female
● New Code   ▲ Revised Code Title   ►◄ Revised Text   NOTES   INCLUDES   EXCLUDES1 Not coded here   EXCLUDES2 Not included here
4th 4th character required   5th 5th character required   6th 6th character required   7th 7th character required   7x Extension 'X' Alert
HAC Hospital-acquired condition (HAC) alert   AHA AHA Coding Clinic®   ☞ Code first alert

T25.42 Corrosion of unspecified degree of foot
  EXCLUDES2 corrosion of unspecified degree of toe(s) (nail) (T25.43-)
    T25.421 Corrosion of unspecified degree of right foot
    T25.422 Corrosion of unspecified degree of left foot
    T25.429 Corrosion of unspecified degree of unspecified foot

T25.43 Corrosion of unspecified degree of toe(s) (nail)
    T25.431 Corrosion of unspecified degree of right toe(s) (nail)
    T25.432 Corrosion of unspecified degree of left toe(s) (nail)
    T25.439 Corrosion of unspecified degree of unspecified toe(s) (nail)

T25.49 Corrosion of unspecified degree of multiple sites of ankle and foot
    T25.491 Corrosion of unspecified degree of multiple sites of right ankle and foot
    T25.492 Corrosion of unspecified degree of multiple sites of left ankle and foot
    T25.499 Corrosion of unspecified degree of multiple sites of unspecified ankle and foot

T25.5 Corrosion of first degree of ankle and foot
  ☛ Code first (T51-T65) to identify chemical and intent
  Use additional external cause code to identify place (Y92)
  T25.51 Corrosion of first degree of ankle
    T25.511 Corrosion of first degree of right ankle
    T25.512 Corrosion of first degree of left ankle
    T25.519 Corrosion of first degree of unspecified ankle
  T25.52 Corrosion of first degree of foot
    EXCLUDES2 corrosion of first degree of toe(s) (nail) (T25.53-)
    T25.521 Corrosion of first degree of right foot
    T25.522 Corrosion of first degree of left foot
    T25.529 Corrosion of first degree of unspecified foot
  T25.53 Corrosion of first degree of toe(s) (nail)
    T25.531 Corrosion of first degree of right toe(s) (nail)
    T25.532 Corrosion of first degree of left toe(s) (nail)
    T25.539 Corrosion of first degree of unspecified toe(s) (nail)
  T25.59 Corrosion of first degree of multiple sites of ankle and foot
    T25.591 Corrosion of first degree of multiple sites of right ankle and foot
    T25.592 Corrosion of first degree of multiple sites of left ankle and foot
    T25.599 Corrosion of first degree of multiple sites of unspecified ankle and foot

T25.6 Corrosion of second degree of ankle and foot
  ☛ Code first (T51-T65) to identify chemical and intent
  Use additional external cause code to identify place (Y92)
  T25.61 Corrosion of second degree of ankle
    T25.611 Corrosion of second degree of right ankle
    T25.612 Corrosion of second degree of left ankle
    T25.619 Corrosion of second degree of unspecified ankle
  T25.62 Corrosion of second degree of foot
    EXCLUDES2 corrosion of second degree of toe(s) (nail) (T25.63-)
    T25.621 Corrosion of second degree of right foot
    T25.622 Corrosion of second degree of left foot
    T25.629 Corrosion of second degree of unspecified foot

T25.63 Corrosion of second degree of toe(s) (nail)
    T25.631 Corrosion of second degree of right toe(s) (nail)
    T25.632 Corrosion of second degree of left toe(s) (nail)
    T25.639 Corrosion of second degree of unspecified toe(s) (nail)

T25.69 Corrosion of second degree of multiple sites of ankle and foot
    T25.691 Corrosion of second degree of right ankle and foot
    T25.692 Corrosion of second degree of left ankle and foot
    T25.699 Corrosion of second degree of unspecified ankle and foot

T25.7 Corrosion of third degree of ankle and foot
  ☛ Code first (T51-T65) to identify chemical and intent
  Use additional external cause code to identify place (Y92)
  T25.71 Corrosion of third degree of ankle
    T25.711 Corrosion of third degree of right ankle
    T25.712 Corrosion of third degree of left ankle
    T25.719 Corrosion of third degree of unspecified ankle
  T25.72 Corrosion of third degree of foot
    EXCLUDES2 corrosion of third degree of toe(s) (nail) (T25.73-)
    T25.721 Corrosion of third degree of right foot
    T25.722 Corrosion of third degree of left foot
    T25.729 Corrosion of third degree of unspecified foot
  T25.73 Corrosion of third degree of toe(s) (nail)
    T25.731 Corrosion of third degree of right toe(s) (nail)
    T25.732 Corrosion of third degree of left toe(s) (nail)
    T25.739 Corrosion of third degree of unspecified toe(s) (nail)
  T25.79 Corrosion of third degree of multiple sites of ankle and foot
    T25.791 Corrosion of third degree of multiple sites of right ankle and foot
    T25.792 Corrosion of third degree of multiple sites of left ankle and foot
    T25.799 Corrosion of third degree of multiple sites of unspecified ankle and foot

Burns and corrosions confined to eye and internal organs (T26-T28)

👁 See Official Guidelines "Coding of Burns and Corrosions" I.C.19.d

T26 Burn and corrosion confined to eye and adnexa
  The appropriate 7th character is to be added to each code from category T26
    A = initial encounter
    D = subsequent encounter
    S = sequela
  T26.0 Burn of eyelid and periocular area
    Use additional external cause code to identify the source, place and intent of the burn (X00-X19, X75-X77, X96-X98, Y92)
    T26.00 Burn of unspecified eyelid and periocular area
    T26.01 Burn of right eyelid and periocular area
    T26.02 Burn of left eyelid and periocular area
  T26.1 Burn of cornea and conjunctival sac
    Use additional external cause code to identify the source, place and intent of the burn (X00-X19, X75-X77, X96-X98, Y92)

PDₓ Unacceptable principal diagnosis symbol per Medicare code edits ✎ Code exempt from diagnosis present on admission requirement
❓ Questionable admission cc Complication or comorbidity mcc Major complication or comorbidity cc/mcc Exc CC/MCC exclusion
HCC HCC diagnosis code RxHCC RxHCC diagnosis code MACRA MACRA code **DEFINITION** Describes condition/terminology
TIP Coding guidance 👁 Official Guideline Reference Z1 Z code as first-listed diagnosis

⑦ T26.10 Burn of cornea and conjunctival sac, unspecified eye POA

⑦ T26.11 Burn of cornea and conjunctival sac, right eye POA

⑦ T26.12 Burn of cornea and conjunctival sac, left eye POA

⑤ T26.2 Burn with resulting rupture and destruction of eyeball
Use additional external cause code to identify the source, place and intent of the burn (X00-X19, X75-X77, X96-X98, Y92)

⑦ T26.20 Burn with resulting rupture and destruction of unspecified eyeball CC POA HAC

⑦ T26.21 Burn with resulting rupture and destruction of right eyeball CC POA HAC

⑦ T26.22 Burn with resulting rupture and destruction of left eyeball CC POA HAC

⑤ T26.3 Burns of other specified parts of eye and adnexa
Use additional external cause code to identify the source, place and intent of the burn (X00-X19, X75-X77, X96-X98, Y92)

⑦ T26.30 Burns of other specified parts of unspecified eye and adnexa POA

⑦ T26.31 Burns of other specified parts of right eye and adnexa POA

⑦ T26.32 Burns of other specified parts of left eye and adnexa POA

⑤ T26.4 Burn of eye and adnexa, part unspecified
Use additional external cause code to identify the source, place and intent of the burn (X00-X19, X75-X77, X96-X98, Y92)

⑦ T26.40 Burn of unspecified eye and adnexa, part unspecified POA

⑦ T26.41 Burn of right eye and adnexa, part unspecified POA

⑦ T26.42 Burn of left eye and adnexa, part unspecified POA

⑤ T26.5 Corrosion of eyelid and periocular area
☞ Code first (T51-T65) to identify chemical and intent
Use additional external cause code to identify place (Y92)

⑦ T26.50 Corrosion of unspecified eyelid and periocular area POA

⑦ T26.51 Corrosion of right eyelid and periocular area POA

⑦ T26.52 Corrosion of left eyelid and periocular area POA

⑤ T26.6 Corrosion of cornea and conjunctival sac
☞ Code first (T51-T65) to identify chemical and intent
Use additional external cause code to identify place (Y92)

⑦ T26.60 Corrosion of cornea and conjunctival sac, unspecified eye POA

⑦ T26.61 Corrosion of cornea and conjunctival sac, right eye POA

⑦ T26.62 Corrosion of cornea and conjunctival sac, left eye POA

⑤ T26.7 Corrosion with resulting rupture and destruction of eyeball
☞ Code first (T51-T65) to identify chemical and intent
Use additional external cause code to identify place (Y92)

⑦ T26.70 Corrosion with resulting rupture and destruction of unspecified eyeball CC POA HAC

⑦ T26.71 Corrosion with resulting rupture and destruction of right eyeball CC POA HAC

⑦ T26.72 Corrosion with resulting rupture and destruction of left eyeball CC POA HAC

⑤ T26.8 Corrosions of other specified parts of eye and adnexa
☞ Code first (T51-T65) to identify chemical and intent
Use additional external cause code to identify place (Y92)

⑦ T26.80 Corrosions of other specified parts of unspecified eye and adnexa POA

⑦ T26.81 Corrosions of other specified parts of right eye and adnexa POA

⑦ T26.82 Corrosions of other specified parts of left eye and adnexa POA

⑤ T26.9 Corrosion of eye and adnexa, part unspecified
☞ Code first (T51-T65) to identify chemical and intent
Use additional external cause code to identify place (Y92)

⑦ T26.90 Corrosion of unspecified eye and adnexa, part unspecified POA

⑦ T26.91 Corrosion of right eye and adnexa, part unspecified POA

⑦ T26.92 Corrosion of left eye and adnexa, part unspecified POA

④ T27 Burn and corrosion of respiratory tract
Use additional external cause code to identify the source and intent of the burn (X00-X19, X75-X77, X96-X98)
Use additional external cause code to identify place (Y92)
The appropriate 7th character is to be added to each code from category T27
A = initial encounter
D = subsequent encounter
S = sequela

⑦ T27.0 Burn of larynx and trachea CC POA HAC CC/MCC Exc

⑦ T27.1 Burn involving larynx and trachea with lung CC POA HAC CC/MCC Exc

⑦ T27.2 Burn of other parts of respiratory tract CC POA HAC CC/MCC Exc
Burn of thoracic cavity

⑦ T27.3 Burn of respiratory tract, part unspecified CC POA HAC CC/MCC Exc

⑦ T27.4 Corrosion of larynx and trachea CC POA HAC CC/MCC Exc
☞ Code first (T51-T65) to identify chemical and intent

⑦ T27.5 Corrosion involving larynx and trachea with lung CC POA HAC CC/MCC Exc
☞ Code first (T51-T65) to identify chemical and intent

⑦ T27.6 Corrosion of other parts of respiratory tract CC POA HAC CC/MCC Exc
☞ Code first (T51-T65) to identify chemical and intent

⑦ T27.7 Corrosion of respiratory tract, part unspecified CC POA HAC CC/MCC Exc
☞ Code first (T51-T65) to identify chemical and intent

④ T28 Burn and corrosion of other internal organs
Use additional external cause code to identify the source and intent of the burn (X00-X19, X75-X77, X96-X98)
Use additional external cause code to identify place (Y92)
The appropriate 7th character is to be added to each code from category T28
A = initial encounter
D = subsequent encounter
S = sequela

⑦ T28.0 Burn of mouth and pharynx POA

⑦ T28.1 Burn of esophagus CC POA HAC CC/MCC Exc

⑦ T28.2 Burn of other parts of alimentary tract CC POA HAC CC/MCC Exc

⑦ T28.3 Burn of internal genitourinary organs POA

⑤ T28.4 Burns of other and unspecified internal organs

⑦ T28.40 Burn of unspecified internal organ POA

⑥ T28.41 Burn of ear drum

⑦ T28.411 Burn of right ear drum POA

⑦ T28.412 Burn of left ear drum POA

⑦ T28.419 Burn of unspecified ear drum POA

⑦ T28.49 Burn of other internal organ POA

⑦ T28.5 Corrosion of mouth and pharynx POA
☞ Code first (T51-T65) to identify chemical and intent

⑦ T28.6 Corrosion of esophagus CC POA HAC CC/MCC Exc
☞ Code first (T51-T65) to identify chemical and intent

⑦ T28.7 Corrosion of other parts of alimentary tract CC POA HAC CC/MCC Exc
☞ Code first (T51-T65) to identify chemical and intent

⑦ T28.8 Corrosion of internal genitourinary organs POA
☞ Code first (T51-T65) to identify chemical and intent

⑤ T28.9 Corrosions of other and unspecified internal organs
☞ Code first (T51-T65) to identify chemical and intent

⑦ T28.90 Corrosions of unspecified internal organs POA

⑥ T28.91 Corrosions of ear drum

⑦ T28.911 Corrosions of right ear drum POA

⑦ T28.912 Corrosions of left ear drum POA

⑦ T28.919 Corrosions of unspecified ear drum POA

⑦ T28.99 Corrosions of other internal organs POA

Burns and corrosions of multiple and unspecified body regions (T30-T32)

④ T30 Burn and corrosion, body region unspecified

T30.0 Burn of unspecified body region, unspecified degree
This code is not for inpatient use. Code to specified site and degree of burns
Burn NOS
Multiple burns NOS

Unspecified Code   Other Specified Code   Manifestation Code   Ⓝ Newborn   Ⓟ Pediatric   Ⓜ Maternity   Ⓐ Adult   ♂ Male   ♀ Female
● New Code   ▲ Revised Code Title   ▶◀ Revised Text   NOTES   INCLUDES   EXCLUDES1 Not coded here   EXCLUDES2 Not included here
④ 4th character required   ⑤ 5th character required   ⑥ 6th character required   ⑦ 7th character required   ⑦ Extension 'X' Alert
HAC Hospital-acquired condition (HAC) alert   AHA AHA Coding Clinic©   ☞ Code first alert

2020 ICD-10-CM   When symbols appear on a code that requires a 7th character extension, refer to Appendix B to identify applicable 7th character codes.   **1117**

T30.4 Corrosion of unspecified body region, unspecified degree
This code is not for inpatient use. Code to specified site and degree of corrosion
Corrosion NOS
Multiple corrosion NOS

4ᵗʰ T31 Burns classified according to extent of body surface involved (Figure 19.3)

👁 **See Official Guidelines** "Burns and Corrosions Classified According to Extent of Body Surface Involved" I.C.19.d.6

NOTES This category is to be used as the primary code only when the site of the burn is unspecified. It should be used as a supplementary code with categories T20-T25 when the site is specified.

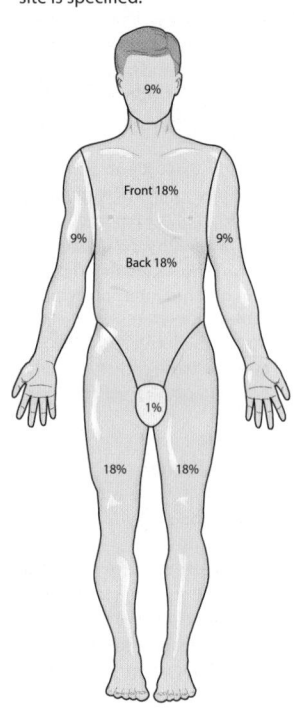

9%

Front 18%

9%   9%

Back 18%

1%

18%   18%

Figure 19.3 Rule of Nines: Percentage of Burn Areas

T31.0 Burns involving less than 10% of body surface
5ᵗʰ T31.1 Burns involving 10-19% of body surface
   T31.10 Burns involving 10-19% of body surface with 0% to 9% third degree burns cc⊘ HAC CC/MCC Exc⊘
      Burns involving 10-19% of body surface NOS
   T31.11 Burns involving 10-19% of body surface with 10-19% third degree burns cc⊘ HAC HCC CC/MCC Exc⊘
5ᵗʰ T31.2 Burns involving 20-29% of body surface
   T31.20 Burns involving 20-29% of body surface with 0% to 9% third degree burns cc⊘ HAC CC/MCC Exc⊘
      Burns involving 20-29% of body surface NOS
   T31.21 Burns involving 20-29% of body surface with 10-19% third degree burns HAC HCC cc⊘ CC/MCC Exc⊘
   T31.22 Burns involving 20-29% of body surface with 20-29% third degree burns HAC HCC cc⊘ CC/MCC Exc⊘
5ᵗʰ T31.3 Burns involving 30-39% of body surface
   T31.30 Burns involving 30-39% of body surface with 0% to 9% third degree burns cc⊘ HAC CC/MCC Exc⊘
      Burns involving 30-39% of body surface NOS
   T31.31 Burns involving 30-39% of body surface with 10-19% third degree burns HAC HCC cc⊘ CC/MCC Exc⊘
   T31.32 Burns involving 30-39% of body surface with 20-29% third degree burns HAC HCC Mcc⊘ CC/MCC Exc⊘
   T31.33 Burns involving 30-39% of body surface with 30-39% third degree burns HAC HCC Mcc⊘ CC/MCC Exc⊘
5ᵗʰ T31.4 Burns involving 40-49% of body surface
   T31.40 Burns involving 40-49% of body surface with 0% to 9% third degree burns cc⊘ HAC CC/MCC Exc⊘
      Burns involving 40-49% of body surface NOS

T31.41 Burns involving 40-49% of body surface with 10-19% third degree burns HAC HCC Mcc⊘ CC/MCC Exc⊘
T31.42 Burns involving 40-49% of body surface with 20-29% third degree burns HAC HCC Mcc⊘ CC/MCC Exc⊘
T31.43 Burns involving 40-49% of body surface with 30-39% third degree burns HAC HCC Mcc⊘ CC/MCC Exc⊘
T31.44 Burns involving 40-49% of body surface with 40-49% third degree burns HAC HCC Mcc⊘ CC/MCC Exc⊘
5ᵗʰ T31.5 Burns involving 50-59% of body surface
   T31.50 Burns involving 50-59% of body surface with 0% to 9% third degree burns cc⊘ HAC CC/MCC Exc⊘
      Burns involving 50-59% of body surface NOS
   T31.51 Burns involving 50-59% of body surface with 10-19% third degree burns HAC HCC Mcc⊘ CC/MCC Exc⊘
   T31.52 Burns involving 50-59% of body surface with 20-29% third degree burns HAC HCC Mcc⊘ CC/MCC Exc⊘
   T31.53 Burns involving 50-59% of body surface with 30-39% third degree burns HAC HCC Mcc⊘ CC/MCC Exc⊘
   T31.54 Burns involving 50-59% of body surface with 40-49% third degree burns HAC HCC Mcc⊘ CC/MCC Exc⊘
   T31.55 Burns involving 50-59% of body surface with 50-59% third degree burns HAC HCC Mcc⊘ CC/MCC Exc⊘
5ᵗʰ T31.6 Burns involving 60-69% of body surface
   T31.60 Burns involving 60-69% of body surface with 0% to 9% third degree burns cc⊘ HAC CC/MCC Exc⊘
      Burns involving 60-69% of body surface NOS
   T31.61 Burns involving 60-69% of body surface with 10-19% third degree burns HAC HCC Mcc⊘ CC/MCC Exc⊘
   T31.62 Burns involving 60-69% of body surface with 20-29% third degree burns HAC HCC Mcc⊘ CC/MCC Exc⊘
   T31.63 Burns involving 60-69% of body surface with 30-39% third degree burns HAC HCC Mcc⊘ CC/MCC Exc⊘
   T31.64 Burns involving 60-69% of body surface with 40-49% third degree burns HAC HCC Mcc⊘ CC/MCC Exc⊘
   T31.65 Burns involving 60-69% of body surface with 50-59% third degree burns HAC HCC Mcc⊘ CC/MCC Exc⊘
   T31.66 Burns involving 60-69% of body surface with 60-69% third degree burns HAC HCC Mcc⊘ CC/MCC Exc⊘
5ᵗʰ T31.7 Burns involving 70-79% of body surface
   T31.70 Burns involving 70-79% of body surface with 0% to 9% third degree burns cc⊘ HAC CC/MCC Exc⊘
      Burns involving 70-79% of body surface NOS
   T31.71 Burns involving 70-79% of body surface with 10-19% third degree burns HAC HCC Mcc⊘ CC/MCC Exc⊘
   T31.72 Burns involving 70-79% of body surface with 20-29% third degree burns HAC HCC Mcc⊘ CC/MCC Exc⊘
   T31.73 Burns involving 70-79% of body surface with 30-39% third degree burns HAC HCC Mcc⊘ CC/MCC Exc⊘
   T31.74 Burns involving 70-79% of body surface with 40-49% third degree burns HAC HCC Mcc⊘ CC/MCC Exc⊘
   T31.75 Burns involving 70-79% of body surface with 50-59% third degree burns HAC HCC Mcc⊘ CC/MCC Exc⊘
   T31.76 Burns involving 70-79% of body surface with 60-69% third degree burns HAC HCC Mcc⊘ CC/MCC Exc⊘
   T31.77 Burns involving 70-79% of body surface with 70-79% third degree burns HAC HCC Mcc⊘ CC/MCC Exc⊘
5ᵗʰ T31.8 Burns involving 80-89% of body surface
   T31.80 Burns involving 80-89% of body surface with 0% to 9% third degree burns cc⊘ HAC CC/MCC Exc⊘
      Burns involving 80-89% of body surface NOS
   T31.81 Burns involving 80-89% of body surface with 10-19% third degree burns HAC HCC Mcc⊘ CC/MCC Exc⊘
   T31.82 Burns involving 80-89% of body surface with 20-29% third degree burns HAC HCC Mcc⊘ CC/MCC Exc⊘
   T31.83 Burns involving 80-89% of body surface with 30-39% third degree burns HAC HCC Mcc⊘ CC/MCC Exc⊘
   T31.84 Burns involving 80-89% of body surface with 40-49% third degree burns HAC HCC Mcc⊘ CC/MCC Exc⊘
   T31.85 Burns involving 80-89% of body surface with 50-59% third degree burns HAC HCC Mcc⊘ CC/MCC Exc⊘
   T31.86 Burns involving 80-89% of body surface with 60-69% third degree burns HAC HCC Mcc⊘ CC/MCC Exc⊘
   T31.87 Burns involving 80-89% of body surface with 70-79% third degree burns HAC HCC Mcc⊘ CC/MCC Exc⊘
   T31.88 Burns involving 80-89% of body surface with 80-89% third degree burns HAC HCC Mcc⊘ CC/MCC Exc⊘

5ᵗʰ **T31.9** Burns involving 90% or more of body surface

T31.90 Burns involving 90% or more of body surface with 0% to 9% third degree **burns** CC⁰ HAC CC/MCC
Burns involving 90% or more of body surface NOS

T31.91 Burns involving 90% or more of body surface with 10-19% third degree **burns** HAC HCC McC⁰ CC/MCC

T31.92 Burns involving 90% or more of body surface with 20-29% third degree **burns** HAC HCC McC⁰ CC/MCC

T31.93 Burns involving 90% or more of body surface with 30-39% third degree **burns** HAC HCC McC⁰ CC/MCC

T31.94 Burns involving 90% or more of body surface with 40-49% third degree **burns** HAC HCC McC⁰ CC/MCC

T31.95 Burns involving 90% or more of body surface with 50-59% third degree **burns** HAC HCC McC⁰ CC/MCC

T31.96 Burns involving 90% or more of body surface with 60-69% third degree **burns** HAC HCC McC⁰ CC/MCC

T31.97 Burns involving 90% or more of body surface with 70-79% third degree **burns** HAC HCC McC⁰ CC/MCC

T31.98 Burns involving 90% or more of body surface with 80-89% third degree **burns** HAC HCC McC⁰ CC/MCC

T31.99 Burns involving 90% or more of body surface with 90% or more third degree burns HAC HCC McC⁰ CC/MCC

4ᵗʰ **T32** Corrosions **classified** according to extent of body surface involved

👁 **See Official Guidelines** "Burns and Corrosions Classified According to Extent of Body Surface Involved" I.C.19.d.6

NOTES This category is to be used as the primary code only when the site of the corrosion is unspecified. It may be used as a supplementary code with categories T20-T25 when the site is specified.

T32.0 Corrosions involving less than 10% of body surface

5ᵗʰ **T32.1** Corrosions involving 10-19% of body surface

T32.10 Corrosions involving 10-19% of body surface with 0% to 9% third degree **corrosion** CC⁰ HAC CC/MCC
Corrosions involving 10-19% of body surface NOS

T32.11 Corrosions involving 10-19% of body surface with 10-19% third degree **corrosion** CC⁰ HAC HCC CC/MCC

5ᵗʰ **T32.2** Corrosions involving 20-29% of body surface

T32.20 Corrosions involving 20-29% of body surface with 0% to 9% third degree **corrosion** CC⁰ HAC CC/MCC

T32.21 Corrosions involving 20-29% of body surface with 10-19% third degree **corrosion** HAC HCC McC⁰ CC/MCC

T32.22 Corrosions involving 20-29% of body surface with 20-29% third degree **corrosion** HAC HCC McC⁰ CC/MCC

5ᵗʰ **T32.3** Corrosions involving 30-39% of body surface

T32.30 Corrosions involving 30-39% of body surface with 0% to 9% third degree **corrosion** CC⁰ HAC CC/MCC

T32.31 Corrosions involving 30-39% of body surface with 10-19% third degree **corrosion** HAC HCC McC⁰ CC/MCC

T32.32 Corrosions involving 30-39% of body surface with 20-29% third degree **corrosion** HAC HCC McC⁰ CC/MCC

T32.33 Corrosions involving 30-39% of body surface with 30-39% third degree **corrosion** HAC HCC McC⁰ CC/MCC

5ᵗʰ **T32.4** Corrosions involving 40-49% of body surface

T32.40 Corrosions involving 40-49% of body surface with 0% to 9% third degree **corrosion** CC⁰ HAC CC/MCC

T32.41 Corrosions involving 40-49% of body surface with 10-19% third degree **corrosion** HAC HCC McC⁰ CC/MCC

T32.42 Corrosions involving 40-49% of body surface with 20-29% third degree **corrosion** HAC HCC McC⁰ CC/MCC

T32.43 Corrosions involving 40-49% of body surface with 30-39% third degree **corrosion** HAC HCC McC⁰ CC/MCC

T32.44 Corrosions involving 40-49% of body surface with 40-49% third degree **corrosion** HAC HCC McC⁰ CC/MCC

5ᵗʰ **T32.5** Corrosions involving 50-59% of body surface

T32.50 Corrosions involving 50-59% of body surface with 0% to 9% third degree **corrosion** CC⁰ HAC CC/MCC

T32.51 Corrosions involving 50-59% of body surface with 10-19% third degree **corrosion** HAC HCC McC⁰ CC/MCC

T32.52 Corrosions involving 50-59% of body surface with 20-29% third degree **corrosion** HAC HCC McC⁰ CC/MCC

T32.53 Corrosions involving 50-59% of body surface with 30-39% third degree **corrosion** HAC HCC McC⁰ CC/MCC

T32.54 Corrosions involving 50-59% of body surface with 40-49% third degree **corrosion** HAC HCC McC⁰ CC/MCC

T32.55 Corrosions involving 50-59% of body surface with 50-59% third degree **corrosion** HAC HCC McC⁰ CC/MCC

5ᵗʰ **T32.6** Corrosions involving 60-69% of body surface

T32.60 Corrosions involving 60-69% of body surface with 0% to 9% third degree **corrosion** CC⁰ HAC CC/MCC

T32.61 Corrosions involving 60-69% of body surface with 10-19% third degree **corrosion** HAC HCC McC⁰ CC/MCC

T32.62 Corrosions involving 60-69% of body surface with 20-29% third degree **corrosion** HAC HCC McC⁰ CC/MCC

T32.63 Corrosions involving 60-69% of body surface with 30-39% third degree **corrosion** HAC HCC McC⁰ CC/MCC

T32.64 Corrosions involving 60-69% of body surface with 40-49% third degree **corrosion** HAC HCC McC⁰ CC/MCC

T32.65 Corrosions involving 60-69% of body surface with 50-59% third degree **corrosion** HAC HCC McC⁰ CC/MCC

T32.66 Corrosions involving 60-69% of body surface with 60-69% third degree **corrosion** HAC HCC McC⁰ CC/MCC

5ᵗʰ **T32.7** Corrosions involving 70-79% of body surface

T32.70 Corrosions involving 70-79% of body surface with 0% to 9% third degree **corrosion** CC⁰ HAC CC/MCC

T32.71 Corrosions involving 70-79% of body surface with 10-19% third degree **corrosion** HAC HCC McC⁰ CC/MCC

T32.72 Corrosions involving 70-79% of body surface with 20-29% third degree **corrosion** HAC HCC McC⁰ CC/MCC

T32.73 Corrosions involving 70-79% of body surface with 30-39% third degree **corrosion** HAC HCC McC⁰ CC/MCC

T32.74 Corrosions involving 70-79% of body surface with 40-49% third degree **corrosion** HAC HCC McC⁰ CC/MCC

T32.75 Corrosions involving 70-79% of body surface with 50-59% third degree **corrosion** HAC HCC McC⁰ CC/MCC

T32.76 Corrosions involving 70-79% of body surface with 60-69% third degree **corrosion** HAC HCC McC⁰ CC/MCC

T32.77 Corrosions involving 70-79% of body surface with 70-79% third degree **corrosion** HAC HCC McC⁰ CC/MCC

5ᵗʰ **T32.8** Corrosions involving 80-89% of body surface

T32.80 Corrosions involving 80-89% of body surface with 0% to 9% third degree **corrosion** CC⁰ HAC CC/MCC

T32.81 Corrosions involving 80-89% of body surface with 10-19% third degree **corrosion** HAC HCC McC⁰ CC/MCC

T32.82 Corrosions involving 80-89% of body surface with 20-29% third degree **corrosion** HAC HCC McC⁰ CC/MCC

T32.83 Corrosions involving 80-89% of body surface with 30-39% third degree **corrosion** HAC HCC McC⁰ CC/MCC

T32.84 Corrosions involving 80-89% of body surface with 40-49% third degree **corrosion** HAC HCC McC⁰ CC/MCC

T32.85 Corrosions involving 80-89% of body surface with 50-59% third degree **corrosion** HAC HCC McC⁰ CC/MCC

T32.86 Corrosions involving 80-89% of body surface with 60-69% third degree **corrosion** HAC HCC McC⁰ CC/MCC

T32.87 Corrosions involving 80-89% of body surface with 70-79% third degree **corrosion** HAC HCC McC⁰ CC/MCC

T32.88 Corrosions involving 80-89% of body surface with 80-89% third degree **corrosion** HAC HCC McC⁰ CC/MCC

5ᵗʰ **T32.9** Corrosions involving 90% or more of body surface

T32.90 Corrosions involving 90% or more of body surface with 0% to 9% third degree **corrosion** CC⁰ HAC CC/MCC

T32.91 Corrosions involving 90% or more of body surface with 10-19% third degree **corrosion** HAC HCC McC⁰ CC/MCC

T32.92 Corrosions involving 90% or more of body surface with 20-29% third degree **corrosion** HAC HCC McC⁰ CC/MCC

T32.93 Corrosions involving 90% or more of body surface with 30-39% third degree **corrosion** HAC HCC McC⁰ CC/MCC

T32.94 Corrosions involving 90% or more of body surface with 40-49% third degree **corrosion** HAC HCC McC⁰ CC/MCC

T32.95 Corrosions involving 90% or more of body surface with 50-59% third degree **corrosion** HAC HCC McC⁰ CC/MCC

T32.96 Corrosions involving 90% or more of body surface with 60-69% third degree **corrosion** HAC HCC McC⁰ CC/MCC

T32.97 Corrosions involving 90% or more of body surface with 70-79% third degree **corrosion** HAC HCC McC⁰ CC/MCC

T32.98 Corrosions involving 90% or more of body surface with 80-89% third degree **corrosion** HAC HCC McC⁰ CC/MCC

T32.99 Corrosions involving 90% or more of body surface with 90% or more third degree **corrosion** HAC HCC McC⁰ CC/MCC

CHAPTER 19: INJURY, POISONING, AND CERTAIN OTHER CONSEQUENCES OF EXTERNAL CAUSES (S00-T88)

T33 - T34.521

Frostbite (T33-T34)

EXCLUDES2 hypothermia and other effects of reduced temperature (T68, T69.-)

T33 Superficial frostbite
  INCLUDES frostbite with partial thickness skin loss
  The appropriate 7th character is to be added to each code from category T33
    A = initial encounter
    D = subsequent encounter
    S = sequela

  T33.0 Superficial frostbite of head
    T33.01 Superficial frostbite of ear
      T33.011 Superficial frostbite of right ear
      T33.012 Superficial frostbite of left ear
      T33.019 Superficial frostbite of unspecified ear
    T33.02 Superficial frostbite of nose
    T33.09 Superficial frostbite of other part of head
  T33.1 Superficial frostbite of neck
  T33.2 Superficial frostbite of thorax
  T33.3 Superficial frostbite of abdominal wall, lower back and pelvis
  T33.4 Superficial frostbite of arm
    EXCLUDES2 superficial frostbite of wrist and hand (T33.5-)
    T33.40 Superficial frostbite of unspecified arm
    T33.41 Superficial frostbite of right arm
    T33.42 Superficial frostbite of left arm
  T33.5 Superficial frostbite of wrist, hand, and fingers
    T33.51 Superficial frostbite of wrist
      T33.511 Superficial frostbite of right wrist
      T33.512 Superficial frostbite of left wrist
      T33.519 Superficial frostbite of unspecified wrist
    T33.52 Superficial frostbite of hand
      EXCLUDES2 superficial frostbite of fingers (T33.53-)
      T33.521 Superficial frostbite of right hand
      T33.522 Superficial frostbite of left hand
      T33.529 Superficial frostbite of unspecified hand
    T33.53 Superficial frostbite of finger(s)
      T33.531 Superficial frostbite of right finger(s)
      T33.532 Superficial frostbite of left finger(s)
      T33.539 Superficial frostbite of unspecified finger(s)
  T33.6 Superficial frostbite of hip and thigh
    T33.60 Superficial frostbite of unspecified hip and thigh
    T33.61 Superficial frostbite of right hip and thigh
    T33.62 Superficial frostbite of left hip and thigh
  T33.7 Superficial frostbite of knee and lower leg
    EXCLUDES2 superficial frostbite of ankle and foot (T33.8-)
    T33.70 Superficial frostbite of unspecified knee and lower leg
    T33.71 Superficial frostbite of right knee and lower leg
    T33.72 Superficial frostbite of left knee and lower leg
  T33.8 Superficial frostbite of ankle, foot, and toe(s)

  T33.81 Superficial frostbite of ankle
    T33.811 Superficial frostbite of right ankle
    T33.812 Superficial frostbite of left ankle
    T33.819 Superficial frostbite of unspecified ankle
  T33.82 Superficial frostbite of foot
    T33.821 Superficial frostbite of right foot
    T33.822 Superficial frostbite of left foot
    T33.829 Superficial frostbite of unspecified foot
  T33.83 Superficial frostbite of toe(s)
    T33.831 Superficial frostbite of right toe(s)
    T33.832 Superficial frostbite of left toe(s)
    T33.839 Superficial frostbite of unspecified toe(s)
  T33.9 Superficial frostbite of other and unspecified sites
    T33.90 Superficial frostbite of unspecified sites
      Superficial frostbite NOS
    T33.99 Superficial frostbite of other sites
      Superficial frostbite of leg NOS
      Superficial frostbite of trunk NOS

T34 Frostbite with tissue necrosis
  The appropriate 7th character is to be added to each code from category T34
    A = initial encounter
    D = subsequent encounter
    S = sequela

  T34.0 Frostbite with tissue necrosis of head
    T34.01 Frostbite with tissue necrosis of ear
      T34.011 Frostbite with tissue necrosis of right ear
      T34.012 Frostbite with tissue necrosis of left ear
      T34.019 Frostbite with tissue necrosis of unspecified ear
    T34.02 Frostbite with tissue necrosis of nose
    T34.09 Frostbite with tissue necrosis of other part of head
  T34.1 Frostbite with tissue necrosis of neck
  T34.2 Frostbite with tissue necrosis of thorax
  T34.3 Frostbite with tissue necrosis of abdominal wall, lower back and pelvis
  T34.4 Frostbite with tissue necrosis of arm
    EXCLUDES2 frostbite with tissue necrosis of wrist and hand (T34.5-)
    T34.40 Frostbite with tissue necrosis of unspecified arm
    T34.41 Frostbite with tissue necrosis of right arm
    T34.42 Frostbite with tissue necrosis of left arm
  T34.5 Frostbite with tissue necrosis of wrist, hand, and finger(s)
    T34.51 Frostbite with tissue necrosis of wrist
      T34.511 Frostbite with tissue necrosis of right wrist
      T34.512 Frostbite with tissue necrosis of left wrist
      T34.519 Frostbite with tissue necrosis of unspecified wrist
    T34.52 Frostbite with tissue necrosis of hand
      EXCLUDES2 frostbite with tissue necrosis of finger(s) (T34.53-)
      T34.521 Frostbite with tissue necrosis of right hand

PDx Unacceptable principal diagnosis symbol per Medicare code edits   Code exempt from diagnosis present on admission requirement
? Questionable admission   Complication or comorbidity   MCC Major complication or comorbidity   CC/MCC Exc CC/MCC exclusion
HCC HCC diagnosis code   RxHCC RxHCC diagnosis code   MACRA code   **DEFINITION** Describes condition/terminology
TIP Coding guidance   Official Guideline Reference   Z1 Z code as first-listed diagnosis

7ᵗʰ T34.522 Frostbite with tissue necrosis of left hand · CC POA HAC CC/MCC Exc

7ᵗʰ T34.529 Frostbite with tissue necrosis of unspecified hand · POA HAC CC/MCC Exc

6ᵗʰ T34.53 Frostbite with tissue necrosis of finger(s)

  7ᵗʰ T34.531 Frostbite with tissue necrosis of right finger(s) · CC POA HAC CC/MCC Exc

  7ᵗʰ T34.532 Frostbite with tissue necrosis of left finger(s) · CC POA HAC CC/MCC Exc

  7ᵗʰ T34.539 Frostbite with tissue necrosis of unspecified finger(s) · CC POA HAC CC/MCC Exc

5ᵗʰ T34.6 Frostbite with tissue necrosis of hip and thigh

  7ᵗʰ T34.60 Frostbite with tissue necrosis of unspecified hip and thigh · CC POA HAC CC/MCC Exc

  7ᵗʰ T34.61 Frostbite with tissue necrosis of right hip and thigh · CC POA HAC CC/MCC Exc

  7ᵗʰ T34.62 Frostbite with tissue necrosis of left hip and thigh · CC POA HAC CC/MCC Exc

5ᵗʰ T34.7 Frostbite with tissue necrosis of knee and lower leg

  EXCLUDES2 frostbite with tissue necrosis of ankle and foot (T34.8-)

  7ᵗʰ T34.70 Frostbite with tissue necrosis of unspecified knee and lower leg · CC POA HAC CC/MCC Exc

  7ᵗʰ T34.71 Frostbite with tissue necrosis of right knee and lower leg · CC POA HAC CC/MCC Exc

  7ᵗʰ T34.72 Frostbite with tissue necrosis of left knee and lower leg · CC POA HAC CC/MCC Exc

5ᵗʰ T34.8 Frostbite with tissue necrosis of ankle, foot, and toe(s)

  6ᵗʰ T34.81 Frostbite with tissue necrosis of ankle

    7ᵗʰ T34.811 Frostbite with tissue necrosis of right ankle · CC POA HAC CC/MCC Exc

    7ᵗʰ T34.812 Frostbite with tissue necrosis of left ankle · CC POA HAC CC/MCC Exc

    7ᵗʰ T34.819 Frostbite with tissue necrosis of unspecified ankle · CC POA HAC CC/MCC Exc

  6ᵗʰ T34.82 Frostbite with tissue necrosis of foot

    7ᵗʰ T34.821 Frostbite with tissue necrosis of right foot · CC POA HAC CC/MCC Exc

    7ᵗʰ T34.822 Frostbite with tissue necrosis of left foot · CC POA HAC CC/MCC Exc

    7ᵗʰ T34.829 Frostbite with tissue necrosis of unspecified foot · CC POA HAC CC/MCC Exc

  6ᵗʰ T34.83 Frostbite with tissue necrosis of toe(s)

    7ᵗʰ T34.831 Frostbite with tissue necrosis of right toe(s) · CC POA HAC CC/MCC Exc

    7ᵗʰ T34.832 Frostbite with tissue necrosis of left toe(s) · CC POA HAC CC/MCC Exc

    7ᵗʰ T34.839 Frostbite with tissue necrosis of unspecified toe(s) · CC POA HAC CC/MCC Exc

5ᵗʰ T34.9 Frostbite with tissue necrosis of other and unspecified sites

  7ᵗʰ T34.90 Frostbite with tissue necrosis of unspecified sites · CC POA HAC CC/MCC Exc

      Frostbite with tissue necrosis NOS

  7ᵗʰ T34.99 Frostbite with tissue necrosis of other sites · CC POA HAC CC/MCC Exc

      Frostbite with tissue necrosis of leg NOS
      Frostbite with tissue necrosis of trunk NOS

Poisoning by, adverse effects of and underdosing of drugs, medicaments and biological substances (T36-T50)

👁 **See Official Guidelines** "Poisoning" I.C.19.e.5.b, "Underdosing" I.C.19.e.5.c, "Adverse Effects, Poisoning, Underdosing and Toxic Effects" I.C.19.e

INCLUDES adverse effect of correct substance properly administered
    poisoning by overdose of substance
    poisoning by wrong substance given or taken in error
    underdosing by (inadvertently) (deliberately) taking less substance than prescribed or instructed

☞ **Code first,** for adverse effects, the nature of the adverse effect, such as:
    adverse effect NOS (T88.7)
    aspirin gastritis (K29.-)
    blood disorders (D56-D76)
    contact dermatitis (L23-L25)
    dermatitis due to substances taken internally (L27.-)
    nephropathy (N14.0-N14.2)

NOTES The drug giving rise to the adverse effect should be identified by use of codes from categories T36-T50 with fifth or sixth character 5.

Use additional code(s) to specify:
manifestations of poisoning
underdosing or failure in dosage during medical and surgical care (Y63.6, Y63.8-Y63.9)
underdosing of medication regimen (Z91.12-, Z91.13-)

EXCLUDES1 toxic reaction to local anesthesia in pregnancy (O29.3-)

EXCLUDES2 abuse and dependence of psychoactive substances (F10-F19)
    abuse of non-dependence-producing substances (F55.-)
    drug reaction and poisoning affecting newborn (P00-P96)
    pathological drug intoxication (inebriation) (F10-F19)

4ᵗʰ T36 Poisoning by, adverse effect of and underdosing of systemic antibiotics

  EXCLUDES1 antineoplastic antibiotics (T45.1-)
      locally applied antibiotic NEC (T49.0)
      topically used antibiotic for ear, nose and throat (T49.6)
      topically used antibiotic for eye (T49.5)

The appropriate 7th character is to be added to each code from category T36
    A = initial encounter
    D = subsequent encounter
    S = sequela

5ᵗʰ T36.0 Poisoning by, adverse effect of and underdosing of penicillins

  6ᵗʰ T36.0X Poisoning by, adverse effect of and underdosing of penicillins

    7ᵗʰ T36.0X1 Poisoning by penicillins, accidental (unintentional) · POA
        Poisoning by penicillins NOS

    7ᵗʰ T36.0X2 Poisoning by penicillins, intentional self-harm · POA HCC

    7ᵗʰ T36.0X3 Poisoning by penicillins, assault · POA

    7ᵗʰ T36.0X4 Poisoning by penicillins, undetermined · POA

    7ᵗʰ T36.0X5 Adverse effect of penicillins · POA PDxIn

    7ᵗʰ T36.0X6 Underdosing of penicillins · POA PDxIn

5ᵗʰ T36.1 Poisoning by, adverse effect of and underdosing of cephalosporins and other beta-lactam antibiotics

  6ᵗʰ T36.1X Poisoning by, adverse effect of and underdosing of cephalosporins and other beta-lactam antibiotics

    7ᵗʰ T36.1X1 Poisoning by cephalosporins and other beta-lactam antibiotics, accidental (unintentional) · POA
        Poisoning by cephalosporins and other beta-lactam antibiotics NOS

    7ᵗʰ T36.1X2 Poisoning by cephalosporins and other beta-lactam antibiotics, intentional self-harm · POA HCC

    7ᵗʰ T36.1X3 Poisoning by cephalosporins and other beta-lactam antibiotics, assault · POA

    7ᵗʰ T36.1X4 Poisoning by cephalosporins and other beta-lactam antibiotics, undetermined · POA

    7ᵗʰ T36.1X5 Adverse effect of cephalosporins and other beta-lactam antibiotics · POA PDxIn

    7ᵗʰ T36.1X6 Underdosing of cephalosporins and other beta-lactam antibiotics · POA PDxIn

5ᵗʰ T36.2 Poisoning by, adverse effect of and underdosing of chloramphenicol group

  6ᵗʰ T36.2X Poisoning by, adverse effect of and underdosing of chloramphenicol group

    7ᵗʰ T36.2X1 Poisoning by chloramphenicol group, accidental (unintentional) · POA
        Poisoning by chloramphenicol group NOS

    7ᵗʰ T36.2X2 Poisoning by chloramphenicol group, intentional self-harm · POA HCC

    7ᵗʰ T36.2X3 Poisoning by chloramphenicol group, assault · POA

    7ᵗʰ T36.2X4 Poisoning by chloramphenicol group, undetermined · POA

Unspecified Code Other Specified Code Manifestation Code N Newborn P Pediatric M Maternity A Adult ♂ Male ♀ Female
● New Code ▲ Revised Code Title ►◄ Revised Text NOTES INCLUDES EXCLUDES1 Not coded here EXCLUDES2 Not included here
4ᵗʰ 4ᵗʰ character required 5ᵗʰ 5ᵗʰ character required 6ᵗʰ 6ᵗʰ character required 7ᵗʰ 7ᵗʰ character required X Extension 'X' Alert
HAC Hospital-acquired condition (HAC) alert AHA AHA Coding Clinic© ☞ Code first alert

[7th] **T36.2X5** Adverse effect of chloramphenicol group [POA] [PDx]
[7th] **T36.2X6** Underdosing of chloramphenicol group [POA] [PDx]

[5th] **T36.3 Poisoning by, adverse effect of and underdosing of macrolides**
[6th] **T36.3X Poisoning by, adverse effect of and underdosing of macrolides**
[7th] **T36.3X1** Poisoning by macrolides, accidental (unintentional) [POA]
Poisoning by macrolides NOS
[7th] **T36.3X2** Poisoning by macrolides, intentional self-harm [POA] [HCC]
[7th] **T36.3X3** Poisoning by macrolides, assault [POA]
[7th] **T36.3X4** Poisoning by macrolides, undetermined [POA]
[7th] **T36.3X5** Adverse effect of macrolides [POA] [PDx]
[7th] **T36.3X6** Underdosing of macrolides [POA] [PDx]

[5th] **T36.4 Poisoning by, adverse effect of and underdosing of tetracyclines**
[6th] **T36.4X Poisoning by, adverse effect of and underdosing of tetracyclines**
[7th] **T36.4X1** Poisoning by tetracyclines, accidental (unintentional) [POA]
Poisoning by tetracyclines NOS
[7th] **T36.4X2** Poisoning by tetracyclines, intentional self-harm [POA] [HCC]
[7th] **T36.4X3** Poisoning by tetracyclines, assault [POA]
[7th] **T36.4X4** Poisoning by tetracyclines, undetermined [POA]
[7th] **T36.4X5** Adverse effect of tetracyclines [POA] [PDx]
[7th] **T36.4X6** Underdosing of tetracyclines [POA] [PDx]

[5th] **T36.5 Poisoning by, adverse effect of and underdosing of aminoglycosides**
Poisoning by, adverse effect of and underdosing of streptomycin
[6th] **T36.5X Poisoning by, adverse effect of and underdosing of aminoglycosides**
[7th] **T36.5X1** Poisoning by aminoglycosides, accidental (unintentional) [POA]
Poisoning by aminoglycosides NOS
[7th] **T36.5X2** Poisoning by aminoglycosides, intentional self-harm [POA] [HCC]
[7th] **T36.5X3** Poisoning by aminoglycosides, assault [POA]
[7th] **T36.5X4** Poisoning by aminoglycosides, undetermined [POA]
[7th] **T36.5X5** Adverse effect of aminoglycosides [POA] [PDx]
[7th] **T36.5X6** Underdosing of aminoglycosides [POA] [PDx]

[5th] **T36.6 Poisoning by, adverse effect of and underdosing of rifampicins**
[6th] **T36.6X Poisoning by, adverse effect of and underdosing of rifampicins**
[7th] **T36.6X1** Poisoning by rifampicins, accidental (unintentional) [POA]
Poisoning by rifampicins NOS
[7th] **T36.6X2** Poisoning by rifampicins, intentional self-harm [POA] [HCC]
[7th] **T36.6X3** Poisoning by rifampicins, assault [POA]
[7th] **T36.6X4** Poisoning by rifampicins, undetermined [POA]
[7th] **T36.6X5** Adverse effect of rifampicins [POA] [PDx]
[7th] **T36.6X6** Underdosing of rifampicins [POA] [PDx]

[5th] **T36.7 Poisoning by, adverse effect of and underdosing of antifungal antibiotics, systemically used**
[6th] **T36.7X Poisoning by, adverse effect of and underdosing of antifungal antibiotics, systemically used**
[7th] **T36.7X1** Poisoning by antifungal antibiotics, systemically used, accidental (unintentional) [POA]
Poisoning by antifungal antibiotics, systemically used NOS
[7th] **T36.7X2** Poisoning by antifungal antibiotics, systemically used, intentional self-harm [POA] [HCC]
[7th] **T36.7X3** Poisoning by antifungal antibiotics, systemically used, assault [POA]
[7th] **T36.7X4** Poisoning by antifungal antibiotics, systemically used, undetermined [POA]
[7th] **T36.7X5** Adverse effect of antifungal antibiotics, systemically used [POA] [PDx]
[7th] **T36.7X6** Underdosing of antifungal antibiotics, systemically used [POA] [PDx]

[5th] **T36.8 Poisoning by, adverse effect of and underdosing of other systemic antibiotics**
[6th] **T36.8X Poisoning by, adverse effect of and underdosing of other systemic antibiotics**
[7th] **T36.8X1** Poisoning by other systemic antibiotics, accidental (unintentional) [POA]
Poisoning by other systemic antibiotics NOS
[7th] **T36.8X2** Poisoning by other systemic antibiotics, intentional self-harm [POA] [HCC]
[7th] **T36.8X3** Poisoning by other systemic antibiotics, assault [POA]
[7th] **T36.8X4** Poisoning by other systemic antibiotics, undetermined [POA]
[7th] **T36.8X5** Adverse effect of other systemic antibiotics [POA] [PDx]
AHA: Q1 2017
[7th] **T36.8X6** Underdosing of other systemic antibiotics [POA] [PDx]

[5th] **T36.9 Poisoning by, adverse effect of and underdosing of unspecified systemic antibiotic**
[7th] **T36.91** Poisoning by unspecified systemic antibiotic, accidental (unintentional) [POA]
Poisoning by systemic antibiotic NOS
[7th] **T36.92** Poisoning by unspecified systemic antibiotic, intentional self-harm [POA] [HCC]
[7th] **T36.93** Poisoning by unspecified systemic antibiotic, assault [POA]
[7th] **T36.94** Poisoning by unspecified systemic antibiotic, undetermined [POA]
[7th] **T36.95** Adverse effect of unspecified systemic antibiotic [POA] [PDx]
[7th] **T36.96** Underdosing of unspecified systemic antibiotic [POA] [PDx]

[4th] **T37 Poisoning by, adverse effect of and underdosing of other systemic anti-infectives and antiparasitics**
[EXCLUDES1] *anti-infectives topically used for ear, nose and throat (T49.6-)*
anti-infectives topically used for eye (T49.5-)
locally applied anti-infectives NEC (T49.0-)

The appropriate 7th character is to be added to each code from category T37
A = initial encounter
D = subsequent encounter
S = sequela

[5th] **T37.0 Poisoning by, adverse effect of and underdosing of sulfonamides**
[6th] **T37.0X Poisoning by, adverse effect of and underdosing of sulfonamides**
[7th] **T37.0X1** Poisoning by sulfonamides, accidental (unintentional) [POA]
Poisoning by sulfonamides NOS
[7th] **T37.0X2** Poisoning by sulfonamides, intentional self-harm [POA] [HCC]
[7th] **T37.0X3** Poisoning by sulfonamides, assault [POA]
[7th] **T37.0X4** Poisoning by sulfonamides, undetermined [POA]
[7th] **T37.0X5** Adverse effect of sulfonamides [POA] [PDx]
[7th] **T37.0X6** Underdosing of sulfonamides [POA] [PDx]

[5th] **T37.1 Poisoning by, adverse effect of and underdosing of antimycobacterial drugs**
[EXCLUDES1] *rifampicins (T36.6-)*
streptomycin (T36.5-)
[6th] **T37.1X Poisoning by, adverse effect of and underdosing of antimycobacterial drugs**

[PDx] Unacceptable principal diagnosis symbol per Medicare code edits [POA] Code exempt from diagnosis present on admission requirement
[?] Questionable admission [CC] Complication or comorbidity [MCC] Major complication or comorbidity [CC/MCC Excl] CC/MCC exclusion
[HCC] HCC diagnosis code [RxHCC] RxHCC diagnosis code MACRA code **DEFINITION** Describes condition/terminology
TIP Coding guidance [Official Guideline Reference] Official Guideline Reference [Z1] Z code as first-listed diagnosis

7️⃣ **T37.1X1** Poisoning by antimycobacterial drugs, accidental (unintentional) POA
Poisoning by antimycobacterial drugs NOS

7️⃣ **T37.1X2** Poisoning by antimycobacterial drugs, intentional self-harm POA HCC

7️⃣ **T37.1X3** Poisoning by antimycobacterial drugs, assault POA

7️⃣ **T37.1X4** Poisoning by antimycobacterial drugs, undetermined POA

7️⃣ **T37.1X5** Adverse effect of antimycobacterial drugs POA PDxIn

7️⃣ **T37.1X6** Underdosing of antimycobacterial drugs POA PDxIn

5️⃣ **T37.2** Poisoning by, adverse effect of and underdosing of antimalarials and drugs acting on other blood protozoa
EXCLUDES1 hydroxyquinoline derivatives (T37.8-)

6️⃣ **T37.2X** Poisoning by, adverse effect of and underdosing of antimalarials and drugs acting on other blood protozoa

7️⃣ **T37.2X1** Poisoning by antimalarials and drugs acting on other blood protozoa, accidental (unintentional) POA
Poisoning by antimalarials and drugs acting on other blood protozoa NOS

7️⃣ **T37.2X2** Poisoning by antimalarials and drugs acting on other blood protozoa, intentional self-harm POA HCC

7️⃣ **T37.2X3** Poisoning by antimalarials and drugs acting on other blood protozoa, assault POA

7️⃣ **T37.2X4** Poisoning by antimalarials and drugs acting on other blood protozoa, undetermined POA

7️⃣ **T37.2X5** Adverse effect of antimalarials and drugs acting on other blood protozoa POA PDxIn

7️⃣ **T37.2X6** Underdosing of antimalarials and drugs acting on other blood protozoa POA PDxIn

5️⃣ **T37.3** Poisoning by, adverse effect of and underdosing of other antiprotozoal drugs

6️⃣ **T37.3X** Poisoning by, adverse effect of and underdosing of other antiprotozoal drugs

7️⃣ **T37.3X1** Poisoning by other antiprotozoal drugs, accidental (unintentional) POA
Poisoning by other antiprotozoal drugs NOS

7️⃣ **T37.3X2** Poisoning by other antiprotozoal drugs, intentional self-harm POA HCC

7️⃣ **T37.3X3** Poisoning by other antiprotozoal drugs, assault POA

7️⃣ **T37.3X4** Poisoning by other antiprotozoal drugs, undetermined POA

7️⃣ **T37.3X5** Adverse effect of other antiprotozoal drugs POA PDxIn

7️⃣ **T37.3X6** Underdosing of other antiprotozoal drugs POA PDxIn

5️⃣ **T37.4** Poisoning by, adverse effect of and underdosing of anthelminthics

6️⃣ **T37.4X** Poisoning by, adverse effect of and underdosing of anthelminthics

7️⃣ **T37.4X1** Poisoning by anthelminthics, accidental (unintentional) POA
Poisoning by anthelminthics NOS

7️⃣ **T37.4X2** Poisoning by anthelminthics, intentional self-harm POA HCC

7️⃣ **T37.4X3** Poisoning by anthelminthics, assault POA

7️⃣ **T37.4X4** Poisoning by anthelminthics, undetermined POA

7️⃣ **T37.4X5** Adverse effect of anthelminthics POA PDxIn

7️⃣ **T37.4X6** Underdosing of anthelminthics POA PDxIn

5️⃣ **T37.5** Poisoning by, adverse effect of and underdosing of antiviral drugs
EXCLUDES1 amantadine (T42.8-)
cytarabine (T45.1-)

6️⃣ **T37.5X** Poisoning by, adverse effect of and underdosing of antiviral drugs

7️⃣ **T37.5X1** Poisoning by antiviral drugs, accidental (unintentional) POA
Poisoning by antiviral drugs NOS

7️⃣ **T37.5X2** Poisoning by antiviral drugs, intentional self-harm POA HCC

7️⃣ **T37.5X3** Poisoning by antiviral drugs, assault POA

7️⃣ **T37.5X4** Poisoning by antiviral drugs, undetermined POA

7️⃣ **T37.5X5** Adverse effect of antiviral drugs POA PDxIn

7️⃣ **T37.5X6** Underdosing of antiviral drugs POA PDxIn

5️⃣ **T37.8** Poisoning by, adverse effect of and underdosing of other specified systemic anti-infectives and antiparasitics
Poisoning by, adverse effect of and underdosing of hydroxyquinoline derivatives
EXCLUDES1 antimalarial drugs (T37.2-)

6️⃣ **T37.8X** Poisoning by, adverse effect of and underdosing of other specified systemic anti-infectives and antiparasitics

7️⃣ **T37.8X1** Poisoning by other specified systemic anti-infectives and antiparasitics, accidental (unintentional) POA
Poisoning by other specified systemic anti-infectives and antiparasitics NOS

7️⃣ **T37.8X2** Poisoning by other specified systemic anti-infectives and antiparasitics, intentional self-harm POA HCC

7️⃣ **T37.8X3** Poisoning by other specified systemic anti-infectives and antiparasitics, assault POA

7️⃣ **T37.8X4** Poisoning by other specified systemic anti-infectives and antiparasitics, undetermined POA

7️⃣ **T37.8X5** Adverse effect of other specified systemic anti-infectives and antiparasitics POA PDxIn

7️⃣ **T37.8X6** Underdosing of other specified systemic anti-infectives and antiparasitics POA PDxIn

5️⃣ **T37.9** Poisoning by, adverse effect of and underdosing of unspecified systemic anti-infective and antiparasitics

7️⃣ **T37.91** Poisoning by unspecified systemic anti-infective and antiparasitics, accidental (unintentional) POA
Poisoning by, adverse effect of and underdosing of systemic anti-infective and antiparasitics NOS

7️⃣ **T37.92** Poisoning by unspecified systemic anti-infective and antiparasitics, intentional self-harm POA HCC

7️⃣ **T37.93** Poisoning by unspecified systemic anti-infective and antiparasitics, assault POA

7️⃣ **T37.94** Poisoning by unspecified systemic anti-infective and antiparasitics, undetermined POA

7️⃣ **T37.95** Adverse effect of unspecified systemic anti-infective and antiparasitic POA PDxIn

7️⃣ **T37.96** Underdosing of unspecified systemic anti-infectives and antiparasitics POA PDxIn

4️⃣ **T38** Poisoning by, adverse effect of and underdosing of hormones and their synthetic substitutes and antagonists, not elsewhere classified
EXCLUDES1 mineralocorticoids and their antagonists (T50.0-)
oxytocic hormones (T48.0-)
parathyroid hormones and derivatives (T50.9-)

The appropriate 7th character is to be added to each code from category T38
A = initial encounter
D = subsequent encounter
S = sequela

5️⃣ **T38.0** Poisoning by, adverse effect of and underdosing of glucocorticoids and synthetic analogues
EXCLUDES1 glucocorticoids, topically used (T49.-)

6️⃣ **T38.0X** Poisoning by, adverse effect of and underdosing of glucocorticoids and synthetic analogues

7️⃣ **T38.0X1** Poisoning by glucocorticoids and synthetic analogues, accidental (unintentional) POA
Poisoning by glucocorticoids and synthetic analogues NOS

Unspecified Code	Other Specified Code	Manifestation Code	N Newborn	P Pediatric	M Maternity	A Adult	♂ Male	♀ Female

● New Code ▲ Revised Code Title ▶◀ Revised Text **NOTES** *INCLUDES* EXCLUDES1 Not coded here EXCLUDES2 Not included here
4️⃣ 4th character required 5️⃣ 5th character required 6️⃣ 6th character required 7️⃣ 7th character required 7️⃣ Extension 'X' Alert
HAC Hospital-acquired condition (HAC) alert **AHA** AHA Coding Clinic© 📢 Code first alert

[7th] **T38.0X2 Poisoning by glucocorticoids and synthetic analogues, intentional self-harm** [POA] [HCC]
[7th] **T38.0X3 Poisoning by glucocorticoids and synthetic analogues, assault** [POA]
[7th] **T38.0X4 Poisoning by glucocorticoids and synthetic analogues, undetermined** [POA]
[7th] **T38.0X5 Adverse effect of glucocorticoids and synthetic analogues** [POA] [PDx]
[7th] **T38.0X6 Underdosing of glucocorticoids and synthetic analogues** [POA] [PDx]

[5th] **T38.1 Poisoning by, adverse effect of and underdosing of thyroid hormones and substitutes**
[6th] **T38.1X Poisoning by, adverse effect of and underdosing of thyroid hormones and substitutes**
[7th] **T38.1X1 Poisoning by thyroid hormones and substitutes, accidental (unintentional)** [POA]
Poisoning by thyroid hormones and substitutes NOS
[7th] **T38.1X2 Poisoning by thyroid hormones and substitutes, intentional self-harm** [POA] [HCC]
[7th] **T38.1X3 Poisoning by thyroid hormones and substitutes, assault** [POA]
[7th] **T38.1X4 Poisoning by thyroid hormones and substitutes, undetermined** [POA]
[7th] **T38.1X5 Adverse effect of thyroid hormones and substitutes** [POA] [PDx]
[7th] **T38.1X6 Underdosing of thyroid hormones and substitutes** [POA] [PDx]

[5th] **T38.2 Poisoning by, adverse effect of and underdosing of antithyroid drugs**
[6th] **T38.2X Poisoning by, adverse effect of and underdosing of antithyroid drugs**
[7th] **T38.2X1 Poisoning by antithyroid drugs, accidental (unintentional)** [POA]
Poisoning by antithyroid drugs NOS
[7th] **T38.2X2 Poisoning by antithyroid drugs, intentional self-harm** [POA] [HCC]
[7th] **T38.2X3 Poisoning by antithyroid drugs, assault** [POA]
[7th] **T38.2X4 Poisoning by antithyroid drugs, undetermined** [POA]
[7th] **T38.2X5 Adverse effect of antithyroid drugs** [POA] [PDx]
[7th] **T38.2X6 Underdosing of antithyroid drugs** [POA] [PDx]

[5th] **T38.3 Poisoning by, adverse effect of and underdosing of insulin and oral hypoglycemic [antidiabetic] drugs**
[6th] **T38.3X Poisoning by, adverse effect of and underdosing of insulin and oral hypoglycemic [antidiabetic] drugs**
[7th] **T38.3X1 Poisoning by insulin and oral hypoglycemic [antidiabetic] drugs, accidental (unintentional)** [POA]
👁 **See Official Guidelines** "Overdose of insulin due to insulin pump failure" I.C.4.a.5.b
Poisoning by insulin and oral hypoglycemic [antidiabetic] drugs NOS
[7th] **T38.3X2 Poisoning by insulin and oral hypoglycemic [antidiabetic] drugs, intentional self-harm** [POA] [HCC]
[7th] **T38.3X3 Poisoning by insulin and oral hypoglycemic [antidiabetic] drugs, assault** [POA]
[7th] **T38.3X4 Poisoning by insulin and oral hypoglycemic [antidiabetic] drugs, undetermined** [POA]
[7th] **T38.3X5 Adverse effect of insulin and oral hypoglycemic [antidiabetic] drugs** [POA] [PDx]
[7th] **T38.3X6 Underdosing of insulin and oral hypoglycemic [antidiabetic] drugs** [POA] [PDx]
👁 **See Official Guidelines** "Underdose of insulin due to insulin pump failure" I.C.4.a.5.a

[5th] **T38.4 Poisoning by, adverse effect of and underdosing of oral contraceptives**
Poisoning by, adverse effect of and underdosing of multiple- and single-ingredient oral contraceptive preparations
[6th] **T38.4X Poisoning by, adverse effect of and underdosing of oral contraceptives**
[7th] **T38.4X1 Poisoning by oral contraceptives, accidental (unintentional)** [POA]
Poisoning by oral contraceptives NOS
[7th] **T38.4X2 Poisoning by oral contraceptives, intentional self-harm** [POA] [HCC]
[7th] **T38.4X3 Poisoning by oral contraceptives, assault** [POA]
[7th] **T38.4X4 Poisoning by oral contraceptives, undetermined** [POA]
[7th] **T38.4X5 Adverse effect of oral contraceptives** [POA] [PDx]
[7th] **T38.4X6 Underdosing of oral contraceptives** [POA] [PDx]

[5th] **T38.5 Poisoning by, adverse effect of and underdosing of other estrogens and progestogens**
Poisoning by, adverse effect of and underdosing of estrogens and progestogens mixtures and substitutes
[6th] **T38.5X Poisoning by, adverse effect of and underdosing of other estrogens and progestogens**
[7th] **T38.5X1 Poisoning by other estrogens and progestogens, accidental (unintentional)** [POA]
Poisoning by other estrogens and progestogens NOS
[7th] **T38.5X2 Poisoning by other estrogens and progestogens, intentional self-harm** [POA] [HCC]
[7th] **T38.5X3 Poisoning by other estrogens and progestogens, assault** [POA]
[7th] **T38.5X4 Poisoning by other estrogens and progestogens, undetermined** [POA]
[7th] **T38.5X5 Adverse effect of other estrogens and progestogens** [POA] [PDx]
[7th] **T38.5X6 Underdosing of other estrogens and progestogens** [POA] [PDx]

[5th] **T38.6 Poisoning by, adverse effect of and underdosing of antigonadotrophins, antiestrogens, antiandrogens, not elsewhere classified**
Poisoning by, adverse effect of and underdosing of tamoxifen
[6th] **T38.6X Poisoning by, adverse effect of and underdosing of antigonadotrophins, antiestrogens, antiandrogens, not elsewhere classified**
[7th] **T38.6X1 Poisoning by antigonadotrophins, antiestrogens, antiandrogens, not elsewhere classified, accidental (unintentional)** [POA]
Poisoning by antigonadotrophins, antiestrogens, antiandrogens, not elsewhere classified NOS
[7th] **T38.6X2 Poisoning by antigonadotrophins, antiestrogens, antiandrogens, not elsewhere classified, intentional self-harm** [POA] [HCC]
[7th] **T38.6X3 Poisoning by antigonadotrophins, antiestrogens, antiandrogens, not elsewhere classified, assault** [POA]
[7th] **T38.6X4 Poisoning by antigonadotrophins, antiestrogens, antiandrogens, not elsewhere classified, undetermined** [POA]
[7th] **T38.6X5 Adverse effect of antigonadotrophins, antiestrogens, antiandrogens, not elsewhere classified** [POA] [PDx]
[7th] **T38.6X6 Underdosing of antigonadotrophins, antiestrogens, antiandrogens, not elsewhere classified** [POA] [PDx]

[5th] **T38.7 Poisoning by, adverse effect of and underdosing of androgens and anabolic congeners**
[6th] **T38.7X Poisoning by, adverse effect of and underdosing of androgens and anabolic congeners**
[7th] **T38.7X1 Poisoning by androgens and anabolic congeners, accidental (unintentional)** [POA]
Poisoning by androgens and anabolic congeners NOS
[7th] **T38.7X2 Poisoning by androgens and anabolic congeners, intentional self-harm** [POA] [HCC]

[PDx] Unacceptable principal diagnosis symbol per Medicare code edits [POA] Code exempt from diagnosis present on admission requirement
[?] Questionable admission [CC] Complication or comorbidity [MCC] Major complication or comorbidity [CC/MCC Exc] CC/MCC exclusion
[HCC] HCC diagnosis code [RxHCC] RxHCC diagnosis code MACRA code **DEFINITION** Describes condition/terminology
TIP Coding guidance 👁 Official Guideline Reference [Z1] Z code as first-listed diagnosis

7ᵗʰ T38.7X3 **Poisoning by androgens and anabolic congeners**, assault

7ᵗʰ T38.7X4 **Poisoning by androgens and anabolic congeners**, undetermined

7ᵗʰ T38.7X5 Adverse effect **of androgens and anabolic congeners**

7ᵗʰ T38.7X6 Underdosing **of androgens and anabolic congeners**

5ᵗʰ T38.8 **Poisoning by, adverse effect of and underdosing of other and unspecified hormones and synthetic substitutes**

6ᵗʰ T38.80 **Poisoning by, adverse effect of and underdosing of** unspecified hormones and synthetic substitutes

7ᵗʰ T38.801 **Poisoning by unspecified hormones and synthetic substitutes**, accidental (unintentional)

Poisoning by unspecified hormones and synthetic substitutes NOS

7ᵗʰ T38.802 **Poisoning by unspecified hormones and synthetic substitutes**, intentional self-harm

7ᵗʰ T38.803 **Poisoning by unspecified hormones and synthetic substitutes**, assault

7ᵗʰ T38.804 **Poisoning by unspecified hormones and synthetic substitutes**, undetermined

7ᵗʰ T38.805 Adverse effect **of unspecified hormones and synthetic substitutes**

7ᵗʰ T38.806 Underdosing **of unspecified hormones and synthetic substitutes**

6ᵗʰ T38.81 **Poisoning by, adverse effect of and underdosing of** anterior pituitary [adenohypophyseal] hormones

7ᵗʰ T38.811 **Poisoning by anterior pituitary [adenohypophyseal] hormones**, accidental (unintentional)

Poisoning by anterior pituitary [adenohypophyseal] hormones NOS

7ᵗʰ T38.812 **Poisoning by anterior pituitary [adenohypophyseal] hormones**, intentional self-harm

7ᵗʰ T38.813 **Poisoning by anterior pituitary [adenohypophyseal] hormones**, assault

7ᵗʰ T38.814 **Poisoning by anterior pituitary [adenohypophyseal] hormones**, undetermined

7ᵗʰ T38.815 Adverse effect **of anterior pituitary [adenohypophyseal] hormones**

7ᵗʰ T38.816 Underdosing **of anterior pituitary [adenohypophyseal] hormones**

6ᵗʰ T38.89 **Poisoning by, adverse effect of and underdosing of** other hormones and synthetic substitutes

7ᵗʰ T38.891 **Poisoning by other hormones and synthetic substitutes**, accidental (unintentional)

Poisoning by other hormones and synthetic substitutes NOS

7ᵗʰ T38.892 **Poisoning by other hormones and synthetic substitutes**, intentional self-harm

7ᵗʰ T38.893 **Poisoning by other hormones and synthetic substitutes**, assault

7ᵗʰ T38.894 **Poisoning by other hormones and synthetic substitutes**, undetermined

7ᵗʰ T38.895 Adverse effect **of other hormones and synthetic substitutes**

7ᵗʰ T38.896 Underdosing **of other hormones and synthetic substitutes**

5ᵗʰ T38.9 **Poisoning by, adverse effect of and underdosing of other and unspecified hormone antagonists**

6ᵗʰ T38.90 **Poisoning by, adverse effect of and underdosing of** unspecified hormone antagonists

7ᵗʰ T38.901 **Poisoning by unspecified hormone antagonists**, accidental (unintentional)

Poisoning by unspecified hormone antagonists NOS

7ᵗʰ T38.902 **Poisoning by unspecified hormone antagonists**, intentional self-harm

7ᵗʰ T38.903 **Poisoning by unspecified hormone antagonists**, assault

7ᵗʰ T38.904 **Poisoning by unspecified hormone antagonists**, undetermined

7ᵗʰ T38.905 Adverse effect **of unspecified hormone antagonists**

7ᵗʰ T38.906 Underdosing **of unspecified hormone antagonists**

6ᵗʰ T38.99 **Poisoning by, adverse effect of and underdosing of** other hormone antagonists

7ᵗʰ T38.991 **Poisoning by other hormone antagonists**, accidental (unintentional)

Poisoning by other hormone antagonists NOS

7ᵗʰ T38.992 **Poisoning by other hormone antagonists**, intentional self-harm

7ᵗʰ T38.993 **Poisoning by other hormone antagonists**, assault

7ᵗʰ T38.994 **Poisoning by other hormone antagonists**, undetermined

7ᵗʰ T38.995 Adverse effect **of other hormone antagonists**

7ᵗʰ T38.996 Underdosing **of other hormone antagonists**

4ᵗʰ T39 **Poisoning by, adverse effect of and underdosing of nonopioid analgesics, antipyretics and antirheumatics**

The appropriate 7th character is to be added to each code from category T39

A = initial encounter
D = subsequent encounter
S = sequela

5ᵗʰ T39.0 **Poisoning by, adverse effect of and underdosing of salicylates**

6ᵗʰ T39.01 **Poisoning by, adverse effect of and underdosing of** aspirin

Poisoning by, adverse effect of and underdosing of acetylsalicylic acid

7ᵗʰ T39.011 **Poisoning by aspirin**, accidental (unintentional)

7ᵗʰ T39.012 **Poisoning by aspirin**, intentional self-harm

7ᵗʰ T39.013 **Poisoning by aspirin**, assault
7ᵗʰ T39.014 **Poisoning by aspirin**, undetermined
7ᵗʰ T39.015 Adverse effect **of aspirin**

AHA: Q1 2016

7ᵗʰ T39.016 Underdosing **of aspirin**

6ᵗʰ T39.09 **Poisoning by, adverse effect of and underdosing of** other salicylates

7ᵗʰ T39.091 **Poisoning by salicylates**, accidental (unintentional)

Poisoning by salicylates NOS

7ᵗʰ T39.092 **Poisoning by salicylates**, intentional self-harm

7ᵗʰ T39.093 **Poisoning by salicylates**, assault
7ᵗʰ T39.094 **Poisoning by salicylates**, undetermined
7ᵗʰ T39.095 Adverse effect **of salicylates**
7ᵗʰ T39.096 Underdosing **of salicylates**

5ᵗʰ T39.1 **Poisoning by, adverse effect of and underdosing of 4-Aminophenol derivatives**

6ᵗʰ T39.1X **Poisoning by, adverse effect of and underdosing of** 4-Aminophenol derivatives

7ᵗʰ T39.1X1 **Poisoning by 4-Aminophenol derivatives**, accidental (unintentional)

Poisoning by 4-Aminophenol derivatives NOS

7ᵗʰ T39.1X2 **Poisoning by 4-Aminophenol derivatives**, intentional self-harm

7ᵗʰ T39.1X3 **Poisoning by 4-Aminophenol derivatives**, assault

7️⃣ T39.1X4 Poisoning by 4-Aminophenol derivatives, undetermined POA

7️⃣ T39.1X5 Adverse effect of 4-Aminophenol derivatives POA PDxIn

7️⃣ T39.1X6 Underdosing of 4-Aminophenol derivatives POA PDxIn

5️⃣ T39.2 Poisoning by, adverse effect of and underdosing of pyrazolone derivatives

6️⃣ T39.2X Poisoning by, adverse effect of and underdosing of pyrazolone derivatives

7️⃣ T39.2X1 Poisoning by pyrazolone derivatives, accidental (unintentional) POA
Poisoning by pyrazolone derivatives NOS

7️⃣ T39.2X2 Poisoning by pyrazolone derivatives, intentional self-harm POA HCC

7️⃣ T39.2X3 Poisoning by pyrazolone derivatives, assault POA

7️⃣ T39.2X4 Poisoning by pyrazolone derivatives, undetermined POA

7️⃣ T39.2X5 Adverse effect of pyrazolone derivatives POA PDxIn

7️⃣ T39.2X6 Underdosing of pyrazolone derivatives POA PDxIn

5️⃣ T39.3 Poisoning by, adverse effect of and underdosing of other nonsteroidal anti-inflammatory drugs [NSAID]

6️⃣ T39.31 Poisoning by, adverse effect of and underdosing of propionic acid derivatives
Poisoning by, adverse effect of and underdosing of fenoprofen
Poisoning by, adverse effect of and underdosing of flurbiprofen
Poisoning by, adverse effect of and underdosing of ibuprofen
Poisoning by, adverse effect of and underdosing of ketoprofen
Poisoning by, adverse effect of and underdosing of naproxen
Poisoning by, adverse effect of and underdosing of oxaprozin

7️⃣ T39.311 Poisoning by propionic acid derivatives, accidental (unintentional) POA

7️⃣ T39.312 Poisoning by propionic acid derivatives, intentional self-harm POA HCC

7️⃣ T39.313 Poisoning by propionic acid derivatives, assault POA

7️⃣ T39.314 Poisoning by propionic acid derivatives, undetermined POA

7️⃣ T39.315 Adverse effect of propionic acid derivatives POA PDxIn

7️⃣ T39.316 Underdosing of propionic acid derivatives POA PDxIn

6️⃣ T39.39 Poisoning by, adverse effect of and underdosing of other nonsteroidal anti-inflammatory drugs [NSAID]

7️⃣ T39.391 Poisoning by other nonsteroidal anti-inflammatory drugs [NSAID], accidental (unintentional) POA
Poisoning by other nonsteroidal anti-inflammatory drugs NOS

7️⃣ T39.392 Poisoning by other nonsteroidal anti-inflammatory drugs [NSAID], intentional self-harm POA HCC

7️⃣ T39.393 Poisoning by other nonsteroidal anti-inflammatory drugs [NSAID], assault POA

7️⃣ T39.394 Poisoning by other nonsteroidal anti-inflammatory drugs [NSAID], undetermined POA

7️⃣ T39.395 Adverse effect of other nonsteroidal anti-inflammatory drugs [NSAID] POA PDxIn

7️⃣ T39.396 Underdosing of other nonsteroidal anti-inflammatory drugs [NSAID] POA PDxIn

5️⃣ T39.4 Poisoning by, adverse effect of and underdosing of antirheumatics, not elsewhere classified
EXCLUDES1 poisoning by, adverse effect of and underdosing of glucocorticoids (T38.0-)
poisoning by, adverse effect of and underdosing of salicylates (T39.0-)

6️⃣ T39.4X Poisoning by, adverse effect of and underdosing of antirheumatics, not elsewhere classified

7️⃣ T39.4X1 Poisoning by antirheumatics, not elsewhere classified, accidental (unintentional) POA
Poisoning by antirheumatics, not elsewhere classified NOS

7️⃣ T39.4X2 Poisoning by antirheumatics, not elsewhere classified, intentional self-harm POA HCC

7️⃣ T39.4X3 Poisoning by antirheumatics, not elsewhere classified, assault POA

7️⃣ T39.4X4 Poisoning by antirheumatics, not elsewhere classified, undetermined POA

7️⃣ T39.4X5 Adverse effect of antirheumatics, not elsewhere classified POA PDxIn

7️⃣ T39.4X6 Underdosing of antirheumatics, not elsewhere classified POA PDxIn

5️⃣ T39.8 Poisoning by, adverse effect of and underdosing of other nonopioid analgesics and antipyretics, not elsewhere classified

6️⃣ T39.8X Poisoning by, adverse effect of and underdosing of other nonopioid analgesics and antipyretics, not elsewhere classified

7️⃣ T39.8X1 Poisoning by other nonopioid analgesics and antipyretics, not elsewhere classified, accidental (unintentional) POA
Poisoning by other nonopioid analgesics and antipyretics, not elsewhere classified NOS

7️⃣ T39.8X2 Poisoning by other nonopioid analgesics and antipyretics, not elsewhere classified, intentional self-harm POA HCC

7️⃣ T39.8X3 Poisoning by other nonopioid analgesics and antipyretics, not elsewhere classified, assault POA

7️⃣ T39.8X4 Poisoning by other nonopioid analgesics and antipyretics, not elsewhere classified, undetermined POA

7️⃣ T39.8X5 Adverse effect of other nonopioid analgesics and antipyretics, not elsewhere classified POA PDxIn

7️⃣ T39.8X6 Underdosing of other nonopioid analgesics and antipyretics, not elsewhere classified POA PDxIn

5️⃣ T39.9 Poisoning by, adverse effect of and underdosing of unspecified nonopioid analgesic, antipyretic and antirheumatic

7️⃣ T39.91 Poisoning by unspecified nonopioid analgesic, antipyretic and antirheumatic, accidental (unintentional) POA
Poisoning by nonopioid analgesic, antipyretic and antirheumatic NOS

7️⃣ T39.92 Poisoning by unspecified nonopioid analgesic, antipyretic and antirheumatic, intentional self-harm POA HCC

7️⃣ T39.93 Poisoning by unspecified nonopioid analgesic, antipyretic and antirheumatic, assault POA

7️⃣ T39.94 Poisoning by unspecified nonopioid analgesic, antipyretic and antirheumatic, undetermined POA

7️⃣ T39.95 Adverse effect of unspecified nonopioid analgesic, antipyretic and antirheumatic POA PDxIn

7️⃣ T39.96 Underdosing of unspecified nonopioid analgesic, antipyretic and antirheumatic POA PDxIn

---

When symbols appear on a code that requires a 7th character extension, refer to Appendix B to identify applicable 7th character codes.
2020 ICD-10-CM

4⁹ **T40** Poisoning by, adverse effect of and underdosing of narcotics and psychodysleptics [hallucinogens]

> *EXCLUDES2* *drug dependence and related mental and behavioral disorders due to psychoactive substance use (F10.-F19.-)*

The appropriate 7th character is to be added to each code from category T40

> A = initial encounter
> D = subsequent encounter
> S = sequela

5ᵗʰ **T40.0** Poisoning by, adverse effect of and underdosing of opium

6ᵗʰ **T40.0X** Poisoning by, adverse effect of and underdosing of opium

7ᵗʰ **T40.0X1** Poisoning by opium, accidental (unintentional) POA HCC
> Poisoning by opium NOS

7ᵗʰ **T40.0X2** Poisoning by opium, intentional self-harm POA HCC

7ᵗʰ **T40.0X3** Poisoning by opium, assault POA

7ᵗʰ **T40.0X4** Poisoning by opium, undetermined POA HCC

7ᵗʰ **T40.0X5** Adverse effect of opium POA PDxIn

7ᵗʰ **T40.0X6** Underdosing of opium POA PDxIn

5ᵗʰ **T40.1** Poisoning by and adverse effect of heroin

6ᵗʰ **T40.1X** Poisoning by and adverse effect of heroin

7ᵗʰ **T40.1X1** Poisoning by heroin, accidental (unintentional) POA HCC
> Poisoning by heroin NOS

7ᵗʰ **T40.1X2** Poisoning by heroin, intentional self-harm POA HCC

7ᵗʰ **T40.1X3** Poisoning by heroin, assault POA

7ᵗʰ **T40.1X4** Poisoning by heroin, undetermined POA HCC

5ᵗʰ **T40.2** Poisoning by, adverse effect of and underdosing of other opioids

6ᵗʰ **T40.2X** Poisoning by, adverse effect of and underdosing of other opioids

7ᵗʰ **T40.2X1** Poisoning by other opioids, accidental (unintentional) POA HCC
> Poisoning by other opioids NOS

7ᵗʰ **T40.2X2** Poisoning by other opioids, intentional self-harm POA HCC

7ᵗʰ **T40.2X3** Poisoning by other opioids, assault POA

7ᵗʰ **T40.2X4** Poisoning by other opioids, undetermined POA HCC

7ᵗʰ **T40.2X5** Adverse effect of other opioids POA PDxIn

7ᵗʰ **T40.2X6** Underdosing of other opioids POA PDxIn

5ᵗʰ **T40.3** Poisoning by, adverse effect of and underdosing of methadone

6ᵗʰ **T40.3X** Poisoning by, adverse effect of and underdosing of methadone

7ᵗʰ **T40.3X1** Poisoning by methadone, accidental (unintentional) POA HCC
> Poisoning by methadone NOS

7ᵗʰ **T40.3X2** Poisoning by methadone, intentional self-harm POA HCC

7ᵗʰ **T40.3X3** Poisoning by methadone, assault POA

7ᵗʰ **T40.3X4** Poisoning by methadone, undetermined POA HCC

7ᵗʰ **T40.3X5** Adverse effect of methadone POA PDxIn

7ᵗʰ **T40.3X6** Underdosing of methadone POA PDxIn

5ᵗʰ **T40.4** Poisoning by, adverse effect of and underdosing of other synthetic narcotics

6ᵗʰ **T40.4X** Poisoning by, adverse effect of and underdosing of other synthetic narcotics

7ᵗʰ **T40.4X1** Poisoning by other synthetic narcotics, accidental (unintentional) POA HCC
> Poisoning by other synthetic narcotics NOS

7ᵗʰ **T40.4X2** Poisoning by other synthetic narcotics, intentional self-harm POA HCC

7ᵗʰ **T40.4X3** Poisoning by other synthetic narcotics, assault POA

7ᵗʰ **T40.4X4** Poisoning by other synthetic narcotics, undetermined POA HCC

7ᵗʰ **T40.4X5** Adverse effect of other synthetic narcotics POA PDxIn

7ᵗʰ **T40.4X6** Underdosing of other synthetic narcotics POA PDxIn

5ᵗʰ **T40.5** Poisoning by, adverse effect of and underdosing of cocaine

6ᵗʰ **T40.5X** Poisoning by, adverse effect of and underdosing of cocaine

7ᵗʰ **T40.5X1** Poisoning by cocaine, accidental (unintentional) POA HCC
> **AHA:** Q2 2016
> Poisoning by cocaine NOS

7ᵗʰ **T40.5X2** Poisoning by cocaine, intentional self-harm POA HCC

7ᵗʰ **T40.5X3** Poisoning by cocaine, assault POA

7ᵗʰ **T40.5X4** Poisoning by cocaine, undetermined POA HCC

7ᵗʰ **T40.5X5** Adverse effect of cocaine POA PDxIn

7ᵗʰ **T40.5X6** Underdosing of cocaine POA PDxIn

5ᵗʰ **T40.6** Poisoning by, adverse effect of and underdosing of other and unspecified narcotics

6ᵗʰ **T40.60** Poisoning by, adverse effect of and underdosing of unspecified narcotics

7ᵗʰ **T40.601** Poisoning by unspecified narcotics, accidental (unintentional) POA HCC
> Poisoning by narcotics NOS

7ᵗʰ **T40.602** Poisoning by unspecified narcotics, intentional self-harm POA HCC

7ᵗʰ **T40.603** Poisoning by unspecified narcotics, assault POA

7ᵗʰ **T40.604** Poisoning by unspecified narcotics, undetermined POA HCC

7ᵗʰ **T40.605** Adverse effect of unspecified narcotics POA PDxIn

7ᵗʰ **T40.606** Underdosing of unspecified narcotics POA PDxIn

6ᵗʰ **T40.69** Poisoning by, adverse effect of and underdosing of other narcotics

7ᵗʰ **T40.691** Poisoning by other narcotics, accidental (unintentional) POA HCC
> Poisoning by other narcotics NOS

7ᵗʰ **T40.692** Poisoning by other narcotics, intentional self-harm POA HCC

7ᵗʰ **T40.693** Poisoning by other narcotics, assault POA

7ᵗʰ **T40.694** Poisoning by other narcotics, undetermined POA HCC

7ᵗʰ **T40.695** Adverse effect of other narcotics POA PDxIn

7ᵗʰ **T40.696** Underdosing of other narcotics POA PDxIn

5ᵗʰ **T40.7** Poisoning by, adverse effect of and underdosing of cannabis (derivatives)

6ᵗʰ **T40.7X** Poisoning by, adverse effect of and underdosing of cannabis (derivatives)

7ᵗʰ **T40.7X1** Poisoning by cannabis (derivatives), accidental (unintentional) POA
> Poisoning by cannabis NOS

7ᵗʰ **T40.7X2** Poisoning by cannabis (derivatives), intentional self-harm POA HCC

7ᵗʰ **T40.7X3** Poisoning by cannabis (derivatives), assault POA

7ᵗʰ **T40.7X4** Poisoning by cannabis (derivatives), undetermined POA

7ᵗʰ **T40.7X5** Adverse effect of cannabis (derivatives) POA PDxIn

7ᵗʰ **T40.7X6** Underdosing of cannabis (derivatives) POA PDxIn

5ᵗʰ **T40.8** Poisoning by and adverse effect of lysergide [LSD]

6ᵗʰ **T40.8X** Poisoning by and adverse effect of lysergide [LSD]

7ᵗʰ **T40.8X1** Poisoning by lysergide [LSD], accidental (unintentional) POA HCC
> Poisoning by lysergide [LSD] NOS

7ᵗʰ **T40.8X2** Poisoning by lysergide [LSD], intentional self-harm POA HCC

7ᵗʰ **T40.8X3** Poisoning by lysergide [LSD], assault POA

7ᵗʰ **T40.8X4** Poisoning by lysergide [LSD], undetermined POA HCC

T40.9 Poisoning by, adverse effect of and underdosing of other and unspecified psychodysleptics [hallucinogens]

T40.90 Poisoning by, adverse effect of and underdosing of unspecified psychodysleptics [hallucinogens]

T40.901 Poisoning by unspecified psychodysleptics [hallucinogens], accidental (unintentional) POA HCC

T40.902 Poisoning by unspecified psychodysleptics [hallucinogens], intentional self-harm POA HCC

T40.903 Poisoning by unspecified psychodysleptics [hallucinogens], assault POA

T40.904 Poisoning by unspecified psychodysleptics [hallucinogens], undetermined POA HCC

T40.905 Adverse effect of unspecified psychodysleptics [hallucinogens] POA PDxIn

▲ T40.906 Underdosing of unspecified psychodysleptics ▶[hallucinogens]◀ POA PDxIn

T40.99 Poisoning by, adverse effect of and underdosing of other psychodysleptics [hallucinogens]

T40.991 Poisoning by other psychodysleptics [hallucinogens], accidental (unintentional) POA HCC

Poisoning by other psychodysleptics [hallucinogens] NOS

T40.992 Poisoning by other psychodysleptics [hallucinogens], intentional self-harm POA HCC

T40.993 Poisoning by other psychodysleptics [hallucinogens], assault POA

T40.994 Poisoning by other psychodysleptics [hallucinogens], undetermined POA HCC

T40.995 Adverse effect of other psychodysleptics [hallucinogens] POA PDxIn

▲ T40.996 Underdosing of other psychodysleptics ▶[hallucinogens]◀ POA PDxIn

T41 Poisoning by, adverse effect of and underdosing of anesthetics and therapeutic gases

EXCLUDES1 benzodiazepines (T42.4-)

cocaine (T40.5-)

complications of anesthesia during pregnancy (O29.-)

complications of anesthesia during labor and delivery (O74.-)

complications of anesthesia during the puerperium (O89.-)

opioids (T40.0-T40.2-)

The appropriate 7th character is to be added to each code from category T41

A = initial encounter

D = subsequent encounter

S = sequela

T41.0 Poisoning by, adverse effect of and underdosing of inhaled anesthetics

EXCLUDES1 oxygen (T41.5-)

T41.0X Poisoning by, adverse effect of and underdosing of inhaled anesthetics

T41.0X1 Poisoning by inhaled anesthetics, accidental (unintentional) POA

Poisoning by inhaled anesthetics NOS

T41.0X2 Poisoning by inhaled anesthetics, intentional self-harm POA HCC

T41.0X3 Poisoning by inhaled anesthetics, assault POA

T41.0X4 Poisoning by inhaled anesthetics, undetermined POA

T41.0X5 Adverse effect of inhaled anesthetics POA PDxIn

T41.0X6 Underdosing of inhaled anesthetics POA PDxIn

T41.1 Poisoning by, adverse effect of and underdosing of intravenous anesthetics

Poisoning by, adverse effect of and underdosing of thiobarbiturates

T41.1X Poisoning by, adverse effect of and underdosing of intravenous anesthetics

T41.1X1 Poisoning by intravenous anesthetics, accidental (unintentional) POA

Poisoning by intravenous anesthetics NOS

T41.1X2 Poisoning by intravenous anesthetics, intentional self-harm POA HCC

T41.1X3 Poisoning by intravenous anesthetics, assault POA

T41.1X4 Poisoning by intravenous anesthetics, undetermined POA

T41.1X5 Adverse effect of intravenous anesthetics POA PDxIn

T41.1X6 Underdosing of intravenous anesthetics POA PDxIn

T41.2 Poisoning by, adverse effect of and underdosing of other and unspecified general anesthetics

T41.20 Poisoning by, adverse effect of and underdosing of unspecified general anesthetics

T41.201 Poisoning by unspecified general anesthetics, accidental (unintentional) POA

Poisoning by general anesthetics NOS

T41.202 Poisoning by unspecified general anesthetics, intentional self-harm POA HCC

T41.203 Poisoning by unspecified general anesthetics, assault POA

T41.204 Poisoning by unspecified general anesthetics, undetermined POA

T41.205 Adverse effect of unspecified general anesthetics POA PDxIn

T41.206 Underdosing of unspecified general anesthetics POA PDxIn

T41.29 Poisoning by, adverse effect of and underdosing of other general anesthetics

T41.291 Poisoning by other general anesthetics, accidental (unintentional) POA

Poisoning by other general anesthetics NOS

T41.292 Poisoning by other general anesthetics, intentional self-harm POA HCC

T41.293 Poisoning by other general anesthetics, assault POA

T41.294 Poisoning by other general anesthetics, undetermined POA

T41.295 Adverse effect of other general anesthetics POA PDxIn

T41.296 Underdosing of other general anesthetics POA PDxIn

T41.3 Poisoning by, adverse effect of and underdosing of local anesthetics

Cocaine (topical)

EXCLUDES2 poisoning by cocaine used as a central nervous system stimulant (T40.5X1-T40.5X4)

T41.3X Poisoning by, adverse effect of and underdosing of local anesthetics

T41.3X1 Poisoning by local anesthetics, accidental (unintentional) POA

Poisoning by local anesthetics NOS

T41.3X2 Poisoning by local anesthetics, intentional self-harm POA HCC

T41.3X3 Poisoning by local anesthetics, assault POA

T41.3X4 Poisoning by local anesthetics, undetermined POA

T41.3X5 Adverse effect of local anesthetics POA PDxIn

T41.3X6 Underdosing of local anesthetics POA PDxIn

T41.4 Poisoning by, adverse effect of and underdosing of unspecified anesthetic

T41.41 Poisoning by unspecified anesthetic, accidental (unintentional) POA

Poisoning by anesthetic NOS

T41.42 Poisoning by unspecified anesthetic, intentional self-harm POA HCC

T41.43 Poisoning by unspecified anesthetic, assault POA

PDxIn Unacceptable principal diagnosis symbol per Medicare code edits   POA Code exempt from diagnosis present on admission requirement
❓ Questionable admission   CC Complication or comorbidity   MCC Major complication or comorbidity   CC/MCC Exc CC/MCC exclusion
HCC HCC diagnosis code   RxHCC RxHCC diagnosis code   MACRA code   **DEFINITION** Describes condition/terminology
TIP Coding guidance   👁 Official Guideline Reference   Z1 Z code as first-listed diagnosis

1128   When symbols appear on a code that requires a 7th character extension, refer to Appendix B to identify applicable 7th character codes.   **2020 ICD-10-CM**

T41.44 Poisoning by unspecified anesthetic, undetermined POA

T41.45 Adverse effect of unspecified anesthetic POA PDxIn

T41.46 Underdosing of unspecified anesthetics POA PDxIn

T41.5 Poisoning by, adverse effect of and underdosing of therapeutic gases

T41.5X Poisoning by, adverse effect of and underdosing of therapeutic gases

T41.5X1 Poisoning by therapeutic gases, accidental (unintentional) POA

Poisoning by therapeutic gases NOS

T41.5X2 Poisoning by therapeutic gases, intentional self-harm POA HCC

T41.5X3 Poisoning by therapeutic gases, assault POA

T41.5X4 Poisoning by therapeutic gases, undetermined POA

T41.5X5 Adverse effect of therapeutic gases POA PDxIn

T41.5X6 Underdosing of therapeutic gases POA PDxIn

T42 Poisoning by, adverse effect of and underdosing of antiepileptic, sedative- hypnotic and antiparkinsonism drugs

EXCLUDES2 drug dependence and related mental and behavioral disorders due to psychoactive substance use (F10.--F19.-)

The appropriate 7th character is to be added to each code from category T42

A = initial encounter
D = subsequent encounter
S = sequela

T42.0 Poisoning by, adverse effect of and underdosing of hydantoin derivatives

T42.0X Poisoning by, adverse effect of and underdosing of hydantoin derivatives

T42.0X1 Poisoning by hydantoin derivatives, accidental (unintentional) POA

Poisoning by hydantoin derivatives NOS

T42.0X2 Poisoning by hydantoin derivatives, intentional self-harm POA HCC

T42.0X3 Poisoning by hydantoin derivatives, assault POA

T42.0X4 Poisoning by hydantoin derivatives, undetermined POA

T42.0X5 Adverse effect of hydantoin derivatives POA PDxIn

T42.0X6 Underdosing of hydantoin derivatives POA PDxIn

T42.1 Poisoning by, adverse effect of and underdosing of iminostilbenes

Poisoning by, adverse effect of and underdosing of carbamazepine

T42.1X Poisoning by, adverse effect of and underdosing of iminostilbenes

T42.1X1 Poisoning by iminostilbenes, accidental (unintentional) POA

Poisoning by iminostilbenes NOS

T42.1X2 Poisoning by iminostilbenes, intentional self-harm POA HCC

T42.1X3 Poisoning by iminostilbenes, assault POA

T42.1X4 Poisoning by iminostilbenes, undetermined POA

T42.1X5 Adverse effect of iminostilbenes POA PDxIn

T42.1X6 Underdosing of iminostilbenes POA PDxIn

T42.2 Poisoning by, adverse effect of and underdosing of succinimides and oxazolidinediones

T42.2X Poisoning by, adverse effect of and underdosing of succinimides and oxazolidinediones

T42.2X1 Poisoning by succinimides and oxazolidinediones, accidental (unintentional) POA

Poisoning by succinimides and oxazolidinediones NOS

T42.2X2 Poisoning by succinimides and oxazolidinediones, intentional self-harm POA HCC

T42.2X3 Poisoning by succinimides and oxazolidinediones, assault POA

T42.2X4 Poisoning by succinimides and oxazolidinediones, undetermined POA

T42.2X5 Adverse effect of succinimides and oxazolidinediones POA PDxIn

T42.2X6 Underdosing of succinimides and oxazolidinediones POA PDxIn

T42.3 Poisoning by, adverse effect of and underdosing of barbiturates

EXCLUDES1 poisoning by, adverse effect of and underdosing of thiobarbiturates (T41.1-)

T42.3X Poisoning by, adverse effect of and underdosing of barbiturates

T42.3X1 Poisoning by barbiturates, accidental (unintentional) POA

Poisoning by barbiturates NOS

T42.3X2 Poisoning by barbiturates, intentional self-harm POA HCC

T42.3X3 Poisoning by barbiturates, assault POA

T42.3X4 Poisoning by barbiturates, undetermined POA

T42.3X5 Adverse effect of barbiturates POA PDxIn

T42.3X6 Underdosing of barbiturates POA PDxIn

T42.4 Poisoning by, adverse effect of and underdosing of benzodiazepines

T42.4X Poisoning by, adverse effect of and underdosing of benzodiazepines

T42.4X1 Poisoning by benzodiazepines, accidental (unintentional) POA

Poisoning by benzodiazepines NOS

T42.4X2 Poisoning by benzodiazepines, intentional self-harm POA HCC

T42.4X3 Poisoning by benzodiazepines, assault POA

T42.4X4 Poisoning by benzodiazepines, undetermined POA

T42.4X5 Adverse effect of benzodiazepines POA PDxIn

T42.4X6 Underdosing of benzodiazepines POA PDxIn

T42.5 Poisoning by, adverse effect of and underdosing of mixed antiepileptics

T42.5X Poisoning by, adverse effect of and underdosing of antiepileptics

T42.5X1 Poisoning by mixed antiepileptics, accidental (unintentional) POA

Poisoning by mixed antiepileptics NOS

T42.5X2 Poisoning by mixed antiepileptics, intentional self-harm POA HCC

T42.5X3 Poisoning by mixed antiepileptics, assault POA

T42.5X4 Poisoning by mixed antiepileptics, undetermined POA

T42.5X5 Adverse effect of mixed antiepileptics POA PDxIn

T42.5X6 Underdosing of mixed antiepileptics POA PDxIn

T42.6 Poisoning by, adverse effect of and underdosing of other antiepileptic and sedative-hypnotic drugs

Poisoning by, adverse effect of and underdosing of methaqualone

Poisoning by, adverse effect of and underdosing of valproic acid

EXCLUDES1 poisoning by, adverse effect of and underdosing of carbamazepine (T42.1-)

T42.6X Poisoning by, adverse effect of and underdosing of other antiepileptic and sedative-hypnotic drugs

T42.6X1 Poisoning by other antiepileptic and sedative-hypnotic drugs, accidental (unintentional) POA

Poisoning by other antiepileptic and sedative-hypnotic drugs NOS

T42.6X2 Poisoning by other antiepileptic and sedative-hypnotic drugs, intentional self-harm POA HCC

Unspecified Code   Other Specified Code   Manifestation Code   N Newborn   P Pediatric   M Maternity   A Adult   ♂ Male   ♀ Female
● New Code   ▲ Revised Code Title   ►◄ Revised Text   NOTES   INCLUDES   EXCLUDES1 Not coded here   EXCLUDES2 Not included here
4th character required   5th character required   6th character required   7th character required   Extension 'X' Alert
HAC Hospital-acquired condition (HAC) alert   AHA AHA Coding Clinic©   ☛ Code first alert

[7th] T42.6X3 Poisoning by other antiepileptic and sedative-hypnotic drugs, assault [POA]

[7th] T42.6X4 Poisoning by other antiepileptic and sedative-hypnotic drugs, undetermined [POA]

[7th] T42.6X5 Adverse effect of other antiepileptic and sedative-hypnotic drugs [POA] [PDx]

[7th] T42.6X6 Underdosing of other antiepileptic and sedative-hypnotic drugs [POA] [PDx]

[5th] T42.7 Poisoning by, adverse effect of and underdosing of unspecified antiepileptic and sedative-hypnotic drugs

[7th] T42.71 **Poisoning by unspecified antiepileptic and sedative-hypnotic drugs, accidental (unintentional)** [POA]
Poisoning by antiepileptic and sedative-hypnotic drugs NOS

[7th] T42.72 **Poisoning by unspecified antiepileptic and sedative-hypnotic drugs, intentional self-harm** [POA] [HCC]

[7th] T42.73 **Poisoning by unspecified antiepileptic and sedative-hypnotic drugs, assault** [POA]

[7th] T42.74 **Poisoning by unspecified antiepileptic and sedative-hypnotic drugs, undetermined** [POA]

[7th] T42.75 **Adverse effect of unspecified antiepileptic and sedative-hypnotic drugs** [POA] [PDx]

[7th] T42.76 **Underdosing of unspecified antiepileptic and sedative-hypnotic drugs** [POA] [PDx]

[5th] T42.8 Poisoning by, adverse effect of and underdosing of antiparkinsonism drugs and other central muscle-tone depressants
Poisoning by, adverse effect of and underdosing of amantadine

[6th] T42.8X Poisoning by, adverse effect of and underdosing of antiparkinsonism drugs and other central muscle-tone depressants

[7th] T42.8X1 Poisoning by antiparkinsonism drugs and other central muscle-tone depressants, accidental (unintentional) [POA]
Poisoning by antiparkinsonism drugs and other central muscle-tone depressants NOS

[7th] T42.8X2 Poisoning by antiparkinsonism drugs and other central muscle-tone depressants, intentional self-harm [POA] [HCC]

[7th] T42.8X3 Poisoning by antiparkinsonism drugs and other central muscle-tone depressants, assault [POA]

[7th] T42.8X4 Poisoning by antiparkinsonism drugs and other central muscle-tone depressants, undetermined [POA]

[7th] T42.8X5 Adverse effect of antiparkinsonism drugs and other central muscle-tone depressants [POA] [PDx]

[7th] T42.8X6 Underdosing of antiparkinsonism drugs and other central muscle-tone depressants [POA] [PDx]

[4th] T43 Poisoning by, adverse effect of and underdosing of psychotropic drugs, not elsewhere classified

[EXCLUDES1] *appetite depressants (T50.5-)*
barbiturates (T42.3-)
benzodiazepines (T42.4-)
methaqualone (T42.6-)
psychodysleptics [hallucinogens] (T40.7-T40.9-)

[EXCLUDES2] *drug dependence and related mental and behavioral disorders due to psychoactive substance use (F10.- -F19.-)*

The appropriate 7th character is to be added to each code from category T43
A = initial encounter
D = subsequent encounter
S = sequela

[5th] T43.0 Poisoning by, adverse effect of and underdosing of tricyclic and tetracyclic antidepressants

[6th] T43.01 Poisoning by, adverse effect of and underdosing of tricyclic antidepressants

[7th] T43.011 Poisoning by tricyclic antidepressants, accidental (unintentional) [POA]
Poisoning by tricyclic antidepressants NOS

[7th] T43.012 Poisoning by tricyclic antidepressants, intentional self-harm [POA] [HCC]

[7th] T43.013 Poisoning by tricyclic antidepressants, assault [POA]

[7th] T43.014 Poisoning by tricyclic antidepressants, undetermined [POA]

[7th] T43.015 Adverse effect of tricyclic antidepressants [POA] [PDx]

[7th] T43.016 Underdosing of tricyclic antidepressants [POA] [PDx]

[6th] T43.02 Poisoning by, adverse effect of and underdosing of tetracyclic antidepressants

[7th] T43.021 Poisoning by tetracyclic antidepressants, accidental (unintentional) [POA]
Poisoning by tetracyclic antidepressants NOS

[7th] T43.022 Poisoning by tetracyclic antidepressants, intentional self-harm [POA] [HCC]

[7th] T43.023 Poisoning by tetracyclic antidepressants, assault [POA]

[7th] T43.024 Poisoning by tetracyclic antidepressants, undetermined [POA]

[7th] T43.025 Adverse effect of tetracyclic antidepressants [POA] [PDx]

[7th] T43.026 Underdosing of tetracyclic antidepressants [POA] [PDx]

[5th] T43.1 Poisoning by, adverse effect of and underdosing of monoamine-oxidase-inhibitor antidepressants

[6th] T43.1X Poisoning by, adverse effect of and underdosing of monoamine-oxidase-inhibitor antidepressants

[7th] T43.1X1 Poisoning by monoamine-oxidase-inhibitor antidepressants, accidental (unintentional) [POA]
Poisoning by monoamine-oxidase-inhibitor antidepressants NOS

[7th] T43.1X2 Poisoning by monoamine-oxidase-inhibitor antidepressants, intentional self-harm [POA] [HCC]

[7th] T43.1X3 Poisoning by monoamine-oxidase-inhibitor antidepressants, assault [POA]

[7th] T43.1X4 Poisoning by monoamine-oxidase-inhibitor antidepressants, undetermined [POA]

[7th] T43.1X5 Adverse effect of monoamine-oxidase-inhibitor antidepressants [POA] [PDx]

[7th] T43.1X6 Underdosing of monoamine-oxidase-inhibitor antidepressants [POA] [PDx]

[5th] T43.2 Poisoning by, adverse effect of and underdosing of other and unspecified antidepressants

[6th] T43.20 Poisoning by, adverse effect of and underdosing of unspecified antidepressants

[7th] T43.201 **Poisoning by unspecified antidepressants, accidental (unintentional)** [POA]
Poisoning by antidepressants NOS

[7th] T43.202 **Poisoning by unspecified antidepressants, intentional self-harm** [POA] [HCC]

[7th] T43.203 **Poisoning by unspecified antidepressants, assault** [POA]

[7th] T43.204 **Poisoning by unspecified antidepressants, undetermined** [POA]

[7th] T43.205 **Adverse effect of unspecified antidepressants** [POA] [PDx]
Antidepressant discontinuation syndrome

[7th] T43.206 **Underdosing of unspecified antidepressants** [POA] [PDx]

[6th] T43.21 Poisoning by, adverse effect of and underdosing of selective serotonin and norepinephrine reuptake inhibitors
Poisoning by, adverse effect of and underdosing of SSNRI antidepressants

[PDx] Unacceptable principal diagnosis symbol per Medicare code edits [POA] Code exempt from diagnosis present on admission requirement
[?] Questionable admission [CC] Complication or comorbidity [MCC] Major complication or comorbidity [CC/MCC Exc] CC/MCC exclusion
[HCC] HCC diagnosis code [RxHCC] RxHCC diagnosis code MACRA code **DEFINITION** Describes condition/terminology
TIP Coding guidance 👁 Official Guideline Reference [Z1] Z code as first-listed diagnosis

[7th] T43.211 Poisoning by selective serotonin and norepinephrine reuptake inhibitors, accidental (unintentional) POA

[7th] T43.212 Poisoning by selective serotonin and norepinephrine reuptake inhibitors, intentional self-harm POA HCC

[7th] T43.213 Poisoning by selective serotonin and norepinephrine reuptake inhibitors, assault POA

[7th] T43.214 Poisoning by selective serotonin and norepinephrine reuptake inhibitors, undetermined POA

[7th] T43.215 Adverse effect of selective serotonin and norepinephrine reuptake inhibitors POA PDxIn

[7th] T43.216 Underdosing of selective serotonin and norepinephrine reuptake inhibitors POA PDxIn

[6th] T43.22 Poisoning by, adverse effect of and underdosing of selective serotonin reuptake inhibitors

Poisoning by, adverse effect of and underdosing of SSRI antidepressants

[7th] T43.221 Poisoning by selective serotonin reuptake inhibitors, accidental (unintentional) POA

[7th] T43.222 Poisoning by selective serotonin reuptake inhibitors, intentional self-harm POA HCC

[7th] T43.223 Poisoning by selective serotonin reuptake inhibitors, assault POA

[7th] T43.224 Poisoning by selective serotonin reuptake inhibitors, undetermined POA

[7th] T43.225 Adverse effect of selective serotonin reuptake inhibitors POA PDxIn

[7th] T43.226 Underdosing of selective serotonin reuptake inhibitors POA PDxIn

[6th] T43.29 Poisoning by, adverse effect of and underdosing of other antidepressants

[7th] T43.291 Poisoning by other antidepressants, accidental (unintentional) POA

Poisoning by other antidepressants NOS

[7th] T43.292 Poisoning by other antidepressants, intentional self-harm POA HCC

[7th] T43.293 Poisoning by other antidepressants, assault POA

[7th] T43.294 Poisoning by other antidepressants, undetermined POA

[7th] T43.295 Adverse effect of other antidepressants POA PDxIn

[7th] T43.296 Underdosing of other antidepressants POA PDxIn

[5th] T43.3 Poisoning by, adverse effect of and underdosing of phenothiazine antipsychotics and neuroleptics

[6th] T43.3X Poisoning by, adverse effect of and underdosing of phenothiazine antipsychotics and neuroleptics

[7th] T43.3X1 Poisoning by phenothiazine antipsychotics and neuroleptics, accidental (unintentional) POA

Poisoning by phenothiazine antipsychotics and neuroleptics NOS

[7th] T43.3X2 Poisoning by phenothiazine antipsychotics and neuroleptics, intentional self-harm POA HCC

[7th] T43.3X3 Poisoning by phenothiazine antipsychotics and neuroleptics, assault POA

[7th] T43.3X4 Poisoning by phenothiazine antipsychotics and neuroleptics, undetermined POA

[7th] T43.3X5 Adverse effect of phenothiazine antipsychotics and neuroleptics POA PDxIn

[7th] T43.3X6 Underdosing of phenothiazine antipsychotics and neuroleptics POA PDxIn

[5th] T43.4 Poisoning by, adverse effect of and underdosing of butyrophenone and thiothixene neuroleptics

[6th] T43.4X Poisoning by, adverse effect of and underdosing of butyrophenone and thiothixene neuroleptics

[7th] T43.4X1 Poisoning by butyrophenone and thiothixene neuroleptics, accidental (unintentional) POA

Poisoning by butyrophenone and thiothixene neuroleptics NOS

[7th] T43.4X2 Poisoning by butyrophenone and thiothixene neuroleptics, intentional self-harm POA HCC

[7th] T43.4X3 Poisoning by butyrophenone and thiothixene neuroleptics, assault POA

[7th] T43.4X4 Poisoning by butyrophenone and thiothixene neuroleptics, undetermined POA

[7th] T43.4X5 Adverse effect of butyrophenone and thiothixene neuroleptics POA PDxIn

[7th] T43.4X6 Underdosing of butyrophenone and thiothixene neuroleptics POA PDxIn

[5th] T43.5 Poisoning by, adverse effect of and underdosing of other and unspecified antipsychotics and neuroleptics

[EXCLUDES1] *poisoning by, adverse effect of and underdosing of rauwolfia (T46.5-)*

[6th] T43.50 Poisoning by, adverse effect of and underdosing of unspecified antipsychotics and neuroleptics

[7th] T43.501 Poisoning by unspecified antipsychotics and neuroleptics, accidental (unintentional) POA

Poisoning by antipsychotics and neuroleptics NOS

[7th] T43.502 Poisoning by unspecified antipsychotics and neuroleptics, intentional self-harm POA HCC

[7th] T43.503 Poisoning by unspecified antipsychotics and neuroleptics, assault POA

[7th] T43.504 Poisoning by unspecified antipsychotics and neuroleptics, undetermined POA

[7th] T43.505 Adverse effect of unspecified antipsychotics and neuroleptics POA PDxIn

[7th] T43.506 Underdosing of unspecified antipsychotics and neuroleptics POA PDxIn

[6th] T43.59 Poisoning by, adverse effect of and underdosing of other antipsychotics and neuroleptics

[7th] T43.591 Poisoning by other antipsychotics and neuroleptics, accidental (unintentional) POA

Poisoning by other antipsychotics and neuroleptics NOS

[7th] T43.592 Poisoning by other antipsychotics and neuroleptics, intentional self-harm POA HCC

AHA: Q1 2017

[7th] T43.593 Poisoning by other antipsychotics and neuroleptics, assault POA

[7th] T43.594 Poisoning by other antipsychotics and neuroleptics, undetermined POA

[7th] T43.595 Adverse effect of other antipsychotics and neuroleptics POA PDxIn

[7th] T43.596 Underdosing of other antipsychotics and neuroleptics POA PDxIn

[5th] T43.6 Poisoning by, adverse effect of and underdosing of psychostimulants

[EXCLUDES1] *poisoning by, adverse effect of and underdosing of cocaine (T40.5-)*

[6th] T43.60 Poisoning by, adverse effect of and underdosing of unspecified psychostimulant

[7th] T43.601 Poisoning by unspecified psychostimulants, accidental (unintentional) POA HCC

Poisoning by psychostimulants NOS

[7th] T43.602 Poisoning by unspecified psychostimulants, intentional self-harm POA HCC

[7th] T43.603 Poisoning by unspecified psychostimulants, assault POA

[7th] T43.604 Poisoning by unspecified psychostimulants, undetermined POA HCC

Unspecified Code Other Specified Code Manifestation Code [N] Newborn [P] Pediatric [M] Maternity [A] Adult ♂ Male ♀ Female
● New Code ▲ Revised Code Title ►◄ Revised Text [NOTES] *INCLUDES* [EXCLUDES1] Not coded here [EXCLUDES2] Not included here
[4th] 4th character required [5th] 5th character required [6th] 6th character required [7th] 7th character required [x] Extension 'X' Alert
[HAC] Hospital-acquired condition (HAC) alert AHA AHA Coding Clinic© ☞ Code first alert

7️⃣ **T43.605 Adverse effect of unspecified
psychostimulants** POA PDxIn

7️⃣ **T43.606 Underdosing of unspecified
psychostimulants** POA PDxIn

6️⃣ **T43.61 Poisoning by, adverse effect of and underdosing of
caffeine**

7️⃣ **T43.611 Poisoning by caffeine, accidental
(unintentional)** POA HCC
Poisoning by caffeine NOS

7️⃣ **T43.612 Poisoning by caffeine, intentional
self-harm** POA HCC

7️⃣ **T43.613 Poisoning by caffeine, assault** POA

7️⃣ **T43.614 Poisoning by caffeine, undetermined** POA HCC

7️⃣ **T43.615 Adverse effect of caffeine** POA PDxIn

7️⃣ **T43.616 Underdosing of caffeine** POA PDxIn

6️⃣ **T43.62 Poisoning by, adverse effect of and underdosing of
amphetamines**
Poisoning by, adverse effect of and underdosing of
methamphetamines

7️⃣ **T43.621 Poisoning by amphetamines, accidental
(unintentional)** POA HCC
Poisoning by amphetamines NOS

7️⃣ **T43.622 Poisoning by amphetamines, intentional
self-harm** POA HCC

7️⃣ **T43.623 Poisoning by amphetamines, assault** POA

7️⃣ **T43.624 Poisoning by amphetamines,
undetermined** POA HCC

7️⃣ **T43.625 Adverse effect of amphetamines** POA PDxIn

7️⃣ **T43.626 Underdosing of amphetamines** POA PDxIn

6️⃣ **T43.63 Poisoning by, adverse effect of and underdosing of
methylphenidate**

7️⃣ **T43.631 Poisoning by methylphenidate, accidental
(unintentional)** POA HCC
Poisoning by methylphenidate NOS

7️⃣ **T43.632 Poisoning by methylphenidate,
intentional self-harm** POA HCC

7️⃣ **T43.633 Poisoning by methylphenidate, assault** POA

7️⃣ **T43.634 Poisoning by methylphenidate,
undetermined** POA HCC

7️⃣ **T43.635 Adverse effect of methylphenidate** POA PDxIn

7️⃣ **T43.636 Underdosing of methylphenidate** POA PDxIn

6️⃣ **T43.64 Poisoning by ecstasy**
Poisoning by MDMA
Poisoning by 3,4-methylenedioxymethamphetamine

7️⃣ **T43.641 Poisoning by ecstasy, accidental
(unintentional)** POA HCC
AHA: Q4 2018
Poisoning by ecstasy NOS

7️⃣ **T43.642 Poisoning by ecstasy, intentional
self-harm** POA HCC
AHA: Q4 2018

7️⃣ **T43.643 Poisoning by ecstasy, assault** POA
AHA: Q4 2018

7️⃣ **T43.644 Poisoning by ecstasy, undetermined** POA HCC
AHA: Q4 2018

6️⃣ **T43.69 Poisoning by, adverse effect of and underdosing of
other psychostimulants**

7️⃣ **T43.691 Poisoning by other psychostimulants,
accidental (unintentional)** POA HCC
Poisoning by other psychostimulants NOS

7️⃣ **T43.692 Poisoning by other psychostimulants,
intentional self-harm** POA HCC

7️⃣ **T43.693 Poisoning by other psychostimulants,
assault** POA

7️⃣ **T43.694 Poisoning by other psychostimulants,
undetermined** POA HCC

7️⃣ **T43.695 Adverse effect of other
psychostimulants** POA PDxIn

7️⃣ **T43.696 Underdosing of other
psychostimulants** POA PDxIn

5️⃣ **T43.8 Poisoning by, adverse effect of and underdosing of other
psychotropic drugs**

6️⃣ **T43.8X Poisoning by, adverse effect of and underdosing of
other psychotropic drugs**

7️⃣ **T43.8X1 Poisoning by other psychotropic drugs,
accidental (unintentional)** POA
Poisoning by other psychotropic drugs NOS

7️⃣ **T43.8X2 Poisoning by other psychotropic drugs,
intentional self-harm** POA HCC

7️⃣ **T43.8X3 Poisoning by other psychotropic drugs,
assault** POA

7️⃣ **T43.8X4 Poisoning by other psychotropic drugs,
undetermined** POA

7️⃣ **T43.8X5 Adverse effect of other
psychotropic drugs** POA PDxIn

7️⃣ **T43.8X6 Underdosing of other
psychotropic drugs** POA PDxIn

5️⃣ **T43.9 Poisoning by, adverse effect of and underdosing of
unspecified psychotropic drug**

7️⃣ **T43.91 Poisoning by unspecified psychotropic drug,
accidental (unintentional)** POA
Poisoning by psychotropic drug NOS

7️⃣ **T43.92 Poisoning by unspecified psychotropic drug,
intentional self-harm** POA HCC

7️⃣ **T43.93 Poisoning by unspecified psychotropic drug,
assault** POA

7️⃣ **T43.94 Poisoning by unspecified psychotropic drug,
undetermined** POA

7️⃣ **T43.95 Adverse effect of unspecified
psychotropic drug** POA PDxIn

7️⃣ **T43.96 Underdosing of unspecified
psychotropic drug** POA PDxIn

4️⃣ **T44 Poisoning by, adverse effect of and underdosing of drugs primarily
affecting the autonomic nervous system**

The appropriate 7th character is to be added to each code from
category T44

A = initial encounter
D = subsequent encounter
S = sequela

5️⃣ **T44.0 Poisoning by, adverse effect of and underdosing of
anticholinesterase agents**

6️⃣ **T44.0X Poisoning by, adverse effect of and underdosing of
anticholinesterase agents**

7️⃣ **T44.0X1 Poisoning by anticholinesterase agents,
accidental (unintentional)** POA
Poisoning by anticholinesterase agents NOS

7️⃣ **T44.0X2 Poisoning by anticholinesterase agents,
intentional self-harm** POA HCC

7️⃣ **T44.0X3 Poisoning by anticholinesterase agents,
assault** POA

7️⃣ **T44.0X4 Poisoning by anticholinesterase agents,
undetermined** POA

7️⃣ **T44.0X5 Adverse effect of anticholinesterase
agents** POA PDxIn

7️⃣ **T44.0X6 Underdosing of anticholinesterase
agents** POA PDxIn

5️⃣ **T44.1 Poisoning by, adverse effect of and underdosing of other
parasympathomimetics [cholinergics]**

6️⃣ **T44.1X Poisoning by, adverse effect of and underdosing of
other parasympathomimetics [cholinergics]**

7️⃣ **T44.1X1 Poisoning by other
parasympathomimetics [cholinergics],
accidental (unintentional)** POA
Poisoning by other parasympathomimetics
[cholinergics] NOS

7️⃣ **T44.1X2 Poisoning by other
parasympathomimetics [cholinergics],
intentional self-harm** POA HCC

7️⃣ **T44.1X3 Poisoning by other
parasympathomimetics [cholinergics],
assault** POA

7️⃣ **T44.1X4 Poisoning by other
parasympathomimetics [cholinergics],
undetermined** POA

PDxIn Unacceptable principal diagnosis symbol per Medicare code edits   POA Code exempt from diagnosis present on admission requirement
❓ Questionable admission   CC Complication or comorbidity   MCC Major complication or comorbidity   CC/MCC Exc CC/MCC exclusion
HCC HCC diagnosis code   RxHCC RxHCC diagnosis code   MACRA MACRA code   **DEFINITION** Describes condition/terminology
TIP Coding guidance   👁 Official Guideline Reference   Z1 Z code as first-listed diagnosis

7️⃣ T44.1X5 Adverse effect of other parasympathomimetics [cholinergics] POA PDxIn

▲ 7️⃣ T44.1X6 Underdosing of other parasympathomimetics ►[cholinergics]◄ POA PDxIn

5️⃣ T44.2 Poisoning by, adverse effect of and underdosing of ganglionic blocking drugs

6️⃣ T44.2X Poisoning by, adverse effect of and underdosing of ganglionic blocking drugs

7️⃣ T44.2X1 Poisoning by ganglionic blocking drugs, accidental (unintentional) POA

Poisoning by ganglionic blocking drugs NOS

7️⃣ T44.2X2 Poisoning by ganglionic blocking drugs, intentional self-harm POA HCC

7️⃣ T44.2X3 Poisoning by ganglionic blocking drugs, assault POA

7️⃣ T44.2X4 Poisoning by ganglionic blocking drugs, undetermined POA

7️⃣ T44.2X5 Adverse effect of ganglionic blocking drugs POA PDxIn

7️⃣ T44.2X6 Underdosing of ganglionic blocking drugs POA PDxIn

5️⃣ T44.3 Poisoning by, adverse effect of and underdosing of other parasympatholytics [anticholinergics and antimuscarinics] and spasmolytics

Poisoning by, adverse effect of and underdosing of papaverine

6️⃣ T44.3X Poisoning by, adverse effect of and underdosing of other parasympatholytics [anticholinergics and antimuscarinics] and spasmolytics

7️⃣ T44.3X1 Poisoning by other parasympatholytics [anticholinergics and antimuscarinics] and spasmolytics, accidental (unintentional) POA

Poisoning by other parasympatholytics [anticholinergics and antimuscarinics] and spasmolytics NOS

7️⃣ T44.3X2 Poisoning by other parasympatholytics [anticholinergics and antimuscarinics] and spasmolytics, intentional self-harm POA HCC

7️⃣ T44.3X3 Poisoning by other parasympatholytics [anticholinergics and antimuscarinics] and spasmolytics, assault POA

7️⃣ T44.3X4 Poisoning by other parasympatholytics [anticholinergics and antimuscarinics] and spasmolytics, undetermined POA

7️⃣ T44.3X5 Adverse effect of other parasympatholytics [anticholinergics and antimuscarinics] and spasmolytics POA PDxIn

7️⃣ T44.3X6 Underdosing of other parasympatholytics [anticholinergics and antimuscarinics] and spasmolytics POA PDxIn

5️⃣ T44.4 Poisoning by, adverse effect of and underdosing of predominantly alpha-adrenoreceptor agonists

Poisoning by, adverse effect of and underdosing of metaraminol

6️⃣ T44.4X Poisoning by, adverse effect of and underdosing of predominantly alpha-adrenoreceptor agonists

7️⃣ T44.4X1 Poisoning by predominantly alpha-adrenoreceptor agonists, accidental (unintentional) POA

Poisoning by predominantly alpha-adrenoreceptor agonists NOS

7️⃣ T44.4X2 Poisoning by predominantly alpha-adrenoreceptor agonists, intentional self-harm POA HCC

7️⃣ T44.4X3 Poisoning by predominantly alpha-adrenoreceptor agonists, assault POA

7️⃣ T44.4X4 Poisoning by predominantly alpha-adrenoreceptor agonists, undetermined POA

7️⃣ T44.4X5 Adverse effect of predominantly alpha-adrenoreceptor agonists POA PDxIn

7️⃣ T44.4X6 Underdosing of predominantly alpha-adrenoreceptor agonists POA PDxIn

5️⃣ T44.5 Poisoning by, adverse effect of and underdosing of predominantly beta-adrenoreceptor agonists

EXCLUDES1 poisoning by, adverse effect of and underdosing of beta-adrenoreceptor agonists used in asthma therapy (T48.6-)

6️⃣ T44.5X Poisoning by, adverse effect of and underdosing of predominantly beta-adrenoreceptor agonists

7️⃣ T44.5X1 Poisoning by predominantly beta-adrenoreceptor agonists, accidental (unintentional) POA

Poisoning by predominantly beta-adrenoreceptor agonists NOS

7️⃣ T44.5X2 Poisoning by predominantly beta-adrenoreceptor agonists, intentional self-harm POA HCC

7️⃣ T44.5X3 Poisoning by predominantly beta-adrenoreceptor agonists, assault POA

7️⃣ T44.5X4 Poisoning by predominantly beta-adrenoreceptor agonists, undetermined POA

7️⃣ T44.5X5 Adverse effect of predominantly beta-adrenoreceptor agonists POA PDxIn

7️⃣ T44.5X6 Underdosing of predominantly beta-adrenoreceptor agonists POA PDxIn

5️⃣ T44.6 Poisoning by, adverse effect of and underdosing of alpha-adrenoreceptor antagonists

EXCLUDES1 poisoning by, adverse effect of and underdosing of ergot alkaloids (T48.0)

6️⃣ T44.6X Poisoning by, adverse effect of and underdosing of alpha-adrenoreceptor antagonists

7️⃣ T44.6X1 Poisoning by alpha-adrenoreceptor antagonists, accidental (unintentional) POA

Poisoning by alpha-adrenoreceptor antagonists NOS

7️⃣ T44.6X2 Poisoning by alpha-adrenoreceptor antagonists, intentional self-harm POA HCC

7️⃣ T44.6X3 Poisoning by alpha-adrenoreceptor antagonists, assault POA

7️⃣ T44.6X4 Poisoning by alpha-adrenoreceptor antagonists, undetermined POA

7️⃣ T44.6X5 Adverse effect of alpha-adrenoreceptor antagonists POA PDxIn

7️⃣ T44.6X6 Underdosing of alpha-adrenoreceptor antagonists POA PDxIn

5️⃣ T44.7 Poisoning by, adverse effect of and underdosing of beta-adrenoreceptor antagonists

6️⃣ T44.7X Poisoning by, adverse effect of and underdosing of beta-adrenoreceptor antagonists

7️⃣ T44.7X1 Poisoning by beta-adrenoreceptor antagonists, accidental (unintentional) POA

Poisoning by beta-adrenoreceptor antagonists NOS

7️⃣ T44.7X2 Poisoning by beta-adrenoreceptor antagonists, intentional self-harm POA HCC

7️⃣ T44.7X3 Poisoning by beta-adrenoreceptor antagonists, assault POA

7️⃣ T44.7X4 Poisoning by beta-adrenoreceptor antagonists, undetermined POA

7️⃣ T44.7X5 Adverse effect of beta-adrenoreceptor antagonists POA PDxIn

7️⃣ T44.7X6 Underdosing of beta-adrenoreceptor antagonists POA PDxIn

5️⃣ T44.8 Poisoning by, adverse effect of and underdosing of centrally-acting and adrenergic-neuron- blocking agents

EXCLUDES1 poisoning by, adverse effect of and underdosing of clonidine (T46.5)

poisoning by, adverse effect of and underdosing of guanethidine (T46.5)

6️⃣ T44.8X Poisoning by, adverse effect of and underdosing of centrally-acting and adrenergic- neuron-blocking agents

7️⃣ T44.8X1 Poisoning by centrally-acting and adrenergic-neuron-blocking agents, accidental (unintentional) POA

Poisoning by centrally-acting and adrenergic-neuron-blocking agents NOS

Unspecified Code   Other Specified Code   Manifestation Code   N Newborn   P Pediatric   M Maternity   A Adult   ♂ Male   ♀ Female
● New Code   ▲ Revised Code Title   ►◄ Revised Text   NOTES   INCLUDES   EXCLUDES1 Not coded here   EXCLUDES2 Not included here
4️⃣ 4th character required   5️⃣ 5th character required   6️⃣ 6th character required   7️⃣ 7th character required   Ⓧ Extension 'X' Alert
HAC Hospital-acquired condition (HAC) alert   AHA AHA Coding Clinic©   📖 Code first alert

2020 ICD-10-CM   When symbols appear on a code that requires a 7th character extension, refer to Appendix B to identify applicable 7th character codes.   **1133**

T44.8X2 Poisoning by centrally-acting and adrenergic-neuron-blocking agents, intentional self-harm POA HCC

T44.8X3 Poisoning by centrally-acting and adrenergic-neuron-blocking agents, assault POA

T44.8X4 Poisoning by centrally-acting and adrenergic-neuron-blocking agents, undetermined POA

T44.8X5 Adverse effect of centrally-acting and adrenergic-neuron-blocking agents POA PDxIn

T44.8X6 Underdosing of centrally-acting and adrenergic-neuron-blocking agents POA PDxIn

T44.9 Poisoning by, adverse effect of and underdosing of other and unspecified drugs primarily affecting the autonomic nervous system

Poisoning by, adverse effect of and underdosing of drug stimulating both alpha and beta-adrenoreceptors

T44.90 Poisoning by, adverse effect of and underdosing of unspecified drugs primarily affecting the autonomic nervous system

T44.901 Poisoning by unspecified drugs primarily affecting the autonomic nervous system, accidental (unintentional) POA

Poisoning by unspecified drugs primarily affecting the autonomic nervous system NOS

T44.902 Poisoning by unspecified drugs primarily affecting the autonomic nervous system, intentional self-harm POA HCC

T44.903 Poisoning by unspecified drugs primarily affecting the autonomic nervous system, assault POA

T44.904 Poisoning by unspecified drugs primarily affecting the autonomic nervous system, undetermined POA

T44.905 Adverse effect of unspecified drugs primarily affecting the autonomic nervous system POA PDxIn

T44.906 Underdosing of unspecified drugs primarily affecting the autonomic nervous system POA PDxIn

T44.99 Poisoning by, adverse effect of and underdosing of other drugs primarily affecting the autonomic nervous system

T44.991 Poisoning by other drug primarily affecting the autonomic nervous system, accidental (unintentional) POA

Poisoning by other drugs primarily affecting the autonomic nervous system NOS

T44.992 Poisoning by other drug primarily affecting the autonomic nervous system, intentional self-harm POA HCC

T44.993 Poisoning by other drug primarily affecting the autonomic nervous system, assault POA

T44.994 Poisoning by other drug primarily affecting the autonomic nervous system, undetermined POA

T44.995 Adverse effect of other drug primarily affecting the autonomic nervous system POA PDxIn

T44.996 Underdosing of other drug primarily affecting the autonomic nervous system POA PDxIn

T45 Poisoning by, adverse effect of and underdosing of primarily systemic and hematological agents, not elsewhere classified

The appropriate 7th character is to be added to each code from category T45

A = initial encounter
D = subsequent encounter
S = sequela

T45.0 Poisoning by, adverse effect of and underdosing of antiallergic and antiemetic drugs

EXCLUDES1 poisoning by, adverse effect of and underdosing of phenothiazine-based neuroleptics (T43.3)

T45.0X Poisoning by, adverse effect of and underdosing of antiallergic and antiemetic drugs

T45.0X1 Poisoning by antiallergic and antiemetic drugs, accidental (unintentional) POA

Poisoning by antiallergic and antiemetic drugs NOS

T45.0X2 Poisoning by antiallergic and antiemetic drugs, intentional self-harm POA HCC

T45.0X3 Poisoning by antiallergic and antiemetic drugs, assault POA

T45.0X4 Poisoning by antiallergic and antiemetic drugs, undetermined POA

T45.0X5 Adverse effect of antiallergic and antiemetic drugs POA PDxIn

T45.0X6 Underdosing of antiallergic and antiemetic drugs POA PDxIn

T45.1 Poisoning by, adverse effect of and underdosing of antineoplastic and immunosuppressive drugs

EXCLUDES1 poisoning by, adverse effect of and underdosing of tamoxifen (T38.6)

T45.1X Poisoning by, adverse effect of and underdosing of antineoplastic and immunosuppressive drugs

T45.1X1 Poisoning by antineoplastic and immunosuppressive drugs, accidental (unintentional) POA

Poisoning by antineoplastic and immunosuppressive drugs NOS

T45.1X2 Poisoning by antineoplastic and immunosuppressive drugs, intentional self-harm POA HCC

T45.1X3 Poisoning by antineoplastic and immunosuppressive drugs, assault POA

T45.1X4 Poisoning by antineoplastic and immunosuppressive drugs, undetermined POA

T45.1X5 Adverse effect of antineoplastic and immunosuppressive drugs POA PDxIn

See Official Guidelines "Anemia associated with chemotherapy, immunotherapy and radiation therapy" I.C.2.c.2

AHA: Q1 2019, Q2 2019

T45.1X6 Underdosing of antineoplastic and immunosuppressive drugs POA PDxIn

T45.2 Poisoning by, adverse effect of and underdosing of vitamins

EXCLUDES2 poisoning by, adverse effect of and underdosing of nicotinic acid (derivatives) (T46.7)

poisoning by, adverse effect of and underdosing of iron (T45.4)

poisoning by, adverse effect of and underdosing of vitamin K (T45.7)

T45.2X Poisoning by, adverse effect of and underdosing of vitamins

T45.2X1 Poisoning by vitamins, accidental (unintentional) POA

Poisoning by vitamins NOS

T45.2X2 Poisoning by vitamins, intentional self-harm POA HCC

T45.2X3 Poisoning by vitamins, assault POA

T45.2X4 Poisoning by vitamins, undetermined POA

T45.2X5 Adverse effect of vitamins POA PDxIn

T45.2X6 Underdosing of vitamins POA PDxIn

EXCLUDES1 vitamin deficiencies (E50-E56)

T45.3 Poisoning by, adverse effect of and underdosing of enzymes

T45.3X Poisoning by, adverse effect of and underdosing of enzymes

T45.3X1 Poisoning by enzymes, accidental (unintentional) POA

Poisoning by enzymes NOS

When symbols appear on a code that requires a 7th character extension, refer to Appendix B to identify applicable 7th character codes.

2020 ICD-10-CM

	7ᵗʰ T45.3X2	Poisoning by enzymes, intentional self-harm	POA HCC
	7ᵗʰ T45.3X3	Poisoning by enzymes, assault	POA
	7ᵗʰ T45.3X4	Poisoning by enzymes, undetermined	POA
	7ᵗʰ T45.3X5	Adverse effect of enzymes	POA PDxIn
	7ᵗʰ T45.3X6	Underdosing of enzymes	POA PDxIn

5ᵗʰ **T45.4 Poisoning by, adverse effect of and underdosing of iron and its compounds**

6ᵗʰ **T45.4X Poisoning by, adverse effect of and underdosing of iron and its compounds**

7ᵗʰ T45.4X1 Poisoning by iron and its compounds, accidental (unintentional) POA
Poisoning by iron and its compounds NOS

7ᵗʰ T45.4X2 Poisoning by iron and its compounds, intentional self-harm POA HCC

7ᵗʰ T45.4X3 Poisoning by iron and its compounds, assault POA

7ᵗʰ T45.4X4 Poisoning by iron and its compounds, undetermined POA

7ᵗʰ T45.4X5 Adverse effect of iron and its compounds POA PDxIn

7ᵗʰ T45.4X6 Underdosing of iron and its compounds POA PDxIn
EXCLUDES1 iron deficiency (E61.1)

5ᵗʰ **T45.5 Poisoning by, adverse effect of and underdosing of anticoagulants and antithrombotic drugs**

6ᵗʰ **T45.51 Poisoning by, adverse effect of and underdosing of anticoagulants**

7ᵗʰ T45.511 Poisoning by anticoagulants, accidental (unintentional) POA
Poisoning by anticoagulants NOS

7ᵗʰ T45.512 Poisoning by anticoagulants, intentional self-harm POA HCC

7ᵗʰ T45.513 Poisoning by anticoagulants, assault POA

7ᵗʰ T45.514 Poisoning by anticoagulants, undetermined POA

7ᵗʰ T45.515 Adverse effect of anticoagulants POA PDxIn
AHA: Q1 2016

7ᵗʰ T45.516 Underdosing of anticoagulants POA PDxIn

6ᵗʰ **T45.52 Poisoning by, adverse effect of and underdosing of antithrombotic drugs**
Poisoning by, adverse effect of and underdosing of antiplatelet drugs
EXCLUDES2 poisoning by, adverse effect of and underdosing of aspirin (T39.01-)
poisoning by, adverse effect of and underdosing of acetylsalicylic acid (T39.01-)

7ᵗʰ T45.521 Poisoning by antithrombotic drugs, accidental (unintentional) POA
Poisoning by antithrombotic drug NOS

7ᵗʰ T45.522 Poisoning by antithrombotic drugs, intentional self-harm POA HCC

7ᵗʰ T45.523 Poisoning by antithrombotic drugs, assault POA

7ᵗʰ T45.524 Poisoning by antithrombotic drugs, undetermined POA

7ᵗʰ T45.525 Adverse effect of antithrombotic drugs POA PDxIn
AHA: Q1 2016

7ᵗʰ T45.526 Underdosing of antithrombotic drugs POA PDxIn

5ᵗʰ **T45.6 Poisoning by, adverse effect of and underdosing of fibrinolysis-affecting drugs**

6ᵗʰ **T45.60 Poisoning by, adverse effect of and underdosing of unspecified fibrinolysis-affecting drugs**

7ᵗʰ T45.601 Poisoning by unspecified fibrinolysis-affecting drugs, accidental (unintentional) POA
Poisoning by fibrinolysis-affecting drug NOS

7ᵗʰ T45.602 Poisoning by unspecified fibrinolysis-affecting drugs, intentional self-harm POA HCC

7ᵗʰ T45.603 Poisoning by unspecified fibrinolysis-affecting drugs, assault POA

7ᵗʰ T45.604 Poisoning by unspecified fibrinolysis-affecting drugs, undetermined POA

7ᵗʰ T45.605 Adverse effect of unspecified fibrinolysis-affecting drugs POA PDxIn

7ᵗʰ T45.606 Underdosing of unspecified fibrinolysis-affecting drugs POA PDxIn

6ᵗʰ **T45.61 Poisoning by, adverse effect of and underdosing of thrombolytic drugs**

7ᵗʰ T45.611 Poisoning by thrombolytic drug, accidental (unintentional) POA
Poisoning by thrombolytic drug NOS

7ᵗʰ T45.612 Poisoning by thrombolytic drug, intentional self-harm POA HCC

7ᵗʰ T45.613 Poisoning by thrombolytic drug, assault POA

7ᵗʰ T45.614 Poisoning by thrombolytic drug, undetermined POA

7ᵗʰ T45.615 Adverse effect of thrombolytic drugs POA PDxIn
AHA: Q2 2017

7ᵗʰ T45.616 Underdosing of thrombolytic drugs POA PDxIn

6ᵗʰ **T45.62 Poisoning by, adverse effect of and underdosing of hemostatic drugs**

7ᵗʰ T45.621 Poisoning by hemostatic drug, accidental (unintentional) POA
Poisoning by hemostatic drug NOS

7ᵗʰ T45.622 Poisoning by hemostatic drug, intentional self-harm POA HCC

7ᵗʰ T45.623 Poisoning by hemostatic drug, assault POA

7ᵗʰ T45.624 Poisoning by hemostatic drug, undetermined POA

7ᵗʰ T45.625 Adverse effect of hemostatic drug POA PDxIn

7ᵗʰ T45.626 Underdosing of hemostatic drugs POA PDxIn

6ᵗʰ **T45.69 Poisoning by, adverse effect of and underdosing of other fibrinolysis-affecting drugs**

7ᵗʰ T45.691 Poisoning by other fibrinolysis-affecting drugs, accidental (unintentional) POA
Poisoning by other fibrinolysis-affecting drug NOS

7ᵗʰ T45.692 Poisoning by other fibrinolysis-affecting drugs, intentional self-harm POA HCC

7ᵗʰ T45.693 Poisoning by other fibrinolysis-affecting drugs, assault POA

7ᵗʰ T45.694 Poisoning by other fibrinolysis-affecting drugs, undetermined POA

7ᵗʰ T45.695 Adverse effect of other fibrinolysis-affecting drugs POA PDxIn

7ᵗʰ T45.696 Underdosing of other fibrinolysis-affecting drugs POA PDxIn

5ᵗʰ **T45.7 Poisoning by, adverse effect of and underdosing of anticoagulant antagonists, vitamin K and other coagulants**

6ᵗʰ **T45.7X Poisoning by, adverse effect of and underdosing of anticoagulant antagonists, vitamin K and other coagulants**

7ᵗʰ T45.7X1 Poisoning by anticoagulant antagonists, vitamin K and other coagulants, accidental (unintentional) POA
Poisoning by anticoagulant antagonists, vitamin K and other coagulants NOS

7ᵗʰ T45.7X2 Poisoning by anticoagulant antagonists, vitamin K and other coagulants, intentional self-harm POA HCC

7ᵗʰ T45.7X3 Poisoning by anticoagulant antagonists, vitamin K and other coagulants, assault POA

7ᵗʰ T45.7X4 Poisoning by anticoagulant antagonists, vitamin K and other coagulants, undetermined POA

7ᵗʰ T45.7X5 Adverse effect of anticoagulant antagonists, vitamin K and other coagulants POA PDxIn

7ᵗʰ T45.7X6 Underdosing of anticoagulant antagonist, vitamin K and other coagulants POA PDxIn
EXCLUDES1 vitamin K deficiency (E56.1)

T45.8 Poisoning by, adverse effect of and underdosing of other primarily systemic and hematological agents

Poisoning by, adverse effect of and underdosing of liver preparations and other antianemic agents

Poisoning by, adverse effect of and underdosing of natural blood and blood products

Poisoning by, adverse effect of and underdosing of plasma substitute

EXCLUDES2 *poisoning by, adverse effect of and underdosing of immunoglobulin (T50.Z1)*

poisoning by, adverse effect of and underdosing of iron (T45.4)

transfusion reactions (T80.-)

T45.8X Poisoning by, adverse effect of and underdosing of other primarily systemic and hematological agents

T45.8X1 Poisoning by other primarily systemic and hematological agents, accidental (unintentional)

Poisoning by other primarily systemic and hematological agents NOS

T45.8X2 Poisoning by other primarily systemic and hematological agents, intentional self-harm

T45.8X3 Poisoning by other primarily systemic and hematological agents, assault

T45.8X4 Poisoning by other primarily systemic and hematological agents, undetermined

T45.8X5 Adverse effect of other primarily systemic and hematological agents

AHA: Q4 2016

T45.8X6 Underdosing of other primarily systemic and hematological agents

T45.9 Poisoning by, adverse effect of and underdosing of unspecified primarily systemic and hematological agent

T45.91 Poisoning by unspecified primarily systemic and hematological agent, accidental (unintentional)

Poisoning by primarily systemic and hematological agent NOS

T45.92 Poisoning by unspecified primarily systemic and hematological agent, intentional self-harm

T45.93 Poisoning by unspecified primarily systemic and hematological agent, assault

T45.94 Poisoning by unspecified primarily systemic and hematological agent, undetermined

T45.95 Adverse effect of unspecified primarily systemic and hematological agent

T45.96 Underdosing of unspecified primarily systemic and hematological agent

T46 Poisoning by, adverse effect of and underdosing of agents primarily affecting the cardiovascular system

EXCLUDES1 *poisoning by, adverse effect of and underdosing of metaraminol (T44.4)*

The appropriate 7th character is to be added to each code from category T46

A = initial encounter

D = subsequent encounter

S = sequela

T46.0 Poisoning by, adverse effect of and underdosing of cardiac-stimulant glycosides and drugs of similar action

T46.0X Poisoning by, adverse effect of and underdosing of cardiac-stimulant glycosides and drugs of similar action

T46.0X1 Poisoning by cardiac-stimulant glycosides and drugs of similar action, accidental (unintentional)

Poisoning by cardiac-stimulant glycosides and drugs of similar action NOS

T46.0X2 Poisoning by cardiac-stimulant glycosides and drugs of similar action, intentional self-harm

T46.0X3 Poisoning by cardiac-stimulant glycosides and drugs of similar action, assault

T46.0X4 Poisoning by cardiac-stimulant glycosides and drugs of similar action, undetermined

T46.0X5 Adverse effect of cardiac-stimulant glycosides and drugs of similar action

T46.0X6 Underdosing of cardiac-stimulant glycosides and drugs of similar action

T46.1 Poisoning by, adverse effect of and underdosing of calcium-channel blockers

T46.1X Poisoning by, adverse effect of and underdosing of calcium-channel blockers

T46.1X1 Poisoning by calcium-channel blockers, accidental (unintentional)

Poisoning by calcium-channel blockers NOS

T46.1X2 Poisoning by calcium-channel blockers, intentional self-harm

T46.1X3 Poisoning by calcium-channel blockers, assault

T46.1X4 Poisoning by calcium-channel blockers, undetermined

T46.1X5 Adverse effect of calcium-channel blockers

T46.1X6 Underdosing of calcium-channel blockers

T46.2 Poisoning by, adverse effect of and underdosing of other antidysrhythmic drugs, not elsewhere classified

EXCLUDES1 *poisoning by, adverse effect of and underdosing of beta-adrenoreceptor antagonists (T44.7-)*

T46.2X Poisoning by, adverse effect of and underdosing of other antidysrhythmic drugs

T46.2X1 Poisoning by other antidysrhythmic drugs, accidental (unintentional)

Poisoning by other antidysrhythmic drugs NOS

T46.2X2 Poisoning by other antidysrhythmic drugs, intentional self-harm

T46.2X3 Poisoning by other antidysrhythmic drugs, assault

T46.2X4 Poisoning by other antidysrhythmic drugs, undetermined

T46.2X5 Adverse effect of other antidysrhythmic drugs

T46.2X6 Underdosing of other antidysrhythmic drugs

T46.3 Poisoning by, adverse effect of and underdosing of coronary vasodilators

Poisoning by, adverse effect of and underdosing of dipyridamole

EXCLUDES1 *poisoning by, adverse effect of and underdosing of calcium-channel blockers (T46.1)*

T46.3X Poisoning by, adverse effect of and underdosing of coronary vasodilators

T46.3X1 Poisoning by coronary vasodilators, accidental (unintentional)

Poisoning by coronary vasodilators NOS

T46.3X2 Poisoning by coronary vasodilators, intentional self-harm

T46.3X3 Poisoning by coronary vasodilators, assault

T46.3X4 Poisoning by coronary vasodilators, undetermined

T46.3X5 Adverse effect of coronary vasodilators

T46.3X6 Underdosing of coronary vasodilators

T46.4 Poisoning by, adverse effect of and underdosing of angiotensin-converting-enzyme inhibitors

T46.4X Poisoning by, adverse effect of and underdosing of angiotensin-converting-enzyme inhibitors

---

PDxIn Unacceptable principal diagnosis symbol per Medicare code edits   POA Code exempt from diagnosis present on admission requirement

❓ Questionable admission   CC Complication or comorbidity   MCC Major complication or comorbidity   CC/MCC CC/MCC exclusion

HCC HCC diagnosis code   RxHCC RxHCC diagnosis code   MACRA code   **DEFINITION** Describes condition/terminology

TIP Coding guidance   👁 Official Guideline Reference   Z1 Z code as first-listed diagnosis

[7th] T46.4X1 Poisoning by angiotensin-converting-enzyme inhibitors, accidental (unintentional) POA
Poisoning by angiotensin-converting-enzyme inhibitors NOS
[7th] T46.4X2 Poisoning by angiotensin-converting-enzyme inhibitors, intentional self-harm POA HCC
[7th] T46.4X3 Poisoning by angiotensin-converting-enzyme inhibitors, assault POA
[7th] T46.4X4 Poisoning by angiotensin-converting-enzyme inhibitors, undetermined POA
[7th] T46.4X5 Adverse effect of angiotensin-converting-enzyme inhibitors POA PDxIn
[7th] T46.4X6 Underdosing of angiotensin-converting-enzyme inhibitors POA PDxIn

[5th] T46.5 Poisoning by, adverse effect of and underdosing of other antihypertensive drugs
EXCLUDES2 *poisoning by, adverse effect of and underdosing of beta-adrenoreceptor antagonists (T44.7)*
poisoning by, adverse effect of and underdosing of calcium-channel blockers (T46.1)
poisoning by, adverse effect of and underdosing of diuretics (T50.0-T50.2)
[6th] T46.5X Poisoning by, adverse effect of and underdosing of other antihypertensive drugs
[7th] T46.5X1 Poisoning by other antihypertensive drugs, accidental (unintentional) POA
Poisoning by other antihypertensive drugs NOS
[7th] T46.5X2 Poisoning by other antihypertensive drugs, intentional self-harm POA HCC
[7th] T46.5X3 Poisoning by other antihypertensive drugs, assault POA
[7th] T46.5X4 Poisoning by other antihypertensive drugs, undetermined POA
[7th] T46.5X5 Adverse effect of other antihypertensive drugs POA PDxIn
[7th] T46.5X6 Underdosing of other antihypertensive drugs POA PDxIn

[5th] T46.6 Poisoning by, adverse effect of and underdosing of antihyperlipidemic and antiarteriosclerotic drugs
[6th] T46.6X Poisoning by, adverse effect of and underdosing of antihyperlipidemic and antiarteriosclerotic drugs
[7th] T46.6X1 Poisoning by antihyperlipidemic and antiarteriosclerotic drugs, accidental (unintentional) POA
Poisoning by antihyperlipidemic and antiarteriosclerotic drugs NOS
[7th] T46.6X2 Poisoning by antihyperlipidemic and antiarteriosclerotic drugs, intentional self-harm POA HCC
[7th] T46.6X3 Poisoning by antihyperlipidemic and antiarteriosclerotic drugs, assault POA
[7th] T46.6X4 Poisoning by antihyperlipidemic and antiarteriosclerotic drugs, undetermined POA
[7th] T46.6X5 Adverse effect of antihyperlipidemic and antiarteriosclerotic drugs POA PDxIn
[7th] T46.6X6 Underdosing of antihyperlipidemic and antiarteriosclerotic drugs POA PDxIn

[5th] T46.7 Poisoning by, adverse effect of and underdosing of peripheral vasodilators
Poisoning by, adverse effect of and underdosing of nicotinic acid (derivatives)
EXCLUDES1 *poisoning by, adverse effect of and underdosing of papaverine (T44.3)*
[6th] T46.7X Poisoning by, adverse effect of and underdosing of peripheral vasodilators
[7th] T46.7X1 Poisoning by peripheral vasodilators, accidental (unintentional) POA
Poisoning by peripheral vasodilators NOS
[7th] T46.7X2 Poisoning by peripheral vasodilators, intentional self-harm POA HCC
[7th] T46.7X3 Poisoning by peripheral vasodilators, assault POA
[7th] T46.7X4 Poisoning by peripheral vasodilators, undetermined POA
[7th] T46.7X5 Adverse effect of peripheral vasodilators POA PDxIn
[7th] T46.7X6 Underdosing of peripheral vasodilators POA PDxIn

[5th] T46.8 Poisoning by, adverse effect of and underdosing of antivaricose drugs, including sclerosing agents
[6th] T46.8X Poisoning by, adverse effect of and underdosing of antivaricose drugs, including sclerosing agents
[7th] T46.8X1 Poisoning by antivaricose drugs, including sclerosing agents, accidental (unintentional) POA
Poisoning by antivaricose drugs, including sclerosing agents NOS
[7th] T46.8X2 Poisoning by antivaricose drugs, including sclerosing agents, intentional self-harm POA HCC
[7th] T46.8X3 Poisoning by antivaricose drugs, including sclerosing agents, assault POA
[7th] T46.8X4 Poisoning by antivaricose drugs, including sclerosing agents, undetermined POA
[7th] T46.8X5 Adverse effect of antivaricose drugs, including sclerosing agents POA PDxIn
[7th] T46.8X6 Underdosing of antivaricose drugs, including sclerosing agents POA PDxIn

[5th] T46.9 Poisoning by, adverse effect of and underdosing of other and unspecified agents primarily affecting the cardiovascular system
[6th] T46.90 Poisoning by, adverse effect of and underdosing of unspecified agents primarily affecting the cardiovascular system
[7th] T46.901 Poisoning by unspecified agents primarily affecting the cardiovascular system, accidental (unintentional) POA
[7th] T46.902 Poisoning by unspecified agents primarily affecting the cardiovascular system, intentional self-harm POA HCC
[7th] T46.903 Poisoning by unspecified agents primarily affecting the cardiovascular system, assault POA
[7th] T46.904 Poisoning by unspecified agents primarily affecting the cardiovascular system, undetermined POA
[7th] T46.905 Adverse effect of unspecified agents primarily affecting the cardiovascular system POA PDxIn
[7th] T46.906 Underdosing of unspecified agents primarily affecting the cardiovascular system POA PDxIn
[6th] T46.99 Poisoning by, adverse effect of and underdosing of other agents primarily affecting the cardiovascular system
[7th] T46.991 Poisoning by other agents primarily affecting the cardiovascular system, accidental (unintentional) POA
[7th] T46.992 Poisoning by other agents primarily affecting the cardiovascular system, intentional self-harm POA HCC
[7th] T46.993 Poisoning by other agents primarily affecting the cardiovascular system, assault POA
[7th] T46.994 Poisoning by other agents primarily affecting the cardiovascular system, undetermined POA
[7th] T46.995 Adverse effect of other agents primarily affecting the cardiovascular system POA PDxIn
[7th] T46.996 Underdosing of other agents primarily affecting the cardiovascular system POA PDxIn

T47 **Poisoning by, adverse effect of and underdosing of agents primarily affecting the gastrointestinal system**

The appropriate 7th character is to be added to each code from category T47

A = initial encounter
D = subsequent encounter
S = sequela

T47.0 **Poisoning by, adverse effect of and underdosing of histamine H2-receptor blockers**

T47.0X **Poisoning by, adverse effect of and underdosing of histamine H2-receptor blockers**

T47.0X1 **Poisoning by histamine H2-receptor blockers, accidental (unintentional)**
Poisoning by histamine H2-receptor blockers NOS

T47.0X2 **Poisoning by histamine H2-receptor blockers, intentional self-harm** POA HCC

T47.0X3 **Poisoning by histamine H2-receptor blockers, assault** POA

T47.0X4 **Poisoning by histamine H2-receptor blockers, undetermined** POA

T47.0X5 **Adverse effect of histamine H2-receptor blockers** POA PDxIn

T47.0X6 **Underdosing of histamine H2-receptor blockers** POA PDxIn

T47.1 **Poisoning by, adverse effect of and underdosing of other antacids and anti-gastric-secretion drugs**

T47.1X **Poisoning by, adverse effect of and underdosing of other antacids and anti-gastric-secretion drugs**

T47.1X1 **Poisoning by other antacids and anti-gastric-secretion drugs, accidental (unintentional)** POA
Poisoning by other antacids and anti-gastric-secretion drugs NOS

T47.1X2 **Poisoning by other antacids and anti-gastric-secretion drugs, intentional self-harm** POA HCC

T47.1X3 **Poisoning by other antacids and anti-gastric-secretion drugs, assault** POA

T47.1X4 **Poisoning by other antacids and anti-gastric-secretion drugs, undetermined** POA

T47.1X5 **Adverse effect of other antacids and anti-gastric-secretion drugs** POA PDxIn

T47.1X6 **Underdosing of other antacids and anti-gastric-secretion drugs** POA PDxIn

T47.2 **Poisoning by, adverse effect of and underdosing of stimulant laxatives**

T47.2X **Poisoning by, adverse effect of and underdosing of stimulant laxatives**

T47.2X1 **Poisoning by stimulant laxatives, accidental (unintentional)** POA
Poisoning by stimulant laxatives NOS

T47.2X2 **Poisoning by stimulant laxatives, intentional self-harm** POA HCC

T47.2X3 **Poisoning by stimulant laxatives, assault** POA

T47.2X4 **Poisoning by stimulant laxatives, undetermined** POA

T47.2X5 **Adverse effect of stimulant laxatives** POA PDxIn

T47.2X6 **Underdosing of stimulant laxatives** POA PDxIn

T47.3 **Poisoning by, adverse effect of and underdosing of saline and osmotic laxatives**

T47.3X **Poisoning by and adverse effect of saline and osmotic laxatives**

T47.3X1 **Poisoning by saline and osmotic laxatives, accidental (unintentional)** POA
Poisoning by saline and osmotic laxatives NOS

T47.3X2 **Poisoning by saline and osmotic laxatives, intentional self-harm** POA HCC

T47.3X3 **Poisoning by saline and osmotic laxatives, assault** POA

T47.3X4 **Poisoning by saline and osmotic laxatives, undetermined** POA

T47.3X5 **Adverse effect of saline and osmotic laxatives** POA PDxIn

T47.3X6 **Underdosing of saline and osmotic laxatives** POA PDxIn

T47.4 **Poisoning by, adverse effect of and underdosing of other laxatives**

T47.4X **Poisoning by, adverse effect of and underdosing of other laxatives**

T47.4X1 **Poisoning by other laxatives, accidental (unintentional)** POA
Poisoning by other laxatives NOS

T47.4X2 **Poisoning by other laxatives, intentional self-harm** POA HCC

T47.4X3 **Poisoning by other laxatives, assault** POA

T47.4X4 **Poisoning by other laxatives, undetermined** POA

T47.4X5 **Adverse effect of other laxatives** POA PDxIn

T47.4X6 **Underdosing of other laxatives** POA PDxIn

T47.5 **Poisoning by, adverse effect of and underdosing of digestants**

T47.5X **Poisoning by, adverse effect of and underdosing of digestants**

T47.5X1 **Poisoning by digestants, accidental (unintentional)** POA
Poisoning by digestants NOS

T47.5X2 **Poisoning by digestants, intentional self-harm** POA HCC

T47.5X3 **Poisoning by digestants, assault** POA

T47.5X4 **Poisoning by digestants, undetermined** POA

T47.5X5 **Adverse effect of digestants** POA PDxIn

T47.5X6 **Underdosing of digestants** POA PDxIn

T47.6 **Poisoning by, adverse effect of and underdosing of antidiarrheal drugs**

EXCLUDES2 *poisoning by, adverse effect of and underdosing of systemic antibiotics and other anti-infectives (T36-T37)*

T47.6X **Poisoning by, adverse effect of and underdosing of antidiarrheal drugs**

T47.6X1 **Poisoning by antidiarrheal drugs, accidental (unintentional)** POA
Poisoning by antidiarrheal drugs NOS

T47.6X2 **Poisoning by antidiarrheal drugs, intentional self-harm** POA HCC

T47.6X3 **Poisoning by antidiarrheal drugs, assault** POA

T47.6X4 **Poisoning by antidiarrheal drugs, undetermined** POA

T47.6X5 **Adverse effect of antidiarrheal drugs** POA PDxIn

T47.6X6 **Underdosing of antidiarrheal drugs** POA PDxIn

T47.7 **Poisoning by, adverse effect of and underdosing of emetics**

T47.7X **Poisoning by, adverse effect of and underdosing of emetics**

T47.7X1 **Poisoning by emetics, accidental (unintentional)** POA
Poisoning by emetics NOS

T47.7X2 **Poisoning by emetics, intentional self-harm** POA HCC

T47.7X3 **Poisoning by emetics, assault** POA

T47.7X4 **Poisoning by emetics, undetermined** POA

T47.7X5 **Adverse effect of emetics** POA PDxIn

T47.7X6 **Underdosing of emetics** POA PDxIn

T47.8 **Poisoning by, adverse effect of and underdosing of other agents primarily affecting gastrointestinal system**

T47.8X **Poisoning by, adverse effect of and underdosing of other agents primarily affecting gastrointestinal system**

T47.8X1 **Poisoning by other agents primarily affecting gastrointestinal system, accidental (unintentional)** POA
Poisoning by other agents primarily affecting gastrointestinal system NOS

PDxIn Unacceptable principal diagnosis symbol per Medicare code edits   POA Code exempt from diagnosis present on admission requirement
? Questionable admission   cc Complication or comorbidity   MCC Major complication or comorbidity   cc/MCC Exc CC/MCC exclusion
HCC HCC diagnosis code   RxHCC RxHCC diagnosis code   MACRA MACRA code   **DEFINITION** Describes condition/terminology
TIP Coding guidance   Official Guideline Reference   Z1 Z code as first-listed diagnosis

1138   When symbols appear on a code that requires a 7th character extension, refer to Appendix B to identify applicable 7th character codes.   **2020 ICD-10-CM**

7️⃣ T47.8X2 Poisoning by other agents primarily affecting gastrointestinal system, intentional self-harm POA HCC

7️⃣ T47.8X3 Poisoning by other agents primarily affecting gastrointestinal system, assault POA

7️⃣ T47.8X4 Poisoning by other agents primarily affecting gastrointestinal system, undetermined POA

7️⃣ T47.8X5 Adverse effect of other agents primarily affecting gastrointestinal system POA PDxIn

7️⃣ T47.8X6 Underdosing of other agents primarily affecting gastrointestinal system POA PDxIn

5️⃣ T47.9 Poisoning by, adverse effect of and underdosing of unspecified agents primarily affecting the gastrointestinal system

7️⃣ T47.91 Poisoning by unspecified agents primarily affecting the gastrointestinal system, accidental (unintentional) POA

Poisoning by agents primarily affecting the gastrointestinal system NOS

7️⃣ T47.92 Poisoning by unspecified agents primarily affecting the gastrointestinal system, intentional self-harm POA HCC

7️⃣ T47.93 Poisoning by unspecified agents primarily affecting the gastrointestinal system, assault POA

7️⃣ T47.94 Poisoning by unspecified agents primarily affecting the gastrointestinal system, undetermined POA

7️⃣ T47.95 Adverse effect of unspecified agents primarily affecting the gastrointestinal system POA PDxIn

7️⃣ T47.96 Underdosing of unspecified agents primarily affecting the gastrointestinal system POA PDxIn

4️⃣ T48 Poisoning by, adverse effect of and underdosing of agents primarily acting on smooth and skeletal muscles and the respiratory system

The appropriate 7th character is to be added to each code from category T48

A = initial encounter
D = subsequent encounter
S = sequela

5️⃣ T48.0 Poisoning by, adverse effect of and underdosing of oxytocic drugs

EXCLUDES1 poisoning by, adverse effect of and underdosing of estrogens, progestogens and antagonists (T38.4-T38.6)

6️⃣ T48.0X Poisoning by, adverse effect of and underdosing of oxytocic drugs

7️⃣ T48.0X1 Poisoning by oxytocic drugs, accidental (unintentional) POA

Poisoning by oxytocic drugs NOS

7️⃣ T48.0X2 Poisoning by oxytocic drugs, intentional self-harm POA HCC

7️⃣ T48.0X3 Poisoning by oxytocic drugs, assault POA

7️⃣ T48.0X4 Poisoning by oxytocic drugs, undetermined POA

7️⃣ T48.0X5 Adverse effect of oxytocic drugs POA PDxIn

7️⃣ T48.0X6 Underdosing of oxytocic drugs POA PDxIn

5️⃣ T48.1 Poisoning by, adverse effect of and underdosing of skeletal muscle relaxants [neuromuscular blocking agents]

6️⃣ T48.1X Poisoning by, adverse effect of and underdosing of skeletal muscle relaxants [neuromuscular blocking agents]

7️⃣ T48.1X1 Poisoning by skeletal muscle relaxants [neuromuscular blocking agents], accidental (unintentional) POA

Poisoning by skeletal muscle relaxants [neuromuscular blocking agents] NOS

7️⃣ T48.1X2 Poisoning by skeletal muscle relaxants [neuromuscular blocking agents], intentional self-harm POA HCC

7️⃣ T48.1X3 Poisoning by skeletal muscle relaxants [neuromuscular blocking agents], assault POA

7️⃣ T48.1X4 Poisoning by skeletal muscle relaxants [neuromuscular blocking agents], undetermined POA

7️⃣ T48.1X5 Adverse effect of skeletal muscle relaxants [neuromuscular blocking agents] POA PDxIn

7️⃣ T48.1X6 Underdosing of skeletal muscle relaxants [neuromuscular blocking agents] POA PDxIn

5️⃣ T48.2 Poisoning by, adverse effect of and underdosing of other and unspecified drugs acting on muscles

6️⃣ T48.20 Poisoning by, adverse effect of and underdosing of unspecified drugs acting on muscles

7️⃣ T48.201 Poisoning by unspecified drugs acting on muscles, accidental (unintentional) POA

Poisoning by unspecified drugs acting on muscles NOS

7️⃣ T48.202 Poisoning by unspecified drugs acting on muscles, intentional self-harm POA HCC

7️⃣ T48.203 Poisoning by unspecified drugs acting on muscles, assault POA

7️⃣ T48.204 Poisoning by unspecified drugs acting on muscles, undetermined POA

7️⃣ T48.205 Adverse effect of unspecified drugs acting on muscles POA PDxIn

7️⃣ T48.206 Underdosing of unspecified drugs acting on muscles POA PDxIn

5️⃣ T48.29 Poisoning by, adverse effect of and underdosing of other drugs acting on muscles

7️⃣ T48.291 Poisoning by other drugs acting on muscles, accidental (unintentional) POA

Poisoning by other drugs acting on muscles NOS

7️⃣ T48.292 Poisoning by other drugs acting on muscles, intentional self-harm POA HCC

7️⃣ T48.293 Poisoning by other drugs acting on muscles, assault POA

7️⃣ T48.294 Poisoning by other drugs acting on muscles, undetermined POA

7️⃣ T48.295 Adverse effect of other drugs acting on muscles POA PDxIn

7️⃣ T48.296 Underdosing of other drugs acting on muscles POA PDxIn

5️⃣ T48.3 Poisoning by, adverse effect of and underdosing of antitussives

6️⃣ T48.3X Poisoning by, adverse effect of and underdosing of antitussives

7️⃣ T48.3X1 Poisoning by antitussives, accidental (unintentional) POA

Poisoning by antitussives NOS

7️⃣ T48.3X2 Poisoning by antitussives, intentional self-harm POA HCC

7️⃣ T48.3X3 Poisoning by antitussives, assault POA

7️⃣ T48.3X4 Poisoning by antitussives, undetermined POA

7️⃣ T48.3X5 Adverse effect of antitussives POA PDxIn

7️⃣ T48.3X6 Underdosing of antitussives POA PDxIn

5️⃣ T48.4 Poisoning by, adverse effect of and underdosing of expectorants

6️⃣ T48.4X Poisoning by, adverse effect of and underdosing of expectorants

7️⃣ T48.4X1 Poisoning by expectorants, accidental (unintentional) POA

Poisoning by expectorants NOS

7️⃣ T48.4X2 Poisoning by expectorants, intentional self-harm POA HCC

7️⃣ T48.4X3 Poisoning by expectorants, assault POA

7️⃣ T48.4X4 Poisoning by expectorants, undetermined POA

7️⃣ T48.4X5 Adverse effect of expectorants POA PDxIn

7️⃣ T48.4X6 Underdosing of expectorants POA PDxIn

Unspecified Code   Other Specified Code   Manifestation Code   N Newborn   P Pediatric   M Maternity   A Adult   ♂ Male   ♀ Female
● New Code   ▲ Revised Code Title   ▶◀ Revised Text   NOTES   INCLUDES   EXCLUDES1 Not coded here   EXCLUDES2 Not included here
4️⃣ 4th character required   5️⃣ 5th character required   6️⃣ 6th character required   7️⃣ 7th character required   Extension 'X' Alert
HAC Hospital-acquired condition (HAC) alert   AHA AHA Coding Clinic©   📭 Code first alert

T48.5 - T49.2X

CHAPTER 19: INJURY, POISONING, AND CERTAIN OTHER CONSEQUENCES OF EXTERNAL CAUSES (S00-T88)

T48.5 Poisoning by, adverse effect of and underdosing of other anti-common-cold drugs

Poisoning by, adverse effect of and underdosing of decongestants

EXCLUDES2 *poisoning by, adverse effect of and underdosing of antipyretics, NEC (T39.9-)*

poisoning by, adverse effect of and underdosing of non-steroidal antiinflammatory drugs (T39.3-)

poisoning by, adverse effect of and underdosing of salicylates (T39.0-)

T48.5X Poisoning by, adverse effect of and underdosing of other anti-common-cold drugs

T48.5X1 Poisoning by other anti-common-cold drugs, accidental (unintentional)

Poisoning by other anti-common-cold drugs NOS

T48.5X2 Poisoning by other anti-common-cold drugs, intentional self-harm

T48.5X3 Poisoning by other anti-common-cold drugs, assault

T48.5X4 Poisoning by other anti-common-cold drugs, undetermined

T48.5X5 Adverse effect of other anti-common-cold drugs

T48.5X6 Underdosing of other anti-common-cold drugs

T48.6 Poisoning by, adverse effect of and underdosing of antiasthmatics, not elsewhere classified

Poisoning by, adverse effect of and underdosing of beta-adrenoreceptor agonists used in asthma therapy

EXCLUDES1 *poisoning by, adverse effect of and underdosing of beta-adrenoreceptor agonists not used in asthma therapy (T44.5)*

poisoning by, adverse effect of and underdosing of anterior pituitary [adenohypophyseal] hormones (T38.8)

T48.6X Poisoning by, adverse effect of and underdosing of antiasthmatics

T48.6X1 Poisoning by antiasthmatics, accidental (unintentional)

Poisoning by antiasthmatics NOS

T48.6X2 Poisoning by antiasthmatics, intentional self-harm

T48.6X3 Poisoning by antiasthmatics, assault

T48.6X4 Poisoning by antiasthmatics, undetermined

T48.6X5 Adverse effect of antiasthmatics

T48.6X6 Underdosing of antiasthmatics

T48.9 Poisoning by, adverse effect of and underdosing of other and unspecified agents primarily acting on the respiratory system

T48.90 Poisoning by, adverse effect of and underdosing of unspecified agents primarily acting on the respiratory system

T48.901 Poisoning by unspecified agents primarily acting on the respiratory system, accidental (unintentional)

T48.902 Poisoning by unspecified agents primarily acting on the respiratory system, intentional self-harm

T48.903 Poisoning by unspecified agents primarily acting on the respiratory system, assault

T48.904 Poisoning by unspecified agents primarily acting on the respiratory system, undetermined

T48.905 Adverse effect of unspecified agents primarily acting on the respiratory system

T48.906 Underdosing of unspecified agents primarily acting on the respiratory system

T48.99 Poisoning by, adverse effect of and underdosing of other agents primarily acting on the respiratory system

T48.991 Poisoning by other agents primarily acting on the respiratory system, accidental (unintentional)

T48.992 Poisoning by other agents primarily acting on the respiratory system, intentional self-harm

T48.993 Poisoning by other agents primarily acting on the respiratory system, assault

T48.994 Poisoning by other agents primarily acting on the respiratory system, undetermined

T48.995 Adverse effect of other agents primarily acting on the respiratory system

T48.996 Underdosing of other agents primarily acting on the respiratory system

T49 Poisoning by, adverse effect of and underdosing of topical agents primarily affecting skin and mucous membrane and by ophthalmological, otorhinolaryngological and dental drugs

INCLUDES *poisoning by, adverse effect of and underdosing of glucocorticoids, topically used*

The appropriate 7th character is to be added to each code from category T49

A = initial encounter

D = subsequent encounter

S = sequela

T49.0 Poisoning by, adverse effect of and underdosing of local antifungal, anti-infective and anti-inflammatory drugs

T49.0X Poisoning by, adverse effect of and underdosing of local antifungal, anti-infective and anti-inflammatory drugs

T49.0X1 Poisoning by local antifungal, anti-infective and anti-inflammatory drugs, accidental (unintentional)

Poisoning by local antifungal, anti-infective and anti-inflammatory drugs NOS

T49.0X2 Poisoning by local antifungal, anti-infective and anti-inflammatory drugs, intentional self-harm

T49.0X3 Poisoning by local antifungal, anti-infective and anti-inflammatory drugs, assault

T49.0X4 Poisoning by local antifungal, anti-infective and anti-inflammatory drugs, undetermined

T49.0X5 Adverse effect of local antifungal, anti-infective and anti-inflammatory drugs

T49.0X6 Underdosing of local antifungal, anti-infective and anti-inflammatory drugs

T49.1 Poisoning by, adverse effect of and underdosing of antipruritics

T49.1X Poisoning by, adverse effect of and underdosing of antipruritics

T49.1X1 Poisoning by antipruritics, accidental (unintentional)

Poisoning by antipruritics NOS

T49.1X2 Poisoning by antipruritics, intentional self-harm

T49.1X3 Poisoning by antipruritics, assault

T49.1X4 Poisoning by antipruritics, undetermined

T49.1X5 Adverse effect of antipruritics

T49.1X6 Underdosing of antipruritics

T49.2 Poisoning by, adverse effect of and underdosing of local astringents and local detergents

T49.2X Poisoning by, adverse effect of and underdosing of local astringents and local detergents

---

PDxIn Unacceptable principal diagnosis symbol per Medicare code edits   Code exempt from diagnosis present on admission requirement
? Questionable admission   Complication or comorbidity   MCC Major complication or comorbidity   CC/MCC exclusion
HCC HCC diagnosis code   RxHCC RxHCC diagnosis code   MACRA code   **DEFINITION** Describes condition/terminology
TIP Coding guidance   Official Guideline Reference   Z1 Z code as first-listed diagnosis

7️⃣ T49.2X1 Poisoning by local astringents and local detergents, accidental (unintentional) POA

Poisoning by local astringents and local detergents NOS

7️⃣ T49.2X2 Poisoning by local astringents and local detergents, intentional self-harm POA HCC

7️⃣ T49.2X3 Poisoning by local astringents and local detergents, assault POA

7️⃣ T49.2X4 Poisoning by local astringents and local detergents, undetermined POA

7️⃣ T49.2X5 Adverse effect of local astringents and local detergents POA PDxIn

7️⃣ T49.2X6 Underdosing of local astringents and local detergents POA PDxIn

5️⃣ T49.3 Poisoning by, adverse effect of and underdosing of emollients, demulcents and protectants

6️⃣ T49.3X Poisoning by, adverse effect of and underdosing of emollients, demulcents and protectants

7️⃣ T49.3X1 Poisoning by emollients, demulcents and protectants, accidental (unintentional) POA

Poisoning by emollients, demulcents and protectants NOS

7️⃣ T49.3X2 Poisoning by emollients, demulcents and protectants, intentional self-harm POA HCC

7️⃣ T49.3X3 Poisoning by emollients, demulcents and protectants, assault POA

7️⃣ T49.3X4 Poisoning by emollients, demulcents and protectants, undetermined POA

7️⃣ T49.3X5 Adverse effect of emollients, demulcents and protectants POA PDxIn

7️⃣ T49.3X6 Underdosing of emollients, demulcents and protectants POA PDxIn

5️⃣ T49.4 Poisoning by, adverse effect of and underdosing of keratolytics, keratoplastics, and other hair treatment drugs and preparations

6️⃣ T49.4X Poisoning by, adverse effect of and underdosing of keratolytics, keratoplastics, and other hair treatment drugs and preparations

7️⃣ T49.4X1 Poisoning by keratolytics, keratoplastics, and other hair treatment drugs and preparations, accidental (unintentional) POA

Poisoning by keratolytics, keratoplastics, and other hair treatment drugs and preparations NOS

7️⃣ T49.4X2 Poisoning by keratolytics, keratoplastics, and other hair treatment drugs and preparations, intentional self-harm POA HCC

7️⃣ T49.4X3 Poisoning by keratolytics, keratoplastics, and other hair treatment drugs and preparations, assault POA

7️⃣ T49.4X4 Poisoning by keratolytics, keratoplastics, and other hair treatment drugs and preparations, undetermined POA

7️⃣ T49.4X5 Adverse effect of keratolytics, keratoplastics, and other hair treatment drugs and preparations POA PDxIn

7️⃣ T49.4X6 Underdosing of keratolytics, keratoplastics, and other hair treatment drugs and preparations POA PDxIn

5️⃣ T49.5 Poisoning by, adverse effect of and underdosing of ophthalmological drugs and preparations

6️⃣ T49.5X Poisoning by, adverse effect of and underdosing of ophthalmological drugs and preparations

7️⃣ T49.5X1 Poisoning by ophthalmological drugs and preparations, accidental (unintentional) POA

Poisoning by ophthalmological drugs and preparations NOS

7️⃣ T49.5X2 Poisoning by ophthalmological drugs and preparations, intentional self-harm POA HCC

7️⃣ T49.5X3 Poisoning by ophthalmological drugs and preparations, assault POA

7️⃣ T49.5X4 Poisoning by ophthalmological drugs and preparations, undetermined POA

7️⃣ T49.5X5 Adverse effect of ophthalmological drugs and preparations POA PDxIn

7️⃣ T49.5X6 Underdosing of ophthalmological drugs and preparations POA PDxIn

5️⃣ T49.6 Poisoning by, adverse effect of and underdosing of otorhinolaryngological drugs and preparations

6️⃣ T49.6X Poisoning by, adverse effect of and underdosing of otorhinolaryngological drugs and preparations

7️⃣ T49.6X1 Poisoning by otorhinolaryngological drugs and preparations, accidental (unintentional) POA

Poisoning by otorhinolaryngological drugs and preparations NOS

7️⃣ T49.6X2 Poisoning by otorhinolaryngological drugs and preparations, intentional self-harm POA HCC

7️⃣ T49.6X3 Poisoning by otorhinolaryngological drugs and preparations, assault POA

7️⃣ T49.6X4 Poisoning by otorhinolaryngological drugs and preparations, undetermined POA

7️⃣ T49.6X5 Adverse effect of otorhinolaryngological drugs and preparations POA PDxIn

7️⃣ T49.6X6 Underdosing of otorhinolaryngological drugs and preparations POA PDxIn

5️⃣ T49.7 Poisoning by, adverse effect of and underdosing of dental drugs, topically applied

6️⃣ T49.7X Poisoning by, adverse effect of and underdosing of dental drugs, topically applied

7️⃣ T49.7X1 Poisoning by dental drugs, topically applied, accidental (unintentional) POA

Poisoning by dental drugs, topically applied NOS

7️⃣ T49.7X2 Poisoning by dental drugs, topically applied, intentional self-harm POA HCC

7️⃣ T49.7X3 Poisoning by dental drugs, topically applied, assault POA

7️⃣ T49.7X4 Poisoning by dental drugs, topically applied, undetermined POA

7️⃣ T49.7X5 Adverse effect of dental drugs, topically applied POA PDxIn

7️⃣ T49.7X6 Underdosing of dental drugs, topically applied POA PDxIn

5️⃣ T49.8 Poisoning by, adverse effect of and underdosing of other topical agents

Poisoning by, adverse effect of and underdosing of spermicides

6️⃣ T49.8X Poisoning by, adverse effect of and underdosing of other topical agents

7️⃣ T49.8X1 Poisoning by other topical agents, accidental (unintentional) POA

Poisoning by other topical agents NOS

7️⃣ T49.8X2 Poisoning by other topical agents, intentional self-harm POA HCC

7️⃣ T49.8X3 Poisoning by other topical agents, assault POA

7️⃣ T49.8X4 Poisoning by other topical agents, undetermined POA

7️⃣ T49.8X5 Adverse effect of other topical agents POA PDxIn

7️⃣ T49.8X6 Underdosing of other topical agents POA PDxIn

5️⃣ T49.9 Poisoning by, adverse effect of and underdosing of unspecified topical agent

7️⃣ T49.91 Poisoning by unspecified topical agent, accidental (unintentional) POA

7️⃣ T49.92 Poisoning by unspecified topical agent, intentional self-harm POA HCC

7️⃣ T49.93 Poisoning by unspecified topical agent, assault POA

7️⃣ T49.94 Poisoning by unspecified topical agent, undetermined POA

7️⃣ T49.95 Adverse effect of unspecified topical agent POA PDxIn

7️⃣ T49.96 Underdosing of unspecified topical agent POA PDxIn

---

Unspecified Code   Other Specified Code   Manifestation Code   N Newborn   P Pediatric   M Maternity   A Adult   ♂ Male   ♀ Female
● New Code   ▲ Revised Code Title   ▶◀ Revised Text   NOTES   INCLUDES   EXCLUDES1 Not coded here   EXCLUDES2 Not included here
4️⃣ 4th character required   5️⃣ 5th character required   6️⃣ 6th character required   7️⃣ 7th character required   Ⓧ Extension 'X' Alert
HAC Hospital-acquired condition (HAC) alert   AHA AHA Coding Clinic®   📕 Code first alert

T50 - T50.6X4

CHAPTER 19: INJURY, POISONING, AND CERTAIN OTHER CONSEQUENCES OF EXTERNAL CAUSES (S00-T88)

4ᵗʰ **T50** Poisoning by, adverse effect of and underdosing of diuretics and other and unspecified drugs, medicaments and biological substances

The appropriate 7th character is to be added to each code from category T50

  A = initial encounter
  D = subsequent encounter
  S = sequela

5ᵗʰ **T50.0** Poisoning by, adverse effect of and underdosing of mineralocorticoids and their antagonists

  6ᵗʰ **T50.0X** Poisoning by, adverse effect of and underdosing of mineralocorticoids and their antagonists

    7ᵗʰ **T50.0X1** Poisoning by mineralocorticoids and their antagonists, accidental (unintentional) POA

      Poisoning by mineralocorticoids and their antagonists NOS

    7ᵗʰ **T50.0X2** Poisoning by mineralocorticoids and their antagonists, intentional self-harm POA HCC

    7ᵗʰ **T50.0X3** Poisoning by mineralocorticoids and their antagonists, assault POA

    7ᵗʰ **T50.0X4** Poisoning by mineralocorticoids and their antagonists, undetermined POA

    7ᵗʰ **T50.0X5** Adverse effect of mineralocorticoids and their antagonists POA PDxIn

    7ᵗʰ **T50.0X6** Underdosing of mineralocorticoids and their antagonists POA PDxIn

5ᵗʰ **T50.1** Poisoning by, adverse effect of and underdosing of loop [high-ceiling] diuretics

  6ᵗʰ **T50.1X** Poisoning by, adverse effect of and underdosing of loop [high-ceiling] diuretics

    7ᵗʰ **T50.1X1** Poisoning by loop [high-ceiling] diuretics, accidental (unintentional) POA

      Poisoning by loop [high-ceiling] diuretics NOS

    7ᵗʰ **T50.1X2** Poisoning by loop [high-ceiling] diuretics, intentional self-harm POA HCC

    7ᵗʰ **T50.1X3** Poisoning by loop [high-ceiling] diuretics, assault POA

    7ᵗʰ **T50.1X4** Poisoning by loop [high-ceiling] diuretics, undetermined POA

    7ᵗʰ **T50.1X5** Adverse effect of loop [high-ceiling] diuretics POA PDxIn

    7ᵗʰ **T50.1X6** Underdosing of loop [high-ceiling] diuretics POA PDxIn

5ᵗʰ **T50.2** Poisoning by, adverse effect of and underdosing of carbonic-anhydrase inhibitors, benzothiadiazides and other diuretics

  Poisoning by, adverse effect of and underdosing of acetazolamide

  6ᵗʰ **T50.2X** Poisoning by, adverse effect of and underdosing of carbonic-anhydrase inhibitors, benzothiadiazides and other diuretics

    7ᵗʰ **T50.2X1** Poisoning by carbonic-anhydrase inhibitors, benzothiadiazides and other diuretics, accidental (unintentional) POA

      Poisoning by carbonic-anhydrase inhibitors, benzothiadiazides and other diuretics NOS

    7ᵗʰ **T50.2X2** Poisoning by carbonic-anhydrase inhibitors, benzothiadiazides and other diuretics, intentional self-harm POA HCC

    7ᵗʰ **T50.2X3** Poisoning by carbonic-anhydrase inhibitors, benzothiadiazides and other diuretics, assault POA

    7ᵗʰ **T50.2X4** Poisoning by carbonic-anhydrase inhibitors, benzothiadiazides and other diuretics, undetermined POA

    7ᵗʰ **T50.2X5** Adverse effect of carbonic-anhydrase inhibitors, benzothiadiazides and other diuretics POA PDxIn

    7ᵗʰ **T50.2X6** Underdosing of carbonic-anhydrase inhibitors, benzothiadiazides and other diuretics POA PDxIn

5ᵗʰ **T50.3** Poisoning by, adverse effect of and underdosing of electrolytic, caloric and water-balance agents

  Poisoning by, adverse effect of and underdosing of oral rehydration salts

  6ᵗʰ **T50.3X** Poisoning by, adverse effect of and underdosing of electrolytic, caloric and water-balance agents

    7ᵗʰ **T50.3X1** Poisoning by electrolytic, caloric and water-balance agents, accidental (unintentional) POA

      Poisoning by electrolytic, caloric and water-balance agents NOS

    7ᵗʰ **T50.3X2** Poisoning by electrolytic, caloric and water-balance agents, intentional self-harm POA HCC

    7ᵗʰ **T50.3X3** Poisoning by electrolytic, caloric and water-balance agents, assault POA

    7ᵗʰ **T50.3X4** Poisoning by electrolytic, caloric and water-balance agents, undetermined POA

    7ᵗʰ **T50.3X5** Adverse effect of electrolytic, caloric and water-balance agents POA PDxIn

    7ᵗʰ **T50.3X6** Underdosing of electrolytic, caloric and water-balance agents POA PDxIn

5ᵗʰ **T50.4** Poisoning by, adverse effect of and underdosing of drugs affecting uric acid metabolism

  6ᵗʰ **T50.4X** Poisoning by, adverse effect of and underdosing of drugs affecting uric acid metabolism

    7ᵗʰ **T50.4X1** Poisoning by drugs affecting uric acid metabolism, accidental (unintentional) POA

      Poisoning by drugs affecting uric acid metabolism NOS

    7ᵗʰ **T50.4X2** Poisoning by drugs affecting uric acid metabolism, intentional self-harm POA HCC

    7ᵗʰ **T50.4X3** Poisoning by drugs affecting uric acid metabolism, assault POA

    7ᵗʰ **T50.4X4** Poisoning by drugs affecting uric acid metabolism, undetermined POA

    7ᵗʰ **T50.4X5** Adverse effect of drugs affecting uric acid metabolism POA PDxIn

    7ᵗʰ **T50.4X6** Underdosing of drugs affecting uric acid metabolism POA PDxIn

5ᵗʰ **T50.5** Poisoning by, adverse effect of and underdosing of appetite depressants

  6ᵗʰ **T50.5X** Poisoning by, adverse effect of and underdosing of appetite depressants

    7ᵗʰ **T50.5X1** Poisoning by appetite depressants, accidental (unintentional) POA

      Poisoning by appetite depressants NOS

    7ᵗʰ **T50.5X2** Poisoning by appetite depressants, intentional self-harm POA HCC

    7ᵗʰ **T50.5X3** Poisoning by appetite depressants, assault POA

    7ᵗʰ **T50.5X4** Poisoning by appetite depressants, undetermined POA

    7ᵗʰ **T50.5X5** Adverse effect of appetite depressants POA PDxIn

    7ᵗʰ **T50.5X6** Underdosing of appetite depressants POA PDxIn

5ᵗʰ **T50.6** Poisoning by, adverse effect of and underdosing of antidotes and chelating agents

  Poisoning by, adverse effect of and underdosing of alcohol deterrents

  6ᵗʰ **T50.6X** Poisoning by, adverse effect of and underdosing of antidotes and chelating agents

    7ᵗʰ **T50.6X1** Poisoning by antidotes and chelating agents, accidental (unintentional) POA

      Poisoning by antidotes and chelating agents NOS

    7ᵗʰ **T50.6X2** Poisoning by antidotes and chelating agents, intentional self-harm POA HCC

    7ᵗʰ **T50.6X3** Poisoning by antidotes and chelating agents, assault POA

    7ᵗʰ **T50.6X4** Poisoning by antidotes and chelating agents, undetermined POA

PDxIn Unacceptable principal diagnosis symbol per Medicare code edits   POA Code exempt from diagnosis present on admission requirement
? Questionable admission   cc Complication or comorbidity   mcc Major complication or comorbidity   cc/mcc exc CC/MCC exclusion
HCC HCC diagnosis code   RxHCC RxHCC diagnosis code   MACRA code   **DEFINITION** Describes condition/terminology
TIP Coding guidance   👁 Official Guideline Reference   Z1 Z code as first-listed diagnosis

T50.6X5 Adverse effect of antidotes and chelating agents ⊘POA

T50.6X6 Underdosing of antidotes and chelating agents ⊘POA PDxⓈ

5ᵗʰ T50.7 Poisoning by, adverse effect of and underdosing of analeptics and opioid receptor antagonists

6ᵗʰ T50.7X Poisoning by, adverse effect of and underdosing of analeptics and opioid receptor antagonists

7ᵗʰ T50.7X1 Poisoning by analeptics and opioid receptor antagonists, accidental (unintentional) ⊘POA

Poisoning by analeptics and opioid receptor antagonists NOS

7ᵗʰ T50.7X2 Poisoning by analeptics and opioid receptor antagonists, intentional self-harm ⊘POA HCC

7ᵗʰ T50.7X3 Poisoning by analeptics and opioid receptor antagonists, assault ⊘POA

7ᵗʰ T50.7X4 Poisoning by analeptics and opioid receptor antagonists, undetermined ⊘POA

7ᵗʰ T50.7X5 Adverse effect of analeptics and opioid receptor antagonists ⊘POA PDxⓈ

7ᵗʰ T50.7X6 Underdosing of analeptics and opioid receptor antagonists ⊘POA PDxⓈ

5ᵗʰ T50.8 Poisoning by, adverse effect of and underdosing of diagnostic agents

6ᵗʰ T50.8X Poisoning by, adverse effect of and underdosing of diagnostic agents

7ᵗʰ T50.8X1 Poisoning by diagnostic agents, accidental (unintentional) ⊘POA

Poisoning by diagnostic agents NOS

7ᵗʰ T50.8X2 Poisoning by diagnostic agents, intentional self-harm ⊘POA HCC

7ᵗʰ T50.8X3 Poisoning by diagnostic agents, assault ⊘POA

7ᵗʰ T50.8X4 Poisoning by diagnostic agents, undetermined ⊘POA

7ᵗʰ T50.8X5 Adverse effect of diagnostic agents ⊘POA PDxⓈ

7ᵗʰ T50.8X6 Underdosing of diagnostic agents ⊘POA PDxⓈ

5ᵗʰ T50.A Poisoning by, adverse effect of and underdosing of bacterial vaccines

6ᵗʰ T50.A1 Poisoning by, adverse effect of and underdosing of pertussis vaccine, including combinations with a pertussis component

7ᵗʰ T50.A11 Poisoning by pertussis vaccine, including combinations with a pertussis component, accidental (unintentional) ⊘POA

7ᵗʰ T50.A12 Poisoning by pertussis vaccine, including combinations with a pertussis component, intentional self-harm ⊘POA HCC

7ᵗʰ T50.A13 Poisoning by pertussis vaccine, including combinations with a pertussis component, assault ⊘POA

7ᵗʰ T50.A14 Poisoning by pertussis vaccine, including combinations with a pertussis component, undetermined ⊘POA

7ᵗʰ T50.A15 Adverse effect of pertussis vaccine, including combinations with a pertussis component ⊘POA PDxⓈ

7ᵗʰ T50.A16 Underdosing of pertussis vaccine, including combinations with a pertussis component ⊘POA PDxⓈ

6ᵗʰ T50.A2 Poisoning by, adverse effect of and underdosing of mixed bacterial vaccines without a pertussis component

7ᵗʰ T50.A21 Poisoning by mixed bacterial vaccines without a pertussis component, accidental (unintentional) ⊘POA

7ᵗʰ T50.A22 Poisoning by mixed bacterial vaccines without a pertussis component, intentional self-harm ⊘POA HCC

7ᵗʰ T50.A23 Poisoning by mixed bacterial vaccines without a pertussis component, assault ⊘POA

7ᵗʰ T50.A24 Poisoning by mixed bacterial vaccines without a pertussis component, undetermined ⊘POA

7ᵗʰ T50.A25 Adverse effect of mixed bacterial vaccines without a pertussis component ⊘POA PDxⓈ

7ᵗʰ T50.A26 Underdosing of mixed bacterial vaccines without a pertussis component ⊘POA PDxⓈ

6ᵗʰ T50.A9 Poisoning by, adverse effect of and underdosing of other bacterial vaccines

7ᵗʰ T50.A91 Poisoning by other bacterial vaccines, accidental (unintentional) ⊘POA

7ᵗʰ T50.A92 Poisoning by other bacterial vaccines, intentional self-harm ⊘POA HCC

7ᵗʰ T50.A93 Poisoning by other bacterial vaccines, assault ⊘POA

7ᵗʰ T50.A94 Poisoning by other bacterial vaccines, undetermined ⊘POA

7ᵗʰ T50.A95 Adverse effect of other bacterial vaccines ⊘POA PDxⓈ

7ᵗʰ T50.A96 Underdosing of other bacterial vaccines ⊘POA PDxⓈ

5ᵗʰ T50.B Poisoning by, adverse effect of and underdosing of viral vaccines

6ᵗʰ T50.B1 Poisoning by, adverse effect of and underdosing of smallpox vaccines

7ᵗʰ T50.B11 Poisoning by smallpox vaccines, accidental (unintentional) ⊘POA

7ᵗʰ T50.B12 Poisoning by smallpox vaccines, intentional self-harm ⊘POA HCC

7ᵗʰ T50.B13 Poisoning by smallpox vaccines, assault ⊘POA

7ᵗʰ T50.B14 Poisoning by smallpox vaccines, undetermined ⊘POA

7ᵗʰ T50.B15 Adverse effect of smallpox vaccines ⊘POA PDxⓈ

7ᵗʰ T50.B16 Underdosing of smallpox vaccines ⊘POA PDxⓈ

6ᵗʰ T50.B9 Poisoning by, adverse effect of and underdosing of other viral vaccines

7ᵗʰ T50.B91 Poisoning by other viral vaccines, accidental (unintentional) ⊘POA

7ᵗʰ T50.B92 Poisoning by other viral vaccines, intentional self-harm ⊘POA HCC

7ᵗʰ T50.B93 Poisoning by other viral vaccines, assault ⊘POA

7ᵗʰ T50.B94 Poisoning by other viral vaccines, undetermined ⊘POA

7ᵗʰ T50.B95 Adverse effect of other viral vaccines ⊘POA PDxⓈ

7ᵗʰ T50.B96 Underdosing of other viral vaccines ⊘POA PDxⓈ

5ᵗʰ T50.Z Poisoning by, adverse effect of and underdosing of other vaccines and biological substances

6ᵗʰ T50.Z1 Poisoning by, adverse effect of and underdosing of immunoglobulin

7ᵗʰ T50.Z11 Poisoning by immunoglobulin, accidental (unintentional) ⊘POA

7ᵗʰ T50.Z12 Poisoning by immunoglobulin, intentional self-harm ⊘POA HCC

7ᵗʰ T50.Z13 Poisoning by immunoglobulin, assault ⊘POA

7ᵗʰ T50.Z14 Poisoning by immunoglobulin, undetermined ⊘POA

7ᵗʰ T50.Z15 Adverse effect of immunoglobulin ⊘POA PDxⓈ

7ᵗʰ T50.Z16 Underdosing of immunoglobulin ⊘POA PDxⓈ

6ᵗʰ T50.Z9 Poisoning by, adverse effect of and underdosing of other vaccines and biological substances

7ᵗʰ T50.Z91 Poisoning by other vaccines and biological substances, accidental (unintentional) ⊘POA

7ᵗʰ T50.Z92 Poisoning by other vaccines and biological substances, intentional self-harm ⊘POA HCC

7ᵗʰ T50.Z93 Poisoning by other vaccines and biological substances, assault ⊘POA

7ᵗʰ T50.Z94 Poisoning by other vaccines and biological substances, undetermined ⊘POA

7ᵗʰ T50.Z95 Adverse effect of other vaccines and biological substances ⊘POA PDxⓈ

Unspecified Code   Other Specified Code   Manifestation Code   Ⓝ Newborn   Ⓟ Pediatric   Ⓜ Maternity   Ⓐ Adult   ♂ Male   ♀ Female
● New Code   ▲ Revised Code Title   ▶◀ Revised Text   NOTES   INCLUDES   EXCLUDES1 Not coded here   EXCLUDES2 Not included here
4ᵗʰ character required   5ᵗʰ character required   6ᵗʰ character required   7ᵗʰ character required   Extension 'X' Alert
HAC Hospital-acquired condition (HAC) alert   AHA AHA Coding Clinic©   ☛ Code first alert

T50.Z96   Underdosing of other vaccines and biological substances   POA PDxIn

5ᵗʰ T50.9   Poisoning by, adverse effect of and underdosing of other and unspecified drugs, medicaments and biological substances

6ᵗʰ T50.90   Poisoning by, adverse effect of and underdosing of unspecified drugs, medicaments and biological substances

7ᵗʰ T50.901   Poisoning by unspecified drugs, medicaments and biological substances, accidental (unintentional)   POA

AHA: Q1 2015

7ᵗʰ T50.902   Poisoning by unspecified drugs, medicaments and biological substances, intentional self-harm   POA HCC

7ᵗʰ T50.903   Poisoning by unspecified drugs, medicaments and biological substances, assault   POA

7ᵗʰ T50.904   Poisoning by unspecified drugs, medicaments and biological substances, undetermined   POA

7ᵗʰ T50.905   Adverse effect of unspecified drugs, medicaments and biological substances   POA

7ᵗʰ T50.906   Underdosing of unspecified drugs, medicaments and biological substances   POA

● 6ᵗʰ T50.91   Poisoning by, adverse effect of and underdosing of multiple unspecified drugs, medicaments and biological substances

Multiple drug ingestion NOS

Code also any specific drugs, medicaments and biological substances

● 7ᵗʰ T50.911   Poisoning by multiple unspecified drugs, medicaments and biological substances, accidental (unintentional)

● 7ᵗʰ T50.912   Poisoning by multiple unspecified drugs, medicaments and biological substances, intentional self-harm

● 7ᵗʰ T50.913   Poisoning by multiple unspecified drugs, medicaments and biological substances, assault

● 7ᵗʰ T50.914   Poisoning by multiple unspecified drugs, medicaments and biological substances, undetermined

● 7ᵗʰ T50.915   Adverse effect of multiple unspecified drugs, medicaments and biological substances

● 7ᵗʰ T50.916   Underdosing of multiple unspecified drugs, medicaments and biological substances

6ᵗʰ T50.99   Poisoning by, adverse effect of and underdosing of other drugs, medicaments and biological substances

7ᵗʰ T50.991   Poisoning by other drugs, medicaments and biological substances, accidental (unintentional)   POA

7ᵗʰ T50.992   Poisoning by other drugs, medicaments and biological substances, intentional self-harm   POA HCC

7ᵗʰ T50.993   Poisoning by other drugs, medicaments and biological substances, assault   POA

7ᵗʰ T50.994   Poisoning by other drugs, medicaments and biological substances, undetermined   POA

7ᵗʰ T50.995   Adverse effect of other drugs, medicaments and biological substances   POA

7ᵗʰ T50.996   Underdosing of other drugs, medicaments and biological substances   POA

Toxic effects of substances chiefly nonmedicinal as to source (T51-T65)

👁 **See Official Guidelines** "Adverse Effects, Poisoning, Underdosing and Toxic Effects" I.C.19.e

NOTES   When no intent is indicated code to accidental. Undetermined intent is only for use when there is specific documentation in the record that the intent of the toxic effect cannot be determined.

Use additional code(s):

for all associated manifestations of toxic effect, such as: respiratory conditions due to external agents (J60-J70)

personal history of foreign body fully removed (Z87.821)

to identify any retained foreign body, if applicable (Z18.-)

EXCLUDES1 contact with and (suspected) exposure to toxic substances (Z77.-)

4ᵗʰ T51   **Toxic effect of** alcohol

The appropriate 7th character is to be added to each code from category T51

A = initial encounter

D = subsequent encounter

S = sequela

5ᵗʰ T51.0   **Toxic effect of ethanol**

Toxic effect of ethyl alcohol

EXCLUDES2 acute alcohol intoxication or 'hangover' effects (F10.129, F10.229, F10.929)

drunkenness (F10.129, F10.229, F10.929)

pathological alcohol intoxication (F10.129, F10.229, F10.929)

6ᵗʰ T51.0X   **Toxic effect of** ethanol

7ᵗʰ T51.0X1   **Toxic effect of ethanol,** accidental (unintentional)   POA HCC

Toxic effect of ethanol NOS

7ᵗʰ T51.0X2   **Toxic effect of ethanol,** intentional self-harm   POA HCC

7ᵗʰ T51.0X3   **Toxic effect of ethanol,** assault   POA

7ᵗʰ T51.0X4   **Toxic effect of ethanol,** undetermined   POA HCC

5ᵗʰ T51.1   **Toxic effect of methanol**

Toxic effect of methyl alcohol

6ᵗʰ T51.1X   **Toxic effect of** methanol

7ᵗʰ T51.1X1   **Toxic effect of methanol,** accidental (unintentional)   POA

Toxic effect of methanol NOS

7ᵗʰ T51.1X2   **Toxic effect of methanol,** intentional self-harm   POA HCC

7ᵗʰ T51.1X3   **Toxic effect of methanol,** assault   POA

7ᵗʰ T51.1X4   **Toxic effect of methanol,** undetermined   POA

5ᵗʰ T51.2   **Toxic effect of 2-Propanol**

Toxic effect of isopropyl alcohol

6ᵗʰ T51.2X   **Toxic effect of** 2-Propanol

7ᵗʰ T51.2X1   **Toxic effect of 2-Propanol,** accidental (unintentional)   POA

Toxic effect of 2-Propanol NOS

7ᵗʰ T51.2X2   **Toxic effect of 2-Propanol,** intentional self-harm   POA HCC

7ᵗʰ T51.2X3   **Toxic effect of 2-Propanol,** assault   POA

7ᵗʰ T51.2X4   **Toxic effect of 2-Propanol,** undetermined   POA

5ᵗʰ T51.3   **Toxic effect of fusel oil**

Toxic effect of amyl alcohol

Toxic effect of butyl [1-butanol] alcohol

Toxic effect of propyl [1-propanol] alcohol

6ᵗʰ T51.3X   **Toxic effect of** fusel oil

7ᵗʰ T51.3X1   **Toxic effect of fusel oil,** accidental (unintentional)   POA

Toxic effect of fusel oil NOS

7ᵗʰ T51.3X2   **Toxic effect of fusel oil,** intentional self-harm   POA HCC

7ᵗʰ T51.3X3   **Toxic effect of fusel oil,** assault   POA

7ᵗʰ T51.3X4   **Toxic effect of fusel oil,** undetermined   POA

5ᵗʰ T51.8   **Toxic effect of other alcohols**

6ᵗʰ T51.8X   **Toxic effect of** other alcohols

POA ❓ Unacceptable principal diagnosis symbol per Medicare code edits   POA Code exempt from diagnosis present on admission requirement
❓ Questionable admission   ℅ Complication or comorbidity   MCC Major complication or comorbidity   CC/MCC excl CC/MCC exclusion
HCC HCC diagnosis code   RHCC RxHCC diagnosis code   MACRA code   **DEFINITION** Describes condition/terminology
TIP Coding guidance   👁 Official Guideline Reference   Z1 Z code as first-listed diagnosis

7️⃣ **T51.8X1** Toxic effect of other alcohols, accidental (unintentional) POA
Toxic effect of other alcohols NOS

7️⃣ **T51.8X2** Toxic effect of other alcohols, intentional self-harm POA HCC

7️⃣ **T51.8X3** Toxic effect of other alcohols, assault POA

7️⃣ **T51.8X4** Toxic effect of other alcohols, undetermined POA

5️⃣ **T51.9** Toxic effect of unspecified alcohol

7️⃣ **T51.91** Toxic effect of unspecified alcohol, accidental (unintentional) POA

7️⃣ **T51.92** Toxic effect of unspecified alcohol, intentional self-harm POA HCC

7️⃣ **T51.93** Toxic effect of unspecified alcohol, assault POA

7️⃣ **T51.94** Toxic effect of unspecified alcohol, undetermined POA

4️⃣ **T52** Toxic effect of organic solvents

EXCLUDES1 halogen derivatives of aliphatic and aromatic hydrocarbons (T53.-)

The appropriate 7th character is to be added to each code from category T52
A = initial encounter
D = subsequent encounter
S = sequela

5️⃣ **T52.0** Toxic effects of petroleum products
Toxic effects of gasoline [petrol]
Toxic effects of kerosene [paraffin oil]
Toxic effects of paraffin wax
Toxic effects of ether petroleum
Toxic effects of naphtha petroleum
Toxic effects of spirit petroleum

6️⃣ **T52.0X** Toxic effects of petroleum products

7️⃣ **T52.0X1** Toxic effect of petroleum products, accidental (unintentional) POA
Toxic effects of petroleum products NOS

7️⃣ **T52.0X2** Toxic effect of petroleum products, intentional self-harm POA HCC

7️⃣ **T52.0X3** Toxic effect of petroleum products, assault POA

7️⃣ **T52.0X4** Toxic effect of petroleum products, undetermined POA

5️⃣ **T52.1** Toxic effects of benzene

EXCLUDES1 homologues of benzene (T52.2)
nitroderivatives and aminoderivatives of benzene and its homologues (T65.3)

6️⃣ **T52.1X** Toxic effects of benzene

7️⃣ **T52.1X1** Toxic effect of benzene, accidental (unintentional) POA
Toxic effects of benzene NOS

7️⃣ **T52.1X2** Toxic effect of benzene, intentional self-harm POA HCC

7️⃣ **T52.1X3** Toxic effect of benzene, assault POA

7️⃣ **T52.1X4** Toxic effect of benzene, undetermined POA

5️⃣ **T52.2** Toxic effects of homologues of benzene
Toxic effects of toluene [methylbenzene]
Toxic effects of xylene [dimethylbenzene]

6️⃣ **T52.2X** Toxic effects of homologues of benzene

7️⃣ **T52.2X1** Toxic effect of homologues of benzene, accidental (unintentional) POA
Toxic effects of homologues of benzene NOS

7️⃣ **T52.2X2** Toxic effect of homologues of benzene, intentional self-harm POA HCC

7️⃣ **T52.2X3** Toxic effect of homologues of benzene, assault POA

7️⃣ **T52.2X4** Toxic effect of homologues of benzene, undetermined POA

5️⃣ **T52.3** Toxic effects of glycols

6️⃣ **T52.3X** Toxic effects of glycols

7️⃣ **T52.3X1** Toxic effect of glycols, accidental (unintentional) POA
Toxic effects of glycols NOS

7️⃣ **T52.3X2** Toxic effect of glycols, intentional self-harm POA HCC

7️⃣ **T52.3X3** Toxic effect of glycols, assault POA

7️⃣ **T52.3X4** Toxic effect of glycols, undetermined POA

5️⃣ **T52.4** Toxic effects of ketones

6️⃣ **T52.4X** Toxic effects of ketones

7️⃣ **T52.4X1** Toxic effects of ketones, accidental (unintentional) POA
Toxic effects of ketones NOS

7️⃣ **T52.4X2** Toxic effects of ketones, intentional self-harm POA HCC

7️⃣ **T52.4X3** Toxic effects of ketones, assault POA

7️⃣ **T52.4X4** Toxic effects of ketones, undetermined POA

5️⃣ **T52.8** Toxic effects of other organic solvents

6️⃣ **T52.8X** Toxic effects of other organic solvents

7️⃣ **T52.8X1** Toxic effects of other organic solvents, accidental (unintentional) POA
Toxic effects of other organic solvents NOS

7️⃣ **T52.8X2** Toxic effects of other organic solvents, intentional self-harm POA HCC

7️⃣ **T52.8X3** Toxic effects of other organic solvents, assault POA

7️⃣ **T52.8X4** Toxic effects of other organic solvents, undetermined POA

5️⃣ **T52.9** Toxic effects of unspecified organic solvent

7️⃣ **T52.91** Toxic effect of unspecified organic solvent, accidental (unintentional) POA

7️⃣ **T52.92** Toxic effect of unspecified organic solvent, intentional self-harm POA HCC

7️⃣ **T52.93** Toxic effect of unspecified organic solvent, assault POA

7️⃣ **T52.94** Toxic effect of unspecified organic solvent, undetermined POA

4️⃣ **T53** Toxic effect of halogen derivatives of aliphatic and aromatic hydrocarbons

The appropriate 7th character is to be added to each code from category T53
A = initial encounter
D = subsequent encounter
S = sequela

5️⃣ **T53.0** Toxic effects of carbon tetrachloride
Toxic effects of tetrachloromethane

6️⃣ **T53.0X** Toxic effects of carbon tetrachloride

7️⃣ **T53.0X1** Toxic effect of carbon tetrachloride, accidental (unintentional) POA
Toxic effects of carbon tetrachloride NOS

7️⃣ **T53.0X2** Toxic effect of carbon tetrachloride, intentional self-harm POA HCC

7️⃣ **T53.0X3** Toxic effect of carbon tetrachloride, assault POA

7️⃣ **T53.0X4** Toxic effect of carbon tetrachloride, undetermined POA

5️⃣ **T53.1** Toxic effects of chloroform
Toxic effects of trichloromethane

6️⃣ **T53.1X** Toxic effects of chloroform

7️⃣ **T53.1X1** Toxic effect of chloroform, accidental (unintentional) POA
Toxic effects of chloroform NOS

7️⃣ **T53.1X2** Toxic effect of chloroform, intentional self-harm POA HCC

7️⃣ **T53.1X3** Toxic effect of chloroform, assault POA

7️⃣ **T53.1X4** Toxic effect of chloroform, undetermined POA

5️⃣ **T53.2** Toxic effects of trichloroethylene
Toxic effects of trichloroethene

6️⃣ **T53.2X** Toxic effects of trichloroethylene

7️⃣ **T53.2X1** Toxic effect of trichloroethylene, accidental (unintentional) POA
Toxic effects of trichloroethylene NOS

7️⃣ **T53.2X2** Toxic effect of trichloroethylene, intentional self-harm POA HCC

7️⃣ **T53.2X3** Toxic effect of trichloroethylene, assault POA

Unspecified Code Other Specified Code Manifestation Code Ⓝ Newborn Ⓟ Pediatric Ⓜ Maternity Ⓐ Adult ♂ Male ♀ Female
● New Code ▲ Revised Code Title ▶◀ Revised Text NOTES INCLUDES EXCLUDES1 Not coded here EXCLUDES2 Not included here
4️⃣ 4th character required 5️⃣ 5th character required 6️⃣ 6th character required 7️⃣ 7th character required Extension 'X' Alert
HAC Hospital-acquired condition (HAC) alert AHA AHA Coding Clinic© ☞ Code first alert

[7th] T53.2X4 Toxic effect of trichloroethylene, undetermined [POA]

[5th] T53.3 Toxic effects of tetrachloroethylene
Toxic effects of perchloroethylene
Toxic effect of tetrachloroethene

[6th] T53.3X Toxic effects of tetrachloroethylene

[7th] T53.3X1 Toxic effect of tetrachloroethylene, accidental (unintentional) [POA]
Toxic effects of tetrachloroethylene NOS

[7th] T53.3X2 Toxic effect of tetrachloroethylene, intentional self-harm [POA] [HCC]

[7th] T53.3X3 Toxic effect of tetrachloroethylene, assault [POA]

[7th] T53.3X4 Toxic effect of tetrachloroethylene, undetermined [POA]

[5th] T53.4 Toxic effects of dichloromethane
Toxic effects of methylene chloride

[6th] T53.4X Toxic effects of dichloromethane

[7th] T53.4X1 Toxic effect of dichloromethane, accidental (unintentional) [POA]
Toxic effects of dichloromethane NOS

[7th] T53.4X2 Toxic effect of dichloromethane, intentional self-harm [POA] [HCC]

[7th] T53.4X3 Toxic effect of dichloromethane, assault [POA]

[7th] T53.4X4 Toxic effect of dichloromethane, undetermined [POA]

[5th] T53.5 Toxic effects of chlorofluorocarbons

[6th] T53.5X Toxic effects of chlorofluorocarbons

[7th] T53.5X1 Toxic effect of chlorofluorocarbons, accidental (unintentional) [POA]
Toxic effects of chlorofluorocarbons NOS

[7th] T53.5X2 Toxic effect of chlorofluorocarbons, intentional self-harm [POA] [HCC]

[7th] T53.5X3 Toxic effect of chlorofluorocarbons, assault [POA]

[7th] T53.5X4 Toxic effect of chlorofluorocarbons, undetermined [POA]

[5th] T53.6 Toxic effects of other halogen derivatives of aliphatic hydrocarbons

[6th] T53.6X Toxic effects of other halogen derivatives of aliphatic hydrocarbons

[7th] T53.6X1 Toxic effect of other halogen derivatives of aliphatic hydrocarbons, accidental (unintentional) [POA]
Toxic effects of other halogen derivatives of aliphatic hydrocarbons NOS

[7th] T53.6X2 Toxic effect of other halogen derivatives of aliphatic hydrocarbons, intentional self-harm [POA] [HCC]

[7th] T53.6X3 Toxic effect of other halogen derivatives of aliphatic hydrocarbons, assault [POA]

[7th] T53.6X4 Toxic effect of other halogen derivatives of aliphatic hydrocarbons, undetermined [POA]

[5th] T53.7 Toxic effects of other halogen derivatives of aromatic hydrocarbons

[6th] T53.7X Toxic effects of other halogen derivatives of aromatic hydrocarbons

[7th] T53.7X1 Toxic effect of other halogen derivatives of aromatic hydrocarbons, accidental (unintentional) [POA]
Toxic effects of other halogen derivatives of aromatic hydrocarbons NOS

[7th] T53.7X2 Toxic effect of other halogen derivatives of aromatic hydrocarbons, intentional self-harm [POA] [HCC]

[7th] T53.7X3 Toxic effect of other halogen derivatives of aromatic hydrocarbons, assault [POA]

[7th] T53.7X4 Toxic effect of other halogen derivatives of aromatic hydrocarbons, undetermined [POA]

[5th] T53.9 Toxic effects of unspecified halogen derivatives of aliphatic and aromatic hydrocarbons

[7th] T53.91 Toxic effect of unspecified halogen derivatives of aliphatic and aromatic hydrocarbons, accidental (unintentional) [POA]

[7th] T53.92 Toxic effect of unspecified halogen derivatives of aliphatic and aromatic hydrocarbons, intentional self-harm [POA] [HCC]

[7th] T53.93 Toxic effect of unspecified halogen derivatives of aliphatic and aromatic hydrocarbons, assault [POA]

[7th] T53.94 Toxic effect of unspecified halogen derivatives of aliphatic and aromatic hydrocarbons, undetermined [POA]

[4th] T54 Toxic effect of corrosive substances
The appropriate 7th character is to be added to each code from category T54
A = initial encounter
D = subsequent encounter
S = sequela

[5th] T54.0 Toxic effects of phenol and phenol homologues

[6th] T54.0X Toxic effects of phenol and phenol homologues

[7th] T54.0X1 Toxic effect of phenol and phenol homologues, accidental (unintentional) [POA]
Toxic effects of phenol and phenol homologues NOS

[7th] T54.0X2 Toxic effect of phenol and phenol homologues, intentional self-harm [POA] [HCC]

[7th] T54.0X3 Toxic effect of phenol and phenol homologues, assault [POA]

[7th] T54.0X4 Toxic effect of phenol and phenol homologues, undetermined [POA]

[5th] T54.1 Toxic effects of other corrosive organic compounds

[6th] T54.1X Toxic effects of other corrosive organic compounds

[7th] T54.1X1 Toxic effect of other corrosive organic compounds, accidental (unintentional) [POA]
Toxic effects of other corrosive organic compounds NOS

[7th] T54.1X2 Toxic effect of other corrosive organic compounds, intentional self-harm [POA] [HCC]

[7th] T54.1X3 Toxic effect of other corrosive organic compounds, assault [POA]

[7th] T54.1X4 Toxic effect of other corrosive organic compounds, undetermined [POA]

[5th] T54.2 Toxic effects of corrosive acids and acid-like substances
Toxic effects of hydrochloric acid
Toxic effects of sulfuric acid

[6th] T54.2X Toxic effects of corrosive acids and acid-like substances

[7th] T54.2X1 Toxic effect of corrosive acids and acid-like substances, accidental (unintentional) [POA]
Toxic effects of corrosive acids and acid-like substances NOS

[7th] T54.2X2 Toxic effect of corrosive acids and acid-like substances, intentional self-harm [POA] [HCC]

[7th] T54.2X3 Toxic effect of corrosive acids and acid-like substances, assault [POA]

[7th] T54.2X4 Toxic effect of corrosive acids and acid-like substances, undetermined [POA]

[5th] T54.3 Toxic effects of corrosive alkalis and alkali-like substances
Toxic effects of potassium hydroxide
Toxic effects of sodium hydroxide

[6th] T54.3X Toxic effects of corrosive alkalis and alkali-like substances

[7th] T54.3X1 Toxic effect of corrosive alkalis and alkali-like substances, accidental (unintentional) [POA]
Toxic effects of corrosive alkalis and alkali-like substances NOS

[7th] T54.3X2 Toxic effect of corrosive alkalis and alkali-like substances, intentional self-harm [POA] [HCC]

[7th] T54.3X3 Toxic effect of corrosive alkalis and alkali-like substances, assault [POA]

[PDx] Unacceptable principal diagnosis symbol per Medicare code edits [POA] Code exempt from diagnosis present on admission requirement
[?] Questionable admission [CC] Complication or comorbidity [MCC] Major complication or comorbidity [CC/MCC Exc] CC/MCC exclusion
[HCC] HCC diagnosis code [RxHCC] RxHCC diagnosis code MACRA code **DEFINITION** Describes condition/terminology
TIP Coding guidance 👁 Official Guideline Reference [Z-1] Z code as first-listed diagnosis

[7th] T54.3X4 Toxic effect of corrosive alkalis and alkali-like substances, undetermined [POA]

[5th] T54.9 Toxic effects of unspecified corrosive substance

[7th] T54.91 Toxic effect of unspecified corrosive substance, accidental (unintentional) [POA]

[7th] T54.92 Toxic effect of unspecified corrosive substance, intentional self-harm [POA] [HCC]

[7th] T54.93 Toxic effect of unspecified corrosive substance, assault [POA]

[7th] T54.94 Toxic effect of unspecified corrosive substance, undetermined [POA]

[4th] T55 Toxic effect of soaps and detergents

The appropriate 7th character is to be added to each code from category T55
- A = initial encounter
- D = subsequent encounter
- S = sequela

[5th] T55.0 Toxic effect of soaps

[6th] T55.0X Toxic effect of soaps

[7th] T55.0X1 Toxic effect of soaps, accidental (unintentional) [POA]
Toxic effect of soaps NOS

[7th] T55.0X2 Toxic effect of soaps, intentional self-harm [POA] [HCC]

[7th] T55.0X3 Toxic effect of soaps, assault [POA]

[7th] T55.0X4 Toxic effect of soaps, undetermined [POA]

[5th] T55.1 Toxic effect of detergents

[6th] T55.1X Toxic effect of detergents

[7th] T55.1X1 Toxic effect of detergents, accidental (unintentional) [POA]
Toxic effect of detergents NOS

[7th] T55.1X2 Toxic effect of detergents, intentional self-harm [POA] [HCC]

[7th] T55.1X3 Toxic effect of detergents, assault [POA]

[7th] T55.1X4 Toxic effect of detergents, undetermined [POA]

[4th] T56 Toxic effect of metals

INCLUDES *toxic effects of fumes and vapors of metals*
toxic effects of metals from all sources, except medicinal substances

Use additional code to identify any retained metal foreign body, if applicable (Z18.0-, T18.1-)

EXCLUDES1 *arsenic and its compounds (T57.0)*
manganese and its compounds (T57.2)

The appropriate 7th character is to be added to each code from category T56
- A = initial encounter
- D = subsequent encounter
- S = sequela

[5th] T56.0 Toxic effects of lead and its compounds

[6th] T56.0X Toxic effects of lead and its compounds

[7th] T56.0X1 Toxic effect of lead and its compounds, accidental (unintentional) [POA]
Toxic effects of lead and its compounds NOS

[7th] T56.0X2 Toxic effect of lead and its compounds, intentional self-harm [POA] [HCC]

[7th] T56.0X3 Toxic effect of lead and its compounds, assault [POA]

[7th] T56.0X4 Toxic effect of lead and its compounds, undetermined [POA]

[5th] T56.1 Toxic effects of mercury and its compounds

[6th] T56.1X Toxic effects of mercury and its compounds

[7th] T56.1X1 Toxic effect of mercury and its compounds, accidental (unintentional) [POA]
Toxic effects of mercury and its compounds NOS

[7th] T56.1X2 Toxic effect of mercury and its compounds, intentional self-harm [POA] [HCC]

[7th] T56.1X3 Toxic effect of mercury and its compounds, assault [POA]

[7th] T56.1X4 Toxic effect of mercury and its compounds, undetermined [POA]

[5th] T56.2 Toxic effects of chromium and its compounds

[6th] T56.2X Toxic effects of chromium and its compounds

[7th] T56.2X1 Toxic effect of chromium and its compounds, accidental (unintentional) [POA]
Toxic effects of chromium and its compounds NOS

[7th] T56.2X2 Toxic effect of chromium and its compounds, intentional self-harm [POA] [HCC]

[7th] T56.2X3 Toxic effect of chromium and its compounds, assault [POA]

[7th] T56.2X4 Toxic effect of chromium and its compounds, undetermined [POA]

[5th] T56.3 Toxic effects of cadmium and its compounds

[6th] T56.3X Toxic effects of cadmium and its compounds

[7th] T56.3X1 Toxic effect of cadmium and its compounds, accidental (unintentional) [POA]
Toxic effects of cadmium and its compounds NOS

[7th] T56.3X2 Toxic effect of cadmium and its compounds, intentional self-harm [POA] [HCC]

[7th] T56.3X3 Toxic effect of cadmium and its compounds, assault [POA]

[7th] T56.3X4 Toxic effect of cadmium and its compounds, undetermined [POA]

[5th] T56.4 Toxic effects of copper and its compounds

[6th] T56.4X Toxic effects of copper and its compounds

[7th] T56.4X1 Toxic effect of copper and its compounds, accidental (unintentional) [POA]
Toxic effects of copper and its compounds NOS

[7th] T56.4X2 Toxic effect of copper and its compounds, intentional self-harm [POA] [HCC]

[7th] T56.4X3 Toxic effect of copper and its compounds, assault [POA]

[7th] T56.4X4 Toxic effect of copper and its compounds, undetermined [POA]

[5th] T56.5 Toxic effects of zinc and its compounds

[6th] T56.5X Toxic effects of zinc and its compounds

[7th] T56.5X1 Toxic effect of zinc and its compounds, accidental (unintentional) [POA]
Toxic effects of zinc and its compounds NOS

[7th] T56.5X2 Toxic effect of zinc and its compounds, intentional self-harm [POA] [HCC]

[7th] T56.5X3 Toxic effect of zinc and its compounds, assault [POA]

[7th] T56.5X4 Toxic effect of zinc and its compounds, undetermined [POA]

[5th] T56.6 Toxic effects of tin and its compounds

[6th] T56.6X Toxic effects of tin and its compounds

[7th] T56.6X1 Toxic effect of tin and its compounds, accidental (unintentional) [POA]
Toxic effects of tin and its compounds NOS

[7th] T56.6X2 Toxic effect of tin and its compounds, intentional self-harm [POA] [HCC]

[7th] T56.6X3 Toxic effect of tin and its compounds, assault [POA]

[7th] T56.6X4 Toxic effect of tin and its compounds, undetermined [POA]

[5th] T56.7 Toxic effects of beryllium and its compounds

[6th] T56.7X Toxic effects of beryllium and its compounds

[7th] T56.7X1 Toxic effect of beryllium and its compounds, accidental (unintentional) [POA]
Toxic effects of beryllium and its compounds NOS

[7th] T56.7X2 Toxic effect of beryllium and its compounds, intentional self-harm [POA] [HCC]

[7th] T56.7X3 Toxic effect of beryllium and its compounds, assault [POA]

[7th] T56.7X4 Toxic effect of beryllium and its compounds, undetermined [POA]

- 5ᵗʰ **T56.8** Toxic effects of other metals
  - 6ᵗʰ **T56.81** Toxic effect of thallium
    - 7ᵗʰ **T56.811 Toxic effect of thallium,** accidental **(unintentional)** poₐˢ
      Toxic effect of thallium NOS
    - 7ᵗʰ **T56.812 Toxic effect of thallium,** intentional self-harm poₐˢ HCC
    - 7ᵗʰ **T56.813 Toxic effect of thallium,** assault poₐˢ
    - 7ᵗʰ **T56.814 Toxic effect of thallium,** undetermined poₐˢ
  - 6ᵗʰ **T56.89** Toxic effects of other metals
    - 7ᵗʰ **T56.891 Toxic effect of other metals,** accidental **(unintentional)** poₐˢ
      Toxic effects of other metals NOS
    - 7ᵗʰ **T56.892 Toxic effect of other metals,** intentional self-harm poₐˢ HCC
    - 7ᵗʰ **T56.893 Toxic effect of other metals,** assault poₐˢ
    - 7ᵗʰ **T56.894 Toxic effect of other metals,** undetermined poₐˢ
- 5ᵗʰ **T56.9** Toxic effects of unspecified metal
  - 7ᵗʰ **T56.91 Toxic effect of unspecified metal,** accidental **(unintentional)** poₐˢ
  - 7ᵗʰ **T56.92 Toxic effect of unspecified metal,** intentional self-harm poₐˢ HCC
  - 7ᵗʰ **T56.93 Toxic effect of unspecified metal,** assault poₐˢ
  - 7ᵗʰ **T56.94 Toxic effect of unspecified metal,** undetermined poₐˢ
- 4ᵗʰ **T57** Toxic effect of other inorganic substances

  The appropriate 7th character is to be added to each code from category T57
  A = initial encounter
  D = subsequent encounter
  S = sequela
  - 5ᵗʰ **T57.0** Toxic effect of arsenic and its compounds
    - 6ᵗʰ **T57.0X** Toxic effect of arsenic and its compounds
      - 7ᵗʰ **T57.0X1 Toxic effect of arsenic and its compounds,** accidental **(unintentional)** poₐˢ
        Toxic effect of arsenic and its compounds NOS
      - 7ᵗʰ **T57.0X2 Toxic effect of arsenic and its compounds,** intentional self-harm poₐˢ HCC
      - 7ᵗʰ **T57.0X3 Toxic effect of arsenic and its compounds,** assault poₐˢ
      - 7ᵗʰ **T57.0X4 Toxic effect of arsenic and its compounds,** undetermined poₐˢ
  - 5ᵗʰ **T57.1** Toxic effect of phosphorus and its compounds
    EXCLUDES1 organophosphate insecticides (T60.0)
    - 6ᵗʰ **T57.1X** Toxic effect of phosphorus and its compounds
      - 7ᵗʰ **T57.1X1 Toxic effect of phosphorus and its compounds,** accidental **(unintentional)** poₐˢ
        Toxic effect of phosphorus and its compounds NOS
      - 7ᵗʰ **T57.1X2 Toxic effect of phosphorus and its compounds,** intentional self-harm poₐˢ HCC
      - 7ᵗʰ **T57.1X3 Toxic effect of phosphorus and its compounds,** assault poₐˢ
      - 7ᵗʰ **T57.1X4 Toxic effect of phosphorus and its compounds,** undetermined poₐˢ
  - 5ᵗʰ **T57.2** Toxic effect of manganese and its compounds
    - 6ᵗʰ **T57.2X** Toxic effect of manganese and its compounds
      - 7ᵗʰ **T57.2X1 Toxic effect of manganese and its compounds,** accidental **(unintentional)** poₐˢ
        Toxic effect of manganese and its compounds NOS
      - 7ᵗʰ **T57.2X2 Toxic effect of manganese and its compounds,** intentional self-harm poₐˢ HCC
      - 7ᵗʰ **T57.2X3 Toxic effect of manganese and its compounds,** assault poₐˢ
      - 7ᵗʰ **T57.2X4 Toxic effect of manganese and its compounds,** undetermined poₐˢ
  - 5ᵗʰ **T57.3** Toxic effect of hydrogen cyanide
    - 6ᵗʰ **T57.3X** Toxic effect of hydrogen cyanide

- 7ᵗʰ **T57.3X1 Toxic effect of hydrogen cyanide,** accidental **(unintentional)** poₐˢ
  Toxic effect of hydrogen cyanide NOS
- 7ᵗʰ **T57.3X2 Toxic effect of hydrogen cyanide,** intentional self-harm poₐˢ HCC
- 7ᵗʰ **T57.3X3 Toxic effect of hydrogen cyanide, assault** poₐˢ
- 7ᵗʰ **T57.3X4 Toxic effect of hydrogen cyanide,** undetermined poₐˢ
- 5ᵗʰ **T57.8** Toxic effect of other specified inorganic substances
  - 6ᵗʰ **T57.8X** Toxic effect of other specified inorganic substances
    - 7ᵗʰ **T57.8X1 Toxic effect of other specified inorganic substances,** accidental **(unintentional)** poₐˢ
      Toxic effect of other specified inorganic substances NOS
    - 7ᵗʰ **T57.8X2 Toxic effect of other specified inorganic substances,** intentional self-harm poₐˢ HCC
    - 7ᵗʰ **T57.8X3 Toxic effect of other specified inorganic substances,** assault poₐˢ
    - 7ᵗʰ **T57.8X4 Toxic effect of other specified inorganic substances,** undetermined poₐˢ
- 5ᵗʰ **T57.9** Toxic effect of unspecified inorganic substance
  - 7ᵗʰ **T57.91 Toxic effect of unspecified inorganic substance,** accidental **(unintentional)** poₐˢ
  - 7ᵗʰ **T57.92 Toxic effect of unspecified inorganic substance,** intentional self-harm poₐˢ HCC
  - 7ᵗʰ **T57.93 Toxic effect of unspecified inorganic substance,** assault poₐˢ
  - 7ᵗʰ **T57.94 Toxic effect of unspecified inorganic substance,** undetermined poₐˢ
- 4ᵗʰ **T58** Toxic effect of carbon monoxide

  INCLUDES asphyxiation from carbon monoxide
  toxic effect of carbon monoxide from all sources

  The appropriate 7th character is to be added to each code from category T58
  A = initial encounter
  D = subsequent encounter
  S = sequela
  - 5ᵗʰ **T58.0** Toxic effect of carbon monoxide from motor vehicle exhaust
    Toxic effect of exhaust gas from gas engine
    Toxic effect of exhaust gas from motor pump
    - 7ᵗʰ **T58.01 Toxic effect of carbon monoxide from motor vehicle exhaust,** accidental **(unintentional)** poₐˢ
    - 7ᵗʰ **T58.02 Toxic effect of carbon monoxide from motor vehicle exhaust,** intentional self-harm poₐˢ HCC
    - 7ᵗʰ **T58.03 Toxic effect of carbon monoxide from motor vehicle exhaust,** assault poₐˢ
    - 7ᵗʰ **T58.04 Toxic effect of carbon monoxide from motor vehicle exhaust,** undetermined poₐˢ
  - 5ᵗʰ **T58.1** Toxic effect of carbon monoxide from utility gas
    Toxic effect of acetylene
    Toxic effect of gas NOS used for lighting, heating, cooking
    Toxic effect of water gas
    - 7ᵗʰ **T58.11 Toxic effect of carbon monoxide from utility gas,** accidental **(unintentional)** poₐˢ
    - 7ᵗʰ **T58.12 Toxic effect of carbon monoxide from utility gas,** intentional self-harm poₐˢ HCC
    - 7ᵗʰ **T58.13 Toxic effect of carbon monoxide from utility gas,** assault poₐˢ
    - 7ᵗʰ **T58.14 Toxic effect of carbon monoxide from utility gas,** undetermined poₐˢ
  - 5ᵗʰ **T58.2** Toxic effect of carbon monoxide from incomplete combustion of other domestic fuels
    Toxic effect of carbon monoxide from incomplete combustion of coal, coke, kerosene, wood
    - 6ᵗʰ **T58.2X** Toxic effect of carbon monoxide from incomplete combustion of other domestic fuels
      - 7ᵗʰ **T58.2X1 Toxic effect of carbon monoxide from incomplete combustion of other domestic fuels,** accidental **(unintentional)** poₐˢ
      - 7ᵗʰ **T58.2X2 Toxic effect of carbon monoxide from incomplete combustion of other domestic fuels,** intentional self-harm poₐˢ HCC

---

poₐˢ Unacceptable principal diagnosis symbol per Medicare code edits   ₚₒˢ Code exempt from diagnosis present on admission requirement
❓ Questionable admission   🄲 Complication or comorbidity   ᴹᶜᶜ Major complication or comorbidity   ᶜᶜ/ᴹᶜᶜ ᴱˣᶜ CC/MCC exclusion
HCC HCC diagnosis code   RHCC RxHCC diagnosis code   MACRA code   **DEFINITION** Describes condition/terminology
TIP Coding guidance   👁 Official Guideline Reference   🅩 Z code as first-listed diagnosis

⑦ **T58.2X3** Toxic effect of carbon monoxide from incomplete combustion of other domestic fuels, assault POA

⑦ **T58.2X4** Toxic effect of carbon monoxide from incomplete combustion of other domestic fuels, undetermined POA

⑤ **T58.8** Toxic effect of carbon monoxide from other source
Toxic effect of carbon monoxide from blast furnace gas
Toxic effect of carbon monoxide from fuels in industrial use
Toxic effect of carbon monoxide from kiln vapor

⑥ **T58.8X** Toxic effect of carbon monoxide from other source

⑦ **T58.8X1** Toxic effect of carbon monoxide from other source, accidental (unintentional) POA

⑦ **T58.8X2** Toxic effect of carbon monoxide from other source, intentional self-harm POA HCC

⑦ **T58.8X3** Toxic effect of carbon monoxide from other source, assault POA

⑦ **T58.8X4** Toxic effect of carbon monoxide from other source, undetermined POA

⑤ **T58.9** Toxic effect of carbon monoxide from unspecified source

⑦ **T58.91** Toxic effect of carbon monoxide from unspecified source, accidental (unintentional) POA

⑦ **T58.92** Toxic effect of carbon monoxide from unspecified source, intentional self-harm POA HCC

⑦ **T58.93** Toxic effect of carbon monoxide from unspecified source, assault POA

⑦ **T58.94** Toxic effect of carbon monoxide from unspecified source, undetermined POA

④ **T59** Toxic effect of other gases, fumes and vapors

INCLUDES   aerosol propellants

EXCLUDES1   chlorofluorocarbons (T53.5)

The appropriate 7th character is to be added to each code from category T59
A = initial encounter
D = subsequent encounter
S = sequela

⑤ **T59.0** Toxic effect of nitrogen oxides

⑥ **T59.0X** Toxic effect of nitrogen oxides

⑦ **T59.0X1** Toxic effect of nitrogen oxides, accidental (unintentional) POA
Toxic effect of nitrogen oxides NOS

⑦ **T59.0X2** Toxic effect of nitrogen oxides, intentional self-harm POA HCC

⑦ **T59.0X3** Toxic effect of nitrogen oxides, assault POA

⑦ **T59.0X4** Toxic effect of nitrogen oxides, undetermined POA

⑤ **T59.1** Toxic effect of sulfur dioxide

⑥ **T59.1X** Toxic effect of sulfur dioxide

⑦ **T59.1X1** Toxic effect of sulfur dioxide, accidental (unintentional) POA
Toxic effect of sulfur dioxide NOS

⑦ **T59.1X2** Toxic effect of sulfur dioxide, intentional self-harm POA HCC

⑦ **T59.1X3** Toxic effect of sulfur dioxide, assault POA

⑦ **T59.1X4** Toxic effect of sulfur dioxide, undetermined POA

⑤ **T59.2** Toxic effect of formaldehyde

⑥ **T59.2X** Toxic effect of formaldehyde

⑦ **T59.2X1** Toxic effect of formaldehyde, accidental (unintentional) POA
Toxic effect of formaldehyde NOS

⑦ **T59.2X2** Toxic effect of formaldehyde, intentional self-harm POA HCC

⑦ **T59.2X3** Toxic effect of formaldehyde, assault POA

⑦ **T59.2X4** Toxic effect of formaldehyde, undetermined POA

⑤ **T59.3** Toxic effect of lacrimogenic gas
Toxic effect of tear gas

⑥ **T59.3X** Toxic effect of lacrimogenic gas

⑦ **T59.3X1** Toxic effect of lacrimogenic gas, accidental (unintentional) POA
Toxic effect of lacrimogenic gas NOS

⑦ **T59.3X2** Toxic effect of lacrimogenic gas, intentional self-harm POA HCC

⑦ **T59.3X3** Toxic effect of lacrimogenic gas, assault POA

⑦ **T59.3X4** Toxic effect of lacrimogenic gas, undetermined POA

⑤ **T59.4** Toxic effect of chlorine gas

⑥ **T59.4X** Toxic effect of chlorine gas

⑦ **T59.4X1** Toxic effect of chlorine gas, accidental (unintentional) POA
Toxic effect of chlorine gas NOS

⑦ **T59.4X2** Toxic effect of chlorine gas, intentional self-harm POA HCC

⑦ **T59.4X3** Toxic effect of chlorine gas, assault POA

⑦ **T59.4X4** Toxic effect of chlorine gas, undetermined POA

⑤ **T59.5** Toxic effect of fluorine gas and hydrogen fluoride

⑥ **T59.5X** Toxic effect of fluorine gas and hydrogen fluoride

⑦ **T59.5X1** Toxic effect of fluorine gas and hydrogen fluoride, accidental (unintentional) POA
Toxic effect of fluorine gas and hydrogen fluoride NOS

⑦ **T59.5X2** Toxic effect of fluorine gas and hydrogen fluoride, intentional self-harm POA HCC

⑦ **T59.5X3** Toxic effect of fluorine gas and hydrogen fluoride, assault POA

⑦ **T59.5X4** Toxic effect of fluorine gas and hydrogen fluoride, undetermined POA

⑤ **T59.6** Toxic effect of hydrogen sulfide

⑥ **T59.6X** Toxic effect of hydrogen sulfide

⑦ **T59.6X1** Toxic effect of hydrogen sulfide, accidental (unintentional) POA
Toxic effect of hydrogen sulfide NOS

⑦ **T59.6X2** Toxic effect of hydrogen sulfide, intentional self-harm POA HCC

⑦ **T59.6X3** Toxic effect of hydrogen sulfide, assault POA

⑦ **T59.6X4** Toxic effect of hydrogen sulfide, undetermined POA

⑤ **T59.7** Toxic effect of carbon dioxide

⑥ **T59.7X** Toxic effect of carbon dioxide

⑦ **T59.7X1** Toxic effect of carbon dioxide, accidental (unintentional) POA
Toxic effect of carbon dioxide NOS

⑦ **T59.7X2** Toxic effect of carbon dioxide, intentional self-harm POA HCC

⑦ **T59.7X3** Toxic effect of carbon dioxide, assault POA

⑦ **T59.7X4** Toxic effect of carbon dioxide, undetermined POA

⑤ **T59.8** Toxic effect of other specified gases, fumes and vapors

⑥ **T59.81** Toxic effect of smoke
Smoke inhalation
EXCLUDES2   toxic effect of cigarette (tobacco) smoke (T65.22-)

⑦ **T59.811** Toxic effect of smoke, accidental (unintentional) POA
AHA: Q4 2013
Toxic effect of smoke NOS

⑦ **T59.812** Toxic effect of smoke, intentional self-harm POA HCC

⑦ **T59.813** Toxic effect of smoke, assault POA

⑦ **T59.814** Toxic effect of smoke, undetermined POA

⑥ **T59.89** Toxic effect of other specified gases, fumes and vapors

⑦ **T59.891** Toxic effect of other specified gases, fumes and vapors, accidental (unintentional) POA

⑦ **T59.892** Toxic effect of other specified gases, fumes and vapors, intentional self-harm POA HCC

⑦ **T59.893** Toxic effect of other specified gases, fumes and vapors, assault POA

⑦ **T59.894** Toxic effect of other specified gases, fumes and vapors, undetermined POA

Unspecified Code   Other Specified Code   Manifestation Code   Ⓝ Newborn   Ⓟ Pediatric   Ⓜ Maternity   Ⓐ Adult   ♂ Male   ♀ Female
● New Code   ▲ Revised Code Title   ►◄ Revised Text   NOTES   INCLUDES   EXCLUDES1 Not coded here   EXCLUDES2 Not included here
④ 4th character required   ⑤ 5th character required   ⑥ 6th character required   ⑦ 7th character required   ⑧ Extension 'X' Alert
HAC Hospital-acquired condition (HAC) alert   AHA AHA Coding Clinic®   ☛ Code first alert

- 5ᵗʰ **T59.9 Toxic effect of unspecified gases, fumes and vapors**
  - 7ᵗʰ **T59.91 Toxic effect of unspecified gases, fumes and vapors, accidental (unintentional)** POA
  - 7ᵗʰ **T59.92 Toxic effect of unspecified gases, fumes and vapors, intentional self-harm** POA HCC
  - 7ᵗʰ **T59.93 Toxic effect of unspecified gases, fumes and vapors, assault** POA
  - 7ᵗʰ **T59.94 Toxic effect of unspecified gases, fumes and vapors, undetermined** POA

- 4ᵗʰ **T60 Toxic effect of pesticides**
  - *INCLUDES* toxic effect of wood preservatives
  - The appropriate 7th character is to be added to each code from category T60
    - A = initial encounter
    - D = subsequent encounter
    - S = sequela
  - 5ᵗʰ **T60.0 Toxic effect of organophosphate and carbamate insecticides**
    - 6ᵗʰ **T60.0X Toxic effect of organophosphate and carbamate insecticides**
      - 7ᵗʰ **T60.0X1 Toxic effect of organophosphate and carbamate insecticides, accidental (unintentional)** POA
        Toxic effect of organophosphate and carbamate insecticides NOS
      - 7ᵗʰ **T60.0X2 Toxic effect of organophosphate and carbamate insecticides, intentional self-harm** POA HCC
      - 7ᵗʰ **T60.0X3 Toxic effect of organophosphate and carbamate insecticides, assault** POA
      - 7ᵗʰ **T60.0X4 Toxic effect of organophosphate and carbamate insecticides, undetermined** POA
  - 5ᵗʰ **T60.1 Toxic effect of halogenated insecticides**
    - *EXCLUDES1* chlorinated hydrocarbon (T53.-)
    - 6ᵗʰ **T60.1X Toxic effect of halogenated insecticides**
      - 7ᵗʰ **T60.1X1 Toxic effect of halogenated insecticides, accidental (unintentional)** POA
        Toxic effect of halogenated insecticides NOS
      - 7ᵗʰ **T60.1X2 Toxic effect of halogenated insecticides, intentional self-harm** POA HCC
      - 7ᵗʰ **T60.1X3 Toxic effect of halogenated insecticides, assault** POA
      - 7ᵗʰ **T60.1X4 Toxic effect of halogenated insecticides, undetermined** POA
  - 5ᵗʰ **T60.2 Toxic effect of other insecticides**
    - 6ᵗʰ **T60.2X Toxic effect of other insecticides**
      - 7ᵗʰ **T60.2X1 Toxic effect of other insecticides, accidental (unintentional)** POA
        Toxic effect of other insecticides NOS
      - 7ᵗʰ **T60.2X2 Toxic effect of other insecticides, intentional self-harm** POA HCC
      - 7ᵗʰ **T60.2X3 Toxic effect of other insecticides, assault** POA
      - 7ᵗʰ **T60.2X4 Toxic effect of other insecticides, undetermined** POA
  - 5ᵗʰ **T60.3 Toxic effect of herbicides and fungicides**
    - 6ᵗʰ **T60.3X Toxic effect of herbicides and fungicides**
      - 7ᵗʰ **T60.3X1 Toxic effect of herbicides and fungicides, accidental (unintentional)** POA
        Toxic effect of herbicides and fungicides NOS
      - 7ᵗʰ **T60.3X2 Toxic effect of herbicides and fungicides, intentional self-harm** POA HCC
      - 7ᵗʰ **T60.3X3 Toxic effect of herbicides and fungicides, assault** POA
      - 7ᵗʰ **T60.3X4 Toxic effect of herbicides and fungicides, undetermined** POA
  - 5ᵗʰ **T60.4 Toxic effect of rodenticides**
    - *EXCLUDES1* strychnine and its salts (T65.1)
      - thallium (T56.81-)
    - 6ᵗʰ **T60.4X Toxic effect of rodenticides**
      - 7ᵗʰ **T60.4X1 Toxic effect of rodenticides, accidental (unintentional)** POA
        Toxic effect of rodenticides NOS

- 7ᵗʰ **T60.4X2 Toxic effect of rodenticides, intentional self-harm** POA HCC
- 7ᵗʰ **T60.4X3 Toxic effect of rodenticides, assault** POA
- 7ᵗʰ **T60.4X4 Toxic effect of rodenticides, undetermined** POA
  - 5ᵗʰ **T60.8 Toxic effect of other pesticides**
    - 6ᵗʰ **T60.8X Toxic effect of other pesticides**
      - 7ᵗʰ **T60.8X1 Toxic effect of other pesticides, accidental (unintentional)** POA
        Toxic effect of other pesticides NOS
      - 7ᵗʰ **T60.8X2 Toxic effect of other pesticides, intentional self-harm** POA HCC
      - 7ᵗʰ **T60.8X3 Toxic effect of other pesticides, assault** POA
      - 7ᵗʰ **T60.8X4 Toxic effect of other pesticides, undetermined** POA
  - 5ᵗʰ **T60.9 Toxic effect of unspecified pesticide**
    - 7ᵗʰ **T60.91 Toxic effect of unspecified pesticide, accidental (unintentional)** POA
    - 7ᵗʰ **T60.92 Toxic effect of unspecified pesticide, intentional self-harm** POA HCC
    - 7ᵗʰ **T60.93 Toxic effect of unspecified pesticide, assault** POA
    - 7ᵗʰ **T60.94 Toxic effect of unspecified pesticide, undetermined** POA

- 4ᵗʰ **T61 Toxic effect of noxious substances eaten as seafood**
  - *EXCLUDES1* allergic reaction to food, such as:
    - anaphylactic reaction or shock due to adverse food reaction (T78.0-)
    - bacterial foodborne intoxications (A05.-)
    - dermatitis (L23.6, L25.4, L27.2)
    - food protein-induced enterocolitis syndrome (K52.21)
    - food protein-induced enteropathy (K52.22)
    - gastroenteritis (noninfective) (K52.29)
    - toxic effect of aflatoxin and other mycotoxins (T64)
    - toxic effect of cyanides (T65.0-)
    - toxic effect of harmful algae bloom (T65.82-)
    - toxic effect of hydrogen cyanide (T57.3-)
    - toxic effect of mercury (T56.1-)
    - toxic effect of red tide (T65.82-)
  - The appropriate 7th character is to be added to each code from category T61
    - A = initial encounter
    - D = subsequent encounter
    - S = sequela
  - 5ᵗʰ **T61.0 Ciguatera fish poisoning**
    - 7ᵗʰ **T61.01 Ciguatera fish poisoning, accidental (unintentional)** POA
    - 7ᵗʰ **T61.02 Ciguatera fish poisoning, intentional self-harm** POA HCC
    - 7ᵗʰ **T61.03 Ciguatera fish poisoning, assault** POA
    - 7ᵗʰ **T61.04 Ciguatera fish poisoning, undetermined** POA
  - 5ᵗʰ **T61.1 Scombroid fish poisoning**
    Histamine-like syndrome
    - 7ᵗʰ **T61.11 Scombroid fish poisoning, accidental (unintentional)** POA
    - 7ᵗʰ **T61.12 Scombroid fish poisoning, intentional self-harm** POA HCC
    - 7ᵗʰ **T61.13 Scombroid fish poisoning, assault** POA
    - 7ᵗʰ **T61.14 Scombroid fish poisoning, undetermined** POA
  - 5ᵗʰ **T61.7 Other fish and shellfish poisoning**
    - 6ᵗʰ **T61.77 Other fish poisoning**
      - 7ᵗʰ **T61.771 Other fish poisoning, accidental (unintentional)** POA
      - 7ᵗʰ **T61.772 Other fish poisoning, intentional self-harm** POA HCC
      - 7ᵗʰ **T61.773 Other fish poisoning, assault** POA
      - 7ᵗʰ **T61.774 Other fish poisoning, undetermined** POA
    - 6ᵗʰ **T61.78 Other shellfish poisoning**
      - 7ᵗʰ **T61.781 Other shellfish poisoning, accidental (unintentional)** POA

POA Unacceptable principal diagnosis symbol per Medicare code edits   POA Code exempt from diagnosis present on admission requirement
? Questionable admission   CC Complication or comorbidity   MCC Major complication or comorbidity   CC/MCC CC/MCC exclusion
HCC HCC diagnosis code   RHCC RxHCC diagnosis code   MACRA code   **DEFINITION** Describes condition/terminology
TIP Coding guidance   ⊛ Official Guideline Reference   Z1 Z code as first-listed diagnosis

7️⃣ **T61.782** Other shellfish poisoning, *intentional self-harm* POA HCC

7️⃣ **T61.783** Other shellfish poisoning, *assault* POA

7️⃣ **T61.784** Other shellfish poisoning, *undetermined* POA

5️⃣ **T61.8** Toxic effect of other seafood

6️⃣ **T61.8X** Toxic effect of *other seafood*

7️⃣ **T61.8X1** Toxic effect of other seafood, *accidental (unintentional)* POA

7️⃣ **T61.8X2** Toxic effect of other seafood, *intentional self-harm* POA HCC

7️⃣ **T61.8X3** Toxic effect of other seafood, *assault* POA

7️⃣ **T61.8X4** Toxic effect of other seafood, *undetermined* POA

5️⃣ **T61.9** Toxic effect of unspecified seafood

7️⃣ **T61.91** Toxic effect of unspecified seafood, *accidental (unintentional)* POA

7️⃣ **T61.92** Toxic effect of unspecified seafood, *intentional self-harm* POA HCC

7️⃣ **T61.93** Toxic effect of unspecified seafood, *assault* POA

7️⃣ **T61.94** Toxic effect of unspecified seafood, *undetermined* POA

4️⃣ **T62** Toxic effect of *other noxious substances* eaten as *food*

EXCLUDES1 *allergic reaction to food, such as:*

anaphylactic shock (reaction) due to adverse food reaction (T78.0-)

bacterial food borne intoxications (A05.-)

dermatitis (L23.6, L25.4, L27.2)

food protein-induced enterocolitis syndrome (K52.21)

food protein-induced enteropathy (K52.22)

gastroenteritis (noninfective) (K52.29)

toxic effect of aflatoxin and other mycotoxins (T64)

toxic effect of cyanides (T65.0-)

toxic effect of hydrogen cyanide (T57.3-)

toxic effect of mercury (T56.1-)

The appropriate 7th character is to be added to each code from category T62

A = initial encounter

D = subsequent encounter

S = sequela

5️⃣ **T62.0** Toxic effect of ingested mushrooms

6️⃣ **T62.0X** Toxic effect of *ingested mushrooms*

7️⃣ **T62.0X1** Toxic effect of ingested mushrooms, *accidental (unintentional)* POA
Toxic effect of ingested mushrooms NOS

7️⃣ **T62.0X2** Toxic effect of ingested mushrooms, *intentional self-harm* POA HCC

7️⃣ **T62.0X3** Toxic effect of ingested mushrooms, *assault* POA

7️⃣ **T62.0X4** Toxic effect of ingested mushrooms, *undetermined* POA

5️⃣ **T62.1** Toxic effect of ingested berries

6️⃣ **T62.1X** Toxic effect of *ingested berries*

7️⃣ **T62.1X1** Toxic effect of ingested berries, *accidental (unintentional)* POA
Toxic effect of ingested berries NOS

7️⃣ **T62.1X2** Toxic effect of ingested berries, *intentional self-harm* POA HCC

7️⃣ **T62.1X3** Toxic effect of ingested berries, *assault* POA

7️⃣ **T62.1X4** Toxic effect of ingested berries, *undetermined* POA

5️⃣ **T62.2** Toxic effect of other ingested (parts of) plant(s)

6️⃣ **T62.2X** Toxic effect of *other ingested* (parts of) *plant(s)*

7️⃣ **T62.2X1** Toxic effect of other ingested (parts of) plant(s), *accidental (unintentional)* POA
Toxic effect of other ingested (parts of) plant(s) NOS

7️⃣ **T62.2X2** Toxic effect of other ingested (parts of) plant(s), *intentional self-harm* POA HCC

7️⃣ **T62.2X3** Toxic effect of other ingested (parts of) plant(s), *assault* POA

7️⃣ **T62.2X4** Toxic effect of other ingested (parts of) plant(s), *undetermined* POA

5️⃣ **T62.8** Toxic effect of other specified noxious substances eaten as food

6️⃣ **T62.8X** Toxic effect of *other specified noxious substances eaten as food*

7️⃣ **T62.8X1** Toxic effect of other specified noxious substances eaten as food, *accidental (unintentional)* POA
Toxic effect of other specified noxious substances eaten as food NOS

7️⃣ **T62.8X2** Toxic effect of other specified noxious substances eaten as food, *intentional self-harm* POA HCC

7️⃣ **T62.8X3** Toxic effect of other specified noxious substances eaten as food, *assault* POA

7️⃣ **T62.8X4** Toxic effect of other specified noxious substances eaten as food, *undetermined* POA

5️⃣ **T62.9** Toxic effect of *unspecified noxious substance* eaten as food

7️⃣ **T62.91** Toxic effect of unspecified noxious substance eaten as food, *accidental* (unintentional) POA
Toxic effect of unspecified noxious substance eaten as food NOS

7️⃣ **T62.92** Toxic effect of unspecified noxious substance eaten as food, *intentional self-harm* POA HCC

7️⃣ **T62.93** Toxic effect of unspecified noxious substance eaten as food, *assault* POA

7️⃣ **T62.94** Toxic effect of unspecified noxious substance eaten as food, *undetermined* POA

4️⃣ **T63** Toxic effect of contact with venomous animals and plants

INCLUDES *bite or touch of venomous animal*
pricked or stuck by thorn or leaf

EXCLUDES2 *ingestion of toxic animal or plant (T61.-, T62.-)*

The appropriate 7th character is to be added to each code from category T63

A = initial encounter

D = subsequent encounter

S = sequela

5️⃣ **T63.0** Toxic effect of snake venom

6️⃣ **T63.00** Toxic effect of *unspecified snake* venom

7️⃣ **T63.001** Toxic effect of unspecified snake venom, *accidental (unintentional)* POA
Toxic effect of unspecified snake venom NOS

7️⃣ **T63.002** Toxic effect of unspecified snake venom, *intentional self-harm* POA HCC

7️⃣ **T63.003** Toxic effect of unspecified snake venom, *assault* POA

7️⃣ **T63.004** Toxic effect of unspecified snake venom, *undetermined* POA

6️⃣ **T63.01** Toxic effect of *rattlesnake* venom

7️⃣ **T63.011** Toxic effect of rattlesnake venom, *accidental (unintentional)* POA
Toxic effect of rattlesnake venom NOS

7️⃣ **T63.012** Toxic effect of rattlesnake venom, *intentional self-harm* POA HCC

7️⃣ **T63.013** Toxic effect of rattlesnake venom, *assault* POA

7️⃣ **T63.014** Toxic effect of rattlesnake venom, *undetermined* POA

6️⃣ **T63.02** Toxic effect of *coral snake* venom

7️⃣ **T63.021** Toxic effect of coral snake venom, *accidental (unintentional)* POA
Toxic effect of coral snake venom NOS

7️⃣ **T63.022** Toxic effect of coral snake venom, *intentional self-harm* POA HCC

7️⃣ **T63.023** Toxic effect of coral snake venom, *assault* POA

Unspecified Code   Other Specified Code   Manifestation Code   N Newborn   P Pediatric   M Maternity   A Adult   ♂ Male   ♀ Female
● New Code   ▲ Revised Code Title   ►◄ Revised Text   NOTES   *INCLUDES*   EXCLUDES1 Not coded here   EXCLUDES2 Not included here
4️⃣ 4th character required   5️⃣ 5th character required   6️⃣ 6th character required   7️⃣ 7th character required   Ⓧ Extension 'X' Alert
HAC Hospital-acquired condition (HAC) alert   AHA AHA Coding Clinic©   ☛ Code first alert

CHAPTER 19: INJURY, POISONING, AND CERTAIN OTHER CONSEQUENCES OF EXTERNAL CAUSES (S00-T88)

T63.024 - T63.332

⑦ T63.024 Toxic effect of coral snake venom, undetermined POA

6ᵗʰ T63.03 Toxic effect of taipan venom
- ⑦ T63.031 Toxic effect of taipan venom, accidental (unintentional) POA
  Toxic effect of taipan venom NOS
- ⑦ T63.032 Toxic effect of taipan venom, intentional self-harm POA HCC
- ⑦ T63.033 Toxic effect of taipan venom, assault POA
- ⑦ T63.034 Toxic effect of taipan venom, undetermined POA

6ᵗʰ T63.04 Toxic effect of cobra venom
- ⑦ T63.041 Toxic effect of cobra venom, accidental (unintentional) POA
  Toxic effect of cobra venom NOS
- ⑦ T63.042 Toxic effect of cobra venom, intentional self-harm POA HCC
- ⑦ T63.043 Toxic effect of cobra venom, assault POA
- ⑦ T63.044 Toxic effect of cobra venom, undetermined POA

6ᵗʰ T63.06 Toxic effect of venom of other North and South American snake
- ⑦ T63.061 Toxic effect of venom of other North and South American snake, accidental (unintentional) POA
  Toxic effect of venom of other North and South American snake NOS
- ⑦ T63.062 Toxic effect of venom of other North and South American snake, intentional self-harm POA HCC
- ⑦ T63.063 Toxic effect of venom of other North and South American snake, assault POA
- ⑦ T63.064 Toxic effect of venom of other North and South American snake, undetermined POA

6ᵗʰ T63.07 Toxic effect of venom of other Australian snake
- ⑦ T63.071 Toxic effect of venom of other Australian snake, accidental (unintentional) POA
  Toxic effect of venom of other Australian snake NOS
- ⑦ T63.072 Toxic effect of venom of other Australian snake, intentional self-harm POA HCC
- ⑦ T63.073 Toxic effect of venom of other Australian snake, assault POA
- ⑦ T63.074 Toxic effect of venom of other Australian snake, undetermined POA

6ᵗʰ T63.08 Toxic effect of venom of other African and Asian snake
- ⑦ T63.081 Toxic effect of venom of other African and Asian snake, accidental (unintentional) POA
  Toxic effect of venom of other African and Asian snake NOS
- ⑦ T63.082 Toxic effect of venom of other African and Asian snake, intentional self-harm POA HCC
- ⑦ T63.083 Toxic effect of venom of other African and Asian snake, assault POA
- ⑦ T63.084 Toxic effect of venom of other African and Asian snake, undetermined POA

6ᵗʰ T63.09 Toxic effect of venom of other snake
- ⑦ T63.091 Toxic effect of venom of other snake, accidental (unintentional) POA
  Toxic effect of venom of other snake NOS
- ⑦ T63.092 Toxic effect of venom of other snake, intentional self-harm POA HCC
- ⑦ T63.093 Toxic effect of venom of other snake, assault POA
- ⑦ T63.094 Toxic effect of venom of other snake, undetermined POA

5ᵗʰ T63.1 Toxic effect of venom of other reptiles
6ᵗʰ T63.11 Toxic effect of venom of gila monster
- ⑦ T63.111 Toxic effect of venom of gila monster, accidental (unintentional) POA
  Toxic effect of venom of gila monster NOS

⑦ T63.112 Toxic effect of venom of gila monster, intentional self-harm POA HCC
⑦ T63.113 Toxic effect of venom of gila monster, assault POA
⑦ T63.114 Toxic effect of venom of gila monster, undetermined POA

6ᵗʰ T63.12 Toxic effect of venom of other venomous lizard
- ⑦ T63.121 Toxic effect of venom of other venomous lizard, accidental (unintentional) POA
  Toxic effect of venom of other venomous lizard NOS
- ⑦ T63.122 Toxic effect of venom of other venomous lizard, intentional self-harm POA HCC
- ⑦ T63.123 Toxic effect of venom of other venomous lizard, assault POA
- ⑦ T63.124 Toxic effect of venom of other venomous lizard, undetermined POA

6ᵗʰ T63.19 Toxic effect of venom of other reptiles
- ⑦ T63.191 Toxic effect of venom of other reptiles, accidental (unintentional) POA
  Toxic effect of venom of other reptiles NOS
- ⑦ T63.192 Toxic effect of venom of other reptiles, intentional self-harm POA HCC
- ⑦ T63.193 Toxic effect of venom of other reptiles, assault POA
- ⑦ T63.194 Toxic effect of venom of other reptiles, undetermined POA

5ᵗʰ T63.2 Toxic effect of venom of scorpion
6ᵗʰ T63.2X Toxic effect of venom of scorpion
- ⑦ T63.2X1 Toxic effect of venom of scorpion, accidental (unintentional) POA
  Toxic effect of venom of scorpion NOS
- ⑦ T63.2X2 Toxic effect of venom of scorpion, intentional self-harm POA HCC
- ⑦ T63.2X3 Toxic effect of venom of scorpion, assault POA
- ⑦ T63.2X4 Toxic effect of venom of scorpion, undetermined POA

5ᵗʰ T63.3 Toxic effect of venom of spider
6ᵗʰ T63.30 Toxic effect of unspecified spider venom
- ⑦ T63.301 Toxic effect of unspecified spider venom, accidental (unintentional) POA
- ⑦ T63.302 Toxic effect of unspecified spider venom, intentional self-harm POA HCC
- ⑦ T63.303 Toxic effect of unspecified spider venom, assault POA
- ⑦ T63.304 Toxic effect of unspecified spider venom, undetermined POA

6ᵗʰ T63.31 Toxic effect of venom of black widow spider
- ⑦ T63.311 Toxic effect of venom of black widow spider, accidental (unintentional) POA
- ⑦ T63.312 Toxic effect of venom of black widow spider, intentional self-harm POA HCC
- ⑦ T63.313 Toxic effect of venom of black widow spider, assault POA
- ⑦ T63.314 Toxic effect of venom of black widow spider, undetermined POA

6ᵗʰ T63.32 Toxic effect of venom of tarantula
- ⑦ T63.321 Toxic effect of venom of tarantula, accidental (unintentional) POA
- ⑦ T63.322 Toxic effect of venom of tarantula, intentional self-harm POA HCC
- ⑦ T63.323 Toxic effect of venom of tarantula, assault POA
- ⑦ T63.324 Toxic effect of venom of tarantula, undetermined POA

6ᵗʰ T63.33 Toxic effect of venom of brown recluse spider
- ⑦ T63.331 Toxic effect of venom of brown recluse spider, accidental (unintentional) POA
- ⑦ T63.332 Toxic effect of venom of brown recluse spider, intentional self-harm POA HCC

POA⃠ Unacceptable principal diagnosis symbol per Medicare code edits   POA Code exempt from diagnosis present on admission requirement
❓ Questionable admission   CC Complication or comorbidity   MCC Major complication or comorbidity   CC/MCC EXC CC/MCC exclusion
HCC HCC diagnosis code   RHCC RxHCC diagnosis code   MACRA code   **DEFINITION** Describes condition/terminology
TIP Coding guidance   👁 Official Guideline Reference   Z1 Z code as first-listed diagnosis

1152   When symbols appear on a code that requires a 7th character extension, refer to Appendix B to identify applicable 7th character codes.   **2020 ICD-10-CM**

[7th] T63.333 Toxic effect of venom of brown recluse spider, assault [POA]
[7th] T63.334 Toxic effect of venom of brown recluse spider, undetermined [POA]
[6th] T63.39 Toxic effect of venom of other spider
[7th] T63.391 Toxic effect of venom of other spider, accidental (unintentional) [POA]
[7th] T63.392 Toxic effect of venom of other spider, intentional self-harm [POA] [HCC]
[7th] T63.393 Toxic effect of venom of other spider, assault [POA]
[7th] T63.394 Toxic effect of venom of other spider, undetermined [POA]
[5th] T63.4 Toxic effect of venom of other arthropods
[6th] T63.41 Toxic effect of venom of centipedes and venomous millipedes
[7th] T63.411 Toxic effect of venom of centipedes and venomous millipedes, accidental (unintentional) [POA]
[7th] T63.412 Toxic effect of venom of centipedes and venomous millipedes, intentional self-harm [POA] [HCC]
[7th] T63.413 Toxic effect of venom of centipedes and venomous millipedes, assault [POA]
[7th] T63.414 Toxic effect of venom of centipedes and venomous millipedes, undetermined [POA]
[6th] T63.42 Toxic effect of venom of ants
[7th] T63.421 Toxic effect of venom of ants, accidental (unintentional) [POA]
[7th] T63.422 Toxic effect of venom of ants, intentional self-harm [POA] [HCC]
[7th] T63.423 Toxic effect of venom of ants, assault [POA]
[7th] T63.424 Toxic effect of venom of ants, undetermined [POA]
[6th] T63.43 Toxic effect of venom of caterpillars
[7th] T63.431 Toxic effect of venom of caterpillars, accidental (unintentional) [POA]
[7th] T63.432 Toxic effect of venom of caterpillars, intentional self-harm [POA] [HCC]
[7th] T63.433 Toxic effect of venom of caterpillars, assault [POA]
[7th] T63.434 Toxic effect of venom of caterpillars, undetermined [POA]
[6th] T63.44 Toxic effect of venom of bees
[7th] T63.441 Toxic effect of venom of bees, accidental (unintentional) [POA]
[7th] T63.442 Toxic effect of venom of bees, intentional self-harm [POA] [HCC]
[7th] T63.443 Toxic effect of venom of bees, assault [POA]
[7th] T63.444 Toxic effect of venom of bees, undetermined [POA]
[6th] T63.45 Toxic effect of venom of hornets
[7th] T63.451 Toxic effect of venom of hornets, accidental (unintentional) [POA]
[7th] T63.452 Toxic effect of venom of hornets, intentional self-harm [POA] [HCC]
[7th] T63.453 Toxic effect of venom of hornets, assault [POA]
[7th] T63.454 Toxic effect of venom of hornets, undetermined [POA]
[6th] T63.46 Toxic effect of venom of wasps
Toxic effect of yellow jacket
[7th] T63.461 Toxic effect of venom of wasps, accidental (unintentional) [POA]
[7th] T63.462 Toxic effect of venom of wasps, intentional self-harm [POA] [HCC]
[7th] T63.463 Toxic effect of venom of wasps, assault [POA]
[7th] T63.464 Toxic effect of venom of wasps, undetermined [POA]
[6th] T63.48 Toxic effect of venom of other arthropod
[7th] T63.481 Toxic effect of venom of other arthropod, accidental (unintentional) [POA]
[7th] T63.482 Toxic effect of venom of other arthropod, intentional self-harm [POA] [HCC]
[7th] T63.483 Toxic effect of venom of other arthropod, assault [POA]
[7th] T63.484 Toxic effect of venom of other arthropod, undetermined [POA]
[5th] T63.5 Toxic effect of contact with venomous fish
EXCLUDES2 *poisoning by ingestion of fish (T61.-)*
[6th] T63.51 Toxic effect of contact with stingray
[7th] T63.511 Toxic effect of contact with stingray, accidental (unintentional) [POA]
[7th] T63.512 Toxic effect of contact with stingray, intentional self-harm [POA] [HCC]
[7th] T63.513 Toxic effect of contact with stingray, assault [POA]
[7th] T63.514 Toxic effect of contact with stingray, undetermined [POA]
[6th] T63.59 Toxic effect of contact with other venomous fish
[7th] T63.591 Toxic effect of contact with other venomous fish, accidental (unintentional) [POA]
[7th] T63.592 Toxic effect of contact with other venomous fish, intentional self-harm [POA] [HCC]
[7th] T63.593 Toxic effect of contact with other venomous fish, assault [POA]
[7th] T63.594 Toxic effect of contact with other venomous fish, undetermined [POA]
[5th] T63.6 Toxic effect of contact with other venomous marine animals
EXCLUDES1 *sea-snake venom (T63.09)*
EXCLUDES2 *poisoning by ingestion of shellfish (T61.78-)*
[6th] T63.61 Toxic effect of contact with Portugese Man-o-war
Toxic effect of contact with bluebottle
[7th] T63.611 Toxic effect of contact with Portugese Man-o-war, accidental (unintentional) [POA]
[7th] T63.612 Toxic effect of contact with Portugese Man-o-war, intentional self-harm [POA] [HCC]
[7th] T63.613 Toxic effect of contact with Portugese Man-o-war, assault [POA]
[7th] T63.614 Toxic effect of contact with Portugese Man-o-war, undetermined [POA]
[6th] T63.62 Toxic effect of contact with other jellyfish
[7th] T63.621 Toxic effect of contact with other jellyfish, accidental (unintentional) [POA]
[7th] T63.622 Toxic effect of contact with other jellyfish, intentional self-harm [POA] [HCC]
[7th] T63.623 Toxic effect of contact with other jellyfish, assault [POA]
[7th] T63.624 Toxic effect of contact with other jellyfish, undetermined [POA]
[6th] T63.63 Toxic effect of contact with sea anemone
[7th] T63.631 Toxic effect of contact with sea anemone, accidental (unintentional) [POA]
[7th] T63.632 Toxic effect of contact with sea anemone, intentional self-harm [POA] [HCC]
[7th] T63.633 Toxic effect of contact with sea anemone, assault [POA]
[7th] T63.634 Toxic effect of contact with sea anemone, undetermined [POA]
[6th] T63.69 Toxic effect of contact with other venomous marine animals
[7th] T63.691 Toxic effect of contact with other venomous marine animals, accidental (unintentional) [POA]
[7th] T63.692 Toxic effect of contact with other venomous marine animals, intentional self-harm [POA] [HCC]
[7th] T63.693 Toxic effect of contact with other venomous marine animals, assault [POA]
[7th] T63.694 Toxic effect of contact with other venomous marine animals, undetermined [POA]

Unspecified Code Other Specified Code Manifestation Code [N] Newborn [P] Pediatric [M] Maternity [A] Adult ♂ Male ♀ Female
● New Code ▲ Revised Code Title ►◄ Revised Text NOTES INCLUDES EXCLUDES1 Not coded here EXCLUDES2 Not included here
[4th] 4th character required [5th] 5th character required [6th] 6th character required [7th] 7th character required [X] Extension 'X' Alert
[HAC] Hospital-acquired condition (HAC) alert AHA AHA Coding Clinic© Code first alert

5ᵗʰ **T63.7** **Toxic effect of contact with venomous plant**
 6ᵗʰ **T63.71** **Toxic effect of contact with** venomous marine plant
  7ᵗʰ **T63.711** **Toxic effect of contact with venomous marine plant,** accidental (unintentional) POA
  7ᵗʰ **T63.712** **Toxic effect of contact with venomous marine plant,** intentional self-harm POA HCC
  7ᵗʰ **T63.713** **Toxic effect of contact with venomous marine plant,** assault POA
  7ᵗʰ **T63.714** **Toxic effect of contact with venomous marine plant,** undetermined POA
 6ᵗʰ **T63.79** **Toxic effect of contact with** other venomous plant
  7ᵗʰ **T63.791** **Toxic effect of contact with other venomous plant,** accidental (unintentional) POA
  7ᵗʰ **T63.792** **Toxic effect of contact with other venomous plant,** intentional self-harm POA HCC
  7ᵗʰ **T63.793** **Toxic effect of contact with other venomous plant,** assault POA
  7ᵗʰ **T63.794** **Toxic effect of contact with other venomous plant,** undetermined POA

5ᵗʰ **T63.8** **Toxic effect of** contact with other venomous animals
 6ᵗʰ **T63.81** **Toxic effect of contact with venomous** frog
  EXCLUDES1 *contact with nonvenomous frog (W62.0)*
  7ᵗʰ **T63.811** **Toxic effect of contact with venomous frog,** accidental (unintentional) POA
  7ᵗʰ **T63.812** **Toxic effect of contact with venomous frog,** intentional self-harm POA HCC
  7ᵗʰ **T63.813** **Toxic effect of contact with venomous frog,** assault POA
  7ᵗʰ **T63.814** **Toxic effect of contact with venomous frog,** undetermined POA
 6ᵗʰ **T63.82** **Toxic effect of contact with venomous** toad
  EXCLUDES1 *contact with nonvenomous toad (W62.1)*
  7ᵗʰ **T63.821** **Toxic effect of contact with venomous toad,** accidental (unintentional) POA
  7ᵗʰ **T63.822** **Toxic effect of contact with venomous toad,** intentional self-harm POA HCC
  7ᵗʰ **T63.823** **Toxic effect of contact with venomous toad,** assault POA
  7ᵗʰ **T63.824** **Toxic effect of contact with venomous toad,** undetermined POA
 6ᵗʰ **T63.83** **Toxic effect of contact with** other venomous amphibian
  EXCLUDES1 *contact with nonvenomous amphibian (W62.9)*
  7ᵗʰ **T63.831** **Toxic effect of contact with other venomous amphibian,** accidental (unintentional) POA
  7ᵗʰ **T63.832** **Toxic effect of contact with other venomous amphibian,** intentional self-harm POA HCC
  7ᵗʰ **T63.833** **Toxic effect of contact with other venomous amphibian,** assault POA
  7ᵗʰ **T63.834** **Toxic effect of contact with other venomous amphibian,** undetermined POA
 6ᵗʰ **T63.89** **Toxic effect of contact with** other venomous animals
  7ᵗʰ **T63.891** **Toxic effect of contact with other venomous animals,** accidental (unintentional) POA
  7ᵗʰ **T63.892** **Toxic effect of contact with other venomous animals,** intentional self-harm POA HCC
  7ᵗʰ **T63.893** **Toxic effect of contact with other venomous animals,** assault POA
  7ᵗʰ **T63.894** **Toxic effect of contact with other venomous animals,** undetermined POA

5ᵗʰ **T63.9** **Toxic effect of contact with unspecified venomous animal**
 7ᵗʰ **T63.91** **Toxic effect of contact with unspecified venomous animal,** accidental (unintentional) POA

 7ᵗʰ **T63.92** **Toxic effect of contact with unspecified venomous animal,** intentional self-harm POA HCC
 7ᵗʰ **T63.93** **Toxic effect of contact with unspecified venomous animal,** assault POA
 7ᵗʰ **T63.94** **Toxic effect of contact with unspecified venomous animal,** undetermined POA

4ᵗʰ **T64** **Toxic effect of** aflatoxin and other mycotoxin food contaminants
The appropriate 7th character is to be added to each code from category T64
 A = initial encounter
 D = subsequent encounter
 S = sequela
 5ᵗʰ **T64.0** **Toxic effect of** aflatoxin
  7ᵗʰ **T64.01** **Toxic effect of aflatoxin,** accidental (unintentional) POA
  7ᵗʰ **T64.02** **Toxic effect of aflatoxin,** intentional self-harm POA HCC
  7ᵗʰ **T64.03** **Toxic effect of aflatoxin,** assault POA
  7ᵗʰ **T64.04** **Toxic effect of aflatoxin,** undetermined POA
 5ᵗʰ **T64.8** **Toxic effect of** other mycotoxin food contaminants
  7ᵗʰ **T64.81** **Toxic effect of other mycotoxin food contaminants,** accidental (unintentional) POA
  7ᵗʰ **T64.82** **Toxic effect of other mycotoxin food contaminants,** intentional self-harm POA HCC
  7ᵗʰ **T64.83** **Toxic effect of other mycotoxin food contaminants,** assault POA
  7ᵗʰ **T64.84** **Toxic effect of other mycotoxin food contaminants,** undetermined POA

4ᵗʰ **T65** **Toxic effect of** other and unspecified substances
The appropriate 7th character is to be added to each code from category T65
 A = initial encounter
 D = subsequent encounter
 S = sequela
 5ᵗʰ **T65.0** **Toxic effect of** cyanides
  EXCLUDES1 *hydrogen cyanide (T57.3-)*
  6ᵗʰ **T65.0X** **Toxic effect of** cyanides
   7ᵗʰ **T65.0X1** **Toxic effect of cyanides,** accidental (unintentional) POA
    Toxic effect of cyanides NOS
   7ᵗʰ **T65.0X2** **Toxic effect of cyanides,** intentional self-harm POA HCC
   7ᵗʰ **T65.0X3** **Toxic effect of cyanides,** assault POA
   7ᵗʰ **T65.0X4** **Toxic effect of cyanides,** undetermined POA
 5ᵗʰ **T65.1** **Toxic effect of strychnine and its salts**
  6ᵗʰ **T65.1X** **Toxic effect of** strychnine and its salts
   7ᵗʰ **T65.1X1** **Toxic effect of strychnine and its salts,** accidental (unintentional) POA
    Toxic effect of strychnine and its salts NOS
   7ᵗʰ **T65.1X2** **Toxic effect of strychnine and its salts,** intentional self-harm POA HCC
   7ᵗʰ **T65.1X3** **Toxic effect of strychnine and its salts,** assault POA
   7ᵗʰ **T65.1X4** **Toxic effect of strychnine and its salts,** undetermined POA
 5ᵗʰ **T65.2** **Toxic effect of** tobacco and nicotine
  EXCLUDES2 *nicotine dependence (F17.-)*
  6ᵗʰ **T65.21** **Toxic effect of** chewing tobacco
   7ᵗʰ **T65.211** **Toxic effect of chewing tobacco,** accidental (unintentional) POA
    Toxic effect of chewing tobacco NOS
   7ᵗʰ **T65.212** **Toxic effect of chewing tobacco,** intentional self-harm POA HCC
   7ᵗʰ **T65.213** **Toxic effect of chewing tobacco,** assault POA
   7ᵗʰ **T65.214** **Toxic effect of chewing tobacco,** undetermined POA
  6ᵗʰ **T65.22** **Toxic effect of** tobacco cigarettes
   Toxic effect of tobacco smoke
   Use additional code for exposure to second hand tobacco smoke (Z57.31, Z77.22)
   7ᵗʰ **T65.221** **Toxic effect of tobacco cigarettes,** accidental (unintentional) POA
    Toxic effect of tobacco cigarettes NOS

[7th] T65.222 Toxic effect of tobacco cigarettes, intentional self-harm [POA] [HCC]

[7th] T65.223 Toxic effect of tobacco cigarettes, assault [POA]

[7th] T65.224 Toxic effect of tobacco cigarettes, undetermined [POA]

[6th] T65.29 Toxic effect of other tobacco and nicotine

[7th] T65.291 Toxic effect of other tobacco and nicotine, accidental (unintentional) [POA]
Toxic effect of other tobacco and nicotine NOS

[7th] T65.292 Toxic effect of other tobacco and nicotine, intentional self-harm [POA] [HCC]

[7th] T65.293 Toxic effect of other tobacco and nicotine, assault [POA]

[7th] T65.294 Toxic effect of other tobacco and nicotine, undetermined [POA]

[5th] T65.3 Toxic effect of nitroderivatives and aminoderivatives of benzene and its homologues
Toxic effect of anilin [benzenamine]
Toxic effect of nitrobenzene
Toxic effect of trinitrotoluene

[6th] T65.3X Toxic effect of nitroderivatives and aminoderivatives of benzene and its homologues

[7th] T65.3X1 Toxic effect of nitroderivatives and aminoderivatives of benzene and its homologues, accidental (unintentional) [POA]
Toxic effect of nitroderivatives and aminoderivatives of benzene and its homologues NOS

[7th] T65.3X2 Toxic effect of nitroderivatives and aminoderivatives of benzene and its homologues, intentional self-harm [POA] [HCC]

[7th] T65.3X3 Toxic effect of nitroderivatives and aminoderivatives of benzene and its homologues, assault [POA]

[7th] T65.3X4 Toxic effect of nitroderivatives and aminoderivatives of benzene and its homologues, undetermined [POA]

[5th] T65.4 Toxic effect of carbon disulfide

[6th] T65.4X Toxic effect of carbon disulfide

[7th] T65.4X1 Toxic effect of carbon disulfide, accidental (unintentional) [POA]
Toxic effect of carbon disulfide NOS

[7th] T65.4X2 Toxic effect of carbon disulfide, intentional self-harm [POA] [HCC]

[7th] T65.4X3 Toxic effect of carbon disulfide, assault [POA]

[7th] T65.4X4 Toxic effect of carbon disulfide, undetermined [POA]

[5th] T65.5 Toxic effect of nitroglycerin and other nitric acids and esters
Toxic effect of 1,2,3-Propanetriol trinitrate

[6th] T65.5X Toxic effect of nitroglycerin and other nitric acids and esters

[7th] T65.5X1 Toxic effect of nitroglycerin and other nitric acids and esters, accidental (unintentional) [POA]
Toxic effect of nitroglycerin and other nitric acids and esters NOS

[7th] T65.5X2 Toxic effect of nitroglycerin and other nitric acids and esters, intentional self-harm [POA] [HCC]

[7th] T65.5X3 Toxic effect of nitroglycerin and other nitric acids and esters, assault [POA]

[7th] T65.5X4 Toxic effect of nitroglycerin and other nitric acids and esters, undetermined [POA]

[5th] T65.6 Toxic effect of paints and dyes, not elsewhere classified

[6th] T65.6X Toxic effect of paints and dyes, not elsewhere classified

[7th] T65.6X1 Toxic effect of paints and dyes, not elsewhere classified, accidental (unintentional) [POA]
Toxic effect of paints and dyes NOS

[7th] T65.6X2 Toxic effect of paints and dyes, not elsewhere classified, intentional self-harm [POA] [HCC]

[7th] T65.6X3 Toxic effect of paints and dyes, not elsewhere classified, assault [POA]

[7th] T65.6X4 Toxic effect of paints and dyes, not elsewhere classified, undetermined [POA]

[5th] T65.8 Toxic effect of other specified substances

[6th] T65.81 Toxic effect of latex

[7th] T65.811 Toxic effect of latex, accidental (unintentional) [POA]
Toxic effect of latex NOS

[7th] T65.812 Toxic effect of latex, intentional self-harm [POA] [HCC]

[7th] T65.813 Toxic effect of latex, assault [POA]

[7th] T65.814 Toxic effect of latex, undetermined [POA]

[6th] T65.82 Toxic effect of harmful algae and algae toxins
Toxic effect of (harmful) algae bloom NOS
Toxic effect of blue-green algae bloom
Toxic effect of brown tide
Toxic effect of cyanobacteria bloom
Toxic effect of Florida red tide
Toxic effect of pfiesteria piscicida
Toxic effect of red tide

[7th] T65.821 Toxic effect of harmful algae and algae toxins, accidental (unintentional) [POA]
Toxic effect of harmful algae and algae toxins NOS

[7th] T65.822 Toxic effect of harmful algae and algae toxins, intentional self-harm [POA] [HCC]

[7th] T65.823 Toxic effect of harmful algae and algae toxins, assault [POA]

[7th] T65.824 Toxic effect of harmful algae and algae toxins, undetermined [POA]

[6th] T65.83 Toxic effect of fiberglass

[7th] T65.831 Toxic effect of fiberglass, accidental (unintentional) [POA]
Toxic effect of fiberglass NOS

[7th] T65.832 Toxic effect of fiberglass, intentional self-harm [POA] [HCC]

[7th] T65.833 Toxic effect of fiberglass, assault [POA]

[7th] T65.834 Toxic effect of fiberglass, undetermined [POA]

[6th] T65.89 Toxic effect of other specified substances

[7th] T65.891 Toxic effect of other specified substances, accidental (unintentional) [POA]
AHA: Q1 2018
Toxic effect of other specified substances NOS

[7th] T65.892 Toxic effect of other specified substances, intentional self-harm [POA] [HCC]

[7th] T65.893 Toxic effect of other specified substances, assault [POA]

[7th] T65.894 Toxic effect of other specified substances, undetermined [POA]

[5th] T65.9 Toxic effect of unspecified substance

[7th] T65.91 Toxic effect of unspecified substance, accidental (unintentional) [POA]
Poisoning NOS

[7th] T65.92 Toxic effect of unspecified substance, intentional self-harm [POA] [HCC]

[7th] T65.93 Toxic effect of unspecified substance, assault [POA]

[7th] T65.94 Toxic effect of unspecified substance, undetermined [POA]

Unspecified Code | Other Specified Code | Manifestation Code | [N] Newborn | [P] Pediatric | [M] Maternity | [A] Adult | ♂ Male | ♀ Female
● New Code | ▲ Revised Code Title | ►◄ Revised Text | NOTES | INCLUDES | EXCLUDES1 Not coded here | EXCLUDES2 Not included here
[4th] 4th character required | [5th] 5th character required | [6th] 6th character required | [7th] 7th character required | [7th] Extension 'X' Alert
[HAC] Hospital-acquired condition (HAC) alert | AHA AHA Coding Clinic© | ☞ Code first alert

Other and unspecified effects of external causes (T66-T78)

[7th] **T66 Radiation sickness, unspecified** POA
[EXCLUDES1] *specified adverse effects of radiation, such as:*
burns (T20-T31)
leukemia (C91-C95)
radiation gastroenteritis and colitis (K52.0)
radiation pneumonitis (J70.0)
radiation related disorders of the skin and subcutaneous tissue (L55-L59)
sunburn (L55.-)

The appropriate 7th character is to be added to code T66
A = initial encounter
D = subsequent encounter
S = sequela

[4th] **T67 Effects of heat and light**
[EXCLUDES1] *erythema [dermatitis] ab igne (L59.0)*
malignant hyperpyrexia due to anesthesia (T88.3)
radiation-related disorders of the skin and subcutaneous tissue (L55-L59)
[EXCLUDES2] *burns (T20-T31)*
sunburn (L55.-)
sweat disorder due to heat (L74-L75)

The appropriate 7th character is to be added to each code from category T67
A = initial encounter
D = subsequent encounter
S = sequela

[5th] **T67.0 Heatstroke and sunstroke**
Use additional code(s) to identify any associated complications of heatstroke, such as:
coma and stupor (R40.-)
rhabdomyolysis (M62.82)
systemic inflammatory response syndrome (R65.1-)

● [7th] **T67.01 Heatstroke and sunstroke** CC CC/MCC Exc
Heat apoplexy
Heat pyrexia
Siriasis
Thermoplegia

● [7th] **T67.02 Exertional heatstroke** CC CC/MCC Exc
● [7th] **T67.09 Other heatstroke and sunstroke** CC CC/MCC Exc

[7th] **T67.1 Heat syncope** POA
Heat collapse
[7th] **T67.2 Heat cramp** POA
[7th] **T67.3 Heat exhaustion, anhydrotic** POA
Heat prostration due to water depletion
[EXCLUDES1] *heat exhaustion due to salt depletion (T67.4)*
[7th] **T67.4 Heat exhaustion due to salt depletion** POA
Heat prostration due to salt (and water) depletion
[7th] **T67.5 Heat exhaustion, unspecified** POA
Heat prostration NOS
[7th] **T67.6 Heat fatigue, transient** POA
[7th] **T67.7 Heat edema** POA
[7th] **T67.8 Other effects of heat and light** POA
[7th] **T67.9 Effect of heat and light, unspecified** POA

[7th] **T68 Hypothermia** POA
Accidental hypothermia
Hypothermia NOS
Use additional code to identify source of exposure:
Exposure to excessive cold of man-made origin (W93)
Exposure to excessive cold of natural origin (X31)
[EXCLUDES1] *hypothermia following anesthesia (T88.51)*
hypothermia not associated with low environmental temperature (R68.0)
hypothermia of newborn (P80.-)
[EXCLUDES2] *frostbite (T33-T34)*

The appropriate 7th character is to be added to code T68
A = initial encounter
D = subsequent encounter
S = sequela

[4th] **T69 Other effects of reduced temperature**
Use additional code to identify source of exposure:
Exposure to excessive cold of man-made origin (W93)
Exposure to excessive cold of natural origin (X31)
[EXCLUDES2] *frostbite (T33-T34)*

The appropriate 7th character is to be added to each code from category T69
A = initial encounter
D = subsequent encounter
S = sequela

[5th] **T69.0 Immersion hand and foot**
[6th] **T69.01 Immersion hand**
[7th] **T69.011 Immersion hand, right hand** POA
[7th] **T69.012 Immersion hand, left hand** POA
[7th] **T69.019 Immersion hand, unspecified hand** POA
[6th] **T69.02 Immersion foot**
Trench foot
[7th] **T69.021 Immersion foot, right foot** CC POA HAC CC/MCC Exc
[7th] **T69.022 Immersion foot, left foot** CC POA HAC CC/MCC Exc
[7th] **T69.029 Immersion foot, unspecified foot** CC POA HAC CC/MCC Exc
[7th] **T69.1 Chilblains** POA
[7th] **T69.8 Other specified effects of reduced temperature** POA
[7th] **T69.9 Effect of reduced temperature, unspecified** POA

[4th] **T70 Effects of air pressure and water pressure**

The appropriate 7th character is to be added to each code from category T70
A = initial encounter
D = subsequent encounter
S = sequela

[7th] **T70.0 Otitic barotrauma** POA
Aero-otitis media
Effects of change in ambient atmospheric pressure or water pressure on ears
[7th] **T70.1 Sinus barotrauma** POA
Aerosinusitis
Effects of change in ambient atmospheric pressure on sinuses
[5th] **T70.2 Other and unspecified effects of high altitude**
[EXCLUDES2] *polycythemia due to high altitude (D75.1)*
[7th] **T70.20 Unspecified effects of high altitude** POA
[7th] **T70.29 Other effects of high altitude** POA
Alpine sickness
Anoxia due to high altitude
Barotrauma NOS
Hypobaropathy
Mountain sickness
[7th] **T70.3 Caisson disease [decompression sickness]** CC POA HAC CC/MCC Exc
Compressed-air disease
Diver's palsy or paralysis
[7th] **T70.4 Effects of high-pressure fluids** POA
Hydraulic jet injection (industrial)
Pneumatic jet injection (industrial)
Traumatic jet injection (industrial)
[7th] **T70.8 Other effects of air pressure and water pressure** POA
[7th] **T70.9 Effect of air pressure and water pressure, unspecified** POA

[4th] **T71 Asphyxiation**
Mechanical suffocation
Traumatic suffocation
[EXCLUDES1] *acute respiratory distress (syndrome) (J80)*
anoxia due to high altitude (T70.2)
asphyxia NOS (R09.01)
asphyxia from carbon monoxide (T58.-)
asphyxia from inhalation of food or foreign body (T17.-)
asphyxia from other gases, fumes and vapors (T59.-)
respiratory distress (syndrome) in newborn (P22.-)

PDx Unacceptable principal diagnosis symbol per Medicare code edits · POA Code exempt from diagnosis present on admission requirement
? Questionable admission · CC Complication or comorbidity · MCC Major complication or comorbidity · CC/MCC Exc CC/MCC exclusion
HCC HCC diagnosis code · RxHCC RxHCC diagnosis code · MACRA code · **DEFINITION** Describes condition/terminology
TIP Coding guidance · Official Guideline Reference · Z1 Z code as first-listed diagnosis

The appropriate 7th character is to be added to each code from category T71
- A = initial encounter
- D = subsequent encounter
- S = sequela

🔵 **T71.1** Asphyxiation due to mechanical threat to breathing
Suffocation due to mechanical threat to breathing

🔵 **T71.11** Asphyxiation due to smothering under pillow

🔹 **T71.111** Asphyxiation due to smothering under pillow, accidental `CC` `POA` `HAC` `CC/MCC Exc`
Asphyxiation due to smothering under pillow NOS

🔹 **T71.112** Asphyxiation due to smothering under pillow, intentional self-harm `CC` `POA` `HAC` `HCC` `CC/MCC Exc`

🔹 **T71.113** Asphyxiation due to smothering under pillow, assault `CC` `POA` `HAC` `CC/MCC Exc`

🔹 **T71.114** Asphyxiation due to smothering under pillow, undetermined `CC` `POA` `HAC` `CC/MCC Exc`

🔵 **T71.12** Asphyxiation due to plastic bag

🔹 **T71.121** Asphyxiation due to plastic bag, accidental `CC` `POA` `HAC` `CC/MCC Exc`
Asphyxiation due to plastic bag NOS

🔹 **T71.122** Asphyxiation due to plastic bag, intentional self-harm `CC` `POA` `HAC` `HCC` `CC/MCC Exc`

🔹 **T71.123** Asphyxiation due to plastic bag, assault `CC` `POA` `HAC` `CC/MCC Exc`

🔹 **T71.124** Asphyxiation due to plastic bag, undetermined `CC` `POA` `HAC` `CC/MCC Exc`

🔵 **T71.13** Asphyxiation due to being trapped in bed linens

🔹 **T71.131** Asphyxiation due to being trapped in bed linens, accidental `CC` `POA` `HAC` `CC/MCC Exc`
Asphyxiation due to being trapped in bed linens NOS

🔹 **T71.132** Asphyxiation due to being trapped in bed linens, intentional self-harm `CC` `POA` `HAC` `HCC` `CC/MCC Exc`

🔹 **T71.133** Asphyxiation due to being trapped in bed linens, assault `CC` `POA` `HAC` `CC/MCC Exc`

🔹 **T71.134** Asphyxiation due to being trapped in bed linens, undetermined `CC` `POA` `HAC` `CC/MCC Exc`

🔵 **T71.14** Asphyxiation due to smothering under another person's body (in bed)

🔹 **T71.141** Asphyxiation due to smothering under another person's body (in bed), accidental `CC` `POA` `HAC` `CC/MCC Exc`
Asphyxiation due to smothering under another person's body (in bed) NOS

🔹 **T71.143** Asphyxiation due to smothering under another person's body (in bed), assault `CC` `POA` `HAC` `CC/MCC Exc`

🔹 **T71.144** Asphyxiation due to smothering under another person's body (in bed), undetermined `CC` `POA` `HAC` `CC/MCC Exc`

🔵 **T71.15** Asphyxiation due to smothering in furniture

🔹 **T71.151** Asphyxiation due to smothering in furniture, accidental `CC` `POA` `HAC` `CC/MCC Exc`
Asphyxiation due to smothering in furniture NOS

🔹 **T71.152** Asphyxiation due to smothering in furniture, intentional self-harm `CC` `POA` `HAC` `HCC` `CC/MCC Exc`

🔹 **T71.153** Asphyxiation due to smothering in furniture, assault `CC` `POA` `HAC` `CC/MCC Exc`

🔹 **T71.154** Asphyxiation due to smothering in furniture, undetermined `CC` `POA` `HAC` `CC/MCC Exc`

🔵 **T71.16** Asphyxiation due to hanging
Hanging by window shade cord
Use additional code for any associated injuries, such as:
crushing injury of neck (S17.-)
fracture of cervical vertebrae (S12.0-S12.2-)
open wound of neck (S11.-)

🔹 **T71.161** Asphyxiation due to hanging, accidental `CC` `POA` `HAC` `CC/MCC Exc`
Asphyxiation due to hanging NOS
Hanging NOS

🔹 **T71.162** Asphyxiation due to hanging, intentional self-harm `CC` `POA` `HAC` `HCC` `CC/MCC Exc`

🔹 **T71.163** Asphyxiation due to hanging, assault `CC` `POA` `HAC` `CC/MCC Exc`

🔹 **T71.164** Asphyxiation due to hanging, undetermined `CC` `POA` `HAC` `CC/MCC Exc`

🔵 **T71.19** Asphyxiation due to mechanical threat to breathing due to other causes

🔹 **T71.191** Asphyxiation due to mechanical threat to breathing due to other causes, accidental `CC` `POA` `HAC` `CC/MCC Exc`
AHA: Q4 2016
Asphyxiation due to other causes NOS

🔹 **T71.192** Asphyxiation due to mechanical threat to breathing due to other causes, intentional self-harm `CC` `POA` `HAC` `HCC` `CC/MCC Exc`

🔹 **T71.193** Asphyxiation due to mechanical threat to breathing due to other causes, assault `CC` `POA` `HAC` `CC/MCC Exc`

🔹 **T71.194** Asphyxiation due to mechanical threat to breathing due to other causes, undetermined `CC` `POA` `HAC` `CC/MCC Exc`

🔵 **T71.2** Asphyxiation due to systemic oxygen deficiency due to low oxygen content in ambient air
Suffocation due to systemic oxygen deficiency due to low oxygen content in ambient air

🔹 **T71.20** Asphyxiation due to systemic oxygen deficiency due to low oxygen content in ambient air due to unspecified cause `CC` `POA` `HAC` `CC/MCC Exc`

🔹 **T71.21** Asphyxiation due to cave-in or falling earth `CC` `POA` `HAC` `CC/MCC Exc`
Use additional code for any associated cataclysm (X34-X38)

🔵 **T71.22** Asphyxiation due to being trapped in a car trunk

🔹 **T71.221** Asphyxiation due to being trapped in a car trunk, accidental `CC` `POA` `CC/MCC Exc`

🔹 **T71.222** Asphyxiation due to being trapped in a car trunk, intentional self-harm `CC` `POA` `HCC` `CC/MCC Exc`

🔹 **T71.223** Asphyxiation due to being trapped in a car trunk, assault `CC` `POA` `CC/MCC Exc`

🔹 **T71.224** Asphyxiation due to being trapped in a car trunk, undetermined `CC` `POA` `CC/MCC Exc`

🔵 **T71.23** Asphyxiation due to being trapped in a (discarded) refrigerator

🔹 **T71.231** Asphyxiation due to being trapped in a (discarded) refrigerator, accidental `CC` `POA` `CC/MCC Exc`

🔹 **T71.232** Asphyxiation due to being trapped in a (discarded) refrigerator, intentional self-harm `CC` `POA` `HCC` `CC/MCC Exc`

🔹 **T71.233** Asphyxiation due to being trapped in a (discarded) refrigerator, assault `CC` `POA` `CC/MCC Exc`

🔹 **T71.234** Asphyxiation due to being trapped in a (discarded) refrigerator, undetermined `CC` `POA` `CC/MCC Exc`

🔹 **T71.29** Asphyxiation due to being trapped in other low oxygen environment `CC` `POA` `HAC` `CC/MCC Exc`

🔹 **T71.9** Asphyxiation due to unspecified cause `CC` `POA` `HAC` `CC/MCC Exc`
Suffocation (by strangulation) due to unspecified cause
Suffocation NOS
Systemic oxygen deficiency due to low oxygen content in ambient air due to unspecified cause
Systemic oxygen deficiency due to mechanical threat to breathing due to unspecified cause
Traumatic asphyxia NOS

🔵 **T73** Effects of other deprivation
The appropriate 7th character is to be added to each code from category T73
- A = initial encounter
- D = subsequent encounter
- S = sequela

Unspecified Code Other Specified Code Manifestation Code Ⓝ Newborn Ⓟ Pediatric Ⓜ Maternity Ⓐ Adult ♂ Male ♀ Female
● New Code ▲ Revised Code Title ►◄ Revised Text **NOTES** *INCLUDES* *EXCLUDES1* Not coded here *EXCLUDES2* Not included here
4th character required 5th character required 6th character required 7th character required Extension 'X' Alert
`HAC` Hospital-acquired condition (HAC) alert **AHA** AHA Coding Clinic© ☛ Code first alert

2020 ICD-10-CM   When symbols appear on a code that requires a 7th character extension, refer to Appendix B to identify applicable 7th character codes.   **1157**

7ᵗʰ **T73.0 Starvation**   POA
       Deprivation of food
7ᵗʰ **T73.1 Deprivation of** water   POA
7ᵗʰ **T73.2 Exhaustion due to** exposure   POA
7ᵗʰ **T73.3 Exhaustion due to** excessive exertion   POA
       Exhaustion due to overexertion
7ᵗʰ **T73.8 Other effects of deprivation**   POA
7ᵗʰ **T73.9 Effect of deprivation, unspecified**   POA

4ᵗʰ **T74 Adult and child abuse, neglect and other maltreatment,** confirmed
       👁 **See Official Guidelines** "Factitious Disorder" I.C.5.c, "Adult and
          child abuse, neglect and other maltreatment" I.C.19.f
       Use additional code, if applicable, to identify any associated current
          injury
       Use additional external cause code to identify perpetrator, if known
          (Y07.-)

       EXCLUDES1 abuse and maltreatment in pregnancy (O9A.3-, O9A.4-,
                   O9A.5-)
                   adult and child maltreatment, suspected (T76.-)

       **The appropriate 7th character is to be added to each code from
       category T74**
          A = initial encounter
          D = subsequent encounter
          S = sequela

5ᵗʰ **T74.0 Neglect or abandonment, confirmed**
7ᵗʰ   **T74.01 Adult neglect or abandonment,
                 confirmed**   A CC POA CC/MCC Exc
7ᵗʰ   **T74.02 Child neglect or abandonment,
                 confirmed**   P CC POA CC/MCC Exc
5ᵗʰ **T74.1 Physical abuse, confirmed**
          EXCLUDES2 sexual abuse (T74.2-)
7ᵗʰ   **T74.11 Adult physical abuse, confirmed**   A CC POA CC/MCC Exc
7ᵗʰ   **T74.12 Child physical abuse, confirmed**   P CC POA CC/MCC Exc
          EXCLUDES2 shaken infant syndrome (T74.4)
5ᵗʰ **T74.2 Sexual abuse, confirmed**
          Rape, confirmed
          Sexual assault, confirmed
7ᵗʰ   **T74.21 Adult sexual abuse, confirmed**   A CC POA CC/MCC Exc
7ᵗʰ   **T74.22 Child sexual abuse, confirmed**   P CC POA CC/MCC Exc
5ᵗʰ **T74.3 Psychological abuse, confirmed**
          Bullying and intimidation, confirmed
          Intimidation through social media, confirmed
7ᵗʰ   **T74.31 Adult psychological abuse, confirmed**   A POA
7ᵗʰ   **T74.32 Child psychological abuse, confirmed**   P CC POA CC/MCC Exc
7ᵗʰ **T74.4 Shaken infant syndrome**   P CC POA CC/MCC Exc
5ᵗʰ **T74.5 Forced sexual exploitation, confirmed**
7ᵗʰ   **T74.51 Adult forced sexual exploitation,
                 confirmed**   A CC POA CC/MCC Exc
                 AHA: Q4 2018
7ᵗʰ   **T74.52 Child sexual exploitation, confirmed**   P CC POA CC/MCC Exc
                 AHA: Q4 2018
5ᵗʰ **T74.6 Forced labor exploitation, confirmed**
7ᵗʰ   **T74.61 Adult forced labor exploitation,
                 confirmed**   A CC POA CC/MCC Exc
                 AHA: Q4 2018
7ᵗʰ   **T74.62 Child forced labor exploitation,
                 confirmed**   P CC POA CC/MCC Exc
                 AHA: Q4 2018
5ᵗʰ **T74.9 Unspecified maltreatment, confirmed**
7ᵗʰ   **T74.91 Unspecified adult maltreatment,
                 confirmed**   A CC POA CC/MCC Exc
7ᵗʰ   **T74.92 Unspecified child maltreatment,
                 confirmed**   P CC POA CC/MCC Exc

4ᵗʰ **T75 Other and unspecified effects of other external causes**
          EXCLUDES1 adverse effects NEC (T78.-)
          EXCLUDES2 burns (electric) (T20-T31)

       **The appropriate 7th character is to be added to each code from
       category T75**
          A = initial encounter
          D = subsequent encounter
          S = sequela

5ᵗʰ **T75.0 Effects of** lightning
       Struck by lightning
7ᵗʰ   **T75.00 Unspecified effects of lightning**   POA
                 Struck by lightning NOS
7ᵗʰ   **T75.01 Shock due to being struck by lightning**   POA
7ᵗʰ   **T75.09 Other effects of lightning**   POA
                 Use additional code for other effects of lightning
7ᵗʰ **T75.1 Unspecified effects of drowning and nonfatal
             submersion**   CC POA HAC CC/MCC Exc
       Immersion
          EXCLUDES1 specified effects of drowning- code to effects
5ᵗʰ **T75.2 Effects of** vibration
7ᵗʰ   **T75.20 Unspecified effects of vibration**   POA
7ᵗʰ   **T75.21 Pneumatic hammer syndrome**   POA
7ᵗʰ   **T75.22 Traumatic vasospastic syndrome**   POA
7ᵗʰ   **T75.23 Vertigo from infrasound**   POA
                 EXCLUDES1 vertigo NOS (R42)
7ᵗʰ   **T75.29 Other effects of vibration**   POA
5ᵗʰ **T75.3 Motion sickness**   POA
       Airsickness
       Seasickness
       Travel sickness
       Use additional external cause code to identify vehicle or type
          of motion (Y92.81-, Y93.5-)
7ᵗʰ **T75.4 Electrocution**   POA
       Shock from electric current
       Shock from electroshock gun (taser)
5ᵗʰ **T75.8 Other specified effects of external causes**
7ᵗʰ   **T75.81 Effects of abnormal gravitation [G] forces**   POA
7ᵗʰ   **T75.82 Effects of weightlessness**   POA
7ᵗʰ   **T75.89 Other specified effects of external causes**   POA

4ᵗʰ **T76 Adult and child abuse, neglect and other maltreatment,** suspected
       👁 **See Official Guidelines** "Factitious Disorder" I.C.2.c.2, "Adult and
          child abuse, neglect and other maltreatment" I.C.19.f
       Use additional code, if applicable, to identify any associated current
          injury
       EXCLUDES1 adult and child maltreatment, confirmed (T74.-)
                   suspected abuse and maltreatment in pregnancy (O9A.3-,
                      O9A.4-, O9A.5-)
                   suspected adult physical abuse, ruled out (Z04.71)
                   suspected adult sexual abuse, ruled out (Z04.41)
                   suspected child physical abuse, ruled out (Z04.72)
                   suspected child sexual abuse, ruled out (Z04.42)

       **The appropriate 7th character is to be added to each code from
       category T76**
          A = initial encounter
          D = subsequent encounter
          S = sequela

5ᵗʰ **T76.0 Neglect or abandonment, suspected**
7ᵗʰ   **T76.01 Adult neglect or abandonment,
                 suspected**   A CC POA CC/MCC Exc
7ᵗʰ   **T76.02 Child neglect or abandonment,
                 suspected**   P CC POA CC/MCC Exc
5ᵗʰ **T76.1 Physical abuse, suspected**
7ᵗʰ   **T76.11 Adult physical abuse, suspected**   A CC POA CC/MCC Exc
7ᵗʰ   **T76.12 Child physical abuse, suspected**   P CC POA CC/MCC Exc
5ᵗʰ **T76.2 Sexual abuse, suspected**
       Rape, suspected
          EXCLUDES1 alleged abuse, ruled out (Z04.7)
7ᵗʰ   **T76.21 Adult sexual abuse, suspected**   A CC POA CC/MCC Exc
7ᵗʰ   **T76.22 Child sexual abuse, suspected**   P CC POA CC/MCC Exc
5ᵗʰ **T76.3 Psychological abuse, suspected**
       Bullying and intimidation, suspected
       Intimidation through social media, suspected
7ᵗʰ   **T76.31 Adult psychological abuse, suspected**   A POA
7ᵗʰ   **T76.32 Child psychological abuse, suspected**   P CC POA CC/MCC Exc
5ᵗʰ **T76.5 Forced sexual exploitation, suspected**
7ᵗʰ   **T76.51 Adult forced sexual exploitation,
                 suspected**   A CC POA CC/MCC Exc
                 AHA: Q4 2018

PDₓ Unacceptable principal diagnosis symbol per Medicare code edits   POA Code exempt from diagnosis present on admission requirement
❓ Questionable admission   CC Complication or comorbidity   MCC Major complication or comorbidity   CC/MCC Exc CC/MCC exclusion
HCC HCC diagnosis code   RxHCC RxHCC diagnosis code   MACRA MACRA code   **DEFINITION** Describes condition/terminology
TIP Coding guidance   👁 Official Guideline Reference   Z1 Z code as first-listed diagnosis

[7th] T76.52 Child sexual exploitation, suspected [P] CC POA CC/MCC Exc
AHA: Q4 2018

[5th] T76.6 Forced labor exploitation, suspected

[7th] T76.61 Adult forced labor exploitation, suspected [A] CC POA CC/MCC Exc
AHA: Q4 2018

[7th] T76.62 Child forced labor exploitation, suspected [P] CC POA CC/MCC Exc
AHA: Q4 2018

[5th] T76.9 Unspecified maltreatment, suspected

[7th] T76.91 Unspecified adult maltreatment, suspected [A] CC POA CC/MCC Exc

[7th] T76.92 Unspecified child maltreatment, suspected [P] CC POA CC/MCC Exc

[4th] T78 Adverse effects, not elsewhere classified

EXCLUDES2 *complications of surgical and medical care NEC (T80-T88)*

The appropriate 7th character is to be added to each code from category T78
A = initial encounter
D = subsequent encounter
S = sequela

[5th] T78.0 Anaphylactic reaction due to food
Anaphylactic reaction due to adverse food reaction
Anaphylactic shock or reaction due to nonpoisonous foods
Anaphylactoid reaction due to food

[7th] T78.00 Anaphylactic reaction due to unspecified food CC POA CC/MCC Exc

[7th] T78.01 Anaphylactic reaction due to peanuts CC POA CC/MCC Exc

[7th] T78.02 Anaphylactic reaction due to shellfish (crustaceans) CC POA CC/MCC Exc

[7th] T78.03 Anaphylactic reaction due to other fish CC POA CC/MCC Exc

[7th] T78.04 Anaphylactic reaction due to fruits and vegetables CC POA CC/MCC Exc

[7th] T78.05 Anaphylactic reaction due to tree nuts and seeds CC POA CC/MCC Exc
EXCLUDES2 *anaphylactic reaction due to peanuts (T78.01)*

[7th] T78.06 Anaphylactic reaction due to food additives CC POA CC/MCC Exc

[7th] T78.07 Anaphylactic reaction due to milk and dairy products CC POA CC/MCC Exc

[7th] T78.08 Anaphylactic reaction due to eggs CC POA CC/MCC Exc

[7th] T78.09 Anaphylactic reaction due to other food products CC POA CC/MCC Exc

[7th] T78.1 Other adverse food reactions, not elsewhere classified POA
Use additional code to identify the type of reaction, if applicable
EXCLUDES1 *anaphylactic reaction or shock due to adverse food reaction (T78.0-)*
anaphylactic reaction due to food (T78.0-)
bacterial food borne intoxications (A05.-)
EXCLUDES2 *allergic and dietetic gastroenteritis and colitis (K52.29)*
allergic rhinitis due to food (J30.5)
dermatitis due to food in contact with skin (L23.6, L24.6, L25.4)
dermatitis due to ingested food (L27.2)
food protein-induced enterocolitis syndrome (K52.21)
food protein-induced enteropathy (K52.22)

[7th] T78.2 Anaphylactic shock, unspecified CC POA CC/MCC Exc
Allergic shock
Anaphylactic reaction
Anaphylaxis
EXCLUDES1 *anaphylactic reaction or shock due to adverse effect of correct medicinal substance properly administered (T88.6)*
anaphylactic reaction or shock due to adverse food reaction (T78.0-)
anaphylactic reaction or shock due to serum (T80.5-)

[7th] T78.3 Angioneurotic edema POA
Allergic angioedema
Giant urticaria
Quincke's edema
EXCLUDES1 *serum urticaria (T80.6-)*
urticaria (L50.-)

[5th] T78.4 Other and unspecified allergy
EXCLUDES1 *specified types of allergic reaction such as:*
allergic diarrhea (K52.29)
allergic gastroenteritis and colitis (K52.29)
dermatitis (L23-L25, L27.-)
food protein-induced enterocolitis syndrome (K52.21)
food protein-induced enteropathy (K52.22)
hay fever (J30.1)

[7th] T78.40 Allergy, unspecified POA
Allergic reaction NOS
Hypersensitivity NOS

[7th] T78.41 Arthus phenomenon POA
Arthus reaction

[7th] T78.49 Other allergy POA

[7th] T78.8 Other adverse effects, not elsewhere classified POA

Certain early complications of trauma (T79)

[4th] T79 Certain early complications of trauma, not elsewhere classified

EXCLUDES2 *acute respiratory distress syndrome (J80)*
complications occurring during or following medical procedures (T80-T88)
complications of surgical and medical care NEC (T80-T88)
newborn respiratory distress syndrome (P22.0)

The appropriate 7th character is to be added to each code from category T79
A = initial encounter
D = subsequent encounter
S = sequela

[7th] T79.0 Air embolism (traumatic) POA HCC MCC CC/MCC Exc
EXCLUDES1 *air embolism complicating abortion or ectopic or molar pregnancy (O00-O07, O08.2)*
air embolism complicating pregnancy, childbirth and the puerperium (O88.0)
air embolism following infusion, transfusion, and therapeutic injection (T80.0)
air embolism following procedure NEC (T81.7-)

[7th] T79.1 Fat embolism (traumatic) POA HCC MCC CC/MCC Exc
EXCLUDES1 *fat embolism complicating:*
abortion or ectopic or molar pregnancy (O00-O07, O08.2)
pregnancy, childbirth and the puerperium (O88.8)

[7th] T79.2 Traumatic secondary and recurrent hemorrhage and seroma CC POA HCC CC/MCC Exc

[7th] T79.4 Traumatic shock POA HCC MCC CC/MCC Exc
Shock (immediate) (delayed) following injury
EXCLUDES1 *anaphylactic shock due to adverse food reaction (T78.0-)*
anaphylactic shock due to correct medicinal substance properly administered (T88.6)
anaphylactic shock due to serum (T80.5-)
anaphylactic shock NOS (T78.2)
anesthetic shock (T88.2)
electric shock (T75.4)
nontraumatic shock NEC (R57.-)
obstetric shock (O75.1)
postprocedural shock (T81.1-)
septic shock (R65.21)
shock complicating abortion or ectopic or molar pregnancy (O00-O07, O08.3)
shock due to lightning (T75.01)
shock NOS (R57.9)

- **T79.5 Traumatic** anuria
  Crush syndrome
  Renal failure following crushing
- **T79.6 Traumatic** ischemia of muscle
  Traumatic rhabdomyolysis
  Volkmann's ischemic contracture
  EXCLUDES2 anterior tibial syndrome (M76.8)
  compartment syndrome (traumatic) (T79.A-)
  nontraumatic ischemia of muscle (M62.2-)
- **T79.7 Traumatic** subcutaneous emphysema
  EXCLUDES1 emphysema NOS (J43)
  emphysema (subcutaneous) resulting from a procedure (T81.82)
- **T79.A Traumatic compartment syndrome**
  EXCLUDES1 fibromyalgia (M79.7)
  nontraumatic compartment syndrome (M79.A-)
  EXCLUDES2 traumatic ischemic infarction of muscle (T79.6)
  - **T79.A0 Compartment syndrome, unspecified**
    Compartment syndrome NOS
  - **T79.A1 Traumatic compartment syndrome of** upper extremity
    Traumatic compartment syndrome of shoulder, arm, forearm, wrist, hand, and fingers
    - **T79.A11 Traumatic compartment syndrome of** right upper extremity
    - **T79.A12 Traumatic compartment syndrome of** left upper extremity
    - **T79.A19 Traumatic compartment syndrome of** unspecified upper extremity
  - **T79.A2 Traumatic compartment syndrome of** lower extremity
    Traumatic compartment syndrome of hip, buttock, thigh, leg, foot, and toes
    - **T79.A21 Traumatic compartment syndrome of** right lower extremity
    - **T79.A22 Traumatic compartment syndrome of** left lower extremity
    - **T79.A29 Traumatic compartment syndrome of** unspecified lower extremity
  - **T79.A3 Traumatic compartment syndrome of** abdomen
  - **T79.A9 Traumatic compartment syndrome of** other sites
- **T79.8 Other early complications** of trauma
- **T79.9 Unspecified early complication of trauma**

Complications of surgical and medical care, not elsewhere classified (T80-T88)

Use additional code for adverse effect, if applicable, to identify drug (T36-T50 with fifth or sixth character 5)

Use additional code(s) to identify the specified condition resulting from the complication

Use additional code to identify devices involved and details of circumstances (Y62-Y82)

EXCLUDES2 any encounters with medical care for postprocedural conditions in which no complications are present, such as:
artificial opening status (Z93.-)
closure of external stoma (Z43.-)
fitting and adjustment of external prosthetic device (Z44.-)
burns and corrosions from local applications and irradiation (T20-T32)
complications of surgical procedures during pregnancy, childbirth and the puerperium (O00-O9A)
mechanical complication of respirator [ventilator] (J95.850)
poisoning and toxic effects of drugs and chemicals (T36-T65 with fifth or sixth character 1-4 or 6)
postprocedural fever (R50.82)
specified complications classified elsewhere, such as:

cerebrospinal fluid leak from spinal puncture (G97.0)
colostomy malfunction (K94.0-)
disorders of fluid and electrolyte imbalance (E86-E87)
functional disturbances following cardiac surgery (I97.0-I97.1)
intraoperative and postprocedural complications of specified body systems (D78.-, E36.-, E89.-, G97.3-, G97.4, H59.3-, H59.-, H95.2-, H95.3, I97.4-, I97.5, J95.6-, J95.7, K91.6-, L76.-, M96.-, N99.-)
ostomy complications (J95.0-, K94.-, N99.5-)
postgastric surgery syndromes (K91.1)
postlaminectomy syndrome NEC (M96.1)
postmastectomy lymphedema syndrome (I97.2)
postsurgical blind-loop syndrome (K91.2)
ventilator associated pneumonia (J95.851)

- **T80 Complications following infusion, transfusion and therapeutic injection**
  INCLUDES complications following perfusion
  EXCLUDES2 bone marrow transplant rejection (T86.01)
  febrile nonhemolytic transfusion reaction (R50.84)
  fluid overload due to transfusion (E87.71)
  posttransfusion purpura (D69.51)
  transfusion associated circulatory overload (TACO) (E87.71)
  transfusion (red blood cell) associated hemochromatosis (E83.111)
  transfusion related acute lung injury (TRALI) (J95.84)

  The appropriate 7th character is to be added to each code from category T80
  A = initial encounter
  D = subsequent encounter
  S = sequela

  - **T80.0 Air embolism following infusion, transfusion and therapeutic injection**
  - **T80.1 Vascular complications following infusion, transfusion and therapeutic injection**
    Use additional code to identify the vascular complication
    EXCLUDES2 extravasation of vesicant agent (T80.81-)
    infiltration of vesicant agent (T80.81-)
    vascular complications specified as due to prosthetic devices, implants and grafts (T82.8-, T83.8-, T84.8-, T85.8-)
    postprocedural vascular complications (T81.7-)
  - **T80.2 Infections following infusion, transfusion and therapeutic injection**
    Use additional code to identify the specific infection, such as: sepsis (A41.9)
    Use additional code (R65.2-) to identify severe sepsis, if applicable
    EXCLUDES2 infections specified as due to prosthetic devices, implants and grafts (T82.6-T82.7, T83.5-T83.6, T84.5-T84.7, T85.7)
    postprocedural infections (T81.4-)
    - **T80.21 Infection due to** central venous catheter
      Infection due to pulmonary artery catheter (Swan-Ganz catheter)
      - **T80.211 Bloodstream infection due to central venous catheter**
        AHA: Q1 2019, Q4 2018
        Catheter-related bloodstream infection (CRBSI) NOS
        Central line-associated bloodstream infection (CLABSI)
        Bloodstream infection due to Hickman catheter
        Bloodstream infection due to peripherally inserted central catheter (PICC)
        Bloodstream infection due to portacath (port-a-cath)
        Bloodstream infection due to pulmonary artery catheter
        Bloodstream infection due to triple lumen catheter
        Bloodstream infection due to umbilical venous catheter

PDx Unacceptable principal diagnosis symbol per Medicare code edits   Code exempt from diagnosis present on admission requirement
? Questionable admission   Complication or comorbidity   MCC Major complication or comorbidity   CC/MCC CC/MCC exclusion
HCC HCC diagnosis code   RxHCC RxHCC diagnosis code   MACRA code   **DEFINITION** Describes condition/terminology
TIP Coding guidance   Official Guideline Reference   Z1 Z code as first-listed diagnosis

1160 When symbols appear on a code that requires a 7th character extension, refer to Appendix B to identify applicable 7th character codes.   **2020 ICD-10-CM**

T80.212 Local infection **due to central venous catheter** CC POA HAC CC/MCC Exc
  Exit or insertion site infection
  Local infection due to Hickman catheter
  Local infection due to peripherally inserted central catheter (PICC)
  Local infection due to portacath (port-a-cath)
  Local infection due to pulmonary artery catheter
  Local infection due to triple lumen catheter
  Local infection due to umbilical venous catheter
  Port or reservoir infection
  Tunnel infection

T80.218 Other infection **due to central venous catheter** CC POA HAC CC/MCC Exc
  Other central line-associated infection
  Other infection due to Hickman catheter
  Other infection due to peripherally inserted central catheter (PICC)
  Other infection due to portacath (port-a-cath)
  Other infection due to pulmonary artery catheter
  Other infection due to triple lumen catheter
  Other infection due to umbilical venous catheter

T80.219 **Unspecified infection due to central venous catheter** CC POA HAC CC/MCC Exc
  Central line-associated infection NOS
  Unspecified infection due to Hickman catheter
  Unspecified infection due to peripherally inserted central catheter (PICC)
  Unspecified infection due to portacath (port-a-cath)
  Unspecified infection due to pulmonary artery catheter
  Unspecified infection due to triple lumen catheter
  Unspecified infection due to umbilical venous catheter

T80.22 Acute infection **following transfusion, infusion, or injection of blood and blood products** CC POA CC/MCC Exc

T80.29 **Infection following other infusion, transfusion and therapeutic injection** CC POA CC/MCC Exc

T80.3 ABO incompatibility **reaction due to transfusion of blood or blood products**
  EXCLUDES1 minor blood group antigens reactions (Duffy) (E) (K) (Kell) (Kidd) (Lewis) (M) (N) (P) (S) (T80.A-)

T80.30 **ABO incompatibility reaction due to transfusion of blood or blood products, unspecified** CC POA HAC CC/MCC Exc
  ABO incompatibility blood transfusion NOS
  Reaction to ABO incompatibility from transfusion NOS

T80.31 **ABO incompatibility** with hemolytic transfusion reaction

T80.310 **ABO incompatibility with** acute **hemolytic transfusion reaction** CC POA HAC CC/MCC Exc
  ABO incompatibility with hemolytic transfusion reaction less than 24 hours after transfusion
  Acute hemolytic transfusion reaction (AHTR) due to ABO incompatibility

T80.311 **ABO incompatibility with** delayed **hemolytic transfusion reaction** CC POA HAC CC/MCC Exc
  ABO incompatibility with hemolytic transfusion reaction 24 hours or more after transfusion
  Delayed hemolytic transfusion reaction (DHTR) due to ABO incompatibility

T80.319 **ABO incompatibility with hemolytic transfusion reaction, unspecified** CC POA HAC

  ABO incompatibility with hemolytic transfusion reaction at unspecified time after transfusion
  Hemolytic transfusion reaction (HTR) due to ABO incompatibility NOS

T80.39 Other **ABO incompatibility reaction due to transfusion of blood or blood products** CC POA HAC CC/MCC Exc
  Delayed serologic transfusion reaction (DSTR) from ABO incompatibility
  Other ABO incompatible blood transfusion
  Other reaction to ABO incompatible blood transfusion

T80.4 Rh incompatibility **reaction due to transfusion of blood or blood products**
  Reaction due to incompatibility of Rh antigens (C) (c) (D) (E) (e)

T80.40 **Rh incompatibility reaction due to transfusion of blood or blood products, unspecified** CC POA CC/MCC Exc
  Reaction due to Rh factor in transfusion NOS
  Rh incompatible blood transfusion NOS

T80.41 **Rh incompatibility** with hemolytic transfusion reaction

T80.410 **Rh incompatibility with** acute **hemolytic transfusion reaction** CC POA CC/MCC Exc
  Acute hemolytic transfusion reaction (AHTR) due to Rh incompatibility
  Rh incompatibility with hemolytic transfusion reaction less than 24 hours after transfusion

T80.411 **Rh incompatibility with** delayed **hemolytic transfusion reaction** CC POA CC/MCC Exc
  Delayed hemolytic transfusion reaction (DHTR) due to Rh incompatibility
  Rh incompatibility with hemolytic transfusion reaction 24 hours or more after transfusion

T80.419 **Rh incompatibility with hemolytic transfusion reaction, unspecified** CC POA CC/MCC Exc
  Rh incompatibility with hemolytic transfusion reaction at unspecified time after transfusion
  Hemolytic transfusion reaction (HTR) due to Rh incompatibility NOS

T80.49 Other **Rh incompatibility reaction due to transfusion of blood or blood products** CC POA CC/MCC Exc
  Delayed serologic transfusion reaction (DSTR) from Rh incompatibility
  Other reaction to Rh incompatible blood transfusion

T80.A Non-ABO incompatibility **reaction due to transfusion of blood or blood products**
  Reaction due to incompatibility of minor antigens (Duffy) (Kell) (Kidd) (Lewis) (M) (N) (P) (S)

T80.A0 **Non-ABO incompatibility reaction due to transfusion of blood or blood products, unspecified** CC POA CC/MCC Exc
  Non-ABO antigen incompatibility reaction from transfusion NOS

T80.A1 **Non-ABO incompatibility** with hemolytic transfusion reaction

T80.A10 **Non-ABO incompatibility with** acute **hemolytic transfusion reaction** CC POA CC/MCC Exc
  Acute hemolytic transfusion reaction (AHTR) due to non-ABO incompatibility
  Non-ABO incompatibility with hemolytic transfusion reaction less than 24 hours after transfusion

T80.A11 **Non-ABO incompatibility with** delayed **hemolytic transfusion reaction** CC POA CC/MCC Exc
  Delayed hemolytic transfusion reaction (DHTR) due to non-ABO incompatibility
  Non-ABO incompatibility with hemolytic transfusion reaction 24 or more hours after transfusion

---

Unspecified Code   Other Specified Code   Manifestation Code   N Newborn   P Pediatric   M Maternity   A Adult   ♂ Male   ♀ Female
● New Code   ▲ Revised Code Title   ▶◀ Revised Text   NOTES   INCLUDES   EXCLUDES1 Not coded here   EXCLUDES2 Not included here
4th character required   5th character required   6th character required   7th character required   Extension 'X' Alert
HAC Hospital-acquired condition (HAC) alert   AHA AHA Coding Clinic©   Code first alert

CHAPTER 19: INJURY, POISONING, AND CERTAIN OTHER CONSEQUENCES OF EXTERNAL CAUSES (S00-T88)

T80.A19 - T81.19

T80.A19 Non-ABO incompatibility with hemolytic transfusion reaction, unspecified CC POA CC/MCC Exc

Hemolytic transfusion reaction (HTR) due to non-ABO incompatibility NOS

Non-ABO incompatibility with hemolytic transfusion reaction at unspecified time after transfusion

T80.A9 Other non-ABO incompatibility reaction due to transfusion of blood or blood products CC POA CC/MCC Exc

Delayed serologic transfusion reaction (DSTR) from non-ABO incompatibility

Other reaction to non-ABO incompatible blood transfusion

T80.5 Anaphylactic reaction due to serum

Allergic shock due to serum

Anaphylactic shock due to serum

Anaphylactoid reaction due to serum

Anaphylaxis due to serum

EXCLUDES1 *ABO incompatibility reaction due to transfusion of blood or blood products (T80.3-)*

allergic reaction or shock NOS (T78.2)

anaphylactic reaction or shock NOS (T78.2)

anaphylactic reaction or shock due to adverse effect of correct medicinal substance properly administered (T88.6)

other serum reaction (T80.6-)

T80.51 Anaphylactic reaction due to administration of blood and blood products CC POA CC/MCC Exc

T80.52 Anaphylactic reaction due to vaccination CC POA CC/MCC Exc

T80.59 Anaphylactic reaction due to other serum CC POA CC/MCC Exc

T80.6 Other serum reactions

Intoxication by serum

Protein sickness

Serum rash

Serum sickness

Serum urticaria

EXCLUDES2 *serum hepatitis (B16-B19)*

T80.61 Other serum reaction due to administration of blood and blood products CC POA CC/MCC Exc

T80.62 Other serum reaction due to vaccination CC POA CC/MCC Exc

T80.69 Other serum reaction due to other serum CC POA CC/MCC Exc

Code also, if applicable, arthropathy in hypersensitivity reactions classified elsewhere (M36.4)

T80.8 Other complications following infusion, transfusion and therapeutic injection

T80.81 Extravasation of vesicant agent

Infiltration of vesicant agent

T80.810 Extravasation of vesicant antineoplastic chemotherapy CC POA CC/MCC Exc

Infiltration of vesicant antineoplastic chemotherapy

T80.818 Extravasation of other vesicant agent CC POA CC/MCC Exc

Infiltration of other vesicant agent

T80.89 Other complications following infusion, transfusion and therapeutic injection CC POA CC/MCC Exc

Delayed serologic transfusion reaction (DSTR), unspecified incompatibility

Use additional code to identify graft-versus-host reaction, if applicable, (D89.81-)

T80.9 Unspecified complication following infusion, transfusion and therapeutic injection

T80.90 Unspecified complication following infusion and therapeutic injection POA

T80.91 Hemolytic transfusion reaction, unspecified incompatibility

EXCLUDES1 *ABO incompatibility with hemolytic transfusion reaction (T80.31-)*

Non-ABO incompatibility with hemolytic transfusion reaction (T80.A1-)

Rh incompatibility with hemolytic transfusion reaction (T80.41-)

T80.910 Acute hemolytic transfusion reaction, unspecified incompatibility CC POA CC/MCC Exc

T80.911 Delayed hemolytic transfusion reaction, unspecified incompatibility CC POA CC/MCC Exc

T80.919 Hemolytic transfusion reaction, unspecified incompatibility, unspecified as acute or delayed CC POA CC/MCC Exc

Hemolytic transfusion reaction NOS

T80.92 Unspecified transfusion reaction POA

Transfusion reaction NOS

T81 Complications of procedures, not elsewhere classified

Use additional code for adverse effect, if applicable, to identify drug (T36-T50 with fifth or sixth character 5)

EXCLUDES2 *complications following immunization (T88.0-T88.1)*

complications following infusion, transfusion and therapeutic injection (T80.-)

complications of transplanted organs and tissue (T86.-)

specified complications classified elsewhere, such as:

complication of prosthetic devices, implants and grafts (T82-T85)

dermatitis due to drugs and medicaments (L23.3, L24.4, L25.1, L27.0-L27.1)

endosseous dental implant failure (M27.6-)

floppy iris syndrome (IFIS) (intraoperative) H21.81

intraoperative and postprocedural complications of specific body system (D78.-, E36.-, E89.-, G97.3-, G97.4, H59.3-, H59.-, H95.2-, H95.3, I97.4-, I97.5, J95, K91.-, L76.-, M96.-, N99.-)

ostomy complications (J95.0-, K94.-, N99.5-)

plateau iris syndrome (post-iridectomy) (postprocedural) H21.82

poisoning and toxic effects of drugs and chemicals (T36-T65 with fifth or sixth character 1-4 or 6)

The appropriate 7th character is to be added to each code from category T81

A = initial encounter

D = subsequent encounter

S = sequela

T81.1 Postprocedural shock

Shock during or resulting from a procedure, not elsewhere classified

EXCLUDES1 *anaphylactic shock NOS (T78.2)*

anaphylactic shock due to correct substance properly administered (T88.6)

anaphylactic shock due to serum (T80.5-)

anesthetic shock (T88.2)

electric shock (T75.4)

obstetric shock (O75.1)

septic shock (R65.21)

shock following abortion or ectopic or molar pregnancy (O00-O07, O08.3)

traumatic shock (T79.4)

T81.10 Postprocedural shock unspecified CC POA CC/MCC Exc

Collapse NOS during or resulting from a procedure, not elsewhere classified

Postprocedural failure of peripheral circulation

Postprocedural shock NOS

T81.11 Postprocedural cardiogenic shock POA HCC MCC CC/MCC Exc

T81.12 Postprocedural septic shock POA HCC MCC PDxIn CC/MCC Exc

See Official Guidelines "Septic shock" I.C.1.d.2.a, "Postprocedural infection and postprocedural septic shock" I.C.1.d.5.c

AHA: Q4 2018

Postprocedural endotoxic shock resulting from a procedure, not elsewhere classified

Postprocedural gram-negative shock resulting from a procedure, not elsewhere classified

Code first underlying infection

Use additional code, to identify any associated acute organ dysfunction, if applicable

T81.19 Other postprocedural shock POA MCC CC/MCC Exc

Postprocedural hypovolemic shock

POA Unacceptable principal diagnosis symbol per Medicare code edits   POA Code exempt from diagnosis present on admission requirement

? Questionable admission   CC Complication or comorbidity   MCC Major complication or comorbidity   CC/MCC Exc CC/MCC exclusion

HCC HCC diagnosis code   RHCC RxHCC diagnosis code   MACRA MACRA code   **DEFINITION** Describes condition/terminology

TIP Coding guidance   👁 Official Guideline Reference   Z1 Z code as first-listed diagnosis

[5th] T81.3 Disruption of wound, not elsewhere classified
Disruption of any suture materials or other closure methods
EXCLUDES1 *breakdown (mechanical) of permanent sutures (T85.612)*
displacement of permanent sutures (T85.622)
disruption of cesarean delivery wound (O90.0)
disruption of perineal obstetric wound (O90.1)
mechanical complication of permanent sutures NEC (T85.692)

[7th] T81.30 **Disruption of wound, unspecified** CC POA CC/MCC Exc
Disruption of wound NOS

[7th] T81.31 **Disruption of external operation (surgical) wound, not elsewhere classified** CC POA CC/MCC Exc
AHA: Q1 2015
Dehiscence of operation wound NOS
Disruption of operation wound NOS
Disruption or dehiscence of closure of cornea
Disruption or dehiscence of closure of mucosa
Disruption or dehiscence of closure of skin and subcutaneous tissue
Full-thickness skin disruption or dehiscence
Superficial disruption or dehiscence of operation wound
EXCLUDES1 *dehiscence of amputation stump (T87.81)*

[7th] T81.32 **Disruption of internal operation (surgical) wound, not elsewhere classified** CC POA CC/MCC Exc
Deep disruption or dehiscence of operation wound NOS
Disruption or dehiscence of closure of internal organ or other internal tissue
Disruption or dehiscence of closure of muscle or muscle flap
Disruption or dehiscence of closure of ribs or rib cage
Disruption or dehiscence of closure of skull or craniotomy
Disruption or dehiscence of closure of sternum or sternotomy
Disruption or dehiscence of closure of tendon or ligament
Disruption or dehiscence of closure of superficial or muscular fascia

[7th] T81.33 **Disruption of traumatic injury wound repair** CC POA CC/MCC Exc
Disruption or dehiscence of closure of traumatic laceration (external) (internal)

[5th] T81.4 **Infection following a procedure**
Wound abscess following a procedure
Use additional code to identify infection
Use additional code (R65.2-) to identify severe sepsis, if applicable
EXCLUDES2 *bleb associated endophthalmitis (H59.4-)*
infection due to infusion, transfusion and therapeutic injection (T80.2-)
infection due to prosthetic devices, implants and grafts (T82.6-T82.7, T83.5-T83.6, T84.5-T84.7, T85.7)
obstetric surgical wound infection (O86.0-)
postprocedural fever NOS (R50.82)
postprocedural retroperitoneal abscess (K68.11)

[7th] T81.40 **Infection following a procedure, unspecified** CC POA HAC CC/MCC Exc
See Official Guidelines "Sepsis due to a postprocedural infection" I.C.1.d.5.b
AHA: Q2 2019, Q4 2018

[7th] T81.41 **Infection following a procedure, superficial incisional surgical site** CC POA HAC CC/MCC Exc
See Official Guidelines "Sepsis due to a postprocedural infection" I.C.1.d.5.b
AHA: Q4 2018
Subcutaneous abscess following a procedure
Stitch abscess following a procedure

[7th] T81.42 **Infection following a procedure, deep incisional surgical site** CC POA HAC CC/MCC Exc
See Official Guidelines "Sepsis due to a postprocedural infection" I.C.1.d.5.b
AHA: Q4 2018
Intra-muscular abscess following a procedure

[7th] T81.43 **Infection following a procedure, organ and space surgical site** CC POA HAC CC/MCC Exc
See Official Guidelines "Sepsis due to a postprocedural infection" I.C.1.d.5.b
AHA: Q2 2019, Q4 2018
Intra-abdominal abscess following a procedure
Subphrenic abscess following a procedure

[7th] T81.44 **Sepsis following a procedure** CC POA HAC HCC CC/MCC Exc
See Official Guidelines "Sepsis due to a postprocedural infection" I.C.1.d.5.b
AHA: Q2 2019, Q4 2018
Use additional code to identify the sepsis

[7th] T81.49 **Infection following a procedure, other surgical site** CC POA HAC CC/MCC Exc
AHA: Q4 2018

[5th] T81.5 **Complications of foreign body accidentally left in body following procedure**

[6th] T81.50 **Unspecified complication of foreign body accidentally left in body following procedure**

[7th] T81.500 **Unspecified complication of foreign body accidentally left in body following surgical operation** CC POA HAC CC/MCC Exc

[7th] T81.501 **Unspecified complication of foreign body accidentally left in body following infusion or transfusion** CC POA HAC CC/MCC Exc

[7th] T81.502 **Unspecified complication of foreign body accidentally left in body following kidney dialysis** CC POA HAC HCC RxHCC CC/MCC Exc

[7th] T81.503 **Unspecified complication of foreign body accidentally left in body following injection or immunization** CC POA HAC CC/MCC Exc

[7th] T81.504 **Unspecified complication of foreign body accidentally left in body following endoscopic examination** CC POA HAC CC/MCC Exc

[7th] T81.505 **Unspecified complication of foreign body accidentally left in body following heart catheterization** CC POA HAC CC/MCC Exc

[7th] T81.506 **Unspecified complication of foreign body accidentally left in body following aspiration, puncture or other catheterization** CC POA HAC CC/MCC Exc

[7th] T81.507 **Unspecified complication of foreign body accidentally left in body following removal of catheter or packing** CC POA HAC CC/MCC Exc

[7th] T81.508 **Unspecified complication of foreign body accidentally left in body following other procedure** CC POA HAC CC/MCC Exc

[7th] T81.509 **Unspecified complication of foreign body accidentally left in body following unspecified procedure** CC POA HAC CC/MCC Exc

[6th] T81.51 **Adhesions due to foreign body accidentally left in body following procedure**

[7th] T81.510 Adhesions due to foreign body accidentally left in body following surgical operation CC POA HAC CC/MCC Exc

[7th] T81.511 Adhesions due to foreign body accidentally left in body following infusion or transfusion CC POA HAC CC/MCC Exc

[7th] T81.512 Adhesions due to foreign body accidentally left in body following kidney dialysis CC POA HAC HCC RxHCC CC/MCC Exc

[7th] T81.513 Adhesions due to foreign body accidentally left in body following injection or immunization CC POA HAC CC/MCC Exc

[7th] T81.514 Adhesions due to foreign body accidentally left in body following endoscopic examination CC POA HAC CC/MCC Exc

[7th] T81.515 Adhesions due to foreign body accidentally left in body following heart catheterization CC POA HAC CC/MCC Exc

[7th] T81.516 Adhesions due to foreign body accidentally left in body following aspiration, puncture or other catheterization CC POA HAC CC/MCC Exc

Unspecified Code Other Specified Code Manifestation Code [N] Newborn [P] Pediatric [M] Maternity [A] Adult ♂ Male ♀ Female
● New Code ▲ Revised Code Title ►◄ Revised Text NOTES INCLUDES EXCLUDES1 Not coded here EXCLUDES2 Not included here
[4th] 4th character required [5th] 5th character required [6th] 6th character required [7th] 7th character required [X] Extension 'X' Alert
HAC Hospital-acquired condition (HAC) alert AHA AHA Coding Clinic© ☞ Code first alert

7️⃣ **T81.517** **Adhesions due to foreign body accidentally left in body following** removal of catheter or packing 🔄 POA HAC CC/MCC Exc

7️⃣ **T81.518** **Adhesions due to foreign body accidentally left in body following** other procedure 🔄 POA HAC CC/MCC Exc

7️⃣ **T81.519** **Adhesions due to foreign body accidentally left in body following unspecified procedure** 🔄 POA HAC CC/MCC Exc

6️⃣ T81.52 Obstruction **due to foreign body accidentally left in body following procedure**

7️⃣ **T81.520** **Obstruction due to foreign body accidentally left in body following** surgical operation 🔄 POA HAC CC/MCC Exc

7️⃣ **T81.521** **Obstruction due to foreign body accidentally left in body following** infusion or transfusion 🔄 POA HAC CC/MCC Exc

7️⃣ **T81.522** **Obstruction due to foreign body accidentally left in body following** kidney dialysis 🔄 POA HAC HCC RxHCC CC/MCC Exc

7️⃣ **T81.523** **Obstruction due to foreign body accidentally left in body following** injection or immunization 🔄 POA HAC CC/MCC Exc

7️⃣ **T81.524** **Obstruction due to foreign body accidentally left in body following** endoscopic examination 🔄 POA HAC CC/MCC Exc

7️⃣ **T81.525** **Obstruction due to foreign body accidentally left in body following** heart catheterization 🔄 POA HAC CC/MCC Exc

7️⃣ **T81.526** **Obstruction due to foreign body accidentally left in body following** aspiration, puncture or other catheterization 🔄 POA HAC CC/MCC Exc

7️⃣ **T81.527** **Obstruction due to foreign body accidentally left in body following** removal of catheter or packing 🔄 POA HAC CC/MCC Exc

7️⃣ **T81.528** **Obstruction due to foreign body accidentally left in body following** other procedure 🔄 POA HAC CC/MCC Exc

7️⃣ **T81.529** **Obstruction due to foreign body accidentally left in body following unspecified procedure** 🔄 POA HAC CC/MCC Exc

6️⃣ T81.53 Perforation **due to foreign body accidentally left in body following procedure**

7️⃣ **T81.530** **Perforation due to foreign body accidentally left in body following** surgical operation 🔄 POA HAC CC/MCC Exc

7️⃣ **T81.531** **Perforation due to foreign body accidentally left in body following** infusion or transfusion 🔄 POA HAC CC/MCC Exc

7️⃣ **T81.532** **Perforation due to foreign body accidentally left in body following** kidney dialysis 🔄 POA HAC HCC RxHCC CC/MCC Exc

7️⃣ **T81.533** **Perforation due to foreign body accidentally left in body following** injection or immunization 🔄 POA HAC CC/MCC Exc

7️⃣ **T81.534** **Perforation due to foreign body accidentally left in body following** endoscopic examination 🔄 POA HAC CC/MCC Exc

7️⃣ **T81.535** **Perforation due to foreign body accidentally left in body following** heart catheterization 🔄 POA HAC CC/MCC Exc

7️⃣ **T81.536** **Perforation due to foreign body accidentally left in body following** aspiration, puncture or other catheterization 🔄 POA HAC CC/MCC Exc

7️⃣ **T81.537** **Perforation due to foreign body accidentally left in body following** removal of catheter or packing 🔄 POA HAC CC/MCC Exc

7️⃣ **T81.538** **Perforation due to foreign body accidentally left in body following** other procedure 🔄 POA HAC CC/MCC Exc

7️⃣ **T81.539** **Perforation due to foreign body accidentally left in body following unspecified procedure** 🔄 POA HAC CC/MCC Exc

6️⃣ T81.59 Other complications **of foreign body accidentally left in body following procedure**

EXCLUDES2 *obstruction or perforation due to prosthetic devices and implants intentionally left in body (T82.0-T82.5, T83.0-T83.4, T83.7, T84.0-T84.4, T85.0-T85.6)*

7️⃣ **T81.590** **Other complications of foreign body accidentally left in body following** surgical operation 🔄 POA HAC CC/MCC Exc

7️⃣ **T81.591** **Other complications of foreign body accidentally left in body following** infusion or transfusion 🔄 POA HAC CC/MCC Exc

7️⃣ **T81.592** **Other complications of foreign body accidentally left in body following** kidney dialysis 🔄 POA HAC HCC RxHCC CC/MCC Exc

7️⃣ **T81.593** **Other complications of foreign body accidentally left in body following** injection or immunization 🔄 POA HAC CC/MCC Exc

7️⃣ **T81.594** **Other complications of foreign body accidentally left in body following** endoscopic examination 🔄 POA HAC CC/MCC Exc

7️⃣ **T81.595** **Other complications of foreign body accidentally left in body following** heart catheterization 🔄 POA HAC CC/MCC Exc

7️⃣ **T81.596** **Other complications of foreign body accidentally left in body following** aspiration, puncture or other catheterization 🔄 POA HAC CC/MCC Exc

7️⃣ **T81.597** **Other complications of foreign body accidentally left in body following** removal of catheter or packing 🔄 POA HAC CC/MCC Exc

7️⃣ **T81.598** **Other complications of foreign body accidentally left in body following** other procedure 🔄 POA HAC CC/MCC Exc

7️⃣ **T81.599** **Other complications of foreign body accidentally left in body following unspecified procedure** 🔄 POA HAC CC/MCC Exc

5️⃣ T81.6 Acute reaction **to foreign substance accidentally left during a procedure**

EXCLUDES2 *complications of foreign body accidentally left in body cavity or operation wound following procedure (T81.5-)*

7️⃣ **T81.60** **Unspecified acute reaction to foreign substance accidentally left during a procedure** 🔄 POA HAC CC/MCC Exc

7️⃣ **T81.61** Aseptic peritonitis **due to foreign substance accidentally left during a procedure** 🔄 POA HAC CC/MCC Exc
Chemical peritonitis

7️⃣ **T81.69** Other **acute reaction to foreign substance accidentally left during a procedure** 🔄 POA HAC CC/MCC Exc

5️⃣ T81.7 Vascular complications **following a procedure, not elsewhere classified**
Air embolism following procedure NEC
Phlebitis or thrombophlebitis resulting from a procedure

EXCLUDES1 *embolism complicating abortion or ectopic or molar pregnancy (O00-O07, O08.2)*

embolism complicating pregnancy, childbirth and the puerperium (O88.-)

traumatic embolism (T79.0)

EXCLUDES2 *embolism due to prosthetic devices, implants and grafts (T82.8-, T83.81, T84.8-, T85.81-)*

embolism following infusion, transfusion and therapeutic injection (T80.0)

6️⃣ T81.71 Complication of artery **following a procedure, not elsewhere classified**

7️⃣ **T81.710** **Complication of** mesenteric **artery following a procedure, not elsewhere classified** 🔄 POA CC/MCC Exc

---

POA🔄 Unacceptable principal diagnosis symbol per Medicare code edits   POA🔄 Code exempt from diagnosis present on admission requirement
❓ Questionable admission   🔄 Complication or comorbidity   MCC Major complication or comorbidity   CC/MCC Exc CC/MCC exclusion
HCC HCC diagnosis code   RxHCC RxHCC diagnosis code   MACRA code   **DEFINITION** Describes condition/terminology
TIP Coding guidance   👁 Official Guideline Reference   Z1 Z code as first-listed diagnosis

[7th] **T81.711 Complication of renal artery following a procedure, not elsewhere classified** CC POA CC/MCC Exc

[7th] **T81.718 Complication of other artery following a procedure, not elsewhere classified** CC POA CC/MCC Exc
AHA: Q2 2019

[7th] **T81.719 Complication of unspecified artery following a procedure, not elsewhere classified** CC POA CC/MCC Exc

[7th] **T81.72 Complication of vein following a procedure, not elsewhere classified** CC POA CC/MCC Exc
AHA: Q2 2019

[5th] **T81.8 Other complications of procedures, not elsewhere classified**
EXCLUDES2 *hypothermia following anesthesia (T88.51)*
malignant hyperpyrexia due to anesthesia (T88.3)

[7th] **T81.81 Complication of inhalation therapy** POA

[7th] **T81.82 Emphysema (subcutaneous) resulting from a procedure** POA

[7th] **T81.83 Persistent postprocedural fistula** CC POA CC/MCC Exc
AHA: Q3 2017

[7th] **T81.89 Other complications of procedures, not elsewhere classified** POA
Use additional code to specify complication, such as:
postprocedural delirium (F05)

[7th] **T81.9 Unspecified complication of procedure** POA

[4th] **T82 Complications of cardiac and vascular prosthetic devices, implants and grafts**
EXCLUDES2 *failure and rejection of transplanted organs and tissue (T86.-)*
The appropriate 7th character is to be added to each code from category T82
A = initial encounter
D = subsequent encounter
S = sequela

[5th] **T82.0 Mechanical complication of heart valve prosthesis**
Mechanical complication of artificial heart valve
EXCLUDES1 *mechanical complication of biological heart valve graft (T82.22-)*

[7th] **T82.01 Breakdown (mechanical) of heart valve prosthesis** CC POA CC/MCC Exc

[7th] **T82.02 Displacement of heart valve prosthesis** CC POA CC/MCC Exc
Malposition of heart valve prosthesis

[7th] **T82.03 Leakage of heart valve prosthesis** CC POA CC/MCC Exc

[7th] **T82.09 Other mechanical complication of heart valve prosthesis** CC POA CC/MCC Exc
Obstruction (mechanical) of heart valve prosthesis
Perforation of heart valve prosthesis
Protrusion of heart valve prosthesis

[5th] **T82.1 Mechanical complication of cardiac electronic device**

[6th] **T82.11 Breakdown (mechanical) of cardiac electronic device**

[7th] **T82.110 Breakdown (mechanical) of cardiac electrode** CC POA CC/MCC Exc

[7th] **T82.111 Breakdown (mechanical) of cardiac pulse generator (battery)** CC POA CC/MCC Exc

[7th] **T82.118 Breakdown (mechanical) of other cardiac electronic device** CC POA CC/MCC Exc

[7th] **T82.119 Breakdown (mechanical) of unspecified cardiac electronic device** CC POA

[6th] **T82.12 Displacement of cardiac electronic device**
Malposition of cardiac electronic device

[7th] **T82.120 Displacement of cardiac electrode** CC POA CC/MCC Exc

[7th] **T82.121 Displacement of cardiac pulse generator (battery)** CC POA CC/MCC Exc

[7th] **T82.128 Displacement of other cardiac electronic device** CC POA CC/MCC Exc

[7th] **T82.129 Displacement of unspecified cardiac electronic device** CC POA

[6th] **T82.19 Other mechanical complication of cardiac electronic device**
Leakage of cardiac electronic device
Obstruction of cardiac electronic device
Perforation of cardiac electronic device
Protrusion of cardiac electronic device

[7th] **T82.190 Other mechanical complication of cardiac electrode** CC POA CC/MCC Exc

[7th] **T82.191 Other mechanical complication of cardiac pulse generator (battery)** CC POA CC/MCC Exc

[7th] **T82.198 Other mechanical complication of other cardiac electronic device** CC POA CC/MCC Exc

[7th] **T82.199 Other mechanical complication of unspecified cardiac device** CC POA

[5th] **T82.2 Mechanical complication of coronary artery bypass graft and biological heart valve graft**
EXCLUDES1 *mechanical complication of artificial heart valve prosthesis (T82.0-)*

[6th] **T82.21 Mechanical complication of coronary artery bypass graft**

[7th] **T82.211 Breakdown (mechanical) of coronary artery bypass graft** CC POA CC/MCC Exc

[7th] **T82.212 Displacement of coronary artery bypass graft** CC POA CC/MCC Exc
Malposition of coronary artery bypass graft

[7th] **T82.213 Leakage of coronary artery bypass graft** CC POA CC/MCC Exc

[7th] **T82.218 Other mechanical complication of coronary artery bypass graft** CC POA CC/MCC Exc
Obstruction, mechanical of coronary artery bypass graft
Perforation of coronary artery bypass graft
Protrusion of coronary artery bypass graft

[6th] **T82.22 Mechanical complication of biological heart valve graft**

[7th] **T82.221 Breakdown (mechanical) of biological heart valve graft** CC POA CC/MCC Exc

[7th] **T82.222 Displacement of biological heart valve graft** CC POA CC/MCC Exc
Malposition of biological heart valve graft

[7th] **T82.223 Leakage of biological heart valve graft** CC POA CC/MCC Exc

[7th] **T82.228 Other mechanical complication of biological heart valve graft** CC POA CC/MCC Exc
Obstruction of biological heart valve graft
Perforation of biological heart valve graft
Protrusion of biological heart valve graft

[5th] **T82.3 Mechanical complication of other vascular grafts**

[6th] **T82.31 Breakdown (mechanical) of other vascular grafts**

[7th] **T82.310 Breakdown (mechanical) of aortic (bifurcation) graft (replacement)** CC POA HCC CC/MCC Exc

[7th] **T82.311 Breakdown (mechanical) of carotid arterial graft (bypass)** CC POA HCC CC/MCC Exc

[7th] **T82.312 Breakdown (mechanical) of femoral arterial graft (bypass)** CC POA HCC CC/MCC Exc

[7th] **T82.318 Breakdown (mechanical) of other vascular grafts** CC POA HCC CC/MCC Exc

[7th] **T82.319 Breakdown (mechanical) of unspecified vascular grafts** CC POA HCC CC/MCC Exc

[6th] **T82.32 Displacement of other vascular grafts**
Malposition of other vascular grafts

[7th] **T82.320 Displacement of aortic (bifurcation) graft (replacement)** CC POA HCC CC/MCC Exc

[7th] **T82.321 Displacement of carotid arterial graft (bypass)** CC POA HCC CC/MCC Exc

[7th] **T82.322 Displacement of femoral arterial graft (bypass)** CC POA HCC CC/MCC Exc

[7th] **T82.328 Displacement of other vascular grafts** CC POA HCC CC/MCC Exc

[7th] **T82.329 Displacement of unspecified vascular grafts** CC POA HCC CC/MCC Exc

T82.33 Leakage of other vascular grafts
- **T82.330** Leakage of aortic (bifurcation) graft (replacement)
- **T82.331** Leakage of carotid arterial graft (bypass)
- **T82.332** Leakage of femoral arterial graft (bypass)
- **T82.338** Leakage of other vascular grafts
- **T82.339** Leakage of unspecified vascular graft

T82.39 Other mechanical complication of other vascular grafts
Obstruction (mechanical) of other vascular grafts
Perforation of other vascular grafts
Protrusion of other vascular grafts
- **T82.390** Other mechanical complication of aortic (bifurcation) graft (replacement)
- **T82.391** Other mechanical complication of carotid arterial graft (bypass)
- **T82.392** Other mechanical complication of femoral arterial graft (bypass)
- **T82.398** Other mechanical complication of other vascular grafts
- **T82.399** Other mechanical complication of unspecified vascular grafts

T82.4 Mechanical complication of vascular dialysis catheter
Mechanical complication of hemodialysis catheter
EXCLUDES1 mechanical complication of intraperitoneal dialysis catheter (T85.62)

T82.41 Breakdown (mechanical) of vascular dialysis catheter

T82.42 Displacement of vascular dialysis catheter
Malposition of vascular dialysis catheter

T82.43 Leakage of vascular dialysis catheter

T82.49 Other complication of vascular dialysis catheter
Obstruction (mechanical) of vascular dialysis catheter
Perforation of vascular dialysis catheter
Protrusion of vascular dialysis catheter

T82.5 Mechanical complication of other cardiac and vascular devices and implants
EXCLUDES2 mechanical complication of epidural and subdural infusion catheter (T85.61)

T82.51 Breakdown (mechanical) of other cardiac and vascular devices and implants
- **T82.510** Breakdown (mechanical) of surgically created arteriovenous fistula
- **T82.511** Breakdown (mechanical) of surgically created arteriovenous shunt
- **T82.512** Breakdown (mechanical) of artificial heart
- **T82.513** Breakdown (mechanical) of balloon (counterpulsation) device
- **T82.514** Breakdown (mechanical) of infusion catheter
- **T82.515** Breakdown (mechanical) of umbrella device
- **T82.518** Breakdown (mechanical) of other cardiac and vascular devices and implants
- **T82.519** Breakdown (mechanical) of unspecified cardiac and vascular devices and implants

T82.52 Displacement of other cardiac and vascular devices and implants
Malposition of other cardiac and vascular devices and implants

T82.520 Displacement of surgically created arteriovenous fistula
T82.521 Displacement of surgically created arteriovenous shunt
T82.522 Displacement of artificial heart
T82.523 Displacement of balloon (counterpulsation) device
T82.524 Displacement of infusion catheter
T82.525 Displacement of umbrella device
T82.528 Displacement of other cardiac and vascular devices and implants
T82.529 Displacement of unspecified cardiac and vascular devices and implants

T82.53 Leakage of other cardiac and vascular devices and implants
- **T82.530** Leakage of surgically created arteriovenous fistula
- **T82.531** Leakage of surgically created arteriovenous shunt
- **T82.532** Leakage of artificial heart
- **T82.533** Leakage of balloon (counterpulsation) device
- **T82.534** Leakage of infusion catheter
- **T82.535** Leakage of umbrella device
- **T82.538** Leakage of other cardiac and vascular devices and implants
- **T82.539** Leakage of unspecified cardiac and vascular devices and implants

T82.59 Other mechanical complication of other cardiac and vascular devices and implants
Obstruction (mechanical) of other cardiac and vascular devices and implants
Perforation of other cardiac and vascular devices and implants
Protrusion of other cardiac and vascular devices and implants
- **T82.590** Other mechanical complication of surgically created arteriovenous fistula
- **T82.591** Other mechanical complication of surgically created arteriovenous shunt
- **T82.592** Other mechanical complication of artificial heart
- **T82.593** Other mechanical complication of balloon (counterpulsation) device
- **T82.594** Other mechanical complication of infusion catheter
- **T82.595** Other mechanical complication of umbrella device
- **T82.598** Other mechanical complication of other cardiac and vascular devices and implants
- **T82.599** Other mechanical complication of unspecified cardiac and vascular devices and implants

T82.6 Infection and inflammatory reaction due to cardiac valve prosthesis
Use additional code to identify infection

T82.7 Infection and inflammatory reaction due to other cardiac and vascular devices, implants and grafts
AHA: Q1 2019, Q1 2015
Use additional code to identify infection

T82.8 Other specified complications of cardiac and vascular prosthetic devices, implants and grafts
T82.81 Embolism due to cardiac and vascular prosthetic devices, implants and grafts
- **T82.817** Embolism due to cardiac prosthetic devices, implants and grafts
AHA: Q4 2016

1166

When symbols appear on a code that requires a 7th character extension, refer to Appendix B to identify applicable 7th character codes.

2020 ICD-10-CM

7️⃣ **T82.818** Embolism due to vascular prosthetic devices, implants and grafts cc🔵 POA HCC CC/MCC Exc

6️⃣ **T82.82** Fibrosis due to cardiac and vascular prosthetic devices, implants and grafts

  7️⃣ **T82.827** Fibrosis due to cardiac prosthetic devices, implants and grafts cc🔵 POA CC/MCC Exc

  7️⃣ **T82.828** Fibrosis due to vascular prosthetic devices, implants and grafts cc🔵 POA HCC CC/MCC Exc

6️⃣ **T82.83** Hemorrhage due to cardiac and vascular prosthetic devices, implants and grafts

  7️⃣ **T82.837** Hemorrhage due to cardiac prosthetic devices, implants and grafts cc🔵 POA CC/MCC Exc

  7️⃣ **T82.838** Hemorrhage due to vascular prosthetic devices, implants and grafts cc🔵 POA HCC CC/MCC Exc

6️⃣ **T82.84** Pain due to cardiac and vascular prosthetic devices, implants and grafts

  7️⃣ **T82.847** Pain due to cardiac prosthetic devices, implants and grafts cc🔵 POA CC/MCC Exc

  7️⃣ **T82.848** Pain due to vascular prosthetic devices, implants and grafts cc🔵 POA HCC CC/MCC Exc

6️⃣ **T82.85** Stenosis due to cardiac and vascular prosthetic devices, implants and grafts

  7️⃣ **T82.855** Stenosis of coronary artery stent cc🔵 POA CC/MCC Exc

    AHA: Q4 2016
In-stent stenosis (restenosis) of coronary artery stent
Restenosis of coronary artery stent

  7️⃣ **T82.856** Stenosis of peripheral vascular stent cc🔵 POA HCC CC/MCC Exc

    AHA: Q4 2016
In-stent stenosis (restenosis) of peripheral vascular stent
Restenosis of peripheral vascular stent

  7️⃣ **T82.857** Stenosis of other cardiac prosthetic devices, implants and grafts cc🔵 POA CC/MCC Exc

    AHA: Q4 2016

  7️⃣ **T82.858** Stenosis of other vascular prosthetic devices, implants and grafts cc🔵 POA HCC CC/MCC Exc

    AHA: Q4 2016

6️⃣ **T82.86** Thrombosis of cardiac and vascular prosthetic devices, implants and grafts

  7️⃣ **T82.867** Thrombosis due to cardiac prosthetic devices, implants and grafts cc🔵 POA CC/MCC Exc

    AHA: Q2 2019

  7️⃣ **T82.868** Thrombosis due to vascular prosthetic devices, implants and grafts cc🔵 POA HCC CC/MCC Exc

6️⃣ **T82.89** Other specified complication of cardiac and vascular prosthetic devices, implants and grafts

  7️⃣ **T82.897** Other specified complication of cardiac prosthetic devices, implants and grafts cc🔵 POA CC/MCC Exc

    AHA: Q2 2019

  7️⃣ **T82.898** Other specified complication of vascular prosthetic devices, implants and grafts cc🔵 POA HCC CC/MCC Exc

🄿 **T82.9** Unspecified complication of cardiac and vascular prosthetic device, implant and graft 🔵 POA CC/MCC Exc

4️⃣ **T83** Complications of genitourinary prosthetic devices, implants and grafts

  EXCLUDES2 failure and rejection of transplanted organs and tissue (T86.-)

  The appropriate 7th character is to be added to each code from category T83

    A = initial encounter
    D = subsequent encounter
    S = sequela

5️⃣ **T83.0** Mechanical complication of urinary catheter

  EXCLUDES2 complications of stoma of urinary tract (N99.5-)

  6️⃣ **T83.01** Breakdown (mechanical) of urinary catheter

    7️⃣ **T83.010** Breakdown (mechanical) of cystostomy catheter cc🔵 POA HCC CC/MCC Exc

7️⃣ **T83.011** Breakdown (mechanical) of indwelling urethral catheter POA HCC

7️⃣ **T83.012** Breakdown (mechanical) of nephrostomy catheter POA HCC

7️⃣ **T83.018** Breakdown (mechanical) of other urinary catheter POA HCC

  Breakdown (mechanical) of Hopkins catheter
  Breakdown (mechanical) of ileostomy catheter
  Breakdown (mechanical) urostomy catheter

6️⃣ **T83.02** Displacement of urinary catheter

  Malposition of urinary catheter

  7️⃣ **T83.020** Displacement of cystostomy catheter cc🔵 POA HCC CC/MCC Exc

  7️⃣ **T83.021** Displacement of indwelling urethral catheter POA HCC

  7️⃣ **T83.022** Displacement of nephrostomy catheter POA HCC

  7️⃣ **T83.028** Displacement of other urinary catheter POA HCC

    Displacement of Hopkins catheter
    Displacement of ileostomy catheter
    Displacement of urostomy catheter

6️⃣ **T83.03** Leakage of urinary catheter

  7️⃣ **T83.030** Leakage of cystostomy catheter cc🔵 POA HCC CC/MCC Exc

  7️⃣ **T83.031** Leakage of indwelling urethral catheter POA HCC

  7️⃣ **T83.032** Leakage of nephrostomy catheter POA HCC

  7️⃣ **T83.038** Leakage of other urinary catheter POA HCC

    Leakage of Hopkins catheter
    Leakage of ileostomy catheter
    Leakage of urostomy catheter

6️⃣ **T83.09** Other mechanical complication of urinary catheter

  Obstruction (mechanical) of urinary catheter
  Perforation of urinary catheter
  Protrusion of urinary catheter

  7️⃣ **T83.090** Other mechanical complication of cystostomy catheter cc🔵 POA HCC CC/MCC Exc

  7️⃣ **T83.091** Other mechanical complication of indwelling urethral catheter POA HCC

  7️⃣ **T83.092** Other mechanical complication of nephrostomy catheter

  7️⃣ **T83.098** Other mechanical complication of other urinary catheter POA HCC

    Other mechanical complication of Hopkins catheter
    Other mechanical complication of ileostomy catheter
    Other mechanical complication of urostomy catheter

5️⃣ **T83.1** Mechanical complication of other urinary devices and implants

  6️⃣ **T83.11** Breakdown (mechanical) of other urinary devices and implants

    7️⃣ **T83.110** Breakdown (mechanical) of urinary electronic stimulator device cc🔵 POA HCC CC/MCC Exc

      EXCLUDES2 Breakdown (mechanical) of electrode (lead) for sacral nerve neurostimulator (T85.111)
        Breakdown (mechanical) of implanted electronic sacral neurostimulator, pulse generator or receiver (T85.113)

    7️⃣ **T83.111** Breakdown (mechanical) of implanted urinary sphincter cc🔵 POA HCC CC/MCC Exc

    7️⃣ **T83.112** Breakdown (mechanical) of indwelling ureteral stent cc🔵 POA HCC CC/MCC Exc

    7️⃣ **T83.113** Breakdown (mechanical) of other urinary stents cc🔵 HCC CC/MCC Exc

      Breakdown (mechanical) of ileal conduit stent
      Breakdown (mechanical) of nephroureteral stent

Unspecified Code   Other Specified Code   Manifestation Code   N Newborn   P Pediatric   M Maternity   A Adult   ♂ Male   ♀ Female
● New Code   ▲ Revised Code Title   ▶◀ Revised Text   NOTES   INCLUDES   EXCLUDES1 Not coded here   EXCLUDES2 Not included here
4️⃣ 4th character required   5️⃣ 5th character required   6️⃣ 6th character required   7️⃣ 7th character required   🔵 Extension 'X' Alert
HAC Hospital-acquired condition (HAC) alert   AHA AHA Coding Clinic©   📣 Code first alert

2020 ICD-10-CM   When symbols appear on a code that requires a 7th character extension, refer to Appendix B to identify applicable 7th character codes.   **1167**

⑦ᵗʰ **T83.118** **Breakdown (mechanical) of** other urinary devices and implants cc̸ POA HCC CC/MCC Exc

⑥ᵗʰ **T83.12** Displacement **of other urinary devices and implants**
Malposition of other urinary devices and implants

⑦ᵗʰ **T83.120** **Displacement of urinary** electronic stimulator device cc̸ POA HCC CC/MCC Exc

EXCLUDES2 *Displacement of electrode (lead) for sacral nerve neurostimulator (T85.121)*

Displacement of implanted electronic sacral neurostimulator, pulse generator or receiver (T85.123)

⑦ᵗʰ **T83.121** **Displacement of** implanted urinary sphincter cc̸ POA HCC CC/MCC Exc

⑦ᵗʰ **T83.122** **Displacement of** indwelling ureteral stent cc̸ POA HCC CC/MCC Exc

⑦ᵗʰ **T83.123** **Displacement of** other urinary stents cc̸ HCC CC/MCC Exc
Displacement of ileal conduit stent
Displacement of nephroureteral stent

⑦ᵗʰ **T83.128** **Displacement of** other urinary devices and implants cc̸ POA HCC CC/MCC Exc

⑥ᵗʰ **T83.19** Other **mechanical complication of other urinary devices and implants**
Leakage of other urinary devices and implants
Obstruction (mechanical) of other urinary devices and implants
Perforation of other urinary devices and implants
Protrusion of other urinary devices and implants

⑦ᵗʰ **T83.190** **Other mechanical complication of urinary** electronic stimulator device cc̸ POA HCC CC/MCC Exc

EXCLUDES2 *Other mechanical complication of electrode (lead) for sacral nerve neurostimulator (T85.191)*

Other mechanical complication of implanted electronic sacral neurostimulator, pulse generator or receiver (T85.193)

⑦ᵗʰ **T83.191** **Other mechanical complication of** implanted urinary sphincter cc̸ POA HCC CC/MCC Exc

⑦ᵗʰ **T83.192** **Other mechanical complication of** indwelling ureteral stent cc̸ POA HCC CC/MCC Exc

⑦ᵗʰ **T83.193** **Other mechanical complication of** other urinary stent cc̸ POA HCC CC/MCC Exc
Other mechanical complication of ileal conduit stent
Other mechanical complication of nephroureteral stent

⑦ᵗʰ **T83.198** Other **mechanical complication of other urinary devices and implants** cc̸ POA HCC CC/MCC Exc

⑤ᵗʰ **T83.2** **Mechanical complication of** graft of urinary organ

⑦ᵗʰ **T83.21** Breakdown (mechanical) **of graft of urinary organ** cc̸ POA HCC CC/MCC Exc

⑦ᵗʰ **T83.22** Displacement **of graft of urinary organ** cc̸ POA HCC CC/MCC Exc
Malposition of graft of urinary organ

⑦ᵗʰ **T83.23** Leakage **of graft of urinary organ** cc̸ POA HCC CC/MCC Exc

⑦ᵗʰ **T83.24** Erosion **of graft of urinary organ** cc̸ POA HCC CC/MCC Exc
AHA: Q4 2016

⑦ᵗʰ **T83.25** Exposure **of graft of urinary organ** cc̸ POA HCC CC/MCC Exc
AHA: Q4 2016

⑦ᵗʰ **T83.29** Other **mechanical complication of graft of urinary organ** cc̸ POA HCC CC/MCC Exc
Obstruction (mechanical) of graft of urinary organ
Perforation of graft of urinary organ
Protrusion of graft of urinary organ

⑤ᵗʰ **T83.3** **Mechanical complication of** intrauterine contraceptive device

⑦ᵗʰ **T83.31** Breakdown (mechanical) **of intrauterine contraceptive device** POA ♀

⑦ᵗʰ **T83.32** Displacement **of intrauterine contraceptive device** POA ♀
Malposition of intrauterine contraceptive device
Missing string of intrauterine contraceptive device

⑦ᵗʰ **T83.39** Other **mechanical complication of intrauterine contraceptive device** POA ♀
Leakage of intrauterine contraceptive device
Obstruction (mechanical) of intrauterine contraceptive device
Perforation of intrauterine contraceptive device
Protrusion of intrauterine contraceptive device

⑤ᵗʰ **T83.4** **Mechanical complication of** other prosthetic devices, implants and grafts of genital tract

⑥ᵗʰ **T83.41** Breakdown (mechanical) **of other prosthetic devices, implants and grafts of genital tract**

⑦ᵗʰ **T83.410** **Breakdown (mechanical) of** implanted penile prosthesis cc̸ HCC ♂ CC/MCC Exc
Breakdown (mechanical) of penile prosthesis cylinder
Breakdown (mechanical) of penile prosthesis pump
Breakdown (mechanical) of penile prosthesis reservoir

⑦ᵗʰ **T83.411** **Breakdown (mechanical) of implanted** testicular prosthesis cc̸ POA HCC CC/MCC Exc

⑦ᵗʰ **T83.418** **Breakdown (mechanical) of** other **prosthetic devices, implants and grafts of genital tract** cc̸ POA HCC CC/MCC Exc

⑥ᵗʰ **T83.42** Displacement **of other prosthetic devices, implants and grafts of genital tract**
Malposition of other prosthetic devices, implants and grafts of genital tract

⑦ᵗʰ **T83.420** **Displacement of** implanted penile prosthesis cc̸ POA HCC ♂ CC/MCC Exc
Displacement of penile prosthesis cylinder
Displacement of penile prosthesis pump
Displacement of penile prosthesis reservoir

⑦ᵗʰ **T83.421** **Displacement of** implanted testicular prosthesis cc̸ POA HCC CC/MCC Exc

⑦ᵗʰ **T83.428** **Displacement of** other **prosthetic devices, implants and grafts of genital tract** cc̸ POA HCC CC/MCC Exc
AHA: Q1 2018

⑥ᵗʰ **T83.49** Other **mechanical complication of other prosthetic devices, implants and grafts of genital tract**
Leakage of other prosthetic devices, implants and grafts of genital tract
Obstruction, mechanical of other prosthetic devices, implants and grafts of genital tract
Perforation of other prosthetic devices, implants and grafts of genital tract
Protrusion of other prosthetic devices, implants and grafts of genital tract

⑦ᵗʰ **T83.490** **Other mechanical complication of** implanted penile prosthesis cc̸ POA HCC ♂ CC/MCC Exc
Other mechanical complication of penile prosthesis cylinder
Other mechanical complication of penile prosthesis pump
Other mechanical complication of penile prosthesis reservoir

⑦ᵗʰ **T83.491** **Other mechanical complication of** implanted testicular prosthesis cc̸ POA HCC CC/MCC Exc

⑦ᵗʰ **T83.498** **Other mechanical complication of** other **prosthetic devices, implants and grafts of genital tract** cc̸ POA HCC CC/MCC Exc

⑤ᵗʰ **T83.5** Infection and inflammatory reaction **due to prosthetic device, implant and graft in** urinary system
Use additional code to identify infection

⑥ᵗʰ **T83.51** **Infection and inflammatory reaction due to** urinary catheter

EXCLUDES2 *complications of stoma of urinary tract (N99.5-)*

⑦ᵗʰ **T83.510** **Infection and inflammatory reaction due to** cystostomy catheter cc̸ POA HCC CC/MCC Exc

POA̸ Unacceptable principal diagnosis symbol per Medicare code edits POA Code exempt from diagnosis present on admission requirement
❓ Questionable admission cc̸ Complication or comorbidity MCC Major complication or comorbidity CC/MCC Exc CC/MCC exclusion
HCC HCC diagnosis code RxHCC RxHCC diagnosis code MACRA MACRA code **DEFINITION** Describes condition/terminology
TIP Coding guidance 👁 Official Guideline Reference Z1 Z code as first-listed diagnosis

When symbols appear on a code that requires a 7th character extension, refer to Appendix B to identify applicable 7th character codes.

2020 ICD-10-CM

[7th] **T83.511 Infection and inflammatory reaction due to indwelling urethral catheter** [CC] [POA] [HAC] [HCC] [CC/MCC Exc]

[7th] **T83.512 Infection and inflammatory reaction due to nephrostomy catheter** [CC] [POA] [HCC] [CC/MCC Exc]

[7th] **T83.518 Infection and inflammatory reaction due to other urinary catheter** [CC] [POA] [HAC] [HCC] [CC/MCC Exc]
Infection and inflammatory reaction due to Hopkins catheter
Infection and inflammatory reaction due to ileostomy catheter
Infection and inflammatory reaction due to urostomy catheter

[6th] **T83.59 Infection and inflammatory reaction due to prosthetic device, implant and graft in urinary system**

[7th] **T83.590 Infection and inflammatory reaction due to implanted urinary neurostimulation device** [CC] [POA] [HCC] [CC/MCC Exc]
[EXCLUDES2] *Infection and inflammatory reaction due to electrode lead of sacral nerve neurostimulator (T85.732)*
Infection and inflammatory reaction due to pulse generator or receiver of sacral nerve neurostimulator (T85.734)

[7th] **T83.591 Infection and inflammatory reaction due to implanted urinary sphincter** [CC] [POA] [HCC] [CC/MCC Exc]

[7th] **T83.592 Infection and inflammatory reaction due to indwelling ureteral stent** [CC] [POA] [HCC] [CC/MCC Exc]

[7th] **T83.593 Infection and inflammatory reaction due to other urinary stents** [CC] [POA] [HCC] [CC/MCC Exc]
Infection and inflammatory reaction due to ileal conduit stents
Infection and inflammatory reaction due to nephroureteral stent

[7th] **T83.598 Infection and inflammatory reaction due to other prosthetic device, implant and graft in urinary system** [CC] [POA] [HCC] [CC/MCC Exc]

[5th] **T83.6 Infection and inflammatory reaction due to prosthetic device, implant and graft in genital tract**
Use additional code to identify infection

[7th] **T83.61 Infection and inflammatory reaction due to implanted penile prosthesis** [CC] [POA] [HCC] [CC/MCC Exc]
Infection and inflammatory reaction due to penile prosthesis cylinder
Infection and inflammatory reaction due to penile prosthesis pump
Infection and inflammatory reaction due to penile prosthesis reservoir

[7th] **T83.62 Infection and inflammatory reaction due to implanted testicular prosthesis** [CC] [POA] [HCC] [CC/MCC Exc]

[7th] **T83.69 Infection and inflammatory reaction due to other prosthetic device, implant and graft in genital tract** [CC] [POA] [HCC] [CC/MCC Exc]

[5th] **T83.7 Complications due to implanted mesh and other prosthetic materials**

[6th] **T83.71 Erosion of implanted mesh and other prosthetic materials to surrounding organ or tissue**

[7th] **T83.711 Erosion of implanted vaginal mesh to surrounding organ or tissue** [POA] [HCC] ♀
AHA: Q4 2016
Erosion of implanted vaginal mesh into pelvic floor muscles

[7th] **T83.712 Erosion of implanted urethral mesh to surrounding organ or tissue** [CC] [POA] [HCC] [CC/MCC Exc]
Erosion of implanted female urethral sling
Erosion of implanted male urethral sling
Erosion of implanted urethral mesh into pelvic floor muscles

[7th] **T83.713 Erosion of implanted urethral bulking agent to surrounding organ or tissue** [CC] [POA] [HCC] [CC/MCC Exc]

[7th] **T83.714 Erosion of implanted ureteral bulking agent to surrounding organ or tissue** [CC] [POA] [HCC] [CC/MCC Exc]

[7th] **T83.718 Erosion of other implanted mesh to organ or tissue** [CC] [POA] [HCC] [CC/MCC Exc]
AHA: Q4 2016

[7th] **T83.719 Erosion of other prosthetic materials to surrounding organ or tissue** [CC] [POA] [HCC] [CC/MCC Exc]
AHA: Q4 2016

[6th] **T83.72 Exposure of implanted mesh and other prosthetic materials into surrounding organ or tissue**
Extrusion of implanted mesh

[7th] **T83.721 Exposure of implanted vaginal mesh into vagina** [POA] [HCC] ♀
Exposure of implanted vaginal mesh through vaginal wall

[7th] **T83.722 Exposure of implanted urethral mesh into urethra** [CC] [POA] [HCC] [CC/MCC Exc]
Exposure of implanted female urethral sling
Exposure of implanted male urethral sling
Exposure of implanted urethral mesh through urethral wall

[7th] **T83.723 Exposure of implanted urethral bulking agent into urethra** [CC] [POA] [HCC] [CC/MCC Exc]

[7th] **T83.724 Exposure of implanted ureteral bulking agent into ureter** [CC] [POA] [HCC] [CC/MCC Exc]

[7th] **T83.728 Exposure of other implanted mesh into organ or tissue** [CC] [POA] [HCC] [CC/MCC Exc]
AHA: Q4 2016

[7th] **T83.729 Exposure of other prosthetic materials into organ or tissue** [CC] [POA] [HCC] [CC/MCC Exc]
AHA: Q4 2016

[7th] **T83.79 Other specified complications due to other genitourinary prosthetic materials** [CC] [POA] [HCC] [CC/MCC Exc]

[5th] **T83.8 Other specified complications of genitourinary prosthetic devices, implants and grafts**

[7th] **T83.81 Embolism due to genitourinary prosthetic devices, implants and grafts** [CC] [POA] [HCC] [CC/MCC Exc]

[7th] **T83.82 Fibrosis due to genitourinary prosthetic devices, implants and grafts** [CC] [POA] [HCC] [CC/MCC Exc]

[7th] **T83.83 Hemorrhage due to genitourinary prosthetic devices, implants and grafts** [CC] [POA] [HCC] [CC/MCC Exc]

[7th] **T83.84 Pain due to genitourinary prosthetic devices, implants and grafts** [CC] [POA] [HCC] [CC/MCC Exc]

[7th] **T83.85 Stenosis due to genitourinary prosthetic devices, implants and grafts** [CC] [POA] [HCC] [CC/MCC Exc]

[7th] **T83.86 Thrombosis due to genitourinary prosthetic devices, implants and grafts** [CC] [POA] [HCC] [CC/MCC Exc]

[7th] **T83.89 Other specified complication of genitourinary prosthetic devices, implants and grafts** [CC] [POA] [HCC] [CC/MCC Exc]

[7th] **T83.9 Unspecified complication of genitourinary prosthetic device, implant and graft** [CC] [POA] [HCC] [CC/MCC Exc]

[4th] **T84 Complications of internal orthopedic prosthetic devices, implants and grafts**
[EXCLUDES2] *failure and rejection of transplanted organs and tissues (T86.-)*
fracture of bone following insertion of orthopedic implant, joint prosthesis or bone plate (M96.6)

The appropriate 7th character is to be added to each code from category T84
A = initial encounter
D = subsequent encounter
S = sequela

[5th] **T84.0 Mechanical complication of internal joint prosthesis**

[6th] **T84.01 Broken internal joint prosthesis**
Breakage (fracture) of prosthetic joint
Broken prosthetic joint implant
[EXCLUDES1] *periprosthetic joint implant fracture (M97-)*

Unspecified Code | Other Specified Code | Manifestation Code | [N] Newborn | [P] Pediatric | [M] Maternity | [A] Adult | ♂ Male | ♀ Female
● New Code | ▲ Revised Code Title | ►◄ Revised Text | [NOTES] | *INCLUDES* | [EXCLUDES1] Not coded here | [EXCLUDES2] Not included here
[4th] 4th character required | [5th] 5th character required | [6th] 6th character required | [7th] 7th character required | [7th] Extension 'X' Alert
[HAC] Hospital-acquired condition (HAC) alert | AHA AHA Coding Clinic© | ☞ Code first alert

7ᵗʰ **T84.010** **Broken internal** right hip **prosthesis** CC POₐ HCC CC/MCC Exc

7ᵗʰ **T84.011** **Broken internal** left hip **prosthesis** CC POₐ HCC CC/MCC Exc

7ᵗʰ **T84.012** **Broken internal** right knee **prosthesis** CC POₐ HCC CC/MCC Exc

7ᵗʰ **T84.013** **Broken internal** left knee **prosthesis** CC POₐ HCC CC/MCC Exc

7ᵗʰ **T84.018** **Broken internal joint prosthesis,** other site CC POₐ HCC CC/MCC Exc

Use additional code to identify the joint (Z96.6-)

7ᵗʰ **T84.019** **Broken internal joint prosthesis, unspecified site** CC POₐ HCC CC/MCC Exc

6ᵗʰ **T84.02** Dislocation **of internal joint prosthesis**

Instability of internal joint prosthesis
Subluxation of internal joint prosthesis

7ᵗʰ **T84.020** **Dislocation of internal** right hip **prosthesis** CC POₐ HCC CC/MCC Exc

7ᵗʰ **T84.021** **Dislocation of internal** left hip **prosthesis** CC POₐ HCC CC/MCC Exc

AHA: Q2 2019

7ᵗʰ **T84.022** **Instability of internal** right knee **prosthesis** CC POₐ HCC CC/MCC Exc

7ᵗʰ **T84.023** **Instability of internal** left knee **prosthesis** CC POₐ HCC CC/MCC Exc

7ᵗʰ **T84.028** **Dislocation of** other **internal joint prosthesis** CC POₐ HCC CC/MCC Exc

Use additional code to identify the joint (Z96.6-)

7ᵗʰ **T84.029** **Dislocation of unspecified internal joint prosthesis** CC POₐ HCC CC/MCC Exc

6ᵗʰ **T84.03** Mechanical loosening **of internal prosthetic joint**

Aseptic loosening of prosthetic joint

7ᵗʰ **T84.030** **Mechanical loosening of internal** right hip **prosthetic joint** CC POₐ HCC CC/MCC Exc

7ᵗʰ **T84.031** **Mechanical loosening of internal** left hip **prosthetic joint** CC POₐ HCC CC/MCC Exc

7ᵗʰ **T84.032** **Mechanical loosening of internal** right **knee prosthetic joint** CC POₐ HCC CC/MCC Exc

7ᵗʰ **T84.033** **Mechanical loosening of internal** left knee **prosthetic joint** CC POₐ HCC CC/MCC Exc

7ᵗʰ **T84.038** **Mechanical loosening of** other **internal prosthetic joint** CC POₐ HCC CC/MCC Exc

Use additional code to identify the joint (Z96.6-)

7ᵗʰ **T84.039** **Mechanical loosening of unspecified internal prosthetic joint** CC POₐ HCC CC/MCC Exc

6ᵗʰ **T84.05** Periprosthetic osteolysis **of internal prosthetic joint**

Use additional code to identify major osseous defect, if applicable (M89.7-)

7ᵗʰ **T84.050** **Periprosthetic osteolysis of internal** right hip **joint** CC POₐ HCC CC/MCC Exc

7ᵗʰ **T84.051** **Periprosthetic osteolysis of internal prosthetic** left hip **joint** CC POₐ HCC CC/MCC Exc

7ᵗʰ **T84.052** **Periprosthetic osteolysis of internal prosthetic** right knee **joint** CC POₐ HCC CC/MCC Exc

7ᵗʰ **T84.053** **Periprosthetic osteolysis of internal prosthetic** left knee **joint** CC POₐ HCC CC/MCC Exc

7ᵗʰ **T84.058** **Periprosthetic osteolysis of** other **internal prosthetic joint** CC POₐ HCC CC/MCC Exc

Use additional code to identify the joint (Z96.6-)

7ᵗʰ **T84.059** **Periprosthetic osteolysis of unspecified internal prosthetic joint** CC POₐ HCC CC/MCC Exc

6ᵗʰ **T84.06** Wear of articular bearing surface **of internal prosthetic joint**

7ᵗʰ **T84.060** **Wear of articular bearing surface of internal prosthetic** right hip **joint** CC POₐ HCC CC/MCC Exc

7ᵗʰ **T84.061** **Wear of articular bearing surface of internal prosthetic** left hip **joint** CC POₐ HCC CC/MCC Exc

7ᵗʰ **T84.062** **Wear of articular bearing surface of internal prosthetic** right knee **joint** CC POₐ HCC CC/MCC Exc

7ᵗʰ **T84.063** **Wear of articular bearing surface of internal prosthetic** left knee **joint** CC POₐ HCC CC/MCC Exc

7ᵗʰ **T84.068** **Wear of articular bearing surface of** other **internal prosthetic joint** CC POₐ HCC CC/MCC Exc

Use additional code to identify the joint (Z96.6-)

7ᵗʰ **T84.069** **Wear of articular bearing surface of unspecified internal prosthetic joint** CC POₐ HCC CC/MCC Exc

6ᵗʰ **T84.09** Other **mechanical complication of internal joint prosthesis**

Prosthetic joint implant failure NOS

7ᵗʰ **T84.090** **Other mechanical complication of internal** right hip prosthesis CC POₐ HCC CC/MCC Exc

7ᵗʰ **T84.091** **Other mechanical complication of internal** left hip prosthesis CC POₐ HCC CC/MCC Exc

7ᵗʰ **T84.092** **Other mechanical complication of internal** right knee prosthesis CC POₐ HCC CC/MCC Exc

7ᵗʰ **T84.093** **Other mechanical complication of internal** left knee prosthesis CC POₐ HCC CC/MCC Exc

7ᵗʰ **T84.098** **Other mechanical complication of** other **internal joint prosthesis** CC POₐ HCC CC/MCC Exc

Use additional code to identify the joint (Z96.6-)

7ᵗʰ **T84.099** **Other mechanical complication of unspecified internal joint prosthesis** CC POₐ HCC CC/MCC Exc

5ᵗʰ **T84.1** **Mechanical complication of** internal fixation device of bones of limb

EXCLUDES2 *mechanical complication of internal fixation device of bones of feet (T84.2-)*

mechanical complication of internal fixation device of bones of fingers (T84.2-)

mechanical complication of internal fixation device of bones of hands (T84.2-)

mechanical complication of internal fixation device of bones of toes (T84.2-)

6ᵗʰ **T84.11** Breakdown **(mechanical) of internal fixation device of bones of limb**

7ᵗʰ **T84.110** **Breakdown (mechanical) of internal fixation device of** right humerus CC POₐ HCC CC/MCC Exc

7ᵗʰ **T84.111** **Breakdown (mechanical) of internal fixation device of** left humerus CC POₐ HCC CC/MCC Exc

7ᵗʰ **T84.112** **Breakdown (mechanical) of internal fixation device of bone of** right forearm CC POₐ HCC CC/MCC Exc

7ᵗʰ **T84.113** **Breakdown (mechanical) of internal fixation device of bone of** left forearm CC POₐ HCC CC/MCC Exc

7ᵗʰ **T84.114** **Breakdown (mechanical) of internal fixation device of** right femur CC POₐ HCC CC/MCC Exc

7ᵗʰ **T84.115** **Breakdown (mechanical) of internal fixation device of** left femur CC POₐ HCC CC/MCC Exc

7ᵗʰ **T84.116** **Breakdown (mechanical) of internal fixation device of bone of** right lower leg CC POₐ HCC CC/MCC Exc

7ᵗʰ **T84.117** **Breakdown (mechanical) of internal fixation device of bone of** left lower leg CC POₐ HCC CC/MCC Exc

7ᵗʰ **T84.119** **Breakdown (mechanical) of internal fixation device of unspecified bone of limb** CC POₐ HCC CC/MCC Exc

6ᵗʰ **T84.12** Displacement **of internal fixation device of bones of limb**
  Malposition of internal fixation device of bones of limb

  7ᵗʰ **T84.120** **Displacement of internal fixation device of** right humerus   CC POA HCC CC/MCC Exc

  7ᵗʰ **T84.121** **Displacement of internal fixation device of** left humerus   CC POA HCC CC/MCC Exc

  7ᵗʰ **T84.122** **Displacement of internal fixation device of bone of** right forearm   CC POA HCC CC/MCC Exc

  7ᵗʰ **T84.123** **Displacement of internal fixation device of bone of** left forearm   CC POA HCC CC/MCC Exc

  7ᵗʰ **T84.124** **Displacement of internal fixation device of** right femur   CC POA HCC CC/MCC Exc

  7ᵗʰ **T84.125** **Displacement of internal fixation device of** left femur   CC POA HCC CC/MCC Exc

  7ᵗʰ **T84.126** **Displacement of internal fixation device of bone of** right lower leg   CC POA HCC CC/MCC Exc

  7ᵗʰ **T84.127** **Displacement of internal fixation device of bone of** left lower leg   CC POA HCC CC/MCC Exc

  7ᵗʰ **T84.129** **Displacement of internal fixation device of unspecified bone of limb**   CC POA HCC CC/MCC Exc

6ᵗʰ **T84.19** Other **mechanical complication of internal fixation device of bones of limb**
  Obstruction (mechanical) of internal fixation device of bones of limb
  Perforation of internal fixation device of bones of limb
  Protrusion of internal fixation device of bones of limb

  7ᵗʰ **T84.190** **Other mechanical complication of internal fixation device of** right humerus   CC POA HCC CC/MCC Exc

  7ᵗʰ **T84.191** **Other mechanical complication of internal fixation device of** left humerus   CC POA HCC CC/MCC Exc

  7ᵗʰ **T84.192** **Other mechanical complication of internal fixation device of bone of** right forearm   CC POA HCC CC/MCC Exc

  7ᵗʰ **T84.193** **Other mechanical complication of internal fixation device of bone of** left forearm   CC POA HCC CC/MCC Exc

  7ᵗʰ **T84.194** **Other mechanical complication of internal fixation device of** right femur   CC POA HCC CC/MCC Exc

  7ᵗʰ **T84.195** **Other mechanical complication of internal fixation device of** left femur   CC POA HCC CC/MCC Exc

  7ᵗʰ **T84.196** **Other mechanical complication of internal fixation device of bone of** right lower leg   CC POA HCC CC/MCC Exc

  7ᵗʰ **T84.197** **Other mechanical complication of internal fixation device of bone of** left lower leg   CC POA HCC CC/MCC Exc

  7ᵗʰ **T84.199** **Other mechanical complication of internal fixation device of unspecified bone of limb**   CC POA HCC CC/MCC Exc

5ᵗʰ **T84.2** **Mechanical complication of** internal fixation device **of** other bones

  6ᵗʰ **T84.21** Breakdown **(mechanical) of internal fixation device of other bones**

    7ᵗʰ **T84.210** **Breakdown (mechanical) of internal fixation device of bones of** hand and fingers   CC POA HCC CC/MCC Exc

    7ᵗʰ **T84.213** **Breakdown (mechanical) of internal fixation device of bones of** foot and toes   CC POA HCC CC/MCC Exc

    7ᵗʰ **T84.216** **Breakdown (mechanical) of internal fixation device of** vertebrae   CC POA HCC CC/MCC Exc

    7ᵗʰ **T84.218** **Breakdown (mechanical) of internal fixation device of** other bones   CC POA HCC CC/MCC Exc

  6ᵗʰ **T84.22** Displacement **of internal fixation device of other bones**
    Malposition of internal fixation device of other bones

    7ᵗʰ **T84.220** **Displacement of internal fixation device of bones of** hand and fingers   CC POA HCC CC/MCC Exc

    7ᵗʰ **T84.223** **Displacement of internal fixation device of bones of** foot and toes   CC POA HCC CC/MCC Exc

    7ᵗʰ **T84.226** **Displacement of internal fixation device of** vertebrae   CC POA HCC CC/MCC Exc

    7ᵗʰ **T84.228** **Displacement of internal fixation device of** other **bones**   CC POA HCC CC/MCC Exc

  6ᵗʰ **T84.29** Other **mechanical complication of internal fixation device of other bones**
    Obstruction (mechanical) of internal fixation device of other bones
    Perforation of internal fixation device of other bones
    Protrusion of internal fixation device of other bones

    7ᵗʰ **T84.290** **Other mechanical complication of internal fixation device of bones of** hand and fingers   CC POA HCC CC/MCC Exc

    7ᵗʰ **T84.293** **Other mechanical complication of internal fixation device of bones of** foot and toes   CC POA HCC CC/MCC Exc

    7ᵗʰ **T84.296** **Other mechanical complication of internal fixation device of** vertebrae   CC POA HCC CC/MCC Exc

    7ᵗʰ **T84.298** **Other mechanical complication of internal fixation device of** other **bones**   CC POA HCC CC/MCC Exc

5ᵗʰ **T84.3** **Mechanical complication of** other bone devices, implants and grafts
  EXCLUDES2 *other complications of bone graft (T86.83-)*

  6ᵗʰ **T84.31** Breakdown **(mechanical) of other bone devices, implants and grafts**

    7ᵗʰ **T84.310** **Breakdown (mechanical) of** electronic bone stimulator   CC POA HCC CC/MCC Exc

    7ᵗʰ **T84.318** **Breakdown (mechanical) of** other **bone devices, implants and grafts**   CC POA HCC CC/MCC Exc

  6ᵗʰ **T84.32** Displacement **of other bone devices, implants and grafts**
    Malposition of other bone devices, implants and grafts

    7ᵗʰ **T84.320** **Displacement of** electronic bone stimulator   CC POA HCC CC/MCC Exc

    7ᵗʰ **T84.328** **Displacement of** other **bone devices, implants and grafts**   CC POA HCC CC/MCC Exc

  6ᵗʰ **T84.39** Other **mechanical complication of other bone devices, implants and grafts**
    Obstruction (mechanical) of other bone devices, implants and grafts
    Perforation of other bone devices, implants and grafts
    Protrusion of other bone devices, implants and grafts

    7ᵗʰ **T84.390** **Other mechanical complication of** electronic bone stimulator   CC POA HCC CC/MCC Exc

    7ᵗʰ **T84.398** **Other mechanical complication of** other **bone devices, implants and grafts**   CC POA HCC CC/MCC Exc

5ᵗʰ **T84.4** **Mechanical complication of** other internal orthopedic devices, implants and grafts

  6ᵗʰ **T84.41** Breakdown **(mechanical) of other internal orthopedic devices, implants and grafts**

    7ᵗʰ **T84.410** **Breakdown (mechanical) of** muscle and tendon graft   CC POA HCC CC/MCC Exc

    7ᵗʰ **T84.418** **Breakdown (mechanical) of other** internal orthopedic devices, implants and grafts   CC POA HCC CC/MCC Exc

  6ᵗʰ **T84.42** Displacement **of other internal orthopedic devices, implants and grafts**
    Malposition of other internal orthopedic devices, implants and grafts

    7ᵗʰ **T84.420** **Displacement of** muscle and tendon graft   CC POA HCC CC/MCC Exc

    7ᵗʰ **T84.428** **Displacement of** other internal orthopedic devices, implants and grafts   CC POA HCC CC/MCC Exc

---

Unspecified Code   Other Specified Code   Manifestation Code   N Newborn   P Pediatric   M Maternity   A Adult   ♂ Male   ♀ Female
● New Code   ▲ Revised Code Title   ▶◀ Revised Text   **NOTES**   *INCLUDES*   *EXCLUDES1*   Not coded here   *EXCLUDES2*   Not included here
4ᵗʰ 4ᵗʰ character required   5ᵗʰ 5ᵗʰ character required   6ᵗʰ 6ᵗʰ character required   7ᵗʰ 7ᵗʰ character required   Extension 'X' Alert
HAC Hospital-acquired condition (HAC) alert   **AHA** AHA Coding Clinic©   📖 Code first alert

T84.49 Other mechanical complication of other internal orthopedic devices, implants and grafts

Mechanical complication of other internal orthopedic devices, implants and grafts NOS

Obstruction (mechanical) of other internal orthopedic devices, implants and grafts

Perforation of other internal orthopedic devices, implants and grafts

Protrusion of other internal orthopedic devices, implants and grafts

T84.490 Other mechanical complication of muscle and tendon graft

T84.498 Other mechanical complication of other internal orthopedic devices, implants and grafts

T84.5 Infection and inflammatory reaction due to internal joint prosthesis

Use additional code to identify infection

T84.50 Infection and inflammatory reaction due to unspecified internal joint prosthesis

AHA: Q1 2015

T84.51 Infection and inflammatory reaction due to internal right hip prosthesis

AHA: Q4 2015

T84.52 Infection and inflammatory reaction due to internal left hip prosthesis

AHA: Q1 2015

T84.53 Infection and inflammatory reaction due to internal right knee prosthesis

T84.54 Infection and inflammatory reaction due to internal left knee prosthesis

T84.59 Infection and inflammatory reaction due to other internal joint prosthesis

T84.6 Infection and inflammatory reaction due to internal fixation device

Use additional code to identify infection

T84.60 Infection and inflammatory reaction due to internal fixation device of unspecified site

T84.61 Infection and inflammatory reaction due to internal fixation device of arm

T84.610 Infection and inflammatory reaction due to internal fixation device of right humerus

T84.611 Infection and inflammatory reaction due to internal fixation device of left humerus

T84.612 Infection and inflammatory reaction due to internal fixation device of right radius

T84.613 Infection and inflammatory reaction due to internal fixation device of left radius

T84.614 Infection and inflammatory reaction due to internal fixation device of right ulna

T84.615 Infection and inflammatory reaction due to internal fixation device of left ulna

T84.619 Infection and inflammatory reaction due to internal fixation device of unspecified bone of arm

T84.62 Infection and inflammatory reaction due to internal fixation device of leg

T84.620 Infection and inflammatory reaction due to internal fixation device of right femur

T84.621 Infection and inflammatory reaction due to internal fixation device of left femur

T84.622 Infection and inflammatory reaction due to internal fixation device of right tibia

T84.623 Infection and inflammatory reaction due to internal fixation device of left tibia

T84.624 Infection and inflammatory reaction due to internal fixation device of right fibula

T84.625 Infection and inflammatory reaction due to internal fixation device of left fibula

T84.629 Infection and inflammatory reaction due to internal fixation device of unspecified bone of leg

T84.63 Infection and inflammatory reaction due to internal fixation device of spine

T84.69 Infection and inflammatory reaction due to internal fixation device of other site

T84.7 Infection and inflammatory reaction due to other internal orthopedic prosthetic devices, implants and grafts

Use additional code to identify infection

T84.8 Other specified complications of internal orthopedic prosthetic devices, implants and grafts

T84.81 Embolism due to internal orthopedic prosthetic devices, implants and grafts

T84.82 Fibrosis due to internal orthopedic prosthetic devices, implants and grafts

T84.83 Hemorrhage due to internal orthopedic prosthetic devices, implants and grafts

T84.84 Pain due to internal orthopedic prosthetic devices, implants and grafts

T84.85 Stenosis due to internal orthopedic prosthetic devices, implants and grafts

T84.86 Thrombosis due to internal orthopedic prosthetic devices, implants and grafts

T84.89 Other specified complication of internal orthopedic prosthetic devices, implants and grafts

T84.9 Unspecified complication of internal orthopedic prosthetic device, implant and graft

T85 Complications of other internal prosthetic devices, implants and grafts

EXCLUDES2 failure and rejection of transplanted organs and tissue (T86.-)

The appropriate 7th character is to be added to each code from category T85

A = initial encounter

D = subsequent encounter

S = sequela

T85.0 Mechanical complication of ventricular intracranial (communicating) shunt

T85.01 Breakdown (mechanical) of ventricular intracranial (communicating) shunt

T85.02 Displacement of ventricular intracranial (communicating) shunt

Malposition of ventricular intracranial (communicating) shunt

T85.03 Leakage of ventricular intracranial (communicating) shunt

T85.09 Other mechanical complication of ventricular intracranial (communicating) shunt

Obstruction (mechanical) of ventricular intracranial (communicating) shunt

Perforation of ventricular intracranial (communicating) shunt

Protrusion of ventricular intracranial (communicating) shunt

T85.1 Mechanical complication of implanted electronic stimulator of nervous system

T85.11 Breakdown (mechanical) of implanted electronic stimulator of nervous system

T85.110 Breakdown (mechanical) of implanted electronic neurostimulator of brain electrode (lead)

PDX⚕ Unacceptable principal diagnosis symbol per Medicare code edits   ⚕ Code exempt from diagnosis present on admission requirement

❓ Questionable admission   cc Complication or comorbidity   MCC Major complication or comorbidity   cc/mcc Exc CC/MCC exclusion

HCC HCC diagnosis code   RxHCC RxHCC diagnosis code   MACRA MACRA code   DEFINITION Describes condition/terminology

TIP Coding guidance   👁 Official Guideline Reference   Z1 Z code as first-listed diagnosis

7ᵗʰ **T85.111 Breakdown (mechanical) of implanted electronic neurostimulator of** peripheral nerve **electrode (lead)** CC◯ PDX HCC CC/MCC Exc◯
Breakdown of electrode (lead) for cranial nerve neurostimulators
Breakdown of electrode (lead) for gastric neurostimulator
Breakdown of electrode (lead) for sacral nerve neurostimulator
Breakdown of electrode (lead) for vagal nerve neurostimulators

7ᵗʰ **T85.112 Breakdown (mechanical) of implanted electronic neurostimulator of** spinal cord **electrode (lead)** CC◯ PDX HCC CC/MCC Exc◯

7ᵗʰ **T85.113 Breakdown (mechanical) of implanted electronic neurostimulator, generator** CC◯ PDX HCC CC/MCC Exc◯
Breakdown (mechanical) of implanted electronic neurostimulator generator, brain, peripheral, gastric, spinal
Breakdown (mechanical) of implanted electronic sacral neurostimulator, pulse generator or receiver

7ᵗʰ **T85.118 Breakdown (mechanical) of** other **implanted electronic stimulator of nervous system** CC◯ PDX HCC CC/MCC Exc◯

6ᵗʰ **T85.12** Displacement **of implanted electronic stimulator of nervous system**
Malposition of implanted electronic stimulator of nervous system

7ᵗʰ **T85.120 Displacement of implanted electronic neurostimulator of** brain **electrode (lead)** CC◯ PDX HCC CC/MCC Exc◯

7ᵗʰ **T85.121 Displacement of implanted electronic neurostimulator of** peripheral nerve **electrode (lead)** CC◯ PDX HCC CC/MCC Exc◯
Displacement of electrode (lead) for cranial nerve neurostimulators
Displacement of electrode (lead) for gastric neurostimulator
Displacement of electrode (lead) for sacral nerve neurostimulator
Displacement of electrode (lead) for vagal nerve neurostimulators

7ᵗʰ **T85.122 Displacement of implanted electronic neurostimulator of** spinal cord **electrode (lead)** CC◯ PDX HCC CC/MCC Exc◯

7ᵗʰ **T85.123 Displacement of implanted electronic neurostimulator,** generator CC◯ PDX HCC CC/MCC Exc◯
Displacement of implanted electronic neurostimulator generator, brain, peripheral, gastric, spinal
Displacement of implanted electronic sacral neurostimulator, pulse generator or receiver

7ᵗʰ **T85.128 Displacement of** other **implanted electronic stimulator of nervous system** CC◯ PDX HCC CC/MCC Exc◯

6ᵗʰ **T85.19** Other **mechanical complication of implanted electronic stimulator of nervous system**
Leakage of implanted electronic stimulator of nervous system
Obstruction (mechanical) of implanted electronic stimulator of nervous system
Perforation of implanted electronic stimulator of nervous system
Protrusion of implanted electronic stimulator of nervous system

7ᵗʰ **T85.190 Other mechanical complication of implanted electronic neurostimulator of** brain **electrode (lead)** CC◯ PDX HCC CC/MCC Exc◯

7ᵗʰ **T85.191 Other mechanical complication of implanted electronic neurostimulator of** peripheral nerve **electrode (lead)** CC◯ PDX HCC CC/MCC Exc◯

Other mechanical complication of electrode (lead) for cranial nerve neurostimulators
Other mechanical complication of electrode (lead) for gastric neurostimulator
Other mechanical complication of electrode (lead) for sacral nerve neurostimulator
Other mechanical complication of electrode (lead) for vagal nerve neurostimulators

7ᵗʰ **T85.192 Other mechanical complication of implanted electronic neurostimulator of** spinal cord **electrode (lead)** CC◯ PDX HCC CC/MCC Exc◯

7ᵗʰ **T85.193 Other mechanical complication of implanted electronic neurostimulator, generator** CC◯ PDX HCC CC/MCC Exc◯
Other mechanical complication of implanted electronic neurostimulator generator, brain, peripheral, gastric, spinal
Other mechanical complication of implanted electronic sacral neurostimulator, pulse generator or receiver

7ᵗʰ **T85.199 Other mechanical complication of** other **implanted electronic stimulator of nervous system** CC◯ PDX HCC CC/MCC Exc◯

5ᵗʰ **T85.2 Mechanical complication of** intraocular lens

7ᵗʰ **T85.21** Breakdown (mechanical) of **intraocular lens** CC◯ PDX CC/MCC Exc◯

7ᵗʰ **T85.22** Displacement **of intraocular lens** CC◯ PDX CC/MCC Exc◯
Malposition of intraocular lens

7ᵗʰ **T85.29** Other **mechanical complication of intraocular lens** CC◯ PDX CC/MCC Exc◯
Obstruction (mechanical) of intraocular lens
Perforation of intraocular lens
Protrusion of intraocular lens

5ᵗʰ **T85.3 Mechanical complication of** other ocular prosthetic devices, implants and grafts
EXCLUDES2 other complications of corneal graft (T86.84-)

6ᵗʰ **T85.31** Breakdown (mechanical) of other **ocular prosthetic devices, implants and grafts**

7ᵗʰ **T85.310 Breakdown (mechanical) of prosthetic orbit of** right eye CC◯ PDX CC/MCC Exc◯

7ᵗʰ **T85.311 Breakdown (mechanical) of prosthetic orbit of** left eye CC◯ PDX CC/MCC Exc◯

7ᵗʰ **T85.318 Breakdown (mechanical) of** other **ocular prosthetic devices, implants and grafts** PDX

6ᵗʰ **T85.32** Displacement **of other ocular prosthetic devices, implants and grafts**
Malposition of other ocular prosthetic devices, implants and grafts

7ᵗʰ **T85.320 Displacement of prosthetic orbit of** right eye CC◯ PDX CC/MCC Exc◯

7ᵗʰ **T85.321 Displacement of prosthetic orbit of** left eye CC◯ PDX CC/MCC Exc◯

7ᵗʰ **T85.328 Displacement of** other **ocular prosthetic devices, implants and grafts** PDX

6ᵗʰ **T85.39** Other **mechanical complication of other ocular prosthetic devices, implants and grafts**
Obstruction (mechanical) of other ocular prosthetic devices, implants and grafts
Perforation of other ocular prosthetic devices, implants and grafts
Protrusion of other ocular prosthetic devices, implants and grafts

7ᵗʰ **T85.390 Other mechanical complication of prosthetic orbit of** right eye CC◯ PDX CC/MCC Exc◯

7ᵗʰ **T85.391 Other mechanical complication of prosthetic orbit of** left eye CC◯ PDX CC/MCC Exc◯

7ᵗʰ **T85.398 Other mechanical complication of** other **ocular prosthetic devices, implants and grafts** PDX

5ᵗʰ **T85.4 Mechanical complication of** breast prosthesis and implant

7ᵗʰ **T85.41** Breakdown (mechanical) of breast prosthesis and **implant** CC◯ PDX CC/MCC Exc◯

Unspecified Code   Other Specified Code   Manifestation Code   Ⓝ Newborn   Ⓟ Pediatric   Ⓜ Maternity   Ⓐ Adult   ♂ Male   ♀ Female
● New Code   ▲ Revised Code Title   ►◄ Revised Text   **NOTES**   *INCLUDES*   *EXCLUDES1* Not coded here   *EXCLUDES2* Not included here
4ᵗʰ character required   5ᵗʰ character required   6ᵗʰ character required   7ᵗʰ character required   Extension 'X' Alert
HAC Hospital-acquired condition (HAC) alert   **AHA** AHA Coding Clinic©   ☛ Code first alert

7ᵗʰ **T85.42** Displacement **of breast prosthesis and implant** CC POA CC/MCC Exc

Malposition of breast prosthesis and implant

7ᵗʰ **T85.43** Leakage **of breast prosthesis and implant** CC POA CC/MCC Exc

7ᵗʰ **T85.44** Capsular contracture **of breast implant** CC POA CC/MCC Exc

7ᵗʰ **T85.49** Other **mechanical complication of breast prosthesis and implant** CC POA CC/MCC Exc

Obstruction (mechanical) of breast prosthesis and implant

Perforation of breast prosthesis and implant

Protrusion of breast prosthesis and implant

5ᵗʰ **T85.5 Mechanical complication of** gastrointestinal prosthetic devices, implants and grafts

6ᵗʰ **T85.51** Breakdown **(mechanical) of gastrointestinal prosthetic devices, implants and grafts**

7ᵗʰ **T85.510 Breakdown (mechanical) of** bile duct **prosthesis** CC POA CC/MCC Exc

7ᵗʰ **T85.511 Breakdown (mechanical) of** esophageal anti-reflux device CC POA CC/MCC Exc

7ᵗʰ **T85.518 Breakdown (mechanical) of** other **gastrointestinal prosthetic devices, implants and grafts** CC POA CC/MCC Exc

6ᵗʰ **T85.52** Displacement **of gastrointestinal prosthetic devices, implants and grafts**

Malposition of gastrointestinal prosthetic devices, implants and grafts

7ᵗʰ **T85.520 Displacement of** bile duct **prosthesis** CC POA CC/MCC Exc

7ᵗʰ **T85.521 Displacement of** esophageal anti-reflux device CC POA CC/MCC Exc

7ᵗʰ **T85.528 Displacement of** other **gastrointestinal prosthetic devices, implants and grafts** CC POA CC/MCC Exc

6ᵗʰ **T85.59** Other **mechanical complication of gastrointestinal prosthetic devices, implants and**

Obstruction, mechanical of gastrointestinal prosthetic devices, implants and grafts

Perforation of gastrointestinal prosthetic devices, implants and grafts

Protrusion of gastrointestinal prosthetic devices, implants and grafts

7ᵗʰ **T85.590 Other mechanical complication of** bile duct **prosthesis** CC POA CC/MCC Exc

7ᵗʰ **T85.591 Other mechanical complication of** esophageal anti-reflux **device** CC POA CC/MCC Exc

7ᵗʰ **T85.598 Other mechanical complication of** other **gastrointestinal prosthetic devices, implants and grafts** CC POA CC/MCC Exc

5ᵗʰ **T85.6 Mechanical complication of** other specified internal and external prosthetic devices, implants and grafts

👁 **See Official Guidelines** "Underdose of insulin due to insulin pump failure" I.C.4.a.5.a, "Overdose of insulin due to insulin pump failure" I.C.4.a.5.b

6ᵗʰ **T85.61** Breakdown **(mechanical) of other specified internal prosthetic devices, implants and grafts**

7ᵗʰ **T85.610 Breakdown (mechanical) of** cranial or spinal infusion catheter CC POA CC/MCC Exc

Breakdown (mechanical) of epidural infusion catheter

Breakdown (mechanical) of intrathecal infusion catheter

Breakdown (mechanical) of subarachnoid infusion catheter

Breakdown (mechanical) of subdural infusion catheter

7ᵗʰ **T85.611 Breakdown (mechanical) of** intraperitoneal dialysis catheter CC POA HCC RxHCC CC/MCC Exc

EXCLUDES1 mechanical complication of vascular dialysis catheter (T82.4-)

7ᵗʰ **T85.612 Breakdown (mechanical) of** permanent sutures CC POA CC/MCC Exc

EXCLUDES1 mechanical complication of permanent (wire) suture used in bone repair (T84.1-T84.2)

7ᵗʰ **T85.613 Breakdown (mechanical) of** artificial skin graft and decellularized allodermis CC POA CC/MCC Exc

Failure of artificial skin graft and decellularized allodermis

Non-adherence of artificial skin graft and decellularized allodermis

Poor incorporation of artificial skin graft and decellularized allodermis

Shearing of artificial skin graft and decellularized allodermis

7ᵗʰ **T85.614 Breakdown (mechanical) of** insulin pump CC POA CC/MCC Exc

7ᵗʰ **T85.615 Breakdown (mechanical) of** other **nervous system device, implant or graft** HCC CC/MCC Exc

Breakdown (mechanical) of intrathecal infusion pump

7ᵗʰ **T85.618 Breakdown (mechanical) of other specified internal prosthetic devices, implants and grafts**

6ᵗʰ **T85.62** Displacement **of other specified internal prosthetic devices, implants and grafts**

Malposition of other specified internal prosthetic devices, implants and grafts

7ᵗʰ **T85.620 Displacement of** cranial or spinal infusion catheter CC POA CC/MCC Exc

Displacement of epidural infusion catheter

Displacement of intrathecal infusion catheter

Displacement of subarachnoid infusion catheter

Displacement of subdural infusion catheter

7ᵗʰ **T85.621 Displacement of** intraperitoneal dialysis catheter CC POA HCC RxHCC CC/MCC Exc

EXCLUDES1 mechanical complication of vascular dialysis catheter (T82.4-)

7ᵗʰ **T85.622 Displacement of** permanent sutures CC POA CC/MCC Exc

EXCLUDES1 mechanical complication of permanent (wire) suture used in bone repair (T84.1-T84.2)

7ᵗʰ **T85.623 Displacement of** artificial skin graft and decellularized allodermis CC POA CC/MCC Exc

Dislodgement of artificial skin graft and decellularized allodermis

7ᵗʰ **T85.624 Displacement of** insulin pump CC POA CC/MCC Exc

7ᵗʰ **T85.625 Displacement of** other nervous system device, implant or graft CC POA HCC CC/MCC Exc

Displacement of intrathecal infusion pump

7ᵗʰ **T85.628 Displacement of other specified internal prosthetic devices, implants and grafts** CC POA CC/MCC Exc

AHA: Q1 2015

6ᵗʰ **T85.63** Leakage **of other specified internal prosthetic devices, implants and grafts**

7ᵗʰ **T85.630 Leakage of** cranial or spinal infusion catheter CC POA CC/MCC Exc

Leakage of epidural infusion catheter

Leakage of intrathecal infusion catheter infusion catheter

Leakage of subdural infusion catheter

Leakage of subarachnoid infusion catheter

7ᵗʰ **T85.631 Leakage of** intraperitoneal dialysis catheter CC POA HCC RxHCC CC/MCC Exc

EXCLUDES1 mechanical complication of vascular dialysis catheter (T82.4)

PDxⁿ Unacceptable principal diagnosis symbol per Medicare code edits   POA Code exempt from diagnosis present on admission requirement

❓ Questionable admission   CC Complication or comorbidity   MCC Major complication or comorbidity   CC/MCC Exc CC/MCC exclusion

HCC HCC diagnosis code   RxHCC RxHCC diagnosis code   MACRA code   **DEFINITION** Describes condition/terminology

TIP Coding guidance   👁 Official Guideline Reference   Z1 Z code as first-listed diagnosis

When symbols appear on a code that requires a 7th character extension, refer to Appendix B to identify applicable 7th character codes.   **2020 ICD-10-CM**

7ᵗ **T85.633** Leakage of insulin pump CC POA CC/MCC Exc

7ᵗ **T85.635** Leakage of other nervous system **device, implant or graft** CC POA HCC CC/MCC Exc
Leakage of intrathecal infusion pump

7ᵗ **T85.638** Leakage of other specified internal prosthetic devices, implants and grafts CC POA CC/MCC Exc

6ᵗ **T85.69** Other **mechanical complication of other specified internal prosthetic devices, implants and grafts**
Obstruction, mechanical of other specified internal prosthetic devices, implants and grafts
Perforation of other specified internal prosthetic devices, implants and grafts
Protrusion of other specified internal prosthetic devices, implants and grafts

7ᵗ **T85.690** Other mechanical complication of cranial or spinal infusion catheter CC POA CC/MCC Exc
Other mechanical complication of epidural infusion catheter
Other mechanical complication of intrathecal infusion catheter
Other mechanical complication of subarachnoid infusion catheter
Other mechanical complication of subdural infusion catheter

7ᵗ **T85.691** Other mechanical complication of intraperitoneal dialysis catheter CC POA HCC RxHCC CC/MCC Exc
EXCLUDES1 *mechanical complication of vascular dialysis catheter (T82.4)*

7ᵗ **T85.692** Other mechanical complication of permanent sutures CC POA CC/MCC Exc
EXCLUDES1 *mechanical complication of permanent (wire) suture used in bone repair (T84.1-T84.2)*

7ᵗ **T85.693** Other mechanical complication of artificial skin graft and decellularized allodermis CC POA CC/MCC Exc

7ᵗ **T85.694** Other mechanical complication of insulin pump CC POA CC/MCC Exc

7ᵗ **T85.695** Other mechanical complication of other nervous system **device, implant or graft** CC POA HCC CC/MCC Exc
Other mechanical complication of intrathecal infusion pump

7ᵗ **T85.698** Other mechanical complication of other specified internal prosthetic devices, implants and grafts CC POA CC/MCC Exc
Mechanical complication of nonabsorbable surgical material NOS

5ᵗ **T85.7** Infection and inflammatory reaction due to other internal prosthetic devices, implants and grafts
Use additional code to identify infection

7ᵗ **T85.71** Infection and inflammatory reaction due to peritoneal dialysis catheter CC POA HCC RxHCC CC/MCC Exc

7ᵗ **T85.72** Infection and inflammatory reaction due to insulin pump CC POA HCC CC/MCC Exc

6ᵗ **T85.73** Infection and inflammatory reaction due to nervous system **devices, implants and graft**

7ᵗ **T85.730** Infection and inflammatory reaction due to ventricular intracranial (communicating) shunt CC POA HCC CC/MCC Exc

7ᵗ **T85.731** Infection and inflammatory reaction due to implanted electronic neurostimulator of brain, electrode (lead) CC POA HCC CC/MCC Exc

7ᵗ **T85.732** Infection and inflammatory reaction due to implanted electronic neurostimulator of peripheral nerve, electrode (lead) CC POA HCC CC/MCC Exc
Infection and inflammatory reaction due to electrode (lead) for cranial nerve neurostimulators
Infection and inflammatory reaction due to electrode (lead) for gastric neurostimulator
Infection and inflammatory reaction due to electrode (lead) for sacral nerve neurostimulator
Infection and inflammatory reaction due to electrode (lead) for vagal nerve neurostimulators

7ᵗ **T85.733** Infection and inflammatory reaction due to implanted electronic neurostimulator of spinal cord, electrode (lead) CC POA HCC CC/MCC Exc

7ᵗ **T85.734** Infection and inflammatory reaction due to implanted electronic neurostimulator, generator CC POA HCC CC/MCC Exc
Generator pocket infection

7ᵗ **T85.735** Infection and inflammatory reaction due to cranial or spinal infusion catheter CC POA HCC CC/MCC Exc
Infection and inflammatory reaction due to epidural catheter
Infection and inflammatory reaction due to intrathecal infusion catheter
Infection and inflammatory reaction due to subarachnoid catheter
Infection and inflammatory reaction due to subdural catheter

7ᵗ **T85.738** Infection and inflammatory reaction due to other nervous system **device, implant or graft** CC POA HCC CC/MCC Exc
Infection and inflammatory reaction due to intrathecal infusion pump

7ᵗ **T85.79** Infection and inflammatory reaction due to other internal prosthetic devices, implants and grafts CC POA HCC CC/MCC Exc
AHA: Q4 2016

5ᵗ **T85.8** Other specified **complications of internal prosthetic devices, implants and grafts, not elsewhere classified**

6ᵗ **T85.81** Embolism **due to internal prosthetic devices, implants and grafts, not elsewhere classified**

7ᵗ **T85.810** Embolism due to nervous system **prosthetic devices, implants and grafts** CC POA HCC CC/MCC Exc

7ᵗ **T85.818** Embolism due to other internal prosthetic **devices, implants and grafts** POA

6ᵗ **T85.82** Fibrosis **due to internal prosthetic devices, implants and grafts, not elsewhere classified**

7ᵗ **T85.820** Fibrosis due to nervous system **prosthetic devices, implants and grafts** CC POA HCC CC/MCC Exc

7ᵗ **T85.828** Fibrosis due to other internal prosthetic **devices, implants and grafts** POA

6ᵗ **T85.83** Hemorrhage **due to internal prosthetic devices, implants and grafts, not elsewhere classified**

7ᵗ **T85.830** Hemorrhage due to nervous system **prosthetic devices, implants and grafts** CC POA HCC CC/MCC Exc

7ᵗ **T85.838** Hemorrhage due to other internal prosthetic **devices, implants and grafts** POA

6ᵗ **T85.84** Pain **due to internal prosthetic devices, implants and grafts, not elsewhere classified**

7ᵗ **T85.840** Pain due to nervous system **prosthetic devices, implants and grafts** CC POA HCC CC/MCC Exc

7ᵗ **T85.848** Pain due to other internal prosthetic **devices, implants and grafts** POA

[6th] T85.85 Stenosis due to internal prosthetic devices, implants and grafts, not elsewhere classified
- [7th] T85.850 Stenosis due to nervous system prosthetic devices, implants and grafts [CC] [POA] [HCC] [CC/MCC Exc]
- [7th] T85.858 Stenosis due to other internal prosthetic devices, implants and grafts [POA]

[6th] T85.86 Thrombosis due to internal prosthetic devices, implants and grafts, not elsewhere classified
- [7th] T85.860 Thrombosis due to nervous system prosthetic devices, implants and grafts [CC] [POA] [HCC] [CC/MCC Exc]
- [7th] T85.868 Thrombosis due to other internal prosthetic devices, implants and grafts [POA]

[6th] T85.89 Other specified complication of internal prosthetic devices, implants and grafts, not elsewhere classified
Erosion or breakdown of subcutaneous device pocket
- [7th] T85.890 Other specified complication of nervous system prosthetic devices, implants and grafts [CC] [POA] [HCC] [CC/MCC Exc]
- [7th] T85.898 Other specified complication of other internal prosthetic devices, implants and grafts [POA]

[7th] T85.9 Unspecified complication of internal prosthetic device, implant and graft [POA]
Complication of internal prosthetic device, implant and graft NOS

[4th] T86 Complications of transplanted organs and tissue

👁 See Official Guidelines "Transplant complications other than kidney" I.C.19.g.3.a

Use additional code to identify other transplant complications, such as:
- graft-versus-host disease (D89.81-)
- malignancy associated with organ transplant (C80.2)
- post-transplant lymphoproliferative disorders (PTLD) (D47.Z1)

[5th] T86.0 Complications of bone marrow transplant
- T86.00 Unspecified complication of bone marrow transplant [CC] [HCC] [RxHCC] [CC/MCC Exc]
- T86.01 Bone marrow transplant rejection [CC] [HCC] [RxHCC] [CC/MCC Exc]
- T86.02 Bone marrow transplant failure [CC] [HCC] [RxHCC] [CC/MCC Exc]
- T86.03 Bone marrow transplant infection [CC] [HCC] [RxHCC] [CC/MCC Exc]
- T86.09 Other complications of bone marrow transplant [CC] [HCC] [RxHCC] [CC/MCC Exc]

[5th] T86.1 Complications of kidney transplant
👁 See Official Guidelines "Kidney transplant complications" I.C.19.g.3.b
- T86.10 Unspecified complication of kidney transplant [CC] [RxHCC] [CC/MCC Exc]
- T86.11 Kidney transplant rejection [CC] [RxHCC] [CC/MCC Exc]
- T86.12 Kidney transplant failure [CC] [RxHCC] [CC/MCC Exc]
  AHA: Q1 2013
- T86.13 Kidney transplant infection [CC] [RxHCC] [CC/MCC Exc]
  Use additional code to specify infection
- T86.19 Other complication of kidney transplant [CC] [RxHCC] [CC/MCC Exc]
  AHA: Q2 2019

[5th] T86.2 Complications of heart transplant
👁 See Official Guidelines "Status" I.C.21.c.3
[EXCLUDES1] *complication of:*
artificial heart device (T82.5)
heart-lung transplant (T86.3)
- T86.20 Unspecified complication of heart transplant [CC] [HCC] [RxHCC] [CC/MCC Exc]
- T86.21 Heart transplant rejection [CC] [HCC] [RxHCC] [CC/MCC Exc]
- T86.22 Heart transplant failure [CC] [HCC] [RxHCC] [CC/MCC Exc]
- T86.23 Heart transplant infection [CC] [HCC] [RxHCC] [CC/MCC Exc]
  Use additional code to specify infection

[6th] T86.29 Other complications of heart transplant
- T86.290 Cardiac allograft vasculopathy [CC] [HCC] [RxHCC] [CC/MCC Exc]
  [EXCLUDES1] *atherosclerosis of coronary arteries (I25.75-, I25.76-, I25.81-)*
- T86.298 Other complications of heart transplant [CC] [HCC] [RxHCC] [CC/MCC Exc]

[5th] T86.3 Complications of heart-lung transplant
- T86.30 Unspecified complication of heart-lung transplant [CC] [HCC] [RxHCC] [CC/MCC Exc]
- T86.31 Heart-lung transplant rejection [CC] [HCC] [RxHCC] [CC/MCC Exc]
- T86.32 Heart-lung transplant failure [CC] [HCC] [RxHCC] [CC/MCC Exc]
- T86.33 Heart-lung transplant infection [CC] [HCC] [RxHCC] [CC/MCC Exc]
  Use additional code to specify infection
- T86.39 Other complications of heart-lung transplant [CC] [HCC] [RxHCC] [CC/MCC Exc]

[5th] T86.4 Complications of liver transplant
- T86.40 Unspecified complication of liver transplant [CC] [HCC] [RxHCC] [CC/MCC Exc]
- T86.41 Liver transplant rejection [CC] [HCC] [RxHCC] [CC/MCC Exc]
- T86.42 Liver transplant failure [CC] [HCC] [RxHCC] [CC/MCC Exc]
- T86.43 Liver transplant infection [CC] [HCC] [RxHCC] [CC/MCC Exc]
  Use additional code to identify infection, such as:
  Cytomegalovirus (CMV) infection (B25.-)
- T86.49 Other complications of liver transplant [CC] [HCC] [RxHCC] [CC/MCC Exc]

T86.5 Complications of stem cell transplant [CC] [HCC] [RxHCC] [CC/MCC Exc]
Complications from stem cells from peripheral blood
Complications from stem cells from umbilical cord

[5th] T86.8 Complications of other transplanted organs and tissues

[6th] T86.81 Complications of lung transplant
[EXCLUDES1] *complication of heart-lung transplant (T86.3-)*
- T86.810 Lung transplant rejection [CC] [HCC] [RxHCC] [CC/MCC Exc]
- T86.811 Lung transplant failure [CC] [HCC] [RxHCC] [CC/MCC Exc]
- T86.812 Lung transplant infection [CC] [HCC] [RxHCC] [CC/MCC Exc]
  Use additional code to specify infection
- T86.818 Other complications of lung transplant [CC] [HCC] [RxHCC] [CC/MCC Exc]
  AHA: Q2 2019
- T86.819 Unspecified complication of lung transplant [CC] [HCC] [RxHCC] [CC/MCC Exc]

[6th] T86.82 Complications of skin graft (allograft) (autograft)
[EXCLUDES2] *complication of artificial skin graft (T85.693)*
- T86.820 Skin graft (allograft) rejection [CC] [CC/MCC Exc]
- T86.821 Skin graft (allograft) (autograft) failure [CC] [CC/MCC Exc]
- T86.822 Skin graft (allograft) (autograft) infection [CC] [CC/MCC Exc]
  Use additional code to specify infection
- T86.828 Other complications of skin graft (allograft) (autograft) [CC] [CC/MCC Exc]
- T86.829 Unspecified complication of skin graft (allograft) (autograft) [CC] [CC/MCC Exc]

[6th] T86.83 Complications of bone graft
[EXCLUDES2] *mechanical complications of bone graft (T84.3-)*
- T86.830 Bone graft rejection [CC] [CC/MCC Exc]
- T86.831 Bone graft failure [CC] [CC/MCC Exc]
- T86.832 Bone graft infection [CC] [CC/MCC Exc]
  Use additional code to specify infection
- T86.838 Other complications of bone graft [CC] [CC/MCC Exc]
- T86.839 Unspecified complication of bone graft [CC] [CC/MCC Exc]

[6th] T86.84 Complications of corneal transplant
[EXCLUDES2] *mechanical complications of corneal graft (T85.3-)*
- T86.840 Corneal transplant rejection [CC] [CC/MCC Exc]
- T86.841 Corneal transplant failure [CC] [CC/MCC Exc]
- T86.842 Corneal transplant infection [CC] [HCC] [CC/MCC Exc]
  Use additional code to specify infection
- T86.848 Other complications of corneal transplant [CC] [CC/MCC Exc]
- T86.849 Unspecified complication of corneal transplant [CC] [CC/MCC Exc]

[PDx] Unacceptable principal diagnosis symbol per Medicare code edits [POA] Code exempt from diagnosis present on admission requirement
[?] Questionable admission [CC] Complication or comorbidity [MCC] Major complication or comorbidity [CC/MCC Exc] CC/MCC exclusion
[HCC] HCC diagnosis code [RxHCC] RxHCC diagnosis code MACRA code **DEFINITION** Describes condition/terminology
TIP Coding guidance 👁 Official Guideline Reference [Z] Z code as first-listed diagnosis

   T86.85   **Complication of** intestine **transplant**
      T86.850   **Intestine transplant rejection**   cc HCC RxHCC CC/MCC Exc
      T86.851   **Intestine transplant** failure   cc HCC RxHCC CC/MCC Exc
      T86.852   **Intestine transplant infection**   cc HCC RxHCC CC/MCC Exc
        Use additional code to specify infection
      T86.858   Other **complications of intestine transplant**   cc HCC RxHCC CC/MCC Exc
      T86.859   **Unspecified complication of intestine transplant**   cc HCC RxHCC CC/MCC Exc

   T86.89   **Complications of** other **transplanted** tissue
       Transplant failure or rejection of pancreas
      T86.890   **Other transplanted tissue rejection**   cc CC/MCC Exc
      T86.891   **Other transplanted tissue** failure   cc CC/MCC Exc
      T86.892   **Other transplanted tissue infection**   cc CC/MCC Exc
        Use additional code to specify infection
      T86.898   Other **complications of other transplanted tissue**   cc CC/MCC Exc
      T86.899   **Unspecified complication of other transplanted tissue**   cc CC/MCC Exc

  T86.9   **Complication of** unspecified **transplanted organ and tissue**
      T86.90   **Unspecified complication of unspecified transplanted organ and tissue**   cc CC/MCC Exc
      T86.91   **Unspecified transplanted organ and tissue rejection**   cc CC/MCC Exc
      T86.92   **Unspecified transplanted organ and tissue failure**   cc CC/MCC Exc
      T86.93   **Unspecified transplanted organ and tissue infection**   cc CC/MCC Exc
        Use additional code to specify infection
      T86.99   **Other complications of unspecified transplanted organ and tissue**   cc CC/MCC Exc

T87   **Complications peculiar to reattachment and amputation**
  T87.0   **Complications of reattached (part of) upper extremity**
    T87.0X   **Complications of reattached (part of) upper extremity**
      T87.0X1   **Complications of reattached (part of)** right **upper extremity**   cc HCC CC/MCC Exc
      T87.0X2   **Complications of reattached (part of)** left **upper extremity**   cc HCC CC/MCC Exc
      T87.0X9   **Complications of reattached (part of) unspecified upper extremity**   cc HCC CC/MCC Exc

  T87.1   **Complications of reattached (part of) lower extremity**
    T87.1X   **Complications of reattached (part of) lower extremity**
      T87.1X1   **Complications of reattached (part of)** right **lower extremity**   cc HCC CC/MCC Exc
      T87.1X2   **Complications of reattached (part of)** left **lower extremity**   cc HCC CC/MCC Exc
      T87.1X9   **Complications of reattached (part of) unspecified lower extremity**   cc HCC CC/MCC Exc

  T87.2   **Complications of** other **reattached body part**   cc HCC CC/MCC Exc
  T87.3   Neuroma **of amputation stump**
      T87.30   **Neuroma of amputation stump, unspecified extremity**   HCC
      T87.31   **Neuroma of amputation stump,** right upper **extremity**   HCC
      T87.32   **Neuroma of amputation stump,** left upper **extremity**   HCC
      T87.33   **Neuroma of amputation stump,** right lower **extremity**   HCC
      T87.34   **Neuroma of amputation stump,** left lower **extremity**   HCC
  T87.4   Infection **of amputation stump**
      T87.40   **Infection of amputation stump, unspecified extremity**   cc HCC CC/MCC Exc
      T87.41   **Infection of amputation stump,** right upper **extremity**   cc HCC CC/MCC Exc

      T87.42   **Infection of amputation stump,** left upper **extremity**   cc HCC CC/MCC Exc
      T87.43   **Infection of amputation stump,** right lower **extremity**   cc HCC CC/MCC Exc
      T87.44   **Infection of amputation stump,** left lower **extremity**   cc HCC CC/MCC Exc

  T87.5   Necrosis **of amputation stump**
      T87.50   **Necrosis of amputation stump, unspecified extremity**   HCC
      T87.51   **Necrosis of amputation stump,** right upper **extremity**   HCC
      T87.52   **Necrosis of amputation stump,** left upper **extremity**   HCC
      T87.53   **Necrosis of amputation stump,** right lower **extremity**   HCC
      T87.54   **Necrosis of amputation stump,** left lower **extremity**   HCC

  T87.8   Other **complications of amputation stump**
      T87.81   Dehiscence **of amputation stump**   HCC
      T87.89   Other **complications of amputation stump**   HCC
        Amputation stump contracture
        Amputation stump contracture of next proximal joint
        Amputation stump flexion
        Amputation stump edema
        Amputation stump hematoma
        EXCLUDES2   *phantom limb syndrome (G54.6-G54.7)*

  T87.9   **Unspecified complications of amputation stump**   HCC

T88   Other **complications of** surgical and medical care, **not elsewhere classified**
     EXCLUDES2   *complication following infusion, transfusion and therapeutic injection (T80.-)*
        complication following procedure NEC (T81.-)
        complications of anesthesia in labor and delivery (O74.-)
        complications of anesthesia in pregnancy (O29.-)
        complications of anesthesia in puerperium (O89.-)
        complications of devices, implants and grafts (T82-T85)
        complications of obstetric surgery and procedure (O75.4)
        dermatitis due to drugs and medicaments (L23.3, L24.4, L25.1, L27.0-L27.1)
        poisoning and toxic effects of drugs and chemicals (T36-T65 with fifth or sixth character 1-4 or 6)
        specified complications classified elsewhere

    The appropriate 7th character is to be added to each code from category T88
      A = initial encounter
      D = subsequent encounter
      S = sequela

  T88.0   Infection **following** immunization   cc POA CC/MCC Exc
      AHA: Q1 2019, Q4 2018
      Sepsis following immunization

  T88.1   Other **complications following** immunization, **not elsewhere classified**   cc POA CC/MCC Exc
      Generalized vaccinia
      Rash following immunization
     EXCLUDES1   *vaccinia not from vaccine (B08.011)*
     EXCLUDES2   *anaphylactic shock due to serum (T80.5-)*
        other serum reactions (T80.6-)
        postimmunization arthropathy (M02.2)
        postimmunization encephalitis (G04.02)
        postimmunization fever (R50.83)

  T88.2   Shock **due to anesthesia**   cc POA CC/MCC Exc
      Use additional code for adverse effect, if applicable, to identify drug (T41.- with fifth or sixth character 5)
     EXCLUDES1   *complications of anesthesia (in):*
        labor and delivery (O74.-)
        pregnancy (O29.-)
        puerperium (O89.-)
        postprocedural shock NOS (T81.1-)

Unspecified Code   Other Specified Code   Manifestation Code   N Newborn   P Pediatric   M Maternity   A Adult   ♂ Male   ♀ Female
● New Code   ▲ Revised Code Title   ▶◀ Revised Text   **NOTES**   *INCLUDES*   *EXCLUDES1* Not coded here   *EXCLUDES2* Not included here
4ᵗʰ 4th character required   5ᵗʰ 5th character required   6ᵗʰ 6th character required   7ᵗʰ 7th character required   7x Extension 'X' Alert
HAC Hospital-acquired condition (HAC) alert   **AHA** AHA Coding Clinic©   📌 Code first alert

T88.3 Malignant hyperthermia **due to anesthesia**
Use additional code for adverse effect, if applicable, to identify drug (T41.- with fifth or sixth character 5)

T88.4 Failed or difficult intubation

T88.5 Other complications of anesthesia
Use additional code for adverse effect, if applicable, to identify drug (T41.- with fifth or sixth character 5)

　T88.51 Hypothermia following anesthesia

　T88.52 Failed moderate sedation during procedure
Failed conscious sedation during procedure
EXCLUDES2 personal history of failed moderate sedation (Z92.83)

　T88.53 Unintended awareness under general anesthesia during procedure
AHA: Q4 2016
EXCLUDES2 personal history of unintended awareness under general anesthesia (Z92.84)

　T88.59 Other complications of anesthesia

T88.6 Anaphylactic reaction due to adverse effect of correct drug or medicament properly administered
Anaphylactic shock due to adverse effect of correct drug or medicament properly administered
Anaphylactoid reaction NOS
Use additional code for adverse effect, if applicable, to identify drug (T36-T50 with fifth or sixth character 5)
EXCLUDES1 anaphylactic reaction due to serum (T80.5-)
anaphylactic shock or reaction due to adverse food reaction (T78.0-)

T88.7 Unspecified adverse effect of drug or medicament
Drug hypersensitivity NOS
Drug reaction NOS
Use additional code for adverse effect, if applicable, to identify drug (T36-T50 with fifth or sixth character 5)
EXCLUDES1 specified adverse effects of drugs and medicaments (A00-R94 and T80-T88.6, T88.8)

T88.8 Other specified complications of surgical and medical care, not elsewhere classified
Use additional code to identify the complication

T88.9 Complication of surgical and medical care, unspecified
See Official Guidelines "Used with any code in the range of A00.0-T88.9, Z00-Z99" I.C.20.a.1

PDxIn Unacceptable principal diagnosis symbol per Medicare code edits　 Code exempt from diagnosis present on admission requirement
? Questionable admission　 Complication or comorbidity　MCC Major complication or comorbidity　 CC/MCC exclusion
HCC HCC diagnosis code　RHCC RxHCC diagnosis code　MACRA code　DEFINITION Describes condition/terminology
TIP Coding guidance　 Official Guideline Reference　 Z code as first-listed diagnosis

1178　When symbols appear on a code that requires a 7th character extension, refer to Appendix B to identify applicable 7th character codes.　2020 ICD-10-CM

Chapter 20: External Causes of Morbidity (V00-Y99)

External causes of morbidity (V00-Y99)

NOTES This chapter permits the classification of environmental events and circumstances as the cause of injury, and other adverse effects. Where a code from this section is applicable, it is intended that it shall be used secondary to a code from another chapter of the Classification indicating the nature of the condition. Most often, the condition will be classifiable to Chapter 19, Injury, poisoning and certain other consequences of external causes (S00-T88). Other conditions that may be stated to be due to external causes are classified in Chapters I to XVIII. For these conditions, codes from Chapter 20 should be used to provide additional information as to the cause of the condition.

This chapter contains the following blocks:

V00-X58	Accidents
V00-V99	Transport accidents
V00-V09	Pedestrian injured in transport accident
V10-V19	Pedal cycle rider injured in transport accident
V20-V29	Motorcycle rider injured in transport accident
V30-V39	Occupant of three-wheeled motor vehicle injured in transport accident
V40-V49	Car occupant injured in transport accident
V50-V59	Occupant of pick-up truck or van injured in transport accident
V60-V69	Occupant of heavy transport vehicle injured in transport accident
V70-V79	Bus occupant injured in transport accident
V80-V89	Other land transport accidents
V90-V94	Water transport accidents
V95-V97	Air and space transport accidents
V98-V99	Other and unspecified transport accidents
W00-X58	Other external causes of accidental injury
W00-W19	Slipping, tripping, stumbling and falls
W20-W49	Exposure to inanimate mechanical forces
W50-W64	Exposure to animate mechanical forces
W65-W74	Accidental non-transport drowning and submersion
W85-W99	Exposure to electric current, radiation and extreme ambient air temperature and pressure
X00-X08	Exposure to smoke, fire and flames
X10-X19	Contact with heat and hot substances
X30-X39	Exposure to forces of nature
X50	Overexertion and strenuous or repetitive movements
X52-X58	Accidental exposure to other specified factors
X71-X83	Intentional self-harm
X92-Y09	Assault
Y21-Y33	Event of undetermined intent
Y35-Y38	Legal intervention, operations of war, military operations, and terrorism
Y62-Y84	Complications of medical and surgical care
Y62-Y69	Misadventures to patients during surgical and medical care
Y70-Y82	Medical devices associated with adverse incidents in diagnostic and therapeutic use
Y83-Y84	Surgical and other medical procedures as the cause of abnormal reaction of the patient, or of later complication, without mention of misadventure at the time of the procedure
Y90-Y99	Supplementary factors related to causes of morbidity classified elsewhere

Accidents (V00-X58)

Transport accidents (V00-V99)

NOTES This section is structured in 12 groups. Those relating to land transport accidents (V00-V89) reflect the victim's mode of transport and are subdivided to identify the victim's 'counterpart' or the type of event. The vehicle of which the injured person is an occupant is identified in the first two characters since it is seen as the most important factor to identify for prevention purposes. A transport accident is one in which the vehicle involved must be moving or running or in use for transport purposes at the time of the accident.

Use additional code to identify:

Airbag injury (W22.1)

Type of street or road (Y92.4-)

Use of cellular telephone and other electronic equipment at the time of the transport accident (Y93.C-)

EXCLUDES1 *agricultural vehicles in stationary use or maintenance (W31.-)*

assault by crashing of motor vehicle (Y03.-)

automobile or motor cycle in stationary use or maintenance- code to type of accident

crashing of motor vehicle, undetermined intent (Y32)

intentional self-harm by crashing of motor vehicle (X82)

EXCLUDES2 *transport accidents due to cataclysm (X34-X38)*

NOTES Definitions related to transport accidents:

(a) A transport accident (V00-V99) is any accident involving a device designed primarily for, or used at the time primarily for, conveying persons or good from one place to another.

(b) A public highway [trafficway] or street is the entire width between property lines (or other boundary lines) of land open to the public as a matter of right or custom for purposes of moving persons or property from one place to another. A roadway is that part of the public highway designed, improved and customarily used for vehicular traffic.

(c) A traffic accident is any vehicle accident occurring on the public highway [i.e. originating on, terminating on, or involving a vehicle partially on the highway]. A vehicle accident is assumed to have occurred on the public highway unless another place is specified, except in the case of accidents involving only off-road motor vehicles, which are classified as nontraffic accidents unless the contrary is stated.

(d) A nontraffic accident is any vehicle accident that occurs entirely in any place other than a public highway.

(e) A pedestrian is any person involved in an accident who was not at the time of the accident riding in or on a motor vehicle, railway train, streetcar or animal-drawn or other vehicle, or on a pedal cycle or animal. This includes, a person changing a tire, working on a parked car, or a person on foot. It also includes the user of a pedestrian conveyance such as a baby stroller, ice-skates, skis, sled, roller skates, a skateboard, nonmotorized or motorized wheelchair, motorized mobility scooter, or nonmotorized scooter.

(f) A driver is an occupant of a transport vehicle who is operating or intending to operate it.

(g) A passenger is any occupant of a transport vehicle other than the driver, except a person traveling on the outside of the vehicle.

(h) A person on the outside of a vehicle is any person being transported by a vehicle but not occupying the space normally reserved for the driver or passengers, or the space intended for the transport of property. This includes a person travelling on the bodywork, bumper, fender, roof, running board or step of a vehicle, as well as, hanging on the outside of the vehicle.

(i) A pedal cycle is any land transport vehicle operated solely by nonmotorized pedals including a bicycle or tricycle.

(j) A pedal cyclist is any person riding a pedal cycle or in a sidecar or trailer attached to a pedal cycle.

(k) A motorcycle is a two-wheeled motor vehicle with one or two riding saddles and sometimes with a third wheel for the support of a sidecar. The sidecar is considered part of the motorcycle. This includes a moped, motor scooter, or motorized bicycle.

(l) A motorcycle rider is any person riding a motorcycle or in a sidecar or trailer attached to the motorcycle.

(m) A three-wheeled motor vehicle is a motorized tricycle designed primarily for on-road use. This includes a motor-driven tricycle, a motorized rickshaw, or a three-wheeled motor car.

(n) A car [automobile] is a four-wheeled motor vehicle designed primarily for carrying up to 7 persons. A trailer being towed by the car is considered part of the car. It does not include a van or minivan - *see* definition (o)

(o) A pick-up truck or van is a four or six-wheeled motor vehicle designed for carrying passengers as well as property or cargo weighing less than the local limit for classification as a heavy goods vehicle, and not requiring a special driver's license. This includes a minivan and a sport-utility vehicle (SUV).

(p) A heavy transport vehicle is a motor vehicle designed primarily for carrying property, meeting local criteria for classification as a heavy goods vehicle in terms of weight and requiring a special driver's license.

(q) A bus (coach) is a motor vehicle designed or adapted primarily for carrying more than 10 passengers, and requiring a special driver's license.

(r) A railway train or railway vehicle is any device, with or without freight or passenger cars couple to it, designed for traffic on a railway track. This includes subterranean (subways) or elevated trains.

(s) A streetcar, is a device designed and used primarily for transporting passengers within a municipality, running on rails, usually subject to normal traffic control signals, and operated principally on a right-of-way that forms part of the roadway. This includes a tram or trolley that runs on rails. A trailer being towed by a streetcar is considered part of the streetcar.

(t) A special vehicle mainly used on industrial premises is a motor vehicle designed primarily for use within the buildings and premises of industrial or commercial establishments. This includes battery-powered airport passenger vehicles or baggage/mail trucks, forklifts, coal-cars in a coal mine, logging cars and trucks used in mines or quarries.

(u) A special vehicle mainly used in agriculture is a motor vehicle designed specifically for use in farming and agriculture (horticulture), to work the land, tend and harvest crops and transport materials on the farm. This includes harvesters, farm machinery and tractor and trailers.

(v) A special construction vehicle is a motor vehicle designed specifically for use on construction and demolition sites. This includes bulldozers, diggers, earth levellers, dump trucks. backhoes, front-end loaders, pavers, and mechanical shovels.

(w) A special all-terrain vehicle is a motor vehicle of special design to enable it to negotiate over rough or soft terrain, snow or sand. Examples of special design are high construction, special wheels and tires, tracks, and support on a cushion of air. This includes snow mobiles, All-terrain vehicles (ATV), and dune buggies. It does not include passenger vehicle designated as Sport Utility Vehicles. (SUV)

(x) A watercraft is any device designed for transporting passengers or goods on water. This includes motor or sail boats, ships, and hovercraft.

(y) An aircraft is any device for transporting passengers or goods in the air. This includes hot-air balloons, gliders, helicopters and airplanes.

(z) A military vehicle is any motorized vehicle operating on a public roadway owned by the military and being operated by a member of the military.

Pedestrian injured in transport accident (V00-V09)

INCLUDES   person changing tire on transport vehicle

person examining engine of vehicle broken down in (on side of) road

EXCLUDES1   fall due to non-transport collision with other person (W03)

pedestrian on foot falling (slipping) on ice and snow (W00.-)

struck or bumped by another person (W51)

V00   **Pedestrian conveyance accident**

Use additional place of occurrence and activity external cause codes, if known (Y92.-, Y93.-)

EXCLUDES1   collision with another person without fall (W51)

fall due to person on foot colliding with another person on foot (W03)

fall from non-moving wheelchair, nonmotorized scooter and motorized mobility scooter without collision (W05.-)

pedestrian (conveyance) collision with other land transport vehicle (V01-V09)

pedestrian on foot falling (slipping) on ice and snow (W00.-)

The appropriate 7th character is to be added to each code from category V00

A = initial encounter

D = subsequent encounter

S = sequela

V00.0   **Pedestrian on foot injured in collision with pedestrian conveyance**

V00.01   **Pedestrian on foot injured in collision with** roller-skater

V00.02   **Pedestrian on foot injured in collision with** skateboarder

V00.09   **Pedestrian on foot injured in collision with other pedestrian conveyance**

V00.1   **Rolling-type pedestrian conveyance accident**

EXCLUDES1   accident with baby stroller (V00.82-)

accident with wheelchair (powered) (V00.81-)

accident with motorized mobility scooter (V00.83-)

V00.11   In-line roller-skate **accident**

V00.111   Fall from **in-line roller-skates**

V00.112   **In-line roller-skater** colliding with stationary object

V00.118   **Other in-line roller-skate accident**

EXCLUDES1   roller-skater collision with other land transport vehicle (V01-V09 with 5th character 1)

V00.12   Non-in- line roller-skate **accident**

V00.121   Fall from **non-in-line roller-skates**

V00.122   **Non-in-line roller-skater** colliding with stationary object

V00.128   **Other non-in-line roller-skating accident**

EXCLUDES1   roller-skater collision with other land transport vehicle (V01-V09 with 5th character 1)

V00.13   Skateboard **accident**

V00.131   Fall from **skateboard**

V00.132   **Skateboarder** colliding with stationary object

V00.138   **Other skateboard accident**

EXCLUDES1   skateboarder collision with other land transport vehicle (V01-V09 with 5th character 2)

V00.14   Scooter (nonmotorized) **accident**

EXCLUDES1   motor scooter accident (V20-V29)

V00.141   Fall from **scooter (nonmotorized)**

V00.142   **Scooter (nonmotorized)** colliding with stationary object

V00.148   **Other scooter (nonmotorized) accident**

EXCLUDES1   scooter (nonmotorized) collision with other land transport vehicle (V01-V09 with fifth character 9)

V00.15   Heelies **accident**

Rolling shoe

Wheeled shoe

Wheelies accident

V00.151   Fall from **heelies**

V00.152   **Heelies** colliding with stationary object

V00.158   **Other heelies accident**

[6th] V00.18 Accident on other rolling-type pedestrian conveyance
- [7th] V00.181 Fall from other rolling-type pedestrian conveyance [POA]
- [7th] V00.182 Pedestrian on other rolling-type pedestrian conveyance colliding with stationary object [POA]
- [7th] V00.188 Other accident on other rolling-type pedestrian conveyance [POA]

[5th] V00.2 Gliding-type pedestrian conveyance accident

[6th] V00.21 Ice-skates accident
- [7th] V00.211 Fall from ice-skates [POA]
- [7th] V00.212 Ice-skater colliding with stationary object [POA]
- [7th] V00.218 Other ice-skates accident [POA]
  - EXCLUDES1 *ice-skater collision with other land transport vehicle (V01-V09 with 5th character 9)*

[6th] V00.22 Sled accident
- [7th] V00.221 Fall from sled [POA]
- [7th] V00.222 Sledder colliding with stationary object [POA]
- [7th] V00.228 Other sled accident [POA]
  - EXCLUDES1 *sled collision with other land transport vehicle (V01-V09 with 5th character 9)*

[6th] V00.28 Other gliding-type pedestrian conveyance accident
- [7th] V00.281 Fall from other gliding-type pedestrian conveyance [POA]
- [7th] V00.282 Pedestrian on other gliding-type pedestrian conveyance colliding with stationary object [POA]
- [7th] V00.288 Other accident on other gliding-type pedestrian conveyance [POA]
  - EXCLUDES1 *gliding-type pedestrian conveyance collision with other land transport vehicle (V01-V09 with 5th character 9)*

[5th] V00.3 Flat-bottomed pedestrian conveyance accident

[6th] V00.31 Snowboard accident
- [7th] V00.311 Fall from snowboard [POA]
- [7th] V00.312 Snowboarder colliding with stationary object [POA]
- [7th] V00.318 Other snowboard accident [POA]
  - EXCLUDES1 *snowboarder collision with other land transport vehicle (V01-V09 with 5th character 9)*

[6th] V00.32 Snow-ski accident
- [7th] V00.321 Fall from snow-skis [POA]
  - AHA: Q1 2015
- [7th] V00.322 Snow-skier colliding with stationary object [POA]
- [7th] V00.328 Other snow-ski accident [POA]
  - EXCLUDES1 *snow-skier collision with other land transport vehicle (V01-V09 with 5th character 9)*

[6th] V00.38 Other flat-bottomed pedestrian conveyance accident
- [7th] V00.381 Fall from other flat-bottomed pedestrian conveyance [POA]
- [7th] V00.382 Pedestrian on other flat-bottomed pedestrian conveyance colliding with stationary object [POA]
- [7th] V00.388 Other accident on other flat-bottomed pedestrian conveyance [POA]

[5th] V00.8 Accident on other pedestrian conveyance

[6th] V00.81 Accident with wheelchair (powered)
- [7th] V00.811 Fall from moving wheelchair (powered)
  - EXCLUDES1 *fall from non-moving wheelchair (W05.0)*
- [7th] V00.812 Wheelchair (powered) colliding with stationary object
- [7th] V00.818 Other accident with wheelchair (powered)

[6th] V00.82 Accident with baby stroller
- [7th] V00.821 Fall from baby stroller [POA]
- [7th] V00.822 Baby stroller colliding with stationary object [POA]
- [7th] V00.828 Other accident with baby stroller [POA]

[6th] V00.83 Accident with motorized mobility scooter
- [7th] V00.831 Fall from motorized mobility scooter
  - EXCLUDES1 *fall from non-moving motorized mobility scooter (W05.2)*
- [7th] V00.832 Motorized mobility scooter colliding with stationary object
- [7th] V00.838 Other accident with motorized mobility scooter

[6th] V00.89 Accident on other pedestrian conveyance
- [7th] V00.891 Fall from other pedestrian conveyance [POA]
- [7th] V00.892 Pedestrian on other pedestrian conveyance colliding with stationary object [POA]
- [7th] V00.898 Other accident on other pedestrian conveyance [POA]
  - EXCLUDES1 *other pedestrian (conveyance) collision with other land transport vehicle (V01-V09 with 5th character 9)*

[4th] V01 Pedestrian injured in collision with pedal cycle

The appropriate 7th character is to be added to each code from category V01
- A = initial encounter
- D = subsequent encounter
- S = sequela

[5th] V01.0 Pedestrian injured in collision with pedal cycle in nontraffic accident
- [7th] V01.00 Pedestrian on foot injured in collision with pedal cycle in nontraffic accident [POA]
  - Pedestrian NOS injured in collision with pedal cycle in nontraffic accident
- [7th] V01.01 Pedestrian on roller-skates injured in collision with pedal cycle in nontraffic accident [POA]
- [7th] V01.02 Pedestrian on skateboard injured in collision with pedal cycle in nontraffic accident [POA]
- [7th] V01.09 Pedestrian with other conveyance injured in collision with pedal cycle in nontraffic accident [POA]
  - Pedestrian with baby stroller injured in collision with pedal cycle in nontraffic accident
  - Pedestrian on ice-skates injured in collision with pedal cycle in nontraffic accident
  - Pedestrian on nonmotorized scooter injured in collision with pedal cycle in nontraffic accident
  - Pedestrian on sled injured in collision with pedal cycle in nontraffic accident
  - Pedestrian on snowboard injured in collision with pedal cycle in nontraffic accident
  - Pedestrian on snow-skis injured in collision with pedal cycle in nontraffic accident
  - Pedestrian in wheelchair (powered) injured in collision with pedal cycle in nontraffic accident
  - Pedestrian in motorized mobility scooter injured in collision with pedal cycle in nontraffic accident

[5th] V01.1 Pedestrian injured in collision with pedal cycle in traffic accident
- [7th] V01.10 Pedestrian on foot injured in collision with pedal cycle in traffic accident [POA]
  - Pedestrian NOS injured in collision with pedal cycle in traffic accident
- [7th] V01.11 Pedestrian on roller-skates injured in collision with pedal cycle in traffic accident [POA]
- [7th] V01.12 Pedestrian on skateboard injured in collision with pedal cycle in traffic accident [POA]

V01.19 **Pedestrian** with other conveyance **injured in collision with pedal cycle in traffic accident** POA

Pedestrian with baby stroller injured in collision with pedal cycle in traffic accident

Pedestrian on ice-skates injured in collision with pedal cycle in traffic accident

Pedestrian on nonmotorized scooter injured in collision with pedal cycle in traffic accident

Pedestrian on sled injured in collision with pedal cycle in traffic accident

Pedestrian on snowboard injured in collision with pedal cycle in traffic accident

Pedestrian on snow-skis injured in collision with pedal cycle in traffic accident

Pedestrian in wheelchair (powered) injured in collision with pedal cycle in traffic accident

Pedestrian in motorized mobility scooter injured in collision with pedal cycle in traffic accident

V01.9 **Pedestrian injured in collision with pedal cycle,** unspecified whether traffic or nontraffic accident

V01.90 **Pedestrian** on foot **injured in collision with pedal cycle, unspecified whether traffic or nontraffic accident** POA

Pedestrian NOS injured in collision with pedal cycle, unspecified whether traffic or nontraffic accident

V01.91 **Pedestrian** on roller-skates **injured in collision with pedal cycle, unspecified whether traffic or nontraffic accident** POA

V01.92 **Pedestrian** on skateboard **injured in collision with pedal cycle, unspecified whether traffic or nontraffic accident** POA

V01.99 **Pedestrian with other conveyance injured in collision with pedal cycle, unspecified whether traffic or nontraffic accident** POA

Pedestrian with baby stroller injured in collision with pedal cycle, unspecified whether traffic or nontraffic accident

Pedestrian on ice-skates injured in collision with pedal cycle unspecified, whether traffic or nontraffic accident

Pedestrian on nonmotorized scooter injured in collision with pedal cycle, unspecified whether traffic or nontraffic accident

Pedestrian on sled injured in collision with pedal cycle unspecified, whether traffic or nontraffic accident

Pedestrian on snowboard injured in collision with pedal cycle, unspecified whether traffic or nontraffic accident

Pedestrian on snow-skis injured in collision with pedal cycle, unspecified whether traffic or nontraffic accident

Pedestrian in wheelchair (powered) injured in collision with pedal cycle, unspecified whether traffic or nontraffic accident

Pedestrian in motorized mobility scooter injured in collision with pedal cycle, unspecified whether traffic or nontraffic accident

V02 **Pedestrian injured in collision with** two- or three-wheeled motor vehicle

The appropriate 7th character is to be added to each code from category V02

A = initial encounter

D = subsequent encounter

S = sequela

V02.0 **Pedestrian** injured in **collision with two- or three-wheeled motor vehicle** in nontraffic accident

V02.00 **Pedestrian** on foot **injured in collision with two- or three-wheeled motor vehicle in nontraffic accident** POA

Pedestrian NOS injured in collision with two- or three-wheeled motor vehicle in nontraffic accident

V02.01 **Pedestrian** on roller-skates **injured in collision with two- or three-wheeled motor vehicle in nontraffic accident** POA

V02.02 **Pedestrian** on skateboard **injured in collision with two- or three-wheeled motor vehicle in nontraffic accident** POA

V02.09 **Pedestrian with other conveyance injured in collision with two- or three-wheeled motor vehicle in nontraffic accident** POA

Pedestrian with baby stroller injured in collision with two- or three-wheeled motor vehicle in nontraffic accident

Pedestrian on ice-skates injured in collision with two- or three-wheeled motor vehicle in nontraffic accident

Pedestrian on nonmotorized scooter injured in collision with two- or three-wheeled motor vehicle in nontraffic accident

Pedestrian on sled injured in collision with two- or three-wheeled motor vehicle in nontraffic accident

Pedestrian on snowboard injured in collision with two- or three-wheeled motor vehicle in nontraffic accident

Pedestrian on snow-skis injured in collision with two- or three-wheeled motor vehicle in nontraffic accident

Pedestrian in wheelchair (powered) injured in collision with two- or three-wheeled motor vehicle in nontraffic accident

Pedestrian in motorized mobility scooter injured in collision with two- or three-wheeled motor vehicle in nontraffic accident

V02.1 **Pedestrian injured in collision with two- or three-wheeled motor vehicle** in traffic accident

V02.10 **Pedestrian** on foot **injured in collision with two- or three-wheeled motor vehicle in traffic accident** POA

Pedestrian NOS injured in collision with two- or three-wheeled motor vehicle in traffic accident

V02.11 **Pedestrian** on roller-skates **injured in collision with two- or three-wheeled motor vehicle in traffic accident** POA

V02.12 **Pedestrian** on skateboard **injured in collision with two- or three-wheeled motor vehicle in traffic accident** POA

V02.19 **Pedestrian with other conveyance injured in collision with two- or three-wheeled motor vehicle in traffic accident** POA

Pedestrian with baby stroller injured in collision with two- or three-wheeled motor vehicle in traffic accident

Pedestrian on ice-skates injured in collision with two- or three-wheeled motor vehicle in traffic accident

Pedestrian on nonmotorized scooter injured in collision with two- or three-wheeled motor vehicle in traffic accident

Pedestrian on sled injured in collision with two- or three-wheeled motor vehicle in traffic accident

Pedestrian on snowboard injured in collision with two- or three-wheeled motor vehicle in traffic accident

Pedestrian on snow-skis injured in collision with two- or three-wheeled motor vehicle in traffic accident

Pedestrian in wheelchair (powered) injured in collision with two- or three-wheeled motor vehicle in traffic accident

Pedestrian in motorized mobility scooter injured in collision with two- or three-wheeled motor vehicle in traffic accident

V02.9 **Pedestrian injured in collision with two- or three-wheeled motor vehicle,** unspecified whether traffic or nontraffic accident

V02.90 **Pedestrian on foot injured in collision with two- or three-wheeled motor vehicle, unspecified whether traffic or nontraffic accident** POA

Pedestrian NOS injured in collision with two- or three-wheeled motor vehicle, unspecified whether traffic or nontraffic accident

---

[7th] **V02.91 Pedestrian on roller-skates injured in collision with two- or three-wheeled motor vehicle, unspecified whether traffic or nontraffic accident** [POA]

[7th] **V02.92 Pedestrian on skateboard injured in collision with two- or three-wheeled motor vehicle, unspecified whether traffic or nontraffic accident** [POA]

[7th] **V02.99 Pedestrian with other conveyance injured in collision with two- or three-wheeled motor vehicle, unspecified whether traffic or nontraffic accident** [POA]

Pedestrian with baby stroller injured in collision with two- or three-wheeled motor vehicle, unspecified whether traffic or nontraffic accident
Pedestrian on ice-skates injured in collision with two- or three-wheeled motor vehicle, unspecified whether traffic or nontraffic accident
Pedestrian on nonmotorized scooter injured in collision with two- or three-wheeled motor vehicle, unspecified whether traffic or nontraffic accident
Pedestrian on sled injured in collision with two- or three-wheeled motor vehicle, unspecified whether traffic or nontraffic accident
Pedestrian on snowboard injured in collision with two- or three-wheeled motor vehicle, unspecified whether traffic or nontraffic accident
Pedestrian on snow-skis injured in collision with two- or three-wheeled motor vehicle, unspecified whether traffic or nontraffic accident
Pedestrian in wheelchair (powered) injured in collision with two- or three-wheeled motor vehicle, unspecified whether traffic or nontraffic accident
Pedestrian in motorized mobility scooter injured in collision with two- or three-wheeled motor vehicle, unspecified whether traffic or nontraffic accident

[4th] **V03 Pedestrian injured in collision with car, pick-up truck or van**

The appropriate 7th character is to be added to each code from category V03
A = initial encounter
D = subsequent encounter
S = sequela

[5th] **V03.0 Pedestrian injured in collision with car, pick-up truck or van in nontraffic accident**

[7th] **V03.00 Pedestrian on foot injured in collision with car, pick-up truck or van in nontraffic accident** [POA]

Pedestrian NOS injured in collision with car, pick-up truck or van in nontraffic accident

[7th] **V03.01 Pedestrian on roller-skates injured in collision with car, pick-up truck or van in nontraffic accident** [POA]

[7th] **V03.02 Pedestrian on skateboard injured in collision with car, pick-up truck or van in nontraffic accident** [POA]

[7th] **V03.09 Pedestrian with other conveyance injured in collision with car, pick-up truck or van in nontraffic accident** [POA]

Pedestrian with baby stroller injured in collision with car, pick-up truck or van in nontraffic accident
Pedestrian on ice-skates injured in collision with car, pick-up truck or van in nontraffic accident
Pedestrian on nonmotorized scooter injured in collision with car, pick-up truck or van in nontraffic accident
Pedestrian on sled injured in collision with car, pick-up truck or van in nontraffic accident
Pedestrian on snowboard injured in collision with car, pick-up truck or van in nontraffic accident
Pedestrian on snow-skis injured in collision with car, pick-up truck or van in nontraffic accident
Pedestrian in wheelchair (powered) injured in collision with car, pick-up truck or van in nontraffic accident
Pedestrian in motorized mobility scooter injured in collision with car, pick-up truck or van in nontraffic accident

[5th] **V03.1 Pedestrian injured in collision with car, pick-up truck or van in traffic accident**

[7th] **V03.10 Pedestrian on foot injured in collision with car, pick-up truck or van in traffic accident** [POA]

Pedestrian NOS injured in collision with car, pick-up truck or van in traffic accident

[7th] **V03.11 Pedestrian on roller-skates injured in collision with car, pick-up truck or van in traffic accident** [POA]

[7th] **V03.12 Pedestrian on skateboard injured in collision with car, pick-up truck or van in traffic accident** [POA]

[7th] **V03.19 Pedestrian with other conveyance injured in collision with car, pick-up truck or van in traffic accident** [POA]

Pedestrian with baby stroller injured in collision with car, pick-up truck or van in traffic accident
Pedestrian on ice-skates injured in collision with car, pick-up truck or van in traffic accident
Pedestrian on nonmotorized scooter injured in collision with car, pick-up truck or van in traffic accident
Pedestrian on sled injured in collision with car, pick-up truck or van in traffic accident
Pedestrian on snowboard injured in collision with car, pick-up truck or van in traffic accident
Pedestrian on snow-skis injured in collision with car, pick-up truck or van in traffic accident
Pedestrian in wheelchair (powered) injured in collision with car, pick-up truck or van in traffic accident
Pedestrian in motorized mobility scooter injured in collision with car, pick-up truck or van in traffic accident

[5th] **V03.9 Pedestrian injured in collision with car, pick-up truck or van, unspecified whether traffic or nontraffic accident**

[7th] **V03.90 Pedestrian on foot injured in collision with car, pick-up truck or van, unspecified whether traffic or nontraffic accident** [POA]

Pedestrian NOS injured in collision with car, pick-up truck or van, unspecified whether traffic or nontraffic accident

[7th] **V03.91 Pedestrian on roller-skates injured in collision with car, pick-up truck or van, unspecified whether traffic or nontraffic accident** [POA]

[7th] **V03.92 Pedestrian on skateboard injured in collision with car, pick-up truck or van, unspecified whether traffic or nontraffic accident** [POA]

[7th] **V03.99 Pedestrian with other conveyance injured in collision with car, pick-up truck or van, unspecified whether traffic or nontraffic accident** [POA]

Pedestrian with baby stroller injured in collision with car, pick-up truck or van, unspecified whether traffic or nontraffic accident
Pedestrian on ice-skates injured in collision with car, pick-up truck or van, unspecified whether traffic or nontraffic accident
Pedestrian on nonmotorized scooter injured in collision with car, pick-up truck or van, unspecified whether traffic or nontraffic accident
Pedestrian on sled injured in collision with car, pick-up truck or van in nontraffic accident
Pedestrian on snowboard injured in collision with car, pick-up truck or van, unspecified whether traffic or nontraffic accident
Pedestrian on snow-skis injured in collision with car, pick-up truck or van, unspecified whether traffic or nontraffic accident
Pedestrian in wheelchair (powered) injured in collision with car, pick-up truck or van, unspecified whether traffic or nontraffic accident
Pedestrian in motorized mobility scooter injured in collision with car, pick-up truck or van, unspecified whether traffic or nontraffic accident

[4th] **V04 Pedestrian injured in collision with heavy transport vehicle or bus**

[EXCLUDES1] *pedestrian injured in collision with military vehicle (V09.01, V09.21)*

The appropriate 7th character is to be added to each code from category V04
A = initial encounter
D = subsequent encounter
S = sequela

Unspecified Code | Other Specified Code | Manifestation Code | [N] Newborn | [P] Pediatric | [M] Maternity | [A] Adult | ♂ Male | ♀ Female
● New Code | ▲ Revised Code Title | ►◄ Revised Text | [NOTES] | *INCLUDES* | [EXCLUDES1] Not coded here | [EXCLUDES2] Not included here
[4th] 4th character required | [5th] 5th character required | [6th] 6th character required | [7th] 7th character required | [7th] Extension 'X' Alert
[HAC] Hospital-acquired condition (HAC) alert | AHA AHA Coding Clinic© | ☞ Code first alert

5ᵗʰ V04.0 **Pedestrian injured in collision with heavy transport vehicle or bus** in nontraffic accident

7ᵗʰ V04.00 **Pedestrian** on foot **injured in collision with heavy transport vehicle or bus in nontraffic accident** POA

Pedestrian NOS injured in collision with heavy transport vehicle or bus in nontraffic accident

7ᵗʰ V04.01 **Pedestrian** on roller-skates **injured in collision with heavy transport vehicle or bus in nontraffic accident** POA

7ᵗʰ V04.02 **Pedestrian** on skateboard **injured in collision with heavy transport vehicle or bus in nontraffic accident** 🚫

7ᵗʰ V04.09 **Pedestrian with other conveyance injured in collision with heavy transport vehicle or bus in nontraffic accident** 🚫

Pedestrian with baby stroller injured in collision with heavy transport vehicle or bus in nontraffic accident

Pedestrian on ice-skates injured in collision with heavy transport vehicle or bus in nontraffic accident

Pedestrian on nonmotorized scooter injured in collision with heavy transport vehicle or bus in nontraffic accident

Pedestrian on sled injured in collision with heavy transport vehicle or bus in nontraffic accident

Pedestrian on snowboard injured in collision with heavy transport vehicle or bus in nontraffic accident

Pedestrian on snow-skis injured in collision with heavy transport vehicle or bus in nontraffic accident

Pedestrian in wheelchair (powered) injured in collision with heavy transport vehicle or bus in nontraffic accident

Pedestrian in motorized mobility scooter injured in collision with heavy transport vehicle or bus in nontraffic accident

5ᵗʰ V04.1 **Pedestrian injured in collision with heavy transport vehicle or bus** in traffic accident

7ᵗʰ V04.10 **Pedestrian** on foot **injured in collision with heavy transport vehicle or bus in traffic accident** POA

Pedestrian NOS injured in collision with heavy transport vehicle or bus in traffic accident

7ᵗʰ V04.11 **Pedestrian** on roller-skates **injured in collision with heavy transport vehicle or bus in traffic accident** POA

7ᵗʰ V04.12 **Pedestrian** on skateboard **injured in collision with heavy transport vehicle or bus in traffic accident** POA

7ᵗʰ V04.19 **Pedestrian with other conveyance injured in collision with heavy transport vehicle or bus in traffic accident** 🚫

Pedestrian with baby stroller injured in collision with heavy transport vehicle or bus in traffic accident

Pedestrian on ice-skates injured in collision with heavy transport vehicle or bus in traffic accident

Pedestrian on nonmotorized scooter injured in collision with heavy transport vehicle or bus in traffic accident

Pedestrian on sled injured in collision with heavy transport vehicle or bus in traffic accident

Pedestrian on snowboard injured in collision with heavy transport vehicle or bus in traffic accident

Pedestrian on snow-skis injured in collision with heavy transport vehicle or bus in traffic accident

Pedestrian in wheelchair (powered) injured in collision with heavy transport vehicle or bus in traffic accident

Pedestrian in motorized mobility scooter injured in collision with heavy transport vehicle or bus in traffic accident

5ᵗʰ V04.9 **Pedestrian injured in collision with heavy transport vehicle or bus,** unspecified whether traffic or nontraffic accident

7ᵗʰ V04.90 **Pedestrian on foot injured in collision with heavy transport vehicle or bus, unspecified whether traffic or nontraffic accident** POA

Pedestrian NOS injured in collision with heavy transport vehicle or bus, unspecified whether traffic or nontraffic accident

7ᵗʰ V04.91 **Pedestrian on roller-skates injured in collision with heavy transport vehicle or bus, unspecified whether traffic or nontraffic accident** POA

7ᵗʰ V04.92 **Pedestrian on skateboard injured in collision with heavy transport vehicle or bus, unspecified whether traffic or nontraffic accident** 🚫

7ᵗʰ V04.99 **Pedestrian with other conveyance injured in collision with heavy transport vehicle or bus, unspecified whether traffic or nontraffic accident** 🚫

Pedestrian with baby stroller injured in collision with heavy transport vehicle or bus, unspecified whether traffic or nontraffic accident

Pedestrian on ice-skates injured in collision with heavy transport vehicle or bus, unspecified whether traffic or nontraffic accident

Pedestrian on nonmotorized scooter injured in collision with heavy transport vehicle or bus, unspecified whether traffic or nontraffic accident

Pedestrian on sled injured in collision with heavy transport vehicle or bus, unspecified whether traffic or nontraffic accident

Pedestrian on snowboard injured in collision with heavy transport vehicle or bus, unspecified whether traffic or nontraffic accident

Pedestrian on snow-skis injured in collision with heavy transport vehicle or bus, unspecified whether traffic or nontraffic accident

Pedestrian in wheelchair (powered) injured in collision with heavy transport vehicle or bus, unspecified whether traffic or nontraffic accident

Pedestrian in motorized mobility scooter injured in collision with heavy transport vehicle or bus, unspecified whether traffic or nontraffic accident

4ᵗʰ V05 **Pedestrian injured in collision** with railway train or railway vehicle

The appropriate 7th character is to be added to each code from category V05

A = initial encounter
D = subsequent encounter
S = sequela

5ᵗʰ V05.0 **Pedestrian injured in collision with railway train or railway vehicle** in nontraffic accident

7ᵗʰ V05.00 **Pedestrian** on foot **injured in collision with railway train or railway vehicle in nontraffic accident** POA

Pedestrian NOS injured in collision with railway train or railway vehicle in nontraffic accident

7ᵗʰ V05.01 **Pedestrian** on roller-skates **injured in collision with railway train or railway vehicle in nontraffic accident** POA

7ᵗʰ V05.02 **Pedestrian** on skateboard **injured in collision with railway train or railway vehicle in nontraffic accident** POA

7ᵗʰ V05.09 **Pedestrian with other conveyance injured in collision with railway train or railway vehicle in nontraffic accident** POA

Pedestrian with baby stroller injured in collision with railway train or railway vehicle in nontraffic accident

Pedestrian on ice-skates injured in collision with railway train or railway vehicle in nontraffic accident

Pedestrian on nonmotorized scooter injured in collision with railway train or railway vehicle in nontraffic accident

Pedestrian on sled injured in collision with railway train or railway vehicle in nontraffic accident

Pedestrian on snowboard injured in collision with railway train or railway vehicle in nontraffic accident

Pedestrian on snow-skis injured in collision with railway train or railway vehicle in nontraffic accident

Pedestrian in wheelchair (powered) injured in collision with railway train or railway vehicle in nontraffic accident

Pedestrian in motorized mobility scooter injured in collision with railway train or railway vehicle in nontraffic accident

(5ᵗʰ) **V05.1 Pedestrian injured in collision with railway train or railway vehicle** in traffic accident

    (7ᵗʰ) **V05.10 Pedestrian** on foot **injured in collision with railway train or railway vehicle in traffic accident** ᴾᴼᴬ

        Pedestrian NOS injured in collision with railway train or railway vehicle in traffic accident

    (7ᵗʰ) **V05.11 Pedestrian** on roller-skates **injured in collision with railway train or railway vehicle in traffic accident** ᴾᴼᴬ

    (7ᵗʰ) **V05.12 Pedestrian** on skateboard **injured in collision with railway train or railway vehicle in traffic accident** ᴾᴼᴬ

    (7ᵗʰ) **V05.19 Pedestrian with other conveyance injured in collision with railway train or railway vehicle in traffic accident** ᴾᴼᴬ

        Pedestrian with baby stroller injured in collision with railway train or railway vehicle in traffic accident

        Pedestrian on ice-skates injured in collision with railway train or railway vehicle in traffic accident

        Pedestrian on nonmotorized scooter injured in collision with railway train or railway vehicle in traffic accident

        Pedestrian on sled injured in collision with railway train or railway vehicle in traffic accident

        Pedestrian on snowboard injured in collision with railway train or railway vehicle in traffic accident

        Pedestrian on snow-skis injured in collision with railway train or railway vehicle in traffic accident

        Pedestrian in wheelchair (powered) injured in collision with railway train or railway vehicle in traffic accident

        Pedestrian in motorized mobility scooter injured in collision with railway train or railway vehicle in traffic accident

(5ᵗʰ) **V05.9 Pedestrian injured in collision with railway train or railway vehicle, unspecified whether traffic or nontraffic accident**

    (7ᵗʰ) **V05.90 Pedestrian on foot injured in collision with railway train or railway vehicle, unspecified whether traffic or nontraffic accident** ᴾᴼᴬ

        Pedestrian NOS injured in collision with railway train or railway vehicle, unspecified whether traffic or nontraffic accident

    (7ᵗʰ) **V05.91 Pedestrian on roller-skates injured in collision with railway train or railway vehicle, unspecified whether traffic or nontraffic accident** ᴾᴼᴬ

    (7ᵗʰ) **V05.92 Pedestrian on skateboard injured in collision with railway train or railway vehicle, unspecified whether traffic or nontraffic accident** ᴾᴼᴬ

    (7ᵗʰ) **V05.99 Pedestrian with other conveyance injured in collision with railway train or railway vehicle, unspecified whether traffic or nontraffic accident** ᴾᴼᴬ

        Pedestrian with baby stroller injured in collision with railway train or railway vehicle, unspecified whether traffic or nontraffic

        Pedestrian on ice-skates injured in collision with railway train or railway vehicle, unspecified whether traffic or nontraffic

        Pedestrian on nonmotorized scooter injured in collision with railway train or railway vehicle, unspecified whether traffic or nontraffic

        Pedestrian on sled injured in collision with railway train or railway vehicle, unspecified whether traffic or nontraffic

        Pedestrian on snowboard injured in collision with railway train or railway vehicle, unspecified whether traffic or nontraffic

        Pedestrian on snow-skis injured in collision with railway train or railway vehicle, unspecified whether traffic or nontraffic

        Pedestrian in wheelchair (powered) injured in collision with railway train or railway vehicle, unspecified whether traffic or nontraffic

        Pedestrian in motorized mobility scooter injured in collision with railway train or railway vehicle, unspecified whether traffic or nontraffic

(4ᵗʰ) **V06 Pedestrian injured in collision** with other nonmotor vehicle

    INCLUDES collision with animal-drawn vehicle, animal being ridden, nonpowered streetcar

    EXCLUDES1 pedestrian injured in collision with pedestrian conveyance (V00.0-)

    The appropriate 7th character is to be added to each code from category V06

        A = initial encounter

        D = subsequent encounter

        S = sequela

(5ᵗʰ) **V06.0 Pedestrian injured in collision with other nonmotor vehicle** in nontraffic accident

    (7ᵗʰ) **V06.00 Pedestrian** on foot **injured in collision with other nonmotor vehicle in nontraffic accident** ᴾᴼᴬ

        Pedestrian NOS injured in collision with other nonmotor vehicle in nontraffic accident

    (7ᵗʰ) **V06.01 Pedestrian** on roller-skates **injured in collision with other nonmotor vehicle in nontraffic accident** ᴾᴼᴬ

    (7ᵗʰ) **V06.02 Pedestrian** on skateboard **injured in collision with other nonmotor vehicle in nontraffic accident** ᴾᴼᴬ

    (7ᵗʰ) **V06.09 Pedestrian with other conveyance injured in collision with other nonmotor vehicle in nontraffic accident** ᴾᴼᴬ

        Pedestrian with baby stroller injured in collision with other nonmotor vehicle in nontraffic accident

        Pedestrian on ice-skates injured in collision with other nonmotor vehicle in nontraffic accident

        Pedestrian on nonmotorized scooter injured in collision with other nonmotor vehicle in nontraffic accident

        Pedestrian on sled injured in collision with other nonmotor vehicle in nontraffic accident

        Pedestrian on snowboard injured in collision with other nonmotor vehicle in nontraffic accident

        Pedestrian on snow-skis injured in collision with other nonmotor vehicle in nontraffic accident

        Pedestrian in wheelchair (powered) injured in collision with other nonmotor vehicle in nontraffic accident

        Pedestrian in motorized mobility scooter injured in collision with other nonmotor vehicle in nontraffic accident

(5ᵗʰ) **V06.1 Pedestrian injured in collision with other nonmotor vehicle** in traffic accident

    (7ᵗʰ) **V06.10 Pedestrian** on foot **injured in collision with other nonmotor vehicle in traffic accident** ᴾᴼᴬ

        Pedestrian NOS injured in collision with other nonmotor vehicle in traffic accident

    (7ᵗʰ) **V06.11 Pedestrian** on roller-skates **injured in collision with other nonmotor vehicle in traffic accident** ᴾᴼᴬ

    (7ᵗʰ) **V06.12 Pedestrian** on skateboard **injured in collision with other nonmotor vehicle in traffic accident** ᴾᴼᴬ

    (7ᵗʰ) **V06.19 Pedestrian with other conveyance injured in collision with other nonmotor vehicle in traffic accident** ᴾᴼᴬ

        Pedestrian with baby stroller injured in collision with other nonmotor vehicle in nontraffic accident

        Pedestrian on ice-skates injured in collision with other nonmotor vehicle in traffic accident

        Pedestrian on nonmotorized scooter injured in collision with other nonmotor vehicle in traffic accident

        Pedestrian on sled injured in collision with other nonmotor vehicle in traffic accident

        Pedestrian on snowboard injured in collision with other nonmotor vehicle in traffic accident

        Pedestrian on snow-skis injured in collision with other nonmotor vehicle in traffic accident

        Pedestrian in wheelchair (powered) injured in collision with other nonmotor vehicle in traffic accident

        Pedestrian in motorized mobility scooter injured in collision with other nonmotor vehicle in traffic accident

Unspecified Code   Other Specified Code   Manifestation Code   Ⓝ Newborn   Ⓟ Pediatric   Ⓜ Maternity   Ⓐ Adult   ♂ Male   ♀ Female

● New Code   ▲ Revised Code Title   ▶◀ Revised Text   **NOTES**   *INCLUDES*   *EXCLUDES1* Not coded here   *EXCLUDES2* Not included here

4ᵗʰ character required   5ᵗʰ character required   6ᵗʰ character required   7ᵗʰ character required   Extension 'X' Alert

HAC Hospital-acquired condition (HAC) alert   **AHA** AHA Coding Clinic©   📖 Code first alert

2020 ICD-10-CM   When symbols appear on a code that requires a 7th character extension, refer to Appendix B to identify applicable 7th character codes.   **1185**

🔵 V06.9 Pedestrian injured in collision with other nonmotor vehicle, unspecified whether traffic or nontraffic accident

    🔹 V06.90 Pedestrian on foot injured in collision with other nonmotor vehicle, unspecified whether traffic or nontraffic accident *POA*

        Pedestrian NOS injured in collision with other nonmotor vehicle, unspecified whether traffic or nontraffic accident

    🔹 V06.91 Pedestrian on roller-skates injured in collision with other nonmotor vehicle, unspecified whether traffic or nontraffic accident *POA*

    🔹 V06.92 Pedestrian on skateboard injured in collision with other nonmotor vehicle, unspecified whether traffic or nontraffic accident *POA*

    🔹 V06.99 Pedestrian with other conveyance injured in collision with other nonmotor vehicle, unspecified whether traffic or nontraffic accident *POA*

        Pedestrian with baby stroller injured in collision with other nonmotor vehicle, unspecified whether traffic or nontraffic accident

        Pedestrian on ice-skates injured in collision with other nonmotor vehicle, unspecified whether traffic or nontraffic accident

        Pedestrian on nonmotorized scooter injured in collision with other nonmotor vehicle, unspecified whether traffic or nontraffic accident

        Pedestrian on sled injured in collision with other nonmotor vehicle, unspecified whether traffic or nontraffic accident

        Pedestrian on snowboard injured in collision with other nonmotor vehicle, unspecified whether traffic or nontraffic accident

        Pedestrian on snow-skis injured in collision with other nonmotor vehicle, unspecified whether traffic or nontraffic accident

        Pedestrian in wheelchair (powered) injured in collision with other nonmotor vehicle, unspecified whether traffic or nontraffic accident

        Pedestrian in motorized mobility scooter injured in collision with other nonmotor vehicle, unspecified whether traffic or nontraffic accident

🔵 V09 Pedestrian injured in other and unspecified transport accidents

    The appropriate 7th character is to be added to each code from category V09

      A = initial encounter

      D = subsequent encounter

      S = sequela

  🔵 V09.0 Pedestrian injured in nontraffic accident involving other and unspecified motor vehicles

    🔹 V09.00 Pedestrian injured in nontraffic accident involving unspecified motor vehicles *POA*

    🔹 V09.01 Pedestrian injured in nontraffic accident involving military vehicle *POA*

    🔹 V09.09 Pedestrian injured in nontraffic accident involving other motor vehicles *POA*

        Pedestrian injured in nontraffic accident by special vehicle

  🔹 V09.1 Pedestrian injured in unspecified nontraffic accident *POA*

  🔵 V09.2 Pedestrian injured in traffic accident involving other and unspecified motor vehicles

    🔹 V09.20 Pedestrian injured in traffic accident involving unspecified motor vehicles *POA*

    🔹 V09.21 Pedestrian injured in traffic accident involving military vehicle *POA*

    🔹 V09.29 Pedestrian injured in traffic accident involving other motor vehicles *POA*

  🔹 V09.3 Pedestrian injured in unspecified traffic accident *POA*

  🔹 V09.9 Pedestrian injured in unspecified transport accident *POA*

Pedal cycle rider injured in transport accident (V10-V19)

  INCLUDES any non-motorized vehicle, excluding an animal-drawn vehicle, or a sidecar or trailer attached to the pedal cycle

  EXCLUDES2 rupture of pedal cycle tire (W37.0)

🔵 V10 Pedal cycle rider injured in collision with pedestrian or animal

    EXCLUDES1 pedal cycle rider collision with animal-drawn vehicle or animal being ridden (V16.-)

    The appropriate 7th character is to be added to each code from category V10

      A = initial encounter

      D = subsequent encounter

      S = sequela

  🔹 V10.0 Pedal cycle driver injured in collision with pedestrian or animal in nontraffic accident *POA*

  🔹 V10.1 Pedal cycle passenger injured in collision with pedestrian or animal in nontraffic accident *POA*

  🔹 V10.2 Unspecified pedal cyclist injured in collision with pedestrian or animal in nontraffic accident *POA*

  🔹 V10.3 Person boarding or alighting a pedal cycle injured in collision with pedestrian or animal *POA*

  🔹 V10.4 Pedal cycle driver injured in collision with pedestrian or animal in traffic accident *POA*

  🔹 V10.5 Pedal cycle passenger injured in collision with pedestrian or animal in traffic accident *POA*

  🔹 V10.9 Unspecified pedal cyclist injured in collision with pedestrian or animal in traffic accident *POA*

🔵 V11 Pedal cycle rider injured in collision with other pedal cycle

    The appropriate 7th character is to be added to each code from category V11

      A = initial encounter

      D = subsequent encounter

      S = sequela

  🔹 V11.0 Pedal cycle driver injured in collision with other pedal cycle in nontraffic accident *POA*

  🔹 V11.1 Pedal cycle passenger injured in collision with other pedal cycle in nontraffic accident *POA*

  🔹 V11.2 Unspecified pedal cyclist injured in collision with other pedal cycle in nontraffic accident *POA*

  🔹 V11.3 Person boarding or alighting a pedal cycle injured in collision with other pedal cycle *POA*

  🔹 V11.4 Pedal cycle driver injured in collision with other pedal cycle in traffic accident *POA*

  🔹 V11.5 Pedal cycle passenger injured in collision with other pedal cycle in traffic accident *POA*

  🔹 V11.9 Unspecified pedal cyclist injured in collision with other pedal cycle in traffic accident *POA*

🔵 V12 Pedal cycle rider injured in collision with two- or three-wheeled motor vehicle

    The appropriate 7th character is to be added to each code from category V12

      A = initial encounter

      D = subsequent encounter

      S = sequela

  🔹 V12.0 Pedal cycle driver injured in collision with two- or three-wheeled motor vehicle in nontraffic accident *POA*

  🔹 V12.1 Pedal cycle passenger injured in collision with two- or three-wheeled motor vehicle in nontraffic accident *POA*

  🔹 V12.2 Unspecified pedal cyclist injured in collision with two- or three-wheeled motor vehicle in nontraffic accident *POA*

  🔹 V12.3 Person boarding or alighting a pedal cycle injured in collision with two- or three-wheeled motor vehicle *POA*

  🔹 V12.4 Pedal cycle driver injured in collision with two- or three-wheeled motor vehicle in traffic accident *POA*

  🔹 V12.5 Pedal cycle passenger injured in collision with two- or three-wheeled motor vehicle in traffic accident *POA*

  🔹 V12.9 Unspecified pedal cyclist injured in collision with two- or three-wheeled motor vehicle in traffic accident *POA*

PDsm Unacceptable principal diagnosis symbol per Medicare code edits   *POA* Code exempt from diagnosis present on admission requirement

❓ Questionable admission   🔵 Complication or comorbidity   *MCC* Major complication or comorbidity   *CC/MCC Excl* CC/MCC exclusion

HCC HCC diagnosis code   **RxHCC** RxHCC diagnosis code   MACRA code   **DEFINITION** Describes condition/terminology

TIP Coding guidance   👁 Official Guideline Reference   🔲 Z code as first-listed diagnosis

1186   When symbols appear on a code that requires a 7th character extension, refer to Appendix B to identify applicable 7th character codes.   **2020 ICD-10-CM**

V13 Pedal cycle rider injured in collision with car, pick-up truck or van

The appropriate 7th character is to be added to each code from category V13

    A = initial encounter

    D = subsequent encounter

    S = sequela

  V13.0 Pedal cycle driver injured in collision with car, pick-up truck or van in nontraffic accident

  V13.1 Pedal cycle passenger injured in collision with car, pick-up truck or van in nontraffic accident

  V13.2 Unspecified pedal cyclist injured in collision with car, pick-up truck or van in nontraffic accident

  V13.3 Person boarding or alighting a pedal cycle injured in collision with car, pick-up truck or van

  V13.4 Pedal cycle driver injured in collision with car, pick-up truck or van in traffic accident

  V13.5 Pedal cycle passenger injured in collision with car, pick-up truck or van in traffic accident

  V13.9 Unspecified pedal cyclist injured in collision with car, pick-up truck or van in traffic accident

V14 Pedal cycle rider injured in collision with heavy transport vehicle or bus

  EXCLUDES1 pedal cycle rider injured in collision with military vehicle (V19.81)

The appropriate 7th character is to be added to each code from category V14

    A = initial encounter

    D = subsequent encounter

    S = sequela

  V14.0 Pedal cycle driver injured in collision with heavy transport vehicle or bus in nontraffic accident

  V14.1 Pedal cycle passenger injured in collision with heavy transport vehicle or bus in nontraffic accident

  V14.2 Unspecified pedal cyclist injured in collision with heavy transport vehicle or bus in nontraffic accident

  V14.3 Person boarding or alighting a pedal cycle injured in collision with heavy transport vehicle or bus

  V14.4 Pedal cycle driver injured in collision with heavy transport vehicle or bus in traffic accident

  V14.5 Pedal cycle passenger injured in collision with heavy transport vehicle or bus in traffic accident

  V14.9 Unspecified pedal cyclist injured in collision with heavy transport vehicle or bus in traffic accident

V15 Pedal cycle rider injured in collision with railway train or railway vehicle

The appropriate 7th character is to be added to each code from category V15

    A = initial encounter

    D = subsequent encounter

    S = sequela

  V15.0 Pedal cycle driver injured in collision with railway train or railway vehicle in nontraffic accident

  V15.1 Pedal cycle passenger injured in collision with railway train or railway vehicle in nontraffic accident

  V15.2 Unspecified pedal cyclist injured in collision with railway train or railway vehicle in nontraffic accident

  V15.3 Person boarding or alighting a pedal cycle injured in collision with railway train or railway vehicle

  V15.4 Pedal cycle driver injured in collision with railway train or railway vehicle in traffic accident

  V15.5 Pedal cycle passenger injured in collision with railway train or railway vehicle in traffic accident

  V15.9 Unspecified pedal cyclist injured in collision with railway train or railway vehicle in traffic accident

V16 Pedal cycle rider injured in collision with other nonmotor vehicle

  INCLUDES collision with animal-drawn vehicle, animal being ridden, streetcar

The appropriate 7th character is to be added to each code from category V16

    A = initial encounter

    D = subsequent encounter

    S = sequela

  V16.0 Pedal cycle driver injured in collision with other nonmotor vehicle in nontraffic accident

  V16.1 Pedal cycle passenger injured in collision with other nonmotor vehicle in nontraffic accident

  V16.2 Unspecified pedal cyclist injured in collision with other nonmotor vehicle in nontraffic accident

  V16.3 Person boarding or alighting a pedal cycle injured in collision with other nonmotor vehicle in nontraffic accident

  V16.4 Pedal cycle driver injured in collision with other nonmotor vehicle in traffic accident

  V16.5 Pedal cycle passenger injured in collision with other nonmotor vehicle in traffic accident

  V16.9 Unspecified pedal cyclist injured in collision with other nonmotor vehicle in traffic accident

V17 Pedal cycle rider injured in collision with fixed or stationary object

The appropriate 7th character is to be added to each code from category V17

    A = initial encounter

    D = subsequent encounter

    S = sequela

  V17.0 Pedal cycle driver injured in collision with fixed or stationary object in nontraffic accident

  V17.1 Pedal cycle passenger injured in collision with fixed or stationary object in nontraffic accident

  V17.2 Unspecified pedal cyclist injured in collision with fixed or stationary object in nontraffic accident

  V17.3 Person boarding or alighting a pedal cycle injured in collision with fixed or stationary object

  V17.4 Pedal cycle driver injured in collision with fixed or stationary object in traffic accident

  V17.5 Pedal cycle passenger injured in collision with fixed or stationary object in traffic accident

  V17.9 Unspecified pedal cyclist injured in collision with fixed or stationary object in traffic accident

V18 Pedal cycle rider injured in noncollision transport accident

  INCLUDES fall or thrown from pedal cycle (without antecedent collision)

    overturning pedal cycle NOS

    overturning pedal cycle without collision

The appropriate 7th character is to be added to each code from category V18

    A = initial encounter

    D = subsequent encounter

    S = sequela

  V18.0 Pedal cycle driver injured in noncollision transport accident in nontraffic accident

  V18.1 Pedal cycle passenger injured in noncollision transport accident in nontraffic accident

  V18.2 Unspecified pedal cyclist injured in noncollision transport accident in nontraffic accident

  V18.3 Person boarding or alighting a pedal cycle injured in noncollision transport accident

  V18.4 Pedal cycle driver injured in noncollision transport accident in traffic accident

  V18.5 Pedal cycle passenger injured in noncollision transport accident in traffic accident

  V18.9 Unspecified pedal cyclist injured in noncollision transport accident in traffic accident

V19 Pedal cycle rider injured in other and unspecified transport accidents

The appropriate 7th character is to be added to each code from category V19

    A = initial encounter

    D = subsequent encounter

    S = sequela

  V19.0 Pedal cycle driver injured in collision with other and unspecified motor vehicles in nontraffic accident

    V19.00 Pedal cycle driver injured in collision with unspecified motor vehicles in nontraffic accident

    V19.09 Pedal cycle driver injured in collision with other motor vehicles in nontraffic accident

V19.1 Pedal cycle passenger injured in collision with other and unspecified motor vehicles in nontraffic accident

  V19.10 Pedal cycle passenger injured in collision with unspecified motor vehicles in nontraffic accident POA

  V19.19 Pedal cycle passenger injured in collision with other motor vehicles in nontraffic accident POA

V19.2 Unspecified pedal cyclist injured in collision with other and unspecified motor vehicles in nontraffic accident

  V19.20 Unspecified pedal cyclist injured in collision with unspecified motor vehicles in nontraffic accident POA
    Pedal cycle collision NOS, nontraffic

  V19.29 Unspecified pedal cyclist injured in collision with other motor vehicles in nontraffic accident POA

V19.3 Pedal cyclist (driver) (passenger) injured in unspecified nontraffic accident POA
  Pedal cycle accident NOS, nontraffic
  Pedal cyclist injured in nontraffic accident NOS

V19.4 Pedal cycle driver injured in collision with other and unspecified motor vehicles in traffic accident

  V19.40 Pedal cycle driver injured in collision with unspecified motor vehicles in traffic accident POA

  V19.49 Pedal cycle driver injured in collision with other motor vehicles in traffic accident POA

V19.5 Pedal cycle passenger injured in collision with other and unspecified motor vehicles in traffic accident

  V19.50 Pedal cycle passenger injured in collision with unspecified motor vehicles in traffic accident POA

  V19.59 Pedal cycle passenger injured in collision with other motor vehicles in traffic accident POA

V19.6 Unspecified pedal cyclist injured in collision with other and unspecified motor vehicles in traffic accident

  V19.60 Unspecified pedal cyclist injured in collision with unspecified motor vehicles in traffic accident POA
    Pedal cycle collision NOS (traffic)

  V19.69 Unspecified pedal cyclist injured in collision with other motor vehicles in traffic accident POA

V19.8 Pedal cyclist (driver) (passenger) injured in other specified transport accidents

  V19.81 Pedal cyclist (driver) (passenger) injured in transport accident with military vehicle POA

  V19.88 Pedal cyclist (driver) (passenger) injured in other specified transport accidents POA

V19.9 Pedal cyclist (driver) (passenger) injured in unspecified traffic accident POA
  Pedal cycle accident NOS

Motorcycle rider injured in transport accident (V20-V29)

  INCLUDES moped
             motorcycle with sidecar
             motorized bicycle
             motor scooter

  EXCLUDES1 three-wheeled motor vehicle (V30-V39)

V20 Motorcycle rider injured in collision with pedestrian or animal

  EXCLUDES1 motorcycle rider collision with animal-drawn vehicle or animal being ridden (V26.-)

  The appropriate 7th character is to be added to each code from category V20
    A = initial encounter
    D = subsequent encounter
    S = sequela

  V20.0 Motorcycle driver injured in collision with pedestrian or animal in nontraffic accident POA

  V20.1 Motorcycle passenger injured in collision with pedestrian or animal in nontraffic accident POA

  V20.2 Unspecified motorcycle rider injured in collision with pedestrian or animal in nontraffic accident POA

  V20.3 Person boarding or alighting a motorcycle injured in collision with pedestrian or animal POA

  V20.4 Motorcycle driver injured in collision with pedestrian or animal in traffic accident

  V20.5 Motorcycle passenger injured in collision with pedestrian or animal in traffic accident POA

  V20.9 Unspecified motorcycle rider injured in collision with pedestrian or animal in traffic accident POA

V21 Motorcycle rider injured in collision with pedal cycle

  The appropriate 7th character is to be added to each code from category V21
    A = initial encounter
    D = subsequent encounter
    S = sequela

  V21.0 Motorcycle driver injured in collision with pedal cycle in nontraffic accident POA

  V21.1 Motorcycle passenger injured in collision with pedal cycle in nontraffic accident POA

  V21.2 Unspecified motorcycle rider injured in collision with pedal cycle in nontraffic accident POA

  V21.3 Person boarding or alighting a motorcycle injured in collision with pedal cycle POA

  V21.4 Motorcycle driver injured in collision with pedal cycle in traffic accident POA

  V21.5 Motorcycle passenger injured in collision with pedal cycle in traffic accident POA

  V21.9 Unspecified motorcycle rider injured in collision with pedal cycle in traffic accident POA

V22 Motorcycle rider injured in collision with two- or three-wheeled motor vehicle

  The appropriate 7th character is to be added to each code from category V22
    A = initial encounter
    D = subsequent encounter
    S = sequela

  V22.0 Motorcycle driver injured in collision with two- or three-wheeled motor vehicle in nontraffic accident POA

  V22.1 Motorcycle passenger injured in collision with two- or three-wheeled motor vehicle in nontraffic accident POA

  V22.2 Unspecified motorcycle rider injured in collision with two- or three-wheeled motor vehicle in nontraffic accident POA

  V22.3 Person boarding or alighting a motorcycle injured in collision with two- or three-wheeled motor vehicle POA

  V22.4 Motorcycle driver injured in collision with two- or three-wheeled motor vehicle in traffic accident POA

  V22.5 Motorcycle passenger injured in collision with two- or three-wheeled motor vehicle in traffic accident POA

  V22.9 Unspecified motorcycle rider injured in collision with two- or three-wheeled motor vehicle in traffic accident POA

V23 Motorcycle rider injured in collision with car, pick-up truck or van

  The appropriate 7th character is to be added to each code from category V23
    A = initial encounter
    D = subsequent encounter
    S = sequela

  V23.0 Motorcycle driver injured in collision with car, pick-up truck or van in nontraffic accident POA

  V23.1 Motorcycle passenger injured in collision with car, pick-up truck or van in nontraffic accident POA

  V23.2 Unspecified motorcycle rider injured in collision with car, pick-up truck or van in nontraffic accident POA

  V23.3 Person boarding or alighting a motorcycle injured in collision with car, pick-up truck or van POA

  V23.4 Motorcycle driver injured in collision with car, pick-up truck or van in traffic accident POA

  V23.5 Motorcycle passenger injured in collision with car, pick-up truck or van in traffic accident POA

  V23.9 Unspecified motorcycle rider injured in collision with car, pick-up truck or van in traffic accident POA

PDₓ Unacceptable principal diagnosis symbol per Medicare code edits   POA Code exempt from diagnosis present on admission requirement
  ❓ Questionable admission   CC Complication or comorbidity   MCC Major complication or comorbidity   CC/MCC Excl CC/MCC exclusion
  HCC HCC diagnosis code   RxHCC RxHCC diagnosis code   MACRA code   **DEFINITION** Describes condition/terminology
  TIP Coding guidance   👁 Official Guideline Reference   Z1 Z code as first-listed diagnosis

4ᵗʰ V24 **Motorcycle rider injured in** collision with heavy transport vehicle or bus

    EXCLUDES1 *motorcycle rider injured in collision with military vehicle (V29.81)*

    The appropriate 7th character is to be added to each code from category V24

        A = initial encounter

        D = subsequent encounter

        S = sequela

  7ᵗʰ V24.0 **Motorcycle** driver **injured in collision with heavy transport vehicle or bus in** nontraffic accident POA

  7ᵗʰ V24.1 **Motorcycle** passenger **injured in collision with heavy transport vehicle or bus in** nontraffic accident POA

  7ᵗʰ V24.2 **Unspecified motorcycle rider injured in collision with heavy transport vehicle or bus in nontraffic accident** POA

  7ᵗʰ V24.3 Person boarding or alighting **a motorcycle injured in collision with heavy transport vehicle or bus** POA

  7ᵗʰ V24.4 **Motorcycle** driver **injured in collision with heavy transport vehicle or bus in** traffic accident POA

  7ᵗʰ V24.5 **Motorcycle** passenger **injured in collision with heavy transport vehicle or bus in** traffic accident POA

  7ᵗʰ V24.9 **Unspecified motorcycle rider injured in collision with heavy transport vehicle or bus in traffic accident** POA

4ᵗʰ V25 **Motorcycle rider injured in** collision with railway train or railway vehicle

    The appropriate 7th character is to be added to each code from category V25

        A = initial encounter

        D = subsequent encounter

        S = sequela

  7ᵗʰ V25.0 **Motorcycle** driver **injured in collision with railway train or railway vehicle in** nontraffic accident POA

  7ᵗʰ V25.1 **Motorcycle** passenger **injured in collision with railway train or railway vehicle in** nontraffic accident POA

  7ᵗʰ V25.2 **Unspecified motorcycle rider injured in collision with railway train or railway vehicle in nontraffic accident** POA

  7ᵗʰ V25.3 Person boarding or alighting **a motorcycle injured in collision with railway train or railway vehicle** POA

  7ᵗʰ V25.4 **Motorcycle** driver **injured in collision with railway train or railway vehicle in** traffic accident POA

  7ᵗʰ V25.5 **Motorcycle** passenger **injured in collision with railway train or railway vehicle in** traffic accident POA

  7ᵗʰ V25.9 **Unspecified motorcycle rider injured in collision with railway train or railway vehicle in traffic accident** POA

4ᵗʰ V26 **Motorcycle rider injured in** collision with other nonmotor vehicle

    INCLUDES *collision with animal-drawn vehicle, animal being ridden, streetcar*

    The appropriate 7th character is to be added to each code from category V26

        A = initial encounter

        D = subsequent encounter

        S = sequela

  7ᵗʰ V26.0 **Motorcycle** driver **injured in collision with other nonmotor vehicle in** nontraffic accident POA

  7ᵗʰ V26.1 **Motorcycle** passenger **injured in collision with other nonmotor vehicle in** nontraffic accident POA

  7ᵗʰ V26.2 **Unspecified motorcycle rider injured in collision with other nonmotor vehicle in nontraffic accident** POA

  7ᵗʰ V26.3 Person boarding or alighting **a motorcycle injured in collision with other nonmotor vehicle** POA

  7ᵗʰ V26.4 **Motorcycle** driver **injured in collision with other nonmotor vehicle in** traffic accident POA

  7ᵗʰ V26.5 **Motorcycle** passenger **injured in collision with other nonmotor vehicle in** traffic accident POA

  7ᵗʰ V26.9 **Unspecified motorcycle rider injured in collision with other nonmotor vehicle in traffic accident** POA

4ᵗʰ V27 **Motorcycle rider injured in** collision with fixed or stationary object

    The appropriate 7th character is to be added to each code from category V27

        A = initial encounter

        D = subsequent encounter

        S = sequela

  7ᵗʰ V27.0 **Motorcycle** driver **injured in collision with fixed or stationary object in** nontraffic accident POA

  7ᵗʰ V27.1 **Motorcycle** passenger **injured in collision with fixed or stationary object in** nontraffic accident POA

  7ᵗʰ V27.2 **Unspecified motorcycle rider injured in collision with fixed or stationary object in nontraffic accident** POA

  7ᵗʰ V27.3 Person boarding or alighting **a motorcycle injured in collision with fixed or stationary object** POA

  7ᵗʰ V27.4 **Motorcycle** driver **injured in collision with fixed or stationary object in** traffic accident POA

  7ᵗʰ V27.5 **Motorcycle** passenger **injured in collision with fixed or stationary object in** traffic accident POA

  7ᵗʰ V27.9 **Unspecified motorcycle rider injured in collision with fixed or stationary object in traffic accident** POA

4ᵗʰ V28 **Motorcycle rider injured in** noncollision transport accident

    INCLUDES *fall or thrown from motorcycle (without antecedent collision)*

        overturning motorcycle NOS

        overturning motorcycle without collision

    The appropriate 7th character is to be added to each code from category V28

        A = initial encounter

        D = subsequent encounter

        S = sequela

  7ᵗʰ V28.0 **Motorcycle** driver **injured in noncollision transport accident in** nontraffic accident POA

  7ᵗʰ V28.1 **Motorcycle** passenger **injured in noncollision transport accident in** nontraffic accident POA

  7ᵗʰ V28.2 **Unspecified motorcycle rider injured in noncollision transport accident in nontraffic accident** POA

  7ᵗʰ V28.3 Person boarding or alighting **a motorcycle injured in noncollision transport accident** POA

  7ᵗʰ V28.4 **Motorcycle** driver **injured in noncollision transport accident in** traffic accident POA

  7ᵗʰ V28.5 **Motorcycle** passenger **injured in noncollision transport accident in** traffic accident POA

  7ᵗʰ V28.9 **Unspecified motorcycle rider injured in noncollision transport accident in traffic accident** POA

4ᵗʰ V29 **Motorcycle rider injured in** other and unspecified transport accidents

    The appropriate 7th character is to be added to each code from category V29

        A = initial encounter

        D = subsequent encounter

        S = sequela

  5ᵗʰ V29.0 **Motorcycle** driver **injured in collision with other and unspecified motor vehicles in** nontraffic accident

    7ᵗʰ V29.00 **Motorcycle driver injured in collision with unspecified motor vehicles in nontraffic accident** POA

    7ᵗʰ V29.09 **Motorcycle driver injured in collision with other motor vehicles in nontraffic accident** POA

  5ᵗʰ V29.1 **Motorcycle** passenger **injured in collision with other and unspecified motor vehicles in** nontraffic accident

    7ᵗʰ V29.10 **Motorcycle passenger injured in collision with unspecified motor vehicles in nontraffic accident** POA

    7ᵗʰ V29.19 **Motorcycle passenger injured in collision with other motor vehicles in nontraffic accident** POA

  5ᵗʰ V29.2 Unspecified **motorcycle rider injured in collision with other and unspecified motor vehicles in** nontraffic accident

    7ᵗʰ V29.20 **Unspecified motorcycle rider injured in collision with unspecified motor vehicles in nontraffic accident** POA

        Motorcycle collision NOS, nontraffic

    7ᵗʰ V29.29 **Unspecified motorcycle rider injured in collision with other motor vehicles in nontraffic accident** POA

  7ᵗʰ V29.3 **Motorcycle rider (driver) (passenger) injured in unspecified nontraffic accident** POA

    Motorcycle accident NOS, nontraffic

    Motorcycle rider injured in nontraffic accident NOS

  5ᵗʰ V29.4 **Motorcycle** driver **injured in collision with other and unspecified motor vehicles in** traffic accident

---

Unspecified Code   Other Specified Code   Manifestation Code   🆗 Newborn 🅿 Pediatric Ⓜ Maternity 🅰 Adult ♂ Male ♀ Female

● New Code ▲ Revised Code Title ►◄ Revised Text **NOTES** *INCLUDES* *EXCLUDES1* Not coded here *EXCLUDES2* Not included here

4ᵗʰ 4ᵗʰ character required 5ᵗʰ 5ᵗʰ character required 6ᵗʰ 6ᵗʰ character required 7ᵗʰ 7ᵗʰ character required Extension 'X' Alert

HAC Hospital-acquired condition (HAC) alert **AHA** AHA Coding Clinic© 📛 Code first alert

2020 ICD-10-CM   When symbols appear on a code that requires a 7th character extension, refer to Appendix B to identify applicable 7th character codes.   1189

7️⃣ **V29.40** Motorcycle driver injured in collision with unspecified motor vehicles in traffic accident 🚫POA

7️⃣ **V29.49** Motorcycle driver injured in collision with other motor vehicles in traffic accident 🚫POA

5️⃣ᵗʰ **V29.5** Motorcycle passenger injured in collision with other and unspecified motor vehicles in traffic accident

7️⃣ **V29.50** Motorcycle passenger injured in collision with unspecified motor vehicles in traffic accident 🚫POA

7️⃣ **V29.59** Motorcycle passenger injured in collision with other motor vehicles in traffic accident 🚫POA

5️⃣ᵗʰ **V29.6** Unspecified motorcycle rider injured in collision with other and unspecified motor vehicles in traffic accident

7️⃣ **V29.60** Unspecified motorcycle rider injured in collision with unspecified motor vehicles in traffic accident 🚫POA
Motorcycle collision NOS (traffic)

7️⃣ **V29.69** Unspecified motorcycle rider injured in collision with other motor vehicles in traffic accident 🚫POA

5️⃣ᵗʰ **V29.8** Motorcycle rider (driver) (passenger) injured in other specified transport accidents

7️⃣ **V29.81** Motorcycle rider (driver) (passenger) injured in transport accident with military vehicle

7️⃣ **V29.88** Motorcycle rider (driver) (passenger) injured in other specified transport accidents 🚫POA

7️⃣ **V29.9** Motorcycle rider (driver) (passenger) injured in unspecified traffic accident 🚫POA
Motorcycle accident NOS

Occupant of three-wheeled motor vehicle injured in transport accident (V30-V39)

INCLUDES   motorized tricycle
motorized rickshaw
three-wheeled motor car

EXCLUDES1   all-terrain vehicles (V86.-)
motorcycle with sidecar (V20-V29)
vehicle designed primarily for off-road use (V86.-)

4️⃣ᵗʰ **V30** Occupant of three-wheeled motor vehicle injured in collision with pedestrian or animal

EXCLUDES1   three-wheeled motor vehicle collision with animal-drawn vehicle or animal being ridden (V36.-)

The appropriate 7th character is to be added to each code from category V30
A = initial encounter
D = subsequent encounter
S = sequela

7️⃣ **V30.0** Driver of three-wheeled motor vehicle injured in collision with pedestrian or animal in nontraffic accident 🚫POA

7️⃣ **V30.1** Passenger in three-wheeled motor vehicle injured in collision with pedestrian or animal in nontraffic accident 🚫POA

7️⃣ **V30.2** Person on outside of three-wheeled motor vehicle injured in collision with pedestrian or animal in nontraffic accident 🚫POA

7️⃣ **V30.3** Unspecified occupant of three-wheeled motor vehicle injured in collision with pedestrian or animal in nontraffic accident 🚫POA

7️⃣ **V30.4** Person boarding or alighting a three-wheeled motor vehicle injured in collision with pedestrian or animal 🚫POA

7️⃣ **V30.5** Driver of three-wheeled motor vehicle injured in collision with pedestrian or animal in traffic accident 🚫POA

7️⃣ **V30.6** Passenger in three-wheeled motor vehicle injured in collision with pedestrian or animal in traffic accident 🚫POA

7️⃣ **V30.7** Person on outside of three-wheeled motor vehicle injured in collision with pedestrian or animal in traffic accident 🚫POA

7️⃣ **V30.9** Unspecified occupant of three-wheeled motor vehicle injured in collision with pedestrian or animal in traffic accident 🚫POA

4️⃣ᵗʰ **V31** Occupant of three-wheeled motor vehicle injured in collision with pedal cycle

The appropriate 7th character is to be added to each code from category V31
A = initial encounter
D = subsequent encounter
S = sequela

7️⃣ **V31.0** Driver of three-wheeled motor vehicle injured in collision with pedal cycle in nontraffic accident 🚫POA

7️⃣ **V31.1** Passenger in three-wheeled motor vehicle injured in collision with pedal cycle in nontraffic accident 🚫POA

7️⃣ **V31.2** Person on outside of three-wheeled motor vehicle injured in collision with pedal cycle in nontraffic accident 🚫POA

7️⃣ **V31.3** Unspecified occupant of three-wheeled motor vehicle injured in collision with pedal cycle in nontraffic accident 🚫POA

7️⃣ **V31.4** Person boarding or alighting a three-wheeled motor vehicle injured in collision with pedal cycle 🚫POA

7️⃣ **V31.5** Driver of three-wheeled motor vehicle injured in collision with pedal cycle in traffic accident 🚫POA

7️⃣ **V31.6** Passenger in three-wheeled motor vehicle injured in collision with pedal cycle in traffic accident 🚫POA

7️⃣ **V31.7** Person on outside of three-wheeled motor vehicle injured in collision with pedal cycle in traffic accident 🚫POA

7️⃣ **V31.9** Unspecified occupant of three-wheeled motor vehicle injured in collision with pedal cycle in traffic accident 🚫POA

4️⃣ᵗʰ **V32** Occupant of three-wheeled motor vehicle injured in collision with two- or three-wheeled motor vehicle

The appropriate 7th character is to be added to each code from category V32
A = initial encounter
D = subsequent encounter
S = sequela

7️⃣ **V32.0** Driver of three-wheeled motor vehicle injured in collision with two- or three-wheeled motor vehicle in nontraffic accident 🚫POA

7️⃣ **V32.1** Passenger in three-wheeled motor vehicle injured in collision with two- or three-wheeled motor vehicle in nontraffic accident 🚫POA

7️⃣ **V32.2** Person on outside of three-wheeled motor vehicle injured in collision with two- or three-wheeled motor vehicle in nontraffic accident 🚫POA

7️⃣ **V32.3** Unspecified occupant of three-wheeled motor vehicle injured in collision with two- or three-wheeled motor vehicle in nontraffic accident 🚫POA

7️⃣ **V32.4** Person boarding or alighting a three-wheeled motor vehicle injured in collision with two- or three-wheeled motor vehicle 🚫POA

7️⃣ **V32.5** Driver of three-wheeled motor vehicle injured in collision with two- or three-wheeled motor vehicle in traffic accident 🚫POA

7️⃣ **V32.6** Passenger in three-wheeled motor vehicle injured in collision with two- or three-wheeled motor vehicle in traffic accident 🚫POA

7️⃣ **V32.7** Person on outside of three-wheeled motor vehicle injured in collision with two- or three-wheeled motor vehicle in traffic accident 🚫POA

7️⃣ **V32.9** Unspecified occupant of three-wheeled motor vehicle injured in collision with two- or three-wheeled motor vehicle in traffic accident 🚫POA

4️⃣ᵗʰ **V33** Occupant of three-wheeled motor vehicle injured in collision with car, pick-up truck or van

The appropriate 7th character is to be added to each code from category V33
A = initial encounter
D = subsequent encounter
S = sequela

7️⃣ **V33.0** Driver of three-wheeled motor vehicle injured in collision with car, pick-up truck or van in nontraffic accident 🚫POA

7️⃣ **V33.1** Passenger in three-wheeled motor vehicle injured in collision with car, pick-up truck or van in nontraffic accident 🚫POA

7️⃣ **V33.2** Person on outside of three-wheeled motor vehicle injured in collision with car, pick-up truck or van in nontraffic accident 🚫POA

7️⃣ **V33.3** Unspecified occupant of three-wheeled motor vehicle injured in collision with car, pick-up truck or van in nontraffic accident 🚫POA

7️⃣ **V33.4** Person boarding or alighting a three-wheeled motor vehicle injured in collision with car, pick-up truck or van 🚫POA

PDx🚫 Unacceptable principal diagnosis symbol per Medicare code edits   🚫POA Code exempt from diagnosis present on admission requirement
❓ Questionable admission   ℂℂ Complication or comorbidity   MCC Major complication or comorbidity   CC/MCC Exclusion CC/MCC exclusion
HCC HCC diagnosis code   RxHCC RxHCC diagnosis code   MACRA code MACRA code   **DEFINITION** Describes condition/terminology
TIP Coding guidance   👁 Official Guideline Reference   Z1 Z code as first-listed diagnosis

🆖 V33.5 Driver of three-wheeled motor vehicle injured in collision with car, pick-up truck or van in traffic accident 🄟🄾🄰

🆖 V33.6 Passenger in three-wheeled motor vehicle injured in collision with car, pick-up truck or van in traffic accident 🄟🄾🄰

🆖 V33.7 Person on outside of three-wheeled motor vehicle injured in collision with car, pick-up truck or van in traffic accident 🄟🄾🄰

🆖 V33.9 Unspecified occupant of three-wheeled motor vehicle injured in collision with car, pick-up truck or van in traffic accident 🄟🄾🄰

🆖 V34 Occupant of three-wheeled motor vehicle injured in collision with heavy transport vehicle or bus

EXCLUDES1 occupant of three-wheeled motor vehicle injured in collision with military vehicle (V39.81)

The appropriate 7th character is to be added to each code from category V34

A = initial encounter
D = subsequent encounter
S = sequela

🆖 V34.0 Driver of three-wheeled motor vehicle injured in collision with heavy transport vehicle or bus in nontraffic accident 🄟🄾🄰

🆖 V34.1 Passenger in three-wheeled motor vehicle injured in collision with heavy transport vehicle or bus in nontraffic accident 🄟🄾🄰

🆖 V34.2 Person on outside of three-wheeled motor vehicle injured in collision with heavy transport vehicle or bus in nontraffic accident 🄟🄾🄰

🆖 V34.3 Unspecified occupant of three-wheeled motor vehicle injured in collision with heavy transport vehicle or bus in nontraffic accident 🄟🄾🄰

🆖 V34.4 Person boarding or alighting a three-wheeled motor vehicle injured in collision with heavy transport vehicle or bus 🄟🄾🄰

🆖 V34.5 Driver of three-wheeled motor vehicle injured in collision with heavy transport vehicle or bus in traffic accident 🄟🄾🄰

🆖 V34.6 Passenger in three-wheeled motor vehicle injured in collision with heavy transport vehicle or bus in traffic accident 🄟🄾🄰

🆖 V34.7 Person on outside of three-wheeled motor vehicle injured in collision with heavy transport vehicle or bus in traffic accident 🄟🄾🄰

🆖 V34.9 Unspecified occupant of three-wheeled motor vehicle injured in collision with heavy transport vehicle or bus in traffic accident 🄟🄾🄰

🆖 V35 Occupant of three-wheeled motor vehicle injured in collision with railway train or railway vehicle

The appropriate 7th character is to be added to each code from category V35

A = initial encounter
D = subsequent encounter
S = sequela

🆖 V35.0 Driver of three-wheeled motor vehicle injured in collision with railway train or railway vehicle in nontraffic accident 🄟🄾🄰

🆖 V35.1 Passenger in three-wheeled motor vehicle injured in collision with railway train or railway vehicle in nontraffic accident 🄟🄾🄰

🆖 V35.2 Person on outside of three-wheeled motor vehicle injured in collision with railway train or railway vehicle in nontraffic accident 🄟🄾🄰

🆖 V35.3 Unspecified occupant of three-wheeled motor vehicle injured in collision with railway train or railway vehicle in nontraffic accident 🄟🄾🄰

🆖 V35.4 Person boarding or alighting a three-wheeled motor vehicle injured in collision with railway train or railway vehicle 🄟🄾🄰

🆖 V35.5 Driver of three-wheeled motor vehicle injured in collision with railway train or railway vehicle in traffic accident 🄟🄾🄰

🆖 V35.6 Passenger in three-wheeled motor vehicle injured in collision with railway train or railway vehicle in traffic accident 🄟🄾🄰

🆖 V35.7 Person on outside of three-wheeled motor vehicle injured in collision with railway train or railway vehicle in traffic accident 🄟🄾🄰

🆖 V35.9 Unspecified occupant of three-wheeled motor vehicle injured in collision with railway train or railway vehicle in traffic accident 🄟🄾🄰

🆖 V36 Occupant of three-wheeled motor vehicle injured in collision with other nonmotor vehicle

INCLUDES collision with animal-drawn vehicle, animal being ridden, streetcar

The appropriate 7th character is to be added to each code from category V36

A = initial encounter
D = subsequent encounter
S = sequela

🆖 V36.0 Driver of three-wheeled motor vehicle injured in collision with other nonmotor vehicle in nontraffic accident 🄟🄾🄰

🆖 V36.1 Passenger in three-wheeled motor vehicle injured in collision with other nonmotor vehicle in nontraffic accident 🄟🄾🄰

🆖 V36.2 Person on outside of three-wheeled motor vehicle injured in collision with other nonmotor vehicle in nontraffic accident 🄟🄾🄰

🆖 V36.3 Unspecified occupant of three-wheeled motor vehicle injured in collision with other nonmotor vehicle in nontraffic accident 🄟🄾🄰

🆖 V36.4 Person boarding or alighting a three-wheeled motor vehicle injured in collision with other nonmotor vehicle 🄟🄾🄰

🆖 V36.5 Driver of three-wheeled motor vehicle injured in collision with other nonmotor vehicle in traffic accident 🄟🄾🄰

🆖 V36.6 Passenger in three-wheeled motor vehicle injured in collision with other nonmotor vehicle in traffic accident 🄟🄾🄰

🆖 V36.7 Person on outside of three-wheeled motor vehicle injured in collision with other nonmotor vehicle in traffic accident 🄟🄾🄰

🆖 V36.9 Unspecified occupant of three-wheeled motor vehicle injured in collision with other nonmotor vehicle in traffic accident 🄟🄾🄰

🆖 V37 Occupant of three-wheeled motor vehicle injured in collision with fixed or stationary object

The appropriate 7th character is to be added to each code from category V37

A = initial encounter
D = subsequent encounter
S = sequela

🆖 V37.0 Driver of three-wheeled motor vehicle injured in collision with fixed or stationary object in nontraffic accident 🄟🄾🄰

🆖 V37.1 Passenger in three-wheeled motor vehicle injured in collision with fixed or stationary object in nontraffic accident 🄟🄾🄰

🆖 V37.2 Person on outside of three-wheeled motor vehicle injured in collision with fixed or stationary object in nontraffic accident 🄟🄾🄰

🆖 V37.3 Unspecified occupant of three-wheeled motor vehicle injured in collision with fixed or stationary object in nontraffic accident 🄟🄾🄰

🆖 V37.4 Person boarding or alighting a three-wheeled motor vehicle injured in collision with fixed or stationary object 🄟🄾🄰

🆖 V37.5 Driver of three-wheeled motor vehicle injured in collision with fixed or stationary object in traffic accident 🄟🄾🄰

🆖 V37.6 Passenger in three-wheeled motor vehicle injured in collision with fixed or stationary object in traffic accident 🄟🄾🄰

🆖 V37.7 Person on outside of three-wheeled motor vehicle injured in collision with fixed or stationary object in traffic accident 🄟🄾🄰

🆖 V37.9 Unspecified occupant of three-wheeled motor vehicle injured in collision with fixed or stationary object in traffic accident 🄟🄾🄰

🆖 V38 Occupant of three-wheeled motor vehicle injured in noncollision transport accident

INCLUDES fall or thrown from three-wheeled motor vehicle
overturning of three-wheeled motor vehicle NOS
overturning of three-wheeled motor vehicle without collision

The appropriate 7th character is to be added to each code from category V38

A = initial encounter
D = subsequent encounter
S = sequela

Unspecified Code　Other Specified Code　Manifestation Code　Ⓝ Newborn　Ⓟ Pediatric　Ⓜ Maternity　Ⓐ Adult　♂ Male　♀ Female
● New Code　▲ Revised Code Title　▶◀ Revised Text　**NOTES**　*INCLUDES*　*EXCLUDES1* Not coded here　*EXCLUDES2* Not included here
🆖 4th character required　🆖 5th character required　🆖 6th character required　🆖 7th character required　🆖 Extension 'X' Alert
🅗🅐🅒 Hospital-acquired condition (HAC) alert　**AHA** AHA Coding Clinic©　📣 Code first alert

V38.0 **Driver** of three-wheeled motor vehicle injured in noncollision transport accident in nontraffic accident

V38.1 **Passenger** in three-wheeled motor vehicle injured in noncollision transport accident in nontraffic accident

V38.2 **Person on outside** of three-wheeled motor vehicle injured in noncollision transport accident in nontraffic accident

V38.3 Unspecified occupant of three-wheeled motor vehicle injured in noncollision transport accident in nontraffic accident

V38.4 **Person boarding or alighting** a three-wheeled motor vehicle injured in noncollision transport accident

V38.5 **Driver** of three-wheeled motor vehicle injured in noncollision transport accident in traffic accident

V38.6 **Passenger** in three-wheeled motor vehicle injured in noncollision transport accident in traffic accident

V38.7 **Person on outside** of three-wheeled motor vehicle injured in noncollision transport accident in traffic accident

V38.9 Unspecified occupant of three-wheeled motor vehicle injured in noncollision transport accident in traffic accident

V39 Occupant of three-wheeled motor vehicle injured in **other and unspecified** transport accidents

The appropriate 7th character is to be added to each code from category V39
A = initial encounter
D = subsequent encounter
S = sequela

V39.0 **Driver** of three-wheeled motor vehicle injured in collision with other and unspecified motor vehicles in nontraffic accident

V39.00 Driver of three-wheeled motor vehicle injured in collision with unspecified motor vehicles in nontraffic accident

V39.09 Driver of three-wheeled motor vehicle injured in collision with other motor vehicles in nontraffic accident

V39.1 **Passenger** in three-wheeled motor vehicle injured in collision with other and unspecified motor vehicles in nontraffic accident

V39.10 Passenger in three-wheeled motor vehicle injured in collision with unspecified motor vehicles in nontraffic accident

V39.19 Passenger in three-wheeled motor vehicle injured in collision with other motor vehicles in nontraffic accident

V39.2 **Unspecified** occupant of three-wheeled motor vehicle injured in collision with other and unspecified motor vehicles in nontraffic accident

V39.20 Unspecified occupant of three-wheeled motor vehicle injured in collision with unspecified motor vehicles in nontraffic accident
Collision NOS involving three-wheeled motor vehicle, nontraffic

V39.29 Unspecified occupant of three-wheeled motor vehicle injured in collision with other motor vehicles in nontraffic accident

V39.3 Occupant (driver) (passenger) of three-wheeled motor vehicle injured in unspecified nontraffic accident
Accident NOS involving three-wheeled motor vehicle, nontraffic
Occupant of three-wheeled motor vehicle injured in nontraffic accident NOS

V39.4 **Driver** of three-wheeled motor vehicle injured in collision with other and unspecified motor vehicles in traffic accident

V39.40 Driver of three-wheeled motor vehicle injured in collision with unspecified motor vehicles in traffic accident

V39.49 Driver of three-wheeled motor vehicle injured in collision with other motor vehicles in traffic accident

V39.5 **Passenger** in three-wheeled motor vehicle injured in collision with other and unspecified motor vehicles in traffic accident

V39.50 Passenger in three-wheeled motor vehicle injured in collision with unspecified motor vehicles in traffic accident

V39.59 Passenger in three-wheeled motor vehicle injured in collision with other motor vehicles in traffic accident

V39.6 **Unspecified** occupant of three-wheeled motor vehicle injured in collision with other and unspecified motor vehicles in traffic accident

V39.60 Unspecified occupant of three-wheeled motor vehicle injured in collision with unspecified motor vehicles in traffic accident
Collision NOS involving three-wheeled motor vehicle (traffic)

V39.69 Unspecified occupant of three-wheeled motor vehicle injured in collision with other motor vehicles in traffic accident

V39.8 Occupant (driver) (passenger) of three-wheeled motor vehicle injured in other specified transport accidents

V39.81 Occupant (driver) (passenger) of three-wheeled motor vehicle injured in transport accident with military vehicle

V39.89 Occupant (driver) (passenger) of three-wheeled motor vehicle injured in other specified transport accidents

V39.9 Occupant (driver) (passenger) of three-wheeled motor vehicle injured in unspecified traffic accident
Accident NOS involving three-wheeled motor vehicle

Car occupant injured in transport accident (V40-V49)

INCLUDES *a four-wheeled motor vehicle designed primarily for carrying passengers*
automobile (pulling a trailer or camper)

EXCLUDES1 *bus (V50-V59)*
minibus (V50-V59)
minivan (V50-V59)
motorcoach (V70-V79)
pick-up truck (V50-V59)
sport utility vehicle (SUV) (V50-V59)

V40 Car occupant injured in **collision with pedestrian or animal**
EXCLUDES1 *car collision with animal-drawn vehicle or animal being ridden (V46.-)*

The appropriate 7th character is to be added to each code from category V40
A = initial encounter
D = subsequent encounter
S = sequela

V40.0 Car **driver** injured in collision with pedestrian or animal in nontraffic accident

V40.1 Car **passenger** injured in collision with pedestrian or animal in nontraffic accident

V40.2 **Person on outside** of car injured in collision with pedestrian or animal in nontraffic accident

V40.3 Unspecified car occupant injured in collision with pedestrian or animal in nontraffic accident

V40.4 **Person boarding or alighting** a car injured in collision with pedestrian or animal

V40.5 Car **driver** injured in collision with pedestrian or animal in traffic accident

V40.6 Car **passenger** injured in collision with pedestrian or animal in traffic accident

V40.7 **Person on outside** of car injured in collision with pedestrian or animal in traffic accident

V40.9 Unspecified car occupant injured in collision with pedestrian or animal in traffic accident

V41 Car occupant injured in **collision with pedal cycle**
The appropriate 7th character is to be added to each code from category V41
A = initial encounter
D = subsequent encounter
S = sequela

[7th] **V41.0** Car driver injured in collision with pedal cycle in nontraffic accident [POA]

[7th] **V41.1** Car passenger injured in collision with pedal cycle in nontraffic accident [POA]

[7th] **V41.2** Person on outside of car injured in collision with pedal cycle in nontraffic accident [POA]

[7th] **V41.3** Unspecified car occupant injured in collision with pedal cycle in nontraffic accident [POA]

[7th] **V41.4** Person boarding or alighting a car injured in collision with pedal cycle [POA]

[7th] **V41.5** Car driver injured in collision with pedal cycle in traffic accident [POA]

[7th] **V41.6** Car passenger injured in collision with pedal cycle in traffic accident [POA]

[7th] **V41.7** Person on outside of car injured in collision with pedal cycle in traffic accident [POA]

[7th] **V41.9** Unspecified car occupant injured in collision with pedal cycle in traffic accident [POA]

[4th] **V42** Car occupant injured in collision with two- or three-wheeled motor vehicle

The appropriate 7th character is to be added to each code from category V42

A = initial encounter

D = subsequent encounter

S = sequela

[7th] **V42.0** Car driver injured in collision with two- or three-wheeled motor vehicle in nontraffic accident [POA]

[7th] **V42.1** Car passenger injured in collision with two- or three-wheeled motor vehicle in nontraffic accident [POA]

[7th] **V42.2** Person on outside of car injured in collision with two- or three-wheeled motor vehicle in nontraffic accident [POA]

[7th] **V42.3** Unspecified car occupant injured in collision with two- or three-wheeled motor vehicle in nontraffic accident [POA]

[7th] **V42.4** Person boarding or alighting a car injured in collision with two- or three-wheeled motor vehicle [POA]

[7th] **V42.5** Car driver injured in collision with two- or three-wheeled motor vehicle in traffic accident [POA]

[7th] **V42.6** Car passenger injured in collision with two- or three-wheeled motor vehicle in traffic accident [POA]

[7th] **V42.7** Person on outside of car injured in collision with two- or three-wheeled motor vehicle in traffic accident [POA]

[7th] **V42.9** Unspecified car occupant injured in collision with two- or three-wheeled motor vehicle in traffic accident [POA]

[4th] **V43** Car occupant injured in collision with car, pick-up truck or van

The appropriate 7th character is to be added to each code from category V43

A = initial encounter

D = subsequent encounter

S = sequela

[5th] **V43.0** Car driver injured in collision with car, pick-up truck or van in nontraffic accident

[7th] **V43.01** Car driver injured in collision with sport utility vehicle in nontraffic accident [POA]

[7th] **V43.02** Car driver injured in collision with other type car in nontraffic accident [POA]

[7th] **V43.03** Car driver injured in collision with pick-up truck in nontraffic accident [POA]

[7th] **V43.04** Car driver injured in collision with van in nontraffic accident [POA]

[5th] **V43.1** Car passenger injured in collision with car, pick-up truck or van in nontraffic accident

[7th] **V43.11** Car passenger injured in collision with sport utility vehicle in nontraffic accident [POA]

[7th] **V43.12** Car passenger injured in collision with other type car in nontraffic accident [POA]

▲ [7th] **V43.13** Car passenger injured in collision with pick-up ▶truck◀ in nontraffic accident [POA]

[7th] **V43.14** Car passenger injured in collision with van in nontraffic accident [POA]

[5th] **V43.2** Person on outside of car injured in collision with car, pick-up truck or van in nontraffic accident

[7th] **V43.21** Person on outside of car injured in collision with sport utility vehicle in nontraffic accident [POA]

[7th] **V43.22** Person on outside of car injured in collision with other type car in nontraffic accident [POA]

[7th] **V43.23** Person on outside of car injured in collision with pick-up truck in nontraffic accident [POA]

[7th] **V43.24** Person on outside of car injured in collision with van in nontraffic accident [POA]

[5th] **V43.3** Unspecified car occupant injured in collision with car, pick-up truck or van in nontraffic accident

[7th] **V43.31** Unspecified car occupant injured in collision with sport utility vehicle in nontraffic accident [POA]

[7th] **V43.32** Unspecified car occupant injured in collision with other type car in nontraffic accident [POA]

[7th] **V43.33** Unspecified car occupant injured in collision with pick-up truck in nontraffic accident [POA]

[7th] **V43.34** Unspecified car occupant injured in collision with van in nontraffic accident [POA]

[5th] **V43.4** Person boarding or alighting a car injured in collision with car, pick-up truck or van

[7th] **V43.41** Person boarding or alighting a car injured in collision with sport utility vehicle [POA]

[7th] **V43.42** Person boarding or alighting a car injured in collision with other type car [POA]

[7th] **V43.43** Person boarding or alighting a car injured in collision with pick-up truck [POA]

[7th] **V43.44** Person boarding or alighting a car injured in collision with van [POA]

[5th] **V43.5** Car driver injured in collision with car, pick-up truck or van in traffic accident

[7th] **V43.51** Car driver injured in collision with sport utility vehicle in traffic accident [POA]

[7th] **V43.52** Car driver injured in collision with other type car in traffic accident [POA]

[7th] **V43.53** Car driver injured in collision with pick-up truck in traffic accident [POA]

[7th] **V43.54** Car driver injured in collision with van in traffic accident [POA]

[5th] **V43.6** Car passenger injured in collision with car, pick-up truck or van in traffic accident

[7th] **V43.61** Car passenger injured in collision with sport utility vehicle in traffic accident [POA]

AHA: Q1 2015

[7th] **V43.62** Car passenger injured in collision with other type car in traffic accident [POA]

[7th] **V43.63** Car passenger injured in collision with pick-up truck in traffic accident [POA]

[7th] **V43.64** Car passenger injured in collision with van in traffic accident [POA]

[5th] **V43.7** Person on outside of car injured in collision with car, pick-up truck or van in traffic accident

[7th] **V43.71** Person on outside of car injured in collision with sport utility vehicle in traffic accident [POA]

[7th] **V43.72** Person on outside of car injured in collision with other type car in traffic accident [POA]

[7th] **V43.73** Person on outside of car injured in collision with pick-up truck in traffic accident [POA]

[7th] **V43.74** Person on outside of car injured in collision with van in traffic accident [POA]

[5th] **V43.9** Unspecified car occupant injured in collision with car, pick-up truck or van in traffic accident

[7th] **V43.91** Unspecified car occupant injured in collision with sport utility vehicle in traffic accident [POA]

[7th] **V43.92** Unspecified car occupant injured in collision with other type car in traffic accident [POA]

[7th] **V43.93** Unspecified car occupant injured in collision with pick-up truck in traffic accident [POA]

[7th] **V43.94** Unspecified car occupant injured in collision with van in traffic accident [POA]

Unspecified Code Other Specified Code Manifestation Code [N] Newborn [P] Pediatric [M] Maternity [A] Adult ♂ Male ♀ Female
● New Code ▲ Revised Code Title ▶◀ Revised Text NOTES INCLUDES EXCLUDES1 Not coded here EXCLUDES2 Not included here
[4th] 4th character required [5th] 5th character required [6th] 6th character required [7th] 7th character required [x] Extension 'X' Alert
[HAC] Hospital-acquired condition (HAC) alert **AHA** AHA Coding Clinic® ☞ Code first alert

[4th] **V44** Car occupant injured in collision with heavy transport vehicle or bus

[EXCLUDES1] *car occupant injured in collision with military vehicle (V49.81)*

The appropriate 7th character is to be added to each code from category V44
- A = initial encounter
- D = subsequent encounter
- S = sequela

[7th] **V44.0** Car driver injured in collision with heavy transport vehicle or bus in nontraffic accident [POA]
[7th] **V44.1** Car passenger injured in collision with heavy transport vehicle or bus in nontraffic accident [POA]
[7th] **V44.2** Person on outside of car injured in collision with heavy transport vehicle or bus in nontraffic accident [POA]
[7th] **V44.3** Unspecified car occupant injured in collision with heavy transport vehicle or bus in nontraffic accident [POA]
[7th] **V44.4** Person boarding or alighting a car injured in collision with heavy transport vehicle or bus [POA]
[7th] **V44.5** Car driver injured in collision with heavy transport vehicle or bus in traffic accident [POA]
[7th] **V44.6** Car passenger injured in collision with heavy transport vehicle or bus in traffic accident [POA]
[7th] **V44.7** Person on outside of car injured in collision with heavy transport vehicle or bus in traffic accident [POA]
[7th] **V44.9** Unspecified car occupant injured in collision with heavy transport vehicle or bus in traffic accident [POA]

[4th] **V45** Car occupant injured in collision with railway train or railway vehicle

The appropriate 7th character is to be added to each code from category V45
- A = initial encounter
- D = subsequent encounter
- S = sequela

[7th] **V45.0** Car driver injured in collision with railway train or railway vehicle in nontraffic accident [POA]
[7th] **V45.1** Car passenger injured in collision with railway train or railway vehicle in nontraffic accident [POA]
[7th] **V45.2** Person on outside of car injured in collision with railway train or railway vehicle in nontraffic accident [POA]
[7th] **V45.3** Unspecified car occupant injured in collision with railway train or railway vehicle in nontraffic accident [POA]
[7th] **V45.4** Person boarding or alighting a car injured in collision with railway train or railway vehicle [POA]
[7th] **V45.5** Car driver injured in collision with railway train or railway vehicle in traffic accident [POA]
[7th] **V45.6** Car passenger injured in collision with railway train or railway vehicle in traffic accident [POA]
[7th] **V45.7** Person on outside of car injured in collision with railway train or railway vehicle in traffic accident [POA]
[7th] **V45.9** Unspecified car occupant injured in collision with railway train or railway vehicle in traffic accident [POA]

[4th] **V46** Car occupant injured in collision with other nonmotor vehicle

[INCLUDES] *collision with animal-drawn vehicle, animal being ridden, streetcar*

The appropriate 7th character is to be added to each code from category V46
- A = initial encounter
- D = subsequent encounter
- S = sequela

[7th] **V46.0** Car driver injured in collision with other nonmotor vehicle in nontraffic accident [POA]
[7th] **V46.1** Car passenger injured in collision with other nonmotor vehicle in nontraffic accident [POA]
[7th] **V46.2** Person on outside of car injured in collision with other nonmotor vehicle in nontraffic accident [POA]
[7th] **V46.3** Unspecified car occupant injured in collision with other nonmotor vehicle in nontraffic accident [POA]
[7th] **V46.4** Person boarding or alighting a car injured in collision with other nonmotor vehicle [POA]
[7th] **V46.5** Car driver injured in collision with other nonmotor vehicle in traffic accident [POA]
[7th] **V46.6** Car passenger injured in collision with other nonmotor vehicle in traffic accident [POA]
[7th] **V46.7** Person on outside of car injured in collision with other nonmotor vehicle in traffic accident [POA]
[7th] **V46.9** Unspecified car occupant injured in collision with other nonmotor vehicle in traffic accident [POA]

[4th] **V47** Car occupant injured in collision with fixed or stationary object

The appropriate 7th character is to be added to each code from category V47
- A = initial encounter
- D = subsequent encounter
- S = sequela

[7th] **V47.0** Car driver injured in collision with fixed or stationary object in nontraffic accident [POA]
[7th] **V47.1** Car passenger injured in collision with fixed or stationary object in nontraffic accident [POA]
[7th] **V47.2** Person on outside of car injured in collision with fixed or stationary object in nontraffic accident [POA]
[7th] **V47.3** Unspecified car occupant injured in collision with fixed or stationary object in nontraffic accident [POA]
[7th] **V47.4** Person boarding or alighting a car injured in collision with fixed or stationary object [POA]
[7th] **V47.5** Car driver injured in collision with fixed or stationary object in traffic accident [POA]
[7th] **V47.6** Car passenger injured in collision with fixed or stationary object in traffic accident [POA]
[7th] **V47.7** Person on outside of car injured in collision with fixed or stationary object in traffic accident [POA]
[7th] **V47.9** Unspecified car occupant injured in collision with fixed or stationary object in traffic accident [POA]

[4th] **V48** Car occupant injured in noncollision transport accident

[INCLUDES] *overturning car NOS*
overturning car without collision

The appropriate 7th character is to be added to each code from category V48
- A = initial encounter
- D = subsequent encounter
- S = sequela

[7th] **V48.0** Car driver injured in noncollision transport accident in nontraffic accident [POA]
[7th] **V48.1** Car passenger injured in noncollision transport accident in nontraffic accident [POA]
[7th] **V48.2** Person on outside of car injured in noncollision transport accident in nontraffic accident [POA]
[7th] **V48.3** Unspecified car occupant injured in noncollision transport accident in nontraffic accident [POA]
[7th] **V48.4** Person boarding or alighting a car injured in noncollision transport accident [POA]
[7th] **V48.5** Car driver injured in noncollision transport accident in traffic accident [POA]
[7th] **V48.6** Car passenger injured in noncollision transport accident in traffic accident [POA]
[7th] **V48.7** Person on outside of car injured in noncollision transport accident in traffic accident [POA]
[7th] **V48.9** Unspecified car occupant injured in noncollision transport accident in traffic accident [POA]

[4th] **V49** Car occupant injured in other and unspecified transport accidents

The appropriate 7th character is to be added to each code from category V49
- A = initial encounter
- D = subsequent encounter
- S = sequela

[5th] **V49.0** Driver injured in collision with other and unspecified motor vehicles in nontraffic accident
[7th] **V49.00** Driver injured in collision with unspecified motor vehicles in nontraffic accident [POA]
[7th] **V49.09** Driver injured in collision with other motor vehicles in nontraffic accident [POA]
[5th] **V49.1** Passenger injured in collision with other and unspecified motor vehicles in nontraffic accident

[PDx] Unacceptable principal diagnosis symbol per Medicare code edits [POA] Code exempt from diagnosis present on admission requirement
[?] Questionable admission [CC] Complication or comorbidity [MCC] Major complication or comorbidity [CC/MCC Exc] CC/MCC exclusion
[HCC] HCC diagnosis code [RxHCC] RxHCC diagnosis code MACRA code **DEFINITION** Describes condition/terminology
TIP Coding guidance [👁] Official Guideline Reference [Z1] Z code as first-listed diagnosis

V49.10 Passenger injured in collision with unspecified motor vehicles in nontraffic accident

V49.19 Passenger injured in collision with other motor vehicles in nontraffic accident

V49.2 Unspecified car occupant injured in collision with other and unspecified motor vehicles in nontraffic accident

V49.20 Unspecified car occupant injured in collision with unspecified motor vehicles in nontraffic accident
Car collision NOS, nontraffic

V49.29 Unspecified car occupant injured in collision with other motor vehicles in nontraffic accident

V49.3 Car occupant (driver) (passenger) injured in unspecified nontraffic accident
Car accident NOS, nontraffic
Car occupant injured in nontraffic accident NOS

V49.4 Driver injured in collision with other and unspecified motor vehicles in traffic accident

V49.40 Driver injured in collision with unspecified motor vehicles in traffic accident

V49.49 Driver injured in collision with other motor vehicles in traffic accident

V49.5 Passenger injured in collision with other and unspecified motor vehicles in traffic accident

V49.50 Passenger injured in collision with unspecified motor vehicles in traffic accident

V49.59 Passenger injured in collision with other motor vehicles in traffic accident

V49.6 Unspecified car occupant injured in collision with other and unspecified motor vehicles in traffic accident

V49.60 Unspecified car occupant injured in collision with unspecified motor vehicles in traffic accident
Car collision NOS (traffic)

V49.69 Unspecified car occupant injured in collision with other motor vehicles in traffic accident

V49.8 Car occupant (driver) (passenger) injured in other specified transport accidents

V49.81 Car occupant (driver) (passenger) injured in transport accident with military vehicle

V49.88 Car occupant (driver) (passenger) injured in other specified transport accidents

V49.9 Car occupant (driver) (passenger) injured in unspecified traffic accident
AHA: Q1 2015
Car accident NOS

Occupant of pick-up truck or van injured in transport accident (V50-V59)

INCLUDES   a four or six wheel motor vehicle designed primarily for carrying passengers and property but weighing less than the local limit for classification as a heavy goods vehicle
minibus
minivan
sport utility vehicle (SUV)
truck
van

EXCLUDES1 heavy transport vehicle (V60-V69)

V50 Occupant of pick-up truck or van injured in collision with pedestrian or animal

EXCLUDES1 pick-up truck or van collision with animal-drawn vehicle or animal being ridden (V56.-)

The appropriate 7th character is to be added to each code from category V50
A = initial encounter
D = subsequent encounter
S = sequela

V50.0 Driver of pick-up truck or van injured in collision with pedestrian or animal in nontraffic accident

V50.1 Passenger in pick-up truck or van injured in collision with pedestrian or animal in nontraffic accident

V50.2 Person on outside of pick-up truck or van injured in collision with pedestrian or animal in nontraffic accident

V50.3 Unspecified occupant of pick-up truck or van injured in collision with pedestrian or animal in nontraffic accident

V50.4 Person boarding or alighting a pick-up truck or van injured in collision with pedestrian or animal

V50.5 Driver of pick-up truck or van injured in collision with pedestrian or animal in traffic accident

V50.6 Passenger in pick-up truck or van injured in collision with pedestrian or animal in traffic accident

V50.7 Person on outside of pick-up truck or van injured in collision with pedestrian or animal in traffic accident

V50.9 Unspecified occupant of pick-up truck or van injured in collision with pedestrian or animal in traffic accident

V51 Occupant of pick-up truck or van injured in collision with pedal cycle

The appropriate 7th character is to be added to each code from category V51
A = initial encounter
D = subsequent encounter
S = sequela

V51.0 Driver of pick-up truck or van injured in collision with pedal cycle in nontraffic accident

V51.1 Passenger in pick-up truck or van injured in collision with pedal cycle in nontraffic accident

V51.2 Person on outside of pick-up truck or van injured in collision with pedal cycle in nontraffic accident

V51.3 Unspecified occupant of pick-up truck or van injured in collision with pedal cycle in nontraffic accident

V51.4 Person boarding or alighting a pick-up truck or van injured in collision with pedal cycle

V51.5 Driver of pick-up truck or van injured in collision with pedal cycle in traffic accident

V51.6 Passenger in pick-up truck or van injured in collision with pedal cycle in traffic accident

V51.7 Person on outside of pick-up truck or van injured in collision with pedal cycle in traffic accident

V51.9 Unspecified occupant of pick-up truck or van injured in collision with pedal cycle in traffic accident

V52 Occupant of pick-up truck or van injured in collision with two- or three-wheeled motor vehicle

The appropriate 7th character is to be added to each code from category V52
A = initial encounter
D = subsequent encounter
S = sequela

V52.0 Driver of pick-up truck or van injured in collision with two- or three-wheeled motor vehicle in nontraffic accident

V52.1 Passenger in pick-up truck or van injured in collision with two- or three-wheeled motor vehicle in nontraffic accident

V52.2 Person on outside of pick-up truck or van injured in collision with two- or three-wheeled motor vehicle in nontraffic accident

V52.3 Unspecified occupant of pick-up truck or van injured in collision with two- or three-wheeled motor vehicle in nontraffic accident

V52.4 Person boarding or alighting a pick-up truck or van injured in collision with two- or three-wheeled motor vehicle

V52.5 Driver of pick-up truck or van injured in collision with two- or three-wheeled motor vehicle in traffic accident

V52.6 Passenger in pick-up truck or van injured in collision with two- or three-wheeled motor vehicle in traffic accident

V52.7 Person on outside of pick-up truck or van injured in collision with two- or three-wheeled motor vehicle in traffic accident

V52.9 Unspecified occupant of pick-up truck or van injured in collision with two- or three-wheeled motor vehicle in traffic accident

---

Unspecified Code   Other Specified Code   Manifestation Code   N Newborn   P Pediatric   M Maternity   A Adult   ♂ Male   ♀ Female
● New Code   ▲ Revised Code Title   ►◄ Revised Text   NOTES INCLUDES   EXCLUDES1 Not coded here   EXCLUDES2 Not included here
4th character required   5th character required   6th character required   7th character required   Extension 'X' Alert
HAC Hospital-acquired condition (HAC) alert   AHA AHA Coding Clinic©   Code first alert

⚫4️⃣ V53 Occupant of pick-up truck or van injured in collision with car, pick-up truck or van

The appropriate 7th character is to be added to each code from category V53
    A = initial encounter
    D = subsequent encounter
    S = sequela

7️⃣ V53.0 Driver of pick-up truck or van injured in collision with car, pick-up truck or van in nontraffic accident POA

7️⃣ V53.1 Passenger in pick-up truck or van injured in collision with car, pick-up truck or van in nontraffic accident POA

7️⃣ V53.2 Person on outside of pick-up truck or van injured in collision with car, pick-up truck or van in nontraffic accident POA

7️⃣ V53.3 Unspecified occupant of pick-up truck or van injured in collision with car, pick-up truck or van in nontraffic accident POA

7️⃣ V53.4 Person boarding or alighting a pick-up truck or van injured in collision with car, pick-up truck or van POA

7️⃣ V53.5 Driver of pick-up truck or van injured in collision with car, pick-up truck or van in traffic accident POA

7️⃣ V53.6 Passenger in pick-up truck or van injured in collision with car, pick-up truck or van in traffic accident POA

7️⃣ V53.7 Person on outside of pick-up truck or van injured in collision with car, pick-up truck or van in traffic accident POA

7️⃣ V53.9 Unspecified occupant of pick-up truck or van injured in collision with car, pick-up truck or van in traffic accident POA

⚫4️⃣ V54 Occupant of pick-up truck or van injured in collision with heavy transport vehicle or bus

EXCLUDES1 occupant of pick-up truck or van injured in collision with military vehicle (V59.81)

The appropriate 7th character is to be added to each code from category V54
    A = initial encounter
    D = subsequent encounter
    S = sequela

7️⃣ V54.0 Driver of pick-up truck or van injured in collision with heavy transport vehicle or bus in nontraffic accident POA

7️⃣ V54.1 Passenger in pick-up truck or van injured in collision with heavy transport vehicle or bus in nontraffic accident POA

7️⃣ V54.2 Person on outside of pick-up truck or van injured in collision with heavy transport vehicle or bus in nontraffic accident POA

7️⃣ V54.3 Unspecified occupant of pick-up truck or van injured in collision with heavy transport vehicle or bus in nontraffic accident POA

7️⃣ V54.4 Person boarding or alighting a pick-up truck or van injured in collision with heavy transport vehicle or bus POA

7️⃣ V54.5 Driver of pick-up truck or van injured in collision with heavy transport vehicle or bus in traffic accident POA

7️⃣ V54.6 Passenger in pick-up truck or van injured in collision with heavy transport vehicle or bus in traffic accident POA

7️⃣ V54.7 Person on outside of pick-up truck or van injured in collision with heavy transport vehicle or bus in traffic accident POA

7️⃣ V54.9 Unspecified occupant of pick-up truck or van injured in collision with heavy transport vehicle or bus in traffic accident POA

⚫4️⃣ V55 Occupant of pick-up truck or van injured in collision with railway train or railway vehicle

The appropriate 7th character is to be added to each code from category V55
    A = initial encounter
    D = subsequent encounter
    S = sequela

7️⃣ V55.0 Driver of pick-up truck or van injured in collision with railway train or railway vehicle in nontraffic accident POA

7️⃣ V55.1 Passenger in pick-up truck or van injured in collision with railway train or railway vehicle in nontraffic accident POA

7️⃣ V55.2 Person on outside of pick-up truck or van injured in collision with railway train or railway vehicle in nontraffic accident POA

7️⃣ V55.3 Unspecified occupant of pick-up truck or van injured in collision with railway train or railway vehicle in nontraffic accident POA

7️⃣ V55.4 Person boarding or alighting a pick-up truck or van injured in collision with railway train or railway vehicle POA

7️⃣ V55.5 Driver of pick-up truck or van injured in collision with railway train or railway vehicle in traffic accident POA

7️⃣ V55.6 Passenger in pick-up truck or van injured in collision with railway train or railway vehicle in traffic accident POA

7️⃣ V55.7 Person on outside of pick-up truck or van injured in collision with railway train or railway vehicle in traffic accident POA

7️⃣ V55.9 Unspecified occupant of pick-up truck or van injured in collision with railway train or railway vehicle in traffic accident POA

⚫4️⃣ V56 Occupant of pick-up truck or van injured in collision with other nonmotor vehicle

INCLUDES collision with animal-drawn vehicle, animal being ridden, streetcar

The appropriate 7th character is to be added to each code from category V56
    A = initial encounter
    D = subsequent encounter
    S = sequela

7️⃣ V56.0 Driver of pick-up truck or van injured in collision with other nonmotor vehicle in nontraffic accident POA

7️⃣ V56.1 Passenger in pick-up truck or van injured in collision with other nonmotor vehicle in nontraffic accident POA

7️⃣ V56.2 Person on outside of pick-up truck or van injured in collision with other nonmotor vehicle in nontraffic accident POA

7️⃣ V56.3 Unspecified occupant of pick-up truck or van injured in collision with other nonmotor vehicle in nontraffic accident POA

7️⃣ V56.4 Person boarding or alighting a pick-up truck or van injured in collision with other nonmotor vehicle POA

7️⃣ V56.5 Driver of pick-up truck or van injured in collision with other nonmotor vehicle in traffic accident POA

7️⃣ V56.6 Passenger in pick-up truck or van injured in collision with other nonmotor vehicle in traffic accident POA

7️⃣ V56.7 Person on outside of pick-up truck or van injured in collision with other nonmotor vehicle in traffic accident POA

7️⃣ V56.9 Unspecified occupant of pick-up truck or van injured in collision with other nonmotor vehicle in traffic accident POA

⚫4️⃣ V57 Occupant of pick-up truck or van injured in collision with fixed or stationary object

The appropriate 7th character is to be added to each code from category V57
    A = initial encounter
    D = subsequent encounter
    S = sequela

7️⃣ V57.0 Driver of pick-up truck or van injured in collision with fixed or stationary object in nontraffic accident POA

7️⃣ V57.1 Passenger in pick-up truck or van injured in collision with fixed or stationary object in nontraffic accident POA

7️⃣ V57.2 Person on outside of pick-up truck or van injured in collision with fixed or stationary object in nontraffic accident POA

7️⃣ V57.3 Unspecified occupant of pick-up truck or van injured in collision with fixed or stationary object in nontraffic accident POA

7️⃣ V57.4 Person boarding or alighting a pick-up truck or van injured in collision with fixed or stationary object POA

7️⃣ V57.5 Driver of pick-up truck or van injured in collision with fixed or stationary object in traffic accident POA

7️⃣ V57.6 Passenger in pick-up truck or van injured in collision with fixed or stationary object in traffic accident POA

7️⃣ V57.7 Person on outside of pick-up truck or van injured in collision with fixed or stationary object in traffic accident POA

7️⃣ V57.9 Unspecified occupant of pick-up truck or van injured in collision with fixed or stationary object in traffic accident POA

⚫4️⃣ V58 Occupant of pick-up truck or van injured in noncollision transport accident

INCLUDES overturning pick-up truck or van NOS
                  overturning pick-up truck or van without collision

---

POA↓ Unacceptable principal diagnosis symbol per Medicare code edits   POA Code exempt from diagnosis present on admission requirement
  ❓ Questionable admission   cc Complication or comorbidity   MCC Major complication or comorbidity   cc/MCC excl CC/MCC exclusion
  HCC HCC diagnosis code   RxHCC RxHCC diagnosis code   MACRA code   **DEFINITION** Describes condition/terminology
  TIP Coding guidance   👁 Official Guideline Reference   Z Z code as first-listed diagnosis

The appropriate 7th character is to be added to each code from category V58
A = initial encounter
D = subsequent encounter
S = sequela

7th V58.0 Driver of pick-up truck or van injured in noncollision transport accident in nontraffic accident POA

7th V58.1 Passenger in pick-up truck or van injured in noncollision transport accident in nontraffic accident POA

7th V58.2 Person on outside of pick-up truck or van injured in noncollision transport accident in nontraffic accident POA

7th V58.3 Unspecified occupant of pick-up truck or van injured in noncollision transport accident in nontraffic accident POA

7th V58.4 Person boarding or alighting a pick-up truck or van injured in noncollision transport accident POA

7th V58.5 Driver of pick-up truck or van injured in noncollision transport accident in traffic accident POA

7th V58.6 Passenger in pick-up truck or van injured in noncollision transport accident in traffic accident POA

7th V58.7 Person on outside of pick-up truck or van injured in noncollision transport accident in traffic accident POA

7th V58.9 Unspecified occupant of pick-up truck or van injured in noncollision transport accident in traffic accident POA

4th V59 Occupant of pick-up truck or van injured in other and unspecified transport accidents

The appropriate 7th character is to be added to each code from category V59
A = initial encounter
D = subsequent encounter
S = sequela

5th V59.0 Driver of pick-up truck or van injured in collision with other and unspecified motor vehicles in nontraffic accident

7th V59.00 Driver of pick-up truck or van injured in collision with unspecified motor vehicles in nontraffic accident POA

7th V59.09 Driver of pick-up truck or van injured in collision with other motor vehicles in nontraffic accident POA

5th V59.1 Passenger in pick-up truck or van injured in collision with other and unspecified motor vehicles in nontraffic accident

7th V59.10 Passenger in pick-up truck or van injured in collision with unspecified motor vehicles in nontraffic accident POA

7th V59.19 Passenger in pick-up truck or van injured in collision with other motor vehicles in nontraffic accident POA

5th V59.2 Unspecified occupant of pick-up truck or van injured in collision with other and unspecified motor vehicles in nontraffic accident

7th V59.20 Unspecified occupant of pick-up truck or van injured in collision with unspecified motor vehicles in nontraffic accident POA
Collision NOS involving pick-up truck or van, nontraffic

7th V59.29 Unspecified occupant of pick-up truck or van injured in collision with other motor vehicles in nontraffic accident POA

7th V59.3 Occupant (driver) (passenger) of pick-up truck or van injured in unspecified nontraffic accident POA
Accident NOS involving pick-up truck or van, nontraffic
Occupant of pick-up truck or van injured in nontraffic accident NOS

5th V59.4 Driver of pick-up truck or van injured in collision with other and unspecified motor vehicles in traffic accident

7th V59.40 Driver of pick-up truck or van injured in collision with unspecified motor vehicles in traffic accident POA

7th V59.49 Driver of pick-up truck or van injured in collision with other motor vehicles in traffic accident POA

5th V59.5 Passenger in pick-up truck or van injured in collision with other and unspecified motor vehicles in traffic accident

7th V59.50 Passenger in pick-up truck or van injured in collision with unspecified motor vehicles in traffic accident POA

7th V59.59 Passenger in pick-up truck or van injured in collision with other motor vehicles in traffic accident POA

5th V59.6 Unspecified occupant of pick-up truck or van injured in collision with other and unspecified motor vehicles in traffic accident

7th V59.60 Unspecified occupant of pick-up truck or van injured in collision with unspecified motor vehicles in traffic accident
Collision NOS involving pick-up truck or van (traffic)

7th V59.69 Unspecified occupant of pick-up truck or van injured in collision with other motor vehicles in traffic accident POA

5th V59.8 Occupant (driver) (passenger) of pick-up truck or van injured in other specified transport accidents

7th V59.81 Occupant (driver) (passenger) of pick-up truck or van injured in transport accident with military vehicle POA

7th V59.88 Occupant (driver) (passenger) of pick-up truck or van injured in other specified transport accidents POA

7th V59.9 Occupant (driver) (passenger) of pick-up truck or van injured in unspecified traffic accident POA
Accident NOS involving pick-up truck or van

Occupant of heavy transport vehicle injured in transport accident (V60-V69)

INCLUDES   18 wheeler
           armored car
           panel truck

EXCLUDES1 bus
           motorcoach

4th V60 Occupant of heavy transport vehicle injured in collision with pedestrian or animal
EXCLUDES1 heavy transport vehicle collision with animal-drawn vehicle or animal being ridden (V66.-)

The appropriate 7th character is to be added to each code from category V60
A = initial encounter
D = subsequent encounter
S = sequela

7th V60.0 Driver of heavy transport vehicle injured in collision with pedestrian or animal in nontraffic accident POA

7th V60.1 Passenger in heavy transport vehicle injured in collision with pedestrian or animal in nontraffic accident POA

7th V60.2 Person on outside of heavy transport vehicle injured in collision with pedestrian or animal in nontraffic accident POA

7th V60.3 Unspecified occupant of heavy transport vehicle injured in collision with pedestrian or animal in nontraffic accident POA

7th V60.4 Person boarding or alighting a heavy transport vehicle injured in collision with pedestrian or animal POA

7th V60.5 Driver of heavy transport vehicle injured in collision with pedestrian or animal in traffic accident POA

7th V60.6 Passenger in heavy transport vehicle injured in collision with pedestrian or animal in traffic accident POA

7th V60.7 Person on outside of heavy transport vehicle injured in collision with pedestrian or animal in traffic accident POA

7th V60.9 Unspecified occupant of heavy transport vehicle injured in collision with pedestrian or animal in traffic accident POA

4th V61 Occupant of heavy transport vehicle injured in collision with pedal cycle

The appropriate 7th character is to be added to each code from category V61
A = initial encounter
D = subsequent encounter
S = sequela

7th V61.0 Driver of heavy transport vehicle injured in collision with pedal cycle in nontraffic accident POA

7th V61.1 Passenger in heavy transport vehicle injured in collision with pedal cycle in nontraffic accident POA

7th V61.2 Person on outside of heavy transport vehicle injured in collision with pedal cycle in nontraffic accident POA

7th V61.3 Unspecified occupant of heavy transport vehicle injured in collision with pedal cycle in nontraffic accident POA

Unspecified Code   Other Specified Code   Manifestation Code   N Newborn   P Pediatric   M Maternity   A Adult   ♂ Male   ♀ Female
● New Code   ▲ Revised Code Title   ►◄ Revised Text   NOTES   INCLUDES   EXCLUDES1 Not coded here   EXCLUDES2 Not included here
4th 4th character required   5th 5th character required   6th 6th character required   7th 7th character required   X Extension 'X' Alert
HAC Hospital-acquired condition (HAC) alert   AHA AHA Coding Clinic©   📣 Code first alert

🔟 **V61.4** Person boarding or alighting a heavy transport vehicle injured in collision with pedal cycle while boarding or alighting   POA

🔟 **V61.5** Driver of heavy transport vehicle injured in collision with pedal cycle in traffic accident   POA

🔟 **V61.6** Passenger in heavy transport vehicle injured in collision with pedal cycle in traffic accident   POA

🔟 **V61.7** Person on outside of heavy transport vehicle injured in collision with pedal cycle in traffic accident   POA

🔟 **V61.9** Unspecified occupant of heavy transport vehicle injured in collision with pedal cycle in traffic accident   POA

4️⃣ **V62** Occupant of heavy transport vehicle injured in collision with two- or three-wheeled motor vehicle

The appropriate 7th character is to be added to each code from category V62
  A = initial encounter
  D = subsequent encounter
  S = sequela

🔟 **V62.0** Driver of heavy transport vehicle injured in collision with two- or three-wheeled motor vehicle in nontraffic accident   POA

🔟 **V62.1** Passenger in heavy transport vehicle injured in collision with two- or three-wheeled motor vehicle in nontraffic accident   POA

🔟 **V62.2** Person on outside of heavy transport vehicle injured in collision with two- or three-wheeled motor vehicle in nontraffic accident   POA

🔟 **V62.3** Unspecified occupant of heavy transport vehicle injured in collision with two- or three-wheeled motor vehicle in nontraffic accident   POA

🔟 **V62.4** Person boarding or alighting a heavy transport vehicle injured in collision with two- or three-wheeled motor vehicle   POA

🔟 **V62.5** Driver of heavy transport vehicle injured in collision with two- or three-wheeled motor vehicle in traffic accident   POA

🔟 **V62.6** Passenger in heavy transport vehicle injured in collision with two- or three-wheeled motor vehicle in traffic accident   POA

🔟 **V62.7** Person on outside of heavy transport vehicle injured in collision with two- or three-wheeled motor vehicle in traffic accident   POA

🔟 **V62.9** Unspecified occupant of heavy transport vehicle injured in collision with two- or three-wheeled motor vehicle in traffic accident   POA

4️⃣ **V63** Occupant of heavy transport vehicle injured in collision with car, pick-up truck or van

The appropriate 7th character is to be added to each code from category V63
  A = initial encounter
  D = subsequent encounter
  S = sequela

🔟 **V63.0** Driver of heavy transport vehicle injured in collision with car, pick-up truck or van in nontraffic accident   POA

🔟 **V63.1** Passenger in heavy transport vehicle injured in collision with car, pick-up truck or van in nontraffic accident   POA

🔟 **V63.2** Person on outside of heavy transport vehicle injured in collision with car, pick-up truck or van in nontraffic accident   POA

🔟 **V63.3** Unspecified occupant of heavy transport vehicle injured in collision with car, pick-up truck or van in nontraffic accident   POA

🔟 **V63.4** Person boarding or alighting a heavy transport vehicle injured in collision with car, pick-up truck or van   POA

🔟 **V63.5** Driver of heavy transport vehicle injured in collision with car, pick-up truck or van in traffic accident   POA

🔟 **V63.6** Passenger in heavy transport vehicle injured in collision with car, pick-up truck or van in traffic accident   POA

🔟 **V63.7** Person on outside of heavy transport vehicle injured in collision with car, pick-up truck or van in traffic accident   POA

🔟 **V63.9** Unspecified occupant of heavy transport vehicle injured in collision with car, pick-up truck or van in traffic accident   POA

4️⃣ **V64** Occupant of heavy transport vehicle injured in collision with heavy transport vehicle or bus

EXCLUDES1 occupant of heavy transport vehicle injured in collision with military vehicle (V69.81)

The appropriate 7th character is to be added to each code from category V64
  A = initial encounter
  D = subsequent encounter
  S = sequela

🔟 **V64.0** Driver of heavy transport vehicle injured in collision with heavy transport vehicle or bus in nontraffic accident   POA

🔟 **V64.1** Passenger in heavy transport vehicle injured in collision with heavy transport vehicle or bus in nontraffic accident   POA

🔟 **V64.2** Person on outside of heavy transport vehicle injured in collision with heavy transport vehicle or bus in nontraffic accident   POA

🔟 **V64.3** Unspecified occupant of heavy transport vehicle injured in collision with heavy transport vehicle or bus in nontraffic accident   POA

🔟 **V64.4** Person boarding or alighting a heavy transport vehicle injured in collision with heavy transport vehicle or bus while boarding or alighting   POA

🔟 **V64.5** Driver of heavy transport vehicle injured in collision with heavy transport vehicle or bus in traffic accident   POA

🔟 **V64.6** Passenger in heavy transport vehicle injured in collision with heavy transport vehicle or bus in traffic accident   POA

🔟 **V64.7** Person on outside of heavy transport vehicle injured in collision with heavy transport vehicle or bus in traffic accident   POA

🔟 **V64.9** Unspecified occupant of heavy transport vehicle injured in collision with heavy transport vehicle or bus in traffic accident   POA

4️⃣ **V65** Occupant of heavy transport vehicle injured in collision with railway train or railway vehicle

The appropriate 7th character is to be added to each code from category V65
  A = initial encounter
  D = subsequent encounter
  S = sequela

🔟 **V65.0** Driver of heavy transport vehicle injured in collision with railway train or railway vehicle in nontraffic accident   POA

🔟 **V65.1** Passenger in heavy transport vehicle injured in collision with railway train or railway vehicle in nontraffic accident   POA

🔟 **V65.2** Person on outside of heavy transport vehicle injured in collision with railway train or railway vehicle in nontraffic accident   POA

🔟 **V65.3** Unspecified occupant of heavy transport vehicle injured in collision with railway train or railway vehicle in nontraffic accident   POA

🔟 **V65.4** Person boarding or alighting a heavy transport vehicle injured in collision with railway train or railway vehicle   POA

🔟 **V65.5** Driver of heavy transport vehicle injured in collision with railway train or railway vehicle in traffic accident   POA

🔟 **V65.6** Passenger in heavy transport vehicle injured in collision with railway train or railway vehicle in traffic accident   POA

🔟 **V65.7** Person on outside of heavy transport vehicle injured in collision with railway train or railway vehicle in traffic accident   POA

🔟 **V65.9** Unspecified occupant of heavy transport vehicle injured in collision with railway train or railway vehicle in traffic accident   POA

4️⃣ **V66** Occupant of heavy transport vehicle injured in collision with other nonmotor vehicle

INCLUDES collision with animal-drawn vehicle, animal being ridden, streetcar

The appropriate 7th character is to be added to each code from category V66
  A = initial encounter
  D = subsequent encounter
  S = sequela

POA Unacceptable principal diagnosis symbol per Medicare code edits   POA Code exempt from diagnosis present on admission requirement
❓ Questionable admission   cc Complication or comorbidity   mcc Major complication or comorbidity   cc/mcc CC/MCC exclusion
HCC HCC diagnosis code   RxHCC RxHCC diagnosis code   MACRA MACRA code   **DEFINITION** Describes condition/terminology
TIP Coding guidance   👁 Official Guideline Reference   Z1 Z code as first-listed diagnosis

V66.0 Driver of heavy transport vehicle injured in collision with other nonmotor vehicle in nontraffic accident

V66.1 Passenger in heavy transport vehicle injured in collision with other nonmotor vehicle in nontraffic accident

V66.2 Person on outside of heavy transport vehicle injured in collision with other nonmotor vehicle in nontraffic accident

V66.3 Unspecified occupant of heavy transport vehicle injured in collision with other nonmotor vehicle in nontraffic accident

V66.4 Person boarding or alighting a heavy transport vehicle injured in collision with other nonmotor vehicle

V66.5 Driver of heavy transport vehicle injured in collision with other nonmotor vehicle in traffic accident

V66.6 Passenger in heavy transport vehicle injured in collision with other nonmotor vehicle in traffic accident

V66.7 Person on outside of heavy transport vehicle injured in collision with other nonmotor vehicle in traffic accident

V66.9 Unspecified occupant of heavy transport vehicle injured in collision with other nonmotor vehicle in traffic accident

V67 Occupant of heavy transport vehicle injured in collision with fixed or stationary object

The appropriate 7th character is to be added to each code from category V67

A = initial encounter
D = subsequent encounter
S = sequela

V67.0 Driver of heavy transport vehicle injured in collision with fixed or stationary object in nontraffic accident

V67.1 Passenger in heavy transport vehicle injured in collision with fixed or stationary object in nontraffic accident

V67.2 Person on outside of heavy transport vehicle injured in collision with fixed or stationary object in nontraffic accident

V67.3 Unspecified occupant of heavy transport vehicle injured in collision with fixed or stationary object in nontraffic accident

V67.4 Person boarding or alighting a heavy transport vehicle injured in collision with fixed or stationary object

V67.5 Driver of heavy transport vehicle injured in collision with fixed or stationary object in traffic accident

V67.6 Passenger in heavy transport vehicle injured in collision with fixed or stationary object in traffic accident

V67.7 Person on outside of heavy transport vehicle injured in collision with fixed or stationary object in traffic accident

V67.9 Unspecified occupant of heavy transport vehicle injured in collision with fixed or stationary object in traffic accident

V68 Occupant of heavy transport vehicle injured in noncollision transport accident

INCLUDES   overturning heavy transport vehicle NOS
            overturning heavy transport vehicle without collision

The appropriate 7th character is to be added to each code from category V68

A = initial encounter
D = subsequent encounter
S = sequela

V68.0 Driver of heavy transport vehicle injured in noncollision transport accident in nontraffic accident

V68.1 Passenger in heavy transport vehicle injured in noncollision transport accident in nontraffic accident

V68.2 Person on outside of heavy transport vehicle injured in noncollision transport accident in nontraffic accident

V68.3 Unspecified occupant of heavy transport vehicle injured in noncollision transport accident in nontraffic accident

V68.4 Person boarding or alighting a heavy transport vehicle injured in noncollision transport accident

V68.5 Driver of heavy transport vehicle injured in noncollision transport accident in traffic accident

V68.6 Passenger in heavy transport vehicle injured in noncollision transport accident in traffic accident

V68.7 Person on outside of heavy transport vehicle injured in noncollision transport accident in traffic accident

V68.9 Unspecified occupant of heavy transport vehicle injured in noncollision transport accident in traffic accident

V69 Occupant of heavy transport vehicle injured in other and unspecified transport accidents

The appropriate 7th character is to be added to each code from category V69

A = initial encounter
D = subsequent encounter
S = sequela

V69.0 Driver of heavy transport vehicle injured in collision with other and unspecified motor vehicles in nontraffic accident

V69.00 Driver of heavy transport vehicle injured in collision with unspecified motor vehicles in nontraffic accident

V69.09 Driver of heavy transport vehicle injured in collision with other motor vehicles in nontraffic accident

V69.1 Passenger in heavy transport vehicle injured in collision with other and unspecified motor vehicles in nontraffic accident

V69.10 Passenger in heavy transport vehicle injured in collision with unspecified motor vehicles in nontraffic accident

V69.19 Passenger in heavy transport vehicle injured in collision with other motor vehicles in nontraffic accident

V69.2 Unspecified occupant of heavy transport vehicle injured in collision with other and unspecified motor vehicles in nontraffic accident

V69.20 Unspecified occupant of heavy transport vehicle injured in collision with unspecified motor vehicles in nontraffic accident
Collision NOS involving heavy transport vehicle, nontraffic

V69.29 Unspecified occupant of heavy transport vehicle injured in collision with other motor vehicles in nontraffic accident

V69.3 Occupant (driver) (passenger) of heavy transport vehicle injured in unspecified nontraffic accident
Accident NOS involving heavy transport vehicle, nontraffic
Occupant of heavy transport vehicle injured in nontraffic accident NOS

V69.4 Driver of heavy transport vehicle injured in collision with other and unspecified motor vehicles in traffic accident

V69.40 Driver of heavy transport vehicle injured in collision with unspecified motor vehicles in traffic accident

V69.49 Driver of heavy transport vehicle injured in collision with other motor vehicles in traffic accident

V69.5 Passenger in heavy transport vehicle injured in collision with other and unspecified motor vehicles in traffic accident

V69.50 Passenger in heavy transport vehicle injured in collision with unspecified motor vehicles in traffic accident

V69.59 Passenger in heavy transport vehicle injured in collision with other motor vehicles in traffic accident

V69.6 Unspecified occupant of heavy transport vehicle injured in collision with other and unspecified motor vehicles in traffic accident

V69.60 Unspecified occupant of heavy transport vehicle injured in collision with unspecified motor vehicles in traffic accident
Collision NOS involving heavy transport vehicle (traffic)

V69.69 Unspecified occupant of heavy transport vehicle injured in collision with other motor vehicles in traffic accident

V69.8 Occupant (driver) (passenger) of heavy transport vehicle injured in other specified transport accidents

V69.81 Occupant (driver) (passenger) of heavy transport vehicle injured in transport accidents with military vehicle

⑦ V69.88 Occupant (driver) (passenger) of heavy transport vehicle injured in other specified transport accidents 🅟🅞🅐

🄖 V69.9 Occupant (driver) (passenger) of heavy transport vehicle injured in unspecified traffic accident 🅟🅞🅐

Accident NOS involving heavy transport vehicle

Bus occupant injured in transport accident (V70-V79)

INCLUDES   motorcoach

EXCLUDES1   minibus (V50-V59)

🄸 V70   Bus occupant injured in collision with pedestrian or animal

The appropriate 7th character is to be added to each code from category V70

    A = initial encounter
    D = subsequent encounter
    S = sequela

    EXCLUDES1   bus collision with animal-drawn vehicle or animal being ridden (V76.-)

⑦ V70.0   Driver of bus injured in collision with pedestrian or animal in nontraffic accident 🅟🅞🅐

⑦ V70.1   Passenger on bus injured in collision with pedestrian or animal in nontraffic accident 🅟🅞🅐

⑦ V70.2   Person on outside of bus injured in collision with pedestrian or animal in nontraffic accident 🅟🅞🅐

⑦ V70.3   Unspecified occupant of bus injured in collision with pedestrian or animal in nontraffic accident 🅟🅞🅐

⑦ V70.4   Person boarding or alighting from bus injured in collision with pedestrian or animal 🅟🅞🅐

⑦ V70.5   Driver of bus injured in collision with pedestrian or animal in traffic accident 🅟🅞🅐

⑦ V70.6   Passenger on bus injured in collision with pedestrian or animal in traffic accident 🅟🅞🅐

⑦ V70.7   Person on outside of bus injured in collision with pedestrian or animal in traffic accident 🅟🅞🅐

⑦ V70.9   Unspecified occupant of bus injured in collision with pedestrian or animal in traffic accident 🅟🅞🅐

🄸 V71   Bus occupant injured in collision with pedal cycle

The appropriate 7th character is to be added to each code from category V71

    A = initial encounter
    D = subsequent encounter
    S = sequela

⑦ V71.0   Driver of bus injured in collision with pedal cycle in nontraffic accident 🅟🅞🅐

⑦ V71.1   Passenger on bus injured in collision with pedal cycle in nontraffic accident 🅟🅞🅐

⑦ V71.2   Person on outside of bus injured in collision with pedal cycle in nontraffic accident 🅟🅞🅐

⑦ V71.3   Unspecified occupant of bus injured in collision with pedal cycle in nontraffic accident 🅟🅞🅐

⑦ V71.4   Person boarding or alighting from bus injured in collision with pedal cycle 🅟🅞🅐

⑦ V71.5   Driver of bus injured in collision with pedal cycle in traffic accident 🅟🅞🅐

⑦ V71.6   Passenger on bus injured in collision with pedal cycle in traffic accident 🅟🅞🅐

⑦ V71.7   Person on outside of bus injured in collision with pedal cycle in traffic accident 🅟🅞🅐

⑦ V71.9   Unspecified occupant of bus injured in collision with pedal cycle in traffic accident 🅟🅞🅐

🄸 V72   Bus occupant injured in collision with two- or three-wheeled motor vehicle

The appropriate 7th character is to be added to each code from category V72

    A = initial encounter
    D = subsequent encounter
    S = sequela

⑦ V72.0   Driver of bus injured in collision with two- or three-wheeled motor vehicle in nontraffic accident 🅟🅞🅐

⑦ V72.1   Passenger on bus injured in collision with two- or three-wheeled motor vehicle in nontraffic accident 🅟🅞🅐

⑦ V72.2   Person on outside of bus injured in collision with two- or three-wheeled motor vehicle in nontraffic accident 🅟🅞🅐

⑦ V72.3   Unspecified occupant of bus injured in collision with two- or three-wheeled motor vehicle in nontraffic accident 🅟🅞🅐

⑦ V72.4   Person boarding or alighting from bus injured in collision with two- or three-wheeled motor vehicle 🅟🅞🅐

⑦ V72.5   Driver of bus injured in collision with two- or three-wheeled motor vehicle in traffic accident 🅟🅞🅐

⑦ V72.6   Passenger on bus injured in collision with two- or three-wheeled motor vehicle in traffic accident 🅟🅞🅐

⑦ V72.7   Person on outside of bus injured in collision with two- or three-wheeled motor vehicle in traffic accident 🅟🅞🅐

⑦ V72.9   Unspecified occupant of bus injured in collision with two- or three-wheeled motor vehicle in traffic accident 🅟🅞🅐

🄸 V73   Bus occupant injured in collision with car, pick-up truck or van

The appropriate 7th character is to be added to each code from category V73

    A = initial encounter
    D = subsequent encounter
    S = sequela

⑦ V73.0   Driver of bus injured in collision with car, pick-up truck or van in nontraffic accident 🅟🅞🅐

⑦ V73.1   Passenger on bus injured in collision with car, pick-up truck or van in nontraffic accident 🅟🅞🅐

⑦ V73.2   Person on outside of bus injured in collision with car, pick-up truck or van in nontraffic accident 🅟🅞🅐

⑦ V73.3   Unspecified occupant of bus injured in collision with car, pick-up truck or van in nontraffic accident 🅟🅞🅐

⑦ V73.4   Person boarding or alighting from bus injured in collision with car, pick-up truck or van 🅟🅞🅐

⑦ V73.5   Driver of bus injured in collision with car, pick-up truck or van in traffic accident 🅟🅞🅐

⑦ V73.6   Passenger on bus injured in collision with car, pick-up truck or van in traffic accident 🅟🅞🅐

⑦ V73.7   Person on outside of bus injured in collision with car, pick-up truck or van in traffic accident 🅟🅞🅐

⑦ V73.9   Unspecified occupant of bus injured in collision with car, pick-up truck or van in traffic accident 🅟🅞🅐

🄸 V74   Bus occupant injured in collision with heavy transport vehicle or bus

    EXCLUDES1   bus occupant injured in collision with military vehicle (V79.81)

The appropriate 7th character is to be added to each code from category V74

    A = initial encounter
    D = subsequent encounter
    S = sequela

⑦ V74.0   Driver of bus injured in collision with heavy transport vehicle or bus in nontraffic accident 🅟🅞🅐

⑦ V74.1   Passenger on bus injured in collision with heavy transport vehicle or bus in nontraffic accident 🅟🅞🅐

⑦ V74.2   Person on outside of bus injured in collision with heavy transport vehicle or bus in nontraffic accident 🅟🅞🅐

⑦ V74.3   Unspecified occupant of bus injured in collision with heavy transport vehicle or bus in nontraffic accident 🅟🅞🅐

⑦ V74.4   Person boarding or alighting from bus injured in collision with heavy transport vehicle or bus 🅟🅞🅐

⑦ V74.5   Driver of bus injured in collision with heavy transport vehicle or bus in traffic accident 🅟🅞🅐

⑦ V74.6   Passenger on bus injured in collision with heavy transport vehicle or bus in traffic accident 🅟🅞🅐

⑦ V74.7   Person on outside of bus injured in collision with heavy transport vehicle or bus in traffic accident 🅟🅞🅐

⑦ V74.9   Unspecified occupant of bus injured in collision with heavy transport vehicle or bus in traffic accident 🅟🅞🅐

🅟🅞🅐 Unacceptable principal diagnosis symbol per Medicare code edits   🅟🅞🅐 Code exempt from diagnosis present on admission requirement
❓ Questionable admission   ℅ Complication or comorbidity   ℅℠℅ Major complication or comorbidity   ℅℠℅ CC/MCC exclusion
🄷🄲🄲 HCC diagnosis code   🅁🅇🄷🄲🄲 RxHCC diagnosis code   MACRA code   **DEFINITION** Describes condition/terminology
TIP Coding guidance   👁 Official Guideline Reference   🆉 Z code as first-listed diagnosis

4ᵗʰ V75 Bus occupant injured in collision with railway train or railway vehicle

The appropriate 7th character is to be added to each code from category V75

    A = initial encounter
    D = subsequent encounter
    S = sequela

7ᵗʰ V75.0 Driver of bus injured in collision with railway train or railway vehicle in nontraffic accident   POA

7ᵗʰ V75.1 Passenger on bus injured in collision with railway train or railway vehicle in nontraffic accident   POA

7ᵗʰ V75.2 Person on outside of bus injured in collision with railway train or railway vehicle in nontraffic accident   POA

7ᵗʰ V75.3 Unspecified occupant of bus injured in collision with railway train or railway vehicle in nontraffic accident   POA

7ᵗʰ V75.4 Person boarding or alighting from bus injured in collision with railway train or railway vehicle   POA

7ᵗʰ V75.5 Driver of bus injured in collision with railway train or railway vehicle in traffic accident   POA

7ᵗʰ V75.6 Passenger on bus injured in collision with railway train or railway vehicle in traffic accident   POA

7ᵗʰ V75.7 Person on outside of bus injured in collision with railway train or railway vehicle in traffic accident   POA

7ᵗʰ V75.9 Unspecified occupant of bus injured in collision with railway train or railway vehicle in traffic accident   POA

4ᵗʰ V76 Bus occupant injured in collision with other nonmotor vehicle

INCLUDES   collision with animal-drawn vehicle, animal being ridden, streetcar

The appropriate 7th character is to be added to each code from category V76

    A = initial encounter
    D = subsequent encounter
    S = sequela

7ᵗʰ V76.0 Driver of bus injured in collision with other nonmotor vehicle in nontraffic accident   POA

7ᵗʰ V76.1 Passenger on bus injured in collision with other nonmotor vehicle in nontraffic accident   POA

7ᵗʰ V76.2 Person on outside of bus injured in collision with other nonmotor vehicle in nontraffic accident   POA

7ᵗʰ V76.3 Unspecified occupant of bus injured in collision with other nonmotor vehicle in nontraffic accident   POA

7ᵗʰ V76.4 Person boarding or alighting from bus injured in collision with other nonmotor vehicle   POA

7ᵗʰ V76.5 Driver of bus injured in collision with other nonmotor vehicle in traffic accident   POA

7ᵗʰ V76.6 Passenger on bus injured in collision with other nonmotor vehicle in traffic accident   POA

7ᵗʰ V76.7 Person on outside of bus injured in collision with other nonmotor vehicle in traffic accident   POA

7ᵗʰ V76.9 Unspecified occupant of bus injured in collision with other nonmotor vehicle in traffic accident   POA

4ᵗʰ V77 Bus occupant injured in collision with fixed or stationary object

The appropriate 7th character is to be added to each code from category V77

    A = initial encounter
    D = subsequent encounter
    S = sequela

7ᵗʰ V77.0 Driver of bus injured in collision with fixed or stationary object in nontraffic accident   POA

7ᵗʰ V77.1 Passenger on bus injured in collision with fixed or stationary object in nontraffic accident   POA

7ᵗʰ V77.2 Person on outside of bus injured in collision with fixed or stationary object in nontraffic accident   POA

7ᵗʰ V77.3 Unspecified occupant of bus injured in collision with fixed or stationary object in nontraffic accident   POA

7ᵗʰ V77.4 Person boarding or alighting from bus injured in collision with fixed or stationary object   POA

7ᵗʰ V77.5 Driver of bus injured in collision with fixed or stationary object in traffic accident   POA

7ᵗʰ V77.6 Passenger on bus injured in collision with fixed or stationary object in traffic accident   POA

7ᵗʰ V77.7 Person on outside of bus injured in collision with fixed or stationary object in traffic accident   POA

7ᵗʰ V77.9 Unspecified occupant of bus injured in collision with fixed or stationary object in traffic accident   POA

4ᵗʰ V78 Bus occupant injured in noncollision transport accident

INCLUDES   overturning bus NOS
           overturning bus without collision

The appropriate 7th character is to be added to each code from category V78

    A = initial encounter
    D = subsequent encounter
    S = sequela

7ᵗʰ V78.0 Driver of bus injured in noncollision transport accident in nontraffic accident   POA

7ᵗʰ V78.1 Passenger on bus injured in noncollision transport accident in nontraffic accident   POA

7ᵗʰ V78.2 Person on outside of bus injured in noncollision transport accident in nontraffic accident   POA

7ᵗʰ V78.3 Unspecified occupant of bus injured in noncollision transport accident in nontraffic accident   POA

7ᵗʰ V78.4 Person boarding or alighting from bus injured in noncollision transport accident   POA

7ᵗʰ V78.5 Driver of bus injured in noncollision transport accident in traffic accident   POA

7ᵗʰ V78.6 Passenger on bus injured in noncollision transport accident in traffic accident   POA

7ᵗʰ V78.7 Person on outside of bus injured in noncollision transport accident in traffic accident   POA

7ᵗʰ V78.9 Unspecified occupant of bus injured in noncollision transport accident in traffic accident   POA

4ᵗʰ V79 Bus occupant injured in other and unspecified transport accidents

The appropriate 7th character is to be added to each code from category V79

    A = initial encounter
    D = subsequent encounter
    S = sequela

5ᵗʰ V79.0 Driver of bus injured in collision with other and unspecified motor vehicles in nontraffic accident

    7ᵗʰ V79.00 Driver of bus injured in collision with unspecified motor vehicles in nontraffic accident   POA

    7ᵗʰ V79.09 Driver of bus injured in collision with other motor vehicles in nontraffic accident   POA

5ᵗʰ V79.1 Passenger on bus injured in collision with other and unspecified motor vehicles in nontraffic accident

    7ᵗʰ V79.10 Passenger on bus injured in collision with unspecified motor vehicles in nontraffic accident   POA

    7ᵗʰ V79.19 Passenger on bus injured in collision with other motor vehicles in nontraffic accident   POA

5ᵗʰ V79.2 Unspecified bus occupant injured in collision with other and unspecified motor vehicles in nontraffic accident

    7ᵗʰ V79.20 Unspecified bus occupant injured in collision with unspecified motor vehicles in nontraffic accident   POA
         Bus collision NOS, nontraffic

    7ᵗʰ V79.29 Unspecified bus occupant injured in collision with other motor vehicles in nontraffic accident   POA

7ᵗʰ V79.3 Bus occupant (driver) (passenger) injured in unspecified nontraffic accident   POA
     Bus accident NOS, nontraffic
     Bus occupant injured in nontraffic accident NOS

5ᵗʰ V79.4 Driver of bus injured in collision with other and unspecified motor vehicles in traffic accident

    7ᵗʰ V79.40 Driver of bus injured in collision with unspecified motor vehicles in traffic accident   POA

    7ᵗʰ V79.49 Driver of bus injured in collision with other motor vehicles in traffic accident   POA

5ᵗʰ V79.5 Passenger on bus injured in collision with other and unspecified motor vehicles in traffic accident

    7ᵗʰ V79.50 Passenger on bus injured in collision with unspecified motor vehicles in traffic accident   POA

    7ᵗʰ V79.59 Passenger on bus injured in collision with other motor vehicles in traffic accident   POA

🔟 V79.6 Unspecified bus occupant injured in collision with other and unspecified motor vehicles in traffic accident

    7️⃣ V79.60 Unspecified bus occupant injured in collision with unspecified motor vehicles in traffic accident POA
       Bus collision NOS (traffic)

    7️⃣ V79.69 Unspecified bus occupant injured in collision with other motor vehicles in traffic accident POA

🔟 V79.8 Bus occupant (driver) (passenger) injured in other specified transport accidents

    7️⃣ V79.81 Bus occupant (driver) (passenger) injured in transport accidents with military vehicle

    7️⃣ V79.88 Bus occupant (driver) (passenger) injured in other specified transport accidents POA

7️⃣ V79.9 Bus occupant (driver) (passenger) injured in unspecified traffic accident POA
    Bus accident NOS

Other land transport accidents (V80-V89)

4️⃣ V80 Animal-rider or occupant of animal-drawn vehicle injured in transport accident

    The appropriate 7th character is to be added to each code from category V80
    A = initial encounter
    D = subsequent encounter
    S = sequela

🔟 V80.0 Animal-rider or occupant of animal drawn vehicle injured by fall from or being thrown from animal or animal-drawn vehicle in noncollision accident

    6️⃣ V80.01 Animal-rider injured by fall from or being thrown from animal in noncollision accident

       7️⃣ V80.010 Animal-rider injured by fall from or being thrown from horse in noncollision accident POA

       7️⃣ V80.018 Animal-rider injured by fall from or being thrown from other animal in noncollision accident POA

    7️⃣ V80.02 Occupant of animal-drawn vehicle injured by fall from or being thrown from animal-drawn vehicle in noncollision accident POA
       Overturning animal-drawn vehicle NOS
       Overturning animal-drawn vehicle without collision

🔟 V80.1 Animal-rider or occupant of animal-drawn vehicle injured in collision with pedestrian or animal
    EXCLUDES1 animal-rider or animal-drawn vehicle collision with animal-drawn vehicle or animal being ridden (V80.7)

    7️⃣ V80.11 Animal-rider injured in collision with pedestrian or animal POA

    7️⃣ V80.12 Occupant of animal-drawn vehicle injured in collision with pedestrian or animal POA

🔟 V80.2 Animal-rider or occupant of animal-drawn vehicle injured in collision with pedal cycle

    7️⃣ V80.21 Animal-rider injured in collision with pedal cycle POA

    7️⃣ V80.22 Occupant of animal-drawn vehicle injured in collision with pedal cycle POA

🔟 V80.3 Animal-rider or occupant of animal-drawn vehicle injured in collision with two- or three-wheeled motor vehicle

    7️⃣ V80.31 Animal-rider injured in collision with two- or three-wheeled motor vehicle POA

    7️⃣ V80.32 Occupant of animal-drawn vehicle injured in collision with two- or three-wheeled motor vehicle POA

🔟 V80.4 Animal-rider or occupant of animal-drawn vehicle injured in collision with car, pick-up truck, van, heavy transport vehicle or bus
    EXCLUDES1 animal-rider injured in collision with military vehicle (V80.910)
       occupant of animal-drawn vehicle injured in collision with military vehicle (V80.920)

    7️⃣ V80.41 Animal-rider injured in collision with car, pick-up truck, van, heavy transport vehicle or bus POA

    7️⃣ V80.42 Occupant of animal-drawn vehicle injured in collision with car, pick-up truck, van, heavy transport vehicle or bus POA

🔟 V80.5 Animal-rider or occupant of animal-drawn vehicle injured in collision with other specified motor vehicle

    7️⃣ V80.51 Animal-rider injured in collision with other specified motor vehicle POA

    7️⃣ V80.52 Occupant of animal-drawn vehicle injured in collision with other specified motor vehicle POA

🔟 V80.6 Animal-rider or occupant of animal-drawn vehicle injured in collision with railway train or railway vehicle

    7️⃣ V80.61 Animal-rider injured in collision with railway train or railway vehicle POA

    7️⃣ V80.62 Occupant of animal-drawn vehicle injured in collision with railway train or railway vehicle POA

🔟 V80.7 Animal-rider or occupant of animal-drawn vehicle injured in collision with other nonmotor vehicles

    6️⃣ V80.71 Animal-rider or occupant of animal-drawn vehicle injured in collision with animal being ridden

       7️⃣ V80.710 Animal-rider injured in collision with other animal being ridden POA

       7️⃣ V80.711 Occupant of animal-drawn vehicle injured in collision with animal being ridden POA

    6️⃣ V80.72 Animal-rider or occupant of animal-drawn vehicle injured in collision with other animal-drawn vehicle

       7️⃣ V80.720 Animal-rider injured in collision with animal-drawn vehicle POA

       7️⃣ V80.721 Occupant of animal-drawn vehicle injured in collision with other animal-drawn vehicle POA

    6️⃣ V80.73 Animal-rider or occupant of animal-drawn vehicle injured in collision with streetcar

       7️⃣ V80.730 Animal-rider injured in collision with streetcar POA

       7️⃣ V80.731 Occupant of animal-drawn vehicle injured in collision with streetcar POA

    6️⃣ V80.79 Animal-rider or occupant of animal-drawn vehicle injured in collision with other nonmotor vehicles

       7️⃣ V80.790 Animal-rider injured in collision with other nonmotor vehicles POA

       7️⃣ V80.791 Occupant of animal-drawn vehicle injured in collision with other nonmotor vehicles POA

🔟 V80.8 Animal-rider or occupant of animal-drawn vehicle injured in collision with fixed or stationary object

    7️⃣ V80.81 Animal-rider injured in collision with fixed or stationary object POA

    7️⃣ V80.82 Occupant of animal-drawn vehicle injured in collision with fixed or stationary object POA

🔟 V80.9 Animal-rider or occupant of animal-drawn vehicle injured in other and unspecified transport accidents

    6️⃣ V80.91 Animal-rider injured in other and unspecified transport accidents

       7️⃣ V80.910 Animal-rider injured in transport accident with military vehicle POA

       7️⃣ V80.918 Animal-rider injured in other transport accident POA

       7️⃣ V80.919 Animal-rider injured in unspecified transport accident POA
       Animal rider accident NOS

    6️⃣ V80.92 Occupant of animal-drawn vehicle injured in other and unspecified transport accidents

       7️⃣ V80.920 Occupant of animal-drawn vehicle injured in transport accident with military vehicle POA

       7️⃣ V80.928 Occupant of animal-drawn vehicle injured in other transport accident POA

       7️⃣ V80.929 Occupant of animal-drawn vehicle injured in unspecified transport accident POA
       Animal-drawn vehicle accident NOS

POA̶ Unacceptable principal diagnosis symbol per Medicare code edits   POA Code exempt from diagnosis present on admission requirement
❓ Questionable admission   cc Complication or comorbidity   MCC Major complication or comorbidity   cc/mcc exc CC/MCC exclusion
HCC HCC diagnosis code   RxHCC RxHCC diagnosis code   MACRA code   **DEFINITION** Describes condition/terminology
TIP Coding guidance   🔁 Official Guideline Reference   Z1 Z code as first-listed diagnosis

V81 **Occupant of railway train or railway vehicle injured in transport accident**

INCLUDES   derailment of railway train or railway vehicle
person on outside of train

EXCLUDES1 streetcar (V82.-)

The appropriate 7th character is to be added to each code from category V81

A = initial encounter
D = subsequent encounter
S = sequela

V81.0 **Occupant of railway train or railway vehicle injured in collision with motor vehicle** in nontraffic accident

EXCLUDES1 Occupant of railway train or railway vehicle injured due to collision with military vehicle (V81.83)

V81.1 **Occupant of railway train or railway vehicle injured in collision with motor vehicle** in traffic accident

EXCLUDES1 Occupant of railway train or railway vehicle injured due to collision with military vehicle (V81.83)

V81.2 **Occupant of railway train or railway vehicle injured in collision with or** hit by rolling stock

V81.3 **Occupant of railway train or railway vehicle injured in collision with other object**

Railway collision NOS

V81.4 **Person injured** while boarding or alighting **from railway train or railway vehicle**

V81.5 **Occupant of railway train or railway vehicle injured** by fall in railway train or railway vehicle

V81.6 **Occupant of railway train or railway vehicle injured** by fall from railway train or railway vehicle

V81.7 **Occupant of railway train or railway vehicle injured in derailment without antecedent collision**

V81.8 **Occupant of railway train or railway vehicle injured in** other specified **railway accidents**

V81.81 **Occupant of railway train or railway vehicle injured due to** explosion or fire **on train**

V81.82 **Occupant of railway train or railway vehicle injured due to** object falling **onto train**

Occupant of railway train or railway vehicle injured due to falling earth onto train
Occupant of railway train or railway vehicle injured due to falling rocks onto train
Occupant of railway train or railway vehicle injured due to falling snow onto train
Occupant of railway train or railway vehicle injured due to falling trees onto train

V81.83 **Occupant of railway train or railway vehicle injured due to** collision with military vehicle

V81.89 **Occupant of railway train or railway vehicle injured due to other specified railway accident**

V81.9 **Occupant of railway train or railway vehicle injured in unspecified railway accident**

Railway accident NOS

V82 **Occupant of powered streetcar injured in transport accident**

INCLUDES   interurban electric car
person on outside of streetcar
tram (car)
trolley (car)

EXCLUDES1 bus (V70-V79)
motorcoach (V70-V79)
nonpowered streetcar (V76.-)
train (V81.-)

The appropriate 7th character is to be added to each code from category V82

A = initial encounter
D = subsequent encounter
S = sequela

V82.0 **Occupant of streetcar injured in collision with motor vehicle in** nontraffic accident

V82.1 **Occupant of streetcar injured in collision with motor vehicle in** traffic accident

V82.2 **Occupant of streetcar injured in collision with or** hit by rolling stock

V82.3 **Occupant of streetcar injured in collision with other object**

EXCLUDES1 collision with animal-drawn vehicle or animal being ridden (V82.8)

V82.4 **Person injured** while boarding or alighting **from streetcar**

V82.5 **Occupant of streetcar injured by** fall in streetcar

EXCLUDES1 fall in streetcar:
while boarding or alighting (V82.4)
with antecedent collision (V82.0-V82.3)

V82.6 **Occupant of streetcar injured by** fall from streetcar

EXCLUDES1 fall from streetcar:
while boarding or alighting (V82.4)
with antecedent collision (V82.0-V82.3)

V82.7 **Occupant of streetcar injured in** derailment without antecedent collision

EXCLUDES1 occupant of streetcar injured in derailment with antecedent collision (V82.0-V82.3)

V82.8 **Occupant of streetcar injured in other specified transport accidents**

Streetcar collision with military vehicle
Streetcar collision with train or nonmotor vehicles

V82.9 **Occupant of streetcar injured in unspecified traffic accident**

Streetcar accident NOS

V83 **Occupant of special vehicle mainly used on industrial premises injured in transport accident**

INCLUDES   battery-powered airport passenger vehicle
battery-powered truck (baggage) (mail)
coal-car in mine
forklift (truck)
logging car
self-propelled industrial truck
station baggage truck (powered)
tram, truck, or tub (powered) in mine or quarry

EXCLUDES1 special construction vehicles (V85.-)
special industrial vehicle in stationary use or maintenance (W31.-)

The appropriate 7th character is to be added to each code from category V83

A = initial encounter
D = subsequent encounter
S = sequela

V83.0 Driver **of special industrial vehicle injured in** traffic accident

V83.1 Passenger **of special industrial vehicle injured in** traffic accident

V83.2 Person on outside **of special industrial vehicle injured in** traffic accident

V83.3 **Unspecified occupant of special industrial vehicle injured in traffic accident**

V83.4 **Person injured** while boarding or alighting **from special industrial vehicle**

V83.5 Driver **of special industrial vehicle injured in** nontraffic accident

V83.6 Passenger **of special industrial vehicle injured in** nontraffic accident

V83.7 Person on outside **of special industrial vehicle injured in** nontraffic accident

V83.9 **Unspecified occupant of special industrial vehicle injured in** nontraffic accident

Special-industrial-vehicle accident NOS

V84 **Occupant of special vehicle mainly used in agriculture injured in transport accident**

INCLUDES   self-propelled farm machinery
tractor (and trailer)

EXCLUDES1 animal-powered farm machinery accident (W30.8-)
contact with combine harvester (W30.0)
special agricultural vehicle in stationary use or maintenance (W30.-)

The appropriate 7th character is to be added to each code from category V84
- A = initial encounter
- D = subsequent encounter
- S = sequela

[7th] **V84.0** Driver **of special agricultural vehicle injured in** traffic accident [POA]

[7th] **V84.1** Passenger **of special agricultural vehicle injured in** traffic accident [POA]

[7th] **V84.2** Person on outside **of special agricultural vehicle injured in** traffic accident [POA]

[7th] **V84.3** **Unspecified occupant of special agricultural vehicle injured in traffic accident** [POA]

[7th] **V84.4** **Person injured** while boarding or alighting **from special agricultural vehicle** [POA]

[7th] **V84.5** Driver **of special agricultural vehicle injured in** nontraffic accident [POA]

[7th] **V84.6** Passenger **of special agricultural vehicle injured in** nontraffic accident [POA]

[7th] **V84.7** Person on outside **of special agricultural vehicle injured in** nontraffic accident [POA]

[7th] **V84.9** **Unspecified occupant of special agricultural vehicle injured in nontraffic accident** [POA]
Special-agricultural vehicle accident NOS

[4th] **V85 Occupant of special construction vehicle injured in transport accident**

INCLUDES *bulldozer*
digger
dump truck
earth-leveller
mechanical shovel
road-roller

EXCLUDES1 *special industrial vehicle (V83.-)*
special construction vehicle in stationary use or maintenance (W31.-)

The appropriate 7th character is to be added to each code from category V85
- A = initial encounter
- D = subsequent encounter
- S = sequela

[7th] **V85.0** Driver **of special construction vehicle injured in** traffic accident [POA]

[7th] **V85.1** Passenger **of special construction vehicle injured in** traffic accident [POA]

[7th] **V85.2** Person on outside **of special construction vehicle injured in** traffic accident [POA]

[7th] **V85.3** **Unspecified occupant of special construction vehicle injured in traffic accident** [POA]

[7th] **V85.4** **Person injured** while boarding or alighting **from special construction vehicle** [POA]

[7th] **V85.5** Driver **of special construction vehicle injured in** nontraffic accident [POA]

[7th] **V85.6** Passenger **of special construction vehicle injured in** nontraffic accident [POA]

[7th] **V85.7** Person on outside **of special construction vehicle injured in** nontraffic accident [POA]

[7th] **V85.9** **Unspecified occupant of special construction vehicle injured in nontraffic accident** [POA]
Special-construction-vehicle accident NOS

[4th] **V86 Occupant of special all-terrain or other off-road motor vehicle, injured in transport accident**

EXCLUDES1 *special all-terrain vehicle in stationary use or maintenance (W31.-)*
sport-utility vehicle (V50-V59)
three-wheeled motor vehicle designed for on-road use (V30-V39)

The appropriate 7th character is to be added to each code from category V86
- A = initial encounter
- D = subsequent encounter
- S = sequela

[5th] **V86.0** Driver **of special all-terrain or other off-road motor vehicle injured in** traffic accident

[7th] **V86.01** **Driver of** ambulance or fire engine **injured in traffic accident** [POA]

[7th] **V86.02** **Driver of** snowmobile **injured in traffic accident** [POA]

[7th] **V86.03** **Driver of** dune buggy **injured in traffic accident** [POA]

[7th] **V86.04** **Driver of** military vehicle **injured in traffic accident** [POA]

[7th] **V86.05** **Driver of** 3- or 4- wheeled all-terrain vehicle (ATV) **injured in traffic accident** [POA]

[7th] **V86.06** **Driver of** dirt bike or motor/cross bike **injured in traffic accident** [POA]

[7th] **V86.09** **Driver of other special all-terrain or other off-road motor vehicle injured in traffic accident** [POA]
Driver of go cart injured in traffic accident
Driver of golf cart injured in traffic accident

[5th] **V86.1** Passenger **of special all-terrain or other off-road motor vehicle injured in** traffic accident

[7th] **V86.11** **Passenger of** ambulance or fire engine **injured in traffic accident** [POA]

[7th] **V86.12** **Passenger of** snowmobile **injured in traffic accident** [POA]

[7th] **V86.13** **Passenger of** dune buggy **injured in traffic accident** [POA]

[7th] **V86.14** **Passenger of** military vehicle **injured in traffic accident** [POA]

[7th] **V86.15** **Passenger of** 3- or 4- wheeled all-terrain vehicle (ATV) **injured in traffic accident** [POA]

[7th] **V86.16** **Passenger of** dirt bike or motor/cross bike **injured in traffic accident** [POA]

[7th] **V86.19** **Passenger of other special all-terrain or other off-road motor vehicle injured in traffic accident** [POA]
Passenger of go cart injured in traffic accident
Passenger of golf cart injured in traffic accident

[5th] **V86.2** Person on outside **of special all-terrain or other off-road motor vehicle injured in** traffic accident

[7th] **V86.21** **Person on outside of** ambulance or fire engine **injured in traffic accident** [POA]

[7th] **V86.22** **Person on outside of** snowmobile **injured in traffic accident** [POA]

[7th] **V86.23** **Person on outside of** dune buggy **injured in traffic accident** [POA]

[7th] **V86.24** **Person on outside of** military vehicle **injured in traffic accident** [POA]

[7th] **V86.25** **Person on outside of** 3- or 4- wheeled all-terrain vehicle (ATV) **injured in traffic accident** [POA]

[7th] **V86.26** **Person on outside of** dirt bike or motor/cross bike **injured in traffic accident** [POA]

[7th] **V86.29** **Person on outside of other special all-terrain or other off-road motor vehicle injured in traffic accident** [POA]
Person on outside of go cart in traffic accident
Person on outside of golf cart injured in traffic accident

[5th] **V86.3** Unspecified **occupant of special all-terrain or other off-road motor vehicle injured in** traffic accident

[7th] **V86.31** **Unspecified occupant of ambulance or fire engine injured in traffic accident** [POA]

[7th] **V86.32** **Unspecified occupant of snowmobile injured in traffic accident** [POA]

[7th] **V86.33** **Unspecified occupant of dune buggy injured in traffic accident** [POA]

[7th] **V86.34** **Unspecified occupant of military vehicle injured in traffic accident** [POA]

[7th] **V86.35** **Unspecified occupant of 3- or 4- wheeled** all-terrain vehicle **(ATV) injured in traffic accident** [POA]

[7th] **V86.36** **Unspecified occupant of dirt** bike or motor/cross **bike injured in traffic accident** [POA]

[7th] **V86.39** **Unspecified occupant of other special all-terrain or other off-road motor vehicle injured in traffic accident** [POA]
Unspecified occupant of go cart injured in traffic accident
Unspecified occupant of golf cart injured in traffic accident

[PDx] Unacceptable principal diagnosis symbol per Medicare code edits [POA] Code exempt from diagnosis present on admission requirement
[?] Questionable admission [CC] Complication or comorbidity [MCC] Major complication or comorbidity [CC/MCC Exc] CC/MCC exclusion
[HCC] HCC diagnosis code [RxHCC] RxHCC diagnosis code MACRA code **DEFINITION** Describes condition/terminology
TIP Coding guidance 👁 Official Guideline Reference [Z] Z code as first-listed diagnosis

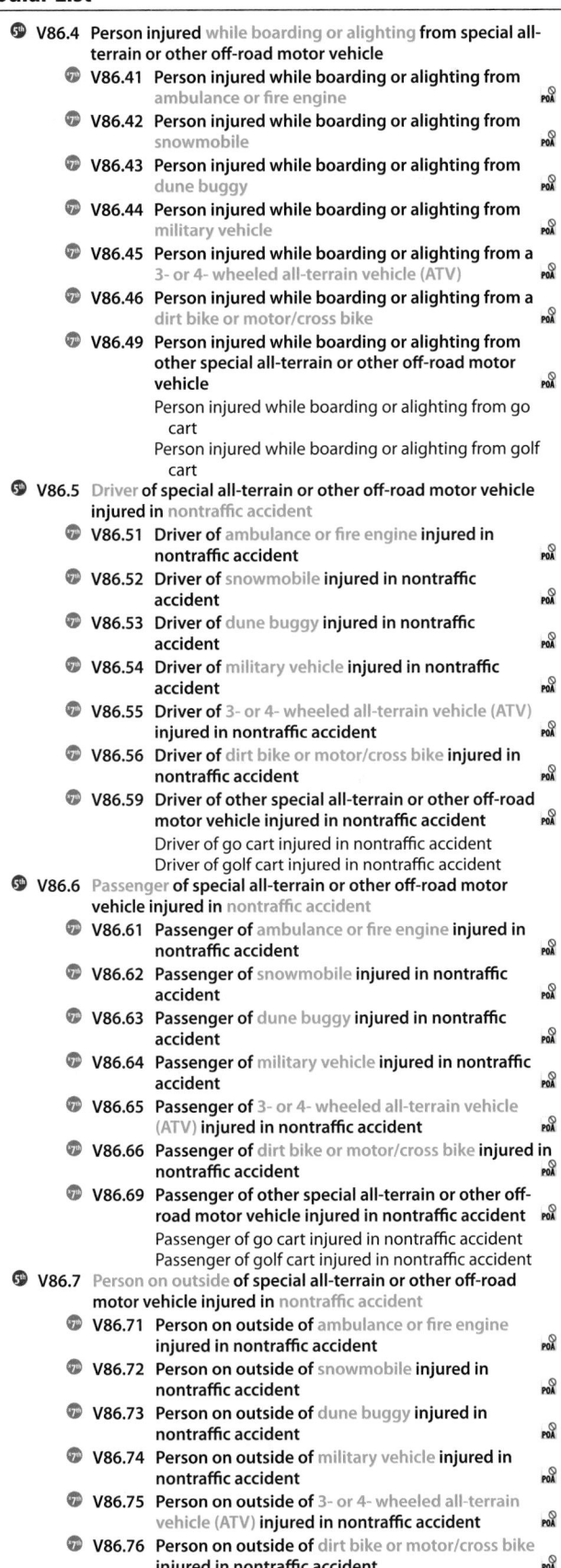

🔶 **V86.4** Person injured while boarding or alighting from special all-terrain or other off-road motor vehicle

🔹 **V86.41** Person injured while boarding or alighting from ambulance or fire engine POA

🔹 **V86.42** Person injured while boarding or alighting from snowmobile POA

🔹 **V86.43** Person injured while boarding or alighting from dune buggy POA

🔹 **V86.44** Person injured while boarding or alighting from military vehicle POA

🔹 **V86.45** Person injured while boarding or alighting from a 3- or 4- wheeled all-terrain vehicle (ATV) POA

🔹 **V86.46** Person injured while boarding or alighting from a dirt bike or motor/cross bike POA

🔹 **V86.49** Person injured while boarding or alighting from other special all-terrain or other off-road motor vehicle POA

Person injured while boarding or alighting from go cart

Person injured while boarding or alighting from golf cart

🔶 **V86.5** Driver of special all-terrain or other off-road motor vehicle injured in nontraffic accident

🔹 **V86.51** Driver of ambulance or fire engine injured in nontraffic accident POA

🔹 **V86.52** Driver of snowmobile injured in nontraffic accident POA

🔹 **V86.53** Driver of dune buggy injured in nontraffic accident POA

🔹 **V86.54** Driver of military vehicle injured in nontraffic accident POA

🔹 **V86.55** Driver of 3- or 4- wheeled all-terrain vehicle (ATV) injured in nontraffic accident POA

🔹 **V86.56** Driver of dirt bike or motor/cross bike injured in nontraffic accident POA

🔹 **V86.59** Driver of other special all-terrain or other off-road motor vehicle injured in nontraffic accident POA

Driver of go cart injured in nontraffic accident

Driver of golf cart injured in nontraffic accident

🔶 **V86.6** Passenger of special all-terrain or other off-road motor vehicle injured in nontraffic accident

🔹 **V86.61** Passenger of ambulance or fire engine injured in nontraffic accident POA

🔹 **V86.62** Passenger of snowmobile injured in nontraffic accident POA

🔹 **V86.63** Passenger of dune buggy injured in nontraffic accident POA

🔹 **V86.64** Passenger of military vehicle injured in nontraffic accident POA

🔹 **V86.65** Passenger of 3- or 4- wheeled all-terrain vehicle (ATV) injured in nontraffic accident POA

🔹 **V86.66** Passenger of dirt bike or motor/cross bike injured in nontraffic accident POA

🔹 **V86.69** Passenger of other special all-terrain or other off-road motor vehicle injured in nontraffic accident POA

Passenger of go cart injured in nontraffic accident

Passenger of golf cart injured in nontraffic accident

🔶 **V86.7** Person on outside of special all-terrain or other off-road motor vehicle injured in nontraffic accident

🔹 **V86.71** Person on outside of ambulance or fire engine injured in nontraffic accident POA

🔹 **V86.72** Person on outside of snowmobile injured in nontraffic accident POA

🔹 **V86.73** Person on outside of dune buggy injured in nontraffic accident POA

🔹 **V86.74** Person on outside of military vehicle injured in nontraffic accident POA

🔹 **V86.75** Person on outside of 3- or 4- wheeled all-terrain vehicle (ATV) injured in nontraffic accident POA

🔹 **V86.76** Person on outside of dirt bike or motor/cross bike injured in nontraffic accident POA

🔹 **V86.79** Person on outside of other special all-terrain or other off-road motor vehicles injured in nontraffic accident POA

Person on outside of go cart injured in nontraffic accident

Person on outside of golf cart injured in nontraffic accident

🔶 **V86.9** Unspecified occupant of special all-terrain or other off-road motor vehicle injured in nontraffic accident

🔹 **V86.91** Unspecified occupant of ambulance or fire engine injured in nontraffic accident POA

🔹 **V86.92** Unspecified occupant of snowmobile injured in nontraffic accident POA

🔹 **V86.93** Unspecified occupant of dune buggy injured in nontraffic accident POA

🔹 **V86.94** Unspecified occupant of military vehicle injured in nontraffic accident POA

🔹 **V86.95** Unspecified occupant of 3- or 4- wheeled all-terrain vehicle (ATV) injured in nontraffic accident POA

🔹 **V86.96** Unspecified occupant of dirt bike or motor/cross bike injured in nontraffic accident POA

🔹 **V86.99** Unspecified occupant of other special all-terrain or other off-road motor vehicle injured in nontraffic accident POA

Off-road motor-vehicle accident NOS

Other motor-vehicle accident NOS

Unspecified occupant of go cart injured in nontraffic accident

Unspecified occupant of golf cart injured in nontraffic accident

🔷 **V87** Traffic accident of specified type but victim's mode of transport unknown

EXCLUDES1 collision involving:

pedal cycle (V10-V19)

pedestrian (V01-V09)

The appropriate 7th character is to be added to each code from category V87

A = initial encounter

D = subsequent encounter

S = sequela

🔹 **V87.0** Person injured in collision between car and two- or three-wheeled powered vehicle (traffic) POA

🔹 **V87.1** Person injured in collision between other motor vehicle and two- or three-wheeled motor vehicle (traffic) POA

🔹 **V87.2** Person injured in collision between car and pick-up truck or van (traffic) POA

🔹 **V87.3** Person injured in collision between car and bus (traffic) POA

🔹 **V87.4** Person injured in collision between car and heavy transport vehicle (traffic) POA

🔹 **V87.5** Person injured in collision between heavy transport vehicle and bus (traffic) POA

🔹 **V87.6** Person injured in collision between railway train or railway vehicle and car (traffic) POA

🔹 **V87.7** Person injured in collision between other specified motor vehicles (traffic) POA

🔹 **V87.8** Person injured in other specified noncollision transport accidents involving motor vehicle (traffic) POA

🔹 **V87.9** Person injured in other specified (collision)(noncollision) transport accidents involving nonmotor vehicle (traffic) POA

🔷 **V88** Nontraffic accident of specified type but victim's mode of transport unknown

EXCLUDES1 collision involving:

pedal cycle (V10-V19)

pedestrian (V01-V09)

The appropriate 7th character is to be added to each code from category V88

A = initial encounter

D = subsequent encounter

S = sequela

🔹 **V88.0** Person injured in collision between car and two- or three-wheeled motor vehicle, nontraffic POA

🔟 **V88.1** **Person injured in collision between other motor vehicle and two- or three-wheeled motor vehicle, nontraffic** 🅿🅾🅰

🔟 **V88.2** **Person injured in collision between** car and pick-up truck or van, **nontraffic** 🅿🅾🅰

🔟 **V88.3** **Person injured in collision between** car and bus, **nontraffic** 🅿🅾🅰

🔟 **V88.4** **Person injured in collision between** car and heavy transport vehicle, **nontraffic** 🅿🅾🅰

🔟 **V88.5** **Person injured in collision between** heavy transport vehicle and bus, **nontraffic** 🅿🅾🅰

🔟 **V88.6** **Person injured in collision between** railway train or railway vehicle and car, **nontraffic** 🅿🅾🅰

🔟 **V88.7** **Person injured in collision between other specified motor vehicle, nontraffic** 🅾

🔟 **V88.8** **Person injured in other specified noncollision transport accidents involving motor vehicle, nontraffic** 🅾

🔟 **V88.9** **Person injured in other specified (collision)(noncollision) transport accidents involving nonmotor vehicle, nontraffic** 🅾

4️⃣ **V89** **Motor- or nonmotor-vehicle accident, type of vehicle unspecified**

The appropriate 7th character is to be added to each code from category V89

    A = initial encounter
    D = subsequent encounter
    S = sequela

🔟 **V89.0** **Person injured in unspecified motor-vehicle accident, nontraffic** 🅿🅾🅰

    Motor-vehicle accident NOS, nontraffic

🔟 **V89.1** **Person injured in unspecified nonmotor-vehicle accident, nontraffic** 🅾

    Nonmotor-vehicle accident NOS (nontraffic)

🔟 **V89.2** **Person injured in unspecified motor-vehicle accident, traffic** 🅿🅾🅰

    Motor-vehicle accident [MVA] NOS
    Road (traffic) accident [RTA] NOS

🔟 **V89.3** **Person injured in unspecified nonmotor-vehicle accident, traffic** 🅾

    Nonmotor-vehicle traffic accident NOS

🔟 **V89.9** **Person injured in unspecified vehicle accident** 🅿🅾🅰

    Collision NOS

Water transport accidents (V90-V94)

4️⃣ **V90** **Drowning and submersion due to accident to watercraft**

    EXCLUDES1 *civilian water transport accident involving military watercraft (V94.81-)*

        fall into water not from watercraft (W16.-)

        military watercraft accident in military or war operations (Y36.0-, Y37.0-)

        water-transport-related drowning or submersion without accident to watercraft (V92.-)

The appropriate 7th character is to be added to each code from category V90

    A = initial encounter
    D = subsequent encounter
    S = sequela

5️⃣ **V90.0** **Drowning and submersion due to** watercraft overturning

🔟 **V90.00** **Drowning and submersion due to** merchant ship **overturning** 🅿🅾🅰

🔟 **V90.01** **Drowning and submersion due to** passenger ship **overturning** 🅿🅾🅰

    Drowning and submersion due to Ferry-boat overturning
    Drowning and submersion due to Liner overturning

🔟 **V90.02** **Drowning and submersion due to** fishing boat **overturning** 🅾

🔟 **V90.03** **Drowning and submersion due to** other powered watercraft **overturning** 🅾

    Drowning and submersion due to Hovercraft (on open water) overturning
    Drowning and submersion due to Jet ski overturning

🔟 **V90.04** **Drowning and submersion due to** sailboat **overturning** 🅾

🔟 **V90.05** **Drowning and submersion due to** canoe or kayak **overturning** 🅾

🔟 **V90.06** **Drowning and submersion due to** (nonpowered) inflatable craft **overturning** 🅾

🔟 **V90.08** **Drowning and submersion due to other unpowered watercraft overturning** 🅾

    Drowning and submersion due to windsurfer overturning

🔟 **V90.09** **Drowning and submersion due to unspecified watercraft overturning** 🅾

    Drowning and submersion due to boat NOS overturning
    Drowning and submersion due to ship NOS overturning
    Drowning and submersion due to watercraft NOS overturning

5️⃣ **V90.1** **Drowning and submersion due to** watercraft sinking

🔟 **V90.10** **Drowning and submersion due to** merchant ship **sinking** 🅿🅾🅰

🔟 **V90.11** **Drowning and submersion due to** passenger ship **sinking** 🅿🅾🅰

    Drowning and submersion due to Ferry-boat sinking
    Drowning and submersion due to Liner sinking

🔟 **V90.12** **Drowning and submersion due to** fishing boat **sinking** 🅿🅾🅰

🔟 **V90.13** **Drowning and submersion due to other powered watercraft sinking** 🅿🅾🅰

    Drowning and submersion due to Hovercraft (on open water) sinking
    Drowning and submersion due to Jet ski sinking

🔟 **V90.14** **Drowning and submersion due to** sailboat **sinking** 🅾

🔟 **V90.15** **Drowning and submersion due to** canoe or kayak **sinking** 🅾

🔟 **V90.16** **Drowning and submersion due to** (nonpowered) inflatable craft **sinking** 🅾

🔟 **V90.18** **Drowning and submersion due to other unpowered watercraft sinking** 🅾

🔟 **V90.19** **Drowning and submersion due to unspecified watercraft sinking** 🅾

    Drowning and submersion due to boat NOS sinking
    Drowning and submersion due to ship NOS sinking
    Drowning and submersion due to watercraft NOS sinking

5️⃣ **V90.2** **Drowning and submersion due to** falling or jumping from burning watercraft

🔟 **V90.20** **Drowning and submersion due to falling or jumping from burning** merchant ship 🅿🅾🅰

🔟 **V90.21** **Drowning and submersion due to falling or jumping from burning** passenger ship 🅿🅾🅰

    Drowning and submersion due to falling or jumping from burning Ferry-boat
    Drowning and submersion due to falling or jumping from burning Liner

🔟 **V90.22** **Drowning and submersion due to falling or jumping from burning** fishing boat 🅾

🔟 **V90.23** **Drowning and submersion due to falling or jumping from** other burning powered watercraft 🅾

    Drowning and submersion due to falling and jumping from burning Hovercraft (on open water)
    Drowning and submersion due to falling and jumping from burning Jet ski

🔟 **V90.24** **Drowning and submersion due to falling or jumping from burning** sailboat 🅾

🔟 **V90.25** **Drowning and submersion due to falling or jumping from burning** canoe or kayak 🅾

🔟 **V90.26** **Drowning and submersion due to falling or jumping from burning** (nonpowered) inflatable craft 🅾

🔟 **V90.27** **Drowning and submersion due to falling or jumping from burning** water-skis 🅾

[7th] **V90.28 Drowning and submersion due to falling or jumping from other burning unpowered watercraft** [POA]
Drowning and submersion due to falling and jumping from burning surf-board
Drowning and submersion due to falling and jumping from burning windsurfer

[7th] **V90.29 Drowning and submersion due to falling or jumping from unspecified burning watercraft** [POA]
Drowning and submersion due to falling or jumping from burning boat NOS
Drowning and submersion due to falling or jumping from burning ship NOS
Drowning and submersion due to falling or jumping from burning watercraft NOS

[5th] **V90.3 Drowning and submersion due to falling or jumping from crushed watercraft**

[7th] **V90.30 Drowning and submersion due to falling or jumping from crushed merchant ship** [POA]

[7th] **V90.31 Drowning and submersion due to falling or jumping from crushed passenger ship** [POA]
Drowning and submersion due to falling and jumping from crushed Ferry boat
Drowning and submersion due to falling and jumping from crushed Liner

[7th] **V90.32 Drowning and submersion due to falling or jumping from crushed fishing boat** [POA]

[7th] **V90.33 Drowning and submersion due to falling or jumping from other crushed powered watercraft** [POA]
Drowning and submersion due to falling and jumping from crushed Hovercraft
Drowning and submersion due to falling and jumping from crushed Jet ski

[7th] **V90.34 Drowning and submersion due to falling or jumping from crushed sailboat** [POA]

[7th] **V90.35 Drowning and submersion due to falling or jumping from crushed canoe or kayak** [POA]

[7th] **V90.36 Drowning and submersion due to falling or jumping from crushed (nonpowered) inflatable craft** [POA]

[7th] **V90.37 Drowning and submersion due to falling or jumping from crushed water-skis** [POA]

[7th] **V90.38 Drowning and submersion due to falling or jumping from other crushed unpowered watercraft** [POA]
Drowning and submersion due to falling and jumping from crushed surf-board
Drowning and submersion due to falling and jumping from crushed windsurfer

[7th] **V90.39 Drowning and submersion due to falling or jumping from crushed unspecified watercraft** [POA]
Drowning and submersion due to falling and jumping from crushed boat NOS
Drowning and submersion due to falling and jumping from crushed ship NOS
Drowning and submersion due to falling and jumping from crushed watercraft NOS

[5th] **V90.8 Drowning and submersion due to other accident to watercraft**

[7th] **V90.80 Drowning and submersion due to other accident to merchant ship** [POA]

[7th] **V90.81 Drowning and submersion due to other accident to passenger ship** [POA]
Drowning and submersion due to other accident to Ferry-boat
Drowning and submersion due to other accident to Liner

[7th] **V90.82 Drowning and submersion due to other accident to fishing boat** [POA]

[7th] **V90.83 Drowning and submersion due to other accident to other powered watercraft** [POA]
Drowning and submersion due to other accident to Hovercraft (on open water)
Drowning and submersion due to other accident to Jet ski

[7th] **V90.84 Drowning and submersion due to other accident to sailboat** [POA]

[7th] **V90.85 Drowning and submersion due to other accident to canoe or kayak** [POA]

[7th] **V90.86 Drowning and submersion due to other accident to (nonpowered) inflatable craft** [POA]

[7th] **V90.87 Drowning and submersion due to other accident to water-skis** [POA]

[7th] **V90.88 Drowning and submersion due to other accident to other unpowered watercraft** [POA]
Drowning and submersion due to other accident to surf-board
Drowning and submersion due to other accident to windsurfer

[7th] **V90.89 Drowning and submersion due to other accident to unspecified watercraft** [POA]
Drowning and submersion due to other accident to boat NOS
Drowning and submersion due to other accident to ship NOS
Drowning and submersion due to other accident to watercraft NOS

[4th] **V91 Other injury due to accident to watercraft**

INCLUDES *any injury except drowning and submersion as a result of an accident to watercraft*

EXCLUDES1 *civilian water transport accident involving military watercraft (V94.81-)*
military watercraft accident in military or war operations (Y36, Y37.-)

EXCLUDES2 *drowning and submersion due to accident to watercraft (V90.-)*

The appropriate 7th character is to be added to each code from category V91
A = initial encounter
D = subsequent encounter
S = sequela

[5th] **V91.0 Burn due to watercraft on fire**

EXCLUDES1 *burn from localized fire or explosion on board ship without accident to watercraft (V93.-)*

[7th] **V91.00 Burn due to merchant ship on fire** [POA]

[7th] **V91.01 Burn due to passenger ship on fire** [POA]
Burn due to Ferry-boat on fire
Burn due to Liner on fire

[7th] **V91.02 Burn due to fishing boat on fire** [POA]

[7th] **V91.03 Burn due to other powered watercraft on fire** [POA]
Burn due to Hovercraft (on open water) on fire
Burn due to Jet ski on fire

[7th] **V91.04 Burn due to sailboat on fire** [POA]

[7th] **V91.05 Burn due to canoe or kayak on fire** [POA]

[7th] **V91.06 Burn due to (nonpowered) inflatable craft on fire** [POA]

[7th] **V91.07 Burn due to water-skis on fire** [POA]

[7th] **V91.08 Burn due to other unpowered watercraft on fire** [POA]

[7th] **V91.09 Burn due to unspecified watercraft on fire** [POA]
Burn due to boat NOS on fire
Burn due to ship NOS on fire
Burn due to watercraft NOS on fire

[5th] **V91.1 Crushed between watercraft and other watercraft or other object due to collision**
Crushed by lifeboat after abandoning ship in a collision

NOTES Select the specified type of watercraft that the victim was on at the time of the collision.

[7th] **V91.10 Crushed between merchant ship and other watercraft or other object due to collision** [POA]

[7th] **V91.11 Crushed between passenger ship and other watercraft or other object due to collision** [POA]
Crushed between Ferry-boat and other watercraft or other object due to collision
Crushed between Liner and other watercraft or other object due to collision

Unspecified Code Other Specified Code Manifestation Code [N] Newborn [P] Pediatric [M] Maternity [A] Adult ♂ Male ♀ Female
● New Code ▲ Revised Code Title ►◄ Revised Text NOTES *INCLUDES* *EXCLUDES1* Not coded here *EXCLUDES2* Not included here
[4th] 4th character required [5th] 5th character required [6th] 6th character required [7th] 7th character required [X] Extension 'X' Alert
[HAC] Hospital-acquired condition (HAC) alert **AHA** AHA Coding Clinic© Code first alert

[7th] **V91.12 Crushed between fishing boat and other watercraft or other object due to collision** [POA]

[7th] **V91.13 Crushed between other powered watercraft and other watercraft or other object due to collision** [POA]
Crushed between Hovercraft (on open water) and other watercraft or other object due to collision
Crushed between Jet ski and other watercraft or other object due to collision

[7th] **V91.14 Crushed between sailboat and other watercraft or other object due to collision** [POA]

[7th] **V91.15 Crushed between canoe or kayak and other watercraft or other object due to collision** [POA]

[7th] **V91.16 Crushed between (nonpowered) inflatable craft and other watercraft or other object due to collision** [POA]

[7th] **V91.18 Crushed between other unpowered watercraft and other watercraft or other object due to collision** [POA]
Crushed between surfboard and other watercraft or other object due to collision
Crushed between windsurfer and other watercraft or other object due to collision

[7th] **V91.19 Crushed between unspecified watercraft and other watercraft or other object due to collision** [POA]
Crushed between boat NOS and other watercraft or other object due to collision
Crushed between ship NOS and other watercraft or other object due to collision
Crushed between watercraft NOS and other watercraft or other object due to collision

[5th] **V91.2 Fall due to collision between watercraft and other watercraft or other object**
Fall while remaining on watercraft after collision
[NOTES] Select the specified type of watercraft that the victim was on at the time of the collision.
[EXCLUDES1] *crushed between watercraft and other watercraft and other object due to collision (V91.1-)*
drowning and submersion due to falling from crushed watercraft (V90.3-)

[7th] **V91.20 Fall due to collision between merchant ship and other watercraft or other object** [POA]

[7th] **V91.21 Fall due to collision between passenger ship and other watercraft or other object** [POA]
Fall due to collision between Ferry-boat and other watercraft or other object
Fall due to collision between Liner and other watercraft or other object

[7th] **V91.22 Fall due to collision between fishing boat and other watercraft or other object** [POA]

[7th] **V91.23 Fall due to collision between other powered watercraft and other watercraft or other object** [POA]
Fall due to collision between Hovercraft (on open water) and other watercraft or other object
Fall due to collision between Jet ski and other watercraft or other object

[7th] **V91.24 Fall due to collision between sailboat and other watercraft or other object** [POA]

[7th] **V91.25 Fall due to collision between canoe or kayak and other watercraft or other object** [POA]

[7th] **V91.26 Fall due to collision between (nonpowered) inflatable craft and other watercraft or other object** [POA]

[7th] **V91.29 Fall due to collision between unspecified watercraft and other watercraft or other object** [POA]
Fall due to collision between boat NOS and other watercraft or other object
Fall due to collision between ship NOS and other watercraft or other object
Fall due to collision between watercraft NOS and other watercraft or other object

[5th] **V91.3 Hit or struck by falling object due to accident to watercraft**
Hit or struck by falling object (part of damaged watercraft or other object) after falling or jumping from damaged watercraft
[EXCLUDES2] *drowning or submersion due to fall or jumping from damaged watercraft (V90.2-, V90.3-)*

[7th] **V91.30 Hit or struck by falling object due to accident to merchant ship** [POA]

[7th] **V91.31 Hit or struck by falling object due to accident to passenger ship** [POA]
Hit or struck by falling object due to accident to Ferry-boat
Hit or struck by falling object due to accident to Liner

[7th] **V91.32 Hit or struck by falling object due to accident to fishing boat** [POA]

[7th] **V91.33 Hit or struck by falling object due to accident to other powered watercraft** [POA]
Hit or struck by falling object due to accident to Hovercraft (on open water)
Hit or struck by falling object due to accident to Jet ski

[7th] **V91.34 Hit or struck by falling object due to accident to sailboat** [POA]

[7th] **V91.35 Hit or struck by falling object due to accident to canoe or kayak** [POA]

[7th] **V91.36 Hit or struck by falling object due to accident to (nonpowered) inflatable craft** [POA]

[7th] **V91.37 Hit or struck by falling object due to accident to water-skis** [POA]
Hit by water-skis after jumping off of waterskis

[7th] **V91.38 Hit or struck by falling object due to accident to other unpowered watercraft** [POA]
Hit or struck by surf-board after falling off damaged surf-board
Hit or struck by object after falling off damaged windsurfer

[7th] **V91.39 Hit or struck by falling object due to accident to unspecified watercraft** [POA]
Hit or struck by falling object due to accident to boat NOS
Hit or struck by falling object due to accident to ship NOS
Hit or struck by falling object due to accident to watercraft NOS

[5th] **V91.8 Other injury due to other accident to watercraft**

[7th] **V91.80 Other injury due to other accident to merchant ship** [POA]

[7th] **V91.81 Other injury due to other accident to passenger ship** [POA]
Other injury due to other accident to Ferry-boat
Other injury due to other accident to Liner

[7th] **V91.82 Other injury due to other accident to fishing boat** [POA]

[7th] **V91.83 Other injury due to other accident to other powered watercraft** [POA]
Other injury due to other accident to Hovercraft (on open water)
Other injury due to other accident to Jet ski

[7th] **V91.84 Other injury due to other accident to sailboat** [POA]

[7th] **V91.85 Other injury due to other accident to canoe or kayak** [POA]

[7th] **V91.86 Other injury due to other accident to (nonpowered) inflatable craft** [POA]

[7th] **V91.87 Other injury due to other accident to water-skis** [POA]

[7th] **V91.88 Other injury due to other accident to other unpowered watercraft** [POA]
Other injury due to other accident to surf-board
Other injury due to other accident to windsurfer

[7th] **V91.89 Other injury due to other accident to unspecified watercraft** [POA]
Other injury due to other accident to boat NOS
Other injury due to other accident to ship NOS
Other injury due to other accident to watercraft NOS

[4th] **V92 Drowning and submersion due to accident on board watercraft, without accident to watercraft**
[EXCLUDES1] *civilian water transport accident involving military watercraft (V94.81-)*
drowning or submersion due to accident to watercraft (V90-V91)
drowning or submersion of diver who voluntarily jumps from boat not involved in an accident (W16.711, W16.721)

[PDx] Unacceptable principal diagnosis symbol per Medicare code edits [POA] Code exempt from diagnosis present on admission requirement
[?] Questionable admission [CC] Complication or comorbidity [MCC] Major complication or comorbidity [CC/MCC Exc] CC/MCC exclusion
[HCC] HCC diagnosis code [RxHCC] RxHCC diagnosis code MACRA code **DEFINITION** Describes condition/terminology
TIP Coding guidance 👁 Official Guideline Reference [Z1] Z code as first-listed diagnosis

fall into water without watercraft (W16.-)

military watercraft accident in military or war operations (Y36, Y37)

The appropriate 7th character is to be added to each code from category V92

A = initial encounter
D = subsequent encounter
S = sequela

5ᵗʰ **V92.0 Drowning and submersion due to** fall off watercraft

Drowning and submersion due to fall from gangplank of watercraft

Drowning and submersion due to fall overboard watercraft

EXCLUDES2 *hitting head on object or bottom of body of water due to fall from watercraft (V94.0-)*

7ᵗʰ **V92.00 Drowning and submersion due to fall off** merchant ship

7ᵗʰ **V92.01 Drowning and submersion due to fall off** passenger ship

Drowning and submersion due to fall off Ferry-boat
Drowning and submersion due to fall off Liner

7ᵗʰ **V92.02 Drowning and submersion due to fall off** fishing boat

7ᵗʰ **V92.03 Drowning and submersion due to fall off other powered watercraft**

Drowning and submersion due to fall off Hovercraft (on open water)
Drowning and submersion due to fall off Jet ski

7ᵗʰ **V92.04 Drowning and submersion due to fall off** sailboat

7ᵗʰ **V92.05 Drowning and submersion due to fall off** canoe or kayak

7ᵗʰ **V92.06 Drowning and submersion due to fall off (nonpowered)** inflatable craft

7ᵗʰ **V92.07 Drowning and submersion due to fall off** water-skis

EXCLUDES1 *drowning and submersion due to falling off burning water-skis (V90.27)*

drowning and submersion due to falling off crushed water-skis (V90.37)

hit by boat while water-skiing NOS (V94.X)

7ᵗʰ **V92.08 Drowning and submersion due to fall off other unpowered watercraft**

Drowning and submersion due to fall off surf-board
Drowning and submersion due to fall off windsurfer

EXCLUDES1 *drowning and submersion due to fall off burning unpowered watercraft (V90.28)*

drowning and submersion due to fall off crushed unpowered watercraft (V90.38)

drowning and submersion due to fall off damaged unpowered watercraft (V90.88)

drowning and submersion due to rider of nonpowered watercraft being hit by other watercraft (V94.-)

other injury due to rider of nonpowered watercraft being hit by other watercraft (V94.-)

7ᵗʰ **V92.09 Drowning and submersion due to fall off unspecified watercraft**

Drowning and submersion due to fall off boat NOS
Drowning and submersion due to fall off ship NOS
Drowning and submersion due to fall off watercraft NOS

5ᵗʰ **V92.1 Drowning and submersion due to being** thrown overboard by motion **of watercraft**

EXCLUDES1 *drowning and submersion due to fall off surf-board (V92.08)*

drowning and submersion due to fall off water-skis (V92.07)

drowning and submersion due to fall off windsurfer (V92.08)

7ᵗʰ **V92.10 Drowning and submersion due to being thrown overboard by motion of** merchant ship

7ᵗʰ **V92.11 Drowning and submersion due to being thrown overboard by motion of** passenger ship

Drowning and submersion due to being thrown overboard by motion of Ferry-boat
Drowning and submersion due to being thrown overboard by motion of Liner

7ᵗʰ **V92.12 Drowning and submersion due to being thrown overboard by motion of** fishing boat

7ᵗʰ **V92.13 Drowning and submersion due to being thrown overboard by motion of other powered watercraft**

Drowning and submersion due to being thrown overboard by motion of Hovercraft

7ᵗʰ **V92.14 Drowning and submersion due to being thrown overboard by motion of** sailboat

7ᵗʰ **V92.15 Drowning and submersion due to being thrown overboard by motion of** canoe or kayak

7ᵗʰ **V92.16 Drowning and submersion due to being thrown overboard by motion of (nonpowered)** inflatable craft

7ᵗʰ **V92.19 Drowning and submersion due to being thrown overboard by motion of unspecified watercraft**

Drowning and submersion due to being thrown overboard by motion of boat NOS
Drowning and submersion due to being thrown overboard by motion of ship NOS
Drowning and submersion due to being thrown overboard by motion of watercraft NOS

5ᵗʰ **V92.2 Drowning and submersion due to being** washed overboard **from watercraft**

Code first any associated cataclysm (X37.0-)

7ᵗʰ **V92.20 Drowning and submersion due to being washed overboard from** merchant ship

7ᵗʰ **V92.21 Drowning and submersion due to being washed overboard from** passenger ship

Drowning and submersion due to being washed overboard from Ferry-boat
Drowning and submersion due to being washed overboard from Liner

7ᵗʰ **V92.22 Drowning and submersion due to being washed overboard from** fishing boat

7ᵗʰ **V92.23 Drowning and submersion due to being washed overboard from other powered watercraft**

Drowning and submersion due to being washed overboard from Hovercraft (on open water)
Drowning and submersion due to being washed overboard from Jet ski

7ᵗʰ **V92.24 Drowning and submersion due to being washed overboard from** sailboat

7ᵗʰ **V92.25 Drowning and submersion due to being washed overboard from** canoe or kayak

7ᵗʰ **V92.26 Drowning and submersion due to being washed overboard from (nonpowered)** inflatable craft

7ᵗʰ **V92.27 Drowning and submersion due to being washed overboard from** water-skis

EXCLUDES1 *drowning and submersion due to fall off water-skis (V92.07)*

7ᵗʰ **V92.28 Drowning and submersion due to being washed overboard from other unpowered watercraft**

Drowning and submersion due to being washed overboard from surf-board
Drowning and submersion due to being washed overboard from windsurfer

7ᵗʰ **V92.29 Drowning and submersion due to being washed overboard from unspecified watercraft**

Drowning and submersion due to being washed overboard from boat NOS
Drowning and submersion due to being washed overboard from ship NOS
Drowning and submersion due to being washed overboard from watercraft NOS

Unspecified Code   Other Specified Code   Manifestation Code   N Newborn   P Pediatric   M Maternity   A Adult   ♂ Male   ♀ Female
● New Code   ▲ Revised Code Title   ▶◀ Revised Text   NOTES   INCLUDES   EXCLUDES1 Not coded here   EXCLUDES2 Not included here
4ᵗʰ 4ᵗʰ character required   5ᵗʰ 5ᵗʰ character required   6ᵗʰ 6ᵗʰ character required   7ᵗʰ 7ᵗʰ character required   Extension 'X' Alert
HAC Hospital-acquired condition (HAC) alert   AHA AHA Coding Clinic©   Code first alert

V93 Other **injury due to accident on board watercraft,** without accident to watercraft

EXCLUDES1 *civilian water transport accident involving military watercraft (V94.81-)*

other injury due to accident to watercraft (V91.-)

military watercraft accident in military or war operations (Y36, Y37.-)

EXCLUDES2 *drowning and submersion due to accident on board watercraft, without accident to watercraft (V92.-)*

The appropriate 7th character is to be added to each code from category V93

A = initial encounter

D = subsequent encounter

S = sequela

V93.0 **Burn due to localized** fire on board **watercraft**

EXCLUDES1 *burn due to watercraft on fire (V91.0-)*

V93.00 **Burn due to localized fire on board** merchant vessel

V93.01 **Burn due to localized fire on board** passenger vessel

Burn due to localized fire on board Ferry-boat

Burn due to localized fire on board Liner

V93.02 **Burn due to localized fire on board** fishing boat

V93.03 **Burn due to localized fire on board other powered watercraft**

Burn due to localized fire on board Hovercraft

Burn due to localized fire on board Jet ski

V93.04 **Burn due to localized fire on board** sailboat

V93.09 **Burn due to localized fire on board unspecified watercraft**

Burn due to localized fire on board boat NOS

Burn due to localized fire on board ship NOS

Burn due to localized fire on board watercraft NOS

V93.1 Other **burn on board watercraft**

Burn due to source other than fire on board watercraft

EXCLUDES1 *burn due to watercraft on fire (V91.0-)*

V93.10 **Other burn on board** merchant vessel

V93.11 **Other burn on board** passenger vessel

Other burn on board Ferry-boat

Other burn on board Liner

V93.12 **Other burn on board** fishing boat

V93.13 **Other burn on board** other powered watercraft

Other burn on board Hovercraft

Other burn on board Jet ski

V93.14 **Other burn on board** sailboat

V93.19 **Other burn on board unspecified watercraft**

Other burn on board boat NOS

Other burn on board ship NOS

Other burn on board watercraft NOS

V93.2 Heat exposure **on board watercraft**

EXCLUDES1 *exposure to man-made heat not aboard watercraft (W92)*

exposure to natural heat while on board watercraft (X30)

exposure to sunlight while on board watercraft (X32)

EXCLUDES2 *burn due to fire on board watercraft (V93.0-)*

V93.20 **Heat exposure on board** merchant ship

V93.21 **Heat exposure on board** passenger ship

Heat exposure on board Ferry-boat

Heat exposure on board Liner

V93.22 **Heat exposure on board** fishing boat

V93.23 **Heat exposure on board other powered watercraft**

Heat exposure on board hovercraft

V93.24 **Heat exposure on board** sailboat

V93.29 **Heat exposure on board unspecified watercraft**

Heat exposure on board boat NOS

Heat exposure on board ship NOS

Heat exposure on board watercraft NOS

V93.3 Fall **on board watercraft**

EXCLUDES1 *fall due to collision of watercraft (V91.2-)*

V93.30 **Fall on board** merchant ship

V93.31 **Fall on board** passenger ship

Fall on board Ferry-boat

Fall on board Liner

V93.32 **Fall on board** fishing boat

V93.33 **Fall on board other powered watercraft**

Fall on board Hovercraft (on open water)

Fall on board Jet ski

V93.34 **Fall on board** sailboat

V93.35 **Fall on board** canoe or kayak

V93.36 **Fall on board (nonpowered)** inflatable craft

V93.38 **Fall on board other unpowered watercraft**

V93.39 **Fall on board unspecified watercraft**

Fall on board boat NOS

Fall on board ship NOS

Fall on board watercraft NOS

V93.4 Struck **by falling object on board watercraft**

Hit by falling object on board watercraft

EXCLUDES1 *struck by falling object due to accident to watercraft (V91.3)*

V93.40 **Struck by falling object on** merchant ship

V93.41 **Struck by falling object on** passenger ship

Struck by falling object on Ferry-boat

Struck by falling object on Liner

V93.42 **Struck by falling object on** fishing boat

V93.43 **Struck by falling object on other powered watercraft**

Struck by falling object on Hovercraft

V93.44 **Struck by falling object on** sailboat

V93.48 **Struck by falling object on other unpowered watercraft**

V93.49 **Struck by falling object on unspecified watercraft**

V93.5 Explosion **on board watercraft**

Boiler explosion on steamship

EXCLUDES2 *fire on board watercraft (V93.0-)*

V93.50 **Explosion on board** merchant ship

V93.51 **Explosion on board** passenger ship

Explosion on board Ferry-boat

Explosion on board Liner

V93.52 **Explosion on board** fishing boat

V93.53 **Explosion on board other powered watercraft**

Explosion on board Hovercraft

Explosion on board Jet ski

V93.54 **Explosion on board** sailboat

V93.59 **Explosion on board unspecified watercraft**

Explosion on board boat NOS

Explosion on board ship NOS

Explosion on board watercraft NOS

V93.6 Machinery accident **on board watercraft**

EXCLUDES1 *machinery explosion on board watercraft (V93.4-)*

machinery fire on board watercraft (V93.0-)

V93.60 **Machinery accident on board** merchant ship

V93.61 **Machinery accident on board** passenger ship

Machinery accident on board Ferry-boat

Machinery accident on board Liner

V93.62 **Machinery accident on board** fishing boat

V93.63 **Machinery accident on board other powered watercraft**

Machinery accident on board Hovercraft

V93.64 **Machinery accident on board** sailboat

V93.69 **Machinery accident on board unspecified watercraft**

Machinery accident on board boat NOS

Machinery accident on board ship NOS

Machinery accident on board watercraft NOS

V93.8 Other **injury due to other accident on board watercraft**

Accidental poisoning by gases or fumes on watercraft

V93.80 **Other injury due to other accident on board** merchant ship

---

[7th] **V93.81 Other injury due to other accident on board passenger ship** [POA]
Other injury due to other accident on board Ferry-boat
Other injury due to other accident on board Liner

[7th] **V93.82 Other injury due to other accident on board fishing boat** [POA]

[7th] **V93.83 Other injury due to other accident on board other powered watercraft** [POA]
Other injury due to other accident on board Hovercraft
Other injury due to other accident on board Jet ski

[7th] **V93.84 Other injury due to other accident on board sailboat** [POA]

[7th] **V93.85 Other injury due to other accident on board canoe or kayak** [POA]

[7th] **V93.86 Other injury due to other accident on board (nonpowered) inflatable craft** [POA]

[7th] **V93.87 Other injury due to other accident on board water-skis** [POA]
Hit or struck by object while waterskiing

[7th] **V93.88 Other injury due to other accident on board other unpowered watercraft** [POA]
Hit or struck by object while surfing
Hit or struck by object while on board windsurfer

[7th] **V93.89 Other injury due to other accident on board unspecified watercraft** [POA]
Other injury due to other accident on board boat NOS
Other injury due to other accident on board ship NOS
Other injury due to other accident on board watercraft NOS

[4th] **V94 Other and unspecified water transport accidents**
[EXCLUDES1] *military watercraft accidents in military or war operations (Y36, Y37)*
The appropriate 7th character is to be added to each code from category V94
A = initial encounter
D = subsequent encounter
S = sequela

[7th] **V94.0 Hitting object or bottom of body of water due to fall from watercraft** [POA]
[EXCLUDES2] *drowning and submersion due to fall from watercraft (V92.0-)*

[5th] **V94.1 Bather struck by watercraft**
Swimmer hit by watercraft

[7th] **V94.11 Bather struck by powered watercraft** [POA]

[7th] **V94.12 Bather struck by nonpowered watercraft** [POA]

[5th] **V94.2 Rider of nonpowered watercraft struck by other watercraft**

[7th] **V94.21 Rider of nonpowered watercraft struck by other nonpowered watercraft** [POA]
Canoer hit by other nonpowered watercraft
Surfer hit by other nonpowered watercraft
Windsurfer hit by other nonpowered watercraft

[7th] **V94.22 Rider of nonpowered watercraft struck by powered watercraft** [POA]
Canoer hit by motorboat
Surfer hit by motorboat
Windsurfer hit by motorboat

[5th] **V94.3 Injury to rider of (inflatable) watercraft being pulled behind other watercraft**

[7th] **V94.31 Injury to rider of (inflatable) recreational watercraft being pulled behind other watercraft** [POA]
Injury to rider of inner-tube pulled behind motor boat

[7th] **V94.32 Injury to rider of non-recreational watercraft being pulled behind other watercraft** [POA]
Injury to occupant of dingy being pulled behind boat or ship
Injury to occupant of life-raft being pulled behind boat or ship

[7th] **V94.4 Injury to barefoot water-skier** [POA]
Injury to person being pulled behind boat or ship

[5th] **V94.8 Other water transport accident**

[6th] **V94.81 Water transport accident involving military watercraft**

[7th] **V94.810 Civilian watercraft involved in water transport accident with military watercraft** [POA]
Passenger on civilian watercraft injured due to accident with military watercraft

[7th] **V94.811 Civilian in water injured by military watercraft** [POA]

[7th] **V94.818 Other water transport accident involving military watercraft** [POA]

[7th] **V94.89 Other water transport accident** [POA]

[7th] **V94.9 Unspecified water transport accident** [POA]
Water transport accident NOS

Air and space transport accidents (V95-V97)

[EXCLUDES1] *military aircraft accidents in military or war operations (Y36, Y37)*

[4th] **V95 Accident to powered aircraft causing injury to occupant**
The appropriate 7th character is to be added to each code from category V95
A = initial encounter
D = subsequent encounter
S = sequela

[5th] **V95.0 Helicopter accident injuring occupant**

[7th] **V95.00 Unspecified helicopter accident injuring occupant** [POA]

[7th] **V95.01 Helicopter crash injuring occupant** [POA]

[7th] **V95.02 Forced landing of helicopter injuring occupant** [POA]

[7th] **V95.03 Helicopter collision injuring occupant** [POA]
Helicopter collision with any object, fixed, movable or moving

[7th] **V95.04 Helicopter fire injuring occupant** [POA]

[7th] **V95.05 Helicopter explosion injuring occupant** [POA]

[7th] **V95.09 Other helicopter accident injuring occupant** [POA]

[5th] **V95.1 Ultralight, microlight or powered-glider accident injuring occupant**

[7th] **V95.10 Unspecified ultralight, microlight or powered-glider accident injuring occupant** [POA]

[7th] **V95.11 Ultralight, microlight or powered-glider crash injuring occupant** [POA]

[7th] **V95.12 Forced landing of ultralight, microlight or powered-glider injuring occupant** [POA]

[7th] **V95.13 Ultralight, microlight or powered-glider collision injuring occupant** [POA]
Ultralight, microlight or powered-glider collision with any object, fixed, movable or moving

[7th] **V95.14 Ultralight, microlight or powered-glider fire injuring occupant** [POA]

[7th] **V95.15 Ultralight, microlight or powered-glider explosion injuring occupant** [POA]

[7th] **V95.19 Other ultralight, microlight or powered-glider accident injuring occupant** [POA]

[5th] **V95.2 Other private fixed-wing aircraft accident injuring occupant**

[7th] **V95.20 Unspecified accident to other private fixed-wing aircraft, injuring occupant** [POA]

[7th] **V95.21 Other private fixed-wing aircraft crash injuring occupant** [POA]

[7th] **V95.22 Forced landing of other private fixed-wing aircraft injuring occupant** [POA]

[7th] **V95.23 Other private fixed-wing aircraft collision injuring occupant** [POA]
Other private fixed-wing aircraft collision with any object, fixed, movable or moving

[7th] **V95.24 Other private fixed-wing aircraft fire injuring occupant** [POA]

[7th] **V95.25 Other private fixed-wing aircraft explosion injuring occupant** [POA]

[7th] **V95.29 Other accident to other private fixed-wing aircraft injuring occupant** [POA]

[5th] **V95.3 Commercial fixed-wing aircraft accident injuring occupant**

[7th] **V95.30 Unspecified accident to commercial fixed-wing aircraft injuring occupant** [POA]

V95.31 Commercial fixed-wing aircraft crash injuring occupant

V95.32 Forced landing of commercial fixed-wing aircraft injuring occupant

V95.33 Commercial fixed-wing aircraft collision injuring occupant

Commercial fixed-wing aircraft collision with any object, fixed, movable or moving

V95.34 Commercial fixed-wing aircraft fire injuring occupant

V95.35 Commercial fixed-wing aircraft explosion injuring occupant

V95.39 Other accident to commercial fixed-wing aircraft injuring occupant

V95.4 Spacecraft accident injuring occupant

V95.40 Unspecified spacecraft accident injuring occupant

V95.41 Spacecraft crash injuring occupant

V95.42 Forced landing of spacecraft injuring occupant

V95.43 Spacecraft collision injuring occupant

Spacecraft collision with any object, fixed, moveable or moving

V95.44 Spacecraft fire injuring occupant

V95.45 Spacecraft explosion injuring occupant

V95.49 Other spacecraft accident injuring occupant

V95.8 Other powered aircraft accidents injuring occupant

V95.9 Unspecified aircraft accident injuring occupant

Aircraft accident NOS
Air transport accident NOS

V96 Accident to nonpowered aircraft causing injury to occupant

The appropriate 7th character is to be added to each code from category V96

A = initial encounter
D = subsequent encounter
S = sequela

V96.0 Balloon accident injuring occupant

V96.00 Unspecified balloon accident injuring occupant

V96.01 Balloon crash injuring occupant

V96.02 Forced landing of balloon injuring occupant

V96.03 Balloon collision injuring occupant

Balloon collision with any object, fixed, moveable or moving

V96.04 Balloon fire injuring occupant

V96.05 Balloon explosion injuring occupant

V96.09 Other balloon accident injuring occupant

V96.1 Hang-glider accident injuring occupant

V96.10 Unspecified hang-glider accident injuring occupant

V96.11 Hang-glider crash injuring occupant

V96.12 Forced landing of hang-glider injuring occupant

V96.13 Hang-glider collision injuring occupant

Hang-glider collision with any object, fixed, moveable or moving

V96.14 Hang-glider fire injuring occupant

V96.15 Hang-glider explosion injuring occupant

V96.19 Other hang-glider accident injuring occupant

V96.2 Glider (nonpowered) accident injuring occupant

V96.20 Unspecified glider (nonpowered) accident injuring occupant

V96.21 Glider (nonpowered) crash injuring occupant

V96.22 Forced landing of glider (nonpowered) injuring occupant

V96.23 Glider (nonpowered) collision injuring occupant

Glider (nonpowered) collision with any object, fixed, moveable or moving

V96.24 Glider (nonpowered) fire injuring occupant

V96.25 Glider (nonpowered) explosion injuring occupant

V96.29 Other glider (nonpowered) accident injuring occupant

V96.8 Other nonpowered-aircraft accidents injuring occupant

Kite carrying a person accident injuring occupant

V96.9 Unspecified nonpowered-aircraft accident injuring occupant

Nonpowered-aircraft accident NOS

V97 Other specified air transport accidents

The appropriate 7th character is to be added to each code from category V97

A = initial encounter
D = subsequent encounter
S = sequela

V97.0 Occupant of aircraft injured in other specified air transport accidents

Fall in, on or from aircraft in air transport accident

EXCLUDES1 accident while boarding or alighting aircraft (V97.1)

V97.1 Person injured while boarding or alighting from aircraft

V97.2 Parachutist accident

V97.21 Parachutist entangled in object

Parachutist landing in tree

V97.22 Parachutist injured on landing

V97.29 Other parachutist accident

V97.3 Person on ground injured in air transport accident

V97.31 Hit by object falling from aircraft

Hit by crashing aircraft
Injured by aircraft hitting house
Injured by aircraft hitting car

V97.32 Injured by rotating propeller

V97.33 Sucked into jet engine

V97.39 Other injury to person on ground due to air transport accident

V97.8 Other air transport accidents, not elsewhere classified

EXCLUDES1 aircraft accident NOS (V95.9)

exposure to changes in air pressure during ascent or descent (W94.-)

V97.81 Air transport accident involving military aircraft

V97.810 Civilian aircraft involved in air transport accident with military aircraft

Passenger in civilian aircraft injured due to accident with military aircraft

V97.811 Civilian injured by military aircraft

V97.818 Other air transport accident involving military aircraft

V97.89 Other air transport accidents, not elsewhere classified

Injury from machinery on aircraft

Other and unspecified transport accidents (V98-V99)

EXCLUDES1 vehicle accident, type of vehicle unspecified (V89.-)

V98 Other specified transport accidents

The appropriate 7th character is to be added to each code from category V98

A = initial encounter
D = subsequent encounter
S = sequela

V98.0 Accident to, on or involving cable-car, not on rails

Caught or dragged by cable-car, not on rails
Fall or jump from cable-car, not on rails
Object thrown from or in cable-car, not on rails

V98.1 Accident to, on or involving land-yacht

V98.2 Accident to, on or involving ice yacht

V98.3 Accident to, on or involving ski lift

Accident to, on or involving ski chair-lift
Accident to, on or involving ski-lift with gondola

V98.8 Other specified transport accidents

V99 Unspecified transport accident

The appropriate 7th character is to be added to code V99

A = initial encounter
D = subsequent encounter
S = sequela

Other external causes of accidental injury (W00-X58)

Slipping, tripping, stumbling and falls (W00-W19)

EXCLUDES1 *assault involving a fall (Y01-Y02)*

fall from animal (V80.-)

fall (in) (from) machinery (in operation) (W28-W31)

fall (in) (from) transport vehicle (V01-V99)

intentional self-harm involving a fall (X80-X81)

EXCLUDES2 *at risk for fall (history of fall) Z91.81*

fall (in) (from) burning building (X00.-)

fall into fire (X00-X04, X08)

4ᵗʰ **W00 Fall due to** ice and snow

INCLUDES *pedestrian on foot falling (slipping) on ice and snow*

EXCLUDES1 *fall on (from) ice and snow involving pedestrian conveyance (V00.-)*

fall from stairs and steps not due to ice and snow (W10.-)

The appropriate 7th character is to be added to each code from category W00

A = initial encounter

D = subsequent encounter

S = sequela

7ᵗʰ **W00.0 Fall on** same level **due to ice and snow**

AHA: Q2 2016

7ᵗʰ **W00.1 Fall from** stairs and steps **due to ice and snow**

7ᵗʰ **W00.2 Other fall from one level to another due to ice and snow**

7ᵗʰ **W00.9 Unspecified fall due to ice and snow**

4ᵗʰ **W01 Fall on same level from** slipping, tripping and stumbling

INCLUDES *fall on moving sidewalk*

EXCLUDES1 *fall due to bumping (striking) against object (W18.0-)*

fall in shower or bathtub (W18.2-)

fall on same level NOS (W18.30)

fall on same level from slipping, tripping and stumbling due to ice or snow (W00.0)

fall off or from toilet (W18.1-)

slipping, tripping and stumbling NOS (W18.40)

slipping, tripping and stumbling without falling (W18.4-)

The appropriate 7th character is to be added to each code from category W01

A = initial encounter

D = subsequent encounter

S = sequela

7ᵗʰ **W01.0 Fall on same level from slipping, tripping and stumbling** without subsequent striking against object

Falling over animal

5ᵗʰ **W01.1 Fall on same level from slipping, tripping and stumbling** with subsequent striking against object

7ᵗʰ **W01.10 Fall on same level from slipping, tripping and stumbling with subsequent striking against unspecified object**

6ᵗʰ **W01.11 Fall on same level from slipping, tripping and stumbling with subsequent striking against** sharp object

7ᵗʰ **W01.110 Fall on same level from slipping, tripping and stumbling with subsequent striking against** sharp glass

7ᵗʰ **W01.111 Fall on same level from slipping, tripping and stumbling with subsequent striking against** power tool or machine

7ᵗʰ **W01.118 Fall on same level from slipping, tripping and stumbling with subsequent striking against other sharp object**

7ᵗʰ **W01.119 Fall on same level from slipping, tripping and stumbling with subsequent striking against unspecified sharp object**

6ᵗʰ **W01.19 Fall on same level from slipping, tripping and stumbling with subsequent striking against** other object

7ᵗʰ **W01.190 Fall on same level from slipping, tripping and stumbling with subsequent striking against** furniture

7ᵗʰ **W01.198 Fall on same level from slipping, tripping and stumbling with subsequent striking against other object**

4ᵗʰ **W03 Other fall on same level due to collision with another person**

AHA: Q1 2015

Fall due to non-transport collision with other person

EXCLUDES1 *collision with another person without fall (W51)*

crushed or pushed by a crowd or human stampede (W52)

fall involving pedestrian conveyance (V00-V09)

fall due to ice or snow (W00)

fall on same level NOS (W18.30)

The appropriate 7th character is to be added to code W03

A = initial encounter

D = subsequent encounter

S = sequela

7ᵗʰ **W04 Fall while being carried or supported by other persons**

Accidentally dropped while being carried

The appropriate 7th character is to be added to code W04

A = initial encounter

D = subsequent encounter

S = sequela

4ᵗʰ **W05 Fall from** non-moving **wheelchair, nonmotorized scooter and motorized mobility scooter**

EXCLUDES1 *fall from moving wheelchair (powered) (V00.811)*

fall from moving motorized mobility scooter (V00.831)

fall from nonmotorized scooter (V00.141)

The appropriate 7th character is to be added to each code from category W05

A = initial encounter

D = subsequent encounter

S = sequela

7ᵗʰ **W05.0 Fall from non-moving** wheelchair

AHA: Q2 2019

7ᵗʰ **W05.1 Fall from non-moving** nonmotorized scooter

7ᵗʰ **W05.2 Fall from non-moving** motorized mobility scooter

7ᵗʰ **W06 Fall from** bed

The appropriate 7th character is to be added to code W06

A = initial encounter

D = subsequent encounter

S = sequela

7ᵗʰ **W07 Fall from** chair

The appropriate 7th character is to be added to code W07

A = initial encounter

D = subsequent encounter

S = sequela

7ᵗʰ **W08 Fall from other furniture**

The appropriate 7th character is to be added to code W08

A = initial encounter

D = subsequent encounter

S = sequela

4ᵗʰ **W09 Fall on and from playground equipment**

EXCLUDES1 *fall involving recreational machinery (W31)*

The appropriate 7th character is to be added to each code from category W09

A = initial encounter

D = subsequent encounter

S = sequela

7ᵗʰ **W09.0 Fall on or from** playground slide

7ᵗʰ **W09.1 Fall from** playground swing

7ᵗʰ **W09.2 Fall on or from** jungle gym

7ᵗʰ **W09.8 Fall on or from** other playground equipment

Unspecified Code   Other Specified Code   Manifestation Code   Ⓝ Newborn   Ⓟ Pediatric   Ⓜ Maternity   Ⓐ Adult   ♂ Male   ♀ Female

● New Code   ▲ Revised Code Title   ▶◀ Revised Text   NOTES   INCLUDES   EXCLUDES1 Not coded here   EXCLUDES2 Not included here

4ᵗʰ 4ᵗʰ character required   5ᵗʰ 5ᵗʰ character required   6ᵗʰ 6ᵗʰ character required   7ᵗʰ 7ᵗʰ character required   7ˣ Extension 'X' Alert

HAC Hospital-acquired condition (HAC) alert   AHA AHA Coding Clinic©   ☛ Code first alert

2020 ICD-10-CM   When symbols appear on a code that requires a 7th character extension, refer to Appendix B to identify applicable 7th character codes.   **1213**

W10 Fall on and from stairs and steps

> EXCLUDES1 *Fall from stairs and steps due to ice and snow (W00.1)*

> The appropriate 7th character is to be added to each code from category W10
> > A = initial encounter
> > D = subsequent encounter
> > S = sequela

- W10.0 Fall (on)(from) escalator
- W10.1 Fall (on)(from) sidewalk curb
- W10.2 Fall (on)(from) incline
  > Fall (on) (from) ramp
- W10.8 Fall (on) (from) other stairs and steps
- W10.9 Fall (on) (from) unspecified stairs and steps

W11 Fall on and from ladder

> The appropriate 7th character is to be added to code W11
> > A = initial encounter
> > D = subsequent encounter
> > S = sequela

W12 Fall on and from scaffolding

> The appropriate 7th character is to be added to code W12
> > A = initial encounter
> > D = subsequent encounter
> > S = sequela

W13 Fall from, out of or through building or structure

> The appropriate 7th character is to be added to each code from category W13
> > A = initial encounter
> > D = subsequent encounter
> > S = sequela

- W13.0 Fall from, out of or through balcony
  > Fall from, out of or through railing
- W13.1 Fall from, out of or through bridge
- W13.2 Fall from, out of or through roof
- W13.3 Fall through floor
- W13.4 Fall from, out of or through window
  > EXCLUDES2 *fall with subsequent striking against sharp glass (W01.110)*
- W13.8 Fall from, out of or through other building or structure
  > Fall from, out of or through viaduct
  > Fall from, out of or through wall
  > Fall from, out of or through flag-pole
- W13.9 Fall from, out of or through building, not otherwise specified
  > EXCLUDES1 *collapse of a building or structure (W20.-)*
  > > *fall or jump from burning building or structure (X00.-)*

W14 Fall from tree

> The appropriate 7th character is to be added to code W14
> > A = initial encounter
> > D = subsequent encounter
> > S = sequela

W15 Fall from cliff

> The appropriate 7th character is to be added to code W15
> > A = initial encounter
> > D = subsequent encounter
> > S = sequela

W16 Fall, jump or diving into water

> EXCLUDES1 *accidental non-watercraft drowning and submersion not involving fall (W65-W74)*
> > *effects of air pressure from diving (W94.-)*
> > *fall into water from watercraft (V90-V94)*
> > *hitting an object or against bottom when falling from watercraft (V94.0)*
> EXCLUDES2 *striking or hitting diving board (W21.4)*

> The appropriate 7th character is to be added to each code from category W16
> > A = initial encounter
> > D = subsequent encounter
> > S = sequela

- W16.0 Fall into swimming pool
  > Fall into swimming pool NOS
  > EXCLUDES1 *fall into empty swimming pool (W17.3)*
  - W16.01 Fall into swimming pool striking water surface
    - W16.011 Fall into swimming pool striking water surface causing drowning and submersion
      > EXCLUDES1 *drowning and submersion while in swimming pool without fall (W67)*
    - W16.012 Fall into swimming pool striking water surface causing other injury
  - W16.02 Fall into swimming pool striking bottom
    - W16.021 Fall into swimming pool striking bottom causing drowning and submersion
      > EXCLUDES1 *drowning and submersion while in swimming pool without fall (W67)*
    - W16.022 Fall into swimming pool striking bottom causing other injury
  - W16.03 Fall into swimming pool striking wall
    - W16.031 Fall into swimming pool striking wall causing drowning and submersion
      > EXCLUDES1 *drowning and submersion while in swimming pool without fall (W67)*
    - W16.032 Fall into swimming pool striking wall causing other injury
- W16.1 Fall into natural body of water
  > Fall into lake
  > Fall into open sea
  > Fall into river
  > Fall into stream
  - W16.11 Fall into natural body of water striking water surface
    - W16.111 Fall into natural body of water striking water surface causing drowning and submersion
      > EXCLUDES1 *drowning and submersion while in natural body of water without fall (W69)*
    - W16.112 Fall into natural body of water striking water surface causing other injury
  - W16.12 Fall into natural body of water striking bottom
    - W16.121 Fall into natural body of water striking bottom causing drowning and submersion
      > EXCLUDES1 *drowning and submersion while in natural body of water without fall (W69)*
    - W16.122 Fall into natural body of water striking bottom causing other injury
  - W16.13 Fall into natural body of water striking side
    - W16.131 Fall into natural body of water striking side causing drowning and submersion
      > EXCLUDES1 *drowning and submersion while in natural body of water without fall (W69)*
    - W16.132 Fall into natural body of water striking side causing other injury
- W16.2 Fall in (into) filled bathtub or bucket of water
  - W16.21 Fall in (into) filled bathtub
    > EXCLUDES1 *fall into empty bathtub (W18.2)*
    - W16.211 Fall in (into) filled bathtub causing drowning and submersion
      > EXCLUDES1 *drowning and submersion while in filled bathtub without fall (W65)*
    - W16.212 Fall in (into) filled bathtub causing other injury
  - W16.22 Fall in (into) bucket of water
    - W16.221 Fall in (into) bucket of water causing drowning and submersion
    - W16.222 Fall in (into) bucket of water causing other injury

---

POA Unacceptable principal diagnosis symbol per Medicare code edits   POA Code exempt from diagnosis present on admission requirement
? Questionable admission   CC Complication or comorbidity   MCC Major complication or comorbidity   CC/MCC Exc CC/MCC exclusion
HCC HCC diagnosis code   RxHCC RxHCC diagnosis code   MACRA code   **DEFINITION** Describes condition/terminology
TIP Coding guidance   Official Guideline Reference   Z1 Z code as first-listed diagnosis

1214   When symbols appear on a code that requires a 7th character extension, refer to Appendix B to identify applicable 7th character codes.   **2020 ICD-10-CM**

[5th] W16.3 Fall into other water
Fall into fountain
Fall into reservoir
[6th] W16.31 Fall into other water striking water surface
[7th] W16.311 Fall into other water striking water surface causing drowning and submersion [POA]
EXCLUDES1 drowning and submersion while in other water without fall (W73)
[7th] W16.312 Fall into other water striking water surface causing other injury [POA]
[6th] W16.32 Fall into other water striking bottom
[7th] W16.321 Fall into other water striking bottom causing drowning and submersion [POA]
EXCLUDES1 drowning and submersion while in other water without fall (W73)
[7th] W16.322 Fall into other water striking bottom causing other injury [POA]
[6th] W16.33 Fall into other water striking wall
[7th] W16.331 Fall into other water striking wall causing drowning and submersion [POA]
EXCLUDES1 drowning and submersion while in other water without fall (W73)
[7th] W16.332 Fall into other water striking wall causing other injury [POA]
[5th] W16.4 Fall into unspecified water
[7th] W16.41 Fall into unspecified water causing drowning and submersion [POA]
[7th] W16.42 Fall into unspecified water causing other injury [POA]
[5th] W16.5 Jumping or diving into swimming pool
[6th] W16.51 Jumping or diving into swimming pool striking water surface
[7th] W16.511 Jumping or diving into swimming pool striking water surface causing drowning and submersion [POA]
EXCLUDES1 drowning and submersion while in swimming pool without jumping or diving (W67)
[7th] W16.512 Jumping or diving into swimming pool striking water surface causing other injury [POA]
[6th] W16.52 Jumping or diving into swimming pool striking bottom
[7th] W16.521 Jumping or diving into swimming pool striking bottom causing drowning and submersion [POA]
EXCLUDES1 drowning and submersion while in swimming pool without jumping or diving (W67)
[7th] W16.522 Jumping or diving into swimming pool striking bottom causing other injury [POA]
[6th] W16.53 Jumping or diving into swimming pool striking wall
[7th] W16.531 Jumping or diving into swimming pool striking wall causing drowning and submersion [POA]
EXCLUDES1 drowning and submersion while in swimming pool without jumping or diving (W67)
[7th] W16.532 Jumping or diving into swimming pool striking wall causing other injury [POA]
[5th] W16.6 Jumping or diving into natural body of water
Jumping or diving into lake
Jumping or diving into open sea
Jumping or diving into river
Jumping or diving into stream
[6th] W16.61 Jumping or diving into natural body of water striking water surface
[7th] W16.611 Jumping or diving into natural body of water striking water surface causing drowning and submersion [POA]
EXCLUDES1 drowning and submersion while in natural body of water without jumping or diving (W69)
[7th] W16.612 Jumping or diving into natural body of water striking water surface causing other injury [POA]
[6th] W16.62 Jumping or diving into natural body of water striking bottom
[7th] W16.621 Jumping or diving into natural body of water striking bottom causing drowning and submersion [POA]
EXCLUDES1 drowning and submersion while in natural body of water without jumping or diving (W69)
[7th] W16.622 Jumping or diving into natural body of water striking bottom causing other injury [POA]
[5th] W16.7 Jumping or diving from boat
EXCLUDES1 Fall from boat into water -see watercraft accident (V90-V94)
[6th] W16.71 Jumping or diving from boat striking water surface
[7th] W16.711 Jumping or diving from boat striking water surface causing drowning and submersion [POA]
[7th] W16.712 Jumping or diving from boat striking water surface causing other injury [POA]
[6th] W16.72 Jumping or diving from boat striking bottom
[7th] W16.721 Jumping or diving from boat striking bottom causing drowning and submersion [POA]
[7th] W16.722 Jumping or diving from boat striking bottom causing other injury [POA]
[5th] W16.8 Jumping or diving into other water
Jumping or diving into fountain
Jumping or diving into reservoir
[6th] W16.81 Jumping or diving into other water striking water surface
[7th] W16.811 Jumping or diving into other water striking water surface causing drowning and submersion [POA]
EXCLUDES1 drowning and submersion while in other water without jumping or diving (W73)
[7th] W16.812 Jumping or diving into other water striking water surface causing other injury [POA]
[6th] W16.82 Jumping or diving into other water striking bottom
[7th] W16.821 Jumping or diving into other water striking bottom causing drowning and submersion [POA]
EXCLUDES1 drowning and submersion while in other water without jumping or diving (W73)
[7th] W16.822 Jumping or diving into other water striking bottom causing other injury [POA]
[6th] W16.83 Jumping or diving into other water striking wall
[7th] W16.831 Jumping or diving into other water striking wall causing drowning and submersion [POA]
EXCLUDES1 drowning and submersion while in other water without jumping or diving (W73)
[7th] W16.832 Jumping or diving into other water striking wall causing other injury [POA]
[5th] W16.9 Jumping or diving into unspecified water
[7th] W16.91 Jumping or diving into unspecified water causing drowning and submersion [POA]
[7th] W16.92 Jumping or diving into unspecified water causing other injury [POA]

Unspecified Code Other Specified Code Manifestation Code [N] Newborn [P] Pediatric [M] Maternity [A] Adult ♂ Male ♀ Female
● New Code ▲ Revised Code Title ►◄ Revised Text NOTES INCLUDES EXCLUDES1 Not coded here EXCLUDES2 Not included here
[4th] 4th character required [5th] 5th character required [6th] 6th character required [7th] 7th character required [7th] Extension 'X' Alert
[HAC] Hospital-acquired condition (HAC) alert AHA AHA Coding Clinic© ☛ Code first alert

W17 **Other fall from** one level to another
The appropriate 7th character is to be added to each code from category W17
> A = initial encounter
> D = subsequent encounter
> S = sequela
- W17.0 **Fall into** well
- W17.1 **Fall into** storm drain or manhole
- W17.2 **Fall into** hole
> Fall into pit
- W17.3 **Fall into** empty swimming pool
> EXCLUDES1 *fall into filled swimming pool (W16.0-)*
- W17.4 **Fall from** dock
- W17.8 **Other fall from** one level to another
  - W17.81 **Fall down** embankment (hill)
  - W17.82 **Fall from (out of)** grocery cart
  > Fall due to grocery cart tipping over
  - W17.89 **Other fall from** one level to another
  > **AHA:** Q2 2015
  > Fall from cherry picker
  > Fall from lifting device
  > Fall from mobile elevated work platform [MEWP]
  > Fall from sky lift

W18 **Other** slipping, tripping and stumbling and falls
The appropriate 7th character is to be added to each code from category W18
> A = initial encounter
> D = subsequent encounter
> S = sequela
- W18.0 **Fall due to** bumping against object
> Striking against object with subsequent fall
> EXCLUDES1 *fall on same level due to slipping, tripping, or stumbling with subsequent striking against object (W01.1-)*
  - W18.00 **Striking against** unspecified object with subsequent fall
  - W18.01 **Striking against** sports equipment with subsequent fall
  - W18.02 **Striking against** glass with subsequent fall
  - W18.09 **Striking against** other object with subsequent fall
- W18.1 **Fall from or off** toilet
  - W18.11 **Fall from or off toilet** without subsequent striking against object
  > Fall from (off) toilet NOS
  - W18.12 **Fall from or off toilet** with subsequent striking against object
- W18.2 **Fall in (into)** shower or empty bathtub
> EXCLUDES1 *fall in full bathtub causing drowning or submersion (W16.21-)*
- W18.3 **Other and unspecified** fall on same level
  - W18.30 **Fall on same level, unspecified**
  - W18.31 **Fall on same level due to** stepping on an object
  > Fall on same level due to stepping on an animal
  > EXCLUDES1 *slipping, tripping and stumbling without fall due to stepping on animal (W18.41)*
  - W18.39 **Other fall on same level**
- W18.4 **Slipping, tripping and stumbling** without falling
> EXCLUDES1 *collision with another person without fall (W51)*
  - W18.40 **Slipping, tripping and stumbling without falling, unspecified**
  - W18.41 **Slipping, tripping and stumbling without falling due to** stepping on object
  > Slipping, tripping and stumbling without falling due to stepping on animal
  > EXCLUDES1 *slipping, tripping and stumbling with fall due to stepping on animal (W18.31)*
  - W18.42 **Slipping, tripping and stumbling without falling due to** stepping into hole or opening
  - W18.43 **Slipping, tripping and stumbling without falling due to** stepping from one level to another

- W18.49 **Other slipping, tripping and stumbling without falling**

W19 **Unspecified fall**
AHA: Q4 2012
Accidental fall NOS
The appropriate 7th character is to be added to code W19
> A = initial encounter
> D = subsequent encounter
> S = sequela

Exposure to inanimate mechanical forces (W20-W49)

> EXCLUDES1 *assault (X92-Y09)*
> *contact or collision with animals or persons (W50-W64)*
> *exposure to inanimate mechanical forces involving military or war operations (Y36.-, Y37.-)*
> *intentional self-harm (X71-X83)*

W20 **Struck by thrown, projected or falling object**
☞ Code first any associated:
cataclysm (X34-X39)
lightning strike (T75.00)
> EXCLUDES1 *falling object in machinery accident (W24, W28-W31)*
> *falling object in transport accident (V01-V99)*
> *object set in motion by explosion (W35-W40)*
> *object set in motion by firearm (W32-W34)*
> *struck by thrown sports equipment (W21.-)*

The appropriate 7th character is to be added to each code from category W20
> A = initial encounter
> D = subsequent encounter
> S = sequela
- W20.0 **Struck by** falling object in cave-in
> EXCLUDES2 *asphyxiation due to cave-in (T71.21)*
- W20.1 **Struck by** object due to collapse of building
> EXCLUDES1 *struck by object due to collapse of burning building (X00.2, X02.2)*
- W20.8 **Other cause of strike by** thrown, projected or falling object
> EXCLUDES1 *struck by thrown sports equipment (W21.-)*

W21 **Striking against or struck by** sports equipment
> EXCLUDES1 *assault with sports equipment (Y08.0-)*
> *striking against or struck by subsequent fall (W18.01)*

The appropriate 7th character is to be added to each code from category W21
> A = initial encounter
> D = subsequent encounter
> S = sequela
- W21.0 **Struck by** hit or thrown ball
  - W21.00 **Struck by hit or thrown ball, unspecified type**
  - W21.01 **Struck by** football
  - W21.02 **Struck by** soccer ball
  - W21.03 **Struck by** baseball
  - W21.04 **Struck by** golf ball
  - W21.05 **Struck by** basketball
  - W21.06 **Struck by** volleyball
  - W21.07 **Struck by** softball
  - W21.09 **Struck by** other hit or thrown ball
- W21.1 **Struck by** bat, racquet or club
  - W21.11 **Struck by** baseball bat
  - W21.12 **Struck by** tennis racquet
  - W21.13 **Struck by** golf club
  - W21.19 **Struck by** other bat, racquet or club
- W21.2 **Struck by** hockey stick or puck
  - W21.21 **Struck by** hockey stick
    - W21.210 **Struck by** ice hockey stick
    - W21.211 **Struck by** field hockey stick
  - W21.22 **Struck by** hockey puck
    - W21.220 **Struck by** ice hockey puck
    - W21.221 **Struck by** field hockey puck

PDxR Unacceptable principal diagnosis symbol per Medicare code edits   POA Code exempt from diagnosis present on admission requirement
? Questionable admission   cc Complication or comorbidity   MCC Major complication or comorbidity   cc-MCC Excl CC/MCC exclusion
HCC HCC diagnosis code   RxHCC RxHCC diagnosis code   MACRA code   **DEFINITION** Describes condition/terminology
TIP Coding guidance   ◉ Official Guideline Reference   Z Z code as first-listed diagnosis

1216   When symbols appear on a code that requires a 7th character extension, refer to Appendix B to identify applicable 7th character codes.   **2020 ICD-10-CM**

5ᵗʰ W21.3 Struck by sports foot wear

   7ᵗʰ W21.31 Struck by shoe cleats   POA

     Stepped on by shoe cleats

   7ᵗʰ W21.32 Struck by skate blades   POA

     Skated over by skate blades

   7ᵗʰ W21.39 Struck by other sports foot wear   POA

7ᵗʰ W21.4 Striking against diving board   POA

   Use additional code for subsequent falling into water, if applicable (W16.-)

5ᵗʰ W21.8 Striking against or struck by other sports equipment

   7ᵗʰ W21.81 Striking against or struck by football helmet   POA

   7ᵗʰ W21.89 Striking against or struck by other sports equipment   POA

7ᵗʰ W21.9 Striking against or struck by unspecified sports equipment   POA

4ᵗʰ W22 Striking against or struck by other objects

   EXCLUDES1 striking against or struck by object with subsequent fall (W18.09)

   The appropriate 7th character is to be added to each code from category W22

     A = initial encounter

     D = subsequent encounter

     S = sequela

  5ᵗʰ W22.0 Striking against stationary object

   EXCLUDES1 striking against stationary sports equipment (W21.8)

   7ᵗʰ W22.01 Walked into wall   POA

   7ᵗʰ W22.02 Walked into lamppost   POA

   7ᵗʰ W22.03 Walked into furniture   POA

   6ᵗʰ W22.04 Striking against wall of swimming pool

     7ᵗʰ W22.041 Striking against wall of swimming pool causing drowning and submersion   POA

       EXCLUDES1 drowning and submersion while swimming without striking against wall (W67)

     7ᵗʰ W22.042 Striking against wall of swimming pool causing other injury   POA

   7ᵗʰ W22.09 Striking against other stationary object   POA

  5ᵗʰ W22.1 Striking against or struck by automobile airbag

   7ᵗʰ W22.10 Striking against or struck by unspecified automobile airbag   POA

   7ᵗʰ W22.11 Striking against or struck by driver side **automobile airbag**   POA

   7ᵗʰ W22.12 Striking against or struck by front passenger side **automobile airbag**   POA

   7ᵗʰ W22.19 Striking against or struck by other automobile airbag   POA

  7ᵗʰ W22.8 Striking against or struck by other objects   POA

   Striking against or struck by object NOS

   EXCLUDES1 struck by thrown, projected or falling object (W20.-)

4ᵗʰ W23 Caught, crushed, jammed or pinched in or between objects

   EXCLUDES1 injury caused by cutting or piercing instruments (W25-W27)

     injury caused by firearms malfunction (W32.1, W33.1-, W34.1-)

     injury caused by lifting and transmission devices (W24.-)

     injury caused by machinery (W28-W31)

     injury caused by nonpowered hand tools (W27.-)

     injury caused by transport vehicle being used as a means of transportation (V01-V99)

     injury caused by struck by thrown, projected or falling object (W20.-)

   The appropriate 7th character is to be added to each code from category W23

     A = initial encounter

     D = subsequent encounter

     S = sequela

  7ᵗʰ W23.0 Caught, crushed, jammed, or pinched between moving objects

  7ᵗʰ W23.1 Caught, crushed, jammed, or pinched between stationary objects

4ᵗʰ W24 Contact with lifting and transmission devices, not elsewhere classified

   EXCLUDES1 transport accidents (V01-V99)

   The appropriate 7th character is to be added to each code from category W24

     A = initial encounter

     D = subsequent encounter

     S = sequela

  7ᵗʰ W24.0 Contact with lifting **devices, not elsewhere classified**   POA

   Contact with chain hoist

   Contact with drive belt

   Contact with pulley (block)

  7ᵗʰ W24.1 Contact with transmission **devices, not elsewhere classified**   POA

   Contact with transmission belt or cable

7ᵗʰ W25 Contact with sharp glass

  ☛ **Code first** any associated:

   injury due to flying glass from explosion or firearm discharge (W32-W40)

   transport accident (V00-V99)

   EXCLUDES1 fall on same level due to slipping, tripping and stumbling with subsequent striking against sharp glass ▶(W01.110)◀

     striking against sharp glass with subsequent fall (W18.02)

   EXCLUDES2 glass embedded in skin (W45)

   The appropriate 7th character is to be added to code W25

     A = initial encounter

     D = subsequent encounter

     S = sequela

4ᵗʰ W26 Contact with other sharp objects

   EXCLUDES2 sharp object(s) embedded in skin (W45)

   The appropriate 7th character is to be added to each code from category W26

     A = initial encounter

     D = subsequent encounter

     S = sequela

  7ᵗʰ W26.0 Contact with knife

   EXCLUDES1 contact with electric knife (W29.1)

  7ᵗʰ W26.1 Contact with sword or dagger   POA

  7ᵗʰ W26.2 Contact with edge of stiff paper   POA

   AHA: Q4 2016

   Paper cut

  7ᵗʰ W26.8 Contact with other sharp object(s), not elsewhere classified   POA

   AHA: Q4 2016

   Contact with tin can lid

  7ᵗʰ W26.9 Contact with unspecified sharp object(s)   POA

   AHA: Q4 2016

4ᵗʰ W27 Contact with nonpowered hand tool

   The appropriate 7th character is to be added to each code from category W27

     A = initial encounter

     D = subsequent encounter

     S = sequela

  7ᵗʰ W27.0 Contact with workbench tool   POA

   Contact with auger

   Contact with axe

   Contact with chisel

   Contact with handsaw

   Contact with screwdriver

  7ᵗʰ W27.1 Contact with garden tool   POA

   Contact with hoe

   Contact with nonpowered lawn mower

   Contact with pitchfork

   Contact with rake

  7ᵗʰ W27.2 Contact with scissors   POA

  7ᵗʰ W27.3 Contact with needle (sewing)   POA

   EXCLUDES1 contact with hypodermic needle (W46.-)

  7ᵗʰ W27.4 Contact with kitchen utensil   POA

   Contact with fork

   Contact with ice-pick

   Contact with can-opener NOS

Unspecified Code   Other Specified Code   Manifestation Code   **N** Newborn   **P** Pediatric   **M** Maternity   **A** Adult   ♂ Male   ♀ Female
● New Code   ▲ Revised Code Title   ▶◀ Revised Text   **NOTES**   *INCLUDES*   *EXCLUDES1* Not coded here   *EXCLUDES2* Not included here
   4ᵗʰ 4ᵗʰ character required   **5ᵗʰ** 5ᵗʰ character required   **6ᵗʰ** 6ᵗʰ character required   **7ᵗʰ** 7ᵗʰ character required   Extension 'X' Alert
   HAC Hospital-acquired condition (HAC) alert   **AHA** AHA Coding Clinic©   ☛ Code first alert

[7th] **W27.5 Contact with paper-cutter** [POA]

[7th] **W27.8 Contact with other nonpowered hand tool** [POA]
Contact with nonpowered sewing machine
Contact with shovel

[7th] **W28 Contact with powered lawn mower** [POA]
Powered lawn mower (commercial) (residential)
[EXCLUDES1] *contact with nonpowered lawn mower (W27.1)*
[EXCLUDES2] *exposure to electric current (W86.-)*
The appropriate 7th character is to be added to code W28
A = initial encounter
D = subsequent encounter
S = sequela

[4th] **W29 Contact with other powered hand tools and household machinery**
[EXCLUDES1] *contact with commercial machinery (W31.82)*
contact with hot household appliance (X15)
contact with nonpowered hand tool (W27.-)
exposure to electric current (W86)
The appropriate 7th character is to be added to each code from category W29
A = initial encounter
D = subsequent encounter
S = sequela

[7th] **W29.0 Contact with powered kitchen appliance** [POA]
Contact with blender
Contact with can-opener
Contact with garbage disposal
Contact with mixer

[7th] **W29.1 Contact with electric knife** [POA]

[7th] **W29.2 Contact with other powered household machinery** [POA]
Contact with electric fan
Contact with powered dryer (clothes) (powered) (spin)
Contact with washing-machine
Contact with sewing machine

[7th] **W29.3 Contact with powered garden and outdoor hand tools and machinery** [POA]
Contact with chainsaw
Contact with edger
Contact with garden cultivator (tiller)
Contact with hedge trimmer
Contact with other powered garden tool
[EXCLUDES1] *contact with powered lawn mower (W28)*

[7th] **W29.4 Contact with nail gun** [POA]

[7th] **W29.8 Contact with other powered hand tools and household machinery** [POA]
Contact with do-it-yourself tool NOS

[4th] **W30 Contact with agricultural machinery**
[INCLUDES] *animal-powered farm machine*
[EXCLUDES1] *agricultural transport vehicle accident (V01-V99)*
explosion of grain store (W40.8)
exposure to electric current (W86.-)
The appropriate 7th character is to be added to each code from category W30
A = initial encounter
D = subsequent encounter
S = sequela

[7th] **W30.0 Contact with combine harvester** [POA]
Contact with reaper
Contact with thresher

[7th] **W30.1 Contact with power take-off devices (PTO)** [POA]

[7th] **W30.2 Contact with hay derrick** [POA]

[7th] **W30.3 Contact with grain storage elevator** [POA]
[EXCLUDES1] *explosion of grain store (W40.8)*

[5th] **W30.8 Contact with other specified agricultural machinery**

[7th] **W30.81 Contact with agricultural transport vehicle in stationary use** [POA]
Contact with agricultural transport vehicle under repair, not on public roadway
[EXCLUDES1] *agricultural transport vehicle accident (V01-V99)*

[7th] **W30.89 Contact with other specified agricultural machinery** [POA]

[7th] **W30.9 Contact with unspecified agricultural machinery** [POA]
Contact with farm machinery NOS

[4th] **W31 Contact with other and unspecified machinery**
[EXCLUDES1] *contact with agricultural machinery (W30.-)*
contact with machinery in transport under own power or being towed by a vehicle (V01-V99)
exposure to electric current (W86)
The appropriate 7th character is to be added to each code from category W31
A = initial encounter
D = subsequent encounter
S = sequela

[7th] **W31.0 Contact with mining and earth-drilling machinery** [POA]
Contact with bore or drill (land) (seabed)
Contact with shaft hoist
Contact with shaft lift
Contact with undercutter

[7th] **W31.1 Contact with metalworking machines** [POA]
Contact with abrasive wheel
Contact with forging machine
Contact with lathe
Contact with mechanical shears
Contact with metal drilling machine
Contact with milling machine
Contact with power press
Contact with rolling-mill
Contact with metal sawing machine

[7th] **W31.2 Contact with powered woodworking and forming machines** [POA]
Contact with band saw
Contact with bench saw
Contact with circular saw
Contact with molding machine
Contact with overhead plane
Contact with powered saw
Contact with radial saw
Contact with sander
[EXCLUDES1] *nonpowered woodworking tools (W27.0)*

[7th] **W31.3 Contact with prime movers** [POA]
Contact with gas turbine
Contact with internal combustion engine
Contact with steam engine
Contact with water driven turbine

[5th] **W31.8 Contact with other specified machinery**

[7th] **W31.81 Contact with recreational machinery** [POA]
Contact with roller coaster

[7th] **W31.82 Contact with other commercial machinery** [POA]
Contact with commercial electric fan
Contact with commercial kitchen appliances
Contact with commercial powered dryer (clothes) (powered) (spin)
Contact with commercial washing-machine
Contact with commercial sewing machine
[EXCLUDES1] *contact with household machinery (W29.-)*
contact with powered lawn mower (W28)

[7th] **W31.83 Contact with special construction vehicle in stationary use** [POA]
Contact with special construction vehicle under repair, not on public roadway
[EXCLUDES1] *special construction vehicle accident (V01-V99)*

[7th] **W31.89 Contact with other specified machinery** [POA]

[7th] **W31.9 Contact with unspecified machinery** [POA]
Contact with machinery NOS

[4th] **W32 Accidental handgun discharge and malfunction**
[INCLUDES] *accidental discharge and malfunction of gun for single hand use*
accidental discharge and malfunction of pistol
accidental discharge and malfunction of revolver
Handgun discharge and malfunction NOS

[PDx] Unacceptable principal diagnosis symbol per Medicare code edits [POA] Code exempt from diagnosis present on admission requirement
[?] Questionable admission [CC] Complication or comorbidity [MCC] Major complication or comorbidity [CC/MCC Exc] CC/MCC exclusion
[HCC] HCC diagnosis code [RxHCC] RxHCC diagnosis code MACRA code **DEFINITION** Describes condition/terminology
TIP Coding guidance 👁 Official Guideline Reference [Z] Z code as first-listed diagnosis

 When symbols appear on a code that requires a 7th character extension, refer to Appendix B to identify applicable 7th character codes.

EXCLUDES1 *accidental airgun discharge and malfunction (W34.010, W34.110)*

accidental BB gun discharge and malfunction (W34.010, W34.110)

accidental pellet gun discharge and malfunction (W34.010, W34.110)

accidental shotgun discharge and malfunction (W33.01, W33.11)

assault by handgun discharge (X93)

handgun discharge involving legal intervention (Y35.0-)

handgun discharge involving military or war operations (Y36.4-)

intentional self-harm by handgun discharge (X72)

Very pistol discharge and malfunction (W34.09, W34.19)

The appropriate 7th character is to be added to each code from category W32

    A = initial encounter

    D = subsequent encounter

    S = sequela

- W32.0 **Accidental handgun** discharge   POA
- W32.1 **Accidental handgun** malfunction   POA
  - Injury due to explosion of handgun (parts)
  - Injury due to malfunction of mechanism or component of handgun
  - Injury due to recoil of handgun
  - Powder burn from handgun

W33 **Accidental** rifle, shotgun and larger firearm **discharge and malfunction**

    INCLUDES   *rifle, shotgun and larger firearm discharge and malfunction NOS*

    EXCLUDES1 *accidental airgun discharge and malfunction (W34.010, W34.110)*

accidental BB gun discharge and malfunction (W34.010, W34.110)

accidental handgun discharge and malfunction (W32.-)

accidental pellet gun discharge and malfunction (W34.010, W34.110)

assault by rifle, shotgun and larger firearm discharge (X94)

firearm discharge involving legal intervention (Y35.0-)

firearm discharge involving military or war operations (Y36.4-)

intentional self-harm by rifle, shotgun and larger firearm discharge (X73)

The appropriate 7th character is to be added to each code from category W33

    A = initial encounter

    D = subsequent encounter

    S = sequela

- W33.0 **Accidental rifle, shotgun and larger firearm** discharge
  - W33.00 **Accidental discharge of unspecified larger firearm**   POA
    - Discharge of unspecified larger firearm NOS
  - W33.01 **Accidental discharge of** shotgun   POA
    - Discharge of shotgun NOS
  - W33.02 **Accidental discharge of** hunting rifle   POA
    - Discharge of hunting rifle NOS
  - W33.03 **Accidental discharge of** machine gun   POA
    - Discharge of machine gun NOS
  - W33.09 **Accidental discharge of other larger firearm**   POA
    - Discharge of other larger firearm NOS
- W33.1 **Accidental rifle, shotgun and larger firearm** malfunction
  - Injury due to explosion of rifle, shotgun and larger firearm (parts)
  - Injury due to malfunction of mechanism or component of rifle, shotgun and larger firearm
  - Injury due to piercing, cutting, crushing or pinching due to (by) slide trigger mechanism, scope or other gun part
  - Injury due to recoil of rifle, shotgun and larger firearm
  - Powder burn from rifle, shotgun and larger firearm
  - W33.10 **Accidental malfunction of unspecified larger firearm**   POA
    - Malfunction of unspecified larger firearm NOS

- W33.11 **Accidental malfunction of** shotgun   POA
  - Malfunction of shotgun NOS
- W33.12 **Accidental malfunction of** hunting rifle   POA
  - Malfunction of hunting rifle NOS
- W33.13 **Accidental malfunction of** machine gun   POA
  - Malfunction of machine gun NOS
- W33.19 **Accidental malfunction of other larger firearm**   POA
  - Malfunction of other larger firearm NOS

W34 **Accidental discharge and malfunction from** other and unspecified **firearms and guns**

The appropriate 7th character is to be added to each code from category W34

    A = initial encounter

    D = subsequent encounter

    S = sequela

- W34.0 **Accidental discharge from other and unspecified** firearms and guns
  - W34.00 **Accidental discharge from unspecified firearms or gun**   POA
    - **AHA:** Q1 2015
    - Discharge from firearm NOS
    - Gunshot wound NOS
    - Shot NOS
  - W34.01 **Accidental discharge of** gas, air or spring-operated guns
    - W34.010 **Accidental discharge of** airgun   POA
      - Accidental discharge of BB gun
      - Accidental discharge of pellet gun
    - W34.011 **Accidental discharge of** paintball gun   POA
      - Accidental injury due to paintball discharge
    - W34.018 **Accidental discharge of other gas, air or spring-operated gun**   POA
  - W34.09 **Accidental discharge from other specified firearms**   POA
    - Accidental discharge from Very pistol [flare]
- W34.1 **Accidental** malfunction **from** other and unspecified **firearms and guns**
  - W34.10 **Accidental malfunction from unspecified firearms or gun**   POA
    - Firearm malfunction NOS
  - W34.11 **Accidental malfunction of** gas, air or spring-operated guns
    - W34.110 **Accidental malfunction of airgun**   POA
      - Accidental malfunction of BB gun
      - Accidental malfunction of pellet gun
    - W34.111 **Accidental malfunction of** paintball gun   POA
      - Accidental injury due to paintball gun malfunction
    - W34.118 **Accidental malfunction of other gas, air or spring-operated gun**   POA
  - W34.19 **Accidental malfunction from other specified firearms**   POA
    - Accidental malfunction from Very pistol [flare]

W35 **Explosion and rupture of** boiler   POA

    EXCLUDES1 *explosion and rupture of boiler on watercraft (V93.4)*

The appropriate 7th character is to be added to code W35

    A = initial encounter

    D = subsequent encounter

    S = sequela

W36 **Explosion and rupture of** gas cylinder

The appropriate 7th character is to be added to each code from category W36

    A = initial encounter

    D = subsequent encounter

    S = sequela

- W36.1 **Explosion and rupture of** aerosol can   POA
- W36.2 **Explosion and rupture of** air tank   POA
- W36.3 **Explosion and rupture of** pressurized-gas tank   POA
- W36.8 **Explosion and rupture of** other gas cylinder   POA
- W36.9 **Explosion and rupture of** unspecified gas cylinder   POA

Unspecified Code   Other Specified Code   Manifestation Code   N Newborn   P Pediatric   M Maternity   A Adult   ♂ Male   ♀ Female

● New Code   ▲ Revised Code Title   ►◄ Revised Text   NOTES   INCLUDES   EXCLUDES1 Not coded here   EXCLUDES2 Not included here

4th character required   5th character required   6th character required   7th character required   Extension 'X' Alert

HAC Hospital-acquired condition (HAC) alert   AHA AHA Coding Clinic©   📖 Code first alert

🔟 W37 **Explosion and rupture of** pressurized tire, pipe or hose
  The appropriate 7th character is to be added to each code from category W37
    A = initial encounter
    D = subsequent encounter
    S = sequela
  7️⃣ W37.0 **Explosion of** bicycle tire   POA
  7️⃣ W37.8 **Explosion and rupture of other pressurized tire,
       pipe or hose**   POA

7️⃣ W38 **Explosion and rupture of other specified pressurized devices**   POA
  The appropriate 7th character is to be added to code W38
    A = initial encounter
    D = subsequent encounter
    S = sequela

🔟 W39 **Discharge of** firework   POA
  The appropriate 7th character is to be added to code W39
    A = initial encounter
    D = subsequent encounter
    S = sequela

🔟 W40 **Explosion of** other materials
  EXCLUDES1 *assault by explosive material (X96)*
              explosion involving legal intervention (Y35.1-)
              explosion involving military or war operations (Y36.0-, Y36.2-)
              intentional self-harm by explosive material (X75)
  The appropriate 7th character is to be added to each code from category W40
    A = initial encounter
    D = subsequent encounter
    S = sequela
  7️⃣ W40.0 **Explosion of** blasting material   POA
       Explosion of blasting cap
       Explosion of detonator
       Explosion of dynamite
       Explosion of explosive (any) used in blasting operations
  7️⃣ W40.1 **Explosion of** explosive gases   POA
       Explosion of acetylene
       Explosion of butane
       Explosion of coal gas
       Explosion in mine NOS
       Explosion of explosive gas
       Explosion of fire damp
       Explosion of gasoline fumes
       Explosion of methane
       Explosion of propane
  7️⃣ W40.8 **Explosion of other specified explosive materials**   POA
       Explosion in dump NOS
       Explosion in factory NOS
       Explosion in grain store
       Explosion in munitions
       EXCLUDES1 *explosion involving legal intervention (Y35.1-)*
                   *explosion involving military or war operations
                   (Y36.0-, Y36.2-)*
  7️⃣ W40.9 **Explosion of unspecified explosive materials**   POA
       Explosion NOS

🔟 W42 **Exposure to** noise
  The appropriate 7th character is to be added to each code from category W42
    A = initial encounter
    D = subsequent encounter
    S = sequela
  7️⃣ W42.0 **Exposure to** supersonic waves   POA
  7️⃣ W42.9 **Exposure to other noise**   POA
       Exposure to sound waves NOS

🔟 W45 **Foreign body or object** entering through skin
  INCLUDES *foreign body or object embedded in skin*
             nail embedded in skin
  EXCLUDES2 *contact with hand tools (nonpowered) (powered) (W27-W29)*
              contact with other sharp object(s) (W26.-)
              contact with sharp glass (W25.-)
              struck by objects (W20-W22)

The appropriate 7th character is to be added to each code from category W45
    A = initial encounter
    D = subsequent encounter
    S = sequela
  7️⃣ W45.0 **Nail** entering through skin   POA
  7️⃣ W45.8 **Other foreign body or object entering through skin**
       Splinter in skin NOS

🔟 W46 **Contact with hypodermic needle**
  The appropriate 7th character is to be added to each code from category W46
    A = initial encounter
    D = subsequent encounter
    S = sequela
  7️⃣ W46.0 **Contact with** hypodermic **needle**
       Hypodermic needle stick NOS
  7️⃣ W46.1 **Contact with** contaminated hypodermic **needle**

🔟 W49 **Exposure to** other inanimate mechanical forces
  INCLUDES *exposure to abnormal gravitational [G] forces*
             exposure to inanimate mechanical forces NEC
  EXCLUDES1 *exposure to inanimate mechanical forces involving military
              or war operations (Y36.-, Y37.-)*
  The appropriate 7th character is to be added to each code from category W49
    A = initial encounter
    D = subsequent encounter
    S = sequela
  5️⃣ W49.0 Item **causing external constriction**
    7️⃣ W49.01 Hair **causing external constriction**   POA
    7️⃣ W49.02 String or thread **causing external constriction**   POA
    7️⃣ W49.03 Rubber band **causing external constriction**   POA
    7️⃣ W49.04 **Ring or other jewelry causing external
         constriction**   POA
    7️⃣ W49.09 **Other specified item causing external
         constriction**   POA
  7️⃣ W49.9 **Exposure to other inanimate mechanical forces**   POA

Exposure to animate mechanical forces (W50-W64)

  EXCLUDES1 *Toxic effect of contact with venomous animals and plants (T63.-)*
🔟 W50 **Accidental hit, strike, kick, twist, bite or scratch by another person**
  INCLUDES *hit, strike, kick, twist, bite, or scratch by another person NOS*
  EXCLUDES1 *assault by bodily force (Y04)*
              struck by objects (W20-W22)
  The appropriate 7th character is to be added to each code from category W50
    A = initial encounter
    D = subsequent encounter
    S = sequela
  7️⃣ W50.0 **Accidental** hit or strike **by another person**
       Hit or strike by another person NOS
  7️⃣ W50.1 **Accidental** kick **by another person**
       Kick by another person NOS
  7️⃣ W50.2 **Accidental** twist **by another person**
       AHA: Q1 2015
       Twist by another person NOS
  7️⃣ W50.3 **Accidental** bite **by another person**
       Human bite
       Bite by another person NOS
  7️⃣ W50.4 **Accidental** scratch **by another person**
       Scratch by another person NOS
🔟 W51 **Accidental** striking against or bumped **into by another person**
  EXCLUDES1 *assault by striking against or bumping into by another
              person (Y04.2)*
              fall due to collision with another person (W03)
  The appropriate 7th character is to be added to code W51
    A = initial encounter
    D = subsequent encounter
    S = sequela

PDXN Unacceptable principal diagnosis symbol per Medicare code edits   POA Code exempt from diagnosis present on admission requirement
❓ Questionable admission   CC Complication or comorbidity   MCC Major complication or comorbidity   CC/MCC Ex CC/MCC exclusion
HCC HCC diagnosis code   RXHCC RxHCC diagnosis code   MACRA code   **DEFINITION** Describes condition/terminology
TIP Coding guidance   👁 Official Guideline Reference   Z Z code as first-listed diagnosis

7th W52 **Crushed, pushed or stepped on by crowd or human stampede** POA
  Crushed, pushed or stepped on by crowd or human stampede with or without fall
  The appropriate 7th character is to be added to code W52
    A = initial encounter
    D = subsequent encounter
    S = sequela

4th W53 **Contact with** rodent
  INCLUDES   *contact with saliva, feces or urine of rodent*
  The appropriate 7th character is to be added to each code from category W53
    A = initial encounter
    D = subsequent encounter
    S = sequela
  5th W53.0 **Contact with** mouse
    7th W53.01 Bitten **by mouse** POA
    7th W53.09 **Other contact with mouse** POA
  5th W53.1 **Contact with** rat
    7th W53.11 Bitten **by rat** POA
    7th W53.19 **Other contact with rat** POA
  5th W53.2 **Contact with** squirrel
    7th W53.21 Bitten **by squirrel** POA
    7th W53.29 **Other contact with squirrel** POA
  5th W53.8 **Contact with** other rodent
    7th W53.81 **Bitten by other rodent** POA
    7th W53.89 **Other contact with other rodent** POA

4th W54 **Contact with** dog
  INCLUDES   *contact with saliva, feces or urine of dog*
  The appropriate 7th character is to be added to each code from category W54
    A = initial encounter
    D = subsequent encounter
    S = sequela
  7th W54.0 Bitten **by dog** POA
    AHA: Q4 2018
  7th W54.1 Struck **by dog** POA
    Knocked over by dog
  7th W54.8 **Other contact with dog** POA

4th W55 **Contact with** other mammals
  INCLUDES   *contact with saliva, feces or urine of mammal*
  EXCLUDES1 *animal being ridden- see transport accidents*
    bitten or struck by dog (W54)
    bitten or struck by rodent (W53.-)
    contact with marine mammals (W56.-)
  The appropriate 7th character is to be added to each code from category W55
    A = initial encounter
    D = subsequent encounter
    S = sequela
  5th W55.0 **Contact with** cat
    7th W55.01 Bitten **by cat** POA
    7th W55.03 Scratched **by cat** POA
    7th W55.09 **Other contact with cat** POA
  5th W55.1 **Contact with** horse
    7th W55.11 Bitten **by horse** POA
    7th W55.12 Struck **by horse** POA
    7th W55.19 **Other contact with horse** POA
  5th W55.2 **Contact with** cow
    Contact with bull
    7th W55.21 Bitten **by cow** POA
    7th W55.22 Struck **by cow** POA
      Gored by bull
    7th W55.29 **Other contact with cow** POA
  5th W55.3 **Contact with** other hoof stock
    Contact with goats
    Contact with sheep
    7th W55.31 Bitten **by other hoof stock** POA

7th W55.32 Struck **by other hoof stock** POA
  Gored by goat
  Gored by ram
7th W55.39 **Other contact with other hoof stock** POA
5th W55.4 **Contact with** pig
  7th W55.41 Bitten **by pig** POA
  7th W55.42 Struck **by pig** POA
  7th W55.49 **Other contact with pig** POA
5th W55.5 **Contact with** raccoon
  7th W55.51 Bitten **by raccoon** POA
  7th W55.52 Struck **by raccoon** POA
  7th W55.59 **Other contact with raccoon** POA
5th W55.8 **Contact with** other mammals
  7th W55.81 Bitten **by other mammals** POA
  7th W55.82 Struck **by other mammals** POA
  7th W55.89 **Other contact with other mammals** POA

4th W56 **Contact with** nonvenomous marine animal
  EXCLUDES1 *contact with venomous marine animal (T63.-)*
  The appropriate 7th character is to be added to each code from category W56
    A = initial encounter
    D = subsequent encounter
    S = sequela
  5th W56.0 **Contact with** dolphin
    7th W56.01 Bitten **by dolphin** POA
    7th W56.02 Struck **by dolphin** POA
    7th W56.09 **Other contact with dolphin** POA
  5th W56.1 **Contact with** sea lion
    7th W56.11 Bitten **by sea lion** POA
    7th W56.12 Struck **by sea lion** POA
    7th W56.19 **Other contact with sea lion** POA
  5th W56.2 **Contact with** orca
    Contact with killer whale
    7th W56.21 Bitten **by orca** POA
    7th W56.22 Struck **by orca** POA
    7th W56.29 **Other contact with orca** POA
  5th W56.3 **Contact with** other marine mammals
    7th W56.31 Bitten **by other marine mammals** POA
    7th W56.32 Struck **by other marine mammals** POA
    7th W56.39 **Other contact with other marine mammals** POA
  5th W56.4 **Contact with** shark
    7th W56.41 Bitten **by shark** POA
    7th W56.42 Struck **by shark** POA
    7th W56.49 **Other contact with shark** POA
  5th W56.5 **Contact with** other fish
    7th W56.51 Bitten **by other fish** POA
    7th W56.52 Struck **by other fish** POA
    7th W56.59 **Other contact with other fish** POA
  5th W56.8 **Contact with** other nonvenomous marine animals
    7th W56.81 Bitten **by other nonvenomous marine animals** POA
    7th W56.82 Struck **by other nonvenomous marine animals** POA
    7th W56.89 **Other contact with other nonvenomous marine animals** POA

7th W57 **Bitten or stung by nonvenomous** insect and other nonvenomous arthropods POA
  EXCLUDES1 *contact with venomous insects and arthropods (T63.2-, T63.3-, T63.4-)*
  The appropriate 7th character is to be added to code W57
    A = initial encounter
    D = subsequent encounter
    S = sequela

4th W58 **Contact with** crocodile or alligator
  The appropriate 7th character is to be added to each code from category W58
    A = initial encounter
    D = subsequent encounter
    S = sequela
  5th W58.0 **Contact with** alligator
    7th W58.01 Bitten **by alligator** POA

Unspecified Code   Other Specified Code   Manifestation Code   N Newborn   P Pediatric   M Maternity   A Adult   ♂ Male   ♀ Female
● New Code   ▲ Revised Code Title   ►◄ Revised Text   **NOTES**   *INCLUDES*   *EXCLUDES1* Not coded here   *EXCLUDES2* Not included here
4th 4th character required   5th 5th character required   6th 6th character required   7th 7th character required   Extension 'X' Alert
HAC Hospital-acquired condition (HAC) alert   **AHA** AHA Coding Clinic©   ☛ Code first alert

W58.02 Struck by alligator POA

W58.03 Crushed by alligator POA

W58.09 Other contact with alligator POA

W58.1 Contact with crocodile

W58.11 Bitten by crocodile POA

W58.12 Struck by crocodile POA

W58.13 Crushed by crocodile POA

W58.19 Other contact with crocodile POA

W59 Contact with other nonvenomous reptiles

EXCLUDES1 contact with venomous reptile (T63.0-, T63.1-)

The appropriate 7th character is to be added to each code from category W59

A = initial encounter

D = subsequent encounter

S = sequela

W59.0 Contact with nonvenomous lizards

W59.01 Bitten by nonvenomous lizards POA

W59.02 Struck by nonvenomous lizards POA

W59.09 Other contact with nonvenomous lizards POA

Exposure to nonvenomous lizards

W59.1 Contact with nonvenomous snakes

W59.11 Bitten by nonvenomous snake POA

W59.12 Struck by nonvenomous snake POA

W59.13 Crushed by nonvenomous snake POA

W59.19 Other contact with nonvenomous snake POA

W59.2 Contact with turtles

EXCLUDES1 contact with tortoises (W59.8-)

W59.21 Bitten by turtle POA

W59.22 Struck by turtle POA

W59.29 Other contact with turtle POA

Exposure to turtles

W59.8 Contact with other nonvenomous reptiles

W59.81 Bitten by other nonvenomous reptiles POA

W59.82 Struck by other nonvenomous reptiles POA

W59.83 Crushed by other nonvenomous reptiles POA

W59.89 Other contact with other nonvenomous reptiles POA

W60 Contact with nonvenomous plant thorns and spines and sharp leaves POA

EXCLUDES1 Contact with venomous plants (T63.7-)

The appropriate 7th character is to be added to code W60

A = initial encounter

D = subsequent encounter

S = sequela

W61 Contact with birds (domestic) (wild)

INCLUDES contact with excreta of birds

The appropriate 7th character is to be added to each code from category W61

A = initial encounter

D = subsequent encounter

S = sequela

W61.0 Contact with parrot

W61.01 Bitten by parrot POA

W61.02 Struck by parrot POA

W61.09 Other contact with parrot POA

Exposure to parrots

W61.1 Contact with macaw

W61.11 Bitten by macaw POA

W61.12 Struck by macaw POA

W61.19 Other contact with macaw POA

Exposure to macaws

W61.2 Contact with other psittacines

W61.21 Bitten by other psittacines POA

W61.22 Struck by other psittacines POA

W61.29 Other contact with other psittacines POA

Exposure to other psittacines

W61.3 Contact with chicken

W61.32 Struck by chicken POA

W61.33 Pecked by chicken POA

W61.39 Other contact with chicken POA

Exposure to chickens

W61.4 Contact with turkey

W61.42 Struck by turkey POA

W61.43 Pecked by turkey POA

W61.49 Other contact with turkey POA

W61.5 Contact with goose

W61.51 Bitten by goose POA

W61.52 Struck by goose POA

W61.59 Other contact with goose POA

W61.6 Contact with duck

W61.61 Bitten by duck POA

W61.62 Struck by duck POA

W61.69 Other contact with duck POA

W61.9 Contact with other birds

W61.91 Bitten by other birds POA

W61.92 Struck by other birds POA

W61.99 Other contact with other birds POA

Contact with bird NOS

W62 Contact with nonvenomous amphibians

EXCLUDES1 contact with venomous amphibians (T63.81-R63.83)

The appropriate 7th character is to be added to each code from category W62

A = initial encounter

D = subsequent encounter

S = sequela

W62.0 Contact with nonvenomous frogs POA

W62.1 Contact with nonvenomous toads POA

W62.9 Contact with other nonvenomous amphibians POA

W64 Exposure to other animate mechanical forces

INCLUDES exposure to nonvenomous animal NOS

EXCLUDES1 contact with venomous animal (T63.-)

The appropriate 7th character is to be added to code W64

A = initial encounter

D = subsequent encounter

S = sequela

Accidental non-transport drowning and submersion (W65-W74)

EXCLUDES1 accidental drowning and submersion due to fall into water (W16.-)

accidental drowning and submersion due to water transport accident (V90.-, V92.-)

EXCLUDES2 accidental drowning and submersion due to cataclysm (X34-X39)

W65 Accidental drowning and submersion while in bath-tub POA

EXCLUDES1 accidental drowning and submersion due to fall in (into) bathtub (W16.211)

The appropriate 7th character is to be added to code W65

A = initial encounter

D = subsequent encounter

S = sequela

W67 Accidental drowning and submersion while in swimming-pool POA

EXCLUDES1 accidental drowning and submersion due to fall into swimming pool (W16.011, W16.021, W16.031)

accidental drowning and submersion due to striking into wall of swimming pool (W22.041)

The appropriate 7th character is to be added to code W67

A = initial encounter

D = subsequent encounter

S = sequela

W69 Accidental drowning and submersion while in natural water POA

Accidental drowning and submersion while in lake

Accidental drowning and submersion while in open sea

Accidental drowning and submersion while in river

Accidental drowning and submersion while in stream

EXCLUDES1 accidental drowning and submersion due to fall into natural body of water (W16.111, W16.121, W16.131)

The appropriate 7th character is to be added to code W69

A = initial encounter

D = subsequent encounter

S = sequela

POA Unacceptable principal diagnosis symbol per Medicare code edits   POA Code exempt from diagnosis present on admission requirement
? Questionable admission   CC Complication or comorbidity   MCC Major complication or comorbidity   CC/MCC CC/MCC exclusion
HCC HCC diagnosis code   RxHCC RxHCC diagnosis code   MACRA MACRA code   DEFINITION Describes condition/terminology
TIP Coding guidance   👁 Official Guideline Reference   Z Z code as first-listed diagnosis

[7th] **W73 Other specified cause of accidental non-transport drowning and submersion** [POA]
Accidental drowning and submersion while in quenching tank
Accidental drowning and submersion while in reservoir
EXCLUDES1 *accidental drowning and submersion due to fall into other water (W16.311, W16.321, W16.331)*
The appropriate 7th character is to be added to code W73
A = initial encounter
D = subsequent encounter
S = sequela

[7th] **W74 Unspecified cause of accidental drowning and submersion** [POA]
Drowning NOS
The appropriate 7th character is to be added to code W74
A = initial encounter
D = subsequent encounter
S = sequela

Exposure to electric current, radiation and extreme ambient air temperature and pressure (W85-W99)

EXCLUDES1 *exposure to:*
failure in dosage of radiation or temperature during surgical and medical care (Y63.2-Y63.5)
lightning (T75.0-)
natural cold (X31)
natural heat (X30)
natural radiation NOS (X39)
radiological procedure and radiotherapy (Y84.2)
sunlight (X32)

[7th] **W85 Exposure to electric transmission lines** [POA]
Broken power line
The appropriate 7th character is to be added to code W85
A = initial encounter
D = subsequent encounter
S = sequela

[4th] **W86 Exposure to other specified electric current**
The appropriate 7th character is to be added to each code from category W86
A = initial encounter
D = subsequent encounter
S = sequela

[7th] **W86.0 Exposure to domestic wiring and appliances** [POA]
[7th] **W86.1 Exposure to industrial wiring, appliances and electrical machinery** [POA]
Exposure to conductors
Exposure to control apparatus
Exposure to electrical equipment and machinery
Exposure to transformers
[7th] **W86.8 Exposure to other electric current** [POA]
Exposure to wiring and appliances in or on farm (not farmhouse)
Exposure to wiring and appliances outdoors
Exposure to wiring and appliances in or on public building
Exposure to wiring and appliances in or on residential institutions
Exposure to wiring and appliances in or on schools

[4th] **W88 Exposure to ionizing radiation**
EXCLUDES1 *exposure to sunlight (X32)*
The appropriate 7th character is to be added to each code from category W88
A = initial encounter
D = subsequent encounter
S = sequela

[7th] **W88.0 Exposure to X-rays** [POA]
[7th] **W88.1 Exposure to radioactive isotopes** [POA]
[7th] **W88.8 Exposure to other ionizing radiation** [POA]

[4th] **W89 Exposure to man-made visible and ultraviolet light**
INCLUDES *exposure to welding light (arc)*
EXCLUDES1 *exposure to sunlight (X32)*
The appropriate 7th character is to be added to each code from category W89
A = initial encounter
D = subsequent encounter
S = sequela

[7th] **W89.0 Exposure to welding light (arc)** [POA]
[7th] **W89.1 Exposure to tanning bed** [POA]
[7th] **W89.8 Exposure to other man-made visible and ultraviolet light** [POA]
[7th] **W89.9 Exposure to unspecified man-made visible and ultraviolet light** [POA]

[4th] **W90 Exposure to other nonionizing radiation**
EXCLUDES1 *exposure to sunlight (X32)*
The appropriate 7th character is to be added to each code from category W90
A = initial encounter
D = subsequent encounter
S = sequela

[7th] **W90.0 Exposure to radiofrequency** [POA]
[7th] **W90.1 Exposure to infrared radiation** [POA]
[7th] **W90.2 Exposure to laser radiation** [POA]
[7th] **W90.8 Exposure to other nonionizing radiation** [POA]

[7th] **W92 Exposure to excessive heat of man-made origin** [POA]
The appropriate 7th character is to be added to code W92
A = initial encounter
D = subsequent encounter
S = sequela

[4th] **W93 Exposure to excessive cold of man-made origin**
The appropriate 7th character is to be added to each code from category W93
A = initial encounter
D = subsequent encounter
S = sequela

[5th] **W93.0 Contact with or inhalation of dry ice**
[7th] **W93.01 Contact with dry ice** [POA]
[7th] **W93.02 Inhalation of dry ice** [POA]
[5th] **W93.1 Contact with or inhalation of liquid air**
[7th] **W93.11 Contact with liquid air** [POA]
Contact with liquid hydrogen
Contact with liquid nitrogen
[7th] **W93.12 Inhalation of liquid air** [POA]
Inhalation of liquid hydrogen
Inhalation of liquid nitrogen
[7th] **W93.2 Prolonged exposure in deep freeze unit or refrigerator** [POA]
[7th] **W93.8 Exposure to other excessive cold of man-made origin** [POA]

[4th] **W94 Exposure to high and low air pressure and changes in air pressure**
The appropriate 7th character is to be added to each code from category W94
A = initial encounter
D = subsequent encounter
S = sequela

[7th] **W94.0 Exposure to prolonged high air pressure** [POA]
[5th] **W94.1 Exposure to prolonged low air pressure**
[7th] **W94.11 Exposure to residence or prolonged visit at high altitude** [POA]
[7th] **W94.12 Exposure to other prolonged low air pressure** [POA]
[5th] **W94.2 Exposure to rapid changes in air pressure during ascent**
[7th] **W94.21 Exposure to reduction in atmospheric pressure while surfacing from deep-water diving** [POA]
[7th] **W94.22 Exposure to reduction in atmospheric pressure while surfacing from underground** [POA]
[7th] **W94.23 Exposure to sudden change in air pressure in aircraft during ascent** [POA]
[7th] **W94.29 Exposure to other rapid changes in air pressure during ascent** [POA]

Unspecified Code Other Specified Code Manifestation Code [N] Newborn [P] Pediatric [M] Maternity [A] Adult ♂ Male ♀ Female
● New Code ▲ Revised Code Title ►◄ Revised Text NOTES INCLUDES EXCLUDES1 Not coded here EXCLUDES2 Not included here
[4th] 4th character required [5th] 5th character required [6th] 6th character required [7th] 7th character required [x] Extension 'X' Alert
[HAC] Hospital-acquired condition (HAC) alert AHA AHA Coding Clinic© ☞ Code first alert

🔟 W94.3 Exposure to rapid changes in air pressure during descent
    7️⃣ W94.31 Exposure to sudden change in air pressure in aircraft during descent ᴘᴏᴬ
    7️⃣ W94.32 Exposure to high air pressure from rapid descent in water ᴘᴏᴬ
    7️⃣ W94.39 Exposure to other rapid changes in air pressure during descent ᴘᴏᴬ

7️⃣ W99 Exposure to other man-made environmental factors
The appropriate 7th character is to be added to code W99
  A = initial encounter
  D = subsequent encounter
  S = sequela

Exposure to smoke, fire and flames (X00-X08)

EXCLUDES1 arson (X97)
EXCLUDES2 explosions (W35-W40)
    lightning (T75.0-)
    transport accident (V01-V99)

4️⃣ X00 Exposure to uncontrolled fire in building or structure
  INCLUDES conflagration in building or structure
  ☞ Code first any associated cataclysm
  EXCLUDES2 Exposure to ignition or melting of nightwear (X05)
    Exposure to ignition or melting of other clothing and apparel (X06.-)
    Exposure to other specified smoke, fire and flames (X08.-)
The appropriate 7th character is to be added to each code from category X00
  A = initial encounter
  D = subsequent encounter
  S = sequela
  7️⃣ X00.0 Exposure to flames in uncontrolled fire in building or structure
    AHA: Q2 2016, Q1 2015
  7️⃣ X00.1 Exposure to smoke in uncontrolled fire in building or structure
  7️⃣ X00.2 Injury due to collapse of burning building or structure in uncontrolled fire
    EXCLUDES1 injury due to collapse of building not on fire (W20.1)
  7️⃣ X00.3 Fall from burning building or structure in uncontrolled fire
  7️⃣ X00.4 Hit by object from burning building or structure in uncontrolled fire
  7️⃣ X00.5 Jump from burning building or structure in uncontrolled fire
  7️⃣ X00.8 Other exposure to uncontrolled fire in building or structure

4️⃣ X01 Exposure to uncontrolled fire, not in building or structure
  INCLUDES exposure to forest fire
The appropriate 7th character is to be added to each code from category X01
  A = initial encounter
  D = subsequent encounter
  S = sequela
  7️⃣ X01.0 Exposure to flames in uncontrolled fire, not in building or structure
  7️⃣ X01.1 Exposure to smoke in uncontrolled fire, not in building or structure
  7️⃣ X01.3 Fall due to uncontrolled fire, not in building or structure
  7️⃣ X01.4 Hit by object due to uncontrolled fire, not in building or structure
  7️⃣ X01.8 Other exposure to uncontrolled fire, not in building or structure

4️⃣ X02 Exposure to controlled fire in building or structure
  INCLUDES exposure to fire in fireplace
    exposure to fire in stove
The appropriate 7th character is to be added to each code from category X02
  A = initial encounter
  D = subsequent encounter
  S = sequela
  7️⃣ X02.0 Exposure to flames in controlled fire in building or structure ᴘᴏᴬ

7️⃣ X02.1 Exposure to smoke in controlled fire in building or structure ᴘᴏᴬ
7️⃣ X02.2 Injury due to collapse of burning building or structure in controlled fire ᴘᴏᴬ
  EXCLUDES1 injury due to collapse of building not on fire (W20.1)
7️⃣ X02.3 Fall from burning building or structure in controlled fire ᴘᴏᴬ
7️⃣ X02.4 Hit by object from burning building or structure in controlled fire ᴘᴏᴬ
7️⃣ X02.5 Jump from burning building or structure in controlled fire ᴘᴏᴬ
7️⃣ X02.8 Other exposure to controlled fire in building or structure ᴘᴏᴬ

4️⃣ X03 Exposure to controlled fire, not in building or structure
  INCLUDES exposure to bon fire
    exposure to camp-fire
    exposure to trash fire
The appropriate 7th character is to be added to each code from category X03
  A = initial encounter
  D = subsequent encounter
  S = sequela
  7️⃣ X03.0 Exposure to flames in controlled fire, not in building or structure ᴘᴏᴬ
    AHA: Q1 2015
  7️⃣ X03.1 Exposure to smoke in controlled fire, not in building or structure ᴘᴏᴬ
  7️⃣ X03.3 Fall due to controlled fire, not in building or structure ᴘᴏᴬ
  7️⃣ X03.4 Hit by object due to controlled fire, not in building or structure ᴘᴏᴬ
  7️⃣ X03.8 Other exposure to controlled fire, not in building or structure ᴘᴏᴬ

7️⃣ X04 Exposure to ignition of highly flammable material ᴘᴏᴬ
  AHA: Q2 2017
  Exposure to ignition of gasoline
  Exposure to ignition of kerosene
  Exposure to ignition of petrol
  EXCLUDES2 exposure to ignition or melting of nightwear (X05)
    exposure to ignition or melting of other clothing and apparel (X06)
The appropriate 7th character is to be added to code X04
  A = initial encounter
  D = subsequent encounter
  S = sequela

7️⃣ X05 Exposure to ignition or melting of nightwear
  EXCLUDES2 exposure to uncontrolled fire in building or structure (X00.-)
    exposure to uncontrolled fire, not in building or structure (X01.-)
    exposure to controlled fire in building or structure (X02.-)
    exposure to controlled fire, not in building or structure (X03.-)
    exposure to ignition of highly flammable materials (X04.-)
The appropriate 7th character is to be added to code X05
  A = initial encounter
  D = subsequent encounter
  S = sequela

4️⃣ X06 Exposure to ignition or melting of other clothing and apparel
  EXCLUDES2 exposure to uncontrolled fire in building or structure (X00.-)
    exposure to uncontrolled fire, not in building or structure (X01.-)
    exposure to controlled fire in building or structure (X02.-)
    exposure to controlled fire, not in building or structure (X03.-)
    exposure to ignition of highly flammable materials (X04.-)
The appropriate 7th character is to be added to each code from category X06
  A = initial encounter
  D = subsequent encounter
  S = sequela
  7️⃣ X06.0 Exposure to ignition of plastic jewelry
  7️⃣ X06.1 Exposure to melting of plastic jewelry
  7️⃣ X06.2 Exposure to ignition of other clothing and apparel
  7️⃣ X06.3 Exposure to melting of other clothing and apparel

---

ᴘᴏᴬ Unacceptable principal diagnosis symbol per Medicare code edits   ᴘᴏᴬ Code exempt from diagnosis present on admission requirement
❓ Questionable admission   ᶜᶜ Complication or comorbidity   ᴹᶜᶜ Major complication or comorbidity   ᶜᶜ/ᴹᶜᶜ ᴇˣᶜ CC/MCC exclusion
HCC HCC diagnosis code   RxHCC RxHCC diagnosis code   MACRA code   **DEFINITION** Describes condition/terminology
TIP Coding guidance   👁 Official Guideline Reference   Z1 Z code as first-listed diagnosis

[4th] **X08 Exposure to other specified smoke, fire and flames**
The appropriate 7th character is to be added to each code from category X08
A = initial encounter
D = subsequent encounter
S = sequela

[5th] **X08.0 Exposure to bed fire**
Exposure to mattress fire
[7th] **X08.00 Exposure to bed fire due to unspecified burning material**
[7th] **X08.01 Exposure to bed fire due to burning cigarette**
AHA: Q1 2015
[7th] **X08.09 Exposure to bed fire due to other burning material**

[5th] **X08.1 Exposure to sofa fire**
[7th] **X08.10 Exposure to sofa fire due to unspecified burning material**
[7th] **X08.11 Exposure to sofa fire due to burning cigarette**
[7th] **X08.19 Exposure to sofa fire due to other burning material**

[5th] **X08.2 Exposure to other furniture fire**
[7th] **X08.20 Exposure to other furniture fire due to unspecified burning material**
[7th] **X08.21 Exposure to other furniture fire due to burning cigarette**
[7th] **X08.29 Exposure to other furniture fire due to other burning material**

[7th] **X08.8 Exposure to other specified smoke, fire and flames**

Contact with heat and hot substances (X10-X19)

[EXCLUDES1] *exposure to excessive natural heat (X30)*
exposure to fire and flames (X00-X08)

[4th] **X10 Contact with hot drinks, food, fats and cooking oils**
The appropriate 7th character is to be added to each code from category X10
A = initial encounter
D = subsequent encounter
S = sequela
[7th] **X10.0 Contact with hot drinks**
[7th] **X10.1 Contact with hot food**
[7th] **X10.2 Contact with fats and cooking oils**

[4th] **X11 Contact with hot tap-water**
[INCLUDES] *contact with boiling tap-water*
contact with boiling water NOS
[EXCLUDES1] *contact with water heated on stove (X12)*
The appropriate 7th character is to be added to each code from category X11
A = initial encounter
D = subsequent encounter
S = sequela
[7th] **X11.0 Contact with hot water in bath or tub**
[EXCLUDES1] *contact with running hot water in bath or tub (X11.1)*
[7th] **X11.1 Contact with running hot water**
Contact with hot water running out of hose
Contact with hot water running out of tap
[7th] **X11.8 Contact with other hot tap-water**
Contact with hot water in bucket
Contact with hot tap-water NOS

[7th] **X12 Contact with other hot fluids**
Contact with water heated on stove
[EXCLUDES1] *hot (liquid) metals (X18)*
The appropriate 7th character is to be added to code X12
A = initial encounter
D = subsequent encounter
S = sequela

[4th] **X13 Contact with steam and other hot vapors**
The appropriate 7th character is to be added to each code from category X13
A = initial encounter
D = subsequent encounter
S = sequela
[7th] **X13.0 Inhalation of steam and other hot vapors**
[7th] **X13.1 Other contact with steam and other hot vapors**

[4th] **X14 Contact with hot air and other hot gases**
The appropriate 7th character is to be added to each code from category X14
A = initial encounter
D = subsequent encounter
S = sequela
[7th] **X14.0 Inhalation of hot air and gases**
[7th] **X14.1 Other contact with hot air and other hot gases**

[4th] **X15 Contact with hot household appliances**
[EXCLUDES1] *contact with heating appliances (X16)*
contact with powered household appliances (W29.-)
exposure to controlled fire in building or structure due to household appliance (X02.8)
exposure to household appliances electrical current (W86.0)
The appropriate 7th character is to be added to each code from category X15
A = initial encounter
D = subsequent encounter
S = sequela
[7th] **X15.0 Contact with hot stove (kitchen)**
[7th] **X15.1 Contact with hot toaster**
[7th] **X15.2 Contact with hotplate**
[7th] **X15.3 Contact with hot saucepan or skillet**
[7th] **X15.8 Contact with other hot household appliances**
Contact with cooker
Contact with kettle
Contact with light bulbs

[7th] **X16 Contact with hot heating appliances, radiators and pipes**
[EXCLUDES1] *contact with powered appliances (W29.-)*
exposure to controlled fire in building or structure due to appliance (X02.8)
exposure to industrial appliances electrical current (W86.1)
The appropriate 7th character is to be added to code X16
A = initial encounter
D = subsequent encounter
S = sequela

[7th] **X17 Contact with hot engines, machinery and tools**
[EXCLUDES1] *contact with hot heating appliances, radiators and pipes (X16)*
contact with hot household appliances (X15)
The appropriate 7th character is to be added to code X17
A = initial encounter
D = subsequent encounter
S = sequela

[7th] **X18 Contact with other hot metals**
Contact with liquid metal
The appropriate 7th character is to be added to code X18
A = initial encounter
D = subsequent encounter
S = sequela

[7th] **X19 Contact with other heat and hot substances**
[EXCLUDES1] *objects that are not normally hot, e.g., an object made hot by a house fire (X00-X08)*
The appropriate 7th character is to be added to code X19
A = initial encounter
D = subsequent encounter
S = sequela

Exposure to forces of nature (X30-X39)

[7th] **X30 Exposure to excessive natural heat** [POA]
👁 **See Official Guidelines** "Other External Causes of Morbidity Code Issues" I.B.19.c
AHA: Q4 2018
Exposure to excessive heat as the cause of sunstroke
Exposure to heat NOS

EXCLUDES1 *excessive heat of man-made origin (W92)*
      exposure to man-made radiation (W89)
      exposure to sunlight (X32)
      exposure to tanning bed (W89)

The appropriate 7th character is to be added to code X30
  A = initial encounter
  D = subsequent encounter
  S = sequela

X31 Exposure to excessive natural cold
  See Official Guidelines "Use of Z codes" I.B.19.d
  AHA: Q4 2018
  Excessive cold as the cause of chilblains NOS
  Excessive cold as the cause of immersion foot or hand
  Exposure to cold NOS
  Exposure to weather conditions
  EXCLUDES1 *cold of man-made origin (W93.-)*
      contact with or inhalation of dry ice (W93.-)
      contact with or inhalation of liquefied gas (W93.-)

The appropriate 7th character is to be added to code X31
  A = initial encounter
  D = subsequent encounter
  S = sequela

X32 Exposure to sunlight
  EXCLUDES1 *man-made radiation (tanning bed) (W89)*
  EXCLUDES2 *radiation-related disorders of the skin and subcutaneous tissue (L55-L59)*

The appropriate 7th character is to be added to code X32
  A = initial encounter
  D = subsequent encounter
  S = sequela

X34 Earthquake
  EXCLUDES2 *tidal wave (tsunami) due to earthquake (X37.41)*

The appropriate 7th character is to be added to code X34
  A = initial encounter
  D = subsequent encounter
  S = sequela

X35 Volcanic eruption
  EXCLUDES2 *tidal wave (tsunami) due to volcanic eruption (X37.41)*

The appropriate 7th character is to be added to code X35
  A = initial encounter
  D = subsequent encounter
  S = sequela

X36 Avalanche, landslide and other earth movements
  INCLUDES *victim of mudslide of cataclysmic nature*
  EXCLUDES1 *earthquake (X34)*
  EXCLUDES2 *transport accident involving collision with avalanche or landslide not in motion (V01-V99)*

The appropriate 7th character is to be added to each code from category X36
  A = initial encounter
  D = subsequent encounter
  S = sequela

  X36.0 Collapse of dam or man-made structure causing earth movement
    See Official Guidelines "Sequencing of External Causes of Morbidity Codes" I.B.19.b
    AHA: Q4 2018
  X36.1 Avalanche, landslide, or mudslide

X37 Cataclysmic storm
The appropriate 7th character is to be added to each code from category X37
  A = initial encounter
  D = subsequent encounter
  S = sequela

  X37.0 Hurricane
    See Official Guidelines "Sequencing of External Causes of Morbidity Codes" I.B.19.b, "Other External Causes of Morbidity Code Issues" I.B.19.c
    AHA: Q4 2018
    Storm surge
    Typhoon

  X37.1 Tornado
    Cyclone
    Twister
  X37.2 Blizzard (snow)(ice)
  X37.3 Dust storm
  X37.4 Tidal wave
    X37.41 Tidal wave due to earthquake or volcanic eruption
      Tidal wave NOS
      Tsunami
    X37.42 Tidal wave due to storm
    X37.43 Tidal wave due to landslide
  X37.8 Other cataclysmic storms
    Cloudburst
    Torrential rain
    EXCLUDES2 *flood (X38)*
  X37.9 Unspecified cataclysmic storm
    Storm NOS
    EXCLUDES1 *collapse of dam or man-made structure causing earth movement (X36.0)*

X38 Flood
  See Official Guidelines "Sequencing of External Causes of Morbidity Codes" I.B.19.b
  AHA: Q4 2018
  Flood arising from remote storm
  Flood of cataclysmic nature arising from melting snow
  Flood resulting directly from storm
  EXCLUDES1 *collapse of dam or man-made structure causing earth movement (X36.0)*
      tidal wave NOS (X37.41)
      tidal wave caused by storm (X37.42)

The appropriate 7th character is to be added to code X38
  A = initial encounter
  D = subsequent encounter
  S = sequela

X39 Exposure to other forces of nature
The appropriate 7th character is to be added to each code from category X39
  A = initial encounter
  D = subsequent encounter
  S = sequela

  X39.0 Exposure to natural radiation
    EXCLUDES1 *contact with and (suspected) exposure to radon and other naturally occurring radiation (Z77.123)*
      exposure to man-made radiation (W88-W90)
      exposure to sunlight (X32)
    X39.01 Exposure to radon
    X39.08 Exposure to other natural radiation
  X39.8 Other exposure to forces of nature

Overexertion and strenuous or repetitive movements (X50)

X50 Overexertion and strenuous or repetitive movements
The appropriate 7th character is to be added to each code from category X50
  A = initial encounter
  D = subsequent encounter
  S = sequela

  X50.0 Overexertion from strenuous movement or load
    AHA: Q4 2016
    Lifting heavy objects
    Lifting weights
  X50.1 Overexertion from prolonged static or awkward postures
    Prolonged bending
    Prolonged kneeling
    Prolonged reaching
    Prolonged sitting
    Prolonged standing
    Prolonged twisting
    Static bending
    Static kneeling

Unacceptable principal diagnosis symbol per Medicare code edits   Code exempt from diagnosis present on admission requirement
? Questionable admission   Complication or comorbidity   MCC Major complication or comorbidity   CC/MCC CC/MCC exclusion
HCC HCC diagnosis code   RxHCC RxHCC diagnosis code   MACRA code   **DEFINITION** Describes condition/terminology
TIP Coding guidance   Official Guideline Reference   Z Z code as first-listed diagnosis

Static reaching
Static sitting
Static standing
Static twisting

🗇 **X50.3 Overexertion from** repetitive **movements** POA
AHA: Q4 2016
Use of hand as hammer
EXCLUDES2 *Overuse from prolonged static or awkward postures (X50.1)*

🗇 **X50.9 Other and unspecified overexertion or strenuous movements or** postures POA
Contact pressure
Contact stress

Accidental exposure to other specified factors (X52-X58)

🗇 **X52 Prolonged stay in weightless environment** POA
Weightlessness in spacecraft (simulator)
The appropriate 7th character is to be added to code X52
A = initial encounter
D = subsequent encounter
S = sequela

🗇 **X58 Exposure to other specified factors**
Accident NOS
Exposure NOS
The appropriate 7th character is to be added to code X58
A = initial encounter
D = subsequent encounter
S = sequela

Intentional self-harm (X71-X83)

Purposely self-inflicted injury
Suicide (attempted)

🔵 **X71 Intentional self-harm by** drowning and submersion
The appropriate 7th character is to be added to each code from category X71
A = initial encounter
D = subsequent encounter
S = sequela

🗇 **X71.0 Intentional self-harm by drowning and submersion** while in bathtub HCC

🗇 **X71.1 Intentional self-harm by drowning and submersion** while in swimming pool POA HCC

🗇 **X71.2 Intentional self-harm by drowning and submersion** after jump into swimming pool POA HCC

🗇 **X71.3 Intentional self-harm by drowning and submersion in** natural water POA HCC

🗇 **X71.8 Other intentional self-harm by drowning and submersion** POA HCC

🗇 **X71.9 Intentional self-harm by drowning and submersion, unspecified** POA HCC

🗇 **X72 Intentional self-harm by** handgun discharge POA HCC
Intentional self-harm by gun for single hand use
Intentional self-harm by pistol
Intentional self-harm by revolver
EXCLUDES1 *Very pistol (X74.8)*
The appropriate 7th character is to be added to code X72
A = initial encounter
D = subsequent encounter
S = sequela

🔵 **X73 Intentional self-harm by rifle, shotgun and larger firearm discharge**
EXCLUDES1 *airgun (X74.01)*
The appropriate 7th character is to be added to each code from category X73
A = initial encounter
D = subsequent encounter
S = sequela

🗇 **X73.0 Intentional self-harm by** shotgun discharge POA HCC
🗇 **X73.1 Intentional self-harm by** hunting rifle discharge POA HCC
🗇 **X73.2 Intentional self-harm by** machine gun discharge POA HCC

🗇 **X73.8 Intentional self-harm by other larger firearm discharge** POA HCC
🗇 **X73.9 Intentional self-harm by unspecified larger firearm discharge** POA HCC

🔵 **X74 Intentional self-harm by** other and unspecified **firearm and gun discharge**
The appropriate 7th character is to be added to each code from category X74
A = initial encounter
D = subsequent encounter
S = sequela

🔵 **X74.0 Intentional self-harm by** gas, air or spring-operated guns

🗇 **X74.01 Intentional self-harm by** airgun POA HCC
Intentional self-harm by BB gun discharge
Intentional self-harm by pellet gun discharge

🗇 **X74.02 Intentional self-harm by** paintball gun POA HCC

🗇 **X74.09 Intentional self-harm by other gas, air or spring-operated gun** POA HCC

🗇 **X74.8 Intentional self-harm by other firearm discharge** POA HCC
Intentional self-harm by Very pistol [flare] discharge

🗇 **X74.9 Intentional self-harm by unspecified firearm discharge** POA HCC

🔵 **X75 Intentional self-harm by** explosive material POA HCC
The appropriate 7th character is to be added to code X75
A = initial encounter
D = subsequent encounter
S = sequela

🔵 **X76 Intentional self-harm by** smoke, fire and flames POA HCC
The appropriate 7th character is to be added to code X76
A = initial encounter
D = subsequent encounter
S = sequela

🔵 **X77 Intentional self-harm by** steam, hot vapors and hot objects
The appropriate 7th character is to be added to each code from category X77
A = initial encounter
D = subsequent encounter
S = sequela

🗇 **X77.0 Intentional self-harm by** steam or hot vapors POA HCC
🗇 **X77.1 Intentional self-harm by** hot tap water POA HCC
🗇 **X77.2 Intentional self-harm by other hot fluids** POA HCC
🗇 **X77.3 Intentional self-harm by** hot household appliances POA HCC
🗇 **X77.8 Intentional self-harm by other hot objects** POA HCC
🗇 **X77.9 Intentional self-harm by unspecified hot objects** POA HCC

🔵 **X78 Intentional self-harm by** sharp object
The appropriate 7th character is to be added to each code from category X78
A = initial encounter
D = subsequent encounter
S = sequela

🗇 **X78.0 Intentional self-harm by** sharp glass HCC
🗇 **X78.1 Intentional self-harm by** knife HCC
🗇 **X78.2 Intentional self-harm by** sword or dagger HCC
🗇 **X78.8 Intentional self-harm by other sharp object** HCC
🗇 **X78.9 Intentional self-harm by unspecified sharp object** HCC

🔵 **X79 Intentional self-harm by** blunt object HCC
The appropriate 7th character is to be added to code X79
A = initial encounter
D = subsequent encounter
S = sequela

🗇 **X80 Intentional self-harm by** jumping from a high place HCC
Intentional fall from one level to another
The appropriate 7th character is to be added to code X80
A = initial encounter
D = subsequent encounter
S = sequela

🔵 **X81 Intentional self-harm by** jumping or lying in front of moving object
The appropriate 7th character is to be added to each code from category X81
A = initial encounter
D = subsequent encounter
S = sequela

Unspecified Code Other Specified Code Manifestation Code N Newborn P Pediatric M Maternity A Adult ♂ Male ♀ Female
● New Code ▲ Revised Code Title ▶◀ Revised Text **NOTES** *INCLUDES* *EXCLUDES1* Not coded here *EXCLUDES2* Not included here
4️⃣ 4th character required 5️⃣ 5th character required 6️⃣ 6th character required 7️⃣ 7th character required 🗇 Extension 'X' Alert
HAC Hospital-acquired condition (HAC) alert **AHA** AHA Coding Clinic© 📌 Code first alert

🔹 X81.0 Intentional self-harm by jumping or lying in front of motor vehicle POA HCC

🔹 X81.1 Intentional self-harm by jumping or lying in front of (subway) train POA HCC

🔹 X81.8 Intentional self-harm by jumping or lying in front of other moving object POA HCC

🔹 X82 Intentional self-harm by crashing of motor vehicle

The appropriate 7th character is to be added to each code from category X82
    A = initial encounter
    D = subsequent encounter
    S = sequela

🔹 X82.0 Intentional collision of motor vehicle with other motor vehicle POA HCC

🔹 X82.1 Intentional collision of motor vehicle with train POA HCC

🔹 X82.2 Intentional collision of motor vehicle with tree POA HCC

🔹 X82.8 Other intentional self-harm by crashing of motor vehicle POA HCC

🔹 X83 Intentional self-harm by other specified means

EXCLUDES1 intentional self-harm by poisoning or contact with toxic substance- See Table of Drugs and Chemicals

The appropriate 7th character is to be added to each code from category X83
    A = initial encounter
    D = subsequent encounter
    S = sequela

🔹 X83.0 Intentional self-harm by crashing of aircraft POA HCC

🔹 X83.1 Intentional self-harm by electrocution POA HCC

🔹 X83.2 Intentional self-harm by exposure to extremes of cold POA HCC

🔹 X83.8 Intentional self-harm by other specified means POA HCC

Assault (X92-Y09)

INCLUDES homicide
    injuries inflicted by another person with intent to injure or kill, by any means

EXCLUDES1 injuries due to legal intervention (Y35.-)
    injuries due to operations of war (Y36.-)
    injuries due to terrorism (Y38.-)

🔹 X92 Assault by drowning and submersion

The appropriate 7th character is to be added to each code from category X92
    A = initial encounter
    D = subsequent encounter
    S = sequela

🔹 X92.0 Assault by drowning and submersion while in bathtub POA

🔹 X92.1 Assault by drowning and submersion while in swimming pool POA

🔹 X92.2 Assault by drowning and submersion after push into swimming pool POA

🔹 X92.3 Assault by drowning and submersion in natural water POA

🔹 X92.8 Other assault by drowning and submersion POA

🔹 X92.9 Assault by drowning and submersion, unspecified POA

🔹 X93 Assault by handgun discharge
    Assault by discharge of gun for single hand use
    Assault by discharge of pistol
    Assault by discharge of revolver
    EXCLUDES1 Very pistol (X95.8)

The appropriate 7th character is to be added to code X93
    A = initial encounter
    D = subsequent encounter
    S = sequela

🔹 X94 Assault by rifle, shotgun and larger firearm discharge
    EXCLUDES1 airgun (X95.01)

The appropriate 7th character is to be added to each code from category X94
    A = initial encounter
    D = subsequent encounter
    S = sequela

🔹 X94.0 Assault by shotgun POA

🔹 X94.1 Assault by hunting rifle POA

🔹 X94.2 Assault by machine gun POA

🔹 X94.8 Assault by other larger firearm discharge POA

🔹 X94.9 Assault by unspecified larger firearm discharge POA

🔹 X95 Assault by other and unspecified firearm and gun discharge

The appropriate 7th character is to be added to each code from category X95
    A = initial encounter
    D = subsequent encounter
    S = sequela

🔹 X95.0 Assault by gas, air or spring-operated guns

🔹 X95.01 Assault by airgun discharge POA
    Assault by BB gun discharge
    Assault by pellet gun discharge

🔹 X95.02 Assault by paintball gun discharge POA

🔹 X95.09 Assault by other gas, air or spring-operated gun POA

🔹 X95.8 Assault by other firearm discharge POA
    Assault by very pistol [flare] discharge

🔹 X95.9 Assault by unspecified firearm discharge POA
    AHA: Q3 2016

🔹 X96 Assault by explosive material

EXCLUDES1 incendiary device (X97)
    terrorism involving explosive material (Y38.2-)

The appropriate 7th character is to be added to each code from category X96
    A = initial encounter
    D = subsequent encounter
    S = sequela

🔹 X96.0 Assault by antipersonnel bomb POA
    EXCLUDES1 antipersonnel bomb use in military or war (Y36.2-)

🔹 X96.1 Assault by gasoline bomb POA

🔹 X96.2 Assault by letter bomb POA

🔹 X96.3 Assault by fertilizer bomb POA

🔹 X96.4 Assault by pipe bomb POA

🔹 X96.8 Assault by other specified explosive POA

🔹 X96.9 Assault by unspecified explosive POA

🔹 X97 Assault by smoke, fire and flames POA
    Assault by arson
    Assault by cigarettes
    Assault by incendiary device

The appropriate 7th character is to be added to code X97
    A = initial encounter
    D = subsequent encounter
    S = sequela

🔹 X98 Assault by steam, hot vapors and hot objects

The appropriate 7th character is to be added to each code from category X98
    A = initial encounter
    D = subsequent encounter
    S = sequela

🔹 X98.0 Assault by steam or hot vapors POA

🔹 X98.1 Assault by hot tap water POA

🔹 X98.2 Assault by hot fluids POA

🔹 X98.3 Assault by hot household appliances POA

🔹 X98.8 Assault by other hot objects POA

🔹 X98.9 Assault by unspecified hot objects POA

🔹 X99 Assault by sharp object

EXCLUDES1 assault by strike by sports equipment (Y08.0-)

The appropriate 7th character is to be added to each code from category X99
    A = initial encounter
    D = subsequent encounter
    S = sequela

🔹 X99.0 Assault by sharp glass POA

🔹 X99.1 Assault by knife POA

🔹 X99.2 Assault by sword or dagger POA

🔹 X99.8 Assault by other sharp object POA

🔹 X99.9 Assault by unspecified sharp object POA
    Assault by stabbing NOS

POA Unacceptable principal diagnosis symbol per Medicare code edits   POA Code exempt from diagnosis present on admission requirement
❓ Questionable admission   CC Complication or comorbidity   MCC Major complication or comorbidity   CC/MCC Excl. CC/MCC exclusion
HCC HCC diagnosis code   RxHCC RxHCC diagnosis code   MACRA code   DEFINITION Describes condition/terminology
TIP Coding guidance   👁 Official Guideline Reference   Z Z code as first-listed diagnosis

[7th] **Y00 Assault by blunt object** [POA]
[EXCLUDES1] *assault by strike by sports equipment (Y08.0-)*
The appropriate 7th character is to be added to code Y00
A = initial encounter
D = subsequent encounter
S = sequela

[7th] **Y01 Assault by pushing from high place** [POA]
The appropriate 7th character is to be added to code Y01
A = initial encounter
D = subsequent encounter
S = sequela

[4th] **Y02 Assault by pushing or placing victim in front of moving object**
The appropriate 7th character is to be added to each code from category Y02
A = initial encounter
D = subsequent encounter
S = sequela
[7th] **Y02.0 Assault by pushing or placing victim in front of motor vehicle** [POA]
[7th] **Y02.1 Assault by pushing or placing victim in front of (subway) train** [POA]
[7th] **Y02.8 Assault by pushing or placing victim in front of other moving object** [POA]

[4th] **Y03 Assault by crashing of motor vehicle**
The appropriate 7th character is to be added to each code from category Y03
A = initial encounter
D = subsequent encounter
S = sequela
[7th] **Y03.0 Assault by being hit or run over by motor vehicle** [POA]
[7th] **Y03.8 Other assault by crashing of motor vehicle** [POA]

[4th] **Y04 Assault by bodily force**
[EXCLUDES1] *assault by:*
submersion (X92.-)
use of weapon (X93-X95, X99, Y00)
The appropriate 7th character is to be added to each code from category Y04
A = initial encounter
D = subsequent encounter
S = sequela
[7th] **Y04.0 Assault by unarmed brawl or fight** [POA]
[7th] **Y04.1 Assault by human bite** [POA]
[7th] **Y04.2 Assault by strike against or bumped into by another person** [POA]
[7th] **Y04.8 Assault by other bodily force** [POA]
Assault by bodily force NOS

[4th] **Y07 Perpetrator of assault, maltreatment and neglect**
👁 **See Official Guidelines** "Child and Adult Abuse Guideline" I.C.20.g
[NOTES] Codes from this category are for use only in cases of confirmed abuse (T74.-)
Selection of the correct perpetrator code is based on the relationship between the perpetrator and the victim
INCLUDES *perpetrator of abandonment*
perpetrator of emotional neglect
perpetrator of mental cruelty
perpetrator of physical abuse
perpetrator of physical neglect
perpetrator of sexual abuse
perpetrator of torture

[5th] **Y07.0 Spouse or partner, perpetrator of maltreatment and neglect**
Spouse or partner, perpetrator of maltreatment and neglect against spouse or partner
Y07.01 Husband, perpetrator of maltreatment and neglect [POA]
Y07.02 Wife, perpetrator of maltreatment and neglect [POA]
Y07.03 Male partner, perpetrator of maltreatment and neglect [POA]
Y07.04 Female partner, perpetrator of maltreatment and neglect [POA]

[5th] **Y07.1 Parent (adoptive) (biological), perpetrator of maltreatment and neglect**
Y07.11 Biological father, perpetrator of maltreatment and neglect [POA]
Y07.12 Biological mother, perpetrator of maltreatment and neglect [POA]
Y07.13 Adoptive father, perpetrator of maltreatment and neglect [POA]
Y07.14 Adoptive mother, perpetrator of maltreatment and neglect [POA]

[5th] **Y07.4 Other family member, perpetrator of maltreatment and neglect**
[6th] **Y07.41 Sibling, perpetrator of maltreatment and neglect**
[EXCLUDES1] *stepsibling, perpetrator of maltreatment and neglect (Y07.435, Y07.436)*
Y07.410 Brother, perpetrator of maltreatment and neglect [POA]
Y07.411 Sister, perpetrator of maltreatment and neglect [POA]
[6th] **Y07.42 Foster parent, perpetrator of maltreatment and neglect**
Y07.420 Foster father, perpetrator of maltreatment and neglect [POA]
Y07.421 Foster mother, perpetrator of maltreatment and neglect [POA]
[6th] **Y07.43 Stepparent or stepsibling, perpetrator of maltreatment and neglect**
Y07.430 Stepfather, perpetrator of maltreatment and neglect [POA]
Y07.432 Male friend of parent (co-residing in household), perpetrator of maltreatment and neglect [POA]
Y07.433 Stepmother, perpetrator of maltreatment and neglect [POA]
Y07.434 Female friend of parent (co-residing in household), perpetrator of maltreatment and neglect [POA]
Y07.435 Stepbrother, perpetrator or maltreatment and neglect [POA]
Y07.436 Stepsister, perpetrator of maltreatment and neglect [POA]
[6th] **Y07.49 Other family member, perpetrator of maltreatment and neglect**
Y07.490 Male cousin, perpetrator of maltreatment and neglect [POA]
Y07.491 Female cousin, perpetrator of maltreatment and neglect [POA]
Y07.499 Other family member, perpetrator of maltreatment and neglect [POA]

[5th] **Y07.5 Non-family member, perpetrator of maltreatment and neglect**
Y07.50 Unspecified non-family member, perpetrator of maltreatment and neglect [POA]
[6th] **Y07.51 Daycare provider, perpetrator of maltreatment and neglect**
Y07.510 At-home childcare provider, perpetrator of maltreatment and neglect [POA]
Y07.511 Daycare center childcare provider, perpetrator of maltreatment and neglect [POA]
Y07.512 At-home adultcare provider, perpetrator of maltreatment and neglect [POA]
Y07.513 Adultcare center provider, perpetrator of maltreatment and neglect [POA]
Y07.519 Unspecified daycare provider, perpetrator of maltreatment and neglect [POA]
[6th] **Y07.52 Healthcare provider, perpetrator of maltreatment and neglect**
Y07.521 Mental health provider, perpetrator of maltreatment and neglect [POA]

Unspecified Code Other Specified Code Manifestation Code [N] Newborn [P] Pediatric [M] Maternity [A] Adult ♂ Male ♀ Female
● New Code ▲ Revised Code Title ►◄ Revised Text [NOTES] *INCLUDES* [EXCLUDES1] Not coded here [EXCLUDES2] Not included here
[4th] 4th character required [5th] 5th character required [6th] 6th character required [7th] 7th character required [X] Extension 'X' Alert
[HAC] Hospital-acquired condition (HAC) alert AHA AHA Coding Clinic© ☞ Code first alert

Y07.528 Other therapist or healthcare provider, **perpetrator of maltreatment and neglect** POA

Nurse perpetrator of maltreatment and neglect

Occupational therapist perpetrator of maltreatment and neglect

Physical therapist perpetrator of maltreatment and neglect

Speech therapist perpetrator of maltreatment and neglect

Y07.529 **Unspecified** healthcare provider, **perpetrator of maltreatment and neglect** POA

Y07.53 Teacher or instructor, **perpetrator of maltreatment and neglect** POA

Coach, perpetrator of maltreatment and neglect

Y07.59 Other **non-family member, perpetrator of maltreatment and neglect** POA

Y07.6 Multiple **perpetrators of maltreatment and neglect** POA

AHA: Q4 2018

Y07.9 **Unspecified perpetrator of maltreatment and neglect** POA

Y08 **Assault by** other specified **means**

The appropriate 7th character is to be added to each code from category Y08
A = initial encounter
D = subsequent encounter
S = sequela

Y08.0 **Assault by** strike by sport equipment

Y08.01 **Assault by strike by** hockey stick POA

Y08.02 **Assault by strike by** baseball bat POA

Y08.09 **Assault by strike by other specified type of sport equipment** POA

Y08.8 **Assault by** other specified **means**

Y08.81 **Assault by** crashing of aircraft POA

Y08.89 **Assault by other specified means** POA

Y09 **Assault by unspecified means**

AHA: Q4 2016

Assassination (attempted) NOS
Homicide (attempted) NOS
Manslaughter (attempted) NOS
Murder (attempted) NOS

Event of undetermined intent (Y21-Y33)

Undetermined intent is only for use when there is specific documentation in the record that the intent of the injury cannot be determined. If no such documentation is present, code to accidental (unintentional)

Y21 **Drowning and submersion, undetermined intent**

The appropriate 7th character is to be added to each code from category Y21
A = initial encounter
D = subsequent encounter
S = sequela

Y21.0 **Drowning and submersion** while in bathtub, **undetermined intent** POA

Y21.1 **Drowning and submersion** after fall into bathtub, **undetermined intent** POA

Y21.2 **Drowning and submersion** while in swimming pool, **undetermined intent** POA

Y21.3 **Drowning and submersion** after fall into swimming pool, **undetermined intent** POA

Y21.4 **Drowning and submersion** in natural water, **undetermined intent** POA

Y21.8 **Other drowning and submersion, undetermined intent** POA

Y21.9 **Unspecified drowning and submersion, undetermined intent** POA

Y22 Handgun **discharge, undetermined intent** POA

Discharge of gun for single hand use, undetermined intent
Discharge of pistol, undetermined intent
Discharge of revolver, undetermined intent
EXCLUDES2 very pistol (Y24.8)

The appropriate 7th character is to be added to code Y22
A = initial encounter
D = subsequent encounter
S = sequela

Y23 Rifle, shotgun and larger firearm **discharge, undetermined intent**

EXCLUDES2 airgun (Y24.0)

The appropriate 7th character is to be added to each code from category Y23
A = initial encounter
D = subsequent encounter
S = sequela

Y23.0 Shotgun **discharge, undetermined intent** POA

Y23.1 Hunting rifle **discharge, undetermined intent** POA

Y23.2 Military firearm **discharge, undetermined intent** POA

Y23.3 Machine gun **discharge, undetermined intent** POA

Y23.8 **Other larger firearm discharge, undetermined intent** POA

Y23.9 **Unspecified larger firearm discharge, undetermined intent** POA

Y24 Other and unspecified **firearm discharge, undetermined intent**

The appropriate 7th character is to be added to each code from category Y24
A = initial encounter
D = subsequent encounter
S = sequela

Y24.0 Airgun **discharge, undetermined intent** POA

BB gun discharge, undetermined intent
Pellet gun discharge, undetermined intent

Y24.8 **Other firearm discharge, undetermined intent** POA

Paintball gun discharge, undetermined intent
Very pistol [flare] discharge, undetermined intent

Y24.9 **Unspecified firearm discharge, undetermined intent** POA

Y25 **Contact with explosive material, undetermined intent**

The appropriate 7th character is to be added to code Y25
A = initial encounter
D = subsequent encounter
S = sequela

Y26 **Exposure to smoke, fire and flames, undetermined intent**

The appropriate 7th character is to be added to code Y26
A = initial encounter
D = subsequent encounter
S = sequela

Y27 **Contact with steam, hot vapors and hot objects, undetermined intent**

The appropriate 7th character is to be added to each code from category Y27
A = initial encounter
D = subsequent encounter
S = sequela

Y27.0 **Contact with** steam and hot vapors, **undetermined intent**

Y27.1 **Contact with** hot tap water, **undetermined intent**

Y27.2 **Contact with** hot fluids, **undetermined intent**

Y27.3 **Contact with** hot household appliance, **undetermined intent**

Y27.8 **Contact with other hot objects, undetermined intent**

Y27.9 **Contact with unspecified hot objects, undetermined intent**

Y28 **Contact with** sharp object, **undetermined intent**

The appropriate 7th character is to be added to each code from category Y28
A = initial encounter
D = subsequent encounter
S = sequela

Y28.0 **Contact with** sharp glass, **undetermined intent**

Y28.1 **Contact with** knife, **undetermined intent**

Y28.2 **Contact with** sword or dagger, **undetermined intent**

Y28.8 **Contact with other sharp object, undetermined intent**

Y28.9 **Contact with unspecified sharp object, undetermined intent**

Y29 **Contact with** blunt object, **undetermined intent**

The appropriate 7th character is to be added to code Y29
A = initial encounter
D = subsequent encounter
S = sequela

POA Unacceptable principal diagnosis symbol per Medicare code edits   POA Code exempt from diagnosis present on admission requirement
❓ Questionable admission   �"Complication or comorbidity   MCC Major complication or comorbidity   CC/MCC CC/MCC exclusion
HCC HCC diagnosis code   RHCC RxHCC diagnosis code   MACRA code   **DEFINITION** Describes condition/terminology
TIP Coding guidance   ◈ Official Guideline Reference   Z1 Z code as first-listed diagnosis

Y30 **Falling, jumping or pushed from a high place, undetermined intent**
Victim falling from one level to another, undetermined intent
The appropriate 7th character is to be added to code Y30
  A = initial encounter
  D = subsequent encounter
  S = sequela

Y31 **Falling, lying or running before or into moving object, undetermined intent**
The appropriate 7th character is to be added to code Y31
  A = initial encounter
  D = subsequent encounter
  S = sequela

Y32 **Crashing of motor vehicle, undetermined intent**
The appropriate 7th character is to be added to code Y32
  A = initial encounter
  D = subsequent encounter
  S = sequela

Y33 **Other specified events, undetermined intent**
The appropriate 7th character is to be added to code Y33
  A = initial encounter
  D = subsequent encounter
  S = sequela

Legal intervention, operations of war, military operations, and terrorism (Y35-Y38)

Y35 **Legal intervention**
  INCLUDES *any injury sustained as a result of an encounter with any law enforcement official, serving in any capacity at the time of the encounter, whether on-duty or off-duty. Includes: injury to law enforcement official, suspect and bystander*
The appropriate 7th character is to be added to each code from category Y35
  A = initial encounter
  D = subsequent encounter
  S = sequela

  Y35.0 **Legal intervention involving** firearm discharge
    Y35.00 **Legal intervention involving** unspecified **firearm discharge**
      Legal intervention involving gunshot wound
      Legal intervention involving shot NOS
      Y35.001 **Legal intervention involving unspecified firearm discharge, law enforcement official injured**
      Y35.002 **Legal intervention involving unspecified firearm discharge, bystander injured**
      Y35.003 **Legal intervention involving unspecified firearm discharge, suspect injured**
    ● Y35.009 **Legal intervention involving unspecified firearm discharge, unspecified person injured**
    Y35.01 **Legal intervention involving injury by** machine gun
      Y35.011 **Legal intervention involving injury by machine gun,** law enforcement official injured
      Y35.012 **Legal intervention involving injury by machine gun,** bystander injured
      Y35.013 **Legal intervention involving injury by machine gun,** suspect injured
    ● Y35.019 **Legal intervention involving injury by machine gun, unspecified person injured**
    Y35.02 **Legal intervention involving injury by** handgun
      Y35.021 **Legal intervention involving injury by handgun,** law enforcement official injured
      Y35.022 **Legal intervention involving injury by handgun,** bystander injured
      Y35.023 **Legal intervention involving injury by handgun,** suspect injured

● Y35.029 **Legal intervention involving injury by handgun, unspecified person injured**
Y35.03 **Legal intervention involving injury by** rifle pellet
  Y35.031 **Legal intervention involving injury by rifle pellet,** law enforcement official injured
  Y35.032 **Legal intervention involving injury by rifle pellet,** bystander injured
  Y35.033 **Legal intervention involving injury by rifle pellet,** suspect injured
● Y35.039 **Legal intervention involving injury by rifle pellet, unspecified person injured**
Y35.04 **Legal intervention involving injury by** rubber bullet
  Y35.041 **Legal intervention involving injury by rubber bullet,** law enforcement official injured
  Y35.042 **Legal intervention involving injury by rubber bullet,** bystander injured
  Y35.043 **Legal intervention involving injury by rubber bullet,** suspect injured
● Y35.049 **Legal intervention involving injury by rubber bullet, unspecified person injured**
Y35.09 **Legal intervention involving** other firearm discharge
  Y35.091 **Legal intervention involving other firearm discharge, law enforcement official injured**
  Y35.092 **Legal intervention involving other firearm discharge, bystander injured**
  Y35.093 **Legal intervention involving other firearm discharge, suspect injured**
● Y35.099 **Legal intervention involving other firearm discharge, unspecified person injured**
Y35.1 **Legal intervention involving** explosives
  Y35.10 **Legal intervention involving** unspecified **explosives**
    Y35.101 **Legal intervention involving unspecified explosives, law enforcement official injured**
    Y35.102 **Legal intervention involving unspecified explosives, bystander injured**
    Y35.103 **Legal intervention involving unspecified explosives, suspect injured**
  ● Y35.109 **Legal intervention involving unspecified explosives, unspecified person injured**
  Y35.11 **Legal intervention involving injury by** dynamite
    Y35.111 **Legal intervention involving injury by dynamite,** law enforcement official injured
    Y35.112 **Legal intervention involving injury by dynamite,** bystander injured
    Y35.113 **Legal intervention involving injury by dynamite,** suspect injured
  ● Y35.119 **Legal intervention involving injury by dynamite, unspecified person injured**
  Y35.12 **Legal intervention involving injury by** explosive shell
    Y35.121 **Legal intervention involving injury by explosive shell,** law enforcement official injured
    Y35.122 **Legal intervention involving injury by explosive shell,** bystander injured
    Y35.123 **Legal intervention involving injury by explosive shell,** suspect injured
  ● Y35.129 **Legal intervention involving injury by explosive shell, unspecified person injured**
  Y35.19 **Legal intervention involving** other explosives
    Legal intervention involving injury by grenade
    Legal intervention involving injury by mortar bomb
    Y35.191 **Legal intervention involving other explosives, law enforcement official injured**
    Y35.192 **Legal intervention involving other explosives, bystander injured**

Unspecified Code   Other Specified Code   Manifestation Code   N Newborn   P Pediatric   M Maternity   A Adult   ♂ Male   ♀ Female
● New Code   ▲ Revised Code Title   ►◄ Revised Text   **NOTES**   *INCLUDES*   *EXCLUDES1* Not coded here   *EXCLUDES2* Not included here
4th character required   5th character required   6th character required   7th character required   Extension 'X' Alert
HAC Hospital-acquired condition (HAC) alert   **AHA** AHA Coding Clinic©   ☛ Code first alert

2020 ICD-10-CM   When symbols appear on a code that requires a 7th character extension, refer to Appendix B to identify applicable 7th character codes.   **1231**

[7th] Y35.193 Legal intervention involving other explosives, suspect injured [POA]

● [7th] Y35.199 Legal intervention involving other explosives, unspecified person injured

[5th] Y35.2 Legal intervention involving gas
Legal intervention involving asphyxiation by gas
Legal intervention involving poisoning by gas

[6th] Y35.20 Legal intervention involving unspecified gas

[7th] Y35.201 Legal intervention involving unspecified gas, law enforcement official injured [POA]

[7th] Y35.202 Legal intervention involving unspecified gas, bystander injured [POA]

[7th] Y35.203 Legal intervention involving unspecified gas, suspect injured [POA]

● [7th] Y35.209 Legal intervention involving unspecified gas, unspecified person injured

[6th] Y35.21 Legal intervention involving injury by tear gas

[7th] Y35.211 Legal intervention involving injury by tear gas, law enforcement official injured [POA]

[7th] Y35.212 Legal intervention involving injury by tear gas, bystander injured [POA]

[7th] Y35.213 Legal intervention involving injury by tear gas, suspect injured [POA]

● [7th] Y35.219 Legal intervention involving injury by tear gas, unspecified person injured

[6th] Y35.29 Legal intervention involving other gas

[7th] Y35.291 Legal intervention involving other gas, law enforcement official injured [POA]

[7th] Y35.292 Legal intervention involving other gas, bystander injured [POA]

[7th] Y35.293 Legal intervention involving other gas, suspect injured [POA]

● [7th] Y35.299 Legal intervention involving other gas, unspecified person injured

[5th] Y35.3 Legal intervention involving blunt objects
Legal intervention involving being hit or struck by blunt object

[6th] Y35.30 Legal intervention involving unspecified blunt objects

[7th] Y35.301 Legal intervention involving unspecified blunt objects, law enforcement official injured [POA]

[7th] Y35.302 Legal intervention involving unspecified blunt objects, bystander injured [POA]

[7th] Y35.303 Legal intervention involving unspecified blunt objects, suspect injured [POA]

● [7th] Y35.309 Legal intervention involving unspecified blunt objects, unspecified person injured

[6th] Y35.31 Legal intervention involving baton

[7th] Y35.311 Legal intervention involving baton, law enforcement official injured [POA]

[7th] Y35.312 Legal intervention involving baton, bystander injured [POA]

[7th] Y35.313 Legal intervention involving baton, suspect injured [POA]

● [7th] Y35.319 Legal intervention involving baton, unspecified person injured

[6th] Y35.39 Legal intervention involving other blunt objects

[7th] Y35.391 Legal intervention involving other blunt objects, law enforcement official injured [POA]

[7th] Y35.392 Legal intervention involving other blunt objects, bystander injured [POA]

[7th] Y35.393 Legal intervention involving other blunt objects, suspect injured [POA]

● [7th] Y35.399 Legal intervention involving other blunt objects, unspecified person injured

[5th] Y35.4 Legal intervention involving sharp objects
Legal intervention involving being cut by sharp objects
Legal intervention involving being stabbed by sharp objects

[6th] Y35.40 Legal intervention involving unspecified sharp objects

[7th] Y35.401 Legal intervention involving unspecified sharp objects, law enforcement official injured [POA]

[7th] Y35.402 Legal intervention involving unspecified sharp objects, bystander injured [POA]

[7th] Y35.403 Legal intervention involving unspecified sharp objects, suspect injured [POA]

● [7th] Y35.409 Legal intervention involving unspecified sharp objects, unspecified person injured

[6th] Y35.41 Legal intervention involving bayonet

[7th] Y35.411 Legal intervention involving bayonet, law enforcement official injured [POA]

[7th] Y35.412 Legal intervention involving bayonet, bystander injured [POA]

[7th] Y35.413 Legal intervention involving bayonet, suspect injured [POA]

● [7th] Y35.419 Legal intervention involving bayonet, unspecified person injured

[6th] Y35.49 Legal intervention involving other sharp objects

[7th] Y35.491 Legal intervention involving other sharp objects, law enforcement official injured [POA]

[7th] Y35.492 Legal intervention involving other sharp objects, bystander injured [POA]

[7th] Y35.493 Legal intervention involving other sharp objects, suspect injured [POA]

● [7th] Y35.499 Legal intervention involving other sharp objects, unspecified person injured

[5th] Y35.8 Legal intervention involving other specified means

[6th] Y35.81 Legal intervention involving manhandling

[7th] Y35.811 Legal intervention involving manhandling, law enforcement official injured [POA]

[7th] Y35.812 Legal intervention involving manhandling, bystander injured [POA]

[7th] Y35.813 Legal intervention involving manhandling, suspect injured [POA]

● [7th] Y35.819 Legal intervention involving manhandling, unspecified person injured

● [6th] Y35.83 Legal intervention involving a conducted energy device
Electroshock device (taser)
Stun gun

● [7th] Y35.831 Legal intervention involving a conducted energy device, law enforcement official injured

● [7th] Y35.832 Legal intervention involving a conducted energy device, bystander injured

● [7th] Y35.833 Legal intervention involving a conducted energy device, suspect injured

● [7th] Y35.839 Legal intervention involving a conducted energy device, unspecified person injured

[6th] Y35.89 Legal intervention involving other specified means

[7th] Y35.891 Legal intervention involving other specified means, law enforcement official injured [POA]

[7th] Y35.892 Legal intervention involving other specified means, bystander injured [POA]

[7th] Y35.893 Legal intervention involving other specified means, suspect injured [POA]
AHA: Q1 2018

[5th] Y35.9 Legal intervention, means unspecified

[7th] Y35.91 Legal intervention, means unspecified, law enforcement official injured [POA]

[7th] Y35.92 Legal intervention, means unspecified, bystander injured [POA]

[7th] Y35.93 Legal intervention, means unspecified, suspect injured [POA]

● [7th] Y35.99 Legal intervention, means unspecified, unspecified person injured

[PDx] Unacceptable principal diagnosis symbol per Medicare code edits [POA] Code exempt from diagnosis present on admission requirement
[?] Questionable admission [CC] Complication or comorbidity [MCC] Major complication or comorbidity [CC/MCC Exc] CC/MCC exclusion
[HCC] HCC diagnosis code [RxHCC] RxHCC diagnosis code MACRA code **DEFINITION** Describes condition/terminology
TIP Coding guidance 👁 Official Guideline Reference [Z1] Z code as first-listed diagnosis

Y36 **Operations of war**

INCLUDES injuries to military personnel and civilians caused by war, civil insurrection, and peacekeeping missions

EXCLUDES1 injury to military personnel occurring during peacetime military operations (Y37.-)

military vehicles involved in transport accidents with non-military vehicle during peacetime (V09.01, V09.21, V19.81, V29.81, V39.81, V49.81, V59.81, V69.81, V79.81)

The appropriate 7th character is to be added to each code from category Y36

A = initial encounter
D = subsequent encounter
S = sequela

Y36.0 **War operations involving** explosion of marine weapons

Y36.00 **War operations involving explosion of** unspecified marine weapon

War operations involving underwater blast NOS

Y36.000 **War operations involving explosion of unspecified marine weapon, military personnel**

Y36.001 **War operations involving explosion of unspecified marine weapon, civilian**

Y36.01 **War operations involving explosion of** depth-charge

Y36.010 **War operations involving explosion of depth-charge,** military personnel

Y36.011 **War operations involving explosion of depth-charge,** civilian

Y36.02 **War operations involving explosion of** marine mine

War operations involving explosion of marine mine, at sea or in harbor

Y36.020 **War operations involving explosion of marine mine,** military personnel

Y36.021 **War operations involving explosion of marine mine,** civilian

Y36.03 **War operations involving explosion of** sea-based artillery shell

Y36.030 **War operations involving explosion of sea-based artillery shell,** military personnel

Y36.031 **War operations involving explosion of sea-based artillery shell,** civilian

Y36.04 **War operations involving explosion of** torpedo

Y36.040 **War operations involving explosion of torpedo,** military personnel

Y36.041 **War operations involving explosion of torpedo,** civilian

Y36.05 **War operations involving** accidental detonation of onboard marine weapons

Y36.050 **War operations involving accidental detonation of onboard marine weapons, military personnel**

Y36.051 **War operations involving accidental detonation of onboard marine weapons, civilian**

Y36.09 **War operations involving explosion of** other marine weapons

Y36.090 **War operations involving explosion of other marine weapons, military personnel**

Y36.091 **War operations involving explosion of other marine weapons, civilian**

Y36.1 **War operations involving destruction of aircraft**

Y36.10 **War operations involving** unspecified destruction of aircraft

Y36.100 **War operations involving unspecified destruction of aircraft, military personnel**

Y36.101 **War operations involving unspecified destruction of aircraft, civilian**

Y36.11 **War operations involving destruction of aircraft due to** enemy fire or explosives

War operations involving destruction of aircraft due to air to air missile

War operations involving destruction of aircraft due to explosive placed on aircraft

War operations involving destruction of aircraft due to rocket propelled grenade [RPG]

War operations involving destruction of aircraft due to small arms fire

War operations involving destruction of aircraft due to surface to air missile

Y36.110 **War operations involving destruction of aircraft due to enemy fire or explosives,** military personnel

Y36.111 **War operations involving destruction of aircraft due to enemy fire or explosives,** civilian

Y36.12 **War operations involving destruction of aircraft due to** collision with other aircraft

Y36.120 **War operations involving destruction of aircraft due to collision with other aircraft,** military personnel

Y36.121 **War operations involving destruction of aircraft due to collision with other aircraft,** civilian

Y36.13 **War operations involving destruction of aircraft due to** onboard fire

Y36.130 **War operations involving destruction of aircraft due to onboard fire,** military personnel

Y36.131 **War operations involving destruction of aircraft due to onboard fire,** civilian

Y36.14 **War operations involving destruction of aircraft due to** accidental detonation of onboard munitions and explosives

Y36.140 **War operations involving destruction of aircraft due to accidental detonation of onboard munitions and explosives,** military personnel

Y36.141 **War operations involving destruction of aircraft due to accidental detonation of onboard munitions and explosives,** civilian

Y36.19 **War operations involving** other destruction of aircraft

Y36.190 **War operations involving other destruction of aircraft, military personnel**

Y36.191 **War operations involving other destruction of aircraft, civilian**

Y36.2 **War operations involving** other explosions and fragments

EXCLUDES1 war operations involving explosion of aircraft (Y36.1-)

war operations involving explosion of marine weapons (Y36.0-)

war operations involving explosion of nuclear weapons (Y36.5-)

war operations involving explosion occurring after cessation of hostilities (Y36.8-)

Y36.20 **War operations involving** unspecified explosion and fragments

War operations involving air blast NOS
War operations involving blast NOS
War operations involving blast fragments NOS
War operations involving blast wave NOS
War operations involving blast wind NOS
War operations involving explosion NOS
War operations involving explosion of bomb NOS

Y36.200 **War operations involving unspecified explosion and fragments, military personnel**

Y36.201 **War operations involving unspecified explosion and fragments, civilian**

Y36.21 **War operations involving explosion of** aerial bomb

Y36.210 **War operations involving explosion of aerial bomb,** military personnel

Unspecified Code   Other Specified Code   Manifestation Code   N Newborn   P Pediatric   M Maternity   A Adult   ♂ Male   ♀ Female
● New Code   ▲ Revised Code Title   ►◄ Revised Text   NOTES   INCLUDES   EXCLUDES1 Not coded here   EXCLUDES2 Not included here
4th character required   5th character required   6th character required   7th character required   Extension 'X' Alert
HAC Hospital-acquired condition (HAC) alert   AHA AHA Coding Clinic©   ☞ Code first alert

Y36.211 **War operations involving explosion of aerial bomb**, civilian POA

6ᵗʰ Y36.22 **War operations involving explosion of** guided missile

7ᵗʰ Y36.220 **War operations involving explosion of guided missile**, military personnel POA

7ᵗʰ Y36.221 **War operations involving explosion of guided missile**, civilian POA

6ᵗʰ Y36.23 **War operations involving explosion of** improvised explosive device [IED]

War operations involving explosion of person-borne improvised explosive device [IED]
War operations involving explosion of vehicle-borne improvised explosive device [IED]
War operations involving explosion of roadside improvised explosive device [IED]

7ᵗʰ Y36.230 **War operations involving explosion of improvised explosive device [IED]**, military personnel POA

7ᵗʰ Y36.231 **War operations involving explosion of improvised explosive device [IED]**, civilian POA

6ᵗʰ Y36.24 **War operations involving explosion due to** accidental detonation and discharge of own munitions or munitions launch device

7ᵗʰ Y36.240 **War operations involving explosion due to accidental detonation and discharge of own munitions or munitions launch device**, military personnel POA

7ᵗʰ Y36.241 **War operations involving explosion due to accidental detonation and discharge of own munitions or munitions launch device**, civilian POA

6ᵗʰ Y36.25 **War operations involving** fragments from munitions

7ᵗʰ Y36.250 **War operations involving fragments from munitions**, military personnel POA

7ᵗʰ Y36.251 **War operations involving fragments from munitions**, civilian POA

6ᵗʰ Y36.26 **War operations involving fragments of** improvised explosive device [IED]

War operations involving fragments of person-borne improvised explosive device [IED]
War operations involving fragments of vehicle-borne improvised explosive device [IED]
War operations involving fragments of roadside improvised explosive device [IED]

7ᵗʰ Y36.260 **War operations involving fragments of improvised explosive device [IED]**, military personnel POA

7ᵗʰ Y36.261 **War operations involving fragments of improvised explosive device [IED]**, civilian POA

6ᵗʰ Y36.27 **War operations involving** fragments from weapons

7ᵗʰ Y36.270 **War operations involving fragments from weapons**, military personnel POA

7ᵗʰ Y36.271 **War operations involving fragments from weapons**, civilian POA

6ᵗʰ Y36.29 **War operations involving** other explosions and fragments

War operations involving explosion of grenade
War operations involving explosions of land mine
War operations involving shrapnel NOS

7ᵗʰ Y36.290 **War operations involving other explosions and fragments, military personnel** POA

7ᵗʰ Y36.291 **War operations involving other explosions and fragments, civilian** POA

5ᵗʰ Y36.3 **War operations involving** fires, conflagrations and hot substances

War operations involving smoke, fumes, and heat from fires, conflagrations and hot substances

EXCLUDES1 war operations involving fires and conflagrations aboard military aircraft (Y36.1-)

war operations involving fires and conflagrations aboard military watercraft (Y36.0-)

war operations involving fires and conflagrations caused indirectly by conventional weapons (Y36.2-)

war operations involving fires and thermal effects of nuclear weapons (Y36.53-)

6ᵗʰ Y36.30 **War operations involving** unspecified **fire, conflagration and hot substance**

7ᵗʰ Y36.300 **War operations involving unspecified fire, conflagration and hot substance, military personnel** POA

7ᵗʰ Y36.301 **War operations involving unspecified fire, conflagration and hot substance, civilian** POA

6ᵗʰ Y36.31 **War operations involving** gasoline bomb

War operations involving incendiary bomb
War operations involving petrol bomb

7ᵗʰ Y36.310 **War operations involving gasoline bomb**, military personnel POA

7ᵗʰ Y36.311 **War operations involving gasoline bomb**, civilian POA

6ᵗʰ Y36.32 **War operations involving** incendiary bullet

7ᵗʰ Y36.320 **War operations involving incendiary bullet**, military personnel POA

7ᵗʰ Y36.321 **War operations involving incendiary bullet**, civilian POA

6ᵗʰ Y36.33 **War operations involving** flamethrower

7ᵗʰ Y36.330 **War operations involving flamethrower**, military personnel POA

7ᵗʰ Y36.331 **War operations involving flamethrower**, civilian POA

6ᵗʰ Y36.39 **War operations involving other fires**, conflagrations and hot substances

7ᵗʰ Y36.390 **War operations involving other fires, conflagrations and hot substances, military personnel** POA

7ᵗʰ Y36.391 **War operations involving other fires, conflagrations and hot substances, civilian** POA

5ᵗʰ Y36.4 **War operations involving firearm discharge and other forms of conventional warfare**

6ᵗʰ Y36.41 **War operations involving** rubber bullets

7ᵗʰ Y36.410 **War operations involving rubber bullets**, military personnel POA

7ᵗʰ Y36.411 **War operations involving rubber bullets**, civilian POA

6ᵗʰ Y36.42 **War operations involving** firearms pellets

7ᵗʰ Y36.420 **War operations involving firearms pellets**, military personnel POA

7ᵗʰ Y36.421 **War operations involving firearms pellets**, civilian POA

6ᵗʰ Y36.43 **War operations involving** other **firearms discharge**

War operations involving bullets NOS

EXCLUDES1 war operations involving munitions fragments (Y36.25-)

war operations involving incendiary bullets (Y36.32-)

7ᵗʰ Y36.430 **War operations involving other firearms discharge, military personnel** POA

7ᵗʰ Y36.431 **War operations involving other firearms discharge, civilian** POA

6ᵗʰ Y36.44 **War operations involving** unarmed hand to hand combat

EXCLUDES1 war operations involving combat using blunt or piercing object (Y36.45-)

war operations involving intentional restriction of air and airway (Y36.46-)

war operations involving unintentional restriction of air and airway (Y36.47-)

7ᵗʰ Y36.440 **War operations involving unarmed hand to hand combat**, military personnel POA

PDxⁿ Unacceptable principal diagnosis symbol per Medicare code edits   ⦸ Code exempt from diagnosis present on admission requirement
❓ Questionable admission   cc Complication or comorbidity   MCC Major complication or comorbidity   CC/MCC CC/MCC exclusion
HCC HCC diagnosis code   RxHCC RxHCC diagnosis code   MACRA code   **DEFINITION** Describes condition/terminology
TIP Coding guidance   👁 Official Guideline Reference   Z1 Z code as first-listed diagnosis

1234   When symbols appear on a code that requires a 7th character extension, refer to Appendix B to identify applicable 7th character codes.   **2020 ICD-10-CM**

[7th] Y36.441 War operations involving unarmed hand to hand combat, civilian [POA]

[6th] Y36.45 War operations involving combat using blunt or piercing object

[7th] Y36.450 War operations involving combat using blunt or piercing object, military personnel [POA]

[7th] Y36.451 War operations involving combat using blunt or piercing object, civilian [POA]

[6th] Y36.46 War operations involving intentional restriction of air and airway

[7th] Y36.460 War operations involving intentional restriction of air and airway, military personnel [POA]

[7th] Y36.461 War operations involving intentional restriction of air and airway, civilian [POA]

[6th] Y36.47 War operations involving unintentional restriction of air and airway

[7th] Y36.470 War operations involving unintentional restriction of air and airway, military personnel [POA]

[7th] Y36.471 War operations involving unintentional restriction of air and airway, civilian [POA]

[6th] Y36.49 War operations involving other forms of conventional warfare

[7th] Y36.490 War operations involving other forms of conventional warfare, military personnel [POA]

[7th] Y36.491 War operations involving other forms of conventional warfare, civilian [POA]

[5th] Y36.5 War operations involving nuclear weapons

War operations involving dirty bomb NOS

[6th] Y36.50 War operations involving unspecified effect of nuclear weapon

[7th] Y36.500 War operations involving unspecified effect of nuclear weapon, military personnel [POA]

[7th] Y36.501 War operations involving unspecified effect of nuclear weapon, civilian [POA]

[6th] Y36.51 War operations involving direct blast effect of nuclear weapon

War operations involving blast pressure of nuclear weapon

[7th] Y36.510 War operations involving direct blast effect of nuclear weapon, military personnel [POA]

[7th] Y36.511 War operations involving direct blast effect of nuclear weapon, civilian [POA]

[6th] Y36.52 War operations involving indirect blast effect of nuclear weapon

War operations involving being thrown by blast of nuclear weapon

War operations involving being struck or crushed by blast debris of nuclear weapon

[7th] Y36.520 War operations involving indirect blast effect of nuclear weapon, military personnel [POA]

[7th] Y36.521 War operations involving indirect blast effect of nuclear weapon, civilian [POA]

[6th] Y36.53 War operations involving thermal radiation effect of nuclear weapon

War operations involving direct heat from nuclear weapon

War operation involving fireball effects from nuclear weapon

[7th] Y36.530 War operations involving thermal radiation effect of nuclear weapon, military personnel [POA]

[7th] Y36.531 War operations involving thermal radiation effect of nuclear weapon, civilian [POA]

[6th] Y36.54 War operation involving nuclear radiation effects of nuclear weapon

War operation involving acute radiation exposure from nuclear weapon

War operation involving exposure to immediate ionizing radiation from nuclear weapon

War operation involving fallout exposure from nuclear weapon

War operation involving secondary effects of nuclear weapons

[7th] Y36.540 War operation involving nuclear radiation effects of nuclear weapon, military personnel [POA]

[7th] Y36.541 War operation involving nuclear radiation effects of nuclear weapon, civilian [POA]

[6th] Y36.59 War operation involving other effects of nuclear weapons

[7th] Y36.590 War operation involving other effects of nuclear weapons, military personnel [POA]

[7th] Y36.591 War operation involving other effects of nuclear weapons, civilian [POA]

[5th] Y36.6 War operations involving biological weapons

[6th] Y36.6X War operations involving biological weapons

[7th] Y36.6X0 War operations involving biological weapons, military personnel [POA]

[7th] Y36.6X1 War operations involving biological weapons, civilian [POA]

[5th] Y36.7 War operations involving chemical weapons and other forms of unconventional warfare

[EXCLUDES1] *war operations involving incendiary devices (Y36.3-, Y36.5-)*

[6th] Y36.7X War operations involving chemical weapons and other forms of unconventional warfare

[7th] Y36.7X0 War operations involving chemical weapons and other forms of unconventional warfare, military personnel [POA]

[7th] Y36.7X1 War operations involving chemical weapons and other forms of unconventional warfare, civilian [POA]

[5th] Y36.8 War operations occurring after cessation of hostilities

War operations classifiable to categories Y36.0-Y36.8 but occurring after cessation of hostilities

[6th] Y36.81 Explosion of mine placed during war operations but exploding after cessation of hostilities

[7th] Y36.810 Explosion of mine placed during war operations but exploding after cessation of hostilities, military personnel [POA]

[7th] Y36.811 Explosion of mine placed during war operations but exploding after cessation of hostilities, civilian [POA]

[6th] Y36.82 Explosion of bomb placed during war operations but exploding after cessation of hostilities

[7th] Y36.820 Explosion of bomb placed during war operations but exploding after cessation of hostilities, military personnel [POA]

[7th] Y36.821 Explosion of bomb placed during war operations but exploding after cessation of hostilities, civilian [POA]

[6th] Y36.88 Other war operations occurring after cessation of hostilities

[7th] Y36.880 Other war operations occurring after cessation of hostilities, military personnel [POA]

[7th] Y36.881 Other war operations occurring after cessation of hostilities, civilian [POA]

[6th] Y36.89 Unspecified war operations occurring after cessation of hostilities

[7th] Y36.890 Unspecified war operations occurring after cessation of hostilities, military personnel [POA]

[7th] Y36.891 Unspecified war operations occurring after cessation of hostilities, civilian [POA]

- **Y36.9** Other and unspecified war operations
  - **Y36.90** War operations, unspecified ⊷
  - **Y36.91** War operations involving unspecified weapon of mass destruction [WMD] ⊷
  - **Y36.92** War operations involving friendly fire ⊷
- **Y37** Military operations
  - INCLUDES *injuries to military personnel and civilians occurring during peacetime on military property and during routine military exercises and operations*
  - EXCLUDES1 *military aircraft involved in aircraft accident with civilian aircraft (V97.81-)*
    - *military vehicles involved in transport accident with civilian vehicle (V09.01, V09.21, V19.81, V29.81, V39.81, V49.81, V59.81, V69.81, V79.81)*
    - *military watercraft involved in water transport accident with civilian watercraft (V94.81-)*
    - *war operations (Y36.-)*

  The appropriate 7th character is to be added to each code from category Y37
  A = initial encounter
  D = subsequent encounter
  S = sequela

  - **Y37.0** Military operations involving explosion of marine weapons
    - **Y37.00** Military operations involving explosion of unspecified marine weapon
      - Military operations involving underwater blast NOS
      - **Y37.000** Military operations involving explosion of unspecified marine weapon, military personnel ⊷
      - **Y37.001** Military operations involving explosion of unspecified marine weapon, civilian ⊷
    - **Y37.01** Military operations involving explosion of depth-charge
      - **Y37.010** Military operations involving explosion of depth-charge, military personnel ⊷
      - **Y37.011** Military operations involving explosion of depth-charge, civilian ⊷
    - **Y37.02** Military operations involving explosion of marine mine
      - Military operations involving explosion of marine mine, at sea or in harbor
      - **Y37.020** Military operations involving explosion of marine mine, military personnel ⊷
      - **Y37.021** Military operations involving explosion of marine mine, civilian ⊷
    - **Y37.03** Military operations involving explosion of sea-based artillery shell
      - **Y37.030** Military operations involving explosion of sea-based artillery shell, military personnel ⊷
      - **Y37.031** Military operations involving explosion of sea-based artillery shell, civilian ⊷
    - **Y37.04** Military operations involving explosion of torpedo
      - **Y37.040** Military operations involving explosion of torpedo, military personnel ⊷
      - **Y37.041** Military operations involving explosion of torpedo, civilian ⊷
    - **Y37.05** Military operations involving accidental detonation of onboard marine weapons
      - **Y37.050** Military operations involving accidental detonation of onboard marine weapons, military personnel ⊷
      - **Y37.051** Military operations involving accidental detonation of onboard marine weapons, civilian ⊷
    - **Y37.09** Military operations involving explosion of other marine weapons
      - **Y37.090** Military operations involving explosion of other marine weapons, military personnel ⊷
      - **Y37.091** Military operations involving explosion of other marine weapons, civilian ⊷
  - **Y37.1** Military operations involving destruction of aircraft
    - **Y37.10** Military operations involving unspecified destruction of aircraft
      - **Y37.100** Military operations involving unspecified destruction of aircraft, military personnel ⊷
      - **Y37.101** Military operations involving unspecified destruction of aircraft, civilian ⊷
    - **Y37.11** Military operations involving destruction of aircraft due to enemy fire or explosives
      - Military operations involving destruction of aircraft due to air to air missile
      - Military operations involving destruction of aircraft due to explosive placed on aircraft
      - Military operations involving destruction of aircraft due to rocket propelled grenade [RPG]
      - Military operations involving destruction of aircraft due to small arms fire
      - Military operations involving destruction of aircraft due to surface to air missile
      - **Y37.110** Military operations involving destruction of aircraft due to enemy fire or explosives, military personnel ⊷
      - **Y37.111** Military operations involving destruction of aircraft due to enemy fire or explosives, civilian ⊷
    - **Y37.12** Military operations involving destruction of aircraft due to collision with other aircraft
      - **Y37.120** Military operations involving destruction of aircraft due to collision with other aircraft, military personnel ⊷
      - **Y37.121** Military operations involving destruction of aircraft due to collision with other aircraft, civilian ⊷
    - **Y37.13** Military operations involving destruction of aircraft due to onboard fire
      - **Y37.130** Military operations involving destruction of aircraft due to onboard fire, military personnel ⊷
      - **Y37.131** Military operations involving destruction of aircraft due to onboard fire, civilian ⊷
    - **Y37.14** Military operations involving destruction of aircraft due to accidental detonation of onboard munitions and explosives
      - **Y37.140** Military operations involving destruction of aircraft due to accidental detonation of onboard munitions and explosives, military personnel ⊷
      - **Y37.141** Military operations involving destruction of aircraft due to accidental detonation of onboard munitions and explosives, civilian ⊷
    - **Y37.19** Military operations involving other destruction of aircraft
      - **Y37.190** Military operations involving other destruction of aircraft, military personnel ⊷
      - **Y37.191** Military operations involving other destruction of aircraft, civilian ⊷
  - **Y37.2** Military operations involving other explosions and fragments
    - EXCLUDES1 *military operations involving explosion of aircraft (Y37.1-)*
      - *military operations involving explosion of marine weapons (Y37.0-)*
      - *military operations involving explosion of nuclear weapons (Y37.5-)*
    - **Y37.20** Military operations involving unspecified explosion and fragments
      - Military operations involving air blast NOS
      - Military operations involving blast NOS

Military operations involving blast fragments NOS
Military operations involving blast wave NOS
Military operations involving blast wind NOS
Military operations involving explosion NOS
Military operations involving explosion of bomb NOS

- Y37.200 **Military operations involving unspecified explosion and fragments, military personnel** POA
- Y37.201 **Military operations involving unspecified explosion and fragments, civilian** POA

Y37.21 **Military operations involving explosion of** aerial bomb
- Y37.210 **Military operations involving explosion of aerial bomb,** military personnel POA
- Y37.211 **Military operations involving explosion of aerial bomb,** civilian POA

Y37.22 **Military operations involving** explosion of guided missile
- Y37.220 **Military operations involving explosion of guided missile,** military personnel POA
- Y37.221 **Military operations involving explosion of guided missile,** civilian POA

Y37.23 **Military operations involving** explosion of improvised explosive device [IED]
Military operations involving explosion of person-borne improvised explosive device [IED]
Military operations involving explosion of vehicle-borne improvised explosive device [IED]
Military operations involving explosion of roadside improvised explosive device [IED]
- Y37.230 **Military operations involving explosion of improvised explosive device [IED],** military personnel POA
- Y37.231 **Military operations involving explosion of improvised explosive device [IED],** civilian POA

Y37.24 **Military operations involving explosion** due to accidental detonation and discharge of own munitions or munitions launch device
- Y37.240 **Military operations involving explosion due to accidental detonation and discharge of own munitions or munitions launch device,** military personnel POA
- Y37.241 **Military operations involving explosion due to accidental detonation and discharge of own munitions or munitions launch device,** civilian POA

Y37.25 **Military operations involving** fragments from munitions
- Y37.250 **Military operations involving fragments from munitions,** military personnel POA
- Y37.251 **Military operations involving fragments from munitions,** civilian POA

Y37.26 **Military operations involving fragments of** improvised explosive device [IED]
Military operations involving fragments of person-borne improvised explosive device [IED]
Military operations involving fragments of vehicle-borne improvised explosive device [IED]
Military operations involving fragments of roadside improvised explosive device [IED]
- Y37.260 **Military operations involving fragments of improvised explosive device [IED],** military personnel POA
- Y37.261 **Military operations involving fragments of improvised explosive device [IED],** civilian POA

Y37.27 **Military operations involving fragments from** weapons
- Y37.270 **Military operations involving fragments from weapons,** military personnel POA
- Y37.271 **Military operations involving fragments from weapons,** civilian POA

- Y37.29 **Military operations involving** other explosions and fragments
Military operations involving explosion of grenade
Military operations involving explosions of land mine
Military operations involving shrapnel NOS
- Y37.290 **Military operations involving other explosions and fragments, military personnel** POA
- Y37.291 **Military operations involving other explosions and fragments, civilian** POA

Y37.3 **Military operations involving** fires, conflagrations and hot substances
Military operations involving smoke, fumes, and heat from fires, conflagrations and hot substances
EXCLUDES1 *military operations involving fires and conflagrations aboard military aircraft (Y37.1-)*
military operations involving fires and conflagrations aboard military watercraft (Y37.0-)
military operations involving fires and conflagrations caused indirectly by conventional weapons (Y37.2-)
military operations involving fires and thermal effects of nuclear weapons (Y36.53-)

Y37.30 **Military operations involving** unspecified fire, conflagration and hot substance
- Y37.300 **Military operations involving unspecified fire, conflagration and hot substance, military personnel** POA
- Y37.301 **Military operations involving unspecified fire, conflagration and hot substance, civilian** POA

Y37.31 **Military operations involving** gasoline bomb
Military operations involving incendiary bomb
Military operations involving petrol bomb
- Y37.310 **Military operations involving gasoline bomb,** military personnel POA
- Y37.311 **Military operations involving gasoline bomb,** civilian POA

Y37.32 **Military operations involving** incendiary bullet
- Y37.320 **Military operations involving incendiary bullet,** military personnel POA
- Y37.321 **Military operations involving incendiary bullet,** civilian POA

Y37.33 **Military operations involving** flamethrower
- Y37.330 **Military operations involving flamethrower,** military personnel POA
- Y37.331 **Military operations involving flamethrower,** civilian POA

Y37.39 **Military operations involving** other fires, conflagrations and hot substances
- Y37.390 **Military operations involving other fires, conflagrations and hot substances, military personnel** POA
- Y37.391 **Military operations involving other fires, conflagrations and hot substances, civilian** POA

Y37.4 **Military operations involving firearm discharge and other forms of conventional warfare**
Y37.41 **Military operations involving** rubber bullets
- Y37.410 **Military operations involving rubber bullets,** military personnel POA
- Y37.411 **Military operations involving rubber bullets,** civilian POA

Y37.42 **Military operations involving** firearms pellets
- Y37.420 **Military operations involving firearms pellets,** military personnel POA
- Y37.421 **Military operations involving firearms pellets,** civilian POA

Y37.43 **Military operations involving** other firearms discharge
Military operations involving bullets NOS
EXCLUDES1 *military operations involving munitions fragments (Y37.25-)*
military operations involving incendiary bullets (Y37.32-)

Unspecified Code   Other Specified Code   Manifestation Code   N Newborn   P Pediatric   M Maternity   A Adult   ♂ Male   ♀ Female
● New Code   ▲ Revised Code Title   ▶◀ Revised Text   NOTES   INCLUDES   EXCLUDES1 Not coded here   EXCLUDES2 Not included here
4th character required   5th character required   6th character required   7th character required   Extension 'X' Alert
HAC Hospital-acquired condition (HAC) alert   AHA AHA Coding Clinic©   Code first alert

2020 ICD-10-CM   When symbols appear on a code that requires a 7th character extension, refer to Appendix B to identify applicable 7th character codes.   **1237**

[7th] Y37.430 Military operations involving other firearms discharge, military personnel [POA]

[7th] Y37.431 Military operations involving other firearms discharge, civilian [POA]

[6th] Y37.44 Military operations involving unarmed hand to hand combat

[EXCLUDES1] *military operations involving combat using blunt or piercing object (Y37.45-)*

military operations involving intentional restriction of air and airway (Y37.46-)

military operations involving unintentional restriction of air and airway (Y37.47-)

[7th] Y37.440 Military operations involving unarmed hand to hand combat, military personnel [POA]

[7th] Y37.441 Military operations involving unarmed hand to hand combat, civilian [POA]

[6th] Y37.45 Military operations involving combat using blunt or piercing object

[7th] Y37.450 Military operations involving combat using blunt or piercing object, military personnel [POA]

[7th] Y37.451 Military operations involving combat using blunt or piercing object, civilian [POA]

[6th] Y37.46 Military operations involving intentional restriction of air and airway

[7th] Y37.460 Military operations involving intentional restriction of air and airway, military personnel [POA]

[7th] Y37.461 Military operations involving intentional restriction of air and airway, civilian [POA]

[6th] Y37.47 Military operations involving unintentional restriction of air and airway

[7th] Y37.470 Military operations involving unintentional restriction of air and airway, military personnel [POA]

[7th] Y37.471 Military operations involving unintentional restriction of air and airway, civilian [POA]

[6th] Y37.49 Military operations involving other forms of conventional warfare

[7th] Y37.490 Military operations involving other forms of conventional warfare, military personnel [POA]

[7th] Y37.491 Military operations involving other forms of conventional warfare, civilian [POA]

[5th] Y37.5 Military operations involving nuclear weapons

Military operation involving dirty bomb NOS

[6th] Y37.50 Military operations involving unspecified effect of nuclear weapon

[7th] Y37.500 Military operations involving unspecified effect of nuclear weapon, military personnel [POA]

[7th] Y37.501 Military operations involving unspecified effect of nuclear weapon, civilian [POA]

[6th] Y37.51 Military operations involving direct blast effect of nuclear weapon

Military operations involving blast pressure of nuclear weapon

[7th] Y37.510 Military operations involving direct blast effect of nuclear weapon, military personnel [POA]

[7th] Y37.511 Military operations involving direct blast effect of nuclear weapon, civilian [POA]

[6th] Y37.52 Military operations involving indirect blast effect of nuclear weapon

Military operations involving being thrown by blast of nuclear weapon

Military operations involving being struck or crushed by blast debris of nuclear weapon

[7th] Y37.520 Military operations involving indirect blast effect of nuclear weapon, military personnel [POA]

[7th] Y37.521 Military operations involving indirect blast effect of nuclear weapon, civilian [POA]

[6th] Y37.53 Military operations involving thermal radiation effect of nuclear weapon

Military operations involving direct heat from nuclear weapon

Military operation involving fireball effects from nuclear weapon

[7th] Y37.530 Military operations involving thermal radiation effect of nuclear weapon, military personnel [POA]

[7th] Y37.531 Military operations involving thermal radiation effect of nuclear weapon, civilian [POA]

[6th] Y37.54 Military operation involving nuclear radiation effects of nuclear weapon

Military operation involving acute radiation exposure from nuclear weapon

Military operation involving exposure to immediate ionizing radiation from nuclear weapon

Military operation involving fallout exposure from nuclear weapon

Military operation involving secondary effects of nuclear weapons

[7th] Y37.540 Military operation involving nuclear radiation effects of nuclear weapon, military personnel [POA]

[7th] Y37.541 Military operation involving nuclear radiation effects of nuclear weapon, civilian [POA]

[6th] Y37.59 Military operation involving other effects of nuclear weapons

[7th] Y37.590 Military operation involving other effects of nuclear weapons, military personnel [POA]

[7th] Y37.591 Military operation involving other effects of nuclear weapons, civilian [POA]

[5th] Y37.6 Military operations involving biological weapons

[6th] Y37.6X Military operations involving biological weapons

[7th] Y37.6X0 Military operations involving biological weapons, military personnel [POA]

[7th] Y37.6X1 Military operations involving biological weapons, civilian [POA]

[5th] Y37.7 Military operations involving chemical weapons and other forms of unconventional warfare

[EXCLUDES1] *military operations involving incendiary devices (Y36.3-, Y36.5-)*

[6th] Y37.7X Military operations involving chemical weapons and other forms of unconventional warfare

[7th] Y37.7X0 Military operations involving chemical weapons and other forms of unconventional warfare, military personnel [POA]

[7th] Y37.7X1 Military operations involving chemical weapons and other forms of unconventional warfare, civilian [POA]

[5th] Y37.9 Other and unspecified military operations

[7th] Y37.90 Military operations, unspecified [POA]

[7th] Y37.91 Military operations involving unspecified weapon of mass destruction [WMD] [POA]

[7th] Y37.92 Military operations involving friendly fire [POA]

[4th] Y38 Terrorism

See Official Guidelines "Cause of injury identified by the FBI as terrorism" I.C.20. j.1

These codes are for use to identify injuries resulting from the unlawful use of force or violence against persons or property to intimidate or coerce a Government, the civilian population, or any segment thereof, in furtherance of political or social objective

Use additional code for place of occurrence (Y92.-)

[PDx] Unacceptable principal diagnosis symbol per Medicare code edits [POA] Code exempt from diagnosis present on admission requirement
[?] Questionable admission [CC] Complication or comorbidity [MCC] Major complication or comorbidity [CC/MCC Exc] CC/MCC exclusion
[HCC] HCC diagnosis code [RxHCC] RxHCC diagnosis code MACRA code **DEFINITION** Describes condition/terminology
TIP Coding guidance Official Guideline Reference [Z1] Z code as first-listed diagnosis

 When symbols appear on a code that requires a 7th character extension, refer to Appendix B to identify applicable 7th character codes.

The appropriate 7th character is to be added to each code from category Y38
- A = initial encounter
- D = subsequent encounter
- S = sequela

[5th] **Y38.0 Terrorism involving explosion of marine weapons**
Terrorism involving depth-charge
Terrorism involving marine mine
Terrorism involving mine NOS, at sea or in harbor
Terrorism involving sea-based artillery shell
Terrorism involving torpedo
Terrorism involving underwater blast

[6th] **Y38.0X Terrorism involving explosion of marine weapons**

[7th] **Y38.0X1 Terrorism involving explosion of marine weapons, public safety official injured** [POA]

[7th] **Y38.0X2 Terrorism involving explosion of marine weapons, civilian injured** [POA]

[7th] **Y38.0X3 Terrorism involving explosion of marine weapons, terrorist injured** [POA]

[5th] **Y38.1 Terrorism involving destruction of aircraft**
Terrorism involving aircraft burned
Terrorism involving aircraft exploded
Terrorism involving aircraft being shot down
Terrorism involving aircraft used as a weapon

[6th] **Y38.1X Terrorism involving destruction of aircraft**

[7th] **Y38.1X1 Terrorism involving destruction of aircraft, public safety official injured** [POA]

[7th] **Y38.1X2 Terrorism involving destruction of aircraft, civilian injured** [POA]

[7th] **Y38.1X3 Terrorism involving destruction of aircraft, terrorist injured** [POA]

[5th] **Y38.2 Terrorism involving other explosions and fragments**
Terrorism involving antipersonnel (fragments) bomb
Terrorism involving blast NOS
Terrorism involving explosion NOS
Terrorism involving explosion of breech block
Terrorism involving explosion of cannon block
Terrorism involving explosion (fragments) of artillery shell
Terrorism involving explosion (fragments) of bomb
Terrorism involving explosion (fragments) of grenade
Terrorism involving explosion (fragments) of guided missile
Terrorism involving explosion (fragments) of land mine
Terrorism involving explosion of mortar bomb
Terrorism involving explosion of munitions
Terrorism involving explosion (fragments) of rocket
Terrorism involving explosion (fragments) of shell
Terrorism involving shrapnel
Terrorism involving mine NOS, on land

EXCLUDES1 *terrorism involving explosion of nuclear weapon (Y38.5)*
terrorism involving suicide bomber (Y38.81)

[6th] **Y38.2X Terrorism involving other explosions and fragments**

[7th] **Y38.2X1 Terrorism involving other explosions and fragments, public safety official injured** [POA]

[7th] **Y38.2X2 Terrorism involving other explosions and fragments, civilian injured** [POA]

[7th] **Y38.2X3 Terrorism involving other explosions and fragments, terrorist injured** [POA]

[5th] **Y38.3 Terrorism involving fires, conflagration and hot substances**
Terrorism involving conflagration NOS
Terrorism involving fire NOS
Terrorism involving petrol bomb

EXCLUDES1 *terrorism involving fire or heat of nuclear weapon (Y38.5)*

[6th] **Y38.3X Terrorism involving fires, conflagration and hot substances**

[7th] **Y38.3X1 Terrorism involving fires, conflagration and hot substances, public safety official injured** [POA]

[7th] **Y38.3X2 Terrorism involving fires, conflagration and hot substances, civilian injured** [POA]

[7th] **Y38.3X3 Terrorism involving fires, conflagration and hot substances, terrorist injured** [POA]

[5th] **Y38.4 Terrorism involving firearms**
Terrorism involving carbine bullet
Terrorism involving machine gun bullet
Terrorism involving pellets (shotgun)
Terrorism involving pistol bullet
Terrorism involving rifle bullet
Terrorism involving rubber (rifle) bullet

[6th] **Y38.4X Terrorism involving firearms**

[7th] **Y38.4X1 Terrorism involving firearms, public safety official injured** [POA]

[7th] **Y38.4X2 Terrorism involving firearms, civilian injured** [POA]

[7th] **Y38.4X3 Terrorism involving firearms, terrorist injured** [POA]

[5th] **Y38.5 Terrorism involving nuclear weapons**
Terrorism involving blast effects of nuclear weapon
Terrorism involving exposure to ionizing radiation from nuclear weapon
Terrorism involving fireball effect of nuclear weapon
Terrorism involving heat from nuclear weapon

[6th] **Y38.5X Terrorism involving nuclear weapons**

[7th] **Y38.5X1 Terrorism involving nuclear weapons, public safety official injured** [POA]

[7th] **Y38.5X2 Terrorism involving nuclear weapons, civilian injured** [POA]

[7th] **Y38.5X3 Terrorism involving nuclear weapons, terrorist injured** [POA]

[5th] **Y38.6 Terrorism involving biological weapons**
Terrorism involving anthrax
Terrorism involving cholera
Terrorism involving smallpox

[6th] **Y38.6X Terrorism involving biological weapons**

[7th] **Y38.6X1 Terrorism involving biological weapons, public safety official injured** [POA]

[7th] **Y38.6X2 Terrorism involving biological weapons, civilian injured** [POA]

[7th] **Y38.6X3 Terrorism involving biological weapons, terrorist injured** [POA]

[5th] **Y38.7 Terrorism involving chemical weapons**
Terrorism involving gases, fumes, chemicals
Terrorism involving hydrogen cyanide
Terrorism involving phosgene
Terrorism involving sarin

[6th] **Y38.7X Terrorism involving chemical weapons**

[7th] **Y38.7X1 Terrorism involving chemical weapons, public safety official injured** [POA]

[7th] **Y38.7X2 Terrorism involving chemical weapons, civilian injured** [POA]

[7th] **Y38.7X3 Terrorism involving chemical weapons, terrorist injured** [POA]

[5th] **Y38.8 Terrorism involving other and unspecified means**

[7th] **Y38.80 Terrorism involving unspecified means** [POA]
Terrorism NOS

[6th] **Y38.81 Terrorism involving suicide bomber**

[7th] **Y38.811 Terrorism involving suicide bomber, public safety official injured** [POA]

[7th] **Y38.812 Terrorism involving suicide bomber, civilian injured** [POA]

[6th] **Y38.89 Terrorism involving other means**
Terrorism involving drowning and submersion
Terrorism involving lasers
Terrorism involving piercing or stabbing instruments

[7th] **Y38.891 Terrorism involving other means, public safety official injured** [POA]

[7th] **Y38.892 Terrorism involving other means, civilian injured** [POA]

[7th] **Y38.893 Terrorism involving other means, terrorist injured** [POA]

Unspecified Code   Other Specified Code   Manifestation Code   [N] Newborn   [P] Pediatric   [M] Maternity   [A] Adult   ♂ Male   ♀ Female
● New Code   ▲ Revised Code Title   ►◄ Revised Text   NOTES   INCLUDES   EXCLUDES1 Not coded here   EXCLUDES2 Not included here
[4th] 4th character required   [5th] 5th character required   [6th] 6th character required   [7th] 7th character required   [7th] Extension 'X' Alert
[HAC] Hospital-acquired condition (HAC) alert   AHA AHA Coding Clinic©   ☛ Code first alert

When symbols appear on a code that requires a 7th character extension, refer to Appendix B to identify applicable 7th character codes.

Y38.9 Terrorism, secondary effects
👁 See Official Guidelines "Code Y38.9, Terrorism, secondary effects" I.C.20. j.3
NOTES This code identifies conditions occurring subsequent to a terrorist attack not those that are due to the initial terrorist attack.
Y38.9X Terrorism, secondary effects
Y38.9X1 Terrorism, secondary effects, public safety official injured
Y38.9X2 Terrorism, secondary effects, civilian injured

Complications of medical and surgical care (Y62-Y84)

INCLUDES   complications of medical devices
surgical and medical procedures as the cause of abnormal reaction of the patient, or of later complication, without mention of misadventure at the time of the procedure

Misadventures to patients during surgical and medical care (Y62-Y69)

EXCLUDES1   surgical and medical procedures as the cause of abnormal reaction of the patient, without mention of misadventure at the time of the procedure (Y83-Y84)

EXCLUDES2   breakdown or malfunctioning of medical device (during procedure) (after implantation) (ongoing use) (Y70-Y82)

Y62 Failure of sterile precautions during surgical and medical care
Y62.0 Failure of sterile precautions during surgical operation
Y62.1 Failure of sterile precautions during infusion or transfusion
Y62.2 Failure of sterile precautions during kidney dialysis and other perfusion
Y62.3 Failure of sterile precautions during injection or immunization
Y62.4 Failure of sterile precautions during endoscopic examination
Y62.5 Failure of sterile precautions during heart catheterization
Y62.6 Failure of sterile precautions during aspiration, puncture and other catheterization
Y62.8 Failure of sterile precautions during other surgical and medical care
Y62.9 Failure of sterile precautions during unspecified surgical and medical care

Y63 Failure in dosage during surgical and medical care
EXCLUDES2   accidental overdose of drug or wrong drug given in error (T36-T50)
Y63.0 Excessive amount of blood or other fluid given during transfusion or infusion
Y63.1 Incorrect dilution of fluid used during infusion
Y63.2 Overdose of radiation given during therapy
Y63.3 Inadvertent exposure of patient to radiation during medical care
Y63.4 Failure in dosage in electroshock or insulin-shock therapy
Y63.5 Inappropriate temperature in local application and packing
Y63.6 Underdosing and nonadministration of necessary drug, medicament or biological substance
👁 See Official Guidelines "Underdosing" I.C.19.e.5.c
AHA: Q4 2018
Y63.8 Failure in dosage during other surgical and medical care
👁 See Official Guidelines "Underdosing" I.C.19.e.5.c
AHA: Q4 2018
Y63.9 Failure in dosage during unspecified surgical and medical care
👁 See Official Guidelines "Underdosing" I.C.19.e.5.c
AHA: Q4 2018

Y64 Contaminated medical or biological substances
Y64.0 Contaminated medical or biological substance, transfused or infused
Y64.1 Contaminated medical or biological substance, injected or used for immunization
Y64.8 Contaminated medical or biological substance administered by other means

Y64.9 Contaminated medical or biological substance administered by unspecified means
Administered contaminated medical or biological substance NOS

Y65 Other misadventures during surgical and medical care
Y65.0 Mismatched blood in transfusion
Y65.1 Wrong fluid used in infusion
Y65.2 Failure in suture or ligature during surgical operation
Y65.3 Endotracheal tube wrongly placed during anesthetic procedure
Y65.4 Failure to introduce or to remove other tube or instrument
Y65.5 Performance of wrong procedure (operation)
Y65.51 Performance of wrong procedure (operation) on correct patient
Wrong device implanted into correct surgical site
EXCLUDES1 performance of correct procedure (operation) on wrong side or body part (Y65.53)
Y65.52 Performance of procedure (operation) on patient not scheduled for surgery
Performance of procedure (operation) intended for another patient
Performance of procedure (operation) on wrong patient
Y65.53 Performance of correct procedure (operation) on wrong side or body part
Performance of correct procedure (operation) on wrong side
Performance of correct procedure (operation) on wrong site
Y65.8 Other specified misadventures during surgical and medical care
AHA: Q2 2019
Y66 Nonadministration of surgical and medical care
Premature cessation of surgical and medical care
EXCLUDES1 DNR status (Z66)
palliative care (Z51.5)
Y69 Unspecified misadventure during surgical and medical care

Medical devices associated with adverse incidents in diagnostic and therapeutic use (Y70-Y82)

INCLUDES   breakdown or malfunction of medical devices (during use) (after implantation) (ongoing use)

EXCLUDES2   later complications following use of medical devices without breakdown or malfunctioning of device (Y83-Y84)
misadventure to patients during surgical and medical care, classifiable to (Y62-Y69)
surgical and other medical procedures as the cause of abnormal reaction of the patient, or of later complication, without mention of misadventure at the time of the procedure (Y83-Y84)

Y70 Anesthesiology devices associated with adverse incidents
Y70.0 Diagnostic and monitoring anesthesiology devices associated with adverse incidents
Y70.1 Therapeutic (nonsurgical) and rehabilitative anesthesiology devices associated with adverse incidents
Y70.2 Prosthetic and other implants, materials and accessory anesthesiology devices associated with adverse incidents
Y70.3 Surgical instruments, materials and anesthesiology devices (including sutures) associated with adverse incidents
Y70.8 Miscellaneous anesthesiology devices associated with adverse incidents, not elsewhere classified
Y71 Cardiovascular devices associated with adverse incidents
Y71.0 Diagnostic and monitoring cardiovascular devices associated with adverse incidents
Y71.1 Therapeutic (nonsurgical) and rehabilitative cardiovascular devices associated with adverse incidents
Y71.2 Prosthetic and other implants, materials and accessory cardiovascular devices associated with adverse incidents
Y71.3 Surgical instruments, materials and cardiovascular devices (including sutures) associated with adverse incidents

---

Y71.8 Miscellaneous **cardiovascular devices associated with adverse incidents, not elsewhere classified**

⁴ᵗʰ Y72 Otorhinolaryngological **devices associated with adverse incidents**

Y72.0 Diagnostic and monitoring **otorhinolaryngological devices associated with adverse incidents**

Y72.1 Therapeutic (nonsurgical) and rehabilitative **otorhinolaryngological devices associated with adverse incidents**

Y72.2 Prosthetic and other implants, **materials and accessory otorhinolaryngological devices associated with adverse incidents**

Y72.3 Surgical instruments, **materials and otorhinolaryngological devices (including sutures) associated with adverse incidents**

Y72.8 Miscellaneous **otorhinolaryngological devices associated with adverse incidents, not elsewhere classified**

⁴ᵗʰ Y73 Gastroenterology and urology **devices associated with adverse incidents**

Y73.0 Diagnostic and monitoring **gastroenterology and urology devices associated with adverse incidents**

Y73.1 Therapeutic (nonsurgical) and rehabilitative **gastroenterology and urology devices associated with adverse incidents**

Y73.2 Prosthetic and other implants, **materials and accessory gastroenterology and urology devices associated with adverse incidents**

Y73.3 Surgical instruments, **materials and gastroenterology and urology devices (including sutures) associated with adverse incidents**

Y73.8 Miscellaneous **gastroenterology and urology devices associated with adverse incidents, not elsewhere classified**

⁴ᵗʰ Y74 General hospital **and personal-use devices associated with adverse incidents**

Y74.0 Diagnostic and monitoring **general hospital and personal-use devices associated with adverse incidents**

Y74.1 Therapeutic (nonsurgical) and rehabilitative **general hospital and personal-use devices associated with adverse incidents**

Y74.2 Prosthetic and other implants, **materials and accessory general hospital and personal-use devices associated with adverse incidents**

Y74.3 Surgical instruments, **materials and general hospital and personal-use devices (including sutures) associated with adverse incidents**

Y74.8 Miscellaneous **general hospital and personal-use devices associated with adverse incidents, not elsewhere classified**

⁴ᵗʰ Y75 Neurological **devices associated with adverse incidents**

Y75.0 Diagnostic and monitoring **neurological devices associated with adverse incidents**

Y75.1 Therapeutic (nonsurgical) and rehabilitative **neurological devices associated with adverse incidents**

Y75.2 Prosthetic and other implants, **materials and neurological devices associated with adverse incidents**

Y75.3 Surgical instruments, **materials and neurological devices (including sutures) associated with adverse incidents**

Y75.8 Miscellaneous **neurological devices associated with adverse incidents, not elsewhere classified**

⁴ᵗʰ Y76 Obstetric and gynecological **devices associated with adverse incidents**

Y76.0 Diagnostic and monitoring **obstetric and gynecological devices associated with adverse incidents** ♀

Y76.1 Therapeutic (nonsurgical) and rehabilitative **obstetric and gynecological devices associated with adverse incidents** ♀

Y76.2 Prosthetic and other implants, **materials and accessory obstetric and gynecological devices associated with adverse incidents** ♀

Y76.3 Surgical instruments, **materials and obstetric and gynecological devices (including sutures) associated with adverse incidents** ♀

Y76.8 Miscellaneous **obstetric and gynecological devices associated with adverse incidents, not elsewhere classified** ♀

⁴ᵗʰ Y77 Ophthalmic **devices associated with adverse incidents**

Y77.0 Diagnostic and monitoring **ophthalmic devices associated with adverse incidents**

Y77.1 Therapeutic (nonsurgical) and rehabilitative **ophthalmic devices associated with adverse incidents**

Y77.2 Prosthetic and other implants, **materials and accessory ophthalmic devices associated with adverse incidents**

Y77.3 Surgical instruments, **materials and ophthalmic devices (including sutures) associated with adverse incidents**

Y77.8 Miscellaneous **ophthalmic devices associated with adverse incidents, not elsewhere classified**

⁴ᵗʰ Y78 Radiological **devices associated with adverse incidents**

Y78.0 Diagnostic and monitoring **radiological devices associated with adverse incidents**

Y78.1 Therapeutic (nonsurgical) and rehabilitative **radiological devices associated with adverse incidents**

Y78.2 Prosthetic and other implants, **materials and accessory radiological devices associated with adverse incidents**

Y78.3 Surgical instruments, **materials and radiological devices (including sutures) associated with adverse incidents**

Y78.8 Miscellaneous **radiological devices associated with adverse incidents, not elsewhere classified**

⁴ᵗʰ Y79 Orthopedic **devices associated with adverse incidents**

Y79.0 Diagnostic and monitoring **orthopedic devices associated with adverse incidents**

Y79.1 Therapeutic (nonsurgical) and rehabilitative **orthopedic devices associated with adverse incidents**

Y79.2 Prosthetic and other implants, **materials and accessory orthopedic devices associated with adverse incidents**

Y79.3 Surgical instruments, **materials and orthopedic devices (including sutures) associated with adverse incidents**

Y79.8 Miscellaneous **orthopedic devices associated with adverse incidents, not elsewhere classified**

⁴ᵗʰ Y80 Physical medicine **devices associated with adverse incidents**

Y80.0 Diagnostic and monitoring **physical medicine devices associated with adverse incidents**

Y80.1 Therapeutic (nonsurgical) and rehabilitative **physical medicine devices associated with adverse incidents**

Y80.2 Prosthetic and other implants, **materials and accessory physical medicine devices associated with adverse incidents**

Y80.3 Surgical instruments, **materials and physical medicine devices (including sutures) associated with adverse incidents**

Y80.8 Miscellaneous **physical medicine devices associated with adverse incidents, not elsewhere classified**

⁴ᵗʰ Y81 General- and plastic-surgery **devices associated with adverse incidents**

Y81.0 Diagnostic and monitoring **general- and plastic-surgery devices associated with adverse incidents**

Y81.1 Therapeutic (nonsurgical) and rehabilitative **general- and plastic-surgery devices associated with adverse incidents**

Y81.2 Prosthetic and other implants, **materials and accessory general- and plastic-surgery devices associated with adverse incidents**

Y81.3 Surgical instruments, **materials and general- and plastic-surgery devices (including sutures) associated with adverse incidents**

Y81.8 Miscellaneous **general- and plastic-surgery devices associated with adverse incidents, not elsewhere classified**

⁴ᵗʰ Y82 Other and unspecified **medical devices associated with adverse incidents**

Y82.8 **Other medical devices associated with adverse incidents**

Y82.9 **Unspecified medical devices associated with adverse incidents**

Unspecified Code   Other Specified Code   Manifestation Code   Ⓝ Newborn   Ⓟ Pediatric   Ⓜ Maternity   Ⓐ Adult   ♂ Male   ♀ Female
● New Code   ▲ Revised Code Title   ▶◀ Revised Text   **NOTES**   *INCLUDES*   *EXCLUDES1* Not coded here   *EXCLUDES2* Not included here
④ 4ᵗʰ character required   ⑤ 5ᵗʰ character required   ⑥ 6ᵗʰ character required   ⑦ 7ᵗʰ character required   Ⓧ Extension 'X' Alert
HAC Hospital-acquired condition (HAC) alert   **AHA** AHA Coding Clinic©   📖 Code first alert

2020 ICD-10-CM   When symbols appear on a code that requires a 7th character extension, refer to Appendix B to identify applicable 7th character codes.   **1241**

Surgical and other medical procedures as the cause of abnormal reaction of the patient, or of later complication, without mention of misadventure at the time of the procedure (Y83-Y84)

EXCLUDES1 misadventures to patients during surgical and medical care, classifiable to (Y62-Y69)

EXCLUDES2 breakdown or malfunctioning of medical device (after implantation) (during procedure) (ongoing use) (Y70-Y82)

Y83 Surgical operation and other surgical procedures as the cause of abnormal reaction of the patient, or of later complication, without mention of misadventure at the time of the procedure

Y83.0 **Surgical operation** with transplant of whole organ **as the cause of abnormal reaction of the patient, or of later complication, without mention of misadventure at the time of the procedure**

Y83.1 **Surgical operation** with implant of artificial internal device **as the cause of abnormal reaction of the patient, or of later complication, without mention of misadventure at the time of the procedure**

Y83.2 **Surgical operation** with anastomosis, bypass or graft **as the cause of abnormal reaction of the patient, or of later complication, without mention of misadventure at the time of the procedure**

Y83.3 **Surgical operation** with formation of external stoma **as the cause of abnormal reaction of the patient, or of later complication, without mention of misadventure at the time of the procedure**

Y83.4 Other reconstructive surgery **as the cause of abnormal reaction of the patient, or of later complication, without mention of misadventure at the time of the procedure**

Y83.5 Amputation of limb(s) **as the cause of abnormal reaction of the patient, or of later complication, without mention of misadventure at the time of the procedure**

Y83.6 Removal of other organ (partial) (total) **as the cause of abnormal reaction of the patient, or of later complication, without mention of misadventure at the time of the procedure**

Y83.8 **Other surgical procedures as the cause of abnormal reaction of the patient, or of later complication, without mention of misadventure at the time of the procedure**

Y83.9 **Surgical procedure, unspecified as the cause of abnormal reaction of the patient, or of later complication, without mention of misadventure at the time of the procedure**

Y84 Other medical procedures **as the cause of abnormal reaction of the patient, or of later complication, without mention of misadventure at the time of the procedure**

Y84.0 Cardiac catheterization **as the cause of abnormal reaction of the patient, or of later complication, without mention of misadventure at the time of the procedure**

Y84.1 Kidney dialysis **as the cause of abnormal reaction of the patient, or of later complication, without mention of misadventure at the time of the procedure**

Y84.2 Radiological procedure and radiotherapy **as the cause of abnormal reaction of the patient, or of later complication, without mention of misadventure at the time of the procedure**

See Official Guidelines "Anemia associated with chemotherapy, immunotherapy and radiation therapy" I.C.2.c.2

AHA: Q1 2019, Q1 2017

Y84.3 Shock therapy **as the cause of abnormal reaction of the patient, or of later complication, without mention of misadventure at the time of the procedure**

Y84.4 Aspiration of fluid **as the cause of abnormal reaction of the patient, or of later complication, without mention of misadventure at the time of the procedure**

Y84.5 Insertion of gastric or duodenal sound **as the cause of abnormal reaction of the patient, or of later complication, without mention of misadventure at the time of the procedure**

Y84.6 Urinary catheterization **as the cause of abnormal reaction of the patient, or of later complication, without mention of misadventure at the time of the procedure**

Y84.7 Blood-sampling **as the cause of abnormal reaction of the patient, or of later complication, without mention of misadventure at the time of the procedure**

Y84.8 **Other medical procedures as the cause of abnormal reaction of the patient, or of later complication, without mention of misadventure at the time of the procedure**

Y84.9 **Medical procedure, unspecified as the cause of abnormal reaction of the patient, or of later complication, without mention of misadventure at the time of the procedure**

Supplementary factors related to causes of morbidity classified elsewhere (Y90-Y99)

NOTES These categories may be used to provide supplementary information concerning causes of morbidity. They are not to be used for single-condition coding.

Y90 **Evidence of alcohol involvement determined by blood alcohol level**

Code first any associated alcohol related disorders (F10)

Y90.0 **Blood alcohol level of** less than 20 mg/100 ml

Y90.1 **Blood alcohol level of** 20-39 mg/100 ml

Y90.2 **Blood alcohol level of** 40-59 mg/100 ml

Y90.3 **Blood alcohol level of** 60-79 mg/100 ml

Y90.4 **Blood alcohol level of** 80-99 mg/100 ml

Y90.5 **Blood alcohol level of** 100-119 mg/100 ml

Y90.6 **Blood alcohol level of** 120-199 mg/100 ml

Y90.7 **Blood alcohol level of** 200-239 mg/100 ml

Y90.8 **Blood alcohol level of** 240 mg/100 ml or more

Y90.9 **Presence of alcohol in blood, level not specified**

Y92 **Place of occurrence of the external cause**

See Official Guidelines "Place of Occurrence Guideline" I.C.20.b

The following category is for use, when relevant, to identify the place of occurrence of the external cause. Use in conjunction with an activity code.

Place of occurrence should be recorded only at the initial encounter for treatment

Y92.0 Non-institutional (private) residence **as the place of occurrence of the external cause**

EXCLUDES1 abandoned or derelict house (Y92.89)

home under construction but not yet occupied (Y92.6-)

institutional place of residence (Y92.1-)

Y92.00 Unspecified **non-institutional (private) residence as the place of occurrence of the external cause**

Y92.000 Kitchen **of unspecified non-institutional (private) residence as the place of occurrence of the external cause**

Y92.001 Dining room **of unspecified non-institutional (private) residence as the place of occurrence of the external cause**

Y92.002 Bathroom **of unspecified non-institutional (private) residence single-family (private) house as the place of occurrence of the external cause**

Y92.003 Bedroom **of unspecified non-institutional (private) residence as the place of occurrence of the external cause**

Y92.007 Garden or yard **of unspecified non-institutional (private) residence as the place of occurrence of the external cause**

Y92.008 Other place **in unspecified non-institutional (private) residence as the place of occurrence of the external cause**

Y92.009 **Unspecified** place **in unspecified non-institutional (private) residence as the** place **of occurrence of the external cause**

Home (NOS) as the place of occurrence of the external cause

Unacceptable principal diagnosis symbol per Medicare code edits   Code exempt from diagnosis present on admission requirement

? Questionable admission   Complication or comorbidity   MCC Major complication or comorbidity   CC/MCC exclusion

HCC HCC diagnosis code   RxHCC RxHCC diagnosis code   MACRA code   **DEFINITION** Describes condition/terminology

TIP Coding guidance   Official Guideline Reference   Z Z code as first-listed diagnosis

1242   When symbols appear on a code that requires a 7th character extension, refer to Appendix B to identify applicable 7th character codes.   **2020 ICD-10-CM**

6⁶ᵗʰ **Y92.01** Single-family non-institutional (private) house as the place of occurrence of the external cause
Farmhouse as the place of occurrence of the external cause
EXCLUDES1 barn (Y92.71)
chicken coop or hen house (Y92.72)
farm field (Y92.73)
orchard (Y92.74)
single family mobile home or trailer (Y92.02-)
slaughter house (Y92.86)

Y92.010 Kitchen of single-family (private) house as the place of occurrence of the external cause POA

Y92.011 Dining room of single-family (private) house as the place of occurrence of the external cause

Y92.012 Bathroom of single-family (private) house as the place of occurrence of the external cause POA

Y92.013 Bedroom of single-family (private) house as the place of occurrence of the external cause POA

Y92.014 Private driveway to single-family (private) house as the place of occurrence of the external cause POA

Y92.015 Private garage of single-family (private) house as the place of occurrence of the external cause POA

Y92.016 Swimming-pool in single-family (private) house or garden as the place of occurrence of the external cause POA

Y92.017 Garden or yard in single-family (private) house as the place of occurrence of the external cause POA

Y92.018 Other place in single-family (private) house as the place of occurrence of the external cause POA

Y92.019 Unspecified place in single-family (private) house as the place of occurrence of the external cause POA

6⁶ᵗʰ **Y92.02** Mobile home as the place of occurrence of the external cause

Y92.020 Kitchen in mobile home as the place of occurrence of the external cause POA

Y92.021 Dining room in mobile home as the place of occurrence of the external cause POA

Y92.022 Bathroom in mobile home as the place of occurrence of the external cause POA

Y92.023 Bedroom in mobile home as the place of occurrence of the external cause POA

Y92.024 Driveway of mobile home as the place of occurrence of the external cause POA

Y92.025 Garage of mobile home as the place of occurrence of the external cause POA

Y92.026 Swimming-pool of mobile home as the place of occurrence of the external cause POA

Y92.027 Garden or yard of mobile home as the place of occurrence of the external cause POA

Y92.028 Other place in mobile home as the place of occurrence of the external cause POA

Y92.029 Unspecified place in mobile home as the place of occurrence of the external cause POA

6⁶ᵗʰ **Y92.03** Apartment as the place of occurrence of the external cause
Condominium as the place of occurrence of the external cause
Co-op apartment as the place of occurrence of the external cause

Y92.030 Kitchen in apartment as the place of occurrence of the external cause POA

Y92.031 Bathroom in apartment as the place of occurrence of the external cause POA

Y92.032 Bedroom in apartment as the place of occurrence of the external cause POA

Y92.038 Other place in apartment as the place of occurrence of the external cause POA

Y92.039 Unspecified place in apartment as the place of occurrence of the external cause

6⁶ᵗʰ **Y92.04** Boarding-house as the place of occurrence of the external cause

Y92.040 Kitchen in boarding-house as the place of occurrence of the external cause POA

Y92.041 Bathroom in boarding-house as the place of occurrence of the external cause POA

Y92.042 Bedroom in boarding-house as the place of occurrence of the external cause POA

Y92.043 Driveway of boarding-house as the place of occurrence of the external cause POA

Y92.044 Garage of boarding-house as the place of occurrence of the external cause POA

Y92.045 Swimming-pool of boarding-house as the place of occurrence of the external cause POA

Y92.046 Garden or yard of boarding-house as the place of occurrence of the external cause POA

Y92.048 Other place in boarding-house as the place of occurrence of the external cause POA

Y92.049 Unspecified place in boarding-house as the place of occurrence of the external cause POA

6⁶ᵗʰ **Y92.09** Other non-institutional residence as the place of occurrence of the external cause

Y92.090 Kitchen in other non-institutional residence as the place of occurrence of the external cause POA

Y92.091 Bathroom in other non-institutional residence as the place of occurrence of the external cause POA

Y92.092 Bedroom in other non-institutional residence as the place of occurrence of the external cause POA

Y92.093 Driveway of other non-institutional residence as the place of occurrence of the external cause POA

Y92.094 Garage of other non-institutional residence as the place of occurrence of the external cause POA

Y92.095 Swimming-pool of other non-institutional residence as the place of occurrence of the external cause POA

Y92.096 Garden or yard of other non-institutional residence as the place of occurrence of the external cause POA

Y92.098 Other place in other non-institutional residence as the place of occurrence of the external cause POA
AHA: Q2 2017

Y92.099 Unspecified place in other non-institutional residence as the place of occurrence of the external cause POA
AHA: Q2 2017

5⁵ᵗʰ **Y92.1** Institutional (nonprivate) residence as the place of occurrence of the external cause

Y92.10 Unspecified residential institution as the place of occurrence of the external cause POA

6⁶ᵗʰ **Y92.11** Children's home and orphanage as the place of occurrence of the external cause

Unspecified Code   Other Specified Code   Manifestation Code   N Newborn   P Pediatric   M Maternity   A Adult   ♂ Male   ♀ Female
● New Code   ▲ Revised Code Title   ▶◀ Revised Text   NOTES   INCLUDES   EXCLUDES1 Not coded here   EXCLUDES2 Not included here
4ᵗʰ 4ᵗʰ character required   5ᵗʰ 5ᵗʰ character required   6ᵗʰ 6ᵗʰ character required   7ᵗʰ 7ᵗʰ character required   7ᵗʰˣ Extension 'X' Alert
HAC Hospital-acquired condition (HAC) alert   AHA AHA Coding Clinic©   ☞ Code first alert

2020 ICD-10-CM   When symbols appear on a code that requires a 7th character extension, refer to Appendix B to identify applicable 7th character codes.   1243

Y92.110 Kitchen in children's home and orphanage as the place of occurrence of the external cause POA

Y92.111 Bathroom in children's home and orphanage as the place of occurrence of the external cause POA

Y92.112 Bedroom in children's home and orphanage as the place of occurrence of the external cause POA

Y92.113 Driveway of children's home and orphanage as the place of occurrence of the external cause POA

Y92.114 Garage of children's home and orphanage as the place of occurrence of the external cause POA

Y92.115 Swimming-pool of children's home and orphanage as the place of occurrence of the external cause POA

Y92.116 Garden or yard of children's home and orphanage as the place of occurrence of the external cause POA

Y92.118 Other place in children's home and orphanage as the place of occurrence of the external cause POA

Y92.119 Unspecified place in children's home and orphanage as the place of occurrence of the external cause POA

Y92.12 Nursing home as the place of occurrence of the external cause

Home for the sick as the place of occurrence of the external cause

Hospice as the place of occurrence of the external cause

Y92.120 Kitchen in nursing home as the place of occurrence of the external cause POA

Y92.121 Bathroom in nursing home as the place of occurrence of the external cause POA

Y92.122 Bedroom in nursing home as the place of occurrence of the external cause POA

Y92.123 Driveway of nursing home as the place of occurrence of the external cause POA

Y92.124 Garage of nursing home as the place of occurrence of the external cause POA

Y92.125 Swimming-pool of nursing home as the place of occurrence of the external cause POA

Y92.126 Garden or yard of nursing home as the place of occurrence of the external cause POA

Y92.128 Other place in nursing home as the place of occurrence of the external cause POA

Y92.129 Unspecified place in nursing home as the place of occurrence of the external cause POA

AHA: Q2 2017

Y92.13 Military base as the place of occurrence of the external cause

EXCLUDES1 military training grounds (Y92.83)

Y92.130 Kitchen on military base as the place of occurrence of the external cause POA

Y92.131 Mess hall on military base as the place of occurrence of the external cause POA

Y92.133 Barracks on military base as the place of occurrence of the external cause POA

Y92.135 Garage on military base as the place of occurrence of the external cause POA

Y92.136 Swimming-pool on military base as the place of occurrence of the external cause POA

Y92.137 Garden or yard on military base as the place of occurrence of the external cause POA

Y92.138 Other place on military base as the place of occurrence of the external cause POA

Y92.139 Unspecified place military base as the place of occurrence of the external cause POA

Y92.14 Prison as the place of occurrence of the external cause

Y92.140 Kitchen in prison as the place of occurrence of the external cause POA

Y92.141 Dining room in prison as the place of occurrence of the external cause POA

Y92.142 Bathroom in prison as the place of occurrence of the external cause POA

Y92.143 Cell of prison as the place of occurrence of the external cause POA

Y92.146 Swimming-pool of prison as the place of occurrence of the external cause POA

Y92.147 Courtyard of prison as the place of occurrence of the external cause POA

Y92.148 Other place in prison as the place of occurrence of the external cause POA

Y92.149 Unspecified place in prison as the place of occurrence of the external cause POA

Y92.15 Reform school as the place of occurrence of the external cause

Y92.150 Kitchen in reform school as the place of occurrence of the external cause POA

Y92.151 Dining room in reform school as the place of occurrence of the external cause POA

Y92.152 Bathroom in reform school as the place of occurrence of the external cause POA

Y92.153 Bedroom in reform school as the place of occurrence of the external cause POA

Y92.154 Driveway of reform school as the place of occurrence of the external cause POA

Y92.155 Garage of reform school as the place of occurrence of the external cause POA

Y92.156 Swimming-pool of reform school as the place of occurrence of the external cause POA

Y92.157 Garden or yard of reform school as the place of occurrence of the external cause POA

Y92.158 Other place in reform school as the place of occurrence of the external cause POA

Y92.159 Unspecified place in reform school as the place of occurrence of the external cause POA

Y92.16 School dormitory as the place of occurrence of the external cause

EXCLUDES1 reform school as the place of occurrence of the external cause (Y92.15-)

school buildings and grounds as the place of occurrence of the external cause (Y92.2-)

school sports and athletic areas as the place of occurrence of the external cause (Y92.3-)

Y92.160 Kitchen in school dormitory as the place of occurrence of the external cause POA

Y92.161 Dining room in school dormitory as the place of occurrence of the external cause POA

Y92.162 Bathroom in school dormitory as the place of occurrence of the external cause POA

Y92.163 Bedroom in school dormitory as the place of occurrence of the external cause POA

Y92.168 Other place in school dormitory as the place of occurrence of the external cause POA

Y92.169 Unspecified place in school dormitory as the place of occurrence of the external cause POA

POA Unacceptable principal diagnosis symbol per Medicare code edits   POA Code exempt from diagnosis present on admission requirement
? Questionable admission   CC Complication or comorbidity   MCC Major complication or comorbidity   CC:MCC:EXC CC/MCC exclusion
HCC HCC diagnosis code   RXHCC RxHCC diagnosis code   MACRA MACRA code   DEFINITION Describes condition/terminology
TIP Coding guidance   ◉ Official Guideline Reference   Z1 Z code as first-listed diagnosis

Y92.19 Other specified residential institution as the place of occurrence of the external cause

Y92.190 Kitchen in other specified residential institution as the place of occurrence of the external cause

Y92.191 Dining room in other specified residential institution as the place of occurrence of the external cause

Y92.192 Bathroom in other specified residential institution as the place of occurrence of the external cause

Y92.193 Bedroom in other specified residential institution as the place of occurrence of the external cause

Y92.194 Driveway of other specified residential institution as the place of occurrence of the external cause

Y92.195 Garage of other specified residential institution as the place of occurrence of the external cause

Y92.196 Pool of other specified residential institution as the place of occurrence of the external cause

Y92.197 Garden or yard of other specified residential institution as the place of occurrence of the external cause

Y92.198 Other place in other specified residential institution as the place of occurrence of the external cause

Y92.199 Unspecified place in other specified residential institution as the place of occurrence of the external cause

AHA: Q2 2017

Y92.2 School, other institution and public administrative area as the place of occurrence of the external cause

Building and adjacent grounds used by the general public or by a particular group of the public

EXCLUDES1 building under construction as the place of occurrence of the external cause (Y92.6)

residential institution as the place of occurrence of the external cause (Y92.1)

school dormitory as the place of occurrence of the external cause (Y92.16-)

sports and athletics area of schools as the place of occurrence of the external cause (Y92.3-)

Y92.21 School (private) (public) (state) as the place of occurrence of the external cause

Y92.210 Daycare center as the place of occurrence of the external cause

Y92.211 Elementary school as the place of occurrence of the external cause

Kindergarten as the place of occurrence of the external cause

Y92.212 Middle school as the place of occurrence of the external cause

Y92.213 High school as the place of occurrence of the external cause

AHA: Q4 2012

Y92.214 College as the place of occurrence of the external cause

University as the place of occurrence of the external cause

Y92.215 Trade school as the place of occurrence of the external cause

Y92.218 Other school as the place of occurrence of the external cause

Y92.219 Unspecified school as the place of occurrence of the external cause

Y92.22 Religious institution as the place of occurrence of the external cause

Church as the place of occurrence of the external cause

Mosque as the place of occurrence of the external cause

Synagogue as the place of occurrence of the external cause

Y92.23 Hospital as the place of occurrence of the external cause

EXCLUDES1 ambulatory (outpatient) health services establishments (Y92.53-)

home for the sick as the place of occurrence of the external cause (Y92.12-)

hospice as the place of occurrence of the external cause (Y92.12-)

nursing home as the place of occurrence of the external cause (Y92.12-)

Y92.230 Patient room in hospital as the place of occurrence of the external cause

Y92.231 Patient bathroom in hospital as the place of occurrence of the external cause

Y92.232 Corridor of hospital as the place of occurrence of the external cause

Y92.233 Cafeteria of hospital as the place of occurrence of the external cause

Y92.234 Operating room of hospital as the place of occurrence of the external cause

Y92.238 Other place in hospital as the place of occurrence of the external cause

Y92.239 Unspecified place in hospital as the place of occurrence of the external cause

Y92.24 Public administrative building as the place of occurrence of the external cause

Y92.240 Courthouse as the place of occurrence of the external cause

Y92.241 Library as the place of occurrence of the external cause

Y92.242 Post office as the place of occurrence of the external cause

Y92.243 City hall as the place of occurrence of the external cause

Y92.248 Other public administrative building as the place of occurrence of the external cause

Y92.25 Cultural building as the place of occurrence of the external cause

Y92.250 Art Gallery as the place of occurrence of the external cause

Y92.251 Museum as the place of occurrence of the external cause

Y92.252 Music hall as the place of occurrence of the external cause

Y92.253 Opera house as the place of occurrence of the external cause

Y92.254 Theater (live) as the place of occurrence of the external cause

Y92.258 Other cultural public building as the place of occurrence of the external cause

Y92.26 Movie house or cinema as the place of occurrence of the external cause

Y92.29 Other specified public building as the place of occurrence of the external cause

Assembly hall as the place of occurrence of the external cause

Clubhouse as the place of occurrence of the external cause

Y92.3 Sports and athletics area as the place of occurrence of the external cause

Y92.31 Athletic court as the place of occurrence of the external cause

EXCLUDES1 tennis court in private home or garden (Y92.09)

Y92.310 Basketball court as the place of occurrence of the external cause

Y92.311 Squash court as the place of occurrence of the external cause POA

Y92.312 Tennis court as the place of occurrence of the external cause POA

Y92.318 Other athletic court as the place of occurrence of the external cause POA

[6th] Y92.32 Athletic field as the place of occurrence of the external cause

Y92.320 Baseball field as the place of occurrence of the external cause POA

Y92.321 Football field as the place of occurrence of the external cause POA

Y92.322 Soccer field as the place of occurrence of the external cause POA

Y92.328 Other athletic field as the place of occurrence of the external cause POA
Cricket field as the place of occurrence of the external cause
Hockey field as the place of occurrence of the external cause

[6th] Y92.33 Skating rink as the place of occurrence of the external cause

Y92.330 Ice skating rink (indoor) (outdoor) as the place of occurrence of the external cause POA

Y92.331 Roller skating rink as the place of occurrence of the external cause POA

Y92.34 Swimming pool (public) as the place of occurrence of the external cause POA
EXCLUDES1 *swimming pool in private home or garden (Y92.016)*

Y92.39 Other specified sports and athletic area as the place of occurrence of the external cause POA
Golf-course as the place of occurrence of the external cause
Gymnasium as the place of occurrence of the external cause
Riding-school as the place of occurrence of the external cause
Stadium as the place of occurrence of the external cause

[5th] Y92.4 Street, highway and other paved roadways as the place of occurrence of the external cause
EXCLUDES1 *private driveway of residence (Y92.014, Y92.024, Y92.043, Y92.093, Y92.113, Y92.123, Y92.154, Y92.194)*

[6th] Y92.41 Street and highway as the place of occurrence of the external cause

Y92.410 Unspecified street and highway as the place of occurrence of the external cause POA
Road NOS as the place of occurrence of the external cause

Y92.411 Interstate highway as the place of occurrence of the external cause POA
Freeway as the place of occurrence of the external cause
Motorway as the place of occurrence of the external cause

Y92.412 Parkway as the place of occurrence of the external cause POA

Y92.413 State road as the place of occurrence of the external cause POA

Y92.414 Local residential or business street as the place of occurrence of the external cause POA

Y92.415 Exit ramp or entrance ramp of street or highway as the place of occurrence of the external cause POA

[6th] Y92.48 Other paved roadways as the place of occurrence of the external cause

Y92.480 Sidewalk as the place of occurrence of the external cause POA

Y92.481 Parking lot as the place of occurrence of the external cause POA

Y92.482 Bike path as the place of occurrence of the external cause POA

Y92.488 Other paved roadways as the place of occurrence of the external cause POA

[5th] Y92.5 Trade and service area as the place of occurrence of the external cause
EXCLUDES1 *garage in private home (Y92.015)*
schools and other public administration buildings (Y92.2-)

[6th] Y92.51 Private commercial establishments as the place of occurrence of the external cause

Y92.510 Bank as the place of occurrence of the external cause POA

Y92.511 Restaurant or café as the place of occurrence of the external cause POA

Y92.512 Supermarket, store or market as the place of occurrence of the external cause POA

Y92.513 Shop (commercial) as the place of occurrence of the external cause POA

[6th] Y92.52 Service areas as the place of occurrence of the external cause

Y92.520 Airport as the place of occurrence of the external cause POA

Y92.521 Bus station as the place of occurrence of the external cause POA

Y92.522 Railway station as the place of occurrence of the external cause POA

Y92.523 Highway rest stop as the place of occurrence of the external cause POA

Y92.524 Gas station as the place of occurrence of the external cause POA
Petroleum station as the place of occurrence of the external cause
Service station as the place of occurrence of the external cause

[6th] Y92.53 Ambulatory health services establishments as the place of occurrence of the external cause

Y92.530 Ambulatory surgery center as the place of occurrence of the external cause
Outpatient surgery center, including that connected with a hospital as the place of occurrence of the external cause
Same day surgery center, including that connected with a hospital as the place of occurrence of the external cause

Y92.531 Health care provider office as the place of occurrence of the external cause POA
Physician office as the place of occurrence of the external cause

Y92.532 Urgent care center as the place of occurrence of the external cause POA

Y92.538 Other ambulatory health services establishments as the place of occurrence of the external cause
AHA: Q1 2019

Y92.59 Other trade areas as the place of occurrence of the external cause POA
Office building as the place of occurrence of the external cause
Casino as the place of occurrence of the external cause
Garage (commercial) as the place of occurrence of the external cause
Hotel as the place of occurrence of the external cause
Radio or television station as the place of occurrence of the external cause
Shopping mall as the place of occurrence of the external cause
Warehouse as the place of occurrence of the external cause

PDx Unacceptable principal diagnosis symbol per Medicare code edits; POA Code exempt from diagnosis present on admission requirement
[?] Questionable admission; CC Complication or comorbidity; MCC Major complication or comorbidity; CC/MCC Exc CC/MCC exclusion
[HCC] HCC diagnosis code; [RxHCC] RxHCC diagnosis code; MACRA code; **DEFINITION** Describes condition/terminology
TIP Coding guidance; 👁 Official Guideline Reference; [Z1] Z code as first-listed diagnosis

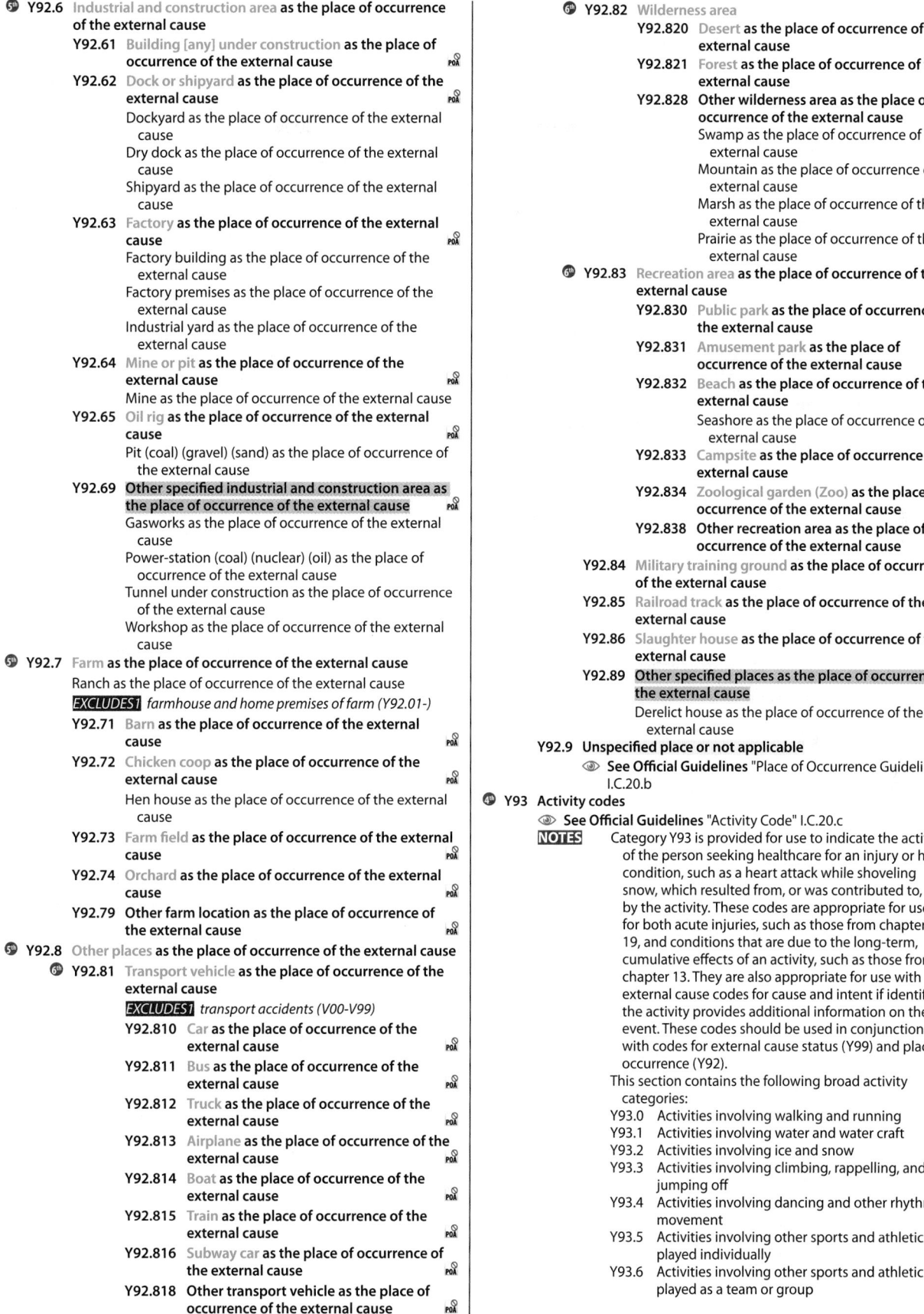

Y92.6 Industrial and construction area as the place of occurrence of the external cause

Y92.61 Building [any] under construction as the place of occurrence of the external cause

Y92.62 Dock or shipyard as the place of occurrence of the external cause

Dockyard as the place of occurrence of the external cause

Dry dock as the place of occurrence of the external cause

Shipyard as the place of occurrence of the external cause

Y92.63 Factory as the place of occurrence of the external cause

Factory building as the place of occurrence of the external cause

Factory premises as the place of occurrence of the external cause

Industrial yard as the place of occurrence of the external cause

Y92.64 Mine or pit as the place of occurrence of the external cause

Mine as the place of occurrence of the external cause

Y92.65 Oil rig as the place of occurrence of the external cause

Pit (coal) (gravel) (sand) as the place of occurrence of the external cause

Y92.69 Other specified industrial and construction area as the place of occurrence of the external cause

Gasworks as the place of occurrence of the external cause

Power-station (coal) (nuclear) (oil) as the place of occurrence of the external cause

Tunnel under construction as the place of occurrence of the external cause

Workshop as the place of occurrence of the external cause

Y92.7 Farm as the place of occurrence of the external cause

Ranch as the place of occurrence of the external cause

EXCLUDES1 farmhouse and home premises of farm (Y92.01-)

Y92.71 Barn as the place of occurrence of the external cause

Y92.72 Chicken coop as the place of occurrence of the external cause

Hen house as the place of occurrence of the external cause

Y92.73 Farm field as the place of occurrence of the external cause

Y92.74 Orchard as the place of occurrence of the external cause

Y92.79 Other farm location as the place of occurrence of the external cause

Y92.8 Other places as the place of occurrence of the external cause

Y92.81 Transport vehicle as the place of occurrence of the external cause

EXCLUDES1 transport accidents (V00-V99)

Y92.810 Car as the place of occurrence of the external cause

Y92.811 Bus as the place of occurrence of the external cause

Y92.812 Truck as the place of occurrence of the external cause

Y92.813 Airplane as the place of occurrence of the external cause

Y92.814 Boat as the place of occurrence of the external cause

Y92.815 Train as the place of occurrence of the external cause

Y92.816 Subway car as the place of occurrence of the external cause

Y92.818 Other transport vehicle as the place of occurrence of the external cause

Y92.82 Wilderness area

Y92.820 Desert as the place of occurrence of the external cause

Y92.821 Forest as the place of occurrence of the external cause

Y92.828 Other wilderness area as the place of occurrence of the external cause

Swamp as the place of occurrence of the external cause

Mountain as the place of occurrence of the external cause

Marsh as the place of occurrence of the external cause

Prairie as the place of occurrence of the external cause

Y92.83 Recreation area as the place of occurrence of the external cause

Y92.830 Public park as the place of occurrence of the external cause

Y92.831 Amusement park as the place of occurrence of the external cause

Y92.832 Beach as the place of occurrence of the external cause

Seashore as the place of occurrence of the external cause

Y92.833 Campsite as the place of occurrence of the external cause

Y92.834 Zoological garden (Zoo) as the place of occurrence of the external cause

Y92.838 Other recreation area as the place of occurrence of the external cause

Y92.84 Military training ground as the place of occurrence of the external cause

Y92.85 Railroad track as the place of occurrence of the external cause

Y92.86 Slaughter house as the place of occurrence of the external cause

Y92.89 Other specified places as the place of occurrence of the external cause

Derelict house as the place of occurrence of the external cause

Y92.9 Unspecified place or not applicable

See Official Guidelines "Place of Occurrence Guideline" I.C.20.b

Y93 Activity codes

See Official Guidelines "Activity Code" I.C.20.c

NOTES Category Y93 is provided for use to indicate the activity of the person seeking healthcare for an injury or health condition, such as a heart attack while shoveling snow, which resulted from, or was contributed to, by the activity. These codes are appropriate for use for both acute injuries, such as those from chapter 19, and conditions that are due to the long-term, cumulative effects of an activity, such as those from chapter 13. They are also appropriate for use with external cause codes for cause and intent if identifying the activity provides additional information on the event. These codes should be used in conjunction with codes for external cause status (Y99) and place of occurrence (Y92).

This section contains the following broad activity categories:

Y93.0 Activities involving walking and running

Y93.1 Activities involving water and water craft

Y93.2 Activities involving ice and snow

Y93.3 Activities involving climbing, rappelling, and jumping off

Y93.4 Activities involving dancing and other rhythmic movement

Y93.5 Activities involving other sports and athletics played individually

Y93.6 Activities involving other sports and athletics played as a team or group

Y93.7 Activities involving other specified sports and athletics

Y93.A Activities involving other cardiorespiratory exercise

Y93.B Activities involving other muscle strengthening exercises

Y93.C Activities involving computer technology and electronic devices

Y93.D Activities involving arts and handcrafts

Y93.E Activities involving personal hygiene and interior property and clothing maintenance

Y93.F Activities involving caregiving

Y93.G Activities involving food preparation, cooking and grilling

Y93.H Activities involving exterior property and land maintenance, building and construction

Y93.I Activities involving roller coasters and other types of external motion

Y93.J Activities involving playing musical instrument

Y93.K Activities involving animal care

Y93.8 Activities, other specified

Y93.9 Activity, unspecified

Y93.0 Activities involving walking and running

EXCLUDES1 activity, walking an animal (Y93.K1)
activity, walking or running on a treadmill (Y93.A1)

Y93.01 Activity, walking, marching and hiking
Activity, walking, marching and hiking on level or elevated terrain
EXCLUDES1 activity, mountain climbing (Y93.31)

Y93.02 Activity, running

Y93.1 Activities involving water and water craft

EXCLUDES1 activities involving ice (Y93.2-)

Y93.11 Activity, swimming

Y93.12 Activity, springboard and platform diving

Y93.13 Activity, water polo

Y93.14 Activity, water aerobics and water exercise

Y93.15 Activity, underwater diving and snorkeling
Activity, SCUBA diving

Y93.16 Activity, rowing, canoeing, kayaking, rafting and tubing
Activity, canoeing, kayaking, rafting and tubing in calm and turbulent water

Y93.17 Activity, water skiing and wake boarding

Y93.18 Activity, surfing, windsurfing and boogie boarding
Activity, water sliding

Y93.19 Activity, other involving water and watercraft
Activity involving water NOS
Activity, parasailing
Activity, water survival training and testing

Y93.2 Activities involving ice and snow

EXCLUDES1 activity, shoveling ice and snow (Y93.H1)

Y93.21 Activity, ice skating
Activity, figure skating (singles) (pairs)
Activity, ice dancing
EXCLUDES1 activity, ice hockey (Y93.22)

Y93.22 Activity, ice hockey

Y93.23 Activity, snow (alpine) (downhill) skiing, snow boarding, sledding, tobogganing and snow tubing
EXCLUDES1 activity, cross country skiing (Y93.24)

Y93.24 Activity, cross country skiing
Activity, nordic skiing

Y93.29 Activity, other involving ice and snow
Activity involving ice and snow NOS

Y93.3 Activities involving climbing, rappelling and jumping off

EXCLUDES1 activity, hiking on level or elevated terrain (Y93.01)
activity, jumping rope (Y93.56)
activity, trampoline jumping (Y93.44)

Y93.31 Activity, mountain climbing, rock climbing and wall climbing

Y93.32 Activity, rappelling

Y93.33 Activity, BASE jumping
Activity, Building, Antenna, Span, Earth jumping

Y93.34 Activity, bungee jumping

Y93.35 Activity, hang gliding

Y93.39 Activity, other involving climbing, rappelling and jumping off

Y93.4 Activities involving dancing and other rhythmic movement

EXCLUDES1 activity, martial arts (Y93.75)

Y93.41 Activity, dancing
AHA: Q4 2012

Y93.42 Activity, yoga

Y93.43 Activity, gymnastics
Activity, rhythmic gymnastics
EXCLUDES1 activity, trampolining (Y93.44)

Y93.44 Activity, trampolining

Y93.45 Activity, cheerleading

Y93.49 Activity, other involving dancing and other rhythmic movements

Y93.5 Activities involving other sports and athletics played individually

EXCLUDES1 activity, dancing (Y93.41)
activity, gymnastic (Y93.43)
activity, trampolining (Y93.44)
activity, yoga (Y93.42)

Y93.51 Activity, roller skating (inline) and skateboarding

Y93.52 Activity, horseback riding

Y93.53 Activity, golf

Y93.54 Activity, bowling

Y93.55 Activity, bike riding

Y93.56 Activity, jumping rope

Y93.57 Activity, non-running track and field events
EXCLUDES1 activity, running (any form) (Y93.02)

Y93.59 Activity, other involving other sports and athletics played individually
EXCLUDES1 activities involving climbing, rappelling, and jumping (Y93.3-)
activities involving ice and snow (Y93.2-)
activities involving walking and running (Y93.0-)
activities involving water and watercraft (Y93.1-)

Y93.6 Activities involving other sports and athletics played as a team or group

EXCLUDES1 activity, ice hockey (Y93.22)
activity, water polo (Y93.13)

Y93.61 Activity, american tackle football
Activity, football NOS

Y93.62 Activity, american flag or touch football

Y93.63 Activity, rugby

Y93.64 Activity, baseball
Activity, softball

Y93.65 Activity, lacrosse and field hockey
AHA: Q1 2015

Y93.66 Activity, soccer

Y93.67 Activity, basketball

Y93.68 Activity, volleyball (beach) (court)

Y93.6A Activity, physical games generally associated with school recess, summer camp and children
Activity, capture the flag
Activity, dodge ball
Activity, four square
Activity, kickball

Y93.69 Activity, other involving other sports and athletics played as a team or group
Activity, cricket

Y93.7 Activities involving other specified sports and athletics

Y93.71 Activity, boxing

Y93.72 Activity, wrestling

Y93.73 **Activity, racquet and hand sports** [POA]
Activity, handball
Activity, racquetball
Activity, squash
Activity, tennis
Y93.74 **Activity, frisbee** [POA]
Activity, ultimate frisbee
Y93.75 **Activity, martial arts** [POA]
Activity, combatives
Y93.79 **Activity, other specified sports and athletics** [POA]
EXCLUDES1 *sports and athletics activities specified in categories Y93.0-Y93.6*

[5th] Y93.A **Activities involving other cardiorespiratory exercise**
Activities involving physical training
Y93.A1 **Activity, exercise machines primarily for cardiorespiratory conditioning** [POA]
Activity, elliptical and stepper machines
Activity, stationary bike
Activity, treadmill
Y93.A2 **Activity, calisthenics** [POA]
Activity, jumping jacks
Activity, warm up and cool down
Y93.A3 **Activity, aerobic and step exercise** [POA]
Y93.A4 **Activity, circuit training** [POA]
Y93.A5 **Activity, obstacle course** [POA]
Activity, challenge course
Activity, confidence course
Y93.A6 **Activity, grass drills** [POA]
Activity, guerilla drills
Y93.A9 **Activity, other involving cardiorespiratory exercise** [POA]
EXCLUDES1 *activities involving cardiorespiratory exercise specified in categories Y93.0-Y93.7*

[5th] Y93.B **Activities involving other muscle strengthening exercises**
Y93.B1 **Activity, exercise machines primarily for muscle strengthening** [POA]
Y93.B2 **Activity, push-ups, pull-ups, sit-ups** [POA]
Y93.B3 **Activity, free weights** [POA]
Activity, barbells
Activity, dumbbells
Y93.B4 **Activity, pilates** [POA]
Y93.B9 **Activity, other involving muscle strengthening exercises** [POA]
EXCLUDES1 *activities involving muscle strengthening specified in categories Y93.0-Y93.A*

[5th] Y93.C **Activities involving computer technology and electronic devices**
EXCLUDES1 *activity, electronic musical keyboard or instruments (Y93.J-)*
Y93.C1 **Activity, computer keyboarding** [POA]
Activity, electronic game playing using keyboard or other stationary device
Y93.C2 **Activity, hand held interactive electronic device** [POA]
Activity, cellular telephone and communication device
Activity, electronic game playing using interactive device
EXCLUDES1 *activity, electronic game playing using keyboard or other stationary device (Y93.C1)*
Y93.C9 **Activity, other involving computer technology and electronic devices** [POA]

[5th] Y93.D **Activities involving arts and handcrafts**
EXCLUDES1 *activities involving playing musical instrument (Y93.J-)*
Y93.D1 **Activity, knitting and crocheting** [POA]
Y93.D2 **Activity, sewing** [POA]
Y93.D3 **Activity, furniture building and finishing** [POA]
Activity, furniture repair
Y93.D9 **Activity, other involving arts and handcrafts** [POA]

[5th] Y93.E **Activities involving personal hygiene and interior property and clothing maintenance**
EXCLUDES1 *activities involving cooking and grilling (Y93.G-)*
activities involving exterior property and land maintenance, building and construction (Y93.H-)
activities involving caregiving (Y93.F-)
activity, dishwashing (Y93.G1)
activity, food preparation (Y93.G1)
activity, gardening (Y93.H2)
Y93.E1 **Activity, personal bathing and showering** [POA]
Y93.E2 **Activity, laundry** [POA]
Y93.E3 **Activity, vacuuming** [POA]
Y93.E4 **Activity, ironing** [POA]
Y93.E5 **Activity, floor mopping and cleaning** [POA]
Y93.E6 **Activity, residential relocation** [POA]
Activity, packing up and unpacking involved in moving to a new residence
Y93.E8 **Activity, other personal hygiene** [POA]
Y93.E9 **Activity, other interior property and clothing maintenance** [POA]

[5th] Y93.F **Activities involving caregiving**
Activity involving the provider of caregiving
Y93.F1 **Activity, caregiving, bathing** [POA]
Y93.F2 **Activity, caregiving, lifting** [POA]
AHA: Q4 2016
Y93.F9 **Activity, other caregiving** [POA]

[5th] Y93.G **Activities involving food preparation, cooking and grilling**
Y93.G1 **Activity, food preparation and clean up** [POA]
Activity, dishwashing
Y93.G2 **Activity, grilling and smoking food** [POA]
Y93.G3 **Activity, cooking and baking** [POA]
Activity, use of stove, oven and microwave oven
Y93.G9 **Activity, other involving cooking and grilling** [POA]

[5th] Y93.H **Activities involving exterior property and land maintenance, building and construction**
Y93.H1 **Activity, digging, shoveling and raking** [POA]
Activity, dirt digging
Activity, raking leaves
Activity, snow shoveling
Y93.H2 **Activity, gardening and landscaping** [POA]
Activity, pruning, trimming shrubs, weeding
Y93.H3 **Activity, building and construction** [POA]
Y93.H9 **Activity, other involving exterior property and land maintenance, building and construction** [POA]

[5th] Y93.I **Activities involving roller coasters and other types of external motion**
Y93.I1 **Activity, roller coaster riding** [POA]
Y93.I9 **Activity, other involving external motion** [POA]

[5th] Y93.J **Activities involving playing musical instrument**
Activity involving playing electric musical instrument
Y93.J1 **Activity, piano playing** [POA]
Activity, musical keyboard (electronic) playing
Y93.J2 **Activity, drum and other percussion instrument playing** [POA]
Y93.J3 **Activity, string instrument playing** [POA]
Y93.J4 **Activity, winds and brass instrument playing** [POA]

[5th] Y93.K **Activities involving animal care**
EXCLUDES1 *activity, horseback riding (Y93.52)*
Y93.K1 **Activity, walking an animal** [POA]
Y93.K2 **Activity, milking an animal** [POA]
Y93.K3 **Activity, grooming and shearing an animal** [POA]
Y93.K9 **Activity, other involving animal care** [POA]

[5th] Y93.8 **Activities, other specified**
Y93.81 **Activity, refereeing a sports activity** [POA]
Y93.82 **Activity, spectator at an event** [POA]
Y93.83 **Activity, rough housing and horseplay** [POA]
AHA: Q1 2015
Y93.84 **Activity, sleeping** [POA]

Unspecified Code Other Specified Code Manifestation Code [N] Newborn [P] Pediatric [M] Maternity [A] Adult ♂ Male ♀ Female
● New Code ▲ Revised Code Title ►◄ Revised Text NOTES INCLUDES EXCLUDES1 Not coded here EXCLUDES2 Not included here
[4th] 4th character required [5th] 5th character required [6th] 6th character required [7th] 7th character required [x7th] Extension 'X' Alert
[HAC] Hospital-acquired condition (HAC) alert **AHA** AHA Coding Clinic© ☞ Code first alert

Y93.85 **Activity,** choking game ⬚POA
       AHA: Q4 2016
       Activity, blackout game
       Activity, fainting game
       Activity, pass out game
Y93.89 **Activity, other specified** ⬚POA
Y93.9 **Activity, unspecified** ⬚POA
       👁 **See Official Guidelines** "Activity Code" I.C.20.c

Y95 **Nosocomial condition**
       AHA: Q4 2013

🔵 Y99 **External cause status**
       👁 **See Official Guidelines** "External cause status" I.C.20.k
       NOTES   A single code from category Y99 should be used in conjunction with the external cause code(s) assigned to a record to indicate the status of the person at the time the event occurred.

Y99.0 Civilian **activity done for income or pay** ⬚POA
       Civilian activity done for financial or other compensation
       EXCLUDES1 *military activity (Y99.1)*
                   volunteer activity (Y99.2)

Y99.1 Military **activity** ⬚POA
       EXCLUDES1 *activity of off duty military personnel (Y99.8)*

Y99.2 Volunteer **activity** ⬚POA
       EXCLUDES1 *activity of child or other family member assisting in compensated work of other family member (Y99.8)*

Y99.8 **Other external cause status** ⬚POA
       Activity NEC
       Activity of child or other family member assisting in compensated work of other family member
       Hobby not done for income
       Leisure activity
       Off-duty activity of military personnel
       Recreation or sport not for income or while a student
       Student activity
       EXCLUDES1 *civilian activity done for income or compensation (Y99.0)*
                   military activity (Y99.1)

Y99.9 **Unspecified external cause status** ⬚POA

PDₓ🚫 Unacceptable principal diagnosis symbol per Medicare code edits   POA🚫 Code exempt from diagnosis present on admission requirement
   ❓ Questionable admission   cc🚫 Complication or comorbidity   mcc🚫 Major complication or comorbidity   cc/mcc🚫 CC/MCC exclusion
      HCC HCC diagnosis code   RxHCC RxHCC diagnosis code   MACRA code   **DEFINITION** Describes condition/terminology
         TIP Coding guidance   👁 Official Guideline Reference   Z1 Z code as first-listed diagnosis

1250   When symbols appear on a code that requires a 7th character extension, refer to Appendix B to identify applicable 7th character codes.   **2020 ICD-10-CM**

Chapter 21: Factors Influencing Health Status and Contact with Health Services (Z00-Z99)

Factors influencing health status and contact with health services (Z00-Z99)

👁 **See Official Guidelines** "Code or codes from A00.0 through T88.9, Z00-Z99.8" I.B3

NOTES Z codes represent reasons for encounters. A corresponding procedure code must accompany a Z code if a procedure is performed. Categories Z00-Z99 are provided for occasions when circumstances other than a disease, injury or external cause classifiable to categories A00-Y89 are recorded as 'diagnoses' or 'problems'. This can arise in two main ways:

(a) When a person who may or may not be sick encounters the health services for some specific purpose, such as to receive limited care or service for a current condition, to donate an organ or tissue, to receive prophylactic vaccination (immunization), or to discuss a problem which is in itself not a disease or injury.

(b) When some circumstance or problem is present which influences the person's health status but is not in itself a current illness or injury.

This chapter contains the following blocks:

Z00-Z13	Persons encountering health services for examinations
Z14-Z15	Genetic carrier and genetic susceptibility to disease
Z16	Resistance to antimicrobial drugs
Z17	Estrogen receptor status
Z18	Retained foreign body fragments
Z19	Hormone sensitivity malignancy status
Z20-Z29	Persons with potential health hazards related to communicable diseases
Z30-Z39	Persons encountering health services in circumstances related to reproduction
Z40-Z53	Encounters for other specific health care
Z55-Z65	Persons with potential health hazards related to socioeconomic and psychosocial circumstances
Z66	Do not resuscitate status
Z67	Blood type
Z68	Body mass index (BMI)
Z69-Z76	Persons encountering health services in other circumstances
Z77-Z99	Persons with potential health hazards related to family and personal history and certain conditions influencing health status

Persons encountering health services for examinations (Z00-Z13)

NOTES Nonspecific abnormal findings disclosed at the time of these examinations are classified to categories R70-R94.

EXCLUDES1 examinations related to pregnancy and reproduction (Z30-Z36, Z39.-)

4️⃣ **Z00 Encounter for general examination without complaint, suspected or reported diagnosis**

👁 **See Official Guidelines** "Routine and administrative examinations" I.C.21.c.13, "Z Codes That May Only be Principal/First-listed Diagnosis" I.C.21.c.16

EXCLUDES1 encounter for examination for administrative purposes (Z02.-)

EXCLUDES2 encounter for pre-procedural examinations (Z01.81-)

special screening examinations (Z11-Z13)

5️⃣ **Z00.0 Encounter for general adult medical examination**

👁 **See Official Guidelines** "Encounters for general medical examinations with abnormal findings" IV.P

Encounter for adult periodic examination (annual) (physical) and any associated laboratory and radiologic examinations

EXCLUDES1 encounter for examination of sign or symptom- code to sign or symptom

general health check-up of infant or child (Z00.12.-)

Z00.00 Encounter for general adult medical examination without abnormal findings A 🅿 PDxIn Z1

AHA: Q4 2017, Q1 2016

Encounter for adult health check-up NOS

Z00.01 Encounter for general adult medical examination with abnormal findings A 🅿 PDxIn Z1

AHA: Q1 2016

Use additional code to identify abnormal findings

5️⃣ **Z00.1 Encounter for newborn, infant and child health examinations**

👁 **See Official Guidelines** "Newborns and Infants" I.C.21.c.12

6️⃣ **Z00.11 Newborn health examination**

Health check for child under 29 days old

Use additional code to identify any abnormal findings

EXCLUDES1 health check for child over 28 days old (Z00.12-)

Z00.110 Health examination for newborn under 8 days old N 🅿 PDxIn Z1

Health check for newborn under 8 days old

Z00.111 Health examination for newborn 8 to 28 days old N 🅿 PDxIn Z1

Health check for newborn 8 to 28 days old

Newborn weight check

6️⃣ **Z00.12 Encounter for routine child health examination**

👁 **See Official Guidelines** "Encounters for general medical examinations with abnormal findings" IV.P

Health check (routine) for child over 28 days old

Immunizations appropriate for age

Routine developmental screening of infant or child

Routine vision and hearing testing

EXCLUDES1 health check for child under 29 days old (Z00.11-)

health supervision of foundling or other healthy infant or child (Z76.1-Z76.2)

newborn health examination (Z00.11-)

Z00.121 Encounter for routine child health examination with abnormal findings P 🅿 PDxIn Z1

AHA: Q4 2017, Q1 2016

Use additional code to identify abnormal findings

Z00.129 Encounter for routine child health examination without abnormal findings P 🅿 PDxIn Z1

AHA: Q1 2016

Encounter for routine child health examination NOS

Z00.2 Encounter for examination for period of rapid growth in childhood P 🅿 PDxIn Z1

Z00.3 Encounter for examination for adolescent development state P 🅿 PDxIn Z1

Encounter for puberty development state

Z00.5 Encounter for examination of potential donor of organ and tissue 🅿 PDxIn Z1

Z00.6 Encounter for examination for normal comparison and control in clinical research program 🅿

Examination of participant or control in clinical research program

5️⃣ **Z00.7 Encounter for examination for period of delayed growth in childhood**

Z00.70 Encounter for examination for period of delayed growth in childhood without abnormal findings P 🅿 PDxIn Z1

Z00.71 Encounter for examination for period of delayed growth in childhood with abnormal findings P 🅿 PDxIn Z1

Use additional code to identify abnormal findings

Z00.8 Encounter for other general examination 🅿 PDxIn Z1

Encounter for health examination in population surveys

Z01 Encounter for other special examination without complaint, suspected or reported diagnosis

👁 **See Official Guidelines** "Routine and administrative examinations" I.C.21.c.13, "Z Codes That May Only be Principal/ First-listed Diagnosis" I.C.21.c.16

INCLUDES routine examination of specific system

NOTES Codes from category Z01 represent the reason for the encounter. A separate procedure code is required to identify any examinations or procedures performed.

EXCLUDES1 encounter for examination for administrative purposes (Z02.-)

encounter for examination for suspected conditions, proven not to exist (Z03.-)

encounter for laboratory and radiologic examinations as a component of general medical examinations (Z00.0-)

encounter for laboratory, radiologic and imaging examinations for sign(s) and symptom(s) - code to the sign(s) or symptom(s)

EXCLUDES2 screening examinations (Z11-Z13)

Z01.0 Encounter for examination of eyes and vision

EXCLUDES1 examination for driving license (Z02.4)

Z01.00 Encounter for examination of eyes and vision without abnormal findings

Encounter for examination of eyes and vision NOS

Z01.01 Encounter for examination of eyes and vision with abnormal findings

AHA: Q4 2016

Use additional code to identify abnormal findings

Z01.02 Encounter for examination of eyes and vision following failed vision screening

EXCLUDES1 examination for examination of eyes and vision with abnormal findings (Z01.01)

examination for examination of eyes and vision without abnormal findings (Z01.00)

Z01.020 Encounter for examination of eyes and vision following failed vision screening without abnormal findings

Z01.021 Encounter for examination of eyes and vision following failed vision screening with abnormal findings

Use additional code to identify abnormal findings

Z01.1 Encounter for examination of ears and hearing

Z01.10 Encounter for examination of ears and hearing without abnormal findings

AHA: Q4 2016

Encounter for examination of ears and hearing NOS

Z01.11 Encounter for examination of ears and hearing with abnormal findings

Z01.110 Encounter for hearing examination following failed hearing screening

AHA: Q3 2016

Z01.118 Encounter for examination of ears and hearing with other abnormal findings

AHA: Q3 2016

Use additional code to identify abnormal findings

Z01.12 Encounter for hearing conservation and treatment

Z01.2 Encounter for dental examination and cleaning

Z01.20 Encounter for dental examination and cleaning without abnormal findings

Encounter for dental examination and cleaning NOS

Z01.21 Encounter for dental examination and cleaning with abnormal findings

Use additional code to identify abnormal findings

Z01.3 Encounter for examination of blood pressure

Z01.30 Encounter for examination of blood pressure without abnormal findings

Encounter for examination of blood pressure NOS

Z01.31 Encounter for examination of blood pressure with abnormal findings

Use additional code to identify abnormal findings

Z01.4 Encounter for gynecological examination

EXCLUDES2 pregnancy examination or test (Z32.0-)

routine examination for contraceptive maintenance (Z30.4-)

Z01.41 Encounter for routine gynecological examination

Encounter for general gynecological examination with or without cervical smear

Encounter for gynecological examination (general) (routine) NOS

Encounter for pelvic examination (annual) (periodic)

Use additional code:

for screening for human papillomavirus, if applicable, (Z11.51)

for screening vaginal pap smear, if applicable (Z12.72)

to identify acquired absence of uterus, if applicable (Z90.71-)

EXCLUDES1 gynecologic examination status-post hysterectomy for malignant condition (Z08)

screening cervical pap smear not a part of a routine gynecological examination (Z12.4)

Z01.411 Encounter for gynecological examination (general) (routine) with abnormal findings

Use additional code to identify abnormal findings

Z01.419 Encounter for gynecological examination (general) (routine) without abnormal findings

Z01.42 Encounter for cervical smear to confirm findings of recent normal smear following initial abnormal smear

Z01.8 Encounter for other specified special examinations

Z01.81 Encounter for preprocedural examinations

Encounter for preoperative examinations

Encounter for radiological and imaging examinations as part of preprocedural examination

Z01.810 Encounter for preprocedural cardiovascular examination

Z01.811 Encounter for preprocedural respiratory examination

Z01.812 Encounter for preprocedural laboratory examination

Blood and urine tests prior to treatment or procedure

Z01.818 Encounter for other preprocedural examination

Encounter for preprocedural examination NOS

Encounter for examinations prior to antineoplastic chemotherapy

Z01.82 Encounter for allergy testing

EXCLUDES1 encounter for antibody response examination (Z01.84)

Z01.83 Encounter for blood typing

Encounter for Rh typing

Z01.84 Encounter for antibody response examination

Encounter for immunity status testing

EXCLUDES1 encounter for allergy testing (Z01.82)

Z01.89 Encounter for other specified special examinations

👁 **See Official Guidelines** "Patients receiving diagnostic services only" IV.K

[4th] **Z02 Encounter for administrative examination**

See Official Guidelines "Routine and administrative examinations" I.C.21.c.13, "Z Codes That May Only be Principal/ First-listed Diagnosis" I.C.21.c.16

Z02.0 Encounter for examination for admission to educational institution POA PDxIn Z-1
Encounter for examination for admission to preschool (education)
Encounter for examination for re-admission to school following illness or medical treatment

Z02.1 Encounter for pre-employment examination POA Z-1

Z02.2 Encounter for examination for admission to residential institution POA PDxIn Z-1
EXCLUDES1 *examination for admission to prison (Z02.89)*

Z02.3 Encounter for examination for recruitment to armed forces POA Z-1

Z02.4 Encounter for examination for driving license POA PDxIn Z-1

Z02.5 Encounter for examination for participation in sport POA PDxIn Z-1
EXCLUDES1 *blood-alcohol and blood-drug test (Z02.83)*

Z02.6 Encounter for examination for insurance purposes POA PDxIn Z-1

[5th] **Z02.7 Encounter for issue of medical certificate**
EXCLUDES1 *encounter for general medical examination (Z00-Z01, Z02.0-Z02.6, Z02.8-Z02.9)*

Z02.71 Encounter for disability determination POA PDxIn Z-1
Encounter for issue of medical certificate of incapacity
Encounter for issue of medical certificate of invalidity

Z02.79 Encounter for issue of other medical certificate POA PDxIn Z-1

[5th] **Z02.8 Encounter for other administrative examinations**

Z02.81 Encounter for paternity testing POA Z-1

Z02.82 Encounter for adoption services POA PDxIn Z-1

Z02.83 Encounter for blood-alcohol and blood-drug test POA Z-1
Use additional code for findings of alcohol or drugs in blood (R78.-)

Z02.89 Encounter for other administrative examinations POA PDxIn Z-1
Encounter for examination for admission to prison
Encounter for examination for admission to summer camp
Encounter for immigration examination
Encounter for naturalization examination
Encounter for premarital examination
EXCLUDES1 *health supervision of foundling or other healthy infant or child (Z76.1-Z76.2)*

Z02.9 Encounter for administrative examinations, unspecified POA PDxIn Z-1
See Official Guidelines "Nonspecific Z codes" I.C.21.c.15

[4th] **Z03 Encounter for medical observation for suspected diseases and conditions ruled out**

See Official Guidelines "Observation" I.C.21.c.6, "Z Codes That May Only be Principal/First-listed Diagnosis" I.C.21.c.16

This category is to be used when a person without a diagnosis is suspected of having an abnormal condition, without signs or symptoms, which requires study, but after examination and observation, is ruled out. This category is also for use for administrative and legal observation status.

EXCLUDES1 *contact with and (suspected) exposures hazardous to health (Z77.-)*
encounter for observation and evaluation of newborn for suspected diseases and conditions ruled out (Z05.-)
person with feared complaint in whom no diagnosis is made (Z71.1)
signs or symptoms under study- code to signs or symptoms

Z03.6 Encounter for observation for suspected toxic effect from ingested substance ruled out POA Z-1
Encounter for observation for suspected adverse effect from drug
Encounter for observation for suspected poisoning

[5th] **Z03.7 Encounter for suspected maternal and fetal conditions ruled out**
Encounter for suspected maternal and fetal conditions not found
EXCLUDES1 *known or suspected fetal anomalies affecting management of mother, not ruled out (O26.-, O35.-, O36.-, O40.-, O41.-)*

Z03.71 Encounter for suspected problem with amniotic cavity and membrane ruled out [M] POA ♀ PDxIn Z-1
Encounter for suspected oligohydramnios ruled out
Encounter for suspected polyhydramnios ruled out

Z03.72 Encounter for suspected placental problem ruled out [M] POA ♀ PDxIn Z-1

Z03.73 Encounter for suspected fetal anomaly ruled out [M] POA ♀ PDxIn Z-1
AHA: Q4 2016

Z03.74 Encounter for suspected problem with fetal growth ruled out [M] POA ♀ PDxIn Z-1

Z03.75 Encounter for suspected cervical shortening ruled out [M] POA ♀ PDxIn Z-1

Z03.79 Encounter for other suspected maternal and fetal conditions ruled out [M] POA ♀ PDxIn Z-1

[5th] **Z03.8 Encounter for observation for other suspected diseases and conditions ruled out**

[6th] **Z03.81 Encounter for observation for suspected exposure to biological agents ruled out**

Z03.810 Encounter for observation for suspected exposure to anthrax ruled out POA Z-1

Z03.818 Encounter for observation for suspected exposure to other biological agents ruled out POA Z-1

Z03.89 Encounter for observation for other suspected diseases and conditions ruled out POA Z-1

[4th] **Z04 Encounter for examination and observation for other reasons**

See Official Guidelines "Observation" I.C.21.c.6, "Z Codes That May Only be Principal/First-listed Diagnosis" I.C.21.c.16

INCLUDES *encounter for examination for medicolegal reasons*

This category is to be used when a person without a diagnosis is suspected of having an abnormal condition, without signs or symptoms, which requires study, but after examination and observation, is ruled-out. This category is also for use for administrative and legal observation status.

Z04.1 Encounter for examination and observation following transport accident Z-1
AHA: Q2 2019, Q2 2018
EXCLUDES1 *encounter for examination and observation following work accident (Z04.2)*

Z04.2 Encounter for examination and observation following work accident Z-1

Z04.3 Encounter for examination and observation following other accident Z-1
AHA: Q2 2018

[5th] **Z04.4 Encounter for examination and observation following alleged rape**
Encounter for examination and observation of victim following alleged rape
Encounter for examination and observation of victim following alleged sexual abuse

Z04.41 Encounter for examination and observation following alleged adult rape [A] Z-1
See Official Guidelines "Adult and child abuse, neglect and other maltreatment" I.C.19.f
AHA: Q4 2018, Q4 2016
Suspected adult rape, ruled out
Suspected adult sexual abuse, ruled out

Z04.42 Encounter for examination and observation following alleged child rape [P] Z-1
See Official Guidelines "Adult and child abuse, neglect and other maltreatment" I.C.19.f
AHA: Q4 2018, Q4 2016
Suspected child rape, ruled out
Suspected child sexual abuse, ruled out

Z04.6 Encounter for general psychiatric examination, requested by authority Z-1

[5th] **Z04.7 Encounter for examination and observation following alleged physical abuse**

Unspecified Code | Other Specified Code | Manifestation Code | [N] Newborn | [P] Pediatric | [M] Maternity | [A] Adult | ♂ Male | ♀ Female
● New Code | ▲ Revised Code Title | ►◄ Revised Text | NOTES | INCLUDES | EXCLUDES1 Not coded here | EXCLUDES2 Not included here
[4th] 4th character required | [5th] 5th character required | [6th] 6th character required | [7th] 7th character required | [7x] Extension 'X' Alert
[HAC] Hospital-acquired condition (HAC) alert | AHA AHA Coding Clinic© | Code first alert

Z04.71 Encounter for examination and observation following alleged adult physical abuse 🅐 🆉

   👁 **See Official Guidelines** "Adult and child abuse, neglect and other maltreatment" I.C.19.f

   Suspected adult physical abuse, ruled out

   EXCLUDES1 *confirmed case of adult physical abuse (T74.-)*

      encounter for examination and observation following alleged adult sexual abuse (Z04.41)

      suspected case of adult physical abuse, not ruled out (T76.-)

Z04.72 Encounter for examination and observation following alleged child physical abuse 🅿 🆉

   👁 **See Official Guidelines** "Adult and child abuse, neglect and other maltreatment" I.C.19.f

   Suspected child physical abuse, ruled out

   EXCLUDES1 *confirmed case of child physical abuse (T74.-)*

      encounter for examination and observation following alleged child sexual abuse (Z04.42)

      suspected case of child physical abuse, not ruled out (T76.-)

🔟 **Z04.8 Encounter for examination and observation for other specified reasons**

   Encounter for examination and observation for request for expert evidence

Z04.81 Encounter for examination and observation of victim following forced sexual exploitation POA 🆉

   AHA: Q4 2018

Z04.82 Encounter for examination and observation of victim following forced labor exploitation POA 🆉

   👁 **See Official Guidelines** "Adult and child abuse, neglect and other maltreatment" I.C.19.f

   AHA: Q4 2018

Z04.89 Encounter for examination and observation for other specified reasons POA 🆉

   AHA: Q4 2018

Z04.9 Encounter for examination and observation for unspecified reason PDxIn 🆉

   👁 **See Official Guidelines** "Nonspecific Z codes" I.C.21.c.15

   Encounter for observation NOS

🔟 **Z05 Encounter for observation and evaluation of newborn for suspected diseases and conditions ruled out**

   👁 **See Official Guidelines** "Use of Z05 codes" I.C.16.b.1, "Observation and Evaluation of Newborns for Suspected Conditions not Found" I.C.16.b.1-3, "Observation" I.C.21.c.6

   This category is to be used for newborns, within the neonatal period (the first 28 days of life), who are suspected of having an abnormal condition, but without signs or symptoms, and which, after examination and observation, is ruled out.

Z05.0 Observation and evaluation of newborn for suspected cardiac condition ruled out N POA

   AHA: Q4 2016

Z05.1 Observation and evaluation of newborn for suspected infectious condition ruled out N POA

   AHA: Q2 2019, Q4 2016

Z05.2 Observation and evaluation of newborn for suspected neurological condition ruled out N POA

   AHA: Q4 2016

Z05.3 Observation and evaluation of newborn for suspected respiratory condition ruled out N POA

   AHA: Q4 2016

🔟 **Z05.4 Observation and evaluation of newborn for suspected genetic, metabolic or immunologic condition ruled out**

Z05.41 Observation and evaluation of newborn for suspected genetic condition ruled out N POA

   AHA: Q4 2016

Z05.42 Observation and evaluation of newborn for suspected metabolic condition ruled out N POA

   AHA: Q4 2016

Z05.43 Observation and evaluation of newborn for suspected immunologic condition ruled out N POA

   AHA: Q4 2016

Z05.5 Observation and evaluation of newborn for suspected gastrointestinal condition ruled out N POA

   AHA: Q4 2016

Z05.6 Observation and evaluation of newborn for suspected genitourinary condition ruled out N POA

   AHA: Q4 2016

🔟 **Z05.7 Observation and evaluation of newborn for suspected skin, subcutaneous, musculoskeletal and connective tissue condition ruled out**

Z05.71 Observation and evaluation of newborn for suspected skin and subcutaneous tissue condition ruled out N POA

   AHA: Q4 2016

Z05.72 Observation and evaluation of newborn for suspected musculoskeletal condition ruled out N POA

   AHA: Q4 2016

Z05.73 Observation and evaluation of newborn for suspected connective tissue condition ruled out N POA

   AHA: Q4 2016

Z05.8 Observation and evaluation of newborn for other specified suspected condition ruled out N POA

   AHA: Q4 2016

Z05.9 Observation and evaluation of newborn for unspecified suspected condition ruled out N POA

   AHA: Q4 2016

Z08 Encounter for follow-up examination after completed treatment for malignant neoplasm POA PDxIn

   👁 **See Official Guidelines** "Follow-up" I.C.21.c.8

   Medical surveillance following completed treatment

   Use additional code to identify any acquired absence of organs (Z90.-)

   Use additional code to identify the personal history of malignant neoplasm (Z85.-)

   EXCLUDES1 *aftercare following medical care (Z43-Z49, Z51)*

Z09 Encounter for follow-up examination after completed treatment for conditions other than malignant neoplasm POA PDxIn

   👁 **See Official Guidelines** "Follow-up" I.C.21.c.8

   AHA: Q1 2017, Q1 2015

   Medical surveillance following completed treatment

   Use additional code to identify any applicable history of disease code (Z86.-. Z87.-)

   EXCLUDES1 *aftercare following medical care (Z43-Z49, Z51)*

      surveillance of contraception (Z30.4-)

      surveillance of prosthetic and other medical devices (Z44-Z46)

🔟 **Z11 Encounter for screening for infectious and parasitic diseases**

   👁 **See Official Guidelines** "Screening" I.C.21.c.5

   Screening is the testing for disease or disease precursors in asymptomatic individuals so that early detection and treatment can be provided for those who test positive for the disease.

   EXCLUDES1 *encounter for diagnostic examination-code to sign or symptom*

Z11.0 Encounter for screening for intestinal infectious diseases POA PDxIn

Z11.1 Encounter for screening for respiratory tuberculosis POA PDxIn

   Encounter for screening for active tuberculosis disease

Z11.2 Encounter for screening for other bacterial diseases POA PDxIn

Z11.3 Encounter for screening for infections with a predominantly sexual mode of transmission POA PDxIn

   EXCLUDES2 *encounter for screening for human immunodeficiency virus [HIV] (Z11.4)*

      encounter for screening for human papillomavirus (Z11.51)

Z11.4 Encounter for screening for human immunodeficiency virus [HIV] POA PDxIn

   👁 **See Official Guidelines** "Encounters for testing for HIV" I.C.1.a.2.h

🔟 **Z11.5 Encounter for screening for other viral diseases**

   EXCLUDES2 *encounter for screening for viral intestinal disease (Z11.0)*

Z11.51 Encounter for screening for human papillomavirus (HPV) POA PDxIn

---

PDxIn Unacceptable principal diagnosis symbol per Medicare code edits   POA Code exempt from diagnosis present on admission requirement

❓ Questionable admission   cc Complication or comorbidity   MCC Major complication or comorbidity   CC/MCC CC/MCC exclusion

HCC HCC diagnosis code   RxHCC RxHCC diagnosis code   MACRA MACRA code   **DEFINITION** Describes condition/terminology

TIP Coding guidance   👁 Official Guideline Reference   🆉 Z code as first-listed diagnosis

Z11.59 Encounter for screening for other viral diseases `POA` `PDxIn`

Z11.6 Encounter for screening for other protozoal diseases and helminthiases `POA` `PDxIn`

EXCLUDES2 *encounter for screening for protozoal intestinal disease (Z11.0)*

● **Z11.7** Encounter for testing for latent tuberculosis infection `POA`

Z11.8 Encounter for screening for other infectious and parasitic diseases `POA` `PDxIn`

Encounter for screening for chlamydia
Encounter for screening for rickettsial
Encounter for screening for spirochetal
Encounter for screening for mycoses

Z11.9 Encounter for screening for infectious and parasitic diseases, unspecified `POA` `PDxIn`

4ᵗʰ **Z12** Encounter for screening for malignant neoplasms

👁 **See Official Guidelines** "Screening" I.C.21.c.5

Screening is the testing for disease or disease precursors in asymptomatic individuals so that early detection and treatment can be provided for those who test positive for the disease.

Use additional code to identify any family history of malignant neoplasm (Z80.-)

EXCLUDES1 *encounter for diagnostic examination-code to sign or symptom*

Z12.0 Encounter for screening for malignant neoplasm of stomach `POA` `PDxIn`

5ᵗʰ **Z12.1** Encounter for screening for malignant neoplasm of intestinal tract

Z12.10 Encounter for screening for malignant neoplasm of intestinal tract, unspecified `POA` `PDxIn`

Z12.11 Encounter for screening for malignant neoplasm of colon

AHA: Q1 2018, Q1 2017

Encounter for screening colonoscopy NOS

Z12.12 Encounter for screening for malignant neoplasm of rectum `POA` `PDxIn`

Z12.13 Encounter for screening for malignant neoplasm of small intestine `POA` `PDxIn`

Z12.2 Encounter for screening for malignant neoplasm of respiratory organs `POA` `PDxIn`

5ᵗʰ **Z12.3** Encounter for screening for malignant neoplasm of breast

Z12.31 Encounter for screening mammogram for malignant neoplasm of breast `POA` `PDxIn`

AHA: Q1 2015

EXCLUDES1 *inconclusive mammogram (R92.2)*

Z12.39 Encounter for other screening for malignant neoplasm of breast `POA` `PDxIn`

Z12.4 Encounter for screening for malignant neoplasm of cervix `POA` ♀ `PDxIn`

Encounter for screening pap smear for malignant neoplasm of cervix

EXCLUDES1 *when screening is part of general gynecological examination (Z01.4-)*

EXCLUDES2 *encounter for screening for human papillomavirus (Z11.51)*

Z12.5 Encounter for screening for malignant neoplasm of prostate `POA` ♂

Z12.6 Encounter for screening for malignant neoplasm of bladder `POA` `PDxIn`

5ᵗʰ **Z12.7** Encounter for screening for malignant neoplasm of other genitourinary organs

Z12.71 Encounter for screening for malignant neoplasm of testis `POA` ♂ `PDxIn`

Z12.72 Encounter for screening for malignant neoplasm of vagina `POA` ♀ `PDxIn`

Vaginal pap smear status-post hysterectomy for non-malignant condition

Use additional code to identify acquired absence of uterus (Z90.71-)

EXCLUDES1 *vaginal pap smear status-post hysterectomy for malignant conditions (Z08)*

Z12.73 Encounter for screening for malignant neoplasm of ovary `POA` ♀ `PDxIn`

Z12.79 Encounter for screening for malignant neoplasm of other genitourinary organs `POA` `PDxIn`

5ᵗʰ **Z12.8** Encounter for screening for malignant neoplasm of other sites

Z12.81 Encounter for screening for malignant neoplasm of oral cavity `POA` `PDxIn`

Z12.82 Encounter for screening for malignant neoplasm of nervous system `POA` `PDxIn`

Z12.83 Encounter for screening for malignant neoplasm of skin `POA` `PDxIn`

Z12.89 Encounter for screening for malignant neoplasm of other sites `POA` `PDxIn`

Z12.9 Encounter for screening for malignant neoplasm, site unspecified `POA` `PDxIn`

4ᵗʰ **Z13** Encounter for screening for other diseases and disorders

👁 **See Official Guidelines** "Screening" I.C.21.c.5

Screening is the testing for disease or disease precursors in asymptomatic individuals so that early detection and treatment can be provided for those who test positive for the disease.

EXCLUDES1 *encounter for diagnostic examination-code to sign or symptom*

Z13.0 Encounter for screening for diseases of the blood and blood-forming organs and certain disorders involving the immune mechanism `POA` `PDxIn`

Z13.1 Encounter for screening for diabetes mellitus `POA` `PDxIn`

5ᵗʰ **Z13.2** Encounter for screening for nutritional, metabolic and other endocrine disorders

Z13.21 Encounter for screening for nutritional disorder `POA` `PDxIn`

6ᵗʰ **Z13.22** Encounter for screening for metabolic disorder

Z13.220 Encounter for screening for lipoid disorders `POA` `PDxIn`

Encounter for screening for cholesterol level
Encounter for screening for hypercholesterolemia
Encounter for screening for hyperlipidemia

Z13.228 Encounter for screening for other metabolic disorders `POA` `PDxIn`

Z13.29 Encounter for screening for other suspected endocrine disorder `POA` `PDxIn`

EXCLUDES1 *encounter for screening for diabetes mellitus (Z13.1)*

5ᵗʰ **Z13.3** Encounter for screening examination for mental health and behavioral disorders

Z13.30 Encounter for screening examination for mental health and behavioral disorders, unspecified `POA` `PDxIn`

AHA: Q4 2018

Z13.31 Encounter for screening for depression `POA` `PDxIn`

AHA: Q4 2018

Encounter for screening for depression, adult
Encounter for screening for depression for child or adolescent

Z13.32 Encounter for screening for maternal depression `POA` ♀ `PDxIn`

AHA: Q4 2018

Encounter for screening for perinatal depression

Z13.39 Encounter for screening examination for other mental health and behavioral disorders `POA` `PDxIn`

AHA: Q4 2018

Encounter for screening for alcoholism
Encounter for screening for intellectual disabilities

5ᵗʰ **Z13.4** Encounter for screening for certain developmental disorders in childhood

Encounter for development testing of infant or child
Encounter for screening for developmental handicaps in early childhood

EXCLUDES2 *encounter for routine child health examination (Z00.12-)*

Z13.40 Encounter for screening for unspecified developmental delays `POA` `PDxIn`

AHA: Q4 2018

Z13.41 Encounter for autism **screening** POA PDxIn
AHA: Q4 2018

Z13.42 Encounter for screening for global **developmental delays** (milestones) POA PDxIn
AHA: Q4 2018
Encounter for screening for developmental handicaps in early childhood

Z13.49 Encounter for screening for other **developmental delays** POA PDxIn
AHA: Q4 2018

Z13.5 Encounter for screening for eye and ear **disorders** POA PDxIn
AHA: Q3 2016
EXCLUDES2 *encounter for general hearing examination (Z01.1-)*
encounter for general vision examination (Z01.0-)

Z13.6 Encounter for screening for cardiovascular **disorders** POA PDxIn

Z13.7 Encounter for screening for genetic and chromosomal **anomalies**
EXCLUDES1 *genetic testing for procreative management (Z31.4-)*

Z13.71 Encounter for nonprocreative screening for genetic disease carrier status POA PDxIn

Z13.79 Encounter for other screening for genetic and chromosomal anomalies POA PDxIn

Z13.8 Encounter for screening for other **specified diseases and disorders**
EXCLUDES2 *screening for malignant neoplasms (Z12.-)*

Z13.81 Encounter for screening for digestive system **disorders**

Z13.810 Encounter for screening for upper gastrointestinal **disorder** POA PDxIn

Z13.811 Encounter for screening for lower gastrointestinal **disorder** POA PDxIn
EXCLUDES1 *encounter for screening for intestinal infectious disease (Z11.0)*

Z13.818 Encounter for screening for other digestive system disorders POA PDxIn

Z13.82 Encounter for screening for musculoskeletal **disorder**

Z13.820 Encounter for screening for osteoporosis POA PDxIn

Z13.828 Encounter for screening for other musculoskeletal disorder POA PDxIn

Z13.83 Encounter for screening for respiratory **disorder NEC** POA PDxIn
EXCLUDES1 *encounter for screening for respiratory tuberculosis (Z11.1)*

Z13.84 Encounter for screening for dental **disorders** POA PDxIn

Z13.85 Encounter for screening for nervous system **disorders**

Z13.850 Encounter for screening for traumatic brain injury POA PDxIn

Z13.858 Encounter for screening for other nervous system disorders POA PDxIn

Z13.88 Encounter for screening for disorder due to exposure to contaminants POA PDxIn
EXCLUDES1 *those exposed to contaminants without suspected disorders (Z57.-, Z77.-)*

Z13.89 Encounter for screening for other disorder POA PDxIn
Encounter for screening for genitourinary disorders

Z13.9 Encounter for screening, unspecified POA PDxIn
See Official Guidelines "Nonspecific Z codes" I.C.21.c.15

Genetic carrier and genetic susceptibility to disease (Z14-Z15)

Z14 Genetic carrier
See Official Guidelines "Status" I.C.21.c.3

Z14.0 Hemophilia A carrier

Z14.01 Asymptomatic hemophilia A carrier POA PDxIn

Z14.02 Symptomatic hemophilia A carrier POA PDxIn

Z14.1 Cystic fibrosis carrier POA PDxIn

Z14.8 Genetic carrier of other disease POA PDxIn

Z15 Genetic susceptibility to disease
See Official Guidelines "Status" I.C.21.c.3
INCLUDES *confirmed abnormal gene*
Use additional code, if applicable, for any associated family history of the disease (Z80-Z84)
EXCLUDES1 *chromosomal anomalies (Q90-Q99)*

Z15.0 Genetic susceptibility to malignant neoplasm
See Official Guidelines "Chapter 2: Neoplasms (C00-D49)" I.C.2
☞ Code first, if applicable, any current malignant neoplasm (C00-C75, C81-C96)
Use additional code, if applicable, for any personal history of malignant neoplasm (Z85.-)

Z15.01 Genetic susceptibility to malignant neoplasm of breast POA PDxIn

Z15.02 Genetic susceptibility to malignant neoplasm of ovary POA ♀ PDxIn

Z15.03 Genetic susceptibility to malignant neoplasm of prostate POA ♂ PDxIn

Z15.04 Genetic susceptibility to malignant neoplasm of endometrium POA ♀ PDxIn

Z15.09 Genetic susceptibility to other malignant neoplasm POA PDxIn

Z15.8 Genetic susceptibility to other disease

Z15.81 Genetic susceptibility to multiple endocrine neoplasia [MEN] POA PDxIn
EXCLUDES1 *multiple endocrine neoplasia [MEN] syndromes (E31.2-)*

Z15.89 Genetic susceptibility to other disease POA PDxIn

Resistance to antimicrobial drugs (Z16)

Z16 Resistance to antimicrobial **drugs**
See Official Guidelines "Infections resistant to antibiotics" I.C.1.c, "Status" I.C.21.c.3
NOTES The codes in this category are provided for use as additional codes to identify the resistance and non-responsiveness of a condition to antimicrobial drugs.
☞ Code first the infection
EXCLUDES1 *Methicillin resistant Staphylococcus aureus infection (A49.02)*
Methicillin resistant Staphylococcus aureus pneumonia (J15.212)
Sepsis due to Methicillin resistant Staphylococcus aureus (A41.02)

Z16.1 Resistance to beta lactam **antibiotics**

Z16.10 Resistance to unspecified beta lactam antibiotics PDxIn

Z16.11 Resistance to penicillins PDxIn
See Official Guidelines "Combination codes for MRSA infection" I.C.1.e.1.a, "Other codes for MRSA infection" I.C.1.e.1.b
Resistance to amoxicillin
Resistance to ampicillin

Z16.12 Extended spectrum beta lactamase (ESBL) resistance CC PDxIn CC/MCC Exc
EXCLUDES2 *Methicillin resistant Staphylococcus aureus infection in diseases classified elsewhere (B95.62)*

Z16.19 Resistance to other specified beta lactam antibiotics PDxIn
Resistance to cephalosporins

Z16.2 Resistance to other **antibiotics**

Z16.20 Resistance to unspecified antibiotic PDxIn
Resistance to antibiotics NOS

Z16.21 Resistance to vancomycin CC PDxIn CC/MCC Exc

Z16.22 Resistance to vancomycin related **antibiotics** PDxIn

Z16.23 Resistance to quinolones and fluoroquinolones PDxIn

Z16.24 Resistance to multiple **antibiotics** CC PDxIn CC/MCC Exc

Z16.29 Resistance to other single specified **antibiotic** PDxIn
Resistance to aminoglycosides
Resistance to macrolides
Resistance to sulfonamides
Resistance to tetracyclines

PDxIn Unacceptable principal diagnosis symbol per Medicare code edits   POA Code exempt from diagnosis present on admission requirement
❓ Questionable admission   Complication or comorbidity   MCC Major complication or comorbidity   CC/MCC Exc CC/MCC exclusion
HCC HCC diagnosis code   RxHCC RxHCC diagnosis code   MACRA MACRA code   **DEFINITION** Describes condition/terminology
TIP Coding guidance   👁 Official Guideline Reference   Z code as first-listed diagnosis

[5th] Z16.3 Resistance to other antimicrobial drugs
[EXCLUDES1] *resistance to antibiotics (Z16.1-, Z16.2-)*
- Z16.30 **Resistance to unspecified antimicrobial drugs** [PDx]
  Drug resistance NOS
- Z16.31 **Resistance to antiparasitic drug(s)** [PDx]
  Resistance to quinine and related compounds
- Z16.32 **Resistance to antifungal drug(s)** [PDx]
- Z16.33 **Resistance to antiviral drug(s)** [PDx]
- [6th] Z16.34 **Resistance to antimycobacterial drug(s)**
  Resistance to tuberculostatics
  - Z16.341 **Resistance to single antimycobacterial drug** [PDx]
    Resistance to antimycobacterial drug NOS
  - Z16.342 **Resistance to multiple antimycobacterial drugs** [PDx]
- Z16.35 **Resistance to multiple antimicrobial drugs** [PDx]
  [EXCLUDES1] *Resistance to multiple antibiotics only (Z16.24)*
- Z16.39 **Resistance to other specified antimicrobial drug** [CC] [PDx] [CC/MCC Exc]

Estrogen receptor status (Z17)

[4th] Z17 **Estrogen receptor status**
👁 **See Official Guidelines** "Status" I.C.21.c.3
☞ **Code first** malignant neoplasm of breast (C50.-)
- Z17.0 **Estrogen receptor positive status [ER+]** [POA] [PDx]
- Z17.1 **Estrogen receptor negative status [ER-]** [POA] [PDx]

Retained foreign body fragments (Z18)

[4th] Z18 **Retained foreign body fragments**
👁 **See Official Guidelines** "Status" I.C.21.c.3
[INCLUDES] *embedded fragment (status)*
embedded splinter (status)
retained foreign body status
[EXCLUDES1] *artificial joint prosthesis status (Z96.6-)*
foreign body accidentally left during a procedure (T81.5-)
foreign body entering through orifice (T15-T19)
in situ cardiac device (Z95.-)
organ or tissue replaced by means other than transplant (Z96.-, Z97.-)
organ or tissue replaced by transplant (Z94.-)
personal history of retained foreign body fully removed Z87.821
superficial foreign body (non-embedded splinter) - code to superficial foreign body, by site

[5th] Z18.0 **Retained radioactive fragments**
- Z18.01 **Retained depleted uranium fragments** [POA] [PDx]
- Z18.09 **Other retained radioactive fragments** [POA] [PDx]
  Other retained depleted isotope fragments
  Retained nontherapeutic radioactive fragments

[5th] Z18.1 **Retained metal fragments**
[EXCLUDES1] *retained radioactive metal fragments (Z18.01-Z18.09)*
- Z18.10 **Retained metal fragments, unspecified** [POA] [PDx]
  Retained metal fragment NOS
- Z18.11 **Retained magnetic metal fragments** [POA] [PDx]
- Z18.12 **Retained nonmagnetic metal fragments** [POA] [PDx]

Z18.2 **Retained plastic fragments** [POA] [PDx]
Acrylics fragments
Diethylhexyl phthalates fragments
Isocyanate fragments

[5th] Z18.3 **Retained organic fragments**
- Z18.31 **Retained animal quills or spines** [POA] [PDx]
- Z18.32 **Retained tooth** [POA] [PDx]
- Z18.33 **Retained wood fragments** [POA] [PDx]
- Z18.39 **Other retained organic fragments** [POA] [PDx]

[5th] Z18.8 **Other specified retained foreign body**
- Z18.81 **Retained glass fragments** [POA] [PDx]
- Z18.83 **Retained stone or crystalline fragments** [POA] [PDx]
  Retained concrete or cement fragments
- Z18.89 **Other specified retained foreign body fragments** [POA] [PDx]
  AHA: Q3 2016

Z18.9 **Retained foreign body fragments, unspecified material** [POA] [PDx]

Hormone sensitivity malignancy status (Z19)

[4th] Z19 **Hormone sensitivity malignancy status**
👁 **See Official Guidelines** "Status" I.C.21.c.3
☞ **Code first** malignant neoplasm - *see Table of Neoplasms, by site, malignant*
- Z19.1 **Hormone sensitive malignancy status** [POA] [PDx]
  AHA: Q4 2016
- Z19.2 **Hormone resistant malignancy status** [POA] [PDx]
  AHA: Q4 2016
  Castrate resistant prostate malignancy status

Persons with potential health hazards related to communicable diseases (Z20-Z29)

[4th] Z20 **Contact with and (suspected) exposure to communicable diseases**
👁 **See Official Guidelines** "Contact/Exposure" I.C.21.c.1
[EXCLUDES1] *carrier of infectious disease (Z22.-)*
diagnosed current infectious or parasitic disease -see Alphabetic Index
[EXCLUDES2] *personal history of infectious and parasitic diseases (Z86.1-)*

[5th] Z20.0 **Contact with and (suspected) exposure to intestinal infectious diseases**
- Z20.01 **Contact with and (suspected) exposure to intestinal infectious diseases due to Escherichia coli (E. coli)**
- Z20.09 **Contact with and (suspected) exposure to other intestinal infectious diseases** [PDx]

Z20.1 **Contact with and (suspected) exposure to tuberculosis** [PDx]
Z20.2 **Contact with and (suspected) exposure to infections with a predominantly sexual mode of transmission** [PDx]
Z20.3 **Contact with and (suspected) exposure to rabies** [PDx]
Z20.4 **Contact with and (suspected) exposure to rubella** [PDx]
Z20.5 **Contact with and (suspected) exposure to viral hepatitis**
Z20.6 **Contact with and (suspected) exposure to human immunodeficiency virus [HIV]**
[EXCLUDES1] *asymptomatic human immunodeficiency virus [HIV] HIV infection status (Z21)*
Z20.7 **Contact with and (suspected) exposure to pediculosis, acariasis and other infestations** [PDx]

[5th] Z20.8 **Contact with and (suspected) exposure to other communicable diseases**
- [6th] Z20.81 **Contact with and (suspected) exposure to other bacterial communicable diseases**
  - Z20.810 **Contact with and (suspected) exposure to anthrax** [PDx]
  - Z20.811 **Contact with and (suspected) exposure to meningococcus**
  - Z20.818 **Contact with and (suspected) exposure to other bacterial communicable diseases** [PDx]
    AHA: Q2 2019
- [6th] Z20.82 **Contact with and (suspected) exposure to other viral communicable diseases**
  - Z20.820 **Contact with and (suspected) exposure to varicella**
  - Z20.821 **Contact with and (suspected) exposure to Zika virus** [POA] [PDx]
    👁 **See Official Guidelines** "Code only confirmed cases" I.C.1.f.1
    AHA: Q4 2018
  - Z20.828 **Contact with and (suspected) exposure to other viral communicable diseases**
    AHA: Q4 2018, Q4 2016
- Z20.89 **Contact with and (suspected) exposure to other communicable diseases** [PDx]

Unspecified Code | Other Specified Code | Manifestation Code | [N] Newborn | [P] Pediatric | [M] Maternity | [A] Adult | ♂ Male | ♀ Female
● New Code | ▲ Revised Code Title | ►◄ Revised Text | [NOTES] | [INCLUDES] | [EXCLUDES1] Not coded here | [EXCLUDES2] Not included here
[4th] 4th character required | [5th] 5th character required | [6th] 6th character required | [7th] 7th character required | [X] Extension 'X' Alert
[HAC] Hospital-acquired condition (HAC) alert | AHA AHA Coding Clinic© | ☞ Code first alert

Z20.9 Contact with and (suspected) exposure to unspecified communicable disease   POA PDxIn

Z21 Asymptomatic **human immunodeficiency virus [HIV] infection status**   HCC ? RxHCC

    👁 **See Official Guidelines** "Asymptomatic human immunodeficiency virus" I.C.1.a.2.d, "Previously diagnosed HIV-related illness" I.C.1.a.2.f, "HIV Infection in Pregnancy, Childbirth and the Puerperium" I.C.1.a.2.g, "Status" I.C.21.c.3

    AHA: Q1 2019

    HIV positive NOS

    ☛ **Code first** Human immunodeficiency virus [HIV] disease complicating pregnancy, childbirth and the puerperium, if applicable (O98.7-)

    EXCLUDES1 acquired immunodeficiency syndrome (B20)

        contact with human immunodeficiency virus [HIV] (Z20.6)

        exposure to human immunodeficiency virus [HIV] (Z20.6)

        human immunodeficiency virus [HIV] disease (B20)

        inconclusive laboratory evidence of human immunodeficiency virus [HIV] (R75)

Z22 **Carrier of infectious disease**

    👁 **See Official Guidelines** "Status" I.C.21.c.3

    INCLUDES colonization status

        suspected carrier

    EXCLUDES2 carrier of viral hepatitis (B18.-)

    Z22.0 **Carrier of** typhoid   POA PDxIn

    Z22.1 **Carrier of other** intestinal **infectious diseases**   POA PDxIn

    Z22.2 **Carrier of** diphtheria   POA PDxIn

    Z22.3 **Carrier of** other **specified bacterial diseases**

        Z22.31 **Carrier of bacterial disease due to** meningococci   POA PDxIn

        Z22.32 **Carrier of bacterial disease due to** staphylococci

            Z22.321 **Carrier or suspected carrier of** Methicillin **susceptible Staphylococcus aureus**   POA PDxIn

                👁 **See Official Guidelines** "MSSA and MRSA colonization" I.C.1.e.1.c

                MSSA colonization

            Z22.322 **Carrier or suspected carrier of** Methicillin **resistant Staphylococcus aureus**   POA PDxIn

                👁 **See Official Guidelines** "MSSA and MRSA colonization" I.C.1.e.1.c, "MRSA colonization and infection" I.C.1.e.1.d

                MRSA colonization

        Z22.33 **Carrier of bacterial disease due to** streptococci

            Z22.330 **Carrier of** Group B **streptococcus**   POA PDxIn

                EXCLUDES1 Carrier of streptococcus group B (GBS) complicating pregnancy, childbirth and the puerperium (O99.82-)

            Z22.338 **Carrier of other streptococcus**   POA PDxIn

        Z22.39 Carrier of other specified bacterial diseases   POA PDxIn

    Z22.4 **Carrier of infections with a** predominantly sexual mode **of transmission**   POA PDxIn

    Z22.6 **Carrier of** human T-lymphotropic virus type-1 **[HTLV-1] infection**   POA PDxIn

    ● **Z22.7** **Latent** tuberculosis   POA

        Latent tuberculosis infection (LTBI)

        EXCLUDES1 nonspecific reaction to cell mediated immunity measurement of gamma interferon antigen response without active tuberculosis (R76.12)

            nonspecific reaction to tuberculin skin test without active tuberculosis (R76.11)

    Z22.8 **Carrier of other infectious diseases**   POA PDxIn

    Z22.9 **Carrier of infectious disease, unspecified**   POA PDxIn

Z23 **Encounter for immunization**

    👁 **See Official Guidelines** "Inoculations and vaccinations" I.C.21.c.2

    ☛ **Code first** any routine childhood examination

    NOTES Procedure codes are required to identify the types of immunizations given.

Z28 **Immunization not carried out and underimmunization status**

    👁 **See Official Guidelines** "Status" I.C.21.c.3, "Miscellaneous Z codes" I.C.21.c.14

    INCLUDES vaccination not carried out

Z28.0 **Immunization not carried out because of** contraindication

    Z28.01 **Immunization not carried out because of** acute illness **of patient**   POA PDxIn

    Z28.02 **Immunization not carried out because of** chronic illness **or condition of patient**   POA PDxIn

    Z28.03 **Immunization not carried out because of** immune compromised state **of patient**   POA PDxIn

    Z28.04 **Immunization not carried out because of patient** allergy to vaccine or component   POA PDxIn

    Z28.09 **Immunization not carried out because of other** contraindication   POA PDxIn

Z28.1 **Immunization not carried out because of patient decision for** reasons of belief or group pressure   POA PDxIn

    Immunization not carried out because of religious belief

Z28.2 **Immunization not carried out because of patient decision for** other and unspecified **reason**

    Z28.20 **Immunization not carried out because of patient decision for unspecified reason**   POA PDxIn

    Z28.21 **Immunization not carried out because of patient** refusal   POA PDxIn

    Z28.29 **Immunization not carried out because of patient decision for other reason**   POA PDxIn

Z28.3 Underimmunization **status**   POA PDxIn

    Delinquent immunization status

    Lapsed immunization schedule status

Z28.8 **Immunization not carried out for other reason**

    Z28.81 **Immunization not carried out due to** patient having had the disease   POA PDxIn

    Z28.82 **Immunization not carried out because of** caregiver refusal   POA PDxIn

        Immunization not carried out because of guardian refusal

        Immunization not carried out because of parent refusal

        EXCLUDES1 immunization not carried out because of caregiver refusal because of religious belief (Z28.1)

    Z28.83 **Immunization not carried out due to** unavailability **of vaccine**   POA PDxIn

        AHA: Q4 2018

        Delay in delivery of vaccine

        Lack of availability of vaccine

        Manufacturer delay of vaccine

    Z28.89 **Immunization not carried out for other reason**   POA PDxIn

Z28.9 **Immunization not carried out for unspecified reason**   POA PDxIn

Z29 **Encounter for other** prophylactic **measures**

    👁 **See Official Guidelines** "Miscellaneous Z codes" I.C.21.c.14

    EXCLUDES1 desensitization to allergens (Z51.6)

        prophylactic surgery (Z40.-)

Z29.1 **Encounter for prophylactic** immunotherapy

    Encounter for administration of immunoglobulin

    Z29.11 **Encounter for prophylactic immunotherapy for** respiratory syncytial virus (RSV)   POA PDxIn

        AHA: Q4 2016

    Z29.12 **Encounter for prophylactic** antivenin   POA PDxIn

        AHA: Q4 2016

    Z29.13 **Encounter for prophylactic** Rho(D) immune globulin   POA PDxIn

        AHA: Q4 2016

    Z29.14 **Encounter for prophylactic** rabies immune globin   POA PDxIn

        AHA: Q4 2016

Z29.3 **Encounter for prophylactic** fluoride administration   POA PDxIn

    AHA: Q4 2016

Z29.8 Encounter for other specified prophylactic measures   POA PDxIn

    AHA: Q4 2016

Z29.9 **Encounter for prophylactic measures, unspecified**   POA PDxIn

    AHA: Q4 2016

POA Unacceptable principal diagnosis symbol per Medicare code edits   POA Code exempt from diagnosis present on admission requirement   ? Questionable admission   CC Complication or comorbidity   MCC Major complication or comorbidity   CC/MCC CC/MCC exclusion   HCC HCC diagnosis code   RxHCC RxHCC diagnosis code   MACRA code   **DEFINITION** Describes condition/terminology   **TIP** Coding guidance   👁 Official Guideline Reference   Z1 Z code as first-listed diagnosis

Persons encountering health services in circumstances related to reproduction (Z30-Z39)

4️⃣ **Z30** Encounter for contraceptive management
👁 **See Official Guidelines** "Encounters for Obstetrical and Reproductive Services" I.C.21.c.11

5️⃣ **Z30.0** Encounter for general counseling and advice on contraception
👁 **See Official Guidelines** "Counseling" I.C.21.c.10

6️⃣ **Z30.01** Encounter for initial prescription of contraceptives
EXCLUDES1 *encounter for surveillance of contraceptives (Z30.4-)*

Z30.011 Encounter for initial prescription of contraceptive pills POA ♀ PDxIn

Z30.012 Encounter for prescription of emergency contraception POA ♀ PDxIn
Encounter for postcoital contraception

Z30.013 Encounter for initial prescription of injectable contraceptive POA ♀ PDxIn

Z30.014 Encounter for initial prescription of intrauterine contraceptive device POA ♀ PDxIn
EXCLUDES1 *encounter for insertion of intrauterine contraceptive device (Z30.430, Z30.432)*

Z30.015 Encounter for initial prescription of vaginal ring hormonal contraceptive POA ♀ PDxIn
AHA: Q4 2016

Z30.016 Encounter for initial prescription of transdermal patch hormonal contraceptive device POA ♀ PDxIn
AHA: Q4 2016

Z30.017 Encounter for initial prescription of implantable subdermal contraceptive POA ♀ PDxIn
AHA: Q4 2016

Z30.018 Encounter for initial prescription of other contraceptives POA ♀ PDxIn
Encounter for initial prescription of barrier contraception
Encounter for initial prescription of diaphragm

Z30.019 Encounter for initial prescription of contraceptives, unspecified POA ♀ PDxIn

Z30.02 Counseling and instruction in natural family planning to avoid pregnancy POA PDxIn

Z30.09 Encounter for other general counseling and advice on contraception POA PDxIn
Encounter for family planning advice NOS

Z30.2 Encounter for sterilization POA

5️⃣ **Z30.4** Encounter for surveillance of contraceptives

Z30.40 Encounter for surveillance of contraceptives, unspecified POA PDxIn

Z30.41 Encounter for surveillance of contraceptive pills POA ♀ PDxIn
Encounter for repeat prescription for contraceptive pill

Z30.42 Encounter for surveillance of injectable contraceptive POA ♀ PDxIn

6️⃣ **Z30.43** Encounter for surveillance of intrauterine contraceptive device

Z30.430 Encounter for insertion of intrauterine contraceptive device POA ♀ PDxIn

Z30.431 Encounter for routine checking of intrauterine contraceptive device POA ♀ PDxIn

Z30.432 Encounter for removal of intrauterine contraceptive device POA ♀ PDxIn

Z30.433 Encounter for removal and reinsertion of intrauterine contraceptive device POA ♀ PDxIn
Encounter for replacement of intrauterine contraceptive device

Z30.44 Encounter for surveillance of vaginal ring hormonal contraceptive device POA ♀ PDxIn
AHA: Q4 2016

Z30.45 Encounter for surveillance of transdermal patch hormonal contraceptive device POA ♀ PDxIn
AHA: Q4 2016

Z30.46 Encounter for surveillance of implantable subdermal contraceptive POA ♀ PDxIn
AHA: Q4 2016
Encounter for checking, reinsertion or removal of implantable subdermal contraceptive

Z30.49 Encounter for surveillance of other contraceptives POA ♀ PDxIn
Encounter for surveillance of barrier contraception
Encounter for surveillance of diaphragm

Z30.8 Encounter for other contraceptive management POA PDxIn
Encounter for postvasectomy sperm count
Encounter for routine examination for contraceptive maintenance
EXCLUDES1 *sperm count following sterilization reversal (Z31.42)*
sperm count for fertility testing (Z31.41)

Z30.9 Encounter for contraceptive management, unspecified POA PDxIn

4️⃣ **Z31** Encounter for procreative management
👁 **See Official Guidelines** "Encounters for Obstetrical and Reproductive Services" I.C.21.c.11
EXCLUDES1 *complications associated with artificial fertilization (N98.-)*
female infertility (N97.-)
male infertility (N46.-)

Z31.0 Encounter for reversal of previous sterilization POA

5️⃣ **Z31.4** Encounter for procreative investigation and testing
EXCLUDES1 *postvasectomy sperm count (Z30.8)*

Z31.41 Encounter for fertility testing POA PDxIn
Encounter for fallopian tube patency testing
Encounter for sperm count for fertility testing

Z31.42 Aftercare following sterilization reversal POA PDxIn
Sperm count following sterilization reversal

6️⃣ **Z31.43** Encounter for genetic testing of female for procreative management
Use additional code for recurrent pregnancy loss, if applicable (N96, O26.2-)
EXCLUDES1 *nonprocreative genetic testing (Z13.7-)*

Z31.430 Encounter of female for testing for genetic disease carrier status for procreative management POA ♀ PDxIn

Z31.438 Encounter for other genetic testing of female for procreative management POA ♀ PDxIn

6️⃣ **Z31.44** Encounter for genetic testing of male for procreative management
EXCLUDES1 *nonprocreative genetic testing (Z13.7-)*

Z31.440 Encounter of male for testing for genetic disease carrier status for procreative management POA ♂ PDxIn

Z31.441 Encounter for testing of male partner of patient with recurrent pregnancy loss A POA ♂ PDxIn

Z31.448 Encounter for other genetic testing of male for procreative management A POA ♂ PDxIn

Z31.49 Encounter for other procreative investigation and testing POA PDxIn

Z31.5 Encounter for procreative genetic counseling POA PDxIn
👁 **See Official Guidelines** "Counseling" I.C.21.c.10
AHA: Q4 2017

5️⃣ **Z31.6** Encounter for general counseling and advice on procreation
👁 **See Official Guidelines** "Counseling" I.C.21.c.10

Z31.61 Procreative counseling and advice using natural family planning POA PDxIn

Z31.62 Encounter for fertility preservation counseling POA PDxIn
Encounter for fertility preservation counseling prior to cancer therapy
Encounter for fertility preservation counseling prior to surgical removal of gonads

Z31.69 Encounter for other general counseling and advice on procreation POA PDxIn

Z31.7 Encounter for procreative management and counseling for gestational carrier POA ♀ PDxIn
AHA: Q4 2016
EXCLUDES1 *pregnant state, gestational carrier (Z33.3)*

Unspecified Code   Other Specified Code   Manifestation Code   N Newborn   P Pediatric   M Maternity   A Adult   ♂ Male   ♀ Female
● New Code   ▲ Revised Code Title   ▶◀ Revised Text   **NOTES**   *INCLUDES*   EXCLUDES1 Not coded here   EXCLUDES2 Not included here
4️⃣ 4th character required   5️⃣ 5th character required   6️⃣ 6th character required   7️⃣ 7th character required   ❌ Extension 'X' Alert
HAC Hospital-acquired condition (HAC) alert   **AHA** AHA Coding Clinic©   📌 Code first alert

Z31.8 Encounter for other procreative management

Z31.81 Encounter for male factor infertility in female patient

> See Official Guidelines "Z Codes That May Only be Principal/First-listed Diagnosis" I.C.21.c.16

Z31.82 Encounter for Rh incompatibility status

AHA: Q3 2015

Z31.83 Encounter for assisted reproductive fertility procedure cycle

> See Official Guidelines "Z Codes That May Only be Principal/First-listed Diagnosis" I.C.21.c.16

Patient undergoing in vitro fertilization cycle
Use additional code to identify the type of infertility
EXCLUDES1 pre-cycle diagnosis and testing - code to reason for encounter

Z31.84 Encounter for fertility preservation procedure

> See Official Guidelines "Z Codes That May Only be Principal/First-listed Diagnosis" I.C.21.c.16

Encounter for fertility preservation procedure prior to cancer therapy
Encounter for fertility preservation procedure prior to surgical removal of gonads

Z31.89 Encounter for other procreative management

Z31.9 Encounter for procreative management, unspecified

Z32 Encounter for pregnancy test and childbirth and childcare instruction

Z32.0 Encounter for pregnancy test

> See Official Guidelines "Routine and administrative examinations" I.C.21.c.13

Z32.00 Encounter for pregnancy test, result unknown
Encounter for pregnancy test NOS

Z32.01 Encounter for pregnancy test, result positive

Z32.02 Encounter for pregnancy test, result negative

Z32.2 Encounter for childbirth instruction

> See Official Guidelines "Counseling" I.C.21.c.10, "Encounters for Obstetrical and Reproductive Services" I.C.21.c.11

Z32.3 Encounter for childcare instruction

> See Official Guidelines "Counseling" I.C.21.c.10, "Encounters for Obstetrical and Reproductive Services" I.C.21.c.11

Encounter for prenatal or postpartum childcare instruction

Z33 Pregnant state

> See Official Guidelines "Encounters for Obstetrical and Reproductive Services" I.C.21.c.11

Z33.1 Pregnant state, incidental

> See Official Guidelines "Codes from chapter 15 and sequencing priority" I.C.15.a.1, "Status" I.C.21.c.3

Pregnant state NOS
EXCLUDES1 complications of pregnancy (O00-O9A)
pregnant state, gestational carrier (Z33.3)

Z33.2 Encounter for elective termination of pregnancy

> See Official Guidelines "Abortion with Liveborn Fetus" I.C.15.q.1, "Z Codes That May Only be Principal/First-listed Diagnosis" I.C.21.c.16

EXCLUDES1 early fetal death with retention of dead fetus (O02.1)
late fetal death (O36.4)
spontaneous abortion (O03)

Z33.3 Pregnant state, gestational carrier

AHA: Q4 2016
EXCLUDES1 encounter for procreative management and counseling for gestational carrier (Z31.7)

Z34 Encounter for supervision of normal pregnancy

> See Official Guidelines "Routine outpatient prenatal visits" I.C.15.b.1, "Encounters for Obstetrical and Reproductive Services" I.C.21.c.11, "Z Codes That May Only be Principal/First-listed Diagnosis" I.C.21.c.16

EXCLUDES1 any complication of pregnancy (O00-O9A)
encounter for pregnancy test (Z32.0-)
encounter for supervision of high risk pregnancy (O09.-)

Z34.0 Encounter for supervision of normal first pregnancy

Z34.00 Encounter for supervision of normal first pregnancy, unspecified trimester

Z34.01 Encounter for supervision of normal first pregnancy, first trimester

Z34.02 Encounter for supervision of normal first pregnancy, second trimester

Z34.03 Encounter for supervision of normal first pregnancy, third trimester

Z34.8 Encounter for supervision of other normal pregnancy

Z34.80 Encounter for supervision of other normal pregnancy, unspecified trimester

Z34.81 Encounter for supervision of other normal pregnancy, first trimester

Z34.82 Encounter for supervision of other normal pregnancy, second trimester

Z34.83 Encounter for supervision of other normal pregnancy, third trimester

Z34.9 Encounter for supervision of normal pregnancy, unspecified

Z34.90 Encounter for supervision of normal pregnancy, unspecified, unspecified trimester

Z34.91 Encounter for supervision of normal pregnancy, unspecified, first trimester

Z34.92 Encounter for supervision of normal pregnancy, unspecified, second trimester

Z34.93 Encounter for supervision of normal pregnancy, unspecified, third trimester

Z36 Encounter for antenatal screening of mother

> See Official Guidelines "Screening" I.C.21.c.5, "Encounters for Obstetrical and Reproductive Services" I.C.21.c.11

INCLUDES Encounter for placental sample (taken vaginally)
Screening is the testing for disease or disease precursors in asymptomatic individuals so that early detection and treatment can be provided for those who test positive for the disease.
EXCLUDES1 diagnostic examination- code to sign or symptom
encounter for suspected maternal and fetal conditions ruled out (Z03.7-)
suspected fetal condition affecting management of pregnancy - code to condition in Chapter 15
EXCLUDES2 abnormal findings on antenatal screening of mother (O28.-)
genetic counseling and testing (Z31.43-, Z31.5)
routine prenatal care (Z34)

Z36.0 Encounter for antenatal screening for chromosomal anomalies

AHA: Q4 2017

Z36.1 Encounter for antenatal screening for raised alphafetoprotein level

AHA: Q4 2017
Encounter for antenatal screening for elevated maternal serum alphafetoprotein level

Z36.2 Encounter for other antenatal screening follow-up

AHA: Q4 2017
Non-visualized anatomy on a previous scan

Z36.3 Encounter for antenatal screening for malformations

AHA: Q4 2017
Screening for a suspected anomaly

Z36.4 Encounter for antenatal screening for fetal growth retardation

AHA: Q4 2017
Intrauterine growth restriction (IUGR)/small-for-dates

Z36.5 Encounter for antenatal screening for isoimmunization

AHA: Q4 2017

Z36.8 Encounter for other antenatal screening

Z36.81 Encounter for antenatal screening for hydrops fetalis

AHA: Q4 2017

Z36.82 Encounter for antenatal screening for nuchal translucency

AHA: Q4 2017

1st 1st trimester   **2nd** 2nd trimester   **3rd** 3rd trimester   Unacceptable principal diagnosis symbol per Medicare code edits   Code exempt from diagnosis present on admission requirement   ❓ Questionable admission   Complication or comorbidity   Major complication or comorbidity   CC/MCC exclusion   HCC diagnosis code   RxHCC diagnosis code   MACRA code   **DEFINITION** Describes condition/terminology   **TIP** Coding guidance   Official Guideline Reference   Z code as first-listed diagnosis

Z36.83	Encounter for fetal screening for congenital cardiac abnormalities	M POA ♀
	AHA: Q4 2017	
Z36.84	Encounter for antenatal screening for fetal lung maturity	M POA ♀
	AHA: Q4 2017	
Z36.85	Encounter for antenatal screening for Streptococcus B	M POA ♀
	AHA: Q4 2017	
Z36.86	Encounter for antenatal screening for cervical length	M POA ♀
	AHA: Q4 2017	
	Screening for risk of pre-term labor	
Z36.87	Encounter for antenatal screening for uncertain dates	M POA ♀
	AHA: Q4 2017	
Z36.88	Encounter for antenatal screening for fetal macrosomia	M POA ♀
	AHA: Q4 2017	
	Screening for large-for-dates	
Z36.89	Encounter for other specified antenatal screening	M POA ♀
	AHA: Q4 2017	
Z36.8A	Encounter for antenatal screening for other genetic defects	M POA ♀
	AHA: Q4 2017	
Z36.9	**Encounter for antenatal screening, unspecified**	M POA ♀
	AHA: Q4 2017	

4th Z3A Weeks of gestation

👁 See Official Guidelines "Encounters for Obstetrical and Reproductive Services" I.C.21.c.11

NOTES Codes from category Z3A are for use, only on the maternal record, to indicate the weeks of gestation of the pregnancy, if known.

📌 Code first complications of pregnancy, childbirth and the puerperium (O09-O9A)

5th Z3A.0 Weeks of gestation of pregnancy, unspecified or less than 10 weeks

Z3A.00	Weeks of gestation of pregnancy not specified	M POA ♀ PDxln
Z3A.01	Less than 8 weeks gestation of pregnancy	1st M POA ♀ PDxln
Z3A.08	8 weeks gestation of pregnancy	1st M POA ♀ PDxln
Z3A.09	9 weeks gestation of pregnancy	1st M POA ♀ PDxln

5th Z3A.1 Weeks of gestation of pregnancy, weeks 10-19

Z3A.10	10 weeks gestation of pregnancy	1st M POA ♀ PDxln
Z3A.11	11 weeks gestation of pregnancy	1st M POA ♀ PDxln
Z3A.12	12 weeks gestation of pregnancy	1st M POA ♀ PDxln
Z3A.13	13 weeks gestation of pregnancy	1st M POA ♀ PDxln
Z3A.14	14 weeks gestation of pregnancy	2nd M POA ♀ PDxln
Z3A.15	15 weeks gestation of pregnancy	2nd M POA ♀ PDxln
Z3A.16	16 weeks gestation of pregnancy	2nd M POA ♀ PDxln
	AHA: Q4 2016	
Z3A.17	17 weeks gestation of pregnancy	2nd M POA ♀ PDxln
Z3A.18	18 weeks gestation of pregnancy	2nd M POA ♀ PDxln
Z3A.19	19 weeks gestation of pregnancy	2nd M POA ♀ PDxln

5th Z3A.2 Weeks of gestation of pregnancy, weeks 20-29

Z3A.20	20 weeks gestation of pregnancy	2nd M POA ♀ PDxln
	AHA: Q4 2016	
Z3A.21	21 weeks gestation of pregnancy	2nd M POA ♀ PDxln
Z3A.22	22 weeks gestation of pregnancy	2nd M POA ♀ PDxln
	AHA: Q4 2016	
Z3A.23	23 weeks gestation of pregnancy	2nd M POA ♀ PDxln
Z3A.24	24 weeks gestation of pregnancy	2nd M POA ♀ PDxln
Z3A.25	25 weeks gestation of pregnancy	2nd M POA ♀ PDxln
Z3A.26	26 weeks gestation of pregnancy	2nd M POA ♀ PDxln
Z3A.27	27 weeks gestation of pregnancy	2nd M POA ♀ PDxln
Z3A.28	28 weeks gestation of pregnancy	3rd M POA ♀ PDxln
Z3A.29	29 weeks gestation of pregnancy	3rd M POA ♀ PDxln

5th Z3A.3 Weeks of gestation of pregnancy, weeks 30-39

Z3A.30	30 weeks gestation of pregnancy	3rd M POA ♀ PDxln
Z3A.31	31 weeks gestation of pregnancy	3rd M POA ♀ PDxln
Z3A.32	32 weeks gestation of pregnancy	3rd M POA ♀ PDxln
	AHA: Q4 2016	
Z3A.33	33 weeks gestation of pregnancy	3rd M POA ♀ PDxln
Z3A.34	34 weeks gestation of pregnancy	3rd M POA ♀ PDxln
Z3A.35	35 weeks gestation of pregnancy	3rd M POA ♀ PDxln
Z3A.36	36 weeks gestation of pregnancy	3rd M POA ♀ PDxln
Z3A.37	37 weeks gestation of pregnancy	3rd M POA ♀ PDxln
Z3A.38	38 weeks gestation of pregnancy	3rd M POA ♀
	AHA: Q2 2016	
Z3A.39	39 weeks gestation of pregnancy	3rd M POA ♀

5th Z3A.4 Weeks of gestation of pregnancy, weeks 40 or greater

Z3A.40	40 weeks gestation of pregnancy	3rd M POA ♀
Z3A.41	41 weeks gestation of pregnancy	3rd M POA ♀
Z3A.42	42 weeks gestation of pregnancy	3rd M POA ♀
Z3A.49	Greater than 42 weeks gestation of pregnancy	3rd M POA ♀ PDxln

4th Z37 Outcome of delivery

👁 See Official Guidelines "Outcome of delivery" I.C.15.b.5, "Abortion with Liveborn Fetus" I.C.15.q.1, "Encounters for Obstetrical and Reproductive Services" I.C.21.c.11

This category is intended for use as an additional code to identify the outcome of delivery on the mother's record. It is not for use on the newborn record.

EXCLUDES1 stillbirth (P95)

Z37.0	**Single live birth**	M POA ♀ PDxln
	👁 See Official Guidelines "Outcome of delivery for O80" I.C.15.n.3	
	AHA: Q2 2016	
Z37.1	**Single stillbirth**	M POA ♀ PDxln
Z37.2	**Twins, both liveborn**	M POA ♀ PDxln
Z37.3	**Twins, one liveborn and one stillborn**	M POA ♀ PDxln
Z37.4	**Twins, both stillborn**	M POA ♀ PDxln

5th Z37.5 Other multiple births, all liveborn

Z37.50	Multiple births, unspecified, all liveborn	M POA ♀ PDxln
Z37.51	Triplets, all liveborn	M POA ♀ PDxln
Z37.52	Quadruplets, all liveborn	M POA ♀ PDxln
Z37.53	Quintuplets, all liveborn	M POA ♀ PDxln
Z37.54	Sextuplets, all liveborn	M POA ♀ PDxln
Z37.59	Other multiple births, all liveborn	M POA ♀ PDxln

5th Z37.6 Other multiple births, some liveborn

Z37.60	Multiple births, unspecified, some liveborn	M POA ♀ PDxln
Z37.61	Triplets, some liveborn	M POA ♀ PDxln
Z37.62	Quadruplets, some liveborn	M POA ♀ PDxln
Z37.63	Quintuplets, some liveborn	M POA ♀ PDxln
Z37.64	Sextuplets, some liveborn	M POA ♀ PDxln
Z37.69	Other multiple births, some liveborn	M POA ♀ PDxln

Z37.7	**Other multiple births, all stillborn**	M POA ♀ PDxln
Z37.9	**Outcome of delivery, unspecified**	M POA ♀ PDxln
	Multiple birth NOS	
	Single birth NOS	

4th Z38 Liveborn infants according to place of birth and type of delivery

👁 See Official Guidelines "Principal Diagnosis for Birth Record" I.C.16.a.2, "Use of Z05 on birth record and on other than birth record" I.C.16.b.2-3, "Observation" I.C.21.c.6, "Newborns and Infants" I.C.21.c.12, "Z Codes That May Only be Principal/First-listed Diagnosis" I.C.21.c.16

This category is for use as the principal code on the initial record of a newborn baby. It is to be used for the initial birth record only. It is not to be used on the mother's record.

5th Z38.0 Single liveborn infant, born in hospital

Single liveborn infant, born in birthing center or other health care facility

Z38.00	Single liveborn infant, delivered vaginally	N POA Z1
	AHA: Q4 2018, Q2 2017, Q4 2016	
Z38.01	Single liveborn infant, delivered by cesarean	N POA Z1
	AHA: Q2 2017, Q3 2016	

Z38.1	**Single liveborn infant, born outside hospital**	N POA Z1
Z38.2	**Single liveborn infant, unspecified as to place of birth**	N POA Z1
	Single liveborn infant NOS	

Unspecified Code   Other Specified Code   Manifestation Code   N Newborn   P Pediatric   M Maternity   A Adult   ♂ Male   ♀ Female
● New Code   ▲ Revised Code Title   ►◄ Revised Text   **NOTES**   *INCLUDES*   *EXCLUDES1* Not coded here   *EXCLUDES2* Not included here
4th 4th character required   5th 5th character required   6th 6th character required   7th 7th character required   7th Extension 'X' Alert
HAC Hospital-acquired condition (HAC) alert   **AHA** AHA Coding Clinic©   📌 Code first alert

Z38.3 Twin liveborn infant, born in hospital
- **Z38.30 Twin liveborn infant,** delivered vaginally N POA Z1
- **Z38.31 Twin liveborn infant,** delivered by cesarean N POA Z1

Z38.4 Twin liveborn infant, born outside hospital N POA Z1

Z38.5 Twin liveborn infant, unspecified as to place of birth N POA Z1

Z38.6 Other multiple liveborn infant, born in hospital
- **Z38.61 Triplet liveborn infant,** delivered vaginally N POA Z1
- **Z38.62 Triplet liveborn infant,** delivered by cesarean N POA Z1
- **Z38.63 Quadruplet liveborn infant,** delivered vaginally N POA Z1
- **Z38.64 Quadruplet liveborn infant,** delivered by cesarean N POA Z1
- **Z38.65 Quintuplet liveborn infant,** delivered vaginally N POA Z1
- **Z38.66 Quintuplet liveborn infant,** delivered by cesarean N POA Z1
- **Z38.68 Other multiple liveborn infant,** delivered vaginally N POA Z1
- **Z38.69 Other multiple liveborn infant,** delivered by cesarean N POA Z1

Z38.7 Other multiple liveborn infant, born outside hospital N POA Z1

Z38.8 Other multiple liveborn infant, unspecified as to place of birth N POA Z1

Z39 Encounter for maternal postpartum care and examination
- See Official Guidelines "Encounters for Obstetrical and Reproductive Services" I.C.21.c.11, "Z Codes That May Only be Principal/First-listed Diagnosis" I.C.21.c.16, "Follow-up" I.C.21.c.8

Z39.0 Encounter for care and examination of mother immediately after delivery M POA ♀ Z1
- See Official Guidelines Admission for routine postpartum care following delivery outside hospital" I.C.15.o.4
- Care and observation in uncomplicated cases when the delivery occurs outside a healthcare facility
- EXCLUDES1 care for postpartum complication- see Alphabetic index

Z39.1 Encounter for care and examination of lactating mother M POA ♀ PDxIn Z1
- Encounter for supervision of lactation
- EXCLUDES1 disorders of lactation (O92.-)

Z39.2 Encounter for routine postpartum **follow-up** M POA ♀ PDxIn Z1

Encounters for other specific health care (Z40-Z53)

Categories Z40-Z53 are intended for use to indicate a reason for care. They may be used for patients who have already been treated for a disease or injury, but who are receiving aftercare or prophylactic care, or care to consolidate the treatment, or to deal with a residual state

EXCLUDES2 follow-up examination for medical surveillance after treatment (Z08-Z09)

Z40 Encounter for prophylactic surgery
- See Official Guidelines "Miscellaneous Z codes" I.C.21.c.14, "Z Codes That May Only be Principal/First-listed Diagnosis" I.C.21.c.16
- EXCLUDES1 organ donations (Z52.-)
  - therapeutic organ removal-code to condition

Z40.0 Encounter for prophylactic surgery for risk factors related to malignant neoplasms
- Admission for prophylactic organ removal
- Use additional code to identify risk factor
- **Z40.00 Encounter for prophylactic removal of unspecified organ** Z1
- **Z40.01 Encounter for prophylactic removal of** breast Z1
- **Z40.02 Encounter for prophylactic removal of** ovary(s) ♀ Z1
  - AHA: Q4 2017
  - Encounter for prophylactic removal of ovary(s) and fallopian tube(s)
- **Z40.03 Encounter for prophylactic removal of** fallopian tube(s) POA ♀ Z1
  - AHA: Q4 2017
- **Z40.09 Encounter for prophylactic removal of other organ** Z1

Z40.8 Encounter for other prophylactic **surgery** PDxIn Z1

Z40.9 Encounter for prophylactic surgery, unspecified PDxIn Z1

Z41 Encounter for procedures for purposes other than remedying health state
- See Official Guidelines "Miscellaneous Z codes" I.C.21.c.14
- **Z41.1 Encounter for** cosmetic surgery POA
  - Encounter for cosmetic breast implant
  - Encounter for cosmetic procedure
  - EXCLUDES1 encounter for plastic and reconstructive surgery following medical procedure or healed injury (Z42.-)
    - encounter for post-mastectomy breast implantation (Z42.1)
- **Z41.2 Encounter for routine and** ritual male circumcision POA ♂
  - AHA: Q3 2018
- **Z41.3 Encounter for** ear piercing POA PDxIn
- **Z41.8 Encounter for other procedures for purposes other than remedying health state** POA
- **Z41.9 Encounter for procedure for purposes other than remedying health state, unspecified** POA PDxIn
  - See Official Guidelines "Nonspecific Z codes" I.C.21.c.15

Z42 Encounter for plastic and reconstructive surgery **following medical procedure or healed injury**
- See Official Guidelines "Aftercare" I.C.21.c.7, "Z Codes That May Only be Principal/First-listed Diagnosis" I.C.21.c.16
- EXCLUDES1 encounter for cosmetic plastic surgery (Z41.1)
  - encounter for plastic surgery for treatment of current injury - code to relevant injury
- **Z42.1 Encounter for breast reconstruction following** mastectomy A POA Z1
  - EXCLUDES1 deformity and disproportion of reconstructed breast (N65.1-)
- **Z42.8 Encounter for other plastic and reconstructive surgery following** medical procedure or healed injury POA Z1
  - AHA: Q1 2017

Z43 Encounter for attention to artificial openings
- See Official Guidelines "Aftercare" I.C.21.c.7
- INCLUDES closure of artificial openings
  - passage of sounds or bougies through artificial openings
  - reforming artificial openings
  - removal of catheter from artificial openings
  - toilet or cleansing of artificial openings
- EXCLUDES1 complications of external stoma (J95.0-, K94.-, N99.5-)
- EXCLUDES2 fitting and adjustment of prosthetic and other devices (Z44-Z46)
- **Z43.0 Encounter for attention to** tracheostomy POA HCC
- **Z43.1 Encounter for attention to** gastrostomy POA HCC
  - EXCLUDES2 artificial opening status only, without need for care (Z93.-)
- **Z43.2 Encounter for attention to** ileostomy POA HCC
  - AHA: Q3 2016
- **Z43.3 Encounter for attention to** colostomy POA HCC
- **Z43.4 Encounter for attention to other artificial** openings of digestive tract POA HCC
- **Z43.5 Encounter for attention to** cystostomy POA HCC
- **Z43.6 Encounter for attention to other artificial** openings of urinary tract POA HCC
  - Encounter for attention to nephrostomy
  - Encounter for attention to ureterostomy
  - Encounter for attention to urethrostomy
- **Z43.7 Encounter for attention to artificial** vagina POA
- **Z43.8 Encounter for attention to other artificial openings** POA HCC
- **Z43.9 Encounter for attention to unspecified artificial opening** POA HCC PDxIn

Z44 Encounter for fitting and adjustment of external prosthetic device
- See Official Guidelines "Aftercare" I.C.21.c.7
- INCLUDES removal or replacement of external prosthetic device
- EXCLUDES1 malfunction or other complications of device - see Alphabetical Index
  - presence of prosthetic device (Z97.-)

POA Unacceptable principal diagnosis symbol per Medicare code edits   POA Code exempt from diagnosis present on admission requirement
? Questionable admission   CC Complication or comorbidity   MCC Major complication or comorbidity   CC/MCC CC/MCC exclusion
HCC HCC diagnosis code   RxHCC RxHCC diagnosis code   MACRA MACRA code   **DEFINITION** Describes condition/terminology
TIP Coding guidance   Official Guideline Reference   Z1 Z code as first-listed diagnosis

Z44.0 Encounter for fitting and adjustment of artificial arm
  Z44.00 Encounter for fitting and adjustment of unspecified artificial arm
    Z44.001 Encounter for fitting and adjustment of unspecified right artificial arm
    Z44.002 Encounter for fitting and adjustment of unspecified left artificial arm
    Z44.009 Encounter for fitting and adjustment of unspecified artificial arm, unspecified arm
  Z44.01 Encounter for fitting and adjustment of complete artificial arm
    Z44.011 Encounter for fitting and adjustment of complete right artificial arm
    Z44.012 Encounter for fitting and adjustment of complete left artificial arm
    Z44.019 Encounter for fitting and adjustment of complete artificial arm, unspecified arm
  Z44.02 Encounter for fitting and adjustment of partial artificial arm
    Z44.021 Encounter for fitting and adjustment of partial artificial right arm
    Z44.022 Encounter for fitting and adjustment of partial artificial left arm
    Z44.029 Encounter for fitting and adjustment of partial artificial arm, unspecified arm
Z44.1 Encounter for fitting and adjustment of artificial leg
  Z44.10 Encounter for fitting and adjustment of unspecified artificial leg
    Z44.101 Encounter for fitting and adjustment of unspecified right artificial leg
    Z44.102 Encounter for fitting and adjustment of unspecified left artificial leg
    Z44.109 Encounter for fitting and adjustment of unspecified artificial leg, unspecified leg
  Z44.11 Encounter for fitting and adjustment of complete artificial leg
    Z44.111 Encounter for fitting and adjustment of complete right artificial leg
    Z44.112 Encounter for fitting and adjustment of complete left artificial leg
    Z44.119 Encounter for fitting and adjustment of complete artificial leg, unspecified leg
  Z44.12 Encounter for fitting and adjustment of partial artificial leg
    Z44.121 Encounter for fitting and adjustment of partial artificial right leg
    Z44.122 Encounter for fitting and adjustment of partial artificial left leg
    Z44.129 Encounter for fitting and adjustment of partial artificial leg, unspecified leg
Z44.2 Encounter for fitting and adjustment of artificial eye
  EXCLUDES1 mechanical complication of ocular prosthesis (T85.3)
  Z44.20 Encounter for fitting and adjustment of artificial eye, unspecified
  Z44.21 Encounter for fitting and adjustment of artificial right eye
  Z44.22 Encounter for fitting and adjustment of artificial left eye
Z44.3 Encounter for fitting and adjustment of external breast prosthesis
  EXCLUDES1 complications of breast implant (T85.4-)
    encounter for adjustment or removal of breast implant (Z45.81-)
    encounter for initial breast implant insertion for cosmetic breast augmentation (Z41.1)
    encounter for breast reconstruction following mastectomy (Z42.1)
  Z44.30 Encounter for fitting and adjustment of external breast prosthesis, unspecified breast

Z44.31 Encounter for fitting and adjustment of external right breast prosthesis
Z44.32 Encounter for fitting and adjustment of external left breast prosthesis
Z44.8 Encounter for fitting and adjustment of other external prosthetic devices
Z44.9 Encounter for fitting and adjustment of unspecified external prosthetic device

Z45 Encounter for adjustment and management of implanted device
  See Official Guidelines "Aftercare" I.C.21.c.7
  INCLUDES removal or replacement of implanted device
  EXCLUDES1 malfunction or other complications of device - see Alphabetical Index
  EXCLUDES2 encounter for fitting and adjustment of non-implanted device (Z46.-)
  Z45.0 Encounter for adjustment and management of cardiac device
    Z45.01 Encounter for adjustment and management of cardiac pacemaker
    Encounter for adjustment and management of cardiac resynchronization therapy pacemaker (CRT-P)
    EXCLUDES1 encounter for adjustment and management of automatic implantable cardiac defibrillator with synchronous cardiac pacemaker (Z45.02)
      Z45.010 Encounter for checking and testing of cardiac pacemaker pulse generator [battery]
      Encounter for replacing cardiac pacemaker pulse generator [battery]
      Z45.018 Encounter for adjustment and management of other part of cardiac pacemaker
      EXCLUDES1 presence of other part of cardiac pacemaker (Z95.0)
      EXCLUDES2 presence of prosthetic and other devices ▶(Z95.1-Z95.5, Z95.811-Z97)◄
    Z45.02 Encounter for adjustment and management of automatic implantable cardiac defibrillator
    Encounter for adjustment and management of automatic implantable cardiac defibrillator with synchronous cardiac pacemaker
    Encounter for adjustment and management of cardiac resynchronization therapy defibrillator (CRT-D)
    Z45.09 Encounter for adjustment and management of other cardiac device
  Z45.1 Encounter for adjustment and management of infusion pump
  Z45.2 Encounter for adjustment and management of vascular access device
    AHA: Q3 2018
    Encounter for adjustment and management of vascular catheters
    EXCLUDES1 encounter for adjustment and management of renal dialysis catheter (Z49.01)
  Z45.3 Encounter for adjustment and management of implanted devices of the special senses
    Z45.31 Encounter for adjustment and management of implanted visual substitution device
    Z45.32 Encounter for adjustment and management of implanted hearing device
    EXCLUDES1 Encounter for fitting and adjustment of hearing aid (Z46.1)
      Z45.320 Encounter for adjustment and management of bone conduction device
      Z45.321 Encounter for adjustment and management of cochlear device
      Z45.328 Encounter for adjustment and management of other implanted hearing device

[5th] **Z45.4 Encounter for adjustment and management of implanted nervous system device**

- **Z45.41 Encounter for adjustment and management of cerebrospinal fluid drainage device** [POA]
  - Encounter for adjustment and management of cerebral ventricular (communicating) shunt
- ▲ **Z45.42 Encounter for adjustment and management of ▶neurostimulator◀** [POA]
  - Encounter for adjustment and management of brain neurostimulator
  - Encounter for adjustment and management of gastric neurostimulator
  - Encounter for adjustment and management of peripheral nerve neurostimulator
  - Encounter for adjustment and management of sacral nerve neurostimulator
  - Encounter for adjustment and management of spinal cord neurostimulator
  - Encounter for adjustment and management of vagus nerve neurostimulator
- **Z45.49 Encounter for adjustment and management of other implanted nervous system device** [POA]

[5th] **Z45.8 Encounter for adjustment and management of other implanted devices**

- [6th] **Z45.81 Encounter for adjustment or removal of breast implant**
  - Encounter for elective implant exchange (different material) (different size)
  - Encounter removal of tissue expander ▶with or◀ without synchronous insertion of permanent implant
  - EXCLUDES1 *complications of breast implant (T85.4-)*
    - *encounter for initial breast implant insertion for cosmetic breast augmentation (Z41.1)*
    - *encounter for breast reconstruction following mastectomy (Z42.1)*
  - **Z45.811 Encounter for adjustment or removal of right breast implant** [POA]
  - **Z45.812 Encounter for adjustment or removal of left breast implant** [POA]
  - **Z45.819 Encounter for adjustment or removal of unspecified breast implant** [POA]
- **Z45.82 Encounter for adjustment or removal of myringotomy device (stent) (tube)** [POA] [PDx]
- **Z45.89 Encounter for adjustment and management of other implanted devices** [POA] [PDx]

Z45.9 Encounter for adjustment and management of unspecified implanted device [POA] [PDx]

[4th] **Z46 Encounter for fitting and adjustment of other devices**

👁 **See Official Guidelines** "Aftercare" I.C.21.c.7

INCLUDES *removal or replacement of other device*

EXCLUDES1 *malfunction or other complications of device - see Alphabetical Index*

EXCLUDES2 *encounter for fitting and management of implanted devices (Z45.-)*
- *issue of repeat prescription only (Z76.0)*
- *presence of prosthetic and other devices (Z95-Z97)*

Z46.0 Encounter for fitting and adjustment of spectacles and contact lenses [POA] [PDx]

Z46.1 Encounter for fitting and adjustment of hearing aid [POA] [PDx]
- EXCLUDES1 *encounter for adjustment and management of implanted hearing device (Z45.32-)*

Z46.2 Encounter for fitting and adjustment of other devices related to nervous system and special senses [POA]
- EXCLUDES2 *encounter for adjustment and management of implanted nervous system device (Z45.4-)*
  - *encounter for adjustment and management of implanted visual substitution device (Z45.31)*

Z46.3 Encounter for fitting and adjustment of dental prosthetic device [POA]
- Encounter for fitting and adjustment of dentures

Z46.4 Encounter for fitting and adjustment of orthodontic device [POA] [PDx]

[5th] **Z46.5 Encounter for fitting and adjustment of other gastrointestinal appliance and device**

- EXCLUDES1 *encounter for attention to artificial openings of digestive tract (Z43.1-Z43.4)*
- **Z46.51 Encounter for fitting and adjustment of gastric lap band** [POA] [PDx]
- **Z46.59 Encounter for fitting and adjustment of other gastrointestinal appliance and device** [POA] [PDx]

Z46.6 Encounter for fitting and adjustment of urinary device [POA] [PDx]
- EXCLUDES2 *attention to artificial openings of urinary tract (Z43.5, Z43.6)*

[5th] **Z46.8 Encounter for fitting and adjustment of other specified devices**

- **Z46.81 Encounter for fitting and adjustment of insulin pump** [POA] [PDx]
  - Encounter for insulin pump instruction and training
  - Encounter for insulin pump titration
- **Z46.82 Encounter for fitting and adjustment of non-vascular catheter** [POA]
- **Z46.89 Encounter for fitting and adjustment of other specified devices** [POA] [PDx]
  - Encounter for fitting and adjustment of wheelchair

Z46.9 Encounter for fitting and adjustment of unspecified device [POA] [PDx]

[4th] **Z47 Orthopedic aftercare**

👁 **See Official Guidelines** "Aftercare" I.C.21.c.7

EXCLUDES1 *aftercare for healing fracture-code to fracture with 7th character D*

Z47.1 Aftercare following joint replacement surgery [POA]
- 👁 **See Official Guidelines** "Admissions/Encounters for Rehabilitation" II.K
- **AHA:** Q4 2017
- **Use additional** code to identify the joint (Z96.6-)

Z47.2 Encounter for removal of internal fixation device [POA]
- EXCLUDES1 *encounter for adjustment of internal fixation device for fracture treatment- code to fracture with appropriate 7th character*
  - *encounter for removal of external fixation device-code to fracture with 7th character D*
  - *infection or inflammatory reaction to internal fixation device (T84.6-)*
  - *mechanical complication of internal fixation device (T84.1-)*

[5th] **Z47.3 Aftercare following explantation of joint prosthesis**

Aftercare following explantation of joint prosthesis, staged procedure

Encounter for joint prosthesis insertion following prior explantation of joint prosthesis

- **Z47.31 Aftercare following explantation of shoulder joint prosthesis** [POA]
  - EXCLUDES1 *acquired absence of shoulder joint following prior explantation of shoulder joint prosthesis (Z89.23-)*
    - *shoulder joint prosthesis explantation status (Z89.23-)*
- **Z47.32 Aftercare following explantation of hip joint prosthesis** [POA]
  - **AHA:** Q1 2015
  - EXCLUDES1 *acquired absence of hip joint following prior explantation of hip joint prosthesis (Z89.62-)*
    - *hip joint prosthesis explantation status (Z89.62-)*
- **Z47.33 Aftercare following explantation of knee joint prosthesis** [POA]
  - EXCLUDES1 *acquired absence of knee joint following prior explantation of knee prosthesis (Z89.52-*
    - *knee joint prosthesis explantation status (Z89.52-)*

[PDx] Unacceptable principal diagnosis symbol per Medicare code edits [POA] Code exempt from diagnosis present on admission requirement
[?] Questionable admission [CC] Complication or comorbidity [MCC] Major complication or comorbidity [CC/MCC Excl] CC/MCC exclusion
[HCC] HCC diagnosis code [RxHCC] RxHCC diagnosis code MACRA code **DEFINITION** Describes condition/terminology
TIP Coding guidance 👁 Official Guideline Reference [Z1] Z code as first-listed diagnosis

Z47.8 Encounter for other orthopedic aftercare
   Z47.81 Encounter for orthopedic aftercare following surgical amputation
     Use additional code to identify the limb amputated (Z89.-)
   Z47.82 Encounter for orthopedic aftercare following scoliosis surgery
   Z47.89 Encounter for other orthopedic aftercare
     AHA: Q1 2015

Z48 Encounter for other postprocedural aftercare
  See Official Guidelines "Aftercare" I.C.21.c.7
  EXCLUDES1 encounter for follow-up examination after completed treatment (Z08-Z09)
     encounter for aftercare following injury - code to Injury, by site, with appropriate 7th character for subsequent encounter
  EXCLUDES2 encounter for attention to artificial openings (Z43.-)
     encounter for fitting and adjustment of prosthetic and other devices (Z44-Z46)

Z48.0 Encounter for attention to dressings, sutures and drains
  EXCLUDES1 encounter for planned postprocedural wound closure (Z48.1)
   Z48.00 Encounter for change or removal of nonsurgical wound dressing
     Encounter for change or removal of wound dressing NOS
   Z48.01 Encounter for change or removal of surgical wound dressing
     AHA: Q2 2019, Q4 2015
   Z48.02 Encounter for removal of sutures
     AHA: Q1 2015
     Encounter for removal of staples
   Z48.03 Encounter for change or removal of drains
Z48.1 Encounter for planned postprocedural wound closure
  EXCLUDES1 encounter for attention to dressings and sutures (Z48.0-)
Z48.2 Encounter for aftercare following organ transplant
   Z48.21 Encounter for aftercare following heart transplant
   Z48.22 Encounter for aftercare following kidney transplant
   Z48.23 Encounter for aftercare following liver transplant
   Z48.24 Encounter for aftercare following lung transplant
   Z48.28 Encounter for aftercare following multiple organ transplant
     Z48.280 Encounter for aftercare following heart-lung transplant
     Z48.288 Encounter for aftercare following multiple organ transplant
   Z48.29 Encounter for aftercare following other organ transplant
     Z48.290 Encounter for aftercare following bone marrow transplant
     Z48.298 Encounter for aftercare following other organ transplant
Z48.3 Aftercare following surgery for neoplasm
     Use additional code to identify the neoplasm
Z48.8 Encounter for other specified postprocedural aftercare
   Z48.81 Encounter for surgical aftercare following surgery on specified body systems
     These codes identify the body system requiring aftercare. They are for use in conjunction with other aftercare codes to fully explain the aftercare encounter. The condition treated should also be coded if still present.
     EXCLUDES1 aftercare for injury- code the injury with 7th character D
      aftercare following surgery for neoplasm (Z48.3)

EXCLUDES2 aftercare following organ transplant (Z48.2-)
     orthopedic aftercare (Z47.-)
   Z48.810 Encounter for surgical aftercare following surgery on the sense organs
   Z48.811 Encounter for surgical aftercare following surgery on the nervous system
     EXCLUDES2 encounter for surgical aftercare following surgery on the sense organs (Z48.810)
   Z48.812 Encounter for surgical aftercare following surgery on the circulatory system
     AHA: Q4 2012
   Z48.813 Encounter for surgical aftercare following surgery on the respiratory system
     AHA: Q2 2019
   Z48.814 Encounter for surgical aftercare following surgery on the teeth or oral cavity
   Z48.815 Encounter for surgical aftercare following surgery on the digestive system
     AHA: Q4 2015
   Z48.816 Encounter for surgical aftercare following surgery on the genitourinary system
     EXCLUDES1 encounter for aftercare following sterilization reversal (Z31.42)
   Z48.817 Encounter for surgical aftercare following surgery on the skin and subcutaneous tissue
     AHA: Q1 2015
   Z48.89 Encounter for other specified surgical aftercare

Z49 Encounter for care involving renal dialysis
  See Official Guidelines "Aftercare" I.C.21.c.7
  Code also associated end stage renal disease (N18.6)
Z49.0 Preparatory care for renal dialysis
     Encounter for dialysis instruction and training
   Z49.01 Encounter for fitting and adjustment of extracorporeal dialysis catheter
     Removal or replacement of renal dialysis catheter
     Toilet or cleansing of renal dialysis catheter
   Z49.02 Encounter for fitting and adjustment of peritoneal dialysis catheter
Z49.3 Encounter for adequacy testing for dialysis
   Z49.31 Encounter for adequacy testing for hemodialysis
   Z49.32 Encounter for adequacy testing for peritoneal dialysis
     Encounter for peritoneal equilibration test

Z51 Encounter for other aftercare and medical care
  See Official Guidelines "Aftercare" I.C.21.c.7, "Treatment directed at the malignancy" I.C.2. a
  Code also condition requiring care
  EXCLUDES1 follow-up examination after treatment (Z08-Z09)
Z51.0 Encounter for antineoplastic radiation therapy
  See Official Guidelines "Patient admission/encounter solely for administration of chemotherapy, immunotherapy and radiation therapy" I.C.2.e.2, "Patient admitted for radiation therapy, chemotherapy or immunotherapy and develops complications" I.C.2.e.3, "Aftercare" I.C.21.c.7, "Z Codes That May Only be Principal/First-listed Diagnosis" I.C.21.c.16
  AHA: Q4 2017
Z51.1 Encounter for antineoplastic chemotherapy and immunotherapy
  See Official Guidelines "Patient admission/encounter solely for administration of chemotherapy, immunotherapy and radiation therapy" I.C.2.e.2, "Patient admitted for radiation therapy, chemotherapy or immunotherapy and develops complications" I.C.2.e.3, "Aftercare" I.C.21.c.7, "Z Codes That May Only be Principal/First-listed Diagnosis" I.C.21.c.16
  EXCLUDES2 encounter for chemotherapy and immunotherapy for nonneoplastic condition - code to condition

Unspecified Code   Other Specified Code   Manifestation Code   N Newborn   P Pediatric   M Maternity   A Adult   ♂ Male   ♀ Female
● New Code   ▲ Revised Code Title   ▶◀ Revised Text   NOTES   INCLUDES   EXCLUDES1 Not coded here   EXCLUDES2 Not included here
4th character required   5th character required   6th character required   7th character required   Extension 'X' Alert
HAC Hospital-acquired condition (HAC) alert   AHA AHA Coding Clinic©   Code first alert

Z51.11 Encounter for antineoplastic chemotherapy 🔲 Z1
  AHA: Q4 2017, Q3 2015

Z51.12 Encounter for antineoplastic immunotherapy 🔲 Z1
  AHA: Q4 2017

Z51.5 Encounter for palliative care
  AHA: Q1 2017

Z51.6 Encounter for desensitization to allergens 🔲 PDxIn
  AHA: Q4 2016

🔵 **Z51.8** Encounter for other specified aftercare
  EXCLUDES1 holiday relief care (Z75.5)

  Z51.81 Encounter for therapeutic drug level monitoring 🔲
    Code also any long-term (current) drug therapy (Z79.-)
    EXCLUDES1 encounter for blood-drug test for administrative or medicolegal reasons (Z02.83)

  Z51.89 Encounter for other specified aftercare 🔲 PDxIn
    AHA: Q4 2012

🔵 **Z52** Donors of organs and tissues
  👁 See Official Guidelines "Donor" I.C.21.c.9, "Z Codes That May Only be Principal/First-listed Diagnosis" I.C.21.c.16
  INCLUDES autologous and other living donors
  EXCLUDES1 cadaveric donor - omit code
    examination of potential donor (Z00.5)

🔵 **Z52.0** Blood donor
  🔵 **Z52.00** Unspecified blood donor
    Z52.000 Unspecified donor, whole blood 🔲 PDxIn Z1
    Z52.001 Unspecified donor, stem cells 🔲 PDxIn Z1
    Z52.008 Unspecified donor, other blood 🔲 PDxIn Z1

  🔵 **Z52.01** Autologous blood donor
    Z52.010 Autologous donor, whole blood 🔲 PDxIn Z1
    Z52.011 Autologous donor, stem cells 🔲 PDxIn Z1
    Z52.018 Autologous donor, other blood 🔲 PDxIn Z1

  🔵 **Z52.09** Other blood donor
    Volunteer donor
    Z52.090 Other blood donor, whole blood 🔲 PDxIn Z1
    Z52.091 Other blood donor, stem cells 🔲 PDxIn Z1
    Z52.098 Other blood donor, other blood 🔲 PDxIn Z1

🔵 **Z52.1** Skin donor
  Z52.10 Skin donor, unspecified 🔲 Z1
  Z52.11 Skin donor, autologous 🔲 Z1
  Z52.19 Skin donor, other 🔲 Z1

🔵 **Z52.2** Bone donor
  Z52.20 Bone donor, unspecified 🔲 Z1
  Z52.21 Bone donor, autologous 🔲 Z1
  Z52.29 Bone donor, other 🔲 Z1

Z52.3 Bone marrow donor 🔲 Z1
Z52.4 Kidney donor 🔲 Z1
Z52.5 Cornea donor 🔲 Z1
Z52.6 Liver donor 🔲 Z1

🔵 **Z52.8** Donor of other specified organs or tissues
  🔵 **Z52.81** Egg (Oocyte) donor
    Z52.810 Egg (Oocyte) donor under age 35, anonymous recipient 🔲 ♀ PDxIn Z1
      Egg donor under age 35 NOS
    Z52.811 Egg (Oocyte) donor under age 35, designated recipient 🔲 ♀ PDxIn Z1
    Z52.812 Egg (Oocyte) donor age 35 and over, anonymous recipient 🔲 ♀ PDxIn Z1
      Egg donor age 35 and over NOS
    Z52.813 Egg (Oocyte) donor age 35 and over, designated recipient 🔲 ♀ PDxIn Z1
    Z52.819 Egg (Oocyte) donor, unspecified 🔲 ♀ PDxIn Z1

  Z52.89 Donor of other specified organs or tissues 🔲 Z1

Z52.9 Donor of unspecified organ or tissue 🔲
  👁 See Official Guidelines "Nonspecific Z codes" I.C.21.c.15
  Donor NOS

🔵 **Z53** Persons encountering health services for specific procedures and treatment, not carried out
  👁 See Official Guidelines "Miscellaneous Z codes" I.C.21.c.14

🔵 **Z53.0** Procedure and treatment not carried out because of contraindication
  Z53.01 Procedure and treatment not carried out due to patient smoking PDxIn
  Z53.09 Procedure and treatment not carried out because of other contraindication PDxIn

Z53.1 Procedure and treatment not carried out because of patient's decision for reasons of belief and group pressure PDxIn

🔵 **Z53.2** Procedure and treatment not carried out because of patient's decision for other and unspecified reasons
  Z53.20 Procedure and treatment not carried out because of patient's decision for unspecified reasons PDxIn
  Z53.21 Procedure and treatment not carried out due to patient leaving prior to being seen by health care provider PDxIn
  Z53.29 Procedure and treatment not carried out because of patient's decision for other reasons PDxIn

🔵 **Z53.3** Procedure converted to open procedure
  Z53.31 Laparoscopic surgical procedure converted to open procedure 🔲 PDxIn
    AHA: Q4 2016
  Z53.32 Thoracoscopic surgical procedure converted to open procedure 🔲 PDxIn
    AHA: Q4 2016
  Z53.33 Arthroscopic surgical procedure converted to open procedure 🔲 PDxIn
    AHA: Q4 2016
  Z53.39 Other specified procedure converted to open procedure 🔲 PDxIn
    AHA: Q4 2016

Z53.8 Procedure and treatment not carried out for other reasons PDxIn

Z53.9 Procedure and treatment not carried out, unspecified reason PDxIn

Persons with potential health hazards related to socioeconomic and psychosocial circumstances (Z55-Z65)

👁 See Official Guidelines "Documentation by Clinicians Other than the Patient's Provider" I.B.14

🔵 **Z55** Problems related to education and literacy
  👁 See Official Guidelines "Miscellaneous Z codes" I.C.21.c.14
  EXCLUDES1 disorders of psychological development (F80-F89)

  Z55.0 Illiteracy and low-level literacy 🔲 PDxIn
    AHA: Q1 2018, Q4 2018
  Z55.1 Schooling unavailable and unattainable 🔲 PDxIn
    AHA: Q1 2018, Q4 2018
  Z55.2 Failed school examinations 🔲 PDxIn
    AHA: Q1 2018, Q4 2018
  Z55.3 Underachievement in school 🔲 PDxIn
    AHA: Q1 2018, Q4 2018
  Z55.4 Educational maladjustment and discord with teachers and classmates 🔲 PDxIn
    AHA: Q1 2018, Q4 2018
  Z55.8 Other problems related to education and literacy 🔲 PDxIn
    AHA: Q1 2018, Q4 2018
    Problems related to inadequate teaching
  Z55.9 Problems related to education and literacy, unspecified 🔲 PDxIn
    AHA: Q1 2018, Q4 2018
    Academic problems NOS

🔵 **Z56** Problems related to employment and unemployment
  👁 See Official Guidelines "Miscellaneous Z codes" I.C.21.c.14
  EXCLUDES2 occupational exposure to risk factors (Z57.-)
    problems related to housing and economic circumstances (Z59.-)

  Z56.0 Unemployment, unspecified 🔲 PDxIn
    AHA: Q1 2018, Q4 2018
  Z56.1 Change of job 🅰 🔲 PDxIn
    AHA: Q1 2018, Q4 2018
  Z56.2 Threat of job loss 🔲 PDxIn
    AHA: Q1 2018, Q4 2018

PDxIn Unacceptable principal diagnosis symbol per Medicare code edits   🔲 Code exempt from diagnosis present on admission requirement
❓ Questionable admission   🆑 Complication or comorbidity   MCC Major complication or comorbidity   cc/mcc excl CC/MCC exclusion
HCC HCC diagnosis code   RHCC RxHCC diagnosis code   MACRA code   **DEFINITION** Describes condition/terminology
TIP Coding guidance   👁 Official Guideline Reference   Z1 Z code as first-listed diagnosis

Z56.3 Stressful **work schedule**
    AHA: Q1 2018, Q4 2018

Z56.4 Discord with boss **and** workmates
    AHA: Q1 2018, Q4 2018

Z56.5 Uncongenial **work environment**
    AHA: Q1 2018, Q4 2018
    Difficult conditions at work

Z56.6 **Other** physical and mental strain **related to work**
    AHA: Q1 2018, Q4 2018

Z56.8 Other **problems related to employment**
    Z56.81 Sexual harassment **on the job**
      AHA: Q1 2018, Q4 2018
    Z56.82 Military deployment **status**
      AHA: Q1 2018, Q4 2018
      Individual (civilian or military) currently deployed in theater or in support of military war, peacekeeping and humanitarian operations
    Z56.89 Other problems related to employment
      AHA: Q1 2018, Q4 2018

Z56.9 Unspecified problems related to employment
    AHA: Q1 2018, Q4 2018
    Occupational problems NOS

Z57 Occupational exposure **to risk factors**
    See Official Guidelines "Miscellaneous Z codes" I.C.21.c.14

Z57.0 **Occupational exposure to** noise
    AHA: Q1 2018, Q4 2018

Z57.1 **Occupational exposure to** radiation
    AHA: Q1 2018, Q4 2018

Z57.2 **Occupational exposure to** dust
    AHA: Q1 2018, Q4 2018

Z57.3 **Occupational exposure to** other air contaminants
    Z57.31 **Occupational exposure to environmental** tobacco smoke
      AHA: Q1 2018, Q4 2018
      EXCLUDES2 exposure to environmental tobacco smoke (Z77.22)
    Z57.39 **Occupational exposure to other** air contaminants
      AHA: Q1 2018, Q4 2018

Z57.4 **Occupational exposure to** toxic agents in agriculture
    AHA: Q1 2018, Q4 2018
    Occupational exposure to solids, liquids, gases or vapors in agriculture

Z57.5 **Occupational exposure to** toxic agents in other industries
    AHA: Q1 2018, Q4 2018
    Occupational exposure to solids, liquids, gases or vapors in other industries

Z57.6 **Occupational exposure to** extreme temperature
    AHA: Q1 2018, Q4 2018

Z57.7 **Occupational exposure to** vibration
    AHA: Q1 2018, Q4 2018

Z57.8 **Occupational exposure to** other risk factors
    AHA: Q1 2018, Q4 2018

Z57.9 **Occupational exposure to unspecified risk factor**
    AHA: Q1 2018, Q4 2018

Z59 Problems related to housing and economic circumstances
    See Official Guidelines "Miscellaneous Z codes" I.C.21.c.14
    EXCLUDES2 problems related to upbringing (Z62.-)

Z59.0 **Homelessness**
    See Official Guidelines "Use of Z codes" I.B.19.d
    AHA: Q1 2018, Q4 2018, Q4 2017

Z59.1 **Inadequate housing**
    See Official Guidelines "Use of Z codes" I.B.19.d
    AHA: Q1 2018, Q4 2018, Q4 2017
    Lack of heating
    Restriction of space
    Technical defects in home preventing adequate care
    Unsatisfactory surroundings
    EXCLUDES1 problems related to the natural and physical environment (Z77.1-)

Z59.2 **Discord with neighbors, lodgers and landlord**
    AHA: Q1 2018, Q4 2018

Z59.3 **Problems related to living in residential institution**
    AHA: Q1 2018, Q4 2018
    Boarding-school resident
    EXCLUDES1 institutional upbringing (Z62.2)

Z59.4 **Lack of adequate food and safe drinking water**
    Inadequate drinking water supply
    EXCLUDES1 effects of hunger (T73.0)
      inappropriate diet or eating habits (Z72.4)
      malnutrition (E40-E46)

Z59.5 **Extreme poverty**
    AHA: Q1 2018, Q4 2018, Q4 2017

Z59.6 **Low income**
    AHA: Q1 2018, Q4 2018

Z59.7 **Insufficient social insurance and welfare support**
    AHA: Q1 2018, Q4 2018

Z59.8 **Other problems related to housing and economic circumstances**
    AHA: Q1 2018, Q4 2018
    Foreclosure on loan
    Isolated dwelling
    Problems with creditors

Z59.9 **Problem related to housing and economic circumstances, unspecified**
    AHA: Q1 2018, Q4 2018

Z60 Problems related to social environment
    See Official Guidelines "Miscellaneous Z codes" I.C.21.c.14

Z60.0 **Problems of adjustment to** life-cycle transitions
    AHA: Q1 2018, Q4 2018
    Empty nest syndrome
    Phase of life problem
    Problem with adjustment to retirement [pension]

Z60.2 **Problems related to** living alone
    AHA: Q1 2018, Q4 2018

Z60.3 Acculturation **difficulty**
    AHA: Q1 2018, Q4 2018
    Problem with migration
    Problem with social transplantation

Z60.4 **Social** exclusion and rejection
    AHA: Q1 2018, Q4 2018
    Exclusion and rejection on the basis of personal characteristics, such as unusual physical appearance, illness or behavior.
    EXCLUDES1 target of adverse discrimination such as for racial or religious reasons (Z60.5)

Z60.5 **Target of (perceived)** adverse discrimination **and** persecution
    AHA: Q1 2018, Q4 2018
    EXCLUDES1 social exclusion and rejection (Z60.4)

Z60.8 Other problems **related to social environment**
    AHA: Q1 2018, Q4 2018

Z60.9 **Problem related to social environment, unspecified**
    AHA: Q1 2018, Q4 2018

Z62 Problems related to upbringing
    See Official Guidelines "Miscellaneous Z codes" I.C.21.c.14
    INCLUDES current and past negative life events in childhood
      current and past problems of a child related to upbringing
    EXCLUDES2 maltreatment syndrome (T74.-)
      problems related to housing and economic circumstances (Z59.-)

Z62.0 Inadequate **parental supervision and control**
    AHA: Q1 2018, Q4 2018

Z62.1 **Parental** overprotection
    AHA: Q1 2018, Q4 2018

Z62.2 **Upbringing** away from parents
    EXCLUDES1 problems with boarding school (Z59.3)
    Z62.21 **Child in** welfare custody
      AHA: Q1 2018, Q4 2018
      Child in care of non-parental family member
      Child in foster care
      EXCLUDES2 problem for parent due to child in welfare custody (Z63.5)

Z62.22 Institutional upbringing   PDxIn
    AHA: Q1 2018, Q4 2018
    Child living in orphanage or group home

Z62.29 Other upbringing away from parents   PDxIn
    AHA: Q1 2018, Q4 2018

Z62.3 Hostility towards and scapegoating of child   P PDxIn
    AHA: Q1 2018, Q4 2018

Z62.6 Inappropriate (excessive) parental pressure   PDxIn
    AHA: Q1 2018, Q4 2018

Z62.8 Other specified problems related to upbringing
   Z62.81 Personal history of abuse in childhood
     Z62.810 Personal history of physical and sexual abuse in childhood   PDxIn
      AHA: Q1 2018, Q4 2018
      EXCLUDES1 current child physical abuse (T74.12, T76.12)
         current child sexual abuse (T74.22, T76.22)

     Z62.811 Personal history of psychological abuse in childhood   PDxIn
      AHA: Q1 2018, Q4 2018
      EXCLUDES1 current child psychological abuse (T74.32, T76.32)

     Z62.812 Personal history of neglect in childhood   PDxIn
      AHA: Q1 2018, Q4 2018
      EXCLUDES1 current child neglect (T74.02, T76.02)

     Z62.813 Personal history of forced labor or sexual exploitation in childhood   POA PDxIn
      AHA: Q4 2018

     Z62.819 Personal history of unspecified abuse in childhood   PDxIn
      AHA: Q1 2018, Q4 2018
      EXCLUDES1 current child abuse NOS (T74.92, T76.92)

   Z62.82 Parent-child conflict
     Z62.820 Parent-biological child conflict   PDxIn
      AHA: Q1 2018, Q4 2018
      Parent-child problem NOS
     Z62.821 Parent-adopted child conflict   PDxIn
      AHA: Q1 2018, Q4 2018
     Z62.822 Parent-foster child conflict   PDxIn
      AHA: Q1 2018, Q4 2018

   Z62.89 Other specified problems related to upbringing
     Z62.890 Parent-child estrangement NEC   PDxIn
      AHA: Q1 2018, Q4 2018
     Z62.891 Sibling rivalry   PDxIn
      AHA: Q1 2018, Q4 2018
     Z62.898 Other specified problems related to upbringing   PDxIn
      AHA: Q1 2018, Q4 2018

Z62.9 Problem related to upbringing, unspecified   PDxIn
    AHA: Q1 2018, Q4 2018

Z63 Other problems related to primary support group, including family circumstances
   ◉ See Official Guidelines "Miscellaneous Z codes" I.C.21.c.14
   EXCLUDES2 maltreatment syndrome (T74.-, T76)
     parent-child problems (Z62.-)
     problems related to negative life events in childhood (Z62.-)
     problems related to upbringing (Z62.-)

Z63.0 Problems in relationship with spouse or partner   POA PDxIn
    AHA: Q1 2018, Q4 2018
    Relationship distress with spouse or intimate partner
    EXCLUDES1 counseling for spousal or partner abuse problems (Z69.1)
      counseling related to sexual attitude, behavior, and orientation (Z70.-)

Z63.1 Problems in relationship with in-laws   POA PDxIn
    AHA: Q1 2018, Q4 2018

Z63.3 Absence of family member   5th
    EXCLUDES1 absence of family member due to disappearance and death (Z63.4)
      absence of family member due to separation and divorce (Z63.5)
   Z63.31 Absence of family member due to military deployment   POA PDxIn
     AHA: Q1 2018, Q4 2018
     Individual or family affected by other family member being on military deployment
     EXCLUDES1 family disruption due to return of family member from military deployment (Z63.71)
   Z63.32 Other absence of family member   POA PDxIn
     AHA: Q1 2018, Q4 2018

Z63.4 Disappearance and death of family member   POA PDxIn
    AHA: Q1 2018, Q4 2018
    Assumed death of family member
    Bereavement

Z63.5 Disruption of family by separation and divorce   POA PDxIn
    AHA: Q1 2018, Q4 2018
    Marital estrangement

Z63.6 Dependent relative needing care at home   POA PDxIn
    AHA: Q1 2018, Q4 2018

Z63.7 Other stressful life events affecting family and household   5th
   Z63.71 Stress on family due to return of family member from military deployment   POA PDxIn
     AHA: Q1 2018, Q4 2018
     Individual or family affected by family member having returned from military deployment (current or past conflict)
   Z63.72 Alcoholism and drug addiction in family   POA PDxIn
     AHA: Q1 2018, Q4 2018
   Z63.79 Other stressful life events affecting family and household   POA PDxIn
     AHA: Q1 2018, Q4 2018
     Anxiety (normal) about sick person in family
     Health problems within family
     Ill or disturbed family member
     Isolated family

Z63.8 Other specified problems related to primary support group   POA PDxIn
    AHA: Q1 2018, Q4 2018
    Family discord NOS
    Family estrangement NOS
    High expressed emotional level within family
    Inadequate family support NOS
    Inadequate or distorted communication within family

Z63.9 Problem related to primary support group, unspecified   POA PDxIn
    AHA: Q1 2018, Q4 2018
    Relationship disorder NOS

Z64 Problems related to certain psychosocial circumstances
   ◉ See Official Guidelines "Miscellaneous Z codes" I.C.21.c.14
   Z64.0 Problems related to unwanted pregnancy   POA ♀ PDxIn
     AHA: Q1 2018, Q4 2018
   Z64.1 Problems related to multiparity   POA ♀ PDxIn
     AHA: Q1 2018, Q4 2018
   Z64.4 Discord with counselors   POA PDxIn
     Discord with probation officer
     Discord with social worker

Z65 Problems related to other psychosocial circumstances
   ◉ See Official Guidelines "Miscellaneous Z codes" I.C.21.c.14
   Z65.0 Conviction in civil and criminal proceedings without imprisonment   POA PDxIn
     AHA: Q1 2018, Q4 2018
   Z65.1 Imprisonment and other incarceration   POA PDxIn
     AHA: Q1 2018, Q4 2018
   Z65.2 Problems related to release from prison   POA PDxIn
     AHA: Q1 2018, Q4 2018

PDxIn Unacceptable principal diagnosis symbol per Medicare code edits   POA Code exempt from diagnosis present on admission requirement
❓ Questionable admission   ᴄᴄ Complication or comorbidity   MCC Major complication or comorbidity   cc/mcc exc CC/MCC exclusion
HCC HCC diagnosis code   RxHCC RxHCC diagnosis code   MACRA code   **DEFINITION** Describes condition/terminology
TIP Coding guidance   ◉ Official Guideline Reference   1st Z code as first-listed diagnosis

Z65.3 Problems related to other legal circumstances POA PDxIn
  AHA: Q1 2018, Q4 2018
  Arrest
  Child custody or support proceedings
  Litigation
  Prosecution
Z65.4 Victim of crime and terrorism POA PDxIn
  AHA: Q1 2018, Q4 2018
  Victim of torture
Z65.5 Exposure to disaster, war and other hostilities POA PDxIn
  AHA: Q1 2018, Q4 2018
  EXCLUDES1 target of perceived discrimination or persecution
    (Z60.5)
Z65.8 Other specified problems related to psychosocial
  circumstances POA PDxIn
  AHA: Q1 2018, Q4 2018
  Religious or spiritual problem
Z65.9 Problem related to unspecified psychosocial
  circumstances POA PDxIn
  AHA: Q1 2018, Q4 2018

Do not resuscitate status (Z66)

Z66 Do not resuscitate PDxIn
  👁 See Official Guidelines "Status" I.C.21.c.3
  DNR status

Blood type (Z67)

⁴ᵗʰ **Z67** Blood type
  👁 See Official Guidelines "Status" I.C.21.c.3
  ⁵ᵗʰ **Z67.1** Type A blood
    Z67.10 Type A blood, Rh positive POA PDxIn
    Z67.11 Type A blood, Rh negative POA PDxIn
  ⁵ᵗʰ **Z67.2** Type B blood
    Z67.20 Type B blood, Rh positive POA PDxIn
    Z67.21 Type B blood, Rh negative POA PDxIn
  ⁵ᵗʰ **Z67.3** Type AB blood
    Z67.30 Type AB blood, Rh positive POA PDxIn
    Z67.31 Type AB blood, Rh negative POA PDxIn
  ⁵ᵗʰ **Z67.4** Type O blood
    Z67.40 Type O blood, Rh positive POA PDxIn
    Z67.41 Type O blood, Rh negative POA PDxIn
  ⁵ᵗʰ **Z67.9** Unspecified blood type
    Z67.90 Unspecified blood type, Rh positive POA PDxIn
    Z67.91 Unspecified blood type, Rh negative POA PDxIn
      AHA: Q3 2015

Body mass index [BMI] (Z68)

⁴ᵗʰ **Z68** Body mass index [BMI]
  👁 See Official Guidelines "Status" I.C.21.c.3
  Kilograms per meters squared
  NOTES BMI adult codes are for use for persons ▶20◀ years of age
    or older.
    BMI pediatric codes are for use for persons 2-▶19◀ years
    of age.
    These percentiles are based on the growth charts
    published by the Centers for Disease Control and
    Prevention (CDC).
  Z68.1 Body mass index (BMI) 19.9 or less, adult A POA PDxIn
  ⁵ᵗʰ **Z68.2** Body mass index (BMI) 20-29, adult
    Z68.20 Body mass index (BMI) 20.0-20.9, adult A POA PDxIn
    Z68.21 Body mass index (BMI) 21.0-21.9, adult A POA PDxIn
    Z68.22 Body mass index (BMI) 22.0-22.9, adult A POA PDxIn
    Z68.23 Body mass index (BMI) 23.0-23.9, adult A POA PDxIn
    Z68.24 Body mass index (BMI) 24.0-24.9, adult A POA PDxIn
    Z68.25 Body mass index (BMI) 25.0-25.9, adult A POA PDxIn
    Z68.26 Body mass index (BMI) 26.0-26.9, adult A POA PDxIn
    Z68.27 Body mass index (BMI) 27.0-27.9, adult A POA PDxIn
    Z68.28 Body mass index (BMI) 28.0-28.9, adult A POA PDxIn
    Z68.29 Body mass index (BMI) 29.0-29.9, adult A POA PDxIn

⁵ᵗʰ **Z68.3** Body mass index (BMI) 30-39, adult
  Z68.30 Body mass index (BMI) 30.0-30.9, adult A POA PDxIn
  Z68.31 Body mass index (BMI) 31.0-31.9, adult A POA PDxIn
  Z68.32 Body mass index (BMI) 32.0-32.9, adult A POA PDxIn
  Z68.33 Body mass index (BMI) 33.0-33.9, adult A POA PDxIn
  Z68.34 Body mass index (BMI) 34.0-34.9, adult A POA PDxIn
  Z68.35 Body mass index (BMI) 35.0-35.9, adult A POA PDxIn
  Z68.36 Body mass index (BMI) 36.0-36.9, adult A POA PDxIn
  Z68.37 Body mass index (BMI) 37.0-37.9, adult A POA PDxIn
  Z68.38 Body mass index (BMI) 38.0-38.9, adult A POA PDxIn
  Z68.39 Body mass index (BMI) 39.0-39.9, adult A POA PDxIn
⁵ᵗʰ **Z68.4** Body mass index (BMI) 40 or greater, adult
  Z68.41 Body mass index (BMI) 40.0-44.9,
    adult A POA HCC RxHCC PDxIn
  Z68.42 Body mass index (BMI) 45.0-49.9,
    adult A POA HCC RxHCC PDxIn
▲ **Z68.43** Body mass index (BMI) ▶50.0-59.9,◀
    adult A CC POA HCC RxHCC PDxIn CC/MCC Exc
  Z68.44 Body mass index (BMI) 60.0-69.9,
    adult A CC POA HCC RxHCC PDxIn CC/MCC Exc
  Z68.45 Body mass index (BMI) 70 or greater,
    adult A CC POA HCC RxHCC PDxIn CC/MCC Exc
⁵ᵗʰ **Z68.5** Body mass index (BMI) pediatric
  Z68.51 Body mass index (BMI) pediatric, less than 5th
    percentile for age POA PDxIn
  Z68.52 Body mass index (BMI) pediatric, 5th percentile to
    less than 85th percentile for age POA PDxIn
  Z68.53 Body mass index (BMI) pediatric, 85th percentile to
    less than 95th percentile for age POA PDxIn
  Z68.54 Body mass index (BMI) pediatric, greater than or
    equal to 95th percentile for age POA PDxIn

Persons encountering health services in other circumstances (Z69-Z76)

⁴ᵗʰ **Z69** Encounter for mental health services for victim and perpetrator of
  abuse
  👁 See Official Guidelines "Counseling" I.C.21.c.10
  INCLUDES counseling for victims and perpetrators of abuse
  ⁵ᵗʰ **Z69.0** Encounter for mental health services for child abuse
    problems
    ⁶ᵗʰ **Z69.01** Encounter for mental health services for parental
      child abuse
      Z69.010 Encounter for mental health services for
        victim of parental child abuse P POA
        Encounter for mental health services for
          victim of child abuse by parent
        Encounter for mental health services for
          victim of child neglect by parent
        Encounter for mental health services for
          victim of child psychological abuse by
          parent
        Encounter for mental health services for
          victim of child sexual abuse by parent
      Z69.011 Encounter for mental health services for
        perpetrator of parental child abuse POA PDxIn
        Encounter for mental health services for
          perpetrator of parental child neglect
        Encounter for mental health services
          for perpetrator of parental child
          psychological abuse
        Encounter for mental health services for
          perpetrator of parental child sexual abuse
        EXCLUDES1 encounter for mental health
          services for non-parental child
          abuse (Z69.02-)
    ⁶ᵗʰ **Z69.02** Encounter for mental health services for non-
      parental child abuse
      Z69.020 Encounter for mental health services for
        victim of non-parental child abuse P POA
        Encounter for mental health services for
          victim of non-parental child neglect

Encounter for mental health services for victim of non-parental child psychological abuse

Encounter for mental health services for victim of non-parental child sexual abuse

Z69.021 Encounter for mental health services for perpetrator **of non-parental child abuse** POA PDxIn

Encounter for mental health services for perpetrator of non-parental child neglect

Encounter for mental health services for perpetrator of non-parental child psychological abuse

Encounter for mental health services for perpetrator of non-parental child sexual abuse

Z69.1 Encounter for mental health services for spousal or partner **abuse problems**

Z69.11 Encounter for mental health services for victim of **spousal or partner abuse** POA PDxIn

Encounter for mental health services for victim of spouse or partner neglect

Encounter for mental health services for victim of spouse or partner psychological abuse

Encounter for mental health services for victim of spouse or partner violence, physical

Z69.12 Encounter for mental health services for perpetrator **of spousal or partner abuse** POA PDxIn

Encounter for mental health services for perpetrator of spouse or partner neglect

Encounter for mental health services for perpetrator of spouse or partner psychological abuse

Encounter for mental health services for perpetrator of spouse or partner violence, physical

Encounter for mental health services for perpetrator of spouse or partner violence, sexual

Z69.8 Encounter for mental health services for victim or perpetrator of other **abuse**

Z69.81 Encounter for mental health services for victim of **other abuse** POA PDxIn

Encounter for mental health services for victim of non-spousal adult abuse

Encounter for mental health services for victim of spouse or partner violence, sexual

Encounter for rape victim counseling

Z69.82 Encounter for mental health services for perpetrator **of other abuse** POA PDxIn

Encounter for mental health services for perpetrator of non-spousal adult abuse

Z70 Counseling related to sexual attitude, behavior and orientation

👁 **See Official Guidelines** "Counseling" I.C.21.c.10

INCLUDES encounter for mental health services for sexual attitude, behavior and orientation

EXCLUDES2 contraceptive or procreative counseling (Z30-Z31)

Z70.0 Counseling related to sexual attitude POA PDxIn

Z70.1 Counseling related to patient's sexual behavior and orientation POA PDxIn

Patient concerned regarding impotence

Patient concerned regarding non-responsiveness

Patient concerned regarding promiscuity

Patient concerned regarding sexual orientation

Z70.2 Counseling related to sexual behavior and orientation of third party POA PDxIn

Advice sought regarding sexual behavior and orientation of child

Advice sought regarding sexual behavior and orientation of partner

Advice sought regarding sexual behavior and orientation of spouse

Z70.3 Counseling related to combined concerns **regarding sexual attitude, behavior and orientation** POA PDxIn

Z70.8 Other sex counseling POA PDxIn

Encounter for sex education

Z70.9 Sex counseling, unspecified POA PDxIn

Z71 Persons encountering health services for other counseling and medical advice, not elsewhere classified

👁 **See Official Guidelines** "Counseling" I.C.21.c.10

EXCLUDES2 contraceptive or procreation counseling (Z30-Z31)

sex counseling (Z70.-)

Z71.0 Person encountering health services to consult on behalf of another person POA PDxIn

Person encountering health services to seek advice or treatment for non-attending third party

EXCLUDES2 anxiety (normal) about sick person in family (Z63.7)

expectant (adoptive) parent(s) pre-birth pediatrician visit (Z76.81)

Z71.1 Person with feared health complaint in whom no diagnosis is made POA PDxIn

AHA: Q4 2016

Person encountering health services with feared condition which was not demonstrated

Person encountering health services in which problem was normal state

'Worried well'

EXCLUDES1 medical observation for suspected diseases and conditions proven not to exist (Z03.-)

Z71.2 Person consulting for explanation of examination or test findings POA PDxIn

Z71.3 Dietary counseling and surveillance

Use additional code for any associated underlying medical condition

Use additional code to identify body mass index (BMI), if known (Z68.-)

Z71.4 Alcohol abuse **counseling and surveillance**

Use additional code for alcohol abuse or dependence (F10.-)

Z71.41 Alcohol abuse counseling and surveillance of alcoholic POA PDxIn

Z71.42 Counseling for family member of alcoholic POA PDxIn

Counseling for significant other, partner, or friend of alcoholic

Z71.5 Drug abuse **counseling and surveillance**

Use additional code for drug abuse or dependence (F11-F16, F18-F19)

Z71.51 Drug abuse counseling and surveillance of drug abuser POA PDxIn

Z71.52 Counseling for family member of drug abuser POA PDxIn

Counseling for significant other, partner, or friend of drug abuser

Z71.6 Tobacco **abuse counseling** POA PDxIn

Use additional code for nicotine dependence (F17.-)

Z71.7 Human immunodeficiency virus **[HIV] counseling** POA PDxIn

👁 **See Official Guidelines** "Encounters for testing for HIV" I.C.1.a.2.h

Z71.8 Other specified **counseling**

EXCLUDES2 counseling for contraception (Z30.0-)

Z71.81 Spiritual or religious **counseling** POA PDxIn

Z71.82 Exercise **counseling** POA PDxIn

AHA: Q4 2017

Z71.83 Encounter for nonprocreative genetic **counseling** POA

AHA: Q4 2017

EXCLUDES1 counseling for procreative genetics (Z31.5)

counseling for procreative management (Z31.6)

● **Z71.84 Encounter for health counseling** related to travel POA

Encounter for health risk and safety counseling for (international) travel

Code also, if applicable, encounter for immunization (Z23)

EXCLUDES2 encounter for administrative examination (Z02.-)

encounter for other special examination without complaint, suspected or reported diagnosis (Z01.-)

Z71.89 Other specified counseling POA PDxIn

PDxIn Unacceptable principal diagnosis symbol per Medicare code edits   POA Code exempt from diagnosis present on admission requirement

❓ Questionable admission   cc Complication or comorbidity   MCC Major complication or comorbidity   CC/MCC Exx CC/MCC exclusion

HCC HCC diagnosis code   RxHCC RxHCC diagnosis code   MACRA code   **DEFINITION** Describes condition/terminology

TIP Coding guidance   👁 Official Guideline Reference   Z1 Z code as first-listed diagnosis

Z71.9 Counseling, unspecified POA PDxIn
Encounter for medical advice NOS

4️⃣ **Z72 Problems related to lifestyle**
👁 See Official Guidelines "Miscellaneous Z codes" I.C.21.c.14
EXCLUDES2 problems related to life-management difficulty (Z73.-)
problems related to socioeconomic and psychosocial circumstances (Z55-Z65)

Z72.0 Tobacco use POA PDxIn
Tobacco use NOS
EXCLUDES1 history of tobacco dependence (Z87.891)
nicotine dependence (F17.2-)
tobacco dependence (F17.2-)
tobacco use during pregnancy (O99.33-)

Z72.3 Lack of physical exercise POA PDxIn

Z72.4 Inappropriate diet and eating habits POA PDxIn
EXCLUDES1 behavioral eating disorders of infancy or childhood (F98.2.-F98.3)
eating disorders (F50.-)
lack of adequate food (Z59.4)
malnutrition and other nutritional deficiencies (E40-E64)

5️⃣ **Z72.5 High risk sexual behavior**
Promiscuity
EXCLUDES1 paraphilias (F65)
Z72.51 High risk heterosexual behavior POA PDxIn
Z72.52 High risk homosexual behavior POA PDxIn
Z72.53 High risk bisexual behavior POA PDxIn

Z72.6 Gambling and betting
EXCLUDES1 compulsive or pathological gambling (F63.0)

5️⃣ **Z72.8 Other problems related to lifestyle**
6️⃣ **Z72.81 Antisocial behavior**
EXCLUDES1 conduct disorders (F91.-)
Z72.810 Child and adolescent antisocial behavior P POA
Antisocial behavior (child) (adolescent) without manifest psychiatric disorder
Delinquency NOS
Group delinquency
Offenses in the context of gang membership
Stealing in company with others
Truancy from school
Z72.811 Adult antisocial behavior A POA
Adult antisocial behavior without manifest psychiatric disorder

6️⃣ **Z72.82 Problems related to sleep**
Z72.820 Sleep deprivation POA
Lack of adequate sleep
EXCLUDES1 insomnia (G47.0-)
Z72.821 Inadequate sleep hygiene POA PDxIn
Bad sleep habits
Irregular sleep habits
Unhealthy sleep wake schedule
EXCLUDES1 insomnia (F51.0-, G47.0-)
Z72.89 Other problems related to lifestyle POA PDxIn
Self-damaging behavior

Z72.9 Problem related to lifestyle, unspecified POA PDxIn

4️⃣ **Z73 Problems related to life management difficulty**
👁 See Official Guidelines "Miscellaneous Z codes" I.C.21.c.14
EXCLUDES2 problems related to socioeconomic and psychosocial circumstances (Z55-Z65)

Z73.0 Burn-out POA PDxIn
Z73.1 Type A behavior pattern POA PDxIn
Z73.2 Lack of relaxation and leisure POA PDxIn
Z73.3 Stress, not elsewhere classified POA PDxIn
Physical and mental strain NOS
EXCLUDES1 stress related to employment or unemployment (Z56.-)

Z73.4 Inadequate social skills, not elsewhere classified POA PDxIn
Z73.5 Social role conflict, not elsewhere classified POA PDxIn
Z73.6 Limitation of activities due to disability POA PDxIn
EXCLUDES1 care-provider dependency (Z74.-)

5️⃣ **Z73.8 Other problems related to life management difficulty**
6️⃣ **Z73.81 Behavioral insomnia of childhood**
Z73.810 Behavioral insomnia of childhood, sleep-onset association type P POA PDxIn
Z73.811 Behavioral insomnia of childhood, limit setting type P POA PDxIn
Z73.812 Behavioral insomnia of childhood, combined type P POA PDxIn
Z73.819 Behavioral insomnia of childhood, unspecified type P POA PDxIn
Z73.82 Dual sensory impairment POA PDxIn
Z73.89 Other problems related to life management difficulty POA PDxIn

Z73.9 Problem related to life management difficulty, unspecified POA PDxIn

4️⃣ **Z74 Problems related to care provider dependency**
👁 See Official Guidelines "Miscellaneous Z codes" I.C.21.c.14
EXCLUDES2 dependence on enabling machines or devices NEC (Z99.-)

5️⃣ **Z74.0 Reduced mobility**
Z74.01 Bed confinement status POA PDxIn
👁 See Official Guidelines "Status" I.C.21.c.3
Bedridden
Z74.09 Other reduced mobility PDxIn
Chairridden
Reduced mobility NOS
EXCLUDES2 wheelchair dependence (Z99.3)
Z74.1 Need for assistance with personal care PDxIn
Z74.2 Need for assistance at home and no other household member able to render care PDxIn
Z74.3 Need for continuous supervision PDxIn
Z74.8 Other problems related to care provider dependency PDxIn
Z74.9 Problem related to care provider dependency, unspecified PDxIn

4️⃣ **Z75 Problems related to medical facilities and other health care**
👁 See Official Guidelines "Miscellaneous Z codes" I.C.21.c.14
Z75.0 Medical services not available in home POA PDxIn
EXCLUDES1 no other household member able to render care (Z74.2)
Z75.1 Person awaiting admission to adequate facility elsewhere POA PDxIn
👁 See Official Guidelines "Use of Z codes" I.B.19.d
AHA: Q4 2018, Q4 2017
Z75.2 Other waiting period for investigation and treatment POA PDxIn
Z75.3 Unavailability and inaccessibility of health-care facilities POA PDxIn
👁 See Official Guidelines "Use of Z codes" I.B.19.d
AHA: Q4 2018, Q4 2017
EXCLUDES1 bed unavailable (Z75.1)
Z75.4 Unavailability and inaccessibility of other helping agencies POA PDxIn
👁 See Official Guidelines "Use of Z codes" I.B.19.d
AHA: Q4 2018, Q4 2017
Z75.5 Holiday relief care POA PDxIn
Z75.8 Other problems related to medical facilities and other health care POA PDxIn
Z75.9 Unspecified problem related to medical facilities and other health care POA PDxIn

4️⃣ **Z76 Persons encountering health services in other circumstances**
Z76.0 Encounter for issue of repeat prescription POA PDxIn
👁 See Official Guidelines "Miscellaneous Z codes" I.C.21.c.14
Encounter for issue of repeat prescription for appliance
Encounter for issue of repeat prescription for medicaments
Encounter for issue of repeat prescription for spectacles
EXCLUDES2 issue of medical certificate (Z02.7)
repeat prescription for contraceptive (Z30.4-)

Unspecified Code   Other Specified Code   Manifestation Code   N Newborn   P Pediatric   M Maternity   A Adult   ♂ Male   ♀ Female
● New Code   ▲ Revised Code Title   ▶◀ Revised Text   NOTES   *INCLUDES*   *EXCLUDES1* Not coded here   *EXCLUDES2* Not included here
4️⃣ 4th character required   5️⃣ 5th character required   6️⃣ 6th character required   7️⃣ 7th character required   👁 Extension 'X' Alert
HAC Hospital-acquired condition (HAC) alert   AHA AHA Coding Clinic©   📖 Code first alert

Z76.1 Encounter for health supervision and care of foundling ⚕🔲
  👁 **See Official Guidelines** "Newborns and Infants" I.C.21.c.12, "Z Codes That May Only be Principal/First-listed Diagnosis" I.C.21.c.16

Z76.2 Encounter for health supervision and care of other healthy infant and child P ⚕ PDxIn 🔲
  👁 **See Official Guidelines** "Use of Z codes" I.B.19.d, "Z Codes That May Only be Principal/First-listed Diagnosis" I.C.21.c.16
  AHA: Q4 2018, Q4 2017
Encounter for medical or nursing care or supervision of healthy infant under circumstances such as adverse socioeconomic conditions at home
Encounter for medical or nursing care or supervision of healthy infant under circumstances such as awaiting foster or adoptive placement
Encounter for medical or nursing care or supervision of healthy infant under circumstances such as maternal illness
Encounter for medical or nursing care or supervision of healthy infant under circumstances such as number of children at home preventing or interfering with normal care

Z76.3 Healthy person accompanying sick person ⚕
  👁 **See Official Guidelines** "Miscellaneous Z codes" I.C.21.c.14

Z76.4 Other boarder to healthcare facility ⚕
  👁 **See Official Guidelines** "Miscellaneous Z codes" I.C.21.c.14
  EXCLUDES1 homelessness (Z59.0)

Z76.5 Malingerer [conscious simulation] ⚕
  👁 **See Official Guidelines** "Miscellaneous Z codes" I.C.21.c.14
  Person feigning illness (with obvious motivation)
  EXCLUDES1 factitious disorder (F68.1-, F68.A)
    peregrinating patient (F68.1-)

5ᵗʰ Z76.8 Persons encountering health services in other specified circumstances
  Z76.81 Expectant parent(s) prebirth pediatrician visit ⚕ PDx⚕
    👁 **See Official Guidelines** "Counseling" I.C.21.c.10, "Encounters for Obstetrical and Reproductive Services" I.C.21.c.11
    Pre-adoption pediatrician visit for adoptive parent(s)
  Z76.82 Awaiting organ transplant status ⚕ PDxIn
    👁 **See Official Guidelines** "Status" I.C.21.c.3
    Patient waiting for organ availability
  Z76.89 Persons encountering health services in other specified circumstances ⚕ PDxIn
    Persons encountering health services NOS

Persons with potential health hazards related to family and personal history and certain conditions influencing health status (Z77-Z99)

Code also any follow-up examination (Z08-Z09)

4ᵗʰ Z77 Other contact with and (suspected) exposures hazardous to health
  INCLUDES contact with and (suspected) exposures to potential hazards to health
  EXCLUDES2 contact with and (suspected) exposure to communicable diseases (Z20.-)
    exposure to (parental) (environmental) tobacco smoke in the perinatal period (P96.81)
    newborn affected by noxious substances transmitted via placenta or breast milk (P04.-)
    occupational exposure to risk factors (Z57.-)
    retained foreign body (Z18.-)
    retained foreign body fully removed (Z87.821)
    toxic effects of substances chiefly nonmedicinal as to source (T51-T65)

5ᵗʰ Z77.0 Contact with and (suspected) exposure to hazardous, chiefly nonmedicinal, chemicals
  6ᵗʰ Z77.01 Contact with and (suspected) exposure to hazardous metals

Z77.010 Contact with and (suspected) exposure to arsenic PDxIn
Z77.011 Contact with and (suspected) exposure to lead PDxIn
Z77.012 Contact with and (suspected) exposure to uranium PDxIn
  EXCLUDES1 retained depleted uranium fragments (Z18.01)
Z77.018 Contact with and (suspected) exposure to other hazardous metals PDxIn
  Contact with and (suspected) exposure to chromium compounds
  Contact with and (suspected) exposure to nickel dust

6ᵗʰ Z77.02 Contact with and (suspected) exposure to hazardous aromatic compounds
Z77.020 Contact with and (suspected) exposure to aromatic amines PDxIn
Z77.021 Contact with and (suspected) exposure to benzene PDxIn
Z77.028 Contact with and (suspected) exposure to other hazardous aromatic compounds PDxIn
  Aromatic dyes NOS
  Polycyclic aromatic hydrocarbons

6ᵗʰ Z77.09 Contact with and (suspected) exposure to other hazardous, chiefly nonmedicinal, chemicals
Z77.090 Contact with and (suspected) exposure to asbestos PDxIn
Z77.098 Contact with and (suspected) exposure to other hazardous, chiefly nonmedicinal, chemicals PDxIn
  Dyes NOS

5ᵗʰ Z77.1 Contact with and (suspected) exposure to environmental pollution and hazards in the physical environment
6ᵗʰ Z77.11 Contact with and (suspected) exposure to environmental pollution
Z77.110 Contact with and (suspected) exposure to air pollution ⚕ PDxIn
Z77.111 Contact with and (suspected) exposure to water pollution ⚕ PDxIn
Z77.112 Contact with and (suspected) exposure to soil pollution ⚕ PDxIn
Z77.118 Contact with and (suspected) exposure to other environmental pollution ⚕ PDxIn

6ᵗʰ Z77.12 Contact with and (suspected) exposure to hazards in the physical environment
Z77.120 Contact with and (suspected) exposure to mold (toxic) ⚕ PDxIn
Z77.121 Contact with and (suspected) exposure to harmful algae and algae toxins ⚕ PDxIn
  Contact with and (suspected) exposure to (harmful) algae bloom NOS
  Contact with and (suspected) exposure to blue-green algae bloom
  Contact with and (suspected) exposure to brown tide
  Contact with and (suspected) exposure to cyanobacteria bloom
  Contact with and (suspected) exposure to Florida red tide
  Contact with and (suspected) exposure to pfiesteria piscicida
  Contact with and (suspected) exposure to red tide
Z77.122 Contact with and (suspected) exposure to noise ⚕ PDxIn
Z77.123 Contact with and (suspected) exposure to radon and other naturally occurring radiation ⚕ PDxIn
  EXCLUDES2 radiation exposure as the cause of a confirmed condition (W88-W90, X39.0-)
    radiation sickness NOS (T66)

PDx⚕ Unacceptable principal diagnosis symbol per Medicare code edits ⚕ Code exempt from diagnosis present on admission requirement
❓ Questionable admission 🄲 Complication or comorbidity MCC Major complication or comorbidity cc/mcc exc CC/MCC exclusion
HCC HCC diagnosis code RxHCC RxHCC diagnosis code MACRA code **DEFINITION** Describes condition/terminology
TIP Coding guidance 👁 Official Guideline Reference 🔲 Z code as first-listed diagnosis

1272   When symbols appear on a code that requires a 7th character extension, refer to Appendix B to identify applicable 7th character codes.   **2020 ICD-10-CM**

Z77.128 Contact with and (suspected) exposure to other hazards in the physical environment POA PDxIn

[5th] Z77.2 Contact with and (suspected) exposure to other hazardous substances

Z77.21 Contact with and (suspected) exposure to potentially hazardous body fluids PDxIn

Z77.22 Contact with and (suspected) exposure to environmental tobacco smoke (acute) (chronic) PDxIn

Exposure to second hand tobacco smoke (acute) (chronic)

Passive smoking (acute) (chronic)

EXCLUDES1 *nicotine dependence (F17.-)*

tobacco use (Z72.0)

EXCLUDES2 *occupational exposure to environmental tobacco smoke (Z57.31)*

Z77.29 Contact with and (suspected) exposure to other hazardous substances PDxIn

AHA: Q2 2016

Z77.9 Other contact with and (suspected) exposures hazardous to health PDxIn

[4th] Z78 Other specified health status

See Official Guidelines "Status" I.C.21.c.3

EXCLUDES2 *asymptomatic human immunodeficiency virus [HIV] infection status (Z21)*

postprocedural status (Z93-Z99)

sex reassignment status (Z87.890)

Z78.0 Asymptomatic menopausal state [A] POA ♀ PDxIn

Menopausal state NOS

Postmenopausal status NOS

EXCLUDES2 *symptomatic menopausal state (N95.1)*

Z78.1 Physical restraint status POA PDxIn

EXCLUDES1 *physical restraint due to a procedure - omit code*

Z78.9 Other specified health status POA PDxIn

[4th] Z79 Long term (current) drug therapy

See Official Guidelines "Diabetes mellitus and the use of insulin and oral hypoglycemics" I.C.4.a.3, "Secondary diabetes mellitus and the use of insulin or oral hypoglycemic drugs" I.C.4.a.6.a, "Status" I.C.21.c.3

INCLUDES *long term (current) drug use for prophylactic purposes*

Code also any therapeutic drug level monitoring (Z51.81)

EXCLUDES2 *drug abuse and dependence (F11-F19)*

drug use complicating pregnancy, childbirth, and the puerperium (O99.32-)

long term (current) use of oral antidiabetic drugs (Z79.84)

long term (current) use of oral hypoglycemic drugs (Z79.84)

[5th] Z79.0 Long term (current) use of anticoagulants and antithrombotics/antiplatelets

EXCLUDES2 *long term (current) use of aspirin (Z79.82)*

Z79.01 Long term (current) use of anticoagulants POA

Z79.02 Long term (current) use of antithrombotics/antiplatelets POA PDxIn

Z79.1 Long term (current) use of non-steroidal anti-inflammatories (NSAID) POA PDxIn

EXCLUDES2 *long term (current) use of aspirin (Z79.82)*

Z79.2 Long term (current) use of antibiotics POA PDxIn

Z79.3 Long term (current) use of hormonal contraceptives POA

Long term (current) use of birth control pill or patch

Z79.4 Long term (current) use of insulin POA HCC RxHCC

See Official Guidelines "Diabetes mellitus and the use of insulin and oral hypoglycemics" I.C.4.a.3, "Secondary diabetes mellitus and the use of insulin or oral hypoglycemic drugs" I.C.4.a.6.a, "Gestational (pregnancy induced) diabetes" I.C.15.i

AHA: Q4 2017, Q4 2016

[5th] Z79.5 Long term (current) use of steroids

Z79.51 Long term (current) use of inhaled steroids POA PDxIn

Z79.52 Long term (current) use of systemic steroids POA PDxIn

[5th] Z79.8 Other long term (current) drug therapy

[6th] Z79.81 Long term (current) use of agents affecting estrogen receptors and estrogen levels

☛ Code first, if applicable:

malignant neoplasm of breast (C50.-)

malignant neoplasm of prostate (C61)

Use additional code, if applicable, to identify:

estrogen receptor positive status (Z17.0)

family history of breast cancer (Z80.3)

genetic susceptibility to malignant neoplasm (cancer) (Z15.0-)

personal history of breast cancer (Z85.3)

personal history of prostate cancer (Z85.46)

postmenopausal status (Z78.0)

EXCLUDES1 *hormone replacement therapy (Z79.890)*

Z79.810 Long term (current) use of selective estrogen receptor modulators (SERMs) POA PDxIn

Long term (current) use of raloxifene (Evista)

Long term (current) use of tamoxifen (Nolvadex)

Long term (current) use of toremifene (Fareston)

Z79.811 Long term (current) use of aromatase inhibitors POA PDxIn

Long term (current) use of anastrozole (Arimidex)

Long term (current) use of exemestane (Aromasin)

Long term (current) use of letrozole (Femara)

Z79.818 Long term (current) use of other agents affecting estrogen receptors and estrogen levels POA PDxIn

Long term (current) use of estrogen receptor downregulators

Long term (current) use of fulvestrant (Faslodex)

Long term (current) use of gonadotropin-releasing hormone (GnRH) agonist

Long term (current) use of goserelin acetate (Zoladex)

Long term (current) use of leuprolide acetate (leuprorelin) (Lupron)

Long term (current) use of megestrol acetate (Megace)

Z79.82 Long term (current) use of aspirin POA

Z79.83 Long term (current) use of bisphosphonates POA PDxIn

AHA: Q4 2016

Z79.84 Long term (current) use of oral hypoglycemic drugs POA PDxIn

AHA: Q4 2016

Long term (current) use of oral antidiabetic drugs

EXCLUDES2 *long term (current) use of insulin (Z79.4)*

[6th] Z79.89 Other long term (current) drug therapy

Z79.890 Hormone replacement therapy POA PDxIn

Z79.891 Long term (current) use of opiate analgesic POA

Long term (current) use of methadone for pain management

EXCLUDES1 *methodone use NOS (F11.9-)*

use of methodone for treatment of heroin addiction (F11.2-)

Z79.899 Other long term (current) drug therapy POA

AHA: Q3 2015, Q4 2015

[4th] Z80 Family history of primary malignant neoplasm

See Official Guidelines "History (of)" I.C.21.c.4

Z80.0 Family history of malignant neoplasm of digestive organs POA PDxIn

AHA: Q1 2018

Conditions classifiable to C15-C26

Z80.1 Family history of malignant neoplasm of trachea, bronchus and lung POA PDxIn

Conditions classifiable to C33-C34

Z80.2 **Family history of malignant neoplasm of other** respiratory and intrathoracic organs
Conditions classifiable to C30-C32, C37-C39

Z80.3 **Family history of malignant neoplasm of** breast
Conditions classifiable to C50.-

Z80.4 **Family history of malignant neoplasm of** genital organs
Conditions classifiable to C51-C63

  Z80.41 **Family history of malignant neoplasm of** ovary

  Z80.42 **Family history of malignant neoplasm of** prostate

  Z80.43 **Family history of malignant neoplasm of** testis

  Z80.49 **Family history of malignant neoplasm of other** genital organs

Z80.5 **Family history of malignant neoplasm of urinary tract**
Conditions classifiable to C64-C68

  Z80.51 **Family history of malignant neoplasm of** kidney

  Z80.52 **Family history of malignant neoplasm of** bladder

  Z80.59 **Family history of malignant neoplasm of other** urinary tract organ

Z80.6 **Family history of** leukemia
Conditions classifiable to C91-C95

Z80.7 **Family history of other malignant neoplasms of** lymphoid, hematopoietic and related tissues
Conditions classifiable to C81-C90, C96.-

Z80.8 **Family history of malignant neoplasm of other** organs or systems
Conditions classifiable to C00-C14, C40-C49, C69-C79

Z80.9 **Family history of malignant neoplasm, unspecified**
Conditions classifiable to C80.1

Z81 **Family history of mental and behavioral disorders**
  ◉ See Official Guidelines "History (of)" I.C.21.c.4

Z81.0 **Family history of** intellectual disabilities
Conditions classifiable to F70-F79

Z81.1 **Family history of** alcohol abuse and dependence
Conditions classifiable to F10.-

Z81.2 **Family history of** tobacco abuse and dependence
Conditions classifiable to F17.-

Z81.3 **Family history of other** psychoactive substance abuse and dependence
Conditions classifiable to F11-F16, F18-F19

Z81.4 **Family history of other substance abuse and dependence**
Conditions classifiable to F55

Z81.8 **Family history of other** mental and behavioral disorders
Conditions classifiable elsewhere in F01-F99

Z82 **Family history of certain disabilities and chronic diseases (leading to disablement)**
  ◉ See Official Guidelines "History (of)" I.C.21.c.4

Z82.0 **Family history of** epilepsy **and** other **diseases of the nervous system**
Conditions classifiable to G00-G99

Z82.1 **Family history of** blindness and visual loss
Conditions classifiable to H54.-

Z82.2 **Family history of** deafness and hearing loss
Conditions classifiable to H90-H91

Z82.3 **Family history of** stroke
Conditions classifiable to I60-I64

Z82.4 **Family history of ischemic heart disease and other diseases of the circulatory system**
Conditions classifiable to I00-I52, I65-I99

  Z82.41 **Family history of** sudden cardiac death

  Z82.49 **Family history of** ischemic heart disease **and other diseases of the circulatory system**

Z82.5 **Family history of** asthma **and** other **chronic lower respiratory diseases**
Conditions classifiable to J40-J47
EXCLUDES2 family history of other diseases of the respiratory system (Z83.6)

Z82.6 **Family history of arthritis and other diseases of the musculoskeletal system and connective tissue**
Conditions classifiable to M00-M99

  Z82.61 **Family history of** arthritis

  Z82.62 **Family history of** osteoporosis

  Z82.69 **Family history of other diseases of the musculoskeletal system and connective tissue**

Z82.7 **Family history of congenital malformations, deformations and chromosomal abnormalities**
Conditions classifiable to Q00-Q99

  Z82.71 **Family history of** polycystic kidney

  Z82.79 **Family history of other congenital malformations, deformations and chromosomal abnormalities**

Z82.8 **Family history of** other disabilities and chronic diseases leading to disablement, **not elsewhere classified**

Z83 **Family history of other specific disorders**
  ◉ See Official Guidelines "History (of)" I.C.21.c.4
  EXCLUDES2 contact with and (suspected) exposure to communicable disease in the family (Z20.-)

Z83.0 **Family history of** human immunodeficiency virus [HIV] disease
Conditions classifiable to B20

Z83.1 **Family history of other** infectious and parasitic diseases
Conditions classifiable to A00-B19, B25-B94, B99

Z83.2 **Family history of diseases of the** blood and blood-forming organs **and certain disorders involving the immune mechanism**
Conditions classifiable to D50-D89

Z83.3 **Family history of** diabetes mellitus
Conditions classifiable to E08-E13

Z83.4 **Family history of other endocrine, nutritional and metabolic diseases**
Conditions classifiable to E00-E07, E15-E88

  Z83.41 **Family history of** multiple endocrine neoplasia [MEN] syndrome

  Z83.42 **Family history of** familial hypercholesterolemia
  AHA: Q4 2016

  Z83.43 **Family history of other disorder of** lipoprotein metabolism **and other lipidemias**

    Z83.430 **Family history of elevated** lipoprotein(a)
    AHA: Q4 2018
    Family history of elevated Lp(a)

    Z83.438 **Family history of** other **disorder of lipoprotein metabolism and** other **lipidemia**
    AHA: Q4 2018
    Family history of familial combined hyperlipidemia

  Z83.49 **Family history of other endocrine, nutritional and metabolic diseases**

Z83.5 **Family history of eye and ear disorders**

  Z83.51 **Family history of** eye disorders
  Conditions classifiable to H00-H53, H55-H59
  EXCLUDES2 family history of blindness and visual loss (Z82.1)

    Z83.511 **Family history of** glaucoma

    Z83.518 **Family history of other specified eye disorder**

  Z83.52 **Family history of** ear disorders
  Conditions classifiable to H60-H83, H92-H95
  EXCLUDES2 family history of deafness and hearing loss (Z82.2)

Z83.6 **Family history of other diseases of the respiratory system**
Conditions classifiable to J00-J39, J60-J99
EXCLUDES2 family history of asthma and other chronic lower respiratory diseases (Z82.5)

Z83.7 **Family history of diseases of the** digestive system
Conditions classifiable to K00-K93

Z83.71 Family history of colonic polyps POA PDxIn
    EXCLUDES2 family history of malignant neoplasm of digestive organs (Z80.0)
Z83.79 Family history of other diseases of the digestive system POA PDxIn

Z84 Family history of other conditions
  See Official Guidelines "History (of)" I.C.21.c.4
Z84.0 Family history of diseases of the skin and subcutaneous tissue POA PDxIn
    Conditions classifiable to L00-L99
Z84.1 Family history of disorders of kidney and ureter POA PDxIn
    Conditions classifiable to N00-N29
Z84.2 Family history of other diseases of the genitourinary system POA PDxIn
    Conditions classifiable to N30-N99
Z84.3 Family history of consanguinity POA PDxIn
Z84.8 Family history of other specified conditions
  Z84.81 Family history of carrier of genetic disease POA PDxIn
  Z84.82 Family history of sudden infant death syndrome POA PDxIn
    AHA: Q4 2016
    Family history of SIDS
  Z84.89 Family history of other specified conditions POA PDxIn

Z85 Personal history of malignant neoplasm
  See Official Guidelines "Primary malignancy previously excised" I.C.2.d, "Current malignancy vs. personal history of malignancy" I.C.2.m "History (of)" I.C.21.c.4
  Code first any follow-up examination after treatment of malignant neoplasm (Z08)
  Use additional code to identify:
    alcohol use and dependence (F10.-)
    exposure to environmental tobacco smoke (Z77.22)
    history of tobacco dependence (Z87.891)
    occupational exposure to environmental tobacco smoke (Z57.31)
    tobacco dependence (F17.-)
    tobacco use (Z72.0)
  EXCLUDES2 personal history of benign neoplasm (Z86.01-)
    personal history of carcinoma-in-situ (Z86.00-)
Z85.0 Personal history of malignant neoplasm of digestive organs
  Z85.00 Personal history of malignant neoplasm of unspecified digestive organ POA PDxIn
    AHA: Q4 2018
  Z85.01 Personal history of malignant neoplasm of esophagus POA PDxIn
    AHA: Q4 2018
    Conditions classifiable to C15
  Z85.02 Personal history of malignant neoplasm of stomach
    Z85.020 Personal history of malignant carcinoid tumor of stomach POA PDxIn
      AHA: Q4 2018
      Conditions classifiable to C7A.092
    Z85.028 Personal history of other malignant neoplasm of stomach POA PDxIn
      AHA: Q4 2018
      Conditions classifiable to C16
  Z85.03 Personal history of malignant neoplasm of large intestine
    Z85.030 Personal history of malignant carcinoid tumor of large intestine POA PDxIn
      AHA: Q4 2018
      Conditions classifiable to C7A.022-C7A.025, C7A.029
    Z85.038 Personal history of other malignant neoplasm of large intestine POA PDxIn
      AHA: Q4 2018
      Conditions classifiable to C18
  Z85.04 Personal history of malignant neoplasm of rectum, rectosigmoid junction, and anus
    Z85.040 Personal history of malignant carcinoid tumor of rectum POA PDxIn
      AHA: Q4 2018
      Conditions classifiable to C7A.026

    Z85.048 Personal history of other malignant neoplasm of rectum, rectosigmoid junction, and anus POA PDxIn
      AHA: Q4 2018
      Conditions classifiable to C19-C21
  Z85.05 Personal history of malignant neoplasm of liver POA PDxIn
    AHA: Q4 2018
    Conditions classifiable to C22
  Z85.06 Personal history of malignant neoplasm of small intestine
    Z85.060 Personal history of malignant carcinoid tumor of small intestine POA PDxIn
      AHA: Q4 2018
      Conditions classifiable to C7A.01-
    Z85.068 Personal history of other malignant neoplasm of small intestine POA PDxIn
      AHA: Q4 2018
      Conditions classifiable to C17
  Z85.07 Personal history of malignant neoplasm of pancreas POA PDxIn
    AHA: Q4 2018
    Conditions classifiable to C25
  Z85.09 Personal history of malignant neoplasm of other digestive organs POA PDxIn
    AHA: Q4 2018
Z85.1 Personal history of malignant neoplasm of trachea, bronchus and lung
  Z85.11 Personal history of malignant neoplasm of bronchus and lung
    Z85.110 Personal history of malignant carcinoid tumor of bronchus and lung POA PDxIn
      AHA: Q4 2018
      Conditions classifiable to C7A.090
    Z85.118 Personal history of other malignant neoplasm of bronchus and lung POA PDxIn
      AHA: Q4 2018
      Conditions classifiable to C34
  Z85.12 Personal history of malignant neoplasm of trachea POA PDxIn
    AHA: Q4 2018
    Conditions classifiable to C33
Z85.2 Personal history of malignant neoplasm of other respiratory and intrathoracic organs
  Z85.20 Personal history of malignant neoplasm of unspecified respiratory organ POA PDxIn
    AHA: Q4 2018
  Z85.21 Personal history of malignant neoplasm of larynx POA PDxIn
    AHA: Q4 2018
    Conditions classifiable to C32
  Z85.22 Personal history of malignant neoplasm of nasal cavities, middle ear, and accessory sinuses POA PDxIn
    AHA: Q4 2018
    Conditions classifiable to C30-C31
  Z85.23 Personal history of malignant neoplasm of thymus
    Z85.230 Personal history of malignant carcinoid tumor of thymus POA PDxIn
      AHA: Q4 2018
      Conditions classifiable to C7A.091
    Z85.238 Personal history of other malignant neoplasm of thymus POA PDxIn
      AHA: Q4 2018
      Conditions classifiable to C37
  Z85.29 Personal history of malignant neoplasm of other respiratory and intrathoracic organs POA PDxIn
    AHA: Q4 2018
Z85.3 Personal history of malignant neoplasm of breast POA PDxIn
  AHA: Q4 2018
  Conditions classifiable to C50.-
Z85.4 Personal history of malignant neoplasm of genital organs
  Conditions classifiable to C51-C63
  Z85.40 Personal history of malignant neoplasm of unspecified female genital organ POA ♀ PDxIn
    AHA: Q4 2018

Z85.41 Personal history of malignant neoplasm of cervix uteri POA ♀ PDxIn
AHA: Q4 2018

Z85.42 Personal history of malignant neoplasm of other parts of uterus POA ♀ PDxIn
AHA: Q4 2018

Z85.43 Personal history of malignant neoplasm of ovary POA ♀ PDxIn
AHA: Q4 2018

Z85.44 Personal history of malignant neoplasm of other female genital organs POA ♀ PDxIn
AHA: Q4 2018

Z85.45 Personal history of malignant neoplasm of unspecified male genital organ POA ♂ PDxIn
AHA: Q4 2018

Z85.46 Personal history of malignant neoplasm of prostate POA ♂ PDxIn
AHA: Q4 2018

Z85.47 Personal history of malignant neoplasm of testis POA ♂ PDxIn
AHA: Q4 2018

Z85.48 Personal history of malignant neoplasm of epididymis POA ♂ PDxIn
AHA: Q4 2018

Z85.49 Personal history of malignant neoplasm of other male genital organs POA ♂ PDxIn
AHA: Q4 2018

5th **Z85.5** Personal history of malignant neoplasm of urinary tract
Conditions classifiable to C64-C68

Z85.50 Personal history of malignant neoplasm of unspecified urinary tract organ POA PDxIn
AHA: Q4 2018

Z85.51 Personal history of malignant neoplasm of bladder POA PDxIn
AHA: Q4 2018

6th **Z85.52** Personal history of malignant neoplasm of kidney
EXCLUDES1 personal history of malignant neoplasm of renal pelvis (Z85.53)

Z85.520 Personal history of malignant carcinoid tumor of kidney POA PDxIn
AHA: Q4 2018
Conditions classifiable to C7A.093

Z85.528 Personal history of other malignant neoplasm of kidney POA PDxIn
AHA: Q4 2018
Conditions classifiable to C64

Z85.53 Personal history of malignant neoplasm of renal pelvis POA PDxIn
AHA: Q4 2018

Z85.54 Personal history of malignant neoplasm of ureter POA PDxIn
AHA: Q4 2018

Z85.59 Personal history of malignant neoplasm of other urinary tract organ POA PDxIn
AHA: Q4 2018

Z85.6 Personal history of leukemia POA PDxIn
AHA: Q4 2018
Conditions classifiable to C91-C95
EXCLUDES1 leukemia in remission C91.0-C95.9 with 5th character 1

5th **Z85.7** Personal history of other malignant neoplasms of lymphoid, hematopoietic and related tissues

Z85.71 Personal history of Hodgkin lymphoma POA PDxIn
AHA: Q4 2018
Conditions classifiable to C81

Z85.72 Personal history of non-Hodgkin lymphomas POA PDxIn
AHA: Q4 2018
Conditions classifiable to C82-C85

Z85.79 Personal history of other malignant neoplasms of lymphoid, hematopoietic and related tissues POA PDxIn
👁 See Official Guidelines "Leukemia, Multiple Myeloma, and Malignant Plasma Cell Neoplasms in remission vs. personal history" I.C.2.n
AHA: Q4 2018
Conditions classifiable to C88-C90, C96

EXCLUDES1 multiple myeloma in remission (C90.01)
plasma cell leukemia in remission (C90.11)
plasmacytoma in remission (C90.21)

5th **Z85.8** Personal history of malignant neoplasms of other organs and systems
Conditions classifiable to C00-C14, C40-C49, C69-C75, C7A.098, C76-C79

6th **Z85.81** Personal history of malignant neoplasm of lip, oral cavity, and pharynx

Z85.810 Personal history of malignant neoplasm of tongue POA PDxIn

Z85.818 Personal history of malignant neoplasm of other sites of lip, oral cavity, and pharynx POA PDxIn

Z85.819 Personal history of malignant neoplasm of unspecified site of lip, oral cavity, and pharynx POA PDxIn

6th **Z85.82** Personal history of malignant neoplasm of skin

Z85.820 Personal history of malignant melanoma of skin POA PDxIn
Conditions classifiable to C43

Z85.821 Personal history of Merkel cell carcinoma POA PDxIn
Conditions classifiable to C4A

Z85.828 Personal history of other malignant neoplasm of skin POA PDxIn
Conditions classifiable to C44

6th **Z85.83** Personal history of malignant neoplasm of bone and soft tissue

Z85.830 Personal history of malignant neoplasm of bone POA PDxIn

Z85.831 Personal history of malignant neoplasm of soft tissue POA PDxIn
EXCLUDES2 personal history of malignant neoplasm of skin (Z85.82-)

6th **Z85.84** Personal history of malignant neoplasm of eye and nervous tissue

Z85.840 Personal history of malignant neoplasm of eye POA PDxIn

Z85.841 Personal history of malignant neoplasm of brain POA PDxIn

Z85.848 Personal history of malignant neoplasm of other parts of nervous tissue POA PDxIn

6th **Z85.85** Personal history of malignant neoplasm of endocrine glands

Z85.850 Personal history of malignant neoplasm of thyroid POA PDxIn

Z85.858 Personal history of malignant neoplasm of other endocrine glands POA PDxIn

Z85.89 Personal history of malignant neoplasm of other organs and systems POA PDxIn

Z85.9 Personal history of malignant neoplasm, unspecified POA PDxIn
Conditions classifiable to C7A.00, C80.1

4th **Z86** Personal history of certain other diseases
👁 See Official Guidelines "History (of)" I.C.21.c.4
☛ Code first any follow-up examination after treatment (Z09)

5th **Z86.0** Personal history of in-situ and benign neoplasms and neoplasms of uncertain behavior
EXCLUDES2 personal history of malignant neoplasms (Z85.-)

6th **Z86.00** Personal history of in-situ neoplasm
Conditions classifiable to D00-D09

Z86.000 Personal history of in-situ neoplasm of breast POA PDxIn
Conditions classifiable to D05

Z86.001 Personal history of in-situ neoplasm of cervix uteri POA ♀ PDxIn
Conditions classifiable to D06
Personal history of cervical intraepithelial neoplasia III [CIN III]

PDxIn Unacceptable principal diagnosis symbol per Medicare code edits   POA Code exempt from diagnosis present on admission requirement
❓ Questionable admission   cc Complication or comorbidity   MCC Major complication or comorbidity   cc/mcc exc CC/MCC exclusion
HCC HCC diagnosis code   RxHCC RxHCC diagnosis code   MACRA code   **DEFINITION** Describes condition/terminology
TIP Coding guidance   👁 Official Guideline Reference   Z1 Z code as first-listed diagnosis

● **Z86.002** **Personal history of in-situ neoplasm of other and unspecified genital organs** POA
  Conditions classifiable to D07
  Personal history of high-grade prostatic intraepithelial neoplasia III [HGPIN III]
  Personal history of vaginal intraepithelial neoplasia III [VAIN III]
  Personal history of vulvar intraepithelial neoplasia III [VIN III]

● **Z86.003** **Personal history of in-situ neoplasm of** oral cavity, esophagus **and** stomach POA
  Conditions classifiable to D00

● **Z86.004** **Personal history of in-situ neoplasm of other and unspecified digestive organs** POA
  Conditions classifiable to D01
  Personal history of anal intraepithelial neoplasia (AIN III)

● **Z86.005** **Personal history of in-situ neoplasm of** middle ear **and** respiratory system POA
  Conditions classifiable to D02

● **Z86.006** **Personal history of** melanoma in-situ POA
  Conditions classifiable to D03
  EXCLUDES2 *sites other than skin - code to personal history of in-situ neoplasm of the site*

● **Z86.007** **Personal history of** in-situ neoplasm of skin POA
  Conditions classifiable to D04
  Personal history of carcinoma in situ of skin

Z86.008 **Personal history of in-situ neoplasm of other site** POA PDxIn
  Conditions classifiable to D09

⑥ **Z86.01** **Personal history of** benign neoplasm

Z86.010 **Personal history of** colonic polyps POA PDxIn
  AHA: Q1 2017

Z86.011 **Personal history of benign neoplasm of the** brain POA PDxIn

Z86.012 **Personal history of benign** carcinoid tumor POA PDxIn

Z86.018 **Personal history of other benign neoplasm** POA PDxIn
  AHA: Q1 2017

Z86.03 **Personal history of** neoplasm of uncertain behavior POA PDxIn

⑤ **Z86.1** **Personal history of** infectious and parasitic diseases
  Conditions classifiable to A00-B89, B99
  EXCLUDES1 *personal history of infectious diseases specific to a body system*
    sequelae of infectious and parasitic diseases (B90-B94)

Z86.11 **Personal history of** tuberculosis POA PDxIn

Z86.12 **Personal history of** poliomyelitis POA PDxIn

Z86.13 **Personal history of** malaria POA PDxIn

Z86.14 **Personal history of** Methicillin resistant Staphylococcus aureus **infection** POA PDxIn
  Personal history of MRSA infection

● **Z86.15** **Personal history of** latent tuberculosis **infection** POA

Z86.19 **Personal history of other infectious and parasitic diseases** POA PDxIn

Z86.2 **Personal history of diseases of the** blood and blood-forming organs **and certain disorders involving the** immune mechanism POA PDxIn
  Conditions classifiable to D50-D89

⑤ **Z86.3** **Personal history of** endocrine, nutritional and metabolic diseases
  Conditions classifiable to E00-E88

Z86.31 **Personal history of** diabetic foot ulcer POA PDxIn
  EXCLUDES2 *current diabetic foot ulcer (E08.621, E09.621, E10.621, E11.621, E13.621)*

Z86.32 **Personal history of** gestational diabetes POA ♀ PDxIn
  Personal history of conditions classifiable to O24.4-

  EXCLUDES1 *gestational diabetes mellitus in current pregnancy (O24.4-)*

Z86.39 **Personal history of other endocrine, nutritional and metabolic disease** POA PDxIn

⑤ **Z86.5** **Personal history of** mental and behavioral **disorders**
  Conditions classifiable to F40-F59

Z86.51 **Personal history of** combat and operational stress reaction A POA PDxIn

Z86.59 **Personal history of other mental and behavioral disorders** POA PDxIn
  ◉ **See Official Guidelines** "Nonspecific Z codes" I.C.21.c.15

⑤ **Z86.6** **Personal history of diseases of the** nervous system and sense organs
  Conditions classifiable to G00-G99, H00-H95

Z86.61 **Personal history of** infections of the central nervous system POA PDxIn
  Personal history of encephalitis
  Personal history of meningitis

Z86.69 **Personal history of other diseases of the nervous system and sense organs** POA PDxIn
  AHA: Q4 2016

⑤ **Z86.7** **Personal history of diseases of the** circulatory system
  Conditions classifiable to I00-I99
  EXCLUDES2 *old myocardial infarction (I25.2)*
    personal history of anaphylactic shock (Z87.892)
    postmyocardial infarction syndrome (I24.1)

⑥ **Z86.71** **Personal history of** venous thrombosis and embolism

Z86.711 **Personal history of** pulmonary embolism POA PDxIn

Z86.718 **Personal history of other venous thrombosis and embolism** POA PDxIn

Z86.72 **Personal history of** thrombophlebitis POA PDxIn

Z86.73 **Personal history of** transient ischemic attack **(TIA), and cerebral infarction without residual deficits** POA PDxIn
  Personal history of prolonged reversible ischemic neurological deficit (PRIND)
  Personal history of stroke NOS without residual deficits
  EXCLUDES1 *personal history of traumatic brain injury (Z87.820)*
    sequelae of cerebrovascular disease (I69.-)

Z86.74 **Personal history of** sudden cardiac arrest POA PDxIn
  Personal history of sudden cardiac death successfully resuscitated

Z86.79 **Personal history of other diseases of the circulatory system** POA PDxIn

④ **Z87** **Personal history of other diseases and conditions**
  ◉ **See Official Guidelines** "History (of)" I.C.21.c.4
  ☞ **Code first** any follow-up examination after treatment (Z09)

⑤ **Z87.0** **Personal history of diseases of the** respiratory system
  Conditions classifiable to J00-J99

Z87.01 **Personal history of** pneumonia **(recurrent)** POA PDxIn

Z87.09 **Personal history of other diseases of the respiratory system** POA PDxIn

⑤ **Z87.1** **Personal history of diseases of the** digestive system
  Conditions classifiable to K00-K93

Z87.11 **Personal history of** peptic ulcer **disease** POA PDxIn

Z87.19 **Personal history of other diseases of the digestive system** POA PDxIn
  AHA: Q1 2017

Z87.2 **Personal history of diseases of the** skin and subcutaneous tissue POA PDxIn
  Conditions classifiable to L00-L99
  EXCLUDES2 *personal history of diabetic foot ulcer (Z86.31)*

⑤ **Z87.3** **Personal history of diseases of the** musculoskeletal system and connective tissue
  Conditions classifiable to M00-M99
  EXCLUDES2 *personal history of (healed) traumatic fracture (Z87.81)*

Unspecified Code   Other Specified Code   Manifestation Code   N Newborn   P Pediatric   M Maternity   A Adult   ♂ Male   ♀ Female
● New Code   ▲ Revised Code Title   ►◄ Revised Text   **NOTES**   *INCLUDES*   *EXCLUDES1* Not coded here   *EXCLUDES2* Not included here
④ 4th character required   ⑤ 5th character required   ⑥ 6th character required   ⑦ 7th character required   ⑦ Extension 'X' Alert
HAC Hospital-acquired condition (HAC) alert   **AHA** AHA Coding Clinic©   ☞ Code first alert

Z87.31 **Personal history of (healed)** nontraumatic fracture

Z87.310 **Personal history of (healed)** osteoporosis fracture POA PDxIn

👁 **See Official Guidelines** "Osteoporosis without pathological fracture" I.C.13.d.1

Personal history of (healed) fragility fracture

Personal history of (healed) collapsed vertebra due to osteoporosis

Z87.311 **Personal history of (healed) other pathological fracture** POA PDxIn

Personal history of (healed) collapsed vertebra NOS

EXCLUDES2 personal history of osteoporosis fracture (Z87.310)

Z87.312 **Personal history of (healed)** stress fracture POA PDxIn

Personal history of (healed) fatigue fracture

Z87.39 **Personal history of other diseases of the musculoskeletal system and connective tissue** POA PDxIn

Z87.4 **Personal history of diseases of** genitourinary system

Conditions classifiable to N00-N99

Z87.41 **Personal history of** dysplasia of the female genital tract

EXCLUDES1 personal history of intraepithelial neoplasia III of female genital tract (Z86.001, Z86.008)

personal history of malignant neoplasm of female genital tract (Z85.40-Z85.44)

Z87.410 **Personal history of** cervical dysplasia POA ♀ PDxIn

Z87.411 **Personal history of** vaginal dysplasia POA ♀ PDxIn

Z87.412 **Personal history of** vulvar dysplasia POA ♀ PDxIn

Z87.42 **Personal history of other diseases of the** female genital tract POA ♀ PDxIn

Z87.43 **Personal history of diseases of** male genital organs

Z87.430 **Personal history of prostatic dysplasia** POA ♂ PDxIn

EXCLUDES1 personal history of malignant neoplasm of prostate (Z85.46)

Z87.438 **Personal history of other diseases of** male genital organs POA ♂ PDxIn

Z87.44 **Personal history of diseases of** urinary system

EXCLUDES1 personal history of malignant neoplasm of cervix uteri (Z85.41)

Z87.440 **Personal history of urinary (tract) infections** POA PDxIn

Z87.441 **Personal history of** nephrotic syndrome POA PDxIn

Z87.442 **Personal history of urinary** calculi POA PDxIn

Personal history of kidney stones

Z87.448 **Personal history of other diseases of urinary system** POA PDxIn

Z87.5 **Personal history of complications of** pregnancy, childbirth and the puerperium

Conditions classifiable to O00-O9A

EXCLUDES2 recurrent pregnancy loss (N96)

Z87.51 **Personal history of** pre-term labor POA ♀ PDxIn

EXCLUDES1 current pregnancy with history of pre-term labor (O09.21-)

Z87.59 **Personal history of other** complications of **pregnancy, childbirth and the puerperium** POA ♀ PDxIn

Personal history of trophoblastic disease

Z87.7 **Personal history of (corrected)** congenital malformations

Conditions classifiable to Q00-Q89 that have been repaired or corrected

EXCLUDES1 congenital malformations that have been partially corrected or repair but which still require medical treatment - code to condition

EXCLUDES2 other postprocedural states (Z98.-)

personal history of medical treatment (Z92.-)

presence of cardiac and vascular implants and grafts (Z95.-)

presence of other devices (Z97.-)

presence of other functional implants (Z96.-)

transplanted organ and tissue status (Z94.-)

Z87.71 **Personal history of (corrected) congenital malformations of** genitourinary system

Z87.710 **Personal history of (corrected)** hypospadias POA ♂ PDxIn

Z87.718 **Personal history of other specified (corrected) congenital malformations of genitourinary system** POA PDxIn

Z87.72 **Personal history of (corrected) congenital malformations of** nervous system and sense organs

Z87.720 **Personal history of (corrected) congenital malformations of** eye POA PDxIn

Z87.721 **Personal history of (corrected) congenital malformations of** ear POA PDxIn

Z87.728 **Personal history of other specified (corrected) congenital malformations of nervous system and sense organs** POA PDxIn

Z87.73 **Personal history of (corrected) congenital malformations of** digestive system

Z87.730 **Personal history of (corrected)** cleft lip and palate POA PDxIn

Z87.738 **Personal history of other specified (corrected) congenital malformations of digestive system** POA PDxIn

Z87.74 **Personal history of (corrected) congenital malformations of** heart and circulatory system POA PDxIn

Z87.75 **Personal history of (corrected) congenital malformations of** respiratory system POA PDxIn

Z87.76 **Personal history of (corrected) congenital malformations of** integument, limbs and musculoskeletal system POA PDxIn

Z87.79 **Personal history of** other (corrected) congenital malformations

Z87.790 **Personal history of (corrected) congenital malformations of** face and neck POA PDxIn

Z87.798 **Personal history of other (corrected) congenital malformations** POA PDxIn

Z87.8 **Personal history of other specified conditions**

EXCLUDES2 personal history of self harm (Z91.5)

Z87.81 **Personal history of (healed)** traumatic fracture POA PDxIn

EXCLUDES2 personal history of (healed) nontraumatic fracture (Z87.31-)

Z87.82 **Personal history of other (healed)** physical injury and trauma

Conditions classifiable to S00-T88, except traumatic fractures

Z87.820 **Personal history of traumatic brain injury** POA PDxIn

EXCLUDES1 personal history of transient ischemic attack (TIA), and cerebral infarction without residual deficits (Z86.73)

Z87.821 **Personal history of** retained foreign body fully removed POA PDxIn

Z87.828 **Personal history of other (healed) physical injury and trauma** POA PDxIn

Z87.89 **Personal history of** other specified **conditions**

Z87.890 **Personal history of sex reassignment** POA

Z87.891 **Personal history of nicotine dependence** POA PDxIn

AHA: Q2 2017

EXCLUDES1 current nicotine dependence (F17.2-)

POA Unacceptable principal diagnosis symbol per Medicare code edits   POA Code exempt from diagnosis present on admission requirement

❓ Questionable admission   cc Complication or comorbidity   mcc Major complication or comorbidity   cc/mcc CC/MCC exclusion

HCC HCC diagnosis code   RxHCC RxHCC diagnosis code   MACRA MACRA code   **DEFINITION** Describes condition/terminology

TIP Coding guidance   👁 Official Guideline Reference   Z1 Z code as first-listed diagnosis

1278

When symbols appear on a code that requires a 7th character extension, refer to Appendix B to identify applicable 7th character codes.

2020 ICD-10-CM

Z87.892 Personal history of anaphylaxis [POA] [PDx]
Code also allergy status such as:
allergy status to drugs, medicaments and biological substances (Z88.-)
allergy status, other than to drugs and biological substances (Z91.0-)

Z87.898 Personal history of other specified conditions [POA] [PDx]
AHA: Q1 2013

[4th] Z88 Allergy status to drugs, medicaments and biological substances
See Official Guidelines "Status" I.C.21.c.3
[EXCLUDES2] *Allergy status, other than to drugs and biological substances (Z91.0-)*

Z88.0 Allergy status to penicillin [POA] [PDx]
Z88.1 Allergy status to other antibiotic agents status [POA] [PDx]
Z88.2 Allergy status to sulfonamides status [POA] [PDx]
AHA: Q3 2015
Z88.3 Allergy status to other anti-infective agents status [POA] [PDx]
Z88.4 Allergy status to anesthetic agent status [POA] [PDx]
Z88.5 Allergy status to narcotic agent status [POA] [PDx]
Z88.6 Allergy status to analgesic agent status [POA] [PDx]
Z88.7 Allergy status to serum and vaccine status [POA] [PDx]
Z88.8 Allergy status to other drugs, medicaments and biological substances status [POA] [PDx]
Z88.9 Allergy status to unspecified drugs, medicaments and biological substances status [POA] [PDx]
See Official Guidelines "Nonspecific Z codes" I.C.21.c.15

[4th] Z89 Acquired absence of limb
See Official Guidelines "Status" I.C.21.c.3
[INCLUDES] *amputation status*
postprocedural loss of limb
post-traumatic loss of limb
[EXCLUDES1] *acquired deformities of limbs (M20-M21)*
congenital absence of limbs (Q71-Q73)

[5th] Z89.0 Acquired absence of thumb and other finger(s)
[6th] Z89.01 Acquired absence of thumb
Z89.011 Acquired absence of right thumb [POA] [PDx]
Z89.012 Acquired absence of left thumb [POA] [PDx]
Z89.019 Acquired absence of unspecified thumb [POA] [PDx]
[6th] Z89.02 Acquired absence of other finger(s)
[EXCLUDES2] *acquired absence of thumb (Z89.01-)*
Z89.021 Acquired absence of right finger(s) [POA] [PDx]
Z89.022 Acquired absence of left finger(s) [POA] [PDx]
Z89.029 Acquired absence of unspecified finger(s) [POA] [PDx]

[5th] Z89.1 Acquired absence of hand and wrist
[6th] Z89.11 Acquired absence of hand
Z89.111 Acquired absence of right hand [POA] [PDx]
Z89.112 Acquired absence of left hand [POA] [PDx]
Z89.119 Acquired absence of unspecified hand [POA] [PDx]
[6th] Z89.12 Acquired absence of wrist
Disarticulation at wrist
Z89.121 Acquired absence of right wrist [POA] [PDx]
Z89.122 Acquired absence of left wrist [POA] [PDx]
Z89.129 Acquired absence of unspecified wrist [POA] [PDx]

[5th] Z89.2 Acquired absence of upper limb above wrist
[6th] Z89.20 Acquired absence of upper limb, unspecified level
Z89.201 Acquired absence of right upper limb, unspecified level [POA] [PDx]
Z89.202 Acquired absence of left upper limb, unspecified level [POA] [PDx]
Z89.209 Acquired absence of unspecified upper limb, unspecified level [POA] [PDx]
Acquired absence of arm NOS
[6th] Z89.21 Acquired absence of upper limb below elbow
Z89.211 Acquired absence of right upper limb below elbow [POA] [PDx]
Z89.212 Acquired absence of left upper limb below elbow [POA] [PDx]
Z89.219 Acquired absence of unspecified upper limb below elbow [POA] [PDx]
[6th] Z89.22 Acquired absence of upper limb above elbow
Disarticulation at elbow
Z89.221 Acquired absence of right upper limb above elbow [POA] [PDx]
Z89.222 Acquired absence of left upper limb above elbow [POA] [PDx]
Z89.229 Acquired absence of unspecified upper limb above elbow [POA] [PDx]
[6th] Z89.23 Acquired absence of shoulder
Acquired absence of shoulder joint following explantation of shoulder joint prosthesis, with or without presence of antibiotic-impregnated cement spacer
Z89.231 Acquired absence of right shoulder [POA] [PDx]
Z89.232 Acquired absence of left shoulder [POA] [PDx]
Z89.239 Acquired absence of unspecified shoulder [POA] [PDx]

[5th] Z89.4 Acquired absence of toe(s), foot, and ankle
[6th] Z89.41 Acquired absence of great toe
Z89.411 Acquired absence of right great toe [POA] [HCC] [PDx]
Z89.412 Acquired absence of left great toe [POA] [HCC] [PDx]
Z89.419 Acquired absence of unspecified great toe [POA] [HCC] [PDx]
[6th] Z89.42 Acquired absence of other toe(s)
[EXCLUDES2] *acquired absence of great toe (Z89.41-)*
Z89.421 Acquired absence of other right toe(s) [POA] [HCC] [PDx]
Z89.422 Acquired absence of other left toe(s) [POA] [HCC] [PDx]
Z89.429 Acquired absence of other toe(s), unspecified side [POA] [HCC] [PDx]
[6th] Z89.43 Acquired absence of foot
Z89.431 Acquired absence of right foot [POA] [HCC] [PDx]
Z89.432 Acquired absence of left foot [POA] [HCC] [PDx]
Z89.439 Acquired absence of unspecified foot [POA] [HCC] [PDx]
[6th] Z89.44 Acquired absence of ankle
Disarticulation of ankle
Z89.441 Acquired absence of right ankle [POA] [HCC] [PDx]
Z89.442 Acquired absence of left ankle [POA] [HCC] [PDx]
Z89.449 Acquired absence of unspecified ankle [POA] [HCC] [PDx]

[5th] Z89.5 Acquired absence of leg below knee
[6th] Z89.51 Acquired absence of leg below knee
Z89.511 Acquired absence of right leg below knee [POA] [HCC] [PDx]
Z89.512 Acquired absence of left leg below knee [POA] [HCC] [PDx]
Z89.519 Acquired absence of unspecified leg below knee [POA] [HCC] [PDx]
[6th] Z89.52 Acquired absence of knee
Acquired absence of knee joint following explantation of knee joint prosthesis, with or without presence of antibiotic-impregnated cement spacer
Z89.521 Acquired absence of right knee [POA] [PDx]
Z89.522 Acquired absence of left knee [POA] [PDx]
Z89.529 Acquired absence of unspecified knee [POA] [PDx]

[5th] Z89.6 Acquired absence of leg above knee
[6th] Z89.61 Acquired absence of leg above knee
Acquired absence of leg NOS
Disarticulation at knee
Z89.611 Acquired absence of right leg above knee [POA] [HCC] [PDx]

Unspecified Code | Other Specified Code | Manifestation Code | [N] Newborn | [P] Pediatric | [M] Maternity | [A] Adult | ♂ Male | ♀ Female
● New Code | ▲ Revised Code Title | ►◄ Revised Text | [NOTES] | [INCLUDES] | [EXCLUDES1] Not coded here | [EXCLUDES2] Not included here
[4th] 4th character required | [5th] 5th character required | [6th] 6th character required | [7th] 7th character required | [X] Extension 'X' Alert
[HAC] Hospital-acquired condition (HAC) alert | AHA AHA Coding Clinic© | Code first alert

Z89.612 Acquired absence of left leg above knee POA HCC PDxIn

Z89.619 Acquired absence of unspecified leg above knee POA HCC PDxIn

6️⃣ Z89.62 Acquired absence of hip

Acquired absence of hip joint following explantation of hip joint prosthesis, with or without presence of antibiotic-impregnated cement spacer

Disarticulation at hip

Z89.621 Acquired absence of right hip joint POA PDxIn

Z89.622 Acquired absence of left hip joint POA PDxIn

Z89.629 Acquired absence of unspecified hip joint POA PDxIn

Z89.9 Acquired absence of limb, unspecified POA PDxIn

4️⃣ Z90 Acquired absence of organs, not elsewhere classified

👁 See Official Guidelines "Status" I.C.21.c.3

INCLUDES postprocedural or post-traumatic loss of body part NEC

EXCLUDES1 congenital absence - see Alphabetical Index

EXCLUDES2 postprocedural absence of endocrine glands (E89.-)

5️⃣ Z90.0 Acquired absence of part of head and neck

Z90.01 Acquired absence of eye POA PDxIn

Z90.02 Acquired absence of larynx POA PDxIn

Z90.09 Acquired absence of other part of head and neck

Acquired absence of nose

EXCLUDES2 teeth (K08.1)

5️⃣ Z90.1 Acquired absence of breast and nipple

Z90.10 Acquired absence of unspecified breast and nipple POA

Z90.11 Acquired absence of right breast and nipple POA

Z90.12 Acquired absence of left breast and nipple POA

Z90.13 Acquired absence of bilateral breasts and nipples POA

Z90.2 Acquired absence of lung [part of] POA PDxIn

Z90.3 Acquired absence of stomach [part of] POA PDxIn

5️⃣ Z90.4 Acquired absence of other specified parts of digestive tract

6️⃣ Z90.41 Acquired absence of pancreas

👁 See Official Guidelines "Assigning and sequencing secondary diabetes codes and its causes" I.C.4.a.6.b.i

Code also exocrine pancreatic insufficiency (K86.81)

Use additional code to identify any associated:
diabetes mellitus, postpancreatectomy (E13.-)
insulin use (Z79.4)

Z90.410 Acquired total absence of pancreas POA PDxIn
Acquired absence of pancreas NOS

Z90.411 Acquired partial absence of pancreas POA PDxIn

Z90.49 Acquired absence of other specified parts of digestive tract POA PDxIn

Z90.5 Acquired absence of kidney POA PDxIn

Z90.6 Acquired absence of other parts of urinary tract POA PDxIn
Acquired absence of bladder

5️⃣ Z90.7 Acquired absence of genital organ(s)

EXCLUDES1 personal history of sex reassignment (Z87.890)

EXCLUDES2 female genital mutilation status (N90.81-)

6️⃣ Z90.71 Acquired absence of cervix and uterus

Z90.710 Acquired absence of both cervix and uterus POA ♀ PDxIn
Acquired absence of uterus NOS
Status post total hysterectomy

Z90.711 Acquired absence of uterus with remaining cervical stump POA ♀ PDxIn
Status post partial hysterectomy with remaining cervical stump

Z90.712 Acquired absence of cervix with remaining uterus POA ♀ PDxIn

6️⃣ Z90.72 Acquired absence of ovaries

Z90.721 Acquired absence of ovaries, unilateral POA ♀ PDxIn

Z90.722 Acquired absence of ovaries, bilateral POA ♀ PDxIn

Z90.79 Acquired absence of other genital organ(s) POA PDxIn

5️⃣ Z90.8 Acquired absence of other organs

Z90.81 Acquired absence of spleen POA PDxIn

Z90.89 Acquired absence of other organs POA PDxIn

4️⃣ Z91 Personal risk factors, not elsewhere classified

EXCLUDES2 contact with and (suspected) exposures hazardous to health (Z77.-)

exposure to pollution and other problems related to physical environment (Z77.1-)

female genital mutilation status (N90.81-)

personal history of physical injury and trauma (Z87.81, Z87.82-)

occupational exposure to risk factors (Z57.-)

5️⃣ Z91.0 Allergy status, other than to drugs and biological substances

👁 See Official Guidelines "Status" I.C.21.c.3

EXCLUDES2 Allergy status to drugs, medicaments, and biological substances (Z88.-)

6️⃣ Z91.01 Food allergy status

EXCLUDES2 food additives allergy status (Z91.02)

Z91.010 Allergy to peanuts POA PDxIn

Z91.011 Allergy to milk products POA PDxIn

EXCLUDES1 lactose intolerance (E73.-)

Z91.012 Allergy to eggs POA PDxIn

Z91.013 Allergy to seafood POA PDxIn
Allergy to shellfish
Allergy to octopus or squid ink

Z91.018 Allergy to other foods POA PDxIn
Allergy to nuts other than peanuts

Z91.02 Food additives allergy status POA PDxIn

6️⃣ Z91.03 Insect allergy status

Z91.030 Bee allergy status POA PDxIn

Z91.038 Other insect allergy status POA PDxIn

6️⃣ Z91.04 Nonmedicinal substance allergy status

Z91.040 Latex allergy status POA PDxIn
Latex sensitivity status

Z91.041 Radiographic dye allergy status POA PDxIn
Allergy status to contrast media used for diagnostic X-ray procedure

Z91.048 Other nonmedicinal substance allergy status POA PDxIn

Z91.09 Other allergy status, other than to drugs and biological substances POA PDxIn

5️⃣ Z91.1 Patient's noncompliance with medical treatment and regimen

👁 See Official Guidelines "Miscellaneous Z codes" I.C.21.c.14

Z91.11 Patient's noncompliance with dietary regimen POA PDxIn

6️⃣ Z91.12 Patient's intentional underdosing of medication regimen

👁 See Official Guidelines "Underdosing" I.C.19.e.5.c

☞ Code first underdosing of medication (T36-T50) with fifth or sixth character 6

EXCLUDES1 adverse effect of prescribed drug taken as directed- code to adverse effect

poisoning (overdose) -code to poisoning

Z91.120 Patient's intentional underdosing of medication regimen due to financial hardship POA PDxIn

Z91.128 Patient's intentional underdosing of medication regimen for other reason POA PDxIn

6️⃣ Z91.13 Patient's unintentional underdosing of medication regimen

👁 See Official Guidelines "Underdosing" I.C.19.e.5.c

☞ Code first underdosing of medication (T36-T50) with fifth or sixth character 6

EXCLUDES1 adverse effect of prescribed drug taken as directed- code to adverse effect

poisoning (overdose) -code to poisoning

Z91.130 Patient's unintentional underdosing of medication regimen due to age-related debility POA PDxIn

PDxIn Unacceptable principal diagnosis symbol per Medicare code edits   POA Code exempt from diagnosis present on admission requirement

❓ Questionable admission   CC Complication or comorbidity   MCC Major complication or comorbidity   CC/MCC EXC CC/MCC exclusion

HCC HCC diagnosis code   RxHCC RxHCC diagnosis code   MACRA MACRA code   DEFINITION Describes condition/terminology

TIP Coding guidance   👁 Official Guideline Reference   Z1 Z code as first-listed diagnosis

1280

When symbols appear on a code that requires a 7th character extension, refer to Appendix B to identify applicable 7th character codes.

2020 ICD-10-CM

Z91.138 **Patient's unintentional underdosing of medication regimen for other reason** POA PDxIn

Z91.14 **Patient's other noncompliance with medication regimen** POA PDxIn

👁 **See Official Guidelines** "Underdosing" I.C.19.e.5.c

AHA: Q4 2018

Patient's underdosing of medication NOS

Z91.15 **Patient's noncompliance with** renal dialysis POA HCC HxHCC PDxIn

Z91.19 **Patient's noncompliance with other medical treatment and regimen** POA PDxIn

Nonadherence to medical treatment

5ᵗʰ Z91.4 **Personal history of psychological trauma, not elsewhere classified**

👁 **See Official Guidelines** "History (of)" I.C.21.c.4

6ᵗʰ Z91.41 **Personal history of** adult abuse

EXCLUDES2 personal history of abuse in childhood (Z62.81-)

Z91.410 **Personal history of adult** physical and sexual **abuse** A POA PDxIn

EXCLUDES1 current adult physical abuse (T74.11, T76.11)

current adult sexual abuse (T74.21, T76.11)

Z91.411 **Personal history of adult** psychological **abuse** A POA PDxIn

Z91.412 **Personal history of** adult neglect A POA PDxIn

EXCLUDES1 current adult neglect (T74.01, T76.01)

Z91.419 **Personal history of unspecified adult abuse** A POA PDxIn

Z91.42 **Personal history of** forced labor **or** sexual **exploitation** POA PDxIn

AHA: Q4 2018

Z91.49 **Other personal history of psychological trauma, not elsewhere classified** POA PDxIn

Z91.5 **Personal history of self-harm** POA PDxIn

👁 **See Official Guidelines** "History (of)" I.C.21.c.4

Personal history of parasuicide

Personal history of self-poisoning

Personal history of suicide attempt

5ᵗʰ Z91.8 **Other specified** personal risk factors, **not elsewhere classified**

Z91.81 **History of** falling POA PDxIn

👁 **See Official Guidelines** "Repeated falls" I.C.18.d, "History (of)" I.C.21.c.4

AHA: Q4 2017

At risk for falling

Z91.82 **Personal history of** military deployment A POA PDxIn

👁 **See Official Guidelines** "History (of)" I.C.21.c.4

AHA: Q4 2017

Individual (civilian or military) with past history of military war, peacekeeping and humanitarian deployment (current or past conflict)

Returned from military deployment

Z91.83 **Wandering in diseases classified elsewhere** POA

👁 **See Official Guidelines** "Miscellaneous Z codes" I.C.21.c.14

📌 **Code first** underlying disorder such as:

Alzheimer's disease (G30.-)

autism or pervasive developmental disorder (F84.-)

intellectual disabilities (F70-F79)

unspecified dementia with behavioral disturbance (F03.9-)

6ᵗʰ Z91.84 Oral health risk factors

👁 **See Official Guidelines** "Miscellaneous Z codes" I.C.21.c.14

Z91.841 **Risk for dental caries,** low POA PDxIn

AHA: Q4 2017

Z91.842 **Risk for dental caries,** moderate POA PDxIn

AHA: Q4 2017

Z91.843 **Risk for dental caries,** high POA PDxIn

AHA: Q4 2017

Z91.849 **Unspecified risk for dental caries** POA PDxIn

AHA: Q4 2017

Z91.89 **Other specified personal risk factors, not elsewhere classified** POA PDxIn

👁 **See Official Guidelines** "Miscellaneous Z codes" I.C.21.c.14

AHA: Q4 2018, Q1 2017

4ᵗʰ Z92 **Personal history of medical treatment**

👁 **See Official Guidelines** "History (of)" I.C.21.c.4

EXCLUDES2 postprocedural states (Z98.-)

Z92.0 **Personal history of** contraception POA PDxIn

EXCLUDES1 counseling or management of current contraceptive practices (Z30.-)

long term (current) use of contraception (Z79.3)

presence of (intrauterine) contraceptive device (Z97.5)

5ᵗʰ Z92.2 **Personal history of** drug therapy

EXCLUDES2 long term (current) drug therapy (Z79.-)

Z92.21 **Personal history of** antineoplastic **chemotherapy** POA PDxIn

Z92.22 **Personal history of** monoclonal drug **therapy** POA PDxIn

Z92.23 **Personal history of** estrogen **therapy** POA PDxIn

6ᵗʰ Z92.24 **Personal history of** steroid **therapy**

Z92.240 **Personal history of** inhaled steroid **therapy** POA PDxIn

Z92.241 **Personal history of** systemic steroid **therapy** POA PDxIn

Personal history of steroid therapy NOS

Z92.25 **Personal history of** immunosupression **therapy** POA PDxIn

EXCLUDES2 personal history of steroid therapy (Z92.24)

Z92.29 **Personal history of other drug therapy** POA PDxIn

Z92.3 **Personal history of** irradiation POA PDxIn

Personal history of exposure to therapeutic radiation

EXCLUDES1 exposure to radiation in the physical environment (Z77.12)

occupational exposure to radiation (Z57.1)

5ᵗʰ Z92.8 **Personal history of other medical treatment**

Z92.81 **Personal history of** extracorporeal membrane oxygenation (ECMO) POA PDxIn

Z92.82 **Status post administration of tPA (rtPA) in a different facility within the last 24 hours prior to admission to current facility** POA PDxIn

👁 **See Official Guidelines** "Status" I.C.21.c.3

AHA: Q4 2013

📌 **Code first** condition requiring tPA administration, such as:

acute cerebral infarction (I63.-)

acute myocardial infarction (I21.-, I22.-)

Z92.83 **Personal history of** failed moderate sedation POA PDxIn

Personal history of failed conscious sedation

EXCLUDES2 failed moderate sedation during procedure (T88.52)

Z92.84 **Personal history of** unintended awareness under general anesthesia POA PDxIn

AHA: Q4 2016

EXCLUDES2 unintended awareness under general anesthesia during procedure (T88.53)

Z92.89 **Personal history of other medical treatment** POA PDxIn

4ᵗʰ Z93 **Artificial opening status**

👁 **See Official Guidelines** "Status" I.C.21.c.3

EXCLUDES1 artificial openings requiring attention or management (Z43.-)

complications of external stoma (J95.0-, K94.-, N99.5-)

Z93.0 Tracheostomy **status** POA HCC PDxIn

👁 **See Official Guidelines** "Aftercare" I.C.21.c.7

AHA: Q4 2013

Unspecified Code • Other Specified Code • Manifestation Code • N Newborn • P Pediatric • M Maternity • A Adult • ♂ Male • ♀ Female
● New Code • ▲ Revised Code Title • ►◄ Revised Text • **NOTES** • *INCLUDES* • *EXCLUDES1* Not coded here • *EXCLUDES2* Not included here
4ᵗʰ 4ᵗʰ character required • 5ᵗʰ 5ᵗʰ character required • 6ᵗʰ 6ᵗʰ character required • 7ᵗʰ 7ᵗʰ character required • Extension 'X' Alert
HAC Hospital-acquired condition (HAC) alert • **AHA** AHA Coding Clinic© • 📌 Code first alert

Z93.1 Gastrostomy **status** [POA] [HCC] [PDx]
Z93.2 Ileostomy **status** [POA] [HCC] [PDx]
Z93.3 Colostomy **status** [POA] [HCC] [PDx]
Z93.4 **Other artificial openings of gastrointestinal tract status** [POA] [HCC] [PDx]
[5th] **Z93.5** Cystostomy **status**
Z93.50 **Unspecified cystostomy status** [POA] [HCC] [PDx]
Z93.51 Cutaneous-vesicostomy **status** [POA] [HCC] [PDx]
Z93.52 Appendico-vesicostomy **status** [POA] [HCC] [PDx]
Z93.59 **Other cystostomy status** [POA] [HCC] [PDx]
Z93.6 **Other artificial openings of** urinary tract **status** [POA] [HCC] [PDx]
Nephrostomy status
Ureterostomy status
Urethrostomy status
Z93.8 **Other artificial opening status** [POA] [HCC] [PDx]
Z93.9 **Artificial opening status, unspecified** [POA] [HCC] [PDx]

[4th] **Z94** **Transplanted organ and tissue status**
👁 **See Official Guidelines** "Status" I.C.21.c.3
[INCLUDES] *organ or tissue replaced by heterogenous or homogenous transplant*
[EXCLUDES1] *complications of transplanted organ or tissue - see Alphabetical Index*
[EXCLUDES2] *presence of vascular grafts (Z95.-)*
Z94.0 Kidney **transplant status** [POA] [RxHCC] [PDx]
👁 **See Official Guidelines** "Chronic kidney disease and kidney transplant status" I.C.14.a.2
Z94.1 Heart **transplant status** [POA] [HCC] [RxHCC] [PDx]
[EXCLUDES1] *artificial heart status (Z95.812)*
heart-valve replacement status (Z95.2-Z95.4)
Z94.2 Lung **transplant status** [POA] [HCC] [RxHCC] [PDx]
Z94.3 Heart and lungs **transplant status** [POA] [HCC] [RxHCC] [PDx]
Z94.4 Liver **transplant status** [POA] [HCC] [RxHCC] [PDx]
Z94.5 Skin **transplant status** [POA] [PDx]
Autogenous skin transplant status
Z94.6 Bone **transplant status** [POA] [PDx]
Z94.7 Corneal **transplant status** [POA] [PDx]
[5th] **Z94.8** **Other transplanted organ and tissue status**
Z94.81 Bone marrow **transplant status** [POA] [HCC] [RxHCC] [PDx]
Z94.82 Intestine **transplant status** [POA] [HCC] [RxHCC] [PDx]
Z94.83 Pancreas **transplant status** [POA] [HCC] [RxHCC] [PDx]
Z94.84 Stem cells **transplant status** [POA] [HCC] [RxHCC] [PDx]
Z94.89 **Other transplanted organ and tissue status** [POA] [PDx]
Z94.9 **Transplanted organ and tissue status, unspecified** [POA] [PDx]

[4th] **Z95** **Presence of cardiac and vascular implants and grafts**
👁 **See Official Guidelines** "Status" I.C.21.c.3
[EXCLUDES2] *complications of cardiac and vascular devices, implants and grafts (T82.-)*
Z95.0 **Presence of** cardiac pacemaker [POA] [PDx]
AHA: Q1 2019
Presence of cardiac resynchronization therapy (CRT-P) pacemaker
[EXCLUDES1] *adjustment or management of cardiac device (Z45.0-)*
adjustment or management of cardiac pacemaker (Z45.0)
presence of automatic (implantable) cardiac defibrillator with synchronous cardiac pacemaker (Z95.810)
Z95.1 **Presence of** aortocoronary bypass graft [POA] [PDx]
👁 **See Official Guidelines** "Aftercare" I.C.21.c.7
Presence of coronary artery bypass graft
Z95.2 **Presence of** prosthetic heart valve [POA] [PDx]
Presence of heart valve NOS
Z95.3 **Presence of** xenogenic heart valve [POA] [PDx]
Z95.4 **Presence of other heart-valve replacement** [POA] [PDx]
Z95.5 **Presence of** coronary angioplasty **implant and graft** [POA] [PDx]
[EXCLUDES1] *coronary angioplasty status without implant and graft (Z98.61)*
[5th] **Z95.8** **Presence of other cardiac and vascular implants and grafts**
[6th] **Z95.81** **Presence of** other **cardiac implants and grafts**
Z95.810 **Presence of** automatic (implantable) cardiac defibrillator [POA] [PDx]
Presence of automatic (implantable) cardiac defibrillator with synchronous cardiac pacemaker
Presence of cardiac resynchronization therapy defibrillator (CRT-D)
Presence of cardioverter-defibrillator (ICD)
Z95.811 **Presence of** heart assist **device** [POA] [HCC] [PDx]
Z95.812 **Presence of** fully implantable artificial heart [POA] [HCC] [PDx]
Z95.818 **Presence of other cardiac implants and grafts** [POA] [PDx]
[6th] **Z95.82** **Presence of other vascular implants and grafts**
Z95.820 **Peripheral** vascular angioplasty status **with implants and grafts** [POA] [PDx]
[EXCLUDES1] *peripheral vascular angioplasty without implant and graft (Z98.62)*
Z95.828 **Presence of other vascular implants and grafts** [POA] [PDx]
Presence of intravascular prosthesis NEC
Z95.9 **Presence of cardiac and vascular implant and graft, unspecified** [POA] [PDx]

[4th] **Z96** **Presence of other functional implants**
👁 **See Official Guidelines** "Status" I.C.21.c.3
[EXCLUDES2] *complications of internal prosthetic devices, implants and grafts (T82-T85)*
fitting and adjustment of prosthetic and other devices (Z44-Z46)
Z96.0 **Presence of** urogenital **implants** [PDx]
Z96.1 **Presence of** intraocular lens [PDx]
Presence of pseudophakia
[5th] **Z96.2** **Presence of** otological and audiological **implants**
Z96.20 **Presence of otological and audiological implant, unspecified** [PDx]
Z96.21 Cochlear implant **status** [PDx]
Z96.22 Myringotomy tube(s) **status** [PDx]
Z96.29 **Presence of other otological and audiological implants** [PDx]
Presence of bone-conduction hearing device
Presence of eustachian tube stent
Stapes replacement
Z96.3 **Presence of** artificial larynx [PDx]
[5th] **Z96.4** **Presence of** endocrine **implants**
Z96.41 **Presence of** insulin pump **(external) (internal)** [PDx]
Z96.49 **Presence of other endocrine implants** [PDx]
Z96.5 **Presence of** tooth-root and mandibular **implants** [PDx]
[5th] **Z96.6** **Presence of** orthopedic joint **implants**
Z96.60 **Presence of unspecified orthopedic joint implant** [PDx]
[6th] **Z96.61** **Presence of** artificial shoulder joint
Z96.611 **Presence of** right **artificial shoulder joint** [PDx]
Z96.612 **Presence of** left **artificial shoulder joint** [PDx]
Z96.619 **Presence of unspecified artificial shoulder joint** [PDx]
[6th] **Z96.62** **Presence of** artificial elbow joint
Z96.621 **Presence of** right **artificial elbow joint** [PDx]
Z96.622 **Presence of** left **artificial elbow joint** [PDx]
Z96.629 **Presence of unspecified artificial elbow joint** [PDx]
[6th] **Z96.63** **Presence of** artificial wrist joint
Z96.631 **Presence of** right **artificial wrist joint** [PDx]
Z96.632 **Presence of** left **artificial wrist joint** [PDx]
Z96.639 **Presence of unspecified artificial wrist joint** [PDx]
[6th] **Z96.64** **Presence of** artificial hip joint
Hip-joint replacement (partial) (total)
Z96.641 **Presence of** right **artificial hip joint** [PDx]
AHA: Q3 2016
Z96.642 **Presence of** left **artificial hip joint** [PDx]
AHA: Q1 2015

[PDx] Unacceptable principal diagnosis symbol per Medicare code edits [POA] Code exempt from diagnosis present on admission requirement
[?] Questionable admission [CC] Complication or comorbidity [MCC] Major complication or comorbidity [CC/MCC Exc] CC/MCC exclusion
[HCC] HCC diagnosis code [RxHCC] RxHCC diagnosis code MACRA code **DEFINITION** Describes condition/terminology
TIP Coding guidance 👁 Official Guideline Reference [Z1] Z code as first-listed diagnosis

	Z96.643	Presence of artificial hip joint, bilateral PDxIn
	Z96.649	Presence of unspecified artificial hip joint PDxIn
6ᵗʰ **Z96.65**		Presence of artificial knee joint
	Z96.651	Presence of right artificial knee joint PDxIn
	Z96.652	Presence of left artificial knee joint PDxIn
	Z96.653	Presence of artificial knee joint, bilateral PDxIn
	Z96.659	Presence of unspecified artificial knee joint PDxIn
6ᵗʰ **Z96.66**		Presence of artificial ankle joint
	Z96.661	Presence of right artificial ankle joint PDxIn
	Z96.662	Presence of left artificial ankle joint PDxIn
	Z96.669	Presence of unspecified artificial ankle joint PDxIn
6ᵗʰ **Z96.69**		Presence of other orthopedic joint implants
	Z96.691	Finger-joint replacement of right hand PDxIn
	Z96.692	Finger-joint replacement of left hand PDxIn
	Z96.693	Finger-joint replacement, bilateral PDxIn
	Z96.698	Presence of other orthopedic joint implants PDxIn

Z96.7 Presence of other bone and tendon implants PDxIn
Presence of skull plate

5ᵗʰ **Z96.8** Presence of other specified functional implants

	Z96.81	Presence of artificial skin PDxIn
●	**Z96.82**	Presence of neurostimulator POA

Presence of brain neurostimulator
Presence of gastric neurostimulator
Presence of peripheral nerve neurostimulator
Presence of sacral nerve neurostimulator
Presence of spinal cord neurostimulator
Presence of vagus nerve neurostimulator

	Z96.89	Presence of other specified functional implants PDxIn

Z96.9 Presence of functional implant, unspecified PDxIn

4ᵗʰ **Z97** Presence of other devices

👁 **See Official Guidelines "Status" I.C.21.c.3**

EXCLUDES1 complications of internal prosthetic devices, implants and grafts (T82-T85)

EXCLUDES2 fitting and adjustment of prosthetic and other devices (Z44-Z46)

presence of cerebrospinal fluid drainage device (Z98.2)

Z97.0 Presence of artificial eye POA PDxIn

5ᵗʰ **Z97.1** Presence of artificial limb (complete) (partial)

	Z97.10	Presence of artificial limb (complete) (partial), unspecified POA PDxIn
	Z97.11	Presence of artificial right arm (complete) (partial) POA PDxIn
	Z97.12	Presence of artificial left arm (complete) (partial) POA PDxIn
	Z97.13	Presence of artificial right leg (complete) (partial) POA PDxIn
	Z97.14	Presence of artificial left leg (complete) (partial) POA PDxIn
	Z97.15	Presence of artificial arms, bilateral (complete) (partial) POA PDxIn
	Z97.16	Presence of artificial legs, bilateral (complete) (partial) POA PDxIn

Z97.2 Presence of dental prosthetic device (complete) (partial) POA PDxIn
Presence of dentures (complete) (partial)

Z97.3 Presence of spectacles and contact lenses POA PDxIn

Z97.4 Presence of external hearing-aid POA PDxIn

Z97.5 Presence of (intrauterine) contraceptive device POA ♀ PDxIn

EXCLUDES1 checking, reinsertion or removal of implantable subdermal contraceptive (Z30.46)

checking, reinsertion or removal of intrauterine contraceptive device (Z30.43-)

Z97.8 Presence of other specified devices POA PDxIn

4ᵗʰ **Z98** Other postprocedural states

👁 **See Official Guidelines "Status" I.C.21.c.3**

EXCLUDES2 aftercare (Z43-Z49, Z51)

follow-up medical care (Z08-Z09)

postprocedural complication - see Alphabetical Index

Z98.0 Intestinal bypass and anastomosis status POA PDxIn

EXCLUDES2 bariatric surgery status (Z98.84)

gastric bypass status (Z98.84)

obesity surgery status (Z98.84)

Z98.1 Arthrodesis status POA PDxIn

Z98.2 Presence of cerebrospinal fluid drainage device POA PDxIn
Presence of CSF shunt

Z98.3 Post therapeutic collapse of lung status POA PDxIn

🖝 **Code first** underlying disease

5ᵗʰ **Z98.4** Cataract extraction status

Use additional code to identify intraocular lens implant status (Z96.1)

EXCLUDES1 aphakia (H27.0)

	Z98.41	Cataract extraction status, right eye POA PDxIn
	Z98.42	Cataract extraction status, left eye POA PDxIn
	Z98.49	Cataract extraction status, unspecified eye POA PDxIn

5ᵗʰ **Z98.5** Sterilization status

EXCLUDES1 female infertility (N97.-)

male infertility (N46.-)

	Z98.51	Tubal ligation status POA ♀ PDxIn
	Z98.52	Vasectomy status A POA ♂ PDxIn

5ᵗʰ **Z98.6** Angioplasty status

	Z98.61	Coronary angioplasty status POA PDxIn

EXCLUDES1 coronary angioplasty status with implant and graft (Z95.5)

	Z98.62	Peripheral vascular angioplasty status POA PDxIn

EXCLUDES1 peripheral vascular angioplasty status with implant and graft (Z95.820)

5ᵗʰ **Z98.8** Other specified postprocedural states

6ᵗʰ **Z98.81** Dental procedure status

	Z98.810	Dental sealant status POA PDxIn
	Z98.811	Dental restoration status POA PDxIn

Dental crown status
Dental fillings status

	Z98.818	Other dental procedure status POA PDxIn

Z98.82 Breast implant status POA PDxIn

EXCLUDES1 breast implant removal status (Z98.86)

Z98.83 Filtering (vitreous) bleb after glaucoma surgery status POA PDxIn

EXCLUDES1 Inflammation (infection) of postprocedural bleb (H59.4-)

Z98.84 Bariatric surgery status POA PDxIn
Gastric banding status
Gastric bypass status for obesity
Obesity surgery status

EXCLUDES1 bariatric surgery status complicating pregnancy, childbirth, or the puerperium (O99.84)

EXCLUDES2 intestinal bypass and anastomosis status (Z98.0)

Z98.85 Transplanted organ removal status POA PDxIn
Transplanted organ previously removed due to complication, failure, rejection or infection

EXCLUDES1 encounter for removal of transplanted organ -code to complication of transplanted organ (T86.-)

Z98.86 Personal history of breast implant removal POA PDxIn

6ᵗʰ **Z98.87** Personal history of in utero procedure

	Z98.870	Personal history of in utero procedure during pregnancy POA ♀ PDxIn

EXCLUDES2 complications from in utero procedure for current pregnancy (O35.7)

supervision of current pregnancy with history of in utero procedure during previous pregnancy (O09.82-)

Unspecified Code	Other Specified Code	Manifestation Code	Ⓝ Newborn	Ⓟ Pediatric	Ⓜ Maternity	Ⓐ Adult	♂ Male	♀ Female
● New Code	▲ Revised Code Title	▶◀ Revised Text	**NOTES**	*INCLUDES*	*EXCLUDES1* Not coded here	*EXCLUDES2* Not included here		

4ᵗʰ 4ᵗʰ character required 5ᵗʰ 5ᵗʰ character required 6ᵗʰ 6ᵗʰ character required 7ᵗʰ 7ᵗʰ character required ⑦ Extension 'X' Alert
HAC Hospital-acquired condition (HAC) alert **AHA** AHA Coding Clinic© 🖝 Code first alert

Z98.871 **Personal history of in utero procedure while a fetus** [POA] [PDx]

[6th] **Z98.89 Other specified postprocedural states**

Z98.890 **Other specified postprocedural states** [POA] [PDx]
AHA: Q4 2016
Personal history of surgery, not elsewhere classified

Z98.891 **History of uterine scar from previous surgery** [POA] ♀ [PDx]
AHA: Q4 2016
EXCLUDES1 *Maternal care due to uterine scar from previous surgery (O34.2-)*

[4th] **Z99 Dependence on enabling machines and devices, not elsewhere classified**
👁 **See Official Guidelines** "Status" I.C.21.c.3
EXCLUDES1 *cardiac pacemaker status (Z95.0)*

Z99.0 **Dependence on aspirator** [POA] [PDx]

[5th] **Z99.1 Dependence on respirator**
Dependence on ventilator

Z99.11 **Dependence on respirator [ventilator] status** [POA] [HCC]
👁 **See Official Guidelines** "Status" I.C.21.c.3
AHA: Q1 2018, Q1 2015

Z99.12 **Encounter for respirator [ventilator] dependence during power failure** [POA] [HCC] [Z-1]
👁 **See Official Guidelines** "Z Codes Than May Only be Principal/First-Listed Diagnosis" I.C.21.c.16, "Use of Z codes" I.B.19.d
AHA: Q4 2018, Q4 2017
EXCLUDES1 *mechanical complication of respirator [ventilator] (J95.850)*

Z99.2 **Dependence on renal dialysis** [POA] [HCC] [RxHCC] [PDx]
AHA: Q1 2016
Hemodialysis status
Peritoneal dialysis status
Presence of arteriovenous shunt for dialysis
Renal dialysis status NOS
EXCLUDES1 *encounter for fitting and adjustment of dialysis catheter (Z49.0-)*
EXCLUDES2 *noncompliance with renal dialysis (Z91.15)*

Z99.3 **Dependence on wheelchair** [POA] [PDx]
Wheelchair confinement status
☛ **Code first** cause of dependence, such as:
muscular dystrophy (G71.0-)
obesity (E66.-)

[5th] **Z99.8 Dependence on other enabling machines and devices**

Z99.81 **Dependence on supplemental oxygen** [POA] [PDx]
AHA: Q4 2013
Dependence on long-term oxygen

Z99.89 **Dependence on other enabling machines and devices** [POA] [PDx]
Dependence on machine or device NOS

[PDx] Unacceptable principal diagnosis symbol per Medicare code edits [POA] Code exempt from diagnosis present on admission requirement
[?] Questionable admission [CC] Complication or comorbidity [MCC] Major complication or comorbidity [CC/MCC Exc] CC/MCC exclusion
[HCC] HCC diagnosis code [RxHCC] RxHCC diagnosis code MACRA code **DEFINITION** Describes condition/terminology
TIP Coding guidance 👁 Official Guideline Reference [Z-1] Z code as first-listed diagnosis

Appendix A: Z Codes for Long-term Use of Drugs

The following Z codes/categories may only be reported as the principal/first-listed diagnosis, except when there are multiple encounters on the same day and the medical records for the encounters are combined. This list is based on 2019 CMS data, which was the most current available at the time of printing. Please visit the CMS website at www.cms.gov for further updates.

Drug Name	Code	Code Descriptor
A-G Profen®	Z79.1	Long term (current) use of non-steroidal anti-inflammatories (NSAID)
Abstral®	Z79.891	Long term (current) use of opiate analgesic
acarbose	Z79.84	Long term (current) use of oral hypoglycemic drugs
acetaminophen	Z79.899	Other long term (current) drug therapy
acetaminophen and hydrocodone	Z79.891	Long term (current) use of opiate analgesic
acetaminophen and oxycodone	Z79.891	Long term (current) use of opiate analgesic
acetaminophen/codine	Z79.891	Long term (current) use of opiate analgesic
acetylsalicylic acid	Z79.82	Long term (current) use of aspirin
Achromycin V®	Z79.2	Long term (current) use of antibiotics
Aclasta®	Z79.83	Long term (current) use of bisphosphonates
Acova®	Z79.02	Long term (current) use of antithrombotics/antiplatelets
Acticlate®	Z79.2	Long term (current) use of antibiotics
Actimmune®	Z79.899	Other long term (current) drug therapy
Actiprofen®	Z79.1	Long term (current) use of non-steroidal anti-inflammatories (NSAID)
Actiq®	Z79.891	Long term (current) use of opiate analgesic
Activella®	Z79.890	Hormone replacement therapy (postmenopausal)
Actonel®	Z79.83	Long term (current) use of bisphosphonates
Actoplus Met®	Z79.84	Long term (current) use of oral hypoglycemic drugs
Actos®	Z79.84	Long term (current) use of oral hypoglycemic drugs
Addaprin®	Z79.1	Long term (current) use of non-steroidal anti-inflammatories (NSAID)
Admelog®	Z79.4	Long term (current) use of insulin
Adoxa®	Z79.2	Long term (current) use of antibiotics
Advair HFA®	Z79.51	Long term (current) use of inhaled steroids
Advil Infants Concentrated Drops®	Z79.1	Long term (current) use of non-steroidal anti-inflammatories (NSAID)
Advil Liqui-Gels®	Z79.1	Long term (current) use of non-steroidal anti-inflammatories (NSAID)
Advil®	Z79.1	Long term (current) use of non-steroidal anti-inflammatories (NSAID)
Aerospan HFA®	Z79.51	Long term (current) use of inhaled steroids
Aflaxen®	Z79.1	Long term (current) use of non-steroidal anti-inflammatories (NSAID)
Afrezza®	Z79.4	Long term (current) use of insulin
Aggrastat®	Z79.02	Long term (current) use of antithrombotics/antiplatelets
Aggrenox®	Z79.02	Long term (current) use of antithrombotics/antiplatelets
Agrylin®	Z79.02	Long term (current) use of antithrombotics/antiplatelets
alendronate	Z79.83	Long term (current) use of bisphosphonates
Aleve®	Z79.1	Long term (current) use of non-steroidal anti-inflammatories (NSAID)
All Day Pain Relief®	Z79.1	Long term (current) use of non-steroidal anti-inflammatories (NSAID)
All Day Relief®	Z79.1	Long term (current) use of non-steroidal anti-inflammatories (NSAID)
Alodox®	Z79.2	Long term (current) use of antibiotics
alogliptin and metformin	Z79.84	Long term (current) use of oral hypoglycemic drugs
alogliptin and pioglitazone	Z79.84	Long term (current) use of oral hypoglycemic drugs
Alora®	Z79.890	Hormone replacement therapy (postmenopausal)
Altabax®	Z79.2	Long term (current) use of antibiotics
Altavera®	Z79.3	Long term (current) use of hormonal contraceptives
Alvesco®	Z79.51	Long term (current) use of inhaled steroids
Alyacen 1/35®	Z79.3	Long term (current) use of hormonal contraceptives
Alyacen 1/35®	Z79.890	Hormone replacement therapy (postmenopausal)
Amaryl®	Z79.84	Long term (current) use of oral hypoglycemic drugs
Amethia Lo®	Z79.3	Long term (current) use of hormonal contraceptives
Amethia®	Z79.3	Long term (current) use of hormonal contraceptives
Amethyst®	Z79.3	Long term (current) use of hormonal contraceptives
amoxicillin	Z79.2	Long term (current) use of antibiotics
amoxicillin and clavulanate potassium	Z79.2	Long term (current) use of antibiotics
Amoxil®	Z79.2	Long term (current) use of antibiotics
ampicillin/sulbactam	Z79.2	Long term (current) use of antibiotics
anagrelide	Z79.02	Long term (current) use of antithrombotics/antiplatelets
Anaprox-DS®	Z79.1	Long term (current) use of non-steroidal anti-inflammatories (NSAID)

Drug Name	Code	Code Descriptor
Anaprox®	Z79.1	Long term (current) use of non-steroidal anti-inflammatories (NSAID)
anastrozole	Z79.811	Long term (current) use of aromatase inhibitors
Ancef®	Z79.2	Long term (current) use of antibiotics
Angeliq®	Z79.890	Hormone replacement therapy (postmenopausal)
Angiomax®	Z79.02	Long term (current) use of antithrombotics/antiplatelets
Ansaid®	Z79.1	Long term (current) use of non-steroidal anti-inflammatories (NSAID)
Antibiotic Plus Pain Relief®	Z79.2	Long term (current) use of antibiotics
antineoplastic/chemotherapy	Z79.899	Other long term (current) drug therapy
Apidra SoloStar®	Z79.4	Long term (current) use of insulin
Apidra®	Z79.4	Long term (current) use of insulin
apixaban	Z79.01	Long term (current) use of anticoagulants
Apri®	Z79.3	Long term (current) use of hormonal contraceptives
Aranelle®	Z79.3	Long term (current) use of hormonal contraceptives
Aranelle®	Z79.890	Hormone replacement therapy (postmenopausal)
Aredia®	Z79.83	Long term (current) use of bisphosphonates
argatroban	Z79.02	Long term (current) use of antithrombotics/antiplatelets
Arimidex®	Z79.811	Long term (current) use of aromatase inhibitors
Aristospan®	Z79.52	Long term (current) use of systemic steroids
Arixtra®	Z79.01	Long term (current) use of anticoagulants
ArmonAir RespiClick®	Z79.51	Long term (current) use of inhaled steroids
Arnuity Ellipta®	Z79.51	Long term (current) use of inhaled steroids
Aromasin®	Z79.811	Long term (current) use of aromatase inhibitors
Arthritis Pain Relief®	Z79.82	Long term (current) use of aspirin
Arthrotec®	Z79.1	Long term (current) use of non-steroidal anti-inflammatories (NSAID)
Ascriptin®	Z79.82	Long term (current) use of aspirin
Ashlyna®	Z79.3	Long term (current) use of hormonal contraceptives
Asmanex HFA®	Z79.51	Long term (current) use of inhaled steroids
Asmanex Twisthaler®	Z79.51	Long term (current) use of inhaled steroids
Aspir 81®	Z79.82	Long term (current) use of aspirin
Aspir-Low®	Z79.82	Long term (current) use of aspirin
aspirin	Z79.82	Long term (current) use of aspirin
aspirin and dipyridamole	Z79.02	Long term (current) use of antithrombotics/antiplatelets
Astagraf XL®	Z79.899	Other long term (current) drug therapy
Astramorph PF®	Z79.891	Long term (current) use of opiate analgesic
Atelvia®	Z79.83	Long term (current) use of bisphosphonates
atovaquone	Z79.2	Long term (current) use of antibiotics
Aubra®	Z79.3	Long term (current) use of hormonal contraceptives
Augmentin®	Z79.2	Long term (current) use of antibiotics
Avandia®	Z79.84	Long term (current) use of oral hypoglycemic drugs
Avar Cleanser®	Z79.2	Long term (current) use of antibiotics
Avar-E Green®	Z79.2	Long term (current) use of antibiotics
Avar-E LS®	Z79.2	Long term (current) use of antibiotics
Avar-E®	Z79.2	Long term (current) use of antibiotics
Avar®	Z79.2	Long term (current) use of antibiotics
Avelox®	Z79.2	Long term (current) use of antibiotics
Aviane®	Z79.3	Long term (current) use of hormonal contraceptives
Avidoxy®	Z79.2	Long term (current) use of antibiotics
Avonex®	Z79.899	Other long term (current) drug therapy
Aygestin®	Z79.3	Long term (current) use of hormonal contraceptives
Azactam®	Z79.2	Long term (current) use of antibiotics
azathioprine	Z79.899	Other long term (current) drug therapy
azithromycin	Z79.2	Long term (current) use of antibiotics
aztreonam	Z79.2	Long term (current) use of antibiotics
Azurette®	Z79.3	Long term (current) use of hormonal contraceptives
BACiiM®	Z79.2	Long term (current) use of antibiotics
bacitracin	Z79.2	Long term (current) use of antibiotics
bacitracin/hydrocortisone/neomycin/polymyxin B	Z79.2	Long term (current) use of antibiotics
bacitracin/polymyxin b	Z79.2	Long term (current) use of antibiotics
Bactrim®	Z79.2	Long term (current) use of antibiotics
Bactroban Nasal®	Z79.2	Long term (current) use of antibiotics

Drug Name	Code	Code Descriptor
Bactroban®	Z79.2	Long term (current) use of antibiotics
Balziva®	Z79.890	Hormone replacement therapy (postmenopausal)
Basaglar®	Z79.4	Long term (current) use of insulin
basiliximab	Z79.899	Other long term (current) drug therapy
Bayer Children's Aspirin®	Z79.82	Long term (current) use of aspirin
Bayer® Aspirin	Z79.82	Long term (current) use of aspirin
bazedoxifene/conjugated estrogens	Z79.890	Hormone replacement therapy (postmenopausal)
beclomethasone	Z79.51	Long term (current) use of inhaled steroids
Bekyree®	Z79.3	Long term (current) use of hormonal contraceptives
betamethasone	Z79.52	Long term (current) use of systemic steroids
Beyaz®	Z79.3	Long term (current) use of hormonal contraceptives
Bicillin L-A®	Z79.2	Long term (current) use of antibiotics
Binosto®	Z79.83	Long term (current) use of bisphosphonates
bivalirudin	Z79.02	Long term (current) use of antithrombotics/antiplatelets
Blisovi 24 Fe®	Z79.3	Long term (current) use of hormonal contraceptives
Boniva®	Z79.83	Long term (current) use of bisphosphonates
BP 10-Wash®	Z79.2	Long term (current) use of antibiotics
Brevicon 28®	Z79.890	Hormone replacement therapy (postmenopausal)
Briellyn®	Z79.3	Long term (current) use of hormonal contraceptives
Briellyn®	Z79.890	Hormone replacement therapy (postmenopausal)
Brilinta®	Z79.02	Long term (current) use of antithrombotics/antiplatelets
budesonide	Z79.52	Long term (current) use of systemic steroids
budesonide and formoterol	Z79.51	Long term (current) use of inhaled steroids
Bufferin Low Dose®	Z79.82	Long term (current) use of aspirin
Bufferin®	Z79.82	Long term (current) use of aspirin
Buprenex®	Z79.891	Long term (current) use of opiate analgesic
buprenorphine	Z79.891	Long term (current) use of opiate analgesic
butorphanol	Z79.891	Long term (current) use of opiate analgesic
Butrans®	Z79.891	Long term (current) use of opiate analgesic
Caldolor®	Z79.1	Long term (current) use of non-steroidal anti-inflammatories (NSAID)
Cambia®	Z79.1	Long term (current) use of non-steroidal anti-inflammatories (NSAID)
Camila®	Z79.3	Long term (current) use of hormonal contraceptives
Camrese®	Z79.3	Long term (current) use of hormonal contraceptives
CamreseLo®	Z79.3	Long term (current) use of hormonal contraceptives
canagliflozin and metformin	Z79.84	Long term (current) use of oral hypoglycemic drugs
Cataflam®	Z79.1	Long term (current) use of non-steroidal anti-inflammatories (NSAID)
Caziant®	Z79.3	Long term (current) use of hormonal contraceptives
cefaclor	Z79.2	Long term (current) use of antibiotics
cefazolin	Z79.2	Long term (current) use of antibiotics
cefdinir	Z79.2	Long term (current) use of antibiotics
cefepime	Z79.2	Long term (current) use of antibiotics
cefixime	Z79.2	Long term (current) use of antibiotics
cefoxitin	Z79.2	Long term (current) use of antibiotics
cefpodoxime	Z79.2	Long term (current) use of antibiotics
ceftaroline	Z79.2	Long term (current) use of antibiotics
ceftazidime	Z79.2	Long term (current) use of antibiotics
Ceftin®	Z79.2	Long term (current) use of antibiotics
ceftolozane/tazobactam	Z79.2	Long term (current) use of antibiotics
ceftriaxone	Z79.2	Long term (current) use of antibiotics
cefuroxime	Z79.2	Long term (current) use of antibiotics
Celebrex®	Z79.1	Long term (current) use of non-steroidal anti-inflammatories (NSAID)
celecoxib	Z79.1	Long term (current) use of non-steroidal anti-inflammatories (NSAID)
Celestone Soluspan®	Z79.52	Long term (current) use of systemic steroids
CellCept®	Z79.899	Other long term (current) drug therapy
Centany AT Kit®	Z79.2	Long term (current) use of antibiotics
Centany®	Z79.2	Long term (current) use of antibiotics
cephalexin	Z79.2	Long term (current) use of antibiotics
Cerisa Wash®	Z79.2	Long term (current) use of antibiotics
Cesia®	Z79.3	Long term (current) use of hormonal contraceptives
Chateal®	Z79.3	Long term (current) use of hormonal contraceptives

Drug Name	Code	Code Descriptor
Children's Advil®	Z79.1	Long term (current) use of non-steroidal anti-inflammatories (NSAID)
Children's Motrin®	Z79.1	Long term (current) use of non-steroidal anti-inflammatories (NSAID)
chlorpropamide	Z79.84	Long term (current) use of oral hypoglycemic drugs
ciclesonide	Z79.51	Long term (current) use of inhaled steroids
Cidomycin®	Z79.2	Long term (current) use of antibiotics
cilostazol	Z79.02	Long term (current) use of antithrombotics/antiplatelets
Cipro®	Z79.2	Long term (current) use of antibiotics
ciprofloxacin	Z79.2	Long term (current) use of antibiotics
Clarifoam EF®	Z79.2	Long term (current) use of antibiotics
clarithromycin	Z79.2	Long term (current) use of antibiotics
Clenia Emollient Cream®	Z79.2	Long term (current) use of antibiotics
Cleocin HCl®	Z79.2	Long term (current) use of antibiotics
Clexane®	Z79.01	Long term (current) use of anticoagulants
Climara Pro®	Z79.890	Hormone replacement therapy (postmenopausal)
Climara®	Z79.890	Hormone replacement therapy (postmenopausal)
Clinacort®	Z79.52	Long term (current) use of systemic steroids
clindamycin	Z79.2	Long term (current) use of antibiotics
Clinoril®	Z79.1	Long term (current) use of non-steroidal anti-inflammatories (NSAID)
clopidogrel bisulfate	Z79.02	Long term (current) use of antithrombotics/antiplatelets
codeine	Z79.891	Long term (current) use of opiate analgesic
Colocort®	Z79.52	Long term (current) use of systemic steroids
CombiPatch®	Z79.890	Hormone replacement therapy (postmenopausal)
conjugated estrogens	Z79.890	Hormone replacement therapy (postmenopausal)
conjugated estrogens/medroxyprogesterone	Z79.890	Hormone replacement therapy (postmenopausal)
ConZip®	Z79.891	Long term (current) use of opiate analgesic
Cortef®	Z79.52	Long term (current) use of systemic steroids
Cortenema®	Z79.52	Long term (current) use of systemic steroids
Cortifoam®	Z79.52	Long term (current) use of systemic steroids
cortisone	Z79.52	Long term (current) use of systemic steroids
cortisone acetate	Z79.52	Long term (current) use of systemic steroids
Cortone Acetate®	Z79.52	Long term (current) use of systemic steroids
Coumadin®	Z79.01	Long term (current) use of anticoagulants
Covaryx HS®	Z79.890	Hormone replacement therapy (postmenopausal)
Covaryx®	Z79.890	Hormone replacement therapy (postmenopausal)
Cryselle 28®	Z79.3	Long term (current) use of hormonal contraceptives
Cyclafem 1/35®	Z79.3	Long term (current) use of hormonal contraceptives
Cyclafem 1/35®	Z79.890	Hormone replacement therapy (postmenopausal)
Cyclafem 7/7/7®	Z79.3	Long term (current) use of hormonal contraceptives
Cyclafem 7/7/7®	Z79.890	Hormone replacement therapy (postmenopausal)
Cyclessa®	Z79.3	Long term (current) use of hormonal contraceptives
cycloserine	Z79.2	Long term (current) use of antibiotics
cyclosporine	Z79.899	Other long term (current) drug therapy
Cyred®	Z79.3	Long term (current) use of hormonal contraceptives
dabigatran	Z79.02	Long term (current) use of antithrombotics/antiplatelets
dalfopristin/quinupristin	Z79.2	Long term (current) use of antibiotics
dalteparin	Z79.01	Long term (current) use of anticoagulants
dapagliflozin and metformin	Z79.84	Long term (current) use of oral hypoglycemic drugs
dapagliflozin and saxagliptin	Z79.84	Long term (current) use of oral hypoglycemic drugs
daptomycin	Z79.2	Long term (current) use of antibiotics
Dasetta 1/35®	Z79.890	Hormone replacement therapy (postmenopausal)
Dasetta 7/7/7®	Z79.890	Hormone replacement therapy (postmenopausal)
Daxbia®	Z79.2	Long term (current) use of antibiotics
Daypro®	Z79.1	Long term (current) use of non-steroidal anti-inflammatories (NSAID)
Daysee®	Z79.3	Long term (current) use of hormonal contraceptives
De-Sone LA®	Z79.52	Long term (current) use of systemic steroids
Delestrogen®	Z79.890	Hormone replacement therapy (postmenopausal)
Delyla®	Z79.3	Long term (current) use of hormonal contraceptives
Demerol®	Z79.891	Long term (current) use of opiate analgesic
Depo-Medrol®	Z79.52	Long term (current) use of systemic steroids
Depo-Provera®	Z79.3	Long term (current) use of hormonal contraceptives

Drug Name	Code	Code Descriptor
Depo-SubQ Provera 104®	Z79.3	Long term (current) use of hormonal contraceptives
desirudin	Z79.02	Long term (current) use of antithrombotics/antiplatelets
Desogen®	Z79.3	Long term (current) use of hormonal contraceptives
dexamethasone	Z79.52	Long term (current) use of systemic steroids
Dexamethasone Intensol®	Z79.52	Long term (current) use of systemic steroids
Dexpak Taperpak®	Z79.52	Long term (current) use of systemic steroids
DiaBeta®	Z79.84	Long term (current) use of oral hypoglycemic drugs
Diabinese®	Z79.84	Long term (current) use of oral hypoglycemic drugs
diclofenac	Z79.1	Long term (current) use of non-steroidal anti-inflammatories (NSAID)
diclofenac/misoprostol	Z79.1	Long term (current) use of non-steroidal anti-inflammatories (NSAID)
dicloxacillin	Z79.2	Long term (current) use of antibiotics
dienogest/estradiol	Z79.3	Long term (current) use of hormonal contraceptives
Dificid®	Z79.2	Long term (current) use of antibiotics
diflunisal	Z79.1	Long term (current) use of non-steroidal anti-inflammatories (NSAID)
Dilaudid®	Z79.891	Long term (current) use of opiate analgesic
dipyridamole	Z79.02	Long term (current) use of antithrombotics/antiplatelets
Divigel®	Z79.890	Hormone replacement therapy (postmenopausal)
Dolobid®	Z79.1	Long term (current) use of non-steroidal anti-inflammatories (NSAID)
Dolophine®	Z79.891	Long term (current) use of opiate analgesic
Doryx®	Z79.2	Long term (current) use of antibiotics
doxycycline	Z79.2	Long term (current) use of antibiotics
drospirenone/estradiol	Z79.890	Hormone replacement therapy (postmenopausal)
drospirenone/ethinyl estradiol	Z79.3	Long term (current) use of hormonal contraceptives
drospirenone/ethinyl estradiol/levomefolate calcium	Z79.3	Long term (current) use of hormonal contraceptives
Duavee®	Z79.890	Hormone replacement therapy (postmenopausal)
Duetact®	Z79.84	Long term (current) use of oral hypoglycemic drugs
Duexis®	Z79.1	Long term (current) use of non-steroidal anti-inflammatories (NSAID)
Dulera®	Z79.51	Long term (current) use of inhaled steroids
Duospore®	Z79.2	Long term (current) use of antibiotics
Duragesic®	Z79.891	Long term (current) use of opiate analgesic
Duramorph®	Z79.891	Long term (current) use of opiate analgesic
Durlaza®	Z79.82	Long term (current) use of aspirin
Dycill®	Z79.2	Long term (current) use of antibiotics
Dynacin®	Z79.2	Long term (current) use of antibiotics
Dynapen®	Z79.2	Long term (current) use of antibiotics
E.E.S. 400 Filmtab®	Z79.2	Long term (current) use of antibiotics
E.E.S. Granules®	Z79.2	Long term (current) use of antibiotics
EC-Naprosyn®	Z79.1	Long term (current) use of non-steroidal anti-inflammatories (NSAID)
Ecotrin®	Z79.82	Long term (current) use of aspirin
Ecpirin®	Z79.82	Long term (current) use of aspirin
edoxaban	Z79.01	Long term (current) use of anticoagulants
EEMT DS®	Z79.890	Hormone replacement therapy (postmenopausal)
EEMT HS®	Z79.890	Hormone replacement therapy (postmenopausal)
EEMT®	Z79.890	Hormone replacement therapy (postmenopausal)
Effient®	Z79.02	Long term (current) use of antithrombotics/antiplatelets
Elestrin®	Z79.890	Hormone replacement therapy (postmenopausal)
Eligard®	Z79.818	Long term (current) use of other agents affecting estrogen receptors and estrogen levels
Elinest®	Z79.3	Long term (current) use of hormonal contraceptives
Eliquis®	Z79.01	Long term (current) use of anticoagulants
Embeda®	Z79.891	Long term (current) use of opiate analgesic
Emcin Clear®	Z79.2	Long term (current) use of antibiotics
Emoquette®	Z79.3	Long term (current) use of hormonal contraceptives
empagliflozin and metformin	Z79.84	Long term (current) use of oral hypoglycemic drugs
Ena®	Z79.890	Hormone replacement therapy (postmenopausal)
enoxaparin	Z79.01	Long term (current) use of anticoagulants
Enpresse®	Z79.3	Long term (current) use of hormonal contraceptives
Enskyce®	Z79.3	Long term (current) use of hormonal contraceptives
Entocort EC®	Z79.52	Long term (current) use of systemic steroids
Envarsus XR®	Z79.899	Other long term (current) drug therapy
eptifibatide	Z79.02	Long term (current) use of antithrombotics/antiplatelets

Drug Name	Code	Code Descriptor
Errin®	Z79.3	Long term (current) use of hormonal contraceptives
ertapenem	Z79.2	Long term (current) use of antibiotics
Ery Pads®	Z79.2	Long term (current) use of antibiotics
Ery-Tab®	Z79.2	Long term (current) use of antibiotics
Eryc®	Z79.2	Long term (current) use of antibiotics
Erygel®	Z79.2	Long term (current) use of antibiotics
EryPed®	Z79.2	Long term (current) use of antibiotics
Erythrocin Stearate Filmtab®	Z79.2	Long term (current) use of antibiotics
erythromycin	Z79.2	Long term (current) use of antibiotics
esomeprazole/naproxen	Z79.1	Long term (current) use of non-steroidal anti-inflammatories (NSAID)
Essian H.S.®	Z79.890	Hormone replacement therapy (postmenopausal)
Essian®	Z79.890	Hormone replacement therapy (postmenopausal)
Estarylla®	Z79.3	Long term (current) use of hormonal contraceptives
esterified estrogens/methyltestosterone	Z79.890	Hormone replacement therapy (postmenopausal)
Estrace®	Z79.890	Hormone replacement therapy (postmenopausal)
Estraderm®	Z79.890	Hormone replacement therapy (postmenopausal)
estradiol valerate	Z79.890	Hormone replacement therapy (postmenopausal)
estradiol, oral	Z79.890	Hormone replacement therapy (postmenopausal)
estradiol, topical emulsion	Z79.890	Hormone replacement therapy (postmenopausal)
estradiol, vaginal	Z79.890	Hormone replacement therapy (postmenopausal)
estradiol/drospirenone	Z79.890	Hormone replacement therapy (postmenopausal)
estradiol/levonorgestrel	Z79.890	Hormone replacement therapy (postmenopausal)
estradiol/norethindrone	Z79.890	Hormone replacement therapy (postmenopausal)
Estratest H.S.®	Z79.890	Hormone replacement therapy (postmenopausal)
Estratest®	Z79.890	Hormone replacement therapy (postmenopausal)
Estring® Vaginal Ring	Z79.890	Hormone replacement therapy (postmenopausal)
EstroGel®	Z79.890	Hormone replacement therapy (postmenopausal)
estropipate	Z79.890	Hormone replacement therapy (postmenopausal)
Estrostep Fe®	Z79.3	Long term (current) use of hormonal contraceptives
Estrostep Fe®	Z79.890	Hormone replacement therapy (postmenopausal)
ethinyl estradiol/desogestrel	Z79.3	Long term (current) use of hormonal contraceptives
ethinyl estradiol/ethynodiol diacetate	Z79.3	Long term (current) use of hormonal contraceptives
ethinyl estradiol/etonogestrel	Z79.3	Long term (current) use of hormonal contraceptives
ethinyl estradiol/levonorgestrel	Z79.3	Long term (current) use of hormonal contraceptives
ethinyl estradiol/norethindrone	Z79.3	Long term (current) use of hormonal contraceptives
ethinyl estradiol/norethindrone	Z79.890	Hormone replacement therapy (postmenopausal)
ethinyl estradiol/norgestimate	Z79.3	Long term (current) use of hormonal contraceptives
ethinyl estradiol/norgestrel	Z79.3	Long term (current) use of hormonal contraceptives
etidronate	Z79.83	Long term (current) use of bisphosphonates
etodolac	Z79.1	Long term (current) use of non-steroidal anti-inflammatories (NSAID)
etonogestrel	Z79.3	Long term (current) use of hormonal contraceptives
Evamist®	Z79.890	Hormone replacement therapy (postmenopausal)
Evista®	Z79.810	Long term (current) use of selective estrogen receptor modulators (SERMs)
exemestane	Z79.811	Long term (current) use of aromatase inhibitors
Factive®	Z79.2	Long term (current) use of antibiotics
Falmina®	Z79.3	Long term (current) use of hormonal contraceptives
famotidine/ibuprofen	Z79.1	Long term (current) use of non-steroidal anti-inflammatories (NSAID)
Fareston®	Z79.810	Long term (current) use of selective estrogen receptor modulators (SERMs)
Faslodex®	Z79.818	Long term (current) use of other agents affecting estrogen receptors and estrogen levels
Fasprin®	Z79.82	Long term (current) use of aspirin
Fayosim®	Z79.3	Long term (current) use of hormonal contraceptives
Feldene®	Z79.1	Long term (current) use of non-steroidal anti-inflammatories (NSAID)
Femara®	Z79.811	Long term (current) use of aromatase inhibitors
Femcon Fe®	Z79.890	Hormone replacement therapy (postmenopausal)
Femhrt®	Z79.890	Hormone replacement therapy (postmenopausal)
Femring®	Z79.890	Hormone replacement therapy (postmenopausal)
Femynor®	Z79.3	Long term (current) use of hormonal contraceptives
fenoprofen	Z79.1	Long term (current) use of non-steroidal anti-inflammatories (NSAID)
Fenortho®	Z79.1	Long term (current) use of non-steroidal anti-inflammatories (NSAID)
fentanyl	Z79.891	Long term (current) use of opiate analgesic

Drug Name	Code	Code Descriptor
Fentora®	Z79.891	Long term (current) use of opiate analgesic
Fiasp®	Z79.4	Long term (current) use of insulin
fidaxomicin	Z79.2	Long term (current) use of antibiotics
Fioricet with Codeine®	Z79.891	Long term (current) use of opiate analgesic
Flagyl 375®	Z79.2	Long term (current) use of antibiotics
Flagyl®	Z79.2	Long term (current) use of antibiotics
Flanax Pain Reliever®	Z79.1	Long term (current) use of non-steroidal anti-inflammatories (NSAID)
Florinef Acetate®	Z79.52	Long term (current) use of systemic steroids
Flovent Diskus®	Z79.51	Long term (current) use of inhaled steroids
Flovent HFA®	Z79.51	Long term (current) use of inhaled steroids
Flovent Rotadisk®	Z79.51	Long term (current) use of inhaled steroids
fludrocortisone	Z79.52	Long term (current) use of systemic steroids
flunisolide	Z79.51	Long term (current) use of inhaled steroids
flurbiprofen sodium	Z79.1	Long term (current) use of non-steroidal anti-inflammatories (NSAID)
fluticasone	Z79.51	Long term (current) use of inhaled steroids
fluticasone and salmeterol	Z79.51	Long term (current) use of inhaled steroids
fondaparinux	Z79.01	Long term (current) use of anticoagulants
formoterol and mometasone	Z79.51	Long term (current) use of inhaled steroids
Fortamet®	Z79.84	Long term (current) use of oral hypoglycemic drugs
Fortaz®	Z79.2	Long term (current) use of antibiotics
Fosamax®	Z79.83	Long term (current) use of bisphosphonates
fosfomycin	Z79.2	Long term (current) use of antibiotics
Fragmin®	Z79.01	Long term (current) use of anticoagulants
fulvestrant	Z79.818	Long term (current) use of other agents affecting estrogen receptors and estrogen levels
Fyavolv®	Z79.890	Hormone replacement therapy (postmenopausal)
Garamycin®	Z79.2	Long term (current) use of antibiotics
Garimide®	Z79.2	Long term (current) use of antibiotics
gemifloxacin	Z79.2	Long term (current) use of antibiotics
Generess Fe®	Z79.3	Long term (current) use of hormonal contraceptives
Generess Fe®	Z79.890	Hormone replacement therapy (postmenopausal)
Gengraf®	Z79.899	Other long term (current) drug therapy
Genpril®	Z79.1	Long term (current) use of non-steroidal anti-inflammatories (NSAID)
gentamicin	Z79.2	Long term (current) use of antibiotics
Gianvi®	Z79.3	Long term (current) use of hormonal contraceptives
Gildagia®	Z79.890	Hormone replacement therapy (postmenopausal)
Gildess 1.5/30®	Z79.3	Long term (current) use of hormonal contraceptives
Gildess 1.5/30®	Z79.890	Hormone replacement therapy (postmenopausal)
Gildess 1/20®	Z79.3	Long term (current) use of hormonal contraceptives
Gildess 1/20®	Z79.890	Hormone replacement therapy (postmenopausal)
Gildess Fe 1.5/30®	Z79.3	Long term (current) use of hormonal contraceptives
Gildess Fe 1.5/30®	Z79.890	Hormone replacement therapy (postmenopausal)
Gildess Fe 1/20®	Z79.3	Long term (current) use of hormonal contraceptives
Gildess Fe 1/20®	Z79.890	Hormone replacement therapy (postmenopausal)
glimepiride	Z79.84	Long term (current) use of oral hypoglycemic drugs
glimepiride and pioglitazone	Z79.84	Long term (current) use of oral hypoglycemic drugs
glipizide	Z79.84	Long term (current) use of oral hypoglycemic drugs
GlipiZIDE XL®	Z79.84	Long term (current) use of oral hypoglycemic drugs
Glucophage XR®	Z79.84	Long term (current) use of oral hypoglycemic drugs
Glucophage®	Z79.84	Long term (current) use of oral hypoglycemic drugs
Glucotrol XL®	Z79.84	Long term (current) use of oral hypoglycemic drugs
Glucotrol®	Z79.84	Long term (current) use of oral hypoglycemic drugs
Glucovance®	Z79.84	Long term (current) use of oral hypoglycemic drugs
Glumetza®	Z79.84	Long term (current) use of oral hypoglycemic drugs
glyburide	Z79.84	Long term (current) use of oral hypoglycemic drugs
glyburide and metformin	Z79.84	Long term (current) use of oral hypoglycemic drugs
Glycron®	Z79.84	Long term (current) use of oral hypoglycemic drugs
Glynase PresTab®	Z79.84	Long term (current) use of oral hypoglycemic drugs
Glynase®	Z79.84	Long term (current) use of oral hypoglycemic drugs
Glyset®	Z79.84	Long term (current) use of oral hypoglycemic drugs
goserelin	Z79.818	Long term (current) use of other agents affecting estrogen receptors and estrogen levels

Drug Name	Code	Code Descriptor
Halfprin®	Z79.82	Long term (current) use of aspirin
Haltran®	Z79.1	Long term (current) use of non-steroidal anti-inflammatories (NSAID)
Hep-Lock®	Z79.01	Long term (current) use of anticoagulants
heparin	Z79.01	Long term (current) use of anticoagulants
Heparin Sodium ADD-Vantage®	Z79.01	Long term (current) use of anticoagulants
histrelin	Z79.818	Long term (current) use of other agents affecting estrogen receptors and estrogen levels
HumaLOG KwikPen®	Z79.4	Long term (current) use of insulin
HumaLOG Mix 50/50 KwikPen®	Z79.4	Long term (current) use of insulin
HumaLOG Mix 50/50®	Z79.4	Long term (current) use of insulin
HumaLOG Mix 75/25 KwikPen®	Z79.4	Long term (current) use of insulin
HumaLOG Mix 75/25®	Z79.4	Long term (current) use of insulin
HumaLOG®	Z79.4	Long term (current) use of insulin
Humulin 70/30 Pen®	Z79.4	Long term (current) use of insulin
Humulin 70/30®	Z79.4	Long term (current) use of insulin
HumuLIN N®	Z79.4	Long term (current) use of insulin
HumuLIN R®	Z79.4	Long term (current) use of insulin
hydrocodone	Z79.891	Long term (current) use of opiate analgesic
hydrocodone and ibuprofen	Z79.891	Long term (current) use of opiate analgesic
hydrocodone bitartrate and acetaminophen	Z79.891	Long term (current) use of opiate analgesic
hydrocortisone	Z79.52	Long term (current) use of systemic steroids
hydromorphone	Z79.891	Long term (current) use of opiate analgesic
hydromorphone hydrochloride extended-release	Z79.891	Long term (current) use of opiate analgesic
Hysingla ER®	Z79.891	Long term (current) use of opiate analgesic
ibandronate	Z79.83	Long term (current) use of bisphosphonates
Ibu-4®	Z79.1	Long term (current) use of non-steroidal anti-inflammatories (NSAID)
Ibu-6®	Z79.1	Long term (current) use of non-steroidal anti-inflammatories (NSAID)
Ibu-8®	Z79.1	Long term (current) use of non-steroidal anti-inflammatories (NSAID)
Ibu-Tab®	Z79.1	Long term (current) use of non-steroidal anti-inflammatories (NSAID)
ibuprofen	Z79.1	Long term (current) use of non-steroidal anti-inflammatories (NSAID)
imipenem/cilastatin	Z79.2	Long term (current) use of antibiotics
Imuran®	Z79.899	Other long term (current) drug therapy
Indocin SR®	Z79.1	Long term (current) use of non-steroidal anti-inflammatories (NSAID)
Indocin®	Z79.1	Long term (current) use of non-steroidal anti-inflammatories (NSAID)
indomethacin	Z79.1	Long term (current) use of non-steroidal anti-inflammatories (NSAID)
Infumorph®	Z79.891	Long term (current) use of opiate analgesic
insulin aspart	Z79.4	Long term (current) use of insulin
insulin aspart/insulin aspart protamine	Z79.4	Long term (current) use of insulin
insulin aspart/insulin degludec	Z79.4	Long term (current) use of insulin
insulin degludec	Z79.4	Long term (current) use of insulin
insulin detemir	Z79.4	Long term (current) use of insulin
insulin glargine	Z79.4	Long term (current) use of insulin
insulin glulisine	Z79.4	Long term (current) use of insulin
insulin inhalation, rapid acting	Z79.4	Long term (current) use of insulin
insulin isophane	Z79.4	Long term (current) use of insulin
insulin isophane/insulin regular	Z79.4	Long term (current) use of insulin
insulin lispro	Z79.4	Long term (current) use of insulin
insulin lispro/insulin lispro protamine	Z79.4	Long term (current) use of insulin
insulin regular	Z79.4	Long term (current) use of insulin
Integrilin®	Z79.02	Long term (current) use of antithrombotics/antiplatelets
interferon alfa-2b	Z79.899	Other long term (current) drug therapy
interferon beta-1a	Z79.899	Other long term (current) drug therapy
interferon gamma-1b	Z79.899	Other long term (current) drug therapy
Intron A®	Z79.899	Other long term (current) drug therapy
Introvale®	Z79.3	Long term (current) use of hormonal contraceptives
INVanz®	Z79.2	Long term (current) use of antibiotics
Invokamet®	Z79.84	Long term (current) use of oral hypoglycemic drugs
Ionsys®	Z79.891	Long term (current) use of opiate analgesic
Iprivask®	Z79.02	Long term (current) use of antithrombotics/antiplatelets
Isibloom®	Z79.3	Long term (current) use of hormonal contraceptives
Isoject Permapen®	Z79.2	Long term (current) use of antibiotics

Drug Name	Code	Code Descriptor
isoniazid	Z79.2	Long term (current) use of antibiotics
Jantoven®	Z79.01	Long term (current) use of anticoagulants
Janumet®	Z79.84	Long term (current) use of oral hypoglycemic drugs
Januvia®	Z79.84	Long term (current) use of oral hypoglycemic drugs
Jencycla®	Z79.3	Long term (current) use of hormonal contraceptives
Jentadueto®	Z79.84	Long term (current) use of oral hypoglycemic drugs
Jevantique Lo (HRT)®	Z79.890	Hormone replacement therapy (postmenopausal)
Jinteli®	Z79.890	Hormone replacement therapy (postmenopausal)
Jolessa®	Z79.3	Long term (current) use of hormonal contraceptives
Jolivette®	Z79.3	Long term (current) use of hormonal contraceptives
Juleber®	Z79.3	Long term (current) use of hormonal contraceptives
Junel 1.5/30®	Z79.3	Long term (current) use of hormonal contraceptives
Junel 1.5/30®	Z79.890	Hormone replacement therapy (postmenopausal)
Junel 1/20®	Z79.3	Long term (current) use of hormonal contraceptives
Junel 1/20®	Z79.890	Hormone replacement therapy (postmenopausal)
Kadian®	Z79.891	Long term (current) use of opiate analgesic
Kaitlib Fe®	Z79.3	Long term (current) use of hormonal contraceptives
Kariva®	Z79.3	Long term (current) use of hormonal contraceptives
Kazano®	Z79.84	Long term (current) use of oral hypoglycemic drugs
Keflex®	Z79.2	Long term (current) use of antibiotics
Kefurox®	Z79.2	Long term (current) use of antibiotics
Kefzol®	Z79.2	Long term (current) use of antibiotics
Kelnor®	Z79.3	Long term (current) use of hormonal contraceptives
Kenalog-10®	Z79.52	Long term (current) use of systemic steroids
Kenalog-40®	Z79.52	Long term (current) use of systemic steroids
ketoprofen	Z79.1	Long term (current) use of non-steroidal anti-inflammatories (NSAID)
ketorolac	Z79.1	Long term (current) use of non-steroidal anti-inflammatories (NSAID)
Kimidess®	Z79.3	Long term (current) use of hormonal contraceptives
Kisqali®	Z79.811	Long term (current) use of aromatase inhibitors
Kitabis Pak®	Z79.2	Long term (current) use of antibiotics
Klaron®	Z79.2	Long term (current) use of antibiotics
Kombiglyze XR®	Z79.84	Long term (current) use of oral hypoglycemic drugs
Kurvelo®	Z79.3	Long term (current) use of hormonal contraceptives
Lantus SoloStar®	Z79.4	Long term (current) use of insulin
Lantus®	Z79.4	Long term (current) use of insulin
Larin Fe 1.5/30®	Z79.3	Long term (current) use of hormonal contraceptives
Larin Fe 1.5/30®	Z79.890	Hormone replacement therapy (postmenopausal)
Larin Fe 1/20®	Z79.3	Long term (current) use of hormonal contraceptives
Larin Fe 1/20®	Z79.890	Hormone replacement therapy (postmenopausal)
Larissia®	Z79.3	Long term (current) use of hormonal contraceptives
Lazanda®	Z79.891	Long term (current) use of opiate analgesic
Leena®	Z79.3	Long term (current) use of hormonal contraceptives
Leena®	Z79.890	Hormone replacement therapy (postmenopausal)
Lessina®	Z79.3	Long term (current) use of hormonal contraceptives
letrozole	Z79.811	Long term (current) use of aromatase inhibitors
leuprolide	Z79.818	Long term (current) use of other agents affecting estrogen receptors and estrogen levels
Levaquin®	Z79.2	Long term (current) use of antibiotics
Levemir®	Z79.4	Long term (current) use of insulin
Levlen®	Z79.3	Long term (current) use of hormonal contraceptives
levofloxacin	Z79.2	Long term (current) use of antibiotics
Levonest®	Z79.3	Long term (current) use of hormonal contraceptives
levonorgestrel	Z79.3	Long term (current) use of hormonal contraceptives
Levora®	Z79.3	Long term (current) use of hormonal contraceptives
levorphanol	Z79.891	Long term (current) use of opiate analgesic
Liletta®	Z79.3	Long term (current) use of hormonal contraceptives
Lillow®	Z79.3	Long term (current) use of hormonal contraceptives
linagliptin and metformin	Z79.84	Long term (current) use of oral hypoglycemic drugs
Lincocin®	Z79.2	Long term (current) use of antibiotics
lincomycin	Z79.2	Long term (current) use of antibiotics
linezolid	Z79.2	Long term (current) use of antibiotics

Drug Name	Code	Code Descriptor
Lo Loestrin Fe®	Z79.3	Long term (current) use of hormonal contraceptives
Lo Loestrin Fe®	Z79.890	Hormone replacement therapy (postmenopausal)
Loestrin 1/20®	Z79.3	Long term (current) use of hormonal contraceptives
Loestrin 1/20®	Z79.890	Hormone replacement therapy (postmenopausal)
Loestrin 21 1.5/30®	Z79.3	Long term (current) use of hormonal contraceptives
Loestrin 21 1.5/30®	Z79.890	Hormone replacement therapy (postmenopausal)
Loestrin 24 Fe®	Z79.3	Long term (current) use of hormonal contraceptives
Loestrin 24 Fe®	Z79.890	Hormone replacement therapy (postmenopausal)
Loestrin Fe 1/20®	Z79.890	Hormone replacement therapy (postmenopausal)
Loryna®	Z79.3	Long term (current) use of hormonal contraceptives
LoSeasonique®	Z79.3	Long term (current) use of hormonal contraceptives
Lovenox®	Z79.01	Long term (current) use of anticoagulants
Low-Ogestrel®	Z79.3	Long term (current) use of hormonal contraceptives
Lupron Depot-PED®	Z79.818	Long term (current) use of other agents affecting estrogen receptors and estrogen levels
Lupron Depot®	Z79.818	Long term (current) use of other agents affecting estrogen receptors and estrogen levels
Lupron®	Z79.818	Long term (current) use of other agents affecting estrogen receptors and estrogen levels
Lutera®	Z79.3	Long term (current) use of hormonal contraceptives
Lyza®	Z79.3	Long term (current) use of hormonal contraceptives
Macrobid®	Z79.2	Long term (current) use of antibiotics
mafenide	Z79.2	Long term (current) use of antibiotics
Marlissa®	Z79.3	Long term (current) use of hormonal contraceptives
Maxipime®	Z79.2	Long term (current) use of antibiotics
meclofenamate	Z79.1	Long term (current) use of non-steroidal anti-inflammatories (NSAID)
Meclomen®	Z79.1	Long term (current) use of non-steroidal anti-inflammatories (NSAID)
Medrol Dosepak®	Z79.52	Long term (current) use of systemic steroids
Medrol®	Z79.52	Long term (current) use of systemic steroids
medroxyprogesterone	Z79.3	Long term (current) use of hormonal contraceptives
mefenamic acid	Z79.1	Long term (current) use of non-steroidal anti-inflammatories (NSAID)
Mefoxin®	Z79.2	Long term (current) use of antibiotics
Megace ES®	Z79.818	Long term (current) use of other agents affecting estrogen receptors and estrogen levels
megestrol	Z79.818	Long term (current) use of other agents affecting estrogen receptors and estrogen levels
meloxicam	Z79.1	Long term (current) use of non-steroidal anti-inflammatories (NSAID)
Menest®	Z79.890	Hormone replacement therapy (postmenopausal)
Menogen®	Z79.890	Hormone replacement therapy (postmenopausal)
Menostar®	Z79.890	Hormone replacement therapy (postmenopausal)
meperidine	Z79.891	Long term (current) use of opiate analgesic
Mepron®	Z79.2	Long term (current) use of antibiotics
meropenem	Z79.2	Long term (current) use of antibiotics
Merrem®	Z79.2	Long term (current) use of antibiotics
metformin	Z79.84	Long term (current) use of oral hypoglycemic drugs
metformin and pioglitazone	Z79.84	Long term (current) use of oral hypoglycemic drugs
metformin and repaglinide	Z79.84	Long term (current) use of oral hypoglycemic drugs
metformin and saxagliptin	Z79.84	Long term (current) use of oral hypoglycemic drugs
metformin and sitagliptin	Z79.84	Long term (current) use of oral hypoglycemic drugs
methadone hydrochloride	Z79.891	Long term (current) use of opiate analgesic
Methadose®	Z79.891	Long term (current) use of opiate analgesic
methylprednisolone	Z79.52	Long term (current) use of systemic steroids
MethylPREDNISolone Dose Pack®	Z79.52	Long term (current) use of systemic steroids
Metro®	Z79.2	Long term (current) use of antibiotics
Metrogel®	Z79.2	Long term (current) use of antibiotics
metronidazole	Z79.2	Long term (current) use of antibiotics
Mexar®	Z79.2	Long term (current) use of antibiotics
Microgestin 1.5/30®	Z79.890	Hormone replacement therapy (postmenopausal)
Microgestin 1/20®	Z79.890	Hormone replacement therapy (postmenopausal)
Microgestin Fe 1/20®	Z79.3	Long term (current) use of hormonal contraceptives
Microgestin Fe 1/20®	Z79.890	Hormone replacement therapy (postmenopausal)
Midol Extended Relief®	Z79.1	Long term (current) use of non-steroidal anti-inflammatories (NSAID)
Midol®	Z79.1	Long term (current) use of non-steroidal anti-inflammatories (NSAID)
miglitol	Z79.84	Long term (current) use of oral hypoglycemic drugs
Millipred DP®	Z79.52	Long term (current) use of systemic steroids

Drug Name	Code	Code Descriptor
Millipred®	Z79.52	Long term (current) use of systemic steroids
Mimvey®	Z79.890	Hormone replacement therapy (postmenopausal)
Minastrin 24 Fe®	Z79.890	Hormone replacement therapy (postmenopausal)
Miniprin®	Z79.82	Long term (current) use of aspirin
Minivelle®	Z79.890	Hormone replacement therapy (postmenopausal)
Minocin®	Z79.2	Long term (current) use of antibiotics
minocycline	Z79.2	Long term (current) use of antibiotics
Mirena®	Z79.3	Long term (current) use of hormonal contraceptives
Mobic®	Z79.1	Long term (current) use of non-steroidal anti-inflammatories (NSAID)
Modicon®	Z79.890	Hormone replacement therapy (postmenopausal)
mometasone	Z79.51	Long term (current) use of inhaled steroids
Mono-Linyah®	Z79.3	Long term (current) use of hormonal contraceptives
monoclonal antibodies	Z79.899	Other long term (current) drug therapy
Monodox®	Z79.2	Long term (current) use of antibiotics
Monurol®	Z79.2	Long term (current) use of antibiotics
Morgidox®	Z79.2	Long term (current) use of antibiotics
MorphaBond ER®	Z79.891	Long term (current) use of opiate analgesic
morphine	Z79.891	Long term (current) use of opiate analgesic
morphine sulfate and naltrexone	Z79.891	Long term (current) use of opiate analgesic
morphine sulfate extended-release	Z79.891	Long term (current) use of opiate analgesic
Motrin IB®	Z79.1	Long term (current) use of non-steroidal anti-inflammatories (NSAID)
Motrin Junior Strength®	Z79.1	Long term (current) use of non-steroidal anti-inflammatories (NSAID)
Motrin®	Z79.1	Long term (current) use of non-steroidal anti-inflammatories (NSAID)
moxifloxacin	Z79.2	Long term (current) use of antibiotics
Moxilin®	Z79.2	Long term (current) use of antibiotics
MS Contin®	Z79.891	Long term (current) use of opiate analgesic
mupirocin	Z79.2	Long term (current) use of antibiotics
My Way®	Z79.3	Long term (current) use of hormonal contraceptives
Mycobutin®	Z79.2	Long term (current) use of antibiotics
mycophenolate mofetil	Z79.899	Other long term (current) drug therapy
Myrac®	Z79.2	Long term (current) use of antibiotics
Myzilra®	Z79.3	Long term (current) use of hormonal contraceptives
nabumetone	Z79.1	Long term (current) use of non-steroidal anti-inflammatories (NSAID)
nafarelin nasal	Z79.818	Long term (current) use of other agents affecting estrogen receptors and estrogen levels
nafcillin	Z79.2	Long term (current) use of antibiotics
nalbuphine	Z79.891	Long term (current) use of opiate analgesic
Nalfon®	Z79.1	Long term (current) use of non-steroidal anti-inflammatories (NSAID)
Nallpen®	Z79.2	Long term (current) use of antibiotics
naltrexone	Z79.899	Other long term (current) drug therapy
Naprelan®	Z79.1	Long term (current) use of non-steroidal anti-inflammatories (NSAID)
Naprosyn®	Z79.1	Long term (current) use of non-steroidal anti-inflammatories (NSAID)
naproxen	Z79.1	Long term (current) use of non-steroidal anti-inflammatories (NSAID)
Natazia®	Z79.3	Long term (current) use of hormonal contraceptives
nateglinide	Z79.84	Long term (current) use of oral hypoglycemic drugs
Nebupent®	Z79.2	Long term (current) use of antibiotics
Necon 1/35®	Z79.890	Hormone replacement therapy (postmenopausal)
Necon 1/50®	Z79.3	Long term (current) use of hormonal contraceptives
Necon 7/7/7®	Z79.3	Long term (current) use of hormonal contraceptives
Necon 7/7/7®	Z79.890	Hormone replacement therapy (postmenopausal)
Neo-Tab®	Z79.2	Long term (current) use of antibiotics
neomycin	Z79.2	Long term (current) use of antibiotics
neomycin/polymyxin b/pramoxine	Z79.2	Long term (current) use of antibiotics
NeoProfen®	Z79.1	Long term (current) use of non-steroidal anti-inflammatories (NSAID)
Neoral®	Z79.899	Other long term (current) drug therapy
Neosporin®	Z79.2	Long term (current) use of antibiotics
Nexplanon®	Z79.3	Long term (current) use of hormonal contraceptives
Next Choice®	Z79.3	Long term (current) use of hormonal contraceptives
Nikki®	Z79.3	Long term (current) use of hormonal contraceptives
nitrofurantoin	Z79.2	Long term (current) use of antibiotics
Nor-QD®	Z79.3	Long term (current) use of hormonal contraceptives

Drug Name	Code	Code Descriptor
Nora-Be®	Z79.3	Long term (current) use of hormonal contraceptives
Norco®	Z79.891	Long term (current) use of opiate analgesic
norethindrone	Z79.3	Long term (current) use of hormonal contraceptives
norethindrone acetate and ethinyl estradiol	Z79.3	Long term (current) use of hormonal contraceptives
norethindrone acetate/ethinyl estradiol/ferrous fumarate	Z79.3	Long term (current) use of hormonal contraceptives
norethindrone/mestranol	Z79.3	Long term (current) use of hormonal contraceptives
Norinyl 1+50®	Z79.3	Long term (current) use of hormonal contraceptives
Nortrel 1/35®	Z79.3	Long term (current) use of hormonal contraceptives
Nortrel 1/35®	Z79.890	Hormone replacement therapy (postmenopausal)
NovoLIN 70/30®	Z79.4	Long term (current) use of insulin
NovoLIN N®	Z79.4	Long term (current) use of insulin
NovoLIN R®	Z79.4	Long term (current) use of insulin
NovoLOG FlexPen®	Z79.4	Long term (current) use of insulin
NovoLOG Mix 70/30 FlexPen®	Z79.4	Long term (current) use of insulin
NovoLOG Mix 70/30®	Z79.4	Long term (current) use of insulin
NovoLOG PenFill®	Z79.4	Long term (current) use of insulin
NovolOG®	Z79.4	Long term (current) use of insulin
Nucynta ER®	Z79.891	Long term (current) use of opiate analgesic
Nucynta®	Z79.891	Long term (current) use of opiate analgesic
Nuprin®	Z79.1	Long term (current) use of non-steroidal anti-inflammatories (NSAID)
NuvaRing®	Z79.3	Long term (current) use of hormonal contraceptives
Nydrazid®	Z79.2	Long term (current) use of antibiotics
Ocella®	Z79.3	Long term (current) use of hormonal contraceptives
Ocudox®	Z79.2	Long term (current) use of antibiotics
Ogen®	Z79.890	Hormone replacement therapy (postmenopausal)
Ogestrel-28®	Z79.3	Long term (current) use of hormonal contraceptives
Onglyza®	Z79.84	Long term (current) use of oral hypoglycemic drugs
Opana ER®	Z79.891	Long term (current) use of opiate analgesic
Opana®	Z79.891	Long term (current) use of opiate analgesic
Oracea®	Z79.2	Long term (current) use of antibiotics
Orapred ODT®	Z79.52	Long term (current) use of systemic steroids
Oraxyl®	Z79.2	Long term (current) use of antibiotics
Orbactiv®	Z79.2	Long term (current) use of antibiotics
oritavancin	Z79.2	Long term (current) use of antibiotics
Orsythia®	Z79.3	Long term (current) use of hormonal contraceptives
Ortho Micronor®	Z79.3	Long term (current) use of hormonal contraceptives
Ortho Micronor®	Z79.3	Long term (current) use of hormonal contraceptives
Ortho-Novum 1/35®	Z79.3	Long term (current) use of hormonal contraceptives
Ortho-Novum 1/35®	Z79.890	Hormone replacement therapy (postmenopausal)
Ortho-Novum 7/7/7®	Z79.890	Hormone replacement therapy (postmenopausal)
Oseni®	Z79.84	Long term (current) use of oral hypoglycemic drugs
ospemifene	Z79.810	Long term (current) use of selective estrogen receptor modulators (SERMs)
Osphena®	Z79.810	Long term (current) use of selective estrogen receptor modulators (SERMs)
Ovace Plus®	Z79.2	Long term (current) use of antibiotics
Ovace®	Z79.2	Long term (current) use of antibiotics
oxaprozin	Z79.1	Long term (current) use of non-steroidal anti-inflammatories (NSAID)
Oxaydo®	Z79.891	Long term (current) use of opiate analgesic
oxycodone	Z79.891	Long term (current) use of opiate analgesic
OxyContin®	Z79.891	Long term (current) use of opiate analgesic
oxymorphone hydrochloride	Z79.891	Long term (current) use of opiate analgesic
pamidronate	Z79.83	Long term (current) use of bisphosphonates
Panixine®	Z79.2	Long term (current) use of antibiotics
paromomycin	Z79.2	Long term (current) use of antibiotics
Paromycin®	Z79.2	Long term (current) use of antibiotics
PCE Dispertab®	Z79.2	Long term (current) use of antibiotics
PediaPred®	Z79.52	Long term (current) use of systemic steroids
peginterferon alfa-2b	Z79.899	Other long term (current) drug therapy
PegIntron®	Z79.899	Other long term (current) drug therapy
penicillin G benzathine	Z79.2	Long term (current) use of antibiotics
penicillin G potassium	Z79.2	Long term (current) use of antibiotics

Drug Name	Code	Code Descriptor
penicillin V potassium	Z79.2	Long term (current) use of antibiotics
Penicillin-VK®	Z79.2	Long term (current) use of antibiotics
Pentam 300®	Z79.2	Long term (current) use of antibiotics
pentamidine	Z79.2	Long term (current) use of antibiotics
Percocet®	Z79.891	Long term (current) use of opiate analgesic
Persantine®	Z79.02	Long term (current) use of antithrombotics/antiplatelets
Pfizerpen®	Z79.2	Long term (current) use of antibiotics
Philith®	Z79.3	Long term (current) use of hormonal contraceptives
Philith®	Z79.890	Hormone replacement therapy (postmenopausal)
Pimtrea®	Z79.3	Long term (current) use of hormonal contraceptives
pioglitazone hydrochloride	Z79.84	Long term (current) use of oral hypoglycemic drugs
piperacillin/tazobactam	Z79.2	Long term (current) use of antibiotics
Pirmella 1/35®	Z79.3	Long term (current) use of hormonal contraceptives
Pirmella 1/35®	Z79.890	Hormone replacement therapy (postmenopausal)
Pirmella 7/7/7®	Z79.3	Long term (current) use of hormonal contraceptives
Pirmella 7/7/7®	Z79.890	Hormone replacement therapy (postmenopausal)
piroxicam	Z79.1	Long term (current) use of non-steroidal anti-inflammatories (NSAID)
Plan B One-Step®	Z79.3	Long term (current) use of hormonal contraceptives
Plavix®	Z79.02	Long term (current) use of antithrombotics/antiplatelets
Pletal®	Z79.02	Long term (current) use of antithrombotics/antiplatelets
Plexion Cleanser®	Z79.2	Long term (current) use of antibiotics
Plexion SCT®	Z79.2	Long term (current) use of antibiotics
Plexion TS®	Z79.2	Long term (current) use of antibiotics
polymyxin b	Z79.2	Long term (current) use of antibiotics
Polysporin®	Z79.2	Long term (current) use of antibiotics
Ponstel®	Z79.1	Long term (current) use of non-steroidal anti-inflammatories (NSAID)
Portia®	Z79.3	Long term (current) use of hormonal contraceptives
Pradaxa®	Z79.02	Long term (current) use of antithrombotics/antiplatelets
pramoxine	Z79.2	Long term (current) use of antibiotics
Prandin®	Z79.84	Long term (current) use of oral hypoglycemic drugs
Prascion Cleanser®	Z79.2	Long term (current) use of antibiotics
Prascion FC Cloths®	Z79.2	Long term (current) use of antibiotics
Prascion RA®	Z79.2	Long term (current) use of antibiotics
prasugrel	Z79.02	Long term (current) use of antithrombotics/antiplatelets
Precose®	Z79.84	Long term (current) use of oral hypoglycemic drugs
prednisolone	Z79.52	Long term (current) use of systemic steroids
prednisone	Z79.52	Long term (current) use of systemic steroids
Prelone®	Z79.52	Long term (current) use of systemic steroids
Premarin Intravenous®	Z79.890	Hormone replacement therapy (postmenopausal)
Premarin Vaginal Cream®	Z79.890	Hormone replacement therapy (postmenopausal)
Premphase®	Z79.890	Hormone replacement therapy (postmenopausal)
Prempro®	Z79.890	Hormone replacement therapy (postmenopausal)
Previfem®	Z79.3	Long term (current) use of hormonal contraceptives
Priftin®	Z79.2	Long term (current) use of antibiotics
Primaxin IV®	Z79.2	Long term (current) use of antibiotics
Primsol®	Z79.2	Long term (current) use of antibiotics
Probuphine®	Z79.891	Long term (current) use of opiate analgesic
procaine penicillin	Z79.2	Long term (current) use of antibiotics
ProFeno®	Z79.1	Long term (current) use of non-steroidal anti-inflammatories (NSAID)
progesterone	Z79.890	Hormone replacement therapy (postmenopausal)
Prograf®	Z79.899	Other long term (current) drug therapy
Prometrium®	Z79.890	Hormone replacement therapy (postmenopausal)
Proprinal®	Z79.1	Long term (current) use of non-steroidal anti-inflammatories (NSAID)
Provera®	Z79.3	Long term (current) use of hormonal contraceptives
Pulmicort Flexhaler®	Z79.51	Long term (current) use of inhaled steroids
Pulmicort Nebuamp®	Z79.51	Long term (current) use of inhaled steroids
Pulmicort Respules®	Z79.51	Long term (current) use of inhaled steroids
Pulmicort Turbuhaler®	Z79.51	Long term (current) use of inhaled steroids
Pulmicort®	Z79.51	Long term (current) use of inhaled steroids
Q-Profen®	Z79.1	Long term (current) use of non-steroidal anti-inflammatories (NSAID)

Drug Name	Code	Code Descriptor
Qtern®	Z79.84	Long term (current) use of oral hypoglycemic drugs
Quartette®	Z79.3	Long term (current) use of hormonal contraceptives
Quasense®	Z79.3	Long term (current) use of hormonal contraceptives
Qvar®	Z79.51	Long term (current) use of inhaled steroids
raloxifene	Z79.810	Long term (current) use of selective estrogen receptor modulators (SERMs)
Rapamune®	Z79.899	Other long term (current) drug therapy
Rayos®	Z79.52	Long term (current) use of systemic steroids
Rebetol®	Z79.2	Long term (current) use of antibiotics
Rebif®	Z79.899	Other long term (current) drug therapy
Reclast®	Z79.83	Long term (current) use of bisphosphonates
Reclipsen®	Z79.3	Long term (current) use of hormonal contraceptives
Relafen®	Z79.1	Long term (current) use of non-steroidal anti-inflammatories (NSAID)
Relenza®	Z79.2	Long term (current) use of antibiotics
Relion NovoLIN 70/30 Innolet®	Z79.4	Long term (current) use of insulin
remifentanil	Z79.891	Long term (current) use of opiate analgesic
repaglinide	Z79.84	Long term (current) use of oral hypoglycemic drugs
Reprexain®	Z79.891	Long term (current) use of opiate analgesic
retapamulin	Z79.2	Long term (current) use of antibiotics
RibaPak®	Z79.899	Other long term (current) drug therapy
Ribasphere®	Z79.899	Other long term (current) drug therapy
RibaTab®	Z79.899	Other long term (current) drug therapy
ribavirin	Z79.2	Long term (current) use of antibiotics
ribociclib	Z79.811	Long term (current) use of aromatase inhibitors
rifabutin	Z79.2	Long term (current) use of antibiotics
Rifadin IV®	Z79.2	Long term (current) use of antibiotics
Rifadin®	Z79.2	Long term (current) use of antibiotics
rifampin	Z79.2	Long term (current) use of antibiotics
rifapentine	Z79.2	Long term (current) use of antibiotics
rifaximin	Z79.2	Long term (current) use of antibiotics
Rimactane®	Z79.2	Long term (current) use of antibiotics
Riomet®	Z79.84	Long term (current) use of oral hypoglycemic drugs
risedronate	Z79.83	Long term (current) use of bisphosphonates
rivaroxaban	Z79.01	Long term (current) use of anticoagulants
Rivelsa®	Z79.3	Long term (current) use of hormonal contraceptives
Romycin®	Z79.2	Long term (current) use of antibiotics
Rosaderm Cleanser®	Z79.2	Long term (current) use of antibiotics
Rosanil Cleanser®	Z79.2	Long term (current) use of antibiotics
rosiglitazone maleate	Z79.84	Long term (current) use of oral hypoglycemic drugs
Rosula Cleanser®	Z79.2	Long term (current) use of antibiotics
Rosula CLK®	Z79.2	Long term (current) use of antibiotics
Rosula NS®	Z79.2	Long term (current) use of antibiotics
Rosula Wash®	Z79.2	Long term (current) use of antibiotics
Rosula®	Z79.2	Long term (current) use of antibiotics
Roxicet®	Z79.891	Long term (current) use of opiate analgesic
Roxicodone®	Z79.891	Long term (current) use of opiate analgesic
Ryzodeg 70/30 FlexTouch®	Z79.4	Long term (current) use of insulin
Safyral®	Z79.3	Long term (current) use of hormonal contraceptives
SandIMMUNE®	Z79.899	Other long term (current) drug therapy
Savaysa®	Z79.01	Long term (current) use of anticoagulants
saxagliptin	Z79.84	Long term (current) use of oral hypoglycemic drugs
Seasonale®	Z79.3	Long term (current) use of hormonal contraceptives
Seasonique®	Z79.3	Long term (current) use of hormonal contraceptives
Seb-Prev®	Z79.2	Long term (current) use of antibiotics
Sebizon®	Z79.2	Long term (current) use of antibiotics
Septra DS®	Z79.2	Long term (current) use of antibiotics
Septra®	Z79.2	Long term (current) use of antibiotics
Seromycin®	Z79.2	Long term (current) use of antibiotics
Setlakin®	Z79.3	Long term (current) use of hormonal contraceptives
Sharobel®	Z79.3	Long term (current) use of hormonal contraceptives
Silvadene®	Z79.2	Long term (current) use of antibiotics

Drug Name	Code	Code Descriptor
silver sulfadiazine	Z79.2	Long term (current) use of antibiotics
Simulect®	Z79.899	Other long term (current) drug therapy
sirolimus	Z79.899	Other long term (current) drug therapy
Sitagliptin®	Z79.84	Long term (current) use of oral hypoglycemic drugs
Sivextro®	Z79.2	Long term (current) use of antibiotics
Skyla®	Z79.3	Long term (current) use of hormonal contraceptives
SMZ-TMP DS®	Z79.2	Long term (current) use of antibiotics
Solodyn®	Z79.2	Long term (current) use of antibiotics
Soltamox®	Z79.810	Long term (current) use of selective estrogen receptor modulators (SERMs)
Solu-Cortef®	Z79.52	Long term (current) use of systemic steroids
Solu-Medrol®	Z79.52	Long term (current) use of systemic steroids
Sprintec®	Z79.3	Long term (current) use of hormonal contraceptives
Sprix®	Z79.1	Long term (current) use of non-steroidal anti-inflammatories (NSAID)
Sronyx®	Z79.3	Long term (current) use of hormonal contraceptives
SSD AF®	Z79.2	Long term (current) use of antibiotics
SSD®	Z79.2	Long term (current) use of antibiotics
Starlix®	Z79.84	Long term (current) use of oral hypoglycemic drugs
streptomycin	Z79.2	Long term (current) use of antibiotics
Sublimaze®	Z79.891	Long term (current) use of opiate analgesic
Subsys®	Z79.891	Long term (current) use of opiate analgesic
Sufenta®	Z79.891	Long term (current) use of opiate analgesic
sufentanil	Z79.891	Long term (current) use of opiate analgesic
sulfacetamide sodium	Z79.2	Long term (current) use of antibiotics
sulfacetamide sodium/sulfur	Z79.2	Long term (current) use of antibiotics
sulfacetamide sodium/urea	Z79.2	Long term (current) use of antibiotics
sulfamethoxazole/trimethoprim	Z79.2	Long term (current) use of antibiotics
Sulfamylon®	Z79.2	Long term (current) use of antibiotics
Sulfatrim Pediatric®	Z79.2	Long term (current) use of antibiotics
sulindac	Z79.1	Long term (current) use of non-steroidal anti-inflammatories (NSAID)
Sumadan®	Z79.2	Long term (current) use of antibiotics
Sumaxin CP®	Z79.2	Long term (current) use of antibiotics
Sumaxin TS®	Z79.2	Long term (current) use of antibiotics
Sumaxin®	Z79.2	Long term (current) use of antibiotics
Suphera®	Z79.2	Long term (current) use of antibiotics
Supprelin LA®	Z79.818	Long term (current) use of other agents affecting estrogen receptors and estrogen levels
Suprax®	Z79.2	Long term (current) use of antibiotics
Syeda®	Z79.3	Long term (current) use of hormonal contraceptives
Sylatron®	Z79.899	Other long term (current) drug therapy
Symbicort®	Z79.51	Long term (current) use of inhaled steroids
Synarel®	Z79.818	Long term (current) use of other agents affecting estrogen receptors and estrogen levels
Synercid®	Z79.2	Long term (current) use of antibiotics
Synjardy®	Z79.84	Long term (current) use of oral hypoglycemic drugs
synthetic conjugated estrogens, A	Z79.890	Hormone replacement therapy (postmenopausal)
synthetic conjugated estrogens, B	Z79.890	Hormone replacement therapy (postmenopausal)
tacrolimus	Z79.899	Other long term (current) drug therapy
tamoxifen	Z79.810	Long term (current) use of selective estrogen receptor modulators (SERMs)
tapentadol	Z79.891	Long term (current) use of opiate analgesic
Targadox®	Z79.2	Long term (current) use of antibiotics
Taytulla®	Z79.3	Long term (current) use of hormonal contraceptives
Tazicef®	Z79.2	Long term (current) use of antibiotics
tedizolid	Z79.2	Long term (current) use of antibiotics
Teflaro®	Z79.2	Long term (current) use of antibiotics
telavancin	Z79.2	Long term (current) use of antibiotics
temsirolimus	Z79.899	Other long term (current) drug therapy
tetracycline hydrochloride	Z79.2	Long term (current) use of antibiotics
Theramycin Z®	Z79.2	Long term (current) use of antibiotics
Thermazene®	Z79.2	Long term (current) use of antibiotics
ticagrelor	Z79.02	Long term (current) use of antithrombotics/antiplatelets
Ticlid®	Z79.02	Long term (current) use of antithrombotics/antiplatelets
ticlopidine	Z79.02	Long term (current) use of antithrombotics/antiplatelets

Drug Name	Code	Code Descriptor
tigecycline	Z79.2	Long term (current) use of antibiotics
Tilia Fe®	Z79.3	Long term (current) use of hormonal contraceptives
Tilia Fe®	Z79.890	Hormone replacement therapy (postmenopausal)
tirofiban	Z79.02	Long term (current) use of antithrombotics/antiplatelets
Tivorbex®	Z79.1	Long term (current) use of non-steroidal anti-inflammatories (NSAID)
Tobi Podhaler®	Z79.2	Long term (current) use of antibiotics
Tobi®	Z79.2	Long term (current) use of antibiotics
tobramycin	Z79.2	Long term (current) use of antibiotics
tolmetin	Z79.1	Long term (current) use of non-steroidal anti-inflammatories (NSAID)
Topisulf®	Z79.2	Long term (current) use of antibiotics
Toradol®	Z79.1	Long term (current) use of non-steroidal anti-inflammatories (NSAID)
toremifene	Z79.810	Long term (current) use of selective estrogen receptor modulators (SERMs)
Torisel®	Z79.899	Other long term (current) drug therapy
Toujeo SoloStar®	Z79.4	Long term (current) use of insulin
tramadol	Z79.891	Long term (current) use of opiate analgesic
Trelstar Depot®	Z79.818	Long term (current) use of other agents affecting estrogen receptors and estrogen levels
Trelstar LA®	Z79.818	Long term (current) use of other agents affecting estrogen receptors and estrogen levels
Trelstar®	Z79.818	Long term (current) use of other agents affecting estrogen receptors and estrogen levels
Tresiba®	Z79.4	Long term (current) use of insulin
Tri-Estarylla®	Z79.3	Long term (current) use of hormonal contraceptives
Tri-Legest Fe®	Z79.3	Long term (current) use of hormonal contraceptives
Tri-Legest Fe®	Z79.890	Hormone replacement therapy (postmenopausal)
Tri-Legest®	Z79.890	Hormone replacement therapy (postmenopausal)
Tri-Linyah®	Z79.3	Long term (current) use of hormonal contraceptives
Tri-Lo-Estarylla®	Z79.3	Long term (current) use of hormonal contraceptives
Tri-Lo-Marzia®	Z79.3	Long term (current) use of hormonal contraceptives
Tri-Norinyl®	Z79.3	Long term (current) use of hormonal contraceptives
Tri-Norinyl®	Z79.890	Hormone replacement therapy (postmenopausal)
Tri-Previfem®	Z79.3	Long term (current) use of hormonal contraceptives
Tri-Sprintec®	Z79.3	Long term (current) use of hormonal contraceptives
triamcinolone	Z79.52	Long term (current) use of systemic steroids
trimethoprim	Z79.2	Long term (current) use of antibiotics
Triphasil®	Z79.3	Long term (current) use of hormonal contraceptives
Triple Antibiotic®	Z79.2	Long term (current) use of antibiotics
Triptodur®	Z79.818	Long term (current) use of other agents affecting estrogen receptors and estrogen levels
triptorelin	Z79.818	Long term (current) use of other agents affecting estrogen receptors and estrogen levels
Trivora-28®	Z79.3	Long term (current) use of hormonal contraceptives
Tygacil®	Z79.2	Long term (current) use of antibiotics
Tylenol with Codeine®	Z79.891	Long term (current) use of opiate analgesic
Tylenol®	Z79.899	Other long term (current) drug therapy
Uceris®	Z79.52	Long term (current) use of systemic steroids
Ultiva®	Z79.891	Long term (current) use of opiate analgesic
Ultram®	Z79.891	Long term (current) use of opiate analgesic
Unasyn®	Z79.2	Long term (current) use of antibiotics
Vagifem®	Z79.890	Hormone replacement therapy (postmenopausal)
Vancocin HCl Pulvules®	Z79.2	Long term (current) use of antibiotics
Vancocin®	Z79.2	Long term (current) use of antibiotics
vancomycin	Z79.2	Long term (current) use of antibiotics
Vantas®	Z79.818	Long term (current) use of other agents affecting estrogen receptors and estrogen levels
Velivet®	Z79.3	Long term (current) use of hormonal contraceptives
Veripred 20®	Z79.52	Long term (current) use of systemic steroids
Vestura®	Z79.3	Long term (current) use of hormonal contraceptives
Viadur®	Z79.818	Long term (current) use of other agents affecting estrogen receptors and estrogen levels
Vibativ®	Z79.2	Long term (current) use of antibiotics
Vibramycin®	Z79.2	Long term (current) use of antibiotics
Vicodin®	Z79.891	Long term (current) use of opiate analgesic
Vicoprofen®	Z79.891	Long term (current) use of opiate analgesic
Vienva®	Z79.3	Long term (current) use of hormonal contraceptives
Vimovo®	Z79.1	Long term (current) use of non-steroidal anti-inflammatories (NSAID)
Viorele®	Z79.3	Long term (current) use of hormonal contraceptives

Drug Name	Code	Code Descriptor
Virazole®	Z79.899	Other long term (current) drug therapy
Virti-Sulf®	Z79.2	Long term (current) use of antibiotics
Vivelle-Dot®	Z79.890	Hormone replacement therapy (postmenopausal)
Vivelle®	Z79.890	Hormone replacement therapy (postmenopausal)
Vivlodex®	Z79.1	Long term (current) use of non-steroidal anti-inflammatories (NSAID)
Voltaren®	Z79.1	Long term (current) use of non-steroidal anti-inflammatories (NSAID)
vorapaxar	Z79.02	Long term (current) use of antithrombotics/antiplatelets
warfarin	Z79.01	Long term (current) use of anticoagulants
Wera®	Z79.3	Long term (current) use of hormonal contraceptives
Wera®	Z79.890	Hormone replacement therapy (postmenopausal)
Wymzya Fe®	Z79.3	Long term (current) use of hormonal contraceptives
Xarelto®	Z79.01	Long term (current) use of anticoagulants
Xifaxan®	Z79.2	Long term (current) use of antibiotics
Xigduo XR®	Z79.84	Long term (current) use of oral hypoglycemic drugs
Ximino®	Z79.2	Long term (current) use of antibiotics
Xtampza ER®	Z79.891	Long term (current) use of opiate analgesic
Yasmin®	Z79.3	Long term (current) use of hormonal contraceptives
Yaz®	Z79.3	Long term (current) use of hormonal contraceptives
zanamivir	Z79.2	Long term (current) use of antibiotics
Zarah®	Z79.3	Long term (current) use of hormonal contraceptives
Zenchent Fe®	Z79.3	Long term (current) use of hormonal contraceptives
Zenchent Fe®	Z79.890	Hormone replacement therapy (postmenopausal)
Zenchent®	Z79.3	Long term (current) use of hormonal contraceptives
Zenchent®	Z79.890	Hormone replacement therapy (postmenopausal)
Zencia Wash®	Z79.2	Long term (current) use of antibiotics
Zeosa®	Z79.3	Long term (current) use of hormonal contraceptives
Zeosa®	Z79.890	Hormone replacement therapy (postmenopausal)
Zerbaxa®	Z79.2	Long term (current) use of antibiotics
Zetacet®	Z79.2	Long term (current) use of antibiotics
Zilretta®	Z79.52	Long term (current) use of systemic steroids
Zinacef®	Z79.2	Long term (current) use of antibiotics
Zipsor®	Z79.1	Long term (current) use of non-steroidal anti-inflammatories (NSAID)
Zithromax Z-Pak®	Z79.2	Long term (current) use of antibiotics
Zithromax®	Z79.2	Long term (current) use of antibiotics
Zmax®	Z79.2	Long term (current) use of antibiotics
Zohydro ER®	Z79.891	Long term (current) use of opiate analgesic
Zoladex®	Z79.818	Long term (current) use of other agents affecting estrogen receptors and estrogen levels
zoledronic acid	Z79.83	Long term (current) use of bisphosphonates
Zometa®	Z79.83	Long term (current) use of bisphosphonates
Zontivity®	Z79.02	Long term (current) use of antithrombotics/antiplatelets
Zorvolex®	Z79.1	Long term (current) use of non-steroidal anti-inflammatories (NSAID)
Zosyn®	Z79.2	Long term (current) use of antibiotics
Zovia 1/35®	Z79.3	Long term (current) use of hormonal contraceptives
Zyvox®	Z79.2	Long term (current) use of antibiotics
N/A	Z79.899	Other long term (current) drug therapy

Note: This list of brand name and generic drugs correspond by drug class to Z codes for long-term use of drugs. This comprehensive but not exhaustive list is provided solely as a reference and does not imply a guarantee of reimbursement. Check with individual payers to determine their billing, coding, and reimbursement guidelines.

This page intentionally left blank

Appendix B: Symbols for 7th-Character Codes

Adult - Age range is 18–124 years inclusive (e.g., senile delirium, mature cataract); based on Medicare's Outpatient Code Editor (OCE).

H35.3110	H35.3190	H35.3232	M80.011K	M80.021A	M80.029K	M80.039K	M80.042K	M80.052A	M80.061K	M80.071A	M80.079K	T74.21XA	T76.01XA	T76.61XA
H35.3111	H35.3191	H35.3233	M80.011P	M80.021D	M80.029P	M80.039D	M80.042P	M80.052D	M80.061P	M80.071D	M80.079P	T74.21XD	T76.01XD	T76.61XD
H35.3112	H35.3192	H35.3290	M80.011S	M80.021G	M80.029S	M80.039G	M80.042S	M80.052G	M80.061S	M80.071G	M80.079S	T74.21XS	T76.01XS	T76.61XS
H35.3113	H35.3193	H35.3291	M80.012A	M80.021K	M80.031A	M80.039K	M80.049A	M80.052K	M80.062A	M80.071K	M80.08XA	T74.31XA	T76.11XA	T76.91XA
H35.3114	H35.3194	H35.3292	M80.012D	M80.021P	M80.031D	M80.039P	M80.049D	M80.052P	M80.062D	M80.071P	M80.08XD	T74.31XD	T76.11XD	T76.91XD
H35.3120	H35.3210	H35.3293	M80.012G	M80.021S	M80.031G	M80.039S	M80.049G	M80.052S	M80.062G	M80.071S	M80.08XG	T74.31XS	T76.11XS	T76.91XS
H35.3121	H35.3211	M80.00XA	M80.012K	M80.022A	M80.031K	M80.041A	M80.049K	M80.059A	M80.062K	M80.072A	M80.08XK	T74.51XA	T76.21XA	
H35.3122	H35.3212	M80.00XD	M80.012P	M80.022D	M80.031P	M80.041D	M80.049P	M80.059D	M80.062P	M80.072D	M80.08XP	T74.51XD	T76.21XD	
H35.3123	H35.3213	M80.00XG	M80.012S	M80.022G	M80.031S	M80.041G	M80.049S	M80.059G	M80.062S	M80.072G	M80.08XS	T74.51XS	T76.21XS	
H35.3124	H35.3220	M80.00XK	M80.019A	M80.022K	M80.032A	M80.041K	M80.051A	M80.059K	M80.069A	M80.072K	T74.01XA	T74.61XA	T76.31XA	
H35.3130	H35.3221	M80.00XP	M80.019D	M80.022P	M80.032D	M80.041P	M80.051D	M80.059P	M80.069D	M80.072P	T74.01XD	T74.61XD	T76.31XD	
H35.3131	H35.3222	M80.00XS	M80.019G	M80.022S	M80.032G	M80.041S	M80.051G	M80.059S	M80.069G	M80.072S	T74.01XS	T74.61XS	T76.31XS	
H35.3132	H35.3223	M80.011A	M80.019K	M80.029A	M80.032K	M80.042A	M80.051K	M80.061A	M80.069K	M80.079A	T74.11XA	T74.91XA	T76.51XA	
H35.3133	H35.3230	M80.011D	M80.019P	M80.029D	M80.032P	M80.042D	M80.051P	M80.061D	M80.069P	M80.079D	T74.11XD	T74.91XD	T76.51XD	
H35.3134	H35.3231	M80.011G	M80.019S	M80.029G	M80.032S	M80.042G	M80.051S	M80.061G	M80.069S	M80.079G	T74.11XS	T74.91XS	T76.51XS	

AHA Coding Clinic®

C44.1021	C44.1922	R40.2113	R40.2210	R40.2242	R40.2324	R40.2361	S36.031A	S82.251D	S92.333A	S92.335G	S99.112S	T59.811A	T81.718A	W03.XXXD
C44.1022	C44.1991	R40.2114	R40.2211	R40.2243	R40.2330	R40.2362	S39.012A	S83.232A	S92.333B	S92.335K	T20.25XS	T65.891A	T82.7XXA	W05.0XXA
C44.1091	C44.1992	R40.2120	R40.2212	R40.2244	R40.2331	R40.2363	S42.295A	S83.511D	S92.333D	S92.335P	T20.312S	T71.191A	T82.867A	W17.89XD
C44.1092	H35.3112	R40.2121	R40.2213	R40.2250	R40.2332	R40.2364	S51.001A	S92.331A	S92.333G	S92.335S	T21.31XD	T80.211A	T82.897A	W19.XXXD
C44.1121	H35.3121	R40.2122	R40.2214	R40.2251	R40.2333	S01.02XA	S52.532D	S92.331B	S92.333K	S92.336A	T23.301S	T81.31XA	T83.428A	W34.00XS
C44.1122	H40.1110	R40.2123	R40.2220	R40.2252	R40.2334	S01.02XD	S53.031A	S92.331D	S92.333P	S92.336B	T23.302S	T81.40XA	T84.021A	W50.2XXA
C44.1191	M80.051A	R40.2124	R40.2221	R40.2253	R40.2340	S01.21XA	S53.031D	S92.331G	S92.333S	S92.336D	T24.391A	T81.40XD	T84.50XA	W50.2XXD
C44.1192	M84.454A	R40.2130	R40.2222	R40.2254	R40.2341	S01.21XD	S53.114A	S92.331K	S92.334A	S92.336G	T24.392A	T81.40XS	T84.51XA	X00.0XXD
C44.1221	M97.01XA	R40.2131	R40.2223	R40.2310	R40.2342	S01.411A	S62.002A	S92.331P	S92.334B	S92.336K	T36.8X5A	T81.41XA	T84.52XA	X00.0XXS
C44.1222	O35.3XX0	R40.2132	R40.2224	R40.2311	R40.2343	S01.411D	S62.102D	S92.331S	S92.334D	S92.336P	T39.015A	T81.41XD	T85.628A	X03.0XXS
C44.1291	O36.80X0	R40.2133	R40.2230	R40.2312	R40.2344	S06.1X0A	S72.002D	S92.332A	S92.334G	S92.336S	T40.5X1A	T81.41XS	T88.53XA	X04.XXXA
C44.1292	O60.14X0	R40.2134	R40.2231	R40.2313	R40.2350	S06.340A	S72.002S	S92.332B	S92.334K	S99.112A	T43.592A	T81.42XA	V00.321A	X08.01XS
C44.1321	O60.14X1	R40.2140	R40.2232	R40.2314	R40.2351	S06.5X0A	S72.141D	S92.332D	S92.334P	S99.112B	T45.1X5A	T81.42XD	V43.61XA	X50.0XXA
C44.1322	O60.14X2	R40.2141	R40.2233	R40.2320	R40.2352	S06.5X0S	S72.401A	S92.332G	S92.334S	S99.112D	T45.525A	T81.42XS	V43.61XD	X95.9XXA
C44.1391	R40.2110	R40.2142	R40.2234	R40.2321	R40.2353	S06.6X0A	S81.841A	S92.332K	S92.335A	S99.112G	T45.615A	T81.43XA	V49.9XXA	Y35.893A
C44.1392	R40.2111	R40.2143	R40.2240	R40.2322	R40.2354	S31.613A	S82.234A	S92.332P	S92.335B	S99.112K	T45.8X5A	T81.43XD	W00.0XXD	
C44.1921	R40.2112	R40.2144	R40.2241	R40.2323	R40.2360	S36.029A	S82.234D	S92.332S	S92.335D	S99.112P	T50.901S	T81.43XS	W03.XXXA	

Complication or Comorbidity (CC) - Based on CMS data

H34.8110	M80.021A	M80.059A	M80.819A	M80.852A	M84.319K	M84.351P	M84.379K	M84.433P	M84.453P	M84.474P	M84.521P	M84.550P	M84.572P	M84.622P
H34.8111	M80.021K	M80.059K	M80.819K	M80.852K	M84.319P	M84.352K	M84.379P	M84.434A	M84.454A	M84.475A	M84.522A	M84.551A	M84.573A	M84.629A
H34.8112	M80.021P	M80.059P	M80.819P	M80.852P	M84.321K	M84.352P	M84.38XK	M84.434K	M84.454K	M84.475K	M84.522K	M84.551K	M84.573K	M84.629K
H34.8120	M80.022A	M80.061A	M80.821A	M80.859A	M84.321P	M84.353K	M84.38XP	M84.434P	M84.454P	M84.475P	M84.522P	M84.551P	M84.573P	M84.629P
H34.8121	M80.022K	M80.061K	M80.821K	M80.859K	M84.322K	M84.353P	M84.40XA	M84.439A	M84.459A	M84.476A	M84.529A	M84.552A	M84.574A	M84.631A
H34.8122	M80.022P	M80.061P	M80.821P	M80.859P	M84.322P	M84.359K	M84.40XK	M84.439K	M84.459K	M84.476K	M84.529K	M84.552K	M84.574K	M84.631K
H34.8130	M80.029A	M80.062A	M80.822A	M80.861A	M84.329K	M84.359P	M84.40XP	M84.439P	M84.459P	M84.476P	M84.529P	M84.552P	M84.574P	M84.631P
H34.8131	M80.029K	M80.062K	M80.822K	M80.861K	M84.329P	M84.361K	M84.411A	M84.441A	M84.461A	M84.477A	M84.531A	M84.553A	M84.575A	M84.632A
H34.8132	M80.029P	M80.062P	M80.822P	M80.861P	M84.331K	M84.361P	M84.411K	M84.441K	M84.461K	M84.477K	M84.531K	M84.553K	M84.575K	M84.632K
H34.8190	M80.031A	M80.069A	M80.829A	M80.862A	M84.331P	M84.362K	M84.411P	M84.441P	M84.461P	M84.477P	M84.531P	M84.553P	M84.575P	M84.632P
H34.8191	M80.031K	M80.069K	M80.829K	M80.862K	M84.332K	M84.362P	M84.412A	M84.442A	M84.462A	M84.478A	M84.532A	M84.559A	M84.576A	M84.633A
H34.8192	M80.031P	M80.069P	M80.829P	M80.862P	M84.332P	M84.363K	M84.412K	M84.442K	M84.462K	M84.478K	M84.532K	M84.559K	M84.576K	M84.633K
M48.50XA	M80.032A	M80.071A	M80.831A	M80.869A	M84.333K	M84.363P	M84.412P	M84.442P	M84.462P	M84.478P	M84.532P	M84.559P	M84.576P	M84.633P
M48.51XA	M80.032K	M80.071K	M80.831K	M80.869K	M84.333P	M84.364K	M84.419A	M84.443A	M84.463A	M84.479A	M84.533A	M84.561A	M84.58XA	M84.634A
M48.52XA	M80.032P	M80.071P	M80.831P	M80.869P	M84.334K	M84.364P	M84.419K	M84.443K	M84.463K	M84.479K	M84.533K	M84.561K	M84.58XK	M84.634K
M48.53XA	M80.039A	M80.072A	M80.832A	M80.871A	M84.334P	M84.369K	M84.419P	M84.443P	M84.463P	M84.479P	M84.533P	M84.561P	M84.58XP	M84.634P
M48.54XA	M80.039K	M80.072K	M80.832K	M80.871K	M84.339K	M84.369P	M84.421A	M84.444A	M84.464A	M84.48XA	M84.534A	M84.562A	M84.60XA	M84.639A
M48.55XA	M80.039P	M80.072P	M80.832P	M80.871P	M84.339P	M84.371K	M84.421K	M84.444K	M84.464K	M84.48XK	M84.534K	M84.562K	M84.60XK	M84.639K
M48.56XA	M80.041A	M80.079A	M80.839A	M80.872A	M84.341K	M84.371P	M84.421P	M84.444P	M84.464P	M84.48XP	M84.534P	M84.562P	M84.60XP	M84.639P
M48.57XA	M80.041K	M80.079K	M80.839K	M80.872K	M84.341P	M84.372K	M84.422A	M84.445A	M84.469A	M84.50XA	M84.539A	M84.563A	M84.611A	M84.641A
M48.58XA	M80.041P	M80.079P	M80.839P	M80.872P	M84.342K	M84.372P	M84.422K	M84.445K	M84.469K	M84.50XK	M84.539K	M84.563K	M84.611K	M84.641K
M80.00XA	M80.042A	M80.08XA	M80.841A	M80.879A	M84.342P	M84.373K	M84.422P	M84.445P	M84.469P	M84.50XP	M84.539P	M84.563P	M84.611P	M84.641P
M80.00XK	M80.042K	M80.08XK	M80.841K	M80.879K	M84.343K	M84.373P	M84.429A	M84.446A	M84.471A	M84.511A	M84.541A	M84.564A	M84.612A	M84.642A
M80.00XP	M80.042P	M80.08XP	M80.841P	M80.879P	M84.343P	M84.374K	M84.429K	M84.446K	M84.471K	M84.511K	M84.541K	M84.564K	M84.612K	M84.642K
M80.011A	M80.049A	M80.80XA	M80.842A	M80.88XA	M84.344K	M84.374P	M84.429P	M84.446P	M84.471P	M84.511P	M84.541P	M84.564P	M84.612P	M84.642P
M80.011K	M80.049K	M80.80XK	M80.842K	M80.88XK	M84.344P	M84.375K	M84.431A	M84.451A	M84.472A	M84.512A	M84.542A	M84.569A	M84.619A	M84.649A
M80.011P	M80.049P	M80.80XP	M80.842P	M80.88XP	M84.345K	M84.375P	M84.431K	M84.451K	M84.472K	M84.512K	M84.542K	M84.569K	M84.619K	M84.649K
M80.012A	M80.051A	M80.811A	M80.849A	M84.30XK	M84.345P	M84.376K	M84.431P	M84.451P	M84.472P	M84.512P	M84.542P	M84.569P	M84.619P	M84.649P
M80.012K	M80.051K	M80.811K	M80.849K	M84.30XP	M84.346K	M84.376P	M84.432A	M84.452A	M84.473A	M84.519A	M84.549A	M84.571A	M84.621A	M84.650A
M80.012P	M80.051P	M80.811P	M80.849P	M84.311K	M84.346P	M84.377K	M84.432K	M84.452K	M84.473K	M84.519K	M84.549K	M84.571K	M84.621K	M84.650K
M80.019A	M80.052A	M80.812A	M80.851A	M84.311P	M84.350K	M84.377P	M84.432P	M84.452P	M84.473P	M84.519P	M84.549P	M84.571P	M84.621P	M84.650P
M80.019K	M80.052K	M80.812K	M80.851K	M84.312K	M84.350P	M84.378K	M84.433A	M84.453A	M84.474A	M84.521A	M84.550A	M84.572A	M84.622A	M84.651A
M80.019P	M80.052P	M80.812P	M80.851P	M84.312P	M84.351K	M84.378P	M84.433K	M84.453K	M84.474K	M84.521K	M84.550K	M84.572K	M84.622K	M84.651K

Complication or Comorbidity (CC) (cont.) - Based on CMS data

M84.651P	M84.759K	O36.0934	S02.11CA	S02.601A	S02.81XK	S05.40XA	S09.302A	S12.230K	S12.631K	S15.319A	S22.039A	S22.49XK	S32.008K	S32.131K
M84.652A	M84.759P	O36.0935	S02.11CK	S02.601B	S02.82XA	S05.41XA	S09.309A	S12.231A	S12.64XA	S15.321A	S22.039K	S22.5XXK	S32.009A	S32.132A
M84.652K	M97.01XA	O36.0939	S02.11DA	S02.601K	S02.82XB	S05.42XA	S09.311A	S12.231K	S12.64XK	S15.322A	S22.040A	S22.9XXA	S32.009K	S32.132K
M84.652P	M97.02XA	O36.1910	S02.11DK	S02.602A	S02.82XK	S05.50XA	S09.312A	S12.24XA	S12.650A	S15.329A	S22.040K	S22.9XXK	S32.010A	S32.139A
M84.653A	M97.11XA	O36.1911	S02.11EA	S02.602B	S02.831A	S05.51XA	S09.313A	S12.24XK	S12.650K	S15.391A	S22.041A	S25.501A	S32.010K	S32.139K
M84.653K	M97.12XA	O36.4XX0	S02.11EK	S02.602K	S02.831B	S05.52XA	S09.319A	S12.250A	S12.651A	S15.392A	S22.041K	S25.502A	S32.011A	S32.14XA
M84.653P	M97.21XA	O36.4XX1	S02.11FA	S02.609A	S02.831K	S05.70XA	S09.391A	S12.250K	S12.651K	S15.399A	S22.042A	S25.509A	S32.011K	S32.14XK
M84.659A	M97.22XA	O36.4XX2	S02.11FK	S02.609B	S02.832A	S05.71XA	S09.392A	S12.251A	S12.690A	S15.8XXA	S22.042K	S25.511A	S32.012A	S32.15XA
M84.659K	M97.31XA	O36.4XX3	S02.11GA	S02.609K	S02.832B	S05.72XA	S09.399A	S12.251K	S12.690K	S15.9XXA	S22.048A	S25.512A	S32.012K	S32.15XK
M84.659P	M97.32XA	O36.4XX4	S02.11GK	S02.610A	S02.832K	S05.8X1A	S11.10XA	S12.290A	S12.691A	S17.0XXA	S22.048K	S25.519A	S32.018A	S32.16XA
M84.661A	M97.41XA	O36.4XX5	S02.11HA	S02.610B	S02.839A	S05.8X2A	S11.11XA	S12.290K	S12.691K	S17.8XXA	S22.049A	S25.591A	S32.018K	S32.16XK
M84.661K	M97.42XA	O36.4XX9	S02.11HK	S02.610K	S02.839B	S05.8X9A	S11.12XA	S12.291A	S12.9XXA	S17.9XXA	S22.049K	S25.592A	S32.019A	S32.17XA
M84.661P	M97.8XXA	O41.01X0	S02.121A	S02.611A	S02.839K	S05.91XA	S11.13XA	S12.291K	S13.0XXA	S21.101A	S22.050A	S25.599A	S32.019K	S32.17XK
M84.662A	M97.9XXA	O41.01X1	S02.121K	S02.611B	S02.841A	S05.92XA	S11.14XA	S12.300A	S13.100A	S21.102A	S22.050K	S25.801A	S32.020A	S32.19XA
M84.662K	O31.8X10	O41.01X2	S02.122A	S02.611K	S02.841B	S06.0X0A	S11.15XA	S12.300K	S13.101A	S21.109A	S22.051A	S25.802A	S32.020K	S32.19XK
M84.662P	O31.8X11	O41.01X3	S02.122K	S02.612A	S02.841K	S06.0X1A	S11.20XA	S12.301A	S13.110A	S21.111A	S22.051K	S25.809A	S32.021A	S32.2XXA
M84.663A	O31.8X12	O41.01X4	S02.129A	S02.612B	S02.842A	S06.0X9A	S11.21XA	S12.301K	S13.111A	S21.112A	S22.052A	S25.811A	S32.021K	S32.2XXK
M84.663K	O31.8X13	O41.01X5	S02.129K	S02.612K	S02.842B	S06.2X1A	S11.22XA	S12.330A	S13.120A	S21.119A	S22.052K	S25.812A	S32.022A	S32.301A
M84.663P	O31.8X14	O41.01X9	S02.19XA	S02.620A	S02.842K	S06.2X2A	S11.23XA	S12.330K	S13.121A	S21.121A	S22.058A	S25.819A	S32.022K	S32.301K
M84.664A	O31.8X15	O41.02X0	S02.19XK	S02.620B	S02.849A	S06.2X3A	S11.24XA	S12.331A	S13.130A	S21.122A	S22.058K	S25.891A	S32.028A	S32.302A
M84.664K	O31.8X19	O41.02X1	S02.2XXB	S02.620K	S02.849B	S06.2X4A	S11.25XA	S12.331K	S13.131A	S21.129A	S22.059A	S25.892A	S32.028K	S32.302K
M84.664P	O31.8X20	O41.02X2	S02.2XXK	S02.621A	S02.849K	S06.2X5A	S12.000A	S12.34XA	S13.140A	S21.131A	S22.059K	S25.899A	S32.029A	S32.309A
M84.669A	O31.8X21	O41.02X3	S02.30XA	S02.621B	S02.85XA	S06.2X9A	S12.000K	S12.34XK	S13.141A	S21.132A	S22.060A	S25.90XA	S32.029K	S32.309K
M84.669K	O31.8X22	O41.02X4	S02.30XB	S02.621K	S02.85XB	S06.301A	S12.001A	S12.350A	S13.150A	S21.139A	S22.060K	S25.91XA	S32.030A	S32.311A
M84.669P	O31.8X23	O41.02X5	S02.30XK	S02.622A	S02.85XK	S06.302A	S12.001K	S12.350K	S13.151A	S21.141A	S22.061A	S25.99XA	S32.030K	S32.311K
M84.671A	O31.8X24	O41.02X9	S02.31XA	S02.622B	S02.91XA	S06.303A	S12.01XA	S12.351A	S13.160A	S21.142A	S22.061K	S26.00XA	S32.031A	S32.312A
M84.671K	O31.8X25	O41.03X0	S02.31XB	S02.622K	S02.91XK	S06.304A	S12.01XK	S12.351K	S13.161A	S21.149A	S22.062A	S26.01XA	S32.031K	S32.312K
M84.671P	O31.8X29	O41.03X1	S02.31XK	S02.630A	S02.92XA	S06.305A	S12.02XA	S12.390A	S13.170A	S21.151A	S22.062K	S26.09XA	S32.032A	S32.313A
M84.672A	O31.8X30	O41.03X2	S02.32XA	S02.630B	S02.92XB	S06.309A	S12.02XK	S12.390K	S13.171A	S21.152A	S22.068A	S26.10XA	S32.032K	S32.313K
M84.672K	O31.8X31	O41.03X3	S02.32XB	S02.630K	S02.92XK	S06.371A	S12.030A	S12.391A	S13.180A	S21.159A	S22.068K	S26.11XA	S32.038A	S32.314A
M84.672P	O31.8X32	O41.03X4	S02.32XK	S02.631A	S04.011A	S06.372A	S12.030K	S12.391K	S13.181A	S21.90XA	S22.069A	S26.19XA	S32.038K	S32.314K
M84.673A	O31.8X33	O41.03X5	S02.400A	S02.631B	S04.012A	S06.373A	S12.031A	S12.400A	S13.20XA	S21.91XA	S22.069K	S26.90XA	S32.039A	S32.315A
M84.673K	O31.8X34	O41.03X9	S02.400B	S02.631K	S04.019A	S06.374A	S12.031K	S12.400K	S13.29XA	S21.92XA	S22.070A	S26.91XA	S32.039K	S32.315K
M84.673P	O31.8X35	O60.10X0	S02.400K	S02.632A	S04.02XA	S06.375A	S12.040A	S12.401A	S15.001A	S21.93XA	S22.070K	S26.99XA	S32.040A	S32.316A
M84.674A	O31.8X39	O60.10X1	S02.401A	S02.632B	S04.031A	S06.379A	S12.040K	S12.401K	S15.002A	S21.94XA	S22.071A	S27.0XXA	S32.040K	S32.316K
M84.674K	O36.0110	O60.10X2	S02.401B	S02.632K	S04.032A	S06.381A	S12.041A	S12.430A	S15.009A	S21.95XA	S22.071K	S27.301A	S32.041A	S32.391A
M84.674P	O36.0111	O60.10X3	S02.401K	S02.640A	S04.039A	S06.382A	S12.041K	S12.430K	S15.011A	S22.000A	S22.072A	S27.302A	S32.041K	S32.391K
M84.675A	O36.0112	O60.10X4	S02.402A	S02.640B	S04.041A	S06.383A	S12.090A	S12.431A	S15.012A	S22.000K	S22.072K	S27.309A	S32.042A	S32.392A
M84.675K	O36.0113	O60.10X5	S02.402B	S02.640K	S04.042A	S06.384A	S12.090K	S12.431K	S15.019A	S22.001A	S22.078A	S27.311A	S32.042K	S32.392K
M84.675P	O36.0114	O60.10X9	S02.402K	S02.641A	S04.049A	S06.385A	S12.091A	S12.44XA	S15.021A	S22.001K	S22.078K	S27.312A	S32.048A	S32.399A
M84.676A	O36.0115	O60.20X0	S02.40AA	S02.641B	S04.10XA	S06.389A	S12.091K	S12.44XK	S15.022A	S22.002A	S22.079A	S27.319A	S32.048K	S32.399K
M84.676K	O36.0119	O60.20X1	S02.40AB	S02.641K	S04.11XA	S06.811A	S12.100A	S12.450A	S15.029A	S22.002K	S22.079K	S27.321A	S32.049A	S32.401A
M84.676P	O36.0120	O60.20X2	S02.40AK	S02.642A	S04.12XA	S06.812A	S12.100K	S12.450K	S15.091A	S22.008A	S22.080A	S27.322A	S32.049K	S32.401K
M84.68XA	O36.0121	O60.20X3	S02.40BA	S02.642B	S04.20XA	S06.813A	S12.101A	S12.451A	S15.092A	S22.008K	S22.080K	S27.329A	S32.050A	S32.402A
M84.68XK	O36.0122	O60.20X4	S02.40BB	S02.642K	S04.21XA	S06.814A	S12.101K	S12.451K	S15.099A	S22.009A	S22.081A	S27.391A	S32.050K	S32.402K
M84.68XP	O36.0123	O60.20X5	S02.40BK	S02.650A	S04.22XA	S06.815A	S12.110A	S12.490A	S15.101A	S22.009K	S22.081K	S27.392A	S32.051A	S32.409A
M84.750A	O36.0124	O60.20X9	S02.40CA	S02.650B	S04.30XA	S06.819A	S12.110K	S12.490K	S15.102A	S22.010A	S22.082A	S27.399A	S32.051K	S32.409K
M84.750K	O36.0125	S01.101A	S02.40CB	S02.650K	S04.31XA	S06.821A	S12.111A	S12.491A	S15.109A	S22.010K	S22.082K	S27.50XA	S32.052A	S32.411K
M84.750P	O36.0129	S01.102A	S02.40CK	S02.651A	S04.32XA	S06.822A	S12.111K	S12.491K	S15.111A	S22.011A	S22.088A	S27.51XA	S32.052K	S32.412K
M84.751A	O36.0130	S01.109A	S02.40DA	S02.651B	S04.40XA	S06.823A	S12.112A	S12.500A	S15.112A	S22.011K	S22.088K	S27.52XA	S32.058A	S32.413K
M84.751K	O36.0131	S02.0XXA	S02.40DB	S02.651K	S04.41XA	S06.824A	S12.112K	S12.500K	S15.119A	S22.012A	S22.089A	S27.53XA	S32.058K	S32.414K
M84.751P	O36.0132	S02.0XXK	S02.40DK	S02.652A	S04.42XA	S06.825A	S12.120A	S12.501A	S15.121A	S22.012K	S22.089K	S27.59XA	S32.059A	S32.415K
M84.752A	O36.0133	S02.101A	S02.40EA	S02.652B	S04.50XA	S06.829A	S12.120K	S12.501K	S15.122A	S22.018A	S22.20XK	S27.60XA	S32.059K	S32.416K
M84.752K	O36.0134	S02.101K	S02.40EB	S02.652K	S04.51XA	S06.891A	S12.121A	S12.530A	S15.129A	S22.018K	S22.21XA	S27.63XA	S32.10XA	S32.421K
M84.752P	O36.0135	S02.102A	S02.40EK	S02.66XA	S04.52XA	S06.892A	S12.121K	S12.530K	S15.191A	S22.019A	S22.21XK	S27.69XA	S32.10XK	S32.422K
M84.753A	O36.0139	S02.102K	S02.40FA	S02.66XB	S04.60XA	S06.893A	S12.130A	S12.531A	S15.192A	S22.019K	S22.22XA	S27.802A	S32.110A	S32.423K
M84.753K	O36.0910	S02.109A	S02.40FB	S02.66XK	S04.61XA	S06.894A	S12.130K	S12.531K	S15.199A	S22.020A	S22.22XK	S27.803A	S32.110K	S32.424K
M84.753P	O36.0911	S02.109K	S02.40FK	S02.670A	S04.62XA	S06.895A	S12.131A	S12.54XA	S15.201A	S22.020K	S22.23XA	S27.808A	S32.111A	S32.425K
M84.754A	O36.0912	S02.110A	S02.411A	S02.670B	S04.70XA	S06.899A	S12.131K	S12.54XK	S15.202A	S22.021A	S22.23XK	S27.809A	S32.111K	S32.426K
M84.754K	O36.0913	S02.110K	S02.411B	S02.670K	S04.71XA	S06.9X1A	S12.14XA	S12.550A	S15.209A	S22.021K	S22.24XA	S27.892A	S32.112A	S32.431K
M84.754P	O36.0914	S02.111A	S02.411K	S02.671A	S04.72XA	S06.9X2A	S12.14XK	S12.550K	S15.211A	S22.022A	S22.24XK	S27.893A	S32.112K	S32.432K
M84.755A	O36.0915	S02.111K	S02.412A	S02.671B	S04.811A	S06.9X3A	S12.150A	S12.551A	S15.212A	S22.022K	S22.31XA	S27.898A	S32.119A	S32.433K
M84.755K	O36.0919	S02.112A	S02.412B	S02.671K	S04.812A	S06.9X4A	S12.150K	S12.551K	S15.219A	S22.028A	S22.31XK	S27.899A	S32.119K	S32.434K
M84.755P	O36.0920	S02.112K	S02.412K	S02.672A	S04.819A	S06.9X5A	S12.151A	S12.590A	S15.221A	S22.028K	S22.32XA	S27.9XXA	S32.120A	S32.435K
M84.756A	O36.0921	S02.113A	S02.413A	S02.672B	S04.891A	S06.9X9A	S12.151K	S12.590K	S15.222A	S22.029A	S22.32XK	S28.1XXA	S32.120K	S32.436K
M84.756K	O36.0922	S02.113K	S02.413B	S02.672K	S04.892A	S07.0XXA	S12.190A	S12.591A	S15.229A	S22.029K	S22.39XA	S29.021A	S32.121A	S32.441K
M84.756P	O36.0923	S02.118A	S02.413K	S02.69XA	S04.899A	S07.1XXA	S12.190K	S12.591K	S15.291A	S22.030A	S22.39XK	S29.029A	S32.121K	S32.442K
M84.757A	O36.0924	S02.118K	S02.42XA	S02.69XB	S04.9XXA	S07.8XXA	S12.191A	S12.600A	S15.292A	S22.030K	S22.41XA	S32.000A	S32.122A	S32.443K
M84.757K	O36.0925	S02.119A	S02.42XB	S02.69XK	S05.20XA	S07.9XXA	S12.191K	S12.600K	S15.299A	S22.031A	S22.41XK	S32.000K	S32.122K	S32.444K
M84.757P	O36.0929	S02.119K	S02.42XK	S02.80XA	S05.21XA	S09.0XXA	S12.200A	S12.601A	S15.301A	S22.031K	S22.42XA	S32.001A	S32.129A	S32.445K
M84.758A	O36.0930	S02.11AA	S02.5XXK	S02.80XB	S05.22XA	S09.20XA	S12.200K	S12.601K	S15.302A	S22.032A	S22.42XK	S32.001K	S32.129K	S32.446K
M84.758K	O36.0931	S02.11AK	S02.600A	S02.80XK	S05.30XA	S09.21XA	S12.201A	S12.630A	S15.309A	S22.032K	S22.43XA	S32.002A	S32.130A	S32.451K
M84.758P	O36.0932	S02.11BA	S02.600B	S02.81XA	S05.31XA	S09.22XA	S12.201K	S12.630K	S15.311A	S22.038A	S22.43XK	S32.002K	S32.130K	S32.452K
M84.759A	O36.0933	S02.11BK	S02.600K	S02.81XB	S05.32XA	S09.301A	S12.230A	S12.631A	S15.312A	S22.038K	S22.49XA	S32.008A	S32.131A	S32.453K

S32.454K - S52.033K

Complication or Comorbidity (CC) (cont.) - Based on CMS data

S32.454K	S36.030A	S36.522A	S37.93XA	S42.101B	S42.144P	S42.225K	S42.293A	S42.343P	S42.414K	S42.452A	S42.495P	S45.992A	S49.041A	S52.001N
S32.455K	S36.039A	S36.523A	S37.99XA	S42.101K	S42.145B	S42.225P	S42.293K	S42.344A	S42.414P	S42.452K	S42.496A	S45.999A	S49.041K	S52.001P
S32.456K	S36.09XA	S36.528A	S42.001B	S42.101P	S42.145K	S42.226A	S42.293P	S42.344K	S42.415A	S42.452P	S42.496K	S46.021A	S49.041P	S52.001Q
S32.461K	S36.112A	S36.529A	S42.001K	S42.102B	S42.145P	S42.226K	S42.294A	S42.344P	S42.415K	S42.453A	S42.496P	S46.022A	S49.042A	S52.001R
S32.462K	S36.113A	S36.530A	S42.001P	S42.102K	S42.146B	S42.226P	S42.294K	S42.345A	S42.415P	S42.453K	S42.90XA	S46.029A	S49.042K	S52.002K
S32.463K	S36.114A	S36.531A	S42.002B	S42.102P	S42.146K	S42.231A	S42.294P	S42.345K	S42.416A	S42.453P	S42.90XK	S46.121A	S49.042P	S52.002M
S32.464K	S36.118A	S36.532A	S42.002K	S42.109B	S42.146P	S42.231K	S42.295A	S42.345P	S42.416K	S42.454A	S42.90XP	S46.122A	S49.049A	S52.002N
S32.465K	S36.119A	S36.533A	S42.002P	S42.109K	S42.151B	S42.231P	S42.295K	S42.346A	S42.416P	S42.454K	S42.91XA	S46.129A	S49.049K	S52.002P
S32.466K	S36.122A	S36.538A	S42.009B	S42.109P	S42.151K	S42.232A	S42.295P	S42.346K	S42.421A	S42.454P	S42.91XK	S46.221A	S49.049P	S52.002Q
S32.471K	S36.123A	S36.539A	S42.009K	S42.111B	S42.151P	S42.232K	S42.296A	S42.346P	S42.421K	S42.455A	S42.91XP	S46.222A	S49.091A	S52.002R
S32.472K	S36.128A	S36.590A	S42.009P	S42.111K	S42.152B	S42.232P	S42.296K	S42.351A	S42.421P	S42.455K	S42.92XA	S46.229A	S49.091K	S52.009K
S32.473K	S36.129A	S36.591A	S42.011B	S42.111P	S42.152K	S42.239A	S42.296P	S42.351K	S42.422A	S42.455P	S42.92XK	S46.321A	S49.091P	S52.009M
S32.474K	S36.13XA	S36.592A	S42.011K	S42.112B	S42.152P	S42.239K	S42.301A	S42.351P	S42.422K	S42.456A	S42.92XP	S46.322A	S49.092A	S52.009N
S32.475K	S36.200A	S36.593A	S42.011P	S42.112K	S42.153B	S42.239P	S42.301K	S42.352A	S42.422P	S42.456K	S43.201A	S46.329A	S49.092K	S52.009P
S32.476K	S36.201A	S36.598A	S42.012B	S42.112P	S42.153K	S42.241A	S42.301P	S42.352K	S42.423A	S42.456P	S43.202A	S46.821A	S49.092P	S52.009Q
S32.481K	S36.202A	S36.599A	S42.012K	S42.113B	S42.153P	S42.241K	S42.302A	S42.352P	S42.423K	S42.461A	S43.203A	S46.822A	S49.099A	S52.009R
S32.482K	S36.209A	S36.60XA	S42.012P	S42.113K	S42.154B	S42.241P	S42.302K	S42.353A	S42.423P	S42.461K	S43.204A	S46.829A	S49.099K	S52.011A
S32.483K	S36.220A	S36.61XA	S42.013B	S42.113P	S42.154K	S42.242A	S42.302P	S42.353K	S42.424A	S42.461P	S43.205A	S46.921A	S49.099P	S52.011K
S32.484K	S36.221A	S36.62XA	S42.013K	S42.114B	S42.154P	S42.242K	S42.309A	S42.353P	S42.424K	S42.462A	S43.206A	S46.922A	S49.101A	S52.011P
S32.485K	S36.222A	S36.63XA	S42.013P	S42.114K	S42.155B	S42.242P	S42.309K	S42.354A	S42.424P	S42.462K	S43.211A	S46.929A	S49.101K	S52.012A
S32.486K	S36.229A	S36.69XA	S42.014B	S42.114P	S42.155K	S42.249A	S42.309P	S42.354K	S42.425A	S42.462P	S43.212A	S48.011A	S49.101P	S52.012K
S32.491K	S36.230A	S36.81XA	S42.014K	S42.115B	S42.155P	S42.249K	S42.311A	S42.354P	S42.425K	S42.463A	S43.213A	S48.012A	S49.102A	S52.012P
S32.492K	S36.231A	S36.892A	S42.014P	S42.115K	S42.156B	S42.249P	S42.311K	S42.355A	S42.425P	S42.463K	S43.214A	S48.019A	S49.102K	S52.019A
S32.499K	S36.232A	S36.893A	S42.015B	S42.115P	S42.156K	S42.251A	S42.311P	S42.355K	S42.426A	S42.463P	S43.215A	S48.021A	S49.102P	S52.019K
S32.601A	S36.239A	S36.898A	S42.015K	S42.116B	S42.156P	S42.251K	S42.312A	S42.355P	S42.426K	S42.464A	S43.216A	S48.022A	S49.109A	S52.019P
S32.601K	S36.240A	S36.899A	S42.015P	S42.116K	S42.191B	S42.251P	S42.312K	S42.356A	S42.426P	S42.464K	S43.221A	S48.029A	S49.109K	S52.021K
S32.602A	S36.241A	S36.90XA	S42.016B	S42.116P	S42.191K	S42.252A	S42.312P	S42.356K	S42.431A	S42.464P	S43.222A	S48.111A	S49.109P	S52.021M
S32.602K	S36.242A	S36.92XA	S42.016K	S42.121B	S42.191P	S42.252K	S42.319A	S42.356P	S42.431K	S42.465A	S43.223A	S48.112A	S49.111A	S52.021N
S32.609A	S36.249A	S36.93XA	S42.016P	S42.121K	S42.192B	S42.252P	S42.319K	S42.361A	S42.431P	S42.465K	S43.224A	S48.119A	S49.111K	S52.021P
S32.609K	S36.250A	S36.99XA	S42.017B	S42.121P	S42.192K	S42.253A	S42.319P	S42.361K	S42.432A	S42.465P	S43.225A	S48.121A	S49.111P	S52.021Q
S32.611A	S36.251A	S37.001A	S42.017K	S42.122B	S42.192P	S42.253K	S42.321A	S42.361P	S42.432K	S42.466A	S43.226A	S48.122A	S49.112A	S52.021R
S32.611K	S36.252A	S37.002A	S42.017P	S42.122K	S42.199B	S42.253P	S42.321K	S42.362A	S42.432P	S42.466K	S45.101A	S48.129A	S49.112K	S52.022K
S32.612A	S36.259A	S37.009A	S42.018B	S42.122P	S42.199K	S42.254A	S42.321P	S42.362K	S42.433A	S42.466P	S45.102A	S48.911A	S49.112P	S52.022M
S32.612K	S36.260A	S37.011A	S42.018K	S42.123B	S42.199P	S42.254K	S42.322A	S42.362P	S42.433K	S42.471A	S45.109A	S48.912A	S49.119A	S52.022N
S32.613A	S36.261A	S37.012A	S42.018P	S42.123K	S42.201A	S42.254P	S42.322K	S42.363A	S42.433P	S42.471K	S45.111A	S48.919A	S49.119K	S52.022P
S32.613K	S36.262A	S37.019A	S42.019B	S42.123P	S42.201K	S42.255A	S42.322P	S42.363K	S42.434A	S42.471P	S45.112A	S48.921A	S49.119P	S52.022Q
S32.614A	S36.269A	S37.021A	S42.019K	S42.124B	S42.201P	S42.255K	S42.323A	S42.363P	S42.434K	S42.472A	S45.119A	S48.922A	S49.121A	S52.022R
S32.614K	S36.290A	S37.022A	S42.019P	S42.124K	S42.202A	S42.255P	S42.323K	S42.364A	S42.434P	S42.472K	S45.191A	S48.929A	S49.121K	S52.023K
S32.615A	S36.291A	S37.029A	S42.021B	S42.124P	S42.202K	S42.256A	S42.323P	S42.364K	S42.435A	S42.472P	S45.192A	S49.001A	S49.121P	S52.023M
S32.615K	S36.292A	S37.031A	S42.021K	S42.125B	S42.202P	S42.256K	S42.324A	S42.364P	S42.435K	S42.473A	S45.199A	S49.001K	S49.122A	S52.023N
S32.616A	S36.299A	S37.032A	S42.021P	S42.125K	S42.209A	S42.256P	S42.324K	S42.365A	S42.435P	S42.473K	S45.201A	S49.001P	S49.122K	S52.023P
S32.616K	S36.30XA	S37.039A	S42.022B	S42.125P	S42.209K	S42.261A	S42.324P	S42.365K	S42.436A	S42.473P	S45.202A	S49.002A	S49.122P	S52.023Q
S32.691A	S36.32XA	S37.041A	S42.022K	S42.126B	S42.209P	S42.261K	S42.325A	S42.365P	S42.436K	S42.474A	S45.209A	S49.002K	S49.129A	S52.023R
S32.691K	S36.33XA	S37.042A	S42.022P	S42.126K	S42.211A	S42.261P	S42.325K	S42.366A	S42.436P	S42.474K	S45.211A	S49.002P	S49.129K	S52.024K
S32.692A	S36.39XA	S37.049A	S42.023B	S42.126P	S42.211K	S42.262A	S42.325P	S42.366K	S42.441A	S42.474P	S45.212A	S49.009A	S49.129P	S52.024M
S32.692K	S36.400A	S37.051A	S42.023K	S42.131B	S42.211P	S42.262K	S42.326A	S42.366P	S42.441K	S42.475A	S45.219A	S49.009K	S49.131A	S52.024N
S32.699A	S36.408A	S37.052A	S42.023P	S42.131K	S42.212A	S42.262P	S42.326K	S42.391A	S42.441P	S42.475K	S45.291A	S49.009P	S49.131K	S52.024P
S32.699K	S36.409A	S37.059A	S42.024B	S42.131P	S42.212K	S42.263A	S42.326P	S42.391K	S42.442A	S42.475P	S45.292A	S49.011A	S49.131P	S52.024Q
S32.810A	S36.410A	S37.10XA	S42.024K	S42.132B	S42.212P	S42.263K	S42.331A	S42.391P	S42.442K	S42.476A	S45.299A	S49.011K	S49.132A	S52.024R
S32.810K	S36.418A	S37.12XA	S42.024P	S42.132K	S42.213A	S42.263P	S42.331K	S42.392A	S42.442P	S42.476K	S45.301A	S49.011P	S49.132K	S52.025K
S32.811A	S36.419A	S37.13XA	S42.025B	S42.132P	S42.213K	S42.264A	S42.331P	S42.392K	S42.443A	S42.476P	S45.302A	S49.012A	S49.132P	S52.025M
S32.811K	S36.420A	S37.19XA	S42.025K	S42.133B	S42.213P	S42.264K	S42.332A	S42.392P	S42.443K	S42.481A	S45.309A	S49.012K	S49.139A	S52.025N
S32.82XA	S36.428A	S37.20XA	S42.025P	S42.133K	S42.214A	S42.264P	S42.332K	S42.399A	S42.443P	S42.481K	S45.311A	S49.012P	S49.139K	S52.025P
S32.82XK	S36.429A	S37.22XA	S42.026B	S42.133P	S42.214K	S42.265A	S42.332P	S42.399K	S42.444A	S42.481P	S45.312A	S49.019A	S49.139P	S52.025Q
S32.89XA	S36.430A	S37.23XA	S42.026K	S42.134B	S42.214P	S42.265K	S42.333A	S42.399P	S42.444K	S42.482A	S45.319A	S49.019K	S49.141A	S52.025R
S32.89XK	S36.438A	S37.29XA	S42.026P	S42.134K	S42.215A	S42.265P	S42.333K	S42.401A	S42.444P	S42.482K	S45.391A	S49.019P	S49.141K	S52.026K
S32.9XXA	S36.439A	S37.30XA	S42.031B	S42.134P	S42.215K	S42.266A	S42.333P	S42.401K	S42.445A	S42.482P	S45.392A	S49.021A	S49.141P	S52.026M
S32.9XXK	S36.490A	S37.32XA	S42.031K	S42.135B	S42.215P	S42.266K	S42.334A	S42.401P	S42.445K	S42.489A	S45.399A	S49.021K	S49.142A	S52.026N
S35.531A	S36.498A	S37.33XA	S42.031P	S42.135K	S42.216A	S42.266P	S42.334K	S42.402A	S42.445P	S42.489K	S45.801A	S49.021P	S49.142K	S52.026P
S35.532A	S36.499A	S37.39XA	S42.032B	S42.135P	S42.216K	S42.271A	S42.334P	S42.402K	S42.446A	S42.489P	S45.802A	S49.022A	S49.142P	S52.026Q
S35.533A	S36.500A	S37.60XA	S42.032K	S42.136B	S42.216P	S42.271K	S42.335A	S42.402P	S42.446K	S42.491A	S45.809A	S49.022K	S49.149A	S52.026R
S35.534A	S36.501A	S37.62XA	S42.032P	S42.136K	S42.221A	S42.271P	S42.335K	S42.409A	S42.446P	S42.491K	S45.811A	S49.022P	S49.149K	S52.031K
S35.535A	S36.502A	S37.63XA	S42.033B	S42.136P	S42.221K	S42.272A	S42.335P	S42.409K	S42.447A	S42.491P	S45.812A	S49.029A	S49.149P	S52.031M
S35.536A	S36.503A	S37.69XA	S42.033K	S42.141B	S42.221P	S42.272K	S42.336A	S42.409P	S42.447K	S42.492A	S45.819A	S49.029K	S49.191A	S52.031N
S35.8X1A	S36.508A	S37.812A	S42.033P	S42.141K	S42.222A	S42.272P	S42.336K	S42.411A	S42.447P	S42.492K	S45.891A	S49.029P	S49.191K	S52.031P
S35.8X8A	S36.509A	S37.813A	S42.034B	S42.141P	S42.222K	S42.279A	S42.336P	S42.411K	S42.448A	S42.492P	S45.892A	S49.031A	S49.191P	S52.031Q
S35.8X9A	S36.510A	S37.818A	S42.034K	S42.142B	S42.222P	S42.279K	S42.341A	S42.411P	S42.448K	S42.493A	S45.899A	S49.031K	S49.192A	S52.031R
S35.90XA	S36.511A	S37.819A	S42.034P	S42.142K	S42.223A	S42.279P	S42.341K	S42.412A	S42.448P	S42.493K	S45.901A	S49.031P	S49.192K	S52.032K
S35.91XA	S36.512A	S37.892A	S42.035B	S42.142P	S42.223K	S42.291A	S42.341P	S42.412K	S42.449A	S42.493P	S45.902A	S49.032A	S49.192P	S52.032M
S35.99XA	S36.513A	S37.893A	S42.035K	S42.143B	S42.223P	S42.291K	S42.342A	S42.412P	S42.449K	S42.494A	S45.909A	S49.032K	S49.199A	S52.032N
S36.00XA	S36.518A	S37.898A	S42.035P	S42.143K	S42.224A	S42.291P	S42.342K	S42.413A	S42.449P	S42.494K	S45.911A	S49.032P	S49.199K	S52.032P
S36.020A	S36.519A	S37.899A	S42.036B	S42.143P	S42.224K	S42.292A	S42.342P	S42.413K	S42.451A	S42.494P	S45.912A	S49.039A	S49.199P	S52.032Q
S36.021A	S36.520A	S37.90XA	S42.036K	S42.144B	S42.224P	S42.292K	S42.343A	S42.413P	S42.451K	S42.495A	S45.919A	S49.039K	S52.001K	S52.032R
S36.029A	S36.521A	S37.92XA	S42.036P	S42.144K	S42.225A	S42.292P	S42.343K	S42.414A	S42.451P	S42.495K	S45.991A	S49.039P	S52.001M	S52.033K

APPENDIX B: SYMBOLS FOR 7TH-CHARACTER CODES

Complication or Comorbidity (CC) (cont.) - Based on CMS data

S52.033M	S52.099P	S52.132N	S52.219K	S52.235M	S52.253R	S52.272Q	S52.312A	S52.334Q	S52.353M	S52.371M	S52.509N	S52.539Q	S52.572M	S52.613R
S52.033N	S52.099Q	S52.132P	S52.219P	S52.235N	S52.254A	S52.272R	S52.312K	S52.334R	S52.353P	S52.372A	S52.509P	S52.539R	S52.572N	S52.614A
S52.033P	S52.099R	S52.132Q	S52.221A	S52.235P	S52.254K	S52.279K	S52.312P	S52.335A	S52.353Q	S52.372K	S52.509R	S52.541A	S52.572P	S52.614K
S52.033Q	S52.101K	S52.132R	S52.221K	S52.235Q	S52.254M	S52.279M	S52.319A	S52.335K	S52.353R	S52.372M	S52.511A	S52.541K	S52.572Q	S52.614M
S52.033R	S52.101M	S52.133K	S52.221M	S52.235R	S52.254N	S52.279N	S52.319K	S52.335M	S52.354A	S52.372N	S52.511K	S52.541M	S52.572R	S52.614N
S52.034K	S52.101N	S52.133M	S52.221N	S52.236A	S52.254P	S52.279P	S52.319P	S52.335N	S52.354K	S52.372P	S52.511M	S52.541N	S52.579A	S52.614P
S52.034M	S52.101P	S52.133N	S52.221P	S52.236K	S52.254Q	S52.279Q	S52.321A	S52.335P	S52.354M	S52.372Q	S52.511N	S52.541P	S52.579K	S52.614Q
S52.034N	S52.101Q	S52.133P	S52.221Q	S52.236M	S52.254R	S52.279R	S52.321K	S52.335Q	S52.354P	S52.372R	S52.511P	S52.541Q	S52.579M	S52.614R
S52.034P	S52.101R	S52.133R	S52.222A	S52.236N	S52.255A	S52.281A	S52.321N	S52.335R	S52.354Q	S52.379A	S52.511Q	S52.541R	S52.579R	S52.615A
S52.034Q	S52.102K	S52.134K	S52.222K	S52.236P	S52.255K	S52.281K	S52.321P	S52.336A	S52.354R	S52.379K	S52.511R	S52.542A	S52.591A	S52.615K
S52.034R	S52.102M	S52.134M	S52.222M	S52.236Q	S52.255M	S52.281N	S52.321Q	S52.336K	S52.355A	S52.379M	S52.512A	S52.542K	S52.591K	S52.615M
S52.035K	S52.102N	S52.134N	S52.222N	S52.236R	S52.255N	S52.281P	S52.321R	S52.336M	S52.355K	S52.379N	S52.512K	S52.542M	S52.591M	S52.615N
S52.035M	S52.102P	S52.134P	S52.222P	S52.241A	S52.255P	S52.281Q	S52.322A	S52.336N	S52.355P	S52.379P	S52.512M	S52.542N	S52.591N	S52.615P
S52.035N	S52.102Q	S52.134Q	S52.222Q	S52.241K	S52.255Q	S52.281R	S52.322K	S52.336P	S52.355Q	S52.379Q	S52.512Q	S52.542P	S52.591P	S52.615Q
S52.035P	S52.102R	S52.134R	S52.222R	S52.241N	S52.255R	S52.282A	S52.322M	S52.336Q	S52.355R	S52.379R	S52.512R	S52.542Q	S52.591Q	S52.615R
S52.035Q	S52.109K	S52.135K	S52.223A	S52.241P	S52.256A	S52.282K	S52.322N	S52.336R	S52.356A	S52.381A	S52.513A	S52.549A	S52.592A	S52.616A
S52.035R	S52.109M	S52.135M	S52.223K	S52.241Q	S52.256K	S52.282M	S52.322P	S52.341A	S52.356K	S52.381K	S52.513K	S52.549K	S52.592K	S52.616K
S52.036K	S52.109N	S52.135N	S52.223M	S52.241R	S52.256M	S52.282N	S52.322Q	S52.341K	S52.356M	S52.381M	S52.513M	S52.549M	S52.592M	S52.616M
S52.036M	S52.109P	S52.135P	S52.223N	S52.242A	S52.256N	S52.282P	S52.322R	S52.341M	S52.356P	S52.381N	S52.513N	S52.549N	S52.592N	S52.616N
S52.036N	S52.109Q	S52.135Q	S52.223P	S52.242K	S52.256P	S52.282Q	S52.323A	S52.341N	S52.356Q	S52.381P	S52.513P	S52.549P	S52.592P	S52.616P
S52.036P	S52.109R	S52.135R	S52.223Q	S52.242N	S52.256Q	S52.282R	S52.323K	S52.341P	S52.356R	S52.381Q	S52.513Q	S52.549Q	S52.592Q	S52.616Q
S52.036Q	S52.111A	S52.136K	S52.223R	S52.242P	S52.256R	S52.283A	S52.323M	S52.341Q	S52.361A	S52.381R	S52.513R	S52.549R	S52.599A	S52.616R
S52.036R	S52.111K	S52.136M	S52.224A	S52.242Q	S52.261A	S52.283K	S52.323N	S52.341R	S52.361K	S52.382A	S52.514A	S52.551A	S52.599K	S52.621A
S52.041K	S52.111P	S52.136N	S52.224K	S52.242R	S52.261K	S52.283M	S52.323P	S52.342A	S52.361M	S52.382K	S52.514K	S52.551K	S52.599M	S52.621K
S52.041M	S52.112A	S52.136P	S52.224M	S52.243A	S52.261N	S52.283N	S52.323Q	S52.342K	S52.361P	S52.382M	S52.514M	S52.551M	S52.599P	S52.621P
S52.041N	S52.112K	S52.136Q	S52.224N	S52.243K	S52.261P	S52.283P	S52.323R	S52.342M	S52.361Q	S52.382P	S52.514N	S52.551N	S52.599R	S52.622A
S52.041P	S52.112P	S52.136R	S52.224P	S52.243M	S52.261Q	S52.283Q	S52.324A	S52.342N	S52.361R	S52.382Q	S52.514P	S52.551P	S52.601A	S52.622K
S52.041Q	S52.119A	S52.181K	S52.224Q	S52.243N	S52.261R	S52.283R	S52.324K	S52.342P	S52.362A	S52.382R	S52.514R	S52.551Q	S52.601K	S52.622P
S52.041R	S52.119K	S52.181M	S52.224R	S52.243P	S52.262A	S52.291A	S52.324M	S52.342Q	S52.362K	S52.389A	S52.515A	S52.552A	S52.601M	S52.629A
S52.042K	S52.121K	S52.181N	S52.225A	S52.243Q	S52.262K	S52.291K	S52.324N	S52.342R	S52.362M	S52.389K	S52.515K	S52.552K	S52.601P	S52.629K
S52.042M	S52.121M	S52.181P	S52.225K	S52.243R	S52.262M	S52.291M	S52.324P	S52.343A	S52.362P	S52.389M	S52.515M	S52.552M	S52.601Q	S52.629N
S52.042N	S52.121N	S52.181Q	S52.225M	S52.244A	S52.262N	S52.291N	S52.324Q	S52.343K	S52.362Q	S52.389N	S52.515P	S52.552N	S52.601R	S52.629P
S52.042P	S52.121P	S52.181R	S52.225N	S52.244K	S52.262P	S52.291P	S52.324R	S52.343M	S52.362R	S52.389P	S52.515R	S52.552P	S52.602A	S52.691A
S52.042Q	S52.121Q	S52.182K	S52.225P	S52.244M	S52.262Q	S52.291Q	S52.325A	S52.343N	S52.363A	S52.389Q	S52.516A	S52.552Q	S52.602K	S52.691K
S52.042R	S52.121R	S52.182M	S52.225Q	S52.244N	S52.262R	S52.291R	S52.325K	S52.343P	S52.363K	S52.389R	S52.516K	S52.552R	S52.602M	S52.691M
S52.043K	S52.122A	S52.182N	S52.225R	S52.244P	S52.263A	S52.292A	S52.325N	S52.343Q	S52.363M	S52.391A	S52.516M	S52.559A	S52.602P	S52.691N
S52.043M	S52.122K	S52.182P	S52.226A	S52.244Q	S52.263K	S52.292K	S52.325P	S52.343R	S52.363P	S52.391K	S52.516P	S52.559K	S52.602Q	S52.691P
S52.043N	S52.122M	S52.182Q	S52.226K	S52.244R	S52.263M	S52.292M	S52.325Q	S52.344A	S52.363Q	S52.391M	S52.516R	S52.559M	S52.602R	S52.691Q
S52.043P	S52.122N	S52.182R	S52.226M	S52.245A	S52.263N	S52.292N	S52.325R	S52.344K	S52.363R	S52.391N	S52.521A	S52.559N	S52.609A	S52.692A
S52.043Q	S52.122P	S52.189K	S52.226N	S52.245K	S52.263P	S52.292P	S52.326A	S52.344M	S52.364A	S52.391P	S52.521K	S52.559P	S52.609K	S52.692K
S52.043R	S52.122Q	S52.189M	S52.226P	S52.245M	S52.263Q	S52.292Q	S52.326K	S52.344N	S52.364K	S52.391Q	S52.521P	S52.559Q	S52.609M	S52.692M
S52.044K	S52.122R	S52.189N	S52.226Q	S52.245N	S52.263R	S52.292R	S52.326M	S52.344P	S52.364M	S52.391R	S52.522A	S52.561A	S52.609P	S52.692N
S52.044M	S52.123K	S52.189P	S52.226R	S52.245P	S52.264A	S52.299A	S52.326N	S52.344Q	S52.364N	S52.392A	S52.522K	S52.561K	S52.609Q	S52.692P
S52.044N	S52.123M	S52.189R	S52.231A	S52.245Q	S52.264K	S52.299K	S52.326P	S52.344R	S52.364P	S52.392K	S52.522P	S52.561M	S52.609R	S52.692Q
S52.044P	S52.123N	S52.201A	S52.231K	S52.245R	S52.264M	S52.299M	S52.326Q	S52.345A	S52.364Q	S52.392M	S52.529A	S52.561N	S52.611A	S52.692R
S52.044Q	S52.123P	S52.201K	S52.231M	S52.246A	S52.264N	S52.299N	S52.326R	S52.345K	S52.364R	S52.392N	S52.529K	S52.561P	S52.611K	S52.699A
S52.044R	S52.123Q	S52.201M	S52.231N	S52.246K	S52.264P	S52.299P	S52.331A	S52.345M	S52.365A	S52.392P	S52.529P	S52.561Q	S52.611M	S52.699K
S52.045K	S52.123R	S52.201N	S52.231P	S52.246M	S52.264Q	S52.299Q	S52.331K	S52.345N	S52.365K	S52.392Q	S52.531A	S52.562A	S52.611P	S52.699P
S52.045M	S52.124K	S52.201P	S52.231Q	S52.246N	S52.264R	S52.299R	S52.331N	S52.345P	S52.365N	S52.392R	S52.531K	S52.562K	S52.611Q	S52.699Q
S52.045N	S52.124M	S52.201Q	S52.231R	S52.246P	S52.265A	S52.301A	S52.331P	S52.345Q	S52.365P	S52.399A	S52.531N	S52.562M	S52.611R	S52.90XA
S52.045P	S52.124N	S52.201R	S52.232A	S52.246Q	S52.265K	S52.301K	S52.331Q	S52.345R	S52.365Q	S52.399K	S52.531P	S52.562N	S52.612A	S52.90XK
S52.045Q	S52.124P	S52.202A	S52.232K	S52.246R	S52.265M	S52.301M	S52.331R	S52.346A	S52.365R	S52.399M	S52.531Q	S52.562P	S52.612K	S52.90XM
S52.045R	S52.124Q	S52.202K	S52.232M	S52.251A	S52.265N	S52.301N	S52.332A	S52.346K	S52.366A	S52.399N	S52.531R	S52.562Q	S52.612M	S52.90XN
S52.046K	S52.124R	S52.202M	S52.232N	S52.251K	S52.265P	S52.301P	S52.332K	S52.346M	S52.366K	S52.399P	S52.532A	S52.569A	S52.612P	S52.90XP
S52.046M	S52.125K	S52.202N	S52.232P	S52.251M	S52.265Q	S52.301Q	S52.332M	S52.346N	S52.366N	S52.399Q	S52.532K	S52.569K	S52.612Q	S52.90XR
S52.046N	S52.125M	S52.202P	S52.232Q	S52.251N	S52.265R	S52.301R	S52.332N	S52.346P	S52.366P	S52.399R	S52.532M	S52.569M	S52.612R	S52.91XA
S52.046P	S52.125N	S52.202Q	S52.232R	S52.251P	S52.266A	S52.302A	S52.332P	S52.346Q	S52.366Q	S52.501A	S52.532N	S52.569N	S52.613A	S52.91XK
S52.046Q	S52.125P	S52.202R	S52.233A	S52.251Q	S52.266K	S52.302K	S52.332Q	S52.346R	S52.366R	S52.501K	S52.532P	S52.569P	S52.613K	S52.91XM
S52.046R	S52.125Q	S52.209A	S52.233K	S52.251R	S52.266M	S52.302M	S52.332R	S52.351A	S52.371A	S52.501M	S52.532Q	S52.569Q	S52.613M	S52.91XN
S52.091K	S52.125R	S52.209K	S52.233M	S52.252A	S52.266N	S52.302N	S52.333A	S52.351K	S52.371K	S52.501N	S52.532R	S52.571A	S52.613P	S52.91XP
S52.091M	S52.126K	S52.209M	S52.233N	S52.252K	S52.266P	S52.302P	S52.333K	S52.351M	S52.371N	S52.501P	S52.539A	S52.571K	S52.613Q	S52.91XR
S52.091N	S52.126M	S52.209N	S52.233P	S52.252M	S52.266Q	S52.302Q	S52.333N	S52.351N	S52.371P	S52.501Q	S52.539K	S52.571M		S52.92XA
S52.091P	S52.126N	S52.209P	S52.233R	S52.252N	S52.266R	S52.302R	S52.333P	S52.351P	S52.371Q	S52.501R	S52.539N	S52.571N		S52.92XK
S52.091Q	S52.126P	S52.209Q	S52.234A	S52.252P	S52.271K	S52.309A	S52.333Q	S52.351R		S52.502A	S52.539P	S52.571P		S52.92XM
S52.092K	S52.126Q	S52.209R	S52.234K	S52.252Q	S52.271M	S52.309K	S52.333R	S52.352A		S52.502K		S52.571Q		S52.92XN
S52.092M	S52.126R	S52.211A	S52.234M	S52.252R	S52.271N	S52.309M	S52.334A	S52.352K		S52.502M		S52.572A		S52.92XP
S52.092N	S52.131K	S52.211K	S52.234N	S52.253A	S52.271P	S52.309N	S52.334K	S52.352M		S52.502P		S52.572K		S52.92XR
S52.092P	S52.131M	S52.211P	S52.234P	S52.253K	S52.271Q	S52.309P	S52.334N	S52.352N		S52.502Q				S55.001A
S52.092Q	S52.131N	S52.212A	S52.234R	S52.253N	S52.271R	S52.309Q	S52.334P	S52.352P		S52.502R				
S52.099K	S52.131P	S52.212K	S52.235A	S52.253P	S52.272M	S52.309R		S52.352Q		S52.509K				
S52.099M	S52.131Q	S52.212P	S52.235K	S52.253Q	S52.272N	S52.311A		S52.352R		S52.509M				
S52.099N	S52.131R	S52.219A			S52.272P	S52.311K		S52.353A						
	S52.132K					S52.311P		S52.353K						
	S52.132M													

Complication or Comorbidity (CC) (cont.) - Based on CMS data

S55.002A	S56.821A	S59.092P	S59.239K	S62.034B	S62.141P	S62.182P	S62.243P	S62.311P	S62.336K	S62.361B	S62.513P	S62.615K	S62.640B	S62.664P
S55.009A	S56.822A	S59.099A	S59.239P	S62.034K	S62.142B	S62.183B	S62.244B	S62.312B	S62.336P	S62.361K	S62.514B	S62.615P	S62.640K	S62.665B
S55.011A	S56.829A	S59.099K	S59.241A	S62.034P	S62.142K	S62.183K	S62.244K	S62.312K	S62.337B	S62.361P	S62.514K	S62.616B	S62.640P	S62.665K
S55.012A	S56.921A	S59.099P	S59.241K	S62.035B	S62.142P	S62.183P	S62.244P	S62.312P	S62.337K	S62.362B	S62.514P	S62.616K	S62.641B	S62.665P
S55.019A	S56.922A	S59.101K	S59.241P	S62.035K	S62.143B	S62.184B	S62.245B	S62.313B	S62.337K	S62.362K	S62.515B	S62.616P	S62.641K	S62.666B
S55.091A	S56.929A	S59.101P	S59.242A	S62.035P	S62.143P	S62.184K	S62.245K	S62.313K	S62.337K	S62.362P	S62.515K	S62.617B	S62.641P	S62.666K
S55.092A	S58.011A	S59.102A	S59.242K	S62.036B	S62.144B	S62.184P	S62.245P	S62.313P	S62.338B	S62.363B	S62.515P	S62.617K	S62.642B	S62.666P
S55.099A	S58.012A	S59.102P	S59.242P	S62.036K	S62.144K	S62.185B	S62.246B	S62.314B	S62.338K	S62.363K	S62.516B	S62.617P	S62.642K	S62.667B
S55.101A	S58.019A	S59.109K	S59.249A	S62.036P	S62.144P	S62.185K	S62.246K	S62.314K	S62.338P	S62.363P	S62.516K	S62.618B	S62.642P	S62.667K
S55.102A	S58.021A	S59.109P	S59.249K	S62.101B	S62.145B	S62.185P	S62.246P	S62.314P	S62.339B	S62.364B	S62.516P	S62.618K	S62.643B	S62.667P
S55.109A	S58.022A	S59.111P	S59.249P	S62.101K	S62.145K	S62.186B	S62.251B	S62.315B	S62.339K	S62.364K	S62.521B	S62.618P	S62.643K	S62.668B
S55.111A	S58.029A	S59.112K	S59.291A	S62.101P	S62.145P	S62.186K	S62.251K	S62.315K	S62.339K	S62.364P	S62.521K	S62.619B	S62.643P	S62.668K
S55.112A	S58.111A	S59.112P	S59.291K	S62.102B	S62.146B	S62.186P	S62.251P	S62.315P	S62.340B	S62.365B	S62.521P	S62.619K	S62.644B	S62.668P
S55.119A	S58.112A	S59.119K	S59.291P	S62.102K	S62.146K	S62.201B	S62.252B	S62.316B	S62.340K	S62.365K	S62.522B	S62.619P	S62.644K	S62.669B
S55.191A	S58.119A	S59.119P	S59.292A	S62.102P	S62.146P	S62.201K	S62.252K	S62.316K	S62.340P	S62.365P	S62.522K	S62.620B	S62.644P	S62.669K
S55.192A	S58.121A	S59.121K	S59.292K	S62.109B	S62.151B	S62.201P	S62.252P	S62.316P	S62.341B	S62.366B	S62.522P	S62.620K	S62.645B	S62.669P
S55.199A	S58.122A	S59.121P	S59.292P	S62.109K	S62.151K	S62.202B	S62.253B	S62.317B	S62.341K	S62.366K	S62.523B	S62.620P	S62.645K	S62.90XB
S55.201A	S58.129A	S59.122K	S59.299A	S62.109P	S62.151P	S62.202K	S62.253K	S62.317K	S62.341P	S62.366P	S62.523K	S62.621B	S62.645P	S62.90XK
S55.202A	S58.911A	S59.122P	S59.299K	S62.111A	S62.152B	S62.202P	S62.253P	S62.317P	S62.342B	S62.367B	S62.523P	S62.621K	S62.646B	S62.90XP
S55.209A	S58.912A	S59.129K	S59.299P	S62.111K	S62.152K	S62.209B	S62.254B	S62.318B	S62.342K	S62.367K	S62.524B	S62.621P	S62.646K	S62.91XB
S55.211A	S58.919A	S59.129P	S62.001B	S62.111P	S62.152P	S62.209K	S62.254K	S62.318K	S62.342P	S62.367P	S62.524K	S62.622B	S62.646P	S62.91XK
S55.212A	S58.921A	S59.131K	S62.001K	S62.112B	S62.153B	S62.209P	S62.254P	S62.318P	S62.343B	S62.368B	S62.524P	S62.622K	S62.647B	S62.91XP
S55.219A	S58.922A	S59.131P	S62.001P	S62.112K	S62.153K	S62.211B	S62.255B	S62.319B	S62.343K	S62.368K	S62.525B	S62.622P	S62.647K	S62.92XB
S55.291A	S58.929A	S59.132K	S62.002B	S62.112P	S62.153P	S62.211K	S62.255K	S62.319K	S62.343P	S62.368P	S62.525K	S62.623B	S62.647P	S62.92XK
S55.292A	S59.001A	S59.132P	S62.002K	S62.113B	S62.154B	S62.211P	S62.255P	S62.319P	S62.344B	S62.369B	S62.525P	S62.623K	S62.648B	S62.92XP
S55.299A	S59.001K	S59.139K	S62.002P	S62.113K	S62.154K	S62.212B	S62.256B	S62.320B	S62.344K	S62.369K	S62.526B	S62.623P	S62.648K	S65.001A
S55.801A	S59.001P	S59.139P	S62.009B	S62.113P	S62.154P	S62.212K	S62.256K	S62.320K	S62.344P	S62.369P	S62.526K	S62.624B	S62.648P	S65.002A
S55.802A	S59.002A	S59.141K	S62.009K	S62.114B	S62.155B	S62.212P	S62.256P	S62.320P	S62.345B	S62.390B	S62.526P	S62.624K	S62.649B	S65.009A
S55.809A	S59.002K	S59.141P	S62.009P	S62.114K	S62.155K	S62.213B	S62.291B	S62.321B	S62.345K	S62.390K	S62.600B	S62.624P	S62.649K	S65.011A
S55.811A	S59.002P	S59.142K	S62.011B	S62.114P	S62.155P	S62.213K	S62.291K	S62.321K	S62.345P	S62.390P	S62.600K	S62.625B	S62.649P	S65.012A
S55.812A	S59.009A	S59.142P	S62.011K	S62.115B	S62.156B	S62.213P	S62.291P	S62.321P	S62.346B	S62.391B	S62.600P	S62.625K	S62.650B	S65.019A
S55.819A	S59.009K	S59.149K	S62.011P	S62.115K	S62.156K	S62.221B	S62.292B	S62.322B	S62.346K	S62.391K	S62.601B	S62.625P	S62.650K	S65.091A
S55.891A	S59.009P	S59.149P	S62.012B	S62.115P	S62.156P	S62.221K	S62.292K	S62.322K	S62.346P	S62.391P	S62.601K	S62.626B	S62.650P	S65.092A
S55.892A	S59.011A	S59.191K	S62.012K	S62.116B	S62.161B	S62.221P	S62.292P	S62.322P	S62.347B	S62.392B	S62.601P	S62.626K	S62.651B	S65.099A
S55.899A	S59.011K	S59.191P	S62.012P	S62.116K	S62.161K	S62.222B	S62.299B	S62.323B	S62.347K	S62.392K	S62.602B	S62.626P	S62.651K	S65.101A
S55.901A	S59.011P	S59.192K	S62.013B	S62.116P	S62.161P	S62.222K	S62.299K	S62.323K	S62.347P	S62.392P	S62.602K	S62.627B	S62.651P	S65.102A
S55.902A	S59.012A	S59.192P	S62.013K	S62.121B	S62.162B	S62.222P	S62.299P	S62.323P	S62.348B	S62.393B	S62.602P	S62.627K	S62.652B	S65.109A
S55.909A	S59.012K	S59.199K	S62.013P	S62.121K	S62.162K	S62.223B	S62.300B	S62.324B	S62.348K	S62.393K	S62.603B	S62.627P	S62.652K	S65.111A
S55.911A	S59.012P	S59.199P	S62.014B	S62.121P	S62.162P	S62.223K	S62.300K	S62.324K	S62.348P	S62.393P	S62.603K	S62.628B	S62.652P	S65.112A
S55.912A	S59.019A	S59.201A	S62.014K	S62.122B	S62.163B	S62.223P	S62.300P	S62.324P	S62.349B	S62.394B	S62.603P	S62.628K	S62.653B	S65.119A
S55.919A	S59.019K	S59.201K	S62.014P	S62.122K	S62.163K	S62.224B	S62.301B	S62.325B	S62.349K	S62.394K	S62.604B	S62.628P	S62.653K	S65.191A
S55.991A	S59.019P	S59.201P	S62.015B	S62.122P	S62.163P	S62.224K	S62.301K	S62.325K	S62.349P	S62.394P	S62.604K	S62.629B	S62.653P	S65.192A
S55.992A	S59.021A	S59.202A	S62.015K	S62.123B	S62.164B	S62.224P	S62.301P	S62.325P	S62.350B	S62.395B	S62.604P	S62.629K	S62.654B	S65.199A
S55.999A	S59.021K	S59.202K	S62.015P	S62.123K	S62.164K	S62.225B	S62.302B	S62.326B	S62.350K	S62.395K	S62.605B	S62.629P	S62.654K	S65.201A
S56.021A	S59.021P	S59.202P	S62.016B	S62.123P	S62.164P	S62.225K	S62.302K	S62.326K	S62.350P	S62.395P	S62.605K	S62.630B	S62.654P	S65.202A
S56.022A	S59.022A	S59.209K	S62.016K	S62.124B	S62.165B	S62.225P	S62.302P	S62.326P	S62.351B	S62.396B	S62.605P	S62.630K	S62.655B	S65.209A
S56.029A	S59.022K	S59.209P	S62.016P	S62.124K	S62.165K	S62.226B	S62.303B	S62.327B	S62.351K	S62.396K	S62.606B	S62.630P	S62.655K	S65.211A
S56.121A	S59.022P	S59.209K	S62.021B	S62.124P	S62.165P	S62.226K	S62.303K	S62.327K	S62.351P	S62.396P	S62.606K	S62.631B	S62.655P	S65.212A
S56.122A	S59.029A	S59.209P	S62.021K	S62.125B	S62.166B	S62.226P	S62.303P	S62.327P	S62.352B	S62.397B	S62.606P	S62.631K	S62.656B	S65.219A
S56.123A	S59.029K	S59.211A	S62.021P	S62.125K	S62.166K	S62.231B	S62.303P	S62.328B	S62.352K	S62.397K	S62.607B	S62.631P	S62.656K	S65.291A
S56.124A	S59.029P	S59.211K	S62.022B	S62.125P	S62.166P	S62.231K	S62.304B	S62.328K	S62.352P	S62.397P	S62.607K	S62.632B	S62.656P	S65.292A
S56.125A	S59.031A	S59.211P	S62.022K	S62.126B	S62.171B	S62.231P	S62.304K	S62.328P	S62.353B	S62.398B	S62.607P	S62.632K	S62.657B	S65.299A
S56.126A	S59.031K	S59.212A	S62.022P	S62.126K	S62.171K	S62.232B	S62.304P	S62.329B	S62.353K	S62.398K	S62.608B	S62.632P	S62.657K	S65.301A
S56.127A	S59.031P	S59.212K	S62.023B	S62.126P	S62.171P	S62.232K	S62.305B	S62.329K	S62.353P	S62.398P	S62.608K	S62.633B	S62.657P	S65.302A
S56.128A	S59.032A	S59.212P	S62.023K	S62.131B	S62.172B	S62.232P	S62.305K	S62.329P	S62.354B	S62.399B	S62.608P	S62.633K	S62.658B	S65.309A
S56.129A	S59.032K	S59.219A	S62.023P	S62.131K	S62.172K	S62.233B	S62.305P	S62.330B	S62.354K	S62.399K	S62.609B	S62.633P	S62.658K	S65.311A
S56.221A	S59.032P	S59.219K	S62.024B	S62.131P	S62.172P	S62.233K	S62.306B	S62.330K	S62.354P	S62.399P	S62.609K	S62.634B	S62.658P	S65.312A
S56.222A	S59.039A	S59.219P	S62.024K	S62.132B	S62.173B	S62.233P	S62.306K	S62.330P	S62.355B	S62.501B	S62.609P	S62.634K	S62.659B	S65.319A
S56.229A	S59.039K	S59.221A	S62.024P	S62.132K	S62.173K	S62.234B	S62.306P	S62.331B	S62.355K	S62.501K	S62.610B	S62.634P	S62.659K	S65.391A
S56.321A	S59.039P	S59.221K	S62.025B	S62.132P	S62.173P	S62.234K	S62.307B	S62.331K	S62.355P	S62.501P	S62.610K	S62.635B	S62.659P	S65.392A
S56.322A	S59.041A	S59.221P	S62.025K	S62.133B	S62.174B	S62.234P	S62.307K	S62.331P	S62.356B	S62.502B	S62.610P	S62.635K	S62.660B	S65.399A
S56.329A	S59.041K	S59.222A	S62.025P	S62.133K	S62.174K	S62.235B	S62.307P	S62.332B	S62.356K	S62.502K	S62.611B	S62.635P	S62.660K	S65.401A
S56.421A	S59.041P	S59.222K	S62.026B	S62.133P	S62.174P	S62.235K	S62.308B	S62.332K	S62.356P	S62.502P	S62.611K	S62.636B	S62.660P	S65.402A
S56.422A	S59.042A	S59.222P	S62.026K	S62.134B	S62.175B	S62.235P	S62.308K	S62.332P	S62.357B	S62.509B	S62.611P	S62.636K	S62.661B	S65.409A
S56.423A	S59.042K	S59.229A	S62.026P	S62.134K	S62.175K	S62.236B	S62.308P	S62.333B	S62.357K	S62.509K	S62.612B	S62.636P	S62.661K	S65.411A
S56.424A	S59.042P	S59.229K	S62.031B	S62.134P	S62.175P	S62.236K	S62.309B	S62.333K	S62.357P	S62.509P	S62.612K	S62.637B	S62.661P	S65.412A
S56.425A	S59.049A	S59.229P	S62.031K	S62.135B	S62.176B	S62.236P	S62.309K	S62.333P	S62.358B	S62.511B	S62.612P	S62.637K	S62.662B	S65.419A
S56.426A	S59.049K	S59.231A	S62.031P	S62.135K	S62.176K	S62.241B	S62.309P	S62.334B	S62.358K	S62.511K	S62.613B	S62.637P	S62.662K	S65.491A
S56.427A	S59.049P	S59.231K	S62.032B	S62.135P	S62.176P	S62.241K	S62.310B	S62.334K	S62.358P	S62.511P	S62.613K	S62.638B	S62.662P	S65.492A
S56.428A	S59.091A	S59.231P	S62.032K	S62.136B	S62.181B	S62.241P	S62.310K	S62.334P	S62.359B	S62.512B	S62.613P	S62.638K	S62.663B	S65.499A
S56.429A	S59.091K	S59.232A	S62.032P	S62.136K	S62.181K	S62.242B	S62.310P	S62.335B	S62.359K	S62.512K	S62.614B	S62.638P	S62.663K	S65.500A
S56.521A	S59.091P	S59.232K	S62.033B	S62.136P	S62.181P	S62.242K	S62.311B	S62.335K	S62.359P	S62.512P	S62.614K	S62.639B	S62.663P	S65.501A
S56.522A	S59.092A	S59.232P	S62.033K	S62.141B	S62.182B	S62.242P	S62.311K	S62.336B	S62.360B	S62.513B	S62.614P	S62.639K	S62.664B	S65.502A
S56.529A	S59.092K	S59.239A	S62.033P	S62.141K	S62.182B	S62.242P	S62.311K	S62.336B	S62.360P	S62.513K	S62.615B	S62.639P	S62.664K	S65.503A

Complication or Comorbidity (CC) (cont.) - Based on CMS data

S65.504A	S66.521A	S72.022N	S72.042Q	S72.066K	S72.115P	S72.134K	S72.22XQ	S72.324R	S72.345M	S72.365P	S72.414Q	S72.433M	S72.451R	S72.466N
S65.505A	S66.522A	S72.022P	S72.042R	S72.066M	S72.115Q	S72.134M	S72.22XR	S72.325K	S72.345N	S72.365Q	S72.414R	S72.433N	S72.452A	S72.466P
S65.506A	S66.523A	S72.022Q	S72.043K	S72.066N	S72.115R	S72.134N	S72.23XA	S72.325M	S72.345P	S72.365R	S72.415A	S72.433P	S72.452K	S72.466Q
S65.507A	S66.524A	S72.022R	S72.043M	S72.066P	S72.116A	S72.134P	S72.23XK	S72.325N	S72.345Q	S72.366K	S72.415K	S72.433Q	S72.452M	S72.466R
S65.508A	S66.525A	S72.023K	S72.043N	S72.066Q	S72.116K	S72.134Q	S72.23XM	S72.325P	S72.345R	S72.366M	S72.415M	S72.433R	S72.452N	S72.471A
S65.509A	S66.526A	S72.023M	S72.043P	S72.066R	S72.116M	S72.134R	S72.23XN	S72.325Q	S72.346K	S72.366N	S72.415N	S72.434A	S72.452P	S72.471K
S65.510A	S66.527A	S72.023N	S72.043Q	S72.091K	S72.116N	S72.135A	S72.23XP	S72.325R	S72.346M	S72.366P	S72.415P	S72.434K	S72.452Q	S72.471P
S65.511A	S66.528A	S72.023P	S72.043R	S72.091M	S72.116P	S72.135K	S72.23XQ	S72.326K	S72.346N	S72.366Q	S72.415Q	S72.434M	S72.452R	S72.472A
S65.512A	S66.529A	S72.023Q	S72.044K	S72.091N	S72.116Q	S72.135M	S72.23XR	S72.326M	S72.346P	S72.366R	S72.415R	S72.434N	S72.453A	S72.472K
S65.513A	S66.821A	S72.023R	S72.044M	S72.091P	S72.116R	S72.135N	S72.24XA	S72.326N	S72.346Q	S72.391K	S72.416A	S72.434P	S72.453K	S72.472P
S65.514A	S66.822A	S72.024K	S72.044N	S72.091Q	S72.121A	S72.135P	S72.24XK	S72.326P	S72.346R	S72.391M	S72.416K	S72.434Q	S72.453M	S72.479A
S65.515A	S66.829A	S72.024M	S72.044P	S72.091R	S72.121K	S72.135Q	S72.24XM	S72.326Q	S72.351K	S72.391N	S72.416M	S72.434R	S72.453N	S72.479K
S65.516A	S66.921A	S72.024N	S72.044Q	S72.092K	S72.121M	S72.135R	S72.24XN	S72.326R	S72.351M	S72.391P	S72.416N	S72.435A	S72.453P	S72.479P
S65.517A	S66.922A	S72.024P	S72.044R	S72.092M	S72.121N	S72.136A	S72.24XP	S72.331K	S72.351N	S72.391Q	S72.416P	S72.435K	S72.453Q	S72.491A
S65.518A	S66.929A	S72.024Q	S72.045K	S72.092N	S72.121P	S72.136K	S72.24XQ	S72.331M	S72.351P	S72.391R	S72.416Q	S72.435M	S72.453R	S72.491K
S65.519A	S68.411A	S72.024R	S72.045M	S72.092P	S72.121Q	S72.136M	S72.24XR	S72.331N	S72.351Q	S72.392K	S72.416R	S72.435N	S72.454A	S72.491M
S65.590A	S68.412A	S72.025K	S72.045N	S72.092Q	S72.121R	S72.136N	S72.25XA	S72.331P	S72.351R	S72.392M	S72.421A	S72.435P	S72.454K	S72.491N
S65.591A	S68.419A	S72.025M	S72.045P	S72.092R	S72.122A	S72.136P	S72.25XK	S72.331Q	S72.352K	S72.392N	S72.421K	S72.435Q	S72.454M	S72.491P
S65.592A	S68.421A	S72.025N	S72.045Q	S72.099K	S72.122K	S72.136Q	S72.25XM	S72.331R	S72.352M	S72.392P	S72.421M	S72.435R	S72.454N	S72.491Q
S65.593A	S68.422A	S72.025P	S72.045R	S72.099M	S72.122M	S72.136R	S72.25XN	S72.332K	S72.352N	S72.392Q	S72.421N	S72.436A	S72.454P	S72.491R
S65.594A	S68.429A	S72.025Q	S72.046K	S72.099N	S72.122N	S72.141A	S72.25XP	S72.332M	S72.352P	S72.392R	S72.421P	S72.436K	S72.454Q	S72.492A
S65.595A	S68.711A	S72.025R	S72.046M	S72.099P	S72.122P	S72.141K	S72.25XQ	S72.332N	S72.352Q	S72.399K	S72.421Q	S72.436M	S72.454R	S72.492K
S65.596A	S68.712A	S72.026K	S72.046N	S72.099Q	S72.122Q	S72.141M	S72.25XR	S72.332P	S72.352R	S72.399M	S72.421R	S72.436N	S72.455A	S72.492M
S65.597A	S68.719A	S72.026M	S72.046P	S72.099R	S72.122R	S72.141N	S72.26XA	S72.332Q	S72.353K	S72.399N	S72.422A	S72.436P	S72.455K	S72.492N
S65.598A	S68.721A	S72.026N	S72.046Q	S72.101K	S72.123A	S72.141P	S72.26XK	S72.332R	S72.353M	S72.399P	S72.422K	S72.436Q	S72.455M	S72.492P
S65.599A	S68.722A	S72.026P	S72.046R	S72.101M	S72.123K	S72.141Q	S72.26XM	S72.333K	S72.353N	S72.399Q	S72.422M	S72.436R	S72.455N	S72.492Q
S65.801A	S68.729A	S72.026Q	S72.051K	S72.101N	S72.123M	S72.141R	S72.26XN	S72.333M	S72.353P	S72.399R	S72.422N	S72.441A	S72.455P	S72.492R
S65.802A	S72.001K	S72.026R	S72.051M	S72.101P	S72.123N	S72.142A	S72.26XP	S72.333N	S72.353Q	S72.401A	S72.422P	S72.441K	S72.455Q	S72.499A
S65.809A	S72.001M	S72.031K	S72.051N	S72.101Q	S72.123P	S72.142K	S72.26XQ	S72.333P	S72.353R	S72.401K	S72.422Q	S72.441M	S72.455R	S72.499K
S65.811A	S72.001N	S72.031M	S72.051P	S72.101R	S72.123Q	S72.142M	S72.26XR	S72.333Q	S72.354K	S72.401M	S72.422R	S72.441N	S72.456A	S72.499M
S65.812A	S72.001P	S72.031N	S72.051Q	S72.102K	S72.123R	S72.142N	S72.301A	S72.333R	S72.354M	S72.401N	S72.423A	S72.441P	S72.456K	S72.499N
S65.819A	S72.001Q	S72.031P	S72.051R	S72.102M	S72.124A	S72.142P	S72.301K	S72.334K	S72.354N	S72.401P	S72.423K	S72.441Q	S72.456M	S72.499P
S65.891A	S72.001R	S72.031Q	S72.052K	S72.102N	S72.124K	S72.142Q	S72.301M	S72.334M	S72.354P	S72.401Q	S72.423M	S72.441R	S72.456N	S72.499Q
S65.892A	S72.002K	S72.031R	S72.052M	S72.102P	S72.124M	S72.142R	S72.301N	S72.334N	S72.354Q	S72.401R	S72.423N	S72.442A	S72.456P	S72.499R
S65.899A	S72.002M	S72.032K	S72.052N	S72.102Q	S72.124N	S72.143A	S72.301P	S72.334P	S72.354R	S72.402A	S72.423P	S72.442K	S72.456Q	S72.8X1K
S65.901A	S72.002N	S72.032M	S72.052P	S72.102R	S72.124P	S72.143K	S72.301Q	S72.334Q	S72.355K	S72.402K	S72.423Q	S72.442M	S72.456R	S72.8X1M
S65.902A	S72.002P	S72.032N	S72.052Q	S72.109K	S72.124Q	S72.143M	S72.301R	S72.334R	S72.355M	S72.402M	S72.423R	S72.442N	S72.461A	S72.8X1N
S65.909A	S72.002Q	S72.032P	S72.052R	S72.109M	S72.124R	S72.143N	S72.302A	S72.335K	S72.355N	S72.402N	S72.424A	S72.442P	S72.461K	S72.8X1P
S65.911A	S72.002R	S72.032Q	S72.059K	S72.109N	S72.125A	S72.143P	S72.302K	S72.335M	S72.355P	S72.402P	S72.424K	S72.442Q	S72.461M	S72.8X1Q
S65.912A	S72.009K	S72.032R	S72.059M	S72.109P	S72.125K	S72.143Q	S72.302M	S72.335N	S72.355Q	S72.402Q	S72.424M	S72.442R	S72.461N	S72.8X1R
S65.919A	S72.009M	S72.033K	S72.059N	S72.109Q	S72.125M	S72.143R	S72.302N	S72.335P	S72.355R	S72.402R	S72.424N	S72.443A	S72.461P	S72.8X2K
S65.991A	S72.009N	S72.033M	S72.059P	S72.109R	S72.125N	S72.144A	S72.302P	S72.335Q	S72.356K	S72.409A	S72.424P	S72.443K	S72.461Q	S72.8X2M
S65.992A	S72.009P	S72.033N	S72.059Q	S72.111A	S72.125P	S72.144K	S72.302Q	S72.335R	S72.356M	S72.409K	S72.424Q	S72.443M	S72.461R	S72.8X2N
S65.999A	S72.009Q	S72.033P	S72.059R	S72.111K	S72.125Q	S72.144M	S72.302R	S72.336K	S72.356N	S72.409M	S72.424R	S72.443N	S72.462A	S72.8X2P
S66.021A	S72.009R	S72.033Q	S72.061K	S72.111M	S72.125R	S72.144N	S72.309A	S72.336M	S72.356P	S72.409N	S72.425A	S72.443P	S72.462K	S72.8X2Q
S66.022A	S72.011A	S72.033R	S72.061M	S72.111N	S72.126A	S72.144P	S72.309K	S72.336N	S72.356Q	S72.409P	S72.425K	S72.443Q	S72.462M	S72.8X2R
S66.029A	S72.011K	S72.034K	S72.061N	S72.111P	S72.126K	S72.144Q	S72.309M	S72.336P	S72.356R	S72.409Q	S72.425M	S72.443R	S72.462N	S72.8X9K
S66.120A	S72.011M	S72.034M	S72.061P	S72.111Q	S72.126M	S72.144R	S72.309N	S72.336Q	S72.361K	S72.409R	S72.425N	S72.444A	S72.462P	S72.8X9M
S66.121A	S72.011N	S72.034N	S72.061Q	S72.111R	S72.126N	S72.145A	S72.309P	S72.336R	S72.361M	S72.411A	S72.425P	S72.444K	S72.462Q	S72.8X9N
S66.122A	S72.011P	S72.034P	S72.061R	S72.112A	S72.126P	S72.145K	S72.309Q	S72.341K	S72.361N	S72.411K	S72.425Q	S72.444M	S72.462R	S72.8X9P
S66.123A	S72.011Q	S72.034Q	S72.062K	S72.112K	S72.126Q	S72.145M	S72.309R	S72.341M	S72.361P	S72.411M	S72.425R	S72.444N	S72.463A	S72.8X9Q
S66.124A	S72.011R	S72.034R	S72.062M	S72.112M	S72.126R	S72.145N	S72.321K	S72.341N	S72.361Q	S72.411N	S72.426A	S72.444P	S72.463K	S72.8X9R
S66.125A	S72.012A	S72.035K	S72.062N	S72.112N	S72.131A	S72.145P	S72.321M	S72.341P	S72.361R	S72.411P	S72.426K	S72.444Q	S72.463M	S72.90XK
S66.126A	S72.012K	S72.035M	S72.062P	S72.112P	S72.131K	S72.145Q	S72.321N	S72.341Q	S72.362K	S72.411Q	S72.426M	S72.444R	S72.463N	S72.90XM
S66.127A	S72.012M	S72.035N	S72.062Q	S72.112Q	S72.131M	S72.145R	S72.321P	S72.341R	S72.362M	S72.411R	S72.426N	S72.445A	S72.463P	S72.90XN
S66.128A	S72.012N	S72.035P	S72.062R	S72.112R	S72.131N	S72.146A	S72.321Q	S72.342K	S72.362N	S72.412A	S72.426P	S72.445K	S72.463Q	S72.90XP
S66.129A	S72.012P	S72.035Q	S72.063K	S72.113A	S72.131P	S72.146K	S72.321R	S72.342M	S72.362P	S72.412K	S72.426Q	S72.445M	S72.463R	S72.90XQ
S66.221A	S72.012Q	S72.035R	S72.063M	S72.113K	S72.131Q	S72.146M	S72.322K	S72.342N	S72.362Q	S72.412M	S72.426R	S72.445N	S72.464A	S72.90XR
S66.222A	S72.012R	S72.036K	S72.063N	S72.113M	S72.131R	S72.146N	S72.322M	S72.342P	S72.362R	S72.412N	S72.431A	S72.445P	S72.464K	S72.91XK
S66.229A	S72.019A	S72.036M	S72.063P	S72.113N	S72.132A	S72.146P	S72.322N	S72.342Q	S72.363K	S72.412P	S72.431K	S72.445Q	S72.464M	S72.91XM
S66.320A	S72.019K	S72.036N	S72.063Q	S72.113P	S72.132K	S72.146Q	S72.322P	S72.342R	S72.363M	S72.412Q	S72.431M	S72.445R	S72.464N	S72.91XN
S66.321A	S72.019M	S72.036P	S72.063R	S72.113Q	S72.132M	S72.146R	S72.322Q	S72.343K	S72.363N	S72.412R	S72.431N	S72.446A	S72.464P	S72.91XP
S66.322A	S72.019N	S72.036Q	S72.064K	S72.113R	S72.132N	S72.21XA	S72.322R	S72.343M	S72.363P	S72.413A	S72.431P	S72.446K	S72.464Q	S72.91XQ
S66.323A	S72.019P	S72.036R	S72.064M	S72.114A	S72.132P	S72.21XK	S72.323K	S72.343N	S72.363Q	S72.413K	S72.431Q	S72.446M	S72.464R	S72.91XR
S66.324A	S72.019Q	S72.041K	S72.064N	S72.114K	S72.132Q	S72.21XM	S72.323M	S72.343P	S72.363R	S72.413M	S72.431R	S72.446N	S72.465A	S72.92XK
S66.325A	S72.019R	S72.041M	S72.064P	S72.114M	S72.132R	S72.21XN	S72.323N	S72.343Q	S72.364K	S72.413N	S72.432A	S72.446P	S72.465K	S72.92XM
S66.326A	S72.021K	S72.041N	S72.064Q	S72.114N	S72.133A	S72.21XP	S72.323P	S72.343R	S72.364M	S72.413P	S72.432K	S72.446Q	S72.465M	S72.92XN
S66.327A	S72.021M	S72.041P	S72.064R	S72.114P	S72.133K	S72.21XQ	S72.323Q	S72.344K	S72.364N	S72.413Q	S72.432M	S72.446R	S72.465N	S72.92XP
S66.328A	S72.021N	S72.041Q	S72.065K	S72.114Q	S72.133M	S72.21XR	S72.323R	S72.344M	S72.364P	S72.413R	S72.432N	S72.451A	S72.465P	S72.92XQ
S66.329A	S72.021P	S72.041R	S72.065M	S72.114R	S72.133N	S72.22XA	S72.324K	S72.344N	S72.364Q	S72.414A	S72.432P	S72.451K	S72.465Q	S72.92XR
S66.421A	S72.021Q	S72.042K	S72.065N	S72.115A	S72.133P	S72.22XK	S72.324M	S72.344P	S72.364R	S72.414K	S72.432Q	S72.451M	S72.465R	S73.001A
S66.422A	S72.021R	S72.042M	S72.065P	S72.115K	S72.133Q	S72.22XM	S72.324N	S72.344Q	S72.365K	S72.414M	S72.432R	S72.451N	S72.466A	S73.002A
S66.429A	S72.022K	S72.042N	S72.065Q	S72.115M	S72.133R	S72.22XN	S72.324P	S72.344R	S72.365M	S72.414N	S72.433A	S72.451P	S72.466K	S73.003A
S66.520A	S72.022M	S72.042P	S72.065R	S72.115N	S72.134A	S72.22XP	S72.324Q	S72.345K	S72.365N	S72.414P	S72.433K	S72.451Q	S72.466M	S73.004A

Complication or Comorbidity (CC) (cont.) - Based on CMS data

S73.005A	S77.00XA	S79.132P	S82.013Q	S82.026A	S82.042C	S82.101P	S82.123K	S82.141Q	S82.156M	S82.223P	S82.242K	S82.256Q	S82.302C	S82.422N
S73.006A	S77.01XA	S79.139A	S82.013R	S82.026B	S82.042K	S82.101Q	S82.123M	S82.141R	S82.156N	S82.223Q	S82.242M	S82.256R	S82.302K	S82.422P
S73.011A	S77.02XA	S79.139K	S82.014A	S82.026C	S82.042M	S82.101R	S82.123N	S82.142A	S82.156P	S82.223R	S82.242N	S82.261A	S82.302M	S82.422Q
S73.012A	S77.10XA	S79.139P	S82.014B	S82.026K	S82.042N	S82.102A	S82.123P	S82.142K	S82.156Q	S82.224A	S82.242P	S82.261K	S82.302N	S82.422R
S73.013A	S77.11XA	S79.141A	S82.014C	S82.026M	S82.042P	S82.102K	S82.123Q	S82.142M	S82.156R	S82.224K	S82.242Q	S82.261M	S82.302P	S82.423K
S73.014A	S77.12XA	S79.141K	S82.014K	S82.026N	S82.042Q	S82.102M	S82.123R	S82.142N	S82.161A	S82.224M	S82.242R	S82.261N	S82.302Q	S82.423M
S73.015A	S78.011A	S79.141P	S82.014M	S82.026P	S82.042R	S82.102N	S82.124A	S82.142P	S82.161K	S82.224N	S82.243A	S82.261P	S82.302R	S82.423N
S73.016A	S78.012A	S79.142A	S82.014N	S82.026Q	S82.043A	S82.102P	S82.124K	S82.142Q	S82.161P	S82.224P	S82.243K	S82.261Q	S82.309B	S82.423P
S73.021A	S78.019A	S79.142K	S82.014P	S82.026R	S82.043B	S82.102Q	S82.124M	S82.142R	S82.162A	S82.224Q	S82.243M	S82.261R	S82.309C	S82.423Q
S73.022A	S78.021A	S79.142P	S82.014Q	S82.031A	S82.043C	S82.102R	S82.124N	S82.143A	S82.162K	S82.224R	S82.243N	S82.262A	S82.309K	S82.423R
S73.023A	S78.022A	S79.149A	S82.014R	S82.031B	S82.043K	S82.109A	S82.124P	S82.143K	S82.162P	S82.225A	S82.243P	S82.262K	S82.309M	S82.424K
S73.024A	S78.029A	S79.149K	S82.015A	S82.031C	S82.043M	S82.109K	S82.124Q	S82.143M	S82.169A	S82.225K	S82.243Q	S82.262M	S82.309N	S82.424M
S73.025A	S78.111A	S79.149P	S82.015B	S82.031K	S82.043N	S82.109M	S82.124R	S82.143N	S82.169K	S82.225M	S82.243R	S82.262N	S82.309P	S82.424N
S73.026A	S78.112A	S79.191A	S82.015C	S82.031M	S82.043P	S82.109N	S82.125A	S82.143P	S82.169P	S82.225N	S82.244A	S82.262P	S82.309Q	S82.424P
S73.031A	S78.119A	S79.191K	S82.015K	S82.031N	S82.043Q	S82.109P	S82.125K	S82.143Q	S82.191A	S82.225P	S82.244K	S82.262Q	S82.309R	S82.424Q
S73.032A	S78.121A	S79.191P	S82.015M	S82.031P	S82.043R	S82.109Q	S82.125M	S82.143R	S82.191K	S82.225Q	S82.244M	S82.262R	S82.311A	S82.424R
S73.033A	S78.122A	S79.192A	S82.015N	S82.031Q	S82.044A	S82.109R	S82.125N	S82.144A	S82.191M	S82.225R	S82.244N	S82.263A	S82.311K	S82.425K
S73.034A	S78.129A	S79.192K	S82.015P	S82.031R	S82.044B	S82.111A	S82.125P	S82.144K	S82.191N	S82.226A	S82.244P	S82.263K	S82.311P	S82.425M
S73.035A	S78.911A	S79.192P	S82.015Q	S82.032A	S82.044C	S82.111K	S82.125Q	S82.144M	S82.191P	S82.226K	S82.244Q	S82.263M	S82.312A	S82.425N
S73.036A	S78.912A	S79.199A	S82.015R	S82.032B	S82.044K	S82.111M	S82.125R	S82.144N	S82.191Q	S82.226M	S82.244R	S82.263N	S82.312K	S82.425P
S73.041A	S78.919A	S79.199K	S82.016A	S82.032C	S82.044M	S82.111N	S82.126A	S82.144P	S82.191R	S82.226N	S82.245A	S82.263P	S82.312P	S82.425Q
S73.042A	S78.921A	S79.199P	S82.016B	S82.032K	S82.044N	S82.111P	S82.126K	S82.144Q	S82.192A	S82.226P	S82.245K	S82.263Q	S82.319A	S82.425R
S73.043A	S78.922A	S82.001A	S82.016C	S82.032M	S82.044P	S82.111Q	S82.126M	S82.144R	S82.192K	S82.226Q	S82.245M	S82.263R	S82.319K	S82.426K
S73.044A	S78.929A	S82.001B	S82.016K	S82.032N	S82.044Q	S82.111R	S82.126N	S82.145A	S82.192M	S82.226R	S82.245N	S82.264A	S82.319P	S82.426M
S73.045A	S79.001K	S82.001C	S82.016M	S82.032P	S82.044R	S82.112A	S82.126P	S82.145K	S82.192N	S82.231A	S82.245P	S82.264K	S82.391B	S82.426N
S73.046A	S79.001P	S82.001K	S82.016N	S82.032Q	S82.045A	S82.112K	S82.126Q	S82.145M	S82.192P	S82.231K	S82.245Q	S82.264M	S82.391C	S82.426P
S75.201A	S79.002K	S82.001M	S82.016P	S82.032R	S82.045B	S82.112M	S82.126R	S82.145N	S82.192Q	S82.231M	S82.245R	S82.264N	S82.391K	S82.426Q
S75.202A	S79.002P	S82.001N	S82.016Q	S82.033A	S82.045C	S82.112N	S82.131A	S82.145P	S82.192R	S82.231N	S82.246A	S82.264P	S82.391M	S82.426R
S75.209A	S79.009K	S82.001P	S82.016R	S82.033B	S82.045K	S82.112P	S82.131K	S82.145Q	S82.199A	S82.231P	S82.246K	S82.264Q	S82.391N	S82.431K
S75.211A	S79.009P	S82.001Q	S82.021A	S82.033C	S82.045M	S82.112Q	S82.131M	S82.145R	S82.199K	S82.231Q	S82.246M	S82.264R	S82.391P	S82.431M
S75.212A	S79.011K	S82.001R	S82.021B	S82.033K	S82.045N	S82.112R	S82.131N	S82.146A	S82.199M	S82.231R	S82.246N	S82.265A	S82.391Q	S82.431N
S75.219A	S79.011P	S82.002A	S82.021C	S82.033M	S82.045P	S82.113A	S82.131P	S82.146K	S82.199N	S82.232A	S82.246P	S82.265K	S82.391R	S82.431P
S75.221A	S79.012K	S82.002B	S82.021K	S82.033N	S82.045Q	S82.113K	S82.131Q	S82.146M	S82.199P	S82.232K	S82.246Q	S82.265M	S82.392B	S82.431Q
S75.222A	S79.012P	S82.002C	S82.021M	S82.033P	S82.045R	S82.113M	S82.131R	S82.146N	S82.199Q	S82.232M	S82.246R	S82.265N	S82.392C	S82.431R
S75.229A	S79.019K	S82.002K	S82.021N	S82.033Q	S82.046A	S82.113N	S82.132A	S82.146P	S82.199R	S82.232N	S82.251A	S82.265P	S82.392K	S82.432K
S75.291A	S79.019P	S82.002M	S82.021P	S82.033R	S82.046B	S82.113P	S82.132K	S82.146Q	S82.201A	S82.232P	S82.251K	S82.265Q	S82.392M	S82.432M
S75.292A	S79.091K	S82.002N	S82.021Q	S82.034A	S82.046C	S82.113Q	S82.132M	S82.146R	S82.201K	S82.232Q	S82.251M	S82.265R	S82.392N	S82.432N
S75.299A	S79.091P	S82.002P	S82.021R	S82.034B	S82.046K	S82.113R	S82.132N	S82.151A	S82.201M	S82.232R	S82.251N	S82.266A	S82.392P	S82.432P
S75.801A	S79.092K	S82.002Q	S82.022A	S82.034C	S82.046M	S82.114A	S82.132P	S82.151K	S82.201N	S82.233A	S82.251P	S82.266K	S82.392Q	S82.432Q
S75.802A	S79.092P	S82.002R	S82.022B	S82.034K	S82.046N	S82.114K	S82.132Q	S82.151M	S82.201P	S82.233K	S82.251Q	S82.266M	S82.392R	S82.432R
S75.809A	S79.099K	S82.009A	S82.022C	S82.034M	S82.046P	S82.114M	S82.132R	S82.151N	S82.201Q	S82.233M	S82.251R	S82.266N	S82.399B	S82.433K
S75.811A	S79.099P	S82.009B	S82.022K	S82.034N	S82.046Q	S82.114N	S82.133A	S82.151P	S82.201R	S82.233N	S82.252A	S82.266P	S82.399C	S82.433M
S75.812A	S79.101A	S82.009C	S82.022M	S82.034P	S82.046R	S82.114P	S82.133K	S82.151Q	S82.202A	S82.233P	S82.252K	S82.266Q	S82.399K	S82.433N
S75.819A	S79.101K	S82.009K	S82.022N	S82.034Q	S82.091A	S82.114Q	S82.133M	S82.151R	S82.202K	S82.233Q	S82.252M	S82.266R	S82.399M	S82.433P
S75.891A	S79.101P	S82.009M	S82.022P	S82.034R	S82.091B	S82.114R	S82.133N	S82.152A	S82.202M	S82.233R	S82.252N	S82.291A	S82.399N	S82.433Q
S75.892A	S79.102A	S82.009N	S82.022Q	S82.035A	S82.091C	S82.115A	S82.133P	S82.152K	S82.202N	S82.234A	S82.252P	S82.291K	S82.399P	S82.433R
S75.899A	S79.102K	S82.009P	S82.022R	S82.035B	S82.091K	S82.115K	S82.133Q	S82.152M	S82.202P	S82.234K	S82.252Q	S82.291M	S82.399Q	S82.434K
S75.901A	S79.102P	S82.009Q	S82.023A	S82.035C	S82.091M	S82.115M	S82.133R	S82.152N	S82.202Q	S82.234M	S82.252R	S82.291N	S82.399R	S82.434M
S75.902A	S79.109A	S82.009R	S82.023B	S82.035K	S82.091N	S82.115N	S82.134A	S82.152P	S82.202R	S82.234N	S82.253A	S82.291P	S82.401K	S82.434N
S75.909A	S79.109K	S82.011A	S82.023C	S82.035M	S82.091P	S82.115P	S82.134K	S82.152Q	S82.209A	S82.234P	S82.253K	S82.291Q	S82.401M	S82.434P
S75.911A	S79.109P	S82.011B	S82.023K	S82.035N	S82.091Q	S82.115Q	S82.134M	S82.152R	S82.209K	S82.234Q	S82.253M	S82.291R	S82.401N	S82.434Q
S75.912A	S79.111A	S82.011C	S82.023M	S82.035P	S82.091R	S82.115R	S82.134N	S82.153A	S82.209M	S82.234R	S82.253N	S82.292A	S82.401P	S82.434R
S75.919A	S79.111K	S82.011K	S82.023N	S82.035Q	S82.092A	S82.116A	S82.134P	S82.153K	S82.209N	S82.235A	S82.253P	S82.292K	S82.401Q	S82.435K
S75.991A	S79.111P	S82.011M	S82.023P	S82.035R	S82.092B	S82.116K	S82.134Q	S82.153M	S82.209P	S82.235K	S82.253Q	S82.292M	S82.401R	S82.435M
S75.992A	S79.112A	S82.011N	S82.023Q	S82.036A	S82.092C	S82.116M	S82.134R	S82.153N	S82.209Q	S82.235M	S82.253R	S82.292N	S82.402K	S82.435N
S75.999A	S79.112K	S82.011P	S82.023R	S82.036B	S82.092K	S82.116N	S82.135A	S82.153P	S82.209R	S82.235N	S82.254A	S82.292P	S82.402M	S82.435P
S76.021A	S79.112P	S82.011Q	S82.024A	S82.036C	S82.092M	S82.116P	S82.135K	S82.153Q	S82.221A	S82.235P	S82.254K	S82.292Q	S82.402N	S82.435Q
S76.022A	S79.119A	S82.011R	S82.024B	S82.036K	S82.092N	S82.116Q	S82.135M	S82.153R	S82.221K	S82.235Q	S82.254M	S82.292R	S82.402P	S82.435R
S76.029A	S79.119K	S82.012A	S82.024C	S82.036M	S82.092P	S82.116R	S82.135N	S82.154A	S82.221M	S82.235R	S82.254N	S82.299A	S82.402Q	S82.436K
S76.121A	S79.119P	S82.012B	S82.024K	S82.036N	S82.092Q	S82.121A	S82.135P	S82.154K	S82.221N	S82.236A	S82.254P	S82.299K	S82.402R	S82.436M
S76.122A	S79.121A	S82.012C	S82.024M	S82.036P	S82.092R	S82.121K	S82.135Q	S82.154M	S82.221P	S82.236K	S82.254Q	S82.299M	S82.409K	S82.436N
S76.129A	S79.121K	S82.012K	S82.024N	S82.036Q	S82.099A	S82.121M	S82.135R	S82.154N	S82.221Q	S82.236M	S82.254R	S82.299N	S82.409M	S82.436P
S76.221A	S79.121P	S82.012M	S82.024P	S82.036R	S82.099B	S82.121N	S82.136A	S82.154P	S82.221R	S82.236N	S82.255A	S82.299P	S82.409N	S82.436Q
S76.222A	S79.122A	S82.012N	S82.024Q	S82.041A	S82.099C	S82.121P	S82.136K	S82.154Q	S82.222A	S82.236P	S82.255K	S82.299Q	S82.409P	S82.436R
S76.229A	S79.122K	S82.012P	S82.024R	S82.041B	S82.099K	S82.121Q	S82.136M	S82.154R	S82.222K	S82.236Q	S82.255M	S82.299R	S82.409Q	S82.441K
S76.321A	S79.122P	S82.012Q	S82.025A	S82.041C	S82.099M	S82.121R	S82.136N	S82.155A	S82.222M	S82.236R	S82.255N	S82.301B	S82.409R	S82.441M
S76.322A	S79.129A	S82.012R	S82.025B	S82.041K	S82.099N	S82.122A	S82.136P	S82.155K	S82.222N	S82.241A	S82.255P	S82.301C	S82.421K	S82.441N
S76.329A	S79.129K	S82.013A	S82.025C	S82.041M	S82.099P	S82.122K	S82.136Q	S82.155M	S82.222P	S82.241K	S82.255Q	S82.301K	S82.421M	S82.441P
S76.821A	S79.129P	S82.013B	S82.025K	S82.041N	S82.099Q	S82.122M	S82.136R	S82.155N	S82.222Q	S82.241M	S82.255R	S82.301M	S82.421N	S82.441Q
S76.822A	S79.131A	S82.013C	S82.025M	S82.041P	S82.099R	S82.122N	S82.141A	S82.155P	S82.222R	S82.241N	S82.256A	S82.301N	S82.421P	S82.441R
S76.829A	S79.131K	S82.013K	S82.025N	S82.041Q	S82.101A	S82.122P	S82.141K	S82.155Q	S82.223A	S82.241P	S82.256K	S82.301P	S82.421Q	S82.442K
S76.921A	S79.131P	S82.013M	S82.025P	S82.041R	S82.101K	S82.122Q	S82.141M	S82.155R	S82.223K	S82.241Q	S82.256M	S82.301Q	S82.421R	S82.442M
S76.922A	S79.132A	S82.013N	S82.025Q	S82.042A	S82.101M	S82.122R	S82.141N	S82.156A	S82.223M	S82.241R	S82.256N	S82.301R	S82.422K	S82.442N
S76.929A	S79.132K	S82.013P	S82.025R	S82.042B	S82.101N	S82.123A	S82.141P	S82.156K	S82.223N	S82.242A	S82.256P	S82.302B	S82.422M	S82.442P

Complication or Comorbidity (CC) (cont.) - Based on CMS data

S82.442Q	S82.463K	S82.55XB	S82.829K	S82.851Q	S82.866N	S82.899Q	S85.411A	S89.012P	S89.199K	S92.016B	S92.056P	S92.134K	S92.215B	S92.255P
S82.442R	S82.463M	S82.55XC	S82.829P	S82.851R	S82.866P	S82.899R	S85.412A	S89.019A	S89.199P	S92.016K	S92.061B	S92.134P	S92.215K	S92.256B
S82.443K	S82.463N	S82.55XK	S82.831K	S82.852B	S82.866Q	S82.90XB	S85.419A	S89.019K	S89.201K	S92.016P	S92.061K	S92.135B	S92.215P	S92.256K
S82.443M	S82.463P	S82.55XM	S82.831M	S82.852C	S82.866R	S82.90XC	S85.491A	S89.019P	S89.201P	S92.021B	S92.061P	S92.135K	S92.216B	S92.256P
S82.443N	S82.463Q	S82.55XN	S82.831N	S82.852K	S82.871B	S82.90XK	S85.492A	S89.021A	S89.202K	S92.021K	S92.062B	S92.135P	S92.216K	S92.301B
S82.443P	S82.463R	S82.55XP	S82.831P	S82.852M	S82.871C	S82.90XM	S85.499A	S89.021K	S89.202P	S92.021P	S92.062K	S92.136B	S92.216P	S92.301K
S82.443Q	S82.464K	S82.55XQ	S82.831Q	S82.852N	S82.871K	S82.90XN	S85.801A	S89.021P	S89.209K	S92.022B	S92.062P	S92.136K	S92.221B	S92.301P
S82.443R	S82.464M	S82.55XR	S82.831R	S82.852P	S82.871M	S82.90XP	S85.802A	S89.022A	S89.209P	S92.022K	S92.063B	S92.136P	S92.221K	S92.302B
S82.444K	S82.464N	S82.56XB	S82.832K	S82.852Q	S82.871N	S82.90XQ	S85.809A	S89.022K	S89.211K	S92.022P	S92.063K	S92.141B	S92.221P	S92.302K
S82.444M	S82.464P	S82.56XC	S82.832M	S82.852R	S82.871P	S82.90XR	S85.811A	S89.022P	S89.211P	S92.023B	S92.063P	S92.141K	S92.222B	S92.302P
S82.444N	S82.464Q	S82.56XK	S82.832N	S82.853B	S82.871Q	S82.91XB	S85.812A	S89.029A	S89.212K	S92.023K	S92.064B	S92.141P	S92.222K	S92.309B
S82.444P	S82.464R	S82.56XM	S82.832P	S82.853C	S82.871R	S82.91XC	S85.819A	S89.029K	S89.212P	S92.023P	S92.064K	S92.142B	S92.222P	S92.309K
S82.444Q	S82.465K	S82.56XN	S82.832Q	S82.853K	S82.872B	S82.91XK	S85.891A	S89.029P	S89.219K	S92.024B	S92.064P	S92.142K	S92.223B	S92.309P
S82.444R	S82.465M	S82.56XP	S82.832R	S82.853M	S82.872C	S82.91XM	S85.892A	S89.031A	S89.219P	S92.024K	S92.065B	S92.142P	S92.223K	S92.311B
S82.445K	S82.465N	S82.56XQ	S82.839K	S82.853N	S82.872K	S82.91XN	S85.899A	S89.031K	S89.221K	S92.024P	S92.065K	S92.143B	S92.223P	S92.311K
S82.445M	S82.465P	S82.56XR	S82.839M	S82.853P	S82.872M	S82.91XP	S85.901A	S89.031P	S89.221P	S92.025B	S92.065P	S92.143K	S92.224B	S92.311P
S82.445N	S82.465Q	S82.61XB	S82.839N	S82.853Q	S82.872N	S82.91XQ	S85.902A	S89.032A	S89.222K	S92.025K	S92.066B	S92.143P	S92.224K	S92.312B
S82.445P	S82.465R	S82.61XC	S82.839P	S82.853R	S82.872P	S82.91XR	S85.909A	S89.032K	S89.222P	S92.025P	S92.066K	S92.144B	S92.224P	S92.312K
S82.445Q	S82.466K	S82.61XK	S82.839Q	S82.854B	S82.872Q	S82.92XB	S85.911A	S89.032P	S89.229K	S92.026B	S92.066P	S92.144K	S92.225B	S92.312P
S82.445R	S82.466M	S82.61XM	S82.839R	S82.854C	S82.872R	S82.92XC	S85.912A	S89.039A	S89.229P	S92.026K	S92.101B	S92.144P	S92.225K	S92.313B
S82.446K	S82.466N	S82.61XN	S82.841B	S82.854K	S82.873B	S82.92XK	S85.919A	S89.039K	S89.291K	S92.026P	S92.101K	S92.145B	S92.225P	S92.313K
S82.446M	S82.466P	S82.61XP	S82.841C	S82.854M	S82.873C	S82.92XM	S85.991A	S89.039P	S89.291P	S92.031B	S92.101P	S92.145K	S92.226B	S92.313P
S82.446N	S82.466Q	S82.61XQ	S82.841K	S82.854N	S82.873K	S82.92XN	S85.992A	S89.041A	S89.292K	S92.031K	S92.102B	S92.145P	S92.226K	S92.314B
S82.446P	S82.466R	S82.61XR	S82.841M	S82.854P	S82.873M	S82.92XP	S85.999A	S89.041K	S89.292P	S92.031P	S92.102K	S92.146B	S92.226P	S92.314K
S82.446Q	S82.491K	S82.62XB	S82.841N	S82.854Q	S82.873N	S82.92XQ	S86.021A	S89.041P	S89.299K	S92.032B	S92.102P	S92.146K	S92.231B	S92.314P
S82.446R	S82.491M	S82.62XC	S82.841P	S82.854R	S82.873P	S82.92XR	S86.022A	S89.042A	S89.299P	S92.032K	S92.109B	S92.146P	S92.231K	S92.315B
S82.451K	S82.491N	S82.62XK	S82.841Q	S82.855B	S82.873Q	S85.101A	S86.029A	S89.042K	S89.301K	S92.032P	S92.109K	S92.151B	S92.231P	S92.315K
S82.451M	S82.491P	S82.62XM	S82.841R	S82.855C	S82.873R	S85.102A	S86.121A	S89.042P	S89.301P	S92.033B	S92.109P	S92.151K	S92.232B	S92.315P
S82.451N	S82.491Q	S82.62XN	S82.842B	S82.855K	S82.874B	S85.109A	S86.122A	S89.049A	S89.302K	S92.033K	S92.111B	S92.151P	S92.232K	S92.316B
S82.451P	S82.491R	S82.62XP	S82.842C	S82.855M	S82.874C	S85.111A	S86.129A	S89.049K	S89.302P	S92.033P	S92.111K	S92.152B	S92.232P	S92.316K
S82.451Q	S82.492K	S82.62XQ	S82.842K	S82.855N	S82.874K	S85.112A	S86.221A	S89.049P	S89.309K	S92.034B	S92.111P	S92.152K	S92.233B	S92.316P
S82.451R	S82.492M	S82.62XR	S82.842M	S82.855P	S82.874M	S85.119A	S86.222A	S89.091A	S89.309P	S92.034K	S92.112B	S92.152P	S92.233K	S92.321B
S82.452K	S82.492N	S82.63XB	S82.842N	S82.855Q	S82.874N	S85.121A	S86.229A	S89.091K	S89.311K	S92.034P	S92.112K	S92.153B	S92.233P	S92.321K
S82.452M	S82.492P	S82.63XC	S82.842P	S82.855R	S82.874P	S85.122A	S86.321A	S89.091P	S89.311P	S92.035B	S92.112P	S92.153K	S92.234B	S92.321P
S82.452N	S82.492Q	S82.63XK	S82.842Q	S82.856B	S82.874Q	S85.129A	S86.322A	S89.092A	S89.312K	S92.035K	S92.113B	S92.153P	S92.234K	S92.322B
S82.452P	S82.492R	S82.63XM	S82.842R	S82.856C	S82.874R	S85.131A	S86.329A	S89.092K	S89.312P	S92.035P	S92.113K	S92.154B	S92.234P	S92.322K
S82.452Q	S82.499K	S82.63XN	S82.843B	S82.856K	S82.875B	S85.132A	S86.821A	S89.092P	S89.319K	S92.036B	S92.113P	S92.154K	S92.235B	S92.322P
S82.452R	S82.499M	S82.63XP	S82.843C	S82.856M	S82.875C	S85.139A	S86.822A	S89.099A	S89.319P	S92.036K	S92.114B	S92.154P	S92.235K	S92.323B
S82.453K	S82.499N	S82.63XQ	S82.843K	S82.856N	S82.875K	S85.141A	S86.829A	S89.099K	S89.321K	S92.036P	S92.114K	S92.155B	S92.235P	S92.323K
S82.453M	S82.499P	S82.63XR	S82.843M	S82.856P	S82.875M	S85.142A	S86.921A	S89.099P	S89.321P	S92.041B	S92.114P	S92.155K	S92.236B	S92.323P
S82.453N	S82.499Q	S82.64XB	S82.843N	S82.856Q	S82.875N	S85.149A	S86.922A	S89.101K	S89.322K	S92.041K	S92.115B	S92.155P	S92.236K	S92.324B
S82.453P	S82.499R	S82.64XC	S82.843P	S82.856R	S82.875P	S85.151A	S86.929A	S89.101P	S89.322P	S92.041P	S92.115K	S92.156B	S92.236P	S92.324K
S82.453Q	S82.51XB	S82.64XK	S82.843Q	S82.861K	S82.875Q	S85.152A	S88.011A	S89.102K	S89.329K	S92.042B	S92.115P	S92.156K	S92.241B	S92.324P
S82.453R	S82.51XC	S82.64XM	S82.843R	S82.861M	S82.875R	S85.159A	S88.012A	S89.102P	S89.329P	S92.042K	S92.116B	S92.156P	S92.241K	S92.325B
S82.454K	S82.51XK	S82.64XN	S82.844B	S82.861N	S82.876B	S85.161A	S88.019A	S89.109K	S89.391K	S92.042P	S92.116K	S92.191B	S92.241P	S92.325K
S82.454M	S82.51XM	S82.64XP	S82.844C	S82.861P	S82.876C	S85.162A	S88.021A	S89.109P	S89.391P	S92.043B	S92.116P	S92.191K	S92.242B	S92.325P
S82.454N	S82.51XN	S82.64XQ	S82.844K	S82.861Q	S82.876K	S85.169A	S88.022A	S89.111K	S89.392K	S92.043K	S92.121B	S92.191P	S92.242K	S92.326B
S82.454P	S82.51XP	S82.64XR	S82.844M	S82.861R	S82.876M	S85.171A	S88.029A	S89.111P	S89.392P	S92.043P	S92.121K	S92.192B	S92.242P	S92.326K
S82.454Q	S82.51XQ	S82.65XB	S82.844N	S82.862K	S82.876N	S85.172A	S88.111A	S89.112K	S89.399K	S92.044B	S92.121P	S92.192K	S92.243B	S92.326P
S82.454R	S82.51XR	S82.65XC	S82.844P	S82.862M	S82.876P	S85.179A	S88.112A	S89.112P	S89.399P	S92.044K	S92.122B	S92.192P	S92.243K	S92.331B
S82.455K	S82.52XB	S82.65XK	S82.844Q	S82.862N	S82.876Q	S85.181A	S88.119A	S89.119K	S92.001B	S92.044P	S92.122K	S92.199B	S92.243P	S92.331K
S82.455M	S82.52XC	S82.65XM	S82.844R	S82.862P	S82.876R	S85.182A	S88.121A	S89.119P	S92.001K	S92.045B	S92.122P	S92.199K	S92.244B	S92.331P
S82.455N	S82.52XK	S82.65XN	S82.845B	S82.862Q	S82.891B	S85.189A	S88.122A	S89.121K	S92.001P	S92.045K	S92.123B	S92.199P	S92.244K	S92.332B
S82.455P	S82.52XM	S82.65XP	S82.845C	S82.862R	S82.891C	S85.201A	S88.129A	S89.121P	S92.002B	S92.045P	S92.123K	S92.201B	S92.244P	S92.332K
S82.455Q	S82.52XN	S82.65XQ	S82.845K	S82.863K	S82.891K	S85.202A	S88.911A	S89.122K	S92.002K	S92.046B	S92.123P	S92.201K	S92.245B	S92.332P
S82.455R	S82.52XP	S82.65XR	S82.845M	S82.863M	S82.891M	S85.209A	S88.912A	S89.122P	S92.002P	S92.046K	S92.124B	S92.201P	S92.245K	S92.333B
S82.456K	S82.52XQ	S82.66XB	S82.845N	S82.863N	S82.891N	S85.211A	S88.919A	S89.129K	S92.009B	S92.046P	S92.124K	S92.202B	S92.245P	S92.333K
S82.456M	S82.52XR	S82.66XC	S82.845P	S82.863P	S82.891P	S85.212A	S88.921A	S89.129P	S92.009K	S92.051B	S92.124P	S92.202K	S92.246B	S92.333P
S82.456N	S82.53XB	S82.66XK	S82.845Q	S82.863Q	S82.891Q	S85.219A	S88.922A	S89.131K	S92.009P	S92.051K	S92.125B	S92.202P	S92.246K	S92.334B
S82.456P	S82.53XC	S82.66XM	S82.845R	S82.863R	S82.891R	S85.291A	S88.929A	S89.131P	S92.011B	S92.051P	S92.125K	S92.209B	S92.246P	S92.334K
S82.456Q	S82.53XK	S82.66XN	S82.846B	S82.864K	S82.892B	S85.292A	S89.001A	S89.132K	S92.011K	S92.052B	S92.125P	S92.209K	S92.251B	S92.334P
S82.456R	S82.53XM	S82.66XP	S82.846C	S82.864M	S82.892C	S85.299A	S89.001K	S89.132P	S92.011P	S92.052K	S92.126B	S92.209P	S92.251K	S92.335B
S82.461K	S82.53XN	S82.66XQ	S82.846K	S82.864N	S82.892K	S85.301A	S89.001P	S89.139K	S92.012B	S92.052P	S92.126K	S92.211B	S92.251P	S92.335K
S82.461M	S82.53XP	S82.66XR	S82.846M	S82.864P	S82.892M	S85.302A	S89.002A	S89.139P	S92.012K	S92.053B	S92.126P	S92.211K	S92.252B	S92.335P
S82.461N	S82.53XQ	S82.811K	S82.846N	S82.864Q	S82.892N	S85.309A	S89.002K	S89.141K	S92.012P	S92.053K	S92.131B	S92.211P	S92.252K	S92.336B
S82.461P	S82.53XR	S82.811P	S82.846P	S82.864R	S82.892P	S85.311A	S89.002P	S89.141P	S92.013B	S92.053P	S92.131K	S92.212B	S92.252P	S92.336K
S82.461Q	S82.54XB	S82.812K	S82.846Q	S82.865K	S82.892Q	S85.312A	S89.009A	S89.142K	S92.013K	S92.054B	S92.131P	S92.212K	S92.253B	S92.336P
S82.461R	S82.54XC	S82.812P	S82.846R	S82.865M	S82.892R	S85.319A	S89.009K	S89.142P	S92.013P	S92.054K	S92.132B	S92.212P	S92.253K	S92.341B
S82.462K	S82.54XK	S82.819K	S82.851B	S82.865N	S82.899B	S85.391A	S89.009P	S89.149K	S92.014B	S92.054P	S92.132K	S92.213B	S92.253P	S92.341K
S82.462M	S82.54XM	S82.819P	S82.851C	S82.865P	S82.899C	S85.392A	S89.011A	S89.149P	S92.014K	S92.055B	S92.132P	S92.213K	S92.254B	S92.341P
S82.462N	S82.54XN	S82.821K	S82.851K	S82.865Q	S82.899K	S85.399A	S89.011K	S89.191K	S92.014P	S92.055K	S92.133B	S92.213P	S92.254K	S92.342B
S82.462P	S82.54XP	S82.821P	S82.851M	S82.865R	S82.899M	S85.401A	S89.011P	S89.191P	S92.015B	S92.055P	S92.133K	S92.214B	S92.254P	S92.342K
S82.462Q	S82.54XQ	S82.822K	S82.851N	S82.866K	S82.899N	S85.402A	S89.012A	S89.192K	S92.015K	S92.056B	S92.133P	S92.214K	S92.255B	S92.342P
S82.462R	S82.54XR	S82.822P	S82.851P	S82.866M	S82.899P	S85.409A	S89.012K	S89.192P	S92.015P	S92.056K	S92.134B	S92.214P	S92.255K	S92.343B

Complication or Comorbidity (CC) (cont.) - Based on CMS data

S92.343K	S92.503K	S95.002A	S98.922A	T22.319A	T23.722A	T26.21XA	T34.61XA	T74.92XA	T81.33XA	T82.121A	T82.827A	T83.84XA	T84.228A	T85.390A
S92.343P	S92.503P	S95.009A	S98.929A	T22.321A	T23.729A	T26.22XA	T34.62XA	T75.1XXA	T81.40XA	T82.128A	T82.828A	T83.85XA	T84.290A	T85.391A
S92.344B	S92.504K	S95.011A	T17.400A	T22.322A	T23.731A	T26.70XA	T34.70XA	T76.01XA	T81.41XA	T82.129A	T82.837A	T83.86XA	T84.293A	T85.41XA
S92.344K	S92.504P	S95.012A	T17.408A	T22.329A	T23.732A	T26.71XA	T34.71XA	T76.02XA	T81.42XA	T82.190A	T82.838A	T83.89XA	T84.296A	T85.42XA
S92.344P	S92.505K	S95.019A	T17.410A	T22.331A	T23.739A	T26.72XA	T34.72XA	T76.11XA	T81.43XA	T82.191A	T82.847A	T83.9XXA	T84.298A	T85.43XA
S92.345B	S92.505P	S95.091A	T17.418A	T22.332A	T23.741A	T27.0XXA	T34.811A	T76.12XA	T81.44XA	T82.198A	T82.848A	T84.010A	T84.310A	T85.44XA
S92.345K	S92.506K	S95.092A	T17.420A	T22.339A	T23.742A	T27.1XXA	T34.812A	T76.21XA	T81.49XA	T82.199A	T82.855A	T84.011A	T84.318A	T85.49XA
S92.345P	S92.506P	S95.099A	T17.428A	T22.341A	T23.749A	T27.2XXA	T34.819A	T76.22XA	T81.500A	T82.211A	T82.856A	T84.012A	T84.320A	T85.510A
S92.346B	S92.511K	S95.101A	T17.490A	T22.342A	T23.751A	T27.3XXA	T34.821A	T76.32XA	T81.501A	T82.212A	T82.857A	T84.013A	T84.328A	T85.511A
S92.346K	S92.511P	S95.102A	T17.498A	T22.349A	T23.752A	T27.4XXA	T34.822A	T76.51XA	T81.502A	T82.213A	T82.858A	T84.018A	T84.390A	T85.518A
S92.346P	S92.512K	S95.109A	T17.500A	T22.351A	T23.759A	T27.5XXA	T34.829A	T76.52XA	T81.503A	T82.218A	T82.867A	T84.019A	T84.398A	T85.520A
S92.351B	S92.512P	S95.111A	T17.508A	T22.352A	T23.761A	T27.6XXA	T34.831A	T76.61XA	T81.504A	T82.221A	T82.868A	T84.020A	T84.410A	T85.521A
S92.351K	S92.513K	S95.112A	T17.510A	T22.359A	T23.762A	T27.7XXA	T34.832A	T76.62XA	T81.505A	T82.222A	T82.897A	T84.021A	T84.418A	T85.528A
S92.351P	S92.513P	S95.119A	T17.518A	T22.361A	T23.769A	T28.1XXA	T34.839A	T76.91XA	T81.506A	T82.223A	T82.898A	T84.022A	T84.420A	T85.590A
S92.352B	S92.514K	S95.191A	T17.520A	T22.362A	T23.771A	T28.2XXA	T34.90XA	T76.92XA	T81.507A	T82.228A	T82.9XXA	T84.023A	T84.428A	T85.591A
S92.352K	S92.514P	S95.192A	T17.528A	T22.369A	T23.772A	T28.6XXA	T34.99XA	T78.00XA	T81.508A	T82.310A	T83.010A	T84.028A	T84.490A	T85.598A
S92.352P	S92.515K	S95.199A	T17.590A	T22.391A	T23.779A	T28.7XXA	T67.01XA	T78.01XA	T81.509A	T82.311A	T83.020A	T84.029A	T84.498A	T85.610A
S92.353B	S92.515P	S95.201A	T17.598A	T22.392A	T23.791A	T33.011A	T67.02XA	T78.02XA	T81.510A	T82.312A	T83.030A	T84.030A	T84.50XA	T85.611A
S92.353K	S92.516K	S95.202A	T17.800A	T22.399A	T23.792A	T33.012A	T67.09XA	T78.03XA	T81.511A	T82.318A	T83.090A	T84.031A	T84.51XA	T85.612A
S92.353P	S92.516P	S95.209A	T17.808A	T22.70XA	T23.799A	T33.019A	T69.021A	T78.04XA	T81.512A	T82.319A	T83.110A	T84.032A	T84.52XA	T85.613A
S92.354B	S92.521K	S95.211A	T17.810A	T22.711A	T24.301A	T33.02XA	T69.022A	T78.05XA	T81.513A	T82.320A	T83.111A	T84.033A	T84.53XA	T85.614A
S92.354K	S92.521P	S95.212A	T17.818A	T22.712A	T24.302A	T33.09XA	T69.029A	T78.06XA	T81.514A	T82.321A	T83.112A	T84.038A	T84.54XA	T85.615A
S92.354P	S92.522K	S95.219A	T17.820A	T22.719A	T24.309A	T33.1XXA	T70.3XXA	T78.07XA	T81.515A	T82.322A	T83.113A	T84.039A	T84.59XA	T85.618A
S92.355B	S92.522P	S95.291A	T17.828A	T22.721A	T24.311A	T33.2XXA	T71.111A	T78.08XA	T81.516A	T82.328A	T83.118A	T84.050A	T84.60XA	T85.620A
S92.355K	S92.523K	S95.292A	T17.890A	T22.722A	T24.312A	T33.3XXA	T71.112A	T78.09XA	T81.517A	T82.329A	T83.120A	T84.051A	T84.610A	T85.621A
S92.355P	S92.523P	S95.299A	T17.898A	T22.729A	T24.319A	T33.40XA	T71.113A	T78.2XXA	T81.518A	T82.330A	T83.121A	T84.052A	T84.611A	T85.622A
S92.356B	S92.524K	S95.801A	T17.900A	T22.731A	T24.321A	T33.41XA	T71.114A	T79.2XXA	T81.519A	T82.331A	T83.122A	T84.053A	T84.612A	T85.623A
S92.356K	S92.524P	S95.802A	T17.910A	T22.732A	T24.322A	T33.42XA	T71.121A	T79.7XXA	T81.520A	T82.332A	T83.123A	T84.058A	T84.613A	T85.624A
S92.356P	S92.525K	S95.809A	T17.920A	T22.739A	T24.329A	T33.511A	T71.122A	T79.A0XA	T81.521A	T82.338A	T83.128A	T84.059A	T84.614A	T85.625A
S92.401K	S92.525P	S95.811A	T17.990A	T22.741A	T24.331A	T33.512A	T71.123A	T79.A11A	T81.522A	T82.339A	T83.190A	T84.060A	T84.615A	T85.628A
S92.401P	S92.526K	S95.812A	T18.190A	T22.742A	T24.332A	T33.519A	T71.124A	T79.A12A	T81.523A	T82.390A	T83.191A	T84.061A	T84.619A	T85.630A
S92.402K	S92.526P	S95.819A	T18.2XXA	T22.749A	T24.339A	T33.521A	T71.131A	T79.A19A	T81.524A	T82.391A	T83.192A	T84.062A	T84.620A	T85.631A
S92.402P	S92.531K	S95.891A	T20.30XA	T22.751A	T24.391A	T33.522A	T71.132A	T79.A21A	T81.525A	T82.392A	T83.193A	T84.063A	T84.621A	T85.633A
S92.403K	S92.531P	S95.892A	T20.311A	T22.752A	T24.392A	T33.529A	T71.133A	T79.A22A	T81.526A	T82.398A	T83.198A	T84.068A	T84.622A	T85.635A
S92.403P	S92.532K	S95.899A	T20.312A	T22.759A	T24.399A	T33.531A	T71.134A	T79.A29A	T81.527A	T82.399A	T83.21XA	T84.069A	T84.623A	T85.638A
S92.404K	S92.532P	S95.901A	T20.319A	T22.761A	T24.701A	T33.532A	T71.141A	T79.A3XA	T81.528A	T82.41XA	T83.22XA	T84.090A	T84.624A	T85.690A
S92.404P	S92.533K	S95.902A	T20.32XA	T22.762A	T24.702A	T33.539A	T71.143A	T79.A9XA	T81.529A	T82.42XA	T83.23XA	T84.091A	T84.625A	T85.691A
S92.405K	S92.533P	S95.909A	T20.33XA	T22.769A	T24.709A	T33.60XA	T71.144A	T80.1XXA	T81.530A	T82.43XA	T83.24XA	T84.092A	T84.629A	T85.692A
S92.405P	S92.534K	S95.911A	T20.34XA	T22.791A	T24.711A	T33.61XA	T71.151A	T80.211A	T81.531A	T82.49XA	T83.25XA	T84.093A	T84.63XA	T85.693A
S92.406K	S92.534P	S95.912A	T20.35XA	T22.792A	T24.712A	T33.62XA	T71.152A	T80.212A	T81.532A	T82.510A	T83.29XA	T84.098A	T84.69XA	T85.694A
S92.406P	S92.535K	S95.919A	T20.36XA	T22.799A	T24.719A	T33.70XA	T71.153A	T80.218A	T81.533A	T82.511A	T83.410A	T84.099A	T84.7XXA	T85.695A
S92.411K	S92.535P	S95.991A	T20.37XA	T23.301A	T24.721A	T33.71XA	T71.154A	T80.219A	T81.534A	T82.512A	T83.411A	T84.110A	T84.81XA	T85.698A
S92.411P	S92.536K	S95.992A	T20.39XA	T23.302A	T24.722A	T33.72XA	T71.161A	T80.22XA	T81.535A	T82.513A	T83.418A	T84.111A	T84.82XA	T85.71XA
S92.412K	S92.536P	S95.999A	T20.70XA	T23.309A	T24.729A	T33.811A	T71.162A	T80.29XA	T81.536A	T82.514A	T83.420A	T84.112A	T84.83XA	T85.72XA
S92.412P	S92.591K	S96.021A	T20.711A	T23.311A	T24.731A	T33.812A	T71.163A	T80.30XA	T81.537A	T82.515A	T83.421A	T84.113A	T84.84XA	T85.730A
S92.413K	S92.591P	S96.022A	T20.712A	T23.312A	T24.732A	T33.819A	T71.164A	T80.310A	T81.538A	T82.518A	T83.428A	T84.114A	T84.85XA	T85.731A
S92.413P	S92.592K	S96.029A	T20.719A	T23.319A	T24.739A	T33.821A	T71.191A	T80.311A	T81.539A	T82.519A	T83.490A	T84.115A	T84.86XA	T85.732A
S92.414K	S92.592P	S96.121A	T20.72XA	T23.321A	T24.791A	T33.822A	T71.192A	T80.319A	T81.590A	T82.520A	T83.491A	T84.116A	T84.89XA	T85.733A
S92.414P	S92.599K	S96.122A	T20.73XA	T23.322A	T24.792A	T33.829A	T71.193A	T80.39XA	T81.591A	T82.521A	T83.498A	T84.117A	T84.9XXA	T85.734A
S92.415K	S92.599P	S96.129A	T20.74XA	T23.329A	T24.799A	T33.831A	T71.194A	T80.40XA	T81.592A	T82.522A	T83.510A	T84.119A	T85.01XA	T85.735A
S92.415P	S92.811B	S96.221A	T20.75XA	T23.331A	T25.311A	T33.832A	T71.20XA	T80.410A	T81.593A	T82.523A	T83.511A	T84.120A	T85.02XA	T85.738A
S92.416K	S92.811K	S96.222A	T20.76XA	T23.332A	T25.312A	T33.839A	T71.21XA	T80.411A	T81.594A	T82.524A	T83.512A	T84.121A	T85.03XA	T85.79XA
S92.416P	S92.811P	S96.229A	T20.77XA	T23.339A	T25.319A	T33.90XA	T71.221A	T80.419A	T81.595A	T82.525A	T83.518A	T84.122A	T85.09XA	T85.810A
S92.421K	S92.812B	S96.821A	T20.79XA	T23.341A	T25.321A	T33.99XA	T71.222A	T80.49XA	T81.596A	T82.528A	T83.590A	T84.123A	T85.110A	T85.810D
S92.421P	S92.812K	S96.822A	T21.30XA	T23.342A	T25.322A	T34.011A	T71.223A	T80.51XA	T81.597A	T82.529A	T83.591A	T84.124A	T85.111A	T85.820A
S92.422K	S92.812P	S96.829A	T21.31XA	T23.349A	T25.329A	T34.012A	T71.224A	T80.52XA	T81.598A	T82.530A	T83.592A	T84.125A	T85.112A	T85.820D
S92.422P	S92.819B	S96.921A	T21.32XA	T23.351A	T25.331A	T34.019A	T71.231A	T80.59XA	T81.599A	T82.531A	T83.593A	T84.126A	T85.113A	T85.830A
S92.423K	S92.819K	S96.922A	T21.33XA	T23.352A	T25.332A	T34.02XA	T71.232A	T80.61XA	T81.60XA	T82.532A	T83.598A	T84.127A	T85.118A	T85.830D
S92.423P	S92.819P	S96.929A	T21.34XA	T23.359A	T25.339A	T34.09XA	T71.233A	T80.62XA	T81.61XA	T82.533A	T83.61XA	T84.129A	T85.120A	T85.840A
S92.424K	S92.901B	S98.011A	T21.35XA	T23.361A	T25.391A	T34.1XXA	T71.234A	T80.69XA	T81.69XA	T82.534A	T83.62XA	T84.190A	T85.121A	T85.840D
S92.424P	S92.901K	S98.012A	T21.36XA	T23.362A	T25.392A	T34.2XXA	T71.29XA	T80.810A	T81.710A	T82.535A	T83.69XA	T84.191A	T85.122A	T85.850A
S92.425K	S92.901P	S98.019A	T21.37XA	T23.369A	T25.399A	T34.3XXA	T71.9XXA	T80.818A	T81.711A	T82.538A	T83.712A	T84.192A	T85.123A	T85.850D
S92.425P	S92.902B	S98.021A	T21.39XA	T23.371A	T25.711A	T34.40XA	T74.01XA	T80.89XA	T81.718A	T82.539A	T83.713A	T84.193A	T85.128A	T85.860A
S92.426K	S92.902K	S98.022A	T21.70XA	T23.372A	T25.712A	T34.41XA	T74.02XA	T80.910A	T81.719A	T82.590A	T83.714A	T84.194A	T85.190A	T85.860D
S92.426P	S92.902P	S98.029A	T21.71XA	T23.379A	T25.719A	T34.42XA	T74.11XA	T80.911A	T81.72XA	T82.591A	T83.718A	T84.195A	T85.191A	T85.890A
S92.491K	S92.909B	S98.311A	T21.72XA	T23.391A	T25.721A	T34.511A	T74.12XA	T80.919A	T81.83XA	T82.592A	T83.719A	T84.196A	T85.192A	T85.890D
S92.491P	S92.909K	S98.312A	T21.73XA	T23.392A	T25.722A	T34.512A	T74.21XA	T80.A0XA	T82.01XA	T82.593A	T83.722A	T84.197A	T85.193A	T88.0XXA
S92.492K	S92.909P	S98.319A	T21.74XA	T23.399A	T25.729A	T34.519A	T74.22XA	T80.A10A	T82.02XA	T82.594A	T83.723A	T84.199A	T85.199A	T88.1XXA
S92.492P	S92.911K	S98.321A	T21.75XA	T23.701A	T25.731A	T34.521A	T74.32XA	T80.A11A	T82.03XA	T82.595A	T83.724A	T84.210A	T85.21XA	T88.2XXA
S92.499K	S92.911P	S98.322A	T21.76XA	T23.702A	T25.732A	T34.522A	T74.4XXA	T80.A19A	T82.09XA	T82.598A	T83.728A	T84.213A	T85.22XA	T88.3XXA
S92.499P	S92.912K	S98.329A	T21.77XA	T23.709A	T25.739A	T34.529A	T74.51XA	T80.A9XA	T82.110A	T82.599A	T83.729A	T84.216A	T85.29XA	T88.6XXA
S92.501K	S92.912P	S98.911A	T21.79XA	T23.711A	T25.791A	T34.531A	T74.52XA	T81.10XA	T82.111A	T82.6XXA	T83.79XA	T84.218A	T85.310A	
S92.501P	S92.919K	S98.912A	T22.30XA	T23.712A	T25.792A	T34.532A	T74.61XA	T81.30XA	T82.118A	T82.7XXA	T83.81XA	T84.220A	T85.311A	
S92.502K	S92.919P	S98.919A	T22.311A	T23.719A	T25.799A	T34.539A	T74.62XA	T81.31XA	T82.119A	T82.817A	T83.82XA	T84.223A	T85.320A	
S92.502P	S95.001A	S98.921A	T22.312A	T23.721A	T26.20XA	T34.60XA	T74.91XA	T81.32XA	T82.120A	T82.818A	T83.83XA	T84.226A	T85.321A	

Complications or Comorbidities/Major Complications or Comorbidities (CC/MCC) Exclusions - Based on CMS data

H34.8110	M80.062P	M80.871K	M84.374P	M84.453K	M84.531A	M84.58XP	M84.669K	O31.8X22	O41.02X4	O60.10X1	R40.2321	S02.129K	S02.612B	S02.842A
H34.8111	M80.069A	M80.871P	M84.375K	M84.453P	M84.531K	M84.60XA	M84.669P	O31.8X23	O41.02X5	O60.10X2	R40.2322	S02.19XA	S02.612K	S02.842B
H34.8112	M80.069K	M80.872A	M84.375P	M84.454A	M84.531P	M84.60XK	M84.671A	O31.8X24	O41.02X9	O60.10X3	R40.2323	S02.19XB	S02.620A	S02.842K
H34.8120	M80.069P	M80.872K	M84.376K	M84.454K	M84.532A	M84.60XP	M84.671K	O31.8X25	O41.03X0	O60.10X4	R40.2324	S02.19XK	S02.620B	S02.849A
H34.8121	M80.071A	M80.872P	M84.376P	M84.454P	M84.532K	M84.611A	M84.671P	O31.8X29	O41.03X1	O60.10X5	R40.2340	S02.2XXB	S02.620K	S02.849B
H34.8122	M80.071K	M80.879A	M84.377K	M84.459A	M84.532P	M84.611K	M84.672A	O31.8X30	O41.03X2	O60.10X9	R40.2341	S02.2XXK	S02.621A	S02.849K
H34.8130	M80.071P	M80.879K	M84.377P	M84.459K	M84.533A	M84.611P	M84.672K	O31.8X31	O41.03X3	O60.12X0	R40.2342	S02.30XA	S02.621B	S02.85XA
H34.8131	M80.072A	M80.879P	M84.378K	M84.459P	M84.533K	M84.612A	M84.672P	O31.8X32	O41.03X4	O60.12X1	R40.2343	S02.30XB	S02.621K	S02.85XB
H34.8132	M80.072K	M80.88XA	M84.378P	M84.461A	M84.533P	M84.612K	M84.673A	O31.8X33	O41.03X5	O60.12X2	R40.2344	S02.30XK	S02.622A	S02.85XK
H34.8190	M80.072P	M80.88XK	M84.379K	M84.461K	M84.534A	M84.612P	M84.673K	O31.8X34	O41.03X9	O60.12X3	S01.101A	S02.31XA	S02.622B	S02.91XA
H34.8191	M80.079A	M80.88XP	M84.379P	M84.461P	M84.534K	M84.619A	M84.673P	O31.8X35	O41.1010	O60.12X4	S01.102A	S02.31XB	S02.622K	S02.91XB
H34.8192	M80.079K	M84.30XK	M84.38XK	M84.462A	M84.534P	M84.619K	M84.674A	O31.8X39	O41.1011	O60.12X5	S01.109A	S02.31XK	S02.630A	S02.91XK
M48.50XA	M80.079P	M84.30XP	M84.38XP	M84.462K	M84.539A	M84.619P	M84.674K	O36.0110	O41.1012	O60.12X9	S02.0XXA	S02.32XA	S02.630B	S02.92XA
M48.51XA	M80.08XA	M84.311K	M84.40XA	M84.462P	M84.539K	M84.621A	M84.674P	O36.0111	O41.1013	O60.13X0	S02.0XXB	S02.32XB	S02.630K	S02.92XB
M48.52XA	M80.08XK	M84.311P	M84.40XK	M84.463A	M84.539P	M84.621K	M84.675A	O36.0112	O41.1014	O60.13X1	S02.0XXK	S02.32XK	S02.631A	S02.92XK
M48.53XA	M80.08XP	M84.312K	M84.40XP	M84.463K	M84.541A	M84.621P	M84.675K	O36.0113	O41.1015	O60.13X2	S02.101A	S02.400A	S02.631B	S04.011A
M48.54XA	M80.80XA	M84.312P	M84.411A	M84.463P	M84.541K	M84.622A	M84.675P	O36.0114	O41.1019	O60.13X3	S02.101B	S02.400B	S02.631K	S04.012A
M48.55XA	M80.80XK	M84.319K	M84.411K	M84.464A	M84.541P	M84.622K	M84.676A	O36.0115	O41.1020	O60.13X4	S02.101K	S02.400K	S02.632A	S04.019A
M48.56XA	M80.80XP	M84.319P	M84.411P	M84.464K	M84.542A	M84.622P	M84.676K	O36.0119	O41.1021	O60.13X5	S02.102A	S02.401A	S02.632B	S04.02XA
M48.57XA	M80.811A	M84.321K	M84.412A	M84.464P	M84.542K	M84.629A	M84.676P	O36.0120	O41.1022	O60.13X9	S02.102B	S02.401B	S02.632K	S04.031A
M48.58XA	M80.811K	M84.321P	M84.412K	M84.469A	M84.542P	M84.629K	M84.68XA	O36.0121	O41.1023	O60.14X0	S02.102K	S02.401K	S02.640A	S04.032A
M80.00XA	M80.811P	M84.322K	M84.412P	M84.469K	M84.549A	M84.629P	M84.68XK	O36.0122	O41.1024	O60.14X1	S02.109A	S02.402A	S02.640B	S04.039A
M80.00XK	M80.812A	M84.322P	M84.419A	M84.469P	M84.549K	M84.631A	M84.68XP	O36.0123	O41.1025	O60.14X2	S02.109B	S02.402B	S02.640K	S04.041A
M80.00XP	M80.812K	M84.329K	M84.419K	M84.471A	M84.549P	M84.631K	M84.750A	O36.0124	O41.1029	O60.14X3	S02.109K	S02.402K	S02.641A	S04.042A
M80.011A	M80.812P	M84.329P	M84.419P	M84.471K	M84.550A	M84.631P	M84.750K	O36.0125	O41.1030	O60.14X4	S02.110A	S02.40AA	S02.641B	S04.049A
M80.011K	M80.819A	M84.331K	M84.421A	M84.471P	M84.550K	M84.632A	M84.750P	O36.0129	O41.1031	O60.14X5	S02.110B	S02.40AB	S02.641K	S04.10XA
M80.011P	M80.819K	M84.331P	M84.421K	M84.472A	M84.550P	M84.632K	M84.751A	O36.0130	O41.1032	O60.14X9	S02.110K	S02.40AK	S02.642A	S04.11XA
M80.012A	M80.819P	M84.332K	M84.421P	M84.472K	M84.551A	M84.632P	M84.751K	O36.0131	O41.1033	O60.20X0	S02.111A	S02.40BA	S02.642B	S04.12XA
M80.012K	M80.821A	M84.332P	M84.422A	M84.472P	M84.551K	M84.633A	M84.751P	O36.0132	O41.1034	O60.20X1	S02.111B	S02.40BB	S02.642K	S04.20XA
M80.012P	M80.821K	M84.333K	M84.422K	M84.473A	M84.551P	M84.633K	M84.752A	O36.0133	O41.1035	O60.20X2	S02.111K	S02.40BK	S02.650A	S04.21XA
M80.019A	M80.821P	M84.333P	M84.422P	M84.473K	M84.552A	M84.633P	M84.752K	O36.0134	O41.1039	O60.20X3	S02.112A	S02.40CA	S02.650B	S04.22XA
M80.019K	M80.822A	M84.334K	M84.429A	M84.473P	M84.552K	M84.634A	M84.752P	O36.0135	O41.1210	O60.20X4	S02.112B	S02.40CB	S02.650K	S04.30XA
M80.019P	M80.822K	M84.334P	M84.429K	M84.474A	M84.552P	M84.634K	M84.753A	O36.0139	O41.1211	O60.20X5	S02.112K	S02.40CK	S02.651A	S04.31XA
M80.021A	M80.822P	M84.339K	M84.429P	M84.474K	M84.553A	M84.634P	M84.753K	O36.0910	O41.1212	O60.20X9	S02.113A	S02.40DA	S02.651B	S04.32XA
M80.021K	M80.829A	M84.339P	M84.431A	M84.474P	M84.553K	M84.639A	M84.753P	O36.0911	O41.1213	O60.22X0	S02.113B	S02.40DB	S02.651K	S04.40XA
M80.021P	M80.829K	M84.341K	M84.431K	M84.475A	M84.553P	M84.639K	M84.754A	O36.0912	O41.1214	O60.22X1	S02.113K	S02.40DK	S02.652A	S04.41XA
M80.022A	M80.829P	M84.341P	M84.431P	M84.475K	M84.559A	M84.639P	M84.754K	O36.0913	O41.1215	O60.22X2	S02.118A	S02.40EA	S02.652B	S04.42XA
M80.022K	M80.831A	M84.342K	M84.432A	M84.475P	M84.559K	M84.641A	M84.754P	O36.0914	O41.1219	O60.22X3	S02.118B	S02.40EB	S02.652K	S04.50XA
M80.022P	M80.831K	M84.342P	M84.432K	M84.476A	M84.559P	M84.641K	M84.755A	O36.0915	O41.1220	O60.22X4	S02.118K	S02.40EK	S02.66XA	S04.51XA
M80.029A	M80.831P	M84.343K	M84.432P	M84.476K	M84.561A	M84.641P	M84.755K	O36.0919	O41.1221	O60.22X5	S02.119A	S02.40FA	S02.66XB	S04.52XA
M80.029K	M80.832A	M84.343P	M84.433A	M84.476P	M84.561K	M84.642A	M84.755P	O36.0920	O41.1222	O60.22X9	S02.119B	S02.40FB	S02.66XK	S04.60XA
M80.029P	M80.832K	M84.344K	M84.433K	M84.477A	M84.561P	M84.642K	M84.756A	O36.0921	O41.1223	O60.23X0	S02.119K	S02.40FK	S02.670A	S04.61XA
M80.031A	M80.832P	M84.344P	M84.433P	M84.477K	M84.562A	M84.642P	M84.756K	O36.0922	O41.1224	O60.23X1	S02.11AA	S02.411A	S02.670B	S04.62XA
M80.031K	M80.839A	M84.345K	M84.434A	M84.477P	M84.562K	M84.649A	M84.756P	O36.0923	O41.1225	O60.23X2	S02.11AB	S02.411B	S02.670K	S04.70XA
M80.031P	M80.839K	M84.345P	M84.434K	M84.478A	M84.562P	M84.649K	M84.757A	O36.0924	O41.1229	O60.23X3	S02.11AK	S02.411K	S02.671A	S04.71XA
M80.032A	M80.839P	M84.346K	M84.434P	M84.478K	M84.563A	M84.649P	M84.757K	O36.0925	O41.1230	O60.23X4	S02.11BA	S02.412A	S02.671B	S04.72XA
M80.032K	M80.841A	M84.346P	M84.439A	M84.478P	M84.563K	M84.650A	M84.757P	O36.0929	O41.1231	O60.23X5	S02.11BB	S02.412B	S02.671K	S04.811A
M80.032P	M80.841K	M84.350K	M84.439K	M84.479A	M84.563P	M84.650K	M84.758A	O36.0930	O41.1232	O60.23X9	S02.11BK	S02.412K	S02.672A	S04.812A
M80.039A	M80.841P	M84.350P	M84.439P	M84.479K	M84.564A	M84.650P	M84.758K	O36.0931	O41.1233	R40.2110	S02.11CA	S02.413A	S02.672B	S04.819A
M80.039K	M80.842A	M84.351K	M84.441A	M84.479P	M84.564K	M84.651A	M84.758P	O36.0932	O41.1234	R40.2111	S02.11CB	S02.413B	S02.672K	S04.891A
M80.039P	M80.842K	M84.351P	M84.441K	M84.48XA	M84.564P	M84.651K	M84.759A	O36.0933	O41.1235	R40.2112	S02.11CK	S02.413K	S02.69XA	S04.892A
M80.041A	M80.842P	M84.352K	M84.441P	M84.48XK	M84.569A	M84.651P	M84.759K	O36.0934	O41.1239	R40.2113	S02.11DA	S02.42XA	S02.69XB	S04.899A
M80.041K	M80.849A	M84.352P	M84.442A	M84.48XP	M84.569K	M84.652A	M84.759P	O36.0935	O41.1410	R40.2114	S02.11DB	S02.42XB	S02.69XK	S04.9XXA
M80.041P	M80.849K	M84.353K	M84.442K	M84.50XA	M84.569P	M84.652K	M97.01XA	O36.0939	O41.1411	R40.2120	S02.11DK	S02.42XK	S02.80XA	S05.20XA
M80.042A	M80.849P	M84.353P	M84.442P	M84.50XK	M84.571A	M84.652P	M97.02XA	O36.1910	O41.1412	R40.2121	S02.11EA	S02.5XXK	S02.80XB	S05.21XA
M80.042K	M80.851A	M84.359K	M84.443A	M84.50XP	M84.571K	M84.653A	M97.11XA	O36.1911	O41.1413	R40.2122	S02.11EB	S02.600A	S02.80XK	S05.22XA
M80.042P	M80.851K	M84.359P	M84.443K	M84.511A	M84.571P	M84.653K	M97.12XA	O36.4XX0	O41.1414	R40.2123	S02.11EK	S02.600B	S02.81XA	S05.30XA
M80.049A	M80.851P	M84.361K	M84.443P	M84.511K	M84.572A	M84.653P	M97.21XA	O36.4XX1	O41.1415	R40.2124	S02.11FA	S02.600K	S02.81XB	S05.31XA
M80.049K	M80.852A	M84.361P	M84.444A	M84.511P	M84.572K	M84.659A	M97.22XA	O36.4XX2	O41.1419	R40.2210	S02.11FB	S02.601A	S02.81XK	S05.32XA
M80.049P	M80.852K	M84.362K	M84.444K	M84.512A	M84.572P	M84.659K	M97.31XA	O36.4XX3	O41.1420	R40.2211	S02.11FK	S02.601B	S02.82XA	S05.40XA
M80.051A	M80.852P	M84.362P	M84.444P	M84.512K	M84.573A	M84.659P	M97.32XA	O36.4XX4	O41.1421	R40.2212	S02.11GA	S02.601K	S02.82XB	S05.41XA
M80.051K	M80.859A	M84.363K	M84.445A	M84.512P	M84.573K	M84.661A	M97.41XA	O36.4XX5	O41.1422	R40.2213	S02.11GB	S02.602A	S02.82XK	S05.42XA
M80.051P	M80.859K	M84.363P	M84.445K	M84.519A	M84.573P	M84.661K	M97.42XA	O36.4XX9	O41.1423	R40.2214	S02.11GK	S02.602B	S02.831A	S05.50XA
M80.052A	M80.859P	M84.364K	M84.445P	M84.519K	M84.574A	M84.661P	M97.8XXA	O41.01X0	O41.1424	R40.2220	S02.11HA	S02.602K	S02.831B	S05.51XA
M80.052K	M80.861A	M84.364P	M84.446A	M84.519P	M84.574K	M84.662A	M97.9XXA	O41.01X1	O41.1425	R40.2221	S02.11HB	S02.609A	S02.831K	S05.52XA
M80.052P	M80.861K	M84.369K	M84.446K	M84.521A	M84.574P	M84.662K	O31.8X10	O41.01X2	O41.1429	R40.2222	S02.11HK	S02.609B	S02.832A	S05.70XA
M80.059A	M80.861P	M84.369P	M84.446P	M84.521K	M84.575A	M84.662P	O31.8X11	O41.01X3	O41.1430	R40.2223	S02.121A	S02.609K	S02.832B	S05.71XA
M80.059K	M80.862A	M84.371K	M84.451A	M84.521P	M84.575K	M84.663A	O31.8X12	O41.01X4	O41.1431	R40.2224	S02.121B	S02.610A	S02.832K	S05.72XA
M80.059P	M80.862K	M84.371P	M84.451K	M84.522A	M84.575P	M84.663K	O31.8X13	O41.01X5	O41.1432	R40.2310	S02.121K	S02.610B	S02.839A	S05.8X1A
M80.061A	M80.862P	M84.372K	M84.451P	M84.522K	M84.576A	M84.663P	O31.8X14	O41.01X9	O41.1433	R40.2311	S02.122A	S02.610K	S02.839B	S05.8X2A
M80.061K	M80.869A	M84.372P	M84.452A	M84.522P	M84.576K	M84.664A	O31.8X15	O41.02X0	O41.1434	R40.2312	S02.122B	S02.611A	S02.839K	S05.8X9A
M80.061P	M80.869K	M84.373K	M84.452K	M84.529A	M84.576P	M84.664K	O31.8X19	O41.02X1	O41.1435	R40.2313	S02.122K	S02.611B	S02.841A	S05.91XA
M80.062A	M80.869P	M84.373P	M84.452P	M84.529K	M84.58XA	M84.664P	O31.8X20	O41.02X2	O41.1439	R40.2314	S02.129A	S02.611K	S02.841B	S05.92XA
M80.062K	M80.871A	M84.374K	M84.453A	M84.529P	M84.58XK	M84.669A	O31.8X21	O41.02X3	O60.10X0	R40.2320	S02.129B	S02.612A	S02.841K	S06.0X0A

Complications or Comorbidities/Major Complications or Comorbidities (CC/MCC) Exclusions (cont.) - Based on CMS data

S06.0X1A	S06.354A	S06.822A	S12.000A	S12.200K	S12.490B	S13.160A	S15.119A	S21.409A	S22.032B	S22.082A	S25.09XA	S26.92XA	S31.612A	S32.028K
S06.0X9A	S06.355A	S06.823A	S12.000B	S12.201A	S12.490K	S13.161A	S15.121A	S21.411A	S22.032K	S22.082B	S25.101A	S26.99XA	S31.613A	S32.029A
S06.1X0A	S06.356A	S06.824A	S12.000K	S12.201B	S12.491A	S13.170A	S15.122A	S21.412A	S22.038A	S22.082K	S25.102A	S27.0XXA	S31.614A	S32.029B
S06.1X1A	S06.357A	S06.825A	S12.001A	S12.201K	S12.491B	S13.171A	S15.129A	S21.419A	S22.038B	S22.088A	S25.109A	S27.1XXA	S31.615A	S32.029K
S06.1X2A	S06.358A	S06.826A	S12.001B	S12.230A	S12.491K	S13.180A	S15.191A	S21.421A	S22.038K	S22.088B	S25.111A	S27.2XXA	S31.619A	S32.030A
S06.1X3A	S06.359A	S06.827A	S12.001K	S12.230B	S12.500A	S13.181A	S15.192A	S21.422A	S22.039A	S22.088K	S25.112A	S27.301A	S31.620A	S32.030B
S06.1X4A	S06.360A	S06.828A	S12.01XA	S12.230K	S12.500B	S13.20XA	S15.199A	S21.429A	S22.039B	S22.089A	S25.119A	S27.302A	S31.621A	S32.030K
S06.1X5A	S06.361A	S06.829A	S12.01XB	S12.231A	S12.500K	S13.29XA	S15.201A	S21.431A	S22.039K	S22.089B	S25.121A	S27.309A	S31.622A	S32.031A
S06.1X6A	S06.362A	S06.891A	S12.01XK	S12.231B	S12.501A	S14.0XXA	S15.202A	S21.432A	S22.040A	S22.089K	S25.122A	S27.311A	S31.623A	S32.031B
S06.1X7A	S06.363A	S06.892A	S12.02XA	S12.231K	S12.501B	S14.101A	S15.209A	S21.439A	S22.040B	S22.20XA	S25.129A	S27.312A	S31.624A	S32.031K
S06.1X8A	S06.364A	S06.893A	S12.02XB	S12.24XA	S12.501K	S14.102A	S15.211A	S21.441A	S22.040K	S22.20XB	S25.191A	S27.319A	S31.625A	S32.032A
S06.1X9A	S06.365A	S06.894A	S12.02XK	S12.24XB	S12.530A	S14.103A	S15.212A	S21.442A	S22.041A	S22.20XK	S25.192A	S27.321A	S31.629A	S32.032B
S06.2X1A	S06.366A	S06.895A	S12.030A	S12.24XK	S12.530B	S14.104A	S15.219A	S21.449A	S22.041B	S22.21XA	S25.199A	S27.322A	S31.630A	S32.032K
S06.2X2A	S06.367A	S06.896A	S12.030B	S12.250A	S12.530K	S14.105A	S15.221A	S21.451A	S22.041K	S22.21XB	S25.20XA	S27.329A	S31.631A	S32.038A
S06.2X3A	S06.368A	S06.897A	S12.030K	S12.250B	S12.531A	S14.106A	S15.222A	S21.452A	S22.042A	S22.21XK	S25.21XA	S27.331A	S31.632A	S32.038B
S06.2X4A	S06.369A	S06.898A	S12.031A	S12.250K	S12.531B	S14.107A	S15.229A	S21.459A	S22.042B	S22.22XA	S25.22XA	S27.332A	S31.633A	S32.038K
S06.2X5A	S06.371A	S06.899A	S12.031B	S12.251A	S12.531K	S14.108A	S15.291A	S21.90XA	S22.042K	S22.22XB	S25.29XA	S27.339A	S31.634A	S32.039A
S06.2X6A	S06.372A	S06.9X1A	S12.031K	S12.251B	S12.54XA	S14.111A	S15.292A	S21.91XA	S22.048A	S22.22XK	S25.301A	S27.391A	S31.635A	S32.039B
S06.2X7A	S06.373A	S06.9X2A	S12.040A	S12.251K	S12.54XB	S14.112A	S15.299A	S21.92XA	S22.048B	S22.23XA	S25.302A	S27.392A	S31.639A	S32.039K
S06.2X8A	S06.374A	S06.9X3A	S12.040B	S12.290A	S12.54XK	S14.113A	S15.301A	S21.93XA	S22.048K	S22.23XB	S25.309A	S27.399A	S31.640A	S32.040A
S06.2X9A	S06.375A	S06.9X4A	S12.040K	S12.290B	S12.550A	S14.114A	S15.302A	S21.94XA	S22.049A	S22.23XK	S25.311A	S27.401A	S31.641A	S32.040B
S06.301A	S06.376A	S06.9X5A	S12.041A	S12.290K	S12.550B	S14.115A	S15.309A	S21.95XA	S22.049B	S22.24XA	S25.312A	S27.402A	S31.642A	S32.040K
S06.302A	S06.377A	S06.9X6A	S12.041B	S12.291A	S12.550K	S14.116A	S15.311A	S22.000A	S22.049K	S22.24XB	S25.319A	S27.409A	S31.643A	S32.041A
S06.303A	S06.378A	S06.9X7A	S12.041K	S12.291B	S12.551A	S14.117A	S15.312A	S22.000B	S22.050A	S22.24XK	S25.321A	S27.411A	S31.644A	S32.041B
S06.304A	S06.379A	S06.9X8A	S12.090A	S12.291K	S12.551B	S14.118A	S15.319A	S22.000K	S22.050B	S22.31XA	S25.322A	S27.412A	S31.645A	S32.041K
S06.305A	S06.381A	S06.9X9A	S12.090B	S12.300A	S12.551K	S14.121A	S15.321A	S22.001A	S22.050K	S22.31XB	S25.329A	S27.419A	S31.649A	S32.042A
S06.306A	S06.382A	S07.0XXA	S12.090K	S12.300B	S12.590A	S14.122A	S15.322A	S22.001B	S22.051A	S22.31XK	S25.391A	S27.421A	S31.650A	S32.042B
S06.307A	S06.383A	S07.1XXA	S12.091A	S12.300K	S12.590B	S14.123A	S15.329A	S22.001K	S22.051B	S22.32XA	S25.392A	S27.422A	S31.651A	S32.042K
S06.308A	S06.384A	S07.8XXA	S12.091B	S12.301A	S12.590K	S14.124A	S15.391A	S22.002A	S22.051K	S22.32XB	S25.399A	S27.429A	S31.652A	S32.048A
S06.309A	S06.385A	S07.9XXA	S12.091K	S12.301B	S12.591A	S14.125A	S15.392A	S22.002B	S22.052A	S22.32XK	S25.401A	S27.431A	S31.653A	S32.048B
S06.310A	S06.386A	S09.0XXA	S12.100A	S12.301K	S12.591B	S14.126A	S15.399A	S22.002K	S22.052B	S22.39XA	S25.402A	S27.432A	S31.654A	S32.048K
S06.311A	S06.387A	S09.20XA	S12.100B	S12.330A	S12.591K	S14.127A	S15.8XXA	S22.008A	S22.052K	S22.39XB	S25.409A	S27.439A	S31.655A	S32.049A
S06.312A	S06.388A	S09.21XA	S12.100K	S12.330B	S12.600A	S14.128A	S15.9XXA	S22.008B	S22.058A	S22.39XK	S25.411A	S27.491A	S31.659A	S32.049B
S06.313A	S06.389A	S09.22XA	S12.101A	S12.330K	S12.600B	S14.131A	S17.0XXA	S22.008K	S22.058B	S22.41XA	S25.412A	S27.492A	S32.000A	S32.049K
S06.314A	S06.4X0A	S09.301A	S12.101B	S12.331A	S12.600K	S14.132A	S17.8XXA	S22.009A	S22.058K	S22.41XB	S25.419A	S27.499A	S32.000B	S32.050A
S06.315A	S06.4X1A	S09.302A	S12.101K	S12.331B	S12.601A	S14.133A	S17.9XXA	S22.009B	S22.059A	S22.41XK	S25.421A	S27.50XA	S32.000K	S32.050B
S06.316A	S06.4X2A	S09.309A	S12.110A	S12.331K	S12.601B	S14.134A	S21.101A	S22.009K	S22.059B	S22.42XA	S25.422A	S27.51XA	S32.001A	S32.050K
S06.317A	S06.4X3A	S09.311A	S12.110B	S12.34XA	S12.601K	S14.135A	S21.102A	S22.010A	S22.059K	S22.42XB	S25.429A	S27.52XA	S32.001B	S32.051A
S06.318A	S06.4X4A	S09.312A	S12.110K	S12.34XB	S12.630A	S14.136A	S21.109A	S22.010B	S22.060A	S22.42XK	S25.491A	S27.53XA	S32.001K	S32.051B
S06.319A	S06.4X5A	S09.313A	S12.111A	S12.34XK	S12.630B	S14.137A	S21.111A	S22.010K	S22.060B	S22.43XA	S25.492A	S27.59XA	S32.002A	S32.051K
S06.320A	S06.4X6A	S09.319A	S12.111B	S12.350A	S12.630K	S14.138A	S21.112A	S22.011A	S22.060K	S22.43XB	S25.499A	S27.60XA	S32.002B	S32.052A
S06.321A	S06.4X7A	S09.391A	S12.111K	S12.350B	S12.631A	S14.141A	S21.119A	S22.011B	S22.061A	S22.43XK	S25.501A	S27.63XA	S32.002K	S32.052B
S06.322A	S06.4X8A	S09.392A	S12.112A	S12.350K	S12.631B	S14.142A	S21.121A	S22.011K	S22.061B	S22.49XA	S25.502A	S27.69XA	S32.008A	S32.052K
S06.323A	S06.4X9A	S09.399A	S12.112B	S12.351A	S12.631K	S14.143A	S21.122A	S22.012A	S22.061K	S22.49XK	S25.509A	S27.802A	S32.008B	S32.058A
S06.324A	S06.5X0A	S11.011A	S12.112K	S12.351B	S12.64XA	S14.144A	S21.129A	S22.012B	S22.062A	S22.5XXA	S25.511A	S27.803A	S32.008K	S32.058B
S06.325A	S06.5X1A	S11.012A	S12.120A	S12.351K	S12.64XB	S14.145A	S21.131A	S22.012K	S22.062B	S22.5XXB	S25.512A	S27.808A	S32.009A	S32.058K
S06.326A	S06.5X2A	S11.013A	S12.120B	S12.390A	S12.64XK	S14.146A	S21.132A	S22.018A	S22.062K	S22.5XXK	S25.519A	S27.809A	S32.009B	S32.059A
S06.327A	S06.5X3A	S11.014A	S12.120K	S12.390B	S12.650A	S14.147A	S21.139A	S22.018B	S22.068A	S22.9XXA	S25.591A	S27.812A	S32.009K	S32.059B
S06.328A	S06.5X4A	S11.015A	S12.121A	S12.390K	S12.650B	S14.148A	S21.141A	S22.018K	S22.068B	S22.9XXB	S25.592A	S27.813A	S32.010A	S32.059K
S06.329A	S06.5X5A	S11.019A	S12.121B	S12.391A	S12.650K	S14.151A	S21.142A	S22.019A	S22.068K	S22.9XXK	S25.599A	S27.818A	S32.010B	S32.10XA
S06.330A	S06.5X6A	S11.021A	S12.121K	S12.391B	S12.651A	S14.152A	S21.149A	S22.019B	S22.069A	S24.0XXA	S25.801A	S27.819A	S32.010K	S32.10XB
S06.331A	S06.5X7A	S11.022A	S12.130A	S12.391K	S12.651B	S14.153A	S21.151A	S22.019K	S22.069B	S24.101A	S25.802A	S27.892A	S32.011A	S32.10XK
S06.332A	S06.5X8A	S11.023A	S12.130B	S12.400A	S12.651K	S14.154A	S21.152A	S22.020A	S22.069K	S24.102A	S25.809A	S27.893A	S32.011B	S32.110A
S06.333A	S06.5X9A	S11.024A	S12.130K	S12.400B	S12.690A	S14.155A	S21.159A	S22.020B	S22.070A	S24.103A	S25.811A	S27.898A	S32.011K	S32.110B
S06.334A	S06.6X0A	S11.025A	S12.131A	S12.400K	S12.690B	S14.156A	S21.301A	S22.020K	S22.070B	S24.104A	S25.812A	S27.899A	S32.012A	S32.110K
S06.335A	S06.6X1A	S11.029A	S12.131B	S12.401A	S12.690K	S14.157A	S21.302A	S22.021A	S22.070K	S24.111A	S25.819A	S27.9XXA	S32.012B	S32.111A
S06.336A	S06.6X2A	S11.031A	S12.131K	S12.401B	S12.691A	S14.158A	S21.309A	S22.021B	S22.071A	S24.112A	S25.891A	S28.1XXA	S32.012K	S32.111B
S06.337A	S06.6X3A	S11.032A	S12.14XA	S12.401K	S12.691B	S15.001A	S21.311A	S22.021K	S22.071B	S24.113A	S25.892A	S29.021A	S32.018A	S32.111K
S06.338A	S06.6X4A	S11.033A	S12.14XB	S12.430A	S12.691K	S15.002A	S21.312A	S22.022A	S22.071K	S24.114A	S25.899A	S29.029A	S32.018B	S32.112A
S06.339A	S06.6X5A	S11.034A	S12.14XK	S12.430B	S12.8XXA	S15.009A	S21.319A	S22.022B	S22.072A	S24.131A	S25.90XA	S31.001A	S32.018K	S32.112B
S06.340A	S06.6X6A	S11.035A	S12.150A	S12.430K	S12.9XXA	S15.011A	S21.321A	S22.022K	S22.072B	S24.132A	S25.91XA	S31.011A	S32.019A	S32.112K
S06.341A	S06.6X7A	S11.039A	S12.150B	S12.431A	S13.0XXA	S15.012A	S21.322A	S22.028A	S22.072K	S24.133A	S25.99XA	S31.021A	S32.019B	S32.119A
S06.342A	S06.6X8A	S11.10XA	S12.150K	S12.431B	S13.100A	S15.019A	S21.329A	S22.028B	S22.078A	S24.134A	S26.00XA	S31.031A	S32.019K	S32.119B
S06.343A	S06.6X9A	S11.11XA	S12.151A	S12.431K	S13.101A	S15.021A	S21.331A	S22.028K	S22.078B	S24.141A	S26.01XA	S31.041A	S32.020A	S32.119K
S06.344A	S06.811A	S11.12XA	S12.151B	S12.44XA	S13.110A	S15.022A	S21.332A	S22.029A	S22.078K	S24.142A	S26.020A	S31.051A	S32.020B	S32.120A
S06.345A	S06.812A	S11.13XA	S12.151K	S12.44XB	S13.111A	S15.029A	S21.339A	S22.029B	S22.079A	S24.143A	S26.021A	S31.600A	S32.020K	S32.120B
S06.346A	S06.813A	S11.14XA	S12.190A	S12.44XK	S13.120A	S15.091A	S21.341A	S22.029K	S22.079B	S24.144A	S26.022A	S31.601A	S32.021A	S32.120K
S06.347A	S06.814A	S11.15XA	S12.190B	S12.450A	S13.121A	S15.092A	S21.342A	S22.030A	S22.079K	S24.151A	S26.09XA	S31.602A	S32.021B	S32.121A
S06.348A	S06.815A	S11.20XA	S12.190K	S12.450B	S13.130A	S15.099A	S21.349A	S22.030B	S22.080A	S24.152A	S26.10XA	S31.603A	S32.021K	S32.121B
S06.349A	S06.816A	S11.21XA	S12.191A	S12.450K	S13.131A	S15.101A	S21.351A	S22.030K	S22.080B	S24.153A	S26.11XA	S31.604A	S32.022A	S32.121K
S06.350A	S06.817A	S11.22XA	S12.191B	S12.451A	S13.140A	S15.102A	S21.352A	S22.031A	S22.080K	S24.154A	S26.12XA	S31.605A	S32.022B	S32.122A
S06.351A	S06.818A	S11.23XA	S12.191K	S12.451B	S13.141A	S15.109A	S21.359A	S22.031B	S22.081A	S25.00XA	S26.19XA	S31.609A	S32.022K	S32.122B
S06.352A	S06.819A	S11.24XA	S12.200A	S12.451K	S13.150A	S15.111A	S21.401A	S22.031K	S22.081B	S25.01XA	S26.90XA	S31.610A	S32.028A	S32.122K
S06.353A	S06.821A	S11.25XA	S12.200B	S12.490A	S13.151A	S15.112A	S21.402A	S22.032A	S22.081K	S25.02XA	S26.91XA	S31.611A	S32.028B	S32.129A

Complications or Comorbidities/Major Complications or Comorbidities (CC/MCC) Exclusions (cont.) - Based on CMS data

S32.129B	S32.409A	S32.446K	S32.491B	S34.105A	S35.512A	S36.410A	S37.061A	S42.022K	S42.126B	S42.209A	S42.249K	S42.294P	S42.336A	S42.366K
S32.129K	S32.409B	S32.451A	S32.491K	S34.109A	S35.513A	S36.418A	S37.062A	S42.022P	S42.126K	S42.209B	S42.249P	S42.295A	S42.336B	S42.366P
S32.130A	S32.409K	S32.451B	S32.492A	S34.111A	S35.514A	S36.419A	S37.069A	S42.023B	S42.126P	S42.209K	S42.251A	S42.295B	S42.336K	S42.391A
S32.130B	S32.411A	S32.451K	S32.492B	S34.112A	S35.515A	S36.420A	S37.091A	S42.023K	S42.131B	S42.209P	S42.251B	S42.295K	S42.336P	S42.391B
S32.130K	S32.411B	S32.452A	S32.492K	S34.113A	S35.516A	S36.428A	S37.092A	S42.023P	S42.131K	S42.211A	S42.251K	S42.295P	S42.341A	S42.391K
S32.131A	S32.411K	S32.452B	S32.499A	S34.114A	S35.531A	S36.429A	S37.099A	S42.024B	S42.131P	S42.211B	S42.251P	S42.296A	S42.341B	S42.391P
S32.131B	S32.412A	S32.452K	S32.499B	S34.115A	S35.532A	S36.430A	S37.10XA	S42.024K	S42.132B	S42.211K	S42.252A	S42.296B	S42.341K	S42.392A
S32.131K	S32.412B	S32.453A	S32.499K	S34.119A	S35.533A	S36.438A	S37.12XA	S42.024P	S42.132K	S42.211P	S42.252B	S42.296K	S42.341P	S42.392B
S32.132A	S32.412K	S32.453B	S32.501B	S34.121A	S35.534A	S36.439A	S37.13XA	S42.025B	S42.132P	S42.212A	S42.252K	S42.296P	S42.342A	S42.392K
S32.132B	S32.413A	S32.453K	S32.502B	S34.122A	S35.535A	S36.490A	S37.19XA	S42.025K	S42.133B	S42.212B	S42.252P	S42.301A	S42.342B	S42.392P
S32.132K	S32.413B	S32.454A	S32.509B	S34.123A	S35.536A	S36.498A	S37.20XA	S42.025P	S42.133K	S42.212K	S42.253A	S42.301B	S42.342K	S42.399A
S32.139A	S32.413K	S32.454B	S32.511B	S34.124A	S35.59XA	S36.499A	S37.22XA	S42.026B	S42.133P	S42.212P	S42.253B	S42.301K	S42.342P	S42.399B
S32.139B	S32.414A	S32.454K	S32.512B	S34.125A	S35.8X1A	S36.500A	S37.23XA	S42.026K	S42.134B	S42.213A	S42.253K	S42.301P	S42.343A	S42.399K
S32.139K	S32.414B	S32.455A	S32.519B	S34.129A	S35.8X8A	S36.501A	S37.29XA	S42.026P	S42.134K	S42.213B	S42.253P	S42.302A	S42.343B	S42.399P
S32.14XA	S32.414K	S32.455B	S32.591B	S34.131A	S35.8X9A	S36.502A	S37.30XA	S42.031B	S42.134P	S42.213K	S42.254A	S42.302B	S42.343K	S42.401A
S32.14XB	S32.415A	S32.455K	S32.592B	S34.132A	S35.90XA	S36.503A	S37.32XA	S42.031K	S42.135B	S42.213P	S42.254B	S42.302K	S42.343P	S42.401B
S32.14XK	S32.415B	S32.456A	S32.599B	S34.139A	S35.91XA	S36.508A	S37.33XA	S42.031P	S42.135K	S42.214A	S42.254K	S42.302P	S42.344A	S42.401K
S32.15XA	S32.415K	S32.456B	S32.601A	S34.3XXA	S35.99XA	S36.509A	S37.39XA	S42.032B	S42.135P	S42.214B	S42.254P	S42.309A	S42.344B	S42.401P
S32.15XB	S32.416A	S32.456K	S32.601B	S35.00XA	S36.00XA	S36.510A	S37.60XA	S42.032K	S42.136B	S42.214K	S42.255A	S42.309B	S42.344K	S42.402A
S32.15XK	S32.416B	S32.461A	S32.601K	S35.01XA	S36.020A	S36.511A	S37.62XA	S42.032P	S42.136K	S42.214P	S42.255B	S42.309K	S42.344P	S42.402B
S32.16XA	S32.416K	S32.461B	S32.602A	S35.02XA	S36.021A	S36.512A	S37.63XA	S42.033B	S42.136P	S42.215A	S42.255K	S42.309P	S42.345A	S42.402K
S32.16XB	S32.421A	S32.461K	S32.602B	S35.09XA	S36.029A	S36.513A	S37.69XA	S42.033K	S42.141B	S42.215B	S42.255P	S42.311A	S42.345B	S42.402P
S32.16XK	S32.421B	S32.462A	S32.602K	S35.10XA	S36.030A	S36.518A	S37.812A	S42.033P	S42.141K	S42.215K	S42.256A	S42.311K	S42.345K	S42.409A
S32.17XA	S32.421K	S32.462B	S32.609A	S35.11XA	S36.031A	S36.519A	S37.813A	S42.034B	S42.141P	S42.215P	S42.256B	S42.311P	S42.345P	S42.409B
S32.17XB	S32.422A	S32.462K	S32.609B	S35.12XA	S36.032A	S36.520A	S37.818A	S42.034K	S42.142B	S42.216A	S42.256K	S42.312A	S42.346A	S42.409K
S32.17XK	S32.422B	S32.463A	S32.609K	S35.19XA	S36.039A	S36.521A	S37.819A	S42.034P	S42.142K	S42.216B	S42.256P	S42.312K	S42.346B	S42.409P
S32.19XA	S32.422K	S32.463B	S32.611A	S35.211A	S36.09XA	S36.522A	S37.892A	S42.035B	S42.142P	S42.216K	S42.261A	S42.312P	S42.346K	S42.411A
S32.19XB	S32.423A	S32.463K	S32.611B	S35.212A	S36.112A	S36.523A	S37.893A	S42.035K	S42.143B	S42.216P	S42.261B	S42.319A	S42.346P	S42.411B
S32.19XK	S32.423B	S32.464A	S32.611K	S35.218A	S36.113A	S36.528A	S37.898A	S42.035P	S42.143K	S42.221A	S42.261K	S42.319K	S42.351A	S42.411K
S32.2XXA	S32.423K	S32.464B	S32.612A	S35.219A	S36.114A	S36.529A	S37.899A	S42.036B	S42.143P	S42.221B	S42.261P	S42.319P	S42.351B	S42.411P
S32.2XXB	S32.424A	S32.464K	S32.612B	S35.221A	S36.115A	S36.530A	S37.90XA	S42.036K	S42.144B	S42.221K	S42.262A	S42.321A	S42.351K	S42.412A
S32.2XXK	S32.424B	S32.465A	S32.612K	S35.222A	S36.116A	S36.531A	S37.92XA	S42.036P	S42.144K	S42.221P	S42.262B	S42.321B	S42.351P	S42.412B
S32.301A	S32.424K	S32.465B	S32.613A	S35.228A	S36.118A	S36.532A	S37.93XA	S42.101B	S42.144P	S42.222A	S42.262K	S42.321K	S42.352A	S42.412K
S32.301B	S32.425A	S32.465K	S32.613B	S35.229A	S36.119A	S36.533A	S37.99XA	S42.101K	S42.145B	S42.222B	S42.262P	S42.321P	S42.352B	S42.412P
S32.301K	S32.425B	S32.466A	S32.613K	S35.231A	S36.122A	S36.538A	S42.001B	S42.101P	S42.145K	S42.222K	S42.263A	S42.322A	S42.352K	S42.413A
S32.302A	S32.425K	S32.466B	S32.614A	S35.232A	S36.123A	S36.539A	S42.001K	S42.102B	S42.145P	S42.222P	S42.263B	S42.322B	S42.352P	S42.413B
S32.302B	S32.426A	S32.466K	S32.614B	S35.238A	S36.128A	S36.590A	S42.001P	S42.102K	S42.146B	S42.223A	S42.263K	S42.322K	S42.353A	S42.413K
S32.302K	S32.426B	S32.471A	S32.614K	S35.239A	S36.129A	S36.591A	S42.002B	S42.102P	S42.146K	S42.223B	S42.263P	S42.322P	S42.353B	S42.413P
S32.309A	S32.426K	S32.471B	S32.615A	S35.291A	S36.13XA	S36.592A	S42.002K	S42.109B	S42.146P	S42.223K	S42.264A	S42.323A	S42.353K	S42.414A
S32.309B	S32.431A	S32.471K	S32.615B	S35.292A	S36.200A	S36.593A	S42.002P	S42.109K	S42.151B	S42.223P	S42.264B	S42.323B	S42.353P	S42.414B
S32.309K	S32.431B	S32.472A	S32.615K	S35.298A	S36.201A	S36.598A	S42.009B	S42.109P	S42.151K	S42.224A	S42.264K	S42.323K	S42.354A	S42.414K
S32.311A	S32.431K	S32.472B	S32.616A	S35.299A	S36.202A	S36.599A	S42.009K	S42.111B	S42.151P	S42.224B	S42.264P	S42.323P	S42.354B	S42.414P
S32.311B	S32.432A	S32.472K	S32.616B	S35.311A	S36.209A	S36.60XA	S42.009P	S42.111K	S42.152B	S42.224K	S42.265A	S42.324A	S42.354K	S42.415A
S32.311K	S32.432B	S32.473A	S32.616K	S35.318A	S36.220A	S36.61XA	S42.011B	S42.111P	S42.152K	S42.224P	S42.265B	S42.324B	S42.354P	S42.415B
S32.312A	S32.432K	S32.473B	S32.691A	S35.319A	S36.221A	S36.62XA	S42.011K	S42.112B	S42.152P	S42.225A	S42.265K	S42.324K	S42.355A	S42.415K
S32.312B	S32.433A	S32.473K	S32.691B	S35.321A	S36.222A	S36.63XA	S42.011P	S42.112K	S42.153B	S42.225B	S42.265P	S42.324P	S42.355B	S42.415P
S32.312K	S32.433B	S32.474A	S32.691K	S35.328A	S36.229A	S36.69XA	S42.012B	S42.112P	S42.153K	S42.225K	S42.266A	S42.325A	S42.355K	S42.416A
S32.313A	S32.433K	S32.474B	S32.692A	S35.329A	S36.230A	S36.81XA	S42.012K	S42.113B	S42.153P	S42.225P	S42.266B	S42.325B	S42.355P	S42.416B
S32.313B	S32.434A	S32.474K	S32.692B	S35.331A	S36.231A	S36.892A	S42.012P	S42.113K	S42.154B	S42.226A	S42.266K	S42.325K	S42.356A	S42.416K
S32.313K	S32.434B	S32.475A	S32.692K	S35.338A	S36.232A	S36.893A	S42.013B	S42.113P	S42.154K	S42.226B	S42.266P	S42.325P	S42.356B	S42.416P
S32.314A	S32.434K	S32.475B	S32.699A	S35.339A	S36.239A	S36.898A	S42.013K	S42.114B	S42.154P	S42.226K	S42.271A	S42.326A	S42.356K	S42.421A
S32.314B	S32.435A	S32.475K	S32.699B	S35.341A	S36.240A	S36.899A	S42.013P	S42.114K	S42.155B	S42.226P	S42.271K	S42.326B	S42.356P	S42.421B
S32.314K	S32.435B	S32.476A	S32.699K	S35.348A	S36.241A	S36.90XA	S42.014B	S42.114P	S42.155K	S42.231A	S42.271P	S42.326K	S42.361A	S42.421K
S32.315A	S32.435K	S32.476B	S32.810A	S35.349A	S36.242A	S36.92XA	S42.014K	S42.115B	S42.155P	S42.231B	S42.272A	S42.326P	S42.361B	S42.421P
S32.315B	S32.436A	S32.476K	S32.810B	S35.401A	S36.249A	S36.93XA	S42.014P	S42.115K	S42.156B	S42.231K	S42.272K	S42.331A	S42.361K	S42.422A
S32.315K	S32.436B	S32.481A	S32.810K	S35.402A	S36.250A	S36.99XA	S42.015B	S42.115P	S42.156K	S42.231P	S42.272P	S42.331B	S42.361P	S42.422B
S32.316A	S32.436K	S32.481B	S32.811A	S35.403A	S36.251A	S37.001A	S42.015K	S42.116B	S42.156P	S42.232A	S42.279A	S42.331K	S42.362A	S42.422K
S32.316B	S32.441A	S32.481K	S32.811B	S35.404A	S36.252A	S37.002A	S42.015P	S42.116K	S42.191B	S42.232B	S42.279K	S42.331P	S42.362B	S42.422P
S32.316K	S32.441B	S32.482A	S32.811K	S35.405A	S36.259A	S37.009A	S42.016B	S42.116P	S42.191K	S42.232K	S42.279P	S42.332A	S42.362K	S42.423A
S32.391A	S32.441K	S32.482B	S32.82XA	S35.406A	S36.260A	S37.011A	S42.016K	S42.121B	S42.191P	S42.232P	S42.291A	S42.332B	S42.362P	S42.423B
S32.391B	S32.442A	S32.482K	S32.82XB	S35.411A	S36.261A	S37.012A	S42.016P	S42.121K	S42.192B	S42.239A	S42.291B	S42.332K	S42.363A	S42.423K
S32.391K	S32.442B	S32.483A	S32.82XK	S35.412A	S36.262A	S37.019A	S42.017B	S42.121P	S42.192K	S42.239B	S42.291K	S42.332P	S42.363B	S42.423P
S32.392A	S32.442K	S32.483B	S32.89XA	S35.413A	S36.269A	S37.021A	S42.017K	S42.122B	S42.192P	S42.239K	S42.291P	S42.333A	S42.363K	S42.424A
S32.392B	S32.443A	S32.483K	S32.89XB	S35.414A	S36.290A	S37.022A	S42.017P	S42.122K	S42.199B	S42.239P	S42.292A	S42.333B	S42.363P	S42.424B
S32.392K	S32.443B	S32.484A	S32.89XK	S35.415A	S36.291A	S37.029A	S42.018B	S42.122P	S42.199K	S42.241A	S42.292B	S42.333K	S42.364A	S42.424K
S32.399A	S32.443K	S32.484B	S32.9XXA	S35.416A	S36.292A	S37.031A	S42.018K	S42.123B	S42.199P	S42.241B	S42.292K	S42.333P	S42.364B	S42.424P
S32.399B	S32.444A	S32.484K	S32.9XXB	S35.491A	S36.299A	S37.032A	S42.018P	S42.123K	S42.201A	S42.241K	S42.292P	S42.334A	S42.364K	S42.425A
S32.399K	S32.444B	S32.485A	S32.9XXK	S35.492A	S36.30XA	S37.039A	S42.019B	S42.123P	S42.201B	S42.241P	S42.293A	S42.334B	S42.364P	S42.425B
S32.401A	S32.444K	S32.485B	S34.01XA	S35.493A	S36.32XA	S37.041A	S42.019K	S42.124B	S42.201K	S42.242A	S42.293B	S42.334K	S42.365A	S42.425K
S32.401B	S32.445A	S32.485K	S34.02XA	S35.494A	S36.33XA	S37.042A	S42.019P	S42.124K	S42.201P	S42.242B	S42.293K	S42.334P	S42.365B	S42.425P
S32.401K	S32.445B	S32.486A	S34.101A	S35.495A	S36.39XA	S37.049A	S42.021B	S42.124P	S42.202A	S42.242K	S42.293P	S42.335A	S42.365K	S42.426A
S32.402A	S32.445K	S32.486B	S34.102A	S35.496A	S36.400A	S37.051A	S42.021K	S42.125B	S42.202B	S42.242P	S42.294A	S42.335B	S42.365P	S42.426B
S32.402B	S32.446A	S32.486K	S34.103A	S35.50XA	S36.408A	S37.052A	S42.021P	S42.125K	S42.202K	S42.249A	S42.294B	S42.335K	S42.366A	S42.426K
S32.402K	S32.446B	S32.491A	S34.104A	S35.511A	S36.409A	S37.059A	S42.022B	S42.125P	S42.202P	S42.249B	S42.294K	S42.335P	S42.366B	S42.426P

Complications or Comorbidities/Major Complications or Comorbidities (CC/MCC) Exclusions (cont.) - Based on CMS data

S42.431A
S42.431B
S42.431K
S42.431P
S42.432A
S42.432B
S42.432K
S42.432P
S42.433A
S42.433B
S42.433K
S42.433P
S42.434A
S42.434B
S42.434K
S42.434P
S42.435A
S42.435B
S42.435K
S42.435P
S42.436A
S42.436B
S42.436K
S42.436P
S42.441A
S42.441B
S42.441K
S42.441P
S42.442A
S42.442B
S42.442K
S42.442P
S42.443A
S42.443B
S42.443K
S42.443P
S42.444A
S42.444B
S42.444K
S42.444P
S42.445A
S42.445B
S42.445K
S42.445P
S42.446A
S42.446B
S42.446K
S42.446P
S42.447A
S42.447B
S42.447K
S42.447P
S42.448A
S42.448B
S42.448K
S42.448P
S42.449A
S42.449B
S42.449K
S42.449P
S42.451A
S42.451B
S42.451K
S42.451P
S42.452A
S42.452B
S42.452K
S42.452P
S42.453A
S42.453B
S42.453K
S42.453P
S42.454A
S42.454B
S42.454K
S42.454P
S42.455A
S42.455B
S42.455K
S42.455P
S42.456A
S42.456B
S42.456K
S42.456P
S42.461A
S42.461B
S42.461K
S42.461P
S42.462A
S42.462B
S42.462K
S42.462P
S42.463A
S42.463B
S42.463K
S42.463P
S42.464A
S42.464B
S42.464K
S42.464P
S42.465A
S42.465B
S42.465K
S42.465P
S42.466A
S42.466B
S42.466K
S42.466P
S42.471A
S42.471B
S42.471K
S42.471P
S42.472A
S42.472B
S42.472K
S42.472P
S42.473A
S42.473B
S42.473K
S42.473P
S42.474A
S42.474B
S42.474K
S42.474P
S42.475A
S42.475B
S42.475K
S42.475P
S42.476A
S42.476B
S42.476K
S42.476P
S42.481A
S42.481K
S42.481P
S42.482A
S42.482K
S42.482P
S42.489A
S42.489K
S42.489P
S42.491A
S42.491B
S42.491K
S42.491P
S42.492A
S42.492B
S42.492K
S42.492P
S42.493A
S42.493B
S42.493K
S42.493P
S42.494A
S42.494B
S42.494K
S42.494P
S42.495A
S42.495B
S42.495K
S42.495P
S42.496A
S42.496B
S42.496K
S42.496P
S42.90XA
S42.90XB
S42.90XK
S42.90XP
S42.91XA
S42.91XB
S42.91XK
S42.91XP
S42.92XA
S42.92XB
S42.92XK
S42.92XP
S43.201A
S43.202A
S43.203A
S43.204A
S43.205A
S43.206A
S43.211A
S43.212A
S43.213A
S43.214A
S43.215A
S43.216A
S43.221A
S43.222A
S43.223A
S43.224A
S43.225A
S43.226A
S45.001A
S45.002A
S45.009A
S45.011A
S45.012A
S45.019A
S45.091A
S45.092A
S45.099A
S45.101A
S45.102A
S45.109A
S45.111A
S45.112A
S45.119A
S45.191A
S45.192A
S45.199A
S45.201A
S45.202A
S45.209A
S45.211A
S45.212A
S45.219A
S45.291A
S45.292A
S45.299A
S45.301A
S45.302A
S45.309A
S45.311A
S45.312A
S45.319A
S45.391A
S45.392A
S45.399A
S45.801A
S45.802A
S45.809A
S45.811A
S45.812A
S45.819A
S45.891A
S45.892A
S45.899A
S45.901A
S45.902A
S45.909A
S45.911A
S45.912A
S45.919A
S45.991A
S45.992A
S45.999A
S46.021A
S46.022A
S46.029A
S46.121A
S46.122A
S46.129A
S46.221A
S46.222A
S46.229A
S46.321A
S46.322A
S46.329A
S46.821A
S46.822A
S46.829A
S46.921A
S46.922A
S46.929A
S48.011A
S48.012A
S48.019A
S48.021A
S48.022A
S48.029A
S48.111A
S48.112A
S48.119A
S48.121A
S48.122A
S48.129A
S48.911A
S48.912A
S48.919A
S48.921A
S48.922A
S48.929A
S49.001A
S49.001K
S49.001P
S49.002A
S49.002K
S49.002P
S49.009A
S49.009K
S49.009P
S49.011A
S49.011K
S49.011P
S49.012A
S49.012K
S49.012P
S49.019A
S49.019K
S49.019P
S49.021A
S49.021K
S49.021P
S49.022A
S49.022K
S49.022P
S49.029A
S49.029K
S49.029P
S49.031A
S49.031K
S49.031P
S49.032A
S49.032K
S49.032P
S49.039A
S49.039K
S49.039P
S49.041A
S49.041K
S49.041P
S49.042A
S49.042K
S49.042P
S49.049A
S49.049K
S49.049P
S49.091A
S49.091K
S49.091P
S49.092A
S49.092K
S49.092P
S49.099A
S49.099K
S49.099P
S49.101A
S49.101K
S49.101P
S49.102A
S49.102K
S49.102P
S49.109A
S49.109K
S49.109P
S49.111A
S49.111K
S49.111P
S49.112A
S49.112K
S49.112P
S49.119A
S49.119K
S49.119P
S49.121A
S49.121K
S49.121P
S49.122A
S49.122K
S49.122P
S49.129A
S49.129K
S49.129P
S49.131A
S49.131K
S49.131P
S49.132A
S49.132K
S49.132P
S49.139A
S49.139K
S49.139P
S49.141A
S49.141K
S49.141P
S49.142A
S49.142K
S49.142P
S49.149A
S49.149K
S49.149P
S49.191A
S49.191K
S49.191P
S49.192A
S49.192K
S49.192P
S49.199A
S49.199K
S49.199P
S52.001B
S52.001C
S52.001K
S52.001M
S52.001N
S52.001P
S52.001Q
S52.001R
S52.002B
S52.002C
S52.002K
S52.002M
S52.002N
S52.002P
S52.002Q
S52.002R
S52.009B
S52.009C
S52.009K
S52.009M
S52.009N
S52.009P
S52.009Q
S52.009R
S52.011A
S52.011K
S52.011P
S52.012A
S52.012K
S52.012P
S52.019A
S52.019K
S52.019P
S52.021B
S52.021C
S52.021K
S52.021M
S52.021N
S52.021P
S52.021Q
S52.021R
S52.022B
S52.022C
S52.022K
S52.022M
S52.022N
S52.022P
S52.022Q
S52.022R
S52.023B
S52.023C
S52.023K
S52.023M
S52.023N
S52.023P
S52.023Q
S52.023R
S52.024B
S52.024C
S52.024K
S52.024M
S52.024N
S52.024P
S52.024Q
S52.024R
S52.025B
S52.025C
S52.025K
S52.025M
S52.025N
S52.025P
S52.025Q
S52.025R
S52.026B
S52.026C
S52.026K
S52.026M
S52.026N
S52.026P
S52.026Q
S52.026R
S52.031B
S52.031C
S52.031K
S52.031M
S52.031N
S52.031P
S52.031Q
S52.031R
S52.032B
S52.032C
S52.032K
S52.032M
S52.032N
S52.032P
S52.032Q
S52.032R
S52.033B
S52.033C
S52.033K
S52.033M
S52.033N
S52.033P
S52.033Q
S52.033R
S52.034B
S52.034C
S52.034K
S52.034M
S52.034N
S52.034P
S52.034Q
S52.034R
S52.035B
S52.035C
S52.035K
S52.035M
S52.035N
S52.035P
S52.035Q
S52.035R
S52.036B
S52.036C
S52.036K
S52.036M
S52.036N
S52.036P
S52.036Q
S52.036R
S52.041B
S52.041C
S52.041K
S52.041M
S52.041N
S52.041P
S52.041Q
S52.041R
S52.042B
S52.042C
S52.042K
S52.042M
S52.042N
S52.042P
S52.042Q
S52.042R
S52.043B
S52.043C
S52.043K
S52.043M
S52.043N
S52.043P
S52.043Q
S52.043R
S52.044B
S52.044C
S52.044K
S52.044M
S52.044N
S52.044P
S52.044Q
S52.044R
S52.045B
S52.045C
S52.045K
S52.045M
S52.045N
S52.045P
S52.045Q
S52.045R
S52.046B
S52.046C
S52.046K
S52.046M
S52.046N
S52.046P
S52.046Q
S52.046R
S52.091B
S52.091C
S52.091K
S52.091M
S52.091N
S52.091P
S52.091Q
S52.091R
S52.092B
S52.092C
S52.092K
S52.092M
S52.092N
S52.092P
S52.092Q
S52.092R
S52.099B
S52.099C
S52.099K
S52.099M
S52.099N
S52.099P
S52.099Q
S52.099R
S52.101B
S52.101C
S52.101K
S52.101M
S52.101N
S52.101P
S52.101Q
S52.101R
S52.102B
S52.102C
S52.102K
S52.102M
S52.102N
S52.102P
S52.102Q
S52.102R
S52.109B
S52.109C
S52.109K
S52.109M
S52.109N
S52.109P
S52.109Q
S52.109R
S52.111A
S52.111K
S52.111P
S52.112A
S52.112K
S52.112P
S52.119A
S52.119K
S52.119P
S52.121B
S52.121C
S52.121K
S52.121M
S52.121N
S52.121P
S52.121Q
S52.121R
S52.122B
S52.122C
S52.122K
S52.122M
S52.122N
S52.122P
S52.122Q
S52.122R
S52.123B
S52.123C
S52.123K
S52.123M
S52.123N
S52.123P
S52.123Q
S52.123R
S52.124B
S52.124C
S52.124K
S52.124M
S52.124N
S52.124P
S52.124Q
S52.124R
S52.125B
S52.125C
S52.125K
S52.125M
S52.125N
S52.125P
S52.125Q
S52.125R
S52.126B
S52.126C
S52.126K
S52.126M
S52.126N
S52.126P
S52.126Q
S52.126R
S52.131B
S52.131C
S52.131K
S52.131M
S52.131N
S52.131P
S52.131Q
S52.131R
S52.132B
S52.132C
S52.132K
S52.132M
S52.132N
S52.132P
S52.132Q
S52.132R
S52.133B
S52.133C
S52.133K
S52.133M
S52.133N
S52.133P
S52.133Q
S52.133R
S52.134B
S52.134C
S52.134K
S52.134M
S52.134N
S52.134P
S52.134Q
S52.134R
S52.135B
S52.135C
S52.135K
S52.135M
S52.135N
S52.135P
S52.135Q
S52.135R
S52.136B
S52.136C
S52.136K
S52.136M
S52.136N
S52.136P
S52.136Q
S52.136R
S52.181B
S52.181C
S52.181K
S52.181M
S52.181N
S52.181P
S52.181Q
S52.181R
S52.182B
S52.182C
S52.182K
S52.182M
S52.182N
S52.182P
S52.182Q
S52.182R
S52.189B
S52.189C
S52.189K
S52.189M
S52.189N
S52.189P
S52.189Q
S52.189R
S52.201A
S52.201B
S52.201C
S52.201K
S52.201M
S52.201N
S52.201P
S52.201Q
S52.201R
S52.202A
S52.202B
S52.202C
S52.202K
S52.202M
S52.202N
S52.202P
S52.202Q
S52.202R
S52.209A
S52.209B
S52.209C
S52.209K
S52.209M
S52.209N
S52.209P
S52.209Q
S52.209R
S52.211A
S52.211K
S52.211P
S52.212A
S52.212K
S52.212P
S52.219A
S52.219K
S52.219P
S52.221A
S52.221B
S52.221C
S52.221K
S52.221M
S52.221N
S52.221P
S52.221Q
S52.221R
S52.222A
S52.222B
S52.222C
S52.222K
S52.222M
S52.222N
S52.222P
S52.222Q
S52.222R
S52.223A
S52.223B
S52.223C
S52.223K
S52.223M
S52.223N
S52.223P
S52.223Q
S52.223R
S52.224A
S52.224B
S52.224C
S52.224K
S52.224M
S52.224N
S52.224P
S52.224Q
S52.224R
S52.225A
S52.225B
S52.225C
S52.225K
S52.225M
S52.225N
S52.225P
S52.225Q
S52.225R
S52.226A
S52.226B
S52.226C
S52.226K
S52.226M
S52.226N
S52.226P
S52.226Q
S52.226R
S52.231A
S52.231B
S52.231C
S52.231K
S52.231M
S52.231N
S52.231P
S52.231Q
S52.231R
S52.232A
S52.232B
S52.232C
S52.232K
S52.232M
S52.232N
S52.232P
S52.232Q
S52.232R
S52.233A
S52.233B
S52.233C
S52.233K
S52.233M
S52.233N
S52.233P
S52.233Q
S52.233R
S52.234A
S52.234B
S52.234C
S52.234K
S52.234M
S52.234N
S52.234P
S52.234Q
S52.234R
S52.235A
S52.235B
S52.235C
S52.235K
S52.235M
S52.235N
S52.235P
S52.235Q
S52.235R
S52.236A
S52.236B
S52.236C
S52.236K
S52.236M
S52.236N
S52.236P
S52.236Q
S52.236R
S52.241A
S52.241B
S52.241C
S52.241K
S52.241M
S52.241N
S52.241P
S52.241Q
S52.241R
S52.242A
S52.242B
S52.242C
S52.242K
S52.242M
S52.242N
S52.242P
S52.242Q
S52.242R
S52.243A
S52.243B
S52.243C
S52.243K
S52.243M
S52.243N
S52.243P
S52.243Q
S52.243R
S52.244A
S52.244B
S52.244C
S52.244K
S52.244M
S52.244N
S52.244P
S52.244Q
S52.244R
S52.245A
S52.245B
S52.245C
S52.245K
S52.245M
S52.245N
S52.245P
S52.245Q
S52.245R
S52.246A
S52.246B
S52.246C
S52.246K
S52.246M
S52.246N
S52.246P
S52.246Q
S52.246R
S52.251A
S52.251B
S52.251C
S52.251K
S52.251M
S52.251N
S52.251P
S52.251Q
S52.251R
S52.252A
S52.252B
S52.252C
S52.252K
S52.252M
S52.252N
S52.252P
S52.252Q
S52.252R
S52.253A
S52.253B
S52.253C
S52.253K
S52.253M
S52.253N
S52.253P
S52.253Q
S52.253R
S52.254A
S52.254B
S52.254C
S52.254K
S52.254M
S52.254N
S52.254P
S52.254Q
S52.254R
S52.255A
S52.255B
S52.255C
S52.255K
S52.255M
S52.255N
S52.255P
S52.255Q
S52.255R
S52.256A
S52.256B
S52.256C
S52.256K
S52.256M
S52.256N
S52.256P
S52.256Q
S52.256R
S52.261A
S52.261B
S52.261C
S52.261K
S52.261M
S52.261N
S52.261P
S52.261Q
S52.261R
S52.262A
S52.262B
S52.262C
S52.262K
S52.262M
S52.262N
S52.262P
S52.262Q
S52.262R
S52.263A
S52.263B
S52.263C
S52.263K
S52.263M
S52.263N
S52.263P
S52.263Q
S52.263R
S52.264A
S52.264B
S52.264C
S52.264K
S52.264M
S52.264N
S52.264P
S52.264Q
S52.264R
S52.265A
S52.265B
S52.265C
S52.265K
S52.265M
S52.265N
S52.265P
S52.265Q
S52.265R
S52.266A
S52.266B
S52.266C
S52.266K
S52.266M
S52.266N
S52.266P
S52.266Q
S52.266R
S52.271B
S52.271C
S52.271K
S52.271M
S52.271N
S52.271P
S52.271Q
S52.271R
S52.272B
S52.272C
S52.272K
S52.272M
S52.272N
S52.272P
S52.272Q
S52.272R
S52.279B
S52.279C
S52.279K
S52.279M
S52.279N
S52.279P
S52.279Q
S52.279R
S52.281A
S52.281B
S52.281C
S52.281K
S52.281M
S52.281N
S52.281P
S52.281Q
S52.281R
S52.282A
S52.282B
S52.282C
S52.282K
S52.282M
S52.282N
S52.282P
S52.282Q
S52.282R
S52.283A
S52.283B
S52.283C
S52.283K
S52.283M
S52.283N
S52.283P
S52.283Q
S52.283R
S52.291A
S52.291B
S52.291C
S52.291K
S52.291M
S52.291N

Complications or Comorbidities/Major Complications or Comorbidities (CC/MCC) Exclusions (cont.) - Based on CMS data

The codes below are arranged in a 15-column grid read top-to-bottom, then left-to-right.

Column 1: S52.291P, S52.291Q, S52.291R, S52.292A, S52.292B, S52.292C, S52.292K, S52.292M, S52.292N, S52.292P, S52.292Q, S52.292R, S52.299A, S52.299B, S52.299C, S52.299M, S52.299N, S52.299P, S52.299Q, S52.299R, S52.301A, S52.301B, S52.301C, S52.301K, S52.301M, S52.301N, S52.301P, S52.301Q, S52.301R, S52.302A, S52.302B, S52.302C, S52.302K, S52.302M, S52.302N, S52.302P, S52.302Q, S52.302R, S52.309A, S52.309B, S52.309C, S52.309K, S52.309M, S52.309N, S52.309P, S52.309Q, S52.309R, S52.311A, S52.311K, S52.311P, S52.312A, S52.312K, S52.312P, S52.319A, S52.319K, S52.319P, S52.321A, S52.321B, S52.321C, S52.321K, S52.321M, S52.321N, S52.321P, S52.321Q, S52.321R, S52.322A, S52.322B, S52.322C, S52.322K, S52.322M, S52.322N, S52.322P, S52.322Q

Column 2: S52.322R, S52.323A, S52.323B, S52.323C, S52.323K, S52.323M, S52.323N, S52.323P, S52.323Q, S52.323R, S52.324A, S52.324B, S52.324C, S52.324K, S52.324M, S52.324N, S52.324P, S52.324Q, S52.324R, S52.325A, S52.325B, S52.325C, S52.325K, S52.325M, S52.325N, S52.325P, S52.325Q, S52.325R, S52.326A, S52.326B, S52.326C, S52.326K, S52.326M, S52.326N, S52.326P, S52.326Q, S52.326R, S52.331A, S52.331B, S52.331C, S52.331K, S52.331M, S52.331N, S52.331Q, S52.331R, S52.332A, S52.332B, S52.332C, S52.332K, S52.332M, S52.332N, S52.332P, S52.332Q, S52.332R, S52.333A, S52.333B, S52.333C, S52.333K, S52.333M, S52.333N, S52.333P, S52.333Q, S52.333R, S52.334A, S52.334B, S52.334C, S52.334K, S52.334M, S52.334N, S52.334P, S52.334Q, S52.334R, S52.335A

Column 3: S52.335B, S52.335C, S52.335K, S52.335M, S52.335N, S52.335P, S52.335Q, S52.335R, S52.336A, S52.336B, S52.336C, S52.336K, S52.336M, S52.336N, S52.336P, S52.336Q, S52.336R, S52.341A, S52.341B, S52.341C, S52.341K, S52.341N, S52.341P, S52.341Q, S52.341R, S52.342A, S52.342C, S52.342K, S52.342M, S52.342N, S52.342P, S52.342Q, S52.343A, S52.343B, S52.343C, S52.343K, S52.343M, S52.343N, S52.343P, S52.343Q, S52.343R, S52.344A, S52.344B, S52.344C, S52.344K, S52.344M, S52.344N, S52.344P, S52.344Q, S52.344R, S52.345A, S52.345B, S52.345C, S52.345K, S52.345M, S52.345N, S52.345P, S52.345Q, S52.345R, S52.346A, S52.346B, S52.346C, S52.346K, S52.346M, S52.346N, S52.346P, S52.346Q, S52.351A, S52.351B, S52.351C

Column 4: S52.351K, S52.351M, S52.351N, S52.351P, S52.351Q, S52.351R, S52.352A, S52.352B, S52.352C, S52.352K, S52.352M, S52.352N, S52.352P, S52.352Q, S52.352R, S52.353A, S52.353B, S52.353C, S52.353K, S52.353M, S52.353N, S52.353Q, S52.353R, S52.354A, S52.354B, S52.354C, S52.354K, S52.354M, S52.354N, S52.354P, S52.354Q, S52.354R, S52.355A, S52.355B, S52.355C, S52.355M, S52.355N, S52.355P, S52.355Q, S52.355R, S52.356A, S52.356B, S52.356C, S52.356K, S52.356M, S52.356N, S52.356P, S52.356R, S52.361A, S52.361B, S52.361C, S52.361K, S52.361M, S52.361N, S52.361P, S52.361Q, S52.361R, S52.362A, S52.362B, S52.362C, S52.362K, S52.362M, S52.362N, S52.362P, S52.362Q, S52.362R, S52.363A, S52.363B, S52.363C, S52.363K, S52.363M

Column 5: S52.363N, S52.363P, S52.363Q, S52.363R, S52.364A, S52.364B, S52.364C, S52.364K, S52.364M, S52.364N, S52.364P, S52.364Q, S52.364R, S52.365A, S52.365B, S52.365C, S52.365K, S52.365M, S52.365N, S52.365P, S52.365Q, S52.366A, S52.366B, S52.366C, S52.366K, S52.366M, S52.366N, S52.366P, S52.366Q, S52.366R, S52.371A, S52.371B, S52.371C, S52.371K, S52.371M, S52.371N, S52.371P, S52.371Q, S52.371R, S52.372A, S52.372B, S52.372C, S52.372K, S52.372M, S52.372N, S52.372P, S52.372Q, S52.372R, S52.379A, S52.379B, S52.379C, S52.379K, S52.379M, S52.379N, S52.379P, S52.379Q, S52.381A, S52.381B, S52.381C, S52.381K, S52.381M, S52.381N, S52.381P, S52.381Q, S52.381R, S52.382A, S52.382B, S52.382C, S52.382K, S52.382M, S52.382N

Column 6: S52.382P, S52.382Q, S52.382R, S52.389A, S52.389B, S52.389C, S52.389K, S52.389M, S52.389N, S52.389P, S52.389Q, S52.389R, S52.391A, S52.391B, S52.391C, S52.391K, S52.391M, S52.391N, S52.391P, S52.391Q, S52.391R, S52.392A, S52.392B, S52.392K, S52.392M, S52.392N, S52.392P, S52.392Q, S52.392R, S52.399A, S52.399B, S52.399C, S52.399K, S52.399M, S52.399N, S52.399P, S52.399Q, S52.399R, S52.501A, S52.501B, S52.501C, S52.501K, S52.501M, S52.501N, S52.501P, S52.501Q, S52.501R, S52.502A, S52.502B, S52.502C, S52.502K, S52.502M, S52.502N, S52.502P, S52.502Q, S52.502R, S52.509A, S52.509B, S52.509C, S52.509K, S52.509M, S52.509N, S52.509P, S52.509Q, S52.509R, S52.511A, S52.511B, S52.511C, S52.511K, S52.511M, S52.511N, S52.511P, S52.511Q, S52.511R

Column 7: S52.512A, S52.512B, S52.512C, S52.512K, S52.512M, S52.512N, S52.512P, S52.512Q, S52.512R, S52.513A, S52.513B, S52.513C, S52.513K, S52.513M, S52.513N, S52.513P, S52.513Q, S52.513R, S52.514A, S52.514B, S52.514C, S52.514K, S52.514M, S52.514N, S52.514P, S52.514Q, S52.514R, S52.515A, S52.515B, S52.515C, S52.515K, S52.515M, S52.515N, S52.515P, S52.515Q, S52.516A, S52.516B, S52.516C, S52.516K, S52.516M, S52.516N, S52.516Q, S52.516R, S52.521A, S52.521K, S52.521P, S52.522A, S52.522K, S52.522P, S52.529A, S52.529K, S52.529P, S52.531A, S52.531B, S52.531C, S52.531K, S52.531M, S52.531N, S52.531P, S52.531Q, S52.531R, S52.532A, S52.532B, S52.532C, S52.532K, S52.532M, S52.532N, S52.532P, S52.532Q, S52.532R, S52.539A, S52.539B

Column 8: S52.539C, S52.539K, S52.539M, S52.539N, S52.539P, S52.539Q, S52.539R, S52.541A, S52.541C, S52.541K, S52.541M, S52.541N, S52.541P, S52.541Q, S52.541R, S52.542A, S52.542B, S52.542C, S52.542K, S52.542M, S52.542P, S52.542Q, S52.542R, S52.549A, S52.549B, S52.549C, S52.549M, S52.549N, S52.549P, S52.549Q, S52.549R, S52.551A, S52.551C, S52.551K, S52.551M, S52.551P, S52.551Q, S52.552A, S52.552B, S52.552C, S52.552K, S52.552M, S52.552N, S52.552P, S52.552Q, S52.552R, S52.559A, S52.559B, S52.559C, S52.559K, S52.559M, S52.559N, S52.559P, S52.559Q, S52.559R, S52.561A, S52.561B, S52.561C, S52.561K, S52.561M, S52.561N, S52.561P, S52.561Q, S52.562A, S52.562B, S52.562C, S52.562K

Column 9: S52.562M, S52.562N, S52.562P, S52.562Q, S52.562R, S52.569A, S52.569B, S52.569C, S52.569K, S52.569M, S52.569N, S52.569P, S52.569Q, S52.569R, S52.571A, S52.571C, S52.571K, S52.571M, S52.571N, S52.571P, S52.571Q, S52.571R, S52.572A, S52.572B, S52.572C, S52.572K, S52.572M, S52.572N, S52.572P, S52.572Q, S52.572R, S52.579A, S52.579B, S52.579C, S52.579K, S52.579M, S52.579N, S52.579P, S52.579Q, S52.579R, S52.591A, S52.591C, S52.591K, S52.591M, S52.591N, S52.591P, S52.591Q, S52.591R, S52.592A, S52.592B, S52.592C, S52.592K, S52.592M, S52.592N, S52.592P, S52.592Q, S52.592R, S52.599A, S52.599B, S52.599C, S52.599K, S52.599M, S52.599N, S52.599P, S52.599Q, S52.599R, S52.601A, S52.601B, S52.601C, S52.601K, S52.601M, S52.601N

Column 10: S52.601P, S52.601Q, S52.601R, S52.602A, S52.602B, S52.602C, S52.602K, S52.602M, S52.602P, S52.602Q, S52.602R, S52.609A, S52.609B, S52.609C, S52.609K, S52.609M, S52.609N, S52.609P, S52.609Q, S52.609R, S52.611A, S52.611B, S52.611C, S52.611K, S52.611N, S52.611P, S52.611Q, S52.611R, S52.612A, S52.612B, S52.612C, S52.612K, S52.612M, S52.612Q, S52.612R, S52.613A, S52.613B, S52.613C, S52.613K, S52.613N, S52.613R, S52.614A, S52.614B, S52.614C, S52.614M, S52.614N, S52.614P, S52.614Q, S52.614R, S52.615A, S52.615B, S52.615C, S52.615K, S52.615M, S52.615N, S52.615Q, S52.616A, S52.616B, S52.616C, S52.616K, S52.616M, S52.616P, S52.616Q

Column 11: S52.616R, S52.621A, S52.621K, S52.621P, S52.622A, S52.622K, S52.622P, S52.629A, S52.629B, S52.629K, S52.629P, S52.629Q, S52.629R, S52.691A, S52.691B, S52.691C, S52.691K, S52.691M, S52.691P, S52.691Q, S52.691R, S52.692A, S52.692B, S52.692C, S52.692M, S52.692N, S52.692P, S52.692Q, S52.699A, S52.699B, S52.699C, S52.699K, S52.699M, S52.699N, S52.699P, S52.699Q, S52.699R, S52.90XA, S52.90XB, S52.90XC, S52.90XK, S52.90XM, S52.90XN, S52.90XP, S52.90XQ, S52.90XR, S52.91XA, S52.91XB, S52.91XC, S52.91XK, S52.91XM, S52.91XN, S52.91XP, S52.91XQ, S52.91XR, S52.92XA, S52.92XB, S52.92XC, S52.92XK, S52.92XM, S52.92XN, S52.92XP, S52.92XQ, S52.92XR, S55.001A, S55.002A, S55.009A, S55.011A, S55.012A, S55.019A, S55.091A, S55.099A, S55.101A

Column 12: S55.102A, S55.109A, S55.111A, S55.112A, S55.119A, S55.191A, S55.192A, S55.199A, S55.201A, S55.202A, S55.209A, S55.211A, S55.212A, S55.219A, S55.291A, S55.292A, S55.299A, S55.801A, S55.802A, S55.809A, S55.811A, S55.812A, S55.819A, S55.891A, S55.892A, S55.899A, S55.901A, S55.902A, S55.909A, S55.911A, S55.912A, S55.919A, S55.991A, S55.992A, S55.999A, S56.021A, S56.022A, S56.029A, S56.121A, S56.122A, S56.123A, S56.124A, S56.125A, S56.126A, S56.127A, S56.128A, S56.129A, S56.221A, S56.222A, S56.229A, S56.321A, S56.322A, S56.329A, S56.421A, S56.422A, S56.423A, S56.424A, S56.425A, S56.426A, S56.427A, S56.428A, S56.429A, S56.521A, S56.522A, S56.529A, S56.821A, S56.822A, S56.829A, S56.921A, S56.922A, S56.929A, S58.011A, S58.012A, S58.019A

Column 13: S58.021A, S58.022A, S58.029A, S58.111A, S58.112A, S58.119A, S58.121A, S58.122A, S58.129A, S58.911A, S58.912A, S58.919A, S58.921A, S58.922A, S58.929A, S59.001A, S59.001K, S59.001P, S59.002A, S59.002K, S59.002P, S59.009A, S59.009K, S59.009P, S59.011A, S59.011K, S59.011P, S59.012A, S59.012K, S59.012P, S59.019A, S59.019K, S59.019P, S59.021A, S59.021K, S59.021P, S59.022A, S59.022K, S59.022P, S59.029A, S59.029K, S59.029P, S59.031A, S59.031K, S59.031P, S59.032A, S59.032K, S59.032P, S59.039A, S59.039K, S59.039P, S59.041A, S59.041K, S59.041P, S59.042A, S59.042K, S59.042P, S59.049A, S59.049K, S59.091A, S59.091K, S59.091P, S59.092A, S59.092K, S59.092P, S59.099A, S59.099K, S59.099P, S59.101K, S59.101P, S59.102A, S59.102K, S59.102P, S59.109K

Column 14: S59.109P, S59.111K, S59.111P, S59.112K, S59.112P, S59.119K, S59.119P, S59.121K, S59.121P, S59.122K, S59.122P, S59.129K, S59.129P, S59.131K, S59.131P, S59.132K, S59.132P, S59.139K, S59.139P, S59.141K, S59.141P, S59.142K, S59.142P, S59.149K, S59.149P, S59.191K, S59.191P, S59.192K, S59.192P, S59.199K, S59.199P, S59.201A, S59.201K, S59.201P, S59.202A, S59.202K, S59.202P, S59.209A, S59.209K, S59.209P, S59.211A, S59.211K, S59.211P, S59.212A, S59.212K, S59.212P, S59.219A, S59.219K, S59.219P, S59.221A, S59.221K, S59.222A, S59.222K, S59.222P, S59.229A, S59.229K, S59.229P, S59.231A, S59.231K, S59.231P, S59.232A, S59.232K, S59.232P, S59.239A, S59.239K, S59.239P, S59.241A, S59.241K, S59.241P, S59.242A, S59.242K, S59.242P, S59.249A

Column 15: S59.249K, S59.249P, S59.291A, S59.291K, S59.291P, S59.292A, S59.292K, S59.292P, S59.299K, S59.299P, S62.001B, S62.001K, S62.001P, S62.002B, S62.002K, S62.002P, S62.009B, S62.009K, S62.009P, S62.011B, S62.011K, S62.011P, S62.012B, S62.012K, S62.012P, S62.013B, S62.013K, S62.013P, S62.014B, S62.014K, S62.014P, S62.015B, S62.015K, S62.015P, S62.016B, S62.016K, S62.016P, S62.021B, S62.021K, S62.021P, S62.022B, S62.022K, S62.022P, S62.023B, S62.023K, S62.023P, S62.024B, S62.024K, S62.024P, S62.025B, S62.025K, S62.025P, S62.026B, S62.026K, S62.026P, S62.031B, S62.031K, S62.032B, S62.032K, S62.032P, S62.033B, S62.033K, S62.034B, S62.034K, S62.034P, S62.035B, S62.035K, S62.035P, S62.036B, S62.036K, S62.036P

Complications or Comorbidities/Major Complications or Comorbidities (CC/MCC) Exclusions (cont.) - Based on CMS data

S62.101B	S62.144P	S62.185K	S62.246B	S62.314P	S62.339K	S62.364B	S62.516P	S62.618K	S62.643B	S62.667P	S65.513A	S66.821A	S72.021C	S72.033M
S62.101K	S62.145B	S62.185P	S62.246K	S62.315B	S62.339P	S62.364K	S62.521B	S62.618P	S62.643K	S62.668B	S65.514A	S66.822A	S72.021K	S72.033N
S62.101P	S62.145K	S62.186B	S62.246P	S62.315K	S62.340B	S62.364P	S62.521K	S62.619B	S62.643P	S62.668K	S65.515A	S66.829A	S72.021M	S72.033P
S62.102B	S62.145P	S62.186K	S62.251B	S62.315P	S62.340K	S62.365B	S62.521P	S62.619K	S62.644B	S62.668P	S65.516A	S66.921A	S72.021N	S72.033Q
S62.102K	S62.146B	S62.186P	S62.251K	S62.316B	S62.340P	S62.365K	S62.522B	S62.619P	S62.644K	S62.669B	S65.517A	S66.922A	S72.021P	S72.033R
S62.102P	S62.146K	S62.201B	S62.251P	S62.316K	S62.341B	S62.365P	S62.522K	S62.620B	S62.644P	S62.669K	S65.518A	S66.929A	S72.021Q	S72.034A
S62.109B	S62.146P	S62.201K	S62.252B	S62.316P	S62.341K	S62.366B	S62.522P	S62.620K	S62.645B	S62.669P	S65.519A	S68.411A	S72.021R	S72.034B
S62.109K	S62.151B	S62.201P	S62.252K	S62.317B	S62.341P	S62.366K	S62.523B	S62.620P	S62.645K	S62.90XB	S65.590A	S68.412A	S72.022A	S72.034C
S62.109P	S62.151K	S62.202B	S62.252P	S62.317K	S62.342B	S62.366P	S62.523K	S62.621B	S62.645P	S62.90XK	S65.591A	S68.419A	S72.022B	S72.034K
S62.111B	S62.151P	S62.202K	S62.253B	S62.317P	S62.342K	S62.367B	S62.523P	S62.621K	S62.646B	S62.90XP	S65.592A	S68.421A	S72.022C	S72.034M
S62.111K	S62.152B	S62.202P	S62.253K	S62.318B	S62.342P	S62.367K	S62.524B	S62.621P	S62.646K	S62.91XB	S65.593A	S68.422A	S72.022K	S72.034N
S62.111P	S62.152K	S62.209B	S62.253P	S62.318K	S62.343B	S62.367P	S62.524K	S62.622B	S62.646P	S62.91XK	S65.594A	S68.429A	S72.022M	S72.034P
S62.112B	S62.152P	S62.209K	S62.254B	S62.318P	S62.343K	S62.368B	S62.524P	S62.622K	S62.647B	S62.91XP	S65.595A	S68.711A	S72.022N	S72.034Q
S62.112K	S62.153B	S62.209P	S62.254K	S62.319B	S62.343P	S62.368K	S62.525B	S62.622P	S62.647K	S62.92XB	S65.596A	S68.712A	S72.022P	S72.034R
S62.112P	S62.153K	S62.211B	S62.254P	S62.319K	S62.344B	S62.368P	S62.525K	S62.623B	S62.647P	S62.92XK	S65.597A	S68.719A	S72.022Q	S72.035A
S62.113B	S62.153P	S62.211K	S62.255B	S62.319P	S62.344K	S62.369B	S62.525P	S62.623K	S62.648B	S62.92XP	S65.598A	S68.721A	S72.022R	S72.035B
S62.113K	S62.154B	S62.211P	S62.255K	S62.320B	S62.344P	S62.369K	S62.526B	S62.623P	S62.648K	S65.001A	S65.599A	S68.722A	S72.023A	S72.035C
S62.113P	S62.154K	S62.212B	S62.255P	S62.320K	S62.345B	S62.369P	S62.526K	S62.624B	S62.648P	S65.002A	S65.801A	S68.729A	S72.023B	S72.035K
S62.114B	S62.154P	S62.212K	S62.256B	S62.320P	S62.345K	S62.390B	S62.526P	S62.624K	S62.649B	S65.009A	S65.802A	S72.001A	S72.023C	S72.035M
S62.114K	S62.155B	S62.212P	S62.256K	S62.321B	S62.345P	S62.390K	S62.600B	S62.624P	S62.649K	S65.011A	S65.809A	S72.001B	S72.023K	S72.035N
S62.114P	S62.155K	S62.213B	S62.256P	S62.321K	S62.346B	S62.390P	S62.600K	S62.625B	S62.649P	S65.012A	S65.811A	S72.001C	S72.023M	S72.035P
S62.115B	S62.155P	S62.213K	S62.291B	S62.321P	S62.346K	S62.391B	S62.600P	S62.625K	S62.650B	S65.019A	S65.812A	S72.001K	S72.023N	S72.035Q
S62.115K	S62.156B	S62.213P	S62.291K	S62.322B	S62.346P	S62.391K	S62.601B	S62.625P	S62.650K	S65.091A	S65.819A	S72.001M	S72.023P	S72.035R
S62.115P	S62.156K	S62.221B	S62.291P	S62.322K	S62.347B	S62.391P	S62.601K	S62.626B	S62.650P	S65.092A	S65.891A	S72.001N	S72.023Q	S72.036A
S62.116B	S62.156P	S62.221K	S62.292B	S62.322P	S62.347K	S62.392B	S62.601P	S62.626K	S62.651B	S65.099A	S65.892A	S72.001P	S72.023R	S72.036B
S62.116K	S62.161B	S62.221P	S62.292K	S62.323B	S62.347P	S62.392K	S62.602B	S62.626P	S62.651K	S65.101A	S65.899A	S72.001Q	S72.024A	S72.036C
S62.116P	S62.161K	S62.222B	S62.292P	S62.323K	S62.348B	S62.392P	S62.602K	S62.627B	S62.651P	S65.102A	S65.901A	S72.001R	S72.024B	S72.036K
S62.121B	S62.161P	S62.222K	S62.299B	S62.323P	S62.348K	S62.393B	S62.602P	S62.627K	S62.652B	S65.109A	S65.902A	S72.002A	S72.024C	S72.036M
S62.121K	S62.162B	S62.222P	S62.299K	S62.324B	S62.348P	S62.393K	S62.603B	S62.627P	S62.652K	S65.111A	S65.909A	S72.002B	S72.024K	S72.036N
S62.121P	S62.162K	S62.223B	S62.299P	S62.324K	S62.349B	S62.393P	S62.603K	S62.628B	S62.652P	S65.112A	S65.911A	S72.002C	S72.024M	S72.036P
S62.122B	S62.162P	S62.223K	S62.300B	S62.324P	S62.349K	S62.394B	S62.603P	S62.628K	S62.653B	S65.119A	S65.912A	S72.002K	S72.024N	S72.036Q
S62.122K	S62.163B	S62.223P	S62.300K	S62.325B	S62.349P	S62.394K	S62.604B	S62.628P	S62.653K	S65.191A	S65.919A	S72.002M	S72.024P	S72.036R
S62.122P	S62.163K	S62.224B	S62.300P	S62.325K	S62.350B	S62.394P	S62.604K	S62.629B	S62.653P	S65.192A	S65.991A	S72.002N	S72.024Q	S72.041A
S62.123B	S62.163P	S62.224K	S62.301B	S62.325P	S62.350K	S62.395B	S62.604P	S62.629K	S62.654B	S65.199A	S65.992A	S72.002P	S72.024R	S72.041B
S62.123K	S62.164B	S62.224P	S62.301K	S62.326B	S62.350P	S62.395K	S62.605B	S62.629P	S62.654K	S65.201A	S65.999A	S72.002Q	S72.025A	S72.041C
S62.123P	S62.164K	S62.225B	S62.301P	S62.326K	S62.351B	S62.395P	S62.605K	S62.630B	S62.654P	S65.202A	S66.021A	S72.002R	S72.025B	S72.041K
S62.124B	S62.164P	S62.225K	S62.302B	S62.326P	S62.351K	S62.396B	S62.605P	S62.630K	S62.655B	S65.209A	S66.022A	S72.009A	S72.025C	S72.041M
S62.124K	S62.165B	S62.225P	S62.302K	S62.327B	S62.351P	S62.396K	S62.606B	S62.630P	S62.655K	S65.211A	S66.029A	S72.009B	S72.025K	S72.041N
S62.124P	S62.165K	S62.226B	S62.302P	S62.327K	S62.352B	S62.396P	S62.606K	S62.631B	S62.655P	S65.212A	S66.120A	S72.009C	S72.025M	S72.041P
S62.125B	S62.165P	S62.226K	S62.303B	S62.327P	S62.352K	S62.397B	S62.606P	S62.631K	S62.656B	S65.219A	S66.121A	S72.009K	S72.025N	S72.041Q
S62.125K	S62.166B	S62.226P	S62.303K	S62.328B	S62.352P	S62.397K	S62.607B	S62.631P	S62.656K	S65.291A	S66.122A	S72.009M	S72.025P	S72.041R
S62.125P	S62.166K	S62.231B	S62.303P	S62.328K	S62.353B	S62.397P	S62.607K	S62.632B	S62.656P	S65.292A	S66.123A	S72.009N	S72.025Q	S72.042A
S62.126B	S62.166P	S62.231K	S62.304B	S62.328P	S62.353K	S62.398B	S62.607P	S62.632K	S62.657B	S65.299A	S66.124A	S72.009P	S72.025R	S72.042B
S62.126K	S62.171B	S62.231P	S62.304K	S62.329B	S62.353P	S62.398K	S62.608B	S62.632P	S62.657K	S65.301A	S66.125A	S72.009Q	S72.026A	S72.042C
S62.126P	S62.171K	S62.232B	S62.304P	S62.329K	S62.354B	S62.398P	S62.608K	S62.633B	S62.657P	S65.302A	S66.126A	S72.009R	S72.026B	S72.042K
S62.131B	S62.171P	S62.232K	S62.305B	S62.329P	S62.354K	S62.399B	S62.608P	S62.633K	S62.658B	S65.309A	S66.127A	S72.011A	S72.026C	S72.042M
S62.131K	S62.172B	S62.232P	S62.305K	S62.330B	S62.354P	S62.399K	S62.609B	S62.633P	S62.658K	S65.311A	S66.128A	S72.011B	S72.026K	S72.042N
S62.131P	S62.172K	S62.233B	S62.305P	S62.330K	S62.355B	S62.399P	S62.609K	S62.634B	S62.658P	S65.312A	S66.129A	S72.011C	S72.026M	S72.042P
S62.132B	S62.172P	S62.233K	S62.306B	S62.330P	S62.355K	S62.501B	S62.609P	S62.634K	S62.659B	S65.319A	S66.221A	S72.011K	S72.026N	S72.042Q
S62.132K	S62.173B	S62.233P	S62.306K	S62.331B	S62.355P	S62.501K	S62.610B	S62.634P	S62.659K	S65.391A	S66.222A	S72.011M	S72.026P	S72.042R
S62.132P	S62.173K	S62.234B	S62.306P	S62.331K	S62.356B	S62.501P	S62.610K	S62.635B	S62.659P	S65.392A	S66.229A	S72.011N	S72.026Q	S72.043A
S62.133B	S62.173P	S62.234K	S62.307B	S62.331P	S62.356K	S62.502B	S62.610P	S62.635K	S62.660B	S65.399A	S66.320A	S72.011P	S72.026R	S72.043B
S62.133K	S62.174B	S62.234P	S62.307K	S62.332B	S62.356P	S62.502K	S62.611B	S62.635P	S62.660K	S65.401A	S66.321A	S72.011Q	S72.031A	S72.043C
S62.133P	S62.174K	S62.235B	S62.307P	S62.332K	S62.357B	S62.502P	S62.611K	S62.636B	S62.660P	S65.402A	S66.322A	S72.011R	S72.031B	S72.043K
S62.134B	S62.174P	S62.235K	S62.308B	S62.332P	S62.357K	S62.509B	S62.611P	S62.636K	S62.661B	S65.409A	S66.323A	S72.012A	S72.031C	S72.043M
S62.134K	S62.175B	S62.235P	S62.308K	S62.333B	S62.357P	S62.509K	S62.612B	S62.636P	S62.661K	S65.411A	S66.324A	S72.012B	S72.031K	S72.043N
S62.134P	S62.175K	S62.236B	S62.308P	S62.333K	S62.358B	S62.509P	S62.612K	S62.637B	S62.661P	S65.412A	S66.325A	S72.012C	S72.031M	S72.043P
S62.135B	S62.175P	S62.236K	S62.309B	S62.333P	S62.358K	S62.511B	S62.612P	S62.637K	S62.662B	S65.419A	S66.326A	S72.012K	S72.031N	S72.043Q
S62.135K	S62.176B	S62.236P	S62.309K	S62.334B	S62.358P	S62.511K	S62.613B	S62.637P	S62.662K	S65.491A	S66.327A	S72.012M	S72.031P	S72.043R
S62.135P	S62.176K	S62.241B	S62.309P	S62.334K	S62.359B	S62.511P	S62.613K	S62.638B	S62.662P	S65.492A	S66.328A	S72.012N	S72.031Q	S72.044A
S62.136B	S62.176P	S62.241K	S62.310B	S62.334P	S62.359K	S62.512B	S62.613P	S62.638K	S62.663B	S65.499A	S66.329A	S72.012P	S72.031R	S72.044B
S62.136K	S62.181B	S62.241P	S62.310K	S62.335B	S62.359P	S62.512K	S62.614B	S62.638P	S62.663K	S65.500A	S66.421A	S72.012Q	S72.032A	S72.044C
S62.136P	S62.181K	S62.242B	S62.310P	S62.335K	S62.360B	S62.512P	S62.614K	S62.639B	S62.663P	S65.501A	S66.422A	S72.012R	S72.032B	S72.044K
S62.141B	S62.181P	S62.242K	S62.311B	S62.335P	S62.360K	S62.513B	S62.614P	S62.639K	S62.664B	S65.502A	S66.429A	S72.019A	S72.032C	S72.044M
S62.141K	S62.182B	S62.242P	S62.311K	S62.336B	S62.360P	S62.513K	S62.615B	S62.639P	S62.664K	S65.503A	S66.520A	S72.019B	S72.032K	S72.044N
S62.141P	S62.182K	S62.243B	S62.311P	S62.336K	S62.361B	S62.513P	S62.615K	S62.640B	S62.664P	S65.504A	S66.521A	S72.019C	S72.032M	S72.044P
S62.142B	S62.182P	S62.243K	S62.312B	S62.336P	S62.361K	S62.514B	S62.615P	S62.640K	S62.665B	S65.505A	S66.522A	S72.019K	S72.032N	S72.044Q
S62.142K	S62.183B	S62.243P	S62.312K	S62.337B	S62.361P	S62.514K	S62.616B	S62.640P	S62.665K	S65.506A	S66.523A	S72.019M	S72.032P	S72.044R
S62.142P	S62.183K	S62.244B	S62.312P	S62.337K	S62.362B	S62.514P	S62.616K	S62.641B	S62.665P	S65.507A	S66.524A	S72.019N	S72.032Q	S72.045A
S62.143B	S62.183P	S62.244K	S62.313B	S62.337P	S62.362K	S62.515B	S62.616P	S62.641K	S62.666B	S65.508A	S66.525A	S72.019P	S72.032R	S72.045B
S62.143K	S62.184B	S62.244P	S62.313K	S62.338B	S62.362P	S62.515K	S62.617B	S62.641P	S62.666K	S65.509A	S66.526A	S72.019Q	S72.033A	S72.045C
S62.143P	S62.184K	S62.245B	S62.313P	S62.338K	S62.363B	S62.515P	S62.617K	S62.642B	S62.666P	S65.510A	S66.527A	S72.019R	S72.033B	S72.045K
S62.144B	S62.184P	S62.245K	S62.314B	S62.338P	S62.363K	S62.516B	S62.617P	S62.642K	S62.667B	S65.511A	S66.528A	S72.021A	S72.033C	S72.045M
S62.144K	S62.185B	S62.245P	S62.314K	S62.339B	S62.363P	S62.516K	S62.618B	S62.642P	S62.667K	S65.512A	S66.529A	S72.021B	S72.033K	S72.045N

Complications or Comorbidities/Major Complications or Comorbidities (CC/MCC) Exclusions (cont.) - Based on CMS data

S72.045P	S72.064R	S72.111B	S72.123K	S72.135N	S72.21XQ	S72.321A	S72.333C	S72.345M	S72.361P	S72.399R	S72.416B	S72.432K	S72.444N	S72.456Q
S72.045Q	S72.065A	S72.111C	S72.123M	S72.135P	S72.21XR	S72.321B	S72.333K	S72.345N	S72.361Q	S72.401A	S72.416C	S72.432M	S72.444P	S72.456R
S72.045R	S72.065B	S72.111K	S72.123N	S72.135Q	S72.22XA	S72.321C	S72.333M	S72.345P	S72.361R	S72.401B	S72.416K	S72.432N	S72.444Q	S72.461A
S72.046A	S72.065C	S72.111M	S72.123P	S72.135R	S72.22XB	S72.321K	S72.333N	S72.345Q	S72.362A	S72.401C	S72.416M	S72.432P	S72.444R	S72.461B
S72.046B	S72.065K	S72.111N	S72.123Q	S72.136A	S72.22XC	S72.321M	S72.333P	S72.345R	S72.362B	S72.401K	S72.416N	S72.432Q	S72.445A	S72.461C
S72.046C	S72.065M	S72.111P	S72.123R	S72.136B	S72.22XK	S72.321N	S72.333Q	S72.346A	S72.362C	S72.401M	S72.416P	S72.432R	S72.445B	S72.461K
S72.046K	S72.065N	S72.111Q	S72.124A	S72.136C	S72.22XM	S72.321P	S72.333R	S72.346B	S72.362K	S72.401N	S72.416Q	S72.433A	S72.445C	S72.461M
S72.046M	S72.065P	S72.111R	S72.124B	S72.136K	S72.22XN	S72.321Q	S72.334A	S72.346C	S72.362M	S72.401P	S72.416R	S72.433B	S72.445K	S72.461N
S72.046N	S72.065Q	S72.112A	S72.124C	S72.136M	S72.22XP	S72.321R	S72.334B	S72.346K	S72.362N	S72.401Q	S72.421A	S72.433C	S72.445M	S72.461P
S72.046P	S72.065R	S72.112B	S72.124K	S72.136N	S72.22XQ	S72.322A	S72.334C	S72.346M	S72.362P	S72.401R	S72.421B	S72.433K	S72.445N	S72.461Q
S72.046Q	S72.066A	S72.112C	S72.124M	S72.136P	S72.22XR	S72.322B	S72.334K	S72.346N	S72.362Q	S72.402A	S72.421C	S72.433M	S72.445P	S72.461R
S72.046R	S72.066B	S72.112K	S72.124N	S72.136Q	S72.23XA	S72.322C	S72.334M	S72.346P	S72.362R	S72.402B	S72.421K	S72.433N	S72.445Q	S72.462A
S72.051A	S72.066C	S72.112M	S72.124P	S72.136R	S72.23XB	S72.322K	S72.334N	S72.346Q	S72.363A	S72.402C	S72.421M	S72.433P	S72.445R	S72.462B
S72.051B	S72.066K	S72.112N	S72.124Q	S72.141A	S72.23XC	S72.322M	S72.334P	S72.346R	S72.363B	S72.402K	S72.421N	S72.433Q	S72.446A	S72.462C
S72.051C	S72.066M	S72.112P	S72.124R	S72.141B	S72.23XK	S72.322N	S72.334Q	S72.351A	S72.363C	S72.402M	S72.421P	S72.433R	S72.446B	S72.462K
S72.051K	S72.066N	S72.112Q	S72.125A	S72.141C	S72.23XM	S72.322P	S72.334R	S72.351B	S72.363K	S72.402N	S72.421Q	S72.434A	S72.446C	S72.462M
S72.051M	S72.066P	S72.112R	S72.125B	S72.141K	S72.23XN	S72.322Q	S72.335A	S72.351C	S72.363M	S72.402P	S72.421R	S72.434B	S72.446K	S72.462N
S72.051N	S72.066Q	S72.113A	S72.125C	S72.141M	S72.23XP	S72.322R	S72.335B	S72.351K	S72.363N	S72.402Q	S72.422A	S72.434C	S72.446M	S72.462P
S72.051P	S72.066R	S72.113B	S72.125K	S72.141N	S72.23XQ	S72.323A	S72.335C	S72.351M	S72.363P	S72.402R	S72.422B	S72.434K	S72.446N	S72.462Q
S72.051Q	S72.091A	S72.113C	S72.125M	S72.141P	S72.23XR	S72.323B	S72.335K	S72.351N	S72.363Q	S72.409A	S72.422C	S72.434M	S72.446P	S72.462R
S72.051R	S72.091B	S72.113K	S72.125N	S72.141Q	S72.24XA	S72.323C	S72.335M	S72.351P	S72.363R	S72.409B	S72.422K	S72.434N	S72.446Q	S72.463A
S72.052A	S72.091C	S72.113M	S72.125P	S72.141R	S72.24XB	S72.323K	S72.335N	S72.351Q	S72.364A	S72.409C	S72.422M	S72.434P	S72.446R	S72.463B
S72.052B	S72.091K	S72.113N	S72.125Q	S72.142A	S72.24XC	S72.323M	S72.335P	S72.351R	S72.364B	S72.409K	S72.422N	S72.434Q	S72.451A	S72.463C
S72.052C	S72.091M	S72.113P	S72.125R	S72.142B	S72.24XK	S72.323N	S72.335Q	S72.352A	S72.364C	S72.409M	S72.422P	S72.434R	S72.451B	S72.463K
S72.052K	S72.091N	S72.113Q	S72.126A	S72.142C	S72.24XM	S72.323P	S72.335R	S72.352B	S72.364K	S72.409N	S72.422Q	S72.435A	S72.451C	S72.463M
S72.052M	S72.091P	S72.113R	S72.126B	S72.142K	S72.24XN	S72.323Q	S72.336A	S72.352C	S72.364M	S72.409P	S72.422R	S72.435B	S72.451K	S72.463N
S72.052N	S72.091Q	S72.114A	S72.126C	S72.142M	S72.24XP	S72.323R	S72.336B	S72.352K	S72.364N	S72.409Q	S72.423A	S72.435C	S72.451M	S72.463P
S72.052P	S72.091R	S72.114B	S72.126K	S72.142N	S72.24XQ	S72.324A	S72.336C	S72.352M	S72.364P	S72.409R	S72.423B	S72.435K	S72.451N	S72.463Q
S72.052Q	S72.092A	S72.114C	S72.126M	S72.142P	S72.24XR	S72.324B	S72.336K	S72.352N	S72.364Q	S72.411A	S72.423C	S72.435M	S72.451P	S72.463R
S72.052R	S72.092B	S72.114K	S72.126N	S72.142Q	S72.25XA	S72.324C	S72.336M	S72.352P	S72.364R	S72.411B	S72.423K	S72.435N	S72.451Q	S72.464A
S72.059A	S72.092C	S72.114M	S72.126P	S72.142R	S72.25XB	S72.324K	S72.336N	S72.352Q	S72.365A	S72.411C	S72.423M	S72.435P	S72.451R	S72.464B
S72.059B	S72.092K	S72.114N	S72.126Q	S72.143A	S72.25XC	S72.324M	S72.336P	S72.352R	S72.365B	S72.411K	S72.423N	S72.435Q	S72.452A	S72.464C
S72.059C	S72.092M	S72.114P	S72.126R	S72.143B	S72.25XK	S72.324N	S72.336Q	S72.353A	S72.365C	S72.411M	S72.423P	S72.435R	S72.452B	S72.464K
S72.059K	S72.092N	S72.114Q	S72.131A	S72.143C	S72.25XM	S72.324P	S72.336R	S72.353B	S72.365K	S72.411N	S72.423Q	S72.436A	S72.452C	S72.464M
S72.059M	S72.092P	S72.114R	S72.131B	S72.143K	S72.25XN	S72.324Q	S72.341A	S72.353C	S72.365M	S72.411P	S72.423R	S72.436B	S72.452K	S72.464N
S72.059N	S72.092Q	S72.115A	S72.131C	S72.143M	S72.25XP	S72.324R	S72.341B	S72.353K	S72.365N	S72.411Q	S72.424A	S72.436C	S72.452M	S72.464P
S72.059P	S72.092R	S72.115B	S72.131K	S72.143N	S72.25XQ	S72.325A	S72.341C	S72.353M	S72.365P	S72.411R	S72.424B	S72.436K	S72.452N	S72.464Q
S72.059Q	S72.099A	S72.115C	S72.131M	S72.143P	S72.25XR	S72.325B	S72.341K	S72.353N	S72.365Q	S72.412A	S72.424C	S72.436M	S72.452P	S72.464R
S72.059R	S72.099B	S72.115K	S72.131N	S72.143Q	S72.26XA	S72.325C	S72.341M	S72.353P	S72.365R	S72.412B	S72.424K	S72.436N	S72.452Q	S72.465A
S72.061A	S72.099C	S72.115M	S72.131P	S72.143R	S72.26XB	S72.325K	S72.341N	S72.353Q	S72.366A	S72.412C	S72.424M	S72.436P	S72.452R	S72.465B
S72.061B	S72.099K	S72.115N	S72.131Q	S72.144A	S72.26XC	S72.325M	S72.341P	S72.353R	S72.366B	S72.412K	S72.424N	S72.436Q	S72.453A	S72.465C
S72.061C	S72.099M	S72.115P	S72.131R	S72.144B	S72.26XK	S72.325N	S72.341Q	S72.354A	S72.366C	S72.412M	S72.424P	S72.436R	S72.453B	S72.465K
S72.061K	S72.099N	S72.115Q	S72.132A	S72.144C	S72.26XM	S72.325P	S72.341R	S72.354B	S72.366K	S72.412N	S72.424Q	S72.441A	S72.453C	S72.465M
S72.061M	S72.099P	S72.115R	S72.132B	S72.144K	S72.26XN	S72.325Q	S72.342A	S72.354C	S72.366M	S72.412P	S72.424R	S72.441B	S72.453K	S72.465N
S72.061N	S72.099Q	S72.116A	S72.132C	S72.144M	S72.26XP	S72.325R	S72.342B	S72.354K	S72.366N	S72.412Q	S72.425A	S72.441C	S72.453M	S72.465P
S72.061P	S72.099R	S72.116B	S72.132K	S72.144N	S72.26XQ	S72.326A	S72.342C	S72.354M	S72.366P	S72.412R	S72.425B	S72.441K	S72.453N	S72.465Q
S72.061Q	S72.101A	S72.116C	S72.132M	S72.144P	S72.26XR	S72.326B	S72.342K	S72.354N	S72.366Q	S72.413A	S72.425C	S72.441M	S72.453P	S72.465R
S72.061R	S72.101B	S72.116K	S72.132N	S72.144Q	S72.301A	S72.326C	S72.342M	S72.354P	S72.366R	S72.413B	S72.425K	S72.441N	S72.453Q	S72.466A
S72.062A	S72.101C	S72.116M	S72.132P	S72.144R	S72.301B	S72.326K	S72.342N	S72.354Q	S72.391A	S72.413C	S72.425M	S72.441P	S72.453R	S72.466B
S72.062B	S72.101K	S72.116N	S72.132Q	S72.145A	S72.301C	S72.326M	S72.342P	S72.354R	S72.391B	S72.413K	S72.425N	S72.441Q	S72.454A	S72.466C
S72.062C	S72.101M	S72.116P	S72.132R	S72.145B	S72.301K	S72.326N	S72.342Q	S72.355A	S72.391C	S72.413M	S72.425P	S72.441R	S72.454B	S72.466K
S72.062K	S72.101N	S72.116Q	S72.133A	S72.145C	S72.301M	S72.326P	S72.342R	S72.355B	S72.391K	S72.413N	S72.425Q	S72.442A	S72.454C	S72.466M
S72.062M	S72.101P	S72.116R	S72.133B	S72.145K	S72.301N	S72.326Q	S72.343A	S72.355C	S72.391M	S72.413P	S72.425R	S72.442B	S72.454K	S72.466N
S72.062N	S72.101Q	S72.121A	S72.133C	S72.145M	S72.301P	S72.326R	S72.343B	S72.355K	S72.391N	S72.413Q	S72.426A	S72.442C	S72.454M	S72.466P
S72.062P	S72.101R	S72.121B	S72.133K	S72.145N	S72.301Q	S72.331A	S72.343C	S72.355M	S72.391P	S72.413R	S72.426B	S72.442K	S72.454N	S72.466Q
S72.062Q	S72.102A	S72.121C	S72.133M	S72.145P	S72.301R	S72.331B	S72.343K	S72.355N	S72.391Q	S72.414A	S72.426C	S72.442M	S72.454P	S72.466R
S72.062R	S72.102B	S72.121K	S72.133N	S72.145Q	S72.302A	S72.331C	S72.343M	S72.355P	S72.391R	S72.414B	S72.426K	S72.442N	S72.454Q	S72.471A
S72.063A	S72.102C	S72.121M	S72.133P	S72.145R	S72.302B	S72.331K	S72.343N	S72.355Q	S72.392A	S72.414C	S72.426M	S72.442P	S72.454R	S72.471K
S72.063B	S72.102K	S72.121N	S72.133Q	S72.146A	S72.302C	S72.331M	S72.343P	S72.355R	S72.392B	S72.414K	S72.426N	S72.442Q	S72.455A	S72.471P
S72.063C	S72.102M	S72.121P	S72.133R	S72.146B	S72.302K	S72.331N	S72.343Q	S72.356A	S72.392C	S72.414M	S72.426P	S72.442R	S72.455B	S72.472A
S72.063K	S72.102N	S72.121Q	S72.134A	S72.146C	S72.302M	S72.331P	S72.343R	S72.356B	S72.392K	S72.414N	S72.426Q	S72.443A	S72.455C	S72.472K
S72.063M	S72.102P	S72.121R	S72.134B	S72.146K	S72.302N	S72.331Q	S72.344A	S72.356C	S72.392M	S72.414P	S72.426R	S72.443B	S72.455K	S72.472P
S72.063N	S72.102Q	S72.122A	S72.134C	S72.146M	S72.302P	S72.331R	S72.344B	S72.356K	S72.392N	S72.414Q	S72.431A	S72.443C	S72.455M	S72.479A
S72.063P	S72.102R	S72.122B	S72.134K	S72.146N	S72.302Q	S72.332A	S72.344C	S72.356M	S72.392P	S72.414R	S72.431B	S72.443K	S72.455N	S72.479K
S72.063Q	S72.109A	S72.122C	S72.134M	S72.146P	S72.302R	S72.332B	S72.344K	S72.356N	S72.392Q	S72.415A	S72.431C	S72.443M	S72.455P	S72.479P
S72.063R	S72.109B	S72.122K	S72.134N	S72.146Q	S72.309A	S72.332C	S72.344M	S72.356P	S72.392R	S72.415B	S72.431K	S72.443N	S72.455Q	S72.491A
S72.064A	S72.109C	S72.122M	S72.134P	S72.146R	S72.309B	S72.332K	S72.344N	S72.356Q	S72.399A	S72.415C	S72.431M	S72.443P	S72.455R	S72.491B
S72.064B	S72.109K	S72.122N	S72.134Q	S72.21XA	S72.309C	S72.332M	S72.344P	S72.356R	S72.399B	S72.415K	S72.431N	S72.443Q	S72.456A	S72.491C
S72.064C	S72.109M	S72.122P	S72.134R	S72.21XB	S72.309K	S72.332N	S72.344Q	S72.361A	S72.399C	S72.415M	S72.431P	S72.443R	S72.456B	S72.491K
S72.064K	S72.109N	S72.122Q	S72.135A	S72.21XC	S72.309M	S72.332P	S72.344R	S72.361B	S72.399K	S72.415N	S72.431Q	S72.444A	S72.456C	S72.491M
S72.064M	S72.109P	S72.122R	S72.135B	S72.21XK	S72.309N	S72.332Q	S72.345A	S72.361C	S72.399M	S72.415P	S72.431R	S72.444B	S72.456K	S72.491N
S72.064N	S72.109Q	S72.123A	S72.135C	S72.21XM	S72.309P	S72.332R	S72.345B	S72.361K	S72.399N	S72.415Q	S72.432A	S72.444C	S72.456M	S72.491P
S72.064P	S72.109R	S72.123B	S72.135K	S72.21XN	S72.309Q	S72.333A	S72.345C	S72.361M	S72.399P	S72.415R	S72.432B	S72.444K	S72.456N	S72.491Q
S72.064Q	S72.111A	S72.123C	S72.135M	S72.21XP	S72.309R	S72.333B	S72.345K	S72.361N	S72.399Q	S72.416A	S72.432C	S72.444M	S72.456P	S72.491R

Complications or Comorbidities/Major Complications or Comorbidities (CC/MCC) Exclusions (cont.) - Based on CMS data

S72.492A	S73.003A	S75.902A	S79.099A	S82.002R	S82.022B	S82.034K	S82.046N	S82.112Q	S82.125A	S82.141C	S82.153M	S82.201P	S82.226R	S82.243B
S72.492B	S73.004A	S75.909A	S79.099K	S82.009A	S82.022C	S82.034M	S82.046P	S82.112R	S82.125B	S82.141K	S82.153N	S82.201Q	S82.231A	S82.243C
S72.492C	S73.005A	S75.911A	S79.099P	S82.009B	S82.022K	S82.034N	S82.046Q	S82.113A	S82.125C	S82.141M	S82.153P	S82.201R	S82.231B	S82.243K
S72.492K	S73.006A	S75.912A	S79.101A	S82.009C	S82.022M	S82.034P	S82.046R	S82.113B	S82.125K	S82.141N	S82.153Q	S82.202A	S82.231C	S82.243M
S72.492M	S73.011A	S75.919A	S79.101K	S82.009K	S82.022N	S82.034Q	S82.091A	S82.113C	S82.125M	S82.141P	S82.153R	S82.202B	S82.231K	S82.243N
S72.492N	S73.012A	S75.991A	S79.101P	S82.009M	S82.022P	S82.034R	S82.091B	S82.113K	S82.125N	S82.141Q	S82.154A	S82.202C	S82.231M	S82.243P
S72.492P	S73.013A	S75.992A	S79.102A	S82.009N	S82.022Q	S82.035A	S82.091C	S82.113M	S82.125P	S82.141R	S82.154B	S82.202K	S82.231N	S82.243Q
S72.492Q	S73.014A	S75.999A	S79.102K	S82.009P	S82.022R	S82.035B	S82.091K	S82.113N	S82.125Q	S82.142A	S82.154C	S82.202M	S82.231P	S82.243R
S72.492R	S73.015A	S76.021A	S79.102P	S82.009Q	S82.023A	S82.035C	S82.091M	S82.113P	S82.125R	S82.142B	S82.154K	S82.202N	S82.231Q	S82.244A
S72.499A	S73.016A	S76.022A	S79.109A	S82.009R	S82.023B	S82.035K	S82.091N	S82.113Q	S82.126A	S82.142C	S82.154M	S82.202P	S82.231R	S82.244B
S72.499B	S73.021A	S76.029A	S79.109K	S82.011A	S82.023C	S82.035M	S82.091P	S82.113R	S82.126B	S82.142K	S82.154N	S82.202Q	S82.232A	S82.244C
S72.499C	S73.022A	S76.121A	S79.109P	S82.011B	S82.023K	S82.035N	S82.091Q	S82.114A	S82.126C	S82.142M	S82.154P	S82.202R	S82.232B	S82.244K
S72.499K	S73.023A	S76.122A	S79.111A	S82.011C	S82.023M	S82.035P	S82.091R	S82.114B	S82.126K	S82.142N	S82.154Q	S82.209A	S82.232C	S82.244M
S72.499M	S73.024A	S76.129A	S79.111K	S82.011K	S82.023N	S82.035Q	S82.092A	S82.114C	S82.126M	S82.142P	S82.154R	S82.209B	S82.232K	S82.244N
S72.499N	S73.025A	S76.221A	S79.111P	S82.011M	S82.023P	S82.035R	S82.092B	S82.114K	S82.126N	S82.142Q	S82.155A	S82.209C	S82.232M	S82.244P
S72.499P	S73.026A	S76.222A	S79.112A	S82.011N	S82.023Q	S82.036A	S82.092C	S82.114M	S82.126P	S82.142R	S82.155B	S82.209K	S82.232N	S82.244Q
S72.499Q	S73.031A	S76.229A	S79.112K	S82.011P	S82.023R	S82.036B	S82.092K	S82.114N	S82.126Q	S82.143A	S82.155C	S82.209M	S82.232P	S82.244R
S72.499R	S73.032A	S76.321A	S79.112P	S82.011Q	S82.024A	S82.036C	S82.092M	S82.114P	S82.126R	S82.143B	S82.155K	S82.209N	S82.232Q	S82.245A
S72.8X1A	S73.033A	S76.322A	S79.119A	S82.011R	S82.024B	S82.036K	S82.092N	S82.114Q	S82.131A	S82.143C	S82.155M	S82.209P	S82.232R	S82.245B
S72.8X1B	S73.034A	S76.329A	S79.119K	S82.012A	S82.024C	S82.036M	S82.092P	S82.114R	S82.131B	S82.143K	S82.155N	S82.209Q	S82.233A	S82.245C
S72.8X1C	S73.035A	S76.821A	S79.119P	S82.012B	S82.024K	S82.036N	S82.092Q	S82.115A	S82.131C	S82.143M	S82.155P	S82.209R	S82.233B	S82.245K
S72.8X1K	S73.036A	S76.822A	S79.121A	S82.012C	S82.024M	S82.036P	S82.092R	S82.115B	S82.131K	S82.143N	S82.155Q	S82.221A	S82.233C	S82.245M
S72.8X1M	S73.041A	S76.829A	S79.121K	S82.012K	S82.024N	S82.036Q	S82.099A	S82.115C	S82.131M	S82.143P	S82.155R	S82.221B	S82.233K	S82.245N
S72.8X1N	S73.042A	S76.921A	S79.121P	S82.012M	S82.024P	S82.036R	S82.099B	S82.115K	S82.131N	S82.143Q	S82.156A	S82.221C	S82.233M	S82.245P
S72.8X1P	S73.043A	S76.922A	S79.122A	S82.012N	S82.024Q	S82.041A	S82.099C	S82.115M	S82.131P	S82.143R	S82.156B	S82.221K	S82.233N	S82.245Q
S72.8X1Q	S73.044A	S76.929A	S79.122K	S82.012P	S82.024R	S82.041B	S82.099K	S82.115N	S82.131Q	S82.144A	S82.156C	S82.221M	S82.233P	S82.245R
S72.8X1R	S73.045A	S77.00XA	S79.122P	S82.012Q	S82.025A	S82.041C	S82.099M	S82.115P	S82.131R	S82.144B	S82.156K	S82.221N	S82.233Q	S82.246A
S72.8X2A	S73.046A	S77.01XA	S79.129A	S82.012R	S82.025B	S82.041K	S82.099N	S82.115Q	S82.132A	S82.144C	S82.156M	S82.221P	S82.233R	S82.246B
S72.8X2B	S75.001A	S77.02XA	S79.129K	S82.013A	S82.025C	S82.041M	S82.099P	S82.115R	S82.132B	S82.144K	S82.156N	S82.221Q	S82.234A	S82.246C
S72.8X2C	S75.002A	S77.10XA	S79.129P	S82.013B	S82.025K	S82.041N	S82.099Q	S82.116A	S82.132C	S82.144M	S82.156P	S82.221R	S82.234B	S82.246K
S72.8X2K	S75.009A	S77.11XA	S79.131A	S82.013C	S82.025M	S82.041P	S82.099R	S82.116B	S82.132K	S82.144N	S82.156Q	S82.222A	S82.234C	S82.246M
S72.8X2M	S75.011A	S77.12XA	S79.131K	S82.013K	S82.025N	S82.041Q	S82.101A	S82.116C	S82.132M	S82.144P	S82.156R	S82.222B	S82.234K	S82.246N
S72.8X2N	S75.012A	S78.011A	S79.131P	S82.013M	S82.025P	S82.041R	S82.101B	S82.116K	S82.132N	S82.144Q	S82.161A	S82.222C	S82.234M	S82.246P
S72.8X2P	S75.019A	S78.012A	S79.132A	S82.013N	S82.025Q	S82.042A	S82.101C	S82.116M	S82.132P	S82.144R	S82.161K	S82.222K	S82.234N	S82.246Q
S72.8X2Q	S75.021A	S78.019A	S79.132K	S82.013P	S82.025R	S82.042B	S82.101K	S82.116N	S82.132Q	S82.145A	S82.161P	S82.222M	S82.234P	S82.246R
S72.8X2R	S75.022A	S78.021A	S79.132P	S82.013Q	S82.026A	S82.042C	S82.101M	S82.116P	S82.132R	S82.145B	S82.162A	S82.222N	S82.234Q	S82.251A
S72.8X9A	S75.029A	S78.022A	S79.139A	S82.013R	S82.026B	S82.042K	S82.101N	S82.116Q	S82.133A	S82.145C	S82.162K	S82.222P	S82.234R	S82.251B
S72.8X9B	S75.091A	S78.029A	S79.139K	S82.014A	S82.026C	S82.042M	S82.101P	S82.116R	S82.133B	S82.145K	S82.162P	S82.222Q	S82.235A	S82.251C
S72.8X9C	S75.092A	S78.111A	S79.139P	S82.014B	S82.026K	S82.042N	S82.101Q	S82.121A	S82.133C	S82.145M	S82.169A	S82.222R	S82.235B	S82.251K
S72.8X9K	S75.099A	S78.112A	S79.141A	S82.014C	S82.026M	S82.042P	S82.101R	S82.121B	S82.133K	S82.145N	S82.169K	S82.223A	S82.235C	S82.251M
S72.8X9M	S75.101A	S78.119A	S79.141K	S82.014K	S82.026N	S82.042Q	S82.102A	S82.121C	S82.133M	S82.145P	S82.169P	S82.223B	S82.235K	S82.251N
S72.8X9N	S75.102A	S78.121A	S79.141P	S82.014M	S82.026P	S82.042R	S82.102B	S82.121K	S82.133N	S82.145Q	S82.191A	S82.223C	S82.235M	S82.251P
S72.8X9P	S75.109A	S78.122A	S79.142A	S82.014N	S82.026Q	S82.043A	S82.102C	S82.121M	S82.133P	S82.145R	S82.191B	S82.223K	S82.235N	S82.251Q
S72.8X9Q	S75.111A	S78.129A	S79.142K	S82.014P	S82.026R	S82.043B	S82.102K	S82.121N	S82.133Q	S82.146A	S82.191C	S82.223M	S82.235P	S82.251R
S72.8X9R	S75.112A	S78.911A	S79.142P	S82.014Q	S82.031A	S82.043C	S82.102M	S82.121P	S82.133R	S82.146B	S82.191K	S82.223N	S82.235Q	S82.252A
S72.90XA	S75.119A	S78.912A	S79.149A	S82.014R	S82.031B	S82.043K	S82.102N	S82.121Q	S82.134A	S82.146C	S82.191M	S82.223P	S82.235R	S82.252B
S72.90XB	S75.121A	S78.919A	S79.149K	S82.015A	S82.031C	S82.043M	S82.102P	S82.121R	S82.134B	S82.146K	S82.191N	S82.223Q	S82.236A	S82.252C
S72.90XC	S75.122A	S78.921A	S79.149P	S82.015B	S82.031K	S82.043N	S82.102Q	S82.122A	S82.134C	S82.146M	S82.191P	S82.223R	S82.236B	S82.252K
S72.90XK	S75.129A	S78.922A	S79.191A	S82.015C	S82.031M	S82.043P	S82.102R	S82.122B	S82.134K	S82.146N	S82.191Q	S82.224A	S82.236C	S82.252M
S72.90XM	S75.191A	S78.929A	S79.191K	S82.015K	S82.031N	S82.043Q	S82.109A	S82.122C	S82.134M	S82.146P	S82.191R	S82.224B	S82.236K	S82.252N
S72.90XN	S75.192A	S79.001A	S79.191P	S82.015M	S82.031P	S82.043R	S82.109B	S82.122K	S82.134N	S82.146Q	S82.192A	S82.224C	S82.236M	S82.252P
S72.90XP	S75.199A	S79.001K	S79.192A	S82.015N	S82.031Q	S82.044A	S82.109C	S82.122M	S82.134P	S82.146R	S82.192B	S82.224K	S82.236N	S82.252Q
S72.90XQ	S75.201A	S79.001P	S79.192K	S82.015P	S82.031R	S82.044B	S82.109K	S82.122N	S82.134Q	S82.151A	S82.192C	S82.224M	S82.236P	S82.252R
S72.90XR	S75.202A	S79.002A	S79.192P	S82.015Q	S82.032A	S82.044C	S82.109M	S82.122P	S82.134R	S82.151B	S82.192K	S82.224N	S82.236Q	S82.253A
S72.91XA	S75.209A	S79.002K	S79.199A	S82.015R	S82.032B	S82.044K	S82.109N	S82.122Q	S82.135A	S82.151C	S82.192M	S82.224P	S82.236R	S82.253B
S72.91XB	S75.211A	S79.002P	S79.199K	S82.016A	S82.032C	S82.044M	S82.109P	S82.122R	S82.135B	S82.151K	S82.192N	S82.224Q	S82.241A	S82.253C
S72.91XC	S75.212A	S79.009A	S79.199P	S82.016B	S82.032K	S82.044N	S82.109Q	S82.123A	S82.135C	S82.151M	S82.192P	S82.224R	S82.241B	S82.253K
S72.91XK	S75.219A	S79.009K	S82.001A	S82.016C	S82.032M	S82.044P	S82.109R	S82.123B	S82.135K	S82.151N	S82.192Q	S82.225A	S82.241C	S82.253M
S72.91XM	S75.221A	S79.009P	S82.001B	S82.016K	S82.032N	S82.044Q	S82.111A	S82.123C	S82.135M	S82.151P	S82.192R	S82.225B	S82.241K	S82.253N
S72.91XN	S75.222A	S79.011A	S82.001C	S82.016M	S82.032P	S82.044R	S82.111B	S82.123K	S82.135N	S82.151Q	S82.199A	S82.225C	S82.241M	S82.253P
S72.91XP	S75.229A	S79.011K	S82.001K	S82.016N	S82.032Q	S82.045A	S82.111C	S82.123M	S82.135P	S82.151R	S82.199B	S82.225K	S82.241N	S82.253Q
S72.91XQ	S75.291A	S79.011P	S82.001M	S82.016P	S82.032R	S82.045B	S82.111K	S82.123N	S82.135Q	S82.152A	S82.199C	S82.225M	S82.241P	S82.253R
S72.91XR	S75.292A	S79.012A	S82.001N	S82.016Q	S82.033A	S82.045C	S82.111M	S82.123P	S82.135R	S82.152B	S82.199K	S82.225N	S82.241Q	S82.254A
S72.92XA	S75.299A	S79.012K	S82.001P	S82.016R	S82.033B	S82.045K	S82.111N	S82.123Q	S82.136A	S82.152C	S82.199M	S82.225P	S82.241R	S82.254B
S72.92XB	S75.801A	S79.012P	S82.001Q	S82.021A	S82.033C	S82.045M	S82.111P	S82.123R	S82.136B	S82.152K	S82.199N	S82.225Q	S82.242A	S82.254C
S72.92XC	S75.802A	S79.019A	S82.001R	S82.021B	S82.033K	S82.045N	S82.111Q	S82.124A	S82.136C	S82.152M	S82.199P	S82.225R	S82.242B	S82.254K
S72.92XK	S75.809A	S79.019K	S82.002A	S82.021C	S82.033M	S82.045P	S82.111R	S82.124B	S82.136K	S82.152N	S82.199Q	S82.226A	S82.242C	S82.254M
S72.92XM	S75.811A	S79.019P	S82.002B	S82.021K	S82.033N	S82.045Q	S82.112A	S82.124C	S82.136M	S82.152P	S82.199R	S82.226B	S82.242K	S82.254N
S72.92XN	S75.812A	S79.091A	S82.002C	S82.021M	S82.033P	S82.045R	S82.112B	S82.124K	S82.136N	S82.152Q	S82.201A	S82.226C	S82.242M	S82.254P
S72.92XP	S75.819A	S79.091K	S82.002K	S82.021N	S82.033Q	S82.046A	S82.112C	S82.124M	S82.136P	S82.152R	S82.201B	S82.226K	S82.242N	S82.254Q
S72.92XQ	S75.891A	S79.091P	S82.002M	S82.021P	S82.033R	S82.046B	S82.112K	S82.124N	S82.136Q	S82.153A	S82.201C	S82.226M	S82.242P	S82.254R
S72.92XR	S75.892A	S79.092A	S82.002N	S82.021Q	S82.034A	S82.046C	S82.112M	S82.124P	S82.136R	S82.153B	S82.201K	S82.226N	S82.242Q	S82.255A
S73.001A	S75.899A	S79.092K	S82.002P	S82.021R	S82.034B	S82.046K	S82.112N	S82.124Q	S82.141A	S82.153C	S82.201M	S82.226P	S82.242R	S82.255B
S73.002A	S75.901A	S79.092P	S82.002Q	S82.022A	S82.034C	S82.046M	S82.112P	S82.124R	S82.141B	S82.153K	S82.201N	S82.226Q	S82.243A	S82.255C

Complications or Comorbidities/Major Complications or Comorbidities (CC/MCC) Exclusions (cont.) - Based on CMS data

S82.255K	S82.291N	S82.399M	S82.426P	S82.443R	S82.461C	S82.51XM	S82.64XP	S82.843M	S82.856P	S82.873R	S85.002A	S85.811A	S89.022P	S89.211P
S82.255M	S82.291P	S82.399N	S82.426Q	S82.444B	S82.461K	S82.51XN	S82.64XQ	S82.843N	S82.856Q	S82.874B	S85.009A	S85.812A	S89.029A	S89.212K
S82.255N	S82.291Q	S82.399P	S82.426R	S82.444C	S82.461M	S82.51XP	S82.64XR	S82.843P	S82.856R	S82.874C	S85.011A	S85.819A	S89.029K	S89.212P
S82.255P	S82.291R	S82.399Q	S82.431B	S82.444K	S82.461N	S82.51XQ	S82.65XB	S82.843Q	S82.861B	S82.874K	S85.012A	S85.891A	S89.029P	S89.219K
S82.255Q	S82.292A	S82.399R	S82.431C	S82.444M	S82.461P	S82.51XR	S82.65XC	S82.843R	S82.861C	S82.874M	S85.019A	S85.892A	S89.031A	S89.219P
S82.255R	S82.292B	S82.401B	S82.431K	S82.444N	S82.461Q	S82.52XB	S82.65XK	S82.844B	S82.861K	S82.874N	S85.091A	S85.899A	S89.031K	S89.221K
S82.256A	S82.292C	S82.401C	S82.431M	S82.444P	S82.461R	S82.52XC	S82.65XM	S82.844C	S82.861M	S82.874P	S85.092A	S85.901A	S89.031P	S89.221P
S82.256B	S82.292K	S82.401K	S82.431N	S82.444Q	S82.462B	S82.52XK	S82.65XN	S82.844K	S82.861N	S82.874Q	S85.099A	S85.902A	S89.032A	S89.222K
S82.256C	S82.292M	S82.401M	S82.431P	S82.444R	S82.462C	S82.52XM	S82.65XP	S82.844M	S82.861P	S82.874R	S85.101A	S85.909A	S89.032K	S89.222P
S82.256K	S82.292N	S82.401N	S82.431Q	S82.445B	S82.462K	S82.52XN	S82.65XQ	S82.844N	S82.861Q	S82.875B	S85.102A	S85.911A	S89.032P	S89.229K
S82.256M	S82.292P	S82.401P	S82.431R	S82.445C	S82.462M	S82.52XP	S82.65XR	S82.844P	S82.861R	S82.875C	S85.109A	S85.912A	S89.039A	S89.229P
S82.256N	S82.292Q	S82.401Q	S82.432B	S82.445K	S82.462N	S82.52XQ	S82.66XB	S82.844Q	S82.862B	S82.875K	S85.111A	S85.919A	S89.039K	S89.291K
S82.256P	S82.292R	S82.401R	S82.432C	S82.445M	S82.462P	S82.52XR	S82.66XC	S82.844R	S82.862C	S82.875M	S85.112A	S85.991A	S89.039P	S89.291P
S82.256Q	S82.299A	S82.402B	S82.432K	S82.445N	S82.462Q	S82.53XB	S82.66XK	S82.845B	S82.862K	S82.875N	S85.119A	S85.992A	S89.041A	S89.292K
S82.256R	S82.299B	S82.402C	S82.432M	S82.445P	S82.462R	S82.53XC	S82.66XM	S82.845C	S82.862M	S82.875P	S85.121A	S85.999A	S89.041K	S89.292P
S82.261A	S82.299C	S82.402K	S82.432N	S82.445Q	S82.463B	S82.53XK	S82.66XN	S82.845K	S82.862N	S82.875Q	S85.122A	S86.021A	S89.041P	S89.299K
S82.261B	S82.299K	S82.402M	S82.432P	S82.445R	S82.463C	S82.53XM	S82.66XP	S82.845M	S82.862P	S82.875R	S85.129A	S86.022A	S89.042A	S89.299P
S82.261C	S82.299M	S82.402N	S82.432Q	S82.446B	S82.463K	S82.53XN	S82.66XQ	S82.845N	S82.862Q	S82.876B	S85.131A	S86.029A	S89.042K	S89.301K
S82.261K	S82.299N	S82.402P	S82.432R	S82.446C	S82.463M	S82.53XP	S82.66XR	S82.845P	S82.862R	S82.876C	S85.132A	S86.121A	S89.042P	S89.301P
S82.261M	S82.299P	S82.402Q	S82.433B	S82.446K	S82.463N	S82.53XQ	S82.811K	S82.845Q	S82.863B	S82.876K	S85.139A	S86.122A	S89.049A	S89.302K
S82.261N	S82.299Q	S82.402R	S82.433C	S82.446M	S82.463P	S82.53XR	S82.811P	S82.845R	S82.863C	S82.876M	S85.141A	S86.129A	S89.049K	S89.302P
S82.261P	S82.299R	S82.409B	S82.433K	S82.446N	S82.463Q	S82.54XB	S82.812K	S82.846B	S82.863K	S82.876N	S85.142A	S86.221A	S89.049P	S89.309K
S82.261Q	S82.301B	S82.409C	S82.433M	S82.446P	S82.463R	S82.54XC	S82.812P	S82.846C	S82.863M	S82.876P	S85.149A	S86.222A	S89.091A	S89.309P
S82.261R	S82.301C	S82.409K	S82.433N	S82.446Q	S82.464B	S82.54XK	S82.819K	S82.846K	S82.863N	S82.876Q	S85.151A	S86.229A	S89.091K	S89.311K
S82.262A	S82.301K	S82.409M	S82.433P	S82.446R	S82.464C	S82.54XM	S82.819P	S82.846M	S82.863P	S82.876R	S85.152A	S86.321A	S89.091P	S89.311P
S82.262B	S82.301M	S82.409N	S82.433Q	S82.451B	S82.464K	S82.54XN	S82.821K	S82.846N	S82.863Q	S82.891B	S85.159A	S86.322A	S89.092A	S89.312K
S82.262C	S82.301N	S82.409P	S82.433R	S82.451C	S82.464M	S82.54XP	S82.821P	S82.846P	S82.863R	S82.891C	S85.161A	S86.329A	S89.092K	S89.312P
S82.262K	S82.301P	S82.409Q	S82.434B	S82.451K	S82.464N	S82.54XQ	S82.822K	S82.846Q	S82.864B	S82.891K	S85.162A	S86.821A	S89.092P	S89.319K
S82.262M	S82.301Q	S82.409R	S82.434C	S82.451M	S82.464P	S82.54XR	S82.822P	S82.846R	S82.864C	S82.891M	S85.169A	S86.822A	S89.099A	S89.319P
S82.262N	S82.301R	S82.421B	S82.434K	S82.451N	S82.464Q	S82.55XB	S82.829K	S82.851B	S82.864K	S82.891N	S85.171A	S86.829A	S89.099K	S89.321K
S82.262P	S82.302B	S82.421C	S82.434M	S82.451P	S82.464R	S82.55XC	S82.829P	S82.851C	S82.864M	S82.891P	S85.172A	S86.921A	S89.099P	S89.321P
S82.262Q	S82.302C	S82.421K	S82.434N	S82.451Q	S82.465B	S82.55XK	S82.831B	S82.851K	S82.864N	S82.891Q	S85.179A	S86.922A	S89.101K	S89.322K
S82.262R	S82.302K	S82.421M	S82.434P	S82.451R	S82.465C	S82.55XM	S82.831C	S82.851M	S82.864P	S82.891R	S85.181A	S86.929A	S89.101P	S89.322P
S82.263A	S82.302M	S82.421N	S82.434Q	S82.452B	S82.465K	S82.55XN	S82.831K	S82.851N	S82.864Q	S82.892B	S85.182A	S88.011A	S89.102K	S89.329K
S82.263B	S82.302N	S82.421P	S82.434R	S82.452C	S82.465M	S82.55XP	S82.831M	S82.851P	S82.864R	S82.892C	S85.189A	S88.012A	S89.102P	S89.329P
S82.263C	S82.302P	S82.421Q	S82.435B	S82.452K	S82.465N	S82.55XQ	S82.831N	S82.851Q	S82.865B	S82.892K	S85.201A	S88.019A	S89.109K	S89.391K
S82.263K	S82.302Q	S82.421R	S82.435C	S82.452M	S82.465P	S82.55XR	S82.831P	S82.851R	S82.865C	S82.892M	S85.202A	S88.021A	S89.109P	S89.391P
S82.263M	S82.302R	S82.422B	S82.435K	S82.452N	S82.465Q	S82.56XB	S82.831Q	S82.852B	S82.865K	S82.892N	S85.209A	S88.022A	S89.111K	S89.392K
S82.263N	S82.309B	S82.422C	S82.435M	S82.452P	S82.465R	S82.56XC	S82.831R	S82.852C	S82.865M	S82.892P	S85.211A	S88.029A	S89.111P	S89.392P
S82.263P	S82.309C	S82.422K	S82.435N	S82.452Q	S82.466B	S82.56XK	S82.832B	S82.852K	S82.865N	S82.892Q	S85.212A	S88.111A	S89.112K	S89.399K
S82.263Q	S82.309K	S82.422M	S82.435P	S82.452R	S82.466C	S82.56XM	S82.832C	S82.852M	S82.865P	S82.892R	S85.219A	S88.112A	S89.112P	S89.399P
S82.263R	S82.309M	S82.422N	S82.435Q	S82.453B	S82.466K	S82.56XN	S82.832K	S82.852N	S82.865Q	S82.899B	S85.291A	S88.119A	S89.119K	S92.001B
S82.264A	S82.309N	S82.422P	S82.435R	S82.453C	S82.466M	S82.56XP	S82.832M	S82.852P	S82.865R	S82.899C	S85.292A	S88.121A	S89.119P	S92.001K
S82.264B	S82.309P	S82.422Q	S82.436B	S82.453K	S82.466N	S82.56XQ	S82.832N	S82.852Q	S82.866B	S82.899K	S85.299A	S88.122A	S89.121K	S92.001P
S82.264C	S82.309Q	S82.422R	S82.436C	S82.453M	S82.466P	S82.56XR	S82.832P	S82.852R	S82.866C	S82.899M	S85.301A	S88.129A	S89.121P	S92.002B
S82.264K	S82.309R	S82.423B	S82.436K	S82.453N	S82.466Q	S82.61XB	S82.832Q	S82.853B	S82.866K	S82.899N	S85.302A	S88.911A	S89.122K	S92.002K
S82.264M	S82.311A	S82.423C	S82.436M	S82.453P	S82.466R	S82.61XC	S82.832R	S82.853C	S82.866M	S82.899P	S85.309A	S88.912A	S89.122P	S92.002P
S82.264N	S82.311K	S82.423K	S82.436N	S82.453Q	S82.491B	S82.61XK	S82.839B	S82.853K	S82.866N	S82.899Q	S85.311A	S88.919A	S89.129K	S92.009B
S82.264P	S82.311P	S82.423M	S82.436P	S82.453R	S82.491C	S82.61XM	S82.839C	S82.853M	S82.866P	S82.899R	S85.312A	S88.921A	S89.129P	S92.009K
S82.264Q	S82.312A	S82.423N	S82.436Q	S82.454B	S82.491K	S82.61XN	S82.839K	S82.853N	S82.866Q	S82.90XB	S85.319A	S88.922A	S89.131K	S92.009P
S82.264R	S82.312K	S82.423P	S82.436R	S82.454C	S82.491M	S82.61XP	S82.839M	S82.853P	S82.866R	S82.90XC	S85.391A	S88.929A	S89.131P	S92.011B
S82.265A	S82.312P	S82.423Q	S82.441B	S82.454K	S82.491N	S82.61XQ	S82.839N	S82.853Q	S82.871B	S82.90XK	S85.392A	S89.001A	S89.132K	S92.011K
S82.265B	S82.319A	S82.423R	S82.441C	S82.454M	S82.491P	S82.61XR	S82.839P	S82.853R	S82.871C	S82.90XM	S85.399A	S89.001K	S89.132P	S92.011P
S82.265C	S82.319K	S82.424B	S82.441K	S82.454N	S82.491Q	S82.62XB	S82.839Q	S82.854B	S82.871K	S82.90XN	S85.401A	S89.001P	S89.139K	S92.012B
S82.265K	S82.319P	S82.424C	S82.441M	S82.454P	S82.491R	S82.62XC	S82.839R	S82.854C	S82.871M	S82.90XP	S85.402A	S89.002A	S89.139P	S92.012K
S82.265M	S82.391B	S82.424K	S82.441N	S82.454Q	S82.492B	S82.62XK	S82.841B	S82.854K	S82.871N	S82.90XQ	S85.409A	S89.002K	S89.141K	S92.012P
S82.265N	S82.391C	S82.424M	S82.441P	S82.454R	S82.492C	S82.62XM	S82.841C	S82.854M	S82.871P	S82.90XR	S85.411A	S89.002P	S89.141P	S92.013B
S82.265P	S82.391K	S82.424N	S82.441Q	S82.455B	S82.492K	S82.62XN	S82.841K	S82.854N	S82.871Q	S82.91XB	S85.412A	S89.009A	S89.142K	S92.013K
S82.265Q	S82.391M	S82.424P	S82.441R	S82.455C	S82.492M	S82.62XP	S82.841M	S82.854P	S82.871R	S82.91XC	S85.419A	S89.009K	S89.142P	S92.013P
S82.265R	S82.391N	S82.424Q	S82.442B	S82.455K	S82.492N	S82.62XQ	S82.841N	S82.854Q	S82.872B	S82.91XK	S85.491A	S89.009P	S89.149K	S92.014B
S82.266A	S82.391P	S82.424R	S82.442C	S82.455M	S82.492P	S82.62XR	S82.841P	S82.854R	S82.872C	S82.91XM	S85.492A	S89.011A	S89.149P	S92.014K
S82.266B	S82.391Q	S82.425B	S82.442K	S82.455N	S82.492Q	S82.63XB	S82.841Q	S82.855B	S82.872K	S82.91XN	S85.499A	S89.011K	S89.191K	S92.014P
S82.266C	S82.391R	S82.425C	S82.442M	S82.455P	S82.492R	S82.63XC	S82.841R	S82.855C	S82.872M	S82.91XP	S85.501A	S89.011P	S89.191P	S92.015B
S82.266K	S82.392B	S82.425K	S82.442N	S82.455Q	S82.499B	S82.63XK	S82.842B	S82.855K	S82.872N	S82.91XQ	S85.502A	S89.012A	S89.192K	S92.015K
S82.266M	S82.392C	S82.425M	S82.442P	S82.455R	S82.499C	S82.63XM	S82.842C	S82.855M	S82.872P	S82.91XR	S85.509A	S89.012K	S89.192P	S92.015P
S82.266N	S82.392K	S82.425N	S82.442Q	S82.456B	S82.499K	S82.63XN	S82.842K	S82.855N	S82.872Q	S82.92XB	S85.511A	S89.012P	S89.199K	S92.016B
S82.266P	S82.392M	S82.425P	S82.442R	S82.456C	S82.499M	S82.63XP	S82.842M	S82.855P	S82.872R	S82.92XC	S85.512A	S89.019A	S89.199P	S92.016K
S82.266Q	S82.392N	S82.425Q	S82.443B	S82.456K	S82.499N	S82.63XQ	S82.842N	S82.855Q	S82.873B	S82.92XK	S85.519A	S89.019K	S89.201K	S92.016P
S82.266R	S82.392P	S82.425R	S82.443C	S82.456M	S82.499P	S82.63XR	S82.842P	S82.855R	S82.873C	S82.92XM	S85.591A	S89.019P	S89.201P	S92.021B
S82.291A	S82.392Q	S82.426B	S82.443K	S82.456N	S82.499Q	S82.64XB	S82.842Q	S82.856B	S82.873K	S82.92XN	S85.592A	S89.021A	S89.202K	S92.021K
S82.291B	S82.392R	S82.426C	S82.443M	S82.456P	S82.499R	S82.64XC	S82.842R	S82.856C	S82.873M	S82.92XP	S85.599A	S89.021K	S89.202P	S92.021P
S82.291C	S82.399B	S82.426K	S82.443N	S82.456Q	S82.51XB	S82.64XK	S82.843B	S82.856K	S82.873N	S82.92XQ	S85.801A	S89.021P	S89.209K	S92.022B
S82.291K	S82.399C	S82.426M	S82.443P	S82.456R	S82.51XC	S82.64XM	S82.843C	S82.856M	S82.873P	S82.92XR	S85.802A	S89.022A	S89.209P	S92.022K
S82.291M	S82.399K	S82.426N	S82.443Q	S82.461B	S82.51XK	S82.64XN	S82.843K	S82.856N	S82.873Q	S85.001A	S85.809A	S89.022K	S89.211K	S92.022P

Complications or Comorbidities/Major Complications or Comorbidities (CC/MCC) Exclusions (cont.) - Based on CMS data

S92.023B	S92.063P	S92.141K	S92.222B	S92.302P	S92.346K	S92.511K	S95.099A	T17.420A	T22.332A	T23.739A	T27.4XXA	T34.821A	T76.22XA	T81.31XA
S92.023K	S92.064B	S92.141P	S92.222K	S92.309B	S92.346P	S92.511P	S95.101A	T17.428A	T22.339A	T23.741A	T27.5XXA	T34.822A	T76.32XA	T81.32XA
S92.023P	S92.064K	S92.142B	S92.222P	S92.309K	S92.351B	S92.512K	S95.102A	T17.490A	T22.341A	T23.742A	T27.6XXA	T34.829A	T76.51XA	T81.33XA
S92.024B	S92.064P	S92.142K	S92.223B	S92.309P	S92.351K	S92.512P	S95.109A	T17.498A	T22.342A	T23.749A	T27.7XXA	T34.831A	T76.52XA	T81.40XA
S92.024K	S92.065B	S92.142P	S92.223K	S92.311B	S92.351P	S92.513K	S95.111A	T17.500A	T22.349A	T23.751A	T28.1XXA	T34.832A	T76.61XA	T81.41XA
S92.024P	S92.065K	S92.143B	S92.223P	S92.311K	S92.352B	S92.513P	S95.112A	T17.508A	T22.351A	T23.752A	T28.2XXA	T34.839A	T76.62XA	T81.42XA
S92.025B	S92.065P	S92.143K	S92.224B	S92.311P	S92.352K	S92.514K	S95.119A	T17.510A	T22.352A	T23.759A	T28.6XXA	T34.90XA	T76.91XA	T81.43XA
S92.025K	S92.066B	S92.143P	S92.224K	S92.312B	S92.352P	S92.514P	S95.191A	T17.518A	T22.359A	T23.761A	T28.7XXA	T34.99XA	T76.92XA	T81.44XA
S92.025P	S92.066K	S92.144B	S92.224P	S92.312K	S92.353B	S92.515K	S95.192A	T17.520A	T22.361A	T23.762A	T33.011A	T67.01XA	T78.00XA	T81.49XA
S92.026B	S92.066P	S92.144K	S92.225B	S92.312P	S92.353K	S92.515P	S95.199A	T17.528A	T22.362A	T23.769A	T33.012A	T67.02XA	T78.01XA	T81.500A
S92.026K	S92.101B	S92.144P	S92.225K	S92.313B	S92.353P	S92.516K	S95.201A	T17.590A	T22.369A	T23.771A	T33.019A	T67.09XA	T78.02XA	T81.501A
S92.026P	S92.101K	S92.145B	S92.225P	S92.313K	S92.354B	S92.516P	S95.202A	T17.598A	T22.391A	T23.772A	T33.02XA	T69.021A	T78.03XA	T81.502A
S92.031B	S92.101P	S92.145K	S92.226B	S92.313P	S92.354K	S92.521K	S95.209A	T17.800A	T22.392A	T23.779A	T33.09XA	T69.022A	T78.04XA	T81.503A
S92.031K	S92.102B	S92.145P	S92.226K	S92.314B	S92.354P	S92.521P	S95.211A	T17.808A	T22.399A	T23.791A	T33.1XXA	T69.029A	T78.05XA	T81.504A
S92.031P	S92.102K	S92.146B	S92.226P	S92.314K	S92.355B	S92.522K	S95.212A	T17.810A	T22.70XA	T23.792A	T33.2XXA	T70.3XXA	T78.06XA	T81.505A
S92.032B	S92.102P	S92.146K	S92.231B	S92.314P	S92.355K	S92.522P	S95.219A	T17.818A	T22.711A	T23.799A	T33.3XXA	T71.111A	T78.07XA	T81.506A
S92.032K	S92.109B	S92.146P	S92.231K	S92.315B	S92.355P	S92.523K	S95.291A	T17.820A	T22.712A	T24.301A	T33.40XA	T71.112A	T78.08XA	T81.507A
S92.032P	S92.109K	S92.151B	S92.231P	S92.315K	S92.356B	S92.523P	S95.292A	T17.828A	T22.719A	T24.302A	T33.41XA	T71.113A	T78.09XA	T81.508A
S92.033B	S92.109P	S92.151K	S92.232B	S92.315P	S92.356K	S92.524K	S95.299A	T17.890A	T22.721A	T24.309A	T33.42XA	T71.114A	T78.2XXA	T81.509A
S92.033K	S92.111B	S92.151P	S92.232K	S92.316B	S92.356P	S92.524P	S95.801A	T17.898A	T22.722A	T24.311A	T33.511A	T71.121A	T79.0XXA	T81.510A
S92.033P	S92.111K	S92.152B	S92.232P	S92.316K	S92.401K	S92.525K	S95.802A	T17.900A	T22.729A	T24.312A	T33.512A	T71.122A	T79.1XXA	T81.511A
S92.034B	S92.111P	S92.152K	S92.233B	S92.316P	S92.401P	S92.525P	S95.809A	T17.910A	T22.731A	T24.319A	T33.519A	T71.123A	T79.2XXA	T81.512A
S92.034K	S92.112B	S92.152P	S92.233K	S92.321B	S92.402K	S92.526K	S95.811A	T17.920A	T22.732A	T24.321A	T33.521A	T71.124A	T79.4XXA	T81.513A
S92.034P	S92.112K	S92.153B	S92.233P	S92.321K	S92.402P	S92.526P	S95.812A	T17.990A	T22.739A	T24.322A	T33.522A	T71.131A	T79.5XXA	T81.514A
S92.035B	S92.112P	S92.153K	S92.234B	S92.321P	S92.403K	S92.531K	S95.819A	T18.190A	T22.741A	T24.329A	T33.529A	T71.132A	T79.7XXA	T81.515A
S92.035K	S92.113B	S92.153P	S92.234K	S92.322B	S92.403P	S92.531P	S95.891A	T18.2XXA	T22.742A	T24.331A	T33.531A	T71.133A	T79.A0XA	T81.516A
S92.035P	S92.113K	S92.154B	S92.234P	S92.322K	S92.404K	S92.532K	S95.892A	T20.30XA	T22.749A	T24.332A	T33.532A	T71.134A	T79.A11A	T81.517A
S92.036B	S92.113P	S92.154K	S92.235B	S92.322P	S92.404P	S92.532P	S95.899A	T20.311A	T22.751A	T24.339A	T33.539A	T71.141A	T79.A12A	T81.518A
S92.036K	S92.114B	S92.154P	S92.235K	S92.323B	S92.405K	S92.533K	S95.901A	T20.312A	T22.752A	T24.391A	T33.60XA	T71.143A	T79.A19A	T81.519A
S92.036P	S92.114K	S92.155B	S92.235P	S92.323K	S92.405P	S92.533P	S95.902A	T20.319A	T22.759A	T24.392A	T33.61XA	T71.144A	T79.A21A	T81.520A
S92.041B	S92.114P	S92.155K	S92.236B	S92.323P	S92.406K	S92.534K	S95.909A	T20.32XA	T22.761A	T24.399A	T33.62XA	T71.151A	T79.A22A	T81.521A
S92.041K	S92.115B	S92.155P	S92.236K	S92.324B	S92.406P	S92.534P	S95.911A	T20.33XA	T22.762A	T24.701A	T33.70XA	T71.152A	T79.A29A	T81.522A
S92.041P	S92.115K	S92.156B	S92.236P	S92.324K	S92.411K	S92.535K	S95.912A	T20.34XA	T22.769A	T24.702A	T33.71XA	T71.153A	T79.A3XA	T81.523A
S92.042B	S92.115P	S92.156K	S92.241B	S92.324P	S92.411P	S92.535P	S95.919A	T20.35XA	T22.791A	T24.709A	T33.72XA	T71.154A	T79.A9XA	T81.524A
S92.042K	S92.116B	S92.156P	S92.241K	S92.325B	S92.412K	S92.536K	S95.991A	T20.36XA	T22.792A	T24.711A	T33.811A	T71.161A	T80.0XXA	T81.525A
S92.042P	S92.116K	S92.191B	S92.241P	S92.325K	S92.412P	S92.536P	S95.992A	T20.37XA	T22.799A	T24.712A	T33.812A	T71.162A	T80.1XXA	T81.526A
S92.043B	S92.116P	S92.191K	S92.242B	S92.325P	S92.413K	S92.591K	S95.999A	T20.39XA	T23.301A	T24.719A	T33.819A	T71.163A	T80.211A	T81.527A
S92.043K	S92.121B	S92.191P	S92.242K	S92.326B	S92.413P	S92.591P	S96.021A	T20.70XA	T23.302A	T24.721A	T33.821A	T71.164A	T80.212A	T81.528A
S92.043P	S92.121K	S92.192B	S92.242P	S92.326K	S92.414K	S92.592K	S96.022A	T20.711A	T23.309A	T24.722A	T33.822A	T71.191A	T80.218A	T81.529A
S92.044B	S92.121P	S92.192K	S92.243B	S92.326P	S92.414P	S92.592P	S96.029A	T20.712A	T23.311A	T24.729A	T33.829A	T71.192A	T80.219A	T81.530A
S92.044K	S92.122B	S92.192P	S92.243K	S92.331B	S92.415K	S92.599K	S96.121A	T20.719A	T23.312A	T24.731A	T33.831A	T71.193A	T80.22XA	T81.531A
S92.044P	S92.122K	S92.199B	S92.243P	S92.331K	S92.415P	S92.599P	S96.122A	T20.72XA	T23.319A	T24.732A	T33.832A	T71.194A	T80.29XA	T81.532A
S92.045B	S92.122P	S92.199K	S92.244B	S92.331P	S92.416K	S92.811B	S96.129A	T20.73XA	T23.321A	T24.739A	T33.839A	T71.20XA	T80.30XA	T81.533A
S92.045K	S92.123B	S92.199P	S92.244K	S92.332B	S92.416P	S92.811K	S96.221A	T20.74XA	T23.322A	T24.791A	T33.90XA	T71.21XA	T80.310A	T81.534A
S92.045P	S92.123K	S92.201B	S92.244P	S92.332K	S92.421K	S92.811P	S96.222A	T20.75XA	T23.329A	T24.792A	T33.99XA	T71.221A	T80.311A	T81.535A
S92.046B	S92.123P	S92.201K	S92.245B	S92.332P	S92.421P	S92.812B	S96.229A	T20.76XA	T23.331A	T24.799A	T34.011A	T71.222A	T80.319A	T81.536A
S92.046K	S92.124B	S92.201P	S92.245K	S92.333B	S92.422K	S92.812K	S96.821A	T20.77XA	T23.332A	T25.311A	T34.012A	T71.223A	T80.39XA	T81.537A
S92.046P	S92.124K	S92.202B	S92.245P	S92.333K	S92.422P	S92.812P	S96.822A	T20.79XA	T23.339A	T25.312A	T34.019A	T71.224A	T80.40XA	T81.538A
S92.051B	S92.124P	S92.202K	S92.246B	S92.333P	S92.423K	S92.819B	S96.829A	T21.30XA	T23.341A	T25.319A	T34.02XA	T71.231A	T80.410A	T81.539A
S92.051K	S92.125B	S92.202P	S92.246K	S92.334B	S92.423P	S92.819K	S96.921A	T21.31XA	T23.342A	T25.321A	T34.09XA	T71.232A	T80.411A	T81.590A
S92.051P	S92.125K	S92.209B	S92.246P	S92.334K	S92.424K	S92.819P	S96.922A	T21.32XA	T23.349A	T25.322A	T34.1XXA	T71.233A	T80.419A	T81.591A
S92.052B	S92.125P	S92.209K	S92.251B	S92.334P	S92.424P	S92.901B	S96.929A	T21.33XA	T23.351A	T25.329A	T34.2XXA	T71.234A	T80.49XA	T81.592A
S92.052K	S92.126B	S92.209P	S92.251K	S92.335B	S92.425K	S92.901K	S98.011A	T21.34XA	T23.352A	T25.331A	T34.3XXA	T71.29XA	T80.51XA	T81.593A
S92.052P	S92.126K	S92.211B	S92.251P	S92.335K	S92.425P	S92.901P	S98.012A	T21.35XA	T23.359A	T25.332A	T34.40XA	T71.9XXA	T80.52XA	T81.594A
S92.053B	S92.126P	S92.211K	S92.252B	S92.335P	S92.426K	S92.902B	S98.019A	T21.36XA	T23.361A	T25.339A	T34.41XA	T74.01XA	T80.59XA	T81.595A
S92.053K	S92.131B	S92.211P	S92.252K	S92.336B	S92.426P	S92.902K	S98.021A	T21.37XA	T23.362A	T25.391A	T34.42XA	T74.02XA	T80.61XA	T81.596A
S92.053P	S92.131K	S92.212B	S92.252P	S92.336K	S92.491K	S92.902P	S98.022A	T21.39XA	T23.369A	T25.392A	T34.511A	T74.11XA	T80.62XA	T81.597A
S92.054B	S92.131P	S92.212K	S92.253B	S92.336P	S92.491P	S92.909B	S98.029A	T21.70XA	T23.371A	T25.399A	T34.512A	T74.12XA	T80.69XA	T81.598A
S92.054K	S92.132B	S92.212P	S92.253K	S92.341B	S92.492K	S92.909K	S98.311A	T21.71XA	T23.372A	T25.711A	T34.519A	T74.21XA	T80.810A	T81.599A
S92.054P	S92.132K	S92.213B	S92.253P	S92.341K	S92.492P	S92.909P	S98.312A	T21.72XA	T23.379A	T25.712A	T34.521A	T74.22XA	T80.818A	T81.60XA
S92.055B	S92.132P	S92.213K	S92.254B	S92.341P	S92.499K	S92.911K	S98.319A	T21.73XA	T23.391A	T25.719A	T34.522A	T74.32XA	T80.89XA	T81.61XA
S92.055K	S92.133B	S92.213P	S92.254K	S92.342B	S92.499P	S92.911P	S98.321A	T21.74XA	T23.392A	T25.721A	T34.529A	T74.4XXA	T80.910A	T81.69XA
S92.055P	S92.133K	S92.214B	S92.254P	S92.342K	S92.501K	S92.912K	S98.322A	T21.75XA	T23.399A	T25.722A	T34.531A	T74.51XA	T80.911A	T81.710A
S92.056B	S92.133P	S92.214K	S92.255B	S92.342P	S92.501P	S92.912P	S98.329A	T21.76XA	T23.701A	T25.729A	T34.532A	T74.52XA	T80.919A	T81.711A
S92.056K	S92.134B	S92.214P	S92.255K	S92.343B	S92.502K	S92.919K	S98.911A	T21.77XA	T23.702A	T25.731A	T34.539A	T74.61XA	T80.A0XA	T81.718A
S92.056P	S92.134K	S92.215B	S92.255P	S92.343K	S92.502P	S92.919P	S98.912A	T21.79XA	T23.709A	T25.732A	T34.60XA	T74.62XA	T80.A10A	T81.719A
S92.061B	S92.134P	S92.215K	S92.256B	S92.343P	S92.503K	S95.001A	S98.919A	T22.30XA	T23.711A	T25.739A	T34.61XA	T74.91XA	T80.A11A	T81.72XA
S92.061K	S92.135B	S92.215P	S92.256K	S92.344B	S92.503P	S95.002A	S98.921A	T22.311A	T23.712A	T25.791A	T34.62XA	T74.92XA	T80.A19A	T81.83XA
S92.061P	S92.135K	S92.216B	S92.256P	S92.344K	S92.504K	S95.009A	S98.922A	T22.312A	T23.719A	T25.792A	T34.70XA	T75.1XXA	T80.A9XA	T82.01XA
S92.062B	S92.135P	S92.216K	S92.301B	S92.344P	S92.504P	S95.011A	S98.929A	T22.319A	T23.721A	T25.799A	T34.71XA	T76.01XA	T81.10XA	T82.02XA
S92.062K	S92.136B	S92.216P	S92.301K	S92.345B	S92.505K	S95.012A	T17.400A	T22.321A	T23.722A	T27.0XXA	T34.72XA	T76.02XA	T81.11XA	T82.03XA
S92.062P	S92.136K	S92.221B	S92.301P	S92.345K	S92.505P	S95.019A	T17.408A	T22.322A	T23.729A	T27.1XXA	T34.811A	T76.11XA	T81.12XA	T82.09XA
S92.063B	S92.136P	S92.221K	S92.302B	S92.345P	S92.506K	S95.091A	T17.410A	T22.329A	T23.731A	T27.2XXA	T34.812A	T76.12XA	T81.19XA	T82.110A
S92.063K	S92.141B	S92.221P	S92.302K	S92.346B	S92.506P	S95.092A	T17.418A	T22.331A	T23.732A	T27.3XXA	T34.819A	T76.21XA	T81.30XA	T82.111A

Complications or Comorbidities/Major Complications or Comorbidities (CC/MCC) Exclusions (cont.) - Based on CMS data

T82.118A	T82.330A	T82.523A	T82.827A	T83.121A	T83.511A	T83.84XA	T84.052A	T84.120A	T84.228A	T84.611A	T85.02XA	T85.390A	T85.622A	T85.738A
T82.120A	T82.331A	T82.524A	T82.828A	T83.122A	T83.512A	T83.85XA	T84.053A	T84.121A	T84.290A	T84.612A	T85.03XA	T85.391A	T85.623A	T85.79XA
T82.121A	T82.332A	T82.525A	T82.837A	T83.123A	T83.518A	T83.86XA	T84.058A	T84.122A	T84.293A	T84.613A	T85.09XA	T85.41XA	T85.624A	T85.810A
T82.128A	T82.338A	T82.528A	T82.838A	T83.128A	T83.590A	T83.89XA	T84.059A	T84.123A	T84.296A	T84.614A	T85.110A	T85.42XA	T85.625A	T85.810D
T82.190A	T82.339A	T82.529A	T82.847A	T83.190A	T83.591A	T83.9XXA	T84.060A	T84.124A	T84.298A	T84.615A	T85.111A	T85.43XA	T85.628A	T85.820A
T82.191A	T82.390A	T82.530A	T82.848A	T83.191A	T83.592A	T84.010A	T84.061A	T84.125A	T84.310A	T84.619A	T85.112A	T85.44XA	T85.630A	T85.820D
T82.198A	T82.391A	T82.531A	T82.855A	T83.192A	T83.593A	T84.011A	T84.062A	T84.126A	T84.318A	T84.620A	T85.113A	T85.49XA	T85.631A	T85.830A
T82.211A	T82.392A	T82.532A	T82.856A	T83.193A	T83.598A	T84.012A	T84.063A	T84.127A	T84.320A	T84.621A	T85.118A	T85.510A	T85.633A	T85.830D
T82.212A	T82.398A	T82.533A	T82.857A	T83.198A	T83.61XA	T84.013A	T84.068A	T84.129A	T84.328A	T84.622A	T85.120A	T85.511A	T85.635A	T85.840A
T82.213A	T82.399A	T82.534A	T82.858A	T83.21XA	T83.62XA	T84.018A	T84.069A	T84.190A	T84.390A	T84.623A	T85.121A	T85.518A	T85.638A	T85.840D
T82.218A	T82.41XA	T82.535A	T82.867A	T83.22XA	T83.69XA	T84.019A	T84.090A	T84.191A	T84.398A	T84.624A	T85.122A	T85.520A	T85.690A	T85.850A
T82.221A	T82.42XA	T82.538A	T82.868A	T83.23XA	T83.712A	T84.020A	T84.091A	T84.192A	T84.410A	T84.625A	T85.123A	T85.521A	T85.691A	T85.850D
T82.222A	T82.43XA	T82.539A	T82.897A	T83.24XA	T83.713A	T84.021A	T84.092A	T84.193A	T84.418A	T84.629A	T85.128A	T85.528A	T85.692A	T85.860A
T82.223A	T82.49XA	T82.590A	T82.898A	T83.25XA	T83.714A	T84.022A	T84.093A	T84.194A	T84.420A	T84.63XA	T85.190A	T85.590A	T85.693A	T85.860D
T82.228A	T82.510A	T82.591A	T82.9XXA	T83.29XA	T83.718A	T84.023A	T84.098A	T84.195A	T84.428A	T84.69XA	T85.191A	T85.591A	T85.694A	T85.890A
T82.310A	T82.511A	T82.592A	T83.010A	T83.410A	T83.719A	T84.028A	T84.099A	T84.196A	T84.490A	T84.7XXA	T85.192A	T85.598A	T85.695A	T85.890D
T82.311A	T82.512A	T82.593A	T83.020A	T83.411A	T83.722A	T84.029A	T84.110A	T84.197A	T84.498A	T84.81XA	T85.193A	T85.610A	T85.698A	T88.0XXA
T82.312A	T82.513A	T82.594A	T83.030A	T83.418A	T83.723A	T84.030A	T84.111A	T84.199A	T84.50XA	T84.82XA	T85.199A	T85.611A	T85.71XA	T88.1XXA
T82.318A	T82.514A	T82.595A	T83.090A	T83.420A	T83.724A	T84.031A	T84.112A	T84.210A	T84.51XA	T84.83XA	T85.21XA	T85.612A	T85.72XA	T88.2XXA
T82.319A	T82.515A	T82.598A	T83.110A	T83.421A	T83.728A	T84.032A	T84.113A	T84.213A	T84.52XA	T84.84XA	T85.22XA	T85.613A	T85.730A	T88.3XXA
T82.320A	T82.518A	T82.599A	T83.111A	T83.428A	T83.729A	T84.033A	T84.114A	T84.216A	T84.53XA	T84.85XA	T85.29XA	T85.614A	T85.731A	T88.6XXA
T82.321A	T82.519A	T82.6XXA	T83.112A	T83.490A	T83.79XA	T84.038A	T84.115A	T84.218A	T84.54XA	T84.86XA	T85.310A	T85.615A	T85.732A	
T82.322A	T82.520A	T82.7XXA	T83.113A	T83.491A	T83.81XA	T84.039A	T84.116A	T84.220A	T84.59XA	T84.89XA	T85.311A	T85.618A	T85.733A	
T82.328A	T82.521A	T82.817A	T83.118A	T83.498A	T83.82XA	T84.050A	T84.117A	T84.223A	T84.60XA	T84.9XXA	T85.320A	T85.620A	T85.734A	
T82.329A	T82.522A	T82.818A	T83.120A	T83.510A	T83.83XA	T84.051A	T84.119A	T84.226A	T84.610A	T85.01XA	T85.321A	T85.621A	T85.735A	

Female - Based on Medicare's Outpatient Code Editor (OCE)

O31.00X0	O31.12X4	O31.31X1	O31.8X95	O32.8XX2	O33.7XX9	O35.6XX3	O36.0190	O36.1124	O36.20X1	O36.5125	O36.60X2	O36.72X9	O36.8223	O36.8910
O31.00X1	O31.12X5	O31.31X2	O31.8X99	O32.8XX3	O35.0XX0	O35.6XX4	O36.0191	O36.1125	O36.20X2	O36.5129	O36.60X3	O36.73X0	O36.8224	O36.8911
O31.00X2	O31.12X9	O31.31X3	O32.0XX0	O32.8XX4	O35.0XX1	O35.6XX5	O36.0192	O36.1129	O36.20X3	O36.5130	O36.60X4	O36.73X1	O36.8225	O36.8912
O31.00X3	O31.13X0	O31.31X4	O32.0XX1	O32.8XX5	O35.0XX2	O35.6XX9	O36.0193	O36.1130	O36.20X4	O36.5131	O36.60X5	O36.73X2	O36.8229	O36.8913
O31.00X4	O31.13X1	O31.31X5	O32.0XX2	O32.8XX9	O35.0XX3	O35.7XX0	O36.0194	O36.1131	O36.20X5	O36.5132	O36.60X9	O36.73X3	O36.8230	O36.8914
O31.00X5	O31.13X2	O31.31X9	O32.0XX3	O32.9XX0	O35.0XX4	O35.7XX1	O36.0195	O36.1132	O36.20X9	O36.5133	O36.61X0	O36.73X4	O36.8231	O36.8915
O31.00X9	O31.13X3	O31.32X0	O32.0XX4	O32.9XX1	O35.0XX5	O35.7XX2	O36.0199	O36.1133	O36.21X0	O36.5134	O36.61X1	O36.73X5	O36.8232	O36.8919
O31.01X0	O31.13X4	O31.32X1	O32.0XX5	O32.9XX2	O35.0XX9	O35.7XX3	O36.0910	O36.1134	O36.21X1	O36.5135	O36.61X2	O36.73X9	O36.8233	O36.8920
O31.01X1	O31.13X5	O31.32X2	O32.0XX9	O32.9XX3	O35.1XX0	O35.7XX4	O36.0911	O36.1135	O36.21X2	O36.5139	O36.61X3	O36.80X0	O36.8234	O36.8921
O31.01X2	O31.13X9	O31.32X3	O32.1XX0	O32.9XX4	O35.1XX1	O35.7XX5	O36.0912	O36.1139	O36.21X3	O36.5190	O36.61X4	O36.80X1	O36.8235	O36.8922
O31.01X3	O31.20X0	O31.32X4	O32.1XX1	O32.9XX5	O35.1XX2	O35.7XX9	O36.0913	O36.1190	O36.21X4	O36.5191	O36.61X5	O36.80X2	O36.8239	O36.8923
O31.01X4	O31.20X1	O31.32X5	O32.1XX2	O32.9XX9	O35.1XX3	O35.8XX0	O36.0914	O36.1191	O36.21X5	O36.5192	O36.61X9	O36.80X3	O36.8290	O36.8924
O31.01X5	O31.20X2	O31.32X9	O32.1XX3	O33.3XX0	O35.1XX4	O35.8XX1	O36.0915	O36.1192	O36.21X9	O36.5193	O36.62X0	O36.80X4	O36.8291	O36.8925
O31.01X9	O31.20X3	O31.33X0	O32.1XX4	O33.3XX1	O35.1XX5	O35.8XX2	O36.0919	O36.1193	O36.22X0	O36.5194	O36.62X1	O36.80X5	O36.8292	O36.8929
O31.02X0	O31.20X4	O31.33X1	O32.1XX5	O33.3XX2	O35.1XX9	O35.8XX3	O36.0920	O36.1194	O36.22X1	O36.5195	O36.62X2	O36.80X9	O36.8293	O36.8930
O31.02X1	O31.20X5	O31.33X2	O32.1XX9	O33.3XX3	O35.2XX0	O35.8XX4	O36.0921	O36.1195	O36.22X2	O36.5199	O36.62X3	O36.8120	O36.8294	O36.8931
O31.02X2	O31.20X9	O31.33X3	O32.2XX0	O33.3XX4	O35.2XX1	O35.8XX5	O36.0922	O36.1199	O36.22X3	O36.5910	O36.62X4	O36.8121	O36.8295	O36.8932
O31.02X3	O31.21X0	O31.33X4	O32.2XX1	O33.3XX5	O35.2XX2	O35.8XX9	O36.0923	O36.1910	O36.22X4	O36.5911	O36.62X5	O36.8122	O36.8299	O36.8933
O31.02X4	O31.21X1	O31.33X5	O32.2XX2	O33.3XX9	O35.2XX3	O35.9XX0	O36.0924	O36.1911	O36.22X5	O36.5912	O36.62X9	O36.8123	O36.8310	O36.8934
O31.02X5	O31.21X2	O31.33X9	O32.2XX3	O33.4XX0	O35.2XX4	O35.9XX1	O36.0925	O36.1912	O36.22X9	O36.5913	O36.63X0	O36.8124	O36.8311	O36.8935
O31.02X9	O31.21X3	O31.8X10	O32.2XX4	O33.4XX1	O35.2XX5	O35.9XX2	O36.0929	O36.1913	O36.23X0	O36.5914	O36.63X1	O36.8125	O36.8312	O36.8939
O31.03X0	O31.21X4	O31.8X11	O32.2XX5	O33.4XX2	O35.2XX9	O35.9XX3	O36.0930	O36.1914	O36.23X1	O36.5915	O36.63X2	O36.8129	O36.8313	O36.8990
O31.03X1	O31.21X5	O31.8X12	O32.2XX9	O33.4XX3	O35.3XX0	O35.9XX4	O36.0931	O36.1915	O36.23X2	O36.5919	O36.63X3	O36.8130	O36.8314	O36.8991
O31.03X2	O31.21X9	O31.8X13	O32.3XX0	O33.4XX4	O35.3XX1	O35.9XX5	O36.0932	O36.1919	O36.23X3	O36.5920	O36.63X4	O36.8131	O36.8315	O36.8992
O31.03X3	O31.22X0	O31.8X14	O32.3XX1	O33.4XX5	O35.3XX2	O35.9XX9	O36.0933	O36.1920	O36.23X4	O36.5921	O36.63X5	O36.8132	O36.8319	O36.8993
O31.03X4	O31.22X1	O31.8X15	O32.3XX2	O33.4XX9	O35.3XX3	O36.0110	O36.0934	O36.1921	O36.23X5	O36.5922	O36.63X9	O36.8133	O36.8320	O36.8994
O31.03X5	O31.22X2	O31.8X19	O32.3XX3	O33.5XX0	O35.3XX4	O36.0111	O36.0935	O36.1922	O36.23X9	O36.5923	O36.70X0	O36.8134	O36.8321	O36.8995
O31.03X9	O31.22X3	O31.8X20	O32.3XX4	O33.5XX1	O35.3XX5	O36.0112	O36.0939	O36.1923	O36.4XX0	O36.5924	O36.70X1	O36.8135	O36.8322	O36.8999
O31.10X0	O31.22X4	O31.8X21	O32.3XX5	O33.5XX2	O35.3XX9	O36.0113	O36.0990	O36.1924	O36.4XX1	O36.5925	O36.70X2	O36.8139	O36.8323	O36.90X0
O31.10X1	O31.22X5	O31.8X22	O32.3XX9	O33.5XX3	O35.4XX0	O36.0114	O36.0991	O36.1925	O36.4XX2	O36.5929	O36.70X3	O36.8190	O36.8324	O36.90X1
O31.10X2	O31.22X9	O31.8X23	O32.4XX0	O33.5XX4	O35.4XX1	O36.0115	O36.0992	O36.1929	O36.4XX3	O36.5930	O36.70X4	O36.8191	O36.8325	O36.90X2
O31.10X3	O31.23X0	O31.8X24	O32.4XX1	O33.5XX5	O35.4XX2	O36.0119	O36.0993	O36.1930	O36.4XX4	O36.5931	O36.70X5	O36.8192	O36.8329	O36.90X3
O31.10X4	O31.23X1	O31.8X25	O32.4XX2	O33.5XX9	O35.4XX3	O36.0120	O36.0994	O36.1931	O36.4XX5	O36.5932	O36.70X9	O36.8193	O36.8330	O36.90X4
O31.10X5	O31.23X2	O31.8X29	O32.4XX3	O33.6XX0	O35.4XX4	O36.0121	O36.0995	O36.1932	O36.4XX9	O36.5933	O36.71X0	O36.8194	O36.8331	O36.90X5
O31.10X9	O31.23X3	O31.8X30	O32.4XX4	O33.6XX1	O35.4XX5	O36.0122	O36.0999	O36.1933	O36.5110	O36.5934	O36.71X1	O36.8195	O36.8332	O36.90X9
O31.11X0	O31.23X4	O31.8X31	O32.4XX5	O33.6XX2	O35.4XX9	O36.0123	O36.1110	O36.1934	O36.5111	O36.5935	O36.71X2	O36.8199	O36.8333	O36.91X0
O31.11X1	O31.23X5	O31.8X32	O32.4XX9	O33.6XX3	O35.5XX0	O36.0124	O36.1111	O36.1935	O36.5112	O36.5939	O36.71X3	O36.8210	O36.8334	O36.91X1
O31.11X2	O31.23X9	O31.8X33	O32.6XX0	O33.6XX4	O35.5XX1	O36.0125	O36.1112	O36.1939	O36.5113	O36.5990	O36.71X4	O36.8211	O36.8335	O36.91X2
O31.11X3	O31.30X0	O31.8X34	O32.6XX1	O33.6XX5	O35.5XX2	O36.0129	O36.1113	O36.1990	O36.5114	O36.5991	O36.71X5	O36.8212	O36.8339	O36.91X3
O31.11X4	O31.30X1	O31.8X35	O32.6XX2	O33.6XX9	O35.5XX3	O36.0130	O36.1114	O36.1991	O36.5115	O36.5992	O36.71X9	O36.8213	O36.8390	O36.91X4
O31.11X5	O31.30X2	O31.8X39	O32.6XX3	O33.7XX0	O35.5XX4	O36.0131	O36.1115	O36.1992	O36.5119	O36.5993	O36.72X0	O36.8214	O36.8391	O36.91X5
O31.11X9	O31.30X3	O31.8X90	O32.6XX4	O33.7XX1	O35.5XX5	O36.0132	O36.1119	O36.1993	O36.5120	O36.5994	O36.72X1	O36.8215	O36.8392	O36.91X9
O31.12X0	O31.30X4	O31.8X91	O32.6XX5	O33.7XX2	O35.5XX9	O36.0133	O36.1120	O36.1994	O36.5121	O36.5995	O36.72X2	O36.8219	O36.8393	O36.92X0
O31.12X1	O31.30X5	O31.8X92	O32.6XX9	O33.7XX3	O35.6XX0	O36.0134	O36.1121	O36.1995	O36.5122	O36.5999	O36.72X3	O36.8220	O36.8394	O36.92X1
O31.12X2	O31.30X9	O31.8X93	O32.8XX0	O33.7XX4	O35.6XX1	O36.0135	O36.1122	O36.1999	O36.5123	O36.60X0	O36.72X4	O36.8221	O36.8395	O36.92X2
O31.12X3	O31.31X0	O31.8X94	O32.8XX1	O33.7XX5	O35.6XX2	O36.0139	O36.1123	O36.20X0	O36.5124	O36.60X1	O36.72X5	O36.8222	O36.8399	O36.92X3

Female (cont.) - Based on Medicare's Outpatient Code Editor (OCE)

O36.92X4	O41.00X5	O41.1039	O41.1420	O41.8X91	O60.12X2	O64.0XX3	O64.8XX4	O69.4XX5	S30.814A	S31.40XD	S35.533S	S37.499A	S37.592D	T21.27XS
O36.92X5	O41.00X9	O41.1090	O41.1421	O41.8X92	O60.12X3	O64.0XX4	O64.8XX5	O69.4XX9	S30.814D	S31.40XS	S35.534A	S37.499D	S37.592S	T21.37XA
O36.92X9	O41.01X0	O41.1091	O41.1422	O41.8X93	O60.12X4	O64.0XX5	O64.8XX9	O69.5XX0	S30.814S	S31.41XA	S35.534D	S37.499S	S37.599A	T21.37XD
O36.93X0	O41.01X1	O41.1092	O41.1423	O41.8X94	O60.12X5	O64.0XX9	O64.9XX0	O69.5XX1	S30.816A	S31.41XD	S35.534S	S37.501A	S37.599D	T21.37XS
O36.93X1	O41.01X2	O41.1093	O41.1424	O41.8X95	O60.12X9	O64.1XX0	O64.9XX1	O69.5XX2	S30.816D	S31.41XS	S35.535A	S37.501D	S37.599S	T21.47XA
O36.93X2	O41.01X3	O41.1094	O41.1425	O41.8X99	O60.13X0	O64.1XX1	O64.9XX2	O69.5XX3	S30.816S	S31.42XA	S35.535D	S37.501S	S37.60XA	T21.47XD
O36.93X3	O41.01X4	O41.1095	O41.1429	O41.90X0	O60.13X1	O64.1XX2	O64.9XX3	O69.5XX4	S30.824A	S31.42XD	S35.535S	S37.502A	S37.60XD	T21.47XS
O36.93X4	O41.01X5	O41.1099	O41.1430	O41.90X1	O60.13X2	O64.1XX3	O64.9XX4	O69.5XX5	S30.824D	S31.42XS	S35.536A	S37.502D	S37.60XS	T21.57XA
O36.93X5	O41.01X9	O41.1210	O41.1431	O41.90X2	O60.13X3	O64.1XX4	O64.9XX5	O69.5XX9	S30.824S	S31.43XA	S35.536D	S37.502S	S37.62XA	T21.57XD
O36.93X9	O41.02X0	O41.1211	O41.1432	O41.90X3	O60.13X4	O64.1XX5	O64.9XX9	O69.81X0	S30.826A	S31.43XD	S35.536S	S37.509A	S37.62XD	T21.57XS
O40.1XX0	O41.02X1	O41.1212	O41.1433	O41.90X4	O60.13X5	O64.1XX9	O69.0XX0	O69.81X1	S30.826D	S31.43XS	S37.401A	S37.509D	S37.62XS	T21.67XA
O40.1XX1	O41.02X2	O41.1213	O41.1434	O41.90X5	O60.13X9	O64.2XX0	O69.0XX1	O69.81X2	S30.826S	S31.44XA	S37.401D	S37.509S	S37.63XA	T21.67XD
O40.1XX2	O41.02X3	O41.1214	O41.1435	O41.90X9	O60.14X0	O64.2XX1	O69.0XX2	O69.81X3	S30.844A	S31.44XD	S37.401S	S37.511A	S37.63XD	T21.67XS
O40.1XX3	O41.02X4	O41.1215	O41.1439	O41.91X0	O60.14X1	O64.2XX2	O69.0XX3	O69.81X4	S30.844D	S31.44XS	S37.402A	S37.511D	S37.63XS	T21.77XA
O40.1XX4	O41.02X5	O41.1219	O41.1490	O41.91X1	O60.14X2	O64.2XX3	O69.0XX4	O69.81X5	S30.844S	S31.45XA	S37.402D	S37.511S	S37.69XA	T21.77XD
O40.1XX5	O41.02X9	O41.1220	O41.1491	O41.91X2	O60.14X3	O64.2XX4	O69.0XX5	O69.81X9	S30.846A	S31.45XD	S37.402S	S37.512A	S37.69XD	T21.77XS
O40.1XX9	O41.03X0	O41.1221	O41.1492	O41.91X3	O60.14X4	O64.2XX5	O69.0XX9	O69.82X0	S30.846D	S31.45XS	S37.409A	S37.512D	S37.69XS	T83.31XA
O40.2XX0	O41.03X1	O41.1222	O41.1493	O41.91X4	O60.14X5	O64.2XX9	O69.1XX0	O69.82X1	S30.846S	S31.502A	S37.409D	S37.512S	S38.002A	T83.31XD
O40.2XX1	O41.03X2	O41.1223	O41.1494	O41.91X5	O60.14X9	O64.3XX0	O69.1XX1	O69.82X2	S30.854A	S31.502D	S37.409S	S37.519A	S38.002D	T83.31XS
O40.2XX2	O41.03X3	O41.1224	O41.1495	O41.91X9	O60.20X0	O64.3XX1	O69.1XX2	O69.82X3	S30.854D	S31.502S	S37.421A	S37.519D	S38.002S	T83.32XA
O40.2XX3	O41.03X4	O41.1225	O41.1499	O41.92X0	O60.20X1	O64.3XX2	O69.1XX3	O69.82X4	S30.854S	S31.512A	S37.421D	S37.519S	S38.03XA	T83.32XD
O40.2XX4	O41.03X5	O41.1229	O41.8X10	O41.92X1	O60.20X2	O64.3XX3	O69.1XX4	O69.82X5	S30.856A	S31.512D	S37.421S	S37.521A	S38.03XD	T83.32XS
O40.2XX5	O41.03X9	O41.1230	O41.8X11	O41.92X2	O60.20X3	O64.3XX4	O69.1XX5	O69.82X9	S30.856D	S31.512S	S37.422A	S37.521D	S38.03XS	T83.39XA
O40.2XX9	O41.1010	O41.1231	O41.8X12	O41.92X3	O60.20X4	O64.3XX5	O69.1XX9	O69.89X0	S30.856S	S31.522A	S37.422D	S37.521S	S38.211A	T83.39XD
O40.3XX0	O41.1011	O41.1232	O41.8X13	O41.92X4	O60.20X5	O64.3XX9	O69.2XX0	O69.89X1	S30.864A	S31.522D	S37.422S	S37.522A	S38.211D	T83.39XS
O40.3XX1	O41.1012	O41.1233	O41.8X14	O41.92X5	O60.20X9	O64.4XX0	O69.2XX1	O69.89X2	S30.864D	S31.522S	S37.429A	S37.522D	S38.211S	T83.711A
O40.3XX2	O41.1013	O41.1234	O41.8X15	O41.92X9	O60.22X0	O64.4XX1	O69.2XX2	O69.89X3	S30.864S	S31.532A	S37.429D	S37.522S	S38.212A	T83.711D
O40.3XX3	O41.1014	O41.1235	O41.8X19	O41.93X0	O60.22X1	O64.4XX2	O69.2XX3	O69.89X4	S30.866A	S31.532D	S37.429S	S37.529A	S38.212D	T83.711S
O40.3XX4	O41.1015	O41.1239	O41.8X20	O41.93X1	O60.22X2	O64.4XX3	O69.2XX4	O69.89X5	S30.866D	S31.532S	S37.431A	S37.529D	S38.212S	T83.721A
O40.3XX5	O41.1019	O41.1290	O41.8X21	O41.93X2	O60.22X3	O64.4XX4	O69.2XX5	O69.89X9	S30.866S	S31.542A	S37.431D	S37.529S	T19.2XXA	T83.721D
O40.3XX9	O41.1020	O41.1291	O41.8X22	O41.93X3	O60.22X4	O64.4XX5	O69.2XX9	O69.9XX0	S30.874A	S31.542D	S37.431S	S37.531A	T19.2XXD	T83.721S
O40.9XX0	O41.1021	O41.1292	O41.8X23	O41.93X4	O60.22X5	O64.4XX9	O69.3XX0	O69.9XX1	S30.874D	S31.542S	S37.432A	S37.531D	T19.2XXS	
O40.9XX1	O41.1022	O41.1293	O41.8X24	O41.93X5	O60.22X9	O64.5XX0	O69.3XX1	O69.9XX2	S30.874S	S31.552A	S37.432D	S37.531S	T19.3XXA	
O40.9XX2	O41.1023	O41.1294	O41.8X25	O41.93X9	O60.23X0	O64.5XX1	O69.3XX2	O69.9XX3	S30.876A	S31.552D	S37.432S	S37.532A	T19.3XXD	
O40.9XX3	O41.1024	O41.1295	O41.8X29	O60.10X0	O60.23X1	O64.5XX2	O69.3XX3	O69.9XX4	S30.876D	S31.552S	S37.439A	S37.532D	T19.3XXS	
O40.9XX4	O41.1025	O41.1299	O41.8X30	O60.10X1	O60.23X2	O64.5XX3	O69.3XX4	O69.9XX5	S30.876S	S35.531A	S37.439D	S37.532S	T21.07XA	
O40.9XX5	O41.1029	O41.1410	O41.8X31	O60.10X2	O60.23X3	O64.5XX4	O69.3XX5	O69.9XX9	S30.95XA	S35.531D	S37.439S	S37.539A	T21.07XD	
O40.9XX9	O41.1030	O41.1411	O41.8X32	O60.10X3	O60.23X4	O64.5XX5	O69.3XX9	S30.202A	S30.95XD	S35.531S	S37.491A	S37.539D	T21.07XS	
O41.00X0	O41.1031	O41.1412	O41.8X33	O60.10X4	O60.23X5	O64.5XX9	O69.4XX0	S30.202D	S30.95XS	S35.532A	S37.491D	S37.539S	T21.17XA	
O41.00X1	O41.1032	O41.1413	O41.8X34	O60.10X5	O60.23X9	O64.8XX0	O69.4XX1	S30.202S	S30.97XA	S35.532D	S37.491S	S37.591A	T21.17XD	
O41.00X2	O41.1033	O41.1414	O41.8X35	O60.10X9	O64.0XX0	O64.8XX1	O69.4XX2	S30.23XA	S30.97XD	S35.532S	S37.492A	S37.591D	T21.17XS	
O41.00X3	O41.1034	O41.1415	O41.8X39	O60.12X0	O64.0XX1	O64.8XX2	O69.4XX3	S30.23XD	S30.97XS	S35.533A	S37.492D	S37.591S	T21.27XA	
O41.00X4	O41.1035	O41.1419	O41.8X90	O60.12X1	O64.0XX2	O64.8XX3	O69.4XX4	S30.23XS	S31.40XA	S35.533D	S37.492S	S37.592A	T21.27XD	

Hospital-acquired Condition (HAC) - Based on CMS data

S02.0XXA	S02.11EA	S02.40CB	S02.612B	S02.670B	S06.2X1A	S06.320A	S06.348A	S06.376A	S06.5X4A	S06.824A	S12.000A	S12.112A	S12.24XA	S12.400A
S02.0XXB	S02.11EB	S02.40DA	S02.620A	S02.671A	S06.2X2A	S06.321A	S06.349A	S06.377A	S06.5X5A	S06.825A	S12.000B	S12.112B	S12.24XB	S12.400B
S02.101A	S02.11FA	S02.40DB	S02.620B	S02.671B	S06.2X3A	S06.322A	S06.350A	S06.378A	S06.5X6A	S06.826A	S12.001A	S12.120A	S12.250A	S12.401A
S02.101B	S02.11FB	S02.40EA	S02.621A	S02.672A	S06.2X4A	S06.323A	S06.351A	S06.379A	S06.5X7A	S06.827A	S12.001B	S12.120B	S12.250B	S12.401B
S02.102A	S02.11GA	S02.40EB	S02.621B	S02.672B	S06.2X5A	S06.324A	S06.352A	S06.380A	S06.5X8A	S06.828A	S12.01XA	S12.121A	S12.251A	S12.430A
S02.102B	S02.11GB	S02.40FA	S02.622A	S02.69XA	S06.2X6A	S06.325A	S06.353A	S06.381A	S06.5X9A	S06.829A	S12.01XB	S12.121B	S12.251B	S12.430B
S02.109A	S02.11HA	S02.40FB	S02.622B	S02.69XB	S06.2X7A	S06.326A	S06.354A	S06.382A	S06.6X0A	S06.891A	S12.02XA	S12.130A	S12.290A	S12.431A
S02.109B	S02.11HB	S02.411A	S02.630A	S02.80XA	S06.2X8A	S06.327A	S06.355A	S06.383A	S06.6X1A	S06.892A	S12.02XB	S12.130B	S12.290B	S12.431B
S02.110A	S02.19XA	S02.411B	S02.630B	S02.80XB	S06.2X9A	S06.328A	S06.356A	S06.384A	S06.6X2A	S06.893A	S12.030A	S12.131A	S12.291A	S12.44XA
S02.110B	S02.19XB	S02.412A	S02.631A	S02.81XA	S06.301A	S06.329A	S06.357A	S06.385A	S06.6X3A	S06.894A	S12.030B	S12.131B	S12.291B	S12.44XB
S02.111A	S02.2XXB	S02.412B	S02.631B	S02.81XB	S06.302A	S06.330A	S06.358A	S06.386A	S06.6X4A	S06.895A	S12.031A	S12.14XA	S12.300A	S12.450A
S02.111B	S02.30XA	S02.413A	S02.632A	S02.82XA	S06.303A	S06.331A	S06.359A	S06.387A	S06.6X5A	S06.896A	S12.031B	S12.14XB	S12.300B	S12.450B
S02.112A	S02.30XB	S02.413B	S02.632B	S02.82XB	S06.304A	S06.332A	S06.360A	S06.388A	S06.6X6A	S06.897A	S12.040A	S12.150A	S12.301A	S12.451A
S02.112B	S02.31XA	S02.42XA	S02.640A	S02.91XA	S06.305A	S06.333A	S06.361A	S06.389A	S06.6X7A	S06.898A	S12.040B	S12.150B	S12.301B	S12.451B
S02.113A	S02.31XB	S02.42XB	S02.640B	S02.91XB	S06.306A	S06.334A	S06.362A	S06.4X0A	S06.6X8A	S06.899A	S12.041A	S12.151A	S12.330A	S12.490A
S02.113B	S02.32XA	S02.600A	S02.641A	S02.92XA	S06.307A	S06.335A	S06.363A	S06.4X1A	S06.6X9A	S06.9X1A	S12.041B	S12.151B	S12.330B	S12.490B
S02.118A	S02.32XB	S02.600B	S02.641B	S02.92XB	S06.308A	S06.336A	S06.364A	S06.4X2A	S06.811A	S06.9X2A	S12.090A	S12.190A	S12.331A	S12.491A
S02.118B	S02.400A	S02.601A	S02.642A	S06.0X1A	S06.309A	S06.337A	S06.365A	S06.4X3A	S06.812A	S06.9X3A	S12.090B	S12.190B	S12.331B	S12.491B
S02.119A	S02.400B	S02.601B	S02.642B	S06.0X9A	S06.310A	S06.338A	S06.366A	S06.4X4A	S06.813A	S06.9X4A	S12.091A	S12.191A	S12.34XA	S12.500A
S02.119B	S02.401A	S02.602A	S02.650A	S06.1X1A	S06.311A	S06.339A	S06.367A	S06.4X5A	S06.814A	S06.9X5A	S12.091B	S12.191B	S12.34XB	S12.500B
S02.11AA	S02.401B	S02.602B	S02.650B	S06.1X2A	S06.312A	S06.340A	S06.368A	S06.4X6A	S06.815A	S06.9X6A	S12.100A	S12.200A	S12.350A	S12.501A
S02.11AB	S02.402A	S02.609A	S02.651A	S06.1X3A	S06.313A	S06.341A	S06.369A	S06.4X7A	S06.816A	S06.9X7A	S12.100B	S12.200B	S12.350B	S12.501B
S02.11BA	S02.402B	S02.609B	S02.651B	S06.1X4A	S06.314A	S06.342A	S06.370A	S06.4X8A	S06.817A	S06.9X8A	S12.101A	S12.201A	S12.351A	S12.530A
S02.11BB	S02.40AA	S02.610A	S02.652A	S06.1X5A	S06.315A	S06.343A	S06.371A	S06.4X9A	S06.818A	S06.9X9A	S12.101B	S12.201B	S12.351B	S12.530B
S02.11CA	S02.40AB	S02.610B	S02.652B	S06.1X6A	S06.316A	S06.344A	S06.372A	S06.5X0A	S06.819A	S07.0XXA	S12.110A	S12.230A	S12.390A	S12.531A
S02.11CB	S02.40BA	S02.611A	S02.66XA	S06.1X7A	S06.317A	S06.345A	S06.373A	S06.5X1A	S06.821A	S07.1XXA	S12.110B	S12.230B	S12.390B	S12.531B
S02.11DA	S02.40BB	S02.611B	S02.66XB	S06.1X8A	S06.318A	S06.346A	S06.374A	S06.5X2A	S06.822A	S07.8XXA	S12.111A	S12.231A	S12.391A	S12.54XA
S02.11DB	S02.40CA	S02.612A	S02.670A	S06.1X9A	S06.319A	S06.347A	S06.375A	S06.5X3A	S06.823A	S07.9XXA	S12.111B	S12.231B	S12.391B	S12.54XB

Hospital-acquired Condition (HAC) (cont.) - Based on CMS data

S12.550A	S14.134A	S22.059B	S24.153A	S32.120B	S32.423A	S32.483B	S34.113A	S42.199B	S42.292B	S42.364B	S42.452A	S49.001A	S52.043B	S52.223C
S12.550B	S14.135A	S22.060A	S24.154A	S32.121A	S32.423B	S32.484A	S34.114A	S42.201A	S42.293A	S42.365A	S42.452B	S49.002A	S52.043C	S52.224A
S12.551A	S14.136A	S22.060B	S32.000A	S32.121B	S32.424A	S32.484B	S34.115A	S42.201B	S42.293B	S42.365B	S42.453A	S49.009A	S52.044B	S52.224B
S12.551B	S14.137A	S22.061A	S32.000B	S32.122A	S32.424B	S32.485A	S34.119A	S42.202A	S42.294A	S42.366A	S42.453B	S49.011A	S52.044C	S52.224C
S12.590A	S14.151A	S22.061B	S32.001A	S32.122B	S32.425A	S32.485B	S34.121A	S42.202B	S42.294B	S42.366B	S42.454A	S49.012A	S52.045B	S52.225A
S12.590B	S14.152A	S22.062A	S32.001B	S32.129A	S32.425B	S32.486A	S34.122A	S42.209A	S42.295A	S42.391A	S42.454B	S49.019A	S52.045C	S52.225B
S12.591A	S14.153A	S22.062B	S32.002A	S32.129B	S32.426A	S32.486B	S34.123A	S42.209B	S42.295B	S42.391B	S42.455A	S49.021A	S52.046B	S52.225C
S12.591B	S14.154A	S22.068A	S32.002B	S32.130A	S32.426B	S32.491A	S34.124A	S42.211A	S42.296A	S42.392A	S42.455B	S49.022A	S52.046C	S52.226A
S12.600A	S14.155A	S22.068B	S32.008A	S32.130B	S32.431A	S32.491B	S34.125A	S42.211B	S42.296B	S42.392B	S42.456A	S49.029A	S52.091B	S52.226B
S12.600B	S14.156A	S22.069A	S32.008B	S32.131A	S32.431B	S32.492A	S34.129A	S42.212A	S42.301A	S42.399A	S42.456B	S49.031A	S52.091C	S52.226C
S12.601A	S14.157A	S22.069B	S32.009A	S32.131B	S32.432A	S32.492B	S34.131A	S42.212B	S42.301B	S42.399B	S42.461A	S49.032A	S52.092B	S52.231A
S12.601B	S17.0XXA	S22.070A	S32.009B	S32.132A	S32.432B	S32.499A	S34.132A	S42.213A	S42.302A	S42.401A	S42.461B	S49.039A	S52.092C	S52.231B
S12.630A	S17.8XXA	S22.070B	S32.010A	S32.132B	S32.433A	S32.499B	S34.139A	S42.213B	S42.302B	S42.401B	S42.462A	S49.041A	S52.099B	S52.231C
S12.630B	S17.9XXA	S22.071A	S32.010B	S32.139A	S32.433B	S32.501A	S34.3XXA	S42.214A	S42.309A	S42.402A	S42.462B	S49.042A	S52.099C	S52.232A
S12.631A	S22.000A	S22.071B	S32.011A	S32.139B	S32.434A	S32.501B	S42.001B	S42.214B	S42.309B	S42.402B	S42.463A	S49.049A	S52.101B	S52.232B
S12.631B	S22.000B	S22.072A	S32.011B	S32.14XA	S32.434B	S32.502A	S42.002B	S42.215A	S42.311A	S42.409A	S42.463B	S49.091A	S52.101C	S52.232C
S12.64XA	S22.001A	S22.072B	S32.012A	S32.14XB	S32.435A	S32.502B	S42.009B	S42.215B	S42.312A	S42.409B	S42.464A	S49.092A	S52.102B	S52.233A
S12.64XB	S22.001B	S22.078A	S32.012B	S32.15XA	S32.435B	S32.509A	S42.011B	S42.216A	S42.319A	S42.411A	S42.464B	S49.099A	S52.102C	S52.233B
S12.650A	S22.002A	S22.078B	S32.018A	S32.15XB	S32.436A	S32.509B	S42.012B	S42.216B	S42.321A	S42.411B	S42.465A	S49.101A	S52.109B	S52.233C
S12.650B	S22.002B	S22.079A	S32.018B	S32.16XA	S32.436B	S32.511A	S42.013B	S42.221A	S42.321B	S42.412A	S42.465B	S49.102A	S52.109C	S52.234A
S12.651A	S22.008A	S22.079B	S32.019A	S32.16XB	S32.441A	S32.511B	S42.014B	S42.221B	S42.322A	S42.412B	S42.466A	S49.109A	S52.111A	S52.234B
S12.651B	S22.008B	S22.080A	S32.019B	S32.17XA	S32.441B	S32.512A	S42.015B	S42.222A	S42.322B	S42.413A	S42.466B	S49.111A	S52.112A	S52.234C
S12.690A	S22.009A	S22.080B	S32.020A	S32.17XB	S32.442A	S32.512B	S42.016B	S42.222B	S42.323A	S42.413B	S42.471A	S49.112A	S52.119A	S52.235A
S12.690B	S22.009B	S22.081A	S32.020B	S32.19XA	S32.442B	S32.519A	S42.017B	S42.223A	S42.323B	S42.414A	S42.471B	S49.119A	S52.121B	S52.235B
S12.691A	S22.010A	S22.081B	S32.021A	S32.19XB	S32.443A	S32.519B	S42.018B	S42.223B	S42.324A	S42.414B	S42.472A	S49.121A	S52.121C	S52.235C
S12.691B	S22.010B	S22.082A	S32.021B	S32.2XXA	S32.443B	S32.591A	S42.019B	S42.224A	S42.324B	S42.415A	S42.472B	S49.122A	S52.122B	S52.236A
S12.8XXA	S22.011A	S22.082B	S32.022A	S32.2XXB	S32.444A	S32.591B	S42.021B	S42.224B	S42.325A	S42.415B	S42.473A	S49.129A	S52.122C	S52.236B
S12.9XXA	S22.011B	S22.088A	S32.022B	S32.301A	S32.444B	S32.592A	S42.022B	S42.225A	S42.325B	S42.416A	S42.473B	S49.131A	S52.123B	S52.236C
S13.0XXA	S22.012A	S22.088B	S32.028A	S32.301B	S32.445A	S32.592B	S42.023B	S42.225B	S42.326A	S42.416B	S42.474A	S49.132A	S52.123C	S52.241A
S13.100A	S22.012B	S22.089A	S32.028B	S32.302A	S32.445B	S32.599A	S42.024B	S42.226A	S42.326B	S42.421A	S42.474B	S49.139A	S52.124B	S52.241B
S13.101A	S22.018A	S22.089B	S32.029A	S32.302B	S32.446A	S32.599B	S42.025B	S42.226B	S42.331A	S42.421B	S42.475A	S49.141A	S52.124C	S52.241C
S13.110A	S22.018B	S22.20XA	S32.029B	S32.309A	S32.446B	S32.601A	S42.026B	S42.231A	S42.331B	S42.422A	S42.475B	S49.142A	S52.125B	S52.242A
S13.111A	S22.019A	S22.20XB	S32.030A	S32.309B	S32.451A	S32.601B	S42.031B	S42.231B	S42.332A	S42.422B	S42.476A	S49.149A	S52.125C	S52.242B
S13.120A	S22.019B	S22.21XA	S32.030B	S32.311A	S32.451B	S32.602A	S42.032B	S42.232A	S42.332B	S42.423A	S42.476B	S49.191A	S52.126B	S52.242C
S13.121A	S22.020A	S22.21XB	S32.031A	S32.311B	S32.452A	S32.602B	S42.033B	S42.232B	S42.333A	S42.423B	S42.481A	S49.192A	S52.126C	S52.243A
S13.130A	S22.020B	S22.22XA	S32.031B	S32.312A	S32.452B	S32.609A	S42.034B	S42.239A	S42.333B	S42.424A	S42.482A	S49.199A	S52.131B	S52.243B
S13.131A	S22.021A	S22.22XB	S32.032A	S32.312B	S32.453A	S32.609B	S42.035B	S42.239B	S42.334A	S42.424B	S42.489A	S52.001B	S52.131C	S52.243C
S13.140A	S22.021B	S22.23XA	S32.032B	S32.313A	S32.453B	S32.611A	S42.036B	S42.241A	S42.334B	S42.425A	S42.491A	S52.001C	S52.132B	S52.244A
S13.141A	S22.022A	S22.23XB	S32.038A	S32.313B	S32.454A	S32.611B	S42.101B	S42.241B	S42.335A	S42.425B	S42.491B	S52.002B	S52.132C	S52.244B
S13.150A	S22.022B	S22.24XA	S32.038B	S32.314A	S32.454B	S32.612A	S42.102B	S42.242A	S42.335B	S42.426A	S42.492A	S52.002C	S52.133B	S52.244C
S13.151A	S22.028A	S22.24XB	S32.039A	S32.314B	S32.455A	S32.612B	S42.109B	S42.242B	S42.336A	S42.426B	S42.492B	S52.009B	S52.133C	S52.245A
S13.160A	S22.028B	S22.31XA	S32.039B	S32.315A	S32.455B	S32.613A	S42.111B	S42.249A	S42.336B	S42.431A	S42.493A	S52.009C	S52.134B	S52.245B
S13.161A	S22.029A	S22.31XB	S32.040A	S32.315B	S32.456A	S32.613B	S42.112B	S42.249B	S42.341A	S42.431B	S42.493B	S52.011A	S52.134C	S52.245C
S13.170A	S22.029B	S22.32XA	S32.040B	S32.316A	S32.456B	S32.614A	S42.113B	S42.251A	S42.341B	S42.432A	S42.494A	S52.012A	S52.135B	S52.246A
S13.171A	S22.030A	S22.32XB	S32.041A	S32.316B	S32.461A	S32.614B	S42.114B	S42.251B	S42.342A	S42.432B	S42.494B	S52.019A	S52.135C	S52.246B
S13.180A	S22.030B	S22.39XA	S32.041B	S32.391A	S32.461B	S32.615A	S42.115B	S42.252A	S42.342B	S42.433A	S42.495A	S52.021B	S52.136B	S52.246C
S13.181A	S22.031A	S22.39XB	S32.042A	S32.391B	S32.462A	S32.615B	S42.116B	S42.252B	S42.343A	S42.433B	S42.495B	S52.021C	S52.136C	S52.251A
S13.20XA	S22.031B	S22.41XA	S32.042B	S32.392A	S32.462B	S32.616A	S42.121B	S42.253A	S42.343B	S42.434A	S42.496A	S52.022B	S52.181B	S52.251B
S13.29XA	S22.032A	S22.41XB	S32.048A	S32.392B	S32.463A	S32.616B	S42.122B	S42.253B	S42.344A	S42.434B	S42.496B	S52.022C	S52.181C	S52.251C
S14.101A	S22.032B	S22.42XA	S32.048B	S32.399A	S32.463B	S32.691A	S42.123B	S42.254A	S42.344B	S42.435A	S42.90XA	S52.023B	S52.182B	S52.252A
S14.102A	S22.038A	S22.42XB	S32.049A	S32.399B	S32.464A	S32.691B	S42.124B	S42.254B	S42.345A	S42.435B	S42.90XB	S52.023C	S52.182C	S52.252B
S14.103A	S22.038B	S22.43XA	S32.049B	S32.401A	S32.464B	S32.692A	S42.125B	S42.255A	S42.345B	S42.436A	S42.91XA	S52.024B	S52.189B	S52.252C
S14.104A	S22.039A	S22.43XB	S32.050A	S32.401B	S32.465A	S32.692B	S42.126B	S42.255B	S42.346A	S42.436B	S42.91XB	S52.024C	S52.189C	S52.253A
S14.105A	S22.039B	S22.49XA	S32.050B	S32.402A	S32.465B	S32.699A	S42.131B	S42.256A	S42.346B	S42.441A	S42.92XA	S52.025B	S52.201A	S52.253B
S14.106A	S22.040A	S22.49XB	S32.051A	S32.402B	S32.466A	S32.699B	S42.132B	S42.256B	S42.351A	S42.441B	S42.92XB	S52.025C	S52.201B	S52.253C
S14.107A	S22.040B	S22.5XXA	S32.051B	S32.409A	S32.466B	S32.810A	S42.133B	S42.261A	S42.351B	S42.442A	S43.201A	S52.026B	S52.201C	S52.254A
S14.111A	S22.041A	S22.5XXB	S32.052A	S32.409B	S32.471A	S32.810B	S42.134B	S42.261B	S42.352A	S42.442B	S43.202A	S52.026C	S52.202A	S52.254B
S14.112A	S22.041B	S22.9XXA	S32.052B	S32.411A	S32.471B	S32.811A	S42.135B	S42.262A	S42.352B	S42.443A	S43.203A	S52.031B	S52.202B	S52.254C
S14.113A	S22.042A	S22.9XXB	S32.058A	S32.411B	S32.472A	S32.811B	S42.136B	S42.262B	S42.353A	S42.443B	S43.204A	S52.031C	S52.202C	S52.255A
S14.114A	S22.042B	S24.101A	S32.058B	S32.412A	S32.472B	S32.82XA	S42.141B	S42.263A	S42.353B	S42.444A	S43.205A	S52.032B	S52.209A	S52.255B
S14.115A	S22.048A	S24.102A	S32.059A	S32.412B	S32.473A	S32.82XB	S42.142B	S42.263B	S42.354A	S42.444B	S43.206A	S52.032C	S52.209B	S52.255C
S14.116A	S22.048B	S24.103A	S32.059B	S32.413A	S32.473B	S32.89XA	S42.143B	S42.264A	S42.354B	S42.445A	S43.211A	S52.033B	S52.209C	S52.256A
S14.117A	S22.049A	S24.104A	S32.10XA	S32.413B	S32.474A	S32.89XB	S42.144B	S42.264B	S42.355A	S42.445B	S43.212A	S52.033C	S52.211A	S52.256B
S14.121A	S22.049B	S24.111A	S32.10XB	S32.414A	S32.474B	S32.9XXA	S42.145B	S42.265A	S42.355B	S42.446A	S43.213A	S52.034B	S52.212A	S52.256C
S14.122A	S22.050A	S24.112A	S32.110A	S32.414B	S32.475A	S32.9XXB	S42.146B	S42.265B	S42.356A	S42.446B	S43.214A	S52.034C	S52.219A	S52.261A
S14.123A	S22.050B	S24.113A	S32.110B	S32.415A	S32.475B	S34.101A	S42.151B	S42.266A	S42.356B	S42.447A	S43.215A	S52.035B	S52.221A	S52.261B
S14.124A	S22.051A	S24.114A	S32.111A	S32.415B	S32.476A	S34.102A	S42.152B	S42.266B	S42.361A	S42.447B	S43.216A	S52.035C	S52.221B	S52.261C
S14.125A	S22.051B	S24.131A	S32.111B	S32.416A	S32.476B	S34.103A	S42.153B	S42.271A	S42.361B	S42.448A	S43.221A	S52.036B	S52.221C	S52.262A
S14.126A	S22.052A	S24.132A	S32.112A	S32.416B	S32.481A	S34.104A	S42.154B	S42.272A	S42.362A	S42.448B	S43.222A	S52.036C	S52.222A	S52.262B
S14.127A	S22.052B	S24.133A	S32.112B	S32.421A	S32.481B	S34.105A	S42.155B	S42.279A	S42.362B	S42.449A	S43.223A	S52.041B	S52.222B	S52.262C
S14.131A	S22.058A	S24.134A	S32.119A	S32.421B	S32.482A	S34.109A	S42.156B	S42.291A	S42.363A	S42.449B	S43.224A	S52.041C	S52.222C	S52.263A
S14.132A	S22.058B	S24.151A	S32.119B	S32.422A	S32.482B	S34.111A	S42.191B	S42.291B	S42.363B	S42.451A	S43.225A	S52.042B	S52.223A	S52.263B
S14.133A	S22.059A	S24.152A	S32.120A	S32.422B	S32.483A	S34.112A	S42.192B	S42.292A	S42.364A	S42.451B	S43.226A	S52.042C	S52.223B	S52.263C

Hospital-acquired Condition (HAC) (cont.) - Based on CMS data

S52.264A	S52.334B	S52.381C	S52.561A	S52.92XB	S62.126B	S62.303B	S62.396B	S62.654B	S72.041A	S72.114B	S72.24XC	S72.352A	S72.422B	S72.462C
S52.264B	S52.334C	S52.382A	S52.561B	S52.92XC	S62.131B	S62.304B	S62.397B	S62.655B	S72.041B	S72.114C	S72.25XA	S72.352B	S72.422C	S72.463A
S52.264C	S52.335A	S52.382B	S52.561C	S59.001A	S62.132B	S62.305B	S62.398B	S62.656B	S72.041C	S72.115A	S72.25XB	S72.352C	S72.423A	S72.463B
S52.265A	S52.335B	S52.382C	S52.562A	S59.002A	S62.133B	S62.306B	S62.399B	S62.657B	S72.042A	S72.115B	S72.25XC	S72.353A	S72.423B	S72.463C
S52.265B	S52.335C	S52.389A	S52.562B	S59.009A	S62.134B	S62.307B	S62.501B	S62.658B	S72.042B	S72.115C	S72.26XA	S72.353B	S72.423C	S72.464A
S52.265C	S52.336A	S52.389B	S52.562C	S59.011A	S62.135B	S62.308B	S62.502B	S62.659B	S72.042C	S72.116A	S72.26XB	S72.353C	S72.424A	S72.464B
S52.266A	S52.336B	S52.389C	S52.569A	S59.012A	S62.136B	S62.309B	S62.509B	S62.660B	S72.043A	S72.116B	S72.26XC	S72.354A	S72.424B	S72.464C
S52.266B	S52.336C	S52.391A	S52.569B	S59.019A	S62.141B	S62.310B	S62.511B	S62.661B	S72.043B	S72.116C	S72.301A	S72.354B	S72.424C	S72.465A
S52.266C	S52.341A	S52.391B	S52.569C	S59.021A	S62.142B	S62.311B	S62.512B	S62.662B	S72.043C	S72.121A	S72.301B	S72.354C	S72.425A	S72.465B
S52.271B	S52.341B	S52.391C	S52.571A	S59.022A	S62.143B	S62.312B	S62.513B	S62.663B	S72.044A	S72.121B	S72.301C	S72.355A	S72.425B	S72.465C
S52.271C	S52.341C	S52.392A	S52.571B	S59.029A	S62.144B	S62.313B	S62.514B	S62.664B	S72.044B	S72.121C	S72.302A	S72.355B	S72.425C	S72.466A
S52.272B	S52.342A	S52.392B	S52.571C	S59.031A	S62.145B	S62.314B	S62.515B	S62.665B	S72.044C	S72.122A	S72.302B	S72.355C	S72.426A	S72.466B
S52.272C	S52.342B	S52.392C	S52.572A	S59.032A	S62.146B	S62.315B	S62.516B	S62.666B	S72.045A	S72.122B	S72.302C	S72.356A	S72.426B	S72.466C
S52.279B	S52.342C	S52.399A	S52.572B	S59.039A	S62.151B	S62.316B	S62.521B	S62.667B	S72.045B	S72.122C	S72.309A	S72.356B	S72.426C	S72.471A
S52.279C	S52.343A	S52.399B	S52.572C	S59.041A	S62.152B	S62.317B	S62.522B	S62.668B	S72.045C	S72.123A	S72.309B	S72.356C	S72.431A	S72.472A
S52.281A	S52.343B	S52.399C	S52.579A	S59.042A	S62.153B	S62.318B	S62.523B	S62.669B	S72.046A	S72.123B	S72.309C	S72.361A	S72.431B	S72.479A
S52.281B	S52.343C	S52.501A	S52.579B	S59.049A	S62.154B	S62.319B	S62.524B	S62.90XB	S72.046B	S72.123C	S72.321A	S72.361B	S72.431C	S72.491A
S52.281C	S52.344A	S52.501B	S52.579C	S59.091A	S62.155B	S62.320B	S62.525B	S62.91XB	S72.046C	S72.124A	S72.321B	S72.361C	S72.432A	S72.491B
S52.282A	S52.344B	S52.501C	S52.591A	S59.092A	S62.156B	S62.321B	S62.526B	S62.92XB	S72.051A	S72.124B	S72.321C	S72.362A	S72.432B	S72.491C
S52.282B	S52.344C	S52.502A	S52.591B	S59.099A	S62.161B	S62.322B	S62.600B	S72.001A	S72.051B	S72.124C	S72.322A	S72.362B	S72.432C	S72.492A
S52.282C	S52.345A	S52.502B	S52.591C	S59.201A	S62.162B	S62.323B	S62.601B	S72.001B	S72.051C	S72.125A	S72.322B	S72.362C	S72.433A	S72.492B
S52.283A	S52.345B	S52.502C	S52.592A	S59.202A	S62.163B	S62.324B	S62.602B	S72.001C	S72.052A	S72.125B	S72.322C	S72.363A	S72.433B	S72.492C
S52.283B	S52.345C	S52.509A	S52.592B	S59.209A	S62.164B	S62.325B	S62.603B	S72.002A	S72.052B	S72.125C	S72.323A	S72.363B	S72.433C	S72.499A
S52.283C	S52.346A	S52.509B	S52.592C	S59.211A	S62.165B	S62.326B	S62.604B	S72.002B	S72.052C	S72.126A	S72.323B	S72.363C	S72.434A	S72.499B
S52.291A	S52.346B	S52.509C	S52.599A	S59.212A	S62.166B	S62.327B	S62.605B	S72.002C	S72.059A	S72.126B	S72.323C	S72.364A	S72.434B	S72.499C
S52.291B	S52.346C	S52.511A	S52.599B	S59.219A	S62.171B	S62.328B	S62.606B	S72.009A	S72.059B	S72.126C	S72.324A	S72.364B	S72.434C	S72.8X1A
S52.291C	S52.351A	S52.511B	S52.599C	S59.221A	S62.172B	S62.329B	S62.607B	S72.009B	S72.059C	S72.131A	S72.324B	S72.364C	S72.435A	S72.8X1B
S52.292A	S52.351B	S52.511C	S52.601A	S59.222A	S62.173B	S62.330B	S62.608B	S72.009C	S72.061A	S72.131B	S72.324C	S72.365A	S72.435B	S72.8X1C
S52.292B	S52.351C	S52.512A	S52.601B	S59.229A	S62.174B	S62.331B	S62.609B	S72.011A	S72.061B	S72.131C	S72.325A	S72.365B	S72.435C	S72.8X2A
S52.292C	S52.352A	S52.512B	S52.601C	S59.231A	S62.175B	S62.332B	S62.610B	S72.011B	S72.061C	S72.132A	S72.325B	S72.365C	S72.436A	S72.8X2B
S52.299A	S52.352B	S52.512C	S52.602A	S59.232A	S62.176B	S62.333B	S62.611B	S72.011C	S72.062A	S72.132B	S72.325C	S72.366A	S72.436B	S72.8X2C
S52.299B	S52.352C	S52.513A	S52.602B	S59.239A	S62.181B	S62.334B	S62.612B	S72.012A	S72.062B	S72.132C	S72.326A	S72.366B	S72.436C	S72.8X9A
S52.299C	S52.353A	S52.513B	S52.602C	S59.241A	S62.182B	S62.335B	S62.613B	S72.012B	S72.062C	S72.133A	S72.326B	S72.366C	S72.441A	S72.8X9B
S52.301A	S52.353B	S52.513C	S52.609A	S59.242A	S62.183B	S62.336B	S62.614B	S72.012C	S72.063A	S72.133B	S72.326C	S72.391A	S72.441B	S72.8X9C
S52.301B	S52.353C	S52.514A	S52.609B	S59.249A	S62.184B	S62.337B	S62.615B	S72.019A	S72.063B	S72.133C	S72.331A	S72.391B	S72.441C	S72.90XA
S52.301C	S52.354A	S52.514B	S52.609C	S59.291A	S62.185B	S62.338B	S62.616B	S72.019B	S72.063C	S72.134A	S72.331B	S72.391C	S72.442A	S72.90XB
S52.302A	S52.354B	S52.514C	S52.611A	S59.292A	S62.186B	S62.339B	S62.617B	S72.019C	S72.064A	S72.134B	S72.331C	S72.392A	S72.442B	S72.90XC
S52.302B	S52.354C	S52.515A	S52.611B	S59.299A	S62.201B	S62.340B	S62.618B	S72.021A	S72.064B	S72.134C	S72.332A	S72.392B	S72.442C	S72.91XA
S52.302C	S52.355A	S52.515B	S52.611C	S62.001B	S62.202B	S62.341B	S62.619B	S72.021B	S72.064C	S72.135A	S72.332B	S72.392C	S72.443A	S72.91XB
S52.309A	S52.355B	S52.515C	S52.612A	S62.002B	S62.209B	S62.342B	S62.620B	S72.021C	S72.065A	S72.135B	S72.332C	S72.399A	S72.443B	S72.91XC
S52.309B	S52.355C	S52.516A	S52.612B	S62.009B	S62.211B	S62.343B	S62.621B	S72.022A	S72.065B	S72.135C	S72.333A	S72.399B	S72.443C	S72.92XA
S52.309C	S52.356A	S52.516B	S52.612C	S62.011B	S62.212B	S62.344B	S62.622B	S72.022B	S72.065C	S72.136A	S72.333B	S72.399C	S72.444A	S72.92XB
S52.311A	S52.356B	S52.516C	S52.613A	S62.012B	S62.213B	S62.345B	S62.623B	S72.022C	S72.066A	S72.136B	S72.333C	S72.401A	S72.444B	S72.92XC
S52.312A	S52.356C	S52.521A	S52.613B	S62.013B	S62.221B	S62.346B	S62.624B	S72.023A	S72.066B	S72.136C	S72.334A	S72.401B	S72.444C	S73.001A
S52.319A	S52.361A	S52.522A	S52.613C	S62.014B	S62.222B	S62.347B	S62.625B	S72.023B	S72.066C	S72.141A	S72.334B	S72.401C	S72.445A	S73.002A
S52.321A	S52.361B	S52.529A	S52.614A	S62.015B	S62.223B	S62.348B	S62.626B	S72.023C	S72.091A	S72.141B	S72.334C	S72.402A	S72.445B	S73.003A
S52.321B	S52.361C	S52.531A	S52.614B	S62.016B	S62.224B	S62.349B	S62.627B	S72.024A	S72.091B	S72.141C	S72.335A	S72.402B	S72.445C	S73.004A
S52.321C	S52.362A	S52.531B	S52.614C	S62.021B	S62.225B	S62.350B	S62.628B	S72.024B	S72.091C	S72.142A	S72.335B	S72.402C	S72.446A	S73.005A
S52.322A	S52.362B	S52.531C	S52.615A	S62.022B	S62.226B	S62.351B	S62.629B	S72.024C	S72.092A	S72.142B	S72.335C	S72.409A	S72.446B	S73.006A
S52.322B	S52.362C	S52.532A	S52.615B	S62.023B	S62.231B	S62.352B	S62.630B	S72.025A	S72.092B	S72.142C	S72.336A	S72.409B	S72.446C	S73.011A
S52.322C	S52.363A	S52.532B	S52.615C	S62.024B	S62.232B	S62.353B	S62.631B	S72.025B	S72.092C	S72.143A	S72.336B	S72.409C	S72.451A	S73.012A
S52.323A	S52.363B	S52.532C	S52.616A	S62.025B	S62.233B	S62.354B	S62.632B	S72.025C	S72.099A	S72.143B	S72.336C	S72.411A	S72.451B	S73.013A
S52.323B	S52.363C	S52.539A	S52.616B	S62.026B	S62.234B	S62.355B	S62.633B	S72.026A	S72.099B	S72.143C	S72.341A	S72.411B	S72.451C	S73.014A
S52.323C	S52.364A	S52.539B	S52.616C	S62.031B	S62.235B	S62.356B	S62.634B	S72.026B	S72.099C	S72.144A	S72.341B	S72.411C	S72.452A	S73.015A
S52.324A	S52.364B	S52.539C	S52.621A	S62.032B	S62.236B	S62.357B	S62.635B	S72.026C	S72.101A	S72.144B	S72.341C	S72.412A	S72.452B	S73.016A
S52.324B	S52.364C	S52.541A	S52.622A	S62.033B	S62.241B	S62.358B	S62.636B	S72.031A	S72.101B	S72.144C	S72.342A	S72.412B	S72.452C	S73.021A
S52.324C	S52.365A	S52.541B	S52.629A	S62.034B	S62.242B	S62.359B	S62.637B	S72.031B	S72.101C	S72.145A	S72.342B	S72.412C	S72.453A	S73.022A
S52.325A	S52.365B	S52.541C	S52.691A	S62.035B	S62.243B	S62.360B	S62.638B	S72.031C	S72.102A	S72.145B	S72.342C	S72.413A	S72.453B	S73.023A
S52.325B	S52.365C	S52.542A	S52.691B	S62.036B	S62.244B	S62.361B	S62.639B	S72.032A	S72.102B	S72.145C	S72.343A	S72.413B	S72.453C	S73.024A
S52.325C	S52.366A	S52.542B	S52.691C	S62.101B	S62.245B	S62.362B	S62.640B	S72.032B	S72.102C	S72.146A	S72.343B	S72.413C	S72.454A	S73.025A
S52.326A	S52.366B	S52.542C	S52.692A	S62.102B	S62.246B	S62.363B	S62.641B	S72.032C	S72.109A	S72.146B	S72.343C	S72.414A	S72.454B	S73.026A
S52.326B	S52.366C	S52.549A	S52.692B	S62.109B	S62.251B	S62.364B	S62.642B	S72.033A	S72.109B	S72.146C	S72.344A	S72.414B	S72.454C	S73.031A
S52.326C	S52.371A	S52.549B	S52.692C	S62.111B	S62.252B	S62.365B	S62.643B	S72.033B	S72.109C	S72.21XA	S72.344B	S72.414C	S72.455A	S73.032A
S52.331A	S52.371B	S52.549C	S52.699A	S62.112B	S62.253B	S62.366B	S62.644B	S72.033C	S72.111A	S72.21XB	S72.344C	S72.415A	S72.455B	S73.033A
S52.331B	S52.371C	S52.551A	S52.699B	S62.113B	S62.254B	S62.367B	S62.645B	S72.034A	S72.111B	S72.21XC	S72.345A	S72.415B	S72.455C	S73.034A
S52.331C	S52.372A	S52.551B	S52.699C	S62.114B	S62.255B	S62.368B	S62.646B	S72.034B	S72.111C	S72.22XA	S72.345B	S72.415C	S72.456A	S73.035A
S52.332A	S52.372B	S52.551C	S52.90XA	S62.115B	S62.256B	S62.369B	S62.647B	S72.034C	S72.112A	S72.22XB	S72.345C	S72.416A	S72.456B	S73.036A
S52.332B	S52.372C	S52.552A	S52.90XB	S62.116B	S62.291B	S62.390B	S62.648B	S72.035A	S72.112B	S72.22XC	S72.346A	S72.416B	S72.456C	S73.041A
S52.332C	S52.379A	S52.552B	S52.90XC	S62.121B	S62.292B	S62.391B	S62.649B	S72.035B	S72.112C	S72.23XA	S72.346B	S72.416C	S72.461A	S73.042A
S52.333A	S52.379B	S52.552C	S52.91XA	S62.122B	S62.299B	S62.392B	S62.650B	S72.035C	S72.113A	S72.23XB	S72.346C	S72.421A	S72.461B	S73.043A
S52.333B	S52.379C	S52.559A	S52.91XB	S62.123B	S62.300B	S62.393B	S62.651B	S72.036A	S72.113B	S72.23XC	S72.351A	S72.421B	S72.461C	S73.044A
S52.333C	S52.381A	S52.559B	S52.91XC	S62.124B	S62.301B	S62.394B	S62.652B	S72.036B	S72.113C	S72.24XA	S72.351B	S72.421C	S72.462A	S73.045A
S52.334A	S52.381B	S52.559C	S52.92XA	S62.125B	S62.302B	S62.395B	S62.653B	S72.036C	S72.114A	S72.24XB	S72.351C	S72.422A	S72.462B	S73.046A

Hospital-acquired Condition (HAC) (cont.) - Based on CMS data

S77.00XA	S82.025B	S82.115C	S82.156A	S82.245B	S82.422B	S82.55XC	S82.899B	S92.116B	S92.324B	T22.329A	T23.729A	T26.20XA	T34.532A	T81.502A
S77.01XA	S82.025C	S82.116A	S82.156B	S82.245C	S82.422C	S82.56XB	S82.899C	S92.121B	S92.325B	T22.331A	T23.731A	T26.21XA	T34.539A	T81.503A
S77.02XA	S82.026A	S82.116B	S82.156C	S82.246A	S82.423B	S82.56XC	S82.90XB	S92.122B	S92.326B	T22.332A	T23.732A	T26.22XA	T34.60XA	T81.504A
S77.10XA	S82.026B	S82.116C	S82.161A	S82.246B	S82.423C	S82.61XB	S82.90XC	S92.123B	S92.331B	T22.339A	T23.739A	T26.70XA	T34.61XA	T81.505A
S77.11XA	S82.026C	S82.121A	S82.162A	S82.246C	S82.424B	S82.61XC	S82.91XB	S92.124B	S92.332B	T22.341A	T23.741A	T26.71XA	T34.62XA	T81.506A
S77.12XA	S82.031A	S82.121B	S82.169A	S82.251A	S82.424C	S82.62XB	S82.91XC	S92.125B	S92.333B	T22.342A	T23.742A	T26.72XA	T34.70XA	T81.507A
S79.001A	S82.031B	S82.121C	S82.191A	S82.251B	S82.425B	S82.62XC	S82.92XB	S92.126B	S92.334B	T22.349A	T23.749A	T27.0XXA	T34.71XA	T81.508A
S79.002A	S82.031C	S82.122A	S82.191B	S82.251C	S82.425C	S82.63XB	S82.92XC	S92.131B	S92.335B	T22.351A	T23.751A	T27.1XXA	T34.72XA	T81.509A
S79.009A	S82.032A	S82.122B	S82.191C	S82.252A	S82.426B	S82.63XC	S89.001A	S92.132B	S92.336B	T22.352A	T23.752A	T27.2XXA	T34.811A	T81.510A
S79.011A	S82.032B	S82.122C	S82.192A	S82.252B	S82.426C	S82.64XB	S89.002A	S92.133B	S92.341B	T22.359A	T23.759A	T27.3XXA	T34.812A	T81.511A
S79.012A	S82.032C	S82.123A	S82.192B	S82.252C	S82.431B	S82.64XC	S89.009A	S92.134B	S92.342B	T22.361A	T23.761A	T27.4XXA	T34.819A	T81.512A
S79.019A	S82.033A	S82.123B	S82.192C	S82.253A	S82.431C	S82.65XB	S89.011A	S92.135B	S92.343B	T22.362A	T23.762A	T27.5XXA	T34.821A	T81.513A
S79.091A	S82.033B	S82.123C	S82.199A	S82.253B	S82.432B	S82.65XC	S89.012A	S92.136B	S92.344B	T22.369A	T23.769A	T27.6XXA	T34.822A	T81.514A
S79.092A	S82.033C	S82.124A	S82.199B	S82.253C	S82.432C	S82.66XB	S89.019A	S92.141B	S92.345B	T22.391A	T23.771A	T27.7XXA	T34.829A	T81.515A
S79.099A	S82.034A	S82.124B	S82.199C	S82.254A	S82.433B	S82.66XC	S89.021A	S92.142B	S92.346B	T22.392A	T23.772A	T28.1XXA	T34.831A	T81.516A
S79.101A	S82.034B	S82.124C	S82.201A	S82.254B	S82.433C	S82.831B	S89.022A	S92.143B	S92.351B	T22.399A	T23.779A	T28.2XXA	T34.832A	T81.517A
S79.102A	S82.034C	S82.125A	S82.201B	S82.254C	S82.434B	S82.831C	S89.029A	S92.144B	S92.352B	T22.70XA	T23.791A	T28.6XXA	T34.839A	T81.518A
S79.109A	S82.035A	S82.125B	S82.201C	S82.255A	S82.434C	S82.832B	S89.031A	S92.145B	S92.353B	T22.711A	T23.792A	T28.7XXA	T34.90XA	T81.519A
S79.111A	S82.035B	S82.125C	S82.202A	S82.255B	S82.435B	S82.832C	S89.032A	S92.146B	S92.354B	T22.712A	T23.799A	T33.011A	T34.99XA	T81.520A
S79.112A	S82.035C	S82.126A	S82.202B	S82.255C	S82.435C	S82.839B	S89.039A	S92.151B	S92.355B	T22.719A	T24.301A	T33.012A	T69.021A	T81.521A
S79.119A	S82.036A	S82.126B	S82.202C	S82.256A	S82.436B	S82.839C	S89.041A	S92.152B	S92.356B	T22.721A	T24.302A	T33.019A	T69.022A	T81.522A
S79.121A	S82.036B	S82.126C	S82.209A	S82.256B	S82.436C	S82.841B	S89.042A	S92.153B	S92.811B	T22.722A	T24.309A	T33.02XA	T69.029A	T81.523A
S79.122A	S82.036C	S82.131A	S82.209B	S82.256C	S82.441B	S82.841C	S89.049A	S92.154B	S92.812B	T22.729A	T24.311A	T33.09XA	T70.3XXA	T81.524A
S79.129A	S82.041A	S82.131B	S82.209C	S82.261A	S82.441C	S82.842B	S89.091A	S92.155B	S92.819B	T22.731A	T24.312A	T33.1XXA	T71.111A	T81.525A
S79.131A	S82.041B	S82.131C	S82.221A	S82.261B	S82.442B	S82.842C	S89.092A	S92.156B	S92.901B	T22.732A	T24.319A	T33.2XXA	T71.112A	T81.526A
S79.132A	S82.041C	S82.132A	S82.221B	S82.261C	S82.442C	S82.843B	S89.099A	S92.191B	S92.902B	T22.739A	T24.321A	T33.3XXA	T71.113A	T81.527A
S79.139A	S82.042A	S82.132B	S82.221C	S82.262A	S82.443B	S82.843C	S92.001B	S92.192B	S92.909B	T22.741A	T24.322A	T33.40XA	T71.114A	T81.528A
S79.141A	S82.042B	S82.132C	S82.222A	S82.262B	S82.443C	S82.844B	S92.002B	S92.199B	T20.30XA	T22.742A	T24.329A	T33.41XA	T71.121A	T81.529A
S79.142A	S82.042C	S82.133A	S82.222B	S82.262C	S82.444B	S82.844C	S92.009B	S92.201B	T20.311A	T22.749A	T24.331A	T33.42XA	T71.122A	T81.530A
S79.149A	S82.043A	S82.133B	S82.222C	S82.263A	S82.444C	S82.845B	S92.011B	S92.202B	T20.312A	T22.751A	T24.332A	T33.511A	T71.123A	T81.531A
S79.191A	S82.043B	S82.133C	S82.223A	S82.263B	S82.445B	S82.845C	S92.012B	S92.209B	T20.319A	T22.752A	T24.339A	T33.512A	T71.124A	T81.532A
S79.192A	S82.043C	S82.134A	S82.223B	S82.263C	S82.445C	S82.846B	S92.013B	S92.211B	T20.32XA	T22.759A	T24.391A	T33.519A	T71.131A	T81.533A
S79.199A	S82.044A	S82.134B	S82.223C	S82.264A	S82.446B	S82.846C	S92.014B	S92.212B	T20.33XA	T22.761A	T24.392A	T33.521A	T71.132A	T81.534A
S82.001A	S82.044B	S82.134C	S82.224A	S82.264B	S82.446C	S82.851B	S92.015B	S92.213B	T20.34XA	T22.762A	T24.399A	T33.522A	T71.133A	T81.535A
S82.001B	S82.044C	S82.135A	S82.224B	S82.264C	S82.451B	S82.851C	S92.016B	S92.214B	T20.35XA	T22.769A	T24.701A	T33.529A	T71.134A	T81.536A
S82.001C	S82.045A	S82.135B	S82.224C	S82.265A	S82.451C	S82.852B	S92.021B	S92.215B	T20.36XA	T22.791A	T24.702A	T33.531A	T71.141A	T81.537A
S82.002A	S82.045B	S82.135C	S82.225A	S82.265B	S82.452B	S82.852C	S92.022B	S92.216B	T20.37XA	T22.792A	T24.709A	T33.532A	T71.143A	T81.538A
S82.002B	S82.045C	S82.136A	S82.225B	S82.265C	S82.452C	S82.853B	S92.023B	S92.221B	T20.39XA	T22.799A	T24.711A	T33.539A	T71.144A	T81.539A
S82.002C	S82.046A	S82.136B	S82.225C	S82.266A	S82.453B	S82.853C	S92.024B	S92.222B	T20.70XA	T23.301A	T24.712A	T33.60XA	T71.151A	T81.590A
S82.009A	S82.046B	S82.136C	S82.226A	S82.266B	S82.453C	S82.854B	S92.025B	S92.223B	T20.711A	T23.302A	T24.719A	T33.61XA	T71.152A	T81.591A
S82.009B	S82.046C	S82.141A	S82.226B	S82.266C	S82.454B	S82.854C	S92.026B	S92.224B	T20.712A	T23.309A	T24.721A	T33.62XA	T71.153A	T81.592A
S82.009C	S82.091A	S82.141B	S82.226C	S82.291A	S82.454C	S82.855B	S92.031B	S92.225B	T20.719A	T23.311A	T24.722A	T33.70XA	T71.154A	T81.593A
S82.011A	S82.091B	S82.141C	S82.231A	S82.291B	S82.455B	S82.855C	S92.032B	S92.226B	T20.72XA	T23.312A	T24.729A	T33.71XA	T71.161A	T81.594A
S82.011B	S82.091C	S82.142A	S82.231B	S82.291C	S82.455C	S82.856B	S92.033B	S92.231B	T20.73XA	T23.319A	T24.731A	T33.72XA	T71.162A	T81.595A
S82.011C	S82.092A	S82.142B	S82.231C	S82.292A	S82.456B	S82.856C	S92.034B	S92.232B	T20.74XA	T23.321A	T24.732A	T33.811A	T71.163A	T81.596A
S82.012A	S82.092B	S82.142C	S82.232A	S82.292B	S82.456C	S82.861B	S92.035B	S92.233B	T20.75XA	T23.322A	T24.739A	T33.812A	T71.164A	T81.597A
S82.012B	S82.092C	S82.143A	S82.232B	S82.292C	S82.461B	S82.861C	S92.036B	S92.234B	T20.76XA	T23.329A	T24.791A	T33.819A	T71.191A	T81.598A
S82.012C	S82.099A	S82.143B	S82.232C	S82.299A	S82.461C	S82.862B	S92.041B	S92.235B	T20.77XA	T23.331A	T24.792A	T33.821A	T71.192A	T81.599A
S82.013A	S82.099B	S82.143C	S82.233A	S82.299B	S82.462B	S82.862C	S92.042B	S92.236B	T20.79XA	T23.332A	T24.799A	T33.822A	T71.193A	T81.60XA
S82.013B	S82.099C	S82.144A	S82.233B	S82.299C	S82.462C	S82.863B	S92.043B	S92.241B	T21.30XA	T23.339A	T25.311A	T33.829A	T71.194A	T81.61XA
S82.013C	S82.101A	S82.144B	S82.233C	S82.301B	S82.463B	S82.863C	S92.044B	S92.242B	T21.31XA	T23.341A	T25.312A	T33.831A	T71.20XA	T81.69XA
S82.014A	S82.101B	S82.144C	S82.234A	S82.301C	S82.463C	S82.864B	S92.045B	S92.243B	T21.32XA	T23.342A	T25.319A	T33.832A	T71.21XA	T82.6XXA
S82.014B	S82.101C	S82.145A	S82.234B	S82.302B	S82.464B	S82.864C	S92.046B	S92.244B	T21.33XA	T23.349A	T25.321A	T33.839A	T71.29XA	T82.7XXA
S82.014C	S82.102A	S82.145B	S82.234C	S82.302C	S82.464C	S82.865B	S92.051B	S92.245B	T21.34XA	T23.351A	T25.322A	T33.90XA	T71.9XXA	T83.511A
S82.015A	S82.102B	S82.145C	S82.235A	S82.309B	S82.465B	S82.865C	S92.052B	S92.246B	T21.35XA	T23.352A	T25.329A	T33.99XA	T75.1XXA	T83.518A
S82.015B	S82.102C	S82.146A	S82.235B	S82.309C	S82.465C	S82.866B	S92.053B	S92.251B	T21.36XA	T23.359A	T25.331A	T34.011A	T80.0XXA	T84.60XA
S82.015C	S82.109A	S82.146B	S82.235C	S82.311A	S82.466B	S82.866C	S92.054B	S92.252B	T21.37XA	T23.361A	T25.332A	T34.012A	T80.211A	T84.610A
S82.016A	S82.109B	S82.146C	S82.236A	S82.312A	S82.466C	S82.871B	S92.055B	S92.253B	T21.39XA	T23.362A	T25.339A	T34.019A	T80.212A	T84.611A
S82.016B	S82.109C	S82.151A	S82.236B	S82.319A	S82.491B	S82.871C	S92.056B	S92.254B	T21.70XA	T23.369A	T25.391A	T34.02XA	T80.218A	T84.612A
S82.016C	S82.111A	S82.151B	S82.236C	S82.391B	S82.491C	S82.872B	S92.061B	S92.255B	T21.71XA	T23.371A	T25.392A	T34.09XA	T80.219A	T84.613A
S82.021A	S82.111B	S82.151C	S82.241A	S82.391C	S82.492B	S82.872C	S92.062B	S92.256B	T21.72XA	T23.372A	T25.399A	T34.1XXA	T80.30XA	T84.614A
S82.021B	S82.111C	S82.152A	S82.241B	S82.392B	S82.492C	S82.873B	S92.063B	S92.301B	T21.73XA	T23.379A	T25.711A	T34.2XXA	T80.310A	T84.615A
S82.021C	S82.112A	S82.152B	S82.241C	S82.392C	S82.499B	S82.873C	S92.064B	S92.302B	T21.74XA	T23.391A	T25.712A	T34.3XXA	T80.311A	T84.619A
S82.022A	S82.112B	S82.152C	S82.242A	S82.399B	S82.499C	S82.874B	S92.065B	S92.309B	T21.75XA	T23.392A	T25.719A	T34.40XA	T80.319A	T84.63XA
S82.022B	S82.112C	S82.153A	S82.242B	S82.399C	S82.51XB	S82.874C	S92.066B	S92.311B	T21.76XA	T23.399A	T25.721A	T34.41XA	T80.39XA	T84.69XA
S82.022C	S82.113A	S82.153B	S82.242C	S82.401B	S82.51XC	S82.875B	S92.101B	S92.312B	T21.77XA	T23.701A	T25.722A	T34.42XA	T81.40XA	T84.7XXA
S82.023A	S82.113B	S82.153C	S82.243A	S82.401C	S82.52XB	S82.875C	S92.102B	S92.313B	T21.79XA	T23.702A	T25.729A	T34.511A	T81.41XA	
S82.023B	S82.113C	S82.154A	S82.243B	S82.402B	S82.52XC	S82.876B	S92.109B	S92.314B	T22.30XA	T23.709A	T25.731A	T34.512A	T81.42XA	
S82.023C	S82.114A	S82.154B	S82.243C	S82.402C	S82.53XB	S82.876C	S92.111B	S92.315B	T22.311A	T23.711A	T25.732A	T34.519A	T81.43XA	
S82.024A	S82.114B	S82.154C	S82.244A	S82.409B	S82.53XC	S82.891B	S92.112B	S92.316B	T22.312A	T23.712A	T25.739A	T34.521A	T81.44XA	
S82.024B	S82.114C	S82.155A	S82.244B	S82.409C	S82.54XB	S82.891C	S92.113B	S92.321B	T22.319A	T23.719A	T25.791A	T34.522A	T81.49XA	
S82.024C	S82.115A	S82.155B	S82.244C	S82.421B	S82.54XC	S82.892B	S92.114B	S92.322B	T22.321A	T23.721A	T25.792A	T34.529A	T81.500A	
S82.025A	S82.115B	S82.155C	S82.245A	S82.421C	S82.55XB	S82.892C	S92.115B	S92.323B	T22.322A	T23.722A	T25.799A	T34.531A	T81.501A	

HCC - Based on CMS data

E08.3211	E09.3493	E10.3591	E13.3393	M84.459A	S02.110A	S02.40DS	S02.652B	S06.303S	S06.350S	S06.4X5S	S06.892S	S12.191B	S12.600B	S14.119D
E08.3212	E09.3499	E10.3592	E13.3399	M84.551A	S02.110B	S02.40EA	S02.652S	S06.304A	S06.351A	S06.4X6A	S06.893A	S12.200A	S12.601A	S14.119S
E08.3213	E09.3511	E10.3593	E13.3411	M84.552A	S02.110S	S02.40EB	S02.66XA	S06.304S	S06.351S	S06.4X6S	S06.893S	S12.200B	S12.601B	S14.121A
E08.3219	E09.3512	E10.3599	E13.3412	M84.553A	S02.111A	S02.40ES	S02.66XB	S06.305A	S06.352A	S06.4X9A	S06.894A	S12.201A	S12.630A	S14.121D
E08.3291	E09.3513	E10.37X1	E13.3413	M84.559A	S02.111B	S02.40FA	S02.66XS	S06.305S	S06.352S	S06.4X9S	S06.894S	S12.201B	S12.630B	S14.121S
E08.3292	E09.3519	E10.37X2	E13.3419	M84.651A	S02.111S	S02.40FB	S02.670A	S06.306A	S06.353A	S06.5X0A	S06.895A	S12.230A	S12.631A	S14.122A
E08.3293	E09.3521	E10.37X3	E13.3491	M84.652A	S02.112A	S02.40FS	S02.670B	S06.306S	S06.353S	S06.5X0S	S06.895S	S12.230B	S12.631B	S14.122D
E08.3299	E09.3522	E10.37X9	E13.3492	M84.653A	S02.112B	S02.411A	S02.670S	S06.309A	S06.354A	S06.5X1A	S06.896A	S12.231A	S12.64XA	S14.122S
E08.3311	E09.3523	E11.3211	E13.3493	M84.659A	S02.112S	S02.411B	S02.671A	S06.309S	S06.354S	S06.5X1S	S06.896S	S12.231B	S12.64XB	S14.123A
E08.3312	E09.3529	E11.3212	E13.3499	M84.754A	S02.113A	S02.411S	S02.671B	S06.310A	S06.355A	S06.5X2A	S06.899A	S12.24XA	S12.650A	S14.123D
E08.3313	E09.3531	E11.3213	E13.3511	M84.755A	S02.113B	S02.412A	S02.671S	S06.310S	S06.355S	S06.5X2S	S06.899S	S12.24XB	S12.650B	S14.123S
E08.3319	E09.3532	E11.3219	E13.3512	M84.756A	S02.113S	S02.412B	S02.672A	S06.311A	S06.356A	S06.5X3A	S06.9X0A	S12.250A	S12.651A	S14.124A
E08.3391	E09.3533	E11.3291	E13.3513	M84.757A	S02.118A	S02.412S	S02.672B	S06.311S	S06.356S	S06.5X3S	S06.9X0S	S12.250B	S12.651B	S14.124D
E08.3392	E09.3539	E11.3292	E13.3519	M84.758A	S02.118B	S02.413A	S02.672S	S06.312A	S06.359A	S06.5X4A	S06.9X1A	S12.251A	S12.690A	S14.124S
E08.3393	E09.3541	E11.3293	E13.3521	M84.759A	S02.118S	S02.413B	S02.69XA	S06.312S	S06.359S	S06.5X4S	S06.9X1S	S12.251B	S12.690B	S14.125A
E08.3399	E09.3542	E11.3299	E13.3522	M97.01XA	S02.119A	S02.413S	S02.69XB	S06.313A	S06.360A	S06.5X5A	S06.9X2A	S12.290A	S12.691A	S14.125D
E08.3411	E09.3543	E11.3311	E13.3523	M97.02XA	S02.119B	S02.42XA	S02.69XS	S06.313S	S06.360S	S06.5X5S	S06.9X2S	S12.290B	S12.691B	S14.125S
E08.3412	E09.3549	E11.3312	E13.3529	R40.2110	S02.119S	S02.42XB	S02.80XA	S06.314A	S06.361A	S06.5X6A	S06.9X3A	S12.291A	S12.8XXA	S14.126A
E08.3413	E09.3551	E11.3313	E13.3531	R40.2111	S02.11AA	S02.42XS	S02.80XB	S06.314S	S06.361S	S06.5X6S	S06.9X3S	S12.291B	S12.9XXA	S14.126D
E08.3419	E09.3552	E11.3319	E13.3532	R40.2112	S02.11AB	S02.600A	S02.80XS	S06.315A	S06.362A	S06.5X9A	S06.9X4A	S12.300A	S14.0XXA	S14.126S
E08.3491	E09.3553	E11.3391	E13.3533	R40.2113	S02.11AS	S02.600B	S02.81XA	S06.315S	S06.362S	S06.5X9S	S06.9X4S	S12.300B	S14.0XXD	S14.127A
E08.3492	E09.3559	E11.3392	E13.3539	R40.2114	S02.11BA	S02.600S	S02.81XB	S06.316A	S06.363A	S06.6X0A	S06.9X5A	S12.301A	S14.0XXS	S14.127D
E08.3493	E09.3591	E11.3393	E13.3541	R40.2120	S02.11BB	S02.601A	S02.81XS	S06.316S	S06.363S	S06.6X0S	S06.9X5S	S12.301B	S14.101A	S14.127S
E08.3499	E09.3592	E11.3399	E13.3542	R40.2121	S02.11BS	S02.601B	S02.82XA	S06.319A	S06.364A	S06.6X1A	S06.9X6A	S12.330A	S14.101D	S14.128A
E08.3511	E09.3593	E11.3411	E13.3543	R40.2122	S02.11CA	S02.601S	S02.82XB	S06.319S	S06.364S	S06.6X1S	S06.9X6S	S12.330B	S14.101S	S14.128D
E08.3512	E09.3599	E11.3412	E13.3549	R40.2123	S02.11CB	S02.602A	S02.82XS	S06.320A	S06.365A	S06.6X2A	S06.9X9A	S12.331A	S14.102A	S14.128S
E08.3513	E09.37X1	E11.3413	E13.3551	R40.2124	S02.11CS	S02.602B	S02.91XA	S06.320S	S06.365S	S06.6X2S	S06.9X9S	S12.331B	S14.102D	S14.129A
E08.3519	E09.37X2	E11.3419	E13.3552	R40.2210	S02.11DA	S02.602S	S02.91XB	S06.321A	S06.366A	S06.6X3A	S12.000A	S12.34XA	S14.102S	S14.129D
E08.3521	E09.37X3	E11.3491	E13.3553	R40.2211	S02.11DB	S02.609A	S02.91XS	S06.321S	S06.366S	S06.6X3S	S12.000B	S12.34XB	S14.103A	S14.129S
E08.3522	E09.37X9	E11.3492	E13.3559	R40.2212	S02.11DS	S02.609B	S02.92XA	S06.322A	S06.369A	S06.6X4A	S12.001A	S12.350A	S14.103D	S14.131A
E08.3523	E10.3211	E11.3493	E13.3591	R40.2213	S02.11EA	S02.609S	S02.92XB	S06.322S	S06.369S	S06.6X4S	S12.001B	S12.350B	S14.103S	S14.131D
E08.3529	E10.3212	E11.3499	E13.3592	R40.2214	S02.11EB	S02.610A	S02.92XS	S06.323A	S06.370A	S06.6X5A	S12.01XA	S12.351A	S14.104A	S14.131S
E08.3531	E10.3213	E11.3511	E13.3593	R40.2220	S02.11ES	S02.610B	S06.0X0S	S06.323S	S06.370S	S06.6X5S	S12.01XB	S12.351B	S14.104D	S14.132A
E08.3532	E10.3219	E11.3512	E13.3599	R40.2221	S02.11FA	S02.610S	S06.0X1S	S06.324A	S06.371A	S06.6X6A	S12.02XA	S12.390A	S14.104S	S14.132D
E08.3533	E10.3291	E11.3513	E13.37X1	R40.2222	S02.11FB	S02.611A	S06.0X9S	S06.324S	S06.371S	S06.6X6S	S12.02XB	S12.390B	S14.105A	S14.132S
E08.3539	E10.3292	E11.3519	E13.37X2	R40.2223	S02.11FS	S02.611B	S06.1X0A	S06.325A	S06.372A	S06.6X9A	S12.030A	S12.391A	S14.105D	S14.133A
E08.3541	E10.3293	E11.3521	E13.37X3	R40.2224	S02.11GA	S02.611S	S06.1X0S	S06.325S	S06.372S	S06.6X9S	S12.030B	S12.391B	S14.105S	S14.133D
E08.3542	E10.3299	E11.3522	E13.37X9	R40.2310	S02.11GB	S02.612A	S06.1X1A	S06.326A	S06.373A	S06.810A	S12.031A	S12.400A	S14.106A	S14.133S
E08.3543	E10.3311	E11.3523	H35.3210	R40.2311	S02.11GS	S02.612B	S06.1X1S	S06.326S	S06.373S	S06.810S	S12.031B	S12.400B	S14.106D	S14.134A
E08.3549	E10.3312	E11.3529	H35.3211	R40.2312	S02.11HA	S02.612S	S06.1X2A	S06.329A	S06.374A	S06.811A	S12.040A	S12.401A	S14.106S	S14.134D
E08.3551	E10.3313	E11.3531	H35.3212	R40.2313	S02.11HB	S02.620A	S06.1X2S	S06.329S	S06.374S	S06.811S	S12.040B	S12.401B	S14.107A	S14.134S
E08.3552	E10.3319	E11.3532	H35.3213	R40.2314	S02.11HS	S02.620B	S06.1X3A	S06.330A	S06.375A	S06.812A	S12.041A	S12.430A	S14.107D	S14.135A
E08.3553	E10.3391	E11.3533	H35.3220	R40.2320	S02.19XA	S02.620S	S06.1X3S	S06.330S	S06.375S	S06.812S	S12.041B	S12.430B	S14.107S	S14.135D
E08.3559	E10.3392	E11.3539	H35.3221	R40.2321	S02.19XB	S02.621A	S06.1X4A	S06.331A	S06.376A	S06.813A	S12.090A	S12.431A	S14.108A	S14.135S
E08.3591	E10.3393	E11.3541	H35.3222	R40.2322	S02.19XS	S02.621B	S06.1X4S	S06.331S	S06.376S	S06.813S	S12.090B	S12.431B	S14.108D	S14.136A
E08.3592	E10.3399	E11.3542	H35.3223	R40.2323	S02.30XA	S02.621S	S06.1X5A	S06.332A	S06.379A	S06.814A	S12.091A	S12.44XA	S14.108S	S14.136D
E08.3593	E10.3411	E11.3543	H35.3230	R40.2324	S02.30XB	S02.622A	S06.1X5S	S06.332S	S06.379S	S06.814S	S12.091B	S12.44XB	S14.109A	S14.136S
E08.3599	E10.3412	E11.3549	H35.3231	R40.2340	S02.30XS	S02.622B	S06.1X6A	S06.333A	S06.380A	S06.815A	S12.100A	S12.450A	S14.109D	S14.137A
E08.37X1	E10.3413	E11.3551	H35.3232	R40.2341	S02.31XA	S02.622S	S06.1X6S	S06.333S	S06.380S	S06.815S	S12.100B	S12.450B	S14.109S	S14.137D
E08.37X2	E10.3419	E11.3552	H35.3233	R40.2342	S02.31XB	S02.630A	S06.1X9A	S06.334A	S06.381A	S06.816A	S12.101A	S12.451A	S14.111A	S14.137S
E08.37X3	E10.3491	E11.3553	H35.3290	R40.2343	S02.31XS	S02.630B	S06.1X9S	S06.334S	S06.381S	S06.816S	S12.101B	S12.451B	S14.111D	S14.138A
E08.37X9	E10.3492	E11.3559	H35.3291	R40.2344	S02.32XA	S02.630S	S06.2X0A	S06.335A	S06.382A	S06.819A	S12.110A	S12.490A	S14.111S	S14.138D
E09.3211	E10.3493	E11.3591	H35.3292	R40.2430	S02.32XB	S02.631A	S06.2X0S	S06.335S	S06.382S	S06.819S	S12.110B	S12.490B	S14.112A	S14.138S
E09.3212	E10.3499	E11.3592	H35.3293	R40.2431	S02.32XS	S02.631B	S06.2X1A	S06.336A	S06.383A	S06.820A	S12.111A	S12.491A	S14.112D	S14.139A
E09.3213	E10.3511	E11.3593	M48.50XA	R40.2432	S02.400A	S02.631S	S06.2X1S	S06.336S	S06.383S	S06.820S	S12.111B	S12.491B	S14.112S	S14.139D
E09.3219	E10.3512	E11.3599	M48.51XA	R40.2433	S02.400B	S02.632A	S06.2X2A	S06.339A	S06.384A	S06.821A	S12.112A	S12.500A	S14.113A	S14.139S
E09.3291	E10.3513	E11.37X1	M48.52XA	R40.2434	S02.400S	S02.632B	S06.2X2S	S06.339S	S06.384S	S06.821S	S12.112B	S12.500B	S14.113D	S14.141A
E09.3292	E10.3519	E11.37X2	M48.53XA	R40.2440	S02.401A	S02.632S	S06.2X3A	S06.340A	S06.385A	S06.822A	S12.120A	S12.501A	S14.113S	S14.141D
E09.3293	E10.3521	E11.37X3	M48.54XA	R40.2441	S02.401B	S02.640A	S06.2X3S	S06.340S	S06.385S	S06.822S	S12.120B	S12.501B	S14.114A	S14.141S
E09.3299	E10.3522	E11.37X9	M48.55XA	R40.2442	S02.401S	S02.640B	S06.2X4A	S06.341A	S06.386A	S06.823A	S12.121A	S12.530A	S14.114D	S14.142A
E09.3311	E10.3523	E13.3211	M48.56XA	R40.2443	S02.402A	S02.640S	S06.2X4S	S06.341S	S06.386S	S06.823S	S12.121B	S12.530B	S14.114S	S14.142D
E09.3312	E10.3529	E13.3212	M48.57XA	R40.2444	S02.402B	S02.641A	S06.2X5A	S06.342A	S06.389A	S06.824A	S12.130A	S12.531A	S14.115A	S14.142S
E09.3313	E10.3531	E13.3213	M48.58XA	S02.0XXA	S02.402S	S02.641B	S06.2X5S	S06.342S	S06.389S	S06.824S	S12.130B	S12.531B	S14.115D	S14.143A
E09.3319	E10.3532	E13.3219	M80.051A	S02.0XXB	S02.40AA	S02.641S	S06.2X6A	S06.343A	S06.4X0A	S06.825A	S12.131A	S12.54XA	S14.115S	S14.143D
E09.3391	E10.3533	E13.3291	M80.052A	S02.0XXS	S02.40AB	S02.642A	S06.2X6S	S06.343S	S06.4X0S	S06.825S	S12.131B	S12.54XB	S14.116A	S14.143S
E09.3392	E10.3539	E13.3292	M80.059A	S02.101A	S02.40AS	S02.642B	S06.2X9A	S06.344A	S06.4X1A	S06.826A	S12.14XA	S12.550A	S14.116D	S14.144A
E09.3393	E10.3541	E13.3293	M80.08XA	S02.101B	S02.40BA	S02.642S	S06.2X9S	S06.344S	S06.4X1S	S06.826S	S12.14XB	S12.550B	S14.116S	S14.144D
E09.3399	E10.3542	E13.3299	M80.851A	S02.101S	S02.40BB	S02.650A	S06.300A	S06.345A	S06.4X2A	S06.829A	S12.150A	S12.551A	S14.117A	S14.144S
E09.3411	E10.3543	E13.3311	M80.852A	S02.102A	S02.40BS	S02.650B	S06.300S	S06.345S	S06.4X2S	S06.829S	S12.150B	S12.551B	S14.117D	S14.145A
E09.3412	E10.3549	E13.3312	M80.859A	S02.102B	S02.40CA	S02.650S	S06.301A	S06.346A	S06.4X3A	S06.890A	S12.151A	S12.590A	S14.117S	S14.145D
E09.3413	E10.3551	E13.3313	M80.88XA	S02.102S	S02.40CB	S02.651A	S06.301S	S06.346S	S06.4X3S	S06.890S	S12.151B	S12.590B	S14.118A	S14.145S
E09.3419	E10.3552	E13.3319	M84.451A	S02.109A	S02.40CS	S02.651B	S06.302A	S06.349A	S06.4X4A	S06.891A	S12.190A	S12.591A	S14.118D	S14.146A
E09.3491	E10.3553	E13.3391	M84.452A	S02.109B	S02.40DA	S02.651S	S06.302S	S06.349S	S06.4X4S	S06.891S	S12.190B	S12.591B	S14.118S	S14.146D
E09.3492	E10.3559	E13.3392	M84.453A	S02.109S	S02.40DB	S02.652A	S06.303A	S06.350A	S06.4X5A	S06.892A	S12.191A	S12.600A	S14.119A	S14.146S

HCC (cont.) - Based on CMS data

S14.147A	S22.039A	S24.112D	S32.019A	S32.17XA	S32.442A	S32.519A	S34.113S	S58.011A	S68.511S	S72.031A	S72.101C	S72.145B	S72.343A	S72.413C
S14.147D	S22.039B	S24.112S	S32.019B	S32.17XB	S32.442B	S32.519B	S34.114A	S58.011S	S68.512S	S72.031B	S72.102A	S72.145C	S72.343B	S72.414A
S14.147S	S22.040A	S24.113A	S32.020A	S32.19XA	S32.443A	S32.591A	S34.114D	S58.012A	S68.519S	S72.031C	S72.102B	S72.146A	S72.343C	S72.414B
S14.148A	S22.040B	S24.113D	S32.020B	S32.19XB	S32.443B	S32.591B	S34.114S	S58.012S	S68.521S	S72.032A	S72.102C	S72.146B	S72.344A	S72.414C
S14.148D	S22.041A	S24.113S	S32.021A	S32.2XXA	S32.444A	S32.592A	S34.115A	S58.019A	S68.522S	S72.032B	S72.109A	S72.146C	S72.344B	S72.415A
S14.148S	S22.041B	S24.114A	S32.021B	S32.2XXB	S32.444B	S32.592B	S34.115D	S58.019S	S68.529S	S72.032C	S72.109B	S72.21XA	S72.344C	S72.415B
S14.149A	S22.042A	S24.114D	S32.022A	S32.301A	S32.445A	S32.599A	S34.115S	S58.021A	S68.610S	S72.033A	S72.109C	S72.21XB	S72.345A	S72.415C
S14.149D	S22.042B	S24.114S	S32.022B	S32.301B	S32.445B	S32.599B	S34.119A	S58.021S	S68.611S	S72.033B	S72.111A	S72.21XC	S72.345B	S72.416A
S14.149S	S22.048A	S24.119A	S32.028A	S32.302A	S32.446A	S32.601A	S34.119D	S58.022A	S68.612S	S72.033C	S72.111B	S72.22XA	S72.345C	S72.416B
S14.151A	S22.048B	S24.119D	S32.028B	S32.302B	S32.446B	S32.601B	S34.119S	S58.022S	S68.613S	S72.034A	S72.111C	S72.22XB	S72.346A	S72.416C
S14.151D	S22.049A	S24.119S	S32.029A	S32.309A	S32.451A	S32.602A	S34.121A	S58.029A	S68.614S	S72.034B	S72.112A	S72.22XC	S72.346B	S72.421A
S14.151S	S22.049B	S24.131A	S32.029B	S32.309B	S32.451B	S32.602B	S34.121D	S58.029S	S68.615S	S72.034C	S72.112B	S72.23XA	S72.346C	S72.421B
S14.152A	S22.050A	S24.131D	S32.030A	S32.311A	S32.452A	S32.609A	S34.121S	S58.111A	S68.616S	S72.035A	S72.112C	S72.23XB	S72.351A	S72.421C
S14.152D	S22.050B	S24.131S	S32.030B	S32.311B	S32.452B	S32.609B	S34.122A	S58.111S	S68.617S	S72.035B	S72.113A	S72.23XC	S72.351B	S72.422A
S14.152S	S22.051A	S24.132A	S32.031A	S32.312A	S32.453A	S32.611A	S34.122D	S58.112A	S68.618S	S72.035C	S72.113B	S72.24XA	S72.351C	S72.422B
S14.153A	S22.051B	S24.132D	S32.031B	S32.312B	S32.453B	S32.611B	S34.122S	S58.112S	S68.619S	S72.036A	S72.113C	S72.24XB	S72.352A	S72.422C
S14.153D	S22.052A	S24.132S	S32.032A	S32.313A	S32.454A	S32.612A	S34.123A	S58.119A	S68.620S	S72.036B	S72.114A	S72.24XC	S72.352B	S72.423A
S14.153S	S22.052B	S24.133A	S32.032B	S32.313B	S32.454B	S32.612B	S34.123D	S58.119S	S68.621S	S72.036C	S72.114B	S72.25XA	S72.352C	S72.423B
S14.154A	S22.058A	S24.133D	S32.038A	S32.314A	S32.455A	S32.613A	S34.123S	S58.121A	S68.622S	S72.041A	S72.114C	S72.25XB	S72.353A	S72.423C
S14.154D	S22.058B	S24.133S	S32.038B	S32.314B	S32.455B	S32.613B	S34.124A	S58.121S	S68.623S	S72.041B	S72.115A	S72.25XC	S72.353B	S72.424A
S14.154S	S22.059A	S24.134A	S32.039A	S32.315A	S32.456A	S32.614A	S34.124D	S58.122A	S68.624S	S72.041C	S72.115B	S72.26XA	S72.353C	S72.424B
S14.155A	S22.059B	S24.134D	S32.039B	S32.315B	S32.456B	S32.614B	S34.124S	S58.122S	S68.625S	S72.042A	S72.115C	S72.26XB	S72.354A	S72.424C
S14.155D	S22.060A	S24.134S	S32.040A	S32.316A	S32.461A	S32.615A	S34.125A	S58.129A	S68.626S	S72.042B	S72.116A	S72.26XC	S72.354B	S72.425A
S14.155S	S22.060B	S24.139A	S32.040B	S32.316B	S32.461B	S32.615B	S34.125D	S58.129S	S68.627S	S72.042C	S72.116B	S72.301A	S72.354C	S72.425B
S14.156A	S22.061A	S24.139D	S32.041A	S32.391A	S32.462A	S32.616A	S34.125S	S58.911A	S68.628S	S72.043A	S72.116C	S72.301B	S72.355A	S72.425C
S14.156D	S22.061B	S24.139S	S32.041B	S32.391B	S32.462B	S32.616B	S34.129A	S58.911S	S68.629S	S72.043B	S72.121A	S72.301C	S72.355B	S72.426A
S14.156S	S22.062A	S24.141A	S32.042A	S32.392A	S32.463A	S32.691A	S34.129D	S58.912A	S68.711A	S72.043C	S72.121B	S72.302A	S72.355C	S72.426B
S14.157A	S22.062B	S24.141D	S32.042B	S32.392B	S32.463B	S32.691B	S34.129S	S58.912S	S68.711S	S72.044A	S72.121C	S72.302B	S72.356A	S72.426C
S14.157D	S22.068A	S24.141S	S32.048A	S32.399A	S32.464A	S32.692A	S34.131A	S58.919A	S68.712A	S72.044B	S72.122A	S72.302C	S72.356B	S72.431A
S14.157S	S22.068B	S24.142A	S32.048B	S32.399B	S32.464B	S32.692B	S34.131D	S58.919S	S68.712S	S72.044C	S72.122B	S72.309A	S72.356C	S72.431B
S14.158A	S22.069A	S24.142D	S32.049A	S32.401A	S32.465A	S32.699A	S34.131S	S58.921A	S68.719A	S72.045A	S72.122C	S72.309B	S72.361A	S72.431C
S14.158D	S22.069B	S24.142S	S32.049B	S32.401B	S32.465B	S32.699B	S34.132A	S58.921S	S68.719S	S72.045B	S72.123A	S72.309C	S72.361B	S72.432A
S14.158S	S22.070A	S24.143A	S32.050A	S32.402A	S32.466A	S32.810A	S34.132D	S58.922A	S68.721A	S72.045C	S72.123B	S72.321A	S72.361C	S72.432B
S14.159A	S22.070B	S24.143D	S32.050B	S32.402B	S32.466B	S32.810B	S34.132S	S58.922S	S68.721S	S72.046A	S72.123C	S72.321B	S72.362A	S72.432C
S14.159D	S22.071A	S24.143S	S32.051A	S32.409A	S32.471A	S32.811A	S34.139A	S58.929A	S68.722A	S72.046B	S72.124A	S72.321C	S72.362B	S72.433A
S14.159S	S22.071B	S24.144A	S32.051B	S32.409B	S32.471B	S32.811B	S34.139D	S58.929S	S68.722S	S72.046C	S72.124B	S72.322A	S72.362C	S72.433B
S22.000A	S22.072A	S24.144D	S32.052A	S32.411A	S32.472A	S32.82XA	S34.139S	S68.011S	S68.729A	S72.051A	S72.124C	S72.322B	S72.363A	S72.433C
S22.000B	S22.072B	S24.144S	S32.052B	S32.411B	S32.472B	S32.82XB	S34.3XXA	S68.012S	S68.729S	S72.051B	S72.125A	S72.322C	S72.363B	S72.434A
S22.001A	S22.078A	S24.149A	S32.058A	S32.412A	S32.473A	S32.89XA	S48.011A	S68.019S	S72.001A	S72.051C	S72.125B	S72.323A	S72.363C	S72.434B
S22.001B	S22.078B	S24.149D	S32.058B	S32.412B	S32.473B	S32.89XB	S48.011S	S68.021S	S72.001B	S72.052A	S72.125C	S72.323B	S72.364A	S72.434C
S22.002A	S22.079A	S24.149S	S32.059A	S32.413A	S32.474A	S32.9XXA	S48.012A	S68.022S	S72.001C	S72.052B	S72.126A	S72.323C	S72.364B	S72.435A
S22.002B	S22.079B	S24.151A	S32.059B	S32.413B	S32.474B	S32.9XXB	S48.012S	S68.029S	S72.002A	S72.052C	S72.126B	S72.324A	S72.364C	S72.435B
S22.008A	S22.080A	S24.151D	S32.10XA	S32.414A	S32.475A	S34.01XA	S48.019A	S68.110S	S72.002B	S72.059A	S72.126C	S72.324B	S72.365A	S72.435C
S22.008B	S22.080B	S24.151S	S32.10XB	S32.414B	S32.475B	S34.01XD	S48.019S	S68.111S	S72.002C	S72.059B	S72.131A	S72.324C	S72.365B	S72.436A
S22.009A	S22.081A	S24.152A	S32.110A	S32.415A	S32.476A	S34.01XS	S48.021A	S68.112S	S72.009A	S72.059C	S72.131B	S72.325A	S72.365C	S72.436B
S22.009B	S22.081B	S24.152D	S32.110B	S32.415B	S32.476B	S34.02XA	S48.021S	S68.113S	S72.009B	S72.061A	S72.131C	S72.325B	S72.366A	S72.436C
S22.010A	S22.082A	S24.152S	S32.111A	S32.416A	S32.481A	S34.02XD	S48.022A	S68.114S	S72.009C	S72.061B	S72.132A	S72.325C	S72.366B	S72.441A
S22.010B	S22.082B	S24.153A	S32.111B	S32.416B	S32.481B	S34.02XS	S48.022S	S68.115S	S72.011A	S72.061C	S72.132B	S72.326A	S72.366C	S72.441B
S22.011A	S22.088A	S24.153D	S32.112A	S32.421A	S32.482A	S34.101A	S48.029A	S68.116S	S72.011B	S72.062A	S72.132C	S72.326B	S72.391A	S72.441C
S22.011B	S22.088B	S24.153S	S32.112B	S32.421B	S32.482B	S34.101D	S48.029S	S68.117S	S72.011C	S72.062B	S72.133A	S72.326C	S72.391B	S72.442A
S22.012A	S22.089A	S24.154A	S32.119A	S32.422A	S32.483A	S34.101S	S48.111A	S68.118S	S72.012A	S72.062C	S72.133B	S72.331A	S72.391C	S72.442B
S22.012B	S22.089B	S24.154D	S32.119B	S32.422B	S32.483B	S34.102A	S48.111S	S68.119S	S72.012B	S72.063A	S72.133C	S72.331B	S72.392A	S72.442C
S22.018A	S24.0XXA	S24.154S	S32.120A	S32.423A	S32.484A	S34.102D	S48.112A	S68.120S	S72.012C	S72.063B	S72.134A	S72.331C	S72.392B	S72.443A
S22.018B	S24.0XXD	S24.159A	S32.120B	S32.423B	S32.484B	S34.102S	S48.112S	S68.121S	S72.019A	S72.063C	S72.134B	S72.332A	S72.392C	S72.443B
S22.019A	S24.0XXS	S24.159D	S32.121A	S32.424A	S32.485A	S34.103A	S48.119A	S68.122S	S72.019B	S72.064A	S72.134C	S72.332B	S72.399A	S72.443C
S22.019B	S24.101A	S24.159S	S32.121B	S32.424B	S32.485B	S34.103D	S48.119S	S68.123S	S72.019C	S72.064B	S72.135A	S72.332C	S72.399B	S72.444A
S22.020A	S24.101D	S32.000A	S32.122A	S32.425A	S32.486A	S34.103S	S48.121A	S68.124S	S72.021A	S72.064C	S72.135B	S72.333A	S72.399C	S72.444B
S22.020B	S24.101S	S32.000B	S32.122B	S32.425B	S32.486B	S34.104A	S48.121S	S68.125S	S72.021B	S72.065A	S72.135C	S72.333B	S72.401A	S72.444C
S22.021A	S24.102A	S32.001A	S32.129A	S32.426A	S32.491A	S34.104D	S48.122A	S68.126S	S72.021C	S72.065B	S72.136A	S72.333C	S72.401B	S72.445A
S22.021B	S24.102D	S32.001B	S32.129B	S32.426B	S32.491B	S34.104S	S48.122S	S68.127S	S72.022A	S72.065C	S72.136B	S72.334A	S72.401C	S72.445B
S22.022A	S24.102S	S32.002A	S32.130A	S32.431A	S32.492A	S34.105A	S48.129A	S68.128S	S72.022B	S72.066A	S72.136C	S72.334B	S72.402A	S72.445C
S22.022B	S24.103A	S32.002B	S32.130B	S32.431B	S32.492B	S34.105D	S48.129S	S68.129S	S72.022C	S72.066B	S72.141A	S72.334C	S72.402B	S72.446A
S22.028A	S24.103D	S32.008A	S32.131A	S32.432A	S32.499A	S34.105S	S48.911A	S68.411A	S72.023A	S72.066C	S72.141B	S72.335A	S72.402C	S72.446B
S22.028B	S24.103S	S32.008B	S32.131B	S32.432B	S32.499B	S34.109A	S48.911S	S68.411S	S72.023B	S72.091A	S72.141C	S72.335B	S72.409A	S72.446C
S22.029A	S24.104A	S32.009A	S32.132A	S32.433A	S32.501A	S34.109D	S48.912A	S68.412A	S72.023C	S72.091B	S72.142A	S72.335C	S72.409B	S72.451A
S22.029B	S24.104D	S32.009B	S32.132B	S32.433B	S32.501B	S34.109S	S48.912S	S68.412S	S72.024A	S72.091C	S72.142B	S72.336A	S72.409C	S72.451B
S22.030A	S24.104S	S32.010A	S32.139A	S32.434A	S32.502A	S34.111A	S48.919A	S68.419A	S72.024B	S72.092A	S72.142C	S72.336B	S72.411A	S72.451C
S22.030B	S24.109A	S32.010B	S32.139B	S32.434B	S32.502B	S34.111D	S48.919S	S68.419S	S72.024C	S72.092B	S72.143A	S72.336C	S72.411B	S72.452A
S22.031A	S24.109D	S32.011A	S32.14XA	S32.435A	S32.509A	S34.111S	S48.921A	S68.421A	S72.025A	S72.092C	S72.143B	S72.341A	S72.411C	S72.452B
S22.031B	S24.109S	S32.011B	S32.14XB	S32.435B	S32.509B	S34.112A	S48.921S	S68.421S	S72.025B	S72.099A	S72.143C	S72.341B	S72.412A	S72.452C
S22.032A	S24.111A	S32.012A	S32.15XA	S32.436A	S32.511A	S34.112D	S48.922A	S68.422A	S72.025C	S72.099B	S72.144A	S72.341C	S72.412B	S72.453A
S22.032B	S24.111D	S32.012B	S32.15XB	S32.436B	S32.511B	S34.112S	S48.922S	S68.422S	S72.026A	S72.099C	S72.144B	S72.342A	S72.412C	S72.453B
S22.038A	S24.111S	S32.018A	S32.16XA	S32.441A	S32.512A	S34.113A	S48.929A	S68.429A	S72.026B	S72.101A	S72.144C	S72.342B	S72.413A	S72.453C
S22.038B	S24.112A	S32.018B	S32.16XB	S32.441B	S32.512B	S34.113D	S48.929S	S68.429S	S72.026C	S72.101B	S72.145A	S72.342C	S72.413B	S72.454A

HCC (cont.) - Based on CMS data

S72.454B	S73.031A	S79.099A	S98.011D	S98.312A	T38.1X2A	T40.7X2A	T43.612S	T46.1X2A	T49.7X2A	T53.2X2A	T59.1X2A	T63.112A	T65.4X2A	T82.321A
S72.454C	S73.032A	S79.101A	S98.011S	S98.312D	T38.1X2S	T40.7X2S	T43.614A	T46.1X2S	T49.7X2S	T53.2X2S	T59.1X2S	T63.112S	T65.4X2S	T82.322A
S72.455A	S73.033A	S79.102A	S98.012A	S98.312S	T38.2X2A	T40.8X1A	T43.621A	T46.2X2A	T49.8X2A	T53.3X2A	T59.2X2A	T63.122A	T65.5X2A	T82.328A
S72.455B	S73.034A	S79.109A	S98.012D	S98.319A	T38.2X2S	T40.8X2A	T43.622A	T46.2X2S	T49.8X2S	T53.3X2S	T59.2X2S	T63.122S	T65.5X2S	T82.329A
S72.455C	S73.035A	S79.111A	S98.012S	S98.319D	T38.3X2A	T40.8X2S	T43.622S	T46.3X2A	T49.92XA	T53.4X2A	T59.3X2A	T63.192A	T65.6X2A	T82.330A
S72.456A	S73.036A	S79.112A	S98.019A	S98.319S	T38.3X2S	T40.8X4A	T43.624A	T46.3X2S	T49.92XS	T53.4X2S	T59.3X2S	T63.192S	T65.6X2S	T82.331A
S72.456B	S73.041A	S79.119A	S98.019D	S98.321A	T38.4X2A	T40.901A	T43.631A	T46.4X2A	T50.0X2A	T53.5X2A	T59.4X2A	T63.2X2A	T65.812A	T82.332A
S72.456C	S73.042A	S79.121A	S98.019S	S98.321D	T38.4X2S	T40.902A	T43.632A	T46.4X2S	T50.0X2S	T53.5X2S	T59.4X2S	T63.2X2S	T65.812S	T82.338A
S72.461A	S73.043A	S79.122A	S98.021A	S98.321S	T38.5X2A	T40.902S	T43.632S	T46.5X2A	T50.1X2A	T53.6X2A	T59.5X2A	T63.302A	T65.822A	T82.339A
S72.461B	S73.044A	S79.129A	S98.021D	S98.322A	T38.5X2S	T40.904A	T43.634A	T46.5X2S	T50.1X2S	T53.6X2S	T59.5X2S	T63.302S	T65.822S	T82.390A
S72.461C	S73.045A	S79.131A	S98.021S	S98.322D	T38.6X2A	T40.991A	T43.641A	T46.6X2A	T50.2X2A	T53.7X2A	T59.6X2A	T63.312A	T65.832A	T82.391A
S72.462A	S73.046A	S79.132A	S98.022A	S98.322S	T38.6X2S	T40.992A	T43.642A	T46.6X2S	T50.2X2S	T53.7X2S	T59.6X2S	T63.312S	T65.832S	T82.392A
S72.462B	S78.011A	S79.139A	S98.022D	S98.329A	T38.7X2A	T40.992S	T43.642S	T46.7X2A	T50.3X2A	T53.92XA	T59.7X2A	T63.322A	T65.892A	T82.398A
S72.462C	S78.011D	S79.141A	S98.022S	S98.329D	T38.7X2S	T40.994A	T43.644A	T46.7X2S	T50.3X2S	T53.92XS	T59.7X2S	T63.322S	T65.892S	T82.399A
S72.463A	S78.011S	S79.142A	S98.029A	S98.329S	T38.802A	T41.0X2A	T43.691A	T46.8X2A	T50.4X2A	T54.0X2A	T59.812A	T63.332A	T65.92XA	T82.41XA
S72.463B	S78.012A	S79.149A	S98.029D	S98.911A	T38.802S	T41.0X2S	T43.692A	T46.8X2S	T50.4X2S	T54.0X2S	T59.812S	T63.332S	T65.92XS	T82.41XD
S72.463C	S78.012D	S79.191A	S98.029S	S98.911D	T38.812A	T41.1X2A	T43.692S	T46.902A	T50.5X2A	T54.1X2A	T59.892A	T63.392A	T71.112A	T82.41XS
S72.464A	S78.012S	S79.192A	S98.111A	S98.911S	T38.812S	T41.1X2S	T43.694A	T46.902S	T50.5X2S	T54.1X2S	T59.892S	T63.392S	T71.112S	T82.42XA
S72.464B	S78.019A	S79.199A	S98.111D	S98.912A	T38.892A	T41.202A	T43.8X2A	T46.992A	T50.6X2A	T54.2X2A	T59.92XA	T63.412A	T71.122A	T82.42XD
S72.464C	S78.019D	S88.011A	S98.111S	S98.912D	T38.892S	T41.202S	T43.8X2S	T46.992S	T50.6X2S	T54.2X2S	T59.92XS	T63.412S	T71.122S	T82.42XS
S72.465A	S78.019S	S88.011D	S98.112A	S98.912S	T38.902A	T41.292A	T43.92XA	T47.0X2A	T50.7X2A	T54.3X2A	T60.0X2A	T63.422A	T71.132A	T82.43XA
S72.465B	S78.021A	S88.011S	S98.112D	S98.919A	T38.902S	T41.292S	T43.92XS	T47.0X2S	T50.7X2S	T54.3X2S	T60.0X2S	T63.422S	T71.132S	T82.43XD
S72.465C	S78.021D	S88.012A	S98.112S	S98.919D	T38.992A	T41.3X2A	T44.0X2A	T47.1X2A	T50.8X2A	T54.92XA	T60.1X2A	T63.432A	T71.152A	T82.43XS
S72.466A	S78.021S	S88.012D	S98.119A	S98.919S	T38.992S	T41.3X2S	T44.0X2S	T47.1X2S	T50.8X2S	T54.92XS	T60.1X2S	T63.432S	T71.152S	T82.49XA
S72.466B	S78.022A	S88.012S	S98.119D	S98.921A	T39.012A	T41.42XA	T44.1X2A	T47.2X2A	T50.902A	T55.0X2A	T60.2X2A	T63.442A	T71.162A	T82.49XD
S72.466C	S78.022D	S88.019A	S98.119S	S98.921D	T39.012S	T41.42XS	T44.1X2S	T47.2X2S	T50.902S	T55.0X2S	T60.2X2S	T63.442S	T71.162S	T82.49XS
S72.471A	S78.022S	S88.019D	S98.121A	S98.921S	T39.092A	T41.5X2A	T44.2X2A	T47.3X2A	T50.992A	T55.1X2A	T60.3X2A	T63.452A	T71.192A	T82.510A
S72.472A	S78.029A	S88.019S	S98.121D	S98.922A	T39.092S	T41.5X2S	T44.2X2S	T47.3X2S	T50.992S	T55.1X2S	T60.3X2S	T63.452S	T71.192S	T82.511A
S72.479A	S78.029D	S88.021A	S98.121S	S98.922D	T39.1X2A	T42.0X2A	T44.3X2A	T47.4X2A	T50.A12A	T56.0X2A	T60.4X2A	T63.462A	T71.222A	T82.513A
S72.491A	S78.029S	S88.021D	S98.122A	S98.922S	T39.1X2S	T42.0X2S	T44.3X2S	T47.4X2S	T50.A12S	T56.0X2S	T60.4X2S	T63.462S	T71.222S	T82.514A
S72.491B	S78.111A	S88.021S	S98.122D	S98.929A	T39.2X2A	T42.1X2A	T44.4X2A	T47.5X2A	T50.A22A	T56.1X2A	T60.8X2A	T63.482A	T71.232A	T82.515A
S72.491C	S78.111D	S88.022A	S98.122S	S98.929D	T39.2X2S	T42.1X2S	T44.4X2S	T47.5X2S	T50.A22S	T56.1X2S	T60.8X2S	T63.482S	T71.232S	T82.518A
S72.492A	S78.111S	S88.022D	S98.129A	S98.929S	T39.312A	T42.2X2A	T44.5X2A	T47.6X2A	T50.A92A	T56.2X2A	T60.92XA	T63.512A	T79.0XXA	T82.520A
S72.492B	S78.112A	S88.022S	S98.129D	T14.91XA	T39.312S	T42.2X2S	T44.5X2S	T47.6X2S	T50.A92S	T56.2X2S	T60.92XS	T63.512S	T79.1XXA	T82.521A
S72.492C	S78.112D	S88.029A	S98.129S	T14.91XD	T39.392A	T42.3X2A	T44.6X2A	T47.7X2A	T50.B12A	T56.3X2A	T61.02XA	T63.592A	T79.2XXA	T82.523A
S72.499A	S78.112S	S88.029D	S98.131A	T14.91XS	T39.392S	T42.3X2S	T44.6X2S	T47.7X2S	T50.B12S	T56.3X2S	T61.02XS	T63.592S	T79.4XXA	T82.524A
S72.499B	S78.119A	S88.029S	S98.131D	T36.0X2A	T39.4X2A	T42.4X2A	T44.7X2A	T47.8X2A	T50.B92A	T56.4X2A	T61.12XA	T63.612A	T79.5XXA	T82.525A
S72.499C	S78.119D	S88.111A	S98.131S	T36.0X2S	T39.4X2S	T42.4X2S	T44.7X2S	T47.8X2S	T50.B92S	T56.4X2S	T61.12XS	T63.612S	T79.6XXA	T82.528A
S72.8X1A	S78.119S	S88.111D	S98.132A	T36.1X2A	T39.8X2A	T42.5X2A	T44.8X2A	T47.92XA	T50.Z12A	T56.5X2A	T61.772A	T63.622A	T79.7XXA	T82.530A
S72.8X1B	S78.121A	S88.111S	S98.132D	T36.1X2S	T39.8X2S	T42.5X2S	T44.8X2S	T47.92XS	T50.Z12S	T56.5X2S	T61.772S	T63.622S	T79.8XXA	T82.531A
S72.8X1C	S78.121D	S88.112A	S98.132S	T36.2X2A	T39.92XA	T42.6X2A	T44.902A	T48.0X2A	T50.Z92A	T56.6X2A	T61.782A	T63.632A	T79.9XXA	T82.533A
S72.8X2A	S78.121S	S88.112D	S98.139A	T36.2X2S	T39.92XS	T42.6X2S	T44.902S	T48.0X2S	T50.Z92S	T56.6X2S	T61.782S	T63.632S	T79.A0XA	T82.534A
S72.8X2B	S78.122A	S88.112S	S98.139D	T36.3X2A	T40.0X1A	T42.72XA	T44.992A	T48.1X2A	T51.0X1A	T56.7X2A	T61.8X2A	T63.692A	T79.A11A	T82.535A
S72.8X2C	S78.122D	S88.119A	S98.139S	T36.3X2S	T40.0X2A	T42.72XS	T44.992S	T48.1X2S	T51.0X2A	T56.7X2S	T61.8X2S	T63.692S	T79.A12A	T82.538A
S72.8X9A	S78.122S	S88.119D	S98.141A	T36.4X2A	T40.0X2S	T42.8X2A	T45.0X2A	T48.202A	T51.0X2S	T56.812A	T61.92XA	T63.712A	T79.A19A	T82.590A
S72.8X9B	S78.129A	S88.119S	S98.141D	T36.4X2S	T40.0X4A	T42.8X2S	T45.0X2S	T48.202S	T51.0X4A	T56.812S	T61.92XS	T63.712S	T79.A21A	T82.591A
S72.8X9C	S78.129D	S88.121A	S98.141S	T36.5X2A	T40.1X1A	T43.012A	T45.1X2A	T48.292A	T51.1X2A	T56.892A	T62.0X2A	T63.792A	T79.A22A	T82.593A
S72.90XA	S78.129S	S88.121D	S98.142A	T36.5X2S	T40.1X2A	T43.012S	T45.1X2S	T48.292S	T51.1X2S	T56.892S	T62.0X2S	T63.792S	T79.A29A	T82.594A
S72.90XB	S78.911A	S88.121S	S98.142D	T36.6X2A	T40.1X2S	T43.022A	T45.2X2A	T48.3X2A	T51.2X2A	T56.92XA	T62.1X2A	T63.812A	T79.A3XA	T82.595A
S72.90XC	S78.911D	S88.122A	S98.142S	T36.6X2S	T40.1X4A	T43.022S	T45.2X2S	T48.3X2S	T51.2X2S	T56.92XS	T62.1X2S	T63.812S	T79.A9XA	T82.598A
S72.91XA	S78.911S	S88.122D	S98.149A	T36.7X2A	T40.2X1A	T43.1X2A	T45.3X2A	T48.4X2A	T51.3X2A	T57.0X2A	T62.2X2A	T63.822A	T81.11XA	T82.6XXA
S72.91XB	S78.912A	S88.122S	S98.149D	T36.7X2S	T40.2X2A	T43.1X2S	T45.3X2S	T48.4X2S	T51.3X2S	T57.0X2S	T62.2X2S	T63.822S	T81.12XA	T82.7XXA
S72.91XC	S78.912D	S88.129A	S98.149S	T36.8X2A	T40.2X2S	T43.202A	T45.4X2A	T48.5X2A	T51.8X2A	T57.1X2A	T62.8X2A	T63.832A	T81.44XA	T82.818A
S72.92XA	S78.912S	S88.129D	S98.211A	T36.8X2S	T40.2X4A	T43.202S	T45.4X2S	T48.5X2S	T51.8X2S	T57.1X2S	T62.8X2S	T63.832S	T81.502A	T82.828A
S72.92XB	S78.919A	S88.129S	S98.211D	T36.92XA	T40.3X1A	T43.212A	T45.512A	T48.6X2A	T51.92XA	T57.2X2A	T62.92XA	T63.892A	T81.502D	T82.838A
S72.92XC	S78.919D	S88.911A	S98.211S	T36.92XS	T40.3X2A	T43.212S	T45.512S	T48.6X2S	T51.92XS	T57.2X2S	T62.92XS	T63.892S	T81.502S	T82.848A
S73.001A	S78.919S	S88.911D	S98.212A	T37.0X2A	T40.3X2S	T43.222A	T45.522A	T48.902A	T52.0X2A	T57.3X2A	T63.002A	T63.92XA	T81.512A	T82.856A
S73.002A	S78.921A	S88.911S	S98.212D	T37.0X2S	T40.3X4A	T43.222S	T45.522S	T48.902S	T52.0X2S	T57.3X2S	T63.002S	T63.92XS	T81.512D	T82.858A
S73.003A	S78.921D	S88.912A	S98.212S	T37.1X2A	T40.4X1A	T43.292A	T45.602A	T48.992A	T52.1X2A	T57.8X2A	T63.012A	T64.02XA	T81.512S	T82.868A
S73.004A	S78.921S	S88.912D	S98.219A	T37.1X2S	T40.4X2A	T43.292S	T45.602S	T48.992S	T52.1X2S	T57.8X2S	T63.012S	T64.02XS	T81.522A	T82.898A
S73.005A	S78.922A	S88.912S	S98.219D	T37.2X2A	T40.4X2S	T43.3X2A	T45.612A	T49.0X2A	T52.2X2A	T57.92XA	T63.022A	T64.82XA	T81.522D	T83.010A
S73.006A	S78.922D	S88.919A	S98.219S	T37.2X2S	T40.4X4A	T43.3X2S	T45.612S	T49.0X2S	T52.2X2S	T57.92XS	T63.022S	T64.82XS	T81.522S	T83.011A
S73.011A	S78.922S	S88.919D	S98.221A	T37.3X2A	T40.5X1A	T43.4X2A	T45.622A	T49.1X2A	T52.3X2A	T58.02XA	T63.032A	T65.0X2A	T81.532A	T83.012A
S73.012A	S78.929A	S88.919S	S98.221D	T37.3X2S	T40.5X2A	T43.4X2S	T45.622S	T49.1X2S	T52.3X2S	T58.02XS	T63.032S	T65.0X2S	T81.532D	T83.018A
S73.013A	S78.929D	S88.921A	S98.221S	T37.4X2A	T40.5X2S	T43.502A	T45.692A	T49.2X2A	T52.4X2A	T58.12XA	T63.042A	T65.1X2A	T81.532S	T83.020A
S73.014A	S78.929S	S88.921D	S98.222A	T37.4X2S	T40.5X4A	T43.502S	T45.692S	T49.2X2S	T52.4X2S	T58.12XS	T63.042S	T65.1X2S	T81.592A	T83.021A
S73.015A	S79.001A	S88.921S	S98.222D	T37.5X2A	T40.601A	T43.592A	T45.7X2A	T49.3X2A	T52.8X2A	T58.2X2A	T63.062A	T65.212A	T81.592D	T83.022A
S73.016A	S79.002A	S88.922A	S98.222S	T37.5X2S	T40.602A	T43.592S	T45.7X2S	T49.3X2S	T52.8X2S	T58.2X2S	T63.062S	T65.212S	T81.592S	T83.028A
S73.021A	S79.009A	S88.922D	S98.229A	T37.8X2A	T40.602S	T43.601A	T45.8X2A	T49.4X2A	T52.92XA	T58.8X2A	T63.072A	T65.222A	T82.310A	T83.030A
S73.022A	S79.011A	S88.922S	S98.229D	T37.8X2S	T40.604A	T43.602A	T45.8X2S	T49.4X2S	T52.92XS	T58.8X2S	T63.072S	T65.222S	T82.311A	T83.031A
S73.023A	S79.012A	S88.929A	S98.229S	T37.92XA	T40.691A	T43.602S	T45.92XA	T49.5X2A	T53.0X2A	T58.92XA	T63.082A	T65.292A	T82.312A	T83.032A
S73.024A	S79.019A	S88.929D	S98.311A	T37.92XS	T40.692A	T43.604A	T45.92XS	T49.5X2S	T53.0X2S	T58.92XS	T63.082S	T65.292S	T82.318A	T83.038A
S73.025A	S79.091A	S88.929S	S98.311D	T38.0X2A	T40.692S	T43.611A	T46.0X2A	T49.6X2A	T53.1X2A	T59.0X2A	T63.092A	T65.3X2A	T82.319A	T83.090A
S73.026A	S79.092A	S98.011A	S98.311S	T38.0X2S	T40.694A	T43.612A	T46.0X2S	T49.6X2S	T53.1X2S	T59.0X2S	T63.092S	T65.3X2S	T82.320A	T83.091A

HCC (cont.) - Based on CMS data

T83.092A	T83.418A	T83.721A	T84.028A	T84.099A	T84.196A	T84.490A	T84.7XXA	T85.192A	T85.732A	X71.8XXA	X74.01XD	X77.1XXS	X78.9XXA	X82.2XXD
T83.098A	T83.420A	T83.722A	T84.029A	T84.110A	T84.197A	T84.498A	T84.81XA	T85.197A	T85.733A	X71.8XXD	X74.01XS	X77.2XXA	X78.9XXD	X82.2XXS
T83.110A	T83.421A	T83.723A	T84.030A	T84.111A	T84.199A	T84.50XA	T84.82XA	T85.199A	T85.734A	X71.8XXS	X74.02XA	X77.2XXD	X78.9XXS	X82.8XXA
T83.111A	T83.428A	T83.724A	T84.031A	T84.112A	T84.210A	T84.51XA	T84.83XA	T85.611A	T85.735A	X71.9XXA	X74.02XD	X77.2XXS	X79.XXXA	X82.8XXD
T83.112A	T83.490A	T83.728A	T84.032A	T84.113A	T84.213A	T84.52XA	T84.84XA	T85.611D	T85.738A	X71.9XXD	X74.02XS	X77.3XXA	X79.XXXD	X82.8XXS
T83.113A	T83.491A	T83.729A	T84.033A	T84.114A	T84.216A	T84.53XA	T84.85XA	T85.611S	T85.79XA	X71.9XXS	X74.09XA	X77.3XXD	X79.XXXS	X83.0XXA
T83.118A	T83.498A	T83.79XA	T84.038A	T84.115A	T84.218A	T84.54XA	T84.86XA	T85.615A	T85.810A	X72.XXXA	X74.09XD	X77.3XXS	X80.XXXA	X83.0XXD
T83.120A	T83.510A	T83.81XA	T84.039A	T84.116A	T84.220A	T84.59XA	T84.89XA	T85.621A	T85.820A	X72.XXXD	X74.09XS	X77.8XXA	X80.XXXD	X83.0XXS
T83.121A	T83.511A	T83.82XA	T84.050A	T84.117A	T84.223A	T84.60XA	T84.9XXA	T85.621D	T85.830A	X72.XXXS	X74.8XXA	X77.8XXD	X80.XXXS	X83.1XXA
T83.122A	T83.512A	T83.83XA	T84.051A	T84.119A	T84.226A	T84.610A	T85.01XA	T85.621S	T85.840A	X73.0XXA	X74.8XXD	X77.8XXS	X81.0XXA	X83.1XXD
T83.123A	T83.518A	T83.84XA	T84.052A	T84.120A	T84.228A	T84.611A	T85.02XA	T85.625A	T85.850A	X73.0XXD	X74.8XXS	X77.9XXA	X81.0XXD	X83.1XXS
T83.128A	T83.590A	T83.85XA	T84.053A	T84.121A	T84.290A	T84.612A	T85.03XA	T85.631A	T85.860A	X73.0XXS	X74.9XXA	X77.9XXD	X81.0XXS	X83.2XXA
T83.190A	T83.591A	T83.86XA	T84.058A	T84.122A	T84.293A	T84.613A	T85.09XA	T85.631D	T85.890A	X73.1XXA	X74.9XXD	X77.9XXS	X81.1XXA	X83.2XXD
T83.191A	T83.592A	T83.89XA	T84.059A	T84.123A	T84.296A	T84.614A	T85.110A	T85.631S	X71.0XXA	X73.1XXD	X74.9XXS	X78.0XXA	X81.1XXD	X83.2XXS
T83.192A	T83.593A	T83.9XXA	T84.060A	T84.124A	T84.298A	T84.615A	T85.111A	T85.635A	X71.0XXD	X73.1XXS	X75.XXXA	X78.0XXD	X81.1XXS	X83.8XXA
T83.193A	T83.598A	T84.010A	T84.061A	T84.125A	T84.310A	T84.619A	T85.112A	T85.691A	X71.0XXS	X73.2XXA	X75.XXXD	X78.0XXS	X81.8XXA	X83.8XXD
T83.198A	T83.61XA	T84.011A	T84.062A	T84.126A	T84.318A	T84.620A	T85.113A	T85.691D	X71.1XXA	X73.2XXD	X75.XXXS	X78.1XXA	X81.8XXD	X83.8XXS
T83.21XA	T83.62XA	T84.012A	T84.063A	T84.127A	T84.320A	T84.621A	T85.118A	T85.691S	X71.1XXD	X73.2XXS	X76.XXXA	X78.1XXD	X81.8XXS	
T83.22XA	T83.69XA	T84.013A	T84.068A	T84.129A	T84.328A	T84.622A	T85.120A	T85.695A	X71.1XXS	X73.8XXA	X76.XXXD	X78.1XXS	X82.0XXA	
T83.23XA	T83.711A	T84.018A	T84.069A	T84.190A	T84.390A	T84.623A	T85.121A	T85.71XA	X71.2XXA	X73.8XXD	X76.XXXS	X78.2XXA	X82.0XXD	
T83.24XA	T83.712A	T84.019A	T84.090A	T84.191A	T84.398A	T84.624A	T85.122A	T85.71XD	X71.2XXD	X73.8XXS	X77.0XXA	X78.2XXD	X82.0XXS	
T83.25XA	T83.713A	T84.020A	T84.091A	T84.192A	T84.410A	T84.625A	T85.123A	T85.71XS	X71.2XXS	X73.9XXA	X77.0XXD	X78.2XXS	X82.1XXA	
T83.29XA	T83.714A	T84.021A	T84.092A	T84.193A	T84.418A	T84.629A	T85.128A	T85.72XA	X71.3XXA	X73.9XXD	X77.0XXS	X78.8XXA	X82.1XXD	
T83.410A	T83.718A	T84.022A	T84.093A	T84.194A	T84.420A	T84.63XA	T85.190A	T85.730A	X71.3XXD	X73.9XXS	X77.1XXA	X78.8XXD	X82.1XXS	
T83.411A	T83.719A	T84.023A	T84.098A	T84.195A	T84.428A	T84.69XA	T85.191A	T85.731A	X71.3XXS	X74.01XA	X77.1XXD	X78.8XXS	X82.2XXA	

MACRA - Based on CMS data

C44.1021	E08.3551	E09.37X2	E10.3591	E11.3543	E13.3531	H35.3123	H40.1222	H40.2213	H40.51X4	H54.1225	M80.029A	M80.051P	M80.079G	M80.829A
C44.1022	E08.3552	E09.37X3	E10.3592	E11.3549	E13.3532	H35.3124	H40.1223	H40.2214	H40.52X0	M48.40XA	M80.029D	M80.051S	M80.079K	M80.829D
C44.1091	E08.3553	E10.3211	E10.3593	E11.3551	E13.3533	H35.3130	H40.1224	H40.2220	H40.52X1	M48.41XA	M80.029G	M80.052A	M80.079P	M80.829G
C44.1092	E08.3591	E10.3212	E10.3599	E11.3552	E13.3539	H35.3131	H40.1230	H40.2221	H40.52X2	M48.42XA	M80.029K	M80.052D	M80.079S	M80.829K
C44.1121	E08.3592	E10.3213	E10.37X1	E11.3553	E13.3541	H35.3132	H40.1231	H40.2222	H40.52X3	M48.43XA	M80.029P	M80.052G	M80.08XA	M80.829P
C44.1122	E08.3593	E10.3219	E10.37X2	E11.3559	E13.3542	H35.3133	H40.1232	H40.2223	H40.52X4	M48.44XA	M80.029S	M80.052K	M80.08XD	M80.829S
C44.1191	E08.37X1	E10.3291	E10.37X3	E11.3591	E13.3543	H35.3134	H40.1233	H40.2224	H40.53X0	M48.45XA	M80.031A	M80.052P	M80.08XG	M80.831A
C44.1192	E08.37X2	E10.3292	E10.37X9	E11.3592	E13.3549	H35.3210	H40.1234	H40.2230	H40.53X1	M48.46XA	M80.031D	M80.052S	M80.08XK	M80.831D
C44.1221	E08.37X3	E10.3293	E11.3211	E11.3593	E13.3551	H35.3211	H40.1310	H40.2231	H40.53X2	M48.47XA	M80.031G	M80.059A	M80.08XP	M80.831G
C44.1222	E09.3211	E10.3299	E11.3212	E11.3599	E13.3552	H35.3212	H40.1311	H40.2232	H40.53X3	M48.48XA	M80.031K	M80.059D	M80.08XS	M80.831K
C44.1291	E09.3212	E10.3311	E11.3213	E11.37X1	E13.3553	H35.3213	H40.1312	H40.2233	H40.53X4	M80.00XA	M80.031P	M80.059G	M80.80XA	M80.831P
C44.1292	E09.3213	E10.3312	E11.3219	E11.37X2	E13.3559	H35.3220	H40.1313	H40.2234	H40.61X0	M80.00XD	M80.031S	M80.059K	M80.80XD	M80.831S
C44.1921	E09.3291	E10.3313	E11.3291	E11.37X3	E13.3591	H35.3221	H40.1314	H40.31X0	H40.61X1	M80.00XG	M80.032A	M80.059P	M80.80XG	M80.832A
C44.1922	E09.3292	E10.3319	E11.3292	E11.37X9	E13.3592	H35.3222	H40.1320	H40.31X1	H40.61X2	M80.00XK	M80.032D	M80.059S	M80.80XK	M80.832D
C44.1991	E09.3293	E10.3391	E11.3293	E13.3211	E13.3593	H35.3223	H40.1321	H40.31X2	H40.61X3	M80.00XP	M80.032G	M80.061A	M80.80XP	M80.832G
C44.1992	E09.3311	E10.3392	E11.3299	E13.3212	E13.3599	H35.3230	H40.1322	H40.31X3	H40.61X4	M80.00XS	M80.032K	M80.061D	M80.80XS	M80.832K
E08.3211	E09.3312	E10.3393	E11.3311	E13.3213	E13.37X1	H35.3231	H40.1323	H40.31X4	H40.62X0	M80.011A	M80.032P	M80.061G	M80.811A	M80.832P
E08.3212	E09.3313	E10.3399	E11.3312	E13.3219	E13.37X2	H35.3232	H40.1324	H40.32X0	H40.62X1	M80.011D	M80.032S	M80.061K	M80.811D	M80.832S
E08.3213	E09.3391	E10.3411	E11.3313	E13.3291	E13.37X3	H35.3233	H40.1330	H40.32X1	H40.62X2	M80.011G	M80.039A	M80.061P	M80.811G	M80.839A
E08.3291	E09.3392	E10.3412	E11.3319	E13.3292	E13.37X9	H40.10X0	H40.1331	H40.32X2	H40.62X3	M80.011K	M80.039D	M80.061S	M80.811K	M80.839D
E08.3292	E09.3393	E10.3413	E11.3391	E13.3293	H34.8110	H40.10X1	H40.1332	H40.32X3	H40.62X4	M80.011P	M80.039G	M80.062A	M80.811P	M80.839G
E08.3293	E09.3411	E10.3419	E11.3392	E13.3299	H34.8111	H40.10X2	H40.1333	H40.32X4	H40.63X0	M80.011S	M80.039K	M80.062D	M80.811S	M80.839K
E08.3311	E09.3412	E10.3491	E11.3393	E13.3311	H34.8112	H40.10X3	H40.1334	H40.33X0	H40.63X1	M80.012A	M80.039P	M80.062G	M80.812A	M80.839P
E08.3312	E09.3413	E10.3492	E11.3399	E13.3312	H34.8120	H40.10X4	H40.1410	H40.33X1	H40.63X2	M80.012D	M80.039S	M80.062K	M80.812D	M80.839S
E08.3313	E09.3491	E10.3493	E11.3411	E13.3313	H34.8121	H40.1110	H40.1411	H40.33X2	H40.63X3	M80.012G	M80.041A	M80.062P	M80.812G	M80.841A
E08.3391	E09.3492	E10.3499	E11.3412	E13.3319	H34.8122	H40.1111	H40.1412	H40.33X3	H40.63X4	M80.012K	M80.041D	M80.062S	M80.812K	M80.841D
E08.3392	E09.3493	E10.3511	E11.3413	E13.3391	H34.8130	H40.1112	H40.1413	H40.33X4	H54.0X33	M80.012P	M80.041G	M80.069A	M80.812P	M80.841G
E08.3393	E09.3511	E10.3512	E11.3419	E13.3392	H34.8131	H40.1113	H40.1414	H40.41X0	H54.0X34	M80.012S	M80.041K	M80.069D	M80.812S	M80.841K
E08.3411	E09.3512	E10.3513	E11.3491	E13.3393	H34.8132	H40.1114	H40.1420	H40.41X1	H54.0X35	M80.019A	M80.041P	M80.069G	M80.819A	M80.841P
E08.3412	E09.3513	E10.3519	E11.3492	E13.3399	H34.8310	H40.1120	H40.1421	H40.41X2	H54.0X43	M80.019D	M80.041S	M80.069K	M80.819D	M80.841S
E08.3413	E09.3521	E10.3521	E11.3493	E13.3411	H34.8311	H40.1121	H40.1422	H40.41X3	H54.0X44	M80.019G	M80.042A	M80.069P	M80.819G	M80.842A
E08.3491	E09.3522	E10.3522	E11.3499	E13.3412	H34.8312	H40.1122	H40.1423	H40.41X4	H54.0X45	M80.019K	M80.042D	M80.069S	M80.819K	M80.842D
E08.3492	E09.3523	E10.3523	E11.3511	E13.3413	H34.8320	H40.1123	H40.1424	H40.42X0	H54.0X53	M80.019P	M80.042G	M80.071A	M80.819P	M80.842G
E08.3493	E09.3531	E10.3529	E11.3512	E13.3419	H34.8321	H40.1124	H40.1430	H40.42X1	H54.0X54	M80.019S	M80.042K	M80.071D	M80.819S	M80.842K
E08.3511	E09.3532	E10.3531	E11.3513	E13.3491	H34.8322	H40.1130	H40.1431	H40.42X2	H54.0X55	M80.021A	M80.042P	M80.071G	M80.821A	M80.842P
E08.3512	E09.3533	E10.3532	E11.3519	E13.3492	H34.8330	H40.1131	H40.1432	H40.42X3	H54.1131	M80.021D	M80.042S	M80.071K	M80.821D	M80.842S
E08.3513	E09.3541	E10.3533	E11.3521	E13.3493	H34.8331	H40.1132	H40.1433	H40.42X4	H54.1132	M80.021G	M80.049A	M80.071P	M80.821G	M80.849A
E08.3521	E09.3542	E10.3539	E11.3522	E13.3499	H34.8332	H40.1133	H40.1434	H40.43X0	H54.1141	M80.021K	M80.049D	M80.071S	M80.821K	M80.849D
E08.3522	E09.3543	E10.3541	E11.3523	E13.3511	H35.3110	H40.1134	H40.20X0	H40.43X1	H54.1142	M80.021P	M80.049G	M80.072A	M80.821P	M80.849G
E08.3523	E09.3551	E10.3542	E11.3529	E13.3512	H35.3111	H40.1210	H40.20X1	H40.43X2	H54.1151	M80.021S	M80.049K	M80.072D	M80.821S	M80.849K
E08.3531	E09.3552	E10.3543	E11.3531	E13.3513	H35.3112	H40.1211	H40.20X2	H40.43X3	H54.1152	M80.022A	M80.049P	M80.072G	M80.822A	M80.849P
E08.3532	E09.3553	E10.3549	E11.3532	E13.3519	H35.3113	H40.1212	H40.20X3	H40.43X4	H54.1213	M80.022D	M80.049S	M80.072K	M80.822D	M80.849S
E08.3533	E09.3591	E10.3551	E11.3533	E13.3521	H35.3114	H40.1213	H40.20X4	H40.51X0	H54.1214	M80.022G	M80.051A	M80.072P	M80.822G	M80.851A
E08.3541	E09.3592	E10.3552	E11.3539	E13.3522	H35.3120	H40.1214	H40.2210	H40.51X1	H54.1215	M80.022K	M80.051D	M80.072S	M80.822K	M80.851D
E08.3542	E09.3593	E10.3553	E11.3541	E13.3523	H35.3121	H40.1220	H40.2211	H40.51X2	H54.1223	M80.022P	M80.051G	M80.079A	M80.822P	M80.851G
E08.3543	E09.37X1	E10.3559	E11.3542	E13.3529	H35.3122	H40.1221	H40.2212	H40.51X3	H54.1224	M80.022S	M80.051K	M80.079D	M80.822S	M80.851K

MACRA (cont.) - Based on CMS data

M80.851P	M84.359A	S02.402A	S06.2X2A	S09.90XA	S12.301A	S22.001A	S22.078A	S32.031A	S32.312A	S32.453A	S32.611A	S42.036A	S42.201A	S42.293B
M80.851S	M84.361A	S02.40AA	S06.2X3A	S09.92XA	S12.301B	S22.001B	S22.078B	S32.031B	S32.312B	S32.453B	S32.611B	S42.036B	S42.201B	S42.294A
M80.852A	M84.362A	S02.40BA	S06.2X4A	S09.93XA	S12.330A	S22.002A	S22.079A	S32.032A	S32.313A	S32.454A	S32.612A	S42.101A	S42.202A	S42.294B
M80.852D	M84.363A	S02.40CA	S06.2X9A	S10.0XXA	S12.330B	S22.002B	S22.079B	S32.032B	S32.313B	S32.454B	S32.612B	S42.101B	S42.202B	S42.295A
M80.852G	M84.364A	S02.40DA	S06.300A	S10.83XA	S12.331A	S22.008A	S22.080A	S32.038A	S32.314A	S32.455A	S32.613A	S42.102A	S42.209A	S42.295B
M80.852K	M84.369A	S02.40EA	S06.301A	S10.93XA	S12.331B	S22.008B	S22.080B	S32.038B	S32.314B	S32.455B	S32.613B	S42.102B	S42.209B	S42.296A
M80.852P	M84.371A	S02.40FA	S06.302A	S12.000A	S12.34XA	S22.009A	S22.081A	S32.039A	S32.315A	S32.456A	S32.614A	S42.109A	S42.211A	S42.296B
M80.852S	M84.372A	S02.411A	S06.303A	S12.000B	S12.34XB	S22.009B	S22.081B	S32.039B	S32.315B	S32.456B	S32.614B	S42.109B	S42.211B	S42.301A
M80.859A	M84.373A	S02.412A	S06.304A	S12.001A	S12.350A	S22.010A	S22.082A	S32.040A	S32.316A	S32.461A	S32.615A	S42.111A	S42.212A	S42.301B
M80.859D	M84.374A	S02.413A	S06.309A	S12.001B	S12.350B	S22.010B	S22.082B	S32.040B	S32.316B	S32.461B	S32.615B	S42.111B	S42.212B	S42.302A
M80.859G	M84.375A	S02.42XA	S06.340A	S12.01XA	S12.351A	S22.011A	S22.088A	S32.041A	S32.391A	S32.462A	S32.616A	S42.112A	S42.213A	S42.302B
M80.859K	M84.376A	S02.600A	S06.341A	S12.01XB	S12.351B	S22.011B	S22.088B	S32.041B	S32.391B	S32.462B	S32.616B	S42.112B	S42.213B	S42.309A
M80.859P	M84.38XA	S02.601A	S06.342A	S12.02XA	S12.390A	S22.012A	S22.089A	S32.042A	S32.392A	S32.463A	S32.691A	S42.113A	S42.214A	S42.309B
M80.859S	M84.750A	S02.602A	S06.343A	S12.02XB	S12.390B	S22.012B	S22.089B	S32.042B	S32.392B	S32.463B	S32.691B	S42.113B	S42.214B	S42.311A
M80.861A	M84.751A	S02.609A	S06.344A	S12.030A	S12.391A	S22.018A	S22.20XA	S32.048A	S32.399A	S32.464A	S32.692A	S42.114A	S42.215A	S42.312A
M80.861D	M84.752A	S02.610A	S06.349A	S12.030B	S12.391B	S22.018B	S22.20XB	S32.048B	S32.399B	S32.464B	S32.692B	S42.114B	S42.215B	S42.319A
M80.861G	M84.753A	S02.611A	S06.350A	S12.031A	S12.400A	S22.019A	S22.21XA	S32.049A	S32.401A	S32.465A	S32.699A	S42.115A	S42.216A	S42.321A
M80.861K	M84.754A	S02.612A	S06.351A	S12.031B	S12.400B	S22.019B	S22.21XB	S32.049B	S32.401B	S32.465B	S32.699B	S42.115B	S42.216B	S42.321B
M80.861P	M84.755A	S02.620A	S06.352A	S12.040A	S12.401A	S22.020A	S22.22XA	S32.050A	S32.402A	S32.466A	S32.810A	S42.116A	S42.221A	S42.322A
M80.861S	M84.756A	S02.621A	S06.353A	S12.040B	S12.401B	S22.020B	S22.22XB	S32.050B	S32.402B	S32.466B	S32.810B	S42.116B	S42.221B	S42.322B
M80.862A	M84.757A	S02.622A	S06.354A	S12.041A	S12.430A	S22.021A	S22.23XA	S32.051A	S32.409A	S32.471A	S32.811A	S42.121A	S42.222A	S42.323A
M80.862D	M84.759A	S02.630A	S06.359A	S12.041B	S12.430B	S22.021B	S22.23XB	S32.051B	S32.409B	S32.471B	S32.811B	S42.121B	S42.222B	S42.323B
M80.862G	M97.01XA	S02.631A	S06.360A	S12.090A	S12.431A	S22.022A	S22.24XA	S32.052A	S32.411A	S32.472A	S32.82XA	S42.122A	S42.223A	S42.324A
M80.862K	M97.02XA	S02.632A	S06.361A	S12.090B	S12.431B	S22.022B	S22.24XB	S32.052B	S32.411B	S32.472B	S32.82XB	S42.122B	S42.223B	S42.324B
M80.862P	M97.11XA	S02.640A	S06.362A	S12.091A	S12.44XA	S22.028A	S22.31XA	S32.058A	S32.412A	S32.473A	S32.89XA	S42.123A	S42.224A	S42.325A
M80.862S	M97.12XA	S02.641A	S06.363A	S12.091B	S12.44XB	S22.028B	S22.31XB	S32.058B	S32.412B	S32.473B	S32.89XB	S42.123B	S42.224B	S42.325B
M80.869A	M97.21XA	S02.642A	S06.364A	S12.100A	S12.450A	S22.029A	S22.32XA	S32.059A	S32.413A	S32.474A	S32.9XXA	S42.124A	S42.225A	S42.326A
M80.869D	M97.22XA	S02.650A	S06.369A	S12.100B	S12.450B	S22.029B	S22.32XB	S32.059B	S32.413B	S32.474B	S32.9XXB	S42.124B	S42.225B	S42.326B
M80.869G	M97.31XA	S02.651A	S06.4X0A	S12.101A	S12.451A	S22.030A	S22.39XA	S32.10XA	S32.414A	S32.475A	S42.001A	S42.125A	S42.226A	S42.331A
M80.869K	M97.32XA	S02.652A	S06.4X1A	S12.101B	S12.451B	S22.030B	S22.39XB	S32.10XB	S32.414B	S32.475B	S42.001B	S42.125B	S42.226B	S42.331B
M80.869P	M97.41XA	S02.66XA	S06.4X2A	S12.110A	S12.490A	S22.031A	S22.41XA	S32.110A	S32.415A	S32.476A	S42.002A	S42.126A	S42.231A	S42.332A
M80.869S	M97.42XA	S02.670A	S06.4X3A	S12.110B	S12.490B	S22.031B	S22.41XB	S32.110B	S32.415B	S32.476B	S42.002B	S42.126B	S42.231B	S42.332B
M80.871A	O36.0110	S02.671A	S06.4X4A	S12.111A	S12.491A	S22.032A	S22.42XA	S32.111A	S32.416A	S32.481A	S42.009A	S42.131A	S42.232A	S42.333A
M80.871D	O36.0111	S02.672A	S06.4X9A	S12.111B	S12.491B	S22.032B	S22.42XB	S32.111B	S32.416B	S32.481B	S42.009B	S42.131B	S42.232B	S42.333B
M80.871G	O36.0190	S02.69XA	S06.5X0A	S12.112A	S12.500A	S22.038A	S22.43XA	S32.112A	S32.421A	S32.482A	S42.011A	S42.132A	S42.239A	S42.334A
M80.871K	O36.0191	S02.80XA	S06.5X1A	S12.112B	S12.500B	S22.038B	S22.43XB	S32.112B	S32.421B	S32.482B	S42.011B	S42.132B	S42.239B	S42.334B
M80.871P	O36.0910	S02.81XA	S06.5X2A	S12.120A	S12.501A	S22.039A	S22.49XA	S32.119A	S32.422A	S32.483A	S42.012A	S42.133A	S42.241A	S42.335A
M80.871S	O36.0911	S02.82XA	S06.5X3A	S12.120B	S12.501B	S22.039B	S22.49XB	S32.119B	S32.422B	S32.483B	S42.012B	S42.133B	S42.241B	S42.335B
M80.872A	O36.0990	S02.91XA	S06.5X4A	S12.121A	S12.530A	S22.040A	S22.5XXA	S32.120A	S32.423A	S32.484A	S42.013A	S42.134A	S42.242A	S42.336A
M80.872D	O36.0991	S02.92XA	S06.5X9A	S12.121B	S12.530B	S22.040B	S22.5XXB	S32.120B	S32.423B	S32.484B	S42.013B	S42.134B	S42.242B	S42.336B
M80.872G	S00.03XA	S04.011A	S06.6X0A	S12.130A	S12.531A	S22.041A	S22.9XXA	S32.121A	S32.424A	S32.485A	S42.014A	S42.135A	S42.249A	S42.341A
M80.872K	S00.33XA	S04.012A	S06.6X1A	S12.130B	S12.531B	S22.041B	S22.9XXB	S32.121B	S32.424B	S32.485B	S42.014B	S42.135B	S42.249B	S42.341B
M80.872P	S00.431A	S04.02XA	S06.6X2A	S12.131A	S12.54XA	S22.042A	S32.000A	S32.122A	S32.425A	S32.486A	S42.015A	S42.136A	S42.251A	S42.342A
M80.872S	S00.432A	S04.031A	S06.6X3A	S12.131B	S12.54XB	S22.042B	S32.000B	S32.122B	S32.425B	S32.486B	S42.015B	S42.136B	S42.251B	S42.342B
M80.879A	S00.439A	S04.032A	S06.6X4A	S12.14XA	S12.550A	S22.048A	S32.001A	S32.129A	S32.426A	S32.491A	S42.016A	S42.141A	S42.252A	S42.343A
M80.879D	S00.531A	S04.041A	S06.6X9A	S12.14XB	S12.550B	S22.048B	S32.001B	S32.129B	S32.426B	S32.491B	S42.016B	S42.141B	S42.252B	S42.343B
M80.879G	S00.532A	S04.042A	S06.810A	S12.150A	S12.551A	S22.049A	S32.002A	S32.130A	S32.431A	S32.492A	S42.017A	S42.142A	S42.253A	S42.344A
M80.879K	S00.83XA	S05.11XA	S06.811A	S12.150B	S12.551B	S22.049B	S32.002B	S32.130B	S32.431B	S32.492B	S42.017B	S42.142B	S42.253B	S42.344B
M80.879P	S00.93XA	S05.12XA	S06.812A	S12.151A	S12.590A	S22.050A	S32.008A	S32.131A	S32.432A	S32.499A	S42.018A	S42.143A	S42.254A	S42.345A
M80.879S	S02.0XXA	S05.21XA	S06.813A	S12.151B	S12.590B	S22.050B	S32.008B	S32.131B	S32.432B	S32.499B	S42.018B	S42.143B	S42.254B	S42.345B
M80.88XA	S02.101A	S05.22XA	S06.814A	S12.190A	S12.591A	S22.051A	S32.009A	S32.132A	S32.433A	S32.501A	S42.019A	S42.144A	S42.255A	S42.346A
M80.88XD	S02.102A	S05.31XA	S06.819A	S12.190B	S12.591B	S22.051B	S32.009B	S32.132B	S32.433B	S32.501B	S42.019B	S42.144B	S42.255B	S42.346B
M80.88XG	S02.109A	S05.32XA	S06.820A	S12.191A	S12.600A	S22.052A	S32.010A	S32.139A	S32.434A	S32.502A	S42.021A	S42.145A	S42.256A	S42.351A
M80.88XK	S02.110A	S05.51XA	S06.821A	S12.191B	S12.600B	S22.052B	S32.010B	S32.139B	S32.434B	S32.502B	S42.021B	S42.145B	S42.256B	S42.351B
M80.88XP	S02.111A	S05.52XA	S06.822A	S12.200A	S12.601A	S22.058A	S32.011A	S32.14XA	S32.435A	S32.509A	S42.022A	S42.146A	S42.261A	S42.352A
M80.88XS	S02.112A	S05.61XA	S06.823A	S12.200B	S12.601B	S22.058B	S32.011B	S32.14XB	S32.435B	S32.509B	S42.022B	S42.146B	S42.261B	S42.352B
M84.311A	S02.113A	S05.62XA	S06.824A	S12.201A	S12.630A	S22.059A	S32.012A	S32.15XA	S32.436A	S32.511A	S42.023A	S42.151A	S42.262A	S42.353A
M84.312A	S02.118A	S05.71XA	S06.829A	S12.201B	S12.630B	S22.059B	S32.012B	S32.15XB	S32.436B	S32.511B	S42.023B	S42.151B	S42.262B	S42.353B
M84.319A	S02.119A	S05.72XA	S06.890A	S12.230A	S12.631A	S22.060A	S32.018A	S32.16XA	S32.441A	S32.512A	S42.024A	S42.152A	S42.263A	S42.354A
M84.321A	S02.11AA	S05.8X1A	S06.891A	S12.230B	S12.631B	S22.060B	S32.018B	S32.16XB	S32.441B	S32.512B	S42.024B	S42.152B	S42.263B	S42.354B
M84.322A	S02.11BA	S05.8X2A	S06.892A	S12.231A	S12.64XA	S22.061A	S32.019A	S32.17XA	S32.442A	S32.519A	S42.025A	S42.153A	S42.264A	S42.355A
M84.329A	S02.11CA	S05.91XA	S06.893A	S12.231B	S12.64XB	S22.061B	S32.019B	S32.17XB	S32.442B	S32.519B	S42.025B	S42.153B	S42.264B	S42.355B
M84.331A	S02.11DA	S05.92XA	S06.894A	S12.24XA	S12.650A	S22.062A	S32.020A	S32.19XA	S32.443A	S32.591A	S42.026A	S42.154A	S42.265A	S42.356A
M84.332A	S02.11EA	S06.0X0A	S06.899A	S12.24XB	S12.650B	S22.062B	S32.020B	S32.19XB	S32.443B	S32.591B	S42.026B	S42.154B	S42.265B	S42.356B
M84.333A	S02.11FA	S06.0X1A	S06.9X0A	S12.250A	S12.651A	S22.068A	S32.021A	S32.2XXA	S32.444A	S32.592A	S42.031A	S42.155A	S42.266A	S42.361A
M84.334A	S02.11GA	S06.0X9A	S06.9X1A	S12.250B	S12.651B	S22.068B	S32.021B	S32.2XXB	S32.444B	S32.592B	S42.031B	S42.155B	S42.266B	S42.361B
M84.339A	S02.11HA	S06.1X0A	S06.9X2A	S12.251A	S12.690A	S22.069A	S32.022A	S32.301A	S32.445A	S32.599A	S42.032A	S42.156A	S42.271A	S42.362A
M84.341A	S02.19XA	S06.1X1A	S06.9X3A	S12.251B	S12.690B	S22.069B	S32.022B	S32.301B	S32.445B	S32.599B	S42.032B	S42.156B	S42.272A	S42.362B
M84.342A	S02.2XXA	S06.1X2A	S06.9X4A	S12.290A	S12.691A	S22.070A	S32.028A	S32.302A	S32.446A	S32.601A	S42.033A	S42.191A	S42.279A	S42.363A
M84.343A	S02.30XA	S06.1X3A	S06.9X9A	S12.290B	S12.691B	S22.070B	S32.028B	S32.302B	S32.446B	S32.601B	S42.033B	S42.191B	S42.291A	S42.363B
M84.350A	S02.31XA	S06.1X4A	S09.10XA	S12.291A	S12.8XXA	S22.071A	S32.029A	S32.309A	S32.451A	S32.602A	S42.034A	S42.192A	S42.291B	S42.364A
M84.351A	S02.32XA	S06.1X9A	S09.11XA	S12.291B	S12.9XXA	S22.071B	S32.029B	S32.309B	S32.451B	S32.602B	S42.034B	S42.192B	S42.292A	S42.364B
M84.352A	S02.400A	S06.2X0A	S09.19XA	S12.300A	S22.000A	S22.072A	S32.030A	S32.311A	S32.452A	S32.609A	S42.035A	S42.199A	S42.292B	S42.365A
M84.353A	S02.401A	S06.2X1A	S09.8XXA	S12.300B	S22.000B	S22.072B	S32.030B	S32.311B	S32.452B	S32.609B	S42.035B	S42.199B	S42.293A	S42.365B

MACRA (cont.) - Based on CMS data

S42.366A	S42.454A	S49.119A	S52.045B	S52.202A	S52.254C	S52.324B	S52.365A	S52.541C	S52.691B	S62.002B	S62.133B	S62.211B	S62.307B	S62.344B
S42.366B	S42.454B	S49.121A	S52.045C	S52.202B	S52.255A	S52.324C	S52.365B	S52.542A	S52.691C	S62.009A	S62.134A	S62.212A	S62.308A	S62.345A
S42.391A	S42.455A	S49.122A	S52.046A	S52.202C	S52.255B	S52.325A	S52.365C	S52.542B	S52.692A	S62.009B	S62.134B	S62.212B	S62.308B	S62.345B
S42.391B	S42.455B	S49.129A	S52.046B	S52.209A	S52.255C	S52.325B	S52.366A	S52.542C	S52.692B	S62.011A	S62.135A	S62.213A	S62.309A	S62.346A
S42.392A	S42.456A	S49.131A	S52.046C	S52.209B	S52.256A	S52.325C	S52.366B	S52.549A	S52.692C	S62.011B	S62.135B	S62.213B	S62.309B	S62.346B
S42.392B	S42.456B	S49.132A	S52.091A	S52.209C	S52.256B	S52.326A	S52.366C	S52.549B	S52.699A	S62.012A	S62.136A	S62.221A	S62.310A	S62.347A
S42.399A	S42.461A	S49.139A	S52.091B	S52.211A	S52.256C	S52.326B	S52.371A	S52.549C	S52.699B	S62.012B	S62.136B	S62.221B	S62.310B	S62.347B
S42.399B	S42.461B	S49.141A	S52.091C	S52.212A	S52.261A	S52.326C	S52.371B	S52.551A	S52.699C	S62.013A	S62.141A	S62.222A	S62.311A	S62.348A
S42.401A	S42.462A	S49.142A	S52.092A	S52.219A	S52.261B	S52.331A	S52.371C	S52.551B	S52.90XA	S62.013B	S62.141B	S62.222B	S62.311B	S62.348B
S42.401B	S42.462B	S49.149A	S52.092B	S52.221A	S52.261C	S52.331B	S52.372A	S52.551C	S52.90XB	S62.014A	S62.142A	S62.223A	S62.312A	S62.349A
S42.402A	S42.463A	S49.191A	S52.092C	S52.221B	S52.262A	S52.331C	S52.372B	S52.552A	S52.90XC	S62.014B	S62.142B	S62.223B	S62.312B	S62.349B
S42.402B	S42.463B	S49.192A	S52.099A	S52.221C	S52.262B	S52.332A	S52.372C	S52.552B	S52.91XA	S62.015A	S62.143A	S62.224A	S62.313A	S62.350A
S42.409A	S42.464A	S49.199A	S52.099B	S52.222A	S52.262C	S52.332B	S52.379A	S52.552C	S52.91XB	S62.015B	S62.143B	S62.224B	S62.313B	S62.350B
S42.409B	S42.464B	S52.001A	S52.099C	S52.222B	S52.263A	S52.332C	S52.379B	S52.559A	S52.91XC	S62.016A	S62.144A	S62.225A	S62.314A	S62.351A
S42.411A	S42.465A	S52.001B	S52.101A	S52.222C	S52.263B	S52.333A	S52.379C	S52.559B	S52.92XA	S62.016B	S62.144B	S62.225B	S62.314B	S62.351B
S42.411B	S42.465B	S52.001C	S52.101B	S52.223A	S52.263C	S52.333B	S52.381A	S52.559C	S52.92XB	S62.021A	S62.145A	S62.226A	S62.315A	S62.352A
S42.412A	S42.466A	S52.002A	S52.101C	S52.223B	S52.264A	S52.333C	S52.381B	S52.561A	S52.92XC	S62.021B	S62.145B	S62.226B	S62.315B	S62.352B
S42.412B	S42.466B	S52.002B	S52.102A	S52.223C	S52.264B	S52.334A	S52.381C	S52.561B	S59.001A	S62.022A	S62.146A	S62.231A	S62.316A	S62.353A
S42.413A	S42.471A	S52.002C	S52.102B	S52.224A	S52.264C	S52.334B	S52.382A	S52.561C	S59.002A	S62.022B	S62.146B	S62.231B	S62.316B	S62.353B
S42.413B	S42.471B	S52.009A	S52.102C	S52.224B	S52.265A	S52.334C	S52.382B	S52.562A	S59.009A	S62.023A	S62.151A	S62.232A	S62.317A	S62.354A
S42.414A	S42.472A	S52.009B	S52.109A	S52.224C	S52.265B	S52.335A	S52.382C	S52.562B	S59.011A	S62.023B	S62.151B	S62.232B	S62.317B	S62.354B
S42.414B	S42.472B	S52.009C	S52.109B	S52.225A	S52.265C	S52.335B	S52.389A	S52.562C	S59.012A	S62.024A	S62.152A	S62.233A	S62.318A	S62.355A
S42.415A	S42.473A	S52.011A	S52.109C	S52.225B	S52.266A	S52.335C	S52.389B	S52.569A	S59.019A	S62.024B	S62.152B	S62.233B	S62.318B	S62.355B
S42.415B	S42.473B	S52.012A	S52.111A	S52.225C	S52.266B	S52.336A	S52.389C	S52.569B	S59.021A	S62.025A	S62.153A	S62.234A	S62.319A	S62.356A
S42.416A	S42.474A	S52.019A	S52.112A	S52.226A	S52.266C	S52.336B	S52.391A	S52.569C	S59.022A	S62.025B	S62.153B	S62.234B	S62.319B	S62.356B
S42.416B	S42.474B	S52.021A	S52.119A	S52.226B	S52.271A	S52.336C	S52.391B	S52.571A	S59.029A	S62.026A	S62.154A	S62.235A	S62.320A	S62.357A
S42.421A	S42.475A	S52.021B	S52.121A	S52.226C	S52.271B	S52.341A	S52.391C	S52.571B	S59.031A	S62.026B	S62.154B	S62.235B	S62.320B	S62.357B
S42.421B	S42.475B	S52.021C	S52.121B	S52.231A	S52.271C	S52.341B	S52.392A	S52.571C	S59.032A	S62.031A	S62.155A	S62.236A	S62.321A	S62.358A
S42.422A	S42.476A	S52.022A	S52.121C	S52.231B	S52.272A	S52.341C	S52.392B	S52.572A	S59.039A	S62.031B	S62.155B	S62.236B	S62.321B	S62.358B
S42.422B	S42.476B	S52.022B	S52.122A	S52.231C	S52.272B	S52.342A	S52.392C	S52.572B	S59.041A	S62.032A	S62.156A	S62.241A	S62.322A	S62.359A
S42.423A	S42.481A	S52.022C	S52.122B	S52.232A	S52.272C	S52.342B	S52.399A	S52.572C	S59.042A	S62.032B	S62.156B	S62.241B	S62.322B	S62.359B
S42.423B	S42.482A	S52.023A	S52.122C	S52.232B	S52.279A	S52.342C	S52.399B	S52.579A	S59.049A	S62.033A	S62.161A	S62.242A	S62.323A	S62.360A
S42.424A	S42.489A	S52.023B	S52.123A	S52.232C	S52.279B	S52.343A	S52.399C	S52.579B	S59.091A	S62.033B	S62.161B	S62.242B	S62.323B	S62.360B
S42.424B	S42.491A	S52.023C	S52.123B	S52.233A	S52.279C	S52.343B	S52.501A	S52.579C	S59.092A	S62.034A	S62.162A	S62.243A	S62.324A	S62.361A
S42.425A	S42.491B	S52.024A	S52.123C	S52.233B	S52.281A	S52.343C	S52.501B	S52.591A	S59.099A	S62.034B	S62.162B	S62.243B	S62.324B	S62.361B
S42.425B	S42.492A	S52.024B	S52.124A	S52.233C	S52.281B	S52.344A	S52.501C	S52.591B	S59.101A	S62.035A	S62.163A	S62.244A	S62.325A	S62.362A
S42.426A	S42.492B	S52.024C	S52.124B	S52.234A	S52.281C	S52.344B	S52.502A	S52.591C	S59.102A	S62.035B	S62.163B	S62.244B	S62.325B	S62.362B
S42.426B	S42.493A	S52.025A	S52.124C	S52.234B	S52.282A	S52.344C	S52.502B	S52.592A	S59.109A	S62.036A	S62.164A	S62.245A	S62.326A	S62.363A
S42.431A	S42.493B	S52.025B	S52.125A	S52.234C	S52.282B	S52.345A	S52.502C	S52.592B	S59.111A	S62.036B	S62.164B	S62.245B	S62.326B	S62.363B
S42.431B	S42.494A	S52.025C	S52.125B	S52.235A	S52.282C	S52.345B	S52.509A	S52.592C	S59.112A	S62.101A	S62.165A	S62.246A	S62.327A	S62.364A
S42.432A	S42.494B	S52.026A	S52.125C	S52.235B	S52.283A	S52.345C	S52.509B	S52.599A	S59.119A	S62.101B	S62.165B	S62.246B	S62.327B	S62.364B
S42.432B	S42.495A	S52.026B	S52.126A	S52.235C	S52.283B	S52.346A	S52.509C	S52.599B	S59.121A	S62.102A	S62.166A	S62.251A	S62.328A	S62.365A
S42.433A	S42.495B	S52.026C	S52.126B	S52.236A	S52.283C	S52.346B	S52.511A	S52.599C	S59.122A	S62.102B	S62.166B	S62.251B	S62.328B	S62.365B
S42.433B	S42.496A	S52.031A	S52.126C	S52.236B	S52.291A	S52.346C	S52.511B	S52.601A	S59.129A	S62.109A	S62.171A	S62.252A	S62.329A	S62.366A
S42.434A	S42.496B	S52.031B	S52.131A	S52.236C	S52.291B	S52.351A	S52.511C	S52.601B	S59.131A	S62.109B	S62.171B	S62.252B	S62.329B	S62.366B
S42.434B	S42.90XA	S52.031C	S52.131B	S52.241A	S52.291C	S52.351B	S52.512A	S52.601C	S59.132A	S62.111A	S62.172A	S62.253A	S62.330A	S62.367A
S42.435A	S42.90XB	S52.032A	S52.131C	S52.241B	S52.292A	S52.351C	S52.512B	S52.602A	S59.139A	S62.111B	S62.172B	S62.253B	S62.330B	S62.367B
S42.435B	S42.91XA	S52.032B	S52.132A	S52.241C	S52.292B	S52.352A	S52.512C	S52.602B	S59.141A	S62.112A	S62.173A	S62.254A	S62.331A	S62.368A
S42.436A	S42.91XB	S52.032C	S52.132B	S52.242A	S52.292C	S52.352B	S52.513A	S52.602C	S59.142A	S62.112B	S62.173B	S62.254B	S62.331B	S62.368B
S42.436B	S42.92XA	S52.033A	S52.132C	S52.242B	S52.299A	S52.352C	S52.513B	S52.609A	S59.149A	S62.113A	S62.174A	S62.255A	S62.332A	S62.369A
S42.441A	S42.92XB	S52.033B	S52.133A	S52.242C	S52.299B	S52.353A	S52.513C	S52.609B	S59.191A	S62.113B	S62.174B	S62.255B	S62.332B	S62.369B
S42.441B	S49.001A	S52.033C	S52.133B	S52.243A	S52.299C	S52.353B	S52.514A	S52.609C	S59.192A	S62.114A	S62.175A	S62.256A	S62.333A	S62.390A
S42.442A	S49.002A	S52.034A	S52.133C	S52.243B	S52.301A	S52.353C	S52.514B	S52.611A	S59.199A	S62.114B	S62.175B	S62.256B	S62.333B	S62.390B
S42.442B	S49.009A	S52.034B	S52.134A	S52.243C	S52.301B	S52.354A	S52.514C	S52.611B	S59.201A	S62.115A	S62.176A	S62.291A	S62.334A	S62.391A
S42.443A	S49.011A	S52.034C	S52.134B	S52.244A	S52.301C	S52.354B	S52.515A	S52.611C	S59.202A	S62.115B	S62.176B	S62.291B	S62.334B	S62.391B
S42.443B	S49.012A	S52.035A	S52.134C	S52.244B	S52.302A	S52.354C	S52.515B	S52.612A	S59.209A	S62.116A	S62.181A	S62.292A	S62.335A	S62.392A
S42.444A	S49.019A	S52.035B	S52.135A	S52.244C	S52.302B	S52.355A	S52.515C	S52.612B	S59.211A	S62.116B	S62.181B	S62.292B	S62.335B	S62.392B
S42.444B	S49.021A	S52.035C	S52.135B	S52.245A	S52.302C	S52.355B	S52.516A	S52.612C	S59.212A	S62.121A	S62.182A	S62.299A	S62.336A	S62.393A
S42.445A	S49.022A	S52.036A	S52.135C	S52.245B	S52.309A	S52.355C	S52.516B	S52.613A	S59.219A	S62.121B	S62.182B	S62.299B	S62.336B	S62.393B
S42.445B	S49.029A	S52.036B	S52.136A	S52.245C	S52.309B	S52.356A	S52.516C	S52.613B	S59.221A	S62.122A	S62.183A	S62.300A	S62.337A	S62.394A
S42.446A	S49.031A	S52.036C	S52.136B	S52.246A	S52.309C	S52.356B	S52.521A	S52.613C	S59.222A	S62.122B	S62.183B	S62.300B	S62.337B	S62.394B
S42.446B	S49.032A	S52.041A	S52.136C	S52.246B	S52.311A	S52.356C	S52.522A	S52.614A	S59.229A	S62.123A	S62.184A	S62.301A	S62.338A	S62.395A
S42.447A	S49.039A	S52.041B	S52.181A	S52.246C	S52.312A	S52.361A	S52.529A	S52.614B	S59.231A	S62.123B	S62.184B	S62.301B	S62.338B	S62.395B
S42.447B	S49.041A	S52.041C	S52.181B	S52.251A	S52.319A	S52.361B	S52.531A	S52.614C	S59.232A	S62.124A	S62.185A	S62.302A	S62.339A	S62.396A
S42.448A	S49.042A	S52.042A	S52.181C	S52.251B	S52.321A	S52.361C	S52.531B	S52.615A	S59.239A	S62.124B	S62.185B	S62.302B	S62.339B	S62.396B
S42.448B	S49.049A	S52.042B	S52.182A	S52.251C	S52.321B	S52.362A	S52.531C	S52.615B	S59.241A	S62.125A	S62.186A	S62.303A	S62.340A	S62.397A
S42.449A	S49.091A	S52.042C	S52.182B	S52.252A	S52.321C	S52.362B	S52.532A	S52.615C	S59.242A	S62.125B	S62.186B	S62.303B	S62.340B	S62.397B
S42.449B	S49.092A	S52.043A	S52.182C	S52.252B	S52.322A	S52.362C	S52.532B	S52.616A	S59.249A	S62.126A	S62.201A	S62.304A	S62.341A	S62.398A
S42.451A	S49.099A	S52.043B	S52.189A	S52.252C	S52.322B	S52.363A	S52.532C	S52.616B	S59.291A	S62.126B	S62.201B	S62.304B	S62.341B	S62.398B
S42.451B	S49.101A	S52.043C	S52.189B	S52.253A	S52.322C	S52.363B	S52.539A	S52.616C	S59.292A	S62.131A	S62.202A	S62.305A	S62.342A	S62.399A
S42.452A	S49.102A	S52.044A	S52.189C	S52.253B	S52.323A	S52.363C	S52.539B	S52.621A	S59.299A	S62.131B	S62.202B	S62.305B	S62.342B	S62.399B
S42.452B	S49.109A	S52.044B	S52.201A	S52.253C	S52.323B	S52.364A	S52.539C	S52.622A	S62.001A	S62.132A	S62.209A	S62.306A	S62.343A	S62.90XA
S42.453A	S49.111A	S52.044C	S52.201B	S52.254A	S52.323C	S52.364B	S52.541A	S52.629A	S62.001B	S62.132B	S62.209B	S62.306B	S62.343B	S62.90XB
S42.453B	S49.112A	S52.045A	S52.201C	S52.254B	S52.324A	S52.364C	S52.541B	S52.691A	S62.002A	S62.133A	S62.211A	S62.307A	S62.344A	S62.91XA

MACRA (cont.) - Based on CMS data

S62.91XB	S72.046C	S72.124B	S72.322A	S72.362C	S72.433B	S72.499A	S82.016C	S82.111B	S82.152A	S82.241C	S82.391B	S82.452A	S82.65XC	S82.871B
S62.92XA	S72.051A	S72.124C	S72.322B	S72.363A	S72.433C	S72.499B	S82.021A	S82.111C	S82.152B	S82.242A	S82.391C	S82.452B	S82.66XA	S82.871C
S62.92XB	S72.051B	S72.125A	S72.322C	S72.363B	S72.434A	S72.499C	S82.021B	S82.112A	S82.152C	S82.242B	S82.392A	S82.452C	S82.66XB	S82.872A
S72.001A	S72.051C	S72.125B	S72.323A	S72.363C	S72.434B	S72.8X1A	S82.021C	S82.112B	S82.153A	S82.242C	S82.392B	S82.453A	S82.66XC	S82.872B
S72.001B	S72.052A	S72.125C	S72.323B	S72.364A	S72.434C	S72.8X1B	S82.022A	S82.112C	S82.153B	S82.243A	S82.392C	S82.453B	S82.811A	S82.872C
S72.001C	S72.052B	S72.126A	S72.323C	S72.364B	S72.435A	S72.8X1C	S82.022B	S82.113A	S82.153C	S82.243B	S82.399A	S82.453C	S82.812A	S82.873A
S72.002A	S72.052C	S72.126B	S72.324A	S72.364C	S72.435B	S72.8X2A	S82.022C	S82.113B	S82.154A	S82.243C	S82.399B	S82.454A	S82.819A	S82.873B
S72.002B	S72.059A	S72.126C	S72.324B	S72.365A	S72.435C	S72.8X2B	S82.023A	S82.113C	S82.154B	S82.244A	S82.399C	S82.454B	S82.821A	S82.873C
S72.002C	S72.059B	S72.131A	S72.324C	S72.365B	S72.436A	S72.8X2C	S82.023B	S82.114A	S82.154C	S82.244B	S82.401A	S82.454C	S82.822A	S82.874A
S72.009A	S72.059C	S72.131B	S72.325A	S72.365C	S72.436B	S72.8X9A	S82.023C	S82.114B	S82.155A	S82.244C	S82.401B	S82.455A	S82.829A	S82.874B
S72.009B	S72.061A	S72.131C	S72.325B	S72.366A	S72.436C	S72.8X9B	S82.024A	S82.114C	S82.155B	S82.245A	S82.401C	S82.455B	S82.831A	S82.874C
S72.009C	S72.061B	S72.132A	S72.325C	S72.366B	S72.441A	S72.8X9C	S82.024B	S82.115A	S82.155C	S82.245B	S82.402A	S82.455C	S82.831B	S82.875A
S72.011A	S72.061C	S72.132B	S72.326A	S72.366C	S72.441B	S72.90XA	S82.024C	S82.115B	S82.156A	S82.245C	S82.402B	S82.456A	S82.831C	S82.875B
S72.011B	S72.062A	S72.132C	S72.326B	S72.391A	S72.441C	S72.90XB	S82.025A	S82.115C	S82.156B	S82.246A	S82.402C	S82.456B	S82.832A	S82.875C
S72.011C	S72.062B	S72.133A	S72.326C	S72.391B	S72.442A	S72.90XC	S82.025B	S82.116A	S82.156C	S82.246B	S82.409A	S82.456C	S82.832B	S82.876A
S72.012A	S72.062C	S72.133B	S72.331A	S72.391C	S72.442B	S72.91XA	S82.025C	S82.116B	S82.161A	S82.246C	S82.409B	S82.461A	S82.832C	S82.876B
S72.012B	S72.063A	S72.133C	S72.331B	S72.392A	S72.442C	S72.91XB	S82.026A	S82.116C	S82.162A	S82.251A	S82.409C	S82.461B	S82.839A	S82.876C
S72.012C	S72.063B	S72.134A	S72.331C	S72.392B	S72.443A	S72.91XC	S82.026B	S82.121A	S82.169A	S82.251B	S82.421A	S82.461C	S82.839B	S82.891A
S72.019A	S72.063C	S72.134B	S72.332A	S72.392C	S72.443B	S72.92XA	S82.026C	S82.121B	S82.191A	S82.251C	S82.421B	S82.462A	S82.839C	S82.891B
S72.019B	S72.064A	S72.134C	S72.332B	S72.399A	S72.443C	S72.92XB	S82.031A	S82.121C	S82.191B	S82.252A	S82.421C	S82.462B	S82.841A	S82.891C
S72.019C	S72.064B	S72.135A	S72.332C	S72.399B	S72.444A	S72.92XC	S82.031B	S82.122A	S82.191C	S82.252B	S82.422A	S82.462C	S82.841B	S82.892A
S72.021A	S72.064C	S72.135B	S72.333A	S72.399C	S72.444B	S79.001A	S82.031C	S82.122B	S82.192A	S82.252C	S82.422B	S82.463A	S82.841C	S82.892B
S72.021B	S72.065A	S72.135C	S72.333B	S72.401A	S72.444C	S79.002A	S82.032A	S82.122C	S82.192B	S82.253A	S82.422C	S82.463B	S82.842A	S82.892C
S72.021C	S72.065B	S72.136A	S72.333C	S72.401B	S72.445A	S79.009A	S82.032B	S82.123A	S82.192C	S82.253B	S82.423A	S82.463C	S82.842B	S82.899A
S72.022A	S72.065C	S72.136B	S72.334A	S72.401C	S72.445B	S79.011A	S82.032C	S82.123B	S82.199A	S82.253C	S82.423B	S82.464A	S82.842C	S82.899B
S72.022B	S72.066A	S72.136C	S72.334B	S72.402A	S72.445C	S79.012A	S82.033A	S82.123C	S82.199B	S82.254A	S82.423C	S82.464B	S82.843A	S82.899C
S72.022C	S72.066B	S72.141A	S72.334C	S72.402B	S72.446A	S79.019A	S82.033B	S82.124A	S82.199C	S82.254B	S82.424A	S82.464C	S82.843B	S82.90XA
S72.023A	S72.066C	S72.141B	S72.335A	S72.402C	S72.446B	S79.091A	S82.033C	S82.124B	S82.201A	S82.254C	S82.424B	S82.465A	S82.843C	S82.90XB
S72.023B	S72.091A	S72.141C	S72.335B	S72.409A	S72.446C	S79.092A	S82.034A	S82.124C	S82.201B	S82.255A	S82.424C	S82.465B	S82.844A	S82.90XC
S72.023C	S72.091B	S72.142A	S72.335C	S72.409B	S72.451A	S79.099A	S82.034B	S82.125A	S82.201C	S82.255B	S82.425A	S82.465C	S82.844B	S82.91XA
S72.024A	S72.091C	S72.142B	S72.336A	S72.409C	S72.451B	S79.101A	S82.034C	S82.125B	S82.202A	S82.255C	S82.425B	S82.466A	S82.844C	S82.91XB
S72.024B	S72.092A	S72.142C	S72.336B	S72.411A	S72.451C	S79.102A	S82.035A	S82.125C	S82.202B	S82.256A	S82.425C	S82.466B	S82.845A	S82.91XC
S72.024C	S72.092B	S72.143A	S72.336C	S72.411B	S72.452A	S79.109A	S82.035B	S82.126A	S82.202C	S82.256B	S82.426A	S82.466C	S82.845B	S82.92XA
S72.025A	S72.092C	S72.143B	S72.341A	S72.411C	S72.452B	S79.111A	S82.035C	S82.126B	S82.209A	S82.256C	S82.426B	S82.491A	S82.845C	S82.92XB
S72.025B	S72.099A	S72.143C	S72.341B	S72.412A	S72.452C	S79.112A	S82.036A	S82.126C	S82.209B	S82.261A	S82.426C	S82.491B	S82.846A	S82.92XC
S72.025C	S72.099B	S72.144A	S72.341C	S72.412B	S72.453A	S79.119A	S82.036B	S82.131A	S82.209C	S82.261B	S82.431A	S82.491C	S82.846B	S89.001A
S72.026A	S72.099C	S72.144B	S72.342A	S72.412C	S72.453B	S79.121A	S82.036C	S82.131B	S82.221A	S82.261C	S82.431B	S82.492A	S82.846C	S89.002A
S72.026B	S72.101A	S72.144C	S72.342B	S72.413A	S72.453C	S79.122A	S82.041A	S82.131C	S82.221B	S82.262A	S82.431C	S82.492B	S82.851A	S89.009A
S72.026C	S72.101B	S72.145A	S72.342C	S72.413B	S72.454A	S79.129A	S82.041B	S82.132A	S82.221C	S82.262B	S82.432A	S82.492C	S82.851B	S89.011A
S72.031A	S72.101C	S72.145B	S72.343A	S72.413C	S72.454B	S79.131A	S82.041C	S82.132B	S82.222A	S82.262C	S82.432B	S82.499A	S82.851C	S89.012A
S72.031B	S72.102A	S72.145C	S72.343B	S72.414A	S72.454C	S79.132A	S82.042A	S82.132C	S82.222B	S82.263A	S82.432C	S82.499B	S82.852A	S89.019A
S72.031C	S72.102B	S72.146A	S72.343C	S72.414B	S72.455A	S79.139A	S82.042B	S82.133A	S82.222C	S82.263B	S82.433A	S82.499C	S82.852B	S89.021A
S72.032A	S72.102C	S72.146B	S72.344A	S72.414C	S72.455B	S79.141A	S82.042C	S82.133B	S82.223A	S82.263C	S82.433B	S82.51XA	S82.852C	S89.022A
S72.032B	S72.109A	S72.146C	S72.344B	S72.415A	S72.455C	S79.142A	S82.043A	S82.133C	S82.223B	S82.264A	S82.433C	S82.51XB	S82.853A	S89.029A
S72.032C	S72.109B	S72.21XA	S72.344C	S72.415B	S72.456A	S79.149A	S82.043B	S82.134A	S82.223C	S82.264B	S82.434A	S82.51XC	S82.853B	S89.031A
S72.033A	S72.109C	S72.21XB	S72.345A	S72.415C	S72.456B	S79.191A	S82.043C	S82.134B	S82.224A	S82.264C	S82.434B	S82.52XA	S82.853C	S89.032A
S72.033B	S72.111A	S72.21XC	S72.345B	S72.416A	S72.456C	S79.192A	S82.044A	S82.134C	S82.224B	S82.265A	S82.434C	S82.52XB	S82.854A	S89.039A
S72.033C	S72.111B	S72.22XA	S72.345C	S72.416B	S72.461A	S79.199A	S82.044B	S82.135A	S82.224C	S82.265B	S82.435A	S82.52XC	S82.854B	S89.041A
S72.034A	S72.111C	S72.22XB	S72.346A	S72.416C	S72.461B	S82.001A	S82.044C	S82.135B	S82.225A	S82.265C	S82.435B	S82.53XA	S82.854C	S89.042A
S72.034B	S72.112A	S72.22XC	S72.346B	S72.421A	S72.461C	S82.001B	S82.045A	S82.135C	S82.225B	S82.266A	S82.435C	S82.53XB	S82.855A	S89.049A
S72.034C	S72.112B	S72.23XA	S72.346C	S72.421B	S72.462A	S82.001C	S82.045B	S82.136A	S82.225C	S82.266B	S82.436A	S82.53XC	S82.855B	S89.091A
S72.035A	S72.112C	S72.23XB	S72.351A	S72.421C	S72.462B	S82.002A	S82.045C	S82.136B	S82.226A	S82.266C	S82.436B	S82.54XA	S82.855C	S89.092A
S72.035B	S72.113A	S72.23XC	S72.351B	S72.422A	S72.462C	S82.002B	S82.046A	S82.136C	S82.226B	S82.291A	S82.436C	S82.54XB	S82.856A	S89.099A
S72.035C	S72.113B	S72.24XA	S72.351C	S72.422B	S72.463A	S82.002C	S82.046B	S82.141A	S82.226C	S82.291B	S82.441A	S82.54XC	S82.856B	S89.101A
S72.036A	S72.113C	S72.24XB	S72.352A	S72.422C	S72.463B	S82.009A	S82.046C	S82.141B	S82.231A	S82.291C	S82.441B	S82.55XA	S82.856C	S89.102A
S72.036B	S72.114A	S72.24XC	S72.352B	S72.423A	S72.463C	S82.009B	S82.091A	S82.141C	S82.231B	S82.292A	S82.441C	S82.55XB	S82.861A	S89.109A
S72.036C	S72.114B	S72.25XA	S72.352C	S72.423B	S72.464A	S82.009C	S82.091B	S82.142A	S82.231C	S82.292B	S82.442A	S82.55XC	S82.861B	S89.111A
S72.041A	S72.114C	S72.25XB	S72.353A	S72.423C	S72.464B	S82.011A	S82.091C	S82.142B	S82.232A	S82.292C	S82.442B	S82.56XA	S82.861C	S89.112A
S72.041B	S72.115A	S72.25XC	S72.353B	S72.424A	S72.464C	S82.011B	S82.092A	S82.142C	S82.232B	S82.299A	S82.442C	S82.56XB	S82.862A	S89.119A
S72.041C	S72.115B	S72.26XA	S72.353C	S72.424B	S72.465A	S82.011C	S82.092B	S82.143A	S82.232C	S82.299B	S82.443A	S82.56XC	S82.862B	S89.121A
S72.042A	S72.115C	S72.26XB	S72.354A	S72.424C	S72.465B	S82.012A	S82.092C	S82.143B	S82.233A	S82.299C	S82.443B	S82.61XA	S82.862C	S89.122A
S72.042B	S72.116A	S72.26XC	S72.354B	S72.425A	S72.465C	S82.012B	S82.099A	S82.143C	S82.233B	S82.301A	S82.443C	S82.61XB	S82.863A	S89.129A
S72.042C	S72.116B	S72.301A	S72.354C	S72.425B	S72.466A	S82.012C	S82.099B	S82.144A	S82.233C	S82.301B	S82.444A	S82.61XC	S82.863B	S89.131A
S72.043A	S72.116C	S72.301B	S72.355A	S72.425C	S72.466B	S82.013A	S82.099C	S82.144B	S82.234A	S82.301C	S82.444B	S82.62XA	S82.863C	S89.132A
S72.043B	S72.121A	S72.301C	S72.355B	S72.426A	S72.466C	S82.013B	S82.101A	S82.144C	S82.234B	S82.302A	S82.444C	S82.62XB	S82.864A	S89.139A
S72.043C	S72.121B	S72.302A	S72.355C	S72.426B	S72.471A	S82.013C	S82.101B	S82.145A	S82.234C	S82.302B	S82.445A	S82.62XC	S82.864B	S89.141A
S72.044A	S72.121C	S72.302B	S72.356A	S72.426C	S72.472A	S82.014A	S82.101C	S82.145B	S82.235A	S82.302C	S82.445B	S82.63XA	S82.864C	S89.142A
S72.044B	S72.122A	S72.302C	S72.356B	S72.431A	S72.479A	S82.014B	S82.102A	S82.145C	S82.235B	S82.309A	S82.445C	S82.63XB	S82.865A	S89.149A
S72.044C	S72.122B	S72.309A	S72.356C	S72.431B	S72.491A	S82.014C	S82.102B	S82.146A	S82.235C	S82.309B	S82.446A	S82.63XC	S82.865B	S89.191A
S72.045A	S72.122C	S72.309B	S72.361A	S72.431C	S72.491B	S82.015A	S82.102C	S82.146B	S82.236A	S82.309C	S82.446B	S82.64XA	S82.865C	S89.192A
S72.045B	S72.123A	S72.309C	S72.361B	S72.432A	S72.491C	S82.015B	S82.109A	S82.146C	S82.236B	S82.311A	S82.446C	S82.64XB	S82.866A	S89.199A
S72.045C	S72.123B	S72.321A	S72.361C	S72.432B	S72.492A	S82.015C	S82.109B	S82.151A	S82.236C	S82.312A	S82.451A	S82.64XC	S82.866B	S89.201A
S72.046A	S72.123C	S72.321B	S72.362A	S72.432C	S72.492B	S82.016A	S82.109C	S82.151B	S82.241A	S82.319A	S82.451B	S82.65XA	S82.866C	S89.202A
S72.046B	S72.124A	S72.321C	S72.362B	S72.433A	S72.492C	S82.016B	S82.111A	S82.151C	S82.241B	S82.391A	S82.451C	S82.65XB	S82.871A	S89.209A

MACRA (cont.) - Based on CMS data

S89.211A	S92.011B	S92.033B	S92.055B	S92.114B	S92.136B	S92.192B	S92.224B	S92.246B	S92.315B	S92.341B	S92.819B	S99.032B	S99.121B	T26.22XA
S89.212A	S92.012A	S92.034A	S92.056A	S92.115A	S92.141A	S92.199A	S92.225A	S92.251A	S92.316A	S92.342A	S92.901A	S99.039A	S99.122A	T26.31XA
S89.219A	S92.012B	S92.034B	S92.056B	S92.115B	S92.141B	S92.199B	S92.225B	S92.251B	S92.316B	S92.342B	S92.901B	S99.039B	S99.122B	T26.32XA
S89.221A	S92.013A	S92.035A	S92.061A	S92.116A	S92.142A	S92.201A	S92.226A	S92.252A	S92.321A	S92.343A	S92.902A	S99.041A	S99.129A	T26.41XA
S89.222A	S92.013B	S92.035B	S92.061B	S92.116B	S92.142B	S92.201B	S92.226B	S92.252B	S92.321B	S92.343B	S92.902B	S99.041B	S99.129B	T26.42XA
S89.229A	S92.014A	S92.036A	S92.062A	S92.121A	S92.143A	S92.202A	S92.231A	S92.253A	S92.322A	S92.344A	S92.909A	S99.042A	S99.131A	T26.51XA
S89.291A	S92.014B	S92.036B	S92.062B	S92.121B	S92.143B	S92.202B	S92.231B	S92.253B	S92.322B	S92.344B	S92.909B	S99.042B	S99.131B	T26.52XA
S89.292A	S92.015A	S92.041A	S92.063A	S92.122A	S92.144A	S92.209A	S92.232A	S92.254A	S92.323A	S92.345A	S99.001A	S99.049A	S99.132A	T26.61XA
S89.299A	S92.015B	S92.041B	S92.063B	S92.122B	S92.144B	S92.209B	S92.232B	S92.254B	S92.323B	S92.345B	S99.001B	S99.049B	S99.132B	T26.62XA
S89.301A	S92.016A	S92.042A	S92.064A	S92.123A	S92.145A	S92.211A	S92.233A	S92.255A	S92.324A	S92.346A	S99.002A	S99.091A	S99.139A	T26.71XA
S89.302A	S92.016B	S92.042B	S92.064B	S92.123B	S92.145B	S92.211B	S92.233B	S92.255B	S92.324B	S92.346B	S99.002B	S99.091B	S99.139B	T26.72XA
S89.309A	S92.021A	S92.043A	S92.065A	S92.124A	S92.146A	S92.212A	S92.234A	S92.256A	S92.325A	S92.351A	S99.009A	S99.092A	S99.141A	T26.81XA
S89.311A	S92.021B	S92.043B	S92.065B	S92.124B	S92.146B	S92.212B	S92.234B	S92.256B	S92.325B	S92.351B	S99.009B	S99.092B	S99.141B	T26.82XA
S89.312A	S92.022A	S92.044A	S92.066A	S92.125A	S92.151A	S92.213A	S92.235A	S92.301A	S92.326A	S92.352A	S99.011A	S99.099A	S99.142A	T26.91XA
S89.319A	S92.022B	S92.044B	S92.066B	S92.125B	S92.151B	S92.213B	S92.235B	S92.301B	S92.326B	S92.352B	S99.011B	S99.099B	S99.142B	T26.92XA
S89.321A	S92.023A	S92.045A	S92.101A	S92.126A	S92.152A	S92.214A	S92.236A	S92.302A	S92.331A	S92.353A	S99.012A	S99.101A	S99.149A	T44.7X5A
S89.322A	S92.023B	S92.045B	S92.101B	S92.126B	S92.152B	S92.214B	S92.236B	S92.302B	S92.331B	S92.353B	S99.012B	S99.101B	S99.149B	T44.7X5D
S89.329A	S92.024A	S92.046A	S92.102A	S92.131A	S92.153A	S92.215A	S92.241A	S92.309A	S92.332A	S92.354A	S99.019A	S99.102A	S99.191A	T44.7X5S
S89.391A	S92.024B	S92.046B	S92.102B	S92.131B	S92.153B	S92.215B	S92.241B	S92.309B	S92.332B	S92.354B	S99.019B	S99.102B	S99.191B	T85.44XA
S89.392A	S92.025A	S92.051A	S92.109A	S92.132A	S92.154A	S92.216A	S92.242A	S92.311A	S92.333A	S92.355A	S99.021A	S99.109A	S99.192A	T85.44XD
S89.399A	S92.025B	S92.051B	S92.109B	S92.132B	S92.154B	S92.216B	S92.242B	S92.311B	S92.333B	S92.355B	S99.021B	S99.109B	S99.192B	T85.44XS
S92.001A	S92.026A	S92.052A	S92.111A	S92.133A	S92.155A	S92.221A	S92.243A	S92.312A	S92.334A	S92.356A	S99.022A	S99.111A	S99.199A	
S92.001B	S92.026B	S92.052B	S92.111B	S92.133B	S92.155B	S92.221B	S92.243B	S92.312B	S92.334B	S92.356B	S99.022B	S99.111B	S99.199B	
S92.002A	S92.031A	S92.053A	S92.112A	S92.134A	S92.156A	S92.222A	S92.244A	S92.313A	S92.335A	S92.811A	S99.029A	S99.112A	T26.01XA	
S92.002B	S92.031B	S92.053B	S92.112B	S92.134B	S92.156B	S92.222B	S92.244B	S92.313B	S92.335B	S92.811B	S99.029B	S99.112B	T26.02XA	
S92.009A	S92.032A	S92.054A	S92.113A	S92.135A	S92.191A	S92.223A	S92.245A	S92.314A	S92.336A	S92.812A	S99.031A	S99.119A	T26.11XA	
S92.009B	S92.032B	S92.054B	S92.113B	S92.135B	S92.191B	S92.223B	S92.245B	S92.314B	S92.336B	S92.812B	S99.031B	S99.119B	T26.12XA	
S92.011A	S92.033A	S92.055A	S92.114A	S92.136A	S92.192A	S92.224A	S92.246A	S92.315A	S92.341A	S92.819A	S99.032A	S99.121A	T26.21XA	

Major Complication or Comorbidity (MCC) - Based on CMS data

O41.1010	O41.1411	O60.22X2	R40.2341	S06.310A	S06.353A	S06.5X8A	S12.001B	S12.430B	S14.121A	S21.339A	S22.038B	S24.0XXA	S25.309A	S27.439A
O41.1011	O41.1412	O60.22X3	R40.2342	S06.311A	S06.354A	S06.5X9A	S12.01XB	S12.431B	S14.122A	S21.341A	S22.039B	S24.101A	S25.311A	S27.491A
O41.1012	O41.1413	O60.22X4	R40.2343	S06.312A	S06.355A	S06.6X0A	S12.02XB	S12.44XB	S14.123A	S21.342A	S22.040B	S24.102A	S25.312A	S27.492A
O41.1013	O41.1414	O60.22X5	R40.2344	S06.313A	S06.356A	S06.6X1A	S12.030B	S12.450B	S14.124A	S21.349A	S22.041B	S24.103A	S25.319A	S27.499A
O41.1014	O41.1415	O60.22X9	S02.0XXB	S06.314A	S06.357A	S06.6X2A	S12.031B	S12.451B	S14.125A	S21.351A	S22.042B	S24.104A	S25.321A	S27.812A
O41.1015	O41.1419	O60.23X0	S02.101B	S06.315A	S06.358A	S06.6X3A	S12.040B	S12.490B	S14.126A	S21.352A	S22.048B	S24.111A	S25.322A	S27.813A
O41.1019	O41.1420	O60.23X1	S02.102B	S06.316A	S06.359A	S06.6X4A	S12.041B	S12.491B	S14.127A	S21.359A	S22.049B	S24.112A	S25.329A	S27.818A
O41.1020	O41.1421	O60.23X2	S02.109B	S06.317A	S06.360A	S06.6X5A	S12.090B	S12.500B	S14.128A	S21.401A	S22.050B	S24.113A	S25.391A	S27.819A
O41.1021	O41.1422	O60.23X3	S02.110B	S06.318A	S06.361A	S06.6X6A	S12.091B	S12.501B	S14.131A	S21.402A	S22.051B	S24.114A	S25.392A	S31.001A
O41.1022	O41.1423	O60.23X4	S02.111B	S06.319A	S06.362A	S06.6X7A	S12.100B	S12.530B	S14.132A	S21.409A	S22.052B	S24.131A	S25.399A	S31.011A
O41.1023	O41.1424	O60.23X5	S02.112B	S06.320A	S06.363A	S06.6X8A	S12.101B	S12.531B	S14.133A	S21.411A	S22.058B	S24.132A	S25.401A	S31.021A
O41.1024	O41.1425	O60.23X9	S02.113B	S06.321A	S06.364A	S06.6X9A	S12.110B	S12.54XB	S14.134A	S21.412A	S22.059B	S24.133A	S25.402A	S31.031A
O41.1025	O41.1429	R40.2110	S02.118B	S06.322A	S06.365A	S06.816A	S12.111B	S12.550B	S14.135A	S21.419A	S22.060B	S24.134A	S25.409A	S31.041A
O41.1029	O41.1430	R40.2111	S02.119B	S06.323A	S06.366A	S06.817A	S12.112B	S12.551B	S14.136A	S21.421A	S22.061B	S24.141A	S25.411A	S31.051A
O41.1030	O41.1431	R40.2112	S02.11AB	S06.324A	S06.367A	S06.818A	S12.120B	S12.590B	S14.137A	S21.422A	S22.062B	S24.142A	S25.412A	S31.600A
O41.1031	O41.1432	R40.2113	S02.11BB	S06.325A	S06.368A	S06.826A	S12.121B	S12.591B	S14.138A	S21.429A	S22.068B	S24.143A	S25.419A	S31.601A
O41.1032	O41.1433	R40.2114	S02.11CB	S06.326A	S06.369A	S06.827A	S12.130B	S12.600B	S14.141A	S21.431A	S22.069B	S24.144A	S25.421A	S31.602A
O41.1033	O41.1434	R40.2120	S02.11DB	S06.327A	S06.370A	S06.828A	S12.131B	S12.601B	S14.142A	S21.432A	S22.070B	S24.151A	S25.422A	S31.603A
O41.1034	O41.1435	R40.2121	S02.11EB	S06.328A	S06.376A	S06.896A	S12.14XB	S12.630B	S14.143A	S21.439A	S22.071B	S24.152A	S25.429A	S31.604A
O41.1035	O41.1439	R40.2122	S02.11FB	S06.329A	S06.377A	S06.897A	S12.150B	S12.631B	S14.144A	S21.441A	S22.072B	S24.153A	S25.491A	S31.605A
O41.1039	O60.12X0	R40.2123	S02.11GB	S06.330A	S06.378A	S06.898A	S12.151B	S12.64XB	S14.145A	S21.442A	S22.078B	S24.154A	S25.492A	S31.609A
O41.1210	O60.12X1	R40.2124	S02.11HB	S06.331A	S06.380A	S06.9X6A	S12.190B	S12.650B	S14.146A	S21.449A	S22.079B	S25.00XA	S25.499A	S31.610A
O41.1211	O60.12X2	R40.2210	S02.121B	S06.332A	S06.386A	S06.9X7A	S12.191B	S12.651B	S14.147A	S21.451A	S22.080B	S25.01XA	S26.020A	S31.611A
O41.1212	O60.12X3	R40.2211	S02.122B	S06.333A	S06.387A	S06.9X8A	S12.200B	S12.690B	S14.148A	S21.452A	S22.081B	S25.02XA	S26.021A	S31.612A
O41.1213	O60.12X4	R40.2212	S02.129B	S06.334A	S06.388A	S11.011A	S12.201B	S12.691B	S14.151A	S21.459A	S22.082B	S25.09XA	S26.022A	S31.613A
O41.1214	O60.12X5	R40.2213	S02.19XB	S06.335A	S06.4X0A	S11.012A	S12.230B	S12.8XXA	S14.152A	S22.000B	S22.088B	S25.101A	S26.12XA	S31.614A
O41.1215	O60.12X9	R40.2214	S02.91XB	S06.336A	S06.4X1A	S11.013A	S12.231B	S14.0XXA	S14.153A	S22.001B	S22.089B	S25.102A	S26.92XA	S31.615A
O41.1219	O60.13X0	R40.2220	S06.1X0A	S06.337A	S06.4X2A	S11.014A	S12.24XB	S14.101A	S14.154A	S22.002B	S22.20XA	S25.109A	S27.1XXA	S31.619A
O41.1220	O60.13X1	R40.2221	S06.1X1A	S06.338A	S06.4X3A	S11.015A	S12.250B	S14.102A	S14.155A	S22.008B	S22.20XB	S25.111A	S27.2XXA	S31.620A
O41.1221	O60.13X2	R40.2222	S06.1X2A	S06.339A	S06.4X4A	S11.019A	S12.251B	S14.103A	S14.156A	S22.009B	S22.21XB	S25.112A	S27.331A	S31.621A
O41.1222	O60.13X3	R40.2223	S06.1X3A	S06.340A	S06.4X5A	S11.021A	S12.290B	S14.104A	S14.157A	S22.010B	S22.22XB	S25.119A	S27.332A	S31.622A
O41.1223	O60.13X4	R40.2224	S06.1X4A	S06.341A	S06.4X6A	S11.022A	S12.291B	S14.105A	S14.158A	S22.011B	S22.23XB	S25.121A	S27.339A	S31.623A
O41.1224	O60.13X5	R40.2310	S06.1X5A	S06.342A	S06.4X7A	S11.023A	S12.300B	S14.106A	S21.301A	S22.012B	S22.24XB	S25.122A	S27.401A	S31.624A
O41.1225	O60.13X9	R40.2311	S06.1X6A	S06.343A	S06.4X8A	S11.024A	S12.301B	S14.107A	S21.302A	S22.018B	S22.31XB	S25.129A	S27.402A	S31.625A
O41.1229	O60.14X0	R40.2312	S06.1X7A	S06.344A	S06.4X9A	S11.025A	S12.330B	S14.108A	S21.309A	S22.019B	S22.32XB	S25.191A	S27.409A	S31.629A
O41.1230	O60.14X1	R40.2313	S06.1X8A	S06.345A	S06.5X0A	S11.029A	S12.331B	S14.111A	S21.311A	S22.020B	S22.39XB	S25.192A	S27.411A	S31.630A
O41.1231	O60.14X2	R40.2314	S06.1X9A	S06.346A	S06.5X1A	S11.031A	S12.34XB	S14.112A	S21.312A	S22.021B	S22.41XB	S25.199A	S27.412A	S31.631A
O41.1232	O60.14X3	R40.2320	S06.2X6A	S06.347A	S06.5X2A	S11.032A	S12.350B	S14.113A	S21.319A	S22.022B	S22.42XB	S25.20XA	S27.419A	S31.632A
O41.1233	O60.14X4	R40.2321	S06.2X7A	S06.348A	S06.5X3A	S11.033A	S12.351B	S14.114A	S21.321A	S22.028B	S22.43XB	S25.21XA	S27.421A	S31.633A
O41.1234	O60.14X5	R40.2322	S06.2X8A	S06.349A	S06.5X4A	S11.034A	S12.390B	S14.115A	S21.322A	S22.029B	S22.49XB	S25.22XA	S27.422A	S31.634A
O41.1235	O60.14X9	R40.2323	S06.306A	S06.350A	S06.5X5A	S11.035A	S12.391B	S14.116A	S21.329A	S22.030B	S22.5XXA	S25.29XA	S27.429A	S31.635A
O41.1239	O60.22X0	R40.2324	S06.307A	S06.351A	S06.5X6A	S11.039A	S12.400B	S14.117A	S21.331A	S22.031B	S22.5XXB	S25.301A	S27.431A	S31.639A
O41.1410	O60.22X1	R40.2340	S06.308A	S06.352A	S06.5X7A	S12.000B	S12.401B	S14.118A	S21.332A	S22.032B	S22.9XXB	S25.302A	S27.432A	S31.640A

Major Complication or Comorbidity (MCC) (cont.) - Based on CMS data

S31.641A	S32.402B	S32.471B	S34.131A	S37.099A	S42.399B	S52.022B	S52.189C	S52.282B	S52.366C	S52.602B	S72.035C	S72.115B	S72.326C	S72.391C
S31.642A	S32.409B	S32.472A	S34.132A	S42.201B	S42.401B	S52.022C	S52.201B	S52.282C	S52.371B	S52.602C	S72.036A	S72.115C	S72.331A	S72.392A
S31.643A	S32.411A	S32.472B	S34.139A	S42.202B	S42.402B	S52.023B	S52.201C	S52.283B	S52.371C	S52.609B	S72.036B	S72.116B	S72.331B	S72.392B
S31.644A	S32.411B	S32.473A	S34.3XXA	S42.209B	S42.409B	S52.023C	S52.202B	S52.283C	S52.372B	S52.609C	S72.036C	S72.116C	S72.331C	S72.392C
S31.645A	S32.412A	S32.473B	S35.00XA	S42.211B	S42.411B	S52.024B	S52.202C	S52.291B	S52.372C	S52.611B	S72.041A	S72.121B	S72.332A	S72.399A
S31.649A	S32.412B	S32.474A	S35.01XA	S42.212B	S42.412B	S52.024C	S52.209B	S52.291C	S52.379B	S52.611C	S72.041B	S72.121C	S72.332B	S72.399B
S31.650A	S32.413A	S32.474B	S35.02XA	S42.213B	S42.413B	S52.025B	S52.209C	S52.292B	S52.379C	S52.612B	S72.041C	S72.122B	S72.332C	S72.399C
S31.651A	S32.413B	S32.475A	S35.09XA	S42.214B	S42.414B	S52.025C	S52.221B	S52.292C	S52.381B	S52.612C	S72.042A	S72.122C	S72.333A	S72.401B
S31.652A	S32.414A	S32.475B	S35.10XA	S42.215B	S42.415B	S52.026B	S52.221C	S52.299B	S52.381C	S52.613B	S72.042B	S72.123B	S72.333B	S72.401C
S31.653A	S32.414B	S32.476A	S35.11XA	S42.216B	S42.416B	S52.026C	S52.222B	S52.299C	S52.382B	S52.613C	S72.042C	S72.123C	S72.333C	S72.402B
S31.654A	S32.415A	S32.476B	S35.12XA	S42.221B	S42.421B	S52.031B	S52.222C	S52.301B	S52.382C	S52.614B	S72.043A	S72.124B	S72.334A	S72.402C
S31.655A	S32.415B	S32.481A	S35.19XA	S42.222B	S42.422B	S52.031C	S52.223B	S52.301C	S52.389B	S52.614C	S72.043B	S72.124C	S72.334B	S72.409B
S31.659A	S32.416A	S32.481B	S35.211A	S42.223B	S42.423B	S52.032B	S52.223C	S52.302B	S52.389C	S52.615B	S72.043C	S72.125B	S72.334C	S72.409C
S32.000B	S32.416B	S32.482A	S35.212A	S42.224B	S42.424B	S52.032C	S52.224B	S52.302C	S52.391B	S52.615C	S72.044A	S72.125C	S72.335A	S72.411B
S32.001B	S32.421A	S32.482B	S35.218A	S42.225B	S42.425B	S52.033B	S52.224C	S52.309B	S52.391C	S52.616B	S72.044B	S72.126B	S72.335B	S72.411C
S32.002B	S32.421B	S32.483A	S35.219A	S42.226B	S42.426B	S52.033C	S52.225B	S52.309C	S52.392B	S52.616C	S72.044C	S72.126C	S72.335C	S72.412B
S32.008B	S32.422A	S32.483B	S35.221A	S42.231B	S42.431B	S52.034B	S52.225C	S52.321B	S52.392C	S52.691B	S72.045A	S72.131B	S72.336A	S72.412C
S32.009B	S32.422B	S32.484A	S35.222A	S42.232B	S42.432B	S52.034C	S52.226B	S52.321C	S52.399B	S52.691C	S72.045B	S72.131C	S72.336B	S72.413B
S32.010B	S32.423A	S32.484B	S35.228A	S42.239B	S42.433B	S52.035B	S52.226C	S52.322B	S52.399C	S52.692B	S72.045C	S72.132B	S72.336C	S72.413C
S32.011B	S32.423B	S32.485A	S35.229A	S42.241B	S42.434B	S52.035C	S52.231B	S52.322C	S52.501B	S52.692C	S72.046A	S72.132C	S72.341A	S72.414B
S32.012B	S32.424A	S32.485B	S35.231A	S42.242B	S42.435B	S52.036B	S52.231C	S52.323B	S52.501C	S52.699B	S72.046B	S72.133B	S72.341B	S72.414C
S32.018B	S32.424B	S32.486A	S35.232A	S42.249B	S42.436B	S52.036C	S52.232B	S52.323C	S52.502B	S52.699C	S72.046C	S72.133C	S72.341C	S72.415B
S32.019B	S32.425A	S32.486B	S35.238A	S42.251B	S42.441B	S52.041B	S52.232C	S52.324B	S52.502C	S52.90XB	S72.051A	S72.134B	S72.342A	S72.415C
S32.020B	S32.425B	S32.491A	S35.239A	S42.252B	S42.442B	S52.041C	S52.233B	S52.324C	S52.509B	S52.90XC	S72.051B	S72.134C	S72.342B	S72.416B
S32.021B	S32.426A	S32.491B	S35.291A	S42.253B	S42.443B	S52.042B	S52.233C	S52.325B	S52.509C	S52.91XB	S72.051C	S72.135B	S72.342C	S72.416C
S32.022B	S32.426B	S32.492A	S35.292A	S42.254B	S42.444B	S52.042C	S52.234B	S52.325C	S52.511B	S52.91XC	S72.052A	S72.135C	S72.343A	S72.421B
S32.028B	S32.431A	S32.492B	S35.298A	S42.255B	S42.445B	S52.043B	S52.234C	S52.326B	S52.511C	S52.92XB	S72.052B	S72.136B	S72.343B	S72.421C
S32.029B	S32.431B	S32.499A	S35.299A	S42.256B	S42.446B	S52.043C	S52.235B	S52.326C	S52.512B	S52.92XC	S72.052C	S72.136C	S72.343C	S72.422B
S32.030B	S32.432A	S32.499B	S35.311A	S42.261B	S42.447B	S52.044B	S52.235C	S52.331B	S52.512C	S72.001A	S72.059A	S72.141B	S72.344A	S72.422C
S32.031B	S32.432B	S32.501B	S35.318A	S42.262B	S42.448B	S52.044C	S52.236B	S52.331C	S52.513B	S72.001B	S72.059B	S72.141C	S72.344B	S72.423B
S32.032B	S32.433A	S32.502B	S35.319A	S42.263B	S42.449B	S52.045B	S52.236C	S52.332B	S52.513C	S72.001C	S72.059C	S72.142B	S72.344C	S72.423C
S32.038B	S32.433B	S32.509B	S35.321A	S42.264B	S42.451B	S52.045C	S52.241B	S52.332C	S52.514B	S72.002A	S72.061A	S72.142C	S72.345A	S72.424B
S32.039B	S32.434A	S32.511B	S35.328A	S42.265B	S42.452B	S52.046B	S52.241C	S52.333B	S52.514C	S72.002B	S72.061B	S72.143B	S72.345B	S72.424C
S32.040B	S32.434B	S32.512B	S35.329A	S42.266B	S42.453B	S52.046C	S52.242B	S52.333C	S52.515B	S72.002C	S72.061C	S72.143C	S72.345C	S72.425B
S32.041B	S32.435A	S32.519B	S35.331A	S42.291B	S42.454B	S52.091B	S52.242C	S52.334B	S52.515C	S72.009A	S72.062A	S72.144B	S72.346A	S72.425C
S32.042B	S32.435B	S32.591B	S35.338A	S42.292B	S42.455B	S52.091C	S52.243B	S52.334C	S52.516B	S72.009B	S72.062B	S72.144C	S72.346B	S72.426B
S32.048B	S32.436A	S32.592B	S35.339A	S42.293B	S42.456B	S52.092B	S52.243C	S52.335B	S52.516C	S72.009C	S72.062C	S72.145B	S72.346C	S72.426C
S32.049B	S32.436B	S32.599B	S35.341A	S42.294B	S42.461B	S52.092C	S52.244B	S52.335C	S52.531B	S72.011B	S72.063A	S72.145C	S72.351A	S72.431B
S32.050B	S32.441A	S32.601B	S35.348A	S42.295B	S42.462B	S52.099B	S52.244C	S52.336B	S52.531C	S72.011C	S72.063B	S72.146B	S72.351B	S72.431C
S32.051B	S32.441B	S32.602B	S35.349A	S42.296B	S42.463B	S52.099C	S52.245B	S52.336C	S52.532B	S72.012B	S72.063C	S72.146C	S72.351C	S72.432B
S32.052B	S32.442A	S32.609B	S35.401A	S42.301B	S42.464B	S52.101B	S52.245C	S52.341B	S52.532C	S72.012C	S72.064A	S72.21XB	S72.352A	S72.432C
S32.058B	S32.442B	S32.611B	S35.402A	S42.302B	S42.465B	S52.101C	S52.246B	S52.341C	S52.539B	S72.019B	S72.064B	S72.21XC	S72.352B	S72.433B
S32.059B	S32.443A	S32.612B	S35.403A	S42.309B	S42.466B	S52.102B	S52.246C	S52.342B	S52.539C	S72.019C	S72.064C	S72.22XB	S72.352C	S72.433C
S32.10XB	S32.443B	S32.613B	S35.404A	S42.321B	S42.471B	S52.102C	S52.251B	S52.342C	S52.541B	S72.021A	S72.065A	S72.22XC	S72.353A	S72.434B
S32.110B	S32.444A	S32.614B	S35.405A	S42.322B	S42.472B	S52.109B	S52.251C	S52.343B	S52.541C	S72.021B	S72.065B	S72.23XB	S72.353B	S72.434C
S32.111B	S32.444B	S32.615B	S35.406A	S42.323B	S42.473B	S52.109C	S52.252B	S52.343C	S52.542B	S72.021C	S72.065C	S72.23XC	S72.353C	S72.435B
S32.112B	S32.445A	S32.616B	S35.411A	S42.324B	S42.474B	S52.121B	S52.252C	S52.344B	S52.542C	S72.022A	S72.066A	S72.24XB	S72.354A	S72.435C
S32.119B	S32.445B	S32.691B	S35.412A	S42.325B	S42.475B	S52.121C	S52.253B	S52.344C	S52.549B	S72.022B	S72.066B	S72.24XC	S72.354B	S72.436B
S32.120B	S32.446A	S32.692B	S35.413A	S42.326B	S42.476B	S52.122B	S52.253C	S52.345B	S52.549C	S72.022C	S72.066C	S72.25XB	S72.354C	S72.436C
S32.121B	S32.446B	S32.699B	S35.414A	S42.331B	S42.491B	S52.122C	S52.254B	S52.345C	S52.551B	S72.023A	S72.091A	S72.25XC	S72.355A	S72.441B
S32.122B	S32.451A	S32.810B	S35.415A	S42.332B	S42.492B	S52.123B	S52.254C	S52.346B	S52.551C	S72.023B	S72.091B	S72.26XB	S72.355B	S72.441C
S32.129B	S32.451B	S32.811B	S35.416A	S42.333B	S42.493B	S52.123C	S52.255B	S52.346C	S52.552B	S72.023C	S72.091C	S72.26XC	S72.355C	S72.442B
S32.130B	S32.452A	S32.82XB	S35.491A	S42.334B	S42.494B	S52.124B	S52.255C	S52.351B	S52.552C	S72.024A	S72.092A	S72.301B	S72.356A	S72.442C
S32.131B	S32.452B	S32.89XB	S35.492A	S42.335B	S42.495B	S52.124C	S52.256B	S52.351C	S52.559B	S72.024B	S72.092B	S72.301C	S72.356B	S72.443B
S32.132B	S32.453A	S32.9XXB	S35.493A	S42.336B	S42.496B	S52.125B	S52.256C	S52.352B	S52.559C	S72.024C	S72.092C	S72.302B	S72.356C	S72.443C
S32.139B	S32.453B	S34.01XA	S35.494A	S42.341B	S42.90XB	S52.125C	S52.261B	S52.352C	S52.561B	S72.025A	S72.099A	S72.302C	S72.361A	S72.444B
S32.14XB	S32.454A	S34.02XA	S35.495A	S42.342B	S42.91XB	S52.126B	S52.261C	S52.353B	S52.561C	S72.025B	S72.099B	S72.309B	S72.361B	S72.444C
S32.15XB	S32.454B	S34.101A	S35.496A	S42.343B	S42.92XB	S52.126C	S52.262B	S52.353C	S52.562B	S72.025C	S72.099C	S72.309C	S72.361C	S72.445B
S32.16XB	S32.455A	S34.102A	S35.50XA	S42.344B	S45.001A	S52.131B	S52.262C	S52.354B	S52.562C	S72.026A	S72.101A	S72.321A	S72.362A	S72.445C
S32.17XB	S32.455B	S34.103A	S35.511A	S42.345B	S45.002A	S52.131C	S52.263B	S52.354C	S52.569B	S72.026B	S72.101B	S72.321B	S72.362B	S72.446B
S32.19XB	S32.456A	S34.104A	S35.512A	S42.346B	S45.009A	S52.132B	S52.263C	S52.355B	S52.569C	S72.026C	S72.101C	S72.321C	S72.362C	S72.446C
S32.2XXB	S32.456B	S34.105A	S35.513A	S42.351B	S45.011A	S52.132C	S52.264B	S52.355C	S52.571B	S72.031A	S72.102A	S72.322A	S72.363A	S72.451B
S32.301B	S32.461A	S34.109A	S35.514A	S42.352B	S45.012A	S52.133B	S52.264C	S52.356B	S52.571C	S72.031B	S72.102B	S72.322B	S72.363B	S72.451C
S32.302B	S32.461B	S34.111A	S35.515A	S42.353B	S45.019A	S52.133C	S52.265B	S52.356C	S52.572B	S72.031C	S72.102C	S72.322C	S72.363C	S72.452B
S32.309B	S32.462A	S34.112A	S35.516A	S42.354B	S45.091A	S52.134B	S52.265C	S52.361B	S52.572C	S72.032A	S72.109A	S72.323A	S72.364A	S72.452C
S32.311B	S32.462B	S34.113A	S35.59XA	S42.355B	S45.092A	S52.134C	S52.266B	S52.361C	S52.579B	S72.032B	S72.109B	S72.323B	S72.364B	S72.453B
S32.312B	S32.463A	S34.114A	S36.031A	S42.356B	S45.099A	S52.135B	S52.266C	S52.362B	S52.579C	S72.032C	S72.109C	S72.323C	S72.364C	S72.453C
S32.313B	S32.463B	S34.115A	S36.032A	S42.361B	S52.001B	S52.135C	S52.271B	S52.362C	S52.591B	S72.033A	S72.111B	S72.324A	S72.365A	S72.454B
S32.314B	S32.464A	S34.119A	S36.115A	S42.362B	S52.001C	S52.136B	S52.271C	S52.363B	S52.591C	S72.033B	S72.111C	S72.324B	S72.365B	S72.454C
S32.315B	S32.464B	S34.121A	S36.116A	S42.363B	S52.002B	S52.136C	S52.272B	S52.363C	S52.592B	S72.033C	S72.112B	S72.324C	S72.365C	S72.455B
S32.316B	S32.465A	S34.122A	S37.061A	S42.364B	S52.002C	S52.181B	S52.272C	S52.364B	S52.592C	S72.034A	S72.112C	S72.325A	S72.366A	S72.455C
S32.391B	S32.465B	S34.123A	S37.062A	S42.365B	S52.009B	S52.181C	S52.279B	S52.364C	S52.599B	S72.034B	S72.113B	S72.325B	S72.366B	S72.456B
S32.392B	S32.466A	S34.124A	S37.069A	S42.366B	S52.009C	S52.182B	S52.279C	S52.365B	S52.599C	S72.034C	S72.113C	S72.325C	S72.366C	S72.456C
S32.399B	S32.466B	S34.125A	S37.091A	S42.391B	S52.021B	S52.182C	S52.281B	S52.365C	S52.601B	S72.035A	S72.114B	S72.326A	S72.391A	S72.461B
S32.401B	S32.471A	S34.129A	S37.092A	S42.392B	S52.021C	S52.189B	S52.281C	S52.366B	S52.601C	S72.035B	S72.114C	S72.326B	S72.391B	S72.461C

(side tab) S72.462B - O36.1133 · APPENDIX B: SYMBOLS FOR 7TH-CHARACTER CODES

Major Complication or Comorbidity (MCC) (cont.) - Based on CMS data

S72.462B	S72.8X9A	S75.092A	S79.099A	S82.122C	S82.141C	S82.156C	S82.225C	S82.244C	S82.263C	S82.422C	S82.441C	S82.456C	S82.832C	S85.092A
S72.462C	S72.8X9B	S75.099A	S82.101B	S82.123B	S82.142B	S82.191B	S82.226B	S82.245B	S82.264B	S82.423B	S82.442B	S82.461B	S82.839B	S85.099A
S72.463B	S72.8X9C	S75.101A	S82.101C	S82.123C	S82.142C	S82.191C	S82.226C	S82.245C	S82.264C	S82.423C	S82.442C	S82.461C	S82.839C	S85.501A
S72.463C	S72.90XA	S75.102A	S82.102B	S82.124B	S82.143B	S82.192B	S82.231B	S82.246B	S82.265B	S82.424B	S82.443B	S82.462B	S82.861B	S85.502A
S72.464B	S72.90XB	S75.109A	S82.102C	S82.124C	S82.143C	S82.192C	S82.231C	S82.246C	S82.265C	S82.424C	S82.443C	S82.462C	S82.861C	S85.509A
S72.464C	S72.90XC	S75.111A	S82.109B	S82.125B	S82.144B	S82.199B	S82.232B	S82.251B	S82.266B	S82.425B	S82.444B	S82.463B	S82.862B	S85.511A
S72.465B	S72.91XA	S75.112A	S82.109C	S82.125C	S82.144C	S82.199C	S82.232C	S82.251C	S82.266C	S82.425C	S82.444C	S82.463C	S82.862C	S85.512A
S72.465C	S72.91XB	S75.119A	S82.111B	S82.126B	S82.145B	S82.201B	S82.233B	S82.252B	S82.291B	S82.426B	S82.445B	S82.464B	S82.863B	S85.519A
S72.466B	S72.91XC	S75.121A	S82.111C	S82.126C	S82.145C	S82.201C	S82.233C	S82.252C	S82.291C	S82.426C	S82.445C	S82.464C	S82.863C	S85.591A
S72.466C	S72.92XA	S75.122A	S82.112B	S82.131B	S82.146B	S82.202B	S82.234B	S82.253B	S82.292B	S82.431B	S82.446B	S82.465B	S82.864B	S85.592A
S72.491B	S72.92XB	S75.129A	S82.112C	S82.131C	S82.146C	S82.202C	S82.234C	S82.253C	S82.292C	S82.431C	S82.446C	S82.465C	S82.864C	S85.599A
S72.491C	S72.92XC	S75.191A	S82.113B	S82.132B	S82.151B	S82.209B	S82.235B	S82.254B	S82.299B	S82.432B	S82.451B	S82.466B	S82.865B	T79.0XXA
S72.492B	S75.001A	S75.192A	S82.113C	S82.132C	S82.151C	S82.209C	S82.235C	S82.254C	S82.299C	S82.432C	S82.451C	S82.466C	S82.865C	T79.1XXA
S72.492C	S75.002A	S75.199A	S82.114B	S82.133B	S82.152B	S82.221B	S82.236B	S82.255B	S82.401B	S82.433B	S82.452B	S82.491B	S82.866B	T79.4XXA
S72.499B	S75.009A	S79.001A	S82.114C	S82.133C	S82.152C	S82.221C	S82.236C	S82.255C	S82.401C	S82.433C	S82.452C	S82.491C	S82.866C	T79.5XXA
S72.499C	S75.011A	S79.002A	S82.115B	S82.134B	S82.153B	S82.222B	S82.241B	S82.256B	S82.402B	S82.434B	S82.453B	S82.492B	S85.001A	T80.0XXA
S72.8X1A	S75.012A	S79.009A	S82.115C	S82.134C	S82.153C	S82.222C	S82.241C	S82.256C	S82.402C	S82.434C	S82.453C	S82.492C	S85.002A	T81.11XA
S72.8X1B	S75.019A	S79.011A	S82.116B	S82.135B	S82.154B	S82.223B	S82.242B	S82.261B	S82.409B	S82.435B	S82.454B	S82.499B	S85.009A	T81.12XA
S72.8X1C	S75.021A	S79.012A	S82.116C	S82.135C	S82.154C	S82.223C	S82.242C	S82.261C	S82.409C	S82.435C	S82.454C	S82.499C	S85.011A	T81.19XA
S72.8X2A	S75.022A	S79.019A	S82.121B	S82.136B	S82.155B	S82.224B	S82.243B	S82.262B	S82.421B	S82.436B	S82.455B	S82.831B	S85.012A	
S72.8X2B	S75.029A	S79.091A	S82.121C	S82.136C	S82.155C	S82.224C	S82.243C	S82.262C	S82.421C	S82.436C	S82.455C	S82.831C	S85.019A	
S72.8X2C	S75.091A	S79.092A	S82.122B	S82.141B	S82.156B	S82.225B	S82.244B	S82.263B	S82.422B	S82.441B	S82.456B	S82.832B	S85.091A	

Male - Based on Medicare's Outpatient Code Editor (OCE)

S30.201A	S30.813S	S30.842D	S30.855A	S30.872S	S30.96XD	S31.24XA	S31.32XS	S31.511D	S37.822A	S38.001S	S38.231D	T21.16XA	T21.56XS	T83.490D
S30.201D	S30.815A	S30.842S	S30.855D	S30.873A	S30.96XS	S31.24XD	S31.33XA	S31.511S	S37.822D	S38.01XD	S38.231S	T21.16XD	T21.66XA	T83.490S
S30.201S	S30.815D	S30.843A	S30.855S	S30.873D	S31.20XA	S31.24XS	S31.33XD	S31.521A	S37.822S	S38.01XS	S38.232A	T21.16XS	T21.66XD	
S30.21XA	S30.815S	S30.843D	S30.862A	S30.873S	S31.20XD	S31.25XA	S31.33XS	S31.521D	S37.823A	S38.02XA	S38.232D	T21.26XA	T21.66XS	
S30.21XD	S30.822A	S30.843S	S30.862D	S30.875A	S31.20XS	S31.25XD	S31.34XA	S31.521S	S37.823D	S38.02XD	S38.232S	T21.26XD	T21.76XA	
S30.21XS	S30.822D	S30.845A	S30.862S	S30.875D	S31.21XA	S31.25XS	S31.34XD	S31.531A	S37.823S	S38.02XS	S39.840A	T21.26XS	T21.76XD	
S30.22XA	S30.822S	S30.845D	S30.863A	S30.875S	S31.21XD	S31.30XA	S31.34XS	S31.531D	S37.828A	S38.221A	S39.840D	T21.36XA	T21.76XS	
S30.22XD	S30.823A	S30.845S	S30.863D	S30.93XA	S31.21XS	S31.30XD	S31.35XA	S31.531S	S37.828D	S38.221D	S39.840S	T21.36XD	T83.410A	
S30.22XS	S30.823D	S30.852A	S30.863S	S30.93XD	S31.22XA	S31.30XS	S31.35XD	S31.541A	S37.828S	S38.221S	T19.4XXA	T21.36XS	T83.410D	
S30.812A	S30.823S	S30.852D	S30.865A	S30.93XS	S31.22XD	S31.31XA	S31.35XS	S31.541D	S37.829A	S38.222A	T19.4XXD	T21.46XA	T83.420A	
S30.812D	S30.825A	S30.852S	S30.865D	S30.94XA	S31.22XS	S31.31XD	S31.501A	S31.541S	S37.829D	S38.222D	T19.4XXS	T21.46XD	T83.420D	
S30.812S	S30.825D	S30.853A	S30.865S	S30.94XD	S31.23XA	S31.31XS	S31.501D	S31.551A	S37.829S	S38.222S	T21.06XA	T21.46XS	T83.420S	
S30.813A	S30.825S	S30.853D	S30.872A	S30.94XS	S31.23XD	S31.32XA	S31.501S	S31.551D	S38.001A	S38.231A	T21.06XD	T21.56XA	T83.490A	
S30.813D	S30.842A	S30.853S	S30.872D	S30.96XA	S31.23XS	S31.32XD	S31.511A	S31.551S	S38.001D		T21.06XS	T21.56XD		

Manifestation - Based on CMS data

E08.3211	E08.3291	E08.3311	E08.3391	E08.3411	E08.3491	E08.3511	E08.3521	E08.3531	E08.3541	E08.3551	E08.3591	E08.37X1
E08.3212	E08.3292	E08.3312	E08.3392	E08.3412	E08.3492	E08.3512	E08.3522	E08.3532	E08.3542	E08.3552	E08.3592	E08.37X2
E08.3213	E08.3293	E08.3313	E08.3393	E08.3413	E08.3493	E08.3513	E08.3523	E08.3533	E08.3543	E08.3553	E08.3593	E08.37X3
E08.3219	E08.3299	E08.3319	E08.3399	E08.3419	E08.3499	E08.3519	E08.3529	E08.3539	E08.3549	E08.3559	E08.3599	E08.37X9

Maternity - Based on Medicare's Outpatient Code Editor (OCE)

O31.00X0	O31.03X4	O31.13X1	O31.22X5	O31.32X2	O31.8X29	O32.1XX3	O32.6XX0	O33.3XX4	O33.7XX1	O35.2XX5	O35.6XX2	O35.9XX9	O36.0193	O36.0990
O31.00X1	O31.03X5	O31.13X2	O31.22X9	O31.32X3	O31.8X30	O32.1XX4	O32.6XX1	O33.3XX5	O33.7XX2	O35.3XX0	O35.6XX3	O36.0110	O36.0194	O36.0991
O31.00X2	O31.03X9	O31.13X3	O31.23X0	O31.32X4	O31.8X31	O32.1XX5	O32.6XX2	O33.3XX9	O33.7XX3	O35.3XX1	O35.6XX4	O36.0111	O36.0195	O36.0992
O31.00X3	O31.10X0	O31.13X4	O31.23X1	O31.32X5	O31.8X32	O32.1XX9	O32.6XX3	O33.4XX0	O33.7XX4	O35.3XX2	O35.6XX5	O36.0112	O36.0199	O36.0993
O31.00X4	O31.10X1	O31.13X5	O31.23X2	O31.33X0	O31.8X33	O32.2XX0	O32.6XX4	O33.4XX1	O33.7XX5	O35.3XX3	O35.6XX9	O36.0113	O36.0910	O36.0994
O31.00X5	O31.10X2	O31.13X9	O31.23X3	O31.33X1	O31.8X34	O32.2XX1	O32.6XX5	O33.4XX2	O35.0XX0	O35.3XX4	O35.7XX0	O36.0114	O36.0911	O36.0995
O31.00X9	O31.10X3	O31.20X0	O31.23X4	O31.33X2	O31.8X35	O32.2XX2	O32.6XX9	O33.4XX3	O35.0XX1	O35.3XX5	O35.7XX1	O36.0115	O36.0912	O36.0999
O31.01X0	O31.10X4	O31.20X1	O31.23X5	O31.33X3	O31.8X39	O32.2XX3	O32.8XX0	O33.4XX4	O35.0XX2	O35.3XX9	O35.7XX2	O36.0119	O36.0913	O36.1110
O31.01X1	O31.10X5	O31.20X2	O31.23X9	O31.33X4	O31.8X90	O32.2XX4	O32.8XX1	O33.4XX5	O35.0XX3	O35.4XX0	O35.7XX3	O36.0120	O36.0914	O36.1111
O31.01X2	O31.10X9	O31.20X3	O31.30X0	O31.33X5	O31.8X91	O32.2XX5	O32.8XX2	O33.4XX9	O35.0XX4	O35.4XX1	O35.7XX4	O36.0121	O36.0915	O36.1112
O31.01X3	O31.11X0	O31.20X4	O31.30X1	O31.33X9	O31.8X92	O32.2XX9	O32.8XX3	O33.5XX0	O35.0XX5	O35.4XX2	O35.7XX5	O36.0122	O36.0919	O36.1113
O31.01X4	O31.11X1	O31.20X5	O31.30X2	O31.8X10	O31.8X93	O32.3XX0	O32.8XX4	O33.5XX1	O35.1XX0	O35.4XX3	O35.7XX9	O36.0123	O36.0920	O36.1114
O31.01X5	O31.11X2	O31.20X9	O31.30X3	O31.8X11	O31.8X94	O32.3XX1	O32.8XX5	O33.5XX2	O35.1XX1	O35.4XX4	O35.8XX0	O36.0124	O36.0921	O36.1115
O31.01X9	O31.11X3	O31.21X0	O31.30X4	O31.8X12	O31.8X95	O32.3XX2	O32.8XX9	O33.5XX3	O35.1XX2	O35.4XX5	O35.8XX1	O36.0125	O36.0922	O36.1119
O31.02X0	O31.11X4	O31.21X1	O31.30X5	O31.8X13	O31.8X99	O32.3XX3	O32.9XX0	O33.5XX4	O35.1XX3	O35.4XX9	O35.8XX2	O36.0129	O36.0923	O36.1120
O31.02X1	O31.11X5	O31.21X2	O31.30X9	O31.8X14	O32.0XX0	O32.3XX4	O32.9XX1	O33.5XX5	O35.1XX4	O35.5XX0	O35.8XX3	O36.0130	O36.0924	O36.1121
O31.02X2	O31.11X9	O31.21X3	O31.31X0	O31.8X15	O32.0XX1	O32.3XX5	O32.9XX2	O33.5XX9	O35.1XX5	O35.5XX1	O35.8XX4	O36.0131	O36.0925	O36.1122
O31.02X3	O31.12X0	O31.21X4	O31.31X1	O31.8X16	O32.0XX2	O32.3XX9	O32.9XX3	O33.6XX0	O35.1XX9	O35.5XX2	O35.8XX5	O36.0132	O36.0929	O36.1123
O31.02X4	O31.12X1	O31.21X5	O31.31X2	O31.8X20	O32.0XX3	O32.4XX0	O32.9XX4	O33.6XX1	O35.2XX0	O35.5XX3	O35.8XX9	O36.0133	O36.0930	O36.1124
O31.02X5	O31.12X2	O31.21X9	O31.31X3	O31.8X21	O32.0XX4	O32.4XX1	O32.9XX5	O33.6XX2	O35.2XX1	O35.5XX4	O35.9XX0	O36.0134	O36.0931	O36.1125
O31.02X9	O31.12X3	O31.22X0	O31.31X4	O31.8X22	O32.0XX5	O32.4XX2	O32.9XX9	O33.6XX3	O35.2XX2	O35.5XX5	O35.9XX1	O36.0135	O36.0932	O36.1129
O31.03X0	O31.12X4	O31.22X1	O31.31X5	O31.8X23	O32.0XX9	O32.4XX3	O33.3XX0	O33.6XX4	O35.2XX3	O35.6XX0	O35.9XX2	O36.0139	O36.0933	O36.1130
O31.03X1	O31.12X5	O31.22X2	O31.31X9	O31.8X24	O32.1XX0	O32.4XX4	O33.3XX1	O33.6XX5	O35.2XX4	O35.6XX1	O35.9XX3	O36.0190	O36.0934	O36.1131
O31.03X2	O31.12X9	O31.22X3	O31.32X0	O31.8X25	O32.1XX1	O32.4XX5	O33.3XX2	O33.7XX0			O35.9XX4	O36.0191	O36.0935	O36.1132
O31.03X3	O31.13X0	O31.22X4	O31.32X1		O32.1XX2	O32.4XX9	O33.3XX3				O35.9XX5	O36.0192	O36.0939	O36.1133

Maternity (cont.) - Based on Medicare's Outpatient Code Editor (OCE)

O36.1134	O36.21X2	O36.5190	O36.61X5	O36.80X3	O36.8291	O36.8929	O40.1XX4	O41.03X2	O41.1230	O41.8X15	O41.93X3	O60.23X1	O64.5XX9	O69.4XX4
O36.1135	O36.21X3	O36.5191	O36.61X9	O36.80X4	O36.8292	O36.8930	O40.1XX5	O41.03X3	O41.1231	O41.8X19	O41.93X4	O60.23X2	O64.8XX0	O69.4XX5
O36.1139	O36.21X4	O36.5192	O36.62X0	O36.80X5	O36.8293	O36.8931	O40.1XX9	O41.03X4	O41.1232	O41.8X20	O41.93X5	O60.23X3	O64.8XX1	O69.4XX9
O36.1190	O36.21X5	O36.5193	O36.62X1	O36.80X9	O36.8294	O36.8932	O40.2XX0	O41.03X5	O41.1233	O41.8X21	O41.93X9	O60.23X4	O64.8XX2	O69.5XX0
O36.1191	O36.21X9	O36.5194	O36.62X2	O36.8120	O36.8295	O36.8933	O40.2XX1	O41.03X9	O41.1234	O41.8X22	O60.10X0	O60.23X5	O64.8XX3	O69.5XX1
O36.1192	O36.22X0	O36.5195	O36.62X3	O36.8121	O36.8299	O36.8934	O40.2XX2	O41.1010	O41.1235	O41.8X23	O60.10X1	O60.23X9	O64.8XX4	O69.5XX2
O36.1193	O36.22X1	O36.5199	O36.62X4	O36.8122	O36.8310	O36.8935	O40.2XX3	O41.1011	O41.1239	O41.8X24	O60.10X2	O64.0XX0	O64.8XX5	O69.5XX3
O36.1194	O36.22X2	O36.5910	O36.62X5	O36.8123	O36.8311	O36.8939	O40.2XX4	O41.1012	O41.1290	O41.8X25	O60.10X3	O64.0XX1	O64.8XX9	O69.5XX4
O36.1195	O36.22X3	O36.5911	O36.62X9	O36.8124	O36.8312	O36.8990	O40.2XX5	O41.1013	O41.1291	O41.8X29	O60.10X4	O64.0XX2	O64.9XX0	O69.5XX5
O36.1199	O36.22X4	O36.5912	O36.63X0	O36.8125	O36.8313	O36.8991	O40.2XX9	O41.1014	O41.1292	O41.8X31	O60.10X5	O64.0XX3	O64.9XX1	O69.5XX9
O36.1910	O36.22X5	O36.5913	O36.63X1	O36.8129	O36.8314	O36.8992	O40.3XX0	O41.1015	O41.1293	O41.8X32	O60.12X0	O64.0XX4	O64.9XX2	O69.81X0
O36.1911	O36.23X0	O36.5914	O36.63X2	O36.8130	O36.8315	O36.8993	O40.3XX1	O41.1019	O41.1294	O41.8X33	O60.12X1	O64.0XX5	O64.9XX3	O69.81X1
O36.1912	O36.23X0	O36.5915	O36.63X3	O36.8131	O36.8319	O36.8994	O40.3XX2	O41.1020	O41.1295	O41.8X34	O60.12X3	O64.0XX9	O64.9XX4	O69.81X2
O36.1913	O36.23X1	O36.5919	O36.63X4	O36.8132	O36.8320	O36.8995	O40.3XX3	O41.1021	O41.1299	O41.8X35	O60.12X4	O64.1XX0	O64.9XX5	O69.81X3
O36.1914	O36.23X2	O36.5920	O36.63X5	O36.8133	O36.8321	O36.8999	O40.3XX4	O41.1022	O41.1410	O41.8X39	O60.12X5	O64.1XX1	O64.9XX9	O69.81X4
O36.1915	O36.23X3	O36.5921	O36.63X9	O36.8134	O36.8322	O36.90X0	O40.3XX5	O41.1023	O41.1411	O41.8X90	O60.12X9	O64.1XX2	O69.0XX0	O69.81X5
O36.1919	O36.23X4	O36.5922	O36.70X0	O36.8135	O36.8323	O36.90X1	O40.3XX9	O41.1024	O41.1412	O41.8X91	O60.13X0	O64.1XX3	O69.0XX1	O69.81X9
O36.1920	O36.23X5	O36.5923	O36.70X1	O36.8139	O36.8324	O36.90X2	O40.9XX0	O41.1025	O41.1413	O41.8X92	O60.13X0	O64.1XX4	O69.0XX2	O69.82X0
O36.1921	O36.4XX0	O36.5924	O36.70X2	O36.8190	O36.8325	O36.90X3	O40.9XX1	O41.1029	O41.1414	O41.8X93	O60.13X1	O64.1XX5	O69.0XX3	O69.82X1
O36.1922	O36.4XX0	O36.5925	O36.70X3	O36.8191	O36.8329	O36.90X4	O40.9XX2	O41.1030	O41.1415	O41.8X94	O60.13X2	O64.1XX9	O69.0XX4	O69.82X2
O36.1923	O36.4XX1	O36.5929	O36.70X4	O36.8192	O36.8330	O36.90X5	O40.9XX3	O41.1031	O41.1419	O41.8X95	O60.13X3	O64.2XX0	O69.0XX5	O69.82X3
O36.1924	O36.4XX2	O36.5930	O36.70X5	O36.8193	O36.8331	O36.90X9	O40.9XX4	O41.1032	O41.1420	O41.8X99	O60.13X4	O64.2XX1	O69.0XX9	O69.82X4
O36.1925	O36.4XX3	O36.5931	O36.70X9	O36.8194	O36.8332	O36.91X0	O40.9XX5	O41.1033	O41.1421	O41.90X0	O60.13X5	O64.2XX2	O69.1XX0	O69.82X5
O36.1929	O36.4XX4	O36.5932	O36.71X0	O36.8195	O36.8333	O36.91X1	O40.9XX9	O41.1034	O41.1422	O41.90X1	O60.13X9	O64.2XX3	O69.1XX1	O69.82X9
O36.1930	O36.4XX5	O36.5933	O36.71X1	O36.8199	O36.8334	O36.91X2	O41.00X0	O41.1035	O41.1423	O41.90X3	O60.14X0	O64.2XX4	O69.1XX2	O69.89X0
O36.1931	O36.4XX9	O36.5934	O36.71X2	O36.8210	O36.8335	O36.91X3	O41.00X1	O41.1039	O41.1424	O41.90X4	O60.14X1	O64.2XX5	O69.1XX3	O69.89X1
O36.1932	O36.5110	O36.5935	O36.71X3	O36.8211	O36.8339	O36.91X4	O41.00X2	O41.1090	O41.1425	O41.90X5	O60.14X2	O64.2XX9	O69.1XX4	O69.89X2
O36.1933	O36.5111	O36.5939	O36.71X4	O36.8212	O36.8390	O36.91X5	O41.00X3	O41.1091	O41.1429	O41.90X9	O60.14X3	O64.3XX0	O69.1XX5	O69.89X3
O36.1934	O36.5112	O36.5990	O36.71X5	O36.8213	O36.8391	O36.91X9	O41.00X4	O41.1092	O41.1430	O41.91X0	O60.14X4	O64.3XX1	O69.1XX9	O69.89X4
O36.1935	O36.5113	O36.5991	O36.71X9	O36.8214	O36.8392	O36.92X0	O41.00X5	O41.1093	O41.1431	O41.91X0	O60.14X5	O64.3XX2	O69.2XX0	O69.89X5
O36.1939	O36.5114	O36.5992	O36.72X0	O36.8215	O36.8393	O36.92X1	O41.00X9	O41.1094	O41.1432	O41.91X1	O60.20X0	O64.3XX3	O69.2XX1	O69.89X9
O36.1990	O36.5115	O36.5993	O36.72X1	O36.8219	O36.8394	O36.92X2	O41.01X0	O41.1095	O41.1433	O41.91X1	O60.20X1	O64.3XX4	O69.2XX2	O69.9XX0
O36.1991	O36.5119	O36.5994	O36.72X2	O36.8220	O36.8395	O36.92X3	O41.01X1	O41.1099	O41.1434	O41.91X3	O60.20X2	O64.3XX5	O69.2XX3	O69.9XX1
O36.1992	O36.5120	O36.5995	O36.72X3	O36.8221	O36.8399	O36.92X4	O41.01X2	O41.1210	O41.1435	O41.91X4	O60.20X2	O64.3XX9	O69.2XX4	O69.9XX2
O36.1993	O36.5121	O36.5999	O36.72X4	O36.8222	O36.8910	O36.92X5	O41.01X3	O41.1211	O41.1439	O41.91X5	O60.20X2	O64.4XX0	O69.2XX5	O69.9XX3
O36.1994	O36.5122	O36.60X0	O36.72X5	O36.8223	O36.8911	O36.92X9	O41.01X4	O41.1212	O41.1490	O41.91X9	O60.20X3	O64.4XX1	O69.2XX9	O69.9XX4
O36.1995	O36.5123	O36.60X1	O36.72X9	O36.8224	O36.8912	O36.93X0	O41.01X5	O41.1213	O41.1491	O41.92X0	O60.20X4	O64.4XX2	O69.3XX0	O69.9XX5
O36.1999	O36.5124	O36.60X2	O36.73X0	O36.8225	O36.8913	O36.93X1	O41.01X9	O41.1214	O41.1492	O41.92X1	O60.20X5	O64.4XX3	O69.3XX1	O69.9XX9
O36.20X0	O36.5125	O36.60X3	O36.73X1	O36.8229	O36.8914	O36.93X2	O41.02X0	O41.1215	O41.1493	O41.92X1	O60.20X9	O64.4XX4	O69.3XX2	
O36.20X1	O36.5129	O36.60X4	O36.73X2	O36.8230	O36.8915	O36.93X3	O41.02X1	O41.1219	O41.1494	O41.92X1	O60.22X0	O64.4XX5	O69.3XX3	
O36.20X2	O36.5130	O36.60X5	O36.73X3	O36.8231	O36.8919	O36.93X4	O41.02X2	O41.1220	O41.1495	O41.92X3	O60.22X1	O64.4XX9	O69.3XX4	
O36.20X3	O36.5131	O36.60X9	O36.73X4	O36.8232	O36.8920	O36.93X5	O41.02X3	O41.1221	O41.1499	O41.92X4	O60.22X2	O64.5XX0	O69.3XX5	
O36.20X4	O36.5132	O36.61X0	O36.73X5	O36.8233	O36.8921	O36.93X9	O41.02X4	O41.1222	O41.8X10	O41.92X5	O60.22X3	O64.5XX1	O69.3XX9	
O36.20X5	O36.5133	O36.61X1	O36.73X9	O36.8234	O36.8922	O40.1XX0	O41.02X5	O41.1223	O41.8X11	O41.92X9	O60.22X4	O64.5XX2	O69.4XX0	
O36.20X9	O36.5134	O36.61X2	O36.80X0	O36.8235	O36.8923	O40.1XX1	O41.02X9	O41.1224	O41.8X12	O41.93X0	O60.22X5	O64.5XX3	O69.4XX1	
O36.21X0	O36.5135	O36.61X3	O36.80X1	O36.8239	O36.8924	O40.1XX2	O41.03X0	O41.1225	O41.8X13	O41.93X1	O60.22X9	O64.5XX4	O69.4XX2	
O36.21X1	O36.5139	O36.61X4	O36.80X2	O36.8290	O36.8925	O40.1XX3	O41.03X1	O41.1229	O41.8X14	O41.93X2	O60.23X0	O64.5XX5	O69.4XX3	

Pediatrics - For patients 0-17 years of age; based on Medicare's Outpatient Code Editor (OCE)

T74.02XA	T74.12XA	T74.22XA	T74.32XA	T74.4XXA	T74.52XA	T74.62XA	T74.92XA	T76.02XA	T76.12XA	T76.22XA	T76.32XA	T76.52XA	T76.62XA	T76.92XA
T74.02XD	T74.12XD	T74.22XD	T74.32XD	T74.4XXD	T74.52XD	T74.62XD	T74.92XD	T76.02XD	T76.12XD	T76.22XD	T76.32XD	T76.52XD	T76.62XD	T76.92XD
T74.02XS	T74.12XS	T74.22XS	T74.32XS	T74.4XXS	T74.52XS	T74.62XS	T74.92XS	T76.02XS	T76.12XS	T76.22XS	T76.32XS	T76.52XS	T76.62XS	T76.92XS

RxHCC - Based on CMS data

E08.3211	E08.3419	E08.3543	E09.3292	E09.3511	E09.3559	E10.3313	E10.3522	E10.37X1	E11.3399	E11.3533	E13.3212	E13.3491	E13.3549	H40.1111
E08.3212	E08.3491	E08.3549	E09.3293	E09.3512	E09.3591	E10.3319	E10.3523	E10.37X2	E11.3411	E11.3539	E13.3213	E13.3492	E13.3551	H40.1112
E08.3213	E08.3492	E08.3551	E09.3299	E09.3513	E09.3592	E10.3391	E10.3529	E10.37X3	E11.3412	E11.3541	E13.3219	E13.3493	E13.3552	H40.1113
E08.3219	E08.3493	E08.3552	E09.3311	E09.3519	E09.3593	E10.3392	E10.3531	E10.37X9	E11.3413	E11.3542	E13.3291	E13.3499	E13.3553	H40.1114
E08.3291	E08.3499	E08.3553	E09.3312	E09.3521	E09.3599	E10.3393	E10.3532	E11.3211	E11.3419	E11.3543	E13.3292	E13.3511	E13.3559	H40.1120
E08.3292	E08.3511	E08.3559	E09.3313	E09.3522	E09.37X1	E10.3399	E10.3533	E11.3212	E11.3491	E11.3549	E13.3293	E13.3513	E13.3591	H40.1121
E08.3293	E08.3512	E08.3591	E09.3319	E09.3523	E09.37X2	E10.3411	E10.3539	E11.3213	E11.3492	E11.3551	E13.3299	E13.3513	E13.3592	H40.1122
E08.3299	E08.3513	E08.3592	E09.3391	E09.3529	E09.37X3	E10.3412	E10.3541	E11.3219	E11.3493	E11.3552	E13.3311	E13.3519	E13.3593	H40.1123
E08.3311	E08.3519	E08.3593	E09.3392	E09.3531	E09.37X9	E10.3413	E10.3542	E11.3291	E11.3499	E11.3553	E13.3312	E13.3521	E13.3599	H40.1124
E08.3312	E08.3521	E08.3599	E09.3393	E09.3532	E10.3211	E10.3419	E10.3543	E11.3292	E11.3511	E11.3559	E13.3313	E13.3522	E13.37X1	H40.1130
E08.3313	E08.3522	E08.37X1	E09.3399	E09.3533	E10.3212	E10.3491	E10.3549	E11.3293	E11.3512	E11.3591	E13.3319	E13.3523	E13.37X2	H40.1131
E08.3319	E08.3523	E08.37X2	E09.3411	E09.3539	E10.3213	E10.3492	E10.3551	E11.3299	E11.3513	E11.3592	E13.3391	E13.3529	E13.37X3	H40.1132
E08.3391	E08.3529	E08.37X3	E09.3412	E09.3541	E10.3219	E10.3493	E10.3552	E11.3311	E11.3519	E11.3593	E13.3392	E13.3531	E13.37X9	H40.1133
E08.3392	E08.3531	E08.37X9	E09.3413	E09.3542	E10.3291	E10.3499	E10.3553	E11.3312	E11.3521	E11.3599	E13.3393	E13.3532	H40.10X0	H40.1134
E08.3393	E08.3532	E09.3211	E09.3419	E09.3543	E10.3292	E10.3511	E10.3559	E11.3313	E11.3522	E11.37X1	E13.3399	E13.3533	H40.10X1	H40.1190
E08.3399	E08.3533	E09.3212	E09.3491	E09.3549	E10.3293	E10.3512	E10.3591	E11.3319	E11.3523	E11.37X2	E13.3411	E13.3539	H40.10X2	H40.1191
E08.3411	E08.3539	E09.3213	E09.3492	E09.3551	E10.3299	E10.3513	E10.3592	E11.3391	E11.3529	E11.37X3	E13.3412	E13.3541	H40.10X3	H40.1192
E08.3412	E08.3541	E09.3219	E09.3493	E09.3552	E10.3311	E10.3519	E10.3593	E11.3392	E11.3531	E11.37X9	E13.3413	E13.3542	H40.10X4	H40.1193
E08.3413	E08.3542	E09.3291	E09.3499	E09.3553	E10.3312	E10.3521	E10.3599	E11.3393	E11.3532	E13.3211	E13.3419	E13.3543	H40.1110	H40.1194

RxHCC (cont.) - Based on CMS data

H40.1210	H40.1291	H40.1332	M48.58XA	M80.059A	M80.832A	M84.411A	M84.446A	M84.476A	M84.539A	M84.573A	M84.639A	M84.673A	T81.532S	T85.611A
H40.1211	H40.1292	H40.1333	M80.00XA	M80.061A	M80.839A	M84.412A	M84.451A	M84.477A	M84.541A	M84.574A	M84.641A	M84.674A	T81.592A	T85.611D
H40.1212	H40.1293	H40.1334	M80.011A	M80.062A	M80.841A	M84.419A	M84.452A	M84.478A	M84.542A	M84.575A	M84.642A	M84.675A	T81.592D	T85.611S
H40.1213	H40.1294	H40.1390	M80.012A	M80.069A	M80.842A	M84.421A	M84.453A	M84.479A	M84.549A	M84.576A	M84.649A	M84.676A	T81.592S	T85.621A
H40.1214	H40.1310	H40.1391	M80.019A	M80.071A	M80.849A	M84.422A	M84.454A	M84.48XA	M84.550A	M84.58XA	M84.650A	M84.68XA	T82.41XA	T85.621D
H40.1220	H40.1311	H40.1392	M80.021A	M80.072A	M80.851A	M84.429A	M84.459A	M84.50XA	M84.551A	M84.60XA	M84.651A	T81.502A	T82.41XD	T85.621S
H40.1221	H40.1312	H40.1393	M80.022A	M80.079A	M80.852A	M84.431A	M84.461A	M84.511A	M84.552A	M84.611A	M84.652A	T81.502D	T82.41XS	T85.631A
H40.1222	H40.1313	H40.1394	M80.029A	M80.08XA	M80.859A	M84.432A	M84.462A	M84.512A	M84.553A	M84.612A	M84.653A	T81.502S	T82.42XA	T85.631D
H40.1223	H40.1314	M48.50XA	M80.031A	M80.80XA	M80.861A	M84.433A	M84.463A	M84.519A	M84.559A	M84.619A	M84.659A	T81.512A	T82.42XD	T85.631S
H40.1224	H40.1320	M48.51XA	M80.032A	M80.811A	M80.862A	M84.434A	M84.464A	M84.521A	M84.561A	M84.621A	M84.661A	T81.512D	T82.42XS	T85.691A
H40.1230	H40.1321	M48.52XA	M80.039A	M80.812A	M80.869A	M84.439A	M84.469A	M84.522A	M84.562A	M84.622A	M84.662A	T81.512S	T82.43XA	T85.691D
H40.1231	H40.1322	M48.53XA	M80.041A	M80.819A	M80.871A	M84.441A	M84.471A	M84.529A	M84.563A	M84.629A	M84.663A	T81.522A	T82.43XD	T85.691S
H40.1232	H40.1323	M48.54XA	M80.042A	M80.821A	M80.872A	M84.442A	M84.472A	M84.531A	M84.564A	M84.631A	M84.664A	T81.522D	T82.43XS	T85.71XA
H40.1233	H40.1324	M48.55XA	M80.049A	M80.822A	M80.879A	M84.443A	M84.473A	M84.532A	M84.569A	M84.632A	M84.669A	T81.522S	T82.49XA	T85.71XD
H40.1234	H40.1330	M48.56XA	M80.051A	M80.829A	M80.88XA	M84.444A	M84.474A	M84.533A	M84.571A	M84.633A	M84.671A	T81.532A	T82.49XD	T85.71XS
H40.1290	H40.1331	M48.57XA	M80.052A	M80.831A	M84.40XA	M84.445A	M84.475A	M84.534A	M84.572A	M84.634A	M84.672A	T81.532D	T82.49XS	

Unacceptable Principal Diagnosis - Based on Medicare code edits

H40.1210	R40.2124	R40.2350	T36.4X5S	T37.3X6D	T38.5X5A	T39.095S	T40.2X6D	T41.1X5A	T42.3X5S	T43.206D	T43.625A	T44.4X5S	T45.2X6D	T45.8X5A
H40.1211	R40.2130	R40.2351	T36.4X6A	T37.3X6S	T38.5X5D	T39.096A	T40.2X6S	T41.1X5D	T42.3X6A	T43.206S	T43.625D	T44.4X6A	T45.2X6S	T45.8X5D
H40.1212	R40.2131	R40.2352	T36.4X6D	T37.4X5A	T38.5X5S	T39.096D	T40.3X5A	T41.1X5S	T42.3X6D	T43.215A	T43.625S	T44.4X6D	T45.3X5A	T45.8X5S
H40.1213	R40.2132	R40.2353	T36.4X6S	T37.4X5D	T38.5X6A	T39.096S	T40.3X5D	T41.1X6A	T42.3X6S	T43.215D	T43.626A	T44.4X6S	T45.3X5D	T45.8X6A
H40.1214	R40.2133	R40.2354	T36.5X5A	T37.4X5S	T38.5X6D	T39.1X5A	T40.3X5S	T41.1X6D	T42.4X5A	T43.215S	T43.626D	T44.5X5A	T45.3X5S	T45.8X6D
H40.1220	R40.2134	R40.2360	T36.5X5D	T37.4X6A	T38.5X6S	T39.1X5D	T40.3X6A	T41.1X6S	T42.4X5D	T43.216A	T43.626S	T44.5X5D	T45.3X6A	T45.8X6S
H40.1221	R40.2140	R40.2361	T36.5X5S	T37.4X6D	T38.6X5A	T39.1X5S	T40.3X6D	T41.205A	T42.4X5S	T43.216D	T43.635A	T44.5X5S	T45.3X6D	T45.95XA
H40.1222	R40.2141	R40.2362	T36.5X6A	T37.4X6S	T38.6X5D	T39.1X6A	T40.3X6S	T41.205D	T42.4X6A	T43.216S	T43.635D	T44.5X6A	T45.3X6S	T45.95XD
H40.1223	R40.2142	R40.2363	T36.5X6D	T37.5X5A	T38.6X5S	T39.1X6D	T40.4X5A	T41.205S	T42.4X6D	T43.225A	T43.635S	T44.5X6D	T45.4X5A	T45.95XS
H40.1224	R40.2143	R40.2364	T36.5X6S	T37.5X5D	T38.6X6A	T39.1X6S	T40.4X5D	T41.206A	T42.4X6S	T43.225D	T43.636A	T44.5X6S	T45.4X5D	T45.96XA
H40.1230	R40.2144	R40.2410	T36.6X5A	T37.5X5S	T38.6X6D	T39.2X5A	T40.4X5S	T41.206D	T42.5X5A	T43.225S	T43.636D	T44.6X5A	T45.4X5S	T45.96XD
H40.1231	R40.2210	R40.2411	T36.6X5D	T37.5X6A	T38.6X6S	T39.2X5D	T40.4X6A	T41.206S	T42.5X5D	T43.226A	T43.636S	T44.6X5D	T45.4X6A	T45.96XS
H40.1232	R40.2211	R40.2412	T36.6X5S	T37.5X6D	T38.7X5A	T39.2X5S	T40.4X6D	T41.295A	T42.5X5S	T43.226D	T43.695A	T44.6X5S	T45.4X6D	T46.0X5A
H40.1233	R40.2212	R40.2413	T36.6X6A	T37.5X6S	T38.7X5D	T39.2X6A	T40.4X6S	T41.295D	T42.5X6A	T43.226S	T43.695D	T44.6X6A	T45.4X6S	T46.0X5D
H40.1234	R40.2213	R40.2414	T36.6X6D	T37.8X5A	T38.7X5S	T39.2X6D	T40.5X5A	T41.295S	T42.5X6D	T43.295A	T43.695S	T44.6X6D	T45.515A	T46.0X5S
H40.1290	R40.2214	R40.2420	T36.6X6S	T37.8X5D	T38.7X6A	T39.2X6S	T40.5X5D	T41.296A	T42.5X6S	T43.295D	T43.696A	T44.6X6S	T45.515D	T46.0X6A
H40.1291	R40.2220	R40.2421	T36.7X5A	T37.8X5S	T38.7X6D	T39.315A	T40.5X5S	T41.296D	T42.6X5A	T43.295S	T43.696D	T44.7X5A	T45.515S	T46.0X6D
H40.1292	R40.2221	R40.2422	T36.7X5D	T37.8X6A	T38.7X6S	T39.315D	T40.5X6A	T41.296S	T42.6X5D	T43.296A	T43.696S	T44.7X5D	T45.516A	T46.0X6S
H40.1293	R40.2222	R40.2423	T36.7X5S	T37.8X6D	T38.805A	T39.315S	T40.5X6D	T41.3X5A	T42.6X5S	T43.296D	T43.8X5A	T44.7X5S	T45.516D	T46.1X5A
H40.1294	R40.2223	R40.2424	T36.7X6A	T37.8X6S	T38.805D	T39.316A	T40.5X6S	T41.3X5D	T42.6X6A	T43.296S	T43.8X5D	T44.7X6A	T45.516S	T46.1X5D
H40.1310	R40.2224	R40.2430	T36.7X6D	T37.95XA	T38.805S	T39.316D	T40.605A	T41.3X5S	T42.6X6D	T43.3X5A	T43.8X5S	T44.7X6D	T45.525A	T46.1X5S
H40.1311	R40.2230	R40.2431	T36.7X6S	T37.95XD	T38.806A	T39.316S	T40.605D	T41.3X6A	T42.6X6S	T43.3X5D	T43.8X6A	T44.7X6S	T45.525D	T46.1X6A
H40.1312	R40.2231	R40.2432	T36.8X5A	T37.95XS	T38.806D	T39.395A	T40.605S	T41.3X6D	T42.75XA	T43.3X5S	T43.8X6D	T44.8X5A	T45.525S	T46.1X6D
H40.1313	R40.2232	R40.2433	T36.8X5D	T37.96XA	T38.806S	T39.395D	T40.606A	T41.3X6S	T42.75XD	T43.3X6A	T43.8X6S	T44.8X5D	T45.526A	T46.1X6S
H40.1314	R40.2233	R40.2434	T36.8X5S	T37.96XD	T38.815A	T39.395S	T40.606D	T41.45XA	T42.75XS	T43.3X6D	T43.95XA	T44.8X5S	T45.526D	T46.2X5A
H40.1320	R40.2234	R40.2440	T36.8X6A	T37.96XS	T38.815D	T39.396A	T40.606S	T41.45XD	T42.76XA	T43.3X6S	T43.95XD	T44.8X6A	T45.526S	T46.2X5D
H40.1321	R40.2240	R40.2441	T36.8X6D	T38.0X5A	T38.815S	T39.396D	T40.695A	T41.45XS	T42.76XD	T43.4X5A	T43.95XS	T44.8X6D	T45.605A	T46.2X5S
H40.1322	R40.2241	R40.2442	T36.8X6S	T38.0X5D	T38.816A	T39.396S	T40.695D	T41.46XA	T42.76XS	T43.4X5D	T43.96XA	T44.8X6S	T45.605D	T46.2X6A
H40.1323	R40.2242	R40.2443	T36.95XA	T38.0X5S	T38.816D	T39.4X5A	T40.695S	T41.46XD	T42.8X5A	T43.4X5S	T43.96XD	T44.905A	T45.605S	T46.2X6D
H40.1324	R40.2243	R40.2444	T36.95XD	T38.0X6A	T38.816S	T39.4X5D	T40.696A	T41.46XS	T42.8X5D	T43.4X6A	T43.96XS	T44.905D	T45.606A	T46.2X6S
H40.1330	R40.2244	T36.0X5A	T36.95XS	T38.0X6D	T38.895A	T39.4X5S	T40.696D	T41.5X5A	T42.8X5S	T43.4X6D	T44.0X5A	T44.905S	T45.606D	T46.3X5A
H40.1331	R40.2250	T36.0X5D	T36.96XA	T38.0X6S	T38.895D	T39.4X6A	T40.696S	T41.5X5D	T42.8X6A	T43.4X6S	T44.0X5D	T44.906A	T45.606S	T46.3X5D
H40.1332	R40.2251	T36.0X5S	T36.96XD	T38.1X5A	T38.895S	T39.4X6D	T40.7X5A	T41.5X5S	T42.8X6D	T43.505A	T44.0X5S	T44.906D	T45.615A	T46.3X5S
H40.1333	R40.2252	T36.0X6A	T36.96XS	T38.1X5D	T38.896A	T39.4X6S	T40.7X5D	T41.5X6A	T42.8X6S	T43.505D	T44.0X6A	T44.906S	T45.615D	T46.3X6A
H40.1334	R40.2253	T36.0X6D	T37.0X5A	T38.1X5S	T38.896D	T39.8X5A	T40.7X5S	T41.5X6D	T43.015A	T43.505S	T44.0X6D	T44.995A	T45.615S	T46.3X6D
H40.1390	R40.2254	T36.0X6S	T37.0X5D	T38.1X6A	T38.896S	T39.8X5D	T40.7X6A	T41.5X6S	T43.015D	T43.506A	T44.0X6S	T44.995D	T45.616A	T46.3X6S
H40.1391	R40.2310	T36.1X5A	T37.0X5S	T38.1X6D	T38.905A	T39.8X5S	T40.7X6D	T42.0X5A	T43.015S	T43.506D	T44.1X5A	T44.995S	T45.616D	T46.4X5A
H40.1392	R40.2311	T36.1X5D	T37.0X6A	T38.1X6S	T38.905D	T39.8X6A	T40.7X6S	T42.0X5D	T43.016A	T43.506S	T44.1X5D	T44.996A	T45.616S	T46.4X5D
H40.1393	R40.2312	T36.1X5S	T37.0X6D	T38.2X5A	T38.905S	T39.8X6D	T40.905A	T42.0X5S	T43.016D	T43.595A	T44.1X5S	T44.996D	T45.625A	T46.4X5S
H40.1394	R40.2313	T36.1X6A	T37.0X6S	T38.2X5D	T38.906A	T39.8X6S	T40.905D	T42.0X6A	T43.016S	T43.595D	T44.1X6A	T44.996S	T45.625D	T46.4X6A
O36.80X0	R40.2314	T36.1X6D	T37.1X5A	T38.2X5S	T38.906D	T39.95XA	T40.905S	T42.0X6D	T43.025A	T43.595S	T44.1X6D	T45.0X5A	T45.625S	T46.4X6D
O36.80X1	R40.2320	T36.1X6S	T37.1X5D	T38.2X6A	T38.906S	T39.95XD	T40.906A	T42.0X6S	T43.025D	T43.596A	T44.1X6S	T45.0X5D	T45.626A	T46.4X6S
O36.80X2	R40.2321	T36.2X5A	T37.1X5S	T38.2X6D	T38.995A	T39.95XS	T40.906D	T42.1X5A	T43.025S	T43.596D	T44.2X5A	T45.0X5S	T45.626D	T46.5X5A
O36.80X3	R40.2322	T36.2X5D	T37.1X6A	T38.2X6S	T38.995D	T39.96XA	T40.906S	T42.1X5D	T43.026A	T43.596S	T44.2X5D	T45.0X6A	T45.626S	T46.5X5D
O36.80X4	R40.2323	T36.2X5S	T37.1X6D	T38.3X5A	T38.995S	T39.96XD	T40.995A	T42.1X5S	T43.026D	T43.605A	T44.2X5S	T45.0X6D	T45.695A	T46.5X5S
O36.80X5	R40.2324	T36.2X6A	T37.1X6S	T38.3X5D	T38.996A	T39.96XS	T40.995D	T42.1X6A	T43.026S	T43.605D	T44.2X6A	T45.0X6S	T45.695D	T46.5X6A
O36.80X9	R40.2330	T36.2X6D	T37.2X5A	T38.3X5S	T38.996D	T40.0X5A	T40.995S	T42.1X6D	T43.1X5A	T43.605S	T44.2X6D	T45.1X5A	T45.695S	T46.5X6D
R40.2110	R40.2331	T36.2X6S	T37.2X5D	T38.3X6A	T38.996S	T40.0X5D	T40.996A	T42.1X6S	T43.1X5D	T43.606A	T44.2X6S	T45.1X5D	T45.696A	T46.5X6S
R40.2111	R40.2332	T36.3X5A	T37.2X5S	T38.3X6D	T39.015A	T40.0X5S	T40.996D	T42.2X5A	T43.1X5S	T43.606D	T44.3X5A	T45.1X5S	T45.696D	T46.6X5A
R40.2112	R40.2333	T36.3X5D	T37.2X6A	T38.3X6S	T39.015D	T40.0X6A	T40.996S	T42.2X5D	T43.1X6A	T43.606S	T44.3X5D	T45.1X6A	T45.696S	T46.6X5D
R40.2113	R40.2334	T36.3X5S	T37.2X6D	T38.4X5A	T39.015S	T40.0X6D	T41.0X5A	T42.2X5S	T43.1X6D	T43.615A	T44.3X5S	T45.1X6D	T45.7X5A	T46.6X5S
R40.2114	R40.2340	T36.3X6A	T37.2X6S	T38.4X5D	T39.016A	T40.0X6S	T41.0X5D	T42.2X6A	T43.1X6S	T43.615D	T44.3X6A	T45.1X6S	T45.7X5D	T46.6X6A
R40.2120	R40.2341	T36.3X6D	T37.3X5A	T38.4X5S	T39.016D	T40.2X5A	T41.0X5S	T42.2X6D	T43.205A	T43.615S	T44.3X6D	T45.2X5A	T45.7X5S	T46.6X6D
R40.2121	R40.2342	T36.3X6S	T37.3X5D	T38.4X6A	T39.016S	T40.2X5D	T41.0X6A	T42.2X6S	T43.205D	T43.616A	T44.3X6S	T45.2X5D	T45.7X6A	T46.6X6S
R40.2122	R40.2343	T36.4X5A	T37.3X5S	T38.4X6D	T39.095A	T40.2X5S	T41.0X6D	T42.3X5A	T43.205S	T43.616D	T44.4X5A	T45.2X5S	T45.7X6D	T46.7X5A
R40.2123	R40.2344	T36.4X5D	T37.3X6A	T38.4X6S	T39.095D	T40.2X6A	T41.0X6S	T42.3X5D	T43.206A	T43.616S	T44.4X5D	T45.2X6A	T45.7X6S	T46.7X5D

Unacceptable Principal Diagnosis (cont.) - Based on Medicare code edits

T46.7X5S	T46.996S	T47.3X5S	T47.6X6S	T48.0X5S	T48.296S	T48.6X5S	T49.0X6S	T49.4X5S	T49.7X6S	T50.1X5S	T50.4X6S	T50.8X5S	T50.A96S	T50.Z95S
T46.7X6A	T47.0X5A	T47.3X6A	T47.7X5A	T48.0X6A	T48.3X5A	T48.6X6A	T49.1X5A	T49.4X6A	T49.8X5A	T50.1X6A	T50.5X5A	T50.8X6A	T50.B15A	T50.Z96A
T46.7X6D	T47.0X5D	T47.3X6D	T47.7X5D	T48.0X6D	T48.3X5D	T48.6X6D	T49.1X5D	T49.4X6D	T49.8X5D	T50.1X6D	T50.5X5D	T50.8X6D	T50.B15D	T50.Z96D
T46.7X6S	T47.0X5S	T47.3X6S	T47.7X5S	T48.0X6S	T48.3X5S	T48.6X6S	T49.1X5S	T49.4X6S	T49.8X5S	T50.1X6S	T50.5X5S	T50.8X6S	T50.B15S	T50.Z96S
T46.8X5A	T47.0X6A	T47.4X5A	T47.7X6A	T48.1X5A	T48.3X6A	T48.905A	T49.1X6A	T49.5X5A	T49.8X6A	T50.2X5A	T50.5X6A	T50.A15A	T50.B16A	T81.12XA
T46.8X5D	T47.0X6D	T47.4X5D	T47.7X6D	T48.1X5D	T48.3X6D	T48.905D	T49.1X6D	T49.5X5D	T49.8X6D	T50.2X5D	T50.5X6D	T50.A15D	T50.B16D	T81.12XD
T46.8X5S	T47.0X6S	T47.4X5S	T47.7X6S	T48.1X5S	T48.3X6S	T48.905S	T49.1X6S	T49.5X5S	T49.8X6S	T50.2X5S	T50.5X6S	T50.A15S	T50.B16S	T81.12XS
T46.8X6A	T47.1X5A	T47.4X6A	T47.8X5A	T48.1X6A	T48.4X5A	T48.906A	T49.2X5A	T49.5X6A	T49.95XA	T50.2X6A	T50.6X5A	T50.A16A	T50.B95A	
T46.8X6D	T47.1X5D	T47.4X6D	T47.8X5D	T48.1X6D	T48.4X5D	T48.906D	T49.2X5D	T49.5X6D	T49.95XD	T50.2X6D	T50.6X5D	T50.A16D	T50.B95D	
T46.8X6S	T47.1X5S	T47.4X6S	T47.8X5S	T48.1X6S	T48.4X5S	T48.906S	T49.2X5S	T49.5X6S	T49.95XS	T50.2X6S	T50.6X5S	T50.A16S	T50.B95S	
T46.905A	T47.1X6A	T47.5X5A	T47.8X6A	T48.205A	T48.4X6A	T48.995A	T49.2X6A	T49.6X5A	T49.96XA	T50.3X5A	T50.6X6A	T50.A25A	T50.B96A	
T46.905D	T47.1X6D	T47.5X5D	T47.8X6D	T48.205D	T48.4X6D	T48.995D	T49.2X6D	T49.6X5D	T49.96XD	T50.3X5D	T50.6X6D	T50.A25D	T50.B96D	
T46.905S	T47.1X6S	T47.5X5S	T47.8X6S	T48.205S	T48.4X6S	T48.995S	T49.2X6S	T49.6X5S	T49.96XS	T50.3X5S	T50.6X6S	T50.A25S	T50.B96S	
T46.906A	T47.2X5A	T47.5X6A	T47.95XA	T48.206A	T48.5X5A	T48.996A	T49.3X5A	T49.6X6A	T50.0X5A	T50.3X6A	T50.7X5A	T50.A26A	T50.Z15A	
T46.906D	T47.2X5D	T47.5X6D	T47.95XD	T48.206D	T48.5X5D	T48.996D	T49.3X5D	T49.6X6D	T50.0X5D	T50.3X6D	T50.7X5D	T50.A26D	T50.Z15D	
T46.906S	T47.2X5S	T47.5X6S	T47.95XS	T48.206S	T48.5X5S	T48.996S	T49.3X5S	T49.6X6S	T50.0X5S	T50.3X6S	T50.7X5S	T50.A26S	T50.Z15S	
T46.995A	T47.2X6A	T47.6X5A	T47.96XA	T48.295A	T48.5X6A	T49.0X5A	T49.3X6A	T49.7X5A	T50.0X6A	T50.4X5A	T50.7X6A	T50.A95A	T50.Z16A	
T46.995D	T47.2X6D	T47.6X5D	T47.96XD	T48.295D	T48.5X6D	T49.0X5D	T49.3X6D	T49.7X5D	T50.0X6D	T50.4X5D	T50.7X6D	T50.A95D	T50.Z16D	
T46.995S	T47.2X6S	T47.6X5S	T47.96XS	T48.295S	T48.5X6S	T49.0X5S	T49.3X6S	T49.7X5S	T50.0X6S	T50.4X5S	T50.7X6S	T50.A95S	T50.Z16S	
T46.996A	T47.3X5A	T47.6X6A	T48.0X5A	T48.296A	T48.6X5A	T49.0X6A	T49.4X5A	T49.7X6A	T50.1X5A	T50.4X6A	T50.8X5A	T50.A96A	T50.Z95A	
T46.996D	T47.3X5D	T47.6X6D	T48.0X5D	T48.296D	T48.6X5D	T49.0X6D	T49.4X5D	T49.7X6D	T50.1X5D	T50.4X6D	T50.8X5D	T50.A96D	T50.Z95D	

1st Trimester - Based on CMS data

O31.01X0	O31.11X5	O31.31X3	O36.0111	O36.0919	O36.1914	O36.5112	O36.61X0	O36.71X5	O36.8313	O36.91X1	O40.1XX9	O41.1014	O41.1412	O41.91X0
O31.01X1	O31.11X9	O31.31X4	O36.0112	O36.1110	O36.1915	O36.5113	O36.61X1	O36.71X9	O36.8314	O36.91X2	O41.01X0	O41.1015	O41.1413	O41.91X1
O31.01X2	O31.21X0	O31.31X5	O36.0113	O36.1111	O36.1919	O36.5114	O36.61X2	O36.8210	O36.8315	O36.91X3	O41.01X1	O41.1019	O41.1414	O41.91X2
O31.01X3	O31.21X1	O31.31X9	O36.0114	O36.1112	O36.21X0	O36.5115	O36.61X3	O36.8211	O36.8319	O36.91X4	O41.01X2	O41.1210	O41.1415	O41.91X3
O31.01X4	O31.21X2	O31.8X10	O36.0115	O36.1113	O36.21X1	O36.5119	O36.61X4	O36.8212	O36.8910	O36.91X5	O41.01X3	O41.1211	O41.1419	O41.91X4
O31.01X5	O31.21X3	O31.8X11	O36.0119	O36.1114	O36.21X2	O36.5910	O36.61X5	O36.8213	O36.8911	O36.91X9	O41.01X4	O41.1212	O41.8X10	O41.91X5
O31.01X9	O31.21X4	O31.8X12	O36.0910	O36.1115	O36.21X3	O36.5911	O36.61X6	O36.8214	O36.8912	O40.1XX0	O41.01X5	O41.1213	O41.8X11	O41.91X9
O31.11X0	O31.21X5	O31.8X13	O36.0911	O36.1119	O36.21X4	O36.5912	O36.71X0	O36.8215	O36.8913	O40.1XX1	O41.01X9	O41.1214	O41.8X12	
O31.11X1	O31.21X9	O31.8X14	O36.0912	O36.1910	O36.21X5	O36.5913	O36.71X1	O36.8219	O36.8914	O40.1XX2	O41.1010	O41.1215	O41.8X13	
O31.11X2	O31.31X0	O31.8X15	O36.0913	O36.1911	O36.21X9	O36.5914	O36.71X2	O36.8310	O36.8915	O40.1XX3	O41.1011	O41.1219	O41.8X14	
O31.11X3	O31.31X1	O31.8X19	O36.0914	O36.1912	O36.5110	O36.5915	O36.71X3	O36.8311	O36.8919	O40.1XX4	O41.1012	O41.1410	O41.8X15	
O31.11X4	O31.31X2	O36.0110	O36.0915	O36.1913	O36.5111	O36.5919	O36.71X4	O36.8312	O36.91X0	O40.1XX5	O41.1013	O41.1411	O41.8X19	

2nd Trimester - Based on CMS data

O31.02X0	O31.22X0	O31.8X20	O36.0920	O36.1920	O36.5120	O36.62X0	O36.8120	O36.8320	O36.92X0	O41.02X0	O41.1220	O41.8X20	O60.12X0	O60.22X0
O31.02X1	O31.22X1	O31.8X21	O36.0921	O36.1921	O36.5121	O36.62X1	O36.8121	O36.8321	O36.92X1	O41.02X1	O41.1221	O41.8X21	O60.12X1	O60.22X1
O31.02X2	O31.22X2	O31.8X22	O36.0922	O36.1922	O36.5122	O36.62X2	O36.8122	O36.8322	O36.92X2	O41.02X2	O41.1222	O41.8X22	O60.12X2	O60.22X2
O31.02X3	O31.22X3	O31.8X23	O36.0923	O36.1923	O36.5123	O36.62X3	O36.8123	O36.8323	O36.92X3	O41.02X3	O41.1223	O41.8X23	O60.12X3	O60.22X3
O31.02X4	O31.22X4	O31.8X24	O36.0924	O36.1924	O36.5124	O36.62X4	O36.8124	O36.8324	O36.92X4	O41.02X4	O41.1224	O41.8X24	O60.12X4	O60.22X4
O31.02X5	O31.22X5	O31.8X25	O36.0925	O36.1925	O36.5125	O36.62X5	O36.8125	O36.8325	O36.92X5	O41.02X5	O41.1225	O41.8X25	O60.12X5	O60.22X5
O31.02X9	O31.22X9	O31.8X29	O36.0929	O36.1929	O36.5129	O36.62X9	O36.8129	O36.8329	O36.92X9	O41.02X9	O41.1229	O41.8X29	O60.12X9	O60.22X9
O31.12X0	O31.32X0	O36.0120	O36.1120	O36.22X0	O36.5920	O36.72X0	O36.8220	O36.8920	O40.2XX0	O41.1020	O41.1420	O41.92X0	O60.13X0	
O31.12X1	O31.32X1	O36.0121	O36.1121	O36.22X1	O36.5921	O36.72X1	O36.8221	O36.8921	O40.2XX1	O41.1021	O41.1421	O41.92X1	O60.13X1	
O31.12X2	O31.32X2	O36.0122	O36.1122	O36.22X2	O36.5922	O36.72X2	O36.8222	O36.8922	O40.2XX2	O41.1022	O41.1422	O41.92X2	O60.13X2	
O31.12X3	O31.32X3	O36.0123	O36.1123	O36.22X3	O36.5923	O36.72X3	O36.8223	O36.8923	O40.2XX3	O41.1023	O41.1423	O41.92X3	O60.13X3	
O31.12X4	O31.32X4	O36.0124	O36.1124	O36.22X4	O36.5924	O36.72X4	O36.8224	O36.8924	O40.2XX4	O41.1024	O41.1424	O41.92X4	O60.13X4	
O31.12X5	O31.32X5	O36.0125	O36.1125	O36.22X5	O36.5925	O36.72X5	O36.8225	O36.8925	O40.2XX5	O41.1025	O41.1425	O41.92X5	O60.13X5	
O31.12X9	O31.32X9	O36.0129	O36.1129	O36.22X9	O36.5929	O36.72X9	O36.8229	O36.8929	O40.2XX9	O41.1029	O41.1429	O41.92X9	O60.13X9	

3rd Trimester - Based on CMS data

O31.03X0	O31.23X0	O31.8X30	O36.0930	O36.1930	O36.5130	O36.63X0	O36.8130	O36.8330	O36.93X0	O41.03X0	O41.1230	O41.8X30	O60.13X0	O60.23X0
O31.03X1	O31.23X1	O31.8X31	O36.0931	O36.1931	O36.5131	O36.63X1	O36.8131	O36.8331	O36.93X1	O41.03X1	O41.1231	O41.8X31	O60.13X1	O60.23X1
O31.03X2	O31.23X2	O31.8X32	O36.0932	O36.1932	O36.5132	O36.63X2	O36.8132	O36.8332	O36.93X2	O41.03X2	O41.1232	O41.8X32	O60.13X2	O60.23X2
O31.03X3	O31.23X3	O31.8X33	O36.0933	O36.1933	O36.5133	O36.63X3	O36.8133	O36.8333	O36.93X3	O41.03X3	O41.1233	O41.8X33	O60.13X3	O60.23X3
O31.03X4	O31.23X4	O31.8X34	O36.0934	O36.1934	O36.5134	O36.63X4	O36.8134	O36.8334	O36.93X4	O41.03X4	O41.1234	O41.8X34	O60.13X4	O60.23X4
O31.03X5	O31.23X5	O31.8X35	O36.0935	O36.1935	O36.5135	O36.63X5	O36.8135	O36.8335	O36.93X5	O41.03X5	O41.1235	O41.8X35	O60.13X5	O60.23X5
O31.03X9	O31.23X9	O31.8X39	O36.0939	O36.1939	O36.5139	O36.63X9	O36.8139	O36.8339	O36.93X9	O41.03X9	O41.1239	O41.8X39	O60.13X9	O60.23X9
O31.13X0	O31.33X0	O36.0130	O36.1130	O36.23X0	O36.5930	O36.73X0	O36.8230	O36.8930	O40.3XX0	O41.1030	O41.1430	O41.93X0	O60.14X0	
O31.13X1	O31.33X1	O36.0131	O36.1131	O36.23X1	O36.5931	O36.73X1	O36.8231	O36.8931	O40.3XX1	O41.1031	O41.1431	O41.93X1	O60.14X1	
O31.13X2	O31.33X2	O36.0132	O36.1132	O36.23X2	O36.5932	O36.73X2	O36.8232	O36.8932	O40.3XX2	O41.1032	O41.1432	O41.93X2	O60.14X2	
O31.13X3	O31.33X3	O36.0133	O36.1133	O36.23X3	O36.5933	O36.73X3	O36.8233	O36.8933	O40.3XX3	O41.1033	O41.1433	O41.93X3	O60.14X3	
O31.13X4	O31.33X4	O36.0134	O36.1134	O36.23X4	O36.5934	O36.73X4	O36.8234	O36.8934	O40.3XX4	O41.1034	O41.1434	O41.93X4	O60.14X4	
O31.13X9	O31.33X9	O36.0139	O36.1139	O36.23X9	O36.5939	O36.73X9	O36.8239	O36.8939	O40.3XX9	O41.1039	O41.1439	O41.93X9	O60.14X5	

Code exempt from diagnosis present on admission requirement

CMS includes thousands of codes that are exempt. Please go to the CMS site for the most updated Present on Admission (POA) Exempt List (https://www.cms.gov/Medicare/Medicare-Fee-for-Service-Payment/HospitalAcqCond/Coding.html - Go to downloads).

Editor's Note: At press time, the most updated list on the CMS site was FY 2020.

NOTES

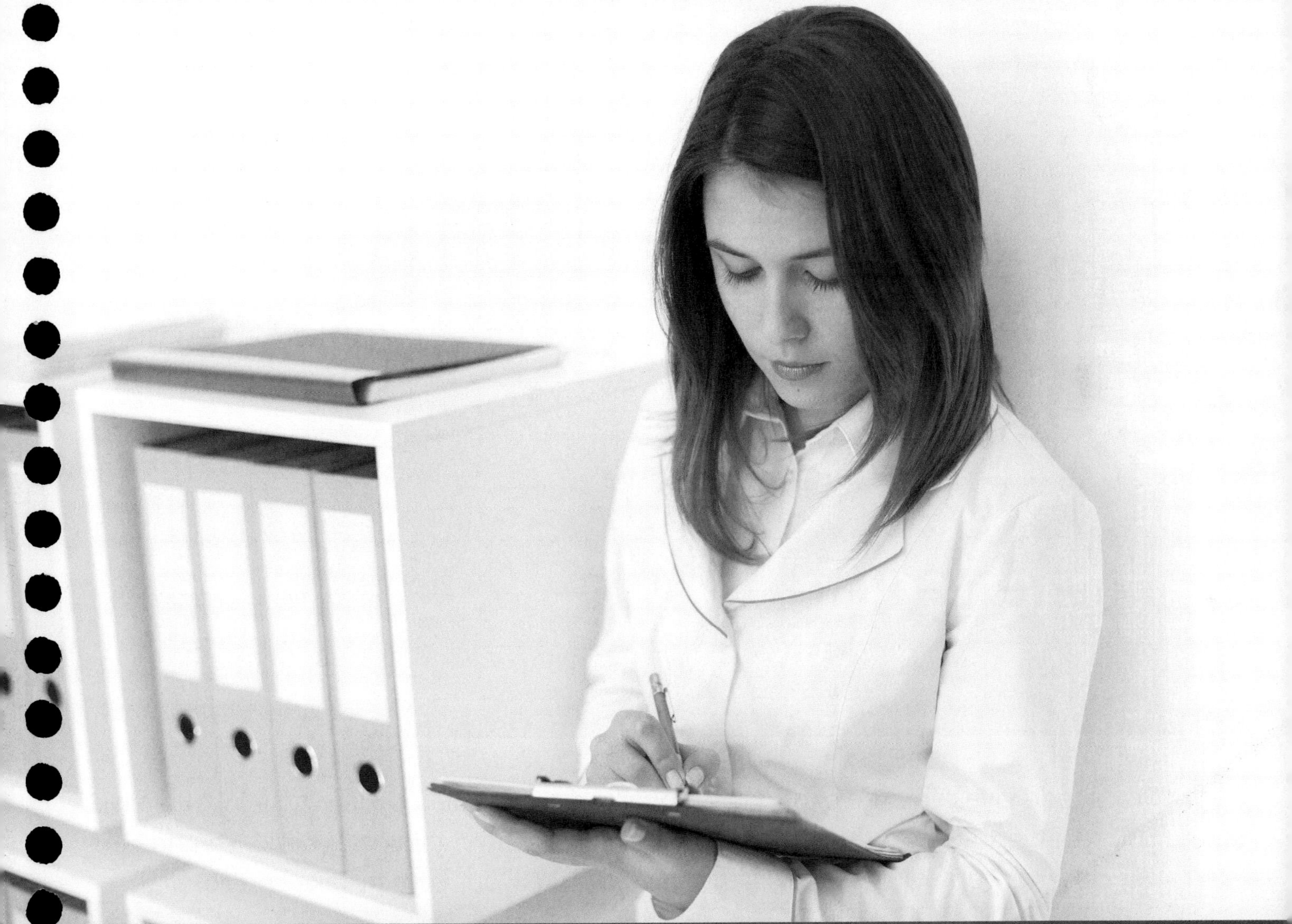

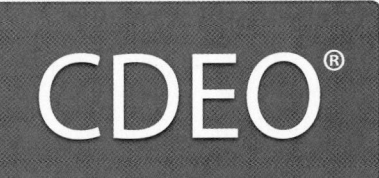
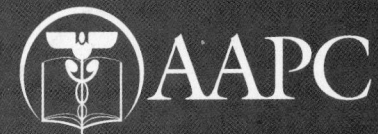

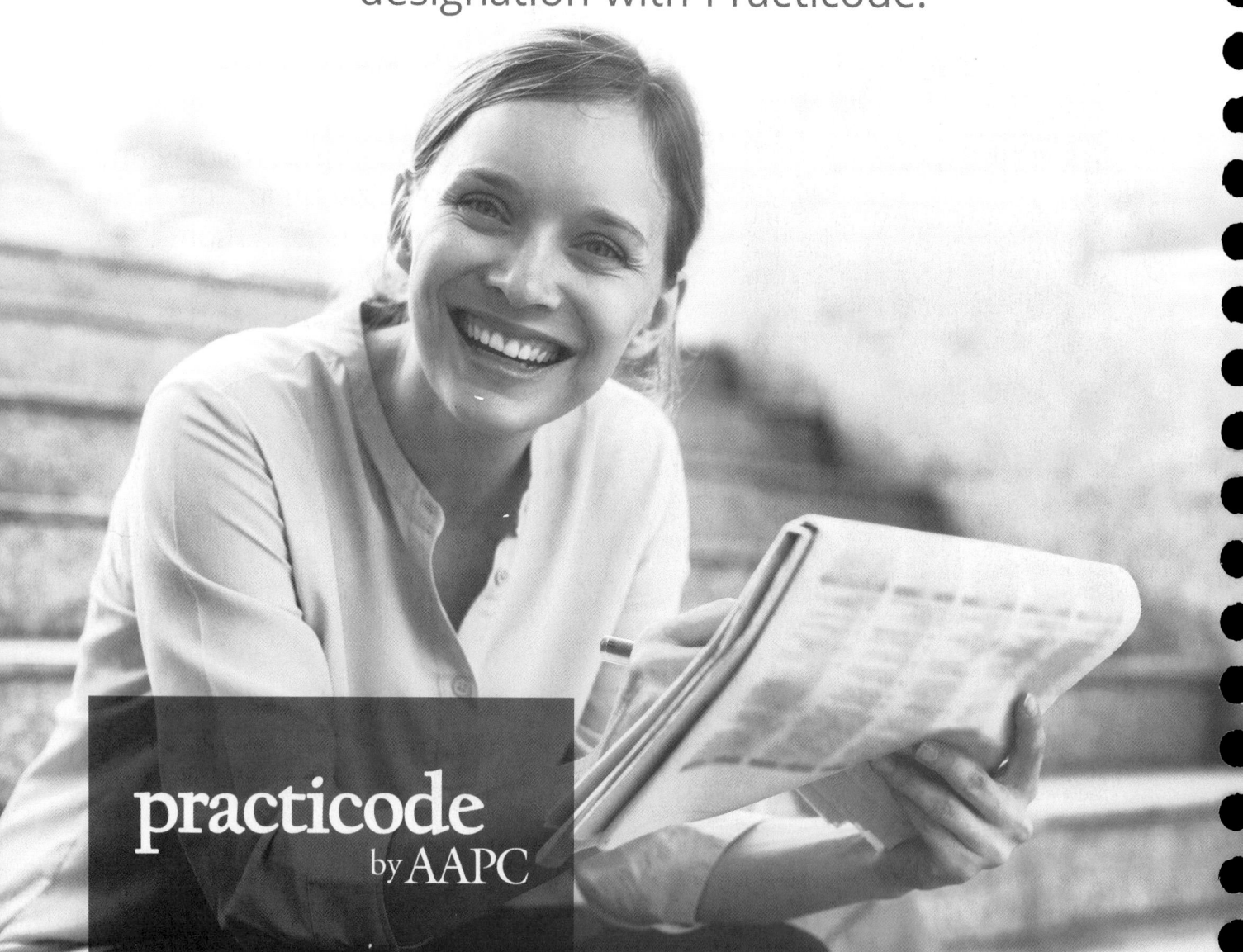

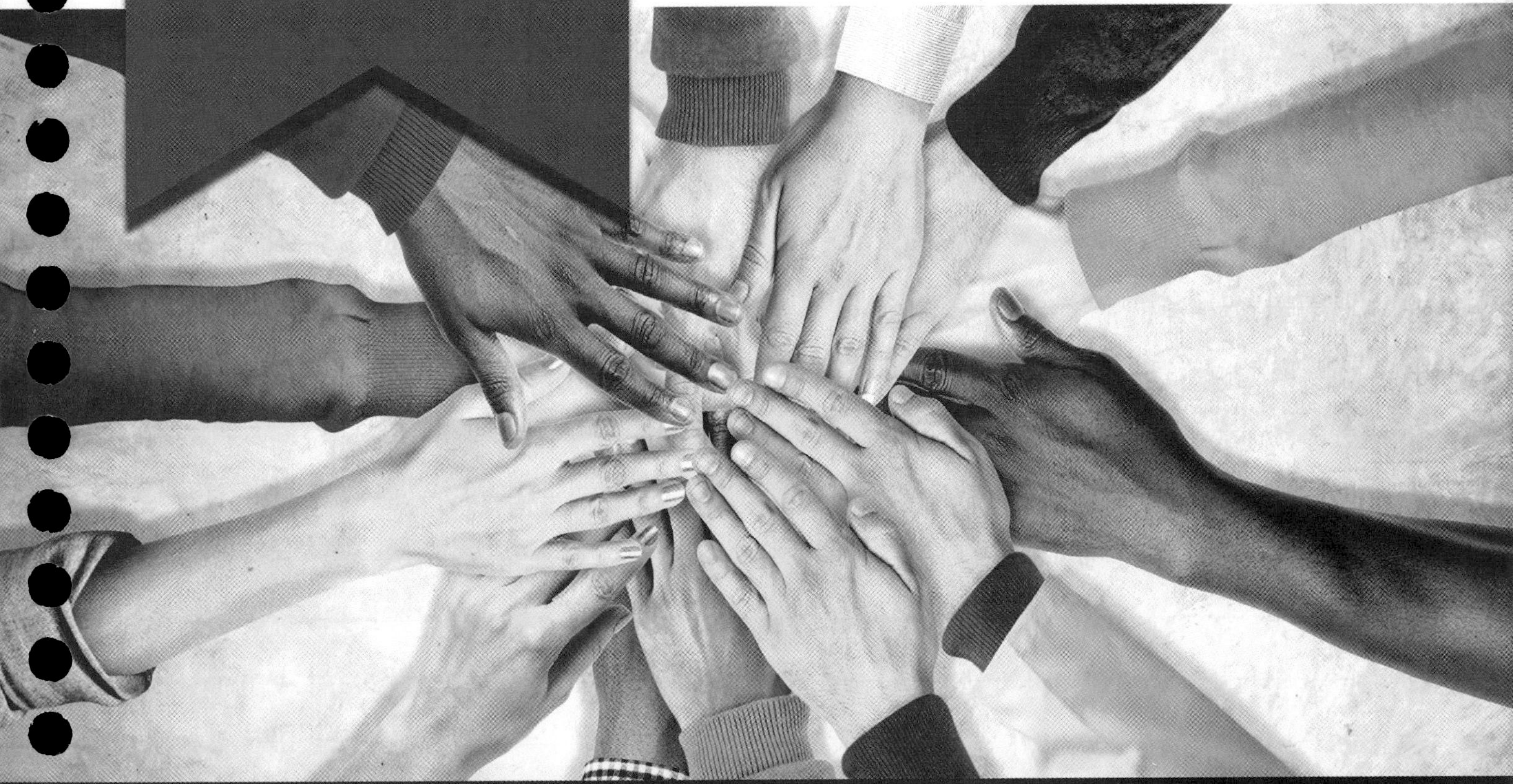

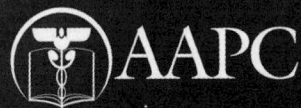

NOTES

NOTES

NOTES

NOTES

NOTES